KELLEY'S TEXTBOOK OF INTERNAL MEDICINE

KELLEY'S TEXTBOOK OF INTERNAL MEDICINE

FOURTH EDITION

Editor-in-Chief

H. David Humes, MD

Editors

Herbert L. DuPont, MD
Laurence B. Gardner, MD
John W. Griffin, MD
Edward D. Harris, Jr, MD
William R. Hazzard, MD
Talmadge E. King, Jr., MD
D. Lynn Loriaux, MD, PhD
Elizabeth G. Nabel, MD
Robert F. Todd, III, MD, PhD
Peter G. Traber, MD

LIPPINCOTT WILLIAMS & WILKINS
A **Wolters Kluwer** Company

Philadelphia • Baltimore • New York • London
Buenos Aires • Hong Kong • Sydney • Tokyo

Acquisitions Editor: Richard Winters
Developmental Editor: Mary Beth Murphy
Production Editor: Patrick Carr
Manufacturing Manager: Colin Warnock
Cover Designer: Karen Quigley
Compositor: Maryland Composition
Printer: Quebecor World Color

© **2000 by LIPPINCOTT WILLIAMS & WILKINS**
530 Walnut Street
Philadelphia, PA 19106 USA
LWW.com

Printed in the USA

Library of Congress Cataloging-in-Publication Data

Kelley's textbook of internal medicine.—4th ed. / editor-in-chief, H. David Humes; editors, Herbert L. DuPont . . . [et al.].
   p. ; cm.
  Includes bibliographical references and index.
  ISBN 0-7817-1787-6
  1. Internal medicine. I. Title: Textbook of internal medicine. II. Humes, H. David. III. Textbook of internal medicine.
  [DNLM: 1. Internal Medicine. WB 115 K29 2000]
  RC46.T329 2000
  616—dc21

                                                   00-033094

---

10 9 8 7 6 5 4 3 2 1

CONTENTS

CONTRIBUTORS

Keith D. Aaronson, MD Assistant Professor of Internal Medicine, University of Michigan Medical Center, Ann Arbor, Michigan

Janet L. Abrahm, MD Associate Professor of Medicine, University of Pennsylvania School of Medicine, Attending Physician, Medicine/Hematology-Oncology, Hospital of the University of Pennsylvania, Philadelphia, Pennsylvania

Jonathan Abrams, MD Professor of Medicine, University of New Mexico, Albuquerque, New Mexico

Norman E. Adair, MD Wake Forest University Baptist Medical Center, Pulmonary/Critical Care, Winston-Salem, North Carolina

David H. Adams, MD Assistant Professor of Surgery, Harvard Medical School, Associate Chief, Cardiac Surgery, Bringham and Women's Hospital, Boston, Massachusetts

Dennis J. Ahnen, MD Professor of Medicine, University of Colorado, Staff Physician, Department of Veteran Affairs Medical Center, Denver, Colorado

Moira L. Aitken, MD, FRCP Associate Professor of Medicine, University of Washington Medical Center, Director, Adult Cystic Fibrosis Program, University of Washington Medical Center, Seattle, Washington

George J. Alangaden, MD Assistant Professor of Medicine, Division of Infectious Diseases, Wayne State University School of Medicne, Detroit, Michigan

Thomas K. Aldrich, MD Professor of Medicine, Director, Unified Pulmonary Medicine, Albert Einstein College of Medicine and Montefiore Medical Center, Bronx, New York

Richard M. Allman, MD Professor of Medicine, Director, Center for Aging and Division of Gerontology and Geriatric Medicine, University of Alabama at Birmingham, Birmingham VA Medical Center, Birmingham, Virginia

David H. Alpers, MD William B. Kountz Professor of Medicine, Division of Gastroenterology, Washington University School of Medicine, St. Louis, Missouri

Joseph H. Antin, MD Associate Professor of Medicine, Harvard Medical School, Chief, Adult Oncology Stem Cell Transplantation, Dana-Farber Cancer Institute, Boston, Massachusetts

Frederick R. Appelbaum, MD Member and Director, Clinical Research Division, Fred Hutchinson Cancer Research Center, Professor and Head, Division of Medical Oncology, University of Washington School of Medicine, Seattle, Washington

William B. Applegate, MD, MPH Professor and Chairman, Department of Internal Medicine, Wake Forest University, Winston-Salem, North Carolina

Roberto C. Arduino, MD Assistant Professor of Medicine, Department of Internal Medicine, Division of Infectious Diseases, The University of Texas Health Science Center at Houston, Houston, Texas

James O. Armitage, MD James O. Armitage, M.D., Professor and Chairman, Department of Internal Medicine, University of Nebraska Medical Center, Omaha, Nebraska

Donald Armstrong, MD Professor of Medicine, Cornell University Medical College, Consultant, Infectious Disease/Medicine, Memorial Sloan-Kettering Cancer Center, New York, New York

William F. Armstrong, MD Professor of Internal Medicine, Associate Chair for Network Development, Internal Medicine, Director, Echocardiology Laboratory, Associate Clinical Chief, Division of Cardiology, University of Michigan Health System, Ann Arbor, Michigan

Frank C. Arnett, MD Professor, Department of Internal Medicine, University of Texas-Houston Medical School, Chief of Rheumatology, Memorial Hermann Hospital, Houston, Texas

William J. Arnold, MD, FACP, FACR Executive Vice President and Chief Medical Officer, Advanced Bio-Surfaces, Inc., Minnetonka, Minnesota, Rheumatologist, Illinois Bone and Joint Institute, LTD, Lutheran General Hospital, Park Ridge, Illinois

Robert L. Atmar, MD Associate Professor, Department of Medicine- Infectious Disease, Baylor College of Medicine, Houston, Texas

George F. Atweh, MD Lillian & Henry Stratton Professor, Department of Medicine, Chief, Division of Hematology, Mount Sinai Medical Center, New York, New York

David S. Bach, MD Clinical Associate Professor of Medicine, Director, Intraoperative Echocardiography, Associate Director, Echocardiography Laboratory, University of Michigan Medical Center, Ann Arbor, Michigan

Bruce R. Bacon, MD James F. King Professor of Internal Medicine, Director, Division of Gastroenterology and Hepatology, Saint Louis University School of Medicine, St. Louis, Missouri

Laurence H. Baker, DO Professor, Department of Medicine, Director, Clinical Research, University of Michigan Comprehensive Cancer Center, Ann Arbor, Michigan

Kresimir Banovac, MD, PhD Professor of Medicine, Orthopaedics and Rehabilitation, University of Miami School of Medicine, Jackson Memorial Center, Miami, Florida

Robert L. Barbieri, MD Kate Macy Ladd Professor of Obstetrics, Gynecology and Reproductive Biology, Harvard Medical School, Chief, Ostetrics and Gynecology, Brigham and Women's Hospital, Boston, Massachusetts

Ariel L. Barkan, MD Professor of Medicine and Surgery, Co-Director, Pituitary and Neuroendocrine Center, University of Michigan Medical Center, Ann Arbor, Michigan

Alan F. Barker, MD Professor of Medicine, Internal Medicine in Pulmonary & Critical Care Division, Oregon Health Sciences University, Portland, Oregon

Christopher M. Barnard, MD Clinical Assistant Professor, Department of Dermatology, Stanford University School of Medicine, Stanford, California

Jeffrey L. Barnett, MD Associate Professor of Internal Medicine, Gastroenterology Division, Director, Medical Procedures Unit, University of Michigan Medical Center, Ann Arbor, Michigan

Craig Basson, MD, PhD Assistant Professor of Cardiology and Medicine, Director, Molecular Cardiology, Weill Medical College of Cornell University, Assistant Attending Physician, Cardiology and Medicine, The New York Presyterian Hospital- Cornell Medical Center, New York, New York

E. Joseph Bauerlein, MD, FACC Associate Professor of Clinical Medicine, University of Miami School of Medicine, Medical Director, Cardiac Transplantation Program, Jackson Memorial Medical Center, Miami, Florida

Kenneth Lee Baughman, MD Professor of Medicine, Chief of Cardiology, The Johns Hopkins University School of Medicine, Baltimore, Maryland

Thomas H. Belhorn, MD, PhD Visiting Assistant Professor of Pediatrics- Infectious Diseases, University of North Carolina, Pediatrician, University of North Carolina Hospitals, Chapel Hill, North Carolina

Michele F. Bellantoni, MD Associate Professor of Medicine, Johns Hopkins University School of Medicine, Division of Geriatric Medicine and Gerontology, Baltimore, Maryland

Elise M. Beltrami, MD HIV Infections Branch, Hospital Infections Program, National Center for Infectious Diseases, Centers for Disease Control and Prevention, Atlanta, Georgia

Ivor Benjamin, MD Assistant Professor, Department of Obstetrics and Gynecology, Hospital of the University of Pennsylvania, Philadelphia, Pennsylvania

Joel S. Bennett, MD Professor of Medicine and Pharmacology, Hematology-Oncology Division, Department of Medicine, University of Pennsylvania School of Medicine, Philadelphia, Pennsylvania

Edward M. Bernard, BA Associate Senior Investigator, Memorial Sloan-Kettering Cancer Center, New York, New York

Kenneth Berry, MD Clinical Professor of Pathology, University of British Columbia, St. Paul's Hospital, Division of Neuropathology, Vancouver, British Columbia, Canada

Michael Alfred Bettmann, MD Professor of Radiology, Dartmouth Medical School, Chief, Cardiovascular and Interventional Radiology, Dartmouth-Hitchcock Medical Center, Lebanon, New Hampshire

Jia Bi, MD Fellow in Medical Oncology, USC Norris Comprehensive Cancer Center, Los Angeles, California

J. Sybil Bierman, MD Assistant Professor of Orthopaedic Surgery, Director, Orthopaedic Oncology, Comprehensive Cancer Center, University of Michigan, Ann Arbor, Michigan

Barbara B. Biesecker, MS National Institutes of Health, Bethesda, Maryland

Leslie G. Biesecker, MD Head, Human Development Section, Genetic Diseases Research Branch, Investigator, National Human Genome Research Institute, National Institutes of Health, Bethesda, Maryland

William C. Black, MD Associate Professor of Radiology and Community and Family Medicine, Dartmouth-Hitchcock Medical Center, Lebanon, New Hampshire

Jorge D. Blanco, MD Clinical Professor of Obstetrics and Gynecology, University of Florida College of Medicine, Director, Residency Support Services, Sacred Heart Women's Hospital, Pensacola, Florida

Ronald Blanton, MD Associate Professor of Medicine and International Health, Case Western Reserve University School of Medicine, Cleveland, Ohio

William A. Blattner, MD Professor of Medicine, Associate Director, Institute of Human Virology, University of Maryland, Baltimore, Maryland

Dan German Blazer, MD, PhD J.P. Gibbons Professor of Psychiatry and Behavioral Sciences, Department of Psychiatry, Dean of Medical Education, Duke University Medical Center, Durham, North Carolina

R. Gregory Bociek, MD, MSc Department of Internal Medicine, Section of Hematology/Oncology, Universityof Nebraska Medical Center, Omaha, Nebraska

Gerald P. Bodey, MD Professor Emeritus, Infectious Diseases, The University of Texas M.D. Anderson Cancer Center, Houston, Texas

C. Richard Boland, MD Professor of Medicine, Chief, Gastroenterology, University of California, San Diego, San Diego, California

William Bonnez, MD Associate Professor of Medicine, Infectious Diseases Unit, University of Rochester School of Medicine and Dentistry, Attending Physician, Strong Memorial Hospital, Rochester, New York

Robert O. Bonow, MD Goldberg Distinguished Professor of Cardiology, Professor of Medicine, Chief, Division of Cardiology, Northwesten University, Chicago, Illinois

Teresa A. Borkowski, MD Assistant Professor of Dematology, Johns Hopkins School of Medicine, Baltimore, Maryland

George J. Bosl, MD Professor of Medicine, Weill Medical College of Cornell University, Chairman, Department of Medicine, Memorial Sloan-Kettering Cancer Center, New York, New York

Laurence A. Boxer, MD Professor and Director, Division of Pediatric Hematology/Oncology, University of Michigan Medical Center, Ann Arbor, Michigan

Christopher R. Braden, MD Centers for Disease Control and Prevention, National Center for HIV, STD, TB Prevention, Division of TB Elimination, Atlanta, Georgia

D. Craig Brater, MD Chairman, Department of Medicine, Director of Clinical Pharmacology, Indiana University School of Medicine, Indianapolis, Indiaina

Glenn D. Braunstein, MD Chairman, Department of Medicine, Cedars-Sinai Medical Center, Professor of Medicine, UCLA School of Medicine, Los Angeles, California

Peter C. Brazy, MD Professor of Medicine, University of Wisconsin, Chief of Nephrology, Vice Chair, Department of Medicine, University of Wisconsin Hospital and Clinics, Madison, Wisconsin

Kenneth R. Bridges, MD Associate Professor of Medicine, Harvard Medical School, Director, Joint Center for Sickle Cell and Thalassemic Disorders, Brigham & Women's Hospital, Boston, Massachusetts

Michael R. Bristow, MD, PhD Head, Division of Cardiology, University of Colorado Health Sciences Center, Denver, Colorado

Geo. F. Brooks, MD Professor of Laboratory Medicine, University of California- San Francisco, San Francisco, California

Patrick Brophy, MD Fellow, Division of Nephrology, Department of Pediatrics and Communicable Diseases, University of Michigan School of Medicine, Ann Arbor, Michigan

Frank C. Brosius, MD Associate Professor of Internal Medicine, University of Michigan, Director, Nephrology Training Program, Nephrology Division, University of Michigan Hospitals, Ann Arbor, Michigan

Roger J. Broughton, MD, PhD, FRCP(C) Professor of Neurology, University of Ottawa, Medical Director, Sleep Medicine Center, Ottawa Hospital (General Campus), Ottawa, Ontario, Canada

Kevin K. Brown, MD Assistant Professor of Medicine, Division of Pulmonary Services, University of Colorado Health Sciences Center, Director, Clinical Interstitial Lung Disease Program, National Jewish Medical and Research Center, Denver, Colorado

Kenneth Brummel-Smith, MD Associate Professor of Medicine and Family Medicine, Oregon Health Sciences University, Bain Chair, Providence Center on Aging, Providence Health System, Portland, Oregon

Warner Burch, MD Associate Professor of Medicine, Duke University Medical Center, Durham, North Carolina

Susan J. Burgert, MD, FACP Clinical Instructor of Medicine, Baylor College of Medicine, Section of Infectious Disease, St. Luke's Episcopal Hospital, Houston, Texas

Kenneth D. Burman, MD Professor of Medicine, The Uniformed Services University of the Health Services, Bethesda, Maryland, Clinical Professor of Medicine, Georgetown and George Washington Universities, Director, Section of Endocrinology, Washington Hospital Center, Washington, D.C.

David A. Bushinsky, MD Professor of Medicine and of Pharmacology and Physiology, University of Rchester School of Medicine, Chief, Nephrology Unit, Strong Memerial Hospital, Rochester, New York

Thomas Butler, MD Professor of Internal Medicine, Chief of Infectious Diseases, Texas Tech University Health Sciences Center, Chief of Infectious Diseases, University Medical Center, Lubbock, Texas

John G. Byrne, MD Assistant Professor of Surgery, Harvard School of Medicine, Bringham and Women's Hospital, Boston, Massachusetts

J. Gregory Cairncross, MD CEO, London Regional Cancer Center, Chair, Division of Neurosciences, University of Western Ontario, London, Ontario, Canada

Preston Calvert, MD Assistant Professor of Neurology and Ophthomology, Johns Hopkins University School of Medicine, Director, Neurology Outpatient Consultation Center, Johns Hopkins Outpatient Center, Baltimore, Maryland

George P. Canellos, MD, FACP, FRCP William Rosenberg Professor of Medicine, Harvard Medical School, Dana-Farber Cancer Institute, Boston, Massachusetts

Juan J. Canoso, MD Adjunct Professor of Medicine, Tufts University School of Medicine, Lomas de Chapultepec, Mexico

Arthur L. Caplan, PhD Director, Center for Bioethics, University of Pennsylvania, Philadelphia, Pennsylvania

Denise M. Cardo, MD HIV Infections Branch, Hospital Infections Program, National Center for Infectious Disease, Centers for Disease Control and Prevention, Atlanta, Georgia

Ralph Carmel, MD Director of Research, Department of Medicine, New York Methodist Hospital, Professor of Medicine, Cornell University Medical College, New York, New York

John J. Caronna, MD Professor of Clinical Neurology, Department of Neurology and Neuroscience, Weill Medical College of Cornell University, Attending Neurologist, The New York-Presbyterian Hospital, New York, New York

Christine K. Cassel, MD Professor and Chairman, The Henry L. Schwartz Department of Geriatrics and Adult Development, Professor, Department of Geriatrics and Internal Medicine, Mount Sinai/NYU Health, New York, New York

Ronald A. Castellino, MD Professor of Radiology, Cornell University Medical School, Chairman, Department of Radiology, Memorial Sloan Kettering Cancer Center, New York, New York

Joseph P. Catlett, MD, FACP Attending Physician, Section of Hematology/Oncology, Washington Hospital Center, Assistant Professor of Medicine, Uniformed Services University, of the Health Sciences, Washington, DC

Bruce A. Chabner, MD Professor of Medicine, Harvard Medical School, Clinical Director, MGH Cancer Center, Massachusetts General Hospital, Boston, Massachusetts

Eugene B. Chang, MD Department of Medicine, University of Chicago, Chicago, Illinois

Cynthia L. Chappell, PhD Associate Professor, Center for Infectious Diseases, University of Texas School of Public Health, Houston, Texas

Sarah H. Cheeseman, MD Professor of Medicine, Pediatrics, Molecular Genetics and Microbiology, University of Massachusetts Medical School, Worcester, Massachusetts

Robert T. Chen, MD, MA Chief, Vaccine Safety and Development Branch, National Immunization Program, Centers for Disease Control and Prevention, Atlanta, Georgia

Raymond H. Chen, MD, PhD Clinical Fellow in Surgery, Harvard School of Medicine, Bringham and Women's Hospital, Boston, Massachusetts

Anthony W. Chow, MD, FRCPC, FACP Professor of Medicine, Division of Infectious Diseases, Department of Medicine, Director MD/PhD Program, University of British Columbia, Vancouver, British Columbia

Kian Fan Chung, MD, FRCP Professor of Respiratory Medicine, National Heart and Lung Institute, Imperial College School of Medicine, Consultant Physician, Royal Brompton Hospital, London, England

Marianne Cinat, MD Assistant Professor of Surgery UCI Medical Center, Orange, California

Douglas B. Cines, MD Professor, Department of Pathology and Laboratory Medicine, Director, Hematology and Coagulation Laboratories and Medicine, Hospital of the University of Pennsylvania, Philadelphia, Pennsylvania

Christopher M. Clark, MD Associate Professor of Neurology, Director, Memory Disorders Program, Hospital of the University of Pennsylvania, Philadelphia, Pennsylvania

Jack L. Clausen, MD Clinical Professor of Medicine, School of Medicine, University of California, San Diego, San Diego, California

C. Glenn Cobbs, MD Professor Emeritus and Vice Chairman for VA Affairs, UAB, Chief, Medical Service, VAMC, Birmingham, Alabama

Barbara A. Cockrill, MD Assistant Physician, Pulmonary and Critical Care, Director, Partners Asthma Center, Massachusetts General Hospital, Boston, Massachusetts

Robert J. Cody, MD Professor of Medicine, Associate Chief, Division of Cardiology, Director, Heart Failure and Transplant Management, University of Michigan Medical Center, Ann Arbor, Michigan

Peter Cole, MD Host Defense Unit/Thoracic Medicine, National Heart & Institute, London, England

Francis S. Collins, MD, PhD Director, National Human Genome Research Institute, Bethesda, Maryland

Robert E. Condon, MD Department of Surgery, Medical College of Wisconsin, Milwaukee, Wisconsin

Kimberly A. Cook, Esq. Fowler-White, Miami, Florida

Paul Michael Copeland, MD Assistant Clinical Professor of Medicine, Harvard Medical School, Endocrine Unit, Massachusetts General Hospital, Boston, Massachusetts, Co-Director, Eating Disorders Program, Salem Hospital, Salem, Massachusetts

Tom Corbridge, MD Director, Medical Intensive Care Unit, Northwestern Mermorial Hospital, Chicago, Illinois

Andrea M. Corse, MD Assistant Professor of Neurology, Johns Hopkins University School of Medicine, Attending Neurologist, Johns Hopkins Hospital, Baltimore, Maryland

Malcolm Cox, MD Professor of Medicine, Associate Dean, Network and Primary Care Education, University of Pennsylvania School of Medicine, Philadelphia, Pennsylvania

David W. Crabb, MD Professor and Vice Chair for Research, Department of Medicine, Indiana University, Indianapolis, Indiana

William A. Craig, MD Professor of Medicine, University of Wisconsin, Madison, Wisconsin

Mark A. Creager, MD Associate Professor of Medicine, Cardiovascular Division, Brigham & Women's Hospital, Boston, Massachusetts

William F. Crowley, Jr., MD Professor of Medicine, Harvard School of Medicine, Boston, Massachusetts

Mark R. Cullen, MD Professor of Medicine and Public Health, Yale University School of Medicine, Occupational and Environmental Medicine Program, New Haven, Connecticut

Burke A. Cunha, MD, FACP Chief, Infectious Disease Division, Winthrop-University Hospital, Mineola, New York, Professor of Medicine, State University of New York at Stony Brook, Stony Brook, New York

Glenn R. Cunningham, MD Professor of Medicine and Cell Biology, Vice Chairman for Research, Baylor College of Medicine, ACOS, Research & Development, Veterans Affairs Medical Center, Houston, Texas

Albert J. Czaja, MD Professor of Medicine, Mayo Medical School, Consultant, Gastroenterology and Hepatology, Mayo Clinic, Rochester, Minnesota

Charles L. Daley, MD Assistant Professor of Medicine, University of California, San Francisco, Chief, Chest Clinic, San Francisco General Hospital, Medical Director, Training Center, F.J. Curry National Tuberculosis Center, San Francisco, California

John M. Daly, MD, FACS Lewis Atterbury Stimson Professor and Chairman, Department of Surgery, Weill Medical College of Cornell University, Surgeon-in-Chief, New York Presbyterian Hospital- Cornell Campus, New York, New York

Gary L. Darmstadt, MD Assistant Professor, Divisions of Dermatology and Infectious Diseases, Departments of Pediatrics and Medicine, University of Washington School of Medicine, Seattle, Washington; Adjunct Assistant Professor, Department of International Health, School of Hygiene and Public Health, The Johns Hopkins Medical Institutions, Baltimore, Maryland

Lisa M. DeAngelis, MD Chairman, Department of Neurology, Memorial Sloan Kettering Cancer Center, Professor of Clinical Neurology, Weill Medical College of Cornell University, New York, New York

Albert B. Deisseroth, MD, PhD Ensign Professor of Medicine, Chief, Section of Medical Oncology, Department of Internal Medicine, Yale University School of Medicine, New Haven, Connecticut

Antonio V. Delgado-Escueta, MD Professor of Neurology, West Los Angeles Healthcare Center, Los Angeles, California

E. Patchen Dellinger, MD Professor and Vice-Chairman, Department of Surgery, University of Washington School of Medicine, Associate Medical Director, University of Washington Medical Center, Seattle, Washington

Peter Densen, MD Professor of Internal Medicine, University of Iowa, Iowa City, Iowa

Paul M. Dorinsky, MD Clinical Associate Professor of Medicine, University of North Carolina, Chapel Hill, North Carolina

Marc K. Drezner, MD Professor of Medicine, Head, Section of Endocrinology, Diabetes and Metabolism, University of Wisconsin Medical School, Madison, Wisconsin

Douglas A. Drossman, MD Professor of Medicine and Psychiatry, Division of Digestive Diseases, Co-Director, UNC Funcional Gastrointestinal Disorder Center, University of North Caronlina, Chapel Hill, North Carolina

Thomas D. DuBose, Jr., MD Peter T. Bohan Professor and Chairman, Department of Internal Medicine, Kansas University Medical Center, Kansas City, Kansas

Thomas P. Duffy, MD Professor of Medicine, Yale University School of Medicine, Attending Physician, Yale-New Haven Hospital, New Haven, Connecticut

Richard J. Duma, MD, PhD Director of Infectious Diseases, Halifax Medical Center, Daytona Beach, Florida

Janice P. Dutcher, MD Professor, New York Medical College, Associate Director for Clinical, Affairs, Our Lady of Mercy Cancer Center, New York, New York

Kim A. Eagle, MD Albion Walter Hewlett Professor of Internal Medicine, Senior Associate Chair, Department of Internal Medicine, Chief, Clinical Cardiology, University of Michigan Medical Center, Ann Arbor, Michigan

George C. Ebers, MD University Department of Clinical Neurology, Radcliffe Infirmary, Oxford, United Kingdom

John E. Edwards, Jr., MD Chief, Division of Infectious Diseases, Harbor-UCLA Medical Center, Professor of Medicine, UCLA School of Medicine, Torrance, California

Theodore C. Eickhoff, MD Professor of Medicine, Division of Infectious Disease, University of Colorado Health Sciences Center, Denver, Colorado

Andrew A. Eisen, MD Neuromuscular Diseases Unit, Vancouver Hospital, Vancouver, British Columbia, Canada

Wafaa El-Sadr, MD, MPH Director, Infectious Diseases, Columbia University, New York, New York

Charles O. Elson, MD Basil I. Hirschowitz Chair in Gastroenterology, Professor of Medicine, University of Alabama at Birmingham, Birmingham, Alabama

Grace H. Elta, MD Professor of Medicine, University of Michigan School of Medicine, Ann Arbor, Michigan

Stephen G. Emerson, MD, PhD Professor of Medicine, University of Pennsylvania School of Medicine, Chief, Hematology-Oncology Division, Hospital of the University of Pennsylvania, Philadelphia, Pennsylvania

Richard W. Erbe, MD Chief, Division of Genetics, Children's Hospital of Buffalo, Professor of Pediatrics and Medicine, School of Medicine and Biomedical Sciences, State University of New York at Buffalo

Walter H. Ettinger, Jr., MD, MBA Executive Vice-President for Physicians' Services, Virtua Health, Marlton, New Jersey

Michael D. Ezekowitz, MB, ChB Professor of Medicine, Yale University School of Medicine, New Haven, Connecticut

James A. Fagin, MD Heady Professor of Medicine, Director, Division of Endocrinology and Metabolism, University of Cincinnati Medical Center, Cincinnati, Ohio

Ronald J. Falk, MD Professor of Medicine, University of North Caroline at Chapel Hill, Department of Medicine, Division of Nephrology and Hypertension, Chapel Hill, North Carolina

Monica M. Farley, MD Veterans Affairs Medical Center, Decatur, Georgia

Timmothy M. Farrell, MD Department of Surgery, Emory University school of Medicine, Atlanta, Georgia

Thomas E. Feasby, MD Department of Clinical Neurosciences, University of Calgary, Calgary, Alberta, CANADA

Jerome M. Feldman, MD Professor of Medicine, Division of Endocrinology and Metabolism, Duke University Medical Center, Durham, North Carolina

G. Michael Felker, MD Fellow, Division of Cardiology, The Johns Hopkins University School of Medicine, Baltimore, Maryland

Debbie Fertel, MD Department of Medicine, University of Miami School of Medicine, Miami, Florida

Stuart L. Fine, MD William F. Norris and George E. de Schweinitz Professor of Ophthalmology, Chairman, Department of Ophthalmology, Director, Scheie Eye Institute, University of Pennsylvania, Philadelphia, Pennsylvania

Sydney M. Finegold, MD Staff Physician, Infectious Disease Section, Wadsworth Veterans Medical Center, Los Angeles, California

Gary S. Firestein, MD Division of Rheumatology, University of California, San Diego School of Medicine, La Jolla, California

Charles Fisch, MD Distinguished Professor Emeritus of Medicine, Indiana University School of Medicine, Krannert Institute of Cardiology, Indianapolis, Indiana

Daniel B. Fishbein, MD Senior Medical Epidemiologist, Division of International Health, Epidemiology Program Office, Centers for Disease Control and Prevention, Atlanta, Georgia

Faith T. Fitzgerald, MD Professor of Internal Medicine, University of California, Davis Medical Center, Sacramento, California

Lisa Fitzpatrick, MD Centers for Disease Control and Prevention, National Center for HIV, STD, TB Prevention, Division of TB Elimination, Atlanta, Georgia

Alan M. Fogelman, MD   Professor, Executive Chairman of Medicine, UCLA School of Medicine, Los Angeles, California

Kevin R. Fox, MD   Associate Professor of Medicine, Attending Physician, Hemotology/Oncology Division, University of Pennsylvania School of Medicine, Philadelphia, Pennsylvania

Uta Francke, MD   Professor of Genetics, Stanford University School of Medicine, Stanford, California

David O. Freedman, MD   Director, UAB Travelers Health Clinic, Associate Professor of Medicine and Epidemiology/International Health, Division of Geographic Medicine, University of Alabama at Birmingham, Birmingham, Alabama

Eugene P. Frenkel, MD   Professor of Internal Medicine and Radiology, Patsy R and Raymond D. Nasher, Distinguished Chair in Cancer Research, A. Kenneth Pye Professorship in Cancer Research, University of Texas Southwestern Medical Center at Dallas, Dallas, Texas

Linda P. Fried, MD, MPH   Professor, Medicine and Epidemiology, Director, Center on Aging and Health, Deputy Director, Department of Medicine, for Clinical Epidemiology and Health Services Research, The Johns Hopkins Medical Institutions, Baltimore, Maryland

Michael A. Friedman, MD   Deputy Commissioner for Operations, Food and Drug Administration, Rockville, Maryland

Lawrence S. Friedman, MD   Associate Professor of Medicine, Harvard Medical School, Physician, Gastrointestinal Unit and Chief, Walter Bauer Firm (Medical Services), Massachusetts General Hospital, Boston, Massachusetts

Victor F. Froelicher, MD   Professor of Medicine, Stanford University, Director, ECG/Cardiology Laboratory, PA-VAHCS, Palo Alto, California

Bruce Furie, MD   Professor of Medicine, Harvard Medical School, Director, Beth Israel Deaconess Cancer Center, Boston, Massachusetts

John H. Galla, MD   Professor of Medicine, Director, Division of Nephrology and Hypertension, University of Cincinnati College of Medicine, Cincinnati, Ohio

Suzette Garofano, MD, FCCP   Clinical Assistant Professor, Department of Medicine, NYU School of Medicine, Assistant Attending, Tisch Hospital, New York, New York

Layne O. Gentry, MD   Infectious Diseases, St. Luke's Episcopal Hospital, Houston, Texas

W. Lance George, MD   Professor of Medicine, UCLA School of Medicine, Los Angeles, California

Anne A. Gershon, MD   Professor of Pediatrics, Attending Physician, Babies and Childrens Hospital, New York, New York

Alan M. Gewirtz, MD   Professor of Medicine and Pathology, Leader, Stem Cell Biology/Transplantation Program, University of Pennsylvania Cancer Center, University of Pennsylvania Medical Center, Philadelphia, Pennsylvania

Mihai Gheorghiade, MD   Professor of Medicine, Associate Chief, Division of Cardiology, Northwestern University Medical School, Chicago, Illinois

Amit K. Ghosh   Professor, Materials Science & Engineering, College of Engineering, University of Michigan, Ann Arbor, Michigan

Teresa Gilewski, MD   Memorial-Sloan Kettering Cancer Center, New York, New York

Gregory G. Ginsberg, MD   Associate Professor of Medicine, Gastroentrology Division, Director of Endoscopic Services, University of Pennsylvania Health System, Philadelphia, Pennsylvania

David Ginsburg, MD   Professor of Internal Medicine and Human Genetics, Chief, Division of Medical Genetics, University of Michigan Medical School, Ann Arbor, Michigan

Roger I. Glass, MD, PhD   Chief, Viral Gastroenteritus Section, Centers for Disease Control and Prevention, Atlanta, Georgia

Michael G. Glenn, MD   Clinical Associate Professor of Otolaryngology- Head and Neck Surgery, University of Washington, Seattle, Washington

John K. Gohagan, PhD, FACE   Chief, Early Detection Research Group, Division of Cancer Prevention, National Cancer Institute, Rockville, Maryland

Andrew P. Goldberg, MD   Chief, Division of Gerontology and GRECC Director, University of Maryland, Baltimore, Baltimore VA Maryland Health Care System, Baltimore, Maryland

Jorge T. Gonzalez, MD   Neurology, Alpena General Hospital, Alpena, Michigan

David Y. Graham, MD   Professor of Medicine and Molecular Virology, Chief, Gastroenterology, Department of Medicine, Baylor College of Medicine and Veterans Medical Center, Houston, Texas

Richard J. Gralla, MD   Director, Oshner Cancer Institute, New Orleans, Louisiana

Daryl K. Granner, MD   Director, Vanderbilt Diabetes Center, Vanderbilt University Medical Center, Nashville, Tennessee

Frank Anthony Greco, MD   Medical Director, Sarah Cannon-Minnie Pearl Cancer Center, Centennial Medical Center, Nashville, Tennessee

Stephen B. Greenberg, MD   Professor of Medicine, Baylor College of Medicine, Houston, Texas

Jack O. Greenberg, MD   Clinical Professor of Neurology, MCP-Hahneman, School of Medicine, Philadelphia, Pennsylvania

Peter Greenwald, MD, DrPH   Director, Division of Cancer Prevention, National Cancer Institute, Bethesda, Maryland

Martin C. Gregory, BM, D. Phil   Professor of Medicine, Divisions of General Internal Medicine and Nephrology, Department of Medicine, University of Utah Health Sciences Center, Salt Lake City, Utah

James H. Grendell, MD   Professor of Medicine, Weill Medical College of Cornell University, Attending Physician, New York Presbyterian Hospital, New York, New York

Phillip R. Griepp, MD   Professor of Medicine, Professor of Laboratory Medicine and Pathology, Department of Internal Medicine, Division of Hematology, Mayo Clinic, Rochester, Minnesota

David E. Griffith, MD   Professor of Medicine, Director of Tuberculosis Services, Director of Medical Affairs, Center for Pulmonary, Infectious Disease Control, The University of Texas Health Center at Tyler, Tyler, Texas

Coleman Gross, MD   Assistant Professor of Medicine, Department of Medicine, University of California, San Francisco, Staff Physician, Department of Veterans Affairs Medical Center, San Francisco, California

John D. Hainsworth, MD   Director, Clinical Research, Sarah Cannon Cancer Center, Centennial Medical Center, Nashville, Tennessee

Daniel G. Haller, MD   Professor of Medicine, Hematology/Oncology Division, University of Pennsylvania, Philadelphia, Pennsylvania

Jeffrey B. Halter, MD   Professor of Internal Medicine, Chief, Division of Geriatric Medicine, Director, Geriatrics Center, University of Michigan, Research Scientist, GRECC, Ann Arbor VAMC, Ann Arbor, Michigan

E. William Hancock, MD   Professor of Medicine (Cardiovascular) (Emeritus), Stanford University School of Medicine, Stanford University Hospital, Stanford, California

Michael E. Hanley, MD   Associate Professor of Medicine, University of Colorado School of Medicine, Denver, Colorado

Edward F. Haponik, MD   Clinical Director, Pulmonary and Critical Care Medicine, Department of Medicine, Johns Hopkins Medical Institutions, Baltimore, Maryland

John A. Hardin, MD   Chair, Department of Medicine, Medical College of Georgia, Augusta, Georgia

Stanley Hashimoto, MD, FRCPC   Clinical Professor of Medicine, Division Neurology, University of British Columbia, Vancouver, British Columbia, Canada

William L. Hasler, MD   Associate Professor of Internal Medicine, University of Michigan Medical Center, Ann Arbor, Michigan

Michael R. Hayden, MB, ChB, DCh, PhD, FRCPC, FRSC   Centre for Molecular Medicine & Therapeutic, University of British Columbia, Vancouver, British Columbia

Frances J. Hayes, MB, MRCPI   Instructor in Medicine at, Harvard Medical School, Assistant in Medicine at Massachusetts General Hospital, Boston, Massachusetts

Curtis W. Hayes, MD   Professor, Radiology Department, University of Michigan Medical Center, Ann Arbor, Michigan

Daniel F. Hayes, MD   Associate Professor of Medicine, Georgetown University Medical Center, Clinical Director, Breast Cancer Program, Lombardi Cancer Center, Washington, DC

William R. Hazzard, MD   Professor of Internal Medicine, Senior Adviser, J. Paul Sticht Center on Aging, Wake Forest University School of Medicine, Winston-Salem, North Carolina

E. Jenny Heathcote, MD, FRCP   Professor of Medicine, University of Toronto, University Health Network, Toronto Western Hospital, Toronto, Ontario, Canada

John E. Heffner, MD   Professor and Vice Chair, Department of Medicine, Medical University of South Carolina, Charleston, South Carolina

Charles M. Helms, MD, PhD   Professor of Medicine, Department of Internal Medicine, The University of Iowa College of Medicine, Iowa City, Iowa

Mark A. Helvie, MD   Associate Professor of Radiology, Director, Division of Breast Imaging, University of Michigan Health System, Ann Arbor, Michigan

William L. Henrich, MD   Professor and Chairman, Department of Medicine, University of Maryland School of Medicine, Baltimore, Maryland

Robert Hernandez, MD   University of Miami School of Medicine, Division of General Medicine, Miami, Florida

L. David Hillis, MD   Vice Chair, Department of Medicine, University of Texas Southwestern Medical Center, Dallas, Texas

Subhash K. Hira, MD, MPH   Professor of Infectious Diseases, The University of Texas-Houston, Director, AIDS Research and Control Centre, Mumbai, Technical Advisor, Ministry of Health, Government of India, Mumbai, India

Max Hirshkowitz, PhD   Associate Professor, Department of Psychiatry, Baylor College of Medicine, Director, Sleep Research Center, Veterans Affairs Medical Center, Houston, Texas

Marc C. Hochberg, MD, MPH   Professor of Medicine, Head, Division of Rheumatology, University of Maryland, Baltimore, Maryland

Gary S. Hoffman, MD, PhD   Chairman, Rheumatic and Immunologic Diseases, Cleveland Clinic Foundation, Professor of Medicine, Ohio State Unioversity

Ahmet Hoke, MD, PhD, FRCP (C)   Assistant Professor, Department of Neurology, Johns Hopkins University School of Medicine, Baltimore, Maryland

Philip C. Hopewell, MD   Professor of Medicine, University of California, San Francisco, Associate Dean, San Francisco General Hospital, San Francisco, California

Sandra J. Horning, MD   Professor of Medicine, Division of Oncology, Department of Medicine, Stanford University Medical Center, Palo Alto, California

Joel D. Howell, MD, PhD   Professor of Internal Medicine, Historyand Health Management, University of Michigan, Ann Arbor, Michigan

Dennis Hsieh,   Deputy Associate Chief of Staff for Geriatrics & Extended Care VA, Philadelphia VA Medical Center, Philadelphia, Pennsylvania

Ging-Yuek Robin Hsiung, MD, FRCPC   Fellow, Movement Disorders and Neurogenetics, Department of Clinical Neurosciences, Foothills Hospital and the University of Calgary, Calgary, Alberta, Canada

Leonard D. Hudson, MD   Professor of Medicine, Head, Pulminary and Critical Care Medicine, University of Washington, Seattle, Washington

Thomas Hyers, MD   Clinical Professor of Internal Medicine, St. Louis University School of Medicine, St. Louis, Missouri

David H. Ingbar, MD   Professor of Medicine and Pediatrics, University of Minnesota School of Medicine, Director, Medical Intensive Care Unit, Fairview University Medical Center, Minneapolis, Minnesota

Sharon K. Inouye, MD, MPH   Sharon K. Inouye, MD, MPH, Associate Professor of Medicine, Department of Internal Medicine, Yale University School of Medicine, New Haven, Connecticut

Ian Irwin, MD   Cemtar Pharmaceuticals, Sunnyvale, California

Richard Jackson, MD   Joslin Diabetes Center, One Joslin Place, Boston, Massachusetts

Robert R. Jacobson, MD, PhD   Director, DNHDP/GWLHDC, Gillis W. Long Hansen's Disease Center, Carville, Louisianna

Sheldon Jacobson, MD   Mt. Sinai Medical Center, New York, New York

Majd I. Jaradat, MD   Division of Nephrology, Indiana University School of Medicine, Indianapolis, Indiana

Robert M. Jasmer, MD   Assistant Professor of Medicine, Division of Pulmonary and Critical Care Medicine, University of California, San Francisco, San Francisco, California

James R. Jett, MD   Professor of Medicine, Consultant in Pulmonary Diseases and Medical Oncology, Mayo Clinic, Rochester, Minnesota

Sarah A. Jewell   Assistant Clinical Professor, Occupational Medicine, University of California San Francisco School of Medicine, San Francisco, California

Theodore M. Johnson, II, MD, MPH   Director, Nursing Home Care Unit, Atlanta VAMC, Decatur, Georgia

Alicia Johnston, MD   Department of Pediatrics, Duke University Medical Center, Durham, North Carolina

Robert B. Jones, MD, PhD   Associate Dean, Clinical Affairs, Indiana University School of Medicine, Indianapolis, Indiana

William D. Kaehny, MD   Profrssor of Medicine, University of Colorado, School of Medicine, Department of Veterans Affairs, Medical Center, Denver, Colorado

Gregory P. Kalemkerian, M.D.   Clinical Associate Professor of Medicine, Co-Director, Thoracic Oncology, University of Michigan Cancer Center, Ann Arbor, Michigan

Adrian I. Katz, MD   Professor of Medicine, The University of Chicago; Attending Physician, University of Chicago Hospitals, Chicago, Illinois

James W. Kazura, MD, PhD   Professor of Medicine and International Health, Case Western Reserve University, School of Medicine, University Hospitals of Cleveland, Cleveland, Ohio

William N. Kelley, MD   Professor of Medicine, University of Pennsylvania School of Medicine, Philadelphia, Pennsylvania

Carolyn J. Kelly, MD   Professor of Medicine, Department of Medicine, University of California San Diego, La Jolla, California; Clinical Investigator, VA San Diego Healthcare System, San Diego, California

David W. Kennedy, MD Professor and Chair, Department of Otorhinolaryngology: Head and Neck Surgery, Hospital of the University of Pennsylvania, Philadelphia, Pennsylvania

Ali S. Khan, MD Epidemiology Section, Special Pathogens Branch, Centers for Disease Control and Prevention, Atlanta, Georgia

Marcia Kielhofner, MD Clinical Associate Professor of Medicine, Baylor College of Medicine, Houston, Texas

John A. Kiernan, MB, ChB, PhD, DSc Professor of Anatomy, The University of Western Ontario, London, Ontario, Canada

Charles H. King, MD Associate Professor of Medicine and International Health, Case Western Reserve University and, University Hospitals of Cleveland, Cleveland, Ohio

Talmadge E. King, Jr., MD Chief, Medical Services, San Francisco General Hospital, Constance B. Wofsy Distinguished Professor and Vice Chairman, Department of Medicine, University of California, San Fransisco, San Fransisco, California

Bradley P. Knight, MD Assistant Professor of Medicine, University of Michigan Health System, Ann Arbor, Michigan

Alisa A. Koch, MD Gallagher Research Professor of Medicine, Northwestern University Medical School, Chicago, Illinios

Michael L. Kochman, MD, FACP Associate Professor of Medicine, Co-Director, Gastrointestinal Oncology, Gastroenterology Division, University of Pennsylvania Medical School, Philadelphia, Pennsylvania

Robert M. Kotloff, MD Associate Professor of Medicine, Director, Program for Advanced Lung Disease and Lung Transplantation, Pulmonary, Allergy and Critical Care Division, University of Pennsylvania Medical Center, Philadelphia, Pennsylvania

Barnett S. Kramer, MD Associate Director, Early Detection and Community Oncology Program, Division of Cancer Prevention and Control, National Cancer Institute, Rockville, Maryland

Donald J. Krogstad, MD Henderson Professor and Chair, Department of Tropical Medicine, Tulane University School of Public Health and Tropical Medicine, Director, Tulane Center for Infectious Diseases, Tulane University Medical Center, New Orleans, Louisiana

Ralph Kuncl, MD, PhD Department of Neurology, Johns Hopkins University, 600 N. Wolfe Street, Meyer 5-119, Baltimore, Maryland

Robert A. Kyle, MD Professor, Medicine & Laboratory Medicine, Mayo Medical School, Rochester, Minnesota

F. Marc LaForce, MD Clinical Professor of Medicine, University of Rochester School of Medicine, Rochester, New York

Christopher J. Lahart, MD Medical Director, Thomas Street Clinic; Assistant Professor of Medicine, Baylor College of Medicine, Houston, Texas

James W. Lance, MD, FRCP, FRACP Institute of Neurological Sciences, Prince of Wales Hospital Medical Centre, Sydney, Australia

Richard A. Lange, MD Jonsson-Rogers Chair in Cardiology, Professor of Internal Medicine, The University of Texas Southwestern Medical Center, Director, Cardiac Catheterization Laboratory, Parkland Mermorial Hospital, Dallas, Texas

J. William Langston, MD The Parkinson's Institute, Sunnyvale, California

Risa J. Lavisso-Mourey, MD University of Pennsylvania, Institute on Aging, Ralston House, Philadelphia, Pennsylvania

Mark A. Lawson, MD Oklahoma Cardiovascular Associates, Oklahoma City, Oklahoma

Blair R. Leavitt, MD University of British Columbia, Vancouver, British Columbia

Sum Ping Lee, MD, PhD Head and Professor, Department of Medicine, Division of Gastroenterology, University of Washington Medical Center, Seattle, Washington

Stephanie J. Lee, MD Assistant Professor of Medicine, Dana-Farber Cancer Institutel, Boston, Massachusetts

Richard S. Legro, MD Associate Professor, Department of OB/GYN, Penn State University College of Medicine, Hershey, Pennsylvania

Lawrence S. Lessin, MD Medical Director, The Washington Cancer Institute at Washington Hospital Center, Washington, DC

Nelson Leung, MD Fellow, Department of Internal Medicine, Mayo Clinic, Rochester, Minnesota

Myron M. Levine, MD, DTPH Professor and Head, Division of Geographic Medicine, Department of Medicine, Professor and Head, Division of Infectious Diseases and Tropical Pediatrics, Department of Pediatrics, Director, Center for Vaccine Development, University of Maryland School of Medicine, Baltimore, Maryland

William C. Levine, MD, MSc Chief, Surveillance and Special Studies Section, Epidemiology and Surveillance Branch, Centers for Disease Control Division of STD Prevention, National Center for HIV, STD, and TB Prevention, Atlanta, Georgia

Sharon Lewin, MD, PhD Post-Doctoral Fellow, Aaron Diamond AIDS Research Center, Rockefeller University, New York, New York

Ronald T. Lewis, MD, MBBS, FRCS Associate Professor of Surgery, McGill University, Montreal, Quebec, Canada

Gary R. Lichtenstein, MD Hospital of the University of Pennsylvania, University of Pennsylvania School of Medicine, Philadelphia, Pennsylvania

Allen S. Lichter, MD Isadore Lampe Professor, Department of Radiation Oncology, University of Michigan Medical Center, Ann Arbor, Michigan

Daniel Lichtstein, MD University of Miami School of Medicine, Division of General Medicine, Miami, Florida

Michael D. Lieberman, MD Division of Pulmonary and Critical Care Medicine, San Francisco General Hospital, San Francisco, California

Marshall D. Lindheimer, MD Professor of Medicine, Ob-Gyn, and Clinical Pharmacology, The University of Chicago, Chicago, Illinois

Lewis A. Lipsitz, MD Associate Professor of Medicine, Harvard Medical School, Vice President of Medical Affairs and Physician-in-Chief, Hebrew Rehabilitation Center for Aged, Boston, Massachusetts

Virginia A. LiVolsi, MD Professor of Pathology and Laboratory Medicine, Vice Chair for Anatomic Pthology, University of Pennsylvania, Philadelphia, Pennsylvania

Maria Llorente, MD Associate Professor, University of Miami School of Medicine, Department of Psychiatry and Behavioral Sciences, Geriatric Research, Evaluation and Clinical Center (GRECC), Miami VA Medical Center, Miami, Florida

Bruce Lobaugh, MD Department of Medicine and Cell Biology, Duke University Medical Center, Durham, North Carolina

Shelly C. Lu, MD Associate Professor of Medicine, USC School of Medicine, Division of Gastrointestinal and Liver Disease, Los Angeles, California

Christopher Y. Lu, MD Professor, Department of Internal Medicine/Nephrology, University of Texas Southwestern Medical Center, and Parkland Memorial Hospital, Dallas, Texas

Bertram H. Lubin, MD Adjunct Professor of Pediatrics, Department of Pediatrics, University of California Medical Center, Director of Medical research, Children's Hospital Oakland Research Institute, Oakland, California

James P. Luby, MD Professor of Internal Medicine, The University of Texas Southwestern Medical Center at Dallas, Parkland Mermorial Hospital, Zale Lipshy University Hospital, Dallas, Texas

John M. Luce, MD Professor of Medicine and Anesthesia, University of California, San Francisco, Associate Director, Medical-Surgical Intensive Care Unit, San Francisco General Hospital, San Francisco, California

Michael R. Lucey, MD Professor of Medicine, Division of Gastroenterology, University of Pennsylvania Medical Center, Philadelphia, Pennsylvania

Benjamin J. Luft, MD Edmund D. Pellegrino Professor, Chairman, Department of Medicine, Stony Brook, New York

Lawrence Lumeng, MD Professor of Medicine and Biochemistry/Molecular Biology, Chief, division of Gastroenterology/Hepatology, Indiana University School of Medicine & VAMC, Indainapolis, Indiana

David Lynch, MD Associate Professor of Radiology and Medicine, University of Colorado Health Sciences Center, Denver, Colorado

Joseph P. Lynch, III, MD Professor of Medicine, University of Michigan Medical Center, Ann Arbor, Michigan

Joanne Lynn, MD, MA, MS Director, The Center to Improve Care of the Dying, George Washington University Medical Center, Washington, DC

David MacDonald, MD Clinical Assistant Professor, University of British Columbia, Vancouver, British Columbia

Phillip A. Mackowiak, MD Chief, Medical Care Clinical Center, VA Maryland Health Care System, Professor and Vice Chairman, Department of Medicine, University of Maryland School of Medicine, Baltimore, Maryland

Adel A.F. Mahmoud, MD, PhD President, Merck Vaccines, Merck & Company, Whitehouse Station, New Jersey

Brian W.J Mahy, PhD, ScD National Center for Infectious Diseases, Adjunct Professor, Emory University, Atlanta, Georgia

Brian F. Mandell, PhD, MD Education Program Director, Rheumatic and Immunologic Diseases, The Cleveland Foundation, Associate Professor of Medicine, Ohio State, University

Erin N. Marcus, MD Assiatant Professor of Medicine, University of Miami School of Medicine, Attending Physician, Jackson Mermorial Hospital, Miami, Florida

Stephen I. Marglin, MD Associate Professor, of Radiology, University of Washington School of Medicine, Seattle, Washington

Russell L Margolis, MD Associate Professor of Psychiatry, Johns Hopkins University School of Medicine, Attending Psychiatrist, Johns Hopkins Hospital, Baltimore, Maryland

John J. Marini, MD   Professor of Medicine, University of Minnesota, Academic Chair of Medicine and Director of Critical Care Programs, Regions Hospital, Minneapolis/St. Paul, Minnesota

Martin Markowitz, MD   Staff Investigator, Aaron Diamond AIDS Research Center, Rockefeller University, New York, New York

John C. Marshall, MD,PhD   Arthur and Margaret Ebbert Professor of Medical Science, Director, Center for Research in Reproduction, University of Virginia Health Sciences Center, Charlottesville, Virginia

Manuel Martinez-Maldonado, MD   President and Dean, Ponce School of Medicine, Ponce, Puerto Rico

Stephen J. Marx, MD   Chief, Genetics abd Endocrinology Section, National Institutes of Health, National Institute of Diabetes and Digestive and Kidney Diseases, Bethesda, Maryland

Henry Masur, MD   Department of Critical Care, National Institutes of Health, Bethesda, Maryland

Gordon O. Matheson, MD, PhD   Associate Professor of Functional Restoration, Stanford Sports Medicine Program, Stanford University School of Medicine, Stanford, California

Michael A. Matthay, MD   Professor of Medicine and Anesthesia, Associate Director, Intensive Care Unit, Senior Associate, Cardiovascular Research Institute, University of California, San Francisco, San Francisco, California

Paul McCaffrey Ford, MD, MS   Assistant Professor of Medicine, Assistant Professor of Functional Restoration (by courtesy), Stanford Sports Medicine Program, Stanford University School of Medicine, Stanford, California

Keith R. McCrae, MD   Associate Professor of Medicine, Hematology/Oncology Division, Case Western Reserve University, School of Medicine, Cleveland, Ohio

Ross E. McKinney, Jr., MD   Associate Professor, Pediatrics, Assistant Professor, Microbiology, Duke University Medical Center, Durham, North Carolina

James A. McLean, MD   Division of Allergy, University of Michigan Medical Center, Ann Arbor, Michigan

Marc McMorris, MD   Clinical Assistant Professor, Division of Allergy/Immunology, Department of Internal Medicine, Department of Pediatrics and Communicable Diseases, The University of Michigan Medical Center, Ann Arbor, Michigan

Robert T. Means, Jr., MD   Professor of Medicine, Associate Chief / Head of Hematology, Medical University of South Carolina; Chief, Hematology/Oncology Section, Ralph H. Johnson VA Medical Center, Charleston, South Carolina

Andrew W. Menzin, MD   Assistant Professor, Obstetrics and Gynecology, New York University School of Medicine, New York, New York

Sofia A. Merajver, MD, PhD   Associate Professor of Internal Medicine, Director, Breast and Ovarian Cancer Risk Evaluation Clinic, University of Michigan Health System, Ann Arbor, Michigan

William W. Merrill, MD   Director, Medicine Service Line, New Orleans VMAC, Professor, Tulane University, New Orleans, Louisiana

Luisa Mestroni, MD, FACC, FESC   Professor of Medicine, Director, Molecular Genetics, University of Colorado Cardiovascular Institute, University of Colorado Health Sciences Center, Aurora, Colorado

David Metz, MD   Assocciate Professor of Medicine, Director, Aeid-Pephe Disease Program, University of Pennsylvania Health Program, Philadelphia, Pennsylvania

Bruce L. Miller, MD   AW & Mary Margaret Clausen Distinguished Professor of Neurology, University of California, San Franscisco, San Francisco, California

Richard A. Miller, MD, PhD   Associate Director, Geriatrics Center, University of Michigan Medical Center, Ann Arbor, Michigan

Alberto A. Mitrani, MD   Associate Professor of Medicine, University of Miami School of Medicine, Miami, Florida

Ronald T. Mitsuyasu, MD   Associate Professor of Medicine, University of California, Los Angeles, Director, UCLA Center for Clinical AIDS Research and Education, Los Angeles, California

Bruce A. Molitoris, MD   Professor of Medicine, Director, Division of Nephrology, Indiana University Medical Center, Indiana, Indiana

Rebeca D. Monk, MD   Assistant Professor of Medicine, University of Rochester School of Medicine, Nephrology Unit, Strong Memorial Hospital, Rochester, New York

James Montie, MD   George F. and Nancy P. Valassis Professor of Urologic Oncology, Section Head, Urology-Surgery Section, University of Michigan, Ann Arbor, Michigan

Malcom A.S. Moore, D.Phil.   Enid A. Haupt Professor of Cell Biology, Head, James Ewing Laboratory of Developemental Hematopoiesis, Memorial Sloan-Kettering Cancer Center, New York, New York

Fred Morady, MD   Division of Cardiology, Department of Internal Medicine, University of Michigan, Ann Arbor, Michigan

Mark A. Morgan, MD   Associate Professor, Division of Gynocologic Oncology, University of Pennsylvania Medical Center, Philadelphia, Pennsylvania

J. Glenn Morris Jr., MD   Professor of Medicine, University of Maryland School of Medicine, Baltimore, Maryland

Lori J. Mosca, MD, MPH, PhD   Assistant Professor, University of Michigan, Director, Preventive Cardiology Research and Educational Programs Medsport, Ann Arbor, Michigan

Richard H. Moseley, MD   Associate Professor of Medicine, University of Michigan Medical School, Chief, Medical Servicer VA Medical Center, Ann Arbor, Michigan

George F. Moxley, MD   Associate Professor of Internal Medicine, Virginia Commonwealth University, Richmond., Chief, Rheumatology Section, McGuire VAMC, Richmond, Virginia

Robert R. Muder, MD   Hospital Epidemiologist, VA Pittsburgh Healthcare System, Associate Professor of Medicine, University of Pittsburgh School of Medicine, Pittsburgh, Pennsylvania

Michael W. Mulholland, PhD   Department of Surgery, University of Michigan Medical Center, Ann Arbor, Michigan

Albert G. Mulley, PhD   Chief, General Medicine Division, Massachusetts General Hospital, Associate Professor of Medicine, Harvard Medical School, Boston, Massachusetts

Mark Multach, MD   Associate Professor and Chief, Division of General Internal Medicine, Vice Chair, Department of Medicine, University of Miami School of Medicine, Miami, Florida

Alfred Munzer, MD   Clinical Assistant Professor of Medicine, Georgetown University School of Medicine, Co-Director, Pulminary Medicine, Washington Adventist Hospital, Takoma Park, Maryland

Jonathan N. Myers, PhD   Clinical Assistant Professor of Medicine, Stanford University, Palo Alto Health Care System, Palo Alto, California

Naiel N. Nassar, MD   Medical Director, Center for AIDS Research, Education and Services (CARES), Assistant Professor of Clinical Medicine, Division of Infectious and Immunologic Diseases, University of California, Davis Medical Center, Sacramento, California

Karl A. Nath, MD   Department of Internal Medicie, Division of Nephrology, Mayo Clinic, Rochester, Minnesota

Eric G. Neilson, MD   Hugh J. Morgan Professor and Chairman, Department of Medicine, Vanderbilt, University Medical Center, Nashville, Tennessee

Lee S. Newman, MD, MA   Head, Division of Environmental and Occupational Health Sciences, National Jewish Medical and Research Center:, Department of Medicine and Department of Preventive Medicine and Biometrics, Division of Pulmonary Medicine, University of Colorado School of Medicine, Denver, Colorado

Michael S. Niederman, MD   Winthrop-University Hospital, SUNY at Stony Brook, Mineola, New York

Larry Norton, MD   Associate Professor, Memorial Sloan-Kettering Cancer Center, New York, New York

Gary Noskin, MD   Associate Professor of Medicine, Northwestern University Medical School, Medical Director, Infection Control, Healthcare Epidemiologist, Northwestern Memorial Hospital, Chicago, Illinois

Sogol Nowbar, MD   Instructor of Medicine, University of Colorado Health Science Center, Denver, Colorado

Peter C. Nowell, MD   Professor of Pathology and Laboratory Medicine, University of Pennsylvania Medical School, Philadelphia, Pennsylvania

Frederick A. Nunes, MD   Gastroenterology Division, University of Pennsylvania Health System, Philadelphia, Pennsylvania

William O'Brian, MD   Chief, AIDS Pathogenesis Research Program, Department of Internal Medicine, The University of Texas Medical Branch, Galveston, Texas

Charles P. O'Brien, MD, PhD   Professor and Vice Chair, Department of Psychiatry, University of Pennsylvania Medical Center, Chief of Psychiatry, Veterans Affairs Medical Center, Philadelphia, Pennsylvania

Mark O'Connell, MD   Associate Professor of Medicine, Division of General Internal Medicine, Senior Associate Dean, Medical Education, University of Miami School of Medicine, Miami, Florida

Patrick T. O'Gara, MD   Director, Clinical Cardiology, Cardiovascular Division, Vice Chairman, Clinical Affairs, Department of Medicine, Assistant Professor of Medicine, Brigham & Women's Hospital, Boston, Massachusetts

Glen S. O'Sullivan, MD   Assistant Professor, Orthopaedic Surgery, Stanford University School of Medicine, Stanford, California

Pablo C. Okhuysen, MD   Division of Infectious Diseases, The University of Texas- Houston Medical School, Houston, Texas

Eric Olson, MD   Assistant Professor of Medicine, Mayo Medical School, Consultant, Division of Pulmonary and Critical Care Medicine, Mayo Clinic, Rochester, Minnesota

Walter A. Orenstein, MD   Director, National Immunization Program, Centers for Disease Control and Prevention, Atlanta, Georgia

Joseph G. Ouslander, MD   Professor of Medicine, Vice President for Professional Affairs, Wesley Woods Center of Emory University, Director, Atlanta VA Rehabilitation Research And Development Center, Atlanta, Georgia

Chung Owyang, MD   Gastroenterology Division, University of Michigan Medical Center, Ann Arbor, Michigan

Michael N. Oxman, MD   Professor of Medicine and Pathology, University of California, San Diego, Staff Physician, Infectious Diseases Section, Veterans Affairs Medical Center, San Diego, California

Emil P. Paganini, MD, FACP, FRCP   Professor of Clinical Medicine, The Cleveland Clinic Foundation, Head, Section of Dialysis and Extracorporeal Therapy, Cleveland, Ohio

Joseph S. Pagano, MD   Lineberger Professor of Cancer Research and Director Emeritus, Lineberger Comprehensive Cancer Center, University of North Carolina School of Medicine, Chapel Hill, North Carolina

Patricia Paredes-Casillas, MD, MTM   Professor of Tropical Diseases, Center for the Health Sciences, University of Guadalajara, Staff Member, Preventive Medicine Service, Antiguo Hospital Civil de Guadalajara, Guadalajara, Jalisco, Mexico

Mario Paredes-Espinoza, MD   Professor of Medicine, Center for the Health Sciences, University of Guadalajara, Chief, Internal Medicine Service, Antiguo Hospital Civil de Guadalajara, Guadalajara, Jalisco, Mexico

Roberta Parillo, MHA   Adjunct Assistant Professor, Department of Medicine, University of Miami, Miami, Florida

Henry P. Parkman, MD   Associate Professor of Medicine and Physiology, Temple University School of Medicine, Philadelphia, Pennsylvania

Helen Pass, MD   Assistant Professor of Surgery, Director, Breast Care Center, University of Michigan Health System, Ann Arbor, Michigan

Thomas F. Patterson, MD   Department of Medicine, UT Health Science Center at San Antoinio, San Antonio, Texas

Jan Evans Patterson, MD   Professor of Medicine (Infectious diseases) and Pathology, University of Texas Health Science Center, Hospital Epidemiologist, University Health System and South Texas Veterans Health Care System, San Antonio, Texas

Donald W. Paty   Division of Neurology, University of British Columbia, Vancouver, British Columbia, Canada

Laurence D. Petz, MD   Professor, Pathology and Laboratory Medicine, University of California, Los Angeles, Co-Director, Division of Transfusion Medicine, UCLA Medical Center, Los Angeles, California

David G. Pfister, MD   Associate Professor, Cornell University-Weill Medical College, Asociate Attending Physician, Memorial Sloan-Kettering Cancer Center, New York, New York

Anne K. Pflieger, MD   Epidemiology Unit, Centers for Disease Control and Prevention, Atlanta, Georgia

John P. Phair, MD   Professor of Medicine, Chief, division of Infectiuos Disease, Director, Comprehensive AIDS Center, Northwestern University Medical School and Northwestern Memorial Hospital, Chicago, Illinois

Michele R. Piccone, MD   Assistant Professor of Ophthalmology, Director of Medical Student Teaching, University of Pennsylvania Health System, Scheie Eye Institute, Philadelphia, Pennsylvania

Kenneth Pienta, MD   Professor, Internal Medicine and Surgery, University of Michigan, Ann Arbor, Michigan

Theodore Pincus, MD   Professor of Medicine and Microbiology, Division of Rheumatology and Immunology, Vanderbilt University School of Medicine, Nashville, Tennessee

Andrew G. Plaut, MD   Staff Physician, Tufts New England Medical Center, Professor of Medicine, Tufts University School of Medicine, Boston, Massachusetts

Daniel K. Podolsky, MD   Mallinckrodt Professor of Medicine, Harvard Medical School, Chief, Gastrointestinal Unit, Massachusetts General Hospital, Boston, Massachusetts

Paula Podrazik, MD   Division of Clinical Pharmacology and Geriatric Medicine, Northwestern University Medical School, Chicago, Illinois

Gerald M. Pohost, MD   Mary Gertrude Waters Professor of Cardiovascular Medicine, University of Alabama at Birmingham, Birmingham, Alabama

Karen M. Prestwood, MD   Assistant Professor of Medicine, Center on Aging, University of Connecticut Health Center, Farmington, Connecticut

Richard W. Price, MD   Professor and Vice-Chair, Department of Neurology, University of California, San Francisco, Chief, Neurology Service, San Francisco General Hospital, San Francisco, California

Daniel J. Rader, MD   Director, Preventive Cardiology, University of Pennsylvania Health System, University of Pennsylvania School of Medicine, Hospital of the University of Pennsylvania, Presbyterian Medical Center, Philadelphia, Pennsylvania

Eric L. Radin, MD   The Breech Chair, Director, Bone and Joint Center, Henry Ford Hospital, Detroit, Michigan

Justin Radolf, MD   Director, Center for Microbial Pathogenesis, Professor of Medicine and Microbiology, University of Connecticut Health Center, Farmington, Connecticut

Derek Raghavan, MD, PhD   USC Norris Comprehensive Cancer Center, Los Angeles, California

Joel S. Raichlen, MD Clinical Professor of Medicine, Jefferson Medical College, Thomas Jefferson University, Director, Noninvasive Cardiology, Thomas Jefferson University Hospital, Philadelphia, Pennsylvania

Joel M. Rappeport, MD Professor of Medicine and Pediatrics, Yale School of Medicine, New Haven, Connecticut

Stephen Reich, MD Associate Professor, Neurology, The Johns Hopkins University School of Medicine, Baltimore, Maryland

David B. Reuben, MD Chief, Division of Geriatrics, Director, Multicampus Program in Geriatric Medicine and Gernontology, Professor of Medicine, UCLA School of Medicine, Los Angeles, California

John H. Rex, MD, FACP Associate Professor of Medicine, Univeristy of Texax Medical School, Houston, Medical Director for Epidemiology, Herman Hospital, Houston, Texas

Juan Reyes, Esq. Fowler-White, Miami, Florida

Robert M. A. Richardson, MD Professor of Medicine, University of Toronto, Director of Hemodialysis, The Toronto Hospital, Toronto, Canada

John R. Richert, MD Professor and Chair, Department of Microbiology and Immunology, Professor of Neurology, Georgetown University Medical Center, Washington, DC

Joel E. Richter, MD, FACP, FACG Chairman, Department of Gastroenterology, The Cleveland Clinic Foundation, Professor of Medicine, The Cleveland Clinic Foundation, Health Sciences Center for the Ohio State University, Cleveland, Ohio

Andrew L. Ries, MD, MPH Professor of Medicine, University of California, San Diego, San Diego, California

Ian R. Rifkin, MD, PhD Assistant Professor of Medicine, Boston University School of Medicine, Renal Section, Boston Medical Center, Boston, Massachusetts

Yehuda Ringel, MD Dpartment of Gastroenterology, Tel-Aviv Soutasky Medical Center, Sacklen School of Medicine, Tel-Aviv University, Tel-Aviv, Israel

Marc L. Rivo, MD, MPH Medical Director for Outpatient Care, AuMed Health Plan of Florida, Clinical Professor of Medicine, University of Miami School of Medicine, Medical Editor, Family Practice Management, Senoir Scholar, Center for the Health Professions University of California, San Francisco

Robert Roberts, MD Don W. Chapman Professor of Medicine, Professor of Cell Biology, Peofessor of Molecular Physiology and Biophysics, Chief of Cardiology, Director, Bugher Foundation Center for Molecular Biology, Houston, Texas

Norbert J. Roberts, Jr., MD Professor of Internal Medicine and Microbiology and Immunology, Director, Division of Infectious Diseases, The University of Texas Medical Branch, Galveston, Texas

Jean E. Robillard, MD Chair, Pediatrics and Communicable Diseases, University of Michigan Medical School, Ann Arbor, Michigan

Alan G. Robinson, MD Vice Provost, Medical Sciences, Executive Associate Dean, UCLA School of Medicine, Los Angeles, California

Kenneth V.I. Rolston, MD The University of Texas, M.D., Anderson Cancer Center, Houston, Texas

Allen R. Ronald, MD, FRCPC, FACP Distinguished Professor Emeritus, The University of Manitoba, Infectious Disease Consultant, St. Boniface Hospital, Winnepeg, Manitoba, Canada

Cecile S. Rose, MD,MPH Division of Environmental and Occupational Health Sciences, National Jewish Medical and Research Center:, Department of Medicine and Department of Preventive Medicine and Biometrics, Division of Pulmonary Medicine, University of Colorado School of Medicine, Denver, Colorado

Linda Rosenstock, MD NIOSH, Washington, DC

Christopher A. Ross, MD, PhD Professor of Psychiatry and Neuroscience, Johns Hopkins University School of Medicine, Attending Psychiatrist, Johns Hopkins Hospital, Baltimore, Maryland

Lewis J. Rubin, MD Professor of Medicine, Director, Division of Pulminary and Critical Care Medicine, Director, Pulminary Vascular Center, University of California, San Diego School of Medicine, San Diego, California

Stephen C. Rubin, MD Professor, Obstetrics and Gynecology, Chief, Division of Gynecologic Oncology, University of Pennsylvania Health System, Philadelphia, Pennsylvania

Charles E. Rupprecht, VMD, MS, PhD Director, World Health Organization, Collaborating Center for Reference and Reasearch on Rabies, Centers for Disease Control and Prevention, Atlanta, Georgia

Anil K. Rustgi, MD T. Grier Miller Associate Professor of Medicine and Genetics, Chief of Gastroenterology, University of Pennsylvania, Philadelphia, Pennsylvania

Thomas Ryan, MD Associate Professor of Medicine, Duke University Medical Center, Durham, North Carolina

Alice S. Ryan, PhD Assistant Professor, University of Maryland School of Medicine, Baltimore VA Medical Center, Baltimore, Maryland

John D. Rybock, MD   Assistant Professor, Neurological Surgery, The Johns Hopkins School of Medicine, Attending Neurosurgeon, The Johns Hopkins Hospital, Baltimore, Maryland

Michael Saccente, MD   Assistant Professor of Medicine, University of Arkansas for Medical Sciences, John L. McClellan Memorial Veterans Hospital, Little Rock, Arkansas

Steven A. Sahn, MD   Professor of Medicine, Director, Division of Pulmonary and Critical Care Medicine, Allergy and Clinical Immunology, Charleston, South Carolina

Paul Sakiewicz, MD   Cleveland Clinic Foundation, Cleveland, Ohio

David J. Salant, MD   Professor of Medicine, Boston University School of Medicine, Chief, Renal Section, Boston Medical Center, Boston, Massachussets

Robert A. Salata, MD   Professor of Medicine, Case Western Reserve University, Chief and Clinical Director, Division of Infectious Diseases, Department of Medicine, University Hospitals of Cleveland, Cleveland, Ohio

Paul W. Sanders, MD   Professor of Medicine, University of Alabama, Chief, Renal Section, Veterans Affairs Medical Center, Birmingham, Alabama

Dennis Schaberg, MD   Professor and Chairman, Department of Medicine, University of Tennessee-Memphis, Memphis, Tennessee

Jeffrey R. Schelling, MD   Assistant Professor of Medicine, Case Western University, Cleveland, Ohio

Charles J. Schleupner, MS, MD   Professor of Internal Medicine, University of North Carolina School of Medicine, Chapel Hill, North Carolina

Alvin H. Schmaier, MD   Professor of Internal Medicine and Pathology, Director, Coagulation Laboratory, Ann Arbor, Michigan

George P. Schmid, MD, MSc   Medical Epidemiologist, Division of STD Prevention, Centers for Disease Control and Prevention, Atlanta, Georgia

Robert B. Schoene, MD   University of Washington School of Medicine, Department of Medicine, Division of Pulmonary and Critical Medicine, Seattle, Washington

Anton C. Schoolwerth, MD, MSHA   Division of Nephrology, Medical College of Virginia, Richmond, Virginia

David Schottenfeld, MD, MSc   John G. Searl Professor of Epidemiology, Professor of Internal Medicine, University of Michigan, Ann Arbor, Michigan

Kathleen S. Schrank, MD   Professor of Medicine, Chief, Division of Emergency Medicine, University of Miami School of Medicine, Emergency Care Center Educational Coordinator and EMS Medical Director, Jackson Memorial Hospital, Miami, Florida

David E. Schteingart, MD   Division of Endocrinology, University of Michigan, Ann Arbor, Michigan

Lynn M. Schuchter, MD   Associate Professor, Department of Medicine, University of Pennsylvania, Department of Hematology/Oncology, Hospital of the University of Pennsylvania, Philadelphia, Pennsylvania

Christopher F. Schutlz, MD   Department of Medicine, University of Pennsylvania School of Medicine, Philadelphia, Pennsylvania

Benjamin Schwartz   Deputy Director, Epidemiology and Surveillance Division, National Immunization Program, Centers for Disease Control and Prevention, Atlanta, Georgia

Janice B. Schwartz, MD   Professor of Medicine, Chief, Clinical Pharmacology and Geriatric Medicine, Northwestern University Medical School, Chicago, Illinois

Robert S. Schwartz, MD   Head, Division of Geriatric Medicine, Goodstein Professor of Medicine and Geriatrics, University of Colorado Health Sciences Center, Denver, Colorado

David A. Schwarz, MD   Professor, University of Iowa, Iowa City, Iowa

Ilias Scotiniotis, MD   Instructor in Medicine, Gastroenterology Division, University of Pennsylvania Health System, Philadelphia, Pennsylvania

John R. Sedor, MD   Professor of Medicine and Physiology & Biophysics, Case Western University, Director, Division of Nephrology, MetroHealth Medical Center, Cleveland, Ohio

Stanton Segal, MD   Professor of Pediatrics and Medicine, Department of Pediatrics and Medicine, University of Pennsylvania, Division of Biochemical Development and Molecular Diseases, The Children's Hospital of Philadelphia, Philadelphia, Pennsylvania

James R. Seibold, MD   Professor and Director, Sclerdoma Program, UMDNJ-Robert Wood Johnson Medical School, New Brunswick, New Jersey

Carol E. Semrad, MD   Columbia University College of Physicians and Surgeons, Department of Medicine, New York, New York

F. John Service, MD, PhD   Professor of Medicine, Mayo Medical School, Rochester, Minnesota

Brahm Shapiro, MB, ChB, PhD Professor of Internal Medicine, Division of Nuclear Medicine, Department of Internal Medicine, University of Michigan Medical Center and Nuclear Medicine Service, Ann Arbor Veterans Affairs Medical Center, Ann Arbor, Michigan

Sanford J. Shattil, MD Professor, Department of Vascular Biology, Scripps Research Institute, La Jolla, California

James A. Shayman, MD Professor of Internal Medicine and Pharmacology, Associate Chair for Research Programs, Department of Internal Medicine, University of Michigan, Ann Arbor, Michigan

Judith A. Shizuru, MD, Ph.D. Assistant Professor of Medicine, Stanford University School of Medicine, Bone Marrow Transplant Program, Stanford, California

Dolores M. Shoback, MD Associate Professor of Medicine, Department of Medicine, University of California, San Francisco, Staff Physician, San Francisco Department of Veterans Affairs Medical Center, San Francisco, California

Edward H. Shortliffe, MD, PhD Professor and Chair, Department of Medical Informatics, Columbia College of Physicians and Surgeons, New York, New York

David J. Shulkin, MD Associate Professor of Medicine, University of Pennsylvania School of Medicine, Philadelphia, Pennsylvania

Mark Siegler, MD University of Chicago Hospital, Chicago, Illinois

Kathy E. Sietsema, MD Associate Professor of Medicine, UCLA School of Medicine, Harbor-UCLA Medical Center, Torrance, California

Leonard H. Sigal, MD Professor and Chief, Division of Rheumatology, Department of Medicine, UMDNJ- Robert Wood Johnson Medical School, Chief, Rheumatology Service, Robert Wood Johnson University Hospital, New Brunswick, New Jersey

Richard Simon, D.Sc. Chief, Biometric Research, National Cancer Institute, Rockville, Maryland

Peter A. Singer, MD University of Pennsylvania, Philadelphia, Pennsylvanis

Jeffrey D. Sklar, MD Department of Pathology, Brigham and Women's Hospital, Boston, Massachussetts

Jay S. Skyler, MD Professor of Medicine, Pediatrics and Psychology, University of Miami, Miami, Florida

Gail B. Slap, MD Rauh Professor of Pediatrics and Internal Medicine, University of Cincinnati College of Medicine, Director, Division of Adolescent Medicine, Children's Hospital Medical Center, Cincinnati, Ohio

Raymond A. Smego, Jr., MD, MPH, FACP, DTM&H The Ibne-e-Sina Professor and Chair, Department of Medicine, Aga Khan University Medical College, Karachi, Pakistan

C. Daniel Smith, MD Associate Professor of Surgery, Chief, General and Gastrointestinal Surgery, Emory University School of Medicine, Atlanta, Georgia

Robert J. Smith, MD Chief, Section on Metabolism, Joslin Diabetes Center, Associate Professor of Medicine, Harvard Medical School, Boston, Massachusetts

David C. Smith, MD Associate Professor, Department of Internal Medicine, University of Michigan School of Medicine, Medical Director, Multidisciplinary Urologic Oncology Clinic, University of Michigan Comprehensive Cancer Center, Ann Arbor, Michigan

John W. Smith, II, MD Chief, Clinical Research, Robert W. Franz Cancer Research Center, Earle A. Chiles Research Institute, Providence Portland Medical Center, Portland, Oregon

Peter J. Snyder, MD Professor of Medicine, Department of Medicine, Division of Endocrinology, Diabetes & Metabolism, University of Pennsylvania Medical Center, Philadelphia, Pennsylvania

Jay Sosenko, MD Professor of Medicine, University of Miami School of Medicine, Miami, Florida

Ulrich Specks, MD Associate Professor of Medicine, Mayo Medical School, Rochester, Minnesota

Martin G. St. John Sutton, MBBS Hospital of the University of Pennsylvania, Philadelphia, Pennsylvania

James C. Stanley, MD Professor of Surgery, Head, Section of Vascular Surgery, University of Michigan Medical Center, Ann Arbor, Michigan

Robert B. Stein, MD Assistant Professor of Medicine, Department of Medicine, Division of Gastroenterology, University of Pennsylvania School of Medicine, Philadelphia, Pennsylvania

Kenneth P. Steinberg, MD University of Washington, Seattle, Washington

William F. Stenson, MD Professor of Medicine, Washington University School of Medicine, St. Louis, Missouri

Charmaine A. Stewart, MD Assistant Professor of Medicine, Division of Gastroenterology, University of Pennsylvania Medical Center, Philadelphia, Pennsylvania

Mary M. Stimmler, MD Associate Professor of Clinical Medicine, Department of Rheumatology and Clinical Immunology, University of Southern California School of Medicine, Los Angeles, California

Andrew Stolz, MD Associate Professor of Medicine, Hoffman Medical Research, Los Angeles, California

Diane E. Stover, MD   Chief of Pulmonary Service, Memorial Sloan Kettering Cancer Center, Professor of Clinical Medicine, Weill Medical College of Cornell University, New York, New York

Albert J. Stunkard, MD   Professor of Psychiatry, University of Pennsylvania, Philadelphia, Pennsylvania

Oksana Suchowersky, MD, FRCPC, FCCMG   Clinical Professor, Departments of Clinical Neurosciences and Medical Genetics, Foothills Hospital and University of Calgary, Calgary, Alberta, Canada

Suzanne K. Swan, MD   Associate Professor of Medicine, Division of Nephrology, Hennepin County Medical Center, University of Minnesota School of Medicine, Minneapolis, Minnesota

Vincent P. Sweeney, MB, ChB, FRCPC   Vancouver Hospital and Health Sciences Center, Vancouver, British Columbia, Canada

Susan M. Swetter, MD   Assistant Professor, Department of Dermatology, Stanford University Medical Center, Assistant Chief, Dermatology Service, VA Palo Alto Health Care System, Stanford, California

Zoltan Szekanecz, MD, PhD   Senior Assistant Professor of Medicine, Immunology, and Rheumatology, Third Department of Medicine, University Medical School of Debrecen, Debrecen, Hungary

Robert D. Tarver, MD   Indiana University School of Medicine, Department of Radiology, Indianapolis, Indiana

Robert V. Tauxe, MD, MPH   Chief, Foodborne and Diarrheal Diseases BranchNational Center for Infectious Diseases, Centers for Disease Control and Prevention, Atlanta, Georgia

J. Lisa Tenover, MD, PhD   Chief of Medicine, Wesley Woods Hospital, Associate Professor, Division of Geriatric Medicine and Gerontology, Department of Medicine, Emory University School of Medicine, Atlanta, Georgia

Abba I. Terr, MD   Clinical Professor of Medicine, Stanford University Medical School, Stanford, California

Erica R. Thaler, MD   Assistant Professor, Department of Otorhinolaryngology: Head and Neck Surgery, Hospital of the University of Pennsylvania, Philadelphia, Pennsylvania

Cheleste Thorpe, MD   Division of Geographic Medicine, New England Medical Center, Boston, Massachussetts

Mary E. Tinetti, MD   Professor, Medicine and Epidemiology and Public Health, Chief, Program in Geriatrics, Yale University School of Medicine, New Haven, Connecticut

Sheldon Tobe, MD, FRCPC   Assistant Professor of Medicine, University of Toronto, Acting Director, Division of Nephrology, Sunnybrook and Women's College Health Sciences Centre, Toronto, Ontario, Canada

Robert F. Todd, III, MD, PhD   Professor of Internal Medicine, Chief, Division of Hematology and Oncology, University of Michigan Medical School, Ann Arbor, Michigan

Galen B. Toews, MD   Professor and Chief of Pulminary& Critical Care Medicine, University of Michigan Pulmonary Division, Ann Arbor, Michigan

John E. Tomaszewski, MD   Professor of Pathology and Labotatory Medicine, University of Pennsylvania School of Medicine, Director of Surgical Pathology, University of Pennsylvania Medical Center, Philadelphia, Pennsylvania

Stephen W. Trenkner, MD   Associate Professor of Radiology, Department of Radiology, University of Minnesota Medical School, Minneapolis, Minnesota

Mark C. Udey, MD, PhD   Senior Investigator, Dermatology Branch, National Cancer Institute, Bethesda, Maryland

Walter J. Urba, MD   Director, Cancer Research, Robert W. Franz Cancer Research Center, Earle A. Chiles Research Institute, Providence Portland Medical Center, Portland, Oregon

Ronald F. van Vollenhoven, MD, PhD   Chief, Inpatient Unit, Department of Rheumatology, Karolinska Hospital, Stockholm, Sweden

Mary Lee Vance, MD   Professor of Medicine, University of Virginia Health System, Charlottesville, Virginia

Carl J. Vaughan, MD   Cardiology Division, Weill Medical College of Cornell University, The New York Presbyterian Hospital-Cornell Medical Center, New York, New York

David J. Vaughn, MD   Associate Professor of Medicine, University of Pennsylvania School of Medicine, Hematology/Oncology Division, Hospital of the University Of Pennsylvania, Philadelphia, Pennsylvania

Martin Vazquez, MD   Department of Dermatology, Palo Alto Veterans Healthcare System, Palo Alto, California

Abraham Verghese, MD   Professor of Medicine, Texas Tech University, El Paso, Texas

Emanuel N. Vergis, MD   Assistant Professor, Department of Medicine, University of Pittsburgh School of Medicine, University of Pittsburgh Medical Center, VA Medical Center, Pittsburgh, Pennsylvania

Julie M. Vose, MD   Professor of Medicine, Department of Internal Medicine, University of Nebraska Medical Center, Omaha, Nebraska

Mark F. Walker, M.D.   Instructor, Department of Neurology and Ophthalmology, Johns Hopkins University School of Medicine, Baltimore, Maryland

Jeffrey I. Wallace, MD, MPH   Assistant Professor, Division of Gerontology and Geriatric Medicine, University of Washington School of Medicine, Seattle, Washington

Richard Wallace, Jr., MD   Chairman, Department of Microbiology, The University of Texas Health Center at Tyler, Tyler, Texas

Ralph O. Wallerstein, MD   Clinical Professor Emeritus, Department of Medicine, UCSF, San Francisco, California

John H. Walsh, MD   Professor of Medicine, UCLA School of Medicine, Los Angeles, California

Jeremy Walston, MD   The Johns Hopkins Medical Institutions, Baltimore, Maryland

Stewart C. Wang, MD, PhD   Assistant Professor of Surgery, Trauma, Burns, and Emergency Surgery, University of Michigan Medical Center, Ann Arbor, Michigan

Michael M. Ward, MD   Assistant Professor Department of Medicine, Stanford University School of Medicine, Stanford, California

Leonard Wartofsky, MD, MPH   Professor of Medicine and Physiology, Uniformed Services University of the Health Sciences, Clinical Professor of Medicine, Georgetown, Howard, and George Washington University Schools of Medicine, Chairman, Department of Medicine, Washington Hospital Center, Washington, DC

Ronald Washburn, MD   Chief, Infectious Diseases University of Nevada School of Medicine and, Reno VA Medical Center, Reno, Nevada

Myron H. Weinberger, MD   Professor of Medicine, Director, Hypertension Research Center, Indiana University Medical Center, Indianapolis, Indiana

Joan Weinryb   Clinical Assistant Professor of Medicine, University of Pennsylvania, Division of Geriatric Medicine, Ralston-Penn Center, Philadelphia, Pennsylvania

Carolyn H. Welsh, MD   Associate Professor of Medicine, Pulmonary Sciences, and Critical Care Medicine, Denver Veterans Affairs Medical Center, University of Colorado Health Sciences Center, Denver, Colorado

Sally Wenzel, MD   Associate Professor of Medicine, National Jewish Medical and Research Center, University of Colorado Health Sciences Center, Denver, Colorado

Ernest A. Weymuller, MD   University of Washington, Seattle, Washington

Melinda Wharton   Centers for Disease Control and Prevention, Atlanta, Georgia

David P. White, MD   Associate Professor of Medicine, Harvard Medical School, Director, Sleep Disorders Program, Brigham and Women's Hospital, Boston, Massachussets

A. Clinton White, Jr., MD   Associate Professor, Baylor College of Medicine, Houston, Texas

Max S. Wicha, MD   Distinguished Professor of Oncology, Professor of Internal Medicine, Director, University of Michigan Comprehensive Cancer Center, Ann Arbor, Michigan

Peter H. Wiernik, MD   Professor Departments of Medicne and Radiation Medicine, New York Medical College, Valhall, New York

Jo Wiggins, BM, BCh, MRCP   Lecturer in Geriatric Medicine, University of Michigan School of Medicine, Ann Arbor, Michigan

Stephen D. Williams, MD, PhD   Director, Indiana University Cancer Center, Indianapolis, Indiana

James M. Wilson, MD, PhD   Director, Institute for Human Gene Therapy, John Herr Musser Professor and Chair, Department of Molecular and Cellular Engineering, Professor of Medicine and Chief, Division of Medical Genetics, University of Pennsylvania Health System, Professor of the Wistar Institute, Philadelphia, Pennsylvania

Robert Winchester, MD   Professorof Pediatrics, Medicine and Pathology, Columbia University, New York, New York

Julie Anne Winfield, BSN, MD   Clinical Professor, Dermatology, Stanford University College of Medicine, Palo Alto, California

Murray Wittner, MD, PhD   Professor, Pathology, Parasitology, Tropical Medicine, Albert Einstein College of Medicine, Attending Physician, Jacobi Medical Center, New York, New York

Jerry S. Wolinsky, MD   Professor of Neurology, University of Texas Health Science Center, Houston, Texas

Judi M. Woolger, MD   Assistant Professor of Medicine, University of Miami, School of Medicine, Director, Medical Consultation Service, Miami, Florida

James O. Woolliscroft, MD   Professor of Internal Medicine, Josiah Macy Jr. Professor of Medical Education, Executive Associate Dean, University of Michigan Medical Center, Ann Arbor, Michigan

Robert L. Wortmann, MD   Professor and Chairman, Department of Internal Medicine, The University of Oklahoma-Tulsa, Tulsa, Oklahoma

Cameron D. Wright, MD   Associate Professor of Surgery, Harvard Medical School, Boston, Massachussets

David J. Wyler, MD   Geographic Medicine/ID Division, New England Medical Center, Boston, Massachussets

Eric W. Young, MD   Associate Professor of Internal Medicine, VA Medical Center, Ann Arbor, Michigan

Edward J. Young, MD   Professor of Medicine, Baylor College of Medicine, Houston, Texas

Victor L. Yu, MD   Division of Infectious Disease, University of Pittsburgh, Pittsburgh, Pennsylvania

David Zee, MD   Departments of Neurology, Ophthalmology, Otolaryngology - Head and Neck Surgery, and Neuroscience, Johns Hopkins University School of Medicine, Baltimore, Maryland

Gillian Zeldin, MD   Assistant Professor of Medicine, Hospital of the University of Pennsylvania, Philadelphia, Pennsylvania

Barry J. Zeluff, MD   The E.L. Wagner, M.D. Volunteer Faculty Professor of Internal Medicine, Baylor College of Medicine, Associate Chief and Program Director, Internal Medicine Service, St. Luke's Episcopal Hospital, Houston, Texas

Leslie H. Zimmerman, MD   Associate Professor of Clinical Medicine, University of California at San Francisco, Medical Director, ICU at the San Francisco Veterans Administration Medical Center, San Francisco, California

Fuad N. Ziyadeh, MD   Professor of Medicine, Renal-Electrolyte and Hypertension Division, Penn Center for Molecular Studies of Kidney Diseases, Philadelphia, Pennsylvania

Clifford W. Zwillich, MD   Professor of Medicine, University of Colorado School of Medicine, Department of Medicine, Vice Chairman, Chief Medical Services, Denver VA Medical Center, Denver, Colorado

PREFACE

In just over ten years, the *Textbook of Internal Medicine* has become widely regarded as a classic medical text, both for its breadth of coverage and ease of use by busy students and practitioners. Hundreds of talented individuals contributed to the success of the first three editions. These include the many leading scientists and scholars who served as editors and authors, and the dozens of supporting staff who met the organizational and logistical challenges associated with so large a publishing endeavor.

In this new 4th edition, the present editorial board has strived to maintain the high standards of excellence set forth by its predecessors. Seven of the eleven section editors are new to this project and have demonstrated the highest degree of professionalism and commitment in their new roles. The new Editors include Laurence B. Gardner, Principles of Medical Practice; Elizabeth G. Nabel, Cardiology; Peter G. Traber, Gastroenterology; Robert F. Todd, III, Oncology and Hematology; Talmadge E. King, Jr., Pulmonary and Critical Care Medicine; Lynn D. Loriaux, Endocrinology; Metabolism, and Genetics; and John W. Griffin, Neurology. With the addition of these new Editors, several sections have been substantially reorganized to improve content and accessibility.

We are proud to add many more new contributors representing a wide range of specialties—their expertise has immensely enriched the *Textbook*. We are greatly indebted to their efforts and to the fine work of the many authors of the present edition who were repeat contributors.

The organization of the *Textbook* continues to emphasize the quick reference needs of the student and clinician seeking cogent solutions to real world medical problems everyday.

Each major section includes a series of "Approach to the Patient" chapters focusing on evaluation and work-up of major presenting problems and clinical syndromes—the problems most often seen by the student or physician on the ward or by the "front-line" physician in a primary care practice.

The descriptions of specific disease entities are complete, to the point, and eminently practical, with "Indications for Referral" and "Indications for Hospitalization" cited wherever relevant for quick reference to these key decision points in pressing situations.

Each major section also includes chapters discussing diagnostic and therapeutic modalities. These technique-oriented chapters focus particularly on cost-effective use of the technology of medicine today.

The *Textbook* is the flagship of a series of products published by Lippincott, Williams & Wilkins designed to be responsive to the changing needs of medical students and practitioners. Related products include the *Rapid Access Guide*, a distillation of the key facts about diseases or conditions commonly encountered in the clinical setting. Conspicuously located at the front of the main volume and indexed on the inside covers, the *Guide* permits the quick retrieval of basic presentation, diagnosis, and other information. It is also separately available in a handy pocket-size format. The new edition, superbly edited by Dr. Paul Fine, contains more comprehensive discussions and many more figures and tables.

A major new feature for the 4th edition is a series of evidence-based "clinical decision guides," which concisely outline the work-up or management protocols for major problems indicated by the most authoritative data available. With these clinical decision guides the *Textbook* brings evidence-based medicine from academic study to direct utility for the student or clinician at the point of care. The clinical decision guides are also separately available as a pocket-sized *Clinical Decision Manual* edited by Dr. Kim A. Eagle.

The *Textbook* is again supported by a companion board review book, *Review of Internal Medicine*, again ably edited in its 2nd edition by Dr. David Schlossberg.

We are pleased to announce that preparations are underway to launch an up-to-date web version of the *Textbook*. This new format will feature ongoing content updates to help keep pace with the latest clinical breakthroughs as well as a highly user-friendly interface designed for clinical efficiency and utility, and links to other key sites. Finally, the 2nd edition of the *Textbook's* condensed version, the *Essentials of Internal Medicine*, will be published in 2001. The *Textbook of Internal Medicine* and its related training and reference tools provide a wealth of information in a variety of formats, improving accessibility and responding to the need for greater flexibility.

Like prior editions, this edition of the *Textbook* would not have been possible without the editorial and production assistance of numerous individuals. The work of the Editors has been greatly facilitated by the excellent editorial and organizational skills of Tom Cichonski. The Editors were fortunate to receive the assistance of many staff members, including

Virginia Benen, Jean Dorean-Matua, Nancy Esajian, Kathryn Eslinger-Lutz, Marianne Incmikoski, Anne Mraunac, Mark Multach, MD, Rene Tesdal, Teri Tyrrell and Nancy Woolard.

Successful completion of the present edition could not have been accomplished without the commitment of Lippincott Williams & Wilkins to publish the most authoritative and the best-formatted textbook of medicine currently available. The Editors give special thanks to our colleagues at Lippincott Williams & Wilkins for their unswerving dedication, professionalism, and organizational talents. Although they are numerous, we especially wish to recognize the tireless efforts of Richard Winters and Mary Beth Murphy.

The person most responsible for the *Textbook's* enthusiastic welcome by the medical community, however, is its founding Editor-in-Chief, Dr. William N. Kelley. Keenly aware of the increasing rate of scientific, technical, economic, and social change faced by the internal medicine practitioner, and of the many difficulties and opportunities this change presents, Dr. Kelley saw the need for a "fresh and pragmatic" approach to the teaching of internal medicine. Training and reference resources, he asserted, must adapt to the vastly expanding body of knowledge and the demands to reduce costs and improve efficiency that characterize today's dynamic health care environment. Thanks to his vision, dedication, and fine stewardship, the *Textbook* is acclaimed for both its encyclopedic depth and its utility in the clinical setting.

H. David Humes
Editor-in-Chief

LIST OF CLINICAL DECISION GUIDES

The Clinical Decision Guides are denoted by category grades appearing below the legends or captions of key decision algorithms and/or tables that are particularly directed at common medical problems. Using these algorithms as guides, a practitioner can quickly sort through a differential diagnosis and/or treatment and formulate options in an evidence-based fashion.

The Clinical Decision Guides have been selected from literally scores of decision algorithms and tables included in the *Textbook*. Each Guide has been graded based on the level of scientific evidence underlying the material so that the user has an appropriate level of confidence surrounding the scientific information. Category "A" tables and figures are based upon national guidelines and/or highly robust clinical trials. Category "B" refers to material which is based upon a limited amount of trial information or large observational studies. Category "C" decision aids are based primarily upon expert consensus. The Category indication appears just below the legend or caption of the Guide.

The Clinical Decision Guides are intended to be used at the patient's bedside. Providers can use this information in real time as they try to create the most appropriate and evidenced-based care possible for their patients.

Kim A. Eagle Editor, Clinical Decision Manual

PRINCIPLES OF MEDICAL PRACTICE

CARDIOLOGY

NEUROLOGY

GERIATRICS

KELLEY'S TEXTBOOK OF
INTERNAL MEDICINE

RAPID ACCESS GUIDE

Paul L. Fine

How to use the Rapid Access Guide to Internal Medicine

The Rapid Access Guide to Internal Medicine is an index of the major disease entities and clinical syndromes described in the *Kelley's Textbook of Internal Medicine, 4th Edition*. It is a quick-reference feature of the *Textbook* that is intended to provide a brief summary of the most important facts regarding a specific disease or syndrome at those times when speed is essential.

The Rapid Access Guide includes 149 of the common diseases and clinical syndromes most likely to be encountered in clinical practice. For greater ease of use, the information in each entry is compartmentalized into the following categories: definition, etiology, epidemiology, clinical features, diagnosis, prognosis, and management. Each entry contains a cross-reference to the chapter(s) in *Kelley's Textbook of Internal Medicine, 4th Edition* in which the disease or syndrome is discussed comprehensively. Figures and tables that are contained within the *Textbook* chapters themselves have not been duplicated. Instead, cross-references have been included to direct readers quickly to the location of the figures and tables in the main text.

In order to achieve the promised rapid access, *The Rapid Access Guide to Internal Medicine* is arranged according to the major sections of *Kelley's Textbook of Internal Medicine, 4th Edition*, with the entries listed alphabetically within each section. Moreover, on the inside covers of the *Textbook*, all of the *Rapid Access Guide* entries are listed alphabetically, accompanied by their page number and the *Textbook* section from which they are derived. Though an attempt has been made to minimize the use of acronyms and abbreviations with which readers may not be familiar, the common acronyms and abbreviations that have been employed are listed for easy reference.

The complete *Rapid Access Guide* is also available separately as a pocket handbook companion to *Kelley's Textbook of Internal Medicine, 4th Edition*.

Paul L. Fine, MD
University of Michigan Medical School

Abbreviations

ABG	arterial blood gas	CSF	cerebrospinal fluid
ACE	angiotensin converting enzyme	CT	computed tomography
ACTH	adrenocorticotropic hormone	CXR	chest x-ray
ADH	antidiuretic hormone	D	day
AIDS	acquired immunodeficiency syndrome	D_LCO	single-breath diffusing capacity for carbon dioxide
ANA	antinuclear antibody	DNA	deoxyribonucleic acid
A_2	aortic component of the second heart sound	DBP	diastolic blood pressure
BID	twice each day	ECG	electrocardiogram
BP	blood pressure	EEG	electroencephalogram
CBC	complete blood count	ELISA	enzyme-linked immunosorbent assay
CDC	Centers for Disease Control and Prevention	EMG	electromyogram
CHF	congestive heart failure	ERCP	endoscopic retrograde cholangiopancreatography
CMV	Cytomegalovirus	ESR	erythrocyte sedimentation rate
COPD	chronic obstructive pulmonary disease	FEV_1	forced expiratory volume in one second
CPK	creatine phosphokinase	FVC	forced vital capacity
CNS	central nervous system	GFR	glomerular filtration rate

ABBREVIATIONS

GH	growth hormone		**PSA**	prostate-specific antigen
GI	gastrointestinal		**PTT**	partial thromboplastin time
GU	genitourinary		**P$_2$**	pulmonic component of the second heart sound
h	hour		**QID**	four times each day
HLA	human leukocyte antigen		**RBC(s)**	red blood cell(s)
Ig	immunoglobulin		**RNA**	ribonucleic acid
INR	international normalized ratio (of the prothrombin time)		**RPR**	rapid plasma reagin
			RV	right ventricular
IVP	intravenous pyelogram		**S$_1$**	first heart sound
JVD	jugular venous distention		**S$_2$**	second heart sound
LDH	lactase dehydrogenase		**S$_3$**	third heart sound
LP	lumbar puncture		**S$_4$**	fourth heart sound
LV	left ventricular		**SBP**	systolic blood pressure
MI	myocardial infarction		**SLE**	systemic lupus erythematosus
MRI	magnetic resonance imaging		**TID**	three times each day
NSAIDs	nonsteroidal antiinflammatory drugs		**TPN**	total parenteral nutrition
PO	orally (per os)		**VDRL**	Venereal Disease Research Laboratory
PFTs	pulmonary function tests		**WBC**	white blood cell count
PND	paroxysmal nocturnal dyspnea		**WBCs**	white blood cells

CARDIOLOGY

■ ACUTE MYOCARDIAL INFARCTION

DEFINITION AND EPIDEMIOLOGY
Acute myocardial infarction (MI) is irreversible ischemic injury to the myocardium. In 1997, about 1.5 million persons in the United States experienced MI.

PATHOPHYSIOLOGY AND CLASSIFICATION
Acute MI is almost always associated with a thrombus superimposed on marked coronary atherosclerosis. It is a regional disease limited to the vascular territory of one of the three major vessels or their branches. Irreversible myocardial injury requires at least 15 to 20 minutes of ischemia; it begins in the subendocardium and spreads to the epicardium. MI is more common from 4 A.M. until noon, which corresponds to a time of decreased adrenergic activity, increased plasma fibrinogen levels, and increased platelet adhesiveness.

MI can be classified as Q-wave or non-Q-wave depending on whether Q waves develop in the relevant leads of the electrocardiogram (ECG). This classification has prognostic and therapeutic importance.

CLINICAL FINDINGS
History: The main symptom is prolonged (more than 30 minutes) chest pain, although patients may refer to it as "chest pressure" or "chest tightness." The pain is generally retrosternal, commonly radiates to the arm and neck, and usually is not relieved by nitroglycerin. Associated symptoms include nausea and vomiting, which are especially common with inferior infarction, diaphoresis, and dyspnea.

Physical examination: The typical patient is anxious, has an ashen face beaded with perspiration, and appears dyspneic. The pulse tends to be increased in anterior MI but decreased in inferior MI. Blood pressure usually is normal. Increased jugular venous pressure may reflect left-sided heart failure but also may be caused by involvement of the right ventricle in inferior MI. Right ventricular dysfunction also causes the Kussmaul sign (lack of the normal decrease in jugular venous pressure on inspiration) among about two-thirds of patients with inferior MI. Within 24 hours, there usually is some abnormality of the precordial pulsations, either a lack of a point of maximal impulse or the presence of a diffuse contraction. An S_4 is heard in almost all patients, and an S_3 in about 25%. The S_3 may be the only manifestation of cardiac decompensation. A systolic murmur from papillary muscle dysfunction occurs at least transiently in most patients within the first 24 hours. Approximately 10% of patients with Q-wave infarction have a pericardial friction rub, generally after about 48 to 72 hours. Patients with previous infarction may come to medical attention with worsening cardiac failure.

DIFFERENTIAL DIAGNOSIS
Conditions that may simulate acute MI include acute pulmonary embolism, acute pericarditis, dissecting aortic aneurysm, esophagitis and esophageal spasm, hiatal hernia, cholecystitis, pancreatitis, and spontaneous pneumothorax.

DIAGNOSIS
Electrocardiographic findings: The ECG findings generally are limited to the leads that reflect a certain anatomic region of the heart (anterior, inferior, posterior, or lateral), although reciprocal changes can occur elsewhere in the ECG. Fewer than one-half of patients have the characteristic profile of ST-segment elevation followed by the development of new Q waves (Q-wave MI). The rest have changes limited to ST-segment elevation or depression or only mild, nonspecific abnormalities (non-Q-wave MI). When the changes are restricted to the ST segment and T waves, confirmation by means of enzymatic and radiologic assessment is essential, because these changes also are associated with ischemia without irreversible injury. The ECG diagnosis of MI is notably difficult among patients with left bundle-branch block or previous MI with residual Q waves, because the development of new Q waves may be masked. When there is suspicion of inferior MI, an ECG with right precordial leads may demonstrate ST elevation that indicates right ventricular infarction.

Cardiac enzymes: Elevations of several myocyte enzymes have been incorporated into the diagnostic approach to MI. The level of plasma total MB isoenzyme of creatine kinase (CK-MB) is elevated (more than 7 ng per milliliter) within 6 to 10 hours of the onset of infarction and peaks between 12 and 28 hours. The level returns to normal after 72 to 96 hours. Troponin T and troponin I

are contractile proteins (normal levels less than 0.1 ng per milliliter and 1.5 ng per milliliter, respectively). They are released within 6 to 10 hours of the onset of MI and peak within 24 to 36 hours. A more gradual return to normal levels (10 to 12 days) makes levels of these substances particularly suitable for the late diagnosis of MI. Of these three enzymes, cardiac troponin I appears to be the most specific for cardiac injury. CK-MB and troponin T levels may be elevated in musculoskeletal disorders and renal failure. Although measurement of these various markers is useful in the diagnosis of MI, delay in release makes them less satisfactory in quickly excluding the diagnosis among patients arrive in an emergency department with chest pain (only 10% of whom have MI). The only markers that offer the sensitivity and specificity for diagnosis within the first 6 hours are myoglobin and CK-MB isoforms. The ratio of the two CK-MB isoforms becomes abnormal (CK-MB-2/CK-MB-1 greater than 1.7) well before the total CK-MB levels rise to diagnostic levels. Once a diagnosis is made, infarct size can be estimated with serial determination of CK-MB levels over 48 to 72 hours.

Noninvasive imaging: These techniques are useful when the diagnosis of MI is unclear. Echocardiography shows infarct-associated regional wall motion abnormalities but cannot help differentiate acute MI from prior myocardial scarring. Echocardiography also shows ventricular dysfunction, aneurysm, or thrombus. Thallium-201 imaging shows regions of decreased tracer uptake but does not allow reliable differentiation between prior and current MI.

PROGNOSIS AND MANAGEMENT
Treatment in a cardiac care unit, which provides constant ECG monitoring and highly trained medical and nursing personnel, has been associated with a decrease in the immediate mortality rate from MI to 10% to 15%. Patients generally stay in the unit for 2 or 3 days, after which the risk of ventricular fibrillation and ventricular tachycardia is much reduced. Most deaths are caused by pump failure from myocardial destruction rather than by arrhythmia. The use of thrombolytic therapy limits myocardial destruction and has been associated with a further lowering of the acute death rate to approximately 6%. Q-wave MI and non-Q-wave MI have distinct natural histories. The former confers a high-risk period of 6 to 12 weeks and is followed by a low mortality in subsequent years. Patients with non-Q-wave MI have a low mortality initially but a prolonged high-risk period of 1 to 2 years thereafter. After this interval, the accumulated mortality rate is similar to that of Q-wave MI. Figure 73.2 provides an overview of the treatment of patients with chest pain believed to be caused by MI.

INITIAL ASSESSMENT
Vital signs are checked and the patient is immediately given intravenous saline solution and aspirin. Morphine is indicated for pain relief and lidocaine for the management of ventricular arrhythmias. Supplemental oxygen is necessary only if hypoxemia is present. Continuous ECG monitoring should be established. All patients should be assessed for eligibility for thrombolytic therapy within the first 30 minutes.

Reperfusion therapy: Patients with chest pain who have new ST-segment elevation or bundle-branch block are candidates for reperfusion; those with ST-segment depression or T-wave inversion are not. Thrombolytic therapy with recombinant tissue plasminogen activator, streptokinase, or anistreplase (APSAC) improves ventricular function and decreases both infarct size and risk of immediate death when administered within the initial 4 to 6 hours. Studies show some benefit even among patients treated up to 12 hours. Contraindications to thrombolysis include bleeding tendency, prior stroke, hypertension, peptic ulcer, or recent (within 6 weeks) surgery. Age is not a contraindication. Patients undergoing thrombolytic therapy should receive heparin and aspirin, but to date there has been insufficient evidence to support routine cardiac catheterization after thrombolysis. Patients with recurrent ischemia or those who exhibit ischemia at stress testing before discharge should undergo catheterization for possible angioplasty or bypass surgery.

Primary angioplasty is associated with a vessel patency rate of more than 90% (consistently better than that of thrombolysis) and is an acceptable alternative to thrombolysis, if it can be performed within 45 minutes of the time the patient arrives at the hospital. The long-term comparative efficacy of primary angioplasty in relation to thrombolytic therapy remains to be determined. Among patients with contraindications to thrombolysis, primary angioplasty is the preferred therapy.

Adjunctive medications: The routine use of calcium channel blockers is not indicated for limitation of infarct size. However, diltiazem has been shown to be effective in preventing death and reinfarction among patients recovering from non-Q-wave MI and is recommended for routine use in the care of these patients. Angiotensin-converting enzyme inhibitors have been shown to prolong life among patients with left ventricular dysfunction or cardiac failure. Patients with an ejection fraction of 45% or less should routinely receive these agents. Four β-blockers (timolol, propranolol, metoprolol, and atenolol) have been shown to prolong life after Q-wave MI. One of these drugs should be given to patients with Q-wave MI who do not have contraindications to use of such a drug, including uncompensated heart failure, asthma, and conduction disturbances, and who meet one or more of the following criteria: age older than 60 years, ischemia demonstrated at exercise testing, ejection fraction less than 45%, concomitant angina or hypertension, or an episode of sustained ventricular tachycardia or fibrillation during the hospital stay. Aspirin therapy (325 mg each day) has been shown to decrease the risk of nonfatal MI or death among patients who have had an MI. Two recent large trials indicated that magnesium has no benefit in the management of acute MI.

ASSOCIATED COMPLICATIONS

Ventricular arrhythmias: These are common in the first 48 hours after MI and include multifocal ventricular extrasystole, runs of 3 or more ectopic ventricular beats, and 5 or more isolated ectopic ventricular beats per minute. Intravenous lidocaine (1 mg per kilogram, then 2 to 4 mg per minute) is recommended as first-line therapy and for prophylactic use before thrombolytic therapy. Persistent arrhythmias may necessitate addition of procainamide or bretylium. Patients in hemodynamically unstable condition need electrical cardioversion or defibrillation.

Atrial arrhythmias: Sinus tachycardia occurs among 20% to 30% of patients. If caused by ventricular failure, sinus tachycardia responds to therapy for that condition. If associated with minimal myocardial damage and normal hemodynamics, sinus tachycardia should be managed with β-blockers to avoid development of ischemia or more severe arrhythmias. Therapy should not be provided for asymptomatic sinus bradycardia.

Conduction disturbances: Type I second-degree heart block may develop, generally in patients with inferior MI. This type of heart block usually is transient and intermittent and rarely progresses to complete block. Type II second-degree heart block is rare, occurring in fewer than 1% of cases. It is almost always associated with anterior MI and a wide QRS complex. This type of heart block often progresses to complete block and always necessitates use of a pacemaker. The associated mortality rate is more than 80% with or without a pacemaker. Complete block necessitates pacing. Intraventricular conduction disturbances occur in as many as 5% of cases. If more than one of the three fascicles (right bundle, left anterior and posterior fascicles) is blocked, temporary pacing is recommended. The need for a permanent pacemaker among such patients is controversial.

Postinfarction angina: Persistent or recurrent chest pain that lasts more than 24 to 48 hours reflects the presence of viable but ischemic myocardium. It is an adverse prognostic indicator and is much more common after non-Q-wave MI. Pericarditis may be the cause of recurrent chest pain and should be excluded. The condition of a patient with postinfarction angina should be stabilized with nitrates and diltiazem, and β-blockers, if necessary. The patient then should undergo catheterization. More than 90% of patients with postinfarction angina and ECG changes have multiple-vessel disease at coronary angiography.

Early reinfarction: The overall incidence of early reinfarction, confirmed with a secondary elevation in plasma CK-MB level, is 10% to 15% after non-Q-wave MI, 5% to 10% after thrombolytic therapy, and less than 5% after Q-wave MI. Patients recovering from non-Q-wave MI should undergo routine plasma CK-MB analysis every 12 hours throughout the hospitalization. Early reinfarction is an indication for coronary angiography.

Cardiac failure: Cardiac failure develops when more than 25% of the left ventricle is involved, but it is often temporary. Because these patients do not have marked sodium and water retention, loss of fluid into the lungs occurs at the expense of vascular volume and may precipitate hypotension and decreased coronary perfusion. Patents with inferior MI, especially if there is also right ventricular involvement, need high filling pressures to maintain cardiac output. Therefore, diuretics should never be given unless central pressures are measured first. Dobutamine and vasodilating agents such as nitroglycerin are considered superior to diuretics in this setting; dopamine is added in the treatment of patients with marked hypotension.

Cardiogenic shock: Cardiogenic shock occurs among 5% to 10% of patients and is the most common cause of death. The only effective therapy is prevention. Clinical criteria include primary cardiac abnormality, a sustained drop in systolic blood pressure to less than 85 mm Hg, a ventricular filling pressure of 16 mm Hg or more, a cardiac index less than 1.5 L per minute per square meter, and peripheral organ involvement (oliguria, altered mentation). Hypovolemia, right ventricular infarction, pulmonary embolism, and cardiac tamponade must be excluded. Treatment includes discontinuation of vasodilators and negative inotropic agents and infusion of dopamine. Mechanical ventilation may be needed. If problems that can be corrected, such as ventricular septal rupture, are found, mechanical assist devices can help to keep patients alive until specific therapies can be undertaken.

Papillary muscle rupture: In rare instances rupture of the papillary muscle occurs 2 to 7 days after onset of MI. It is characterized by the sudden onset of pulmonary edema caused by acute mitral insufficiency. A new, low-pitched, holosystolic murmur radiates to the axilla and frequently is accompanied by an S_3 or an S_4. Pulmonary crackles are present. Swan-Ganz tracings show a large v wave. Echocardiography is useful in the diagnosis. The patient's condition is stabilized with an intra-aortic balloon pump. The mortality rate without surgery is about 90%; early surgery has a mortality rate of about 50%.

Ventricular septal rupture: This is a rare complication, usually occurring between the first and fifth days of recovery among patients with a first anterior MI. Rupture initiates a left-to-right shunt that causes biventricular failure, pulmonary edema, and cardiogenic shock. A harsh holosystolic murmur suddenly appears; jugular venous pressure elevation and conduction defects occur frequently. Monitoring with a Swan-Ganz catheter shows a step-up in oxygen saturation at the right ventricular level.

Pericarditis and Dressler's syndrome: Pericarditis develops in 5% to 10% of patients with Q-wave MI, usually more than 48 hours after infarction. It usually is heralded by the appearance of pleural-pericardial pain and a pericardial friction rub. The treatment is aspirin. Dressler syndrome is characterized by fever and pleural or pericardial chest pain and usually occurs within 2 to 6 weeks after MI. It is believed to be autoimmune in origin. Initial treatment consists of salicylates; glucocorticoids are added if necessary.

POSTINFARCTION MANAGEMENT

Medical therapy: See *Adjunctive medications.*

Postinfarction stratification: Patients at high risk are characterized by an ejection fraction less than 40%, ECG evidence of ischemia at exercise testing, and frequent or complex ventricular arrhythmias. All patients surviving MI should, before discharge, undergo assessment of left ventricular function by means of radionuclide ventriculography or echocardiography. Those who have been treated with thrombolytic agents probably should undergo cardiac catheterization only if there are symptoms of spontaneous or exercise-induced myocardial ischemia. Patients who have not received thrombolytic agents and who have had their first episode of MI, have an ejection fraction less than 40%, or have refractory pain or early reinfarction should undergo coronary angiography. All other patients may be stratified through exercise testing (preferably with thallium imaging), and catheterization can be reserved for those who show considerable ischemia.

Revascularization: Bypass surgery is clearly indicated for left main coronary artery disease or for three-vessel disease associated with decreased ejection fraction (less than 45%). The role of angioplasty is less well defined.

Activity: Patients should stay in bed for the first 24 hours after MI but may use a bedside commode. By the fifth or sixth day, they may walk in the room. After discharge, patients are encouraged to walk daily at home for the next 3 to 6 weeks. They usually can return to work in 6 weeks. Formal cardiac rehabilitation programs sometimes are indicated.

Chapter 73

◼ AORTIC VALVE DISEASE

DEFINITIONS, EPIDEMIOLOGY, AND ETIOLOGY

Aortic Stenosis: Aortic stenosis (AS) implies obstruction of left ventricular (LV) outflow caused by a fixed anatomic abnormality of the aortic valve. In adults, AS may be congenital, rheumatic, or degenerative (calcific). Congenital AS is more common among men and usually is associated with a bicuspid aortic valve.

Rheumatic AS may occur in isolation but is more commonly associated with mitral valve disease. Degenerative AS occurs exclusively among older adults.

Aortic regurgitation: Aortic regurgitation (AR) is a condition of LV volume overload caused by incompetence of the aortic valve. Congenital causes include bicuspid aortic valve. Acquired AR may be caused by rheumatic disease, hypertensive and atherosclerotic diseases, infective endocarditis, and nonpenetrating trauma. Diseases of the ascending aorta, such as aortic aneurysm and dissection, Reiter's syndrome, ankylosing spondylitis, syphilitic aortitis, and cystic medial necrosis, also can cause AR.

PATHOPHYSIOLOGY

Aortic stenosis: Increased afterload causes compensatory LV hypertrophy. LV systolic function is preserved until late in the course, although diastolic function may be impaired earlier by the increased LV mass. The increased LV mass and intracavitary pressures can cause mismatch of myocardial oxygen demand and supply and lead to angina. Because cardiac output is relatively fixed, the peripheral vasodilatation that occurs with exercise may cause hypotension and syncope.

Aortic regurgitation: When AR is chronic, volume overload and increased wall tension trigger compensatory LV dilation and hypertrophy. Ejection fraction remains normal until late in the disease. Myocardial ischemia occurs in advanced disease because of the increased LV mass and low coronary perfusion pressure. In acute AR, tachycardia is the only compensatory mechanism, and patients frequently have pulmonary edema and shock.

CLINICAL FINDINGS

Aortic stenosis: A long latent period precedes the development of the classic symptoms of dyspnea, angina, and exertional syncope. Late in the course, a decrease in cardiac output causes congestive heart failure (CHF), the effects of which are fatigue, weakness, and peripheral cyanosis. Peripheral edema, hepatomegaly, and ascites may occur. The classic physical finding is *pulsus parvus et tardus*, a delayed and prolonged arterial pulse of diminished intensity, typically assessed in the carotid or brachial artery. On auscultation, the aortic component of S_2 is diminished. An S_4 usually is audible, and an S_3 may be heard if the patient has CHF. The murmur is a harsh, low-pitched, crescendo-decrescendo systolic ejection murmur that radiates from the base of the heart into the carotid arteries. With increasing severity of AS, the murmur peaks progressively later in systole. The murmur of end-stage AS may have a softer volume because of decreasing cardiac output.

Aortic regurgitation: Most patients have no symptoms for years or decades. Early symptoms include palpitations. Exertional dyspnea may be the first manifestation of LV decompensation; orthopnea and paroxysmal nocturnal dyspnea develop later. Symptoms of more advanced disease include angina, ascites, and peripheral edema. Most physical findings in chronic AR reflect the combination of increased stroke volume and widened pulse pressure, including bobbing of the head (de Musset sign), water-hammer pulse, visible capillary pulsation in the nail beds with gentle nail compression (Quincke pulse), and a diastolic murmur with pressure over the peripheral arteries (Duroziez sign). The aortic component of S_2 may be diminished. The murmur is a high-pitched, blowing, decrescendo diastolic murmur, loudest at the left or right upper sternal border. It may radiate to the cardiac apex (Austin Flint murmur) as a low-pitched diastolic rumble that mimics mitral stenosis. There may be a loud accompanying systolic murmur caused by the large stroke volume. Many of the physical findings associated with chronic AR are absent among patients with acute AR, because there are no acute increases in stroke volume or pulse pressure.

DIAGNOSTIC STUDIES

Aortic stenosis: The ECG may show evidence of LV hypertrophy. The chest radiograph may be normal or show an enlarged cardiac silhouette. Echocardiography with Doppler technique is an accurate, noninvasive means of establishing the diagnosis and determining cause and severity. It also provides an assessment of LV size, mass, and systolic function. Cardiac catheterization should be reserved for patients who have a discrepancy between clinical and echocardiographic data or those undergoing planned aortic valve operations that may include coronary artery bypass if severe coronary artery disease is found. AS is not usually of hemodynamic importance until the valve area is reduced to one-fourth normal. In general, AS is considered severe when the valve area is 1.0 cm^2 or less and the mean transvalvular pressure gradient is 50 mm Hg or more, although patients with LV dysfunction may have lower gradients because of decreased flow.

Aortic regurgitation: Neither chest radiography nor ECG is very helpful. Echocardiography with Doppler techniques can be used to confirm the diagnosis and determine cause and severity. LV dimensions, mass, and systolic function should

be evaluated, as should the size and anatomic details of the aortic root. Cardiac catheterization with coronary angiography is useful when a planned aortic valve operation may include coronary artery bypass if severe coronary artery disease is demonstrated.

PROGNOSIS AND STRATEGIES FOR MANAGEMENT

Aortic stenosis: Mortality is low as long as patients have no symptoms. With the onset of symptoms, the average survival time without intervention is 2 to 3 years. The worst prognosis is associated with symptoms of CHF. All patients should receive prophylactic antibiotics prior to procedures that are likely to cause bacteremia. There is no suitable medical therapy. Medications that decrease preload (nitrates, diuretics) may reduce the cardiac output of patients with LV hypertrophy and must be used with caution. Agents that decrease afterload (calcium channel blockers, angiotensin-converting enzyme inhibitors) may cause marked hypotension in the setting of fixed cardiac output and are best avoided. Valve replacement is associated with symptomatic improvement and an increased survival rate and should be considered strongly in the care of almost all patients with symptoms, even elderly patients or those with LV systolic dysfunction. Use of a mechanical prosthesis has the advantages of a favorable hemodynamic profile and durability but necessitates long-term anticoagulation because of thrombogenicity. Aortic balloon valvuloplasty is important in delaying the need for valve replacement among younger patients or in palliative treatment of patients who cannot undergo surgical therapy.

Aortic regurgitation: Prognosis worsens with the onset of symptoms; the mortality rate is estimated to be more than 10% per year among patients with severe AR and angina and more than 20% per year among those with symptoms of CHF. LV systolic dysfunction and marked LV dilatation also are associated with a worse prognosis, even if patients continue to have no symptoms. Patients should receive prophylactic antibiotics prior to procedures that are likely to cause bacteremia. Patients with chronic mild or moderate AR do not benefit from any other therapy. However, patients without symptoms who have chronic, severe AR benefit from long-term vasodilating therapy with nifedipine or possibly angiotensin-converting enzyme inhibitors. Drug therapy appears to delay the need for valve replacement and to improve outcomes after surgery. Therapy should be limited to patients with systolic hypertension. Aortic valve replacement is indicated in the care of patients with severe AR and symptoms of angina or CHF and for patient without symptoms who have severe AR and decreased LV systolic function (resting ejection fraction less than 50%) or marked LV dilatation. Severe acute AR can be stabilized with diuretics and aggressive afterload reduction, as with nitroprusside, before urgent valve replacement.

Chapter 77

ATRIAL ARRHYTHMIAS

DEFINITION AND CLINICAL PRESENTATION

Cardiac arrhythmias are disorders of the normal heart rhythm. Most commonly, they cause palpitations, an awareness of the heartbeat because of an abnormally strong ventricular contraction, a pause in normal rhythm, or extra beats. Less commonly, they can produce syncope, near-syncope, angina, congestive heart failure, or death.

SPECIFIC ARRHYTHMIAS

Premature atrial complexes: These manifest as a premature P wave morphologically different from the sinus P wave. They usually discharge the sinus node and are followed by a noncompensatory pause. They occur among healthy persons and can be provoked by drugs, alcohol, caffeine, or tobacco. They usually do not necessitate therapy, but patients without symptoms may be given digitalis, propranolol, or verapamil.

Atrial flutter: This rhythm is recognized on an electrocardiogram (ECG) as sawtooth-shaped atrial complexes, usually at rates of approximately 300 beats per minute, with a 2:1 ventricular response among untreated persons. If the atrioventricular (AV) conduction ratio remains constant, the ventricular rhythm is regular; otherwise it is irregular. Atrial flutter usually is associated with underlying heart disease. Reentry is the most probable cause. Synchronous direct-current cardioversion is the initial therapy of choice; rapid atrial pacing also is effective. Therapy with class IA, IC, or III drugs can be tried (Table 1). Before class I drugs are given, the ventricular rate must be slowed (as described in the section on atrial fibrillation).

TABLE 1.	DRUGS WITH ANTIARRHYTHMIC ACTIVITY

Class I: Drugs That Interact Predominantly with the Fast Sodium Channel

Quinidine-like: quinidine, procainamide, disopyramide
Lidocaine-like: lidocaine, mexiletine, tocainide
Flecainide-like: flecainide, propafenone
Phenytoin

Class II: β-Adrenergic Antagonists

Nonselective: propranolol, nadolol, timolol
Cardioselective: atenolol, metoprolol
Intrinsic sympathomimetic activity
  Nonselective: pindolol
  Cardioselective: acebutolol, carvedilol

Class III: Drugs That Prolong Repolarization

Bietylium
Amiodarone
N-Acetylprocainamide (NAPA) (acecainide)
Sotalol

Class IV: Calcium Channel Antagonists

Verapamil
Diltiazem

Atrial fibrillation: Atrial fibrillation is the most common sustained arrhythmia; the incidence increases with age. It also occurs commonly among patients with hypertension, rheumatic heart disease, atrial septal defect, cardiomyopathy, coronary heart disease, or thyrotoxicosis and among those who have undergone cardiac surgery. It can occur among patients without structural heart disease (lone atrial fibrillation). The rhythm is characterized by totally disorganized atrial depolarization without effective contraction and is most commonly sustained by multiple wavelets of reentry. An ECG shows small, irregular baseline undulations of varying amplitude and morphologic characteristics. Because many of the fibrillatory impulses are blocked in the AV node, the ventricular rhythm is irregularly irregular, although this may be difficult to appreciate when the ventricular response is rapid. Among patients with normal AV conduction, the ventricular rate usually is 100 to 160 beats per minute.

If acute cardiovascular decompensation has occurred, electrical cardioversion is the initial treatment. Otherwise, the therapeutic objective is to slow the ventricular rate and then to restore atrial systole. (Atrial fibrillation accompanying Wolff-Parkinson-White syndrome must be treated differently, however.) Drugs that slow the ventricular response (digitalis, β-blockers, and calcium channel blockers) can be used alone or in combination. The adequacy of rate control must be assessed both at rest and with activity; digitalis is often ineffective during exertion. Inadequate rate control can lead to tachycardia-induced cardiomyopathy. If the ventricular rate proves refractory to medical therapy, or if such therapy is poorly tolerated, radiofrequency ablation of the AV node followed by implantation of a pacemaker may be useful. Conversion to sinus rhythm should be considered in the care of patients with symptoms or when the ventricular rate cannot be controlled. Outpatient electrical cardioversion is the most effective technique. Many oral and intravenous drugs are useful, although pharmacologic conversion for patients with structural heart disease should be performed in a monitored, hospital setting. Amiodarone is ineffective at converting atrial fibrillation but does decrease risk for recurrence. Unlike quinidine and flecainide, amiodarone does not appear to increase mortality due to proarrhythmia when used for long-term treatment of patients with extensive structural heart disease. The strongest predictor of recurrent atrial fibrillation is the duration of arrhythmia before cardioversion. Catheter and surgical techniques are being developed for the management of atrial fibrillation.

Patients with chronic atrial fibrillation are at increased risk of stroke. Risk factors include hypertension, rheumatic heart disease, diabetes, history of previous thromboembolic events, left atrial enlargement, history of congestive heart failure, and age older than 65 years. Long-term anticoagulation with warfarin is effective in reducing this risk. Aspirin can be used to treat patients without

risk factors. Electrical and pharmacologic cardioversion are associated with atrial contractile dysfunction (stunning) and thrombus formation. Therefore, unless a contraindication is present, short-term anticoagulation before and after cardioversion is necessary in the care of all patients with atrial fibrillation that persists for more than 2 days or is of unknown duration. Absence of a left atrial thrombus on a transesophageal echocardiogram has been demonstrated to allow safe cardioversion without prior anticoagulation. However, the cardioversion should be preceded by the initiation of heparin therapy and must be followed by 4 weeks of warfarin therapy. Patients who have undergone AV node ablation and implantation of a pacemaker are still at risk of stroke and should undergo anticoagulation.

Atrial tachycardia: Atrial tachycardia can be caused by enhanced atrial automaticity, reentry, or triggered activity. The atrial rate usually is 150 to 200 beats per minute and can be slightly irregular. Vagal maneuvers usually do not stop the tachycardia, even though they may produce transient AV nodal block. Atrial tachycardia occurs most commonly among patients with structural heart disease, such as coronary artery disease or cor pulmonale, or with digitalis intoxication. If digitalis is not the cause, this drug may be given to slow the ventricular response, as may β-blockers and calcium channel blockers. Recurrent atrial tachycardia can be controlled with antiarrhythmic drugs and often can be cured with catheter ablation.

Multifocal atrial tachycardia (chaotic atrial tachycardia): This type of arrhythmia is characterized on an ECG by atrial rates of 100 to 130 beats per minute, marked variation in P-wave structure, and irregular PP intervals. At least three P-wave shapes usually are found. As in atrial fibrillation, ventricular rhythm usually is irregularly irregular. Multifocal atrial tachycardia occurs commonly among patients with pulmonary disease. Therapy is directed at the underlying disease; antiarrhythmic agents often are ineffective in slowing the atrial rate or the ventricular response. Potassium and magnesium replacement may suppress the tachycardia.

AV nodal reentrant tachycardia: This type of arrhythmia occurs when characteristics of conduction pathways near the AV node allow an impulse to travel slowly along one path and then return in a reverse direction along an initially blocked path to reexcite tissue proximal to the site of the block. AV nodal reentrant tachycardia is characterized by regular tachycardia, usually at rates of 180 to 200 beats per minute, a narrow QRS complex and retrograde P waves at the onset of or immediately after termination of the QRS complex. The onset and termination both are sudden. Examination of the jugular veins may reveal constant cannon *a* waves. This type of tachycardia occurs commonly among patients without structural heart disease. Depending on the duration and rate and the presence of structural heart disease, AV nodal reentrant tachycardia produces symptoms ranging from palpitations, nervousness, and anxiety to angina, heart failure, or syncope. Termination initially involves a vagal maneuver, such as carotid sinus massage, a Valsalva maneuver, or gagging. The drug of first choice is intravenous adenosine (a vagomimetic drug). Alternatives are diltiazem, verapamil or a short-acting β-blocker such as esmolol. Prevention of recurrence with these AV nodal blocking agents may prove more difficult, but radiofrequency catheter ablation of the slow pathway has a high success rate (about 95%) and low risk (less than 2%). The prognosis among patients without heart disease is good.

Chapter 76

APPROACH TO THE PATIENT WITH CHEST PAIN

DIFFERENTIAL DIAGNOSIS

The differential diagnosis of chest pain is extensive (Table 32.5). Rapid assessment is essential to identify whether a patient has acute coronary syndrome and hence is at risk of sudden cardiac death. Most patients with chest pain related to a noncardiac cause have esophageal or anxiety disorders.

HISTORY AND PHYSICAL EXAMINATION

A carefully obtained history is the best initial diagnostic tool (Table 32.1). Patients may not call their problem *pain*. Morning episodes of discomfort and radiation to the arms, neck, or shoulder both are more frequent with myocardial ischemia than with other disorders. The presence of nausea or vomiting and diaphoresis should heighten the suspicion of ischemia. Symptoms occurring at rest or those related to meals, movement, stress, and respiratory pattern are more likely to have a noncardiac than a cardiac cause. A sensation described as "stabbing" or "fleeting" also is less likely to represent myocardial ischemia.

A detailed cardiovascular examination can provide vital clues, but normal findings do not exclude a cardiac disorder. Detection of a murmur of papillary muscle insufficiency, S_3 or S_4, loud P_2, abnormal precordial impulse, jugular venous distention, rales, or lower extremity edema is associated with organic heart disease and may indicate ischemia or infarction. A diminished A_2 with a crescendo-decrescendo systolic murmur and decreased carotid upstroke suggests hemodynamically significant aortic stenosis. Unequal pulses or blood pressures should be a warning of possible aortic dissection. Detection of a pericardial friction rub, tachycardia, and pulsus paradoxus suggest pericarditis and possible tamponade. A pleural friction rub, evidence of consolidation, and absent or abnormal breath sounds may indicate a pulmonary cause. Persistent sinus tachycardia with tachypnea, a pleural rub, and localized wheezing can indicate pulmonary embolization. Atypical pain that is reproducible with cervical motion probably is caused by C6-7 radiculopathy.

DIAGNOSTIC TESTS

An ECG is essential. About 50% to 60% of patients with acute myocardial infarction have ECG changes that suggest the diagnosis. Normal ECG findings make the diagnosis less likely but do not exclude it. Pericarditis, pulmonary embolism, pulmonary hypertension, and esophageal spasm also can be associated with ECG abnormalities. A rational approach to biochemical testing includes both creatine kinase-MB and troponin I, which is found only in myocardial muscle and can be detected for up to 10 days after myocardial injury. Exercise ECG testing may be useful in the care of patients with a stable pattern of chest pain but is contraindicated in the care of patients at high risk. The addition of imaging techniques, such as thallium 201 or sestamibi scanning and echocardiography, to ECG monitoring is advisable in the care of patients with abnormal resting ECGs and women younger than 40 years. Pharmacologic testing with adenosine, dipyridamole, or dobutamine is helpful in evaluations of patients who cannot exercise adequately.

For patients whose signs and symptoms suggest pain unrelated to myocardial ischemia or whose evaluation does not prove the presence of myocardial ischemia, other specific tests may be warranted. In many cases, however, the diagnosis, such as gastroesophageal reflux disease or panic disorder, can be made clinically.

Chapter 65

■ CORONARY ARTERY DISEASE

EPIDEMIOLOGY

In the United States, atherosclerotic coronary artery disease (CAD) is the leading cause of death among both men and women and is a clinically significant process in about 11 million people. Risk factors include cigarette smoking, hypercholesterolemia, hypertension, diabetes mellitus, male sex, menopause, and family history. Recent studies also implicate elevated levels of plasma homocysteine or lipoprotein(a) and dormant infection with *Chlamydia* or cytomegalovirus organisms.

DEFINITIONS AND PATHOPHYSIOLOGY

Chronic coronary disease: The most common cause of CAD is stenosis of the proximal segments of the left anterior descending (LAD), right, or circumflex coronary arteries by atherosclerotic plaque. For most patients, myocardial ischemia occurs during stress, when progressive increases in myocardial oxygen demand exceed the ability of the coronary circulation to increase blood flow. Endothelial dysfunction of the coronary arteries, even those with plaques that are not themselves flow limiting, contributes to this imbalance. The chief mechanism is a decrease in the production of nitrous oxide, a potent endogenous vasodilator that also inhibits smooth-muscle proliferation and platelet aggregation.

Acute coronary syndrome: Acute coronary syndrome (ACS) is characterized by an increase in the intensity or frequency of angina and is associated with an increased risk of myocardial infarction (MI) and cardiac death. Examples include prolonged rest angina (more than 20 minutes), new onset of angina (pain of less than 2 months' duration), and acceleration of angina. ACS and non-Q-wave MI generally result from the formation of thrombus after rupture of an atherosclerotic plaque, often one that is angiographically insignificant.

Variant angina: Prinzmetal's angina is a syndrome of angina that usually occurs at rest and is associated with reversible ST-segment elevation without enzymatic evidence of acute MI. It is caused by coronary vasospasm and is associated with heavy smoking, migraine headaches, and Raynaud's phenomenon.

CLINICAL FEATURES

Chronic coronary disease: Stable angina is characterized by poorly localized discomfort in the chest or left arm associated with physical exertion or emotional stress and relieved promptly with rest or sublingual nitroglycerin. The pain also can involve the neck, jaw, and teeth. Dyspnea, diaphoresis, nausea, and dizziness may be present. Many patients have no chest discomfort; the only symptoms may be a combination of dyspnea and pain in the neck, shoulder, or arm. An anginal episode may last a few minutes to 15 to 20 minutes. Common precipitants include exercise, sexual activity, and emotional distress. The anginal threshold may be lowered by mental stress, exposure to cold temperatures, meals, cigarette smoking, anemia, and hyperthyroidism. For reasons that are not clear, most ischemic episodes among patients with stable angina are painless, or "silent." The physical examination helps to exclude valvular heart disease or obstructive hypertrophic cardiomyopathy as the cause of chest pain. Some patients with prior MI may show evidence of LV dysfunction. Vascular bruits suggest diffuse atherosclerotic disease. During an attack of angina, an S_3, an S_4, or the murmur of mitral regurgitation may be present.

Acute coronary syndrome: The chest discomfort of ACS is similar to that of stable angina but is usually more severe and protracted. The discomfort often is associated with diaphoresis, an S_3 or S_4, and a systolic murmur. Electrocardiographic (ECG) findings during a symptomatic attack may show ST-segment depression or elevation or T-wave abnormalities. If they persist for several hours, these abnormalities often are associated with elevation of creatine kinase-MB and the diagnosis of non-Q-wave MI. Elevation of troponin T and troponin I levels is associated with increased risk of death.

Variant angina: Most patients have angiographically significant atherosclerotic CAD and therefore are at risk of MI and sudden death. The chest discomfort usually occurs at rest, although the vasospasm can be triggered by exercise. The duration is somewhat longer than that of stable angina.

DIFFERENTIAL DIAGNOSIS

Several conditions may produce an anginal syndrome indistinguishable from that caused by atherosclerotic CAD. These include aortic stenosis, aortic insufficiency, hypertrophic cardiomyopathy, dilated cardiomyopathy, pulmonary hypertension, and cocaine use. Microvascular angina, or syndrome X, is caused by a reduction in vasodilator reserve of the coronary vasculature. It is common among women and persons with hypertension and is a common cause of chest pain when coronary arteriograms are normal. Other conditions may cause chest pain unrelated to myocardial ischemia, These include aortic dissection, pulmonary embolism, acute pericarditis, reflux esophagitis, esophageal spasm, peptic ulcer, and biliary disease.

LABORATORY TESTS AND DIAGNOSIS

Chronic coronary disease: Anemia and hyperthyroidism should be excluded, and a serum lipid profile should be obtained. The ECG may be entirely normal or show evidence of prior (possibly silent) MI. Additional diagnostic testing should be reserved for patients with moderate pretest probability of CAD, such as patients with symptoms or several risk factors for CAD. Among patients with a high probability of disease, such as middle-aged men with typical angina and numerous risk factors, the diagnosis is usually well established without further testing. The various noninvasive tests are compared in Table 72.5; cardiac magnetic resonance imaging and electron-beam computed tomography are additional techniques under investigation. Among patients with known or suspected CAD, coronary angiography is performed for diagnosis, for risk stratification, and for the assessment of appropriateness and feasibility of myocardial revascularization with percutaneous transluminal coronary angioplasty (PTCA) or coronary artery bypass grafting (CABG). Angiography is indicated in evaluations of patients classified as being at high risk at noninvasive testing and of patients with stable angina who continue to have evidence of ischemia despite adequate medical therapy.

Acute coronary syndrome: The diagnosis of ACS usually is made on clinical grounds, although additional testing often is helpful in guiding management (see later).

Variant angina: The diagnosis is made on clinical grounds and demonstration of ST-segment elevation during an attack of angina that normalizes with sublingual nitroglycerin. Ambulatory ECG monitoring and exercise testing may be useful in demonstrating ST-segment elevation. All patients should undergo coronary angiography. Intravenous or intracoronary administration of ergonovine in the catheterization laboratory elicits coronary vasospasm in more than 90% of patients with variant angina; a negative test result essentially excludes the diagnosis.

MANAGEMENT

Chronic coronary disease: Acute cardiac events are caused by disruption of atherosclerotic plaques; the plaque need not be stenotic to rupture and cause occlusive thrombosis. The goals of therapy include both improvement of symptoms and prevention of the plaque disruption and growth that can lead to progression and acute cardiac events. Risk factor modification is essential and includes smoking cessation, control of hyperglycemia, and aggressive management of hypertension. The total cholesterol level should be reduced to less than 200 mg per deciliter, the low-density lipoprotein cholesterol level decreased to less than 100 mg per deciliter, and the high-density lipoprotein cholesterol level increased to more than 35 mg per deciliter. HMG-CoA reductase inhibitors have been shown to be particularly beneficial in this setting. Reducing homocysteine levels with folic acid and vitamins B_6 and B_{12} has not yet been demonstrated to improve clinical outcomes. Correction of contributing conditions (such as anemia, thyrotoxicosis, fever, and hypoxemia) should be undertaken.

Aspirin (81 to 324 mg per day) reduces the risk of MI and sudden death and should be used to treat all patients unless contraindicated. Clopidogrel and ticlopidine also block platelet activation and may be used in place of aspirin.

Nitrates are potent systemic venous and coronary arterial vasodilators that may be used to abort (0.4-mg sublingual capsules or spray) or prevent (long-acting tablets and transdermal patches) attacks of angina. Tolerance develops to the long-acting forms unless there is an 8 to 12 hour nitrate-free period each day. The most common side effects are headache and hypotension.

β-Blockers are among the most important therapies for CAD. These agents decrease the frequency of attacks of angina and improve exercise tolerance. They are at least relatively contraindicated in the care of patients with asthma, atrioventricular conduction defects, profound bradycardia, severe hypotension, peripheral artery disease, and Raynaud's phenomenon. They must be used with extreme caution by patients with overt heart failure, although use of these agents does improve survival in such cases. These drugs should be discontinued gradually over several weeks, if possible, to avoid rebound effects.

Calcium channel blockers relax vascular smooth muscle in the arterial and coronary circulation. The different agents depress myocardial contractility to varying degrees (most with verapamil, least with dihydropyradines such as nifedipine and amlodipine). They may reduce the frequency of angina and increase exercise tolerance and are generally well tolerated. Calcium channel blockers must be used with extreme caution by patients with systolic heart failure. The use of short-acting agents, particularly by patients with hypertension, has been associated with an increased risk of MI. β-Blockers are preferred over calcium channel blockers in the management of stable angina.

Percutaneous coronary revascularization (PCR) is a nonsurgical procedure on a stenotic artery in which the coronary lumen is dilated with a balloon catheter or other intracoronary device. PCR is technically successful about 90% of the time. Indications include a considerable stenosis of a major epicardial artery (other than the left main) in patients with angina that does not respond to medical therapy or with evidence of myocardial ischemia in the territory of the artery to be dilated. The main limitation of angioplasty is coronary restenosis, which occurs among 30% to 50% of patients within the first 6 months after the procedure. Stents and platelet glycoprotein IIb/IIIA receptor blockers may reduce the rate of restenosis. Bypass surgery with saphenous veins and the internal mammary artery is used primarily to treat patients with symptoms that are not responsive to medical therapy or PTCA. Unlike medical therapy, CABG improves the survival rate among patients with left main coronary artery disease, three-vessel disease, or two-vessel disease when one of the two vessels involved is a large LAD artery with severe proximal stenosis. This benefit is particularly evident among patients who have LV systolic dysfunction. Among selected patients with multivessel CAD, PCR and CABG have similar clinical outcomes, although patients undergoing PCR are more likely to have persistent angina and have a greater need for additional revascularization procedures. Patients with diabetes have a significantly lower mortality rate with CABG than with PCR. For patients with disease of the left main coronary artery, multivessel disease involving the proximal LAD, or three-vessel disease with impaired LV systolic function, CABG is preferred over PCR.

Acute coronary syndrome: Patients with suspected ACS should undergo initial risk stratification (Table 72.11). Patients at low risk can undergo outpatient evaluation. Therapy should consist of aspirin, sublingual nitroglycerin as needed, oral β-blockers, and long-acting topical or oral nitrates. Patients at intermediate or high risk should be admitted to the hospital and undergo serial cardiac enzyme measurements and ECG to exclude acute MI. These patients should be treated with aspirin, intravenous heparin or low-molecular-weight heparin, glycoprotein IIb/IIIa antagonists, nitrates, and β-blockers. Calcium channel blockers should be reserved for patients with hypertension or ischemia refractory to the other agents. Intravenous thrombolytic therapy is not indicated unless there is prolonged rest pain and either elevation of the ST segments in two consecutive leads or a left bundle-branch block. Patients who continue to have ischemia despite medical therapy or who have marked ischemia at stress testing should undergo coronary angiography. Indications for CABG are the same as those mentioned earlier. Treatment of patients with two-vessel or one-vessel disease remains controversial, but revascularization usually is recommended.

Variant angina: Nitrates and calcium channel blockers are extremely effective in preventing coronary artery spasm. β-Blockers should not be used unless there is extensive concomitant atherosclerotic disease. High doses of aspirin may increase the severity of vasospasm. The indications for revascularization among patients with variant angina and significant multivessel atherosclerotic disease are the same as for other patients with chronic CAD.

Chapter 72

■ HEART BLOCK

DEFINITION AND CLINICAL PRESENTATION

Heart block is a disturbance of impulse conduction that can occur at any site but is recognized commonly between the sinus node and the atrium (SA block), between the atrium and ventricle (AV block), or within the ventricles (intraventricular or bundle-branch block). The symptoms are those of bradycardia—syncope, near-syncope, angina, and congestive heart failure.

SPECIFIC ARRHYTHMIAS

First-degree atrioventricular block: In this block, the PR interval exceeds 200 milliseconds, but all P waves conduct to the ventricles. The prolonged PR interval can be caused by a conduction delay in the AV node or in the His–Purkinje system. It is almost always asymptomatic.

Second-degree atrioventricular block: Second-degree AV block is divided into type I (Wenckebach) and type II. During type I AV block, there is a regular PP interval, and progressive PR interval prolongation precedes a nonconducted P wave. Because the increment in PR interval conduction delay decreases after the first cycle, the RR interval progressively decreases. In type II, the PR interval remains constant before one or more nonconducted P waves. If the QRS complex is normal, the block is more likely to be type I; almost always, type II AV block occurs in the setting of a bundle-branch block. As a rule, type I AV block is a more benign conduction disturbance and can occur among healthy persons. Often it produces no symptoms and requires no pacemaker therapy. Type II block usually is located in the His–Purkinje system and is associated more often with syncope and the need for pacemaker therapy. A transient type I block occurs in some patients with inferior wall MI; type II block more often accompanies severe anterior infarction.

Complete atrioventricular block: Complete AV block, or third-degree AV block, occurs when no atrial activity conducts to the ventricles and, therefore, independent pacemakers control the atria and ventricles. When the block occurs at the level of the AV node, usually a congenital condition, the QRS complex is normal and the ventricular rate usually is 40 to 60 beats per minute. Atropine and exercise increase the ventricular rate. Children most often have no symptoms. Acquired complete AV block occurs most commonly distal to the bundle of His. The QRS complexes are abnormal, and the ventricular rate usually is less than 40 beats per minute and fails to increase with administration of atropine or with exercise. Complete AV block can be associated with electrolyte disturbances, endocarditis, tumors, rheumatoid nodules, calcific aortic stenosis, infiltrative processes, drug toxicity, coronary artery disease, and degenerative processes. The patients usually have Adams-Stokes syncope and need pacemaker implantation.

Chapter 76

■ APPROACH TO THE PATIENT WITH HEART FAILURE

ETIOLOGY AND PATHOPHYSIOLOGY

Heart failure is not a disease. It is a wide-ranging expression of left ventricular (LV) dysfunction attributable to diverse etiologic factors. The most common form, systolic LV dysfunction, represents failure of the heart as a pump. It usually is caused by myocardial infarction or hypertension. The clinical expression of heart failure also can be seen without systolic dysfunction among patients with valvular or pericardial disease, abnormalities of cardiac rhythm, or impaired diastolic filling (diastolic dysfunction). Heart failure stimulates a cascade of compensatory responses, including activation of the renin–angiotensin system, increases in sympathetic tone, and enhanced production of antidiuretic hormone. These responses enhance renal sodium and water retention and contribute to the formation of edema.

CLINICAL FINDINGS

History: Most patients seek medical attention because of breathlessness or exercise-induced fatigue. Sometimes the first recognized manifestation of heart failure is orthopnea or paroxysmal nocturnal dyspnea. For other patients, pedal edema may be the first concern.

Physical examination: Tachycardia usually represents chronotropic compensation for the reduced cardiac output. If irregular, the tachycardia most typically reflects atrial fibrillation, the most common atrial arrhythmia in this population. Blood pressure is often low among patients with chronic heart failure. A narrow pulse pressure is consistent with low stroke volume or inadequate diastolic filling time. The magnitude of jugular venous distention provides an estimate of cardiac filling pressure. Pulmonary examination may reveal tachypnea, dyspnea with speech, or crackles. In general, the height of the crackles in the posterior fields is proportional to the severity of LV decompensation. Crackles may be obscured by the presence of pleural effusion, which is more often a marker of chronic decompensation. A diffuse apical impulse displaced away from the midsternal line suggests ventricular enlargement and is typical of heart failure. Cardiac auscultation may show murmurs (mitral regurgitation is common), an accentuated P_2, an S_3, which indicates ventricular dysfunction or decompensation, and an S_4, which indicates abnormal atrioventricular filling characteristics. Abdominal examination findings suggest the presence of hepatomegaly or ascites. Pitting edema of the lower extremities is common.

LABORATORY FINDINGS AND DIAGNOSTIC TESTS

Chest radiograph The cardiothoracic ratio, which is measured on a conventional posteroanterior radiograph, provides an estimate of overall heart enlargement. Pulmonary blood volume often is redistributed to the upper lobes on an upright image, producing cephalization. Perihilar infiltrates suggest cardiogenic pulmonary edema.

Electrocardiogram: The presence of Q waves indicates prior myocardial infarction. The increased voltage of LV hypertrophy may be seen. Various arrhythmias (atrial, ventricular, heart block) are common among patients with heart failure.

Specialized cardiac studies: Ventricular performance can be quantified by means of echocardiography or radionuclide blood pool scanning. An LV ejection fraction less than 45% at rest is considered abnormal. Echocardiography also provides information about valvular function, wall thickness, and regional wall motion. Doppler flow measurements are used to assess the functional significance of observed stenotic and regurgitant valvular lesions. Coronary angiography often is necessary to clarify the cause of heart failure (ischemic or nonischemic). Direct measurement of right atrial, right ventricular and pulmonary artery wedge pressures confirms the diagnosis of heart failure. In difficult cases, an exercise test with monitoring of ECG and gas exchange can help differentiate cardiac, pulmonary, deconditioning, and nonmotivational disability.

PROGNOSIS AND MANAGEMENT

General strategies: The overall 5-year survival of heart failure is less than 50%. Management goals include identification of causes that can be corrected, prevention of disease progression, maintenance of physical activity, reversal of sodium retention, and reduction of the risk of death. Moderation of sodium intake (2 to 3 g per day) helps counteract the tendency toward sodium retention and edema. Dynamic, not isometric, exercise should be encouraged within the limits of tolerance. Associated conditions, such as cardiac arrhythmia, hypertension, chronic lung disease, and diabetes should be managed aggressively. Overweight patients should be encouraged to lose weight.

"Standard" pharmacologic therapy: Angiotensin-converting enzyme (ACE) inhibitors are recommended for all stages of heart failure. By decreasing systemic vascular resistance, these agents improve symptoms, limit progression of LV dysfunction, and reduce mortality. The dosage should be small at first and gradually escalated (e.g., to 40 mg lisinopril per day or 20 mg enalapril twice a day). Diuretic dosage should be reduced if hypotension (symptomatic or systolic pressure less than 80 to 85 mm Hg) or clinically significant azotemia develops. Transient reduction of renal function may occur but should not discourage continued therapy in most cases. Side effects include dry cough, hyperkalemia, and skin rash. Other vasodilators, such as the combination of hydralazine and isosorbide dinitrate, may be given to patients who cannot tolerate ACE inhibitors. Because of a lack of benefit in most trials, no calcium channel blocker has been approved for the management of heart failure.

Loop diuretics reduce intravascular volume and allow reabsorption of edema fluid. The response is monitored by assessing of symptoms, signs of fluid overload, daily weights, and changes in blood urea nitrogen and creatinine levels. Among patients who seem to be resistant to high doses of a loop diuretic, the addition of a thiazide diuretic (which acts at a different location within the nephron) can be helpful. Hypokalemia is a common problem and may contribute to arrhythmia, especially among patients receiving digoxin. Replacement may be difficult if there is a coexisting magnesium deficiency. Digoxin has been shown to have some benefits, including a decreased rate of hospitalization, in the care of patients with normal sinus rhythm. No effect on mortality has been demonstrated.

Supplemental therapy: Angiotensin II antagonists are not approved for the management of heart failure but have been beneficial in some trials. Some clinicians have substituted them for ACE inhibitors when ACE inhibitors were suspected of causing a bothersome cough. In the recent RALES trial, the aldosterone antagonist spironolactone produced a highly significant reduction in mortality when added to standard therapy (ACE inhibitor, diuretic, and digoxin). The effective dose was 25 mg per day, much lower than the historical dosage.

β-Blockers have emerged as important therapy despite initial concerns about their negative inotropic effect. β-Blockers exert favorable effects through reduction of heart rate, suppression of the renin–angiotensin system, and resetting of abnormal sympathetic nervous system abnormalities. Trials of three different agents all showed significant reductions in mortality when β-blockers were added to standard therapy. One should start with the lowest possible does and gradually advance over 1 to 3 months, as tolerated, to target doses (e.g., 100 mg metoprolol twice a day and 25 mg carvedilol twice a day).

Because sudden death accounts for 35% to 70% of the mortality in published studies of heart failure, the use of antiarrhythmic agents has been investigated. A mortality benefit with amiodarone has been reported but not conclusively established. For patients with symptomatic ventricular arrhythmia, implantation of a cardiac defibrillator has been shown to be most effective in preventing sudden death.

Advanced heart failure: "Refractory" heart failure is progressive decompensation despite optimal medical therapy. In some cases, patients may respond to intravenous diuretics or intravenous dobutamine. Ventricular assist devices are being used as a bridge to cardiac transplantation, which is now a practical option limited chiefly by a shortage of donor hearts.

Chapter 66

■ APPROACH TO THE PATIENT WITH HYPOTENSION AND SHOCK

DEFINITIONS AND PATHOPHYSIOLOGY

Hypotension is the reduction of systemic blood pressure below the usual range. It becomes clinically important only when it elicits symptoms of decreased organ perfusion or when it is a manifestation of an underlying disease, such as hemorrhage or myocardial infarction. *Orthostatic hypotension* is defined as a reduction in systolic blood pressure of at least 20 mm Hg within 3 minutes of standing. It represents a failure of the usual circulatory compensations to upright posture (increases in heart rate, myocardial contractility, and vasoconstriction). *Shock* is a syndrome of inadequate organ and tissue perfusion due to extreme circulatory failure. The pathophysiologic mechanism may be hypovolemia, increased vascular capacitance, cardiac failure, or obstruction of blood flow. If the condition remains uncontrolled or progresses despite the maximal recruitment of compensatory mechanisms (those noted above, as well as an increase in renal salt and water retention), the patient enters a stage of tissue dysfunction, which eventually leads to cell injury and death.

CLINICAL FEATURES AND DIFFERENTIAL DIAGNOSIS

Orthostatic hypotension: Patients often have postural symptoms such as light-headedness, dizziness, blurred vision, or headache. Common causes include dehydration, effects of medications (such as phenothiazines, tricyclic antidepressants, diuretics, and antihypertensive drugs), autonomic dysfunction, blood loss and anemia, hypokalemia, deconditioning, and malnutrition. The history should focus on prior medical problems, medications use, alcohol consumption, and dietary habits. Patients with autonomic dysfunction also may have a history of constipation, urinary difficulties, sexual dysfunction, or night blindness. The physical examination should include evaluation of positional changes in heart rate. Patients whose pulse does not increase when they stand may have autonomic dysfunction. Careful cardiac and neurologic examinations also are essential.

Shock: The pulse may be rapid and faint. Because systemic hypoperfusion provokes intense dermal vasoconstriction, the skin appears pale to light blue and becomes cool to the touch. The palms are frequently moist. Myocardial ischemia is likely to occur. Ventilation–perfusion mismatches reduce the arterial oxygen content; hypoxemia is markedly exacerbated if adult respiratory distress syndrome develops. Cardiogenic forms of shock may cause pulmonary edema due to high left ventricular filling pressure. Renal hypoperfusion decreases urine output and increases the blood urea nitrogen (BUN) to creatinine ratio to more than $10:1$. If acute tubular necrosis develops, the urine output decreases further (less than 20 mL per hour), the BUN to creatinine ratio decreases to less than $10:1$, and the urine sodium concentration usually exceeds 40 mEq per liter. Gastritis and stress ulcers are common. Intestinal infarction can occur. Hepatic hypoperfusion increases serum liver enzyme levels. The liver injury may evolve into hepatic necrosis in severe cases. Icterus is common. The patient's mental status may range from anxiety in mild shock to confusion, disorientation, and somnolence in moderate cases to obtundation and coma in prolonged or severe shock. Disseminated intravascular coagulation commonly accompanies terminal stages. Metabolic acidosis usually is caused by lactate production by underperfused muscle. A classification of shock according to causative factors is presented in Table 71.2.

STRATEGIES FOR MANAGEMENT

Orthostatic hypotension: Reversible causes should be treated. Patients should be counseled to rise slowly and to perform isometric exercises of the extremities beforehand. Increasing dietary salt intake may improve symptoms by expanding intravascular volume. If these measures fail, salt tablets or fludrocortisone acetate may be effective in increasing intravascular volume. Patients with supine hypertension and orthostatic hypotension may respond to nonselective β-blockers, such as propranolol, which reduce the vasodilating effect of β-adrenergic stimulation.

Shock: The evaluation and management of shock are outlined in Fig. 71.1. The physician must perform the initial evaluation and the initial treatment simultaneously. The choice among the possible diagnostic and therapeutic options is guided by the evolving clinical suspicion.

Chapter 71

◾ MITRAL VALVE DISEASE

DEFINITIONS, EPIDEMIOLOGY, AND ETIOLOGY

Mitral Stenosis: Mitral stenosis (MS) implies valvular obstruction of left ventricular (LV) inflow. MS among adults is predominantly of rheumatic origin. Women are affected more than men.

Mitral regurgitation: Mitral regurgitation (MR) is an acute or chronic process of LV volume overload caused by incompetence of the mitral valve. Regurgitation due to abnormal leaflet anatomy can be caused by congenital or rheumatic disease, myxomatous degeneration, connective tissue disease, or infective endocarditis. Ischemic MR is caused by incomplete coaptation of the mitral leaflets due to ischemic changes in the function or geometric features of the LV. Any myopathic process that causes LV dilatation can cause MR by a similar mechanism. Acute, severe MR is caused by infective endocarditis, acute myocardial infarction with papillary muscle rupture, or prosthetic valve dysfunction.

Mitral valve prolapse: Mitral valve prolapse (MVP) is a fairly common syndrome of myxomatous degeneration of the mitral valve that produces redundant

leaflets and elongation of the chordae tendineae. It occurs in 2% to 6% of the adult population, more commonly in women. There is evidence of an autosomal dominant inheritance pattern and an association with connective tissue diseases.

PATHOPHYSIOLOGY

Mitral Stenosis: The normal mitral valve area is 4.0 to 5.0 cm^2. Symptoms occur with exercise or tachycardia when the area is approximately 2.0 to 2.5 cm^2 but do not usually occur at rest until the area is 1.5 cm^2 or smaller. Obstruction to LV inflow causes left atrial (LA) dilatation, pulmonary venous and arterial hypertension, and right ventricular (RV) hypertrophy.

Mitral regurgitation: Blood is ejected from the LV into both the low-pressure LA and the high-pressure aorta. LV volume overload results. Forward cardiac output is maintained by means of compensatory LV dilation. The volume overload eventually leads to LV systolic dysfunction and pulmonary congestion. Because LV emptying does not rely on overcoming high aortic pressure, the stroke volume and ejection fraction remain normal despite progressive systolic dysfunction.

Mitral valve prolapse: Patients with MVP have a propensity to premature valve degeneration, leaflet flail, and mitral regurgitation. There is prolapse of the mitral valve into the left atrium during ventricular systole.

CLINICAL FINDINGS

Mitral stenosis: The first symptoms of rheumatic MS typically occur decades after an episode of rheumatic fever that may have been unrecognized or forgotten. There is usually another long period during which symptoms are present but mild. Early symptoms include fatigue or dyspnea precipitated by events with associated tachycardia (such as exercise, emotional stress, fever, pregnancy, or surgery). Later, dyspnea occurs with less strenuous activity and eventually at rest. Pulmonary edema may lead to orthopnea and paroxysmal nocturnal dyspnea and the production of frothy, pink sputum. Patients may notice palpitations caused by ectopic beats, paroxysmal atrial tachycardia, or atrial fibrillation. Late symptoms include hemoptysis (caused by rupture of small bronchial vessels in the setting of pulmonary hypertension) and peripheral edema, ascites, and pleural effusion (from RV failure).

Neck vein distention is found at physical examination. The LV apical impulse is diminished or nonpalpable. Auscultation reveals accentuation of S_1 and usually an increase in P_2. The classic high-pitched opening snap occurs soon after the A_2. A low-pitched diastolic rumble occurs after the opening snap and is heard best at the LV apex with the patient in the left lateral decubitus position. Presystolic accentuation occurs in sinus rhythm. As the severity of MS increases, the opening snap occurs sooner after A_2, and the duration of the murmur increases. Late findings include hepatomegaly, ascites, pleural effusion, and peripheral edema.

Mitral regurgitation: Chronic MR remains asymptomatic for an extended period. Fatigue and exertional dyspnea eventually develop, followed by more overt symptoms of congestive heart failure, including orthopnea and paroxysmal nocturnal dyspnea. Patients with acute, severe MR almost always have fulminant symptoms of pulmonary edema. At examination, patients with chronic MR have a hyperactive precordium and a displaced LV apical impulse. An S_3 is often present and is not necessarily indicative of ventricular failure. The classic murmur is a loud, blowing, holosystolic murmur that may obliterate S_1 and S_2. It usually is loudest at the apex, and there is radiation to the axilla or back. The large volume of blood crossing the mitral valve in diastole may cause a diastolic rumble in the absence of mitral stenosis. In acute MR, the systolic murmur may be decrescendo rather than holosystolic because of early equilibration of LA and LV pressures in the presence of an LA of normal size.

Mitral valve prolapse: MVP can remain asymptomatic. Some patients have palpitations, usually from isolated ectopic beats or supraventricular tachycardia, or atypical, nonexertional chest pain. There are controversial associations between MVP and both transient ischemic attacks and panic attacks. The symptoms of MR also may be present. Patients with MVP classically have a thin body habitus, and there is an association with pectus excavatum. Auscultation reveals one or more high-pitched mid-to-late systolic nonejection clicks. If the patient has MR, the murmur begins in systole after the click.

DIAGNOSTIC STUDIES

Mitral stenosis: MS is associated with broadened, notched P waves in the inferior leads are caused by enlargement of the LA (P mitrale). Atrial fibrillation is common, and right axis deviation and RV hypertrophy may be evident. A chest radiograph shows apical redistribution and prominent vascularity in the lung parenchyma, interstitial edema, and peribronchial and perivascular cuffing. The cardiac silhouette has prominent pulmonary arteries. LA enlargement straightens the left heart border and splays the bronchi with elevation of the left main stem bronchus. The diagnosis is confirmed with echocardiography, including Doppler techniques. This modality also can be used to assess severity and associated cardiac abnormalities, such as LA and RV hypertrophy and pulmonary hypertension. Cardiac catheterization with coronary angiography is useful when a planned mitral valve operation may also include coronary artery bypass if severe coronary artery disease is demonstrated.

Mitral regurgitation: For patients with chronic MR, the ECG and chest radiograph may contain show evidence of LA or LV enlargement. Echocardiography with Doppler technique is the diagnostic test of choice and can be used to define severity and causation. Cardiac catheterization is useful for assessment of coronary anatomy in the care of patients at risk of coronary disease who are undergoing a mitral valve operation and in the care of patients with MR believed to be ischemic in origin.

Mitral valve prolapse: Echocardiography with Doppler techniques is the preferred diagnostic test.

PROGNOSIS AND STRATEGIES FOR MANAGEMENT

Mitral stenosis: The 10-year survival rate is more than 80% among patients with MS who are asymptomatic or have mild symptoms. Once debilitating symptoms occur, usually with associated pulmonary hypertension, prognosis is poor. The estimated survival rate becomes less than 3 years among patients who do not undergo surgical treatment. Mortality is related to progressive heart failure, pulmonary embolization, and infection. Patients should receive prophylaxis against endocarditis prior to procedures likely to cause bacteremia. Those with evidence of rheumatic heart disease should receive secondary prophylaxis against recurrent infection, usually with monthly intramuscular injections of 1.2 million units of penicillin G benzathine. Patients in sinus rhythm with symptoms at rapid heart rates may benefit from calcium channel blockers or β-blockers. Pulmonary congestion is treated with salt restriction and diuretics. Patients with atrial fibrillation or a history of prior embolization should receive long-term anticoagulation.

Mitral valve surgery is indicated for patients with moderate or severe MS along with intolerable symptoms, pulmonary hypertension regardless of symptoms, or recurrent thromboembolism despite adequate anticoagulation. Mitral valve replacement is indicated only for patients who should not undergo percutaneous valvotomy or open commissurotomy, such as those with marked mitral regurgitation, left atrial thrombus, or extensive fibrosis of the mitral valve leaflets. Mechanical prostheses have greater durability but high thrombogenicity. Tissue prostheses have lower thrombogenicity, and thus no independent requirement for anticoagulation, but more limited durability than do mechanical prostheses.

Mitral regurgitation: Appropriate antibiotic prophylaxis should be used prior to procedures likely to cause bacteremia. Afterload-reducing agents my decrease the severity of MR by reducing the resistance to anterograde flow from the LV. Mitral valve surgery is indicated to treat patients with severe MR and either symptoms of heart failure or evidence of LV systolic dysfunction. Because preoperative LV systolic function is an important predictor of postoperative survival, patients without symptoms should be evaluated with echocardiography once a year and be referred for surgical intervention before the onset of systolic dysfunction. (Stroke volume and ejection fraction are poor markers of systolic function, however, because regurgitant flow allows LV emptying to be maintained despite progressive systolic dysfunction). The choice of surgical procedure includes mitral valve repair and mitral valve replacement with or without chordal preservation. Repair minimizes the use of prosthetic material and is associated with more favorable hemodynamics and a lower mortality rate, but it is a more technically demanding procedure and may not be feasible for all valves.

Mitral valve prolapse: Patients who have associated MR or leaflet thickening at echocardiography should receive antibiotic prophylaxis prior to undergoing procedures likely to cause bacteremia. Patients without symptoms need no additional therapy. β-Blockers often are useful for the management of palpitations. Patients who have had focal neurologic events who are in sinus rhythm and have no LA thrombus should receive antiplatelet therapy with aspirin. Long-term anticoagulation with warfarin is recommended for patients with no contraindications who have had a stroke or who have recurrent transient ischemic attacks while receiving aspirin.

Chapter 77

▄ PERICARDIAL DISEASES

CLASSIFICATION

There are three broad pericardial syndromes—acute pericarditis, pericardial effusion and tamponade, and constrictive pericarditis.

PATHOPHYSIOLOGY AND DIFFERENTIAL DIAGNOSIS

Acute pericarditis: Most cases are of unknown origin and are assumed to be related to an unidentified viral infection. Bacterial, mycobacterial, fungal, and parasitic infections are relatively rare in the United States. Many cases are noninfective and occur after surgery (postpericardiotomy syndrome), myocardial infarction (Dressler syndrome), irradiation, or trauma. Other associations are with renal failure, collagen vascular disease, especially lupus erythematosus, and myxedema.

Pericardial effusion tamponade: Pericardial effusion often occurs as part of a general increase in extracellular fluid volume, as in congestive heart failure and nephrotic syndrome. It also occurs as a feature of almost every form of pericardial disease. Neoplasm accounts for about one-half of cases. The clinical consequences depend on the quantity of fluid and rate of accumulation. Cardiac tamponade occurs when the increased pressure within a pericardial effusion is sufficient to compress the heart and impede its diastolic filling. Acute tamponade is caused most frequently by hemopericardium associated with trauma, cardiac surgery, aortic dissection, or myocardial rupture.

Constrictive pericarditis: In constrictive pericarditis, the heart is compressed by solid tissue surrounding the heart. The solid tissue is usually scar tissue but can be malignant solid tumors and organizing blood. Any of the causes of pericardial disease can produce sufficient scarring to cause constriction. The most common causes are irradiation therapy and cardiac surgery.

CLINICAL FEATURES AND DIAGNOSTIC EVALUATION

Acute pericarditis: Idiopathic or viral acute pericarditis often is preceded by a low-grade fever, sore throat, and myalgia. Anterior chest pain is the most prominent symptom. It is classically substernal and pleuritic, often sudden in onset and severe, and is partially relieved by sitting up. The corresponding finding at examination is pericardial friction rub. Definite pericardial rubs have both systolic and diastolic components, and the classic rub also has a third component in late diastole that is caused by atrial contraction. The characteristic ECG abnormalities are diffuse ST-segment elevation from subepicardial inflammation without reciprocal ST-segment depression and PQ-segment depression. Creatine kinase levels generally remain normal unless there is accompanying myocarditis. Erythrocyte sedimentation rate and white blood cell count often are elevated. Initial diagnostic studies should focus on ruling out bacterial infection. A tuberculin skin test usually is indicated. Cultures of blood and other tissue are indicated when the degree of fever and leukocytosis and the severity of the illness suggest that purulent pericarditis is a reasonable possibility. Screening tests for rheumatic conditions, hypothyroidism, and renal failure may prove useful.

Cardiac tamponade: Hemopericardium generally manifests with sudden hypotension and elevation of venous pressure. Tamponade associated with medical conditions such as idiopathic or infective pericarditis, neoplasm, renal failure, or collagen vascular disease usually manifests in a less acute manner. The principal symptom is dyspnea, which occurs despite clear lungs. Pleural effusion often is present. Jugular venous pressure is nearly always elevated. The other key finding is the paradoxical pulse, an inspiratory decline of more than 10 mm Hg in systolic blood pressure. An electrocardiogram (ECG) often shows low amplitude of the complexes. Beat-to-beat alternation in the amplitude of the QRS complexes (electrical alternans) often is a specific sign. Except in very acute cases, a chest radiograph shows enlargement of the cardiomediastinal silhouette. Echocardiography is the most valuable diagnostic procedure for detecting pericardial effusion. Specific findings, such as collapse of the right atrium and ventricle in early diastole, also suggest tamponade.

Constrictive pericarditis: Patients usually have at least mild dyspnea and impaired exercise tolerance. Ankle edema, ascites, congestive hepatomegaly, and pleural effusion may occur. Because these patients often are younger and have less venous insufficiency, they frequently have less ankle edema than patients with more common forms of heart disease. Examination reveals elevated jugular venous pressure in almost every case. The venous pulsation shows a prominent brief dip in early diastole and an increase with inspiration (Kussmaul sign). Auscultation shows a pericardial knock, an abnormal extra heart sound in early diastole. Paradoxical pulse is not prominent in most patients. The ECG findings are not distinctive. The chest radiograph usually shows normal heart size and clear lungs.

Echocardiography is helpful chiefly in excluding cardiac disease or pericardial effusion. Computed tomography and magnetic resonance imaging have better resolution than echocardiography and provide a more accurate assessment of the thickness of the pericardium. Findings at cardiac catheterization can support the diagnosis and indicate severity. The classic finding is diastolic pressure equalization in all cardiac chambers and dip-plateau pressure waveforms in the right ventricle. Some patients with amyloidosis or idiopathic restrictive cardiomyopathy have findings at cardiac catheterization and angiography that closely resemble those of constrictive pericarditis. A myocardial biopsy or exploratory thoracotomy may be necessary.

MANAGEMENT

Acute pericarditis: Idiopathic or viral pericarditis usually is self-limited. Treatment is directed primarily at symptom relief. After initial use of narcotics to relieve the pain, aspirin should be prescribed for its analgesic and anti-inflammatory effects. In severe cases, glucocorticoids may be necessary. Bacterial forms must be managed with antibiotics and surgical drainage. Cases associated with uremia, malignant tumors, and rheumatic disease respond to specific therapies for the underlying condition.

Pericardial tamponade: Although the circulation may be supported temporarily by fluid infusion, only removal of pericardial fluid is consistently effective. Needle pericardiocentesis is less traumatic than surgical drainage, but surgical drainage is more likely to be effective and provides a specimen for pericardial biopsy.

Constrictive pericarditis: In mild cases, fluid retention can be controlled with diuretics alone. In general, however, surgical pericardiectomy is the only effective treatment. It can be a difficult operation with high morbidity and mortality.

Chapter 79

PULMONARY HYPERTENSION AND COR PULMONALE

DEFINITIONS

Pulmonary hypertension is defined as a mean pulmonary artery pressure exceeding 25 mm Hg at rest or 30 mm Hg during exercise. Cor pulmonale is best defined as pulmonary hypertension in the setting of chronic respiratory disease. Right-sided heart failure is a late manifestation.

ETIOLOGY AND DIFFERENTIAL DIAGNOSIS

The causes of pulmonary hypertension can be categorized according to the primary circulatory site affected. Postcapillary pulmonary hypertension is caused by obstruction of pulmonary venous return (e.g., left ventricular failure, mitral or aortic valve disease, left atrial myxoma, and pulmonary veno-occlusive disease). Precapillary pulmonary hypertension is caused by obstruction, constriction, or obliteration of a substantial component of the pulmonary arterial tree (e.g., parenchymal lung diseases, sleep apnea and hypoventilation syndromes, high altitude disease, intracardiac septal defects, massive or chronic pulmonary embolism, pulmonary vasculitis, and primary pulmonary hypertension). Primary pulmonary hypertension is a rare disease in which there are substantial elevations in pulmonary artery pressure in the absence of known causative factors. It is characterized by a spectrum of vascular lesions, from medial hypertrophy of small pulmonary arteries and intimal proliferation of pulmonary arteries to more severe destructive vascular abnormalities such as fibrinoid necrosis. Primary pulmonary hypertension occurs with greater frequency among women, particularly during the childbearing years, and in some families. An association with the diet drugs fenfluramine and dexfenfluramine has been demonstrated.

CLINICAL FEATURES

Symptoms: The symptoms of pulmonary hypertension usually are nonspecific. Patients with chronic respiratory disease in whom cor pulmonale develops may come to medical attention merely with a worsening of their previous symptoms. Exertional dyspnea, tachypnea, chest pain, and light-headedness are common and are related to the increase in right ventricular (RV) work. Syncope, pedal edema, and ascites are indicative of more critical impairments in RV function. Hemoptysis, from small-vessel rupture, occurs occasionally among patients with precapillary pulmonary hypertension but is more common among those with postcapillary pulmonary hypertension. Hoarseness can be caused by compression of the left recurrent laryngeal nerve by enlarged proximal pulmonary arteries. Some patients with connective tissue disease or primary pulmonary hypertension have Raynaud's phenomenon.

Physical examination: There may be findings referable to underlying diseases. Jugular venous distention may be present (a prominent *cv* wave indicates tricuspid insufficiency). RV enlargement may cause a parasternal lift. The P_2 is loud, and there may be a pulmonic ejection click. An S_3 may be heard at the left parasternal region in RV failure and an S_4 in severe pulmonary hypertension. The murmur of tricuspid insufficiency frequently is audible, as is the Graham Steell murmur of pulmonic insufficiency. Venous congestion may cause tender hepatomegaly. Ascites and lower extremity edema indicate overt RV failure in the absence of other causes. Digital clubbing is common among patients with chronic obstructive lung disease, pulmonary fibrosis, cystic fibrosis, and congenital heart disease but is uncommon in primary pulmonary hypertension and thromboembolism.

DIAGNOSIS

The diagnostic approach involves establishing the presence and severity of pulmonary vascular disease and clarifying its cause. Primary pulmonary hypertension may be diagnosed when pulmonary hypertension exists in the absence of significant parenchymal lung disease, thromboembolic disease, or congenital or left-sided cardiac disease.

Cardiac testing: The ECG usually shows RV hypertrophy and P pulmonale, though the latter (a P wave greater than 2.5 mm in amplitude in inferior leads) is not specific for pulmonary hypertension. Echocardiography is a useful noninvasive procedure. Chamber size and wall motion can be assessed, and Doppler technique allows accurate evaluation of the function of the tricuspid and pulmonic valves. It also provides information about left ventricular and mitral valve function. A right-to-left shunt can be found with a bubble study. Pulmonary artery systolic pressure can be estimated with Doppler techniques, but these measurements are not consistently reliable.

Pulmonary testing: The chest radiographic findings of pulmonary veno-occlusive disease include signs of pulmonary edema and Kerley B lines. Pulmonary function tests and assessment of arterial blood gases are useful in detecting unsuspected or worsening respiratory disease. Sleep studies can be used to exclude sleep apnea syndromes. Ventilation–perfusion scanning is critical. The perfusion scan is essentially normal in primary pulmonary hypertension but may show patchy abnormalities in veno-occlusive disease or multiple defects in recurrent or unresolved thromboembolism. Patients with suspected thromboembolism should undergo pulmonary arteriography to clarify the diagnosis and determine the extent and site of the clot. The role of lung biopsy in the evaluation of unexplained pulmonary hypertension is controversial. Biopsy findings can establish the presence of subclinical interstitial disease, pulmonary vasculitis, or small-vessel thromboembolism.

Laboratory tests: A low titer of antinuclear antibody occurs among about 25% of patients with primary pulmonary hypertension. The presence of polycythemia suggests hypoxemia. Detailed coagulation studies should be performed for patients with recurrent or unresolved thromboembolism.

PROGNOSIS AND MANAGEMENT

Coexisting pulmonary hypertension in the setting of chronic respiratory disease is a poor prognostic sign; death commonly occurs within 3 to 5 years of the onset of disease. The median survival time from the initial diagnosis of primary pulmonary hypertension is 2 to 3 years. It depends more on RV function than on pulmonary artery pressure.

Underlying conditions should be treated with agents such as bronchodilators, mucolytics, and glucocorticoids. Supplemental oxygen may be indicated for patients with resting or exertional hypoxemia. Chronic hypoxemia can cause polycythemia and worsening of pulmonary hypertension. Isovolumic phlebotomy is recommended if the hematocrit exceeds 50%. Digitalis is of limited value in isolated RV dysfunction but may be useful therapy for biventricular failure or control of supraventricular tachyarrhythmias. Diuretics must be used cautiously, because the RV is sensitive to reductions in preload. Unless use of anticoagulants is contraindicated, patients with pulmonary hypertension due to thromboembolism and primary pulmonary hypertension should be treated with anticoagulants, usually warfarin, for life. The use of anticoagulants to manage other causes of pulmonary hypertension is controversial.

Vasodilators: A variety of vasodilators have been used cautiously with mixed results. They usually increase cardiac output but produce little change in pulmonary artery pressure. Most patients notice improvement in symptoms when cardiac output increases. Therapy must be discontinued if systemic hypotension, an increase in pulmonary artery pressure, or worsened hypoxemia develops. Prostaglandin I_2 (PGI_2) is a potent, short-acting, titratable vasodilator that is administered intravenously. Patients who respond to PGI_2 infusion with decreases in pulmonary artery pressure or pulmonary vascular resistance seem to have similar responses to therapy with orally active drugs such as nifedipine and diltiazem. PGI_2 has been used in continuous infusion for the management of severe pulmonary hypertension and may be particularly useful as a bridge to transplantation. Inhaled nitrous oxide, the endothelium-derived relaxing factor, has been used to test vascular reactivity initially and to treat patients with severe pulmonary hypertension for brief periods.

Transplantation: Combined heart–lung transplantation has been performed successfully on patients with primary pulmonary hypertension or Eisenmenger syndrome. Single- or double-lung transplantation has been performed successfully on patients with less severe impairment of RV function.

Chapter 80

▪ APPROACH TO THE PATIENT WITH SYNCOPE

DEFINITION AND PATHOPHYSIOLOGY

Syncope is a sudden transient loss of consciousness associated with a loss of postural tone and a spontaneous recovery. Most episodes are the result of reduced blood flow to the brain centers responsible for the maintenance of consciousness. Decreased cerebral blood flow is usually the result of one of four physiologic abnormalities: disorders of vascular tone or blood volume, cardiopulmonary mechanical disorders, cardiac arrhythmias, and cerebrovascular disease. Syncope can occur with normal cerebral blood flow when there is a lack of essential nutrients required for cerebral metabolism (e.g., hypoglycemia and hypoxemia). Some of the causes of syncope are presented in Table 69.1. Vasovagal syncope, a common cause of syncope among otherwise healthy persons, is thought to be caused by inappropriate bradycardia and vasodilation in the face of declining arterial pressure.

DIFFERENTIAL DIAGNOSIS

Seizures can mimic syncope. They account for loss of consciousness among 5% to 10% of patients in most studies. Seizures often can be differentiated from syncope by the presence of an aura, the maintenance of muscular tone during the episode, and the presence of drowsiness and confusion after an episode. Tongue-biting may occur. Hysterical fainting and other neuropsychiatric disorders also can mimic syncope. These episodes usually occur in the presence of observers, typically in emotionally charged situations, and rarely result in physical injury. Anxiety with hyperventilation may decrease cerebral blood flow owing to hypocapnea. Diagnostic clues include digital and circumoral numbness and tingling and lack of relief from light-headedness with recumbency. Unlike most patients with syncope, those with metabolic disorders such as hypoglycemia, hypoxemia, and hypercapnea typically have both a gradual onset of symptoms and a gradual recovery.

CLINICAL FEATURES

The interview is the cornerstone of the evaluation. Specific historical issues and key elements of the physical examination are summarized in Table 69.4.

Vasovagal syncope: Vasovagal syncope often is preceded by a prodromal period that lasts for as long as a few minutes. The person, who is almost always sitting or standing, experiences weakness, nausea, diaphoresis, light-headedness, and often a sense of impending darkness. Tachycardia, decreased blood pressure, and pallor usually occur at the beginning of the episode. Cardiac slowing ensues, as does diaphoresis, pupillary constriction, and syncope. The duration of unconsciousness rarely is longer than a few minutes. A variety of factors may precipitate vasovagal syncope, including a hot or crowded environment, the effects of alcohol consumption, extreme fatigue, hunger, long-term recumbency, prolonged standing, and emotional or stressful situations.

Cardiac arrhythmias: Syncope is uncommon unless the heart rate drops to less than 30 beats per minute or exceeds 180 beats per minute. Syncope associated with tachyarrhythmia or bradyarrhythmia often occurs with little or no warning. Supraventricular arrhythmia rarely causes syncope in the absence of associated cardiovascular disease.

DIAGNOSTIC EVALUATION

Laboratory findings: Serum electrolyte and plasma glucose levels and the hematocrit sometimes help to establish the cause of syncope. The presence of hypokalemia makes arrhythmia more likely. Cardiac enzymes should be evaluated for patients with a history that suggests myocardial infarction. Blood and urine toxicology screens may reveal the presence of alcohol or other drugs.

Electrocardiogram: The electrocardiogram (ECG) at the time of evaluation may reveal arrhythmia, but it more commonly shows a sinus rhythm. Nevertheless, an ECG may provide clues such as a prolonged QT interval or Q waves. Hospitalized patients should undergo continuous ECG monitoring unless the suspicion of cardiac arrhythmias is very low. Holter monitoring is appropriate for patients undergoing outpatient evaluation, although the diagnostic yield diminishes dramatically after the first 24 to 48 hours of monitoring. It is important to correlate any arrhythmias with a diary of the patient's symptoms. Event recorders are small ECG monitors that the patient can carry for weeks, if necessary. The recorder can be activated by the patient when symptoms of palpitation or light-headedness occur.

Other tests: Other diagnostic tests may be indicated for selected patients. A signal-averaged ECG can help identify electrical signals that indicate a substrate for ventricular tachycardia; it is most useful in the care of patients with a history of myocardial infarction. Exercise testing may help detect ischemia or exercise-induced arrhythmias but should not be used in the care of patients who may have aortic stenosis or hypertrophic cardiomyopathy. Electrophysiologic studies are invasive tests that can provide diagnostic and prognostic information about sinus and atrioventricular node function, conduction pathways, and a variety of types of arrhythmia. Depending on the group studied, electrophysiologic studies can help identify the cause of syncope in 12% to 70% of cases. Echocardiography with Doppler examination is useful for diagnosing or excluding many cardiac mechanical causes of syncope, such as valvular and pericardial disease, atrial myxoma, and hypertrophic cardiomyopathy. Patients with regional wall motion abnormalities and diminished left ventricular function are at higher risk of ventricular arrhythmias than those with normal echocardiograms. The upright tilt-table test often induces syncope among patients with vasovagal events (sensitivity 75%, specificity 93%). The addition of intravenous isoproterenol increases the sensitivity of the test at the cost of some of its specificity. Cardiac catheterization is necessary in the care of some patients to determine the presence and severity of coronary artery disease or the anatomic basis for an abnormality detected by noninvasive means. Electroencephalography, carotid ultrasonography, and computed tomography of the head rarely are helpful.

OPTIMAL MANAGEMENT

Treatment depends on the specific cause of the syncope and the frequency and severity of the episodes. Until it is clear that the syncope has been effectively controlled, patients should avoid operating automobiles or heavy mechanical equipment. Therapy for vasovagal syncope includes β-blockers and disopyramide, which are thought to act by decreasing myocardial contractility. Other agents that have been used include theophylline, scopolamine, and ephedrine. Mineralocorticoids, salt loading, and support stockings may be effective for patients in whom hypovolemia or venous pooling initiates vasovagal syncope.

Chapter 69

▪ SYSTEMIC HYPERTENSION

DEFINITION

Chronic elevations in blood pressure to more than 140/90 mm Hg are regarded as hypertension. However, the relation between blood pressure and morbidity is continuous rather than dichotomous, and the optimal blood pressure has not been established conclusively.

EPIDEMIOLOGY

The prevalence of hypertension ranges from about 20% among white Americans to almost 40% among blacks. Blood pressure increases with age; more than 60% of Americans older than 65 years have hypertension.

ETIOLOGY

Genetic and environmental factors may interact to increase blood pressure. A hereditary risk has been well demonstrated. Some persons also seem to have a sensitivity to high sodium intake, alcohol consumption, oral contraceptives, nonsteroidal anti-inflammatory agents, exogenous glucocorticoids, and the sympathomimetic agents in decongestants and appetite suppressants.

PATHOGENESIS AND PATHOPHYSIOLOGY

Primary, or essential, hypertension: Primary hypertension accounts for more than 90% of cases. It results from an alteration in one or more of the following: extracellular fluid volume, renal function, vasoactive factors and peripheral resistance, and cardiac output.

Secondary hypertension: Uncommon, but potentially curable, causes of hypertension include two forms of renal vascular hypertension: an atherosclerotic narrowing of one or both renal arteries (common among older patients) and stenosis from fibromuscular dysplasia (more common among young women). Decreased renal perfusion stimulates renin release, raises peripheral resistance, and prompts reabsorption of sodium and water. Primary aldosteronism, usually from an adrenal adenoma or hyperplasia, also induces salt and water retention. In pheochromocytoma, hypertension is caused by increased production of catecholamines, usually norepinephrine, and consequent increased cardiac output and peripheral vasoconstriction. Cushing's syndrome is produced by excessive adrenal corticosteroid production. Secondary hypertension also can be produced by coarctation of the aorta, hyperthyroidism, and the medications listed earlier.

CLINICAL FINDINGS

Most patients have no symptoms, and the only finding is the elevated blood pressure reading itself. The major effects of chronic hypertension can be separated into those caused directly by the increased pressure (cerebral hemorrhage, retinopathy, vascular rupture, left ventricular hypertrophy, and congestive heart failure), those caused by atherosclerosis (increased coronary, cerebral, and renal vascular resistance), and those caused by decreased blood flow and ischemia (myocardial and cerebral infarction and renal nephrosclerosis). A physical examination therefore may reveal nicking of retinal arterioles, a loud A_2, and an S_4. Malignant hypertension is rarely encountered at levels less than 160/110 mm Hg. Manifestations can include central nervous system effects (headaches, blurred vision, altered mental status, hemiparesis, seizures, and papilledema), cardiac effects (angina or acute pulmonary edema), and acute renal failure. The various forms of secondary hypertension should be considered when a patient has severe hypertension in an accelerated phase or when blood pressure control is difficult despite appropriate combination therapy and patient compliance. Paroxysmal headaches, sweating, and tachycardia suggest pheochromocytoma. Thyromegaly, cushingoid appearance, and midepigastric bruit also suggest secondary forms of hypertension.

LABORATORY FINDINGS

Screening tests include urinalysis and measurement of blood urea nitrogen and creatinine to detect renal disease, fasting glucose because diabetes often coexists with hypertension, serum potassium when the patient is not taking diuretics (low value suggests hyperaldosteronism or renal artery stenosis), and electrocardiography (left ventricular hypertrophy suggests long-standing hypertension). Specific imaging studies and laboratory tests are used to diagnose the secondary forms of hypertension.

MANAGEMENT

Nonpharmacologic therapy: The most recent recommendations of the Joint National Committee on High Blood Pressure are to use nonpharmacologic interventions, including weight loss, exercise, and reduction of sodium and alcohol intake, when blood pressure reaches a persistent level of 140 mm Hg systolic or 85 mm Hg diastolic. In the absence of target-organ damage, concomitant cardiovascular disease, or diabetes mellitus, these interventions also can be used to manage mild hypertension (diastolic pressure 90 to 95 mm Hg).

Pharmacologic Therapy: One approach to the initiation of antihypertensive therapy is presented in Fig. 30.1. Because some side effects are dose dependent, it often is wise to add a second drug before reaching the maximum dose of the initial agent. Combination therapy is more effective when drugs of different classes are used. Diuretics are the first choice for patients who are sensitive to sodium, particularly blacks and elderly persons. The starting dose of hydrochlorothiazide is usually 12.5 to 25 mg per day. Potassium or a potassium-sparing agent can be added. β-Blockers reduce blood pressure by reducing cardiac output and are most useful in the treatment of young patients with hyperdynamic circulation. Labetalol combines α- and β-blockade and is particularly useful in the emergency management of hypertension. Centrally acting sympatholytic agents such as α-methyldopa and clonidine can be useful adjuncts but are used infrequently because of side effects such as fatigue, depression, sleepiness, and dry mouth. Calcium channel blockers, angiotensin-converting enzyme (ACE) inhibitors, angiotensin receptor blockers, and peripheral α-blockers reduce vascular resistance, usually without promoting tachycardia or fluid retention. Direct-acting vasodilators, including minoxidil and hydralazine, are used chiefly to manage refractory hypertension owing to their tendency to induce salt and water retention.

Special situations: Secondary forms of hypertension have specific therapies. Recent evidence supports reduction of blood pressure to levels at or below 130/85 mm Hg among patients with diabetes for preservation of renal function. For

pregnant women with preexisting hypertension, dosages may have to be reduced because blood pressure normally drops in the first two trimesters. Pregnancy-induced hypertension usually occurs among young primigravidas after the twenty-seventh week. Centrally acting sympatholytic agents, peripheral α-blockers, and short-acting β-blockers can be used. ACE inhibitors and angiotensin receptor blockers are contraindicated during pregnancy.

Chapter 30

■ VENTRICULAR ARRHYTHMIAS

DEFINITION AND CLINICAL PRESENTATION

Cardiac arrhythmias are disorders of the normal heart rhythm. Most commonly, they cause palpitations, an awareness of the heartbeat caused by abnormally strong ventricular contraction, a pause in normal rhythm, or extra beats. Less commonly, they can produce syncope, near-syncope, angina, congestive heart failure, or death.

SPECIFIC ARRHYTHMIAS

Premature ventricular complexes: A premature ventricular complex (PVC) is characterized by occurrence of a QRS complex that is bizarre in shape and has a duration usually exceeding the dominant QRS complex (typically more than 120 milliseconds). A large T wave opposite in direction to the major deflection of the QRS is present. A premature P wave does not precede the QRS, but a sinus P wave that occurs at its usual time may be present. A PVC usually does not discharge the atria and sinus node; therefore a fully compensatory pause follows it (a pause that exactly makes up for the prematurity of the PVC so that the R wave of the following, normal QRS falls when it otherwise would have). An aberrantly conducted supraventricular complex can mimic a PVC. PVCs with different contours are called *multiform* or *polymorphic.*

The prevalence of PVCs increases with age. Symptoms include palpitations, discomfort in the neck or chest from the supranormal contractile force of the postextrasystolic beat, or the feeling that the heart has stopped during the compensatory pause. PVCs can be produced by direct mechanical, electrical, and chemical stimulation of the heart. Coronary artery disease, myocarditis, medications, electrolyte imbalance, tension states, caffeine, tobacco, alcohol, and autonomic stimulation all can provoke PVCs. In the absence of underlying heart disease, PVCs have little importance, and patients do not have to be treated. Among patients with known heart disease, PVCs are a marker for higher mortality. Despite this fact, antiarrhythmic therapy with flecainide and encainide has been shown to increase mortality even as it suppresses PVCs. Thus PVCs may be only a marker for risk and not themselves the cause of the risk. When they produce intolerable symptoms, PVCs can be controlled with radiofrequency ablation or the medications used to manage ventricular tachycardia (VT).

Ventricular tachycardia: VT arises distal to the bifurcation of the His bundle. It is defined as three or more consecutive PVCs. The rate and duration of VT and the presence of associated heart disease help determine the symptoms, as does the location of impulse formation. Ischemic heart disease is the most common cause. VT can be nonsustained (stopping spontaneously in less than 30 seconds) or sustained. Atrioventricular dissociation may be present, during which atrial activity is independent of the VT, or the atria may be activated by retrograde conduction through the AV node. QRS complexes can be uniform or vary. The finding of wide-QRS tachycardia is not specific for VT; supraventricular tachycardia with aberrance (bundle-branch blocks and conduction over accessory pathways) is another cause. Table 76.2 lists several electrocardiographic features that are useful in differentiating these two diagnoses. Prior probabilities must be considered; a wide QRS tachycardia occurring for the first time in a middle-aged man with a history of myocardial infarction has a greater than 90% chance of being VT. Torsades de pointes is a form of VT characterized by prolonged QT intervals and QRS complexes of changing amplitude that appear to twist about the isoelectric line and occur at rates of 200 to 250 beats per minute. Predisposing factors include severe bradycardia, potassium depletion, and use of class IA and IC antiarrhythmic agents.

VT that does not cause hemodynamic decompensation can be controlled with intravenous administration of lidocaine. Intravenous procainamide or bretylium can be administered next. Amiodarone is effective when given intravenously. Hypokalemia, ischemia, and hypomagnesemia should be corrected. If pharmacologic therapy is unsuccessful or hemodynamic decompensation is present, prompt direct-current electrical cardioversion is indicated. Competitive pacing also can be effective. Recurrent episodes usually are controlled with class I drugs (see *Atrial Arrhythmias*), sotalol, or amiodarone. Combinations of drugs with different mechanisms of action can be successful when single agents fail. Implantable defibrillators have been shown to be more effective than antiarrhythmic drugs for improving survival among patients who have had cardiac arrest or sustained VT. For selected patients, radiofrequency catheter ablation may be indicated. Management of VT with a polymorphic pattern is influenced by whether the QT interval is prolonged. If it is, the VT may be torsades de pointes, which is managed effectively by means of accelerating the ventricular rate, usually with pacing or isoproterenol. Magnesium infusions also are helpful.

Ventricular fibrillation: Ventricular fibrillation (VF) is severe derangement of the heartbeat that usually leads to death within 3 to 5 minutes unless it is terminated. VF probably accounts for more than 75% of sudden cardiac deaths (bradycardia and asystole account for the rest). VF is recognized by the presence of irregular undulations of varying contour and amplitude without distinct QRS complexes, ST segments, or T waves. Sometimes the fibrillatory waves are so small they simulate asystole. VF causes immediate loss of consciousness, seizures, apnea, and death. It occurs most commonly in association with coronary artery disease, administration of antiarrhythmic drugs, hypoxemia, and atrial fibrillation. Immediate nonsynchronized electrical shock with 200 to 360 J is mandatory treatment. Time should not be wasted with cardiopulmonary resuscitation if electrical defibrillation can be done promptly.

Chapter 76

◼ WOLFF–PARKINSON–WHITE SYNDROME

DEFINITION AND PATHOPHYSIOLOGY

Wolff–Parkinson–White (WPW) syndrome is a symptomatic preexcitation disorder in which muscular connections of working myocardial fibers exist outside the specialized conduction tissue and connect the atrium and ventricle. The atrial impulse travels through this tissue and activates the ventricle earlier than would be expected if the impulse traveled through the normal conduction pathway. In some cases, the pathway can conduct impulses only retrograde, from the ventricle to the atrium.

Preexcitation is associated with a variety of tachyarrhythmias. The most common is orthodromic reciprocating tachycardia, which occurs when a premature atrial complex conducts to the ventricle over the normal pathway and then returns to the atrium over a previously blocked accessory pathway to cause eccentric reactivation of the atria. Less commonly, the tachycardia can be antidromic, during which anterograde conduction occurs over the accessory pathway and retrograde conduction over the atrioventricular (AV) node. Approximately 15% to 30% of patients have atrial fibrillation.

EPIDEMIOLOGY

It is probable that acquisition of an accessory pathway is congenital. The prevalence is about 0.15% but is higher among relatives with WPW syndrome. WPW syndrome occurs in all age groups, has a higher prevalence among boys and men, and decreases in prevalence with age. Most adults with preexcitation syndrome have normal hearts.

CLINICAL MANIFESTATIONS

The clinical manifestations of these types of tachycardia range from palpitations and light-headedness to syncope, angina, and congestive heart failure. When the atrial impulse prematurely activates the ventricle, two major electrocardiographic (ECG) changes result: (a) the PR interval is less than 120 milliseconds during sinus rhythm and (b) the QRS complex lasts longer than 120 milliseconds and has a slurred, slowly rising QRS onset in some leads (delta waves). These abnormalities are not present, however, in patients who have concealed accessory pathways that are not capable of anterograde conduction. In orthodromic tachycardia, the QRS complex appears normal, but the retrograde P waves may have an unusual contour. In antidromic forms of tachycardia, the QRS complex is abnormal (as described earlier) owing to ventricular activation over the accessory pathway. Patients with atrial fibrillation have the characteristic ECG abnormalities of that rhythm, although conduction over the accessory pathway usually broadens the QRS and increases the ventricular rate.

PROGNOSIS AND MANAGEMENT

The prognosis is excellent among patients without tachycardia or an associated cardiac abnormality. For these patients, no therapy is indicated. For most patients with tachycardia, the prognosis is good, but sudden death does occur. Termination of the acute episode of orthodromic tachycardia should be as for AV nodal reentry (vagal maneuvers, adenosine, calcium channel blockers, or short-acting β-blockers). For atrial flutter or atrial fibrillation conducted over the accessory pathway, drugs that prolong refractoriness in that pathway (class 1A, 1C, and amiodarone) must be used. For some patients with very rapid ventricular rates, electrical cardioversion should be the initial treatment of choice. Verapamil, digitalis, and lidocaine may increase the ventricular rate during atrial fibrillation in a patient with WPW syndrome, and intravenous verapamil can precipitate ventricular tachycardia. Atrial fibrillation among patients with a concealed accessory pathway is managed in the same manner as if the pathway were not present, because anterograde conduction is preceding only over the AV node and not the accessory pathway. Radiofrequency catheter ablation usually is the initial treatment of choice for patients with symptoms because it has an excellent success rate (95%) and a low complication rate (less than 2%).

Chapter 88

GASTROENTEROLOGY

◼ APPROACH TO THE PATIENT WITH ABDOMINAL PAIN

CLASSIFICATION

There are three major types of abdominal pain—visceral, parietal, and referred. Visceral pain (e.g., pain from intestinal or ureteral obstruction or biliary colic) is perceived as dull, gnawing, or burning pain that is poorly localized. It may be elicited by numerous stimuli, such as muscle contractions or spasms, mural distention, ischemia, or necrosis. It is often described as an uncomfortable feeling rather than as pain and is frequently accompanied by autonomic disturbances such as nausea, vomiting, pallor, and diaphoresis. Patients often feel restless and attempt to move about to relieve the discomfort. Parietal pain (e.g., pain from peritonitis) is sharp, well-localized, and more intense. It is not usually associated with autonomic disturbances. Patients attempt to lie still, because even small movements often exacerbate the pain. Referred pain combines features of both visceral and parietal pain and is felt at sites distant to the involved organ. It is usually well localized and increases in intensity as organ damage progresses.

DIFFERENTIAL DIAGNOSIS

A list of causes of acute and chronic abdominal pain is presented in Table 96.3. Disorders of the chest can mimic abdominal disorders and must be considered.

Upper abdominal pain is common among persons with cholecystitis, pancreatitis, or peptic ulcer disease. Midabdominal pain may represent appendicitis, intestinal obstruction, or mesenteric vascular occlusion. Lower abdominal pain is commonly caused by appendicitis, diverticulitis, ureteral colic, ectopic pregnancy, or ovarian cyst torsion.

HISTORY

A carefully obtained history is the best initial diagnostic tool. Table 96.2 characterizes some of the important types of acute abdominal pain. The presence of other symptoms also is useful for diagnosis. Acute viral gastroenteritis usually is accompanied by nausea and vomiting early in its course. Patients with small-bowel obstruction often vomit only after the onset of abdominal pain. Anorexia is an early symptom of appendicitis. Patients with mesenteric ischemia often have persistent anorexia and subsequent weight loss. Diarrhea often accompanies gastroenteritis and colitis. Bloody diarrhea usually suggests severe colitis caused by infection, ischemia, nonsteroidal anti-inflammatory drugs (NSAIDs), or inflammatory bowel disease. Alternating diarrhea and constipation is a classic presentation of irritable bowel syndrome. Lower abdominal pain and constipation together may be a sign of colonic neoplasm. Fever occurs with gastroenteritis, abscesses, cholangitis, and diverticulitis. Jaundice suggests biliary tract disease or hepatitis. Neurologic disturbances and photosensitivity occur with porphyria.

Nephrolithiasis may cause gross hematuria. Careful attention should be paid to menstrual history, family history, travel history, and the use of medications.

PHYSICAL EXAMINATION

The general examination may disclose findings that suggest certain etiologies factors. Such findings include fever, hypotension, jaundice, atrial fibrillation, and weak distal pulses. The abdominal examination begins with inspection for hernias, surgical scars, and distention. Diffuse peritonitis usually obliterates bowel sounds, whereas early intestinal obstruction produces tinkling, high-pitched sounds. A succussion splash may be detectable in patients with gastric outlet obstruction. A midabdominal bruit may be audible in patients with an aortic aneurysm.

Palpation should begin lightly at an area distant from the region of greatest pain. It is important to increase pressure slowly and not abruptly. Rebound tenderness suggests peritoneal irritation, as does guarding. Percussion is useful to detect fluid or gas within the abdominal cavity and can be used to estimate the size of the liver and spleen.

Rectal and pelvic examinations always should be included in evaluations of acute abdominal pain. Intraabdominal disorders such as appendicitis may not initially involve the anterior abdominal wall and may first be detected during rectal examination. Stool should be tested for occult blood. Among women, a pelvic examination may reveal ovarian cysts or the cervical motion tenderness characteristic of pelvic inflammatory disease.

DIAGNOSTIC TESTS

The presence of anemia often suggests gastrointestinal bleeding, which may be occult. A complete blood cell count with differential should be obtained. The finding of leukocytosis with immature forms suggests infection, and eosinophilia suggests an allergic reaction or a parasitic infection. Urinalysis may suggest pyelonephritis or renal calculi. A urine pregnancy test should be performed for all women of childbearing age who have acute abdominal pain. Serum levels of electrolytes should be measured, and renal function tests should be performed. Amylase, lipase, and liver enzymes should be measured selectively. Elevated amylase and lipase levels suggest pancreatitis, whereas marked elevation of liver enzyme levels occurs with biliary obstruction and hepatocellular injury. Patients with ascites who have abdominal pain should undergo diagnostic paracentesis to determine whether they have spontaneous bacterial peritonitis.

Radiographic evaluation should be guided by the clinical signs and symptoms and the laboratory results. A series of plain abdominal radiographs is essential in the care of all patients with an acute presentation. These radiographs can depict abnormal gas patterns, as in small-bowel obstruction, and the presence of intraperitoneal free air caused by perforation of a viscus. Most renal calculi can be seen, but gallstones usually are radiolucent. An upright chest radiograph adds sensitivity to the detection of free intraperitoneal air and may depict signs of pneumonia or pleural effusion. Ultrasonography is particularly helpful in the diagnosis of cholelithiasis, biliary ductal dilatation, ovarian cyst, and ectopic pregnancy. Abdominal computed tomography is more expensive than ultrasonography but is the preferred method of detecting many intra-abdominal disorders, such as appendicitis and pancreatic cancer. It can also demonstrate changes that occur within the mesentery (e.g., fat stranding due to diverticulitis) or intestinal wall (e.g., ischemia).

Endoscopy should be used selectively. It is appropriate in the evaluation of chronic epigastric pain or lower abdominal pain accompanied by rectal bleeding. Cholangitis caused by an obstructing gallstone or mass may best be managed with emergency endoscopic retrograde cholangiopancreatography with stone extraction or biliary stenting. Diagnostic laparoscopy can be performed as an emergency procedure on extremely ill patients or an elective procedure on patients with chronic abdominal pain when the diagnosis remains elusive despite all noninvasive testing.

MANAGEMENT

Therapy for chronic abdominal pain of known causation is focused on management of the underlying pathologic condition and relief of the pain with medications, nerve block (e.g., celiac plexus block), or nerve stimulation. NSAIDs are less effective in the management of chronic abdominal pain than they are in that of musculoskeletal pain. Antidepressants and opioids have been used successfully. For patients who have chronic functional abdominal pain (no identifiable cause despite appropriate evaluation), the goal should be to improve quality of

life, not necessarily to eliminate pain. A multidisciplinary approach is recommended. Continued diagnostic evaluation is unlikely to be fruitful.

Chapter 96

APPROACH TO THE PATIENT WITH ABNORMAL LIVER CHEMISTRIES

DEFINITIONS

Liver disease can be categorized into four main types—cholestatic, immunologic, hepatocellular, and infiltrative. Cholestasis can be categorized further as either a functional defect in bile formation at the level of the hepatocyte (intrahepatic cholestasis) or a structural impairment in bile secretion and flow (extrahepatic cholestasis). Depending on the target of the immune response, immunologic injury causes either cholestasis (the bile ducts are involved preferentially, as in primary biliary cirrhosis) or a hepatocellular form of injury (the primary insult is to the hepatocyte membrane, as in viral and autoimmune hepatitis).

There are three categories of liver tests. *Hepatic function tests* reflect the synthetic and excretory capabilities of the liver. They include measurement of albumin, immunoglobulins, clotting factors, bilirubin, and serum bile acids. *Serum markers* of hepatobiliary dysfunction serve as markers of hepatocellular necrosis, cholestasis, or infiltrative processes. They include measurement of transaminases (aspartate aminotransferase [AST] and alanine aminotransferase [ALT]), lactate dehydrogenase (LDH), alkaline phosphatase (AP), and other enzyme markers of cholestasis (γ-glutamyl transpeptidase [GGTP] and serum leucine aminopeptidase [SLAP]). Evaluation of *disease-specific markers*, such as viral serologic testing, immunologic testing, measurement of ceruloplasmin, assessment of iron storage characteristics, measurement of α_1-antitrypsin, and liver biopsy, helps determine the specific cause of any laboratory abnormalities.

MARKERS OF HEPATOBILIARY DYSFUNCTION

Transaminases: The AST and ALT are important markers of hepatocellular injury, but the levels are not predictive of histologic findings. AST is present in various tissues (Table 104.3), but ALT is limited to the liver, and elevation of the level of this enzyme therefore is a more specific indicator of hepatic injury. The highest levels of these enzymes are present in patients with viral, toxin-induced, or ischemic hepatitis. Smaller elevations (less than 300 U) occur with alcoholic hepatitis. As a rule, transaminase levels greater than 400 U indicate hepatocellular injury. In contrast, milder degrees of elevation are of little diagnostic benefit; they occur with cholestatic disorders as often as with acute and chronic hepatocellular disease. An AST/ALT ratio greater than 2 is highly suggestive of the existence of alcoholic liver disease. In most other conditions, a ratio less than 1 is typical.

Lactate dehydrogenase: Total LDH level has limited specificity for liver disease. Moderate elevations in LDH level often occur with hepatocellular disorders such as viral hepatitis and cirrhosis and are less common in cholestatic disorders. Fractionation of LDH to determine levels of the hepatic isoenzyme (LDH-5) is occasionally useful.

Alkaline phosphatase: In the liver, AP is produced by cells that line the bile canaliculi. Hepatocellular injury causes increases in AP level, but elevations more than four times normal are typical with cholestatic syndromes. AP activity is not specific to the liver; the enzyme also is produced in bone, placenta, intestine, kidney, and leukocytes. However, liver and bone are the predominant sources among healthy persons.

Other markers of cholestasis: Although AP isoenzymes can be separated, alternative approaches are useful in clinical practice. Elevated serum levels of GGTP or SLAP generally establish the hepatic origin of an elevated AP level. These enzymes are produced in biliary tract cells but not in bone. Alcohol consumption increases GGTP level independently of any liver disease.

GENERAL APPROACH

Nonhepatic causes must be considered first (Table 104.3). Each type of liver disease is characteristically associated with a particular pattern of liver test abnormalities. Hepatocellular necrosis usually is characterized by marked elevations in transaminase levels, a normal or mildly increased level of AP, a normal to markedly increased bilirubin level, prolonged prothrombin time, and a decrease in albumin level if the condition is chronic. Cholestasis usually is associated with normal or mildly elevated transaminase levels, marked elevations in AP level, normal to markedly increased bilirubin level, prolonged prothrombin time responsive to vitamin K, and a normal albumin level. Infiltrative processes generally affect AP, though transaminase and bilirubin levels can be mildly elevated. The diagnosis of selected hepatobiliary disorders is reviewed in Table 104.5. The most direct approach to the differential diagnosis of cholestasis is the use of abdominal ultrasonography to assess bile duct size followed by endoscopic retrograde cholangiopancreatography if biliary ductal dilatation is present. If the presence of infiltrative disease is suspected, imaging with abdominal ultrasound or abdominal computed tomography is an appropriate first step, although liver biopsy may eventually be necessary.

Chapter 104

ACUTE AND CHRONIC PANCREATITIS

DEFINITIONS

Acute pancreatitis is an acute inflammatory process that starts in the pancreas and variably involves peripancreatic tissues or remote organ systems. Chronic pancreatitis is an inflammatory process involving the pancreas that results in irreversible fibrosis of the gland and atrophy of both exocrine and endocrine tissue.

ETIOLOGY AND PATHOGENESIS

Acute pancreatitis: Gallstone disease and excessive alcohol use account for 70% to 80% of cases in industrialized countries. Other etiologic factors are listed in Table 117.2. Acute pancreatitis is believed to begin as an autodigestive process within the gland that is caused by premature activation of digestive enzyme precursors. The result is acinar cell damage and necrosis and pancreatic edema and inflammation. Extension of the inflammatory process beyond the pancreas leads to local complications (e.g., inflammatory phlegmon, peripancreatic effusion, abscess formation, ileus) or systemic effects (e.g., hypovolemia, hypotension, respiratory failure, azotemia and oliguria, hypercalcemia, metabolic acidosis, and disseminated intravascular coagulation).

Chronic pancreatitis: In industrialized nations, alcohol consumption accounts for about 70% of cases. Other etiologic factors are chronic obstruction of the pancreatic duct, genetic hyperlipidemia, pancreatic trauma, hyperparathyroidism, and cystic fibrosis. The pathogenesis remains uncertain. Gland fibrosis and atrophy often lead to malabsorption and diabetes mellitus. Other complications include pancreatic cancer (10-fold increased risk), splenic venous thrombosis, bile duct or duodenal obstruction, pancreatic ascites and pleural effusion, and pseudocysts.

CLINICAL FEATURES

Acute pancreatitis: Abdominal pain is present in 95% of cases. It is usually epigastric, radiates to the back, and is worsened by ingesting food or alcohol or by vomiting. Cessation of eating and drinking and leaning forward may provide some relief. Nausea, vomiting, and abdominal distention are frequent. Hematemesis, melena, and diarrhea occur infrequently. At examination, abdominal tenderness usually is present; it may be mild and limited to the epigastrium or severe and accompanied by abdominal rigidity and rebound tenderness. An uncommon finding is dissection of blood along fascial planes to subcutaneous tissues, which can cause bluish discoloration of the skin of the periumbilical region (Cullen sign) or flanks (Grey Turner sign). The patient may have fever, tachycardia, tachypnea, hypotension, and other manifestations of the systemic complications listed earlier.

Chronic pancreatitis: Pain is the most common presenting symptom; it is similar to that of acute pancreatitis. Nausea and vomiting may occur. About half of patients have episodes lasting several days, the other have symptoms almost constantly. For some patients, the pain diminishes or resolves over 5 to 15 years, coincident with the appearance of pancreatic calcifications, steatorrhea, and diabetes ("burnout" of the gland). Patients typically lose weight because of decreased caloric intake, malabsorption due to pancreatic exocrine insufficiency, and poorly controlled diabetes mellitus. Physical examination usually shows abdominal tenderness of a degree less impressive than the amount of abdominal pain.

LABORATORY TESTING AND DIAGNOSIS

Acute pancreatitis: Serum amylase levels are the traditional diagnostic test but are neither fully sensitive nor specific for acute pancreatitis. Serum lipase level is as sensitive as amylase level and has greater specificity. A threefold or greater elevation in serum alanine aminotransferase level suggests gallstones as the etiologic factor. Computed tomography (CT) of the gland almost always has abnormal findings in moderate to severe disease. Dynamic CT has been used, but the criteria have not been standardized. After the diagnosis is established, the Ranson and the modified Glasgow criteria can be used to estimate severity and assess prognosis (Table 117.4).

Chronic pancreatitis: Chronic pancreatitis should be suspected when a patient has with the typical pattern and character of abdominal pain, particularly if accompanied by symptoms suggestive of steatorrhea or diabetes. Calcifications in the region of the pancreas are depicted on plain abdominal radiographs in about one-third of cases and can establish the diagnosis. Abdominal ultrasonography, CT, and endoscopic retrograde cholangiopancreatography (ERCP), in increasing order of sensitivity, cost, and invasiveness, can be used to confirm the diagnosis for patients without calcifications. The typical findings are tiny calcifications, dilatation of the pancreatic duct, and pancreatic pseudocysts. Endoscopic ultrasonography is the only modality that allows detailed evaluation of both the duct system and the parenchyma. Therefore it can be used to identify subtle changes in early disease not seen with other modalities. An alternative approach is assessment of pancreatic exocrine function by means of measuring the bicarbonate concentration in pancreatic juice collected before and after secretin infusion.

DIFFERENTIAL DIAGNOSIS

Acute pancreatitis: Various intra-abdominal processes may manifest similarly to acute pancreatitis and may even elevate serum amylase levels. These include penetrating duodenal ulcer, perforated gastric or duodenal ulcer, cholangitis, intestinal ischemia or infarction, and ruptured ectopic pregnancy. Ruptured abdominal aortic aneurysm may present with similar symptoms and signs.

Chronic pancreatitis: The differential diagnosis includes peptic ulcer disease, gastric or pancreatic cancer, chronic partial obstruction of the small intestine, and functional abdominal pain syndromes. Steatorrhea from pancreatic insufficiency must be differentiated from that caused by diseases of the small intestine.

MANAGEMENT

Acute pancreatitis: Most patients have a mild, self-limited course that necessitates only bed rest, cessation of oral intake, intravenous hydration, and analgesia (usually with narcotics such as meperidine). Nasogastric suction does not shorten the course but may relieve nausea, vomiting, and abdominal distention. Patients may be fed cautiously once abdominal pain and tenderness have abated and serum amylase and lipase levels have begun to return to normal. In severe cases, vigorous resuscitation with intravenous hydration and electrolytes may be necessary.

Patients with presumed gallstone pancreatitis should undergo urgent ERCP if cholangitis is suspected because of the presence of right upper quadrant pain, fever, or a leukocyte count greater than 20,000 per milliliter. There is no consensus currently on whether urgent ERCP should be performed within 24 to 72 hours of admission for patients with presumed gallstone pancreatitis of moderate to severe degree who do not have cholangitis. Agents that inactivate pancreatic enzymes, decrease pancreatic secretion (e.g., atropine or somatostatin), or reduce inflammation (e.g., glucocorticoids) have not been shown to be beneficial. Prophylactic administration of antibiotics is controversial; current evidence best supports the use of a combination of ciprofloxacin and metronidazole in the care of patients with predicted severe pancreatitis or suspected cholangitis. Pancreatic necrosis or abscess usually manifests more than 1 week after admission with worsening pain or vomiting, fever, or leukocytosis. After confirmation of disease by means of CT, such patients should undergo extensive debridement and drainage. About 10% to 15% of patients have a pseudocyst—an encapsulated collection of inflammatory fluid and pancreatic juice. If they cause only mild symptoms, pseudocysts may be followed with ultrasonography or CT for at least 6 weeks to determine whether they will resolve (about half do) or shrink without surgical intervention.

Chronic pancreatitis: Oral analgesics, including potent narcotics, often are needed for pain relief. Pancreatic enzyme supplementation sometimes reduces pain, presumably by inhibiting pancreatic secretion. Results of celiac plexus and splanchnic nerve blocks have generally been disappointing. Surgical resection usually improves pain but worsens pancreatic exocrine and endocrine insufficiency. Malabsorption is managed with a low-fat diet and pancreatic enzyme supplementation. Symptomatic pseudocysts and expanding pseudocysts larger than 6 cm in diameter should be managed with internal or percutaneous drainage.

Chapter 117

ALCOHOLIC LIVER DISEASE

DEFINITIONS, EPIDEMIOLOGY, AND ETIOLOGY

Alcohol abuse is one of the most important causes of chronic liver disease. Alcoholic liver disease (ALD) includes three major histologic stages—fatty liver (or steatosis), hepatitis, and cirrhosis. Two or more of these stages often coincide. The peak incidence of ALD is at 40 to 55 years of age; the male to female ratio is about 3 : 1. Only about 35% of heavy drinkers contract alcoholic hepatitis and only about 20% develop cirrhosis. Both the amount of ethanol ingested and the duration of intake are important factors; the pattern of drinking and the type of beverage are not. Other factors postulated to increase susceptibility to ALD include female sex and an enhanced sensitivity of cytokine metabolism to the effects of alcohol. There is also a high prevalence of hepatitis B and C infections among persons with alcoholism and cirrhosis, suggesting an interaction between viral infection and the effects of ethanol.

PATHOGENESIS AND PATHOLOGY

The development of alcoholic fatty liver occurs largely because alcohol alters the hepatic NADH/NAD ratio and inhibits fatty acid oxidation. The effect is most pronounced on perivenous cells. The accumulation of fat is accompanied by an induction of microsomal proteins and fatty acid–binding protein and by the retention of secretory proteins and water. This causes the hepatocytes to swell (ballooning degeneration) and interferes with blood flow to the perivenous zone. The decreased flow coupled with increased oxygen consumption may induce perivenular hypoxia and thus pericentral necrosis and fibrosis. The development of alcoholic hepatitis and cirrhosis has been linked to a number of other pathophysiologic events as well.

The fatty liver is enlarged and firm. Microscopic examination shows great variation in the number of fat droplets found, and there is a distinct tendency toward fat accumulation in the perivenous and middle zones. There generally is little inflammation or necrosis. In alcoholic hepatitis, ballooning degeneration and focal hepatocyte necrosis occur, and a neutrophilic inflammatory infiltrate develops. About 30% of patients have alcoholic hyaline, which is aggregates of perinuclear, eosinophilic, amorphous material. The final stage is cirrhosis, which is characterized by fibrous bands connecting portal triads with central veins and by regenerating nodules, which are typically small and uniform in size.

CLINICAL FINDINGS

Alcoholic fatty liver: Hepatomegaly may be the only initial finding; however, signs of alcoholism (e.g., Dupuytren's contractures, testicular atrophy, loss of the male pattern of body hair, palmar erythema, spider angiomas, and gynecomastia) may be present. More advanced disease, most likely representing incipient progression to alcoholic hepatitis, may be associated with some of the symptoms and signs of alcoholic hepatitis.

Alcoholic hepatitis: Although a few patients have no symptoms, most have anorexia, nausea, malaise, weakness, abdominal pain, icterus, weight loss, and fever. Common physical findings include hepatomegaly, hepatic tenderness, splenomegaly, ascites, jaundice, and fever. Some patients have severe jaundice, ascites, azotemia, and hepatic encephalopathy.

Alcoholic cirrhosis: Alcoholic cirrhosis may be asymptomatic as much 20% of the time, but it more commonly manifests the complications of chronic liver disease—cachexia, coagulopathy, ascites, spontaneous bacterial peritonitis, hepatorenal syndrome, hepatic encephalopathy, hepatocellular carcinoma, and gastrointestinal (GI) bleeding from esophageal and gastric varices. The physical findings associated with chronic liver disease and alcoholism may be present.

LABORATORY EVALUATION

Alcoholic fatty liver: Serum aspartate aminotransferase (AST) and alanine aminotransferase (ALT) levels usually are less than 300 IU per liter. The ratio of AST to ALT is 2 or more in 80% of cases. In the absence of cholestasis, alkaline phosphatase (AP) level is only modestly elevated (less than 300 IU per deciliter). A γ-glutamyl transpeptidase to AP ratio greater than 5 is characteristic of ALD. The serum albumin level usually is normal. Macrocytosis is common among persons with alcoholism.

Alcoholic hepatitis: The laboratory abnormalities are more severe in alcoholic hepatitis. Anemia develops in 50% to 70% of cases and is caused by the toxic effects of alcohol on bone marrow, impaired vitamin B_6 metabolism, folic acid deficiency, iron deficiency from blood loss, or hypersplenism. Leukocytosis occurs in 25% to 75% of cases. Leukopenia and thrombocytopenia are present in 10% to 15%. Serum AST and ALT levels are elevated but rarely exceed 300 IU per liter. AP level is elevated in 80% of cases. Serum albumin level usually is decreased and the prothrombin time often is prolonged. Electrolyte abnormalities may include hyponatremia, hyperchloremia, hypokalemia, hypomagnesemia, and respiratory alkalosis.

Alcoholic cirrhosis: Liver enzyme abnormalities are less pronounced than those of alcoholic hepatitis. With compensated cirrhosis, many of the test results are nearly normal. Abnormalities include mild elevations in AST, ALT and AP levels; depression of serum albumin level; prolongation of prothrombin time; leukopenia; thrombocytopenia; and anemia.

DIAGNOSIS AND MANAGEMENT

There are two pitfalls in the diagnosis of ALD. The first is failure to consider the diagnosis when a patient does not fit the stereotype of a skid-row denizen with alcoholism; the second is the assumption that when an alcoholic patient has abnormalities in liver tests, these results are invariably due to ALD. Alcoholism should be considered for any patient with liver disease, and the interview should include either the CAGE questions or the MAST test as a means of screening for alcohol abuse. A liver biopsy is necessary to reliably differentiate among fatty liver, alcoholic hepatitis, and cirrhosis. Appropriate blood tests (see *Approach to the Patient with Abnormal Liver Chemistries*) and biopsy should be performed to exclude nonalcoholic causes of liver disease and to define the severity of the disease. If tense ascites, severe thrombocytopenia, or a prolonged prothrombin time precludes percutaneous needle biopsy, transjugular liver biopsy may be done.

Alcoholic fatty liver: This condition is benign unless accompanied by perivenular fibrosis or foamy degeneration. If the patient abstains from alcohol and nutritional deficits are corrected, the fatty changes usually regress within 6 weeks.

Alcoholic hepatitis: The early mortality rate varies from about 20% to about 80%. Those who have severe jaundice, encephalopathy, renal failure, ascites, and variceal bleeding have a worse prognosis. Certain laboratory abnormalities are prognostic indicators. For example, patients with Maddrey discriminant function (4.6 × [prothrombin time in seconds − control time] + serum bilirubin in milligrams per deciliter) greater than 32 have a 50% risk of death within 1 month. Other studies indicate that the presence of hepatic encephalopathy is equally predictive. Supportive treatment consists of cessation of alcohol consumption and a nutritious diet. Parenteral amino acid therapy or enteral amino acid–protein therapy have been shown to be beneficial for malnourished patients. Glucocorticoids (e.g., prednisone, 40 to 80 mg every day for 4 to 6 weeks) are indicated in the treatment of patients with hepatic encephalopathy or a Maddrey score greater than 32, excluding those with GI bleeding, active infection, or renal failure.

Alcoholic cirrhosis: The prognosis depends on whether the patient continues to drink, the coexistence of alcoholic hepatitis, and the severity of the disease. In one study, the 5-year survival ranged from 85% among abstainers without jaundice, ascites, or GI bleeding to only 20% among drinkers with GI bleeding. Therapy with glucocorticoids has no effect on survival. Prophylactic nonselective portacaval shunting merely shifts the cause of death from GI bleeding to hepatic coma. Colchicine therapy improved survival in one study and is under investigation. Advanced alcoholic cirrhosis can be managed by means of liver transplantation and now accounts for approximately 25% of liver transplantation procedures performed on adults in the United States.

Chapter 121

APPROACH TO THE PATIENT WITH CHRONIC LIVER DISEASE

DEFINITIONS

Hepatic cirrhosis is a diffuse pathologic process in which the normal structure of the liver is replaced by regenerative nodules of hepatocytes separated by bands of fibrosis. It may result from various hepatic diseases (Table 105.1).

PATHOGENESIS

The clinical features of cirrhosis occur as a consequence of portal hypertension, hepatocellular insufficiency, and cholestasis. Portal hypertension occurs when resistance to flow causes an increase in blood pressure within the portal vein; the level of the resistance may be presinusoidal, sinusoidal, or postsinusoidal. Hepatocellular insufficiency is a pathologic deficiency of hepatic protein synthesis coupled with the disordered metabolism of certain endogenous proteins and xenobiotics. Cholestasis is caused by impairment of bile secretion and specific defects in the secretion of anions.

CLINICAL FINDINGS

Portal hypertension: When portal pressure increases, collateral vessels (varices) in the lower esophagus, stomach, or rectum may dilate and become prone to hemorrhage. Portal hypertension also causes splenomegaly and hypersplenism, with a consequent sequestration of white blood cells and platelets. Ascites is the accumulation of serous fluid in the peritoneal cavity. Portal hypertension plays a role in the development of ascites, but other factors, such as altered renal sodium handling and a reduction in plasma oncotic pressure from diminished albumin secretion, also play a role. Ascites increases abdominal girth and causes rapid weight gain and occasionally dyspnea and early satiety. It is detected clinically when percussion of the abdominal flanks elicits dullness that moves as the patient changes position (shifting dullness) and when a fluid wave is detected. Small volumes of ascites (less than 1,500 mL) often are clinically undetectable. In such cases, an imaging study such as computed tomography (CT) or ultrasonography is needed for diagnosis. Hepatic encephalopathy occurs because of the transmission of portal blood to the right side of the heart through intra- or extrahepatic shunts. Although patients with encephalopathy often have elevated serum ammonia levels, it is still uncertain which substances are the actual mediators of the syndrome. Patients have a broad range of neuropsychological syndromes up to and including coma.

Hepatocellular insufficiency: Clinical manifestations include coagulopathy and hypoalbuminemia. The clinical manifestations of coagulopathy include easy bruising, bleeding from the gums and nose, and minor degrees of anorectal bleeding. Coagulopathy also may contribute to variceal hemorrhage. Hypoalbuminemia develops because of diminished hepatic synthesis, but malnutrition may play a role for some patients. The clinical consequences of hypoalbuminemia include ascites, cirrhotic hydrothorax, and peripheral edema. The reduced albumin concentration of ascites among patients with cirrhosis is thought to be an important factor in the pathogenesis of spontaneous bacterial peritonitis (SBP). Men may have both androgenic failure and feminization (e.g., gynecomastia); women often have anovulation and amenorrhea. Spider angiomas and palmar erythema are thought to be endocrine features of hepatocellular insufficiency.

Cholestasis: Cholestasis is characterized by pruritus, jaundice, and elevated levels of alkaline phosphatase. Hyperlipidemia occurs because of impaired excretion of cholesterol and phospholipids into bile. Fat malabsorption and steatorrhea may be caused by impaired bile acid delivery. Deficiencies of the fat-soluble vitamins (A, D, E, and K) may occur and cause altered vision, osteoporosis, and worsened coagulopathy.

Miscellaneous complications: Many forms of liver disease are complicated by disorders of bone metabolism. Hepatic osteodystrophy is particularly common in chronic cholestatic disorders such as primary biliary cirrhosis. Patients with cirrhosis also have a higher rate of infection; SBP is the most important among patients with ascites. SBP, which is usually caused by gram-negative aerobes or *Streptococcus pneumoniae*, must be suspected whenever a patient with cirrhosis has a sudden deterioration in hepatic or renal function, worsening malaise, encephalopathy, or unexplained leukocytosis, even in the absence of fever and abdominal pain. The diagnosis is confirmed when more than 250 neutrophils are found per microliter of ascitic fluid; demonstration of an organism is not required. Patients with cirrhosis are at risk of hepatocellular carcinoma.

APPROACH TO CARE OF THE PATIENT WITH LIVER DISEASE

A careful history and physical examination may allow differentiation of acute from chronic liver disease and should allow the physician to form diagnostic hypotheses (Table 105.6).

LABORATORY EVALUATION

Profiles of serum transaminases, bilirubin, and alkaline phosphatase are not specific for diagnosis but indicate broader categories of liver injury, such as hepatocellular injury or cholestasis, which often coexist in a given patient. Specific serum tests exist for many of the hepatic diseases that can lead to cirrhosis (see *Approach to the Patient with Abnormal Liver Chemistries*). Liver imaging

studies include sonography with Doppler technique, CT, magnetic resonance imaging, angiography, and CT angiography. All patients with putative chronic liver disease should undergo at least one baseline structural imaging study. Endoscopic retrograde cholangiopancreatography is the best method to differentiate primary sclerosing cholangitis from other chronic cholestatic processes. Histopathologic examination of liver tissue can be helpful in confirming the presence of cirrhosis or estimating the degree of activity of chronic hepatitis. It also may be helpful in making the diagnosis of specific conditions such as hemochromatosis, Wilson's disease, α_1 antitrypsin deficiency, autoimmune chronic hepatitis, and primary biliary cirrhosis.

MANAGEMENT

Acute gastrointestinal hemorrhage, bacterial infection, and multisystem failure (particularly the combination of hepatic and renal failure) are the most common modes of death. Although therapy may control the initial decompensating event (e.g., sclerotherapy for bleeding varices or antibiotics for SBP), the measures do not change the long-term risk of death unless liver failure is corrected. Therapies that reverse liver failure include abstinence from alcohol for patients with alcoholic liver disease, glucocorticoids for autoimmune hepatitis, and specific therapies for metabolic disorders such as hemochromatosis and Wilson's disease. Liver transplantation has become the therapy of choice for end-stage liver disease, but use of this procedure has been limited by cost and by an inadequate supply of donor organs.

Bleeding esophageal varices: Patients with cirrhosis and features of portal hypertension should undergo endoscopy, because prophylactic therapy with noncardioselective β-blockade reduces portal pressure and the incidence of first or recurrent variceal hemorrhage among patients at high risk. Active variceal hemorrhage is always an emergency. Endoscopic ligation banding and injection sclerotherapy are the standard therapies, although balloon tamponade often is used to control persistent bleeding. Intravenous vasopressin (usually given with glyceryl trinitrate to limit cardiac effects) and IV octreotide produce splanchnic vasoconstriction and can help control hemorrhage. If bleeding persists or recurs, a transjugular intrahepatic portosystemic shunt (TIPS) is the treatment of choice.

Ascites: Management is directed at controlling fluid overload without precipitating renal failure and, for selected patients, at providing prophylaxis against SBP. Sodium intake should be limited to 2 g per day. Furosemide and spironolactone (usually in combination) are the diuretics most commonly used. Use of these agents necessitates careful monitoring of results of renal function tests and serum sodium and potassium levels. Intractable ascites is managed by means of intermittent. large-volume paracentesis. Albumin replacement (12.5 g for each liter of ascites removed) is controversial but is probably a reasonable precaution in the care of patients with an elevated serum creatinine levels. It has been shown that a functioning TIPS improves the control of ascites. Prophylactic therapy against SBP with quinolones and trimethoprim–sulfamethoxazole has been studied; a reasonable plan is to limit prophylaxis to patients who are awaiting liver transplantation, are considered to be at high risk of a first episode of SBP (e.g., have an ascites protein content less than 1 g per deciliter), or who have had a previous episode of SBP.

Hepatic encephalopathy: Acute exacerbations should always prompt a search for a precipitating cause, such as gastrointestinal bleeding, new-onset renal failure or electrolyte disturbance, infection, intracranial hemorrhage, or the administration of benzodiazepines and other central nervous system depressants. Lactulose is the mainstay of management. The dose should be titrated to produce two or three soft bowel movements a day. Metronidazole may be useful if lactulose is insufficient. Protein restriction should be reserved for management of disabling, severe encephalopathy.

Chapter 105

◼ COLORECTAL CANCER

EPIDEMIOLOGY AND ETIOLOGY

Cancer of the large intestine (adenocarcinoma in 95% of cases) is the most frequent neoplasm of the gastrointestinal tract and the second most common cause of death from cancer in the United States. It occurs at some time in the lives of 5% to 6% of the population. Colorectal cancer is slightly more common among men than in women but is equal in frequency between blacks and whites. The incidence is very low before 40 years of age; thereafter the risk increases as an exponential function of age. The age-adjusted risk is higher among persons with affected first-degree relatives, especially if the relative had cancer before 45 years of age. That a relatives had colorectal cancer after 60 years of age does not add substantial risk. There are many familial colorectal cancer syndromes, including familial adenomatous polyposis, hereditary nonpolyposis colorectal cancer (Lynch syndrome), and Peutz–Jeghers syndrome.

ETIOLOGY, PATHOGENESIS, AND STAGING

Colorectal cancer develops through a multistep accumulation of critical mutations in genes that regulate growth, such as the p53 gene. The tumors probably always evolve from adenomas, although not necessarily from polyps. Diets high in fat and low in fiber have been implicated as a factor in the high incidence of colon cancer in industrialized nations. The incidence is lower among persons who frequently use aspirin and nonsteroidal anti-inflammatory drugs than among persons who do not use these agents. The prognosis is directly related to the penetration depth of the malignant tumor rather than to the total tumor bulk. Colon cancers spread by direct extension through the wall of the intestine into the pericolic fat and mesentery, to the mesenteric lymph nodes, and through the portal vein to the liver. Additional spread may be evident throughout the peritoneal cavity, to the lungs, and to other distant sites. Rectal carcinoma spreads by means of direct extension into the perirectal fat and to the regional lymph nodes. It metastasizes to the liver or other distant sites somewhat less frequently. A number of different staging schemes of colorectal cancer have been used, including the Dukes classification, the Astler–Coller modification, and the tumor-nodes-metastasis (TNM) system.

CLINICAL FINDINGS

Early cancers produce no symptoms. Symptomatic colorectal neoplasia has three characteristic modes of presentation—lower intestinal obstruction (usually tumors of the sigmoid colon or rectum), hematochezia (usually distal tumors), and iron deficiency anemia (most often with cancers of the cecum or ascending colon). At physical examination, an abdominal mass or enlarged liver is found only when the patient has advanced disease. Occult bleeding may be detected by means of rectal examination. In rare instances, colon cancer perforates spontaneously and causes acute abdominal pain.

LABORATORY EVALUATION

Most early colorectal cancers are not associated with any laboratory abnormalities. Advanced cancer, especially from the cecum or proximal colon, may cause anemia. Adenocarcinoma can elevate the level of plasma carcinoembryonic antigen. This finding may help in assessment of residual or recurrent tumor burden, but it is not an effective screening test because it is neither sensitive nor specific for colorectal cancer.

PROGNOSIS AND OPTIMAL MANAGEMENT

Surgical therapy: Some colorectal tumors, particularly those found in adenomatous polyps, can be excised colonoscopically. Most necessitate surgical resection. Cancer of the cecum, ascending colon, and hepatic flexure is best managed with right hemicolectomy and ileocolonic anastomosis. Cancer of the distal transverse colon, splenic flexure, or proximal descending colon can be managed by means of extended right hemicolectomy or segmental resection. Cancer of the distal descending colon or sigmoid colon is managed by means of segmental resection and primary colonic anastomosis. Therapy for rectal cancer is more complex and depends on the location, depth, and size of the lesion. Cancer in the lower rectum may necessitate proctocolectomy and sigmoid colostomy.

Adjuvant therapy: Adjuvant therapy is used to prevent tumor recurrence among patients who have undergone successful resection. It is not indicated in the care of patients with stage I or II tumors (those limited to the colonic wall and not associated with lymph node metastasis), because the cancer-free survival rate is already more than 80% and is not significantly improved by chemotherapy. Patients with regional lymph node involvement (stage III) should be treated with adjuvant chemotherapy, usually 5-fluorouracil combined with either levamisole or leucovorin. Such regimens improve the disease-free survival rate from about 50% to about 65% and delay the time to recurrence. Rectal cancer are more likely to be associated with the presence of progressive local disease after initial resection, especially resection of high rectal lesions when tumor is left behind in an attempt to preserve the rectum. Radiation therapy has been shown to decrease the recurrence rate in such cases. In some instances, preoperative chemoradiation therapy can be used to convert an apparently nonresectable tumor into one that can be removed surgically.

Metastatic colorectal cancer: If an isolated focus of metastatic disease is found in the liver, it is best managed by means of surgical resection. There are no successful modalities for management of widespread metastatic disease. Chemotherapy with 5-fluorouracil and other drugs may produce partial tumor shrinkage in 15% to 25% of patients but has not been shown to prolong survival. Radiation therapy may also be palliative in some cases.

SCREENING AND SURVEILLANCE

There is evidence that periodic screening with fecal occult blood tests (every 1 to 2 years) and sigmoidoscopy (every 3 to 5 years) decreases the incidence of fatal colorectal cancer. The optimal screening program for persons with a family history of sporadic colon cancer is not known. Annual or frequent colonoscopy for such patients, particularly in those with a single affected relative, has a low yield and a high cost per detected neoplastic lesion. Surveillance of patients who have undergone removal of adenomatous polyps is controversial. It is most important to initiate a follow-up program for patients who have had larger (more than 1 cm in diameter), multiple, or more dysplastic lesions removed. Such patients may benefit from colonoscopic examinations every 3 years.

Chapter 116

■ APPROACH TO THE PATIENT WITH CONSTIPATION

DEFINITION AND PATHOPHYSIOLOGY

Constipation is the most frequent digestive disorder in the United States. Patients may use the term to describe infrequent defecation (less than 2 to 3 bowel movements a week), dry stools, excessive straining, or a sense of incomplete evacuation. Constipation is caused by obstruction of the flow of luminal contents or by poor colonic propulsion.

DIFFERENTIAL DIAGNOSIS

Causes of constipation are listed in Table 100.1.

HISTORY AND PHYSICAL EXAMINATION

Symptoms of hypothyroidism, collagen vascular disease, or diabetes may be uncovered. A careful medication history is essential. Examination includes anorectal examination for tumors, hemorrhoids, and fissures and assessment of rectal tone.

LABORATORY STUDIES AND DIAGNOSTIC TESTS

Results of laboratory studies can confirm the existence of electrolyte or metabolic disturbances. If the results of initial evaluation suggest obstruction, a barium radiographic study or colonoscopy is performed. Once obstruction is excluded, treatment is attempted. Most patients improve, and no additional evaluation is necessary. Special studies are indicated for the minority of patients with severe constipation. These include marker transit studies, anal manometry, and defecography.

COMPLICATIONS AND MANAGEMENT

Chronic constipation plays a role in the development of rectal prolapse, anal fissures, hemorrhoids, ischemic colitis, and fecal incontinence. Contributing metabolic and pharmacologic influences must be removed; daily exercise should be encouraged. Patients should allocate a limited amount of time for defecation after a chosen meal. Daily fiber supplements taken with water should be tried for 2 to 3 weeks, although flatus and bloating may worsen temporarily. The next step is intermittent or short-term use of saline (magnesium citrate), lubricant (mineral oil), or osmotic (lactulose, polyethylene glycol) laxatives. Stool softeners are of marginal benefit. Stimulant laxatives (bisacodyl, senna) should be used for brief periods if at all, because they can damage myenteric neurons and cause dependency.

Chapter 100

■ APPROACH TO THE PATIENT WITH DIARRHEA

DEFINITIONS AND PATHOPHYSIOLOGY

Diarrhea can be defined as a stool output of more than 200 g per day. However, patients may use the term to describe bowel movements of increased frequency or that are loose in consistency. It is important, therefore, to differentiate true diarrhea from conditions, such as fecal incontinence or functional bowel disease, in which stools may be frequent or loose but are of normal total daily weight. Diarrhea is caused by two basic mechanisms—increased active anion secretion and decreased absorption of water and electrolytes. The former is caused by bacterial enterotoxins, hormones, neuropeptides, inflammatory mediators, bile salts, laxatives, and medications. The latter is caused by bacterial enterotoxins; ingestion of poorly absorbed, osmotically active solute, such as magnesium or lactose among persons with lactase deficiency; decreased absorptive surface from mucosal damage or intestinal resection; hypermotility and decreased contact time between luminal fluid and the mucosal surface; and impairment of mucosal barrier function that causes back flux of water and electrolytes into the intestinal lumen.

DIFFERENTIAL DIAGNOSIS

Acute diarrhea in normal hosts: Acute diarrhea (less than 2 to 3 weeks' duration) usually is caused by infection or ingestion of toxins, medications, or dietary products. The most common cause is infection due to viruses and food-borne toxins. Viral diarrhea usually occurs among children and their family members, whereas diarrhea due to food poisoning usually occurs within several hours of the meal. Pathogens that cause traveler's diarrhea usually are acquired though the fecal-oral route; these include enterotoxigenic bacteria (*Escherichia coli, Vibrio cholerae*), bacteria of genuses *Campylobacter, Shigella,* and *Salmonella,* viruses, and parasites. Giardiasis is the most common parasitic infection in the United States. Sporadic waterborne outbreaks of cryptosporidiosis have occurred on farms and in cities. Bloody stool has a limited differential diagnosis that includes invasive bacterial enteritis (*Campylobacter, Shigella,* or *Yersinia* organisms), *Entamoeba histolytica* infection, exposure to cytopathic toxins (*Clostridium difficile, E. coli,* or Shiga toxin), inflammatory bowel disease, and ischemic bowel.

A number of drugs and dietary products cause acute diarrhea. Antibiotics are the most common. Only about 25% of cases of antibiotic-associated diarrhea are caused by *C. difficile* toxin; in the remaining cases, the cause is unknown. Other drugs commonly implicated include antacids, prokinetic agents such as cisapride and metoclopramide, and prostaglandins. Dietary substances that cause diarrhea include lactose (among persons with lactase deficiency), sorbitol (elixirs, dietetic candies, gum), fructose (pears, prunes, apple juice), and Olestra indigestible fat substitute.

Acute diarrhea is other settings: Immunocompromised hosts, such as patients with HIV infection and a CD4 cell count less than 150 per microliter, can acquire any of the infections mentioned earlier and are at risk of infection with cytomegalovirus (CMV), and organisms of *Mycobacterium avium* complex, *Cryptosporidium, Isospora belli, Microsporida,* and *Cyclospora.* Diarrhea is common among patients treated with chemotherapy or abdominal radiation. Direct intestinal toxicity is the most common cause. Diarrhea occurs among 30% to 50% of patients in intensive care units and can be caused by antibiotics, other medications, fecal impaction, tube feedings, or the underlying disease. *C. difficile* infection is the most common cause of diarrhea among hospitalized patients; viral infections are the most common cause among nursing home residents.

Chronic diarrhea: Chronic diarrhea can be caused by malabsorption of nutrients or poorly absorbable solute, deranged water and electrolyte transport, or inflammatory disease of the intestine. Table 99.6 lists some of the etiologic factors. Diarrhea due to malabsorption of nutrients or poorly absorbable solute usually is low in volume (less than 1 L per day) and diminishes with fasting. Secretory diarrhea usually is high in volume (more than 1 L per day) and does not improve with fasting. Inflammatory diarrhea with mucosal destruction is associated with the presence of blood and pus in the stool.

HISTORICAL FEATURES

One must first determine whether the patient truly has diarrhea and, if so, whether it is acute or chronic. Persons with irritable bowel syndrome or fecal incontinence often have frequent small stools of normal weight rather than diarrhea. Diarrhea usually is caused by organic illness if it is of recent onset, occurs daily or at night, or is associated with metabolic disturbances.

Associated symptoms: Low-grade fever occurs with viral or toxigenic diarrhea; high-grade fever may complicate invasive bacterial infection, amebiasis, CMV colitis, and inflammatory bowel disease. The existence of orthostatic light-headedness or weakness suggests that the patient has high-volume diarrhea. Weight loss in the setting of acute diarrhea implies fluid loss; in chronic diarrhea, it usually indicates nutrient malabsorption. Nausea and vomiting are associated most often with viral infection or food poisoning. Abdominal cramps can be caused by infection or by carbohydrate malabsorption. Severe abdominal pain occurs with invasive or cytopathic bacterial infection and intestinal ischemia. Blood in the stool indicates an infectious, inflammatory, or ischemic process. Associated neurologic symptoms occur with botulism and exposure to marine toxins (scromboid, ciguatera). Systemic manifestations of enteric bacterial infection include arthritis, urethritis, and conjunctivitis (*Salmonella, Shigella, Campylobacter, Yersinia*) and hemolytic-uremic syndrome (hemorrhagic *E. coli, Shigella*).

Setting: The setting in which diarrhea occurs provides important clues. Recent travel, restaurant dining, change in drinking water, or ingestion of imported or poorly cooked foods may point to an infectious cause. Diarrhea may occur with use of new medications, over-the-counter medications, herbal products, or changes in the diet. Associations with particular foods should be identified. Diarrhea due to *C. difficile* infection is common among hospitalized patients and nursing home residents and persons with a history of antibiotic use. Persons with compromised immune function may have diarrhea caused by common organisms or those unique to the impaired host. Among the elderly and persons predisposed to thrombosis, diarrhea with pain out of proportion to physical findings suggests the existence of intestinal ischemia. Questions should be asked routinely about previous abdominal operations, chemotherapy, or radiation therapy.

PHYSICAL EXAMINATION

Attention should be paid to vital signs, volume status, and the abdominal and rectal examinations. High fever raises the suspicion of the presence of invasive organisms. Hyperventilation may be a consequence of metabolic acidosis caused by the loss of bicarbonate in the stool. Patients with chronic diarrhea should be evaluated for signs of malnutrition and evidence of vitamin or mineral deficiency. These include weight loss, muscle wasting, tetany, oral and skin lesions, peripheral neuropathy, ataxia, and edema. The abdomen should be examined for distention, bowel sounds, tenderness, and masses. A stool swab for culture, when necessary, should be obtained before the rectal examination because lubricants contain bacteriostatic agents that can interfere with bacterial growth. The rectum should be examined for stool texture, masses, and sphincter tone. Stool should be tested for occult blood.

LABORATORY FINDINGS

Stool studies for the presence of intestinal inflammation include microscopic examination for fecal leukocytes and evaluation of the stool for occult blood; the former is less sensitive but more specific for inflammatory causes. Results of stool cultures are only positive among 40% to 60% of persons with dysentery; special culture techniques are needed for some pathogens. Stool can be examined for ova and parasites and tested for *C. difficile* toxin. Sudan staining is a qualitative test for fat in the stool; the results are valid only if the patient consumes a high-fat diet. The test is 90% sensitive for fat malabsorption greater than 10 g per day. Measurement of electrolytes in the stool is useful in differentiating secretory from osmotic diarrhea. The stool osmotic gap is calculated as follows: Stool osmotic gap = Stool osmolarity − 2 × (stool [Na] + stool [K]). Because stool osmolarity can be falsely elevated by laboratory processing delays, plasma osmolarity, which is the same, usually is substituted.

Secretory diarrhea is characterized by high stool sodium (more than 90 mmol per liter) and bicarbonate concentrations and the absence of a stool osmotic gap. Osmotic diarrhea, in contrast, is characterized by low stool sodium concentration (less than 50 mmol per liter) and the presence of a stool osmotic gap greater than 100 mOsm per kilogram water. Measurement of stool volume over 24 to 48 hours while the patient fasts also provides useful information about whether the diarrhea is functional (less than 250 mL per day), osmotic (250 to 1,000 mL per day), or secretory (more than 1 L per day). Fluids should be administered intravenously during the fast. A stool pH less than 7.0 can indicate carbohydrate malabsorption or gastrinoma. A 72-hour stool collection for fat while the patient is consuming 70 to 100 g fat per day should be performed if there is a high suspicion of malabsorption despite a negative Sudan stain result. For patients with high-volume secretory diarrhea of undetermined origin, serum levels of gastrin, vasoactive intestinal polypeptide, somatostatin, cortisol, neurokinins, and calcitonin can be considered. For suspected carcinoid syndrome, serotonin and urine 5-hydroxyindoleacetic acid should be measured.

EVALUATION

Acute diarrhea in normal hosts: In cases of uncomplicated acute diarrhea in a normal host, no evaluation is necessary. Stool for ova and parasites should be obtained only when the history suggests exposure to parasites or when diarrhea does not resolve. When diarrhea is associated with fever, a screening test should be used to differentiate inflammatory from noninflammatory causes. A stool occult blood test is the easiest to perform. If there is a high suspicion that the patient has invasive bacterial enteritis, a stool culture should be obtained regardless of the result of stool screening studies. If the patient has bloody diarrhea, a stool culture should be obtained. If the result is negative, colonoscopy with biopsy is the next diagnostic procedure.

Acute diarrhea in other settings: For patients with compromised immune systems, stool should be obtained for culture and detection of parasites and *C. difficile* toxin. If fever is present, blood cultures for bacteria and fungus also should be obtained. When the patient has both blood in the stool and fever, and the result of initial stool studies are negative, full colonoscopy should be performed that includes collection of biopsy specimens of the colon and a stool aspirate for culture, detection of *C. difficile* toxin, and parasite examination. If the stool is watery, upper gastrointestinal endoscopy with duodenal aspiration and biopsy should be performed. Among hospitalized patients, *C. difficile* infection should be excluded and the medication list examined carefully. For patients with blood in the stool and negative results of *C. difficile* toxin tests, flexible sigmoidoscopy can be used to look for pseudomembranes. Stool culture and parasite examination are generally not recommended for patients who contract diarrhea in the hospital.

Chronic diarrhea: An informative history can provide the diagnosis (e.g., lactose intolerance or sorbitol ingestion) or can help streamline the evaluation. Initial tests include measurement of serum electrolytes and serum albumin, complete blood cell count, and the erythrocyte sedimentation rate. Stool should be tested for occult blood, ova and parasites, *Giardia* antigen, fat (Sudan stain), and phenolphthalein (to detect surreptitious laxative use). Flexible sigmoidoscopy with biopsy can be useful in detecting inflammatory (inflammatory bowel disease, microscopic colitis), infectious (shistosomiasis), infiltrative (amyloidosis), and cathartic (anthracene laxatives) lesions. If the diagnosis is still obscure, additional tests are necessary. These may include measurement of fasting stool volume, quantitative fecal fat determination, and colonoscopy with biopsy. One can differentiate osmotic from secretory diarrhea by calculating the stool osmotic gap. If the fecal fat levels are elevated, specific diagnostic tests should be performed on the basis of suspicion of pancreatic disease, bacterial overgrowth, mucosal disease, or lymphatic obstruction. Blood tests for thyroid function and hormone levels (see earlier) may be helpful.

MANAGEMENT

Acute diarrhea: Fluid therapy is most important, especially for infants and the elderly. When large diarrheal losses are replaced with water or oral solutions low in sodium content (e.g., juice, soda, sports drinks), hyponatremia results. Oral rehydration solutions are preferable. In some cases, intravenous saline solution may be necessary. Patients with acute infectious diarrhea should not be treated with antibiotics unless they are travelers or are likely to have invasive bacterial enteritis. Single doses of a quinolone and an antimotility agent at the onset of symptoms relieve traveler's diarrhea in most cases. Patients with severe diarrhea, a high fever, or bloody stools should be given a quinolone to take orally for 3 days. Antimotility agents should not be given to these patients (see later). For patients with *C. difficile* infection, the offending antibiotic should be discontinued (if possible) and metronidazole therapy begun. Oral vancomycin should be reserved for patients with severe or refractory infection.

Chronic diarrhea: Treatment consists of fluid repletion and specific therapy for the underlying condition. Lactase deficiency is managed with a lactose-free diet, pancreatic insufficiency with pancreatic enzyme replacement, and celiac disease with a gluten-free diet. Bacterial overgrowth and tropical sprue respond to antibiotics. Patients with a limited ileal resection are treated with cholestyramine.

Antidiarrheal agents: These can be grouped into four categories: bismuth subsalicylate, antimotility agents, antisecretory agents, and anti-inflammatory agents. Bismuth has both antimicrobial and antisecretory properties and is used most often in the prevention of traveler's diarrhea. Antimotility agents such as loperamide slow intestinal transit and increase contact time for fluid reabsorption. These agents usually are reserved for patients with mild to moderate diarrhea who do not have fever or blood in the stool. They should not be used or should be used with caution to manage high-volume diarrhea (can lead to underestimation of fluid losses), invasive bacterial enteritis (can delay clearance), or ulcerative colitis (can precipitate toxic megacolon). No agent specifically inhibits intestinal

fluid secretion. Octreotide, the long-acting somatostatin analogue, inhibits all gastrointestinal secretions and is effective in decreasing secretory diarrhea from any cause. Steroids and 5-aminosalicylic acid decrease prostaglandin and leukotriene production and are effective in the management of inflammatory bowel disease and microscopic colitis Indomethacin may decrease diarrhea caused by radiation enteritis.

Chapter 99

APPROACH TO THE PATIENT WITH DYSPHAGIA

DEFINITION

Dysphagia means either difficulty initiating a swallow (oropharyngeal dysphagia) or the sensation that foods, liquids, or both are hindered in their passage from mouth to stomach (esophageal dysphagia). It is important to differentiate dysphagia from odynophagia (pain with swallowing).

HISTORY AND PHYSICAL EXAMINATION

Oropharyngeal dysphagia: Because patients have difficulty initiating swallowing, symptoms occur within 1 second of swallowing. Patients identify the cervical esophagus as the problem area. Associated symptoms include nasal regurgitation, coughing, choking, dysarthria, and nasal speech. Examination usually reveals that a neuromuscular condition is contributing to the symptoms. Oropharyngeal dysphagia should not be confused with globus, a constant sensation of a lump or tightness in the throat that does not interfere with swallowing.

Esophageal dysphagia: The patient describes the problem as food "hanging up" somewhere behind the sternum. Localized to the lower sternum or epigastrium, the lesion is most likely in the distal esophagus. Localization to the lower part of the neck may indicate dysfunction in this area, but often the symptoms are referred from a more distal blockage. It is important to determine whether the symptoms are progressive or intermittent and whether they occur with solids only or with both liquids and solids. Historical features of gastroesophageal reflux, chest pain, and weight loss should be sought. Examination is of limited value. Patients with esophageal cancer may have lymphadenopathy; those with scleroderma may have features of the CREST syndrome.

DIFFERENTIAL DIAGNOSIS

Oropharyngeal dysphagia: Neuromuscular disease, especially stroke, is responsible for about 80% of cases. Other causes are listed in Table 94.1.

Esophageal dysphagia: Causes are listed in Table 94.1. Figure 94.1 shows an algorithm for the evaluation of dysphagia.

LABORATORY STUDIES AND DIAGNOSTIC TESTS

Barium esophagography, preferably with video technique, is the initial diagnostic test for oropharyngeal or esophageal dysphagia. For patients with the former, administration of various consistencies of barium and food products helps ascertain who can swallow safely without aspiration. For patients with esophageal dysphagia, the test outlines irregularities in the esophageal lumen, defines sites of obstruction, and provides information about liquid transit through the esophagus. If there is an obstructing lesion, endoscopy with biopsy can confirm the diagnosis. Endoscopy should not be the initial study, however, because a narrow endoscope tends to miss rings and strictures. If results of barium studies are normal or suggest a motility disorder, esophageal manometry is the next step. This study can help diagnose achalasia and spastic motility disorders, and the findings may suggest scleroderma esophagus.

MANAGEMENT

Modification of diet and instruction in swallowing techniques may benefit patients with oropharyngeal dysphagia. Therapy for contributing conditions such as Parkinson's disease, polymyositis, and myasthenia gravis is indicated. Strictures and webs often can be managed during endoscopy by the use of dilators. Proton pump inhibitors and promotility agents may be helpful to manage strictures and webs associated with gastroesophageal reflux.

Chapter 94

GALLSTONES AND CHOLECYSTITIS

INCIDENCE AND EPIDEMIOLOGY

Cholelithiasis is a common disorder in the United States, particularly among women. By the age of 75 years, approximately 35% of women and 20% of men have gallstones, most of which are asymptomatic. Native Americans and Northern Europeans have particularly high rates of gallstone formation, Asians and Africans much lower rates.

ETIOLOGY AND PATHOGENESIS

In the United States, at least 75% of all gallstones are cholesterol stones. Risk factors for cholesterol stones include obesity, rapid weight loss, spinal cord injury, female sex (risk ratio 2:1), ileal resection or disease, pregnancy, and estrogen use. The presence of biliary sludge (also called *microcrystalline disease*) is believed to be a precursor stage of lithogenesis and is associated with many of the same risk factors. Although it may resolve spontaneously or cause macroscopic stone formation, biliary sludge has been implicated convincingly as a cause of classic biliary pain, acute cholecystitis, and acute pancreatitis.

The spontaneous formation of biliary sludge or cholesterol gallstones is a multistep process. The precipitation of solid cholesterol crystals from supersaturated bile is called *nucleation*. The cholesterol concentration must exceed the capacity of bile salts and phospholipids to hold it in solution. As the bile is progressively concentrated, biliary vesicles aggregate and fuse into larger multi-lammelar vesicles. Crystals begin to emerge when the balance of nucleator and antinucleator activity favors solid crystal formation. Cholesterol crystals and calcium bilirubinate pigment if sequestered within the gallbladder, may form a stone over time.

About 25% of all gallstones are pigment stones. These stones are categorized as either black or brown depending on their chemical composition and appearance. Risk factors for black pigment stones include chronic hemolysis, cirrhosis, and total parenteral nutrition. The risk factors for brown pigment stones are biliary stasis and chronic biliary infection. Although the pathogenesis of pigment stones is incompletely understood, some degree of elevation in the level of biliary unconjugated bilirubin appears to be important.

PATHOPHYSIOLOGY AND CLINICAL FINDINGS

Asymptomatic stones: Most gallstones remain clinically silent. The frequency of symptomatic stone disease is approximately 1% to 2% per year in the period after the diagnosis of cholelithiasis; this frequency decreases over time.

Biliary Colic: Classic biliary colic is caused by mechanical obstruction of the gallbladder neck by a stone and a resultant increase in intraluminal pressure. It is a discrete episode of a steady, severe pain, typically located in the epigastrium or right upper quadrant. It may radiate to the back or right shoulder region, but the intensity does not usually fluctuate in the manner that the term *colic* implies. The pain usually comes on rapidly, lasts 30 minutes to 3 hours, and then gradually subsides. The pain is not associated with fever, leukocytosis, or acute peritoneal signs. The presence of these findings or biliary pain lasting longer than 4 to 6 hours should raise the suspicion of acute cholecystitis. True attacks of biliary pain should be differentiated from dyspeptic symptoms such as belching, epigastric burning, bloating, heartburn, flatulence, and intolerance of fatty foods. Abdominal discomfort that is chronically present or fleeting in nature (less than 10 to 15 minutes) should not be attributed to the presence of gallstones.

Chronic cholecystitis: Chronic cholecystitis is a consequence of repeated attacks of discrete biliary pain or acute cholecystitis. These episodes induce a chronic inflammatory process that may be mild and patchy or quite severe and extensive. Over time, the gallbladder wall may become thick and fibrotic, and the gallbladder becomes contracted and nonfunctional. When this is the case, the gallbladder does not opacify during oral cholecystography.

Acute cholecystitis: Acute obstruction of the cystic duct by a stone leads to gallbladder distention and can eventually cause inflammation of the gallbladder. The histologic findings range from edema, erythema, and mild mucosal inflammation to gross infiltration of the wall with neutrophils and evidence of necrosis and perforation. Superimposed bacterial infection may occur and is critical in the development of complications such as empyema, emphysematous cholecystitis, perforation, and the formation of a cholecystenteric fistula, which can lead to gallstone ileus if a large gallstone passes through the fistula and causes small-intestinal obstruction. Patients with acute cholecystitis report continuous upper abdominal pain and a history of similar but self-limited attacks in the past. They may have nausea but generally cannot relieve the pain by vomiting or changing

position. Low-grade fever and right subcostal tenderness are typical findings at examination. A classic Murphy's sign may be elicited when the patient's inspiration is abruptly halted because of pain during palpation of the right upper quadrant. Generalized rebound tenderness suggests perforation.

Acalculous cholecystitis (cholecystitis in the absence of stone obstruction) accounts for 5% to 10% of cases of acute cholecystitis. It is most commonly associated with critical illness, major surgery, extensive trauma, or burn-related injury. Elderly men with peripheral vascular disease and patients receiving total parenteral nutrition appear to be at greater risk than other patients. The pathophysiologic mechanism involves a combination of gallbladder stasis, inflammation, and ischemia. Gallbladder infection, such as cytomegalovirus infection in a patient with AIDS, also may be responsible. Patients may not manifest the typical signs and symptoms of acute cholecystitis.

Choledocholithiasis: Stones are found in the common bile duct (CBD) in approximately 10% to 15% of patients with symptomatic gallstones. Obstruction by stones in the distal duct or ampulla may cause jaundice, gallstone pancreatitis, or cholangitis. Cholangitis is bacterial infection of an obstructed bile duct. Patients have biliary pain, fever with chills, and jaundice (Charcot's triad). The infecting organisms commonly include gram-negative aerobic bacteria, enterococci, and intestinal anaerobic bacteria.

DIAGNOSTIC EVALUATION

Laboratory findings: The results of laboratory evaluation of uncomplicated biliary colic usually are unremarkable. In contrast, acute cholecystitis often is associated with mild elevations in peripheral white blood cell count and bilirubin levels. Bilirubin levels of 2 to 10 mg per deciliter, however, suggest obstructive choledocholithiasis. Acute obstruction of the CBD also can elevate serum transaminase levels; if amylase and lipase levels also are increased, gallstone-induced pancreatitis is likely.

Imaging studies: Ultrasonography is the preferred imaging study in the evaluation of acute or recurrent biliary pain. It can accurately depict the presence or absence or gallstones and can show evidence of acute cholecystitis (gallbladder wall thickening more than 3 mm, pericholecystic fluid, and gallbladder tenderness with transducer pressure). Although dilatation of the CBD suggests biliary obstruction due to choledocholithiasis, ultrasonography depicts only about 50% of nonobstructing CBD stones. Radionuclide scanning of the biliary system is helpful in demonstrating cystic duct obstruction in selected patients with symptoms and signs of acute cholecystitis and normal or inconclusive results of ultrasound examinations. Direct cholangiography with either endoscopic retrograde cholangiopancreatography (ERCP) or percutaneous transhepatic cholangiography is performed when additional delineation of the biliary tree is needed or when therapy such as CBD stone extraction or biliary stent placement is being considered.

MANAGEMENT

Asymptomatic stones: Adults with silent or incidental stones should be observed and treated expectantly regardless of age or sex. The course of gallstones in such patients usually is benign, and warning symptoms of biliary pain usually arise before a serious complication occurs.

Symptomatic stones: A patient with an episode of uncomplicated biliary pain has a 30% to 50% chance of having another attack within 1 to 2 years and a 3% per year risk for development of a complication. The decision to proceed with cholecystectomy, usually a laparoscopic procedure, depends on the patient's desires and ability to tolerate a surgical procedure. Nonsurgical intervention, such as bile acid dissolution therapy, plays a limited role and is best reserved for patients with symptoms who decline surgery or have a high operative risk.

Acute cholecystitis: Early laparoscopic cholecystectomy is indicated once the diagnosis is secure and the patient's condition has been optimized, usually with intravenous fluids and antibiotics for 24 to 48 hours. Patients with a major complication such as perforation undergo urgent open laparotomy. Percutaneous cholecystostomy is considered for patients with acute cholecystitis who are deemed to be at excessive risk of a poor surgical outcome, such as many critically ill patients with acalculous cholecystitis.

Common duct stones: When a patient with known gallbladder stones has signs and symptoms of concomitant choledocholithiasis, a number of treatment options exist. The presence of obstructive jaundice with or without fever and abdominal pain generally leads to a preoperative ERCP examination with sphincterotomy and stone extraction, followed by routine laparoscopic cholecystectomy. Patients also can go directly to laparoscopic surgery and undergo intraoperative cholangiography to determine whether a CBD stone is present. If a stone is present, it may be possible to remove it through the cystic duct. Otherwise, the CBD can be opened and then closed over a T tube, or the surgeon can convert the procedure to open CBD exploration or arrange for postoperative ERCP.

Chapter 124

GASTRODUODENAL ULCER DISEASE

DEFINITION AND EPIDEMIOLOGY
Peptic ulcers are defects in the mucosal lining of the stomach or duodenum that extend through the submucosa into the muscle layer. Duodenal ulcers are common, affecting about 10% of the population at some time in their lives. Women are now affected as often as men.

ETIOLOGY AND PATHOGENESIS
Peptic ulcer disease requires the presence of aggressive noxious substances such as acid and pepsin but rarely is caused solely by excessive acid secretion. Most cases result from a combination of exposure to these noxious substances and factors that undermine mucosal integrity. Chronic gastric infection with *Helicobacter pylori* is the most important predisposing factor to both gastric (70% of cases) and duodenal (90% of cases) ulcers. It has effects on both gastric acid secretion and gastric mucosal integrity. About 15% to 20% of persons with *H. pylori* infection have ulcers during their lifetime. About 75% infected of patients with a single episode of gastric or duodenal ulcer experience repeated ulceration if *H. pylori* is not eradicated. The second most common cause of ulcers is ingestion of nonsteroidal anti-inflammatory drugs (NSAIDs), which undermine mucosal integrity by depleting gastric mucosal prostaglandins. Cigarette smoking has been implicated as a risk factor for duodenal ulcer. Gastrinoma (Zollinger–Ellison syndrome) is a rare cause of peptic ulcer disease.

CLINICAL FINDINGS
Symptoms: Although the characteristic pain is a dull ache in the epigastrium relieved by ingestion of food or antacids, there are many variations, including pain in the right and left upper quadrants. Bleeding ulcers may be painless and manifest as hematemesis, melena, anemia, or even hematochezia. Perforated ulcers typically manifest as severe generalized abdominal pain associated with signs of peritonitis. Patients with ulcer-induced gastric outlet obstruction may have repeated episodes of vomiting. It usually is impossible to differentiate duodenal and gastric ulcers according to symptoms alone. Duodenal ulcer pain usually is episodic, typically occurs at night, and often is relieved by ingestion of food. Gastric ulcer (or gastric cancer) is suggested by pain that occurs within 30 minutes after eating, continuous rather than episodic pain, anorexia, nausea, vomiting, and weight loss.

Physical examination: Midepigastric tenderness is common but nonspecific. The examination may reveal evidence of other causes of epigastric pain, such as musculoskeletal tenderness, neuropathy, or abdominal masses. Succussion splash, a sign that the stomach contains excessive air and fluid, suggests gastric outlet obstruction. Patients with free ulcer perforation usually have abdominal rigidity and signs of generalized peritonitis.

DIFFERENTIAL DIAGNOSIS
The differential diagnosis includes nonulcer dyspepsia, gastroesophageal reflux disease, drug-induced dyspepsia and gastropathy, gastric or duodenal tumors (benign or malignant), Crohn's disease of the stomach or duodenum, pancreatic disease (benign or malignant), hepatobiliary disease, and neuromuscular pain. The diagnosis of nonulcer dyspepsia is made when a patient has epigastric symptoms for more than 4 weeks and diagnostic evaluation reveals no obvious cause. Though nonulcer dyspepsia cannot reliably be differentiated from peptic ulcer disease with the history or examination findings, it is suggested by earlier age at onset, female sex, precipitation by ingestion of food, daily occurrence, impaired sleep pattern, and worsening of symptoms during periods of stress.

LABORATORY FINDINGS AND DIAGNOSTIC EVALUATION
Diagnostic studies: During upper gastrointestinal endoscopy, ulcers are seen as depressions with white or yellow bases, often with erythematous or edematous edges surrounded by normal mucosa. Other structural diseases can be excluded, such as erosive esophagitis or gastric cancer, and biopsy and culture specimens may be obtained. Therapy for bleeding ulcers can be administered directly. Most gastric and duodenal ulcers can be diagnosed with barium radiography, especially when double-contrast technique is used, although this method does not allow biopsy, culture, or therapy. Radiography is especially useful for identifying infiltrative diseases, such as lymphoma or linitis plastica, and extrinsic compression of the stomach or duodenum by mass lesions.

Ancillary studies: Routine laboratory studies generally are not useful in establishing the diagnosis, but they can help define the cause. In selected cases, fasting gastrin and acid secretory measurements are useful in excluding gastrinoma. Testing for *H. pylori* is essential for all patients with documented ulceration. This can be done by invasive (histologic identification or rapid urease testing of biopsy specimens) or noninvasive (serum antibody testing or urea breath testing) means. Serologic tests are highly sensitive and specific but cannot help differentiate a previously treated infection from a currently active one. Serologic testing therefore cannot be used to document eradication of the infection after therapy, which is a role well suited to urea breath testing.

MANAGEMENT
Nonspecific measures: Dietary manipulations are not of proven benefit. Because smoking is associated with poor healing and increased recurrence rates, smoking cessation is a reasonable adjunct. The role of alcohol restriction is controversial. Discontinuation of aspirin and NSAIDs is important both for healing and for reducing recurrence rates. If these drugs cannot be discontinued, an NSAID with low ulcerogenic potential, such as ibuprofen, should be used. Studies are currently underway to evaluate specific cyclooxygenase II inhibitors, which are likely to carry a lower risk of peptic ulcer complications than NSAIDs do. Other measures that may decrease ulcer formation in patients who need NSAIDs are eradication of *H. pylori* and long-term therapy with misoprostol or acid-inhibiting drugs.

Cure of H. pylori infection: Eradication of *H. pylori* accelerates the healing of *H. pylori*–associated ulcers, greatly diminishes the likelihood of ulcer relapse, and may decrease the frequency of complications. The optimal treatment regimen is not yet established, but consensus is emerging that triple-therapy combinations should be used to ensure adequate cure rates. A 2-week course of standard triple therapy with metronidazole (250 mg three times a day), a bismuth compound (e.g., 2 chewable bismuth subsalicylate tablets four times a day), and tetracycline (500 mg four times a day) with standard doses of antisecretory therapy provides excellent results but is poorly tolerated. Proton pump inhibitor–based triple-therapy regimens are therefore the current regimens of choice. The U.S. Food and Drug Administration has approved 7- to 14-day regimens consisting of lansoprazole (30 mg twice a day) or omeprazole (20 mg twice a day) combined with two of the following three antibiotics: amoxicillin (1 g twice a day), clarithromycin (500 mg twice a day), or metronidazole (500 mg twice a day).

Medical Management: Several drugs are effective for healing active ulcers, and some of these may decrease the rate of recurrence when used for long-term therapy after healing. These drugs work by inhibiting acid secretion, neutralizing acid secretion, or improving cytoprotection in the ulcer environment. Administration of a single daily dose of histamine-2 receptor antagonists (e.g., 300 mg ranitidine or nizatidine, 40 mg famotidine) at bedtime heals 90% of duodenal ulcers within 6 weeks. Gastric ulcers ulcers heal more slowly and respond better to 6 to 8 weeks of therapy. Maintenance therapy usually is given as half of the treatment dose. Proton pump inhibitors (20 mg omeprazole or 30 mg lansoprazole each morning) produce more rapid healing than do histamine-2 receptor antagonists and have a better side effect profile. They are the agents of choice for patients with gastrinoma. Low doses of antacids (e.g., 2 tablets four times a day) can heal ulcers effectively at a low cost. Prostaglandins such as misoprostol have cytoprotective properties and may inhibit acid production. They may have a special protective action on damage produced by NSAIDs. Use of prostaglandins is limited by side effects such as abdominal cramps and diarrhea and the ability to cause uterine contraction and abortion. Sucralfate is an aluminum sulfate disaccharide that acts locally on the gastric and duodenal mucosa. It has no specific side effects and produces healing rates comparable to those of the histamine-2 receptor antagonists.

Surgical management: Some complications of ulcer disease necessitate surgical treatment, such as hemorrhage unresponsive to medical management, including endoscopic hemostasis, gastric outlet obstruction not reversed by medical management, perforation, and malignant tumors. The most effective operation for gastric ulcer is simple antrectomy. Partial gastric resection with vagotomy is effective in the management of duodenal ulcer. The procedure may be performed with a Billroth I (gastroduodenal) or Billroth II (gastrojejunal) anastomosis. Perforated ulcers may necessitate only simple closure with an omental patch.

Surgical complications include bile gastritis, anastomotic ulcer, dumping syndrome, and malabsorption.

Chapter 107

GASTROESOPHAGEAL REFLUX DISEASE

DEFINITION, EPIDEMIOLOGY AND PATHOPHYSIOLOGY

Gastroesophageal reflux disease (GERD) is the pathologic manifestation of the movement of gastroduodenal contents into the esophagus. It is probably the most common condition affecting the gastrointestinal tract. More than 40% of adults in the United States experience its primary symptom, heartburn, at least once a month. Pregnant women have the highest prevalence. The pathophysiologic mechanism is a complex interplay of numerous factors, but the common denominator is the development of a common cavity that represents equilibration of intragastric and intraesophageal pressures. Transient lower esophageal sphincter (LES) relaxation is the main mechanism that promotes free reflux of gastric contents. Delayed gastric emptying, increases in intra-abdominal pressure, and dysfunction of esophageal acid clearance are factors in some patients. Most patients with esophagitis have a sliding hiatal hernia, but many persons with hiatal hernias do not have GERD. The mechanism of mucosal damage involves the action of pepsin and the direct effects of acid.

CLINICAL FINDINGS

Heartburn is the classic symptom; it is generally described as retrosternal burning pain that also may be felt in the epigastrium, neck, and throat. It often occurs after meals and is exacerbated by recumbency or bending over. Patients may have dysphagia, odynophagia, water brash, and belching. Dysphagia suggests the presence of a peptic esophageal stricture or severe esophagitis. Water brash is the sudden appearance in the mouth of slightly sour or salty fluid from the salivary glands in response to intraesophageal acid exposure. GERD also can manifest with extraesophageal symptoms such as hoarseness, chronic cough, and wheezing.

COMPLICATIONS

Peptic strictures represent the end stage of ongoing reflux, mucosal damage, healing, and fibrosis. They manifest as slowly progressive dysphagia for solids. Barrett's esophagus results when severe esophagitis induces a unique reparative process in which the original squamous epithelium is replaced by metaplastic columnar epithelium. The prevalence is 5% to 10% among patients with symptomatic GERD; higher rates occur among patients with esophagitis or peptic strictures. The diagnosis is made by means of endoscopy and biopsy. The main concern is a markedly increased risk of esophageal adenocarcinoma.

DIAGNOSIS

In most cases, the history is sufficiently typical to allow a trial of therapy without diagnostic testing. Early investigation should be undertaken when a patient has an atypical presentation of GERD, when symptoms are unresponsive to medical therapy, or when there is clinical evidence of the complications of GERD, such as dysphagia.
Endoscopy: All patients with persistent symptoms or frequent relapses after medical therapy should undergo endoscopy to ascertain the presence of esophagitis or other complications of GERD. Such patients need biopsy to exclude malignant disease and Barrett's esophagus. However, most patients with GERD have no evidence of esophagitis at endoscopy.
Other tests: Barium esophagography is the best first test in the care of patients with dysphagia. It can demonstrate reflux fluoroscopically and depicts signs of erosive esophagitis and peptic strictures. It is less sensitive for mild esophagitis. Prolonged esophageal pH monitoring is the best test for diagnosing GERD. It is helpful when the disease has an atypical presentation, such as noncardiac chest pain or pulmonary symptoms, or causes intractable symptoms in association with normal endoscopic findings. Esophageal pH monitoring has essentially replaced the acid perfusion Bernstein test. Manometric assessment of LES pressure is not sensitive; it is reserved for instances in which another diagnosis, such as achalasia, is suspected.

PROGNOSIS AND MANAGEMENT

In the care of patients who do not have esophagitis, the goal is simply to relieve symptoms. For patients with esophagitis, the goal is to eliminate the inflammation and prevent further complications such as strictures and Barrett's metaplasia.

Strategies include lifestyle modifications (Table 106.3), antacid therapy; administration of prokinetic drugs (of which cisapride is the best for controlling symptoms and healing mild esophagitis), histamine-2 antagonists, or proton pump inhibitors; and antireflux surgery. A general approach is outlined in Table 106.2. Patients with peptic strictures often need dilation of the narrowing with blunt bougies. For patients with Barrett's esophagus, endoscopic surveillance with biopsy is recommended to detect high-grade dysplasia or early cancer and to allow curative resection.

Chapter 106

APPROACH TO THE PATIENT WITH GASTROINTESTINAL BLEEDING

DEFINITIONS

Gastrointestinal (GI) bleeding may be chronic (manifesting as iron-deficiency anemia or occult fecal blood) or acute. Bleeding from the upper GI tract often manifests as hematemesis (bloody vomitus). This may reflect recent (bright-red vomitus) or previous (coffee-ground vomitus) hemorrhage. Melena consists of black, tarry, malodorous stool caused by the presence of degraded blood in the intestine. Melena generally indicates an upper GI source but can originate in the right colon. Other causes of black stool (iron or bismuth ingestion) must be excluded. Hematochezia is the passage of bright red blood from the rectum; it generally indicates a lower GI lesion. Lower GI bleeding is defined as hemorrhage from below the ligament of Treitz. Occult GI bleeding is bleeding of which the patient is unaware; it manifests as guaiac-positive stools or iron deficiency anemia.

DIFFERENTIAL DIAGNOSIS

Upper GI Bleeding: The three major causes are peptic ulcer disease, gastropathy or gastric erosions, and esophageal varices. Other causes include Mallory–Weiss tears, esophagitis, erosive duodenitis, and neoplasms. Patients with no endoscopic diagnosis (10% to 15%) have an excellent prognosis.
Lower GI Bleeding: Seventy percent to 80% of lower GI hemorrhage is from the right colon. The two major causes of acute lower GI hemorrhage are diverticulosis and angiodysplasia. Diverticular hemorrhage occurs when an artery ruptures into the diverticular sac; therefore diverticulosis is not thought to be a cause of occult GI bleeding or slow bleeding. Other causes include neoplasia, radiation or ischemic colitis, and inflammatory bowel disease. Hemorrhoids and colonic neoplasia are the most common causes of chronic lower GI bleeding.
Occult GI Bleeding: In Western countries, acid-peptic disease accounts for 30% to 70% of cases of occult bleeding (aspirin and other nonsteroidal anti-inflammatory drugs [NSAIDs] often are implicated); however, when the stool occult blood test is used for screening among patients older than 50 years, the goal is early detection of colonic polyps and colon cancer. The specificity of the test for these lesions is quite low. Therefore many positive results must be investigated, usually with colonoscopy, to find one polyp or instance of cancer.

HISTORY AND PHYSICAL EXAMINATION

Upper GI Bleeding: A history of peptic disease or dyspeptic symptoms suggests ulcers; a history of cirrhosis suggests variceal bleeding, although 30% to 60% of patients with cirrhosis have a nonvariceal source of bleeding. Use of aspirin, NSAIDs, and alcohol must be ascertained, and the patient should be asked about recent nose bleeds. Physical examination should focus on signs and symptoms of cirrhosis or evidence of underlying malignant disease, such as lymphadenopathy. Epigastric tenderness is common in peptic disease. Maroon or melenic stool found at rectal examination indicates severe bleeding. In severe cases, the patient may be in a state of shock.
Lower GI Bleeding: A recent history of anorexia or weight loss may indicate malignant disease. Symptoms such as abdominal pain or diarrhea suggest inflammatory bowel disease and ischemic or infectious colitis. In severe cases, the patient may be in a state of shock.

LABORATORY STUDIES AND DIAGNOSTIC TESTS

Serial hemoglobin determinations help determine severity. In the presence of acute hemorrhage, the initial hematocrit is a poor reflection of the amount of hemorrhage.
Upper GI Bleeding: Nasogastric lavage can be used to assess the rate of ongoing blood loss and confirm an upper GI source, although a negative result does not

exclude duodenal hemorrhage. Diagnostic endoscopy is the procedure of choice. Angiography and radionuclide scans are used to localize the site of hemorrhage only when endoscopy does not.

Lower GI Bleeding: All patients need a diagnostic evaluation (Fig. 102.2). When bleeding is rapid, the colonoscopic view may be obscured by blood, and the patient should undergo immediate angiography. Before angiography, nasogastric lavage and even upper GI endoscopy should be considered to rule out an upper GI source.

Bleeding from unknown source: About 5% of patients have no identifiable source despite extensive examination. In most instances, the cause is thought to be vascular ectasia. In the care of young patients, a radionuclide scan for Meckel's diverticulum is valuable. Enteroclysis may identify small-bowel sources. If these modalities are not revealing and the severity of the bleeding is sufficient to warrant transfusion, visceral angiography or small-bowel enteroscopy is indicated.

Occult GI bleeding: In the absence of anemia or GI symptoms, a patient older than 40 years should undergo colonoscopy or the combination of air-contrast barium enema radiographic examination and sigmoidoscopy. A patient younger than 40 years can be observed with repeat hemoglobin levels and stool samples. If the patient has iron deficiency or has upper GI symptoms and is older than 40 years, colonoscopy should be performed first but should be followed by upper endoscopy if the colonoscopic findings are not revealing. If both studies have normal findings, enteroclysis may help identify small-bowel sources. If the severity of bleeding is sufficient to warrant transfusion, visceral angiography or small-bowel enteroscopy is indicated.

PROGNOSIS AND MANAGEMENT

Upper GI Bleeding: About 80% of episodes are self-limited and necessitate only supportive care. The mortality rate is about 10% and increases to about 30% to 40% with continued or recurrent bleeding. Management begins with resuscitation (saline infusion with or without red blood cell transfusion). Acid-reducing therapy often is started empirically, although conclusive evidence of benefit has been lacking. For variceal hemorrhage, intravenous somatostatin and the combination of intravenous vasopressin and nitroglycerin are helpful. Endoscopic therapies include thermal coagulation of bleeding vessels and sclerotherapy or band ligation of varices. Massive variceal hemorrhage may necessitate balloon tamponade. Bleeding refractory to all of these interventions may necessitate urgent surgery.

Lower GI Bleeding: Episodes resolve spontaneously in 80% of patients. Unlike upper GI bleeding, most lower GI bleeding is slow and intermittent and does not necessitate hospitalization. Management begins with resuscitation (saline infusion with or without red blood cell transfusion). Most patients with bleeding that ceases or is slow need elective treatment of the underlying disorder, such as colonoscopic electrocoagulation techniques for angiodysplasia. Urgent therapy is indicated when a patient needs more than three units of red blood cells. Intra-arterial vasopressin (0.2 unit per minute) after selective catheterization of the bleeding vessels is the best initial therapy; subtotal colectomy and intra-arterial embolization are next in order of effectiveness.

Bleeding from unknown source: A therapeutic trial of estrogen–progesterone therapy for possible vascular ectasia may be worthwhile.

Chapter 102

GIARDIASIS

DEFINITION AND EPIDEMIOLOGY

Giardia lamblia is the organism that causes most instances of protozoal infection of the intestinal tract worldwide. Prevalence varies from 2% to 5% in industrialized nations to 20% to 30% in the developing world. The illness usually is acquired by means of consuming water contaminated with the feces of humans or animals. Streams and wells are common sources. Transmission also is common in day care centers, in institutions for the mentally ill and retarded, and among homosexual men.

CLINICAL FEATURES

Clinical giardiasis ranges from asymptomatic carriage to severe chronic diarrhea and malabsorption. Acute illness is characterized by abdominal cramps, nausea

and vomiting, and watery diarrhea. Many cases are short-lived and resolve without therapy. However, giardiasis often becomes chronic and can then manifest as a nonspecific chronic diarrheal syndrome or as a malabsorptive syndrome characterized by abdominal distress, gas bloating, and malaise without much diarrhea. Urticaria and arthralgia also have been reported.

DIAGNOSIS

Diagnosis is made by means of finding trophozoites or cysts in stool or intestinal fluid or tissue. Examination of the stool has a sensitivity of 35% to 50% at best. Duodenal contents can be aspirated directly or by means of a string test. A stool antigen test also is available.

MANAGEMENT

Treatment is with 250 mg metronidazole three times a day for 5 days.

Chapter 113

HEPATIC NEOPLASMS

DEFINITION, EPIDEMIOLOGY, AND PATHOGENESIS

Primary hepatocellular carcinoma (HCC) is a malignant transformation of hepatocytes and is a well-recognized complication of long-standing liver disease of numerous causes. The incidence worldwide is correlated with the prevalence of chronic hepatitis B virus infection. Other risk factors include male sex, hemochromatosis, α_1-antitrypsin deficiency, Wilson's disease, exposure to aflatoxin B (a by-product of *Aspergillus* infection of grains, rice, and peanuts), androgens, estrogen, and vinyl chloride exposure. Chronic inflammation is thought to expose the liver to genotoxic free radicals that lead to mutations and formation of HCC. Fibrolamellar HCC is a distinct variant that usually occurs among patients who do not have cirrhosis and is associated with a better prognosis.

There are several types of benign hepatic tumors. Hepatic adenoma and focal nodular hyperplasia (FNH) are the most common. The true incidence is unknown. Women are at increased risk of hepatic adenoma, especially during the reproductive years and with the use of oral contraceptives. Hepatic adenoma is made up of normal-appearing hepatocytes without portal triad elements. FNH is composed of all cell populations normally present in the liver and appears as a central vascular scar with fibrous septa radiating form it. The liver is a preferential site for the deposition of tumor metastases, especially from cancers of the pancreas, gallbladder, colon, or breast; malignant melanoma; and neuroendocrine tumors.

CLINICAL FINDINGS

Hepatocellular carcinoma: The presentation depends in part on the presence of associated liver disease, which may cause fatigue, jaundice, weight loss, pain in the right upper quadrant, ascites, or hepatomegaly. HCC should be sought in evaluation of patients with chronic liver disease who have hepatic decompensation with no identifiable precipitating factor.

Benign neoplasms: Patients with hepatic adenoma are of childbearing age and have histories of oral contraceptive use. Symptoms, including abdominal mass or pain, are present in 80% of cases. Patients with FNH are in their fifth to sixth decades of life. The lesion often is found in patients without symptoms during radiographic evaluation of the liver. Only 10% of patients have pain or an asymptomatic hepatic mass at the time of diagnosis.

Metastatic disease: Patients may notice weight loss, anorexia, or right upper quadrant pain. About 50% of patients have hepatomegaly and 15% have jaundice. Ascites occurs among 50% of patients with metastatic gastric, ovarian, or gallbladder carcinoma. Patients with metastasis from primary tumors in the pancreas, stomach, or lung often have no symptoms. At examination, firm, distinct nodules may be felt.

LABORATORY FINDINGS AND DIAGNOSTIC EVALUATION

Hepatocellular carcinoma: Routine laboratory tests should be performed for the evaluation of liver injury and function. Assessment of serum markers for specific diseases should be performed; these include serologic testing for viruses, measurement of ceruloplasmin, calculation of iron-binding ratio, and measurement of ferritin. Serum HCC tumor markers, most notably α-fetoprotein (AFP), can be measured. AFP levels are elevated in 60% to 70% of cases (not in fibrolamellar HCC). Values greater than 400 ng per milliliter are highly specific for HCC. Imaging by means of ultrasonography and computed tomography (CT) is used to identify and characterize the features of the liver tumor, to direct percutaneous biopsy, and to assess the extent of disease. Helical CT facilitates detection of small nodules. Magnetic resonance imaging is especially useful for detection of hemangioma and fatty liver infiltrates.

Benign neoplasms: AFP levels are normal. Hepatic imaging and biopsy are the primary tools used to differentiate benign from malignant disease. If hepatic adenoma is suspected, radiologic evaluation should be performed first, because biopsy carries a significant risk of bleeding. Biopsy is safe in the evaluation of FNH.

Metastatic disease: An elevated alkaline phosphatase level is common. Increased serum bilirubin levels may be a sign of large-duct obstruction. AFP levels are normal. CT can be used to define the location and number of lesions and to identify the presence of a primary, extrahepatic tumor in the abdomen. Percutaneous biopsy may be necessary to confirm the diagnosis.

PROGNOSIS AND MANAGEMENT

Hepatocellular carcinoma: Early detection and resection of HCC nodules smaller than 2 cm in diameter followed by resection, for patients with adequate hepatic reserve, is the optimum approach to definitive cure. The 5-year survival rates range from 30% to 85%. Ultrasound screening every 6 months for patients with long-standing cirrhosis is essential for early detection. When resection is not feasible because of widespread disease, poor hepatic reserve, or evidence of metastases, other noncurative options can be used. These include intra-arterial chemoembolization, percutaneous injection of alcohol, and cryosurgical ablation. Orthotopic liver transplantation has been used to manage HCC.

Benign neoplasms: When a woman is found to have a hepatic mass, discontinuation of any estrogen is the first priority. Large hepatic adenomas occasionally shrink or resolve in the absence of hormone. If hepatic adenoma is suspected because of clinical and radiologic features, surgical resection is the preferred treatment because of the risk of rupture or hemorrhage and the documented potential for malignant transformation. For FNH, no risk of bleeding or malignant transformation exists, and tumors can be removed by means of enucleation or wedge resection to release compression on normal liver tissue or to ameliorate pain.

Metastatic disease: Resection of metastatic lesions from noncolorectal tumors has a dismal prognosis. For selected patients with colorectal carcinoma, resection of metastatic lesions improves prognosis. Favorable factors include the presence of three or fewer lesions, an interval of more than 1 year between bowel and liver resection, and a greater margin of normal resected liver around the tumor.

Chapter 126

■ HEREDITARY HEMOCHROMATOSIS

DEFINITION, EPIDEMIOLOGY, AND PATHOGENESIS

Hereditary hemochromatosis is a common disorder of iron metabolism that affects approximately 1 in 200 to 400 persons of Northern European descent. It is caused by an increase in absorption of iron from the proximal intestine and deposition of iron in the liver, pancreas, heart, joints, skin, and endocrine organs. Affected individuals have two copies of the mutant hemochromatosis gene (*HFE*).

CLINICAL FEATURES

Hereditary hemochromatosis is increasingly being identified during the evaluations conducted because routine chemistry panels show abnormal iron levels or because screening iron studies are performed on persons with a family history of hereditary hemochromatosis. Cases diagnosed in this way usually are asymptomatic. Symptomatic cases often manifest as fatigue, right upper quadrant abdominal pain, arthralgia, impotence, decreased libido, symptoms of heart failure, or diabetes. Physical examination findings include hepatomegaly, cirrhosis, extrahepatic manifestations of chronic liver disease, testicular atrophy, signs of congestive heart failure, skin pigmentation, and arthritis.

LABORATORY FINDINGS AND DIAGNOSTIC EVALUATION

Fasting transferrin saturation (serum iron divided by total iron binding capacity) should be calculated. If the ratio is 45% or more, *HFE* mutation analysis should be performed to confirm the diagnosis. Patients with symptoms also typically have elevated levels of serum ferritin. Patients older than 40 years or with abnormal liver tests, regardless of *HFE* test results should undergo percutaneous liver

biopsy quantitative iron studies for histologic interpretation. Patients with symptoms typically have elevated levels of serum ferritin.

MANAGEMENT

Treatment is weekly therapeutic phlebotomy of 500 mL of whole blood. Phlebotomy typically is continued until the transferring saturation is less than 50% or serum ferritin levels are less than 50 ng per milliliter. Once excess iron stores are depleted, maintenance phlebotomy continues every 2 to 3 months for the duration of the patient's life. If treatment is initiated before complications of liver disease develop, the prognosis is excellent. All first-degree relatives should be offered genetic screening.

Chapter 123

■ INFLAMMATORY BOWEL DISEASE

DEFINITION AND EPIDEMIOLOGY

Inflammatory bowel disease (IBD) encompasses at least two forms of idiopathic intestinal inflammation—ulcerative colitis and Crohn's disease (also known as regional enteritis). Ulcerative colitis and Crohn's disease are at least partially distinct in initial pathogenic events, but they have many key pathophysiologic processes in common. Men and women are affected equally, but the prevalence is higher among the U.S. white than the U.S. black and U.S. Hispanic populations. Onset is usually in the second and third decades of life; there is a small increase in incidence in the fifth and sixth decades.

ETIOLOGY AND PATHOPHYSIOLOGY

The precise causes are unknown. Both environmental and genetic factors seem to contribute to the pathogenesis. The clinical manifestations depend on a series of immunologic and inflammatory events. Activation of inflammatory cells produces reactive oxygen metabolites that may serve as the final common pathway of tissue damage.

PATHOLOGY

Ulcerative colitis: The inflammatory process in ulcerative colitis is confined to the mucosa and superficial submucosa of the colon and rectum (neutrophilic microabcesses within the lamina propria and crypts). The inflammatory process typically extends in a continuous manner proximally from the rectum, the length of proximal extension varying among patients.

Crohn's disease: Crohn's disease is much more varied in its manifestations. Active disease is characterized by an infiltrate in which macrophages and lymphocytes predominate. Noncaseating granulomas are found in most patients. Extension of the inflammatory process into the deeper layers of the bowel wall is a distinguishing feature. Transmural involvement is common and may lead to fistula formation and serosal adherence to adjacent structures. Although Crohn's disease may affect any region of the gastrointestinal tract, involvement of the terminal ileum or colon is most common. The inflammation can be patchy, and segmental involvement of different areas is typical.

CLINICAL FEATURES

Ulcerative colitis: The cardinal symptom is bloody diarrhea. Bowel movements are frequent but often small in volume. Additional symptoms can include crampy lower abdominal pain, rectal pain, tenesmus, and fecal urgency. With more extensive colonic inflammation, fatigue, fever, and weight loss are common. Ulcerative colitis typically follows a chronic relapsing course characterized by intermittent acute attacks interspersed with periods of remission. Local complications include colonic perforation or stricture. Toxic megacolon is the most serious complication of acute ulcerative colitis. Extension of the inflammatory process into the muscularis leads to impairment of contraction and colonic distention along with fever, tachycardia, and leukocytosis. Patients with long-standing ulcerative colitis have a markedly increased risk of colon cancer.

Crohn's disease: Crohn's disease is more varied than ulcerative colitis in clinical course, owing to its diversity of anatomic involvement and the presence of transmural inflammation. Patients most often have the triad of diarrhea, abdominal pain, and weight loss. The onset can be insidious; most patients have had symptoms for months before medical evaluation. Among patients with colonic disease, diarrhea is often small in volume and associated with rectal urgency and tenesmus. Among patients with disease confined to the small intestine, stool volume is larger, especially if disease of the terminal ileum causes secretory diarrhea from bile salt malabsorption. Weight loss may be caused by diffuse intestinal inflammation, malabsorption, or decreased intake of food. Colonic Crohn's disease is more likely than small-intestinal Crohn's disease to be associated with rectal bleeding. Physical examination may reveal evidence of weight loss and muscle wasting. The abdomen often is tender. Laboratory findings include anemia (from chronic inflammation, blood loss, or deficiencies of iron, folate, or vitamin B_{12}), leukocytosis, elevated erythrocyte sedimentation rate, and hypoalbuminemia. Complications include fistulas, usually enterocutaneous or enteroenteric, intra-abdominal abscesses, small-bowel obstruction, and perianal abscesses or fistulas. Free intestinal perforation is rare. Patients have an increased incidence of cholesterol gallstones and calcium oxalate nephrolithiasis. As in ulcerative colitis, the risk of colon cancer is increased among patients with Crohn's colitis.

EXTRAINTESTINAL MANIFESTATIONS

Both ulcerative colitis and Crohn's disease are associated with a variety of extraintestinal manifestations. The most common is arthritis (25% of cases). Pauciarticular (fewer than five joints) peripheral arthritis tends to be acute and self-limited and correlates with bowel disease activity. Polyarticular (more than five joints) peripheral arthritis may be independent of the activity of IBD and is associated with uveitis. Sacroiliitis with or without ankylosing spondylitis also can occur and tends to pursue a relentlessly progressive course independent of the bowel disease. Hepatic complications include fatty liver, primary sclerosing cholangitis (more common with ulcerative colitis than in Crohn's disease), chronic hepatitis, and cirrhosis. Dermal complications include erythema nodosum, pyoderma gangrenosum, and rare instances of neutrophilic dermatosis. The principal ocular complications are episcleritis and uveitis.

DIFFERENTIAL DIAGNOSIS AND DIAGNOSTIC STUDIES

The differential diagnosis includes acute infectious colitis, giardiasis, ischemic colitis (among the elderly), diverticulitis, hemorrhoids or anal fissures, irritable bowel syndrome, medication-induced colitis (e.g., nonsteroidal anti-inflammatory drugs and allopurinol) and lymphocytic or collagenous colitis.

In most cases, the diagnosis of IBD is strongly suspected on the basis of a clinical presentation of diarrhea, bloody diarrhea, abdominal pain, or perianal disease. For patients with diarrhea, stool cultures for enteric pathogens and examination for ova and parasites should be performed. The principal techniques to confirm the diagnosis and monitor progression disease are endoscopy (sigmoidoscopy and colonoscopy) and contrast radiography. Endoscopy is useful in defining the extent of mucosal inflammation, detecting mild inflammation, obtaining biopsy specimens, and conducting surveillance examinations for dysplasia. Air contrast radiography is useful in assessing colonic distensibility and detecting fistulas and strictures. Barium enema radiographic studies and colonoscopy are contraindicated in the evaluation of patients with severe ulcerative colitis or Crohn's colitis because of the possibility of precipitating toxic megacolon or colonic perforation. Computed tomography is particularly useful in the evaluation of patients with Crohn's disease because it depicts abscesses and thickening of the bowel wall.

PROGNOSIS AND MANAGEMENT

Supportive therapy includes antidiarrheal agents such as loperamide and diphenoxylate (contraindicated in moderate or severe colitis because of the risk of toxic megacolon), repletion of fluids and electrolytes, and blood transfusions. The value of elemental diets as primary therapy is controversial. Surveillance colonoscopic examinations to detect dysplasia are recommended for patients with chronic ulcerative colitis or Crohn's colitis. There is no specific curative drug therapy for IBD; therapy must be individualized (Table 111.7). Patients with ulcerative colitis who do not respond to aggressive medical therapy can be cured with colectomy. Most patients with Crohn's disease ultimately undergo operative treatment for indications such as intestinal obstruction, symptomatic fistulas, abscesses, toxic dilatation, perforation, and cancer. The extraintestinal manifestations may necessitate specific therapies.

Chapter 111

◼ IRRITABLE BOWEL SYNDROME

DEFINITION

Irritable bowel syndrome (IBS) is a group of functional bowel disorders in which abdominal discomfort is associated with features of disordered defecation.

EPIDEMIOLOGY

IBS affects about 10% to 20% of adults in western countries. No ethnic differences have been reported; the prevalence appears to decrease among older persons. Although only 30% those with IBS seek medical attention, it is still one of the most frequently seen disorders in medical settings.

ETIOLOGY AND PATHOPHYSIOLOGY

No unique pathophysiologic mechanism for IBS has been identified. Patients with IBS often have abnormalities of gastrointestinal motility, but the findings are not unique to IBS and correlate poorly with symptoms. Several studies have shown that patients with IBS have lower pain thresholds to rectal distention and experience the urge to defecate at lower rectal volume. Psychological distress can cause prolonged motor abnormalities and a reduction in the threshold at which people experience afferent gastrointestinal symptoms. Patients with IBS have a higher prevalence of comorbid affective disorders, personality disturbances, and psychiatric illnesses. As many as 50% of women evaluated in a gastroenterology referral practice report a history of physical or sexual abuse.

CLINICAL FEATURES

Abdominal pain associated with a change in the consistency or frequency of stools and relieved with defecation is the hallmark of IBS. The pain is often poorly localized and may be migratory and variable. However, it often occurs after a meal, during psychological stress, or at the time of menses. Associated symptoms may include bloating or feeling of distention, presence of mucus in stool, urgency, and a feeling of incomplete evacuation. IBS may be diarrhea predominant, constipation predominant, or a combination of both at different times. The physical examination findings usually are unremarkable, although mild to moderate abdominal tenderness may be elicited.

LABORATORY FINDINGS AND DIAGNOSIS

The diagnosis is made clinically. The initial evaluation to exclude other disorders should include complete blood cell count; erythrocyte sedimentation rate (ESR); blood chemistries; stool examination for ova, parasites, and blood; and sigmoidoscopy. Colonoscopy or barium enema with sigmoidoscopy is recommended if the patient is older than 50 years. The following signs should alert the clinician to other diagnoses and lower the threshold for obtaining additional studies: history of weight loss; onset of symptoms at an older age; nocturnal symptoms; family history of carcinoma of the colon or inflammatory bowel disease; fever; abnormal physical findings, such as abdominal mass or hepatomegaly; or abnormal laboratory results, such as occult blood in stool, anemia, leukocytosis, elevated ESR, or abnormal results of blood chemical analysis. If any of these abnormal results is present, or if an initial therapeutic trial fails, additional testing is necessary. For patients with constipation-predominant IBS, the additional studies may include colonic transit time and anal manometry. For those with diarrhea the additional studies include stool tests (volume, electrolytes, fat, leukocyte count), small-bowel radiography, breath tests to exclude bacterial overgrowth, and colonic biopsy to exclude collagenous or lymphocytic colitis. For patients with bloating and pain, abdominal radiographs to exclude partial obstruction and abdominal ultrasonography may be indicated.

MANAGEMENT

Once the diagnosis has been made, the patient should receive education and reassurance about the condition and its consequences. A specific treatment strategy is based on the nature and severity of the symptoms. Referral for psychological treatment usually is recommended for patients with disabling symptoms or associated psychiatric disorders.

Dietary modifications: Identifying and eliminating offending dietary substances can be useful. These may include lactose for persons with lactose intolerance, caffeine, fatty foods, alcohol, sorbitol, and gas-producing foods such as cabbage and beans.

Pharmacotherapy: Most patients need no medications. When used, the choice of medication should be based on the predominant symptom. Pain and bloating respond to anticholinergic agents such as dicyclomine hydrochloride or hyoscyamine sulfate, preferably before meals. In severe cases, low doses of tricyclic antidepressants (50 to 150 mg desipramine; 25 to 100 mg amitriptyline) should be considered for their neuromodulatory and analgesic properties and for their psychotropic effects. Fluoxetine or paroxetine may be better tolerated by older patients. When diarrhea is the predominant symptom, agents such as loperamide (4 to 8 mg per day) may help to decrease urgency and stool frequency. For patients with constipation, an increase in dietary fiber (25 g per day) may be effective. If not, osmotic laxatives such as milk of magnesia, sorbitol, or lactulose may be added. Use of stimulant laxatives such as senna should not be prolonged. Promotility agents such as cisapride may be helpful only to patients with milder symptoms.

Chapter 109

APPROACH TO THE PATIENT WITH MALABSORPTION

PATHOPHYSIOLOGY AND DIFFERENTIAL DIAGNOSIS

Generalized maldigestion and malabsorption: Generalized maldigestion may be caused by a deficiency of pancreatic digestive enzyme secretion. Among adults, the two most common are chronic pancreatitis and pancreatic carcinoma. Among children, cystic fibrosis is the most common cause. Because solubilization of fatty acids requires bile acids, moderate fat malabsorption (steatorrhea) can occur with bile duct obstruction, intrahepatic cholestasis, and diseases or resection of the terminal ileum, which is responsible for bile acid reabsorption. Mucosal diseases such as celiac sprue, tropical sprue, Whipple's disease, radiation enteritis, amyloidosis, and giardiasis can cause generalized malabsorption, as can resection of the small intestine and protein-wasting enteropathy. A combination of maldigestion and malabsorption may occur with Zollinger–Ellison syndrome and with intestinal bacterial overgrowth caused by achlorhydria, small-intestinal strictures, the presence of blind loops of intestine, ileal resection, and motility disorders.

Disorders of specific nutrient assimilation: These disorders are caused by an isolated defect in an enzyme or transport system and are not associated with generalized malabsorption or malnutrition. The most common of these disorders is lactase deficiency, which causes malabsorption of the disaccharide lactose. The deficiency may be primary but is also commonly caused by mucosal diseases or the lingering effects of acute enteritis.

CLINICAL FEATURES

Generalized malabsorption: The major symptoms are caused by loss of calories into the stool (weight loss), an increase in stool volume (diarrhea), colonic fermentation of unabsorbed carbohydrates (abdominal bloating and distention, flatulence), and deficiency of dietary nutrients (a combination of anemia, dehydration, and hypokalemia). The weight loss often occurs despite a normal, or even enhanced, appetite. Although abdominal discomfort is common, severe abdominal pain is unusual. Among patients with steatorrhea, oil or undigested food particles may be present in the stool, which is commonly pale, yellow, sponge-like, and difficult to flush down the toilet. Deficiency of iron, folate, or cobalamin may cause anemia. Excessive bruising or bleeding (vitamin K deficiency), paresthesia or tetany (hypocalcemia or hypomagnesemia), and pathologic fractures due to osteoporosis or osteomalacia (calcium and protein deficiency) are the common initial manifestations of specific nutrient deficiencies.

Clinical examination often reveals pallor, muscle wasting, and hair loss. Follicular hyperkeratosis, cheilosis, and glossitis are common signs of nutritional deficits. The abdomen may have a doughy consistency because loops of small intestine become dilated and filled with fluid. Peripheral edema occurs as the result of hypoalbuminemia.

Deficiency of specific nutrients: Isolated malabsorption of specific nutrients usually produces a narrower clinical spectrum than does generalized malabsorption. Lactose malabsorption, for example, causes osmotic diarrhea but is not associated with weight loss and malnutrition.

LABORATORY TESTS

In generalized malabsorption, the stool usually is semiformed or watery and has an increased volume. It may appear greasy. Anemia is common and may be microcytic, normocytic, or macrocytic depending on the underlying deficiency. Prothrombin time may be elevated because of vitamin K deficiency. Profound electrolyte depletion with hyponatremia, hypokalemia, and a metabolic acidosis may occur with severe disease. Decreases in serum levels of calcium, magnesium, zinc, and phosphorus are common. Hypoalbuminemia and hypocholesterolemia are typical in moderate to severe disease.

DIAGNOSTIC EVALUATION

Generalized malabsorption and steatorrhea: Serum levels of carotene, cholesterol, and albumin are routinely low and can therefore be useful as a screening

battery, although these findings are not specific for malabsorption. Measurement of stool pH and total reducing substances is useful to screen for carbohydrate malabsorption. The quantification of fat in a 72-hour stool collection (more than 6 g per day after the patient ingests 70 to 100 g fat per day for at least 3 days) is considered the standard of reference for the diagnosis of steatorrhea. Sudan staining of a single stool specimen has 85% sensitivity for severe steatorrhea (more than 15 g per day) but a low sensitivity for mild to moderate disease. Blunted carbon 14 oxygen production after ingestion of carbon 14 C triolein also suggests fat malabsorption. Once generalized malabsorption is established, the D-[^{14}C]xylose test is helpful in identifying the pathophysiologic mechanism. D-[^{14}C]Xylose is normally absorbed passively in the jejunum; its absorption decreases in diffuse mucosal diseases but is typically normal in luminal causes of maldigestion such as pancreatic or bile acid deficiency. Small-bowel radiographs and small-bowel biopsy are useful in differentiating luminal and mucosal causes. The presence of pancreatic secretory insufficiency can be established directly with pancreatic function testing or indirectly by measurement in the urine, plasma, or breath of the pancreatic hydrolytic products of orally administered substrates, such as bentiromide. Patients with protein-wasting enteropathy have α_1-antitrypsin leakage into the stool. A simplified approach to the diagnosis of generalized malabsorption is shown in Fig. 110.7.

Tests for bacterial overgrowth and specific nutrient malabsorption: Jejunal cultures are the standard for documenting small-intestinal bacterial overgrowth. Owing to bacterial fermentation, patients with bacterial overgrowth also usually have a prompt increase in breath carbon 14 oxygen after ingestion of D-[^{14}C]xylose or the radiolabeled bile acid cholyl–L–carbon 14 C glycine. Several breath hydrogen tests can be used to detect fermentation of undigested carbohydrates such as lactose. Cobalamin absorption is classically measured with a dual-labeled Schilling test.

MANAGEMENT

Patients with specific diseases should be treated with therapies such as a gluten-free diet for celiac sprue; antibiotic therapy for Whipple's disease, giardiasis, and bacterial overgrowth; and pancreatic enzyme supplements for pancreatic insufficiency. If the specific cause cannot be adequately controlled, parenteral nutrition may be necessary. Patients with lactase deficiency can discontinue the consumption of milk, ice cream, cheeses, and other dairy products or can take these foods with supplemental lactase.

Chapter 110

APPROACH TO THE PATIENT WITH NAUSEA AND VOMITING

DEFINITIONS

Nausea and vomiting are nonspecific responses to a variety of conditions. Nausea is the sensation of an impending urge to vomit; vomiting is the forceful ejection from the mouth of contents of the upper gastrointestinal (GI) tract.

PATHOPHYSIOLOGY

Vomiting is caused by a coordinated interaction of neural, somatic muscular, and gastrointestinal myoelectric and muscular phenomena. Although the mechanisms that cause nausea are less well understood than those that cause vomiting, activation of selected cerebral cortical sites seems to be necessary.

DIFFERENTIAL DIAGNOSIS

The differential diagnosis of nausea and vomiting is extensive and includes a broad range of conditions that affect the GI tract, the peritoneal cavity, the central nervous system, and endocrine and metabolic functions (Table 98.1).

HISTORY AND PHYSICAL EXAMINATION

Duration of symptoms: Acute vomiting (1 to 2 days) is most often caused by infection, ingestion of a medication or toxin, or accumulation of endogenous toxins, as in uremia or diabetic ketoacidosis. Vomiting for more than 1 week usually is caused by a long-standing medical or psychiatric condition.

Timing of symptoms: Vomiting soon after a meal may occur with gastric outlet obstruction or psychogenic vomiting. Nausea and vomiting from inflammatory conditions such as cholecystitis or pancreatitis may occur in the first hour after a meal. Vomiting more than 1 hour after eating occurs in gastroparesis. Vomiting before breakfast is typical of early pregnancy, uremia, and alcoholism. Nausea from peptic ulcer disease and esophagitis may be improved by ingestion of food.

Character of the vomitus: Vomiting of undigested food suggests achalasia or a Zenker's diverticulum. Vomiting of partially digested food long after ingestion suggests gastroparesis or gastric outlet obstruction. The presence of bile excludes obstruction proximal to the ampulla of Vater. Blood indicates a process causing mucosal damage, such as an ulcer or malignant tumor, or Mallory–Weiss tear caused by the vomiting itself. Feculent emesis occurs in obstruction of the distal small intestine or colon.

Associated symptoms: Abdominal pain occurs with peptic ulcer disease, small-intestinal obstruction, and inflammatory disorders such as cholecystitis and pancreatitis. Vomiting may relieve the pain of the first two but has no effect on inflammatory conditions. The occurrence of diarrhea and fever suggests gastroenteritis. Weight loss is common for many patients, but not those with a psychogenic cause. Central nervous system lesions and meningitis are associated with headaches, neurologic deficits, or neck stiffness. In these disorders, vomiting may be effortless and are not associated with nausea. Specific symptoms can occur with many of the other conditions listed in Table 98.1, such as pregnancy, hyperthyroidism, and labyrinthine disorders.

Physical Examination: The existence of orthostatic hypotension suggests hypovolemia and the need for intravenous fluids. The absence of bowel sounds signifies ileus, whereas the presence of high-pitched, hyperactive bowel sounds and abdominal distention is consistent with intestinal obstruction. A succussion splash may occur with gastric outlet obstruction. Abdominal tenderness or occult fecal blood are present in many of the disorders listed in Table 98.1.

LABORATORY STUDIES AND DIAGNOSTIC TESTS
A through history and physical examination are sufficient in most instances. Figure 98.2 shows a suspicion-based algorithm for the evaluation of nausea and vomiting.

MANAGEMENT
Dietary therapy: Frequent small liquid meals should be prescribed to minimize gastric distention. Fats delay gastric emptying and tend to worsen nausea.

Medical therapy: Specific therapies should be directed at the underlying disorder, such as acid suppression for peptic ulcer disease, hydrocortisone for Addison's disease, and surgery for cholecystitis and small-bowel obstruction. For chronic nausea and vomiting, antiemetic medications provide relief. Dopamine receptor antagonists such as prochlorperazine are the most commonly prescribed. The side effects include drowsiness, dystonic reactions, and hyperprolactinemia-induced galactorrhea and sexual dysfunction. Patients with motor dysfunction of the upper GI tract may benefit from use of prokinetic agents that promote gastric emptying and intestinal transit; these include metoclopramide, domperidone, and cisapride. For the emesis caused by cancer chemotherapy, combination approaches are necessary. Serotonin antagonists such as ondansetron have become mainstays. Benzodiazepines, glucocorticoids, and dopamine receptor antagonists are used frequently.

Chapter 98

PRIMARY SCLEROSING CHOLANGITIS

DEFINITION AND EPIDEMIOLOGY
Primary sclerosing cholangitis (PSC) is a probably autoimmune disease that causes multiple strictures of the extra- and intrahepatic bile ducts. The onset usually is in the fourth or fifth decade of life, and there is a 2 : 1 male predominance. Between 50% and 70% of patients with PSC also have inflammatory bowel disease, predominantly ulcerative colitis.

PATHOGENESIS
The pathogenesis is unclear, although an association with certain HLA patterns suggests an autoimmune basis. PSC is characterized by progressive, irreversible fibrosis of the bile ducts. Eventually the small intrahepatic ducts become obliterated and the larger ducts strictured and narrowed. There is an approximately 10% lifetime risk of cholangiocarcinoma.

CLINICAL PRESENTATION
Symptoms, when present, include fatigue, right upper quadrant pain, and pruritus. Episodes of fever and chills suggest the presence of complicating bacterial cholangitis. Osteoporosis is frequent. The clinical course tends to be one of either recurrent episodes of cholangitis or of slow, silent progression of cholestasis and liver fibrosis with eventual cirrhosis and liver failure. Portal hypertension occurs early in the disease and may be present before the onset of cirrhosis.

LABORATORY STUDIES AND DIAGNOSTIC TESTS
Results of liver biochemical tests generally reflect cholestasis (increased alkaline phosphatase and bilirubin levels). There are no biochemical or serologic tests specific for PSC. Until recently, the diagnostic standard was endoscopic retrograde cholangiopancreatography, but magnetic resonance cholangiography is now equally reliable. Liver biopsy is not helpful in diagnosis but is used to determine whether cirrhosis is present. A complete blood cell count may reveal leukocytosis among patients with cholangitis.

MANAGEMENT
Progression of the disease is slow. The 10-year survival rate is 85% among patients without symptoms and 65% among those with symptoms. Trials have shown that ursodeoxycholic acid, a bile acid, improves biochemical values without improving survival. The only cure is liver transplantation. Though the disease can recur, the survival rate after transplantation is higher than that for any other chronic liver disease. Other measures include pharmacologic prophylaxis of variceal bleeding for patients with esophageal varices, therapy for osteoporosis, and the use of cholestyramine to control pruritus.

Chapter 125

VIRAL GASTROENTERITIS

DEFINITION AND EPIDEMIOLOGY
Viral gastroenteritis is a common cause of acute infectious diarrhea. The usual pathogens are the rotaviruses (the most important cause of serious diarrhea among children worldwide) and the calciviruses (including the Norwalk agent). In the Untied States, rotavirus infection is most common in the winter. Although person-to-person spread can occur, the Norwalk agent usually is transmitted through ingestion of contaminated water or foods such as shellfish and salads.

CLINICAL FEATURES
The typical illness is characterized by fever, nausea, vomiting, cramps, and watery diarrhea. The diarrhea is not inflammatory; leukocytes and blood are only infrequently present in the stool. Bloody diarrhea should direct attention instead to bacterial or protozoan pathogens. There usually are no long-term sequelae.

DIAGNOSIS
Presumptive diagnosis of either infection can be confirmed with an increase in serum antibody titer or detection of viral antigens in stool.

MANAGEMENT
Treatment is limited to adequate fluid replacement and supportive care.

Chapter 113

VIRAL HEPATITIS

INTRODUCTION AND GENERAL CLINICAL FINDINGS
Viral hepatitis is a major cause of acute and chronic liver disease in the United States and worldwide. Five viruses (hepatitis viruses A, B, C, D, and E) are known chiefly to affect hepatic tissue. A hepatitis G virus has been described but has not yet been shown to cause clinical hepatitis. All five viruses cause acute hepatitis. The viruses associated with hepatitis B (HBV), hepatitis C (HCV), and hepatitis D (HDV) also cause chronic inflammation. HDV can infect only in the presence of HBV infection. It tends to worsen the acute hepatitis associated with HBV and to increase the risk of severe chronic disease. Hepatitis E virus is transmitted through the fecal–oral route. Endemic areas include India, Bangladesh, and Central and South America. The case–fatality rate is 1% to 3% overall, but 15% to 25% among pregnant women. Therapy is supportive.

The clinical presentation of acute viral hepatitis is the same regardless of the specific infecting virus. Many cases are subclinical or manifest with a flulike illness that may not be recognized as viral hepatitis unless liver chemistry blood tests are performed. Serum transaminase levels often are more than 20 times the normal limit. Some patients have the classic pattern of a viral prodrome followed by the development of overt jaundice.

EPIDEMIOLOGY, ETIOLOGY, AND PATHOGENESIS

Hepatitis A: Hepatitis A has a worldwide distribution and is transmitted almost exclusively through the fecal–oral route. Outbreaks may be caused by fecal contamination of food or drinking water. HAV contains RNA and is not cytopathic; the mechanisms by which it leads to cellular injury remain unclear. The incubation period ranges from 15 to 45 days.

Hepatitis B: The prevalence of HBV infection varies greatly throughout the world and is particularly high in certain parts of Africa, Asia, and the Mediterranean basin. The virus is transmitted mainly by means of percutaneous exposure or inapparent skin or mucosal exposure. The incubation period ranges from a few weeks to 6 months. Sexual and perinatal transmission rates are high. The likelihood of chronic infection declines with advancing age, such that fewer than 5% of healthy adults have chronic hepatitis after infection. HBV is a DNA-containing virus that is generally not cytopathic. The damaging effects of infection are thought to be caused by the immune response of the host to virally encoded proteins. Portions of the HBV genome may integrate into the genome of the host.

Hepatitis C: Hepatitis C has a high prevalence throughout the world. It is transmitted chiefly through the percutaneous route. Risk factors include blood transfusion before 1992, intravenous drug use, tattooing, hemodialysis, and occupational exposure to blood products. Sexual transmission is rare. Maternal–fetal transmission occurs occasionally at the time of birth. Alcohol use appears to increase HCV replication, and there is a high prevalence of hepatitis C infection among alcoholic patients with liver disease. HCV is an RNA-containing virus of the Flaviviridae family and has at least six distinct genotypes worldwide. The incubation period ranges from 2 weeks to 2 months.

CLINICAL FINDINGS

Hepatitis A: The infection is most often a subclinical disorder among children, but adults usually have symptoms. Unlike infection with the other hepatitis viruses, hepatitis A may cause serious cholestasis. Most cases are self-limited. In rare instances, fulminant hepatitis occurs and leads to death. Persons with underlying chronic liver disease are at increased risk of severe hepatitis A infection.

Hepatitis B: Most patients have no symptoms or have mild, flulike symptoms. Jaundice occurs among fewer than one-third of patients. A prodrome of fever, arthralgia, and rash occurs in 10% to 20% of cases of acute infection and is caused by circulating antigen–antibody complexes that activate complement after becoming deposited in synovium and cutaneous blood vessels.

Hepatitis C: Most acute and chronic HCV infections are asymptomatic. If symptoms occur as a result of acute infection, they generally last 2 to 12 weeks. A small number of persons with chronic HCV infection have signs and symptoms of liver disease, such as fatigue, mild right upper quadrant discomfort, nausea, anorexia, myalgia, or arthralgia. Extrahepatic manifestations develop among 1% to 2% of patients with chronic infection. The most important are essential mixed cryoglobulinemia, membranoproliferative glomerulonephritis, and porphyria cutanea tarda. Cirrhosis develops among at least 20% of patients older than 10 to 20 years.

DIAGNOSTIC EVALUATION

Hepatitis A: An anti-HAV IgM antibody response occurs with acute infection. It occurs early and usually lasts 3 to 6 months after the onset of clinical disease. As IgM antibody titer decreases, IgG anti-HAV emerges and persists for life.

Hepatitis B: Detection of HBV surface antigen (HBsAg) in serum establishes the diagnosis of HBV infection. HBsAg appears in the blood about 6 weeks after infection and usually is cleared within 3 months among patients with transient disease. Persistence beyond 6 months implies chronic infection. Antibody to HBV surface antigen (anti-HBs) generally can be detected 3 months after infection and implies recovery and immunity. Absence of anti-HBs suggests chronic infection. HbsAg usually can no longer be detected by the time anti-HBs appears. In some patients, however, both can be detected simultaneously. The presence of IgM antibody to HBV core antigen (anti-HBc IgM) signifies the presence of acute or reactivated chronic infection. Assessment of HBV DNA is a sensitive measure of viral replication and infectivity, as is detection of HBe antigen (HBeAg) in the bloodstream. Among patients with chronic infection, liver biopsy can assist in assessment of the degree of scar and inflammation and in the detection of viral antigens.

Hepatitis C: Serum alanine aminotransferase (ALT) level usually is less than five times the upper limit of normal. As many as 25% of carriers may have normal levels. Prothrombin time and levels of alkaline phosphatase, albumin, and serum bilirubin are normal until advanced liver disease develops. Iron and ferritin levels may be slightly elevated. The diagnosis is based on results of serologic tests to detect anti-HCV antibody and molecular tests to identify the presence of viral RNA. The initial serologic test usually is an immunoassay. Because of a risk of false-positive results, positive test results require confirmation with a second-generation recombinant immunoblot assay (RIBA-2). Anti-HCV antibody titers are present in almost all patients within 1 month after the onset of acute infection but may never become detectable among persons with compromised immune systems. Anti-HCV antibody is not neutralizing and does not confer immunity. Testing for the presence of HCV in serum or liver tissue is the standard for the diagnosis of active HCV infection. Liver biopsy is not necessary for diagnosis but assists in determining the degree of inflammation and scarring and in excluding other causes of liver disease. In general, there is a poor correlation between serum ALT level and liver disease activity determined at histologic examination.

PREVENTION AND OPTIMAL MANAGEMENT

Hepatitis A: HAV vaccine is effective for pre-exposure prophylaxis and is recommended for persons travelling to endemic areas, day care workers, sewage workers, homosexual men, and residents of communities experiencing hepatitis A outbreaks. Immune globulin is effective as postexposure prophylaxis if given to household and sexual contacts within 2 weeks of exposure. Treatment is supportive. Liver transplantation may be indicated for the rare patient with fulminant hepatic failure.

Hepatitis B: Transmission of HBV can be prevented by means of pre-exposure prophylaxis with HBV vaccine or, after exposure, with a combination of vaccination and HBV immune globulin. Pre-exposure vaccination is recommended for all infants at birth, children 11 to 12 years of age if not previously vaccinated, and persons of any age who are at high risk, including health care workers.

Table 119.5 lists indications for treatment. Interferon alfa-2B, given at a dose of 5 million units subcutaneously daily or 10 million units subcutaneously 3 times a week for 4 to 6 months, clears HBV DNA and brings about disease remission for approximately one-third of treated persons. Patients with normal serum aminotransferase levels and those with decompensated cirrhosis are generally not candidates for interferon therapy. Lamivudine, a reverse transcriptase inhibitor, is approved for the management of chronic hepatitis B associated with viral replication and active inflammation. Orthotopic liver transplantation with HBV immunoglobulin given to block graft infection is accepted therapy for end-stage liver disease due to chronic hepatitis B.

Hepatitis C: There is no effective vaccine. Postexposure prophylaxis with immunoglobulin is not effective. Indications for treatment are listed in Table 119.5. Patients with normal serum aminotransferase levels and those with decompensated cirrhosis are generally not candidates for therapy. Long-term response, defined as persistently normal serum HCV RNA levels for at least 6 months after completion of treatment, occurs among only 10% to 15% of patients treated with interferon-alfa monotherapy for 6 to 12 months. Side effects of treatment include acute flulike symptoms and chronic malaise and depression. The addition of ribavirin to interferon therapy produces a higher rate of sustained response (30% to 40%) but can cause hemolytic anemia. Liver transplantation is accepted therapy for end-stage liver disease due to hepatitis C.

Chapter 119

▋ WILSON'S DISEASE

DEFINITION, EPIDEMIOLOGY, AND PATHOGENESIS

Wilson's disease is an uncommon autosomal recessive inherited disorder that affects 1 in 30,000 persons. In Wilson's disease, a defect in biliary copper excretion causes accumulation of copper in the liver and brain in excess of normal metabolic needs.

CLINICAL FEATURES

Wilson's disease can manifest in childhood or early adulthood with abnormal liver enzyme levels, complications of chronic liver disease, hemolytic anemia, or a variety of neurologic and neuropsychiatric disturbances. A small number of patients have fulminant hepatic failure. Copper deposition in Descemet's membrane in the periphery of the cornea produces characteristic Kayser–Fleisher rings.

LABORATORY FINDINGS AND DIAGNOSTIC EVALUATION

The diagnosis is established with a combination of clinical and biochemical findings. Laboratory studies show increased urinary copper excretion, and a low level of serum ceruloplasmin occurs among approximately 85% of patients. Liver enzyme levels are typically elevated and there may be laboratory evidence of chronic liver disease, such as hypoalbuminemia, thrombocytopenia, and elevated prothrombin time. Liver biopsy shows an increase in hepatic copper level and is necessary for definitive diagnosis. The gene for Wilson's disease has been identified, but routine genetic testing is impractical because more than 60 different mutations have been identified.

MANAGEMENT

Treatment usually is initiated with the copper chelator, D-penicillamine. Patients with side effects of this medication can be treated with trientine, another copper-chelating agent. Zinc supplementation can impair absorption of copper and can induce the synthesis of metallothionein, which binds copper in the intestine. If Wilson's disease is diagnosed before hepatic and neurologic complications have developed, the prognosis is excellent with lifelong copper chelation therapy. Hepatic transplantation has been used successfully to treat patients with fulminant or severe Wilson's disease. All first-degree relatives should be screened for the disorder.

Chapter 123

NEPHROLOGY

■ APPROACH TO THE PATIENT WITH ACIDEMIA

DEFINITION

Arterial pH is determined by serum bicarbonate levels and arterial carbon dioxide tension (P_aCO_2). Acidemia is a systemic arterial pH less than 7.35.

PATHOPHYSIOLOGY

Respiratory acidosis is an increase in respiratory acid measured with P_aCO_2 and caused by a reduction in alveolar ventilation. The basis may be severe pulmonary disease, a respiratory muscle disorder or fatigue, or depression of ventilatory control.

Metabolic acidosis is characterized by a decline in bicarbonate level. It is caused by a marked increase in endogenous production of acid, such as lactic acid and ketoacids, loss of bicarbonate stores (diarrhea or renal tubular acidosis [RTA]), or progressive accumulation of endogenous acids in renal insufficiency. The three main types of RTA reflect different defects in urine acidification. The hallmark finding in distal RTA (type I) is inability of the distal tubule to acidify the urine appropriately. Acid retention then decreases bicarbonate level. Although inherited forms of RTA exist, most patients with distal RTA have a systemic illness, such as an autoimmune disorder, hyperthyroidism, hypercalciuria, pyelonephritis, or obstructive uropathy, or a side-effect of a drug such as amphotericin B or lithium.

In proximal RTA (type II), the tubule fails to reabsorb the normal amount of filtered bicarbonate. Metabolic acidosis often occurs in association with Fanconi syndrome, which is generalized dysfunction of the proximal tubule manifested by glycosuria, aminoaciduria, and phosphaturia. Associated systemic conditions include multiple myeloma and Wilson's disease. In both proximal and distal RTA, renal potassium excretion increases, and hypokalemia develops. Type IV RTA, which occurs among patients with diabetes mellitus and tubulointerstitial disease, is caused by a failure of the distal nephron to excrete normal amounts of acid and potassium. The cause usually is hypoaldosteronism or reduction in sensitivity to aldosterone. Unlike proximal and distal RTA, type IV RTA causes hyperkalemia.

Each form of acidosis provokes a compensatory response that tends to offset the change in pH. If the degree of compensation is either more or less than predicted (Table 149.2), an additional acid–base disturbance is present. In acute respiratory acidosis, an immediate compensatory increase in serum bicarbonate levels is caused by cellular buffering mechanisms. After 24 hours, an increase in renal bicarbonate reabsorption accomplishes an even greater increase in bicarbonate level. In metabolic acidosis, stimulation of medullary chemoreceptors increases ventilation and decreases P_aCO_2 so that acidosis is partially ameliorated.

CLINICAL CONSEQUENCES

Respiratory acidosis: A rapid increase in P_aCO_2 can cause a state of anxiety, dyspnea, confusion, psychosis, and hallucinations that can progress to coma. Lesser degrees of dysfunction in chronic hypercapnia include headaches, sleep disturbances, loss of memory, daytime somnolence, and personality changes.
Metabolic acidosis: Respiratory compensation triggers hyperventilation, which often is perceived by patients as dyspnea. Cardiac effects include reduced contrac-

tility and ventricular arrhythmia. Lethargy and coma may occur. RTA can cause symptoms and signs of intravascular volume loss and potassium imbalance. In distal RTA, chronic positive acid balance leads to calcium mobilization from bone, metabolic bone disease, hypercalciuria, urinary stone formation, and nephrocalcinosis. Proximal RTA is not associated with bone disease or nephrolithiasis, but acquired forms may have features of Fanconi syndrome.

DIFFERENTIAL DIAGNOSIS, LABORATORY STUDIES, AND DIAGNOSTIC TESTS

Respiratory acidosis: The differential diagnosis includes central causes (sedating drugs, stroke, central nervous system infection), airway obstruction (foreign body, bronchospasm), parenchymal disease (emphysema, chronic bronchitis, pneumoconiosis, adult respiratory distress syndrome), obesity, and neuromuscular disorders (muscular dystrophy, myositis, cord injuries, myasthenia gravis). Patients stimulated to hyperventilate by metabolic acidosis may experience respiratory fatigue if the metabolic abnormality is not controlled promptly. Pulmonary function testing, including measurement of lung volume and diffusing capacity, arterial oxygen levels, and neuromuscular studies, including electromyography, all may be useful.

Metabolic acidosis: The serum anion gap is used to differentiate high anion gap acidosis from hyperchloremic acidosis. The anion gap, defined as sodium ion concentration plus potassium ion concentration minus bicarbonate ion concentration, represents unmeasured anions normally present in plasma. When acid anions such as acetoacetate and lactate accumulate, the anion gap increases to higher than the normal range of 10 to 12 mEq per liter.

Disorders associated with an elevated anion gap include advanced renal failure, toxin ingestion (ethylene glycol, methanol, salicylates, and paraldehyde), ketoacidosis (alcoholic, diabetic, and starvation), and lactic acidosis. Measurement of serum levels of lactate and acetoacetate can be helpful. Other clinical features associated with high anion gap acidosis are listed in Table 2.

Hyperchloremic (normal anion gap) disorders include gastrointestinal bicarbonate loss (diarrhea, ureterosigmoidostomy), RTA types I, II, and IV, early renal insufficiency, rapid administration of saline solution, acid loads, and the posthypocapneic state. Laboratory evidence of distal RTA can be found by calculating the urinary net charge, $Cl^-_u - (Na^+ + K^+)_u$, which becomes abnormally negative owing to a decline in urinary ammonium excretion. Proximal RTA can be diagnosed from an increased urine bicarbonate concentration response to administration of bicarbonate. Hyperkalemia suggests the existence of type IV RTA.

MANAGEMENT

Respiratory acidosis: Treatment depends on severity and rate of onset. Acute respiratory acidosis can be life threatening and may necessitate mechanical ventilation if the underlying cause cannot be reversed quickly. Supplemental oxygen must be carefully titrated in the treatment of patients with severe chronic obstructive disease who retain carbon dioxide at baseline, because it may worsen the respiratory acidosis. Chronic respiratory acidosis often is difficult to control, but

TABLE 2.	HIGH ANION GAP METABOLIC ACIDOSIS	

Acidosis	Retained Anions	Associated Findings
Ketosis	Acetoacetate, β-hydroxybutyrate	Hyperglycemia, history of diabetes, starvation or alcohol intake
Uremic	Phosphate, sulfate, organic	Elevated BUN and serum creatinine concentration
Salicylate	Mixed organic	Associated respiratory alkalosis
Methanol	Formate	Elevated osmolal gap, retinitis
Lactic	Lactate	Presence of shock, hypoxia
Ethylene glycol	Glycolate, oxalate	Mildly elevated osmolal gap, hypocalcemia, calcium oxalate crystals in urine, acute renal failure

general measures, such as smoking cessation, use of bronchodilators, glucocorticoids, and diuretics, and physiotherapy, to manage underlying conditions may be helpful. Respiratory stimulants are used only in selected cases.

Metabolic acidosis: Table 149.9 outlines the therapy for the various forms of metabolic acidosis. Mild-to-moderate acidemia (pH greater than 7.20) often requires no specific therapy, especially if the underlying cause can be controlled. Proximal RTA is difficult to manage, because administered bicarbonate is rapidly filtered and lost. High doses therefore are necessary when treatment is needed. High doses of potassium supplements also are needed because of the kaliuresis induced by the high rate of distal delivery of bicarbonate.

Chapter 149

APPROACH TO ACUTE RENAL FAILURE

DEFINITION
Acute renal failure (ARF) is a clinical syndrome characterized by an abrupt decline in renal function.

PATHOPHYSIOLOGY
ARF can have prerenal, intrarenal, and postrenal causes. Prerenal ARF is caused by a decrease in renal blood flow. Intrarenal ARF is caused by a sudden, severe renal parenchymal insult, which most often is due to acute tubular necrosis (ATN) from ischemia or exposure to a nephrotoxic agent. Postrenal ARF is caused by obstruction at a site along the urinary tract.

CLINICAL FEATURES, DIFFERENTIAL DIAGNOSIS, AND DIAGNOSTIC TESTS
Prerenal: The causes are outlined in Table 140.1; myocardial failure and intravascular volume depletion are most common. Important historical features and physical examination findings are presented in Table 140.4. The urinalysis is usually unremarkable, though the urine tends to be highly concentrated (more than 450 mOsm per kilogram) and low in sodium (fractional excretion of sodium [FENa] less than 1%). Reabsorption of blood urea nitrogen (BUN) with sodium raises the ratio of BUN to creatinine (often more than 20:1).

Intrarenal: The causes include ischemic ATN, nephrotoxic ATN (aminoglycosides, amphotericin B, heavy metals, cisplatin, radiocontrast agents, and endogenous toxins such as myoglobin, hemoglobin, and myeloma light chains), vascular processes (atheroembolic disease, renal artery occlusion, and vasculitis), acute glomerulonephritis, and acute tubulointerstitial nephritis. Distinguishing clinical features are presented in Table 140.4 and also include the following: (a) Hypertension, proteinuria, and hematuria, especially red blood cell casts, suggest acute glomerulonephritis. The urine has low sodium, low FENa, and is isotonic. (b) Skin rash, fever, eosinophilia, and eosinophiluria suggest acute interstitial nephritis when there is a history of exposure to a causative drug. Only biopsy provides enough information for a definitive diagnosis. (c) Anuria (less than 100 mL per 24 hours) can be caused by urinary tract obstruction or bilateral renal cortical necrosis, vascular occlusion, or overwhelming acute glomerulonephritis. (d) Myoglobinuric rhabdomyolytic ARF is associated with a high plasma level of creatine kinase and a urine dipstick test result positive for blood in the absence

of red blood cells in the spun urinary sediment. Serum creatinine concentration often rises rapidly. Thus the BUN to creatinine ratio is often less than 10:1. Hyperkalemia often is severe. (e) Hemoglobinuric ATN is suggested when a hemolytic event is followed by excretion of dark urine, often with chills and hypotension.

Postrenal: Urine flow can be obstructed either in the kidney, as in crystal formation, methotrexate precipitation, and uric acid nephropathy after therapy for leukemia or lymphoma, or outside the kidney, as in ureteral compression or blockage. Acute ureteral obstruction typically causes severe colicky pain in the back and flank. Chronic obstruction can cause vague aching or no discomfort. Good urine output can be maintained in partial obstruction. A postvoid residual urine volume of more than 100 mL suggests infravesical obstruction. Renal ultrasonography reveals hydronephrosis and can also show polycystic or scarred kidneys but is less useful in showing the exact location and cause of obstruction. Computed tomography is useful in detecting extrinsic compression of the urinary tract. Intravenous pyelography remains the radiologic procedure of choice in the care of patients with normal renal function.

Figure 140.1 demonstrates the use of urinary indexes and findings in the diagnosis of ARF.

TREATMENT
Prerenal: If ARF is caused by volume depletion, treatment involves saline and volume expanders. For patients in hemodynamically unstable condition, Swan–Ganz monitoring provides better measurement of effective intravascular volume. In hepatorenal syndrome, improvement depends on improved liver function.

Intrarenal: The underlying disease should be controlled, and nephrotoxic drugs should be discontinued. In ATN, fluid and electrolyte balance and adequate nutrition must be maintained, and infection should be managed. In early oliguric ARF, a trial of 80 to 400 mg intravenous furosemide or 12.5 to 25 mg mannitol may reduce the need for dialysis. Diuretics should be discontinued if urine flow does not improve. There are no clinical data to support the efficacy of low-dose dopamine. Uremic symptoms, volume overload, intractable acidosis, hyperkalemia, or oliguria with steadily rising creatinine concentration to 8 to 10 mg per deciliter are indications for dialysis.

Postrenal: The goals are to (a) decompress the urinary tract and (b) establish long-term drainage. Decompression may be followed by a large diuresis, hence hydration status and electrolytes must be monitored carefully. Uric acid nephropathy may be minimized by increasing urine pH with sodium bicarbonate infusion and acetazolamide. Patients receiving chemotherapy for leukemia should be pretreated with allopurinol for 1 to 3 days.

CLINICAL COURSE AND OUTCOME
Possible clinical problems include volume overload, hyponatremia, hyperkalemia, hyperphosphatemia, hypocalcemia, acidemia, and uremia (pericarditis, lethargy, vomiting, infection). Nonoliguric ATN has a better prognosis. Renal failure from ATN usually lasts 7 to 21 days; renal function then may return to baseline. The mortality rate for ATN after surgery or trauma is more than 40%. For nephrotoxic ATN, it is less than 10%.

Chapter 140

APPROACH TO THE PATIENT WITH ALKALEMIA

DEFINITION
Arterial pH is determined by the serum bicarbonate levels and arterial carbon dioxide tension (P_aCO_2). Alkalemia is a systemic arterial pH greater than 7.45.

PATHOPHYSIOLOGY
Respiratory alkalosis is a decrease in respiratory acid reflected by a decreased serum P_aCO_2 level and caused by alveolar hyperventilation. *Metabolic alkalosis* is characterized by an increase in bicarbonate level; it is caused by bicarbonate administration, loss of acid from the upper gastrointestinal tract, or failure of the kidneys to eliminate bicarbonate in the usual manner. Accompanying hypovolemia may enhance reabsorption of bicarbonate in the proximal tubule. Each form of alkalosis provokes a compensatory response that tends to offset the change in pH. If the degree of compensation is either more or less than predicted (Table 149.2), an additional acid–base disturbance is present. In respiratory alkalosis, the kidney begins to respond within several hours by decreasing bicarbonate reabsorption and acid production. The consequent decline in bicarbonate levels tends to bring the pH toward normal. Full compensation may take several days and depends on normal volume status and renal function. In metabolic alkalosis, compensatory respiratory hypoventilation increases P_aCO_2 and lowers pH.

CLINICAL CONSEQUENCES
Respiratory alkalosis: Effects vary according to duration and severity but are generally those of the underlying condition. A rapid decline in P_aCO_2 can cause dizziness, confusion, and seizures as a consequence of reduced cerebral blood flow.
Metabolic alkalosis: Effects are generally those of the underlying condition.

DIFFERENTIAL DIAGNOSIS, LABORATORY STUDIES, AND DIAGNOSTIC TESTS
Respiratory alkalosis: The differential diagnosis includes various cardiopulmonary conditions, especially those associated with dyspnea, central nervous system lesions, pregnancy, endotoxemia, presence of salicylates, hepatic failure, hypoxemia, sepsis, anxiety, and pain.
Metabolic alkalosis: Diuretics and vomiting are the most common causes. Figure 149.2 shows the differential diagnosis and an approach based on urinary levels of chloride and potassium.

MANAGEMENT
Respiratory alkalosis: Treatment is directed at alleviating the underlying disorder. Patients with hyperventilation syndrome may benefit from reassurance and paper bag rebreathing during attacks.
Metabolic alkalosis: Treatment is directed at removing the underlying stimulus for bicarbonate generation. Chloride-responsive alkalosis (Fig. 149.2) is associated with volume contraction and generally is corrected with administration of saline solution, which eliminates the hypovolemic stimulus for enhanced renal bicarbonate reabsorption. Management of underlying problems such as vomiting also is helpful. If the vomiting is refractory to therapy, proton-pump inhibitors can be used to decrease the gastric acid loss. Alkalosis unresponsive to chloride is managed by means of control of the underlying condition, such as an excess of mineralocorticoid. Ongoing diuretic use should be discontinued, if possible. Accelerated renal bicarbonate loss can be achieved with acetazolamide, a carbonic anhydrase inhibitor. Hemodialysis can be effective when renal function is impaired.

Chapter 149

BLADDER CANCER

EPIDEMIOLOGY, ETIOLOGY, AND PATHOGENESIS
Bladder cancer accounts for more than 90% of malignant tumors of the urinary tract. The incidence increases with age and peaks during the seventh decade of life. The male-to-female ratio is about 4:1. Cigarette smoking is by far the leading risk factor. Others include occupational exposure to carcinogenic compounds in dyes, rubber, and paint; chronic infection of the lower urinary tract; history of external beam radiation to the pelvis; and use of cyclophosphamide. In the United States, about 90% of bladder cancers are transitional cell carcinoma

(TCC); squamous cell carcinoma accounts for about 7%. In the Mediterranean basin, schistosomiasis is the main causative agent and is associated with squamous cell carcinoma.

CLINICAL FINDINGS
Most bladder cancers manifest as painless, gross or microscopic hematuria, which can occur suddenly and intermittently. Urinary frequency and urgency can be caused by bladder wall irritation or volume loss. Invasive bladder cancer may extend into the prostate, rectum, uterus or vagina, and sacral vertebrae. It spreads through the lymphatic and blood vessels to distant lymph nodes, lungs, liver, and bones. About 5% to 20% of patients have symptoms caused by metastatic lesions. Constitutional symptoms can occur with disseminated disease, but paraneoplastic syndromes are rare.

DIAGNOSTIC STUDIES
Routine urinalysis almost invariably shows hematuria, the degree of which does not correlate with the extent of the lesion. Intravenous pyelography reveals an intravesical filling defect in 60% of cases. Ultrasonography sometimes is used to assess the bladder wall and to evaluate the kidneys and ureters. Urine cytologic examination has a sensitivity and specificity of 80% for grade III tumors but relatively low sensitivity for grade I and II tumors. Direct visualization and biopsy of the tumor usually are performed by means of cystoscopy. Staging should include a complete blood cell count, hepatic and renal chemical analysis, chest radiography, and abdominal and pelvic computed tomography.

PROGNOSIS AND MANAGEMENT
The most significant prognostic factor in transitional cell carcinoma is the depth of tumor invasion; tumor grade also is important. For superficial papillary bladder cancer, the initial treatment is endoscopic resection. Intravesicular administration of Bacile Calmette Guerin (BCG) vaccine is adjuvant treatment of patients at high risk of recurrence. Patients with invasive cancer confined to the bladder organ usually are treated with radical cystectomy, which results in a 60% to 75% 5-year survival rate for T2 disease and a 20% to 40% survival rate with more invasive (T3 or T4) disease. Continent reservoirs such as the Koch pouch have been used to improve patient self-image after radical cystectomy. Postoperative combination chemotherapy has shown some promise. For patients with localized invasive disease who are not surgical candidates, radiation is alternative therapy. The role of neoadjuvant (first-line) systemic chemotherapy is being investigated. For patients with metastatic disease, combination chemotherapy is the treatment of choice, although therapy with even the best agents is associated with a median survival period of only 12.5 months.

Chapter 160

APPROACH TO THE PATIENT WITH CHRONIC RENAL FAILURE

DEFINITION
Chronic renal failure (CRF) is a slowly progressive and irreversible reduction in glomerular filtration rate (GFR). *Chronic renal insufficiency* is a term used to describe a mild to moderate reduction in GFR, usually less than 25 to 30 mL per minute, that has not reached the point at which symptoms of uremia appear.

PATHOPHYSIOLOGY
A characteristic of most forms of CRF is progressive deterioration of renal function long after the initial insult. The pathogenesis has not been fully explained but likely involves mesangial cytokine production and the adverse effects of chronic proteinuria. The rate of loss of GFR varies with the type of renal disease but tends to be constant for any given patient. Two major mechanisms account for uremic syndrome—accumulation of ill-defined toxins normally eliminated by the kidney and defects in the function of specific organs.

CLINICAL FEATURES
The manifestations of CRF depend on severity and on the rapidity with which the reduction in GFR develops. In general, uremic symptoms develop when GFR decreases to less than 10 to 15 mL per minute. The initial symptoms may be so insidious that the patient is aware of them only in retrospect, after effective management has been implemented.
History: Uremia usually develops as the blood urea nitrogen (BUN) level ex-

ceeds 90 mg per deciliter. Generalized manifestations include fatigue and malaise. Gastrointestinal symptoms are common, including anorexia, nausea, vomiting, and hiccups. Cardiovascular symptoms consist of dyspnea, orthopnea, edema, and pericardial chest pain. Neuromuscular manifestations include impaired mentation and concentration, insomnia, irritability, headache, muscle cramps, restless legs, and twitching. Severe encephalopathy may develop and progress to confusion, stupor, seizures, and coma. Peripheral neuropathy may manifest initially as paresthesia with subsequent disturbances of motor function, including muscle weakness and atrophy. Autonomic neuropathy, especially among diabetic patients, may impair bowel and bladder function. Skin manifestations include itching and bruising. Genitourinary symptoms include nocturia, amenorrhea, and loss of libido.

Physical examination: The signs usually do not appear until late in the course. The patient may appear chronically ill with weight loss and muscle wasting. Dermal manifestations include pallor, yellow-brown discoloration, hyperpigmentation, ecchymosis, and petechiae. Inspection of the head may reveal hypertensive retinopathy or epistaxis. Cardiovascular findings include hypertension, cardiomegaly, edema, and in the preterminal stages, a pericardial friction rub. Kussmaul's respirations reflect the severity of the underlying metabolic acidosis. Mental status findings include confusion, drowsiness, stupor, or coma. Myoclonic twitches and asterixis are typical of advanced uremia. Sensory abnormalities may include loss of vibratory and position sense. Loss of deep tendon reflexes and foot drop may occur. Severe renal osteodystrophy may give rise to bone tenderness and fractures.

LABORATORY DATA

The diagnosis is established with documentation of an elevation in BUN and creatinine levels, typically in a ratio of 10:1 to 15:1. The BUN level is disproportionately elevated with urinary obstruction, cardiac decompensation, high protein intake, gastrointestinal bleeding, and catabolism associated with sepsis or glucocorticoid therapy. The creatinine level is disproportionately elevated with liver disease or malnutrition. When the GFR falls to less than 25 to 30 mL per minute, other laboratory abnormalities may occur, including normocytic anemia, metabolic acidosis, hyperphosphatemia, hypocalcemia, and hyperuricemia. Hyperkalemia is a late manifestation.

PATIENT EVALUATION

A primary question in the evaluation of renal failure is whether it is acute or chronic. Chronic failure implies stability and thus presents a less immediate threat. The best evidence that renal failure is chronic is a prior documented elevation in BUN and creatinine levels. Also valuable are findings of long-standing renal failure, such as renal osteodystrophy or small kidneys at ultrasonography (although normal or even large kidneys may be associated with CRF caused by polycystic kidney disease, myeloma, amyloidosis, and diabetic nephropathy). Anemia, hyperphosphatemia, hypocalcemia, and acidosis are relatively poor indicators that renal failure is chronic; the presence of these disorders often correlates better with the severity of renal failure.

A second question is whether potentially reversible factors contribute to or aggravate the renal failure, such as hypovolemia, hypertension, reflux nephropathy, congestive heart failure, nephrotoxins, sepsis, hypercalcemia, pericarditis, or pericardial tamponade. Definitive diagnosis should then be attempted in which specific diseases that might be remediable are considered, such as malignant hypertension, renal artery stenosis, Wegener's granulomatosis, systemic lupus erythematosus, multiple myeloma, obstruction, reflux, hypercalcemic nephropathy, interstitial nephritis, cholesterol emboli, and lead nephropathy.

DIFFERENTIAL DIAGNOSIS

CRF can have numerous causes (Table 141.1). The history and examination may reflect abnormalities of the underlying cause. The results of urinalysis typically are abnormal in most stages of renal failure and may show variable degrees of proteinuria, hematuria, pyuria, and casts. However, in many forms of CRF, such as hypertensive nephrosclerosis, obstructive uropathy, and polycystic kidney disease, urinalysis shows few abnormalities. Broad and waxy casts occur with CRF of almost any cause. The presence of heavy proteinuria or red blood cell casts suggests glomerulonephritis. Abnormal findings at serum and urine electrophoresis may occur with multiple myeloma. Serum and urine culture results may be positive in the presence of endocarditis or renal tuberculosis. Depressed serum complement levels and positive test results for antinuclear and anti-DNA antibodies are important clues to the presence of lupus nephritis. Antibodies

for glomerular basement membrane are present in Goodpasture's syndrome or antiglomerular basement membrane nephritis. The presence of antineutrophil cytoplasmic antibodies is helpful in the diagnosis of Wegener's granulomatosis and other systemic types of vasculitis.

Renal ultrasonography provides valuable data about cystic disease, renal calculi, or a dilated pelvicalyceal system. Unfortunately, renal biopsy is of limited value in establishing the cause of renal failure, because the histologic findings may be too unspecific to disclose the cause of the original insult. Nevertheless, in some forms of renal failure associated with normal-sized kidneys, renal biopsy may be useful.

CONSERVATIVE MANAGEMENT

Even after causes of renal failure that can be treated are ruled out, many factors may still require intervention. Control of blood pressure (systolic less than 125 to 130 mm Hg, diastolic less than 80 mm Hg) is essential to limit progression of CRF and development of atherosclerosis. Another therapeutic goal is to maintain near-normal values of serum calcium, phosphate, and parathyroid hormone. This is accomplished by means of restricting phosphate intake (less than 0.8 g per day), prescribing phosphate binders such as calcium carbonate (long-term administration of aluminum hydroxide has detrimental side effects) when the serum phosphate level exceeds 5.0 to 5.5 mg per deciliter, and adding calcium and calcitriol supplements if the serum calcium level is less than 8.5 mg per deciliter despite normal phosphate levels.

Patient without symptoms should be instructed to follow a diet that contains 4 to 6 g per day of sodium; this should be reduced to 2 to 3 g per day in the presence of edema or hypertension and expanded if hypotension or an acute decline in GFR ensues. If hyperkalemia is present, patients should follow a low-potassium diet and avoid medications that increase serum potassium level, such as angiotensin-converting enzyme inhibitors and spironolactone. The potassium binder sodium polystyrene sulfonate (Kayexalate) may be necessary in refractory cases. Sodium bicarbonate or citrate may be given when the serum bicarbonate level falls to less than 18 to 20 mEq per liter. The dosages of medications that are excreted by the kidney, including digoxin, insulin, and many antibiotics, must be adjusted. Magnesium-containing compounds, nonsteroidal antiinflammatory drugs, and radiographic contrast materials are particularly dangerous and should be avoided altogether. A low-protein diet can reduce symptoms and retard progression of CRF, but care must be taken to avoid malnutrition. Recombinant erythropoietin and iron supplements are used to control anemia.

INDICATIONS FOR DIALYSIS

Objective findings that indicate the need for renal replacement therapy include progressive peripheral neuropathy, pericarditis, inadequate nutrition, congestive heart failure, severe hypertension, extreme and refractory hyperkalemia, metabolic acidosis, and general malaise and weakness that interfere with the ability to work. Long-term dialysis ideally should be started when there is an expectation that uremic symptoms soon will develop. A creatinine clearance of less than 10 mL per minute often is used as a guideline. Long-term options include hemodialysis, peritoneal dialysis, and renal transplantation.

Chapter 141

APPROACH TO THE PATIENT WITH EDEMA

DEFINITION AND PATHOPHYSIOLOGY

Edema is the excessive accumulation of fluid within the interstitial space. Edema is caused by four primary abnormalities—increased mean capillary hydrostatic pressure, decreased capillary oncotic pressure, increased capillary permeability to protein, or obstruction of lymphatic flow. Most disorders associated with edema are initiated by an alteration in oncotic or hydrostatic forces and are perpetuated by renal sodium retention.

DIFFERENTIAL DIAGNOSIS

Common disorders associated with either generalized or localized edema are categorized according to primary pathophysiologic mechanism (Table 143.1). Some conditions, including primary aldosteronism, acute glomerulonephritis, and estrogen administration, appear to produce edema by causing inappropriate retention of sodium by the kidney independent of a primary alteration in Starling forces.

CLINICAL FEATURES

Sodium retention that causes a generalized edematous state may be associated with pulmonary edema, peripheral edema, or ascites. Patients with pulmonary edema often report dyspnea and orthopnea. Physical examination shows tachypnea and pulmonary crackles. The chest radiograph shows interstitial edema or alveolar fluid accumulation. Peripheral edema is associated with swollen legs or presacral accumulation of fluid in a patient at bed rest. Pitting edema is the persistence of a depression in the skin after 10 seconds of pressure applied with the fingers and usually occurs when at least 10 lb (4.5 kg) of fluid has accumulated. Patients with ascites have increased abdominal girth. The demonstration of shifting dullness or a fluid wave at physical examination suggests the presence of ascites. Ascites can be confirmed with abdominal ultrasonography.

MANAGEMENT

Diuretics: Several classes are available. There are two groups of sulfonamide diuretics—the thiazides, such as hydrochlorothiazide, and the nonthiazides, such as chlorthalidone and metolazone. These agents act primarily at the distal tubule to inhibit the transport of sodium and chloride. Loop diuretics, such as furosemide, bumetanide, and ethacrynic acid, act at the thick ascending limb of the loop of Henle to inhibit the Na–K–2Cl transporter. These potent agents may increase urinary sodium excretion to more than 20% of the filtered sodium load. Potassium-sparing diuretics, such as spironolactone, triamterene, and amiloride, act in the distal tubule to induce natriuresis and to inhibit potassium excretion. If mild diuresis is needed, sulfonamide diuretics often are the agents of choice. They have poor efficacy in the setting of renal insufficiency. If more potent diuresis is needed, a loop diuretic is chosen. Loop diuretics bind to plasma proteins, and the effectiveness of these agents depends on the concentration of unbound drug. Therefore a single dose is more likely to be effective than the same amount administered in divided doses. Secondary hyperaldosteronism is common with cirrhosis. The diuretic of choice therefore is spironolactone, a competitive antagonist of aldosterone.

Diuretics alone often cannot eliminate generalized edema because of secondary physiologic changes that they induce. They may cause intravascular volume depletion, cardiovascular compromise, and untoward metabolic effects such as hypokalemia (except for potassium-sparing agents), hyponatremia, and hyperglycemia.

Adjunctive therapy: Restriction of dietary sodium and water intake is important. In general, this restriction limits the development of additional edema but has little effect on the resolution of existing edema. Bed rest or elevation of the lower extremities often improves the response to diuretics by increasing renal perfusion and blood return to the heart. The use of elastic stockings over edematous areas helps mobilize interstitial fluid and often promotes natriuresis and diuresis.

Disease-specific treatments: Among patients with cirrhosis, the use of high-volume paracentesis to manage ascites has become popular. Because this procedure can decrease effective arterial blood volume, concomitant colloid expansion, usually with albumin, is indicated. In the care of patients with congestive heart failure, the goal is to lower intravascular volume to the lowest level compatible with optimal cardiac output. This may necessitate monitoring of cardiac filling pressures in an intensive care unit. In the outpatient setting, the physician must rely on measurements of central venous pressure, assessed by measurement of jugular venous distention or hepatojugular reflux. For patients receiving an optimal drug regimen, daily weight is perhaps the best indicator of volume status. Increasing cardiac output with inotropic agents or vasodilators augments diuresis.

Chapter 143

◼ APPROACH TO THE PATIENT WITH HEMATURIA

DEFINITION

Hematuria is the presence of excessive numbers of red blood cells (RBCs) in the urine and can be gross or microscopic. Finding more than 3 to 5 RBCs per high-power field is considered abnormal. A urine dipstick test result positive for blood in the absence of microscopic hematuria suggests the presence of hemoglobin or myoglobin in the urine.

DIFFERENTIAL DIAGNOSIS

Some causes of hematuria are listed in Table 134.2. Among adults, infection is most common, followed by renal calculi, cancer, and prostatic hypertrophy.

HISTORY AND PHYSICAL EXAMINATION

Urothelial tumors are rare before the age of 40 years. Hematuria coincident with menses suggests endometriosis. Clots occur more often with nonglomerular lesions. Frequency, urgency, or dysuria suggests bladder or urethral involvement. Flank pain occurs with stones, acute obstruction, and IgA nephropathy. Systemic symptoms suggest lupus erythematosus or vasculitis. Use of oral contraceptives has been associated with loin pain–hematuria syndrome. Examination may reveal findings of a specific systemic illness.

LABORATORY STUDIES AND DIAGNOSTIC TESTS

Initial studies include urinalysis, which confirms the presence of hematuria and may show RBC casts and proteinuria (glomerulonephritis) or pyuria and bacteria (infection). Marked proteinuria suggests intrinsic renal disease. Helpful blood studies include complete blood cell count, coagulation times, and serum measurement of blood urea nitrogen and creatinine. Other tests are outlined in Fig. 134.1.

MANAGEMENT

Management is directed at the identified cause.

Chapter 134

◼ HEMOLYTIC-UREMIC SYNDROME

DEFINITION

Hemolytic-uremic syndrome (HUS), a disease closely related to thrombotic thrombocytopenic purpura, is characterized by renal failure, thrombocytopenia, and microangiopathic hemolytic anemia.

ETIOLOGY, PATHOGENESIS, AND CLINICAL FEATURES

HUS may occur after infection with veracytotoxin-producing *Escherichia coli* strains or other bacteria, such as *Shigella* species, *Salmonella typhi*, *Campylobacter* species, *Yersinia* species, *Streptococcus pneumoniae*, or *Legionella* species. It also occurs among patients using oral contraceptives and among postpartum women. There is an association with some collagen vascular diseases, such as lupus erythematosus and scleroderma. The pathogenesis is thought to involve vascular endothelial cell damage, but thrombocytopenia, enhanced platelet aggregation, and an abnormal factor VIII level also contribute. HUS among adults has a varied presentation. Renal function may decline subacutely in association with minimal hemolysis and thrombocytopenia. There also is an acute presentation with rapidly developing renal insufficiency and severe hemolysis and thrombocytopenia. A blood smear shows fragmented red blood cells. Renal biopsy shows widespread capillary wall thickening and capillary thrombi. Adults can have arteriolar necrosis and interlobular arterial thrombosis.

MANAGEMENT

Supportive therapy is critical. It includes vigorous control of blood pressure, fluids and electrolytes, and hemorrhage. Dialysis may be necessary. Therapy with exchange transfusions, plasmapheresis, and glucocorticoids has been associated with remission of the disease, although there have been no large, prospective trials of therapy.

Chapter 152

◼ APPROACH TO THE PATIENT WITH HYPERKALEMIA

DEFINITION

Hyperkalemia is a serum potassium value greater than 5.0 mEq per liter.

PATHOPHYSIOLOGY

Hyperkalemia can be caused by a spurious laboratory value, redistribution from the intracellular to the extracellular compartment, or potassium retention. Chronic hyperkalemia is always the result of a defect in renal potassium excretion.

CLINICAL CONSEQUENCES

Depolarization of cell membranes leads to dysfunction of cardiac and skeletal muscle. An early manifestation is peaking of T waves on an electrocardiogram

(ECG) that is most prominent with a potassium concentration greater than 6 mEq per liter. More severe cases cause widening of the QRS complex. Ventricular fibrillation and cardiac arrest may follow. Neurologic effects such as tingling, weakness, and even flaccid paralysis can occur when potassium concentration is greater than 8 mEq per liter. Respiratory muscles are spared.

DIFFERENTIAL DIAGNOSIS, LABORATORY STUDIES, AND DIAGNOSTIC TESTS
Figure 147.1 outlines the differential diagnosis and the diagnostic approach to hyperkalemia.

MANAGEMENT
Acute hyperkalemia is a life-threatening abnormality. The higher the plasma level and more severe the ECG alterations, the more urgent is the need for treatment. Table 147.1 lists therapies for hyperkalemia. The goals are to stabilize the myocardial membranes with calcium and to lower serum potassium level by means of redistribution and either gastrointestinal or renal potassium excretion.

Chapter 147

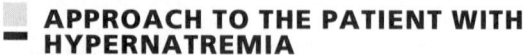

APPROACH TO THE PATIENT WITH HYPERNATREMIA

DEFINITION
Hypernatremia is a serum sodium concentration greater than 145 mEq per liter. Because body fluid tonicity is tightly regulated in healthy persons, hypernatremia is generally a disorder of the very old, very young, or very ill.

PATHOPHYSIOLOGY AND DIFFERENTIAL DIAGNOSIS
Sodium is the major extracellular cation, accounting for almost all of the osmolarity of this body fluid compartment. Therefore, hypernatremia always implies hypertonicity and a shift of water from the intracellular to the extracellular compartment. This cell shrinkage, especially that in the brain, is responsible for the clinical manifestations. Hypernatremia can be caused by a gain of solute in excess of water or by loss of water in excess of solute. Because hypertonicity is a potent stimulus to thirst, sustained hypernatremia always implies inadequate water intake. Figure 145.2 outlines the differential diagnosis and the diagnostic approach to hypernatremia.

CLINICAL CONSEQUENCES
Because adaptive responses exist, the clinical manifestations depend on the rapidity of the increase in serum sodium level as well as the absolute level attained. When symptomatic, hypernatremia typically manifests as altered sensorium. Symptoms can range from agitation, restlessness, confusion, and lethargy to seizures, stupor, and coma. Reductions in brain volume can lead to intracranial hemorrhage from rupture of cerebral blood vessels. Changes in extracellular fluid volume may dominate the clinical findings. For example, hypernatremia due to excess salt often is associated with symptoms of volume overload such as edema, whereas hypernatremia caused by loss of hypotonic fluids is associated with signs of volume depletion. A patient with a pure water deficit generally appears clinically euvolemic, because only one-twelfth of a pure water deficit is derived from the intravascular compartment.

LABORATORY STUDIES AND DIAGNOSTIC TESTS
The important laboratory studies are presented in Figure 145.2. In addition, elevations in levels of blood urea nitrogen, creatinine, and uric acid support volume depletion and therefore suggest hypotonic fluid losses.

MANAGEMENT
Initial therapy should be directed at normalizing intravascular volume. When volume depletion is evident, isotonic (0.9%) saline solution should be infused. When pulmonary edema is present, initial therapy must include removal of the excess sodium with potent diuretics. Once intravascular volume is corrected, attention can be turned to the management of hypernatremia itself. Because of the danger that accompanies rapid correction of chronic hypertonicity (cerebral edema), aggressive therapy should never be used unless the hypertonicity can be ascertained to be acute in origin. Chronic hypernatremia always should be corrected over a period of several days.
Estimation of water deficit: The magnitude of an isolated free water deficit

can be estimated as follows because total body solute has not changed from baseline in this situation. Current total body water (TBW) multiplied by serum sodium level equals normal TBW (roughly 60% of mass in kilograms) multiplied by normal serum sodium level. Therefore, for a 60 kg patient with a sodium level of 160 mEq per liter, the current TBW is $(0.6 \times 60) \times 140/160 = 31.5$ L, and the water deficit is 36 L − 31.5 L, or 4.5 L. The same calculation can be used to estimate the water deficit of patients with hypernatremia caused by loss of hypotonic fluids. The calculation, however, underestimates true water deficit if performed before the total body sodium deficit has been corrected with intravenous saline solution.
Correction of acute hypernatremia: No more than half of the estimated water deficit should be replaced during the first 24 hours. Neurologic status and serum sodium levels should be monitored carefully. The rest can be replaced over the ensuing 24 to 48 hours. The oral route is always preferable, if the patient is alert. Otherwise, 5% dextrose in water should be administered intravenously.

Chapter 145

APPROACH TO THE PATIENT WITH HYPOKALEMIA

DEFINITION
Hypokalemia is a serum potassium value less than 3.5 mEq per liter.

PATHOPHYSIOLOGY
Most total body potassium exists within cells. Hypokalemia results either from (a) a shift of extracellular potassium to the intracellular compartment, usually associated with metabolic alkalosis and use of insulin or sympathomimetic agents, (b) renal or gastrointestinal loss of potassium, or (c) inadequate potassium intake.

CLINICAL CONSEQUENCES
The most important effects of hypokalemia, usually at values less than 3 mEq per liter, are on the myocardium. Severe hypokalemia may lead to prolongation of the PR interval and widening of the QRS complex. Atrioventricular block and supraventricular tachycardia can occur, and the risk of digitalis toxicity increases. Symptoms include malaise, muscular weakness, and muscle cramps. Constipation and ileus can occur. Hyperglycemia can be caused by defective insulin secretion, polyuria by impaired renal concentrating ability.

DIFFERENTIAL DIAGNOSIS, LABORATORY STUDIES, AND DIAGNOSTIC TESTS
Figures 146.2 and 146.3 outline the differential diagnosis and the diagnostic approach to hypokalemia. Gastrointestinal fluid loss through diarrhea or vomiting and diuretic use are particularly common. Little potassium is lost in vomitus itself, but the loss of hydrochloric acid causes metabolic alkalosis and increases renal potassium excretion.

MANAGEMENT
The magnitude of potassium depletion can be inferred from the plasma level—300 mEq per 70 kg body weight leads to a reduction in plasma potassium of 1 mEq per liter. Severe weakness or serious cardiac dysrhythmia necessitates rapid correction. Otherwise, slow intravenous or oral therapy is preferable to lower the risk of hyperkalemia. Potassium chloride is available as a liquid and as a slow-release tablet.

Chapter 146

APPROACH TO THE PATIENT WITH HYPONATREMIA

DEFINITION
Hyponatremia is a serum sodium concentration less than 135 mEq per liter. It is one of the most common electrolyte disorders.

PATHOPHYSIOLOGY AND DIFFERENTIAL DIAGNOSIS
Sodium is the main extracellular cation, accounting, along with its companion anions, for almost all of the osmolarity of this body fluid compartment. There-

fore, hypotonicity always implies hyponatremia. In contrast, hyponatremia can coexist with low, normal, or high levels of plasma tonicity. Hypotonic hyponatremia always reflects inability of the kidney to excrete enough electrolyte-free water to match water intake. Isotonic hyponatremia is a laboratory artifact caused by hypertriglyceridemia or paraproteinemia. Hypertonic hyponatremia is caused by the presence in extracellular fluid of abnormal amounts of osmotically active solutes other than sodium, such as glucose. These solutes draw water from the intra- to the extracellular compartment, causing cellular dehydration and hypernatremia. Figure 144.1 shows the differential diagnosis and diagnostic approach to hyponatremia. The syndrome of inappropriate secretion of antidiuretic hormone (SIADH) deserves special mention. It is characterized by persistently elevated levels of antidiuretic hormone in the absence of physiologically appropriate stimuli such as intravascular volume depletion. It is associated with numerous medications and various intrathoracic and intracranial processes.

CLINICAL CONSEQUENCES

Clinical manifestations occur chiefly with hypotonic types of hyponatremia, because these disorders are associated with cellular edema. This intracellular volume expansion is of greatest importance in the brain, where it is translated into increased intracranial pressure. Because adaptive mechanisms exist, morbidity and mortality are related not only to magnitude of hypotonicity but also to rate of development. (For example, patients with a very gradual decline in serum sodium level to 120 mEq per liter may have no symptoms at all.) Elderly patients, persons with alcoholism, and premenopausal women have more severe neurologic consequences for any given degree of hypotonicity. The symptoms usually do not occur until serum sodium level falls to less than 125 mEq per liter, at which time the patient may have anorexia, nausea, and malaise. Between 120 and 110 mEq per liter, headache, lethargy, confusion, agitation, and obtundation may occur. Seizures and coma may occur as levels decrease to less than 110 mEq per liter. Focal neurologic findings are unusual but do occur.

LABORATORY STUDIES AND DIAGNOSTIC TESTS

The laboratory evaluation is detailed in Figure 144.1. Once isotonic and hypertonic disorders are excluded, urine osmolarity is the discriminating factor between excessive water intake and impaired renal diluting ability. For patients with the latter problem, measurement of urine sodium and physical examination can categorize patients according to extracellular volume status (hypovolemic, euvolemic, and hypervolemic). SIADH can be diagnosed when the urine is not maximally dilute (tonicity is greater than 100 mOsm per kilogram), there is no evidence of extracellular volume depletion, hypothyroidism and glucocorticoid insufficiency have been excluded, and the urine sodium level is greater than 20 mEq per liter. Decreased serum uric acid levels are common in SIADH. A water load test may be used in challenging cases but must be avoided in the care of patients with severe hyponatremia because of the risk of precipitating neurologic symptoms.

MANAGEMENT

Only hypotonic hyponatremia requires therapy directed at the sodium level. Therapy is directed at raising extracellular fluid tonicity to shift water out of the intracellular space and reduce cerebral edema. The rate of correction must be carefully regulated, however. Overly rapid correction can produce the irreversible neurologic deficits of central pontine myelinolysis. In most circumstances, the sodium level should be raised by no more than 10 mEq per liter in the first 24 hours and no more than 18 mEq per liter in the first 48 hours. Severe, symptomatic hypotonicity should be managed with 3% saline solution along with a loop diuretic to prevent complications of excessive extracellular volume. The management of chronic, asymptomatic hypotonicity should be directed at the underlying cause. Hypovolemic hyponatremia is managed by means of restoration of intravascular volume and correction of the cause of hypovolemia. Because euvolemic hyponatremia represents pure water excess, treatment depends on restricting water intake to less than daily water output. If the cause of SIADH cannot be corrected and water restriction is ineffective or poorly tolerated, demeclocycline can be used to inhibit vasopressin-mediated renal water reabsorption. Management of hypervolemic hyponatremia is difficult. Salt and water restriction is the mainstay of therapy. Diuretics help reduce the volume excess but may trigger vasopressin secretion and further water retention.

Chapter 144

IMMUNE-MEDIATED GLOMERULOPATHIES

PRESENTATION

Two broad categories of immune-mediated glomerulopathy are recognized. Acute nephritic syndrome includes some or all of the following: hematuria with red blood cell casts, oliguria, azotemia, hypertension, mild-to-moderate proteinuria (1 to 3 g per day), and moderate edema. The underlying glomerular disease usually is inflammatory in nature. A subgroup of patients with rapidly progressive glomerulonephritis have a course that leads to end-stage renal disease in weeks to months unless it is halted with treatment.

Nephrotic syndrome is defined by heavy proteinuria (more than 3 g per day), severe edema, and hypoalbuminemia, often accompanied by hyperlipidemia and hypercoagulability. Hematuria may be present but is not a major feature, and there is frequently only minimal impairment of glomerular filtration rate (GFR) at initial presentation. The underlying glomerular abnormality usually is not inflammatory.

PATHOLOGY

Immune-mediated glomerulopathy comprises a disparate group of diseases in which glomerular injury is thought to be caused directly by immunologic mechanisms. The decrease in glomerular filtration rate may lead to renal failure with accumulation of metabolic waste products (azotemia) and derangement in fluid and electrolyte balance. An alteration in permeability also leads to egress of cells or protein into the urine. The term *diffuse* implies that all or most glomeruli are affected more or less uniformly; *focal* and *segmental* mean that some glomeruli are only partly abnormal. *Proliferative lesion* refers to a hypercellular inflammatory process involving infiltrating leukocytes and proliferation of intrinsic glomerular cells. *Sclerosis* describes a degenerative process in which an increase in extracellular matrix accompanies the loss of glomerular cells and collapse of capillary loops.

DIFFERENTIAL DIAGNOSIS

Table 150.1 lists clinical syndromes and histologic lesions caused by immunologic glomerular diseases. The immunopathologic classification of necrotizing and crescentic glomerulonephritis is outlined in Fig. 150.3. IgA nephropathy is the most common form of primary glomerulonephritis. Certain nonimmune glomerulopathies may manifest as clinical syndromes indistinguishable from immune-mediated diseases, including diabetic nephropathy, hemolytic-uremia syndrome, amyloidosis, the paraproteinemia, and hereditary nephritis.

LABORATORY STUDIES AND DIAGNOSTIC TESTS

The presence of various types of glomerulopathy often is suggested by historical data (e.g., recent pharyngitis with post-streptococcal glomerulonephritis, hemoptysis in Wegener's disease or Goodpasture syndrome, or the various systemic manifestations of systemic lupus erythematosus). Table 150.2 outlines the serum complement profiles and serologic results associated with glomerular diseases. The specific diagnosis and therapy often are guided by the results of renal biopsy including immunofluorescence microscopic examination, which gives diagnostic information and an indication of the relative amounts of inflammation and fibrosis.

MANAGEMENT

The various conditions are managed different ways, although patients with nephrotic syndrome of any cause generally benefit from therapy with angiotensin-converting enzyme inhibitors, reduction of hyperlipidemia, and control of edema with sodium restriction and diuretics. For post-streptococcal glomerulonephritis, spontaneous resolution is the norm, and management is predominantly supportive. Other types of postinfectious glomerulonephritis are managed with appropriate antibiotics. Rapidly progressive glomerulonephritis generally requires immunosuppressive medications with or without plasma exchange (for anti–glomerular basement membrane disease). Patients with IgA nephropathy need no treatment as long as they have normal renal function and no hypertension or proteinuria. Those with more serious disease may respond to glucocorticoids, immunosuppressive agents, or omega-3 fatty acid products. Glucocorticoids are particularly effective in the management of minimal change disease, in which the overall prognosis is excellent.

The management of idiopathic membranous nephropathy with immunosuppressive medication is controversial. A reasonable approach is to reserve cytotoxic agents, in combination with glucocorticoids, for patients at high risk with progressive renal dysfunction or a debilitating nephrotic syndrome unresponsive to conservative therapy. The cornerstone of therapy for secondary membranous nephropathy is management of the associated disease or discontinuation of the offending drug. Primary focal segmental glomerulosclerosis (FSGS) is managed with prednisone or cytotoxic agents; cyclosporin A effectively reduces proteinuria. Secondary FSGS is best managed by removing the cause, if possible, and by lowering intraglomerular pressure with angiotensin-converting enzyme inhibitors.

Secondary causes of membranoproliferative glomerulonephritis (MPGN) type I should be diligently sought and controlled if possible. Idiopathic MPGN and MPGN type II are managed with a prolonged course of prednisone if either nephrotic syndrome or renal insufficiency is present. Because the World Health Organization classification recognizes six histologic classes of lupus nephritis, treatment decisions are based largely on the result of renal biopsy. Glucocorticoids with or without immunosuppressive agents such as cyclophosphamide or azathioprine are indicated for most patients.

Chapter 150

■ APPROACH TO THE PATIENT WITH NEPHROLITHIASIS

EPIDEMIOLOGY AND PRESENTATION
The lifetime risk of development of stone disease in industrial nations approaches 20% among men, a rate 3 to 5 times greater than among women. The peak age at onset for both groups is the twenties. The typical patient has severe pain that generally originates in the flank and radiates anteriorly toward the groin as the stone moves along the ureter to the bladder. Dysuria, gross hematuria, urgency, and frequency may be present. Passage of the stone confers almost instant relief. Associated urinary tract infection or obstruction contributes to morbidity, but death is rare. Stones in the renal pelvis may be asymptomatic or cause hematuria alone.

ETIOLOGY AND PATHOPHYSIOLOGY
Stones develop from urine that is oversaturated with respect to the ionic components of the stone. This may happen because of low urine volume, excessive excretion of the components, or other factors that determine solubility (such as urine pH and the presence of inhibitors of crystallization such as citrate). About 70% of all stones contain calcium (about 25% calcium oxalate, 5% calcium phosphate, and 40% both). Magnesium ammonium phosphate (struvite) stones account for approximately 15%, uric acid stones for 5%, and cystine for 2%.
Calcium stones: Calcium oxalate stones may be associated with hypercalciuria or hyperoxaluria. Hypercalciuria is associated with use of loop diuretics, distal renal tubular acidosis, and disorders that cause hypercalcemia. Hyperoxaluria is associated with fat malabsorption and high oxalate intake (see later). Calcium phosphate stones tend to occur in the setting of a high urinary pH, often in association with distal renal tubular acidosis.
Uric acid stones: The three cardinal features of uric acid nephrolithiasis are low urine volume, low urinary pH, and elevated urinary uric acid level. Disorders associated with increased serum and urine uric acid levels include leukemia and lymphoma, (especially after chemotherapy), gout, and renal failure. Patients with chronic diarrhea are particularly at risk, because they tend to have both low urine output (because of dehydration) and acidic urine (to compensate for the metabolic acidosis of diarrhea).
Struvite stones: These form only when the urinary tract is infected with urea-splitting bacteria such as *Proteus* and *Providentia* species. The stones grow rapidly and can fill the renal collecting system, resulting in a staghorn calculus.
Cystine stones: These result from a rare hereditary disorder in which a tubular defect enhances excretion of dibasic amino acids, including cystine. They are more likely to form in acidic urine.

HISTORY AND PHYSICAL EXAMINATION
All patients, even those with stones for the first time, should undergo a thorough interview and physical examination. There may be evidence of one or more of the disorders that predispose to stone formation. A history of frequent urinary tract infections suggests the possibility of struvite stones. Medications may be implicated: acetazolamide raises urinary pH and predisposes to calcium phosphate stone precipitation. Calcium-containing antacids, excessive vitamin D ingestion, and loop diuretics can increase calcium excretion. Excessive ingestion of vitamin C may cause hyperoxaluria. Information about a patient's fluid intake

and diet is essential. Meats and other purine-containing foods augment uric acid excretion; foods rich in oxalate include spinach, kale, mustard greens, tea, chocolate, and nuts. The physical examination findings for patients who do not have renal colic usually are normal.

LABORATORY STUDIES AND DIAGNOSTIC TESTS
Analysis of stone composition allows therapy to focus on measures that can decrease the urinary levels of the constituents. Elevated urinary pH (greater than 7) is associated with struvite and calcium phosphate stones; uric acid stones tend to form in acidic urine (pH less than 6). Microscopic urinalysis may show bacteria and leukocytes (the presence of which suggest infection), characteristic crystals, or hematuria that connotes active stone disease. For all patients, even those with a single stone, the following laboratory evaluation is warranted: serum electrolytes, creatinine, calcium, phosphorus, and uric acid levels. If serum calcium is high, parathyroid hormone level should be measured. Qualitative cystine screening of the urine should be performed in each case. For patients with a second stone or a growing stone, a 24-hour urine specimen collected while the patient continues eating his or her usual diet should be analyzed for volume, pH, calcium, phosphate, sodium, uric acid, oxalate, citrate, and creatinine. Radiologic studies are important in diagnosis and management. If the stones are radiopaque (those containing calcium and cystine), size, location, and number can be ascertained with radiography of the kidneys, ureter, and bladder. Intravenous urography can provide additional information, such as the presence of radiolucent stones (those containing uric acid), anatomic abnormalities, medullary sponge kidney, and obstruction. Ultrasonography may miss ureteral calculi.

DIFFERENTIAL DIAGNOSIS
Acute renal colic must be differentiated from other conditions that cause severe pain in either the costovertebral angle (CVA) or the upper and lower quadrants of the abdomen. Pain due to appendicitis often occurs in the right lower quadrant, but it usually originates in the periumbilical area rather than the CVA. Musculoskeletal pain or pain due to disc disease generally does not cause pain as severe as that due to renal colic and is not associated with dysuria or urgency. The presence of hematuria, crystalluria, or radiologic evidence of calculus further assists in making the correct diagnosis. Patients with stone disease may have hematuria even when not experiencing acute renal colic. If no urinary crystals are present, one must exclude other causes of painless hematuria, such as a malignant tumor, infection, or glomerulonephritis.

MANAGEMENT
Most stones less than 5 mm in diameter pass spontaneously. Larger stones, however, rarely pass through the narrow ureters without urologic intervention. The specific intervention, such as extracorporeal shock wave lithotripsy (ESWL), endoscopic removal, percutaneous nephrostomy, or open surgical removal, is selected on the basis of size, number, and location of the stone or stones. Medical management is used to prevent further stone occurrence or growth. Nonspecific therapies include an increase in fluid intake to more than 2 L per day and dietary adjustments. A low-sodium diet decreases both sodium and calcium excretion, and a reduction in dietary protein decreases calcium excretion and increases citrate excretion. Specific therapy is guided by stone analysis or is based on a strong diagnostic suspicion afforded by the serum and urine test results.
Calcium stones: Any underlying disease should be controlled. For patients with hypercalciuria (more than 300 mg per day for men and more than 250 mg per day for women), thiazide diuretics with potassium supplements decrease calcium excretion. A low-calcium diet is not recommended. It leads to negative calcium balance and bone demineralization and may enhance oxalate absorption and excretion. Citrate tablets may be useful to patients with hypocitraturia. Patients with excessive oxalate excretion (more than 100 mg per day) due to malabsorption should consume a low-fat diet and supplemental calcium with meals to bind oxalate. Cholestyramine chelates bile salts, fatty acids, and oxalate. Excessive urinary urate (more than 800 mg per day for men and more than 750 mg per day for women) can provide nuclei for calcium oxalate aggregation. Purine restriction or allopurinol may be needed to decrease urinary excretion of uric acid.
Uric acid stones: Therapy includes oral hydration to increase urine volume to more than 3 L per day and alkalinization of the urine (with oral bicarbonate, potassium citrate, or acetazolamide) to a pH of 6.5 (a higher pH can cause calcium phosphate precipitation). With a urine pH of 6.5, even uric acid levels as high as 1,000 mg per day may be soluble. Higher levels of excretion require dietary purine restriction or the use of allopurinol.

Struvite stones: After appropriate antibiotic therapy is instituted, ESWL or percutaneous nephrolithotomy usually is needed, because the stones are large and frequently form staghorns. Long-term use of suppressive antibiotics may be needed.

Cystine stones: Therapy consists of sufficient water intake to lower the urinary cystine concentration to less than 300 mg per day. Large volumes (more than 4 L per day) may be needed, however, and may be poorly tolerated. Urinary pH should be higher than 7.5. Medications such as D-penicillamine and tiopronin form soluble complexes with cysteine and decrease excretion of cystine. Cystine stones do not crush well with ESWL and when large have to be removed by means of percutaneous nephrolithotomy.

Chapter 139

APPROACH TO THE PATIENT WITH PROTEINURIA AND NEPHROTIC SYNDROME

DEFINITION
Proteinuria often is the first evidence of renal disease and usually is discovered at routine screening urinalysis. The incidence in population-based studies ranges from 0.6% to 10.7%. The quantity of urine protein has diagnostic and prognostic significance. Nephrotic proteinuria (more than 3.5 g per 24 hours) usually is caused by glomerular disease and is a risk factor for progression of underlying renal disease. Most patients, however, have non-nephrotic proteinuria (less than 3.5 g per 24 hours and usually less than 1 g per 24 hours), which is more typically associated with tubulointerstitial or glomerular diseases that have a more benign clinical course. Abnormally increased albumin excretion that cannot be detected with standard reagent strips is defined as *microalbuminuria*. It is common among patients with diabetes or hypertension, appears to be a marker of cardiovascular risk, and is predictive of development of diabetic nephropathy.

PATHOPHYSIOLOGY
Protein filtration is normally restrained by ionic charge and molecular size. The proximal tubule reabsorbs and catabolizes almost all filtered protein, so less than 150 mg per day is excreted. Glomerular damage eliminates charge or size selectivity. Leakage of protein then overwhelms the tubular reabsorptive capacity. Loss of glomerular basement membrane charge selectivity alone, usually in minimal change nephropathy, results in albuminuria and little loss of larger proteins such as globulins. Tubular disorders reduce reabsorptive capacity and can cause secretion of uroepithelial mucoproteins and IgA in response to inflammation. Immunoglobulin light chains (Bence Jones protein) are freely filtered by the normal kidney. Patients with excessive production have increased proteinuria but no albuminuria and hence a negative result of a urine dipstick test for protein.

HISTORY AND PHYSICAL EXAMINATION
Symptoms and signs of systemic diseases that cause proteinuria (Table 135.1) may be evident. The use of medications and street drugs should be documented. Hypertension is common in focal segmental glomerulosclerosis and proliferative glomerulonephritis but is uncommon with minimal change disease or membranous nephropathy. Signs of intravascular volume depletion or edema suggest hypoalbuminemia from nephrotic syndrome.

LABORATORY STUDIES AND DIAGNOSTIC TESTS
Initial evaluation is limited to dipstick and microscopic urinalysis and measurement of urinary protein and serum blood urea nitrogen and creatinine. Fasting blood sugar or antinuclear antibody (ANA) titers may be obtained to screen for undiagnosed diabetes or systemic lupus erythematosus. Other diagnostic tests should be performed selectively on the basis of clinical suspicion. For patients with nephrotic range proteinuria, serum protein, albumin, triglycerides, cholesterol, calcium, and phosphate can be measured to assess for associated metabolic abnormalities (see later).

Measurement of urinary protein: Urine dipstick results are reliable in the detection of albuminuria that exceeds 20 to 30 mg per deciliter but are insensitive for detection of other proteins, such as Bence Jones protein. These proteins can be measured with protein precipitation techniques. In concentrated urine, dipstick protein may be falsely elevated. When the dipstick test is twice positive, urine protein should be quantified with 24-hour collection or the protein to creatinine ratio of an early morning specimen, which approximates the daily protein excretion rate in grams per 24 hours.

Microscopic urinalysis: The presence of red blood cell (RBC) casts indicates glomerulonephritis. Oval fat bodies and fatty casts accompany nephrotic glomerular proteinuria. Mild proteinuria with white blood cells but no hematuria is characteristic of tubulointerstitial disease.

Biopsy: Renal biopsy is indicated for unexplained nephrotic syndrome. Biopsy should be strongly considered in the care of a patient with non-nephrotic proteinuria who has azotemia, whose urine sediment contains RBCs or RBC casts, or who has a systemic disease that has eluded diagnosis.

DIFFERENTIAL DIAGNOSIS
Non-nephrotic proteinuria: Patients are more likely to have a normal glomerular filtration rate (GFR), normal results of urinalysis, and no associated systemic disease, although some systemic diseases such as vasculitis or incipient diabetes mellitus manifest as non-nephrotic proteinuria. Patients without serious systemic disease may have transient proteinuria that resolves without sequelae (associated with strenuous exercise, fever, acute illness, and congestive heart failure but may be idiopathic) or orthostatic proteinuria that occurs only when the patient is in the upright position (diagnosed by means of quantifying both daytime and nighttime protein excretion) and resolves spontaneously in 80% of cases. About 90% of young men with proteinuria have this condition. Persistent proteinuria occurs with either glomerular or tubulointerstitial disease. If no other abnormalities are found at urinalysis, the course often is indolent, although renal failure and hypertension may develop.

Nephrotic syndrome: This is caused by primary glomerulopathy or occurs as a manifestation of a systemic disorder (Table 135.1). Fifty percent to 70% of adults have an associated systemic illness, most commonly diabetes mellitus, systemic lupus erythematosus and other collagen vascular diseases, and amyloidosis. Chronic hepatitis C may be the most common infectious cause. Carcinoma can be associated with the histologic changes of membranous glomerulopathy, leukemia and lymphoma with those of minimal change disease. Between 30% and 50% of adult patients have idiopathic nephrotic syndrome without a systemic disorder. Biopsy usually reveals one of four pathologic entities—membranous glomerulopathy (30% to 40% of cases), focal segmental glomerulosclerosis (20% to 30%), minimal change disease (10% to 20%), or membranoproliferative glomerulonephritis (10% to 20%). Minimal change disease accounts for more than 80% of cases of nephrotic syndrome among children.

CLINICAL MANIFESTATIONS OF NEPHROTIC SYNDROME
Hypoalbuminemia is caused by a failure of hepatic synthesis to compensate for increased urinary losses. Some patients have edema because of reduced plasma oncotic pressure, but for others the cause may be increased blood volume from enhanced renal sodium reabsorption. Transudative pleural effusions and ascites may occur, but pulmonary edema is unusual in the absence of concomitant heart or renal failure. Hypoalbuminemia leads to increased hepatic synthesis of apolipoprotein B and hyperlipidemia (low-density lipoprotein cholesterol and triglyceride levels). Lipiduria is caused by increased glomerular permeability to low-molecular-weight proteins. Both arterial and venous thrombosis may occur, especially renal vein thrombosis. Urinary loss of antithrombin III may play a role, but numerous other potential mechanisms have been identified. Loss of vitamin D–binding globulin in the urine may lead to hypocalcemia, osteomalacia, and secondary hyperparathyroidism. Loss of immunoglobulins may contribute to the increased rate of infection among patients with nephrotic syndrome.

MANAGEMENT
There are specific therapies for particular glomerular and tubulointerstitial diseases. Supportive treatment of patients with proteinuria includes vigorous control of hypertension, which reduces the rate of decline in GFR. Angiotensin-converting enzyme inhibitors slow progression of renal disease independent of their antihypertensive effect, probably by means of reducing proteinuria and the toxic effects of filtered protein on the tubule cells. Aggressive blood glucose control among patients with diabetes has been shown to delay progression of nephropathy. Adequate protein intake is necessary to offset urinary losses. Restriction of dietary protein to delay progression of renal disease is controversial. Edema is treated with dietary sodium restriction (2 to 3 g per day) and judicious use of diuretics with or without low-dose dopamine. Overzealous diuresis of patients with edema who have intravascular volume depletion can precipitate acute renal failure. HMG-CoA reductase inhibitors are the most effective therapy for hyper-

of patients with acute pyelonephritis; urine white blood cell casts are present among two-thirds of such patients.

Differentiation of upper- from lower-tract UTI may be clinically difficult. The absence of upper-tract signs is unreliable in excluding renal infection. As many as 30% of patients with "cystitis" have subclinical pyelonephritis as documented with localization studies. Despite its low sensitivity in the diagnosis of renal infection (30% to 70%), failure to respond to short-course antibiotic therapy may be the more practical way to diagnose upper UTI among women with only lower-tract symptoms.

Because anatomic abnormalities are present in about 25% of men with UTI, imaging studies such as helical computed tomography, renal ultrasonography, or intravenous pyelography usually are recommended. For women, these studies are necessary only with renal infections that relapse after a 2-week course of therapy. Radiographic and cystoscopic examination of women with reinfection who have no evidence of upper-tract involvement rarely helps identify important abnormalities.

MANAGEMENT

Lower-tract infection: The mainstay of treatment is antimicrobial therapy. Supporting measures such as hydration and urinary analgesia play only a minor role. Conventional therapy is a 7 to 14 day course of trimethoprim-sulfamethoxazole (TMP-SMX), amoxicillin, cephalexin, or a fluoroquinolone. For young, healthy women, several single-dose or 3-day treatment regimens cure 90% of lower-tract infections, a rate equivalent to that of longer conventional regimens. Therapy with TMP-SMX or ciprofloxacin is preferred for this purpose because of an increased incidence of amoxicillin resistance of community-acquired *E. coli* infection.

Upper-tract infection: All men and women with symptoms suggestive of upper-tract involvement should be treated with at least 14 days of antibiotics. Patients who are only moderately ill may be treated initially with oral antibiotics such as TMP-SMX or a fluoroquinolone. For sicker patients, the standard approach has been to start intravenous ampicillin plus an aminoglycoside while awaiting urine and blood culture data. Monotherapy with various agents, including cefotaxime, ceftazidime, piperacillin-tazobactam, ciprofloxacin, and TMP-SMX, has also been shown to be effective. Most patients are afebrile with minimal flank tenderness after 48 hours of therapy. If a patient is slow to respond, investigations are needed to exclude obstruction or abscess. Once the patient is afebrile for 24 hours, therapy can be switched to oral medication.

Asymptomatic UTI: Treatment may be indicated among certain subgroups at risk of increased morbidity, including patients undergoing urinary tract manipulation, those with diabetes mellitus, those who are pregnant, and those who have suppressed immune systems. Elderly patients and those who must stay in bed should not be treated because of the futility of maintaining sterile urine and because of the emergence of resistant organisms with therapy.

Recurrent infection: Relapses usually can be managed effectively with longer courses of the original antibiotic. For recurrent infection, prevention with single daily doses of TMP-SMX or fluoroquinolones is cost-effective among women who have more than two infections per year. An alternative strategy is prophylaxis only after intercourse. Women with sporadic infections may choose to self-diagnose and manage the infection themselves. Among postmenopausal women, intravaginal administration of estrogen alters the vaginal flora and reduces the rate of recurrent UTI.

Chapter 271

RHEUMATOLOGY

◼ BACTERIAL ARTHRITIS

DEFINITION

Bacterial arthritis can be classified as gonococcal, nongonococcal, or mycobacterial.

EPIDEMIOLOGY, ETIOLOGY, AND PATHOPHYSIOLOGY

Gonococcal arthritis: *Neisseria gonorrhoeae* is the most common organism causing bacterial arthritis, accounting for almost 75% of infections among healthy, sexually active adults. Disseminated gonococcal infection follows spread of infection from mucosal surfaces and is more common among women, especially during pregnancy, the immediately postpartum period, and within 1 week of menses. Also at risk are those with deficiencies of terminal complement components.

Nongonococcal infections: Most patients have one of the following risk factors: extremes of age, recent manipulation of or injury to a joint, chronic debilitating disease, a disease that alters joint integrity, immunosuppression, intravenous drug use, or prosthetic joints. Most organisms reach the joint through hematogenous spread, although extension from local soft tissue or bone can occur. Gram-positive cocci predominate in healthy adults, the elderly, and those with suppressed immune systems. Polyarticular infection usually is caused by *Staphylococcus aureus* and occurs most often with rheumatoid arthritis, hemophilia, and immunocompromising states. Gram-negative bacilli are present in patients with neutropenia and those who use intravenous drugs. *Staphylococcus epidermidis* is present in early postoperative prosthetic joint infection. Patients with sickle cell disease often are infected with *Salmonella* organisms.

CLINICAL FEATURES

Gonococcal infection: Two forms have been described. The bacteremic form, resembling serum sickness, occurs in about two-thirds of patients and consists of polyarthralgia, tenosynovitis, and dermatitis. It begins with migratory polyarthralgia, fever, chills, and constitutional symptoms. Tendonitis or tenosynovitis may affect the wrists, fingers, ankles, or toes. The skin lesions are papular or pustular, usually on the torso and extremities. Genitourinary symptoms usually

are absent. The second form is nonerosive, suppurative arthritis that usually is monarticular and affects the knees, feet, and ankles. The patient may have a fever, but rash and tenosynovitis usually are absent. Synovial fluid is inflammatory (white blood cell [WBC] count 30,000 to 100,000 cells per microliter). Either form can be associated with mild leukocytosis and a mild to moderate increase in erythrocyte sedimentation rate (ESR). The diagnosis is made through demonstration of the organism on a culture of mucosal surfaces (urethra, endocervix, rectum, or pharynx), blood, and synovial fluid. Blood culture results are positive in as many as 30% of cases in the bacteremic phase. Synovial fluid culture results are positive in about 50% of cases of purulent arthritis. The yield is higher on urogenital cultures, especially cervical cultures (80% to 90%).

Nongonococcal infection: Patients have an acute decrease in range of motion in a painful, warm, swollen joint. Signs of inflammation may be less impressive among patients with chronic disease. Most infections are monarticular and involve the knees (42%), hips (13%), and ankles and shoulders (10% to 12%). Fibrocartilaginous joints of the axial skeleton are involved in intravenous drug users. Signs of systemic infection are common but may be absent among persons with diabetes, the elderly, and persons with compromised immune systems. Infection should be suspected in rheumatoid arthritis when one or two joints are more inflamed than the other joints. The peripheral WBC count is normal in 40% to 50% of cases, but C-reactive protein level and ESR usually are strikingly elevated. Radiographs usually are normal but should be obtained to rule out underlying osteomyelitis. Blood culture results are positive in 30% to 50% of cases. All suspect joints should be aspirated before antibiotics are started. The synovial WBC count typically is more than 50,000 per microliter with more than 90% neutrophils. A Gram stain is positive in about 50% of cases, bacterial cultures in as many as 95%.

MANAGEMENT

Gonococcal infection: Patients improve dramatically within 48 hours of beginning treatment with antibiotics. Therapy is initiated with intravenous antibiotics until the fever has resolved and the symptoms are controlled (typically 3 to 4 days in the bacteremic form and 7 to 10 days in the suppurative form) followed by a week of oral antibiotics. Because of increasing antibiotic resistance, intravenous therapy with ceftriaxone (1 g per day) is recommended initially, with a switch to penicillin if the strain is susceptible. Oral therapy consists of cefuroxime or ciprofloxacin (500 mg twice a day), and should be accompanied by doxycycline (100 mg twice a day), because genitourinary coinfection with *Chlamydia trachomatis* occurs in as many as 40% of cases. Daily aspiration may be needed for the first few days to ensure adequate response to therapy.

Nongonococcal infection: Treatment consists of parenteral antibiotics and drainage of the affected joint. Initial antibiotic therapy is directed at the most likely organism and may be modified when culture results are available. Intravenous therapy for 2 to 4 weeks is recommended to be followed by 2 to 4 weeks of oral therapy. Drainage is accomplished by means of daily joint aspiration, although immediate surgical intervention is needed for infection of the hip and shoulder and for unresponsive organisms in a damaged joint. The mortality rate is 5% to 10%; complete function is recovered by 50% to 70% of patients. Rheumatoid arthritis is associated with a worse prognosis.

Chapter 182

CHRONIC FATIGUE SYNDROME

DEFINITION
Chronic fatigue syndrome (CFS) is characterized by debilitating fatigue and a variety of other systemic symptoms.

EPIDEMIOLOGY, PATHOGENESIS, AND PATHOPHYSIOLOGY
CFS predominantly affects young women. The reported prevalence of chronic fatigue in the general population is 1% to 3%. Because CFS often follows a viral illness and shows some laboratory evidence of immune system activation, some investigators consider it to be a host response to triggering or persistent viral infection. However, studies of viruses, including Epstein–Barr virus, have been disappointing. Another view is that CFS and fibromyalgia are clinical correlates of a shared sleep disturbance.

CLINICAL FINDINGS
The onset of CFS is abrupt, often in the aftermath of a viral illness. Profound fatigue, sore throat, tender adenopathy found through the history rather than documented at examination, headache, and an array of neurologic symptoms, such as mild memory impairment or sensory disturbances, characterize the condition. Unrefreshing sleep, depression, and fibromyalgic tender points often are present. The diagnostic criteria for CFS are shown in Table 185.2.

DIFFERENTIAL DIAGNOSIS AND LABORATORY FINDINGS
Medical conditions to be ruled out include anemia, chronic infection, including HIV infection, liver disease, hypothyroidism, chronic adrenal insufficiency, and systemic lupus erythematosus. Laboratory investigation should include a complete blood cell count, erythrocyte sedimentation rate, liver enzyme levels, thyroid-stimulating antibody, antinuclear antibody, and a chest radiograph. For selected patients, HIV screening and cortisol levels before and after adrenal stimulation are indicated. In CFS, all results should be normal.

PROGNOSIS AND MANAGEMENT
Therapy for CFS is similar to that for fibromyalgia—reassurance, physical exercise, aerobic conditioning, and tricyclic antidepressants. Acyclovir is ineffective.

Chapter 185

CHURG–STRAUSS SYNDROME (ALLERGIC ANGIITIS AND GRANULOMATOSIS)

DEFINITION, EPIDEMIOLOGY, AND PATHOPHYSIOLOGY
Churg–Strauss syndrome (CSS) is a rare hypereosinophilic, granulomatous disorder that affects small and medium-sized vessels. It has a predilection for smaller arteries, arterioles, capillaries, and venules. There is no clear sex preference, and persons of any age may be affected. Pathologic studies reveal intra- or extravascular granulomas and inflammatory lesions rich in eosinophils.

CLINICAL FEATURES
Systemic vasculitis occurs in the setting of asthma or allergic rhinitis. Asthma usually precedes the features of vasculitis by months to years, but both processes may begin simultaneously. Apart from asthma and eosinophilia, CSS is similar to Wegener's granulomatosis (WG) in that it can affect the upper and lower airways and kidneys. However, the allergic nasal and sinus disease of CSS generally is not destructive, and the pulmonary manifestations are more likely to be fleeting infiltrates and less likely to be nodules. The degree of blood and tissue eosinophilia in CSS usually is more marked than in WG, and the renal involvement usually is milder. Coronary arteritis, myocarditis, and gastrointestinal involvement are more frequent in CSS than in WG.

DIAGNOSTIC EVALUATION
There are no specific serologic tests. Erythrocyte sedimentation rate often is elevated. Diagnosis is best achieved with a combination of clinical findings and biopsy of symptomatic or abnormal structures.

MANAGEMENT
The response to high doses of prednisone (about 1 mg per kilogram per day) often is prompt. Cytotoxic agents such as cyclophosphamide should be reserved for patients with severe or progressive disease.

Chapter 374

FIBROMYALGIA

DEFINITION
Fibromyalgia is a clinical syndrome characterized by fatigue and widespread musculoskeletal pain and stiffness in the setting of normal laboratory and radiologic findings.

EPIDEMIOLOGY, PATHOGENESIS, AND PATHOPHYSIOLOGY
Fibromyalgia predominantly affects women. It is believed to be a self-maintained neuropsychiatric disturbance in which environmental or endogenous stress affects nonrapid eye movement during sleep. This disturbance in sleep causes pain amplification, depression, and fatigue. It may be associated with a variety of systemic illnesses, such as systemic lupus erythematosus, hypothyroidism, and Lyme disease.

CLINICAL FINDINGS
A typical patient reports fatigue, widespread pain, and stiffness. Sleep disturbance involves repeated awakening and greater fatigue on rising in the morning than on retiring at night. The patient may have symptoms of associated conditions, such as depression, migraine, irritable bowel syndrome, orthostatic intolerance, and temporomandibular joint pain. The examination reveals multiple, symmetric tender points (Table 185.1). In contrast to normal tenderness, the tenderness of fibromyalgia is characterized by an exaggerated emotional response, withdrawal of the tender part, and worsening of pain after examination. Examination often reveals the presence of previously unknown tender areas.

LABORATORY FINDINGS
Laboratory and radiographic findings are normal unless an associated disease causes an abnormality.

PROGNOSIS AND MANAGEMENT
Low doses of amitriptyline (25 mg at night) tend to improve the sleep pattern and diminish the pain. To decrease the pain further and restore endurance, a structured exercise program, particularly involving swimming or rhythmic dance, is recommended. Sympathetic support is helpful; patients need to understand that the condition is not crippling. Tender points often persist despite symptomatic improvement.

Chapter 185

GIANT CELL ARTERITIS

DEFINITION, EPIDEMIOLOGY, AND PATHOPHYSIOLOGY
Giant cell arteritis (GCA) is sterile granulomatous inflammation of large and medium-sized arteries. It is diagnosed among persons older than 50 years; the mean age is 70 years in most series. Women are affected 2 to 3 times more than men. There is an association with polymyalgia rheumatica (PMR); between 30% and 50% of patients with GCA also have features of PMR.

CLINICAL FEATURES

GCA most often involves the temporal artery. New onset of severe headaches, scalp or temporal artery tenderness, acute monocular visual loss, and claudication of the muscles of mastication are among the common features. Systemic symptoms, such as fever, also are common, as are manifestations of PMR (discomfort of the hip and shoulder girdles). Some patients have inflammatory arthritis of the peripheral joints.

DIAGNOSTIC EVALUATION

There are no specific serologic tests. The erythrocyte sedimentation rate (ESR) usually is markedly elevated. The combination of typical clinical findings and an elevated ESR allows a clinical diagnosis, even without temporal artery biopsy. However, because it generally does not cause considerable morbidity, biopsy often is performed when clinical features are not entirely classic. Positive biopsy results occur among only 50% to 80% of patients considered likely to have GCA, depending on the size of the biopsy specimen, the clinical features of the illness, and whether bilateral samples have been obtained. A biopsy specimen that provides enough information for a diagnosis can be obtained even after more than 1 week of glucocorticoid therapy. A clinical diagnosis should be questioned if dramatic improvement does not occur within 72 hours after the initiation of glucocorticoid therapy.

MANAGEMENT

Prednisone (0.7 to 1.0 mg per kilogram per day) reduces symptoms within 1 to 2 days and often eliminates symptoms within 1 week. After about 1 month, a slow taper usually can be initiated. Unfortunately, the ESR does not always normalize with disease control, so it should not be relied on as the only measure of disease activity. Patients with disease that responds incompletely to glucocorticoids or that relapses with glucocorticoid taper often are treated with cytotoxic or immunosuppressive agents, although the efficacy of this approach has not been demonstrated in controlled trials.

Chapter 181

▮ GOUT

DEFINITION AND EPIDEMIOLOGY

Gout is a heterogeneous group of disorders characterized by hyperuricemia, recurrent acute arthritis, joint destruction, tophi (painless, firm masses of urate crystals in and around joints or in soft tissue), renal damage, and uric acid urolithiasis. Acute gouty arthritis primarily affects middle-aged and elderly men and less commonly affects elderly women.

ETIOLOGY AND PATHOPHYSIOLOGY

Only about 20% of patients with hyperuricemia (serum urate level greater than 7 mg per deciliter for men and greater than 6 mg per deciliter for women) ever have gout. Nevertheless, a high serum level of uric acid, the end product of purine metabolism, is a prerequisite for the development of gout. Increased urate production (responsible for less than 10% of cases of gout) can be primary (idiopathic, genetic), secondary to elevated degradation of adenosine triphosphate (ethanol intake, tissue hypoxia, exercise, glycogen storage disease), secondary to increased nucleic acid turnover (blood dyscrasia, malignant tumor, psoriasis), or secondary to excessive purine intake. Decreased renal excretion (responsible for about 90% of cases of gout) can be caused by increased tubular reabsorption (diabetes insipidus, dehydration, diuretics) or decreased tubular secretion (inherited defect, acute ethanol intoxication, ketoacidosis, starvation, lead toxicity, and drugs such as salicylates, diuretics, ethambutol, and cyclosporine). Hyperuricemia leads to crystal deposition in joints and eventually (e.g., after 20 to 30 years of sustained hyperuricemia) may incite acute local inflammation. Local trauma and sudden increases or decreases in serum urate levels are known precipitating factors.

CLINICAL FEATURES

Acute and chronic gout: The basic pattern is one of acute attacks of exquisitely painful arthritis. At first, such attacks typically are monarticular and associated with few constitutional symptoms. Later the attacks may be polyarticular and associated with fever. Attacks eventually recur at shorter intervals and resolve incompletely. In at least one-half of initial attacks, the first metatarsophalangeal joint is affected (podagra); 90% of persons with gout have acute attacks in the great toe at some time. Next in order of frequency as sites of initial involvement are the insteps, ankles, heels, wrists, finger, and elbows. The first attack commonly begins at night. Within a few hours, the affected joint becomes hot, dusky red, and extremely tender, and the symptoms may progress to resemble those of bacterial cellulitis. Symptoms usually peak within 24 hours.

Between attacks, there typically is complete remission of symptoms. About 75% of patients have a second attack within 2 years. When the patient has no symptoms, the diagnosis can be uncertain. After many years, a stage of chronic gout develops. Deposits of monosodium urate around the joints increase and cause erosive changes, chronic swelling, and pain. Visible tophi occur after an average of 12 years of gout and may be located in the helix of the ear; on the ulnar surface of the forearm; in the fingers, hands, knees, and feet; or in the olecranon bursa. Eventually there may be severe joint destruction and deformation.

Renal disease: Urate nephropathy is attributed to the deposition of monosodium urate crystals in the interstitium of the medulla and is associated with chronic hyperuricemia. It is rarely associated with clinically significant renal disease. Acute uric acid nephropathy is acute renal failure related to the formation of uric acid crystals in the collecting tubules, pelvis, or ureter. It is associated with markedly elevated urinary uric acid levels, most commonly in conditions of high cell turnover, such as leukemia, lymphoma, or the tumor lysis syndrome that sometimes accompanies chemotherapy. Uric acid calculi account for about 10% of all stones and occur in 10% to 25% of all patients with gout.

LABORATORY FINDINGS

During episodes of acute gout, serum urate levels may be spuriously normal or low and are unreliable for diagnosis. The condition is best diagnosed by means of examination of synovial fluid from the acutely inflamed joint under a polarizing microscope for negatively birefringent monosodium urate crystals in neutrophils. The crystals appear as needles with blunted ends. The synovial fluid leukocyte count ranges from 5,000 per microliter to 100,000 per microliter. With chronic disease tophi accumulate and produce soft-tissue densities on radiographs. Bony erosions typically consist of a round or oval shape, a sclerotic border, a punched-out appearance, and an overhanging edge of bone. Urinary uric acid excretion more than 800 to 1,000 mg per day while a normal diet is being consumed clearly shows that uric acid overproduction as the cause of hyperuricemia.

MANAGEMENT

Acute gout can be controlled with indomethacin or another nonsteroidal anti-inflammatory agent (NSAID), although these agents should be avoided by patients with renal failure. Oral colchicine also is effective but commonly causes diarrhea, abdominal pain, and vomiting. Intra-articular or oral glucocorticoids are used to manage polyarticular attacks. With treatment, attacks may last 2 to 7 days; uncontrolled attacks may last several weeks. Therapy for hyperuricemia (to lower urate level to less than 6.8 mg per deciliter) is beneficial in preventing recurrent attacks, chronic gout, and renal complications. However, because such treatment can aggravate acute attacks, it is prudent to wait 4 to 6 weeks after an attack to initiate therapy and to use NSAIDs or daily colchicine concurrently for a few weeks. A uricosuric drug such as probenecid or a xanthine oxidase inhibitor such as allopurinol provides good long-term control. Allopurinol is preferred for patients known to overproduce urate, for those who undergo unsuccessful treatment with uricosuric agents, for those with a creatinine clearance of less than 60 mL per minute, and for those with uric acid nephrolithiasis or tophi. Asymptomatic hyperuricemia less than 13 mg per deciliter does not require therapy, although prophylaxis with allopurinol is indicated before chemotherapy among patients at risk for acute uric acid nephropathy due to tumor lysis syndrome.

Chapter 177

▮ HENOCH–SCHÖNLEIN PURPURA

DEFINITION, EPIDEMIOLOGY, AND PATHOPHYSIOLOGY

Henoch–Schönlein purpura is a type of systemic, small-vessel vasculitis that predominantly affects postcapillary venules. Children of any age can be affected; adults are affected less often. There is no sex preference. IgA is the predominant immunoglobulin in circulating and tissue-deposited immune complexes.

CLINICAL FEATURES

In almost 70% of cases among children, upper respiratory infection precedes Henoch–Schönlein purpura by 1 to 3 weeks. Among adults, there usually is no association. The syndrome is characterized by an urticarial or purpuric rash that is most striking in gravity-dependent areas. Other common features include fever (75%), gastrointestinal pain or bleeding (70%), musculoskeletal symptoms (68%), and glomerulonephritis (45%). Gastrointestinal manifestations are less common among adults.

DIAGNOSTIC EVALUATION

There are no specific serologic tests. The diagnosis usually can be made on the basis of signs and symptoms, although skin or renal biopsy sometimes is necessary. IgA and complement deposition is characteristic.

MANAGEMENT

Most patients do well without glucocorticoid or immunosuppressive treatment. These agents should be used, however, if a patient has severe abdominal pain, peritoneal inflammation, gastrointestinal bleeding, or aggressive glomerulonephritis.

Chapter 150

■ INFLAMMATORY MYOPATHIES

DEFINITIONS

Idiopathic inflammatory myopathy is a group of conditions characterized by symmetric proximal muscle weakness and evidence of nonsuppurative inflammation in skeletal muscle. The group includes polymyositis, dermatomyositis, myositis with associated connective tissue disease, myositis with associated malignant disease, inclusion body myositis, and focal myositis.

ETIOLOGY AND PATHOGENESIS

The cause is unknown, but these disorders are believed to develop in genetically susceptible persons as a result of immune-mediated processes that might be triggered by environmental factors such as viral infections.

PREVALENCE AND EPIDEMIOLOGY

These are uncommon diseases. The age at onset for the group as a whole has a bimodal distribution, with a peak at 10 to 15 years of age and another at about 50 years of age. Myositis associated with malignant disease and inclusion body myositis are more common after 50 years of age. Blacks are affected more than whites, and women twice as often as men (in inclusion body myositis, however, the ratio is reversed).

CLINICAL FEATURES

Symmetric proximal muscle weakness is the dominant feature. It can be accompanied by myalgia and tenderness. Atrophy may develop over time. Systemic symptoms include malaise, fatigue, morning stiffness, arthralgia, anorexia, weight loss, and low-grade fever.

Polymyositis: The onset usually is insidious. Involvement of the proximal shoulder and pelvic girdles is most common; the neck flexors and pharyngeal muscles also may be involved. Facial and bulbar muscle weakness is rare, and ocular muscle involvement does not occur. Cardiac involvement is uncommon, but heart block, supraventricular arrhythmia, or cardiomyopathy may develop and cause palpitations, syncope, or heart failure. Interstitial pulmonary fibrosis, arthralgia, and Raynaud's phenomenon are more common among patients with a myositis-specific autoantibody.

Dermatomyositis: Patients have all the features of polymyositis and also have cutaneous features, which may predate the onset of weakness by as much as 4 years. The classic changes are Gottron's papules (violaceous scaly areas over the knuckles, elbows, and knees) and heliotrope discoloration of the eyelids or periorbital regions. Other rashes also occur. Among some patients, the rash and muscle weakness tend to remit and flare up together; among others, there is no apparent connection.

Myositis with other connective tissue diseases: Muscle weakness may accompany systemic lupus erythematosus, scleroderma, mixed connective tissue disease, Wegener's granulomatosis, polyarteritis nodosa, and giant cell arteritis. The myopathic features may be indistinguishable from those of polymyositis.

Myositis with malignant disease: The association is somewhat controversial but seems more likely with dermatomyositis than with polymyositis. With the exception of ovarian cancer among women with dermatomyositis, the sites and types of tumors are the same as those among other patients of the same age and sex.

Inclusion body myositis: Lower extremity weakness tends to predominate; the distinctive clinical feature is involvement of distal muscles. Myalgia and muscle tenderness are uncommon. Dysphagia occurs among about one-third of patients.

DIFFERENTIAL DIAGNOSIS

Conditions that can mimic idiopathic inflammatory myopathy include neurologic disorders (muscular dystrophy, myasthenia gravis, amyotrophic lateral sclerosis, Eaton–Lambert syndrome), infectious disease (toxoplasmosis, viral infection, trichinosis), electrolyte disorders (hyponatremia, hypocalcemia, hypokalemia, hypophosphatemia, hypomagnesemia), exposure to toxins and medications, inborn errors of metabolism (mitochondrial myopathy, carnitine deficiency, glycogen storage diseases), sarcoidosis, and chronic fatigue syndrome.

LABORATORY STUDIES AND DIAGNOSTIC TESTS

Serum levels of muscle enzymes (creatine kinase, aldolase) are elevated and can be used to gauge disease activity and the response to therapy. The erythrocyte sedimentation rate is mildly increased in about 50% of patients. Anemia is uncommon. Most patients have circulating autoantibodies such as Jo-1 and SRP. Electromyographic changes suggestive of inflammatory myopathy include the triad of increased insertional activity, fibrillations, and sharp positive waves. Patients with inclusion body myositis also may have neuropathic features. In 10% of cases, the electromyogram is normal. Magnetic resonance imaging can be used to establish the extent of disease and to localize sites for biopsy. The characteristic changes at biopsy include degenerating and regenerating fibers, fibrosis, and an endomysial inflammatory infiltrate with lymphocytes surrounding and invading nonnecrotic fibers. Inclusion body myositis also shows lined vacuoles on histologic examination and filamentous inclusions at electron microscopic examination.

PROGNOSIS AND MANAGEMENT

Treatment involves physical therapy, glucocorticoids, and early detection of pulmonary fibrosis and swallowing abnormalities. Prednisone is given in a single morning dose of about 1 mg per kilogram (2 mg per kilogram in severe cases). It is continued until strength improves, usually over weeks to months. The medication is then tapered gradually over many months. Glucocorticoids produce a response among 90% of patients and complete remission among 50% to 75%. If there has been no remission after 6 to 12 weeks, a second agent such as azathioprine or methotrexate should be added. The cutaneous manifestations of dermatomyositis may respond to hydroxychloroquine. Myositis associated with malignant disease or connective tissue disease generally responds to therapy for the associated condition. Inclusion body myositis can be refractory to therapy.

Chapter 180

■ LYME DISEASE

DEFINITION AND EPIDEMIOLOGY

Lyme disease (LD) is a multisystem inflammatory condition caused by spirochetes known collectively as *Borrelia burgdorferi* and spread by *Ixodes* ticks. About 90% of cases in the United States occur in the following states: Massachusetts, Connecticut, Rhode Island, New York, New Jersey, Pennsylvania, Minnesota, Wisconsin, and California. Most cases occur during the late spring, summer, and early fall. It takes 48 hours or more after tick attachment for LD to be spread; even in areas where 40% of adult *Ixodes* ticks carry *B. burgdorferi*, LD develops among only about 1% of people who are bitten. Only about 30% of patients recall being bitten by a tick.

CLINICAL FEATURES

Early, localized disease: Erythema migrans occurs among 50% to 80% of patients, usually less than 1 month after the tick bite. It expands over a few days, often with central clearing, and is most often found in or near the axilla or groin. Half of all patients have multiple lesions caused by spirochetemia. Patients also may have fatigue, malaise, headache, myalgia, arthralgia, and lymphadenopathy.

Early, disseminated disease: This stage occurs days to months after the tick bite and can occur with no antecedent erythema migrans or documented tick bite. Musculoskeletal symptoms are common and include migratory polyarthritis or arthralgia and fibromyalgia. Neurologic findings, which occur among 10% of untreated patients, include lymphocytic meningitis, cranial nerve palsy (especially of the seventh cranial nerve), and radiculoneuritis. About 8% of untreated patients have carditis, including mild myopericarditis and any degree of heart block, which usually begins to resolve during or even before the initiation of therapy.

Chronic or late disease: Late disease occurs months to years after infection and may not be preceded by other features of LD. About 80% of untreated patients have musculoskeletal symptoms, including arthralgia, intermittent arthritis, and chronic monarthritis, usually in the knee. The other feature is tertiary neuroborreliosis, which is characterized by encephalopathy, cognitive dysfunction, and peripheral neuropathy. Acrodermatitis chronica atrophicans may occur.

DIAGNOSIS

Enzyme-linked immunosorbent assay (ELISA) and Western blot techniques are used to detect antibodies to *B. burgdorferi.* The results suggest exposure but alone do not provide enough information for a diagnosis. The diagnosis is made on clinical grounds, and the test results are used only for confirmation. False-positive ELISA results can occur with other spirochetal diseases (e.g., syphilis), rheumatologic diseases (e.g., rheumatoid arthritis), and other infections (e.g., endocarditis, Epstein–Barr disease). Positive and equivocal ELISA results therefore necessitate corroboration with Western blot results. The ELISA result may not become positive for 6 to 8 weeks and may never become positive if the patient receives antibiotic therapy early in the course. Antibody levels may stay elevated for years after successful treatment.

MANAGEMENT

Timely antibiotic therapy prevents progression to later stages of disease, although it may not decrease the duration or severity of many of the features of early LD. Early, localized disease can be controlled with 3 to 4 weeks of oral doxycycline or amoxicillin. The later stages require intravenous therapy for 2 to 4 weeks; third-generation cephalosporins, penicillin G, and chloramphenicol can be used. There is no evidence that prolonged therapy or oral therapy after intravenous therapy is helpful. Fewer than 10% of patients with early LD have a Jarisch–Herxheimer reaction within the first days of therapy (a worsening of many of the signs and symptoms). This usually lasts for less than a day and is never fatal. Because studies suggest that the risk of contracting LD from a known tick bite is small, prophylactic therapy is not recommended.

Chapter 183

■ OSTEOARTHRITIS

DEFINITION AND EPIDEMIOLOGY

Osteoarthritis (OA) is a joint disease characterized by progressive loss of articular cartilage and reactive changes in the underlying bone. OA is the most common form of arthritis. Risk factors include increasing age, female sex, African-American race, obesity, trauma, abnormal joint biomechanics, prior inflammatory joint disease, and metabolic disorders such as hemochromatosis and acromegaly.

PATHOPHYSIOLOGY

OA is thought to be primarily a disease of the articular cartilage and subchondral bone with mild secondary inflammation in the synovial membrane. Proliferation of cartilage at the margins of the joint and subsequent endochondral ossification lead to formation of the osteophytes, the radiologic hallmark of OA.

CLINICAL FEATURES

History: The typical patient with OA is middle-aged or elderly and has a gradual onset of pain and stiffness accompanied by loss of function. The joints most commonly involved include the distal and proximal interphalangeal joints of the hands, first carpometacarpal, cervical or lumbar intervertebral joints, first metatarsophalangeal, knees, and hips. The pain usually is mild, is worsened by use of the involved joints, and improves or is relieved with rest. Pain at rest and nocturnal pain are features of severe disease or of local inflammation. Morning stiffness is common, but the duration is considerably shorter (often less than 30 minutes) than in active rheumatoid arthritis. Gel phenomenon, stiffness after inactivity, is common and resolves within several minutes. In many instances,

pain and stiffness are modified by weather changes, generally worsening with damp, cool, rainy weather.

Physical examination: Bony enlargement with tenderness at the joint margins and periarticular tendons is common. Limitation of motion of the affected joint usually is related to osteophyte formation or severe cartilage loss. Heberden's and Bouchard's nodes are bony enlargements of the distal and proximal interphalangeal joints, respectively. Mild signs of local inflammation may be present, but a hot, erythematous, markedly swollen joint suggests superimposed crystalline or infectious arthritis. Crepitus, present among more than 90% of patients with OA of the knee, is caused by irregularity of the opposing cartilage surfaces.

LABORATORY FINDINGS

The diagnosis usually is confirmed with radiographs. The classic finding is marginal osteophyte formation. With disease progression, radiographs show subchondral sclerosis of the bone and asymmetric joint space narrowing caused by loss of articular cartilage. Bone demineralization and marginal erosions do not occur. The presence of these findings strongly suggests inflammatory arthritis. The complete blood cell count and erythrocyte sedimentation rate usually are normal. Because as many as 20% of elderly patients have a low titer of rheumatoid factor, the presence of this factor does not exclude a diagnosis of OA. Synovial fluid analysis usually reveals noninflammatory fluid. The leukocyte count rarely exceeds 2,000 per microliter.

MANAGEMENT

Nonpharmacologic approaches include patient education, physical and occupational therapy, range of motion and strengthening exercises, aerobic conditioning, and weight loss. The main indication for drug therapy is pain relief. Simple analgesics, such as acetaminophen, are the drugs of choice. Several studies have demonstrated that the short-term efficacy of acetaminophen is comparable with that of nonsteroidal anti-inflammatory drugs (NSAIDs). Patients who do not respond to acetaminophen should be treated with an NSAID. The various NSAIDs are approximately equal in efficacy, although cyclooxygenase-2–specific inhibitors have the lowest incidence of adverse upper gastrointestinal side effects. Although there is no indication for systemic glucocorticoid therapy, intra-articular glucocorticoid injections have a role in the care of patients with effusion in the joints and signs of local inflammation. The frequency of injections should be limited to fewer than 4 per year. Topical analgesic creams, such as capsaicin, sometimes are useful. Patients are candidates for reconstructive joint surgery if the symptoms are not adequately controlled with medical therapy and if they have moderate to severe pain and functional impairment.

Chapter 175

■ OSTEOPOROSIS IN OLDER ADULTS

DEFINITION

Osteoporosis is a disease characterized by low bone mass, microarchitectural deterioration of bone tissue, enhanced bone fragility, and an increase in the risk of fractures.

EPIDEMIOLOGY, ETIOLOGY, AND PATHOPHYSIOLOGY

Each year in the United States, approximately 1 million persons sustain fragility fractures. Among women, the incidence of vertebral fractures begins to increase near the time of menopause; the incidence of hip fracture accelerates approximately 10 years later. Older women have an incidence of hip fracture twice that of older men; the female to male ratio for vertebral fractures is 8:1. The pathogenesis is multifactorial and may involve increased bone resorption (due to hypogonadism and secondary hyperparathyroidism from calcium deficiency) and diminished osteoblast activity.

RISK FACTORS

Primary osteoporosis: Risk factors for primary osteoporotic fracture that can be modified include cigarette smoking, low body weight, estrogen deficiency, lifelong low calcium intake, alcoholism, impaired eyesight, recurrent falls, inadequate physical activity, and poor health. Risk factors that cannot be modified include a personal history of fracture, advanced age, female sex, dementia, and having a first-degree relative with a history of fracture.

Secondary causes: Osteoporosis can be associated with primary hyperparathyroidism (detected with an increased level of ionized calcium), multiple myeloma (serum and urine electrophoresis), Paget's disease (increased alkaline phosphatase level), osteomalacia (increased alkaline phosphatase and decreased vitamin D levels), hyperthyroidism (decreased level of thyroid-stimulating hormone, increased level of thyronine), and hypogonadism among men (decreased free testosterone level). Implicated medications include glucocorticoids, excess thyroid supplementation, anticonvulsants, methotrexate, cyclosporine, and heparin.

DIAGNOSIS

The diagnosis is made by means of bone mineral density (BMD) measurement before fracture or with the occurrence of a fracture. According to World Health Organization criteria, BMD is evaluated in relation to that of young adult women who are at the age of peak bone mass. For each standard deviation below peak bone mass (called a 1 unit decrease in t score), a women's risk of fracture approximately doubles. Osteopenia is defined as a t score between (-1) and (-2.5), osteoporosis as a t score of -2.5 or less. The use of biochemical markers of bone density, such as urinary deoxypyridinoline cross links and serum or urine N telopeptides of type I collagen, is under study; they may be useful in monitoring response to treatment.

Measurement of BMD (best obtained with dual-energy x-ray absorptiometry) should be considered for: (a) all postmenopausal women younger than 65 years with one or more additional risk factors; (b) all women older than 65 years; (c) all postmenopausal women with fractures; (d) women considering therapy for osteoporosis, if BMD testing would facilitate the decision; and (e) women who have been using hormone replacement therapy (HRT) for a long time. BMD determination also can be used to establish the diagnosis and severity of osteoporosis among men.

PREVENTION AND MANAGEMENT

Prevention begins with risk factor modification and calcium (1,500 mg per day) and vitamin D (400 to 800 IU per day) supplements. If HRT is contraindicated or unacceptable to the patient, raloxifene (60 mg per day) or alendronate (5 mg per day) should be considered. BMD measurement should be repeated every 2 to 3 years. If more than 4% of BMD has been lost, one should consider combination therapy (e.g., HRT plus alendronate or alendronate plus raloxifene).

An algorithm for the treatment of postmenopausal women with osteoporosis is presented in Fig. 465.4.

Chapter 465

◾ POLYARTERITIS NODOSA

DEFINITION, EPIDEMIOLOGY, AND PATHOPHYSIOLOGY

Polyarteritis nodosa is an inflammatory disease of medium-sized or small arteries. It affects patients of any age with no sex preference.

CLINICAL FEATURES

Patients may have fever, musculoskeletal symptoms, neurologic symptoms (peripheral more than central), cardiac disease, gastrointestinal vasculitis, and a variety of skin lesions, including livedo, nodules, ulcers, and gangrene but not palpable purpura. The peripheral neuropathy often is mononeuritis multiplex but may be symmetric polyneuropathy. Glomerulonephritis is not a feature, but patients may have renal failure or hypertension due to involvement of the renal arteries.

DIAGNOSTIC EVALUATION

There are no specific serologic tests. The erythrocyte sedimentation rate often is elevated. Diagnosis is best achieved by means of biopsy of symptomatic or abnormal structures. If this approach is impossible or unrevealing and visceral or systemic symptoms are present, angiography should be considered. To maximize the diagnostic yield, a complete study should include the celiac artery and its principal branches, the superior and inferior mesenteric arteries, and the renal arteries.

MANAGEMENT

Uncontrolled polyarteritis nodosa has a 5-year mortality rate higher than 85%. Treatment with high-dose glucocorticoids may improve this rate to 48%, and the combination of glucocorticoids and an immunosuppressive agent, usually cyclophosphamide, may further reduce it to approximately 20%.

Chapter 181

◾ RHEUMATOID ARTHRITIS

DEFINITION AND EPIDEMIOLOGY

Rheumatoid arthritis (RA) is chronic, symmetric polyarthritis of the small joints of the hands and feet and of the larger appendicular joints. It is the most common form of inflammatory arthritis, affecting 1% of the population. Women are affected 2 to 3 times more often than men. The disease can begin at any age, but the peak onset is in the fifth decade of life.

ETIOLOGY AND PATHOGENESIS

Susceptibility to RA has a genetic component. There is some evidence of both infectious and autoimmune causes, but a definite connection has yet to be proved. In RA, the synovium is transformed into a hyperplastic, chronically inflamed tissue. The change is caused by local proliferation of fibroblast-like cells, an increase in the number of macrophage-like synoviocytes, and a prominent mononuclear cell infiltrate comprising mainly T cells, B cells, and macrophages.

CLINICAL FEATURES

Articular manifestations: Although many patterns occur, RA typically begins insidiously with symmetric polyarticular arthritis involving the small joints of the hands and feet. In some cases, there is an abrupt onset of polyarthritis associated with constitutional signs such as fever and weight loss. Morning stiffness lasting greater than 30 minutes is particularly prominent and can persist for several hours. A similar gel phenomenon occurs when patients remain in a single position for a prolonged period. The proximal interphalangeal (PIP) and metacarpophalangeal (MCP) joints usually are tender and swollen. Prominent distal interphalangeal joint involvement is more characteristic of psoriatic arthritis or osteoarthritis. Wrist disease is common. Deformities of the hand include radial deviation at the MCP joints. Swan neck and boutonniere deformities of the hands and feet are common later in the course. Larger proximal joints such as the elbows, shoulders, knees, and hips may be affected. Cervical spine disease is another frequent complication. In long-standing disease, the odontoid process can become severely eroded, predisposing the patient to subluxation of the atlantoaxial joint and resultant myelopathy. Rheumatoid joints are at high risk of bacterial infection.

Extra-articular manifestations: Rheumatoid nodules are present in about 20% of patients (almost all of whom have rheumatoid factor that can be detected) and are caused by the formulation of extra-articular granulation tissue. They can appear anywhere but are most common on bony prominences and tendon sheaths. They tend to wax and wane over time. Pleuropulmonary manifestations include asymptomatic effusions, interstitial lung disease, and parenchymal rheumatoid nodules. Other complications include pericardial effusion, carpal tunnel syndrome, popliteal (Baker's) cysts, episcleritis or scleritis, amyloidosis, and sicca syndrome. A vasculitic syndrome similar to idiopathic polyarteritis nodosa can occur among patients with rheumatoid factor and cause complications such as mononeuritis multiplex and palpable purpura. Felty's syndrome is RA with splenomegaly and hypersplenism.

LABORATORY STUDIES

Characteristic findings include mild normocytic, normochromic anemia, a normal leukocyte count, and an elevated erythrocyte sedimentation rate. Rheumatoid factors are antibodies, usually IgM, that bind to the Fc portion of immunoglobulin. About 85% of patients with RA have positive serologic results for rheumatoid factor and are prone to having more aggressive disease. Despite its name, the test is relatively nonspecific. A positive result occurs among 1% to 5% of healthy persons and among patients with endocarditis, tuberculosis, other connective tissue diseases, sarcoidosis, and hepatic cirrhosis. The white blood cell count in the synovial fluid usually is moderately elevated (2,000 to 20,000 cells per microliter) with about 50% to 75% neutrophils. Synovial biopsy provides little useful information. Bone radiographs can help with the diagnosis and can be used to follow response to therapy. The first changes in the hand usually are periarticular osteopenia and soft-tissue swelling, especially of the PIP and MCP joints. With progression of the disease, cartilage loss causes joint-space narrowing, and bone erosions appear in the recesses of joints where bone is not protected from synovial fluid by cartilage. In advanced disease, the erosions and joint-space narrowing become more prominent, intra-osseous cysts can occur, and a variety of deformities can be visualized.

DIAGNOSIS

There are no specific diagnostic tests. The American College of Rheumatology revised 1987 criteria require four or more of the following for at least 6 weeks: morning stiffness (more than 1 hour before maximal improvement), arthritis of three or more joint areas observed by a physician (e.g., MCP joints, wrists, knees), arthritis of the hands, symmetric arthritis, rheumatoid nodules, serum rheumatoid factor, or radiographic changes typical of RA (e.g., marginal erosions, periarticular osteopenia).

MANAGEMENT

A typical paradigm for treating patients is shown in Fig. 174.2.

Chapter 174

SCLERODERMA AND RAYNAUD'S PHENOMENON

DEFINITIONS

Systemic sclerosis (scleroderma) is characterized by thickening and fibrosis of the skin (scleroderma) and by distinctive forms of involvement of the internal organs. Scleroderma can be grouped into two principal syndromes of prognostic and therapeutic importance. Patients with diffuse or generalized scleroderma are at risk of rapidly progressive and widespread skin involvement and the early development of the full complement of abnormalities of the internal organs. A nearly equal number have slowly progressive skin changes that usually are restricted to the fingers, hands, and face and may have an extended course before the development of visceral abnormalities. This group has limited scleroderma, historically termed the *CREST syndrome* variant (subcutaneous calcinosis, Raynaud's phenomenon, esophageal dysmotility, sclerodactyly, telangiectasia). Raynaud's phenomenon (RP) is the clinical syndrome of episodic color changes of the digits in response to cold or, for some patients, emotional stress. The typical sequence is pallor (arterial constriction) followed by cyanosis (venospasm and oxygen desaturation) followed by reactive hyperemia.

ETIOLOGY AND PATHOGENESIS

Early tissue lesions feature inflammatory cells such as T lymphocytes, monocytes, and mast cells. Fibroblast stimulation leads to excessive production of collagen. A complex array of cells and signal factors leads to accumulation of extracellular matrix in addition to the collagen, including glycoaminoglycan, fibronectin, adherence molecules, and tissue water. RP may be caused by one of three following mechanisms: vasospasm (associated with primary or idiopathic RP, migraine, pheochromocytoma, and use of β-blockers or ergots), narrowing of digital arteries caused by intimal accumulation of ground substance and collagen (connective tissue diseases, vibration syndrome, arteriosclerosis, thromboangiitis obliterans), or increased blood viscosity (cryoglobulinemia, paraproteinemia, polycythemia).

INCIDENCE AND EPIDEMIOLOGY

The annual incidence of scleroderma is 1 to 2 cases per 100,000 persons. The onset is highest in the fourth and fifth decades of life and is four times more common among women. There is no consistent link to race or geographic region. The link between silicone gel breast implants and scleroderma that has been described in case reports has not been supported in formal studies. RP occurs among as many as 10% of premenopausal women. Primary RP typically begins in the teens to early twenties; secondary forms begin later in life. Among men RP usually is a secondary form.

CLINICAL FEATURES

Raynaud's phenomenon and skin involvement: The typical sequence in all forms of scleroderma is RP, followed by finger and hand edema, which typically is painless, followed by tightening and thickening of the skin. In limited scleroderma, unlike the diffuse variant, patients may have RP alone for years before other manifestations develop.

Musculoskeletal features: As skin thickening worsens, underlying joints become tethered and restricted. Symptoms of arthritis are common. Weakness and atrophy may occur. Skin tightening on the face may restrict the ability to open the mouth and may impair adequate oral hygiene.

Gastrointestinal involvement: Atrophy of the muscularis and submucosal fibrosis occur in all forms of scleroderma. Weakness of the lower esophageal sphincter causes chronic reflux esophagitis. Hypomotility of the lower esophagus causes dysphagia for solid foods. Small-bowel involvement manifests as intermittent abdominal cramping and diarrhea. Bacterial overgrowth and malabsorption from intraluminal stagnation may occur. Colonic involvement manifests as constipation. Hepatic disease is uncommon, although patients with limited scleroderma may have primary biliary cirrhosis.

Cardiac involvement: Patchy fibrosis of the myocardium occurs among as many as 80% of patients. Supraventricular and ventricular arrhythmias occur among 60% to 70% of patients. Involvement of the conduction system is less frequent.

Pulmonary involvement: Lung disease combining interstitial inflammation, fibrosis, and vascular injury is a major cause of morbidity and mortality. Patients with diffuse scleroderma are more likely to have interstitial lung disease (basilar rales, abnormal findings on chest radiographs, loss of lung volume), whereas those with limited scleroderma are at risk of progressive pulmonary hypertension and a disproportionate loss of diffusing capacity.

Renal involvement: Scleroderma renal crisis is the sudden onset of accelerated to malignant hypertension and progressive renal insufficiency. It usually is accompanied by microangiopathic hemolytic anemia. It is caused by obliterative vasculopathy and occurs most often in the first 2 to 3 years after the diagnosis of the diffuse form of scleroderma.

LABORATORY STUDIES AND DIAGNOSTIC TESTS

Nonspecific serologic abnormalities are common, including antinuclear antibodies (usually nucleolar in pattern) in 90% of patients and rheumatoid factor in 30%. Many have a moderate elevation in erythrocyte sedimentation rate. Anticentromere antibody is found in 50% to 60% of patients with limited scleroderma but rarely in those with diffuse disease. Antibodies to DNA topoisomerase I and RNA polymerases I and III have low sensitivity but excellent specificity.

PROGNOSIS AND MANAGEMENT

Raynaud's phenomenon: Cessation of cigarette smoking is a necessity. Warm mittens and footwear are helpful. Medications that may be useful include calcium channel blockers, such as nifedipine and amlodipine, and sympatholytic agents, such as prazosin. When digits are compromised by ischemia, which is more common in secondary forms of RP, angiographic localization of the occlusion and prompt therapy are needed.

Scleroderma: Morbidity and mortality are related chiefly to visceral involvement. The early accrual of visceral disease in diffuse scleroderma is responsible for a 5-year survival rate of 60%. There are no proven, effective therapies for the basic fibrotic features of scleroderma and none that can be described as disease-modifying. Prolonged therapy with D-penicillamine has been used because this agent inhibits cross linking of collagen. However, a multicenter dosage comparison of 1 g per day and 125 mg every other day did not demonstrate an effect on survival rate, skin thickening, or internal organ status. Numerous studies of immunosuppressants have proved their lack of benefit.

Visceral involvement: Nonsteroidal anti-inflammatory drugs and physical therapy are useful for musculoskeletal disorders. Symptoms of gastroesophageal reflux and esophagitis respond to gastric acid suppression and changes in lifestyle. Patients with diarrhea and cramping often are treated with antibiotics for presumed bacterial overgrowth. Little is known about effective therapy for cardiac and pulmonary disease. Pulmonary hypertension may respond to prostacyclin preparations. Early management of renal crisis with angiotensin-converting enzyme inhibitors can arrest the progressive renal insufficiency and ameliorate the hypertension.

Chapter 179

SMALL-VESSEL VASCULITIS (HYPERSENSITIVITY VASCULITIS)

DEFINITION AND PATHOPHYSIOLOGY

Vasculitis that exclusively involves arterioles and predominantly postcapillary venules can occur as a limited cutaneous disease or be part of a more severe systemic vasculitic process. Limited cutaneous vasculitis has been called *hypersensitivity vasculitis* even though a triggering antigen usually cannot be identified. Biopsy of the skin usually demonstrates leukocytoclastic angiitis with or without immune complex deposition.

CLINICAL FEATURES AND DIFFERENTIAL DIAGNOSIS

Cutaneous vasculitis most often manifests as palpable purpura. Urticarial lesions are less common. Cutaneous vasculitis can occur in association with infection (endocarditis, hepatitis B and C, or caused by *Neisseria, Rickettsia,* cytomegalovirus, or HIV), malignant disease (predominantly myelo- or lymphoproliferative diseases but also solid-tissue carcinoma), allergic reactions to drugs, cryoglobulinemia, and systemic autoimmune disorders, such as rheumatoid arthritis, lupus erythematosus, or Sjögren's syndrome. Nonvasculitic causes of purpura include Kaposi's sarcoma, bacterial and fungal emboli, steroid therapy, amyloidosis, senile purpura, warfarin necrosis, calciphylaxis, and trauma.

DIAGNOSTIC EVALUATION

Clinical examination often is sufficient to make the diagnosis, although biopsy may be necessary in some contexts to differentiate vasculitis from nonvasculitic causes of purpura.

MANAGEMENT

If cutaneous vasculitis is mild and of recent onset without compromise of skin integrity, and a controllable etiologic factor is not identified, only careful observation may be necessary. However, progression or visceral involvement necessitates treatment. Therapy with nonsteroidal anti-inflammatory drugs, colchicine, dapsone, or pentoxifylline may be tried, although these agents are inconsistently helpful. Glucocorticoids should be used sparingly, and cytotoxic therapy for non-necrotizing, isolated cutaneous disease should be avoided. If extremely high levels of cryoglobulins are present, apheresis may be of benefit, although results of controlled studies are not available.

Chapter 181

◼ SPONDYLARTHROPATHIES

DEFINITIONS

Spondylarthropathy encompasses a family of chronic inflammatory disorders primarily affecting peripheral and axial joints. Members of this family include ankylosing spondylitis, a predominantly axial form of arthritis usually beginning in the sacroiliac joints and slowly progressing to spinal fusion; Reiter's syndrome, or reactive arthritis, an acute peripheral type of arthritis associated with nongonococcal urethritis, conjunctivitis, or other mucocutaneous features, which typically occurs after enteric or genitourinary infection; psoriatic arthritis, a slowly progressive peripheral type of arthritis, with or without axial disease, that occurs in the setting of cutaneous psoriasis; and enteropathic arthritis, a peripheral or axial arthropathy accompanying ulcerative colitis and Crohn's disease.

ETIOLOGY AND EPIDEMIOLOGY

An atypical immune response to certain bacteria, mediated by HLA-B27 and other class I major histocompatibility complex genes, is believed to underlie most forms of spondyloarthropathy. The prevalence of these disorders, especially ankylosing spondylitis and reactive arthritis, generally parallels the frequency of HLA-B27 in different populations. American and European whites are affected more often than other racial groups.

CLINICAL FEATURES

Unifying features of the forms of spondylarthropathy include (a) a tendency for involvement of sacroiliac and other spinal joints (sacroiliitis and spondylitis); (b) peripheral arthritis, typically asymmetric and oligoarticular; (c) inflammatory lesions of tendon and fascial insertions (enthesopathy) at peripheral and axial sites; (d) extra-articular complications affecting the eye (anterior uveitis) or heart (aortitis and conduction disturbance); (e) disease onset among young adults, especially men; (f) absence of rheumatoid factor and other autoantibodies; and (g) strong associations with class I histocompatibility antigens, especially HLA-B27. Despite these common characteristics, each of the disorders manifests unique clinical features.

LABORATORY STUDIES AND DIAGNOSTIC TESTS

Laboratory abnormalities are few. Mild normocytic, normochromic anemia and elevation in erythrocyte sedimentation rate can occur in all types. Modest leukocytosis and thrombocytosis are most common in acute Reiter's syndrome and enteropathic arthritis. Serum rheumatoid factor and antinuclear antibody tests results are uniformly negative. Synovial fluid findings include leukocyte counts ranging from 5,000 to 50,000 per microliter (the highest counts occurring in Reiter's syndrome), elevated protein levels, normal glucose levels, and an absence of organisms on Gram stain and culture. Radiologic abnormalities occur in all forms of spondylarthropathy, depending on the involved joints.

PROGNOSIS AND MANAGEMENT

Death occurs in fewer than 5% of cases and is caused primarily by vertebral fractures, especially of the cervical vertebrae, cardiac complications, and amyloidosis. Therapy involves pharmacologic suppression of joint inflammation in conjunction with physical therapy to preserve axial and peripheral joint function and to prevent deformity. Unlike rheumatoid arthritis, this type of arthritis usually does not respond to salicylates, propionic acids, glucocorticoids, or long-acting drugs such as gold salts, D-penicillamine, or hydroxychloroquine. Instead, the nonsteroidal anti-inflammatory drugs indomethacin, tolmetin, piroxicam, and others are more effective in suppressing symptoms of pain and stiffness and signs of inflammation. Sulfasalazine (2 to 3 g per day) has been shown to be effective in relieving joint symptoms and signs in all of these conditions.

For all patients with reactive arthritis, an attempt should be made to identify the causative microorganism so that appropriate antibiotics can be prescribed. Immunosuppressants such as methotrexate or azathioprine sometimes are needed, but they should be used sparingly by patients with reactive arthritis in view of the possibility of promoting bacterial persistence. The presence of peripheral arthritis among patients with inflammatory bowel disease indicates active bowel inflammation. Treatment of the bowel with glucocorticoids or other medications, or colectomy for ulcerative colitis, results in resolution of the peripheral, but not the axial, joint disease.

Chapter 176

◼ SYSTEMIC LUPUS ERYTHEMATOSUS

DEFINITION AND EPIDEMIOLOGY

Systemic lupus erythematosus (SLE) is a chronic, multisystem disease of unknown causation. The estimated prevalence in the United States is 0.05% to 0.1% of the population; African-Americans and other minorities appear to be at higher risk. Disease onset is most common in the second and third decades of life; women of childbearing age are affected disproportionately.

ETIOLOGY AND PATHOGENESIS

Although the cause is unknown, genetic (e.g., inherited complement deficiencies and some HLA haplotypes), environmental (e.g., ultraviolet light, aromatic amines, and certain medications), and hormonal (high estrogen to androgen ratio) factors have been implicated. The pathologic features are those of an inflammatory disorder with evidence of autoimmunity, immune complex deposition, complement activation, and chronic lymphocytic inflammation. Thromboembolic phenomena can result from the binding of antibodies to coagulation factors or cofactors, platelets, or endothelium.

CLINICAL FEATURES

The American College of Rheumatism (ACR) classification criteria are listed in Table 178.1; other manifestations are included in Table 178.2. Most patients have mild to moderate disease with chronic, smoldering symptoms punctuated by gradual or sudden increases in disease activity (flare-ups). Drug-induced SLE (most strongly associated with hydralazine and procainamide) tends to cause skin manifestations, arthralgia, and serositis and to spare the kidneys and central nervous system (CNS).

LABORATORY STUDIES AND DIAGNOSTIC TESTS

Common laboratory abnormalities are listed in Table 178.1. The erythrocyte sedimentation rate may be markedly elevated but can be normal even in active disease. The antinuclear antibody (ANA) test result almost always is positive but is not specific for SLE. Demonstration of antibodies against double-stranded DNA is the most helpful confirmatory test; unlike the ANA test, anti-DNA titers may reflect disease activity and even be predictive of impending flare-ups. Anti-Smith antibodies also are very specific for SLE but are found infrequently. Anti-ribosomal P and anti-neuronal antibodies support a diagnosis of CNS lupus. Anti-histone antibodies are present in almost all cases of drug-induced SLE. Anti-Ro (SSA) and anti-La (SSB) antibodies are found in as many as half of patients and indicate a greater likelihood of cutaneous manifestations, photosensitivity, and neonatal lupus among the offspring of female patients. Low complement levels (particularly of C3, C4, and total hemolytic complement) are important both in diagnosis and in monitoring disease activity. Various tests can indicate a thrombotic tendency, including anti-cardiolipin antibodies and the so-called lupus anticoagulant.

Ancillary studies for selected patients include radiographs of affected joints, echocardiography for patients with myocardial or pericardial disease, high-resolution computed tomography of the lungs to define parenchymal lung disease, and magnetic resonance imaging of the CNS to evaluate patients for suspected CNS lupus. Biopsy is invaluable in the evaluation of skin and kidney disease. The results of renal biopsy can be classified into World Health Organization classes I through VI, higher classes reflecting more serious disease.

DIAGNOSIS

There is no single diagnostic test. The diagnosis should be considered only when clinical suspicion is aroused by an appropriate set of symptoms. For such patients, a positive ANA test result can further strengthen the suspicion. A negative test result generally directs the evaluation elsewhere. A positive ANA result also opens up the possibility of finding more SLE-specific autoantibodies, such as anti-DNA. Although the ACR criteria provide a useful frame of reference, the diagnosis for an individual patient does depends not on meeting these criteria but on a consistent diagnostic impression by a qualified clinician. A large number of symptoms and signs not included in the ACR criteria may be present or absent in patients under evaluation.

MANAGEMENT

Although the mainstay of therapy for active SLE is glucocorticoids, the medications chosen must be tailored to the organs involved and the activity of the disease in these organs (Table 178.2). Antimalarial agents, such as 200 to 400 mg hydroxychloroquine every day, are very useful in long-term management, particularly the prevention of flare-ups.

Chapter 178

■ TAKAYASU'S ARTERITIS

DEFINITION, EPIDEMIOLOGY, AND PATHOPHYSIOLOGY

Takayasu's arteritis is large-vessel vasculitis that involves the aorta and its main branches. It chiefly affects young women. The cause is unknown. Stenotic lesions are characteristic, but aneurysms can form, particularly in the aortic root.

CLINICAL FEATURES

Morbidity is caused by organ ischemia. Common syndromes include extremity claudication, cerebral ischemia, renal artery hypertension, coronary syndromes, and mesenteric vascular insufficiency. In about 20% of patients, aortic root involvement may cause valvular insufficiency and congestive heart failure. Fever may be present, but skin lesions, pulmonary infiltrates, and glomerulonephritis are unusual. Examination may disclose vascular bruits, particularly of the upper extremities, and asymmetric peripheral pulses or blood pressures.

DIAGNOSTIC EVALUATION

There are no specific serologic tests. The erythrocyte sedimentation rate often is elevated. Angiography can establish the initial diagnosis and can be repeated to assess the degree of disease progression. The utility of other imaging techniques, such as ultrasonography and magnetic resonance imaging, is under investigation.

MANAGEMENT

Approximately 60% of patients achieve remission with glucocorticoid therapy (e.g., 1 mg prednisone per kilogram per day). Patients with disease that is resistant or relapses on tapering of drug therapy can be treated with low doses of cyclo-

phosphamide or weekly doses of methotrexate. Whenever feasible, anatomic correction of clinically significant lesions should be considered, especially in the setting of renal artery stenosis and hypertension. Adequate blood pressure control is critical. When peripheral blood pressures does not accurately reflect aortic root pressure because of extensive arterial stenosis, intravascular pressure recordings can be obtained during angiography.

Chapter 181

■ WEGENER'S GRANULOMATOSIS

DEFINITION, EPIDEMIOLOGY, AND PATHOPHYSIOLOGY

Wegener's granulomatosis (WG) is a multisystem necrotizing vasculitis. It is an uncommon disease, equally frequent in men and women, with a mean age at diagnosis of about 40–45 years. Disease manifestations are caused by aseptic inflammation with necrosis, granuloma formation, and vasculitis of the upper and lower respiratory tract, ears, eyes, kidneys, skin, or nervous system. Biopsy shows geographic necrosis with giant cells and vessel necrosis.

CLINICAL FEATURES

Most patients first seek medical attention because of upper or lower airway disease. The finding of recurrent epistaxis, mucosal ulceration, nasal septal perforation, nasal deformity, or hearing loss suggests WG. About 80% of patients do not have renal involvement at the time of diagnosis, and about 50% do not have overt lung disease. Over the course of the illness, however, more than 80% have pulmonary or renal disease. Pulmonary involvement may cause coughing, hemoptysis, dyspnea, or pleuritis. Computed tomography of the chest is more sensitive than radiography of the chest in demonstrating nodules and infiltrates. Renal involvement manifests as glomerulonephritis associated with hematuria, red blood cell casts, azotemia, or uremia. Musculoskeletal features are common, but joint deformity or destruction are rare. About 25% of patients have peripheral or central nervous system disease.

DIAGNOSTIC EVALUATION

Approximately 90% of patients with active disease have an immunofluorescence test result positive for antineutrophil cytoplasmic antibodies (ANCA), usually in a cytoplasmic (C-ANCA) rather than a perinuclear pattern (P-ANCA). Antibody titers correlate loosely with disease activity. A positive ANCA test result is not entirely specific for WG, however. A suspected diagnosis of WG ideally should be confirmed by means of biopsy. Open lung biopsy is the most likely to yield an unequivocal diagnosis. Transbronchial specimens often are inadequate but are useful in excluding infection. Nasal biopsy may not provide enough information for a diagnosis. Renal biopsy usually shows a glomerulonephritis with little evidence of immune complex deposition.

MANAGEMENT

Management of severe, generalized WG should include initial glucocorticoid therapy in conjunction with cyclophosphamide. After substantial improvement has occurred, usually within 1 month, high-doses of glucocorticoids can be tapered over several months. Cytotoxic therapy should be continued for at least 1 year after the induction of remission. For patients with less severe disease, weekly doses of methotrexate can be used in place of cyclophosphamide. Daily treatment with trimethoprim-sulfamethoxazole has been shown to decrease the frequency of upper airway flare-ups in WG without influencing the course of renal or pulmonary disease.

Chapter 181

ONCOLOGY AND HEMATOLOGY

■ ACUTE LEUKEMIA

DEFINITIONS AND PATHOPHYSIOLOGY

Acute leukemia is caused by uncontrolled proliferation of a malignant clone of hematopoietic cells that does not differentiate and mature normally. Leukemic cells are introduced into the blood from the bone marrow. They may divide in

the blood or infiltrate an organ, such as the spleen, liver, or lymph nodes, where they may also divide and then reenter the blood. In acute lymphocytic leukemia (ALL), the abnormal clone has characteristics of lymphoid cells. All other types of acute leukemia are classified as acute myeloid leukemia (AML). AML is subdivided according to cell type—myelocytic, promyelocytic, myelomonocytic, monocytic, erythroleukemic, and megakaryocytic.

EPIDEMIOLOGY

Acute lymphocytic leukemia: Most patients are younger than 15 years. The median age of adult patients is 42 years. Men are affected more often than women.

Acute myeloid leukemia: The average patient is older than 55 years at diagnosis. The incidence increases with age. Ionizing radiation and some chemotherapeutic agents, especially alkylating agents, are associated with an increased incidence of AML.

CLINICAL FINDINGS

Acute lymphocytic leukemia: Adults usually have the subacute onset of fatigue, lethargy, and anorexia. Petechiae or easy bruising may be found. An expanding bone marrow mass can cause bone pain. Most patients have palpable lymphadenopathy; the spleen is palpable in 50% of patients. About 15% of patients have a fever, which may be caused by occult infection. Signs of increased intracranial pressure or cranial nerve dysfunction caused by leukemic infiltration of the central nervous system may be evident. Anemia, granulocytopenia, and thrombocytopenia are almost always present at the time of diagnosis. For 85% of patients, the blood smear reveals lymphoblasts. The bone marrow biopsy specimen almost always is hypercellular with lymphoblastic predominance and a reduction in normal elements. Cerebrospinal fluid should be examined for leukemic cells. Serum lactate dehydrogenase and uric acid levels usually are elevated.

Acute myeloid leukemia: The features vary somewhat among the different subtypes. Adults usually have a vague history of progressive lethargy. However, as many as one-third of patients may come to medical attention with an acute illness due to infection. The patients usually have petechiae. Lymphadenopathy, splenomegaly, and hepatomegaly are unusual. The white blood cell (WBC) count is normal, elevated, or depressed with equal frequencies at diagnosis, although granulocytopenia is essentially universal. Anemia and thrombocytopenia usually are present. Blast cells are initially absent from the peripheral blood in about 15% of cases. The bone marrow usually is markedly hypercellular and has at least 50% to 75% leukemic cells. Uric acid levels generally are elevated.

DIAGNOSTIC EVALUATION

Morphologic examination, histochemical reaction, cytogenetic and enzymologic studies and cell surface antigen identification are the principal laboratory tools for differentiating ALL from AML and for identifying clinically important subtypes of both.

PROGNOSIS AND MANAGEMENT

Acute lymphocytic leukemia: Prognosis is influenced adversely by advanced age, B-cell phenotype, greatly elevated WBC count at diagnosis, and a complex, abnormal karyotype. Most adults respond well to initial therapy, but unlike children with ALL, most adults ultimately die of the disease. Before chemotherapy is started, active infection must be controlled with antibiotics, and hyperuricemia with hydration and allopurinol. The standard induction regimens include drugs such as vincristine, prednisone, daunorubicin, and L-asparaginase. After the patient has achieved a complete remission and recovered from induction therapy, intensive postremission therapy with drugs not used during induction or with bone marrow transplantation is necessary to maximize the duration of the response. The median duration is 1 to 2 years; most relapses occur within 3 years. About 30% to 40% of patients live disease free for 5 years after treatment. Central nervous system involvement can be managed effectively with intrathecal methotrexate.

Acute myeloid leukemia: Remission therapy usually consists of only two drugs, cytarabine and daunorubicin or idarubicin. Almost all patients need prophylactic platelet transfusions and at least 90% need empiric broad-spectrum antibiotic therapy for fever while granulocytopenic. Complete remission is obtained among 70% or more of adults. All-*trans* retinoic acid induces remission of acute promyelocytic leukemia through induction of maturation and differentiation rather than by means of cytotoxicity. Intensive postremission therapy prolongs remission to a mean of 12 to 24 months. About 30% to 50% of patients with a complete response live disease free for at least 5 years after treatment. Late relapses occur but are rare.

Chapter 227

■ AMYLOIDOSIS

DEFINITION

Amyloidosis refers to a group of protein deposition diseases. Amyloid is a substance that consists of protein fibrils. Stained with Congo red and viewed with polarized light, it produces an apple-green birefringence.

EPIDEMIOLOGY AND ETIOLOGY

Approximately 2,500 cases occur annually in the United States; only 1% of patients are younger than 40 years. In primary amyloidosis, the fibrils consist of monoclonal κ or λ light chains. The condition is closely related to multiple myeloma. Secondary amyloidosis is associated with inflammatory processes such as rheumatoid arthritis and Crohn's disease. The fibrils consist of protein A. Other varieties include familial amyloidosis, senile amyloidosis, and a β_2 microglobulin amyloidosis associated with renal dialysis.

CLINICAL FINDINGS

Primary amyloidosis: Weakness, fatigue, and weight loss are common, as are light-headedness, syncope, change in voice or tongue, dyspnea, and edema. Nephrotic syndrome, hepatomegaly, macroglossia, congestive heart failure, carpal tunnel syndrome, peripheral neuropathy, and orthostatic hypotension occur in 10% to 30% of cases.

Secondary amyloidosis: At diagnosis, more than 90% of patients have renal insufficiency or nephrotic syndrome. Gastrointestinal involvement often manifests as a malabsorption syndrome. Unlike primary amyloidosis, secondary amyloidosis rarely involves the heart and peripheral nerves.

LABORATORY STUDIES AND DIAGNOSTIC TESTS

Primary amyloidosis: Findings are those suggested by pattern of organ involvement. They may include azotemia and an echocardiogram that demonstrates increased ventricular wall thickness and an abnormal myocardial texture. Monoclonal protein is found in the serum and the urine of more than 70% of patients. The diagnosis depends on the demonstration of amyloid deposits. Findings at examination of an abdominal fat aspirate or rectal biopsy are abnormal more than 90% of the time.

Secondary amyloidosis: Most patients have azotemia and proteinuria. The diagnosis is made by means of biopsy of an affected organ.

PROGNOSIS AND MANAGEMENT

Primary amyloidosis: The median survival period ranges from 1 to 2 years. Therapy is unsatisfactory, but melphalan and prednisone prolong survival several months.

Secondary amyloidosis: The median survival time is approximately 2 years. Treatment depends on the underlying disease. Renal transplantation is helpful.

Chapter 235

■ APPROACH TO THE PATIENT WITH ANEMIA

DEFINITION

Anemia represents a reduction in the normal red blood cell (RBC) mass within the body as measured with peripheral blood hemoglobin level and hematocrit. The hematocrit of healthy men is 47% ± 7%; that of healthy women is 42% ± 5%.

PATHOPHYSIOLOGY

The normal cycle of erythropoiesis requires coordination of erythropoietin stimulation with the necessary precursor cells and building blocks in a conducive microenvironment. RBC structure and extramedullary circumstances then determine the life span of the erythrocyte. Lesions in any component of this cycle can cause anemia.

DIFFERENTIAL DIAGNOSIS

Hyporegenerative versus hyperregenerative anemia: If shortened RBC survival causes anemia, as in bleeding or hemolysis, an erythropoietin surge leads to the release of increased numbers of reticulocytes (immature RBC precursors). An elevated reticulocyte count (more than 100,000 per microliter) thus indicates that the marrow is attempting to compensate for an extramedullary abnormality. A lower reticulocyte count suggests an abnormality within the marrow.

Categorization of anemia according to size of red blood cells: Anemia can be classified as microcytic, normocytic, or macrocytic (Table 211.2). Microcytic anemia originates in an iron or hemoglobin deficiency. Most cases of macrocytic anemia are caused by folate and vitamin B_{12} deficiencies. Normocytic anemia is a more heterogeneous group that includes most hemolytic disorders (Table 211.3).

HISTORY AND PHYSICAL EXAMINATION

Anemia often is asymptomatic unless it is severe, develops rapidly, or occurs in a patient with an underlying cardiopulmonary disorder. The symptoms include dyspnea on exertion, angina, and fatigue. Physical examination may reveal conjunctival and palmar pallor, tachycardia, and a systolic flow murmur.

Microcytic anemia: Patients with an iron deficiency may have overt hemorrhage or symptoms that suggest a source of occult bleeding. Result of stool tests for occult blood may be positive. Family history and ethnic background are useful in the diagnosis of thalassemia. History or examination findings of chronic inflammatory disease such as osteomyelitis or rheumatoid arthritis suggest anemia of chronic disease.

Normocytic hyporegenerative anemia: Findings of chronic inflammation suggest anemia of chronic disease. The symptoms of uremia may be elicited. Pancytopenia is suggested by a history of easy bruising or frequent infection. Hematologic malignant disease may be associated with fever, weight loss, lymphadenopathy, or splenomegaly.

Normocytic hyperregenerative anemia: The history may suggest hemolytic anemia (e.g., malaria among travelers or autoimmune hemolysis among patients with other symptoms of systemic lupus erythematosus). The history and physical examination may suggest a source of hemorrhage. However, hemorrhage causes a hyperproliferative anemia only if it has not caused a concomitant iron deficiency.

Macrocytic anemia: Hypothyroidism, alcoholism, and chronic liver disease may be apparent. Patients with vitamin B_{12} deficiency, but not those with folate deficiency, often have a loss of vibratory and positional sense in the lower extremities.

LABORATORY STUDIES AND DIAGNOSTIC TESTS

In addition to reticulocyte count and cell size determination, the initial approach includes examination of a peripheral blood smear, white blood cell and platelet counts, and measurement of RBC distribution width (RDW), an indicator of the range of RBC sizes. An overall approach is outlined in Fig. 211.1.

Microcytic anemia: Iron deficiency is suggested by low serum levels of ferritin, a storage form of iron. The absence of bone marrow iron stores is considered the diagnostic gold standard, but a trial of iron therapy can be useful. In thalassemia, the RBCs are particularly microcytic for the degree of anemia; hemoglobin electrophoresis may help establish a diagnosis. Sideroblastic anemia shows iron accumulation in the mitochondria of developing RBCs within the marrow (ringed sideroblasts).

Normocytic hyporegenerative anemia: Results of bone marrow biopsy often are definitive. The anemia of renal failure has low erythropoietin levels; blood urea nitrogen and creatinine levels are elevated. Aplastic or hypoplastic processes affect the WBC and platelet counts. Marrow infiltration produces myelophthisis, in which the peripheral blood smear shows nucleated and teardrop-shaped RBCs and immature WBCs that have been extruded from the marrow.

Normocytic hyperregenerative anemia: Hemolysis may be associated with hyperbilirubinemia, low haptoglobin levels, and production of RBC autoantibodies. The peripheral blood smear may provide many diagnostic clues (e.g., schistocytes in microangiopathic processes that fragment RBCs and spherocytes in immune-mediated processes or hereditary spherocytosis).

Macrocytic anemia: Megaloblastic anemia is associated with exaggerated macrocytosis (mean corpuscular volume [MCV] more than 115 fL), a reduction in platelet and WBC counts, high levels of lactate dehydrogenase (LDH), and hypersegmentation of polymorphonuclear leukocytes on the peripheral blood smear. Serum vitamin B_{12} and RBC folate tests help identify the specific deficiency. The coexistence of iron deficiency anemia and megaloblastic anemias may yield a normal MCV but an elevated RDW. Nonmegaloblastic macrocytic anemia does not cause pancytopenia.

MANAGEMENT

Anemia frequently is not the primary concern but is instead a clue to the presence of an underlying disorder that must be identified and treated (e.g., iron deficiency as a first manifestation of colon cancer). Management of the underlying disorder

improves or resolves the anemia. If the degree of improvement is insufficient or there are acute symptoms of anemia, RBC transfusions can be performed.

Chapter 211

APLASTIC ANEMIA

DEFINITION, EPIDEMIOLOGY, AND ETIOLOGY

Aplastic anemia is a syndrome of bone marrow failure characterized by pancytopenia of the peripheral blood and hypocellularity of the bone marrow. Patients of all ages and both sexes are affected. It is caused by various pathophysiologic processes that affect the pluripotent stem cells. Most cases appear to be acquired, but approximately 50% have no identifiable cause and are called *idiopathic*. Recognized causes are listed in Table 230.1.

CLINICAL FEATURES

Two types of presentation are possible depending on the severity of pancytopenia. Some patients have a gradual onset of signs and symptoms of anemia, including fatigue, dyspnea, and pallor. Laboratory evaluation reveals variable but often mild pancytopenia and hypoplastic bone marrow. Other patients have signs and symptoms of thrombocytopenia and leukopenia in addition to those of anemia. They may have a sudden onset of high-spiking fevers and spontaneous petechiae and ecchymosis. In more severe cases, patients may have retinal hemorrhage, epistaxis, or oral mucosal bleeding. Except for evidence of bleeding, the physical examination findings generally are unremarkable. Lymphadenopathy and splenomegaly are not seen. In the absence of granulocytes, the findings associated with infection, such as pneumonia, may be minimal.

LABORATORY STUDIES

Laboratory evaluation should include studies that attempt to identify the cause of the aplasia, including tests for paroxysmal nocturnal hemoglobinuria, systemic lupus erythematosus, hepatitis, infectious mononucleosis, and pregnancy. Deficiency of vitamin B_{12} or folate should be excluded. Cytogenetic analysis may be helpful in identifying myelodysplastic syndromes and those with underlying chromosomal fragility states, such as Fanconi's anemia.

PROGNOSIS AND MANAGEMENT

General supportive management: Drugs that interfere with platelet function should be avoided. Women of childbearing age should undergo menstrual suppression. Because of the need for frequent phlebotomy and transfusions, indwelling vascular catheters may be necessary. Fever and potential infection should be managed promptly and aggressively with cultures and antibiotics. Transfusions should be used judiciously. Active bleeding should be controlled with platelet transfusion if the platelet count is less than 20,000 per microliter. Prophylactic platelet transfusions need not be given until the platelet count is less than 5,000 to 10,000 per microliter. Transfusions should be leukocyte depleted, and family-derived transfusions should be avoided if bone marrow transplantation is being considered. Cytomegalovirus (CMV) antibody-negative patients should receive transfusions only from CMV antibody-negative donors.

Definitive treatment: Any possible offending exposures should be discontinued. Specific therapies include marrow stimulation (androgens, cytokines), immunosuppression (antithymocyte globulin, glucocorticoids, cyclophosphamide, cyclosporine), and bone marrow transplantation. The last should be considered primary treatment of patients younger than 40 to 45 years.

Chapter 230

BREAST CANCER

EPIDEMIOLOGY AND ETIOLOGY

The term *breast cancer* usually refers to adenocarcinoma, the most common malignant neoplasm of mammary tissue and, with lung cancer, one of the two most common cancers of women in the developed world. Risk factors include advanced age, history of breast cancer in a first-degree relative (especially if the lesions are bilateral or the relative is premenopausal), early onset of menarche (12 years of age or earlier), nulliparity or first pregnancy after 35 years of age, alcohol consumption, and prior radiation exposure. Current evidence suggests that use of oral contraceptives or postmenopausal estrogen replacement is associated with a slight increase in risk. Use of newer estrogens such as raloxifene may actually reduce risk. Germ-line mutations of the genes *BRCA1* and *BRCA2* are associated with a higher risk of both breast and ovarian cancer. Benign lesions such as cysts, mastitis, and most fibroadenomas are not predisposing conditions. The incidence of breast cancer among men is about 1% of the incidence among women.

PATHOPHYSIOLOGY, CLASSIFICATION, AND STAGING

Most adenocarcinomas of the breast are thought to arise from ductal epithelial cells. These cancers may be in situ or infiltrating (also called *invasive*). The in situ carcinomas are further classified as lobular carcinoma in situ (LCIS) or ductal carcinoma in situ (DCIS). LCIS and DCIS do not invade the parenchyma or stroma and have a very low potential for generating metastasis. DCIS lesions are usually regarded as a unilateral, very early, preinvasive form of true breast cancer. LCIS, in contrast, often is considered a marker of carcinogenic potential (equally shared with the uninvolved breast) rather than true cancer. Invasive adenocarcinoma, which does infiltrate into surrounding normal tissue, also has ductal and lobular types, the ductal types predominating. The most common sites of metastasis are the axillary lymph nodes. The number of nodes containing cancer is a good indicator of the propensity of the tumor to metastasize to more distant anatomic sites such as bone, lung, liver, and brain. About 15% of breast cancers have special histopathologic patterns, including mucinous and papillary types. Inflammatory breast cancer is an especially aggressive form of the disease characterized by diffuse breast swelling, erythema and warmth of the skin, breast pain, and peau d'orange edema of the skin.

Breast cancer is staged through assessment of tumor size (T), nodal involvement (N), and the presence or absence of distant metastases (M) and subsequent classification of the stage as 0, I, IIA, IIB, IIIA, IIIB, or IV. Proper staging requires pathologic examination of the breast tissue and axillary nodes, physical examination, chest radiograph, and measurement of serum markers such as liver transaminases and alkaline phosphatase. Physical examination is not a reliable way of assessing axillary nodal involvement. With sentinel lymph node mapping, a radioactive tracer or a dye is introduced into the breast at tumor resection, and only the nodes that first take up the substance are dissected. If these nodes are free of cancer, it is extremely likely that the other axillary nodes will be free as well.

CLINICAL FINDINGS

A review of breast symptoms is essential. The rest of the history should focus on indications of possible metastasis, such as bone pain and respiratory difficulties. The physical examination should include special emphasis on the breast, axilla, and supraclavicular areas. The presence of a supraclavicular node is an indication of metastatic disease and therefore alters prognosis and treatment.

LABORATORY EVALUATION

A preoperative mammogram is useful in evaluating the rest of the abnormal breast and the contralateral breast for masses or calcifications before definitive surgery. A normal mammogram does not exclude the presence of a malignant lesion, however. A biopsy must be performed on a persistent mass regardless of the mammographic findings. Bone and liver scans are not performed routinely if laboratory values are normal. A complete blood cell count (CBC) and chemistry panel are recommended. After surgical treatment, a yearly mammogram is obligatory, and many oncologists obtain CBCs, hepatic enzymes, and alkaline phosphatase levels on a routine basis.

PROGNOSIS AND MANAGEMENT

DCIS and LCIS: DCIS can manifest as a mass, but it is more commonly found by means of biopsy of abnormal calcifications detected with a mammogram. Optimal management is not yet established. Most patients undergo radiation therapy after local excision. Although there is no established role for systemic chemotherapy because of the very small likelihood of metastasis, tamoxifen may decrease the risk of invasive breast cancer among patients treated with lumpectomy and radiation. Because LCIS usually is not palpable and is invisible at mammography, the diagnosis is commonly incidental to breast biopsy performed for another reason. Because the presence of LCIS is an indicator of a propensity for development of breast cancer and because both breasts are at equal risk, treatment options include observation alone or bilateral simple, prophylactic mastectomy. There is no role for radiation therapy. Recent data have demonstrated a 50% reduction in the risk of infiltrating breast cancer among patients with a history of LCIS who are treated with tamoxifen.

Infiltrating tumors: Adverse prognostic factors include a greater number of positive axillary nodes, larger tumor size, poorly differentiated histologic features, and the absence of receptors for estrogen and progesterone in the cancer cells. Most patients with stage I cancers, many with stage II cancers, and some with stage III cancers can be cured with local therapy. Patients with more advanced stage III cancers and with stage IV disease cannot be cured with surgery alone and need systemic therapy. Local therapy consists of surgery (now often breast sparing rather than mastectomy or radical mastectomy), axillary dissection, and radiation therapy. Adverse effects include disfigurement (breast reconstruction can be performed) and lymphedema (which may occur less often when sentinel lymph node–mapping techniques are used). Systemic drug therapy is used in the following three settings: (a) as an adjunct to local therapy to limit micrometastatic disease, (b) in the management of overt metastatic disease, and (c) as primary therapy for locally advanced breast cancer to render the local disease amenable to surgical and radiotherapeutic approaches. Cyclophosphamide, methotrexate, 5-fluorouracil, paclitaxel, and docetaxel are the chemotherapeutic drugs used most commonly. The first three often are combined into the CMF regimen. The drug most commonly used in hormonal therapy for breast cancer is tamoxifen (usually 20 mg by mouth per day), which acts as an antiestrogen in breast tissue. Tumor estrogen receptors are required. The most common toxicities are hot flashes, irregular menses, and depressed mood. Increased risk of uterine cancer has also been found.

Metastatic disease: In addition to systemic treatment, some metastatic processes may necessitate special therapy. For example, bony metastases leading to intractable pain or to skeletal instability may necessitate radiation therapy or even surgery. Malignant pleural effusions may necessitate repeated thoracentesis or pleurodesis with a sclerosing agent. Morbidity from central nervous system metastasis can be minimized by use of glucocorticoids and radiation therapy. Hypercalcemia generally responds to immediate intravenous hydration followed by the administration of a biphosphonate such as pamidronate.

Chapter 220

CHRONIC LEUKEMIA

DEFINITIONS

Chronic leukemia is a group of heterogeneous proliferative disorders involving lymphoid or myeloid cells that retain some capability of differentiation and maturation. The group includes chronic lymphocytic leukemia (CLL), chronic myelocytic leukemia (CML), and hairy cell leukemia (HCL).

EPIDEMIOLOGY AND PATHOPHYSIOLOGY

Chronic lymphocytic leukemia: CLL is caused by malignant expansion of a clone of lymphocytes. Most patients in the United States have the B-cell subtype. T-cell CLL is more common in Japan. CLL occurs primarily among older persons and is equally distributed between men and women.

Chronic myelocytic leukemia: CML is a myeloproliferative disorder of the stem cells common to bone marrow cells and B lymphocytes. Abnormalities of red blood cell (RBC) and platelet production accompany the increase in granulocytes. All of the cells have the Philadelphia (Ph) chromosome, which reflects reciprocal translocation of material between chromosomes 9 and 22. The key event is translocation of the *ABL* gene. CML usually is diagnosed in midlife or later.

CLINICAL FINDINGS AND DIAGNOSIS

Chronic lymphocytic leukemia: About half of patients come to medical attention with lymphadenopathy in addition to lymphocytosis (usually more than 15,000 cells per microliter). Splenomegaly also may be present. Anemia and thrombocytopenia usually are late features unless an autoimmune process has supervened. Fever and painful lymphadenopathy are uncommon and suggest infection. The bone marrow usually is diffusely displaced by small, mature lymphocytes. A few patients have abdominal tumors with the histologic features of large cell lymphoma (Richter's syndrome). Associated autoimmune phenomena, such as hemolytic anemia, can develop at any time and do not influence prognosis. Death usually is related to infection. The T-cell variety tends to involve the skin and to respond less well to therapy.

Chronic myelocytic leukemia: Initially, patients are asymptomatic, though complaints related to splenomegaly may be offered. The WBC count usually is 2 to 4 times the upper limit of normal, and the blood smear discloses the immaturity of the granulocyte series (myelocytes, metamyelocytes). The platelet count is normal or elevated, and anemia does not occur early in the course. Leukocyte alkaline phosphatase activity is low or absent and helps to differentiate CML from other causes of granulocytosis, such as infection and polycythemia vera. The bone marrow is hypercellular, primarily because the granulocyte compartment is expanded and immature (but not blastic). There often is an accelerated phase or blastic phase within 3 to 4 years of presentation.

PROGNOSIS AND MANAGEMENT

Chronic lymphocytic leukemia: CLL usually is an indolent disease with a median survival period of 3 to 10 years, depending on presenting stage. Therapy is palliative and does not influence survival. No therapy is needed for asymptomatic lymphocytosis with minimal lymphadenopathy and normal RBC and platelet counts. In time, progressive lymphadenopathy or hepatosplenomegaly may necessitate therapy with an alkylating agent such as chlorambucil with or without prednisone. Splenectomy or splenic irradiation may benefit patients with hypersplenism. Lymphomatous transformation necessitates parenteral combination chemotherapy.

Chronic myelocytic leukemia: An adverse prognosis is associated with higher degrees of leukocytosis, the presence of blasts in the peripheral blood, and greater splenomegaly and thrombocytosis. Oral hydoxyurea is used to treat the chronic form of the disease. Recombinant interferon-α also is effective. These treatments are palliative, and it is uncertain that they delay the blastic phase, which may necessitate intensive antileukemic chemotherapy. Allogeneic bone marrow transplantation in the chronic phase can cure about half of patients.

Chapter 228

■ HODGKIN'S DISEASE

DEFINITION AND PATHOPHYSIOLOGY
Hodgkin's disease is a B-cell lymphoid neoplasm. The diagnosis is based on the recognition of Reed–Sternberg cells interspersed among a reactive mixed-cell population of lymphocytes, eosinophils, histiocytes, plasma cells, and neutrophils.

EPIDEMIOLOGY AND ETIOLOGY
The incidence of Hodgkin's disease is higher among men than women and higher among blacks than whites. The rate increases through early life, peaks in the third decade, declines until 45 years of age, and steadily increases thereafter. There is evidence of both an infectious cause (Epstein–Barr viral genomes are found in 18% to 50% of persons with Hodgkin's disease) and a genetic susceptibility. The disease also is associated with a variety of defects in cellular immunity.

CLASSIFICATION
Four histologic types have been described, based on the appearance and relative proportions of Reed–Sternberg cells and the histologic background—lymphocyte predominance, nodular sclerosis, mixed cellularity, and lymphocyte depletion. The nodular sclerosis type is most common among young adults. The mixed cellularity type predominates among children and the elderly.

CLINICAL FINDINGS
The most common presentation is an unexplained mass or swelling in the superficial lymph nodes, especially in the neck. The nodes are characteristically nontender and have a rubbery consistency. About two-thirds of patients have intrathoracic disease at diagnosis. Mediastinal lymphadenopathy and splenic involvement are common. Constitutional symptoms, called *B symptoms,* include fever in excess of 38°C, drenching night sweats, and weight loss exceeding 10%. The presence of the rare Pel–Ebstein fever (a cyclic pattern of high fevers for 1 to 2 weeks alternating with afebrile periods of similar lengths) almost confirms the diagnosis of Hodgkin's disease. Unexplained, generalized pruritus may occur. Pain in involved lymph nodes immediately after the ingestion of alcohol is almost pathognomonic for Hodgkin's disease.

LABORATORY STUDIES, DIAGNOSTIC TESTS, AND STAGING
The diagnosis of Hodgkin's disease is made by means of biopsy. Baseline studies should include a complete blood cell count, liver and renal chemical analysis, and measurement of calcium. Cytopenia may occur as a result of marrow involvement, hypersplenism, or autoimmune destruction. An elevated erythrocyte sedi-

TABLE 3.	ANN ARBOR STAGING CLASSIFICATION FOR HODGKIN'S DISEASE
Stage	**Description**
I	Involvement of a single lymph node region or localized involvement of a single extranodal organ or site (IE)
II	Involvement of more than one lymph node region on the same side of the diaphragm or of one or more lymph node regions and localized involvement of an extralymphatic organ or site (IIE) on the same side of the diaphragm
III	Involvement of lymph node regions on both sides of the diaphragm, which may be accompanied by involvement of the spleen (IIIS) or by localized involvement of an extralymphatic organ or site (IIIE) or both (IIIS/E)
IV	Diffuse or disseminated involvement of one or more extralymphatic organs or sites with or without lymph node involvement
A	Asymptomatic
B	Fever, sweats, unexplained weight loss of more than 10% of body weight

mentation rate correlates with advanced disease and a worse prognosis. The evaluation also includes computed tomography of the chest, abdomen, and pelvis. Bone marrow biopsy is not a routine procedure. The use of staging laparotomy and splenectomy has become increasingly selective. The anatomic distribution of Hodgkin's disease in contiguous lymphatic structures is predictable and nonrandom. These patterns form the basis for the Ann Arbor staging classification (Table 3), which has been shown to correlate well with prognosis.

PROGNOSIS AND MANAGEMENT
Hodgkin's disease is one of the most highly curable malignant diseases. About 80% of patients with newly diagnosed disease are cured, and fewer than 10% will die directly of the disease. Tumor burden and older age are adverse prognostic factors. Additional prognostic variables include histologic type, sex, the presence of B symptoms, the number of disease sites, and the presence of bone marrow involvement.

Primary therapy: Stage I or II supradiaphragmatic disease is controlled with extended-field radiation therapy, chemotherapy, or both. Cure rates greater than 90% have been reported with combination therapy, such as radiation therapy and chemotherapy with doxorubicin, bleomycin, vinblastine, and dacarbazine. For extensive mediastinal disease, a combination of radiation therapy and chemotherapy can cure 70% to 80% of patients. Sixty-five percent to 70% of patients with stage III or IV disease treated with chemotherapy regimens containing doxorubicin hydrochloride (Adriamycin) are free of disease after 5 years.

Relapse: Relapse after radiation therapy responds very well to chemotherapy. Relapse after primary chemotherapy or combination therapy has a less favorable outcome. The initial remission duration after primary chemotherapy greatly affects response to subsequent treatment. High-dose therapy with stem cell rescue is the favored treatment when primary induction fails or when there is a brief initial remission.

Complications of therapy: Acute effects such as nausea can be managed effectively. Of greater concern are later effects, including second malignant diseases (acute leukemia, non-Hodgkin's lymphoma, and solid tumors such as breast cancer), and sterility. Mediastinal and neck irradiation are associated with cardiac disease and hypothyroidism, respectively.

Chapter 232

cholesterolemia. Thrombotic complications are managed with anticoagulants, although the risk to benefit ratio of long-term anticoagulation has not been established. Finally, doses of all drugs tightly bound to albumin may have to be reduced to avoid toxicity.

Chapter 135

RENAL CELL CARCINOMA

PATHOGENESIS, EPIDEMIOLOGY, AND ETIOLOGY
Renal cell carcinoma (RCC) originates from the proximal convoluted tubular cells. It usually manifests during the fifth to seventh decades of life. The median age at diagnosis is 60 years. Men are affected twice as frequently as women, but there is no racial predilection. About 2% of cases occur as part of autosomal dominant von Hippel–Lindau syndrome. Risk factors include smoking among men, obesity, and hypertension but not polycystic kidney disease.

CLINICAL FINDINGS
About 20% to 30% of lesions are found incidentally as small tumors in a clinically asymptomatic stage. The classic triad of hematuria, flank pain, and palpable mass occurs in fewer than 10% of patients. However, presentation with one or two of these symptoms is common. The tumor may extend and invade into surrounding structures, such as the inferior vena cava, ureter, adrenal gland, spleen, liver, or pancreas. Only 40% of patients have disease confined to the kidney at diagnosis; 20% have symptoms of metastatic lesions. The common sites of distant metastasis include the lungs, lymph nodes, liver, bone, and brain. Tumor secretion of parathyroid hormone–like protein, erythropoietin, antidiuretic hormone, or corticotropin may cause hypercalcemia, erythrocytosis, hyponatremia, or Cushing's syndrome, respectively.

DIAGNOSTIC STUDIES
For a patient believed to have RCC, initial characterization of a mass lesion may be achieved with intravenous pyelography or ultrasonography. Computed tomography (CT) is the technique of choice for diagnosis and staging. Magnetic resonance imaging (MRI) may have additional benefit in detecting tumors less than 2 cm in diameter and in delineating local anatomy more clearly. Angiography should be used only for tumors in a solitary kidney, for vascular mapping before surgery, and for instances in which tumor angioinfarction is planned. Additional staging procedures include basic laboratory tests, chest radiography, and a bone scan. Patients with neurologic symptoms or signs should undergo CT or MRI of the brain. If the tumor appears to be confined to the kidney, the patient probably should undergo surgical resection without biopsy; a normal biopsy result would not prove conclusively the absence of cancer. In contrast, if there is extrarenal tumor involvement, CT-guided biopsy of the primary lesion may be indicated.

PROGNOSIS AND MANAGEMENT
The pathologic stage of RCC is the most important prognostic factor. Stage I (tumor confined within the capsule) has a 5-year survival rate of 65% to 85%; stage II (tumor invading through the capsule but confined within Gerota's fascia), 45% to 80%; stage III (tumor invading the renal vein, inferior vena cava, or regional lymph node), 15% to 35%; and stage IV (distant metastases), zero to 10%. For stages I to III, standard treatment is surgical resection. For some patients, partial nephrectomy may replace conventional radical nephrectomy. Radiation therapy does not add any benefit. The outcome among patients with stage IV disease is very poor, because RCC is resistant to chemotherapy in general. The role of immunomodulators such as interleukin-2 and interferon-α is being defined. For patients with stage IV disease, nephrectomy should be considered only for palliation of local symptoms such as pain and hematuria. Radiation therapy may improve symptoms of metastasis to bone or brain.

Chapter 160

URINARY TRACT INFECTIONS

DEFINITIONS
Urinary tract infection (UTI) is one of the most common forms of infection. *Bacteriuria* is the presence of bacteria in the urine. The term *significant bacteriuria*

was introduced to differentiate contaminated from infected urine. The criterion has been more than 10^5 colony-forming units per milliliter of urine, although urine from patients with symptomatic UTI may have lower colony counts. *Acute cystitis* is bacterial infection of the bladder epithelium or urethra. *Acute pyelonephritis* is a clinical syndrome of flank pain, fever, and chills due to bacterial invasion of the renal parenchyma. *Asymptomatic bacteriuria* is the presence of significant bacteriuria in the absence of any symptoms of infection. *Complicated UTI* is that which occurs among patients with functionally or anatomically abnormal urinary tracts and is more difficult to manage than other types of UTI. Recurrent infections are categorized as relapse or reinfection. *Relapse* is the recurrence of bacteriuria with the original infecting organism within 2 weeks of cessation of therapy. *Reinfection* is recurrence of bacteriuria with a new organism.

EPIDEMIOLOGY
Among women, the prevalence of bacteriuria is 3% to 7% but rises to 10% to 25% among women older than 60 years. Among men, the prevalence in much lower but increases in later years. Risk factors for women include sexual intercourse, diabetes mellitus, and the use of spermicides for contraception. Risk factors for men include lack of circumcision and homosexual intercourse. Risk factors for both sexes include interruption of normal urine flow, renal calculi, bladder catheterization, and vesicoureteral reflux.

PATHOPHYSIOLOGY AND MICROBIOLOGY
Although infection by the hematogenous route (usually due to *Candida albicans* or *Staphylococcus aureus*) can occur, the ascending route is the most important. Migration of pathogens from the fecal-perineal reservoir causes colonization of the distal urethra, and the infection ascends to the proximal urethra and bladder or through the ureter to the kidney. The interaction between host defenses, including normal urine flow, and the organism determines whether infection occurs.

Urine is normally sterile. About 80% of community-acquired infections are caused by *Escherichia coli*; another 10% can be attributed to other gram-negative organisms, including *Klebsiella* species, *Proteus mirabilis*, and *Enterobacter* species. *P. mirabilis* is of particular importance because it predisposes to the formation of struvite calculi. *Staphylococcus saprophyticus* is the second most common cause of acute cystitis among young, sexually active women. *Enterococcus faecalis* is an important pathogen among the elderly and among patients who have undergone urinary tract instrumentation. *S. aureus* bacteriuria is less common and is frequently caused by bacteremic seeding of the kidneys during hematogenous infection. Nosocomial infection is more often caused by less susceptible strains of Enterobacteriaceae, *Pseudomonas aeruginosa*, yeast, and *E. faecalis*.

CLINICAL FEATURES AND DIFFERENTIAL DIAGNOSIS
Patients with acute cystitis have dysuria, urgency, and frequency sometimes accompanied by suprapubic discomfort or gross hematuria. Fever rarely exceeds 38°C (100.4°F) if infection is confined to the lower tract. The presentation of acute pyelonephritis consists of fever–usually greater than 38.5°C (101.2°F)–chills, and flank pain. Radiation of the pain to the groin suggests ureteral obstruction. Constitutional symptoms include malaise, anorexia, nausea, vomiting, diarrhea, myalgia, and headache. Fewer than 30% of patients have concomitant lower-tract symptoms. Physical examination findings may be normal, but there is often percussion tenderness in the costovertebral angle. Among the elderly, flank tenderness is less common and confusion is more common. The presentation of acute pyelonephritis can be confused with that of conditions such as bacterial pneumonia, myocardial infarction, acute hepatitis, cholecystitis, and acute pelvic inflammatory disease. Early varicella-zoster infection also can mimic renal pain.

LABORATORY STUDIES AND DIAGNOSTIC TESTS
Diagnosis requires positive urine culture results, as defined earlier. The best criterion for infection with gram-negative aerobes among women with symptoms is 10^2 or more bacteria per milliliter with pyuria. Pyuria is the presence of more than 5 white blood cells per high-power field in centrifuged urine sediment. The leukocyte esterase dipstick test is less sensitive than is microscopic examination but is an acceptable, simple alternative. Pretherapy cultures do not improve outcomes among healthy women with acute cystitis and may be unnecessary. Urine Gram stain is useful in predicting the presence of bacteriuria and may narrow the etiologic spectrum. Blood culture results are positive among 20%

INHERITED DISORDERS OF BLOOD COAGULATION

EPIDEMIOLOGY, ETIOLOGY, AND PATHOPHYSIOLOGY

Hemophilia is the most frequent cause of a clinically severe hemorrhagic diathesis. Deficiency in factor VIII causes hemophilia A (classic hemophilia, 80% to 90% of cases) and deficiency of factor IX causes hemophilia B. The genes for both factors are located on the X chromosome, accounting for the X-linked inheritance of the disorders. The specific genetic defect can be either a point mutation or a deletion. The severity of bleeding is directly correlated with the level of residual clotting factor activity; most patients have undetectable levels. Von Willebrand's disease (VWD) is the most common inherited (autosomal dominant pattern) bleeding disorder. It is caused by a deficiency of von Willebrand's factor (VWF), a large plasma glycoprotein that serves as a carrier of factor VIII and as an adhesive bridge between platelets and the vessel wall. There are three subtypes of VWD. Type I and type III are produced by mutations that completely disrupt the function of VWF. The type II variants are usually caused by single amino acid substitutions that cause mildly decreased or altered function, particularly loss of the largest and most functionally active VWF multimers. Type IIB is accompanied by thrombocytopenia.

CLINICAL FEATURES

Hemophilia: The presentations of the two forms of hemophilia are essentially indistinguishable. The diagnosis should be suspected for any man or boy with a severe congenital bleeding disorder and for older men with mild bleeding. The bleeding is primarily localized to soft tissues or joints. The most serious complication is central nervous system hemorrhage, which can follow even minor trauma. Mildly affected patients may show only easy bruising and excessive bleeding after trauma or surgery. The bleeding manifestations have been overshadowed by the profound infectious complications (HIV infection and hepatitis) that have developed among patients who received blood products before 1984.

Von Willebrand's disease: Unlike that in hemophilia, bleeding in VWD is immediate and most prominent from mucosal surfaces. Symptoms usually are mild, except in type III disease. Nosebleeds are a common presentation, as are easy bruising, gastrointestinal bleeding, and excessive menstrual bleeding. Bleeding into joints or deep tissue usually does not occur except in type III WVD, in which severe VWF deficiency engenders a critical deficiency of factor VIII.

LABORATORY FINDINGS

Hemophilia: Bleeding time and prothrombin time (PT) are normal. The activated partial thromboplastin time (aPTT) is at least mildly prolonged. The critical diagnostic tests are specific assays for factor VIII and factor IX procoagulation activity. Levels in excess of 25% generally are associated with normal hemostasis.

Von Willebrand's disease: The PT and aPTT generally are normal, except among patients with type III disease, in whom a marked reduction in factor VIII can lead to a prolongation of the aPTT. The bleeding time typically is prolonged. The standard VWD evaluation consists of three laboratory tests—VWF activity (based on platelet aggregation induced by the antibody ristocetin in the presence of VWF), factor VIII coagulation activity, and VWF antigen level. In typical type I VWD, levels of all substances are similarly decreased to the range of 20% to 50% of normal.

MANAGEMENT

Hemophilia: The foundation is replacement of the missing clotting factor. Because the available products are rapidly changing, consultation with a hemophilia specialist may be helpful. Most patients with newly diagnosed hemophilia are treated with recombinant factor VIII or factor IX, although high cost and limited availability restrict use to short-term management of profuse hemorrhage or prophylactic treatment before a surgical procedure. Unfortunately, inhibitory factor VIII antibodies develop in 10% to 20% of patients. Mild-to-moderate hemophilia A sometimes can be successfully managed with desmopressin (DDAVP), which can produce a two- to fivefold increase in factor VIII that lasts for several hours. The fibrinolytic inhibitor ϵ-aminocaproic acid can be effective in the control of dental or superficial bleeding.

Von Willebrand's disease: Desmopressin can produce a two- to threefold increase in plasma levels of VWF and factor VIII that can last for 4 to 12 hours. It can be administered intravenously or in a nasal spray. Use of this agent is relatively contraindicated in type IIB VWD, because it can exacerbate thrombocytopenia. Patients with severe type III VWD often need treatment with factor replacement. Because a recombinant VWF product is not currently available, treatment is limited to selected factor VIII concentrates prepared from pooled plasma that contain large amounts of VWF. Patients also can be treated with fresh frozen plasma or cryoprecipitate, although use of these products carries risk of infection. ϵ-Aminocaproic acid can be effective in the control of dental or mucosal bleeding. Estrogen and oral contraceptives increase VWF levels and are particularly useful in managing menorrhagia.

Chapter 237

APPROACH TO THE PATIENT WITH LEUKOCYTOSIS

DEFINITIONS

Leukocytosis is elevation of the white blood cell (WBC) count above the normal range. An elevated total WBC count can be attributed to an elevation in one or more of the individual classes of leukocytes: neutrophils (more than approximately 8,000 cells per microliter), eosinophils (more than 450 cells per microliter), basophils (more than 100 cells per microliter), monocytes (more than 1,000 cells per microliter), and lymphocytes (more than 6,000 cells per microliter). Each of these cell types makes an important contribution to host defense and repair. The degree of elevation is important; normal ranges are really the mean and two units of standard deviation in a large population sampling. The higher the WBC count, the less likely it is that it is a normal gaussian variation.

DIFFERENTIAL DIAGNOSIS

The differential diagnosis of leukocytosis depends on the class of leukocyte affected and the duration of the elevation, if that can be determined. The causes of neutrophilia and eosinophilia are listed in Tables 216.1 and 216.2. Basophilia is rare and should prompt consideration of the existence of myeloproliferative disease, such as chronic myelogenous leukemia (CML) or polycythemia vera, and many of the disorders associated with eosinophilia. Monocytosis is most often a sign of acute bacterial, viral, protozoan, or rickettsial infection. Monocytosis without neutrophilia occurs especially with tuberculosis, syphilis, brucellosis, and typhoid fever. Lymphocytosis most commonly occurs with acute viral infection. However, persistent lymphocytosis is more commonly a sign of clonal lymphoproliferative disease, especially chronic lymphocytic lymphoma (CLL), than of infection.

HISTORY AND PHYSICAL EXAMINATION

Leukocytosis itself usually is asymptomatic, and the clinical presentation is determined instead by the underlying etiologic factors. Signs and symptoms of infection, inflammatory disease, and hematologic malignant disease are particularly relevant.

DIAGNOSTIC EVALUATION

The findings depend on the condition underlying the leukocytosis. The leukocyte alkaline phosphatase score is useful in evaluating persistent neutrophilia. The result is near zero in CML but is normal to elevated in reactive, secondary neutrophilia and polycythemia vera. If the result is low, examination of a bone marrow aspirate may detect the t(9:22) translocation associated with CML. Unexplained, persistent basophilia or monocytosis should prompt bone marrow aspiration for morphologic and karyotyping studies. The blood smear of a patient with persistent lymphocytosis may reveal smudge cells, a sign of B-cell CLL, or large lymphocytes with fine granules, a sign of T-cell CLL. Flow cytometric analysis of the blood may show patterns of lymphocyte cell surface proteins diagnostic of either form of CLL.

MANAGEMENT

The underlying disease should be managed, if possible.

Chapter 216

APPROACH TO THE PATIENT WITH LYMPHADENOPATHY

PATHOPHYSIOLOGY

Lymph node enlargement may be caused by infiltration of inflammatory cells into the lymph node (infection), malignant transformation and proliferation of cells indigenous to the node (lymphoma), infiltration of the node by metastatic malignant cells (leukemia and cancer of epithelial and sarcomatous origin), or accumulation of benign cells or substances in the node parenchyma (lipid-storage disease and amyloidosis).

HISTORY AND PHYSICAL EXAMINATION

Age: Among persons younger than 30 years, most cases are benign and caused by infection. Among patients older than 50 years, only 40% of cases are benign, so malignancy must be excluded.

Other symptoms and signs: Fever is common with infection and malignant disease. Symptoms and signs of localized infection may be present. Night sweats or weight loss suggest lymphoma, HIV infection, or tuberculosis.

Characteristics of nodes: In acute infection, the nodes may be tender, asymmetric, or matted. In chronic infection, they may be less tender and more symmetric. In lymphoma, they often are large, rubbery, and nontender. Metastatic carcinoma produces hard, fixed, asymmetric nodes.

Location of nodes: See Table 201.1.

Examination of spleen: Tender enlargement occurs in mononucleosis. Lymphoma, leukemia, lipid storage disease, and amyloidosis also may cause splenomegaly.

DIAGNOSTIC TESTS

There is no routine battery of laboratory tests. Complete blood cell count and blood smear may be helpful when infection or malignant disease is suspected. Monospot, throat culture, serologic testing for HIV, and autoimmune antibody testing are used in appropriate settings. Serologic titers for cytomegalovirus or toxoplasmosis may be helpful. Radiographs often are unnecessary in the presence of superficial lymphadenopathy. Chest radiographs and computed tomography of the chest, abdomen, and pelvis reveal deeper nodes and are especially useful if lymphoma is suspected. Aspiration is particularly useful in diagnosing metastatic carcinoma or infectious lymphadenitis but does not provide tissue for the histopathologic review critical in classification of lymphoma. Biopsy is appropriate for (a) persistent, unexplained, localized or generalized lymphadenopathy, especially if the node is firm, rubbery, or fixed; (b) lymphadenopathy accompanied by fevers, night sweats, and weight loss but no clear infectious source; or (c) staging for patients with known malignant disease. The largest accessible node should be selected. Biopsy provides enough information for diagnosis in only about 50% of cases. When biopsy does not provide enough diagnostic information, the patient must be observed closely with repeated biopsy to find persistent lymphadenopathy and repeated examination to find constitutional symptoms.

DIFFERENTIAL DIAGNOSIS

See Table 201.3.

MANAGEMENT

If a specific infection is suspected, a period of observation or trial of antimicrobial therapy may be instituted. Empiric use of antibiotics or glucocorticoids should be avoided. HIV testing should be considered for those with persistent generalized lymphadenopathy. If nodes have characteristics that suggest malignancy or if unexplained lymphadenopathy persists, biopsy should be performed. However, biopsy should be avoided in the evaluation of patients who may have infectious mononucleosis, because the pathologic findings may mimic those of malignant lymphoma.

Chapter 201

◼ MULTIPLE MYELOMA

DEFINITION

Multiple myeloma (MM) is a malignant disease of plasma cells. It is associated with the production of monoclonal immunoglobulin (M protein).

EPIDEMIOLOGY

The annual incidence of MM in the United States is 3 to 4 cases per 100,000 persons. The median age at diagnosis is 75 years. Blacks have twice the risk of whites and men twice the risk of women. The cause is unknown.

CLINICAL FINDINGS

Most patients have anemia, and many have pallor, fatigue, and dyspnea. Most also have lytic, punched-out bone lesions and pain. In most instances the pain

ceases when the patient is at rest. Bone tenderness or pathologic fractures may occur, especially in the vertebrae, ribs, and sternum. About 5% of patients have spinal cord compression during the course of disease. Symptoms and signs include unremitting back pain, especially radicular pain, unilateral or bilateral numbness of the lower extremities, paresis or paralysis, urinary or bowel incontinence, hyperreflexia, and pathologic reflexes. Hypercalcemia may cause anorexia, somnolence, nausea, vomiting, constipation, or dehydration. Recurrent infection with encapsulated organisms occurs among about 10% of patients, owing to decreased production of polyclonal antibody. Infection with gram-negative pathogens is common if there is neutropenia. Hypercalcemia and the production of nephrotoxic light chains (Bence Jones proteinuria) often lead to renal impairment. Bleeding generally occurs late in the disease and is caused by thrombocytopenia and interference of the M protein with clotting factors. Amyloidosis, usually asymptomatic, complicates as many as 10% of cases.

LABORATORY STUDIES

Serum and urine immunoelectrophoresis always is performed. A monoclonal protein is present in the serum of 85% of patients and in the urine of 75%. About 1% to 2% have neither and therefore have nonsecretory disease. A skeletal radiographic survey shows characteristic lytic lesions in almost 70% of patients (bone scintigraphy is less reliable). Magnetic resonance imaging or computed tomography of suspected areas may be needed to demonstrate bone lesions. Hypercalcemia and renal insufficiency occur among 10% to 15% of patients. One-half have an elevated β_2-microglobulin level.

DIAGNOSIS AND STAGING

Many disorders are associated with monoclonal gammopathy, including MM, monoclonal gammopathy of undetermined significance (MGUS), primary amyloidosis, and cryoglobulinemia. For a patient with no symptoms and less than 2 g per deciliter of monoclonal protein, the most likely diagnosis is MGUS. The diagnostic criteria for MM are (a) M protein in the serum or urine, (b) more than 10% plasma cells in the marrow aspirate, and (c) demonstration of bone lesions, anemia, hypercalcemia, or renal failure. Stage is based on hemoglobin concentration, calcium level, the presence or absence of bone lesions or renal insufficiency, and the quantities of monoclonal immunoglobulin in the blood and urine. The level of β_2-microglobulin also is predictive of outcome.

PROGNOSIS AND MANAGEMENT

The typical course lasts 3 to 4 years, but there is a wide variation in survival periods. The cause of death usually is infection or bleeding. The goal of therapy is control, not cure. Therapy with melphalan and prednisone produces a response for about 50% of patients. Combination chemotherapy may be advantageous for rapidly lowering tumor burden but has not been shown to increase survival time. Interferon can prolong the plateau phase after discontinuation of chemotherapy but also fails to improve survival time. Peripheral stem cell transplantation is gaining prominence, especially for younger, healthier patients. Radiation therapy is used for bone lesions that pose a threat to life or that may cause long-term disability. Antibiotic prophylaxis with trimethoprim-sulfamethoxazole or ciprofloxacin may improve outcome. Renal function may be preserved by means of minimizing risk of infection, dehydration, and exposure to contrast dyes and nephrotoxic antibiotics. Hypercalcemia should be controlled.

Chapter 234

◼ NON-HODGKIN'S LYMPHOMA

DEFINITION AND PATHOPHYSIOLOGY

Non-Hodgkin's lymphoma (NHL) is a heterogeneous group of malignant tumors that begin as a clonal malignant expansion of B or T lymphocytes. NHL is caused by transformation of normal lymphoid cells at various stages of differentiation. Numerous chromosomal translocations have been found.

EPIDEMIOLOGY AND ETIOLOGY

NHL is the fifth most common cause of cancer death in the United States. The incidence increases with age, although Burkitt's and lymphoblastic lymphoma are more common among children. There is an association with HIV infection, chronic immunosuppressive therapy, certain autoimmune diseases (such as Hashimoto's thyroiditis and Sjögren's syndrome), and infection with HTLV-1, Epstein–Barr virus, and *Helicobacter pylori*. Most cases have no identifiable etiologic factor.

CLASSIFICATION

The Working Formulation (Table 233.1) classifies NHL into three prognostic grades based on the appearance of the disease within the node (follicular versus diffuse) and on the principal size of the lymphoma cells (small, cleaved cells versus large, noncleaved cells versus mixed populations). A Revised European–American Classification is gaining favor. Follicular lymphoma (low grade) accounts for 30% to 40% of cases.

CLINICAL FINDINGS

NHL generally manifests as progressive lymphadenopathy. Patients may have constitutional symptoms (fever, night sweats, unexplained weight loss), fatigue, early satiety due to splenomegaly, or regional pain from enlarging tumor masses. Bone marrow involvement may produce anemia, thrombocytopenia, or predisposition to atypical or recurrent infection. Intermediate- and high-grade NHL more often is associated with rapidly progressive (weeks or months) lymphadenopathy, constitutional symptoms, and central nervous system (CNS) involvement.

LABORATORY STUDIES, DIAGNOSTIC TESTS, AND STAGING

The diagnosis is made by means of biopsy. Clinicians who suspect lymphoma should inform the pathologist so that special studies can be added to routine histologic examination. Histologic subtype determines the type and speed of staging procedures. Baseline studies should include a complete blood cell count, liver and renal chemical analysis, and measurement of calcium, lactate dehydrogenase (LDH), and β_2 microglobulin. The evaluation also usually includes bone marrow biopsy and computed tomography of the chest, abdomen, and pelvis. Patients with high-grade lymphoma or CNS symptoms should undergo diagnostic lumbar puncture. The Ann Arbor staging system is used (see Table 3). Spread is hematogenous and unpredictable.

PROGNOSIS AND MANAGEMENT

Adverse outcome is associated with advanced age, the presence of systemic symptoms, CNS or marrow involvement, elevated LDH and β_2 microglobulin levels, and certain cytogenetic markers. Histologic type and stage also are important. The International Prognostic Index was devised to stratify patients by risk and to guide choice of therapy.

Low grade: Although the course is generally indolent, transformation to higher-grade illness occurs at a rate of about 6% per year. Localized disease is managed with radiation therapy; about 50% of patients are disease-free at 10 years. Stage III or IV disease is incurable with standard therapy; watchful waiting and single-agent or combination chemotherapeutic regimens can be used. Autologous stem cell transplantation and monoclonal antibodies have been used for refractory or relapse cases.

Intermediate grade: Combination chemotherapy (most commonly CHOP) can be curative. Radiation therapy can be added for localized disease. Localized disease has 70% to 80% long-term disease-free survival rate. Advanced-stage disease has a 5-year survival rate of 30% to 50%.

High grade: Intensive combination regimens produce the best results. Complete responses occur among 20% to 30% of patients, but less than 5% of patients survive long term. CNS prophylaxis (intrathecal chemotherapy and craniospinal irradiation) is routine. If the prognostic score is poor, autologous stem cell transplantation can be used as consolidation therapy.

Chapter 233

POLYCYTHEMIA VERA

DEFINITIONS AND EPIDEMIOLOGY

Polycythemia vera (PV), a myeloproliferative disorder, is autonomous clonal proliferation of multipotential stem cells that results in generalized hyperplasia of the bone marrow, increased production of red blood cells (RBCs), and an absolute increase in the number of circulating RBCs. PV is most often diagnosed among persons between 50 and 70 years of age. There is a slight male predominance.

CLINICAL FEATURES AND COURSE OF DISEASE

The preerythocytotic phase of PV often is unrecognized. RBC mass is normal, and the only abnormalities may be pruritus after bathing or splenomegaly. This phase lasts for a few months to 1 to 2 years. The erythrocytotic phase often is first recognized when the patient sustains an occlusive arterial or venous lesion, such as cerebral or myocardial infarction or ischemia, portal venous obstruction, or peripheral venous thrombosis. The expanded RBC mass produces symptoms of hyperviscosity such as headaches, dizziness, and visual disturbances. Plethora and conjunctival or oral mucosal suffusion are common. Some patients have epistaxis, ecchymosis, or gastrointestinal or genitourinary hemorrhage. Gastrointestinal symptoms and peptic ulcer disease are frequent. Episodes of acute gout associated with overproduction of urate occur among about 5% of patients. The most common physical finding is splenomegaly, which occurs among almost 90% of these patients. Hepatomegaly occurs among about half. The erythrocytotic phase may last 5 to 10 years if treatment is given.

A proliferative phase follows and usually is characterized by thrombocytosis, leukocytosis, and increasing splenomegaly. It usually lasts a few years. Evolution into the postpolycythemic myeloid metaplasia phase is gradual and occurs among 20% of patients. Asthenia is the most common symptom. Weight loss, generalized wasting, myelofibrosis, and cytopenia develop. Most patients with disease in this phase have a shortened survival period, dying either of complications or of evolution to acute nonlymphocytic leukemia.

LABORATORY STUDIES AND DIAGNOSTIC TESTS

PV usually is recognized by an increase in RBC count, hemoglobin concentration, and hematocrit. Early in the disease, the RBCs are of normal size. Because mucosal bleeding is common, iron deficiency may develop and lead to microcytosis and normalization of the RBC count. Thrombocytosis and increased numbers of granulocytes and basophils are common. There is an increase in leukocyte alkaline phosphate activity and in serum levels of vitamin B_{12} (from augmented production of cobalamin-binding proteins). The bone marrow is diffusely hypercellular, with an increase in all hematopoietic elements but without pathognomonic histologic changes. In later phases, marrow fibrosis and pancytopenia develop. Diagnostic criteria are presented in Table 231.1.

PROGNOSIS AND MANAGEMENT

The median survival rate improves with therapy from 18 months to 9 to 14 years. In the preerythrocytotic phase, therapy with H_1 and H_2 blockers may ameliorate pruritus. During the erythrocytotic phase, phlebotomy is the treatment of choice. Because the likelihood of thrombotic events increases during the first 2 to 3 years of phlebotomy treatment, treatment with hydroxyurea or recombinant interferon-alfa (rIFN-α) often is added. Low-dose aspirin may be beneficial. Myelosuppressive therapy is indicated for young patients requiring phlebotomy of more than 6 units per year or for anyone with features of the proliferative phase, such as thrombocytosis or splenomegaly. Hydroxyurea is the drug of choice, and rIFN-α is emerging as an alternative. Anagrelide is particularly effective in improving thrombocytosis. Therapy during the postpolycythemic myeloid metaplasia phase is supportive. Erythropoietin has reduced transfusion requirements. Recurrent painful splenic infarctions or symptomatic congestive splenomegaly may necessitate splenectomy. Transition to leukemia is associated with a poor response to therapy.

Chapter 231

PROSTATE CANCER

DEFINITION

Prostate cancer generally refers to adenocarcinoma of the prostate, which accounts for more than 98% of all cases of prostate cancer.

INCIDENCE AND EPIDEMIOLOGY

Prostate cancer is the most common cancer among men and the second leading cause of cancer-related deaths of men. In 1998, an estimated 184,500 new cases were diagnosed. Prevalence increases with age.

ETIOLOGY

A hereditary risk has been demonstrated; incidence varies with race and ethnic background (highest for African Americans). Vasectomy, smoking, infection, and level of sexual activity are not considered risk factors. Prostate cancer is an androgen-sensitive disease.

PATHOGENESIS AND PATHOPHYSIOLOGY

The prostate is situated at the base of the bladder. Most tumors originate in the peripheral zone. The prominent grading system is that of Gleason (scores from 2 to 10). It reflects aberrations in glandular architecture. Patients with higher Gleason scores have shorter survival periods. Staging paradigms include the American (ABCD) and tumor–node–metastasis (TNM) systems; the latter is more accurate. The most common site of distant metastasis is bone. The spine is most commonly affected, and the metastases generally are osteoblastic.

CLINICAL FINDINGS

Localized prostate cancer is asymptomatic. Urinary symptoms, such as frequency, dysuria, or decreased force, can occur but are much more common with benign prostatic hyperplasia. Microscopic or gross hematuria is more representative of a urinary tract infection, urinary tract stones, or a tumor of the bladder or kidney. Metastatic disease can cause bone pain, weight loss, or fatigue. Approximately 75% of patients have clinically localized disease at diagnosis, mainly owing to the use of measurement of prostate-specific antigen (PSA) as a screening tool. There are few physical findings. Digital rectal examination is not a sufficiently sensitive or specific test for detection.

LABORATORY FINDINGS

Levels of prostate-specific antigen: PSA determination has taken a central role in the diagnosis of prostate cancer. PSA is not specific to prostate cancer, however. Elevations can occur with benign prostatic hyperplasia and in infected normal tissue. A normal value of 4.0 ng per milliliter has been established, but a level from 4 to 10 ng per milliliter has only a 20% chance of being associated with prostate cancer. Conversely, 20% to 35% of clinically detectable prostate cancers are associated with a PSA level less than 4.0 ng per milliliter. A number of techniques for improving the test characteristics of PSA measurement have been proposed, including age-specific normal ranges, determination of the PSA level per unit volume of prostatic tissue, and measurement of the rate of change in PSA levels over time. Once prostate cancer is diagnosed, PSA measurements are an excellent way to monitor response to therapy and detect treatment failure. *Other studies:* The diagnosis is almost always made by means of transrectal ultrasound (TRUS)–guided needle biopsy. A bone scan is the most sensitive method to detect osseous metastasis, but abnormal findings may reflect injury or arthritis. Computed tomography (CT) of the pelvis depicts regional lymphadenopathy. For patients with a PSA level less than 10 ng per milliliter, the diagnostic yield of an evaluation for metastasis, which includes CT and a bone scan, is very low.

PROGNOSIS AND MANAGEMENT

Localized disease: Without treatment, the average survival period for stage A and B disease is 8 to 10 years. Radical prostatectomy is considered a standard of care for men younger than 70 years who have an expected survival time of more than 10 years. The principal morbidities are urinary incontinence (less than 5%) and erectile dysfunction (more than 50%). Patients with localized disease have a 5-year disease-free survival rate of 95%. External beam radiation is considered an equivalent treatment and is the preferred therapy for clinical stage C or T3 disease. Patients older than 70 years are commonly referred for radiation therapy. Complications include erectile dysfunction (20% to 80%), rectal bleeding or diarrhea (less than 5%), and urinary incontinence (less than 1%). Active observation, with androgen ablation reserved for palliative use at the time of progression, is a reasonable option for patients with a low-grade tumor or less than a 10-year expected survival period.
Metastatic disease: Patients with disease in the lymph nodes but no osseous disease are generally treated with some form of androgen ablation. Pelvic irradiation often is used to treat younger patients. The 5-year overall survival rate is 70% to 85%. Patients with distant metastatic disease usually are treated with androgen deprivation, which results in tumor regression in more than 80% of cases. It is accomplished either through surgical castration or the administration of luteinizing hormone–releasing hormone agonists (such as leuprolide or goserelin), with or without an anti-androgen such as flutamide. Chemotherapy has previously been unsuccessful in the management of hormone-refractory prostate cancer, although recent results are encouraging.

Chapter 223

■ SICKLE CELL DISEASE

DEFINITIONS AND ETIOLOGY

Sickle cell disease (SCD) is a hereditary hemoglobin disorder in which sickling of red blood cells (RBCs) causes chronic hemolytic anemia, vascular occlusion, and progressive organ damage. In SCD, both of the β-globin chains have a substitution of valine for glutamic acid in the sixth position. Sickle cell trait occurs when there is one normal gene and one sickle cell gene. Hybrid types of hemoglobinopathy exist that combines one sickle cell gene with either a hemoglobin C gene (SC disease) or a gene for β-thalassemia (sickle β-thalassemia).

EPIDEMIOLOGY

The estimated frequency among newborn African Americans is 1 in 600. Because persons with sickle cell trait have a greater chance of surviving severe malaria, the distribution of the sickle cell gene throughout the world parallels that of *Plasmodium falciparum.*

PATHOPHYSIOLOGY

The mutation in the β-globin chain causes deoxygenated hemoglobin to polymerize, making it relatively insoluble and rigid. The kidney, spleen, retina, and bone marrow often are affected because conditions are sufficiently hypoxic and acidotic to induce sickling.

CLINICAL FEATURES

The clinical manifestations are those of anemia and vaso-occlusion. The anemia includes chronic hemolysis, aplastic crisis, and splenic sequestration. The vaso-occlusive complications (called *crises*) include pain and organ impairment, such as splenic infarction, stroke, aseptic necrosis of the hip, and acute chest syndrome. Almost every organ system can be affected (Table 245.1).

LABORATORY TESTS AND DIAGNOSTIC STUDIES

Laboratory evaluation for SCD includes examination of the peripheral blood smear, which demonstrates sickle cells. The presence of nuclear remnants (Howell–Jolly bodies) within the red cell indicates functional asplenia. The mean corpuscular volume is high because of the presence of young red blood cells. The numbers of granulocytes and platelets increases. Definitive diagnosis can be made with hemoglobin electrophoresis and a solubility test (which confirms that a hemoglobin migrating in the S position on electrophoresis is S and not D or G).

PROGNOSIS AND MANAGEMENT

Among patients receiving care in designated SCD programs, 50% are alive at 45 years of age. Therapy should first be directed at the elimination of hypertonicity, dehydration, acidosis, and hypoxemia. RBC transfusions are indicated for cardiac decompensation, severe acute anemia, erythroid hypoplasia with a hemoglobin concentration less than 5.0 g per deciliter, stroke and transient ischemic attacks, multiorgan failure syndrome, acute chest syndrome, and preoperative preparation for surgery. Transfusions should not be used in the management of chronic steady-state anemia, acute painful episodes, or infection. Hydroxyurea can increase fetal hemoglobin level and decrease the frequency of painful crises. Bone marrow transplantation and gene therapy are under investigation.

Painful crises should be managed with adequate analgesia once surgical causes have been excluded. Severe pain necessitates parenteral administration of morphine, preferably with patient-controlled methods. With improvement, the dose and route of administration can be modified. Because of the frequency and consequences of bacteremia, unexplained fever should be considered an emergency. Prompt antibiotic therapy is required while the diagnostic evaluation is undertaken. The presence of encapsulated organisms must be considered strongly if a patient has functional asplenia.

Chapter 245

■ APPROACH TO THE PATIENT WITH SPLENOMEGALY

PATHOPHYSIOLOGY

The spleen is the largest lymphoid organ in the body. It consists of a fibrous capsule and radiating fibrous trabeculae that enclose the white and red pulp.

Splenomegaly can be caused by infiltration of the organ by reactive lymphoid cells or proliferating macrophages (infection or inflammation), neoplastic cells (hematologic malignant disease), or abnormal material (amyloidosis, Gaucher's disease). Vascular congestion or space-occupying lesions also can cause splenomegaly. Splenomegaly often is associated with hypersplenism, a pathologic increase in the normal splenic sequestration and destruction of circulating blood elements.

DIFFERENTIAL DIAGNOSIS

Systemic infections such as mononucleosis are the most common cause of moderate and transient splenomegaly. Massive splenomegaly usually is caused by lymphoma or a myeloproliferative disorder (Table 202.1).

HISTORY AND PHYSICAL EXAMINATION

The presentation depends on the underlying disease. The most common symptom directly related to the spleen is pain in the left upper quadrant from capsular stretching or splenic infarction. The patient also may have early satiety. The interview should be focused on symptoms and predispositions that suggest infectious or hematologic malignant disease. If a patient has a long history of splenomegaly, a neoplastic process often is implicated; infectious splenomegaly more commonly develops over days. A history of alcoholism or previous liver disease suggests portal hypertension from hepatic cirrhosis. The examination reveals evidence of splenomegaly. The larger the spleen, the greater is the likelihood of a serious underlying medical problem. As the organ enlarges, dullness may be detected at percussion of the ninth intercostal space in the left anterior axillary line. Palpation of the spleen during inspiration usually signifies enlargement. However, patients can have marked splenomegaly in the absence of a palpable spleen. The enlarged spleen generally is not tender in infiltrative and malignant diseases. It may be tender in the presence of acute infection. Examination for lymphadenopathy and chronic liver disease is particularly important.

DIAGNOSTIC TESTS

A palpable spleen in an adult always necessitates evaluation. Testing of the spleen itself often is unnecessary, but computed tomography, magnetic resonance imaging, ultrasonography, and radioisotope scanning all have a place in determining shape, size, and the presence of parenchymal abnormalities. The most valuable laboratory tests are the complete blood cell count (hypersplenism causes cytopenia), blood smear, and measurement of liver enzymes. For patients with fever, blood cultures and specific viral serologic tests often are useful. Bone marrow aspiration and biopsy are often useful in the diagnosis of malignant disease, lipid storage disorders, and disseminated fungal and mycobacterial infection. Biopsy of enlarged lymph nodes often discloses the diagnosis.

MANAGEMENT

Medical indications for splenectomy include two broad categories—diagnostic splenectomy and splenectomy to alleviate the consequences of splenomegaly, chiefly cytopenia. The main complication is the risk of serious infection, particularly by encapsulated bacterial organisms such as *Streptococcus pneumoniae*, *Neisseria meningitidis*, and *Haemophilus influenzae*. All patients undergoing splenectomy should receive vaccinations against these organisms at least 10 days before the procedure, if possible.

Chapter 203

■ APPROACH TO THE PATIENT WITH THROMBOCYTOPENIA

DEFINITIONS

Thrombocytopenia is a reduction in the number of circulating platelets. Automated blood counting has allowed frequent detection of mild to moderate thrombocytopenia.

PATHOPHYSIOLOGY AND DIFFERENTIAL DIAGNOSIS

Thrombocytopenia develops when there is a profound dysequilibrium between platelet production, distribution, and destruction. Impairment of production usually is part of a multilineage process and may be congenital or acquired (Table 213.1). Any disorder that causes splenomegaly increases splenic sequestration of platelets. Some of these processes also accelerate splenic destruction of platelets.

Platelet destruction has an immunologic or a nonimmunologic basis (Table 213.2). The differential diagnosis of simultaneous thrombosis and thrombocytopenia includes heparin-induced thrombocytopenia, thrombotic thrombocytopenic purpura (TTP), hemolytic-uremic syndrome (HUS), systemic lupus erythematosus, and disseminated intravascular coagulation.

HISTORY AND PHYSICAL EXAMINATION

Spontaneous bleeding is rare at platelet counts more than 30,000 per microliter. As counts decrease to less than 20,000 per microliter, patients may have easy bruisability, gingival bleeding after brushing, menorrhagia, and epistaxis. As counts decrease to less than 5,000 per microliter, persistent gastrointestinal bleeding and spontaneous intracranial hemorrhage may occur. Evidence of chronicity may be obtained from prior platelet counts or a history of excessive bleeding. Attention should be given to medications, alcohol use, recent infections, and family history. Symptoms and signs of a multisystem disorder may be elicited. Examination should include a thorough eye examination, stool testing for occult blood, and special attention to the liver, spleen, and lymphatic tissue.

LABORATORY STUDIES AND DIAGNOSTIC TESTS

No single paradigm fits all cases. A complete blood cell count and peripheral blood smear should be routinely performed, however. Platelet clumping can cause underestimation of the actual count and can be caused by EDTA, the anticoagulant in which blood is routinely collected. Examination of the blood smear shows the clumps. The smear also may provide clues such as schistocytes (in HUS and TTP), hypersegmented neutrophils (megaloblastic anemia), and leukemic cells. Mean platelet volume commonly is increased in processes that accelerate peripheral destruction of platelets. The utility of testing for antibodies to platelet glycoproteins is not well established. Bone marrow aspiration and biopsy may be indicated when the cause remains uncertain.

MANAGEMENT

If possible, the underlying disease should be managed. The risk of bleeding may be reduced by avoidance of trauma, control of medical problems that predispose to bleeding (hypertension, peptic ulcer disease), and avoidance of medications that interfere with platelet function (such as aspirin). For patients with active bleeding, platelet transfusion to achieve a level of at least 20,000 cells per microliter is indicated. Counts of 50,000 cells per microliter to 100,000 cells per microliter generally are required for surgical procedures. For patients in clinically stable condition who do not need an invasive procedure, there is no absolute level of thrombocytopenia at which a platelet transfusion is mandatory. Platelet transfusion is associated with a higher risk of allergic, pyogenic, and infectious complications than is red blood cell transfusion; moreover, in about 40% of patients alloantibodies develop that ultimately render transfusions (even of HLA-matched platelets) futile. Platelet transfusions are contraindicated in TTP and HUS in the absence of severe hemorrhage, because they can worsen the thrombosis.

Chapter 217

■ APPROACH TO THE PATIENT WITH THROMBOSIS AND PULMONARY EMBOLISM

PRESENTATION AND ETIOLOGY

Thrombosis is among the most common problems encountered by physicians. Arterial thrombosis is principally a complication of arteriosclerosis and most often presents with coronary ischemia and as cerebrovascular and peripheral vascular disease. Other conditions associated with arterial thrombosis include homozygous and heterozygous homocysteinemia, arteritis, myeloproliferative disorders, thrombotic thrombocytopenic purpura (TTP), heparin-induced thrombocytopenia, and the antiphospholipid antibody syndrome. Venous thrombosis occurs most often in the veins of the lower extremities, where it presents with pain and swelling. Venous thrombi may also dislodge and cause pulmonary embolism (PE). Inherited disorders predisposing to venous thrombosis include deficiencies of antithrombin III, protein C, protein S, and plasminogen; factor V Leiden; prothrombin G20210A; homocysteinemia; and dysfibrinogenemia. Acquired disorders that increase the risk of venous thrombosis include malignancy, immobilization, pregnancy, oral contraceptive and estrogen use, nephrotic syndrome, antiphospholipid antibody syndrome, and paroxysmal nocturnal hemoglobinuria.

Pathophysiology:

Arterial thrombi are composed primarily of aggregated platelets (white thrombi) and form when the endothelial lining of the artery is breached, allowing platelets to interact with subendothelial connective tissue. Thrombi may form on the surface of an atherosclerotic plaque when its surface is denuded or disrupted and platelets are exposed to thrombogenic material in the plaque interior. Venous thrombi are composed primarily of fibrin and trapped RBCs (red thrombi). Venous thrombi can form in regions of venous stasis, especially when coagulability is enhanced by conditions such as those listed earlier.

History and Physical Examination:

Arterial thrombi: When arterial thombosis complicates a myeloproliferative disorder such as polycythemia rubra vera or essential thrombocytosis, it is likely to occur in arteries involved by atherosclerosis and thus lead to acute MI or stroke. In contrast, the hyaline thrombi characteristic of TTP obstruct normal arterioles.

Venous thrombi: The symptoms result from obstruction of venous outflow and from accompanying local inflammation. Most often, symptomatic deep venous thrombosis (DVT) presents as calf discomfort or tenderness or as unexplained leg edema. Larger thrombi rarely lyse completely and may instead organize and recanalize. The resultant venous obstruction and venous valve destruction can produce the post-phlebitic syndrome of chronic calf pain associated with brawny edema, hyperpigmentation, induration, and ulceration of the lower leg. Less commonly, significant thrombosis can also involve the axillary, mesenteric, hepatic, renal, and cerebral veins. Hepatic vein thrombosis (Budd-Chiari syndrome) is a feature of the myeloproliferative disorders and paroxysmal nocturnal hemoglobinuria. Acute and chronic renal vein thrombosis occurs in the nephrotic syndrome, especially that associated with membranous glomerulonephritis.

Pulmonary embolism: Venous thrombi that lead to PE are almost invariably located in the proximal veins of the legs, but may begin as calf vein thrombi that extend proximally. Patients with PE most often complain of dyspnea, pleuritic chest pain, or hemoptysis; the examination most commonly reveals tachypnea or tachycardia. Of note, asymptomatic DVT has been found in 70% of patients with confirmed PE and asymptomatic PE has been detected in about 50% of patients with proximal DVT.

Differential Diagnosis:

Conditions confused with DVT of the legs include muscle strains and tears, swelling related to paralysis, lymphatic obstruction, Baker's cyst, cellulitis, internal derangements of the knee, and the postphlebitic syndrome. The symptoms of PE are nonspecific; the differential diagnosis includes panic attacks and a broad range of cardiopulmonary conditions.

Diagnostic Evaluation:

Venous thrombi: A diagnosis of DVT is difficult on clinical grounds alone and should be based on objective tests. The standard is venogram, but it is invasive and associated with a 2%-3% incidence of chemical phlebitis. Real-time B-mode ultrasonography is reported to be 97% sensitive and specific for proximal DVT in symptomatic patients. The most sensitive finding is failure of a vein to collapse under gentle pressure. The test is not as sensitive for calf vein or pelvic vein thrombi or for thrombi in asymptomatic patients. Nevertheless, most recent studies suggest that it is safe to withhold anticoagulant therapy in the face of normal serial real-time B-mode ultrasound examinations. Impedance plethysmography (IPG) measures changes in electrical impedence in the calf following deflation of a pressure cuff around the thigh; it detects impairment in venous outflow from the leg. It is far less sensitive than previously thought and cannot be recommended as a test to rule out DVT. The roles of plasma D-dimer levels, CT, and magnetic resonance venography remain to be determined.

Pulmonary embolism: Unless contraindicated, anticoagulation should be initiated while the results of the diagnostic evaluation are pending. The CXR may show non-specific findings of hemidiaphragmatic elevation, small pleural effusions, or ill-defined parenchymal infiltrates. The ABG usually reveals widening of the alveolar-to-arterial oxygen gradient, often with a low PO_2. The ECG most often shows tachycardia with nonspecific ST segment and T-wave changes. The most commonly used initial initial diagnostic test for PE is ventilation and perfusion lung scanning (V/Q scans). PE is highly unlikely if the scans are entirely normal. In contrast, PE is very likely if the scans show a normal ventilation pattern with two or more large perfusion defects (>25% of an anatomic lung segment). Unfortunately, most patients with suspected PE have abnormal but non-diagnostic scans and require further testing. Figure 378.2 shows a step-wise initial diagnostic approach that incorporates clinical probability, V/Q scans, and lower extremity ultrasound studies. Pulmonary arteriography is considered the diagnostic gold standard, but is expensive, invasive, and not always available. Recently, spiral CT scanning has shown promise in the diagnosis of PE, particularly emboli that lodge in segmental or larger pulmonary vessels.

Evaluation for Hypercoagulability:

Arterial thrombi: Because most cases of arterial thrombosis result from atherosclerosis, and not from abnormalities of platelet function or blood coagulation, studies should focus on the extent of the atherosclerosis and on factors that might contribute to its progression. When arterial thrombosis occurs in the absence of significant atherosclerosis, hemostatic abnormalities should be sought.

Venous thromboembolism: Because tests to detect specific causes of thrombosis are expensive and are unlikely to change the management of patients following the first episode of thrombosis, such testing should be restricted to patients with recurrent thrombosis, unless the patient has a family history strongly suggestive of a hereditary disorder. It is important to remember that measurement of proteins associated with familial thrombosis (antithrombin III, proteins C and S) may not be reliable until several weeks after an acute thrombotic episode and may be affected by warfarin therapy (proteins C and S are vitamin K-dependent). On occasion, venous thrombosis is a presenting symptom of malignancy, particularly when patients have mucin-producing carcinomas (Trousseau's syndrome). Malignancy has been found in 3%-10% of patients presenting with venous thrombosis and in 7%-11% of patients during the subsequent 6-24 months. It is found most often in patients without an obvious cause for venous thrombosis, in those with recurrent idiopathic thrombosis, and in those older than 60 years. However, there is no evidence that an extensive workup to detect malignancy is beneficial. A reasonable approach is to supplement routine studies with multiple fecal samples for occult blood, PSA measurements in men, and mammography in women.

Prevention:

Arterial thrombi: Drugs that inhibit platelet function (e.g. aspirin, ticolpidine, and clopidogrel) have been shown to be beneficial in preventing thrombosis in patients with atherosclerotic vascular disease.

Venous thromboembolism: Prophylactic heparin given at a dose of 5,000 units every 12 hours decreases the incidence of DVT and PE in general surgical patients. It is less effective for prophylaxis following orthopedic surgery or trauma, however. In these circumstances, more effective approaches include subcutaneous heparin adjusted to maintain a top normal PTT or the use of low molecular weight heparin (LMWH) or moderate-dose warfarin therapy.

Treatment:

Arterial thrombi: Except for specific circumstances such as unstable angina, early acute MI, and selected cases of peripheral arterial thrombosis, the goal for patients with arterial thrombi is prevention of recurrence with anti-platelet agents.

Venous thromboembolism: The treatment of choice for venous thromboembolism (including symptomatic calf vein thrombi and PE) is heparin (either intravenous or subcutaneous) at a dose sufficient to prolong the PTT to 1.5-2.5 times the mean of the control PTT. Achieving this dose within the first 24 hours of treatment has been found to minimize treatment failure and recurrence. Generally, an initial intravenous bolus of 5,000 units followed by >30,000 units/24 hours is required. LMWH preferentially catalyzes the inhibition of factor Xa over the inhibition of thrombin. When given at a fixed dosage subcutaneously once or twice daily and without laboratory monitoring, LMWH has been found to be at least as effective as standard heparin. It is particularly advantageous in the outpatient setting, where its higher cost is outweighed by the saved costs of hospitalization. Current practice is to treat with heparin for at least 5 days, starting warfarin on day #1. Once the warfarin effect is adequate (INR = 2.0-3.0), an overlap of 2 days is recommended to insure that patients are adequately anticoagulated when the heparin is stopped and to prevent the rare occurrence of warfarin-induced skin necrosis. The duration of warfarin therapy depends on the inciting cause of the DVT. In patients with reversible risk factors such as recent surgery, 6-12 weeks may be sufficient. However, in patients with idiopathic thrombosis, a longer course of therapy is necessary. Although the optimal duration of therapy remains to be established, a recent study revealed a recurrence rate of 27%/patient-year in a group treated for 3 months compared to 1.3%/patient-year in those treated for an average of 12 months, suggesting that treatment for only 3 months is inadequate. Patients with ongoing risk factors or recurrent venous thromboembolism should be treated indefinitely. When there are containdications to the use of anticoagulant drugs (such as active bleeding) or if thrombosis recurs despite adequate anticoagulation, vena caval interruption may be indicated to reduce the risk of PE. Surgical thrombectomy and thrombolutic agents such as streptokinase and tissue plasminogen activator are usually reserved for patients with life-threatening pulmonary embolism or massive ileofemoral thrombosis where compromise of the adjacent arterial circulation seems imminent.

Chapter 219, 378

INFECTIOUS DISEASES

■ BACTERIAL MENINGITIS

DEFINITION, EPIDEMIOLOGY AND ETIOLOGY
Meningitis develops when the cerebrospinal fluid (CSF) in the subarachnoid space becomes infected, usually because of hematogenous spread. Community-acquired meningitis is particularly common among children, young adults, and the elderly. Among children and young adults, the most common pathogens are *Streptococcus pneumoniae, Neisseria meningitidis,* and *Haemophilus influenzae* type B, although the incidence of *H. influenzae* infection has decreased dramatically because of the wide use of vaccine. Elderly patients are infected most often by gram-negative bacilli, *S. pneumoniae,* and *Listeria monocytogenes.* Patients who have undergone splenectomy or who have sickle cell disease are particularly susceptible to *S. pneumoniae* and *H. influenzae* infection. Bacterial meningitis due to head trauma, craniotomy, CSF leak, or congenital defects such as spina bifida is most frequently caused by *Staphylococcus aureus* and *S. pneumoniae* and less frequently by *Pseudomonas aeruginosa* or other Enterobacteriaceae. Patients undergoing cancer chemotherapy and those with underlying immunodeficiency are prone to infection with a variety of pathogens, including *L. monocytogenes,* Enterobacteriaceae, mycobacteria, and fungi. An increasing proportion of cases are nosocomially acquired, and approximately one-third of such cases are caused by gram-negative bacteria other than *H. influenzae.*

CLINICAL FEATURES
The cardinal features are fever, headache, and nuchal rigidity. Other signs of cerebral dysfunction vary depending on the onset and clinical course of the illness. They include confusion, cranial nerve palsy, and seizures. In acute purulent meningitis caused by *S. pneumoniae, N. meningitidis,* and *H. influenzae* type B, progression from confusion and lethargy to coma can occur within 24 hours. Other common symptoms include weakness, anorexia, shaking chills, profuse sweats, photophobia, vomiting, and myalgia of the lower extremities. At examination, neck stiffness may be subtle or marked. Kernig's and Brudzinski's signs suggest meningeal inflammation. Cranial nerve palsy, principally of the third, fourth, sixth, and seventh nerves, occurs among 10% to 20% of patients. Focal neurologic findings such as hemiparesis, visual field defects, papilledema, and dysphasia suggest the coexistence of a brain abscess, subdural empyema, or septic thrombophlebitis.

DIFFERENTIAL DIAGNOSIS AND DIAGNOSTIC TESTS
The typical CSF profiles in bacterial and nonbacterial meningitis are shown in Table 431.3. Partially controlled bacterial meningitis typically is associated with lymphocytic predominance in the CSF. Patients with viral meningitis have polymorphonuclear pleocytosis in the CSF early in the course of disease. In bacterial meningitis, the yield of both Gram stain and culture is reduced by prior administration of antimicrobial agents. There are several techniques for the rapid detection of specific microbial antigens in the CSF. Blood culture results are positive in at least 50% of cases.

MANAGEMENT
Table 431.4 lists choices for initial empiric antimicrobial therapy in various age groups. The final antibiotic selection should be guided by culture results and susceptibility data. Penicillin G remains the drug of choice for meningococcal meningitis. A third-generation cephalosporin such as ceftriaxone or cefotaxime is best for *H. influenzae* type B and penicillin-resistant *S. pneumoniae,* though vancomycin should be used if there is high-level penicillin resistance and an elevated minimum inhibitory concentration to third-generation cephalosporins. Newer quinolones such as trovafloxacin are effective against high-level penicillin-resistant pneumococcal meningitis in experimental models, but clinical experi-

ence is limited. Meningitis caused by *P. aeruginosa* should be managed with the combination of an antipseudomonal β-lactam plus a fluoroquinolone or an aminoglycoside. Ampicillin or penicillin G plus an aminoglycoside should be used to control *L. monocytogenes* infection.

There is no consensus regarding the use of glucocorticoids as adjunctive therapy for acute bacterial meningitis among adults. It is also unclear whether therapy with monoclonal antibodies or other agents directed at blocking the effect of inflammatory cytokines in the CSF can prevent hearing loss, seizure disorders, or other chronic neurologic sequelae.

Chapter 279

■ CANDIDAL INFECTIONS

EPIDEMIOLOGY AND PATHOGENESIS
Candida organisms are ubiquitous and are normal commensal organisms of humans and certain animals. *Candida albicans* is the most prominent of the eight species that infect humans with frequency. Most species exist in three forms—yeast (which may bud), hyphae, and pseudohyphae. Severe infections usually are iatrogenic. The two most important predisposing factors are neutropenia and exposure to broad-spectrum antibiotics. *Candida* organisms are the third most common pathogen in blood cultures of hospitalized patients.

CLINICAL FEATURES
Skin and mucous membranes: Intertrigo on the warm, moist areas of the skin occurs among obese and diabetic patients. Chronic mucocutaneous candidiasis is a long-standing, severe disease associated with lymphocyte-mediated immunodeficiency. Thrush is manifest by white plaques in the oral cavity. It occurs among patients who have taken antibiotics or used inhaled steroids and among those who are severely debilitated or immunocompromised, such as patients with AIDS. Candidal esophagitis causes odynophagia and white plaques on the esophageal mucosa. It occurs frequently among patients receiving cytotoxic chemotherapy and among patients with AIDS.
Genitourinary system: Although *Candida* species are found in the urine of 8% of healthy men and 12% of healthy women, candiduria may signify cystitis, pyelonephritis, papillary necrosis, or perinephric abscess. A common problem is prolonged colonization of the bladders of patients with indwelling Foley catheters.
Intravascular infection: About 2% of cases of endocarditis are caused by *Candida* organisms, and 50% of these are complications of cardiac surgery. The hallmarks of candidal endocarditis are large vegetations and occlusion of large vessels. Infection at sites of peripheral indwelling intravascular catheters is another common cause of persistent candidemia.
Disseminated Candidiasis: Widespread disseminated candidiasis occurs most frequently among patients with neutropenia and those experiencing prolonged, complicated postoperative courses of disease. Other predisposing factors include use of antibiotics, neutropenia, the presence of an indwelling intravascular catheter, and exposure to hyperalimentation fluid and steroids.

LABORATORY STUDIES AND DIAGNOSTIC TESTS
Intravascular infection is associated with positive results of blood cultures. Mucosal membrane infections can be diagnosed on the basis of the clinical appearance of the lesions and recovery of the organism from scrapings of the infected area. The diagnosis of candidal infection of deep organs requires biopsy evidence of the organism invading the tissue. There are no reliable serologic tests for invasive candidiasis.

MANAGEMENT

Mucocutaneous infection is successfully controlled with azole antifungal agent such as fluconazole, itraconazole, and ketoconazole. For most patients, candiduria is self-limited, but some may need an amphotericin B bladder washout or treatment with oral fluconazole. All patients with candidemia should be treated with an antifungal agent. Removal of an infected intravenous catheter is necessary but not sufficient. Fluconazole has been demonstrated to be as effective as amphotericin B in the management of candidemia among patients with and without neutropenia. Until further studies are completed, therapy for life-threatening candidal infections is amphotericin B.

Chapter 203

■ CELLULITIS

DEFINITIONS

Cellulitis is a spreading acute infection of the skin and subcutaneous tissues characterized by erythema, warmth, swelling, and tenderness. It may be classified as mild and uncomplicated, severe, high risk, or necrotizing.

ETIOLOGY AND CLINICAL FEATURES

Most cases of cellulitis are mild and uncomplicated. They are caused by group A streptococci or *Staphylococcus aureus.* Diffuse erythema, swelling, and tenderness develop over 2 to 4 days. In an extremity, a red line along the course of lymphatic vessels indicates accompanying lymphangitis. Enlargement and tenderness of regional lymph nodes are common. Fever, malaise, and chills often are present.

    Orbital cellulitis is a rare complication of sinusitis and carries a risk of blindness, brain abscess, and meningitis. Erysipelas usually follows a streptococcal sore throat and usually affects the young and the elderly. The infection involves the dermis and the lymphatic vessels and manifests as pain and bright-red peau d'orange lesions with advancing red borders that are sharply demarcated from normal skin. Erysipeloid is a form of cellulitis that occurs among workers who handle fish, meat, and poultry. It is caused by the gram-positive bacillus *Erysipelothrix rhusiopathiae.* About 1 week after a minor injury to the hand, a violaceous painful area appears. As the central area clears, the lesion spreads outward with distinct raised borders. Animal and human bites of the hands are potentially dangerous because of tissue damage and secondary infection. *Pasteurella multocida* often infects dog and cat bites, and *Eikenella corrodens* often is implicated in human bites. Deep infections such as tenosynovitis are particularly common after human bites. Necrotizing cellulitis is a serious gangrenous soft-tissue infection often associated with the presence of anaerobic bacteria, tissue toxins, and bacterial synergy. It should be suspected when a patient has edema out of proportion to erythema, skin vesicles, crepitus on palpation or air in the tissues on a radiograph, local anesthesia, or patchy gangrene of the skin.

MANAGEMENT

Most cases of cellulitis can be managed simply on an outpatient basis. Severe, complicated, or high-risk infections necessitate aggressive inpatient antibiotic therapy and often surgery. Patients with necrotizing infections must be treated surgically. Uncomplicated mild cellulitis, commonly caused by *Streptococcus pyogenes* or *S. aureus,* responds well to oral cloxacillin or cephalexin (500 mg every 6 hours for 7 to 10 days). For patients allergic to penicillin, erythromycin (500 mg every 6 hours for 7 to 10 days) is an alternative. Local therapy includes cleansing the area and resting the extremity. In severe cellulitis, treatment should start with intravenous cloxacillin (1 g every 6 hours). Intravenous vancomycin (500 mg every 8 hours if renal function is normal) and teicoplanin (1 g daily) are alternatives for patients allergic to penicillin. An aminoglycoside may be added when the clinical setting suggests that gram-negative bacilli may play a role (e.g., perianal cellulitis, neutropenia, glucocorticoid therapy, and diabetes mellitus), although monotherapy with second- or third-generation cephalosporins is an alternative in these situations.

    Erysipelas usually responds to intravenous penicillin G (1 million units every 6 hours). Orbital cellulitis is managed with broad-spectrum antibiotics. Computed tomographic evidence of an abscess or intracranial involvement and failure to respond to antibiotics within 48 hours are indications for prompt exploration and decompression of the orbit. Erysipeloid responds to amoxicillin–clavulanate or erythromycin. Animal and human bites necessitate therapy with oral amoxicilin-clavulanate and local debridement.

Chapter 263

■ INFECTIONS CAUSED BY DIMORPHIC FUNGI

DEFINITION

The dimorphic fungi are soil-growing organisms that exist in a mycelian form in the environment but grow as yeast at body temperature. Infections caused by these fungi include histoplasmosis, coccidioidomycosis, blastomycosis, and sporotrichosis. The clinical manifestations depend on the immune status of the host; normal hosts may have minimal symptoms, but those with immunocompromise may develop overwhelming, disseminated infection.

EPIDEMIOLOGY, CLINICAL FEATURES, AND DIAGNOSIS

Histoplasmosis: *Histoplasma capsulatum* is the etiologic agent of histoplasmosis, a disease endemic to the Ohio River and Mississippi River valleys. The organism is found in soil contaminated with droppings from fowl. The clinical manifestations depend on underlying host defense, intensity of exposure, and previous immunity. The acute self-limited illness is characterized by flulike symptoms of fever, chills, headache, myalgia, anorexia, nonproductive cough, and chest pain. A chest radiograph may show enlarged hilar and mediastinal lymph nodes with patchy infiltrates. After heavy inoculation, more extensive pulmonary disease may develop. Inflammatory complications such as arthritis and erythema nodosum occur among about 10% of patients with symptomatic infection. Dissemination is most likely among patients with advanced AIDS, organ transplant recipients, and patients receiving steroids or chemotherapy. The manifestations include fever, weight loss, gastrointestinal lesions, skin lesions, oropharyngeal ulceration, adrenal insufficiency, meningitis, endocarditis, hepatomegaly, lymphadenopathy, and pancytopenia from bone marrow involvement. The diagnosis is established by means of culture, histopathologic examination, or serologic testing. Skin tests are not useful because most persons in endemic zones have reactive skin tests, and cross reactions with other fungi are common.

Coccidioidomycosis: Coccidioidomycosis is caused by *Coccidioides immitis,* a soil organism endemic to the southwestern United States, Mexico, and South America. Infection is asymptomatic for 60% of infected persons and is indicated by a positive skin test result. For the remaining 40%, a self-limited, flulike illness develops 1 to 3 weeks after exposure. It is characterized by a dry cough, pleuritic chest pain, myalgia, arthralgia, fever, sweats, anorexia, and weakness. Immune complex complications can include an erythematous macular rash, erythema multiforme, and erythema nodosum. Acute infection usually resolves without therapy. Approximately 5% of persons with the infection have pulmonary residua, which include nodules and cavities. Chronic progressive pulmonary infection is characterized, particularly among immunocompromised patients, by the development of extensive thin-walled cavities that may be complicated by cavity rupture, bronchopleural fistula, and empyema. Extrapulmonary disease develops in 1 in 200 patients and typically involves the skin and soft tissues, bones, and meninges. The diagnosis can be established by means of identification of spherules in histopathologic specimens or by means of culture. Serologic tests can be performed, although skin tests are of limited utility.

Blastomycosis: Most cases of blastomycosis, which is caused by *Blastomyces dermatitidis,* occur in the midwestern and southeastern United States and the Canadian provinces of Ontario, Quebec, and Alberta. About 50% of infected persons have symptoms such as fever, chills, cough, myalgia, and arthralgia. A chest radiograph may show lobar or segmental consolidation, although a nodular pattern may be seen with chronic infection. The acute pulmonary symptoms usually resolve, but patients may have progressive pulmonary disease or disseminated infection. The skin is the most frequent site of dissemination; the verrucous or ulcerative lesions may be mistaken for squamous cell carcinoma. Other extrapulmonary sites include subcutaneous tissue, bones, the genitourinary tract (prostate and epididymis), and the central nervous system. The diagnosis is established by means of demonstration the organism on wet preparations or histopathologic study. The organism can be cultured, but the presence of the mycelian form before conversion to a yeast does not confirm the diagnosis. Serologic studies are less reliable.

Sporotrichosis: Sporotrichosis is caused by the soil fungus *Sporothrix schenckii,* usually by means of direct inoculation from contaminated soil or plants, especially thorny plants such as roses. After an incubation period of 1 to 10 weeks, reddish-purple, nodular, cutaneous lesions appear that follow the lymphatic vessels and frequently ulcerate. Direct spread to bone or joints sometimes occurs. Pulmonary infection and disseminated infection are uncommon.

MANAGEMENT

Guidelines for selection of an antifungal agent are given in Table 336.1. In general, amphotericin B is preferred as initial treatment of profoundly ill patients. Side effects include fever, chills, and hypotension during initiation of therapy; malaise; anemia; azotemia, renal tubular acidosis; hypokalemia; and hypomagnesemia. Lipid-associated formulations cause less nephrotoxicty but are very expensive. They are most appropriate for patients who are intolerant of therapy with standard amphotericin B. The azoles (ketoconazole, itraconazole, and fluconazole) are used as primary treatment of less acutely ill patients and as long-term therapy after a brief course of amphotericin B. All have oral formulations and have a potential for pharmacokinetic interaction with many other agents. The chief side effect is hepatotoxicity.

Chapter 302

■ INFECTIVE ENDOCARDITIS

DEFINITIONS AND PATHOGENESIS

Infective endocarditis (IE) is microbial invasion of the endocardium, usually involving valvular surfaces. Disruption of the endocardial surface exposes collagen and promotes adherence of platelets and fibrin. IE occurs when circulating microorganisms colonize the injured endocardial surface. Bacteria invade the blood through local barriers, such as skin and mucous membranes, or are directly inoculated into capillaries and venules, as in dental surgery.

EPIDEMIOLOGY AND MICROBIOLOGY

The epidemiologic pattern of IE is a function of the frequency of bloodstream invasion by pathogens and the prevalence of predisposing endocardial disease. The mean age of patients with IE has increased and is now about 55 years. Risk factors include valvular heart disease (including mitral valve prolapse), intravenous drug abuse (IVDA), and use of intravascular or intracardiac devices.

Streptococci are the most commonly reported cause of native valve endocarditis (NVE), *Streptococcus viridans* species predominating (about 35% of all cases). About 80% of patients have underlying cardiac disease and are infected when the bacteria, which are normal oral flora, gain access to the bloodstream. Enterococcal IE accounts for about 10% of all cases. About 40% of patients have no known underlying heart disease. Older men undergoing urologic procedures, women undergoing gynecologic procedures, and parenteral drug users are at particular risk. *Streptococcus bovis* IE is associated with bowel lesions, including colon cancer. Staphylococci cause 25% of cases of NVE; 90% are caused by *Staphylococcus aureus*. No prior valve abnormality is recognized in one-third of these patients. Aerobic gram-negative bacteria cause 5% to 10% of cases; risk factors include IVDA and the presence of prosthetic valves. For another 5% to 10% of patients with presumed IE, no etiologic microorganism is isolated from the blood, most commonly because of prior antibiotic use. Coagulase-negative staphylococci are the most common cause of prosthetic valve endocarditis (PVE).

CLINICAL FEATURES

History: There may be known underlying heart disease and a preceding bacteremic event such as dental work, IVDA, or instrumentation of the gastrointestinal or genitourinary tracts. Fever is present in more than 90% of cases. Most patients with subacute IE have nonspecific symptoms such as malaise, arthralgia, myalgia, and fatigue. Symptoms of congestive heart failure are present among about 50% of those with NVE. Emboli to the lungs or abdominal organs can cause chest or abdominal pain.

Physical examination: Most patients with left-sided valvular disease have murmurs at some point but may not initially. Classic peripheral signs include petechiae, Roth's spots (oval retinal hemorrhages), splenomegaly, clubbing, Osler's nodes (painful, purple to red nodules on the pads of the fingers or toes), linear splinter hemorrhages beneath the fingernails or toenails, and red, macular Janeway lesions on the palms or soles.

Special situations: IE associated with IVDA most commonly involves *S. aureus* infection of the tricuspid valve. Such patients typically have an acute onset of fever, pleuritic chest pain, dyspnea, and cough. A murmur of tricuspid regurgitation usually is heard. The initial chest radiograph is abnormal in most cases and may show nodular opacities, abscesses with cavitation, patchy pneumonitis, or pleural effusions. Gram-negative infections are frequent. Infection with *Pseudomonas aeruginosa* is associated with high mortality.

Prosthetic valve IE occurs among about 2% of patients after valve replacement, one-third of these cases occurring within 2 months of surgery. Infection by staphylococci (both *S. aureus* and coagulase-negative species) is the most common cause, but gram-negative bacilli and fungi are more common than in NVE. Patients come to medical attention in much the same manner as those with NVE, although a higher frequency of a new or changed murmur reflects a higher rate of local suppurative complications, such as valve ring abscess.

LABORATORY STUDIES AND DIAGNOSTIC TESTS

The blood culture is the most important laboratory test. Bacteremia is typically low grade and constant. One of the first two sets yields the etiologic bacteria in 90% of cases. At least three sets should be obtained within the first 24 hours for patients with suspected IE. Nonspecific laboratory abnormalities include anemia and an elevated erythrocyte sedimentation rate. Leukocytosis is unusual in subacute IE but is more likely in acute IE caused by staphylococci, pneumococci, or gonococci. Hematuria, proteinuria, and detectable rheumatoid factor are present in about one-half of cases. Echocardiography is the most useful imaging study. Transthoracic echocardiography reveals vegetations in about 50% to 60% of patients. Transesophageal echocardiography is more accurate and has a sensitivity approaching 90%. Echocardiography is useful for defining the severity of valvular destruction, detecting complications such as abscess or aortic mycotic aneurysm, and assessing the hemodynamic effects of IE. The Duke criteria for IE are listed in Table 270.2.

COMPLICATIONS

Cardiac: Valvular dysfunction, usually insufficiency, is the most important complication. Extension of a paravalvular abscess in the conduction system may cause varying degrees of atrioventricular block and bundle branch block. This is most common in aortic valve IE. Pericarditis is especially frequent with staphylococcal disease. Heart failure is the most common cause of death. Valvular dysfunction is the usual basis, but embolic myocardial infarction, myocarditis, and conduction disturbances can contribute.

Noncardiac: Emboli, which occur among about one-third of patients, may be bland (uninfected) or septic and are most common with *S. aureus* and fungal IE. In left-sided IE, the spleen, kidney, brain, and heart are most commonly affected. Mycotic aneurysms complicate 15% to 25% of cases; they occur most frequently in the central nervous system and abdominal aorta. The main risk is rupture with bleeding, sometimes months to years after the infection has resolved. Renal failure from immune-complex glomerulonephritis occurs among 10% of patients.

MANAGEMENT

Antibiotics: Therapy must include bactericidal drugs given parenterally for a prolonged time (2 to 6 weeks, depending on the clinical circumstances). Antimicrobial therapy should be started without delay in the following four situations: when the clinical diagnosis seems certain, although blood culture results are not yet available; when the diagnosis seems likely and the patient is seriously ill; when antimicrobial therapy for another condition is necessary; and when the patient may have IE, and blood culture results are positive. Empiric therapy must include agents likely to be effective against enterococci. Antistaphylococcal agents should be considered in the treatment of patients with PVE; those with a rapidly progressive illness that suggests acute IE; those with aortic valve involvement but without prior valvular abnormality; those with IVDA; those with a previously infected intravenous catheter; and those undergoing long-term hemodialysis. Once the infecting pathogen is identified, a more specific antibiotic regimen is administered.

Surgery: Indications include severe or refractory heart failure, valvular obstruction, fungal endocarditis, ineffective antimicrobial therapy, and instability of a prosthetic valve. Relative indications in NVE include nonstreptococcal IE, recurrent IE, intracardiac extension of infection, the presence of two or more emboli, and echocardiographic detection of vegetations or mitral valve preclosure. Relative indications in PVE include early infection, nonstreptococcal late PVE, and periprosthetic leak. Tricuspid valve IE is generally well tolerated hemodynamically; persistent infection with resistant bacteria or fungi is the most common surgical indication.

PROPHYLAXIS

Although the use of prophylactic antibiotics to prevent IE is recommended in certain situations, no randomized, controlled trials addressing this issue have been performed, and most cases if IE do not occur in association with an invasive procedure. The risk of bacteremia is highest for some dental and oral procedures, intermediate for urologic procedures, and lowest for most gastrointestinal procedures (with the exception of esophageal dilation and variceal sclerotherapy), including those that involve biopsy. According to the American Heart Association, high-risk cardiac conditions include the presence of prosthetic valves, prior IE, complex cyanotic congenital defects, and the presence of surgically constructed systemic-pulmonary shunts. Rheumatic heart disease and mitral valve prolapse with valvular regurgitation are classified as moderate risk. Antibiotic selection is directed against *S. viridans* for dental, oral, respiratory, and esophageal procedures (2 g amoxicillin before the procedure is the preferred antibiotic) and against enterococci for other gastrointestinal and urologic procedures (amoxicillin or ampicillin with or without gentamicin, depending on risk).

Chapter 270

EPSTEIN–BARR VIRUS INFECTION AND INFECTIOUS MONONUCLEOSIS

DEFINITION
Epstein–Barr virus (EBV) is a DNA human herpesvirus associated with infectious mononucleosis (IM) and a number of malignant diseases, such as Hodgkin's disease, Burkitt's lymphoma in Africa, and nasopharyngeal carcinoma in China. It is also the causative agent of hairy leukoplakia of the tongue among immunocompromised patients.

EPIDEMIOLOGY AND PATHOPHYSIOLOGY
EBV occurs worldwide and spreads from person to person by close contact and exchange of oral secretions. IM typically occurs in adolescence and the early third decade of life. The incubation period is 4 to 6 weeks. The virus infects lymphocytes and the oropharyngeal epithelium. Like other herpesviruses, EBV causes infections with three phases—primary, latent, and reactivated. Reactivation is associated with the malignant conditions.

CLINICAL FEATURES
Primary EBV infection causes about 90% of cases of IM. The onset is insidious, and acute pharyngitis often is the primary symptom. The classic findings are fever lasting up to 3 weeks or more, lymphadenopathy, splenomegaly, and florid atypical lymphocytosis, with malaise that may be slow to resolve. Coupled with a positive heterophil antibody reaction or Monospot test, these findings are sufficient for diagnosis in most cases. The diagnosis is made definite by the finding of EBV antibodies. Complications include acute hepatitis that usually is mild and transient, neurologic syndromes such as encephalitis, neuritis, transverse myelitis, and Guillain–Barré syndrome, and hematologic abnormalities such as agranulocytosis, aplastic anemia, and thrombocytopenia. These usually resolve without therapy. A rare complication is splenic rupture. Acute IM sometimes seems to lapse into a chronic phase that lasts as long as a year or more and is marked by persistent fatigue, low-grade fevers, malaise, and a labile emotional state. IM caused by cytomegalovirus mimics that caused by EBV, although sore throat and atypical lymphocytosis may not be as prominent.

LABORATORY FINDINGS
For IM, the diagnosis is confirmed by finding antibodies to EBV viral capsid antigen (CVA) (both IgG and IgM in primary infection) and, ideally, EBV early antigen (EA-D) but not EBV nuclear antigen (EBNA) antibodies. Antibodies to EA-D are transient and indicate recent or reactivated infection, whereas antibodies to EBNA often cannot be detected in primary infection, and appear only months later. The characteristic pattern of past infection would be a moderate titer of IgG VCA antibodies and a low titer of EBNA antibodies, both persistent for life.

PROGNOSIS AND MANAGEMENT
Most cases are mild and resolve within 2 to 3 weeks. Treatment is supportive. Controlled trials of acyclovir for IM have disclosed marginal benefit, in part because many of the symptoms are caused by secondary immunopathologic processes unaffected by antiviral therapy. There is also no evidence that so-called chronic mononucleosis responds to antiviral drugs.

Chapter 314

APPROACH TO THE PATIENT WITH FEVER OF UNKNOWN ORIGIN

DEFINITION
Fever is a complex physiologic process characterized clinically by a body temperature higher than 37.7°C (100°F). The temperatures of the rectum, mouth, and tympanic membrane all can be used to estimate core temperature. On average, rectal readings exceed oral readings by 0.4°C (0.7°F) and exceed tympanic membrane readings by 0.8°C (1.4°F).

PATHOPHYSIOLOGY AND CLINICAL MANIFESTATIONS
Fever is a process in which the thermoregulatory set point is altered by the action of various cytokines on the anterior hypothalamus. Hyperthermia, in contrast, is an increase in body temperature not mediated by such cytokines. Hyperthermia is not regulated, is not defended by physiologic mechanisms, and does not respond to standard antipyretic agents. Disorders associated with hyperthermia include malignant hyperthermia, neuroleptic malignant syndrome, pheochromocytoma, and thyrotoxicosis, all of which increase heat production, and dehydration and heatstroke, which decrease heat loss. Experiments with animals have shown that fever enhances survival during some infections. However, when fever is extreme, the beneficial effect is reversed, and febrile convulsions can occur.

DIFFERENTIAL DIAGNOSIS
Most fevers either resolve spontaneously or are diagnosed quickly, usually in association with an infection. Fevers that persist for 2 to 3 weeks and defy intensive diagnostic scrutiny (fevers of unknown origin) occur more often with common diseases that have unusual manifestations than they do with exotic disorders. The three most common causes of the syndrome are infection, malignant neoplasia, and connective tissue disorders (Table 266.4). Familial Mediterranean fever is a hereditary disorder characterized by recurrent episodes of unexplained fever, frequently accompanied by peritonitis, pleuritis, or monarticular arthritis. Long-term colchicine therapy reportedly decreases the incidence of attacks and complications. Many medications have been reported to cause drug fever. Quinidine, α-methyldopa, and penicillins have been implicated most frequently. The various medications differ in the average duration of therapy that precedes the fever. For antibiotics, the median time lag between initiation of therapy and the onset of drug fever is 6 days. The fever generally abates within 48 to 72 hours of discontinuation of the offending agent.

HISTORY AND PHYSICAL EXAMINATION
A detailed history and careful examination are crucial. Important historical features include occupation, recent travel, exposure to a pet, and food consumption. When performing the physical examination, one should not overlook the fundoscopic examination, the less prominent chains of lymph nodes, and the prostate, epididymis, and testicles.

LABORATORY STUDIES AND DIAGNOSTIC TESTS
Initial studies should include a complete blood cell count, urinalysis, biochemical tests, serologic tests for fungal infection and connective tissue disorders, examination of the stool for occult blood, and bacterial cultures of urine, sputum, and blood. Chest radiography, electrocardiography, lumbar puncture, tuberculin skin test, and thyroid function tests also are performed. Abnormalities detected with one of these studies should be pursued with more specific investigations. If the initial studies are not revealing, more specialized studies are ordered, such as computed tomography of the brain, chest, and abdomen, oral cholecystography, gallium scintigraphy, intravenous pyelography, and gastrointestinal endoscopy. Biopsies of the liver, bone marrow, and skin may follow.

MANAGEMENT
Antipyretic therapy: In most clinical settings, antipyretics alone are sufficient to reduce fever. Studies comparing the efficacy of acetaminophen and aspirin have not found substantial differences. The two are equally effective in relieving the malaise, headache, and myalgia that often accompany fever. Salicylates should be avoided by those with peptic ulcer disease and bleeding disorders, and acetaminophen by patients with underlying liver disease. During extreme pyrexia, physical methods such as sponging and application of cooling blankets are combined with use of antipyretic agents to lower temperature. In hyperthermia, such measures may be the only effective antipyretic therapy.

Specific therapy: If an etiologic factor is identified, therapy for that disorder is initiated. If all of the diagnostic studies listed earlier fail to yield a diagnosis, the physician has three options, as follows: (a) repeat the entire evaluation in the hope that abnormalities may have developed in a previously normal test result; (b) direct a therapeutic trial against a probable but unproven diagnosis such as occult tuberculosis; (c) observe the patient for new signs or symptoms that merit further investigation and plan for a systematic reevaluation in 6 to 8 weeks.

Chapter 266

▇ GONOCOCCAL INFECTIONS

DEFINITION AND EPIDEMIOLOGY

Infection with the gram-negative diplococcal bacteria *Neisseria gonorrhoeae,* is transmitted by means of sexual contact. In the United States, the incidence of infection is highest among adolescents and young adults, particularly the urban poor and minority ethnic groups. Coexistent chlamydial infection is common. The most common infection among men is urethritis. Among women, endocervicitis is most common, but the complication of pelvic inflammatory disease (PID) is most important. Because most infected women have no symptoms, uncontrolled endocervical infection is an important bacterial reservoir. A man's likelihood of infection after a single exposure to an infected woman is about 25%. The incubation period is 3 to 4 days.

CLINICAL FEATURES

Infection among women: Urethritis may cause dysuria and a urethral discharge. Symptoms of endocervical infection are recognized by only about 25% of women. Patients typically have an unusual or purulent vaginal discharge and may have irregular or abnormal menstrual periods. For about 20% of women with endocervical gonorrhea, the infection spreads to involve the endometrium, fallopian tubes, and peritoneum, causing PID. The symptoms and signs of PID include fever, pelvic pain, adnexal masses, and pain with cervical motion. Perihepatitis (Fitz-Hugh and Curtis syndrome) often manifests as right upper quadrant pain and elevated liver enzyme levels and may occur after retrograde spread of infection.

Infections among men: Between 60% and 95% of men with urethritis have symptoms, typically urethral discharge and dysuria. *N. gonorrhoeae,* along with *Chlamydia trachomatis,* is also a common cause of epididymitis among men younger than 35 years.

Infections among women and men: Conjunctivitis can occur among adults whose fingers are contaminated with infected genital secretions. Pharyngeal infection is acquired through oral-genital sex; transmission by means of kissing or through oral secretions is rare. Isolation of the organism from the anal canal is common among women who have endocervical infection. Anorectal infection among men occurs in those who engage in receptive anal intercourse with an infected partner. Symptoms (most often absent) include pruritus, tenesmus, purulent discharge, and bloody diarrhea. Disseminated gonococcal infection (DGI) occurs in less than 1% of genital infections, usually among menstruating women. The symptoms variably include fever, skin rash, joint or tendon pain, and migratory polyarthritis. Gonococcal infection is the most common cause of septic arthritis among young adults.

LABORATORY FINDINGS

Among men with symptomatic urethritis, the diagnosis can be made when a Gram stain of the urethral discharge reveals gram-negative diplococci within neutrophils. The sensitivity is more than 90%, and the specificity is 98% to 99%. Therefore, cultures are not indicated if the stain result is positive. The diagnosis of gonococcal infection among women and at all anatomic sites in men except the urethra is best made by means of culture. In DGI, blood culture results are positive in only 25% of cases and joint fluid cultures in only 10%. A presumptive diagnosis can be made when a young adult with typical clinical findings has *N. gonorrhoeae* isolated from a mucosal surface and responds rapidly to antibiotic therapy directed at the gonococcus. An enzyme immunoassay can be performed to diagnose genital infection for men and women. However, it offers no advantage over Gram stain for men and is less sensitive and specific than culture for women.

PROGNOSIS AND MANAGEMENT

Effective antibiotic therapy eradicates gonococcal infection. Resolution of symptoms indicates cure; follow-up cultures are unnecessary. Controlled gonococcal arthritis usually has no sequelae, but gonococcal salpingitis may lead to infertility, ectopic pregnancy, or recurrent PID. Guidelines for management of gonococcal infection reflect the emergence of antibiotic resistance, the frequency of coexisting chlamydial infections, and the potentially serious complications.

Uncomplicated infection: Options for infection of the urethra, cervix, and rectum include cefixime (400 mg by mouth in a single dose), ceftriaxone (125 mg intramuscularly [IM] in a single dose), ciprofloxacin (500 mg by mouth in a single dose), or ofloxacin (400 mg by mouth in a single dose). Patients also receive a regimen effective against possible coinfection with *C. trachomatis,* such as azithromycin (1 g by mouth in a single dose) or doxycycline (100 mg by mouth twice a day for 7 days).

Complicated infection: Therapy for PID includes agents active against *N. gonorrhoeae, C. trachomatis,* gram-negative facultative bacteria, streptococci, and anaerobic bacteria. One approach includes either cefotetan (2 g intravenously [IV] every 12 hours) or cefoxitin (2 g IV every 6 hours) plus doxycycline (100 mg IV or by mouth every 12 hours) until 24 hours after the patient improves clinically followed by doxycycline (same dose) to complete 14 days of therapy. An alternative is clindamycin (900 mg IV every 8 hours) plus gentamicin (2 mg per kilogram IV or IM followed by 1.5 mg per kilogram every 8 hours) until clinical improvement occurs, at which time therapy is changed to clindamycin (450 mg by mouth four times a day) or doxycycline (100 mg by mouth twice a day) to complete a total of 14 days of therapy. Patients with DGI should receive ceftriaxone (1 g IM or IV every 24 hours) or cefotaxime (1 g IV every 8 hours) for 1 week. For persons allergic to β-lactam drugs, alternatives include ciprofloxacin (500 mg IV every 12 hours) or ofloxacin (400 mg IV every 12 hours). Reliable patients with uncomplicated cases can be discharged 24 to 48 hours after improvement and may complete therapy with an oral regimen of cefixime (400 mg twice a day), ciprofloxacin (500 mg twice a day), or ofloxacin (400 mg twice a day).

Chapter 280

▇ HIV INFECTION AND AIDS

DEFINITION AND EPIDEMIOLOGY

Acquired immunodeficiency syndrome (AIDS) is a condition of decreased cellular immunity caused by the human immunodeficiency virus (HIV). An estimated 40 million persons worldwide have the infection. HIV is chiefly transmitted through sexual contact, although it also can be transmitted through blood exposure. Increased transmission has been associated with the presence of genital ulcers or other sexually transmitted diseases. The mean time from infection to clinical expression of AIDS is 8 to 10 years. Persons at high risk include homosexual and bisexual men, users of injected drugs, persons with hemophilia, recipients of blood products, and the sexual partners of these persons. The probability of transmission from an infected pregnant woman to her infant is about 25%.

PATHOPHYSIOLOGY

HIV is a retrovirus composed of single-stranded RNA surrounded by a protein envelope. It primarily infects cells with a CD4 + cell-membrane glycoprotein. Once the virus enters cells, uncoating occurs, and a reverse transcriptase enzyme transcribes viral RNA into double-stranded DNA, which is then inserted into the host genome. When the cell is activated by antigenic or viral stimulation, DNA transcription occurs, and new viral particles are assembled at the cell surface. The infected cell then dies. After the initial infection of monocytes, macrophages, and dendritic cells, the virus disseminates to the germinal center of lymph nodes.

CLINICAL DEFINITION OF HIV INFECTION

Depending on the stage, HIV infection can be asymptomatic or cause severe opportunistic infections or cancer. A revised Centers for Disease Control and Prevention (CDC) classification identifies three clinical categories.

Category A: Patients have asymptomatic HIV infection, persistent generalized lymphadenopathy, or acute (primary) HIV illness.

Category B: Patients have symptoms but do not have the conditions in categories A or C. Associated conditions include bacillary angiomatosis, vulvovaginal or oropharyngeal candidiasis, cervical dysplasia or carcinoma in situ, unexplained fever, and diarrhea lasting longer than 1 month.

Category C: Patients have symptoms and a combination of any of the following: candidiasis (esophageal, tracheal, bronchial); extrapulmonary coccidioidomycosis; extrapulmonary cryptococcosis; invasive cervical cancer; chronic intestinal cryptosporidiosis; cytomegalovirus (CMV) retinitis or CMV infection in organs other than liver, spleen, or nodes; HIV encephalopathy; herpes simplex with chronic mucocutaneous ulcer, bronchitis, or pneumonia; disseminated histoplasmosis; chronic isosporiasis; Kaposi's sarcoma; Burkitt's lymphoma; extrapulmonary *Mycobacterium avium* or *Mycobacterium kansasii* infection; pulmonary or extrapulmonary *Mycobacterium tuberculosis* infection; *Pneumocystis carinii* pneumonia (PCP); recurrent pneumonia; progressive multifocal leukoencephalopathy (PML); recurrent *Salmonella* bacteremia; cerebral toxoplasmosis; or HIV wasting syndrome.

CD4 + cell count Because progression of HIV infection yields a decline in CD4 + cell population that predisposes patients to infection, the CDC classification scheme includes CD4 + cell count as a marker of disease progression, as follows: category 1, 500 or more cells per microliter; category 2, 200 to 499 cells per microliter; and category 3, fewer than 200 cells per microliter. Categories A3, B3, and C are AIDS. No CDC definitions currently include HIV RNA levels.

CLINICAL PRESENTATION

There is a typical relation between clinical manifestations of HIV infection and CD4 + cell count (Fig. 341.1).

Acute HIV infection: Approximately 20% of patients have acute seroconversion syndrome, typically a mononucleosis-like illness of sudden onset. Fever, lethargy, headaches, lymphadenopathy, sore throat, and macular rash are the most common symptoms and signs.

Fever: The most common symptom among persons with HIV infection is fever. Common etiologic factors include PCP, *M. avium-intracellulare* (MAC) infection, bacterial pneumonia, sinusitis, lymphoma, catheter infection, drug allergy, and occasionally CMV infection.

Lymphadenopathy: Diffuse lymphadenopathy involving the axillary, inguinal, and cervical areas is common. Generalized lymphadenopathy can occur with acute HIV infection, mycobacterial or fungal infection, lymphoma, Kaposi's sarcoma, syphilis, toxoplasmosis, and infection with Epstein–Barr virus (EBV) or CMV.

Cutaneous manifestations: The most commonly reported maculopapular rashes include molluscum contagiosum, secondary syphilis, cryptococcosis, histoplasmosis, candidiasis, atypical mycobacteria, and warts. The most common causes of nodular lesions include bacillary angiomatosis, MAC infection, and Kaposi's sarcoma. Vesicopustular lesions are typical of herpes simplex and varicella-zoster infection. The most common noninfectious skin disorder is seborrheic dermatitis.

Nervous system manifestations: AIDS dementia complex is diagnosed among one-third of adult patients. Other causes of declining mental activity include depression and the early stages of PML. Cognitive impairment with altered consciousness most commonly is caused by advanced AIDS dementia complex, cryptococcal meningitis, *Toxoplasma* encephalitis, CMV encephalitis, tuberculous meningitis, and herpes simplex encephalitis. Drugs, hypoxemia, and metabolic abnormalities also can depress consciousness. Focal neurologic signs developing over several days suggest *Toxoplasma* encephalitis, primary CNS lymphoma, tuberculosis, or cryptococcoma. PML is caused by a papovavirus (the JC virus), manifests slowly among patients with AIDS and CD4 + counts of 100 or more cells per microliter, and causes altered mentation with or without limb weakness, visual defects, or seizures.

Visual loss: Acute loss of vision is most commonly caused by CMV papillitis, varicella-zoster virus retinitis, secondary syphilis, cryptococcal meningitis, and bacterial or fungal endophthalmitis.

Gastrointestinal signs and symptoms: The most common cause of oral and pharyngeal lesions is candidiasis (thrush). Oral ulcers may be caused by herpes simplex virus or CMV. Oral hairy leukoplakia is a painless Epstein–Barr infection of the epithelium of the tongue. The most common cause of dysphagia and odynophagia is candidiasis. CMV esophagitis usually manifests as odynophagia with little dysphagia. Chronic watery diarrhea and enteritis are common with infection by *Cryptosporidium, Cyclospora, Giardia, Isospora belli, Microsporida,* and MAC organisms. Weight loss is a common manifestation of AIDS.

Respiratory tract signs and symptoms: Bacterial sinusitis is common. The causes of cough and fever vary in different settings. If the CD4 + count is 200 or more cells per microliter and the chest radiograph is clear, acute sinusitis and bronchitis are likely. If the CD4 + count is less than 200 cells per microliter

and the chest radiograph is clear, one must also consider PCP, tuberculosis, cryptococcosis, and MAC infection. If infiltrates are found on the chest radiograph, the differential diagnosis expands to include infection with the bacteria associated with community-acquired pneumonia. The most common cause of dyspnea is PCP, although bacterial pneumonia and infection with fungi and mycobacteria also can cause this symptom. Noninfectious causes include pulmonary lymphoma, Kaposi's sarcoma of the lung, primary pulmonary hypertension, and cardiomyopathy.

Musculoskeletal signs and symptoms: Although of low incidence, septic arthritis is the most common infection of the musculoskeletal system. *Staphylococcus aureus* is the most commonly isolated organism. Reiter's syndrome is more prevalent among patients with HIV infection. Other musculoskeletal infections include osteomyelitis, pyomyositis, and septic bursitis.

LABORATORY ABNORMALITIES

Results of routine laboratory tests often are abnormal among patients with HIV infection (Table 346.4). The CD4 + lymphocyte count reflects the degree of immunocompromise and is predictive of susceptibility to particular infections (Fig. 341.1). The level of plasma HIV RNA correlates to total viral burden and is the best prognostic indicator of HIV infection. Higher levels, especially those greater than 30,000 to 55,000 copies per milliliter, are associated with more rapid disease progression, more rapid CD4 + lymphocyte depletion, and higher risk for AIDS or death.

MANAGEMENT

Anti-retroviral medications: Currently available agents can be divided into two categories: inhibitors of HIV protease (such as saquinavir, ritonavir, indinavir, and nelfinavir), and inhibitors of HIV reverse transcriptase. The reverse transcriptase inhibitors are either nucleoside (such as zidovudine, didanosine, zalcitabine, stavudine, lamivudine, and abacavir), or non-nucleoside (such as nevirapine, delavirdine, and efavirenz).

Initial therapy: Anti-retroviral therapy should be initiated for any patient with symptoms, regardless of CD4 + lymphocyte count and plasma HIV RNA level, and for those with either a CD4 + lymphocyte count less than 500 cells per microliter or a plasma HIV RNA level greater than 5,000 copies per milliliter. Current guidelines suggest only two initial approaches to anti-retroviral therapy—two nucleosides with a protease inhibitor (or the ritonavir–saquinavir combination) or two nucleosides with efavirenz (preferred) or nevirapine or delavirdine (alternatives). Other regimens may be selected, however, on the basis of factors such as medication side effects and patient compliance. Within 3 to 6 weeks of the initiation of effective therapy, a three- to tenfold decrease in the HIV RNA level should occur. The assay is repeated on a regular basis to confirm continued efficacy. The most durable responses occur among persons in whom the viral load has declined to less than the limit of detection (fewer than 400 to 500 copies per milliliter in standard testing and fewer than 50 copies per milliliter in highly sensitive assays).

Changing Therapy: If the toxicity of a particular drug is intolerable, that drug can be replaced with an alternative without changing the other components of the regimen. If treatment fails, however, a single drug should never be switched or added. Instead, the entire treatment history should be investigated, and an effort should be made to avoid new drugs with potential for cross resistance. It is not clear how helpful some resistance tests may be. Because information about optimal combinations and sequences is rapidly changing, patients who do not have good results with an initial regimen should be treated by practitioners highly experienced in the care of patients with HIV infection.

Chapters 339, 340, 341, 345, 346

■ APPROACH TO INFECTION IN THE IMMUNOCOMPROMISED HOST

SPECIFIC IMMUNOLOGICAL DEFICITS

Immunocompromised patients pose special challenges because of the wide spectrum of infections encountered, the difficulties in establishing a diagnosis, and the limited efficacy of therapeutic regimens. Management strategies differ with the underlying immunologic deficit. Among patients with severe neutropenia and among those with asplenia, the risk of fulminant infection is so great that empiric antibiotic therapy must be administered promptly. In contrast, among patients with impaired cellular immunity (lymphoma, AIDS), the spectrum of potential pathogens is so great that establishing a specific diagnosis is of paramount importance. Table 267.1 lists many of the important kinds of immunocompromise, examples of diseases associated with them, and the infections frequently associated with them. Although neutropenia is defined as an absolute neutrophil count (ANC) less than 1,000 per microliter, most severe infections occur when the ANC is less than 100 per microliter.

MANAGEMENT OF FEVER IN AN IMMUNOCOMPROMISED HOST

Neutropenia: Fever (101°F or higher) in a neutropenic patient should be considered indicative of infection unless there is another, obvious cause. Patients with neutropenia cannot mount an adequate inflammatory response and can have extensive infection without characteristic symptoms and signs. The physician should obtain appropriate culture specimens and perform a careful examination. If the patient is acutely ill or has signs of infection when the fever is first detected, broad-spectrum antibiotic therapy should be initiated immediately. Otherwise, antibiotic therapy can be delayed until the fever has persisted for at least 2 hours. Current antibiotic regimens of choice include combinations of broad-spectrum β-lactams plus aminoglycosides (with or without vancomycin for the possibility of resistant gram-positive infection) and certain broad-spectrum agents, such as cefepime, imipenem, meropenum, used alone. Alternatives to aminoglycosides include quinolones and trimethoprim–sulfamethoxazole.

If the patient responds to initial therapy and never has signs of local infection, oral therapy can be substituted and the patient discharged. As long as the patient continues to have neutropenia, therapy should be continued for 1 week or for 4 days after the patient becomes afebrile, whichever is longer. If the patient has signs of localized infection, the duration of therapy depends on the clinical response. If patients remain febrile despite therapy with broad-spectrum antibiotics, one must consider drug or transfusion fever, tumor fever, and infection caused by antibiotic-resistant bacteria, viruses, mycobacteria, protozoa, or fungi. Of these, the most common is fungal infection. Because culture specimens often do not provide enough information to confirm a diagnosis, a therapeutic trial of antifungal therapy is appropriate.

Other causes of immunosuppression: Infection among patients with impaired lymphocyte and monocyte function is diverse in causation and usually is indolent. For these reasons, empiric therapy should be deferred in favor of vigorous attempts at diagnosis. Careful history taking is critical, and special attention should be given to possible exposures. Biopsy of infected tissue is the most rapid and reliable diagnostic procedure, although special stains and culture procedures may be needed. Serologic profiles and skin tests may be necessary. Lists of site-specific infections are helpful. Table 267.4 lists some causes of pneumonitis among persons with compromised immune systems.

Chapter 267

INFLUENZA

DEFINITION AND EPIDEMIOLOGY

Influenza viruses are pleomorphic members of the Orthomyxoviridae. Of the three types, only influenza A and B are important causes of morbidity and mortality. Epidemics occur annually in temperate climates during the cold weather months. Minor antigenic changes in the hemagglutinin or neuraminidase lead to decreased reactivity with antibody acquired from previous infection. Influenza is spread through contact with virus-containing respiratory secretions. The incubation period ranges from 1 to 5 days. School-aged children usually are affected disproportionately at the start of an epidemic.

CLINICAL FEATURES

Illness is typically characterized by systemic symptoms such as fever, headache, myalgia, and malaise in association with respiratory symptoms that include sore throat and dry cough. However, 30% of persons with the infection have upper respiratory symptoms without fever and another 20% have no symptoms. With febrile influenza, the systemic symptoms often are more prominent at the onset of illness and subside as the respiratory symptoms worsen. Fever and systemic symptoms usually last 3 to 5 days; the cough may last several weeks. The two principal pulmonary complications are primary viral pneumonia and secondary bacterial pneumonia. Exacerbations of asthma also occur. Nonpulmonary complications include myositis, myocarditis, pericarditis, and neurologic diseases

such as transverse myelitis and Guillain–Barré syndrome. Reye syndrome is a severe complication among children.

LABORATORY STUDIES AND DIAGNOSIS TESTS

A presumptive diagnosis can be made for patients with typical clinical features of febrile influenza when influenza is documented to be in the community. The diagnosis is confirmed by means of detection of the virus in respiratory secretions or a serologic response to the virus. Rapid virus detection tests have good specificity (more than 90%) but low sensitivity (less than 60% among adults).

MANAGEMENT

Antipyretics and analgesics are used for symptom relief, although salicylates should be avoided in the treatment of children because of an association with Reye syndrome. For influenza A infections only, amantadine and rimantadine are effective in reducing the duration of symptoms and viral shedding when administered within 48 hours after the onset of illness. Rimantadine has fewer side effects, such as insomnia, light-headedness, and irritability.

PREVENTION

Inactivated influenza vaccines have been shown to prevent hospitalization and death in high-risk populations. Vaccines should be offered to persons older than 65 years, those with chronic medical illnesses or cardiopulmonary disease, and residents of chronic care facilities and persons who can transmit the virus to them, such as health care workers and household members. Administration of the vaccine to members of the general population who are not at high risk also is acceptable. The composition of the vaccine changes from year to year to reflect the antigenic changes seen in circulating influenza A and B viral isolates. Persons with egg allergies should not be given the vaccine. Amantadine and rimantadine are approved for the prophylaxis of influenza A virus infection and should be considered in the care of persons at high risk who are vaccinated after influenza A virus activity has begun (for up to 2 weeks after vaccination), those with immunodeficiency, and persons for whom the vaccine is contraindicated.

Chapter 310

MALARIA

DEFINITION, EPIDEMIOLOGY, AND PATHOPHYSIOLOGY

Malaria is the sequela of infection with one of four species of plasmodia: *Plasmodium falciparum, P. vivax, P. ovale,* and *P. malariae.* Malaria is endemic in most of the developing tropical world. Transmission depends on the bite of an infected *Anopheles* mosquito, which introduces sporozoites into the human circulation. Within hepatocytes, the parasite matures to a merozoite stage. The merozoites invade red blood cells (RBCs) and mature further through a series of erythrocytic stages. After 48 to 72 hours, the host RBC is lysed, freeing merozoites that can then invade additional RBCs and perpetuate the cycle. *P. vivax* and *P. ovale* have persistent liver stages that may remain dormant in the liver for 6 to 12 months or more.

P. falciparum malaria is the most serious infection, partly because this species, unlike the others, can invade RBCs of any age and can therefore cause greater degrees of parasitemia. In addition, RBCs containing mature *P. falciparum* parasites adhere to the microvascular endothelium and can cause ischemia, hypoglycemia, and acidosis in affected tissues. Pulmonary edema may be caused by capillary leak syndrome.

CLINICAL FEATURES

The cardinal clinical features of malaria are recurring fevers and chills (associated with lysis of RBCs) in the absence of localizing signs. The periodicity of the fevers is typically 48 hours with *P. vivax* or *P. ovale* and 72 hours with *P. malariae.* In contrast, irregular fevers occur with *P. falciparum* infection. In severe *P. falciparum* infection, acute complications include coma, pulmonary edema, acute renal failure, thrombocytopenia, and gastroenteritis. Chronic infection may produce splenomegaly.

DIAGNOSIS

Malaria is diagnosed by means of identification of parasites on a Giemsa-stained blood film. Experienced observers can determine both the degree of the parasitemia and the infecting species of plasmodium. Antigen detection and DNA probes can be useful but are not used routinely.

MANAGEMENT

The Centers for Disease Control and Prevention (CDC) maintains a 24-hour telephone line to help physicians in the treatment of patients with severe and complicated malaria: (888) 232-3228. Similar information is available on the Internet at the CDC site: http://www.cdc.gov/. Infection of a nonimmune patient with *P. falciparum* is considered a medical emergency and generally requires hospitalization. Chloroquine should be used if the patient has come from an area where there is no evidence of chloroquine resistance. Table 322.2 lists alternatives available in the United States for the treatment of patients who may have been exposed to chloroquine-resistant species.

PREVENTION

Although efforts are underway, no safe and effective malaria vaccine exists. Chemoprophylaxis is the most important preventive measure. Chloroquine (500 mg weekly beginning 1 week before exposure and continuing until 4 weeks after exposure) is the agent of choice for persons traveling to areas without chloroquine resistance. Alternatives for travel to areas with documented resistance to chloroquine include mefloquine (250 mg weekly during exposure and for 4 weeks after exposure) and doxycycline (100 mg per day beginning 1 day before exposure and continuing until 4 weeks after exposure). It also is important to reduce vector exposure as much as possible with mosquito netting and mosquito repellents (DEET). A 2-week course of primaquine (15 mg per day) given after the traveler leaves the malaria-endemic area effectively prevents late relapse caused by the hepatic stages of *P. vivax* or *P. ovale*.

Chapter 322

■ OSTEOMYELITIS

DEFINITIONS

Osteomyelitis is defined as inflammation involving the bone marrow, the surrounding cortical bone, and the periosteum. *Acute osteomyelitis* is defined as the first clinical episode, complete with the signs, symptoms, and diagnostic confirmation of bone infection. *Chronic osteomyelitis* is the diagnostic term for bone infections not controlled with one or more treatment attempts.

PATHOPHYSIOLOGY

Pathogens gain access to bone in three ways—hematogenous dissemination, direct inoculation, or extension from contiguous sites. Bone infection among children and intravenous drug users usually is hematogenous. In contrast, direct inoculation at the site of fracture or injury is common among adults. Osteomyelitis extending from contiguous infected sites often occurs among patients with diabetes who have foot infections or among patients with decubitus ulcers. Regardless of the route of entry, the initial bone infection causes inflammation, vascular compromise, local hypoxia, and eventually the death of bone tissue. Infection may result in formation of avascular tissue, or bone sequestrum, which forms a nidus for persistent infection.

ETIOLOGY

Staphylococcus aureus is the most common pathogen among adults, accounting for 50% to 70% of cases. The number of infections with gram-negative bacilli, either as a single infectious agent or as a part of a polymicrobial infection, has increased recently. These organisms have been cultured in as many as 50% of infections in some studies. These bacteria are more likely to cause osteomyelitis among patients with open fractures and prolonged hospitalization, patients who have undergone multiple hospital procedures, and those who have an extended stay in intensive care units. Infection with *Staphylococcus epidermidis* is common after implantation of an orthopedic prosthesis and in poststernotomy osteomyelitis. The presence of anaerobic bacteria should be considered when infection follows a human bite or is contiguous to a dental, intraabdominal, foot, or ear-nose-throat infection. Polymicrobial aerobic and anaerobic infections are common among patients with diabetes and those with decubitus ulcers.

CLINICAL FEATURES

Adults often have localized pain unresponsive to nonsteroidal anti-inflammatory drugs, heat, or rest. Swelling or redness may be present. Patients with vertebral osteomyelitis may have back pain; however, patients with infections of the larger cortical bones or patients with peripheral neuropathy might not have pain. The extremity should be examined for signs of venous stasis, acrocyanosis, edema,

draining sinus tracts, erythema, induration, tenderness, and impaired range of motion or sensory perception. The history should include questions regarding previous illnesses and any conditions that might have contributed to local or systemic host immune deficiencies.

DIAGNOSIS

Diagnosis involves a combination of clinical suspicion, appropriate laboratory tests, and radiographic and radionuclide scanning studies. It should be confirmed by means of histologic examination and microbiologic culture of bone specimens obtained at surgery or percutaneous needle biopsy.

Laboratory tests: The white blood cell count usually is elevated only in the early stages of infection. The erythrocyte sedimentation rate often is elevated.

Radiographs: In the early stages of osteomyelitis, specific signs on conventional radiographs may be absent for as long as 2 weeks. Within 4 weeks, one or more of the following changes should be evident: periosteal elevation, lytic bone destruction, sclerosis, or the presence of sequestrum or an overlying soft-tissue mass. Computed tomography and magnetic resonance imaging (MRI) are useful adjuncts in evaluations of selected patients, particularly in the early stages, when conventional radiographs are normal. MRI has excellent specificity, especially in differentiation of bone tumor and infarction from osteomyelitis. It is the modality of choice for diagnosing and staging spinal infection and for staging the extent of infection in long cortical bones before definitive open debridement. Bone scanning with technetium Tc 99m has excellent sensitivity for the diagnosis of osteomyelitis, especially within the first 2 weeks, but the specificity is relatively low. False-positive results occur among patients with tumors or infarction or patients with bone injury involving the periosteum.

Culture results: Blood cultures may be positive in the acute phase of the disease, but is rare among adults. Swab cultures of sinus tracts usually are not accurate. Therefore, microbiologic diagnosis almost always depends on aerobic and anaerobic culture of a bone biopsy specimen.

MANAGEMENT

Therapy for acute or chronic osteomyelitis requires prolonged antibiotic therapy (4 to 6 weeks) and complete surgical debridement of necrotic bone and soft tissue where there is evidence of residual sequestrum or foreign material. Parenteral administration is generally recommended, although quinolones have been effective given orally. Broader-spectrum agents frequently are necessary for chronic osteomyelitis because polymicrobial infection is more common in such cases. The most effective strategy is the institution of appropriate antimicrobial therapy based on culture and sensitivity results after complete surgical debridement. For *S. aureus,* therapy may include a β-lactamase–resistant penicillin such as nafcillin, a first-generation cephalosporin such as cefazolin, or a fluoroquinolone. Infection with *S. epidermidis* or methicillin-resistant strains of *S. aureus* necessitates use of vancomycin. Enterococcal infections can be managed with ampicillin plus gentamicin. Pseudomonal infections respond best to a combination of an aminoglycoside and a third-generation cephalosporin (such as ceftazidime), ciprofloxacin, or semisynthetic penicillin (such as piperacillin). Other gram-negative organisms can be controlled with ciprofloxacin or the combination of ticarcillin and clavulanic acid. The presence of anaerobic organisms may necessitate therapy with clindamycin or metronidazole.

Chapter 265

■ STREPTOCOCCAL PHARYNGITIS AND RHEUMATIC FEVER

DEFINITION, INCIDENCE, AND EPIDEMIOLOGY

Pharyngitis is the most common clinical manifestation of group A streptococcal infection. Most cases of pharyngitis, however, are caused by respiratory viruses. Most cases of streptococcal pharyngitis occur during winter and spring. Transmission occurs through large respiratory droplets from infected persons; thus the infection is common in crowded settings such as child care centers, schools, and military barracks.

CLINICAL FINDINGS

Characteristic symptoms include the acute onset of fever and sore throat. Headache, abdominal pain, vomiting, and malaise also can occur, especially among children. Physical examination typically reveals pharyngeal erythema and edema. Tonsils are enlarged and may have a grayish-white exudate. Tender anterior cervical lymphadenopathy frequently is present. Signs of upper respiratory infection such as rhinorrhea, cough, and hoarseness suggest a nonstreptococcal cause.

COMPLICATIONS

Suppurative complications: These include direct extension of infection and resultant peritonsillar or retropharyngeal abscess, sinusitis, otitis media, mastoiditis, or cervical lymphadenitis. Bacteremic spread may produce metastatic foci of infection.

Nonsuppurative sequelae: These include acute rheumatic fever and acute glomerulonephritis, although the later more often follows cutaneous streptococcal infection. In acute rheumatic fever, which usually occurs 2 to 3 weeks after the pharyngitis, antibodies to streptococcal M protein epitopes may cross react with myocardial proteins, antigens in the basal ganglia, and antigens in articular cartilage. Major manifestations include carditis, which may lead to mitral and aortic valve stenosis; arthritis, particularly of the ankles, knees, wrists, and elbows; chorea; subcutaneous nodules; and erythema marginatum, which is a serpiginous, erythematous rash on the torso or extremities. Minor manifestations include fever, arthralgia, first-degree heart block, and elevated levels of acute-phase reactants. That there has been preceding group A streptococcal infection can be ascertained with serologic tests and less commonly with culture.

DIAGNOSTIC EVALUATION

The accurate diagnosis of group A streptococcal pharyngitis cannot be made with consistency through clinical findings alone. Throat swab culture remains the standard for diagnosis. Rapid antigen detection tests offer excellent specificity but low sensitivity. For this reason, negative results of such tests should always be followed by a throat culture.

MANAGEMENT

Treatment reduces spread, prevents suppurative and nonsuppurative complications, and may shorten the duration of illness. Penicillin V (250 mg by mouth three times a day for 10 days) or intramuscular benzathine penicillin (600,000 U for patients who weigh less than 27 kg; 1,200,000 U for patients who weigh more than 27 kg) is the treatment of choice. Erythromycin is recommended for treatment of persons with penicillin allergy. Therapy can be initiated for up to 9 days after the onset of symptoms and still prevent the occurrence of rheumatic fever. Repeat throat culture to document cure after therapy is not recommended. Because recurrences of rheumatic fever may follow subsequent group A streptococcal infections, intramuscular benzathine penicillin given every 4 weeks is recommended for at least 5 years after an episode of rheumatic fever.

Chapter 275

■ SYPHILIS

DEFINITION AND EPIDEMIOLOGY

Syphilis is a chronic, systemic, sexually transmitted disease caused by the spirochete *Treponema pallidum* subspecies *pallidum.* Most cases are caused by sexual contact with mucocutaneous lesions that occur in the primary or secondary stages. Late syphilis is considered noninfectious. Throughout the 1990s, rates of primary and secondary syphilis declined 84% in the United States.

PATHOPHYSIOLOGY

Organisms rapidly penetrate intact mucous membranes and microscopically abraded skin and disseminate soon thereafter. Two histopathologic features characterize the syphilitic lesions of all stages of disease—obliterative endarteritis, in which hyperplasia and swelling of endothelial cells completely occlude blood vessels, and a loose perivascular infiltrate consisting of lymphocytes, macrophages, and plasma cells. Granuloma formation is common with more advanced disease.

CLINICAL FINDINGS AND DIFFERENTIAL DIAGNOSIS

Primary syphilis: Although classic syphilis is divided into stages, there is considerable temporal, clinical, and histopathologic overlap among them. The chancre, the primary lesion of syphilis, appears at the incubation site after an incubation period of 10 to 90 days (average, 3 weeks). It begins as an erythematous papule that ulcerates before healing spontaneously within 2 to 4 weeks. The typical chancre is painless, solitary, rounded, and has a raised, discrete border with a rubbery consistency. Approximately 50% of patients with primary syphilis have

painless, nonsuppurative, bilateral regional lymphadenopathy. Primary syphilis must be differentiated from other causes of genital ulceration, including venereal infection (e.g., chancroid, herpes genitalis, lymphogranuloma venereum, and granuloma inguinale), nonvenereal infection (e.g., cat-scratch fever and sporotrichosis), and noninfectious disorders (e.g., trauma and malignant disease).

Secondary syphilis: About 6 to 24 weeks after infection, usually when the chancre is either healing or has disappeared entirely, the secondary, or disseminated, stage of syphilis begins. The cutaneous lesions (syphilids) usually are described as macular or maculopapular and are generally symmetric and widespread, varying from several millimeters to several centimeters in diameter. Some patients have lesions characteristically confined to the distal extremities, especially the palms and the soles. Syphilids may resemble lesions of psoriasis, lichen planus, or pityriasis rosea. Other common mucocutaneous manifestations include patchy alopecia and thinning of the eyebrows and beard; diffuse redness of the tonsils and pharynx; and moist, papular excrescences in the intertriginous areas (condyloma lata) that are highly infectious. Generalized lymphadenopathy often is present, and splenomegaly may occur. Other organ systems that may be involved include the gastrointestinal tract (granulomatous hepatitis associated with a markedly elevated alkaline phosphatase level), the central nervous system (headache and meningism, less commonly basilar meningitis, acute hydrocephalus, optic neuritis, or cerebrovascular syndromes), the eyes (anterior uveitis), the kidneys (rare instances of immune complex glomerulonephritis), and the bones (mild osteitis with bone pain).

Latency: After the manifestations of secondary syphilis subside, untreated patients enter an asymptomatic stage, called *latency.* About 25% of patients experience one or more infectious relapses during the first 4 years of latency; after that, infectious relapses are rare. These relapses may be indistinguishable from the patient's previous secondary episode, but cutaneous lesions tend to be less prominent, and mucosal lesions may predominate. Isolated visceral relapses can occur.

Tertiary syphilis: Approximately 30% of untreated patients with late latent disease have one or more forms of tertiary syphilis years, even decades, after infection. Tertiary syphilis is traditionally divided into three categories—benign tertiary (gummatous), cardiovascular, and neurosyphilis. Gummatous disease is characterized by the development of one or more granulomatous lesions (gummas) 7 to 10 years after initial infection. They can occur anywhere but are most common on mucocutaneous surfaces and in bone. Cardiovascular syphilis is caused by obliterative endarteritis of the vasa vasorum of the large arteries, particularly the proximal ascending aorta, that leads to aneurysmal dilatation. Aortic regurgitation and congestive heart failure can occur. There are four categories of neurosyphilis—asymptomatic (cerebrospinal fluid [CSF] abnormalities only), meningovascular (manifesting as stroke), gummatous (central nervous system mass lesions), and parenchymatous (tabes dorsalis and generalized paresis). Tabes dorsalis is caused by demyelinization of the posterior columns of the spinal cord, dorsal roots, and dorsal root ganglia. Patients experience lancinating pain, pupillary abnormalities, impotence, bladder incontinence, truncal ataxia, lower extremity areflexia, and a profound loss of position and vibratory sensation in the lower extremities that gives rise to chronic traumatic arthritis (Charcot joints). Generalized paresis is an insidious dementia that can include seizures, dramatic and bizarre changes in personality, and intellectual deterioration.

LABORATORY FINDINGS

Diagnosis requires either reactive serologic results or identification of the treponeme in clinical specimens. Serologic tests are the mainstay of diagnosis. Nontreponemal tests (e.g., VDRL and rapid plasma reagin) measure flocculating antibodies to a mixture of cardiolipin, cholesterol, and lecithin. These antibodies presumably arise from the interaction of treponemes with host tissues. Titers tend to be highest in secondary disease and decline gradually thereafter. Approximately 30% of patients with primary, late latent, and tertiary disease have nonreactive test results. Many conditions may give rise to falsely positive results, either acutely (various viral illnesses, malaria, *Mycoplasma pneumoniae* infection) or chronically (autoimmune disorders such as lupus erythematosus, narcotic addiction, leprosy, pregnancy, and normal aging).

Treponemal tests measure antibodies specific to the pathogenic treponemes and are necessary to confirm that reactive nontreponemal serologic results are caused by treponemal infection. The most commonly used are the fluorescent treponemal antibody absorption test (FTA-ABS) and the microhemagglutination assay—*Treponema pallidum* (MHATP). These tests are almost perfectly sensitive for secondary, latent, and tertiary disease but are only about 85% sensitive for primary disease. False-positive results occur among as much as 2% of the general population owing to cross reaction with nonpathogenic treponemes.

The most rapid and direct means of identifying treponemes in clinical specimens is dark-field microscopic examination. Exudates from chancres and moist secondary lesions are most amenable to this procedure. Examination of specimens from mucosal surfaces is not recommended because they are colonized with nonpathogenic treponemes that may be confused with *T. pallidum.* Demonstration of treponemes in tissue may be accomplished by means of silver stain or anti–*T. pallidum* antibodies, the latter being more sensitive and specific.

To diagnose neurosyphilis, CSF examination should be performed on any patient with reactive serologic results and neurologic abnormalities. Active disease usually is accompanied by CSF pleocytosis, usually lymphocytic, and often by an elevated protein level. In the absence of a traumatic lumbar puncture, a reactive CSF-VDRL test result is almost 100% specific for neurosyphilis, although its sensitivity varies from about 60% (tabes dorsalis) to nearly 100% (meningovascular syphilis).

MANAGEMENT

Penicillin is the drug of choice for therapy for all stages of syphilis (Table 297.2). Several hours after receiving therapy, some patients experience a sudden onset of chills, fever, tachycardia, headache, flushing, and headache (Jarisch–Herxheimer reaction). Symptoms usually abate within 24 hours and can be managed with aspirin. When initially reactive, nontreponemal serologic results should be followed at regular intervals, ideally beginning 3 months after therapy, to confirm cure. On average, among successfully treated patients with primary or secondary syphilis, titers decrease fourfold at 6 months and eightfold at 12 months. Patients with early syphilis and nontreponemal test results that remain active at a low, stable titer also may be considered cured.

Chapter 297

■ TUBERCULOSIS

DEFINITION, INCIDENCE, AND EPIDEMIOLOGY

Tuberculosis (TB) is infection by *Mycobacterium tuberculosis.* Asia and Africa currently have more than 70% of reported cases. In the United States, infection rates have declined since 1953, except for a period from 1985 through 1992. Cases tend to cluster in urban areas, where the infection disproportionately affects persons with HIV disease, members of racial and ethnic minorities, and those who are foreign born. *M. tuberculosis* is transmitted through the air by droplet nuclei expelled from the cough of a person with pulmonary or laryngeal TB. The risk is greatest in spaces lacking air volume, fresh air, and natural or ultraviolet light. The best predictors of a patient's contagiousness are the number of bacilli in the pulmonary secretions and the presence and frequency of cough. Persons with latent infection (see later) are not contagious.

PATHOGENESIS

Once inspired, droplet nuclei may lodge in the pulmonary alveoli to establish infection. Among approximately 5% of those infected, bacilli multiply locally over weeks to months to cause primary tuberculosis—hilar or peritracheal lymphadenopathy, lobar pneumonia, usually in the middle or lower lobes, or pleuritis. Infection includes the invasion of alveolar macrophages, within which the mycobacteria can survive and disseminate throughout the body. In response, infected macrophages may combine to form swirls of multinucleated giant cells in a stroma of fibrous inflammatory tissue, the hallmark of tuberculous granuloma. Over a period of years, a granuloma may become relatively large and calcified.

Most persons with *M. tuberculosis* infection have no signs of infection other than development of delayed-type hypersensitivity to tuberculin proteins. In such cases, the infection generally becomes latent and may uncommonly evolve to active disease only after many years, particularly if the person sustains an immunocompromising condition or reaches old age. Reactivation disease is much more common than primary disease. Although it can take place in any tissue, reactivation most often occurs in the apical regions of the lung. Large caseous foci may produce visible cavities in the lung parenchyma and destroy lung tissue over a period of years.

CLINICAL FINDINGS

Pulmonary TB constitutes 80% to 85% of active cases. The other cases are extrapulmonary. Concomitant pulmonary and extrapulmonary disease occurs

among about 7% of patients, and miliary TB accounts for 0.2% of cases. The diagnosis of TB can be elusive, because the disease can masquerade as a variety of pulmonary illnesses, including bacterial or viral pneumonia, interstitial lung disease, and neoplasm. Moreover, among patients with compromised immune systems, such as those with AIDS, symptoms generally are subtle, and chest radiographic findings may be atypical.

Pulmonary disease: About 10% to 20% of persons with active TB have no symptoms, particularly those who are elderly or who have early disease. The most common symptoms include cough with or without sputum production and hemoptysis, fever, night sweats, and weight loss. Other symptoms include pleuritic chest pain, dyspnea, hemoptysis, fatigue, and anorexia. The physical findings are nonspecific and vary depending on the stage of the disease. In early disease, the examination findings may be normal. Later signs include rales, rhonchi, or signs of consolidation such as tubular breath sounds or enhanced tactile fremitus. In advanced disease, generalized wasting may occur.

Extrapulmonary disease: Extrapulmonary TB usually is a consequence of lymphohematogenous dissemination of *M. tuberculosis* organisms during primary infection and is more common among immunocompromised patients. In descending order of frequency, the most common forms are lymphatic (scrofula, usually involving the cervical and supraclavicular chains), pleural (usually unilateral), bone and joint (most often vertebral and also known as Pott's disease), genitourinary, meningeal, peritoneal, and pericardial. Symptoms of local disease generally are limited to the affected site. Symptoms in systemic (miliary) disease are nonspecific and may consist only of constitutional symptoms such as fever, anorexia, and weight loss.

DIAGNOSTIC EVALUATION

A thorough clinical evaluation is essential. It is especially important to obtain accurate information about past TB exposure and immunocompromising conditions or medications. Other important diagnostic elements include a Mantoux tuberculin skin test, which has a positive result among 85% to 90% of immunocompetent patients with pulmonary TB; chest radiography; and smears and cultures for acid-fast bacteria (AFB).

Pulmonary disease: TB may have various manifestations on chest radiographs, but the hallmark is an infiltrate with cavitation, usually in the apical region. Other findings include lymphadenopathy, lobar infiltrates, and interstitial infiltrates. Unless occult pulmonary disease is suspected, computed tomography of the chest is not usually helpful in the initial evaluation. Laboratory abnormalities may include leukocytosis or leukopenia and normocytic anemia.

Extrapulmonary disease: Chest radiography can demonstrate a pleural effusion or a form of cardiomegaly suggestive of pericardial effusion. Effusions from peritoneal, pleural, and pericardial spaces typically are lymphocytic exudates. Fluid glucose level usually is low but may be normal; protein level is elevated. Smears, cultures, and biopsy specimens from these sites are positive in about 65%, 75%, and 85% of cases, respectively. The diagnostic yield from a cerebrospinal fluid smear and culture is disappointingly low (15% and 50%, respectively), but polymerase chain reaction techniques improve rates of detection. In miliary disease, blood cultures can be useful and biopsy specimens from sites such as the liver, bone marrow, lymph nodes, and lung may be examined for evidence of granuloma formation and AFB.

Management when TB is suspected: The diagnosis of TB may be suggested by symptoms and signs or by a positive tuberculin skin test result. It is important to determine the patient's degree of possible contagiousness when making decisions regarding disposition and restrictions in activity. Patients believed to have TB can be hospitalized or be evaluated as outpatients, depending on the severity of illness and the living situation. If patients are hospitalized, prompt isolation in a negative pressure room is critical for preventing transmission. For all persons believed to have TB, sputum specimens should be obtained on three consecutive mornings and sent for AFB smear and culture. If the smear results are negative, the patient is considered noninfectious. All cases of suspected TB must be reported to the local health department.

MANAGEMENT

Pulmonary disease: Hospitalized patients with positive smear results should remain in isolation, and persons being treated as outpatients should remain at home until they have three consecutive negative smears and have demonstrated a clinical response to antituberculous therapy. The course of therapy is divided into two components--the initial intensive phase (usually 2 weeks to 2 months in duration) and the continuation phase (4 months or longer, aimed at killing the few bacilli harbored in intracellular compartments). The three guiding principles of therapy are as follows: (a) regimens must contain at least three drugs to which the organisms are susceptible; (b) the drugs must be taken regularly; and (c) drug therapy must be continued for a sufficient period of time. First-line drugs include isoniazid (INH), rifampin, pyrazinamide (PZA), ethambutol, and streptomycin. Many treatment approaches may be used; one common regimen consists of daily doses of INH (5 mg per kilogram, up to 300 mg), rifampin (10 mg per kilogram, up to 600 mg), and PZA (20 to 35 mg per kilogram, up to 2 g) for the first 2 months and followed by INH and rifampin at the same dosages for another 4 months.

Extrapulmonary disease: Therapy for extrapulmonary TB usually follows the same principles as for pulmonary TB. The same drug regimens are used for the same durations. The exceptions are miliary TB, TB of bone and joints, and TB meningitis, all of which necessitate 12 months of therapy. Management of TB pericarditis and meningitis also includes adjunctive use of glucocorticoids, to lessen the risk of constrictive pericarditis and permanent neurologic sequelae, respectively.

Therapy for drug-resistant TB: Multidrug-resistant TB (MDRTB) is suspected when the source of infection is known to have had drug-resistant disease and when a patient does not respond to adequate therapy. Drug susceptibility of a bacterial isolate can confirm the presence of MDRTB. When a patient is believed to have disease resistant to at least INH and rifampin, the initial regimen should contain at least three drugs to which susceptibility is considered likely and to which the patient is naive. Second-line antituberculous drugs include quinolones, capreomycin, cycloserine, kanamycin, ethionamide, and para-aminosalicylic acid. Medications should be administered under directly observed therapy. In the event of treatment failure, at least two drugs not previously taken by the patient should be added to the regimen simultaneously. Therapy for MDRTB should extend for at least 12 months after culture-negative status has been achieved.

SCREENING

Target groups and technique: Tuberculin skin testing is performed to ascertain who is at high risk of latent infection with *M. tuberculosis* and who would benefit from therapy to prevent reactivation. Current recommendations suggest that the following groups be screened: persons with HIV infection, close contacts of persons with infectious TB, persons with immunocompromising medical conditions, users of injected drugs, foreign-born persons from areas where TB is common, homeless persons, low-income populations, and residents or workers in congregate settings, such as correctional institutions, nursing homes, and mental institutions. The Mantoux tuberculin skin test with 5 units of purified protein derivative (PPD) is the standard method. The PPD is placed subcutaneously into the volar aspect of the forearm, and the result is interpreted 48 to 72 hours later. A positive reaction is determined by the size of the induration (not erythema) in millimeters and varies depending on risk category (Table 294.3). A two-step test, which consists of a second test 1 to 3 weeks after an initially negative test result, is more sensitive, because it may detect cases of latent infection in which the initial immune response is muted but becomes evident owing to a booster phenomenon.

Therapy for latent infection: Persons with a positive tuberculin skin test result should undergo chest radiography and clinical evaluation to exclude active disease. If the findings are normal, latent infection is likely. The decision to treat patients for latent infection depends on the person's circumstances. Treatment is recommended, regardless of age, for the following groups: those who are known or are likely to have HIV infection, close contacts of a person with TB, persons who inject drugs, persons with skin test results that have recently (within 2 years) converted, persons with certain medical conditions (such as diabetes mellitus, chronic renal failure, an organ transplant, hematologic malignant disease, ongoing use of glucocorticoids, and prior gastrectomy), and those who have chest radiographic findings that suggest prior active TB but have not received adequate antituberculous therapy. The following groups should be treated only if younger than 35 years: foreign-born persons from areas where TB is common; medically underserved, low-income populations; and homeless persons. A 9-month course of daily INH therapy is now thought to be the most effective regimen for eradication of latent TB infection. For persons with conditions in which neuropathy is common, such as diabetes, uremia, alcoholism, and HIV infection, pyridoxine also should be administered.

Chapter 294

■ VARICELLA-ZOSTER VIRUS INFECTION

DEFINITION, EPIDEMIOLOGY, AND ETIOLOGY

Varicella-zoster virus (VZV) is a member of the herpesvirus family that causes two diseases, varicella and zoster. Varicella (chickenpox), the primary infection, is mainly a highly contagious disease of young children, but about 5% of adults in the United States are susceptible. The infection tends to be more severe among adults. Zoster, the secondary infection, is caused by reactivation of VZV acquired during varicella that became latent within sensory ganglia. It is mainly a disease of adults with a steady rise in incidence after 50 years of age. Zoster also is more common among persons with compromised cellular immunity.

CLINICAL FINDINGS

Varicella: Varicella manifests as a generalized, pruritic rash after an incubation period ranging from 10 to 21 days. The rash, which is usually accompanied by fever, is most concentrated on the torso and head and consists progressively of maculopapules, vesicles, pustules, and crusts. There are often several crops of lesions, so all forms of the rash may be present on any one area of skin. All vesicles usually crust within 5 to 7 days, at which time the patient is no longer contagious to others. About 5% of adult patients have pulmonary involvement 1 to 6 days after the onset of the rash. Although usually self-limited and benign, varicella can be severe or fatal among pregnant women, those with immunodeficiency or hematologic malignant disease, and those treated with chemotherapeutic agents or high doses of glucocorticoids. Such patients may have hemorrhagic skin lesions, severe pneumonia, and disseminated intravascular coagulation.

Zoster: Zoster manifests as a unilateral rash in a dermatomic distribution; one to three dermatomes usually are involved. Fever may be present. Zoster occurs most commonly in the thoracic region, followed by the facial-cervical area, torso, and extremities. Pain occurs in the acute phase, and patients, particularly those older than 50 years, may have postherpetic neuralgia for many months after the rash has healed. Some patients have only dermatomic pain without a rash, a situation that may lead to considerable diagnostic confusion. Zoster of the face often involves the ophthalmic division of the trigeminal nerve. This commonly is associated with central nervous system involvement such as headache, aphasia, and seizures. Granulomatous angiitis of the cerebral blood vessels occurs occasionally among elderly patients.

DIAGNOSIS

Infections caused by VZV usually are distinctive, so laboratory confirmation often is unnecessary. However, about 10% of cases diagnosed clinically as zoster may actually be caused by herpes simplex virus (HSV). For example, HSV, rather than VZV, is almost always the cause of recurrent dermatomic rashes. A specific diagnosis of VZV infection is best made by means of culturing the skin scrapings of vesicular lesions. Serologic tests also can be performed. The Tzanck smear does not differentiate between VZV and HSV infection.

MANAGEMENT

Local measures, such as application of calamine lotion for varicella and Burow's solution for zoster, often are used.

Varicella: Aspirin should not be given to children and adolescents with varicella because of the risk of Reye syndrome. Acetaminophen can be used to control fever. Antihistamines may be given to reduce itching. Patients with severe or potentially severe infection, such as those with compromised immune systems, should be treated with intravenous acyclovir (30 mg per kilogram per day for adults), although the dosage should be reduced in the treatment of patients with renal insufficiency. In the care of patients with competent immune systems, oral acyclovir (4 g per day in 5 divided doses) started within 24 hours of onset of the rash shortens the course of varicella by about 1 day but does not prevent complications or transmission.

Zoster: Acyclovir is effective even if 3 days have elapsed since the onset of the rash, but the benefit is greater with earlier intervention. Because there is some indication that acyclovir therapy given for 7 days may decrease pain associated with zoster and the incidence of postherpetic neuralgia, it has become customary to treat elderly patients who have early zoster. Famciclovir and valacyclovir have been approved for oral therapy for zoster. Because these agents are administered only 3 times a day, patient compliance may be better with these agents than with acyclovir. The use of glucocorticoids is controversial; these agents have not been shown to improve healing or decrease postherpetic neuralgia, but they may improve quality of life.

PREVENTION AND CONTROL

Passive immunization against varicella may be achieved with varicella-zoster immune globulin (VZIG). It is indicated for prevention or modification of severe varicella among persons at high risk, including those with an underlying malignant disease or immunodeficiency and those receiving high doses of glucocorticoids. Recipients should have had intimate exposure to VZV within the preceding 5 days from a person with either varicella or zoster. A live attenuated varicella vaccine has been approved for use in the care of healthy varicella-susceptible children and adults. Adults should be given two doses 1 month apart.

Chapter 315

PULMONARY MEDICINE

▬ APPROACH TO THE MANAGEMENT OF THE PATIENT WITH ACUTE RESPIRATORY DISTRESS SYNDROME

DEFINITION AND ETIOLOGY

Acute respiratory distress syndrome (ARDS, previously called adult respiratory distress syndrome) represents the abrupt onset of diffuse lung injury characterized by severe hypoxemia and generalized pulmonary infiltrates in the absence of cardiac failure. It has most often been associated with sepsis syndrome and bacterial or viral pneumonia. Other causes include major traumatic injury, aspiration of gastric contents, massive transfusion, inhalation injury, pancreatitis, near-drowning, fat embolism after long bone fractures, and drug overdose.

PATHOPHYSIOLOGY

Structural changes: Inflammatory cells, especially neutrophils, accumulate within the alveolar space and are believed to contribute to lung injury by releasing granular enzymes and oxidants. Type I alveolar epithelial cells undergo cytopathic changes, and the alveolar basement membrane is damaged. Changes in cellular permeability allow interstitial and alveolar edema; hyaline membranes are then produced by aggregation of fibrin and other proteins in the alveolar space. As the process continues, intravascular thrombosis, loss of pulmonary microvasculature, and fibrotic distortion of septal architecture occur.
Physiologic changes: ARDS is associated with impaired gas exchange, altered lung mechanics, and pulmonary vascular changes. Lung compliance and functional residual capacity decrease, and work of breathing increases. The loss of microvasculature in the later stages leads to pulmonary hypertension.

CLINICAL PRESENTATION AND DIAGNOSIS

ARDS develops rapidly, usually within 12 to 72 hours of the predisposing event. Respiratory distress, severe hypoxemia, and generalized pulmonary infiltrates all are necessary for the diagnosis. The most widely accepted definition of hypoxemia in this setting is a ratio of the arterial oxygen tension (P_aO_2) to the fraction of inspired oxygen (FiO_2) less than 200. Congestive heart failure as an alternative diagnosis can be excluded either clinically or by determining that the pulmonary artery occlusion pressure is less than 18 mm Hg. To date, no specific laboratory findings have been described.

PROGNOSIS AND MANAGEMENT

Therapy is primarily supportive. Well-controlled studies have failed to find a benefit for glucocorticoids in the management or prevention of ARDS. The selective pulmonary vasodilator nitric oxide has been shown to improve oxygenation and to reduce pulmonary artery pressures without affecting mortality. Mechanical ventilation is almost always needed, as is positive end-expiratory pressure (PEEP). The assist-control (A/C) ventilator mode is preferred by most experts. Lower ventilator tidal volumes (6 mL per kilogram rather than 10 to 15 mL per kilogram) have been proved to decrease ventilator-associated lung injury, such as barotrauma-induced pneumothorax, and to reduce mortality. Survival rates in the most recent studies have been 60% to 70%. The course is variable, lasting from a few days to several weeks. The average duration of mechanical ventilation is approximately 10 to 12 days. One-third of the deaths of patients with ARDS are related to the underlying disease or injury.

Chapter 357

▬ ASTHMA

DEFINITION, EPIDEMIOLOGY, AND ETIOLOGY

Asthma is defined as intermittent, reversible airway obstruction in association with increased nonspecific bronchial reactivity and airway inflammation. It is one of the most common and expensive chronic illnesses in the United States, affecting 5% to 10% of the population. The incidence follows a bimodal age distribution, with an early peak from 4 to 10 years of age and second peak after 40 years of age. African American and Hispanic populations, particularly those in inner city areas, have both higher incidences and higher mortality rates than other groups. The basis for asthma is poorly understood. Multifactorial genetic factors likely contribute to susceptibility, but environmental exposures also are important. Among children, potential triggers include maternal cigarette smoking, infection with respiratory syncytial virus, and exposure to indoor allergens such as house dust mites, cockroaches, cats, and molds. Among adults, occupational asthma is prevalent in the lumber, plastics, and paint industries and among hospital workers with a sensitivity to latex.

PATHOPHYSIOLOGY

For asthma to develop, a complex immunologic reaction involving inflammatory cells and cytokines must be initiated and maintained. Although many cell types may be involved, lymphocytes, eosinophils, and mast cells predominate. Tissue damage involves the epithelium and the submucosal space, and hyperplasia of the airway smooth muscle occurs. Reversible airflow limitation is present, demonstrated by a reduction in the ratio of forced expiratory volume in 1 second (FEV_1) to forced vital capacity (FVC) (less than 75% among adults) and an improvement in the FEV_1 more than 12% to 15% after inhalation of a β-agonist. Other physiologic changes include hyperinflation (increased residual volume) and increased airway resistance. Airway hyperresponsiveness is demonstrated by methacholine, histamine, or exercise testing. A positive result of a methacholine challenge is defined as a reduction in FEV_1 of 20% or more with 8 mg per milliliter or less of methacholine. However, other diseases can be associated with airway hyperresponsiveness, such as chronic obstructive pulmonary disease (COPD), congestive heart failure (CHF), bronchiectasis, and seasonal allergic rhinitis.

CLINICAL FINDINGS AND DIAGNOSIS

The symptoms of asthma include cough, wheezing, chest tightness, and dyspnea. The diagnosis should be made through documentation of reversible airway obstruction (see earlier) in the setting of symptoms of the disease. Because of the intermittent nature of the disease, however, an occasional patient may have normal spirometric findings. If the history suggests asthma, the patient's peak flow can be monitored at home. Variation in peak flows more than 10% generally is considered diagnostic of asthma. If this sign is not present and the patient still has symptoms, a methacholine challenge may be performed (see earlier). The methacholine challenge is particularly helpful in the evaluation of patients with cough variant asthma, who often have normal spirograms and no symptoms other than cough.

DIFFERENTIAL DIAGNOSIS

Differentiation of COPD from asthma among cigarette smokers can be difficult. COPD usually decreases diffusion capacity, which does not occur in asthma. Vocal cord dysfunction involves involuntary closure of the vocal cords, usually during inspiration but occasionally during expiration as well. The diagnosis is made through laryngoscopic visualization of inappropriate closure of the cords during inspiration or flattening of the inspiratory limb of a flow-volume loop. Upper airway obstruction due to tumors or strictures causes flattening in both the inspiratory and expiratory phases of the flow-volume loops. CHF can cause wheezing known as *cardiac asthma*.

MANAGEMENT

A thorough history should be obtained to determine possible triggers such as exposure to allergens, use of nonsteroidal anti-inflammatory drugs, and occupational exposure to antigens. If indoor allergens are suspected, allergy skin testing should be undertaken to guide avoidance therapy. Exacerbating factors such as sinus disease, gastroesophageal reflux, and stressful life situations should be sought. Table 363.1 outlines the current definitions for asthma severity. Table 363.2 presents the appropriate treatments for each level.

Chronic maintenance therapy: In general, inhalation of glucocorticoids is the cornerstone of the management of all but the most mild asthma. These agents are effective and safe and counter the underlying inflammatory basis of the disease. The side effect of oral thrush can be minimized with the use of a spacer device or by rinsing the mouth after use. Fluticasone, budesonide, and beclomethasone are likely more potent than flunisolide or triamcinolone. Cromones such as nedocromil and cromolyn sodium are considered second-line agents for long-term control among adults. Little is known about the mechanism of action. Although these agents do have mast cell–stabilizing properties, the clinical importance of this effect is unclear.

Theophyllines are nonspecific phosphodiesterase inhibitors with weak bronchodilating effects and some antiinflammatory properties. They are classified as second-line agents for long-term control among patients with mild or moderate persistent asthma. Disadvantages include numerous drug–drug interactions and a narrow therapeutic window that can lead to seizures and arrhythmias with higher serum drug levels. Long-acting inhaled β-agonists include salmeterol and formoterol. These agents provide effective bronchodilation for more than 12 hours and have been shown to prevent nocturnal symptoms and diurnal peak flow fluctuations. They are primarily recommended for use with inhaled glucocorticoids in moderate persistent asthma. Because the pharmacokinetic properties make these drugs poor therapy for acute exacerbations, patients should always have a short-acting inhaled β-agonist to use for acute symptoms.

Leukotriene modulators (zafirlukast, montelukast, zileuton) diminish the production of leukotrienes and have shown efficacy in control of asthma induced by allergens, exercise, or aspirin. The most recent guidelines suggest that these drugs be used to manage mild, persistent asthma as alternatives to inhaled glucocorticoids, theophylline, and cromones.

Quick relief medications: Patients may need quick relief if symptoms worsen acutely. However, because patients' perceptions of airflow limitation do not correlate well with the actual degree of obstruction, home peak flow monitoring should be used to guide therapy. More than a 20% decrease in peak flow should be an indication for attention and treatment by the patient, whereas a 50% decline from baseline always necessitates an aggressive approach by the treating physician. All patients should have an action plan to begin treatment at home. This can include increased use of short-acting inhaled β-agonists, such as albuterol, and initial oral glucocorticoid therapy if there is insufficient response to the β-agonists. Although systemic glucocorticoids are the most effective asthma medications, toxicity necessitates that ongoing use be as limited as possible. The initial daily dose of prednisone for patients with an acute, severe exacerbation is 60 to 120 mg. The dose can be tapered gradually on the basis of clinical response.

Chapter 363

CHRONIC OBSTRUCTIVE PULMONARY DISEASE

DEFINITIONS

Chronic obstructive pulmonary disease (COPD) is a group of disorders that have in common the presence of persistent airflow obstruction. Chronic bronchitis is characterized clinically by chronic cough and sputum production for at least 3 months for 2 successive years without other known causes. Emphysema is a condition with abnormal permanent enlargement of airspaces distal to the terminal bronchioles accompanied by nonfibrotic destruction of walls. Asthma is characterized by reversible airway narrowing and increased responsiveness to

various stimuli. Many patients have features of more than one of these diseases and are given the less specific diagnosis COPD.

INCIDENCE AND EPIDEMIOLOGY

The overall prevalence in the United States is 4% to 6% among men and 1% to 3% among women. COPD is recognized among 10% to 15% of adults older than 55 years. As of 1990, COPD was the fourth leading cause of death in the United States and accounted for more than 13% of all hospitalizations.

ETIOLOGY AND PATHOGENESIS

Cigarette smoking is the most important risk factor and accounts for nearly 90% of all cases of COPD. Current smokers have 10 times the relative risk of nonsmokers. There is, however, marked individual variation in susceptibility; only 10% to 15% of smokers experience COPD. It has not been clearly established that passive smoke exposure causes COPD. The mechanisms by which smoking leads to COPD are not well understood. In the case of emphysema, the disease seems to be caused by an imbalance between lung proteases and antiproteases that leads to increased lung destruction. An inherited deficiency of α_1 protease inhibitor is associated with premature emphysema. In chronic bronchitis, pathologic changes in the airways include an inflammatory cell response, goblet cell proliferation, and an increase in smooth muscle.

CLINICAL FEATURES

COPD typically manifests later in life. The insidious development of dyspnea is the hallmark symptom. A cough is frequent and often is attributed to smoker's cough early in disease. The cough usually is productive of mucoid sputum. There may be a history of frequent respiratory infections. Some patients with COPD have abnormal gas exchange with hypoxemia or hypercapnea. Hypoxemia may be associated with cognitive or personality changes, polycythemia, and cyanosis. Chronic hypercapnea may cause headache.

During the physical examination, it is important to assess maximum expiratory flow for persons at high risk. This can be assessed easily with forced expiratory time (FET). Healthy persons can exhale completely within 4 seconds. An FET longer than 6 seconds signifies substantial obstruction. Other physical signs develop only when the disease is moderate to severe. Overinflation of the lungs can increase the anteroposterior diameter of the thorax, lower and flatten the diaphragm, and reduce respiratory excursion. The accessory breathing muscles (neck and intercostals) contribute more to ventilation. Wheezing with tidal respirations may be evident. With advanced emphysema, the breath sounds are diminished because of a reduction in flow and an increase in lung inflation. Signs of pulmonary hypertension and right-sided heart failure, such as peripheral edema and hepatic congestion, usually represent advanced disease.

LABORATORY STUDIES AND DIAGNOSTIC TESTS

Pulmonary function tests: The central diagnostic feature is reduced expiratory airflow due to airway narrowing. Spirometry is the standard test and is useful for detecting obstruction, staging severity, and following the disease course. A reduction in forced expiratory volume in 1 second (FEV_1) in relation to the forced vital capacity (FVC)—the FEV_1/FVC ratio—is the standard indicator of obstruction. The FEV_1 is the best measure of severity; it correlates with exercise tolerance and survival. Measurements of lung volume reveal increased residual volume, functional residual capacity, and sometimes total lung capacity (TLC). Emphysema causes a greater increase in TLC than do other lung diseases and reduces carbon monoxide diffusing capacity because of the loss of alveolar–capillary surface area.

Radiologic studies: Chest radiography has limited usefulness in diagnosing or staging COPD. The main use of this modality is in detecting other parenchymal lung or cardiovascular diseases that manifest with similar symptoms. With advanced emphysema, a chest radiograph may reveal hyperinflation of the lungs with a low, flat diaphragm and an increase in the retrosternal airspace on the lateral projection. The emphysematous lungs may appear radiolucent because of bullous changes. High-resolution computed tomography may document evidence of emphysema.

Arterial blood gas analysis: The analysis may reveal hypoxemia, particularly with exercise, and hypercapnea, particularly in advanced disease. The relation between gas exchange abnormalities and other measures of lung function is poor. Two characteristic patterns of disease can be defined with blood gas findings. Patients with severe dyspnea, mild hypoxemia, and normal-to-low arterial PCO_2 have been called *pink puffers* (type A COPD), reflecting their color and increased breathing effort. Patients with severe hypoxemia, carbon dioxide retention, right-sided heart failure, but little dyspnea are called *blue bloaters* (type B COPD), reflecting their bloated, cyanotic appearance and low ventilation. These differences may reflect variations in ventilation–perfusion ($\dot{V}/\dot{Q}$) mismatching and central respiratory drive. Most patients, however, fall between these two extremes.

MANAGEMENT

Prevention: Primary and secondary prevention strategies include avoidance or discontinuation of cigarette smoking and α_1 protease inhibitor replacement for persons with both proven genetic deficiency and abnormal lung function. Tertiary prevention to reduce complications of symptomatic disease include smoking cessation, influenza and pneumococcal vaccination, and pulmonary rehabilitation.

Oxygen therapy: Oxygen is the only therapy proven to prolong survival. Studies have justified the long-term use of oxygen therapy for severe resting hypoxemia (arterial PO_2 55 mm Hg or less). For patients with an arterial PO_2 between 56 and 59 mm Hg, oxygen therapy is indicated if erythrocytosis (hematocrit 55% or more) or cor pulmonale is present. The decision for long-term therapy should be made only when the patient has been in stable condition with optimal therapy for at least 30 days.

Symptomatic treatment: Medical treatment is directed at the reversible component of airway obstruction and control of secretions. Bronchodilators used to improve symptoms and increase airway caliber include β_2-agonists, anticholinergics, and methylxanthines such as theophylline. β_2-Agonists are best administered by means of inhalation with an emphasis on proper technique. The most common side effects are tremor and tachycardia. Anticholinergics such as ipratropium bromide have recently gained prominence in the management of COPD. They, too, are best administered by means of inhalation. Oral theophylline improves bronchial tone, diaphragmatic function, respiratory drive, and mucociliary clearance. The target therapeutic level is typically 10 to 20 µg per milliliter. Side effects occur even within this range; they include tremor, insomnia, irritability, and gastrointestinal upset. More serious side effects, including vomiting, arrhythmias, hypotension, and seizures, generally develop at higher blood levels.

Glucocorticoids can be beneficial to some patients with stable symptoms. A limited trial is probably justified for patients who cannot be treated with standard bronchodilators alone. Treatment should be continued only for the minority who have marked improvement in pulmonary function. Inhaled steroids are safer, but their effectiveness has not been as well established. Oral or intravenous steroids are clearly indicated for patients experiencing acute flare-ups of COPD.

Control of secretions is important for patients with a chronic productive cough. These patients should be encouraged to drink several glasses of fluid each day, but excessive hydration is not warranted. The patients also should be taught the technique of controlled coughing, which involves deep inspiration, breath-holding for a few seconds, and then coughing two or three times. The use of mucolytic agents (iodinated glycerol, nebulized acetylcysteine, or recombinant DNase) to thin secretions and promote clearance is controversial. Because cough is an essential protective mechanism, cough suppression therapy is not recommended. For acute exacerbations, when sputum changes color and increases in volume, treatment with antibiotics for 7 to 10 days is indicated. Oral antibiotics such as trimethoprim–sulfamethoxazole, amoxicillin, amoxicillin–clavulanate, tetracycline, or erythromycin are commonly chosen to cover pathogens colonizing the respiratory tract, including *Haemophilus influenzae*, *Streptococcus pneumoniae*, and *Moraxella catarrhalis*.

Chapter 364

■ APPROACH TO THE PATIENT WITH COUGH

EPIDEMIOLOGY AND PATHOPHYSIOLOGY

Coughing is the fifth most common symptom among patients at outpatient clinics in the United States. The cough reflex is subserved by vagal afferent pathways arising from the trachea, intrapulmonary airways, and larynx. Although it is an important natural defense mechanism, excessive coughing generates considerable intrathoracic pressure and may be associated with complications such as pneumothorax, syncope, subconjunctival hemorrhage, cervical disc prolapse, urinary incontinence, and esophageal perforation.

DIFFERENTIAL DIAGNOSIS

The differential diagnosis is extensive (Table 352.2). Acute cough usually is caused by viral or bacterial upper respiratory infection. It also, however, can be a manifestation of more serious conditions such as acute bacterial pneumonia, congestive heart failure, pulmonary embolism, asthma, or aspiration. These conditions usually are accompanied by other symptoms, such as dyspnea or fever. Chronic cough (cough that persists for more than 1 month) is most commonly caused by asthma, gastroesophageal reflux (GER), postnasal drip, chronic bronchitis, or bronchiectasis. Smoking is also a common cause of coughing.

DIAGNOSTIC APPROACH

The best approach is to exclude first the most common conditions associated with chronic dry coughing—postnasal drip, asthma, and GER. Often the history and physical examination are sufficient to suggest one of these diagnoses, and a therapeutic trial can then be undertaken. If further diagnostic evaluation for these conditions is necessary, the tests performed should be based on the initial suspicion, as follows: for possible postnasal drip, allergy tests and sinus computed tomography (CT); for suspected asthma, peak expiratory flow measurements at home and a bronchoprovocation test with histamine or methacholine; and for possible GER, 24-hour pH monitoring and perhaps endoscopic examination of the esophagus. A chest radiograph is recommended for most patients, unless a cause is quickly apparent and the cough improves with therapy. If the diagnosis remains elusive, studies such as full pulmonary function tests, lung CT, and fiberoptic bronchoscopy should be considered.

MANAGEMENT

Specific therapies: Many of the causes of chronic cough have specific therapies. The most straightforward is discontinuation of an offending medication, such as an angiotensin-converting enzyme (ACE) inhibitor, although it may take weeks for the cough to resolve. Postnasal drip is managed with glucocorticoid nasal sprays and an antihistamine with or without a short course of nasal decongestants; an antibiotic is used if purulent sinusitis is suspected. GER is managed with histamine 2 blockers or proton pump inhibitors, asthma with bronchodilators and inhaled glucocorticoids.

Nonspecific therapy: Opiates such as codeine are the most effective antitussive agents, but they cause physical dependence, respiratory depression, nausea and vomiting, and constipation. Non-narcotic antitussives include dextromethorphan, a synthetic morphine derivative with no analgesic or sedative properties. It is a constituent of many nonprescription cough remedies. Mucolytic agents such as acetylcysteine often are used to facilitate expectoration by reducing sputum viscosity in patients with chronic bronchitis, but there is little evidence that these agents are beneficial. Local anesthetics such as aerosolized lidocaine should be reserved for cases of severe, intractable cough, because they remove reflexes that protect the lungs from noxious substances.

Chapter 352

■ CYSTIC FIBROSIS

EPIDEMIOLOGY AND PATHOPHYSIOLOGY

Cystic fibrosis (CF) is an autosomal recessive disorder; it affects 1 in 3,000 U.S. whites, 1 in 15,000 African Americans, and 1 in 90,000 Asian Americans. The CF gene encodes for the CF transmembrane conductance regulator (CFTR). In CF, one of the chloride ion channels of epithelial cells is either absent or dysfunctional. This leads to decreased water content and increased viscosity of various secretions, including those in the lung and the pancreas. In addition, the high sodium concentrations in airway secretions may inactivate the antimicrobial peptides secreted by airway epithelial cells.

CLINICAL FINDINGS

Pulmonary and sinus disease: Symptoms generally begin in childhood. A self-perpetuating destructive inflammatory reaction is manifested by bronchitis, bronchiolitis, bronchiectasis, and a progressive decline in pulmonary function. Infection is predominantly caused by *Staphylococcus aureus*, *Haemophilus influenzae*, and *Pseudomonas aeruginosa* organisms. *P. aeruginosa* eventually becomes the dominant organism in more than 90% of patients; a mucoid strain eventually replaces other pathogens. Acute exacerbations consist of increased coughing, sputum production, and dyspnea. Hemoptysis and pneumothorax are complications of more advanced disease. Clubbing of the fingers and toes is a universal finding. Mechanical obstruction of the sinus ostia by viscous mucus can occur and is followed by bacterial infection. Nasal polyposis is common.

Pancreatic and gastrointestinal disease: Most patients have exocrine pancreatic insufficiency and malabsorption; acute pancreatitis occurs in 10% of cases. Diabetes mellitus occurs among 15% of patients. It is slow in onset and nonketotic. Episodes of complete or partial intestinal obstruction occur among 10% to 20% of adult patients. Other gastrointestinal complications include gastroesophageal reflux, peptic ulceration, Crohn's disease, cholelithiasis, and elevated levels of liver enzymes.

Other complications: Men with CF have obstructive azoospermia and are infertile. Women have normal fertility. Nondestructive, episodic arthritis, most commonly involving the lower limbs and fingers, occurs among some patients. Patients are susceptible to osteopenia and osteoporosis.

LABORATORY FINDINGS

The diagnosis is based on a positive result of a sweat chloride test (more than 60 mEq per liter) or results of genetic tests that demonstrate two CF alleles and symptoms compatible with CF. The sweat test is highly sensitive (96% in adults) and specific for CF, although false-positive results can occur if the patient has hypoadrenalism, hypothyroidism, or nephrogenic diabetes insipidus. Chest radiographs first show overinflation, peribronchial cuffing, and small infiltrates and then show bronchiectasis and diffuse fibrosis, which is most marked in the upper lobes. Almost all patients have panopacification of the paranasal sinuses. Malabsorption is characterized by elevated fecal fat levels and decreased serum levels of fat-soluble vitamins.

PROGNOSIS AND MANAGEMENT

In the United States in 1997, the median survival period was 30.6 years. Prognostic factors include genotype, pulmonary function, results of chest radiographs, and nutritional status. The forced expiratory volume in 1 second (FEV_1) is the single most sensitive predictor of mortality. An FEV_1 less than 30% of predictive is associated with a 45% 2-year mortality risk. About 95% of patients die of pulmonary complications.

Pulmonary and sinus disease: The mainstays of treatment are chest physical therapy and antibiotics, although the bacterial pathogens rarely are eradicated. For exacerbations, intervenous antibiotics are usually given for 2 weeks. The use of prophylactic antibiotics, including aerosolized forms, is controversial. Inhaled bronchodilators such as β_2-agonists and ipratropium bromide are indicated for those who respond. Recombinant human DNase alters the rheologic qualities of the sputum by cutting the size of DNA molecules. Oral glucocorticoids slow the decline in pulmonary function but cause serious side effects. Inhalation of steroids has been less well studied but seems reasonable in the care of patients with an asthmatic component to the disease. Oxygen therapy is given to patients with hypoxemia. A final therapeutic option for a few patients is lung transplantation. Sinus disease is managed with antibiotics, nasal irrigation, nasal steroids, and, if necessary, surgical drainage.

Pancreatic and gastrointestinal disease: Malabsorption is managed with oral pancreatic enzymes. Diabetes necessitates dietary control and insulin; the use of oral hypoglycemic agents is controversial. Intestinal obstruction is treated with rehydration, nasogastric suction, and hyperosmolar enemas. Surgery rarely is needed.

Nutritional management: Nutritional deficiencies are caused by malabsorption, decreases in food intake, and an increase in metabolic requirements due to the disease. Malabsorption must be controlled. Most patients need vitamin A and E supplementation. Enteral feedings should be offered to patients who lose weight despite aggressive dietary measures.

Genetic counseling: Patients and their relatives should be offered nondirective counseling concerning carrier testing and the risks of having a CF-affected child.

Gene therapy: CFTR vectors have been given to CF patients, either to the nose or lungs or both. The efficacy and safety of this intervention are under study.

Chapter 370

■ APPROACH TO THE PATIENT WITH DYSPNEA

DEFINITIONS AND PATHOPHYSIOLOGY

The term *dyspnea* is used to describe a variety of perceptions of difficulty or distress relating to breathing. Several factors may be identified that help determine whether a given pathophysiologic condition is associated with dyspnea. There may be an increased ventilatory requirement or a reduced ventilatory capacity. Even if ventilatory requirements are within a person's capacity, the ventilatory effort may be increased by such factors as abnormal lung mechanics or respiratory muscle fatigue. Finally, for any condition to cause dyspnea, there must be sensory perceptions related to breathing and ventilatory stimuli.

DIFFERENTIAL DIAGNOSIS

Acute dyspnea: Dyspnea developing over minutes to days most often reflects an acute cardiac or pulmonary process. Cardiovascular causes include thromboembolism, pericardial disease, and pulmonary edema due to myocardial or valvular dysfunction. Pulmonary processes likely in this context include diffuse airway obstruction; pneumonia; upper airway obstruction; compression of the lung by chest wall trauma or diaphragmatic or pleural processes; rapidly progressive inflammatory disease; or diffuse lung injury with noncardiogenic pulmonary edema.

Chronic dyspnea: Longstanding dyspnea is more likely to present diagnostic difficulty. Table 351.1 categorizes causes of chronic dyspnea according to pathophysiologic mechanism.

HISTORY AND PHYSICAL EXAMINATION

It is important to establish the acuity of the symptoms and to determine the patient's current and past activity levels. Patients may have unconsciously reduced their activity levels to avoid symptoms of breathlessness. One should identify environmental, temporal, and postural factors that worsen the symptoms and ask about associated symptoms such as chest pain, cough, or syncope. The physical examination has to be comprehensive. Although attention should be directed at cardiorespiratory findings, signs of systemic diseases such as collagen vascular disorders, thyroid disease, or neurologic syndromes also should be sought.

LABORATORY STUDIES AND DIAGNOSTIC TESTS

Acute dyspnea: For acutely ill patients, chest radiography to evaluate for pulmonary infiltrates or edema and arterial blood gas analysis to assess the adequacy of gas exchange are almost always indicated. Peak expiratory flow rates provide an objective measure of the severity of airflow obstruction among patients with airway disease. Electrocardiography (ECG) is indicated whenever cardiac disease is known or suspected. Additional studies that might be indicated on the basis of the initial evaluation include perfusion lung scanning to evaluate for thromboembolism, echocardiography to assess valvular or ventricular dysfunction, and analysis of respiratory secretions or lung tissue to identify infectious agents or noninfectious inflammatory processes.

Chronic dyspnea: The cause often is evident from the results of history, examination, and basic screening tests such as hematocrit and blood chemistries. Additional tests should be selected with specific goals; no set sequence of diagnostic studies can be recommended. The most useful tests usually are measures of pulmonary function, including simple spirometry, lung volume, and diffusing capacity. Chest radiography usually is indicated to demonstrate focal or diffuse disease of the lung parenchyma and to assess cardiac size. Exercise testing may uncover dysfunction of a diseased organ system that had been adequately compensated at rest. A comprehensive exercise test includes measurement of respiratory gas exchange, ventilation, heart rate and blood pressure, ECG, pulse oximetry, and when appropriate, arterial blood gas analysis. The following studies are reserved for selected patients: spirometry with bronchoprovocation when asthma is suspected despite normal results of pulmonary function tests, echocardiography chiefly for identifying valvular lesions and resting or exercise ventricular dysfunction, bronchoscopy for finding focal obstructing lesions of the airways, and computed tomography for confirming the presence of interstitial inflammatory diseases, which may require histologic examination for specific diagnosis.

MANAGEMENT

Treatment is directed at the underlying condition, if possible. For many disorders, however, particularly chronic obstructive pulmonary disease, interstitial lung disease, and pulmonary hypertension, treatment may not reverse the disease or relieve its symptoms fully. Nonspecific interventions include supplemental oxygen, which may relieve dyspnea even for some patients with normal arterial oxygen levels; narcotic analgesics; anxiolytics; and pulmonary rehabilitation.

Chapter 351

IDIOPATHIC PULMONARY FIBROSIS

DEFINITION, EPIDEMIOLOGY, AND PATHOPHYSIOLOGY

Idiopathic pulmonary fibrosis (IPF) is the prototypic interstitial lung disease and is characterized by progressive pulmonary parenchymal inflammation and fibrosis. Most patients receive the diagnosis in the fifth to seventh decades of life. Although no racial, seasonal, or geographic variations have been found, men appear to be at slightly greater risk than women. The true prevalence is unknown. The pathogenesis is highly complex and probably multifactorial; genetic, viral, environmental, and autoimmune factors have been implicated.

PATHOLOGY

The alveolar walls become progressively thickened by fibrosis. Alveolar spaces and vascular beds become obliterated, and the parenchymal architecture becomes distorted into multiple cystic structures surrounded by dense bands of fibrotic tissue. Fibroblasts are prominent, and the lymphocyte and plasma cell populations expand within the alveolar wall.

CLINICAL FEATURES

The symptoms are nonspecific. Most patients notice the insidious development of exertional dyspnea with or without a nonproductive cough. Constitutional symptoms such as fatigue, malaise, and weight loss are less common. With disease progression, patients may have dyspnea at rest and produce sputum. Exertional chest discomfort and peripheral edema are associated with the development of pulmonary hypertension and cor pulmonale. Although the physical findings can be normal in early stages of disease, chest auscultation usually reveals basilar inspiratory crackles. As the disease progresses, the crackles become courser and more widespread, and digital clubbing and cyanosis may develop. The presence of a prominent P_2, palpable pulmonary arterial impulse, or right ventricular heave suggests pulmonary arterial hypertension. Jugular venous distention, hepatomegaly, and peripheral edema signal the development of cor pulmonale.

LABORATORY STUDIES AND DIAGNOSTIC TESTS

Laboratory studies: Rheumatoid factor, antinuclear antibodies, and cryoglobulin may be present in low titer. The complete blood cell count usually is normal.

Chest imaging and pulmonary function tests: A chest radiograph typically shows bibasilar reticular opacities with reduced lung volume. As the disease progresses, the upper lung fields become involved, coarse polygonal markings (honeycombing) become evident, and pulmonary arterial enlargement and cardiomegaly may occur. High-resolution computed tomography is more sensitive than chest radiography in the detection of parenchymal abnormalities. Typical findings include reticular opacities, honeycombing, traction bronchiectasis, architectural distortion, and focal areas of ground-glass opacities. The distribution of these abnormalities usually is peripheral, subpleural, and basal. Static pulmonary function tests reveal the characteristic findings of restrictive lung disease, including reductions in forced expiratory volume at 1 second (FEV_1), forced vital capacity (FVC), and total lung volume with a normal or elevated ratio of FEV_1 to FVC. The diffusing capacity of the lung for carbon dioxide (D_{LCO}) is reduced, reflecting a loss of functional alveolar capillary gas exchange area. The resting arterial blood gas values may be normal but typically reveal some degree of hypoxemia and respiratory alkalosis. Carbon dioxide retention is a late finding. Cardiopulmonary exercise testing reveals diminished maximal oxygen consumption and exercise capacity, elevated physiologic dead space, and oxygen desaturation.

Bronchoalveolar lavage and biopsy: Bronchoalveolar lavage findings are highly variable and nondiagnostic. Transbronchial lung biopsy can help exclude the diagnosis if definitive diagnostic findings are recovered (e.g., infection, granulomatous inflammation, or malignant lesions); however, findings of nonspecific interstitial fibrosis must not be considered diagnostic of IPF because of the sampling error inherent to the technique. Surgical lung biopsy from multiple sites can better confirm the diagnosis and may be predictive of the response to therapy.

PROGNOSIS AND MANAGEMENT

The median survival period after the onset of symptoms is less than 5 years. Most patients experience steadily progressive deterioration. Patients with IPF have a 10% to 15% incidence of lung cancer.

For a few patients, treatment appears to stabilize or retard disease progression. Because patients rarely improve appreciably with glucocorticoid therapy alone, combination therapy with azathioprine or cyclophosphamide has been recommended as initial treatment. In the absence of complications or adverse effects of the medications, therapy should be continued for 6 months, at which time repeat studies should be performed to determine whether there has been objective improvement. Anecdotal reports suggest that methotrexate, D-penicillamine, antioxidants, colchicine, and cyclosporine occasionally are helpful, but there are no data to justify routine use of these agents. For patients who respond to therapy, treatment is continued indefinitely. Lung transplantation is a realistic option for many patients who do not respond to therapy.

Important adjuncts to therapy include smoking cessation, administration of supplemental oxygen to those with resting or exercise-induced hypoxemia, and judicious diuretic therapy for those with cor pulmonale. Pneumococcal and influenza vaccines should be administered to all patients.

Chapter 371

LUNG CANCER

DEFINITION, CLASSIFICATION, AND EPIDEMIOLOGY

The term *lung cancer* usually is applied to neoplasms arising from the respiratory epithelium (bronchogenic carcinoma). Bronchogenic carcinoma is divided into two major groups—small-cell lung cancer (SCLC) and non–small cell lung cancer (NSCLC). SCLC is part of the spectrum of neuroendocrine tumors. NSCLC includes adenocarcinoma, squamous cell carcinoma, large cell carcinoma, and their subtypes. In the United States, lung cancer is the second most common malignant tumor among both men and women. The diagnosis is made most typically between the ages of 55 and 74 years. The incidence among men has declined since peaking in 1984, whereas the incidence among women continues to climb. One-third of all cancer deaths are attributable to lung cancer.

ETIOLOGY AND PATHOGENESIS

Tobacco smoking is estimated to be responsible for 80% to 90% of cases of lung cancer. Exposure to environmental cigarette smoke and the smoking of pipes or cigars increase risk to a lesser degree. Indoor exposure to radon is thought to be responsible for 10% of cases of lung cancer in the United States. Other risk factors include asbestos exposure, chronic obstructive pulmonary disease (COPD), and diets lacking fresh fruits and vegetables. Lung cancer is thought to arise from pluripotent respiratory epithelial stem cells that undergo neoplastic transformation as a result of the accumulation of numerous, carcinogen-induced genetic mutations.

CLINICAL FINDINGS

Local and regional effects: Coughing, or a change in a chronic cough, is the most common symptom and may be caused by bronchial mucosal invasion by tumor, postobstructive pneumonitis or atelectasis, tumor cavitation, or pleural effusion. Dyspnea and hemoptysis, usually blood-streaked sputum, each occur among about 50% of patients, and chest pain among about 40%. Pleural effusions occur among 10% of patients. The malignant effusions usually are exudative, lymphocytic, moderate to large in size, and ipsilateral to the main tumor. Extension of the cancer to the mediastinum can cause phrenic or recurrent laryngeal nerve palsy. Extension to the pericardium can produce effusions, tamponade, or dysrhythmia. Obstruction of venous return in the superior vena cava causes a syndrome of headache, facial fullness, jugular venous congestion, prominent collateral venous channels over the upper chest, and swelling of the face, neck, and upper extremities. Pancoast syndrome is invasion of the chest wall, brachial plexus, and sympathetic ganglion by a tumor in the superior sulcus. The symptoms are pain in the ipsilateral shoulder and scapula, pain in the ulnar nerve distribution, and Horner's syndrome (ptosis, miosis, and ipsilateral facial anhidrosis).

Metastatic effects: Common sites of metastatic spread are the adrenal glands, liver, central nervous system (CNS), and bone. Adrenal metastases usually are asymptomatic and detected as unilateral adrenal enlargement at staging computed tomography (CT) of the chest extended to the upper abdomen. Liver metastases are more common in SCLC (25%) than NSCLC (5%). Brain metastases occur most frequently with SCLC (10% at presentation) and adenocarcinoma, least often with squamous cell carcinoma. Skeletal metastases typically are osteolytic lesions of the vertebral bodies, ribs, and long bones of the extremities. SCLC has the highest propensity for bony metastases (25% of patients at initial staging).

Paraneoplastic effects: Approximately 10% to 20% of patients have paraneoplastic syndromes due to effects of lung cancer apart from the physical presence of the primary or metastatic lesions. Hypercalcemia, usually in association with squamous cell cancer, is the most common of these. It is caused primarily by tumor production of parathyroid hormone–related peptide. The syndrome of inappropriate secretion of antidiuretic hormone (SIADH) causes hyponatremia and inappropriately increased urine osmolarity and is nearly always caused by SCLC. SCLC and pulmonary carcinoid tumors may cause Cushing's syndrome through ectopic production of corticotropin or corticotropin-releasing hormone. The Eaton–Lambert myasthenic syndrome occurs in 1% to 3% of cases of SCLC and is characterized by proximal muscle weakness, hyporeflexia, and autonomic dysfunction. Other autoimmune neurologic syndromes are less common. Cachexia is a common paraneoplastic syndrome of multifactorial causation. Clubbing of the fingers and toes may occur and often is accompanied by hypertrophic osteoarthropathy, painful periosteal inflammation of the lung bones of the arms and legs. Lung cancer can cause a hypercoagulability state and recurrent thrombophlebitis (Trousseau's syndrome).

DIAGNOSIS

The essential aspects of the evaluation are histologic differentiation of SCLC from NSCLC, accurate appraisal of the extent of the disease, and determination of the patient's performance status. Difficulty differentiating SCLC from NSCLC is unusual, but SCLC can be mistaken for carcinoid tumors or lymphoma. Differentiation of primary lung cancer from pulmonary metastatic lesions may necessitate special immunohistochemical tests.

Imaging studies: Chest radiography is 70% to 80% sensitive in detection. Squamous cell carcinoma often manifests as a perihilar mass that may cavitate, adenocarcinoma as a solitary peripheral nodule or mass, large cell carcinoma as a large peripheral mass, and SCLC as a rapidly enlarging central mass with early hilar and mediastinal spread. CT provides further definition of the appearance of the primary lesion; may depict concurrent lymphadenopathy, parenchymal disease, or pleural involvement; and guides diagnostic maneuvers.

Biopsy techniques: The sensitivity of sputum cytologic examination is highest for central squamous cell cancer but less than 20% for peripheral nodules. The yield of cells from thoracentesis of a malignant pleural effusion is 50% to 70%, depending on the number of samples submitted. Diagnostic techniques that can be used during flexible fiberoptic bronchoscopy include forceps biopsy, brushing, and washing. The diagnostic yield is high for central lesions, especially if the tumor is endoscopically visible. For peripheral lesions sampled with fluoroscopic guidance, the yield ranges from about 15% for lesions smaller than 2 cm in greatest dimension to 80% for lesions larger than 4 cm. Transbronchial needle aspiration of paratracheal, subcarinal, and hilar lymph nodes can be helpful in staging, although a negative result does not exclude lymph node metastases. Transthoracic needle aspiration may be used to sample peripheral lesions or those with extension to the mediastinum, pleura, or chest wall. The false-negative rate is 10% to 20%, however, so a negative result cannot be interpreted as a diagnostic end point unless a specific benign diagnosis can be made from the aspirate. The procedure is associated with a 15% to 30% incidence of pneumothorax. Thoracic surgical procedures may be used to exclude metastatic spread to mediastinal lymph nodes. This operation is necessary for any patient with NSCLC who has mediastinal nodes larger than 1 cm in greatest dimension and is considered a candidate for thoracotomy and surgical resection of the primary lesion.

STAGING

Non–small cell lung cancer: Staging is based on the TNM classification, in which T refers to the size and location of the primary tumor, N to the local lymph node involvement, and M to the presence of distant metastasis. There are eight stage groupings: 0, IA, IB, IIA, IIB, IIIA, IIIB, and IV. The 5-year survival rate ranges from 67% for stage IA (tumor smaller than 3 cm in greatest dimension without nodal or distant metastases) to 1% for stage IV (any case with distant metastasis). All patients with NSCLC should undergo a complete blood cell count, serum chemical profile (including liver enzymes), chest radiography, and chest CT to the level of the adrenal glands. If the findings are normal, no further testing in necessary. Liver imaging with contrast CT or ultrasonography is recommended if hepatomegaly is detected or liver test results are abnormal. Radionuclide bone scanning is warranted when the patient has hypercalcemia, focal bony abnormalities, or an increased bone alkaline phosphatase level.

If NSCLC is believed to be resectable, the clinician must determine whether there are medical contraindications to surgery and whether there is adequate pulmonary reserve for a curative lung resection. Between 80% and 90% of patients with lung cancer have COPD. Patients with a forced expiratory volume in 1 second (FEV_1) greater than 1.5 to 2 L (or 60% of predicted value) and a diffusing capacity of the lung for carbon dioxide (D_{LCO}) greater than 60% of predicted value can proceed directly to thoracotomy. Patients with lower values need quantitative ventilation-perfusion lung scanning and arterial blood gas analysis. Either a P_{CO_2} greater than 45 mm Hg or a predicted postoperative FEV_1 less than 0.8 L (or less than 40% of predicted value) indicates high risk of postoperative problems.

Small-cell lung cancer: The TNM staging system usually is not applied to SCLC because of the limited role of surgery and because more than 90% of patients have locally advanced (stage III) or metastatic (stage IV) disease when they come to medical attention. Cases instead are classified as *limited* (tumor confined to one hemithorax and its regional lymph nodes) or *extensive* (everything else) disease. Pretreatment evaluation includes the tests for NSCLC described earlier. In addition, because two-thirds of patients have extensive disease when they come to medical attention, it is prudent to obtain a radionuclide bone scan and perform either CT or magnetic resonance imaging of the brain.

MANAGEMENT

Non–small cell lung cancer stages I and II: Surgical resection with curative intent is the treatment of choice for the 20% to 25% of patients with NSCLC that falls into these stages. The standard operation is thoracotomy with mediastinal lymph node sampling combined with lobectomy, bilobectomy, or pneumonectomy. Less extensive resection should be reserved for patients with a pulmonary status that does not allow lobectomy. Adjuvant chemotherapy has not been shown to improve survival, and postoperative radiation therapy actually worsens outcomes. A follow-up chest radiograph should be obtained every 3 to 4 months for the first 2 years and every 6 to 12 months thereafter.

Non–small cell lung cancer stages III and IV: Studies have suggested that preoperative chemotherapy (with or without radiation therapy) followed by surgery improves survival among patients with stage IIIA disease and carefully selected patients with stage IIIB disease. Thoracic radiation therapy combined with platinum-based chemotherapy is recommended for inoperable stage IIIA and IIIB disease. Palliative radiation therapy alone is an option for patients with limited medical reserve. For the 50% of patients with NSCLC who have metastatic disease (stage IV) when they come to medical attention, there are no curative options. The median survival time is only 5 to 7 months. Radiation therapy can be used for palliation of brain or bone metastasis or to relieve bronchial or superior vena caval obstruction. Chemotherapy provides a modest survival benefit (1.5 months) over supportive care.

Small-cell lung cancer: SCLC is highly responsive to current systemic therapy; the response rate is 80% to 90%. Current therapy for limited disease consists of four cycles of etoposide and either cisplatin or carboplatin, with thoracic radiation therapy administered concurrently with at least two of the cycles. Complete responses can be obtained by 50% of patients. The median survival time is 18 to 20 months, and the 5-year survival rate is 15% to 20%. Extensive disease is managed with the same chemotherapy, but thoracic radiation therapy is not recommended. Complete responses are obtained in 25% of cases; the median survival time is 9 months, and there are almost no 5-year survivors. Prophylactic cranial irradiation is controversial and should not be considered unless the disease is in complete remission. This treatment decreases the rate of CNS relapse but may be associated with the late sequelae of cognitive dysfunction and ataxia.

Chapter 377

■ OBSTRUCTIVE SLEEP APNEA

DEFINITION, PATHOPHYSIOLOGY, AND EPIDEMIOLOGY

Obstructive sleep apnea (OSA) is characterized by the recurrent collapse of the pharyngeal airway during sleep. Most patients have anatomically small pharyngeal airways owing to obesity, small or posteriorly placed mandibles, or tonsillar hypertrophy. During sleep, a substantial decrement in the activity of the pharyngeal dilator muscles leads to the collapse of the airway. Progressive hypoxemia and hypercapnia then stimulate respiratory effort, which awakens the patient. The dilator muscles reactivate, and airway patency and ventilation are restored. When hypoxemia and hypercapnia are corrected, the patient returns to sleep, and the process begins again. Studies have suggested that 4% of men and 2% of women have at least mild OSA.

CLINICAL CONSEQUENCES

Sleep fragmentation causes neurocognitive effects. Patients are sleepy, perform less well at many tasks, and perceive their quality of life to be substantially diminished. The hypoxemia and hypercapnia appear to be linked to cardiovascular consequences, such as systemic hypertension and mild pulmonary hypertension. Cardiac arrhythmia also has been reported. A relation to stroke and myocardial infarction has not been proved.

DIAGNOSTIC APPROACH

Symptoms and signs suggestive of OSA include (a) loud snoring, (b) witnessed apnea or gasping during sleep, (c) neck or collar size more than 16.5 inches (42 cm) for men and more than 15.5 inches (39 cm) for women, and (d) occasional dozing or falling asleep during the day when not busy or active. Snoring alone, unless a social nuisance, rarely necessitates further testing or treatment. The most commonly used diagnostic study for OSA is the in-laboratory split night study. During the initial 2 to 3 hours of the study, polysomnographic monitoring is used to determine the combined number of episodes of apnea and hypopnea per hour of sleep (respiratory disturbance index; RDI). *Apnea* is defined as complete cessation of ventilation for longer than 10 seconds. *Hypopnea* as a decrement in ventilation (generally more than 50%) associated with oxygen desaturation or arousal. Patients with symptoms and an RDI greater than 5 probably need therapy.

MANAGEMENT

Treatment is tailored to the severity of OSA. For patients with mild disease, behavioral approaches such as weight loss, maximizing nasal patency, avoidance of alcohol or sedatives near bedtime, and avoidance of a supine sleeping posture may be beneficial. For severe disease, the main therapeutic options are nasal continuous positive airway pressure (CPAP), dental appliances, and upper airway surgery. Nasal CPAP applies positive pressure through the nose to the pharyngeal airway, pneumatically splinting the airway open. It can be started during the second portion of the in-laboratory split night study and titrated to the pressure that abolishes the disordered breathing. It is highly effective for most patients, but compliance is difficult. Should CPAP prove ineffective or intolerable, dental appliances can be considered. Most are fabricated by a dentist and are used to advance the mandible and pull the tongue apparatus off the posterior pharyngeal wall. Upper airway surgery is aimed at enlarging the pharyngeal airway so that sleep-induced decrements in muscle activity do not lead to airway collapse. Most procedures include removal of the uvula and portions of the soft palate with or without advancement of the tongue or mandible. The success rate varies from 30% to 90% for different procedures. There are no effective methods of determining which patients will respond.

Chapter 382

APPROACH TO THE PATIENT WITH PLEURAL DISEASE

DEFINITIONS AND PATHOPHYSIOLOGY

Pleurisy is inflammation of the pleura with or without pleural effusion, an accumulation of excess fluid in the pleural space. The parietal pleura, unlike the visceral pleura and lung, is a highly sensitive surface. Injury and inflammation therefore cause pain. The presence of pleural effusion signifies that there is a dysequilibrium in the formation and removal of pleural fluid. An effusion may form because of alterations in hydrostatic or oncotic forces that favor the transudation of fluid into the pleural space (transudative effusion) or because of capillary protein leak or decreased removal of protein from the pleural space (exudative effusion).

CLINICAL FEATURES

Pleurisy: The patient has pain on breathing that can be minimal or severe. It is worsened by deep breathing, coughing, and sneezing. It may be relieved by manual pressure against the chest wall. Dyspnea is common. It is partially caused by voluntary and involuntary restriction in respiration. A large associated pleural effusion often contributes as well. Other associated symptoms depend on the cause of pleurisy. Examination shows splinted respiratory movements and a

pleural friction rub (best heard at or near the end of inspiration). There also may be evidence of associated pleural effusion.

Pleural effusion: The patient may have no symptoms, may report pleurisy, or may have painless dyspnea. Examination shows decreased breath sounds and dullness to percussion on the affected side. There may be consolidative findings, such as egophony, in the atelectatic lung adjacent to the effusion.

DIFFERENTIAL DIAGNOSIS

Pleurisy: Pleurisy can be caused by direct trauma to the chest wall but most commonly is caused by viral infection; by extension of localized disease of the lung (pneumonia, pulmonary embolism), mediastinum (esophageal rupture), pericardium (pericarditis, Dressler's syndrome), or abdomen (pancreatitis, subphrenic abscess); or by systemic disease such as systemic lupus erythematosus, rheumatoid arthritis, sarcoidosis, or uremia. The presence or absence of pleural fluid may help differentiate these possibilities: viral, rheumatoid, and sarcoid pleurisy often lack effusions; bacterial pneumonia, lupus erythematosus, and postcardiac injury syndrome usually are associated with accumulation of pleural fluid.

Pleural effusion: Causes of transudative and exudative effusions are listed in Tables 358.4 and 358.5.

LABORATORY STUDIES AND DIAGNOSTIC TESTS

Chest radiographs may show a pleural effusion or evidence of a condition such as pneumonia or pneumothorax. Pleural fluid analysis is the most helpful diagnostic test in establishing the cause of pleurisy or a pleural effusion and should include measurements of cell counts, protein, lactate dehydrogenase (LDH), glucose and amylase concentrations, pH, and appropriate cultures. A definitive diagnosis, such as finding malignant cells or specific organisms, can be established in only 25% of cases, but a presumptive diagnosis based on the clinical impression can be substantiated in an additional 50%. The fluid is characterized as an exudate if it meets any of the following criteria: (a) ratio of pleural fluid protein to serum protein greater than 0.5; (b) ratio of pleural fluid LDH to serum LDH greater than 0.6; or (c) pleural fluid LDH greater than 0.45 multiplied by the upper limit of normal of the serum LDH; (d) ratio of pleural fluid cholesterol to serum cholesterol greater than 0.3; or (e) pleural fluid cholesterol greater than 45 mg per deciliter. Essentially all patients with pleurisy have exudative effusions.

Examination of the aspirate: Straw-colored fluid is typical of all transudates. A milky effusion suggests chylothorax. Bloody effusion in the absence of trauma suggests pulmonary embolism, pleural neoplasm, uremia, postcardiac injury syndrome, or asbestosis. The presence of pus confirms the diagnosis of empyema.

Cell counts: A fluid leukocyte count of more than 10,000 per milliliter with polymorphonuclear predominance suggests bacterial pneumonia, pancreatitis, and lupus pleuritis. A low leukocyte count (less than 5,000 per milliliter) with lymphocyte predominance usually is found with tuberculous pleurisy. Pleural fluid eosinophilia (more than 10% of pleural leukocytes) occurs with pneumothorax, hemothorax, asbestosis, pulmonary embolism, and parasitic and drug-induced disease. It is rarely associated with carcinoma or tuberculosis.

Protein and amylase: When exudative criteria are met with LDH but not protein measurements, malignant disease and parapneumonic effusion should be considered. An increased pleural fluid amylase level is found with pancreatitis, malignant disease, or esophageal rupture.

Glucose and pH: Causes of pleural effusion with low pH (less than 7.30) and a glucose level less than 50 mg per deciliter include empyema, esophageal rupture, rheumatoid pleurisy, lupus pleuritis, malignant disease, and tuberculous pleurisy.

Cytology: Pleural fluid cytology has a positive diagnostic yield among 40% to 90% of patients with malignant pleural tumors (high with adenocarcinoma but low with Hodgkin's disease). Tumors can cause effusions owing to local effects without directly involving the pleural space.

Other tests: The presence of immunologic markers in pleural fluid, such as rheumatoid factor and antinuclear antibody, suggest the presence of the associated diseases but with the exception of lupus erythematosus cells is not enough information for diagnosis. If the cause is unclear after pleural fluid analysis, other studies may be necessary, including ventilation-perfusion lung scanning, abdominal or chest computed tomography, bronchoscopy or thoracoscopy, and pleural biopsy (frequently needed for the diagnosis of tuberculous or malignant pleurisy).

MANAGEMENT

Treatment varies with the underlying disease. Drainage of the pleural space is necessary to manage empyema, esophageal rupture, some cases of pneumothorax, and parapneumonic effusion. Subphrenic abscesses also necessitate drainage. Metastatic pleural disease may respond to chemotherapy, but chemical pleurodesis or pleuroperitoneal shunt may be necessary for palliation. Lupus pleuritis and postcardiac injury syndrome respond rapidly to glucocorticoid therapy, and most patients with pleurisy obtain relief with nonsteroidal anti-inflammatory drugs.

Chapter 358

SARCOIDOSIS

DEFINITION, INCIDENCE, AND EPIDEMIOLOGY

Sarcoidosis is a systemic granulomatous disorder of unknown causation that most commonly affects adults. It occurs worldwide but may be more common in Scandinavian countries, the United Kingdom, Ireland, Japan, and the United States. The estimated prevalence ranges from 1 to 40 per 100,000 population. Within the United States, blacks have three times the incidence of whites.

ETIOLOGY AND PATHOGENESIS

The cause remains unknown. The disease most likely represents a hypersensitivity response to one or many agents (bacteria, fungi, chemicals) by a person with either an inherited or acquired predisposition. However, no infective agent or single antigen has been consistently linked to sarcoidosis. The basic pathologic lesion is noncaseating granuloma made up of radially arranged epithelioid cells with pale nuclei, a few multinucleated giant cells, and lymphocytic infiltration.

CLINICAL FINDINGS

Sarcoidosis may involve one or multiple organ systems. Most patients have nonspecific systemic symptoms such as fatigue, weight loss, fever, anorexia, and, occasionally, chills and night sweats.

Respiratory tract: The respiratory system is involved in more than 90% of cases. Symptoms typically include dyspnea, retrosternal chest discomfort, and nonproductive cough. Hemoptysis is rare. In fewer than 20% of cases, interstitial involvement causes inspiratory crackles in association with restricted lung volume and abnormalities of gas exchange during pulmonary function testing. Bronchial involvement often results in airflow limitation and bronchial hyperreactivity. Sarcoidosis of the upper respiratory tract occurs in 2% to 18% of patients and may produce nasal obstruction, recurrent or persistent sinusitis, and hoarseness. Chest radiographic abnormalities are classified as follows: stage 0, no abnormality; stage I, bilateral hilar adenopathy without parenchymal infiltrates; stage II, hilar adenopathy with parenchymal infiltrates; stage III, parenchymal infiltrates without hilar adenopathy; and stage IV, fibrosis with honeycombing, hilar retraction, bullae, or emphysema. Radiographic evidence of disease does not necessarily progress through all stages.

Lymphatic and hematologic systems: Palpable peripheral lymphadenopathy occurs in 5% to 30% of cases, especially in the cervical, epitrochlear, axillary, and inguinal regions. The nodes are discrete, mobile, and nontender. Splenomegaly occurs in 10% of cases. Peripheral lymphopenia is the most common hematologic manifestation, although mild anemia and thrombocytopenia also can occur.

Cardiac system: Serious cardiac involvement occurs among 5% to 10% of patients. Symptoms may include chest pain, palpitations, and even sudden cardiac death. Half of patients with cardiac sarcoidosis have abnormalities of rhythm, conduction, or repolarization. Other manifestations include pericarditis, papillary muscle dysfunction, and infiltrative cardiomyopathy with congestive heart failure. Echocardiographic findings can suggest the diagnosis; the diagnostic yield of endomyocardial biopsy is low.

Other organ systems: Ocular lesions occur among about 25% of patients, granulomatous uveitis being the most common finding. The symptoms include blurred vision, photophobia, and excessive lacrimation. Approximately 25% of patients have dermal manifestations such as erythema nodosum (painful, 1 to 2 cm, red nodules over the shins), lupus pernio (a violaceous nodular or plaque-like lesion over the nose, cheeks, and ears), and purple-red, indurated annular lesions. Neurologic manifestations, affecting fewer than 10% of patients, may include cranial nerve palsy (particularly unilateral facial nerve palsy), peripheral neuropathy, myopathy, hypopituitarism, and central diabetes insipidus. Headache and confusion, accompanied by cerebrospinal fluid lymphocytosis, reflect leptomeningeal sarcoidosis. Nephrolithiasis is the most common renal manifestation; it stems from the overproduction of calcitriol and consequent hypercalciuria with or without hypercalcemia. Clinically significant hepatic dysfunction is un-

common, even though liver biopsy reveals granulomatous involvement of the liver in most patients. Up to one-third of patients have hepatomegaly or a cholestatic pattern of liver enzyme elevations.

Special syndromes: Symmetric parotid swelling associated with uveitis, with or without facial nerve palsy, is called *Heerfordt's disease.* Lofgren's syndrome, characterized by fever, arthralgia, erythema nodosum, and bilateral hilar lymphadenopathy, generally has a good prognosis.

DIFFERENTIAL DIAGNOSIS

Mimics of sarcoidosis include (a) infections by organisms that commonly trigger a granulomatous host response, such as mycobacteria, fungi, bacteria, and parasites, (b) occupational or lung diseases such as hypersensitivity pneumonitis, chronic beryllium disease, and other metal-induced lung diseases, (c) drug-induced granulomatous vasculitis, and (d) autoimmune disorders associated with granulomatous lesions, such as Wegener's granulomatosis, primary biliary cirrhosis, and Churg–Strauss syndrome.

DIAGNOSTIC EVALUATION

Diagnosis depends on compatible clinical signs and symptoms, histologic findings of noncaseating granuloma in affected organs, and the exclusion of other granulomatous diseases. Transbronchial lung biopsy has a diagnostic yield approaching 90%; other potential biopsy sites in a given patient include the conjunctiva, skin, lip, peripheral lymph nodes, and enlarged mediastinal lymph nodes. The specimens should be carefully examined and cultured for infectious organisms capable of causing granulomatous disease. Serum angiotensin-converting enzyme level is elevated in more than one-half of patients, but this elevation is not specific to sarcoidosis. The recommended baseline evaluation includes a complete blood cell count, liver chemical analysis, renal function tests, measurement of serum calcium and 24-hour urine calcium excretion, chest radiography, pulmonary function tests (including gas exchange), electrocardiography, and a slit-lamp examination of the eyes to exclude subclinical uveitis.

PROGNOSIS AND MANAGEMENT

Without therapy, stage I disease remits in 60% to 80% of cases, stage II in 50% to 60%, and stage III in less than 30%. Factors associated with a poor prognosis include older age at onset, black race, symptoms lasting more than 6 months, splenomegaly, lupus pernio, multiorgan involvement, and extrathoracic disease. Pulmonary infiltration that persists for longer than 2 years is unlikely to remit without therapy.

Glucocorticoids are the mainstay of therapy. In most cases, a 3-month period of observation before treatment allows assessment of disease activity. If there is interval deterioration in lung function or gas exchange, oral glucocorticoids should be started (e.g., 40 mg prednisone daily for 6 to 12 weeks with a gradual taper to 5 to 10 mg daily for 6 to 12 months). If steroids are ineffective or associated with severe side effects, methotrexate can be used (7.5 to 15 orally each week), often in combination with a lower dose of prednisone. Lung transplantation is an option for some patients; however, patients with sarcoidosis may have an abnormally high rate of rejection, and the disease can develop in the pulmonary allograft. Hydroxychloroquine (200 mg by mouth twice a day) is efficacious for cutaneous sarcoidosis and for hypercalcemia. Management of cardiac sarcoidosis may involve antiarrhythmic agents, pacemakers, and implantable defibrillators.

Chapter 373

APPROACH TO THE PATIENT WITH A SOLITARY PULMONARY NODULE

DEFINITION

A solitary pulmonary nodule (SPN) is a single circumscribed nodular density within the lung parenchyma.

DIFFERENTIAL DIAGNOSIS

Infectious granuloma and primary bronchogenic carcinoma each account for between 30% and 60% of SPNs in most series. Hamartoma constitutes about 6%, bronchial adenoma 2%, and metastatic malignant lesions 3% to 5%. Miscellaneous conditions (such as intrapulmonary lymph nodes, pulmonary infarction, and arteriovenous malformations) account for fewer than 5% of SPNs.

FACTORS THAT PREDICT A BENIGN RATHER THAN A MALIGNANT NATURE

Clinical features: The probability that a lesion is malignant increases progressively with increasing age. SPNs in patients younger than 35 years are malignant in fewer than 2% of cases. In contrast, SPNs are malignant in 15% to 30% of patients between the ages of 35 and 45 years and in more than 50% of patients older than 50 years. The presence or absence of symptoms cannot differentiate benign from malignant lesions. Although smoking history has predictive value, the risk of malignancy among nonsmokers older than 35 years is sufficiently high to justify aggressive evaluation.

Radiographic appearance: Various radiologic criteria have been applied to differentiate benign from malignant SPNs, including the size and growth rate of the lesion and the presence or absence of calcification. The likelihood of malignancy increases with increasing size of the lesion. SPNs smaller than 1 cm in diameter are benign in more than 90% of cases. Seventy percent of SPNs exceeding 2 cm and more than 90% of those larger than 3 cm are malignant. Lesions stable in size for 2 or more years are so rarely malignant that they can be followed with radiographs at 6 and 12 months. This approach is helpful when prior radiographs, not only reports, can be obtained. However, obtaining serial radiographs prospectively to assess the rate of growth before confirming the nature of the lesion is not recommended. Calcification within the SPN markedly reduces the chance of malignancy but does not exclude it. The pattern of calcification is of great importance. Dense, central calcification, multiple punctate foci, and a laminated pattern all are reliable signs that a lesion is benign. Large clumps of calcification within the lesion (popcorn pattern) are essentially pathognomonic for hamartoma.

Although these various features are useful in estimating the probability that a lesion is benign or malignant, they can be misleading. The only radiographic criteria that reliably prove that a lesion is benign are distinctive central, laminated, popcorn diffuse calcification within the nodule and lack of growth for at least 2 years.

DIAGNOSTIC TESTS

Computed tomography of the chest: Computed tomography (CT), especially thin-section CT, is far more sensitive than plain chest radiography in detecting calcification and can provide information about the size of the lesion, distribution of calcification, and regularity of the margin. Quantitative determination of the amount of calcification is reported in Hounsfield units (HU). There is a high likelihood of malignancy for lesions larger than 2.5 cm or with an irregular edge. Thus only lesions meeting all of the following CT criteria should be categorized as benign: (a) diffuse calcification (attenuation value more than 164 HU) occupying at least 10% of the cross-sectional area, (b) a smooth margin with no irregularity or spiculation, and (c) diameter less than 2.5 cm.

Other diagnostic studies: Positron emission tomography has been shown to discriminate accurately between benign and malignant lesions more than 2 cm in diameter but is not widely available. Flexible fiberoptic bronchoscopy (FFB) or percutaneous needle aspiration can be helpful, because thoracotomy may be avoided if a specific benign tumor can be established with either technique. Thoracotomy is needed, however, if the biopsy findings are nonspecific or normal. FFB helps establish the diagnosis of 40% to 80% of malignant SPNs but only 5% to 20% of benign SPNs. The diagnostic yield is greatest for lesions larger than 3 cm. Percutaneous needle aspiration has a greater yield but a higher rate of complications such as pneumothorax.

MANAGEMENT

An SPN usually can be resected by means of either video-assisted thoracoscopic (VATS) techniques or minithoracotomy. These techniques have less morbidity than conventional thoracotomy and are ideally suited to identification and resection of benign SPNs. If the lesion proves to be malignant at surgery, many surgeons extend the incision and perform conventional thoracotomy with curative intent. Because of the low risk of surgery for benign lesions, and the potentially fatal outcome if malignant lesions are not promptly resected, the prudent approach is to resect SPNs when there is not clear evidence of calcification on chest radiographs or CT scans and when ancillary studies (such as FFB or needle aspiration) have not supplied enough information to confirm a specific benign diagnosis.

The decision to proceed with surgery depends on many factors, including the likelihood that a lesion is malignant, the patient's overall physical condition and ability to withstand surgery, and the patient's desires. For example, for a patient with an asymptomatic SPN but such severe pulmonary disease that

thoracic resection would be impossible, the clinician could justify following the lesion with serial chest radiographs. In contrast, "watching" a noncalcified SPN of indeterminate causation in a healthy 50-year-old patient cannot be justified. For a 30-year-old nonsmoker with a 1 cm, smooth-margined SPN, the decision to repeat chest radiography in 3 months would be reasonable. This approach would be ill-advised, however, if the same person had a history of heavy smoking, a larger nodule, or a lesion with irregular borders.

Chapter 359

APPROACH TO THE PATIENT WITH SUSPECTED PNEUMONIA

DEFINITION AND EPIDEMIOLOGY

Pneumonia is acute inflammation of the lung parenchyma. Lower respiratory tract infection affects 3 million persons annually in the United States, is the leading cause of death of infection in the United States, and is the sixth most common cause of death overall.

PATHOPHYSIOLOGY

The lungs are repeatedly inoculated with microorganisms from the upper airways and from inhaled aerosols. Inoculum size, bacterial virulence, and the state of host defenses determine the pathogenic potential of a microbial challenge. Host defense mechanisms normally include secretory immunoglobulin A, the epiglottis, bronchial ciliary action, the cough reflex, and a variety of cellular and noncellular host factors at the level of the alveolus.

DIFFERENTIAL DIAGNOSIS

The most common pathogens associated with pneumonia are listed in Table 361.4. Although the clinical presentation does not allow the clinician to make a specific etiologic diagnosis for patients with community-acquired pneumonia, certain pathogens cause pneumonia more commonly among persons with specific risk factors. Pneumococcal pneumonia occurs more commonly among the elderly and among patients with chronic obstructive pulmonary disease (COPD), cardiovascular disease, HIV infection, immunoglobulin deficiency, asplenia, and hematologic malignant disease. *Legionella* is an opportunistic pathogen; it is an important cause of pneumonia among patients with COPD who smoke, patients with renal failure, and organ transplant recipients. *Staphylococcus aureus* pneumonia often occurs among intravenous drug users and among patients in the convalescent phase of influenza. Gram-negative bacilli cause severe pneumonia almost exclusively among patients with COPD, alcoholism, and diabetes mellitus.

CLINICAL FINDINGS

Community-acquired pneumonia syndrome: Symptoms include coughing, with or without sputum production, change in the color of respiratory secretions, dyspnea, chest discomfort, fever or hypothermia, shaking chills, sweats, and pleuritic chest pain. Abdominal pain, anorexia, myalgia, and headache also occur. Physical examination may show fever, tachycardia, and tachypnea. In advanced cases, confusion, cyanosis, splinting, and labored breathing may occur. Localized, fine, crepitant rales are heard initially over the involved portion of the lung, and signs of lobar consolidation (bronchial breath sounds, whispered pectoriloquy, vocal fremitus, and dullness to percussion) may occur as the disease progresses. Extension to pleural surfaces is associated with pleuritic pain and signs of pleural effusion.

Cavitary pneumonia syndrome: Anaerobic infection usually manifests as a 3 to 5 week history of chronic, productive coughing. The sputum commonly smells putrid; the presence of this sign almost always confirms the diagnosis of anaerobic infection. Fever and chest pain occur in 50% of cases, hemoptysis and weight loss in about 30%. About 75% of patients have a risk factor for aspiration of oropharyngeal secretions (alcoholism, seizure disorder, dysphagia, cerebrovascular accident, and undergoing general anesthesia). Poor dental hygiene and periodontal disease often are present. Non-anaerobic infections that can manifest in a similar manner include tuberculosis, blastomycosis, coccidioidomycosis, cryptococcosis, and nocardiosis.

Laboratory and radiographic findings: Most patients have an elevated white blood cell count. Although a localized bronchopneumonia pattern is the most frequent finding, chest radiographs may show multilobar consolidation, cavitation, or large pleural effusions. Although the chest radiograph almost never allows conclusive identification of a specific infectious agent, certain features can be of diagnostic aid. Multiple, bilateral, cavitary infiltrates suggest infection by *S. aureus*. Cavitation also suggests gram-negative, *Streptococcus pneumoniae* type 3, or anaerobic infection. Anaerobic cavitations involve the right lung in 75% of cases and usually are in dependent segments, such as the posterior segment of the right upper lobe.

DIAGNOSTIC EVALUATION

Sputum staining: Sample collection should be directly supervised by a physician; otherwise, there is a 75% chance that the specimen will be of poor quality. Large numbers of epithelial cells (more than 25 per low-power field) reflect contamination with oral secretions. A predominance of gram-positive lancet-shaped diplococci on a Gram stain suggest *S. pneumoniae* infection. The presence of small gram-negative coccobacillary organisms likewise suggests *Haemophilus influenzae* infection. The presence of gram-positive cocci in tetrads and grape-like clusters suggests *S. aureus* infection. An acid-fast smear should be performed whenever a patients has subacute, chronic, or cavitary pneumonia; it may provide the first evidence of tuberculous infection. In these cases, examination of a potassium hydroxide wet-mount preparation may allow rapid diagnosis of blastomycosis, coccidioidomycosis, and cryptococcosis.

Sputum cultures: Culture of expectorated sputum is neither specific nor sensitive. It may be difficult to determine whether an isolated bacterial species is a pulmonary pathogen, a colonizer of the oropharynx, or a contaminant. Sputum cultures are valuable, however, in the diagnosis of certain subacute and cavitary types of pneumonia, such as tuberculosis and fungal pneumonitis.

Other tests: Two specimens for blood culture should be obtained from all patients who need hospitalization. A positive culture result occurs among only about 25% of patients with pneumococcal and gram-negative bacillary pneumonia but does offer definitive identification of the causative organism. A polymerase chain reaction assay for *Mycobacterium tuberculosis* can be performed. Rapid diagnostic tests are being developed in which nucleic acid amplification will be used to detect other microbes.

PROGNOSIS AND MANAGEMENT

Prognosis and indications for hospitalization: A rule to predict 30-day hospital mortality among patients with community-acquired pneumonia has been developed (Table 361.2). The prognosis is sufficiently good in categories I and II to consider outpatient management. Category III patients can be hospitalized briefly or treated as outpatients. Patients in categories IV or V need admission to the hospital.

Antibiotic selection: Selection of antibiotics is straightforward if a causative agent has been identified. However, initial therapy for community-acquired pneumonia is necessarily empiric because clinical and radiographic findings are nonspecific, and diagnostic testing cannot confirm the responsible microbe in most instances. Initial antibiotic therapy must be broad and should be administered promptly after the diagnosis is established. A delay from the time of admission to initiation of antibiotic therapy exceeding 8 hours is associated with an increase in mortality. Therapy can be adjusted to narrow-spectrum agents if an etiologic agent is identified and results of antimicrobial susceptibility tests are available.

A macrolide antibiotic is reasonable empiric treatment of outpatients. Erythromycin (250 mg by mouth every 6 hours for 14 days) provides excellent coverage for *S. pneumoniae, Mycoplasma pneumoniae, Chlamydia pneumoniae,* and *Legionella* organisms but is relatively inactive against *H. influenzae.* Clarithromycin (500 mg by mouth every 12 hours for 14 days) or azithromycin (500 mg by mouth on the first day then 250 mg by mouth each day for 4 days) can be used to treat smokers, who are at greater risk of *H. influenzae* infection, and of patients who experience unacceptable gastrointestinal symptoms with erythromycin. Acceptable alternatives include doxycycline (100 mg by mouth twice a day for 14 days) and levofloxacin (500 mg by mouth daily for 7 to 14 days).

Patients who need hospitalization usually are treated with parenteral antibiotics. Intravenous (IV) therapy with cefuroxime (750 to 1500 mg every 8 hours), ceftriaxone (1 g every 12 hours), or cefotaxime (1 g every 8 hours) plus erythromycin (1 g every 6 hours) is appropriate and has good activity against *S. pneumoniae*, H. influenzae, anaerobic, and *Legionella* organisms and many gram-negative bacilli. IV therapy with levofloxacin (500 mg daily) alone also is appropriate. Among patients with severe community-acquired pneumonia, likely pathogens include *S. pneumoniae* and *Legionella* organisms. *Pseudomonas aeruginosa* infection is rare except among patients with bronchiectasis, those who have received broad-spectrum antibiotics for 1 week, and those with deficient phagocytosis. Patients with one of these risk factors should receive piperacillin–tazobactam (3.375 g IV every 6 hours), imipenem (500 mg IV every 6 hours), or cefepime (1 to 2 g IV every 6 hours) plus erythromycin (1 g IV every 6 hours). An alternative regimen is levofloxacin (500 mg IV daily) plus gentamycin or tobramycin (1.7 mg per kilogram IV every 8 hours). Clindamycin is the drug of choice for anaerobic pulmonary infection. If clinical suspicion of tuberculosis is high, antituberculous therapy should be initiated while culture results are pending.

Chapter 361

ENDOCRINOLOGY

ADRENAL INSUFFICIENCY

DEFINITION, EPIDEMIOLOGY, AND ETIOLOGY

Adrenal insufficiency occurs when there is inadequate production of one or both of the two major adrenocortical hormones, cortisol and aldosterone. It can develop as a consequence of destruction or suppression of the adrenal cortex (primary adrenal insufficiency) or as a result of a failure of pituitary corticotropin production or renal renin secretion (secondary adrenal insufficiency).

Primary adrenal insufficiency usually occurs sporadically; the reported prevalence is 4 to 6 cases per 100,000 population. In the United States, the most common cause is autoimmune adrenalitis, which can be associated with other autoimmune disorders such as Hashimoto's thyroiditis, Graves' disease, type I diabetes mellitus, and pernicious anemia. Other causes include infection (tuberculous, fungal, cytomegalovirus), bilateral adrenal hemorrhage (sepsis, pneumonia, recent abdominal surgery, anticoagulation), infiltrative disease (lymphoma, amyloidosis, metastatic neoplasia), and congenital enzyme deficiencies. The most common cause of secondary adrenal insufficiency is suppression of corticotropin secretion with chronic glucocorticoid therapy. Other causes of decreased corticotropin production include pituitary tumors and pituitary infarction. Renin deficiency occurs with diabetic nephropathy, chronic renal failure, or the administration of indomethacin or angiotensin-converting enzyme inhibitors.

PATHOGENESIS

In primary adrenal insufficiency, there is destruction of the adrenal cortex with resultant inability to synthesize all major adrenal cortical hormones, including cortisol, aldosterone, and androgens. Secondary adrenal insufficiency develops as a consequence of either corticotropin or renin deficiency, leading to an isolated deficiency of either cortisol or aldosterone.

CLINICAL FEATURES

History: Symptoms of cortisol deficiency include fatigue, anorexia, weight loss, generalized muscle and joint aches, and abdominal pain. Patients with primary adrenal insufficiency, owing to the elevated production of corticotropin precursors, may have hyperpigmentation. They also may have postural light-headedness because of the loss of aldosterone production. Patients with secondary adrenal insufficiency from corticotropin deficiency may have symptoms related to the deficiency of other pituitary hormones, such as amenorrhea, erectile dysfunction, dry skin, cold intolerance, and lethargy.

Physical examination: Patients with primary adrenal insufficiency have hyperpigmentation of the skin and mucous membranes, particularly the dorsum of the hands, the palmar creases, the elbows and knees, and the nipples. Orthostatic hypotension can occur. Women have a decrease in body hair. Patients with pituitary corticotropin deficiency appear pale because of a decrease in the pigmentation of the skin. The presence of hypogonadism (decreased sexual hair, mammary gland atrophy among women, decreased testicular size) indicates concomitant deficiency of other pituitary tropic hormones.

LABORATORY STUDIES AND DIAGNOSTIC TESTS

Aldosterone deficiency is associated with hyponatremia, hyperkalemia, metabolic acidosis, and urinary sodium excretion more than 20 mEq per liter. Because of intravascular volume contraction, serum urea and creatinine are increased. Cortisol deficiency is associated with normocytic anemia and leukopenia with relative lymphocytosis and eosinophilia. Fasting hypoglycemia may occur among patients who have been eating poorly.

Patients whose clinical features suggest adrenal insufficiency should undergo biochemical confirmation of the diagnosis. Because these tests can take a long time to process, therapy should be initiated and continued until the results are available. The corticotropin stimulation test serves as a good screening tool. Patients receive 250 µg of synthetic corticotropin, and serum cortisol levels are checked at baseline, 30 minutes, and 60 minutes. Increments of more than 10 µg per deciliter or peak values more than 20 µg per deciliter usually exclude adrenal insufficiency. A diagnosis of primary adrenal insufficiency is based on the finding of low random serum cortisol and aldosterone levels together with high levels of corticotropin and renin. Patients with secondary adrenal insufficiency related to inadequate corticotropin production have low corticotropin and cortisol levels but normal levels of aldosterone and renin. Those with secondary adrenal insufficiency related to diminished renin production have low renin and aldosterone levels but normal levels of corticotropin and cortisol. Additional studies may be useful in the evaluation of adrenal insufficiency, including adrenal computed tomography and tests of pituitary function.

MANAGEMENT

Chronic adrenal insufficiency: Physiologic doses of hydrocortisone usually are administered in a way that mimics the normal circadian rhythm of cortisol secretion (e.g., 10 to 15 mg on arising, 5 to 10 mg in the early afternoon, and 5 mg before bed). The maintenance therapy should be altered under conditions of physical stress (e.g., infection, trauma, or surgical procedures). Systemic infections associated with fever necessitate a doubling of the usual oral dose. Patients undergoing general anesthesia should receive about 300 mg parenteral cortisol in divided doses throughout the day of the procedure. Patients with primary adrenal insufficiency also need therapy with fludrocortisone, which has mineralocorticoid activity similar to that of aldosterone. The usual dose is 0.05 to 0.2 mg daily, adjusted according to serum electrolyte and blood pressure response. During hot, humid weather, a higher dose may be needed.

Acute adrenal insufficiency: Acute adrenal insufficiency is a medical emergency. It may develop as a result of progression of undiagnosed or untreated chronic insufficiency or in patients with chronic insufficiency who undergo acute physical stress without a concomitant increase in hydrocortisone doses. Patients have nausea, vomiting, rapid weight loss, and hypotension. Therapy should begin with an infusion of 5% dextrose in 0.9% saline solution (1 L in the first hour). If adrenal insufficiency has not previously been diagnosed, blood samples for hormone levels should be obtained as outlined earlier. A dose of 100 mg intravenous hydrocortisone should be given immediately and followed by a continuous infusion of 10 mg per hour for the next 5 hours.

Chapters 407, 408

APPROACH TO AMENORRHEA

PATHOGENESIS AND ETIOLOGY

The menstrual cycle is controlled by the interaction of the hypothalamus (pulsatile secretion of gonadotropin-releasing hormone), pituitary (secretion of luteinizing hormone [LH] and follicle-stimulating hormone [FSH]), ovaries (follicular growth, ovulation, and corpus luteum formation), and uterus (cyclic growth and shedding of the endometrium). Abnormalities in any of these systems can cause menstrual abnormalities.

Primary amenorrhea is present when the first menses has not occurred by 16 years of age. It is usually caused by a genetic or congenital defect, particularly gonadal dysgenesis, and often is associated with disorders of puberty. Secondary amenorrhea is present when a woman who has undergone menarche experiences the absence of periods for a time greater than three of her previous cycle intervals. One common cause, of course, is pregnancy. Once that is excluded the causes can be listed as follows: hypothalamic dysfunction (35%, usually related to

stress, poor nutrition, or strenuous exercise), pituitary disease (17%, usually hyperprolactinemia), which is the single most common cause of secondary amenorrhea, ovarian disease (10% with ovarian failure and another 30% with the polycystic ovary syndrome), and uterine disease (7%, often Asherman's syndrome of intrauterine synechiae). Adrenal hyperplasia, hypothyroidism, and ovarian and adrenal tumors also can cause secondary amenorrhea.

DIAGNOSIS

Primary amenorrhea: Evaluation should focus on breast development, the presence or absence of the uterus and cervix, and FSH level. If there is no breast development and the FSH level is elevated, the probable diagnosis is gonadal dysgenesis. If the uterus is absent, the probable diagnosis is müllerian agenesis. Karyotyping is indicated for patients with gonadal dysgenesis.

Secondary amenorrhea: Pregnancy must be excluded. Height and weight should be measured. Women who are more than 10% below their "ideal" body weight should be evaluated for anorexia nervosa. The evaluation includes a measurement of prolactin and FSH levels for all patients and thyroid testing and serum testosterone levels when the there is still diagnostic uncertainty. High levels of prolactin suggest prolactinoma, though hypothyroidism, medications, and renal failure can be responsible. FSH levels are elevated in ovarian failure, which may be caused by premature menopause (women older than 30 years) or chromosomal abnormalities (women younger than 30 years). Patients also should undergo a progestin withdrawal test, which is performed by means of administration of medroxyprogesterone acetate (10 mg a day for 5 days) and monitoring any uterine bleeding. The absence of uterine bleeding suggests that endogenous estrogen levels are particularly low or that Asherman's syndrome is present. Uterine bleeding indicates that Asherman's syndrome is not present.

MANAGEMENT

Primary amenorrhea: In many cases, long-term therapy with estrogen and progesterone is needed to stimulate development of secondary sex characteristics and to protect bone mass. Women with gonadal dysgenesis due to 45X are at high risk of thyroid disease and diabetes mellitus.

Secondary amenorrhea: The underlying cause should be managed when possible (e.g., prolactinomas can be controlled with surgical resection or bromocriptine therapy). Because women with secondary amenorrhea are at risk of osteoporosis, some authorities recommend that all be treated with estrogen–progestin hormone replacement.

Chapter 393

CUSHING'S SYNDROME

DEFINITION AND ETIOLOGY

Cushing's syndrome is the clinical expression of the metabolic effects of persistent, inappropriate hypercortisolism. Exogenous administration of glucocorticoids is the most common cause. Pituitary corticotropin hypersecretion (Cushing's disease), usually from microadenoma, accounts for about 60% of noniatrogenic cases; ectopic production of corticotropin by tumors (most often lung cancer) accounts for an additional 10%. The diseases that cause corticotropin-independent elevations in cortisol secretion (adrenal adenoma, adrenal carcinoma, and adrenal hyperplasia) each account for approximately 10% of noniatrogenic cases.

CLINICAL FEATURES

History: Patients with Cushing's disease usually have had symptoms for 2 to 3 years before diagnosis. The earliest symptoms include weight gain, hypertension, and glucose intolerance. A redistribution of adipose tissue causes facial rounding, increased central adiposity, and thinning of the upper and lower extremities. Patients may have striae, easy bruising, and increased growth of body hair. Women may have irregularities of menses; men may have gynecomastia. Proximal muscle weakness and peripheral edema are common. Back pain and loss of height may occur if osteoporosis and vertebral compression fractures have developed. Cognition and affect may be impaired.

Patients with adrenal adenoma and adrenal hyperplasia have signs and symptoms similar to those of patients with Cushing's disease. Patients with ectopic corticotropin syndrome usually have a shorter duration of symptoms. Some have minimal symptoms of Cushing's syndrome because of the short duration of hypercortisolemia. Among these patients, very high levels of cortisol often are associated with manifestations of mineralocorticoid excess, including weakness from hypokalemia. Symptoms related to the underlying tumor also may be evident. Patients with adrenocortical carcinoma also a shorter duration of symptoms before they seek medical attention. They typically have severe manifestations of androgen excess; for this reason, muscle atrophy may be less prominent. *Physical examination:* The examination reveals plethora, a round face with preauricular fullness, a prominent upper lip, supraclavicular fossa fullness, and a cervicodorsal fat pad (buffalo hump) disproportionate to the degree of obesity. Patients have torso obesity but thin extremities with decreased muscle mass. Peripheral edema may be present. The skin is thin, and there are wide, purple striae over the abdomen and chest. Other skin lesions include tinea versicolor, verruca vulgaris, acne vulgaris, and hirsutism. Patients with ectopic corticotropin production or adrenocortical carcinoma may have abnormalities related to the underlying tumor, such as a palpable mass.

LABORATORY STUDIES AND DIAGNOSTIC TESTS

Laboratory evaluation first requires confirmation of hypercortisolism by means of detection of either an elevated level of free cortisol in a 24-hour urine collection or an abnormal result of an overnight dexamethasone suppression test (the failure of 1 mg of dexamethasone given at 11 P.M. to suppress the serum cortisol level to less than 5 μg per deciliter at 8 A.M. the following day). If the screening test result is abnormal, further testing is needed to determine the cause of hypercortisolism (Fig. 407.3).

MANAGEMENT

Cushing's disease: Transsphenoidal selective resection of the pituitary microadenoma is the most effective therapy for pituitary corticotropin-dependent Cushing's disease. If the operation fails or cannot be performed, pituitary irradiation can be useful. When these treatments have failed, bilateral total adrenalectomy is the preferred treatment. The main disadvantage of this approach is that the pituitary tumor may continue to grow and become locally invasive and difficult to control (Nelson's syndrome). Various inhibitors of adrenal function have been used to suppress cortisol secretion, including aminoglutethimide, ketoconazole, and mitotane.

Other etiologic factors: Management of ectopic corticotropin syndrome entails surgical resection of the primary tumor followed by radiation therapy or chemotherapy if necessary. If the neoplasm cannot be resected, the use of adrenal inhibitors can be considered. Adrenocortical adenoma should be surgically removed. Adrenal hyperplasia can be managed with adrenalectomy or adrenal inhibitors. Adrenocortical carcinoma typically responds poorly to attempts at resection or chemotherapy.

Chapter 407

▬ DIABETES MELLITUS

DEFINITION AND EPIDEMIOLOGY

Diabetes mellitus is a chronic metabolic syndrome caused by a relative or absolute deficiency of insulin. Although the condition is recognized because of hyperglycemia, the metabolism of fats and proteins also is affected. One in every 20 persons in the United States has diabetes. The condition with its complications is the seventh leading cause of death of disease in the United States.

CLASSIFICATION, PATHOPHYSIOLOGY, AND ETIOLOGY

Type I diabetes accounts for 5% to 10% of cases of diabetes in the United States and usually has its onset in the first two decades of life. There is a familial predisposition. The disease is characterized by immune-mediated destruction of pancreatic islet β cells, absolute insulin deficiency, and a dependence on insulin therapy for the preservation of life. These patients are prone to ketosis.

Type II diabetes accounts for 90% to 95% of cases of diabetes in the Untied States and usually begins after 40 years of age. As with type I disease, there is a genetic predisposition. The disease is characterized by altered insulin secretory dynamics but retention of endogenous pancreatic insulin secretion, the absence of ketosis, and insulin resistance in target cells. Most patients are obese. Other associations include a family history of diabetes mellitus, hypertension, dyslipidemia, or a particular ethnic background (African American, Hispanic, Native American).

Secondary diabetes can occur with pancreatic disease or surgery, chronic liver disease, Cushing's syndrome, acromegaly, pregnancy, and the use of glucocorticoids. Women with gestational diabetes usually return to normal glucose tolerance after parturition.

DIAGNOSIS

Diabetes mellitus can be diagnosed when at least one of the following criteria is met: (a) unequivocal symptoms (polyuria, polydipsia, polyphagia, unexplained weight loss) and a random plasma glucose level of 200 mg per deciliter or more; (b) fasting plasma glucose (FBG) level 126 mg per deciliter or more; or (c) 2-hour plasma glucose level 200 mg per deciliter or more after the ingestion of 75 g glucose during an oral glucose tolerance test. In the absence of unequivocal hyperglycemia with acute metabolic decompensation, such as ketoacidosis, these criteria should be confirmed by means of another test on a different day.

COMPLICATIONS

Acute complications include diabetic ketoacidosis and hyperosmolar hyperglycemic nonketotic coma (described in the next entry). Two infections occur almost exclusively among patients with diabetes. Malignant otitis externa is potentially fatal, erosive *Pseudomonas aeruginosa* infection of the soft tissue and cartilage around the external auditory canal. It can cause progressive destruction of the temporal and petrous bones and requires vigorous debridement and prolonged therapy with intravenous (IV) antibiotics. Rhinocerebral mucormycosis is a very rapidly progressive invasive infection caused by the mycelia of *Mucor* and *Rhizopus* fungi. Aggressive surgical debridement and IV amphotericin B are the mainstays of therapy.

Chronic complications include neurologic deficits and accelerated vascular disease. The vascular disease is of two types: microangiopathy, characterized by thickening of capillary basement membranes and manifested principally in the retina and kidney, and macroangiopathy, increased frequency and severity of arterial atherosclerotic disease. The development of diabetic complications is likely multifactorial and caused by a combination of protein glycation, sorbitol accumulation within cells, glycosylation of basement membranes, platelet and endothelial dysfunction, and hemodynamic abnormalities. The Diabetes Control and Complications Trial (DCCT) firmly established the beneficial effects of improved glucose control on the risk of retinopathy, neuropathy, and nephropathy among patients with type I diabetes. Subsequent studies extended these findings to patients with type II disease.

Diabetic retinopathy: Diabetic retinopathy is the leading cause of blindness among working-age adults in the United States. The earliest stage is background retinopathy, which consists of microaneurysms, dot and blot hemorrhages, and exudates. It affects 80% of patients within 5 years of the onset of diabetes. With advancing disease, proliferative retinopathy develops and is characterized by neovascularization. Because laser photocoagulation has a dramatic effect in preventing visual loss among patients with high-risk retinal characteristics, a yearly comprehensive ophthalmologic examination is recommended for all patients who have had diabetes for more than 5 years.

Diabetic nephropathy: Diabetic nephropathy is the leading cause of end-stage renal disease in the United States. The risk increases with the duration of diabetes, although it is rare for nephropathy to develop after 25 to 30 years. The earliest clinical manifestation is a slightly elevated level of urinary albumin excretion (microalbuminuria) of 30 to 300 mg per day. There is associated glomerular hyperfiltration at this stage. With advancing disease, the amount of proteinuria increases to more than 300 mg per day, and the patient eventually has hypertension and a progressive decline in creatinine clearance. The development of nephropathy can be slowed with meticulous blood pressure control and the use of angiotensin-converting enzyme inhibitors by patients whose daily albumin excretion exceeds 30 mg, even if they have normal blood pressure.

Diabetic neuropathy: Diabetic neuropathy manifests as a peripheral neurologic deficit or autonomic dysfunction (Table 411.6). Among patients with distal symmetric neuropathy, neuropathic foot ulceration can necessitate limb amputation. There is no effective means of reducing the risk of neuropathy other than improved glycemic control. The risk of amputation, however, can be reduced by patient education about appropriate foot care, regular inspection of the feet by health care providers and patients, use of appropriate shoes and footwear, appropriate podiatric and pedorthic referral, aggressive early control of foot ulcers, and appropriate use of vascular surgical intervention. Painful neuropathy can be managed with tricyclic antidepressants, gabapentin, carbamazepine, or topical capsaicin cream. Narcotics should be avoided because of the high risk of addiction in this setting and a predictable loss of effectiveness due to tachyphylaxis.

MANAGEMENT

Type I diabetes: There are three major components of therapy—a nutritional plan, exercise, and insulin dosage. Patient education is essential to successful therapy, and the treatment program must be sufficiently flexible to allow highly varied and changing lifestyles without sacrificing careful metabolic control. Dietary protein should contribute about 10% to 20% of the total daily calories, leaving 80% to 90% of the total to be distributed between dietary fat and carbohydrate. Foods that cause rapid increases in blood glucose level should be avoided.

Monitoring consists of measurement of glycosylated hemoglobin every 3 months and patient monitoring of blood glucose level, typically before meals and at bedtime and whenever hypoglycemia is suspected. Therapeutic objectives are listed in Table 399.1. The insulin dosage needed for meticulous glucose control is typically 0.5 to 1.0 U per kilogram per day. During the honeymoon period of relative remission early in the disease, insulin requirements are less. During intercurrent illness, the necessary dosage may increase markedly.

Because patients with type I diabetes lack both basal and prandial insulin secretion, contemporary flexible insulin programs have multiple components. The most precise way to mimic normal insulin secretion is to use an insulin pump in a program of continuous subcutaneous insulin infusion. More commonly, basal therapy, usually about 40% to 50% of the daily insulin dose, is given as either intermediate-acting human insulin (NPH or lente) at bedtime with or without a small morning dose or as two daily injections of long-acting ultralente human insulin. Prandial insulin secretion is best duplicated by giving preprandial injections of rapid-onset regular insulin before each meal. Regular human insulin takes at least 20 minutes to become effective, but lispro insulin acts rapidly enough to be given immediately before a meal. Typically, 50% to 60% of the daily insulin is divided among the meals in proportion to carbohydrate content, although any given dose can be adjusted if the amount of food to be ingested differs from the patient's usual pattern or if the simultaneous blood glucose reading deviates from the target range.

Type II diabetes: The recommended treatment goals are fasting and preprandial glucose levels less than 120 mg per deciliter with glycosylated hemoglobin levels normal or near normal. Differing patient circumstances, however, such as advanced age and comorbid conditions, may dictate that higher degrees of hyperglycemia be tolerated. Normalizing weight among obese patients also is important. Because atherosclerotic risk is substantial among these patients, attention should be given to smoking cessation and meticulous control of hypertension and hyperlipidemia. Glycosylated hemoglobin levels should be obtained quarterly. Patient monitoring of FBG should be performed every day, and preprandial and bedtime levels should be checked periodically.

The treatment program consists of diet and exercise for all patients, and pharmacologic therapy for most. Moderate calorie restriction (250 to 500 calories less than average daily intake) usually is recommended for obese patients. Additional dietary principles include (a) balanced nutrient intake, (b) emphasis on appropriate alterations as necessary to achieve lipid and blood pressure goals, (c) adequate spacing of meals (4 to 5 hours), (d) consideration of consuming additional dietary fiber, and (e) avoidance of intake of rapidly absorbed simple sugars (sucrose, glucose, maltose) unless they are substitutes for other carbohydrates.

Many oral antidiabetic drugs are available. Sulfonylurea drugs such as glipizide and glyburide augment insulin secretion but may cause weight gain and hypoglycemia. Meglitinides such as repaglinide and nateglinide also augment endogenous insulin secretion. Because of their short duration of action, these agents can be given at meals for extra flexibility. They also may cause hypoglycemia and weight gain. Metformin decreases hepatic glucose output and increases peripheral glucose utilization. It does not cause weight gain or hypoglycemia but may cause nausea, abdominal discomfort, and diarrhea. It is contraindicated in the care of patients with elevated serum creatinine levels, hepatic disease, or congestive heart failure, who are at increased risk of lactic acidosis. Metformin should be withheld in the period surrounding the use of intravenous contrast agents.

Thiazolidinediones such as rosiglitazone and pioglitazone enhance insulin sensitivity and augment uptake of glucose in muscle and adipose tissue. They work best in combination with insulin or other oral agents. Because use of troglitazone has been associated with hepatotoxicity, monthly monitoring of liver enzymes is recommended. α-Glucosidase inhibitors such as acarbose compete with carbohydrates for binding to the enzymes in the intestinal brush border that digest complex carbohydrates. They therefore retard gastrointestinal glucose absorption. The primary role of these drugs is in combination with other agents when glycemic targets have not been met. Unabsorbed carbohydrates can cause flatulence, nausea, abdominal pain, and diarrhea.

If diet and exercise do not yield satisfactory glucose control, an oral agent (generally a sulfonylurea, meglitinide, or metformin) usually is chosen as first-line therapy. Glycemic control is then assessed at intervals. The dose of the oral agent can be increased or additional oral agents with different mechanisms of action can be added to achieve optimal control. Because of the number of oral agents that can be used alone or in combination, insulin therapy may be unnecessary for patients with mild disease. For those with moderate disease, a single dose of NPH or lente insulin can be added at bedtime (usually 0.3 to 0.6 U per kilogram per day) to provide basal insulin therapy. For patients with severe disease (those with FBS greater than 250 mg per deciliter), more intensive insulin programs usually are necessary (0.5 to 1.2 U per kilogram per day) to attain glucose control. Options include continuous insulin infusion and the use of twice-daily injections of 70/30 insulin, which contains 70% NPH and 30% regular insulin. Although oral agents have traditionally been discontinued when insulin therapy is initiated, current strategies often combine insulin with one or more oral agents, particularly the agents that enhance the peripheral effects of insulin, such as metformin or the thiazolidinediones.

SCREENING

Because 35% to 40% of cases of type II diabetes mellitus are undiagnosed, screening is considered an important public health measure. Asymptomatic patients older than 45 years should have a FBG determination every 3 years. Screening at a younger age should be considered for persons who are at higher risk.

Chapter 411

DIABETIC KETOACIDOSIS AND HYPEROSMOLAR HYPERGLYCEMIC NONKETOTIC COMA

DEFINITIONS, EPIDEMIOLOGY, AND ETIOLOGY

Diabetic ketoacidosis (DKA) is acute, life-threatening, metabolic acidosis that represents the most extreme result of uncontrolled diabetes mellitus. It occurs most commonly among patients with type I diabetes mellitus but can occur with type II diabetes, particularly when there is a severe intercurrent illness. Hyperosmolar hyperglycemic nonketotic coma (HHNC) is an acute syndrome that occurs with uncontrolled type II diabetes mellitus. It usually affects elderly patients, particularly those with other underlying medical problems and concurrent infections.

PATHOPHYSIOLOGY AND DIAGNOSIS

Diabetic ketoacidosis: DKA develops as a consequence of severe insulin deficiency and an excess of the glucose counterregulatory hormones such as glucagon, cortisol, and the catecholamines. Hyperglycemia is caused by both decreased glucose uptake and utilization and increased hepatic gluconeogenesis. The hyperglycemia causes osmotic diuresis, hypovolemia, and large urinary losses of potassium and phosphate. Uninhibited lipolysis stimulates production of ketones (acetoacetate and β-hydroxybutyrate) from free fatty acids and produces metabolic acidosis and compensatory hyperpnea. The cardinal diagnostic features are hyperglycemia (250 mg per deciliter or more), ketosis (ketonemia or ketonuria), and acidosis (arterial pH less than 7.3 and serum bicarbonate less than 15 mEq per liter). Other features include an elevated anion gap, volume depletion, and Kussmaul's respirations. The degree of hyperglycemia need not be great; a large proportion of patients have a glucose concentration less than 350 mg per deciliter.

Hyperosmolar hyperglycemic nonketotic coma: Because insulin levels are sufficient to suppress lipolysis, ketosis and acidosis do not occur. For this reason, the syndrome tends to last longer than DKA before it is recognized clinically. The severity of hyperglycemia, hyperosmolarity, and dehydration tends to be worse than with DKA because of the more prolonged period of osmotic diuresis. The extreme hyperosmolarity causes dehydration of the brain and altered mental status. The diagnosis is confirmed when a patient with abnormal mental status has severe hyperglycemia (usually 600 to 1,200 mg per deciliter), elevated serum osmolarity (more than 350 mOsm per kilogram), and minimal or absent ketonemia or ketonuria.

MANAGEMENT

Diabetic ketoacidosis: Patients with mild acidemia can be treated at home as long as they can tolerate large amounts of oral fluid. For patients with more severe illness, hospitalization is necessary. Because average fluid losses are 10% of body weight, vigorous fluid supplementation is necessary to restore intravascular volume (1 to 2 L of isotonic saline solution over the first hour, 1 L per hour for the next 3 to 4 hours, then a decrease in rate based on clinical assessment). Insulin administration is initiated rapidly, unless there is evidence of severe hypovolemia or hypokalemia. An initial priming dose of 0.1 units of regular insulin IV per kilogram body weight is followed by a continuous infusion of regular insulin at a rate of 0.1 U per kilogram per hour. Because too rapid a decline in serum glucose levels can lead to cerebral edema, the insulin infusion rate should be adjusted about every 2 hours so that glucose levels decrease at a rate of approximately 100 mg per deciliter per hour.

Hyperglycemia usually resolves more quickly than metabolic acidosis. For this reason, when the glucose level reaches 200 to 300 mg per deciliter, glucose or dextrose is added to the intravenous fluids to allow continuation of the insulin infusion without the risk of hypoglycemia. At the same time, the insulin infusion rate is decreased to 0.05 U per kilogram per hour and maintained for at least 6 hours after the acidosis has resolved.

Serum potassium levels in DKA do not reflect total body levels, which are almost invariably reduced, because the acidosis and insulin deficiency cause a redistribution of potassium from the intracellular to the extracellular compartment. The potassium deficiency therefore becomes more evident as treatment progresses. If the patient is not treated, the deficiency places the patient at risk of cardiac arrhythmia. Potassium supplementation is given immediately unless the patient has anuria, has an initial serum potassium level more than 6.0 mEq per liter, or has hyperkalemic T-wave changes on an electrocardiogram. The recommended rate of potassium infusion ranges from 10 mEq per hour for those with initial levels of 5 to 6 mEq per liter to 40 mEq per hour for patients with initial serum potassium levels less than 3 mEq per liter.

The use of bicarbonate is the management of DKA is controversial. Bicarbonate should probably be restricted to cases of very severe acidemia (pH less than 7.0), although it may be beneficial for patients with marked acidemia (pH 7.0 to 7.1) who have severe underlying medical problems such as myocardial infarction, cardiac arrhythmia, or sepsis.

Hyperosmolar hyperglycemic nonketotic coma: The first priority is to restore intravascular volume. The rate of saline infusion is generally slower than in DKA, because the patients are usually elderly and may have cardiac or renal insufficiency. The initial rate usually is restricted to 1 L per hour until peripheral perfusion is normalized. Then hypotonic fluids are given at a rate that approximates twice urine output. The goal is gradual restoration of the normal metabolic state. Insulin therapy should be withheld until volume status is normalized because the movement of glucose and water from the extracellular to the intracellular compartment can precipitate shock. Even without insulin therapy, the plasma glucose level begins to decrease in response to intravenous fluids owing to hemodilution and improvement in renal blood flow and glucose excretion.

Chapter 149

APPROACH TO THE PATIENT WITH HYPERCALCEMIA AND HYPOCALCEMIA

DEFINITIONS AND PATHOPHYSIOLOGY

The normal range for total serum calcium level is about 8.9 to 10.1 mg per deciliter. Total serum calcium level reflects both bound calcium and ionized, or free, calcium. Only the former is metabolically active; it typically comprises about 50% of the total. Changes in the amount of bound hormone must be excluded as a cause of spurious hypocalcemia or hypercalcemia. For example, hypoalbuminemia decreases total serum calcium level by reducing the amount of bound calcium. The level of ionized calcium can be obtained directly in many laboratories and eliminates this potential source of confusion. Hypercalcemia is caused by disturbances of the calcitropic hormones (parathyroid hormone [PTH], calcitonin, and calcitriol) or from abnormal processes directly affecting bone resorption, intestinal calcium absorption, or mineral excretion. In contrast, defects in PTH secretion or resistance to PTH are the primary causes of permanent hypocalcemia.

DIFFERENTIAL DIAGNOSIS

Hypercalcemia: Many disorders can cause hypercalcemia (Table 402.1), but the most common are primary hyperparathyroidism (PHP) and malignant disease. Malignant hypercalcemia is caused by osteolytic metastasis, such as cancer of the breast, kidney, lung, or thyroid; hematologic malignant disease with skeletal infiltration, such as multiple myeloma; or secretion of humoral agents by non-

parathyroid tumors, such as squamous cell carcinoma, carcinoma of the kidney or bladder, and malignant tumors of the ovary.

Hypocalcemia: The most common disorders are hypoparathyroidism and vitamin D deficiency associated with conditions such as chronic renal failure, malabsorption, or dietary deficiency. Other causes include pseudohypoparathyroidism (end-organ unresponsiveness to PTH), magnesium deficiency, medications (e.g., calcitonin, bisphosphonates, phosphates, foscarnet, pentamidine, citrated blood), osteoblastic metastasis, phosphate excess (e.g., tumor lysis syndrome or rhabdomyolysis), and pancreatitis.

CLINICAL CONSEQUENCES

Hypercalcemia: Because of the widespread use of multiphasic laboratory screening, many patients do not have symptoms at the time of diagnosis. Nephrolithiasis may cause renal colic, hematuria, and the passage of stones or gravel. Bone pain and tenderness may develop. Nonspecific symptoms include muscle weakness, depression, memory impairment, personality changes, pruritus, anorexia, constipation, polyuria, and polydipsia. Associations with peptic ulcers, pancreatitis, and hypertension are controversial. With severe or prolonged hypercalcemia, anemia, weight loss, coma, and death can occur. Symptoms and signs of any underlying disease also occur.

Hypocalcemia: Patients experience paresthesia, particularly in the oral area, muscle spasm, carpopedal spasm, and facial grimacing. In extreme cases, laryngeal spasm and convulsion occur. Central nervous system manifestations include irritability, depression, impaired memory, and psychosis. Cardiovascular effects include arrhythmia, bradycardia, hypotension, and impaired cardiac contractility. At physical examination, the Chvostek or Trousseau signs can be used to confirm latent tetany.

LABORATORY STUDIES AND DIAGNOSTIC TESTS

Hypercalcemia: Current PTH immunoassays reliably confirm or exclude the diagnosis of PHP, although the hypercalcemia associated with use of thiazide diuretics and lithium can be associated with elevated levels. In PHP and malignant hypercalcemia, serum phosphate levels typically are depressed. Serum chloride levels tend to be mildly elevated in PHP but mildly depressed in malignant conditions. Other laboratory tests and imaging studies can be useful for investigating the possibility of malignancy or the other disorders listed in Table 402.1.

Hypocalcemia: Among patients with PTH deficiency, serum phosphorus levels usually are increased, and PTH levels are low or undetectable. Serum vitamin D levels are low in this disorder and in vitamin D deficiency. Other laboratory tests and diagnostic studies can be useful in confirming or excluding other disorders in the differential diagnosis.

MANAGEMENT

Hypercalcemia: The necessity for short-term therapy is signaled by the occurrence of anorexia, nausea, mental status changes, hypertension, or worsening renal function in association with a serum calcium level greater than 13.5 mg per deciliter. Initial therapy is saline hydration, which increases renal calcium clearance. After any volume deficits have been restored, calciuresis can be further enhanced by combining large volumes of saline solution (up to 6 L per day) and intravenous furosemide (in doses up to 100 mg every 2 hours). Careful monitoring is required to prevent hypovolemia, hypervolemia, hyponatremia, or hypokalemia. Biphosphonates inhibit osteoclasts and block mobilization of calcium from bone. Of these, pamidronate is the preferred agent; the effective dose is 30 to 90 mg administered as a single intravenous infusion over 24 hours. Glucocorticoids (40 to 100 mg prednisone in divided doses each day) are useful in treating hypercalcemia from vitamin D intoxication and granulomatous disease. Calcitonin (25 to 50 U parenterally every 6 to 8 hours) is particularly effective in treatment of patients with vitamin D intoxication, thyrotoxicosis, or immobilization. Because of adverse effects and the emergence of other effective therapies, mithramycin is now best reserved for particularly difficult or unusual situations.

Long-term therapy is best directed at the underlying disease. If hypercalcemia persists despite optimal management, options include hydration with or without furosemide, combination therapy with subcutaneous injections of calcitonin and low-dose prednisone, and therapy with bisphosphonates. For patients with PHP, parathyroidectomy is indicated if there is a history of symptomatic or asymptomatic renal stones, substantial or progressive bone loss, symptoms attributable to hypercalcemia, or a serum calcium level more than 11.5 mg per deciliter.

Hypocalcemia: The objectives of short-term therapy for hypocalcemia with tetany are to relieve symptoms and prevent laryngeal obstruction. The serum calcium level is best maintained at more than 7 mg per deciliter. For adults, 10 to 20 mL 10% calcium gluconate is given by means of intravenous push. If a patient can take oral medications, 100 mg calcium should be given every 2 hours with an increase in the dose to 500 mg if necessary. Otherwise, continuous infusion of 10 mL 10% solution added to 500 mL saline solution should be given over 6 hours. Long-term treatment depends on the cause. Vitamin D deficiency is managed with supplementation of that vitamin. In states of parathyroid deficiency or resistance, calcium and vitamin D supplements are used. However, this therapy can cause hypercalciuria owing to the PTH deficiency, and careful monitoring for nephrocalcinosis and nephrolithiasis is critical. Chlorthalidone often is added to decrease urinary calcium excretion.

Chapter 402

APPROACH TO HYPERLIPIDEMIA

PRESENTATION
Elevated total cholesterol and low-density lipoprotein cholesterol (LDL-C) levels, elevated triglyceride levels, and reduced high-density lipoprotein cholesterol (HDL-C) levels all are independently associated with increased risk of atherosclerotic cardiovascular disease (ASCVD). Markedly elevated triglyceride levels (more than 1,000 mg per deciliter) also are associated with risk of acute pancreatitis.

HISTORY AND PHYSICAL EXAMINATION
A complete history should be obtained, including the presence of ASCVD and calculation of the number of cardiovascular risk factors other than total cholesterol and LDL-C. Risk factors include age older than 45 years for men and older than 55 years for women (or premature menopause without estrogen replacement); definite myocardial infarction or sudden death before 55 years of age of a male first-degree relative or before 65 years of age of a female first-degree relative; current cigarette smoking; hypertension; diabetes mellitus; and an HDL-C level less than 35 mg per deciliter. Because an elevated HDL-C level is protective, one risk factor is subtracted from the total if the HDL-C level is more than 60 mg per deciliter. Evidence of the secondary causes of hyperlipidemia (Table 31.3). should be sought. The physical examination should include examination of the eyes for arcus corneae, the eyelids for xanthelasma, the palms for palmar xanthoma, the knuckles and Achilles tendons for tendon xanthoma, and the elbows and knees for cutaneous and tuberoeruptive xanthoma. The thyroid should be palpated and the major arteries should be examined for vascular bruits.

DIFFERENTIAL DIAGNOSIS
Table 31.3 outlines the diagnostic considerations for patients with dyslipidemia.

LABORATORY STUDIES AND DIAGNOSTIC TESTS
All adults older than 20 years should undergo screening for hypercholesterolemia. For adults without established ASCVD, the total and HDL-C cholesterol should be measured in the fasting state. Patients with established ASCVD should undergo a full lipid profile, which consists of triglyceride, total cholesterol, and HDL-C levels after an overnight fast of at least 12 hours. The LDL-C level usually is calculated by means of subtracting the HDL-C level and one-fifth of the triglyceride level from the total cholesterol; however, this formula is not accurate if the triglyceride level exceeds 400 mg per deciliter. Once a lipoprotein disorder has been diagnosed, common secondary causes should be excluded by means of measurement of thyroid-stimulating hormone and fasting glucose; liver enzymes and serum albumin are measured in selected cases.

MANAGEMENT
Secondary causes should be actively sought and controlled. Obese persons should be encouraged to lose weight and sedentary persons to exercise. Every effort should be made to modify other cardiovascular risk factors. Additional management decisions depend on whether ASCVD or other cardiovascular risk factors are present (see Table 31.2). Aggressive management of hypercholesterolemia for patients with established ASCVD (secondary prevention) has been shown to reduce cardiovascular events and total mortality. For patients without ASCVD, primary prevention trials have shown that lowering total or LDL-C cholesterol among patients at high risk reduces the likelihood of cardiovascular events and

mortality. The higher the level of LDL-C and the greater the number of risk factors, the greater is the potential benefit of drug therapy to lower LDL-C levels. Among persons considered to be at lower risk, the emphasis is more on dietary modification and less on drug therapy.

Diet therapy: To lower LDL-C level by means of diet modification, the intake of saturated fats must be restricted. Decreasing the intake of total fats and cholesterol also is beneficial although less important. Useful diet programs include those developed by the American Heart Association and the National Cholesterol Education Program. If therapeutic goals are not reached after 3 months, the patient should be referred to a registered dietitian for more detailed dietary instruction and implementation of a stricter diet (step II). If there is an inadequate response after another 3 months, drug therapy should be strongly considered. For patients with established ASCVD or numerous risk factors, the period of observation with diet alone can be shortened, and the stricter diet can be recommended initially.

Drug therapy: HMG-CoA reductase inhibitors (statins) are considered the drugs of first choice in most settings. They reduce hepatic cholesterol biosynthesis and generally lower LDL-C level by 20% to 30% at initial doses. Patient acceptance is high. Side effects include elevated liver enzyme levels (transaminases should be measured periodically), muscle or joint pain, and gastrointestinal upset. Among the lipid-lowering drugs, nicotinic acid (niacin) has the greatest effect in raising HDL-C level. The mechanism of action is unclear but probably involves a reduction in hepatic production of very low density lipoprotein (VLDL). It is particularly useful in combination with statins in the treatment of patients who cannot achieve LDL-C goals with a statin alone and patients who have combined hyperlipidemia and a persistently elevated triglyceride level or low HDL-C level with statin therapy. Patient acceptance of immediate-release niacin can be limited by the cutaneous flushing and pruritus it causes, although pretreatment with aspirin can relieve these symptoms in many cases. Sustained-release forms are better tolerated but may be more likely to cause hepatotoxicity. Other side effects include hyperglycemia, hyperuricemia, and exacerbation of peptic ulcer disease.

Bile acid sequestrants (resins), including cholestyramine and colestipol, accelerate the loss of bile acids in the stool and promote increased hepatic conversion of cholesterol to bile acids. They are a good choice for young, motivated patients with mild hypercholesterolemia and are useful in combination therapy with niacin or statins. They may aggravate hypertriglyceridemia. Other adverse effects include bloating, constipation, and interference with the absorption of other medications. Fibric acid derivatives, such as gemfibrozil, stimulate lipoprotein lipase activity and may reduce hepatic production of VLDL. They lower triglyceride levels effectively and generally raise HDL-C levels modestly, but they have limited ability to lower LDL-C levels. Their primary use, therefore, is in the management of moderate to severe hypertriglyceridemia. They are generally well tolerated but can cause gastrointestinal upset and muscle pain. The risk of myopathy increases when fibrates are used in combination with statins.

Chapter 31

HYPOGLYCEMIA

PRESENTATION
Symptoms may begin at plasma levels of about 60 mg per deciliter, impairment of brain function at approximately 50 mg per deciliter. The rate of decline in glucose level is not an important factor. Symptoms vary among patients but are usually consistent from episode to episode for each patient. Autonomic symptoms (sweating, trembling, anxiety, nausea, palpitation, hunger, and tingling) do not always precede symptoms of neuroglycopenia (confusion, abnormal behavior, visual disturbance, and seizure) and may not be present at all.

CLASSIFICATION
The long-established classification of hypoglycemia as fasting or nonfasting is less useful than one based on the clinical characteristics of the patient (Table 400.1). Persons who appear healthy are likely to have hypoglycemic disorders different from those experienced by persons who are ill.

DIAGNOSTIC EVALUATION
Healthy-appearing patients: Because the symptoms of hypoglycemia are non-specific, it is necessary to verify a low plasma glucose level when spontaneous symptoms occur and to demonstrate that symptoms are relieved through correc-

tion of the hypoglycemia. Patients with frank hypoglycemia at evaluation should undergo immediate laboratory evaluation (see later); otherwise, a prolonged fast (up to 72 hours) should be undertaken (often starting in the outpatient setting and continuing in the hospital if necessary) until the patient has both symptoms of hypoglycemia and a plasma glucose level less than 45 mg per deciliter. Calorie-free and caffeine-free beverages are permitted during the fast.

The main diagnostic consideration is insulinoma. The diagnosis of endogenous hyperinsulinemic hypoglycemia is made at the end of the fast the laboratory findings are as follows: plasma insulin 6 μU per milliliter or more (radioimmunoassay) or 3 μU per milliliter or more (immunochemiluminescent assay), C-peptide 200 pmol per milliliter or more, proinsulin 5 pmol per milliliter or more, β-hydroxybutyrate 2.7 mmol per liter or less, increment of plasma glucose in response to 1 mg glucagon intravenously 25 mg per deciliter or more, and absence from the plasma of sulfonylureas. The insulin-secreting tumor can be localized with transabdominal ultrasonography, endoscopic ultrasonography, computed tomography, angiography, or a selective arterial calcium stimulation test.

Ill-appearing patients: It may be sufficient to recognize the underlying disease and its association with hypoglycemia and to take action to minimize recurrences of hypoglycemia. Confirmation of the suspected etiologic factor may be sought, such as low insulin and C-peptide levels in ethanol hypoglycemia, elevated insulin-like growth factor II levels in non–β-cell tumor hypoglycemia, low cortisol levels in adrenal insufficiency, and blunted plasma glucose responses to intravenous glucagon in hypoglycemia due to conditions that impair liver function, such as glycogen storage disease, sepsis, and congestive heart failure.

MANAGEMENT

Ultimately, hypoglycemia is managed best by controlling any underlying illnesses. Insulinoma is managed by means of surgical excision.

Chapter 400

HYPOTHYROIDISM

DEFINITIONS, PATHOGENESIS, AND ETIOLOGY

Thyroid deficiency can be caused by a primary defect in the thyroid gland (primary hypothyroidism, 95% of cases) or by inadequate production of thyroid-stimulating hormone (TSH) by the pituitary gland (secondary hypothyroidism, 5% of cases). In the United States, the most common cause is lymphocytic (Hashimoto's) thyroiditis, in which cytotoxic antibodies directed against thyroid follicular cells cause thyroid atrophy and fibrosis. This condition can be associated with other autoimmune diseases and occasionally occurs as part of a polyglandular endocrine deficiency state in which various autoantibodies impair the function of the thyroid, adrenal glands, parathyroid glands, and gonads.

Another variant of autoimmune hypothyroidism is caused by production of TSH-receptor blocking antibodies. Next in frequency is probably iatrogenic hypothyroidism caused by therapy for Graves' disease. Hypothyroidism among adults also can be caused by incomplete forms of hereditary enzymatic defects, medications that induce defects in hormone synthesis (e.g., aminosalicylic acid and lithium), and iodine deficiency. A self-limited interval of hypothyroidism typically occurs during the course of subacute (de Quervain's) thyroiditis, lymphocytic (painless) thyroiditis, and postpartum thyroiditis and among patients with functioning thyroid glands whose suppressive doses of thyroid supplementation are abruptly discontinued. Secondary hypothyroidism may be caused by pituitary tumor, postpartum pituitary necrosis (Sheehan's syndrome), or autoimmune hypophysitis.

CLINICAL PRESENTATION

The signs and symptoms vary greatly depending on the severity and duration of the thyroid deficiency, the patient's age, and the effects of concomitant illnesses. Among adults, early symptoms often are nonspecific and insidious in onset. These may include fatigue, lethargy, constipation, cold intolerance, muscle stiffness and cramping, carpal tunnel syndrome, and menorrhagia. There is a slowing of mental agility and motor activity, reduced memory, and weight gain in spite of a reduced appetite. The skin and hair become dry, and the hair thins and begins to fall out. Edema of the vocal cords may cause deepening of the voice. In severe hypothyroidism (myxedema), the patient appears pallid, depressed, and hypokinetic and has hoarseness, an expressionless face, sparse hair, and a large tongue. The skin is cool to touch, dry, and rough, and there are facial and periorbital puffiness and generalized edema. Goiter may or may not be present,

depending on the cause hypothyroidism. With Hashimoto's thyroiditis, there is usually goiter in the early phases of the disease, but the gland later atrophies and is not palpable. Neurologic findings include a delayed relaxation phase of deep tendon reflexes, muscle weakness, and ataxia.

LABORATORY STUDIES AND DIAGNOSTIC TESTS

The single most important test is measurement of the serum TSH, which is elevated among patients with primary thyroid disease of any kind and is in the low-normal to undetectable range among patients with pituitary or hypothalamic disease. Levels of serum total and free thyronine (T_4) are decreased in all forms of hypothyroidism. Measurement of total triiodothyronine (T_3) is less useful, because it is within the normal range among most patients. Thyroid autoantibodies (anti-thyroglobulin and anti-microsomal) are detectable in most patients with Hashimoto's thyroiditis. Radioiodine uptake studies have little diagnostic utility in this setting. Nonthyroid laboratory abnormalities include hyperlipidemia, anemia, and elevated levels of creatine kinase and lactate dehydrogenase. Electrocardiographic changes include bradycardia, low-amplitude QRS complexes, and flattened or inverted T waves.

MANAGEMENT

Subclinical primary hypothyroidism: Patients with early hypothyroidism often have only mildly elevated TSH levels (between 4 and 10 mU per liter) and T_4 levels within the normal range. The symptoms may be so minimal as to be overlooked, but studies have shown mild hyperlipidemia to be present in such cases. About 50% of such cases progress to overt hypothyroidism within 5 to 7 years. Early initiation of levothyroxine replacement in low dosage has been recommended, because it may eliminate progression from mild to overt disease and may reduce the cardiovascular risks of ongoing atherogenesis.

Overt primary hypothyroidism: Almost all patients can be treated with a single daily dose of synthetic levothyroxine. Because T_4 is converted to T_3, normal serum concentrations of T_3 can be restored with levothyroxine alone. In general, the initial dose is 25 to 50 μg levothyroxine each day, with increments of 25 to 50 μg at 4 to 6 week intervals until a normal metabolic state is attained. This gradual approach to thyroid repletion is especially important for elderly patients and those with heart disease, because a sudden increase in metabolic rate may tax cardiac or coronary reserve. For patients with primary hypothyroidism, the best indication that a normal metabolic state has been achieved is a reduction in serum TSH level to the range of 0.5 to 1.5 mU per liter. On average, this requires a replacement dose of approximately 1.7 μg per kilogram per day for patients with Hashimoto's thyroiditis and 2.1 μg per kilogram per day for those who have undergone total surgical or radioiodine thyroid ablation. Dosage increases may be necessary during pregnancy or with progression of the underlying thyroid disease.

Overt secondary hypothyroidism: For patients with pituitary or hypothalamic disease, measurements of free T_4 usually are an accurate guide to the adequacy of replacement. In such circumstances, because of the theoretical risk of precipitating acute adrenocortical deficiency through augmentation of cortisol metabolism, it is traditional to treat patients with glucocorticoids for the first 10 to 14 days of thyroid replacement.

Myxedema coma: Any patient with long-standing hypothyroidism is at risk of stupor or coma. Patients also may have hypothermia, hypotension, hypoglycemia, hyponatremia, hypoventilation with hypercapnia, and seizures. Even with aggressive management, mortality ranges from 30% to 60%. When this condition is suspected, blood samples for TSH, free T_4, and cortisol should be obtained. Intravenous treatment with thyroid hormones (e.g., 3 to 4 μg per kilogram levothyroxine followed by 100 μg per day thereafter and 10 μg of liothyronine every 8 hours) and hydrocortisone should follow immediately. Supportive care is essential, with special attention to ventilation. The dosages of some medications, such as digoxin, may have to be modified because of the altered distribution and slowed metabolism associated with profound hypothyroidism.

Chapter 406

HYPERTHYROIDISM AND THYROTOXICOSIS

DEFINITIONS, PATHOGENESIS, AND ETIOLOGY

Thyrotoxicosis is the term applied to the clinical and biochemical findings caused by the presence in the body of excess thyroid hormone. Not all patients with thyrotoxicosis have hyperthyroidism, a sustained overproduction of hormone by the thyroid gland. For example, in some types of thyroiditis, an inflammatory process causes leakage of preformed hormone from the gland. The patient has thyrotoxicosis, but the suppression of thyroid-stimulating hormone actually decreases new hormone formation and may cause a period of transient hypothyroidism after the stores are depleted. Thyrotoxicosis without true hyperthyroidism also can be caused by exogenous sources of excess hormone or by thyroid hormone derived from follicular cells outside the thyroid gland, such as functioning metastatic thyroid carcinoma and struma ovarii.

True hyperthyroidism can be caused by a hyperfunctioning autonomous nodule or toxic multinodular goiter, but the most frequent cause is Graves' disease, which occurs most commonly among women in their third or fourth decades. In Graves' disease, it is speculated that infectious factors initiate an immunologic cascade in susceptible individuals that stimulates lymphocytes that secrete immunoglobulins that stimulate the TSH receptor. The pathogenesis of the ophthalmopathic and dermopathic manifestations of Graves' disease is less clear, although pathologic examination shows inflammatory infiltration of the orbital muscles and lymphocytic infiltration of the dermis.

CLINICAL PRESENTATION

Thyrotoxicosis: Common symptoms include anxiety and nervousness, emotional lability, easy fatigability, insomnia, increased perspiration, heat intolerance, palpitations, dyspnea, weakness, hyperdefecation, and weight loss despite increased appetite. Signs common to all patients with thyrotoxicosis include hyperactivity; eye lid retraction; thyroid enlargement; hair thinning; warm, moist skin with a velvety texture; onycholysis; tremor; muscle weakness; hyperreflexia; and tachycardia with or without evidence of atrial fibrillation. The presentation may depend on the age of the patient; irritability, heat intolerance, and increased appetite are more prevalent among younger persons, whereas weight loss and cardiac manifestations are more common among the elderly. Some elderly patients may have paradoxical apathy rather than hyperactivity (apathetic thyrotoxicosis).

Graves' disease: Patients may have any of the manifestations of thyrotoxicosis. Graves' ophthalmopathy is characterized by impaired eye muscle movement and periorbital edema with or without proptosis. When severe, the ophthalmopathy can be associated with corneal ulceration, optic neuritis, and optic atrophy. Infiltrative dermopathy, when present, usually occurs over the dorsum of the leg or feet, and has been called *pretibial myxedema*. The affected area usually is raised, plaque-like, and hyperpigmented and has a peau d'orange appearance.

Thyrotoxic storm: Thyrotoxic storm is a syndrome of exaggerated signs and symptoms of thyrotoxicosis with systemic decompensation likely to be fatal unless the patient is vigorously treated. The diagnosis is made clinically when a patient has proven thyrotoxicosis as well as fever (temperature usually greater than 38.5°C), tachycardia out of proportion to the fever, central nervous system signs (irritability, confusion, delirium or coma), and gastrointestinal disturbances such as nausea, vomiting, and diarrhea. Events known to precipitate thyrotoxic storm include withdrawal of antithyroid drug therapy, sepsis, surgical procedures, use of iodinated contrast agents, hypoglycemia, parturition, emotional stress, diabetic ketoacidosis, burn injury, vigorous palpation of the thyroid, pulmonary thromboembolism, and stroke.

LABORATORY STUDIES AND DIAGNOSTIC TESTS

Thyrotoxicosis usually is associated with inability to detect TSH (when it is measured with a sensitive assay) and with an increase in levels of total and free thyronine (T_4) and triiodothyronine (T_3). Some patients have so-called T_3 thyrotoxicosis, in which only the T_3 level is elevated, or hyperthyroidism due to a TSH-secreting pituitary tumor, in which case the TSH level is normal or elevated. Once thyrotoxicosis is confirmed, the diagnosis of Graves' disease can be made clinically if either ophthalmopathy or dermopathy is present. Otherwise, additional studies are necessary to differentiate the possible etiologic factors. Patients with hyperthyroidism have increased thyroid radioiodine uptake. Patients with nonhyperthyroid thyrotoxicosis have decreased uptake. An ultrasound or radionuclide scan discloses whether there is a hyperfunctioning autonomous nodule or a toxic multinodular goiter. An immeasurably low thyroglobulin level suggests an exogenous source of thyroid hormone. Elevated titers of thyroid-stimulating immunoglobulin in the blood is strong evidence of Graves' disease. It is not possible to differentiate patients with thyrotoxic storm from those with uncomplicated thyrotoxicosis on the basis of routine thyroid studies. Other laboratory abnormalities associated with thyrotoxicosis include hypercalcemia and elevations in lactate dehydrogenase, transaminases, alkaline phosphatase,

and angiotensin-converting enzyme activity. Bone densitometry may show osteopenia or osteoporosis.

MANAGEMENT

Thyrotoxicosis and hyperthyroidism: The adrenergic symptoms of thyrotoxicosis can be managed with β-blockers. Iodine (100 to 200 mg per day) acutely inhibits proteolysis of colloid within the gland and reduces release of hormone. Hyperthyroidism itself requires one of three therapies— antithyroid medications that block hormone synthesis, thyroidectomy, or thyroid ablation with radioactive iodine. Treatment with radioiodine is generally considered to be the most efficient and cost-effective, although it not appropriate for treatment of young patients (younger than 25 years) and pregnant women. Most patients need thyroid supplementation after treatment. Patients with Graves' ophthalmopathy may have an exacerbation after radioiodine therapy; the use of glucocorticoids for several weeks lowers this risk. The primary advantage of antithyroid drugs such as methimazole or propylthiouracil is that patients have an opportunity to remain euthyroid after discontinuation of therapy, if they enter a sustained remission (as sometimes occurs with Graves' disease). Leukopenia is a severe, though uncommon, side effect.

Thyroidectomy is infrequently performed. Candidates for surgery include those who decline radioiodine therapy and have had severe allergic reactions to antithyroid drugs or habitually do not take them; pregnant patients who cannot tolerate antithyroid therapy or who need very large doses; patients with unusually large goiters; and those in whom concomitant malignant disease is suspected. The most important side effect is hypothyroidism; laryngeal nerve injury and hypoparathyroidism also can occur.

Other manifestations of Graves' disease: Eye disease may occur independently of the thyroid disease and it may not improve with therapy for the hyperthyroidism. Initial therapy consists of elevation of the head of the bed, methylcellulose eye drops, nocturnal eye patching, and diuretics. In more severe cases, prednisone or orbital radiation may be needed. Graves' dermopathy may improve with therapy for the thyrotoxicosis. If not, potent topical or injected glucocorticoids may be beneficial.

Thyrotoxic storm: Supportive therapy includes control of dehydration and intravenous administration of glucose, vitamin B complex, and glucocorticoids. Propranolol may be used to suppress the adrenergic effects of thyrotoxicosis but must be given cautiously. Intravenous pressor agents may be needed to control hypotension. Large doses of an antithyroid medication should be given immediately (e.g., 100 mg propylthiouracil every 2 hours). Soon after antithyroid medication is given, potassium iodide is added to block further hormone release from the gland.

Chapter 406

■ PHEOCHROMOCYTOMA

DEFINITION, EPIDEMIOLOGY, AND ETIOLOGY

The term *pheochromocytoma* may be used for all catecholamine-secreting tumors, adrenal or extraadrenal, but is sometimes reserved for adrenal tumors only. Pheochromocytoma may be present in 0.1% to 0.5% of patients with hypertension. Most cases are sporadic and of unknown causation, although associations with some hereditary syndromes have been identified, such as multiple endocrine neoplasia [MEN] and von Hippel–Lindau disease.

PATHOGENESIS

Pheochromocytoma originates in chromaffin tissue. Most tumors (90%) are intraadrenal. The most common extraadrenal site is the organ of Zuckerkandl near the aortic bifurcation. The clinical manifestations vary somewhat depending on the relative proportions of secreted epinephrine and norepinephrine. Manifestations such as hypercalcemia and polycythemia are not explained by catecholamine excess and implicate the secretion of other neuropeptides in some cases.

CLINICAL FEATURES

Hypertension is the cardinal abnormality. In many cases it is sustained. In the others, baseline hypertension is associated with paroxysms of greater severity. Truly intermittent hypertension is unusual. Other features of the hypertension include severity, early onset, resistance to conventional therapy, and exacerbation by β-blockers. Patients have paroxysmal episodes characterized by various combinations of throbbing headache, anxiety, drenching sweats, tachycardia, palpitations, chest and abdominal pain, nausea and vomiting, tremor, and blanching followed by flushing. These episodes may occur spontaneously or after provocation by stimuli such as exercise or meals. Extraadrenal tumors have a greater tendency to metastasize than do adrenal tumors. Metastasis to bones, lymph nodes, and the liver can cause local symptoms and signs. Physical examination may show only hypertension. In some instances, abdominal palpation triggers more severe hypertension. Intravascular volume constriction may cause postural hypertension. Among patients with familial syndromes, the other manifestations of those syndromes may be apparent.

DIFFERENTIAL DIAGNOSIS

The clinical features of pheochromocytoma overlap those of many other disorders, including essential and secondary hypertension, thyrotoxicosis, anxiety states (including panic attacks), carcinoid syndrome, mastocytosis, paroxysmal tachycardia, vasodilatory headaches, intracranial lesions, atypical diencephalic seizures, and hypoglycemia.

LABORATORY STUDIES AND DIAGNOSTIC TESTS

If possible, laboratory studies should be performed when the patient is in a drug-free state. The diagnosis is made with demonstration of excessive catecholamine secretion. Although the choice of biochemical studies is controversial, 24-hour urine collection for measurement of catecholamines or their metabolites (e.g., metanephrines or vanillylmandelic acid) is the most common study. Measurement of plasma catecholamine levels is an alternative, although only 80% of patients have unequivocal elevations. When results of initial testing are ambiguous, a clonidine suppression test can be performed. In this test patients with pheochromocytoma fail to have normal suppression of serum catecholamines with administration of clonidine. Preoperative tumor location is best accomplished with computed tomography (which is less effective for extraadrenal tumors), magnetic resonance imaging, or scintigraphy with metaiodobenzylguanidine.

MANAGEMENT

The only definitive cure is surgical resection of the tumor. Meticulous preoperative preparation is essential to avoid intraoperative hypertensive crisis. Phenoxybenzamine, a noncompetitive α-adrenergic blocker, is given at an initial dose of 10 mg by mouth twice a day with a dose increase of 10 mg every other day. Prazosin is an alternative. After about 2 weeks, this α-blockade allows reexpansion of the contracted plasma volume. β-Blockade is only occasionally necessary to manage tachycardia or tachyarrhythmia. β-Blockers should not be used before α-blockade is well established, because unopposed α-adrenergic agonism can cause a hypertensive crisis. After surgery, as many as one-third of patients have residual hypertension despite normal catecholamine levels, probably because of damage to the renal blood vessels. All patients need long-term follow-up care because metastasis or second primary tumors may become evident after long periods.

Chapter 408

▆ PITUITARY TUMORS

PATHOGENESIS

Pituitary tumors represent at least 10% to 15% of all intracranial tumors. The tumors are almost always benign and expand slowly over years. The most common functioning tumor is prolactinoma, followed by growth hormone (GH)–secreting adenoma and corticotropin-secreting adenoma. Thyroid-stimulating hormone–secreting and gonadotropin-secreting tumors are rare. About 10% to 20% of the tumors secrete more than one hormone; a roughly equal number appear to be nonfunctioning. Pituitary tumors may occur as part multiple endocrine neoplasia type 1 syndrome. A single-cell somatic mutation rather than hypothalamic stimulation is likely to be the initiating event.

CLINICAL FEATURES

Endocrinologic features: The tumors may cause hypopituitarism, hypersecretion of one or more hormones, or both. Patients with nonfunctioning tumors usually have hypopituitarism. Hypogonadism may reflect destruction of pituitary gonadotropes, but more often is caused by suppression of secretion of gonadotropin-releasing hormone because of an elevation in prolactin level. Among women,

hyperprolactinemia causes oligomenorrhea or amenorrhea, infertility, and galactorrhea. Among men, the symptoms are reduced libido, infertility, and erectile dysfunction. Acromegaly is a chronic disorder caused by hypersecretion of GH and secondary overproduction of insulin-like growth factor I (IGF-I). An increase in shoe, glove, or ring size is typical, as is a gradual coarsening of facial features that leads to a large nose, thick lips, and accentuated nasolabial and frontal furrows. Other symptoms include severe snoring, deepening of the voice, skin tags, arthralgia, manifestations of carpal tunnel syndrome, and increased perspiration. Hypertension, cardiac hypertrophy, insulin resistance, and hyperlipidemia are common. Corticotropin-secreting adenoma is discussed with Cushing's syndrome.

Neurologic features: A dull, generalized headache is the most common feature. Visual field defects occur among patients who have large tumors and suprasellar extension. The classic defect is bitemporal hemianopsia from compression of the optic chiasm, but the defects are variable and often asymmetric. Less common problems include cranial nerve palsy, seizures, and cerebrospinal fluid rhinorrhea. Infarction after tumor hemorrhage (pituitary apoplexy) can manifest dramatically with the acute onset of severe headache and meningism, vomiting, and progressive loss of consciousness.

DIFFERENTIAL DIAGNOSIS AND DIAGNOSTIC EVALUATION

Laboratory findings: Basal levels of pituitary hormones should be obtained. Serum prolactin levels greater than 200 ng per milliliter virtually confirm the diagnosis of prolactinoma. The differential diagnosis for lesser elevations includes prolactinoma, severe primary hypothyroidism, hypothalamic or stalk disorders, renal failure, and use of medications that interfere with the synthesis or secretion of dopamine (such as phenothiazines or methyldopa). The diagnosis of acromegaly can be confirmed with the presence of an elevated IGF-I level and failure of plasma GH to be suppressed by an oral glucose load.

Radiologic findings: Plain radiographs of the skull can help identify an enlarged sella, but computed tomography or magnetic resonance imaging is needed to demonstrate intrasellar lesions and to define the extent of suprasellar extension. Failure of a target gland (thyroid, adrenal glands, or gonads) occasionally causes loss of negative feedback and leads to hyperplasia of the corresponding pituitary cells, a situation that can mimic a true pituitary tumor.

MANAGEMENT

Treatment is aimed at reducing any hormonal oversecretion, preventing loss of pituitary function, and halting progression of tumor growth. Medical therapy for prolactinoma with a dopamine agonist such as bromocriptine often is successful, as is therapy with bromocriptine or octreotide in some cases of acromegaly. In most other situations, medical therapy is ineffective and treatment consists of pituitary surgery (usually by the transsphenoidal route) or radiation therapy. In general, good results are obtained for microadenoma, but it is rarely possible to cure large tumors with surgery. Pituitary apoplexy is managed with intravenous fluids and hydrocortisone; urgent surgical decompression may be necessary.

Chapter 403

▆ PRIMARY ALDOSTERONISM

DEFINITION, EPIDEMIOLOGY, AND ETIOLOGY

Primary aldosteronism (Conn's syndrome) is caused by renin-independent inappropriate hypersecretion of aldosterone. It is present in at least 1% to 3% of patients with hypertension. Approximately 60% of patients have a single, benign adrenal adenoma; the others have bilateral adrenal cortical hyperplasia.

PATHOGENESIS

Excessive production of aldosterone increases renal potassium excretion and sodium retention. The consequent volume expansion suppresses plasma renin and decreases generation of angiotensin II.

CLINICAL FEATURES

The principal clinical findings are hypertension and hypokalemia. The hypertension is moderate to severe and may be complicated by stroke or proteinuria. The manifestations of hypokalemia include muscular weakness and tetany, polyuria from nephrogenic diabetes insipidus, and impaired glucose tolerance.

LABORATORY STUDIES AND DIAGNOSTIC TESTS

Laboratory testing reveals hypernatremia, hypokalemia, and metabolic alkalosis. Patients have elevated urine and plasma aldosterone levels and suppressed plasma renin levels. The high ratio of aldosterone to renin (greater than 50) confirms the diagnosis of primary aldosteronism. For patients with equivocal results, one may test for the absence of aldosterone suppression by saline infusion or for an inability to stimulate renin production with captopril. Adenoma can be differentiated from hyperplasia by means of assessment of the response of aldosterone to changes in posture. Patients with adenoma have a decrease in aldosterone level with standing; those with hyperplasia have an increase. Adenoma can be localized with computed tomography or magnetic resonance imaging of the adrenal glands, adrenal scintigraphy, or selective adrenal venous catheterization and sampling.

MANAGEMENT

Patients with a single adenoma should undergo laparoscopic unilateral adrenalectomy. Hypertension is cured in 50% to 70% of cases, the electrolyte abnormalities invariably. Patients with bilateral adrenal hyperplasia do not benefit from bilateral adrenalectomy. Although hypertension improves, most patients continue to be hypertensive. Treatment with high doses of spironolactone, an aldosterone antagonist, is effective.

Chapter 407

▋ APPROACH TO THE PATIENT WITH A THYROID NODULE

DEFINITIONS, EPIDEMIOLOGY, AND ETIOLOGY

Thyroid nodules are discrete swellings within the thyroid gland that are present in about 5% of the adult population. They are more common among women and older persons. Nodules are considered solitary if they are found within a gland that is otherwise normal to palpation. Adenomatous colloid nodules are the most common. These hyperplastic lesions are histologic features of multinodular goiter, which can manifest as a large dominant nodule in an apparently normal gland. Follicular adenoma is a benign neoplasm that is somewhat less common than colloid nodules. Thyroid cancer represents fewer than 10% of all clinically apparent nodules. Papillary carcinoma is the most common type (75%), followed by follicular (15%), medullary, and anaplastic carcinoma. Persons with a history of radiation exposure are at increased risk of papillary thyroid carcinomas; those with a family history of medullary thyroid carcinoma or multiple endocrine neoplasia type 2 are at substantial risk for that cancer. Lymphocytic or subacute thyroiditis occasionally manifests as regional or nodular thyroid enlargement. Additional causes include thyroid lymphoma, thyroid metastasis, abscess, and infiltrative or granulomatous disease.

PRESENTATION

Thyroid nodules usually are asymptomatic and discovered as a visible or palpable neck mass by the physician or patient. A few patients report dysphagia or hoarseness. Pain is infrequent and suggests subacute thyroiditis or spontaneous bleeding into a preexisting nodule. Physical characteristics of the nodule are not usually helpful in differentiating benign from malignant lesions, although the presence of a hard nodule, fixation to adjacent structures, vocal cord paralysis, and regional lymphadenopathy all substantially increase the likelihood of malignancy. A solitary nodule discovered during radiologic imaging of the neck should be evaluated if it exceeds 1 cm in diameter.

DIAGNOSTIC EVALUATION

Thyroid function should be assessed routinely. Measurement of thyroid-stimulating hormone usually is sufficient. If there is a strong suspicion of hypothyroidism or hyperthyroidism, free thyronine and triiodothyronine also should be measured.

Abnormal thyroid function: In a patient with hypothyroidism, a nodule likely represents regional thyromegaly associated with Hashimoto's (lymphocytic) thyroiditis. Measurement of thyroid autoantibodies is helpful in such cases. Patients with hyperthyroidism should undergo radionuclide scanning. A hyperfunctioning, or hot, nodule generally is a benign, autonomously functioning nodule. The presence of a hypofunctioning, or cold, nodule within a gland that otherwise has diffusely increased uptake necessitates fine-needle aspiration (FNA) because it may represent a malignant tumor associated with Graves' disease.

Normal thyroid function: Most patients have normal thyroid function. In these cases, FNA is the initial procedure of choice. Cytologic evaluation of the aspirate can indicate whether the nodule is benign (features consistent with colloid nodules, thyroiditis, or benign cysts), suspicious (hypercellular follicular lesions or Hürthle cell changes), or malignant. The designation of an aspirate as *suspicious* stems from the inability to differentiate benign follicular and Hürthle cell adenomas from their carcinomatous counterparts on the basis of cytologic appearance. If FNA does not provide a specimen adequate for a diagnosis, the procedure must be repeated. Although it is not recommended in the initial evaluation of a thyroid nodule, ultrasonography can be useful in guiding FNA when conventional techniques have not provided a specimen sufficient for diagnosis. Patients with multiple nodules larger than 1 cm in diameter should be treated with near-total thyroidectomy without FNA.

MANAGEMENT

About 65% of patients have a benign aspirate. These patients are best treated expectantly by means of assessment of the nodule over time with or without ultrasonography. Nodules that show considerable growth should be aspirated again. Suppressive therapy with thyroid hormone usually is not indicated for benign nodules. Patients with suspicious or indeterminate aspirates should be referred for surgery, because the possibility of malignancy cannot be excluded. Patients with malignant aspirates are treated surgically, usually with total or near-total thyroidectomy.

Chapter 392

NEUROLOGY

▋ ALZHEIMER'S DISEASE

DEFINITION

Dementia is a progressive decline in intellectual function and clear consciousness. Alzheimer's disease (AD), the most common cause, is a heterogeneous neurodegenerative illness that produces progressive memory loss, changes in behavior and personality, psychotic symptoms, and impairments in insight, judgment, and executive abilities.

DIFFERENTIAL DIAGNOSIS

Late-life dementia can be caused by conditions other than AD, including ischemic vascular dementia, Parkinson dementia, Pick's disease, frontotemporal dementia, and dementia with Lewy bodies.

EPIDEMIOLOGY, ETIOLOGY, AND PATHOPHYSIOLOGY

The prevalence of AD is about 3% among persons between 65 and 74 years of age. This figure climbs to 47% among persons older than 85 years. The pathologic features of AD are extensive neuron loss, numerous amyloid plaques, and abundant neurofibrillary tangles in vulnerable regions of the brain. Risk factors include age, the presence of an ApoE ε4 allele, female sex, a history of head trauma, and having a first-degree relative with AD-like dementia. A small number of patients have an autosomal dominant form of AD.

CLINICAL FEATURES AND DIAGNOSIS

AD is characterized by the insidious onset of memory failure. Symptoms most commonly begin between the ages of 70 and 85 years but can occur as early as 40 years of age and as late as 90 years. During the first several years, patients may have difficulty with problem solving and word finding. They often have subtle personality and behavioral changes. As they withdraw from social situations, they may have symptoms that mimic mild depression. Although they may be aware that their memory is failing, persons with AD usually do not appreciate the extent of the problem. It is almost always a family member who brings the patient to medical attention.

A key diagnostic feature is documentation of memory loss as the earliest manifestation of the illness. Elements that strengthen the diagnosis include a family history of similar late-life dementia, normal results of routine blood studies (including those for thyroid disease and vitamin B_{12} deficiency), the presence of one or more ApoE ε4 alleles, an elevated cerebrospinal fluid τ level, and magnetic resonance images that is either normal for age or shows mild generalized cortical atrophy. Findings that cast doubt on the diagnosis include the following: parkinsonism (slow gait, decreased arm swing, en bloc turning), early prominence of language impairment or confusion, symptoms or signs of frontal lobe involvement (disinhibition, perseveration, delusions, or hallucinations) within the first several years, the finding of any focal neurologic signs at examination, and seizures or myoclonus early in the course.

Diagnostic criteria are used to place patients into one of three categories—definite AD, probable AD, and possible AD. A diagnosis of probable AD requires (a) dementia with onset between 40 and 90 years of age, (b) cognitive deficits in two or more areas, (c) progressive memory and cognitive deterioration, (d) no other illness that could account for the dementia, and (e) no disturbance of consciousness. A definite diagnosis requires neuropathologic examination and the clinical criteria for probable AD.

PROGNOSIS AND MANAGEMENT

AD lasts 6 to 12 years on average. There are several components of treatment. First is education of the primary caregiver about the illness, the need for long-range planning, and how to maintain an appropriate living environment. Donepezil has become the standard symptomatic treatment. Its benefits are modest and do not occur for all patients. High-dose vitamin E (α-tocopherol) has been adopted as the standard disease-slowing treatment. Therapy for the behavioral, psychotic, and mood changes is accomplished through the gentle and short-term use of psychotropic, anti-anxiety, and hypnotic medications.

Chapter 466

■ CEREBROVASCULAR DISEASES

DEFINITIONS

Ischemic cerebrovascular events may be divided into three categories. *Transient ischemic attacks* (TIAs) are ischemic episodes of focal cerebral dysfunction that last less than 24 hours, usually only a few minutes, and are followed by complete recovery. Modern imaging techniques can depict evidence of cerebral infarction in a high percentage of cases. Therefore, TIAs, especially those of long duration, are best considered small strokes with transient signs and symptoms. Stroke in evolution describes signs and symptoms that worsen while the patient is being observed. *Completed stroke* denotes a relatively stable neurologic deficit caused by cerebral infarction. *Lacunar infarctions* are subcortical strokes almost always associated with hypertension.

ETIOLOGY AND PATHOPHYSIOLOGY

Transient ischemic attacks: The cause usually can be limited to one of three broad categories—vascular, cardiologic, or hematologic. The most common mechanism is probably platelet embolization from atherosclerotic extracranial or intracranial cerebral arteries.

Ischemic cerebral infarction: The cause is a reduction in blood flow below the level necessary to maintain tissue viability. Atherosclerotic disease of large arteries is the main cause and can trigger stroke either through occlusion at the site of atherosclerosis (thrombotic stroke) or through embolization to the cerebral vasculature (embolic stroke). Hypertension is the most important risk factor. Others include diabetes mellitus, hyperlipidemia, smoking, family history of vascular disease, and use of oral contraceptives. The extent of infarction is determined by the effectiveness of collateral circulation, possible vasospasm, development of brain edema, hemorrhage from damaged arterioles, and systemic factors such as hyperglycemia and hyperviscosity.

Hypertensive vascular syndromes: Lacunar infarction and hypertensive hemorrhage are caused by hypertensive damage to small arteries deep in the brain. If

cases of trauma and ruptured saccular aneurysm or arteriovenous malformation are excluded, the classic type of intracerebral hemorrhage is almost always caused by hypertension.

CLINICAL FEATURES

Transient ischemic attacks: The most common presentation in the carotid artery territory is sudden onset of weakness, paralysis, or clumsiness in one or both extremities on the same side. Sensory symptoms also may be present. If the TIA involves the hemisphere dominant for language function, dysphasia is present. A transient loss of vision in one eye or part of one visual field may occur. In vertebrobasilar TIAs, the most common symptom is a motor defect such as weakness, clumsiness, or paralysis of any combination of extremities with or without sensory changes. The patient may have an unsteady gait, dysequilibrium, and vertigo. Diplopia or loss of vision (varying from complete blindness to partial blindness in homonymous fields) may occur.

The differential diagnosis includes classic migraine with scotoma, hemiplegic migraine, focal convulsive events, Ménière's disease, and peripheral vestibulopathy. Unlike TIAs, migrainous phenomena generally worsen gradually over several minutes. Headache may accompany TIAs but is generally brief and not severe. Focal seizures generally progress from the distal to the proximal portions of an extremity and may produce persistent neurologic deficits. Isolated vertigo without other motor and sensory symptoms rarely can be attributed to a TIA.

Ischemic cerebral infarction:

Middle cerebral artery: Infarction of the cortex supplied by the superior and inferior divisions of the middle cerebral artery causes contralateral hemiplegia (involving the face, hand, and arm, but sparing the leg), hemisensory deficit, homonymous hemianopsia, and if the dominant hemisphere is affected, both expressive and receptive aphasia. Occlusion of the superior division of the middle cerebral artery produces greater weakness and sensory loss in the face and arm than in the leg, with no visual field defect. If the dominant hemisphere is involved, expressive (Broca's) aphasia is present with impaired speaking, naming, and writing ability but relative preservation of comprehension. With occlusion of the inferior division, contralateral sensory loss predominates, and weakness may be minimal or absent. If the dominant hemisphere is involved, receptive (Wernicke's) aphasia is present with impaired comprehension and fluent speech output with jargon and paraphrasia.

Anterior and posterior cerebral arteries: Involvement of the former produces weakness, clumsiness, and sensory loss affecting mainly the contralateral leg and foot. Occlusion of the latter causes contralateral homonymous hemianopsia and may cause transient disturbance of memory due to infarction of the medial temporal lobe.

Basilar artery: Emboli tend to affect the distal portion, whereas atheromatous occlusion affects the proximal and middle portions. Distal vessel effects include loss of consciousness, unilateral or bilateral palsies of the third cranial nerve, and hemiplegia or quadriplegia with decerebrate or decorticate posturing. Consequences of occlusion of the proximal and middle segments include hemiplegia or quadriplegia and unilateral damage to the sixth cranial nerve or nucleus that causes impairment of horizontal eye movement.

Vertebral artery: Unilateral occlusion causes severe vertigo, nausea and vomiting, nystagmus, and loss of pain and temperature sensation in the ipsilateral face. Damage to the inferior cerebellar peduncle causes ipsilateral ataxia and Horner's syndrome and loss of pain and temperature sensation in the contralateral part of the body. Damage to the ninth and tenth cranial nerves causes hiccups and dysphagia.

Cerebellar infarction: Manifestations include difficulty standing and walking, headache, nausea, vomiting, dizziness, clumsiness, and slurred speech. With progression, most patients have lateral gaze palsy, nystagmus toward the side of the lesion, facial palsy, impaired cognitive function, or depressed consciousness.

Hypertensive vascular syndromes: Lacunar infarctions are the most common cerebrovascular lesions and occur most frequently in the deep nuclei of the brain, the pons, and the posterior limb of the internal capsule. Many are not recognized clinically. The onset usually is gradual, developing over several hours or days. Headache and alterations in consciousness are absent. The four major syndromes are (a) pure motor hemiparesis, with weakness of the face, arm, and leg but no associated sensory, visual or cortical deficits; (b) pure sensory stroke of the face, arm, and leg; (c) homolateral ataxia and crural (distal leg) paresis characterized by weakness of one leg, especially the toes and ankle, with Babinski's sign and striking incoordination of the ipsilateral arm and leg; and (d) lacunar state, a syndrome in which lability of affect, dementia, small-stepped rigid gait, dysarthria, incontinence, and bilateral long-tract signs are present.

Hypertensive hemorrhage most often occurs among persons older than 50 years. It occurs without warning while the patient is awake and often during exertion. Headache may be severe but is absent or trivial in one-half of cases. Vomiting is common; in thrombotic or embolic strokes it is rare. Blood pressure almost always remains elevated after onset. Once hemorrhage has occurred, the patient's condition worsens steadily over a period of minutes to days until the neurologic deficit stabilizes or the patient dies. Because much of the deficit is caused by compression rather than destruction, return of function as swelling subsides can be dramatic. Pontine hemorrhage produces coma, pinpoint pupils, impaired horizontal eye movements, quadriparesis, and hyperthermia. Deep cerebral hemorrhage occurs most commonly in the putamen and thalamus. The motor deficit is more severe in the former and the sensory defect more prominent in the latter. Either may be associated with aphasia if there is pressure on cortical speech areas. Cerebellar hemorrhage is sudden without loss of consciousness. Within several minutes, the patient cannot stand or walk and must vomit repeatedly. Headache and dizziness occur in about 50% of cases. Almost 90% of patients become comatose within 24 hours.

ANCILLARY STUDIES AND DIAGNOSTIC TESTS

Transient ischemic attacks: The evaluation is directed at detection of vascular disease. Risk factor assessment should be performed (see earlier). Abnormalities in the vascular system can be detected noninvasively with Doppler ultrasonography or magnetic resonance angiography, although cerebral angiography remains the most definitive test. Transesophageal echocardiography can help identify intracardiac thrombus or lesions such as patent foramen ovale. Testing for hypercoagulable states (such as factor V Leiden and deficiencies of protein C, protein S, and antithrombin III) may be indicated.

Ischemic cerebral infarction: The evaluation is similar to that described earlier. Computed tomography (CT) or magnetic resonance imaging (MRI) of the brain should be performed as soon as possible to rule out cerebral hemorrhage and tumor. In many instances, the CT findings are normal even when the patient has a severe clinical deficit. For these patients, immediate MRI or additional CT performed within 24 to 48 hours will reveal the area of infarction. Cerebral arteriography is not needed unless vasculitis or a cerebral aneurysm is suspected. Ultrasound evaluation of the cervical and intracranial vessels may be used to define the site of occlusion. In patients without evidence of atherosclerotic disease of the cervical carotid arteries, a thorough search should be made for a cardiac source of emboli.

Hypertensive vascular syndromes: Associated hypertension is present. The diagnosis is made clinically and with imaging studies.

MANAGEMENT

Transient ischemic attacks: Risk factor modification is mandatory. Studies of heparin or warfarin therapy have demonstrated little benefit except among patients with a hypercoagulable state or TIAs due to cardiac-origin emboli. Antiplatelet drugs such as aspirin (one to four 325-mg tablets daily) have been shown to reduce the incidence of TIAs and stroke. Clopidigrel or ticlopidine, antiplatelet agents more potent than aspirin, can be used to treat patients with recurrent TIAs taking aspirin who are not candidates for surgery. Carotid endarterectomy is the treatment of choice of patients with TIAs in the carotid distribution who have ipsilateral high-grade stenosis (greater than 60%) without complete occlusion.

Ischemic cerebral infarction: All patients with acute ischemic stroke who are seen within 3 hours of the time of symptom onset and have no evidence of hemorrhage on CT should be evaluated for treatment with tissue plasminogen activator, a thrombolytic agent. In a recent trial, thrombolytic therapy under these circumstances produced a 12% increase in the number of patients with a good clinical outcome 3 months after the stroke but also resulted in a 6% incidence of cerebral hemorrhage, almost one-half of them fatal. Anticoagulation with heparin may be used to treat patients with acute ischemic cardioembolic strokes. Its use to manage ischemic strokes is controversial owing to the increased risk of intracranial hemorrhage. The mainstay of treatment is good nursing care to prevent pneumonia and deep venous thrombosis in paralyzed or paretic limbs. Medical care is focused on the judicious management of hypertension, arrhythmias, and cardiac failure. Seizures, if present, should be controlled to prevent further cerebral damage.

There is extreme variation in outcome from stroke. The overall mortality rate is about 25% in the first month and approaches 50% at 5 years. Neurologic complications account for most deaths in the first week; later deaths usually are caused by heart disease and intercurrent infection. Most patients show some improvement after 14 to 21 days when the cerebral edema of infarction has resolved. In general, 50% of the potential recovery is attained 1 month from onset, 75% at 3 months, 90% at 6 months, and 100% at 1 year. Rehabilitation should begin early (days after onset).

Hypertensive vascular syndromes: Lacunar stroke syndromes are self-limited and relatively benign. Anticoagulation is not needed and may actually be dangerous because lacunar infarction often is associated with microhemorrhages. The prognosis for almost complete recovery is good; the likelihood of future lacunar strokes is reduced with adequate control of blood pressure. Cerebellar hematoma is managed by means of early surgical decompression, which may be life saving and often leads to complete reversal of the neurologic deficits. Surgery is not indicated for pontine or deep cerebral hypertensive hemorrhage, unless a large superficial hemorrhage has caused midline shift and herniation. There is no effective medical treatment. Glucocorticoids and dehydrating agents have given only temporary benefit. Attempts to lower blood pressure may compromise cerebral blood flow, but continued hypertension may cause cerebral edema. It seems reasonable to lower blood pressure carefully to normal levels with initial small doses of the less potent antihypertensive agents.

Chapter 432

■ DEPRESSION

DEFINITION
Depression is an affective syndrome occurring in unipolar or bipolar forms.

EPIDEMIOLOGY
The incidence of depression is 1% among men and 3% among women. The age at first episode of major depression has steadily decreased, with the mean age now 40 years for both sexes. Concomitant psychiatric conditions are common, including anxiety disorders and alcohol and substance abuse.

ETIOLOGY AND PATHOPHYSIOLOGY
Depression is two to three times more frequent among first-degree relatives of patients with depression. No cause of the disorder is known. Theories include (a) excessive activity of the hypothalamic-pituitary-adrenal axis; (b) disturbed functioning of catecholamines; (c) sleep and circadian rhythm disruptions; and (d) left frontal hypometabolism.

CLINICAL FEATURES AND DIAGNOSIS
Major depression is characterized by at least 2 weeks of a sad mood or loss of interest. The patient also must have four of the following symptoms (remembered with the mnemonic *SIG E CAPS*): *s*leep disturbance (usually early morning awakening); loss of *i*nterest; *g*uilt or worthlessness; *e*nergy loss; impairment of *c*oncentration; change in *a*ppetite, usually a decrease; *p*sychomotor agitation or retardation; *s*uicidal or death wishes. Depressed patients may report irritability, deny sadness, or have vague somatic symptoms. No laboratory tests exist to confirm the diagnosis.

Major depression can be subcategorized as (a) atypical with hypersomnia, appetite increase, and hypersensitivity to rejection; (b) with psychosis (presence of auditory hallucinations and delusions); (c) postpartum, occurring within 4 weeks of delivery; and (d) pseudodementia (abrupt cognitive decline associated with depressive symptoms, primarily among the elderly). Dysthymic disorder is similar to major depression but the symptoms are less severe and are intermittently present for 2 or more years. In adjustment disorder, symptoms of depression or anxiety develop after exposure to an identifiable precipitating stressor. These symptoms typically disappear when the stressor is gone. Seasonal affective disorder is characterized by development of depressive symptoms (often the atypical symptoms described earlier) in fall or winter and a return to baseline in spring and summer. Bipolar disorder is characterized by one or more manic episodes, which consist of an elevated, expansive, or irritable mood and three or four of the following: grandiosity, decreases in sleep, excessive talking, racing thoughts, distractibility, and excessive involvement in pleasurable activities that have high potential for negative consequences, such as spending sprees.

PROGNOSIS AND MANAGEMENT
Suicide risk must be assessed for each patient. As many as 15% of depressed patients die by suicide. Women are three to four times more likely to make an attempt, but men are three times more likely to be successful. Suicide risk factors

include psychosis, absence of social support, chronic medical illness, substance abuse, particularly of alcohol, and an organized plan with little chance of rescue.

Various antidepressants are equally effective, response rates averaging 70%. Patients must be informed that antidepressants are not immediately effective and must be taken daily for at least 2 to 3 weeks before symptoms improve. Drug selection is based on side effect profile and potential drug-drug interactions. Selective serotonin reuptake inhibitors are currently the best initial choice for most patients. The starting dose for fluoxetine or paroxetine is 20 mg per day (maximum 40 mg per day) and for sertraline is 50 mg per day (maximum 200 mg per day).

For patients who have not responded to maximum dosages after 4 to 6 weeks, treatment alternatives include a change to a different agent (e.g., a tricyclic agent such as desipramine or nortriptyline or an agent such as bupropion or venlafaxine), augmentation with lithium or thyroid hormone, consultation with a psychiatrist, or electroconvulsive therapy (ECT). ECT is the most effective therapy for major depression. Once a patient's symptoms have responded, antidepressants should be continued for 4 to 9 months at the same dose. Maintenance treatment for several years or longer is indicated for patients with age at onset younger than 20 years and a family history of bipolar disease, two previous severe episodes with early recurrence, or three or more previous episodes. Patients with bipolar disease can be treated with lithium, sodium valproate, and carbamazepine. Monotherapy with antidepressants may cause a conversion to mania.

Chapter 39

■ APPROACH TO THE PATIENT WITH DIZZINESS AND VERTIGO

PRESENTATION AND PATHOPHYSIOLOGY
"Dizziness" encompasses a variety of symptoms. A feeling of light-headedness or impending fainting may suggest hypotension and a cardiovascular cause. Vertigo is an illusion of motion of self or of the environment. Patients may describe sensations of spinning or tumbling. Vertigo is caused by an acute imbalance in the vestibular inputs from the two labyrinths or in their central connections. Patients with symmetric vestibular lesions (e.g., aminoglycoside toxicity) and those with a slowly developing unilateral lesion (e.g., schwannoma) may not have vertigo. Dysequilibrium is a feeling of imbalance while standing or walking. It may occur among patients with sensory deficits (e.g., blurred vision or bilateral vestibular loss), cerebellar disease, or efferent motor disorders such as Parkinson's disease or stroke. Dizziness that cannot be further characterized often accompanies anxiety, phobias, and panic attacks.

HISTORY AND PHYSICAL EXAMINATION OF A PATIENT WITH THE VERTIGO
The first issue is whether symptoms are acute or chronic and whether they have occurred more than once. If vertigo is episodic, the duration of episodes is important. Brief (less than 1 minute) episodes of vertigo precipitated by a change in the attitude of the head with respect to gravity are typical of benign paroxysmal positional vertigo (BPPV). Vertigo lasting for several minutes up to an hour suggests transient ischemic attacks (TIAs). Longer episodes can be caused by migraine, Ménière's disease, labyrinthitis, or central nervous system infarction. Associated hearing loss, tinnitus, or ear fullness suggests a peripheral vestibular cause, whereas symptoms of brain stem or cerebellar dysfunction implicate a central cause. In general, symptoms provoked by head movements or changes in head position with respect to gravity are the hallmark of a disturbance in the peripheral vestibular system.

A complete neurologic examination must be performed with particular attention to eye movements (nystagmus), hearing, other cranial nerves, coordination, gait, and balance. The eyes must be examined in the absence of visual fixation, which may suppress spontaneous nystagmus. This may be done either with Frenzel lenses or by looking for movement of the optic disc during direct ophthalmoscopy with the opposite eye occluded. Positioning maneuvers may help identify BPPV.

DIAGNOSTIC TESTS
Every patient with vestibular symptoms should undergo an audiogram. Low-frequency hearing loss is characteristic of Ménière's disease. Unilateral hearing loss raises the possibility of a tumor involving the vestibulocochlear nerve, such as vestibular schwannoma. Magnetic resonance imaging of the posterior fossa should be ordered whenever symptoms or signs suggest a brain stem or cerebellar

lesion. Patients believed to have TIAs should undergo magnetic resonance angiography of the head and neck and additional evaluation for stroke as indicated. Specific vestibular tests, including electronystagmography with caloric or rotatory chair testing and posturography, are helpful to a minority of patients.

SELECTED DISORDERS
BPPV is the most common cause of recurrent vertigo. It occurs when calcium carbonate crystals are released from the otolithic membranes and aggregate in a semicircular canal (usually the posterior canal). Many patients can identify a preceding event, such as an episode of labyrinthitis, trauma, or a prolonged period of having the head back. Symptoms are produced when a change in head position, such as looking up or rolling over in bed, causes the debris to move. The resultant shift of endolymph produces vertigo. Symptoms are usually worse in the morning. BPPV is diagnosed with the Dix-Hallpike maneuver. With the head turned 45 degrees to one side, the patient is moved rapidly from a seated to a supine position with the head hanging down. After a latency of several seconds, the patient experiences vertigo and nystagmus; the upper poles of the eyes beat toward the affected (down) ear. Fatiguing of nystagmus occurs with repeated maneuvers. BPPV is managed with a particle repositioning maneuver.

Vestibular migraine is a common cause of recurrent vertigo. Treatment consists of the usual migraine prophylactic agents. Ménière's disease is attributed to endolymphatic hydrops, which increases pressure in the inner ear. Attacks may be difficult to differentiate from vestibular migraine, but characteristic additional features include aural fullness, fluctuating hearing loss in the affected ear, and a low-pitched tinnitus. Evaluation should include screening for syphilis and autoimmune disorders. Treatment is aimed at reducing hydrops and includes a low sodium diet and diuretics. Vestibular suppressants may be helpful during an attack. Refractory cases can be managed with surgical labyrinthectomy.

Labyrinthitis and vestibular neuritis often are attributed to viral infection of the vestibular nerve or labyrinth. Severe vertigo, nausea, and vomiting appear suddenly and improve over several days. Central compensatory mechanisms produce further improvement over several weeks to months. Important differential diagnoses are labyrinthine and cerebellar infarction or hemorrhage. Treatment includes vestibular suppressants and antiemetics.

MANAGEMENT
In general, treatment is directed at the specific diagnosis, described earlier. Vestibular suppressant and antiemetic medications, such as diazepam, lorazepam, promethazine, and meclizine, can be useful in the initial phase of an acute vestibular syndrome (e.g., labyrinthitis) and in the management of recurrent attacks of vertigo that last at least several hours. Brief episodes of vertigo, such as those that occur with BPPV, are not amenable to such treatment. Chronic prophylactic vestibular suppression may be appropriate when attacks are frequent; however, prolonged use after an acute vestibular lesion may impede central adaptation and should be avoided. Vestibular rehabilitation may be beneficial in the management of both acute and chronic vestibular disorders.

Chapter 422

■ APPROACH TO THE PATIENT WITH HEADACHE

PATHOPHYSIOLOGY
Receptors responsible for pain registration are present in the proximal parts of the cerebral and dural arteries, the large veins and venous sinuses, and the extracranial arteries. Distention or displacement of these vessels by inflammation, an aneurysm, a hematoma, a tumor, or ventricular dilatation from obstruction of cerebrospinal pathways causes headache. Migraine and cluster headaches are accompanied by vascular dilatation that contributes to the headache. Pain also may be caused by irritation of the meninges, cranial nerves, or occipital nerves. Some forms of tension headache are associated with overcontraction of muscles.

DIFFERENTIAL DIAGNOSIS
See also History and Physical Examination.

Migraine: Migraine is an episodic cerebral disturbance (aura), headache, or both with intervening periods of relative freedom from headache and without evidence of primary structural abnormality. The headache is usually severe, unilateral, and associated with nausea, vomiting, and photophobia. About one-third of patients have some attacks in which an aura (visual changes, paresthesia, or speech disturbance) precedes the headache by 5 to 60 minutes. Migraine is common (20% of women of reproductive age), and women are affected twice as often as men. Many patients can identify triggers such as noise, perfume, stress, relaxation after stress, particular foods, ingestion of alcohol or other vasodilators, physical exertion, or menses.

Cluster headache: Cluster headache has a prevalence about 3% of that of migraine and tends to recur in bouts or clusters that last weeks or months and are separated by months or years of freedom. During a bout, patients (85% of whom are men) each day or night have one or more attacks of severe pain in and around the eye or adjacent areas of the head and face; these attacks last from 10 minutes to hours at a time. The ipsilateral eye usually becomes red and waters; there is ipsilateral nasal congestion or rhinorrhea. Ocular Horner's syndrome may be present.

Tension headache: This term is applied to the sensation of tightness around the head or pressure at the top of the head that may recur daily in its chronic form. It affects women more commonly than men and may start at any age.

Pain arising from extracranial structures: Temporal arteritis occurs among women more than men and primarily affects persons older than 50 years. It is an immune disorder of the arterial wall associated with a giant cell arteritis. The scalp arteries are most commonly involved but involvement of the ophthalmic arteries may produce sudden blindness. There is an association with polymyalgia rheumatica. The diagnosis is supported when the erythrocyte sedimentation rate (ESR) is greater than 40 mm per hour. Results of temporal artery biopsy confirm the diagnosis; treatment with glucocorticoids should be started before the biopsy if suspicion is high, in order to minimize the risk of blindness. Other extracranial disorders include acute angle-closure glaucoma, sinusitis, dental infection, temporomandibular joint syndrome, occipital neuralgia, and disorders of the cervical spine affecting the C2 and C3 nerve roots.

Pain arising from the cranial nerves: Headache can be caused by excessive stimulation of peripheral branches of the first division of the trigeminal nerve by exposure to cold air, food, or drinks. Herpes zoster or trigeminal neuralgia also cause pain in the distribution of the trigeminal nerve, commonly the first division.

Pain of intracranial origin: Headache is a symptom of many intracranial and systemic disorders and can be caused by meningeal irritation or displacement or dilatation of pain-sensitive blood vessels. Investigation determines whether the patient needs neurosurgical or medical management. Benign intracranial hypertension (pseudotumor cerebri) is chiefly a disorder of overweight young women with menstrual abnormalities. They have symptoms and signs of raised intracranial pressure (headache, vomiting, transient obscuring of vision, and papilledema) with no obvious systemic or local cause. Computed tomography demonstrates small ventricles, and results of lumbar puncture confirm the elevation in cerebrospinal fluid (CSF) pressure.

HISTORY AND PHYSICAL EXAMINATION

Acute headache may be accompanied by neck rigidity when there is meningeal irritation and by elevated temperature when there is systemic infection or meningitis. Aggravation of the headache by jarring, coughing, sneezing, or bending forward suggests an intracranial origin. Drowsiness, changes in mental status, seizures, or any neurologic deficits also increase the likelihood of intracranial abnormality.

The temporal pattern of headaches is of great importance. Sudden onset of pain raises the possibility of a life-threatening condition such as subarachnoid hemorrhage or meningitis. Headache increasing in severity over a period of days, weeks, or months also arouses suspicion of a serious organic disturbance. Recurrent episodic headaches include migraines, cluster headaches, paroxysmal hypertension (pheochromocytoma), post-alcohol hangover, and benign recurrent syndromes (benign only if an intracranial lesion has been excluded) such as headaches associated with coughing, exertion, or orgasm. Causes of chronic continuous headache include tension headache, posttraumatic headache, postherpetic neuralgia, atypical facial pain, and psychogenic headache.

Careful examination of the nervous system and other systems is mandatory. The examiner needs to look for localizing neurologic signs and indications of systemic illness. The examination findings are normal if the patient has migraine, cluster, or tension headaches.

LABORATORY STUDIES AND DIAGNOSTIC TESTS

Only a few patients need more than a careful history and physical examination. A complete blood cell count and ESR should be obtained when systemic infection is suggested or when the headache is of recent onset in a patient older than 50 years. Sudden onset of a headache or a progressive course warrants investigation. If a patient with acute headache has a fever and meningitis is suspected, immediate lumbar puncture may be justified, provided there are no signs of high intracranial pressure. Except for such an emergency, computed tomography (CT) of the brain usually is the first step because it demonstrates hemorrhage and structural causes of headache. Lumbar puncture rarely is necessary. It is used chiefly in the diagnosis of meningitis, for confirmation of subarachnoid hemorrhage if the story is typical but the CT findings are normal, and for measurement of CSF pressure in benign intracranial hypertension. Cerebral angiography and magnetic resonance angiography are reserved for patients with cerebrovascular problems such as cerebral aneurysm.

MANAGEMENT

Migraine: The management of migraine is outlined in Figure 421.2. The treatment has been transformed by the triptans (5-HT$_{1B/D}$ agonists), of which sumatriptan was the first. These agents relieve 50% to 60% of migraine headaches within 2 hours; subcutaneous, oral, and intranasal preparations are available. Because of a vasoconstrictive action, these drugs should not be prescribed for patients with suspected coronary artery disease, Prinzmetal's angina, or uncontrolled hypertension. For the same reason, they should not be administered for 24 hours after ergotamine tartrate.

Cluster headaches: Most episodes can be suppressed with ergotamine preparations. Inhalation of 100% oxygen at 7 L per minute relieves cluster pain within 10 minutes for most patients. Sumatriptan also is effective. Prednisone (40 to 50 mg per day) interrupts the cluster pattern in most cases. The dose can then be lowered progressively to the minimum necessary to control attacks for the rest of the bout. Lithium and verapamil also can provide control of cluster headache.

Tension headache: Management requires psychological counseling, readjustment of physical or emotional stress situations, and muscle relaxation therapy. Amitriptyline and other tricyclic agents are useful.

Headache syndromes with an identifiable cause: Many of the causes of headaches have specific treatments. For example, meningitis responds to intravenous antibiotics, temporal arteritis to prednisone, and benign intracranial hypertension to repeated CSF removal and acetazolamide. Tumors and aneurysms require neurosurgical approaches.

COMPLICATIONS AND PITFALLS

Misinterpretation of the acute or progressive subacute onset of headaches can have serious consequences. The abrupt onset of pain can be migrainous in origin, but it is important to exclude subarachnoid hemorrhage, sentinel headache (enlargement of a cerebral aneurysm without rupture), meningitis, acute obstruction of CSF pathways, or a precipitous increase in blood pressure. Intravenous antibiotics should be given immediately if meningitis is suspected. CT of the brain discloses most cases of subarachnoid hemorrhage. Reassurance that there is no shift of midline structures or other contraindications to lumbar puncture enables safe acquisition of CSF. Temporal arteritis may be overlooked in evaluations of older patients. The ESR is not always elevated, and temporal artery biopsy may be warranted if there is localized scalp tenderness. As with meningitis, specific therapy (glucocorticoids) must be instituted when suspicion is high, even before the definitive diagnostic test is performed.

Chapter 421

APPROACH TO THE PATIENT WITH IMPAIRMENT OF CONSCIOUSNESS

DEFINITIONS

Level of consciousness is defined by both arousal and conscious behavior. Changes in the level of consciousness depend on the activities of a brain stem regulatory system called the *reticular activating system* (RAS). Coma is a pathologic state in which neither arousal nor awareness is present. Stupor resembles coma except that the patient can be aroused if strong external stimulation is provided. In some cases, both cerebral hemispheres are severely damaged, but the brain stem RAS is preserved. In such cases, after a coma, wakefulness returns without evidence of purposeful behaviors or cognition. This is called the *vegetative state.*

PATHOPHYSIOLOGY AND DIFFERENTIAL DIAGNOSIS

All types of coma may be divided into three categories—supratentorial lesions, infratentorial lesions, and metabolic encephalopathy. Mass lesions of the cerebral hemispheres (e.g., deep midline tumor, large edematous hemisphere infarct, subdural hematoma, or an expanding mass in one hemisphere) cause coma by herniating beyond the confines of the supratentorial compartment and compressing the brain stem RAS. Two types of posterior fossa (infratentorial) lesions produce coma—lesions intrinsic to the brain stem that destroy the RAS (e.g., pontine hemorrhage or infarction) and lesions extrinsic to the brain stem that compress and distort it (e.g., cerebellar tumor and hematoma). Unconsciousness also follows direct blows to the RAS, as occurs with cerebral concussion. *Metabolic encephalopathy* refers to changes in levels of consciousness caused by diffuse failure of cerebral metabolism. Examples include anoxia, hypoglycemia, hyperglycemia, severe electrolyte disturbances, uremia, hepatic failure, meningitis, and drug intoxication.

NEUROLOGIC EXAMINATION AND DIAGNOSIS

The key to clinical diagnosis when the history is in doubt is to identify the initial anatomic distribution of the lesion and how it evolves (Table 424.1). Clinical neurologic signs can be correlated with specific anatomic sites to establish the severity and extent of central nervous system dysfunction (Table 424.3).

LABORATORY STUDIES AND DIAGNOSTIC TESTS

Computed tomography or magnetic resonance imaging (MRI) of the brain is best for identifying structural lesions; MRI has the greatest sensitivity for detection of lesions in the posterior fossa. Metabolic abnormalities can be detected with appropriate laboratory studies.

MANAGEMENT

The initial step in the care of a patient in a coma is stabilization. An adequate airway must be ensured, by intubation if necessary. Blood should be collected for measurement of blood glucose, routine chemical analysis, and toxicology studies. Immediately afterward, 25 to 50 g dextrose should be administered intravenously. Bedside glucose measurements are valuable but should never delay the administration of dextrose. Even in cases of hyperosmolar coma, infusion of one ampule of dextrose is not harmful. Naloxone (0.4 to 0.8 mg) and thiamine (100 mg) should be administered intravenously to all patients whether or not opiate or alcohol abuse is suggested. At this point, arterial blood gases should be analyzed to confirm that oxygenation is adequate. Placement of a nasogastric tube may be indicated to remove and examine the stomach contents, but a cuffed endotracheal tube should be in place first to minimize the risk of aspiration. The presence of fever demands lumbar puncture to exclude meningitis, provided mass lesions have been excluded with radiologic imaging. If the diagnostic evaluation has yielded a specific diagnosis for which the patient can be treated, therapy should be instituted without delay.

The mortality rate among all patients in coma for more than 48 hours is 77%. It must be ascertained whether a patient has brain death and cannot benefit from intensive care. Such patients have no cerebral function and no brain stem reflexes for at least 12 hours and have evidence of a structural cerebral lesion. Any possibility that the patient has drug poisoning, hypothermia, or a severe but reversible metabolic abnormality must be excluded. Within a few hours or days after the onset of coma, many patients show neurologic signs that differentiate with a high degree of accuracy the outcome extremes of death or vegetative state and good recovery.

Chapter 424

■ MULTIPLE SCLEROSIS

DEFINITION

Multiple sclerosis (MS) is an inflammatory, demyelinating disease of the central nervous system (CNS).

ETIOLOGY AND PATHOPHYSIOLOGY

Evidence suggests that MS is precipitated by initial exposure of a genetically susceptible host to a relatively common infectious agent in the mid-teenage

years. This exposure ultimately leads to an autoimmune process that pathologically targets CNS myelin, leading to inflammation and demyelination years after the initial exposure. Axonal loss or cerebral atrophy may occur early in the course of the disease.

EPIDEMIOLOGY AND CLINICAL FEATURES

The onset of MS is most common between 20 and 50 years of age. Women outnumber men about 2:1. The disease is somewhat arbitrarily divided into primary progressive (PP) and relapsing-remitting (R-R) forms. Approximately 15% of patients have the PP form, characterized by gradual accumulation of neurologic deficits without clear-cut exacerbations or remissions. About 75% of cases begin with an R-R course. The patients, at least after the initial attacks, tend to not return completely to their previous baseline status after many of the exacerbations, such that the R-R course is superimposed on a progressively worsening baseline. With time, many of these patients have a more gradually progressive course with few or no subsequent exacerbations.

Any region of CNS white matter can be affected. Involvement of the cerebral white matter may produce hemiparesis, a hemisensory deficit, or a cognitive deficit. Various brain stem syndromes may occur; internuclear ophthalmoplegia is common. Cranial nerve deficits may develop. Optic neuritis is common (the optic nerves are myelinated with CNS rather than peripheral nerve myelin) and may produce scotomata, loss of visual acuity, and color desaturation. Cerebellar involvement causes ataxia or intention tremor. Spinal cord disease may produce a spastic paraparesis or paraplegia with neurogenic bowel and bladder and sexual dysfunction.

DIAGNOSIS

The diagnosis rests on well-described criteria for possible, probable, and definite MS. The hallmark is dissemination in time and space, that is, multiple episodes of dysfunction and multiple areas of involvement within the CNS. Thus it is impossible to make the diagnosis with certainty at the onset of neurologic symptoms. The diagnosis of PP MS is difficult to make. Magnetic resonance imaging is superior to computed tomography in the detection of MS lesions, which typically appear as areas of increased signal intensity on T2-weighted and proton density images. Evoked potential studies can help detect slowing of conduction within demyelinated CNS pathways. Cerebrospinal fluid (CSF) abnormalities are present in 90% of patients. Mild mononuclear cell pleocytosis and modest protein elevation are common. CSF oligoclonal IgG bands are common and imply the production of large amounts of immunoglobulin by a small number of CNS plasma cell clones.

DIFFERENTIAL DIAGNOSIS

Other inflammatory diseases that mimic MS from clinical, radiologic, and CSF standpoints include syphilis, neuroborreliosis, CNS vasculitis, and sarcoidosis. Other entities to be considered include multiple infarcts caused by small-vessel atherosclerosis or hypertensive vascular disease, or hypercoagulable states. Vitamin B_{12} deficiency should be excluded.

MANAGEMENT

Symptomatic treatment is used to ameliorate various physiologic abnormalities, such as constipation (fiber), muscle spasticity (baclofen) and bladder spasticity (anticholinergic agents). Amantadine frequently improves the fatigue that commonly accompanies MS. Treatments aimed at reducing inflammation in the CNS have included glucocorticoids, recombinant interferon-β, and glatiramer acetate. Glucocorticoids speed improvement in acute exacerbations but have no demonstrated effect on long-term prognosis. Progressive forms of MS are more difficult to manage; intravenous cyclophosphamide and oral methotrexate have been advocated by some neurologists but are of uncertain value. Mitoxantrone has been reported to be effective.

Chapter 433

■ PARKINSON'S DISEASE

EPIDEMIOLOGY AND PATHOGENESIS

Parkinson's disease is the second most common degenerative disorder among adults, after Alzheimer's disease. It is estimated that more than 1 million Americans are affected. The pathologic hallmarks are degeneration of the dopaminergic neurons of the substantia nigra and the presence of eosinophilic, cytoplasmic inclusions known as *Lewy bodies*. Current hypotheses implicate varying combinations of genetic susceptibility, exogenous or endogenous toxicity, and aging. Drug-induced parkinsonism can occur with the use of neuroleptics, metoclopramide, methyldopa, and reserpine.

CLINICAL FINDINGS

The *sine qua non* of PD is bradykinesia (slowness of movement) with either a rest tremor or cogwheel rigidity. Most patients have all three, but approximately 30% lack the tremor. The symptoms initially affect one side, but they eventually become bilateral within several years. Additional symptoms and signs encountered early in the course include micrographia; impaired dexterity, especially for rapid repetitive movements such as shampooing hair or brushing teeth; slowness when arising from a deep chair, the toilet, or a car; trouble turning in bed; a soft, monotone voice; diminished facial expression and blink rate; and diminished arm swing while walking. Later manifestations include dysequilibrium with falls and progressive difficulty initiating and maintaining movements. Non-motor manifestations include pain and autonomic problems such as constipation, erectile dysfunction, orthostatic hypotension, urinary bladder instability, and impaired thermoregulation. Depression is extremely common. Most patients do not have dementia, although it may appear in the later stages of the disease.

DIAGNOSIS

Parkinson's disease is a clinical diagnosis. It may be confused with essential tremor and parkinsonian syndromes such as progressive supranuclear palsy, multisystem atrophy, corticobasal degeneration, and Lewy body dementia. Alzheimer's disease and normal aging also are accompanied by parkinsonian features. The three most reliable clinical features that differentiate Parkinson's disease from these related disorders are classic rest tremor, unilateral or asymmetric onset, and sustained improvement with levodopa therapy.

PROGNOSIS AND MANAGEMENT

With therapy, most persons with Parkinson's disease have a normal life expectancy and, with some limitation, a fairly good lifestyle. Almost all current therapies are directed at increasing the levels of dopamine in the striatum.

Medical therapy: A patient with minimal symptoms may need no therapy initially. All patients eventually need treatment with levodopa, but it is usually withheld (see later) until there is marked compromise in the activities of daily living. Until that point, there are the following three options: dopamine agonists (including bromocriptine, pergolide and newer agents such as pramipexole and ropinirole); anticholinergics, such as benztropine, which are particularly effective for tremor; and the antiviral agent, amantadine. Amantadine and the dopamine agonists also are useful later in the course of the illness as adjuncts to levodopa.

When it becomes necessary to begin therapy with levodopa, pills containing 100 mg levodopa and 25 mg carbidopa (to reduce nausea) are dispensed, and the patient starts with one-half or 1 tablet each day. The dose is then gradually escalated according to clinical response. Most patients improve with 300 mg levodopa per day. The usual approach is to keep the dosage at a modest level, between 600 and 1,000 mg per day, with the early introduction of a dopamine agonist. Central nervous system side effects may include acute confusion, hallucinations, and delusions. These can be managed with a reduction of the dosage of antiparkinsonian medications or with atypical antipsychotic agents such as clozapine. After several years of therapy, the effectiveness of levodopa wanes, and symptoms, such as dysequilibrium, falls, akinesia, and dysphagia, develop that do not respond to therapy. Moreover, the initial smooth response to levodopa begins to be punctuated by motor fluctuations that progress from being predictable (before the next dose) to unpredictable (the on-off effect). At this point, management should be overseen by a specialist.

Surgical therapy: Surgical options available for the small percentage of patients with a disabling, refractory tremor include thalamotomy or deep brain stimulation (DBS) of the motor thalamus. For other features of advanced disease, particularly motor fluctuations and dyskinesia, options include disruption or DBS of the internal segment of the globus pallidus or subthalamic nucleus. Implantation of fetal nigral tissue has demonstrated promise but is still considered experimental.

Chapter 434

▪ APPROACH TO DISORDERS OF THE PERIPHERAL NERVOUS SYSTEM

CLASSIFICATION

The two common patterns are a symmetric, usually distal, distribution (polyneuropathy) and an asymmetric or multifocal distribution (mononeuropathy). Polyneuropathy can be divided into distal axonopathy and myelinopathy (demyelinating neuropathy). Mononeuropathy can affect one nerve or can be multifocal (mononeuropathy multiplex).

CLINICAL FEATURES

Polyneuropathy: Negative symptoms (loss of function) predominate, such as weakness and numbness. Positive motor symptoms such as cramps and fasciculations can occur, and positive sensory symptoms such as tingling and pain are frequent. Imbalance is common and reflects a loss of proprioception. Signs found at examination correspond closely to the symptoms and are predominantly distal and symmetric. Weakness is common, and wasting, if present, signifies axonal loss. Sensory loss usually is in a glove-and-stocking distribution. Loss of tendon reflexes is common. Autonomic neuropathy can cause postural hypotension, urinary retention and incontinence, constipation, nocturnal diarrhea, impotence, and sweating abnormalities.

Mononeuropathy: Mononeuropathy generally affects the territory of individual nerves and usually is asymmetric. Symptoms are more abrupt in onset. The symptoms can be sensory alone or combined motor and sensory. Pain often is a feature.

DIFFERENTIAL DIAGNOSIS

Table 446.2 lists some causes of polyneuropathy according to temporal course; Table 446.3 lists causes of polyneuropathy multiplex. Mononeuropathy can be caused by nerve entrapment or compression; common examples include carpal tunnel syndrome (median nerve), meralgia paresthetica (lateral femoral cutaneous nerve), and Bell's palsy (facial nerve).

DIAGNOSIS

A thorough history is essential. The onset and progression vary greatly (Table 446.2). Stepwise progression suggests multiple mononeuropathy. A history of infection, travel, diet, toxic exposure, alcohol, and medications must be sought. Occupational factors can be important. The family history often is critical. The history and examination allow categorization of the nerve disorder. Nerve conduction studies and electromyography (EMG) provide a physiologic nerve "biopsy." The main utility is to determine whether the predominant pathologic process is demyelination or axonal loss. The former is characterized chiefly by slowed conduction velocity and conduction block. The latter is associated with modest slowing of conduction and evidence of denervation (e.g., fibrillation potentials) at needle EMG. Nerve biopsy, usually of the sural nerve, is reserved for difficult diagnostic situations, such as the suspicion of vasculitis. It also is valuable in the search for neuropathy due to amyloid, sarcoid, or leprosy. Many hereditary diseases formerly diagnosed in part by means of biopsy can be diagnosed better with genetic analysis.

MANAGEMENT

The management consists largely of therapy for associated diseases, such as hypothyroidism, vitamin B_{12} deficiency, or vasculitis. Guillain-Barré syndrome is best managed with either plasma exchange or intravenous immunoglobulin. There is evidence that strict control of blood sugar for patients with diabetes can delay the development of neuropathy and retard its progression. Any implicated medication should be discontinued, if possible, and toxic exposures should be eliminated. When there are positive sensory symptoms such as pain and tingling, patients may respond to treatment with tricyclic agents (e.g., amitriptyline), gabapentin, or topical capsaicin cream.

Chapter 446

▪ APPROACH TO THE PATIENT WITH SEIZURES

DEFINITION AND CLASSIFICATION

Epilepsy is an abnormal tendency for the brain to produce paroxysmal depolarization shifts within neurons. Clinically, a person may have motor, sensory, or behavioral symptoms, with or without alteration in consciousness. An individual seizure is differentiated from epilepsy. The latter term is reserved for patients with three or more recurrent seizures. Epileptic seizures can be classified as simple partial (focal motor, somatosensory, or psychic symptoms without impairment of consciousness), complex partial (partial seizures with impairment of consciousness at sometime during the event), generalized seizures (either convulsive episodes with tonic-clonic or myoclonic features or nonconvulsive absence seizures), and partial seizures evolving to secondarily generalized seizures.

DIFFERENTIAL DIAGNOSIS

First, seizures must be differentiated from syncope. Epileptic seizures should then be differentiated from nonepileptic convulsive seizures produced by processes such as cerebral ischemia or hypoxia, hypoglycemia, meningitis or encephalitis, cocaine use, and withdrawal from alcohol, barbiturates, and benzodiazepines. Pseudoepileptic behavior produced by conversion hysteria must not be mistaken for true epilepsy.

CLINICAL PRESENTATION AND DIAGNOSTIC EVALUATION

A detailed case history and description of the attacks must be obtained from the patient, friends, and family. Figure 426.1A shows an algorithm for diagnosis and initial management. Electroencephalography (EEG) is indispensable when epilepsy is first suggested. It should be performed with the patient awake and asleep, with photic stimulation and hyperventilation. Brain imaging (magnetic resonance imaging, computed tomography, or both) is recommended in the care of all patients with recurrent, symptomatic partial complex seizures. Seizures associated with fever and meningeal signs suggest meningitis or encephalitis and warrant lumbar puncture.

MANAGEMENT

Whom to treat: Antiepileptic therapy is obligatory for generalized or partial forms of epilepsy but is seldom indicated after a single tonic-clonic seizure. Most of these patients have no risk factors for epilepsy and have normal neurologic and EEG examinations. The seizures often can be attributed to sleep deprivation (more than 36 hours), stress, extreme fatigue, drug or alcohol withdrawal, or use of cocaine. However, patients with a strong family history, an aura, absence or complex partial seizure, abnormal neurologic examination, or epileptiform EEG patterns need immediate evaluation and treatment.

Which drug to use: Treatment should begin with one antiepileptic agent, preferably the drug of choice (Table 426.1). Single-drug management of generalized seizures suppresses attacks among 80% of patients. Single-drug therapy for partial, complex partial, and secondary tonic-clonic seizures results in satisfactory long-term control for 60% to 90% of patients and complete eradication of seizures for 40% to 60%. If seizures persist, the dosage should be increased until seizures stop or toxic side effects develop. If seizure control is still unsatisfactory, a second drug of choice is substituted and the first agent is gradually withdrawn after therapeutic levels of the new drug have been attained. A third agent can be used for monotherapy, if necessary, and then two or three drugs can be given in combination, usually at low doses. Refractory seizures can be managed with epilepsy surgery or implantation of a vagus nerve stimulator.

Status epilepticus: Status epilepticus, a medical emergency, occurs when seizures persist longer than 30 minutes or when convulsions continue without recovery of consciousness. Three options are available as initial therapy: (a) Lorazepam 0.1 mg per kilogram IV bolus (no faster than 2 mg per minute) with a repeat dose in 15 minutes if control is not achieved. Fosphenytoin is then given immediately at a dose of 15 to 20 mg per kilogram IV and a rate of 75 to 150 mg per minute. (b) Diazepam infusion is given (no faster than 2 mg per minute) until seizures stop or a total of 20 mg has been infused. Simultaneously, fosphenytoin infusion 75 to 150 mg per minute is given until a total dose of 15 to 20 mg per kilogram has been achieved. If hypotension develops, the infusion rate is slowed. (c) Phenobarbital is administered at 100 mg per minute IV until seizures stop or a total dose of 10 mg per kilogram has been administered. If seizures continue, the rate is slowed to 50 mg per minute until a total dose of 20 mg per kilogram has been reached. If first-line options do not control seizures, EEG monitoring and endotracheal intubation are undertaken. If seizures continue, general anesthesia, usually pentobarbital, can be administered.

Withdrawal of antiepileptic treatment: Drugs usually can be withdrawn gradually after 4 years of complete control of simple partial epilepsy, complex partial epilepsy, absence associated with tonic-clonic seizures, and grand mal tonic-

clonic seizures. EEG and clinic visits should be scheduled for 6 months and 1 year after treatment.

Chapter 444

APPROACH TO THE ELDERLY PATIENT WITH ACUTE CHANGE IN MENTAL STATUS

DEFINITIONS

Delirium, or acute confusional state, is a change in mental status characterized by inattention, disorganized thinking, acute onset, and a fluctuating course.

EPIDEMIOLOGY

Acutely altered mental status accounts for at least 30% of emergency evaluations of older persons and may be the only manifestation of serious underlying disease. Each year delirium complicates hospital stays for more than 2.3 million older persons in the United States.

ETIOLOGY, PATHOPHYSIOLOGY, AND PATHOGENESIS

Delirium usually involves a complex relation between a vulnerable patient and precipitating factors that culminates in widespread reduction of cerebral oxidative metabolism with resultant impairment of cholinergic transmission. Risk factors include preexisting dementia, severe underlying illness, functional impairment, advanced age, chronic renal insufficiency, dehydration, malnutrition, and impairment of vision or hearing. Medications contribute to more than 40% of cases of delirium; the most commonly implicated are sedative-hypnotics, narcotics, histamine 2 blockers, and those with anticholinergic effects. Other precipitating factors include immobilization, use of indwelling bladder catheters, use of physical restraints, dehydration, malnutrition, iatrogenic events, medical illness, infection, metabolic derangement (e.g. hypernatremia or hyponatremia, hypercalcemia, acid-base disorders, hypoglycemia or hyperglycemia, and thyroid or adrenal disorders), alcohol or drug intoxication or withdrawal, environmental influences, and psychosocial factors. Patients who are highly vulnerable, such as those with cognitive impairment or severe illness, may have delirium with just a single dose of a sedative medication, whereas those who are not vulnerable can tolerate multiple insults.

CLINICAL FEATURES

There is an acute onset, but lucid intervals are characteristic. Inattention is recognized as difficulty focusing, maintaining, or shifting attention. Patients are easily distracted, have difficulty following commands, and often have perseveration with an answer to a previous question. They have difficulty repeating five digits forward or reciting the months backward. Other features include disorganization of thought and altered level of consciousness. A hypoactive form, characterized by lethargy and reduced psychomotor activity, is the most common form among older patients. It is often unrecognized and is associated with a poor prognosis. The hyperactive form, in which the patient is agitated, vigilant, and often hallucinating, is rarely missed.

DIFFERENTIAL DIAGNOSIS AND EVALUATION

The leading differential diagnoses are dementia, depression, and nonorganic psychotic disorders. The most difficult challenge is differentiating dementia. The two conditions are differentiated according to the acuity of onset and the impairment of consciousness and attention seen in dementia. Disorientation and memory impairment may occur with either. A systematic approach to the evaluation of changes in mental status among older adults is presented in Fig. 459.1.

MANAGEMENT

Prevention: Prevention is the most effective strategy. Effective interventions include nonpharmacologic sleep enhancement, early mobilization protocols, and measures to ensure optimal vision and hearing.

Nonpharmacologic management: Room and staff changes should be kept to a minimum. Patients should have access to eyeglasses, hearing aids, clocks, and calendars. Personal contact and communication are vital; patients must be allowed an uninterrupted period for sleep at night. Physical restraints should be avoided because of the adverse effects of immobility and increased agitation, questionable efficacy, and potential for injury.

Drug therapy: Any identified precipitating factors, such as occult infection, should be managed. Otherwise, pharmacologic approaches should be reserved for patients with severe agitation that endangers the patients' own safety or that of the staff. Drugs may further cloud mental status, so should be given in the lowest dose for the shortest time possible. Neuroleptics are the preferred agents. The recommended starting dose of haloperidol is 0.5 to 1.0 mg orally or parenterally, with repeated doses every 20 to 30 minutes (after vital signs have been checked) until sedation has been achieved. The end point should be an awake but manageable patient. A maintenance dose of one-half the loading dose should be administered in divided doses over the next 24 hours with tapering doses over the next few days. Side effects include hypotension, acute dystonia, extrapyramidal effects, and anticholinergic effects such as dry mouth, constipation, and urinary retention. Benzodiazepines are not recommended for the management of delirium, unless the cause is withdrawal from alcohol or sedative drugs, because of the tendency to cause oversedation and exacerbation of the confused state.

Chapter 459

APPROACH TO THE ELDERLY PATIENT WITH URINARY INCONTINENCE

DEFINITION AND EPIDEMIOLOGY
Urinary incontinence (UI) is involuntary loss of urine severe enough to be a social or health problem. As many as one-third of community-dwelling older adults and 50% to 70% of nursing home residents have some degree of UI.

ETIOLOGY AND PATHOPHYSIOLOGY
There are four basic types of UI, although they are not mutually exclusive. The most common type of UI among women younger than 75 years is stress incontinence, in which abnormality of the bladder outlet causes urinary leakage with increases in intra-abdominal pressure. The most common type among men and patients of both sexes older than 75 years is urge incontinence with involuntary bladder contractions (detrusor instability, termed "detrusor hyperreflexia" when associated with a neurologic disorder). Older women commonly have mixed incontinence and have symptoms of both stress and urge UI. Overflow incontinence from urinary retention is less common but is important to recognize because chronic large postvoid residual urine volumes can cause recurrent infection or upper urinary tract damage.

Several potentially reversible factors can cause or contribute to UI. The most common can be remembered with the acronym DRIP (*d*elerium; *r*estricted mobility, *r*etention of urine; *i*nfection of the bladder, *i*nflammation of the lower urinary tract, *i*mpaction of stool; *p*olyuria [hypercalcemia, hyperglycemia, excessive fluid intake], *p*harmaceuticals). Implicated medications include anticholinergic and α-adrenergic drugs (urinary retention and overflow incontinence), psychotropic drugs (sedation and immobility), α-adrenergic antagonists (urethral relaxation and stress UI), and diuretics (increased urine output).

CLINICAL FINDINGS
Among older patients, the most common presenting symptoms are the irritative symptoms of urge incontinence. These include urinary frequency during the day (voiding more frequently than every 2 hours), nocturia (two or more voids during normal sleeping hours), and a precipitant urge to void. Older women also commonly have symptoms of stress incontinence (leakage caused by coughing, laughing, or bending) or a combination of irritative and stress symptoms. Older men often have obstructive symptoms, which include irritative symptoms and hesitancy, a weak or intermittent stream, and straining to void.

DIAGNOSTIC EVALUATION
General approach: All patients with UI undergo a focused history interview and physical examination, postvoid residual measurement, and urinalysis. The history should focus on medications and active medical problems, full characterization of the UI (onset, precipitating factors, timing, frequency, amount of urine loss), and any irritative, stress, or obstructive symptoms. Voiding diaries can be useful. Physical examination should focus on cognitive function, mobility, cardiovascular findings, neurologic status, and pelvic and rectal examinations. The pelvic examination of women can reveal urine loss with stress (e.g., forceful coughing), a cystocele, or atrophic vaginitis. The postvoid residual measurement is performed by means of catheterization or ultrasonography. Volumes greater than 200 mL are abnormal and should lead to additional evaluation.
Further evaluation: Some patients need additional testing (Table 458.3).

MANAGEMENT
Stress incontinence: Women should be instructed to perform pelvic muscle (Kegel) exercises and to void regularly to avoid a full bladder. Factors such as obesity and chronic cough should be addressed. If no contraindications exist, an α-adrenergic agonist (30 to 60 mg pseudoephedrine three times a day, 75 mg phenylpropanolamine twice a day) and estrogen (orally or vaginally) can be tried. If all of these measures fail, the patient needs further evaluation and consideration for bladder neck suspension (for hypermobility of the bladder neck) or periurethral injections of collagen (for urethral sphincter weakness).
Urge incontinence: Patients can be treated with behavioral therapy. Pelvic muscle exercises work because voluntary contraction of the pelvic floor muscles inhibits bladder spasticity and contraction. Other behavioral therapies include bladder training for functional and motivated patients and scheduled toileting or prompted voiding for patients with impaired cognitive or physical functioning. Bladder relaxant therapy with anticholinergic agents can be added as necessary. Dicyclomine, imipramine, oxybutynin, and propantheline all have systemic anticholinergic effects (such as dry mouth) that may limit their use. Newer agents such as tolterodine and extended-release oxybutynin have fewer side effects. Patients who take any bladder relaxant must be observed carefully for evidence of urinary retention, and some patients need periodic postvoid residual measurements. Men with irritative symptoms associated with benign prostatic hyperplasia may benefit from a trial of an α-adrenergic antagonist (e.g., terazosin, tamsulosin) if surgery for obstruction is neither indicated nor desired.
Overflow incontinence: Patients with overflow UI due to anatomic obstruction need surgical intervention unless an operation is contraindicated. Patients who have an acontractile bladder are treated with catheter drainage (intermittent rather than indwelling, if feasible) because pharmacologic treatment with a cholinergic agonist or α-adrenergic antagonist usually is ineffective.

Chapter 458

1

PRINCIPLES OF MEDICAL PRACTICE

Laurence B. Gardner, Editor

HUMANISM AND ETHICS

INTRODUCTION TO INTERNAL MEDICINE AS A DISCIPLINE

WILLIAM N. KELLEY
JOEL D. HOWELL

Internal medicine is a scientific discipline encompassing the study, diagnosis, and treatment of nonsurgical diseases of adolescent and adult patients. Intrinsic to the discipline are the tenets of professionalism and humanistic values. Mastery of internal medicine requires not only comprehensive knowledge of the pathophysiology, epidemiology, and natural history of disease processes but also acquisition of skills in medical interviewing, physical examination, humanistic relations with patients, and procedural competency.

HISTORY

Throughout the 19th century, the idea of specialization was tinged with suspicion, if not outright hostility. Some thought the specialist was a "rattlebrained person, who, having tried general practice for a year or two and miserably failed, immediately takes up some sub-department of medicine which his inclination may point out as alluring, and becomes a specialist" (Van Zant, 1887).

Against the background of such attitudes, those who advocated specialization in the early 20th century attempted to define a method for identifying medical specialists. The structure of undergraduate medical training was becoming standardized and presented an unlikely place to train specialists. Although 70% of graduating medical students elected a 1-year rotating internship, it was not until 1914 that Pennsylvania became the first state to require postgraduate training for licensure. Few physi-

cians pursued formal training beyond that single year of internship.

During World War I, the Surgeon General divided U.S. Army physicians into specialist sections. How those sections were defined illustrates the arbitrary definition of internal medicine. The Army considered cardiovascular disease, tuberculosis, dermatology, neurology, and psychologic disorders to be subspecialties of internal medicine. (The latter three divisions are no longer considered part of internal medicine.) After World War I, various groups debated how to define a specialist. Each definition might well have succeeded, and every alternative would have produced very different results. The definition of internal medicine might have been different, depending on who defined it and when.

Through the early 20th century one point remained clear: American medicine needed a system for defining specialists. The public needed to know whom to trust, physicians needed to be able to identify appropriate colleagues for consultations, and hospital administrators wanted assurance of a physician's ability to perform specialized procedures. As the prestigious Commission on Medical Education reported in 1932, "many specialists are self-named; many are not fully trained even in their limited field and still less well equipped in the broad fundamentals of medicine." The Commission further advised that "a particular identification for those who profess to be specialists should be created" (Wilson, 1940).

That identification came to be certification by a specialty board. In 1917, the American Board of Ophthalmology was the first to offer board certification, and by 1936, 10 specialty boards had been created. During the next 2 years, internal medicine (in 1936) and surgery (in 1937) incorporated their specialty boards.

The founders of the American Board of Internal Medicine (ABIM) did not want every practitioner of internal medicine to be board-certified. Rather they saw the ABIM as a national group designed to recognize only a few outstanding internists. The board examination was designed to test whether the candidate had superb knowledge of the practice of medicine. As originally envisioned, the board-certified internist would be part of a special breed and function as an outstanding consultant. Most of the ABIM's founders thought that a small, highly qualified group of specialists would practice within clearly defined areas, and the rest of medical practice, accounting for 85% of all care, would remain the realm of general physicians. This vision depended on the continued existence of general practitioners who could refer patients to the consulting internists.

Portions of this chapter were previously published in Howell JD. The invention and development of American internal medicine. *J Gen Intern Med* 1989;4:127. Reprinted with permission.

The ABIM was formed just in time to include some nascent subspecialists under the larger umbrella of internal medicine. In 1940, soon after its formation, the ABIM decided to certify candidates as subspecialists in four fields—cardiology, gastroenterology, tuberculosis (later called pulmonary medicine), and allergy—but only if the candidates were first board-certified in general internal medicine.

By 1940, 16 specialty boards had been formed and more than 14,000 physicians had earned the right to call themselves board-certified specialists. However, medicine was soon confronted with World War II, whose impact persisted far longer than the 5 years the United States spent at war. The war changed the shape of American medicine by emphasizing the importance of specialization and by enabling the federal government to become the primary source of support for scientific research. These new conditions transformed the ABIM from the original vision of its founders—that the ABIM should recognize a few exceptional consulting physicians—into an organization more consistent with the large, successful, subspecialized discipline that internal medicine has become.

Additional subspecialties of internal medicine were formally recognized through the ABIM in 1972 with the development of subspecialty examinations in endocrinology and metabolism, hematology, infectious diseases, nephrology, and rheumatology. "Tuberculosis" was changed to "pulmonary medicine." In subsequent years, additional specialties and areas of special competence were added, including oncology, geriatrics, sports medicine, electrophysiology, and others.

THE PRACTICE OF INTERNAL MEDICINE AND ITS SUBSPECIALTIES

The changing nature of internal medicine and its subspecialties can be expected to continue. The internist has been a case manager, a consultant, and a primary care physician. Today there is intensified interest in the role of the general internist as a primary care physician. The essential role of the generalist physician has become apparent to other providers of health care and to payers for health care. The primary care physician sees each patient with a focus on prevention and on management of the patient's health, hoping to minimize the development of disease, and, when disease does occur, to detect it early and manage it effectively.

Other professionals have entered the realm of primary care. The family practitioner has established a major role as a primary care physician, and nurse practitioners are commonly involved in providing primary care in collaboration with primary care physicians and through more independent roles. Occasionally, primary care is provided by subspecialists, and this role may become increasingly common as fewer physicians need to function entirely as subspecialists. One of the major unanswered policy questions is who is best able to provide primary care most efficiently: the subspecialist, the general internist, the family practitioner, or the nurse practitioner?

A second major role of the general internist has been to function as a case manager. Case management may range from appropriate placement of the patient after hospitalization to the management of social issues or management of home care to allow the patient to remain independent and continue to receive good follow-up care at a reasonable cost. As more people need more long-term care for chronic illnesses, case management may become increasingly important. The case manager role commonly is supplemented by others, such as nurse case managers, who focus their efforts on the ancillary aspects of managing the patient in collaboration with the physician, who manages the medical aspects of the patient's illness.

Case management often is critical to achieving good outcomes, particularly with the 5% of the patient population who require 50% of health care dollars. The potential cost savings of this approach has led to aggressive implementation of programs for case management by payer and provider organizations that take full financial risk for patient care. For many years, general internists, particularly those in major academic health centers, served as case managers for patients with complex illnesses requiring the participation of many different specialists. In that setting, it is productive to have one physician who is able to manage the vast array of consultant recommendations. This function is a requirement of some health maintenance organizations (HMOs).

The creators of the ABIM envisioned that the internist could serve as consultant to the generalist physician. The breadth of the internist's role led to important differences between internal medicine and family medicine, which excluded the role of consultant. At a time when virtually all physicians were general practitioners, the role of the consultant internist was quite different from the situation today. However, this function continues to be important in rural settings, where most care is still provided by nurse practitioners or family practitioners and where few subspecialists are available. Furthermore, the generalist as consultant to the surgical practitioner has grown in importance.

With the continued development of integrated delivery systems, a new division of labor is likely to occur among general internists. In urban areas that have heavy market penetration of managed care, the general internist can spend virtually all of his or her time in the ambulatory setting, providing continuity of care as a primary care physician. It becomes extremely inefficient for those physicians also to care for patients who may require hospitalization, and it becomes more practical for another population of general internists, "hospitalists," to care for patients admitted to the hospital. In this capacity, they may serve as the physicians responsible for the patients' overall care, prioritizing the advice and recommendations of the various subspecialty consultants. This function is likely to remain less common in rural areas.

In response to the dramatic and ongoing evolution of specialties within internal medicine, the ABIM has recognized three types of subspecialists. The first is the basic scientist. This individual has training in internal medicine, has clinical training in her or his subspecialty, has spent substantial time in the basic research laboratory, and is able to carry out fundamental research, collaborating and competing with other basic scientists who have no clinical expertise. These individuals can envision the importance of basic research findings in improving human health—a valuable skill in this era of rapidly advancing biomedical research. These individuals often have some continued clinical practice in their subspecialty, and they teach in that subspecialty, but they spend most of their time in the laboratory doing basic research.

The second type of subspecialist is the clinical investigator. This individual has extensive training in internal medicine and in a clinical subspecialty, and has considerable research training involving human subjects. These subspecialists are able to transfer the advances in the laboratory to human subjects. This is perhaps best exemplified in an area such as gene therapy, which requires critical initial studies using selected human subjects before application to larger groups of patients can be carried out.

The third group contains those who serve as subspecialty clinicians. This is the largest group of subspecialists in internal medicine and is perhaps the group in greatest oversupply. This group can be further subdivided. The first subtype encompasses those providing principal care, which is long-term continuity of care for patients with chronic disease; most care is provided by the subspecialist, with some care provided by other members of the team, such as a general internist or nurse practitioner. The second subtype of the subspecialty clinician is the individual who is highly procedure-oriented and spends most of his or her time conducting procedures. An example is the invasive cardiologist who spends a substantial portion of his or her time in the cardiac catheterization laboratory doing coronary angiograms and angioplasties. A continuum of subspecialty practice exists between these two extremes.

All subspecialists in internal medicine must have received full training as general internists before their specialization. In this way, they differ from most other subspecialists in organized medicine because they can function as generalist physicians when that role is appropriate. In an era of an apparent oversupply of subspecialists, this additional training is immensely valuable because it allows these physicians to provide principal or primary care. This is especially valuable in the management of chronic, complex disease.

ROLES OF THE TEXTBOOK OF INTERNAL MEDICINE

Kelley's Textbook of Internal Medicine is designed for the medical student, for the postgraduate trainee, for the practitioner in general internal medicine, and for the subspecialist. Certain sections of the book may appeal more to some individuals than others, but it has been our commitment to make this book useful across this broad range of training. For example, the "Approach to the Patient" sections are probably most useful to the medical student or beginning resident in internal medicine. The sections on the "Approach to Common Primary Care Issues" and "Diagnostic and Therapeutic Modalities" might also be of considerable interest to students and residents. The sections on "Basic Mechanisms of Health and Disease" and on "Disorders" should interest students, residents, and physicians who have been practicing medicine or one of its subspecialties for many years. In this context, *Kelley's Textbook of Internal Medicine* serves as an important device for continuing medical education.

BIBLIOGRAPHY

Advisory Board for Medical Specialists. *Directory of medical specialists.* New York: Columbia University Press, 1940.
Council on Medical Education and Hospitals. *A history of the Council on Medical Education and Hospitals of the American Medical Association.* Chicago: American Medical Association, 1959:21.
Derbyshire RC. *Medical licensure and discipline in the United States.* Baltimore: Johns Hopkins University Press, 1967.
Lynch C, Weed FW, McAfee L. *The Medical Department of the United States Army in the World War,* Vol. 1, *The Surgeon General's Office.* Washington, DC: U.S. Government Printing Office, 1923;1114.
Stevens R. Trends in medical specialization in the United States. *Inquiry* 1971;8:9.
Stevens R. *American medicine and the public interest.* Updated with a new introduction. Berkeley: University of California Press, 1998.
Van Zandt HC. Specialists. *Trans NY State Med Assoc* 1887;4:347.
Wilson LB. The work of the National Board of Medical Examiners during its first quarter century. *Diplomate* 1940;12:161.

Kelley's Textbook of Internal Medicine, fourth edition. Edited by H. David Humes. Lippincott Williams & Wilkins, Philadelphia © 2000.

CHAPTER

2

CLINICAL MEDICINE, CLINICAL ETHICS, AND PHYSICIANS' PROFESSIONALISM

MARK SIEGLER
ARTHUR CAPLAN
PETER SINGER

To practice medicine competently, physicians require both scientific–technical proficiency and knowledge of clinical ethics. They need to manage issues in the areas of informed consent, truth telling, confidentiality, do-not-resuscitate orders, end-of-life decisions, palliative care, proxy decision making, and patient rights. A working knowledge of practical clinical ethics is an addition to, not a substitute for, the traditional standards of character and virtue expected of the good physician: competency, integrity, honesty, compassion, and respect for patients and colleagues. During the past 15 years, the discipline of clinical ethics has emerged as a new and useful component of medical practice and has assisted physicians and patients to reach ethically acceptable decisions.

Clinical ethical issues now occur more frequently in medical practice for a variety of reasons. Scientific advances and new technologies have raised unprecedented ethical problems, e.g., when should efforts to prolong life with ventilators or dialysis machines be stopped and under what circumstances is it permissible to forgo life-prolonging interventions such as artificial hydration? Changes in molecular medicine, genetics, and the neurosciences are generating new and different ethical problems in such traditional areas as informed consent and confidentiality. Changes in the relationship between patients and physicians to a more equal relationship of shared decision making require attention to ethical issues such as honest disclosure, effective communication, and informed consent. Managed care has given rise to new ethical issues such as limitations on decisional freedom for patients and physicians, the need to accurately explain what is available for patients with respect to diagnostic services and treatments, and potential financial conflicts of interest associated with limiting the use of health resources.

Sound ethical analysis in clinical settings rests on a foundation of trust between the patient and physician. Crucial components in the analysis of any ethical issue include an understanding by both parties of the medical and scientific facts; the preferences, values, and goals of both patient and physician; and the external constraints such as cost, limited resources, and legal duties that shape or restrict choices. By communicating clearly with patients about the prognosis and treatment goals, physicians can cement trust and reduce the chances of conflict arising with respect to care decisions, including end-of-life decisions.

The doctor–patient relationship (DPR) is the central and organizing theme in clinical ethics. Most of the routine ethical problems that arise in patient care present in the context of the DPR and most are resolved within this relationship. The field of clinical ethics focuses on how patients and physicians work within existing administrative, economic, and political structures to reach mutual agreement on clinical decisions that affect the patient. In the United States, the DPR has undergone two major changes in the past generation. Initially, in the 1970s and 1980s, the relationship changed from a paternalistic one, in which physicians make choices for patients based on professional values, to a more equal relationship of shared decision making, in which physicians advise patients but patients ultimately make their own health care choices. The second major change in the DPR, which occurred in the 1990s, relates to cost containment and managed care. Private and government payers for health care are effectively limiting the decisional freedom of both patients and physicians, and such actions have given rise to new and recurring ethical concerns within the DPR. This latter change in the DPR has seen a new emphasis on populations rather than individual patients and on attempts to eliminate variations in health care decisions by emphasizing practice guidelines derived from evidence-based medicine, outcomes studies, and clinical trials. These shifts, while laudable in many ways, put new pressures on the traditional patient advocacy that has been at the core of the DPR.

In this chapter, we examine three of the central professional values of physicians: clinical competence, respect for patients, and efforts to minimize conflicts of interest by placing the patient's welfare above other considerations. These three values are then related to three clinical–ethical issues that physicians frequently encounter: (a) providing quality end-of-life care (an application of clinical competence); (b) negotiating informed consent (an application of respect for persons); and (c) working within managed care organizations (an application of minimizing conflicts of interest).

THREE CENTRAL PROFESSIONAL VALUES

In considering three of the central professional values of medicine, we realize that despite scientific developments of the past century the role of the medical profession in human societies has changed surprisingly little since the time of Hippocrates. The DPR has also changed very little, and the encounter of healer and patient has remained the principal means by which medicine achieves its goals. Several reasons explain the extraordinary continuity of the DPR over time: (a) medicine serves a universal and unchanging human need by responding to a patient's sense of illness or "dis-ease"; (b) medicine has an unchanging central goal, which is to help patients; and (c) most medical help is delivered in the direct encounter of patient and physician, that is, in the DPR. In this context, we examine three core professional values: competence, respect for patients, and minimizing of conflicts of interest.

CLINICAL COMPETENCE

Excellent clinical practice has always blended technical proficiency with ethical sensitivity. The physician's relationship to the patient is based on specific technical training and competency and on respect for medicine's ethical standards. This specialized knowledge and proficiency is used to assist patients, sometimes by curing or managing their illness and disease, and sometimes by helping them overcome the fear, pain, and suffering that are often associated with illness. Once sought out by the patient, the physician becomes involved in the patient's problem and never again is a mere observer. Physicians are responsible and personally accountable to their patients if they fail to perform their task adequately because of lack of skill, knowledge, dedication, or clinical judgment, or if, for any other reason, they fail to act in the patient's behalf.

RESPECT FOR PATIENTS

In 1983, a report of the American Board of Internal Medicine defined "respect" as the personal commitment to honor the preferences, choices, and rights of others regarding their medical care and to recognize the dignity and freedom of the patient. Patient preferences are the ethical and legal nucleus of the DPR. In addition, respect for patients and their preferences is a clinical obligation because patients who reach a shared health care decision have greater trust and loyalty in the DPR, cooperate more fully to implement the shared decision, express greater satisfaction with their health care, and, most important, have been shown to have better clinical outcomes in several chronic diseases.

MINIMIZING CONFLICTS OF INTEREST

Conflicts of interest are inevitable. A minimum requirement for a conflict of interest is two human beings, especially when they are involved in a relationship that provides care in return for a fee. Such conflicts have always existed in medicine: in Hippocratic times, under fee-for-service systems of payment, and today, in managed health systems. The central issue is not the existence of conflicts of interest but rather how these conflicts are addressed and minimized within the professional relationships of doctors and patients. Two basic rules offer guidance to physicians: (a) Place the patient's interest first by subordinating financial matters and other self-interests to achieve the central goal of medicine, i.e., helping patients. The American Medical Association's 1994 guidelines on this point are clear: "Under no circumstances may physicians place their own financial interests above the welfare of their patients. If a conflict develops between the physician's financial interest and the physician's responsibilities to the patient, the conflict must be resolved to the patient's benefit." (b) Inform the patient when there are substantial conflicts of interest, such as financial or similar incentives that could influence the physician's recommendations to the patient. The three central professional values will now be related to three specific clinical-ethical issues.

QUALITY END-OF-LIFE CARE

Good-quality care at the end of life, an example of clinical competence, is something that the public is demanding and medicine is committed to deliver. Although media reports on end-of-life care frequently highlight euthanasia or assisted suicide, most of the care provided by internists to dying patients focuses on the control of pain, symptom management, decisions about life-sustaining treatments, and the provision of support to patients and families. While there is increasing expertise among physicians, nurses, and others specializing in palliative care medicine, most end-of-life care is delivered by internists. The training and education available in this area have not always been adequate.

There are some simple steps that physicians can take to ensure the ethical management of terminally ill patients. In approaching patients at the end of life, internists should ask themselves three questions: Have I relieved the patient's pain and other symptoms? Have I addressed the use of life-sustaining treatment? Am I doing what I can to support the patient and family?

HAVE I RELIEVED THE PATIENT'S PAIN AND SYMPTOMS?

Adequate pain and symptom management is the *sine qua non* of ethical end-of-life care. Although most pain can be controlled, unfortunately, many patients still die with uncontrolled pain. Other symptoms experienced by dying patients such as dyspnea, fatigue, depression, and nausea are also often inadequately addressed. The reasons for suboptimal control of pain and other symptoms are complex, but two principal reasons are inadequate education about pain and symptom control in medical school and residency, and physician concerns about the ethics of hastening death. Physicians must seek sources of continuing education on treatment of pain and symptom management in dying patients. If the primary physician cannot control a dying patient's pain or other symptoms, the physician should seek assistance from a palliative care specialist (see Chapter 40).

Physicians sometimes feel that by administering adequate analgesia or sedation they are hastening death. This concern is understandable in light of the opinions advanced in professional codes of ethics such as those of the American Medical Association and the American College of Physicians opposing any form of active euthanasia. There are also serious legal consequences facing anyone participating in euthanasia.

It is important, however, to distinguish appropriate analgesia and sedation of dying patients from euthanasia. Physicians are morally bound to manage pain and suffering aggressively. Legal authorities must be made to understand this duty. For instance, according to guidelines developed by the Chief Coroner of Ontario, an act is considered palliative care, and not euthanasia, if (a) it is intended solely to relieve the person's suffering, (b) it is administered in response to symptoms or signs of the patient's suffering and is commensurate with that suffering, and (c) it is not the deliberate infliction of death. The Supreme Court of the United States and many state courts have endorsed similar considerations in allowing physicians the discretion to pursue aggressive pain control even to the point of terminal sedation.

HAVE I ADEQUATELY ADDRESSED THE USE OF LIFE-SUSTAINING TREATMENTS?

The basic principles applying to use of life-sustaining treatment are those of consent. Patients have the ethical and legal right to decide to not start (withhold) or to stop (withdraw) treatment, including life-sustaining treatment such as cardiopulmonary resuscitation and renal dialysis, even if this refusal results in their death. Valid consent requires adequate disclosure of information and voluntary decision making by a competent patient. If the patient is incompetent, his or her right to accept or refuse treatment is exercised through a process known as substitute decision making, which asks two key questions: (a) Who should make the decision on behalf of the patient? and (b) How should the decision be made? The specific detailed answers to these questions will vary from jurisdiction to jurisdiction. In general, the most appropriate decision maker is (a) someone named by the patient in advance, (b) a family member or loved one, and (c) for those with no other substitute decision maker, a public official such as a public guardian or trustee. The most appropriate basis for the decision is (a) the person's previously expressed wish (either verbal or through a written advanced directive), (b) their known values and beliefs, and (c) their best interests.

Patients and their families may plan in advance for decisions about life-sustaining treatment using a process called *advance care planning*. An advanced directive is a written document in which the patient states who should make the treatment decisions (a durable power of attorney for health care) and what decisions the patient wants made (a living will) if he or she becomes incompetent and can no longer make decisions. The Study to Understand Prognoses and Preferences for Outcomes and Risks of Treatments (known as the SUPPORT study) showed that an advanced care planning intervention had no effect on clinical and administrative outcomes. However, Singer's recent qualitative research suggests that the primary goal of advanced care planning is to help patients prepare for death, which entails facing death, achieving a sense of control, and strengthening relationships.

In contrast to cases in which patients and families refuse life-sustaining treatment proposed by health care providers, a "new" type of case, in which patients and families request treatment that health care providers believe is inappropriate, is becoming increasingly prevalent. These so-called "futility" cases lead to great distress on the part of patients, families, and health care providers since there are few policies and almost no legislation governing this issue. On the one side, some patients and families insist that the decision about treatment is one of values and therefore they have the right to make it. On the other side, health care providers sometimes argue that they should not be forced to provide treatment that will not prolong life or will lead only to prolonged unconsciousness and debility and dependence on medical technology. In such cases, it is important to negotiate a treatment plan based on realistic prognosis and in this way to avoid such conflicts by not raising false hopes of patients and families. It is also important that decisions to end treatment on the grounds of futility not be made individually but rather be undertaken with guidance and consultation from hospital ethics committees and if necessary appropriate administrative and legal bodies.

HAVE I DONE WHAT I CAN TO SUPPORT THE PATIENT AND FAMILY?

Many psychological, social, cultural, and religious issues surface at the end of life. Psychologically, individuals might want to maintain a sense of control over their dying. Socially, individuals might want to strengthen relationships with, or relieve burdens of, their family members. Culturally, death and dying have different meanings and rituals for different cultural groups. People often seek meaning at the end of life through their spiritual beliefs.

Physicians who care for dying patients must help patients and families address these issues. Every death is different, and there is no specific "formula" for assisting patients and families. Nevertheless, the simple, open-ended question "Is there anything else I can do to help you or your family?" might evoke useful clues for physician action. Physicians must be aware of, and offer to dying patients, spiritual, religious, and emotional resources such as chaplaincy, social services, and hospice care.

■ INFORMED CONSENT AND SHARED DECISION MAKING

The process by which physicians and patients make decisions together is often summarized in the phrase *informed consent*. This doctrine, which reflects respect for patients, is at the heart of the DPR and is based on the ethical principles of respect for individual autonomy, dignity, and self-determination. Informed consent has three key components: disclosure, competency, and voluntariness.

Disclosure means that physicians tell patients about the medical diagnosis, prognosis, and risks and benefits associated with possible treatment options. Patients are entitled to enough information to permit them to ask reasonable questions about the diagnosis and the options that are available. *Competency* means that patients are capable of understanding relevant information, appreciate their own needs and values, manipulate information

rationally, and communicate a treatment choice. *Voluntariness* means that a patient chooses freely, ideally without coercion from the physician or anyone else.

Informed consent is not an event, nor does it refer to a patient's signature on a consent form. It is a process of continuous communication and dialogue between doctor and patient. In this process, physicians empower patients to act in an autonomous manner by educating them about the nature of their medical problems and reasonable medical alternatives to resolve or cope with them. Patients are then in a position to choose treatment based on personal preferences, values, and goals.

The outcome of care may be improved by the informed consent process. Empowering patients to participate in decision making has been associated with beneficial outcomes for several chronic diseases. In patients with diabetes, hypertension, and peptic ulcer disease, pilot programs aimed at increasing patient participation in medical care result in improved functional and health outcomes. Compliance is improved by informing patients about their options and maintaining open and full communication with them. And the prospects for conflict around highly charged decisions, such as end-of-life decisions, are minimized when informed consent is managed effectively.

■ THE DOCTOR–PATIENT RELATIONSHIP IN THE AGE OF MANAGED CARE

Efforts at cost containment, which raise the specter of physician conflict of interest, often involve some of the following approaches: using clinical guidelines to standardize care; restricting services seen to be of marginal benefit; rationing some potentially beneficial services; and restricting both patient and physician freedom of choice to make individual clinical decisions. These strategies for achieving cost containment and health reform already have placed enormous stress on the DPR. A recent study of managed care physicians highlights the ways in which physician-respondents believe that financial conflicts of interest interfere with the DPR and with the doctors' ethical obligations to patients.

In order to maintain ethical integrity in clinical practice, particularly in dealing with end-of-life care decisions, physicians must adopt and maintain a patient-centered perspective that makes patients understand that the physician is their advocate, seeking, within the financial and practice limits that exist, to permit patients to make their own health care decisions. Physicians must also insist on patients' rights in developing clinical guidelines and appeal mechanisms for the large number of clinical decisions that, despite research on medical outcomes, will continue to be made in the face of considerable clinical uncertainty.

■ CONCLUSION

In the face of unprecedented changes in the doctor–patient relationship, the question has sometimes been raised regarding whether the relationship will survive in modern medicine and whether it is really necessary. Is there a residual role for the physician within a DPR when practice guidelines and expert consensus statements exist? We believe there is. A vigorous defense of the role of the physician was offered almost a generation ago by Dr. Philip Tumulty: "A clinician is defined as one whose prime function is to manage a sick person with a purpose of alleviating most effectively the total impact of the illness upon that person. ... Managing a sick person is entirely different from diagnosing an illness and prescribing therapy for it. ... Management means that the physician comprehends and is sensitive to the total effects of an illness on the total person." In Tumulty's view, the DPR is essential for determining the diagnosis, communicating effectively with the patient, reaching a joint decision on how to treat the problem, and then proceeding to the management of the disease process with the goal of alleviating most effectively the total impact of the illness on the patient. In our view, the clinical encounter between the patient who seeks help and the physician who is trained to provide help is the *unchanging event in medicine* and has remained relatively constant despite the scientific, social, economic, and political changes that have occurred in medicine during the past 3,000 years. Furthermore, the goals of the encounter have not changed much as physicians have always attempted to help those who ask for help and to improve patients' length and quality of life. Finally, the DPR, with its emphasis on the primary clinical skills of communication, history taking, and physical diagnosis—skills that internists are trained to provide—probably remains the most cost-effective way to provide health care to individuals and populations.

BIBLIOGRAPHY

American Medical Association Council on Ethical and Judicial Affairs. *Code of Medical Ethics,* 1998–1999 edition. Chicago: American Medical Association, 1998; sec. 8.03:118–126.

Benson JA. Humanistic qualities in medicine. In: Kelley WN, editor-in-chief. *Textbook of medicine,* third ed. Philadelphia: Lippincott-Raven Publishers, 1997:4–6.

Carron AT, Lynn J, Keaney P. End-of-life care in medical textbooks. *Ann Intern Med* 1999;130:82–86.

Feldman DS, Novack DN, Gracely R. Effects of managed care on physician–patient relationships, quality of care, and the ethical practice of medicine: a physicians survey. *Arch Intern Med* 1998;158:1626–1632.

Jonsen AR, Siegler M, Winslade WJ. *Clinical ethics,* fourth ed. New York: McGraw-Hill, 1998.

Siegler M. The physician–patient accommodation: a central event in clinical medicine. *Arch Intern Med* 1982;142:1899–1902.

Siegler M, Pellegrino ED, Singer PA. Clinical medical ethics: the first decade. *J Clin Ethics* 1990;1:5–9.

Siegler M. Falling off the pedestal: what is happening to the traditional doctor–patient relationship? *Mayo Clin Proc* 1993;68:1–7.

Singer PA, Martin DK, Kelner MJ. Quality end of life care: patients' perspectives. *JAMA* 1999;281:163–168.

SUPPORT Principal Investigators. A controlled trial to improve care for seriously ill hospitalized patients. The Study to Understand Prognoses and Preferences for Outcomes and Risks of Treatments (SUPPORT). *JAMA* 1995;274:1591–1598.

Tarlov AL, Ware JE, Greenfield S, et al. The Medical Outcomes Study: an application of methods for monitoring the results of medical care. *JAMA* 1989;262:925.

Tumulty PA. What is a clinician and what does he do? *N Engl J Med* 1970; 283:20–24.

Kelley's Textbook of Internal Medicine, fourth edition. Edited by H. David Humes.
Lippincott Williams & Wilkins, Philadelphia © 2000.

BASIC MECHANISMS OF HEALTH AND DISEASE

CHAPTER

3

THE GENOME PROJECT AND MOLECULAR DIAGNOSIS

LESLIE G. BIESECKER
BARBARA B. BIESECKER
FRANCIS S. COLLINS

Advances in molecular biology have begun to transform the practice of clinical medicine in many specialties and subspecialties. The genetic and molecular dissection of pathogenic mechanisms will fundamentally alter medical practice, comparable in scale to the alterations caused by the advent of antibiotics. Adult medical practice that involves genetic testing and counseling will require melding the disciplines of internal medicine and clinical genetics. Primary care internists and subspecialists will need to become familiar with advances in molecular genetics and genetic counseling to effect these changes in their practices.

To understand the magnitude of these advances, it is necessary to consider some of the research sources. The Human Genome Project is an organized effort to create a biologically and medically useful database of genome structure, sequence, and function in humans and experimental animal model systems. Initiated in 1990, the genome project provides resources that allow investigators to rapidly locate and clone disease or susceptibility genes—efforts that previously required years of work. By the year 2003, the entire human DNA sequence encoding 80,000 to 100,000 genes will be determined. In addition to the genome project, medical genetics research is performed in independent laboratories around the world. The melding of information from the large-scale project and the independent research efforts will produce an enormous dataset that will profoundly alter medical practice.

The successes in gene discovery thus far have primarily included single-gene disorders that cause symptoms in a large proportion of persons who have abnormal genotypes (highly penetrant mutations). These include disorders such as cystic fibrosis, neurofibromatosis, muscular dystrophy, Huntington's disease, and many others. These disorders can have variable severities because different mutations lead to various degrees of dysfunction. Although we consider these to be single-gene disorders, the severity of the phenotype also depends on other gene products in a molecular pathway.

In contrast, many diseases result from the interaction of multiple genes with the environment. Because these diseases involve many genes and potentially many possible mutations, an enormous number of combinations of genotypes are possible. These combinations lead to a range of susceptibility and a distribution of phenotypic severity. In addition to causing or predisposing to a disease, genetic variation might also affect a drug's efficacy or its ability to induce side effects. These concepts of disease have the potential to radically alter not only how medicine is practiced but also how medical research trials are designed and conducted. In addition, pharmacogenomics will profoundly alter our approach to therapeutics. Research studies will divine variations in drug efficacy and metabolism among the population and assist in the definition of distinct subject cohorts. Drugs that have significant pharmacogenetic variation will spawn clinical pharmacogenetic tests that will be used before the selection of a drug for a given patient. Such testing will have two profound effects: the ability to maximize drug efficacy and to minimize adverse effects by determining the pharmacogenetic variables of the individual patient.

Determining the molecular pathophysiology of human disease and pharmacogenomics will provide opportunities for diagnosis, prevention, and treatment (Fig. 3.1). However, genetic tests differ from other medical tests in that they have important implications for family members and for reproductive decision making. They often raise issues of privacy, autonomy, voluntariness, and discrimination, and the test results may have significant emotional consequences. Genetic counseling is the process that combines the provision of genetic information with psychosocial counseling. It is generally nondirective in that patients are not advised as to whether to undergo genetic testing. The voluntary and personal nature of decisions about genetic tests, most importantly tests that impact reproductive decisions, are respected.

Genetic counseling should accompany the offer of any genetic test to facilitate informed decision making. This process of genetic counseling includes an explanation of risk, and an exploration of the patient's perceptions of the meaning of the condition and implications of the potential results of testing. In this context, the outcomes of test decisions are anticipated in a manner that supports decision making. While genetic testing is

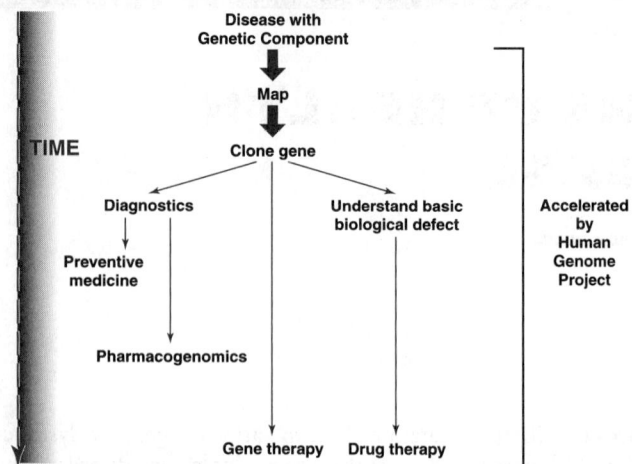

FIGURE 3.1. Flow chart of the course of gene discovery and its implications for clinical medicine.

increasingly used as a tool of medicine, the choice to pursue it remains personal. People may or may not prefer to learn predictive or diagnostic genetic information about their own health. Their interest in the information depends primarily on their perception of what they can do with the information to protect their future health. Furthermore, state-of-the-art genetic testing may produce ambiguous molecular results associated with uncertainty about the susceptibility to, and severity of, the disorder. These technical complexities speak to the importance of providing genetic counseling in follow-up to testing for help with interpretation and risk communication.

Before genetic testing can be offered, the state of the art for the specific disorder must be evaluated. The number and distribution of different mutations are major determinants of the practicality of genetic testing. Disorders that are caused by one or a few mutations (e.g., sickle cell anemia, Huntington's disease) are amenable to the design of simple, sensitive, and reliable molecular diagnostic tests that rarely have false-positive or false-negative results. Disorders with multiple mutations may have none of these desirable features. Along with the technical challenges of designing a genetic test, there are other issues that must be addressed before a test is ready for clinical use. Issues of genotype–phenotype correlation, sensitivity and specificity, proper informed consent, access to genetic counseling, and other concerns must be addressed before test release. For all types of genetic testing, it is important for the medical practitioner to be familiar with the methodologies, strengths, and limitations of all tests that will likely be used in clinical practice.

■ GENETIC TESTING IN MEDICAL PRACTICE

In addition to common tests that have genetic implications (e.g., cholesterol levels for familial hypercholesterolemia, echocardiograms for Marfan's syndrome), there are a host of DNA and cytogenetic diagnostic tests that may be used in a clinical genetics encounter.

DIRECT MUTATION ANALYSIS

It is possible to design a test that can directly detect the causative mutations for a disorder if several conditions are satisfied. The gene must be cloned, and there must be a specific and sensitive method to detect most mutations. The severity of the phenotype associated with the specific mutations must also be determined through analysis of the patient's family or by studies of many other affected individuals. Although the analysis of mutations by the direct method is technically straightforward, the interpretation of results can be challenging. For genes that have multiple alleles, it might be difficult to predict the severity of the disorder from the mutation, especially when the mutation causes amino acid substitutions. Such "mutations" must be carefully analyzed to ensure that they do not represent polymorphisms and are, in effect, false positives. The BRCA1 breast cancer susceptibility gene provides an example of this problem. Mutation detection by whole-gene sequencing has led to the description of more than 600 mutations. The penetrance and severity of some of the mutations are well delineated (e.g., del185AG); however, others are so rare (and some are even unique to single families) that it is difficult or impossible to assess the consequences of having such a mutation. This is an example of a test that has the potential to assist greatly in the management of a patient, yet it also has a significant probability of generating an uninterpretable result.

The complexities of predicting phenotype from genotype suggest that physicians should be skeptical about ordering such tests. Before ordering a test, one should be clear about the prior probability of finding a mutation (a screening study versus a person at 50% risk of inheriting a mutation), the state of knowledge concerning the penetrance of various mutations in the gene under consideration, and how a normal or abnormal result will affect the care of the patient. These considerations are overlaid by many of the factors described above including insurability and employability, self-esteem, anxiety about risks to the offspring of the patient, and so forth. All of these factors must be taken into account before ordering such a test, and they conspire to make such a decision complex and multifaceted.

LINKAGE ANALYSIS

Linkage analysis may be used for a mendelian disorder when mutation detection is impractical because the gene has not yet been cloned or because the mutations are too heterogeneous to be readily identified. This test takes advantage of the fact that markers that are located near certain genes are likely to be inherited together with those genes and can be used to assess the probability that a mutant allele was inherited. The advantages of linkage analysis are that it can be performed before the responsible mutations are discovered and that it can be used on families in whom the responsible mutation is unknown or is undetectable. The disadvantages of linkage analysis are that it requires blood samples on multiple family members and that the results are often limited to maximum confidences of 95% to 98%. This reduced confidence is related to the distance between the marker and the mutation on the chromosome. The uncertainty of a linkage test is in addition to the variables described above for direct mutation analysis because the linkage is being used as a proxy for the actual mutation.

COMPLEX GENETIC DISORDERS

One current major challenge for medical genetics is the elucidation of the molecular etiology of disorders that are caused by alterations in several genes and that have significant variability attributable to environmental influences. Examples of this class of disorders include adult-onset diabetes mellitus, essential hypertension, and schizophrenia, among others. The complexity of identifying each of these genetic and environmental components of disease liability is much greater than that involved in the isolation of a single-gene disorder. It is anticipated that such research will reveal an array of genes, some of which have more than one allele contributing to disease liability. Within that array of genes, some will pose particular susceptibilities to environmental influences. The determination of the cumulative liabilities and susceptibilities of each of these allelic variants will require detailed analyses of large cohorts of subjects.

As of this writing, no significant diseases in this category have been fully or even partially elucidated, though it is expected that some of these will be unraveled in the near future. Beyond the challenges of isolating the genes that predispose to these disorders, the implementation of testing for such disorders will pose a number of technical, logistical, and clinical practice challenges. The technical challenges of such testing will require developing tools to assay one or more alleles of several genes. These technologies, such as microarrays, mass spectroscopy, and gene chips, are already under development and may be mature before the genetic research to find and determine the effects of the genes is complete. It is reasonable to anticipate that such testing will require the input of a small blood sample and entry of a number of clinical parameters (age, sex, weight, etc.) into a computerized testing apparatus. The apparatus will output an assessment not only of the overall risk of the disease but of particular environmental susceptibilities. The melding of this approach with that of pharmacogenomics, described above, will allow prediction of therapeutic options that maximize efficacy and minimize side effects. It should be noted that such testing is not dependent on the presence of any disease symptom, nor is treatment limited to those with symptoms. The ability to diagnose a high susceptibility to adult-onset diabetes mellitus, for example, may allow presymptomatic pharmacologic treatment of insulin resistance and dietary advice about weight control that might delay or even prevent the onset of frank disease.

TREATMENT

Clinical genetics has been historically characterized as a diagnostic specialty because it has traditionally focused on diagnosis, prognosis, and counseling but provided few treatment options. This perception was never entirely correct, and the specialty is changing rapidly in this regard. The dissection of the molecular pathophysiology of disease, the ability to assess individual disease susceptibility, and pharmacogenomics will provide opportunities for treatment of many common and rare genetic disorders. Thus, the molecular dissection of human disease will provide a plethora of therapeutic targets and the design of novel classes of agents to be applied to the treatment and prevention of disease. All of these advances will require internists to expand their current understanding of genetic diagnosis and treatment.

BIBLIOGRAPHY

Gelehrter TD, Collins FS, Ginsburg D. *Principles of medical genetics.* Baltimore: Williams & Wilkins, 1998.

King RA, Rotter JI, Motulsky AG. *The genetic basis of common diseases.* New York: Oxford University Press, 1992.

Scriver CR, Beaudet AL, Sly WS, et al. *The metabolic and molecular bases of inherited disease,* seventh ed. New York: McGraw-Hill, 1995.

Kelley's Textbook of Internal Medicine, fourth edition. Edited by H. David Humes.
Lippincott Williams & Wilkins, Philadelphia © 2000.

C H A P T E R
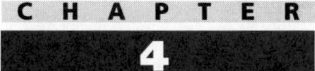

CELL GROWTH, DIFFERENTIATION, AND DEATH

MAX WICHA

In multicellular organisms, the function and fate of cells is tightly regulated. These cells must respond to environmental factors and to each other in a manner that promotes survival and reproduction of the entire organism. The basic mechanisms involved in this complex organization and cellular interdependence have been conserved throughout evolution and are remarkably similar in organisms as diverse as the roundworm, the fruit fly, mice, and humans.

As indicated in Figure 4.1, cell function can be conceptualized as occurring along three pathways: cell growth (division), cell differentiation, and cell death (apoptosis). Although these are depicted as distinct pathways, in actuality they are highly interconnected. The extracellular signals that regulate these cellular behaviors fall into three main classes: soluble signals (hormones and growth factors), extracellular matrix (ECM) signals (e.g., basement membrane), and cell–cell interactions (gap junctions). These extracellular signals act on the cell through specific receptors that transmit this information to the interior cellular machinery through signal transduction pathways. The cell must in turn integrate these complex signals and respond by initiating programs of cell growth, differentiation, or cell death. Our knowledge of the molecular details of these pathways has been greatly expanded in recent years. It has also become clear that disregulation of these pathways results in a variety of pathologic

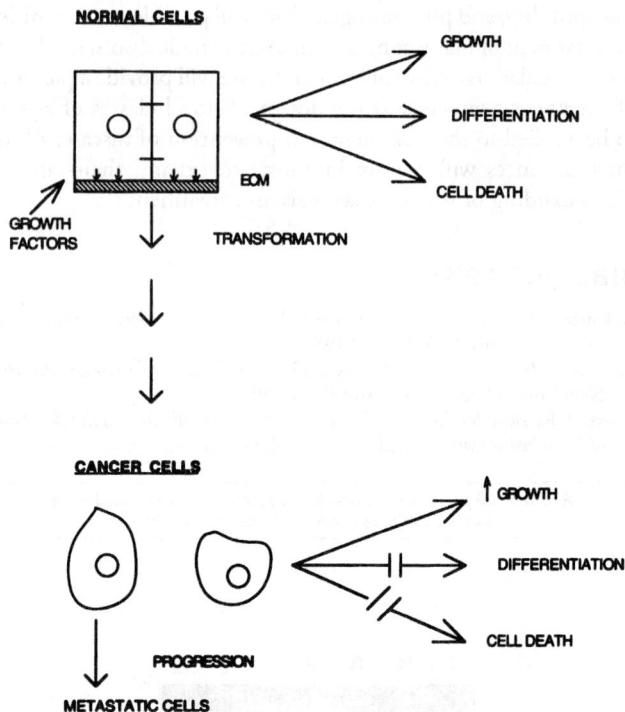

FIGURE 4.1. Regulation of cell growth, differentiation, and death. In normal cells, cell growth, differentiation, and death are regulated by extracellular signals from soluble signals (hormones and growth factors), extracellular matrix components, and cell–cell communication. Defects in these pathways result in neoplastic transformation.

conditions, including cancer formation (Fig. 4.1). Aspects of these pathways are summarized below and discussed in more detail in references.

EXTRACELLULAR SIGNALS

GROWTH FACTORS, HORMONES, AND THEIR RECEPTORS

Growth factors and hormones serve to facilitate intercellular communication to coordinate cellular functions in complex multicellular organisms. Hormones produced in one organ act at distant sites, whereas growth factors and cytokines usually act locally, facilitating interactions between tissues. This interaction manifests itself in such phenomena as stromal epithelial interactions regulating cellular differentiation. Such locally acting factors are said to function in a paracrine fashion.

Both hormones and growth factors act by binding to specific cellular receptors, either on the plasma membrane or in the intracellular compartment. These receptors in turn initiate signal transduction pathways that ultimately regulate gene expression, controlling growth, differentiation, and cell death states. There has been a tremendous increase in our understanding of receptor function. This information has provided important new insights for pharmacologic development. In general, cell receptors can be divided into two classes. "Cargo receptors" (such as the low-density lipoprotein receptor) deliver nutrients, minerals, and

other components directly to cells. Such receptors themselves do not initiate signal transduction pathways. The other major class of receptors are capable of interacting with and triggering intracellular signal transduction molecules. For example, one class of these receptors has intrinsic activity, such as that of tyrosine kinase, and are activated by growth factors. Receptors in this class with tyrosine kinase activity include those for epidermal growth factor and platelet-derived growth factor. Another class of receptors of which several hundred have been described is coupled to large G proteins.

EXTRACELLULAR MATRIX AND INTEGRINS

Extracellular matrix molecules provide a scaffolding to which most cells are anchored. The composition of the ECM differs from tissue to tissue. Epithelial and endothelial cells are anchored to a basement membrane containing mostly type IV collagen, laminin, and heparan sulfate proteoglycans, whereas stromal cells are anchored to an ECM consisting largely of type I and type III collagens and fibronectin. It is now clear that these ECMs are far more than an inert scaffolding; rather, they provide important positional information and cooperate closely with growth factors and hormones to regulate cellular functions. For example, the basement membrane attachment of epithelial cells regulates their decisions to undergo growth, differentiation, or cell death.

The ECM molecules interact with cells through specific receptors, the most important of which are the integrin receptors. These heterodimeric molecules mediate cellular attachment to ECM and are linked to signal transduction pathways. There are important interactions between these ECM-regulated pathways and those for growth factors, allowing cells to integrate complex information from the cell's environment. Furthermore, the interaction between ECM and integrin receptors is bidirectional. The ECM components regulate integrin expression and activation, and integrins function in turn in ECM assembly. Abnormalities in these pathways may contribute to a number of disease states, such as cardiovascular disease and psoriasis.

CELL–CELL INTERACTIONS AND GAP JUNCTION PROTEINS

Cells may communicate directly with each other through proteins that form small channels, termed *gap junctions,* which link cells within tissues. Gap junctions are composed of a family of proteins known as connexins. Most normal cells utilize these channels to transport nutrients and small molecules. At least 13 connexins have been described, and recently, the three-dimensional structure of a recombinant gap junction channel was solved. Mutations in connexin molecules have been described and are believed to play an important role in the etiology of a number of human disease states such as the X-linked form of Charcot–Marie–Tooth syndrome and autosomal recessive deafness, as well as abnormalities in the development of the cardiovascular system. In addition, it has been shown that many if not most cancers show defects in gap junctional communication, which might contribute to their cellular autonomy.

CELL GROWTH, DIFFERENTIATION, AND DEATH

As summarized above, cells receive diverse cues from their environment through interconnecting signal transduction pathways. In turn, cells regulate the expression of genes that determine whether a quiescent cell will enter the cell cycle, differentiate, or die.

CELL CYCLE

Growth factors engaging specific cellular receptors trigger signal transduction pathways that in turn cause quiescent cells in the G_0 phase of the cell cycle to enter the cell cycle G_1 at which time specific protein synthesis begins. In late G_1 the cell reaches a point termed the restriction point R in which the cell makes a commitment to undergo DNA replication and complete the cell cycle. DNA is replicated during the S phase. Following the G_2 phase, the cell divides in the M or mitotic phase. At each stage in the cell cycle, cells must traverse checkpoints that ensure the integrity of the process. Abnormalities in cell cycle control contribute to such disease states as arteriosclerosis and cancer. An understanding of these pathways might lead to new interventions for these diseases.

DIFFERENTIATION

Most cells in tissues and organs are capable of exiting the cell cycle and initiating a program of gene expression specific to these tissues. It is this process, termed *terminal differentiation,* that distinguishes cells in different organs such as those in the liver, brain, or breast. Deregulation of these differentiation pathways might contribute to cancer formation.

CELL SENESCENCE AND DEATH

In 1961, Hayflick showed that normal somatic cells have a limited replicated potential of approximately 50 cell divisions. Furthermore, fibroblasts from younger individuals underwent more cell divisions than those from older individuals, suggesting that a finite number of cell divisions characterizes both in vivo and in vitro growth. Although the mechanisms responsible for this phenomenon have yet to be fully elucidated, there is increasing evidence that shortening of the telomeric ends of chromosomes during each cell division plays an important role in determining cellular age and in triggering cellular senescence. In support of this, expression of the enzyme telomerase, which can block telomere shortening, results in increased replicative life span of cells. The contribution of telomerase to human aging and related diseases remains to be determined; however, many tumor cells express telomerase, thus overcoming replicative senescence.

APOPTOSIS

Another process that limits growth of cells is programmed cell death, or "apoptosis." This process plays a pivotal role in such normal processes as lymphocyte and nervous system development. In addition, it provides a means for multicellular organisms to eliminate cells damaged beyond repair. There has been a tremendous increase in our knowledge of the intracellular pathways that mediate apoptosis. There is substantial evidence that growth factors, hormones, and ECM, regulate apoptotic pathways, ensuring that a cell in an inappropriate environment will "self-destruct." The apoptotic "threshold" of a cell is regulated by the bcl-2 family of proteins, which act by regulating cytochrome c release. These pathways might have evolved as a protection against neoplastic transformation. Indeed, most if not all cancers have defects in cellular apoptotic pathways. In contrast, inappropriate activation of caspases may be important in a variety of neurodegenerative diseases such as Alzheimer's disease.

Apoptotic pathways have been highly conserved in organisms as diverse as worms, flies, mice, and humans. Indeed, valuable insights into these pathways have come from elucidation of apoptosis pathways in the roundworm, *Caenorhabditis elegans.* Apoptotic signals result in cell death through activation of a specific set of proteases, termed caspases, which cleave at aspartic acid residues, and ultimately result in cellular destruction. These caspases may be activated through specific cellular receptors, such as *fas,* or through the sensing of cellular damage. This results in mitochondrial release of cytochrome c, which together with the protein Apaf-1 and dATP initiates caspase activation and triggers cell death.

INTER-RELATIONSHIP OF SIGNAL TRANSDUCTION PATHWAYS

Although signaling mechanisms and signal transduction pathways have been described as distinct pathways, in actuality they are highly interconnected. For instance, appropriate hormones, ECM, and cell–cell contact are necessary for cells to initiate differentiation programs. In addition, both growth factors and ECM closely cooperate in regulating cell growth and apoptosis. Removal of either the appropriate growth factor or ECM molecule triggers a normal cell to undergo apoptosis. In addition, there is evidence that cell growth and death are closely related. This interconnection might have evolved as a mechanism to prevent against cancer formation. The recent development of new DNA array technologies that can simultaneously examine the expression of thousands of genes promises to lead to a better understanding of how these signal transduction pathways interact. Indeed, the picture that is emerging from such technologies is that these pathways are not linear but rather branched networks with numerous interconnections. These new technologies might facilitate our understanding of how defects in these pathways contribute to human diseases. Furthermore, elucidation of these pathways provides a multitude of new targets for therapeutic development.

BIBLIOGRAPHY

Adams JM, Cory S. The Bcl-2 protein family: arbiters of cell survival. *Science* 1998;281(5381):1322–1326.

Bata-Csorgo Z, Cooper KD, Ting KM, et al. Fibronectin and alpha5 integrin regulate keratinocyte cell cycling: a mechanism for increased fibronectin protentiation of T cell lymphokine–driven keratinocyte hyperproliferation in psoriasis. *J Clin Invest* 1998;101(7):1509–1518.

Bergoffen J, Scherer SS, Wang S, et al. Connexin mutations in X-linked Charcot–Marie–Tooth disease. *Science* 1993;262(5142):2039–2042.

Braun-Dullaeus RC, Mann MJ, Dzau VJ. Cell cycle progression: new therapeutic target for vascular proliferative disease. *Circulation* 1999;98(1):82–89.

Evan G, Littlewood T. A matter of life and cell death. *Science* 1998;281(5381):1317–1322.

Fossel M. Telomerase and the aging cell: implications for human health. *JAMA* 1998;279(21):1732–1735.

Iyer VR, Eisen MB, Ross DT, et al. The transcriptional program in the response of human fibroblasts to serum. *Science* 1999;283(5398):83–87.

Makino S, Fukuda K, Kodama H, et al. Expression of cyclins, cyclin-dependent kinases and cell cycle inhibitors in terminal differentiation of cardiomyocytes. *Circulation* 1997;96(8S):513-I.

Ruoslahti E, Engvall E. Integrins and vascular extracellular matrix assembly. *J Clin Invest* 1997;100(11S):53S–56S.

Stergiopoulos K, Taffet SM, Delmar M. Connexin diversity and pH regulation of gap junction channels. *Circulation* 1998;98(17S):8211.

Stone DK. Receptors: structure and function. *Am J Med* 1998;105(3):244–250.

Thornberry NA, Lazebnik Y. Caspases: enemies within. *Science* 1998;281(5381):1312–1316.

Unger VM, Kumar NM, Gilula NB, et al. Three-dimensional structure of a recombinant gap junction membrane channel. *Science* 1999;283(5405):1176–1180.

Kelley's Textbook of Internal Medicine, fourth edition. Edited by H. David Humes. Lippincott Williams & Wilkins, Philadelphia © 2000.

TABLE 5.1. CLASSIFICATION OF DISEASES INVOLVING THE IMMUNE SYSTEM

Disease of immune deficiency (ie, failures to perform one or more surveillance and elimination function)

Disorders of immune recognition and response

  Allergic diseases (ie, misidentification of environmental exogenous molecules as suitable targets for an IgE or cellular immune response)

  Autoimmune diseases (ie, misidentification of endogenous self antigens as targets of an immune response)

    Attack of self by T cells; release of cytokines

    Attack by antibody and immune complex disease

Persistent infections

  Disease may result from viral infection of cells, such as neurons without effective class I surveillance mechanism, by suppression of surveillance mechanisms, or lack of ability of an individual's immune system to recognize appropriate regions of the viral sequence.

  Effector mechanisms of injury may merge with those of autoimmune disease.

Disorders of inappropriate activation of elements of the immune system, such as nephritogenic streptococcal infection that induces C3nef; superantigen activation syndromes, including toxic shock syndrome; and possibly Kawasaki's disease and rheumatic fever

Unregulated proliferation of immune system cells, such as leukemias, lymphomas, and benign monoclonal gammopathy, which each reflect clonal expansion of a lymphoid cell at a particular state of differentiation

Granulomatous and fibrosing disorders of unknown causes in which wound healing, inflammation, and certain immune effector processes are implicated in the mechanisms of disease

CHAPTER 5

PRINCIPLES OF THE IMMUNE RESPONSE

ROBERT WINCHESTER

INTEGRATION OF THE SYSTEMS MEDIATING INFLAMMATION, WOUND HEALING, AND IMMUNITY

The integrated and closely regulated group of diverse processes responsible for the homeostatic maintenance of tissue integrity includes wound healing, inflammation, and the immune response. Two fundamentally distinct systems contribute to the immune response. The first is the adaptive immune system proper, based on recognition of specific unique antigenic structures by different clones of lymphocytes. The function of the adaptive system depends on expansion of particular lymphocyte clones and their subsequent differentiation into effector cells, each separately specific for unique structures. These phenomena account for the acquisition of specific immune recognition and for immune memory. The second is the innate immune system. It is triggered by stereotyped receptors that recognize evolutionarily conserved features of microorganisms or by receptors that recognize cytokines elaborated by activated or injured cells. The innate immune system includes the mononuclear and polymorphonuclear, leukocyte phagocytes, natural killer (NK) cells, and the complement, clotting, and fibrinolysis systems of the plasma. A large number of diseases or pathophysiologic processes may be classified as the direct or indirect result of either the failure of one of these homeostatic mechanisms to maintain tissue integrity or an inappropriately excessive activation of a response system that suggests improper function of a regulatory element (Table 5.1).

The coordination of the immune and inflammatory responses involves the interaction of several cell lineages, including lymphocytes, monocytes, macrophages, dendritic cells, and vascular endothelium. The regulation of these interactions is through the release of cytokines and chemokines as well as cell–cell contact. However, these coordinating molecules have the potential to affect the structure and function of bystander cells that compose the organ in which the response is occurring.

COMPONENTS OF THE INNATE IMMUNE SYSTEM

THE NEUTROPHIL

The terminally differentiated circulating neutrophil has a half-life of 6 hours and is produced at a baseline rate of 10^{11} per day.

Neutrophils have a series of innate immune defense functions initiated by engagement of stereotyped receptors typical of the innate immune system that are shared by neutrophil, macrophage, and monocyte lineage cells. There are receptors that stimulate phagocytosis, such as those binding the immunoglobulin constant region (FcR), and complement receptors that bind to particles opsonized with C3b or C3bi, products of the activated complement system. There are also receptors for stereotyped structures on microorganisms, such as CD14, the receptor that binds bacterial lipopolysaccharide (endotoxin) when complexed to the serum lipopolysaccharide–binding protein and formyl–methionine–leucine–phenylalanine receptors that are directly triggered by the N-terminally modified peptide characteristic of prokaryotes. Other receptors bind the chemotactic and activating anaphylatoxic fragments of certain complement components, such as C3a and C5a. Many of these receptors are G-protein-linked. The response of the neutrophil to engagement of these receptors is rapid activation characterized by multiple events, among which are up-regulation from preformed reserves and subsequent activation of molecules such as the C3bi receptors CR3 (CD11b/CD18) and CR4 (CD11c/CD18), integrin structures that have adhesive and phagocytic functions. The CR3 and CR4 receptors also function in aspects of leukocyte adhesion involving passage of these cells into sites of inflammation from the vasculature, but this depends on interaction with counter-receptors such as intercellular adhesion molecule (ICAM) and not with C3b. The disorder known as leukocyte adhesion deficiency involves a defect in production of the CD18 chain and illustrates the importance of this molecule to inflammation. Other consequences of neutrophil activation include production of reactive oxygen intermediates, discharge of proteolytic enzymes, activation of arachidonic acid cascades, and release of cytokines such as interleukin-1 (IL-1), IL-8, tumor necrosis factor α (TNF-α), and IL-12, which signal to both neutrophils and other cells in the innate and adaptive immune response.

Inappropriate triggering of neutrophil receptors by cytokines or other triggers results in the marked activation of adhesive receptors, especially the CDllb/CD18 integrin molecule. The overexpression of this molecule appears to be implicated in the induction of the pathologic states of homotypic neutrophil–neutrophil adhesion underlying a Schwartzmann response–like reaction in blood vessels and lungs. This response is seen in certain infections, in immune disorders such as systemic lupus erythematosus, and in vasculopathies.

MONONUCLEAR PHAGOCYTES

The mononuclear phagocyte, including monocytes and macrophages, is arguably the central cell lineage in inflammation and immunity, serving as a critical link between the innate and the adaptive immune systems. The relatively long life of this cell and its ability to respond to a variety of stimuli by sustained changes in patterns of gene expression result in its prolonged activation, modulation, or differentiation.

The engagement of one or more of the receptors on the mononuclear phagocytes that are shared with the neutrophil initiates the response of activation that includes the synthesis of a variety of cytokines, including IL-1, IL-6, IL-8, IL-12, and TNF-α. Interleukin-1 and TNF-α act on the vascular endothelium to increase its expression of adhesive receptors and foster an increase in permeability, allowing cells and plasma factors necessary for the inflammatory response to enter the tissue. Interleukins 1 and 6 foster lymphocyte activation. Interleukin-12 causes both activation of NK cells and differentiation of CD4 T cells to a T_h1 phenotype. Interleukin-8 is responsible for neutrophil chemotaxis and, in concert with TNF-α, for neutrophil activation. Interleukin-6 also orchestrates the systemic response of fever by acting on the hypothalamus and the hepatic synthesis of acute phase reactants.

The mononuclear phagocyte is the effector cell for two components of the adaptive immune system. First, it recognizes and phagocytizes targets that have been coated with specific antibody or opsonized with C3b. Second, it is specialized for an intricate interaction with CD4 T cells that involves serving not only as the effector cell of an antigen-activated CD4 T cell, but also as one of the cells capable of presentation of antigen to this T cell. Indeed, some monocytes differentiate into dendritic cells that are particularly specialized for the presentation of peptides to naive CD4 T cells. The activated CD4 T cell in turn elaborates a series of cytokines including IL-1 and interferon-γ (IFN-γ), which bind to receptors present on the monocyte. These cytokines, in concert with cell–cell interactions involving molecules such as CD40L, prompt the monocyte to become activated to a far more destructive functional stage, characterized by more effective phagocytosis and killing. The interaction of the CD4 T cell with the macrophage also influences the potential for the naive CD4 T cell to differentiate into either a T_h1 or a T_h2 effector T cell through the phagocyte's elaboration of cytokines such as IL-12. Another pathway of IFN-γ production is via the NK cell, discussed below.

The tissue macrophage can remain in an activated state for several months, releasing additional cytokines and engaging in cell–cell interactions that result in the accumulation and activation of fibroblasts. This process, if sustained, leads to a granulomatous and fibrotic reaction. Sustained release of cytokines such as IL-1 and TNF-α may alter the pattern of gene expression in the parenchymal cells of the involved organ. Thus, the inappropriately activated monocyte is a key mediator of pathogenic consequences in many diseases apart from those with a typical autoimmune etiology, and agents that block the effects of TNF-α are finding application in various diseases. The activated monocyte may also express tissue factor and plasminogen activator, which serve to initiate clotting and fibrinolysis, respectively. Inappropriate activation of the monocyte by autoantibodies occurs in the antiphospholipid syndrome, resulting in pathologic thrombosis.

NATURAL KILLER CELLS

The NK cell is an unusual member of the lymphocyte lineage that does not have a somatically rearranged T-cell antigen receptor (TCR), but contains several stimulatory and inhibitory receptors that regulate its ability to kill target cells. Different NK subpopulations exist with various combinations of stimulatory and inhibitory receptors. Among these is CD16, an Fc receptor that stimulates the NK cell to kill antibody-coated targets in the antibody-dependent cellular cytotoxicity (ADCC) pathway. The stimulated NK cell produces IL-4, a cytokine that deviated the adaptive CD4 T-cell response toward the production of T_h2 cells. In addition, the NK cell has receptor for cytokines such as IL-12 and TNF-α, and the combination of these two cytokines produced by the macrophage or neutrophil elicits the production of IFN-γ by the NK cell. Interferon-γ acts to activate the macrophage and also causes the CD4 T-cell response to deviate to a T_h1 phenotype.

In addition, the NK cell has several other types of important but less well-defined activating receptors. One of these is a lectin receptor that recognizes cell surface carbohydrate of intracellularly infected cells. Another receptor recognizes self antigens presented by the CD1d molecules. This recognition involves an unusual type of T-cell $\alpha\beta$ receptor that does not undergo somatic junctional diversity and often uses a single Vα and Jα gene segment, Vα24 and JαQ. These two receptors are involved in the recognition of tumor or infected cells. Key to the regulation of the function of these latter self-recognition receptors are two additional receptors with interesting recognition specificities that give an inhibitory signal to the NK cell and prevent its killing a normal cell. One receptor is a heterodimer of two molecules used to define the presence of a cell in the NK lineage (CD94 and NKG2). This molecule recognizes human leukocyte antigen E (HLA-E), a nonclassic major histocompatibility complex (MHC) class I molecule that can usually be expressed only if other typical class I molecules are expressed. Another receptor is the killer inhibitory receptor (KIR), which comes in several varieties that are separately specific for HLA-A, B, or C class I MHC molecules. Thus, normal class I molecules down-regulate a potentially always "on" killing function of NK cells. When class I gene expression is altered by certain intracellular infections with viruses and some other microorganisms, or by malignant transformation, the potential of the NK cell to kill the target cell is released.

COMPLEMENT SYSTEM

The complement system is a tightly regulated cascade of at least 24 interacting molecules found in serum and on cells. It participates in the inflammatory response in three ways. First, it coordinates several elements of the inflammatory response to microorganisms and tissue injury through the generation of potent, biologically active peptides, C3a and C5a, termed anaphylatoxins, derived from cleavage of C3 and C5 that initiate effects such as mononuclear phagocyte or neutrophil activation, chemotaxis, and adhesion. The anaphylatoxins also directly enhance endothelial permeability and cause mast cell degranulation. Second, the system participates in the immune response as a potent amplifier of phagocytosis. It facilitates this function by coating (opsonizing) the target particle with the C3b fragment derived from C3. Third, the complement system has a series of proenzymes and other molecules that form the membrane attack complex capable of lysing the cell membranes of certain bacteria such as *Neisseria* and human cells.

The central event in the complement system is the generation of C3 convertase, which cleaves C3 into C3a and C3b. Three different recognition events and associated pathways initiate the generation of C3 convertase. The classical complement pathway is activated by IgG or IgM immune complexes. The transducing molecule is C1q, a part of the trimolecular first component of the complement system. C1q circulates loosely bound to serum immunoglobulin molecules but, on encountering several immunoglobulin molecules fixed to an antigen, C1q undergoes a conformational change that initiates activation of the classic pathway. It then interacts with C2 and C4 to generate C3 convertase. The classical pathway can also be activated by the binding of C1q to the acute phase protein (C-reactive protein) when the latter has bound to certain bacterial and fungal lipopolysaccharides. A second pathway is initiated by bacterial mannose-containing carbohydrate. The transducing molecule is a plasma protein, mannan-binding lectin (MBL), a calcium-dependent lectin that shares overall structural features with C1q and, like it, activates C2 and C4. This activation occurs via binding of MBL to two proteases, the MBL-associated proteases (MASP-1 and MASP-2). The third, or alternative, pathway is triggered by C3b fragments bound to a substrate that have been generated through either of the preceding pathways and is in many respects an amplification loop. Factors B and D bind to C3b to generate the C3 convertase activity.

A set of circulating proteins and cell-associated molecules regulate the ability of the complement system to injure the individual's own cells. Most act to reduce the generation or effect of C3 convertase. C1 inhibitor, in contrast, acts to inhibit the serine esterase function of C1, and a deficiency of this molecule results in hereditary angioneurotic edema. CD59 acts to prevent the formation of the membrane attack complex on homologous cells. This GPI-anchored protein becomes deficient in some hemopoietic clones in paroxysmal nocturnal hemoglobinuria.

In addition to the complement receptors, CR3 and CR4, discussed previously, another complement receptor on phagocytic leukocytes capable of binding C3b is CR1 (CD21), a member of the immunoglobulin family. CR1 is also highly expressed on erythrocytes where it serves the protective function of binding soluble circulating immune complexes and transporting them to the liver for removal. Erythrocyte CR1 is markedly depleted in immune complex diseases.

THE INNATE IMMUNE SYSTEM IN THE RESPONSE TO EARLY INFECTION

The integration of these systems is seen in the early events of an infection. Almost immediately after entrance of microorganisms into the tissue, the foreign organisms are detected by binding and activation of complement components through the MBL pathway or by binding C-reactive protein. Wandering tissue neutrophils and monocytes initially interact with the microorganism through their stereotyped receptors that recognize characteristic features of microbial structure and are subsequently drawn to the microorganism by complement chemotactic fragments or the presence of bacterial products. The immediate response of the neutrophil is to release cytokines and chemokines that recruit additional neutrophils and monocytes, as well as lymphocytes, into the region through their effects on both the vasculature and the leukocytes. The monocyte reinforces the chemokine release initiated by the neutrophil, and together both phagocytes may interact with NK cells to initiate elaboration of IFN-γ to potentiate monocyte activation—functions also related to the adaptive immune response.

ENTRANCE OF CELLS INTO A SITE OF INFLAMMATION

As discussed above, the presence of inflammation in a region is reflected by alterations in the vascular endothelium that are induced by cytokines such as IL-1, IFN-γ, and TNF-α. These act on the vascular endothelium to increase the expression of adhesive receptors such as ICAM-1 and vascular addressins. At the same time, a gradient of immunoreactants is established. The immunoreactants include chemokines released by neutrophils or monocytes (macrophage inflammatory protein, IL-8) that have had chance encounters with the bacteria or that have been activated by other routes. Other potent chemokines, such as slow death factor–1 (SDF-1), are released by parenchymal cells. Anaphylatoxins such as C3a and C5a are elaborated locally if a microorganism activates the complement system. The intravascular leukocyte that enters this inflammatory environment is diverted from rapid laminar flow motion and begins to roll along the endothelium, interacting weakly with the addressins via its homing receptors. When the leukocyte encounters the gradient of immunoreactants it undergoes prompt activation via G-protein-coupled receptors that activate β₂ integrins such as lymphocyte function–associated antigen–1 (LFA-1, or CD11a) to an adhesive state. This arrests the leukocyte via an interaction with molecules such as ICAM-1. The chemokine receptors are rapidly inactivated, releasing the cell to diapedese through the endothelial junctions to enter the tissue. There it is attracted to the site of inflammation by the chemokinetic gradient of immunoreactants.

◼ THE ADAPTIVE IMMUNE SYSTEM

The adaptive immune system is characterized by the following: (a) the intricate diversity and specificity of the recognition structures employed in the immune response; (b) the somatic genetic processes underlying their development; (c) the clonal nature of the expression of these receptors; (d) the selection of an individually specific repertoire that is efficient and lacking potential for injurious self-recognition; and (e) the selective processes of clonal expansion and the differentiation to effector status that is induced by antigen. The adaptive immune system is closely interrelated to the innate immune system, making a highly antigen-specific way of intensively activating the innate immune system to a higher level of selective destruction that could not be obtained through the use of stereotyped receptors.

ADAPTIVE IMMUNE RESPONSE PROVIDES MULTIPLE TYPES OF IMMUNITY

The inaccurate older division of the adaptive immune system into humoral and cellular components has been replaced by grouping the main protective tasks facing the immune system into three categories that each involve a fundamentally different type of immunity.

CD4 T-CELL SYSTEM

This component of the adaptive immune system deals with recognizing the presence of microorganisms, such as bacteria (e.g., *Mycobacterium tuberculosis*), fungi, and parasites that seek to replicate within the environment of the body and that can be phagocytized by macrophages. The CD4 TCR is specialized to recognize small portions of the amino acid sequence of antigens that have been endocytized and degraded to peptides of 9 to 15 amino acids in the endocytic pathway following phagocytosis (Fig. 5.1). The peptides are bound by the MHC class II molecules in a chaperone-like function. The class II molecules have previously trafficked to the endosome with the aid of a protein, the invariant chain, that both directs the MHC class II molecule to the endosomal compartment and blocks the peptide binding groove. The invariant chain is degraded in the endosome, freeing the MHC molecule to bind peptides derived from ingested proteins. The MHC molecule containing a peptide then travels to the cell surface where antigen presentation occurs. The complex of MHC class II molecule and peptide is recognized by specific TCRs found on CD4 T-cell clones. The CD4 molecule assists in this recognition process by specifically binding to MHC class II molecules.

B-CELL SYSTEM

The second parallel adaptive immune system detects largely the same group of organisms as the CD4 T-cell immune system, but it is able to recognize regions of molecules in their intact state or free in solution prior to phagocytosis and digestion. This system is centered on the properties of the specific B-cell antigen receptors present on the surface of B cells that are capable of recognizing molecular conformations with sufficient affinity such that there is no requirement for an antigen-presenting mol-

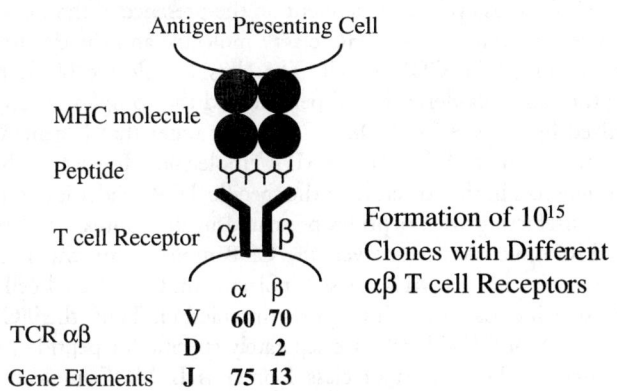

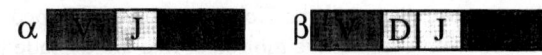

FIGURE 5.1. The molecular elements involved in the somatic generation of an αβ T-cell receptor from germ line elements.

ecule. When a B-cell clone characterized by a specific BCR responds fully to recognition of a specific antigen, the B-cell terminally differentiates into a plasma cell and expresses the recognition portion of the specific B-cell antigen receptor in a soluble form that is the familiar antibody of humoral immunity. We can envision that the requirement to control organisms, such as *Streptococcus pneumoniae,* drove the evolution of this immune system. These organisms are optimally controlled by the formation of antibodies that coat the incoming organism, placing on it a set of recognition signals that activate neutrophil phagocytosis and other effector systems described in the section on innate immunity, leading to clearance and inactivation of the invader.

In the B-cell system, there is another extensive level of diversification of the receptor immunoglobulin molecule involving the constant regions and their potential to interface with various effector systems. IgM and IgD are two surface immunoglobulin isotypes, both expressing the same variable region sequences. Each has a transmembrane domain and sites for cytoplasmic signaling. As the B cell differentiates to an antibody-secreting form (the plasma cell), different exons are used to encode secreted forms of these molecules. With the help of the CD4 T cell, the immunoglobulin class may switch to IgG, IgA, or IgE. IgA-bearing cells often are found in mucosal membranes, and the IgA molecule may be secreted with a supplemental "chaperone" secretory piece that protects the IgA molecule from digestion. The COOH$^-$ terminal portion of the IgE molecule binds to receptors found in high concentration on basophils and mast cells. This serves to passively arm these cells with receptors containing immunoglobulin detection molecules that are, in allergic individuals, directed to a variety of environmental allergens. The allergic symptoms result from the activation and discharge of the potent pathways of acute inflammation initiated by the molecules of these cells.

CD8 T-CELL SYSTEM

The third task is dealing with infection by a virus, whose own genome can commandeer the replicative machinery of a host cell. The recognition of a virally infected cell, especially early in the infectious cycle, is dependent on the presence of the surveillance functions of the MHC class I molecule and the cytotoxic function of the CD8 T cell. The class I molecule binds the cytoplasmically derived viral peptide and the complex is recognized by the specific CD8 TCR in a manner that is generally similar to that of the class II MHC molecule. However, subtle differences in the structure of the specific TCR render it specific for interacting with peptides presented in the context of class I MHC molecules. Moreover, the CD8 molecule on the T cell interacts with the MHC class I molecule on the infected cell to further increase the affinity of the interaction. Thus, the TCRs on CD8 or CD4 T cells are separately specific for peptide presented in the context of class I or class II MHC molecules, respectively. However, unlike the class II molecules, the class I MHCs are synthesized and assembled with β_2-microglobulin in the endoplasmic reticulum and the Golgi apparatus. The peptides are derived from cytoplasmic molecules that are degraded by a complex of enzymes, the proteasome, and the resulting peptides transported to the endoplasmic reticulum compartment

by an ATP-dependent transporter of antigenic peptides (TAP) that spans the endoplasmic reticulum membrane. The peptides enter the class I molecule peptide binding groove and stabilize its interaction with β_2-microglobulin, resulting in the expression of the class I molecule on the cell surface with its bound peptide. The proteasome system degrades a fraction of all cytoplasmic proteins, especially those with anomalous structural features, a property that might increase the representation of virally encoded peptides in this surveillance system. In the case of an influenza virus–laden respiratory epithelial cell, the virally encoded peptides are degraded in the cell's cytoplasm and appear on the cell surface in the context of MHC class I molecules. Each of the 100,000 to 200,000 MHC class I molecules on the epithelial cell surface displays a single peptide, the large majority being from normal self-peptides, but among them a few contain virally encoded peptides. Each T cell sifts through this collection of presented peptides until it identifies a specific peptide. Recognition activates the cytotoxic mechanism of the peptide-specific CD8 T cell, which kills the infected epithelial cell.

The adaptive systems do not function in separate compartments, e.g., antibodies also play a role in virus infection by mediating viral neutralization or by binding to intact virions budding through the cell surface. Similarly, macrophages phagocytize infected cells if triggered by bound antibodies or by innate mechanisms.

CLONAL BASIS OF ADAPTIVE IMMUNE RECOGNITION AND ITS REGULATION

Engagement of the clonal antigen-specific receptor on the lymphocyte initiates a complex series of signaling events that induce the expression of new genes and initiate several developmental consequences. Included among these genes are those that induce the cell to divide and to sustain subsequent proliferation by an autocrine mechanism, which in the case of the T cells involves elaboration of IL-2 and receptors for this cytokine. Each lymphocyte involved in the recognition of a specific antigen is characterized by a single type of antigen-specific receptor. The descendants of a lymphocyte inherit the same receptor genes, making the same specific receptor and thus constituting a clone. The clones proliferate in response to specific antigenic stimulation. This expansion is one of the key elements that confers enhanced responsiveness to the inciting antigen, the fundamental element of adaptive immunity. The signaling events also include the acquisition of new functional properties as a result of the activation and differentiation mediated by this gene expression, the second key element in adaptive immunity. These may be specific effector functions, such as acquiring the mechanism to kill a target by the CD8 T cell, or the secretion of IFN-γ by a CD4 T cell. In the case of the B cell this includes differentiation to antibody-secreting plasma cells. The outcome of the signaling process is not stereotyped and in some instances a proportion of the expanded clone differentiates into long-lived memory cells that remain quiescent until exposed again to the stimulating antigen. This is the third key feature that the response of the lymphocyte provides to the clonal basis of adaptive immunity.

TWO SIGNALS REQUIRED FOR T-CELL ACTIVATION

It is evident that a multiplicity of regulatory steps exist to control this process. While the general process of clonal activation and expansion are common to all lymphocytes, the regulatory steps obviously must be specific to each of the three main lymphocyte lineages to effect their separate control. In the case of the CD4 or CD8 T cell, one or more second signals are required that are provided by the activated antigen-presenting cell. Without these second signals the T cell responds by entering an anergic or tolerized state, presumably to safeguard against stimulation by self-peptides. A dendritic cell, derived from a macrophage precursor, is specially constituted to effectively provide these costimulatory signals. Most CD4 T-cell responses are initiated by antigen presentation by a dendritic cell and then subsequently expanded by subsequent presentation of the same antigen by a macrophage or a B cell, both of which express class II MHC molecules and have the appropriate endocytic processing pathway. In the case of the B cell, internalization of the antigen is mediated by binding to the specific B-cell clonal receptor. The critical second signal is provided by engagement of the CD28 molecule on the T cell with its ligand molecule, B7 (CD80, CD86), that is selectively expressed on the surface of the activated antigen-presenting cell. Activation of the CD4 T cell by this two-signal mechanism also initiates a down-regulatory mechanism in the form of the initiation of synthesis of the molecule CTLA-4 (CD152). This molecule competes with higher affinity to bind to the B7 molecule, making it unavailable to the T cell. Furthermore, engagement of CTLA-4 by B7 activates an additional negative signaling pathway in the T cell.

The expression of several molecules on the surface of the activated T cell serves as clinically useful markers of the presence of T-cell activation. The most frequently measured activation markers are the appearance of MHC class II molecules (HLA-DR), CD69, and CD40 ligand, all of which are undetectable on resting T cells. As the cell continues its response to receptor engagement, the cell surface phenotype changes to reveal the appearance of new molecules such as integrins involved in cell–endothelial adhesion and additional molecules responsible for the trafficking of the cell to particular sites. The problem of getting the lymphocyte that has been activated in a lymph node to the site of inflammation where it is needed is solved by the presence of a variety of homing receptors that are expressed in a combinatorial pattern to give some vascular anatomic specificity. The cells undergo the same sequence of rolling, activation, arrest, and diapedesis discussed above in the section on innate immunity.

CENTRAL ROLE OF THE T_h1 OR T_h2 CD4 T CELL IN REGULATING B-CELL AND CD8 T-CELL RESPONSE TO STIMULATION

The CD4 T cell occupies a central role in the regulation of the response of the B cell to antigen. While the B cell can be fully triggered to activation without involvement of the CD4 T cell, the differentiation of the B cell to a plasma cell, and especially the class switch from IgM to IgG, requires a signal provided by the CD4 T cell. Importantly, the somatic maturation of B-cell affinity, which depends on the induction of mutation in the B-cell receptor and selection of progeny containing the more avidly binding receptors, also requires CD4 T-cell help. The interaction is mediated by a regulatory cell–cell interaction that is somewhat similar to that between CD28 and B7. The B cell constitutively expresses CD40 molecules and stimulation through this molecule by an activated CD4 T cell bearing the CD40 ligand molecule is necessary for induction of these two features of B-cell differentiation. The CD40 ligand molecule is transiently expressed on the CD4 T cell for several hours following activation of the T cell. This requirement for cognate interaction between a B cell and a CD4 T cell responding to the same antigen is an essential mechanism to give specificity to the immune response. While T-cell cytokines such as IL-4 assist in this process, the cell–cell interaction is the biologically relevant control of B-cell differentiation. This interaction between B cell and T cell occurs in the germinal center of the lymph node. It appears that each germinal center is organized around the interaction of a particular clone of CD4 T cells and a clone of B cells undergoing class switching and somatic mutation.

One subset of CD4 T cells, designated the T_h2 T cell, appears particularly specialized to engage in this interaction. The T_h2 T cell is stimulated by peptides presented by MHC class II molecules on the B cell. In turn, it becomes activated, expresses CD40 ligand molecules, and secretes IL-4, IL-5, IL-10, and IL-13, fostering high-affinity IgG antibody production by the B cell. The decay of expression of CD40 ligand on the T_h2 T cell stops the provision of the cognate help activity.

A second subset of CD4 T cells, designated the T_h1 T cell, is primarily involved in either activating macrophages via secretion of IFN-γ or in inducing the differentiation of precursor CD8 T cells to cytolytic effector CD8 T cells. The most characteristic difference between T_h1 and T_h2 CD4 T cells is that T_h1 T cells secrete IFN-γ upon stimulation, while T_h2 T cells secrete IL-4 and related B-cell cytokines. Analogously to the interaction of the T_h2 cell, the T_h1 cell is capable of reacting to antigen presented by the macrophage by in turn fostering further specific activation of the presenting macrophage. T_h1 cells also secrete abundant IL-2. The second role of the CD4 T cell in inducing the differentiation of the CD8 T cell is, however, primarily carried out on the surface of dendritic cells, forming a three-cell complex. The CD40–CD40 ligand system also plays a critical role in these cognate interactions, with the activated CD4 T_h1 cell also transiently expressing the CD40 ligand molecule.

The development of a given CD4 T cell to acquire the T_h1 or T_h2 phenotype is a property of the cytokine milieu and is possibly influenced by the intensity of the signaling through the TCR. Members of a given CD4 T-cell clone can differentiate to either T_h1 or T_h2 status. The presence of IL-12 results in a naive T cell acquiring the T_h1 phenotype, while the presence of IL-4 fosters the development of the T_h2 phenotype. The activation status of the cells of the innate immune system plays a major role in this determination, with activated macrophages or dendritic cells a source of IL-12, whereas NK cells are a source of IL-4.

FORMATION OF THE ADAPTIVE IMMUNE SYSTEM LYMPHOCYTE REPERTOIRES

The enormous size of the initial repertoire of clones bearing different T- and B-cell antigen–specific receptors necessitates that they each be developed by a somatic mechanism in which a limited series of gene elements are joined in a diversification process that produces well in excess of 10^{15} different clones. Otherwise, there is insufficient germ line DNA in a cell to encode these repertoires. The Ig heavy chain and the T-cell β chain are each assembled from four different gene elements: V (variable), D (diversity), J (joining), and C (constant). The Ig light chain and the T-cell α chain are assembled from V, J, and C elements. One level of diversity comes from the selection of various combinations of elements to make up a given receptor chains as shown in Figure 5.1. A second and much greater form of diversification, called junctional diversity, comes about because junctional events that bring together the V, D, and J elements involve nibbling back by exonucleases and addition of nucleotides not encoded in the germ line. This results in chains that differ in size from another by 10 or more amino acids. The somatically created junctional region in the T-cell receptor interacts specifically with the peptide in the MHC molecule.

The B-cell repertoire is formed initially in the bone marrow and subsequently refined to higher affinity interactions during the immune response in the germinal centers. The B-cell tolerance and repertoire formation is less clearly etched and appears far less stringent than T-cell repertoire formation. Indeed, a major form of B-cell clonal regulation is performed by the cognate interaction with CD4 T cells. A large proportion of the receptors of the B-cell repertoire are potentially reactive with self-molecules, as can be demonstrated by the production of autoantibodies by many B cells during infection of the B cell by Epstein–Barr virus. Presumably, this event does not generate a sustained autoimmune disease because T-cell help is not forthcoming.

The T-cell repertoire is generated and stringently selected in the thymus. Somatic mutation is not permitted. Precursor T cells, lacking CD4 and CD8 molecules, begin by rearranging their β chains. If this is successfully done in frame, the β chain pairs with a monomorphic precursor T α chain. This event shuts off the recombination process, excluding the rearrangement of a second β chains (allelic exclusion). The clone expands about 100-fold, at which time α-chain rearrangement is initiated in a successive wave of recombinase activity. At this time, if the rearrangement is successful, the T cell expresses a functional $\alpha\beta$ receptor in association with CD3. The CD4 and CD8 molecules are expressed (double positive) and the cell is subjected to the processes of selection to determine whether the receptor is better suited at recognizing peptides in the context of the individual's class I or class II MHC molecules. If the T cell recognizes a self-peptide in a class I MHC molecule, the cell is signaled to express only CD8 molecules; reciprocally, if it recognizes self-peptides in the context of class II MHC, it will then express only CD4. If the cell is not positively selected by either route, it undergoes apoptosis. Excessively self-reactive T cells are eliminated centrally by negative selection, but this negative selection does not eliminate the potential for all self-reactivity, since the remaining 10^{12} T cells have been selected with a self-peptide.

Subsequently, in the immune response to a microorganism or virus, a number of different T-cell clones are expanded, including ones drawn from different V-region families and characterized by variable junctional patterns. Certain microorganisms contain molecules that bind specific sequences on particular V regions. For example, the staphylococcal exotoxin TSST, which mediated the toxic shock syndrome, binds specifically to all T-cell receptors that have been derived from the V gene designated BV2 (Vβ2). The clinical syndrome is produced by the massive release of a variety of cytokines by all BV2 CD4 and CD8 T cells. Repertoire analysis is proving to give valuable insight into the clonal immune recognition events in immunologic disorders.

AUTOIMMUNE DISEASE

Although the capacity to differentiate self from nonself is considered intrinsic to the formation of the immune system during early development, the phenomenon of positive selection on self-peptides lays the basis for the potential development of overtly autoreactive T cells. It is now clear that autoreactive T cells underlie the development of autoimmune disease by providing help to the switch to IgG isotype and somatic maturation of autoantibody affinity. Thus, autoimmune disease is a reflection of the fact that all T cells used in any immune response have been originally selected on self-peptides. The still unanswered question is what events initiate sustained activation of these T cells in the events leading to the development of an autoimmune disease. The control stage of the two-signal activation requirement and other regulatory check points are bypassed. Two prominent possible mechanisms are activation of a T-cell clone by mimicry of a self-peptide by one in a microorganism and stimulation of a clone by a superantigen. It appears that in all respects the autoimmune response parallels the normal physiologic immune response. The regulatory mechanisms involving CD28 and CD40 ligand appear to be very attractive targets for returning the T cells to a self-tolerant state.

ROLE OF THE MAJOR HISTOCOMPATIBILITY COMPLEX ALLELES IN IMMUNE REGULATION

The alternative allelic forms of the MHC molecules make a critical contribution to diversifying the immune recognition capabilities of a species by endowing each individual with a nearly unique repertoire of T cells that recognizes different peptides. The evolutionary strategy used by the repertoires of immune recognition receptors on CD4 T cells, CD8 T cells, and B cells is to endow each individual with the ability to make any receptor, and before repertoire selection all persons are essentially equivalent. Then this repertoire is selected and edited by events that are dependent on the particular allelic MHC molecules of the individual. The MHC allele differ from one another primarily in a functional sense by the presence of different pockets that preferentially bind different amino acids and hence different peptides. The particular MHC molecules that a person inherits select the particular self-peptides to be bound. The complex of

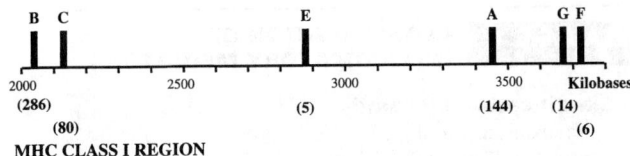

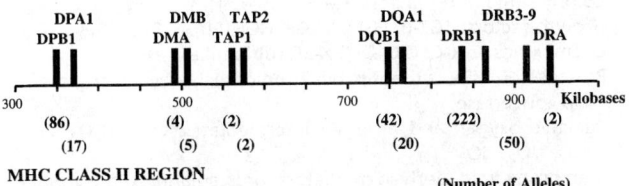

FIGURE 5.2. The organization of class I and II major histocompatibility complex genes. The class II region is centromeric to the class I region on the short arm of the sixth chromosome. The current number of alleles is indicated in parentheses. The genes of the class II region are not shown.

the individual's MHC molecules and self-peptides preferentially bound, in turn, selects the T-cell clones that comprise the CD4 and CD8 T-cell repertoires. Figure 5.2 shows the organization of the class I and II genes of the MHC. The alleles, which are not shown, are numbered and grouped according to the major serologic specificity (e.g., DRI, DR2, B8, B27) that is encoded by the allele. The designation of the allele includes the locus, an asterisk followed by two digits describing the serologic specificity, and an additional two digits referring to the particular allele that reflects the order in which the allele was identified by gene sequencing, e.g., HLA-DRB1*0101 or HLA-B*2705.

As an example, in the class I MHC molecule, the peptide is linearly splayed out, with its NH_2 terminus at the left and COOH terminus to the right. An important pocket in the MHC class I molecule is formed by the polymorphic amino acids that define the different class I alleles. This pocket is located at the upper left portion of the peptide binding grove, under the α-helical portion of the α chain. This pocket, termed the "B" pocket, binds the side chain of what is usually the second amino acid in the antigenic peptide, and it is the major determinant of the specificity of a class I allele for different peptides. For example, this pocket in an HLA-B35 molecule (HLAB*3501) has a narrow hydrophobic shape and preferentially binds peptide antigens with proline at this position. The HLA-B27 (HLAB*2705) molecule has a very hydrophilic pocket with a negative charge at its base, making it likely to bind a peptide with a positively charged lysine or arginine at this position. The universe of peptides seen by T cells in an HLA-B27 molecule nearly all have arginine at position 2, while the very different universe of peptides presented by an HLA-B35 molecule mainly have proline at this position. Other pockets define a second set of specificities for the side chains of the peptide COOH terminus. The positively selected T-cell repertoires of individuals with these two HLA types are, as a result, different. This is the basis of the phenomenon of MHC restriction, which means that the T-cell repertoire selected in an HLA-B27 person is incapable of recognizing a peptide presented in the context of an HLA-B35 molecule and vice versa.

The marked influence that class I or II MHC alleles have on the susceptibility to develop autoimmune disease is a reflection of the repertoire of self-peptides that can be bound and the recognition properties of the T-cell receptors selected by them in the positive selection phase of repertoire formation. For this reason, considerable insight can be gained into a distinctive and potentially pathogenic mechanism by measuring the HLA alleles shared by individuals with a particular disease. There are currently 222 HLA-DRB1 alleles, 286 HLA-B alleles, and 144 HLA-A alleles (Fig. 5.2). In contrast with the situation in the MHC class I molecule, class II MHC molecules have their most important allele-associated binding pockets nearer to the center of the peptide. This point is emphasized by the "shared epitope" susceptibility motif in the region of the fourth amino acid side chain (P4) that confers susceptibility to rheumatoid arthritis. The several alleles (DRB1*0401, 0404, 0101, etc.) that encode positively charged residues in the rim of this pocket on the β chain appear to influence both the T-cell repertoire and the binding of a self-peptide with a negatively charged amino acid in position 4.

If there were no MHC alleles, the resulting state of immunity would be optimized against one set of foreign molecules or peptides. This, from the viewpoint of a microorganism, would be a Maginot line of static defense against which the bacterium or virus would employ its mutational diversity to find a point of vulnerability. For example, a microorganism could mutate to create a peptide sequence that was inefficiently bound or presented by the monomorphic MHC molecule, thus evading recognition and overwhelming the species. Indeed, this unfortunate event does occur in some individuals with chronic HIV infection who are not able to bind functionally critical parts of the virus, leading to the development of escape mutants that can no longer be recognized and controlled by the immune system.

In addition to the use of MHC alleles, another strategy used by the species is to increase the number of different kinds of MHC molecules on the cells of an individual through duplication of class I and II loci. This evolutionary strategy results in the presence on a typical somatic cell of three kinds of classic MHC class I and class II molecules: HLA-A, HLA-B, and HLA-C, and HLA-DR, HLA-DQ, and HLA-DP (Fig. 5-2). The total of 12 to 14 different types of MHC molecules is near the point of diminishing returns for the repertoire. Further numerical increases in different MHC species in an individual would diminish the size of the T-cell receptor repertoire because autoreactivity must be avoided at the price of deleting an increasingly larger proportion of the repertoire.

BIBLIOGRAPHY

Frank M, Austen K, Claman H, et al., eds. *Samter's immunologic diseases*, fifth ed. Two volumes. Boston: Little, Brown and Company, 1995.
Janeway CA, Travers P, Walport M, et al. *Immunobiology: the immune system in health and disease*, fourth ed. New York: Elsevier Science, 1999.

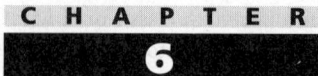

INFLAMMATION: CELLS, CYTOKINES, AND OTHER MEDIATORS

ZOLTAN SZEKANECZ
ALISA E. KOCH

Inflammation is a complex process involving various cell types and inflammatory mediators, such as cytokines, chemokines, growth factors, and proteolytic enzymes, among others. Inflammatory diseases range from hyperacute reactions such as anaphylactic shock to chronic diseases such as rheumatoid arthritis (RA). Cells participating in the inflammatory process include leukocytes (lymphocytes, monocyte/macrophages, neutrophils, eosinophils, basophils, and mast cells) as well as endothelial cells and fibroblasts. The outcome of inflammation depends on the interactions between pro- and anti-inflammatory mediators produced by these cells.

As a clear distinction between acute and chronic inflammation is somewhat artificial due to numerous overlapping patterns, in this chapter we summarize the most important characteristics of the relevant cell types in inflammation, followed by discussion of crucial processes underlying inflammation, including cell adhesion, migration, angiogenesis, and tissue destruction and repair (Table 6.1).

▦ CELLS IN INFLAMMATION

LYMPHOCYTES

T and B cells arise from lymphocyte progenitors in the bone marrow. Both cells are able to recognize the antigen. In addition, T cells interact with other cell types by producing a number of cytokines, as well as by direct cell–cell contact. For example, lymphocyte adhesion to and transmigration through endothelial cells are major events during inflammatory cell infiltration of tissues. Recently, at least two polarized subsets have been distinguished within the $CD4^+$ T-cell population. These subsets have important clinical relevance. Briefly, T_h1-type T cells produce predominantly interferon-γ (IFN-γ), interleukin 2 (IL-2), and IL-12, whereas T_h2-type lymphocytes secrete mostly IL-4, IL-5, IL-6, IL-10, and IL-13. The T_h cell phenotype may determine the function of the T-cell subsets, as T_h1 versus T_h2 cells mediate predominantly cellular versus humoral immune response, respectively. As a clinical example, RA is characterized by T_h1, while systemic lupus erythematosus (SLE), a disease with the production of autoantibodies, has been associated with a T_h2-type response. The T_h1-derived cytokines often inhibit the T_h2-type response and vice versa. T_h2-derived cytokines IL-4, IL-10, and IL-13 have been found to suppress arthritis in animal models.

TABLE 6.1.   CLASSIFICATION OF INFLAMMATORY MEDIATORS

Classification by Family

Interleukins: IL-1 to IL-18
Interferons: IFN-α, IFN-β, IFN-γ
Tumor necrosis factors: TNF-α, TNF-β (LT)
Colony stimulating factors: G-CSF, GM-CSF
Growth factors: TGF-β, FGFs, VEGF, HGF, PDGF, EGF, IGFs
Chemokines: C-X-C, C-C, C, C-X-3C subfamilies
Proteases: MMPs, cathepsin, hyaluronidase, lysozyme, angiotensin convertase
Reactive oxygen and nitrogen intermediates: O_2^-, H_2O_2, OH, NO, NO_2, NO_3
Membrane lipid–derived mediators: prostaglandins, thromboxane, leukotrienes, PAF
Coagulation factors
Components and regulators of the complement cascade
Neuropeptides: substance P, somatostatin, VIP, NGF

Classification by Balance Mechanisms (see text for more details)

Proinflammatory ⇔ anti-inflammatory
T_h1 ⇔ T_h2
Adhesion promoting ⇔ adhesion suppressing
Angiogenic ⇔ angiostatic
Destructive ⇔ destruction-inhibitory
Fibrogenic ⇔ antifibrogenic

EGF, epidermal growth factor; FGF, fibroblast growth factor; G-CSF, granulocyte colony-stimulating factor; GM-CSF, granulocyte-macrophage colony-stimulating factor; HGF, hepatocyte growth factor; IFN, interferon; IGF, insulin-like growth factor; IL, interleukin; LT, lymphotoxin; MMP, matrix metalloproteinase; NGF, nerve growth factor; PAF, platelet-activating factor; PDGF, platelet-derived growth factor; TGF, transforming growth factor; TNF, tumor necrosis factor; VEGF, vascular endothelial growth factor; VIP, vasoactive intestinal peptide.

MONOCYTE/MACROPHAGES

Monocytes are found in the peripheral blood, whereas macrophages are more differentiated monocytes found resident in various tissues including the synovial tissue, the skin, and the internal organs. Some mediators, such as chemokines, are chemotactic for monocytes and may recruit these cells into inflammatory sites. Monocyte/macrophages play a central role in the pathogenesis of chronic inflammation, such as RA. These cells produce proinflammatory cytokines, such as IL-1 and tumor necrosis factor α (TNF-α), as well as granulocyte-monocyte colony-stimulating factor (GM-CSF) in abundance. Macrophages also produce a number of angiogenic mediators and destructive proteolytic enzymes, which play a role in the perpetuation of inflammation. On the other hand, these cells also release inhibitory molecules, such as IL-1 receptor antagonist (IL-1Ra), and reparative mediators, such as transforming growth factor β (TGF-β).

NEUTROPHILS

These cells derive from the myeloid lineage. They are weak producers of IL-1, IL-8, IL-1Ra, TNF-α, and GM-CSF, but the secretion of these cytokines is enhanced in response to TNF-α or GM-CSF. Large numbers of neutrophils are found in certain inflammatory rheumatic diseases, such as in necrotizing vasculitis. A subclass of chemokines stimulate neutrophil accumulation into inflammatory sites. However, while neutrophils play an important role in the development of acute and subacute inflammation, such as reactive arthritis, they may be virtually absent from sites of chronic inflammation, such as the rheumatoid synovial tissue.

EOSINOPHILS, BASOPHILS, AND MAST CELLS

Eosinophils, basophils, and mast cells are key players in immediate hypersensitivity. Basophil-derived mast cells release a number of preformed mediators, such as histamine, neutrophil chemotactic factors (NCF-A), and eosinophil chemotactic factors (ECF-A), as well as neutral proteases and other enzymes. In addition, upon activation they also produce the leukotrienes LTB$_4$, LTC$_4$, and LTD$_4$, thromboxane A$_2$ (TxA$_2$), other lipid products, platelet-activating factor (PAF), adenosine, bradykinin, and several cytokines. Basophils also release histamine, ECF-A, and LTC$_4$. The secretion of these mediators results in vasodilatation, vasopermeability, bronchoconstriction, mucus secretion, edema, and platelet aggregation, which are crucial processes in the pathogenesis of hypersensitivity reactions. In contrast, eosinophils down-regulate these reactions by inactivating histamine, PAF, and leukotrienes. Eosinophils also promote tissue damage in asthma and kill parasites, such as helminths.

ENDOTHELIAL CELLS

These cells themselves probably cannot be considered as "inflammatory cells," although they release a number of cytokines and other mediators. Rather, these cells are targets in systemic inflammation. Resting vascular endothelial cells are not very active, but cytokines such as IL-1, TNF-α, and IFN-γ stimulate endothelia to release vasoactive mediators. Upon activation, endothelial cells also express adhesion molecules and secrete chemokines, thus facilitating leukocyte adhesion and migration into inflammatory sites. Angiogenic mediators, mostly released by macrophages, trigger endothelial cells to form new capillaries. Endothelial activation is also associated with increased vascular permeability. All of these mechanisms lead to increased leukocyte extravasation and thus the perpetuation of inflammation.

FIBROBLASTS

Proinflammatory cytokine-activated fibroblasts produce matrix components including collagen types I and III and fibronectin, and they also release matrix metalloproteinases (MMPs), lipid metabolites, and a variety of cytokines and chemokines. Collagen biosynthesis by fibroblasts is stimulated by TGF-β and inhibited by IFN-γ. The aggressive growth and proliferation of synovial fibroblasts play a key role in pannus formation and joint destruction. Tissue fibrosis is crucial in the pathogenesis of scleroderma, pulmonary fibrosis, and other fibrotic conditions.

INFLAMMATORY MEDIATORS

Cytokines are composed of a broad spectrum of soluble mediators. Apart from interleukins, interferons, and tumor necrosis factors (the first mediators described as cytokines), the discovery of numerous growth factors, colony-stimulating factors, and chemokines (chemotactic cytokines) led to the expansion of the cytokine family (Table 6.1). Mediators of inflammation also contain proteases, reactive oxygen and nitrogen intermediates, membrane lipid–derived mediators, coagulation factors, components and regulators of the complement cascade, and neuropeptides, among others.

INTERLEUKINS

At present, the interleukin family has at least 18 members. Most of them have been associated with inflammation. Interleukins 3, 4, 6, and 11 are involved in neutrophil and monocyte/macrophage development, whereas IL-1, IL-2, IL-4, IL-5, IL-6, IL-7, IL-11, and IL-13 are important for thymocyte/T-lymphocyte differentiation, as well as B- and plasma cell maturation. Interleukins 3 and 5 are also involved in mast cell and eosinophil development, respectively. The role of interleukins in various inflammatory processes will be described later. Briefly, IL-1 and IL-8 are major proinflammatory cytokines. Interleukin 1 exerts a variety of systemic and local proinflammatory effects as it is involved in matrix metabolism by stimulating MMP production, thereby stimulating angiogenesis and cell adhesion molecule expression. IL-8, also a C-X-C chemokine, is chemotactic for neutrophils. In contrast, IL-4, IL-10, and IL-13 inhibit most mechanisms underlying inflammation. Interleukins 6 and 11 have disparate, both pro- and anti-inflammatory effects in chronic inflammation. IL-2 plays a role in T-cell growth and activation. Interleukin 15 exerts IL-2-like activities. The recently described IL-16, IL-17, and IL-18 are involved in T-cell chemotaxis and function.

INTERFERONS

Interferon-γ enhances cell adhesion and activates endothelial cells. Both IFN-α and IFN-γ inhibit neovascularization and fibrosis.

TUMOR NECROSIS FACTOR α

Tumor necrosis factor α plays a central role in inflammation. Tumor necrosis factor α affects leukocyte extravasation, matrix degradation, and angiogenesis in a way similar to that of IL-1. Tumor necrosis factor α induces the production of a number of other proinflammatory cytokines and chemokines, thus up-regulating the inflammatory response.

COLONY-STIMULATING FACTORS

Granulocyte-macrophage colony-stimulating factor and granulocyte colony-stimulating factor (G-CSF) also exert proinflammatory effects. Apart from mediating leukocyte differentiation and growth, these mediators enhance intercellular adhesion and angiogenesis.

GROWTH FACTORS

A number of these mediators are involved in the inflammatory events, mesenchymal cell proliferation and synovial pannus formation. Yet their key functions in inflammation are stimulation of angiogenesis as well as tissue fibrosis and repair. The major angiogenic growth factors are basic and acidic fibroblast growth factors (bFGF and aFGF), as well as vascular endothelial (VEGF), platelet-derived (PDGF), hepatocyte (HGF), epidermal (EGF), insulin-like (IGF-I), and transforming growth factors (TGF-β). Transforming growth factor β, PDGF, IGF-I, FGFs, and EGF are also fibrogenic. These mediators are produced by macrophages and endothelia.

CHEMOKINES

Chemokines constitute the largest cytokine family, consisting of almost 40 members, which has been classified into at least four distinct supergene families based on their structural homology regarding the location of two of four conserved cysteine residues. Some C-X-C chemokines, such as IL-8, epithelial neutrophil-activating protein (ENA) 78, growth-related oncogene α (groα), groβ, and connective tissue–activating protein (CTAP) III are chemotactic for neutrophils, exert proinflammatory effects, and mediate angiogenesis. In contrast, platelet factor 4 (PF4) and IFN-γ-inducible protein-10 (IP-10), which belong to the same subfamily of chemokines, are anti-inflammatory and angiostatic mediators. The C-C chemokines, including monocyte chemoattractant protein-1 (MCP-1), macrophage inflammatory protein–1α (MIP-1α), MIP-1β, and the chemokine termed Regulated upon Activation Normally T cell Expressed and Secreted (RANTES) are monocyte chemoattractants, but they may also be chemotactic for T cells, natural killer cells, basophils, and eosinophils. The role of the recently described additional chemokine families termed C and C-X-C3 chemokines in inflammation is still under investigation.

PROTEOLYTIC ENZYMES

Matrix metalloproteinases, including collagenase, gelatinase, and stomelysin, are crucial mediators of tissue destruction. Proinflammatory cytokines, such as IL-1 and TNF-α, stimulate, whereas anti-inflammatory cytokines, such as IL-4, IL-10, and IL-13, inhibit MMP secretion. Other important enzymes include hyaluronidase, cathepsins, lysozyme, angiotensin convertase, and others.

OTHER INFLAMMATORY MEDIATORS

Reactive oxygen and nitrogen intermediates, such as O_2^-, H_2O_2, OH, NO, NO_2, and NO_3, as well as membrane lipid–derived mediators, such as prostaglandins E_2, $F_{2\alpha}$, leukotrienes, prostacyclin, and PAFs, are produced by macrophages. The activation of the complement system results in the produc-

tion of anaphylatoxins, such as C5a. Neuropeptides including substance P, somatostatin, vasoactive intestinal polypeptide, and nerve growth factor trigger mast cells to secrete histamine. All of these mediators play an important role in tissue destruction and immediate hypersensitivity reactions.

▌ MAJOR BALANCE MECHANISMS IN INFLAMMATION

There is a balance of mediators in inflammation based on feedback mechanisms and the opposing effects of these soluble factors. The net outcome of the inflammatory response depends on the balance or imbalance between these mediators on the levels of cell adhesion, migration, angiogenesis, tissue destruction, and fibrosis (Table 6.1; Fig. 6.1).

INTERCELLULAR ADHESION AND ADHESION MOLECULE EXPRESSION

Leukocyte extravasation into tissues occurs in four distinct steps. The initial, relatively weak adhesion to endothelium termed "rolling," which is mediated by selectins, triggers leukocyte activation due to the interactions between chemokine receptors on leukocytes and proteoglycans on endothelial cells. Then activation-dependent, firm adhesion occurs; this interaction is mediated by integrins. Finally, transendothelial migration or diapedesis occurs when secreted chemokines bind to endothelial proteoglycans. Chemokines attract endothelium-bound neutrophils and mononuclear leukocytes. Among cytokines, IL-1, TNF-α, IL-4, and IFN-γ stimulate the expression of most endothelial adhesion molecules and therefore leukocyte extravasation. Interleukins 12 and 15 have also been found to enhance T-cell recruitment under certain conditions. Cell contact itself may also up-regulate adhesion molecule expression, which is highly TNF-α-dependent. In contrast, anti-inflammatory cytokines,

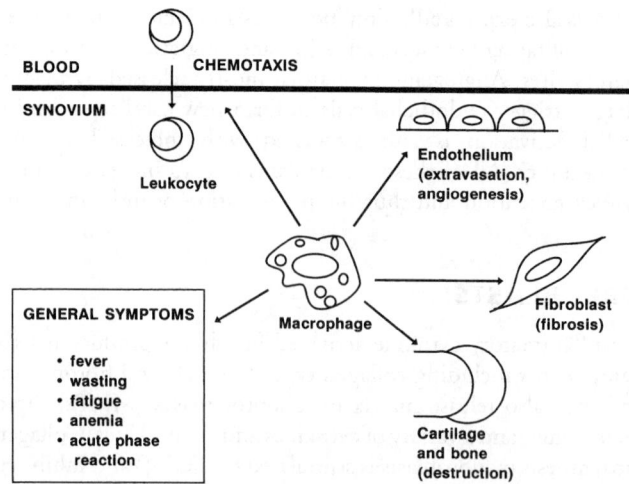

FIGURE 6.1. Interactions between inflammatory cells via mediators in inflammation. This figure represents an example of this intercellular communication existing in the inflamed synovial tissue in rheumatoid arthritis.

such as IL-10 and IL-13, may under various conditions stimulate or inhibit leukocyte-endothelial adhesion and endothelial adhesion molecule expression. Transforming growth factor β also exerts disparate effects on adhesion, as it locally induces integrin expression on leukocytes but may down-regulate adhesion molecule expression on endothelial cells.

PROINFLAMMATORY AND ANTI-INFLAMMATORY MEDIATORS

Interleukin 1, IL-8, and TNF-α have been termed major pro-inflammatory cytokines, as these mediators stimulate most mechanisms in inflammation including cell proliferation and activation, adhesion, chemotaxis, angiogenesis, as well as cartilage and bone destruction. Interleukin 6, the IL-6-like IL-11, and oncostatin M, as well as TGF-β, have both stimulatory and inhibitory effects in inflammation. The T_h2-type cytokines IL-4, IL-10, and IL-13 suppress the T_h1-type response, the production of proinflammatory cytokines, and inflammatory cell emigration. In addition, they increase the synthesis of IL-1Ra, and inhibit the release of proteolytic enzymes. As described above, certain chemokines, such as PF4 and IP-10, may also inhibit crucial events in inflammation.

ANGIOGENESIS

The formation of new vessels leads to the perpetuation of leukocyte emigration. Most growth factors, such as aFGF, bFGF, VEGF, HGF, PDGF, EGF, and IGF-I, the cytokines TNF-α, IL-1, IL-6, and IL-15, as well as some C-X-C chemokines containing the ELR amino acid sequence including IL-8, ENA-78, groα, groβ, and CTAP-III are potent inducers of angiogenesis. In a dose-dependent fashion, TFG-β stimulates or inhibits neovascularization. The major angiostatic mediators are IFN-α, IFN-γ, IL-4, IL-12, and the chemokines PF4 and IP-10.

TISSUE DESTRUCTION

Interleukin 1 and TNF-α are the main proinflammatory and destructive cytokines. Both cytokines stimulate the production of MMPs. Tissue inhibitors of metalloproteinases (TIMPs) oppose the effects of the proteolytic enzymes. Thus, IL-4, IL-10, and IL-13, cytokines stimulating the synthesis of TIMPs, may also prevent tissue injury.

FIBROSIS AND REPAIR

A number of growth factors, such as TGF-β, PDGF, aFGF, bFGF, IGF, and EGF, stimulate fibroblast activation, the transcription of collagen mRNA, and extracellular matrix deposition. Among other "fibrogenic" cytokines, IL-1, IL-4, and TNF-α have been shown to activate fibroblasts, although they are less potent than growth factors. The C-X-C chemokine CTAP-III also stimulates connective tissue metabolism. Cytokines that may directly inhibit collagen production in vitro include EGF, IFN-α, and IFN-γ.

CLINICAL RELEVANCE

Therapeutic intervention targeting these balance mechanisms may influence the outcome of inflammation (Fig. 6.1). There are a number of ongoing trials using agents to suppress the effects of pro-inflammatory mediators or to enhance the anti-inflammatory response.

BIBLIOGRAPHY

Dayer JM, Arend WP. Cytokines and growth factors. In: Kelley WN, Harris ED, Jr., Ruddy S, Sledge CB, eds. *Textbook of rheumatology,* fifth ed. Philadelphia: WB Saunders, 1997:267.
Hermann J, Walmsley M, Brennan FM. Cytokine therapy in rheumatoid arthritis. *Springer Semin Immunopathol* 1998;20:275.
Imhof BA, Dunon D. Leukocyte migration and adhesion. *Adv Immunol* 1995;58:345.
Koch AE. Angiogenesis: implications for rheumatoid arthritis. *Arthritis Rheum* 1998;41:951.
Koch AE, Strieter RM. *Chemokines in disease.* Austin, TX: RG Landes Company, 1996:103.
Mackay CR. Chemokines: what chemokine is that? *Curr Biol* 1997;7:R384.
Szekanecz Z, Strieter RM, Koch AE. Cytokines in rheumatoid arthritis: potential targets for pharmacological intervention. *Drugs Aging* 1998;12:377.
Szekanecz Z, Strieter RM, Kunkel SL, et al. Chemokines in rheumatoid arthritis. *Springer Semin Immunopathol* 1998;20:115.
Szekanecz Z, Szegedi G, Koch AE. Cellular adhesion molecules in rheumatoid arthritis. Regulation by cytokines and possible clinical importance. *J Invest Med* 1996;44:124.
Szekanecz Z, Szegedi G, Koch AE. Angiogenesis in rheumatoid arthritis: pathogenic and clinical significance. *J Invest Med* 1998;46:27.

Kelley's Textbook of Internal Medicine, fourth edition. Edited by H. David Humes. Lippincott Williams & Wilkins, Philadelphia © 2000.

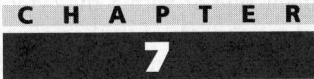

CHAPTER 7

MECHANISMS OF HORMONE ACTION

DARYL K. GRANNER

Multicellular organisms employ intercellular communication mechanisms to coordinate the responses necessary for adjusting to a constantly changing external and internal environment, thereby ensuring their survival. Two convergent systems comprising several highly differentiated tissues have evolved to serve these functions. The nervous system conducts signals or messages through a fixed structural system, although the final mediator may be a neurotransmitter substance released from a nerve ending. The endocrine system uses mobile messages, called *hormones,* to alter cellular function. Neurotransmitters and hormones share certain structural similarities and often have common mechanisms of action; these two systems converge. This chapter briefly describes the concepts and principles necessary for understanding how hormones work.

TARGET CELL CONCEPT

There are approximately 200 types of differentiated cells in humans. Only a few of these produce hormones, but virtually all of the 75 trillion cells in each human being are targets of one or more of the 50 or so known hormones.

The concept of target cells is undergoing redefinition. It was originally thought that hormones affected a single cell type or a few different kinds of cells, and that a hormone elicited a unique biochemical or physiologic action. With the delineation of specific cell surface and intracellular hormone receptors, the definition of a target has been expanded to include any cell in which the hormone binds to its receptor, whether or not a biochemical or physiologic response has been determined. This definition also is imperfect, but it has heuristic merit because it assumes that not all actions of hormones have been elucidated.

The response of a target cell is determined by the differentiated state of the cell, and a cell can respond in several ways to a single hormone. Cells can also respond to a given hormone in an endocrine (i.e., distant regulation), paracrine (i.e., adjacent regulation), or autocrine (i.e., self-regulation) fashion. Several factors determine the overall response of a target cell to a hormone. The concentration of a hormone around the target cell depends on five factors: the rate of synthesis and secretion of the hormone; the proximity of target and source; the association–dissociation constants of the hormone with specific plasma carrier proteins, if the latter exist; the rate of conversion of an inactive or suboptimally active form of the hormone into the active form; and the rate of clearance of the hormone from blood by other tissues or from degradation or excretion. The actual response to the hormone depends on (a) the relative activity or state of occupancy, or both, of the specific hormone receptors on the plasma membrane or within the cytoplasm or nucleus, and (b) the rate of metabolism of the hormone in the target cell and postreceptor desensitization of the cell. Alterations of any of these processes can result in a change of the hormonal activity on a given target cell and must be considered in addition to the classic feedback loops.

HORMONE RECEPTORS

One of the major challenges in making the hormone-based communication system work is that these molecules are present at low concentrations in the extracellular fluid, generally in the range of 10^{-15} to 10^{-9} mol per L. This is much lower than that of the many structurally similar molecules (e.g., sterols, amino acids, peptides, proteins) and a variety of other molecules that circulate at concentrations in the range of 10^{-5} to 10^{-3} mol per L. Target cells must differentiate between different hormones present in small amounts and between a given hormone and the 10^6- to 10^9-fold excess of other molecules. This high degree of discrimination is provided by recognition molecules called *receptors*, which are protein molecules located in the plasma membrane or within the target cell. Hormones initiate their biologic effects by binding to specific receptors, and because any effective control system must also provide a means of stopping

a response, hormone-induced actions begin to terminate when the effector dissociates from the receptor.

RECOGNITION AND COUPLING DOMAINS

All polypeptide and steroid receptors have at least two functional domains, and most have several more. A recognition domain binds the hormone, and a second region generates a signal that couples hormone recognition to some intracellular function. The binding of hormone by receptor implies that some region of the hormone molecule has a conformation that is complementary to a region of the receptor molecule. The degree of similarity, or fit, determines the tightness of the association; this is measured as the affinity of binding *(K)*. If the native hormone has a relative *K* value of 1, other natural molecules range between 0 and 1. In absolute terms, this actually spans a binding affinity range of more than a trillion.

Coupling (i.e., signal transduction) occurs in two general ways. Polypeptide hormones, protein hormones, and catecholamines bind to receptors located in the plasma membrane, and binding generates a signal that regulates various intracellular functions. Steroid, sterol, and thyroid hormones interact with intracellular receptors, and this complex provides the signal. The recognition and coupling functions generally reside in a single molecule, and these dual functions ultimately define a receptor. It is the coupling of hormone binding to signal transduction, the *receptor–effector coupling,* that provides the first step in the amplification of the hormonal response. This dual purpose also differentiates the target cell receptor from the plasma carrier proteins that bind hormone but generally do not generate a signal.

RELATION BETWEEN RECEPTOR OCCUPANCY AND BIOLOGIC EFFECT

The concentrations of hormone required for occupancy of the receptor and for elicitation of a specific biologic response often are similar (Fig. 7.1A), such as steroid hormone induction of enzymes. This is especially true for steroid hormones, but some polypeptide hormones also exhibit this characteristic. This tight coupling is remarkable, considering the many steps that must occur between hormone binding and complex responses such as transport, enzyme induction, cell lysis, or cell replication. When receptor occupancy and biologic effect are tightly coupled, significant changes in the latter occur if receptor occupancy changes. This happens when fewer receptors are available or when the affinity of the receptor changes but the hormone concentration remains constant. In other instances, there is a marked dissociation of binding and effect, producing a maximal biologic effect despite the fact that only a small percentage of the receptors are occupied (Fig. 7.1B, effect 2), as is the case for most aspects of insulin action. Different responses within the same cell can require various degrees of receptor occupancy. For example, successively greater degrees of occupancy of the adipose cell insulin receptor increase, in sequence, lipolysis, glucose oxidation, amino acid transport, and protein synthesis.

Receptors not involved in eliciting a response are said to be *spare receptors.* Spare receptors are observed in the response of

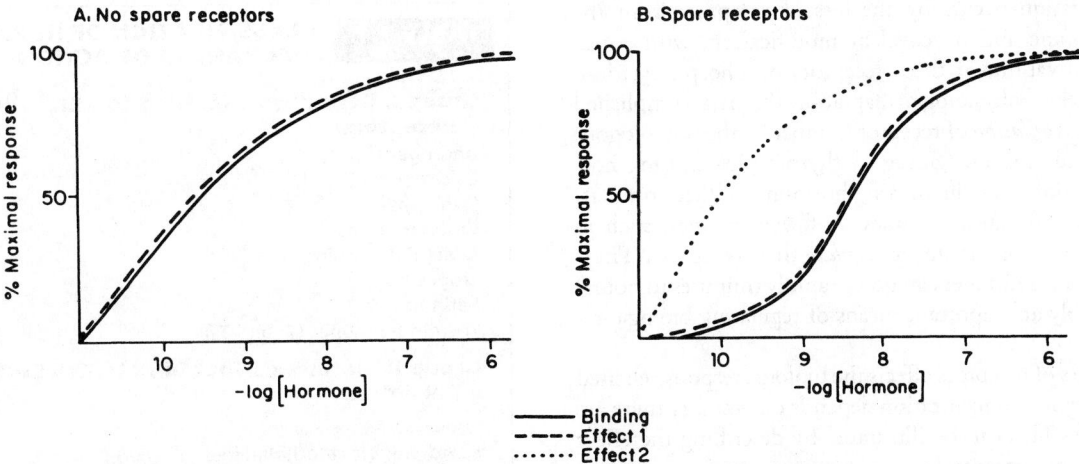

FIGURE 7.1. Hormone binding and biologic effects are compared in the absence **(A)** and presence **(B)** of spare receptors. Some biologic effects in a tissue may be tightly coupled to binding; another effect shows the spare receptor phenomenon (compare effects 1 and 2 in B). (Adapted from Murray RK, Granner DK, Mayes PA, et al. *Harper's biochemistry,* twenty-second ed. East Norwalk, CT: Appleton & Lange, 1990.)

several polypeptide hormones and are thought to provide a means of increasing the sensitivity of a target cell to activation by low concentrations of hormone and to provide a reservoir of receptors. The concept of spare receptors is operational, and it might depend on which aspect of the response is examined and which tissue is involved. For example, there is excellent agreement between luteinizing hormone binding and cAMP production in rat testis and ovarian granulosa cells (there are generally no spare receptors when any hormone activates adenylate cyclase), but steroidogenesis in these tissues, which is cAMP-dependent, occurs when fewer than 1% of the receptors are occupied (compare effect 1 with effect 2 in Fig. 7.1).

AGONIST–ANTAGONIST CONCEPT

Molecules can be divided into four groups with respect to their ability to elicit a given hormone receptor-mediated response: agonists, partial agonists, antagonists, and inactive agents. *Agonists* elicit the maximal response, although different concentrations may be required (Fig. 7.2, line A). *Partial agonists* evoke an incomplete response, even when large concentrations of the hormone are employed (see Fig. 7.2, line B). *Antagonists* generally have no effect themselves, but they competitively inhibit the action of agonists or partial agonists (see Fig. 7.2, line A + C and line B + C). A large group of structurally similar compounds elicit no effect at all and have no effect on the action of the agonists or antagonists. These are classified as *inactive agents* and are represented in Figure 7.2, line D.

Partial agonists also compete with agonists for binding to and activation of the receptor, in which case they become partial antagonists. The extent of the inhibition of agonist activity caused by partial or complete antagonists depends on the relative concentration of the various steroids. Generally, much higher concentrations of the antagonist are required to inhibit an agonist than are necessary for the agonist to exert its maximal effect. Because such concentrations are rarely achieved in vivo, this

phenomenon usually is employed for studies of the mechanism of action of glucocorticoid hormones in vitro.

REGULATION OF RECEPTORS

Receptors are in a dynamic state. They can be regulated physiologically, or they can be influenced by diseases or therapeutic measures. Receptor concentration and the affinity of hormone binding can be regulated. These changes can be acute and can significantly affect hormone responsiveness of the cell. For instance, cells exposed to β-adrenergic agonists for minutes to hours no longer activate adenylate cyclase in response to the addition of agonist, and the biologic response is lost. This partic-

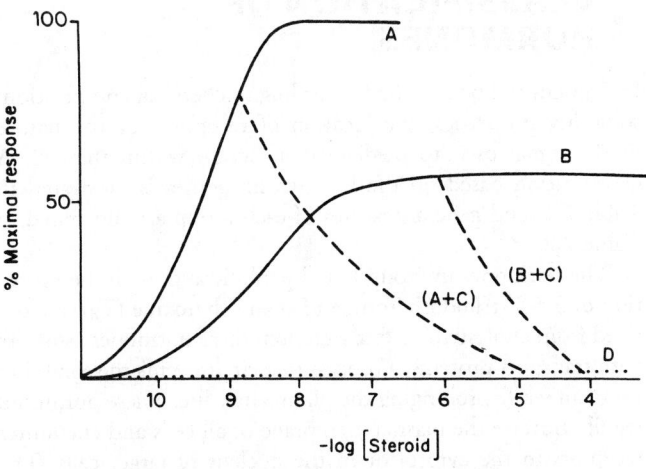

FIGURE 7.2. Classification of hormones according to their biologic activity. Steroids, for example, can be classified as agonists *(line A)*, partial agonists *(line B)*, antagonists *(C in A + C or B + C)*, or inactive agents *(dotted line D)*. (Adapted from Murray RK, Granner DK, Mayes PA, et al. *Harper's biochemistry,* twenty-second ed. East Norwalk, CT: Appleton & Lange, 1990.)

ular desensitization occurs by the loss of receptors from the plasma membrane and by covalent modification, with corresponding inactivation, of these receptors by phosphorylation. Other examples of physiologic adaptation that is accomplished through *down-regulation* of receptor number by the homologous hormone include insulin, glucagon, thyrotropin-releasing hormone, growth hormone, luteinizing hormone, follicle-stimulating hormone, and catecholamines. A few hormones, such as angiotensin II and prolactin, *up-regulate* their receptors. These changes in receptor number can occur rapidly (minutes to hours) and are probably an important means of regulating biologic responses.

How the loss of receptors affects the biologic response elicited at a given hormone concentration depends on whether there are spare receptors. This can be illustrated by describing the effect a fivefold loss of receptor has on the concentration–response curve in both conditions. With no spare receptors, the maximal response obtained is 20% that of control; the effect is on the V_{max}. With spare receptors, the maximal response is obtained, but at five times the originally effective hormone concentration, analogous to a K_m effect.

RECEPTOR MOVEMENT IN TARGET CELLS

There is little evidence to suggest that peptide hormone–receptor complexes must enter the cell to act. Receptor-mediated endocytosis, analogous to the process used to get low-density lipoprotein particles into cells, occurs with hormones. For example, intact insulin is found within the cell, often in association with lysosomes and other organelles, although this probably represents a degradative or down-regulation pathway. The cytoplasmic and nuclear receptors for steroids and thyroid hormones are a different case because they move between compartments within the cell, probably in response to changes in the intracellular concentration of the hormone.

■ CLASSIFICATION OF HORMONES

Hormones can be classified according to chemical composition, solubility properties, the location of receptors, or the nature of the signal used to mediate their action within the cell. A classification based on the last two properties is illustrated in Table 7.1, and general features of each group are illustrated in Table 7.2.

The hormones in group I are lipophilic and, with the exception of 3,5,3′-triiodothyronine (T_3) and thyroxine (T_4), are derived from cholesterol. After secretion, these hormones associate with transport proteins, a process that circumvents the solubility problem while prolonging the plasma half-life. These hormones readily traverse the plasma membrane of all cells and encounter receptors in the cytosol or in the nucleus of target cells. The ligand–receptor complex is assumed to be the intracellular messenger in this group.

The second major group consists of water-soluble hormones that bind to the plasma membrane of the target cell. Such hormones regulate intracellular metabolic processes through inter-

---

TABLE 7.1.	CLASSIFICATION OF HORMONES BY MECHANISM OF ACTION

Group I. Hormones That Bind to Intracellular Receptors

Androgens
Calcitriol
Estrogens
Glucocorticoids
Mineralocorticoids
Progestins
Retinoic acid
Thyroid hormones (T_3 and T_4)

Group II. Hormones That Bind to Cell Surface Receptors

SECOND-MESSENGER cAMP

α_2-Adrenergic catecholamines
β_2-Adrenergic catecholamines
Adrenocorticotropic hormone
Angiotensin II
Antidiuretic hormone
Calcitonin
Chorionic gonadotropin
Corticotropin-releasing hormone
Follicle-stimulating hormone
Glucagon
Lipotropin
Luteinizing hormone
Melanocyte-stimulating hormone
Parathyroid hormone
Somatostatin
Thyroid-stimulating hormone

SECOND MESSENGER cGMP

Atriopeptins

SECOND-MESSENGER CALCIUM OR PHOSPHATIDYLINOSITIDES (OR BOTH)

α_1-Adrenergic catecholamines
Acetylcholine (muscarinic)
Angiotensin II
Antidiuretic hormone
Cholecystokinin
Epidermal growth factor
Gastrin
Gonadotropin-releasing hormone
Oxytocin
Platelet-derived growth factor
Thyrotropin-releasing hormone

INTRACELLULAR MESSENGER INVOLVING A PROTEIN KINASE CASCADE

Chorionic somatomammotropin (CS)
Erythropoietin
Fibroblast growth factor (FGF)
Growth hormone
Insulin
Insulin-like growth peptides
Nerve growth factor
Prolactin

---

mediary molecules, called *second messengers* (the hormone itself is the first messenger), which are generated as a consequence of the ligand–receptor interaction. Hormones that employ cAMP as the second messenger are shown in Table 7.1. The atriopeptins use cGMP as a second messenger, as do other potent nonhormonal substances, including nitric oxide and nitroglycerin. Several hormones use calcium or phosphatidylinositide metabo-

TABLE 7.2.	GENERAL FEATURES OF HORMONE CLASSES	
Feature	Class I	Class II
Types	Steroids	Polypeptides
	Iodothyronines	Proteins
	Calcitriol	Glycoproteins
		Catecholamines
Solubility	Lipophilic	Hydrophilic
Transport proteins	Yes	No
Plasma half-life	Long (hours to days)	Short (min)
Receptor	Intracellular	Plasma membrane
Mediators	Receptor hormone complex	cAMP, Ca^{2+}, phosphatidylinositides, diacylglycerol, cGMP, protein kinase cascade

lites (or both) as the intracellular signal. Several hormones have been found to mediate biologic effects by initiating a protein kinase cascade. A few hormones fit in more than one category; for example, there is increasing evidence that some hormones act through cAMP and Ca^{2+}.

MECHANISM OF ACTION OF GROUP I HORMONES

The lipophilic molecules of group I hormones diffuse through the plasma membrane of all cells but only encounter their specific, high-affinity receptor within target cells. The hormone–receptor complex then undergoes an activation reaction that results in size, conformation, and surface charge changes that allow it to bind to DNA. In some cases—the glucocorticoid receptor for example—this process involves the disruption of a receptor–heat-shock protein complex. Whether the association and activation processes occur in the cytoplasm or the nucleus appears to depend on the specific hormone in question. The hormone–receptor complex binds to specific regions of DNA called hormone response elements (HREs), and this initiates the assembly of a multicomponent complex that regulates the rate of transcription of specific genes. By selectively affecting gene transcription and production of the respective mRNAs, the amounts of specific proteins are changed, and metabolic processes are influenced. The effect of each of these hormones is specific; generally the hormone affects fewer than 1% of the proteins or mRNAs in a target cell.

In recent years it has become apparent that a simple HRE is not sufficient to mediate the effects of a hormone on a specific gene. Genes have at least two separate regulatory regions in the DNA sequence immediately 5′ of the transcription initiation site. The first of these, the basal promoter element (BPE), is generic because it is present in some form in all genes. The BPE generally contains the TATA box and one or more additional DNA elements. The BPE specifies the site of RNA polymerase II attachment to DNA and therefore the accuracy of transcription initiation.

A second regulatory region is located slightly farther upstream than the BPE and this may also consist of several discrete elements. This region modulates the frequency of transcript initiation and is less dependent on position and orientation. In these respects, it resembles the transcription enhancer elements found in other genes. The regulatory region consists of two types of DNA elements in genes that respond to hormones. The HREs described above are short segments of DNA that bind a specific hormone receptor–ligand complex. The GRE binds the ligand–glucocorticoid receptor complex, the ERE binds the ligand–estrogen receptor complex, etc. The HREs are often capable of regulating transcription from test promoter–reporter gene constructs, but in most physiologic circumstances other DNA element–protein complexes are required.

The HRE must interact with other elements (and associated binding proteins) to function optimally. Such assemblies of cis-acting DNA elements and trans-acting factors are called *hormone response units* (HRUs) or *composite elements*. An HRU therefore consists of one or more HREs and one or more DNA elements with associated accessory factors (Fig. 7.3). In complex promoters—regulated by a variety of hormones—certain accessory factor components of one HRU (glucocorticoid) may be part of that for another (cAMP). This arrangement may provide for the hormonal integration of complex metabolic responses.

The communication between an HRU and the basal transcription apparatus is facilitated by coregulator molecules (Fig. 7.3). The first of these described was the CREB-binding protein, so-called CBP. This protein, through an amino terminal domain, binds to phosphorylated serine 137 of CREB and facilitates transactivation in response to cAMP. It thus is described as a coactivator. The CREB-activating protein and its close relative, p300, interact with a number of signaling molecules, including activator protein–1 (AP-1), signal transducers and activators of transcription (STATS), nuclear receptors, and CREB.

The CREB-binding protein/p300 also binds to the p160 family of coactivators described below and to a number of other proteins. Some of the many actions of CBP/p300 appear to depend on intrinsic enzyme activities and the ability of this protein to serve as a scaffold for the binding of other proteins. It is important to note that CBP/p300 also has intrinsic histone acetyltransferase (HAT) activity. The importance of this is described below. Three other families of coactivator molecules, all of about 160 kd, have been described. These members of the p160 family of coactivators include (a) SRC-1 and NCoA-1; (b) GRIP 1, TIF2, and NCoA-2; and (c) p/CIP, ACTR, AIB1, RAC3, and TRAM-1.

The role of these many coactivators is still evolving. It appears that certain combinations are responsible for specific ligand-induced actions through various receptors. The role of HAT is particularly interesting. Mutations of the HAT domain disable many of these transcription factors. Current thinking holds that these HAT activities acetylate histones and result in the remodeling of chromatin into a transcription-efficient environment. In keeping with this hypothesis, histone deacetylation is associated with the inactivation of transcription.

In certain instances, the removal of a corepressor complex through a ligand–receptor interaction results in the activation of transcription. For example, in the absence of hormone, the

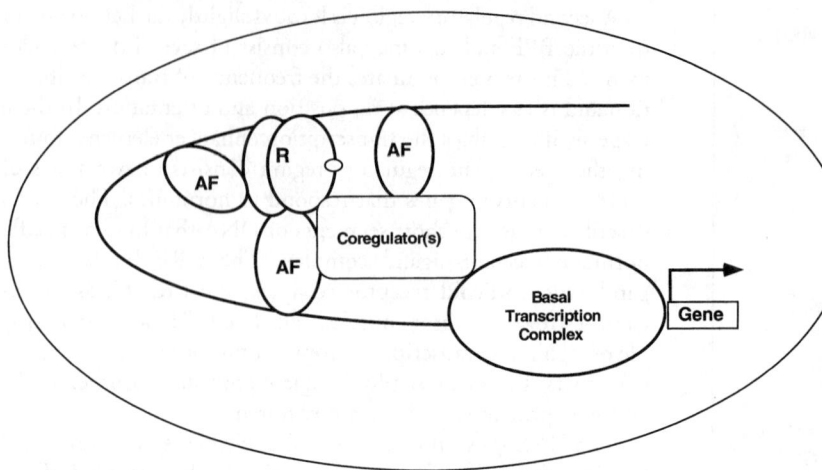

FIGURE 7.3. The hormone response unit, an assembly of DNA elements and bound proteins. An essential component is the hormone response element with ligand-bound receptor. Also important are the accessory factor (AF) elements with bound transcription factors. More than two dozen of these accessory factors have been linked to hormone effects on transcription. The AFs can interact with each other or with the nuclear receptors. The components of the hormone response unit communicate with the basal transcription machinery through a coactivator complex. (Adapted from Murray RK, Granner DK, Mayes PA, et al. *Harper's biochemistry*, twenty-fifth ed. East Norwalk, CT: Appleton & Lange, 1999.)

thyroid or retinoic acid receptors are bound to a corepressor complex containing N-CoR or SMRT and associated proteins, some of which have histone deacetylase activity. The target gene is repressed until the binding of hormone to the thyroid receptor results in the dissociation of this complex, and gene activation then ensues.

The nuclear actions of steroid hormones are reasonably well defined, but direct actions of these hormones in the cytoplasm and on various organelles and membranes have also been described. Although steroid hormones affect nuclear mRNA processing, mRNA degradation rates, and post-translational processing, most evidence suggests that these hormones exert their predominant effect on the transcription of specific genes.

MECHANISM OF ACTION OF GROUP II POLYPEPTIDE HORMONES

The majority of hormones are water-soluble, have no transport proteins (with the exception of insulin-like growth factors IGF-I and IGF-II), and therefore have a short plasma half-life. They initiate a response by binding to a receptor located in the plasma membrane, an interaction that results in the generation of an intracellular signal or messenger that then mediates the action of the hormone (Tables 7.1 and 7.2). The mechanisms of action of this group of hormones can be discussed best in terms of their intracellular messengers.

CYCLIC AMP AS THE SECOND MESSENGER

Cyclic AMP, a ubiquitous nucleotide derived from ATP through the action of the enzyme adenylate cyclase (located on the inner surface of the plasma membrane), plays a crucial role in the action of several hormones. The intracellular level of cAMP is increased or decreased by various hormones that activate or inactivate adenylate cyclase (Table 7.3). This process is mediated by at least two types of GTP-dependent regulatory protein complexes, designated G_s (stimulatory) and G_i (inhibitory). Hormones that bind to receptors coupled to G_s activate adenylate

cyclase and increase cAMP production, and hormones that bind to receptors coupled to G_i decrease cAMP production. G_q is a pertussis-resistant G protein that can activate phosphoinositidase C.

The components of the cyclase system have been purified, revealing a large family of G proteins. The G-protein complexes are heterotrimers consisting of α, β, and γ peptide chain subunits. There are at least 16 α subunits, 6 β subunits, 12 γ subunits, and 8 different adenylate cyclases, so that many different combinations are possible. The α subunit, active when bound to GTP, contains an intrinsic GTPase activity that hydrolyzes GTP to GDP. The α subunit is inactive when bound to GDP, providing a tightly regulated on–off mechanism. The α subunits, in addition to regulating adenylate cyclase activity, can also regulate ion channel activity. Some forms of α_s stimulate K^+ channels and inactivate Ca^{2+} channels, and some α_i iso-

TABLE 7.3.	**SUBCLASSIFICATION OF GROUP II HORMONES FOR WHICH THE SECOND MESSENGER IS cAMP**

Hormones That Stimulate Adenylate Cyclase (H_S)

Adrenocorticotropic hormone
Antidiuretic hormone
β-Adrenergics
Calcitonin
Corticotropin-stimulating hormone
Follicle-stimulating hormone
Glucagon
Human chorionic gonadotropin
Luteinizing hormone
Lipotropin
Melanocyte-stimulating hormone
Parathyroid hormone
Thyroid stimulating hormone

Hormones That Inhibit Adenylate Cyclase (H_I)

α_2-Adrenergics
Acetylcholine (muscarinic)
Angiotensin II
Opioids
Somatostatin

forms inhibit K$^+$ channels and activate Ca^{2+} channels. The G$_q$ heterocomplexes activate phospholipase C. The $\beta\gamma$-subunit complexes have also been shown to activate K$^+$ channels and phospholipase C. In addition to hormone-regulated metabolic processes, such as gluconeogenesis, lipolysis, and glycogenolysis, G proteins are involved in many other important and diverse biologic processes, including neuronal activity, heart rate, blood pressure control, muscle contraction, cell replication, vision, and smell.

In eukaryotic cells, cAMP activates a protein kinase that is a heterotetrameric molecule consisting of two regulatory subunits (R) and two catalytic subunits (C). cAMP binds to the regulatory subunits and results in the following reaction: 4 cAMP + R$_2$C$_2$ $\longleftrightarrow$ R$_2\times$ (4 cAMP) + 2C. The R$_2$C$_2$ complex has no enzymatic activity, but the binding of cAMP by R dissociates R from C, thereby activating the latter. The active C subunit catalyzes the transfer of the γ-phosphate of adenosine triphosphate (ATP) in an Mg^{2+}-dependent reaction to a serine or threonine residue in a variety of proteins, resulting in altered activity of the protein.

Reactions caused by hormones in this class can be terminated in several ways, including the hydrolysis of cAMP by phosphodiesterases. The presence of these hydrolytic enzymes ensures a rapid turnover of the signal (cAMP); termination of the biologic process is rapid after the hormonal stimulus is removed. The cAMP phosphodiesterases are themselves subject to regulation by hormones and by intracellular messengers such as calcium, probably acting through calmodulin. Inhibitors of phosphodiesterase, most notably xanthine derivatives (e.g., caffeine, theophylline), increase intracellular cAMP and mimic or prolong the actions of hormones. Another means of controlling hormone action is the regulation of the protein dephosphorylation reaction. The phosphoprotein phosphatases are themselves subject to regulation by phosphorylation–dephosphorylation reactions and by a variety of other mechanisms, often as a consequence of the action of a hormone.

CYCLIC GMP AS THE SECOND MESSENGER

Cyclic GMP is made from GTP by the enzyme guanylate cyclase, which exists in soluble and membrane-bound forms. Each of these isozymes has unique kinetic, physiochemical, and antigenic properties. The atriopeptins, a family of peptides produced in cardiac atrial tissue, cause natriuresis, diuresis, vasodilatation, and inhibition of aldosterone secretion. These peptides (e.g., atrial natriuretic factor) bind to and activate the membrane-bound form of guanylate cyclase. This action increases the concentration of cGMP, by as much as 50-fold in some cases, which is thought to mediate the effects of these peptides.

Other evidence links cGMP to vasodilatation. A series of compounds, including nitroprusside, nitroglycerin, sodium nitrite, and sodium azide, cause smooth muscle relaxation and are potent vasodilators. These agents activate nitric oxide synthase, which catalyzes the formation of nitric oxide. Nitric oxide activates guanylate cyclase, which produces cGMP. The increased cGMP concentration activates cGMP-dependent protein kinase, which phosphorylates several smooth muscle proteins, including the myosin light chain. Presumably, this mechanism is involved in relaxation of smooth muscle and vasodilatation. This reaction is terminated by a specific cGMP-dependent phosphodiesterase,

PDE type 5. [PDE5 is the target of sildenafil (Viagra), and this accounts for the smooth muscle relaxation effect of this drug and its activity in erectile dysfunction.]

CALCIUM AND PHOSPHATIDYLINOSITIDES AS SECOND MESSENGERS

Ionized calcium is an important regulator of a variety of cellular processes, including muscle contraction, stimulus–secretion coupling, the blood clotting cascade, enzyme activity, and membrane excitability. It also is an intracellular messenger of hormone action.

A role for ionized calcium in hormone action is suggested by several observations. First, the hormone effect is blunted when tested in Ca^{2+}-free media or when intracellular calcium is depleted. Second, the effect can be mimicked by agents that increase cytosolic Ca^{2+}, such as the Ca^{2+} ionophore A23187. Third, the hormonal effect involves changes of cellular calcium movement. These processes have been studied in some detail in cells of the pituitary, smooth muscle, platelets, and salivary gland, but most is known about how vasopressin and α-adrenergic catecholamines regulate glycogen metabolism in liver.

The extracellular calcium concentration of about 1.2 mmol per L is rigidly controlled. The intracellular free concentration of this ion is much lower, about 100 to 200 mmol per L, and the concentration associated with intracellular organelles is in the range of 1 to 20 μmol per L. Despite this 5000- to 10,000-fold concentration gradient and a favorable transmembrane electrical gradient, Ca^{2+} is restrained from entering the cell. There are three ways of changing cytosolic Ca^{2+}. Certain hormones enhance membrane permeability to Ca^{2+} and thereby increase Ca^{2+} influx. This is probably accomplished by a 3Na$^+$/Ca^{2+} exchange mechanism that has a high capacity but a low affinity for Ca^{2+}. There is also a Ca^{2+}/2H$^+$-ATPase-dependent pump that extrudes Ca^{2+} in exchange for H$^+$. This has a high affinity for Ca^{2+} but a low capacity, and the mechanism is probably responsible for fine-tuning cytosolic Ca^{2+} concentrations. Ca^{2+} also can be mobilized from or deposited into the mitochondrial and endoplasmic reticulum pools.

The calcium-dependent regulatory protein is now referred to as *calmodulin,* a protein that is homologous to the muscle protein called troponin C in structure and function. Calmodulin has four Ca^{2+} binding sites, and full occupancy of these leads to a marked conformational change that presumably is linked to the ability of calmodulin to activate or inactivate enzymes. The interaction of Ca^{2+} with calmodulin and the resulting change of activity of the latter is conceptually similar to the binding of cAMP to protein kinase and the subsequent activation of this molecule. The cAMP-mediated and Ca^{2+}-mediated systems are linked because calmodulin is involved in regulating various protein kinases and enzymes of cyclic nucleotide generation and degradation (Fig. 7.4).

In addition to its effects on enzymes and ion transport, Ca^{2+}-calmodulin regulates the activity of many structural elements in cells. These include the actin–myosin complex of smooth muscle, which is under β-adrenergic control, and various microfilament-mediated processes in noncontractile cells, including cell motility, conformation changes, mitotic apparatus, granule release, and endocytosis. Several critical metabolic enzymes, in-

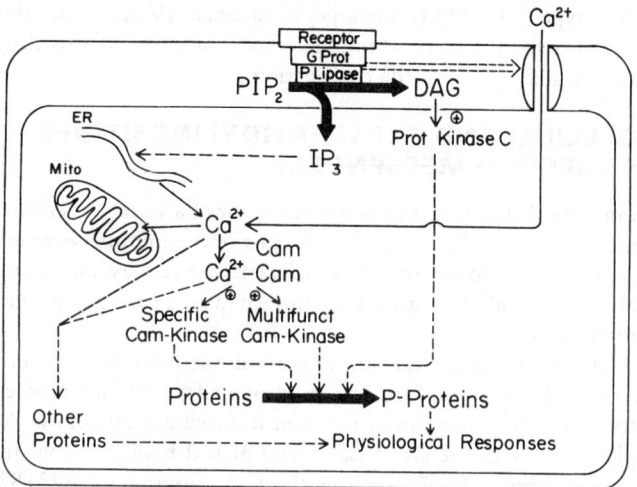

FIGURE 7.4. Mechanisms by which Ca^{2+}-mobilizing agonists exert their effects. G Prot, guanine nucleotide–binding regulatory protein; P Lipase, phospholipase C; PIP_2, phosphatidylinositol 4,5-biphosphate; DAG, 1,2-diacylglycerol; IP_3, myo-inositol 1,4,5-triphosphate; ER, endoplasmic reticulum; Mito, mitochondrion; Cam, calmodulin; Multifunct Cam-Kinase, multifunctional or multisubstrate Ca^{2+}-calmodulin-dependent protein kinase. (Courtesy of J. H. Exton, MD, Vanderbilt University.)

cluding glycogen synthetase, pyruvate kinase, pyruvate carboxylase, glycerol 3-phosphate dehydrogenase, and pyruvate dehydrogenase, are regulated by Ca^{2+}, by phosphorylation, or by both. Many of these effects are mediated through activation of a specific calmodulin-dependent protein kinase, and others are mediated through a multifunctional protein kinase (Fig. 7.4). These kinases phosphorylate specific residues on proteins, but a given protein might be phosphorylated by more than one kinase.

Some signal must provide communication between the hormone receptor on the plasma membrane and the intracellular Ca^{2+} reservoirs. The best candidates appear to be products of phosphatidylinositide metabolism. Phosphatidylinositol 4,5-biphosphate is hydrolyzed to myo-inositol 1,4,5-triphosphate and diacylglycerol through the action of a phospholipase C, which is activated by a member of the G_q family (Fig. 7.4). This reaction occurs within seconds after the addition of vasopressin or epinephrine to hepatocytes. Myo-inositol 1,4,5-triphosphate, at a concentration of 0.1 to 0.4 mmol/L, releases Ca^{2+} from a variety of membrane and organelle preparations with appropriately rapid kinetics. Another product of phosphoinositide hydrolysis, 1,2-diacylglycerol, activates a Ca^{2+}-dependent protein kinase, protein kinase C. The hormones that activate this system generate two intracellular signals: Ca^{2+} and diacylglycerol.

Steroidogenic agents, including adrenocorticotropic hormone (corticotropin; ACTH) and cAMP in the adrenal cortex; angiotensin II, K^+, serotonin, ACTH, and dibutyryl cAMP in the zona glomerulosa of the adrenal; luteinizing hormone in the ovary, and luteinizing hormone and cAMP in the Leydig cells of the testes have been associated with increased amounts of phosphatidic acid, phosphatidylinositol, and polyphosphatidylinositides in the respective target tissues. Other examples of the possible role of phosphatidylinositide metabolites in hormone action can be cited. The addition of thyrotropin-releasing hor-

mone to pituitary cells is followed within 15 seconds by a marked increase of inositol degradation by phospholipase C. The intracellular levels of inositol diphosphates and triphosphates increase markedly, resulting in mobilization of intracellular calcium. This activates protein kinase C, which phosphorylates several proteins, one of which presumably is involved in thyroid-stimulating hormone release. Calcium also appears to be the intracellular mediator of gonadotropin-releasing hormone action on luteinizing hormone release. This reaction probably involves calmodulin.

The roles that Ca^{2+} and phosphoinositide breakdown products might play in hormone action are presented in Figure 7.4. In this scheme, the phosphoinositide products are the second messengers and Ca^{2+} is a tertiary messenger. It is likely that more examples of the complex networking of intracellular messengers will be discovered.

PROTEIN KINASE CASCADES PROVIDE THE SECOND MESSENGER

Phosphorylation is perhaps the most common post-translational modification of proteins. The usual amino acid residues modified by this process are serine or threonine. The phosphorylation of tyrosine residues accounts for only 0.03% of phosphorylated amino acids, but it is extremely important for hormone action. The seminal discovery was that the epidermal growth factor receptor contained an intrinsic tyrosine kinase that was activated when epidermal growth factor was bound. Shortly thereafter, the insulin and IGF-I receptors were shown to contain ligand-activated tyrosine kinases. Many studies, including extensive mutational analysis of these receptors, provided conclusive evidence of the importance of receptor-associated tyrosine kinase in the action of insulin, IGF-I, epidermal growth factor, and other growth factors.

Not explained was how this activity coupled to specific biologic effects, but a clue came from further analysis of insulin action. Activation of the receptor tyrosine kinase results in the phosphorylation of a family of proteins, called the insulin receptor substrates (IRS 1 to 4), on tyrosine residues. For example, phosphorylated IRS-1 associates with so-called docking proteins through Src homology 2 (SH2) domains. One of these SH2 domain–containing docking proteins, GRB-2, results in activation of a kinase cascade, the last member of which is a microtubule-associated protein kinase. This kinase is thought to phosphorylate target proteins on serine and threonine residues and thereby influence biologic processes. In insulin action this pathway is associated with cell growth and replication events. Phosphorylated IRS-2 binds to the SH2 domain of phosphoinositol-3 kinase, linking tyrosine phosphorylation to phosphoinositide metabolism and action. This pathway has been associated with certain metabolic effects of insulin, such as glucose transporter translocation and the regulation of genes involved in metabolism. Many of the components of this complex system remain to be identified and placed in order, and it is not clear as to how hormone specificity is achieved, but a major advance has been made in understanding how this class of hormones works.

Growth hormone, prolactin, erythropoietin, and cytokine receptors do not have intrinsic tyrosine kinase activity, but tyrosine phosphorylation is involved in the action of this group of hormones. The hormone receptor interaction attracts and activates cytoplasmic protein tyrosine kinases, such as Tyk-2, Jak-1, and Jak-2. These activated kinases phosphorylate one or more cytoplasmic proteins that then associate with other proteins through SH2 domains. One target appears to be the signal transduction and activators of transcription (STAT) family of proteins. Activated STAT proteins translocate from the cytoplasm to the nucleus wherein they regulate the transcription of specific genes.

The exact components of these pathways, the docking proteins, kinases, and phosphatases must be established, and it is particularly important to link these pathways to the well-established physiologic and biochemical actions of the hormones.

BIBLIOGRAPHY

Berridge M. Inositol triphosphate and calcium signaling. *Nature* 1993;361: 315.

Cheatum B, Kahn CR. Insulin action and the insulin signaling network. *Endocr Rev* 1995;16:117.

Darnell JE Jr, Kerr IM, Stark GR. Jak-STAT pathways and transcriptional activation in response to IFNs and other extracellular signaling proteins. *Science* 1994;264:1415.

Fantl WJ, Johnson DE, Williams LT. Signaling by receptor tyrosine kinases. *Annu Rev Biochem* 1993;62:453.

Lucas PC, Granner DK. Hormone response domains in gene transcription. *Annu Rev Biochem* 1992;61:1131.

Montminy M. Transcriptional regulation by cyclic AMP. *Annu Rev Biochem* 1997;66:807.

Neer EJ. Heterotrimeric G proteins: organizers of transmembrane signals. *Cell* 1995;80:249.

Taussig R, Gilman AG. Mammalian membrane-bound adenylyl cyclases. *J Biol Chem* 1995;270:1.

Torchia J, Glass C, Rosenfeld MG. Co-activators and co-repressors in the investigation of transcriptional responses. *Curr Opin Cell Biol* 1998;10: 373.

Tsai MJ, O'Malley BW. Molecular mechanisms of action of steroid/thyroid receptor super-family members. *Annu Rev Biochem* 1994;64:451.

Kelley's Textbook of Internal Medicine, fourth edition. Edited by H. David Humes. Lippincott Williams & Wilkins, Philadelphia © 2000.

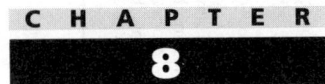

C H A P T E R
8

PRINCIPLES OF NUTRITION

DAVID H. ALPERS

The field of nutrition has been incompletely understood and knowledge about it incompletely used by the practicing physi-

cian. This state of affairs results from the multidisciplinary nature of the field, so that only a portion of the available data is easily accessible to the physician working in any single branch of medicine. In addition, the patient frequently is aware of a large body of information that is not known to the physician, some of it nonscientific but some resulting from public policy statements and positions. One example of such information is the new (1994) food labels and their interpretation. This chapter can only touch on the enormous volume of information in nutrition of which the physician should be aware. For further reading, there are standard texts and manuals listed at the end of the chapter.

Nutritional deficiencies occur commonly in association with many disorders. These involve problems with calorie and protein (macronutrient) intake or with specific vitamin and mineral (micronutrient) deficiencies. The disorders that affect caloric balance are those that lead to decreased intake or increased utilization; those that alter protein balance include disorders that decrease intake, increase loss in urine or stool, or decrease synthesis. Calorie and protein needs are large and are required on a daily basis, and consequently are the most difficult ones to meet. Thus, they are stressed in this chapter. Deriving a simple, efficient, and acceptable plan for nutritional therapy involves a series of steps that require knowledge of the nutritional requirements, how to assess nutritional status, and how to deliver replacement therapy. This chapter discusses the dietary guidelines and recommended daily allowances (RDAs) that define nutrient sufficiency for the population; the nutritional assessment that defines nutrient sufficiency for the individual; the key questions that must be addressed in planning macronutrient replacement therapy; and some practical aspects of delivering such therapy.

■ DIETARY GUIDELINES AND RECOMMENDED DAILY ALLOWANCES

Guidelines for dietary intake to promote good health have been developed by a variety of organizations, federal and private, and the results agree closely (Table 8.1). These guidelines were developed to provide a diet that would minimize the risks of major chronic diseases such as heart disease, cancer, stroke, diabetes mellitus, hypertension, dental caries, alcoholism, and obesity. All diets recommend achieving and maintaining desirable body weight, most commonly defined by the 1983 Metropolitan Life Insurance Height–Weight Tables (Table 8.2). The diets also recommend decreasing saturated fatty acids to less than 10% of total kilocalories per day, increasing complex carbohydrate and fiber intake, and decreasing salt intake. The diets listed in Table 8.1 are designed for general populations in the United States, but somewhat different dietary recommendations may need to be emphasized for African Americans and other minority groups. For example, diets for middle-aged African-American women tend to be lower in calcium, magnesium, iron, folacin, and zinc, and desirable weight may be more difficult to achieve in this group. Hispanic Americans tend to have a diet higher in fiber and lower in animal fat, but obesity is still a major problem in this group. Asian or Pacific Americans have a diet generally higher in fish, shellfish, and fruits and vegetables, but lower in

TABLE 8.1.   DIETARY RECOMMENDATIONS TO THE UNITED STATES PUBLIC

	Maintain Appropriate Body Weight, Exercise	Limit or Reduce Total Fat (% kcal)	Reduce Saturated Fatty Acids (% kcal)	Increase Polyunsaturated Fatty Acids (% kcal)	Limit Cholesterol (mg/d)	Limit Simple Sugars	Increase Complex Carbohydrates (% kcal from total carbohydrates)	Increase Fiber	Restrict Sodium Chloride (g)	Moderate Alcohol Intake
DHHS (1988)	Yes	Yes	Yes	No	Yes	Yes	Yes	Yes	Yes	Yes
USDA/DHHS (1990)	Yes	Yes	Yes	No	Yes	Yes	Choose diet with plenty of fruits, vegetables, and grain products	Yes	Yes	
ADA (1994)	Yes	<30	Yes	Up to 10	<300	No	Variable but not restricted; based on nutritional assessment and treatment goals	20–35 g/d	≤3 g/d of sodium, ≤2.4 g/d sodium if hypertensive	Yes
AHA (1996)	Yes	<30	8–10	Up to 10[a]	<300	NS	55–60	NS	≤2–4 g/d of sodium	1–2 oz ethanol/d
NCI (1987)	Yes	Yes	Yes	No	NC	NC	Yes, more whole grains, fruits, and vegetables	To 20–35 g/d	NC	Yes

NC, no comment; NS, not specified; USDA, U.S. Department of Agriculture; DHHS, U.S. Department of Health and Human Services; ADA, American Diabetes Association; AHA, American Heart Association; NCI, National Cancer Institute.
[a] Up to 15% of total kilocalories from monosaturated fatty acids.
(National Research Council. Diet and health: implications for reducing chronic disease risk. Washington, DC: National Academy Press, 1989. Modified from Alpers DH, Bier DM, Stenson WF. *Manual of nutritional therapeutics*, third ed. Boston: Little, Brown and Company, 1995:38.)

| TABLE 8.2. | HEIGHT-WEIGHT TABLE, 1983 |

Men				Women			
Height (Feet, Inches)	Small Frame	Medium Frame	Large Frame	Height (Feet, Inches)	Small Frame	Medium Frame	Large Frame
5, 2	128–134	131–141	138–150	4, 10	102–111	109–121	118–131
5, 3	130–136	133–143	140–153	4, 11	103–113	111–123	120–134
5, 4	132–138	135–145	142–156	5, 0	104–115	113–126	122–137
5, 5	134–140	137–148	144–160	5, 1	106–118	115–129	125–140
5, 6	136–142	139–151	146–164	5, 2	108–121	118–132	128–143
5, 7	138–145	142–154	149–168	5, 3	111–124	121–135	131–147
5, 8	140–148	145–157	152–172	5, 4	114–127	124–138	134–151
5, 9	142–151	148–160	155–176	5, 5	117–130	127–141	137–155
5, 10	144–154	151–163	158–180	5, 6	120–133	130–144	140–159
5, 11	146–157	154–166	161–184	5, 7	123–136	133–147	143–163
6, 0	149–160	157–170	164–188	5, 8	126–139	136–150	146–167
6, 1	152–164	160–174	168–192	5, 9	129–142	139–153	149–170
6, 2	155–168	164–178	172–197	5, 10	132–145	142–156	152–173
6, 3	158–172	167–182	176–202	5, 11	135–148	145–159	155–176
6, 4	162–176	171–187	181–207	6, 0	138–151	148–162	158–179

Weight according to frame (ages 25 to 59 years) for men wearing indoor clothing weighing 5 lb, shoes with 1-in. heels; for women indoor clothing weighing 3 lb, shoes with 1-in. heels.
(Reprinted with permission from the Metropolitan Life Insurance Company, New York.)

dairy products and calcium. Use of the guidelines in Table 8.1 thus must be tailored to groups as well as to individuals. It is clear that these guidelines are not intended as rigid rules, but as suggestions to form a plan that will be useful for the individual. To discuss the principles involved in these guidelines, the nine points of the report, *Diet and Health* (National Academy of Sciences, National Research Council, 1989) are reviewed:

1. *Balance food intake and physical activity to maintain an appropriate body weight.* To implement this requires knowledge of the person's energy expenditure. Resting energy expenditure (REE, kilocalories per day) for adults can be estimated from body weight (kilograms) using the equations from the RDAs:

- For men 18 to 30 years of age: REE = (15.3 × weight) + 679
- For men 30 to 60 years of age: REE = (11.6 × weight) + 879
- For women 18 to 30 years of age: REE = (14.7 × weight) + 496
- For women 30 to 60 years of age: REE = (8.7 × weight) + 829

The total daily energy requirement = REE + energy expenditure of activity + energy expenditure associated with food ingestion. The last component is relatively small, and for practical purposes only the first two need to be considered. The overall daily energy expenditure for young adults suggested by the RDAs is 1.6 × REE for men and 1.55 × REE for women, although periods of heavy physical activity can use up to 7 × REE. The range of energy of activity is from 1.5 to 8.4 kcal per kg per hour. Thus, for the "average" 79-kg man and 63-kg woman, the average daily energy allowances are 2,900 kcal (37 kcal per kg) and 2,200 kcal (36 kcal per kg), respectively. Because the intersubject variation is about 20%, it is apparent that such estimates must be adjusted to the individual's needs. For patients, additional requirements must be added for disease. These are difficult to estimate, but for outpatients about 10% can be added to energy needs for mild illness (not interfering with normal activity) and up to 25% for moderate disease (interfering with normal activity but not hospitalized). Severe disease requiring hospitalization usually produces a decrease in the energy of activity and thus a decline in total daily energy requirement to close to 2,000 kcal.

2. *Maintain protein intake at moderate levels.* The RDA for protein intake in young adults is 0.8 g per kg per day, or about 10% of dietary energy intake (Table 8.3). This estimate is based on average nitrogen losses incurred in the urine, stool, and skin, coupled with factors to account for the inefficiency of absorption of vegetable protein and for the variable amount of such protein in the Western diet. Increasing the protein intake over this level also increases triglyceride and (in most cases) cholesterol intake. Moreover, if protein intake exceeds the need for new protein synthesis, much of the amino acid is converted by transamination to carbohydrate. At the same time, low protein intake is not recommended for the general population because animal protein is the major source for cobalamin and an excellent source of thiamine, absorbable iron, and zinc. For patients with normal protein synthesis but with increased protein losses, such as from

| TABLE 8.3. | RECOMMENDED ALLOWANCES OF REFERENCE PROTEIN AND U.S. DIETARY PROTEIN |

Category	Age (y) or Condition	Weight (kg)	Derived Allowance of Reference Protein[a]		Recommended Dietary Allowance	
			g/kg	g/d	g/kg[b]	g/d
Both sexes	0–0.5	6	2.20[c]		2.2	13
	0.5–1	9	1.56		1.6	14
	1–3	13	1.14		1.2	16
	4–6	20	1.03		1.1	24
	7–10	28	1.00		1.0	28
Male	11–14	45	0.98		1.0	45
	15–18	66	0.86		0.9	59
	19–24	72	0.75		0.8	58
	25–50	79	0.75		0.8	63
	51+	77	0.75		0.8	63
Female	11–14	46	0.93		1.8	46
	15–18	55	0.81		0.8	44
	19–24	58	0.75		0.8	46
	25–50	63	0.75		0.8	50
	51+[c]	65	0.75		0.8	50
Pregnancy	1st trimester			+1.3		+10
	2nd trimester			+6.1		+10
	3rd trimester			+10.7		+10
Lactation	1st 6 mo			+14.7		+15
	2nd 6 mo			+11.8		+12

[a] Data from WHO (1985).
[b] Amino acid score of typical U.S. diet is 100 for all age groups, except young infants. Digestibility is equal to reference proteins. Values have been rounded upward to 0.1 g/kg.
[c] For infants 0 to 3 months of age, breast-feeding that meets energy needs also meets protein needs. Formula substitutes should have the same amino acid amount and composition as human milk, corrected for digestibility, if appropriate.
(Reprinted with permission from Food and Nutrition Board, National Research Council. *Recommended-dietary allowances,* tenth ed. Washington, DC: National Academy Press, 1989:66.)

skin diseases or inflammatory bowel disease, the protein requirement can be increased by 30% for mild disease and by 50% to 60% for moderate to severe disease.

3. *Reduce total fat intake to 30% or less of calories; reduce saturated fatty acid intake to less than 10% of calories and the intake of cholesterol to less than 300 mg daily.* Dietary intake of saturated fats and cholesterol is associated with risks for atherosclerotic heart disease and possibly certain cancers. Moreover, polyunsaturated fatty acids have a cholesterol-lowering effect. Although these risks are not equal for all people, fatty acids are the largest potential source of calories (9 kcal per g) of the macronutrients. Consequently, limiting their intake is an important principle in maintaining normal weight—a goal for each of the guidelines listed in Table 8.1. Such limitation is difficult to maintain because fat is present in so many foods in concentrated form. For example, even in "extralean" beef, half the calories derive from fat; a single egg yolk contains two-thirds of the cholesterol RDA; 70% of the calories in cheese is from fat. Difficulty in following this recommendation is probably the single most important factor in the development of increasing obesity with age that characterizes populations on a Western diet.

The new food labels contain terms that help establish good eating patterns. First, the calories per serving from fat are listed prominently. Second, terms such as "low-fat" have been given standardized and clear definitions (Table 8.4). For example, "low" now refers to a content such that eating the food frequently will not provide more than the daily value allowed. Low-fat means no more than 3 g of fat per serving. "Less fat" means that the food contains one quarter less fat than the food to which it is compared. Because the most common example of malnutrition in the United States is obesity, education regarding fat sources and intake is crucially important.

4. *Every day eat five or more servings of a combination of vegetables and fruits, especially green and yellow vegetables and citrus fruits.* Also, increase intake of starches and other complex carbohydrates by eating six or more daily servings of a combination of breads, cereals, and legumes. Most vitamins, especially A, C, K, folate niacin, and riboflavin, and the minerals K, Mg, and Mn, and dietary fiber are contained in the foods recommended here. The RDA is the most widely publicized of the definitions of nutrient sufficiency. Table 8.5 lists the RDA for vitamins and minerals, as well as for macronutrients. Remember that water-soluble vitamins are lost in the cooking fluid and that fat-soluble vitamins can be oxidized during cooking. The content of vitamins and minerals listed in many publications usually refers to the raw food. When the cooked food is used as a reference, the

TABLE 8.4.	NUTRIENT CONTENT DESCRIPTORS

Term	Meaning
Free	Contains no or trivial amount "Calorie-free" = <5 kcal; "fat-free" = <0.5 g If natural food is free, the label must so state
Low	Eating the food frequently will not exceed daily values "Low-fat" = <3 g; "low-Na" = <140 mg "Low-calorie" = <40 kcal
Lean, extralean	For meats, poultry, seafood "Lean" = <10 g fat, <4 g saturated fat, <95 mg cholesterol "Extra-lean" = <5 g fat, <2 g saturated fat, <95 mg cholesterol
Reduced	Altered to contain <25% of unaltered product
Less	Contains 25% less than reference food
Light	Altered to contain <one-third calories or <50% fat or sodium
More	Contains ≥10% of daily value of reference food
Enriched, fortified	Altered to contain ≥10% of daily value of reference food
Good source	Contains 10%–19% of daily value
High	Contains ≥20% of daily value

nutrient content is only a rough estimate. There is no RDA for dietary fiber, but the average intake in the United States of 12 g per day is about half of what is considered optimal. Most of the committees establishing guidelines recommend increasing carbohydrate to 55% or more of total energy intake, and this should be accomplished by ingestion of fresh fruits and vegetables and of whole-grain products.

There are many population groups for whom RDAs have been developed (e.g., children, the elderly, men, women), making food labeling an educational problem. The USRDAs were established in 1973, based on the RDAs of 1968, to cover all of the recommendations for adults. By taking the highest RDA recommendation, the USRDAs were more generous than the RDAs because they were meant to cover the needs of 100% of the population. The 1990 Nutrition Labelling and Education Act changed the USRDAs to RDIs (recommended daily intake) to avoid confusion with the RDAs. Although most values remain the same as the USRDAs, after 1995 new values extended the scope and application of previous nutrient guidelines, beginning with Vol. 1 of dietary reference intakes for calcium, phosphorus, magnesium, vitamin D, and fluoride. The 1989 RDAs for micronutrients are shown in Table 8.5. On food labels, these RDIs are called Daily Values (Fig. 8.1). The Daily Values contain recommendations for some components, such as fiber and cholesterol, for which there is no RDI. An understanding of the new food labels should enable patients to maintain more readily an adequate intake of micronutrients; physicians should have the same facility with this information.

5. *Maintain adequate calcium intake.* The principal source of readily available calcium is dairy products. For those people who are lactose-intolerant, intake can be maintained by ingestion of green leafy vegetables or by calcium supplements. As with other nutrients, there is no information that ingestion of excess calcium is beneficial, unless the person has a disease associated with excess nutrient loss or malabsorption.

6. *Limit total daily intake of salt (NaCl) to 6 g or less.* Limit the use of salt in cooking and avoid adding it to food at the table. Salty, highly processed salty, salt-preserved, and salt-pickled foods should be consumed sparingly. The average intake of salt in the United States is 4 g per day. For patients with hypertension or edema, the limitation of salt intake is especially important.

7. *Alcohol consumption is not recommended.* If alcoholic beverages are consumed, they should be limited to less than 1 oz of pure alcohol daily. This is the equivalent of two cans of beer, two small glasses of wine, or two average cocktails. Pregnant women should avoid alcoholic beverages. Alcohol ingestion cannot yet be recommended for prevention of disorders such as coronary artery disease. Even if it could be, many experts believe that the risks of alcohol abuse outweigh the potential benefits of modest consumption. Moreover, alcohol is a concentrated caloric source. To estimate the caloric content (in kilocalories) of an alcoholic beverage, calculate $0.8 \times$ beverage proof (%) $\times$ number of ounces.

8. *Avoid taking dietary supplements in excess of the RDA in any one day.* Most studies show that people who consume vitamin or mineral supplements also consume an adequate diet. For people following the dietary recommendations outlined here, there is no known benefit from nutrient supplementation. Also, for the general population, there is no evidence that pharmacologic doses of nutrients are beneficial. Large amounts of individual nutrients have, however, been useful in some diseases (e.g., vitamin A in promyelocytic leukemia).

9. *Maintain an optimal intake of fluoride, particularly during the years of primary and secondary tooth formation and growth.* Most fluoride is now provided in the water supply.

IMPLEMENTATION OF GUIDELINES

The US Department of Agriculture Food Guide Pyramid (Fig. 8.2) is a schematic diagram designed to reinforce visually the recommendations for dietary health and to aid people in meal planning. The relative sizes of the blocks reflect the relative proportions of the components to overall energy intake. Examples of recommended serving number and portion sizes are as follows:

Breads, cereals (6 to 11 servings per day): 1 slice, 1/2 cup of cooked rice, pasta, or cereal

Vegetables (3 to 5 servings per day): 1/2 cup of chopped raw or cooked vegetables, 1 cup of leafy vegetables

Fruits (2 to 4 servings per day): 1 piece, 3/4 cup of juice, 1/4 cup dried fruit

Dairy products (2 to 3 servings per day): 1 cup milk or yogurt, 1/2 to 2 oz of cheese

TABLE 8.5. FOOD AND NUTRITION BOARD, NATIONAL ACADEMY OF SCIENCES—NATIONAL RESEARCH COUNCIL RECOMMENDED DIETARY ALLOWANCES,[a] REVISED 1989

Category	Age (yr) or Condition	Weight[b] kg	Weight[b] lb	Height[b] cm	Height[b] in.	Protein (g)	Vitamin A (µg RE)[c]	Vitamin D (µg)[d]	Vitamin E (mg α-TE)[e]	Vitamin K (µg)	Vitamin C (mg)	Thiamine (mg)	Riboflavin (mg)	Niacin (mg NE)[f]	Vitamin B6 (mg)	Folate (µg)	Vitamin B12 (µg)	Calcium (mg)	Phosphorus (mg)	Magnesium (mg)	Iron (mg)	Zinc (mg)	Iodine (µg)	Selenium (µg)
Infants	0.0–0.5	6	13	60	24	13	375	7.5	3	5	30	0.3	0.4	5	0.3	25	0.3	400	300	40	6	5	40	10
	0.5–1.0	9	20	71	28	14	375	10	4	10	35	0.4	0.5	6	0.6	35	0.5	600	500	60	10	5	50	15
Children	1–3	13	29	90	35	16	400	10	6	15	40	0.7	0.8	9	1.0	50	0.7	800	800	80	10	10	70	20
	4–6	20	44	112	44	24	500	10	7	20	45	0.9	1.1	12	1.1	75	1.0	800	800	120	10	10	90	20
	7–10	28	62	132	52	28	700	10	7	30	45	1.0	1.2	13	1.4	100	1.4	800	800	170	10	10	120	30
Males	11–14	45	99	157	62	45	1,000	10	10	45	50	1.3	1.5	17	1.7	150	2.0	1,200	1,200	270	12	15	150	40
	15–18	66	145	176	69	59	1,000	10	10	65	60	1.5	1.8	20	2.0	200	2.0	1,200	1,200	400	12	15	150	50
	19–24	72	160	177	70	58	1,000	10	10	70	60	1.5	1.7	19	2.0	200	2.0	1,200	1,200	350	10	15	150	70
	25–50	79	174	176	70	63	1,000	5	10	80	60	1.5	1.7	19	2.0	200	2.0	800	800	350	10	15	150	70
	51+	77	170	173	68	63	1,000	5	10	80	60	1.2	1.4	15	2.0	200	2.0	800	800	350	10	15	150	70
Females	11–14	46	101	157	62	46	800	10	8	45	50	1.1	1.3	15	1.4	150	2.0	1,200	1,200	280	15	12	150	45
	15–18	55	120	163	64	44	800	10	8	55	60	1.1	1.3	15	1.5	180	2.0	1,200	1,200	300	15	12	150	50
	19–24	58	128	164	65	46	800	10	8	60	60	1.1	1.3	15	1.6	180	2.0	1,200	1,200	280	15	12	150	55
	25–50	63	138	163	64	50	800	5	8	65	60	1.1	1.3	15	1.6	180	2.0	800	800	280	15	12	150	55
	51+	65	143	160	63	50	800	5	8	65	60	1.0	1.2	13	1.6	180	2.0	800	800	280	10	12	150	55
Pregnant						60	800	10	10	65	70	1.5	1.6	17	2.2	400	2.2	1,200	1,200	320	30	15	175	65
Lactating	1st 6 mo					65	1,300	10	12	65	95	1.6	1.8	20	2.1	280	2.6	1,200	1,200	355	15	19	200	75
	2nd 6 mo					62	1,200	10	11	65	90	1.6	1.7	20	2.1	260	2.6	1,200	1,200	340	15	16	200	75

[a] The allowances, expressed as average daily intakes over time, are intended to provide for individual variations most normal people as they live in the United States under usual environmental stresses. Diets should be based on a variety of common foods to provide other nutrients for which human requirements have been less well defined.

[b] Weights and heights of Reference Adults are actual medians for the U.S. population of the designated age, as reported by NHANES II. The median weights and heights of those younger than 19 years of age were taken from Hamill and colleagues (Am J Clin Nutr 1979;32:607). The use of these figures does not imply that the height-to-weight ratios are ideal.

[c] Retinol equivalents; 1 retinol equivalent = 1 µg retinol or 6 µg β-carotene. See text for calculation of vitamin A activity of diets as retinol equivalents.

[d] As cholecalciferol, 10 µg cholecalciferol = 400 IU of vitamin D.

[e] α-Tocopherol equivalents; 1 mg/d α-tocopherol = 1 mg α-TE. See text for variation in allowances and calculation of vitamin E activity of the diet as α-tocopherol equivalents.

[f] Niacin equivalents; 1 niacin equivalent = 1 mg of niacin or 60 mg of dietary tryptophan.

(Reprinted with permission from Food and Nutrition Board, National Research Council. Recommended dietary allowances, tenth ed. Washington, DC: National Academy Press, 1989.)

Serving sizes are now more consistent across product lines, stated in both household and metric measures, and reflect the amounts people actuallly eat.

New title signals that the label contains the newly required information.

Calories from fat are now shown on the label to help consumers meet dietary guidelines that recommend people get no more than 30 percent of their calories from fat.

% Daily Value shows how a food fits into the overall daily diet.

The list of nutrients covers those most important to the health of today's consumers, most of whom need to worry about getting *too much* of certain items (fat, for example), rather than too few vitamins or minerals, as in the past.

Daily Values are also something new. Some are maximums, as with fat (65 grams *or less*); others are minimums, as with carbohydrates (300 grams *or more*). The Daily Values on the label are shown for a daily diet of 2,000 and 2,500 calories. Individuals should adjust the values to fit their own calorie intake.

The label will now tell the number of calories per gram of fat, carbohydrates, and protein.

Nutrition Facts

Serving Size: ½ cup (114 g)
Servings Per Container: 4
Calories per serving: 90
Calories per serving from Fat: 30

Amount Per Serving		% Daily Value*
Total Fat	3 g	5%
Saturated Fat	0 g	0%
Cholesterol	0 mg	0%
Sodium	300 mg	13%
Total Carbohydrate	13 g	4%
Dietary Fiber	3 g	12%
Sugars	3 g	
Protein	3 g	
Vitamin A		80%
Vitamin C		60%
Calcium		4%
Iron		4%

*Percent Daily Values are based on a 2,000 calorie diet. Your Daily Values may be higher or lower depending on your calorie needs:

Nutrient		2,000 Calories	2,500 Calories
Total Fat	Less than	65 g	80 g
Sat Fat	Less than	20 g	25 g
Cholesterol	Less than	300 mg	300 mg
Sodium	Less than	2,400 mg	2,400 mg
Total Carbohydrate		300 g	375 g
Fiber		25 g	30 g

1 gram of Fat = 9 calories
1 gram of Carbohydrates = 4 calories
1 gram of Protein = 4 calories

Source: Food and Drug Administration 1992

FIGURE 8.1. Chart of nutrition facts showing how daily values (recommended daily intake) fit into a person's diet. (Reproduced with permission from Bull Publishing Company.)

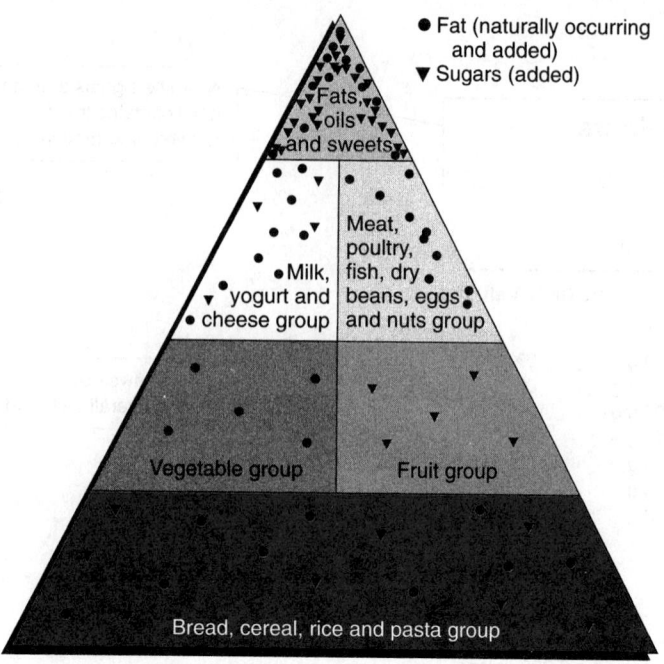

● Fat (naturally occurring and added)
▼ Sugars (added)

FIGURE 8.2. The USDA Food Guide Pyramid.

TABLE 8.6.	DRUG-INDUCED ALTERATION OF FOOD INTAKE	
Drugs Producing Hypophagia	**Drugs Producing Hyperphagia**	**Drugs Producing Hypogeusia/ Dysgeusia**
Alcohol	Amitriptyline hydrochloride	Amphetamines
Amiodarone	Anabolic steroids	Benzodiazepines
Amphetamine	Benzodiazepines	Captopril
		Carbimazole
		Chlorpromazine
Cisplatin	Buclizine hydrochloride	Clofibrate
Cocaine	Chlorpropamide	d-Penicillamine
Diethylpropion hydrochloride		
Fenfluramine hydrochloride	Cyproheptadine hydrochloride	5-Fluorouracil
Hydrazaline		Gold salts
Hydroxyurea		Griseofulvin
		Levodopa
	Glucocorticoids	Lincomycin
Methotrexate	Phenothiazines	Lithium carbonate
Phenethylbiguanide	Reserpine	Methimazole
		Methocarbamol
Phenmetrazine hydrochloride	Tolbutamide	
		Penicillin
		Propranolol
		Quinidine
		Tranquilizers

(Modified from Alpers DH, Bier DM, Stenson WF. *Manual of nutritional therapeutics,* third ed. Boston: Little, Brown and Company, 1995:35.)

Meat, fish, eggs, nuts (2 to 3 servings per day): 2-1/2 to 3 oz cooked lean meat, poultry, fish; 1 egg, 1/2 cup cooked beans, 2 tablespoons (tbsp) peanut butter = 1 oz meat

Fats, oils, sweets: use sparingly

The new food labels (1994) have been developed to assist the consumer (and patient; Fig. 8.1). Nearly all processed foods now carry this label in the United States; the label highlights fat and caloric content, but also protein, carbohydrate, sodium, calcium, iron, and vitamins A and C. The fat content of foods can be decreased by steaming, baking, broiling, or microwaving.

Patients may have difficulty in maintaining nutrient intake because of their underlying illness, which can produce anorexia or nausea. A major cause of altered food intake, either increased or decreased, is prescription medications. Table 8.6 lists some of the drugs producing these effects, including those that alter taste. Other major causes of altered taste include menopause, depression, and local oral factors.

■ NUTRITIONAL ASSESSMENT

Global (energy, protein) or specific (micronutrient) nutrient deficiency is assessed by history, physical examination, and testing for specific deficiencies. The pathophysiology of nutrient deficiency is based on a number of factors important in the physiologic handling of the nutrient; these factors are illustrated for vitamins in Table 8.7. These factors include decreased intake, increased loss, and increased utilization. When taking a history,

questions must be asked that are directed at these physiologic causes, questions that are not routinely asked as part of the general medical history (Table 8.8). Such questions might include those about dental disease, taste disturbances, anorexia-producing effects of medication, and careful assessment of the importance of factors such as diarrhea and fever that would increase nutrient losses or requirements. Not all nutrient deficiencies become apparent at the same time because symptoms and signs do not develop until body stores are depleted. Symptoms develop earliest for those nutrients with the largest fractional turnover rate (i.e., the percentage of total body content that can be lost each day) (Table 8.9).

During the physical examination, particular attention should be paid to the skin, hair, and mucous membranes because these rapidly renewing tissues can reflect deficiency states early (Table 8.10). The neurologic examination should be especially thorough to detect signs of vitamin deficiency, especially those that are more common in the elderly, such as cobalamin. Once a micronutrient deficiency is suspected,

Physiologic Factor	Vitamins Affected	Comments
TABLE 8.7.	**PATHOPHYSIOLOGY OF VITAMIN DEFICIENCY**	
Dietary intake	All except K, B$_6$, biotin	K, B$_6$, and biotin are probably produced by enteric bacteria
Endogenous synthesis	D (skin), K, B$_6$, biotin	
Enterohepatic circulation	A, polar metabolites of vitamin D, folic acid, cobalamin	
Decreased storage capacity	Cobalamin, A	Stored in liver
Increased utilization	Folic acid	Used in increased amounts during pregnancy, hemolysis
Increased loss from body	All	During malabsorption

(Modified from Alpers DH, Bier DM, Stenson WF. *Manual of nutritional therapeutics,* third ed. Boston: Little, Brown and Company, 1995:116.)

24). Weight is a measure of fat and protein mass, and an unintentional weight loss in excess of 10% of body weight is an important sign of serious illness (and in some cases of malnutrition). This finding can be important even when the initial weight is well over normal. Triceps skin fold, another measure of fat stores, is still a research tool because it requires careful attention to detail for accuracy. Somatic protein mass is best determined by the creatinine–height index, which is the actual 24-hour creatinine excretion for an adult of a given height, divided by ideal 24-hour excretion derived from an age- and gender-matched population on a creatinine-free diet. Hepatic protein synthesis is usually estimated by serum albumin levels, but this assumes a steady state, which is often not the case. The long half-life of this protein makes it a poor marker for following rapid changes. Plasma albumin concentration usually reflects transport between intravascular and extravascular pools, but does not necessarily correlate with somatic protein mass, especially in edematous states or in acute illness.

NUTRITIONAL PLANNING FOR PATIENTS WITH PROTEIN AND CALORIE DEFICIENCY

Most vitamins can be easily replaced (parenteral delivery of fat-soluble vitamins can be a problem). Many minerals are also replaced with relative ease, although adequate replacement of minerals with large body stores and low fractional daily retention (e.g., calcium, magnesium) poses a problem. In contrast, protein and calorie requirements are the largest (in mass) and are required on a daily basis; thus, they can be the most difficult to meet. There are certain key questions that can be used to determine whether protein-calorie support is needed (mostly for hospitalized patients) and, if so, how vigorously it should be pursued. Although algorithms are available, they are not recommended for routine use because they cannot show all of the subtleties of decision making, nor can they include all of the possible factors involved in arriving at a decision. For example, social setting and cost of delivering therapy are not usually included in such algorithms. The first key question to be asked illustrates the difficulty in answering even a seemingly straightforward question.

ARE PROTEIN AND CALORIE REQUIREMENTS BEING MET?

Energy and protein requirements can be estimated by standard methods (see equations earlier in the chapter), but these estimates are accurate, and for energy requirements are within 10% to 20%, only for the healthy population of average weight range. For ill or hospitalized patients, as well as for overweight or underweight patients, the estimates are even less accurate. The energy requirement of most hospitalized patients is no more than their resting energy requirement because they are largely inactive. The increased energy requirement that was anticipated to be caused by illness has not been documented; the inflammatory component of illness is less than was initially thought likely. Energy and protein intake can be estimated from documented food

it can be diagnosed by the use of laboratory tests. The appropriate test must be selected; usually it is the one that measures body stores. Some tests correlate only with recent intake and are not very useful for diagnosing deficiency. The most obvious example of this principle is measurement of serum carotenoids, a dietary component for which there is no normal storage in the body. Tables 8.11 and 8.12 list the most commonly used tests for body stores of micronutrients.

For assessment of macronutrient or protein energy status, an entirely different group of tests is available. In general, these tests are more useful as measures of the severity of the illness than as tests for specific deficiency states. This is because protein and energy balance are affected by illness, but it is the non-nutritional and metabolic aspects that affect the usual "nutritional" markers, such as serum albumin or transferrin. In this significant way, tests for macronutrient deficiency differ from tests analyzing body stores of micronutrients. The importance of making this distinction is that there is not much evidence that improving protein or energy balance affects the outcome of most illnesses. History, physical examination, and overall clinical assessment tend to identify most patients with protein-calorie malnutrition.

All tests of fat or protein mass depend on comparison with values for adults having values in the middle range of general populations. The most commonly used and most readily available is body weight. For best use, weight should be actually measured and without outer clothing. Weight should be coupled with height, especially if evaluation for obesity is the concern. Body mass index (weight in kg per height in meters^2) is useful in determining the degree of obesity (normal values are 18 to

TABLE 8.8.   NUTRITIONAL SCREENING HISTORY

Mechanism of Deficiency	If History of	Suspect Deficiency of
Inadequate intake	All foods—ask about alcoholism, weight loss, poverty, dental disease, AIDS, taste disturbance, medications, illegal drugs	Calories, protein, thiamine, niacin, folate, pyridoxine, riboflavin
	Fruit, vegetables, grains	Vitamin C, thiamine, niacin, folate, dietary fiber
	Meat, dairy products, eggs	Protein, vitamin B_{12}
	Food idiosyncracies, allergy	Lactase, fructo-oligosaccharide absorption
Inadequate absorption	Drugs (especially antacids, anticonvulsants, cholestyramine, laxatives, neomycin, alcohol)	Selected vitamins and minerals
	Malabsorption (diarrhea, weight loss, steatorrhea)	Vitamins A, D, K, calories, protein, iron, calcium, magnesium, zinc
	AIDS	Vitamin B_{12}
	Surgery, gastrectomy	Vitamin B_{12}, iron
	Resection of small intestine	Vitamin B_{12}, bile salts (if >100 cm of distal ileum), all others (if jejunal)
Increased losses	Alcohol abuse	Magnesium, zinc, phosphorus
	Blood loss	Iron
	Diabetes, poorly controlled	Calories
	Diarrhea	Protein, zinc, electrolytes
	Draining abscesses, wounds	Protein
	Peritoneal dialysis or hemodialysis	Protein, water-soluble vitamins, zinc
	Drugs (esp. diuretics, laxatives)	Potassium, magnesium
Increased requirements	Fever	Calories
	Increased physiologic demands (infancy, adolescence, pregnancy, lactation)	Various nutrients
	Surgery, trauma, burns, infection	Calories, protein

(Modified from Alpers DH, Bier DM, Stenson WF. *Manual of nutritional therapeutics,* third ed. Boston: Little, Brown and Company, 1995:20.)

TABLE 8.9.   ESTIMATED TIME TO ONSET OF CHRONIC VITAMIN AND MINERAL DEFICIENCIES

Nutrient	Fractional Daily Turnover (Daily Loss/ Body Content)	Estimated Total Body Content	Possible Daily Loss	Usual Cause of Loss	Onset of Symptoms
Sodium	12–14	2,500 mg	300–350 mg	Diarrhea, vomiting	1–2 wk
Folic acid	2	5,000 µg	100 µg	Malabsorption, ↓ intake	3–6 wk
Thiamine	1.4	25 mg	0.35 mg	↓ Intake	2–3 mo
Iron	0.4–0.5	5,000 mg	20–25 mg	Gastrointestinal bleeding, menstruation	4–6 mo
Vitamin A	0.2	500,000 IU	1,000 IU	Malabsorption	1–2 y
Cobalamin	0.1–0.2	5,000 µg	5–10 µg	Malabsorption	1–2 y
Calcium	0.0067	1,500 g	0.1 g	↓ Intake, ↑ urine loss	10–20 y

TABLE 8.10. SIGNS AND SYMPTOMS OF NUTRITIONAL DEFICIENCY IN ADULT PATIENTS	
Sign	**Possible Nutrient Deficiency**
General	
Wasted, skinny (esp. temporal muscles)	Protein-calorie
Abdomen	
Distention	Protein-calorie
Hepatomegaly	Protein-calorie
Extremities	
Edema	Protein, thiamine
Decubitus ulcers, poor wound healing	Protein, vitamin C, zinc
Bone tenderness	Vitamin D
Bone acne, joint pain	Vitamin C
Muscle wasting and weakness	Protein-calorie, vitamin D
Muscle tenderness, muscle pain	Thiamine
Skin	
Pallor	Folate, iron, vitamin B_{12}
Follicular hyperkeratosis	Vitamins A, C
Perifollicular petechiae (esp. after ↑ d venous pressure)	Vitamin C
Flaking dermatitis, scaling	Protein, calories, niacin, riboflavin, zinc, vitamin A
Bruising, purpura	Vitamins C, K, essential fatty acids
Pigmentation changes	Niacin, protein-calorie
Scrotal dermatosis	Riboflavin
Cellophane appearance	Protein (also with corticosteroid use, aging)
Hair	
Sparse and thin	Protein, zinc, biotin
Corkscrew hairs, coiled hair	Vitamins C, A
Nails	
Spooning	Iron
Transverse lines	Protein
Eyes	
History of night blindness (esp. impaired visual recovery after glare)	Vitamin A
Photophobia, blurring, conjunctival inflammation	Riboflavin, vitamin A
Mouth	
Glossitis (slick, red tongue)	Riboflavin, niacin, folic acid, vitamin B_{12}, protein
Gums—bleeding, receding, spongy, ulcers, hypertrophic	Vitamins C, A, K, folic acid, niacin; Vitamin A
Cheilosis (dry, cracking, ulcerated lips)	Riboflavin, pyridoxine, niacin
Angular stomatitis	Riboflavin, pyridoxine, niacin
Hypogeusia	Zinc, vitamin A
Tongue fissuring	Niacin
Burning/sore mouth/tongue	Vitamins B_{12}, B_6, C, niacin, folic acid, iron
Leukoplakia	Vitamins A, B_{12}, B complex, folic acid, niacin
Neck	
Goiter	Iodine
Parotid enlargement	Protein (also alcohol excess, starch chewing)
Neurologic	
Tetany	Calcium, magnesium
Peripheral neuropathy (paresthesias)	Thiamine, pyridoxine, Vitamin B_{12}
Loss of reflexes, wrist drop, foot drop (loss of vibratory and position sense)	Vitamins B_{12}, E
Dementia, disorientation	Niacin, vitamin B_{12}
Confabulation	Thiamine
Ophthalmoplegia	Thiamine, vitamin E
Depression	Biotin, folic acid, vitamin B_{12}

(Modified from Alpers DH, Bier DM, Stenson WF. *Manual of nutritional therapeutics,* third ed. Boston: Little, Brown and Company, 1995:28.)

TABLE 8.11.   CLINICAL LABORATORY TESTS FOR DETECTION OF VITAMIN DEFICIENCY

Vitamin	Test	Method	Reference Range (Units)[a] Marginal	Deficient	Usefulness
B_1	RBC transketolase activity coefficient (serum)	Spectrophotometric	1.23–1.29	>1.29 (ratio)	Advanced deficiency
B_1	Thiamine (serum, blood)	HPLC after enzymatic digestion		<0.33 ± 0.07 (μg/dL) <3.52 ± 0.74 (μg/dL)	Direct measure
B_1	Thiamine (urine)	HPLC	30–65	<30 (μg/g creatinine)	Body stores
B_2	RBC glutathione reductase activity coefficient (serum)	Spectrophotometric	1.2–1.4	>1.4 (ratio)	Long-term status
B_2	Urinary output	Spectrophotometric	27–29	<27 (μg/g creatinine)	Recent intake
B_6	RBC AST activity coefficient (serum)	Spectrophotometric	1.9–2.2	>2.2 (ratio)	Long-term status
B_6	4-Pyridoxic acid (urine) Total B_6 (urine)	HPLC	500–800	<500 (μg/d) <20 (μg/g creatinine)	Recent intake
Niacin	N-methyl-nicotinamide (urine)	HPLC	0.5–2.5	<0.5 (mg/g creatinine)	Recent intake
	2-Pyridone N-methyl-nicotinamide ratio (urine)			<1.0 (ratio)	
Folate	Folic acid (serum) (RBC)	Competitive protein binding	2–5.9 150–300	<2.0 (ng/mL) <150 (ng/mL)	Body stores and recent intake Body stores
B_{12}	Cobalamin (serum)	Competitive protein binding	180–200	<180 (pg/mL)	Body stores
B_{12} or folate	Homocysteine (serum)	HPLC		>20 (μmol/L)	Tests functional block in enzyme activity
B_{12}	Methylmalonic acid (serum)	HPLC, GC	>390–500	>500 (mmol/L)	Tests functional block in enzyme activity
C	Ascorbic acid (serum) (WBC)	Calorimetric	0.2–0.5 8.0–15	<0.2 (mg/dL) <8.0 (mg/dL)	Recent intake Body stores
A	Retinol (serum)	HPLC	35–70	<35 (μg/dL)	Recent intake and body stores
Carotene	Total carotenoids (serum)	Spectrophotometry	50–70	<40–50 (μg/dL)	Dietary intake
	β-Carotene (serum)	HPLC	10–20	<10 (μg/dL)	
D	25-Hydroxy vitamin D (serum)	Ligand-binding	10–20	<8–10 (ng/mL)	Body stores
E	Tocopherol (serum)	HPLC	120–150	<120 (μg/dL)	Body stores
	Tocopherol/total lipid		0.6–1.0	<0.6 (ratio mg/g)	Ratio is preferred
K	Prothrombin time (plasma)	Clotting test	1.5–2	>2.0 (sec. over control)	Not specific for vitamin K
	Vitamin K_1	HPLC	0.1–0.3	<0.1 (nmol/L)	Body stores

[a] Check local laboratory for variations from these ranges, which are composites derived from various sources.
AST, aspartate aminotransferase; GC, gas chromatography; HPLC, high-pressure liquid chromatography; RBC, red blood cell; WBC, white blood cell.
(Modified from Alpers DH, Bier DM, Stenson WF. *Manual of nutritional therapeutics,* third ed. Boston: Little, Brown and Company, 1995:28.)

| TABLE 8.12. | CLINICAL LABORATORY DETECTION OF MICRONUTRIENT MINERAL DEFICIENCY | | | |

Nutrient	Test	Method	Reference Range (Units)[a]	Usefulness
Iron	Iron (serum)	Colorimetry	50–200 (μg/dL)	Poor measure of body stores
	Total iron binding (serum)	Colorimetry	245–400 (μg/dL)	
	Total iron binding capacity	Calculation	15–50 (%)	Insensitive for iron status
	Transferrin (serum)	Immunoturbidimetry	200–400 (μg/dL)	Preferred over total iron binding capacity if available
	Ferritin (serum)	Immunoturbidimetry	12–300 (ng/mL)	Measures body stores: high specificity when low, poor sensitivity
Zn	Zinc (plasma)	Flame atomic absorption	20–130 (μg/dL)	Poor specificity for body stores
Cu	Copper (serum)	Flame atomic absorption	55–175 (μg/dL)	Insensitive for body stores
	Ceruloplasmin (plasma)	Immunoturbidimetry	10–60 (mg/dL)	Independent of body stores
Selenium	Selenium (serum)	Fluorometry	100–340 (ng/mL)	Measures body stores
	Glutathione peroxidase (plasma)	Spectrophotometry	455–800 (U/L)	More sensitive for body stores

[a] Check local laboratory for variation from the ranges.
(Modified from Alpers DH, Bier DM, Stenson WF. *Manual of nutritional therapeutics,* third ed. Boston: Little, Brown and Company, 1995:30.)

intake or from intravenous or enteral feedings. If the hospitalized patient is in negative energy or protein balance, remedial causes of appetite suppression should be addressed, such as medication, upper gastrointestinal disease, or depression. If the patient remains in negative balance, the clinician must decide whether supplementation is needed. This decision is based on the severity of the illness, the estimated length of time for which the negative balance will be present, and the chance of increased intake modifying the clinical outcome of the illness. It makes little sense to insist on a vigorous replacement of calories and protein if there is no evidence to support such a role in disease management. In such a circumstance, a better policy would be simply to prevent further weight loss by maintaining daily requirements. In any case, the patient requires at least 200 to 400 kcal per day in the form of dextrose to minimize protein degradation and conversion by transamination of the mobilized amino acids for the process of gluconeogenesis.

WHAT IS THE CURRENT DEGREE OF BODY PROTEIN AND FAT DEPLETION?

As mentioned, the existing measures correlate better with severity of illness than with precise deficiency states. In the absence of large fluid shifts, however, weight is a good overall measure of caloric deficiency due to decreased intake, increased utilization, or both. The initial degree of depletion is relevant, particularly during a long illness, because most well-nourished patients tolerate negative energy and protein balance fairly well during self-limited illnesses. The cumulative effect of negative calorie balance in pure starvation can be estimated by calculating 3,500

kcal per lb. Thus, in the absence of illness causing marked protein breakdown, a negative calorie balance of 1,000 kcal per day would lead to loss of 2 lb per week. If the amount of weight loss exceeds that estimated by decreased caloric intake alone, the difference might be attributable to underlying illness. Regardless of the cause of the weight loss, this estimate helps to answer the next question.

WHAT IS THE ANTICIPATED LENGTH OF TIME NEEDED FOR NUTRITIONAL SUPPORT?

If the patient is well nourished at the start of the illness, even large caloric deficits can be tolerated for a matter of weeks. If the patient is poorly nourished, the clinician could calculate how many calories would be needed daily to maintain body weight at 90% of ideal weight, for example. The major dangers in planning nutritional support are overestimating need, and trying to recapture lost weight and protein mass during the acute phase of the illness. Delivery of high loads of calories and protein by enteral or parenteral feeding requires the use of large fluid volumes and salt loads. Excessive use of tube feedings may cause diarrhea or pulmonary aspiration. Inappropriate use of total parenteral nutrition (TPN) may lead to all of the potential complications of that technique. The most important decision in providing calorie and protein support is the first one: what is the goal of the therapy, and how vigorously should it be pursued?

IS THE INTESTINAL TRACT AVAILABLE AND ADEQUATE?

If supplementary treatment is needed, the clinician must decide whether to use enteral or parenteral routes. Total parenteral nu-

TABLE 8.13.	MODIFIED DIETS
Diet	**Possible Indications**
Low fat	Steatorrhea of any cause, especially when colon is present; protein-losing enteropathy
Reduced calorie	Obesity, preventive measure for good health
Low lactose	Lactose intolerance
Low fructose	Fructo-oligosaccharide intolerance
High fiber	Prevention of recurrent diverticulitis; irritable bowel syndrome with alternating bowel habits
Low fiber	Acute diarrhea, bowel preparation
Low sodium	Edema-forming conditions, hypertension
Low oxalate	Steatorrhea with hyperoxaluria
Elimination diet	Food allergies

trition is discussed in Chapter 130. Whenever possible, the gastrointestinal tract should be used. Sometimes the oral route can be used, but more often forced enteral feeding is needed if the supplement must be large. If gastric emptying is normal, infusion into the stomach is possible. If the stomach is abnormal, jejunal or duodenal infusion must be used. The presence of diarrhea can make enteral supplementation difficult.

ENTERAL NUTRITION THERAPY

USE OF DIETS IN THE MANAGEMENT OF DISEASE

Modification of the basic diet is needed for management of certain diseases (Table 8.13). Such modifications may or may not use commercial supplements. Diets can be used to alter consistency of the meal (e.g., soft diets for patients with difficulty chewing), to restrict certain elements (e.g., low-lactose or gluten-restricted diets), or to add specific elements (e.g., calcium, fiber, pancreatic enzymes). Discussion of the specific diseases is included in chapters 109–111 and 117.

MICRONUTRIENT DEFICIENCIES

Vitamin and mineral deficiencies are treated by addition of specific nutrients or by use of nutritional supplements that are fortified with vitamins or minerals.

ESSENTIAL FATTY ACID DEFICIENCY

The uncommon disorder known as essential fatty acid deficiency was seen formerly in patients treated with TPN but without fatty acid supplementation. Today three-in-one TPN therapy using intravenous lipid is routine, and fatty acid deficiency is

rarely encountered. When it is, 1 to 2 tbsp of vegetable oil per day by mouth is usually sufficient for treatment.

ORAL SUPPLEMENTATION

Most often, protein and calorie supplements are used to improve diets in a reliable way. The usual sources of protein in table foods that are appropriate for use as supplements include milk products, eggs, peanut butter, fish, and meat. When low fat (triglyceride) content is desirable, skim milk, chicken or turkey without skin, shellfish, and flat fish are useful. The most commonly used commercial supplements add a defined nutrient content and are prescribed as medications. There are a large number of available products, and new ones are introduced frequently. Although the best diet for a given patient provides for individual needs, there is seldom a single product that is "best" for a given patient. Many calorie supplements are lactose free and are available in multiple flavors to improve taste selection over a long period. Milk-based supplements are usually less expensive, but they cannot be used by lactose-intolerant patients, who can tolerate on average less than 8 oz of milk daily. Fiber supplements are commonly used, usually in the form of psyllium extract (hemicellulose) when prescribed alone, but soy polysaccharide is now added to many protein-calorie supplements to increase their fiber content. Hemicellulose has a high water-holding capacity, but other fiber components, such as cellulose and pectins, also retain water. Any of these fiber components is usually included when it is desirable to alter the consistency of the stool, although this is not a consistent benefit of such supplements. Dietary fiber is converted to short-chain fatty acids in the colon, with potential benefits to colonic mucosal integrity; however, such usefulness in critically ill patients has not been demonstrated.

A number of supplements are available that are designed for very special needs (e.g., chronic renal failure, hepatic encephalopathy), but these are expensive and in general are designed for forced enteral feeding. There are several products designed for use in pulmonary failure because high carbohydrate load can lead to excess production of carbon dioxide and, rarely, to worsening hypercapnia. However, the amount of carbon dioxide produced by a person is more a function of the total caloric load than of the macronutrient source of the calories, and hypercapnia is rarely related to dietary intake. Glutamine is a nonessential amino acid that is highly abundant and an important fuel for the intestinal mucosa. Although all enteral protein-calorie supplements contain glutamine, some contain high levels. There are not yet sufficient data demonstrating improved outcome to support the routine use of glutamine supplementation.

ORAL REHYDRATION THERAPY

Although well described for the treatment of dehydrated children and for adults with cholera, oral rehydration therapy has not been widely used for rehydration of adults after or during acute diarrheal or other illness. If signs of dehydration are present (especially postural hypotension) and the patient's clinical status does not require hospitalization, oral rehydration can be effective and rapid. It is based on the concept that coupled sodium-glucose absorption is preserved during diarrheal illness and such absorption carries with it free water. Most of the commercially available rehydration solutions are formulated in pediatric doses, but some (e.g., Pedialyte) are available in liter portions. The World Health Organization has developed an oral rehydration solution that can be made at home and is applicable to adults. To 1 L of water add 3 to 4 (teaspoons) tsp of table salt; 1/2 tsp of baking soda or 1 tsp of baking powder; 1 cup of orange juice; and 4 tbsp of cane or table sugar (sucrose) or 2 tbsp of honey (enriched in fructose). The usual daily dose for adults is 2 to 3 L. Sports drinks (e.g., Gatorade) were designed to provide energy and to replace electrolytes lost in sweat. When fluid loss from vomiting or diarrhea is not severe, such beverages may be well tolerated and are helpful in maintaining fluid volume. However, they are not useful in replacing lost volume because the sodium concentration is too low. Most soft drinks contain only 1 to 4 mEq per L of sodium and 0.1 to 0.6 mEq per L of potassium with 10% carbohydrate, and thus are inadequate for the treatment of dehydration.

FORCED ENTERAL FEEDING

The term *forced enteral feeding* refers to nutritional support using tube feeding techniques. Usually all, or nearly all, nutritional requirements are delivered to the patient in this way. Such diets therefore should be nutritionally complete, providing protein, calories, and other essential nutrients. Patients who are usual candidates for forced enteral feeding have an available and functioning gastrointestinal tract, and have existing protein-calorie malnutrition and some condition that prevents standard oral supplementation. Such conditions would include coma or depressed mental state, anorexia, or oropharyngeal malfunction preventing normal swallowing. When the period for required supplementation is short, nasogastric or nasoduodenal feeding tubes should be used. When nutritional support must be prolonged to maintain the quality of life agreed on by the patient (or patient's family) and the physician, gastrostomy or jejunostomy may be used as the portal of entry into the gastrointestinal tract.

BIBLIOGRAPHY

Alpers DH, Bier DM, Stenson WF. *Manual of nutritional therapeutics*, third ed. Boston: Little, Brown and Company, 1995.

American Society of Parenteral and Enteral Nutrition. Guidelines for the use of parenteral and enteral nutrition in adult and pediatric patients. *J Parenter Enteral Nutr* 1993;17:1S.

Food and Nutrition Board, National Research Council. *Diet and health: implications for reducing chronic disease risk*. Washington, DC: National Academy Press, 1989.

Food and Nutrition Board, National Research Council. *Recommended dietary allowances*, tenth ed. Washington, DC: National Academy Press, 1989.

Food and Nutrition Board, Institute of Medicine, Dietary reference intakes for calcium, phosphorus, magnesium, vitamin D, and fluoride. Washington DC: National Academy Press, 1999.

Hands ES. *Food finder: food sources of vitamins and minerals*, second ed. Salem, OR: ESHA Research, 1990.

Kelley's Textbook of Internal Medicine, fourth edition. Edited by H. David Humes.
Lippincott Williams & Wilkins, Philadelphia © 2000.

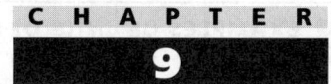

PRINCIPLES OF RENAL REGULATION OF FLUID AND ELECTROLYTES

L. B. GARDNER
H. DAVID HUMES

▪ BASIC CONCEPTS

BODY FLUID COMPARTMENTS

Body fluids, composed predominantly of water, its accompanying electrolytes, and circulating serum proteins and lipoproteins, constitute approximately 60% of total body weight. Thus, in a hypothetical 70-kg individual, total body fluid, or, as commonly referred to, total body water approximates 42 L, with 28 L contained in the intracellular fluid (ICF) and 14 L contained in the extracellular fluid (ECF) compartment as interstitial fluid (that fluid outside cells and outside the capillaries) and as plasma.

The forces that govern the distribution of fluids between the ICF and ECF compartments—the osmotic pressure—are determined by the pressure exerted by the concentration of *effective* osmotic particles in each compartment. In a steady-state condition under virtually all circumstances, the intracellular and extracellular effective osmotic pressures are equal.

In the ECF, different pressures determine the distribution of fluid between the plasma volume and the interstitial fluid volume. Here Starling's forces are the determining factors. Hydrostatic pressure within the capillaries and their accompanying arterioles and venules tends to induce the movement of fluid from the plasma volume to the interstitial volume, whereas oncotic pressure (determined almost exclusively by the concentration of albumin in the plasma) induces the movement from the interstitial compartment to the plasma volume. In reality, these fluids are constantly in motion crossing the capillary membrane. At steady state approximately one-fourth of the ECF volume is contained within the capillaries and three-fourths constitutes the interstitial fluid. This circulation of the interstitial fluid is critically important for the delivery of vital nutrients to the cells and for the removal of waste products from the cellular milieu back into the plasma volume for eventual disposal.

CLINICAL IMPLICATIONS

In a hypothetical patient, it is possible to lose the entire plasma volume iso-osmotically and to be limited to only the interstitial fluid volume to replenish the falling plasma volume (as might happen in severe hemorrhage). Not even 1 mL of intracellular fluid would cross the cellular membrane if there were no change in effective osmotic pressure.

TABLE 9.1.	EXAMPLES OF UNITS OF SOLUTE MEASUREMENT				
Substance	Grams (mol wt)	Moles (6×10^{23} molecules)	Equivalents (6×10^{23} charges) Cation	Anion	Osmoles (6×10^{23} particles)
Ionized					
Na^+	23	1	1	0	1
Cl^-	35.5	1	0	1	1
K^+	39	1	1	0	1
HCO_3^-	61	1	0	1	1
Ca^{2+}	41	1	2	0	1
Nondissociable					
Urea	60	1	0	0	1
Glucose	180	1	0	0	1
Dissociable					
Univalent					
NaCl	58.5	1	1	1	2
KCl	74.5	1	1	1	2
Divalent					
$CaSO_4$	136	1	2	2	2
Mixed					
Na_2SO_4	142	1	2	2	3
$CaCl_2$	111	1	2	2	3
Complex					
$(Ca)_3 (PO_4)_2$	310	1	6	6	5

UNITS OF SOLUTE MEASUREMENT

Solute concentration can be expressed in milligrams per deciliter, millimoles per liter or per kilogram of water, milliequivalents per liter, or milliosmoles per liter or per kilogram of water. For example, in the case of the calcium ion (Ca^{2+}), the values 4 mg per dL, 1 mmol per L, 2 mEq per L, and 1 mOsm per L indicate the same concentration of Ca^{2+}. Because of different concentration units, the amount of any given solute can be expressed in several different ways (Table 9.1).

The simplest way to express the amount of solute is by mass or weight, using gram or kilogram as the unit. More information can be conveyed by employing units based on the molecular weight of the substance. The molecular weight is defined as the quantity (in grams) of any substance that contains 6.023×10^{23} (Avogadro's number) molecules of that substance. This amount is known as 1 mol of the substance. For example, 1 mol of sodium (Na^+) contains the same number of molecules as 1 mol of chloride (Cl^-), although the former weighs 23 g and the latter weighs 35.5 g. Conversely, to convert from mass units, such as grams and milligrams, to moles or millimoles, the weight of the substance is divided by its molecular weight. For example, 1 g of NaCl (molecular weight = 23 + 35.5 = 58.5) contains $1000 \div 58.5 = 17.1$ mmol NaCl.

With electrically charged compounds (electrolytes and ions), it is often most useful to consider the number of positive or negative charges. Positively charged particles are called cations, and negatively charged particles are called anions. When ions combine, they do so according to their ionic charge, or valence, and not according to molecular weight. The unit used to indicate charge is the chemical equivalent. One equivalent of an anion is defined as the amount that combines with, or replaces, 1 mol of hydrogen ion (H^+). Because Na^+ is a univalent ion (charge + 1), 1 mol of Na^+ is equal to 1 equivalent. Because Ca^{2+} is a bivalent ion (charge + 2), 1 mol of Ca^{2+} equals 2 equivalents. To convert from units of moles to equivalents, the following simple formula can be used:

$$Equivalents = moles \times valence$$

The most common term used for expressing concentrations of electrolytes in serum is milliequivalents per liter. There are two advantages in using this unit of concentration. First, it reinforces the principle that ions combine milliequivalent for milliequivalent, not millimole for millimole or milligram for milligram. Second, to maintain electroneutrality, there must be an equal number of cations and anions in each fluid compartment of the body.

Not all ions are easily measured in milliequivalents per liter. For instance, the total calcium concentration in serum is about 10 mg per dL, or 5 mEq per L. Because 50% to 55% of the plasma calcium is bound to albumin, the free ionized (unbound) calcium concentration in plasma is 2.0 to 2.5 mEq per L. For these reasons, the precise concentration of ionized calcium is difficult to determine with present clinical laboratory techniques. Consequently, the total serum calcium is routinely reported in mass units (mg per dL) rather than equivalence units (mEq per L).

A different problem occurs with phosphate because it exists in several different ionic forms: $H_2PO_4^-$, HPO_4^{2-}, and PO_4^{3-}. Although an exact valence cannot be given, an approximate valence of 1.8 can be assigned because roughly 80% of extracellular phosphate exists as HPO_4^{2-} and 20% as $H_2PO_4^-$ in serum at a pH of 7.4. Because of the imprecision of valance and equivalence for this electrolyte, serum phosphorus concentrations are routinely reported in mass units (milligrams per deciliter).

OSMOLALITY

The osmolality of a given body fluid is determined by the concentration of the circulating dissociated ionic and nonionic particles contained in that fluid. In the extracellular fluid volume, since sodium makes up more than 95% of the circulating cationic ionized particles, and glucose and urea account for virtually all of the normally occurring circulating nonionic particles, the total plasma osmolality can be easily approximated by the formula: plasma osmolality = $2 \times$ [plasma sodium concentration] + glucose concentration (mg %) ÷ 18 + BUN ÷ 2.8. This value is referred to as the calculated plasma osmolality and, as mentioned above, equals the osmolality of the entire ECF and the osmolality of the ICF as well. The pathology laboratory confirms the measurement of plasma osmolality by use of a technique that measures the concentration of osmotically active particles through its effect on depressing the freezing point of any given solution. In general, the difference between the calculated plasma osmolality and the measured plasma osmolality is less than 5 to 10 mOsm per L.

While determination of the plasma osmolality is important, it is vital to recognize that not all particles contributing to the plasma osmolality are osmotically effective. The most significant exception is urea. Because of its permeability across cell membranes, intracellular and extracellular urea concentrations are equal; in effect, the osmotic pressure that they would generate across these fluid compartments "cancels itself out." Hence, clinicians are much better served by calculating the *effective plasma osmolality* by the formula noted above with the urea term removed. Effective osmolality is also known as tonicity, a term that many find useful in distinguishing between total osmolality and effective osmolality.

■ TONICITY AND CELL VOLUME

As noted above, when water is added to the body it is distributed between the two major body fluid compartments such that at steady state two-thirds is located in the ICF and one-third in the ECF. Similarly, a pure water deficit is distributed such that at steady state two-thirds of the net loss is derived from the ICF and one-third from the ECF. Because the gain or loss of pure water is shared proportionately by the two major body fluid compartments, it does not alter the relative volumes of these two compartments.

If an effective solute (e.g., sodium, glucose) is added to the ECF, the ECF tonicity increases and water moves out of the cells. The ECF volume increases at the expense of the ICF volume until the tonicity of the two fluid compartments is equal-

ized. Conversely, if an effective solute is removed from the ECF, the ECF tonicity decreases and water moves into the cells. The ICF volume increases at the expense of ECF volume until the tonicity of the two fluid compartments is equalized. In contrast, if an ineffective solute (e.g., urea) is added to or removed from the ECF, the ECF tonicity does not change and cell volume remains constant.

Changes in body fluid tonicity are associated with characteristic alterations in cell volume. Hypertonicity leads to ICF contraction (cell shrinkage or dehydration), while hypotonicity leads to ICF expansion (cell swelling or edema). The major clinical features of disorders of water homeostasis are largely attributable to changes in cell volume.

CLINICAL IMPLICATIONS

As a consequence of these physiologic parameters it becomes relatively easy to assess the effect of intravenous replacement solutions on patients with various body fluid deficits. The administration of 5% dextrose in water, while effectively addressing a water deficit, does little to expand plasma volume in particular. One liter of 5% dextrose in water, for example, in the absence of diabetes, will distribute 667 mL to the ICF and 333 mL to the ECF. Three-fourths of that fluid will be retained in the interstitial compartment, leaving approximately 85 mL of the original liter to distribute to the plasma volume, a poor plasma expander indeed.

Administration of Ringer's lactate, normal saline, or any other isonatric sodium containing solution is far more effective in plasma volume expansion. One liter of normal saline will remain entirely in the extracellular fluid (sodium being limited from entry to the intracellular compartment by active extrusion from virtually all cells). Of the liter retained in the ECF compartment, 250 mL distributes to the plasma volume—a far better effect. For the ultimate volume expander, plasma infusion is theoretically ideal. An entire liter of infused plasma (because of its iso-osmotic and iso-oncotic pressures) remains in the plasma volume and would be most effective in emergency plasma volume expansion.

The converse physiologic circumstance to that noted above is also true. Water loss is well tolerated with regard to hemodynamics; salt loss (with its accompanying water) is more significant; and plasma loss can be fatal.

SERUM SODIUM CONCENTRATION

Sodium salts make up more than 95% of ECF effective solutes, and in most circumstances, the serum sodium concentration (S_{Na}) accurately reflects body fluid tonicity. Because the symptoms and signs of abnormal body fluid tonicity are generally nonspecific, disorders of water homeostasis are often detected clinically by the presence of an abnormal S_{Na}. The features of altered body fluid tonicity relate to changes in tonicity and not to associated changes in S_{Na}. Consequently, tonicity and S_{Na} need not always change concordantly. Although hypernatremia always implies hypertonicity, the converse is not always true; hyponatremia does not always imply hypotonicity.

Hypertonicity can occur in the absence of hypernatremia

when an effective solute other than sodium (e.g., glucose) is present in excessive amounts in the ECF. The osmotic pressure exerted by the nonsodium solute leads to redistribution of water from the ICF to the ECF and consequently leads to hyponatremia and intracellular volume depletion. Hyperglycemic hypertonicity is common in patients with uncontrolled diabetes mellitus.

Hyponatremia can occur in the absence of hypotonicity if an effective solute other than sodium is present in significant quantity in the ECF (hypertonic hyponatremia) or when large amounts of lipids or proteins are present in the plasma (isotonic hyponatremia). The latter circumstance, also known as pseudo-hyponatremia, is discussed in Chapter 144.

WATER BALANCE

Water balance in a normal person is maintained through a series of hemodynamic, hormonal, and molecular mechanisms. Balance is so finely tuned that neither water retention nor water loss will occur despite changes in fluid intake of 10-fold or greater (e.g., 1 L to 10 L per day). One of the characteristics of chronic renal disease (see Chapters 133 and 141) is that this broad range over which water balance can be achieved is narrowed significantly because the homeostatic mechanisms have themselves been compromised by the process, causing injury to the kidney.

The following sequence of events occurs after the ingestion of water in a normal individual (Fig. 9.1). Plasma osmolality is transiently diluted and the effective osmolality falls; extracellular fluid volume is expanded, albeit minimally. This expansion results in a minimal, clinically undetectable increase in glomerular filtration rate and delivery of more sodium to the proximal tubule of the kidney (see below). As a consequence of the dilution of effective plasma osmolality, antidiuretic hormone (ADH; also known as vasopressin) production and release is inhibited at the level of the hypothalamus. This inhibition lowers the level of circulating ADH and decreases its effects on the distal portions of the nephron: the distal cortical tubule, the collecting tubule, and the collecting duct. Also, the increase in extracellular fluid volume and increased perfusion of the hypothalamus sends a signal of hypervolemia to a variety of volume receptors through-

out the body, which further inhibit ADH synthesis and release. The increased sodium delivered to the proximal tubule is for the most part reabsorbed, but a greater absolute amount of the filtered sodium travels down to the prime diluting site in the ascending limb of the loop of Henle, where chloride (with sodium following passively) is removed and water stays behind. This segment of the nephron is unalterably impermeable to water. The increased volume of hypotonic fluid enters the cortical distal tubule, collecting tubule, and collecting duct (these structures are impermeable to water due to the absence of ADH), and increased urine volume accompanied by increased excretion of water results. Subsequently, the plasma osmolality, extracellular fluid volume, and glomerular filtration rate return to normal.

In states of fluid restriction, the opposite sequence of events occurs. Increased plasma osmolality increases ADH release. Decreased extracellular fluid volume results in a decrease in glomerular filtration rate and sodium delivery. In this setting, more water is reabsorbed (conserved). These same homeostatic mechanisms are responsible for minimizing the effect of low fluid intake on plasma osmolality and serum sodium concentration.

SODIUM BALANCE

The kidney increases the excretion of sodium in states of sodium excess and retains sodium in states of sodium deprivation, controlling the extracellular fluid volume (since osmolality is also controlled and the accompanying quantity of water is appropriate for the absolute quantity of sodium) within narrow limits. Regulation of the ECF volume depends upon a number of afferent stimuli by which the kidney senses changes in extracellular or intravascular volume. Furthermore, there are efferent pathways by which the kidney alters the excretion of sodium in response to these volume changes (Fig. 9.2).

AFFERENT PATHWAYS

The receptors that control renal sodium excretion have not all been clearly defined, but there is evidence for the existence of volume receptors in the low-pressure central venous circulation and the high-pressure arterial circulation. The cardiac atria contain the best examined receptors within the low-pressure circulation. Distention of the atria suppresses hypothalamic sympathetic output to the kidney and the sympathetic vasculature, and inhibits ADH release from the neurohypophysis (see above). Besides the neural effects of atrial distention, atrial myocytes contain atrial natriuretic peptide, the release of which is directly proportional to the central venous pressure. Atrial natriuretic peptide is strongly natriuretic.

Volume receptors also exist in the arterial side of the circulation. One such very important receptor is the juxtaglomerular apparatus within the kidney. Secretion of renin by granular cells in the afferent arterial of the juxtaglomerular apparatus is sensitive to ECF volume and renal perfusion pressure. When pressure falls, renin release increases. Renin stimulates angiotensin II production, which promotes an increase in the circulating levels of aldosterone, a hormone that is an important modulator of so-

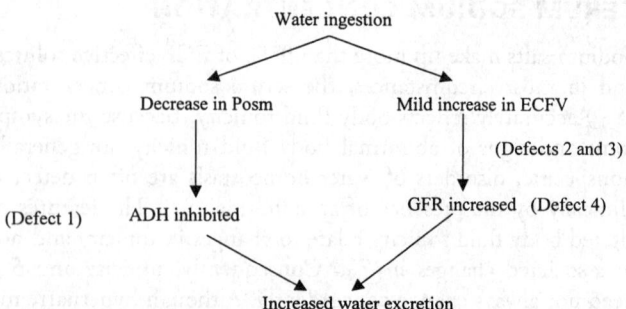

FIGURE 9.1. Water homeostasis and defects producing hyponatremia. 1, defect in SIADH; 2, defect in volume depletion; 3, defect in edematous disorders; 4, defect in renal failure.

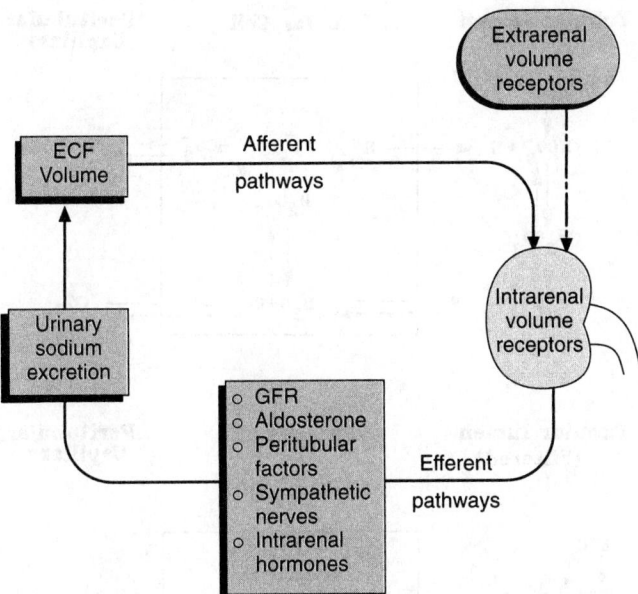

FIGURE 9.2. Afferent and efferent pathways for renal sodium excretion. Renal excretion of sodium is regulated by afferent mechanisms, by which changes in extracellular fluid (ECF) volume are signaled to the kidney, and efferent mechanisms, in which the kidney changes the rate of sodium excretion in response to changes in ECF. The most critical afferent pathways may be intrarenal rather than extrarenal.

dium homeostasis. Although the exact sensing mechanism and precise location of other high-pressure sensors remains unclear, baroreceptors, which respond to wall tension, appear to be located in the carotid arteries and aorta. Stimulation of these receptors results in a natriuresis that depends on intact renal sympathetic innervation. From such data, the concept of effective arterial blood volume (EABV), which is that portion of the arterial blood volume capable of stimulating high-pressure volume receptors, has evolved as a major factor in the regulation of renal sodium excretion. In normal circumstances, EABV and ECF volume are closely and directly related. In disease states, EABV and ECF volume may not change in the same direction. The distinction between the conceptual EABV and the real measurable ECF volume becomes important in understanding the pathogenesis of sodium retention states. These states are discussed in greater detail in Chapter 143. The EABV is a concept with no, or only poorly identified, structural correlates, and extrarenal perception of changes in ECF volume or EABV might not be a prerequisite for alterations in renal sodium handling.

EFFERENT PATHWAYS

Once the kidneys, by whatever afferent pathways, perceive an increase in ECF volume or EABV, a wide variety of efferent mechanisms come into play to modify renal sodium excretion.

Glomerular Filtration Rate

The renal excretion of sodium is ultimately determined by the relation between the glomerular filtration rate (GFR) and the rate of tubular sodium reabsorption. Were there no correlation

between filtration and reabsorption, changes in GFR would result in significant volume expansion or depletion. Instead, a rise in GFR is accompanied by an increase in sodium reabsorption and a fall by a decrease in sodium reabsorption. This association between GFR and tubular reabsorption is called glomerulotubular balance. As a result of glomerulotubular balance, the fractional reabsorption of sodium (the fraction of the filtered load of sodium that undergoes tubular reabsorption) remains relatively constant unless disease processes supervene.

Peritubular Capillary Forces

Peritubular capillary forces, the so-called physical factors, exert an important influence on renal sodium handling, primarily at the level of the proximal tubule. The proximal tubule normally reabsorbs 50% to 65% of the filtered load of sodium. Net sodium transport in the proximal tubule appears to be governed by a pump-leak system. Filtered sodium is actively transported across the renal tubule cell to the intercellular (interstitial) space. Sodium salts and water that accumulate in this space may be taken up into the systemic circulation by the peritubular capillaries or may leak back into the lumen across the tight junctions between epithelial cells. The modulation of proximal tubule sodium reabsorption appears to be governed primarily by changes in the rate of back flux into the lumen and not in the rate of active sodium transport. Factors that increase peritubular capillary oncotic pressure or decrease peritubular capillary hydrostatic pressure favor fluid reabsorption, and factors that produce the opposite changes decrease fluid reabsorption.

The efferent arteriole has a major role in modulating proximal tubular fluid reabsorption. Efferent arteriolar constriction decreases peritubular capillary hydrostatic pressure and, by increasing the fraction of plasma filtered at the glomerulus (filtration fraction), increases peritubular capillary oncotic pressure. Both of these effects favor increased proximal tubular fluid reabsorption. Efferent arteriolar dilatation has the opposite effect and leads to a fall in proximal tubular fluid reabsorption.

The uptake of sodium and water by the peritubular capillaries ultimately controls the net rate of sodium transport by the proximal tubule. As with all capillaries, the movement of fluid from the intercellular space into the peritubular capillary is governed by Starling's forces. These intrarenal physical factors control the rate of fluid reabsorption in the proximal tubule and are responsible for the maintenance of glomerulotubular balance. Because the magnitude of proximal tubular sodium reabsorption alone does not account for the maintenance of sodium balance, other mechanisms must regulate sodium transport in more distal segments of the nephron. Aldosterone, acting at the site of the sodium–potassium exchanger, is one of these mechanisms and can account for up to 1% of the filtered sodium reabsorption.

◼ ACID–BASE BALANCE

DAILY PRODUCTION AND EXCRETION

Each day during the course of metabolism of ingested foodstuffs, two types of acid waste products are produced. The first, so-called volatile acid, in the form of CO_2 gas is produced in large quantities (15,000 to 20,000 mM/day) but is eliminated normally without great difficulty by the lungs. The second type of acid residue, so-called fixed or metabolic acid, is produced in much smaller quantities (1.0 to 1.5 mEq per kg of body weight per day) but requires a much more elaborate and complex mechanism for elimination.

If one were to consider the consequences of 100 mEq of metabolic hydrogen ion in the form of sulfuric acid (H_2SO_4) or phosphoric acid (H_3PO_4) added to the ECF volume each day as a consequence of the metabolism of primarily protein-containing food, the result would be dramatic. While metabolic acid is known to be buffered approximately 50% intracellularly (by the protonation of intracellular proteins), 50 mEq would remain to be buffered extracellularly. Sodium bicarbonate is the circulating extracellular buffer system responsible for protection against body fluid acidity and exists in the ECF in a concentration of approximately 25 mEq per L. Simple arithmetic would demonstrate that the entire quantity of circulating bicarbonate would be consumed in 7 days or less were there not a mechanism to (a) replenish bicarbonate stores and (b) eliminate so-called metabolic hydrogen ion.

RENAL ELIMINATION OF METABOLIC HYDROGEN ION (ACIDIFICATION)

Consider for a moment the challenge the kidney faces in eliminating 100 mEq of metabolic or strong acid in 1 L of urine per day. An elementary knowledge of logarithms would suggest that the pH of that urine would have to be 1.0 (hydrogen ion concentration 10^{-1}) to "contain" 100 mEq of hydrogen ion. The circumstance is not improved greatly even if urine output is increased drastically to 10 L per day. One hundred milliequivalents of free hydrogen ion and 10 L of urine would result in a hydrogen ion concentration of 10^{-2} equivalents per liter and the resultant urine would have a pH of 2.0. It is obvious that the excretion of free metabolic hydrogen ion in the urine in either circumstance is a physiologic impossibility.

Nonetheless, the kidney must eliminate that much hydrogen ion and do so by a series of mechanisms that do not destroy the epithelial lining of the renal tubules. At the same time, the consumed bicarbonate used to buffer the hydrogen ion at its source must be regenerated. As Figure 9.3 clearly illustrates, there are two major processes involved in hydrogen ion elimination and bicarbonate conservation and regeneration. First, virtually all filtered bicarbonate is reclaimed in the proximal tubule. The mechanism is illustrated in the figure and involves the intracellular production of carbonic acid, the passive diffusion down a concentration gradient of hydrogen ion, the interaction of hydrogen ion with bicarbonate in the tubular lumen to form CO_2 and water, and increasing intracellular production of bicarbonate, which is then reabsorbed with sodium as has been discussed earlier in this chapter.

Much more complex is the regeneration of the previously consumed bicarbonate and the simultaneous excretion of hydrogen ion into the urine in a safe and nonreactive form. This is accomplished by two major mechanisms illustrated in Figure 9-

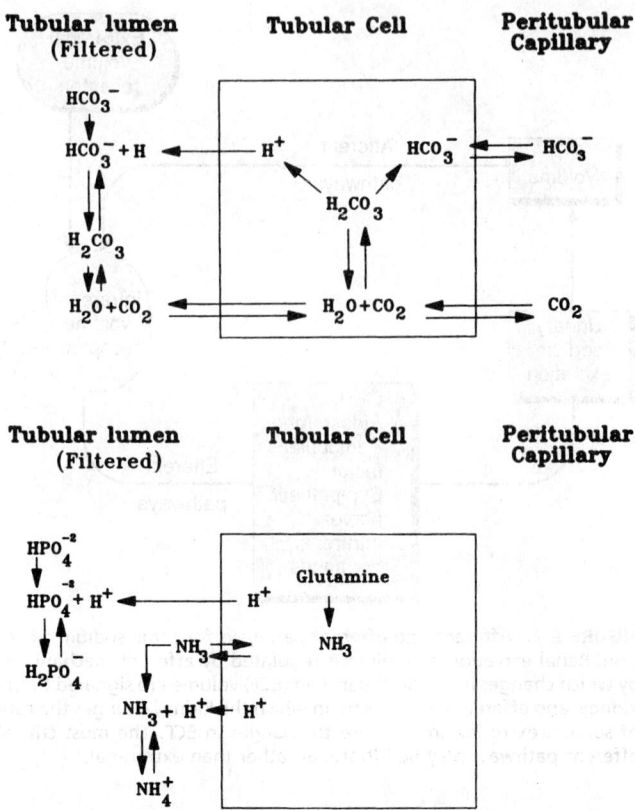

FIGURE 9.3. Cellular and lumenal events in the renal tubular cell resorption of filtered HCO_4^- and formation of titratable acids and NH_4^+.

3. Approximately one-third of the metabolic hydrogen ion (formed inside the cell in a mechanism virtually identical to that referred to above in the proximal tubule) is actively transported against a concentration gradient into the tubular lumen of the distal nephron. This concentration gradient is very important: depending on circumstances, there are between 100 and 1,000 molecules of hydrogen in the tubular lumen for each inside the cell, resulting in a gradient between 100:1 and 1,000:1, or an intracellular pH of 7 to 7.4 and a tubular pH of 4.5 to 5.0. In the face of hydrogen ion concentrations so significant the phosphate moiety of sodium phosphate is able to accept a second hydrogen ion and as long as the urine remains acidic will transport that hydrogen ion from the tubular lumen to the urine and out of the body. Since the hydrogen ion is eliminated in this circumstance, a bicarbonate ion is generated, reabsorbed by the peritubular capillary, and restored to the bicarbonate pool. Two-thirds of the hydrogen ion (or the remaining load) require the manufacture of ammonia and the diffusion of ammonia into the tubular lumen from the distal tubular cell. Once again, a hydrogen ion concentration far in excess of that inside the cell is required to protonate the ammonia gas to form ammonium (NH_4^+). In a process similar to that just described for phosphate, two-thirds of the metabolically produced hydrogen ion is removed from the body and two-thirds of the bicarbonate regeneration is accomplished to maintain acid–base balance. It should be obvious that the higher the hydrogen ion concentra-

tion gradient in the tubular lumen, the more easily the phosphate moiety and ammonia can be protonated and become hydrogen ion receptors.

In states of metabolic acidosis where hydrogen ion production increases beyond that of normal, the ammonia buffering system can increase ammonia production 10-fold to account for that degree of increase in hydrogen ion production. This increase is the circumstance which might obtain, for example, in chronic diabetic ketoacidosis and is one of the reasons for the serum bicarbonate concentrations never reaching zero.

Other consequences of the failure to achieve hydrogen ion gradients in the distal tubule between 1:100 and 1:1000 are discussed in Chapter 155.

HORMONES

The renin–angiotensin–aldosterone system influences renal sodium handling. Renin release and the subsequent generation of angiotensin II have several effects on the ECF volume. Angiotensin II is a potent vasoconstrictor, especially in the volume-depleted state, that helps to maintain blood pressure while decreasing tissue perfusion. Within the kidney, angiotensin II causes efferent arteriolar vasoconstriction disproportionately to any effects it might have on the afferent arteriole. This increases the filtration fraction and serves to maintain GFR in the presence of decreased renal blood flow. By decreasing peritubular capillary hydrostatic pressure and increasing peritubular capillary oncotic pressure, angiotensin II enhances proximal tubular fluid reabsorption.

Angiotensin II also stimulates the synthesis and release of aldosterone, a steroid hormone produced in the adrenal gland. The secretion of this mineralocorticoid hormone is largely controlled by sodium balance. Volume depletion (i.e., increased angiotensin II levels) stimulates aldosterone secretion; volume expansion (i.e., decreased angiotensin II levels) suppresses aldosterone secretion. The sodium-retaining action of the hormone occurs primarily in the distal nephron but also operates in a variety of other transporting tissues, such as gut and skin.

Atrial natriuretic peptide (ANP) is a hormone synthesized in the atrium of the heart. This hormone has potent natriuretic properties. It is secreted into the circulation in proportion to central blood volume (degree of atrial stretch). It may play an important role in normal sodium homeostasis by promoting urinary sodium excretion acutely by virtue of a prominent renal vasodilatation effect and chronically by directly suppressing aldosterone secretion from the adrenal gland. Direct inhibition of medullary and papillary collecting duct sodium reabsorption by ANP may also occur. Atrial natriuretic peptide also inhibits renin release, which may be secondary to a direct effect on juxtaglomerular cells or related to increased salt and water delivery to the macula densa. All of these actions are directed at restoring a more normal volume in response to an overfilled vasculature.

Prostaglandins and the kinin–kallikrein system may also participate in sodium homeostasis. These hormone systems interact with each other and with the renin–angiotensin system. Specific roles for these hormones in sodium homeostasis have yet to be defined.

POTASSIUM BALANCE

Despite its low concentration in the ECF fluid compartment, potassium is the predominant cation in the human body. Total body potassium content is about 3,500 mEq, with only about 60 mEq in the extracellular space. Skeletal muscle has a high potassium content per unit of dry weight and, because of its mass, contains most of the total body potassium stores. Potassium is readily absorbed by the gastrointestinal tract, and less than 10% of the daily ingested load is found in stool under normal circumstances. Potassium balance can be maintained on various diets that contain as little as 30 mEq per day or as much as 700 mEq per day. This ability to maintain potassium balance despite varying oral intake results from the ability of the kidney to greatly adjust potassium excretion.

Under normal circumstances, the kidney accounts for 90% of potassium excretion, although the gastrointestinal tract can be an important excretory route when renal function is severely compromised. The renal handling of potassium begins with glomerular filtration, at which point potassium is freely filterable. Potassium is reabsorbed and secreted along the distal nephron. The dynamic balance of potassium reabsorption and secretion along distal sites determines the amount of potassium excreted in the urine, and several factors can alter secretion along these distal nephron sites. Potassium secretion is increased by elevated serum potassium concentrations, elevated delivery of sodium and water to the distal nephron, and elevated aldosterone levels. Urinary excretion of potassium is further modified by acid–base alterations.

Plasma potassium concentration is determined by dietary intake and renal excretion and by factors that affect internal potassium distribution. The intracellular–extracellular potassium ratio is roughly 30:1. This ratio is critically important for the function of excitable membranes, predominantly muscle and nerve. Of these multiple factors that control internal potassium distribution, insulin and β_2-adrenergic activity stimulate cellular potassium uptake secondary to increases in the activity of the Na^+,K^+-ATPase. Metabolic acidosis induced by mineral acids raises plasma potassium concentration through potassium efflux from cells, but metabolic acidosis induced by organic acids does not seem to affect the plasma potassium concentration.

CALCIUM, PHOSPHORUS, AND MAGNESIUM BALANCE

The daily urinary excretion of calcium varies considerably in normal persons. This excretion is only modestly affected by changes in oral calcium intake. Only the ionized portion of calcium is the plasma is ultrafiltered at the glomerulus. Most calcium is reabsorbed along the proximal tubule, where it is closely linked to sodium transport. The final urinary excretion of calcium is therefore influenced by factors that alter renal sodium handling, including extracellular volume expansion and contraction as well as administration of diuretics. The last 5% to 10% of the filtered load of calcium is reabsorbed along the distal portions of the nephron, where the reabsorption of sodium and calcium are dissociated. It is along these distal segments that the homeostatic regulation of urinary calcium excretion occurs. Various factors alter urinary calcium excretion, including serum calcium level, parathyroid hormone, thiazide diuretics, metabolic acidosis and alkalosis, and phosphate depletion by changing calcium transport along the distal nephron. Of these factors, the most important are the state of the ECF volume, which regulates calcium transport at sites along the proximal tubule, and parathyroid hormone, which controls reabsorption along the distal nephron.

The renal handling of phosphate begins at the glomerulus, where it is freely filterable. Most filtered phosphate is reabsorbed along the proximal tubule. Additional phosphate is reabsorbed by the distal portion of the nephron, with about 10% of filtered phosphate appearing in the final urine. The two most important regulatory factors on renal transport are parathyroid hormone and dietary phosphate intake. Parathyroid hormone reduces phosphate reabsorption along the proximal tubule and produces the well-described phosphaturia of elevated parathyroid hormone activity. The effect of dietary phosphate intake on urinary phosphate excretion is seen acutely when a decrease in dietary phosphate occurs. Normal persons respond with a marked reduction in urinary phosphate excretion. This effect is substantial and may result in a diminution in the phosphaturic response to parathyroid hormone and other phosphaturic maneuvers applied during continuous low dietary phosphate ingestion.

Magnesium is second only to potassium as the most abundant intracellular cation. The kidney is a major regulatory organ for control of serum magnesium concentration. About 80% of magnesium is not protein-bound in plasma and is available for glomerular filtration. Of this filtered magnesium only 20% is reabsorbed in the proximal tubule and most is reabsorbed along the loop of Henle. This transport process is stimulated by parathyroid hormone and inhibited by hypercalcemia or hypermagnesemia and loop diuretics such as furosemide.

BIBLIOGRAPHY

Aronson PS. Mechanisms of active H$^+$ secretion in the proximal tubule. *Am J Physiol* 1983;245:F647.

Reineck HH, Stein JH. Sodium metabolism. In: Maxwell MH, Kleeman CR, Narins RG, eds. *Clinical disorders of fluid and electrolyte metabolism.* New York: McGraw-Hill, 1987:33.

Rose BD. *Clinical physiology of acid–base and electrolyte disorders.* New York: McGraw-Hill, 1984.

Szerlip H, Palevsky P, Cox M. Sodium and water. In: Rock RC, Noe DA, eds. *Laboratory medicine: the selection and interpretation of clinical laboratory studies.* Baltimore: Williams & Wilkins, 1994:692.

Wright FS. Renal potassium handling. *Semin Nephrol* 1987;7:174.

Kelley's Textbook of Internal Medicine, fourth edition. Edited by H. David Humes. Lippincott Williams & Wilkins, Philadelphia © 2000.

CHAPTER

10

PULMONARY GAS EXCHANGE

JOHN J. MARINI
DAVID R. DANTZKER

PULMONARY MECHANICS

STRUCTURE OF THE RESPIRATORY SYSTEM

Chest Wall

Twelve pairs of ribs, actuated by the intercostal muscles and tendons, originate at the thoracic spinal column and attach to the sternum with cartilage (Fig. 10.1). The phrenic nerve (C3–C5) innervates the diaphragm, and the spinal nerves (T2–L4) innervate the muscles of the rib cage and abdomen.

The diaphragm powers ventilation by displacing the abdominal contents and splaying the lower ribs outward and upward. During quiet breathing, inspiratory activity also can be demonstrated among certain muscles of the chest cage (scalenes, parasternals, and upper external intercostals). Changing position alters the relative contributions of the intercostals and the diaphragm, with the diaphragmatic component being greatest in the supine horizontal posture. As breathing effort intensifies,

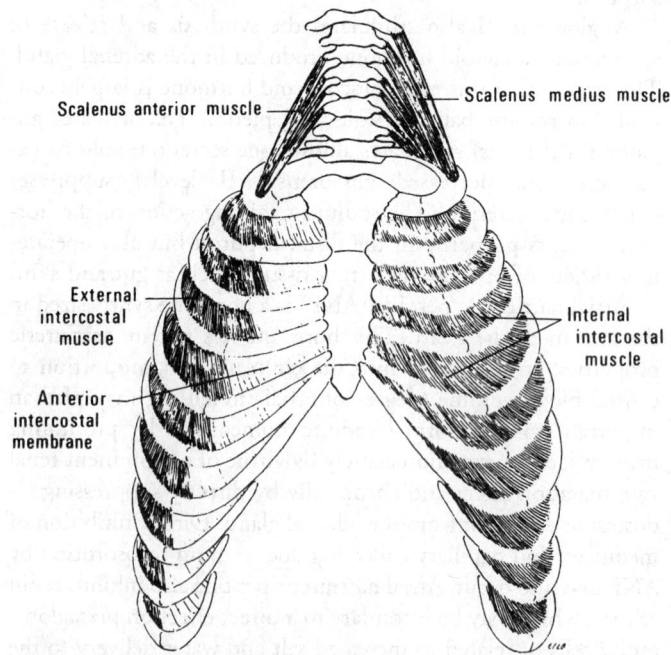

FIGURE 10.1. Intercostal and scalene muscles. On the left side of the chest, the external intercostal muscles and anterior intercostal membrane have been removed to reveal the intercostal muscles, and the left scalenus anterior has been removed to display the scalenus medius. (From Roussos C, Macklem PT. *The thorax,* second ed. New York: Marcel Dekker, 1994:430, with permission.)

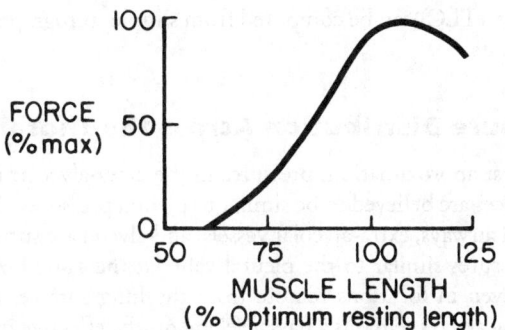

FIGURE 10.2. Stylized force–length (length–tension) curve of normal muscle. Force is expressed as percentage of maximum force (tension) developed during contraction. Length is expressed as percentage of optimum resting length. (From Rochester DF, Arora NS. Respiratory muscle failure. *Med Clin North Am* 1983;67:573, with permission.)

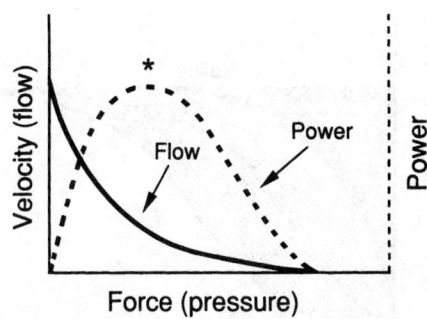

FIGURE 10.3. Relations among pressure, flow, and power. At a given level of neural stimulation, the ventilatory pump has a spectrum of available options for generating pressure and flow, depending on the impedance-to-volume change. From the standpoint of power (rate of performing external work), there is an optimal choice of pressure development and flow (*).

the intercostals and accessory muscles of the chest cage are recruited cephalocaudally. Although exhalation is normally passive, the expiratory muscles and the internal intercostals activate at high levels of minute ventilation (more than 15 to 20 L per minute), during loaded breathing, and during expulsive maneuvers (e.g., coughing or straining).

Skeletal muscle fibers vary in their content of oxidative and glycolytic enzymes. Slow-twitch (type I) motor units consist of fibers that are rich in oxidative enzymes and resistant to fatigue. Their fast-twitch (type II) counterparts show a wide range of fatigability, reflecting varying enzyme composition. Although the diaphragm has a mixed fiber composition, it is relatively resistant to fatigue. As in most skeletal muscles, fatigue-resistant units are recruited first in response to inspiratory efforts of graded severity.

Three fundamental properties of skeletal muscle influence its force-generating behavior: the force–length relation, the force–frequency relation, and the force–velocity relation. The force–length relation (Fig. 10.2) indicates that the maximal force that a muscle fiber can generate is a function of the length from which contraction begins. For the diaphragmatic fibers, maximal inspiratory force can be developed at functional residual capacity (FRC). Force development is a nonlinear function of the frequency with which the fiber is stimulated. As efferent nerve traffic increases, so do firing frequency and the tension developed by the fiber until tetany (sustained maximal contraction) is achieved. Force development is an inverse function of the speed of contraction (Fig. 10.3). Maximal force is developed under static (isometric) conditions, whereas the unloaded fiber develops no tension when it contracts at maximal velocity.

Lung

Airway

A conducting pathway warms and humidifies the inspired air and delivers the gas mixture to the alveoli, where gas exchange occurs. The conducting airway is a network of branching tubes, averaging 10 to 28 generations, depending on the proximity of parenchyma to the hilum. Total cross-sectional area increases by a factor of 1.8 at each branch point, so that airway resistance

and gas velocity fall dramatically at the periphery. Cartilage supports the first seven generations of bronchi. At usual breathing frequencies, bulk flow carries the airstream to the level of the terminal bronchioles, beyond which point gas transport depends on diffusion. Gas-exchanging air sacs bud off the terminal seven generations (the respiratory bronchioles and alveolar ducts).

Parenchyma

The delicate alveolar membrane, composed of juxtaposed epithelial and endothelial cell layers, is draped over a scaffold of fibroelastic connective tissue. This understructure firmly anchors the parenchyma to the hilum and visceral pleura, and is largely responsible for tissue recoil. Most afferent information from the airways and lung parenchyma is conducted through the vagus nerve. Although most efferent signals are believed to flow through the vagus as well, receptors abound for β_2-adrenergic and for noncholinergic, nonadrenergic stimulants.

To achieve the same volume, saline-filled lungs require much less pressure than air-filled lungs, indicating that surface forces at the air–liquid interface add to tissue elastance in determining the total recoil tension (Fig. 10.4). The surface-active material that lines the air–liquid boundary (surfactant) opposes the tendency for expiratory collapse. Surfactant's complex lipoprotein structure changes conformation during different segments of the inflation–deflation cycle, attenuating surface tension at low lung volumes and reducing the tendency for alveolar collapse. Renewal of these unique properties might require periodic stretching.

Pulmonary Vessels

Two distinct vascular networks, the pulmonary and bronchial circulations, perfuse the lung. Within the pulmonary circulation, the arteries conduct blood from the right ventricle to the capillary bed, where gas exchange occurs. Because nearly all cardiac output flows through the lung, the pulmonary circulation filters macroscopic particles (e.g., clot) from the venous blood. Oxygenated postcapillary blood flows to the left atrium in the pulmonary veins. Three types of pulmonary arteries can be distin-

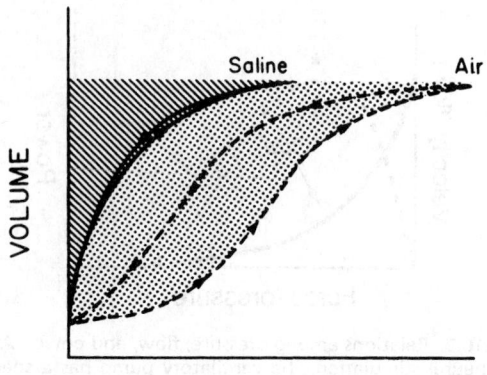

FIGURE 10.4. Relation of static distending pressure to volume for lungs filled with physiologic saline and air. The higher pressure requirement of air-filled lungs indicates the contribution of surface tension to total elastic recoil, an effect that is especially prominent at low lung volumes. The cross-hatched area depicts the elastic mechanical work performed against tissue forces during lung inflation, whereas the stippled area indicates the additional elastic work resulting from the opposition of surface tension forces.

guished: elastic arteries, muscular arteries, and pulmonary arterioles. Unlike the pulmonary veins, they course alongside the airways of similar size, an arrangement that helps to preserve the matching of ventilation to perfusion. Normal pulmonary arteries and veins share a similar structure, consistent with the uniformly low pressures in this circuit. However, the pulmonary veins are more plentiful, providing an effective reservoir to buffer minor variations in right ventricular output.

The bronchial circulation, a lower volume, higher pressure system, normally receives only 1% to 2% of cardiac output. The bronchial arteries vary in number and may arise from the aorta directly or from the intercostal, internal mammary, or subclavian arteries. Like the pulmonary arteries, they distribute with the airways, providing the bulk of nutrient flow to all pulmonary structures other than the parenchyma itself. Communication between the pulmonary and bronchial circulations has been described at both the arterial and the capillary level. Such interconnections can maintain parenchymal nutrition and prevent infarction subsequent to pulmonary artery occlusion.

EVENTS OF THE INFLATION–DEFLATION CYCLE

Subdivisions of Lung Volume

During passive exhalation, the end-expiratory resting position of the lung (FRC) occurs at the volume at which the recoil forces of the lung and chest wall counterbalance. The volume of gas remaining in the chest after a maximal effort to exhale defines the residual volume (RV). Like the FRC, the RV must be measured by techniques other than external gas collection (spirometry). From any known starting point, gas dilution methods (helium equilibration or nitrogen washout), plethysmography, and planimetry of chest radiographs can be used to estimate absolute lung volume. Once the FRC or the RV is known, total lung

capacity (TLC) can be computed from simple spirographic measurements.

Pressure Distribution Across the Thorax

As a first approximation, pressures in the extra-alveolar interstitial spaces are believed to be similar to pleural pressures. At FRC, normal airways, extra-alveolar vessels, and alveoli are surrounded by pressures similar to the pleural value at the same horizontal level, even in locations remote from the lung surface. Because the lung always remains a passive element, the effective transpulmonary pressure is the measured difference between airway (P_{aw}) and intrapleural (P_{pl}) pressures. At any moment, the difference between P_{aw} and the alveolar pressure (P_{alv}) drives gas to or from the alveoli, and the difference between P_{alv} and P_{pl} distends the lung.

Static Pressure–Volume Relations

Under static conditions, the difference between P_{alv} and P_{pl} reflects elastic lung recoil. During inspiration, however, this difference is slightly more than it would be with flow stopped at the same volume because a small pressure increment is needed to overcome tissue resistance. The effective pressure distending the chest wall cannot be directly measured during spontaneous breathing because the relevant forcing pressures are generated within the muscle fibers of the structure itself. Only when the chest wall is passively inflated can its distensibility be assessed.

The lung and chest wall occupy an identical volume, except when air or fluid separates them. The volume of each structure is uniquely determined by its compliance (distensibility) and the trans-structural pressure acting across it (Fig. 10.5). For the lung, tissue elastance and surface tension together determine the static (recoil) pressure corresponding to any specified volume. At low lung volume, surface forces contribute more to total recoil than at high lung volume, where tissue elastance predominates. The

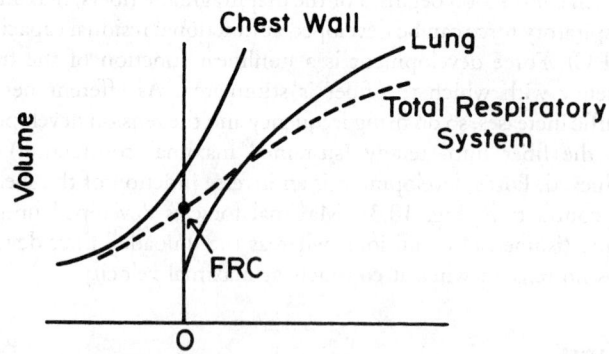

FIGURE 10.5. Static pressure–volume relations for the passive respiratory system. Transmural trans-structural pressures for the lung, chest wall, and total respiratory system are the alveolar–pleural pressure difference, the pleural pressure, and the alveolar pressure, respectively. At rest, the equilibrium volume (functional reserve capacity) occurs when recoil pressures for the lung and chest wall counterbalance. Note that the chest wall has a tendency to spring outward (balanced by a negative transmural pressure) at volumes less than about 60% vital capacity.

limits of distensibility are reached at TLC. Because lung tissue tends to collapse at low volumes, additional pressure must be applied to achieve a given volume on the inflation limb. Processes that deplete surfactant accentuate such hysteresis.

Although nearly linear in the usual tidal volume (V_T) range, the compliance of the lung, defined as the unit change in volume that occurs with any unit change in pressure, is greatest in the midportion of the vital capacity. To reflect tissue recoil properties, compliance should be expressed relative to absolute volume. Specific compliance, defined as the ratio of compliance to absolute volume, compensates for size differences that otherwise render compliance meaningless as a measure of elastic properties. After pneumonectomy, the calculated compliance of the "lungs," for example, would be seriously reduced from the preoperative value, but specific compliance would remain unchanged.

The pressure–volume relation of the chest wall is also curvilinear. Although flexible early in life, the rib cage stiffens with age. The passive chest wall tends to spring outward at volumes less than 60% of vital capacity. Attempts to compress the rib cage to volumes below its equilibrium position meet increasing opposition. The diaphragm also has an elastic limit to cephalad movement.

A thin liquid film seals the lung against the chest wall. Normally, a negative force is created at the lung surface by the opposing actions of lung recoil and chest wall expansion. The elastance (the inverse of compliance) of the lung (C_L) and chest wall (C_W) are additive. Consequently, the inspiratory compliance of the entire respiratory system (C_{RS}) is less than the compliance of either of its individual elements: $1/C_{RS} = (1/C_L) + (1/C_W)$. In the upright position, C_L, C_W, and C_{RS} approximate 200, 200, and 100 mL per cm H_2O, respectively, over the usual V_T range.

Positional Changes in Thoracic Volume

Changing position alters the effective C_W. Lung volume normally increases about 750 to 1,000 mL in moving from the horizontal to the fully upright position, with a major portion gained in peridiaphragmatic regions. Because C_{RS} at 45° averages about 100 mL per cm H_2O, moving from horizontal to upright causes a volume change comparable to about 10 cm H_2O of applied positive end-expiratory pressure (PEEP). This position-related volume increment corresponds roughly to the sine of the angle to the horizontal plane and diminishes with advancing age.

Patients with symptomatic airflow obstruction lose less lung volume than age-matched normal subjects in assuming recumbency, perhaps because normal losses of volume would increase the frictional work of breathing intolerably or because air trapping occurs. Lung volume is marginally lower in the prone versus the supine-horizontal position. Resting lung volume, however, is about 20% greater in the lateral decubitus position than in the supine position. When lateral, the upper lung is held distended at a volume similar to the upright value, whereas the lower lung is compressed.

Relation of Alveolar and Pleural Pressures

Two clinically useful relations relate changes in alveolar and pleural pressures during conditions of passive inflation. Altera-

tions of pleural pressure influence the pressures in the heart chambers and great vessels, thereby affecting venous return and the interpretation of hemodynamic data.

Assuming that equal volume changes occur in the lung (ΔV_L) and chest wall (ΔV_W),

$$\Delta P_{pl} = \Delta P_{alv} * C_L/(C_L + C_W)$$

At end-exhalation, ΔP_{alv} equals $\Delta PEEP$, so that the fractional change in pleural pressure expected from a change in PEEP is $C_L/(C_L + C_W)$. For the normal passive chest, the compliances of the lung and chest wall are about equivalent near FRC, so that about half of a PEEP increment normally transmits to the pleural space. An infinitely stiff chest wall ($C_W = 0$ mL per cm H_2O) would allow no volume change of the lung but would permit complete transmission of alveolar pressure to the pleural space. Conversely, an infinitely stiff lung would transmit none. In either event, no volume increment would result from the PEEP change. The volume change (ΔV) resulting from PEEP applied to the passive thorax can also be estimated:

$$\Delta V = [C_L * C_W/(C_W + C_L)]$$
$$\times \text{ PEEP distribution of pressure along the pleural surface}$$

Local pressures range widely along the pleural surface (Fig. 10.6). Pleural pressures at the top of the lung are more negative than pressures in more dependent areas, normally following a gradient of about 0.2 to 0.3 cm H_2O per centimeter of vertical distance. The weight of the lung exerting lateral pressure at the lower pleural surface may explain this phenomenon. An alternative explanation invokes regional differences in lung recoil. The

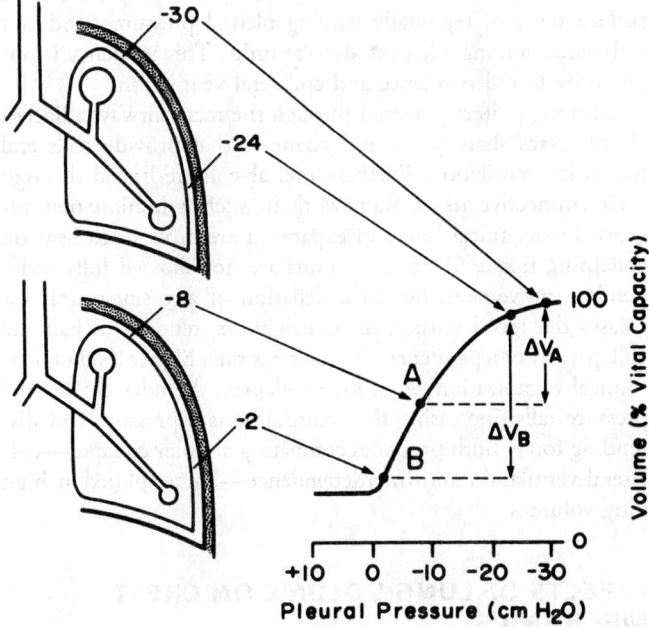

FIGURE 10.6. Vertical distribution of pleural pressure and regional fluctuations of transpulmonary pressure over a major portion of the vital capacity range. Because alveoli in dependent lung regions **(B)** rest on a more highly compliant portion of the pressure–volume relationship than do alveoli located elsewhere **(A)**, they undergo disproportionate shifts in volume (ΔV) for an equivalent change in pleural pressure.

topography of pleural pressure is influenced by the irregular contours of bony and vascular structures in the rib cage and mediastinum. Pleural and pulmonary edema fluid accentuates the gravitational gradient; pneumothorax obliterates it.

Regional compliance of the chest wall varies greatly with position, especially along the surface of the diaphragm. The rib cage is most flexible anteriorly, accounting for the reduction in compliance observed when these regions are braced by the supporting surface in the prone position. In the upright position, the abdominal contents retract from the undersurface of the resting diaphragm, causing reduced and rather uniform pressure in that region. (Abdominal pressures rise during inspiration.) In the supine position, however, the hydrostatic forces of the abdominal contents generate about 1 cm H_2O per centimeter of vertical distance from the anterior abdominal surface, so that pressures in dependent regions exceed those along the anterosuperior surface. As a result, the dependent portion of the diaphragm rises to a position of better mechanical advantage. Therefore, although reduced abdominal pressure in the upper regions allows a higher resting lung volume and better distensibility, regional ventilation is lower during spontaneous efforts. Conversely, higher effective compliance in superior regions of the supine chest enables them to accept a larger than normal fraction of any passive tidal breath delivered by positive pressure or any volume increment resulting from PEEP.

INTERDEPENDENCE AND COLLATERAL VENTILATION

Wherever they are located in the lung, disadvantaged alveolar units tend to collapse when ventilated at uniformly small tidal volumes, a phenomenon partially explained by the effects of surface tension, regionally varying pleural pressures, and size differences among adjacent alveolar units. This tendency is opposed by interdependence and collateral ventilation.

Although directly vented through the main airway, adjacent alveolar sacs share pores and channels that provide collateral routes for ventilation. Furthermore, alveoli are linked through their connective tissue framework in such a fashion that increased mechanical forces of expansion are brought to bear on collapsing tissue. Contiguous units are not allowed fully independent movement. Selective deflation of any single unit increases the recoil tension of its neighbors, tending to halt the collapse. Interdependence also operates on a higher level of anatomical organization. As a lobe collapses, the adjacent pleural pressure falls, increasing the transpulmonary pressure and distending force. Both processes combating alveolar collapse—collateral ventilation and interdependence—are amplified at high lung volumes.

EFFECTS OF LUNG VOLUME ON CHEST MECHANICS

Airway Resistance

Enhanced recoil tethers open the airways and boost the driving pressure for expiratory airflow. Because airway resistance relates inversely to the fourth power of the bronchial radius, airway

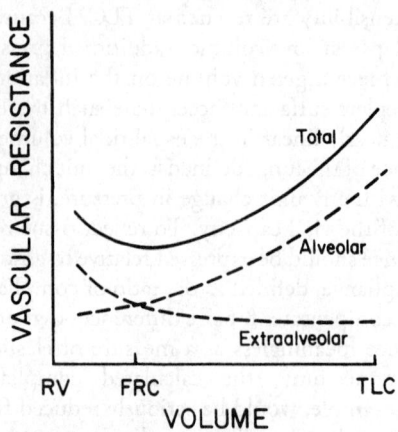

FIGURE 10.7. Relationship of pulmonary vascular resistance to lung volume. Increasing lung volume improves resistance within extra-alveolar vessels but compresses the alveolar capillary bed. Consequently, vascular resistance normally reaches a minimum at a lung volume close to the resting equilibrium (functional reserve capacity).

resistance bears a hyperbolic relation to lung volumes lower than FRC. Above FRC, resistance normally improves only modestly with increasing volume. In severe peripheral airflow obstruction, however, increasing volume well above the equilibrium position may greatly reduce breathing effort.

Pulmonary Vascular Resistance

Increasing volume has a biphasic and largely detrimental impact on pulmonary vascular resistance (Fig. 10.7). As lung volume rises, forces similar to those that affect the airways tether and dilate extra-alveolar vessels. However, increasing wall tension compresses the capillaries embedded in the alveolus. As a result, net pulmonary vascular resistance reaches its nadir near FRC. At volumes above FRC, alveolar vessel compression predominates; below FRC, vascular resistance rises again because of compression of extra-alveolar vessels.

Respiratory Muscle Strength

As with all striated muscles, force generation in the respiratory system depends on the fiber length at which contraction begins. On this basis alone, inspiratory muscles are primed for maximal pressure generation at RV, whereas expiratory force can be maximized at TLC (Fig. 10.8). The geometric configuration of the diaphragm is also optimized at low lung volumes because fiber tension generates its most useful inspiratory force vector with the diaphragm maximally curved. Conversely, near TLC, the flattened diaphragm may actually produce an expiratory action because muscle shortening fails to displace the abdomen and draws the ribs inward at the points of insertion (Hoover's sign). Total lung capacity is the most appropriate volume from which to initiate an effective cough because the expiratory muscles contract best from this position.

EFFECTS OF AIR TRAPPING

Dynamic hyperinflation (air trapping) occurs when lung volume must be maintained above its resting equilibrium position, either

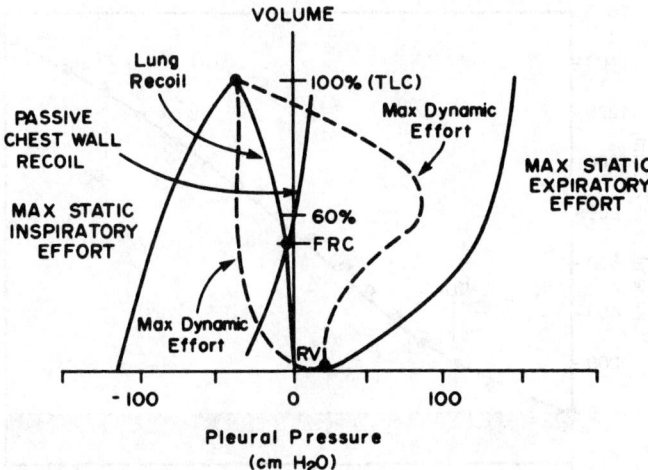

FIGURE 10.8. Relationship of lung volume to maximal inspiratory and expiratory force under isometric *(unbroken lines)* and dynamic *(dashed lines)* conditions in a normal subject. Static inspiratory force is maximized at residual volume, whereas maximal static expiratory pressures are generated at total lung capacity. Maximal values of pleural pressure are greatly attenuated during forceful efforts through an open airway. Pleural pressure values result from the combined actions of the respiratory muscles and the volume-dependent recoil tendency of the passive lung.

lar pressures. This effect increases the elastic work of inspiration and makes it more difficult to trigger machine-aided cycles. Applied PEEP or continuous positive airway pressure (CPAP) can often counterbalance auto-PEEP and reduce breathing effort without causing a major further increase in lung volume.

Pneumothorax and Pleural Effusion

If gas or liquid accumulates under tension, the lung becomes difficult to expand and the muscles are forced into a mechanically inefficient, hyperinflated position. In the setting of pneumothorax, the exact coupling provided by the normal liquid interface is lost, and additional inspiratory pressure dissipates in pleural gas rarefaction. Obliteration of the pleural pressure gradient surrounding the lung worsens ventilation–perfusion mismatching.

In the upright position, large pleural effusions generate hydrostatic pressure that distorts the diaphragm and might even invert it. These effects are reversed when a large effusion is tapped from the pleural space. After the tap, the patient might experience less dyspnea, even though the aerated lung volume is no greater than before.

Atelectasis

At low lung volumes, alveolar instability and airway closure encourage parenchymal collapse, opposed by surfactant and tissue interdependence. As noted, a closing volume can often be identified at which small airways in dependent regions seal (anatomically or functionally) as the lung deflates. Absorption collapse may follow. Airway disease, mucosal edema, and retained secretions raise the closing volume, and recumbency and obesity reduce the resting lung volume. The tendency for closure is countered by deep breathing, which improves collateral ventilation and accentuates tissue interdependence. When the lung is ventilated at unvaryingly small tidal volumes, factors acting to close dependent or regionally compromised alveoli are ineffectively opposed, and widespread microcollapse or platelike atelectasis may develop.

In the postoperative period, numerous factors interact to force the closure of dependent airways. Apart from the nearly 30% decline in FRC that accompanies the supine position, general anesthesia causes an additional loss of resting volume as a result of diaphragmatic relaxation and cephalad displacement of

to minimize breathing effort or to exhale the selected tidal volume in the available time (Fig. 10.9). The usual setting is airflow obstruction and high minute ventilation requirements. Although breathing at an elevated lung volume is costly in terms of elastic work, the savings in frictional work compensates for this. Unfortunately, there is an important additional cost: acute hyperinflation foreshortens inspiratory muscle fibers, compromises the geometric configuration of the diaphragm, and forces the costal and crural portions of the diaphragm to abandon their normal parallel configuration. Moreover, increased pleural pressures and vena caval resistance may impede venous return.

During spontaneous breathing, air trapping implies a background tension in the inspiratory muscle fibers. Expiratory flow continues throughout the exhalation half cycle, and an abrupt inspiratory "braking" pressure to counter the recoil of the thorax must be applied before inhalation can begin. In the setting of mechanical ventilation, this recoil pressure has been variably described as intrinsic, unintentional, inadvertent, or auto-PEEP. Under passive conditions, auto-PEEP elevates pleural and vascu-

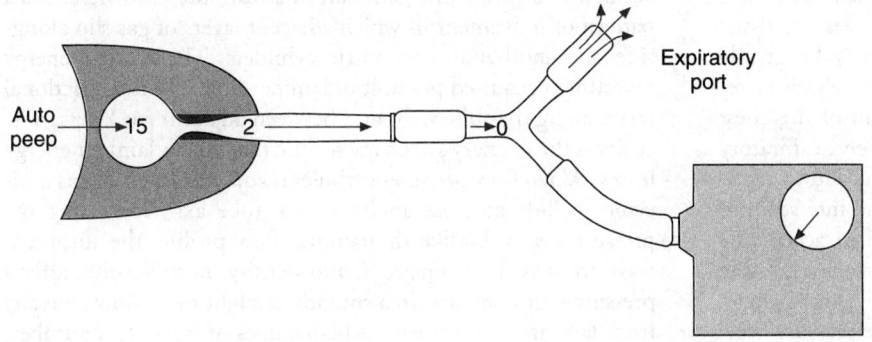

FIGURE 10.9. Dynamic hyperinflation with auto-PEEP (see below). When the respiratory system has insufficient time to empty to its relaxed equilibrium position between inspiratory cycles, the trans-respiratory system pressure remains elevated with respect to airway opening pressure throughout the respiratory cycle. The difference between alveolar pressure at end-expiration and the pressure at the central airway opening at end-expiration is termed *auto-PEEP.* In this instance, 15 cm of water pressure drives airflow through severely narrowed airways at end-expiration.

the relaxed diaphragm. Airway intubation and anesthesia disrupt the function of the mucociliary escalator and may stimulate the outpouring of airway secretions. Thoracic mechanics are severely disturbed by surgical incisions in the chest or abdomen. All lung volumes, including TLC, FRC, and subdivisions of vital capacity, are reduced for at least the first 7 days after upper abdominal surgery. Diaphragmatic dysfunction and the incidence of clinically important atelectasis increase with the proximity of the incision of the diaphragm. Pain and analgesia disrupt the sighing rhythm, whereas coughing and secretion clearance are made inefficient by intubation and pain.

Frequent positional changes are crucial in the treatment and prophylaxis of atelectasis. For example, in the decubitus position, the upper lung is stretched to a greater than normal resting volume and secretions are drained along a gravitational gradient. Conversely, the lower lung may be better ventilated during spontaneous breathing owing to improved diaphragmatic advantage.

Diaphragmatic Paralysis and Quadriplegia: Effects of Volume and Position

Patients with selectively impaired diaphragmatic function have orthopnea when supine but may be comfortable when upright. In the upright position, gravity pulls the diaphragm inferiorly, so that significant negative pressure can be developed by the intercostal and accessory muscles of ventilation. Furthermore, contraction of the expiratory musculature thrusts the diaphragm cephalad, producing a caudal inspiratory action when released.

Conversely, the diaphragm and accessory muscles may be the only ones spared in quadriplegia. In this case, the patient may experience platypnea (intensified dyspnea in the upright position). The diaphragm is flattened and made less efficient when pulled inferiorly by diminished or negative pressures in the abdomen.

Hydrostatic Pulmonary Edema and Adult Respiratory Distress Syndrome

In the early phase of hydrostatic pulmonary edema or adult respiratory distress syndrome (ARDS), alveolar flooding and microatelectasis are the primary abnormalities of mechanics. In the early phase of ARDS, the lung may be viewed as comprising two populations of alveoli: those that are well ventilated and normally compliant (most prevalent in nondependent regions), and those that are consolidated or atelectatic and poorly compliant (most prevalent in dependent regions). Thus, impaired overall compliance in this disease is as much a function of a loss of aeratable lung as a function of an overall increase in tissue elastance. The number of aerated lung units may be greatly reduced (to one-third or less of normal), but their elasticity remains essentially unaffected. The resting position of the chest wall may be normal or even expanded. Positive end-expiratory pressure tends to maintain recruited alveolar units and to redistribute lung water from the alveolar space to the interstitium. In the process, more alveoli are made available to accept the V_T. Without a measurement of absolute lung volume, tissue elastance cannot be deduced from pressure and V_T data alone.

Close inspection of the inspiratory limb of the pressure–vol-

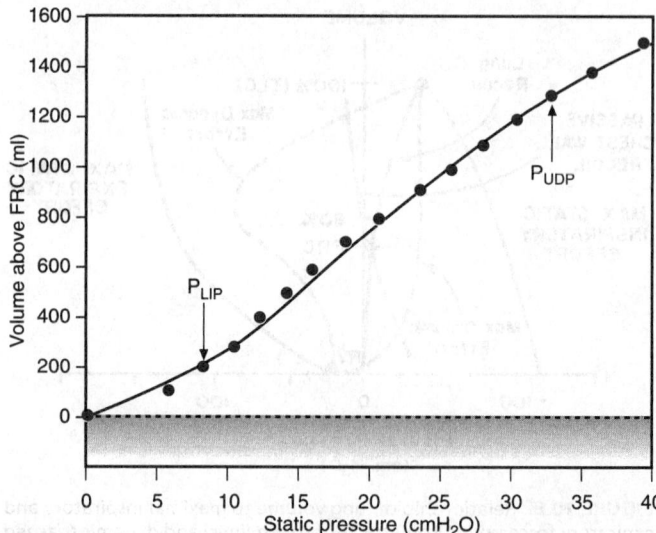

FIGURE 10.10. Static pressure volume curve of the respiratory system in a patient with acute lung injury. The filled circles represent actual measurements of static pressure during inflation from the equilibrium volume. The curved solid line connecting these points represents the third-degree polynomial that best fits the data. Note that the curve is essentially linear in its midportion but demonstrates a lower inflexion point (P_{LIP}) and an upper deflexion point (P_{UDP}).

ume relation of the total respiratory system can give important clues to the presence of potentially recruitable volume that collapses during the tidal cycle. A distinctly biphasic limb of the pressure–volume curve suggests that the effective compliance of the lung improves once a critical "opening pressure" has been surpassed that enlarges the effective size of the aerated lung. Alveoli in dependent regions are the most difficult to keep open. Unless sufficient PEEP prevents reclosure of these difficult-to-recruit units, the process of opening and reclosure is repeated with each ventilatory cycle. Close monitoring of the pressure–volume curve (as well as indexes of gas exchange and oxygen delivery) may aid the clinician greatly in selecting the appropriate level of end-expiratory pressure (Fig. 10.10).

AIRWAY MECHANICS

Airflow and Resistance

Gas flowing in a straight tube can adopt two basic patterns: laminar and turbulent. Laminar, or streamline, flow describes a pattern of movement in which adjacent layers of gas slip alongside one another in concentric cylinders. The modest energy investment required per unit of laminar flow relates to frictional losses along the tube walls and between adjacent gas layers. Viscosity is the primary gas characteristic that affects laminar energy losses. When flow becomes turbulent, adjacent layers of gas molecules collide at cross angles to the tube axis, increasing the pressure losses. Unlike the laminar flow profile, the turbulent wave front is flat ("square"), and density, not viscosity, affects pressure requirements. In a smooth, straight tube, flow converts from laminar to turbulent at high values of Reynold's number, a dimensionless value determined by the quotient: (gas density × velocity × diameter)/gas viscosity. Low gas velocities and narrow airway diameters (the conditions prevailing in small bronchi) favor laminar flow, whereas rapid flows and larger calibers favor turbulence. Turbulence also tends to develop at points of airway irregularity. Reducing gas density (e.g., by using helium to replace nitrogen as a carrier gas for oxygen) can improve breathing effort strikingly in patients with obstructing lesions of the central airways.

Distribution of Airway Resistance

Resistance partitions unevenly along the airway. With the mouth closed, the normal nasal passage accounts for about half of total resistance to airflow (R_{aw}) during quiet breathing and a higher percentage of R_{aw} during forceful efforts, when turbulence accentuates intranasal pressure losses. Under such conditions, opening the mouth greatly lessens the resistance to breathing. With the mouth widely open, the oropharynx and larynx normally account for about 40% of R_{aw} during quiet breathing and a higher percentage as flow increases. Resistance along the normal tracheobronchial tree divides about equally between airways that are smaller and larger than 2 to 3 mm in diameter. Peripheral airway resistance markedly increases in diffuse airflow obstruction (e.g., asthma, chronic bronchitis, emphysema).

Expiratory Airflow

When exhalation is passive, gas empties from the normal lung exponentially, driven by recoil pressure. The product of resistance (R) and compliance (C) is known as the *time constant,* the time required to exhale 63% of the V_T. Increases in R or C delay emptying. Similar principles apply to the rate of lung filling at a constant inflating pressure. In diseased lungs, the time constants of adjacent regions may vary markedly, filling and emptying at different rates when exposed to a common pressure gradient.

If the airways were rigid and resistance were independent of flow, flow would remain proportional to the difference between alveolar and airway opening pressures during both phases of the ventilatory cycle and throughout the effort range. Forceful expiratory efforts raise pleural pressure, adding to recoil pressure and narrowing the compressible intrathoracic airway downstream of what has become known as the equal pressure point (EPP) (Fig. 10.11). At efforts that exceed about two-thirds of maximal, each increment of pleural pressure narrows the airway downstream of the EPP sufficiently to offset the increment in alveolar pressure. The effective driving pressure for flow then becomes alveolar minus pleural pressure, or the recoil pressure itself, which is a volume-dependent quantity. The effective resistance resides in the segment upstream from the critical point of compression. For each lung volume, there is a maximal rate of expiratory airflow that cannot be exceeded, defined by the recoil pressure of the lung and the intrinsic properties of the airway itself. This flow-limiting mechanism does not affect the first 15% to 20% of exhaled volume or any portion of inspiration, which remains dependent on effort.

However attractive the EPP theory may be to explain the

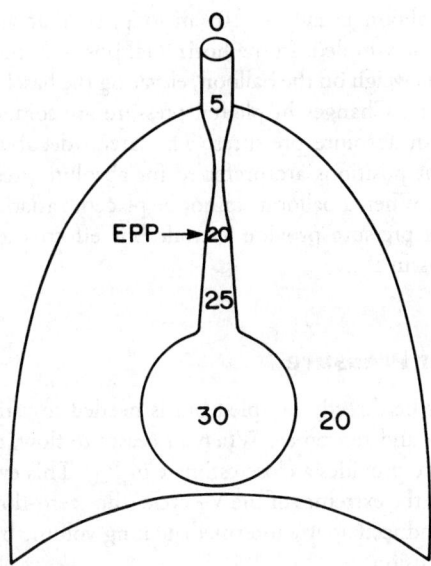

FIGURE 10.11. Dynamics of airway compression and flow limitation during forceful exhalation. At some site along the airway (the equal pressure point), transmural airway pressure becomes zero. Direct compressive forces or wave speed limitations develop at all points closer to the airway opening, offsetting any effort-related boost in alveolar pressure and limiting the maximal rate of airflow achievable at that volume.

phenomenon of flow limitation, the precise mechanism by which flow limitation occurs remains open to debate. For example, whether the point of narrowing occurs precisely at the EPP or at a point determined by a critical transmural pressure further downstream (Starling's resistor model) is unclear. Indeed, the phenomenon of flow limitation (effort independence) may be best explained on another basis entirely—the "wave speed" theory. The speed with which a pressure wave propagates through a compressible tube (the wave speed) is reduced by decreasing the cross-sectional area and by decreasing transmural pressure, two properties that characterize the central airways. Thus, as gas accelerates in approaching the airway opening, it encounters a "choke point" at which its velocity equals the wave speed limit. Further attempts to accelerate gas flow merely compress the downstream segment.

Whatever the actual cause for flow limitation, compression of downstream airway segments produces low-volume, high-velocity gas flow that shears mucus free from the airway walls during coughing. The effort independence of maximal flow also confers reproducibility on the forced spirometric indices of airflow obstruction (e.g., the second forced expiratory volume, FEV_1).

CLINICAL MEASUREMENT OF LUNG MECHANICS

Intrapleural Pressure

The least invasive and most commonly used technique for estimating P_{pl} remains esophageal manometry. A thin latex balloon nearly devoid of air is tied to a multiperforated supporting catheter. The balloon usually is 10 cm long, so that an adequate region can be sampled. In the horizontal position, the mediastinal contents weigh on the balloon, elevating the baseline esophageal pressure. Changes in pleural pressure are somewhat more reliable than absolute pressures. The lateral decubitus, prone, and upright positions are preferred for absolute pressure measurements. When a balloon cannot be placed, variations in central venous pressure provide a crude but effective estimate of fluctuations in P_{pl}.

Alveolar Pressure

P_{alv} cannot be directly sampled but is needed to estimate lung compliance and resistance. When air ceases to flow, central airway pressure provides a close estimate of P_{alv}. This event occurs naturally at the extremes of the V_T cycle (the "zero-flow" points) or can be induced at any intermediate lung volume by transient airway occlusion.

Work of Breathing

Mechanical work (W, the product of force and distance) is performed when a pressure gradient (force/area) moves a passive structure through a volume change (distance * area). For example, when the passive thorax is expanded by a positive-pressure ventilator, the airway is pressurized and the machine performs work. Although mechanical work is done against elastic, frictional, and inertial forces, the inertial component is negligible, except at very high rates of gas flow. The inspiratory work of expanding the lungs or chest wall can be quantified as the integral of the rate of volume change of the structure (flow, $\dot{V}$) and the pressure change that caused it (the trans-structural pressure, P_{TM}). These pressure–volume (work) integrals can be computed electronically by integrating the product of P_{TM} and V, or graphically by plotting cumulated inspired volume against P_{TM}, quantifying the area enclosed by the relevant portion of the resulting figure (Fig. 10.12).

The measurement of external work does not necessarily reflect the energy consumed by the respiratory muscles. The mechanical work of breathing (W_B) is rather easily measured but correlates imprecisely with ventilation-associated oxygen consumption ($\dot{V}O_2$). These two values are interrelated by way of the expression $W_B = \dot{V}O_2 * \omega$, where ω is the efficiency of converting oxygen consumed in the breathing effort to useful mechanical work. Although equal amounts of mechanical work may be done in moving a large volume of air against low resistance or in moving a modest volume of air against high resistance, the latter requires greater oxygen consumption. Furthermore, the timing of contraction and the distribution of force among different muscle groups greatly influence pump efficiency. Therefore, external work relates imprecisely to the total tension developed by the muscle fibers, particularly when loading conditions vary. At the bedside, the product of the external pressure developed by the muscles and the time over which it is generated (the product of pressure and time) may be a preferable index of effort under conditions of changing afterload.

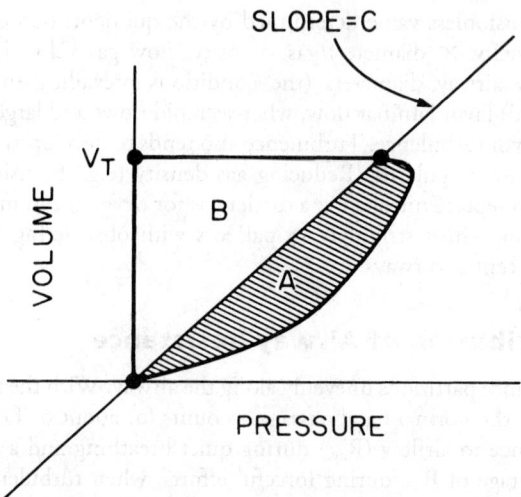

FIGURE 10.12. Calculation of the mechanical work of breathing from the relationship of volume to inflating pressure. In the tidal range, the pressure–volume curve of the lungs and thorax is nearly linear, with a slope equal to compliance, C. The elastic work performed in achieving the tidal volume (V_T) is proportional to area B. The frictional work performed varies with flow rate and resistance and is estimated by area A.

RESPIRATORY MUSCLE WEAKNESS AND FATIGUE

Muscle fatigue must be distinguished from muscle weakness. *Weakness* is the suboptimal generation of force in the resting (and rested) state; *fatigue* is the progressive inability to sustain a targeted force during a single protracted effort or (more commonly) during repeated contractions. Among other causes, muscle weakness can be the result of diminished muscle bulk, ischemia, electrolyte imbalance (e.g., due to K^+, Mg^{2+}, or PO_4^- depletion), hypoxemia, acidemia, acute hypercarbia, systemic illness (e.g., sepsis), neuromuscular disease, or acute hyperinflation (see above). Adequate nutrition and muscle blood flow, correction of electrolyte abnormalities, and reversal of pathogenetic stimuli are essential to improving contractile function.

Fatigue is the result of sustained or repetitive overload and may reflect an imbalance of metabolic energy delivery and consumption. For example, respiratory muscle fatigue may occur in the setting of circulatory shock, even when muscle loads remain within normal limits. Continued overstimulation in the face of fatigue eventually depletes energy reserves and results in irreversible cross bridging of actin-myosin proteins, producing rigor. For this reason, it is believed that neural stimulation to the overloaded muscle spontaneously attenuates well before fatal rigor is produced. (Such a mechanism might help to explain the evolution of respiratory arrest in some critically ill patients.) It has been empirically determined, both for peripheral skeletal muscle and for the intact diaphragm of normal subjects, that force and percentage contraction time influence endurance independently. Thus, the integrative tension–time index correlates well with endurance:

$$(\text{Tension/breath/maximal tension}) * (T_I/T_{TOT})$$

Loads that produce values exceeding 0.20 cannot be sustained indefinitely and result in fatigue. An early (if not infallible) indication of eventual fatigue is provided by electromyographic power spectrum analysis. Shifts to lower values in the centroid frequency or a high/low frequency ratio reliably indicate a fatiguing stress. Physical signs of muscle overload include tachypnea, paradoxical abdominal motion, respiratory alternans, vigorous use of accessory muscles, and dysrhythmic breathing patterns. Once fatigued, a muscle might require 24 hours or more to restore energy reserves and contractile function. Reversal of fatigue requires a reduction in the workload/capacity ratio to a sustainable level. Apart from reducing minute ventilation and pressure generation requirements, improving energy delivery and repleting reserves (nutrition, cardiovascular function), as well as restoring contractile strength (by the measures already noted), are primary clinical objectives.

■ PULMONARY GAS EXCHANGE

Oxygen is required for the efficient production of energy, and carbon dioxide is produced as a by-product. Continuous exchange of these gases between the tissues and the surrounding environment is necessary to maintain concentrations that are consistent with adequate tissue function. The efficiency with which the lungs accomplish this task is reflected in the arterial blood gas analysis, which, when properly interpreted, provides insight into the pathophysiology of lung disease.

NORMAL GAS EXCHANGE

The lung's functional unit of gas exchange is the acinus, which comprises a terminal airway and its surrounding alveoli (about 2,000). There are about 300 million alveoli in the adult lung, each about 0.25 mm in diameter. Because of the way the alveoli are packaged and connected, they can provide an internal surface area of over 100 m^2 (the size of a tennis court). The alveoli are surrounded by a capillary network of similar surface area containing at any one time about 200 mL of blood. The alveolar–capillary interface (the air–blood barrier) is exceedingly thin (only 0.2 mm at some points).

The alveoli are connected to the environment by a series of conducting airways within which no gas exchange takes place. On inspiration, the amount of fresh gas that reaches the alveoli (V_A) is less than the V_T, by the volume of the physiologic dead space (V_{DS}): $V_A = V_T - V_{DS}$. For healthy lungs breathing at normal V_T, the V_{DS} is largely accounted for by the volume of the conducting airways, which approximates 1 mL per pound of lean body weight. In a normal lung, each breath increases the alveolar P_{O_2} ($P_{A}O_2$) and reduces the alveolar P_{CO_2} ($P_{ALV}CO_2$) by 5% to 10%. The small changes are due to the buffering effect of the gas remaining in the lungs at the end of a normal breath (FRC). The normal V_T is about 300 mL, and the normal FRC is about 3,000 mL—a 10-fold difference.

The pulmonary arterial blood (systemic venous) entering the lung has a mixed venous oxygen tension ($P_{\bar{V}}O_2$) and a mixed venous carbon dioxide tension ($P_{\bar{V}}CO_2$) determined by the cardiac output and the metabolic rate of the tissues. The rate at

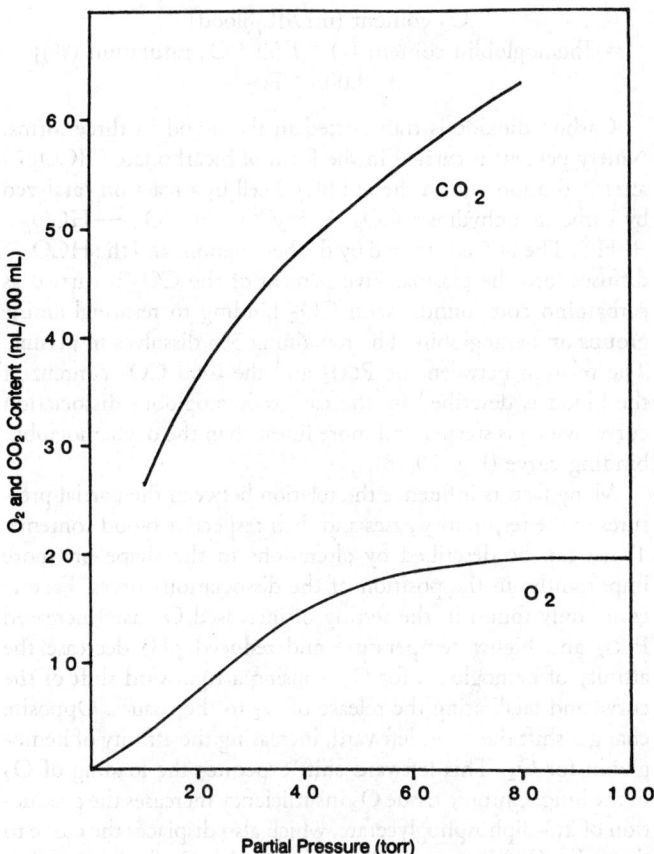

FIGURE 10.13. The oxyhemoglobin and carbon dioxide dissociation curves. The difference in shape of the relationship between partial pressure and content, sigmoid for O_2 and linear for CO_2, has important physiologic consequences. (From Dantzker DR. Pulmonary gas exchange. In: Dantzker DR, ed. *Cardiopulmonary critical care.* Philadelphia: WB Saunders, 1991:34, with permission.)

which gas transfers between the alveolus and the pulmonary arterial blood depends on the inspired gas concentration, the $P_{\bar{V}}O_2$ and $P_{\bar{V}}CO_2$, the ability of the blood and gas phases to equilibrate fully, and the adequacy with which the lung matches alveolar ventilation ($\dot{V}_A$) and blood flow on perfusion ($\dot{Q}$) in each lung unit, the ventilation/perfusion ($\dot{V}/\dot{Q}$) ratio. An abnormality of any of these leads to disordered pulmonary gas exchange.

In the blood, the respiratory gases are carried both dissolved in the plasma and combined with hemoglobin. Hemoglobin is a complex molecule composed of globin folded around heme, an iron-containing O_2 carrier. Each gram of hemoglobin binds 1.39 mL of O_2 when fully saturated. The degree to which the hemoglobin saturates with oxygen depends on the P_{O_2} to which the hemoglobin is exposed. The avidity for binding O_2 decreases as each of the four binding sites on the heme molecule is occupied, resulting in the nonlinear relation between the P_{O_2} and the O_2 saturation described by the oxyhemoglobin dissociation curve (Fig. 10.13). The O_2 is also carried in much smaller amounts dissolved in the plasma (0.003 mL O_2 per mm Hg per dL blood). The total amount of O_2 carried, the O_2 content, can be calculated from the sum of the dissolved and bound forms:

$$O_2 \text{ content (mL/dL blood)}$$
$$= [\text{hemoglobin content (g)} * 1.39 * O_2 \text{ saturation (\%)}]$$
$$+ 0.003 * P_{O_2}$$

Carbon dioxide is transported in the blood in three forms. Ninety percent is carried in the form of bicarbonate (HCO_3^-) after hydration within the red blood cell in a reaction catalyzed by carbonic anhydrase: $CO_2 + H_2O \leftrightarrow H_2CO_3 \leftrightarrow HCO_3^- + H^+$. The H^+ is buffered by the hemoglobin and the HCO_3^- diffuses into the plasma. Five percent of the CO_2 is carried as carbamino compounds, with CO_2 binding to terminal amine groups on hemoglobin. The remaining 5% dissolves in plasma. The relation between the P_{CO_2} and the total CO_2 content of the blood is described by the carboxyhemoglobin dissociation curve, which is steeper and more linear than the oxyhemoglobin binding curve (Fig. 10.13).

Many factors influence the relation between the partial pressures of the respiratory gases and their respective blood contents. These can be described by alterations in the shape or, more importantly, in the position of the dissociation curves. Factors commonly found in the setting of increased O_2 use (increased P_{CO_2} and higher temperature and reduced pH) decrease the affinity of hemoglobin for O_2, causing a rightward shift of the curve and facilitating the release of O_2 to the tissues. Opposite changes shift the curve leftward, increasing the affinity of hemoglobin for O_2. This leftward shift expedites the loading of O_2 in the lung. Chronic tissue O_2 insufficiency increases the production of 2,3-diphosphoglycerate, which also displaces the curve to the right. Carbon monoxide competes with O_2 for hemoglobin binding sites and shifts the curve leftward, impeding the release of O_2. Finally, various genetically determined hemoglobin variants have curves that may be located to the left or the right of normal. The position of the oxyhemoglobin dissociation curve is usually described by calculating the P_{O_2} at which the hemoglobin is 50% saturated (P_{50}). The normal P_{50} is about 27 mm Hg. The position of the carboxyhemoglobin curve is influenced most by the O_2 saturation. Increases in O_2 saturation shift the curve to the right, and the decreased affinity facilitates the unloading of CO_2 in the lungs. The falling O_2 saturation in the tissues shifts it in the opposite direction, making it easier to remove the CO_2 produced by metabolism.

The mature red blood cell is packed with hemoglobin but cannot synthesize protein, making it vulnerable to injury. Its biconcave shape increases the surface area for gas exchange and permits greater deformability, which facilitates its ability to squeeze through capillaries of similar dimension.

PULMONARY MECHANISMS OF ABNORMAL GAS EXCHANGE

Reduction of the Inspired P_{O_2}

During ascent from sea level, the inspired P_{O_2} ($P_{I_{O_2}}$) decreases exponentially with barometric pressure:

$$P_{I_{O_2}} = 0.2093 - (\text{barometric pressure} - \text{water vapor pressure})$$

In the alveolus, water vapor pressure remains at 47 mm Hg when measured at body temperature. The $P_{I_{O_2}}$ is 150 mm Hg

at sea level and falls to about 38 mm Hg on the summit of Mount Everest. Exposure to a reduced $P_{I_{O_2}}$ is quite common in our mobile society. The cabins of commercial aircraft are pressurized to simulate altitudes as high as 8,000 to 10,000 feet, producing a $P_{I_{O_2}}$ as low as 100 mm Hg.

The alveolar gas equation calculates a mean "ideal" alveolar P_{O_2} by considering the lung to be a single homogeneous compartment that receives all ventilation and perfusion. The equation can be simplified as:

$$P_{ALV_{O_2}} = P_{I_{O_2}} - P_{a_{CO_2}}/R$$

where R is the respiratory exchange ratio (CO_2 production divided by O_2 consumption, or $\dot{V}_{CO_2}$ divided by $\dot{V}_{O_2}$). Normally, the difference between the calculated "ideal" $P_{a_{O_2}}$ and the measured $P_{a_{O_2}}$ is small. In patients with lung disease, however, the alveolar–arterial difference for O_2 ($P_{ALV_{O_2}} - P_{a_{O_2}}$) widens. The reduction in $P_{a_{CO_2}}$ that occurs subsequent to hyperventilation increases the alveolar P_{O_2} by 1 to 1.25 mm Hg per mm Hg fall in $P_{a_{CO_2}}$, depending on R. During maximal hypoxic stimulation, a normal subject can maintain $P_{a_{CO_2}}$ as low as 7 mm Hg. Patients with lung disease, however, may not be able to increase minute ventilation ($\dot{V}_E$) to the same degree.

Abnormal Diffusion

The transfer of gas across the alveolar capillary membrane is accomplished by diffusion:

$$\text{Gas transfer} = \text{diffusing capacity of the lung} * (P_A - P_{cap})$$

The diffusing capacity of the lung (D_L) is a lumped parameter encompassing a series of resistances to gas flow. Direct measurements of the D_L for O_2 and CO_2 are difficult to obtain because they require the capillary partial pressures (P_{cap}) of each gas, which are impossible to measure directly.

At rest, an individual blood cell spends about 0.75 second in the pulmonary capillaries but usually can equilibrate fully with alveolar gas within one-third of the time available. This allows for increased diffusion capability when the system is required to transfer increasing amounts of gas, as during exercise. Under certain circumstances, the system may be stressed sufficiently so that diffusion limits gas transfer. Three situations can be hypothesized: an increase in the diffusion pathway, as might be seen subsequent to inflammation or fibrosis; a reduction in the time of contact between alveolar gas and blood, as with a marked increase in cardiac output (such as during exercise) or with a reduction in the cross-sectional area of the vascular bed due to primary vascular disease or diffuse alveolar destruction; and a reduction in the driving pressure ($P_A - P_{cap}$), as would be seen at extreme altitudes or perhaps in individual lung units where the alveolar P_{O_2} is reduced due to $\dot{V}/\dot{Q}$ mismatching. In clinical disease, abnormal diffusion plays only a small role in causing hypoxemia, and even this component is easily overcome by a modest increase in $F_{I_{O_2}}$.

Hypoventilation

Metabolic production of CO_2 ($\dot{V}_{CO_2}$) adds almost 17,000 mEq of acid to the blood each day that must be removed at the same rate at which it is produced. The alveolar, and thus arterial, level of CO_2 depends on the relation between production and excretion:

$$\text{Alveolar } P_{CO_2} \dot{V}_{CO_2}/\dot{V}_A$$

In the normal lung, the $\dot{V}_A$ is a relatively fixed proportion of the $\dot{V}_E$, and it is useful to think of the P_aCO_2 as inversely proportional to the $\dot{V}_E$. Hypoventilation is best defined as a rate of ventilation inadequate to prevent respiratory acidosis. Hyperventilation is the opposite. Because the anatomical dead space is a relatively fixed volume, the proportion of the $\dot{V}_T$ that it comprises varies inversely with the $\dot{V}_T$. Therefore, if the same minute ventilation is achieved with a small $\dot{V}_T$ and increased frequency, the $\dot{V}_A$ decreases and hypoventilation ensues. The $\dot{V}_A$ can also fall in the face of an unchanged (or even increased) $\dot{V}_E$ if an increase in alveolar dead space develops.

Hypoxemia that results from hypoventilation is not due to inefficient O_2 transfer (unless atelectasis supervenes). Normally, $\dot{V}_E$ is closely coupled to $\dot{V}_{CO_2}$. Hypoventilation thus represents an abnormality of ventilatory control or a failure of the respiratory pump to respond to a normal input signal. Such pump failure is most commonly noted in the setting of cerebrovascular accident, deep sedation or narcosis, neuromuscular disease, or skeletal abnormalities of the chest wall such as kyphoscoliosis. Although small increases in F_IO_2 correct hypoventilation-associated hypoxemia, therapy must be directed at the low $\dot{V}_A$ and its underlying, often nonpulmonary, etiology to prevent progressive respiratory acidosis.

Differentiation between pulmonary and nonpulmonary causes of hypoxemia can usually be made by calculating the $P_{ao}O_2 - P_aO_2$. With hypoventilation, the $P_{AO}O_2 - P_aO_2$ remains normal. In patients with $\dot{V}/\dot{Q}$ inequality, the falling P_aO_2 and increasing P_aCO_2 are accompanied by a widening of this index.

Ventilation–Perfusion Inequality

Under ideal conditions, the alveoli would all receive exactly matching amounts of blood flow and ventilation, ensuring maximal transfer of O_2 and CO_2. Even in the normal lung, however, regional differences in the distribution of blood flow and ventilation lead to variability in the $\dot{V}/\dot{Q}$ ratios. Any mismatching of blood flow and ventilation ($\dot{V}/\dot{Q}$ inequality) disrupts pulmonary gas exchange. The $\dot{V}/\dot{Q}$ can vary from 0.0 in shunt units that are perfused but not ventilated to infinity in those that are ventilated but not perfused (dead space).

Influenced by posture and gravity, the $\dot{V}/\dot{Q}$ distribution usually ranges from 0.6 to 3.0, with most units approximating 1.0 (Fig. 10.14). There is also a small shunt (1% to 3%) due to blood flow from the bronchial and thebesian veins that drain directly into the left side of the heart. The normal dead space consists mainly of the non-gas-exchanging airways and during quiet breathing approximates 33% of the $\dot{V}_T$. With increasing age, there is a gradual increase in the degree of $\dot{V}/\dot{Q}$ inequality, which explains the increased $P_{AO}O_2 - P_aO_2$ usually seen in older normal subjects.

In lung disease, units with low or high $\dot{V}/\dot{Q}$ may predominate. Low $\dot{V}/\dot{Q}$ units usually develop as the result of regionally reduced ventilation secondary to airway disease. They may also

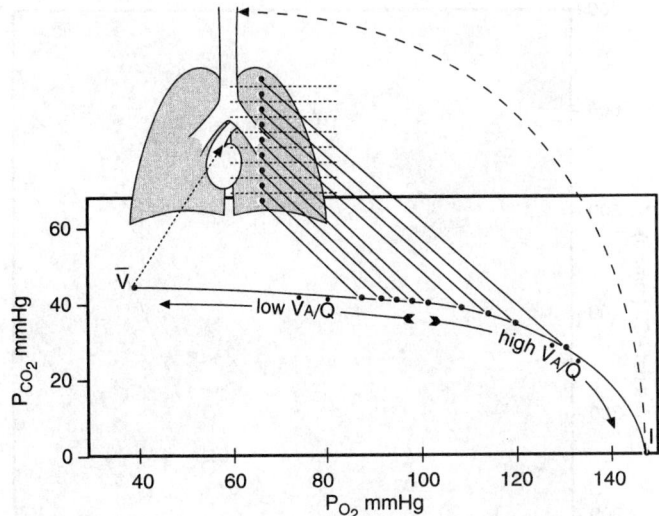

FIGURE 10.14. Composition of pulmonary venous blood leaving different regions of the upright lung. Note the spectrum of ventilation/perfusion ratios and their resultant contributions to the mixture that forms the arterial blood. (From West JB. *Ventilation/blood flow in gas exchange,* fourth ed. Oxford: Blackwell Scientific, 1985, with permission.)

be caused by overperfusion of normally ventilated lung units, as for example after acute pulmonary embolism, when blood flow is suddenly diverted from embolized to nonembolized areas of the lung. The embolized units, by contrast, develop high $\dot{V}/\dot{Q}$ or become dead space, depending on the completeness of occlusion. A more common cause of high $\dot{V}/\dot{Q}$ units is emphysema, a disease in which the loss of blood flow secondary to alveolar wall destruction is even greater than the decrease in $\dot{V}VE$.

Because $\dot{V}/\dot{Q}$ inequality dramatically affects both O_2 and CO_2 transfer, it would invariably lead to both hypoxemia and hypercapnia if $\dot{V}E$ remained unchanged (Fig. 10.14). However, in patients with intact ventilatory drive and muscle function, any increase in the P_aCO_2 due to developing $\dot{V}/\dot{Q}$ inequality leads to an increased $\dot{V}E$ mediated by chemoreceptor drive. To the extent that this increased $\dot{V}E$ can affect lung units with low $\dot{V}/\dot{Q}$, increasing their ratios back toward normal improves both arterial P_O_2 and P_{CO_2}. Noteworthy improvement is possible, however, only when the low $\dot{V}/\dot{Q}$ is caused by overperfusion and the airways are relatively normal. In patients in whom the low $\dot{V}/\dot{Q}$ ratios are caused by significant airway obstruction, any additional ventilation tends to go to the normal, already well-ventilated alveoli. When blood from these units combines with the blood coming from the low $\dot{V}/\dot{Q}$ units, the P_O_2 remains relatively unchanged. Conversely, the carboxyhemoglobin dissociation curve is linear throughout the physiologic range (Fig. 10.13). The low P_aCO_2 in the capillary blood of the well-ventilated units nearly compensates for the decreased removal of CO_2 by the units with low $\dot{V}/\dot{Q}$ ratios. Patients with lung disease often have additional inputs to the respiratory center from stretch and irritant receptors within the lung and airways as well as from hypoxic stimulation, and thus the degree of hyperventilation may exceed the amount required to compensate for the low $\dot{V}/\dot{Q}$

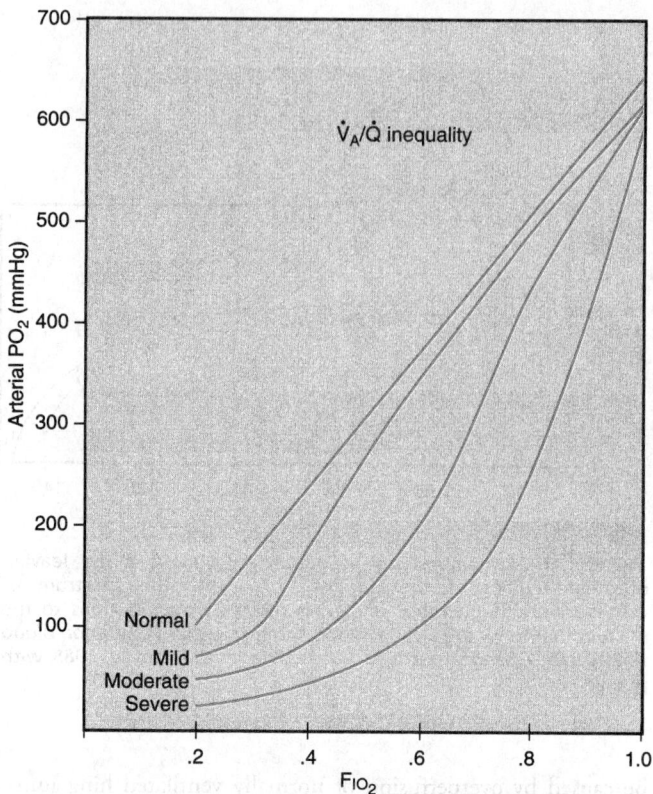

FIGURE 10.15. Effect of increasing ventilation/perfusion inequality on the arterial P_{O_2} at different inspired oxygen fractions ($F_{I_{O_2}}$). Note that an $F_{I_{O_2}}$ of 1.0 essentially eliminates the depression in arterial P_{O_2} caused by any degree of ventilation/perfusion inequality. (From Dantzker DR. *Cardiopulmonary critical care,* second ed. Philadelphia: WB Saunders, 1991:39, with permission.)

units. Raising the inspired fraction of oxygen may dramatically improve arterial P_{O_2}, depending on the severity of $\dot{V}/\dot{Q}$ mismatching and the range over which $F_{I_{O_2}}$ is increased (Fig. 10.15).

As $\dot{V}/\dot{Q}$ inequality increases, however, the work of breathing may rise to the level where further increases in ventilation are impossible, dyspnea becomes intolerable, or the metabolic cost of breathing results in no gain in overall gas exchange. At this point, the only way to eliminate the metabolic CO_2 load is to allow P_aCO_2 to rise. Hypercapnia permits the CO_2 to be cleared at a higher concentration per liter of ventilation, thus making more efficient use of the remaining ventilatory capacity. Two patients with obstructive pulmonary disease might have equal reductions in flow rates and increases in $\dot{V}/\dot{Q}$ inequality, but one might be hypercapnic and the other hypocapnic. The major difference between them is the higher $\dot{V}_E$ in the hypocapnic patient, which is believed to reflect, among other things, a difference in the gain control of the chemoreceptors.

Hypoxic vasoconstriction is a conservative reflex in the lung that minimizes $\dot{V}/\dot{Q}$ inequality when P_aO_2 ranges within 30 to 150 mm Hg. Variations in P_AO_2 result in adjustments of tone within the perfusing arteriole in an attempt to increase the $\dot{V}/\dot{Q}$ ratio. When regional abnormalities are present, hypoxic vasoconstriction can minimize the impact of $\dot{V}/\dot{Q}$ inequality on gas

exchange by diverting blood flow away from these abnormal areas. With generalized hypoxia, however, as is seen with diffuse lung disease or in normal persons exposed to high altitude, any beneficial effect on gas exchange is often overshadowed by the increased pulmonary arterial pressure that develops from global increases in pulmonary vascular resistance. This pulmonary hypertension and sensitivity to hypoxia is particularly intense in patients with a reduced capillary bed (as occurs in emphysema with cor pulmonale). Many drugs interfere with effective hypoxic vasoconstriction, including nitroglycerin, β-adrenergic agonists, calcium channel blockers, various direct arterial vasodilators, and inhalational anesthetics. Because of this, the use of these drugs in patients with lung disease may result in worsened hypoxemia. Nitric oxide is believed to mediate alveolar vasodilatation. Exciting recent work indicates that inhaled nitric oxide preferentially improves blood flow in well-ventilated regions, thereby improving oxygen exchange in acutely diseased lungs.

As the degree of $\dot{V}/\dot{Q}$ inequality worsens, there is an increasing resistance to correct P_aO_2 by raising $F_{I_{O_2}}$. When marked $\dot{V}/\dot{Q}$ inequality is present, as might be seen in the terminal stages of many diffuse pulmonary processes, there may be no substantial rise in P_aO_2 until the $F_{I_{O_2}}$ exceeds 0.40.

Shunt

The shunting of venous blood through non-gas-exchanging units dramatically alters gas exchange. Shunts most commonly result from blood passing through pulmonary capillaries in the walls of alveoli that are atelectatic or filled with edema fluid or inflammatory exudate. Less frequently, right-to-left shunting occurs through atrial or ventricular defects, driven by favorable pressure gradients across them. Rarely, the shunting may be through anatomical arteriovenous channels within the lung such as arteriovenous malformations or the vascular malformations occasionally seen in the lungs of patients with far-advanced hepatic cirrhosis. Whatever the cause, the percentage of cardiac output shunted across the lung tends to parallel cardiac output. The impact on P_aO_2 depends, however, on any simultaneous changes that occur in $P_{\bar{V}}O_2$ and hypoxic vasoconstriction in shunt regions.

Shunt is the cause of hypoxemia in both cardiac and noncardiac pulmonary edema; it constitutes the major abnormality of oxygen exchange seen with pneumonia. The physiologic behavior of shunt demands an approach to therapy that is different from that associated with $\dot{V}/\dot{Q}$ inequality.

Shunt is a potent cause of hypoxemia because of the low saturation of the mixed venous blood. Even a small increase in shunt leads to a significant fall in the P_aO_2. Hypercapnia is not generally seen. A low P_aCO_2 is, in fact, more common because ventilation is usually stimulated in excess of metabolic requirements by the developing hypoxemia as well as by inputs from intrapulmonary stretch receptors.

Unlike $\dot{V}/\dot{Q}$ inequality, the hypoxemia caused by shunt resists correction by increases in $F_{I_{O_2}}$. This feature is often used clinically to differentiate the two mechanisms. As the shunt gets larger, the breathing of even pure O_2 makes only a small impact on the P_aO_2, again unlike the problem of $\dot{V}/\dot{Q}$ inequality. However, even the small increases in P_aO_2 that are seen can be physiologically significant. Small changes in P_aO_2 lead to significant changes in O_2 content because these patients are usually so hypoxemic that P_aO_2 is on the steep portion of the oxyhemoglobin dissociation curve.

Because of the poor response of shunt hypoxemia to supplemental O_2, and considering the risks of exposing the lung to high F_IO_2, other strategies for treatment are required. Recruitment of collapsed lung units or redistribution of lung liquids and blood flow by PEEP, repositioning, or pharmacologic relaxing of the chest wall is often effective. Inhaled vasodilators (prostaglandin or nitric oxide), intensifiers of hypoxic vasoconstriction (almitrine), or measures to improve the O_2 content of the mixed venous blood can also improve P_aO_2 in the setting of acute lung injury.

NONPULMONARY FACTORS AFFECTING GAS EXCHANGE

The degree to which variations in mixed venous P_2 ($P_{\bar{v}}O_2$) alters the end-capillary PO_2 depends on the $\dot{V}/\dot{Q}$ ratio of the unit. For ventilated lung units, the influence of the $P_{\bar{v}}O_2$ is greatest in units with a $\dot{V}/\dot{Q}$ ratio of less than 1.0 and negligible for those with a $\dot{V}/\dot{Q}$ ratio greater than 10. The ability of the $P_{\bar{v}}O_2$ to affect the P_aO_2 increases as the degree of $\dot{V}/\dot{Q}$ inequality or shunt increases.

A low $P_{\bar{v}}O_2$ occurs when there is a disparity between O_2 delivery and the O_2 requirements of the tissues. This is most common in the setting of an inappropriately low cardiac output, O_2 content, and hemoglobin concentration. It is accentuated when the O_2 requirements are increased, as in exercise, fever, vigorous hyperpnea, agitation, or hypermetabolic states.

In normal lung, the effect of a low $P_{\bar{v}}O_2$ on the P_aO_2 can be overcome by increasing $\dot{V}_E$, which effectively increases the $\dot{V}/\dot{Q}$ ratio of all units in the lung. This explains why little or no fall in P_aO_2 occurs in normal subjects during exercise, despite marked venous desaturation. In abnormal lungs, however, this correction is much less effective because the increased $\dot{V}_E$ exerts minimal impact on the poorly ventilated units and no impact on the shunt.

Mixed venous desaturation is the primary cause for the fall in P_aO_2 often noted during exercise in patients with both obstructive and restrictive lung disease when an improving match of ventilation and blood flow cannot compensate for the increased O_2 extraction. It is also a common cause for alterations of P_aO_2 in critically ill patients who are poised at the margin between adequate and inadequate O_2 delivery.

BIBLIOGRAPHY

Dantzker DR, Scharf SM. *Cardiopulmonary critical care*, third ed. Philadelphia: WB Saunders, 1998.

Leach RM, Treacher DF. Oxygen transport. 2. Tissue hypoxia. *Br Med J (Clin Res Ed)* 1998;317:1370–1373.

Marini JJ, Truwit JD. Monitoring the respiratory system. In: Hall J, Schmidt G, Wood LDH, eds. *Principles of critical care medicine*. New York: McGraw-Hill, 1997.

Murray JF. *The normal lung*, second ed. Philadelphia: WB Saunders, 1986.

Roussos C. *The thorax*, second ed. New York: Marcel Dekker, 1995.

Treacher DF, Leach RM. Oxygen transport. 1. Basic principles. *Br Med J (Clin Res Ed)* 1998;317:1302–1306.

West JB. *Ventilation, blood flow, and gas exchange*, fifth ed. London: Blackwell, 1990.

West JB. *Pulmonary pathophysiology—the essentials*. Baltimore: Williams & Wilkins, 1992.

West JB. Mathieu-Costello, O. Structure, strength, failure, and remodeling of the pulmonary blood–gas barrier. *Annu Rev Physiol* 1999;61:543–572.

Zapol WM, Rimar S, Gillis N, et al. Nitric oxide and the lung. *Am J Respir Crit Care Med* 1994;149:1375.

Kelley's Textbook of Internal Medicine, fourth edition. Edited by H. David Humes. Lippincott Williams & Wilkins, Philadelphia © 2000.

CHAPTER

11

VASCULAR BIOLOGY

ELIZABETH G. NABEL

THE NORMAL ARTERY

The normal artery consists of three layers. An intima lined by endothelium is on the inner or luminal aspect of the vessel and is bounded by the internal elastic lamina. The media consists of smooth muscle cells intertwined by elastic fibers. The media is bounded by the internal elastic lamina and by an external elastic lamina. The adventitia is the outer layer of the artery and is bounded by the external elastic lamina and the exterior of the vessel (Fig. 11.1).

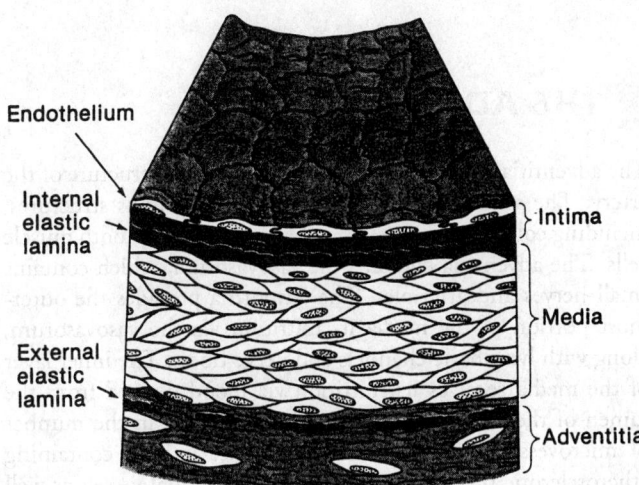

FIGURE 11.1. Structure of a normal muscular artery. (From Ross R, Glomset J. The pathogenesis of atherosclerosis. *N Engl J Med* 1996;295:369, with permission.)

THE INTIMA

In the human being at birth, the intima contains a thin layer of connective tissue and occasional smooth muscle cells. Over time, there is a concentric increase in the number of smooth muscle cells in the intima, referred to as diffuse intimal thickening. The intima is lined by a single layer of endothelial cells that abuts the lumen of the blood vessel.

Atherosclerotic lesions form in the intima. There are several ways in which lesions develop. The typical lesions of atherosclerosis are characterized by an asymmetric thickening of the intima that encroaches on the lumen of the blood vessel, resulting in a decrease in blood flow. A second form of intimal thickening is due to an increase in the intima associated with continued dilatation of the artery such that the actual lumen size does not change. These lesions tend to be concentric and consist of diffuse intimal thickening due to smooth muscle cell hyperplasia, commonly found as a sequela of hypertension.

THE MEDIA

The media is the muscular wall of the artery, bounded by the internal and external elastic lamina. The function of the media is to contract or dilate the blood vessel. Two different types of arteries are present in the human circulation: muscular arteries and elastic arteries. The media of muscular arteries consists of spiraling layers of smooth muscle cells attached to one another. Each smooth muscle cell is surrounded by a discontinuous basement membrane and interspersed collagen fibrils. Elastic arteries contain multiple layers of smooth muscle cells, each equivalent to a single media in a smaller muscular artery. Each layer of smooth muscle cells is bounded by an elastic lamina on its inner and outer aspects. The number of layers or lamellar units in elastic arteries is proportional to the size of the animal and depends on other factors, such as the anatomical position of the artery.

THE ADVENTITIA

The adventitia is the outer layer and the support structure of the artery. The adventitia consists of dense collagenous structures, including collagen fibrils, elastic fibers, and some smooth muscle cells. The adventitia contains the vasovasorum, which contains small nerves and arterioles. The adventitia provides the outermost portion of the media its nutrition via the vasovasorum, along with lymphatic channels and nerve fibers. The inner layer of the media receives its nutrition via blood derived from the lumen of the blood vessel. There is an increase in the number of microvessels in the adventitia opposite intimas containing atherosclerotic plaques. An increase in adventitial vessels as well as an increase in microvessels within the plaque may play important roles in the hemorrhage and thrombosis that follows plaque rupture in unstable atherosclerotic lesions.

CELLS OF THE ARTERY

ENDOTHELIUM

The entire circulatory system is lined by a continuous, single-cell-thick vascular endothelium. In healthy vessels, the vascular endothelium comprises a container for blood within the lumen of the artery and forms the biologic interface between the circulating blood components and all tissues of the artery. Endothelial cells probably represent the largest and most extensive tissue in the body because they line the entire vascular tree. The endothelium is the principal barrier between elements of the blood and the artery wall. In adults, the turnover of endothelial cells is very slow, on the order of 120 days. The endothelium has several very important functions: it forms a highly selective permeability barrier; it provides a nonthrombogenic surface; it is a highly active metabolic tissue; it forms several vasoactive substances; and it participates in the conversion of bloodborne monocytes to tissue-derived macrophages.

Endothelial cells morphologically are very similar throughout the circulatory system. However, there are functional differences in endothelial cells in different anatomical sites. This is important since endothelial cells respond to injury after exposure to various injurious agents in different parts of the arterial tree. This might include infectious agents, which act primarily at the capillary level; or oxidized low-density lipoprotein (LDL) particles that enter the subintima in large elastic and muscular arteries; or the response on the part of the endothelium to sheer stress from systemic hypertension. Endothelial cells are normally attached to each other by gap junctions. They transport substances in both directions across these cells via the process called transcytosis. Transendothelial channels have been observed primarily in capillary endothelium; however, it has been suggested that junctions between endothelial cells serve as potential sites of transendothelial migration by macrophages in large arteries as well.

Endothelial cells rest on a basement membrane that contains type IV collagen. These endothelial cells are capable of synthesis of connective tissue molecules. The basement membrane in addition to the internal elastic lamina serves as a crude type of filter. When the endothelium is removed or the artery is stretched, pores are present in the internal elastic lamina that permit the migration of macromolecules from the lumen to the media or the migration of smooth muscle cells from the media to the intima.

Endothelial cells are highly active cells with multiple functions (Fig. 11.2). Endothelial cells mediate several functions including a selective permeability barrier; hemostasis and thrombosis; vasoconstriction and vasodilatation; regulation of cytokines and growth-regulatory molecules; and transduction of biomechanical forces. These are adaptive processes that contribute to normal homeostasis of the blood vessel. However, when the endothelium is damaged or removed, alterations occur in the blood vessel including enhanced permeability, adhesiveness for leukocytes and other inflammatory molecules, thrombosis, stimulation of smooth muscle cell growth, and disruption of normal regulation of vascular tone, often leading to vasoconstriction. These manifestations are collectively termed endothelial

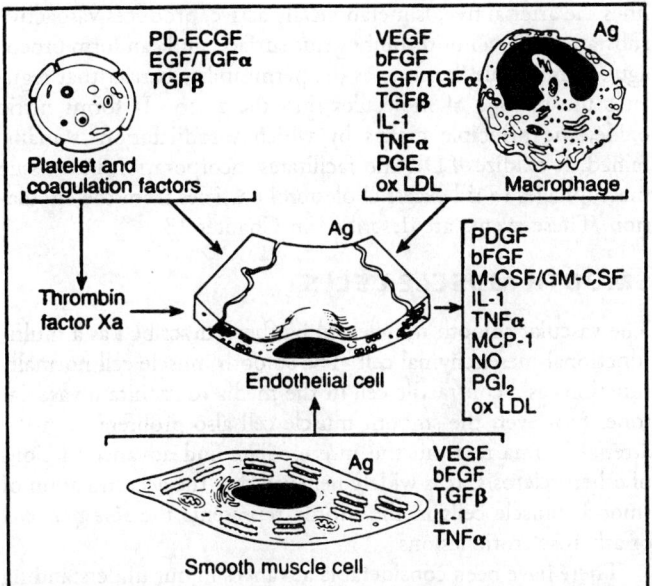

FIGURE 11.2. The endothelial cell presents a barrier to the artery wall, has nonthrombogenic properties, metabolizes vasoactive substances, produces growth factors, and forms connective tissue matrix. (From Ross R. The pathogenesis of atherosclerosis: a perspective for the 1990s. *Nature* 1993;362:108, with permission.)

dysfunction (Fig. 11.3), and they play a critical role in the initiation, progression, and clinical complications of inflammatory and degenerative vascular diseases.

Hemostatic–Thrombotic Balance

Blood normally does not clot inside its endothelial barrier. Failure of the endothelium to activate the coagulation cascade is referred to as nonthrombogenicity. Endothelial cells synthesize an arachidonic metabolite, prostaglandin I_2 (PGI_2; also called

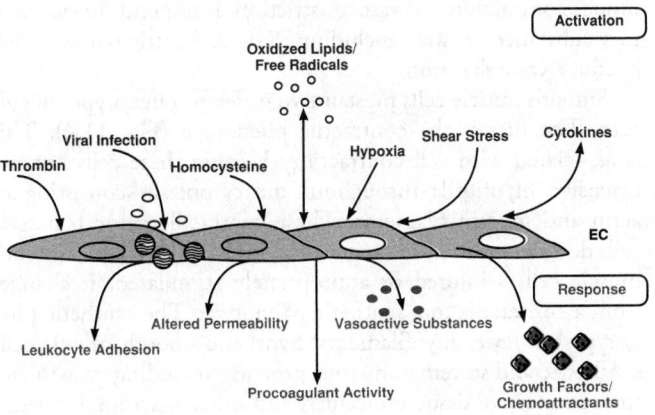

FIGURE 11.3. Generation of a dysfunctional endothelium. Stimulatory or injury provoking agents activate the endothelial cell. In response to injury, endothelial cell function is altered, resulting in a dysfunctional endothelium and leading to progression of vascular disease. (From Dicorleto PE, Gimbrone MA. Vascular endothelium. In: Fuster V, Ross R, Topol EJ, eds. *Atherosclerosis and coronary artery disease.* Philadelphia: Lippincott-Raven Publishers, 1996, with permission.)

prostacyclin) that is an extraordinarily potent inhibitor of platelet aggregation. The discovery of PGI_2 led to the concept that the endothelium plays an active thrombotic role by preventing platelet aggregation on its surface. The endothelium also plays a pivotal role in regulating the coagulation and fibrinolytic systems. Most of these functions are antithrombotic in nature. The endothelium synthesizes a number of natural coagulants including heparin, protein C, thrombomodulin, and tissue plasminogen activator, to name a few. The molecular mechanisms of the coagulation system and its interface with the endothelium are described in greater detail in Chapters 13, 237, and 238.

In contrast to the normal antithrombotic functions that occur in healthy endothelium, dysfunctional endothelial cells are prothrombotic. The endothelium, when damaged, synthesizes adhesive cofactors for platelets, such as von Willebrand's factor, fibronectin, thrombospondin, and procoagulant components like factor V, and is a trigger for the fibrin-generating coagulation cascade. The endothelium also synthesizes an inhibitor of the fibrinolytic pathway, called plasminogen activator inhibitor 1 (PAI-1), which reduces the rate of fibrin breakdown.

Thus, the endothelium functions in a hemostatic and thrombotic manner. This is relevant to maintain normal blood fluidity, stopping hemorrhage at sites of vascular injury, and altering pathologic thrombosis. These endothelium-dependent mechanisms contribute to a dynamic physiological balance between hemostatic and thrombotic factors.

Vasoconstrictor–Vasodilator Balance

The maintenance of arterial tone has traditionally been viewed of a function of the vascular smooth muscle cell within the media that responds to sympathetic or parasympathetic nervous activity. This concept was dramatically altered in the 1980s with the discovery of a potent endothelium-derived relaxing factor (EDRF), subsequently identified as nitric oxide. Landmark experiments performed by Furchgott and Zawadzki identified an EDRF produced by the endothelium that led to dilatation of smooth muscle cells. In the absence of the endothelium, EDRF was not produced, and smooth muscle cells underwent a paradoxical vasoconstriction leading to an increase in arterial tone. This was a new concept in vascular biology; that is, the vascular endothelium locally regulates vascular smooth muscle cells and vascular tone through the synthesis of vasoactive substances. Endothelium-derived relaxing factor was subsequently discovered to be nitric oxide. Studies of its metabolic pathway, the generation of nitric oxide synthase, and the cellular mechanisms of nitric oxide action that result in arterial vasodilatation have added a new dimension to our understanding of the role of endothelial cell–smooth muscle cell interactions and the regulation of vascular function. Nitric oxide along with PGI_2 and other related compounds constitute a class of natural endothelium-derived relaxing substances.

There are also endothelial-derived substances that have vasoconstrictor activity. These include angiotensin II, generated by the conversion of angiotensin I to angiotensin II by angiotensin-converting enzyme at the endothelial surface; platelet-derived growth factor (PDGF), secreted by endothelial cells; and endothelin 1. Endothelin 1 is the most potent vasoconstrictor known. It is generated by the proteolytic cleavage of a larger precursor, big endothelin. There are other prostaglandins that have vasoconstrictor properties.

Cytokines and Growth-Regulatory Molecules

The endothelium synthesizes many cytokines and growth factors that act locally on arteries to promote growth of smooth muscle cells and macrophage as well as mediate inflammatory changes. Thus, the endothelium has often been referred to as an endocrine organ having both paracrine (acting on neighbors) or autocrine (acting on self) functions.

The endothelium maintains a balance between cytokine and growth- regulatory molecules with regard to their primary effect on vascular smooth muscle cell migration and proliferation. Some of the endothelium-derived cytokines include interleukin 1α, IL-1β, IL-6, IL-8, and monocyte chemotactic protein (MCP-1). The endothelium is also the source of growth factors that stimulate smooth muscle cell migration and proliferation. These include PDGF, fibroblast growth factor (FGF), transforming growth factor β (TGF-β), insulin-like growth factor 1 (IGF-1), and heparin-binding epidermal growth factor (EGF). Platelet-derived growth factor is a growth factor for fibroblasts and smooth muscle cells but not endothelial cells. When injured, endothelial cells secrete PDGF that acts as a mitogen and chemoattractant for smooth muscle cells. It stimulates migration of smooth muscle cells from the media into the intima where smooth muscle cells then form atherosclerotic lesions. Another mitogen is FGF, which has angiogenic and growth-promoting effects on endothelium and smooth muscle cells. Transforming growth factor β stimulates smooth muscle cells to synthesize and secrete extracellular matrix, predominantly collagen.

Transducer of Biomechanical Forces

The endothelium is constantly exposed to biomechanical stimuli due to its position in direct contact with flowing blood. These stimuli include mechanical forces generated by pulsatile blood flow, fluid stress, wall tension, and intramural pressure. Some forces are passively transduced across the endothelial layer to other cells and the extracellular matrix, whereas some forces act directly on the endothelial cell to alter its metabolic state and regulate gene expression. Some of the biomechanically induced effects include changes in growth factors, vasoconstrictors, vasodilators, and fibrinolytic factors. For example, a sheer stress response element (SSRE) has been described in the promoter region of PDGF B. Increased sheer stress leads to activation of a promoter element, causing transcription of the PDGF gene and an increase in PDGF protein synthesis by endothelial cells. The PDGF protein stimulates smooth muscle cells to migrate and proliferate. This sheer stress response element is also present in the promoter of some leukocyte adhesion molecules, such as intercellular adhesion molecule 1 (ICAM-1). The role of the endothelium as a transducer of biomechanical forces is important in the context of atherogenesis. It is now appreciated that the early lesions of atherosclerosis arise at sites of increased sheer stress with a predilection for branch points and lesions of curvature. These areas are characterized by disturbed blood flow.

Thus, the endothelium forms an obligate monolayer that lines the arterial tree, is metabolically active, produces vasoactive substances, has a nonthrombogenic surface, and can form procoagulant materials. It serves as the permeability barrier that regulates the passage of molecules into the artery. It forms nitric oxide, the principle means by which vasodilatation is maintained. It oxidizes LDL and facilitates incorporation into tissue macrophages to rid excess cholesterol particles from the circulation. These events are described in Chapter 13.

SMOOTH MUSCLE CELLS

The vascular smooth muscle cell has been described as a multifunctional mesenchymal cell. The smooth muscle cell normally functions as a contractile cell in the media to maintain vascular tone. However, the smooth muscle cell also proliferates in the arterial intima to form the intermediate and advanced lesions of atherosclerosis. It is widely believed that the accumulation of smooth muscle cells in the intima represents the *sine qua non* of atherosclerotic lesions.

There have been considerable advances in our understanding of the biology of smooth muscle cells. Thirty years ago it was widely believed that the only function of smooth muscle cells was to contract within the vessel wall. In the early 1970s it became possible to culture smooth muscle cells. Tissue culture studies then led to a greater understanding of the multiple functions of smooth muscle cells. The smooth muscle cell synthesizes and secretes several forms of collagen, elastic fibers, and proteoglycans. Smooth muscle cells, like fibroblasts, contain high-affinity receptors for a number of ligands. These ligands include LDL, insulin, PDGF, FGF, and TGF-β, to name a few. Smooth muscle cells also synthesize and secrete growth regulatory molecules such as PDGF.

The principal role of the smooth muscle cell in the adult artery is to maintain the tone of the arterial wall. The basic mechanism of contraction involves interaction of the contractile proteins actin and myosin. The contractile force is produced by the sliding of smooth muscle actin and myosin filaments across one another. The smooth muscle cell responds to numerous vasoactive substances, such as epinephrine and angiotensin, that induce contraction and vasoconstriction. It responds to vasodilatory substances as well, including PGI$_2$ and nitric oxide, which produce vasorelaxation.

Smooth muscle cells present two different phenotypes in culture. The first is the contractile phenotype (Fig. 11.4). This is associated with cell contractility because these cells contain extensive myofibrils throughout the cytoplasm consisting of actin and myosin filaments. These contractile smooth muscle cells do not respond to mitogens such as PDGF. When a smooth muscle cell is injured or appropriately stimulated, it changes from a contractile to a synthetic phenotype. The synthetic phenotype has fewer myofilaments. Synthetic smooth muscle cells synthesize and secrete numerous proteins, including growth factors, connective tissue molecules, and other macromolecules.

The phenotypic modulation of smooth muscle cells from a contractile to a synthetic phenotype underlies the pathogenesis of atherosclerotic lesions. Smooth muscle cells in the contractile phenotype are nonresponsive to mitogens, whereas those in the synthetic phenotype are responsive to mitogens. such as PDGF and FGF. For the lesions of atherosclerosis to develop, the

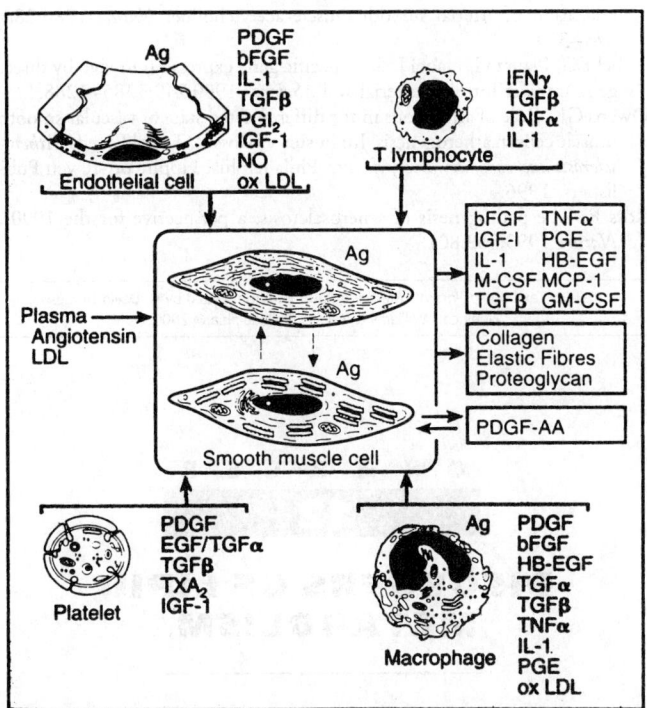

FIGURE 11.4. The smooth muscle cell undergoes phenotypic modulation from a contractile to a synthetic phenotype. In the synthetic phenotype, smooth muscle cells synthesize connective tissue molecules, growth factors, and interact with neighboring T lymphocytes, platelets, and macrophages. The genes that are expressed by each cell type that interacts with the smooth muscle cell are listed to the right of the cell type. (From Ross R. The pathogenesis of atherosclerosis: a perspective for the 1990s. *Nature* 1993;362:801, with permission.)

smooth muscle cell must convert from a contractile to a synthetic phenotype, migrate from the media to the intima, and proliferate in the intima, forming the atherosclerotic lesion. As the smooth muscle cell proliferates within the intima, it also secretes connective tissue macromolecules and metabolizes oxidized LDL, along with macrophages and endothelial cells. Smooth muscle cells are also stimulated to proliferate in the presence of inflammatory cytokines, produced by activated endothelium and macrophages. Consequently, control of the phenotypic state of the smooth muscle cell is critical to understanding and preventing the development of atherosclerosis.

PLATELETS

Platelets are clearly important in the genesis of lesions of atherosclerosis. Platelets are the inciting molecules that adhere and aggregate to the subintima during rupture of the atherosclerotic plaque and formation of an occlusive thrombosis on the platelet-rich clot, leading to unstable angina and myocardial infarction. Platelets are interesting cells in that they synthesize little or no protein. They contain numerous prepackaged, highly potent molecules sequestered in their granules. Among these are a number of factors that are important in the coagulation cascade and are potent growth factors or mitogens. These growth factors include PDGF, FGF, TGF-β, and EGF. The vasoactive substances within platelet granules include serotonin, thromboxane A$_2$, platelet factor IV, and calcium.

When platelets are exposed to a disrupted endothelial surface, they adhere to the subendothelium. Growth factors are released. The coagulation cascade is initiated. Thus, at sites of injury in which collagen exposure, thrombin and fibrin formation, or ADP release occurs, platelet aggregation and thrombosis follow, leading to the release of vasoactive, stimulatory, and proliferative agents carried by the platelets. Thus, platelets also participate in the response to injury and to the pathogenesis of atherosclerosis. During rupture of an atherosclerotic plaque, the subintima is exposed, and platelets adhere to the vasculature via several adhesive molecules, including von Willebrand's factor and tissue factor. Platelets also contain receptors for numerous ligands. The glycoprotein IIB–IIIA receptor plays an essential role in platelet aggregation and adhesion during plaque rupture and the clinical syndromes of unstable angina and myocardial infarction. Inhibitors of the glycoprotein IIB–IIIA receptor have now led to major advances in the treatment of acute coronary syndromes by disruption of platelet adhesion and aggregation.

MACROPHAGES

Macrophages are derived from circulating monocytes. When the monocyte enters the tissue, it takes on characteristics of the host tissue. In most inflammatory sites, the monocyte converts to a tissue macrophage where it acts as a scavenger cell to remove foreign substances by phagocytosis and acts as a second line of defense to neutrophils against microbial organisms. As a scavenger cell, the macrophage removes injurious substances such as oxidized LDL via scavenger receptors. Macrophages also oxidize LDL by 15-lipoxygenase. Macrophages play an important role in the pathogenesis of atherosclerosis and the response to injury. Macrophages act as scavenger cells to ingest oxidized LDL and microbial organisms in the vessel wall. Macrophages secrete a large number of biologically active substances, including leukotrienes, IL-1, oxygen metabolites such as superoxide anion, PDGF, FGF, EGF, TGF-β, and macrophage colony-stimulating factor, a growth factor from monocyte-macrophages. These growth factors then act in an autocrine and paracrine manner to stimulate macrophage and smooth muscle cell replication. Macrophages accumulate in lesions and contribute to the pathogenesis of atherosclerosis. Indeed, plaque rupture commonly occurs at the shoulder region of the plaque at sites of macrophage accumulation and inflammation.

The macrophage is a key cell responsible for promotion of connective tissue proliferation, commonly associated with chronic inflammatory responses. Macrophages are the principal cell in the fatty streak, the initial lesion of atherosclerosis. They accumulate large amounts of lipid in the form of droplets that contain cholesterol ester. Macrophages and smooth muscle cells proliferate in atherosclerotic lesions.

T-LYMPHOCYTES

The CD8$^+$ and CD4$^+$ T lymphocytes have been observed in all phases of atherosclerosis. Their presence in atherosclerotic lesions lends evidence to the hypothesis that atherosclerosis may develop in part as a result of an immune reaction. Also, T lymphocytes are present in transplant atherosclerosis following car-

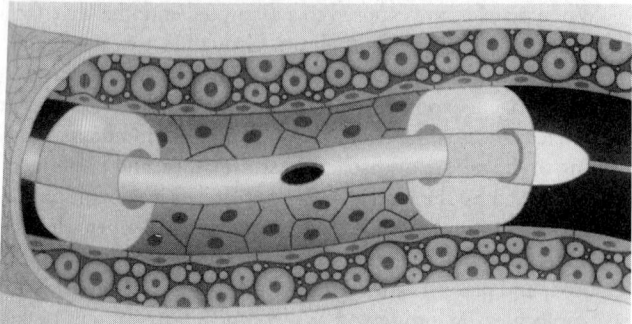

FIGURE 11.5. Gene transfer within an artery. A double-balloon catheter is inserted into an artery. Inflation of the proximal and distal balloon creates an interprotected space into which a vector and recombinant DNA can be introduced into the blood vessel. The gene enters endothelial cells and smooth muscle cells, and recombinant protein is expressed. The recombinant protein can have autocrine and paracrine effects on adjacent endothelial cells, smooth muscle cells, platelets, and macrophages. (From Nabel E. Gene therapy: cardiovascular gene therapy. *Sci Med* 1997:4–5, with permission.)

diac transplantation. While the lesions observed in common atherosclerosis are eccentric in nature, the lesions of transplant atherosclerosis are concentric in nature. The nature of the antigens that play a role in common atherosclerosis have been incompletely characterized; however, *Chlamydia pneumoniae*, cytomegalovirus, and other viral antigens have been proposed. The interactions between T lymphocytes and activated macrophages suggest that antigen presentation and the release of cytokines and growth factors are important steps in the inflammatory reaction. In addition, oxidized LDL may be a potential major antigen that stimulates macrophage–T-cell interactions.

CONCLUSION

Knowledge in the field of vascular biology has exploded in the past decade. The tools of molecular and cellular biology have facilitated rapid expansion of our understanding of the principal cells involved in atherosclerosis: endothelium, smooth muscle, platelets, macrophages, and T cells. Studies in transgenic and knockout mice have increased our understanding of the interaction of these cells and the pathogenesis of vascular diseases. Gene transfer and gene therapy are providing new therapeutic approaches to the treatment of atherosclerosis and other vascular diseases (Fig. 11.5). At present, one of the most critical aspects of vascular disease is the need to understand the basis of genetic susceptibility. A major thrust for future research in vascular biology will focus on the molecular genetics of complex cardiovascular diseases. An understanding of the gene sequences, genetic loci, and complex trait interactions will lend itself to new possibilities for novel therapeutics, including gene therapy.

BIBLIOGRAPHY

Dicorleto PE, Gimbrone MA. Vascular endothelium. In: Fuster V, Ross R, Topol EJ, eds. *Atherosclerosis and coronary artery disease*. Philadelphia: Lippincott-Raven Publishers, 1996.
Furchgott RF, Zawadcki JV. The obligatory role of endothelial cells in the

relaxation of arterial smooth muscle acetylcholine. *Nature* 1980;288: 373–379.
Nabel EG, Plautz G, Nabel J. Site-specific gene expression in vivo by direct gene transfer into the arterial wall. *Science* 1990;249:1285–1288.
Owens GK. Role of alterations in the differentiated state of vascular smooth muscle cells in atherogenesis. In: Fuster V, Ross R, Topol EJ, eds. *Atherosclerosis and coronary artery disease*. Philadelphia: Lippincott-Raven Publishers, 1996.
Ross R. The pathogenesis of atherosclerosis: a perspective for the 1990s. *Nature* 1993;362:801.

Kelley's Textbook of Internal Medicine, fourth edition. Edited by H. David Humes. Lippincott Williams & Wilkins, Philadelphia © 2000.

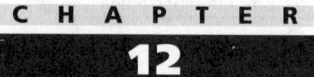

C H A P T E R

12

DISORDERS OF LIPID METABOLISM

DANIEL J. RADER

Lipoproteins are macromolecular complexes that transport nonpolar lipids (primarily triglycerides, cholesteryl esters, and fat-soluble vitamins) through body fluids (lymph, plasma, and interstitial fluid) to tissues that require them for normal metabolic function and from tissues that cannot catabolize them. Therefore, lipoproteins are important for the absorption of dietary cholesterol, long-chain fatty acids, and fat-soluble vitamins; the transport of triglycerides, cholesterol, and vitamin E from the liver to peripheral tissues; and the transport of cholesterol from peripheral tissues to the liver, where it is secreted into bile, converted to bile acids, or recycled into lipoproteins.

LIPOPROTEIN STRUCTURE AND METABOLISM

The general structure of lipoproteins is illustrated in Figure 12.1. Lipoproteins are discoidal or spherical particles that contain a core of nonpolar lipids (triglycerides and cholesteryl esters) sur-

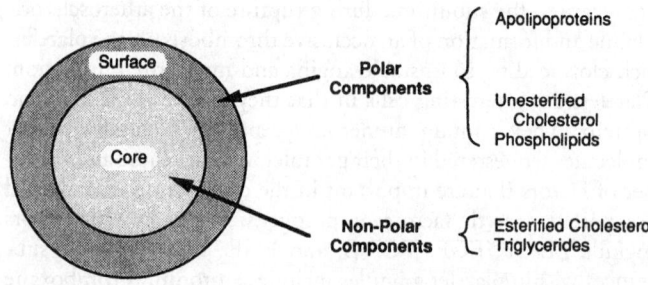

FIGURE 12.1. General structure of a lipoprotein.

TABLE 12.1. CHARACTERISTICS OF THE MAJOR LIPOPROTEINS

Lipoprotein	Density Range (g/mL)	Particle Size (nm)	Electrophoretic Mobility	Major Apolipoprotein
Chylomicrons	0.930	75–1,200	Origin	ApoB-48
Chylomicron remnants	0.930–1.006	30–80	Slow pre-β	ApoB-48
VLDL	0.930–1.006	30–80	Pre-β	ApoB-100
IDL	1.0006–1.019	25–35	Slow pre-β	ApoB-100
LDL	1.019–1.063	18–25	β	ApoB-100
HDL$_2$	1.063–1.125	9–12	α	ApoA-I
HDL$_3$	1.125–1.210	5–9	α	ApoA-I
Lp(a)	1.050–1.120	25	Pre-β	Apo(a)

VLDL, very low density lipoprotein; IDL, intermediate-density lipoprotein; LDL, low-density lipoprotein; HDL, high-density lipoprotein; Lp (a), lipoprotein (a).

rounded by polar components (phospholipids, unesterified cholesterol, and proteins) that interact with body fluids. The plasma lipoproteins are divided into five major families (Table 12.1): chylomicrons, very low density lipoproteins (VLDLs), intermediate-density lipoproteins (IDLs), low-density lipoproteins (LDLs), and high-density lipoproteins (HDLs). Each family contains a spectrum of particles differentiated from one another by their apolipoprotein composition or by certain physicochemical properties such as their density, size, or migration during electrophoresis. The density of a lipoprotein is determined by the ratio of lipid (less dense) to protein (more dense) in the particle. As the lipid content in a lipoprotein decreases relative to protein, the density increases. Chylomicrons and VLDLs are the largest and least dense lipoproteins and contain the greatest amount of lipid per protein. In contrast, HDL particles are the smallest and densest lipoproteins and contain the least amount of lipid per protein.

The proteins of lipoproteins, called apolipoproteins (Table 12.2), are required for important metabolic functions: the assembly and structural integrity of lipoproteins, the activation of enzymes important in lipoprotein metabolism, and the interaction of lipoproteins with cell surface receptors that promote the cellular uptake of lipoproteins. Certain apolipoproteins are markers for specific families of lipoproteins. For example, there are two forms of apolipoprotein B—apoB-48 and apoB-100 (Fig. 12.2)—both derived from the same gene on chromosome 2. In the liver, the full-length apoB mRNA is translated to produce apoB-100, which is found in lipoproteins derived from the liver (VLDLs, IDLs, LDLs). However, in the intestine, the apoB mRNA is "edited" by a complex that introduces a stop codon sequence slightly before the midpoint of the coding sequence, resulting in the synthesis of a smaller protein (apoB-48), which is then found in lipoproteins derived from the intestine (chylomicrons). Apolipoprotein A-I, which is made in both liver and

TABLE 12.2. CHARACTERISTICS OF THE MAJOR APOLIPOPROTEINS

Apolipoprotein	Primary Tissue Source	Lipoprotein Distribution	Physiologic Functions
ApoA-I	Intestine, liver	HDL	Structural protein for HDL / Activator of LCAT
ApoA-II	Liver	HDL	Unknown
ApoA-IV	Intestine	HDL, chylomicrons	Unknown
ApoB-48	Intestine	Chylomicrons	Chylomicron synthesis and secretion
ApoB-100	Liver	VLDL, IDL, LDL, Lp(a)	VLDL synthesis and secretion / Ligand for binding to LDL receptor
ApoC-I	Liver	Chylomicrons, VLDL, HDL	Unknown
ApoC-II	Liver	Chylomicrons, VLDL, HDL	Cofactor for LPL
ApoC-III	Liver	Chylomicrons, VLDL, HDL	Inhibitor of lipoprotein binding to receptors
ApoE	Liver	Chylomicron remnants, VLDL, IDL, HDL	Ligand for binding to LDL receptor and LRP
Apo(a)	Liver	Lp(a)	Unknown

HDL, high-density lipoprotein; VLDL, very low density lipoprotein; IDL, intermediate-density lipoprotein; Lp(a), lipoprotein (a); LRP, LDL receptor-related protein; LPL, lipoprotein lipase.

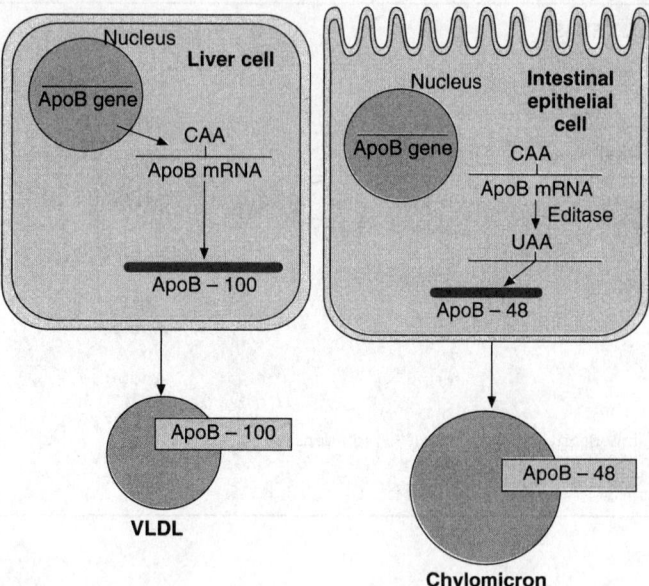

FIGURE 12.2. Synthesis of apoB-100 by the liver and apoB-48 by the intestine from the same gene. In the liver, the apoB mRNA is translated into full-length apoB-100 protein. In the intestine, a CAA codon in the apoB mRNA is edited to a UAA stop codon, resulting in the production of shorter apoB-48.

intestine, is found on virtually all HDL particles and serves as a marker for this lipoprotein family.

EXOGENOUS PATHWAY OF LIPOPROTEIN METABOLISM (FIG. 12.3)

Chylomicrons are synthesized in intestinal epithelial cells in response to the ingestion of dietary fat. The longer chain fatty acids (those with more than 12 to 14 carbons) are converted to triglyceride for incorporation into chylomicrons, whereas shorter chain fatty acids are absorbed directly into the portal circulation. Newly synthesized triglycerides and dietary cholesterol are combined with apoB-48 in a process that requires the microsomal transfer protein (Fig. 12.3). Chylomicrons are secreted into the intestinal lymph and enter the plasma, where they acquire apoC and apoE by exchange from other lipoproteins, especially HDLs. As chylomicrons enter capillaries, they attach to the enzyme lipoprotein lipase (LPL), which is anchored to capillary endothelial cells via proteoglycans (Fig. 12.3). Lipoprotein lipase is activated by apoC-II on the chylomicron surface to hydrolyze the core triglyceride to free fatty acids, which are taken into tissues for oxidation (e.g., muscle) or storage for future use (e.g., adipose tissue). Some of the free fatty acids bind to plasma albumin and are returned to the liver for oxidation or reesterification to triglyceride.

After much of the chylomicron triglyceride core is hydrolyzed, the particle dissociates from LPL as a chylomicron remnant. These remnants are depleted of triglyceride and apoC but retain apoB-48, apoE, and most of the dietary cholesterol. The remnant particles are rapidly removed from the circulation by the liver through the binding of apoE on the remnant particle surface to heparan sulfate proteoglycans and subsequently the LDL receptor or the LDL receptor–related protein (LRP) (Fig. 12.3).

ENDOGENOUS PATHWAY OF LIPOPROTEIN METABOLISM (FIG. 12.4)

Very low density lipoproteins are triglyceride-rich lipoproteins that are smaller and more dense than chylomicrons and are pro-

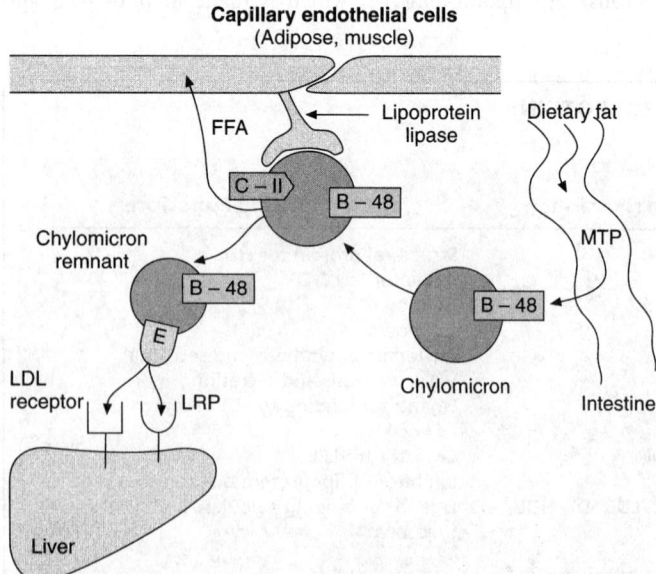

FIGURE 12.3. Exogenous pathway of lipoprotein metabolism. B-48, apoB-48; C-II, apoC-II; E, apoE; FFA, free fatty acids; LRP, LDL receptor–related protein; MTP, microsomal transfer protein.

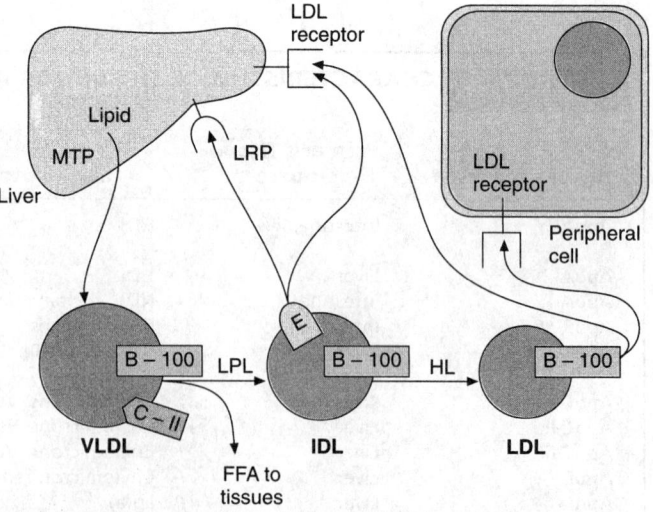

FIGURE 12.4. Endogenous pathway of lipoprotein metabolism. B-100, apoB-100; C-II, apoC-II; E, apoE FFA, free fatty acids; HL, hepatic lipase; LPL, lipoprotein lipase; LRP, LDL receptor–related protein; MTP, microsomal transfer protein.

duced by hepatic parenchymal cells. Hepatic triglycerides and cholesterol are combined with apoB-100 within the endoplasmic reticulum in a process that also requires the microsomal transfer protein (Fig. 12.4). Vitamin E is also packaged into the assembling VLDL particle by a protein known as the tocopherol-binding protein. After secretion into the plasma, VLDLs acquire apoC and apoE by transfer from other lipoproteins, especially HDLs. Like chylomicrons, VLDL triglycerides are hydrolyzed by capillary LPL, especially in muscle and adipose tissue. When VLDL remnants dissociate from LPL, they are called IDLs. The IDL particles may be taken up by receptors on the liver or they may be converted further to LDL (Fig. 12.4). Apolipoprotein E mediates the hepatic uptake of IDL via either the LDL receptor or LR. The IDL particles not catabolized by this route are converted to LDL by a process that involves hepatic lipase (Fig. 12.4).

Low-density lipoproteins are cholesterol-rich lipoproteins that supply cholesterol and vitamin E to cells. The LDL receptors are found in most tissues throughout the body, and apoB-100 serves as the recognition site for binding to the LDL receptor. Approximately 70% to 80% of total clearance of LDL from the plasma is by the liver. Therefore, the amount of LDL receptors expressed by the liver is an important factor in the regulation of plasma levels of LDL.

Knowledge of the normal lipoprotein metabolism allows prediction of the consequences of molecular defects in apolipoproteins, lipolytic enzymes, and lipoprotein receptors. For example, patients with a genetic deficiency of LPL or apoC-II cannot hydolyze triglycerides and therefore have elevated chylomicrons and VLDLs. In contrast, patients with abnormal forms of apoE

cannot clear remnant lipoproteins efficiently and accumulate them in the plasma. Finally, patients with defects in the LDL receptor or in apoB-100 that affect its binding to the LDL receptor have delayed clearance of LDL from the blood and therefore have hypercholesterolemia due to high levels of LDL.

HIGH-DENSITY LIPOPROTEIN METABOLISM (FIG. 12.5)

High-density lipoproteins are believed to participate in a process termed "reverse cholesterol transport" in which excess peripheral cholesterol is acquired by HDLs and returned to the liver for excretion into the bile (Fig. 12.5). Apolipoprotein A-I, the major HDL apolipoprotein, is synthesized by both the intestine and the liver. Nascent HDLs are thought to be discoidal particles that acquire unesterified cholesterol from peripheral tissues, a process facilitated by a cellular protein called ATP-binding cassette protein 1 (ABC1). Unesterified cholesterol is esterified on HDLs by the enzyme lecithin:cholesterol acyltransferase (LCAT), a plasma enzyme associated with HDLs. As nascent HDLs generate more cholesteryl ester, they evolve into spherical particles, which enlarge further as they acquire additional lipid and protein constituents from chylomicrons and VLDLs when the triglyceride core of these lipoproteins is hydrolyzed. The HDL cholesteryl esters can be transferred to the liver through at least two pathways. First, HDL cholesteryl esters can be transferred to apoB-containing lipoproteins in exchange for triglyceride through the action of cholesteryl ester transfer protein (CETP). Some of these apoB-containing lipoproteins are then removed from the plasma by the liver via the LDL receptor or

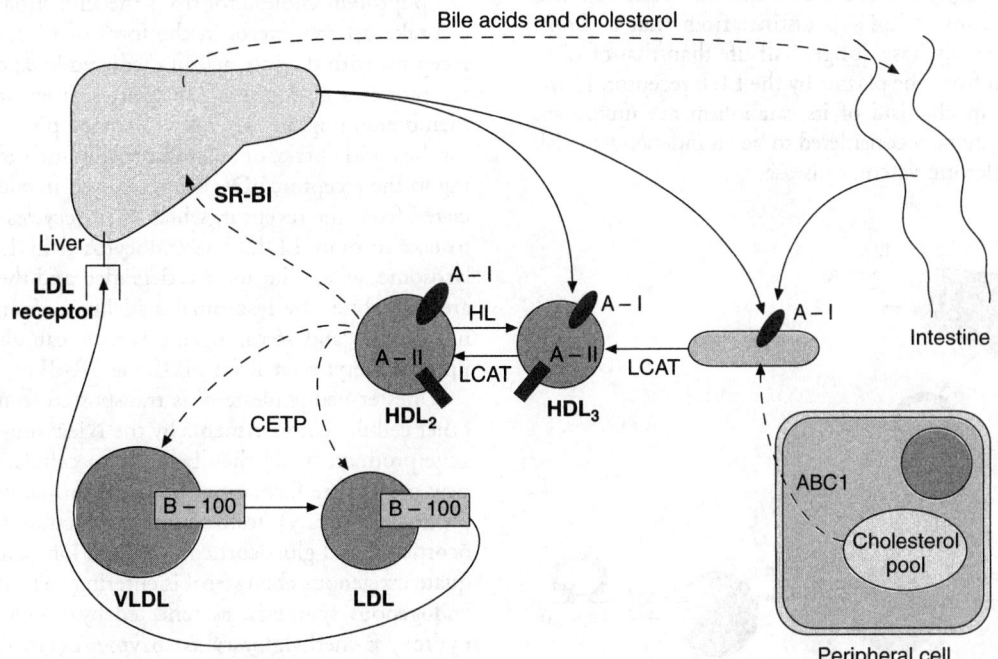

FIGURE 12.5. Pathways of HDL metabolism. Solid lines trace the conversion of lipoprotein particles. Broken lines trace the transfer of free cholesterol or cholesteryl ester between different lipoprotein classes or between lipoprotein and cells. ABC1, ATP-binding cassette protein 1; CETP, cholesteryl ester transfer protein; HL, hepatic lipase; LCAT, lecithin:cholesterol acyltransferase; SR-BI, scavenger receptor class BI.

LRP. Triglyceride-enriched HDL is a substrate for hepatic lipase, which hydrolyzes HDL triglycerides and phospholipids and generates smaller HDL particles. Second, HDL cholesteryl esters can be taken up directly by the liver in a process termed selective cholesterol uptake. This process is mediated by scavenger receptor class BI (SR-BI), a cell surface receptor that facilitates uptake of HDL cholesteryl ester but not of the entire lipoprotein particle. Thus, the metabolism of HDL cholesteryl ester and HDL apoA-I are dissociated. Eventually, apoA-I is removed from the circulation by a process that is not well understood but involves both the kidneys and the liver.

ApoA-II is the second most abundant HDL apolipoprotein. Unlike apoA-I, apoA-II synthesized only by the liver, not by the intestine. Apolipoprotein A-II is found on approximately two-thirds of all HDL particles. This results in two major classes of HDL particles: one containing apoA-I and apoA-II and the other containing apoA-I without apoA-II. These two classes of HDL particles may have different physiologic roles and metabolic pathways, but their significance for human pathophysiology is uncertain.

LIPOPROTEIN(A) (FIG. 12.6)

Lipoprotein(a), or Lp(a), is another lipoprotein found to a variable extent in human plasma. It is related in structure to LDL in that it contains apoB-100 and a core of cholesteryl ester. Lipoprotein(a) is distinguished structurally from LDL by the presence of a unique protein, apolipoprotein(a) [apo(a)], which is linked by a single disulfide bond to the apoB. Apolipoprotein(a) bears a strong resemblance to plasminogen and varies substantially in its molecular weight among different persons. It is synthesized by the liver, and the association of apo(a) with apoB may occur after apo(a) is secreted into the plasma. Once intact, the metabolism of Lp(a) is distinct from that of LDL. Lipoprotein(a) generally has a longer half-life than that of LDL and is not removed from the plasma by the LDL receptor. However, the site and mechanism of its catabolism are unknown. Lipoprotein(a) is generally considered to be an independent risk factor for atherosclerotic vascular disease.

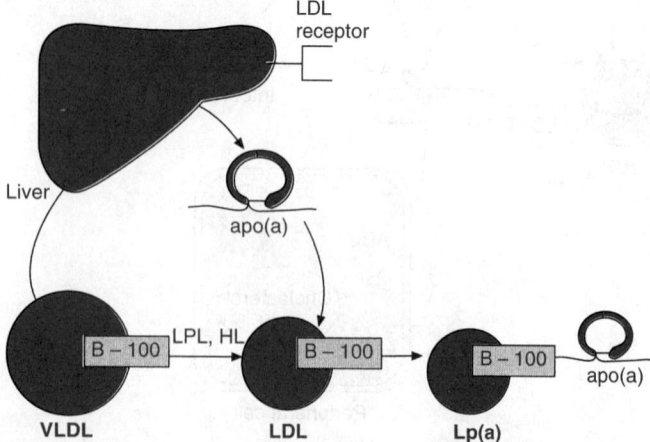

FIGURE 12.6. Pathways of lipoprotein(a) metabolism. Apolipoprotein(a) is secreted by the hepatocyte independently of LDL and subsequently binds to LDL or a precursor to form Lp(a). HL, hepatic lipase; LPL, lipoprotein lipase.

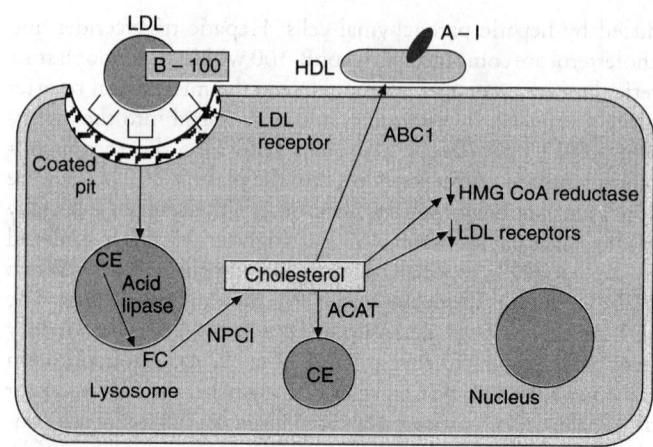

FIGURE 12.7. Intracellular cholesterol metabolism. Low-density lipoprotein (LDL) is targeted to lysosomes by the LDL receptor and LDL cholesteryl esters are hydrolyzed to free cholesterol by the lysosomal acid lipase. The Niemann–Pick C gene 1 is required for transfer of lysosomal free cholesterol to the cytoplasmic pool. Free cholesterol can then be esterified to cholesteryl esters by acyl coenzyme A:cholesterol acyltransferase and stored as lipid droplets or be released to acceptor particles such as HDL. Free cholesterol within the cell down-regulates the expression of genes such as β-hydroxy-β-methylglutaryl-coenzyme A reductase and the LDL receptor. ACAT, acyl coenzyme A:cholesterol acyltransferase; CE, cholesteryl ester; FC, free cholesterol; NPC1, Niemann–Pick C gene 1.

INTRACELLULAR CHOLESTEROL METABOLISM (FIG. 12.7)

Cells require cholesterol for normal function, and they obtain it from two sources: biosynthesis from acetyl CoA and uptake of lipoprotein cholesterol from the interstitial fluid. Most cells can take up cholesterol in the form of LDL through the LDL receptor, with the interaction mediated by apoB-100. The LDL receptor is a glycoprotein that, after insertion into the plasma membrane, migrates laterally to coated pits, regions specialized for the rapid uptake of macromolecules such as LDL. After binding to the receptor, LDL is internalized in endosome and dissociated from the receptor, which then recycles to the cell surface to take in more LDL. The endocytosed LDL is targeted to the lysosome, where the apoB is degraded and the cholesteryl esters are hydrolyzed by lysosomal acid lipase. Some cells, especially hepatocytes and steroidogenic tissues, can also selectively take up cholesteryl ester from HDL via SR-BI.

Unesterified cholesterol is transported from the lysosome to other cellular compartments by the Niemann–Pick C1 (NPC1) gene product. It can then be used for cellular functions such as new membrane formation, bile acid formation (liver), estrogen production (ovary), testosterone production (testis), or mineralocorticoid and glucocorticoid production (adrenal). When adequate exogenous cholesterol is entering cells, they suppress their endogenous synthesis, as reflected by decreased activity of β-hydroxy-β-methylglutaryl coenzyme A (HMG-CoA) reductase, the rate-limiting enzyme in cholesterol biosynthesis. Cells also decrease the number of LDL receptors and increase the activity of acyl coenzyme A:cholesterol acyltransferase (ACAT) to esterify any excess cholesterol for storage as cholesteryl ester droplets.

Cells must also be able to release excess cholesterol, as they lack the enzymes to catabolize the sterol nucleus. The process of cholesterol removal from cells is not completely understood. Spontaneous desorption of unesterified cholesterol from the plasma membrane occurs and is enhanced by the presence of an acceptor of cholesterol, such as HDL. The ATP-binding cassette protein 1 (ABC1) provides a mechanism for the active facilitation of cholesterol removal from cells. High-density lipoprotein has many characteristics consistent with an acceptor particle and probably plays an important role in the efficient removal of excess cholesterol from cells.

DISORDERS OF LIPOPROTEIN METABOLISM

Disorders of lipoprotein metabolism are associated with various clinical features, the most prominent of which are pancreatitis, atherosclerosis, and xanthoma formation. These disorders are usually identified by measuring plasma triglycerides, total cholesterol, and HDL cholesterol after a 12- to 14-hour fast. In the fasting state, chylomicrons are not usually present except in pathologic conditions, and most of the triglycerides are found in VLDL. Because chylomicrons are normally not present in the fasting state, the total cholesterol level is generally equal to the sum of the cholesterol in VLDL, LDL, and HDL. Usually, the cholesterol content of VLDL is about equal to the fasting plasma triglyceride level divided by 5, provided the plasma triglyceride level does not exceed 400 mg per dL. Therefore, the plasma LDL cholesterol level is usually determined by the formula:

$$\text{LDL cholesterol} = \text{total cholesterol} - (\text{triglyceride} \div 5) - \text{HDL cholesterol}$$

This simple calculation usually permits the clinician to estimate the LDL cholesterol level accurately enough. The LDL cholesterol can also be measured directly, and use of these assays is becoming more commonplace in clinical laboratories.

Disorders of lipid metabolism include any disorder that causes substantially elevated or decreased levels of any of the major plasma lipoproteins; such a disorder is often referred to as a dyslipidemia. The term *hyperlipidemia* (or *hyperlipoproteinemia*) is applied when the plasma triglyceride or cholesterol level is increased. The definition of dyslipidemia or hyperlipidemia is based on statistical cutoff points derived from the distribution of lipid and lipoprotein levels found in the general population. These cutoff points are arbitrary, but dyslipidemia is considered to be present when plasma lipid or lipoprotein levels exceed the 90th percentile or fall below the 10th percentile for age and gender. Selected reference values for fasting lipid and lipoprotein levels in adults are listed in Table 12.3.

The statistical norms for LDL cholesterol levels are not considered desirable because significant cardiovascular risk occurs at LDL cholesterol levels considerably lower than the 90th percentile cutoff. The relation of lipid and lipoprotein levels to cardiovascular risk is discussed in Chapter 31.

Dyslipidemia is caused by various disorders, either primary (inherited) or secondary to some other disease process. Lipoprotein disorders have been classified in various ways, but no one system is ideal. A classification based on the type of lipoprotein that is elevated (lipoprotein phenotypes; Table 12.4.) has been used for years but has several shortcomings: the phenotype in a patient may change over time; a phenotype may be primary (genetic) or secondary; a single phenotype may be caused by different genetic defects; and a single genetic defect may be associated with multiple phenotypes.

In this chapter, the lipoprotein disorders are grouped as primary or secondary. The primary disorders are subdivided by the primary lipoprotein that is affected, then further subdivided by the specific gene responsible for the disorder (when known). Some of these disorders cause elevated lipoprotein levels; others cause abnormally low levels of specific lipoproteins.

PRIMARY HYPERLIPOPROTEINEMIAS DUE TO KNOWN SINGLE-GENE DISORDERS

FAMILIAL CHYLOMICRONEMIA SYNDROMES (LIPOPROTEIN LIPASE DEFICIENCY AND APOLIPOPROTEIN C-II DEFICIENCY)

Definition

Familial chylomicronemia syndromes (Table 12.5) are characterized by markedly elevated levels of chylomicrons in fasting plasma. The major clinical features are eruptive xanthomas and recurrent episodes of pancreatitis. These are autosomal recessive disorders caused by mutations in either LPL or its essential cofactor apoC-II.

Incidence and Epidemiology

Familial chylomicronemia syndromes are relatively rare. Lipoprotein lipase deficiency is much more common than apoC-II deficiency. These conditions are found worldwide and are generally diagnosed in childhood.

Etiologic Factors

These are autosomal recessive disorders caused by mutations in either LPL or its essential co-factor apoC-II.

Pathogenesis

The hydrolysis of triglycerides in chylomicrons and VLDL in vivo requires the action of LPL in tissue capillary beds (Figs. 12.3 and 12.4.). Due to mutations in the LPL gene, patients with LPL deficiency cannot produce LPL in their tissues. Lipoprotein lipase requires the presence of the cofactor apoC-II on the lipoprotein for activation (Figs. 12.3. and 12.4.) and therefore deficiency of apoC-II closely resembles LPL deficiency. In both conditions, patients cannot hydrolyze chylomicron triglycerides and therefore develop marked hyperchylomicronemia.

Clinical Findings

Patients with LPL deficiency and apoC-II deficiency usually present in infancy or childhood with recurrent abdominal pain,

TABLE 12.3. SELECTED REFERENCE VALUES FOR FASTING LIPID AND LIPOPROTEIN LEVELS IN ADULTS STRATIFIED BY GENDER, RACE, AND AGE

Age (y)	Total Cholesterol Mean	Total Cholesterol 90th %tile	LDL Cholesterol Mean	LDL Cholesterol 90th %tile	HDL Cholesterol Mean	HDL Cholesterol 10th %tile	HDL Cholesterol 90th %tile	Triglycerides Mean	Triglycerides 90th %tile
Men									
ALL RACES									
20–39	189	244	123	172	47	33	63	119	210
40–59	216	265	140	186	46	29	65	176	309
>60	215	270	137	183	46	30	63	160	263
WHITE									
20–39	193	244	124	172	46	33	61	121	212
40–59	216	265	141	186	45	29	63	184	313
>60	215	270	137	182	45	30	62	162	264
BLACK									
20–39	187	235	117	170	54	36	74	96	163
40–59	210	273	134	204	53	34	76	120	203
>60	214	273	140	195	52	33	72	124	211
Women									
ALL RACES									
20–39	186	232	111	154	55	37	74	106	190
40–59	214	275	131	177	56	38	76	129	221
>60	234	290	147	192	56	37	77	163	264
WHITE									
20–39	186	232	111	152	54	36	73	110	196
40–59	216	277	132	178	56	38	76	133	234
>60	234	290	146	192	56	37	77	164	266
BLACK									
20–39	186	229	113	152	58	40	77	83	131
40–59	212	269	131	176	56	38	76	107	182
>60	233	290	157	210	59	39	84	121	196

(Data from the Third National and Nutrition Examination Survey (NHANES III) 1988–91. Sempos et al. *JAMA* 1993:269:3009)

TABLE 12.4. DEFINITION AND CHARACTERISTICS OF PLASMA LIPOPROTEIN PHENOTYPES

	I	IIa	IIb	III	IV	V
Lipoprotein elevation	Chylomicrons	LDL	LDL, VLDL	Chylomicron and VLDL remnants	VLDL	Chylomicrons and VLDL
Plasma triglycerides	+++	N	+	+	+	+++
Plasma cholesterol	++	++	+	+	N to +	++
Appearance of plasma	Lactescent	Clear	Clear	Turbid	Turbid	Lactescent
Associated xanthomas	Eruptive	Tendon and tuberous	None	Palmar and tuberoeruptive	None	Eruptive
Pancreatitis potential	+++	0	0	0	0	+++
Atherogenic potential	0	+++	+++	++	±	±
Primary molecular defects	Lipoprotein lipase and ApoC-II	LDL receptor and ApoB-100	Unknown	ApoE	Unknown	Unknown

LDL, low-density lipoprotein; VLDL, very low density lipoprotein.

TABLE 12.5.	**PRIMARY HYPERLIPOPROTEINEMIAS CAUSED BY SINGLE-GENE MUTATIONS**					

Genetic Disorder	Molecular Defect	Lipoproteins Elevated	Lipoprotein Phenotype	Clinical Findings	Genetic Transmission	Estimated Incidence
Familial lipoprotein lipase deficiency	LPL deficiency	Chylomicrons	I	Eruptive xanthomas, hepatosplenomegaly, pancreatitis	Autosomal recessive	Rare
Familial apolipoprotein C-II deficiency	ApoC-II deficiency	Chylomicrons	I	Eruptive xanthomas, hepatosplenomegaly, pancreatitis	Autosomal recessive	Rare
Familial dysbetalipoproteinemia	Abnormal apoE (i.e., apoE-2/2)	Chylomicron and VLDL remnants	III	Palmar and tuberoeruptive xanthomas, premature atherosclerosis	Autosomal recessive or autosomal codominant	1/10,000
Familial hepatic lipase deficiency	Hepatic lipase deficiency	VLDL remnants	III	Premature atherosclerosis	Autosomal recessive	Rare
Familial hypercholesterolemia	LDL-receptor deficiency	LDL	IIa	Tendon xanthomas, premature atherosclerosis	Autosomal codominant	1/500
Familial defective apoB-100	Abnormal apoB-100 (i.e., $Arg_{3500} \rightarrow Gln$)	LDL	IIa	Tendon xanthomas, premature atherosclerosis	Autosomal codominant	1/600
Familial hypertriglyceridemia	Unknown	VLDL, occasionally chylomicrons	IV, occasionally V	Usually none	Autosomal dominant	1/500
Familial combined hyperlipidemia	Unknown	VLDL and LDL	IIb, sometimes IIa or IV, rarely V	Premature atherosclerosis	Autosomal dominant	1/200

LPL, lipoprotein lipase; LDL, low-density lipoprotein; VLDL, very low density lipoprotein.

acute pancreatitis, or eruptive xanthomas. The cause of the pancreatitis is not well understood but is clearly secondary to the marked hyperchylomicronemia. Eruptive xanthomas are small papular lesions that occur in showers on the buttocks and back. Lipemia retinalis, a pale appearance to the retinal veins, is due to the lactescent plasma. Patients often have hepatosplenomegaly due to ingestion of chylomicrons by the reticuloendothelial system. Premature atherosclerosis is not a feature of this disease despite the high levels of cholesterol, probably because chylomicrons are too large to enter the arterial intima.

Laboratory Findings

Patients have severe hyperlipidemia from birth. The hyperchylomicronemia produces lactescent plasma, and after overnight refrigeration of plasma the chylomicrons rise to form an easily visible cake. Triglyceride levels are virtually always above 1,000 mg per dL and may reach 10,000 mg per dL or greater. Because chylomicrons contain cholesterol, total cholesterol levels are also extremely elevated and in severe hyperchylomicronemia can approach 1,000 mg per dL. The severe hypertriglyceridemia can render some other laboratory tests inaccurate. Amylase levels during bouts of pancreatitis may be low due to interference with the enzyme assay. Because chylomicrons displace water volume in plasma, other plasma components may be measured as artifac-

tually low. For example, serum sodium levels are artifactually decreased by 2 to 4 mmol per L for each 1,000 mg per dL of plasma triglyceride (pseudohyponatremia). The diagnosis is strongly suggested by the presence of turbidity in the plasma obtained from a child after a 12-hour fast. Triglyceride levels are almost always above 1,000 mg/dL, unless the child has been on a very low fat diet. Lipoprotein electrophoresis demonstrates markedly elevated chylomicrons at the origin. The diagnosis can be confirmed at special centers by the quantitation of LPL in the plasma after intravenous heparin injection (postheparin lipolytic activity). Heparin releases LPL from its capillary endothelial proteoglycan binding sites into the plasma. Patients with familial LPL deficiency have little or no active LPL present in the plasma after heparin injection. If post-heparin LPL activity is normal, the diagnosis of apoC-II deficiency requires a specific immunoassay or two-dimensional gel electrophoresis or plasma.

Optimal Management

Patients with suspected familial hyperchylomicronemia syndrome should be referred to a specialized center for diagnosis and appropriate therapy. The mainstay of therapy for both LPL deficiency and apoC-II deficiency is restriction of total dietary fat. Caloric supplementation with medium-chain triglycerides, which are absorbed directly into the portal vein and therefore do not promote chylomicron formation, is often useful. If dietary fat restriction alone is unsuccessful, some patients may respond to a cautious trial of fish oils. During an attack of severe pancreatitis in a patient with apoC-II deficiency, infusion of fresh-frozen plasma may provide adequate apoC-II to activate the endogenous LPL and improve the hypertriglyceridemia. Plasma exchange could be considered as an acute therapy for a patient with LPL deficiency with severe pancreatitis.

FAMILIAL DYSBETALIPOPROTEINEMIA (TYPE III HYPERLIPOPROTEINEMIA)

Definition

Familial dysbetalipoproteinemia (also known as type III hyperlipoproteinemia and familial broad β disease) is characterized by the accumulation of chylomicron and VLDL remnants in fasting plasma due to mutations in apolipoprotein E, the major ligand for clearance of lipoprotein remnant particles.

Incidence and Epidemiology

Familial dysbetalipoproteinemia occurs in approximately 1 in 10,000 persons and is found worldwide. It is generally diagnosed in adulthood.

Etiologic Factors

Familial dysbetalipoproteinemia is caused by mutations in apoE that impair its ability to bind to lipoprotein receptors. The most common form is autosomal recessive due to homozygosity for the apoE2 allele and has variable penetrance. However, a less common form is autosomal dominant or codominant with a high degree of penetrance and expression of the dyslipidemia in the heterozygous state.

Pathogenesis

The efficient removal of chylomicron and VLDL remnants from the plasma in vivo requires apoE, which binds to both the remnant receptor and the LDL receptor (Figs. 12.3 and 12.4). The most common form of familial dysbetalipoproteinemia, which is autosomal recessive, is related to a common polymorphism of apoE. Three common alleles have been described at the apoE genetic locus: E2, E3, and E4. Allele E3 is the most common, but in North America the E2 allele occurs in approximately 12% and the E4 allele in approximately 25% of persons. The E4 allele is associated with increased LDL cholesterol levels in most populations, and it is also associated independently with premature atherosclerosis and with Alzheimer's disease. In contrast to apoE4, heterozygosity for the E2 allele is associated with lower than average cholesterol and LDL cholesterol levels. However, homozygosity for the E2 allele (the E2/E2 genotype), which has an incidence of about 1 in 200 in North America, is associated with familial dysbetalipoproteinemia. Persons with the E2/E2 genotype develop familial dysbetalipoproteinemia if an additional predisposing factor is also present; some of these factors are obesity, diabetes mellitus, hypothyroidism, renal disease, and

alcohol use, but many patients with familial dysbetalipoproteinemia do not have an obvious predisposing factor in addition to the E2/E2 genotype. The apoE2 protein does not bind adequately to the remnant and LDL receptors, resulting in a defect in the catabolism of chylomicron and VLDL remnants.

The autosomal dominant forms of familial dysbetalipoproteinemia are caused by less common mutations in the apoE gene. These mutations generally result in the synthesis of an apoE protein that is severely defective in its ability to bind to the remnant and LDL receptors, even to the degree that it interferes with the ability of the normal apoE3 from the other allele to bind to the receptors. As a result, patients with "dominant" familial dysbetalipoproteinemia generally do not require other factors for expression of the disease, and often multiple members of a family are affected. Several different mutations in the apoE gene, all in the region of the protein that binds to the receptors, have been described in kindreds with the dominant form of the disease. Finally, several families have been described with complete deficiency of apoE, which causes a severe form of familial dysbetalipoproteinemia.

Clinical Findings

Patients with familial dysbetalipoproteinemia usually present in adulthood, although the dominant form of the disease can present in childhood or adolescence. Patients present with distinctive xanthomas, premature atherosclerosis, or asymptomatic hyperlipidemia. Two forms of xanthomas are observed in this disease and can provide important clues to the diagnosis. Tuberoeruptive xanthomas begin as small papules at pressure points such as elbows, knees, and buttocks, and are yellowish lesions that can grow to several centimeters if the hyperlipidemia is not treated. Palmar xanthomas begin as an orange–yellow discoloration to the creases of the palms and wrists. If the condition goes untreated, small nodules several millimeters in length can develop on the fingers or palms. Premature atherosclerosis is often seen in this disorder and can involve any of the major arterial beds. Compared with other lipid disorders, peripheral vascular disease is particularly common in patients with familial dysbetalipoproteinemia.

Laboratory Findings

Patients have hypertriglyceridemia and hypercholesterolemia, often to relatively similar degrees. Hyperlipidemia can be relatively mild or severe, depending on the presence of other associated metabolic abnormalities. The diagnosis is suggested by the presence of one or both of the characteristic xanthomas or by substantial elevation in both triglyceride and cholesterol levels in relatively similar proportion. In contrast to other conditions associated with elevated triglycerides, HDL cholesterol levels are usually normal in patients with familial dysbetalipoproteinemia. Lipoprotein electrophoresis demonstrates a prominent broad β band due to the presence of remnant lipoproteins. The diagnosis can be supported at special centers by lipoprotein ultracentrifugation demonstrating a ratio of VLDL cholesterol to plasma triglyceride greater than 0.3 (suggesting cholesterol-enriched VLDL particles). The diagnosis is confirmed by documenting the apoE2/E2 phenotype (using isoelectric focusing of plasma) or the apoE2/E2 genotype (using molecular methods). However, because mutations in apoE other than E2 can cause familial dysbetalipoproteinemia, the absence of an E2/E2 pattern does not rule out the diagnosis, which must then be made on clinical grounds.

Optimal Management

A thorough search for other metabolic conditions known to exacerbate hyperlipidemia should be made. General therapeutic measures include diet, weight loss, and discontinuance of alcohol. Postmenopausal women with familial dysbetalipoproteinemia respond favorably to estrogen replacement therapy. Because this disorder is associated with increased cardiovascular risk, drug therapy should be utilized if necessary. Fibric acid derivatives (such as gemfibrozil and fenofibrate) and nicotinic acid are effective in treating this disorder. The HMG-CoA reductase inhibitors have also been used successfully in some patients.

HEPATIC LIPASE DEFICIENCY

Definition

Hepatic lipase deficiency is a rare autosomal recessive disorder characterized by the absence of hepatic lipase activity and the accumulation of lipoprotein remnants in plasma.

Incidence and Epidemiology

Only several kindreds with hepatic lipase deficiency have been described, although because this syndrome can be difficult to recognize it may be more common than currently appreciated.

Etiologic Factors

This disorder is caused by mutations in the hepatic lipase gene.

Pathogenesis

Hepatic lipase is responsible for converting VLDL remnants and IDL to LDL by hydrolysis of triglycerides and phospholipids (Fig. 12.4). Deficiency of hepatic lipase due to mutations in the gene results in a defect in the metabolism of VLDL remnants and IDL, and their subsequent accumulation in the plasma.

Clinical Findings

Patients with hepatic lipase deficiency may present with premature atherosclerosis or asymptomatic hyperlipidemia. Xanthomas are not a consistent feature of this disorder.

Laboratory Findings

Patients have both hypertriglyceridemia and hypercholesterolemia. However, in contrast with most hyperlipidemic patients, HDL cholesterol levels are normal or even elevated—a clue to this diagnosis. The lipoprotein profile can resemble familial dys-

betalipoproteinemia. Lipoprotein electrophoresis demonstrates a broad β band, but the apoE genotype is not the apoE2/E2 pattern characteristic of familial dysbetalipoproteinemia. The diagnosis can be confirmed by measurement of hepatic lipase in postheparin plasma by specialized laboratories. Acquired (usually partial) deficiency in hepatic lipase can be seen in hypothyroidism, chronic renal insufficiency, and chronic liver disease.

Optimal Management

Secondary causes of hepatic lipase deficiency should be excluded. After dietary therapy, a trial of lipid-lowering drug therapy with fibrates, nicotinic acid, or a statin should be considered, but experience in this area is limited.

FAMILIAL HYPERCHOLESTEROLEMIA

Definition

Familial hypercholesterolemia is caused by mutations in the LDL receptor and characterized by elevated LDL cholesterol, tendon xanthomas, and an increased risk of premature atherosclerosis. Familial hypercholesterolemia is an autosomal codominant disorder: heterozygotes have elevated LDL cholesterol levels and increased risk of atherosclerosis as adults, whereas homozygotes have markedly elevated LDL cholesterol levels and develop atherosclerotic cardiovascular disease as children and adolescents.

Incidence and Epidemiology

Familial hypercholesterolemia is found worldwide and is exceptionally common in certain populations, such as Afrikaners, Christian Lebanese, and French Canadians, in which a founder effect is present. Heterozygous familial hypercholesterolemia occurs in about 1 in 500 persons worldwide. Homozygous familial hypercholesterolemia occurs with a frequency of about 1 in a million persons worldwide.

Etiologic Factors

Familial hypercholesterolemia (FH) is caused by mutations in the gene for the LDL receptor that prevent its appearance on the cell surface or impair its ability to bind and internalize LDL. Over 150 different LDL receptor mutations have been described in patients with familial hypercholesterolemia. Familial hypercholesterolemia heterozygotes inherit one normal and one mutant allele for the LDL receptor and therefore produce only about half the normal number of LDL receptors. Homozygotes have two mutant alleles at the LDL receptor locus and therefore produce little or no LDL receptor. Homozygous FH patients are often classified based on the amount of LDL receptor activity measured in their skin fibroblasts as "receptor-negative" (less than 2% of normal activity) or "receptor-defective" (2% to 25% of normal activity). Many apparent familial hypercholesterolemia homozygotes have actually inherited a different mutant allele from each parent and are more properly called compound heterozygotes.

Pathogenesis

The efficient removal of LDL from the plasma requires the LDL receptor (Fig. 12.4). The liver is quantitatively the most important tissue responsible for regulating levels of LDL cholesterol and does so in large part by regulating the expression of the LDL receptor. The elevated LDL cholesterol levels in familial hypercholesterolemia are directly due to the LDL receptor defect causing delayed removal of LDL from the blood as well as increased rates of LDL production in some patients. Elevated LDL cholesterol levels lead to accelerated deposition of cholesterol in the artery wall, cornea, tendons, and skin, producing the manifestations of premature atherosclerosis, corneal arcus, tendon xanthomas, and cutaneous xanthomas. The clinical heterogeneity among familial hypercholesterolemia patients is related at least in part to genetic heterogeneity of the LDL receptor gene mutations.

Clinical Findings

Patients with heterozygous familial hypercholesterolemia have hypercholesterolemia from birth but are often not detected until adulthood, usually due to complications of premature atherosclerosis, tendon xanthomas, or asymptomatic hypercholesterolemia on routine screening. Tendon xanthomas are a major feature of this disease and are found in various locations including the dorsum of the hands, elbows, knees, and especially the Achilles tendons. Arcus cornea is common but not specific for this disorder. Premature atherosclerosis is often seen in this disorder and can involve any of the major arterial beds, usually including the coronary arteries. The age of onset of cardiovascular disease is highly variable and in part depends on other coexisting risk factors. Family history is usually notable for hypercholesterolemia and/or premature cardiovascular disease on one side of the family.

Patients with receptor-negative homozygous familial hypercholesterolemia often present with cutaneous xanthomas as children. These occur in the web spaces between fingers and on the elbows, knees, heels, and buttocks. Patients with receptor-defective homozygous familial hypercholesterolemia often do not have cutaneous xanthomas but develop tuberous or tendon xanthomas on the elbows, knees, or Achilles tendons as older children or adolescents. Arcus cornea is virtually always present to some degree. Atherosclerosis is severe and affects the aortic root as well as all the major arterial beds. A systolic murmur consistent with aortic valvular or supravalvular stenosis is usually present. The coronary artery disease often first involves the coronary ostia. Homozygous familial hypercholesterolemia patients are often asymptomatic despite severe atherosclerotic disease, and when symptoms occur they are often atypical, such as exertional throat pain. Sudden death in the asymptomatic patient with homozygous familial hypercholesterolemia has been described. Survival of the untreated receptor-negative homozygous familial hypercholesterolemia patient into the third decade of life is unusual.

Laboratory Findings

In heterozygous familial hypercholesterolemia, total cholesterol levels are usually above 240 mg per dL and are often above 300 mg per dL, LDL cholesterol levels are generally greater than 190 mg per dL, triglycerides are usually normal, and HDL cholesterol levels are often modestly reduced. In homozygous familial hypercholesterolemia, total cholesterol levels are usually above 600 mg per dL and can be as high as about 1,200 mg per dL. The LDL cholesterol levels are elevated to a similar degree. Receptor-negative patients have higher cholesterol levels than receptor-defective patients. Triglycerides are generally normal. The diagnosis can be confirmed at specialized centers by obtaining a skin biopsy and performing an assay of the LDL receptor activity in skin fibroblasts or by sequencing or other molecular testing of the LDL receptor.

Optimal Management

The diagnosis of heterozygous familial hypercholesterolemia is strongly suggested by hypercholesterolemia above 350 mg per dL in the presence of normal triglyceride levels, but the diagnosis should also be entertained in patients with cholesterol levels above 240 mg per dL, especially if there is a family history of hypercholesterolemia or premature coronary disease. The metacarpophalangeal and Achilles tendons should be examined for the presence of tendon xanthomas, which strongly supports the diagnosis of familial hypercholesterolemia. Hypothyroidism and obstructive liver disease should be excluded as potential secondary causes of hypercholesterolemia. Most heterozygous familial hypercholesterolemia patients require lipid-lowering drug therapy, and statins are the drug class of choice for this disorder (Chapter 31). Many heterozygous familial hypercholesterolemia patients can achieve desired LDL cholesterol goals with statin therapy, but frequently combination drug therapy with the addition of a bile acid sequestrant or nicotinic acid is required. Rarely, heterozygous familial hypercholesterolemia patients cannot be adequately controlled on combination drug therapy or do not tolerate drug therapy. Ileal bypass surgery has been used in some familial hypercholesterolemia heterozygotes; however, it can produce bile salt–induced diarrhea and vitamin B_{12} deficiency, and therefore is not generally recommended. The current optimal approach to heterozygous familial hypercholesterolemia patients with refractory hypercholesterolemia or drug intolerance is LDL apheresis (Chapter 31).

Family screening of relatives, including children, is an important means for detecting other affected persons.

The finding of severe hypercholesterolemia (more than 600 mg per dL) with normal triglycerides in a child without obstructive liver disease strongly suggests homozygous familial hypercholesterolemia and cutaneous, tuberous, or tendon xanthomas support the diagnosis. Further supportive evidence of the diagnosis is derived from the testing of the biologic parents, both of whom have hypercholesterolemia if the diagnosis of homozygous familial hypercholesterolemia is correct. Patients with suspected homozygous familial hypercholesterolemia should be referred to a specialized center for diagnosis and therapy. Careful monitoring for the development of cardiovascular disease is important. A trial of drug therapy with statins is generally attempted and some patients, particularly those who are receptor-defective, may have a modest response. Optimal therapy is LDL apheresis, which can promote regression of xanthomas and retard progression of atherosclerosis. However, venous access is often problematic, especially in young children, and the optimal timing of initiation of LDL apheresis is uncertain. Homozygous familial hypercholesterolemia is a model for the development of liver-directed somatic gene therapy.

FAMILIAL DEFECTIVE APOLIPOPROTEIN B-100

Definition

Familial defective apoB-100 (FDB) is caused by mutations in the receptor-binding region of apolipoprotein B and is characterized by elevated LDL cholesterol and an increased risk of premature atherosclerosis.

Incidence and Epidemiology

Familial defective apoB-100 is a dominantly inherited disorder and occurs in about 1 in 700 persons in Europe and North America.

Etiologic Factors

Familial defective apoB-100 is caused by specific missense mutations in the region of the apoB gene responsible for binding to the LDL receptor. The most common mutation causing FDB is a substitution of glutamine for arginine at position 3500 in apoB, but other mutations have been described as well.

Pathogenesis

These substitutions in the receptor binding region of apoB prevent it from binding effectively to the LDL receptor, resulting in delayed clearance of LDL from the plasma and subsequent hypercholesterolemia. Patients with this condition are generally heterozygotes for the mutation and therefore have both normal and defective LDL; the LDL containing the mutant apoB is present in higher relative amounts in the plasma because it is cleared more slowly.

Clinical Findings

Patients with heterozygous FDB present in adulthood, usually with complications of premature atherosclerosis or with asymptomatic hypercholesterolemia. Premature atherosclerosis is often seen in this disorder and can involve any of the major arterial beds, although coronary artery disease is most prevalent. Tendon xanthomas are sometimes seen in FDB. Therefore, FDB strongly resembles familial hypercholesterolemia clinically and cannot be differentiated on purely clinical grounds.

Laboratory Findings

In FDB, total cholesterol levels are usually above 240 mg per dL and are often above 300 mg per dL, LDL cholesterol levels are generally greater than 190 mg per dL, triglycerides are usually normal, and HDL cholesterol levels are often modestly reduced.

Optimal Management

The diagnosis is suggested by hypercholesterolemia in the presence of normal triglyceride levels. This condition can appear clinically to be very similar to heterozygous familial hypercholesterolemia. However, because it is frequently caused by a single mutation, it can be diagnosed using routine molecular screening techniques available in specialized laboratories. The management of FDB is similar to that of heterozygous familial hypercholesterolemia (Chapter 31).

PRIMARY HYPERLIPOPROTEINEMIAS OF UNKNOWN CAUSE

FAMILIAL HYPERTRIGLYCERIDEMIA

Definition

Familial hypertriglyceridemia (FHTG) is an autosomal dominant trait characterized by elevated triglycerides and VLDL cholesterol (type IV pattern). Some patients may have chylomicronemia and more severe elevations in triglycerides (type V pattern).

Incidence and Epidemiology

Familial hypertriglyceridemia occurs in about 1 in 500 persons. It is inherited but is not usually expressed until adulthood; approximately 10% of children at risk have hypertriglyceridemia.

Etiologic Factors

The genetic cause of FHTG is unknown.

Pathogenesis

The metabolic basis of this disorder is probably heterogeneous and related to impaired catabolism or lipolysis of triglycerides without any obvious defect in LPL or apoC-II. Increased production of VLDL by the liver has been observed in some patients with this phenotype. Very low density lipoprotein or chylomicron overproduction may overload the normal catabolic processes and produce hypertriglyceridemia in some patients. Genetic overproduction of apoC-III could cause this syndrome, but this remains unproven. Obesity, physical inactivity, insulin resistance, alcohol use, and estrogens can all exacerbate the hypertriglyceridemia.

Clinical Findings

No unique clinical features are associated with FHTG. Patients often come to medical attention after hypertriglyceridemia is detected by a routine blood test.

Laboratory Findings

Triglyceride levels usually range from 250 to 1,000 mg per dL, with normal to modestly increased cholesterol levels. The HDL cholesterol levels are usually decreased. Some patients may have more severely elevated triglyceride levels (more than 1,000 mg per dL), indicating the presence of chylomicrons and placing these patients at risk for acute pancreatitis and eruptive xanthomas. The major clinical difference between this severe form of FHTG and the familial chylomicronemia syndrome due to LPL or apoC-II deficiency is that this disorder presents in adulthood, whereas LPL and apoC-II deficiencies present in childhood. The lipid levels alone do not permit the assignment of this diagnosis, which requires data in first-degree relatives demonstrating hypertriglyceridemia without significant hypercholesterolemia. In kindreds with FHTG, hypertriglyceridemia is found in approximately half of adult first-degree relatives. Measurement of the plasma apoB level may help to differentiate FHTG from familial combined hyperlipidemia (FCHL), with a substantially elevated apoB level more suggestive of FCHL (below). Hyperglycemia, hyperinsulinemia, and hyperuricemia are often associated with this syndrome.

Optimal Management

The differential diagnosis of this lipoprotein phenotype includes familial dysbetalipoproteinemia, familial combined hyperlipidemia, sporadic hypertriglyceridemia, and secondary causes. Secondary factors such as diabetes mellitus, hypothyroidism, nephrotic syndrome, and excessive alcohol use should be excluded. Therapy should start with the identification and control of aggravating factors, including obesity, diabetes, alcohol use, and medications such as thiazide diuretics and estrogens. Lipid-lowering drug therapy should be considered in patients who have not responded adequately to diet and control of secondary factors (Chapter 31).

FAMILIAL COMBINED HYPERLIPIDEMIA

Definition

Familial combined hyperlipidemia is an inherited autosomal dominant trait characterized by variably elevated triglyceride or cholesterol levels, elevated plasma apoB levels, and a family history of hyperlipidemia and premature cardiovascular disease.

Incidence and Epidemiology

Familial combined hyperlipidemia occurs in about 1 in 200 persons worldwide and is often not expressed until adulthood. An estimated 15% of patients with premature coronary artery disease have FCHL.

Etiologic Factors

The genetic cause of FCHL is unknown. Some patients with the FCHL phenotype may be heterozygous for LPL deficiency, but this remains to be definitively established. Several different molecular defects can probably produce the phenotype of FCHL.

Pathogenesis

Studies of lipoprotein metabolism in carefully selected persons have indicated that overproduction of VLDL or LDL, or both, may be a common metabolic basis of this condition.

Clinical Findings

No unique clinical features are associated with this disorder. Patients often come to medical attention after hyperlipidemia is detected by a routine blood test or after being diagnosed with premature cardiovascular (usually coronary) disease. Atherosclerotic cardiovascular disease is very common in patients with FCHL and the risk is often out of proportion to the modest degree of hyperlipoproteinemia. Obesity and hypertension are sometimes associated with FCHL but xanthomas are not. The formal diagnosis of FCHL requires the history of dyslipidemia in at least two first-degree relatives; a family history of premature coronary disease supports the diagnosis.

Laboratory Findings

Triglyceride levels usually range from 150 to 500 mg per dL, total cholesterol levels are 200 to 400 mg per dL, and HDL cholesterol levels are almost always decreased. The hallmark biochemical finding is a significantly elevated apoB level, often disproportionate to the degree of hyperlipidemia. This indicates the presence of small dense LDL particles, which are particularly characteristic of this syndrome and are considered highly atherogenic. The term *hyperapobetalipoproteinemia* describes the syndrome of elevated apoB with normal lipid levels and is probably a subset of FCHL. Some specialized assays can specifically detect the presence of increased small dense LDL and a nuclear magnetic resonance (NMR)–based assay can determine the concentration of different types of LDL particles. Greater clinical utilization of such assays may permit more specific diagnoses of FCHL and its subsets. Hyperglycemia, hyperinsulinemia, and hyperuricemia are often, but not invariably, associated with FCHL.

Optimal Management

Secondary disorders are other possible causes of this lipoprotein phenotype. In particular, diabetes mellitus, hypothyroidism, renal disease, alcohol use, and certain medications should be excluded. Patients with FCHL are at significantly increased risk of premature coronary disease. Therefore, once the diagnosis of FCHL has been made, attempts should be made to modify the lipid abnormalities to decrease cardiovascular risk (Chapter 31). General measures include diet, exercise, and weight loss, but most patients with FCHL also require lipid-lowering drug therapy. The HMG-CoA reductase inhibitors are generally the drugs of first choice. Nicotinic acid can be useful in reducing triglycerides and LDL cholesterol, either alone or in combination with statins. Fibric acid derivatives can help control triglycerides but are not as effective as statins in decreasing LDL cholesterol or apoB levels. Bile acid sequestrants can be used together with other drugs, but only after triglyceride levels have been controlled.

POLYGENIC HYPERCHOLESTEROLEMIA

Definition

Polygenic hypercholesterolemia is defined as hypercholesterolemia exceeding the 95th percentile for the population in the absence of a defined genetic or secondary cause.

Incidence and Epidemiology

Polygenic hypercholesterolemia is relatively common, occurring (by definition) in up to 5% of the general population.

Etiologic Factors

Polygenic hypercholesterolemia is attributed to a complex interaction of multiple genetic factors with environmental factors.

Pathogenesis

Genetic differences in metabolic pathways such as cholesterol absorption, cholesterol synthesis, apolipoprotein structure, or rates of bile acid formation may interact with each other and with environmental factors, such as diet, to generate hypercholesterolemia.

Clinical Findings

There are no specific clinical findings. Tendon xanthomas are not observed. The risk of premature atherosclerosis is increased.

Laboratory Findings

Polygenic hypercholesterolemia can usually be differentiated from familial hypercholesterolemia, FDB, and FCHL through laboratory findings. In polygenic hypercholesterolemia, the elevation in total and LDL cholesterol level is milder than in familial hypercholesterolemia and FDB. In FCHL, triglycerides are usually higher and apoB levels are significantly higher relative to the LDL cholesterol level than in polygenic hypercholesterolemia. Family studies are also helpful: only approximately 7% of first-degree relatives of patients with polygenic hypercholesterolemia are hypercholesterolemic, whereas approximately half of relatives with the above disorders have dyslipidemia.

Optimal Management

Treatment of polygenic hypercholesterolemia should start with lifestyle interventions of diet, exercise, and weight loss. Sometimes drug therapy is necessary, and statins, nicotinic acid, or bile acid sequestrants are all reasonable as first-line agents (Chapter 31).

SECONDARY FORMS OF HYPERLIPIDEMIA

The major secondary forms of hyperlipidemia are listed in Table 12.6. Usually the lipid abnormality is relatively mild compared with some of the primary disorders. If the hyperlipidemia is severe, the patient probably has a genetic predisposition to hyperlipidemia that has been aggravated by the secondary disorder. In these cases, correction or control of the secondary disorder may ameliorate, but not fully correct, the lipoprotein abnormality. These patients may then require specific treatment of the hyperlipidemia, especially if they are at risk for pancreatitis or atherosclerosis.

DIETARY INFLUENCES

Epidemiologic evidence indicates that higher cholesterol levels relate directly to a greater consumption of saturated fat and cholesterol. Diets rich in saturated fat and cholesterol suppress hepatic LDL receptor activity and thereby raise the LDL cholesterol level. Substituting polyunsaturated or monounsaturated fats for saturated fats results in lower LDL cholesterol levels. Decreasing total and saturated fat in the diet usually results in a decrease in HDL cholesterol levels as well. Another dietary factor contributing to hyperlipidemia is excess calorie consumption, which promotes increased VLDL production by the liver, both directly and as a result of obesity. This may lead to elevated triglycerides and possibly to elevated LDL cholesterol levels, especially if LDL receptor activity is suppressed. Diets restricted in saturated fats and cholesterol and reduced in calories to maintain ideal body weight often correct mild hyperlipidemia and form the cornerstone of therapy for most forms of hyperlipidemia (Chapter 31).

ALCOHOL

Excess alcohol intake is a common cause of hyperlipidemia. Regular alcohol consumption increases lipid levels in most people, but the response is highly variable. The greatest effects of alcohol are on triglyceride levels. Alcohol consumption stimulates hepatic secretion of VLDL, presumably because hepatic metabolism of ethanol by alcohol dehydrogenase increases levels of nicotinamide adenine dinucleotide, which inhibits oxidation of free fatty acids. The excess free fatty acids in the liver may be used for synthesis of triglyceride, which is then secreted as part of VLDL. The usual lipoprotein pattern with alcohol consumption is type IV (increased VLDL), but persons with an underlying predisposition to defective clearance of triglyceride-rich lipoproteins may develop severe hypertriglyceridemia (type V pattern). Regular alcohol use also raises the HDL cholesterol level by a mechanism that is not completely understood.

DIABETES MELLITUS

Several forms of hyperlipidemia are recognized clinically in patients with diabetes mellitus. Patients with type I diabetes mellitus in diabetic ketoacidosis may have severe hypertriglyceridemia

TABLE 12.6.   DISORDERS ASSOCIATED WITH SECONDARY FORMS OF HYPERLIPIDEMIA

Disorder	Chylomicrons	VLDLs	IDLs	LDLs	Lipoprotein Phenotype	Proposed Mechanism
Endocrine/Metabolic						
Diabetes mellitus (type II)						
Severe, untreated	+	+			IV or V	↓ VLDL and chylomicron metabolism due to decreased lipoprotein lipase activity
Moderate		+			IV	↑ VLDL production
Hypothyroidism		+		+	IIa or IIb	↓ LDL receptor activity
Estrogen or oral contraceptive therapy	+	+			IV or V	↑ VLDL secretion in those predisposed to hypertriglyceridemia
Isolated growth hormone deficiency (ateliotic dwarfism)		+		+	IIb or IV	(?) ↑ VLDL synthesis with enhanced conversion to LDL
Acromegaly		+			IV	↑ VLDL production; ↓ lipoprotein lipase activity
Glucocorticoid therapy or Cushing's syndrome		+		+	IIb or IV	↑ VLDL production, leading to ↑ LDL and ↑ HDL
Lipodysrophy (congenital or acquired)	+	+			IV or V	↑ VLDL secretion
Glycogen storage disease type I	+	+			IV or V	↑ VLDL production and ↓ lipoprotein lipase activity
Anorexia nervosa				+	IIa	(?) Decreased clearance of LDL by liver
Acute intermittent porphyria				+	IIa	Unknown
Werner's syndrome (adult progeria)				+	IIa	Unknown
Renal						
Uremia		+			IV	↓ VLDL clearance due to ↓ lipoprotein lipase activity; remnant particles also accumulate
Nephrotic syndrome		+	+	+	IIa, IIb, or IV	↑ VLDL production and conversion to LDL
Hepatic						
Primary biliary cirrhosis					↑ Cholesterol and phospholipids due to ↑ of lipoprotein X	Lipoproptein X may form as a result of regurgitation of biliary lipids into plasma and because lecithin-cholesterol acyltransferase activity is low
Hepatoma				+	IIa	Cholesterol overproduction due to lack of feedback control in tumor tissue
Acute viral hepatitis		+			IV	Decreased hepatic triglyceride lipase and lecithin-cholesterol acyltransferase activity alter VLDL catabolism
Immunologic/Infectious						
Dyslobulinemia (multiple) myeloma, macroglobulinemia	+	+			III or IV	Immunoglobulin binds to chylomicron remnants and VLDL to impair lipoprotein catabolism
Systemic lupus erythematosus	+				I	Immunoglobulin binds to heparin, a cofactor for lipoprotein lipase, causing decreased activity of this enzyme
HIV Infection	+	+			IV	Cytokine-induced increased VLDL-production
Drug-Related						
Isotretinoin and etretinate		+		+	IV, occasionally IIb	Unknown
Thiazides		+		+	IIa, IIb, or IV	Unknown; effect may be greatest in those genetically predisposed to hypertriglyceridemia
β-Adrenergic blocking drugs		+		+	IIa, IIb, or IV	
Tamoxifen		+			IV	May ↑ VLDL production in those predisposed to hypertriglyceridemia
Cyclosporin				+	IIa	Unknown
HIV protease inhibitors	+	+			IV or V	Unknown

Adapted from Brown MS, Goldstein JL. The hyperlipoproteinemias and other disorders of lipid metabolism. In: Braunwald E et al, eds. *Harrison's Principles of Internal Medicine,* eleventh ed. New York: McGraw Hill, 1987:1650. With permission.)

due to excess release of free fatty acids from adipose tissue, followed by conversion to VLDL triglycerides in the liver. Administration of insulin usually results in the gradual normalization of lipid levels. Patients with type I diabetes mellitus who are under adequate glycemic control do not usually have hyperlipidemia; the presence of hyperlipidemia in such patients suggests an underlying lipoprotein abnormality. In contrast, patients with type II diabetes mellitus often have associated hyperlipidemia. There are at least two causes of the hyperlipidemia: insulin resistance causes decreased LPL activity and reduced capacity to catabolize chylomicrons and VLDL; insulin resistance and obesity itself may stimulate excess VLDL production. Many patients with type II diabetes mellitus have a constellation of lipid abnormalities, including elevated triglyceride (VLDL, lipoprotein remnants), elevated dense LDL, and decreased HDL cholesterol levels. In some diabetic patients who have another underlying lipoprotein abnormality, the triglycerides can be extremely elevated (type V pattern), predisposing to eruptive xanthomas and acute pancreatitis. Significant elevation of LDL cholesterol in the type II diabetic patient often suggests an additional lipoprotein abnormality.

HYPOTHYROIDISM

Hypothyroidism is associated with elevated LDL cholesterol levels due primarily to down-regulation of the LDL receptor and therefore delayed clearance of LDL. Because hypothyroidism can be subtle in its clinical presentation and is eminently treatable, all patients presenting with hypercholesterolemia due to elevated LDL should be screened to rule out hypothyroidism. Thyroid replacement therapy usually results in resolution of the hypercholesterolemia. Hypothyroid patients who remain hypercholesterolemic after adequate replacement probably have an underlying lipoprotein disorder and might require lipid-lowering drug therapy.

RENAL DISEASES

End-stage renal disease (ESRD) is often associated with mild hypertriglyceridemia because of increased VLDL and remnant lipoproteins due to a defect in triglyceride lipolysis and remnant clearance. Plasma levels of Lp(a) are also significantly increased in ESRD. Nephrotic syndrome is always associated with a more pronounced hyperlipoproteinemia involving both elevated triglyceride and cholesterol levels. The mechanism appears to be hepatic overproduction of VLDL with subsequent increased production of LDL. Effective treatment of the nephrotic syndrome normalizes the lipid profile, but patients with chronic nephrotic syndrome may require lipid-lowering drug therapy.

ESTROGENS AND PROGESTINS

In most women, estrogens have relatively little effect on triglyceride and cholesterol levels but result in increased HDL cholesterol levels. In familial dysbetalipoproteinemia (type III), estrogens can result in significant lowering of triglyceride and cholesterol levels. However, in patients with other familial forms of hyper-

lipidemia, such as FCHL, FHTG, and familial type V hyperlipidemia, estrogens may markedly exacerbate the hypertriglyceridemia, predisposing the patient to acute pancreatitis. Therefore, estrogens should be used cautiously in patients with familial disorders causing hypertriglyceridemia. Women being considered for postmenopausal estrogen replacement therapy should be screened with a fasting lipid profile before starting therapy.

▮ ELEVATED LIPOPROTEIN(A)

Definition

Elevated Lp(a) is defined as a plasma Lp(a) level above 30 mg per dL in the absence of metabolic factors (such as ESRD) known to increase Lp(a) levels. It is often associated with a family history of premature atherosclerotic cardiovascular disease.

Incidence and Epidemiology

In the United States, approximately 20% of whites and 50% of blacks have Lp(a) levels above 30 mg per dL.

Etiologic Factors

Lipoprotein(a) levels are highly genetically determined and are inherited as an autosomal codominant trait with expression in childhood.

Pathogenesis

The gene for apo(a) is the major genetic factor controlling the plasma level of Lp(a). The apo(a) gene exhibits a striking size polymorphism, with well over 30 different apo(a) phenotypes described in humans. The apo(a) gene directly affects the production rate of apo(a) by the liver, probably both by transcriptional and post-translational mechanisms. The apo(a) alleles inherited from both parents contribute additively to the Lp(a) concentration in the plasma. Lipoprotein(a) levels correlate with premature atherosclerotic cardiovascular disease, especially in persons with elevated LDL cholesterol levels or a family history of premature atherosclerosis. Lipoprotein(a) is thought to be directly atherogenic, although the mechanism is not well understood. The apo(a) protein is highly homologous to plasminogen, and one major hypothesis holds that Lp(a) inhibits the activation of plasminogen to plasmin at the vessel wall, leading to inadequate fibrinolysis and increasing the likelihood of atherosclerotic plaque development.

Clinical Findings

No unique clinical features are associated with elevated Lp(a) levels. The only clinical consequence of an elevated Lp(a) level is a potentially increased risk of premature atherosclerosis. However, elevated Lp(a) levels may not confer the same degree of increased risk for atherosclerosis in African Americans as in whites.

Laboratory Findings

Many people with elevated Lp(a) levels have normal lipid levels, and therefore Lp(a) must be directly measured if an elevated Lp(a) level is to be diagnosed. Lipoprotein(a) is probably a mild acute- phase reactant and should therefore not be measured in acute inflammatory states or immediately after myocardial infarction or surgical procedures.

Optimal Management

Measurement of Lp(a) is not currently recommended as a general screening tool for cardiovascular risk assessment. It should be reserved for two situations: (a) that involving patients with premature cardiovascular disease or a strong family history who have relatively normal lipid levels, and (b) that involving patients whose LDL cholesterol levels are in a "gray zone" with respect to drug treatment (Chapter 31). In these situations, the finding of an elevated Lp(a) level may influence the clinical approach. If an elevated Lp(a) level is found, renal disease (both chronic renal insufficiency and the nephrotic syndrome) must be excluded as a potential contributing factor. No studies have focused on the clinical benefit of lowering Lp(a) levels, and there is no justification for intervention specifically to lower the Lp(a) level. However, the diagnosis of elevated Lp(a) may influence clinical management in certain situations. Perhaps the most straightforward is in the postmenopausal woman: Lp(a) levels increase after menopause, and this increase can be prevented by estrogen replacement therapy. The postmenopausal woman with an elevated Lp(a) level, especially in the setting of cardiovascular disease, should receive special consideration for estrogen replacement therapy. Elevated Lp(a) levels have been associated with an increased risk of restenosis after balloon angioplasty, and lowering the Lp(a) level in this setting may help prevent restenosis. Finally, measuring the Lp(a) level may be indicated in the patient with an LDL cholesterol level in the gray zone. In this situation, an elevated Lp(a) level may be an additional risk factor to consider in the decision about whether to initiate drug therapy, which should then focus on lowering the LDL cholesterol level. Nicotinic acid is the only lipid-lowering drug that consistently lowers the Lp(a) level, and consequently it should receive extra consideration in the hypercholesterolemic patient who also has an elevated Lp(a) level. However, the major emphasis in this situation must be to lower the LDL cholesterol level.

DISORDERS AFFECTING HDL CHOLESTEROL LEVELS

Because of the strong inverse relation between HDL cholesterol levels and premature coronary artery disease, measurement of HDL cholesterol levels is gaining in clinical importance. The National Cholesterol Education Program recommends that all adults over age 20 years be screened for total and HDL cholesterol levels. Because total and HDL cholesterol levels are not very sensitive to a recent meal, this screening can be done with a random blood draw and does not require a fast. As a result of such widespread screening, patients with low HDL cholesterol levels are being identified at an increasing rate; however, formal guidelines for the approach to the patient with a low HDL cholesterol level have not been developed.

Causes of low HDL cholesterol (hypoalphalipoproteinemia) can be primary or secondary. Lifestyle-related secondary causes of low HDL cholesterol include cigarette smoking, obesity, inactivity, and a very low fat diet. Some medical conditions are associated with low HDL cholesterol levels, such as type II diabetes mellitus, end-stage renal disease, and hypertriglyceridemia from various causes. Certain medications can reduce HDL cholesterol levels, such as β-blockers, thiazide diuretics, androgens, progestins, and probucol. Several genetic disorders produce low HDL cholesterol levels. Some of the genes responsible for these syndromes have been identified, but many families with low HDL levels have no identifiable gene mutation. The clinical and biochemical features of the more well-recognized genetic disorders of HDL metabolism are listed in Table 12.7.

Causes of elevated levels of HDL cholesterol (hyperalphalipoproteinemia) can also be primary or secondary. Secondary causes include vigorous sustained aerobic exercise, regular alcohol consumption, exposure to chlorinated hydrocarbons, and treatment with estrogens, nicotinic acid, or phenytoin. There are also familial syndromes of high HDL cholesterol that in some cases are associated with a decreased risk of coronary heart disease.

PRIMARY CAUSES OF LOW HDL CHOLESTEROL LEVELS

Familial ApoA-I Deficiency and Structural ApoA-I Mutations

Several kindreds have been described in which patients have complete deficiency of apoA-I due to deletions of the apoA-I gene or nonsense mutations that prevent the biosynthesis of apoA-I protein. These patients have virtually undetectable levels of HDL cholesterol and no detectable apoA-I. They have corneal opacities, and many have cutaneous or planar xanthomas. The incidence of premature cardiovascular disease in patients with apoA-I deficiency varies. Some develop coronary disease in the third or fourth decade; others do not develop atherosclerotic disease until the sixth or seventh decade.

Several point mutations in apoA-I have been described that affect apoA-I structure and cause low levels of HDL cholesterol (usually 15 to 30 mg per dL). The first of these mutants to be described was apoA-I$_{Milano}$. Many of these patients develop corneal opacities, and in some cases the apoA-I mutation is associated with other diseases such as systemic amyloidosis. However, premature cardiovascular disease has not been reported in patients with low HDL cholesterol levels due to apoA-I structural mutations. Such mutations are a rare cause of low HDL cholesterol levels in the general population.

Familial Lecithin: Cholesterol Acyltransferase Deficiency

High-density lipoprotein facilitates the removal of excess unesterified cholesterol from peripheral cells, after which the cholesterol is esterified by the lipoprotein-associated enzyme LCAT

TABLE 12.7.   GENETIC DISORDERS CAUSING LOW OR HIGH HDL CHOLESTEROL LEVELS

Genetic Defect	Molecular Defect	Metabolic Defect	Lipoprotein Abnormalities	Clinical Findings	Premature Atherosclerosis	Genetic Transmission
Hypoalphalipoproteinemia (Decreased HDL Cholesterol)						
Familial apoA-I deficiency	ApoA-I deficiency	Absent apoA-I biosynthesis	HDL < 5 mg/dL	Planar xanthomas, corneal opacities	+ +	Autosomal codominant
Familial apoA-I structural mutants	Abnormal apoA-I	Rapid apoA-I catabolism	TG normal HDL 15–30 mg/dL	Often none, sometimes corneal opacities	No	Autosomal dominant
Familial LCAT deficiency	LCAT deficiency (complete)	Rapid HDL catabolism	TG normal to increased HDL < 10 mg/dL	Corneal opacities, anemia, proteinuria, renal insufficiency	No	Autosomal recessive
Fish-eye disease	LCAT deficiency (partial)	Rapid HDL catabolism	TG increased HDL < mg/dL	Corneal opacities	No	Autosomal recessive
Tangier disease	ABC1 mutations	Impaired cholesterol efflux, very rapid HDL catabolism	TG increased HDL < 5 mg/dL	Corneal opacities, enlarged orange tonsils, hepatosplenomegaly, peripheral neuropathy	No or possibly +	Autosomal codominant
Familial hypoalphalipoprotein-emia	Unknown	Usually rapid HDL catabolism	TG usually increased HDL 15–35 mg/dL	Often none, sometimes corneal opacities	No or + +	Autosomal dominant
Hyperalphalipoproteinemia (Increased HDL Cholesterol)						
Familial CETP deficiency	CETP deficiency	Delayed HDL catabolism	HDL > 150 mg/dL	None	No or possibly +	Autosomal recessive
Familial hyperalphalipoprotein-emia	Unknown	Increased apoA-I biosynthesis in one subject	HDL > 80 mg/dL	None	Decreased	Autosomal dominant

LCAT, lecithin:cholesterol acyltransferase; CETP, cholesteryl ester transfer protein; HDL, high-density lipoprotein; TG, triglycerides; ABC1, ATP-binding cassette protein 1.

(Fig. 12.5). Two general types of genetic LCAT deficiency have been described in humans. The first, complete (or classic) LCAT deficiency, is characterized clinically by corneal opacities, anemia, and progressive proteinuria and renal insufficiency. Low plasma levels of HDL cholesterol (less than 10 mg per dL), hypertriglyceridemia, a high fraction of plasma cholesterol in the unesterified form, and virtually complete absence of cholesterol esterification activity in the plasma are the biochemical hallmarks of this disorder. Multiple mutations in the LCAT gene have been described in patients with classic LCAT deficiency.

A second type of LCAT deficiency is a partial enzyme deficiency, also called fish-eye disease. The clinical features are similar to those of classic LCAT deficiency and include corneal opacities and low levels of HDL cholesterol (less than 10 mg per dL). However, patients with fish-eye disease have no anemia or renal disease, the fraction of plasma cholesteryl ester is normal, and there is clearly detectable cholesterol esterification activity in the plasma. The initial patients reported with fish-eye disease had evidence of cholesterol esterification in apoB-containing lipoproteins but not in HDL, but this has not been a consistent finding. Several molecular defects in the LCAT gene have been described in patients with fish-eye disease.

In addition to the low plasma levels of HDL cholesterol, both types of LCAT deficiency are associated with low plasma levels of apoA-I and especially apoA-II due to rapid catabolism. Despite the markedly low levels of HDL cholesterol and apoA-I, there is no apparent increased risk of premature atherosclerotic cardiovascular disease in either complete or partial LCAT deficiency.

Tangier Disease

Tangier disease is a rare autosomal codominant inherited disorder of HDL metabolism. It is caused by mutations in the gene encoding the ATP-binding cassette protein 1, which facilitates the efflux of excess cholesterol from cells, particularly macrophages. Tangier disease homozygotes have HDL cholesterol levels below 5 mg per dL and extremely low levels of apoA-I. The metabolic defect is not failure of apoA-I biosynthesis, as in apoA-I deficiency, but rather markedly accelerated HDL catabolism due to the impaired ability of HDL to acquire lipids from cells. Clinical features include accumulation of cholesterol in the reticuloendothelial system, resulting in hepatosplenomegaly, intestinal mucosal abnormalities, and the pathognomonic enlarged orange tonsils seen in this disease. Intermittent peripheral neuropathy can also be seen due to cholesterol accumulation in Schwann cells. Premature atherosclerotic disease is seen but is not a prominent feature of homozygous Tangier disease. Heterozygotes have moderately reduced HDL cholesterol and apoA-I levels, have no evidence of reticuloendothelial cholesterol accumulation, and may have some increased risk of premature atherosclerosis.

Primary Hypoalphalipoproteinemia

Primary hypoalphalipoproteinemia is the term used for familial low HDL cholesterol levels (below the 10th percentile) in the setting of relatively normal cholesterol and triglyceride levels. High-density lipoprotein cholesterol levels are usually approximately 15 to 35 mg per dL, and patients have no clinical evidence of Tangier disease or LCAT deficiency. Transmission is that of an autosomal dominant trait. The genetic cause in some families may be mutations in ABC1 but in others is unknown. There are no unique clinical features of this disorder other than possibly an increased risk of premature atherosclerotic cardiovascular disease. However, families have been described with familial transmission of low HDL cholesterol levels but no evidence of increased atherosclerosis. Therefore, the direct relationship of primary hypoalphalipoproteinemia to premature coronary disease is uncertain and may depend on the specific nature of the gene defect or metabolic cause of the low HDL cholesterol level.

PRIMARY CAUSES OF HIGH HDL CHOLESTEROL LEVELS

Cholesteryl Ester Transfer Protein Deficiency

Cholesteryl ester transfer protein facilitates the transfer of cholesteryl esters among lipoproteins, especially from HDL to apoB-containing lipoproteins. Homozygous genetic deficiency of CETP results in very high levels of HDL cholesterol (more than 160 mg per dL) due to the accumulation of large, cholesterol-rich HDL particles. The initial reports of homozygous CETP deficiency were in Japanese kindreds all having the same splice site mutation in the CETP gene, but CETP deficiency due to other mutations in the CETP gene have been reported as well. Other than the markedly elevated HDL cholesterol level, there are no distinguishing clinical features and no obvious clinical sequelae of CETP deficiency. Heterozygotes for CETP deficiency have modestly elevated HDL cholesterol levels. Despite the very high levels of HDL cholesterol, homozygous CETP deficiency is not clearly associated with a decreased risk of atherosclerotic cardiovascular disease. In fact, one large epidemiologic study suggested that heterozygosity for CETP deficiency was associated with an increased risk of coronary disease.

Primary Hyperalphalipoproteinemia

Primary hyperalphalipoproteinemia is a term used for familial elevated HDL cholesterol levels (above the 90th percentile). It is inherited as an autosomal dominant trait and is associated with HDL cholesterol levels usually above 80 mg per dL in women and 70 mg per dL in men. The genetic basis is unknown. Some people with familial hyperalphalipoproteinemia may have increased production of apoA-I, but others likely have reduced catabolism of HDL cholesterol and apoA-I. This syndrome has been associated with decreased risk of coronary heart disease and increased longevity.

Primary Hypolipidemias

Some rare genetic disorders of lipoprotein metabolism result in extremely low cholesterol levels (Table 12.8). Although rare, these disorders are important to recognize and diagnose so that appropriate referral and effective therapy can be provided.

Abetalipoproteinemia

Abetalipoproteinemia is a rare autosomal recessive disease characterized clinically by fat malabsorption, spinocerebellar degen-

TABLE 12.8.   GENETIC DISORDERS CAUSING LOW CHOLESTEROL LEVELS

Genetic Disorder	Molecular Defect	Metabolic Defect	Lipoprotein Abnormalities	Clinical Findings	Genetic Transmission
Familial hypobetalipoproteinemia Heterozygous	ApoB-100 truncation mutations	Rapid catabolism of mutant apoB, reduced production of normal apoB-100	Total cholesterol < 120 mg/dL LDL cholesterol < 80 mg/dL Triglycerides normal ApoB-100 25–50% normal	None	Autosomal codominant
Homozygous ("normotriglyceridemic")	ApoB-100 truncation mutations	Rapid catabolism of mutant apoB-100	Total cholesterol < 80 mg/dL LDL cholesterol < 20 mg/dL Triglycerides normal ApoB-100 < 5% of normal	Usually none	Autosomal codominant
Homozygous ("null allele")	ApoB-100 deficiency	Absent apoB-100 biosynthesis	Total cholesterol < 80 mg/dL LDL cholesterol undetectable Triglycerides < 20 mg/dL ApoB-100 undetectable	Fat malabsorption, spinocerebellar degeneration, retinopathy, acanthocytosis	Autosomal codominant
Abetalipoproteinemia	MTP deficiency	Absent chylomicron and VLDL secretion	Total cholesterol < 80 mg/dL LDL cholesterol undetectable Triglycerides < 20 mg/dL ApoB undetectable	Fat malabsorption, spinocerebellar degeneration, retinopathy, acanthocytosis	Autosomal recessive
Chylomicron retention disease (Anderson's disease)	Unknown	Absent chylomicron secretion	Total cholesterol < 100 mg/dL LDL cholesterol < 690 mg/dL Triglycerides normal ApoB 25–50% of normal	Fat malabsorption failure to thrive	Autosomal recessive

MTP, microsomal transfer protein; VLDL, very low density lipoprotein; LDL, low-density lipoprotein.

eration, pigmented retinopathy, and acanthocytosis. The biochemical hallmark is the strikingly abnormal plasma lipid and lipoprotein profile. Total cholesterol and triglyceride levels are extremely low; there are no detectable plasma chylomicrons, VLDLs, or LDLs; and apoB is absent from the plasma. This disease is caused by mutations in the gene for the microsomal transfer protein (MTP), which mediates the intracellular transport of membrane-associated lipids in the intestine and liver and is necessary for the normal formation of chylomicrons in the enterocyte and VLDLs in the hepatocyte.

The most prominent and debilitating symptoms of abetalipoproteinemia are neurologic and ophthalmologic. They usually begin in the second decade of life. The first neurologic sign of disease is usually the loss of deep tendon reflexes, followed by decreased distal lower extremity vibratory and proprioceptive senses and cerebellar signs such as dysmetria, ataxia, and spastic gait. The clinical outcome varies, but the result in untreated patients is often severe ataxia and spasticity by the third or fourth decade. These severe central nervous system effects are the ultimate cause of death in most patients, which often occurs by the fifth decade or earlier. Patients with abetalipoproteinemia also develop a progressive pigmented retinopathy. The first ophthalmic symptoms are decreased night and color vision. Daytime visual acuity usually deteriorates inexorably to virtual blindness by the fourth decade. The presence of spinocerebellar degeneration and pigmented retinopathy in this disease has often resulted in a misdiagnosis of Friedreich's ataxia.

Most of the clinical symptoms of abetalipoproteinemia are the result of defects in the absorption and transport of fat-soluble vitamins, especially vitamin E. Vitamin E is transported from the intestine to the liver, then "repackaged" in the liver and incorporated into the assembling VLDL particle by a specific protein, the tocopherol-binding protein. In the circulation, VLDLs are converted to LDL, and vitamin E is transported by LDL to peripheral tissues and delivered to cells via the LDL receptor. Patients with abetalipoproteinemia are markedly deficient in vitamin E. Vitamin E metabolism is markedly altered in patients with abetalipoproteinemia because the plasma transport of vitamin E requires hepatic secretion of apoB-containing lipoproteins. Most of the major clinical symptoms, especially those of the nervous system and retina, are primarily due to vitamin E deficiency. This concept is supported by the fact that other diseases involving vitamin E deficiency, such as cholestasis and isolated vitamin E deficiency, are characterized by similar symptoms and pathologic changes.

Patients with suspected abetalipoproteinemia should be referred to specialized centers for confirmation of the diagnosis and appropriate therapy.

Obligate heterozygotes (such as the parents of patients with abetalipoproteinemia) have no symptoms and no evidence of reduced plasma lipids. Thus, family studies are important in distinguishing abetalipoproteinemia from clinically similar homozygous hypobetalipoproteinemia (see below), in which obligate heterozygotes have decreased LDL cholesterol and apoB levels.

Hypobetalipoproteinemia

Familial hypobetalipoproteinemia, in contrast to abetalipoproteinemia, is autosomal codominant; heterozygotes' levels of LDL cholesterol and apoB are approximately half of normal or less, whereas homozygotes have very low or absent plasma apoB. Heterozygous familial hypobetalipoproteinemia is not associated with symptoms, but some homozygous patients have symptoms similar to those of patients with abetalipoproteinemia. The gene defect in this disorder resides in most or all cases within the apoB gene itself. Many are nonsense mutations resulting in a truncated apoB protein; at least 25 such mutations have been described. One patient initially described as having "normotriglyceridemic abetalipoproteinemia" was subsequently demonstrated to be homozygous for a truncated apoB and was therefore diagnosed with homozygous hypobetalipoproteinemia.

Clinically, heterozygous hypobetalipoproteinemia is associated with LDL cholesterol levels of approximately 40 to 80 mg per dL, is not associated with clinical sequelae, and requires no specific therapy. However, patients with homozygous hypobetalipoproteinemia have markedly reduced to absent LDL cholesterol and apoB levels, and they might be at risk for many of the sequelae seen in abetalipoproteinemia. Such patients should therefore be referred to specialized centers for confirmation of the diagnosis and appropriate therapy.

Chylomicron Retention Disease

Chylomicron retention disease, or Anderson's disease, is associated with selective inability to secrete apoB from intestinal enterocytes, resulting in fat malabsorption and sometimes neurologic disease similar to that seen in abetalipoproteinemia and homozygous hypobetalipoproteinemia. In contrast to these two disorders, apoB-100 can be detected in the plasma of patients with chylomicron retention disease, as hepatic VLDL secretion is normal. The molecular defect is unknown but appears to be distinct from both the microsomal triglyceride transfer protein and apoB genes.

■ SELECTED GENETIC DISORDERS OF INTRACELLULAR CHOLESTEROL METABOLISM

Several rare genetic disorders of intracellular cholesterol and lipid metabolism exist (Table 12.9). In some of these diseases the molecular cause is established; in other cases it remains unknown. As more of the genes regulating intracellular cholesterol and lipid metabolism are identified, more of these syndromes will undoubtedly be recognized and defined at the molecular level.

CEREBROTENDINOUS XANTHOMATOSIS

Cerebrotendinous xanthomatosis is an autosomal recessive disorder caused by mutations in the gene for sterol 27-hydroxylase, a mitochondrial enzyme involved in the normal biosynthesis of bile acids in the liver. As a result of the deficiency in sterol 27-hydroxylase, bile acid intermediates are shunted into the synthesis of cholestanol, which then accumulates in multiple tissues. Untreated patients develop cataracts, tendon xanthomas, and

| TABLE 12.9. | OTHER RARE GENETIC DISORDERS OF LIPID AND LIPOPROTEIN METABOLISM |

Genetic Disorder	Molecular Defect	Metabolic Defect	Lipid or Lipoprotein Abnormalities	Clinical Findings	Treatment
Cerebrotendinous xanthomatosis	Sterol 27-hydroxlase	Overproduction of cholestanol	Increased plasma cholestanol levels	Tendon and tuberous xanthomas, neurologic dysfunction, cataracts, atherosclerosis, gallstones	Chenodeoxycholic acid
Sitosterolemia	Unknown	Increased intestinal absorption of plant sterols	Increased plasma levels of plant sterols and LDL cholesterol	Tendon xanthomas, atherosclerosis	Bile acid sequestrants
Cholesteryl ester storage disease	Lysosomal acid lipase	Failure to hydrolyze cholesteryl esters and triglycerides in lysosomes	Increased LDL cholesterol	Hepatosplenomegaly in childhood, survival to adulthood	None
Wolman's disease	Lysosomal acid lipase	Failure to hydrolyze cholesteryl esters and triglycerides in lysosomes	Normal	Hepatosplenomegaly in infancy, failure to thrive, death by age 2	None
Niemann–Pick C disease	NPC1	Defect in transport of intracellular cholesterol from lysosome to ACAT	Increased LDL cholesterol	Hepatosplenomegaly, CNS involvement, often death by age 20	None

NPC1, Niemann–Pick (gene.)
ACAT, acyl coenzyme A:cholesterol acyltransferase.
LDL, low-density lipoprotein; CNS, central nervous system.

progressive disease of the central and peripheral nervous system in the second decade of life. Early diagnosis is crucial, as treatment with chenodeoxycholic acid reduces plasma cholestanol levels and prevents the progression of clinical symptoms.

SITOSTEROLEMIA

Sitosterolemia is a rare autosomal recessive disease associated with excess intestinal absorption and tissue accumulation of plant-derived sterols such as sitosterol and cholestanol. The molecular cause is unknown. This disease can present with severe hypercholesterolemia, premature atherosclerosis, and tendon xanthomas similar to those of patients with homozygous or severe heterozygous familial hypercholesterolemia. Sitosterolemia should be ruled out in patients presenting with this constellation of findings. There is no LDL receptor abnormality in sitosterolemia. Patients often benefit from treatment with bile acid sequestrants but generally do not benefit from HMG-CoA reductase inhibition. Patients suspected of having sitosterolemia should be referred to specialized centers for further evaluation.

CHOLESTERYL ESTER STORAGE DISEASE AND WOLMAN'S DISEASE

Cholesteryl ester storage disease is an autosomal recessive disorder caused by mutations in the gene for lysosomal acid lipase, a lysosomal enzyme required for hydrolysis of cholesteryl esters and triglycerides in the lysosome. As a result of the deficiency in acid lipase, cholesteryl esters and triglycerides accumulate in lysosomes. Patients with this disorder present with hepatomegaly and usually hyperlipidemia in childhood. Hepatic dysfunction in childhood can be a consequence of this disease, although some patients have no clinical problems until hepatic fibrosis develops in adulthood. Premature atherosclerosis has been associated with this disease in some patients.

A more severe form of this disease is known as Wolman's disease. Within the first weeks of life, infants develop hepatosplenomegaly, steatorrhea, adrenal calcification, and failure to thrive. This form of the disease is usually fatal by the second year of life. The cause of the phenotypic difference between these two presentations of acid lipase deficiency is unknown but may relate to the specific molecular defects underlying the lipase deficiency.

NIEMANN–PICK C DISEASE

Niemann–Pick C is an autosomal recessive disease characterized by the accumulation of cholesterol and sphingomyelin in tissues, especially the liver, reticuloendothelial system, and central nervous system. It is a disorder of intracellular cholesterol transport caused by mutations in the NPC1 gene, which encodes an intracellular protein that is involved in cholesterol transport and signaling. Niemann–Pick C disease is characterized by hepatosplenomegaly and progressive neurologic disease, often resulting in severe disability and death by the second decade.

BIBLIOGRAPHY

Brewer HB Jr, Zech LA, Gregg RE, et al. Type III hyperlipoproteinemia: diagnosis, molecular defects, pathology, and treatment. *Ann Intern Med* 1983;98:623.

Brown MS, Goldstein JL. A receptor-mediated pathway for cholesterol homeostasis. *Science* 1986;232:34.

Kwiterovich PO. Genetics and molecular biology of familial combined hyperlipidemia. *Curr Opin Lipidol* 1993;4:133.

Rader DJ, Brewer HB Jr. Lipoprotein(a): clinical approach to a unique atherogenic lipoprotein. *JAMA* 1993;267:1109–1112.

Rader DJ, Brewer HB Jr. Abetalipoproteinemia: new insights into lipoprotein assembly and vitamin E metabolism from a rare genetic disease. *JAMA* 1993;270:865.

Rader DJ, Ikewaki K. 1996. Unravelling high density lipoprotein-apolipoprotein metabolism in human mutants and animal models. *Curr Opin Lipidol* 1996;7:117–123.

Scriver CR, Beaudet AL, Sly WS, et al., eds. *The metabolic bases of inherited disease,* sixth ed. New York: McGraw-Hill, 1989.

Sempos CT, Cleeman JI, Carroll MD, et al. Prevalence of high blood cholesterol among US adults. *JAMA* 1993;269:3009.

Tall AR. Plasma high density lipoproteins. Metabolism and relationship to atherogenesis. *J Clin Invest* 1990;86:379–384.

Tybaerg-Hansen AT, Humphries SE. Familial defective apolipoprotein B-100: a single mutation that causes hypercholesterolemia and premature coronary artery disease. *Atherosclerosis* 1992;96:91.

Kelley's Textbook of Internal Medicine, fourth edition. Edited by H. David Humes. Lippincott Williams & Wilkins, Philadelphia © 2000.

C H A P T E R

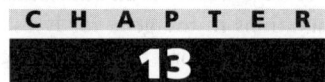

13

PATHOGENESIS OF ATHEROSCLEROSIS

ALAN M. FOGELMAN
FRANKLIN L. MURPHY
PETER A. EDWARDS

■ LESION DEVELOPMENT

The earliest morphologic change in the development of most atherosclerotic lesions is the appearance of mononuclear cells at sites that are destined to become lesions. At least 90% of these cells are blood monocytes. They diapedese between endothelial cells and come to rest in the subendothelial space. Here they convert to macrophages and accumulate lipid droplets rich in cholesteryl esters. Because of the high lipid content, their cytoplasm has a foamy appearance in histologic sections—hence the name *foam cells.* The number of these cells markedly increases in the subendothelial space and deforms the overlying endothelium. With time the endothelial monolayer may develop microscopic separations between cells that expose the underlying foam cells and extracellular matrix. These exposed areas serve as sites of platelet adherence, aggregation, and release.

Mitogenic substances from platelets (e.g., platelet-derived growth factor), endothelial cells, and monocytes stimulate the proliferation of smooth muscle cells that migrate into the subendothelial space. As cells die, their cytoplasmic contents are released, and together with plasma-derived lipoproteins the lipid-rich extracellular matrix increases in size. The cellular and extracellular components are continuously replaced in the subendothelial space, and some foam cells migrate back into the bloodstream. The expanding lesion pushes out from the subendothelial space to the adventitia. In some species, including humans, a compensatory hypertrophy of the artery wall allows further expansion toward the adventitia. If the process continues unabated, however, eventually outward expansion is no longer possible and encroachment on the lumen begins.

The spatial nature of this process is clinically important because it means that normal angiograms may be seen in subjects with extensive lesions that have not yet produced luminal narrowing. It is not rare to see patients with an essentially normal angiogram a year before an angiogram showing extensive three-vessel luminal narrowing. Presumably, the process was present extensively at the time of the first angiogram but was confined to the artery wall. In some cases, the episode of chest pain that led to the first angiogram was induced by vasospasm at the site of such an intramural lesion.

Evidence suggests that the atherosclerotic process impairs the normal ability of the artery wall to generate endothelial-derived relaxing factors. Consequently, instead of the normal response (dilatation) to various stimuli (e.g., exercise), the atherosclerotic artery contracts. Subsequently, in the course of only 1 or 2 years, such intramural lesions may expand into the lumen, particularly in hyperlipidemic subjects.

As the lesion develops, its character can change. Many early lesions contain only macrophage foam cells. These are called fatty streaks and do not cause luminal narrowing. Many fatty streaks do not progress. At predictable sites in the arterial tree, however, these lesions can develop a fibrous cap, and prominent smooth muscle proliferation may occur. Advanced lesions contain a necrotic lipid core and proteins that are associated with calcification. Neovascularization of some advanced lesions is quite extensive, being derived from the adventitia. Thus, in the same subject one can see a wide spectrum of lesions. Some lesions are rich in lipids and others are lipid-poor; some are macrophage-rich and others have only a rare macrophage, and smooth muscle cells are the dominant cell type. Still other lesions are largely acellular. The picture may depend on the stage of lesion development or may even represent different mechanisms of lesion development. Some atherosclerotic plaques contain genetic material similar to oncogenes that may induce a clonal growth of smooth muscle cells; in such lesions, smooth muscle cells would predominate.

More than 90% of all myocardial infarctions are caused by the formation of a thrombus at the site of an atherosclerotic lesion. Most myocardial infarctions occur with clot formation at sites that were narrowed less than that necessary to obstruct flow before the acute event (the average luminal narrowing in infarct arteries is about 50% to 55%). Thrombus formation usually occurs at sites of plaque rupture. Most plaques that rupture are in segments that contain arterial calcification, and the rupture occurs in the shoulder region at the site of intense monocyte infiltration. Arterial calcification has been found to occur as a result of the induction of the same set of genes as those induced in bone formation. Indeed, the calcification that results often cannot be distinguished from bone and may even include bone marrow. Oxidized sterols and transforming growth factor β seem capable of inducing a subset of artery wall cells to undergo osteoblastic differentiation and form bone. As a result of the presence of bone in the lesion, very high shear stress develops at the shoulders of the lesion at sites of inflammation, where monocyte-macrophages release enzymes that destroy the normal arterial matrix. These areas rupture and expose the flowing blood to tissue factor that normally is expressed only in the adventitia but is expressed in atherosclerotic lesions in the intima and media. The result is thrombus formation.

If the thrombus completely occludes the vessel lumen, an infarction occurs, unless collaterals are present to sustain viability. If the thrombus is only partially occlusive, it may contribute to unstable angina, and it can later be incorporated into the plaque, causing further narrowing of the lumen. Unstable angina results from the formation of platelet aggregates at these sites. The aggregates grow and obstruct flow, causing pain and electrocardiographic changes. In unstable angina, however, the platelet plug is washed away before thrombosis is completed, thus averting a myocardial infarction.

ROLE OF LIPIDS AND LIPOPROTEINS

It is rare to find a patient with clinically important atherosclerosis without at least one of the following: a low-density lipoprotein (LDL) cholesterol concentration above 120 mg per dL; a high-density lipoprotein (HDL) cholesterol concentration below 40 mg per dL; triglyceride values above 175 mg per dL on fasting; and a lipoprotein(a) [(Lp(a)] concentration above 30 mg per dL. Occasionally, patients have clinically important atherosclerosis without one of these findings, but almost always, upon questioning, it is learned that the patient has changed his or her diet and lost weight before referral but shortly before or after the onset of symptoms. The mechanisms by which these lipid abnormalities participate in the pathogenesis of atherosclerosis is an area of intense investigation.

Low-density lipoproteins are cholesteryl ester–rich lipoproteins that contain a large protein designated apolipoprotein B-100 (apoB-100). This protein is synthesized in the liver and has a molecular weight of about 500 kd. The gene for this protein has been isolated and sequenced. Portions of this protein mediate the binding of LDL to heparin and to the LDL receptor. Predictably, abnormalities in this protein are being recognized as causes of hypercholesterolemia because of changes in the receptor-binding domain. In most persons with atherosclerosis, LDL binds normally to normal LDL receptors. The concentration of apoB at sites of the arterial tree where lesions are predictably found is substantially greater than the plasma concentration, indicating an accumulation of this protein at these sites. It appears that arterial LDL accumulates at these sites because of an interaction between the extracellular components of the artery wall, such as proteoglycans and glycosaminoglycans that bind LDL. Injection of LDL into a normal rabbit's femoral vein resulted in accumulation of the LDL in the subendothelial space within hours. Ultrastructural studies demonstrated that the LDL was intimately associated with the matrix molecules that constitute the subendothelial space. This indicates that LDL can cross an intact endothelium and bind to the extracellular matrix. The trapped LDL appears to be seeded with oxidative waste products from the artery wall cells. As a consequence, an oxidized phospholipid is generated that induces the expression of the genes and proteins for an endothelial binding protein that binds monocytes but not neutrophils or lymphocytes. This oxidized phospholipid also induces the artery wall cells to express the genes and proteins for monocyte chemoattractant protein 1 (MCP-1) and macrophage colony-stimulating factor (M-CSF). As a result, monocytes bind to the endothelium, migrate down the MCP-1 gradient, and, under the influence of M-CSF, convert to macrophages. The macrophages release oxidative waste and oxidative enzymes that convert the mildly oxidized LDL to highly oxidized LDL. The mildly oxidized LDL is recognized by the normal LDL receptor; the highly oxidized LDL is not but is recognized by scavenger receptors and possibly an oxidized LDL receptor. In contrast to the LDL receptor, these latter receptors are not regulated by the cell's cholesterol content, and the accumulation of cholesterol characteristic of foam cells occurs.

In contrast to LDLs, high-density lipoproteins (HDLs) have no apoB and are not substantially concentrated in the artery wall. The strong inverse relation between HDL levels and atherosclerosis has been thought to be due to the role of HDL in reverse cholesterol transport. Although this hypothesis has many attractive features, it is not proven, and the inverse relation of HDL cholesterol levels to atherosclerosis may be the result of unrelated factors. Some HDL particles (1% to 10%) carry enzymes capable of destroying oxidized lipids; it may be that the content of these enzymes is critical to the protective effect of HDL. Another possibility relates to the formation of HDL during the lipolysis of intestinally derived lipoproteins. High-density lipoproteins are formed as a by-product during the lipolysis of chylomicrons by the enzyme lipoprotein lipase. Thus, in some subjects, low levels of HDL simply may reflect impaired lipolysis. Such subjects have low HDL cholesterol levels and high triglyceride levels. The accelerated atherosclerosis frequently seen in such persons may not be due to a failure of reverse cholesterol transport as much as it is due to the accumulation of chylomicron remnants.

Chylomicrons contain apoB-48. This protein derives from the same gene as apoB-100. However, apoB-48 is synthesized only in the intestine and not to any significant extent in the liver of humans.

In the intestine, an RNA-editing mechanism results in a single nucleotide substitution in the mRNA for apoB, producing a stop codon that results in a truncated protein. This truncated protein contains only 48% of the amino acids found in apoB-100 and hence is known as apoB-48. The truncated protein contains the amino-terminal portion of apoB-100 but lacks the portion necessary for recognition by the LDL receptor. These intestinally derived lipoproteins, however, become enriched in another apolipoprotein that is recognized by the LDL receptor apoE. Apolipoprotein E is recognized by both the LDL receptor and a receptor on liver cells that does not recognize apoB-100.

Normally, these particles are acted on by lipoprotein lipase as the particles circulate through the heart and adipose tissue, where lipoprotein lipase is abundant. The resulting triglyceride-depleted remnants are cleared rapidly in normal subjects by hepatic receptors. Under conditions of impaired lipolysis, however, the metabolism of these particles is slowed, and the remnant lipoproteins can be found even in fasting plasma. Many diabetics are prone to accumulate such chylomicron remnants in their plasma. Considerable evidence suggests that these chylomicron remnants are atherogenic. Thus, the failure of lipolysis in these diabetics results in low HDL levels and the presence of circulating atherogenic particles.

In patients with type III hyperlipoproteinemia (also known as broad β disease), single amino acid substitutions have been found in both alleles of apoE that result in defective binding of the remnant lipoproteins to the E receptor and to the LDL receptor. Consequently, these subjects accumulate remnant particles in their plasma. A required cofactor for lipoprotein lipase is an apolipoprotein designated apoC-II. Homozygotes lacking this apolipoprotein have been found to have impaired lipolysis that is corrected by infusion of apoC-II.

Another lipoprotein that has been associated with increased risk for atherosclerosis is Lp(a). This lipoprotein contains a full copy of apoB-100 that is linked by a disulfide bridge to a remarkable duplication of portions of plasminogen. This lipoprotein contains 37 copies of kringle 4 and one copy of kringle 5 of plasminogen. However, the protease domain differs from plasminogen in such a way that it cannot become proteolytically active on exposure to tissue plasminogen activator. However, Lp(a) competes with plasminogen for the plasminogen binding site with similar affinity and capacity. It has been estimated that at plasma concentrations of 30 mg per dL, plasminogen binding to endothelial cells would be reduced by 20%, thereby decreasing fibrinolysis and favoring a procoagulant state. Lp(a) is found in trace amounts in virtually everyone; it is present in high concentrations in some persons who are at high risk for atherosclerosis.

Free cholesterol exits from cells into plasma, but esterified cholesterol is found as the major form in lipoproteins. The enzyme lecithin:cholesterol acyltransferase is responsible for esterifying free cholesterol entering the plasma compartment. This esterified cholesterol is found initially in the HDL fraction. Subsequently, the esterified cholesterol is transferred to the very low density lipoprotein (VLDL) and LDL fractions by cholesteryl ester transfer proteins in plasma. Abnormalities in the distribution of cholesterol in the plasma compartment have been associated with premature atherosclerosis, particularly in diabetics and in patients on hemodialysis.

Although almost all cells can synthesize cholesterol, most of the circulating plasma cholesterol is synthesized in the liver and intestine. A series of enzymes tightly regulates cholesterol biosynthesis; central among these is 3-hydroxy-3-methylglutaryl coenzyme A (HMG-CoA) reductase. This enzyme is particularly important, as specific inhibitors such as lovastatin are clinically useful.

ROLE OF RECEPTORS

After a person eats, chylomicrons are synthesized in the intestine. These large triglyceride-rich particles are acted on by lipoprotein lipase and are metabolized through particles with the density of VLDL ($d \leq 1.006$ g per mL) to particles of intermediate density ($d = 1.006$ to 1.019 g mL). These particles, called IDLs, are derived from chylomicrons that contain both apoB-48 and apoE. The liver contains two receptors capable of removing these particles: the E receptor and the LDL receptor. The former recognizes apoE; the latter apoB and apoE. After receiving these particles, the liver secretes triglyceride-rich particles that are found in the VLDLs. Unlike those derived from intestinal chylomicrons, these VLDLs contain apoB-100 but not apoB-48.

These hepatic VLDLs are metabolized by lipoprotein lipase to particles in the IDL class, which in turn are converted to LDL ($d = 1.019$ to 1.063 g per mL) by an unknown mechanism that may involve hepatic triglyceride lipase. All of the apoB-100 lipoproteins—VLDL, IDL, and LDL—are recognized and cleared by the hepatic LDL receptor. The apoE receptor appears to be closely related to the LDL receptor. Additionally, there appears to be a VLDL receptor.

In patients with a severe deficiency of the LDL receptor (familial hypercholesterolemia homozygotes), there is some accumulation of remnant particles and a marked accumulation of LDL. The latter results in part because the lack of LDL receptors allows that fraction of VLDL normally cleared by the liver to accumulate, enhancing conversion of VLDL to LDL. Patients with heterozygous familial hypercholesterolemia have one normal and one abnormal LDL receptor allele, resulting in half the number of functional LDL receptors; thus, plasma LDL concentrations are roughly twice normal. Treatment of such patients with bile-sequestering agents or an HMG-CoA reductase inhibitor results in depletion of hepatocyte cholesterol pools. Consequently, there is a compensatory increase in hepatic LDL receptors mediated by the normal allele. This mechanism is largely responsible for the clinical utility of the bile-sequestering agents. Unfortunately, these agents also induce a compensatory increase in the rate-controlling enzymes in the cholesterol biosynthetic pathway (e.g., HMG-CoA reductase), and in more than 50% of cases the plasma LDL concentration returns to

normal after a year's treatment. The addition of a specific agent to block cholesterol biosynthesis (e.g., lovastatin, which blocks HMG-CoA reductase) prevents the compensatory increase in cholesterol biosynthesis and contributes to the induction of hepatic LDL receptors. The combination of a bile-sequestering agent and lovastatin is thus very effective in lowering LDL levels.

The conversion of monocyte-macrophages in the artery wall to foam cells depends on the uptake of cholesterol from plasma lipoproteins. Most lipoprotein cholesterol is carried as the esterified form. After endocytosis, these cholesteryl esters are hydrolyzed and the free cholesterol is re-esterified in the endoplasmic reticulum by the enzyme acyl coenzyme A:cholesterol acyltransferase. Normally, human monocyte-macrophages contain little cholesteryl ester (about 2% of total cellular cholesterol). In foam cells, however, more than half the cellular cholesterol is esterified. Human monocyte-macrophages have normal LDL receptors, but as is the case with LDL receptors elsewhere, these are tightly regulated by the cellular cholesterol content. As the level of cellular cholesterol rises, the synthesis of LDL receptors decreases and the synthesis of the rate-limiting enzymes in cholesterol biosynthesis (e.g., HMG-CoA reductase) also is decreased. Thus, the cell is protected from cholesterol accumulation. Moreover, patients who are receptor-negative (have no detectable LDL receptor) accumulate massive amounts of cholesterol in the monocyte-macrophages of their artery walls.

In the Watanabe heritable hyperlipidemic (WHHL) rabbit, a hypolipidemic agent with antioxidant properties (probucol) has been shown to retard the development of atherosclerosis in the aorta. Moreover, direct examination of the atherosclerotic lesions of these animals disclosed apoB-100, which had been modified by products of lipid peroxidation. The acetyl LDL receptor (or scavenger receptor) is found on macrophages and endothelial cells, but not on smooth muscle cells or fibroblasts. Another high-affinity process for internalizing cholesterol-rich particles is the LDL–dextran sulfate pathway. The LDL complexed to high molecular weight dextran is internalized, causing massive cholesterol accumulation in macrophages. The dextran sulfate pathway may have relevance to LDL bound to proteoglycans or glycosaminoglycans in the artery wall.

Previously it was thought that a macrophage receptor genetically distinct from the LDL receptor recognized β-VLDL (cholesterol ester–rich VLDL found in cholesterol-fed animals and in patients with type III hyperlipoproteinemia). Evidence now suggests that this receptor is immunologically similar, if not identical, to the LDL receptor. Chylomicron remnants and β-VLDL are taken up in cholesterol-loaded human monocyte-macrophages by a lower affinity, high-capacity process—in contrast to LDL, which is taken up by a high-affinity, low-capacity process. Diabetics have increased levels of various glycosylated proteins (e.g., hemoglobin Alc). They also have glycosylated LDL, and some diabetics have antibodies to these glycosylated proteins. In such subjects, LDL–antibody complexes may be taken up by the Fc receptor on human monocyte-macrophages. This receptor is not regulated by cellular cholesterol levels, and consequently this pathway could mediate the cholesteryl ester accumulation seen in arterial foam cells in some diabetics.

Smooth muscle cells also can become foam cells. Although they have a normal LDL receptor pathway, they do not have separate pathways for modified lipoproteins and for remnants. In vitro it has been shown that the cholesteryl ester droplets released from macrophages after they were loaded by the scavenger receptor pathway could be taken up by smooth muscle cells. Presumably, phagocytosis by smooth muscle cells of the lipid droplets released from dying macrophages in the artery wall could explain the origin of smooth muscle cell foam cells.

GENETIC PREDISPOSITION TO ATHEROSCLEROSIS

On average, patients with myocardial infarction are age 65 years or older. Only about 20% of all infarcts occur in patients under age 60 years. Many of these patients have a genetic abnormality in lipid metabolism; indeed, about two-thirds of those with myocardial infarction at age 55 or younger have such a genetic disorder. Abnormalities in HDL levels are common. A rare but informative mutation results in an abnormality in apolipoproteins A-1 and C-III. This is due to an inversion in the DNA sequences for these two proteins, whose genes are adjacent to each other. As a consequence of this mutation, tendon xanthomas, corneal clouding, and severe atherosclerosis result, with total cholesterol levels of less than 200 mg per dL and HDL cholesterol concentrations of less than 10 mg per dL. Early results suggest that restriction fragment length polymorphisms for apoB are also associated with premature coronary atherosclerosis.

Several other disorders are also commonly associated with premature atherosclerosis. Familial hypercholesterolemia is the best understood of the metabolic disorders associated with premature atherosclerosis. This autosomal dominant disorder occurs in both humans and rabbits. Four basic defects in the gene for the LDL receptor have been identified. In some patients, no functional receptor protein or receptor mRNA is observed. These *null* mutants presumably have deletions, insertions, or other mutations in the LDL receptor gene that prevent expression of the receptor. One such abnormality has been recognized as being caused by a 5-kilobase deletion that joins a coding sequence in exon 13 to an *Alu* repetitive element in intron 15. A second defect results in an abnormal protein that is slowly processed in the Golgi apparatus, and 95% of the receptors are destroyed before they can be carried to the cell surface. This defect has been found in the WHHL rabbit and is due to a deletion in the cysteine-rich, ligand-binding domain of the LDL receptor. A third class of defects results from mutations that allow receptor insertion into the cell membrane, but with abnormal receptor binding of ligands. In one family, a deletion due to homologous recombination between repetitive *Alu* sequences in introns 4 and 5 of the LDL receptor gene resulted in a receptor that binds apoE normally but does not bind apoB. This mutant receptor thus binds β-VLDL but not LDL. The fourth class of mutations results in receptors that are inserted into the membrane and can bind LDL normally; however, due to a defect in the cytoplasmic tail of the receptor, the receptor fails to cluster in coated pits. In these mutants there is normal binding of ligand, but there is an abnormality in internalization of the LDL receptor complex into the cell.

Homozygous or compound heterozygous familial hypercholesterolemia is rare, with fewer than 100 cases identified in the United States. In these subjects, LDL levels are elevated at birth and typically are 600 to 1,000 mg of LDL cholesterol per milliliter. These children have palmar, tuberous, and tendon xanthomas, as well as a form of supravalvular aortic stenosis that results from a xanthomatous deposit distal to the aortic valve. They have coronary artery disease and often die before age 20 when left untreated. Treatment includes plasmapheresis, portacaval shunt, and, rarely, liver transplant.

The heterozygous form of familial hypercholesterolemia is common, occurring in as many as 1 in 500 births. About half of affected families have at least one family member with tendon xanthomas. These xanthomas are diagnostic when present, but their absence does not exclude the disease. Typically, LDL cholesterol levels are about twice normal in heterozygotes. The average age for myocardial infarction in male heterozygotes is 40 to 45, and it is 55 years for female heterozygotes unless they smoke cigarettes. Female heterozygotes who smoke have their first infarcts a decade earlier than those who do not. The protective state of the female gender is common to most forms of atherosclerosis, but the cause for this advantage is not well understood. Of particular clinical interest is the high incidence of left main coronary artery disease in patients with familial hypercholesterolemia: about 40% have left main lesions by their fourth decade. This extraordinarily high incidence is not well understood. The treatment of heterozygous familial hypercholesterolemia generally includes a bile-sequestering agent together with niacin or lovastatin.

Nongenetic causes of altered LDL receptor activity are common and probably are important in many cases of hypercholesterolemia and atherosclerosis. Feeding saturated fat decreases LDL receptor activity and increases plasma LDL levels. Hypothyroidism can be associated with a deficiency of LDL receptor activity that mimics homozygous familial hypercholesterolemia; it is reversible with thyroid hormone replacement.

Familial combined hyperlipidemia is an autosomal dominant disorder that has incomplete penetrance in childhood. By age 30, half the members of affected families have hyperlipidemia and the other half are normolipidemic. About one-third of affected family members have elevated cholesterol levels, one-third have elevated triglyceride levels, and another third have both elevated cholesterol and triglyceride levels. Moreover, a person may have one type of abnormality at one time and another type at a later time. Because of this variability, the disorder has also been called *multiple lipoprotein phenotypes*. Tendon xanthomas are not seen. This common disorder is present in up to 1% of the population. The average age of myocardial infarction ranges from 35 to 55 years, depending on the family. No specific cause has been identified, but many affected persons have elevated apoB levels, regardless of whether their cholesterol or triglyceride levels are elevated. Patients with this disorder are sensitive to excess weight. They often appear not to be overweight when in fact they are. For example, a patient may present who is sedentary, is 5 feet 11 inches tall, and weighs 175 pounds at age 50. On taking a history, it is learned that maximal height was achieved by age 18, and at age 22, when he played college basketball, he only weighed 145 pounds. This person thus weighs 30 pounds more than he did at the same height at a time when he was physically fit. Reduction in weight to lean body mass often results in a marked improvement in the metabolic abnormality and even a complete return of lipid levels to normal. In subjects who do not reduce their weight to lean body mass or who do not correct with weight loss, the use of niacin is often helpful in correcting the metabolic abnormality. In some patients, omega-3 fatty acids decrease VLDL levels by suppressing apoB synthesis. This is not the case in all subjects, and careful monitoring is needed.

Type III hyperlipoproteinemia, or broad β disease, is a rare disorder associated with premature peripheral vascular disease and premature coronary artery disease. This disorder is clinically manifested by xanthomas (palmar, tuberous, or tendon), which are found in 75% of patients. A requirement for this disorder is the homozygous apoE2 phenotype (E2:E2). This occurs in about 1 in 100 persons, and yet the clinical disorder of type III hyperlipoproteinemia occurs in no more than 1 in 5,000 persons. Because of amino acid substitutions (usually a single amino acid), apoE in E2:E2 homozygotes binds poorly to the E receptor and poorly to the LDL receptor. Consequently, remnant particles accumulate that are rich in cholesteryl esters (β-VLDL). Most E2:E2 persons are normolipidemic or even hypolipidemic. All have some increase in remnant particles and low LDL levels, however, because of a block in the normal metabolism of hepatic VLDL to LDL. This suggests that apoE binding may be important in hepatic triglyceride lipase conversion of IDL to LDL, as well as in the removal of apoB-48 intestinally derived particles. Clinically significant hyperlipidemia is associated with this disorder when the person gains weight, becomes diabetic, or becomes hypothyroid. These patients are very sensitive to weight reduction and also respond favorably to therapy with niacin. Some female patients also respond to estrogen treatment for reasons that are not entirely clear.

TREATMENT STRATEGIES

A discussion of profiling patients with lipid disorders is presented in Chapter 31. Several general tenets of therapy can be deduced based on the pathogenesis of atherosclerosis. As the pathogenesis becomes better understood, more rational and specific therapies should become available.

The strong link between abnormalities in lipid metabolism and premature atherosclerosis has led to vigorous treatment of lipid abnormalities in patients with a history of atherosclerosis or in patients who are genetically at high risk. Such patients should be treated with dietary modifications, exercise, and, if necessary, hypolipidemic agents. The introduction of specific inhibitors of HMG-CoA reductase, such as lovastatin, has appreciably increased the means of treating hypercholesterolemia. These agents are competitive inhibitors of the major rate-controlling enzyme in cholesterol biosynthesis. They are well tolerated and have few major side effects, other than in a rare to occasional patient who develops elevated levels of liver or muscle enzymes. Lovastatin often lowers plasma cholesterol levels by one-third. When used in combination with a bile-sequestering agent such as cholestyramine, plasma cholesterol levels often are halved. Numerous angiographic studies have demonstrated that vigorously lowering lipids (i.e., lowering LDL cholesterol levels to less than 100 mg per dL and raising HDL levels as much as possible) produces a profound decrease in the number of clinical events without changing the luminal diameter appreciably. Presumably, lowering LDL levels decreases the substrate for the oxidized lipids that induce the continued inflammatory response. With a reduction in the monocyte- macrophage content of the lesions, the lesions stabilize and plaque rupture is averted. Many would argue that all patients who have a myocardial infarction, angioplasty, or coronary artery bypass grafting should be put on LDL-lowering drugs regardless of their initial LDL levels. Because smoking accelerates clinical atherosclerotic events, such patients should be strongly urged to abstain from smoking.

Because platelets play a role in the development and consequences of atherosclerosis, consideration should be given to treating these patients with antiplatelet agents (e.g., aspirin). Epidemiologic evidence suggests that omega-3 fatty acids protect against atherosclerotic events, and some in vitro evidence suggests that omega-3 fatty acids decrease monocyte adherence to endothelial cells. Omega-3 fatty acids prolong the bleeding time. Based on these relatively weak data, it may be reasonable to encourage the use of omega-3 fatty acids in some subjects. In these patients, however, it is important to monitor HDL and LDL levels, as in some patients omega-3 fatty acid feeding leads to a decrease in HDL and an increase in LDL levels.

The reader should refer to Chapters 12 and 29.

BIBLIOGRAPHY

Berliner JA, Navab M, Fogelman AM, et al. Atherosclerosis: basic mechanisms. Oxidation, inflammation, and genetics. *Circulation* 1995;91: 2488.

Brown MS, Goldstein JL. A receptor-mediated pathway for cholesterol homeostasis. *Science* 1986;232:34.

Demer LL, Watson KE, Bostrom K. Mechanism of calcification in atherosclerosis. *Trends Cardiovasc Med* 1994;4:45.

Fuster V, Dadimon L, Badimon JJ, et al. The pathogenesis of coronary artery disease and the acute coronary syndromes. *N Engl J Med* 1992; 326:242.

Lusis AJ, Navab M. Lipoprotein oxidation and gene expression in the artery wall. New opportunities for pharmacologic intervention in atherosclerosis. *Biochem Pharmacol* 1993;46:2119.

Mahley RW. Apolipoprotein E: cholesterol transport protein with expanding role in cell biology. *Science* 1988;240:622.

Ross R. The pathogenesis of atherosclerosis: a perspective for the 1990s. *Nature* 1993;362:801.

Scott J. Lipoprotein(a): thrombogenesis linked to atherogenesis at last? *Nature* 1989;341:22.

van der Wal AC, Becker AE, van der Loos CM, et al. Site of intimal rupture or erosion of thrombosed coronary atherosclerotic plaques is characterized by an inflammatory process irrespective of the dominant plaque morphology. *Circulation* 1994;89:36.

Witztum JL. The oxidation hypothesis of atherosclerosis. *Lancet* 1994;344: 793.

Kelley's Textbook of Internal Medicine, fourth edition. Edited by H. David Humes. Lippincott Williams & Wilkins, Philadelphia © 2000.

C H A P T E R
14

SOME FUNCTIONAL PATHWAYS IN THE CENTRAL NERVOUS SYSTEM

JOHN A. KIERNAN

This chapter reviews the major central pathways for control of movement, somatic sensation, consciousness, memory, and emotion. The localization of functions in the cerebral cortex is also summarized. An understanding of functional connections in the central nervous system (CNS) is needed for the diagnosis of many neurologic disorders.

DESCENDING MOTOR PATHWAYS

The contractions and relaxations of muscles result in movements that occur voluntarily (willed movements) and subconsciously (automatic movements). Even the most skilled movements include major automatic components because the conscious brain does not deliberately stimulate or inhibit individual muscles.

The cells that innervate skeletal muscles are known singly as motor neurons and collectively as "the lower motor neuron." They are in the ventral horn of the spinal gray matter and in the motor nuclei of most of the cranial nerves. The following account applies to the control of motor neurons in the spinal cord and is applicable in modified form to movements mediated by cranial nerves V, VII, IX, X, XI, and XII. Motor neurons do not fire spontaneously; consequently, muscles can contract only when their pathways are intact. The axons that synapse with the dendrites and perikarya of motor neurons are (a) primary sensory fibers, principally proprioceptive, from the dorsal roots; (b) some fibers of some of the descending tracts; and (c) spinal interneurons that fire in response to activity in primary afferents and descending tracts. When motor neurons are deprived of the influence of the descending tracts, they respond excessively to segmental proprioceptive stimulation. A stretch reflex is continuously in operation, so that the muscles are spastic. Contractions in response to additional stretch (the tendon jerk reflexes) or painful stimulation of the limb (withdrawal reflexes) are exaggerated. Movements other than those resulting from spinal reflexes cannot be made.

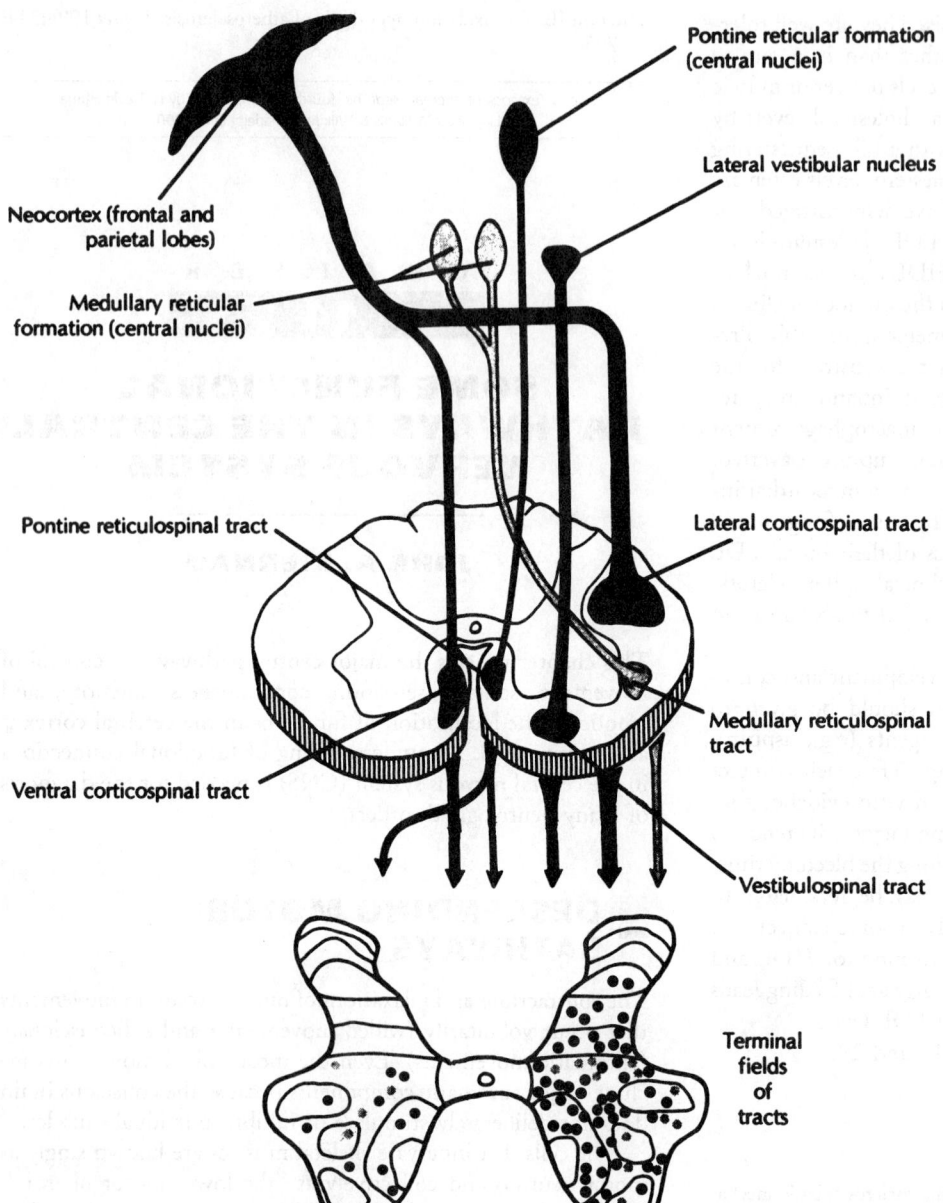

Pontine reticular formation (central nuclei)

Lateral vestibular nucleus

Neocortex (frontal and parietal lobes)

Medullary reticular formation (central nuclei)

Pontine reticulospinal tract

Lateral corticospinal tract

Ventral corticospinal tract

Medullary reticulospinal tract

Vestibulospinal tract

Terminal fields of tracts

FIGURE 14.1. Descending motor tracts in the spinal cord. (From Kiernan JA. *Barr's The Human Nervous System,* seventh ed. Philadelphia: Lippincott-Raven, 1998, with permission.)

In humans, three major motor pathways project from the brain to the spinal cord (Fig. 14.1). Equivalent projections exist for the motor nuclei of cranial nerves V, VII, IX, X, XI, and XII. (The rubrospinal and tectospinal tracts, once considered important, are now believed to be virtually nonexistent in the human CNS. There are also pathways, not considered here, for controlling the oculomotor nuclei, and there are descending tracts that are not concerned with the activities of motor neurons.)

CORTICOSPINAL OR PYRAMIDAL TRACT

The largest descending tract in the spinal cord arises from an area of cortex that extends from the premotor area of the frontal lobe across the central sulcus to the postcentral and nearby gyri. The fibers pass through the posterior limb of the internal capsule into the basis pedunculi of the midbrain. From there, the tract passes through the ventral part of the pons into the medullary pyramids. Most of the pyramidal fibers decussate at the lower end of the medulla. The crossed axons descend in the dorsal half of the lateral funiculus of spinal white matter, whereas the uncrossed axons remain near the ventral sulcus of the cord. In a few persons, most of the pyramidal fibers are uncrossed. The uncrossed corticospinal fibers eventually decussate at segmental levels before terminating in the spinal gray matter alongside the crossed tract. Axons from the somatosensory areas of the parietal lobe end in the dorsal horn, and most of the fibers from the primary motor and premotor areas end in contact with interneurons in the intermediate gray matter. A few pyramidal axons synapse directly with the cell bodies and larger dendrites of motor neurons.

Investigation of those rare cases in which the human pyramidal tract has been selectively transected in the midbrain or medulla confirms experimental studies in monkeys. Such lesions cause a flaccid hemiparesis that, on recovery, leaves residual weakness that is largely confined to the hands. Similar but more localized changes follow small lesions in the primary motor area of the cerebral cortex. The normal function of the motor component of the corticospinal pathway is therefore presumed to be performing skilled (least automatic) movements that need some direct control from the highest levels of the neuraxis. The classical upper motor neuron spastic paralysis results from interruption of more than just the pyramidal system. Lesions involving the premotor cortex cause paresis of muscles that work on the shoulder and hip joints, indicating that a major function of the premotor area may be to bring the distal parts of the limbs into position for the performance of skilled tasks.

RETICULOSPINAL TRACTS

Neurons in the central group of nuclei of the reticular formation give rise to the axons constituting the medullary reticulospinal tract (in the lateral white matter of the spinal cord) and the pontine reticulospinal tract (in the ventral spinal white matter). These tracts terminate bilaterally in the spinal gray matter. Studies in laboratory animals indicate that these pathways mediate control over most movements that do not require dexterity or the maintenance of balance. The central nuclei of the reticular formation receive projections from the spinal cord, the cerebellum, the hypothalamus, and the premotor area of the cerebral cortex. Some parts of the reticular formation serve as pattern generators for frequently performed movements, including those of respiration and locomotion.

The reticulospinal tracts may mediate much of the normal inhibition of spinal reflexes, and spastic paralysis may result from transection either of the tracts themselves or of the fibers that descend through the internal capsule to the reticular formation.

VESTIBULOSPINAL TRACTS

The large neurons of the lateral vestibular nucleus (of Deiters) are in the floor of the lateral part of the fourth ventricle, at the rostral end of the medulla. Their axons descend in the ventral white matter of the cord and end ipsilaterally in the medial zone of the ventral horn among neurons that supply the axial trunk musculature and the postural muscles of the lower limbs. The neurons in Deiters' nucleus, which are driven by the sensory signals from the vestibular nerve, cause contraction of extensors and relaxation of the opposing flexors. Consequently, unilateral destruction of the vestibular labyrinth causes a tendency to fall to the side of the lesion, due to unopposed stimulation of the contralateral antigravity muscles. The vestibular nuclei do not receive descending afferents from the cerebrum.

The motor cortex of the frontal lobe should not be thought of as a command center for willed movements but as part of a larger system. Afferent fibers come to the motor areas from the other cortical regions and from the ventral lateral nucleus of the thalamus. This thalamic nucleus receives the output of the basal ganglia and the cerebellum.

PATHWAYS NECESSARY FOR MOTOR COORDINATION

The parts of the CNS most conspicuously concerned with the production of orderly movement are the basal ganglia and the cerebellum.

BASAL GANGLIA

To the physiologist or clinician, the basal ganglia comprise the corpus striatum (caudate nucleus, putamen, and globus pallidus), the subthalamic nucleus (or corpus Luysii), and the two parts (compacta and reticulata) of the substantia nigra. These structures are in the base of the cerebral hemisphere and nearby parts of the diencephalon and midbrain. Functionally, the system has five components. The striatum consists of the caudate nucleus and the putamen. The lateral pallidum is the lateral division of the globus pallidus. The medial pallidum consists of the medial division of the globus pallidus together with the pars reticulata of the substantia nigra. The other two components are the subthalamic nucleus and the substantia nigra pars compacta. These regions, which are connected with one another and with the thalamus, cerebral cortex, and other parts of the brain, are involved in the automatic execution of learned movements and probably also in cognitive functions. Destruction of neuronal populations in this system results in abnormalities of movement known as dyskinesias. The effects of the basal ganglia on movement are mediated principally through descending pathways from the motor areas of the cerebral cortex, and they affect the contralateral musculature.

The principal connections of the basal ganglia are summarized in Figure 14.2. There it can be seen that the inputs are excitatory, with glutamate as the probable transmitter: first from the whole cerebral cortex to the striatum, second from the intralaminar thalamic nuclei to the striatum, and third from the motor cortical areas to the subthalamic nucleus. The output consists of inhibitory neurons, with their somata in the medial pallidum, which use γ- aminobutyric acid (GABA) as their transmitter. The largest pathway from the medial pallidum is to the anterior division of the ventrolateral nucleus of the thalamus, which projects to the premotor and supplementary motor areas of the cerebral cortex. Thus, the cortex and the basal ganglia can modulate the activity of a large proportion of the motor fibers of the pyramidal system and of the corticoreticulospinal pathway. Pallidal efferents go also to the superior colliculus, the intralaminar thalamic nuclei, and the pedunculopontine nucleus in the reticular formation of the brain stem. The superior colliculus is concerned with the control of eye movements. The intralaminar thalamic nuclei and pedunculopontine nucleus have connections with many parts of the brain and may provide links between the basal ganglia and pathways for consciousness and

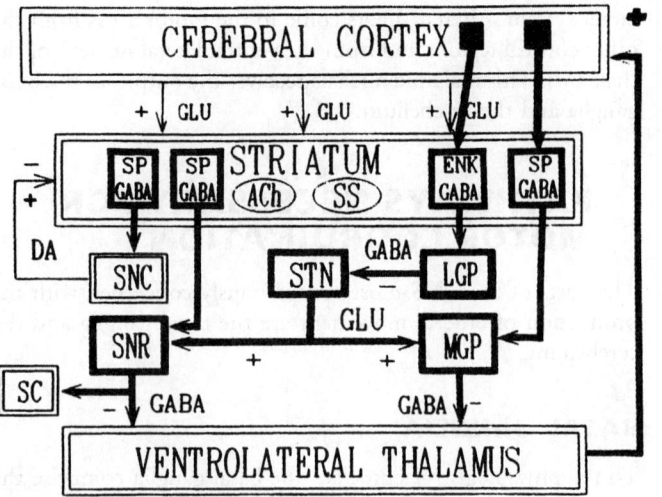

FIGURE 14.2. Connections of the basal ganglia. Shows excitatory (+) and inhibitory (−) synapses and probable neurotransmitters. LGP, lateral pallidum; MGP, medial pallidum; SC, superior colliculus; SNC, substantia nigra pars compacta; SNR, substantia nigra pars reticulata; STN, subthalamic nucleus; ACh, acetylcholine; DA, dopamine; ENK, enkephalins; GABA, γ-aminobutyric acid; GLU, glutamate; SP, substance P; SS, somatostatin. (From Albin RL, Young AB, Penney JB. Functional anatomy of basal ganglia disorders. *Trends Neurosci* 1989;12:366, with permission.)

sensation. Many other known connections of the basal ganglia are not shown in Figure 14.2.

The striatum contains two populations of principal neurons, both causing inhibition at their synapses: those containing GABA and enkephalins that project to the lateral pallidum, and those containing GABA and substance P that project to the medial pallidum and to the substantia nigra pars compacta. The cells of the substantia nigra pars compacta are dopaminergic. Their best known projection is to the striatum, where the two populations of GABAergic cells respond differently to dopamine. The striatal neurons that contain substance P are excited, whereas those that contain enkephalins are inhibited. Knowledge of neurotransmitters and their actions may explain some features of disorders that result from diseases of the basal ganglia, as in the following two examples.

In *hemiballismus*, destruction of the subthalamic nucleus deprives the medial pallidum of excitatory stimuli, resulting in decreased activity of the pallidothalamic neurons and decreased inhibition of the cells in the ventrolateral nucleus of the thalamus. Excessive activity of the ventrolateral nucleus causes excessive stimulation of the premotor cortex, leading to large spontaneous movements at the proximal joints of the contralateral limbs.

In *parkinsonism*, degeneration of nigral dopaminergic neurons leads to decreased activity of striatal neurons containing substance P and increased activity of striatal neurons containing enkephalins. Both types of striatal neuron are inhibitory to pallidal cells (Fig. 14.2). Consequently, in Parkinson's disease, the neurons in the medial pallidum become more active and those in the lateral pallidum become less active. The reduced activity of the lateral pallidum permits a stronger excitatory effect of the subthalamic nucleus on the medial pallidum. The output of the

medial pallidum is therefore increased for two reasons, and the stimulation of the motor cortical areas by the thalamus is suppressed. These events account in a simple way for the reduced motor activity of the parkinsonian patient, but not for the associated tremor and rigidity.

Similar reasoning can be invoked to account for choreiform movements (fragments of learned motor patterns) after degeneration of both types of striatal principal cell in Huntington's disease, and for abnormal saccadic eye movements associated with chorea and parkinsonism.

CEREBELLUM

Some of the circuitry of the cerebellum is summarized in Figure 14.3. All parts of the cerebellum receive input from the inferior olivary complex of nuclei in the contralateral half of the medulla. The olivary nuclei receive their afferents from the motor areas of the cerebral cortex and from the red nucleus. The olivocerebellar system is thought to supply programs of instructions for movement patterns; the programs are stored in the cerebellum. Fibers that reach the cerebellum from other sources, including the vestibular nuclei, the spinal cord, and the pontine nuclei, are active when motor programs are being executed. Another source of fibers to the whole of the cerebellum is the locus ceruleus. This nucleus, in the upper brain stem, contains noradrenergic neurons with greatly branched axons that go to most parts of the CNS. They may have a general modulatory action on the whole cerebellum.

The nonolivary and non-noradrenergic cerebellar afferent fibers are not uniformly distributed. Those from the vestibular system end in the flocculus and nodule, and those from the spinal cord end ipsilaterally in the vermis (cerebellar midline) and paravermal zones. Movements for equilibration and gait, which rely on vestibular and proprioceptive input, are associated with these parts of the cerebellum. The contralateral pontine nuclei, which receive afferent fibers from most of the cerebral cortex, project to the large cerebellar hemispheres and are the source of the largest contingent of afferent fibers. The corticopontocerebellar system controls the force, extent, and timing of muscular contractions and is therefore necessary for performing skilled movements.

The functional deficits that result from damage to the cerebellum vary with the neuroanatomical subdivisions involved in the lesions. Thus, diseases affecting the parts in and around the midline, which receive vestibular and proprioceptive input, cause ataxia. More lateral lesions cause disordered motor coordination that is most pronounced when trying to make precise movements of the hands or feet.

Projections to the vestibular nuclei and the reticular formation enable the cerebellum to influence the vestibulospinal and reticulospinal pathways directly. The largest numbers of cerebellar efferent fibers course rostrally to the posterior division of the ventrolateral nucleus of the contralateral thalamus. The posterior division of the ventrolateral nucleus projects to the primary motor area of the cerebral cortex. In contrast to the cerebral cortex, basal ganglia, and thalamus, the cerebellum has its functional connections with the muscles of the same side of the body.

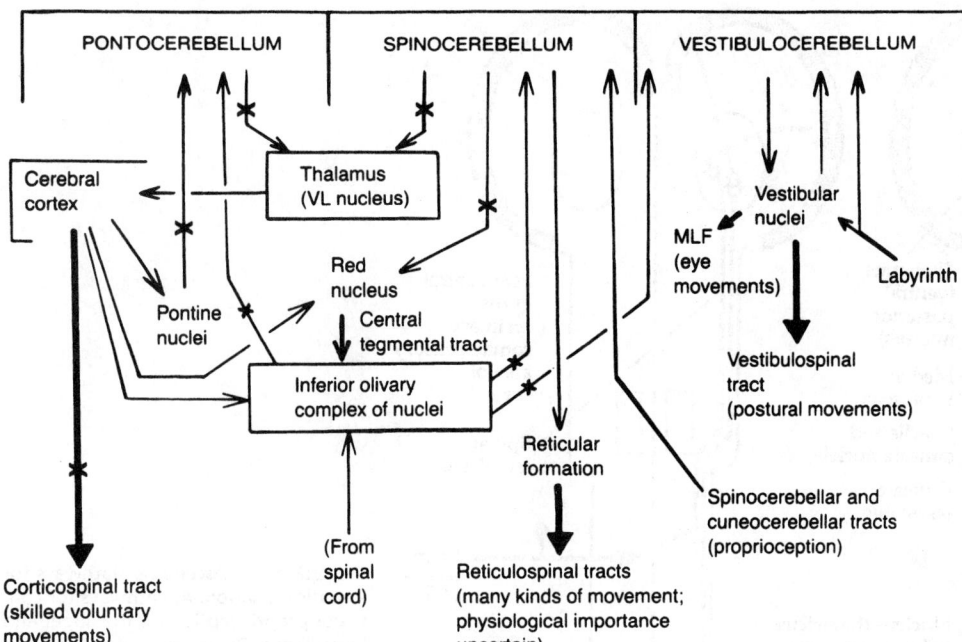

FIGURE 14.3. Major neuronal circuitry of the three functional divisions of the cerebellum. X indicates tracts that cross the midline. (From Kiernan JA. *An introduction to human neuroscience.* Philadelphia: JB Lippincott, 1987, with permission.)

PATHWAYS FOR SOMATIC SENSATION

Receptors in skin, deep connective tissue, skeletal muscle, tendons, and joints transduce mechanical, thermal, and noxious stimuli, sending ordered patterns of impulses through spinal nerves and their dorsal roots to the spinal cord and through cranial nerves to the brain stem. Somatic sensory pathways are traced from peripheral receptors to the postcentral gyrus, which is the primary somatosensory area of the contralateral cerebral cortex. Different routes, each a series of three or four populations of neurons, are followed by the pathways for different kinds of sensation. For all these pathways, the first-order neurons are unipolar, with their cell bodies in dorsal root (or cranial nerve) ganglia. The distal branches of the axons of these cells are directed peripherally, and the central branches enter the CNS. The last neuron in the series is also the same in all pathways, having its cell body and dendrites in the ventroposterior nucleus of the thalamus and an axon that passes through the posterior limb of the internal capsule before ending in the primary somatosensory area. The positions of the cell bodies and axons of the second- and (when present) third-order neurons vary according to the type of sensation.

Distinct ascending pathways exist for pain and temperature, discriminative tactile sensation, and conscious awareness of position and movement of parts of the body (proprioception; Fig. 14.4). Simple (nondiscriminative) touch is served by the pain/temperature sensation pathways. From the positions of the pathways at different levels of the neuraxis, it is possible to predict the effects of lesions on sensation:

1. The pathway for pain and temperature crosses the midline at segmental levels.
2. The pathways for discriminative touch and conscious proprioception cross the midline in the caudal part of the medulla.

3. The spinothalamic tract, for pain and temperature, ascends in the ventral half of the lateral funiculus of spinal white matter and is laterally located in the brain stem.
4. Fibers for discriminative touch ascend in the dorsal spinal white matter and in the medial lemniscus in the brain stem. The medial lemniscus is next to the midline in the medulla and caudal pons. More rostrally, this tract shifts dorsally and laterally, so that in the midbrain it is close to the spinothalamic tract.
5. There are different pathways for conscious proprioception from the upper and lower limbs (Fig. 14.4). At cervical levels, the dorsal funiculus of the spinal cord does not contain proprioceptive fibers from the lower limb.
6. The central branches of the first-order neurons in the pathway for pain and temperature originating in the face, mouth, and head (not shown in Fig. 14.4) descend into the caudal part of the medulla before ending in the spinal trigeminal nucleus. The trigeminothalamic fibers cross the midline before ascending in the trigeminal lemniscus, which is medial to the spinal lemniscus in the caudal half of the pons, and between the spinal and medial lemnisci in the rostral pons and midbrain.
7. The flow of somatosensory information from the spinal cord and brain stem is modulated by activity in descending pathways. These include the corticospinal (pyramidal) tracts; corticobulbar fibers ending in the gracile, cuneate, and trigeminal sensory nuclei; and reticulospinal fibers from various sources. Of the latter, the serotonergic raphe spinal tract from nuclei in the midline of the medulla is best known. These raphe spinal neurons, which can be activated by stimulation of the periaqueductal gray matter of the midbrain, can simulate the analgesic action of morphine and other opiates. The corticospinal and corticobulbar fibers may help to ensure that all peripheral stimuli are not consciously perceived.

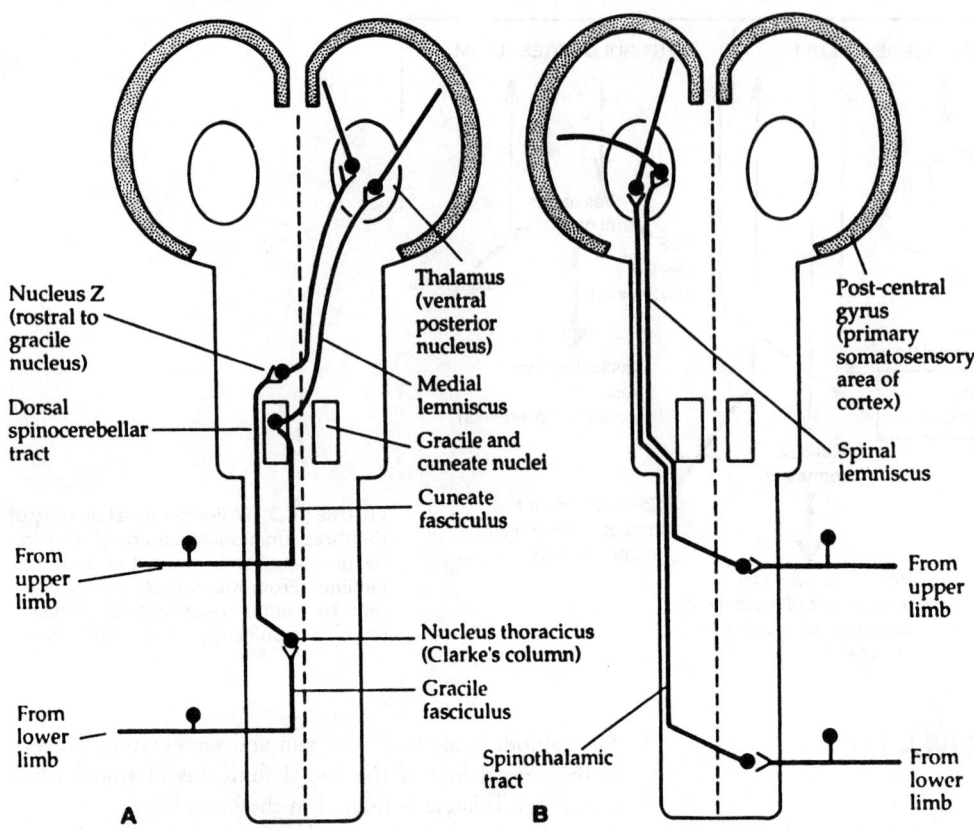

FIGURE 14.4. Ascending pathways for somatic sensation. **A:** Pathways for conscious proprioception for the upper and lower limbs. The pathway shown for the upper limb also conveys discriminative touch sensation. Signals for discriminative touch from the lower limb travel to the medulla in the ipsilateral gracile fasciculus. **B:** Spinothalamic pathway for pain, temperature, and nondiscriminative tactile sensation.

PATHWAYS FOR SLEEP, AROUSAL, AND CONSCIOUSNESS

Two groups of nuclei of the reticular formation of the brain stem are involved in arousal, consciousness, and sleep.

CENTRAL GROUP OF RETICULAR NUCLEI

The central group includes the gigantocellular reticular nucleus in the medulla, the caudal and oral pontine reticular nuclei, and the cuneiform and subcuneiform nuclei in the midbrain. The two latter are laterally located, but their connections and functions place them in the central group. The two pontine reticular nuclei include the neurons constituting the paramedian pontine reticular formation (PPRF), which is involved in eye movements. The nuclei of the central group receive afferent fibers from the spinal cord, the sensory nuclei of the cranial nerves, the vestibulocerebellum, the reticular formation of the midbrain, the tectum, the hypothalamus, and the premotor area of the cerebral cortex (Fig. 14.5). The ascending afferents include collateral branches from the spinothalamic and trigeminothalamic tracts.

Neurons of the central reticular nuclei typically have axons with long ascending and descending branches and numerous

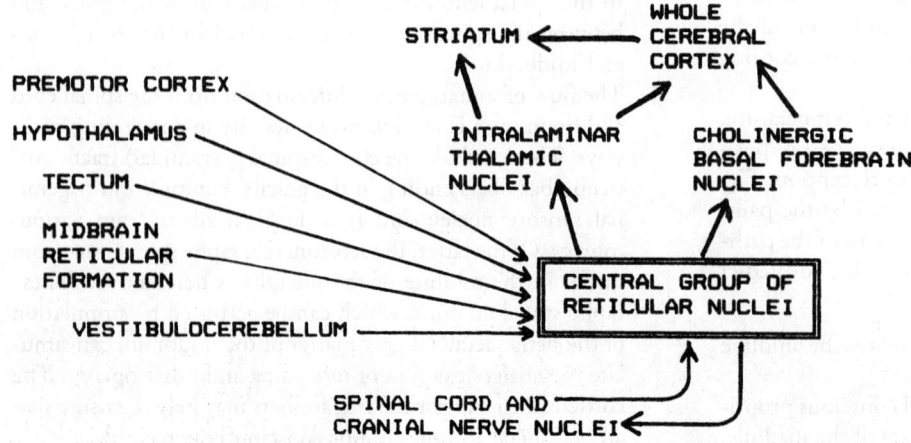

FIGURE 14.5. Some connections of the central group of nuclei of the reticular formation.

collaterals that synapse with other neurons in the brain stem. The long descending fibers constitute the reticulospinal tracts, discussed elsewhere in this chapter. Ascending axons go to the intralaminar thalamic nuclei and the basal cholinergic nuclei of the substantia innominata in the base of the forebrain. The latter cell groups include the nucleus basalis of Meynert, the nucleus of the diagonal band, and certain nuclei of the septal area. The intralaminar and basal forebrain nuclei project diffusely to the whole cerebral cortex, and the intralaminar nuclei also provide a major input to the striatum.

The central or medial group of reticular nuclei was once believed to be the major part of the ascending reticular activating system, conveying to the thalamus and thence to the whole cerebral cortex trains of impulses initiated by all types of sensation. Such a view accords with many experimental and clinical observations, including the irreversible coma that follows bilateral destruction of the medial part of the reticular formation at or above upper pontine levels. The projections of the central group of nuclei are probably also involved in the poorly localized perception of pain that persists after transection of the spinothalamic tracts. In addition, there are neurons that actively induce sleep; these have somata in the serotonergic raphe nuclei, with axons distributed to all parts of the CNS.

RAPHE NUCLEI

Raphe nuclei are groups of neuronal somata that are in or next to the midline, from the caudal medulla to the rostral midbrain. Many of the raphe neurons synthesize and secrete serotonin (5-hydroxytryptamine), and this amine is believed to be their principal synaptic transmitter. The axons of the serotonergic neurons are unmyelinated and greatly branched. They are distributed to gray matter throughout the CNS (Fig. 14.6). The medullary raphe nuclei are involved in the suppression of pain. Those of the pons and midbrain have inhibitory effects on arousal and consciousness.

Afferents to the more rostral raphe nuclei come from the prefrontal cortex, the periaqueductal gray matter, various other nuclei of the reticular formation (including the PPRF), and several components of the limbic system. The latter include the hippocampal formation, the hypothalamus, the interpeduncular nucleus, and the ventral tegmental area (a group of dopaminergic neurons in the rostral midbrain). The axons of the neurons in the rostral raphe nuclei extend to all parts of the forebrain.

The raphe neurons are active in deep sleep, which may be due in part to a widespread inhibitory action of serotonin in the thalamus and cerebral cortex. Occasional release of the PPRF from serotonergic inhibition may account for the eye movements in rapid eye movement (REM) sleep. The dreaming that occurs in this phase of sleep may be due to a similar reduction of the inhibition of telencephalic neurons. Desynchronization of the electroencephalogram in the awake subject and in REM sleep is attributed to the activity of thalamocortical neurons in causing large fluctuations in the membrane potentials of cortical pyramidal neurons. The electroencephalogram recorded from the hippocampus, however, is quiescent in the wakeful state and desynchronized in sleep.

In summary, it seems that the maintenance of a conscious state requires the integrity of projections from the reticular formation to the forebrain. Both the central group of reticular nuclei (active in the alert state) and the serotonergic raphe nuclei (active in sleep) are involved, along with the thalamus, the basal forebrain cholinergic nuclei, and the whole cerebral cortex, including the hippocampal formation.

PATHWAYS FOR MEMORY AND EMOTION

The term *limbic system* embraces the cingulate and parahippocampal gyri, the hippocampal formation, the amygdala, the habenular nuclei, the hypothalamus, and various nuclei of the thalamus and midbrain. The tracts that connect these gray masses include the fornix, stria terminalis, stria medullaris thalami, central tegmental tract, and dorsal longitudinal fasciculus. The exact connections of these structures are known only from tracing experiments in animals, but there is no reason to believe that the connectivity in the human limbic system is different. The limbic structures are larger in the human than in any other species, as would be expected from their involvement in higher behavioral and mental functions.

The connections of the hippocampus, amygdala, and other components of the limbic system are shown in Figure 14.7, which summarizes the circuitry in one hemisphere. The left and right hippocampi are connected by small numbers of fibers that cross in the body of the fornix. Commissural fibers also interconnect the habenular nuclei and at least some of the nuclei in the hypothalamus and midbrain. Furthermore, the neocortical input to the limbic system is from areas connected across the midline by the corpus callosum and anterior commissure. All the func-

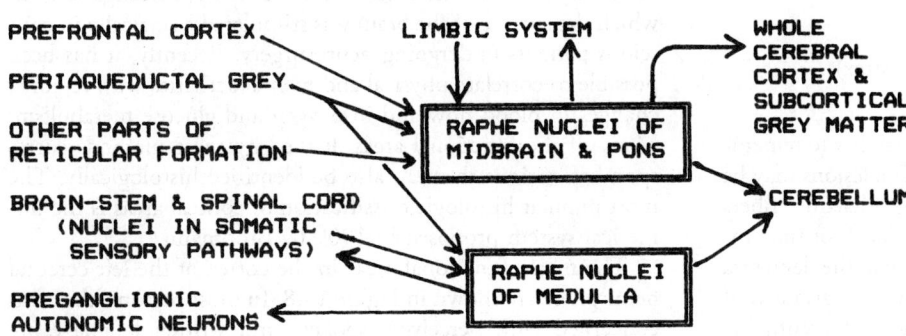

FIGURE 14.6. Some connections of the serotonergic raphe nuclei of the brain stem.

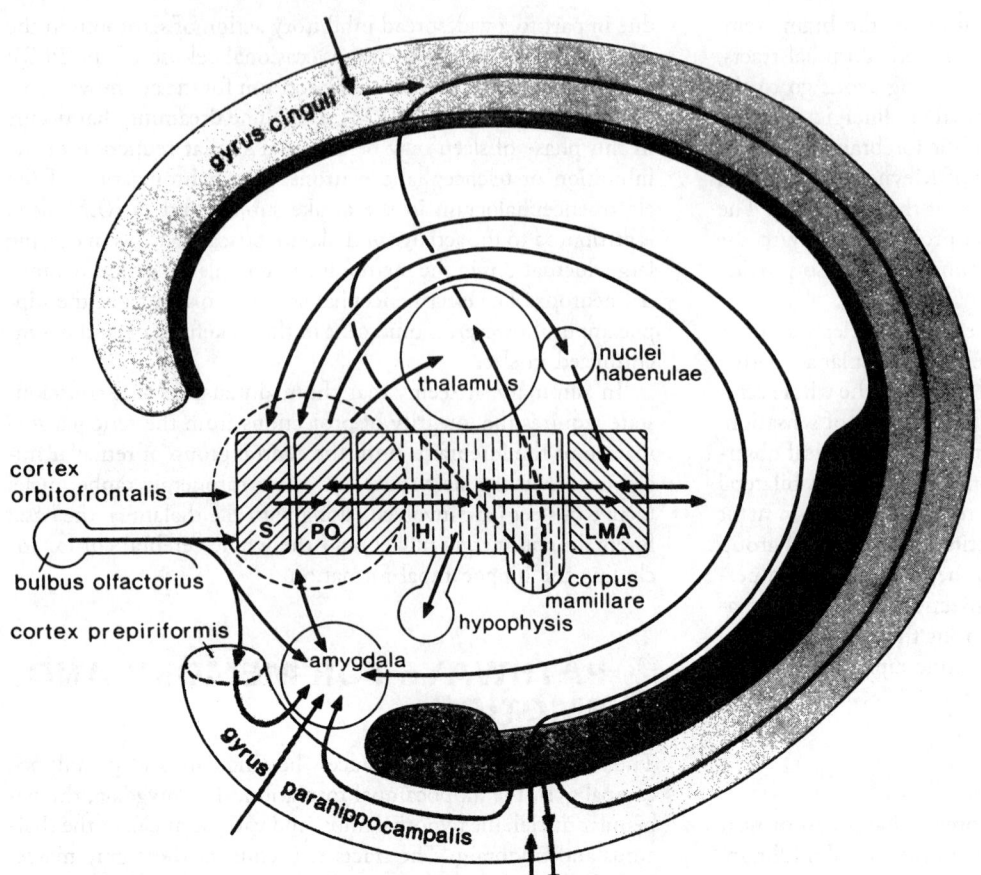

FIGURE 14.7. The limbic system. S, septal area; PO, preoptic area; H, hypothalamus; LMA, limbic midbrain area. (From Niewenhuys R, Voogd J, van Huijzen C. *The human central nervous system: a synopsis and atlas,* third ed. Berlin: Springer-Verlag, 1988, with permission.)

tions of the limbic system are duplicated bilaterally, and destructive lesions on one side do not cause disordered function. Unilateral excitation (an epileptogenic focus in the temporal lobe) can result in abnormal behavior or unreal states of awareness. Such episodes are known as uncinate attacks because hallucinations of smell result from stimulation of the uncus, which is at the anterior end of the parahippocampal gyrus. The uncus is the principal site of termination of the olfactory tract.

The functions of the human limbic system are deduced from clinical studies and by extrapolation from the results of experiments in animals. Traditional teaching emphasizes the "circuit of Papez":

Hippocampus → fornix
　　→ Posterior hypothalamus
　　→ Anterior and lateral-dorsal thalamic nuclei
　　→ Cingulate gyrus
　　→ Cingulum
　　→ Parahippocampal gyrus (= entorhinal cortex)
　　→ Hippocampus

Interruption of this loop bilaterally causes inability to remember recent events or to form new memories. The lesions may be in the mamillary bodies, the thalami (mamillothalamic fibers passing through and near the mediodorsal nucleus), or the hippocampi. Hippocampal damage may contribute to the dementia in Alzheimer's disease, but in this condition there is also loss of neurons in the basal cholinergic forebrain nuclei and, eventually,

throughout the neocortex. Defective memory is only one of the mental derangements associated with limbic lesions. The dopaminergic "mesolimbic" projection from the ventral tegmental area of the midbrain to the limbic structures of the forebrain may function abnormally in schizophrenia. Some thymoleptic drugs block the action of dopamine on postsynaptic cells. Their parkinsonian side effects are due to interference with the other major dopaminergic projection, that from the substantia nigra to the striatum.

FUNCTIONAL LOCALIZATION IN THE CEREBRAL CORTEX

The functions of specific areas of the cerebral cortex were revealed by clinicopathologic studies and by investigations in which the surface of the brain was stimulated electrically in conscious patients undergoing neurosurgery. Recently, it has been possible to correlate physical and mental activities with regional changes in blood flow and in oxygen and glucose metabolism. Many of the functional areas defined by these methods correspond to regions that can also be identified histologically. The most popular histologic classification of cortical areas is the numerical system proposed in 1909 by Brodmann.

The major functional areas in the cortex of the left cerebral hemisphere are shown in Figure 14.8. In most persons, the areas concerned with perceived, spoken, and written language are

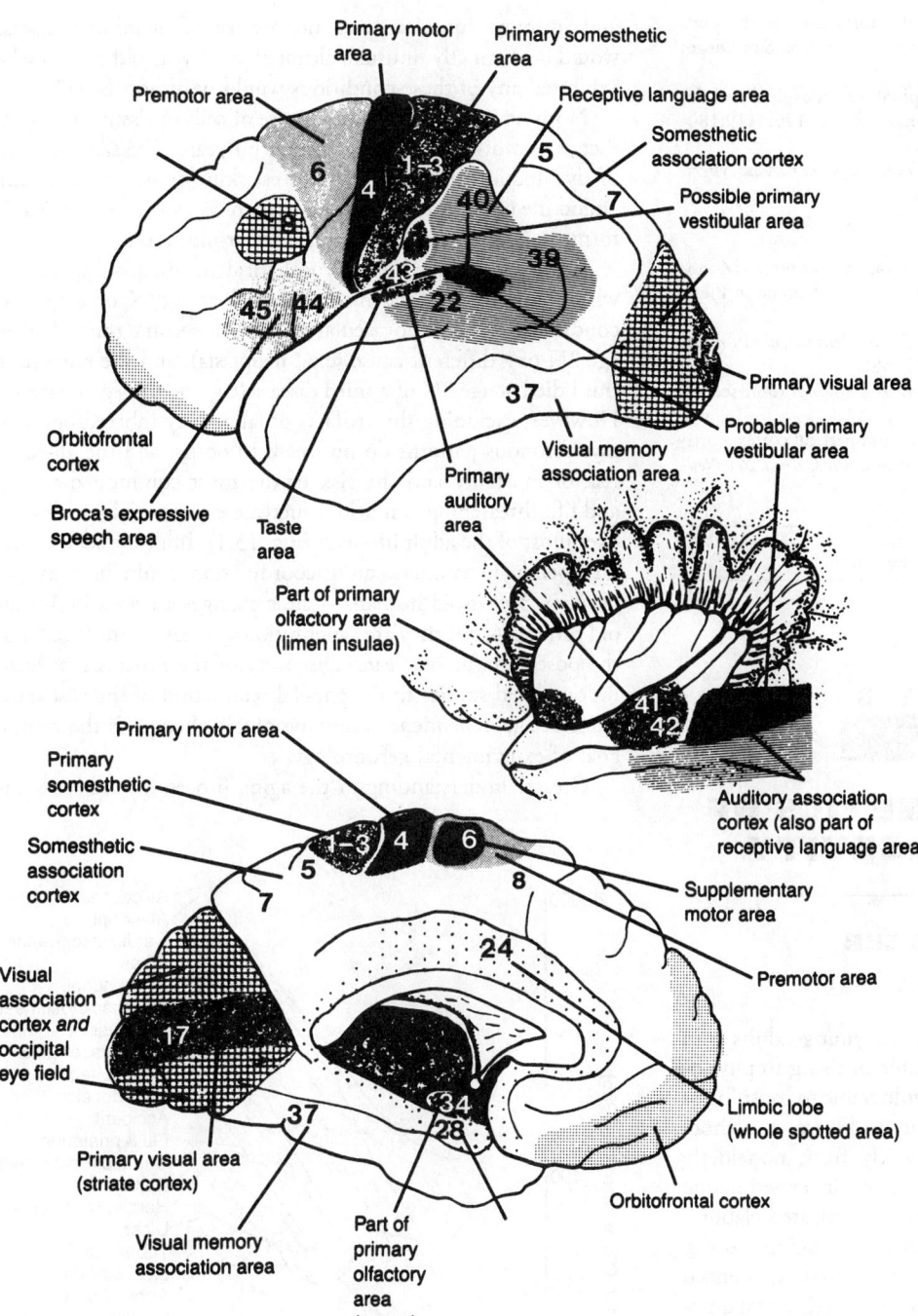

FIGURE 14.8. Functional areas of the cortex of the left cerebral hemisphere. Some of Brodmann's numbers are also shown. In the primary motor and somatosensory area, the contralateral half of the body is represented upside-down, with the mouth and head at the lower end (near the lateral sulcus) and the foot and perineum on the medial surface of the hemisphere. (From Kiernan JA. *An introduction to human neuroscience.* Philadelphia: JB Lippincott, 1987, with permission.)

present only on the left, and the corresponding areas on the right side are concerned with the management of three-dimensional space, including awareness of parts of the body and the tactile recognition of shapes and textures. The cerebral cortex deals with the contralateral side of the body or visual field, except for the auditory system, which is represented bilaterally, the olfactory projection, which is ipsilateral, and the cognitive functions. Symmetric cortical areas are connected by the corpus callosum. An important function of this commissure is to permit the sharing by both hemispheres of sensory and other data received or processed initially on only one side.

Refer to Chapters 432–448, "Disorders of the Nervous System."

BIBLIOGRAPHY

Frackowiak RSF. Functional mapping of verbal memory and language. *Trends Neurosci* 1994;17:109–115.

Hoge CJ, Apkarian AV. The spinothalamic tract. *CRC Crit Rev Neurobiol* 1990;5:363–397.

Kiernan JA. *Barr's The human nervous sytem: an anatomical viewpoint,* seventh ed. Philadelphia: Lippincott-Raven Publishers, 1998.

Lim C, Mufson EJ, Kordower JH, et al. Connections of the hippocampal formation in humans. *J Comp Neurol* 1997;385:325–371.

Martin GF, Holstege G, Mehler WR. Reticular formation of the pons and medulla. In: Paxinos G, ed. *The human nervous system.* San Diego: Academic Press, 1990:203–220.

Nathan PW, Smith M, Deacon P. Vestibulospinal, reticulospinal and descending propriospinal nerve fibres in man. *Brain* 1996;119:180-9–1833.

Nieuwenhuys R, Voogd J, Van Huijzen C. *The human central nervous system. A synopsis and atlas,* third ed. Berlin: Springer-Verlag, 1988.

Parent A, Hazrati LN. Functional anatomy of the basal ganglia. *Brain Res Rev* 1995;20:91–154.

Porter R, Lemon R. *Corticospinal function and voluntary movement.* (Monographs of the Physiological Society, No. 45.) Oxford: Clarendon Press, 1993.

Tranel D. Higher brain functions. In: Conn PM, ed. *Neuroscience in medicine.* Philadelphia: JB Lippincott, 1995:555–580.

Willis WD, Coggeshall RE. *Sensory mechanisms of the spinal cord,* second ed. New York: Plenum Press, 1991.

Wise SP, Boussaoud D, Johnson, et al. Premotor and parietal cortex: corticocortical connectivity and combinatorial computations. *Annu Rev Neurosci* 1997;20:25–42.

Kelley's Textbook of Internal Medicine, fourth edition. Edited by H. David Humes. Lippincott Williams & Wilkins, Philadelphia © 2000.

CHAPTER
15

BIOLOGY AND GENETICS OF AGING AND LONGEVITY

RICHARD A. MILLER

The aging process gradually transforms fit young adults into infirm older ones, progressively less capable of rising to physiologic challenges and progressively more vulnerable to most forms of infectious, neoplastic, and degenerative disease. Preschool children can accurately differentiate elderly from nonelderly adults, and much of the published literature in experimental gerontology has consisted of increasingly sophisticated elaboration of the phenotypic changes of senescence. The aging process, however, is still essentially a mystery in the sense that experienced investigators cannot yet be confident that the experimental questions they are asking are useful steps toward an understanding of the aging process at its most fundamental level.

From one perspective, the most salient feature of aging, its deepest mystery and most promising point for experimental attack, is its species-specific synchrony. Most of the functional deficits seen in elderly persons, whether or not they are diseases considered suitable for treatment by medical professionals, are rare in the reproductive years of adulthood, uncommon in the next two decades, and common thereafter, becoming in the aggregate essentially unavoidable in the longest-lived persons. Very few persons in their 80s or older are entirely free from disabling or life-threatening conditions. An 80-year-old person who exhibited no loss of sight or hearing, no memory deficits, no arthritis, no signs of renal or cardiovascular disorders, no decline in muscle

and immune function, and no history of neoplastic disease would be distinctly unusual, although a 20-year-old person who exhibited any of these conditions would be almost equally rare.

Nothing intrinsic to the structure of cells or tissues or organs dictates a working life of 2 or 20 or 60 years. The same pattern of dysfunction that affects the eyes, skin, brain, muscles, and endocrine organs of 80-year-old humans is seen, in recognizable form, in 2.5-year-old mice and 25-year-old horses.

It is easy to imagine a hypothetical mammalian species in which one-third of the members died at age N of a specific condition (e.g., cardiovascular failure), a second third died at age 2N of a different cause (e.g., neoplasia), and the remaining third died at age 3N of a third disease (e.g., neurodegeneration). However, excluding the artifacts of laboratory inbreeding, such asynchronous patterns do not seem to occur, and the all-cause risk of mortality and the risk of the most common disabling and life-threatening conditions increase exponentially with time over most of the adult life span (Fig. 15.1). Immune senescence, sarcopenia, hepatomas, or discoordination could in principle occur in 3-year-old humans—these changes are seen in 3-year-old rodents—but they are synchronously delayed until well into the postreproductive years. Discovery of the process that leads in long-lived species to the parallel retardation of the vast spectrum of age-dependent pathophysiologic changes is the central goal of experimental gerontology.

Greater understanding of the aging process would have im-

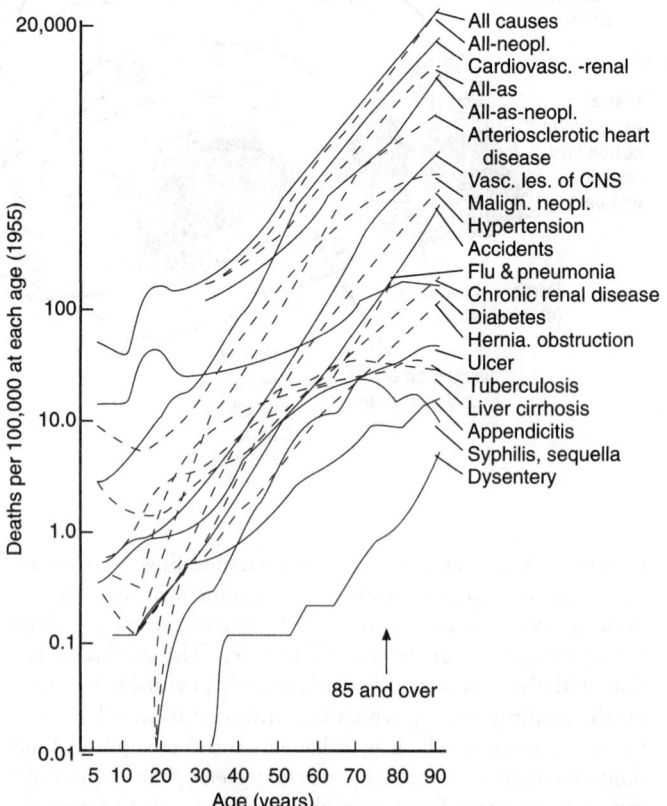

FIGURE 15.1. Parallel, exponential increase in the risk of mortality from selected causes as a function of age in humans.

portant ramifications for the study of and potentially for the prevention or treatment of most late-life diseases. Consider as an example the timing of neoplasia in mice and in humans. The lifelong risk of a potentially lethal neoplastic disease in non-inbred rodents is about the same as in humans—about 25% to 50%. The average human, however, lives about 30 times longer than the average mouse and has approximately 3000 times more cells at risk of undergoing a transformation to a potentially lethal neoplastic clone. If human cells were as susceptible to oncogenesis as mouse cells, very few people would survive to become reproductive. Thus, the evolution of long-lived humans has required an increase of about 90,000 times in antineoplastic defenses (30 × 3000). An understanding of the species-specific defense mechanisms that differentiate long-lived from short-lived species would have provocative implications for our understanding of oncogenesis. Similarly impressive changes have evolved, in parallel, to delay age-dependent deficits in proliferative (e.g., skin), conditionally proliferative (e.g., immune), and essentially nonproliferative (e.g., muscle, nerve) tissues in long-lived animals, changes whose elucidation would have profound implications for medical science and clinical practice.

The extent of our ignorance of aging and the genetic and biochemical processes that regulate the aging rate is still discouragingly vast, although less so than 20 years ago. This chapter discusses some of the methodologic challenges that confront experimental gerontologists, briefly synopsizing some of the most significant findings in biomedical aging research and discussing the status of some popular general theories of aging. It presents a selected catalogue of some research areas that seem most likely to produce impressive progress in the next few decades. Readers who wish to delve more deeply into research on the biology and genetics of aging and longevity are referred to the several excellent monographs and compendia listed in the bibliography.

■ AGING, DEVELOPMENT, AND DISEASE: TERMINOLOGY AND DEFINITIONS

Part of the difficulty in thinking carefully about the biologic basis of aging comes from ambiguities in terminology. In particular, the word *aging* has several overlapping colloquial meanings that can confuse its use as a term for the process that transforms healthy young adults into frail older ones. Cheese, cell clones, and cars "age" in ways that to some extent resemble and suggest hypotheses about aging in adult animals, but that also differ in critical ways from organismic aging. Similarly, the processes that lead to seasonal leaf abscission in plants and that limit the life span of erythrocytes are called *senescence,* but there is little reason to believe that these varieties of senescence resemble closely the processes that limit the life span of intact plants and animals.

The relation between aging and development can also provide a source of confusion and miscommunication. In a colloquial sense, children grow older from birth to and through maturity, and many biologists assert confidently that aging should be considered "just another form of development," likely to yield to the same investigative strategies that are beginning to tease apart the mechanisms of embryogenesis and ontogeny. There are, however, reasons to be cautious about this assumption. The set of events that convert a fertilized egg into a fetus and the fetus into a reproductively mature adult are highly constrained by evolutionary forces, but the processes that lead to the eventual loss of adult function—aging in the sense in which the term is used in this chapter—are characterized chiefly by the dwindling influence of such constraints. A factory designed to convert steel, rubber, and glass into an automobile is unlikely to be ideal for converting new cars to used ones. The forces that mediate senescence are likely to have roots in childhood development, and just as a careful study of automobile factories can provide insights into vehicle durability (e.g., How thick is the steel? Are the workers highly skilled? Is the marketing department aiming for high volume or high quality?), an understanding of developmental biology can only be helpful to experimental gerontologists. Aging itself, however, is likely to involve mechanisms not well modeled by earlier phases of development.

The relation between aging and disease is also a source of much controversy, closely linked to the problem of whether the changes attributed to "normal" aging can be differentiated from those traceable to age-related diseases. Some research questions can be answered intelligently only if the experimenter carefully differentiates between patients who do and do not exhibit signs of one or more specific diseases. An age-related decline in bicycle-exercise tolerance can be interpreted only if one knows whether the elderly group included people with congestive heart failure, osteoarthritis, Alzheimer's disease, and many other potentially limiting conditions. Most studies naturally exclude such patients from analysis, restricting attention to those deemed apparently healthy. A tougher problem is whether to also exclude persons who may not be under clinical care for a treatable condition but who may nonetheless show subtle signs of early illness. Fine distinctions between exclusion criteria designed to differentiate persons who are exceptionally healthy from those who are somewhat less so can lead to major changes in conclusions about the physiologic effects of aging. Some sets of proposed criteria exclude up to 90% of subjects in the oldest age groups; it seems unreasonable to consider such a selected subset of elderly subjects as typical of normal aging. Similar reservations about studies of aged animals are made less salient, although no less serious, by our relative inability to recognize early signs of disease in animal models.

A typical response to the problem of discriminating aging from disease, particularly among research geriatricians, is to deny any distinction between the aging process *per se* and the diseases and disabilities so widely distributed among elderly subjects and to assert that aging is simply the sum of these pathologic conditions. One way to resolve these problems is to consider aging to be the process that operates throughout adult life to mold the elderly individuals who survive to require geriatric care. Many aspects of aging may be more convenient to investigate in middle-aged adults who are old enough to be different from 20-year-old adults but not so old that they exhibit the decompensation and idiosyncrasies that often accompany late-life disease. From this perspective, the normal aged person is chimerical, an intellectual construct as valuable as but ethereal as the sequence of the normal human genome, a sequence none of us actually possesses.

Heterogeneity among the elderly—most dramatically exhibited in the forms of diseases that afflict some elderly persons—should not discourage researchers from seeking common mechanisms, just as the heterogeneity of adult forms, from pygmies to basketball players and from aggressive politicians to shy academics, does not imperil investigation of ontogeny and embryogenesis. This heterogeneity does require careful use of analytic methods that can measure and adjust for the effects of potential confounders, including disease and physiologic idiosyncrasies, and experimental designs that rely more on longitudinal protocols and study of middle-aged subjects than on cross-sectional comparisons of the very oldest with the very youngest adults.

MEASUREMENT OF AGING

A serious obstacle to aging research is the difficulty of measuring aging rates among individuals. Although it is clear that mice, dogs, and humans age at different rates, it is much less clear whether members of the same species exhibit different rates of aging. Evidence based on studies of caloric restriction and genotypic variation suggest that hereditary and noninherited factors can influence aging rate within a species, and it is common in lay and clinical discussions to observe that a certain 60-year-old seems to resemble someone of a younger (or older) chronologic age, but these approaches provide little quantitative guidance for measuring the rate of aging or the *biologic age* of a given subject. This embarrassment has practical and theoretical importance: how would a researcher evaluate the efficacy of a therapeutic maneuver alleged to alter the aging rate?

One traditional strategy has been to rely on life-table analyses. The most influential approach, developed initially by Gompertz, is based on the empirical observation that for humans and for many other species the risk of mortality increases exponentially from an initial nadir at some early stage, typically puberty. Plots of the logarithm of mortality rate as a function of age are linear, with constant slopes, over most of the adult life span for most species for which adequate data exist. This *Gompertz slope* can be taken as a useful measure of the aging rate of the members of the population tested, and demonstrations that two groups exhibit different slopes provide evidence that they are aging at different rates.

An equivalent but more convenient statistic is the *mortality rate doubling time* (MRDT), the period during which the risk of mortality increases twofold. Among mammals, the MRDT varies over a range of at least 25-fold, from 8 or more years in humans and other primates to 0.3 years in rodents; among invertebrates, the MRDT can be as low as 0.005 years. The actual risk of mortality at any age and the mean and maximal life span depend critically on the MRDT and the *initial mortality rate* (IMR), which is the mortality rate at the age at which the mortality risk is lowest. IMRs, like MRDTs, vary widely among species. The MRDT of a species seems to resist alteration by even highly stressful environments; the rate of increase in mortal-

ity risk with age does not differ significantly between concentration camp inmates and unincarcerated residents of highly developed countries.

Although in most studies the maximal life span and the MRDT statistics have served as the standard way to evaluate claims that a genetic or environmental intervention could influence aging rate, these actuarial methods have significant limitations. At least for some populations of invertebrates, including fruit flies and nematode worms, the rate of increase in mortality risk is not constant with age and appears to diminish at ages at which most of the original population has died. A very small subpopulation of fruit flies, for example, may live to ages well beyond those predicted on the basis of the Gompertz law; if a similar subpopulation existed among humans, it would lead to life spans of 300 to 600 years for about 1 person per 1 million. The Gompertz law, which was, to begin with, derived from empirical data rather than from a coherent theory of aging, is best viewed as a useful approximation and summary statistic rather than an indication of a fundamental characteristic of aging in all species.

Life-table analyses can provide information about aging rates in groups of subjects but cannot provide a useful measure of aging in any individual. The reliance on life-table data as the key measure of aging rate also places undue emphasis on death itself as an indirect measure of age. Although the risk of mortality is clearly influenced by age, it is also influenced by a wide range of other factors in humans, including access to health care, as well as genetic predisposition to specific diseases, chance encounters with predators and microbial pathogens, and environmental hazards.

The age at death, which is the end point most widely relied on in experimental aging studies, provides an exceptionally indirect and flawed index of individual aging rate. A few laboratories have tried to overcome this obstacle by suggesting and testing candidate biomarkers of aging, such as tests of age-sensitive characteristics, which can be measured without harm to the animal or human subject and which discriminate among persons who differ in other measures of physiologic aging, including vulnerability to disease. Although it is possible to identify risk factors, such as blood cholesterol, smoking history, avoidance of seat belts, and parental age at death, which together can provide a useful index of remaining life expectancy in humans, it has not yet proved feasible for humans or animal models to generate a useful set of indices that can consistently identify persons whose physiologic and biochemical status resembles those of younger or older chronologic age. Because the mechanism of aging is still thoroughly obscure, a set of such surrogate biomarkers for aging would provide a useful tool for experimental gerontologists in the same sense that stock market indices provide a useful tool for economists.

COMPARATIVE AND EVOLUTIONARY PERSPECTIVES

Important clues about the biology of aging can be gleaned from descriptive studies that seek to determine the distribution, rate, and consequences of aging among species and from theoretical arguments that seek to explain from an evolutionary perspective the near universality of aging among metazoan species. Monographs by Comfort and by Finch provide a wealth of citations to the descriptive literature. In reviewing the mass of field and laboratory data, it is important to notice that the high level of natural attrition for most species in unprotected environments often prevents the accumulation of aged individuals among wild populations. The mortality risks in the wild are frequently so high that age-dependent increases in mortality are comparatively trivial. Determination of whether members of such a species can exhibit aging, measured as a correlated decline in physiologic systems or more usually measured as an exponential increase of mortality risk over time, usually requires removal of the animals from environmental hazards and protection in a laboratory or captive situation arguably less risky than the natural one. Most metazoan species, including flies, worms, reptiles, birds, fish, and the familiar farm, pet, and zoo-housed mammals, exhibit aging when so tested.

Some exceptions to this rule provide more insight into semantic niceties of what we mean by aging than into the mechanism of aging in mammals. Some species of fish, for example, show a high early mortality rate, followed by a period of adult life in which the rate of mortality decreases over time, as the fish grow to sizes that make them progressively less vulnerable to predators. Eventually, a population of such fish at very advanced ages would probably begin to show an acceleration of mortality, but testing such a prediction would be expensive and unrewarding. Other species, such as certain salmon and a species of marsupial mouse, exploit a semelparous life history, during which all reproductive effort is concentrated into a single brief episode immediately followed by physiologic decline and death. It seems mistaken to consider this decline a form of accelerated aging that could offer lessons for the analysis of aging in humans or rodents, because salmon prevented from this reproductive frenzy live for many additional years while showing a typical exponential increase in mortality risk. From this perspective, the semelparous life history pattern seems to prevent the progression of adult individuals to ages at which aging would become physiologically significant and actuarially detectable.

Evolutionary biologists have given much thought to the place of senescence in the theory of selection for life history patterns. A coherent analysis of evolutionary pressures that mold longevity was first produced by Williams and greatly elaborated in a quantitative treatment by Charlesworth. The central points can be summarized qualitatively. Imagine, for example, a species of animal in which aging did not occur, in which the risk of mortality did not increase with age but remained at some constant value throughout life; this constant value would depend on exposure to predators, infectious diseases, and perhaps endogenous processes. In this population, the number of survivors of any starting cohort would decline exponentially over time, just as the amount of a radioisotope decays exponentially at a rate that depends only on the constant half-life of the isotope. If the half-life of our hypothetical species were 5 years, the number of individuals surviving to the age of 25 years would be only 1/32 of the original starting population. The key point is that this unequal

distribution of individuals across age categories leads to differences in the selection pressures for or against genetic mutations whose effects are not equivalent at all ages.

Genetic mutations that lead to deleterious effects (e.g., cardiovascular failure, neoplasia, decline in muscle function) only in persons 25 years of age and older would be subject to much less adverse selective pressure than mutations that cripple or kill 5-year-old children. In particular, mutant alleles that have strong positive effects on survival of 5-year-olds would be favored even if they had negative effects on the survival of 25-year-old adults. In a nonaging species, mutations would inevitably accumulate and lead to ill health and diminished physiologic performance in older, but not younger, members of the species. It is not hard to imagine such alleles: alleles that promote rapid growth of wounded skin but also predispose to skin tumors, alleles that promote rapid calcification of bone but also lead to progressive calcification of arterial walls, and many others with similar pleiotropic effects. The sum of these late-life deleterious effects produces the spectrum of disabilities and disease seen in elderly members of each species and leads to the exponential increase in mortality risk over most of the adult life span.

This theory makes a number of testable predictions and has been confirmed in laboratory and field studies. If severe environmental hazards make it highly unlikely for individual members of a species to continue to breed over an extended interval, the pressures against alleles with late-life deleterious effects are especially relaxed, and genotypes may evolve that tend to produce a burst of early reproduction, even if at the expense of diminished late-life function (i.e., more rapid aging). Environmental changes, such as a decline in predator number, which relax the pressure for early fecundity may encourage the emergence of genotypes that postpone the development of senescent changes to allow continued reproductive effort over a wider time interval. In support of this expectation, Austad showed that island opossums, whose environment is free of significant predation, evolve over a period of not more than 3,000 generations so that they age more slowly than mainland opossums to which they are very closely related. As illustrated in Figure 15.2, members of the island population show decelerated Gompertz curves and do not show the precipitous decline in reproductive success shown by 2-year-old mainland opossums. Aging at the biochemical level also seems to be slowed in the island population, as judged by a measure of collagen cross-linking.

A related prediction is the idea that artificially imposed selection in favor of late-life reproduction ought to select for allele combinations that produce not merely delayed reproduction but also declines in the aging rate. Several groups have confirmed this prediction by showing that fruit flies selected for delayed egg laying do indeed routinely exhibit increased longevity. Physiologic comparisons of the selected, long-lived flies with shorter-lived, unselected flies may provide clues about the mechanisms of augmented longevity in this species. Regardless of whether the pathophysiology of aging in flies has any implications for mammalian senescence, the genetic results provide strong confirmation for the underlying theory and suggest that genetically heterogeneous populations may contain alleles that, in combina-

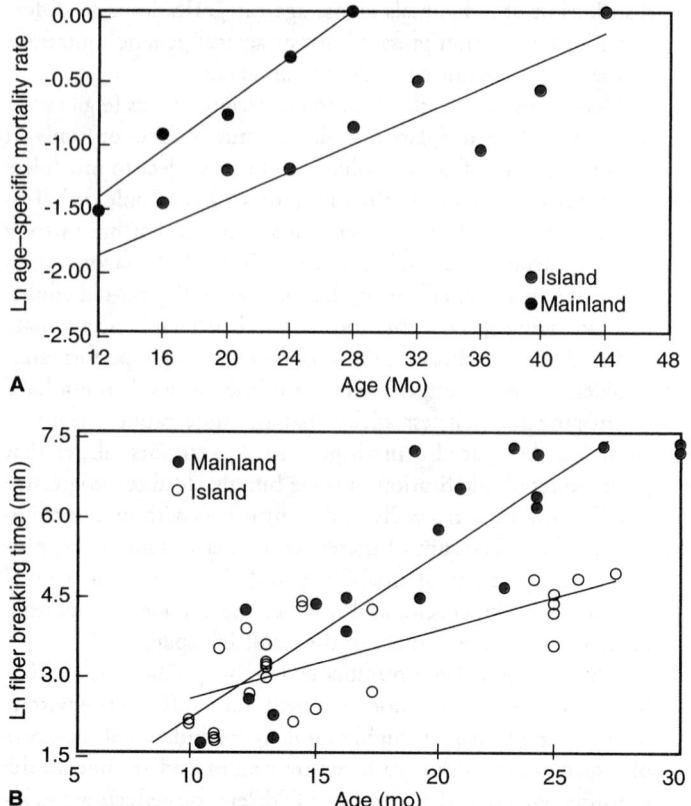

FIGURE 15.2. Diminished rate of aging in opossum populations selected by isolation on a predator-free island for 4,500 years, as predicted by evolutionary genetics. **A:** Gompertz mortality plots; the risk of mortality increases more slowly for island opossums (*open circles*). **B:** Tail tendon fiber breaking time, an index of collagen cross-linking, which increases with age. Island opossums have a lower rate of age-dependent increase in collagen cross-linking.

tion, can lead to substantial increases in mean and maximal longevity. The opossum data previously discussed suggest that mammalian populations also may contain selectable genetic variants that control the aging rate.

A third implication of the evolutionary argument is that the aging rate should vary inversely with environmental hazard. This suggestion has been strongly supported by comparative analyses. After factoring out the effects of body size, different orders of mammals vary widely in maximal longevity, with bats in particular exhibiting life spans that are about 2.5 to 3.0 times greater than those seen in similarly sized nonflying mammals. Nine species of mammals that exhibit "sailing" behavior, such as the flying squirrels, also have maximal life spans that are on average 1.7 times longer than nonsailing mammals of similar size. Birds live about 2.4 times longer than mammals of similar size. The decline in predation risk conveyed by sailing or flying relaxes the pressure for early life reproduction and permits evolution of genotypes in which the effects of late-life deleterious alleles are postponed to increased ages.

These fortuitous evolutionary experiments provide research opportunities that have yet to be adequately exploited by experi-

mental gerontologists. Birds, for example, have high longevity despite high rates of oxygen consumption and high blood glucose levels, and research into their defenses against damage caused from reactive oxygen intermediates and advanced glycosylation end products may yield valuable insights into mammalian aging.

DECELERATION OF AGING BY CALORIC RESTRICTION

Mice and rats given access to diets containing 30% to 40% fewer calories than they would ordinarily consume if given free access to food show a 25% to 40% increase in mean and maximal longevity and a parallel retardation of most age-related physiologic and biochemical changes. Caloric restriction is the only well-substantiated method for increasing maximal longevity and decelerating aging in mammals and has therefore been intensively studied for clues to the physiologic nature of the aging process itself. Its particular value comes from the breadth of the effect: caloric restriction extends the life span not simply by postponement of one or a small number of common diseases, but by parallel retardation of many age-related changes at the molecular, cellular, and organ system levels. Among other effects, caloric restriction impedes the development of cross-linking in extracellular proteins, including collagen and lens crystallins; delays age-related changes in mRNA abundance for many tissue specific genes; interferes with age-associated shifts in T-cell subsets; blocks changes in central nervous system function; and retards development of neoplastic and degenerative disease of all sorts. It seems highly unlikely that separate biochemical mechanisms are involved in each of these cases and the many other caloric restriction–induced modifications in age-dependent pathophysiology; caloric restriction is presumably acting by a modification of a single, underlying aging process of undetermined nature, which is linked to age-dependent changes at multiple levels.

Several hypotheses about the way in which caloric restriction alters aging have been refuted by experimental data. The effect seems not to be caused by any toxic molecule in a dietary component or by limitation of any specific nutrient; it accompanies almost any dietary manipulation that diminishes total caloric intake while providing adequate amounts of micronutrients to avoid malnutrition. The suggestion that caloric restriction works by retarding growth to adult size has been undermined by data showing that caloric restriction is also highly effective when imposed after the attainment of full adult weight. Caloric restriction apparently does not involve a decline in fuel consumption at the level of individual cells, because calorie-restricted rodents are much smaller than control-fed animals, and the number of calories used per gram of lean body mass is unchanged by the caloric restriction protocol. The additional longevity achieved by caloric restriction is not simply a prolongation of the late-life period of disease and disability, because calorie-restricted rodents remain highly active and physically fit at ages at which

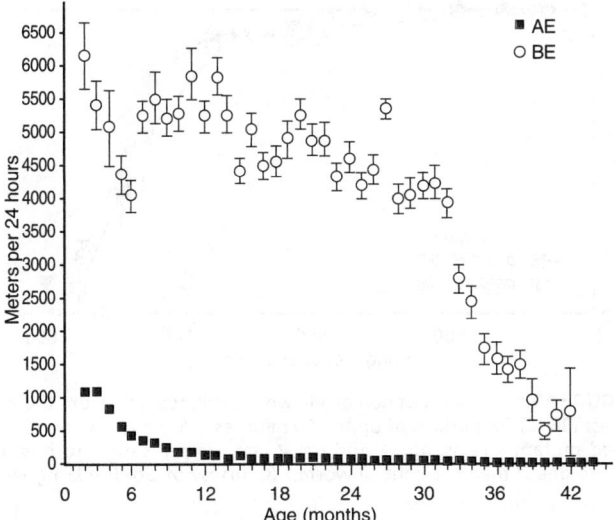

FIGURE 15.3. Spontaneous wheel running by rats on a calorie-restricted diet (*open circles*) compared with rats on a control diet (*squares*). Calorie-restricted rats permitted free access to an exercise wheel run an average of 4 to 5 km per day until the 30th month of life. In contrast, control rats run less than 500 m per day from the sixth month of life. The 50% survival level was 26 months for control rats and 37 months for restricted rats. (Courtesy of Roger J.M. McCarter.)

most members of the control group have already died (Fig. 15.3). The suggestion that control rodents are overfed compared with rodents in the wild and that the benefits of caloric restriction merely represent alleviation of the toxic effects of overfeeding is refuted by the data showing that calorie-restricted rodents have severely impaired early-life fertility; if the natural diet were routinely as severely restricted as the calorie-restricted regimen, it would be incompatible with survival of the species.

The growing body of descriptive data on the physiologic characteristics of calorie-restricted rodents has begun to suggest some mechanistic hypotheses worth further evaluation. Although the amount of fuel used per gram of metabolizing tissue seems not to be altered by caloric restriction, the qualitative properties of fuel use do show provocative changes. Compared with controls, calorie-restricted rats show declines in blood glucose and blood insulin levels, suggesting an increase in sensitivity to insulin action. Changes in the ratio of glucocorticoid hormone to glucocorticoid-binding proteins suggest that calorie-restricted rats are likely to have higher than normal levels of free glucocorticoids. An increase in glucocorticoid tone may contribute to their higher resistance in old age to stressful events. Calorie-restricted rats show less evidence of oxidative damage to macromolecules and higher levels of antioxidant defenses; prevention of damage by oxygen-containing reactants may contribute to the antiaging effects of the calorie-restricted protocol.

Although the effects of caloric restriction establish the important principle that the aging rate can be modified in mammals, it is not yet clear if calorie-restricted diets would achieve similar results in longer-lived species, including humans. At least three research groups have now embarked on a longitudinal study of calorie-restricted diets in nonhuman primates. Preliminary results from one of these studies suggest that caloric restriction may be able to retard the development of age-associated diseases in rhesus monkeys. In a group of 33 control animals, median survival was approximately 20 years, but only one of eight calorie-restricted monkeys had died by 20 years of age. The degree of caloric restriction required for optimal longevity in rodents is too severe to be practical as a human therapeutic maneuver, but some of the studies underway incorporate detailed analysis of the metabolic and physiologic concomitants of food restriction. Further understanding of the mechanism by which caloric restriction works in rodents may suggest more practical interventions for human application.

GENETICS OF LONGEVITY

Experimental gerontologists face two genetic problems: elucidating the basis for interspecies differences in aging and longevity and assessing the role of allelic differences within a species that influence aging and life span. The former problem is hard to approach with current methods, but work on the latter has begun to generate valuable insights. Most of the studies use life span as the sole index of aging rate, and this can present interpretative difficulties, making it difficult to disentangle genetic effects on aging from the effects on specific, common diseases.

The results discussed earlier for selected populations of fruit flies and opossum populations suggest that there may be considerable effects of genotype on maximal longevity and the aging rate within a species. Human twin studies have shown that, for individuals dying after the age of 15 years in modern Denmark, about one-third of the variation in life span can be attributed to genetic effects. Much of the genetic variation was of the nonadditive type; it was attributable to dominance effects and to interactions among alleles at different genetic loci. In some twin pairs, the genetic effects could not be attributed solely to occurrence of diseases that lead to relatively early death (before 60 years of age), because genetic effects were demonstrable even in subsets of twins that lived to older ages.

Screens of a few polymorphic loci have shown that very-long-lived persons (centenarians) have statistically higher probabilities of having inherited the E2 allele of the gene for apolipoprotein E at the expense of the E4 allele, which is associated with atherosclerosis and Alzheimer's disease. It is surprising that centenarians also tend to have inherited in homozygous form the D allele at the angiotensin-converting enzyme locus, even though the D allele is thought to predispose to coronary heart disease. It remains to be seen if these or other human polymorphisms have an effect on age-associated physiologic or pathologic processes unconnected to a specific, common, lethal disease or have predictive value in those who do not live to the age of 100.

Human genetic studies are handicapped by the inability to test the progeny of experimental matings, and much of what is known about the genetic control of aging has emerged from studies of rodents and invertebrates. The most informative study of longevity in mice involved life-span determinations for 360 female mice of 20 different inbred strains, each of which had a different combination of alleles from two parental mouse strains. The mean life span differed substantially between the longest- and shortest-lived strains (904 and 479 days). Genetic variation accounted for only 29% of the total variation in life span, a value consistent with the heritability estimates derived from human twin studies. A surprisingly large proportion, 44%, of the 101 distinguishable genetic markers were significantly correlated with variations in life span when considered individually; this number remains large (16%) even after adjustment for multiple comparison artifacts. Much of the genetic variation could be accounted for by groups of as few as six to seven influential loci.

Analysis of life-span statistics among breeds of dogs are also consistent with the idea that fairly small numbers of genetic alleles may, in concert, lead to significant variation in aging rate within a species. Artificial selection for differences in body size among dog breeds, for example, has led to differences of as much as 50% in mean longevity (Fig. 15.4). Although the number of relevant genetic alleles has not been determined, it is noteworthy that 56% of the variation in breed longevity can be attributed to interbreed variations in size alone, and that the size differences have been shown in some cases to represent differences in production of or response to growth hormone.

Studies of the effects of single genetic loci on aging have progressed most rapidly in invertebrate species, particularly the nematode *Caenorhabditis elegans,* which presents special technical advantages for genetic analysis. Several laboratories have identified single-locus mutations that lead to increased life span in *C. elegans.* The most potent of these lead by themselves to a doubling of life span, and the most potent combinations can lead to a four-fold increase in longevity. Some of the loci have now been cloned and shown to resemble human genes that code, respectively, for the insulin receptor, for a lipid kinase involved in cell activation, and for a transcription factor that is likely to regulate expression of multiple other genes. Three aspects of this work are particularly provocative.

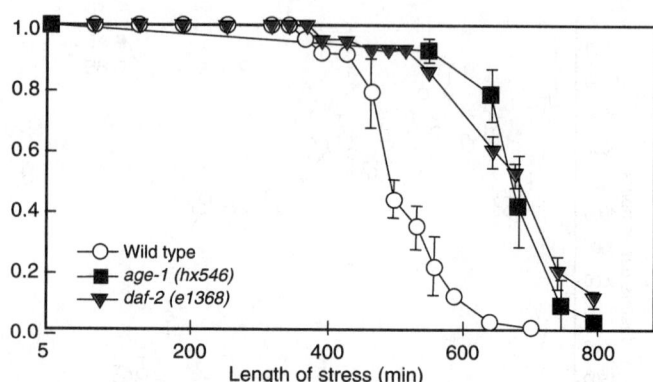

FIGURE 15.5. Survival of nematode worms subjected to acute thermal stress (35° C) for periods of up to 800 minutes. Worms of the two long-lived mutant strains, *age-1* and *daf-2*, are more resistant to heat-induced death than are control worms. (Courtesy of Gordon Lithgow.)

First, it is noteworthy that many, perhaps most, of the genetic alleles that convey extended life span in the worm also render the mutant animals more resistant to a fairly wide range of cellular stresses, such as high temperature, exposure to oxidizing agents, and ultraviolet radiation. It is possible that increased cellular stress resistance is *per se* the common element connecting these genetic changes to life span, and, if so, studies of the molecular basis for stress resistance in mammals might have important implications. Figure 15.5, for example, illustrates the remarkable resistance to heat stress seen in two distinct mutations that extend life span in the nematode. Second, the genetic analysis has shown that normal (nonmutant) worms have a protein, *daf-16,* that ordinarily acts in the adult to turn off a set of genes that would otherwise lead to life span prolongation. Many of the long-lived mutants act by turning off this life-span–shortening gene program in adults. Why this short-life-span *daf-16* gene is helpful to the normal worm, what genes it activates to shorten life span, and whether a similar set of genes lead to late life illness in humans all are important goals for future work. Third, it is interesting to note that several of the life-span–prolonging alleles are arguably related in some way to fuel utilization or food consumption, consistent with the speculation that the pathways they control might be analogous to those used to extend life span in the food-restricted rodent. Thus, it is possible, although still speculative, that analysis of the human or mouse equivalents of these genes and the biochemical pathways that they regulate, might help to tease apart the genetic controls of aging in vertebrates.

There are currently only two examples of mammalian single gene mutations that can extend life span beyond that of nonmutant controls. The "df" (Ames dwarf) and "dw" (Snell dwarf) mutations both prevent normal development of the anterior pituitary, and therefore contribute to the lifelong absence of growth hormone, thyroid hormone, and prolactin. The mutant mice are dwarfs, with an adult weight about one-third of that of their normal siblings, although they become quite obese as adults. Bartke and his colleagues have shown that males of the Ames dwarf genotype live about 50% longer, and females 75% longer, than nonmutant controls, and two groups have similar

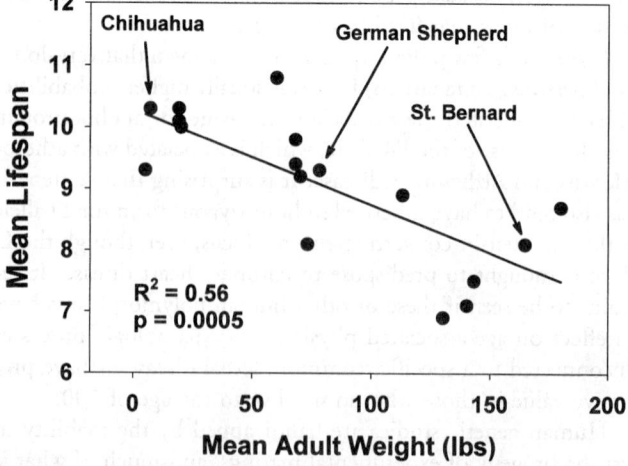

FIGURE 15.4. Big dogs die young: correlation of mean weight with mean longevity for 17 breeds of dogs. Each symbol represents a separate breed. (Data from Y. Li, B. Deeb, W. Pendergrass, and N. Wolf. Cellular proliferative capacity and lifespan in small and large dogs. *J Gerontol Biol Sci* 1996;51:B403–B408, with permission.)

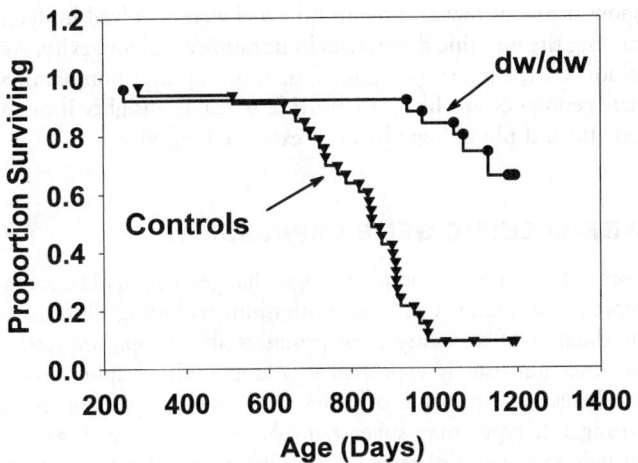

FIGURE 15.6. Extended life span in the *dw/dw* Snell dwarf mutant mice, on the relatively long-lived (DW × C3H)F1 background stock. These mutant mice lack pituitary hormones including growth hormone, prolactin, and thyroid hormone.

unpublished data for the Snell dwarf mice (Fig. 15.6). More work is needed to determine which other aspects of normal aging (aside from mortality risk) are decelerated in these mutant mouse lines, and to learn whether the improvement in life span is due to diminished influences of growth hormone or thyroid hormone *per se*, or rather to some more general effect of small body size.

THEORIES OF AGING

Many authorities have attempted to explain aging in terms of physical, biochemical, or developmental processes, and it is fair to state that none of these theories has yet provided a comprehensive, internally consistent, mechanistic explanation for the phenotype of aged subjects, the differences in aging rates across species, or the timing of aging itself. Incisive experiments and analyses have, however, begun to refute some of the most popular of the proposed ideas.

The *error hypothesis* proposed by Orgel suggested that alterations in the biochemical machinery responsible for fidelity of DNA replication, RNA transcription, and translation of mRNA into protein might become self-amplifying through a form of positive feedback, as changes that led to diminished fidelity (e.g., defects in the genes encoding portions of the ribosomal proteins or transfer RNAs) led to further errors or diminished error-correction capability. Although work to test this idea has led to provocative insights into protein folding and degradation rates in cells from older donors, the hypothesis itself has been disproved by data showing no systematic change with age in the primary amino acid sequences of translated proteins.

The *rate of living theory* proposed by Pearl began by observing that larger animals tended to have lower basal metabolic rates and greater longevity; it suggested in its strongest form that cells had a fixed capacity for metabolism, expressed in calories used per gram of lean tissue, with senescence and death a result of

reaching this intrinsic limit. The weaker form of this theory suggested that high metabolic rates would lead to shorter life spans, perhaps through the effects of toxic byproducts of metabolic pathways, including reactive oxygen intermediates. Detailed analyses of the relation between metabolic rate and longevity, however, fail to support the proposed association. Lifetime energy expenditure per gram varies over a 25-fold range within mammals and over an 8-fold range even among species within a mammalian order. Bats and birds tend to have increased longevity despite metabolic rates that are as high as or higher than nonflying species of similar size. Marsupials, which tend to have metabolic rates about 20% lower than nonmarsupial mammals of similar size, have lower life spans than nonmarsupials, in direct contrast to the prediction of the rate of living idea.

The general relation between metabolic rate and life span now seems well explained on the basis of other considerations: large animals, which tend to be less subject to predation and tend to require more time for development and nurturance of their young, also have a lower ratio of surface area to body mass and need to devote less fuel to maintenance of body temperature. Other provocative ideas, including the proposal that high brain-to-body-weight ratios accompany increased longevity across species, similarly fail when tested against a sufficiently wide range of comparative data.

Despite this progress in testing theories, experimental gerontology is still embarrassed by its rich supply of superficially plausible and largely untested general theories of how aging works. The key timing mechanism has been variously attributed to damage caused by free radicals or other highly reactive oxygen species, to unremovable glycosylation adducts, to changes in the composition and fluidity of plasma membranes, to autoimmune hypersensitivity, to clonal exhaustion by repeated mitosis of proliferative cell populations, to cross-linked extracellular proteins, to deletion of mitochondrial genes, and to alterations in protein synthesis and degradation rates, among numerous others. Each of these ideas is supported by some indirectly supportive circumstantial evidence involving age-associated damage in at least one cell type or tissue in at least one organism.

Critical tests of these notions are difficult to devise and are rarely proposed or carried out. A convincing test of a general theory of aging would need to meet at least two criteria. First, it would need to explain differences between young and old adults in the properties of connective tissues, proliferative cells, nonproliferating cells, and system integration. Second, it would need to account for the wide variations in aging rates among animal species that, like mice and humans, have very similar basic body plans and metabolic pathways.

PROMISING ISSUES IN MODERN BIOGERONTOLOGY

It is impossible to describe here more than a small fraction of the interesting work in progress in experimental gerontology, but a synopsis of a few, highly selected research areas can give some impression of what is underway.

GENETIC MANIPULATION OF THE AGING RATE

Studies of aging have used the nematode *C. elegans* to search for single-gene mutations that extend life span and have selected for delayed reproduction in the fly *Drosophila melanogaster* to generate long-lived lines of fruit flies. Other genetic manipulations designed to test specific theories of aging have begun to produce provocative results. One group, for example, has shown that overexpression of the antioxidant enzyme superoxide dismutase (SOD) in fly motor neurons led to a 40% increase in overall longevity, even though the enzyme was present in only one specific cell type (Fig. 15.7). A second group has suggested that overexpression of both SOD and catalase in flies can lead to improvements in life span that are not seen, in their stocks, when either enzyme is overexpressed by itself. These data support the theory that accumulation of oxidant-mediated damage may limit adult life span, at least in fruit flies.

The idea that diminished immune function might contribute to the development of late-life disease in mammals has been tested by an analysis of mouse lines selectively bred over many generations for high or for low levels of immune responsiveness. Mice bred for high immunity were found to have almost twofold increases in mean and maximal longevity compared with mice bred for low immunity. Within the backcross population, the mice with the highest levels of immunity also tended to have the highest life expectancy. Age-adjusted incidence rates for hematopoietic and solid tumors were lower in the high-immunity animals. Although this study did not include a key control—unselected mice—and may have been complicated by exposure to microorganisms typically present in a conventional mouse colony, the results provide some evidence that selection for high immunity may produce genotypes with extended longevity. Quantitative analyses of the variance among these selected lines

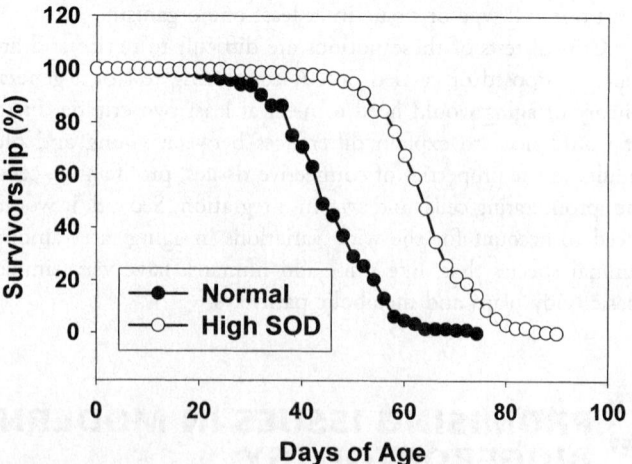

FIGURE 15.7. Increased longevity in transgenic fruit flies overexpressing human superoxide dismutase in motor neuron cells alone. (Courtesy of John Phillips: see *Nature Genetics* 1998;19:171–174.)

showed that as few as three to nine loci were involved in determining the interline differences in immunity and longevity. Additional attempts to manipulate mammalian and nonmammalian genotypes are likely to provide valuable insights into the genetic and physiologic bases of extreme longevity.

AGE-SPECIFIC GENE EXPRESSION

Some of the diseases and physiologic changes seen in old age may represent alterations in gene expression, including diminished production of necessary gene products and ectopic expression of genes not usually expressed in young adults. Exploration of the bases for expression of genes at the wrong times or in the wrong cell types may suggest mechanistic clues, such as age-specific expression of responsible transcriptional regulators.

Invertebrate and mammalian systems have begun to generate interesting results. In fruit flies, for example, enhancer-trap lines can be developed in which cells that express genes of interest can be identified throughout the life span. More than 100 such lines have been developed in some laboratories, and genes whose expression is ordinarily prominent and important in embryogenesis, including those called *engrailed*, hedgehog, and *wingless,* have been found to be expressed with different patterns in adult life, for reasons and with consequences still to be determined. In studies of mouse B lymphocytes, late-life shifts occur in the patterns of antibody gene selection and intersegment gene splicing systems. These shifts could have an impact on antimicrobial defenses, and analysis of their mechanism could throw light on underlying alterations in gene control mechanisms.

Numerous examples can be seen of age-specific alterations in production of mRNA for tissue-specific genes in rodents. Such changes are likely to represent a complex set of intercellular regulatory pathways, compensations for alterations in hormone and cytokine levels, and reactions to early or late stages of diseases, and it is difficult to find in such data indications of primary aging processes. The advent of array-based techniques for automated quantitation of hundreds or thousands of specific mRNA species in tissue samples will soon make it possible to acquire massive amounts of data relevant to age effects on gene expression. These new methods may give useful clues to how aging alters gene expression, and how these changes in gene expression affect tissue and cell function, but the approaches will not by themselves make it easier to deal with the complications of cellular heterogeneity and intercellular interactions, nor make it a simple matter to decide which few of the scores of age-dependent alterations in gene expression are primary or significant for optimal physiologic function and good health.

An alternative to the gene-screening approach involves construction of transgenic mice in which transcription of reporter genes is driven by promoters with interesting age-specific behavior. One group, for example, has shown that transcription from the human transferrin promoter region declines in transgenic mice, reflecting the typical age-dependent decline of human (but not mouse) transferrin expression. This provocative result suggests the promoter complexes may be able to recognize control factors that reflect organismic age and then interpret these signals in a way that reflects the gene and the species of origin. This system also provides an opportunity for examining specific regions of the promoter sequences for effects on the pattern of expression in the aging mice. Similar work based on genes that encode age-sensitive clotting proteins, or proteins involved in late-life diseases, is likely to give useful insights into how aging alters gene expression.

A third research avenue involves genetic engineering, in animal models, to enable the visualization in specific tissues of genes thought to play a role in life-span determination and disease prevention.

CHANGES IN CHROMOSOMAL STRUCTURE

Several lines of evidence suggest age-dependent alterations in higher levels of chromosomal organization with potential implications for gene expression and cellular behavior. One set of investigations showed that cells from female mice can reactivate X-chromosomal loci that had been inactivated early in embryonic life. In one such study, up to 3% of liver cells from older mice were shown to have reactivated the repressed allele of the liver-specific enzyme ornithine carbamoyl transferase. Similar results have emerged from some, but not all, such systems analyzed, and more work is needed to determine the factors that influence age-specific reactivation on the X chromosome to test for possible reactivation of inactivated genes on other chromosomes and to decipher the clinical implications of this heterochronic gene expression.

A second provocative line of research has focused on the effects of aging on the telomeres, which are regions at the tips of the chromosomes. Replication of the ends of DNA molecules requires the activity of an enzyme, telomerase, which is not ordinarily present in somatic cells. Continued cellular replication is accompanied by progressive shortening of the telomeric DNA. There is a reduction with donor age in the length of the telomeric DNA in cell types that are continually generated by mitosis in adult life, including colonic mucosal cells and lymphocytes. It seems plausible—although still speculative—that continued diminution of telomeric DNA may ultimately lead in some cells in old organisms to reexpression of deleterious genes ordinarily repressed in these cell types by their proximity to telomeres or may lead to chromosomal rearrangements that predispose to neoplasia. It is noteworthy, however, that mice genetically engineered to have no functional telomerase appear to be viable, healthy, and fertile, although the decline in telomere length gradually leads to impaired wound healing and lower fertility three to six generations later.

CLONAL SENESCENCE IN CULTURED CELLS

The observation by Hayflick and Moorhead that human diploid fibroblasts are capable of only a limited number of doubling divisions in tissue culture has led to a great deal of further investigation, sparked by the idea that this form of clonal exhaustion might contribute to or at least provide insights into the aging process in intact animals. Most effort has gone into dissection of the changes that prevent further mitosis of the end-stage cells produced at the end of the culture's replicative life span, and a sophisticated picture of changes in gene expression that prevent late passage fibroblasts from dividing in response to mitogenic signals has begun to emerge. It now seems likely that diminished telomere length contributes to the growth cessation seen in late-passage cell lines, because forced expression of telomerase leads (in some cell types) to indefinitely prolonged cellular growth in culture. Many cell types, including human vascular endothelial cells, lymphocytes, and secretory epithelial cells, have only a limited capability for clonal expansion *in vivo,* and it is tempting to speculate that a diminished capacity for continued mitotic growth may contribute to physiologic deficits in elderly individuals, including perhaps alterations in wound healing and tissue remodeling, immune responsiveness, and reendothelialization of denuded vascular surfaces. Much more must be done, however, to establish whether cells with the properties of late-passage fibroblasts are present in the tissues of elderly persons and whether clonal senescence has pathophysiologic consequences. There is at present little or no evidence that clonal senescence of this kind actually occurs to a significant extent in intact organisms, or that this process contributes to late-life disease or dysfunction.

HUMAN DISEASES THAT MIMIC ASPECTS OF ACCELERATED AGING

Certain human diseases involve the development in children or young adults of pathophysiologic changes ordinarily seen in normal elderly persons. George Martin has called these diseases *segmental progeroid* syndromes and championed the idea that analysis of their molecular basis could shed light on the molecular biology of aging itself.

Some of the most dramatic examples are found in the rare genetic diseases of Hutchinson–Gilford progeria syndrome and Werner's syndrome, in which patients in their childhood or young adult years, respectively, exhibit a striking variety of age-related features, including decreased skin elasticity, increased bone fragility, atheroma formation, and other abnormalities. Werner's and progeria victims, however, also exhibit characteristics not seen as a part of normal aging and fail to show many of the features of normal aging. Although neither of these two syndromes can be attributed to a simple acceleration of some hypothetical aging clock, elucidation of their genetic bases could provide valuable insights into the mechanism of age-related changes in tissue structure and function and into how these may be timed to occur at different phases of the life span. The recent cloning of the Werner's syndrome gene *WRN*, and the demonstration that the protein has DNA unwinding and exonuclease activities, has sparked new research on the possible involvement of DNA repair processes in some forms of late-life degenerative disease. Although the mutation that leads to classic Werner's syndrome is extremely rare, there is now some indication that more common alleles of the same genetic locus may increase risk of late-life myocardial infarction in elderly Japanese, with similar studies now underway in other populations. Further study of the molecular pathogenesis of Werner's syndrome could provide information about how aging leads to changes of connective and vascular tissue with clinical significance. In the same way, studies of Down's syndrome and early-onset familial dementias have generated important ideas about age-related changes in cognitive function and their basis in central nervous system architecture.

GERONTOLOGY, GERIATRICS, AND THE PUBLIC HEALTH

Much research has been focused on the major diseases of older persons, including cardiovascular disease, diabetes, neoplasia, arthritis, and other degenerative syndromes. Far less effort has been devoted to understanding the aging process, which seems to time the onset of these clinical entities and the progression of the thousand natural shocks that flesh is heir to but that are considered to lie outside the purview of the modern physician.

Demographic projections show that a complete elimination of the mortality attributable to cancer, adult-onset diabetes, and all cardiovascular diseases would lead to an increase in life expectancy at birth of 21% for male infants and 20% for female infants. By comparison, experimental alteration of aging rate by caloric restriction in rodents can improve life expectancy by 40% or more, with at least as great an impact on a healthy life span. Similarly, single gene changes are now known, which can extend mouse life span by 50% or more and give clues to ways in which alterations of endocrine status may stave off disease late in life. Research into the genetics of aging and the basic biology of the aging process may produce valuable insights into the pathogenesis of late-life illness and perhaps lead to interventions with profound effects on the health and well-being of elderly persons.

Acknowledgment

Preparation of this chapter was supported by grants from the National Institute on Aging, including AG08808, AG09801, and AG11687. I am grateful to many colleagues for allowing me to cite their work before its publication and for instructing me about the implications of their findings.

BIBLIOGRAPHY

Austad SN. Retarded senescence in an insular population of Virginia opossums. *J Zool Lond* 1993;229:695.

Austad SN. *Why we age: what science is discovering about the body's journey through life.* New York: John Wiley & Sons, 1997.

Brown-Borg HM, Borg KE, Meliska CJ, Bartke A. Dwarf mice and the ageing process. *Nature* 1996;384:33.

Comfort A. *The biology of senescence.* New York: Elsevier, 1979.

Finch CE. *Longevity, senescence, and the genome.* Chicago: University of Chicago Press, 1990.

Harrison DE. *Genetic effects on aging, II.* Caldwell, NJ: The Telford Press, 1990.

Masoro EJ. Aging, Section 11. In: *Handbook of physiology.* New York: Oxford University Press, 1995.

Ricklefs RE, Finch CE. *Aging. A natural history.* New York: Scientific American Library, 1995.

Rose MR. *Evolutionary biology of aging.* New York: Oxford University Press, 1991.

Schneider EL, Rowe JW. *Handbook of the biology of aging,* fourth ed. San Diego: Academic Press, 1996.

Kelley's Textbook of Internal Medicine, fourth edition. Edited by H. David Humes. Lippincott Williams & Wilkins, Philadelphia © 2000.

C H A P T E R

16

CLINICAL PHYSIOLOGY OF AGING

LEWIS A. LIPSITZ

Physiology is the integration of a complex network of control systems and feedback loops that enable an organism to perform a variety of functions necessary for survival. The control systems of the human body exist at molecular, subcellular, cellular, organ, and systemic levels of organization. Continuous interplay among the electrical, chemical, and mechanical components of these systems ensures that information is constantly exchanged, even as the organism rests. These dynamic processes give rise to a highly adaptive, resilient organism, which is primed and ready to respond to internal and external perturbations.

Recognition of the dynamic nature of regulatory processes challenges the traditional view of physiology, which was based on Walter B. Cannon's concept of homeostasis. The *principle of homeostasis* states that all healthy cells, tissues, and organs maintain static or steady-state conditions in their internal environment. However, with the introduction of techniques that can acquire continuous data from physiologic processes, such as heart rate, blood pressure, nerve activity, or hormonal secretion, it became apparent that these systems are in constant flux, even under so-called steady-state conditions. Dr. Eugene Yates introduced the term *homeodynamics* to convey the fact that the high level of bodily control required to survive depends on a dynamic interplay of multiple regulatory mechanisms rather than constancy in the internal environment.

Although it is often difficult to separate the effects of aging from those of disease and lifestyle changes such as reduced physical activity, even aging without such confounding, secondary factors (primary aging) appears to have a profound impact on physiologic processes. Because of the progressive degeneration of various tissues and organs and the interruption of communication pathways between them, complex physiologic networks break down, become disconnected, and lose some of their capacity to adapt to stress.

There is considerable redundancy in many of these systems; for example, humans have far more muscle mass, neuronal circuitry, renal nephrons, and hormonal stores than are needed to survive. This *physiologic reserve* allows most persons to compensate effectively for age-related changes. Because the network structure of physiologic systems also enables alternate pathways to be used to achieve the same functions, physiologic changes that result from aging alone usually do not have much impact on everyday life. However, these changes may become manifest at times of increased demand, when the body is subjected to high levels of physiologic stress. For this reason, elderly persons are particularly vulnerable to falls, confusion, or incontinence when exposed to environmental, pharmacologic, or emotional stresses.

The traditional approach to the study of physiology is to divide the topic into separate organ-based systems, such as cardiovascular, respiratory, endocrine, immune, and neurologic systems. However, this approach ignores the integrated, cross-system nature of physiology. This chapter addresses the major functional roles of physiologic processes and how they are affected by normal aging.

■ REGULATION OF OXYGEN AND METABOLIC SUBSTRATE DELIVERY TO VITAL ORGANS

The vitality of all living tissues in the body depends on the delivery of optimal supplies of oxygen and glucose or other metabolic substrates to meet energy requirements during rest and exertion. This critical process relies on a complicated transport system, which picks up oxygen from the lungs and nutrients and metabolic substrates from the gastrointestinal tract or musculature, centrifugally delivers different amounts of these substances to different sites depending on the immediate need, and self-adjusts in response to transient perturbations. In reciprocal centripetal fashion, this system serves to deliver waste products to sites of excretion from the body, notably the kidney and liver. This circulatory system consists of the liquid and cellular components of the blood, vascular tree, cardiac pump, lungs, chemoreceptors, baroreceptors, and neuroendocrine communications between each of these structures. The driving force behind the delivery system is the arterial blood pressure.

AGE-RELATED CHANGES IN BLOOD PRESSURE REGULATION

Blood pressure is the product of heart rate, stroke volume, and systemic vascular resistance. Alterations in the response of any of these parameters may threaten adequate perfusion of vital organs. Normal human aging is associated with several changes that influence these three components of normal blood pressure regulation.

BAROREFLEX SENSITIVITY

The baroreflex maintains a normal blood pressure by increasing heart rate (*cardiovagal baroreflex*) and vascular resistance (*sympathetic vascular baroreflex*) in response to transient reductions in blood pressure and by decreasing these parameters in response to elevations in blood pressure. Reduced sensitivity of the cardiovagal baroreflex is evident in the blunted cardioaccelerator re-

sponse to stimuli (upright posture, nitroprusside infusions, phase II of the Valsalva maneuver, and lower-body negative pressure, for example) that lower blood pressure, and in a reduced bradycardic response to drugs such as phenylephrine or phase IV of the Valsalva that elevate blood pressure. Alteration of the sympathetic baroreflex is manifested as a blunted vasoconstrictor response to sympathetic outflow from the central nervous system. As a result of abnormal baroreflex function, elderly people have increased blood pressure variability, often with potentially dangerous blood pressure reductions during hypotensive stresses, such as upright posture or meal ingestion.

SYMPATHETIC NERVOUS SYSTEM AND END-ORGAN RESPONSE

Studies of sympathetic nervous system activity in healthy humans demonstrate an age-related increase in resting plasma norepinephrine levels and muscle sympathetic nerve activity, as well as the plasma norepinephrine response to upright posture and exercise. The elevation in plasma norepinephrine results primarily from an increased presynaptic norepinephrine secretion rate and secondarily from decreased clearance. Despite apparent elevations in sympathetic nervous system activity with aging, cardiac and vascular responsiveness is diminished. Infusions of β-adrenergic agonists result in smaller increases in heart rate, left ventricular ejection fraction, cardiac output, and vasodilation in older compared with younger men.

CARDIAC RESPONSE

Age effects on the heart have been attributed to multiple molecular and biochemical changes in β-receptor coupling and postreceptor events. The number of β receptors on cardiac myocytes is unchanged with advancing age, but the affinity of β receptors for agonists is reduced. Postreceptor changes that occur with aging include a decrease in the activity of stimulatory G protein (G_s), the adenylate cyclase catalytic unit, and cAMP (cyclic adenosine monophosphate)-dependent phosphokinase-induced protein phosphorylation. As a result of these changes, G-protein—mediated signal transduction is impaired.

The decrease in cardiac contractile response to β-adrenergic stimulation has been studied in rat ventricular myocytes, where it appears to be related to decreased influx of calcium ions through sarcolemmal calcium channels and a reduction in the amplitude of the cytosolic calcium transit. These changes are similar to those seen in receptor desensitization owing to prolonged exposure of myocardial tissue to β-adrenergic agonists. Age-associated alterations in the β-adrenergic response may result from desensitization of the adenylate cyclase system in response to chronic elevations of plasma catecholamine levels.

VASCULAR RESPONSE

The vascular response to sympathetic stimulation has received less attention, but it also appears to be altered by aging. The vasorelaxation response of arteries and veins to infusions of the β-adrenergic agonist isoproterenol is attenuated in elderly people

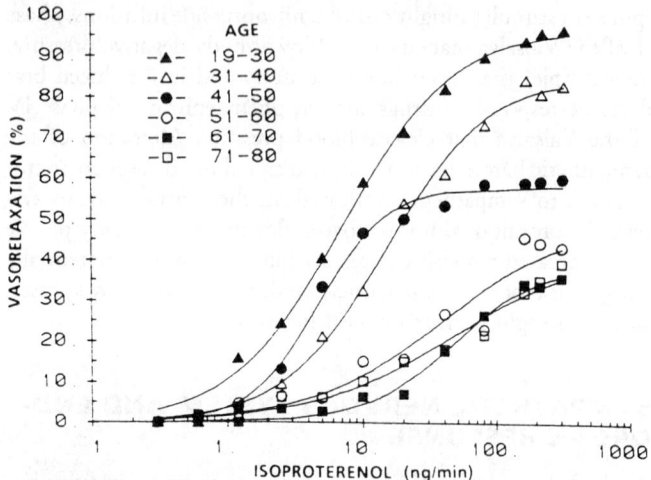

FIGURE 16.1. Effects of isoproterenol infusion in preconstricted dorsal hand veins in the six populations studied. (From Pan HY-M, Hoffman BB, Pershe RA, Blaschke TF. Decline in beta adrenergic receptor-mediated vascular relaxation with aging in man. *J Pharmacol Exp Ther* 1986;239: 802, with permission.)

(Fig. 16.1). α-Adrenergic vasoconstrictor responses to norepinephrine infusion also appear to be reduced in healthy elderly subjects (Fig. 16.2). The fact that this impairment is reversed by suppression of sympathetic nervous system activity with guanadrel suggests that it is also caused by receptor desensitization in response to heightened sympathetic nervous system activity. Thus, some of the physiologic changes associated with aging may be reversible.

AUTONOMIC CONTROL OF HEART RATE

Alterations in sympathetic and parasympathetic influences on the heart may also influence the heart rate response to blood pressure changes. Previous studies demonstrating age-related reductions in overall heart rate variability in response to respiration, cough, and the Valsalva maneuver suggest that aging is associated with impaired vagal control of heart rate. Elderly pa-

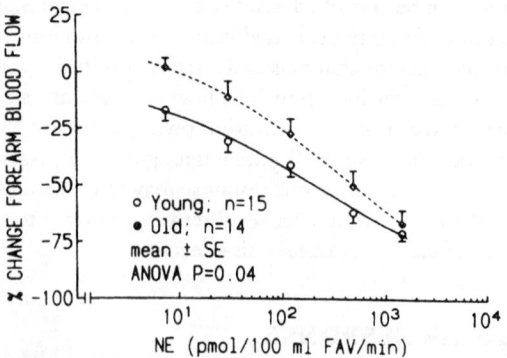

FIGURE 16.2. Group mean data for the percent change in forearm blood flow from the baseline values in response to intra-arterial infusions of norepinephrine (*NE*) in young (—○—) and older (--●--) subjects. (From Hogikyan RV, Supiano MA. Arterial α-adrenergic responsiveness is decreased and SNS activity is increased in older humans. *Am J Physiol* 1994;266:E717, with permission.)

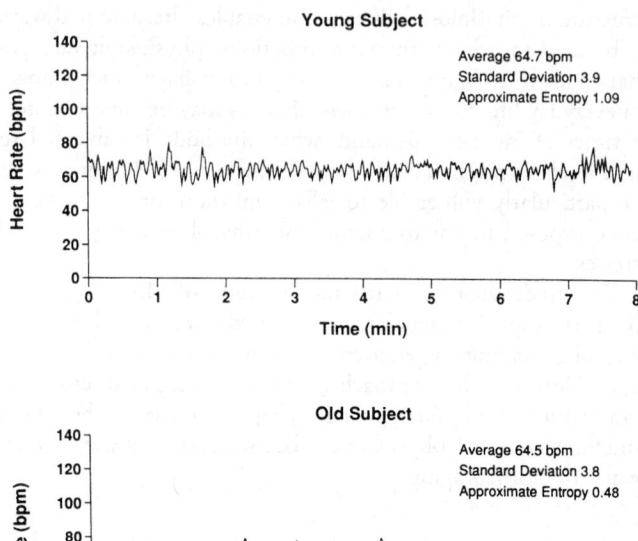

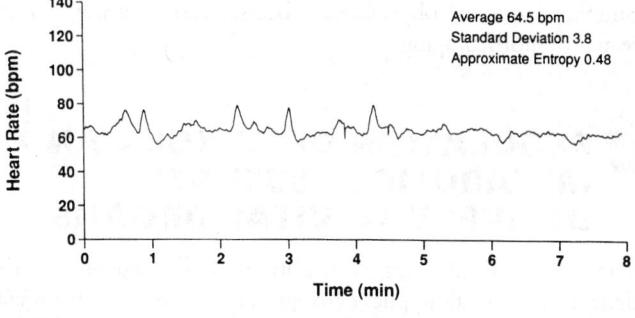

FIGURE 16.3. Heart rate time series for (**A**) a 22-year-old woman and (**B**) a 73-year-old man. Approximate entropy is a measure of "nonlinear complexity." Despite the nearly identical means and standard deviations of heart rate for the two time series, the complexity of the signal from the older subject is markedly reduced. (From Lipsitz LA, Goldberger AL. Loss of "complexity" and aging: potential applications of fractals and chaos theory to senescence. *JAMA* 1992;267:1806, with permission.)

tients with unexplained syncope have even greater impairments in heart rate responses to cough and deep breathing than elderly persons without syncope.

The age-related attenuation of autonomic, neurohumoral, and other influences on heart rate results in a reduction in heart rate variability and in a marked change in the dynamics of beat-to-beat heart rate fluctuations. As shown in Figure 16.3, the highly irregular, complex dynamics of heart rate variability characteristic of healthy young individuals are lost with healthy aging, resulting in a more regular and predictable heart rate time series. This loss of complexity in heart rate dynamics can be generalized to the fluctuating output of many different physiologic processes as they age. For example, measurements of continuous blood pressure, electroencephalographic waves, frequently sampled thyrotropin or luteinizing hormone levels, and center-of-pressure changes during quiet stance all show more regular, less complex behavior with aging. This apparent loss of dynamic range in physiologic functions may reflect fewer regulatory influences as a person ages, leading to an impaired capacity to adapt to stress.

CARDIAC VENTRICULAR FUNCTION

The maintenance of a normal blood pressure also depends on the ability to generate an adequate cardiac output. Cardiac output at rest and during exercise tends to decrease with normal aging because of a reduction in heart rate response to β-adrenergic stimulation and because of changes in systolic and diastolic myocardial performance, which influence stroke volume.

Diastolic Function

As a result of increased cross-linking of myocardial collagen and a prolonged ventricular relaxation time, the aged heart stiffens, and early diastolic ventricular filling becomes impaired (Fig. 16.4). The age-related impairment in early ventricular filling makes the heart depend on adequate preload to fill the ventricle and on atrial contraction during late diastole to maintain stroke volume. Orthostatic hypotension and syncope occur commonly in older persons as a result of volume contraction or venous pooling, which reduces cardiac preload, or as a result of the onset of atrial fibrillation when the atrial contribution to cardiac output is suddenly lost. These changes also render the elderly person more vulnerable to congestive heart failure attributable to diastolic dysfunction.

Systolic Function

With aging, myocardial contractile strength is preserved, but left ventricular ejection fraction in response to exertion decreases

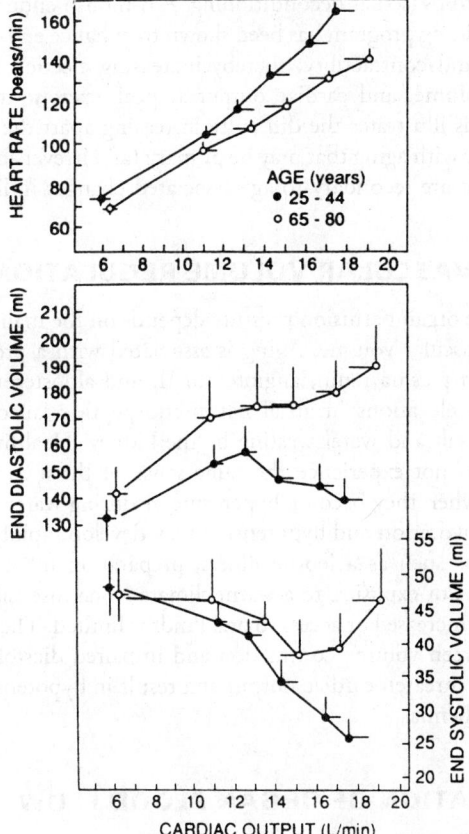

FIGURE 16.5. Heart rate (*top panel*) and cardiac volumes (*bottom panel*) at end diastole and end systole at rest and during graded levels of exercise on a cycle ergometer in older and younger individuals. A blunted heart rate and cardiac dilatation at end diastole and end systole are characteristic features of the exercise response in older persons. (From Rodeheffer RJ, Gerstenblith G, Becker LC, et al. Exercise cardiac output is maintained with advancing age in healthy human subjects: cardiac dilatation and increased stroke volume compensate for a diminished heart rate. *Circulation* 1984;69:203, with permission.)

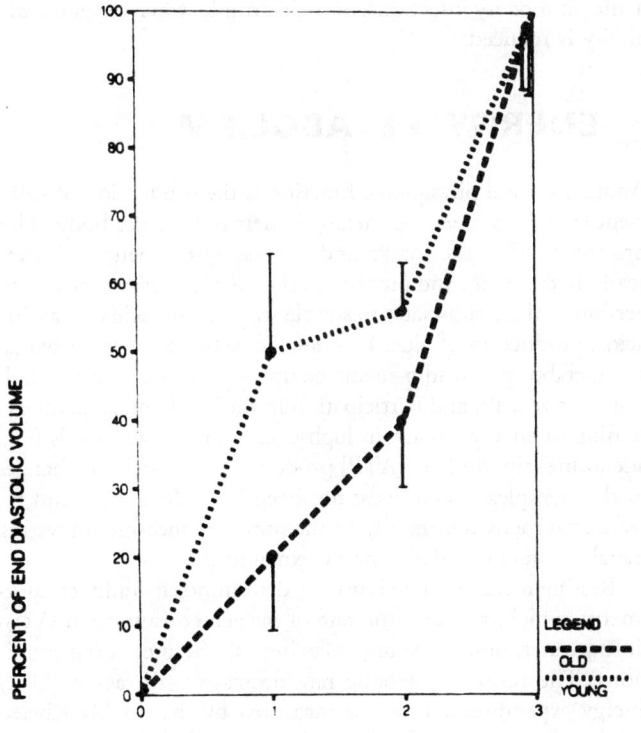

PHASE OF DIASTOLE

FIGURE 16.4. Cumulative percentage of the left ventricular end-diastolic volume filled during each third of diastole for young (*dotted line*) and old (*dashed line*) subjects. Notice the marked reduction in early diastolic filling and greater percentage of filling in late diastole in elderly subjects compared with young persons. (From Lipsitz LA, Jonsson PV, Marks BL, et al. Reduced supine cardiac volumes and diastolic filling rates in elderly patients with chronic medical conditions: implications for postural blood pressure homeostasis. *JAGS* 1990;38:103, with permission.)

because of reduced β-adrenergic responsiveness and an increased afterload. Afterload, which represents opposition to left ventricular ejection, increases progressively with aging because of stiffening of the ascending aorta and narrowing of the peripheral vasculature. These changes result in an increase in systolic blood pressure with aging and a decrease in the maximum cardiac output during exercise.

The cardiac response to exercise is different in healthy young and old subjects (Fig. 16.5). Although the young increase cardiac output by increases in heart rate and decreases in end-systolic volume (greater contractility), the healthy elderly do so by increasing end-diastolic volume (cardiac dilatation). The elderly thus rely on the Frank–Starling relation to achieve an increase in stroke volume during exercise more than do younger persons. A similar mechanism can be demonstrated in young subjects during β-adrenergic blockade, suggesting that the age effect is caused by reduced β-adrenergic responsiveness.

The age-related decrease in maximal cardiac output during exercise may also be related to a sedentary lifestyle and consequent cardiovascular deconditioning. A 6-month endurance exercise training program has been shown to enhance end-diastolic volume and contractility, thereby increasing ejection fraction, stroke volume, and cardiac output at peak exercise in elderly men. This illustrates the difficulty in teasing apart the changes occurring with aging that may be primary (and irreversible) from those that are secondary to age-associated changes in lifestyle.

INTRAVASCULAR VOLUME REGULATION

Adequate organ perfusion pressure depends on the maintenance of intravascular volume. Aging is associated with a progressive decline in plasma renin, angiotensin II, and aldosterone levels and with elevations in atrial natriuretic peptide, all of which promote salt and water wasting by the kidney. Healthy elderly people do not experience the same sense of thirst as younger persons when they become hyperosmolar during water deprivation. Dehydration and hypotension may develop rapidly during conditions such as a febrile illness, preparation for a medical procedure, or exposure to a warm climate when insensible fluid losses are increased or access to oral fluids is limited. The interaction between volume contraction and impaired diastolic function may threaten cardiac output and result in hypotension and organ ischemia.

REGULATION OF ORGAN BLOOD FLOW

The regulation of blood flow to various circulatory beds depends on complex interactions among the endothelium, local vasoactive peptides, neuroendocrine influences, and mechanical forces. In angiographically normal coronary arteries and forearm resistance vessels, the endothelium-dependent vasodilatory response to acetylcholine is reduced with aging.

Normal human aging is also associated with a reduction in cerebral blood flow, which is further compromised by the presence of risk factors for cerebrovascular disease. Although it is not clear whether the decline in cerebral blood flow results from reduced supply or demand, elderly persons, particularly those with cerebrovascular disease, probably have a resting cerebral blood flow that is closer to the threshold for cerebral ischemia. Consequently, relatively small, short-term reductions in blood pressure may produce cerebral ischemic symptoms.

The brain normally maintains a constant blood flow over a wide range of perfusion pressures through the process of autoregulation. During reductions in blood pressure, resistance vessels in the brain dilate to restore blood flow to normal. Although the effects of aging on cerebral autoregulation have received little attention, limited data suggest that the autoregulation of cerebral blood flow is preserved into old age. However, patients with symptomatic orthostatic hypotension appear to have a reduction in cerebral blood flow in response to decreased perfusion pressure.

CONTROL OF RESPIRATION

The delivery of necessary substrates for oxidative metabolism depends on maintaining an optimal tissue perfusion pressure

and on the availability of oxygen from the lungs. Pulmonary and circulatory physiology are closely linked, enabling adjustments in heart rate, cardiac output, blood pressure, and organ flow to be made in response to changing demands for oxygen.

Aging is associated with a reduction in the partial pressure of oxygen in the blood, primarily caused by a mismatch of ventilation and perfusion in the dependent portions of the lungs. This results from a reduction in lung compliance, which causes airways to close prematurely at higher lung volumes (i.e., increased closing volume) within the range of vital capacity. The relative hypoxemia in advanced age was thought to be offset by a reduced tissue demand for oxygen (reduced maximal oxygen uptake). However, much of the reduction in maximum oxygen consumption ($\dot{V}o_2$max) is attributable to reduced muscle mass and is reversible with endurance exercise training.

Chemoreceptors located in brain stem respiratory centers adjust respiratory amplitude and frequency on a moment-to-moment basis to ensure adequate oxygen availability and carbon dioxide clearance in the blood. Longer-term changes in oxygen supply and demand are matched by finely tuned adjustments in the sensitivity (i.e., gain) of chemoreceptors. With advancing age, chemosensitivity to oxygen and carbon dioxide tension declines, resulting in relative hypoventilation in response to hypoxemia or hypercarbia. Therefore, older persons may be more vulnerable to vital organ ischemia during stresses such as surgery, acute pulmonary infections, or high altitude, when oxygen availability is reduced.

ENERGY METABOLISM

Another critical physiologic function is the production of sufficient energy to meet the metabolic demands of the body. This process requires the intake and processing of energy substrate (carbohydrate, fat, and protein) in the gastrointestinal tract; conversion of these substrates to simple sugars, fatty acids, or amino acids; production of glucose or ketoacids by the liver for oxidative metabolism; insulin-mediated uptake of glucose by metabolically active cells; and participation in the biochemical pathways leading to energy storage in high-energy phosphate bonds (i.e., adenosine triphosphate [ATP] production). Age-related changes in this complex system have not been fully elucidated, and research has focused primarily on the summary measures of resting metabolic rate and daily energy expenditure.

Resting metabolic rate is usually determined by indirect calorimetry, which measures the rate of oxygen consumption ($\dot{V}o_2$) during quiet, supine rest under fasting and thermoneutral conditions. The resting metabolic rate decreases with aging. Daily energy expenditure, which is measured by the doubly labeled water technique, includes the resting metabolic rate, the thermic response to feeding, and the energy expenditure of physical activity. Daily energy expenditure also declines with advancing age. However, the resting metabolic rate and daily energy expenditure are strongly influenced by physical fitness and activity, nutritional intake, and body composition, all of which may change over time. Many of the changes in energy metabolism observed in the elderly may reflect altered physical activity and loss of fat-free mass rather than biologic aging.

An exercise program that increases fat-free mass and energy intake can enhance energy expenditure in healthy elderly persons. Because the thermic effect of feeding is higher in physically trained than inactive older men, much of the age-associated reduction in energy expenditure is probably attributable to the adoption of a sedentary lifestyle, with its associated reduction in muscle mass.

Age-related changes in body composition may lead to a variety of disease states in the elderly. If energy intake remains constant despite reductions in physical activity, older individuals accumulate body fat. After a 3-week period of overfeeding, young men develop hypophagia and lose their excess body weight, but older men do not. This impairment in control of food intake and accumulation of body fat may lead to obesity, glucose intolerance, and hypertension.

The decline in glucose tolerance with advancing age has been well documented. It is manifested by modest elevations in fasting plasma glucose levels (approximately 1 mg per deciliter per decade) and marked elevations in 2-hour postprandial glucose levels (approximately 5 mg per liter per decade) during an oral glucose tolerance test. The glucose intolerance of aging is related to peripheral insulin resistance, caused by a postreceptor defect in target tissue insulin action. There is no age-related change in the number or affinity of insulin receptors or in maximal tissue responsiveness to insulin. However, healthy elderly subjects require larger quantities of insulin to achieve a level of glucose uptake similar to that of the young (Fig. 16.6).

Studies of glucose-stimulated insulin secretion in healthy humans have shown impairments in insulin secretory capacity with advancing age. This is balanced by a reduction in insulin clearance, the net result of which is no change in circulating insulin levels. However, the presence of "normal" circulating insulin levels in the face of hyperglycemia suggests that insulin secretion is inappropriately low. Aging thus appears to be associated with insulin resistance and impaired insulin secretion.

Although insulin resistance was once thought to be a natural consequence of biologic aging independent of carbohydrate intake, body composition, or physical activity, studies have shown elevations in body mass index and mean arterial blood pressure to be significant predictors of reduced insulin sensitivity, regardless of age. Insulin resistance can be improved by exercise training. Glucose intolerance may also result from age-associated decreases in physical activity and fat-free mass. Because of the association between chronic hyperglycemia and the development of atherosclerotic cardiovascular disease, renal disease, neuropathy, and retinopathy, the glucose intolerance of advanced age has profound implications in the pathogenesis and prevention of disease in old age. This condition should not be considered a harmless, age-related process; it should be treated as a significant risk factor for disability, which may be preventable through physical exercise and proper nutrition.

DEFENSE SYSTEMS

The ability of the human body to defend itself from external pathogens and to prevent toxic effects of chemical exposures and metabolic by-products relies on the presence of integrated

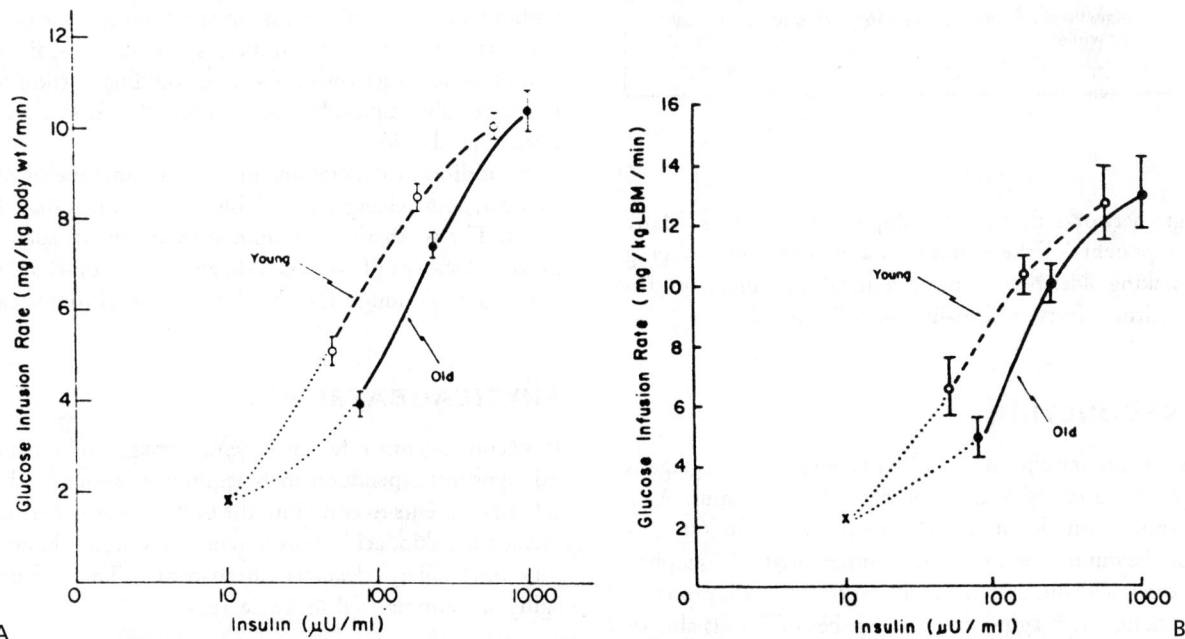

FIGURE 16.6. Dose-response curves for insulin-mediated whole body glucose infusion rates in young (*dashed line*) and old (*solid line*) subjects. **A** (left): Glucose disposal is expressed as milligrams per kilogram of body weight. **B** (right): Glucose infusion rates are normalized for lean body mass. Elderly persons have reduced sensitivity to insulin but no change in maximal glucose disposal. (From Rowe JW, Minaker KL, Pallotta JA. Characterization of the insulin resistance of aging. Reproduced from *J Clin Invest* 1983; 71:1581 by copyright permission of the American Society for Clinical Investigation.)

TABLE 16.1.	PHYSIOLOGIC DEFENSES AND THEIR CHANGES WITH AGE
Defense Mechanism	**Age Change**
Immune Function	
T lymphocytes	Impaired antigen or mitogen response
B lymphocytes	Decreased antigen-specific Ab production
Cytokines	Decreased IL-1, IL-2; increased TNF, interferon, IL-6
Antibody production	Autoantibody formation
Physical Barriers	
Skin	Thinning, loss of subcutaneous fat, decreased blood supply, fewer melanocytes to absorb UV light, decreased collagen and elasticity
Gastrointestinal tract	Hypochlorhydria and gastric atrophy
Respiratory tract	Decreased mucociliary transport and cough (?)
Removal of Toxic Chemicals	
Hepatic metabolism	Decreased first-pass and oxidative metabolism
Renal excretion	Decreased renal blood flow, GFR, and creatinine clearance
Avoidance Reactions	
Sensory awareness	Reduced high-frequency hearing, proprioceptive sensory receptors, visual accommodation, and lens transparency
Reflex motor responses	Increased reflex time and decreased nerve conduction velocity

GFR, glomerular filtration rate; *IL*, interleukin; *TNF*, tumor necrosis factor; *UV*, ultraviolet.

physiologic networks that cross multiple organ systems. Many of the components of these networks are altered by the aging process, making older persons more vulnerable to infectious disease, toxic drug effects, and malignancy (Table 16.1).

IMMUNE FUNCTION

One of the invariant changes that occurs with advancing age is the progressive atrophy and dissolution of the thymus. As a result, thymic hormones are no longer detectable after 60 years of age, and the number of immature, undifferentiated T lymphocytes increases. The number of circulating B and T cells probably does not change with aging, but the number of T cells able to respond to an antigenic challenge or mitogenic stimulus is greatly reduced. Cells that can respond to a stimulus and enter the cell cycle appear to have a decreased ability to divide sequentially in culture.

The defect in T-lymphocyte response may reflect alterations

in various lymphokines, particularly interleukin-2 (IL-2). The production of IL-2 by stimulated CD4 helper cells and the response to IL-2 by proliferating cells are reduced in the elderly, partly because of the loss of thymic hormones that augment IL-2 production by proliferating cells in culture. There appears to be a defect in the ability of lymphocytes to express IL-2 mRNA and in the IL-2 high-affinity receptor (Tac antigen). In addition to alterations in intercellular signaling, many cells lose their intrinsic ability to respond to various stimuli. Alterations in cytoskeletal structures, DNA repair mechanisms, membrane properties, enzyme activity, and protein synthesis all affect cellular responses.

B-cell production of antigen-specific antibodies is reduced with aging, in large part because of a reduction in helper T cells and increased activity of suppressor T cells. It appears as if a breakdown of communication pathways between cells rather than alterations in the intrinsic properties of the cellular components themselves is primarily responsible for immune senescence. Decreased T-cell control of B-cell function also may be responsible for the marked increase in monoclonal immunoglobulin levels seen in the elderly. Elevations of monoclonal immunoglobulins (M components) in the serum may be asymptomatic and benign, or they may be associated with malignancies such as multiple myeloma, Waldenström's macroglobulinemia, primary amyloidosis, or heavy-chain disease. The fact that monoclonal gammopathies can be induced in young mice by ablation of the thymus gland and induction of inflammation by endotoxin lends support to the notion that dysregulation of immune function in the elderly is related in part to loss of thymic hormones.

Aging is also associated with an increase in autoantibodies such as anti-DNA or antithyroglobulin antibodies, although without an associated increase in autoimmune disease. This has been attributed partly to an increase in autoanti-idiotypic antibodies, which react with the antigen-binding portion of the immunoglobulin molecule and suppress the formation of other normal antibodies.

In addition to alterations in cellular components of the immune system, changes in soluble factors other than IL-2 also occur. The synthesis of inflammatory mediators such as tumor necrosis factor-α (TNF-α), IL-6, and interferon-α are increased with aging, although IL-1 has been reported to decrease.

PHYSICAL BARRIERS

Protection against infectious agents, foreign bodies, and chemical exposures depends on an intact immune system and on physical impediments to entry into the body. These defensive barriers include the skin, acid environment in the stomach, and respiratory mucociliary clearance mechanisms. Their changes with aging are summarized in Table 16.1.

CHEMICAL DEFENSES

Several organ systems participate in the metabolism and removal of potentially toxic chemicals and drugs from the body, particularly the liver and kidneys. These organs undergo changes with age that interfere with chemical defense functions. Most important of these are a reduction in hepatic blood flow that reduces first-pass elimination of drugs such as verapamil and propranolol, an impairment in hepatic oxidation and demethylation reactions that metabolize many of the long-acting benzodiazepines, and reduced renal blood flow and glomerular filtration rate, which reduce the clearance of drugs such as digoxin and the aminoglycosides (Chapter 469).

The kidneys participate in defense of the internal chemical environment of the body by maintaining intravascular volume as discussed previously and by excreting excess acid, sodium, potassium, and water. The ability to excrete an acid load is impaired with aging. This may result from a decrease in nephron mass and resultant reduction in the production of urinary ammonium and phosphorus. The ability to excrete an acute sodium load and, probably, a potassium load is reduced with aging, principally because of a decline in the glomerular filtration rate. Elderly persons require almost twice as long as young persons to excrete equivalent amounts of salt.

Normal aging is associated with an impairment in water excretion. After a water load, the elderly have less free water clearance and a higher minimum urine osmolality than middle-aged or young persons. This is largely attributable to an age-related decrease in the glomerular filtration rate, rather than inappropriate vasopressin secretion.

MAINTAINING STRUCTURAL INTEGRITY

Maintaining a skeletal framework sufficiently strong to withstand the stresses of physical activity is an essential physiologic function that depends on the complex interaction of multiple organ systems, hormones, local growth factors, cytokines, osteocytes, and biochemical pathways leading to calcium deposition in bone. The organs that participate in this function include the skin, kidneys, liver, small intestine, parathyroid and thyroid glands, and bone. They produce various hormonal signals that ultimately regulate calcium deposition and mobilization in bone. These hormones are estrogen or testosterone, vitamin D, parathyroid hormone, and calcitonin.

Maintaining skeletal integrity is a dynamic process, characterized by constant bone turnover or remodeling. Periods of bone resorption, mediated by osteoclasts, alternate with bone formation, mediated by osteoblasts. This cyclic process is normally closely coupled, resulting in no net change in bone mass. However, with aging and particularly after menopause in women, there is a relative increase in resorption over formation, resulting in osteoporosis. The acceleration of bone loss after menopause implicates estrogen deficiency as one of the key factors influencing age-related bone loss. However, bone loss also occurs in men, although at a slower rate than in women. Bone loss may be caused by testosterone deficiency in some elderly men or by calcium malabsorption, which is another major determinant of bone loss in both sexes.

Estrogen regulates the production of cytokines and growth factors that control bone remodeling. Stimulation of peripheral blood monocytes by estrogen decreases IL-1 and TNF-α production, inhibiting IL-6 production by osteoblasts and the effect of this cytokine on osteoclast formation and bone resorption. Estrogen decreases granulocyte-macrophage colony-stimulating factor (GM-CSF), which inhibits osteoclast differentiation. Estrogen also stimulates transforming growth factor-β (TGF-β) production by osteoblasts, which decreases osteoclast-mediated bone resorption. Estrogen deficiency results in an increase in IL-1, TNF-α, GM-CSF, and IL-6 and a decrease in TGF-β production, all of which promote osteoclast formation and bone resorption.

In men, testosterone has anabolic effects that normally enhance bone formation, probably through stimulation of TGF-β and insulin-like growth factor I (IGF-I) and inhibition of prostaglandin E_2 production. Reduced levels of testosterone in late life may impair bone formation, leading to unopposed resorption and progressive bone loss.

Several other age-related changes influence bone metabolism in men and women, including decreased cutaneous production of vitamin D_3 by ultraviolet photoconversion of 7-dehydrocholesterol, impaired 1α-hydroxylation of 25-hydroxyvitamin D by the kidney, decreased intestinal absorption of calcium, and increased levels of circulating parathyroid hormone. These changes are interrelated. A decline in 1,25-dihydroxyvitamin D as a result of reduced production of precursors in the skin and impaired 1α-hydroxylation by the kidney, is partly responsible for decreased intestinal calcium absorption. Diminished gastric acid production, which is required for solubilizing and ionizing dietary calcium, and acquired lactase deficiency, which results in avoidance of milk products also contribute to negative calcium balance. The consequent reduction in serum calcium concentration and reduced concentrations of 1,25-dihydroxyvitamin D result in mild, physiologic elevations in parathyroid hormone, which increases osteoclastic bone resorption.

The many age-related changes in calcium and bone metabolism interact with lifestyle and genetic factors to reduce bone volume and predispose elderly persons to fractures. The factors influencing bone loss in the elderly are summarized in Table 16.2.

MOBILITY AND BALANCE

Mobility and balance are essential functions for the performance of activities of daily living. They are subserved by the complex interaction of brain, nerve, muscle, joint, cardiovascular, and sensory organ activity. Without coordinated movement, the human organism cannot acquire energy substrates from food, defend itself from external threats, or reproduce. Many of the changes that impair mobility and balance in advanced age are associated with deconditioning and disease rather than normal physiologic aging. The physiologic changes themselves usually do not impair function under normal circumstances, but they may do so under the demands of more severe stress.

TABLE 16.2.	FACTORS INFLUENCING BONE LOSS IN THE ELDERLY

Sex hormone deficiency
  Estrogen
  Testosterone
Vitamin D deficiency
  Decreased skin production of vitamin D_3
  Decreased α-hydroxylation by the kidney
Calcium malabsorption
  Vitamin D deficiency
  Hypochlorhydria
Calcium regulatory hormone changes
  Increased parathyroid hormone levels
Genetic factors
Lifestyle factors
  Obesity
  Decreased calcium and vitamin D intake and lactase deficiency
  Decreased physical activity (i.e., decreased mechanical loading)
  Smoking
  Decreased sunlight exposure

Healthy aging is associated with several neurologic and sensory changes that may impair postural control. These changes include the degeneration of neurons in the frontal cortex, resulting in difficulty initiating movement; basal ganglion, responsible for parkinsonian features of aging; and the cerebellum, causing ataxia and impaired balance. A gradual loss of peripheral sensory receptors occurs, including mechanoreceptors in the large joints (predominantly ankles, knees, hips, and facet joints of the cervical spine), which send afferent proprioceptive information to the brain stem about how the body is positioned in space. A reduction in proprioceptive information in addition to decreased nerve conduction velocity and consequent prolongation of reflex time impairs the body's ability to correct its position when spatially perturbed. Older persons consequently demonstrate an increase in body sway, which is most evident with the eyes closed because of increased dependence on visual input to maintain balance when other sensory inputs are compromised. Body sway is greatest in elderly people prone to falling.

Aging is also associated with a loss of muscle mass and strength, which to a large degree is related to the adoption of a sedentary lifestyle and resultant deconditioning. The loss of muscle strength is probably partially due to denervation of motor units. Muscle retains its ability to improve performance with resistance training, even well into the tenth decade of life. Gains in quadriceps muscle strength with resistance training exceed changes in muscle mass, suggesting that training results in neural recruitment of additional motor units.

A reduction in growth hormone secretion may also play a role in the age-related loss of muscle mass. Growth hormone is secreted in pulsatile fashion by the anterior pituitary and stimulates skeletal and muscle growth, amino acid uptake, and lipolysis. Its effects are mediated by the somatomedins, most notably IGF-I. The age-related decline in amplitude and frequency of growth hormone secretion occurs particularly during sleep, when this hormone is released in greatest quantity. The reason for this change with age is not fully understood. Low plasma IGF-I levels seen in healthy elderly persons respond to growth hormone replacement. Initial studies of recombinant human growth hormone administration to elderly subjects demonstrated enhancement of lean body mass, lumbar vertebral bone density, and plasma IGF-I levels and a decrease in adipose tissue mass. However, these findings have not been replicated.

 REPRODUCTIVE FUNCTION

Reproduction is another essential physiologic function in all living organisms. In lower-order organisms, the cessation of reproductive function usually coincides with the end of life. In women, reproductive capacity ends in midlife at the time of menopause. This is one of the most striking examples of age-related physiologic changes that subsequently predispose women to the development of pathologic conditions such as cardiovascular disease and osteoporosis. Men do not experience as abrupt a change in reproductive function as women do, but they do undergo gradual alterations in sex steroid metabolism that predispose them to prostate enlargement and bone loss. Although healthy men and women may experience changes in sexual performance with advancing age, their capacity to enjoy sexual activity remains intact.

FEMALE PHYSIOLOGY

In women, normal reproductive physiology is characterized by the following sequence of events, occurring in cyclic fashion:

Pulsatile release of hypothalamic gonadotropin-releasing hormone (GnRH) into the hypophyseal portal system
Pituitary gonadotropin secretion
Gonadotropin stimulation of ovarian follicles to produce estrogen
Ovulation, corpus luteum development, and progesterone production
Negative feedback to hypothalamic and pituitary regulatory centers, resulting in menstruation as estrogen and progesterone are withdrawn

In women between the ages of 45 and 55, the ovary becomes less responsive to gonadotropins; plasma levels of 17β-estradiol, inhibin, and other ovarian hormones decrease; and negative feedback to the hypothalamic-pituitary axis is lost. In response, levels of follicle-stimulating hormone (FSH) and, to a lesser extent, luteinizing hormone (LH) increase. As menopause approaches, the interval between menses lengthens, anovulatory cycles become more common, and menstruation eventually ceases.

After menopause, 17β-estradiol, the predominant circulating estrogen during reproductive life, declines greatly, and estrone becomes the predominant estrogen. Estrone is produced by the peripheral aromatization of adrenal androstenedione in extraglandular tissues, including fat, bone, muscle, skin, and brain.

Estrone levels may be high in obese postmenopausal women, possibly contributing to their reduced risk of osteoporosis. The postmenopausal ovary continues to secrete testosterone under the influence of LH. This may be responsible for the hair growth and virilizing features seen in some women after menopause.

MALE PHYSIOLOGY

In men, normal aging probably results in a modest degree of primary testicular failure, characterized by a decrease in testicular size. There is a decline in numbers of Leydig cells, which make testosterone, and Sertoli cells, which produce sperm and the hormone inhibin. As a result of the decline in circulating testosterone and inhibin, FSH and LH levels increase with age. The age-related decline in testicular function is highly variable, and its clinical implications have not been well established. It may contribute to a decline in the frequency of sexual activity but probably plays a secondary role to social, psychologic, and medical factors that have the greatest influence on sexual dysfunction in late life.

Benign prostatic hypertrophy (BPH) is another consequence of physiologic aging in the male reproductive tract (Chapter 467). Prostatic growth depends on the presence of dihydrotestosterone (DHT). DHT is the active form of testosterone in sexual tissues, produced by the enzyme 5α-reductase. Prostate development does not occur in the absence of DHT. A 5α-reductase inhibitor, finasteride, causes regression of enlarged prostatic tissue. However, levels of DHT do not appear to be increased in men with BPH.

Estrogens and androgens may play a role in the development of prostatic hypertrophy. Estrogen induces *MYC-, RAS,* and *FOS*-encoded mRNA, as well as IGF and epidermal growth factor receptor gene expression. In experimental models, the combination of estrogen and androgen results in greater prostatic growth than androgen alone. As testosterone production declines in advancing age, the decreased androgen/estrogen ratio may promote excessive prostatic growth. However, the exact pathophysiologic mechanism of BPH has not yet been determined.

BIBLIOGRAPHY

Fink RI, Kolterman OG, Griffin J, Olefsky JM. Mechanisms of insulin resistance in aging. *J Clin Invest* 1983;71:1523.

Lakatta EG. Cardiovascular system. In: Masaro EJ, ed. *Handbook of physiology,* Section 11, Aging. New York: Oxford University Press, 1995: 413–474.

MacLaughlin J, Holick MF. Aging decreases the capacity of human skin to produce vitamin D_3. *J Clin Invest* 1985;76:1536.

Meyer BR. Renal function in aging. *J Am Geriatr Soc* 1989;37:791.

Neaves WB, Johnson L, Porter JC, et al. Leydig cell numbers, daily sperm production, and serum gonadotropin levels in aging men. *J Clin Endocrinol Metab* 1984;55:756.

Ng AV, Callister R, Johnson DG, Seals DR. Age and gender influence muscle sympathetic nerve activity at rest in healthy humans. *Hypertension* 1993;21:498.

Roberts SB, Fuss P, Heyman MB, et al. Control of food intake in older men. *JAMA* 1994;272:1601.

Rudman D, Feller AG, Nagraj HS, et al. Effects of human growth hormone in men over 60 years old. *N Engl J Med* 1990;323:1.

Toth MJ, Gardner AW, Ades PA, Poehlman ET. Contribution of body composition and physical activity to age-related decline in peak VO_2 in men and women. *J Appl Physiol* 1994;77:647.

Kelley's Textbook of Internal Medicine, fourth edition. Edited by H. David Humes. Lippincott Williams & Wilkins, Philadelphia © 2000.

C H A P T E R

17

HEALTH CARE IMPLICATIONS OF AN AGING SOCIETY

JOAN WEINRYB
DENNIS HSIEH
RISA LAVIZZO-MOUREY

Changes in the demographics of our society, the aging of the "baby boom" generation, and the fiscal imperative of controlling our society's ever-rising health care costs have increased awareness of the field of geriatrics. Geriatrics does not merely apply the disciplines of internal medicine, surgery, and psychiatry to care of older people. It is a multidisciplinary approach to care, which uses the body of information about biologic and behavioral changes due to aging, in multiple care sites, to minimize the period of dysfunction at the end of life caused by aging and illness.

Geriatricians incorporate the results of current research into clinical practice. Clinical geriatrics combines the age-related effects of biologic and behavioral changes with all the other factors that interact with disease to produce dysfunction. Clinical geriatrics is often challenging because of differences in illness presentation, the presence of multiple diseases or disorders, health-related behaviors of seniors, and limitations of the health care system. Many geriatric patients fail to seek timely treatment. Scarcity of community resources to assist aged persons in avoiding institutionalization impedes care. The geriatrician seeks to apply advances in clinical research to reduce disability, treat modifiable diseases, avoid futile intervention, and promote rational end-of-life decisions. Optimal management of certain recognizable syndromes avoids incomplete medical diagnosis, over- or undermedication, underutilization of rehabilitative or community support services, and inappropriate institutionalization (Table 17.1).

UNDERSTANDING THE ISSUES AND PROBLEMS FACING AN AGING SOCIETY

DEMOGRAPHICS

Older Americans are the fastest-growing segment of the US population. From 1900 to 1997, the percentage of Americans over

TABLE 17.1.	GERIATRIC SYNDROMES OR CONDITIONS THAT MAY BENEFIT FROM OVERSIGHT BY A GERIATRICIAN

- Recurrent falling/gait instability
- Chronic pain
- Functional impairment
- Deconditioning
- Medication noncompliance
- Polypharmacy
- Multiple hospitalizations
- Fecal or urinary incontinence
- Constipation and fecal impaction
- Delirium
- Dementia
- Parkinsons' disease
- Nutritional depletion
- Dehydration
- Depression
- Sleep disorders
- Sexual dysfunction
- Immobility
- Restraints
- Failure to thrive
- Caregiver stress, elder abuse
- Tobacco and alcohol abuse

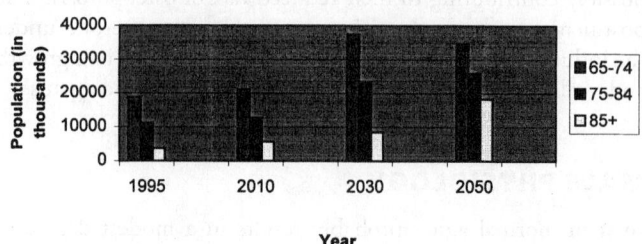

FIGURE 17.1. Projected population growth.

65 has tripled from 4.1% in 1990 to 12.7% in 1997, increasing 11-fold in absolute numbers from 3.1 million in 1900 to 34.1 million in 1997. The term elderly is often used generically to define persons 65 years of age or older, a population, however, manifesting considerable variation in physical, mental, and functional capabilities. Thus, the elderly are extraordinarily heterogeneous, a variance that increases progressively with age. Accordingly, some have segmented this group into subpopulations such as the young-old (those 65 to 74 years), the middle-old (those 75 to 80), the old-old (those 80 to 85), and the oldest-old (those 85 and older). All such classifications reveal a central truth; aging is a continuum. For the population as a whole, age is increasingly associated with an exponential rise in the burden of health problems and, hence, with the cost of health care.

The aging of the baby boom generation will increase the older population rapidly by 2030 to twice the number of older persons in 1997 with a progressive shift to older and older median age. During the period of 1990 to 1997, while the 65- to 74-year-old age group grew eight times, the 75- to 84-year-old cohort grew 16 times, and the over-85 age group multiplied itself 31 times. Although the life expectancy of a person who reached age 65 increased by only 2.4 years between 1900 and 1960, an additional increase of 3.3 years occurred between 1960 and 1997. Thus, a child born in 1997 can expect on average to live 76.5 years, or about 29 years longer than a child born in 1900.

The oldest-old (over 85) is expected to be the fastest-growing group. By 2010, the population of those over 85 is expected to grow 56%, compared with 13% for the 65- to 84-year age group. As the baby boom cohort ages, the over-85 group is expected to grow 116% between 2030 and 2050 (Fig. 17.1).

Minorities are projected to increase from 15.3% to 25% of the older US population by 2030. In absolute terms, while the total population of non-Hispanic whites over age 65 is projected to grow by 78%, the total older minority population is estimated to increase by 238%, that is, the older Hispanic population

by 368%, non-Hispanic Asians and Pacific Islanders by 354%, Native Americans, Inuits, and Aleuts by 159%, and African Americans by 124%.

Although life expectancy is increasing, there are gender differences in the trends: men turning 65 in 1997 have an average additional life expectancy of 15.8 years, and women, an average additional life expectancy of 6 years. Women predominate in each age group of the elderly, with increasing proportions in the oldest groups. This is dramatically different from the previous century, in which a woman was considered fortunate to live until her 48th birthday. Public health improvements, especially in the areas of gynecologic and obstetric care are major contributors to the improved prospects of women. However, a host of chronic health conditions threaten to deprive aging women of good quality of life during these added years.

Although 75% of aging men are married, only 42% of elderly women are married. Because men have shorter life expectancies and on average are older than their wives, the number of widows far outstrips the number of widowers—for example, in 1997, 8.5 million to 2.1 million. In a society in which historically most women worked within their homes, failing to establish savings accounts or pensions of their own and where assets may have been adequate for the life of the marriage but not of the surviving partner, the increasing longevity of women presents problems of poverty and lack of access to health care.

Fifty-two percent of all people over 65 live in just nine states (California, Florida, New York, Texas, Pennsylvania, Ohio, Illinois, Michigan, and New Jersey). Although people over 65 are less likely than their younger counterparts to live in metropolitan areas, about 29% of seniors live in central cities, and another 48% of seniors live in the suburbs. Seniors are less likely to move. In 1997, only 5% of seniors moved in the past year (compared with 18% for those under 65). Those who move tend to stay nearby. Eighty-one percent of seniors who moved in 1997 stayed in the same state. However, states with the most rapid growth in the over-65 population between 1990 and 1997 include Nevada (49%), Alaska (43%), Hawaii (25%), Arizona (25%), Utah (19%), Colorado (19%), and Delaware (17%).

Most noninstitutionalized elderly people live in a family setting. Eight percent of men and 17% of women over age 65 live with children, siblings, or family members other than a spouse. Only 15% of elderly men live alone, whereas 65% of aging women are solitary. The probability of living alone correlates with age. By age 85 or over, 60% of women are solitary dwellers.

Societal contributions to this disparity include the relative youthfulness of wives compared with their husbands and the changes in family composition of the last 50 years. Women now have fewer children than previous generations. In our mobile society, they are less likely to be living near a son or daughter who can provide support. Their female offspring, the traditional caregivers for aging relatives, are more likely to work outside the home and be unavailable for caring for elderly family members.

The percentage of persons living in nursing homes increases with age. Only 1% of those 65 to 74 years old live in a nursing facility, whereas 5% of those 75 to 84 years and 15% of those 85 and over live in nursing homes.

Although they comprise less than 13% of the total population, the elderly accounted for 40% of hospital stays and 49% of inpatient days in 1995. Mortality rates among the oldest-old are declining, but the incidence of disability and chronic illness does not appear to be decreasing or at least not at the same pace as mortality rates. Increasing enrollment in Medicare and increasing use of services threaten to bankrupt the program. Limited resources and a growing elderly population make it imperative that we develop new models of care in which quality and outcome of care are stable or improved and expenditure is stable or decreased. Application of gerontologic research and geriatric management techniques may enable society to assist the elderly in maintaining more vigorous and independent lives. The changes in the demographics of our population and the changes in our society require modification of our medical services and social programs to fulfill the needs of the growing, older population.

ASSOCIATION BETWEEN AGING AND THE MAJOR AGE-RELATED DISEASES

Although recent declines in mortality have led to a increase in life expectancy and proportion of older people in the population, the most common causes of death among the elderly have remained the same over the recent decades.

Over the past century, the leading causes of death have changed. In 1900, the chief cause was influenza and pneumonia. This was followed by tuberculosis, diarrheal diseases, heart disease, and stroke. By the 1980s, the leading cause of death in people over age 65 had become heart disease, followed by cancer, stroke, pulmonary infections, diabetes mellitus, and accidents. The distribution of causes of death does not seem to have changed much since the 1980s, although more people live longer.

A significant proportion of elderly people appear to remain symptom-free and functional until near the time of their death. Others are increasingly disabled, with declining functional status as age increases. Elderly women and African Americans, especially persons with low income, have a higher proportion of functional decrements. There seems to be a bimodal distribution among the elderly of persons who are healthier at advanced ages than their forbears, on the one hand, and significantly disabled persons who because of improved medical care have survived

previously fatal illnesses, on the other hand. The most dramatic reduction in deaths has occurred among women and the oldest-old. Seven out of ten deaths in the United States occur in people 65 or older. Twenty-one percent of deaths occur among those 85 and older and this is expected to rise to 30% by 2050. Chronic disease affects a significant percentage of people. Forty-seven percent of those 65 or older have arthritis, 43% have hypertension, 31% have heart disease, and 10% suffer impaired vision. Thus, the typical older person has multiple disorders.

By self-report, 25% of persons age 65 to 74 who do not live in institutions consider themselves to be in poor or fair health. One-third of those 75 years or older consider their health to be poor or fair. The need for personal assistance increases with age. Only 9% of those 65 to 69 years old require such assistance, whereas, by the decade after the 75th birthday, 20% do need assistance. By age 85 or beyond, 50% of people require personal assistance. Although a reduction in age-specific disability rates may occur, the need for long-term care (including assistance in the home and in other institutional settings) is likely to continue to grow. Currently, 4.7% of the US population requires long-term care services. Most such services are provided informally by family and friends, but the demand for formal services is growing. Public policy must support a two-pronged approach to the problem of expanding numbers of older people and the slower growth of public and private resources. The health system must put forth programs that encourage the development of healthy life habits among the young and middle-aged to forestall disease-related disability in old age. At the same time, programs that integrate health services and expand alternatives to institutional care for the frail elderly must be emphasized.

Regardless of age, heart disease is the leading cause of death in men and women. Men are more likely than women to die of heart disease at an earlier age, and African American men at highest rates in earliest years. After age 75, coronary mortality is nearly equal for men and women. Autopsy series show coronary atherosclerosis in 70% of people between ages 70 and 80. Twenty to 30% of those over age 65 have clinical symptoms and signs of cardiac disease. The American Heart Association estimates that 1.5 million Americans had myocardial infarctions in 1997. One-third of those patients die within a year.

The annual cost of myocardial infarction is $91.7 billion in direct health care costs and $60 billion in lost productivity. The prevalence of congestive heart failure increases with age, with the most patients hospitalized for heart failure being over age 65. Thirty-seven percent of men and 33% of women diagnosed with heart failure die within 2 years. Mortality is age related. Hospitalization for congestive heart failure increases the risk of hospitalization for any reason within the next 3 to 6 months by up to 47% and is associated with significant decline in functional status.

Preferred treatments for medical management of cardiovascular disease, using evidence from randomized trials, supports use of angiotensin-converting enzyme (ACE) inhibitors in patients with left ventricular dysfunction, aspirin and β-blockers after myocardial infarction, and warfarin for stroke prevention in atrial fibrillation. These treatments are applied only at low rates to patients who are elderly. Studies have shown the use of ACE inhibitors in as few as 47% of those eligible, aspirin in only 50%, and β-blockers in only 19% of those who have suffered myocardial infarction. Warfarin use has been shown in only 17% of elderly persons with atrial fibrillation. Some of this is explained by comorbidity, but, overall, it appears that many elderly people are being deprived of useful treatments because of their health care providers' prejudice or misunderstanding.

Reperfusion therapy for ischemia of less than 6 to 12 hours' duration has changed the treatment of anterior myocardial infarction. Pooled data from several large trials indicate that the absolute reduction in mortality is as great in older as in younger patients. Data on patients older than 80 undergoing thrombolytic therapy indicate a 41% reduction in mortality. Intracranial hemorrhage, the most feared complication of thrombolytic therapy, increases with advancing age from a rate of 0.3% in younger patients to a rate of 0.8% in patients older than 75. Coronary angioplasty in older persons appears to carry an increased risk of progression to coronary artery bypass graft, but has a 30-day mortality risk, which compares favorably with thrombolysis. Increasing data about the use of intracoronary stents indicate that these may be the treatment of preference, especially in very old patients.

CANCER

The incidence of many cancers increases with age. Breast, lung, colorectal, prostate, gastric, and head and neck cancers are more common with aging. Lifetime cumulative exposure to carcinogens, age-related alterations in the immune system, and the accumulation of random genetic mutations all have been postulated as causative. Treatments for cancer include surgery, radiation therapy, and chemotherapy, all of which may be less well tolerated in the aged because of suppressed wound healing and reduced organ reserve. Rates of cardiac and gastrointestinal toxicity and neurotoxicity in response to chemotherapy are higher in the elderly. Despite this, many elderly persons have survived cancer treatment surprisingly well. Decisions to forego treatment should not be based on age alone but on functional status, and likelihood that the benefit of treatment outweighs the burden.

The treatment of prostate cancer is an area of considerable dispute. Prostate cancer is present in about 8 million men in the United States and causes 35,000 deaths. Large numbers of men with prostate cancer are unlikely to suffer significant morbidity or mortality from their disease. Aggressive therapy may therefore lead to unnecessary morbidity in this group.

Other factors must be taken into account when treating the elderly cancer patient. Issues of analgesia, community support, and access to treatment may be paramount.

CEREBROVASCULAR DISEASE

Cerebrovascular disease is the third leading cause of death in the United States. The incidence of stroke increases with increasing age. By age 70, stroke occurs in 300 per 10,000 persons per year. The rate of stroke in elderly women is about 25% less than the rate in men. With improved attention to the control of risk factors, such as hypertension, heart disease, diabetes mellitus,

and cigarette smoking, the incidence of stroke is declining in the United States, and with improved treatment, the prevalence of stroke survivors is increasing. The fatality rate within 1 month of an acute stroke is close to one-third across all age groups. However, more than two-thirds of stroke survivors live at least 3 years. Maximal functional recovery is the goal of treatment for stroke victims. Clinical course depends on the type of stroke and its location and size. Complications include aspiration, deep vein thrombosis, contractures, pressure sores, and increased risk of falls and other accidents. Poststroke course can be complicated by depression or reflex sympathetic dystrophy. In terms of best use of societal resources, reliable ways of determining prognosis, therapies to assist recovery and strategies for compensating for disabilities are needed.

PNEUMONIA

Pneumonia remains the fifth leading cause of death, the leading infectious cause of death in people over age 65, and a major reason for hospitalization among elderly people. The incidence and severity of community acquired pneumonia increases with age, with a case rate of 1 to 5 per thousand persons per year in patients aged 5 to 60, and a case rate of 30 per thousand persons per year in patients older than 75. The risk of a complicated course increases after age 65, and advanced age is a significant predictor of hospital mortality. Several studies have confirmed that causative organisms of community acquired pneumonia in adults are similar at any age, and include *Streptococcus pneumoniae, Haemophilus influenzae, Legionella pneumophila, Chlamydia pneumoniae,* and gram-negative bacilli. Eighty percent of influenza deaths occur in people over age 65. Secondary staphylococcal pneumonia is of concern during outbreaks of influenza pneumonia. Outbreaks of respiratory infection in long-term care facilities are common. Aspiration pneumonia, less common among community dwellers than among nursing home residents, remains a significant problem associated with neurodegenerative disorders. The efficacy of pneumococcal and influenza vaccination in preventing mortality and morbidity in elderly patients has been demonstrated repeatedly. These strategies remain underused, with only 10% of eligible elderly persons undergoing pneumococcal vaccination and many remaining at risk from influenza.

DIABETES

Impaired glucose tolerance occurs in 25% of adults over age 65. Nearly 50% of people with type II diabetes mellitus are over age 65. By age 80, the prevalence of diabetes is 20% to 40%, with the diagnosis undiscovered in many. Foot ulcerations are a major cause of morbidity in diabetic patients. Yearly, 50,000 amputations related to diabetes mellitus are performed in the United States, with a direct cost of $1 billion. Renal insufficiency and diabetic retinopathy contribute to the morbidity, mortality, and health care costs of diabetic patients. Health care expenditures to assist in careful control of hyperglycemia through patient education and access to medication and professional evaluation could result in tremendous cost savings. During the past decade, the focus of diabetic care has shifted from the hospital to ambulatory settings. The American Diabetic Association has recommended guidelines for quality of care for individuals with diabetes, hypertension, and hyperlipidemia. Modifications for frail older people are indicated. Outcome studies are needed to guide clinicians in the selection of optimal treatment goals for older diabetics.

FALLS AND ACCIDENTS

Accidents are the seventh most common cause of death among the elderly. Burns cause 41 annual hospitalizations per 100,000 adult age 85 or older, a rate 50% higher than that of the general population. Residential fires kill 10% as many elderly people as renal failure. Two-thirds of accidental deaths in the elderly are caused by falls at an annual rate of 57 per 100,000 persons of age 75 or greater. Falls and injuries cause considerable health care cost and personal suffering. Conditions characterized by impaired sensorimotor processing, such as Alzheimer's dementia, are associated with falls. Central nervous system impairment due to cerebrovascular disease, motor abnormalities due to arthritis, and other conditions associated with chronic pain, neurologic conditions such as Parkinson's disease, all are complicated by high rates of falls and injuries. Falls in persons 65 years and older are estimated to produce medical costs of $3.7 billion per year. Fear of falling may reduce quality of life. Multiple falls are a marker of increased risk of death. Accident prevention through environmental modification and therapies to ameliorate muscular weakness and age-related changes in equilibrium and limb coordination can decrease societal cost and personal suffering.

NEURODEGENERATIVE DISORDERS

In the United States, neurodegenerative disorders cause dementia in about 8% of people over age 65. Rates double every 5 years from about 2% at age 65 to about 30% after age 85. Alzheimer's disease is the most common dementing disorder. Currently, 4 million people in the United States have these diseases, and it is projected to rise to 8 million by the end of the year 2000. Depression is commonly found as a coexisting condition in patients with dementia. More intensive clinical management is often required for patients with both disabilities. As Alzheimer's disease progresses, the level of impairment of affected patients increases, requiring more and more support and services from their families and from society. The economic cost of Alzheimer's disease and related disorders, including medical care, long-term care, and loss of productivity, approaches $100 billion per year. Effective treatment for functional decline, which could delay nursing home placement by even a year, would result in large economic benefit.

▌ PREVENTION AND SCREENING

Disease prevention in elderly persons seeks to render the patient more resistant to illness. Primary prevention includes immuniza-

tion against communicable diseases, blood pressure management, smoking cessation, obesity control, exercise programs, and social support and environmental modifications.

Another aspect of disease prevention is the early detection of asymptomatic disease in the hope of efficacious treatment. Papanicolaou (Pap) smears, breast examinations, tests for fecal occult blood, screening for hypothyroidism, assessment for the presence of depression or of vision, hearing, or dental abnormalities, and testing for tuberculosis all fall under the rubric of screening.

Screening is influenced by physician knowledge of life expectancy and attitude toward aged patients. Published guidelines for screening, immunization, and risk factor counseling are rarely studied for appropriateness in aging populations, especially among those over age 75. Screening for frail elderly patients may consist of identification of problems that will further add to the burden of disability if uncorrected. Most elderly people are active and functional and have much to gain from health screening. Recommendations for this age group must be based on life expectancy and the natural history of the disease for which the screening is done. Controversy exists about the efficacy of screening when doubt exists about the benefit of early intervention. Prostate cancer is one entity for which mass screening for early intervention in elderly men is not yet clearly justified in terms of decreased mortality and morbidity. In contrast, the usefulness of diagnosis and treatment of gait dysfunction to avoid fracture and disability is clear.

Table 17.2 is a compendium of suggestions that attempt to provide a framework for both disease prevention and case finding. Specific guidelines to provide a comprehensive, but economical evaluation have been chosen from among sometimes contradictory recommendations. Identification of active issues by screening allows more intensive intervention. Health promotion and disease prevention are applicable to the elderly, although logistics and frailty mitigate efficacy of some of the recommendations. Attempts to improve care and to avoid complications in the treatment of elderly patients may include geriatric assessment and foot and dental care.

Disability risk assessment and improved management of chronic conditions to modulate the impact of these on function can reduce the burdens and cost of chronic disease. Creative approaches such as in-home geriatric assessment have led to reduction in nursing home placements. Risk factor reduction strategies applied through senior center-based health promotion programs and case management approaches have both resulted in improved status.

▌ FINANCING THE CARE OF OUR AGING POPULATION

Medicare, implemented in 1966 as part of the Social Security Amendments, covers most people over 65, disabled individuals who have received Social Security benefits for at least 2 years, and persons with end-stage renal disease. Traditionally, Medicare Part A covers inpatient hospital services, limited posthospital skilled nursing facility care services, and hospice care, and

TABLE 17.2.   GERIATRIC HEALTH ISSUES BENEFITING FROM PERIODIC REVIEW

Examination	How Frequently	Comment
Mammogram	Yearly	Discontinue when life expectancy <6 years
Pap/pelvic	Yearly	After 3 normal annual exams, they may be performed less frequently at the discretion of the physician
Breast exam	Yearly	Indefinitely
Digital rectal prostate exam/PSA	Yearly	Target men with at least a 10-year life expectancy (American Cancer Society); since benefit of early diagnosis not clear, others discourage screening
Stool for occult blood	Yearly	High false-positive rate with poor sensitivity
Flexible sigmoidoscopy	Every 5 years	If life expectancy ≥13 years
Colonoscopy	Every 10 years	Recommendations changing to performing a screening colonoscopy every 5–10 years after age 50
Heart/lungs/skin	Yearly	—
Hearing	Yearly	Does not require a formal audiogram
Vision	Every 2 years	—
Oral examination	Every 2 years	For tobacco and alcohol users >60
Dental examination	Not established	At entry and with complaint or weight loss
Height	Yearly	—
Weight	Not established	—
Blood pressure	Every visit	USPSTF: every 2 years if normotensive
Feet	Yearly	For diabetics: every visit
Shoulder function	Yearly	Affects driving and personal care and is a common site of reversible dysfunction
Mental status	At entry and periodically	—
Hematocrit and creatinine	At entry and periodically	—
Glucose	Every 3 years	American Diabetes Association recommendations
Thyroid function	Once	For women >age 55.
Urinalysis	No routine indication	—
Total cholesterol	Every 5 years	—
Bone mineral density	As needed to guide treatment of osteoporosis	—
Electrocardiogram	No routine indication	Baseline useful when patient develops symptoms
Chest x-ray	No routine indication	—
Tetanus/diphtheria vaccine	Every 10 years	Tetanus primary series needed if never given
Influenza vaccine	Yearly	—
Pneumococcal vaccine	Once after age 65	—
Nutrition	Periodically	—
Retirement	Periodically, as relevant	—
Living arrangements	Periodically	—
Driving	Periodically	—
Home safety/prevention of falls	Periodically	—
Alcohol	At entry and periodically	—
Smoking	At entry and periodically	—
Advance directives	At entry, periodically, and at change in status	—

Recommendations are modified and adapted after review of the American College of Physicians, American Cancer Society, American Diabetic Association, American Geriatric Society, US Preventive Services Task Force Guide to Clinical Preventive Services, and Mayo Clinic's recommendations. PSA, prostate-specific antigen. They represent the author's current opinion and must be modified as research evolves.

Medicare Part B covers outpatient hospital services (such as outpatient studies and same day surgeries), all physician services, and outpatient services from other disciplines (e.g., physical, occupational, and speech therapy). Some in-home nursing care for acute medical problems is covered by Medicare. Patients are responsible for a portion of the charges. Medicines and custodial care are not covered. Long-term skilled nursing facility services remain the responsibility of the individual until mean test requirements permitting Medicaid reimbursement are met, through "spending down" to poverty levels.

Despite federal budget surpluses in the late 1990s, Medicare is expected to become insolvent by 2012. To control costs, the Medicare Part C plan (commonly called Medicare+Choice) was enacted. Patients can choose to switch out of traditional Medicare into a Medicare Part C plan. Types of plans include health maintenance organizations, provider sponsored organizations, preferred provider organizations, medical savings accounts, and private contracting. Part C plans are privately operated insurance programs to which the government makes a predetermined per-capita payment. Medicare Part C is an attempt to have the private sector assume responsibility for the medical costs of the Medicare population. Some plans offer comprehensive services with low deductibles and copayments but charge the patient additional insurance premiums. In exchange for restricted access to care, other plans offer programs with low deductibles and copayments.

The Part C plan has a fixed amount of money to spend for care, but it is responsible for the needs of the whole group of enrolled patients. When resources are limited, the goal is to maximize the value of services provided to the group, even if it means some persons will receive less service than they would under a fee-for-service system. This may create conflict between the needs of an individual patient and the needs of the group. Insurance and health care organizations perform cost/benefit and cost-effectiveness analyses to find the mix of services that maximizes value for a given amount of money spent. Physicians must participate in deciding on how to allocate health care resources so that individual patient needs, quality of care, economic efficiency, and societal needs are balanced.

Changes in Medicare financing represent challenges for the development of better care models. Nursing home care is now financed by a government-mandated system of per-diem payments, based on patient acuity and regional labor costs, out of which all expenses of care must be paid. House call programs, although time- and labor-intensive, save money. Treating medical problems at home reduces hospital admissions, costly interventions, and hazards of hospitalization in elderly patients. A recent innovation currently spreading nationally, PACE programs (**P**rograms for the **A**ll-inclusive **C**are of the **E**lderly) allow care at home for seniors who would otherwise require nursing home admission. Medicare and Medicaid provide capitated payments to the PACE program, which in turn provides medical services and custodial care. In some hospitals, Acute Care for Elders (ACE) Units minimize hospital-acquired morbidity. Long-term care insurance, privately purchased, can help pay for custodial care in the home or in a nursing facility without pauperizing the patient.

■ THE SOLUTION TO PROVIDING HEALTH CARE TO A GROWING POPULATION OF ELDERS

As the population of elderly people grows, the goals of geriatrics remain to promote independence and optimal functioning, to prevent avoidable decline in health status, and to enhance the elder's quality of life.

For many geriatric patients, the format of a routine office visit is not designed to meet their needs. Their problems are too complex and numerous, their psychosocial and emotional needs too great, and their knowledge of self-care and morbidity prevention too small.

The solution to caring for the increasing numbers of elderly who represent heterogeneous populations is to develop a full

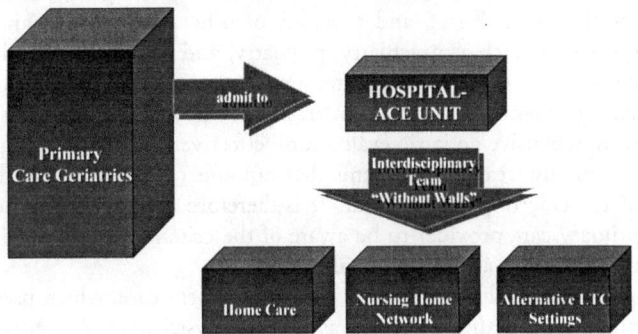

FIGURE 17.2. The continuum of geriatric care.

and coordinated continuum of care in which the different components are linked by teams and disease management guidelines (Fig. 17.2). Each site or component of the continuum–primary care, inpatient care, home care, nursing homes, and alternative arrangements, such as assisted living is essential and presents its own challenges to practice. In the past, life care communities containing all the components in the continuum at a single site were a fast-growing mode of addressing this need but were available and affordable for only a small proportion of the elderly. Increasingly, the growth of managed care is stimulating delivery systems to add components that ensure efficient and more economical access across all parts of the continuum. Clinicians and institutions must develop formal or informal relationships with other providers in the continuum to promote efficient care at the lowest cost.

PRIMARY CARE

The primary care provider focusing on older adults must understand the effects of aging on human physiology and must be knowledgeable about the use of methods that have been shown to improve clinical management of the older adult population. These include risk assessment, comprehensive multidisciplinary assessments and management, proactive use of telephones, health promotion, and preventive services. Because the primary care provider is likely to treat fit, active seniors as well as frail, dependent seniors, screening assessments that allow early identification of persons at risk for disability are effective tools for allocation of scarce, time-consuming, and expensive resources. Many risk assessment instruments have been designed to aid the clinician in the identification of subclinical problems, unreported symptoms, and situations that increase the probability of functional decline or hospitalization. These tools differ in length, mode of administration, and specificity of risk stratification. Patients scoring in high-risk categories during preliminary evaluation can be investigated more comprehensively. Many Medicare managed care programs and some integrated delivery systems have incorporated periodic risk assessments to determine which patients might benefit from case management.

Through simple, office-based screening tools, primary physicians can identify patients who would benefit from comprehensive geriatric assessment. Typically, these assessments are conducted by a team of professionals consisting of a geriatrician, social worker, nurse, and a variety of other professionals and specialties, such as psychiatry, physiatry, and pharmacy. Multidisciplinary evaluations are resource intensive and their cost-saving potential has not been irrefutably proved. Nonetheless, comprehensive geriatric evaluations' effectiveness in identifying potentially treatable problems that can affect the quality of life of the elderly person is clear. It is therefore reasonable for the primary care provider to be aware of the criteria for efficacy of this approach and to use it judiciously.

Creative solutions such as group outpatient care, which uses nursing staff and others to assist the physician in delivering health care information, in providing socialization opportunities, and in allowing frequent clinical assessment, have been shown to reduce acute and specialist visits, decrease hospitalization, increase rates of immunization and of patient satisfaction, and at the same time decrease costs.

The primary care provider must be equally cognizant of the needs of well elderly persons. Here, health promotion and disease–disability prevention are paramount. The importance of health-promoting behaviors such as exercise cannot be overemphasized. The data on the benefit of both aerobic and strength training exercise, even at very advanced ages, are robust. Similarly, the efficacy of some preventive services warrants their inclusion in the primary care for seniors (Table 17.2). The US Preventive Services Task Force is currently reconsidering the recommendations for all age groups, including the elderly and will issue a new report in the first years of the new millennium.

INPATIENT CARE

The elderly account for 40% of inpatient hospital days and experience complications that are uncommon in younger age groups. Avoiding preventable complications and maintaining functional status are at the heart of inpatient geriatrics. Complications such as delirium, deconditioning, pressure ulcers, fluid and electrolyte disorders, and adverse medication reactions are common among hospitalized elderly and often result in extended lengths of stay. Practices aimed at avoiding these complications and improving functional outcome at discharge have resulted in growing numbers of Acute Care for Elders (ACE) hospital units and for the urgency of implementing certain treatments.

ACE units, first conceptualized at Case Western University Hospital, use geriatricians and multidisciplinary teams to create inpatient care plans that maximize the function of the elderly. The underlying principles of care, designed to maintain function in the setting of limited physiologic reserve possessed by the elderly, are important in all hospital settings. As previously noted, physiologic changes with aging alter the immune system, body composition, and metabolism of medications. The rapidity of initiating antibiotic administration, the accuracy of fluid replacement, and the appropriate adjustment of medication doses make enormous differences in the outcome of hospitalization in elderly patients. Even when appropriate attention is paid to these unique aspects of hospital care for the elderly, recovery often cannot be accomplished during the hospital stay alone. Nursing home, home care, and house calls may be critical in facilitating recovery and in maintaining or returning function to elderly patients.

HOME CARE, HOUSE CALLS, AND NURSING HOMES

Nursing homes typically have a bimodal population. There are "short-stayers," who are admitted for rehabilitation or convalescence or for terminal care, and "long-stayers," who are expected to be institutionalized the rest of their lives. The former may be managed in hospital-based "transitional care," "subacute care," or "step-downs" units or in similar facilities in community-based homes. In addition, for every person in a nursing home, there are probably two to four elderly persons living at home with similar levels of frailty and disability. The chronically homebound are perhaps the most neglected subpopulation of elderly. Ambulatory elderly have fewer physician visits per year than many nursing home residents, but homebound elderly claim less than one visit to a physician per year. Despite this, patients frequently express a preference for remaining in their communities, rather than admission to an institutional setting. Many prefer acute illness to be treated in their homes as well. Home care and house calls may allow an elderly person to remain at home. Nursing homes can be used over a broad spectrum of disability to provide a setting for recovery of function and return to the previous living situation. The higher cost of providing the initial therapies and skilled services is often justified by the subsequent lower cost of long-term maintenance in a less skilled setting. The demographic realities illustrate the need for home care, house calls, and nursing homes to be included in the continuum of care for elderly persons.

Treating patients in a nursing home or at home requires a specialized set of skills and knowledge base. The integration of internal medicine and rehabilitation medicine is fundamental to the care of patients in long-term care settings. Mobile diagnostic equipment, such as x-rays, ultrasonography, electrocardiograms, and new medications, have revolutionized the treatment of acute illness in the long-term care or home setting. Simple infections, such as pneumonia, urinary tract infection, and cellulitis, as well as common medical conditions, such as deep venous thrombosis, can now be safely treated either at home or in the nursing home. Despite these advances, much work is needed to move these practice patterns into the mainstream of current medical care.

The dual pressures for the most economical and most effective care will lead to research for better understanding of the unique aspects of *in situ* management, changes in wound care and infection control, new techniques for managing nutritional maladies, and use of computer and telemedicine technologies.

CHRONIC ILLNESS AND PALLIATIVE CARE

Although younger adults tend to have acute and limited illnesses, older adults are more likely to have multiple, chronic illnesses. These illnesses contribute to significant functional limitations, inability to work, and hospitalizations. Congestive heart failure (CHF) and chronic obstructive pulmonary disease (COPD) are the most prevalent of the chronic diseases. More than 3 million

Americans have CHF, and approximately 400,000 new cases are diagnosed annually. Fourteen million Americans have COPD, and 100,000 die because of it each year. These two illnesses account for 25% of deaths in the United States.

The traditional focus on cure does not address many of the needs of our aging population. Patients with advanced heart or lung failure are terminally ill. However, many of these patients do not get adequate medical management, are not provided appropriate education, and are never told that their illness is terminal. The gaps in these patients' care is not due to a lack of concern by providers but to a medical system ill equipped to care for these persons. In addition to receiving care from different physicians and nursing agencies, these patients often receive episodic care from multiple hospitals. Care is often fragmented and treatment recommendations may be contradictory. Although treatment for exacerbation of chronic diseases is essential, no good system exists for providing palliative instead of curative care. Hospice care, traditionally targeted at patients with cancer diagnoses and prognoses measured in months, does not manage well the issues of chronically ill patients with longer prognoses.

The solution lies in improving methods for the transfer of medical information and in developing systems to provide long-term palliative care and multidisciplinary team care. Instead of thinking in terms of cure, with a sudden shift to palliative care (e.g., the transition from chemotherapy to hospice care for many cancer patients), we must learn to plan care that gradually integrates palliative care as illness progresses. Our health system must develop ways to draw on medical and nonmedical disciplines to address the physical, mental, and social needs of our elderly patients. In an era of global access to information, we must improve transfer of medical information between the multiple providers involved in the care of a single patient. Improved access to information and multidisciplinary care, an integrated continuum from acute to chronic care, and smooth transition from independent to institutional care will improve the quality of all our lives and assist in controlling our society's burgeoning health care costs.

FINANCIAL AND POLICY CHALLENGES

With the country facing a growing population living longer, many of whom have chronic medical illnesses, careful examination of our allocation of health care resources is imperative. Postponing the onset of chronic disease and disability to the end of life is as important as delaying death, both in terms of preventing suffering and in reducing the massive outlay of funds for medical care currently occurring in the United States.

In theory, the managed care model can teach us to lower health care costs through active management of resources. Portions of a fixed amount of funding can be designated, not only for acute care of hospitalized patients, but also for care of both acute and chronic diseases in less costly settings, including subacute and transitional units, nursing homes, and other living situations. Funds can also be allocated for the prevention of disability through modification of risk factors. Decreased disability translates to cost savings, despite the initial outlay of funds for risk factor reduction interventions. Experimentation with

innovative service delivery models is possible with capitated reimbursement agreements, because they are not circumscribed by what is reimbursable under classic Medicare.

Medicare Part C, the bulk of it being managed Medicare, was touted as a mechanism to optimize the health outcomes of the enrolled beneficiaries, while also saving the government money. Success in managing a Medicare risk contract requires flexibility in recognizing the special health problems of the elderly, the importance of managing functional deficits, and innovation in the delivery of services. Potentially, managed care can offer geriatric patients coordinated specialty care, avoidance of inappropriately applied technology and pharmacology resulting in iatrogenic illness, and a lowering of costs through better organization of care and management of risk factors. Enthusiasm for this approach has been tempered by the perception that managed Medicare companies have skimmed the healthiest of the population, leaving the cost of caring for the more expensive, frailer patients to fee-for-service Medicare, that covered services are not easily available to participants, and that the quality of those services may be in doubt. Managed Medicare does not seem to reduce costs where specialized planning has not occurred and many for-profit companies have dropped their plans.

The intertwining of many of the medical aspects of health care with the social aspects of health care complicates solving the Medicare finance problem. Many of the elderly live below the poverty level and do not have adequate food, shelter, transportation, and safety. Women, people of color, persons living alone, the very elderly, those living in rural areas, and those with a combination of these characteristics are disproportionately represented. The inadequacies of their lives, combined for many with functional limitations, all affect their health and increase their risk of adverse outcomes. The solution is difficult. It requires compromises and changed expectations from taxpayers, health care providers, and the elderly population.

Society must change its view of medical care. The standard of care for the treatment of acute illness in the elderly may no longer be centralization in technologically advanced hospitals. The most advanced studies and medicines often only add marginal value to the outcome of an aged individual. Medicare beneficiaries and their relatives can be educated to understand that transferring spending from "high-tech" medical services to more basic medical and social services can improve quality of life, simultaneously reducing costs. Flexible approaches to care of acutely ill patients such as ACE units, PACE, and home-based interventions including the home hospital, which brings the physician, nurse, medicines, appropriate diagnostic, and treatment methods to the patient, decrease rates and expense of iatrogenic illness and functional decline. There must be allocation of funds for medications. Many of the elderly with easily treatable illness progress to severe and costly complications because they do not have the money to purchase their medicines. Other elderly persons skimp on food and shelter to purchase their medicines. If we are to avoid a negative impact on the health of the individual, funding to provide adequate nutrition, housing, transportation, and safety must be forthcoming either through universal social insurance programs or through some combination of private insurance and public funding. Custodial services, such as supervision and assistance with the activities of daily living, can improve quality of life and can reduce expensive hospital admissions.

A change in expectations throughout our society is needed if we are to improve our current system. This will require understanding the limits of technology and acceptance of both the reality that unlimited care is not possible and that, through redirecting resources to preventive medicine and to innovative health care solutions, quality of life can be improved. Flexibility is required of both health care providers and their patients and of government officials who have such a prominent place in designing our future society.

BIBLIOGRAPHY

Administration on Aging (http://www.aoa.gov/).

American Geriatric Society. The management of chronic pain in older persons. Clinical practice guidelines. *J Am Geriatr Soc* 1998;46:635–651.

Blazer DG, Hughs DC. Epidemiology of depression in an elderly community population. *Gerontologist* 1987;27:281–287.

Edelberg H, Wei J. Primary care guidelines for community-living older persons. *Clin Geriatr* 1999;7:42–55.

Froelich T, Robison J, Inouye S. Screening for dementia in the outpatient setting: the time and change test. *J Am Geriatr Soc* 1998;46:1506–1511.

Goldberg TH. Preventive medicine and screening in older adults. *J Am Geriatr Soc* 1997;45(3):344–354.

Hazzard WR, Bierman EL, Blass JP, et al, eds. *Principles of geriatric medicine and gerontology*. New York: McGraw-Hill, 1994.

Health Care Financing Administration (http://www.hcfa.gov).

Lavizzo-Mourey R, Forciea MA, ed. *Geriatric secrets*. Philadelphia: Hanley & Belfus, 1996.

Scheitel S, Fleming K. Geriatric Health Maintenance. Symposium on Geriatrics. *Mayo Clin Proc* 1996;71:289–302.

Kelley's Textbook of Internal Medicine, fourth edition. Edited by H. David Humes.
Lippincott Williams & Wilkins, Philadelphia © 2000.

C H A P T E R

18

HOST–MICROBE INTERACTION

HERBERT L. DUPONT
LILIANA RODRIGUEZ

The normal population of microflora in humans is composed of several complex ecosystems. The organisms occupy space and use substrate on external body mucosal surfaces. The endogenous flora are involved in the body's metabolic activity at all levels.

Disease may be caused by resident organisms and other microbial invaders through three mechanisms: their ability to adhere to host tissues, as characteristically seen in the oral cavity; their shear numbers, as found on heavily contaminated mucosal surfaces; and their capacity to produce disease or virulence, as in the case of *Neisseria meningitidis* in the upper respiratory tract

---

TABLE 18.1.	HOST DEFENSES AGAINST MICROBIAL INVADERS

Nonspecific Mechanisms
Use of substrates and antibacterial catabolytes produced by indigenous microflora
Skin and mucous membrane barriers
Lysozymes and lactoferrin
Acid production (e.g., stomach, vagina)
Mucociliary flow apparatus of the respiratory tract
Motility of intestine and urinary system
Macrophages and phagocytes

Specific Mechanisms
Humoral defenses
Cellular defenses

---

or *Salmonella typhi* in the gallbladder and gastrointestinal tract. Host defenses must remain on guard continually, because with altered host resistance, even indigenous flora with normally low pathogenic potential may cause disease. Infection usually can be explained by one or more of the following conditions: presence of a virulent organism to which the host is exposed, a large inoculum of the organism, and reduced resistance (increased susceptibility) of the host.

MECHANISMS OF HOST RESISTANCE TO INFECTION

The body possesses many mechanisms, both nonspecific and specific, designed to deter potential invaders (Table 18.1). Most of the infectious agents encountered are prevented from entering the body by a variety of biochemical and physical barriers. Several critical mechanical barriers to infection include the skin and mucous membranes. The substrate on the skin and the dietary contents of the gastrointestinal tract facilitates the growth of flora that inhibit more hostile organisms in their attempt to gain access to the body. The sebaceous glands on the skin surface produce free fatty acids, which, together with organic acids produced by bacterial flora and locally produced substances such as lysozyme and lactoferrin, inhibit organisms that might otherwise colonize the surfaces. Lysozyme is found in tears, saliva, nasal secretions, and other body fluids. The enzyme lyses the cell wall of certain bacteria. Lactoferrin is an iron-binding protein produced from the granules of polymorphonuclear leukocytes. This substance competes for available iron in the environment, depriving the adjacent microorganisms of a compound essential for their growth.

The acidic environment of the stomach and vagina are not suitable for growth by most bacteria, preventing delivery of important numbers of bacteria to the small bowel, which would result in malabsorption and diarrhea, or to the urethra, which may be important in the pathogenesis of urinary tract infection.

Motility of the gastrointestinal tract and ureters, along with frequent voiding of the urinary bladder, limits colonization of potential pathogens. Exfoliation of skin and cell shedding of the respiratory and intestinal epithelium also helps to limit the extent of local infection.

The lining of the respiratory tract entraps inhaled microorganisms larger than 5 μm in diameter and carries them to the upper respiratory tract from the more sensitive lower parts of the lung by means of the mucociliary flow apparatus. Smaller microorganisms are cleared by alveolar macrophages if they are not too numerous or too virulent. Sneezing and coughing help to clear the respiratory tract of microbial colonizers.

Acute inflammation involving capillary dilatation, movement of leukocytes and plasma proteins into the tissue from the circulation, and subsequent phagocytosis represents a primary defense against most bacterial pathogens. The microbes that escape the nonspecific defenses and multiply in body tissues face a sophisticated immune system mounted to localize the process and eradicate them. Other local host defenses include complement, opsonins, a variety of chemical mediators, and other immune factors of humoral and cellular defenses. Monocytes and macrophages may release cytokines, which are important in modulating the immune system. In the defense against certain viral infections, interferons, natural killer cells, and antibody-dependent cytotoxic cells can limit the infection.

MICROBIAL VIRULENCE

The most successful parasites are those living in harmony with the host. Pathogenic organisms that harm their hosts usually possess well-defined virulence characteristics. However, disease can result from relatively nonpathogenic organisms when abnormally high concentrations of the agent are present, as occurs during antibiotic inhibition of normal flora that allows unchecked growth of resistant organisms, or when the host's immunity is depressed. An increased inoculum of a pathologic agent and immunodepression often participate in infections, such as a gram-negative superinfection (new infection) in a diabetic receiving an antimicrobial agent.

Two parameters to measure microbial virulence in experimental animal models are infectious dose (ID) and lethal dose (LD). The ID_{25} is the dose of a microbial strain that infects 25% of the exposed animals (often mice). The LD_{25} is the dose that results in death of 25% of the exposed animals. These measures are used to compare the relative virulence of various bacterial isolates. Specific virulence mechanisms are discussed in a subsequent section.

MICROBIAL ASSAULTS AND EVASION TACTICS

Potential pathogens may attack the body by the oral route through ingestion (e.g., *Shigella*, *Salmonella*, *Brucella*, poliovirus, hepatitis A and E), after inhalation (e.g., *Mycobacterium tuberculosis*, *Legionella pneumophila*, *Histoplasma capsulatum*), or by direct penetration of intact barriers (e.g., *Clostridium tetani*, *Rickettsia*, sexually transmitted diseases). How a microorganism infects humans is often determined by the organism's resistance to stomach acid, its ability to directly invade tissues, the presence of an insect vector, the finding of the organism in the respiratory tract of carriers, a potential for the organism to grow in respiratory equipment or air-conditioning systems, and the fragility of the organism in the environment. Most of the frankly pathogenic organisms possess one or more well-defined virulence mechanisms (Table 18.2).

NUMBERS OF ORGANISMS

Restriction of the number of organisms colonizing the body is an important factor in preventing invasion. When body surfaces are injured or when growth of commensal organisms reaches very high levels, colonizing flora may obtain access to normally microbe-free deeper structures of the host tissues. In this situation, even without special virulence characteristics, colonization of tissues serves as prelude to infection. Organisms normally colonizing the body may produce infection when they are introduced into normally sterile environments by the respiratory route, during surgery, or when fluids are administered intravenously. A few organisms (e.g., *Shigella* spp, *Cryptosporidium parvum*, *Giardia lamblia*) are capable of producing disease by means of a small inoculum in otherwise healthy persons.

ADHERENCE

A fundamental property of disease production for most pathogenic microbes is attachment to host tissues and cells. High counts of coagulase-negative *Staphylococcus* are usually found on the skin surface. These organisms may colonize plastic intravenous lines, intraventricular shunts, prosthetic heart valves, and joint prostheses during their insertion and subsequently produce low-grade infection. In the oropharynx, bacterial strains attach to mucosal and dental surfaces. Oral streptococci are particularly suited to adherence partly because of the synthesized proteinaceous levans or dextrans that facilitate attachment. Their sticky nature facilitates attachment to the vascular endothelium as well as to dental structures, explaining why these strains are associated with infective endocarditis and dental caries. Similarly, nasal colonization by adherent *Staphylococcus aureus* occurs in about 15% of persons. In these individuals, secondary staphylococcal infections are more likely prone to develop.

The adhesive capacity of certain bacteria results from specialized adhesion molecules that attach to host cell carbohydrates (e.g., glycoproteins, glycolipids). Adherent bacteria in the gut represent important causes of infection. In some of the exogenously acquired diarrhea-producing *Escherichia coli* (enterotoxigenic *E. coli* and enteropathogenic *E. coli*), the organisms possess specialized capsular structures that allow them to attach to receptors in the lining of the intestine. Other intestinal strains of *E. coli* possess different attachment fimbriae, which belong to a certain number of O-antigen serogroups and have a predilection for uroepithelium. These organisms are important causes of pyelonephritis. The fimbriae (pili) attach to a carbohydrate moiety of the P blood group substance on erythrocytes and uroepithelial cells. Persons who lack P blood group antigens have a natural resistance to infection by these strains.

Initial attachment of gonococci to mucosal surfaces also appears to be mediated by pili. Rapid phase shifts between piliated and nonpiliated variants allow the organism to first detach from

TABLE 18.2.	MICROBIAL FACTORS IMPORTANT IN THE PATHOGENESIS OF INFECTION
Factor	**Mechanism**
Numbers of organisms	Impaired clearing mechanism of the gut, ureter, respiratory tract; reduced acid production in the stomach or vagina; elimination of competing organisms during antimicrobial therapy; major body burn; on entry of bacteria into the body by intravenous or by respiratory route from a contaminated source
Adherence	Nonspecific attachment or colonizing properties such as coagulase-negative *Staphylococcus* on the skin surface, *Staphylococcus aureus* in the anterior nose, *Streptococcus viridans* in the mouth, *Giardia* attachment to the small bowel mucosa and *Neisseria gonorrhoeae* in the genitourinary tract. Highly specialized adhesions that bind to host cell receptors in a receptor–ligand interaction (e.g., ETEC, EPEC, P-fimbriate *Escherichia coli* important in pyelonephritis)
Resistance to phagocytosis	Capsular structures resistant to phagocytosis in the absence of opsonins (e.g., M protein for *Streptococcus pyogenes*, capsule of *S. pneumoniae*, K1 antigen of *E. coli* in neonates), or the organisms (e.g., *S. pyogenes*, *Clostridium perfringens*) may elaborate excellular proteins that lyse phagocytes
Exotoxin production	Exotoxin production is important in cholera and ETEC diarrhea, botulism, gas gangrene, toxic shock syndrome due to *S. aureus* or *S. pyogenes* infection, *S. aureus* food poisoning, *Bacillus anthracis*, *Corynebacterium diphtheriae*, *Bordetella pertussis*, and *Pseudomonas aeruginosa* infection
Extracellular proteins	Production of hyaluronidase, collagenase, streptokinase by *S. pyogenes* that facilitate dissemination through tissues; *S. aureus* production of coagulase, promoting coagulation of adjacent vessels, leading to a walled-off abscess (boil)
Microbial antigen shift	Influenza virus, *N. gonorrhoeae*, and the HIV can alter their antigenic makeup, facilitating escape from body immunity
Invasiveness	Some organisms (papillomavirus, dermatophytes, *B. anthracis*) can invade directly through healthy skin or mucous membrane barriers; the invasive enteric bacteria (e.g., *Shigella*, *Salmonella*, *Campylobacter jejuni*) can invade the gut wall if ingested in sufficient numbers
Siderophore elaboration	Many bacteria possess structures that can compete with host binding proteins for available iron

EPEC, enteropathogenic *E. coli*; ETEC, enterotoxigenic *E. coli*.

infected mucosal surfaces and subsequently attach to mucosal surfaces of susceptible hosts.

RESISTANCE TO PHAGOCYTOSIS

Microbes that breech the epithelial surface barrier encounter many phagocytic cells. These cells require alteration of the surface of the organism by immunoglobulins (IgG and IgM) to coat, or opsonize, the surface of bacteria. This defense process is particularly important for the eradication of encapsulated organisms such as *Streptococcus pneumoniae*, *Haemophilus influenzae*, and *N. meningitidis*. Persons who lack these immunoglobulins develop severe and recurrent infections by these organisms and by *S. aureus*. Patients who do not have a spleen (e.g., patients with sickle cell anemia or who have had splenectomy) also lack coating antibodies (i.e., opsonic activity is deficient) and may present with overwhelming infections by one of the encapsulated organisms, particularly *S. pneumoniae*.

During systemic bacterial infection, complement is activated through the classic pathway when stimulated by microbial antigens or through the alternate pathway as a result of stimulation by microbial lipopolysaccharide. Complement participates in the phagocytosis process through its opsonic properties, or it may participate in the direct lysis of certain organisms. A deficiency in plasma complement components C6, C7, or C8 can be found in one-third of patients with meningococcal meningitis, reflecting the importance of complement in the defense against this organism. Deficiency of the terminal components of comple-

ment also predispose patients to bacteremic *N. gonorrhoeae* disease.

Bacteria inhibit phagocytosis through various mechanisms. Some bacteria possess capsular structures that serve as armor, such as K1 antigen of *E. coli* in neonatal meningitis, M proteins of *Streptococcus pyogenes*, and the carbohydrate capsule of *S. pneumoniae*. As a result of previous exposure, the host may opsonize the invader, coating the organism and its antiphagocytic moiety with immunoglobulin and complement, allowing phagocytosis to occur. In the case of *S. pyogenes*, outer surface structures may mimic host tissues, helping to hide the organism from phagocytic cells. Other bacteria produce enzymes that lyse phagocytic cells (e.g., streptolysin produced by *S. pyogenes*, α-toxin elaborated by *Clostridium perfringens*) or inhibit leukocyte chemotaxis (e.g., protein A from metabolically active *S. aureus*).

EXOTOXINS, EXTRACELLULAR PROTEINS, SIDEROPHORES, AND ENDOTOXINS

Strains of *S. aureus* produce several exotoxins that are important in disease expression. One of these is toxic shock toxin-1, a relatively low-molecular-weight, single-peptide-chain protein, important in the pathogenesis of toxic shock syndrome. Other exotoxins produced by *S. aureus* are enterotoxins A through D (implicated in food poisoning). *S. aureus* strains may also produce exfoliative toxins A and B, which may cause severe systemic infection associated with the scalded skin syndrome in neonates and young children and other exfoliative reactions in adults.

In tetanus, neurotoxins produced by *Clostridium tetani* bind to neural cells to produce spastic paralysis in tetanus. Several enzymes, including streptolysin (produced by *S. pyogenes*) and α-toxin (produced by *C. perfringens*), are capable of lysing phagocytic cells. *S. pyogenes* strains produce other pyrogenic exotoxins and are virulent by their ability to multiply rapidly and to excrete a variety of extracellular products that facilitate spreading through tissues planes. *S. pyogenes* grows with a doubling time of 30 minutes in log phase and produces DNAses, hyaluronidase, streptokinase, and proteinases, all of which prevent the host inflammatory response from localizing the infection at the site of bacterial implantation. The propensity of *S. pyogenes* to spread through lymphatics, the subcutaneous tissues, and the bloodstream, resulting in cellulitis, lymphangitis, and bacteremia, appears to be related to these spreading factors.

S. aureus also is a rapidly growing organism with a generation time similar to group A β-hemolytic streptococci. However, *S. aureus* characteristically produces a localized abscess (a boil) as its primary disease manifestation, perhaps because of the elaborated enzyme, coagulase, which leads to capillary thrombosis in the adjacent tissue. The organism is able to avoid phagocytosis by anatomical separation from the circulating host cells.

All living forms require iron for growth. Because tissue iron is normally bound to body proteins, it is necessary for bacteria to compete for iron binding. Some bacteria have siderophores to bind to available iron, or the organisms may induce hemolysis to gain access to iron freed from host tissue.

Endotoxins are complexes of polysaccharide, protein, and lipid composing part of the cell wall structure of gram-negative bacilli and gram-negative cocci. Endotoxin participates in certain septicemic infections through its effects on host factors. In bacteremic disease, the lysis of gram-negative organisms (e.g., Enterobacteriaceae, *Pseudomonas* spp, *N. meningitidis*) releases endotoxin, leading to myriad host responses involving macrophage cytokines (e.g., tumor necrosis factor, interleukin-1), the complement cascade, the intrinsic coagulation system (e.g., Hageman factor), platelet-activating factor, arachidonic acid metabolites, the humoral defense system (e.g., complement, kinins), vascular endothelium, and myocardium. If the responses are generalized and extreme, they result in shock and end-organ failure due to poor tissue perfusion by blood. The types of organ failure and tissue damage include the adult respiratory distress syndrome, renal failure, disseminated intravascular coagulation, altered sensorium, and death. The sequence of metabolic and vascular complications of endotoxemia is known as the *sepsis cascade*.

INVASIVENESS

All viruses must gain access to an intracellular environment to replicate. This also is true for several pathogenic bacteria, fungi, and protozoa. These organisms have developed mechanisms that facilitate attachment and internalization to enhance their chances for survival and replication within the intracellular milieu. Some microorganisms can benefit from binding to phagocytes and lymphocytes; the host cells transport the microbe from an extracellular location to a preferred intracellular environment. For example, the Epstein–Barr virus infects B lymphocytes by attachment to a B-cell–specific membrane protein, CR2. Similarly, HIV gains access to CD4 T lymphocytes by forming a complex between the viral envelop glycoprotein, gp120, and the surface of the T lymphocyte. Other intracellular pathogens such as *H. capsulatum* can bind to the CR3 immune receptor on phagocytic cells to gain access to a protective intracellular environment. *Plasmodium vivax* penetrates human red cells after first attaching to the Duffy blood group determinant by a nonimmune, lectin–carbohydrate interaction.

Once ingested by phagocytic cells, intracellular organisms can bypass host defenses by a variety of mechanisms. One such mechanism is inhibition of phagosome–lysosome fusion (e.g., *Legionella pneumophila*, *M. tuberculosis*, *Toxoplasma gondii*); another is escape from the phagosome into the cytoplasm of macrophages, which lack a specialized mechanism for killing microbial pathogens (e.g., *Trypanosoma cruzi*).

Other organisms, although remaining extracellular, have the capacity to penetrate host tissues as part of their pathogenic mechanisms. *Shigella* species possess the capacity to invade epithelial cells because of chromosomal genes and a large (120 to 140 Md) enteroinvasive plasmid. The plasmid is necessary for the expression of several outer membrane proteins and invasion plasmid antigens, which assist the bacteria in gaining entry into the enterocyte.

MICROBIAL ANTIGENIC PHASE SHIFTS

Pathogens such as *N. gonorrhoeae*, influenza virus, and HIV undergo shifts in their antigenic expression and are able to avoid immune clearance that depends on specific antibody production. For example, hemagglutinin is an antigen on the surface of the influenza virus used to adhere to cells before infection. Significant changes in the antigenicity of the hemagglutinin occur through swapping genetic material with different viruses in other hosts. When the accrued alterations in hemagglutinin are sufficient to render previous lines of immunity ineffective, a new influenza epidemic is inaugurated. Such microbial alterations add complexity to the concept of immunity.

MICROBIAL PERSISTENCE AND LATENCY

Certain organisms undergo metabolic changes and resist host phagocytic effects and antimicrobials while remaining susceptible in vitro to the antibiotics used. Microbial persistence is clinically relevant in chronic bacterial infections. In these cases, pathogens may be cultured from the sites of purulent or granulomatous inflammation even after prolonged therapy with bactericidal antibiotics. *S. aureus* and some species of *Mycobacterium* are examples of organisms that may persist under these conditions.

Many viruses, including herpesviruses, adenoviruses, hepadnaviruses, papillomaviruses, and retroviruses, characteristically undergo a condition of latency after the initial or primary infection. Within the herpesvirus family, cytomegalovirus and Epstein–Barr virus cause a primary mononucleosis syndrome, after which the viruses remain latent in lymphoid tissues. Primary infection by the varicella-zoster virus or by herpes simplex types 1 and 2 is followed by establishment of latency within sensory nerve ganglion cells. Clinically apparent reactivation of these viruses is manifested by vesicular skin eruptions in dermatome distribution (varicella-zoster) or in the oral (herpes simplex 1) or genital (herpes simplex 2) regions.

Factors that trigger reactivation of latent infections are emotional or physical stress and immunodeficiency secondary to underlying disease or to immunosuppressive therapy. Neither free virus nor viral antigens can be detected in tissues during latency. A virally encoded RNA of herpes simplex has been identified within latently infected neurons, although a protein product has not been detected. The precise function of this latency-associated gene has not been determined, but it is almost certainly related to the capacities of latency and reactivation. The propensity of an organism to establish a latent state may be related to its capacity to undergo malignant transformation through a prolonged relation between the virus and host cell.

HOST GENETICS AND INFECTIOUS DISEASES

Persons differ in terms of susceptibility to microbial infection. Studies of the attachment of enterotoxigenic *E. coli* (ETEC) in the natural porcine host has revealed that certain strains of pigs do not possess the intestinal membrane receptors specific for the organism's attachment fimbriae. These animals are naturally resistant to ETEC infection by the organism containing these adherence ligands. Undoubtedly, the same sort of genetic resistance occurs in humans.

Many infectious diseases are correlated with blood type. The antigenic association between the pathogen and the host erythrocyte membrane may facilitate the microorganism's escape from immune surveillance in persons possessing certain blood types. Alternatively, the association may result from the presence or absence of specific receptors important in the interaction of receptor and infectious agent in those with specific blood types.

The geographic distribution of blood groups appears to influence the susceptibility of populations to many epidemic infectious diseases, including cholera, smallpox, plague, tuberculosis, typhoid fever, bartonellosis, leprosy, hepatitis, and echinococcosis. Patients with blood group type O experience more severe cases of cholera in endemic areas. It seems likely that receptor structures on target cells are related in part to the blood group. Patients with genes of the human leukocyte antigen HLA-B27 may develop Reiter's syndrome (hypersensitivity reaction associated with reactive arthritis, conjunctivitis, and uveitis) after infection by certain pathogens such as *Shigella flexneri*, *Shigella dysenteriae*, and *Campylobacter jejuni*. Major histocompatibility complex molecules strongly influence resistance to a variety of parasitic infections, including malaria, trypanosomiasis, onchocerciasis, and tapeworm infestation. The important interplay between host genetics and the infectious organisms is just now being explored.

CLINICAL MANIFESTATIONS OF HOST–MICROBE INTERACTIONS

When a host is exposed to a microbe, several consequences are possible (Table 18.3). No interaction may occur after exposure if the organism fails to propagate or to become established in any fashion. Another possibility is that the organism colonizes host tissues and serves as a commensal, living off available substrate. The organism may provide benefits to the host in return for the use of space and substrate. For example, microbial production of vitamin K facilitates clotting, and colonization with hospitable flora prevents the acquisition of more hostile microbes. The agent may produce a covert infection in which an immune response can be elicited but there is no clinical illness.

Overt disease may result when the host is exposed to the organism. Certain potential pathogens (e.g., smallpox) characteristically produce clinical illness when a susceptible person is exposed to the agent, although the typical response is for most susceptible and exposed persons to develop subclinical infection, with only a minority becoming ill. Epstein–Barr virus infection is a good example of the more typical type of host–parasite response. Perhaps only 5 of 1,000 infected persons experience

TABLE 18.3.	CLINICAL ASPECTS OF HOST–MICROBE INTERACTIONS
Host–Parasite Interaction	**Conditions**
Colonization, transient	During travel to international regions, hospitalization, and confinement in close quarters with multiple persons, the host may be colonized transiently with abnormal flora. During the incubation of certain infections and during convalescence from other infections, transient carriage of virulent organisms occurs.
Colonization, chronic	Some infectious agents (e.g., typhoid, hepatitis B) produce chronic infection that may not be associated with symptoms.
Subclinical infection	Most infectious agents more commonly produce subclinical infection than overt illness. In these cases, studies of antibody development or cell-mediated immunity confirm an infection.
Clinical disease	Some organisms (e.g., smallpox, *Shigella* infection, brucellosis) commonly cause illness when infection occurs. The organisms that characteristically produce subclinical infection less commonly produce overt disease.
Persistence and latency	The herpesvirus family members (e.g., herpes simplex, cytomegalovirus, varicella-zoster virus, Epstein–Barr virus) cause persistent infection. Although there is no evidence of active infection after the primary infection has resolved, relapses or recurrences of illness occur, often with a change in immunity or other factor.

infectious mononucleosis. Most adults have been exposed to the virus and have serologic evidence of past infection. Microbial persistence and latency characterizes infection by one of the herpesviruses.

An important concept in the epidemiology of infectious diseases is organism carriage. Humans often represent the important reservoir and vehicle of transmission for subsequent infection. There are at least four types of carriers. The *inapparent carrier* has an asymptomatic infection; the infectious particles are shed without any clinical illness. The *incubatory carrier* is a person incubating an infectious disease who is transmitting the organism before experiencing symptomatic illness. The *convalescent carrier* has recovered from an infection and is shedding the organism, potentially to other susceptible persons. The *chronic carrier* is clinically well, but for prolonged periods (years to lifetime) is capable of transmitting the virulent organism.

Important examples associated with inapparent carriage include poliovirus and meningococcus; with incubatory carriage, chickenpox, measles, and hepatitis A; with convalescent carriage, diphtheria and hepatitis B; and with chronic carriage, *S. typhi* and hepatitis B.

IMMUNOPATHOLOGY AND IMMUNOSUPPRESSION DURING INFECTION

Many viruses that infect cells of the immune system exert direct immunosuppressive effects. These effects may be severe enough to render the host susceptible to opportunistic infection or malignant transformation of host cells. The measles virus may lead to a loss in delayed hypersensitivity to *M. tuberculosis* antigen during active infection. The loss of allergic reactivity, known as anergy, manifests a few days before onset of the rash and may persist for 6 weeks after recovery from measles. Disseminated *M. tuberculosis*, *Coccidioides immitis*, or *Mycobacterium leprae* infections are associated with anergy in a high percentage of cases. Except for leprosy, antimicrobial therapy of the disseminated infection usually reverses the anergy.

A striking impairment of immunity is seen in HIV infection. The virus causes numeric depletion and dysfunction of CD4 T lymphocytes. HIV also infects and damages macrophages, leading to reduced capacity of these cells to present antigens to T cells and to elaborate cytokines. HIV-infected persons experience infection by a variety of opportunistic pathogens, such as *Pneumocystis carinii*, a commensal of the normal lung.

Other infectious agents produce variable degrees of immunosuppression. Cytomegalovirus is commonly associated with immunosuppression, probably as a consequence of infection of lymphocytes by the virus. Influenza viruses primarily attack columnar epithelial cells of the respiratory tract, monocytes, and macrophages, leading to reduced bactericidal activity. This virus-induced impairment of macrophage function in influenza may contribute to the secondary pulmonary infection by bacteria, including *S. aureus*, *S. pneumoniae*, and *H. influenzae*.

BIBLIOGRAPHY

Ellner PD, Neu HC. *Understanding infectious disease.* St. Louis: Mosby-Year Book, Inc., 1992.

Murray PR, Rosenthal KS, Kobayashi GS, Pfaller MA. *Medical microbiology,* third ed. St. Louis: Mosby-Year Book, Inc., 1998.
Ryan KJ. *Sherris medical microbiology,* third ed. Stamford, CT: Appleton & Lange, 1994.

Kelley's Textbook of Internal Medicine, fourth edition. Edited by H. David Humes.
Lippincott Williams & Wilkins, Philadelphia © 2000.

C H A P T E R
19

ETIOLOGY OF MALIGNANT DISEASE

WILLIAM A. BLATTNER

Over the last 20 years, public awareness of environmental factors, personal habits and lifestyle, and genetic predisposition associated with heightened cancer risk has translated into increased activism reflected in legislation, litigation, and personal commitment to a prevention-oriented lifestyle. Following the lead of AIDS activists, the demand for increased research funding, legislation to improve worker conditions and the environment at large, the "tobacco settlement" for health-related outcomes of tobacco use, and increased attention to diet and exercise are manifestations of this activism. The practicing clinician and subspecialist are called on to be the arbiter of an informed and balanced perspective on these issues.

Recent advances in molecular biology have improved our understanding of the genetic basis of cancer as a complex series of diseases involving multiple steps and multiple pathways involving genes at the center of cell signaling, DNA repair, and other vital check points of cellular function. Beginning with an initiation event that renders a tissue premalignant, followed by a number of promotional steps that increase the potential for an initiated cell to become malignant, cancer is a multistage process. Opportunities for early detection have increased with the emergence of screening approaches such as prostate-specific antigen (PSA), improved imaging techniques, and less invasive sampling such as fine-needle biopsy. These and improved therapies have started to make an impact on the morbidity and mortality of some tumors. With 70% of all deaths caused by cancer and cardiovascular disease in persons over age 65, declines in deaths due to cardiovascular disease and stroke are occurring at a rate faster than those for cancer. With the specter that cancer will become the leading cause of death in this age group in the United States and other developed countries in the next 5 to 10 years, identification of preventable exposures and strategies to reduce or reverse the risk for cancer remains a high priority.

LIFESTYLE FACTORS

In their 1981 monograph, Doll and Peto estimated that at least 30% to 40% of all cancer deaths could be avoided by applying the knowledge we have of the known causes of cancer. Effecting behavioral changes to reduce cancer risk is complex (Chapter 22), although major national campaigns in the areas of diet, physical exercise, and antismoking have achieved some success in changing behavior among targeted populations.

TOBACCO

In the United States, tobacco use accounts for about 40% of all cancers among men and 20% of all cancers among women. Lung cancer is the major tobacco-associated cancer site, with 90% of cases among men and 79% of cases among women attributed to tobacco exposure. The epidemic of lung cancer in the United States emerged among men in the 1930s and among women in the mid-1960s—approximately 20 years after the widespread introduction of cigarette smoking in each of these groups. Since then, an overwhelming body of evidence has amassed that shows that cigarette smoking causes a variety of malignancies of the respiratory, gastrointestinal, and genitourinary systems. For lung cancer, the risk from heavy cigarette smoking (more than two packs per day) is 20 times higher than among nonsmokers. Filter-tipped cigarettes, which decrease the tar and nicotine levels, reduce the risk for smokers, but the rates are still much higher than among nonsmokers.

Nonsmokers exposed to environmental tobacco smoke, *passive smoking,* experience excess risk and present with patterns of tumors similar to that of smokers. Heavily exposed passive smokers have risk estimates similar to that of light smokers. Former smokers experience a reduction in risk compared with active smokers; this is detectable within a few years of cessation.

Other malignancies associated with cigarette smoking are by system: respiratory (lip, oral cavity, pharynx, larynx, trachea, bronchus, and lung); gastrointestinal (esophagus and pancreas); genitourinary (bladder, kidney, and ureter); reproductive (uterus, cervix); and hematologic (myelogenous leukemia). The risk of cancers of the lip, mouth, tongue, pharynx, larynx, and esophagus is further amplified by heavy alcohol consumption.

Smokeless tobacco usage, tobacco chewing, and particularly snuff dipping is of increasing concern, because the practice has become popular among teenagers and young adults. Rates of mouth and throat cancer are increased up to 50 times in longtime snuff users. In general, a dose-response relationship governs mouth and throat cancer; risks increase with the amount and duration of tobacco use.

ALCOHOL

Alcohol consumption synergistically enhances the risk for several tobacco-related neoplasms. Combined exposure to alcohol and smoking account for about 75% of all oral and pharyngeal cancers. Alcohol alone is estimated to contribute to about 3% of cancers and has been associated with colon cancer and colorectal adenomatous polyps and with esophageal, pancreatic, nasopharyngeal, prostate, and breast cancers. Ethanol is not carcinogenic in laboratory animal studies but may enhance carcinogenicity by making carcinogens more soluble or by facilitating tissue penetration. Alcohol is associated with heightened risk for liver cancer, and tissue injury resulting from cirrhosis may contribute

to the carcinogenic process. Nutritional deficiencies among black men who are heavy drinkers have been linked to high rates of cancer of the esophagus. Several analyses suggest that even moderate use of alcohol enhances female breast cancer by a factor of 50%. Although the basis for this determination is unknown, effects on hormonal metabolism have been postulated.

DIET AND NUTRITION

Establishing clear links between diet and cancer is complicated by methodologic issues, such as differential recall bias and the long latency between putative dietary exposures and subsequent cancer risk. Observational studies, such as those among migrants from areas with low colon cancer risk who adopt a Western diet, thus heightening their risk for this tumor in their lifetime, demonstrate the importance of diet in cancer risk. Interventional studies, including one that used vitamin A supplementation to effect reversal of preneoplastic lesions of the esophagus in a high-risk Chinese population, mirror results in experimental animal studies in which supplemental vitamin administration reversed preneoplastic lesions. For cancers with a suspected dietary component, some have estimated that 35% of cancer has a dietary factor involved in the cause, but with a wide range for this attribution. Current public health guidelines suggest that a prudent diet, which emphasizes reduction in total animal fat consumption, increase in intake of fruits and vegetables, good food preservation and healthy preparation, moderation in alcohol consumption, and avoidance of obesity, may reduce cancer rates by as much as one-third while reducing risk of cardiovascular disease as well.

The mechanism or mechanisms by which diet may influence cancer risk—either by increasing or decreasing it, are complex, and it is difficult to distinguish which nutrients are the active agents and how much daily intake is required to have a desired effect. Obesity is strongly linked to risk of endometrial cancer and cancer of the biliary system, colon cancer in men, and possibly renal cell cancer. Higher mortality for breast cancer among obese postmenopausal women may result from delayed detection. However, high fat intake is associated with increased risk for breast cancer in correlational but less clearly in analytic studies. Prostate and colon cancers are more strongly associated with dietary fat and meat consumption, and some studies also suggest a role in ovarian cancer as well.

Sir Dennis Burkitt popularized consumption of high dietary grain fiber as a means of reducing colon cancer risk, but a recent study, while showing benefit of increased fiber intake for cardiovascular disease, did not make a favorable impact on colon cancer. However, high vegetable and fruit intake is beneficial, but the effect may result from vitamins or other nutrients (e.g., vitamin C, indoles, and other nutrients) in reducing cancer risk. Vitamin A, carotenoids, vitamin C, vitamin E, and selenium have been implicated in a variety of studies as having a beneficial effect in reducing cancer risk. These dietary adjuncts have been used in interventional studies in varying combinations or alone with mixed results, including the finding in one Finnish study in which men at high risk of lung cancer experienced increased rates of lung cancer when given vitamin A supplements. In this same trial, those receiving vitamin E did not experience an increased risk of lung cancer, but a modest reduction in prostate cancer was observed.

In vitro studies of carcinogens and mutagens detected as a result of food preparation (e.g., high-temperature cooking) raised questions about the role of these factors in human cancers. But epidemiologic studies in human populations have not linked such factors, except for salt-preserved foods that may heighten risk for stomach cancer and nasopharyngeal cancer in China. Several natural products are themselves carcinogenic, such as aflatoxin, a carcinogenic metabolic product of the fungus *Aspergillus flavus,* which is associated with high rates of liver cancer.

Compelling data from many sources document that diet may modify cancer risk by years. As a fuller understanding of these complex interactions develops and accumulated supportive evidence increases, acceleration of educational campaigns on the health benefits derived from improved nutritional practices may lead to substantial reduction in cancer rates.

THERAPEUTIC FACTORS

The major classes of medically prescribed drugs linked to heightened risk for cancer are hormones, anticancer drugs, and immunosuppressive agents. Despite these associations, drugs are believed to account for less than 2% of all cancers.

EXOGENOUS HORMONES

In the late 1960s, an epidemic of vaginal and cervical adenocarcinoma in young women was linked to prior exposure in utero to diethylstilbestrol, which was used as an adjunct to preventing miscarriage. The use of synthetic conjugated estrogens alone for menopausal symptoms has been linked to the development of endometrial cancer, but low-dose estrogen replacement in combination with progesterone-containing hormonal replacement regimens is not associated with increased endometrial cancer risk. The relation of hormonal replacement therapy and risk for breast cancer is complex, with a number of studies conducted in the 1990s demonstrating modest increases in risk but with several studies suggesting that the associated subtype of breast cancer has a good prognosis. So the impact of such therapy on mortality is not known. Some have argued that the benefits of hormonal replacement outweigh the risks because of reduction in heart disease and osteoporosis. Decisions about hormonal replacement therapy depend on the individual circumstance of the patient and her medical needs as well as results of further studies that can help to refine our understanding of this complex paradigm.

There are conflicting data on oral contraceptives as a risk factor for breast cancer; early, prolonged use in persons with a predisposition is implicated. Other studies of oral contraceptives suggest that they may decrease the risk of ovarian and endometrial cancer, although an association with invasive cervical cancer was suggested in one study.

IMMUNOSUPPRESSIVE AGENTS

The concept of immunosurveillance in cause of cancer, first proposed in the early 1960s, suggested that cancer emerges be-

cause of a loss of immunologic recognition of tumor-associated antigens. Studies of immunodeficiency in various settings have documented a limited repertoire of tumor types. One of the first settings evaluated involved the study of tumors among patients receiving immunosuppressive therapies to suppress rejection of organ transplants. In this setting, non-Hodgkin's lymphomas, especially of the brain, are the most prominent manifestation. The emergence of such tumors within months of transplantation contrasts with the longer duration for cancer induction associated with environmental carcinogens. An infectious agent, Epstein–Barr virus (EBV) is linked to such transplant lymphomas.

Other cancers associated with immunosuppressive therapy include Kaposi's sarcoma and cervical, vulvar, and anal (all human papillomavirus–associated) cancers. Squamous cell carcinoma of the skin and malignant melanoma are also increased in this setting. This pattern of tumors has also been observed in acquired and congenital immunodeficiency, with some additional tumor types linked to specific congenital immunodeficiency states such as ovarian dysgerminomas, and stomach and liver cancers in ataxia telangiectasia, probably associated with this disorder's chromosomal changes. The stomach cancer observed in common variable immunodeficiency is probably a result of the common occurrence of achlorhydria in that disorder.

OTHER DRUGS

With the exception of hormones and several medicinal agents, most drugs as they are ordinarily used clinically pose no risk for cancer. Arsenicals are no longer used in clinical practice but are associated with some risk for skin cancer. Diphenylhydantoin is linked to a slightly increased risk for non-Hodgkin's lymphomas. Phenacetin used in high dosages is linked to renal cancer, whereas nonsteroidal anti-inflammatory drugs, including aspirin, have been shown to reduce the risk of colon cancer. Some anticancer drugs, particularly alkylating agents, which have radiation-like effects, are associated with increased cancer risk, particularly leukemia. However, their use is justified when treating otherwise incurable cancers. Studies of patients treated with alkylating agents for Hodgkin's and non-Hodgkin's lymphoma, multiple myeloma, and ovarian, gastric, and colorectal cancers have shown a 16- to several hundred-fold increase in risk for acute nonlymphocytic leukemia emerging after 3 to 5 years and peaking after 10 to 15 years.

ENVIRONMENTAL FACTORS

IONIZING RADIATION

Ionizing radiation produces its carcinogenic effects by direct damage to the genetic material of the cell. Radiogenic cancers are most prominent in the breast, brain, thyroid, and bone marrow, with excesses of some other tumors associated with particularly heavy local exposure to a particular site, such as with osteosarcomas and bone-seeking radionuclides.

Most data on the carcinogenic potential of ionizing radiation are derived from moderate to high exposure levels; extrapolations from these data suggest the importance of the cumulative effect of exposure. It is unlikely that a threshold dose exists below which there is no carcinogenic effect.

Radiogenic leukemia differs from most radiation-induced cancers in that the latent period is relatively short. Cases occur within a few years of exposure, peak at 6 to 8 years, and are followed by a decline to normal rates within 25 years. Radiogenic carcinomas have much longer latent periods. In the prospective follow-up of the children exposed to radiation after the atomic bomb blasts in Japan, prepubertal girls exposed to moderate doses were at high risk for breast cancers 20 to 30 years later. Even modest doses of prenatal radiation are associated with heightened risk for leukemia and other childhood cancers. Cancers have also developed in sites where radionuclides are concentrated. Some examples include osteosarcoma (radium 224), leukemia (phosphorus 32), and liver angiosarcoma (Thorotrast).

Although ionizing radiation appears to account for no more than 3% of all cancers, there is considerable public concern about this risk factor. Increased public awareness of radon in ground water and its potential for household contamination and the publicity surrounding the general population exposure from the nuclear accident in Chernobyl, intensify this concern.

ULTRAVIOLET RADIATION

Solar radiation causes up to 90% of nonmelanoma skin cancer, and its effects are linked to skin melanoma as well. The link between sunlight exposure and squamous and basal cell carcinomas was determined from the high rates among persons with outdoor occupations (e.g., sailors, farmers), among persons residing in southern latitudes, and among fair-skinned people with lower levels of protective melanin pigment.

Skin cancers tend to occur most prominently in sun-exposed areas. For nonmelanoma skin cancer, risk is related to annual cumulative lifetime ultraviolet-B exposure; for melanoma skin cancer, a history of repeated sunburn, especially in youth, is associated with heightened risk for subsequent skin melanoma years later. Behavioral modification, such as avoidance of excessive sunlight exposure and the use of readily available and highly protective sunscreens, could have a major preventive impact on cancers of the skin.

■ OCCUPATION

Exposures to potential carcinogens in the workplace have led to the recognition of several compounds as human carcinogens, such as asbestos, which causes mesothelioma, and vinyl chloride, which causes liver angiosarcoma. Workers exposed to aromatic amines in dye, rubber, and coal gas manufacture and some chemical workers are at increased risk for bladder cancer.

Respiratory carcinogens include bis-(chloromethyl)-ether (causes oat cell carcinoma of the lung), chromium manufacture (lung cancer), mustard gas exposure (lung, larynx, and nasal sinuses cancer), nickel dust exposure (tumors of lung and nasal sinuses), isopropyl alcohol production (tumors of nasal sinuses), polycyclic hydrocarbons (lung cancer), and wood dust in furniture manufacture (tumors of nasal sinuses). Benzene exposure in leather, petroleum, and other industries is linked to non-

lymphocytic leukemia. Herbicide exposures among foresters and farmers are linked to lymphoproliferative and soft-tissue neoplasms. Cadmium exposure is associated with a heightened risk for prostate cancer, and formaldehyde exposure has been linked to nasopharyngeal cancer. Although occupational exposures account for as much as 5% of all cancer deaths, cancer prevention has been significantly advanced through the identification and elimination of hazardous exposures in the workplace.

POLLUTION

The level of cancer risk attributable to air and water polluted with known carcinogens remains controversial. Results from studies of air pollution by specific manufacturing processes, such as smelter emissions of arsenic, are associated with localized increased risk for lung cancer. Although rates of lung cancer are higher in urban than in rural areas, studies that control for smoking and occupational risk factors and those based on estimates of higher exposure rates in the workplace do not indicate a major risk for air pollution. Between 1% and 2% of cancers are estimated to be due to past exposures, whereas based on existing data, less than 1% of future cancers will result from current air pollution levels.

Water pollution was identified as a potential source of cancer risk, recognizing that the process of chlorination produces trihalomethanes, which are carcinogenic and mutagenic. Results are inconclusive, but excessive levels of these substances have been shown to correlate with bladder, colon, and rectum cancer rates. Analyses suggest a significant correlation between volume of water ingested and risk for cancer. Ground water contamination from local toxic waste disposal and dumping has been implicated in some cancer clusters, but aside from drinking water containing unusually high levels of carcinogens, little substantive evidence suggests that drinking water contributes substantially to cancer risk.

■ INFECTIOUS AGENTS

The contribution of infectious agents to the pathogenesis of cancer varies considerably by geographic area and population, with approximately 10% to 15% of all cancers associated with infectious agents. In developed countries, the contribution made by infectious causes to the overall cancer burden is relatively low; in the populations of some developing countries of Africa and Asia, more than 50% of the cancers are linked to a viral agent.

VIRUSES

The major infectious carcinogens worldwide are the hepatitis B and C viruses, which are strongly linked to hepatocellular carcinoma, the leading cause of cancer mortality in many areas where early life exposure confers a substantial risk. EBV, a herpesvirus, has been linked to Hodgkin's and some non-Hodgkin's lymphomas, especially Burkitt's lymphoma and nasopharyngeal carcinoma (NPC). In southern China, a specific immunogenetic marker identifies persons at high risk for NPC. A variety of cofactors associated with altered immunity, particularly bouts of malaria, are thought to be necessary to trigger the endemic form of Burkitt's lymphoma in Africa. EBV has also been identified in approximately 7% of gastric carcinomas but its etiologic role is not established.

A newly discovered gamma herpesvirus—HHV-8, also known as Kaposi's sarcoma associated virus (KSHV)—is linked to Kaposi's sarcoma in AIDS and in an AIDS-associated form of extranodal (i.e., body cavity) non-Hodgkin's lymphoma as well as the premalignant lymphoproliferative disorder, Castleman's disease.

Cervical and vulvar cancer in women and penile cancer and anal carcinoma in men are linked to some subtypes of human papillomavirus (HPV). Prospective studies demonstrate that high levels of HPV in prediagnostic Papanicolaou (Pap) smears are elevated in some cases decades before the emergence of cervical cancer. This is consistent with the hypothesis that inability to down-regulate papillomavirus expression predisposes to subsequent cervical cancer risk.

The first human RNA retrovirus, human T-cell lymphotrophic virus type I (HTLV-I), is associated with a distinctive clinical pathologic entity, adult T-cell leukemia-lymphoma (ATL). Rarely, in persons who have had early-life exposure, a clonally integrated neoplasm occurs. The disease and virus cluster in southern Japan, the Caribbean basin, and surrounding countries; in these geographic areas, ATL is responsible for more than 50% of all lymphomas, which account for 1% to 2% of all malignancies in these countries.

Because of its immunosuppressive effects, HIV-1, the causal agent of AIDS, is associated with an increased risk for Kaposi's sarcoma, non-Hodgkin's lymphoma, Hodgkin's lymphoma, and anal and possibly cervical carcinomas. With the advent of highly active antiretroviral therapy, the incidence of Kaposi's sarcoma has dramatically declined and regressions of existing lesions noted. The impact of such therapy on non-Hodgkin lymphoma is less certain.

OTHER PATHOGENS

Certain nonviral parasites are also carcinogenic. Schistosomiasis is associated with squamous cell carcinoma of the bladder in the Middle East and North Africa, and liver flukes that cause clonorchiasis and opisthorchiasis are associated with cholangiocarcinoma in Asia.

Some bacterial agents, such as *Helicobacter pylori,* have been linked to gastric carcinoma and mucosa-associated lymphoid tissue lymphoma (MALT).

◼ HOST FACTORS

Although the role for environmental factors in producing cancer is beyond dispute, genetic factors are also consequential. Studies of human populations confirm a wide range of variability in inherent sensitivities to carcinogenesis. The role of individual variation is advanced by the disparity in cancer rates among distinct racial and ethnic populations in which environmental

influences cannot account for the differences. For example, chronic lymphocytic leukemia is consistently absent in Asian populations, regardless of geographic locale; testicular cancer and Ewing's sarcoma occur rarely in blacks, whether they reside in Africa or in the United States.

Molecular epidemiologic techniques are being applied to high-risk groups (a) to examine individual genetic variations that may be identified with increased risk, including variations in the pathways for metabolizing endogenous and exogenous, carcinogenic compounds; (b) to evaluate chromosomal instability; and (c) to investigate oncogenes and suppressor genes. Specific genetic changes have been identified as critical molecular events in the initiation and development of many cancers. Some of these structural changes include activation of oncogenes, inactivation of tumor suppressor genes such as *P53* and the retinoblastoma gene *(RB1)*, and chromosome deletions (Table 19.1).

Over 200 single-gene disorders have been recognized, which confer a cancer-prone genetic predisposition. Studies of such high-risk patients with these predispositions have yielded important insights concerning the fundamental biology of cancer. Hereditary neoplasms are best exemplified by autosomal dominant gene disorders, which result in the development of specific neoplasms or constellations of tumors. Approximately 40% of all retinoblastomas occurring in childhood are of the hereditary type. A deletion involving the long arm of chromosome 13 has been recognized in some cases, and molecular analyses with genetic probes have identified a specific gene region called a *suppressor gene,* which acts by modulating specific cell-cycling regulators. The absence of this down-regulation results in increased and unregulated cell proliferation. Thus, mutations in such genes—and in the case of retinoblastoma a specific gene, *RB1,* a DNA-binding nuclear protein—confer a high risk for tumor formation. For such suppressor genes to lose activity, both alleles of the gene must be mutated. In the case of hereditary retinoblastoma, in which patients are also prone to osteosarcoma of the leg and radiogenic sarcoma of the orbit, susceptible patients are born with an inherited constitutional rearrangement or deletion of chromosome 13q14, where the *RB1* gene resides. A single mutation of the remaining intact *RB1* gene allele results in tumor formation.

Studies of sporadic oat cell carcinoma of the lung and renal carcinoma also suggest a mechanism similar to retinoblastoma that involves a gene on the long arm of chromosome 3. Other cancer genes are the targets of gene-mapping studies applied to a variety of cancer-prone disorders. Table 19.1 lists some of the cancers for which studies of genetic or familial syndromes have contributed to understanding their molecular basis. The practice of oncology will be significantly influenced by these discoveries as these markers are applied to the diagnosis and staging of a wide range of common cancers.

A variety of preneoplastic states have been recognized. Hamartomatous syndromes are typified by autosomal dominant disorders in which faulty embryonic development results in localized abnormal growth in mixed component tissues and heightened risk for various cancers. The genodermatoses are autosomal recessive disorders linked primarily to skin cancers, particularly of sun-exposed areas. Defects in the repair of ultraviolet-induced DNA damage in xeroderma pigmentosum have pro-

TABLE 19.1.	MOLECULAR BASIS OF SELECTED CANCERS AND SYNDROMES	
Condition	**Cancer**	**Genetic Defect**
Retinoblastoma	Secondary primary tumors, including osteosarcoma of leg, radiogenic sarcoma of orbit (loss of *RB1* observed in sporadic breast, lung and other sites)	Chromosome deletion 13q14, site of the *RB1* gene. *RB1* acts at cyclin checkpoint for progression through G1 phase of mitosis.
Li–Fraumeni syndrome	Breast (early onset) plus several neoplasms of soft-tissue sarcoma, osteosarcoma, leukemia, brain tumor, lung, laryngeal, and adrenocortical cancers	*P53* mutation in germ cell line
Familial adenomatous polyposis (FAP)	Colorectal	*APC* gene: long arm of chromosome 5; other genes involved in colon cancer but no FAP; *MCC* gene: long arm chromosome 5; *DCC* gene: chromosome 18: *ras* oncogene; p53
Hereditary nonpolyposis colorectal cancer (HNPCC)	Colorectal, endometrial, stomach, gallbladder	*MSH2* gene: DNA mismatch repair gene on chromosome 2; *MLH1, PMS1, PMS2*
Multiple primary adenocarcinomas (Lynch syndrome)	Colon, endometrial, breast, brain, pancreas, and urinary tract	*HPMS2*: mismatch repair gene defect
Site-specific breast tumor	Breast	*BRCA1*: long arm of chromosome 17 (17q21); *BRACA2*: long arm of chromosome 13
Renal carcinoma	Kidney cancer	*FHIT*
Multiple endocrine neoplasia, type 2	Pheochomocytoma, medullary thyroid carcinoma	*RET*: oncogene transmitted via germline mutation
Familial malignant melanoma	Malignant melanoma	*P16*: suppressor gene; *CDK4*

vided insights into the types of metabolic pathways by which the body repairs solar radiation-induced damage.

The dysplastic nevus syndrome predisposes to malignant melanoma, and because it occurs as a heritable and sporadic condition, it is an important precancerous condition that practitioners are likely to see, diagnose, and cure.

Congenital immune deficiency states predispose to a variety of cancers, especially of the lymphoreticular system. Ataxia telangiectasia, an immune deficiency syndrome, also shares a defect in chromosome fragility. Tissue from these patients is usually susceptible to γ-radiation exposure in vitro and in vivo. Patients with this autosomal recessive disorder are prone to lymphoma, lymphocytic leukemia, stomach cancer, and other cancers; heterozygous relatives are said to be at heightened risk for leukemia, lymphoma, and carcinoma of the biliary tract and a variety of other cancers.

The finding of cancer in close relatives is not unusual, and the risk for a particular cancer has been consistently reported to be about two- to threefold if a close family member has that tumor. Familial cancer family syndrome patients are often distinguished by a tendency for multiple primary cancers in the same person and often by a younger than usual age of onset. Site-specific familial cancer aggregations are the most common, with familial breast and colon clusters observed most frequently. In other instances, multiple types of cancer occur in the same family. Examples include the multiple adenocarcinoma syndrome (colon, endometrial and breast carcinoma); Turcot's syndrome (brain and colon cancer); and the Li–Fraumeni syndrome (bony and soft tissue sarcomas, breast, brain, lung, larynx and adrenocortical neoplasms, and leukemia).

CONCLUSION

Cancer is a complex disease involving multistep molecular and cellular processes. Because no single genetic factor is sufficient to predict risk, the ultimate goal of epidemiology is to understand the environmental factors, lifestyles, and individual risk profiles that can facilitate population-based and individually targeted prevention approaches.

Some cancers are already declining as a result of efforts to eliminate exposures such as cigarette smoking. Nonetheless, more research is needed to identify the risk factors for common cancers, particularly those that are increasing, such as breast cancers in young women and non-Hodgkin's lymphomas.

BIBLIOGRAPHY

Collaborative Group on Hormonal Factors in Breast Cancer. Breast cancer and hormonal replacement therapy: collaborative reanalysis of data from 51 epidemiologic studies of 52,705 women with breast cancer. *Lancet* 1997;350:1484.

Doll R, Peto R. *The cause of cancer.* New York, Oxford University Press, 1981.

Evans A, Kaslow R, eds. *Viral infections of man.* New York: Plenum Press, 1995.

Gapstur S, Morrow M, Sellers T. Hormone replacement therapy and risk of breast cancer with a favorable histology. *JAMA* 1999;281:2091.

Perera F. Environment and cancer: who are susceptible? *Science* 1997;278: 1068.

Ron E. Ionizing radiation and cancer risk: evidence from epidemiology. *Radiat Res* 1998;150(5 Suppl):S30.

Schottenfeld D, Fraumeni JF Jr, eds. *Cancer epidemiology and prevention.* New York: Oxford University Press, 1996.

Vessey MP, Gray M. *Cancer risks and prevention.* Oxford: Oxford University Press, 1985.

Willett W, Colditz G, Mueller N. Strategies for minimizing cancer risk. *Sci Am* 1996;375:88.

Kelley's Textbook of Internal Medicine, fourth edition. Edited by H. David Humes. Lippincott Williams & Wilkins, Philadelphia © 2000.

CHAPTER 20

MOLECULAR AND CELL BIOLOGY OF NEOPLASIA

PETER C. NOWELL

It is now widely accepted that most tumors (neoplasms) are a cellular mass that represents the progeny of a single cell in which one or more mutations resulted in a growth and/or survival advantage over normal cells. It also appears that in most cases, a number of sequential mutations within the expanding cell clone are necessary for it to develop into a clinical neoplasm. If these mutations involve only a growth advantage and the tumor remains localized, it is termed *benign.* If additional changes occur in other genes that allow a subpopulation of the tumor to successfully invade adjacent tissues and metastasize to distant sites, the neoplasm is considered *malignant* (cancer). Typically, malignant tumors at this stage are also less well differentiated and grow more aggressively, but the ability to invade and to metastasize is the critical biologic and clinical difference between benign and malignant neoplasms.

Since the mid-1980s, much progress has been made in identifying the multiple genes and proteins involved in the pathways of normal growth regulation; there has also been the recognition that a wide variety of genes may be altered through somatic mutations or as inherited defects and that they contribute to the development of many kind of tumors. Similarly, numerous genes and proteins associated with invasiveness and metastasis are being identified, along with specific gene defects that confer instability on the tumor cell genome, thus increasing the frequency of further mutational events within such cells.

In some circumstances, these findings are already being applied usefully in clinical diagnosis and prognosis, and new therapies are beginning to be developed, targeting specific genetic alterations in particular neoplasms. At the same time, the enormous amount of new information about normal and abnormal growth regulation has made it clear that no single answer to cancer will be forthcoming and that our clinical progress in dealing with this disease will necessarily be incremental.

The following sections summarize the current state of knowledge about tumor molecular and cell biology.

GROWTH REGULATION IN NORMAL AND NEOPLASTIC CELLS

NORMAL GROWTH REGULATION

Many aspects of growth regulation in normal cells are summarized in Chapter 4; however, before considering neoplastic growth, it is important to reiterate just how much has been learned about the complexity of normal growth-regulatory mechanisms. Although efforts continue to define common pathways, significant differences exist among various types of normal cells as well as a wide spectrum of alternative pathways and redundancies within every cell. We have characterized numerous stimulatory and inhibitory local growth factors, such as epidermal growth factor, platelet-derived growth factor, and transforming growth factor-β, and we continue to learn more about the growth-modulating effects of circulating hormones. Specific receptors have been identified for these various growth-regulatory molecules—many on the cell surface and some within the cytoplasm or nucleus. Researchers have also characterized a variety of kinases and other second messengers that transmit receptor-mediated signals from the cell surface to the nucleus, often through several intermediary proteins. Additional regulatory proteins have been identified in the nucleus, transcription factors that directly interact with DNA and other proteins that represent a further intermediary in the signaling pathway.

Besides the multiple steps involved in triggering a cell to enter the cell cycle and ultimately divide, and inhibitors of these signals, there are a variety of proteins that regulate progression through every phase of the cell cycle and significantly influence cellular proliferation in different organs. Moreover, within the broad context of maintaining homeostasis, considerable information has been developed about genes and proteins involved in signaling cells to enter pathways alternative to cell division, specifically terminal differentiation or programmed cell death (apoptosis). For example, retinoic acids play a key role in signaling certain cells to leave the cell cycle and terminally differentiate, and other proteins, such as *BCL2* and *P53,* are important regulators of apoptosis in many cell lineages.

ABNORMAL GROWTH REGULATION IN NEOPLASIA

Since the mid-1980s, molecular studies in many different human tumors have indicated that alteration in the function of growth-regulatory genes, with or without structural change in the gene, is the mechanism whereby nearly all tumors are initiated and by which their clonal expansion progresses. These genes may code for proteins involved in *growth-stimulatory pathways* (and in their altered state are often called *oncogenes*) or may act within *inhibitory pathways,* such that loss of function results in abnormal growth. The latter genes have been termed *tumor suppressor genes.*

A number of these stimulatory and inhibitory "cancer genes"

have been identified in a variety of human tumors, and the proteins for which they code function at every level of the growth-regulatory pathways. There are several examples in human malignancies of genetic changes leading to altered production of a stimulatory or an inhibitory growth factor, with resultant effect on proliferation through autocrine mechanisms. Even more common are changes in the structure or expression of growth factor receptors as a result of mutation or amplification of genes, such as *EGFR* (previously designated *ERBB*) and *ERBB2*. Aberrant regulatory signals transmitted by these modified receptors appear to play an important role in the pathogenesis of many common epithelial malignancies, including those of the breast and lung.

Similarly, mutations in second messengers, such as the RAS family of proteins and the NF1 gene product, have been demonstrated in a significant proportion of human tumors, also contributing to their altered growth. Particularly within the nucleus, a large number of gene products that either bind directly to DNA or interact with such proteins have been shown to be altered either in structure or expression in many human malignancies. These include both stimulatory molecules, such as *MYC,* and those that have an important growth inhibitory function, such as *RB1* and *P53.*

A few of the better characterized human cancer genes are listed in Table 20.1, with an indication of their function or functions and the associated tumors. Although a few of the genes known to be important in human cancer were originally identified from experimental studies with RNA tumor viruses (e.g., *MYC, RAS, ABL, EGFR*), nearly 100 additional human cancer genes have been recognized through other investigative approaches. Most of these previously unknown growth-regulatory loci are not shown in Table 20.1, in part because their oncogenic effect is often limited to a specific cell type or stage of differentiation so that each is typically associated with only a very small subset of human malignancies.

Furthermore, in addition to this complexity, at least five to ten different oncogenes and tumor suppressor genes appear to be usually altered in every fully developed cancer, and there is also evidence that genes substantially involved in differentiation, such as the retinoic acid receptor-α (*RARA)*, or in apoptosis,

TABLE 20.1.   SOME HUMAN CANCER GENES

Gene	Function	Tumor
EGFR	Growth factor receptor	Carcinomas
ERBB2	Growth factor receptor	Carcinomas
RAS	Cytoplasmic signaling	Diverse tumors
NF1	Cytoplasmic signaling	Neural tumors
ABL	Cytoplasmic signaling	Leukemia
MYC	Regulates transcription	Diverse tumors
RB1	Regulates transcription	Diverse tumors
P53	Multiple	Diverse tumors
BRCA1	Multiple	Breast carcinoma
RARA	Differentiation	Leukemia
BCL2	Apoptosis	Lymphoma
MSH2	DNA repair	Colon carcinoma

such as the *BCL2* gene family, are frequently defective in certain tumors and contribute to the expanding clonal mass. Also under investigation is telomerase activity in many tumors, which may be prolonging cell survival by preventing normal chromosome telomere shortening.

The mutagenic agents that mediate these critical genetic events in human tumor cells, such as ionizing and ultraviolet radiation as well as a variety of chemicals, are discussed in detail in other chapters. Similarly, the inherited gene defects that contribute to this process in a proportion of both childhood and adult tumors are covered elsewhere. It is worth noting, however, that we are increasingly aware that many of these mutations involved in human cancer do not necessarily represent the effects of genotoxic agents in the environment or of inherited genes. Often, particularly in older persons, they may simply represent the accumulation of spontaneous errors in DNA replication or repair that occur in all of our tissues throughout life. Also, inflammatory processes and other types of nonspecific injury that generate in our tissues both increased mitotic activity and endogenous mutagenic agents, such as oxygen radicals, may be important contributory factors.

The specific types of alterations that occur in our growth-regulatory genes and lead to tumor development are also variable. Where there is a structural change in the genome, involving gains or losses of all or part of a chromosome or translocations between chromosomes, many of these alterations are visible at the level of the light microscope. In hematopoietic tumors, for example, several dozen specific reciprocal translocations that characterize different subgroups of leukemias and lymphomas have been identified. Typically, these involve the translocation of a growth-regulatory gene into association with a gene on another chromosome, with resultant critical alteration in function. There may be a structural change in the growth-regulatory gene, as in the formation of a fused *BCR/ABL* locus from the translocation between chromosomes 9 and 22 that characterizes chronic myelogenous leukemia, or aberrant expression, as when an intact *MYC* gene is translocated next to a transcriptionally active immunoglobulin locus in the t(8:14) translocation of Burkitt's lymphoma.

In many of the common solid tumors, such as carcinomas of the lung, breast, and colon, there are frequently *deletions* of particular chromosomes, some of which have been shown to involve a loss of function of specific tumor suppressor genes, such as *RB1* or *P53,* within the tumor cell. In some neoplasms, amplification of a critical oncogene, such as *MYC* or *ERBB2,* in which the gene is duplicated many times with resultant overexpression, is also visible as a karyotypic abnormality.

Of course, many circumstances exist in which the alterations in cancer genes are submicroscopic. With the *RAS* gene family, for example, these usually involve point mutations, and this is also true in some circumstances as a mechanism for loss of function of *P53.* Submicroscopic deletions and other types of rearrangements have been demonstrated by molecular techniques, resulting in alteration of oncogene or suppressor gene function. In a few cases, some potentially reversible changes in gene function, resulting, for example, from altered methylation of particular DNA sequences, appears to play an important role in the multiple genetic events leading to the full development of colon cancer and other malignancies.

The introduction of foreign genetic material by a *tumor virus* is a relatively unimportant aspect of human carcinogenesis. The concept of oncogenes was first developed in experimental systems in which it was shown that an RNA tumor virus could introduce an altered mammalian or avian gene into a normal cell and initiate neoplasia. However, this mechanism does not appear to be a significant factor in human malignancy, and many of the important human growth-regulatory genes (e.g., *SRC, SIS, JUN, FOS*) originally identified in these viral studies appear to have little, if any, direct involvement in human tumors.

Most viruses associated with human cancer, such as the Epstein–Barr virus in B-cell tumors and the hepatitis B virus in liver cancer, act primarily by causing nonspecific cell damage, stimulating polyclonal hyperplasia of the target tissue. Only when other mechanisms lead to a specific mutation in one of these hyperplastic cells, such as the t(8:14) translocation in a B lymphocyte, does a clonal neoplasm develop. The papilloma family of DNA viruses does appear to initiate human genital tumors by introducing viral genes (e.g., *A6, A7*) into the recipient cells, but the products of these genes do not appear to act directly within a growth-stimulatory pathway, as with the classic RNA virus oncogenes, but rather by interacting with and down-regulating the function of the protein products of cellular tumor suppressor genes, specifically *RB1* and *P53*.

It is now clear that many different genes and mechanisms are involved in the specific growth-regulatory defects and related cellular alterations that ultimately lead to the development of an expanding clonal mass that we identify in humans as a neoplasm.

EFFECTS OF ALTERED GROWTH REGULATION

The actual rate at which a tumor enlarges, like every other aspect of neoplastic development, is the result of a number of different factors. First, the initial mutated cell must divide for its acquired growth advantage to be significant. If the mutated cell is in an actively proliferating population, this occurs promptly; but in a tissue such as the liver, kidney, or prostate, there may be a lengthy period before some nonspecific growth stimulus, such as injury, inflammation, or a hormonal change, triggers mitotic activity. This aspect of tumorigenesis, sometimes called *promotion,* is one factor in the long *latent period* frequently observed between exposure to a known carcinogen and the subsequent appearance of a clinical neoplasm.

After the tumor begins to grow, its rate of expansion is primarily determined by the proportion of cells that are in the cell cycle ("growth fraction"), rather than by any change in the length of the cycle itself. The growth fraction at any stage of tumor development is the result of the combined effects of the various specific genetic changes in that particular neoplastic clone.

Although it is common to refer to cancer as uncontrolled growth, most tumors, in fact, remain responsive to some degree to normal growth-regulatory mechanisms. For the clone to begin expanding, it requires only enough alteration in responsiveness to allow a slightly increased proportion of the cells to remain in the cycle and gain a selective growth advantage over adjacent normal cells. In early stages, this advantage may be small enough that local changes in growth factors or other regulators could lead to tumor regression. Later, with the acquisition of additional genetic changes over time within the clone, most neoplasms become decreasingly responsive to normal growth regulation, have an increasing growth fraction, and expand more rapidly.

Other variables also contribute, of course. In addition to a change in response to signals for cell cycling as such, altered signals for differentiation or for apoptosis may also help to determine the number of viable cells within the clone over time. In some circumstances, as in certain slow-growing lymphoid tumors, a lack of apoptosis, resulting from overexpression of the *BCL2* gene, appears to be a much more important factor in the slowly expanding neoplastic clone than an increase in cellular proliferation.

Another extremely important variable, and one that is extracellular, is the ability of the expanding tumor mass to stimulate an adequate blood supply. Tumors that successfully grow and metastasize often secrete increased amounts of various angiogenic factors (e.g., VEGF, bFGF) that stimulate the development of new microvasculature to provide sufficient oxygenation for the neoplasm. It is a common observation, in fact, that rapidly growing tumors outstrip their blood supply and may be largely a mass of dead and dying cells, except at the periphery. Just as with the genes and proteins involved in altered growth regulation, the actual rate at which a tumor mass expands either locally or at a metastatic site is typically the result of many variables.

TUMOR PROGRESSION AND HOST RESPONSE

Many tumors have a tendency to demonstrate much more aggressive growth over time, both locally and at distant sites. Histologically, this is frequently associated with greater loss of differentiation in the tumor cells, often accompanied by more mitotic activity and nuclear atypia. It has also been demonstrated that some tumors at this late stage of development show decreased antigenicity and evoke less of a host immune response.

Many of the clinical and biologic characteristics that commonly emerge during the course of human tumors have long been recognized and collectively termed *tumor progression.* Molecular studies since the mid-1980s have demonstrated that this phenomenon of progression results from *clonal evolution* within the neoplasm, with the accumulation of sequential genetic alterations and the selection of subpopulations with more and more aggressive characteristics (Fig. 20.1). Typically, a number of subclones continue to coexist in every advanced tumor, accounting for the *heterogeneity* of many properties that is commonly observed. The subclones that come to predominate in a particular patient represent the effect of those specific mutations that allow the cells to grow most effectively in that individual and to resist immunologic, therapeutic, and other inhibitory pressures that may be generated by the host and the physician.

Such a sequence of events in a common human cancer has been best documented in *adenocarcinoma of the colon.* In these tumors, using a combination of molecular and cytogenetic tech-

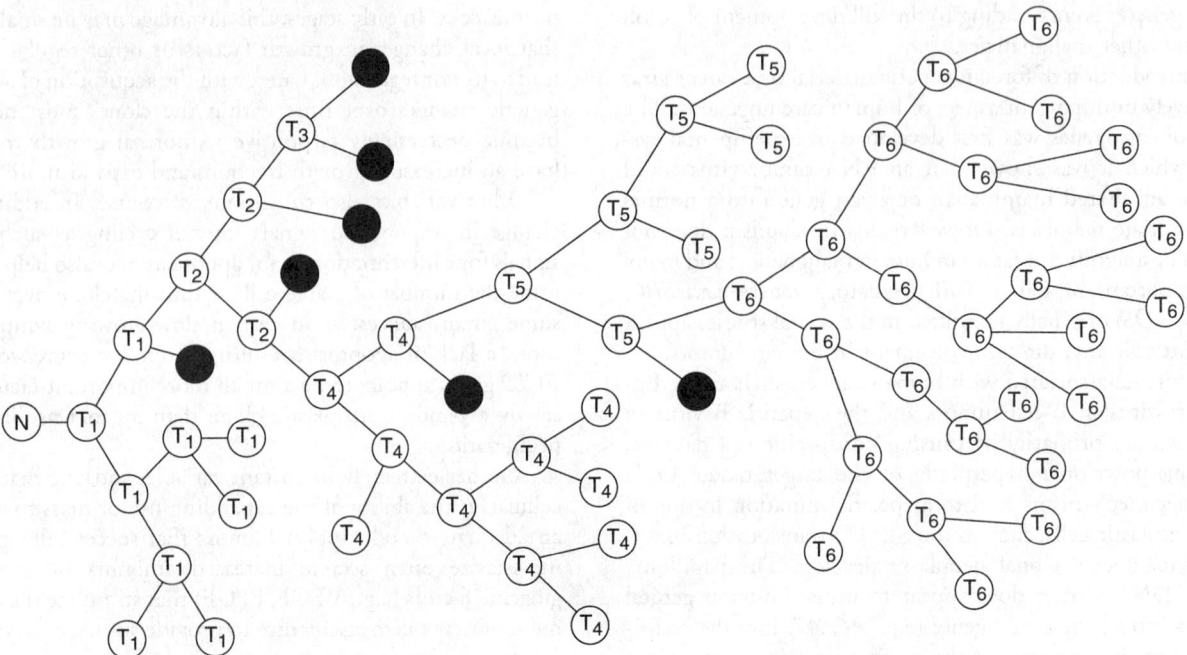

FIGURE 20.1. Model of clonal evolution in neoplasia. A normal cell (N) is converted to a tumor cell (T_1) by mutation in one or more growth-regulatory genes. As the resultant clone expands, additional mutations occur, some lethal (*solid circles*) and some generating subclones (T_2–T_6) with more aggressive biologic and clinical properties. The fully developed malignancy is heterogeneous (coexisting subclones) and has multiple genetic changes in the predominant subclones.

niques, Vogelstein and others demonstrated a series of stepwise genetic alterations associated with the progression from benign colonic polyps to early and late stages of malignancy. For example, they found mutations in a *RAS* oncogene and deletion of a previously unknown tumor suppressor gene, called *APC*, often associated with early lesions, and then, in addition, deletions of two other suppressor genes, *P53* and a newly identified locus called *DCC*, in advanced carcinomas. Although even more genetic changes are usually present and still remain to be defined fully, these findings suggest that the *RAS* and *APC* alterations play an important role in the development of the benign adenomatous polyps, with the loss of *P53* and *DCC* contributing to the subsequent acquisition of more aggressive malignant properties, including the capacity to invade and to metastasize.

Similar sequences of events, involving some of the same genes as well as different genes, are being defined in other common cancers, such as those of the breast and lung. The most critical of the later alterations in terms of clinical significance are those that contribute to local invasion and to the development of distant metastases.

INVASION AND METASTASIS

Studies have indicated that more than half of solid tumors (excluding carcinomas of the skin) have metastasized by the time they are clinically apparent. This represents the most important aspect of tumor progression. Much has been learned concerning the biology and biochemistry of invasion and metastasis, and some of the specific genes directly involved in these phenomena in particular neoplasms are beginning to be identified.

From a variety of studies, it is possible to define rather precisely a sequence of events involved in those malignant properties. The first step involves separation of the neoplastic cells from the primary mass and, in the case of epithelial tumors, the successful invasion of the underlying basement membrane. The cells can then expand within the adjacent extracellular matrix and invade thin-walled vessels—both lymphatics and veins. In many tumors, these early steps involve alterations in cellular adhesion as the result of changes in a variety of membrane proteins (e.g., E-cahedrins, laminin receptors, integrins) and the generation by the tumor cells of a spectrum of proteolytic enzymes (e.g., collagenases, cathepsin B) that permit them to move through cellular and matrix barriers. As with all of the changes associated with invasion and metastasis, such alterations do not represent gains or losses of proteins unique to tumor cells but simply quantitative differences in the amounts being produced, with resultant critical biologic effects. Some of the efforts to control cancer through dietary means have involved agents such as vitamin C and protease inhibitors, which might limit invasiveness by strengthening the extracellular matrix or blocking tumor proteases.

The next step in the systemic dissemination of tumor cells involves moving through circulatory pathways until arrested by a distant capillary bed or comparable microvasculature. There has been much debate over whether the location of metastases is simply a matter of mechanical distribution within the lymphatic and circulatory systems or if certain characteristics of the tumor cells and of the sites where tumor emboli are arrested determine whether metastasis is successful. Current knowledge indicates that both factors are important. Most tumor emboli lodge in lymph nodes or in the first capillary bed that they reach through the venous system. However, there is evidence that not only certain surface molecules but also clotting factors and local growth factors (e.g., insulin-like growth factors) that are associated with particular types of tumor cells and with certain capillary beds may play an important role in the arrest and establishment of a metastatic embolus at a particular location.

Fortunately, most tumor cells that enter the circulation appear to lack the additional characteristics necessary for survival and growth after they arrive at a distant site. Among the properties that have been identified as particularly important to the tumor embolus at this stage of metastasis is the secretion of one or more angiogenic factors (as already mentioned with respect to primary tumors), which are necessary for the local stimulation of endothelial proliferation and the development of new blood vessels to support the nascent metastasis. Also, as with the initial invasion adjacent to the primary tumor, the ability of the embolic tumor cells to grow effectively in their new location depends in part on the secretion of various proteolytic enzymes, such as type IV collagenase, to allow successful escape from the arresting microvasculature and movement into the parenchyma of the lung, liver, or other metastatic site.

A few specific genes that appear to contribute most substantially to this phenomenon of invasion and metastasis have been identified. One is *NM23,* a metastasis-suppressor gene that appears to regulate a number of other genes. Extensive additional studies are underway.

METABOLIC CHANGES IN TUMOR PROGRESSION

Despite repeated efforts, no specific metabolic alteration consistently associated with all cancers has been identified. This is no longer surprising in view of the large number of genes that have been identified as being involved in the development of many different kinds of malignancy. It has long been recognized, however, that as the process of progression occurs, with general reduction in the proportion of differentiated cells within the tumor mass, there does tend to be convergence in the metabolic characteristics of many different cancers. This reflects the metabolic pathways common to actively dividing cells, as opposed to the more variable patterns associated with differentiated populations.

It is true that some neoplasms retain a sufficient degree of differentiation to produce large quantities of specific cellular products (e.g., hormones, epinephrine), which can have clinical effects in the patient, but this is usually associated with relatively early tumors rather than with late-stage malignancies.

In the later stages of tumor progression, as both primary and metastatic tumors grow more aggressively, the tumors often outgrow their blood supply. Not surprisingly, clonal evolution under these circumstances results in the selection of viable subpopulations that are best able to survive in a low-oxygen environment, and increased anaerobic glycolysis is frequently a property of the cells of rapidly growing cancers. At one time, this was thought to represent a specific characteristic of the malignant state, but it is now recognized as another manifestation of the clonal evolution phenomenon.

The same is apparently true of the tendency of many tumors in the later stages of progression to develop drug resistance, particularly after exposure to various therapeutic agents. This also appears to result from the outgrowth of specific subpopulations within the neoplastic clone, in this case under the selective pressure of the particular chemotherapeutic agents being used. The resistant populations have been shown to overexpress one or another drug-resistance genes, often by gene amplification, and, through an effect on the transport or metabolism of particular chemotherapeutic agents, allow a subset of malignant cells to survive and regrow within the patient.

ANTIGENICITY AND THE HOST IMMUNE RESPONSE

A similar phenomenon also appears to prevail with respect to the immunogenicity of many advanced tumors. Since the mid-1950s, through studies in both human populations and experimental animals, it has been extensively demonstrated that neoplasms do evoke a specific immune response from the host and that, through a phenomenon of *immune surveillance,* many incipient tumors are presumably successfully eliminated in healthy persons. Conversely, when a person is in a depressed immune state, either congenital or acquired, tumors grow more readily.

Although many details remain unclear, it appears that most so-called tumor antigens are also present on some normal cells and are only recognized by the host as foreign because of inappropriate location or quantity. A few unique tumor antigens may exist; these are protein products of specific genetic alterations limited to the neoplastic cells. Most tumor-associated antigens are cell-surface proteins, and the host response is similar to that generated against histologically incompatible foreign tissues.

The immune response directed against tumors is primarily T-cell–mediated, with relatively less effect from antitumor antibodies. There is also a subpopulation of small lymphocytes, the natural killer cells, which represent an additional means by which the host generates a cytotoxic effect on tumor cells—in this case one that is immunologically nonspecific. In these various complex pathways, other host cells (e.g., macrophages) and cell products (e.g., interferon, tumor necrosis factor) can also play a critical role.

Unfortunately, with tumor progression, the host's success in controlling the neoplasm through these immunologic mechanisms is frequently reduced. Often, this seems to reflect still another aspect of clonal evolution: the selection of subpopulations that have reduced antigenicity or inhibitory effects on the host response. Some of the difficulties encountered in attempting to develop successful therapeutic approaches to human cancer through immunologic techniques undoubtedly stem from this remarkable ability of the evolving tumor to select for subpopulations that can successfully evade the host's attempts at regulation.

GENETIC INSTABILITY IN TUMOR PROGRESSION

A final aspect of the molecular and cellular biology of neoplasia that plays an important role in the phenomenon of tumor progression is the apparent genetic instability of many neoplastic cell populations. The sequential acquisition of genetic alterations during tumor development seems, in many circumstances, to reflect an increased probability of mutational events in the neoplastic cells compared with normal cells. As with other aspects of tumorigenesis, this appears to result from multiple mechanisms. In the late stages of progression, it is not surprising that cells that have already acquired major cytogenetic alterations may frequently undergo further errors in the course of mitosis. In earlier stages, the mechanisms are not as readily apparent.

It has been postulated that, either as an inherited defect or as an acquired mutation early in tumor development, essentially every neoplastic clone has some abnormality in DNA synthesis, DNA repair, or some other aspect of DNA "housekeeping" that results in increased mutability. A number of candidate *mutator genes,* both inherited and acquired, have been identified in different human tumors. For many years, it has been recognized that the greatly increased risk of cancer associated with certain inherited disorders, such as xeroderma pigmentosum and various chromosomal fragility syndromes (e.g., ataxia telangiectasia, Bloom's syndrome, Fanconi's anemia) results from constitutional defects in various genes necessary for the maintenance of DNA integrity. This concept has now been extended to include a number of genes (e.g., *MSH2, MLH1, PMS1, PMS2*) involved in DNA "mismatch" repair that have been shown to be defective in families prone to hereditary nonpolyposis colorectal cancer. Mutations in several of these genes also have been demonstrated in a variety of sporadic epithelial malignancies, indicating that acquired inactivation of these loci probably represents a basis for the *mutator phenotype* in some nonfamilial human tumors.

Also important is the loss of *P53* gene function, which occurs commonly in almost all types of sporadic human malignancies and is associated, as an inherited defect, with multiple familial cancers in the rare inherited disorder called the Li–Fraumeni syndrome. One normal role of the p53 gene product is to prevent genetically damaged cells from progressing through the cell cycle, and in its absence, the accumulation of such errors is greatly enhanced.

There is still much to be learned about the variety of genes and mechanism that increase the probability of genetic errors occurring and being maintained in tumor cell populations, but enough information has been acquired to support the view that such mutator genes and their defects are of major importance in tumor progression.

Our knowledge is rapidly increasing concerning the complexity of normal growth regulation and how it can be altered in a variety of ways to contribute to the development of an expanding cell clone that we recognize clinically as a tumor. Information is also accumulating on the molecular alterations that lead to the biochemical and biologic changes that allow neoplastic cells to invade and to metastasize successfully, the most critical aspect of the malignant state. And we are beginning to learn more about the molecular mechanisms that make tumor cells more genetically unstable than their normal counterparts and so are more likely to acquire the spectrum of genetic alterations necessary for the full development of the malignant phenotype. All of this information is stimulating a wealth of new approaches to the prevention, diagnosis, monitoring, and specific therapy

of human cancer, and a number of these encouraging developments are discussed in other chapters. It is also clear, however, from our current understanding of the biologic and molecular aspects of human cancer cells, that no single, simple answer to the ultimate control of this disease should be expected.

BIBLIOGRAPHY

Ames B, Gold L. Environmental pollution, pesticides, and the prevention of cancer: misconceptions. *FASEB J* 1997;11:1041.

Fearon E. Human cancer syndromes: clues to the origin and nature of cancer. *Science* 1997;278:1043.

Folkman J. Tumor angiogenesis. In: Holland JF, et al, eds. *Cancer medicine,* fourth ed. Baltimore: Williams & Wilkins, 1997:181.

Hunter T. Oncoprotein networks. *Cell* 1997;88:333.

Kinzler K, Vogelstein B. Lessons from hereditary colorectal cancer. *Cell* 1996;87:159.

Loeb L. Cancer cells manifest a mutator phenotype. *Adv Cancer Res* 1998; 72:25.

Shu S, Plautz G, Krauss J, Chang A. Tumor immunology. *JAMA* 1997; 278:1972.

Woodhouse E, Chuaqui R, Liotta L. General mechanisms of metastasis. *Cancer* 1997;80:1529.

Wylie A. Apoptosis and carcinogenesis. *Eur J Cell Biol* 1997;73:189.

zur Hausen H. Viruses in human tumors. *Adv Cancer Res* 1996;68:1.

Kelley's Textbook of Internal Medicine, fourth edition. Edited by H. David Humes.
Lippincott Williams & Wilkins, Philadelphia © 2000.

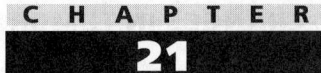

C H A P T E R
21

EPIDEMIOLOGY OF MALIGNANT DISEASE

DAVID SCHOTTENFELD

MAGNITUDE OF CANCER

Cancer is the second leading cause of death in the United States, accounting in 1994 for 534,000 deaths (280,465 in men and 253,845 in women). In 1973, cancer was certified as the underlying cause in 17.7% of all deaths. Although cardiovascular disease mortality continued to decline after 1973 as a competing cause of death, the proportion of all deaths attributed to cancer increased to 23.4% in 1994. An estimated 1,257,800 incident cancer cases occurred in 1997 (about 661,200 occurring in men and 596,600 in women), or a cancer case : death ratio that exceeded 2.0. The estimation of total annual incidence does not include the more than 1 million persons diagnosed with basal cell or squamous cell carcinoma of the skin. Four organ sites—lung and bronchus, colon and rectum, breast, and prostate—accounted for 56% of all incident cancer cases and 53% of all cancer deaths. Based on US mortality and incidence rates for 1992 to 1994, the lifetime probabilities of developing cancer have been estimated to be 46.6% in men and 38.0% in women; the lifetime probabilities of dying of cancer have been estimated at 23.9% in men and 20.6% in women.

Incidence measures the rate of occurrence of newly diagnosed cancer cases over a specified time interval, for example, in 1 year. Similarly, *mortality* is an incidence measure of cancer deaths occurring in a population over a specified time interval. *Prevalence* is a cross-sectional measure of frequency based on the number of existing cancer cases in patients diagnosed in the past and surviving to the point in time of interest. Prevalence is a useful indicator of the impact of cancer on the health care resources in a population. In a population-based survey of adults aged 18 years and older in the United States in 1987, the prevalence of cancer (excluding nonmelanoma skin cancers) in women was estimated to be 4,402 per 100,000 and in men, 1,930 per 100,000. From the sample survey, it was projected that in 1987 there were 5.7 million adults (3.3% of the adult population) who were cancer survivors. The survey also determined that in 1.6% of the adult population with a history of cancer, the cancer had been diagnosed in persons under 15 years of age; the percentage distribution of prevalent cases by age at diagnosis increased with increasing age so that 22% had been diagnosed at age 65 and over.

Increasing incidence rates of site-specific cancers or advances in cancer treatment will almost certainly increase future cancer prevalence rates. Based on cancer incidence and survival rates from the Connecticut Tumor Registry, the prevalence of cancer survivors in the United States was projected to be 8.25 million in 1998. Of this total, patients with breast (24.4%), colorectal (15.0%), and prostate (12.1%) cancers accounted for at least 50% of persons diagnosed and surviving with cancer.

From 1973 to 1990, cancer incidence and mortality rates in the United States for all sites combined have increased by approximately 1.1% and 0.4% per year, respectively. Over the 18-year interval, incidence increased 18.3% and mortality increased 6.7%. The all-cancer mortality rate peaked in 1990, after which it declined on average, from 1990 to 1995, at the rate of 0.6% per year. Forty percent of the decline in the cancer mortality rate was due to a reduction in lung cancer mortality.

AGE AT DIAGNOSIS

In 1994, the percentage of all deaths due to cancer in the US population under age 65 was 26%, which exceeded that attributed to heart disease (20%). For persons aged 65 and over, the proportion attributed to heart disease (37%) exceeded that due to cancer (23%). During the period 1973 to 1990, the average annual percent change in mortality due to cancer at all sites in persons 35 to 64 years decreased 0.6%; in the subsequent 5-year period (1990 to 1995), the average annual decrease was 1.6%. In the population of those 65 to 74 years of age, who currently experience 31% of cancer deaths (Fig. 21.1), the average annual percent change in cancer mortality was an increase of 0.8% during 1973 to 1990 and thereafter a decrease of 0.1% per year.

Major site-specific increases in cancer incidence in those under 65 years of age during 1973 to 1994 were due to prostate,

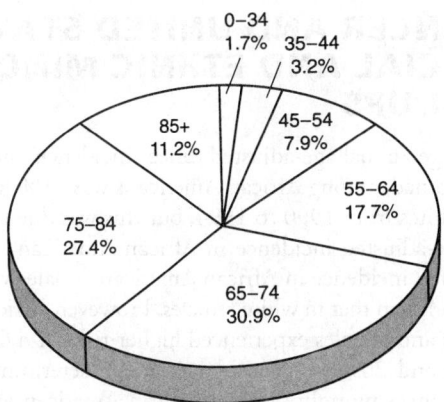

FIGURE 21.1. Percent of cancer deaths in the United States by age group, all sites, 1990–1994. (From SEER Cancer Statistics Review, 1973–1994, with permission.)

melanoma, non-Hodgkin's lymphoma, lung (female), testis, liver (including intrahepatic bile duct), kidney and renal pelvis, and thyroid (female) cancer. Concurrently, there were significantly decreasing incidence trends for cancers of the larynx, stomach, pancreas, cervix uteri (invasive), and corpus uteri. For the subgroup 65 years and older, the significantly increasing cancer incidence trends were exhibited for melanoma, non-Hodgkin's lymphoma, and lung (females), prostate, brain, kidney and renal pelvis, liver (including intrahepatic bile duct), breast, thyroid, and esophagus cancer. Significantly decreasing trends were demonstrated for Hodgkin's lymphoma, stomach, and cervix uteri (invasive) cancer.

An estimated 8,000 children under 15 years of age, less than 1% of total cancer incidence, were diagnosed with cancer in the United States in 1994. The average annual incidence of all cancers in children in 1990 to 1994 was 13.8 per 100,000. The three most common types of cancer in infants under 1 year of age were neuroblastoma (27%), central nervous system tumors (15%), and leukemias (13%). The incidence among white children (14.3 per 100,000) exceeded that in black children (13.0). The most common cancers in children were the leukemias (3.8) and neoplasms of the brain and autonomic and peripheral nervous systems (3.3). This pattern was altered in the 15- to 19-year age group, in whom Hodgkin's disease (3.6) and testicular cancer (3.2) superseded neoplasms of the brain (2.1) as well as the leukemias (2.5). The age-adjusted incidence of primary malignant brain tumors in children increased by 35% during 1973 to 1994. The brain stem and cerebrum were the sites in which the reported incidence increased, in particular, for low-grade gliomas. The observed increase in incidence may have been due to changes in imaging detection practices after 1980. Childhood cancer mortality rates have declined substantially between 1973 (5.5 per 100,000) and 1994 (2.8 per 100,000), particularly for the leukemias, Hodgkin's and non-Hodgkin's lymphomas, and soft-tissue sarcomas. There were 1,571 cancer deaths certified among children in 1994, which represented 10.3% of total deaths; accidents were the leading cause (39.5% of total deaths).

CANCER AND UNITED STATES RACIAL AND ETHNIC MINORITY GROUPS

The average annual age-adjusted cancer incidence, including all sites combined, among African Americans was 11% higher than among whites from 1990 to 1994, but this was due to the 26% higher age-adjusted incidence in African American males. The age-adjusted incidence in African American females was slightly lower (3%) than that in white females. However, African American males and females experienced higher risks of dying of cancer, 49% and 20%, respectively. A major determinant of the elevated cancer mortality rate in African American women was that overall 5-year relative survival rate for persons diagnosed during 1986 to 1993 was significantly lower (47.9%) than that estimated for white women (62.3%). The increased mortality in African American men may be attributed to increased incidence density or risk and inferior survival. Individual sites that involved significant risks for the African Americans included cervix uteri, esophagus, larynx, liver and intrahepatic bile duct, non–small cell lung, multiple myeloma, oral cavity and pharynx, pancreas, prostate, and stomach. It is also instructive to note those sites and cancer types for which African Americans had a significantly reduced risk: corpus uteri, melanoma, non-Hodgkin's lymphoma, ovary, testis, thyroid, and urinary bladder (Table 21.1).

Variations in cancer incidence patterns by race or ethnicity are providing environmental and genetic clues for the epidemiologic and experimental pursuit of complex causal mechanisms. For men, overall cancer risks were highest among African Americans, followed by non-Hispanic whites, Hispanics, and Japanese Americans, whereas for females, the rates were highest for non-Hispanic whites and African Americans. Chinese Americans experienced elevated rates of cancers of the nasopharynx and liver, whereas Japanese Americans had a higher risk of cancers of the stomach and colon (comparable to the rate in non-Hispanic whites). Native Americans experienced about 50% of the overall cancer incidence of non-Hispanic whites but were distinguished by elevated rates of cancers of the liver and bile ducts, gallbladder, stomach, ovary, and cervix uteri.

SOCIAL INEQUALITIES AND CANCER PATTERNS

Poverty and social inequalities may confound patterns of cancer incidence and mortality attributed to racial or ethnic characteristics. Namely, social inequalities may influence access to or quality of medical care; knowledge, attitudes, and behavior with respect to screening and early detection practices; and the distribution of lifestyle risk factors. Studies of social class and health status in industrialized countries have demonstrated in general that persons in the lowest socioeconomic level, as measured by education, income, and occupation, when compared with those in the highest level, incur shorter average life expectancy, higher prevalence of comorbid conditions, and unfavorable distribution of cancer site-specific prognostic factors. The opportunity for providing cost-effective preventive services in the medical care setting appears to be achievable, but consideration is needed of the social context of health and illness and of how to overcome economic, cultural, and medical care systemic barriers.

Social class difference may determine cancer incidence patterns in that the prevalence of consumption of tobacco products and alcoholic beverages, dietary practices, and sexual and reproductive behavior may be highly correlated with socioeconomic status. For men in lower social strata, international studies have described excess risks for respiratory (larynx and lung) and upper

TABLE 21.1. COMPARISON OF FIVE MOST FREQUENTLY DIAGNOSED CANCER SITES IN UNITED STATES WHITES WITH INCIDENCE[a] IN OTHER RACIAL AND ETHNIC GROUPS, 1988–1992

Site	White	African American	Hispanic	Chinese	Japanese	Native American (New Mexico)
Men						
Prostate	134.7	180.6	89.0	46.0	88.0	52.5
Lung and bronchus	76.0	117.0	41.8	52.1	43.0	14.4
Colon and rectum	56.3	60.7	38.3	44.8	64.1	18.6
Urinary bladder	31.7	15.2	15.8	13.0	13.7	[b]
Non-Hodgkin's lymphoma	18.7	13.2	14.1	12.4	11.6	[b]
All sites combined	469	560	319	282	322	196
Women						
Breast	115.7	95.4	69.8	55.0	82.3	31.6
Lung and bronchus	41.5	44.2	19.5	25.3	15.2	[b]
Colon and rectum	39.2	45.5	24.7	33.6	39.5	15.3
Corpus uteri	23.0	14.4	13.7	11.6	14.5	10.7
Ovary	16.2	10.2	11.4	9.3	10.1	17.5
All sites combined	346	326	243	213	241	180

[a] Per 100,000 population, age-adjusted to the 1970 US standard population
[b] Less than 25 cases
(From SEER: Racial/Ethnic Patterns of Cancer in the United States 1988–1992, with permission.)

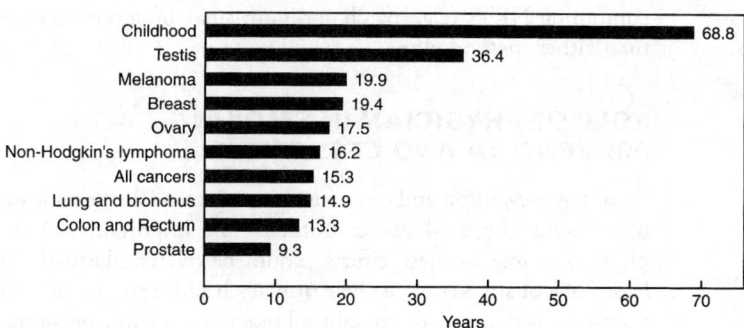

FIGURE 21.2. Average years of life lost from cancer by type of cancer, United States, based on 1990 life tables. (From SEER Cancer Statistics Review, 1973–1994, with permission.)

digestive (including oral cavity, pharynx, stomach, and esophagus) cancers; for women in lower social strata, excess risks are for uterine cervical cancer. For persons in higher social strata, excess risks have been observed for cancers of the colon, brain, breast, endometrium, and ovary and for melanoma of the skin.

EPIDEMIOLOGIC PERSPECTIVE

The year 2000 objectives of the US National Cancer Institute are focused on cancer prevention and control that will achieve substantial reductions in cancer incidence, mortality, and morbidity. Total eradication of cancer by curative and preventive interventions would ultimately result in a gain of about 2.5 years in average life expectancy in the general population. However, for the approximately one in four adult Americans who would have died of cancer, the average gain in life expectancy would be approximately 15 years and would range from 9 years for patients dying of prostate cancer to 36 years for the young adult patients dying of testicular cancer (Fig. 21.2).

The discipline of cancer epidemiology provides the foundation for targeting and assessing cancer prevention and control priorities and practices. Compelling epidemiologic data indicate that a substantial proportion of cancer mortality and morbidity can be prevented, or postponed, by lifestyle choices such as avoiding tobacco products, limiting consumption of alcohol and exposure to ultraviolet radiation, consuming optimal amounts of fresh fruits and vegetables, and controlling dietary energy consumption while increasing physical activity. Globally, infectious agents, such as Epstein–Barr virus (lymphomas and nasopharyngeal carcinoma), hepatitis B and C, human papillomaviruses (anogenital tract cancers), HIV (Kaposi's sarcoma, non-Hodgkin's lymphoma), *Helicobacter pylori* (cofactor in stomach cancer), *Clonorchis sinensis* and other liver trematodes, and *Schistosoma haematobium* (urinary bladder cancer), probably account for 10% to 15% of cancer deaths, which eventually may be avoided by antimicrobial therapy or immunization, as well as targeted surveillance and early detection in high-risk populations. Although 5% to 10% of deaths due to cancer in industrial nations may result from exposures in the workplace, many of the chemical and physical agents currently viewed as environmental carcinogens were originally identified through epidemiologic studies in occupational settings. A relatively smaller proportion of cancers may be attributed to pharmaceutical agents, including sex steroidal hormones, but these established associations have

generated important insights into mechanisms of cancer causation.

BIBLIOGRAPHY

Byrne J, Kessler LG, Devesa SS. The prevalence of cancer among adults in the United States: 1987. *Cancer* 1992;69:2154.

Cole P, Rodu B. Declining cancer mortality in the United States. *Cancer* 1996;78:2045.

Kogevinas M, Pearce N, Susser M, Boffetta P. *Social inequalities and cancer.* International Agency for Research on Cancer Scientific Publications No. 138. Lyon, France, 1997.

Miller BA, Kolonel LN, Bernstein L, et al. *Racial/ethnic patterns of cancer in the United States, 1988–1992.* National Cancer Institute, NIH Publ. No. 96-4104. Bethesda, MD, 1996.

Parkin DM. The global burden of cancer. *Semin Cancer Biol* 1998;8:219.

Polednak AP. Projected number of cancers diagnosed in the US elderly population, 1990 through 2030. *Am J Public Health* 1994;84:1313.

Ries LAG, Kosary CL, Hankey BF, et al. *SEER cancer statistics review: 1973–1994.* National Cancer Institute, NIH Publ. No. 97-2789. Bethesda, MD, 1997.

Schottenfeld D, Fraumeni JF Jr. *Cancer epidemiology and prevention,* second ed. New York: Oxford University Press, 1996.

Kelley's Textbook of Internal Medicine, fourth edition. Edited by H. David Humes. Lippincott Williams & Wilkins, Philadelphia © 2000.

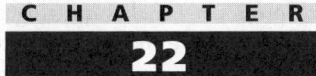

22

PREVENTION OF NEOPLASIA

PETER GREENWALD

Lifestyle factors such as tobacco use and diet are major contributors to cancer risk. Because these lifestyle factors can be controlled, they are a logical focus for cancer prevention strategies. Active participation in developing and carrying out such strategies by the medical community is critical to the success of cancer prevention. The involvement of physicians in recognizing emerging issues (e.g., the increased prevalence of youth smoking) and encouraging patients to undertake a healthier lifestyle (e.g., through adoption of a low-fat, high-fiber diet, decreased consumption of calories, and involvement in a regular exercise program) can result in clear benefits to the individual patient as well as to society.

SMOKING AND CANCER

Developing effective cancer prevention strategies aimed at reducing tobacco use is an enormous public health challenge. Although the total prevalence of smoking has declined in the United States over the past 30 years, tobacco use among adolescents is on the rise. Based on a 1995 survey, approximately 35% of all high school students smoke—an increase of 27% from 1991 through 1995. In the black community, the prevalence of teenage smoking doubled between 1991 (14%) and 1995 (28%). Cigarette smoking is responsible for about one-third of all cancer deaths in the United States. Lung cancer, attributable primarily to cigarette smoking, is the leading cause of cancer deaths among both men and women. Smoking also is a primary cause of cancers of the larynx, oral cavity, and esophagus and contributes to cancers of the pancreas, bladder, kidney, uterine cervix, and renal system. Moreover, consistent evidence indicates that household or occupational exposure of nonsmokers to environmental tobacco smoke (ETS) is associated with increased lung cancer risk. Although this increased risk is modest, the ubiquitous nature of ETS translates into a large number of persons at risk for lung cancer or other respiratory illnesses.

Recent studies indicate that smokers with specific polymorphisms of the *CYP1A1, CYP2D6, GSTM1,* or *MspI* genes may have an increased risk of lung cancer compared with those without these genetic variants. Also, particular alleles of the D2 dopamine receptor (*DRD2*) may play a role in determining nicotine addiction and may thus predispose persons to smoke.

TOBACCO DEPENDENCE

More than 70% of smokers would like to quit, and 60% have tried seriously to do so. However, addiction to nicotine—present in all tobacco products—makes quitting difficult; 50% of smokers who have undergone major surgery for a tobacco-induced disease continue to smoke. Not all smokers exhibit the same degree of nicotine dependence. Increased physical dependence is indicated by a high number of cigarettes smoked per day; frequent smoking in the morning; and smoking while ill. Nicotine dependence must be given serious consideration when developing cancer prevention strategies related to tobacco use. Nicotine replacement therapies (NRTs) should be considered, along with adjuvant behavioral counseling, to facilitate smoking cessation. In an effort to make NRTs more accessible, the nicotine patch and nicotine gum were approved for over-the-counter (OTC) sale in 1996. The change from prescription to OTC use of NRTs resulted in more than twice as many persons attempting smoking cessation in 1997 as in 1995. In addition, nicotine nasal spray, a nicotine inhaler, and buprion hydrochloride are available as prescription medications to assist the smoker in quitting. All available pharmacotherapies appear equally effective;

combining NRTs (e.g., patch and gum) may be more effective than either method alone.

ROLE OF PHYSICIAN IN SMOKING PREVENTION AND CESSATION

Smoking prevention and cessation may represent the best means of reducing the total cancer burden. The importance of the physician's role in these efforts cannot be overemphasized. At least 70% of smokers visit their primary health care provider at least once per year. A recent clinical practice guideline on smoking cessation recommends that every patient who smokes be provided smoking cessation treatment at every office visit. Indeed, patients who smoke expect their physician to inquire into their smoking habits and to advise them in cessation techniques. Studies indicate that 50% of all adult smokers started smoking by age 15, and 90% started by age 18. Thus, early intervention, focused on preteens and teenagers, is critical to reducing the prevalence of adult smoking. Physicians who care for children should anticipate the risk for tobacco use, ask about exposure to tobacco smoke and tobacco use, advise all smoking parents to stop smoking and all children not to use tobacco products, and assist children in resisting tobacco use.

The National Cancer Institute (NCI) has formulated recommendations for physicians, outlined in Table 22.1, to help them institute smoking cessation techniques in their medical practices. These recommendations are discussed in a step-by-step handbook—*How to Help Your Patients Stop Smoking: A National Cancer Institute Manual for Physicians*—which includes resource lists, reprintable materials, and a special section, Clinical Intervention To Prevent Tobacco Use by Children and Adolescents. The handbook is available on the internet at http://rex.nci.nih.gov/PREV_AND_ERLYDETC/PREVED_MAIN_DOC.html. Additional information on smoking prevention, including items designed specifically for youth, is available at the Tobacco Information and Prevention Source (TIPS) Web page of the Centers for Disease Control and Prevention (CDC) at http://www.cdc.gov/nccdphp/osh/.

DIET AND CANCER

A considerable body of evidence supports the hypothesis that dietary factors play a major role in the determination of cancer risk. Illustrating this point are the significant international variations in the incidence of certain cancers as well as the increased risk observed when migrants from countries with a low-fat, high-fiber diet adopt a more Western (high-fat, low-fiber) diet. For colon cancer, the Western diet is associated with increased disease risk in both men and women, especially among those diagnosed before age 67 years. In contrast, consumption of the Mediterranean diet, which emphasizes vegetable, fruits, whole grains, fish, and olive oil (high in monounsaturated fatty acids [MUFAs]), is thought to be cancer-protective, particularly for the digestive and respiratory tracts.

Data from analytic and experimental studies also support a relation between increased intakes of vegetables and fruits, fiber and whole grains, and certain micronutrients and reduced cancer

TABLE 22.1. SYNOPSIS FOR PHYSICIANS: HOW TO HELP YOUR PATIENTS STOP SMOKING

Ask about smoking at every opportunity.
  "Do you smoke?"
  "How much?"
  "How soon after waking do you have your first cigarette?"
  "Are you interested in stopping smoking?"
  "Have you ever tried to stop before?" If yes, "What happened?"

Advise all smokers to stop.
  State your advice clearly, for example: "As your physician, I must advise you to stop smoking now."
  Personalize the message to quit. Refer to the patient's clinical condition, smoking history, family story, personal interests, or social roles.

Assist the patient in stopping.
  Set a quit date. Help the patient pick a date within the next 4 weeks, acknowledging that no time is ideal.
  Provide self-help materials. The smoking cessation coordinator or support staff member can review the materials with the patient if desired (call 1-800-4-CANCER for NCI's *Quit for Good* materials).
  Consider prescribing nicotine gum [or the nicotine patch], especially for highly addicted patients (those who smoke one pack a day or more or who smoke their first cigarette within 30 minutes of waking).
  Consider signing a stop-smoking contract with the patient.
  If the patient is not willing to quit now:
    Provide motivating literature (call 1-800-4-CANCER for NCI's *Why Do You Smoke?* pamphlet).
    Ask again at the next visit.

Arrange follow-up visits.
  Set a follow-up visit within 1 to 2 weeks after the quit date.
  Have a member of the office staff call or write the patient within 7 days after the initial visit, reinforcing the decision to stop and reminding the patient of the quit date.
  At the first follow-up visit, ask about the patient's smoking status to provide support and help prevent relapse. Relapse is common; if it happens, encourage the patient to try again immediately.
  Set a second follow-up visit in 1 to 2 months. For patients who have relapsed, discuss the circumstances of the relapse and other special concerns.

(From Glynn T, Manley M. *How to help your patients stop smoking: a National Cancer Institute manual for physicians.* NIH Publication No. 93-3064. Public Health Service, 1993, with permission.)

risk, whereas increased total caloric intake, body weight, and alcohol consumption are associated with greater risk. Overall risk of developing cancer, however, cannot be separated readily into individual contributions from specific components of diet and diet-related factors, such as body weight and exercise. All may interact to determine cancer risk. Individual genetic susceptibilities also may play an important role. To illustrate, among men who consumed more than one serving of red meat per day, those with rapid acetylator polymorphisms (*NAT1, NAT2,* or both) of the *N*-acetyltransferase gene were at increased risk of colorectal cancer compared with men classified as nonrapid acetylators.

DIETARY FAT

Epidemiologic data suggest a relation between total fat intake or consumption of animal fat and increased cancer risk at several sites (e.g., endometrium, prostate, lung). The association between dietary fat and breast cancer risk is, however, uncertain. This is not surprising, considering that the effects of factors related to dietary fat, including caloric intake, weight gain, obesity, and physical activity, have a high probability of confounding the effect of dietary fat alone. Animal fat from red meat, particularly α-linolenic acid, is associated with an elevated risk of advanced prostate cancer, whereas consumption of polyunsaturated and vegetable fat may be protective. Red meat consumption, possibly independent of total or saturated fat intake, also may increase the risk of both colon and breast cancer. The production of carcinogenic heterocyclic amines in red meat is directly related to the amount of cooking. Data indicate that women consuming red meat at higher levels of doneness are at greater risk of breast cancer than women consuming red meat at lower levels of doneness.

Numerous studies indicate that the type of fat consumed is important to cancer risk. For example, polyunsaturated fats (corn oil, safflower oil, and others) rich in omega-6 fatty acids, primarily linoleic acid, act as tumor promoters in animals and have a direct association with postmenopausal breast cancer. *Trans* fatty acids also may increase breast cancer risk in postmenopausal women. Increasing evidence suggests that consumption of oleic acid—an MUFA that is a major component of olive oil—may decrease a woman's risk of breast cancer. The role of olive oil with regard to other cancers requires further research. Highly unsaturated omega-3 fatty acids, found primarily in fish oils, also may protect against certain types of cancer. The cancer-related effects of dietary fats may be linked to genetic factors. For example, increased consumption of MUFAs (as olive oil) is associated with a decreased frequency of Ki-*ras* wild-type colorectal tumors.

VEGETABLES, FRUITS, AND WHOLE GRAINS

The beneficial effects of vegetables, fruits, and whole grains may be a result of either individual or combined effects of constituents that include fiber, micronutrients, and nonnutritive phytochemicals. A review of more than 200 epidemiologic studies found that increased consumption of vegetables and fruits, particularly allium vegetables, carrots, green vegetables, cruciferous vegetables, tomatoes, total fruits, and citrus fruits, is protective for a variety of cancers. Furthermore, findings indicate that increased consumption of whole grains is associated with a decreased risk of colorectal, gastric, and endometrial cancers. Genetic factors also may influence the cancer-protective effects of plant foods. In one study, consumption of cruciferous vegetables exhibited significant protection against colorectal adenomas only in persons with a particular genetic variant of glutathione transferase.

FIBER

Epidemiologic studies generally endorse the cancer-protective properties of dietary fiber and fiber-rich foods, and some studies indicate that fiber may modulate the risk-enhancing effects of dietary fat. Dietary fiber consumption demonstrates a strong inverse correlation with colon cancer risk in most epidemiologic studies. Epidemiologic evidence regarding the protective effect of fiber consumption on breast cancer risk is mixed, but more rigorously designed studies indicate some beneficial effect, particularly at higher levels of intake.

The type of fiber consumed is important to cancer risk. In one study, the protective effect of fiber consumption against colorectal cancer was strongest for vegetable fiber and less strong for fruit fiber, with no benefit seen for grain fiber. Until more data are available, it is prudent to recommend consumption of a wide variety of vegetables, fruits, and whole grains.

MICRONUTRIENTS

Cancer-protective relations have been demonstrated for foods high in antioxidants (e.g., vitamin C, beta-carotene, vitamin E) as well as the micronutrients vitamin A, calcium, and folate. Epidemiologic studies consistently demonstrate a strong inverse relation between lung cancer risk and foods high in beta-carotene intake but this association could not be confirmed in large-scale clinical trials (discussed in Diet and Cancer Clinical Trials). Significant protective effects of foods containing vitamin C have been found for cancers of the stomach, esophagus, and oral cavity, and moderate protective effects have been found for cancers of the cervix, rectum, breast, and lung. Recent clinical trial data support a possible protective effect of vitamin E for colorectal and prostate cancer. Folate intake appears to be related to reduced risk of cervical and colon cancer, based on a limited number of studies. Although epidemiologic studies on selenium have been inconclusive regarding its potential cancer-protective effect, secondary end-point analyses in a recent clinical trial showed significant reductions in total cancer incidence and mortality as well as incidence of lung, colorectal, and prostate cancers for persons who received a daily 200 μg supplement of selenium.

PHYTOCHEMICALS

Phytochemicals with demonstrated potential for inhibiting cancer include carotenoids, indoles, isothiocyanates, glucosinolates, dithiothiols, coumarins, terpenes, organosulfur compounds, plant sterols, flavonoids, protease inhibitors, and lignans. Although the exact mechanisms of action of many of these phytochemicals are not known, such inhibitors can be classified broadly as carcinogen-blocking compounds, compounds that suppress promotion, and antioxidants. For example, common vegetables and fruits contain approximately 50 carotenoids—a class of compounds that exhibits strong antioxidant activities. Lutein (a component of yellow and orange vegetables and fruits) and lycopene (a component of tomatoes and tomato-based foods) are exceptionally strong antioxidants. Findings from a large prospective epidemiologic study suggested that intake of lycopene and tomato-based foods may be particularly beneficial for reducing prostate cancer risk.

ALCOHOL

Alcohol intake is directly associated with cancers of the esophagus, oral cavity, pharynx, and larynx, in which alcohol acts synergistically with smoking to increase risk. Alcohol also may contribute to increased risk of cancer of the rectum and liver. A pooled analysis of cohort studies that examined incidence of alcohol consumption and breast cancer reported that risk increased linearly with increasing intake, for all types of alcoholic beverages consumed. For total alcohol intake of 30 to 60 g per day (two to five drinks per day), risk of breast cancer increased by an average of 40% compared with nondrinkers after adjustment for other known breast cancer risk factors.

BODY WEIGHT AND PHYSICAL ACTIVITY

A close relation exists between body weight and physical activity—the latter being one of the principal means of maintaining desirable weight. Excessive body weight increases risk for several cancers, including endometrial, renal, colon, and postmenopausal breast cancer. Physical activity reduces the likelihood of colon cancer, perhaps through stimulation of intestinal motility. Some data suggest a protective effect of physical activity on breast cancer. Physical activity, leading to loss of weight and body fat, helps reduce circulating levels of estrogen and progesterone and, thus, possibly breast cancer risk.

DIET AND CANCER CLINICAL TRIALS

Clinical trials are the best means for determining the effectiveness of dietary interventions for reducing cancer risk. Dietary factors being investigated in NCI-sponsored intervention trials include beta-carotene, vitamin E, vitamin C, retinol (vitamin A), folic acid, calcium, selenium, wheat bran, and omega-3 fatty acids. Results from several closed large-scale intervention trials are described here; long-term follow-up is continuing for these trials.

The Physicians' Health Study was conducted among 22,000 male physicians who received a 50-mg supplement of beta-carotene on alternate days. After approximately 12 years of treatment (1982 to December 1995), data showed no significant evidence of either benefit or harm from beta-carotene for either cancer or cardiovascular disease.

The Alpha-Tocopherol, Beta-Carotene Cancer Prevention Study (ATBC) and the Beta-Carotene and Retinol Efficacy Trial (CARET) were carried out in populations at high risk for lung cancer. The ATBC study investigated the efficacy of vitamin E alone, beta-carotene alone, or both on lung cancer among male cigarette smokers. Unexpectedly, this study showed a 16% higher incidence of lung cancer in the beta-carotene group. The adverse effects of beta-carotene were observed at the highest two quartiles of ethanol intake, indicating that alcohol consumption may enhance the actions of beta-carotene. Among men who received vitamin E, 16% fewer cases of colorectal cancer were diagnosed. Recent analysis of ATBC follow-up data found decreases in both prostate cancer incidence (36%) and mortality (41%) among men receiving vitamin E. CARET tested the efficacy of a combination of beta-carotene and retinol (as retinyl

<table>
<tr><td>TABLE 22.2.</td><td>NATIONAL CANCER INSTITUTE DIETARY GUIDELINES</td></tr>
</table>

- Reduce fat intake to ≤30% of calories.
- Increase fiber intake to 20–30 g/day, with an upper limit of 35 g.
- Include a variety of vegetables and fruits in the daily diet.
- Avoid obesity.
- Consume alcoholic beverages in moderation, if at all.
- Minimize consumption of salt-cured, salt-pickled, or smoked foods.

palmitate) in former and current heavy smokers and in men with extensive occupational asbestos exposure. This trial was terminated in January 1996 after 4 years of treatment when data showed an overall 28% higher incidence of lung cancer in participants receiving the beta-carotene/retinyl palmitate combination. Participants with higher serum beta-carotene concentrations, which reflect total intake of vegetables and fruits, at entry into both the ATBC study and CARET developed fewer lung cancers, even among those who received beta-carotene supplements, reaffirming the importance of including an abundance of plant foods in our diets.

ROLE OF PHYSICIAN IN DIET MODIFICATION

An ever-increasing amount of evidence supports a relation between diet and cancer—the clear implication being that modification of behavior has considerable potential for reducing cancer risk. The NCI and various other scientific organizations have developed similar interim dietary guidelines directed at reducing cancer risk while research continues. The NCI's guidelines are outlined in Table 22.2. In addition to reducing cancer risk, these guidelines are likely to benefit overall health. At present, average Americans consume too much fat (more than the 30% or less recommended), the wrong types of fat (too much saturated fat, too little monounsaturated fat), too little fiber, and too few vegetables, fruits, and whole grains. Physicians should take the lead in advising and encouraging patients to adhere to the dietary guidelines. Collaboration with nutritionists and registered dietitians to help patients in modifying their diets is essential.

Information from the Physician Data Query (PDQ) system, a comprehensive database that provides peer-reviewed information on the latest results in cancer prevention, screening, treatment, and supportive care, is available at (800)-4-CANCER as well as online at http://cancernet.nci.nih.gov/market__1.html.

BIBLIOGRAPHY

Dockery DW, Trichopoulos D. Risk of lung cancer from environmental exposures to tobacco smoke. *Cancer Causes Control* 1997;8:333.

Fiore MC, Bailey WC, Cohen SJ, et al. *Smoking cessation: clinical practice guideline.* No. 18. Rockville, MD (USA): US Department of Health and Human Services, Public Health Service, Agency for Health Care Policy and Health Research, April 1996, AHCPR Pub. No. 96-0692.

Hughes JR, Goldstein MG, Hurt RD, Shiffman S. Recent advances in the pharmacotherapy of smoking. *JAMA* 1999;281:72.

Greenwald P. Role of dietary fat in the causation of breast cancer: point. *Cancer Epidemiol Biomarkers Prev* 1999;8:3.

Kviz FJ, Clark MA, Hope H, Davis AM. Patients' perceptions of their physician's role in smoking cessation by age and readiness to stop smoking. *Prev Med* 1997;26:340.

Lipworth L, Martínez ME, Angell J, et al. Olive oil and human cancer: an assessment of the evidence. *Prev Med* 1997;26:181.

Patterson RE, White E, Kristal AR, et al. Vitamin supplements and cancer risk: the epidemiologic evidence. *Cancer Causes Control* 1997;8:786.

Steinmetz KA, Potter JD. Vegetables, fruit, and cancer prevention: a review. *J Am Diet Assoc* 1996;96:1027.

US Department of Health and Human Services. Physical Activity and Health: A Report of the Surgeon General. Atlanta: US Department of Human Services, Centers for Disease Control and Prevention, National Center for Chronic Disease Prevention and Health Promotion, 1996.

World Cancer Research Fund. *Food, nutrition, and the prevention of cancer: a global perspective.* Washington, DC. American Institute for Cancer Research, 1997.

Kelley's Textbook of Internal Medicine, fourth edition. Edited by H. David Humes. Lippincott Williams & Wilkins, Philadelphia © 2000.

CHAPTER 23

TRANSPLANTATION IMMUNOLOGY

JUDITH A. SHIZURU

The transplantation of tissues to replace diseased organs has evolved over the last several decades to become an important therapeutic modality. Success has been possible in transplantation for two reasons: (a) an evolving understanding of how the immune response mediates the recognition and destruction of foreign organisms and (b) the development of multiple classes of drugs that can effectively suppress the immune response.

Although tissue transplantation has been practiced sporadically by a number of civilizations dating back to as early as 700 BC, not until the 1930s did biologists begin systematic study in animals that led to our current understanding of tissue rejection. The most crucial paradigm is that rejection of grafts has an immunologic basis mediated primarily by T cells. Studies of skin graft transplantation between inbred strains of mice revealed the basic rules of rejection: Grafts that are exchanged between different sites on the same animal or person (*autologous*) or exchanged between genetically identical people (twins) or inbred animal strains (*syngeneic*) are accepted 100% of the time. In contrast, when skin grafts are transplanted between genetically disparate humans or animals but within the same species, the graft is initially accepted, but subsequently rejected at about 2 weeks. This donor–recipient combination is termed *allogeneic*. Grafts exchanged between organisms of different species are called *xenografts*.

In the allogeneic and xenogeneic setting, if a second graft is placed from the same donor, but after the first graft is rejected, the tempo of rejection is accelerated, occurring at approximately 6 to 8 days. These responses are called first-set rejection and second-set rejection, respectively, and demonstrate that the reaction against the tissue is specific for antigens on the graft, because transplantation of skin from another unrelated donor results in a first-set rejection. There are special circumstances in which allografts or xenografts are rejected in a very rapid time frame; these are described in the section on hyperacute rejection.

T lymphocytes mediate the rejection of transplanted tissue. This is because T cells, particularly CD4$^+$ T cells, are central to the induction and perpetuation of most antigen-specific immune responses. Experimentally, the role of T cells in tissue rejection was shown by transplantation of skin grafts onto strains of mice that genetically lack T cells. The mice were unable to reject an allogeneic skin graft unless T cells were transferred to them from a genetically matched mouse with a normal immune system.

■ MAJOR HISTOCOMPATIBILITY COMPLEX

Understanding of how tissues are recognized and rejected has occurred in parallel with knowledge of how the immune response functions. The skin graft studies between inbred mouse strains led investigators to discover a gene region that encodes for surface molecules that not only control organ rejection, but also control most T-cell responses. That gene region is generically termed the major histocompatibility complex (MHC) (Fig. 23.1). In mice, the MHC is designated H-2, and in humans it is called the human leukocyte antigen (HLA) complex and is located on the short arm of chromosome 6. The MHC is composed of a stretch of linked genes of three different classes. The class I and class II genes encode proteins that are expressed on the cell surface and whose function it is to bind peptides and present peptides for recognition by a T cell (Fig. 23.2). Thus, the ligand for a T-cell clone's receptor is a composite of an MHC class I or class II molecule plus peptide bound in its antigen-binding groove. The class III MHC–encoded proteins are structurally and functionally distinct from the class I and II molecules.

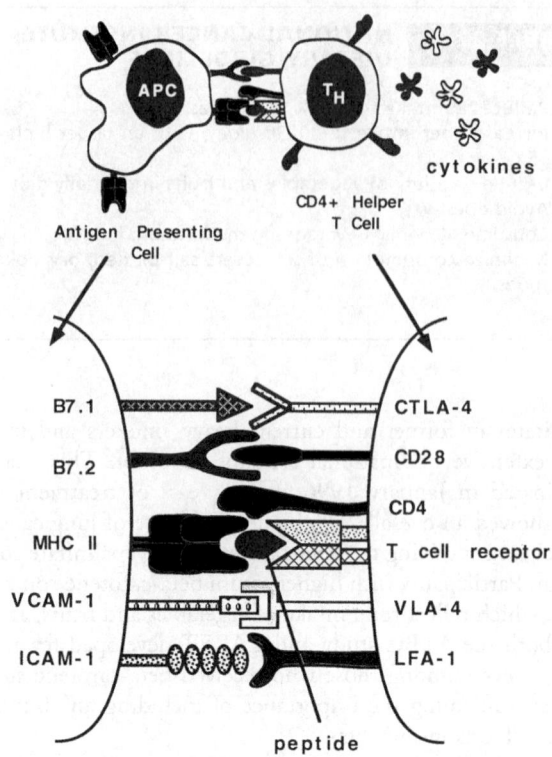

FIGURE 23.2. Schematic representation of the molecular interactions that lead to activation of T lymphocytes. Shown here is the activation of a CD4$^+$ T cell by an antigen-presenting cell. The primary ligand for the antigen-specific T-cell receptor is an MHC class II molecule bound to a peptide antigen. The CD4 molecule stabilizes this interaction. Also shown are some of the known costimulatory and adhesion receptor–ligand pairs that participate in the cellular interaction. *CD*, cluster designation; *VCAM-1*, vascular adhesion molecule-1; *VLA-4*, very late activation antigen-4; *ICAM-1*, intercellular adhesion molecule-1; *LFA-1*, lymphocyte function-related antigen.

These proteins include components of the complement system and certain cytokines, which play a less direct role in transplantation biology. They will not be further discussed as a group in this chapter.

Both class I and class II MHC molecules are cell-surface glycoproteins that resemble one another but have slightly differ-

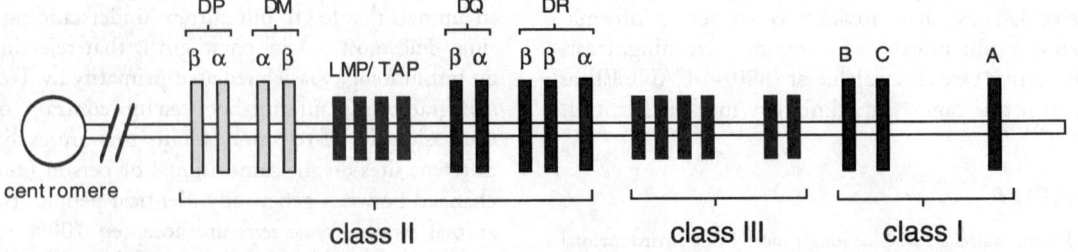

FIGURE 23.1. Genetic organization of the human major histocompatibility complex (MHC). There are separate regions of class I and class II genes, and class III genes are interspersed as indicated. The class I genes are HLA-A, HLA-B, and HLA-C. The class II genes are DR, DQ, and DP. DM genes are related to class II genes and function to catalyze peptide binding to class II MHC molecules. The LMP/TAP genes are class III genes that encode molecules involved in processing and transporting endogenous antigens. Other proteins encoded in the class III region are tumor necrosis factor α and β, and complement factors C2, C4, B, and F.

ent structures. Class MHC I molecules are heterodimers composed of an α chain that is membrane spanning and is associated noncovalently with the molecule β₂-microglobulin. β₂-Microglobulin is not encoded within the MHC complex. Class II MHC molecules are composed of an α and a β chain; both chains are derived from the MHC and both span the plasma membrane. Class I MHC molecules are expressed on virtually all nucleated cells, but their level of expression depends on the cell type. In humans, there are three class I molecules designated A, B, and C. Class I MHC molecules present peptides derived from cytosolic pathogens to CD8⁺ T cells. In contrast to class I molecules, tissue expression of class II molecules is restricted. The cells that express significant amounts of class II molecules include the professional antigen-presenting cells and epithelial cells in the thymus. Class II MHC molecules present peptides that come from pathogens that have been phagocytosed and are thus derived from exogenous antigens. Such antigens are presented by class II molecules primarily to CD4⁺ T cells. In humans, there are three class II molecules that are designated DR, DQ, and DP; in some human haplotypes, the DR region contains an extra β chain whose product can pair with the DRα chain. Thus, three sets of genes give rise to four types of class II MHC molecules. Most mouse strains express two class II molecules designated I-A and I-E.

ROLE OF MHC MOLECULES IN TRANSPLANTATION IMMUNOLOGY

An important feature of the class I and II MHC genes relevant to transplantation immunology is that they are highly polymorphic. Specifically, this means that among individuals in a population, there is great variation in the structure of the gene products encoded at MHC loci. The individual variants of the genes are *alleles*. There are more than 200 alleles of some of the class I and class II loci. Another salient feature of MHC genes is that they are codominantly expressed. Therefore, unlike genes in which only one parental gene is expressed, both paternal and maternal genes are expressed in MHC molecules. This means that an individual human cell can coexpress six class I and eight class II HLA molecules. Together, these variations make it highly unlikely that nonrelated individuals will express identical class I and class II MHC molecules. On the other hand, the likelihood that two siblings will express identical MHC molecules is one in four because molecules within the MHC are tightly linked. Thus, parental MHC molecules are inherited as a group, and the probability of matching at both loci is inherited in a mendelian fashion.

The function of MHC-encoded molecules is to present foreign peptides to T cells to eliminate foreign pathogens by inducing an immune response that results in activation of appropriate effector mechanisms (Fig. 23.2). During T-cell development, T-cell clones that recognize and bind to self-MHC molecules are eliminated. However, T cells that mature and circulate in the blood are capable of recognizing MHC molecules that differ from self-MHC molecules by as little as a single amino acid. Thus, within a population of T cells many clones are capable of recognizing the structural differences that occur between MHC molecules of one individual in contrast to another. It is known

that the frequency of T cells that respond to a single peptide antigen is ~0.001%, whereas the number of T-cell clones that are capable of responding to foreign MHC molecules is between 1% and 10%. The higher frequency of MHC-reactive T-cell clones explains why rejection of foreign tissue elicits such a vigorous immune response.

Thus, it is optimal to attempt to match donor and recipient for MHC type to minimize rejection. But even among those who have identical MHC types, such as MHC-matched siblings, there is still the possibility that rejection can occur, because even siblings have differences in other gene products. The peptide-binding pocket of MHC molecules is often filled with peptides derived from self-antigens; thus, a transplanted organ from a sibling can contain peptides that differ slightly from the recipient, but enough to be recognized by recipient T cells. These other nonhistocompatibility antigens are *minor histocompatibility antigens*. As expected, there are many potential minor histocompatibility antigens, most of which have not been characterized.

THE IMMUNE RESPONSE AND TISSUE REJECTION

Conventional immune responses against bacterial and viral pathogens involve processing and presentation of the bacterial–viral antigens to T cells by professional antigen-presenting cells (APCs). Professional APCs include dendritic cells, macrophages, and B cells and have several important features: (a) They express high levels of class II MHC molecules on their surface and thus interact primarily with CD4⁺ T cells; (b) they synthesize and secrete several cell-activating cytokines such as interleukin-1 and interferon-γ (IFN-γ); and (c) they express cell-surface molecules called *costimulatory molecules* (Fig. 23.2). Among the most well studied of the costimulatory molecules are B71, B72, and the CD40 ligand (CD154). In a T-cell–APC interaction, the primary receptor–ligand pair are the antigen-specific T-cell receptor and the MHC molecule bound to a peptide. However, it is known that unless secondary costimulatory receptors are engaged, the T cell will not become activated and in fact may become refractory to stimulation through its receptor. In addition to the costimulatory molecules, professional APCs express adhesion molecules such as ICAM-1, ICAM-2, LFA-1, and LFA-3.

Activation of CD4⁺ T cells by APCs is a major pathway in the induction and perpetuation of immune responses. Once activated, CD4⁺ T cells stimulate other effector cells either by direct cell–cell contact or by the production and secretion of cytokines. Both antibody-mediated responses (*humoral immunity*) and cellular responses are activated in this way and include the conversion of pre-B cells into antibody-secreting plasma cells, the stimulation of precytotoxic T cells to become mature killer cells, and the activation of antigen-nonspecific inflammatory cells such as macrophages. The effector arms of the immune response ultimately lead to the destruction of the tissue graft.

The central role that CD4⁺ T cells play in rejection of tissue allografts was demonstrated experimentally in animal models. Treatment with monoclonal antibodies directed against the

CD4 molecule in the peri-transplantation phase allows long-term organ graft acceptance without the need for further immunosuppression. The CD4$^+$ T-cell subset can be subdivided into two functional subtypes, T_H1 and T_H2, which activate the cell-mediated versus the humoral arm of the immune response, respectively. Determination of whether a naive T cell becomes a T_H1 or a T_H2 cell is thought to be controlled by the cytokines present locally during the initial phase when a naive T cell is undergoing activation. In vitro experiments have shown that T cells stimulated in the presence of IL-12 and IFN-γ tend to differentiate into T_H1 cells, whereas T cells stimulated in the presence of IL-4 and IL-6 tend to differentiate into T_H2 cells. In addition, activated CD4$^+$ T cells themselves secrete cytokines that further polarize the response so that one TH subtype dominates; T_H1 cells secrete IFN-γ, whereas T_H2 cells secrete IL-4 and IL-10. IFN-γ can prevent the activation of T_H2 cells, and IL-10 can inhibit the development of T_H1 cells.

In the setting of graft rejection, the T-cell subtype that dominates may have important consequences. It is thought that T_H1 responses are ultimately much more damaging to a transplanted organ, whereas T_H2 responses (with the exception of hyperacute rejection, described in the next section) may be protective.

HYPERACUTE REJECTION

For most solid organ transplantations, the rejection and graft destruction ultimately result from a combination of cellular and antibody-mediated effector mechanisms. However, there are special situations when rejection is aggressively mediated by antibodies and leads to a syndrome termed *hyperacute rejection*. This occurs when a recipient has preformed antibodies directed against the graft before its transplantation. The most common reason for this presence is exposure to different MHC alleles as a result of prior blood transfusions. Preformed antibodies can recognize and damage vascular structures. Thus, when anastamoses are made between donor and recipient vessels, a very brisk response ensues; antibody binding to the vascular endothelium of the graft activates the complement and clotting cascades, occluding blood flow to the graft and causing immediate death of the graft. To avoid hyperacute rejection, *cross-matching* is performed between donor and recipient. Cross-matching involves determining whether the recipient has circulating antibodies that react with the white blood cells of the donor. If found, such antibodies are a serious contraindication to transplantation because standard immunosuppressive treatments are ineffective against hyperacute rejection.

XENOGRAFTS

Another scenario in which preformed antibodies appear to play an important role is in transplantations between species (xenografts). Humans are known to naturally produce antibodies that can respond against the antigens on the vascular endothelium of other species and thus cause hyperacute rejection. The pig-to-primate model is perhaps the best-studied xenogeneic system in which the problem of hyperacute rejection has been shown to be further exacerbated because a group of proteins called *complement regulatory proteins* demonstrate species specificity. These regulatory proteins include CD59, decay-accelerating factor (DAF or CD55), and membrane cofactor protein (MCP or CD46); these normally function to protect endothelial cells from damage caused by inadvertent activation of the complement cascade. Because these regulatory proteins are species-specific, the DAF expressed on pig endothelium cannot protect the tissue from attack by primate complement. Recently, transgenic pigs expressing human DAF were produced in attempts to overcome the problems of hyperacute rejection in xenotransplantation.

BONE MARROW TRANSPLANTATION

Transplantation of allogeneic bone marrow (BM) differs from solid organ grafts in several ways. First, the biology of resistance (or rejection) to engraftment differs. From experiments in inbred mouse strains, it is clear that although the MHC molecules and T cells are important in controlling resistance to allogeneic BM, other genes and other immune cells (natural killer cells) also contribute significantly. Second, because BM is a heterogeneous population of cells that contain both mature immune cells and primitive hematopoietic stem cells, the immune cells in the graft have the potential to respond against antigens present on the recipient tissues and cause a syndrome called *graft-versus-host disease* (GVHD). GVHD is a life-threatening complication of allogeneic bone marrow transplantation (BMT); to prevent GVHD (and to prevent BM rejection), BMT patients receive immunosuppressive therapy in the post-transplantation period. Third, the major indications for allogeneic BMTs are hematologic malignancies, and the presence of immune cells contained within the BM graft can have a favorable effect because donor immune cells have been shown to suppress tumor growth. Fourth, BM grafts are unique in that they appear to induce immune tolerance to themselves, as well as to other tissues derived from the BM donor. Thus, most patients who undergo an allogeneic BMT may be eventually tapered off all immunosuppressive therapy. The use of allogeneic BMT to induce tolerance to solid organ grafts is still in the experimental stages and not used clinically. This is because the risks associated with the BMT procedure limit its use primarily to the treatment of malignancies and BM failure states. However, more recently, promising advances have been made in reducing the severity of the BMT conditioning regimens that will likely lead to the more widespread use of BMT for clinical applications that include organ transplantation tolerance induction.

PHARMACOLOGIC SUPPRESSION OF REJECTION OF TRANSPLANTED TISSUES

A major reason why solid organ transplantation and BMT are successful is because pharmacologic agents can effectively suppress the immune system. The drugs currently used to suppress the immune system may be divided into five broad categories: (a) anti-inflammatory drugs of the glucocorticoid family; (b) cytotoxic drugs such as cyclophosphamide; (c) drugs that affect purine metabolism and synthesis required for DNA synthesis, including azathioprine and mycophenolate mofetil; (d) fungal and bacterial derivatives such as cyclosporin A (CSA), FK506, and rapamycin, which inhibit signaling events that occur within T lymphocytes; and (e) monoclonal agents directed against immune cell subsets such as anti-CD3 antibodies or anti-CD25 (anti–IL-2 receptor) antibodies. The current mainstay of immunosuppressive therapy is CSA or its related compounds, which are well tolerated and have powerful effects on T-cell function. These agents are generally used in combination with one or more of the drugs from the other classes. The goal of therapy is to taper the immunosuppressive agents to the lowest effective dose, but most patients who receive a solid organ transplantation remain on one or two of these drugs permanently. Most BMT patients, however, can be withdrawn completely from the immunosuppressive drugs (see above).

CONCLUSIONS

Understanding the way in which organ grafts are recognized and rejected continues to be an active area of research, and newer forms of immunosuppressive therapy are being developed. However, tissue transplantation still involves significant risks. These include infections due to chronic use of immunosuppression, secondary malignancies, metabolic bone disease, hypertension, and, in the case of BMT, GVHD. Additional problems involve the limited availability of organs for transplantation. Moreover, patients who have had prior exposure to alloantigens are at risk of hyperacute rejection, which is poorly treated with currently available immunosuppressive therapies. The ultimate goal still being pursued by transplantation biologists is the induction of immune tolerance. The experimental approaches to achieve this include rendering the grafts nonimmunogenic or alternatively designing recipient immunosuppressive regimens that can be tapered off over a relatively short time. Given the pace of new developments in in vitro and in vivo cellular manipulation, we can look forward to achieving the goal of tissue-specific immune tolerance in the near future.

BIBLIOGRAPHY

Billingham RE. Transplantation: past, present and future. *J Invest Dermatol* 1963;41:165.
Charlton B, Auchincloss H Jr, Fathman CG. Mechanisms of transplantation tolerance. *Ann Rev Immunol* 1994;12:707.
Janeway CA, Bottomly K. Signals and signs for lymphocyte responses. *Cell* 1994;76:275.
Janeway CA, Travers P. *Immunobiology*. New York: Current Biology Ltd/Garland Publishing, 1998.
Kunz J, Jall MN. Cyclosporin A, FK506 and rapamycin: more than just immunosuppression. *Trends Biochem Sci* 1993;18:334.
Mossman TR, Coffman RL. T_H1 and T_H1 cells: Different patterns of lymphkine secretion lead to different functional properties. *Ann Rev Imunol* 1989;7:145.
Steele DJ, Auchincloss H Jr. Xenotransplantation. *Ann Rev Med* 1995;46:345.
Thomas ED, Blume KG, Forman SJ. *Hematopoietic cell transplantation,* second ed. Maldan, MA: Blackwell Science, 1999.
Warrens AN, Lombardi G, Lechler RI. Presentation and recognition of major and minor histocompatibility antigens. *Transpl Immunol* 1994;2:103.

Kelley's Textbook of Internal Medicine, fourth edition. Edited by H. David Humes. Lippincott Williams & Wilkins, Philadelphia © 2000.

APPROACH TO COMMON
PRIMARY CARE ISSUES

PERIODIC HEALTH
EVALUATION

ALBERT G. MULLEY, JR.

More Americans see their physicians for periodic health examinations than for any other reason. Many screening and other preventive measures (e.g., blood pressure measurement, breast examination, testing of stool for occult blood) are performed when patients present with symptoms that are unrelated to the condition that may be prevented or detected. This kind of clinical activity, referred to as *prescriptive screening* or *case finding*, carries with it an ethical imperative for the clinician, who must be certain that the patient is more likely to be helped than harmed by the initiative. The potential for harm and the pressure for cost containment force careful evaluation of the rationale for periodic health evaluation and for specific case-finding procedures.

Several groups, including professional societies and government-sponsored task forces, have examined evidence for and against specific preventive services. Because the evidence is incomplete, resulting recommendations must be made in the face of uncertainty, and they inevitably reflect value judgments about alternative uses of resources. Not surprisingly, such recommendations vary from group to group and change over time. The clinician must know what is recommended and by whom and must understand the rationale for evaluating screening and preventive services. Whether screening results in improved health outcome depends on characteristics of the disease in question and available therapy, characteristics of available screening tests, and characteristics of patients screened (Table 24.1).

■ CRITERIA FOR SCREENING

CHARACTERISTICS OF THE DISEASE

Screening or case finding is performed to identify a condition or disease in a person who is asymptomatic. Without screening, a diagnosis would not be made until and unless signs or symptoms occurred; the effect of screening is to advance the time of diagnosis. Earlier diagnosis is worthwhile when it provides prognostic information that is of value to the patient or when earlier therapeutic intervention produces a better health outcome than would later therapy. In the case of communicable diseases, screening may be warranted to protect potential contacts from infection, regardless of potential benefit to the person already infected.

The relation between natural history of disease and effectiveness of intervention that is critical to the screening decision is illustrated in Figure 24.1. The horizontal line represents the natural history as a function of time, with the biologic onset of disease (e.g., malignant transformation of a cell, infection of a host) at the far left. At some variable point after disease onset, a diagnosis is possible if a screening test is carried out. After another variable period during which the patient remains asymptomatic, symptoms or signs occur that may prompt clinical presentation and subsequent diagnosis. Eventually, after appropriate therapeutic maneuvers, there is an identifiable clinical outcome that can range from cure and complete health to death. At some point in the natural history, the disease may become less amenable to available therapy; an *escape from cure* is said to occur.

TABLE 24.1.   CRITERIA FOR SCREENING

Characteristics of the Disease
Significant effect on the quality and length of life
Prevalence sufficiently high
Acceptable methods of treatment available
Asymptomatic period during which detection and treatment significantly reduce morbidity or mortality
Better therapeutic result with treatment in the asymptomatic phase than with treatment delayed until symptoms appear

Characteristics of the Test
Sufficiently sensitive to detect disease during the asymptomatic period
Sufficiently specific to provide acceptable positive predictive value
Acceptable to patients

Characteristics of the Population Screened
Sufficiently high disease prevalence
Subsequent diagnostic tests and necessary therapy acceptable

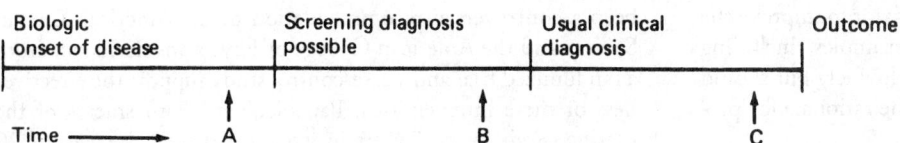

FIGURE 24.1. Relation between screening and natural history of disease. (From Mulley AG Jr. Health maintenance and the role of screening. In: Goroll AH, May LA, Mulley AG Jr, eds. *Primary care medicine: office evaluation and management of the adult patient,* third ed. Philadelphia: JB Lippincott, 1995, with permission.)

Much variability in the natural history of a disease exists among persons with the same disease. Nonetheless, some cautious generalizations about relations illustrated in Figure 24.1 can be useful. If the escape from cure usually occurs before a screening diagnosis is possible (e.g., point A), the value of screening must be questioned; the value of prognostic information must be weighed against the effects of the patient receiving bad news sooner. If the escape from cure regularly occurs after symptoms or signs have pointed the way to a diagnosis (e.g., point C), education of patients or clinicians to ensure early presentation and prompt diagnostic evaluation may be more efficient than screening programs. Diseases for which the escape from cure commonly occur during the asymptomatic detectable period (e.g., point B) are the most promising targets for screening strategies.

Figure 24.1 also is helpful in understanding two methodologic problems that sometimes affect interpretation of evaluations of screening studies: lead time and time-linked bias sampling. *Lead time* is the average time by which diagnosis is advanced by screening. If survival is the outcome measure used to compare screening and nonscreening strategies, longer survival may reflect earlier diagnosis rather than extended life. *Time-linked bias sampling* refers to the potential selection of more indolent cases of a particular disease by means of screening that can occur, because persons with a long asymptomatic detectable period have more opportunity to be detected earlier. Such variability in duration of the asymptomatic period must be kept in mind when screening intervals are chosen. The mean duration of asymptomatic detectable disease is not as important as the distribution of durations or, more specifically, the proportion of asymptomatic detectable periods that are shorter than the designated screening interval.

CHARACTERISTICS OF THE TEST

The validity of a test depends on its ability to differentiate patients with and without a disease or condition, measured by its sensitivity or true-positive rate and its specificity or true-negative rate. The predictive value of the test result depends on these characteristics of the test and on the prior probability of the disease or condition in question (Chapter 42). This relation is particularly important in the screening situation when prior probability of disease (i.e., prevalence in the population tested)

is invariably low. Under these conditions, the positive predictive value is critically influenced by test specificity; even small false-positive rates can generate many false-positive results from the majority of those tested who do not have disease. However, generalizations about which is more important for a screening test—sensitivity or specificity—are hazardous. Any tradeoffs between sensitivity and specificity should be based on the relative value of a true-positive result and the cost of a false-negative result and, conversely, the value of a true-negative result and the cost of a false-positive result.

Before deciding about the appropriateness of a test for the screening situation based on reports of the test's sensitivity and specificity, the clinician should be certain that the reports were generated by studies relevant to the screening situation.

CHARACTERISTICS OF THE PATIENTS

Patients hold widely different views about disease prevention and health promotion activities. How do they feel about the morbidity of a test, whether it is simply a venipuncture or something worse? Given their current level of anxiety and knowledge, how will they respond to a true-positive or true-negative test result? What effect would a false-positive or false-negative result have? Would the patient accept indicated therapy or appropriately change behavior if a disease or condition were identified? The clinician should try to understand these differences and respect the patients' prerogatives.

■ RECOMMENDATIONS FOR THE PERIODIC HEALTH EVALUATION

When criteria such as these are systematically applied, relatively few preventive services are endorsed. The US Preventive Services Task Force examined evidence for and against use of more than 100 interventions, including screening tests, counseling interventions, and immunizations or chemoprophylaxis. The Task Force reports provide specific clinical guidelines, leaving discretion to the clinician when evidence does not justify a definitive judgment. Selectivity in the use of services, based on particular patients' risk factors, is emphasized. Overall, the early recommendations of the Task Force suggest a skepticism about the relative value of screening tests compared with the potential for physician counseling aimed at changing behavior to improve the health of patients. Discussion of specific examples, including some screening tests that should not be used widely but should be used in certain groups, can help clarify the rationale for preventive services.

COMMON CONDITIONS THAT WARRANT INCLUSION

Few conditions meet criteria for screening and are common enough to warrant attention in the periodic health examination of all patients of appropriate age and gender. These appear in Table 24.2.

Hypertension may be the most significant condition for the practitioner concerned about disease prevention and health promotion (Chapters 29 and 30). The prevalence is staggering, and morbidity and mortality attributable to hypertension, as well as benefits of treatment, are well documented. Evidence for benefits derived from treatment of systolic hypertension has produced revisions in treatment guidelines.

Moderate elevations in cholesterol that confer risk are also exceedingly prevalent in most Western societies. Potential benefits to be derived from screening and subsequent treatment have been demonstrated in randomized, controlled trials. Patients younger than 65 years of age should be screened for hypercholesterolemia using total cholesterol and high-density lipoprotein levels. The age at which screening should begin is a matter of controversy. Screening every 5 years after starting at age 18 is the most common recommendation.

Smoking is a major risk factor for coronary and cerebrovascular disease as well as being the primary cause of lung cancer and chronic pulmonary disease and the single largest preventable cause of death in America. Evidence suggests that most clinicians underestimate the effectiveness of counseling and other smoking-cessation interventions. A patient should always be asked whether he or she smokes. Those who smoke must be apprised of the reasons for stopping and of available smoking-cessation resources.

Relatively few screening tests to detect cancer are recommended for patients with no symptoms and without specific risk factors. Annual stool guaiac testing and sigmoidoscopy every 3 to 5 years for men and women older than 50 years of age has

TABLE 24.2.	**CONDITIONS THAT WARRANT PERIODIC EVALUATION IN ALL PATIENTS OF APPROPRIATE AGE AND GENDER**
Disease	**Comments**
Hypertension	See Chapter 29, 30
Hyperlipidemia	See Chapter 12, 28
Breast cancer	See Chapter 22, 28, 220
Colon cancer	See Chapter 22, 28, 102, 116
Cervical cancer	See Chapter 22, 221
Smoking	See Chapter 33
Alcoholism	See Chapter 34

been a controversial recommendation of the American Cancer Society and the American College of Physicians. Evidence from a randomized trial and a case-control study support the effectiveness of these interventions. Papanicolaou (Pap) smears of the uterine cervix every 3 years in women between the ages of 20 and 65 and known risk factors, including early sexual activity and a high number of sexual partners, are indications for screening at yearly intervals.

Annual mammograms in women older than 50 years of age are well supported by evidence and have been endorsed by many expert panels. The recommended age at which screening mammography should begin is controversial. Most professional organizations now advise beginning annual or biannual mammographic screening at age 40. Other groups including the US Task Force recommend starting at age 50, unless there is a history of premenopausal breast cancer in a first-degree relative that warrants mammography at an earlier age. Breast self-examination is complementary, and the technique should be emphasized if the woman is at high risk and has breasts that are suitable for effective self-examination. Physical examination by the physician is also important and should be performed at yearly intervals after the age of 40 or earlier if breast cancer occurred before menopause in a first-degree relative.

A controversial question in cancer screening for men is whether prostate-specific antigen (PSA) should be used to screen for prostate cancer. Prostate cancer is the most common cancer and the second leading cause of cancer death in men. However, most histologically confirmed prostate cancers, which are extremely common among older men, do not produce morbidity and mortality. Screening tests, including PSA, have limited sensitivity and specificity. It is not clear that outcome can be improved significantly for patients with cancers detected by screening. Recommendations vary. Even those most enthusiastic about screening do not advise PSA testing for men with a life expectancy of less than 10 years because it is unlikely that they will survive to see a benefit. PSA should be used only among men who understand and accept the potential harms including the significant morbidity of earlier diagnosis followed by treatment that may not alter outcome.

The rationale behind cancer-screening recommendations is discussed more fully in Chapter 28.

CONDITIONS THAT SHOULD BE SELECTIVELY INCLUDED

Several conditions for which screening cannot be justified in the general population should be sought when risk factors are identified as part of the baseline history or physical examination. Such risk factors should be used to tailor the composition and frequency of the periodic health examination for individual patients. Such an evaluation should include consideration of immunization status (Chapter 26). Conditions that should be addressed in the periodic health examination of some patients appear in Table 24.3. The list is not exhaustive. Inclusions and omissions may be controversial. In considering whether an intervention should be included in the periodic health examination of a particular patient and the frequency of such examinations, the clinician should consider the criteria

TABLE 24.3. **CONDITIONS THAT WARRANT PERIODIC EVALUATION OF SELECTED PATIENTS**

Disease	Risk Factors	Comments
Tuberculosis (PPD reactivity)	Occupation	See Chapter 294
	Exposure	
	HIV Infection	
	High-dose steroids	
Rubella susceptibility	Anticipated pregnancy	See Chapter 311
	Occupation (health care worker)	
Susceptibility to hepatitis B virus	High-risk sexual behavior	See Chapter 119
	Exposure	
	Occupation (health care worker)	
Syphilis	High-risk sexual behavior	See Chapter 297
	Pregnancy	
	Other sexually transmitted disease	
Human immunodeficiency virus (HIV) infection	High-risk sexual behavior	See Chapters 339, 340
	Blood transfusions, 1978–1985	
Chlamydial genitourinary infection	Other sexually transmitted disease	See Chapter 306
	Women of childbearing age	
Endocarditis susceptibility	Valvular heart disease	See Chapter 270
Rheumatic fever susceptibility	Rheumatic fever history	See Chapter 337
Occupational lung disease	Occupational exposure	See Chapter 375
Anemia	Pregnancy	See Chapter 211
Sickle cell trait	African American persons of childbearing age	Genetic counseling must be acceptable; see Chapter 245
Thyroid cancer	Radiation of head and neck	See Chapter 392
Diabetes	Pregnancy	See Chapter 411
	Family history of diabetes	
	Marked obesity	
	History of gestational diabetes	
Endometrial cancer	Exogenous extrogens	See Chapter 221
Vaginal cancer	In utero diethylstilbestrol exposure	
Lower urinary tract cancer	Occupational exposure (aromatic amines, such as dyestuffs, leather tanning, rubber)	See Chapters 50 and 223
Bacteriuria	Pregnancy	See Chapter 271
	Kidney stones	See Chapter 159
Glaucoma	Family history	See Chapter 51
	Advanced age	
Oral cancer	Alcohol	See Chapter 225
	Tobacco	
Skin cancer	Fair skin, sun exposure	See Chapter 198
	Family history	

discussed, including those that relate to characteristics and preferences of the patient.

BIBLIOGRAPHY

Canadian Task Force on the Periodic Health Examination. *Canadian guide to clinical preventive healthcare.* Ottawa: Canada Communication Group, 1994.

Coley CM, Barry MJ, Fleming C, et al. Early detection of prostate cancer: I, Prior probability and effectiveness of tests; II, Estimating the risks, benefits, and costs. *Ann Intern Med* 1997;126:394–406,468–479.

Eddy DM, ed. *Common screening tests.* Philadelphia: American College of Physicians, 1991.

Feinleb M, Zelen M. Some pitfalls in the evaluation of screening programs. *Arch Environ Health* 1969;19:412.

Hayward RSA, Steinberg EP, Ford DE, et al. Preventive care guidelines: 1991. *Ann Intern Med* 1991;114:758 [Erratum, *Ann Intern Med* 1991; 115:332].

Kerlikowske K, Grady D, Rubin SM. Efficiency of screening mammography: a meta-analysis. *JAMA* 1995;273:149–154.

Mulley AG. Health maintenance and the role of screening. In: Goroll AH, May LA, Mulley AG, eds. *Primary care medicine,* third ed. Philadelphia: JB Lippincott, 1995.

Sox HC Jr. Preventive health services in adults. *N Engl J Med* 1994;330: 1589.

US Preventive Services Task Force. *Guide to clinical preventive services,* second ed. Washington, DC: US Department of Health and Human Services, 1996.

Kelley's Textbook of Internal Medicine, fourth edition. Edited by H. David Humes. Lippincott Williams & Wilkins, Philadelphia © 2000.

CHAPTER

25

PREOPERATIVE MEDICAL EVALUATION

JUDI M. WOOLGER

GENERAL APPROACH

As the mortality from general anesthesia continues to decline, the type of patient considered for surgical intervention has expanded to include both older and more medically challenging patients. With an increased willingness to offer surgery to a broader patient base, however, comes an increased need for the internist to be involved in the comprehensive care of the patient, both before and after the surgical procedure. This chapter focuses primarily on the preoperative assessment, although the obligation for care certainly does not end there.

In the preoperative evaluation, the internist is responsible for generating a comprehensive evaluation of all medical problems, with special attention to cardiovascular risk assessment and pulmonary evaluation. Because this may be the only contact the patient has with a generalist, however, it is also important to use this interaction to address preventive health issues and to facilitate follow-up for appropriate screening studies after the surgical issue has been addressed. Furthermore, and often most important, the preoperative evaluation is used to assess risk for specific types of surgical interventions and, when possible, to modify those risks before a patient proceeds to surgery. Recommendations for postoperative care are also made at this time.

Risk assessment is performed much the same as in any patient encounter, focusing on careful history-taking, directed physical examination, and judicious use of laboratory and radiographic evaluation. The medical history needs to focus not only on careful documentation of prior medical problems, but also on prior surgical history and outcomes of prior surgeries. Knowledge of previous complications (i.e., bleeding or reactions to anesthesia) are of paramount importance and dictates a directed search for causes. The review of systems is significant in defining an overall picture of the patient's general state of health and provides insight into potential postoperative issues, such as nutritional status and bowel or urologic issues. This is also the best time to evaluate medication usage of any kind; the surgical team should be aware of potential interactions of any prescription drugs and should recognize the risks for withdrawal in those who abuse alcohol or other nonprescription drugs.

During the physical examination, the physician should pay special attention to the cardiopulmonary system. Likewise, the need for preoperative testing is also directed by needs brought to light during the history and physical examination, still with a focus on the cardiopulmonary systems. Electrocardiograms are indicated for anyone over the age of 45 years or with two or more cardiac risk factors (hypertension, diabetes, hypercholester-

olemia, tobacco use, or family history of accelerated coronary artery disease). Chest radiographs are indicated for any patient with significant respiratory complaints or history, as well as for patients scheduled for intrathoracic or intra-abdominal procedures. The basic laboratory evaluation includes a complete blood cell count and creatinine. Additional studies are based on the patient's overall medical condition, concurrent illnesses, and medications.

CARDIAC EVALUATION

Because of the high prevalence of coronary artery disease and the known cardiovascular stress associated with the induction of general anesthesia, much attention has been focused on the preoperative cardiac assessment of the patient going through

---

TABLE 25.1. CLINICAL PREDICTORS OF CARDIOVASCULAR RISK[a]

Major

Unstable coronary syndromes
  Recent myocardial infarction (MI)[b] with evidence of important ischemic risk by clinical symptoms or noninvasive study
  Unstable or severe angina[c] (Canadian class III or IV)[d]
Decompensated congestive heart failure
Significant arrhythmias
  High-grade atrioventricular block
  Symptomatic ventricular arrhythmias with underlying heart disease
  Supraventricular arrhythmias with uncontrolled ventricular rate
Severe valvular disease

Intermediate

Mild angina pectoris (Canadian class I or II)
Prior MI by history or pathologic Q waves
Significant aortic stenosis
Compensated or prior congestive heart failure
Diabetes mellitus

Minor

Advanced age
Abnormal ECG (left-ventricular hypertrophy, left bundle branch block, ST–T abnormalities)
Rhythm other than sinus (e.g., atrial fibrillation)
Low functional capacity
History of stroke
Uncontrolled systemic hypertension

---

[a] Increased perioperative cardiovascular risk (MI, congestive heart failure, death).
[b] The American College of Cardiology National Database Library defines recent MI as >7 days but ≤1 month (30 days).
[c] May include "stable" angina in patients who are usually sedentary.
[d] Campbeau L. Grading of angina pectoris. *Circulation* 1976;54; 522–525, with permission.
(From Eagle KA, Hertzer NR, Leppo JA, et al. Guidelines for perioperative cardiovascular evaluation for noncardiac surgery. Report of the American College of Cardiology/American Heart Association Task Force on Practice Guidelines. Committee on Perioperative Cardiovascular Evaluation for Noncardiac Surgery. *J Am Coll Cardiol* 1996;27:910–948, with permission.)

TABLE 25.2.	SURGERY-BASED CARDIAC RISK STRATIFICATION FOR NONCARDIAC PROCEDURES[a]

High (Reported Cardiac Risk Often >5%)
Emergent major operations, particularly in the elderly
Aortic and other major vascular
Peripheral vascular
Anticipated prolonged surgical procedures associated with large fluid shifts and/or blood loss

Intermediate (Reported Cardiac Risk <5%)
Carotid endarterectomy
Head and neck
Intraperitoneal and intrathoracic
Orthopedic
Prostate

Low (Reported Cardiac Risk <1%)[b]
Endoscopic procedures
Superficial procedure
Cataract
Breast

---

[a] Combined incidence of cardiac death and nonfatal myocardial infarction.
[b] Generally no further preoperative cardiac testing required.
(From Eagle KA, Hertzer NR, Leppo JA, et al. Guidelines for perioperative cardiovascular evaluation for noncardiac surgery. Report of the American College of Cardiology/American Heart Association Task Force on Practice Guidelines. Committee on Perioperative Cardiovascular Evaluation for Noncardiac Surgery. *J Am Coll Cardiol* 1996;27:910–948, with permission.)

noncardiac surgery. The American Heart Association (AHA), in conjunction with the American College of Cardiology (ACC), and the American College of Physicians (ACP) have outlined evidence-based approaches for determining which subset of at-risk patients for cardiac events needs additional cardiac risk modification before surgery. These algorithmic outlines are fairly similar, although the ACP guidelines place much less emphasis on the functional capacity.

The AHA/ACC approach uses three key components in the patient assessment: (a) cardiac risk factors, (b) exercise capacity, and (c) surgery-specific risk. The cardiac risk factors are divided into low, intermediate, and high risk, as shown in Table 25.1. Exercise capacity is more difficult to quantify and requires careful questioning about both exercise and routine activities of daily living. Surgery-specific risk is based on very broad generalizations taken from historical data and may vary from institution to institution (Table 25.2).

■ OTHER CONSIDERATIONS

Beyond the cardiovascular assessment lies a myriad of issues in the internist's domain. These include pulmonary, renal, hematologic, and nutritional assessments. Complications are best avoided if potential problems are recognized and treated before the patient proceeds to surgery.

Another major area of attention is prevention of deep venous

thrombosis, which is a major risk after many types of surgical intervention. It is appropriate to provide recommendations for postoperative deep vein thrombosis prophylaxis, specific to the patient's concurrent illnesses, type of surgery, and risk of thrombotic event. Available treatments include early ambulation, sequential compression stockings, subcutaneous heparin, and low-molecular-weight heparin (Chapter 378).

Once care has been taken to thoroughly evaluate the patient preoperatively and to have modified any possible risk factors, it is of utmost importance to communicate directly with the surgical or anesthesia team or both. Concise, yet detailed recommendations about the patient need to be transmitted in a timely fashion, and appropriate arrangements should be made for postoperative medical care when warranted.

BIBLIOGRAPHY

American College of Cardiologists/American Heart Association Task Force Report. Guidelines for perioperative cardiovascular evaluation for noncardiac surgery. *J Am Coll Cardiol* 1996;27:910–948.

American College of Chest Physicians Fourth Consensus Conference on Antithrombotic Therapy. Antithrombotic therapy in patients with mechanical and biologic prosthetic heart valves. *Chest* 1995;108:371S.

American College of Physicians. Guidelines for assessing and managing the perioperative risk from coronary artery disease with major noncardiac surgery. *Ann Intern Med* 1997;127:309–312.

Merli G, Weitz H. *Medical management of the surgical patient,* second ed. Philadelphia: WB Saunders, 1998:109–135.

Paul S, Eagle K, Kuntz K, et al. Concordance of preoperative clinical risk with angiographic severity of coronary artery disease in patients undergoing vascular surgery. *Circulation* 1996;94:1561–1566.

Kelley's Textbook of Internal Medicine, fourth edition. Edited by H. David Humes.
Lippincott Williams & Wilkins, Philadelphia © 2000.

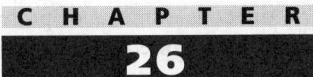

C H A P T E R

26

IMMUNIZATIONS

THEODORE C. EICKHOFF

This chapter deals with immunization of adults, including both normally immunocompetent persons and persons with depressed immunocompetence. Immunizations recommended for all persons are considered first, followed by vaccines recommended under special circumstances. Immunizations to be considered only when international travel is contemplated are discussed in Chapter 27.

■ GENERAL PRINCIPLES OF IMMUNIZATION

An up-to-date immunization history is critically important in determining the need for individual vaccines; this is just as important as any other aspect of a patient's health history and should be reviewed and updated at periodic intervals, for example, annually.

Indicated vaccines should be administered as soon as feasible. If there are contraindications, immunization may need to be deferred, or not given at all if there has been a previous significant adverse reaction to a vaccine. For example, a very small number of persons have true anaphylactic sensitivity to eggs; a number of commonly recommended vaccines, including measles, mumps, and influenza vaccines, are prepared in eggs or in chick embryo cell culture and should not be given to such persons. A significant intercurrent illness may be a sufficient reason to postpone an indicated immunization, but minor illnesses such as a "cold" or other upper respiratory illness, with or without low-grade fever, is not a significant contraindication. Similarly, a previous local reaction such as pain, tenderness, or warmth at the injection site lasting no more than several days is not a contraindication. Moreover, antimicrobial therapy, convalescence from recent illness, recent exposure to an infectious disease, household contact with a pregnant woman, and breast feeding are *not* contraindications.

The most important consideration in determining vaccine contraindication is the immunocompetence of the recipient. Fully immunocompetent persons should, with no other contraindications, receive all routine and special-purpose vaccines that may be indicated. Severely immunocompromised patients, including AIDS patients, on the other hand, should generally not be given live, attenuated vaccines, because such vaccines may pose a lethal risk. The live antigen products that are of concern are measles, mumps, rubella, oral poliomyelitis, varicella, yellow fever, BCG, and typhoid Ty21a vaccines. Killed vaccines may be safely given to such persons, of course, but the immune response may be suboptimal or negligible. Multiple repeated doses may be required to maintain some level of protection, and, with few exceptions, no direct assessments of protective efficacy are possible in immunocompromised patients. Recommendations may differ in persons with lesser degrees of immunocompromise; these issues are discussed in subsequent sections.

Manufacturer's recommendations or comprehensive guides such as the recommendations of the Advisory Committee on Immunization Practices (ACIP), those of the Centers for Disease Control and Prevention (CDC), or the American College of Physicians Guide for Adult Immunization (see bibliography) should be consulted for information on specific doses and schedules, route of administration, and possible adverse effects. Vaccine administration should be noted in the patient's record, including the dose, route of administration, manufacturer, and lot number. Significant adverse reactions that may occur after vaccination should be recorded and reported using the forms and instructions provided in the *FDA Drug Bulletin* or the *Physician's Desk Reference*.

Certain vaccines may be given combined or at the same time without any loss in immunizing effectiveness. For example, measles, mumps, and rubella vaccines are usually given simultaneously as a single product. Influenza and pneumococcal vaccines may be administered together, although at separate sites. Administration of immune globulin within the preceding 3-month interval is a relative contraindication to many live attenuated vac-

cines, because the passively administered antibody may prevent the attenuated infection that is the desired response to the vaccine. Under certain circumstances, for example, hepatitis B and rabies exposures, killed vaccine, and the corresponding hyperimmune globulin may be administered simultaneously to achieve immediate passive and prolonged active protection.

IMMUNIZATIONS ROUTINELY RECOMMENDED FOR ADULTS

The recommended overall schedule for immunization of adults is shown in Table 26.1, and vaccines recommended for routine use are shown in Table 26.2. Additional comments on each vaccine follow.

PNEUMOCOCCAL VACCINE

Pneumococcal vaccine is indicated for all persons over 65 years and for those under 65 years with certain risk factors. Such risk factors are chronic cardiac or pulmonary disease, functional or anatomical asplenia, chronic liver disease, alcoholism, and diabetes mellitus. Patients with chronic renal failure and those on dialysis, patients with hematologic malignancies, those undergoing chemotherapy for carcinoma, and organ transplant recipients are also candidates for the vaccine, but their immunologic response is likely to be diminished. Patients with HIV infection are also at risk and should be vaccinated as soon as possible after HIV seropositivity is recognized. Regardless of the age at which initially vaccinated, a second dose should be given at age 65 unless less than 6 years have elapsed since initial immunization.

Vaccine usage in the target population has been suboptimal, owing in part to concerns about efficacy. In the healthy elderly

TABLE 26.1.	RECOMMENDED IMMUNIZATION SCHEDULE FOR ADULTS
Age	**Recommended Schedule of Vaccines**
Teenagers/ young adults	Completion of all childhood primary immunizations
	Hepatitis B for those not immunized in childhood
	Td booster
	Varicella vaccine for susceptible persons
50 years	Completion of all primary immunizations
	Td booster
	Assess risk factors indicating need for pneumococcal vaccine and annual influenza vaccine
	Varicella vaccine for susceptible high-risk adults
≥65 years	Completion of all primary immunizations
	Annual influenza vaccine
	Pneumococcal vaccine

Td, tetanus–diphtheria toxoid.
(Adapted from: *Guide for adult immunization,* third ed. Philadelphia: American College of Physicians, 1994.)

TABLE 26.2.	VACCINES USED IN ROUTINE IMMUNIZATION OF ADULTS

Vaccine	Recommendation
Pneumococcal	All adults ≥65 years; all younger adults with risk factors; reimmunize at age 65 if ≥6 years has elapsed since prior immunization
Influenza	Yearly for all adults ≥65 years; all younger adults with risk factors; all health care providers; may offer to anyone who wishes to prevent infection
Hepatitis B	Sexually active young adults; high-risk groups; assess serologic response in persons ≥30 years
Measles-mumps-rubella (MMR)	Adults born after 1956 without proof of immunity or documented immunization; two doses for special risk groups
Tetanus–diphtheria toxoids (Td)	Completion of primary (3 doses) immunization, followed by either Td boosters every 10 years or single boosters at about age 15 and again about age 50
Varicella vaccine	All susceptible adults should be vaccinated

(Adapted from *Guide for adult immunization,* third ed. Philadelphia: American College of Physicians, 1994.)

person, efficacy has varied from 67% to 75% and only from 40% to 60% in persons with significant underlying disease. Recent successes with a conjugate pneumococcal vaccine formulated for pediatric use provides hope for a more immunogenic vaccine for adult use in the future.

INFLUENZA VACCINE

Risk factors that indicate the need for annual influenza vaccination before age 65 are virtually identical with those that exist for early use of pneumococcal vaccine, except for asplenia. In addition, persons providing either home care or health care for persons at increased risk for complications of influenza should be vaccinated, because such caretakers could transmit the disease to those at high risk. During epidemic years, persons who provide essential community services should also be vaccinated. It may be prudent to vaccinate immunocompromised persons as well, although efficacy is likely to be lower than in immunocompetent persons.

There have been reports of transient increases in HIV viral loads in persons with AIDS after receipt of influenza vaccine. Such increases have been found after other infections and vaccines and appear to result from a variety of antigenic stimuli. The viral load increases have been transient and not associated with adverse outcomes. For this reason, most physicians caring for AIDS patients continue to provide annual influenza vaccine.

HEPATITIS B VACCINE

The policy goal for hepatitis B vaccine in the United States is universal immunization. Special effort should be made to ensure full immunization of young people as they enter their sexually active years. Older adults at increased risk include health care workers, heterosexual persons with multiple partners, homosexual males, injecting drug users, hemophiliacs and hemodialysis patients, and those with environmental risks, such as household or sexual contacts of hepatitis B surface antigen (HBsAg) carriers, prison inmates, and others. Vaccine response decreases with advancing age, and serologic testing of high-risk individuals over 30 years of age, such as health care workers, is recommended since the protocol for postexposure prophylaxis depends on knowledge of the preexposure immune status. There is no recommendation for booster doses of hepatitis B vaccine after primary immunization in immunocompetent persons, although some health care institutions are providing booster doses to high-risk staff at 7- to 10-year intervals.

MEASLES, MUMPS, AND RUBELLA VACCINE

A two-dose schedule of measles, mumps, and rubella (MMR) vaccine has been recommended since 1989, but until the cohort of children who has already been given two doses of MMR reaches young adulthood, physicians caring for young adults should ensure that a second dose of MMR is given. Although the need for a second dose of this product has been established only for measles, in almost all cases it is simplest to use the existing MMR vaccine, because there is little price advantage to using the monovalent product and there is no adverse effect in giving MMR to persons already immune to one or more of the antigens. It is especially important to ensure that adults born in 1957 and after who may be exposed to measles have received two doses; such persons include students and teachers in educational institutions, health care workers, and travelers to areas in which measles is endemic. Adults born in 1956 and earlier may be considered immune.

Measles has been a special threat in HIV-positive patients and a cause of fatal disseminated infection in susceptible patients with AIDS. Although the data are limited, experience to date suggests that measles vaccine, given as MMR, may be administered safely to patients with asymptomatic or even symptomatic HIV infection. Individual judgment should be exercised in the case of susceptible AIDS patients with extremely low CD4 cell counts (less than 50 per cubic millimeter), depending on the likelihood of exposure. Because vaccine efficacy under such circumstances has not been established, exposed patients with CDC-defined AIDS should be given immune globulin as soon as possible after exposure, even if they have previously received two doses of MMR.

TETANUS AND DIPHTHERIA TOXOIDS

The standard recommendation, after the primary immunization series with tetanus and diphtheria (Td or DTP) has been completed, has been for a booster dose of Td at 10-year intervals throughout the balance of the adult life span. In 1994, the ACP's

Adult Immunization Task Force modified its recommendations. Booster doses every 10 years are still acceptable but may be unnecessary. Alternatively, it is recommended that once primarily immunized, a booster dose be given at adolescence (age 15) and again at age 50; further booster doses are not necessary. The ACIP, however, has not changed its recommendation for booster doses at 10-year intervals, owing to concerns about the adequacy of diphtheria immunity in light of recent outbreaks in Eastern Europe and Asia.

VARICELLA VACCINE

Varicella vaccine is a live, attenuated virus vaccine that has been approved for use since 1995. Since the disease may be severe and even life-threatening in adults, susceptible adults should be immunized. Most adults are immune as a result of childhood chickenpox infection. Adults with a reliable history of chickenpox may therefore be considered immune. Serologic testing may be cost-effective for those with an uncertain history.

The ACIP has defined several groups of adults as being at high risk of being exposed to varicella-zoster virus (VZV). These include (a) persons who live or work in environments where transmission of VZV may occur (e.g., teachers of young children, day care employees, those in institutional settings such as health care workers, college students, military personnel); (b) nonpregnant women of childbearing age; (c) adolescents and adults living in households with children; and (d) international travelers.

Although varicella is a live virus vaccine, it may be given to persons with impaired humoral immunity, but not to persons with severe cellular immunodeficiency. The vaccine has been safely given to patients with asymptomatic or mildly symptomatic HIV infection. It should not generally be given to persons with more advanced AIDS, to persons receiving immunosuppressive therapy, or to those receiving moderate or high-dose corticosteroid therapy.

In spite of years of prelicensure study, there is much yet to be learned about this vaccine and the epidemiologic consequences, if any, of its widespread use. Continuing postlicensure surveillance of varicella and herpes zoster are of critical importance. Whether administration of the vaccine to older adults will decrease the frequency or the severity of subsequent cases of herpes zoster is currently under investigation.

VACCINES FOR USE IN ADULTS UNDER SPECIAL CIRCUMSTANCES

Several vaccines are not recommended for routine use in adults, but are recommended for use in particular circumstances such as occupational risk, unusual epidemiologic circumstances, or exposures. These special-purpose vaccines are summarized in Table 26.3 and include vaccines directed against hepatitis A, poliomyelitis, rabies, meningococcal infection, Lyme disease, typhoid fever, and tuberculosis. Certain other vaccines indicated only for international travel, that is, yellow fever, cholera, plague, and Japanese encephalitis vaccines, will not be discussed further here (Chapter 27).

TABLE 26.3.	VACCINES FOR SPECIAL-PURPOSE IMMUNIZATION OF ADULTS
Vaccine	**Major Indications**
Poliomyelitis (IPV only)	Travelers to endemic/epidemic areas; persons potentially occupationally exposed
Rabies	Postexposure prophylaxis; preexposure prophylaxis for persons with high risk of exposure
Meningococcal	Travelers to endemic areas; outbreak control; consider in certain immunocompromised patients (see text)
Typhoid	Travelers to endemic areas
BCG	Limited settings with unavoidable transmission of tuberculosis (see text)
Hepatitis A	International travelers; persons with occupational or lifestyle exposures; high-risk areas or populations; consider in food handlers
Lyme disease	Persons age 15–70 at high risk of exposure

BCG, Bacille Calmette-Guérin, IPV, inactivated polio vaccine.

HEPATITIS A VACCINE

Hepatitis is an inactivated vaccine that has been approved for use since 1995. It is indicated for the following groups of persons:

- Persons traveling to or living in countries where the endemic incidence of hepatitis A is intermediate or high. In practical terms, this includes all destinations except North America, Western Europe, Japan, and Australia/New Zealand. Thus, any traveler who is a candidate for immune globulin may be considered a candidate for hepatitis A vaccine. For only a single trip of less than 3 months' duration, immune globulin prophylaxis is just as effective and at lower cost.
- Sexually active homosexual males.
- Illegal drug users.
- Persons who have occupational risks, such as workers in infected primate colonies or those working with hepatitis A virus in research settings.
- Persons in whom the consequences of hepatitis A infection might be especially adverse, such as patients with chronic liver disease, including hepatitis B or C, and persons with clotting factor disorders.

Food handlers should be considered for vaccination, depending on state and local circumstances. Restaurants and catering establishments may wish to immunize their employees. The vaccine has also proved useful in controlling several community-wide outbreaks.

Since this is an inactivated vaccine, it poses no risk for immunocompromised patients, although the immune response may be suboptimal.

POLIOMYELITIS VACCINES

Two types of polio vaccines are available: live oral polio vaccine (OPV) and inactivated polio vaccine (IPV). OPV has been until recently the most widely used product in the United States. There is an extremely low (approximately 1 out of 1 million doses) risk of paralytic disease caused by OPV; that fact, combined with the fact that the vaccine has been extremely effective in essentially eradicating natural poliomyelitis from the Western hemisphere, has resulted in the somewhat anomalous circumstance that all the paralytic poliomyelitis occurring in the United States for most of the past decade has been vaccine-induced. The ACIP is currently moving toward exclusive use of IPV in the United States.

After primary immunization has been completed, usually in childhood, the need for subsequent doses is limited to travelers to destinations where polio is occurring and to health care and virology laboratory personnel who, in the course of their occupational duties, may be exposed to wild polio virus. Given the absence of the natural disease from the United States, such circumstances are infrequent.

For primary immunization or booster doses in adults, IPV should be used exclusively. Immunocompromised persons should not be exposed to OPV or to excreted vaccine virus of OPV recipients.

RABIES VACCINE

Present rabies vaccines are inactivated products, prepared from rabies virus grown in human diploid cell culture. Recommended uses are for either preexposure or postexposure prophylaxis of rabies. Preexposure immunization should be considered for persons at high risk for exposure; such persons include veterinarians, animal handlers, those with occupations or hobbies resulting in unavoidable exposure to potentially rabid animals, and laboratory personnel working with wild rabies virus.

Postexposure prophylaxis always includes the use of rabies hyperimmune globulin in addition to the vaccine. Any decision to initiate postexposure prophylaxis should include consideration of the animal species involved, the nature of the bite or other exposure, the vaccination status of the exposed person, and the recent history of presence of rabies in the region. Local or state public health officials should always be consulted whenever questions arise about the need for rabies prophylaxis.

MENINGOCOCCAL VACCINE

The current vaccine is a quadrivalent product containing polysaccharides from serogroup A, C, Y, and W-135 meningococci. No antigen directed against serogroup B meningococci is yet available. Meningococcal vaccine is not recommended for routine use in adults, because the frequency of meningococcal infection in the United States is so low. It is recommended for the small number of high-risk persons who have terminal complement component deficiencies or are asplenic. Meningococcal vaccine is also recommended to be used for travelers to parts of the world where there is an increased frequency of meningococcal infection and for control of outbreaks caused by vaccine

serogroup strains in closed or semiclosed populations, such as those on college campuses.

LYME DISEASE VACCINE

Lyme disease vaccine is a recombinant inactivated vaccine prepared from outer surface protein A (rOspA) of *Borrelia burgdorferi*. It was approved for use in the United States in early 1999. The mechanism of action is unique in that outer surface protein A of the bacterium is expressed only in the gut of the host tick; ingested blood from an immunized human, containing antibody to OspA inactivates the spirochete before it reaches its human host. Once inside humans, OspA is no longer expressed. Thus, the vaccine acts by eliciting antibodies that kill the spirochete in the tick gut, rather than by any direct microbicidal effect within the human host.

Lyme disease vaccine is recommended for persons age 15 to 70 years who are at increased risk of exposure to Lyme disease. The population at risk is thus limited to those who reside in or visit Lyme disease endemic areas and who engage in activities that result in frequent or prolonged exposure to tick-infested areas.

Many questions remain about this vaccine, which could not be addressed in the pivotal field trials leading to licensure. These include, among others, safety and efficacy in children under 15 years of age, safety issues in those with chronic arthritis or autoimmune states, and the need for booster doses. Continuing postlicensure surveillance of the disease and further studies of vaccine are of critical importance.

TYPHOID VACCINE

The administration of typhoid vaccine is not recommended for any persons living in the United States and is generally of no use in areas of natural disaster, such as floods or earthquakes. It is indicated only for travelers who are likely to be exposed in areas of the world in which typhoid fever is endemic.

Three vaccines are available, two inactivated and one live, oral product. Since good alternatives are available, the live attenuated vaccine should not be given to immunocompromised persons.

BACILLE CALMETTE-GUÉRIN VACCINE

Recommendations for the use of Bacille Calmette-Guérin (BCG) vaccine in the United States are extremely limited, in sharp contrast to many other countries where BCG is used widely or even universally in infants. Adults in the United States for whom BCG vaccine might be considered include susceptible adults who are unavoidably exposed and identifiable populations with an excessive rate of new tuberculosis infection (more than 1% per year) that cannot be controlled by the usual public health measures.

Some hospital staff populations in the United States have qualified as having an excessive rate of new tuberculosis infection, and recent hospital outbreaks of multidrug-resistant tuberculosis in AIDS and other immunocompromised patients and hospital staff have also raised questions about a possible role for

BCG vaccine. These situations have usually been amenable to control by implementation of CDC's guidelines for prevention of tuberculosis transmission in health care settings. An expanded role for BCG vaccine, therefore, is not indicated. Furthermore, since it is a live, attenuated vaccine, it is contraindicated in all persons with AIDS as well as in other immunocompromised patients; use in asymptomatic HIV-positive patients should probably be avoided also.

BIBLIOGRAPHY

American College of Physicians and the Infectious Diseases Society of America: Task Force on Adult Immunization. *Guide for adult immunization,* third ed. Philadelphia: American College of Physicians, 1994.

Centers for Disease Control. Recommendations of the Immunization Practices Advisory Committee (ACIP). Update on adult immunization. *MMWR* 1991;40(RR-12):1–94.

Centers for Disease Control and Prevention. Recommendations of the Immunization Practices Advisory Committee (ACIP). General recommendations on immunization. *MMWR* 1994;43(RR-1):1–39.

Centers for Disease Control and Prevention. Prevention of hepatitis A through active or passive immunization. Recommendations of the Advisory Committee on Immunization Practices (ACIP). *MMWR* 1996; 45(RR-15):1–30.

Centers for Disease Control and Prevention. Prevention of varicella. Updated Recommendations of the Advisory Committee on Immunization Practices (ACIP). *MMWR* 1999;48(RR-6):1–5.

Centers for Disease Control and Prevention. Recommendations for the use of Lyme disease vaccine. Recommendations of the Advisory Committee on Immunization Practices (ACIP). *MMWR* 1999;48(RR-7):1–17.

Gardner P, Eickhoff T. Immunization in adults in the 1990s. *Curr Clin Top Infect Dis* 1995;15:271–300.

Gardner P, Schaffner W. Immunization of adults. *N Engl J Med* 1993;328: 1252–1258.

Gellin BG, Curlin GT, Rabinovich NR, LaMontagne JR. Adult immunization: principles and practice. *Adv Intern Med* 1999;44:327–352.

Kelley's Textbook of Internal Medicine, fourth edition. Edited by H. David Humes.
Lippincott Williams & Wilkins, Philadelphia © 2000.

C H A P T E R

27

INFECTIOUS DISEASE PREVENTION IN THE INTERNATIONAL TRAVELER

DAVID O. FREEDMAN

Infectious disease prevention in the international traveler should be based on risk management principles. Prevention strategies and medical interventions must be highly individualized according to both itinerary and traveler-dependent factors. The medical program for travelers to a particular country varies according to specific disease endemic zones visited within that country, urban versus rural travel, previous vaccination history, age, class of travel, duration of stay, and underlying medical history. Essentially all necessary preventive measures, aside from immunization, are behavioral and entirely within the patient's control. Unfortunately, these measures are to be initiated only much later at the destination, making clear printed instructions in lay language mandatory.

■ EPIDEMIOLOGY

Annually, 35 million people travel from industrialized to developing countries. Approximately 5% of US citizens travel by air to the developing world each year. The amount of travel to Central and South America taken together has begun to approach that to Asia. Fewer than 250,000 US citizens travel to Africa each year. A broad range of microbial pathogens present varying degrees of risk to the traveler (Fig. 27.1). Infectious agents account for significant morbidity among travelers but only for 1% of deaths.

Although it is infrequently medically serious, the most common health problem during stays in countries with poor hygiene is traveler's diarrhea. Classic *traveler's diarrhea* is usually defined as three or more unformed stools per day together with one enteric sign such abdominal cramps, fever, nausea, or vomiting. However, milder diarrheal illnesses can make a significant impact on the quality of daily life. The incidence varies from about 7% for travel to developed countries to about 20% in southern Europe, Israel, Japan, South Africa, and some Caribbean islands. In most of Asia, Latin America, Africa, and the Middle East the risk is 25% to 50% in the first 2 weeks abroad and subsides somewhat thereafter. Although there is some regional variation throughout the world, the most common causative agent of diarrhea is enterotoxigenic *Escherichia coli* (6% to 70%). Other types of *E. coli, Salmonella, Shigella,* and *Campylobacter* each account for about 5% to 15%. Parasites such as *Entamoeba histolytica, Giardia lamblia, Cryptosporidium,* and *Cyclospora* account for less than 2% each, and in adults Norwalk virus or rotavirus rarely may be detected.

About 30% of diarrheal episodes remain unexplained but many apparently are of bacterial origin, because they improve with antibacterial agents. *E. coli* and *Cyclospora* are more common during summer months, and *Campylobacter* is more common during cold months. *Campylobacter* and noncholera *Vibrios* are more common in Asia. Nonpediatric travelers showing an above-average incidence of traveler's diarrhea include those taking proton-pump inhibitor drugs (but not those on H_2 blockers), those who are naturally achlorhydric, as well as young adults between 20 and 29 years of age.

Traveler's diarrhea is usually mild and is rarely dehydrating. Only 25% of those affected have more than six bowel movements per day. Fifty percent of affected persons suffer abdominal cramps, and roughly 15% have nausea, vomiting, fever, or blood admixed in the stools. None of the clinical symptoms are pathognomonic for a specific agent. Untreated, the disease is self-limited with an average duration of 4 to 5 days. Persistent diarrhea, that is, diarrhea lasting more than 14 days, occurs in 1% to 2% of travelers and has a different spectrum of causes.

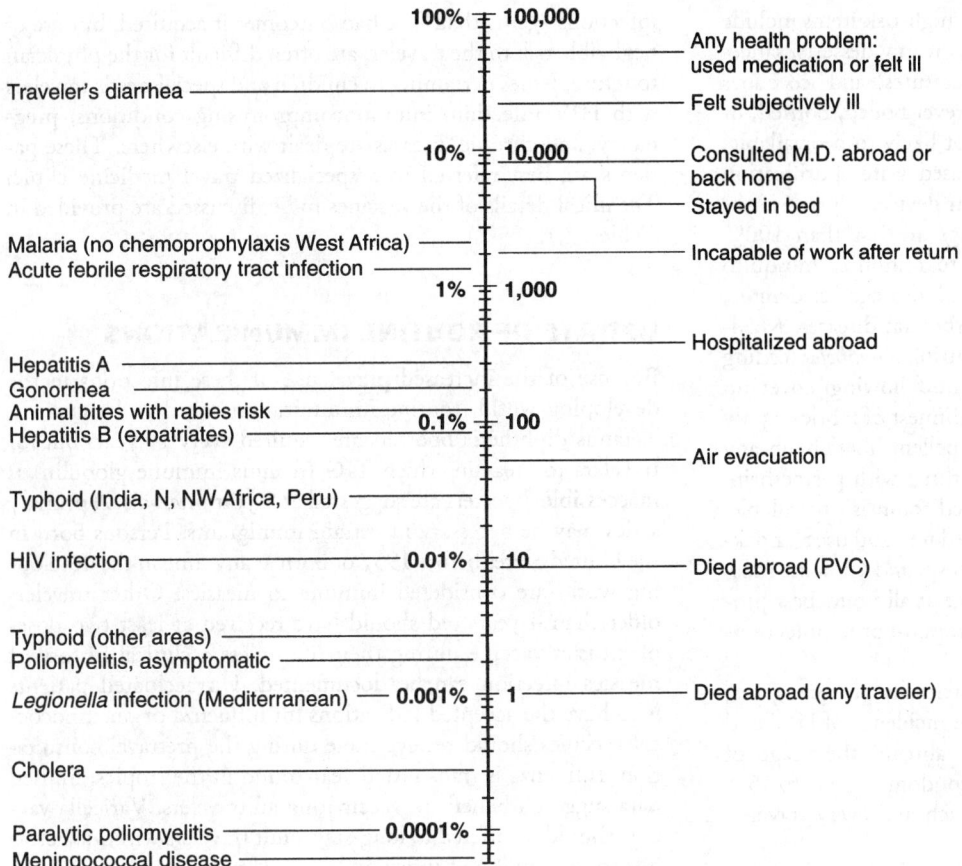

FIGURE 27.1. Incidence (rate/month) of health problems during a stay in developing countries.

Malaria is the most important life-threatening risk for travelers going to endemic areas. Two-thirds of the world's cases occur in Africa, India, Brazil, Sri Lanka, Vietnam, the Solomon Islands, and Colombia. Belize, Nicaragua, and Guatemala have the highest incidence of malaria in Central America. Falciparum malaria has had a recent upsurge in the Amazon regions of Peru, Guyana, and Bolivia. Estimates of risk in travelers not taking chemoprophylaxis vary widely by destination but range from 24 of 1,000 travelers per month in West Africa to 3.5 of 1,000 per month on the Indian subcontinent to 0.5 of 1,000 per month in South America. Most cases of imported malaria in the United States and Europe occur in noncitizen immigrants visiting friends and relatives abroad. Malaria chemoprophylactic drugs are underused by these ethnic minority travelers.

For vaccine-preventable diseases, the monthly incidence in developing countries is most significant for symptomatic hepatitis A (3 of 1,000 travelers per month). The risk of symptomatic hepatitis B is most significant for long-stay travelers and expatriates (0.25 of 1,000 per month). Typhoid fever has a risk of 0.03 per 1,000 per month, but the risk on the Indian subcontinent is ten times higher. Epidemiologic data are scant on the risk of yellow fever, meningococcal meningitis, rabies, cholera, polio, measles, and Japanese encephalitis in travelers. Imported measles occurs with some regularity in nonimmune persons. The risk of the other infections previously listed is real but apparently exceedingly small even for travel to highly endemic areas. In

1996, a fatal case of yellow fever, the first case seen in the United States in over 50 years, occurred in an unvaccinated American traveler to Brazil.

Travel is a disinhibiting experience in itself, and alcohol consumption tends to increase during travel. Between 19% and 26% of all travelers report a new sexual contact during their last trip abroad. Risk factors include younger age, business travel, trip longer than 3 months, previous visits to the same destination, and infection with a sexually transmitted disease (STD) in the past 5 years. Condom use during casual travel sex is uniformly less than 25%, even in those who had received pretravel counseling.

■ PREVENTIVE MEASURES AND RISK MANAGEMENT

The risk of travelers' diarrhea can be reduced but not eliminated by educating the traveler to avoid dietary indiscretions. Nevertheless, increasing evidence suggests surprisingly small differences in the incidence of travelers' diarrhea in persons self-reporting meticulous compared with adventurous eating habits. Less than 3% of all travelers avoid all potentially risky food and drink items. The safest foods include those served steaming hot, fruits that can be peeled, and bread. Hot soup, coffee, or tea, as well as bottled carbonated beverages (preferably multinational brands), beer, and wine are generally safe. Clearly high-risk items include undercooked shellfish and meats, salads, creamy desserts, sauces sitting for long periods at room temperatures, and ice cubes made from contaminated sources. Wherever boiled, bottled, or other safe source of drinking water is not likely to be available, travelers should carry either halogen-based water purification tablets or an iodine resin-based filtration device.

Antimalarial chemoprophylactic drugs are less than 100% effective at many destinations. Efforts to minimize mosquito bites protect not only against malaria but also against dengue, filariasis, and a number of important arboviral diseases. Maximizing personal arthropod protection during *Anopheles* feeding hours (dusk to dawn) should include the following: cover up exposed skin areas with more than the thinnest of fabrics; apply DEET (diethyltoluamide)-containing repellent liberally on any remaining exposed skin; impregnate clothing with permethrin; if an air-conditioned or carefully screened room is unavailable, sleep under a permethrin-impregnated bed net; and use a knockdown insect spray right before bed. *Aedes* sp. and Culicine mosquitoes are usually day biters, so vigilance at all hours best protects against a full spectrum of arthropod-borne infectious agents.

Avoidance of casual travel sex will maximally protect against STDs and HIV. Education regarding the incidence of HIV and STDs among professional sex workers abroad, the usage of condoms, and the failure rate of condoms (3% to 5% breakage/slippage) should be given to each and every traveler, regardless of apparent circumstances.

A predeparture dental checkup reduces the risk of oral infections during travel. A predeparture baseline tuberculin skin test with annual retesting is indicated for long-stay travelers to developing countries. Aggressive treatment of skin-test converters prevents cases of active tuberculosis later. Travelers should carry a compact medical kit. Simple first-aid supplies such as bandages, gauze, antiseptic, antibiotic ointment, and splinter forceps allow early self-treatment of minor wounds before infection ensues. Travelers should be instructed on scrupulous avoidance of recreational (swimming, rafting, wading) or other exposure to fresh water in schistosomiasis endemic areas.

A significant risk of leptospirosis exists in fresh water throughout the developing world owing to excretion of the spirochetes (which can penetrate intact skin) in the urine of rodents and other animals. Walking barefoot in tropical areas predisposes to hookworm, strongyloides, cutaneous larva migrans, and tungiasis. Scabies and lice are prevented by close attention to personal hygiene and careful laundering of clothes. In Africa, all clothes dried outdoors should be ironed to avoid cutaneous myiasis due to the tumbu fly. Long-stay travelers should plug themselves into the local expatriate medical infrastructure immediately after arrival so as to be able to rapidly seek competent care for any ensuing infectious disease early in its course.

■ IMMUNIZATION

Vaccine selection depends on risk evaluation, but travelers differ in their tolerance of risk. Requests for immunization against infectious agents that have bad outcomes if acquired, but are of negligible risk to the traveler, are often difficult for the physician to refuse. Issues pertaining to children and special needs travelers with HIV infection, immunocompromising conditions, pregnancy, and chronic diseases are dealt with elsewhere. These patients are best referred to a specialized travel medicine clinic. Technical details of the vaccines to be discussed are provided in Table 27.1.

UPDATE OF ROUTINE IMMUNIZATIONS

Because of the increased prevalence of these infections in the developing world, routine immunizations need to be current. Tetanus/diphtheria boosters are required every 10 years but for travelers to areas in which TIG (tetanus immune globulin) is inaccessible, boosters are suggested at 5-year intervals. A primary series may be necessary in certain immigrants. Persons born in the United States before 1957 or born at any time in the developing world are considered immune to measles. Other travelers older than 4 years old should have received at least two doses of measles vaccine during their life unless a clinical history of measles infection can be documented. Unvaccinated patients who have the accepted indications for influenza or pneumococcal vaccines should receive these during the pretravel consultation. Influenza is transmitted year-round in the tropics; limited data suggest a benefit to vaccinating all travelers. Varicella vaccine should be offered to long-stay adult travelers without a clear history of childhood infection.

FOR ALL DESTINATIONS IN THE DEVELOPING WORLD

Hepatitis A vaccine is indicated for every nonimmune traveler visiting a developing country. Since even postexposure vaccination has now been shown to be effective in preventing disease, concomitant immune globulin administration for imminent departures is no longer thought necessary. Short-term passive protection with intramuscular immune globulin alone is no longer recommended, and this preparation is increasingly unavailable in the United States. People born in the developing world should be considered immune to hepatitis A. Typhoid vaccine is indicated for those traveling to the developing world under all but the most deluxe and protected of conditions. In distinct contrast to the original whole cell vaccine, the newer preparations (Ty21a, ViCPS) are very well tolerated. Because of the difficulty in controlling transmission-related issues such as sexual transmission, blood transfusions, contaminated medical equipment, and sharing of cooking and bathroom facilities, hepatitis B vaccine is indicated for all long-stay persons who will be residing in endemic areas (in addition to those with the usual indications for this vaccine).

FOR CERTAIN DESTINATIONS

Certain countries in the yellow fever endemic zone (Amazon basin and sub-Saharan Africa) require vaccine certificates from

TABLE 27.1.   SYNOPSIS OF VACCINES FOR USE BY TRAVELERS

Vaccine	Route	Regimen (days)	Efficacy (%)	Effective from Day[a]	Duration of Protection
Cholera					
(WC inactivated)	ID/SC/IM	0/(−28 optional)	30–60	P6, R1	O: 6 mo, E: 3–4 mo
(CVD-103HgR)[b]	PO	0	80	P6, R1	O/E: 6 mo
(WC-BS)[b]	PO	0	80	P7, R1	O/E: 6 mo
Diphtheria	IM	0 (B)	80	15	5(−10) y
Yellow fever	SC	0	>99	P10, R1	O: 10 y, E: >15 y
Hepatitis A					
(Active)	IM	0/180–365	98	<14	10–25 y
(IG, passive)	IM	0	85	2	3–5 mo
Hepatitis B	IM	0/30/180 or 0/30/ 60/365	90	30	Unknown; boosters not recommended
Japanese encephalitis	IM	0,7,B0, or 0/7/14/ 365	90	7	1–4 y
Measles	SC	0 (B)	90	30	Usually >20 y
Meningococcal meningitis	IM	0	70–90	7	1–3 y
Poliomyelitis	PO	0 (B)	>99	30	10 y
	IM		>99	30	5(−10) y
Rabies	IM/ID	0/7/21–28	>99	7	2–3 y
Tetanus	IM	0 (B)	>99	15	10 y
Tuberculosis	ID	0	50	60	10 (?) y
Typhoid fever					
(Ty21a)	PO	0/2/4/6	55–70	15	1(−7) y
(WC inactivated)	IM	0/28	70	15	2–7 y
(Vi CPS)	IM	0	55–70	<28	2–3 y

B, if only a booster shot is needed; *E*, effectively; *ID*, intradermally; *IM*, intramuscularly; *O*, officially; *P*, primary; *PO*, orally; *R*, revaccination; *SC*, subcutaneously.
[a] If more than one dose is necessary, number of days after completion of series.
[b] Not available in the United States.

all visitors, whereas other countries, particularly in Asia and South America, require an official immunization certificate from travelers having transited endemic countries. A special permit is required to administer this vaccine. Paralytic polio is still present in some developing countries outside the Americas, where the disease has now been eradicated. Even with proper previous primary immunization against polio, a one-time adult booster of either oral (if OPV was given previously) or injectable vaccine before travel to these countries should be given. Long-stay travelers to sub-Saharan Africa, short-term travelers to areas with current epidemics, and Haj pilgrims to Saudi Arabia require meningococcal vaccine. A preexposure rabies series is indicated for long-stay travel to endemic areas of Latin America, Asia, and Africa, where the rabies threat is constant and access to adequate postexposure rabies immune globulin and vaccine is likely to be limited.

Cholera vaccination is no longer required by any country, and the risk to typical travelers is insignificant. However, aid workers staying for short periods in disaster areas or refugee camps may consider cholera vaccine. Japanese B encephalitis is endemic to certain uncommonly visited rural areas of Southeast Asia and the Indian subcontinent. Vaccination is recommended only for long-stay travel to an infected area or for short-term travel in the face of a current local epidemic. Plague, BCG, anthrax, and east European tick encephalitis vaccines are, in practice, rarely if ever, used in the United States.

Significant reactions to modern vaccines are uncommon, so that all currently indicated immunizations can and should be given at the same time and in any combination. If two live viral antigens are not administered on the same day, they must be spaced by 1 month. Immune globulin and cholera vaccine, which do have interactions with some other vaccines, are no longer in use except in unusual circumstances. There is no contraindication to athletic activity or alcohol ingestion after any vaccine. Anaphylactic egg allergy precludes administration of yellow fever, influenza, and measles, mumps, and rubella vaccines. No current vaccine contains penicillin.

CHEMOPROPHYLAXIS

No single drug provides optimal protection against malaria in all parts of the world. Chemoprophylactic drug regimens must be individualized to the person's particular itinerary, the duration of travel, medical history, access to medical care abroad, and the traveler's personal tolerance for risk. Not all regions or cities within a malarious country are malarious. In general, malaria is a rural disease, with the cities of Africa and India as exceptions. For malaria prevention, mefloquine (250 mg once weekly) is the drug of choice with two exceptions: (a) the border areas of Thailand, where, because mefloquine resistance, doxycycline (100 mg daily) is indicated; and (b) Central America, Mexico, Haiti, and the Middle East, where chloroquine (500 mg base, once weekly) is still effective. If contraindications to mefloquine exist, daily doxycycline can be used. Chloroquine-resistant *Plasmodium vivax* occurs only in areas where mefloquine is already indicated for prophylaxis because of the concomitant presence of resistant *Plasmodium falciparum*. For long-term residents, a specialized travel clinic should be consulted. Travelers need to be reminded in writing that they should continue antimalarial drugs for 4 weeks after the last possible exposure, that malaria can still occur despite chemoprophylaxis, and that a malaria smear is mandatory for any febrile illness occurring within 3 months of travel. Malaria chemoprophylaxis recommendations are liable to change periodically. Physicians may check the Centers for Disease Control and Prevention Web Page (http://www.cdc.gov/travel/malariadrugs2.htm) or call the CDC physician malaria hotline (770-488-7788) for the latest advice.

Antibiotic prophylaxis for diarrhea is contraindicated for the typical traveler because of potential adverse drug effects while away from medical care and because effective rapid-onset therapy is available for diarrhea if it occurs. However, chemoprophylaxis can be considered for travelers with HIV infection, an underlying chronic medical problem that makes them more prone to adverse consequences from diarrhea and for those on a vital mission for a short period of time (less than 1 week) who cannot tolerate even a day of disability. Bismuth subsalicylate (two tablets four times per day) during travel and for 1 to 2 days after returning may reduce the incidence of diarrhea by up to 60%, but it is inconvenient to take. Antimicrobials are more effective, but they may have significant potential toxicity and may complicate therapy if breakthrough illness occurs. One of the quinolone antibiotics is recommended. These include norfloxacin (400 mg), ciprofloxacin (500 mg), ofloxacin (300 mg), or levofloxacin (500 mg) once daily during travel and for 1 to 3 days after returning home. Antibiotic prophylaxis should be used only for trips of 2 weeks or less. For longer trips, chemoprophylaxis is not advised.

SELF-TREATMENT OF INFECTIOUS DISEASES

All travelers to the developing world should be thoroughly educated in self-therapy for diarrheal disease. All travelers should carry in their medical kit loperamide and a quinolone antibiotic. Diarrhea that does not improve quickly (within a few hours) to loperamide can be treated with a 3-day course of a quinolone (see drugs and dosages above) while loperamide therapy is continued. Eighty percent of patients respond to this regimen within 24 hours. Slower responders may continue therapy for up to 5 days.

Those with dysentery or who don't respond to 5 days of antibacterial agents should seek medical attention, if feasible. A significant increase in quinolone-resistant *Campylobacter* in Southeast Asia is emerging. Bismuth subsalicylate by itself is sometimes curative but is less effective than antibiotics. Traveler's diarrhea is not dehydrating, but those who are going to remote regions should carry packets of oral rehydration salts.

For stays in areas with very low transmission rates of malaria, some physicians, notably in Europe, may advise that only a standby drug be carried, which is to be taken if symptoms suggestive of malaria occur and if there is no access to a physician or facility that can perform a competent malaria smear within 6 to 12 hours. In areas with chloroquine-resistant *P. falciparum,* the drug of choice is mefloquine; 1,250 mg divided in two to three doses separated by an interval of 8 hours. In areas without chloroquine-resistant *P. falciparum,* chloroquine is the drug of choice. Even after a good response, the patient should consult a physician as soon as possible.

The travel medical kit may include an extended-spectrum quinolone, such as levofloxacin, or a macrolide, such as azithromycin, which will allow early self-treatment of respiratory or soft-tissue infections. Antifungal creams or powders alleviate mycotic infections prevalent in humid tropical environments. Travelers to high-risk areas should have a thermometer to document elevations in temperature to determine early the need for antimalarial or antimicrobial drugs or the need to seek medical attention.

BIBLIOGRAPHY

Centers for Disease Control and Prevention. Health information for international travel 1999. Department of Health and Human Services. Atlanta, 1999.
Dupont HL, Steffen R. *Textbook of travel medicine and health,* second ed. Hamilton, Canada: BC Decker, in press.
Freedman DO, Guest Editor. Travel medicine. *Infect Dis Clin North Am* 1998;12:2.
Steffen R, Collard F, Tornieporth N, et al. Epidemiology, etiology, and impact of traveler's diarrhea in Jamaica. *JAMA* 1999;281:811.
Steffen R, Lobel HO. Epidemiologic basis for the practice of travel medicine. *J Wilderness Med* 1994;5:56.
World Health Organization. International travel and health: vaccine requirements and health advice. Geneva: World Health Organization, 1999.

Web Sites

CDC Main Travel Health Information Page. http://www.cdc.gov/travel/index.htm.
WHO Yellow Book. http://www.who.int/ith/.
WHO Outbreak News. http://www.who.int/emc/outbreak news/index.html.
WHO Weekly Epidemiological Record. http://www.who.int/wer/.
EuroSurveillance Weekly. http://www.eurosurv.org.

CHAPTER

28

CANCER SCREENING AND EARLY DETECTION

JOHN K. GOHAGAN
BARNETT S. KRAMER
WILLIAM C. BLACK

PRINCIPLES OF CANCER SCREENING

Several methods of cancer screening have proved effective in decreasing cancer mortality. Dramatic technological advances in imaging and molecular detection during the last two decades have greatly enhanced the opportunities for cancer screening in the future. However, there is much confusion about assessing effectiveness of early detection and the net benefit of specific screening strategies. Experience has shown that arguments for earlier cancer detection based on advances in detection technologies, disease risk, or treatment advances should be treated as plausible hypotheses to be tested with scientific rigor.

Early detection of cancer does not axiomatically confer benefit and may confer harm. For early detection by screening to be appropriate, two consequent conditions must be met:

- Treatment provided at the time of screen detection must be more effective in reducing cause-specific mortality than treatment provided at the usual time of clinical diagnosis.
- The benefits of earlier treatment must outweigh the harms derivative to screening.

The first condition is very difficult to determine. Survival measured in screen detected versus clinically detected cases overestimates effectiveness. The second condition is also very difficult to determine, and the potential for harm is often not recognized by screening advocates. False-positive screening tests often lead to invasive procedures to exclude malignancy. When early detection does not change the course of the disease, the patient suffers the effects of diagnosis and treatment for a longer period of time. This latter harm is particularly relevant to the detection of premalignant lesions and carcinoma *in situ*, many of which might never have become clinically significant.

Some organizations apply categorical quality levels to sources of evidence regarding screening effectiveness. The National Cancer Institute's Physician Data Query system uses a five-level categorization, in declining order of strength, similar to the one listed below. The US Preventive Services Task Force, the Canadian Task Force on the Periodic Health Examination, and the American College of Physicians use similar rating systems.

Randomized controlled trials
Internally controlled trials without randomization (e.g., allocation by birth date)

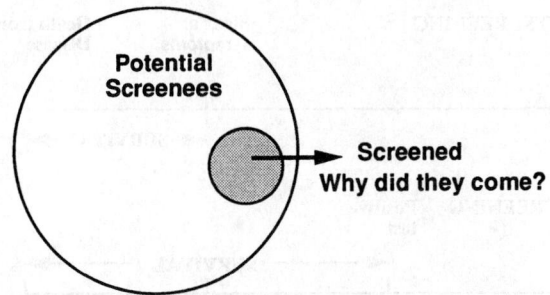

FIGURE 28.1. Selection bias results from the tendency of more health-conscious persons with mortality rates lower than expected to join screening programs. (From Kramer BK, et al. Prostate cancer screening. *Ann Intern Med* 1993;119:917, with permission.)

Cohort or case-control studies
Multiple-time series with or without intervention
Opinions of respected authorities based on clinical experience, descriptive studies, or reports of expert committees

Randomized controlled trials that correct for or eliminate several confounding biases provide the most compelling scientific evidence.

Selection bias can cause either under- or overestimation of screening effectiveness, depending on whether those at higher risk of the disease are more or less likely to undergo screening. *Lead-time bias* pertains to comparisons that are not adjusted for the timing of diagnosis. If screen-detected cases are diagnosed earlier, they will survive longer from the time of diagnosis even if their death is not delayed. *Length bias* pertains to comparisons that are not adjusted for the rate of disease progression. Cases detected by screening are more likely to be slowly progressive than those not detected by screening and ultimately presented clinically. *Overdiagnosis bias* pertains to comparisons that are not adjusted for the detection of pseudodisease, preclinical disease that would not have produced any signs or symptoms before the person would have died from other causes. Overdiagnosis bias, which can be considered an extreme form of length bias, can markedly inflate the survival and cure rates in screen-detected cases (Figs. 28.1 through 28.3).

SCREENING FOR SPECIFIC CANCERS

BREAST CANCER

In 1999, an estimated 176,300 new cases of breast cancer will be detected in the United States. Incidence increased at an annual rate of 1% between 1940 and 1980 and has been increasing at a substantially higher rate since 1980 with the widespread application of screening mammography. Recent data suggest that incidence may be leveling off. In 1999, an estimated 43,700 breast cancer deaths are projected.

Data from the world's eight randomized breast cancer screening trials were reviewed and critiqued at the National Institutes

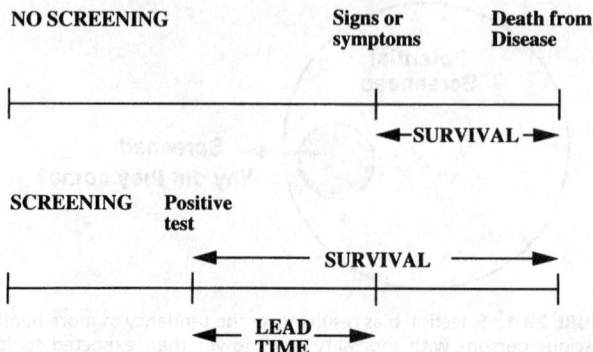

FIGURE 28.2. Lead time bias. Without screening, diagnosis occurs when clinical signs or symptoms develop. With screening, time of diagnosis is advanced by lead time provided by positive test result. If earlier diagnosis has no effect on time of death from disease, then survival with testing is equal to survival without testing plus lead time. (From Black WC, Welch HG. Screening for disease. *Am J Roentgenol* 1997; 168[1]:3–11;www.arrs/org/, with permission.)

of Health (NIH) Consensus Development Conference of January 21–23, 1997. The NIH Consensus Statement on Breast Cancer Screening for Women Ages 40–49 contained two reports. The Majority Report stated, "The Panel concludes that the data currently available do not warrant a universal recommendation for mammography for all women in their forties." Two panel members wrote a Minority Report in which they expressed an opinion that the risks of mammography were overstated by the majority and that current data supported screening mammography for all women ages 40 to 49.

One major concern of the NIH Consensus Panel was the detection of ductal carcinoma in situ (DCIS), which may progress to invasive cancer very slowly or not progress at all. DCIS constitutes about 50% of all mammographically detected

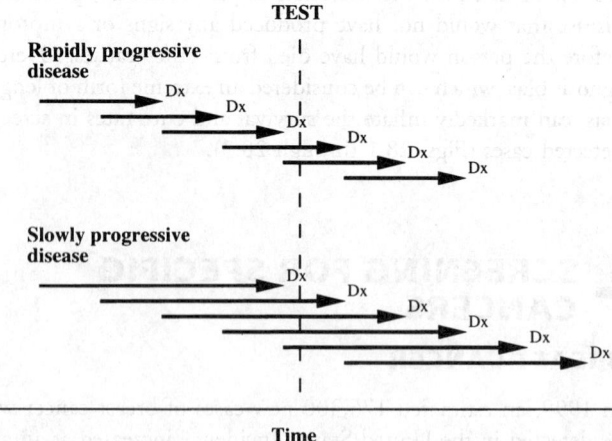

FIGURE 28.3. Length bias. Probability of detection is related to rate of disease progression. The length of each arrow represents length of detectable preclinical phase, from initial detectability to clinical diagnosis (*Dx*). Testing at a single moment in time detects four slowly progressive cases, but only two rapidly progressive cases (*bold arrows*). Cases not detected by test (*gray arrows*) are diagnosed clinically, either before or after time of testing. (From Black WC, Welch HG. Screening for disease. *Am J Roentgenol* 1997;168[1]:3–11;www.arrs/org/, with permission.)

malignancies in women 40 to 49 years of age, and the age-adjusted incidence of DCIS has increased more than threefold since 1983, along with the increased use of mammography.

Controversy continues regarding the appropriateness of periodic mammographic screening of women ages 40 to 49 years.

The Consensus Panel's report did not address the issues of screening mammography for women aged 50 and older. Previously, the National Cancer Institute's International Workshop on Screening for Breast Cancer (February 24–25, 1993) concluded that there is strong evidence from clinical trials that, "between 50 and 69 years of age, screening with mammography alone or in combination with clinical breast examination at 12- to 33-month intervals can reduce mortality by about 30%." The effectiveness of screening beyond 70 years of age is unknown.

PROSTATE CANCER

An estimated 179,300 new cases of prostate cancer and 37,000 prostate cancer-related deaths are projected for 1999 in the United States. It is projected that prostate cancer will account for 29% of all male cancers and 13% of male cancer deaths in the United States in 1999.

The rate of progression of prostate cancer is highly variable and unpredictable. Clinical prostate cancer is rare in men younger than 50 years of age, although occult cancer is common in autopsy series of men who died of causes unrelated to prostate cancer. Incidence rises rapidly after 50 years of age. Age-adjusted incidence among blacks (142.0 cases per 100,000 men) is substantially higher than among whites (108.3 cases per 100,000 men). Men with a family history of prostate cancer are thought to have an increased risk of the disease compared with men without this history.

Widespread prostate cancer screening in the United States has led to dramatic increases in prostate cancers detected in the United States compared with the United Kingdom where screening is less intense. However, prostate cancer mortality in the two countries is nearly identical.

Predictions of the effect of prostate cancer screening from mathematical models range from net benefit to net harm. Opinions based on clinical experience, descriptive studies, or reports of expert committees therefore vary from endorsement to specific recommendations against population screening. Randomized trials designed to ascertain the risk-to-benefit balance will not report results for several years.

COLORECTAL CANCER

Colorectal cancer is the second leading cause of death from cancer in the United States. Approximately 129,400 new cases and 56,600 deaths in the United States are projected for 1999. Incidence is higher among men than women. Both incidence and mortality rates in the United States are declining for reasons that may include dietary changes, improved treatment, and screening.

Screening for colorectal cancer represents a form of primary and secondary prevention, because it can lead to the identification and eradication of preneoplastic lesions such as adenomatous polyps.

Hereditary risk factors, such as familial polyposis, hereditary nonpolyposis syndrome, the cancer family syndrome (autosomal dominant), and hereditary site-specific colon cancer together may account for less than 10% of colorectal cancers. Other risk factors include a personal or first-degree family history of colorectal cancer or adenomas, inflammatory bowel disease (especially ulcerative colitis), and a personal history of ovarian, endometrial, or breast cancer. High-risk groups may account for as much as 23% of all colorectal cancers.

A large percentage of early cancers and precursor adenomas can be detected by screening asymptomatic persons older than 50 years of age using the fecal occult blood test and flexible sigmoidoscopy. It is hypothesized that removal of premalignant adenomatous polyps should decrease mortality, although direct evidence from a randomized clinical trial is not available. The discovery of polyps in the distal colon or rectum or the presence of occult blood mandates colonoscopy to search the entire colon.

Two case-control studies evaluated the association of screening sigmoidoscopy with a decrease in colorectal cancer mortality. One study evaluated rigid sigmoidoscopy; the other evaluated rigid and flexible sigmoidoscopy. Both studies suggested a significantly decreased risk (60% to 80%) of fatal cancer of the distal colon or rectum among persons with a history of one or more sigmoidoscopic examinations compared with nonscreened patients. The decrease in colorectal cancer associated with screening was restricted to cancers that occurred within the reach of a sigmoidoscope.

Several controlled clinical trials are evaluating the efficacy of screening using the fecal occult blood test (FOBT). The Minnesota trial demonstrated that annual FOBT using rehydrated samples decreased mortality from colorectal cancer by 33%; biennial FOBT yielded a 21% reduction. Randomized trials in Denmark and the United Kingdom also report mortality reductions with biennial FOBT screening.

CERVICAL CANCER

In 1999, more than 12,800 new cases of invasive cervical cancer are expected, with about 4,800 women dying of this disease. From 1950 to 1970, the incidence and mortality rates of invasive cervical cancer fell by more than 70%. Since the early 1980s, the rates for incidence and mortality appear to be decreasing more slowly. Mortality rates have actually risen slightly for young white women in recent years. A major aim of cervical cancer screening is to detect and eradicate preneoplastic lesions (carcinoma in situ), making it in large measure a primary prevention practice.

Rates for carcinoma in situ reach a peak for black and white women between 20 and 30 years of age. After the age of 25, however, the incidence of invasive cancer for black women increases rapidly with age, but it rises more slowly for white women. Mortality increases at dramatically different rates for blacks and whites with advancing age.

Substantial evidence exists from numerous observational studies that mortality from cervical cancer is reduced by screening using the Papanicolaou (Pap) test. Data from several large studies show sharp reductions in incidence and mortality rates after the initiation of organized screening programs. Mortality rates fell by 80% over 20 years in Iceland and by 50% and 34%, respectively, in Finland and Sweden. Similar reductions have been found in large populations in the United States and Canada. Reductions in incidence and mortality rates seem to be proportional to the intensity of screening efforts. However, screening every 2 to 3 years has not significantly increased the risk of invasive cervical cancer above the risk expected with annual screening. Cytologic screening of women who have not had a Pap test for several years, usually older women and often of lower socioeconomic status, offers the greatest benefit, because these women have a highest risk of dying of cervical cancer. Pap testing is of little or no value in women who have had a hysterectomy with surgical removal of the uterine cervix.

A randomized, controlled trial of Pap test screening is ruled out by falling cervical cancer mortality rates associated with widespread practice of periodic Pap testing, but the National Cancer Institute is conducting a randomized trial to determine the effectiveness of human papillomavirus testing to discriminate between low- and high-risk cervical intraepithelial lesions.

LUNG CANCER

Cancers of the lung and bronchus are expected to total 171,600 in 1999 and to account for 158,900 deaths. Prevention, especially smoking avoidance, rather than early detection is more likely to favorably affect these statistics. Four randomized lung cancer screening trials have been reported, and none shows any mortality benefit, even in a high-risk population of male smokers. The Memorial Sloan-Kettering Hospital and Johns Hopkins Hospital trials showed no benefit to the addition of sputum cytology to regular chest radiographs for evaluating male smokers. After a prevalence screen for lung cancer, the Mayo Lung Project randomized male smokers to receive regular chest radiographs plus sputum cytology versus routine medical care. However, there was substantial contamination by screening in the control group, which lowered the power of the trial to detect a benefit.

All three trials achieved a stage shift to earlier cancer detection (resulting in more thoracotomies with curative intent) in the screened arms. This was associated with longer survival after diagnosis of screened subjects but no decrease in lung cancer mortality rates. This discrepancy is probably mainly due to lead-time, length, and overdiagnosis biases. A fourth randomized trial in Czechoslovakia of semiannual screening by chest radiograph and sputum cytology versus screening at 3 year intervals also showed no mortality reduction.

However, the issue is not fully settled. Two of the trials screened both study arms with chest radiographs. None was large enough to reliably detect medically important mortality benefits of even 10% to 20%, because even the largest of the trials randomized fewer than 10,000 subjects. It is also important to see whether lung cancer screening with chest radiographs benefits women, who exhibit the most rapidly increasing rate of lung cancer in the United States. The potential for screening with spiral computed tomography and molecular marker is currently under investigation.

OTHER CANCERS

There is no information from clinical trials or even observational studies regarding mortality reduction from screening for other cancers.

ASSESSMENT OF SCREENING EFFECTIVENESS

The National Cancer Institute provides scientific statements through the Physician Data Query system on the state of knowledge regarding cancer screening. The US Agency for Health Care Policy and Research issues periodic organ-specific reviews and policy statements. Many professional organizations issue screening guidelines.

It is firmly established that screening reduces mortality from cervical cancer (Pap tests every few years), breast cancer (mammography with or without clinical breast examination every 1 to 2 years for women 50 to 69 years of age), and colon cancer (rehydrated FOBT annually after 50 years of age). Mortality benefits from flexible sigmoidoscopy (for colon), chest radiograph (lung), transvaginal sonography, and CA125 (ovary), and digital rectal examination and prostate-specific antigen (prostate) are being assessed in the US National Cancer Institute's Prostate, Lung, Colorectal, and Ovarian (PLCO) Cancer Screening Trial. Randomized trials for colon, ovary, and prostate are underway in Europe. Mammographic screening among women ages 40 to 49 years is being studied in the United Kingdom, and a multinational extension of that trial is under consideration elsewhere in Europe.

BIBLIOGRAPHY

Bond JH. Polyp guideline: diagnosis, treatment, and surveillance for patients with nonfamilial colorectal polyps. *Ann Intern Med* 1993;119: 836.

Ernster VL, Barclay J. Increases in ductal carcinoma in situ (DCIS) of the breast in relation to mammography: a dilemma. *J Natl Cancer Inst Monogr* 1997;22:151.

Fleming C, Wasson JH, Albertsen PC, et al. A decision analysis of alternative treatment strategies for clinically localized prostate cancer. *JAMA* 1993; 269:2650.

International Agency for Research on Cancer Working Group on Evaluation of Cervical Cancer Screening Programmes. Screening for squamous cervical cancer: duration of low risk after negative results of cervical cytology and its implication for screening policies. *Br Med J* 1986;293: 659.

Landis SH, Taylor M, Bolden S, Wingo PA. Cancer statistics, 1999. *CA Cancer J Clin* 1999;49:8.

Mandel JS, Church TR, Ederer F, Bond JH. Colorectal cancer mortality: effectiveness of biennial screening for fecal occult blood. *J Natl Cancer Inst* 1999;91:434.

National Institutes of Health Consensus Development Panel, National Institutes of Health Consensus Development Conference Statement: Breast Cancer Screening for Women Ages 40–49, January 21–23, 1997. *J Natl Cancer Inst Monogr* 1997;22:vii–xviii.

Newcomb PA, Norfleet RG, Storer BE, et al. Screening sigmoidoscopy and colorectal cancer mortality. *J Natl Cancer Inst* 1992;84:1572.

Selby JV, Friedman GD, Quesenberry CP, et al. A case-controlled study of screening sigmoidoscopy and mortality from colorectal cancer. *N Engl J Med* 1992;326:653.

Shibata A, Ma J, Whittemore AS. Prostate cancer incidence and mortality in the United States and the United Kingdom. *J Natl Cancer Inst* 1998; 90(16):1230.

Kelley's Textbook of Internal Medicine, fourth edition. Edited by H. David Humes. Lippincott Williams & Wilkins, Philadelphia © 2000.

CHAPTER

29

EPIDEMIOLOGY AND PREVENTION OF CARDIOVASCULAR DISEASE

LORI MOSCA

Cardiovascular disease (CVD) has remained the leading cause of death and a major cause of disability in the United States for nearly a century. Although there has been a decline in the age-adjusted death rate of coronary heart disease (CHD) and stroke exceeding 50% since 1963, there has not been a similar decrease in the actual number of deaths due to CVD relative to the expansion and aging of the US population. For example, between 1986 and 1996, the overall death rate due to CVD decreased 21.3%, with a decline in the actual number of deaths of only 2%. Among women, the absolute number of deaths has increased because more women are living to older ages, when CVD is more common (Fig. 29.1). The decline in the CVD death rate has also been less for women than men and has been smaller for blacks than whites.

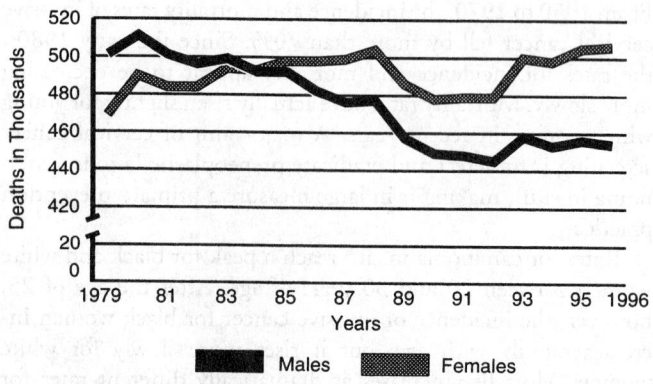

Source: CDC/NCHS and the American Heart Association.

FIGURE 29.1. Cardiovascular disease mortality trends for men and women in the United States, 1979 through 1996.

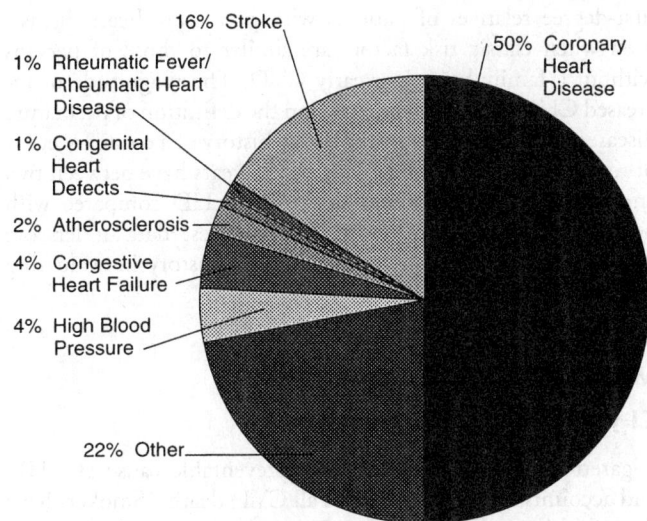

Source: CDC/NCHS and the American Heart Association.

FIGURE 29.2. Breakdown of US deaths from cardiovascular diseases in 1996.

Each year, CVD claims nearly one million lives in the United States, accounting for 40% to 45% of all deaths. This rate is more than for the next seven leading causes of death combined and translates to an average of one death every 33 seconds. Approximately one-sixth of individuals who die from CVD are under age 65 years, and one-third die before the average life expectancy. It is estimated that if CVD were eliminated, the average life expectancy would increase by almost 10 years. CVD is also an important cause of disability. It ranks first among all disease categories in number of hospital discharges. Between 1979 and 1996 there was a 25% increase in discharges from short-stay hospitals, with CVD listed as the first diagnosis. It also accounts for a significant number of physician office visits, hospital outpatient visits, and emergency room visits. According to the American Heart Association, the direct and indirect costs of CVD exceeded $250 billion in 1997. The sheer magnitude of the epidemic of CVD necessitates an emphasis on the prevention of the disease.

Several major forms of CVD, including CHD, stroke, hypertension, and lower-extremity arterial disease, are preventable and have many risk factors in common. CHD accounts for one-half of all CVD deaths and is the principal type of CVD discussed herein (Fig. 29.2). Other kinds of CVD, including rheumatic heart disease, congenital cardiovascular defects, and congestive heart failure, are discussed in subsequent chapters.

EPIDEMIOLOGY OF CORONARY HEART DISEASE

CHD is the single leading cause of death in men and women in the United States. It accounts for nearly a half million deaths each year and an estimated one of every five deaths due to any cause. Approximately every 30 seconds someone suffers a coronary event, and every minute someone dies from one. On the basis of data from the Atherosclerosis Risk in Communities studies, sponsored by the National Heart, Lung, and Blood Institute (NHLBI), it has been estimated that myocardial infarction (MI) is fatal in one-third of the more than one million Americans who experience a new or recurrent episode of MI. A significant proportion of CHD deaths occur within 1 hour of the onset of symptoms and before patients reach the hospital. Over one-half of the men and nearly two-thirds of the women who die suddenly have never had symptoms. Moreover, 80% of CHD deaths in individuals less than 65 years old occur during an initial MI, highlighting the need for prevention of the first coronary event.

The risk of a heart attack is greatest among individuals with a history of MI. Approximately 21% of men and 33% of women have a recurrent heart attack within 6 years of an MI. Of these, 7% experience sudden death, a rate four- to sixfold higher than that of the general population. Another 20% to 30% are disabled with congestive heart failure. CHD accounts for 19% of disability allowances and is the leading cause of premature, permanent disability in the US labor force. Nevertheless, nearly 90% of patients surviving an MI under age 65 years are able to return to their usual work.

Age and gender have an important influence on the occurrence and outcome of CHD. At any given age, women have a lower rate of CHD compared with men. However, because women have a greater likelihood of survival to advanced ages, the number of actual deaths due to CHD is nearly equal in men and women. The onset of CHD is delayed approximately 10 years in women compared with men. The gender gap in the incidence of CHD may reflect the protective effects of endogenous hormones in premenopausal women but is more likely explained by declining levels of testosterone with age and a corresponding slowing of CHD death rates in men. The prognosis for women with CHD is consistently worse than it is for men, and this has been attributed to increased age and severity of initial disease as well as greater comorbidity among women.

Substantial ethnic differences exist in CHD prevalence and mortality rates. The age-adjusted death rate from CHD is nearly 70% higher for black women compared with white women aged 35 to 74 years. On the basis of the NHLBI Cardiovascular Health Study, the rate of new and recurrent MIs per 1,000 people aged 65 to 74 years is 26.3 for nonblack men, 16.3 for black men, 13.3 for black women, and 7.8 for nonblack women. In another study, the prevalence of CHD in adults over the age of 20 years was 7.5% for non-Hispanic whites, 6.9% for non-Hispanic blacks, and 5.6% for Mexican Americans. Among Native Americans aged 65 to 74 years, the rate (per 1,000) of new and recurrent MIs was 25.1 for men and 9.1 for women in the NHLBI Strong Heart Study. During a 19-year follow-up of the NHLBI Honolulu Heart Program, the age-adjusted CHD mortality rate (per 1,000) for middle-aged Japanese-American men living in Hawaii declined from 4.7 to 2.9, which was similar to the decline observed for U.S. white men.

Rates of CHD vary dramatically by state, suggesting that environmental and sociocultural factors are important etiologic elements. The rates of CHD in such states as New Mexico and

Hawaii are about one-half the rates in New York and Oklahoma. Patterns of CHD also differ among nations. European countries tend to have very high rates compared with those of Asian countries and several countries along the Mediterranean. The United States is in the middle of the range. CVD (more specifically, CHD) is the leading cause of death globally, with a majority of deaths occurring in developing nations. Even among those 30 to 69 years old, CVD death exceeds the number of deaths for infectious and parasitic diseases in all populations except those in sub-Saharan Africa, where the death rates are nearly equal. As we begin the new millennium, the rising epidemic of CVD will impart a tremendous burden in terms of death, disability, and health care costs. Fortunately, a substantial proportion of CVD and CHD is preventable through risk factor avoidance and modification.

RISK ASSESSMENT

Evaluation of CHD risk involves measurement and determination of both modifiable and nonmodifiable risk factors. Epidemiologic studies have established several major modifiable risk factors for CHD, including cigarette smoking, hypertension, dyslipidemia, diabetes mellitus, obesity, sedentary lifestyle, and improper nutrition. Age, male gender, and family history of CVD are also independent risk factors, but because they are not modifiable, they are considered more important for predicting risk than for targeted risk factor management.

Data from the Framingham Heart Study have shown that the risk associated with a given risk factor varies as a function of the number and level of other concurrent risk factors. Assessment of risk can involve calculation of the relative risk and/or absolute risk associated with a given factor. The relative risk is a ratio that compares the incidence of disease in a population of individuals with a certain characteristic to a population without the characteristic and is important in understanding causal factors for CHD. Absolute risk is the probability that the disease will develop in an individual with a certain characteristic or set of characteristics during a specified time interval. Quantitative global risk assessment is useful because information about a constellation of risk factors provides better prediction than that for a single factor. Moreover, it allows for identification of a small segment of the population who will experience a large percentage of CHD events. An example of an absolute risk assessment tool derived from Framingham data is shown in Table 29.1. A related concept is attributable risk, which is derived by subtracting the incidence rate of disease in a population without the risk factor from the rate in a population with the risk factor. The attributable risk provides an estimate of how much CHD might be reduced if the risk factor were eliminated; this estimate is important for public health purposes and for prioritizing risk factors.

Assessment of family history of CHD provides valuable information for evaluating an individual's level of risk. Familial aggregation of CHD and antecedent risk factors is well established; contributing further to these risks are genetic influences and shared environmental and cultural factors. About one-half of the variability in quantitative risk factors for CHD are due to genetic factors. The risk of CHD is substantially higher among first-degree relatives of patients with premature heart disease, even when classic risk factors are similar to those of persons without a family history of early CVD. The magnitude of increased CHD risk is dependent upon the definition of premature disease. Persons with a positive family history of a coronary event or revascularization before the age of 55 years have between two and one-half and four times the risk of CHD compared with persons without such a family history. These data underscore the importance of taking a careful family history in evaluating CHD risk.

MAJOR RISK FACTORS

Cigarette Smoking

Cigarette smoking is a completely preventable cause of CHD and accounts for 30% to 40% of all CVD deaths. Smokers have a twofold increase in risk of CHD compared with nonsmokers and a two- to fourfold increase in risk of sudden death. Despite the well-established consequences of smoking, approximately 25% of adults are smokers. Smoking rates have declined 42% since 1965; however, the downward trend has leveled off, and rates are rising among adolescents. Exposure to passive smoke is also a risk factor, and 43% of American children aged 2 months to 11 years are exposed to environmental smoke in the home. Filtered or low-yield cigarettes do not eliminate risk. Cigar and pipe smoking without inhalation do not carry the same risk as cigarette smoking.

Factors proposed to explain the accelerated risk of CHD and precipitation of events among smokers include endothelial damage, dyslipidemia, elevation of blood pressure and heart rate, increased myocardial oxygen demand, reduced oxygen available to the myocardium, vasospasm, increased platelet activation, and increased reactive oxygen species. Smoking cessation has immediate benefits on the cardiovascular system, and after the initial year of cessation, risk drops dramatically. After 5 years of abstinence, risk is nearly equal to that of a nonsmoker. Counseling and nicotine replacement and other forms of pharmacotherapy should be provided in conjunction with behavioral therapy or a formal cessation program, as indicated.

Hypertension

Hypertension is considered a disease entity as well as a risk factor for CHD. High blood pressure is the most prevalent of all CVDs, afflicting 25% of adults. Hypertension is typically defined as systolic blood pressure $\geq$140 mm Hg or diastolic blood pressure $\geq$90 mm Hg or the need for treatment with antihypertensive therapy. The prevalence of high blood pressure is greater in blacks than whites. In hypertensive black men and women, 30% and 20%, respectively, of all deaths are attributable to hypertension. More men than women have high blood pressure until age 55 years, after which the rate in women exceeds that in men. After the age of 45 years, more than one-half of women have elevated blood pressure. Persons living in the southeastern United States also have a high prevalence of hypertension.

The risk of CHD and stroke increases continuously with rising systolic and diastolic blood pressure. For example, the rate

TABLE 29.1. CORONARY HEART DISEASE RISK FACTOR PREDICTION CHART[a]

Find Points for Each Risk Factor

Age (Female)				Age (Male)				HDL Cholesterol		Total Cholesterol		Systolic Blood Pressure		Other	
Age	Pts.	Age	Pts.	Age	Pts.	Age	Pts.	HDLC	Pts.	Total C	Pts.	SBP	Pts.	Other	Pts.
30	−12	47–48	5	30	−2	57–59	13	25–26	7	139–151	−3	98–104	−2	Cigarettes	4
31	−11	49–50	6	31	−1	60–61	14	27–29	6	152–166	−2	105–112	−1	Diabetic male	3
32	−9	51–52	7	32–33	0	62–64	15	30–32	5	167–182	−1	113–120	0	Diabetic female	6
33	−8	53–55	8	34	1	65–67	16	33–35	4	183–199	0	121–129	1	ECG-LVH	9
34	−6	56–60	9	35–36	2	68–70	17	36–38	3	200–219	1	130–139	2		
35	−5	61–67	10	37–38	3	71–73	18	39–42	2	220–239	2	140–149	3	Each NO response	3
36	−4	68–74	11	39	4	74	19	43–46	1	240–262	3	150–160	4		
37	−3			40–41	5			47–50	0	263–288	4	161–172	5		
38	−2			42–43	6			51–55	−1	289–315	5	173–185	6		
39	−1			44–45	7			56–60	−2	316–330	6				
40	0			46–47	8			61–66	−3						
41	1			48–49	9			67–73	−4						
42–43	2			50–51	10			74–80	−5						
44	3			52–54	11			81–87	−6						
45–46	4			55–56	12			88–96	−7						

Sum Points for All Risk Factors

_____ + _____ + _____ + _____ + _____ + _____ + _____ = _____
Age   HDLC   Total C   SBP   Smoker   Diabetes   ECG-LVH   Point Total

Look up Risk Corresponding to Point Total

Compare to Average 10-Year Risk

Probability			Probability			Probability			Probability			Probability		
Pts.	5 Yr.	10 Yr.	Pts.	5 Yr.	10 Yr.	Pts.	5 Yr.	10 Yr.	Pts.	5 Yr.	10 Yr.	Age	Women	Men
≤1	<1%	<2%	10	2%	6%	19	8%	16%	28	19%	33%	30–34	<1%	3%
2	1%	2%	11	3%	6%	20	8%	18%	29	20%	36%	35–39	<1%	5%
3	1%	2%	12	3%	7%	21	9%	19%	30	22%	38%	40–44	2%	6%
4	1%	2%	13	3%	8%	22	11%	21%	31	24%	40%	45–49	5%	10%
5	1%	3%	14	4%	9%	23	12%	23%	32	25%	42%	50–54	8%	14%
6	1%	3%	15	5%	10%	24	13%	25%				55–59	12%	16%
7	1%	4%	16	5%	12%	25	14%	27%				60–64	13%	21%
8	2%	4%	17	6%	13%	26	16%	29%				65–69	9%	30%
9	2%	5%	18	7%	14%	27	17%	31%				70–74	12%	24%

These charts were prepared with the help of William B. Kannel, M.D., Professor of Medicine and Public Health and Ralph D'Agostino, Ph.D., Head, Department of Mathematics, both at Boston University; Keaven Anderson, Ph.D., Statistician, NHLBI, Framingham Study; Daniel McGee, Ph.D., Associate Professor, University of Arizona.
[a] Subtract minus points from total.

---

of coronary events is doubled when the diastolic blood pressure is greater than 105 mm Hg. The sixth report of the Joint National Committee on Detection, Evaluation, and Treatment of High Blood Pressure (JNC VI) defines an optimal blood pressure as less than 120/80 mm Hg and provides a classification system and recommendations for follow-up based on blood pressure measurement (Table 29.2). Blood pressure is strongly influenced by genetics; however, there are many environmental and behav-ioral determinants. Important modifiable contributing factors are excess sodium intake among susceptible individuals, obesity, weight gain, alcohol intake, and sedentary lifestyle. A diet rich in fruits and vegetables has been shown to lower mild to moderately elevated blood pressure effectively.

A meta-analysis of randomized drug-treatment trials has shown a reduction of 14% in nonfatal MIs, 42% in stroke, and 21% in vascular mortality associated with antihypertensive

| TABLE 29.2. | CLASSIFICATION OF BLOOD PRESSURE FOR ADULTS AGE 18 AND OLDER[a] |

Category	Systolic (mm Hg)		Diastolic (mm Hg)	Initial Blood Pressure (mm Hg)*		Followup Recommended†
				Systolic	Diastolic	
Optimal[b]	<120	and	<80	<130	<85	Recheck in 2 years
Normal	<130	and	<85	130–139	85–89	Recheck in 1 year‡
High-normal	130–139	or	85–89	140–159	90–99	Confirm within 2 months‡
Hypertension[c]						
Stage 1	140–159	or	90–99	160–179	100–109	Evaluate or refer to source of care within 1 month
Stage 2	160–179	or	100–109			
Stage 3	≥180	or	≥110	≥180	≥110	Evaluate or refer to source of care immediately or within 1 week depending on clinical situation

[a] Not taking antihypertensive drugs and not acutely ill. When systolic and diastolic blood pressures fall into different categories, the higher category should be selected to classify individual's blood pressure status. For example, 160/92 mm Hg should be classified as stage 2 hypertension, and 174/120 mm Hg should be classified as stage 3 hypertension. Isolated systolic hypertension is defined as systolic blood pressure of 140 mm Hg or greater and diastolic blood pressure as below 90 mm Hg and staged appropriately (e.g., 170/82 mm Hg is defined as stage 2 isolated systolic hypertension). In addition to classifying stages of hypertension on the basis of average blood pressure levels, clinicians should specify presence or absence of target organ disease and additional risk factors. This specificity is important for risk classification and treatment.
[b] Optimal blood pressure with respect to cardiovascular risk is below 120/180 mm Hg. However, unusually low readings should be evaluated for clinical significance.
[c] Based on the average of two or more readings taken at each of two or more visits after an initial screening.
* If systolic and diastolic categories are different, follow recommendations for shorter time followup (e.g., 160/86 mm Hg should be evaluated or referred to source of care within 1 month).
† Modify the scheduling of followup according to reliable information about past blood pressure measurements, other cardiovascular risk factors, or target organ disease.
‡ Provide advice about lifestyle modifications (see Chapter 3).

therapy. The JNC VI recommends that drug therapy be initiated with a diuretic or β-blocker, owing to evidence from clinical trials showing a reduction in morbidity and mortality with these relatively low-cost agents. Comorbid factors, potential drug interactions, patient demographics, quality of life, cost, and compliance issues should also be taken into consideration when choosing an antihypertensive agent.

Dyslipidemia

Increased total serum cholesterol and low-density lipoprotein (LDL) cholesterol are well established causal factors in CHD. Epidemiologic studies have shown that for each 1% increase in total cholesterol, there is a 2% increase in coronary risk. Moreover, several randomized clinical trials have established conclusively that lowering LDL, whether it is high or only moderately elevated in patients with or without CHD, using statin therapy is associated with significant reductions in risk of coronary events and revascularization procedures. Other trials have used a variety of methods to lower cholesterol, including lifestyle approaches, niacin, bile acid resins, and fibric acid derivatives, and have also shown significant reductions in risk. Despite widespread knowledge about the cholesterol link to CHD, 85% of individuals with CHD and more than one-half of those with two or more risk factors for CHD are not receiving treatment or are not treated to target levels of LDL established by the National Cholesterol Education Program (NCEP) of less than 100 mg per deciliter and less than 130 mg per deciliter, respectively. The addition of drug therapy to diet therapy and exercise for the

control of LDL depends on the presence of other risk factors and the level of triglycerides (Tables 29.3 and 29.4).

High-density lipoprotein (HDL) cholesterol, which mediates reverse cholesterol transport, is significantly and inversely correlated with CHD. For each 1 mg per deciliter increase in HDL, the risk of CHD has been found to be reduced 2% to 3% in epidemiologic studies. HDL cholesterol appears to be a stronger predictor of CHD death in older (more than 65 years old) women than in older men. Prospective trials that have evaluated fibrates have found them to be most effective in subgroups of patients with low HDL in conjunction with elevated triglycerides. The value of therapy to raise isolated cases of low HDL cholesterol is not established. Weight loss, smoking cessation, exercise, alcohol, and estrogen replacement therapy have all been shown to increase HDL levels. Oral estrogen favorably affects both LDL and HDL levels; however, combination hormone replacement therapy has not been shown to lower the rate of CHD events in the Heart and Estrogen/Progestin Replacement Study (HERS), the only completed large-scale randomized clinical trial of hormone therapy for postmenopausal women to date.

The role of triglycerides in the development of CHD is not completely understood, but recent data suggest that they are an independent risk factor in both men and women. The relationship is strongest and most consistent in women and in the elderly. Reduction in fat intake (with substitution of monounsaturates and polyunsaturates for saturated fat), restriction of simple carbohydrates and alcohol, and increased physical activity can yield a considerable reduction in triglycerides. Pharmacotherapy with fibric acid derivatives, nicotinic acid, or statins may

TABLE 29.3. PRIMARY PREVENTION OF CARDIOVASCULAR DISEASES	
Risk Intervention	**Recommendations**

Smoking
  Goal: complete
    cessation
	Ask about smoking status as part of routine evaluation. Reinforce nonsmoking status.
	Strongly encourage patients and family to stop smoking.
	Provide counseling, nicotine replacement, and formal cessation programs as appropriate.

Blood pressure control
  Goal: <140/90 mm Hg
    or <130/85 mm Hg
    if heart failure,
    renal insufficiency,
    or diabetes
	Measure blood pressure in all adults at least every 2 yr.
	Promote lifestyle modification: weight control, physical activity, moderation in alcohol intake, and moderate sodium restriction.
	If blood pressure ≥140/90 mm Hg after 6 months of lifestyle modification, or if initial blood pressure >160/100 mm Hg or >130/85 mm Hg with heart failure, renal insufficiency, or diabetes, add blood pressure medication. Individualize therapy to patient's age, race, need for drugs with specific benefits, etc.

Cholesterol
  management
  Primary goal: LDL
    <160 mg/dL if 0–1
    risk factors or LDL
    <130 mg/dL if ≥2
    risk factors
  Secondary goals: HDL
    >35 mg/dL, TG <200
    mg/dL
	Ask about dietary habits as part of routine evaluation.
	Measure total and HDL cholesterol in all adults ≥20 yr old and assess positive and negative risk factors at least every 5 yr.
	For all persons: promote American Heart Association Step 1 diet (≤30% fat, <10% saturated fat, <300 mg/d cholesterol), weight control, and physical activity.
	Measure LDL if total cholesterol ≥240 mg/dL or ≥200 mg/dL with ≥2 risk factors or if HDL <35 mg/dL.

If LDL
  ≥160 mg/dL with 0–1 risk factors or
  ≥130 mg/dL on 2 occasions with ≥2 risk factors, then
  Start Step II diet (≤30% fat, <7% saturated fat, <200 mg/dL cholesterol) and weight control.
  Rule out secondary causes of high LDL (LFTs, TFTs, UA).
If LDL
  ≥160 mg/dL plus 2 risk factors or
  ≥190 mg/dL or
  ≥220 mg/dL in men <35 yr old or in premenopausal women, then consider adding drug therapy to diet therapy for LDL levels >those listed above that persist despite Step II diet.
Suggested drug therapy for high LDL levels (≥160 mg/dL) (drug selection priority modified according to TG level)

Risk factors: age (men ≥45 yr, women ≥55 yr or postmenopausal), hypertension, diabetes, smoking, HDL <35 mg/dL, family history of CHD in first-degree relatives (in male relatives <55 yr, female relatives <65 yr) HDL ≥60 mg/dL, subtract 1 risk factor from the number of positive risk factors.

TG <200 mg/dL	TG 200–400 mg/dL	Tg >400 mg/dL
Statin	Statin	Consider combined
Resin	Niacin	drug therapy
Niacin		(niacin, fibrates, statin)

HDL <35 mg/dL: Emphasize weight management and physical activity, avoidance of cigarette smoking. Niacin raises HDL. Consider niacin if patient has ≥2 risk factors and high LDL (except patients with diabetes).

If LDL goal not achieved, consider combination drug therapy.

Risk Intervention	**Recommendations**

Physical activity
  Goal: Exercise regularly
    3–4 times per week
    for 30–60 min
	Ask about physical activity status and exercise habits as part of routine evaluation.
	Encourage 30 min of vigorous dynamic exercise 3–4 times per week as well as increased physical activity in daily lifestyle activities (e.g., walking breaks at work, gardening, household work).
	Advise medically supervised programs for those with low functional capacity and/or comorbid conditions.

Weight management Goal: BMI 21–25 kg/m²	Measure patient's weight and height. BMI, and waist-to-hip ratio at each visit as part of routine evaluation. Start weight management and physical activity as appropriate. Desirable BMI range: 21–25 kg/m². Desirable waist circumference <40 inches in men and <36 inches in women.

Diabetes management
  Near normal fasting
    plasma glucose and
    near normal HbA1c
    (<7)
	Appropriate hypoglycemic therapy to achieve near-normal fasting plasma glucose as indicated by HbA1c.
	Treatment of other risks (e.g., physical activity, weight management, and blood pressure; for cholesterol management, see recommendations for patients with coronary disease in Table 1.29.4.

Estrogens	Consider estrogen replacement in all postmenopausal women, especially those with multiple CHD risk factors. Individualize recommendation according to other health risks.

TG, triglycerides; LFTs, liver function tests; TFTs, thyroid function tests; UA, uric acid; CHD, coronary heart disease; BMI, body mass index (704.5); HDL, high-density lipoprotein; LDL, low-density lipoprotein.

EVIDENCE LEVEL: A. Reference: Consensus Panel Statement. Guide to primary prevention of cardiovascular diseases. *Circulation* **1997;95:2330.**

TABLE 29.4. COMPREHENSIVE RISK REDUCTION FOR PATIENTS WITH CORONARY AND OTHER VASCULAR DISEASE

Risk Intervention	Recommendations
Smoking Goal: complete cessation	Strongly encourage patient and family to stop smoking. Provide counseling, nicotine replacement, and formal cessation programs as appropriate.
BP control Goal: <140/90 mm Hg or <130/85 mm Hg if heart failure, renal insufficiency, or diabetes	Initiate lifestyle modification—weight control, physical activity, moderation in alcohol intake, and moderate sodium restriction in all patients with blood pressure ≥130 mm Hg systolic or 85 mm Hg diastolic. Add blood pressure medication, individualized to other patient requirements and characteristics (i.e., age, race, need for drugs with specific benefits) if blood pressure is not <140 mm Hg systolic or 90 mm Hg diastolic or if blood pressure is not <130 mm Hg systolic or <85 mm Hg diastolic for individuals with heart failure, renal insufficiency, or diabetes.

Lipid management
  Primary goal: LDL <100 mg/dL
  Secondary goals: HDL >35 mg/dL, TG <200 mg/dL

Start American Heart Association Step II diet in all patients (≤30% fat, <7% saturated fat, <200 mg/d cholesterol) and promote physical activity.
Assess fasting lipid profile. In post-MI patients, lipid profile may take 4 to 6 weeks to stabilize. Add drug therapy according to the following guide.

LDL <100 md/dL	LDL 100–130 mg/dL		LDL >130 mg/dL	HDL <35 mg/dL
No drug therapy	Consider drug therapy to diet, as follows		Add drug therapy to diet, as follows	Emphasize weight management and physical activity. Advise smoking cessation.

	Suggested drug therapy		
TG <200 mg/dL Statin Resin Niacin	TG 200–400 mg/dL Statin Niacin	TG >400 mg/dL Consider combined drug therapy (niacin, fibrates, statin)	If needed to achieve LDL goals, consider niacin, statin, fibrates.

If LDL goal not achieved, consider combination drug therapy.

Risk Intervention	Recommendations
Physical activity Minimum goal: 30 min 3 to 4 times per week	Assess risk, preferably with exercise test, to guide prescription. Encourage minimum of 30–60 min of activity 3–4 times weekly (walking, jogging, cycling, or other aerobic activity) supplemented by an increase in daily lifestyle activities (e.g., walking breaks at work, gardening, household work). Maximun benefit 5 to 6 hours a week. Advise medically supervised programs for moderate- to high-risk patients.
Weight management Goal: BMI 21–25 kg/m²	Measure patient's weight and height, BMI, and waist-to-hip ratio at each visit as part of routine evaluation. Start weight management and physical activity as appropriate. Desirable BMI range: 21–25 kg/m². Desirable waist circumference <40 inches in men and <36 increase in women.
Diabetes management Near normal fasting plasma glucose and near normal HbA1c (<7)	Appropriate hypoglycemic therapy to achieve near-normal fasting plasma glucose as indicated by HbA1c. Treatment of other risks (e.g., physical activity, weight management, and blood pressure; for cholesterol management see earlier recommendations).
Antiplatelet agents/ anticoagulants	Start aspirin 80–325 mg/d if not contraindicated. Manage warfarin to international normalized ratio = 2–3.5 post-MI patients not able to take aspirin.
ACE inhibitors post-MI	Start early post-MI in stable high-risk patients (anterior MI, previous MI, Killip class II [S₃ gallop, rates, radiographic CHF]). Continue indefinitely for all with LV dysfunction (ejection fraction ≤40%) or symptoms of failure. Use as needed to manage blood pressure or symptoms in all other patients.
β-blockers	Start in high-risk post-MI patients (arrhythmia, LV dysfunction, inducible ischemia) at 5–28 days. Continue 6 mo minimum. Observe usual contraindications. Use as needed to manage angina, rhythm, or blood pressure in all other patients.
Estrogens	Estrogen replacement: individualize according to other health risks.

BP, blood pressure; BMI, body mass index; HbA1c,; LD, low-density lipoprotein; HDL, high-density lipoprotein; MI, myocardial infarction; TG, triglycerides; ACE, angiotensin-converting enzyme.

EVIDENCE LEVEL: A. Reference: Consensus Panel Statement. Preventing heart atttack and death in patients with coronary disease. *Circulation* 1995;92:2–4.

be indicated, depending on the level of triglycerides and other lipoproteins (Tables 29.3 and 29.4). Treatment of elevated triglycerides among those with a high ratio of LDL to HDL may be an effective strategy for prevention.

Diabetes Mellitus

Diabetes is associated with a three- to sevenfold increase in CHD risk in women and a two- to threefold increase in men. The difference may be due to the more deleterious effect of diabetes on lipid and blood pressure in women. Approximately two-thirds of diabetics die of heart or vascular disease. The prevalence of diabetes (fasting plasma glucose ≥126 mg per deciliter) ranges from 4.5% of non-Hispanic white women to 10.9% of Mexican American women based on data from the Third National Health and Nutrition Examination Survey. The prevalence of diabetes is extremely high among Native Americans—44% of men and 52% of women aged 45 to 74 have a history of diabetes in the Strong Heart Study. There is also a substantial proportion of unrecognized diabetes and glucose intolerance in many subpopulations.

Only 25% to 50% of the increased CHD risk associated with diabetes is accounted for by traditional risk factors, such as hypercholesterolemia, hypertension, smoking, low HDL cholesterol, and a family history of CHD. Hyperglycemia and hypertriglyceridemia are likely contributors; however, the value of aggressive management of these parameters on clinical CVD end points is not established. National guidelines suggest that the LDL target level for diabetics should be the same as that for patients with established CVD (less than 100 mg per deciliter). Niacin is an effective therapy for patients with low HDL cholesterol and elevated triglycerides, a common pattern in diabetics; however, because niacin may be associated with a worsening of glucose tolerance, statins are often the preferred therapy. Proper nutrition, weight management, and regular exercise are the mainstay of treatment for diabetics, as is control of concomitant risk factors.

Obesity

The number of men and women who are obese is substantial and on the rise. Nearly 60% of white men and 45% of white women aged 20 to 74 years are overweight [body mass index (BMI) between 25 and 30 kg per square meter], and 20% and 22.4%, respectively, are obese (BMI ≥30 kg per square meter). The prevalence of obesity is greater among blacks and is as high as 67% among Mexican Americans. There is a linear relationship between BMI and CHD. Central obesity (intra-abdominal fat) is a stronger predictor than peripherally deposited fat. Measurement of waist circumference is useful as a diagnostic aide. A substantial amount of the risk associated with obesity is mediated through high blood pressure, dyslipidemia, diabetes, and insulin resistance. Gradual (1 to 2 pounds per week) and sustained weight loss in persons whose weight exceeds the ideal for their height should be encouraged through caloric restriction and increased physical activity.

Sedentary Lifestyle

A sedentary lifestyle is associated with a doubling of CHD risk compared with a more active lifestyle, even when other factors are taken into consideration. About 25% of adults report no regular leisure-time activity. Physical inactivity is more common among women than men, greater among older than younger adults, and more prevalent among ethnic minorities and the less educated and less affluent. Physical inactivity increases the risk of high blood pressure 30% to 50%. In contrast, regular physical activity is associated with reduced cholesterol and increased HDL levels, lower triglycerides, enhanced fibrinolysis, improved insulin sensitivity, and a lower incidence of diabetes. Moreover, exercise may slow progression of atherosclerosis, improve myocardial oxygen delivery, enhance myocardial function, and reduce vulnerability to dysrhythmias.

The greatest differential in CHD risk appears to be between those who are completely sedentary and those who exercise moderately on a regular basis. Recent evidence suggests that regular activity of moderate intensity, including brisk walking, is associated with a significant reduction in CHD risk. These data support the 1995 federal exercise guidelines endorsing 30 minutes of moderately intense physical activity most days of the week, a safe and feasible strategy for most of the population. For patients who have experienced cardiovascular events or undergone revascularization procedures, participation in formal cardiac rehabilitation or a physician-guided home exercise program should be encouraged.

Dietary Factors

Diet is a major cause of CHD. Dietary intake of fat, especially saturated fat, and cholesterol is strongly correlated with cholesterol concentrations and CHD risk. Saturated fat intake is also associated with increased thrombogenicity. Intake of *trans* fatty acids has been linked to adverse lipid profiles and increased risk of CHD. Salt and alcohol intake influences blood pressure. Moderate alcohol intake (one to two glasses per day) is associated with increased HDL and reduced CHD risk, but it is not generally recommended as a prevention strategy because of the potential for abuse and increased CVD risk at higher intakes. Increased ingestion of fiber, whole grains, and fruits and vegetables is cardioprotective. Diets rich in antioxidant nutrients, such as vitamin E, asorbic acid, and beta carotene, have been associated with a reduced risk of CHD in epidemiologic studies; however, clinical trials of antioxidant supplementation have been inconsistent. The American Heart Association has recommended that total fat intake not exceed 30%, that saturated fat intake be 8% to 10% of calories, and that cholesterol intake be less than 300 mg per day. Further reductions in saturated fat and cholesterol are indicated in those with CVD or lipid disorders (Tables 29.3 and 29.4). Total dietary fiber intake should be 25 to 30 g per day, salt intake should be limited to 6 g per day, alcohol should be limited to two glasses per day (one glass for women), and five or more servings of fruits and vegetables should be consumed daily.

Pyschosocial Factors

Several psychosocial factors are associated with CHD risk, but there is a paucity of data to verify that improvements in psychosocial parameters lower risk. The type A personality is a good example, with hostility traits also emerging as a consistent factor. Social isolation and features that contribute to it, such as low education level, adverse economic circumstances, and lack of family and social networks, are associated with increased CHD risk. Depression, especially following MI, increases coronary risk. Chronic stress, particularly in situations of "high demand and low control," may double the risk of MI. Acute psychological stress may also trigger MI. Psychosocial risk factors are common and their assessment should be part of a routine screening evaluation for CHD. Intervention may improve quality of life and adherence to medical regimens and potentially lower mortality rates and recurrent CHD events.

New Risk Factors

Well over 200 risk factors have been described for CHD. Only a small fraction of them are classified as major risk factors, because they are not considered independent and causal, because they are modifiable or have a low prevalence, or because there is no reliable screening test or effective intervention. Recently, levels of small, dense LDL particles, insulin, lipoprotein(a), C-reactive protein, *Chlamydia pneumoniae* antibody titers, homocysteine, dehydroepiandrosterone sulfate, oxidative stress, fibrinogen, plasma viscosity, and a number of other thrombotic factors (plasminogen activator inhibitor type 1, tissue-type plasminogen activator antigen, von Willebrand's factor, factor VIIa) have been correlated with CHD risk. The current role of screening for these factors in practice is limited, owing to the reasons cited earlier. Moreover, the added value of measurement of new risk factors over traditional risk factors in identifying individuals at risk of CHD or in developing risk-reduction strategies is not established, but it is unlikely to be substantial. In certain clinical situations or in the case of unexplained or premature CHD, however, selective determination of novel risk factors may be useful to physicians and patients.

■ COMPREHENSIVE PREVENTIVE CARDIOLOGY

A shift in paradigms from a reactive approach to CVD and its side effects to prescribing prevention is necessary to reduce the burden of the disease. Several strategies for prevention are available to guide the physician in determining the type and aggressiveness of interventions in various patients. In healthy patients without known risk factors for CVD, an emphasis should be placed on developing and maintaining healthy lifestyle habits in an effort to prevent the evolution of such risk factors as high blood pressure and hypercholesterolemia. Primary prevention is the term applied to prevention among individuals free of clinical CVD who are susceptible to it because they have a risk factor. Lifestyle modification is also emphasized in this context, as is appropriate treatment of risk factors, especially among individuals with multiple risk factors (Table 29.3). Patients with established CVD (secondary prevention) are at greatest risk of a future event and therefore should be treated most aggressively (Table 29.4).

The risk/benefit ratio of aggressive risk factor management is most favorable among those with the highest level of baseline risk. An overlapping area of risk occurs in patients without clinical manifestations of CVD but with evidence of significant disease based on a screening procedure such as carotid ultrasound or ultrafast computed tomography scanning of the coronary arteries. Because the number of noninvasive tests to identify patients with CVD is increasing and because the predictive value of these tests is often not firmly established, interpretation of the results can present a challenge. Aggressive risk factor management has been shown to prevent the progression of atherosclerosis; therefore, it may be prudent to treat subclinical disease more aggressively than would occur in the context of primary prevention. Because one-third of coronary events are fatal, it is also important to prioritize risk factor management before an event occurs.

There is abundant evidence of missed opportunities to institute the consensus recommendations for the prevention of CVD outlined in Tables 29.3 and 29.4. National data have shown that only a small proportion of patients receive counseling about lifestyle risk factors in ambulatory care settings. As described previously, there are adverse trends in several major risk factors for CHD, and many patients are not being treated to target risk factor levels. Only a small fraction of patients who qualify for cardiac rehabilitation are referred, despite a 25% improvement in survival rates associated with participation. Cardiac rehabilitation is a key step in initiating risk factor management and restoring functional capacity after an MI or revascularization procedure. It is a model for a comprehensive prevention program, yet the reasons for its underutilization are not fully understood. Barriers to the spectrum of prevention strategies may be related to patients, physicians, the lack of organizational structure, or societal factors. Communication, training, infrastructure, and reimbursement for preventive services will undoubtedly help patients achieve risk factor targets that have been shown to reduce the burden of CVD. A multidisciplinary team approach that includes nonphysician health care providers may be an especially cost-effective approach to the prevention of CVD.

BIBLIOGRAPHY

Grundy SM, Balady GJ, Criqui MH, et al. Guide to primary prevention of cardiovascular diseases: a statement for healthcare professionals from the Task Force on Risk Reduction. *Circulation* 1997;95:2329–2331.
1999 Heart and stroke facts: statistical update. Dallas: American Heart Association, 1999.
Miller M, Vogel R. *The practice of coronary disease prevention.* Baltimore: Williams & Wilkins, 1996.
Mosca L, Grundy SM, Judelson D, et al. AHA/ACC scientific statement: guide to preventive cardiology for women. *Circulation* 1999;99:2480–2484.
Pearson TA, Criqui MH, Luepker RV, et al., eds. *Primer in preventive cardiology.* Dallas: American Heart Association, 1994.
Robinson K. *Preventive cardiology: a guide for clinical practice.* xxxxxxxx: Futura Publishing, 1998.
Sixth Report of the Joint National Committee on Prevention, Detection, Evaluation, and Treatment of High Blood Pressure. *Arch Intern Med* 1997;157:2413–2446.
Smith SC, Blair SN, Criqui MH, et al. Preventing heart attack and death in patients with coronary disease: consensus panel statement. *Circulation* 1995;92:2–4.

Summary of the second report of the National Cholesterol Education Program (NCEP) Expert Panel on Detection, Evaluation, and the Treatment of High Blood Cholesterol in Adults (Adults Treatment Panel II). *JAMA* 1996;269:3015–3023.

Twenty-seventh Bethesda Conference. Matching the intensity of risk factor management with the hazard for coronary disease events. *J Am Coll Cardiol* 1996;27(5):957–1047.

Kelley's Textbook of Internal Medicine, fourth edition. Edited by H. David Humes. Lippincott Williams & Wilkins, Philadelphia © 2000.

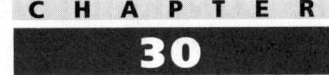

SYSTEMIC HYPERTENSION

MYRON H. WEINBERGER

The definition of hypertension depends on the levels of blood pressure that are associated with vascular damage and increased cardiovascular morbidity and mortality. Actuarial data gathered by the Metropolitan Life Insurance Company confirm the concept that the relationship between blood pressure and life expectancy is continuous rather than dichotomous. Patients with systolic pressures between 130 and 139 mm Hg or with diastolic pressures between 85 and 89 mm Hg are classified as having "high normal" blood pressure levels, since current evidence indicates that fixed hypertension is more likely to develop in these patients with the passage of time; they also have increased morbidity and mortality rates when compared with individuals with lower blood pressure levels.

CONSEQUENCES OF ELEVATED BLOOD PRESSURE

The major effects of blood pressure elevation can be separated into those resulting directly from the increased pressure (cerebral hemorrhage, retinopathy, left ventricular hypertrophy, congestive heart failure, aneurysm, and vascular rupture), those resulting from atherosclerosis (increased coronary, cerebral, and renal vascular resistance), and those resulting from decreased blood flow and ischemia (myocardial infarction, cerebral thrombosis and infarction, renal nephrosclerosis). It has even been suggested that functional cerebral damage and senile dementia may be more common in hypertensive than normotensive persons. The benefits of blood pressure reduction are most immediately observed by a reduction in pressure-related complications, such as stroke, heart failure, retinopathy, and dissecting aneurysm. Those manifestations related to atherosclerosis and ischemia may be more difficult to reverse and thus provide a compelling rationale for primary prevention or for early treatment in the asymptomatic state. Multiple risk factors exist for cardiovascular disease, such as hyperlipidemia, diabetes, cigarette smoking, and left ventricular hypertrophy, and these factors in conjunction with blood pressure have a synergistic impact.

BLOOD PRESSURE MEASUREMENT

Blood pressure is usually measured in an indirect fashion. A standard sphygmomanometer cuff is used to compress the brachial artery from outside the arm by raising pressure to levels that occlude the artery. The examiner then listens carefully as the pressure decreases until the pulse is heard (systolic pressure). Careful auscultation continues during the decline of pressure until the sound completely disappears (Korotkoff's phase V), which is the conventional definition of diastolic pressure. True intra-arterial pressure correlates more closely with the fourth Korotkoff's sound (muffling of the pulse). A rate of cuff deflation of 2 to 4 mm Hg per heartbeat is optimal. The cuff must be wide enough to occlude the artery evenly, thus avoiding the artifact frequently observed when an obese person's blood pressure is measured using a standard-sized cuff. The arm should be at the same level as the heart to avoid artifact. Discrepancies in blood pressure between the right and left arm can be seen in persons with vascular anomalies or compressive lesions involving the aortic arch or distal structures. In addition, in coarctation of the aorta the blood pressure may be substantially lower in the legs than in the arms.

With extreme rigidity of the peripheral vascular system, as is occasionally seen in elderly persons, a phenomenon known as "pseudohypertension" may occur. A marked increase in the external cuff pressure is required to occlude the sclerotic vessel. Generally, such patients have palpably sclerotic peripheral vessels, a primary systolic elevation in pressure without an increase in diastolic pressure, failure of an observable blood pressure response to adequate doses of antihypertensive agents, and, frequently, a positive Osler's maneuver. This indicates that the sclerosis of the vascular wall permits continued palpation of the radial artery after occlusion of the brachial artery by the sphygmomanometer cuff during maximum inflation.

EPIDEMIOLOGY OF HYPERTENSION

In general, elevated blood pressure is more common in industrialized societies. The reasons include variations in levels of stress, nutrient intake, obesity, exercise, and nutritional status. The strongest association between lifestyle and blood pressure is the relationship between dietary intake of sodium and blood pressure. High levels of sodium intake have not always been found to be associated with increased blood pressure, and thus a genetic or physiologic sensitivity to sodium appears to be required for the expression of the effects of sodium on blood pressure. Less consistent inverse relations between blood pressure and the intake of potassium or calcium have also been observed.

Black Americans have an incidence of hypertension approaching 40%, but the incidence among white Americans is between 15% and 20%. Blood pressure also increases with age in acculturated societies, and more than 60% of persons over age 65 in the United States have increased blood pressure. An increased incidence of hypertension is often observed in first-degree relatives of hypertensive subjects. The familial and genetic role of hypertension has been well established.

MECHANISMS FOR BLOOD PRESSURE CONTROL

It is useful to view increased blood pressure as resulting from an alteration in one or more of four major components: extracellular fluid volume, renal function, vasoactive factors and peripheral resistance, and cardiac output. The control of extracellular fluid volume is determined by the intake of sodium, the excretory efficiency of the kidneys, the activity of factors influencing sodium and water metabolism, and the capacitance of the vascular system. Some normotensive persons, such as blacks, older persons, and those with hypertensive first-degree relatives, have a reduced renal excretory capacity for sodium when challenged with an intravenous saline load, which may predispose them to the development of sodium-induced blood pressure elevation. Similarly, enhanced activity of the renin—aldosterone system or an alteration in the renal responsiveness to vasopressin or to atrial natriuretic factor may also increase sodium or water conservation in some persons. Evidence suggests that insulin resistance is common in untreated hypertensives. It has been proposed that interactions among hyperinsulinemia, sodium retention, and increased sympathetic nervous system activity may all contribute to the pathogenesis of essential hypertension.

The kidney plays a pivotal role in the pathogenesis of hypertension. A genetically mediated or acquired abnormality in renal excretion of sodium can increase extracellular fluid volume and blood pressure. The kidney is a source of the enzyme renin, which generates the potent vasoconstrictor peptide angiotensin II. Vasopressin and atrial natriuretic factor can both influence sodium and water handling and may have independent pressor effects in accelerated or malignant forms of hypertension. Other peptides, such as bradykinin and dopamine, have important renal actions that influence blood pressure by various mechanisms of action, including alterations in hemodynamics and sodium handling. The kidney contains catecholamines and adrenergic receptors that influence renal blood flow and resistance as well as sodium reabsorption in the proximal tubule and its subsequent excretion.

Central or local sympathetic nervous system activation can induce constriction and raise resistance and thus blood pressure. An interaction between angiotensin II and norepinephrine release from sympathetic neurons has been identified, and renin release can be stimulated by a β_1-adrenergic mechanism in the kidney. Although prostaglandins and the products of the kallikrein—kinin system are known to be active in promoting contraction and relaxation of vascular smooth muscle, it is likely that these substances act primarily at the local, rather than the systemic, level. Structural abnormalities, such as progressive narrowing of the vasculature or reduction of intraluminal surface area by atherosclerosis or by rarefaction of blood vessels, may also increase peripheral resistance.

Increased blood pressure affects the heart because it causes coronary artery disease by accelerating atherosclerosis, left ventricular hypertrophy, congestive heart failure, and cardiac dysrhythmias. In addition, the heart itself can raise blood pressure by amplifying cardiac output. This happens most often by virtue of an increase in heart rate, in stroke volume, or in the sympathetic responsiveness of the heart. It has also been suggested that there is a direct effect of angiotensin II in terms of increasing cardiac output.

FACTORS CONTRIBUTING TO HYPERTENSION

Current evidence suggests that genetic and environmental factors may interact to raise blood pressure. Other environmental factors, such as stress and alcohol consumption, can produce an acute transitory rise in blood pressure. Generally, the impact of stress is superimposed on a background of predisposition to hypertension and represents an exaggerated vascular response to sympathetic activation induced by stress. It is typically associated with increased cardiac output and intense vasoconstriction. Similarly, alcohol, which has a biphasic effect on blood pressure, can be viewed as producing a depressor effect when used in small doses (less than 2 oz of alcohol or its equivalent per day), which tends to induce peripheral vasodilatation and perhaps enhances the renal excretion of sodium and water. In larger amounts, alcohol acts much as stress does to enhance both sympathetic activity and cardiac output, thus raising blood pressure and increasing resistance.

EXOGENOUS PRESSOR AGENTS

Various agents can raise blood pressure and should be considered in evaluating a hypertensive patient. These include "recreational" drugs, such as amphetamines and cocaine, which can cause marked increases in sympathetic discharge, peripheral resistance, and cardiac output. Proprietary decongestant preparations, cold remedies, and appetite suppressants contain sympathomimetic agents that may raise blood pressure. Thyroid supplements, corticosteroids, and nonsteroidal anti-inflammatory drugs can all raise blood pressure or worsen existing hypertension. Oral contraceptives and conjugated estrogens used to treat menopausal symptoms or to prevent osteoporosis are also a common cause of hypertension in women. It is often necessary to withdraw these agents for 3 months or longer before their effects on blood pressure are seen. Licorice is a rare cause of volume-expansion hypertension.

SECONDARY FORMS OF HYPERTENSION

Occasionally, hypertension is caused by an underlying identifiable abnormality that, if discovered and corrected in a timely fashion, can lead to a cure of the hypertension and the prevention

TABLE 30.1. SECONDARY FORMS OF HYPERTENSION

Disorder	Approximate Incidence (%)
Renal vascular hypertension	5–10
Estrogen-induced hypertension	3–5
Primary aldosteronism	3–5
Pheochromocytoma	<1
Drug-related (corticosteroids, sympathomimetics, "recreation")	<1
Cushing's syndrome	<0.5
Hyperthyroidism	<0.5
Vasculitis	<0.5

There are no definitive studies assessing the incidence of these secondary forms of hypertension in an unselected population of representative American hypertensive subjects. These estimates of incidence are derived from relative incidence data obtained from small, selected samples.

of its side effects (Table 30.1). Clues that can identify persons in whom such a source is likely include hypertension at a young age. This is particularly true if the blood pressure elevation is moderate or severe (diastolic pressure more than 100 mm Hg). When a patient has initial symptoms of severe hypertension in an accelerated or malignant phase, it often indicates a secondary form of hypertension. When blood pressure control is difficult to achieve despite the use of appropriate combination therapy and good patient compliance, a secondary form of hypertension should be sought. When physical examination of the hypertensive patient shows severe hypertensive retinopathy with grade III (hemorrhages, exudates) or grade IV (papilledema) retinal changes, a secondary form of hypertension manifesting in a marked increase in peripheral resistance should be considered (pheochromocytoma, renal vascular hypertension).

RENAL VASCULAR HYPERTENSION

Two forms of renal vascular hypertension are commonly recognized. One form, which occurs predominantly among older persons, is due to atherosclerotic narrowing of one or both renal arteries, reducing renal perfusion. The other form, more common in young persons with hypertension, is the result of fibromuscular dysplasia of the renal arteries. This type is more common in women and is typically found on the right side.

Renal vascular hypertension decreases renal perfusion, stimulating renin release by the involved kidney and raising peripheral resistance. In addition, angiotensin II stimulates aldosterone production, promoting reabsorption of sodium and water and the consequent expansion of the extracellular fluid volume. There is probably a further enhanced effect of angiotensin II on blood pressure in the face of increased total body sodium and fluid content. Suppression of renin secretion is typically seen in the contralateral, uninvolved kidney. Thus, total renin production is at a normal or elevated level in the context of expanded extracellular fluid volume, and a new steady state results, operating

at an elevated blood pressure. The reduction in renin release by the contralateral kidney, if unaffected by the stenotic process, is a protective mechanism to prevent further excessive production of renin and reflects an appropriate response to the increase in volume and pressure.

Clues to renal vascular hypertension include grade III or IV hypertensive retinopathy and a mid-epigastric bruit with both systolic and diastolic characteristics. Some patients may have evidence of secondary aldosteronism caused by increased stimulation of the renin–aldosterone system with consequent potassium loss. Abnormalities of renal blood flow and function can be observed with rapid-sequence intravenous pyelography (films taken at 1, 2, and 3 minutes after dye injection as well as after 5 and 15 minutes) or arteriography. The more costly digital subtraction angiography, particularly if it is combined with rapid-sequence films, can provide information about the size and function of the kidney as well as a direct computer-assisted picture of the renal arteries.

The diagnosis of renal vascular hypertension depends on evidence of the functional significance of the renal arterial lesion and the consequent improvement of hypertension after repair of the obstructive lesion. The use of a competitive antagonist of angiotensin II, such as saralasin (Sarenin), and the blood pressure response to an angiotensin-converting enzyme (ACE) inhibitor that prevents the formation of angiotensin II, though helpful in identifying patients with renal vascular hypertension, are neither sensitive nor specific enough for routine screening purposes. Studies comparing the uptake and excretion of radioisotopes selectively delivered to and filtered by the kidney have been of some benefit in distinguishing renal vascular hypertension. They are generally dependent on cardiac output and can be influenced markedly by renal parenchymal disease as well as by the size of the kidneys and the magnitude of background isotopic uptake. Combining isotopic renography with administration of a short-acting ACE inhibitor (captopril) to enhance detection of significant lesions has proved to be an effective screening test.

A renal vein renin ratio of 1.5:1 or more of the involved over the uninvolved kidney or, in the case of bilateral stenosis, the more involved over the less involved side is helpful in pinpointing functionally significant lesions and predicting the benefit of intervention. More than 92% of such patients improve after effective intervention. Renal vein renin sampling is performed under stimulated conditions using both postural tilting and antihypertensive agents known to stimulate renin release (e.g., diuretics, ACE inhibitors). Furthermore, these observations require that the patient be removed from such drugs as β-adrenergic blockers and antisympathetic agents, which may lower renin production, particularly by the involved kidney. A period of 7 days or more of withdrawal of such renin-suppressing agents may be required to ensure the ability to identify a significant difference between renal vein renin concentrations.

Another valuable clue to the functional significance of a unilateral lesion is the observation that the concentration of renin in the contralateral kidney is equal to or less than that of the inferior vena cava below the level of the renal vein. This observation implies virtually complete suppression of renin release from the contralateral kidney, indicating that the involved kidney is the sole contributor of renin to the circulation. An additional advantage of performing arteriography or digital subtraction angiography before renal vein renin sampling is the identification of segmental renal vascular disease, permitting sampling of the venous drainage from the affected segment when obtaining renal venous samples for renin measurement.

ACE inhibitors, β-adrenergic blocking drugs, and calcium channel blockers have provided an effective array of antihypertensive agents with which to control blood pressure in even the most severe case of renal vascular hypertension. Several studies have suggested that antihypertensive therapy is not a desirable choice for renal vascular hypertension despite adequate blood pressure control, because of the likelihood of progression of renal impairment and the high incidence of diffuse vascular disease seen in such patients.

Various new surgical techniques have expanded the options and approaches available for the repair or reconstruction of renal arterial lesions. The less invasive, less risky angioplastic procedure would appear to be the ideal choice for the patient at relatively high risk with atherosclerotic renal vascular hypertension. Unfortunately, the results of percutaneous angioplasty in such patients have been inconsistent. The atherosclerotic lesions are often located at the ostium of the renal artery, and for this reason, attempts at balloon dilatation may simply displace the plaque into the aortic lumen and may even cause embolization of atheromatous material. Even when angioplasty has been performed successfully in atherosclerotic renal vascular lesions, the recurrence rate has been found to be very high on long-term followup.

Our observations, as well as those of others, suggest that surgical intervention is the most desirable option. Among patients with fibromuscular renal vascular hypertension—typically healthy young women—percutaneous angioplasty has been as effective as surgical intervention in repairing the lesion and improving blood pressure control. Thus, this group often can be effectively treated by percutaneous angioplasty unless fibromuscular disease is present in the segmental branches of the renal artery beyond the reach of the angioplasty catheter.

PRIMARY ALDOSTERONISM

Primary aldosteronism is less common than renal vascular hypertension. Patients with this condition often have severely elevated blood pressure. One clue that a patient may have primary aldosteronism is the relative absence of severe hypertensive retinopathy (grade III or IV) in the context of marked blood pressure elevation of substantial duration. The mechanism of action by which aldosterone induces salt and water retention involves the loss of potassium and hydrogen ions in exchange for sodium by the distal tubule of the kidney. Thus, hypokalemic alkalosis is prevalent in patients with primary aldosteronism. The presence of a normal serum potassium level does not rule out the diagnosis, however. Moreover, hypokalemia in most hypertensive patients results from diuretic therapy or secondary aldosteronism. Because of increased aldosterone production and expanded intravascular volume, there is concomitant suppression of renin production by the kidneys to limit further stimulation of unneeded aldosterone. In the context of normal renal function, therefore, plasma renin activity is markedly suppressed in pa-

tients with primary aldosteronism and cannot be stimulated into the normal range with the usual maneuvers, such as diuretic administration and upright posture.

A useful screening test is the measurement of plasma renin activity and plasma aldosterone in a random blood sample obtained when the patient is not receiving drugs known to suppress the renin–aldosterone system (e.g., β-blockers and centrally acting antisympathetic agents). If the ratio of aldosterone (in nanograms per deciliter) to renin activity (in nanograms per milliliter per 3 hours) on a numeric basis exceeds 30, the diagnosis of primary aldosteronism can be made. The measurement of aldosterone excretion in a 24-hour urine sample is an older way to identify aldosterone excess. It is necessary, however, to administer a high-sodium diet or to provide a sodium load of some sort to differentiate the inappropriate excess of aldosterone excretion in patients with primary aldosteronism from other subjects. A rapid procedure is measurement of plasma aldosterone concentration before and after intravenous administration of 2 L of normal (0.9%) saline given over a 4-hour period in the morning. Normal subjects and patients with hypertension without primary aldosteronism exhibit suppression of plasma aldosterone after intravenous sodium loading to levels of less than 10 ng per deciliter, often to levels below 5 ng per deciliter. Patients with primary aldosteronism, however, fail to suppress their plasma aldosterone levels to that degree.

Once the diagnosis of primary aldosteronism has been made by evidence of nonsuppressible aldosterone production in conjunction with renin levels that cannot be stimulated, the differentiation of unilateral from bilateral forms is required, because surgical removal is usually helpful only when the disease is unilateral. An isotopic scan using I^{131} iodocholesterol has been reported to be useful by some investigators. The benefit of this approach is that it can identify adenomas larger than 1.5 cm in diameter; however, because most tumors producing excessive amounts of aldosterone are smaller than 1 cm in diameter, this approach is not usually effective.

The most useful localizing techniques are adrenal venography and adrenal venous blood sampling during administration of adrenocorticotropic hormone (ACTH). The ratios of aldosterone to cortisol are then compared in venous blood from both adrenals and from the inferior vena cava, below the level of the adrenal veins. In normal subjects, when aldosterone is compared in blood obtained at 8 a.m., after recumbent posture, to that obtained after 4 hours of ambulation at noon, a significant increase in plasma aldosterone is seen. In patients with a unilateral source of hyperaldosteronism, typically from an adenoma, a fall in aldosterone may be seen. This may be related to the primary modulation of aldosterone production in such situations by ACTH. In normal persons as well as in persons with hypertension and in those with hyperaldosteronism due to bilateral adrenal hyperplasia, aldosterone production depends, at least in part, on angiotensin II. If the formation of angiotensin II is rapidly reduced by inhibition of ACE, this major stimulus to aldosterone production is removed, and plasma aldosterone levels decline markedly. In contrast, when primary aldosteronism results from an autonomous adrenal adenoma, the role of angiotensin II in the stimulation of aldosterone production is negligible and, therefore, administration of an ACE inhibitor has little discernible effect on aldosterone levels.

Another rare form of hyperaldosteronism is due to dexamethasone-suppressible hyperaldosteronism. This disorder is typically familial, and evidence of a hypertensive diathesis suggestive of primary aldosteronism with hypokalemia in two or more generations of the same family should be a strong clue to its presence. A trial of treatment with dexamethasone or another glucocorticoid may be useful in establishing this diagnosis. Alternatively, treatment with an aldosterone antagonist (spironolactone) or the use of thiazide diuretics with potassium-sparing components (amiloride or triamterene) may be effective in controlling blood pressure and conserving potassium in these patients. Rare causes of primary aldosteronism include adrenal carcinoma, renin-secreting tumors of the kidney, or an undifferentiated tumor producing various peptides.

PHEOCHROMOCYTOMA

Pheochromocytoma, another secondary form of hypertension, can be fatal if undetected. Hypertension results from enhanced production of catecholamines, usually norepinephrine, causing intense vasoconstriction and increased peripheral resistance in addition to stimulating the β-adrenergic receptors of the heart, intensifying cardiac output. The hypertension in patients with pheochromocytoma is usually sustained, but in 15% of cases it is intermittent. Less often, epinephrine production dominates, which allows localization of the tumor to the adrenal or the organ of Zuckerkandl. With excessive epinephrine production, orthostatic hypotension may occur. Other symptoms of pheochromocytoma include pallor, headache, and nausea. Physical findings may comprise manifestations of intense vasoconstriction, such as grade III or IV hypertensive retinopathy.

The diagnosis of pheochromocytoma depends on evidence of excessive catecholamine production, usually found by measuring the urinary excretion of catecholamines or their major metabolites. These tests can be influenced by various confounding elements. In general, all antihypertensive agents, except for centrally acting antisympathetic drugs (reserpine, clonidine, guanabenz, guanfacine, methyldopa) and ganglionic blocking agents (guanethidine, guanadrel) increase catecholamine excretion. The latter agents tend to lower sympathetic activity and excretion. If a hypertensive patient being treated with an agent that is known to increase catecholamine release is found to have normal values of catecholamines or their metabolites, it is unlikely that pheochromocytoma is present.

By obtaining urine for radioenzymatic measurement of norepinephrine during sleep, the physician can minimize the false-positive and false-negative responses that often accompany 24-hour urine collections. Using this technique, patients with pheochromocytoma can be distinguished from those with hypertension from other causes, including essential hypertension.

Plasma catecholamine levels also can be elevated in patients with hypertension due to pheochromocytoma as well as in those in whom elevated blood pressure results from sympathetic overactivity. The pharmacologic effects of centrally acting antisympathetic agents that suppress sympathetic outflow have been used to advantage in discriminating between hypertension due to

sympathetic overactivity and that due to pheochromocytoma. In normal subjects and hypertensive patients without pheochromocytoma, the administration of clonidine (0.3 mg orally) is associated with at least a 50% decline in plasma catecholamine values within 3 hours. In patients with pheochromocytoma, this degree of suppression is not seen.

Once the diagnosis of pheochromocytoma has been made, it is necessary to provide adequate α-adrenergic receptor blockade before surgery to permit reexpansion of a relatively contracted intravascular volume. It is also important to pinpoint the site of the tumor to enable the surgeon to remove it with a minimum of manipulation. Localizing the tumor is often simplified in patients with pheochromocytoma because it is usually large (more than 3 cm). By obtaining cuts at 0.5-cm increments in both adrenal areas and the organ of Zuckerkandl, computed tomography often identifies these tumors. Intravenous pyelography may find tumors in the adrenal area because of displacement of the kidney. In the case of relatively large tumors, hemorrhagic necrosis and subsequent calcification occasionally permit their identification on a plain abdominal roentgenogram. Most recently, an isotopic scanning technique using a precursor to catecholamine production, meta-iodobenzylguanidine, has been found to be useful in localizing a pheochromocytoma. During surgery, rises in blood pressure induced by anesthesia or manipulation of the tumor can be controlled by intravenous phentolamine, and cardiac dysrhythmias resulting from increased catecholamine production can be controlled by intravenous β-blockade or other antiarrhythmic agents.

CUSHING'S SYNDROME

A less common cause of secondary hypertension is Cushing's syndrome (see Chapter 407). In this condition, the adrenal gland generates excessive amounts of glucocorticoids, predominantly cortisol, either autonomously, because of the presence of an adrenal tumor (usually unilateral), or as the result of increased production of ACTH by pituitary hyperplasia or by an undifferentiated neoplasm producing ACTH-like peptides. In the latter situation, where Cushing's syndrome results from an increase in ACTH production, bilateral adrenal hyperplasia is noted. The hypertension associated with Cushing's syndrome appears to be predominantly the result of increased vasoconstriction and increased peripheral resistance, though cardiac output may also rise. Glucocorticoids can expand renin substrate concentration, thus generating higher levels of angiotensin II, which may contribute to vasoconstriction.

The patient with Cushing's syndrome usually has a characteristic appearance, including truncal obesity; a florid, round facial appearance; a "buffalo hump;" and prominent cervical fat pads. Violaceous striae, often found on the medial aspects of the thighs and knees as well as over the abdomen, also are evident. The diagnosis can be made through evidence of excessive cortisol production by measuring urinary free cortisol in a 24-hour urine sample. Urinary excretion of 17-hydroxysteroids and 17-ketosteroids are weight dependent and are substantially higher in obese persons than in those of normal body weight. Thus, when a patient suspected of having Cushing's syndrome is obese, this must be considered in interpreting 24-hour urinary excretion values. In addition, blood sampling may indicate the absence of the normal diurnal rhythmicity in plasma cortisol concentration, which typically is higher in the morning.

HYPERTHYROIDISM

Another form of secondary hypertension is due to hyperthyroidism (see Chapter 406). In this situation, increased production of thyroid hormone is associated with increased sympathetic nervous system activity, with its attendant peripheral vasoconstriction, enhanced resistance, and amplified cardiac output. The elevated blood pressure frequently resolves with effective treatment of the hyperthyroidism or administration of β-blocking drugs that reduce cardiac output.

ESTROGEN-INDUCED HYPERTENSION

Estrogens, given in the form of birth-control pills or as conjugated estrogen for menopausal symptoms or osteoporosis, can increase blood pressure. In most patients, the rise in blood pressure induced by estrogen therapy is mild and depends on the duration of therapy. In a few normotensive women, however, estrogen administration can be associated with precipitation of overt hypertension and, rarely, with more severe or accelerated forms of blood pressure elevation. Furthermore, when estrogens are given to a hypertensive woman, a further rise in blood pressure may ensue. When a hypertensive patient has a history of estrogen use, it is generally prudent to discontinue the agent and observe carefully for a decline in blood pressure. With oral contraceptives, it may take 6 to 8 weeks for maximum decline; with conjugated estrogens, many months may be required for the decrease in blood pressure to be observed.

MALIGNANT OR ACCELERATED HYPERTENSION

Although no specific numeric level of blood pressure elevation can be used to define malignant or accelerated hypertension, it is rarely encountered at levels below 160/110 mm Hg. The manifestations are directly related to the pressure-induced vascular damage of end-organ structures or to ischemic symptoms resulting from increased vascular resistance. In the brain, these may include severe headache, visual disturbances, changes in mental function or alertness, lethargy, or localizing neurologic features, such as hemiparesis or seizures. These manifestations are usually accompanied by evidence of severe central nervous system involvement by the elevated blood pressure, including grade III or IV hypertensive retinopathy, and, in particular, papilledema.

The presence of accelerated or malignant hypertension mandates rapid blood pressure reduction and simultaneous support of any end-organ dysfunction. When the affected organ is the heart, the manifestations may be acute pulmonary edema, congestive heart failure, or angina. Renal involvement with severe malignant hypertension may manifest as acute renal failure. Physical and laboratory assessments of the status of end-organ function, including chest roentgenogram, electrocardiogram, and evaluation of renal function and electrolyte status, are initiated immediately and followed by the use of antihypertensive agents that are likely to lower blood pressure rapidly and also maintain regional perfusion.

HYPERTENSION IN PREGNANCY

At least two blood pressure problems can be identified in some pregnant women. One is the situation of a hypertensive patient who becomes pregnant. Usually, the hypertension is known to be present before the pregnancy, and when the patient becomes pregnant it is often possible to reduce or eliminate antihypertensive therapy, at least during the first trimester, because of the natural decline in blood pressure that takes place early in gestation. It is desirable to discontinue medication as long as possible during pregnancy, to minimize potentially adverse effects.

Pregnancy-induced hypertension is a unique disorder. It is more common in young primigravidas, is rarely seen before the twenty-seventh week of pregnancy, and is identified by a rise in blood pressure to above 140/90 mm Hg after the twenty-seventh week of gestation in a patient known to be normotensive earlier in pregnancy and, ideally, whose normal blood pressure was documented before pregnancy. The American College of Obstetrics and Gynecology has also identified an increase in blood pressure exceeding 30/15 mm Hg after the first trimester as suggesting the diagnosis of pregnancy-induced hypertension. This syndrome is often associated with pedal edema and proteinuria during the last trimester.

The treatment strategy for hypertension in pregnancy is generally conservative. When hypertension is diagnosed, it is almost invariably the result of increased peripheral resistance and increased sympathetic nervous system activity. Therefore, drugs effective in altering these abnormalities are preferred. In the past, direct-acting vasodilating agents, such as hydralazine, were frequently used. Centrally acting antisympathetic drugs, such as clonidine, guanabenz, and methyldopa, and β-adrenergic blocking drugs have also been used. However, β-blockers can have an effect on labor and can induce fetal and neonatal bradycardia; thus, when β-blockers are used, short-acting agents are preferred and should be eliminated during labor and delivery. The α-blockers (prazosin, terazosin, doxazosin) are also useful in the treatment of pregnancy-related hypertension. The safety and efficacy of calcium channel blockers in the treatment of hypertension in pregnancy has not been established. ACE inhibitors and angiotensin receptor blockers are contraindicated in pregnant women.

After delivery, the elevated blood pressure often declines, and a marked natriuresis is noted. On occasion, blood pressure remains elevated, and there may be no postpartum increase in sodium and water excretion unless diuretics are given. Occasionally, hypertension may occur de novo within 24 hours of delivery; it requires prompt recognition and treatment. Because labor and the fetal effects of drugs are no longer an issue after delivery, the choice of antihypertensive agents is wider, unless the mother is breast-feeding. Rarely, blood pressure elevation is very severe or cannot be adequately controlled with medications, and symptoms of increased neuromuscular irritability may ensue. In these situations, multiple drug therapy for the blood pressure elevation, combining such agents as α-blockers, centrally acting anti-sympathetic drugs, and β-blockers, may be required. Magnesium sulfate given by intramuscular injection is also effective in minimizing the neuromuscular symptoms.

HYPERTENSION AND CONGESTIVE HEART FAILURE

Hypertension and its cardiac side effects, which include left ventricular hypertrophy, are major contributing factors to the development of congestive heart failure (see Chapter 66). The increases in peripheral resistance and extracellular fluid volume often associated with hypertension also are factors aggravating congestive heart failure.

The current approach to the treatment of hypertension and heart failure is to use modest doses of agents that attack both volume and resistance and, preferably, to use indirect-acting vasodilators that reduce preload and afterload. Included in this category are ACE inhibitors, α-adrenergic blocking drugs, β-blockers, angiotensin receptor blockers (ARBs), and long-acting calcium channel blockers. ACE inhibitors can reduce peripheral resistance, limit expansion of intravascular volume, and increase renal blood flow and renal function. When using ACE inhibitors in patients with hypertension and heart failure who are also undergoing diuretic therapy, it is prudent to use a small dose to initiate therapy (see Chapter 66).

HYPERTENSION AND RENAL FAILURE

When choosing drugs to use in the treatment of hypertension associated with renal failure, consideration must be given to the agent's efficacy in the face of impaired kidney function and to the impact of kidney function on its excretion and metabolism. When renal function is impaired, the traditional thiazide diuretics are often ineffective, and loop diuretics must be used. Sometimes these agents alone are inadequate to promote diuresis and natriuresis, and combinations of furosemide and metolazone may be more effective. When there is renal impairment, potassium excretion may also be affected. Thus, serum potassium levels must be monitored carefully, particularly when potassium-sparing agents, potassium supplements, or ACE inhibitors are given.

Many antihypertensive agents can have an adverse impact on renal function, so they should be used cautiously in patients with renal impairment. Some β-adrenergic blocking drugs (propranolol, timolol) not only lower cardiac output, thereby reducing renal blood flow, but may also increase renal vascular resistance. However, nadolol has been shown to enhance renal blood flow and thus may be a safe and effective β-blocker in patients with impaired renal function. Because nadolol is highly water soluble and has a long duration of action, and because the primary route of excretion is renal, it may be necessary to reduce the dose or the frequency of administration of the drug in patients with impaired kidney function.

The centrally acting antisympathetic agents, such as reserpine, methyldopa, clonidine, and guanabenz, do not appear to have adverse effects on renal function, so they can be safely used in patients with renal impairment. Direct-acting vasodilators, such as hydralazine and minoxidil, because of their reflex sympathetic stimulation, may lead to a further increase in renal vascular resistance and a decrease in renal function. This is particularly likely to occur when β-blockers are combined with these agents to enhance blood pressure reduction and to blunt the effects of reflex sympathetic discharge on the heart. Sometimes only such agents as minoxidil are effective in hypertensive patients with renal failure, however; in such cases these agents may be required. The indirect-acting vasodilators, including α-blockers, ACE inhibitors, ARBs, and calcium channel blockers, appear to have a similar beneficial effect on blood pressure and renal function and for this reason are good drugs to use when hypertension is associated with renal impairment.

Hypertension and impaired renal function may be associated with diabetic nephropathy. ACE inhibitors and ARBs, which provide balanced glomerular arteriolar dilatation, appear to be helpful in reducing proteinuria and in limiting the rate of progression of renal impairment. When hypertension and renal impairment are caused by bilateral renal vascular hypertension or by renal vascular hypertension in a solitary functioning kidney, however, the use of ACE inhibitors or ARBs may not be wise because of adverse effects on renal function. In patients with renal impairment associated with collagen vascular disorders (systemic lupus erythematosus, scleroderma, periarteritis nodosa), administration of ACE inhibitors may result in hematologic abnormalities.

HYPERTENSION AND DIABETES

Hypertension and diabetes are both common chronic disorders, but they coexist with a greater frequency than would be predicted from the prevalence of either alone, and they may be pathogenetically related. Hypertension that develops in a previously normotensive diabetic patient is usually associated with a reduction in renal function. Recent observations suggest that hyperinsulinemia and insulin resistance producing carbohydrate intolerance may be pathogenetic features of essential hypertension. Diabetes may also develop in hypertensive patients as a manifestation of diuretic-induced hyperglycemia, perhaps related to potassium loss. The diuretic-associated hyperglycemia and alterations in carbohydrate tolerance can often be corrected by restoring serum potassium levels to normal.

The diagnosis of therapy-related hyperglycemia and diabetes should be suspected when an elevated blood glucose level is encountered in a hypertensive patient receiving diuretic therapy who also manifests hypokalemia. If renal function is normal, it is appropriate to institute a trial of potassium-sparing diuretic agents and reevaluate carbohydrate tolerance after hypokalemia has been corrected. In many of these patients, hyperglycemia remits when the potassium level returns to normal. Hyperglycemia also can be a manifestation of a secondary form of hypertension associated with impairment of carbohydrate tolerance, such as in primary aldosteronism, where the carbohydrate intolerance is often responsive to restoration of normal potassium levels. Hyperglycemia also can be a feature of pheochromocytoma and Cushing's syndrome. Diuretics and β-blockers reduce insulin sensitivity; α-blockers and ACE inhibitors improve it. If the blood glucose abnormality is not corrected after the potassium balance is restored to normal, and if the patient has no evidence of one of the secondary forms of hypertension occasionally associated with hyperglycemia, treatment of carbohydrate intolerance is justified.

If the serum creatinine value is less than 1.8 mg per deciliter, the thiazide diuretics are usually effective and are reasonable initial therapeutic choices. When renal function is more markedly impaired, the use of loop diuretics is often required. Because of carbohydrate intolerance, it is important to avoid hypokalemia when giving diuretics. If renal impairment is severe, potassium loss is often not observed with thiazide or loop diuretics. Furthermore, there is a risk of hyperkalemia with potassium supplementation, potassium-sparing agents, and ACE inhibitors in diabetics with renal impairment, particularly in older subjects with hyporeninemic hypoaldosteronism. Therapy in hypertensive diabetics should thus be initiated with small doses of thiazide or loop agents, and serum potassium levels should be monitored carefully, with supplementation or potassium-sparing agents added only when indicated. This is particularly important when ACE inhibitors are used. Diabetic hypertensive patients often also respond to vasodilators of the indirect-acting category, including α-adrenergic blocking drugs, ACE inhibitors, and calcium channel entry blockers. These agents appear not to have deleterious effects on blood glucose in diabetic subjects and may improve insulin sensitivity. Centrally acting antisympathetic agents also may be used in diabetic hypertensive patients; however, β-adrenergic blocking drugs are generally ineffective and often are relatively contraindicated, particularly in diabetics who require insulin. Recent evidence supports reduction of blood pressure to levels $\leq 130/85$ in diabetic subjects for preservation of renal function.

PREVENTION

Patients known to be at high risk of hypertension because of a high-normal blood pressure, a parental history of blood pressure elevation, black race, or elderly age may be able to reduce the likelihood of hypertension by adopting nutritional and behavioral habits to modify factors known to interact with the predisposition to hypertension. These habits include lowering sodium intake to less than 100 mEq of sodium (2.3 g) per day, adopting a diet low in sodium and high in fruits, vegetables, and low-fat dairy products, losing weight by caloric restriction and a systematic moderate exercise program, restricting alcohol intake to no more than 2 oz per day, quitting cigarette smoking, and avoiding foods high in saturated fat. Increased calcium intake may be of benefit in some susceptible patients: it appears to lower blood pressure in subgroups of normotensive and hypertensive patients. The benefit of increased potassium intake is less well established, but it seems to reduce cerebrovascular disease in hypertension and thus can be recommended as long as the potassium intake is not superimposed on a background of renal impairment that could precipitate dangerous hyperkalemia. The major difficulty with lifestyle modification is in ensuring long-term compliance.

MANAGEMENT

When hypertension is present and no immediate cause is found, the diagnosis of primary or essential hypertension is usually assumed. As previously described, genetic and environmental factors can contribute to blood pressure elevation; there is often a family history of hypertension. Primary hypertension typically begins with a subtle rise in blood pressure in the thirties and forties, progressing to definite and sustained blood pressure elevation in the fifties and older. The most recent recommendations by the Joint National Committee on High Blood Pressure are to use nonpharmacologic interventions when blood pressure reaches a persistent level of 140 mm Hg systolic or 85 mm Hg diastolic or higher. Nondrug therapy (weight loss, reduction of sodium and alcohol intake) is often used for mildly hypertensive patients (90 to 95 mm Hg) as sole therapy in the absence of target-organ disease, concurrent cardiovascular disease, or diabetes mellitus.

BIOFEEDBACK AND OTHER BEHAVIORAL MODIFICATION TECHNIQUES

Studies examining the usefulness of behavioral modification techniques, ranging from transcendental meditation to biofeedback, on blood pressure have verified that relaxation and stress avoidance can be associated with blood pressure reduction in both normotensive persons and hypertensive patients who are successful in achieving these goals. These techniques, which require active conditioning, are often ineffective in maintaining a lower blood pressure level when the patient is busily involved in his or her daily routine, however. There appears to be no holdover effect on blood pressure when these techniques are not being actively applied.

PHARMACOLOGIC THERAPY

Many antihypertensive drugs are available for the treatment of hypertension, and they can be conveniently separated into three general categories on the basis of their mechanism of action: diuretics, antisympathetic agents, and vasodilators.

Diuretics

The short-acting diuretics (furosemide, ethacrynic acid, bumetanide) all act primarily on the loop of Henle of the renal tubule. Their brief duration of action makes them generally unsuitable for routine use in uncomplicated cases of hypertension, because they must be given frequently (three or four times a day) to achieve adequate blood pressure control over a 24-hour period. Torsemide, a long-acting loop diuretic, is an exception. The loop diuretics are generally reserved for use in patients with acute pulmonary edema, congestive heart failure, malignant or accelerated hypertension, or renal failure. For most uncomplicated cases of hypertension requiring diuretic therapy, hydrochlorothiazide can be given once a day because of its 10- to 14-hour duration of action.

Diuretics lower blood pressure primarily by reducing extracellular fluid volume, at the expense of stimulating sympathetic activity and renin activity, increasing heart rate, inducing peripheral and regional vasoconstriction, and increasing vascular resistance as well as raising blood viscosity. In addition, diuretics generally promote potassium and magnesium loss, increasing the risk for ventricular dysrhythmias and sudden death. Furthermore, they increase blood glucose and uric acid levels, catecholamine release, and cholesterol levels (particularly the low-density lipoprotein fraction and triglycerides). All these metabolic changes, which are significant and persist for the duration of diuretic therapy, may increase the risk of coronary artery disease. Long-acting diuretics (chlorthalidone, metolazone, indapamide) have a duration of action of 18 to 30 hours. They often cause nocturia, which may be a cause of noncompliance. In addition, they promote prolonged sodium-for-potassium exchange, causing greater potassium loss for an equivalent pressure-lowering effect than do the intermediate-acting thiazide diuretics.

Potassium-sparing agents (spironolactone, triamterene, amiloride) are generally ineffective in reducing blood pressure when given alone; they usually are administered in combination with thiazide diuretics. Diuretics can be associated with impotence in men, and this appears to be more common with Aldactazide (a combination of spironolactone and hydrochlorothiazide) than with the other potassium-sparing/thiazide combinations. The duration of action of spironolactone and triamterene is only about 60% of that of amiloride, and thus only Moduretic (a combination of hydroclorothiazide and amiloride) is generally effective on a once-daily schedule. It is rarely necessary to exceed a dose of 50 mg per day of hydrochlorothiazide or its equivalent; often, therapy is initiated at 25 or even 12.5 mg per day, particularly in sodium-sensitive and elderly hypertensive patients.

Diuretics remain the drugs of first choice for the treatment of hypertension in sodium-sensitive patients, particularly the elderly, and in black patients. In the context of risk factors for coronary disease, such as left ventricular hypertrophy, diabetes, electrocardiogram abnormalities, gout, hyperuricemia, and hyperlipidemia, diuretics may not be ideal, and effective alternatives that do not increase the risk of cardiovascular disease may be preferable. When combined with other classes of antihypertensive agents, doses of hydrochlorothiazide as low as 6.25 mg per day have been shown to be efficacious. Thus, diuretics, in small doses, have a major role as added therapy when another class of first-step treatment does not lower blood pressure sufficiently.

Antisympathetics

The centrally acting agents reserpine, α-methyldopa, clonidine, guanabenz, and guanfacine are not often used because of their central nervous system side effects, which range from dry mouth and stuffy nose to sleepiness, lethargy, fatigue, depression, and impotence. The β-adrenergic blocking drugs lower blood pressure primarily by diminishing cardiac output. Cardioselectivity is dose dependent and is minimal at higher doses. It appears that the nonselective β-blockers can lessen the likelihood of sudden death, particularly that seen during acute myocardial infarction, by blocking the β_2-receptor. The cardioselective agents, unless used at high doses, do not provide this cardiac protection.

Moreover, this cardioprotective effect of β-blockade is manifest early after myocardial infarction, and continued reduction of mortality rates after 1 year has not been consistently observed.

The combined α- and β-receptor antagonist labetalol lowers blood pressure by diminishing peripheral resistance through α-adrenergic blockade and through reducing cardiac output by β-blockade. Labetalol is very effective in the emergent treatment of hypertension and is efficacious in a broad spectrum of hypertensive patients, particularly those with relatively severe blood pressure elevations. The desirability of routine use of labetalol as initial therapy for mild to moderate hypertension remains to be extensively investigated.

Vasodilators

Direct-acting vasodilators, such as hydralazine and minoxidil, are potent in dilating the vasculature. They are generally reserved for third- or fourth-step antihypertensive therapy because of marked salt and water retention and sympathetic nervous system stimulation. When these direct-acting vasodilators are used, they are generally combined with diuretics and β-blocking agents, thus consigning them to the third or fourth step in the treatment of patients with severe, refractory hypertension. The calcium channel blockers provide peripheral vasodilatation and reduce vascular resistance without promoting expansion of extracellular fluid volume or stimulating reflex sympathetic discharge. The edema seen with some agents is not a reflection of salt and water retention and extracellular volume expansion but rather an effect of capillary dilatation. The increased risk of cardiovascular disease reported with these agents appears to be limited to the short-acting preparations.

Indirect-acting vasodilators include peripheral α-adrenergic blocking agents, such as prazosin, terazosin, and doxazosin; ACE inhibitors; and ARBs. They are effective antihypertensive agents that do not produce volume expansion or stimulate increased sympathetic nervous system activity. Another advantage of the indirect-acting agents is their neutral or beneficial effect on lipid levels and glucose.

ACE inhibitors lower blood pressure by preventing the formation of angiotensin II, the effective vasoconstrictor product of the renin–angiotensin system. ACE inhibitors may have other mechanisms of action involving kinin production and the synthesis of vasodilatory prostaglandins. ACE inhibitors are uniquely devoid of the adverse central nervous system side effects common with other antihypertensive drugs. When ACE inhibitors are given to volume-depleted patients, they may have a pronounced hypotensive action. They may frequently cause an annoying, nonproductive cough, sinusitis, and other respiratory symptoms. A new class of agents, the ARBs, hold the potential for antihypertensive efficacy without many of the side effects of ACE inhibitors, and they may have unique benefits, which are being evaluated in clinical trials currently.

ACE inhibitors have been used in combination with diuretics, calcium channel blockers, β-adrenergic blocking agents, and centrally acting antisympathetic drugs. When combined with diuretics, they appear to blunt or prevent the reactive metabolic responses to diuretic therapy that seem to be related to diuretic-induced stimulation of the renin-angiotensin-aldosterone sys-

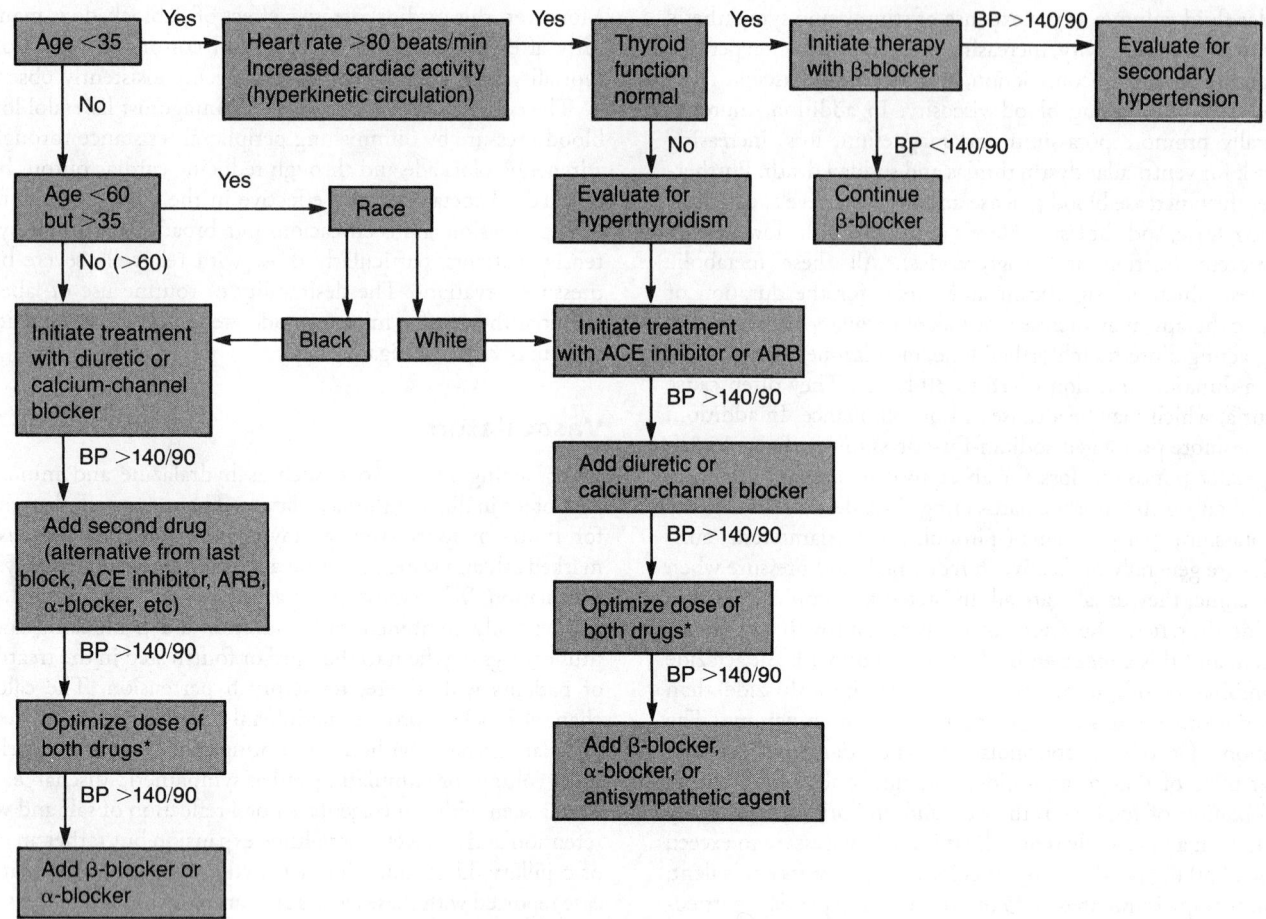

FIGURE 30.1. Beginning antihypertensive therapy.

tem. These responses include hyperuricemia, hypokalemia, hyperglycemia, and hypercholesterolemia. ACE inhibitors have also been shown to improve insulin sensitivity.

CHOOSING INITIAL ANTIHYPERTENSIVE THERAPY

When hypertension develops in white or young patients (less than 60 years of age), it is likely to be responsive to β-adrenergic blocking drugs, ACE inhibitors, or ARBs as initial therapeutic agents. Calcium channel entry blockers and α-blockers have a broader demographic efficacy than do diuretics, β-blockers, ACE inhibitors, or ARBs when used as sole therapy. In black patients, diuretics or calcium channel blockers are usually effective initial agents. In white patients over age 60, diuretics or calcium channel blockers are also good initial therapy. For these reasons, the initial therapy in hypertensives today (Fig. 30.1) is based on the likely pathophysiologic picture, the probability of blood pressure responsiveness to given therapeutic agents, the relative risk of cardiovascular disease, and the presence of other disorders (pulmonary disease, angina, diabetes, gout, hyperlipidemia, peripheral vascular disease). Also, because some side effects of antihypertensive agents are dose dependent, it is often wise to add a second drug before reaching the maximum dose of the initial agent to minimize the dose-dependent adverse effects.

Combination therapy is most likely to be effective if drugs of different classes are used (e.g., diuretics, vasodilators, antisympathetics). Combinations shown to have additive effects include diuretics and β-blockers, diuretics and ACE inhibitors or ARBs, diuretics and α-blockers, diuretics and central sympatholytics, and ACE inhibitors and calcium channel blockers. The combination of a diuretic and a β-blocker produces additive effects on lipids (raising total cholesterol and low-density lipoproteins and lowering high-density lipoproteins) and raises glucose levels. The combination of an ACE inhibitor and a diuretic blunts or prevents the adverse metabolic effects of diuretic therapy on uric acid, potassium, glucose, and cholesterol. The α-blockers also reduce the adverse lipid effects of diuretics. There is little evidence for an additive antihypertensive effect when diuretics are combined with calcium channel entry blockers.

COMPLIANCE WITH ANTIHYPERTENSIVE THERAPY

Hypertension is generally an asymptomatic disease for decades until a cardiovascular complication occurs. Control of blood pressure in the asymptomatic phase significantly reduces overall cardiovascular morbidity and mortality rates. Even in elderly patients with isolated elevation of systolic pressure and normal diastolic pressure, systolic blood pressure reduction has been shown to lower mortality rates, particularly from stroke. Convincing an asymptomatic patient of the need for long-term medical therapy to control blood pressure elevation and to prevent the development of cardiovascular disease is a challenge, however. Thus, patient compliance has been and remains the major deterrent to long-term blood pressure control and prevention of cardiovascular complications. For this reason, it is important to educate the patient that side effects may occur with antihypertensive therapy and to encourage reporting them. It is equally important to be familiar with alternative therapeutic agents that are likely to be effective in a given patient.

Another major challenge in the treatment of the hypertensive patient is to recognize concomitant disorders that may also require treatment and that can complicate the efficacy, side effects, or safety of antihypertensive therapy. The wide variety of effective antihypertensive agents available today, when used alone or in combination with other agents, can provide excellent blood pressure control and can even improve quality of life for a hypertensive patient. The issues of patient well-being and subjective responses to antihypertensive therapy are assuming increasing importance in light of studies addressing this issue as well as the increased awareness of the lay population regarding the variety of agents available for treatment of hypertension.

The asymptomatic nature of uncomplicated hypertension requires a substantial amount of education of the patient regarding the need for continued antihypertensive therapy and periodic blood pressure assessment, end-organ evaluation, and routine laboratory studies. An office reminder system for periodic recall is helpful to maximize follow-up of patients. The issues of compliance with therapy and side effects can be improved by evaluating quality of life through direct questioning of the patient.

BIBLIOGRAPHY

Castelli WP, Anderson K. A population at risk: prevalence of high cholesterol levels in hypertensive patients in the Framingham study. *Am J Med* 1986;80:23–32.

Ganguly A, Henry DP, Yune HY, et al. Diagnosis and localization of pheochromocytoma: detection by measurement of urinary norepinephrine during sleep, plasma norepinephrine concentration and computed axial tomography. *Am J Med* 1979;67:21–26.

Jacob RG, Shapiro AP, Reeves RA, et al. Relaxation therapy for hypertension. *Arch Intern Med* 1986;146:2335–2340.

Sixth report of the Joint National Committee on Prevention, Detection, Evaluation, and Treatment of High Blood Pressure. *Arch Intern Med* 1997;157:2413–2446.

Lyons DF, Kem DC, Brown RD, Hanson CS, Carollo ML. Single-dose captopril as a diagnostic test for primary aldosteronism. *J Clin Endocrinol Metab* 1983;57:892–896.

MacGregor GA. Sodium is more important than calcium in essential hypertension. *Hypertension* 1985;7:628–640.

SHEP Cooperative Research Group. Prevention of stroke by antihypertensive drug treatment in older persons with isolated systolic hypertension. *JAMA* 1991;265:3255–3264.

Weinberger MH. Antihypertensive therapy and lipids: evidence, mechanisms and implications. *Arch Intern Med* 1985;145:1102–1105.

Weinberger MH. Renovascular hypertension: questions, current knowledge and clinical implications. *Am J Kidney Dis* 1985;5:A85–A92.

Weinberger MH, Fineberg NS. The diagnosis of primary aldosteronism and separation of two major subtypes. *Arch Intern Med* 1993;153:2125–2129.

Weinberger MH, Grim CE, Hollifield JW, et al. Primary aldosteronism: diagnosis, localization and treatment. *Ann Intern Med* 1979;90:386–395.

Kelley's Textbook of Internal Medicine, fourth edition. Edited by H. David Humes. Lippincott Williams & Wilkins, Philadelphia © 2000.

CHAPTER

31

APPROACHES TO HYPERCHOLESTEROLEMIA AND OTHER ABNORMAL LIPID PROFILES

DANIEL J. RADER

Elevated total cholesterol and low-density lipoprotein (LDL) cholesterol levels, elevated triglyceride levels, and reduced high-density lipoprotein (HDL) cholesterol levels are all independently associated with a higher risk of atherosclerotic cardiovascular disease. Markedly elevated triglyceride levels (more than 1,000 mg per deciliter) are associated with the risk of acute pancreatitis. The clinical evaluation and treatment of patients with lipid disorders are directed primarily toward preventing atherosclerotic cardiovascular disease (for most patients with lipoprotein disorders) or preventing acute pancreatitis (for patients with severe hypertriglyceridemia).

▍HYPERCHOLESTEROLEMIA

PRESENTATION

The most important clinical consequence of hypercholesterolemia is premature atherosclerotic cardiovascular disease, and any patient with cardiovascular disease should be tested for a potential lipoprotein disorder. In addition, routine screening of asymptomatic adults for potential lipid disorders is also recommended, as described below under "Laboratory Studies and Diagnostic Tests." The subsequent approach to the evaluation and treatment of a patient with an abnormal lipid profile is strongly influenced by the presence of atherosclerotic cardiovascular disease and other risk factors. Treatment in patients with coronary heart disease (CHD) or other forms of atherosclerosis is known as secondary prevention; treatment in patients without CHD is known as primary prevention. A general approach to the screening, diagnosis, and management of hypercholesterolemia has been developed by the Adult Treatment Panel of the National Cholesterol Education Program. The guidelines suggest an approach to management the intensity of which takes into account the presence of CHD or other atherosclerotic cardiovascular disease as well as the presence of other cardiovascular risk factors.

TABLE 31.1.	MAJOR CARDIOVASCULAR RISK FACTORS OTHER THAN LOW-DENSITY LIPOPROTEIN CHOLESTEROL TO CONSIDER IN THE EVALUATION AND TREATMENT OF HYPERCHOLESTEROLEMIA

Positive risk factors

Age, yr
Male >45
Female >55 or premature menopause without estrogen replacement therapy
Family history of premature coronary heart disease (definite myocardial infarction or sudden death before 55 years of age in male first-degree or before 65 years of age in female first-degree relative)
Current cigarette smoking
Hypertension
Diabetes mellitus
Low HDL cholesterol (<35 mg/dL)

Negative risk factors[a]

High HDL cholesterol (>60 mg/dL)

HDL, high-density lipoprotein.
[a] If the HDL cholesterol is >60 mg/dL, subtract one risk factor.
[Adapted from the Summary of the second report of the National Cholesterol Education Program (NCEP) Expert Panel on Detection, Evaluation, and Treatment of High Blood Cholesterol in Adults (Adult Treatment Panel II). *JAMA* 1993;269:3015–3023, with permission.]

PATHOPHYSIOLOGY

The pathophysiologic description of lipoprotein disorders is reviewed extensively in Chapter 12.

HISTORY AND PHYSICAL EXAMINATION

A complete history should be obtained, including a history of atherosclerotic cardiovascular disease and a history of other cardiovascular risk factors (Table 31.1.). The presence of established cardiovascular disease or other risk factors has a significant impact on subsequent evaluation and management. A history of known secondary causes of hyperlipidemia, including medications (see Chapter 12), also should be procured, along with a comprehensive family history of premature cardiovascular disease and hyperlipidemia. The physical examination should include a careful examination of the eyes for arcus corneae, the eyelids for xanthelasmas, the palms for palmar xanthomas, the knuckles and Achilles tendons for tendon xanthomas, and the elbows and knees for cutaneous and tuberoeruptive xanthomas. The thyroid should be palpated and major arteries should be examined for vascular bruits.

LABORATORY STUDIES AND DIAGNOSTIC TESTS

All adults over age 20 should be screened for hypercholesterolemia. In adults without CHD, this screening should be performed by measuring total and HDL cholesterol in the nonfasting state. The initial classification, according to National Cholesterol Education Program guidelines, is described in Table 31.2. A serum cholesterol level below 200 mg per deciliter is desirable and, if the HDL cholesterol level is above 35 mg per deciliter, requires no further evaluation. A serum cholesterol level of 200 to 239 mg per deciliter is borderline high, but if the HDL cholesterol is above 35 mg per deciliter and there is no more than one cardiovascular risk factor, no further evaluation is required. A cholesterol level of 200 to 239 mg per deciliter in the context of two or more risk factors should be evaluated further with a full fasting lipid profile. In addition, a serum cholesterol level above 240 mg per deciliter or an HDL cholesterol level below 35 mg per deciliter are indications for a full fasting lipid profile. Finally, a full fasting lipid profile should be undertaken for patients with established cardiovascular disease.

The full fasting lipid profile includes measurement of the triglyceride, total cholesterol, and HDL cholesterol levels after an overnight fast of at least 12 hours. The LDL cholesterol is usually calculated using the following equation: LDL cholesterol = total cholesterol − (triglycerides/5) − HDL cholesterol. This formula is reasonably accurate if test results are obtained on fasting plasma and if the triglyceride level does not exceed 400 mg per deciliter. The determination of LDL cholesterol levels in patients with triglyceride levels above 400 mg per deciliter usually requires ultracentrifugal techniques in specialized laboratories, though direct assays for LDL measurement have now become available. All further evaluation and treatment should be based on the LDL cholesterol level, not the total cholesterol level. Once a lipoprotein disorder has been diagnosed, the laboratory should rule out potential secondary causes of hyperlipidemia. In practice, this assessment usually includes measurement of fasting glucose to rule out diabetes mellitus, serum thyroid-stimulating hormone (TSH) to rule out hypothyroidism, and serum albumin if the nephrotic syndrome is suspected and liver function tests to assess the possibility of obstructive liver disease.

DIFFERENTIAL DIAGNOSIS

The differential diagnosis of hypercholesterolemia includes primary and secondary causes. The major secondary causes of hypercholesterolemia are listed in Table 31.3. Hypothyroidism should always be ruled out with measurement of the TSH, since this condition can often be subtle and is eminently treatable. Once secondary causes have been excluded, primary causes of elevated LDL cholesterol should be considered. The major inherited conditions that are sources of hypercholesterolemia (see Chapter 12) include familial hypercholesterolemia (FH), familial defective apoB-100 (FDB), familial combined hyperlipidemia (FCHL), familial dysbetalipoproteinemia (type III hyperlipidemia), and polygenic hypercholesterolemia. A few clinical clues and laboratory tests can assist in the diagnosis of these disorders. The presence of tendon xanthomas strongly supports the diagnosis of FH or FDB, though their absence does not rule out these diagnoses. FDB can be pinpointed by molecular screening in specialized laboratories, but heterozygous FH is diagnosed on the basis of clinical features. Elevated triglyceride levels are rarely seen in FH or FDB and are much more suggestive of FCHL.

TABLE 31.2. INITIAL CLASSIFICATION BASED ON TOTAL AND HDL CHOLESTEROL AND TREATMENT DECISIONS BASED ON LDL CHOLESTEROL

Initial Classification and Action Based on Total and HDL Cholesterol (Patients Without CHD Only)

Total Cholesterol	Classification	Action
<200 mg/dL	Desirable	
HDL >35 mg/dL		Repeat in 5 years
HDL <35 mg/dL		Fasting lipoprotein profile
200–240 mg/dL	Borderline high	
HDL >35 *and* fewer than 2 risk factors		Dietary information and repeat in 1 year
HDL <35 *or* 2 other risk factors		Fasting lipoprotein profile
>240 mg/dL	High	Fasting lipoprotein profile

Treatment Decisions Based on LDL Cholesterol Level (All Patients)

Patient Category	Initiate Dietary Therapy	Initiate Drug Therapy	LDL Goal
With CHD or other atherosclerosis	>100 mg/dL	>130 mg/dL	<100 mg/dL
Without CHD and with 2 risk factors	>130 mg/dL	>160 mg/dL	<130 mg/dL
Without CHD and fewer than 2 risk factors	>160 mg/dL	>190 mg/dL	<160 mg/dL
Selected low-risk individuals	>160 mg/dL	>220 mg/dL	<160 mg/dL

LDL, low-density lipoprotein; HDL, high-density lipoprotein; CHD, coronary heart disease.
[Adapted from the Summary of the second report of the National Cholesterol Education Program (NCEP) Expert Panel on Detection, Evaluation, and Treatment of High Blood Cholesterol in Adults (Adult Treatment Panel II). *JAMA* 1993;269: 3015–3023, with permission.]

A family history of hyperlipidemia in at least one first-degree relative is required to support the diagnosis of FCHL. This diagnosis can be established by the measurement of the plasma apoB level. In FCHL, the apoB level is high (usually more than 130 mg per deciliter) and is often elevated disproportionately to the LDL cholesterol level owing to the presence of increased amounts of small, "dense" LDL particles, a biochemical marker for FCHL that is difficult to measure directly. Therefore, a substantially elevated apoB level in the context of modestly elevated LDL and triglyceride levels strongly suggests FCHL.

Familial dysbetalipoproteinemia (type III hyperlipidemia) can masquerade as an apparent cause of elevated LDL cholesterol

TABLE 31.3. DIAGNOSTIC CONSIDERATIONS IN PATIENTS WITH DYSLIPIDEMIA

Type of Dyslipidemia	Lipid Values	Phenotype	Primary Disorders	Secondary Disorders
Elevated LDL cholesterol With normal triglycerides	LDL >160 mg/dL TG <200 mg/dL	IIa	Familial hypercholesterolemia, familial defective apoB-100, polygenic hypercholesterolemia, familial combined hyperlipidemia	Hypothyroidism, nephrotic syndrome, obstructive liver disease
With elevated triglycerides	TG 200–700 mg/dL	IIb	Familial combined hyperlipidemia	Nephrotic syndrome, diabetes mellitus
Elevated remnant lipoproteins	TG 200–800 mg/dL	III	Familial dysbetalipoproteinemia, hepatic lipase deficiency	Dysglobulinemia
Elevated VLDL	TG 200–1,000 mg/dL	IV	Familial hypertriglyceridemia	Diabetes mellitus, alcohol use, estrogen therapy, other drugs
Elevated chylomicrons	TG >1,000 mg/dL	I or V	Lipoprotein lipase deficiency, apoC-II deficiency, familial type V hyperlipidemia	Diabetes mellitus, alcohol use, estrogen therapy, other drugs

LDL, low-density lipoprotein; TG, triglycerides.

(based on the calculated level), but the true LDL cholesterol level is usually low; instead, the level of remnant lipoproteins is elevated. The formula for calculating LDL cholesterol is not accurate in this context because the 5:1 ratio of triglycerides to cholesterol in very low density lipoproteins (VLDLs) is not valid for remnant lipoproteins. Type III hyperlipidemia should be suspected when there is no family history of hyperlipidemia or a secondary cause of hyperlipidemia, when palmar or tuberoeruptive xanthomas are found, or when the total cholesterol and triglyceride levels are both substantially elevated to a similar degree. The diagnosis of type III hyperlipidemia often can be confirmed on laboratory tests. Traditionally, lipoprotein electrophoresis has been used, since the remnant lipoproteins run in the region between beta and prebeta, resulting in the "broad beta" band characteristic of this disorder. Ultracentrifugation has also been used in specialized laboratories to confirm this diagnosis. In many laboratories it is possible to screen for the apoE-2/2 genotype usually associated with this disorder. The finding of an apoE-2/2 genotype in a patient with clinically suspected type III hyperlipidemia confirms the diagnosis, but the absence of this genotype does not rule out rarer forms of type III hyperlipidemia associated with other mutations in apoE.

STRATEGIES FOR OPTIMAL CARE

Management

Secondary causes of hypercholesterolemia should be actively sought and treated. Obese persons should be encouraged to lose weight, sedentary persons to exercise, and those who drink alcohol to minimize their intake. Every attempt should be made to modify other cardiovascular risk factors as well. The decisions in the clinical treatment of patients with hypercholesterolemia are highly dependent on whether established atherosclerotic cardiovascular disease or other cardiovascular risk factors are present (Table 31.2). Aggressive treatment of hypercholesterolemia in patients with established CHD or other atherosclerotic disease (secondary prevention) is well supported by experimental data. Clinical trials have confirmed conclusively that lowering LDL cholesterol levels in patients with established atherosclerotic disease reduces the number of cardiovascular events and total mortality rates. Therefore, aggressive secondary prevention treatment to lower LDL cholesterol levels is clinically indicated and cost-effective. Nevertheless, it is estimated that up to 70% of patients with established CHD are not receiving adequate cholesterol-lowering therapy, according to current guidelines.

In primary prevention, several clinical trials have shown that lowering the total or LDL cholesterol level limits the number of cardiovascular events and mortality rates. Earlier trials were not designed with adequate power to assess the question of the effect on total mortality rates, but one trial has now verified a substantial reduction in total mortality. Therefore, LDL cholesterol lowering in the primary prevention of CHD is indicated for high-risk individuals. The generally accepted approach is that the more cardiovascular risk factors there are, and the higher the absolute LDL cholesterol level, the greater the potential benefit from drug therapy to lower the LDL cholesterol level. In persons considered to be at lower risk, the emphasis is more on dietary modification and less on drug therapy.

The National Cholesterol Education Program provides guidelines for the treatment of patients with elevated LDL cholesterol. A strategy for the management of elevated LDL cholesterol in the patient with established CHD or other atherosclerotic cardiovascular disease (ASCVD) is presented in Figure 31.1. Because patients with diabetes mellitus are at similar very high risk, they should be treated in a similar fashion. The optimal LDL cholesterol level is 100 mg per deciliter or less for patients with established ASCVD or diabetes mellitus. Although dietary therapy should always be instituted as first-line therapy, most patients require drug therapy to reach the optimal LDL cholesterol level. The timing of drug therapy, when indicated, should not be delayed in the context of established CHD.

Primary prevention often divides high-risk and low-risk patients, depending on the presence of other cardiovascular risk factors. A strategy for the management of elevated LDL cholesterol in the patient without CHD but who is at high risk owing to the presence of two or more cardiovascular risk factors is presented in Fig. 31.2. Dietary therapy should be initiated for patients with LDL cholesterol levels above 130 mg per deciliter. It is important to stress weight reduction in overweight patients and increased physical activity in general. After a 3- to 6-month trial of diet therapy, the lipid panel should be repeated and the LDL cholesterol level determined. Drug therapy is indicated in patients with LDL cholesterol levels above 160 mg per deciliter. Patients with LDL cholesterol levels of 130 to 160 mg per deciliter are not usually candidates for drug therapy, but this decision must be individualized in high-risk patients and may be influenced by the HDL cholesterol level and perhaps other blood factors, such as apoB and lipoprotein(a) [Lp(a)].

For patients with no more than one cardiovascular risk factor, an LDL cholesterol level above 190 mg per deciliter is the recommended cutoff point for consideration of drug therapy. In patients at very low risk, with no other cardiovascular risk factors (e.g., men younger than 35 years old and premenopausal women), drug therapy can be reasonably delayed if the LDL cholesterol level is between 190 and 220 mg per deciliter (Table 31.2). All persons with LDL cholesterol levels above 220 mg per deciliter on an optimal dietary and exercise regimen are candidates for drug therapy.

It is often difficult to decide whether to initiate drug therapy in relatively low-risk patients without CHD who have LDL cholesterol levels in the borderline zone between 160 and 220 mg per deciliter. Although it is desirable to avoid drug treatment for patients in whom CHD is unlikely to develop, many patients with premature CHD have LDL cholesterol levels in this range. Therefore, factors that help predict cardiovascular risk may be useful in this population. One such test is the apoB level; if it is elevated, it can suggest the presence of dense LDL, an exceptionally atherogenic form of LDL. LDL particle size can also be determined using specialized gel electrophoresis or NMR methods. Another predictive blood test is the Lp(a) level, which cannot be measured by a standard lipid profile; if it is elevated, however, it points to an increased risk of CHD. Epidemiologic data strongly indicate that the apoE4 genotype is also predictive of increased cardiovascular risk independent of lipid levels. Therefore, these and other tests may assume increased importance in the treatment of patients with borderline LDL cholesterol levels.

Management of Hypercholesterolemia in Patients with ASCVD or Diabetes Mellitus

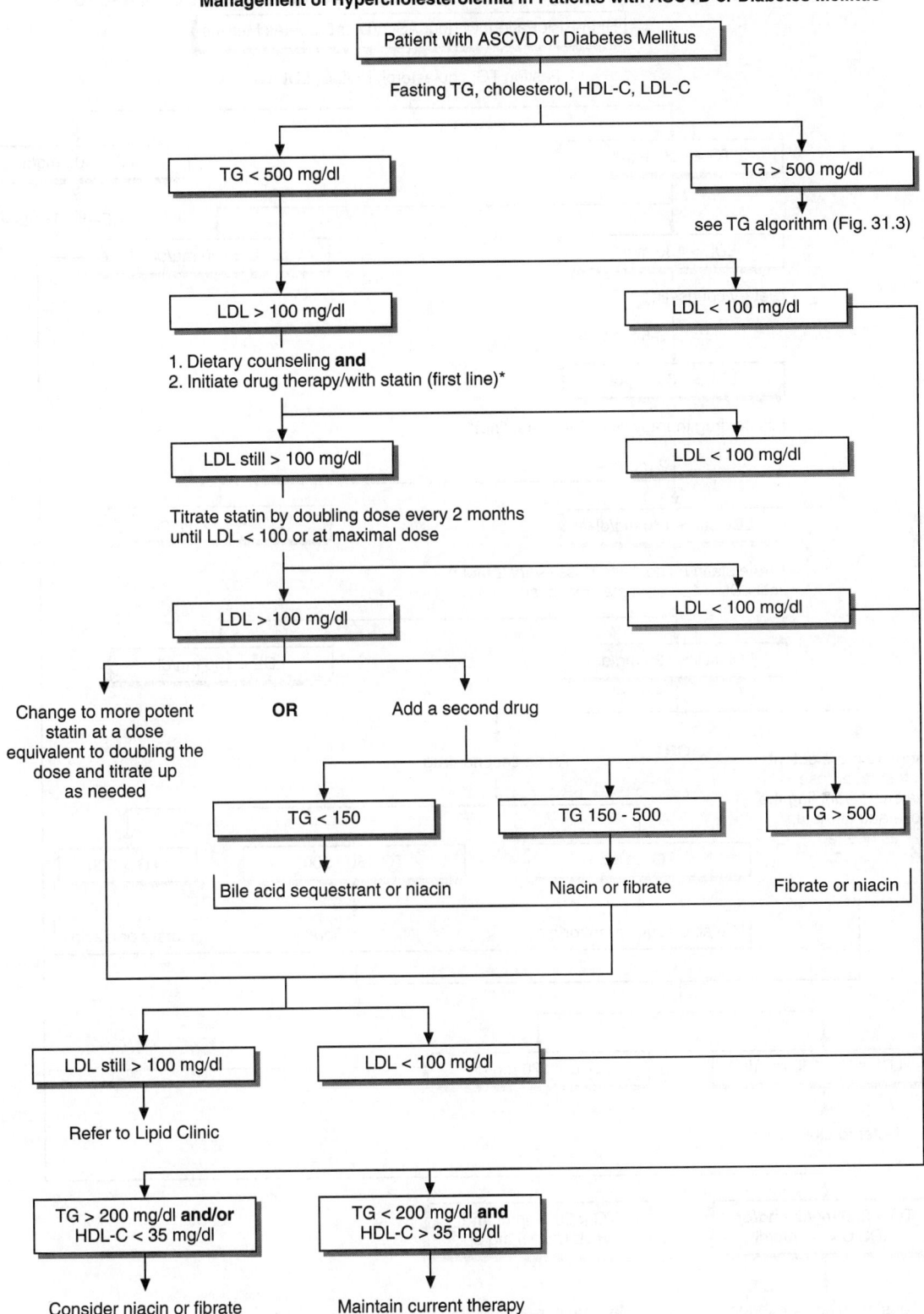

* In patients intolerant of statins, niacin or bile acid sequestrants could be used instead

FIGURE 31.1. Strategy for the management of hypercholesterolemia in the secondary prevention of CHD in patients with established CHD.
EVIDENCE LEVEL: C. Expert Opinion.

Management of Hypercholesterolemia in High-Risk Primary Prevention of ASCVD

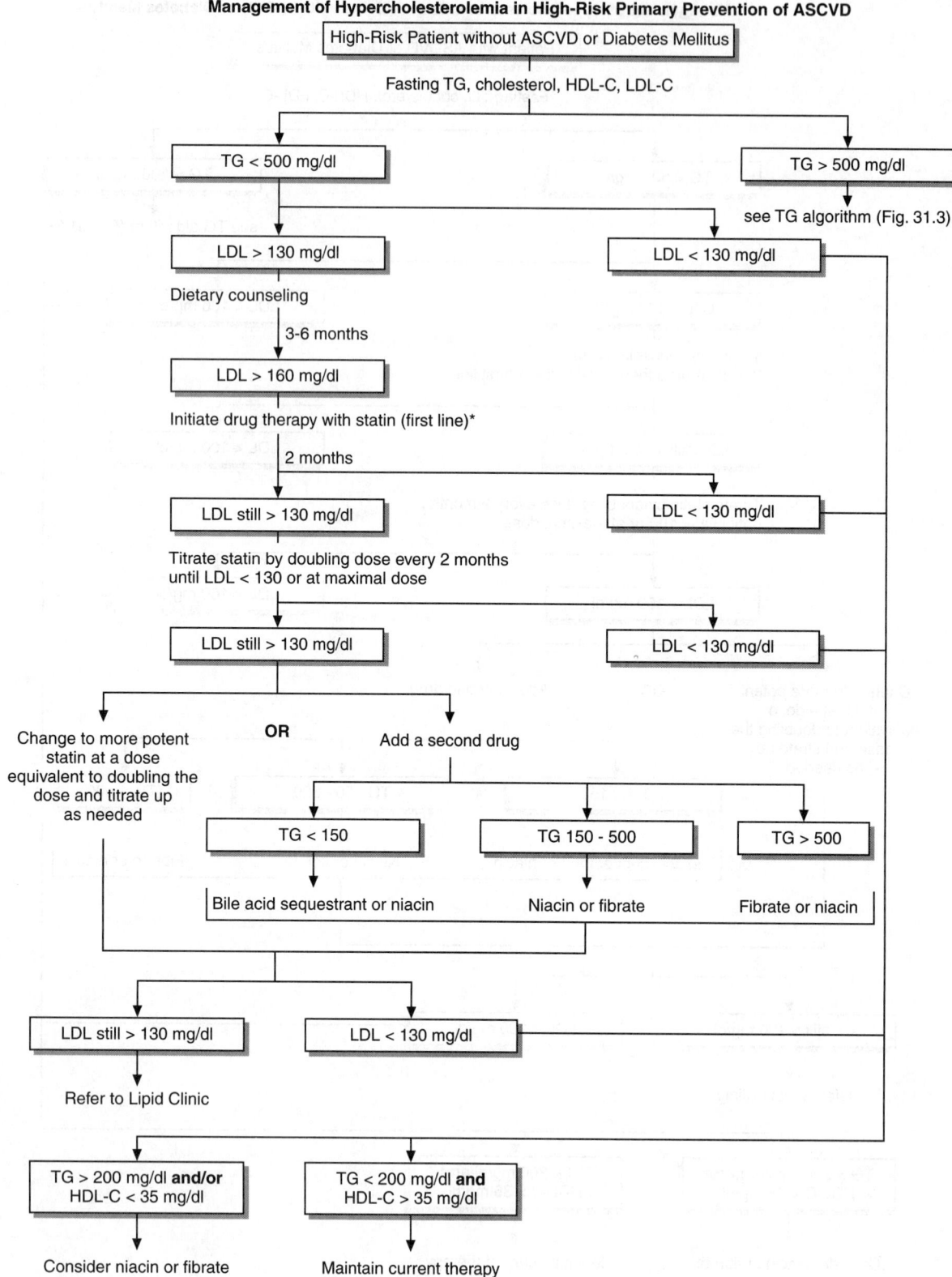

FIGURE 31.2. Strategy for the management of hypercholesterolemia in the primary prevention of CHD in patients with two or more risk factors for CHD.
EVIDENCE LEVEL: C. Expert Opinion.

TABLE 31.4.	DIETARY GUIDELINES FOR THERAPY OF HYPERCHOLESTEROLEMIA	
Dietary Constituent	**Step I Diet**	**Step II Diet**
Total fat	<30% of total calories	<30% of total calories
Saturated fatty acids	<10% of total calories	<7% of total calories
Polyunsaturated fatty acids	<10% of total calories	<10% of total calories
Monounsaturated fatty acids	10–15% of total calories	10–15% of total calories
Carbohydrates	50–60% of total calories	50–60% of total calories
Protein	10–20% of total calories	10–20% of total calories
Cholesterol	<300 mg/day	<200 mg/day
Total calories	To achieve and maintain desirable body weight	To achieve and maintain desirable body weight

[Adapted from the Summary of the second report of the National Cholesterol Education Program (NCEP) Expert Panel on Detection, Evaluation, and Treatment of High Blood Cholesterol in Adults (Adult Treatment Panel II). *JAMA* 1993;269:3015–3023, with permission.]

Diet Therapy

The guidelines for dietary treatment of elevated LDL cholesterol levels are listed in Table 31.4. To lower the LDL cholesterol level by diet modification, the intake of saturated fats must be restricted. Decreasing the intake of total fats and cholesterol is also useful, although less important than the intake of saturated fats. Low-fat, yet palatable diets have been developed; useful diet programs include those suggested by the American Heart Association and the National Cholesterol Education Program. The patient should be instructed in the diet by the physician or a qualified assistant. A second cholesterol measurement should be obtained at 6 weeks and a third at 3 months. If the diet has been successful, the patient can be monitored every 3 months for the first year and every 6 months thereafter. Periodic review of the diet may be needed to reinforce the need for its continued use. If therapeutic goals are not reached after 3 months, the patient should be referred to a registered dietitian for more detailed dietary instruction. The patient may be advanced to a step II diet, which further restricts total and saturated fat (Table 31.4). If the patient does not respond adequately to diet therapy after an additional 3 months and if the LDL cholesterol level remains above the cutoff for drug therapy, drug treatment should be considered (Fig. 31.2).

Patients with established atherosclerotic cardiovascular disease should be instructed concerning a step II diet by a registered dietitian. Diet is important in these high-risk patients, to maximize the chances of achieving the optimal LDL cholesterol level (less than 100 mg per deciliter). The period of observation on diet alone in these patients may be shorter than is the case with primary prevention, however, especially if the LDL cholesterol level is significantly elevated. Responses of total and LDL cholesterol to step I and step II diets vary widely and are greater in controlled studies on metabolic wards than they are among outpatients. In addition, most patients experience a decline in HDL cholesterol when they decrease the amount of total and saturated fats in their diet. It is important to inform patients of this possibility and to reassure them that the diet is nevertheless beneficial in terms of overall cardiovascular risk.

These recommendations do not always apply. For example, patients with significant hypercholesterolemia usually do not respond adequately to diet therapy alone. If the patient already has CHD, it is reasonable to start drug therapy after only 6 weeks of diet therapy or even immediately. In elderly patients with elevated LDL cholesterol levels, the need for dietary therapy should be balanced against the need for adequate nutrition. In pregnant women with hypercholesterolemia, previously initiated dietary therapy may be continued but should be reviewed to ensure adequate nutrient consumption. Pregnancy can be associated with hyperlipidemia in the third trimester, which generally requires no treatment.

Drug Therapy

When diet therapy alone fails to achieve therapeutic goals, drug therapy should be considered. The guidelines for initiating drug treatment based on LDL cholesterol levels are listed in Table 31.2. Table 31.5. summarizes the major drugs used for treating hypercholesterolemia. When drug therapy is started, regular follow-up is necessary to gauge therapeutic effects, to reinforce the need for compliance, and to monitor for side effects. After drug therapy is started, lipids and transaminases should be obtained in 6 to 8 weeks and again in 4 months. If the patient is stable, long-term monitoring can be performed every 6 months. If the initial drug does not reduce LDL cholesterol to the therapeutic goal, a combination of drugs may be used. In these cases, it may be necessary to consult a specialist in lipid disorders. Most of the available lipid-lowering drugs are effective in combination, but patients must be monitored carefully because of the increased potential for complications.

HMG-CoA Reductase Inhibitors (Statins)

Inhibitors of 3-hydroxy-3-methylglutaryl coenzyme A (HMG-CoA reductase) include lovastatin, pravastatin, simvastatin, fluvastatin, atorvastatin, and cerivastatin. HMG-CoA reductase is the rate-limiting step in cholesterol biosynthesis; by reducing

TABLE 31.5.   SUMMARY OF THE MAJOR DRUGS USED FOR THE TREATMENT OF HYPERLIPIDEMIA

Drug	Major Indications	Starting Dose	Maximal Dose	Mechanism	Common Side Effects
Bile acid sequestrants	Elevated LDL			Increased bile acid excretion and increased LDL receptors in liver	Bloating, constipation, elevated triglycerides
Cholestyramine		4 g daily	32 g daily		
Colestipol		5 g daily	40 g daily		
Nicotinic acid	Elevated LDL, VLDL, low HDL			Decreased VLDL synthesis	Cutaneous flushing, GI upset, elevated glucose, uric acid, and liver function tests
Immediate release		100 mg t.i.d. after meals	1 g t.i.d. after meals		
Controlled release (Niaspan)		375 mg q.h.s.	2,000 mg q.h.s.		
HMG-CoA reductase inhibitors	Elevated LDL			Reduced cholesterol synthesis, up-regulated hepatic LDL receptors, reduced VLDL production	Myalgias, arthralgias, GI upset, elevated transaminases, sleep disturbances
Lovastatin		20 mg daily	80 mg daily		
Pravastatin		20 mg q.h.s.	40 mg q.h.s.		
Simvastatin		10 mg q.h.s.	80 mg q.h.s.		
Fluvastatin		20 mg q.h.s.	80 mg q.h.s.		
Atorvastatin		10 mg q.h.s.	80 mg q.h.s.		
Cerivastatin		0.2 mg q.h.s.	0.4 mg q.h.s.		
Fibric acid derivatives	Elevated TG, elevated remnants			Increased lipoprotein lipase, decreased VLDL synthesis	Myositis, GI upset, gallstones, elevated liver function tests
Gemfibrozil		600 mg b.i.d.	600 mg b.i.d.		
Fenofibrate		200 mg q.d.	200 mg q.d.		
Fish oils	Severely elevated TG	3 g daily	12 g daily	Decreased TG synthesis, enhanced TG catabolism	Diarrhea, GI upset, fishy odor to breath

LDL, low-density lipoproteins; VLDL, very low-density lipoproteins; HDL, high-density lipoproteins; TG, triglycerides; HMG-CoA, 3-hydroxy-3-methylglutaryl reductase coenzyme A; GI, gastrointestinal.

hepatic cholesterol biosynthesis, these drugs up-regulate hepatic LDL-receptor activity, leading to increased clearance of plasma LDL. They may also decrease hepatic production of VLDL in some circumstances.

Five major randomized controlled clinical trials of statin monotherapy reported in the 1990s (simvastatin, pravastatin, and lovastatin) found highly significant reductions in fatal and nonfatal myocardial infarction and, in some cases, in stroke and total mortality rates. Three of these trials (4S, CARE, and LIPID) were secondary prevention trials involving patients with established coronary artery disease, and two (WOSCOPS and AF/TexCAPS) were primary prevention trials in persons without known coronary artery disease. Many of the subjects treated in these trials had LDL cholesterol levels that would be considered average with respect to the general population.

The starting dose of each of the statins generally reduces LDL cholesterol by 20% to 30%, though response to the statins is highly variable, and some patients do not respond as well. Statins are generally titrated by doubling the dose, which produces a 6% to 7% further reduction in LDL cholesterol. Patients' acceptance of the statins is high, since they can be taken in tablet form once a day and are well tolerated. Levels of liver transaminases can rise, and they should be monitored during therapy, though the risk to the liver appears to be quite low overall. Other side effects can include muscle or joint pains, gastrointestinal upset, headaches, and sleep disturbance.

Nicotinic Acid (Niacin)

Nicotinic acid, also called niacin, belongs to the vitamin B complex. In doses well above those required as a vitamin, it is a potent lipid-lowering drug useful in the treatment of hypertriglyceridemia and hypercholesterolemia. Among the lipid-lowering drugs, nicotinic acid has the greatest effect in raising HDL cholesterol, and it is the only lipid-lowering drug that consistently lowers Lp(a) levels. Its mechanism of action is uncertain, but it probably reduces hepatic VLDL production. In the Coronary Drug Project, nicotinic acid reduced total mortality rates in patients with established CHD.

The starting dose of immediate-release niacin is 100 mg three times a day at the end of meals. Flushing is to be expected, but this effect improves with continued administration. After 4 to 7 days, the dose can be increased gradually by 100 mg per dose, eventually reaching 500 mg three times a day. After 1 month on this dose, lipids and pertinent blood chemistries should be measured, and, if necessary, the dose can be increased to 1,000 mg three times a day. Rarely, doses of up to 4,500 mg per day are used, but these are not generally recommended. Patients' acceptance of immediate-release nicotinic acid can be limited owing to the cutaneous flushing and pruritus it often causes. Proper education often permits the successful administration of immediate-release nicotinic acid. It may be necessary for some patients to take an aspirin 30 minutes before the dose of niacin, to prevent flushing.

The over-the-counter sustained-release forms of niacin are somewhat better tolerated but may be more likely to cause hepatotoxicity than the regular forms. A controlled-release form of prescription niacin called Niaspan is taken once daily at bedtime, is better tolerated than immediate-release niacin, and is probably safer than over-the-counter sustained-release niacin. Niaspan is titrated over 4 weeks to an initial maintenance dose of 1,000 mg daily at bedtime and can be increased subsequently to 2,000 mg daily.

Other side effects of nicotinic acid include hyperglycemia, hyperuricemia, elevated liver function test results, exacerbation of peptic ulcer disease, and acanthosis nigricans. Successful niacin therapy requires careful education of the patient as to its side effects. Its advantages are its low cost, long-term safety, ability to raise HDL cholesterol levels, and documented benefit in patients with established coronary artery disease. It is particularly useful in combination with statins in patients who cannot achieve LDL cholesterol goals on a statin alone, patients who have combined hyperlipidemia and persistently elevated triglycerides and/or low HDL cholesterol on statin therapy, and patients who require drug therapy to reduce LDL cholesterol but cannot tolerate statins.

Bile Acid Sequestrants (Resins)

Bile acid sequestrants, including cholestyramine and colestipol, interrupt the enterohepatic circulation of bile acids and accelerate the loss of bile acids in the stool. This change promotes increased hepatic conversion of cholesterol to bile acids, followed by stimulation of hepatic LDL-receptor activity and enhanced LDL clearance from the plasma. In the Lipid Research Clinics Coronary Primary Prevention Trial, cholestyramine reduced cardiovascular morbidity and mortality rates in patients without preexisting CHD.

Patients' acceptance of these drugs is limited because they are insoluble resins that must be suspended in liquid and are therefore often inconvenient and unpleasant to take. Colestipol is available in large tablets, which some patients prefer. Because these drugs are not systemically absorbed, major side effects are limited to the gastrointestinal tract (bloating, constipation) but are often dose-limiting. These agents bind many other drugs (digoxin, warfarin) and interfere with their absorption, and for this reason other medications must be taken 1 hour before or 4 hours after the bile acid sequestrants.

These agents are often drugs of first choice because of their safety. They are a particularly good choice for the young, well-motivated patient with mild hypercholesterolemia, but education of patients is critical for acceptance and successful therapy. They should not be prescribed for patients with triglyceride levels above 400 mg per deciliter, because they aggravate hypertriglyceridemia. Bile acid sequestrants are especially effective in combination therapy, and they have an increasingly important clinical role in combination with nicotinic acid or HMG-CoA reductase inhibitors.

Fibric Acid Derivatives (Fibrates)

Fibric acid derivatives include clofibrate, gemfibrozil, and fenofibrate. Fibrates are peroxisome proliferator activated receptor α

(PPARα) agonists, and through this action they stimulate lipoprotein lipase (LPL) activity and may restrict hepatic VLDL production. They lower triglyceride levels effectively and generally raise HDL cholesterol levels modestly, but they have limited ability to lower LDL cholesterol levels. In the World Health Organization study, clofibrate lowered rates of cardiovascular mortality, but the drug was associated on longer follow-up with an increase in total mortality rates. In the Helsinki Heart Study, gemfibrozil reduced the number of major coronary events but had no effect on total mortality rates. Micronized fenofibrate is available for use in the United States and has a somewhat greater LDL cholesterol–reducing effect than gemfibrozil.

Fibrates are generally well tolerated; side effects include gastrointestinal upset and muscle pains. Liver function test results are elevated on rare occasions and should be monitored during therapy. Fibrates potentiate the effect of warfarin and increase the lithogenicity of bile. Fibrates are primarily administered for reduction of triglyceride levels, and their major use is in patients with moderate to severe hypertriglyceridemia.

Combination Drug Therapy

Some patients with severe hypercholesterolemia may require therapy with two and sometimes even three drugs to achieve therapeutic goals. This is especially true in secondary prevention, in which the LDL cholesterol goal of 100 mg per deciliter can be difficult to achieve in many patients. Bile acid sequestrants can be combined successfully with HMG-CoA reductase inhibitors in patients with normal triglyceride levels. Nicotinic acid can be very effective in combination with statins in patients with FH as well as combined hyperlipidemia. Fibrates and statins can be used together successfully in patients with moderate to severe hypertriglyceridemia who also require further LDL cholesterol reduction. This combination should be used with caution, because the risk of myopathy is increased. Patients should be told about the potential for muscle pain. Patients with severe hyperlipidemia requiring combination therapy should be referred to a specialized lipid center.

Low-density Lipoprotein Apheresis

Patients who remain significantly hypercholesterolemic despite combination drug therapy are at high risk of progressive atherosclerotic cardiovascular disease. Patients with drug-refractory hypercholesterolemia who have established CHD or who are high risk should be considered for LDL apheresis. This procedure involves the selective removal of LDL by physically passing plasma over columns containing dextran sulfate or heparin, which binds the LDL; the LDL-depleted plasma is then returned to the patient. LDL apheresis is performed using an automated instrument on a repetitive basis, usually every 2 weeks, because the LDL cholesterol levels rebound over time. This method does not result in HDL lowering and is generally well tolerated. Several studies have indicated that LDL apheresis can retard progression or cause regression of atherosclerosis in patients with severe, drug-resistant hypercholesterolemia. LDL apheresis is the treatment of choice, when possible, for patients with homozygous FH, who respond poorly to drug therapy. Other patients with resistant hypercholesterolemia and CHD are potential candidates for this treatment as well. Patients must be referred to a specialized lipid center for evaluation for LDL apheresis. When LDL apheresis is not available, plasma exchange can be considered. A large volume of plasma is removed and replaced with an albumin/saline solution. This effectively lowers the LDL cholesterol level acutely but also removes many other plasma constituents, including HDL cholesterol. It is generally less well tolerated than selective LDL apheresis.

Partial Ileal Bypass

The partial ileal bypass procedure lowers LDL cholesterol levels by 30% to 40% in reported studies. Its mechanism of action is similar to that of bile acid sequestrants: the enterohepatic circulation of bile acids is interrupted, and the hepatic LDL receptor is up-regulated. One controlled trial of partial ileal bypass in patients with moderate hypercholesterolemia and established CHD showed significantly diminished cardiovascular morbidity and mortality rates in the treated group compared with the control group, which received no lipid-lowering therapy. However, diarrhea is a relatively common side effect, and the incidence of kidney stones, gallstones, and intestinal obstruction is also high. The procedure is relatively ineffective in persons with homozygous FH and in many other patients with severe, drug-refractory hypercholesterolemia. Therefore, its clinical utility is currently limited to those patients with severe hypercholesterolemia with established CHD who cannot tolerate standard lipid-lowering medications and do not have access to LDL apheresis.

Experimental Therapies

Novel therapies for severe, drug-refractory hypercholesterolemia are being developed actively. New molecular targets for the development of lipid-lowering small molecules include the microsomal transfer protein, which is required for assembly and secretion of apoB-containing lipoproteins. Gene therapy is also a consideration for severe conditions, such as homozygous FH. In a pilot study, five patients with homozygous FH were treated in a protocol involving ex vivo retroviral transfer of the LDL receptor gene into autologous hepatocytes, with subsequent reimplantation. LDL cholesterol levels declined modestly in three of five patients. As gene therapy vectors improve, homozygous FH and other conditions of severe, drug-refractory hypercholesterolemia will undoubtedly be targets for the development of gene therapeutic protocols. Patients with severe, resistant hypercholesterolemia should be referred to specialized centers so that they may benefit from experimental therapeutic protocols.

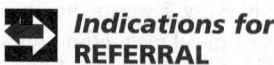

Indications for REFERRAL

Indications for referral to a lipid clinic include the following: inability to reach the LDL cholesterol goal, inability to reduce severely elevated triglyceride levels with a fibrate, intolerance of lipid-lowering medication, abnormal baseline liver transaminase (ALT and/or AST) levels in a patient who requires lipid-lowering drug therapy, increase in liver transaminase levels of greater than three times the upper limit of normal on drug therapy, consideration of LDL apheresis, persistently low HDL cholesterol in a high-risk patient, uncertainty about the need to institute lipid-lowering drug therapy, and suspected rare genetic disorders, such as familial chylomicronemia syndrome, homozygous FH, and abetalipoproteinemia.

COST-EFFECTIVENESS

Drug therapy to reduce LDL cholesterol in secondary prevention is highly cost-effective. The cost-effectiveness of drug therapy in primary prevention is determined by the level of risk of the patient to be treated. The higher the risk, the more cost-effective primary prevention becomes. One rationale for improving methods of risk assessment is to better identify persons who are candidates for lipid lowering in the context of primary prevention and make this intervention more cost-effective.

■ HYPERTRIGLYCERIDEMIA

PRESENTATION

The most important clinical consequence of severe hypertriglyceridemia is acute pancreatitis. In addition, moderate hypertriglyceridemia is frequently, but not invariably, associated with an increased risk of premature atherosclerotic cardiovascular disease. Therefore, any patient with acute pancreatitis or cardiovascular disease should be tested for triglycerides. In contrast to hypercholesterolemia, there are no formal guidelines for the classification and treatment of patients with hypertriglyceridemia. Patients with severe fasting hypertriglyceridemia (triglyceride levels more than 1,000 mg per deciliter) should be treated actively to reduce the risk of acute pancreatitis. For patients with mild to moderate hypertriglyceridemia, treatment should be directed primarily toward the assessment of cardiovascular risk and prevention of atherosclerosis. In general, if LDL cholesterol levels can be determined reliably, patients should be evaluated and treated based on the LDL cholesterol level, as described earlier. A significantly elevated triglyceride level (more than 400 mg per deciliter), however, often makes it difficult to assess the LDL cholesterol level accurately and requires a somewhat different approach to diagnosis and therapy.

PATHOPHYSIOLOGY

The pathophysiologic description of lipoprotein disorders is reviewed extensively in Chapter 12.

HISTORY AND PHYSICAL EXAMINATION

A complete history should be taken, including any record of pancreatitis or recurrent abdominal pain, atherosclerotic cardiovascular disease, other cardiovascular risk factors (Table 31.1), and known secondary causes of hyperlipidemia, including medications (see Chapter 12). A comprehensive family history of pancreatitis, premature cardiovascular disease, and hyperlipidemia should be obtained. The physical examination should include a search of the eyes for arcus corneae and lipemia retinalis, the eyelids for xanthelasmas, the palms for palmar xanthomas, the elbows and knees for tuberoeruptive xanthomas, and the back and buttocks for eruptive xanthomas. The thyroid should be palpated, and major arteries should be examined for vascular bruits. Patients with very high triglyceride levels are at risk of acute pancreatitis.

LABORATORY STUDIES AND DIAGNOSTIC TESTS

Evaluation of triglycerides requires a fasting lipid profile. For assessment purposes, patients with elevated triglyceride levels are often divided into those with borderline high (200 to 400 mg per deciliter), high (400 to 1,000 mg per deciliter), and very high (more than 1,000 mg per deciliter) triglyceride levels. The major concern in patients with borderline and high triglyceride levels is the presence of dyslipidemia, which may increase the risk of CHD. Patients with very high triglycerides are at risk of acute pancreatitis. Once hypertriglyceridemia has been diagnosed, the laboratory should rule out potential secondary causes. In practice, this evaluation usually includes measurement of fasting glucose to eliminate the possibility of diabetes mellitus and measurement of serum albumin if the nephrotic syndrome is suspected. Liver function tests also are undertaken if obstructive liver disease is suspected.

DIFFERENTIAL DIAGNOSIS

The differential diagnosis of hypertriglyceridemia includes primary and secondary causes. Most patients with severe hypertriglyceridemia (more than 1,000 mg per deciliter) probably have an underlying genetic predisposition, which in many cases is exacerbated by another medical condition or a hormonal or environmental factor. Primary genetic causes of severe hypertriglyceridemia (see Chapter 12) include LPL deficiency, apoC-II deficiency, lipodystrophy, type I glycogen storage disease, and familial type V hyperlipidemia (of unknown origin). LPL deficiency can be diagnosed in specialized laboratories by measuring LPL in plasma obtained after the patient has been given a small dose of heparin, but it is unlikely to appear for the first time in an adult. It is much more common for a secondary cause to contribute to severe hypertriglyceridemia (poorly controlled diabetes mellitus, the nephrotic syndrome, heavy alcohol use, or the use of estrogens, isotretinoin, etretinate, or HIV protease inhibitors). In most cases, the secondary cause is probably superimposed on an underlying genetic predisposition to hypertriglyceridemia. Although familial dysbetalipoproteinemia alone normally does not produce triglyceride levels above 1,000 mg per deciliter, when a secondary cause of hypertriglyceridemia is superimposed on the apoE-2/2 genotype, triglyceride levels can be very elevated. Therefore,

consideration should be given to determining the apoE genotype in all patients with severe hypertriglyceridemia.

Primary causes of less severely elevated triglycerides (see Chapter 12) include familial hypertriglyceridemia, FCHL, and familial dysbetalipoproteinemia (type III hyperlipidemia). A few clinical clues and laboratory tests can assist in the diagnosis of these disorders. A family history of hyperlipidemia in at least one first-degree relative is required to support the diagnosis of FCHL. This diagnosis can be corroborated by the measurement of the plasma apoB level. In FCHL, the apoB level is increased (usually more than 130 mg per deciliter) and is often elevated disproportionately to the LDL cholesterol level owing to the presence of increased amounts of small, dense LDL particles, a biochemical marker for FCHL. Therefore, a substantially elevated apoB level in the context of modestly elevated LDL and triglyceride levels strongly suggests FCHL. Familial dysbetalipoproteinemia (type III hyperlipidemia) should be suspected when there is no family history of hyperlipidemia or a secondary cause of hyperlipidemia, when palmar or tuberoeruptive xanthomas are found, or when the total cholesterol and triglyceride levels are both substantially elevated to a similar degree. The diagnosis of type III hyperlipidemia can usually be confirmed by lipoprotein ultracentrifugation or apoE genotyping. The finding of a ratio of VLDL cholesterol to total triglycerides of more than 0.3 or an apoE-2/2 genotype in a patient with clinically suspected type III hyperlipidemia confirms the diagnosis.

STRATEGIES FOR OPTIMAL CARE

Management

Secondary causes of hypertriglyceridemia should be treated. In general, dietary measures are useful in improving hypertriglyceridemia. Alcohol should be avoided. Obese persons should lose weight by restricting caloric intake. Physical exercise can often have a significant impact on triglyceride levels. Restriction of total dietary fat can be effective for patients with severe hypertriglyceridemia. Diabetes should be optimally controlled. Women taking estrogens should consider discontinuing them, especially if the triglyceride level is very high (more than 1,000 mg per deciliter). An algorithm for the management of hypertriglyceridemia is presented in Figure 31.3.

When fasting triglyceride levels remain above 1,000 mg per deciliter despite appropriate dietary and lifestyle measures, drug therapy should be instituted to lessen the risk of acute pancreatitis. There are three major classes of drugs used to lower very high triglyceride levels: fibric acid derivatives, nicotinic acid, and fish oils. The choice must be individualized to the patient. Nicotinic acid and fish oils worsen glucose intolerance, and for this reason fibrates are preferred in patients with diabetes mellitus. Sometimes combinations, particularly a fibrate with fish oils, are necessary for adequate control. When triglyceride levels cannot be reduced to levels below 1,000 mg per deciliter, patients should be referred to a lipid clinic.

Drug therapy also should be considered in the effort to lower triglyceride levels in the patient with established CHD who has a triglyceride level above 400 mg per deciliter. In this context, lowering the triglyceride level is essential for optimal manage-

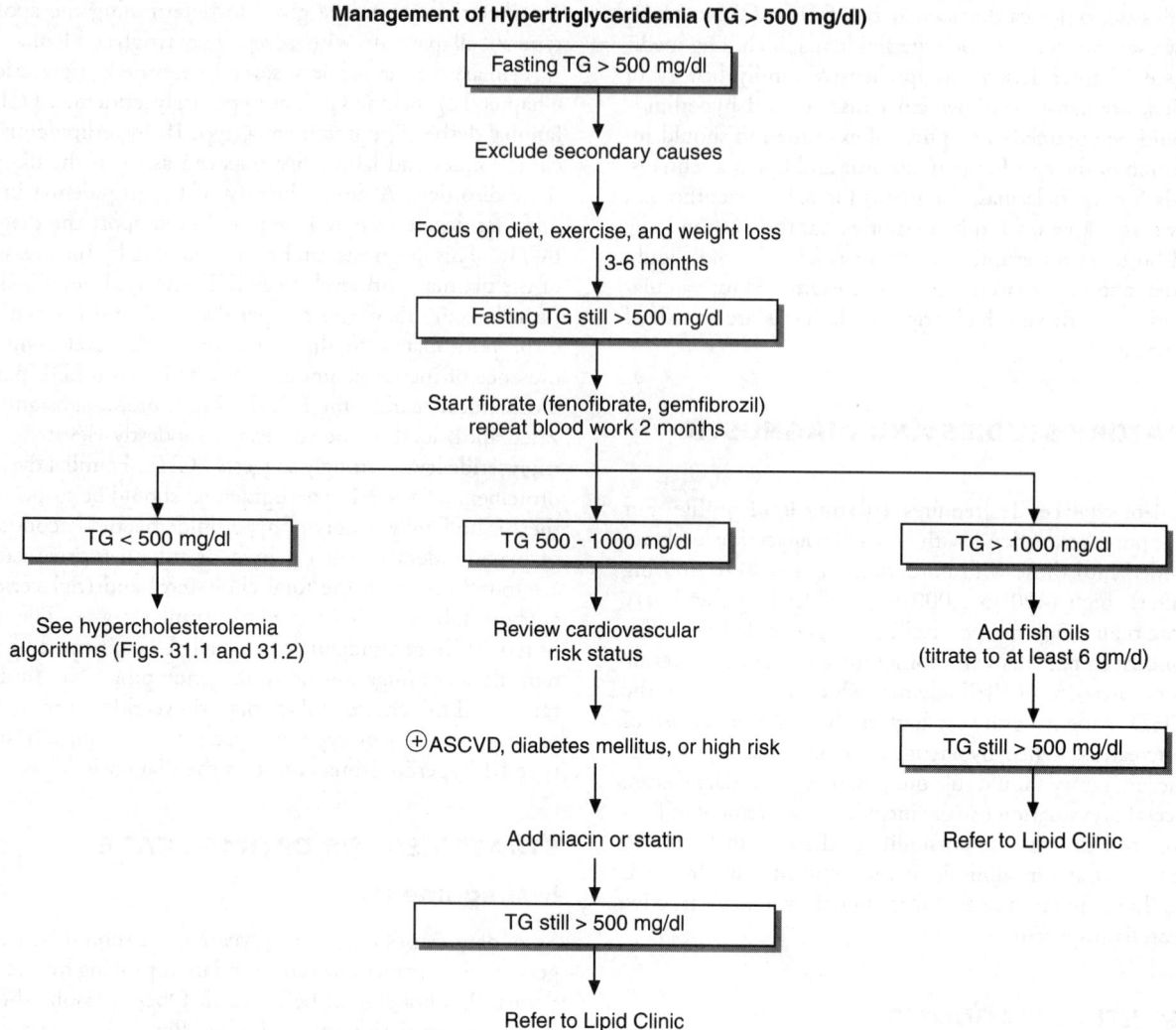

FIGURE 31.3. Strategy for the management of hypertriglyceridemia.
EVIDENCE LEVEL: C. Expert Opinion.

ment of the LDL cholesterol level (which is often difficult to assess when the triglyceride level is more than 400 mg per deciliter). Fibrates and nicotinic acid are the major choices. For triglycerides closer to the 1,000 mg per deciliter range, fish oils can be useful adjunct therapy. For triglycerides closer to the 400 mg per deciliter range in patients who also have elevated LDL cholesterol levels, statins may be helpful in reducing these levels, especially at higher doses. Triglyceride levels in the 200 to 400 mg per deciliter range are associated with increased cardiovascular risk, but little data exist that show that reduction of triglycerides in this range lowers risk. Nevertheless, in patients with established CHD, borderline high triglycerides could be considered a secondary target for intervention after the LDL cholesterol has been lowered to a desirable range. Fibrates and fish oils can cause the LDL cholesterol level to increase; for this reason, nicotinic acid may be preferred in patients with moderate triglyceride elevations and elevated LDL cholesterol levels.

Patients with type III hyperlipoproteinemia respond well to fibrates, but they also respond to nicotinic acid and statins. Type III hyperlipoproteinemia is one of the few hypertriglyceridemic conditions that responds favorably to estrogen replacement therapy.

HYPOALPHALIPOPROTEINEMIA (DECREASED HIGH-DENSITY LIPOPROTEIN CHOLESTEROL)

PRESENTATION

Given the current recommendations for screening of both HDL cholesterol and total cholesterol in all adults, many persons are now being diagnosed with low HDL cholesterol levels. There are no formal guidelines for the classification and treatment of patients with low levels of HDL cholesterol, however, except as an additional risk factor in the management of elevated LDL cholesterol. Many patients with low HDL cholesterol levels have associated hyperlipidemia, in which case they should be evaluated and treated based on the type of hyperlipidemia, as described earlier. Some persons, however, have isolated hypoalphalipoproteinemia (HDL cholesterol level in the bottom tenth percentile) with relatively normal cholesterol and triglyceride levels.

PATHOPHYSIOLOGY

The pathophysiologic description of low HDL cholesterol is reviewed extensively in Chapter 12.

HISTORY AND PHYSICAL EXAMINATION

A complete history should be taken, including any record of atherosclerotic cardiovascular disease, other cardiovascular risk factors (Table 31.1), and known secondary causes of low HDL cholesterol, for example, medications (see Chapter 12). A comprehensive family history of premature cardiovascular disease and lipid disorders should be obtained. The physical examination should include a search of the eyes for arcus corneae. The thyroid should be palpated, and major arteries should be examined for vascular bruits.

LABORATORY STUDIES AND DIAGNOSTIC TESTS

Evaluation of HDL cholesterol can be performed without fasting, but a full evaluation requires a fasting lipid profile. The laboratory should rule out potential secondary causes of low HDL cholesterol.

DIFFERENTIAL DIAGNOSIS

The differential diagnosis and management of isolated low HDL cholesterol levels must distinguish patients with moderately decreased HDL cholesterol levels (15 to 35 mg per deciliter) and those with severely decreased HDL levels (less than 15 mg per deciliter). The major known causes of decreased HDL cholesterol levels are listed in Chapter 12.

Moderately low HDL cholesterol levels often are associated with modestly elevated LDL cholesterol or triglyceride levels. In this context, the low HDL cholesterol level is used in clinical practice as an additional independent cardiovascular risk factor, but it is rarely appropriate to embark on a diagnostic evaluation of the low HDL cholesterol level itself. If the LDL cholesterol and triglyceride levels are relatively normal, the apoB level should be measured. The apoB level is often elevated in patients with moderately low HDL cholesterol levels; this suggests the presence of a form of FCHL often referred to as hyperapobetalipoproteinemia. The syndrome of low HDL cholesterol without accompanying hyperlipidemia has been referred to as primary hypoalphalipoproteinemia. Patients with this disorder may be

at high risk of premature cardiovascular disease. There is no diagnostic test, though a low level of apoA-I can help confirm the low level of HDL cholesterol and supports the diagnosis. Secondary causes of a moderately decreased HDL cholesterol level include smoking, type II diabetes mellitus, obesity, and a sedentary lifestyle.

Severely decreased HDL levels (less than 20 mg per deciliter) often are seen in patients with markedly elevated triglyceride levels (usually more than 1,000 mg per deciliter). When HDL cholesterol levels are in this range in the context of normal to only moderately elevated triglyceride levels, a rare genetic source is virtually always the cause. The major known genetic causes of severely low HDL cholesterol levels (see Chapter 12) include mutations in apoA-I, lecithin:cholesterol acyltransferase, and ATP-binding cassette protein 1 (ATP1; Tangier disease). A patient suspected of having one of these disorders should be referred to a specialized lipid center for further evaluation.

STRATEGIES FOR OPTIMAL CARE

Management

There are no formal guidelines for the treatment of patients with isolated low HDL cholesterol levels. Diabetes should be optimally controlled, smoking should be discontinued, obese persons should lose weight, and sedentary persons should exercise. Postmenopausal women should consider estrogen replacement therapy, which results in a modest increase in HDL cholesterol. Nicotinic acid is the most effective pharmacologic method for raising HDL cholesterol, and fibrates have modest effects, particularly in patients who also have elevated triglycerides. However, there are few clinical data to suggest that raising the HDL cholesterol level protects against the development or progression of atherosclerotic cardiovascular disease. The Veterans Administration HDL Intervention Trial (VA-HIT) trial indicated the benefit of gemfibrozil therapy (which raised HDL cholesterol levels and reduced triglycerides but did not change LDL cholesterol levels) in men with CHD and low HDL cholesterol levels. In practice, in patients with established CHD and low HDL cholesterol levels, LDL cholesterol should be controlled first. If the HDL cholesterol remains low, however, additional consideration may be given to the use of nicotinic acid to raise the HDL level further. In primary prevention it is difficult to recommend drug therapy specifically to raise HDL cholesterol levels, though an individual at very high risk with an isolated low HDL cholesterol level might consider taking niacin despite the absence of clinical trial data. Firm clinical recommendations must await clinical trials designed to address this question.

■ HYPOLIPIDEMIA (DECREASED CHOLESTEROL)

Disorders causing clinically significant low levels of cholesterol are rare. In general, a total cholesterol level above 80 mg per deciliter is not associated with any known clinical signs or symptoms. The two major clinically important disorders of low cholesterol are abetalipoproteinemia and homozygous hypobetalipoproteinemia. Their clinical symptoms include spinocerebellar degeneration, pigmented retinopathy, fat malabsorption, and acanthocytosis (see Chapter 12). They should be suspected only if the total cholesterol level is below 80 mg per deciliter, in which case a full lipid profile should be performed along with quantitation of apoB. The diagnosis is confirmed by extremely low to undetectable levels of LDL cholesterol and apoB.

These disorders are differentiated from each other primarily by family history. Abetalipoproteinemia is autosomal recessive, and obligate heterozygotes (such as the parents) have normal cholesterol levels. Hypobetalipoproteinemia is autosomal codominant, and heterozygotes have about half the normal levels of cholesterol. Patients with either of these disorders should be referred to a specialized center for definitive diagnosis and appropriate therapy. Despite therapy, many patients have slowly progressive neurologic and retinal disease.

BIBLIOGRAPHY

Brown BG, Zhao XQ, Sacco DE, et al. Lipid lowering and plaque regression: new insights into prevention of plaque disruption and clinical events in coronary disease. *Circulation* 1993;87:1781.

Downs JR, Clearfield M, Weis S, et al. Primary prevention of acute coronary events with lovastatin in men and women with average cholesterol levels. *JAMA* 1998;279:1615–1622.

Expert Panel on Detection, Evaluation, and Treatment of High Blood Cholesterol in Adults. Summary of the second report of the National Cholesterol Education Program (NCEP) expert panel on detection, evaluation, and treatment of high blood cholesterol in adults (Adult Treatment Panel II). *JAMA* 1993;269:3015–3023.

Giles WH, Anda RF, Jones DH, et al. Recent trends in the identification and treatment of high blood cholesterol by physicians. *JAMA* 1993; 269:1133–1138.

Gordon BR, Stein E, Jones P, et al. Indications for low-density lipoprotein apheresis. *Am J Cardiol* 1994;74:1109.

Gotto AM. Cholesterol management in theory and practice. *Circulation* 1997;96:4424–4430.

Grundy SM, Balady GJ, Criqui MH, et al. Primary prevention of coronary heart disease: guidance from Framingham. A statement for healthcare professionals from the AHA task force on risk reduction. *Circulation* 1998;97:1876–1887.

Levine GN, Keaney J, Vita JA. Cholesterol reduction in cardiovascular disease: clinical benefits and possible mechanisms. *N Engl J Med* 1995; 332:512–521.

Rader DJ, Hoeg JM, Brewer HB Jr. Quantitation of plasma apolipoproteins in the primary and secondary prevention of coronary artery disease. *Ann Intern Med* 1994;120:1012.

Sacks FM, Pfeffer MA, Moye L, et al. The effect of pravastatin on coronary events after myocardial infarction in patients with average cholesterol levels. *N Engl J Med* 1996;335:1001–1009.

Scandinavian Simvastatin Survival Study Group. Randomised trial of cholesterol lowering in 4444 patients with coronary heart disease: the Scandinavian Simvastatin Survival Study (4S). *Lancet* 1994;344:1383–1389.

Shepherd J, Cobbe SM, Ford I, et al. Prevention of coronary heart disease with pravastatin in men with hypercholesterolemia. *N Engl J Med* 1995; 333:1301–1307.

Smith J, Blair SN, Criqui MH, et al. Preventing heart attack and death in patients with coronary disease. *Circulation* 1995;92:2–4.

Tonkin A, Simes RJ. Prevention of cardiovascular events and death with pravastatin in patients with coronary heart disease and a broad range of initial cholesterol levels. *N Engl J Med* 1998;339:1349–1357.

CHAPTER 32

APPROACH TO THE PATIENT WITH CHEST PAIN (CARDIAC AND NONCARDIAC)

ALBERTO A. MITRANI
MARK MULTACH

The patient with chest pain may suffer from symptoms as trivial as indigestion or have a significant risk of sudden death within minutes. Physicians must be prepared to initiate an evaluation expediently, first differentiating the likelihood of myocardial ischemia or other life-threatening disease from less urgent situations. A rapid assessment is essential to identify the patient who may have an acute coronary syndrome and hence be at risk of sudden cardiac death.

CARDIAC CHEST PAIN

PAIN DUE TO ISCHEMIA

The initial concern is always the possibility of myocardial ischemia. Acute coronary syndromes include myocardial infarction (MI) and the various patterns of unstable angina. The latter is defined as new-onset angina, rest angina, or crescendo-pattern angina (more frequent, prolonged, or severe episodes in a patient with known angina pectoris). Any sustained episode of acute angina should be considered a potential evolving infarction until proved otherwise. These entities should be identified quickly so that immediate treatment to prevent MI or salvage myocardium can be initiated.

Chronic stable angina may stem from coronary artery disease, aortic stenosis, left ventricular hypertrophy, or pulmonary hypertension. The pattern of chest pain is usually related to effort and may become unstable. Owing to the high risk of sudden death with hemodynamically significant aortic stenosis, this diagnosis should be suspected in the patient with concomitant dyspnea or fatigue, transient loss of consciousness, and confirmatory examination results. Prinzmetal's angina typically occurs at rest but may also accompany exertion and other vasospastic phenomena. Aside from its occurrence at rest, the characteristics and associations are similar to those of classic angina.

PAIN NOT DUE TO ISCHEMIA

Pericardial pain results from inflammation and frequently has a pleuritic or positional component, in that it can be relieved in the sitting position. From time to time it is indistinguishable from ischemic pain. Pulmonary embolism (PE) should be suspected when a patient with risk factors for thromboembolism describes pleuritic chest pain. Evaluation with ventilation perfusion lung scanning, pulmonary angiography, or venous imaging of the lower extremities is necessary, since a diagnosis made on

TABLE 32.1.	CHARACTERISTICS OF COMMON CAUSES OF CHEST PAIN				
	Duration	**Quality**	**Provocation**	**Relief**	**Location**
Effort angina	5–15 min	Visceral, pressure	Effort, emotion	Rest, NTG	Substernal, radiates
Rest angina	5–15 min	Visceral, pressure	Spontaneous	NTG	Substernal, radiates
Mitral prolapse	Minutes to hours	Visceral pressure	Spontaneous, no pattern	Time	Left anterior
Esophageal reflux	10–60 min	Visceral	Recumbency, lack of food	Food, antacid, upright position	Substernal, epigastric
Esophageal spasm	5–60 min	Visceral	Spontaneous, cold liquids, exercise	NTG	Substernal, radiates
Peptic ulcer	Hours	Visceral, burning	Lack of foods, "acid" foods	Foods, antacids	Epigastric, substernal
Biliary disease	Hours	Visceral, colic	Spontaneous, foods	Time, analgesics	Epigastric, RUQ, radiates
Cervical disease	Variable	Superficial	Head/neck movement, palpation	Time, analgesics	Chest
Musculoskeletal pain	Variable	Superficial	Movement, palpation	Time, analgesics	Multiple
Pulmonary	30+ min	Visceral, pressure	Often spontaneous	Rest, time, bronchodilator	Multiple

NTG, nitroglycerin; RUQ, right-upper quadrant.
EVIDENCE LEVEL: C. Expert Opinion.

purely clinical grounds is unreliable. The pain of aortic dissection is usually sudden in onset, with radiation to the back. It may be described as an intense or a "tearing" sensation. Rapid confirmation by aortography, computerized tomography, magnetic resonance imaging, or transesophageal echocardiography is crucial for a favorable outcome.

HISTORY AND PHYSICAL EXAMINATION

A careful history is the single best initial diagnostic tool available in assessing chest pain (Table 32.1). In describing symptoms, patients may not refer to their complaint as pain. Any number of descriptive terms can be expected, including tightness, squeezing, crushing, pressure, aching, burning, and "heartburn." Since classic (typical) angina is effort related, any of the previously described sensations that have a consistent association with effort should raise the suspicion of ischemia. Morning episodes of discomfort are more frequent with ischemia. A sensation that radiates to the arms, neck, or shoulder may also be more common in cardiac ischemia. The association of pain with nausea or vomiting and diaphoresis should heighten the suspicion of ischemia. Symptoms occurring at rest or those related to meals, movement, stress, and respiratory pattern are more likely to be from a noncardiac cause. A sensation described as stabbing or fleeting is also less likely to be ischemic. Certain characteristics of symptoms are highly indicative of noncardiac chest pain, including respiratory "tics," obvious sighs, gasping respiration, and short breath-holding time.

A detailed cardiovascular examination can provide vital clues to a cardiac cause, though normal examination results do not rule out a life-threatening process. The detection of a murmur of papillary muscle insufficiency, third or fourth heart sound, loud pulmonic valve component, abnormal precordial impulse,

jugular venous distention, rales, or lower-extremity edema is associated with organic heart disease and may indicate ischemia or infarction. A diminished aortic closure sound, with a crescendo–decrescendo systolic murmur peaking late in systole and accompanied by a decreased carotid upstroke, suggests hemodynamically significant aortic stenosis. Unequal pulses or blood pressures should be a warning of possible aortic dissection. Pericardial friction rub (a rough, leathery sound), tachycardia, and pulsus paradoxus suggest pericarditis and possible tamponade. The presence of a pleural friction rub, evidence of consolidation, absence of or abnormal breath sounds, or Hamman's sign (a crunching sound heard in the precordium) may indicate a pulmonary source. Persistent sinus tachycardia with tachypnea, a pleural rub, and localized wheezing, can reflect pulmonary em-

TABLE 32.2.	SENSITIVITY AND SPECIFICITY FOR THE DIAGNOSIS OF ACUTE MYOCARDIAL INFARCTION WITH REFERENCE TO DIAGNOSTIC CRITERIA[a]

Criteria	Sensitivity	Specificity
ST elevation	49%	92%
ST elevation or depression	61%	71%
ST elevation or depression, Q waves, or LBBB	81%	69%

LBBB, left bundle-branch block.
[a] The sensitivity and specificity will differ, depending on the diagnostic criteria applied. As broader criteria are included, sensitivity rises, while specificity declines.

TABLE 32.3.   SENSITIVITY AND SPECIFICITY AND TEMPORAL APPEARANCE OF BIOCHEMICAL MARKERS FOR INFARCTION/ISCHEMIA[a]

Biochemical Marker	Duration	Peak	Sensitivity	Specificity	Remarks
Glycogen phosphorylase BB	1 hr—unknown	unknown	Probably high	Unknown	May be released in ischemia without necrosis
Myoglobin	1–12 hrs	3–5 hrs	High (near 100%)	Low	Detected within 1 h after onset of infarction, increase with any muscle injury
Myoglobin/CAIII ratio	1–12 hrs	3–5 hrs	Probably high	Probably high	Under evaluation
Myoglobin/FABP ratio	1–12 hrs	3–5 hrs	Probably high	Possibly high	Under evaluation
CKMB/CPK ratio	12–36 hrs	20–28 hrs	High	High	Serial measurement, current WHO reference standard
TnI	8–48+ hrs	12–24 hrs	High (near 100%)	High (near 100%)	Prognostic indicator, no rise in renal failure, no cross-reaction with skeletal Tn
TnT	8–48+ hrs	12–24 hrs	High	High	Rises in renal failure, cross-reactive with skeletal Tn
LDH isoenzymes	36–72+ hrs	36–48 hrs	Low for early diagnosis	Low	Isoenzyme form improves specificity

[a] Biochemical markers for infarction/ischemia differ in temporal appearance and peak after onset of infarction and in sensitivity and specificity.
[b] Duration represented here is the approximate amount of time that a marker is present at a level of twice the upper limit of normal.
Key:–duration of time that a marker is present at a level of twice the upper limit of normal; xx peak and duration of peak; CAIII, carbonic anyhdrase III; FABP, fatty acid binding protein; CPK, creatine phosphokinase; TnI, troponin I; TnT, troponin T; LDH, lactate dehydrogenase.
EVIDENCE LEVEL: C. Expert Opinion.

TABLE 32.4.   IMAGING IN THE EVALUATION OF MYOCARDIAL ISCHEMIA

Method	Advantages	Disadvantages

Echocardiography	High sensitivity in MI
	Sensitive for ischemia
	High negative predictive value
	    With exercise or dobutamine
	    Acute coronary syndrome
	Anatomic and structural information
	Functional assessment
	Estimates intracardiac pressures
	Identifies nonischemic disease
	Pericarditis, pulmonary emboli
	Bedside use
	Sensitivity
	Specificity
		Transmural > nontransmural
		Limited window in obesity and emphysema

Technetium Tc 99m Sestamibi[a]	Sensitive for acute or exercise-induced ischemia Better image quality than thallium Limited redistribution—later imaging possible Less soft-tissue (breast or diaphragm) interference Sensitivity Specificity	Not generally available at the bedside Requires intravenous injection
Thallium 201[a]	Sensitive for acute or exercise-induced ischemia Redistribution necessitates early timing of images Sensitivity Specificity	Soft-tissue interference (breast or diaphragm) Not generally available at the bedside Requires intravenous injection

MI, myocardial infarction.
[a] Single photon emission computed tomography (SPECT) is superior to planar imaging.

bolization. Atypical pain that is reproducible with cervical motion is likely due to a C6-7 radiculopathy.

DIAGNOSTIC TESTS

Electrocardiography (ECG) is essential in the evaluation of chest pain. Some 50% to 60% of patients with acute MI will show ECG changes suggesting the diagnosis. The actual percentage will be influenced by the previous or baseline ECG result, the timing of the study in relation to the onset of pain, the coronary distribution involved, and the specific criteria used. Depending on the diagnostic criteria for MI, sensitivity and specificity of the ECG will vary (Table 32.2). A normal ECG result makes the diagnosis of MI less likely but does not exclude the possibility. The presence of a left bundle-branch block (new or old) is a poor prognostic indicator.

During an acute episode of Prinzmetal's angina, ECG may show ST segment elevation. In pericarditis, pulmonary embolization, and pulmonary hypertension, ECG can be helpful if the clinical findings suggestive of these conditions are evident. ECG interpretation can also be misleading in the case of esophageal spasm, during which T-wave inversion has been observed.

Biochemical markers, such as creatine kinase (CK) and its isoenzymes (CK-MB), have been the standard laboratory test used to evaluate acute coronary syndromes. The mass immunoassay for CK-MB may make it more useful in the early diagnosis of infarction. Troponin inhibitory protein (TnI) is a marker for injury recently introduced into clinical practice. Found only in myocardial muscle, TnI does not rise in the context of renal insufficiency and can be detected for up to 10 days after myocardial injury. Absent in the normal circulation, the presence of TnI must be interpreted as evidence of myocardial injury. A rational approach for biochemical testing presently includes both CK-MB and TnI, the specific choice depending on the time of onset of symptoms relative to the laboratory evaluation. In the future, the ratio of myoglobin to carbonic anhydrase III or human heart fatty acid binding protein is likely to be added to markers currently in use, to aid in earlier infarct detection. Table 32.3 summarizes biochemical markers.

Exercise stress testing may be useful in patients with a stable pattern of chest pain, but it is contraindicated in high-risk patients. The addition of imaging techniques to exercise testing is advisable in patients with abnormal resting electrocardiogram findings and in women under the age of 40, who tend to have a higher incidence of false-positive electrocardiographic study results. Imaging techniques include thallium 201, technetium 99m, sestamibi, and echocardiography (Table 32.4). The use of pharmacologic testing with adenosine, dypiridamole, or dobutamine is helpful in patients who cannot adequately exercise.

CHEST PAIN OF UNCLEAR ORIGIN

Syndrome X may be linked to abnormalities in coronary flow reserve and may be accompanied by insulin resistance. Patients who experience angina are usually, but not exclusively, women in their late forties with a positive stress test. Coronary angiography fails to establish significant occlusion, and life expectancy is not affected. The diagnosis requires exclusion of other causes of chest pain. Current treatment options are limited to nitroglycerin, imipramine, aminophylline, and enalapril, with limited success.

TABLE 32.5.	DIFFERENTIAL DIAGNOSIS OF CHEST PAIN

Cardiac chest pain
  Acute coronary syndromes
  Angina and Prinzmetal's angina
  Valvular heart disease
  Cardiomyopathy
  Mitral valve prolapse
  Aortic dissection
  Pericarditis
  Pulmonary hypertension
  Syndrome X
Noncardiac chest pain
  Pulmonary
    Pulmonary embolus
    Pneumothorax
    Pneumonia
    Thoracic tumors
    Pleurodynia
    Precordial catch syndrome
  Gastrointestinal
    Esophageal spasm
    Esophageal reflux
    Esophagitis
    Peptic ulcer disease
    Gastritis
    Cholecystitis
    Pancreatitis
    Splenic infarction
    Mallory–Weiss syndrome
  Psychiatric
    Panic attack disorder
    Generalized anxiety disorder
    Depression (with one of the previously cited conditions)
    Cocaine use
  Musculoskeletal
    Trauma—recurrent
    Costochondritis (pain without inflammation)
    Tietze's syndrome (inflammation and pain)
    Cervical angina (C6-7) radiculopathy
  Superficial
    Herpes Zoster

NONCARDIAC CHEST PAIN

Once a cardiac source has been deemed unlikely, the differential diagnosis of chest pain is extensive (Table 32.5). In the majority of patients with a noncardiac cause of chest pain, symptoms are related to esophageal and anxiety disorders.

GASTROESOPHAGEAL REFLUX DISEASE

Up to 50% of patients with noncardiac chest pain have an esophageal abnormality that is acid related. Cardiac pain may be indistinguishable from pain of esophageal origin. Nocturnal and/or positional pain is more likely with gastroesophageal reflux disease (GERD). The presence of dysphagia, dyspepsia, or heartburn also suggests GERD. The diagnosis is frequently made on clinical grounds, justifying a trial of proton pump inhibitor or H_2-antagonist therapy. If symptoms do not resolve, diagnostic testing should be pursued. If dysphagia is an initial complaint, imaging with barium swallow or esophagogastroscopy will best iden-

TABLE 32.6.   CRITERIA FOR PANIC ATTACK[a]

A discrete period of intense fear or discomfort in which at least four of the following symptoms develop abruptly.
  Chest pain or discomfort
  Palpitations, cardiac awareness, or accelerated heart rate
  Sweating
  Trembling or shaking
  Sensation of shortness of breath or smothering
  Feeling of choking
  Nausea or abdominal distress
  Feeling dizzy, unsteady, lightheaded, or faint
  Feelings of unreality or detachment from oneself
  Fear of losing control or going crazy
  Fear of dying
  Numbness or tingling sensations
  Chills or hot flashes

[a] Diagnostic and Statistical Manual for Mental Disorders (DSM-IV).
EVIDENCE LEVEL: B. Reference: American Psychiatric Association. *Diagnostic and statistical manual of mental disorders, fourth edition.* **Washington, DC: American Psychiatric Association, 1994.**

tify the stricture, esophagitis, or mass that is most likely to be found in such a patient. In the patient with symptoms suggestive of GERD, evaluation can be individualized and includes barium swallow, pH monitoring, esophageal manometry, motility studies, provocative testing, and esophagogastroscopy.

UNEXPLAINED CHEST PAIN AND PANIC DISORDER

Patients with chest pain and normal coronary angiography have a 30% to 50% likelihood of meeting criteria for panic disorder. Panic attacks are required to establish a diagnosis of panic disorder and frequently include chest pain (Table 32.6). These patients have an excellent cardiac prognosis but continue to seek medical care for recurrent chest pain. Since the patient does not tend to seek psychiatric help, examining physicians must be sensitive to the possibility of panic disorder. The implications of high utilization of limited health care resources in these patients are obvious, and the economic impact is not trivial—a significant proportion of patients with panic disorder will visit an emergency department at least annually complaining of chest pain. The pathophysiologic explanation is not known, but abnormal metabolic activity in the anterior limbic structures has

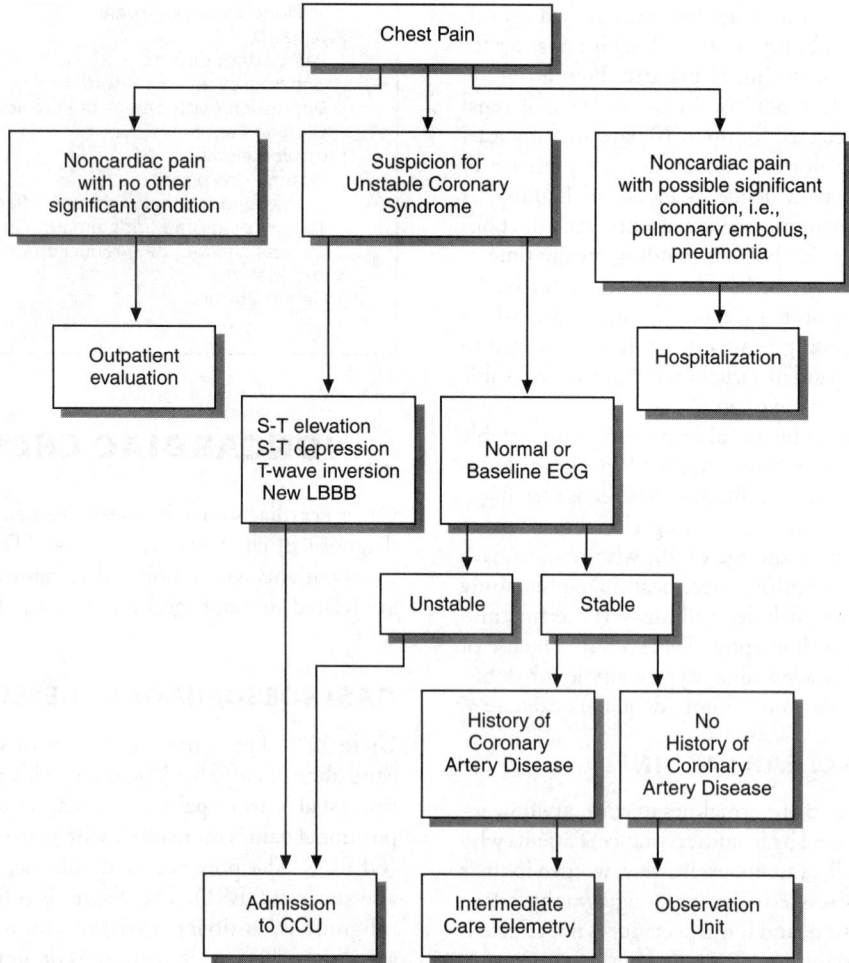

FIGURE 32.1. Potential settings for evaluation of chest pain patients depending on clinical presentation. Unstable defined as hypotension, congestive heart failure, arrythmias, and pain unresponsive to management.

been noted in these patients. A trial of imipramine, other tricyclic antidepressants, or serotonin re-uptake inhibitors is warranted; if not successful, such treatment should be followed by referral to a mental health specialist.

STRATEGIES FOR OPTIMAL COST-EFFECTIVE CARE

The evaluation of patients with chest pain should begin with the initial history, physical examination, and ECG for immediate and appropriate risk stratification. Figure 32.1 categorizes patients by these findings and suggests appropriate contexts for cost-effective evaluation and treatment. Future advances in biochemical markers and imaging techniques may help to distinguish patients with life-threatening conditions requiring hospitalization. The organization and implementation of regional chest pain centers will be studied for their potential to provide high-quality cost-effective care.

BIBLIOGRAPHY

Carter CS, Servan-Schreiber D, Perlstein WM. Anxiety disorders and the syndrome of chest pain with normal coronary arteries: prevalence and pathophysiology. *J Clin Psychiatry* 1997;58(s3):70–75.
Chauban A. Syndrome X-angina and normal coronary angiography. *Postgrad Med J* 1995;71:341–345.
Chen J-W, Lin S-J, Ting CT. Syndrome X: pathophysiology and clinical management. *Chung Hua I Hsueh Tsa Chih (Taipei)* 1997;60:177–183.
Goldman L. Using prediction models and cost-effectiveness analysis to improve clinical decisions: emergency department patients with acute chest pain. *Proc Assoc Am Phys* 1995;107(3):329–333.
Jesse RJ, Kontos MC. Evaluation of chest pain in the emergency department. *Curr Probl Cardiol* 1997;4:149–236.
Katz PO, Codario R, Castell DO. Approach to the patient with unexplained chest pain. *Compr Ther* 1997;23(4):249–253.
Keffer JH. The cardiac profile and proposed practice guideline for acute ischemic heart disease. *Am J Clin Pathol* 1997;107:398–409.
Tueth MJ. Managing recurrent nonischemic chest pain in the emergency department. *Am J Emerg Med* 1997;15:170–172.
Wu AHB. Use of cardia markers as assessed by outcomes analysis. *Clin Biochem* 1997;30(4):339–350.

Kelley's Textbook of Internal Medicine, fourth edition. Edited by H. David Humes. Lippincott Williams & Wilkins, Philadelphia © 2000.

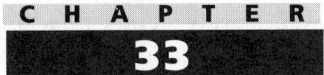

CHAPTER 33

SMOKING AND SMOKING CESSATION

ALFRED MUNZER

Smoking causes dysfunction and disease in virtually every organ of the human body. It is also a source of frustration to the physician, who feels powerless in the face of a habit that is deeply ingrained in the patient and that, despite a massive and largely successful public health campaign, is still condoned and even enshrined by segments of society. This chapter is designed to give an overview of the dimensions of the problem of smoking, to convey an understanding of the nature of tobacco and nicotine, and to provide the foundations for a clinical approach to the smoker.

MAGNITUDE OF THE SMOKING PROBLEM

Smoking remains the most common preventable cause of death in the United States. Smoking claims 450,000 lives annually, as many deaths as are caused by alcohol, cocaine, heroin, suicide, homicide, motor vehicle accidents, fire, and AIDS combined. Smoking doubles the overall mortality rate and is responsible for 30% of all deaths in the United States, including 90% of deaths due to lung cancer, 35% of all cancer deaths, 21% of deaths due to coronary heart disease, and 90% of deaths due to chronic obstructive lung disease. Smoking and the use of smokeless tobacco are also the major cause of cancer of the oral cavity and cancer of the esophagus, and they contribute to the deaths from cancer of the pancreas, cancer of the urinary tract, peripheral vascular disease, and cerebrovascular disease. Smoking also plays a significant role in the development of peptic ulcer disease and infectious respiratory disease and compounds the complications associated with diabetes.

Because women started smoking in large numbers more recently than men, their death rate from smoking has been lower, but the rate is catching up to that of men. Whereas the age-adjusted mortality rate from smoking rose 18% for men from 1973 to 1989, it rose 118% for women. Smoking exposes women to the same risks as men and also increases their risk of cancer of the cervix and osteoporosis. Smoking advances the age of menopause, causes premature aging of the skin, and increases the incidence of complications of stroke associated with the use of oral contraceptives. Smoking in pregnancy leads to premature births, miscarriages, stillbirths, and low-birth-weight babies.

Smoking causes death, disease, and disability not only in smokers but also in those exposed to environmental tobacco smoke. Parental smoking, for example, provokes pneumonia, bronchitis, and middle-ear effusions in children, reduces their lung function, and places them at increased risk of asthma. Smoking by spouses increases the incidence of lung cancer in nonsmoking partners. Environmental tobacco smoke has been estimated to lead to 50,000 deaths due to cancer and coronary heart disease annually in the United States. The direct medical costs associated with smoking have been estimated conservatively at $53 billion annually. The total cost of smoking probably exceeds $100 billion annually.

Despite a massive campaign to inform the public of the hazards of smoking and despite increasing restrictions on smoking in the workplace and in public places, 47 million Americans, or 27.0% of men and 22.6% of women, were still smoking in 1995. In 1965, however, 42.4% of the population smoked, and 50% of all adults who have ever smoked have quit, a success unparalleled in the annals of public health. Furthermore, 70% of smokers responding to a 1994 survey of the Centers for Disease Control and Prevention expressed a desire to quit and have made at least one serious attempt to quit. Unfortunately, the addictive nature of nicotine, the strength of a habit reinforced by a million puffs taken over the career of a smoker, intense marketing by the tobacco industry, and the ready availability of tobacco products conspire to allow only 2.5% of smokers to succeed in quitting in any given year. Even the simplest intervention by the physician can double the success rate. Seventy percent of smokers consult their physicians at least yearly, but 30% of those who consult their physicians are not even advised to stop smoking, and only a few smokers receive the sustained, organized, and appropriately intense counseling and support their devastating habit deserves.

BIOLOGIC BASIS FOR NICOTINE ADDICTION

TOBACCO

The psychoactive properties of tobacco were an important part of the rituals and healing practices of the peoples indigenous to the Americas for millennia. Ancient Mayan manuscripts vividly depict an underworld populated by gods smoking tobacco rolled into cones resembling cigars. Acute intoxication was deemed to have a transcendental purpose and was achieved not only through smoking but also through chewing, drinking, licking, and purging. European discoverers turned tobacco into an important commodity that shaped the economy of the American colonies and laid the foundation for today's giant transnational tobacco companies. The use of tobacco, however, was condemned and even banned for religious and esthetic reasons as early as the sixteenth century.

The advent of the cigarette-making machine in 1884, the invention of the safety match, and the creation of a positive, healthful image associated with smoking broadly popularized the use of tobacco. Acute intoxication was replaced with the problems of long-term addiction and chronic disease. In 1930, lung cancer was listed for the first time as a cause of death in the vital statistics of the United States. Tobacco has undergone many changes. It has been bred into many different varieties that make each specifically suitable to a particular taste or mode of administration. Tobacco is predominantly smoked as cigarettes, but it is also smoked as cigars or in pipes. There has been a resurgence of the use of smokeless, or chewing, tobacco, especially by adolescents.

There are four commonly used types of tobacco: flue-cured, light air-cured, dark, and oriental. Flue-cured tobacco has a high sugar and a low nitrogen content and produces an acidic smoke that prevents the absorption of nicotine in the oral cavity and makes more nicotine available for absorption through the lung. It is therefore a major ingredient of cigarettes. Light air-cured tobacco has a cellular structure that facilitates the absorption of various fillers and flavorings. For this reason it is used as a carrier of additives in cigarettes. Dark tobacco is fermented and thus has a low sugar and a high nitrogen content and produces an alkaline smoke that favors the absorption of nicotine in the oral cavity. Dark tobacco is preferred in pipes and cigars, which are puffed rather than inhaled, and in smokeless tobacco, which is chewed. Oriental tobacco is prized for its aroma.

Tobacco contains an estimated 4,000 compounds, including many that are pharmacologically active, toxic, mutagenic, and carcinogenic. There are several pharmacologically active alkaloids in tobacco, but nicotine is the most important. Among the toxic substances found in tobacco smoke are carbon monoxide, hydrogen cyanide, and ammonia. Forty-three definite carcinogens have been identified in tobacco smoke, including polynuclear aromatic hydrocarbons, *N*-nitrosamines, and inorganic compounds, such as arsenic and chromium. The carcinogens are targeted to the oral cavity when tobacco is chewed, to the oral cavity and the esophagus when pipes or cigars are puffed, and to the lung and remote organs when cigarette smoke is inhaled.

During the manufacture of cigarettes, cigars, and pipe and chewing tobacco, numerous ingredients are added to the tobacco leaf. These include sugars and licorice, which alter the flavor of the cigarette; glycerol and diethylene glycol, which retain moisture; menthol to reduce throat irritation; inorganic salts, which change the burning characteristics of the tobacco; and several oils to enhance the aroma. As a result, there are hundreds of tobacco products on the market targeted to every segment of the population. But all are ultimately designed to deliver nicotine into the system and to reinforce the addictive properties of nicotine.

PSYCHOPHARMACOLOGIC PROPERTIES OF NICOTINE

In the early 1800s, Cerioli and Vauquelin isolated an oily essence of tobacco; they named it "nicotianine" after Jean Nicot, who sent tobacco seeds from Portugal to the French court at the end of the sixteenth century. Nicotine is by far the major, but not the only, psychoactive alkaloid found in tobacco. It is a tertiary amine composed of a pyridine and a pyrrolidine ring. It is a weak base with a pKa of 8.0. In its pure form, it is a clear, volatile, alkaline liquid that has the smell of tobacco and turns brown when exposed to air. The concentration of nicotine varies in different types of tobacco leaves, but after the manufacturing process, the nicotine content of different brands of cigarettes is remarkably constant (about 8.4 mg). The level of nicotine delivered to the smoker, however, varies from 0.1 to 1.9 mg per cigarette, depending on the density of the tobacco in the cigarette and the presence of filters and designs that favor dilution of the smoke that is inhaled.

The temperature at the tip of a burning cigarette is 884°C, allowing for the distillation of nicotine along with other components into a vapor that is easily inhaled and rapidly absorbed across the alveolar surface. After absorption, nicotine is taken up rapidly by the brain and slowly distributed to other tissues. Nicotine is metabolized primarily in the liver to cotinine and nicotine oxide. Nicotine and its metabolites are excreted through the kidney. The half-life of nicotine in blood after tissue uptake is about 120 minutes. This means that during regular smoking, nicotine levels rise over 6 to 8 hours before reaching equilibrium and persist for 8 hours after cessation.

The effects of nicotine felt by the smoker are mediated through both the central and peripheral nervous systems. Nicotine, for example, affects various components of the neuroendocrine system and stimulates the release of anterior and posterior pituitary hormones. It binds to specific receptors in the brain and stimulates the release of acetylcholine in the cerebral cortex. It also causes the release of catecholamines from the adrenal medulla and from sympathetic nerve endings and of acetylcholine in the myenteric plexus of the gastrointestinal tract.

Nicotine, like heroin and cocaine, and far more often than ethanol, causes dependence. Criteria for dependence are the compulsive use of a substance, even when the harmful effects are known; the presence of psychoactive effects; the potential for reinforcement of behavior leading to use of the substance; the presence of physical signs of defense manifested through withdrawal symptoms; and the development of tolerance indicated through the increasing use of the substance to achieve a desired end point. Nicotine meets all these criteria. It is psychoactive because it has effects on mental function and mood. At blood levels most commonly found in smokers, it acts as a euphoriant, an anxiolytic, and a stimulant. More important, nicotine acts as a positive reinforcer, making one dose of nicotine, or one puff, or one cigarette, lead to the next. Abstinence from nicotine leads to a constellation of withdrawal symptoms that together constitute a craving for nicotine. Nicotine, like other psychoactive drugs, produces tolerance. The typical new smoker, therefore, gradually increases cigarette consumption over several years before reaching a plateau.

It was long thought that smokers regulated their smoking to maintain a set level of nicotine in the blood and brain. The basic impetus for maintaining that level was believed to be the avoidance of symptoms of nicotine withdrawal. It is now thought, however, that nicotine use is also governed by a far more complex process of learning and conditioning. A smoker, in other words, learns to smoke in response to specific stimuli, initially because of a perceived benefit and then merely as a conditioned response. These stimuli may be general, such as stress or boredom, or specific, such as the ringing of a telephone, sexual arousal, or completion of a meal. The resulting stereotypical pattern of tobacco use is another important marker of dependence. Treatment of nicotine addiction must be directed to both physical dependence and conditioning.

STAGES IN TOBACCO USE AND SMOKING CESSATION

Tobacco use is often thought of as a career that typically spans decades and runs a circuitous route from experimentation to quitting. No single factor governs the career of tobacco use: it is determined by the complex interaction of the psychopharmacologic properties of nicotine, the psychological makeup of the smoker, and, perhaps most important, the surrounding cultural, social, and economic setting. Several stages have been described in the smoking career: experimentation, initiation, and regular or habitual use. Smoking typically begins during childhood or adolescence. Regular or habitual smoking usually starts during the transition from adolescence to adulthood. Of those who experiment, one-third to one-half go on to smoke habitually. Contrary to the popular belief that early experimentation is merely a rite of passage, it is more likely to lead to habitual smoking than later experimentation. Habitual smoking is more common among persons who are impulsive, extroverted, and subject to depression. Smoking is also more common among those who have a low level of academic achievement and among those whose parents and peers smoke. A higher degree of concordance for smoking status among monozygotic than among heterozygotic twins suggests that there also may be genetic factors involved in establishing the smoking habit.

Tobacco marketing may also be a major influence on smoking initiation and habitual use. The tobacco industry spends an estimated $3.25 billion yearly on advertising and marketing, generally targeted to specific groups. The Joe Camel character, for example, is readily recognized by children. Marlboro cigarettes are the choice of adolescent boys and girls. Virginia Slims, on the other hand, are targeted to young women, many of whom smoke as a means of avoiding weight gain. Much advertising also appears to be directed at those who have quit smoking by emphasizing previous triggers of smoking. Smoking behavior is further complicated by social factors that enhance or deter smoking.

Recent rises in the excise tax on tobacco have shown that the cost of tobacco may be an important deterrent in the use of tobacco, particularly by children and teenagers. Like the development of the smoking habit, it is useful to think of smoking cessation not just as a single event but as a cyclic process with five stages: precontemplation, contemplation, action, maintenance, and relapse. In precontemplation, the smoker is not yet thinking of quitting; he or she may be unwilling, unaware, or discouraged from considering smoking cessation and may be defensive about smoking. Contemplation occurs as the smoker actively considers smoking cessation. At this stage, he or she seeks information and is typically concerned about smoking. Action occurs when the smoker takes steps to stop smoking. The smoker typically develops various strategies to prevent or overcome the temptation to smoke. Maintenance involves ongoing efforts to refrain from smoking after the smoker has achieved abstinence for about 6 months. Relapse, unfortunately the norm in smoking cessation, occurs when the smoker fails to maintain abstinence after quitting. Because smokers typically make many attempts at cessation before succeeding permanently, they may find themselves in various parts of the cycle several times during their smoking careers. Identifying the stages is useful because each requires a different intervention by the health care provider.

EVALUATING THE SMOKER

Because of the devastating impact of smoking on health, determining the smoking status should be as routine a part of every contact with a patient as measuring the vital signs. A more detailed evaluation geared to prescribing a specific smoking-cessation method should include measurement of the duration and severity of the smoking habit, identification of any symptoms

Points

1. How many cigarettes a day do you smoke?

[ ] 0 = 0–15   [ ] 1 = 16–25   [ ] 2 = 26+   _____

2. What brand do you smoke?

[ ] 0 =Low-nicotine   [ ] 1 = Moderate-nicotine   [ ] 2 = High-nicotine   _____

3. Do you inhale?

[ ] 0 = Never   [ ] 1 = Sometimes   [ ] 2 = Always   _____

4. Do you smoke more during the morning than during the rest of the day?

[ ] 0 = No   [ ] 1 = Yes   _____

5. How soon after you wake up do you smoke your first cigarette?

[ ] 1 = Within 30 minutes   _____

6. Which cigarette would you hate to give up?

[ ] 1 = The first cigarette in the morning   _____

7. Do you find it difficult to refrain from smoking in places where it is forbidden, eg, church, movie theater, library?

[ ] 0 = No   [ ] 1 = Yes   _____

8. Do you smoke if you are so ill that you are in bed most of the day?

[ ] 0 = No   [ ] 1 = Yes   _____

Score   0 = Minimal physical dependence
         11 = Maximal physical dependence

FIGURE 33.1. Questionnaire for identifying the addicted smoker. (Modified from Fagerstrom K-O. Measuring degree of physical dependence to tobacco with reference to individualization of treatment. *Addict Behav* 1978;3: 235, with permission.)

or illnesses exhibited by the smoker that may be attributable to smoking, assessment of the smoker's readiness to quit, a history of previous attempts to quit, and identification of personality variables and other internal or external factors that can facilitate or hinder quitting and not relapsing.

DURATION AND SEVERITY OF SMOKING HABIT

The longer and the more packs of cigarettes per day a smoker has smoked, the greater the impact on health, the need for smoking cessation, the likely resistance to quitting and not relapsing, and the necessity for intensive support during cessation. The Fagerstrom Tolerance Questionnaire (Fig. 33.1) is a simple, useful measure of the severity of physical dependence to nicotine. An urgent need to smoke within 30 minutes of waking up appears to be the most important indicator of severe physical dependence.

SYMPTOMS AND ILLNESSES ATTRIBUTABLE TO SMOKING

Evidence of heart disease, in particular, and of other diseases attributable to smoking to a lesser extent are among the most potent motivators for smoking cessation.

READINESS TO QUIT

All smokers should be advised to stop smoking, and all smokers should be told clearly of any adverse effects that smoking has had on their health. Otherwise, it is best to tailor advice to the specific stage the smoker is in. Those in the precontemplation stage, for example, should be given information about the effects of smoking on health, which may motivate them to move to the next stage. They should be asked to read these materials carefully and should be questioned about them at a follow-up visit. Smokers in the contemplation stage should be given information about specific cessation methods and should be encouraged to set a "quit date." Smokers in the action stage should be given maximal support in the form of behavioral techniques and pharmacologic agents to help them withstand the urge to smoke.

Personality Variables and Internal Factors

Rebelliousness, impulsiveness, and "identity assertion" in adolescence and adulthood have traditionally been viewed as major determinants of smoking. They are now seen as modifiers of other forces that favor change. Self-confidence and a sense that one's actions can be effective, or the attribution of success to oneself rather than to others, are important predictors of success in smoking cessation that should be nurtured. A negative attitude or depression may be an obstacle to permanent abstinence from smoking, particularly if the euphoriant properties of nicotine have been used to combat depression.

Fear of weight gain is an important obstacle to smoking cessation and continued abstinence for many smokers. Appetite and hunger are common withdrawal symptoms after smoking cessation. Six months after cessation, men will typically have gained 9 pounds and women 10 pounds; greater weight gains are occasionally encountered. It is important to anticipate changes in weight and to develop appropriate strategies to prevent relapse of smoking. It should be stressed to the patient that the health benefits of smoking cessation far outweigh the risks associated with the usual weight gain.

External Factors

The presence of a nonsmoking environment, beginning in the physician's office and also at home and work and during leisure activities, is an important contributor to success in smoking cessation. Conversely, continued smoking by family and peers can be major obstacles that require specific, predetermined coping strategies.

SMOKING-CESSATION METHODS

Most smokers who have quit have done so without any obvious outside intervention. As the number of smokers in the population declines, however, an increasing number will be highly addicted to nicotine; these are the ones most in need of more intensive support and more specific cessation methods. Smoking-cessation methods can be classified on the basis of the intensity of the intervention and whether pharmacologic agents are used. Every smoker should be individually evaluated to determine the most appropriate smoking-cessation method. The patient's preference and his or her experience of previous attempts at quitting play a key role in choosing a specific cessation method.

MINIMAL INTERVENTION

Helping patients to quit smoking on their own may be the most cost-effective cessation strategy. Only 10% to 15% are likely to remain abstinent from cigarettes at 1 year, but 60% will succeed after repeated attempts. Minimal intervention typically includes providing self-help materials, such as the American Lung Association's Freedom from Smoking self-help manuals; setting a specific quit date; and offering brief counseling and follow-up to identify and deal with any obvious obstacles to smoking cessation.

BEHAVIOR MODIFICATION

More intensive smoking-cessation programs are indicated for smokers who want added support, those who have previously tried to quit and have been unsuccessful, those whose dependence on nicotine and smoking seem more intense, and those who lack sufficient self-confidence and external support. Intensive smoking-cessation programs may take the form of clinics organized by such voluntary health agencies as the American Lung Association, local hospitals, or employers; for-profit smoking-cessation programs; or individual therapy with physicians or other health-care professionals. In addition to providing health information that can motivate the smoker to quit, virtually all rely on behavior-modification techniques, such as the following.

1. Temptation management: careful identification of the time, place, and reason for smoking each cigarette and the development of avoidance and mitigation strategies to reduce the temptation to smoke
2. Cue extinction: deconditioning by purposefully avoiding smoking during exposure to cues that would normally lead to smoking
3. Contingency management: designation of concrete rewards to be earned for achieving specified goals or reaching specified landmarks during the action stage of smoking cessation

Aversive techniques, used in some research and commercial smoking-cessation programs, typically consist of rapid smoking of a series of cigarettes with frequent inhaling and with holding of smoke in the mouth to produce dizziness and nausea. Aversive techniques are effective but are infrequently used because of a fear, probably unfounded, of adverse health effects. In the past, electric shock has been used as an aversive stimulus, but it is applied rarely today. Hypnosis has been the subject of controversy and may or may not be effective. There is also little scientific evidence to support acupuncture as an adjunct to smoking cessation.

PHARMACOLOGIC AGENTS

Pharmacologic agents have been used in the treatment of various forms of substance abuse because they can provide relief of withdrawal symptoms, serve as blockers or replacements, and produce aversion to the ingestion of a substance. Pharmacologic agents increase the likelihood of success in smoking cessation when used in combination with an organized behavior-modification program and should readily be offered to all but very light smokers.

Nicotine substitution in the form of nicotine polacrilex (gum), transdermal nicotine (patch), nicotine inhalers, or nicotine sprays is effective as an adjunct to a behavior-modification program, particularly for smokers who show a high degree of physical dependence to nicotine (as measured, for example, by the Fagerstrom Tolerance Questionnaire). Nicotine gum requires careful instruction in proper use, such as the need to avoid acidic beverages that can prevent absorption of nicotine and a proper way of chewing. Transdermal nicotine has the advantage of once-daily dosing, greater social acceptability than chewing gum, and the availability of various doses that can be tailored to each patient. The nicotine inhaler is said to have the advantage of reproducing the hand-to-mouth ritual of smoking. All forms of nicotine replacement have the potential of causing further nicotine dependence, but the benefits of smoking cessation far outweigh that risk.

Bupropion is an antidepressant that has been shown to decrease the desire for cigarettes. It is an effective alternative to nicotine substitution therapy. Clonidine is effective for the short-term relief of symptoms of nicotine withdrawal. Lobeline is a chemical analogue of nicotine, but its effectiveness as a form of replacement therapy remains unproved. Mecamylamine is a noncompetitive nicotine antagonist that has been tried as an agent to prevent the reinforcing effects of nicotine. Side effects at the high doses that have been used, however, have proved prohibitive. Silver nitrate mixes with a smoker's saliva to produce an unpleasant taste, but it has not been proved effective as a form of aversion therapy in supporting abstinence.

CONCLUSIONS

Smoking has a devastating impact on health. Smoking cessation is difficult because of the addictive nature of nicotine and the continued social acceptance of smoking. The use of behavior-modification techniques and pharmacologic agents greatly increases the likelihood of success in quitting. If every physician and other health care practitioner were familiar with these tools and used them, the number of smokers who quit every year could double.

BIBLIOGRAPHY

Department of Health and Human Services. *The health consequences of smoking: nicotine addiction. A report of the Surgeon General.* Washington D.C.: US Government Printing Office, 1988.

Fiore MC, Wetter DW, Bailey WC, et al. *Smoking cessation clinical practice guideline.* Rockville, Md.: Agency for Health Care Policy and Research, Public Health Service, US Department of Health and Human Services, 1996.

Fisher EB, Haire-Joshu D, Morgan GD, et al. State of the art: smoking and smoking cessation. *Am Rev Respir Dis* 1990;142:702–720.

Orleans CT, Slade J, eds. *Nicotine addiction: principles and management.* New York: Oxford University Press, 1993.

Pomerleau OF, Collins AC, Shiffman S, et al. Why some people smoke and others do not: new perspectives. *J Consult Clin Psychol* 1993;61: 723–731.

Prochaska JO, DiClemente CC. Stages of change in the modification of problem behaviors. *Prog Behav Modif* 1992;28:183–218.

Robbins AS. Pharmacologic approaches to smoking cessation. *Am J Prev Med* 1993;9:31–33.

Kelley's Textbook of Internal Medicine, fourth edition. Edited by H. David Humes. Lippincott Williams & Wilkins, Philadelphia © 2000.

C H A P T E R

34

APPROACH TO THE PROBLEM OF ALCOHOL ABUSE AND DEPENDENCE

CHARLES P. O'BRIEN

DEFINITION

The use of ethyl alcohol as a beverage began before recorded history, and most persons in Western societies at least experi-

TABLE 34.1.	SIGNS OF DEPENDENCE ON ALCOHOL OR ANOTHER DRUG

Regularly consuming more than originally intended
Desire to reduce or regulate use and failure at these attempts
Spending a great deal of time obtaining, consuming, or recovering from the effects of the drug
Important social, occupational, or recreational activities given up or curtailed because of use of the drug
Continuing use despite evidence that the drug is contributing to psychological or physical problems
Tolerance, the need for greatly increased amounts of the drug to achieve the desired effect
Physical dependence, as manifested by a withdrawal syndrome or by the use of more of the drug to prevent the development of withdrawal symptoms

ment with this substance at some time in their lives. Alcohol is a sedative drug, and a high proportion of users find its effects to be quite pleasant. The attractiveness of this beverage leads to excessive use and severe medical problems in about 14% of consumers. Alcohol abuse and alcohol dependence (i.e., alcoholism) are behavioral syndromes that exist along a continuum from minimal use to abuse to addictive use. Alcoholism is a pattern of alcohol use that continues despite significant problems produced by alcohol. There is no specific quantity that is diagnostic of alcoholism, and some alcoholics use ethanol episodically rather than daily. There is no source of alcohol that is more or less toxic than others. One beer (12 ounces) equals approximately one glass of wine (5 ounces), which equals 1.5 ounces of 80-proof liquor (Table 34.1).

As with other sedating drugs, drinkers acquire tolerance to the effects of alcohol. This reduced sensitivity to alcohol is the consequence of an adaptive process that occurs when homeostatic mechanisms are repeatedly perturbed by the stress of alcohol. If alcohol use is discontinued, a rebound occurs as the homeostatic mechanisms adapt to the absence of alcohol. This rebound is seen with many drugs and results in symptoms that are opposite in direction to the effects of the drug itself. This rebound is called a withdrawal syndrome. The state of adaptation to the repeated effects of a drug is called physical dependence, and its presence is determined by the appearance of withdrawal symptoms when the drug is abruptly stopped.

Evidence of increased tolerance and symptoms of withdrawal are frequently found in alcoholics, but neither tolerance nor withdrawal is necessary or sufficient for a diagnosis of alcoholism. Early diagnosis is important, because early treatment is more effective. Unfortunately, at an early stage, alcoholics convincingly deny their excessive drinking, and the physician must obtain a history from family members and look for physical and laboratory evidence to support a clinical suspicion of alcoholism.

An active alcoholic may appear to be a normal and productive person. Too often, physicians fail to recognize alcoholism in prosperous, employed individuals because of the stereotype of the homeless alcoholic who has been unemployed for years. A skilled diagnostician can recognize the signs of early alcoholism and make a referral to a treatment expert. Untreated alcoholism is a progressive disorder, with a downhill course that varies in rate.

INCIDENCE AND EPIDEMIOLOGY

Approximately 70% of American adults consume alcohol occasionally. A US probability sample of noninstitutionalized adults (15 to 54 years of age) conducted from 1990 to 1991 found that about 14% had experienced alcohol dependence at some time in their lives, and approximately 7% met criteria for alcoholism in the past year. This disorder is seen in all socioeconomic groups, including persons who are still gainfully employed.

ETIOLOGY

The development of alcohol abuse and dependence is influenced by a combination of hereditary and environmental factors. Children of alcoholics show an increased likelihood of becoming alcoholics, even when they are adopted at birth and raised by nonalcoholic parents. The studies of genetic influences in this disorder show only an increased risk of alcoholism, not 100% determinism, and this is consistent with the features of a polygenic disorder that has multiple determinants. Even identical twins, who share the same genetic endowment, do not have 100% concordance when one twin is alcoholic. The concordance rate for identical twins, however, is much higher than that of fraternal twins, who share the same environment but have a different genotype.

One of the inherited factors that seems to influence the development of alcoholism is tolerance to alcohol. Although tolerance can be acquired by repeated experience with alcohol, persons vary in the innate tolerance manifested when they first consume alcohol. The sons of alcoholics have reduced sensitivity (i.e., more tolerance) to alcohol than other young men of the same age (22 years) and drinking histories. When reexamined 10 years later, those who tolerated alcohol as young men were the most likely to have become alcoholics during the time since they were first tested. These data suggest that tolerance is partly inherited and that inherited tolerance can increase the probability of developing alcoholism. Having an innate tolerance to alcohol does not make a person an alcoholic, but it seems to enhance significantly the probability that alcoholism will develop.

The opposite influence, a kind of "antialcoholism," also can be inherited. Ethanol is metabolized by alcohol dehydrogenase, producing acetaldehyde, which is itself metabolized by a mitochondrial aldehyde dehydrogenase known as ALDH2. A common mutation occurs in the gene for ALDH2, resulting in a less effective aldehyde dehydrogenase. This allele has a high prevalence in Asian populations and results in excess production of acetaldehyde after the ingestion of alcohol. A person with this allele experiences a very unpleasant facial flushing reaction 5 to 10 minutes after ingesting alcohol. The probability of becoming alcohol dependent is reduced for persons with this heredity pattern, but the risk is not eliminated. Those who are strongly motivated to consume alcoholic beverages can endure the flush-

ing to achieve the other effects of alcohol. There are likely multiple genetic factors that can influence the probability of becoming an alcoholic, but no single factor is determinant. Those who inherit a tolerance to alcohol may avoid alcohol and never become alcoholic. Conversely, those who inherit the gene for a less effective aldehyde dehydrogenase may drink excessively despite the flushing reaction.

PATHOGENESIS

Ethanol is classed as a depressant because it produces sedation and sleep. Nonetheless, the initial effects of alcohol, particularly at lower doses, are often perceived as stimulation and are thought to result from suppression of brain inhibitory systems. The course of alcohol intoxication varies. Early in the drinking period, when blood alcohol levels are rising, reports of expansive mood, increased verbalization, and more assertiveness are common, but the sedative symptoms are dominant for some individuals even at an early stage. Some impairment of psychomotor function is measurable at levels as low as 35 to 50 mg per deciliter, well below the level considered to be legal intoxication in this country. This impairment is not perceptible to the average drinker. With increasing dose, the individual is likely to become progressively more depressed, withdrawn, and cognitively impaired. At very high blood alcohol levels (200 to 300 mg per deciliter), a nontolerant individual is likely to fall asleep and enter the first stage of anesthesia. Higher blood alcohol levels (in excess of 300 to 400 mg per deciliter) can inhibit respiration and pulse and can cause death in nontolerant individuals.

The duration of intoxication depends on how much alcohol was consumed over a given period. In general, the body is able to metabolize approximately one drink per hour, and the blood alcohol level generally declines at a rate of 15 to 20 mg per deciliter per hour. Experience with alcohol can produce greater tolerance (i.e., acquired tolerance) such that extremely high blood levels (300 to 400 mg per deciliter) can be found in alcoholics who do not appear to be grossly sedated. In these cases, the lethal dose does not increase proportionate to the sedating dose, and the margin of safety (i.e., therapeutic index) is dangerously low.

Heavy consumers of alcohol acquire tolerance, and they inevitably develop a state of physical dependence on alcohol. This often leads to drinking in the morning to restore alcohol blood levels diminished during the night. Eventually, alcoholics may awaken during the night and take a drink to avoid the restlessness produced by falling alcohol levels. The withdrawal syndrome generally depends on the size of the average daily dose, and it is usually "treated" by resumption of alcohol ingestion. Withdrawal symptoms are experienced frequently, but they are usually not severe or life-threatening until they occur in conjunction with other medical problems.

Depending on its concentration in tissues, alcohol has effects on brain physiology, varying from specific receptor actions to nonspecific membrane changes. Ethanol enhances the actions of the inhibitory neurotransmitter γ-aminobutyric acid (GABA) at a subpopulation of GABA receptors. One of the effects of ethanol is increased activity of the dopaminergic pathway from the ventral tegmental area (VTA) to the nucleus accumbens (NAc). This activation can be mediated by the effect on GABA receptors through suppression of inhibitory interneurons, but VTA activation results in an increase in extracellular dopamine in the NAc region. This effect can be learned; rats trained to self-administer alcohol begin to show an increase in NAc dopamine levels as soon as they are placed in the chamber where they have previously obtained alcohol. Other drugs of abuse, such as cocaine and heroin, also raise levels of the neurotransmitter dopamine in this brain area.

There is evidence from animal studies that the endogenous opioid system plays a part in alcohol reinforcement, because alcohol self-administration in animals is diminished by opiate receptor antagonists. In human volunteers, alcohol ingestion in the laboratory produced significant increases in peripheral β-endorphin levels in those with a family history of alcoholism, but the levels were not raised in those without such a family history. For alcoholics, data show that the opiate receptor antagonist naltrexone reduces or blocks the ability of alcohol to produce euphoria. Double-blind, placebo-controlled studies have shown that the relapse rate is lower when alcoholics are given naltrexone (50 mg daily) during the rehabilitation process.

CLINICAL FINDINGS

Taking an adequate history from a suspected alcoholic requires diligence and experience. Alcohol abusers typically underestimate the quantity of alcohol they have ingested, but they more often respond truthfully to indirect questions about the effects of their drinking. The CAGE questionnaire (Table 34.2) has been found to be a useful addition to the standard medical history.

Alcohol impairs recent memory and, in high doses, produces the phenomenon of blackouts, after which the drinker has no memory of his or her behavior while intoxicated. The mechanism of the acute memory effects is unclear, but the evidence suggests that reports from patients about their reasons for drinking and their behavior during a binge are not reliable. Alcohol-dependent persons often say that they drink to relieve anxiety or depression. When allowed to drink under observation, however, alcoholics typically become more dysphoric as drinking continues, contradicting the explanation that they drink to relieve ten-

sion. The long-term use of alcohol and other sedatives is associated with the development of depression, and the risk of suicide among alcoholics is one of the highest of any diagnostic category.

Cognitive deficits have been reported in alcoholics tested while sober. These usually improve after weeks to months of abstinence. More severe recent memory impairment is associated with specific brain damage caused by nutritional deficiencies common in alcoholics (see later discussion of Wernicke–Korsakoff syndrome). Contrary to the notions of many physicians, alcohol is not a good treatment for insomnia. Physicians should not recommend a bedtime alcoholic drink as a treatment for complaints of insomnia, because drinking alcohol in the late evening actually impairs sleep. Alcohol ingestion can result in stimulation or sedation, depending on the dose and the experience and metabolism of the individual. When sleep is induced, it tends to be a deep, drugged sleep with disruption of sleep stages and suppression of rapid eye movement sleep. Later in the night, a rebound produces lighter sleep and potential awakenings.

MULTIORGAN SYSTEM EFFECTS OF ALCOHOL

Alcohol is toxic to many organ systems, including the liver, pancreas, hematopoietic system, nervous system, heart, gastrointestinal tract, endocrine glands, and bone. Alcohol may produce mild, otherwise unexplained abnormalities that are noticed on routine laboratory testing. Common findings include signs of hepatotoxicity and hematologic abnormalities (Table 34.3). Although none of these findings is diagnostic of alcoholism, they should alert the clinician to take a more careful history of alcohol intake and look for other signs that would support this diagnosis.

Alcohol is an important cause of treatable hypertension. Physicians should always take a careful history of alcohol intake when evaluating a hypertensive patient. Drinking does not have to be heavy enough to qualify as alcohol abuse or dependence in order to increase blood pressure. Often simply reducing or stopping alcohol will bring the blood pressure of a person with mild hypertension into the normal range, obviating the need for antihypertensive medication.

The gastrointestinal effects of alcohol, including hepatic toxicity, are covered in Chapter 121. Alcoholism also has been associated with an increased rate of cancer of the esophagus, stomach, and other parts of the gastrointestinal tract. Many of

---

TABLE 34.2.	**CAGE QUESTIONNAIRE**[a]

Have you felt that you should **C**ut down on your drinking?
Have you felt **A**nnoyed by people criticizing your drinking?
Have you ever felt **G**uilty about your drinking?
Do you require an "**E**ye-opener" in the morning to steady yourself or get rid of a hangover?

---

[a] A score of two or more positive answers to this screening test correlates highly with alcohol abuse or dependence.

EVIDENCE LEVEL: B. Reference: Bisson J, Nadeau L, Demers A. The validity of the CAGE scale to screen for heavy drinking and drinking problems in a general population survey. Addiction 1999;94:715–722.

TABLE 34.3.	**LABORATORY FINDINGS INDICATING ALCOHOL USE**

Increased mean corpuscular volume
Increased γ-glutamyltransferase
Increased aspartate aminotransferase
Increased alkaline phosphatase
Increased triglycerides
Increased low-density lipoprotein cholesterol
Increased aspartate amino acid transferase
Increased blood pressure

the symptoms and physical findings associated with alcoholism are a consequence of the multiorgan toxicity of this drug. Examples are the dyspepsia, nausea, and bloating that accompany gastritis and the hepatomegaly, esophageal varices, and hemorrhoids associated with alcohol-induced changes in the liver. Other physical signs include tremor, unsteady gait, insomnia, and erectile dysfunction. Individuals with chronic alcoholism may exhibit decreased testicular size and feminizing effects, such as the gynecomastia associated with reduced testosterone levels caused by the endocrine effects of alcohol.

Severe, repeated alcohol intoxication may also suppress immune mechanisms and increase the risk of infections. Meningitis, especially tuberculous meningitis, is greatly overrepresented among alcoholics. Alcohol also impairs judgment and increases the likelihood of unprotected sex. Sexually transmitted infections, such as human immunodeficiency virus infection, syphilis, and gonorrhea, are linked to alcohol use. Spontaneous abortion and fetal alcohol syndrome have been associated with heavy drinking during pregnancy. Alcohol drinking during pregnancy is one of the most common preventable causes of mental retardation. Although the data show a correlation between heavy drinking and fetal alcohol syndrome, it is not clear whether small amounts of alcohol produce any increased risk. Because data from animal models and clinical studies are ambiguous on this point, many physicians advocate complete abstinence from alcohol during pregnancy.

NEUROLOGIC AND OTHER COMPLICATIONS OF ALCOHOL

Alcohol Overdose

Coma due to an overdose of alcohol is a medical emergency. It can occur in someone who rapidly drinks large quantities of alcohol, resulting in a high blood alcohol level. In most overdoses, alcohol is combined with another drug, such as a benzodiazepine. Benzodiazepines are widely prescribed for anxiety, insomnia, and muscle relaxation. Although this class of medication is not dangerous when taken alone, when combined with alcohol, accidental overdoses are common. Blood levels of alcohol and commonly used medications should be obtained when evaluating a comatose patient in the emergency room. For recent ingestion, gastric aspiration can prevent further absorption of toxic agents. Treatment consists mainly of support of vital functions. If opiates are involved, the opiate receptor antagonist naloxone can block opiate effects, but it has no effect on overdose from alcohol or other drugs.

Violence

The potential for violence and antisocial behavior is increased by alcohol. Intoxicated individuals tend to get into fights and commit crimes. Family violence, including spouse abuse and child abuse, is strongly linked to alcohol use.

Trauma

Alcohol is associated with about 50% of all traffic fatalities in the United States each year. Alcohol intoxication may result in falls and accidents that can cause fractures, subdural hematomas, and other forms of brain trauma. Individuals with histories of epilepsy or severe head trauma are more likely to experience alcohol-related seizures.

Alcoholic Blackouts

Alcohol intoxication seriously impairs the storage of memories, and it is not surprising that alcohol abusers and alcoholics frequently have periods of amnesia concerning events that occurred during bouts of heavy drinking. This amnesia facilitates the denial of drinking problems expressed by most alcoholics when confronted by a physician or family member. Even when the patient exhibited outrageous behavior that ordinarily would have been embarrassing, there is no memory of the events, and denial by the patient is facilitated.

Severe Alcoholism and Nutritional Deficiencies

The neurotoxic role of alcohol itself in directly producing chronic neurologic dysfunction is unclear. The neurologic syndromes of alcoholism are seen in a context of chronic nutritional deficiency in heavy drinkers who consume empty calories in the form of ethyl alcohol.

Wernicke–Korsakoff Syndrome

The Wernicke–Korsakoff syndrome is produced by severe nutritional deficiency, especially lack of thiamine. It consists of a persistent inability to encode new memories and specific neurologic signs, including nystagmus, ophthalmoplegia, and ataxia. Wernicke–Korsakoff syndrome usually develops over days and weeks and then suddenly becomes dramatically apparent during a period of stress caused by infection or trauma. The lack of memory often produces confabulation, as patients try to "fill in the gaps." This disorder was called Korsakoff's psychosis, but it was discovered later that confabulation was a behavioral response to the underlying neurologic deficit, known as Wernicke's syndrome. Hemorrhagic lesions of the mamillary bodies, a part of the brain known to be involved in the encoding of recent memories, have been described in cases examined at autopsy. High doses of thiamine partially reverse these deficits, and thiamine should always be given during the acute treatment of alcoholism. Although the Wernicke–Korsakoff syndrome is most often seen in alcoholics, it can be produced by severe nutritional deficiency in the absence of alcohol, as in cases of gastric carcinoma.

Peripheral Neuropathy

Alcoholics have many problems that can lead to peripheral nerve damage, and this is confirmed by reports of a 45% incidence in some alcoholic populations. Pressure palsies, especially affecting the radial or peroneal nerves and sometimes even the brachial plexus (called park bench neuropathy), arise when alcohol produces a deep sleep without the normal position shifts that protect peripheral nerves. Malnutrition probably accounts for most of

TABLE 34.4.	ALCOHOL WITHDRAWAL SYNDROME

Alcohol craving
Tremor, irritability
Nausea
Sleep disturbance
Tachycardia, hypertension
Sweating
Perceptual distortion
Seizures (12–48 h after last drink)
Delirium tremens (rare in uncomplicated withdrawal)
   Severe agitation
   Confusion
   Visual hallucinations
   Fever, tachycardia, profuse sweating, dilated pupils
   Nausea, diarrhea

the neuropathies seen in alcoholics, including those affecting sensorimotor and autonomic nerves. Rare neurologic complications of alcoholism that stem from extreme malnutrition have been described. These include Marchiafava–Bignami syndrome, a primary degeneration of the corpus callosum, and central pontine myelinolysis, which is associated with chronic hyponatremia.

OPTIMAL TREATMENT

DETOXIFICATION

A patient who is seen in a medical setting with an alcohol withdrawal syndrome should be considered to have a potentially lethal condition. Although most mild cases of alcohol withdrawal never come to medical attention, severe cases require general evaluation; attention to hydration and electrolytes; vitamin supplementation, especially high-dose thiamine (100 mg, given intramuscularly daily for 7 days); and a sedating medication that has cross-tolerance with alcohol. Because of the likelihood of liver impairment, a short-acting benzodiazepine, such as oxazepam, can be given at doses sufficient to block or diminish the alcohol withdrawal symptoms described in Table 34.4. A typical alcoholic requires 15 to 30 mg every 6 hours for 48 hours, decreasing the dose by 10% to 20% per day over the next several days. After medical evaluation, uncomplicated alcohol withdrawal can be effectively treated on an outpatient basis. Hospitalization is required for all unstable patients or when there is a history of seizures. The likelihood of alcohol withdrawal seizures is increased by repeated attempts at withdrawal. Adequate treatment of withdrawal symptoms is important for preventing the development of seizures in the current episode of withdrawal and reducing the potential for seizures in the future.

RELAPSE PREVENTION

Detoxification is only the first step of treatment. Complete abstinence is the objective of long-term treatment, and this is accomplished mainly by behavioral approaches. Self-help groups, such

as Alcoholics Anonymous (AA), are a mainstay of the rehabilitation of alcoholics. Physicians should learn about the AA groups in their community and make appropriate referrals. AA is a movement rather than an institution, and each group is different, though they all follow a similar set of principles, called the twelve steps. AA can be an important ally of the physician in the care of alcoholics.

Medications that aid in the rehabilitation process are being sought. Disulfiram blocks the metabolism of alcohol, resulting in the accumulation of acetaldehyde, which produces an unpleasant flushing reaction when alcohol is ingested. This drug has been useful in some programs that focus on behavioral efforts to ensure that the patient ingests the medication. Knowledge of this unpleasant reaction helps the patient resist taking a drink. Although it is pharmacologically quite effective, disulfiram has not been found to be practical in controlled clinical trials, because so many patients have failed to ingest the medication regularly.

Naltrexone is another medication used as an adjunct in the treatment of alcoholism. This opiate antagonist appears to block some of the reinforcing properties of alcohol and has resulted in a decreased rate of relapse to alcohol drinking in double-blind clinical trials. Naltrexone was approved by the Food and Drug Administration for the treatment of opiate dependence in 1983, and in 1995 it received approval for the treatment of alcoholism. Naltrexone has not been shown to be effective when given alone, but in the context of a comprehensive treatment program for alcoholism, it increases the probability of a successful outcome.

LONG-TERM TREATMENT OF ALCOHOLISM

Alcoholism is a chronic, recurring disorder that requires long-term care. Physicians tend to see treatment of addictive disorders as unsuccessful because of their chronic nature. In reality, the course of alcoholism and other addictions is similar to that of hypertension, diabetes, asthma, and other chronic medical conditions. The patient initially responds to fairly intensive intervention, but some type of maintenance treatment is necessary to deal with recurrences and prevent their becoming severe. In this context, the prognosis for alcoholics in treatment is good because their function improves, but complete "cures" are unlikely.

BIBLIOGRAPHY

Anthony JC, Warner LA, Kessler RC. Comparative epidemiology of dependence on tobacco, alcohol, controlled substances, and inhalants: basic findings from the National Comorbidity Survey. *Exp Clin Psychopharmacol* 1994;2:244–268.

Hayashida M, Alterman A, McLellan AT, et al. Comparative effectiveness and costs of inpatient and outpatient detoxification of patients with mild to moderate alcohol withdrawal syndrome. *N Engl J Med* 1989; 320:358–365.

O'Brien CP, McLellan AT. Myths about the treatment of addiction. *Lancet* 1996;347:237–240.

Schuckit MA. Advances in understanding the vulnerability to alcoholism. In: O'Brien CP, Jaffe J, eds. *Addictive states*. New York: Raven Press, 1992:93–108.

Schuckit MA. Low level of response to alcohol as a predictor of future alcoholism. *Am J Psychiatry* 1994;151:184–189.

Volpicelli JR, Rhines KC, Rhines JS, et al. Naltrexone and alcohol dependence. Role of subject compliance. *Arch Gen Psychiatry* 1997;54:737–742.

Weiss F, Lorang MT, Bloom FE, et al. Oral alcohol self-administration stimulates dopamine release in the rat nucleus accumbens: genetic and motivational determinants. *J Pharmacol Exp Ther* 1993;267:250–258.

Kelley's Textbook of Internal Medicine, fourth edition. Edited by H. David Humes. Lippincott Williams & Wilkins, Philadelphia © 2000.

TABLE 35.1.	CLINICAL HINTS REGARDING SUBSTANCE ABUSE

Scarred veins: "needle tracks"
Abscesses or scars from healed abscesses
Nasal septal lesions
Edematous hands or feet
Frequent injuries from falls
Hepatitis
Endocarditis
Respiratory infections

CHAPTER 35

APPROACH TO THE PROBLEM OF SUBSTANCE ABUSE

CHARLES P. O'BRIEN

The most important addicting drugs from the perspective of morbidity and mortality are clearly nicotine (see Chapter 33) and alcohol (see Chapter 34). This chapter addresses other substances that are frequently abused. The definitions of abuse and dependence are consistent across drug categories, and the reader is referred to Chapter 34 on alcoholism for a discussion of terms. It is particularly important that all physicians have a clear understanding of the difference between physical dependence and addiction. Many of the medications that we prescribe produce changes in the body's homeostatic mechanisms; this alteration, in turn, produces an adaptive response to the changes. If the patient abruptly stops taking the drug, the adaptation is unopposed, and there is a rebound, called a withdrawal syndrome. This means that the patient was physically dependent on the drug, but it does not imply that the patient is or was an addict. The diagnosis of addiction (i.e., "substance dependence," as defined in the fourth edition of the *Diagnostic and Statistical Manual of Mental Disorders,* published by the American Psychiatric Association) is mainly a behavioral diagnosis. It is applied when persons engage in drug-seeking behavior that interferes with nor-mal activities and when compulsive drug use continues despite serious social or medical consequences.

Abuse of drugs other than alcohol or nicotine occurs in all socioeconomic groups; general population studies find a lifetime prevalence around 6%. Thus, physicians are likely to encounter such patients in their practice. In some cases involving prescription sedatives and stimulants, the abuse is inadvertent and may be the result of the prescribing physician's ignorance of certain drug effects. In evaluating a patient with substance abuse, a physician should integrate information from all available sources, including the patient's history and information from relatives and the employer, if possible. The physical examination may provide some clues (Table 35.1). Laboratory testing of blood or urine can be useful, but the results require interpretation. The tests, when properly done and confirmed, indicate use within a specific period of time, depending on the drug and its dose (Table 35.2). Such tests give no information about abuse or dependence and must be interpreted in the light of all clinical information.

OPIOIDS

CLINICAL FEATURES

Derivatives of the opium poppy have been used for the treatment of pain, diarrhea, anxiety, and other indications dating back to the third century B.C. Heroin, morphine, and codeine are produced from opium. Synthetic drugs and endogenous peptides that also act at opiate receptors are called opioids. Heroin, the most abused drug in the opiate category, is widely available on

TABLE 35.2.	DRUG SCREENING TESTS		
Drug	**Specimen**	**Metabolite**	**Duration**
Heroin	Urine	Morphine	12–24 hr
Methadone	Urine	Methadone	1–2 d
Cocaine	Urine	Benzoylecognine	3–15 d (10 d after heavy use)
Amphetamine	Urine	Amphetamine	1–2 d
Cannabinoids	Urine	Cannabinoids	2–8 d (14–50 d for long-term use)
Phencyclidine	Urine	Phencyclidine	2–8 d

TABLE 35.3.	OPIOID WITHDRAWAL

Symptoms	Signs
Restlessness, irritability	Sweating, fever
Cramps, diarrhea	Pupillary dilatation
Nausea, vomiting	Piloerection ("gooseflesh")
Anxiety, insomnia	Yawning
Craving for opioids	Increased blood pressure

the illicit market. During the 1990s, the purity of heroin purchased on the street reached an all-time high, and the price per gram was greatly reduced. In the past it was necessary to take heroin via intravenous injections because its potency was so low. In contrast, heroin in a relatively pure state can be smoked, and enough drug survives the heat to be absorbed through the lungs and produce significant pharmacologic effects. It is estimated that there are between 750,000 and one million heroin addicts in the United States.

Heroin produces a calming effect, contentment, and, if the dose is high enough, intense euphoria. The effects wear off in 3 to 5 hours, and heroin addicts may administer the drug two to four times per day. Because of heroin's rapid metabolism, addicts are constantly going in and out of the withdrawal phase, and this creates perturbations of endocrine systems modulated by opiate receptors. Male heroin addicts report many sexual performance problems, and women have irregular menses. Mood varies according to the dose of heroin. Addicts are anxious and irritable during withdrawal and content during periods of adequate heroin effects. Heroin addiction often coexists with a variety of psychiatric disorders, especially depression.

The daily injections of heroin are usually carried out without sterile technique and often with needles previously used by other addicts. The rates of such infections as hepatitis, endocarditis, and human immunodeficiency virus are very high. Intravenous drug abuse, mainly with heroin, has become a major source of new cases of AIDS (see Chapter 349). Heroin addicts become very tolerant to the respiratory effects of opioids, but overdose is still possible when a concentrated supply of heroin unexpectedly becomes available or when street heroin is mixed with a very potent opioid, such as fentanyl (Table 35.3).

TREATMENT

Detoxification refers to the transition from the drug-dependent to the drug-free state. A withdrawal syndrome occurs—although it is unpleasant, opioid withdrawal is rarely life-threatening. Symptoms begin 6 to 12 hours after the last dose of a short-acting opioid such as heroin. Withdrawal symptoms can be treated by giving a long-acting opioid, such as methadone, in a single daily dose or twice daily (Table 35.4). The dose is tailored to the degree of physical dependence. An initial test dose of 20 mg is recommended; if that does not relieve the withdrawal symptoms in 30 minutes, an additional 20 mg can be administered. Higher doses are necessary when the patient has a high degree of physical dependence. After the symptoms are relieved, the dose is gradually reduced over 5 to 10 days. If opioid medication is not available, clonidine, an antihypertensive medication, can be used to block the adrenergic signs of withdrawal. Clonidine is given orally at a dose of 0.1 mg every 6 hours, as needed, depending on the severity of withdrawal signs. Blood pressure must be monitored, because hypotension is a limiting side effect of this treatment. Detoxification on an inpatient basis is usually successful, but it is simply the beginning of treatment. The most difficult aspect of treatment is the prevention of relapse to heroin use.

Because addiction is basically a behavioral disorder, all treatments require counseling or psychotherapy to assist the patient with psychosocial problems. Complete abstinence from opioids is the ultimate goal of treatment, but most drug-free former addicts relapse when they return to neighborhoods where drugs are plentiful. Long-term (months to years) treatment in a therapeutic community can help selected patients remain drug-free, but such treatment is not readily available. The best and most practical treatment is maintenance on methadone.

Daily methadone stabilizes heroin addicts socially and physiologically. Methadone blocks withdrawal and craving while leaving the patient alert and able to work. With this treatment, most patients are able to organize their lives rather than think only of the next dose of heroin. With the help of counseling in a rehabilitation program and, when necessary, psychoactive medi-

TABLE 35.4.	MEDICATIONS HELPFUL IN THE TREATMENT OF OPIOID ADDICTION

Drug	Class	Use
Methadone	Agonist	Analgesia, withdrawal, maintenance
1-α-methadol (LAAM)	Agonist (ultra-long-acting)	Maintenance
Buprenorphine[a]	Partial agonist	Maintenance
Naltrexone	Antagonist	Maintenance
Naloxone	Antagonist (short-acting)	Overdose, diagnosis
Clonidine	α-Adrenergic agonist (autoreceptor)	Withdrawal

[a] Not yet approved for this indication by the Food and Drug Administration.

cation to treat depression or other psychiatric disorders, patients are able to return to employment or school. After months or years without using heroin, patients can be detoxified slowly from methadone.

Another medication that can be used for maintenance is L-alpha-acetyl methadol (LAAM), a long-acting opioid with active metabolites. LAAM can provide good stabilization for 72 hours, thereby requiring administration only three times per week. Both methadone and LAAM are full opiate agonists. Buprenorphine, a partial agonist, is in the final stages of approval for both detoxification and maintenance treatment of heroin addiction. Each medication has advantages and disadvantages, and the clinician can choose based on an individual patient's characteristics. A different approach utilizes naltrexone, an opiate receptor antagonist that prevents relapse by blocking opiate receptors. Naltrexone works well with highly motivated opiate addicts, especially physicians and other medical workers. It has no agonist effects, so it does not relieve anxiety and drug craving and it can be stopped with no withdrawal syndrome.

■ STIMULANTS

COCAINE

Clinical Features

Cocaine is the most important of the abused stimulants. It is widely available at low prices ($3 to $5 per dose in the northeastern United States). Cocaine hydrochloride can be administered in a powdered form through the nasal mucosa, called snorting, or taken intravenously. The alkaloid form, called freebase or crack, can be inhaled after heating. The use of cocaine peaked in the 1980s. Although the number of new users declined during the 1990s, at the turn of the century there are still about 1.3 million Americans who use cocaine.

Cocaine is a short-acting drug that produces intense euphoria, but it may leave the user wanting more cocaine after 20 to 30 minutes. Cocaine can be acutely toxic, even in those who suffered no ill effects from previous use. Acute toxicity is characterized by sympathomimetic effects, including hypertension, tachycardia, hyperthermia, and cardiac arrhythmias. Vasculitis in the cerebral vessels has been observed in persons dying after cocaine ingestion. Clinically, one sees seizures, stroke, coma, and cardiorespiratory collapse as complications of a cocaine binge.

Regular users of cocaine often undergo personality changes, becoming more irritable and suspicious. Continued use and higher doses can produce persecutory delusions and hallucinations. Prolonged psychotic episodes can be provoked in susceptible individuals. Alcohol, sedatives, opioids, and marijuana are often taken to combat the anxiety and irritability experienced by cocaine users. The "crash" after a period of heavy cocaine use constitutes a kind of withdrawal syndrome, reflecting changes in brain chemistry and blood flow. Anxiety and irritability give way to tiredness, sleepiness, lack of energy, and depressive symptoms. This syndrome usually resolves spontaneously over several days. If depression persists, antidepressant medication is indicated.

Treatment

Cocaine-induced psychotic reactions are usually self-limited, but in some cases a neuroleptic, such as haloperidol, may be required for emergency management. When necessary, low-dose, short-term haloperidol (5 to 10 mg daily taken intramuscularly or orally) can be administered. The anxiety reactions and irritability produced by cocaine can be treated with a brief course of benzodiazepines, such as diazepam (5 to 20 mg daily).

As is the case with other addictions, cocaine dependence requires long-term rehabilitation. Counseling and behavioral treatments aimed at reducing the likelihood of return to cocaine use are indicated for at least 1 to 2 years. When a slip occurs, the treatment becomes more intense, and most patients respond. At follow-up, 7 to 12 months after starting treatment, studies found 60% to 70% of former cocaine addicts to be cocaine free and functioning well, though many experienced some slips. No medication consistently improves the psychosocial treatment of cocaine dependence.

OTHER STIMULANTS

Methamphetamine has become an important drug of abuse in the western United States. It can be made in amateur clandestine laboratories, and ephedrine, found in many over-the-counter cold medicines, is often used as starting material. Methamphetamine, which can be smoked, snorted, or taken intravenously, is more neurotoxic than cocaine and has a longer duration of action. Whereas cocaine blocks reuptake of monoamine neurotransmitters, resulting in increased activity of dopamine as well as other transmitters, amphetamine and methamphetamine cause greatly increased neurotransmitter release. Clinical reports suggest that the incidence of psychotic reactions is greater than with cocaine and that psychological deterioration is more rapid.

Prescription stimulants, such as dextroamphetamine and methylphenidate, are used for a variety of conditions, including weight reduction, narcolepsy, and attention deficit hyperactivity disorder in children. For weight reduction, amphetamines have a short-term effect and should be used, if at all, only in conjunction with behavioral interventions. Prescription stimulants have less abuse potential than cocaine, but in susceptible individuals, abuse and dependence occur. Treatment is similar to that for cocaine addiction.

■ PRESCRIPTION SEDATIVES

Sleeping pills and minor tranquilizers can be misused inadvertently because of ignorance of their long-term effects. For example, the symptom of insomnia should not be treated by simply prescribing a sleeping pill. Recurrent insomnia usually signals an underlying problem, such as depression or a primary disorder of sleep physiology. Administration of a sedative produces new problems that begin with changes in sleep patterns and may involve dependence on the medication. A few patients gradually increase their dose, leading to an addiction syndrome.

Benzodiazepines are a large class of drugs referred to as minor tranquilizers. They are a great improvement in terms of safety and efficacy over the medications that they replaced, but tolerance and physical dependence develop when they are used over the long term. Deliberate abuse of benzodiazepines is relatively uncommon and is seen mostly in alcoholics and polydrug abusers. It is common for any patient to show signs of physical dependence when benzodiazepines are prescribed for a long period of time. For example, 20 mg of diazepam daily or the equivalent amount of other benzodiazepines produces physical dependence in about 40% of patients after 4 months of treatment. Physical dependence at even lower doses has been reported in patients receiving benzodiazepines daily for longer periods. For clear-cut indications, such as anxiety disorders, these medications permit the patient to function normally, and long-term use may be justified. The decision to prescribe a benzodiazepine for more than 6 weeks should be considered carefully. Cessation of the medication after it has been taken for several months requires slow detoxification.

CANNABIS: MARIJUANA AND HASHISH

Marijuana, the most commonly used illegal drug, is actually a complex preparation containing many biologically active chemicals. The chemical Δ-9-tetrahydrocannabinol (Δ-9-THC) accounts for most of the psychoactive effects reported by marijuana users. These include a dreamy, so-called stoned feeling and enhanced perceptions of colors, sounds, and tastes. Learning is impaired, and coordination is poor for several hours after the high feeling wears off. The physiologic effects of cannabis are dose related and include tachycardia, conjunctival vascular congestion, decreased intraocular pressure, bronchodilation, increased airway conductance, and peripheral vasodilation. Overdose may produce orthostatic hypotension, fine tremors, ataxia, nystagmus, nausea, and vomiting. Acute panic, paranoid reactions, and frightening distortions of body image are sometimes experienced by marijuana users, especially when a higher dose than expected is taken. Although marijuana is capable of impairing learning and social adjustment in adolescents, few toxic effects have been demonstrated at average use levels. Dependence defined by compulsive frequent use of marijuana occurs in less than 10% of users.

Marijuana is sometimes recommended for its medicinal value in several conditions, including glaucoma, muscle spasm, weight loss of chronic disease, and the nausea produced by cancer chemotherapy. Marijuana as medicine is limited by psychoactive side effects and by the toxic effects of smoking as a means of ingestion. The effects of cannabinoid receptors in the brain, however are just beginning to be understood. These receptors are widespread, and already one endogenous ligand—anandamide—has been isolated. It is likely that useful and specific medications will be developed that interact with this system.

HALLUCINOGENIC DRUGS

CLINICAL FEATURES

Hallucinogenic drugs reliably produce distortions in perception or thinking as a primary effect, even at low doses. They are

TABLE 35.5.	HALLUCINOGENS

Phenethylamines
  Mescaline
  Dimethoxymethylamphetamine (DOM)
  Methylenedioxyamphetamine (MDA)
  5-Methoxy-3,4-methylenedioxyamphetamine (MDM, or "ecstasy")

Anticholinergics
  Atropine
  Benztropine
  Hyoscyamine
  Scopolamine

Indoleamines
  Lysergic acid diethylamide (LSD)
  Psilocybin
  Dimethyltryptamine (DMT)

Phencyclidine (PCP, or "Angel Dust")

ingested for the purpose of inducing hallucinations or because users believe that they will enhance self-understanding. The popularity of this class of drugs has varied from high in the 1960s to low in the 1980s. Surveys among adults in the late 1990s indicated that about 15% of adults have used these drugs during their lifetime.

The main categories of hallucinogens are listed in Table 35.5. Indoles and phenethylamines have high affinity for serotonin receptors and presumably interfere with normal serotonergic transmission. Lysergic acid diethylamide (LSD) is one of the most potent drugs known, in that it produces major changes in visual perception with a total dose as low as 25 to 50 μg. Other signs include pupillary dilation, increased pulse and blood pressure, flushing, salivation, lacrimation, and hyperreflexia. A major factor in the morbidity caused by these drugs is that samples purchased on the illicit market are mislabeled. The dose may be far higher than expected, and phencyclidine (PCP, also called "angel dust") may be sold in place of one of the less dangerous hallucinogens. PCP produces analgesia and amphetamine-like stimulation in addition to hallucinations.

MANAGEMENT

Tolerance develops to some of the effects of LSD, but dependence is not seen. Physicians may be asked to treat the unexpected effects of these drugs, including psychotic episodes, accidental injuries, and suicide attempts during a "trip." Because medications can worsen the situation, counseling and reduction of stimulation are important. For severe agitation, intramuscular lorazepam (2 to 4 mg) or haloperidol (5 to 10 mg) can be helpful. Brief reappearance of the hallucinations or perceptual distortions experienced during the period of acute ingestion that occur days or weeks after the last trip are called "flashbacks." These episodes usually cease without treatment, but in some cases they have persisted for years.

Hallucinogenic drugs tend to be used intermittently rather

than on a daily basis. PCP is an exception. Compulsive, frequent use of PCP qualifies as addiction in some users. Overdose with PCP can progress rapidly from aggressive or psychotic behavior to coma with dilated pupils, muscular rigidity, arrhythmias, elevated blood pressure, and seizures. Support of vital signs, gastric lavage with activated charcoal, and acidification of the urine are part of the acute treatment. Hallucinogenic drugs purchased on the street may contain anticholinergic substances, such as scopolamine. At high doses, these drugs produce visual or tactile hallucinations, acute toxic delirium with confusion, and amnesia for the episode.

INHALANTS

Substances that are volatile at room temperatures may be inhaled to produce changes in mental state. Common substances include toluene (airplane glue), kerosene, gasoline, carbon tetrachloride, amyl nitrite, and nitrous oxide. Solvents found in cleaning fluids, such as aerosol sprays, may be sought for their psychic effects. Frequent use of solvents may result in toxicity affecting the bone marrow, brain, liver, kidney, heart, and peripheral nerves. Fatalities have been reported, probably from cardiac arrhythmias accompanying upper-airway obstruction or exercise. Amyl nitrite causes relaxation of smooth muscle and has been used to treat angina. Adverse effects include postural hypotension, palpitations, and headache progressing to loss of consciousness. Nitrous oxide and halothane are anesthetic gases sometimes used by medical personnel as intoxicants. Specific acute treatments for inhalant intoxication are generally unnecessary. When inhalants are used long term or are associated with other psychiatric diagnoses, specific psychiatric treatment is indicated.

ILLICIT SYNTHETIC DRUGS

Drugs manufactured in illegal laboratories, sometimes called designer drugs, are inherently dangerous, because they vary in composition and purity. Analogs of the potent opioid fentanyl have been synthesized and have resulted in many overdose deaths. Some attempts at synthesis of opioids have produced such toxic compounds as MPTP. This analog of meperidine is a neurotoxin to the substantia nigra of the brain and results in irreversible Parkinson's syndrome.

BIBLIOGRAPHY

Abraham HD, Aldridge A. Adverse consequences of lysergic acid diethylamide. *Addiction* 1993;88:1327–1334.
Anthony JC, Warner LA, Kessler RC. Comparative epidemiology of dependence on tobacco, alcohol, controlled substances, and inhalants: basic findings from the National Comorbidity Survey. *Exp Clin Psychopharmacol* 1994;2:244–268.
Joy JE, Watson SJ, Benson JA, eds. *Marijuana and medicine: assessing the science base.* Washington D.C.: Institute of Medicine, 1999.
Mackler S, O'Brien CP. Cocaine abuse. In: Stollerman G, ed. *Advances in internal medicine.* St. Louis: Mosby–Year Book, 1992;37:21–35.
McLellan AT, Woody GE, O'Brien CP. Development of psychiatric illness in drug abusers. *N Engl J Med* 1979;301:1310–1314.
Metzger DS, Woody GE, McLellan AT, et al. Human immunodeficiency virus seroconversion among in- and out-of-treatment intravenous drug users: an 18-month, prospective follow-up. *J Acquir Immune Defic Syndr* 1993;6:1049–1056.
O'Brien CP. Opioid addiction handbook of experimental pharmacology. In: Herz A, ed. *Opioids II.* Berlin: Springer-Verlag, 1992:104.
O'Brien CP, Jaffe J, eds. *Advances in understanding the addictive states.* New York: Raven Press, 1991.

Kelley's Textbook of Internal Medicine, fourth edition. Edited by H. David Humes. Lippincott Williams & Wilkins, Philadelphia © 2000.

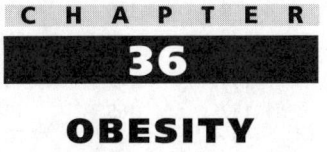

CHAPTER 36

OBESITY

ALBERT J. STUNKARD
THOMAS A. WADDEN

DEFINITION

Obesity is a condition characterized by excessive accumulation of fat in the body. In clinical practice, overweight (weight corrected for height) is used as a surrogate for body fat. This practice is reasonable because body weight and fat are highly correlated, especially at greater degrees of overweight. Traditionally, overweight has been defined in terms of tables of ideal or desirable body weight. It is now defined in terms of the body mass index (BMI = weight in kilograms divided by height in meters squared), with overweight defined as a BMI of greater than 25 and obesity as a BMI greater than 30. Table 36.1 shows the BMI values for different heights and weights in inches and pounds, and Table 36.2 depicts the World Health Organization's classification of obesity. Unlike many "real" diseases and like hypertension, obesity represents one arm of a distribution curve of body weight, with no physiologically defined cutoff point. In the future, diagnosis may be based on newer methods of measuring body fat. Until then, for most practical purposes, the eyeball test is sufficient: if a person looks fat, the person is fat.

INCIDENCE AND EPIDEMIOLOGY

Obesity is one of the most pervasive public health problems in the United States today. One-third of all adults are overweight, and this high prevalence occurs in all ethnic and racial groups at all ages and in both sexes. It is even higher among persons with lower levels of education and certain ethnic or racial groups. Figure 36.1 shows the prevalence of overweight among three racial or ethnic groups by age, separately for men and women. A striking finding is the very high prevalence (almost 60%)

TABLE 36.1.	BODY MASS INDEX			
Body Mass Index				
	Body Weight (lb)			
Height (in)	**20**	**25**	**30**	**40**
58	95	119	143	191
59	99	124	149	198
60	102	127	153	204
61	106	132	159	212
62	109	136	163	217
63	113	141	169	226
64	117	146	176	234
65	120	150	180	240
66	124	156	187	249
67	127	159	191	255
68	132	165	198	264
69	135	169	203	270
70	140	175	210	279
71	143	179	214	286
72	148	185	221	295
73	151	189	226	302
74	156	195	234	312
75	159	199	239	318
76	164	205	246	328

among middle-aged African-American and Mexican-American women; the value for white women is 33.5%.

For men and women, the prevalence of overweight increases with each 10-year increment of age until 50 to 59 years of age, when it begins to fall progressively at older ages. Overweight is also highly correlated with socioeconomic status; increasing body weight is associated with decreasing socioeconomic status, particularly among women. The high prevalence of overweight in the United States is compounded by a striking 30% increase in the past decade. The problem extends across the entire spectrum of body weight. During the past decade, the average American gained 3.6 kg, and the proportion of persons with healthier, lighter weights decreased significantly. Even children have not

TABLE 36.2.	MODIFIED WHO CLASSIFICATION OF OVERWEIGHT AND OBESITY
Classifications	**BMI**
Underweight	<18.50
Normal weight	18.50–24.99
Grade I overweight	25.00–29.99
Grade II overweight	30.00–39.99
Grade III overweight	≥40.00

WHO, World Health Organization; BMI, body mass index. (From Seidell JC, Rissanan AM. Time trends in the worldwide epidemic of obesity. In: Bray GA, Bouchard C, James WPT, eds. *Handbook of obesity.* New York: Marcel Dekker, 1998:79–91.)

been spared the rapid increase in body weight; 25% of American children are overweight.

ETIOLOGY

What causes obesity? In one sense, the answer is simple—consuming more calories than are expended as energy. In another sense, the answer is most elusive. The causes of obesity are to be found in the regulation of body weight (which is primarily the regulation of body fat), and we still have only an imperfect understanding of how this regulation is achieved. We do know that weight is regulated with great precision. During a lifetime, the average person consumes at least 60 million kcal. A gain or loss of 20 lb, or 72,000 kcal, would represent an error of no more than 0.001%. The determinants of obesity or, as we have suggested, an elevated body weight set point can be divided into genetic, environmental, and regulatory factors.

GENETIC DETERMINANTS

The existence of numerous forms of genetic obesity in experimental animals and the ease with which adiposity can be produced by the selective breeding of farm animals suggest that genetic factors can play an important role in human obesity. The stunning advances in our knowledge during the past decade have made it clear that genetic factors do play an important role in human obesity. The first studies, using the classic twin method, estimated very high levels of heritability; the percentage of the variance in body weight accounted for by genetic influences was about 80%. Even studies of identical twins separated at birth, a method that avoided some of the bias in classic twin studies, estimated heritability at 66%. These studies are still widely cited, but there is a growing consensus that they overestimate the influence of heredity.

The results of adoption studies and complex segregation analysis agree on a heritability of BMI of about 33%, a value now viewed as a more reasonable estimate than that of the twin studies. Genetic influences may play a more important part in the determination of regional fat distribution than of total body fat, with a particularly strong influence on the critical visceral fat depot.

Obesity has been considered to be a polygenic disorder. This belief has been challenged by the discovery of major genes responsible for five forms of genetic obesity in mice, and an active search is under way to determine if they participate in human obesity. This dramatic entry of molecular biology into research on the genetics of human obesity will undoubtedly make a major contribution to our understanding of this disorder.

SOCIAL DETERMINANTS

The fact that genetic influences account for only one-third of the variation in body weight means that the environment exerts an enormous influence. One measure of the extent of this influence is the dramatic increase in the prevalence of obesity during the past decade. One surprising aspect of the nature of environ-

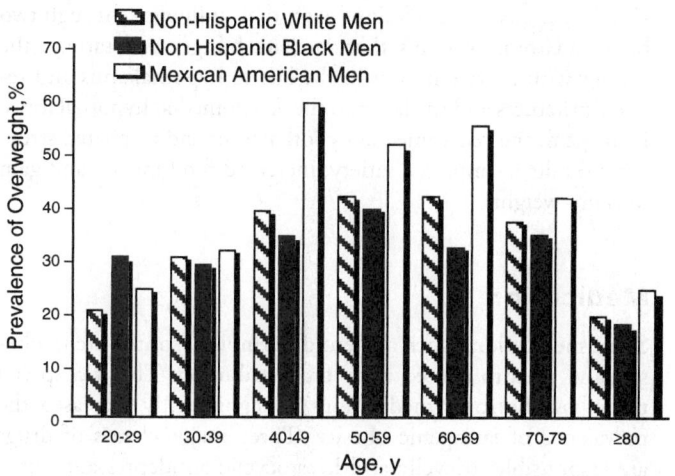
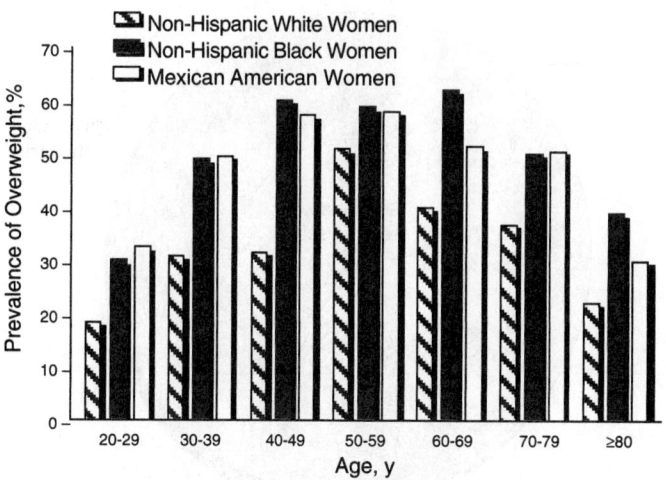

FIGURE 36.1. Prevalence of obesity by gender, age, and ethnic status according to the former criteria of a body mass index greater than 27.8 for men and 27.3 for women. (From Kuczmarski RJ, Flegal KM, Campbell SM, et al. Increasing prevalence of overweight among US adults: the national health and nutrition examination surveys, 1960–1991. *JAMA* 1994;272:205, with permission.)

mental influences has become clear. Adoption studies have revealed that the early home environment, in which children learn their eating habits and which had been blamed for the origins of obesity, plays no role in determining obesity in adult life. The environment in which a person is living, however, makes a profound contribution to body weight.

Some of the most systematic studies of the environmental determinants of obesity are those of socioeconomic status. There is a strong inverse correlation between socioeconomic status and obesity, particularly among women, with lower socioeconomic status apparently favoring the development of obesity. Longitudinal studies on both sides of the Atlantic have shown that growing up in a lower-class environment is a powerful risk factor for the development of obesity, particularly for females.

The social influences on obesity involve energy intake and energy expenditure. Increased food intake plays a major role. After years of uncertainty about the contribution of food intake to the development of obesity, the introduction of doubly labeled water to measure energy expenditure, and so energy intake, has made it clear that obesity is associated with increased food intake. An increase in the fat content of the diet, from 32% in 1910 to 43% in 1985, has mirrored the increase in obesity in the United States. Dietary fat promotes obesity in at least four ways: the greater caloric density of fat (9 kcal versus 4 kcal for carbohydrate and protein); the high palatability of dietary fat; the 25% greater efficiency (compared with carbohydrate and protein) with which dietary fat is converted into body fat; and the likelihood that, unlike carbohydrate and protein, dietary fat is not regulated. Excessive intake of fat at one meal is not followed by decreased intake at the next meal, as is the case with carbohydrate and protein.

The second environmental factor promoting obesity is the sedentary lifestyle so prevalent in the United States today. A decline in physical activity has paralleled the increase in obesity, which is far more prevalent today than it was at the turn of the century. This increase in prevalence has occurred despite a substantial decrease in average food intake. The major drop in energy expenditure reflects a decline in physical activity.

This diminished physical activity has resulted from the proliferation of labor-saving devices that have transformed the nature of work and of leisure activities. It is the rare person today who puts in long hours at heavy labor, and even the home presents fewer opportunities for physical activity. The Bell Telephone Company has estimated that, in the course of a year, an extension phone saves a person 70 miles of walking, the energy equivalent of 2 lb of fat. For genetically predisposed persons, decreased physical activity means increased body weight.

Obese persons are considerably less active than are persons of normal weight. Programs that increase physical activity also decrease body weight, but because some of the decline in body weight in these programs is probably a result of diminished food intake, animal studies provide more direct evidence of the influence of physical activity. As in humans, physical activity is limited in most forms of experimental obesity, and intensifying this activity helps control the obesity. When the tendency toward obesity is strong, as in the obese hyperglycemic mouse (ob/ob) and the Zucker obese rat (fa/fa), exercise can mitigate, but not prevent, the development of obesity. When the tendency toward obesity is weaker, as in the yellow obese mouse (AY) or in rats with small lesions in the ventromedial hypothalamus, exercise can prevent the development of obesity in some cases.

GENES AND ENVIRONMENT

Genetic and environmental determinants of obesity are not in conflict. Neither acts alone to determine a clinical outcome. This outcome is determined instead by the combination of genetic vulnerability and adverse environmental events. This combination is diagrammed in Fig. 36.2, in which the small inner circle represents persons who are genetically predisposed to a disorder. The wedge represents adverse environmental conditions to which these individuals may be exposed. The model indicates

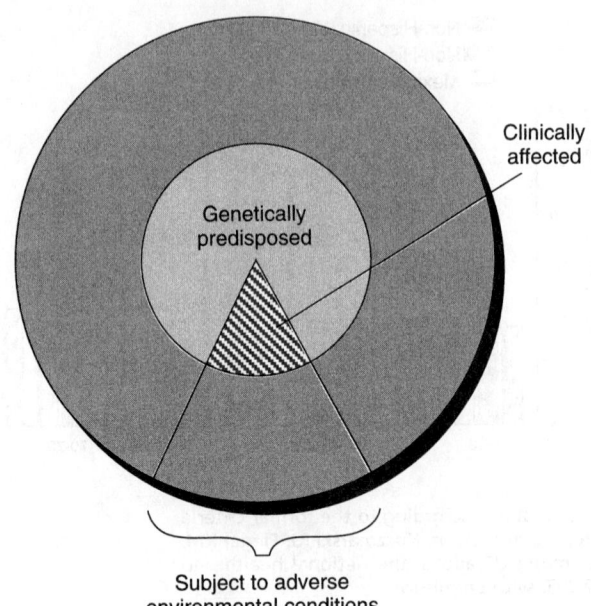

FIGURE 36.2. Model for the interaction of genetic vulnerability and environmental challenge. (From Stunkard AJ. Genetic contributions to human obesity. In: McHugh PR, McKusick VA, eds. *Genes, brain, and behavior.* New York: Raven Press, 1991:205, with permission.)

that only those genetically predisposed persons who are exposed to adverse environmental conditions are clinically affected.

REGULATORY DETERMINANTS

Four determinants of obesity can be classified by their effect on the regulation of body weight: adipose tissue, brain damage, medication, and psychological factors.

Adipose Tissue

Adipose tissue is the organ primarily affected in obesity. Adults of average weight have approximately 25 billion fat cells, and weight gain is associated with an increase in the size of these cells (i.e., hypertrophy) but not in their number (i.e., hyperplasia). Persons who have been obese since childhood usually have hyperplastic and hypertrophic obesity; in those who are 100% or more overweight, the cell number may exceed 150 billion. When weight is lost, it is solely by a decrease in fat cell size; fat cell number appears to be irreversible. As a result, when cell size in hyperplastic obesity is reduced to normal levels by dieting, persons may still have two to five times more fat cells than persons of average weight and, accordingly, a fat mass that is increased by the same amount. This hypercellularity is a major determinant of the elevated body weight (fat) set point of hyperplastic obese persons.

Brain Damage

A small number of persons become obese as a result of brain damage, particularly from tumors (e.g., pharyngeomas), even when they are successfully removed, and from infections (e.g.,

viral infections). These lesions exert their influence through two broad anatomic systems that mediate hunger and satiety, the former with representation in the lateral hypothalamus and related structures and the latter in the ventromedial hypothalamus. Damage to the ventromedial hypothalamus and its related structures results in impaired satiety, increased food intake, and gain in body weight.

Medication

Some medications, such as steroid hormones, contribute to obesity and even to altered body fat distribution. The widespread use of psychotropic medication has significantly increased the prevalence of iatrogenic obesity. Three major classes of drugs are responsible: tricyclic and heterocyclic antidepressants, lithium, and antipsychotic medication.

As many as one-half of all patients on tricyclic antidepressants discontinue desperately needed treatment because of weight gain, which may reach 2 kg per month. A major reason for the popularity of the selective serotonin reuptake inhibitors is that they are associated with far less weight gain. Weight gain with lithium is particularly troublesome, because lithium is usually prescribed for bipolar (manic-depressive) patients on a long-term basis, and weight gains of 10 kg have been reported over 2 to 6 years. Traditional antipsychotic medication also often produces weight gain, and the newer "atypical" neuroleptics may cause even larger weight gains. Since many of these medications are given on a long-term basis, weight gain is a very serious problem. A list of the psychotropic agents that promote weight gain is shown in Table 36.3.

Psychological Factors

Obesity has traditionally been viewed as a disorder with strong psychological determinants, but such determinants are confined to two specific eating disorders, binge-eating disorder and the night-eating syndrome. Binge-eating disorder is characterized by the consumption of large amounts of food in a short period, together with a subjective sense of loss of control during the binge and distress after it. Unlike patients with bulimia nervosa, these patients do not engage in compensatory behaviors, such as vomiting or laxative abuse, to prevent the weight gain after a binge, and the binge accordingly contributes to excessive caloric intake. The disorder is a source of distress, and as many as 50% of obese binge eaters suffer from depression, compared with 5% of obese persons who do not binge. Binge-eating disorder increases in prevalence with increasing body weight and afflicts about 10% to 20% of persons entering treatment programs for obesity. It may interfere with efforts at weight control and be an indication for treatment over and above that for obesity.

The night-eating syndrome, characterized by morning anorexia, evening hyperphagia, and insomnia, appears to be a manifestation of an altered circadian rhythm, precipitated by stressful life circumstances. It increases in prevalence with increasing body weight and may afflict as many as 10% of persons entering treatment programs for obesity.

TABLE 36.3.	**ANTIDEPRESSANT AND ANTIPSYCHOTIC DRUGS AND BODY WEIGHT**		

ANTIDEPRESSANT DRUGS AND BODY WEIGHT
Tendency to increase appetite and body weight

Greatest	*Intermediate*	*Least*
Amitriptyline	Imipramine	Amoxapine
	Trimipramine	Desipramine
	Nortriptyline	Trazodone
	Doxepin	
	Phenelzine (MAO inhibitor)	Tranylcypromine (MAO inhibitor)

May decrease appetite and facilitate weight loss

Fluoxetine
Bupropion

ANTIPSYCHOTIC DRUGS AND BODY WEIGHT
Tendency to increase appetite and body weight

Greatest	*Intermediate*	*Least*
Chlorpromazine	Trifluoperazine	Haloperidol
Thioridazine	Perphenazine	Loxapine
Mesoridazine	Thiothixene	

May decrease appetite and facilitate weight loss

Molindone

(From Bernstein JG. Management of psychotropic drug-induced obesity. In: Bjorntorp P, Brodoff BN, eds. *Obesity.* Philadelphia: JB Lippincott, 1992:445–452.)

CLINICAL FINDINGS

Obesity has been classified on the basis of the nature of the predominant type of adipose tissue as hypertrophic, hyperplastic, or both, and this classification is still recognized. Another classification is based on the age at onset: childhood-onset obesity is characterized by a greater genetic contribution, greater adipose tissue hyperplasia, and a greater body weight than adult-onset obesity.

Body fat distribution has become the basis for a generally accepted classification of obesity. This interest was aroused in the early 1980s by the finding that persons whose fat was located primarily in the upper part of the body suffered far higher mortality and morbidity from ischemic heart disease than persons whose fat was located primarily in the lower part of the body. Body fat distribution has been estimated by the waist-hip ratio, calculated from the waist circumference halfway between the lower rib margin and the iliac crest and the hip circumference at the level of the greater trochanter. Upper-body obesity is defined as a waist-hip ratio of more than 1.0 for men and 0.8 for women. More recently, waist circumference alone has been used, with a value of greater than 100 cm considered to represent upper-body obesity. Risk, however, is directly proportional to the extent of upper-body fat, independent of gender; the mortality and morbidity rates of men are a function of their greater upper-body obesity.

Although the waist circumference is now the most widely used clinical measure of body fat distribution, a major refinement has been introduced by imaging techniques, which have shown that essentially all of the risk of upper-body obesity is conveyed by the visceral fat depot within the abdominal wall. This finding has greatly expanded our understanding of the complications of obesity and has provided a rationale for the metabolic cascade that mediates many of these complications. This rationale suggests that visceral fat, particularly under the influence of steroid hormones, gives rise to an increased free-fatty-acid flux, which leads to decreased hepatic insulin clearance, hyperinsulinemia, insulin resistance, hyperlipidemia, hypertension, and, eventually, cardiovascular disease.

The serious health hazards of obesity have received increasing attention as part of the movement to view obesity as a disease rather than as a biologic variant. McGinnis and Foege estimated that 280,000 deaths per year in the United States are attributable to "overnutrition," making it second only to smoking as a cause of death. Some of the disorders through which this influence is exerted are described in the following sections.

DIABETES

Non-insulin-dependent diabetes (type II) is strongly associated with obesity; 70% of all type II diabetics are overweight or obese, and the prevalence of diabetes increases with advancing age and greater body weight. It occurs in fewer than 1% of young persons of normal weight, rising to 9% of older obese men and 13% of older obese women and to even higher rates in persons with more severe forms of obesity. Risk of diabetes is also amplified by a family history of the disorder and by upper-body-fat distribution. The good news is the remarkable improvement in insulin sensitivity and related abnormalities that is produced by weight reduction.

CORONARY HEART DISEASE

Obesity is responsible for several coronary risk factors and is an independent risk factor for coronary heart disease; compared with other risk factors, however, it is not a particularly strong one. Upper-body obesity is a strong risk factor for coronary heart disease, independent of the overall level of obesity.

HYPERTENSION

Hypertension is one of the indirect measures by which obesity contributes to coronary heart disease. The prevalence of hypertension increases with greater body weight gains, with upper-body-fat distribution, and with advancing age. Weight reduction controls the disorder; the blood pressure values of most obese hypertensive patients fall to normal levels with weight losses of 10 kg. Such weight losses also permit a large percentage of obese hypertensive patients who are receiving antihypertensive medication to cut down or discontinue this medication.

ENDOCRINE ABNORMALITIES

Thyroid problems, which have been invoked in the past as contributing to obesity, are rarely significant. Adrenocortical hyperactivity, which gives rise to the characteristic fat distribution of Cushing's syndrome, is usually readily recognized. Excessive amounts of estrogen, converted from androstenedione and testosterone in adipose tissue, give rise to menstrual irregularities, dysfunctional uterine bleeding, and endometrial carcinoma.

SLEEP APNEA AND THE PICKWICKIAN SYNDROME

Sleep apnea is a greatly underdiagnosed disorder that is characterized by brief periods during sleep when breathing ceases, occurring as often as hundreds of times each night. The resulting impairment in sleep gives rise to daytime somnolence, automobile accidents, cardiovascular mortality and morbidity, and premature death.

Obesity is the most important cause of sleep apnea, and weight reduction is a highly effective therapy. Recognition of sleep apnea requires first becoming aware of the possibility and then enlisting the help of someone who sleeps with the patient. Alerted to the possibility, anyone sleeping with the patient has little difficulty in making a provisional diagnosis that can readily be confirmed by study in a sleep laboratory. The severity of this disorder, the ease of diagnosis, and the effectiveness of treatment cry out for vigorous inquiry into the possibility of sleep apnea in all obese patients.

The obesity-hyperventilation syndrome, also called the pickwickian syndrome, is a sleep-related disorder of greater severity, which is characterized by daytime hypercapnia and cor pulmonale and by a greater risk of premature death.

GALLBLADDER DISEASE

Gallstones occur in about 30% of obese women, compared with 10% of nonobese women. Unlike other obesity-related disorders, weight reduction can exacerbate the problem, presumably because of supersaturation of the bile with cholesterol.

OSTEOARTHRITIS

Obesity is strongly associated with joint symptoms; arthritis of one knee is six times more common and arthritis of both knees is 15 times more common among obese than among nonobese persons. In addition to its association with arthritis of the weight-bearing joints, obesity is also associated with arthritis of non-weight-bearing joints, such as the fingers. Weight loss is remarkably effective in controlling symptoms and in significantly lowering the risk of osteoarthritis.

PSYCHOLOGICAL DISORDERS

Although obesity has been viewed as a result of deep psychological problems, such problems of obese persons are now understood to be a consequence of obesity and of the stigma with which it is associated. In addition to the eating disorders described previously, an emotional problem specific to obesity is disparagement of the body image. Persons with this disturbance feel that their bodies are grotesque and loathsome. The problem most commonly affects middle-class white women, among whom the prevalence of obesity is low and the sanctions against it very high. It is confined to those who have been obese since childhood, in whom neurosis is closely related to their obesity.

■ PHYSICAL EXAMINATION AND LABORATORY FINDINGS

Before weight reduction, significantly obese individuals should undergo a physical examination and routine blood tests (biochemical profile) to rule out the neuroendocrine and other abnormalities described previously. Decreases in medications, such as antihypertensive and antidiabetic agents, that are anticipated with weight loss should be reviewed.

With significantly obese individuals, it is not necessary to assess the body composition with specialized techniques, such as hydrostatic weighing, skinfold measurement, and bioelectric impedance. The patients can be presumed to have excess fat. Such assessment may be useful with athletic, mildly overweight individuals, who may have a surfeit of lean rather than fat tissue. Body composition assessment is commonly available at health clubs and sports medicine clinics.

The resting metabolic rate should be measured for individuals who report weight gain on low-energy intakes. Objective confirmation of low-energy requirements is often reassuring to patients and indicates the desirability of increasing physical activity rather than severely restricting caloric intake. Repudiating the reported low-energy requirements may reveal problems of distortion and denial. The composition of the patient's diet should be assessed by a 3-day food diary, recorded just before the office visit. The objective is to determine the fat content of the diet, the extent to which the patient eats at regular times, and the presence of binge eating.

OPTIMAL TREATMENT

After completing the medical evaluation, the physician should summarize the findings for the patient and then invite questions. They should then discuss the need for weight loss and the goals and methods of treatment.

NEED FOR WEIGHT LOSS

Independent of the degree of obesity, the need for weight loss is greater in overweight persons who have upper-body obesity (particularly increased visceral fat), persons who have one or more obesity-related complications (hypertension, diabetes, hyperlipidemia), those who are younger (20 to 45 years of age), males, and individuals with a family history of an obesity-related illness. The greater the number of these risk factors, the more pressing the need for weight reduction. The absence of these factors minimizes the need for treatment. A goal of weight stability, rather than weight reduction, would seem appropriate for a 60-year-old woman with lower-body obesity who is 15 kg overweight but otherwise in excellent health.

GOALS OF TREATMENT

Persons with health complications from obesity should be encouraged to lose weight—but how much weight loss is necessary? Historically, overweight individuals have been told to reduce to "ideal" weight, as defined by height-weight tables. Obese individuals, however, cannot reach this goal, which has been superseded by a weight-loss goal of as little as 5% to 10% of

their initial weight. Reductions of this magnitude are sufficient to improve or control weight-related complications, including hypertension, diabetes, and hyperlipidemia.

METHODS OF TREATMENT

The review by the Institute of Medicine of the National Academy of Sciences divided methods of treatment into three categories: do-it-yourself programs that include diet books and self-help approaches, such as Overeaters Anonymous; nonclinical (commercial) programs, such as Weight Watchers and Jenny Craig; and clinical programs that provide medical care and more aggressive measures, such as very low calorie diets (VLCDs) and drug therapy.

A primary task of physicians is to manage the health complications of their obese patients. They may also choose to manage their patients' weight-control efforts. Such efforts are most successful with highly motivated, mildly obese individuals who have become obese as adults. Significantly obese persons usually require greater structure and support. The physician should help such patients evaluate the many available treatments and select the most appropriate one. Thereafter, the physician's task is to monitor changes in patients' health and to encourage them to attend treatment sessions and improve their eating and exercise habits.

An overview of current treatments for obesity is provided in Fig. 36.3. The model combines a classification based on body weight with a stepped-care approach and efforts to identify the patient's specific treatment needs. The more obese the individual, the more structured and possibly aggressive is the therapy

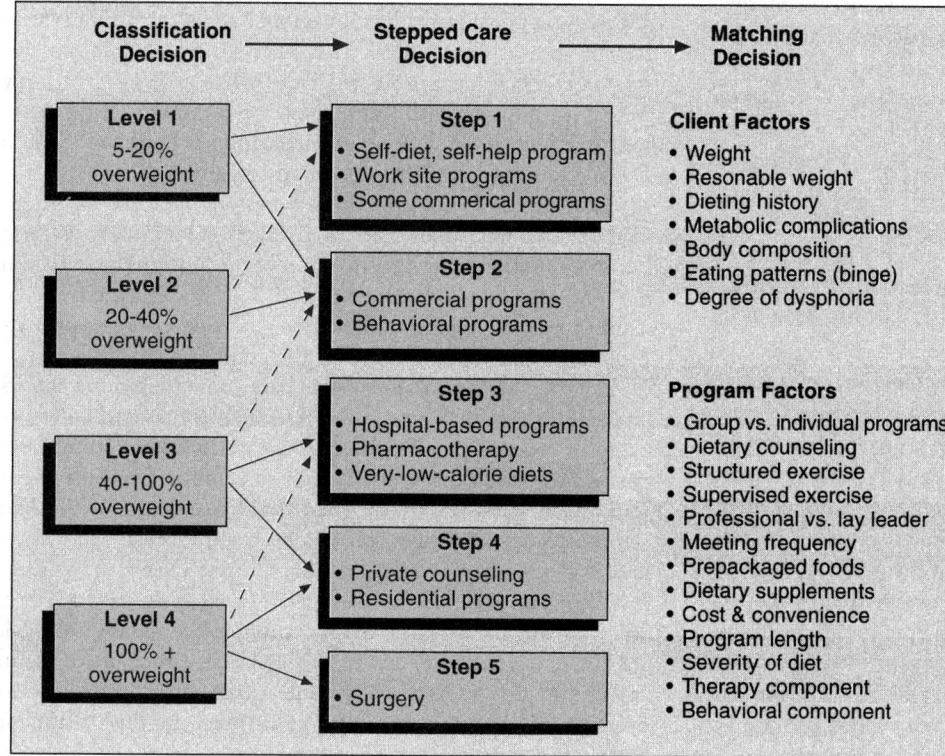

FIGURE 36.3. A conceptual scheme showing a three-stage process for selecting treatment. The first step, the classification decision, divides individuals into four levels, according to their percentage of overweight. These levels dictate which of the five steps would be reasonable in the second stage, the stepped-care decision, which indicates that the least intensive, costly, and risky approach will be selected from among the options. The third stage, the matching decision, is used to make the final selection of a program and is based on client and program variables. The dashed lines with arrows between the classification and stepped-care stages show the lowest level of beneficial treatment, but more intensive treatment is usually necessary for persons at the specified weight level. (From Brownell KD, Wadden TA. The heterogeneity of obesity: fitting treatment to individuals. *Behav Ther* 1991;22:162, with permission.)

required. We think all significantly obese individuals should be treated initially by a 1,200 to 1,800 kcal/day diet of conventional foods combined with a program of behavior modification. Such treatment is provided by Weight Watchers to over two million people a week, at a cost of as little as $12 a week. More intensive and costly versions of this behavioral approach are frequently offered, with better results, by hospital- and university-based programs. If the patient has already received this kind of treatment, the next intervention in the stepped-care model should be considered. The following sections describe behavior therapy, VLCDs, pharmacotherapy, and surgery. Results of nonclinical (commercial and residential) programs are not discussed, because of a lack of adequate data.

Behavior Therapy

As applied to obesity, behavior therapy refers to a set of principles and techniques for the modification of eating and exercise habits. This approach is goal oriented; the objectives and methods of treatment are clearly specified in weekly homework assignments that patients discuss with their counselors each week. The techniques are used to facilitate patients' adherence to any one of a number of dietary regimens. Patients are usually asked to consume their customary foods but to reduce their caloric intake by 500 to 700 kcal/day and their consumption of fat to no more than 30% of total calories. In the initial weeks, patients keep daily records of the types and amounts of foods that they eat. Later, record keeping is expanded to include information about times, places, and feelings associated with eating.

Patients are asked to increase their physical activity by a variety of changes in lifestyle, such as walking more, using stairs rather than escalators, and reducing their dependence on energy-saving devices, for example, extension phones and remote-control devices. Most patients also adopt a structured exercise program, such as walking or swimming, but are cautioned not to make the program heroic or punishing. The behavioral approach is most effective when delivered in groups of 10 to 12 persons in which participants discuss their weekly homework assignments. Individual treatment may also yield adequate weight loss, although it does not usually provide the emotional support of group care. A favorable outcome is facilitated in either case by the use of a structured treatment manual, such as Brownell's *LEARN Program for Weight Control*.

Patients treated by group behavior therapy lose an average of 8 kg in 15 to 20 weeks, equal to a loss of 0.5 kg (1 lb) a week. Longer therapy produces larger losses, but they rarely exceed 15 kg, even when treatment lasts as long as 52 weeks. When patients stop treatment, they regain approximately one-third of their weight loss in the year after therapy, with increasing regain over time. Weight regain can be minimized, if not prevented, if patients maintain frequent, regular contact with their providers after weight loss. Contact can take the form of group meetings, telephone calls, or postcards. Increased physical activity is also a key component of long-term weight control. Persons who engage in regular physical activity for approximately 2 to 3 hours a week are the most likely to maintain reduced weights.

Very Low Calorie Diets

VLCDs, providing 400 to 800 kcal daily, are reserved for patients 30% or more overweight who have failed to lose weight satisfactorily with conventional methods. Candidates for VLCDs should be referred to multidisciplinary centers that provide medical supervision and a comprehensive program of behavior change. In such programs, patients lose an average of 20 to 25 kg and maintain approximately 60% of the weight loss 1 year later. Better results are achieved by combining the diet with a sound exercise program.

Pharmacotherapy

We stand at the threshold of a major new emphasis on the treatment of obesity with medication. This development arises in part out of the growing awareness of limitations of the behavioral programs and in part out of a radical revision of our views on medication that had led to its virtual abandonment in recent years. These views had two sources. The first was the revelation, two decades ago, of the serious abuses of amphetamines by unscrupulous so-called diet doctors. The result was the banning of amphetamines and a concurrent disinclination on the part of physicians to use other safe and effective medications. The second cause for the abandonment of medication was the widespread and mistaken belief that tolerance develops to the effects of appetite-suppressant medication. As a result, state medical boards proscribed their use for periods of longer than 3 months.

This belief was mistaken; appetite-suppressant medication maintains its effectiveness for as long as it is used. As soon as it is discontinued, however, weight, which had been kept down by its use, rapidly rebounds to pretreatment levels. These newer findings reverse the old rationale for treatment and suggest that appetite-suppressant medication should be used on a long-term basis or not at all. Clinical trials have strongly supported this rationale. They have produced weight losses of 10% of body weight within 6 months, and these losses have been generally well maintained for as long as medication is continued; when it is discontinued, weight is promptly regained. Changes in the regulations for use of appetite-suppressant medication are already under way, and it seems likely that long-term use will become standard practice. Other, older medications have proved safe and effective. These agents and their dosages are listed in Table 36.4. Most are noradrenergic, and one of them, phenylpropanolamine, is available over the counter.

In 1997 the most popular medications, fenfluramine and its congener, d-fenfluramine, were removed from the market because of reports of valvular heart disease in a large number of persons who took this agent, usually in combination with phentermine. Since then, sibutramine (Meridia), a noradrenergic and serotonin reuptake inhibitor, has been approved by the FDA, and it is increasingly widely used. Orlistat (Xenecal), a lipase inhibitor that reduces the absorption of fat from the intestine, will probably be approved by the time this volume is published. Its different method of action suggests that it may prove useful in combination therapy. The clinical trials employed diet and exercise; pharmacotherapy was an adjunct to this treatment rather than a replacement for it.

TABLE 36.4.	WEIGHT LOSS MEDICATIONS CURRENTLY APPROVED BY THE FOOD AND DRUG ADMINISTRATION[a]			

Medication Name and Its Mechanism of Action	DEA Schedule	Trade Name	Dosage Size (mg)	Daily Dose Range (mg)
Noradrenergic agents				
Benzphetamine	III	Didrex	25, 50	25–150
Phendimetrazine	III	Anorex and others	35	70–210
Diethylproprion	IV	Tenuate, Tepanol	25, 75 (slow release)	75
Mazindol	IV	Mazanor, Sanorex	1, 2	1–3
Phentermine				
Resin	IV	Ionamin	15, 30	15–30
Hydrochloride	IV	Adipex-P and others	37.5	18.75–35
Hydrochloride	IV	Fastin and others	30	30
Phenylpropanolamine	Over the counter	Dexatrim and others	25, 75	25–75
Noradrenergic/serotonergic agents				
Sibutramine	IV	Meridia	5, 10, 15	5–15

[a] All medications except sibutramine are approved for short-term use only (3 months or less). Sibutramine has been approved for long-term use.
(From Bray GA. Pharmacologic treatment of obesity. In: Bray GA, Bouchard C, James WPT, eds. *Handbook of obesity.* New York: Marcel Dekker, 1998:953–975, with permission.)

Surgery

Surgery is the treatment of choice for severely obese persons—those more than 100 lb or 100% overweight or with a BMI of more than 40 kg per square meter. Surgery may also be indicated for patients with lesser degrees of obesity—those with a BMI between 35 and 40—if they suffer from comorbid conditions. The first widely used operation, jejunoileal bypass, has been replaced by two gastric restriction procedures. In vertical-banded gastroplasty, a small (15 to 30 ml) pouch with a narrow stoma (10 mm in diameter) to the remainder of the stomach is created, which radically reduces the amount of food that can be eaten at any one time. In the gastric bypass, a larger pouch that empties into the jejunum is created. Nutrients bypass much of the stomach and the duodenum. A frequent result is a dumping syndrome, characterized by gastrointestinal distress and other symptoms caused by too-rapid absorption of carbohydrates from the jejunum. Gastric bypass produces somewhat greater weight losses than the vertical banded gastroplasty and is particularly effective with sweets eaters, presumably because of the greater dumping that they experience.

Weight losses after surgery are highly correlated with the extent of overweight and consist of about 50% of the excess weight, usually 40 to 80 kg. Weight loss reaches a nadir at about 2 years, and this loss is reasonably well maintained for another 2 to 3 years. Surgery is surprisingly well tolerated, even by extremely obese persons. In centers that specialize in this treatment, perioperative mortality rates are no more than 1%, and morbidity rates are less than 10%.

Surgery is associated with a striking reduction in physical and psychological complications of obesity. There is a marked decrease in non-insulin-dependent diabetes, hypertension, hyperlipidemia, respiratory distress, and almost all complications of obesity. The most striking indication of improvement is the enhanced life expectancy of operated patients, which approaches actuarial standards of the general population. The psychological benefits of surgery are comparable, with marked improvement in psychosocial functioning, mood, and quality of life. One note of caution is warranted. Surgery should be undertaken only in programs that specialize in this treatment and that have demonstrable records of safety and efficacy.

COMPASSIONATE CARE

One of the most important services that the physician can provide obese individuals is an opportunity to discuss their feelings of sadness and frustration concerning their weight. Moreover, practitioners should be aware that overweight individuals are very sensitive to criticism about their weight, whether from family and friends, passing strangers, or their doctors. It is imperative that the physician, through words and deeds, help patients maintain self-esteem as they struggle with the challenge of weight control.

BIBLIOGRAPHY

Blair SN, Kohl HW, Paffenbarger RS, et al. Physical fitness and all-cause mortality. A prospective study of healthy men and women. *JAMA* 1989; 262:2395–2401.

Bouchard C. *The genetics of obesity.* Boca Raton, FL: CRC Press, 1994.

Bray GA. Use and abuse of appetite-suppressant drugs in the treatment of obesity. *Ann Intern Med* 1993;119:707–713.

Brownell KD. *The LEARN program for weight control.* Dallas: Brownell & Hager, 1990.

Kral JG. Overview of surgical techniques for treating obesity. *Am J Clin Nutr* 1992;55:552s–555s.

McGinnis JM, Foese WH. Actual causes of death in the United States. *JAMA* 1993;270:2207–2212.

National Academy of Sciences, Institute of Medicine. *Weighing the options:*

criteria for evaluating weight-management programs. Washington, D.C.: National Academy Press, 1995.

Pi-Sunyer FX. Medical hazards of obesity. *Ann Intern Med* 1993;119: 655–660.

Ravussin E, Lillioja S, Knowler WC, et al. Reduced rate of energy expenditure as a risk factor for body weight gain. *N Engl J Med* 1988;318: 467–472.

Stunkard AJ, Wadden TA. Psychological aspects of severe obesity. *Am J Clin Nutr* 1992;55:524s–532s.

Wadden TA. Treatment of obesity by moderate and severe caloric restriction: results of clinical research trials. *Ann Intern Med* 1993;119: 688–693.

Kelley's Textbook of Internal Medicine, fourth edition. Edited by H. David Humes. Lippincott Williams & Wilkins, Philadelphia © 2000.

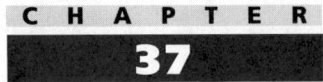

C H A P T E R

37

ANOREXIA NERVOSA AND EATING DISORDERS

PAUL M. COPELAND

DEFINITION

The major eating disorders of anorexia nervosa and bulimia nervosa represent a spectrum of abnormalities with overlapping clinical features. Both disorders are characterized by preoccupation with weight, and about one-half of patients with anorexia nervosa exhibit bulimic behavior. The American Psychiatric Association specifies criteria for the diagnosis of anorexia nervosa that may be summarized as a refusal to maintain weight above 85% of ideal body weight; fear of obesity; distorted body image; and, in females, amenorrhea for at least 3 months. Patients with anorexia nervosa who engage in repeated binge-eating or purging behavior are subcategorized as binge-eating/purging types, and others are classified as restricting types.

Criteria for bulimia nervosa require an average of at least two binge-eating episodes each week for at least 3 months about which the person feels a lack of control. The person has a persistent overconcern with body shape and weight and regularly engages in self-induced vomiting; use of diuretics, laxatives, or enemas; strict dieting or fasting; or vigorous exercise to prevent weight gain. "Eating disorder not otherwise specified" is a category for patients who do not meet full criteria for anorexia nervosa or bulimia nervosa. Amenorrhea, in particular, has been the subject of controversy as a criterion for anorexia nervosa, since the degree of psychopathologic behavior may be as severe in patients who menstruate. Binge-eating disorder, a newly designated diagnosis, shares many characteristics with bulimia nervosa, but patients do not regularly purge or compensate by fasting or excessive exercise. Diagnostic criteria include binge eating at least 2 days per week, on average, for a period of at least 6 months.

INCIDENCE AND EPIDEMIOLOGY

The lifetime prevalence of anorexia nervosa is about 0.5%. Most surveys show a greater preponderance among upper-socioeconomic classes, but later studies suggest that this gap is narrowing. There is a bimodal peak age at onset at 14 and 18 years. Only 4% to 10% of patients are males. Bulimia nervosa occurs in about 1% of young adults; males make up fewer than 10% of the patients. More individuals occasionally engage in bulimic behavior, but do not meet the frequency and duration criteria for bulimia nervosa. About 10% to 19% of young women binge eat and purge. Certain groups are especially vulnerable: eating disorders are more common in women with a history of obesity or diabetes mellitus, models, ballet students, or those in professions that demand high achievement and among men who are homosexual. Binge-eating disorder has a prevalence rate of 0.7% to 4%. Among obese individuals in weight-control programs, the typical prevalence is 30%; females are approximately 1.5 times more likely than males to have this eating pattern.

ETIOLOGY AND PATHOGENESIS

The factors that initiate or perpetuate anorexia nervosa are unknown. Theories include developmental, familial, sociocultural, and biochemical factors. Typically, the person with anorexia nervosa is a perfectionist and may perceive that parents are more concerned with achievements than feelings. Crisp maintained that weight loss also becomes a means of avoiding the characteristics of sexual and psychological maturity. The etiologic importance of a history of sexual abuse is debatable. Fasting has long been associated with asceticism and purity. Although medical reports of anorexia nervosa date to the seventeenth century, the modern societal thin ideal influences choices about weight control. Many patients with anorexia nervosa begin their diets after being teased about the need to lose weight.

Concordance rates of approximately 55% for monozygotic as opposed to 5% for dizygotic twins have suggested a genetic predisposition to anorexia nervosa. Some biochemical theories for the origin of anorexia nervosa have focused on neurotransmitters that affect control of appetite. Defects in central nervous system norepinephrine and serotonin (5-hydroxytryptamine, 5-HT) metabolism have been verified in acutely ill and recovered patients. One difficulty with biochemical theories related to appetite is that anorexia nervosa is not characterized by true anorexia but rather by a willful avoidance of eating, at least in the initial stages. Other genetic data may relate to the behavioral trait of perfectionism; both anorexia nervosa and the frequent comorbid condition of obsessive-compulsive disorder have been associated with polymorphism in the promoter region of the 5-HT_{2A}-receptor gene.

The cause of bulimia nervosa is also unknown, but it typically begins during a diet. The binges often occur during times of stress or depressed mood. Patients describe an initial soothing, albeit frenetic, quality to food ingestion, followed by feelings of guilt and then resolution of the guilt by purging. One-half of those with anorexia nervosa develop bulimic behavior. The stress of chronic dieting may create a breakthrough of binge eating. Keys and co-workers' study of conscientious objectors who volunteered to undergo 6 months of semistarvation toward the end of World War II revealed experiences of uncontrollable binge eating reminiscent of bulimia when the subjects were subsequently allowed unrestricted access to food. As in bulimia nervosa, some patients with binge-eating disorder report episodes triggered by dysphoric moods. Others report binge eating to relieve tension or describe a dissociative "numb" state during episodes.

CLINICAL AND LABORATORY FINDINGS

The behavioral features of anorexia nervosa are most notable for obsessive pursuit of thinness, body image disturbance, and denial of illness. Even those who superficially agree that a problem exists may still not be able to change their behavior. Other characteristic features are hyperactivity, social isolation, food rituals, and hoarding of food that may then be disposed of or eaten in private in small amounts or in binges. Patients with bulimic behavior tend to be more outgoing, more impulsive and more sexually active and have a higher prevalence of alcohol and other drug use than those who purely restrict food intake. Depression is common among patients with anorexia nervosa or bulimia nervosa.

The clinical manifestations of anorexia nervosa are consequences of starvation plus any of the associated behaviors, such as binge eating, vomiting, or abuse of laxatives, diuretics, or ipecac (Table 37.1). Some patients with bulimia nervosa manifest milder consequences of intermittent starvation. Food restriction is typical between binge-eating episodes. Estrogen deficiency and amenorrhea are consequences of diminished hypothalamic gonadotropin-releasing hormone (GnRH) secretion. Leptin deficiency at low weights may lead to decreased GnRH secretion. Gonadotropin secretion is also reduced in males with anorexia nervosa, and low serum testosterone levels may contribute to symptoms of impotence and loss of libido.

About 20% of patients with bulimia nervosa also have amenorrhea, and another 20% to 40% of patients have oligomenorrhea. Reduced luteinizing hormone secretion has been correlated with weight reductions of less than 85% of past high weights. Osteoporosis in anorexia nervosa may lead to vertebral compression fractures and stress fractures. Although osteoporosis is related to the duration of amenorrhea, a lack of estrogen may not be the sole cause. Increased cortisol production rates are correlated with bone loss. Nutritional depletion and resultant low levels of insulin-like growth factor I may also be responsible for bone loss.

Thyroid function in anorexia nervosa resembles that of the euthyroid sick syndrome. Peripheral conversion of thyroxine to triiodothyronine (T_3) is decreased. Bradycardia, hypothermia, cold intolerance, dry skin and hair, slowed relaxation of deep tendon reflexes, and hypercarotenemia may result in part from low T_3 concentrations. Diminished norepinephrine turnover may also contribute to some of these features of slowed metabolic rate.

TABLE 37.1. IMPORTANT CLINICAL AND LABORATORY ABNORMALITIES IN PATIENTS WITH EATING DISORDERS

Organ System	Abnormality	Contributing Factors
Endocrine and metabolic	Amenorrhea	S
	Euthyroid sick syndrome	S
	Osteoporosis	S
	Hypothermia	S
	Hypoglycemia	S
	Hypophosphatemia	B, R
	Hypomagnesemia	S, L
Renal	Hypokalemia	S, V, L
	Hyponatremia	S, V, D, P
	Volume depletion	S, V, L, D
	Renal insufficiency	S, V, L, D
	Renal calculi	S, V, L
	Polyuria	S, D, P
	Peripheral edema	R
Cardiovascular	Bradycardia	S
	Hypotension	S, V, L, D
	Arrhythmia	S, V, L, D, I
	Thinned left ventricle	S
	Mitral valve abnormalities	S
	Cardiomyopathy	S, I
Gastrointestinal	Decreased gastric emptying	S
	Constipation	S
	Cathartic colon	L
	Transaminase elevation	S, I
	Dental erosions	V
	Perimolysis	V
	Oral mucosal trauma	B, V
	Parotid gland swelling	V
	Amylase elevation	S, V
	Pancreatitis	B, D, R
	Esophagitis	V
	Mallory–Weiss tears	V
	Esophageal rupture	V
	Gastric rupture	B
	Superior mesenteric artery syndrome	S
	Necrotizing colitis	S
Pulmonary	Aspiration pneumonia	V
Hematologic	Anemia	S
	Leukopenia	S
	Thrombocytopenia	S
Skin	Lanugo hair	S
	Asteatotic skin	S
	Brittle hair and nails	S
	Carotenodermia	S
	Perniosis	S
Muscular	Myopathy	S, I
	Rhabdomyolysis	V, L, D
Neurologic	Pseudoatrophy on computed tomography scans	S
	Peripheral neuropathy	S

B, binge eating; D, diuretic abuse; I, ipecac use; L, laxative abuse; P, polydipsia; R, refeeding; S, starvation; V, vomiting.

Low serum glucose concentrations are usually well tolerated in fasting; however, hypoglycemia has been associated with coma and death in several patients with anorexia nervosa. Some of these patients had the added stress of an infection, which may have further diminished the gluconeogenic capacity of the liver. Among young women with type 1 diabetes mellitus, approximately 30% intentionally omit insulin to achieve weight control; 8% omit it frequently. Frequent omission is associated with poorer glycemic control and a higher risk of diabetic retinopathy.

Excessive caffeine or water ingestion may cause polyuria. Patients with anorexia nervosa also have diminished or erratic secretion of vasopressin in response to an osmotic challenge. Some patients manifest partial diabetes insipidus. Renal abnormalities largely reflect dehydration and a reduced glomerular filtration rate. Laxative abuse and self-induced vomiting can contribute to hypokalemia, volume depletion, and renal failure. Diuretic abuse can cause hypokalemia and, if coupled with water ingestion and vomiting, hyponatremia. During treatment of severe hyponatremia, too-rapid restoration of serum sodium has led to central pontine myelinolysis.

Patients with anorexia nervosa manifest low blood pressure and diminished cardiac output. Arrhythmia may be lethal. Retrospectively, cardiac deaths have been associated with QT prolongation. Repeated use of ipecac to induce vomiting can cause fatal cardiomyopathy. Hypomagnesemia has been associated with congestive heart failure.

Gastrointestinal changes in anorexia nervosa include decreased gastric emptying and intestinal motility, which are associated with an exaggerated sense of stomach fullness, abdominal pain, and constipation. Metoclopramide and cisapride have been used to enhance gastric emptying. Hepatic transaminases may be elevated in anorexia nervosa because of fatty infiltration of the liver. Vomiting often elevates levels of salivary amylase, and starvation may raise levels of pancreatic amylase. Vomiting during a state of decreased consciousness (with alcohol or other drug use) has resulted in aspiration pneumonia. Low neutrophil counts (less than 1,500 cells per microliter) in patients with anorexia nervosa have been associated with increased risk of infection. A mild elevation of serum creatine phosphokinase and electromyographic changes consistent with myopathy also can be found in patients with anorexia nervosa.

■ OPTIMAL MANAGEMENT

Outcome studies of anorexia nervosa find that 50% of patients totally recover, 30% of patients improve, and 20% remain chronically ill. Studies with up to 20 years of follow-up observation show a 15% mortality rate. Suicide and medical complications each account for one-half of disorder-related deaths. With weight restoration, there may be various degrees of psychological and physical recovery. Most physical manifestations reverse with weight gain, but menstrual disturbances are prone to continue among patients with anxiety disorders or with persistent abnormal eating attitudes. To help improve bone formation, the patient should have a calcium intake of at least 1,500 mg/day and take a vitamin supplement containing 400 IU of vitamin D.

Hormone replacement therapy has improved bone density in patients with ideal body weight less than 70%.

Psychiatric treatment of anorexia nervosa consists of combinations of individual, group, and family therapy. Recovered patients have emphasized the value of a relationship with a therapist or friend. Nutritional counseling and medical follow-up is important. Hospitalization is required for severe cardiovascular or metabolic disturbances, continued or rapid weight loss, or other psychiatric crises. Regular food is given, starting with intakes of 30 to 40 kcal per kilogram per day. Intake may increase up to 70 to 100 kcal per kilogram per day during weight gain and can require as much as 40 to 60 kcal per kilogram per day during weight maintenance. Tube feeding or parenteral hyperalimentation is rarely required and usually should be avoided. Serious volume depletion can be treated with intravenous fluids. Serum phosphorus levels should be assessed.

The course of bulimia nervosa has been less well studied. About 30% to 60% of patients recover. Up to another 20% experience anorexia nervosa. In addition to cognitive-behavioral therapy (also effective in binge-eating disorder) and individual psychotherapy, pharmacotherapy with antidepressant drugs has met with some success. Tricyclic antidepressants, monoamine oxidase inhibitors, and antidepressants that more selectively inhibit serotonin reuptake have reduced binge-eating episodes in double-blind clinical trials. Fluoxetine has been approved for use in cases of bulimia nervosa. The dose of fluoxetine is generally titrated upward from 20 to 60 mg per day.

BIBLIOGRAPHY

Beresin EV. Anorexia nervosa. *Compr Ther* 1997;23:664–671.

Cachelin FM, Maher BA. Is amenorrhea a critical criterion for anorexia nervosa? *J Psychosom Res* 1998;44:435–440.

Copeland PM, Sacks NR, Herzog DB. Longitudinal follow-up of amenorrhea in eating disorders. *Psychosom Med* 1995;57:121–126.

Crisp AH. Some psychological aspects of adolescent growth and their relevance for the fat/thin syndrome anorexia nervosa. *Int J Obes* 1977;1: 231–238.

Enoch M-A, Kaye WH, Rotondo A, et al. 5-HT$_{2A}$ promoter polymorphism-1438G/A, anorexia nervosa, and obsessive-compulsive disorder. *Lancet* 1998;351:1785–1786.

Grinspoon S, Herzog D, Klibanski A. Mechanisms and treatment options for bone loss in anorexia nervosa. *Psychopharmacol Bull* 1997;33: 399–404.

Keys A, Brozek J, Henschel A, et al. *The biology of human starvation.* Minneapolis: University of Minnesota Press, 1950.

Mayer LES, Walsh BT. The use of selective serotonin reuptake inhibitors in eating disorders. *J Clin Psychiatry* 1998;59(suppl 15):28–34.

Nielsen S, Moller-Madsen S, Isager T, et al. Standardized mortality in eating disorders: a quantitative summary of previously published and new evidence. *J Psychosom Res* 1998;44:413–434.

Rydall AC, Rodin GM, Olmsted MP, et al. Disordered eating behavior and microvascular complications in women with insulin-dependent diabetes mellitus. *N Engl J Med* 1997;336:1849–1854.

Stoving RK, Vinten J, Handberg A, et al. Diurnal variation of the serum leptin concentration in patients with anorexia nervosa. *Clin Endocrinol (Oxf)* 1998;48:761–768.

Kelley's Textbook of Internal Medicine, fourth edition. Edited by H. David Humes. Lippincott Williams & Wilkins, Philadelphia © 2000.

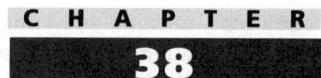

APPROACH TO THE PATIENT WITH UNINTENTIONAL WEIGHT LOSS

DANIEL M. LICHTSTEIN
ROBERT L. HERNANDEZ

Unintentional or involuntary weight loss is a common initial complaint among patients who see primary care physicians, particularly those caring for the elderly. Significant weight loss is generally felt to be a loss of 5 kg or more, or more than 5% of one's usual weight, over a period of 6 months to 1 year. In one study, involuntary weight loss was associated with a 1-year mortality rate of 25%. It has been estimated that in approximately one-half of patients claiming to have lost weight in the recent past, there is no evidence of such weight loss when previous records are reviewed. Therefore, the physician should try to corroborate and accurately quantify weight loss whenever possible. Comparison of the patient's current weight with recordings from previous office visits or with old records from other physicians' offices is the best method of validating weight loss. If this information is not available, speaking with family members of the patient and documenting a change in belt or clothing size can provide evidence of weight loss. Screening for unintentional weight loss, especially in the elderly, should be considered, in light of one study's finding that only one-third of patients found to have significant weight loss related this loss as a chief complaint to the physician.

◼ ETIOLOGY

There have been several published studies examining the origins of unintentional weight loss. Psychiatric illness (depression), malignancy, and benign gastrointestinal diseases are the most common causes of weight loss in these studies. Lung and gastrointestinal tract malignancies are the most common cancers, and esophageal disorders and peptic ulcer disease are typical benign reasons for loss of weight. Despite investigative studies and follow-up, no definitive cause of weight loss could be determined in 25% of the patients studied. There are a large number of causes of unintentional weight loss (Table 38.1). They can be broadly divided into two main categories: those associated with decreased caloric intake and those associated with increased caloric expenditures. Some conditions, such as malignancies and malabsorption, can be related to both.

DECREASED CALORIC INTAKE

Decreases in caloric intake can be due to conditions causing difficulty eating, anorexia, or malabsorption. Difficulty eating

TABLE 38.1.	DIFFERENTIAL DIAGNOSIS OF UNINTENTIONAL WEIGHT LOSS
Decreased Caloric Intake	**Increased Caloric Expenditures**
Psychosocial disorders	Persistent symptoms
Major depression	Fever
Reactive depression (bereavement)	Vomiting
Anxiety disorder	Diarrhea
Anorexia nervosa	Endocrine disorders
Anorexia tardive	Hyperthyroidism
Alcoholism	Poorly controlled
Substance abuse	diabetes mellitus
Poverty	Malignancies
Social isolation	Gastrointestinal
	disorders
	Chronic drainage
	from a fistula
Malignancies	Malabsorption
Lymphoma/leukemia	Stimulants
Solid tumors	(amphetamines,
Gastrointestinal disorders	cocaine)
Dysphagia	
Dysgeusia	
Gastroesophageal reflux disease	
Peptic ulcer disease	
Oropharyngeal disorders	
Poor dentition	
Neurologic disorders	
Dementia (Alzheimer's disease)	
Neuromuscular disorders	
Cardiovascular disorders	
Chronic heart failure	
Pulmonary disorders	
Emphysema/COPD	
Infections	
HIV/AIDS wasting syndrome	
Viral hepatitis	
Mononucleosis	
Tuberculosis	
Rheumatologic disorders	
Metabolic derangements	
Hypokalemia	
Hypercalcemia	
Uremia	
Pharmaceutical agents	
Digoxin	
Quinidine	
Antineoplastic agents	
Cathartics	
Malabsorption syndromes	
Cholestasis	
Pancreatic exocrine insufficiency	
Inflammatory bowel disease	
Parasitic infections	
Viral infections (AIDS)	
Postsurgical changes (gastrectomy)	
Medications (bile acid sequestrants)	

COPD (Chronic Obstructive Pulmonary Disease).

may be caused by oral (poor dentition), oropharyngeal (transfer dysphagia), or gastrointestinal (gastroesophageal reflux) conditions. Anorexia is associated with a wide variety of psychological conditions, including depression, eating disorders, and substance abuse. Social problems, such as poverty and isolation may also lead to a decrease in caloric intake. Appetite can also be suppressed by a large number of acute and chronic medical conditions. The mechanisms of appetite suppression and weight loss are incompletely understood. Circulating tumor-derived factors (tissue necrosis factor), increases in systemic inflammation, chronic activation of the immune system, and decreases in circulating growth factors are some of the mechanisms that have been proposed to explain cancer-related weight loss. Malabsorption syndromes, such as pancreatic exocrine insufficiency and Crohn's disease may cause a decrease in caloric intake, even when the patient ingests a normal amount of calories.

INCREASED CALORIC EXPENDITURES

Weight loss due to increased caloric expenditures may stem from metabolic diseases, such as hyperthyroidism, diabetes, and Addison's disease. Patients with hyperthyroidism may have typical signs and symptoms of the disease, but in the elderly, weight loss and tachycardia may be the only clinical manifestations. The initial signs of poorly controlled or unrecognized diabetes mellitus may be unexplained weight loss and a normal or increased appetite. Loss of calories may occur as a consequence of persistent fever, vomiting, or diarrhea. Some conditions, such as malabsorption, malignancy, and medication side effects, can lead to weight loss in several ways. Malignancies, for example, can suppress appetite while increasing caloric expenditures. Weight loss caused by medications may be the result of vomiting, dysgeusia, gastrointestinal tract involvement, or anorexia.

■ APPROACH TO UNINTENTIONAL WEIGHT LOSS

A detailed history and thorough physical examination should be the cornerstones of the initial evaluation of a patient with unintentional weight loss and will identify most organic causes. Questioning should include a psychosocial history, assessment of alcohol use, and a careful review of all medications. Oropharyngeal symptoms, dysphagia, early satiety, change in bowel pattern, fever, cough, polydypsia, and polyuria should be carefully evaluated. Additional history from family members or caregivers may prove to be valuable.

The physical examination should be comprehensive, starting with observations of the patient's general appearance and mood. A diligent search for lymphadenopathy, thyroid abnormalities, cardiac or pulmonary disease, hepatomegaly, abdominal masses, occult blood in the stool, and neurologic abnormalities (including mental status) should be undertaken. The prostate and genitalia should be examined in men, and a breast and pelvic exam should be performed in women.

Initial laboratory studies should comprise the complete blood count, including platelet count; urinalysis; chemistry panel, in-

cluding liver function tests, calcium, and serum protein levels; ultrasensitive thyroid-stimulating hormone; stool for occult blood; and chest radiography. If risk factors are present for human immunodeficiency virus, appropriate consent for testing should be requested. If the history, physical examination, and laboratory studies yield normal results, it is unlikely that serious organic disease is present. However, cancer screening tests appropriate for the age of the patient should be performed as well (mammography, flexible sigmoidoscopy).

If no source for weight loss is found after the initial evaluation, careful follow-up is indicated. This is preferable to expensive nonfocused laboratory, radiographic, or endoscopic testing. Short-term follow-up allows for confirmation of continued weight loss or the lack of it. In addition, nutritional and psychosocial issues may be pursued further. It can be helpful to have the patient keep a daily record of all food eaten over a period of time to assess true caloric intake. Psychosocial issues, such as depression, alcoholism, and substance abuse may be explored in more depth at follow-up visits. Asking the patient what he or she believes is at the root of the weight loss can be helpful. Some organic diseases provoking unintentional weight loss may show no abnormal findings on history, physical examination, and initial laboratory testing. Pancreatic cancer, Addison's disease, and lymphoma are examples of these conditions. In the absence of symptoms suggestive of such disorders, however, extensive testing of all patients is not justified.

■ CONCLUSION

In summary, the cause of unintentional weight loss usually can be determined after a detailed history, thorough physical examination, and initial laboratory evaluation. More extensive testing should be guided by signs or symptoms or by new information or findings at follow-up visits. Despite appropriate evaluation and close follow-up, no source is established in a significant percentage of patients with unintentional weight loss.

BIBLIOGRAPHY

Evaluation of weight loss. In: Goroll AH, May LA, Mulley AG, eds. *Primary care medicine: office evaluation and management of the adult patient*, third ed. Philadelphia: JB Lippincott, 1995:38–42.

Gazewood JD, Mehr DR. Diagnosis and management of weight loss in the elderly. *J Fam Pract* 1998;47:19–25.

Marton KI, Sox HC, Krupp JR. Involuntary weight loss: diagnostic and prognostic significance. *Ann Intern Med* 1981;95:568–574.

Rabinovitz M, Pitlik SD, Leifer M, et al. Unintentional weight loss: a retrospective analysis of 154 cases. *Arch Intern Med* 1986;146:186–187.

Thompson MP, Morris LK. Unexplained weight loss in the ambulatory elderly. *J Am Geriatr Soc* 1991;39:497–500.

Wallace JI, Schwartz RS, LaCroix AZ, et al. Involuntary weight loss in older populations: incidence and clinical significance. *J Am Geriatr Soc* 1995;43:329–337.

Wise GR, Craig D. Evaluation of weight loss: Where do you start? *Postgrad Med* 1994;95:149–150.

Kelley's Textbook of Internal Medicine, fourth edition. Edited by H. David Humes. Lippincott Williams & Wilkins, Philadelphia © 2000.

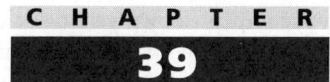

DEPRESSION, ANXIETY, AND OTHER PSYCHIATRIC DISORDERS

MARIA D. LLORENTE

In 1994 alone, psychotropic drugs were prescribed during the course of more than 45 million outpatient visits. Primary care physicians (PCPs) were seen for 55% of antianxiety, 41% of antidepressant, and 30.5% of antipsychotic drug visits. Most unexplained physical symptoms in primary care patients are not associated with organic disease but do correlate with anxiety and depressive disorders. Despite the significant prevalence of mental disorders (Table 39.1), 54% of patients are treated exclusively by generalists. As many as 50% of these disorders, however, are misdiagnosed or inadequately treated. This chapter reviews adult mental disorders commonly seen in primary care practice.

DEFINITION

Psychiatric disorders are classified according to the *Diagnostic and Statistical Manual of Mental Disorders* (DSM-IV). These disorders have characteristic signs and symptoms that lead to impairment in occupational, social, and leisure functioning.

MOOD DISORDERS

INCIDENCE AND EPIDEMIOLOGY

Mood disorders include both depressive (unipolar) and manic-depressive (bipolar) conditions. These disorders represent abnormal clinical syndromes and are not simply normal reactions to stressful situations. The incidence rates of depression and mania are 1% and 1.2% in men and 3% and 1.8% in women, respectively. Age at first episode of major depression has steadily declined in industrialized countries, with mean age at onset of 40 years for men and women. Age at onset for bipolar disorder is 30 years. The majority of patients with depression experience more than one episode in their lifetime. Bipolar disorder is a chronic recurrent illness.

Persons with any mood disorder are 2.6 times more likely than nonaffected individuals to have a comorbid alcohol or substance abuse problem; for example, 56% of bipolar patients have a comorbid substance abuse problem. Additionally, 34% of patients with mood disorders also have anxiety disorders. Seven percent of these patients have mood, anxiety, and substance abuse disorders.

Depressed patients use medical services frequently, with prevalence rates of major depression approaching 8% in outpatient settings and 14.6% on medical inpatient units. Depression is consistently associated with poorer outcomes from coronary artery disease. Patients who have experienced myocardial infarction and who are depressed are 3.5 times more likely to die immediately after a myocardial infarction than nondepressed patients. Depression also has been found to be an independent risk factor for coronary artery disease. While it is still speculative, reasons for this association include altered (decreased) heart rate variability in depressed patients; increased platelet aggregation

TABLE 39.1.	TOTAL LIFETIME AND 12-MO PREVALENCE OF DSM-III-R PSYCHIATRIC DISORDERS PER 100 PERSONS			
	Lifetime		12-Month	
	ECA (wave I)	NCS	ECA (wave II)	NCS
Any disorder[a]	32	48	28.1	29.5
Major depression	5.9	17.1	5.7	10.3
Dysthymic disorder	3.3	6.4	N/A	2.5
Bipolar disorder	1.3	1.6	1.2	1.3
Simple phobia	10.1	11.3	10.9	8.8
Panic disorder	1.6	3.5	1.3	2.3
Generalized anxiety disorder	8.5	5.1	3.8	3.1
Social phobia	2.8	13.3	4.2	7.9
Schizophrenia[b]	1.5	0.7	1.1	0.5

DSM-III-R, *Diagnostic and Statistical Manual of Mental Disorders*; ECA, Epidemiologic Catchment Area Study (n = 20,291, aged 18 yr and older, community and institutionalized samples); NCS, National Comorbidity Survey (n = 8,098, aged 15–54 yr, community samples); N/A, not ascertained.
[a] Including cognitive impairment (2.7), antisocial personality (1.5), and alcohol/substance disorders (9.5).
[b] Includes schizophreniform, schizoaffective, delusional disorders, and atypical psychosis.

in depressed, nonmedicated patients; and poor compliance with medical treatment among depressed patients.

The current suicide rate in the United States is twelve per 100,000 persons. Up to 15% of depressed individuals and 19% of patients with bipolar disorder die by suicide. Women are three to four times more likely than men to make a suicide attempt, but men are three times more likely to be successful; white men older than 65 are at greatest risk. Most persons who commit suicide see their primary care physicians within 1 month of their deaths. Suicide risk factors include psychosis, lack of social support, no spouse, chronic medical illness, substance abuse (particularly alcohol), and an organized plan with little chance of rescue.

ETIOLOGY AND PATHOGENESIS

Family, twin, and adoption studies have consistently found rates of mood disorders to be two to three times higher and 10 times higher in first-degree relatives of unipolar depressed and bipolar patients, respectively. While no cause for these disorders is known, several biologic theories have been postulated: excessive activity of the hypothalamic-pituitary-adrenal axis, disturbed functioning of catecholamines, sleep and circadian rhythm disruptions, and left frontal hypometabolism in depression. Whether the relationship between mood disorders and comorbid psychiatric conditions is causal or secondary remains to be determined.

CLINICAL AND LABORATORY FINDINGS

Four questions are useful in screening for depression and the possibility of suicide:

Has there ever been a period of 2 weeks or more when you

- had trouble falling or staying asleep, woke up too early, or slept too much?
- felt sad, depressed, or lost interest in things you usually care about or enjoy?
- felt worthless, sinful, or guilty?
- felt that life was hopeless?

An affirmative response to any question is followed by a diagnostic clinical interview.

Major depression is characterized by at least 2 weeks of either a sad mood or loss of interest. Moreover, the patient must have four of the following symptoms (remembered with the mnemonic SIG E CAPS): *s*leep disturbance, classically early morning awakening; loss of *i*nterest; feelings of *g*uilt or worthlessness; *e*nergy loss; impaired *c*oncentration; *a*ppetite change, usually decreased; *p*sychomotor agitation or retardation; and *s*uicidal or death wishes. Depressed patients may report irritability, deny sadness, or have vague somatic symptoms. They may also be more anxious than sad, but when the cited symptoms are sought, the symptom criteria for major depression are met.

Major depression can be subcategorized into the following classifications: depression manifesting as atypical hypersomnia, appetite increase, hypersensitivity to rejection, and mood reactivity; depression with psychosis (presence of auditory hallucinations and delusions); postpartum depression (within 4 weeks of delivery, possibly accompanied by psychotic delusions involving the newborn that could lead to infanticide, severe anxiety, initial insomnia, and disinterest in the child); and pseudodementia, represented by abrupt cognitive decline associated with depressive symptoms, primarily in older patients.

Dysthymic disorder is similar to major depression, but symptoms are less severe and are intermittently present for 2 or more years. Approximately one-third of patients with dysthymic disorder experience a superimposed major depressive episode, known as double depression. In adjustment disorder, depressive or anxiety symptoms develop following an identifiable precipitating stressor. These symptoms impair functionality but typically disappear when the stressor is gone.

Bipolar I disorder is characterized by one or more manic episodes. These episodes consist of an elevated, expansive, or irritable mood and three or four of the following features: grandiosity, decreased sleep, excessive talking, racing thoughts, distractibility, or excessive involvement in pleasurable activities that have a high potential for negative consequences (for example, spending sprees). Rapid-cycling patients will experience four or more mood swings in 1 year, are likely to be female (4:1), and have a poorer prognosis. Patients with bipolar II disorder experience major depression and at least one lifetime hypomanic episode (similar symptoms to mania but without marked functional impairment). Bipolar II patients are more likely to be female and have a higher risk of recurrence in the postpartum period.

Seasonal affective disorder (SAD) is characterized by development of depressive symptoms in fall or winter, with a return to baseline or even hypomanic symptoms in spring and summer. SAD shares features with atypical depression (carbohydrate craving with increased appetite, excessive sleep, and hypersensitivity to rejection), is more common in females, and responds to light therapy (2 to 6 hours per day).

When there is clinical evidence that a mood disturbance is due to the physiologic effect of a medical condition, a diagnosis of "mood disorder due to general medical condition" is made. Medical conditions associated with mood disorders and suicide include Parkinson's disease, Huntington's chorea, multiple sclerosis, Alzheimer's disease, hepatitis, pancreatic cancer, HIV, the belief that one has cancer, and pain.

No laboratory tests exist to confirm the diagnosis of any affective disorder. Laboratory abnormalities that have been reported lack sensitivity and specificity. Sleep studies show frequent awakenings with decreased total sleep time in patients with mania. In depression, patients exhibit less stage 4 sleep, diminished rapid eye movement (REM) latency, increased REM density in the first half of sleep, and overall increased REM time. Low levels of serotonin and its metabolite, 5-hydroxyindoleacetic acid, are consistently reported in the brain stem and cerebrospinal fluid of patients who commit suicide.

OPTIMAL MANAGEMENT

The goals of treatment are elimination of disabling symptoms, restoration of functioning, and prevention of relapse/recurrence. Suicidal risk must be assessed in all affective disorders. Antidepressants are equally effective, with response rates averaging

TABLE 39.2.	DOSAGE RANGES FOR NEWER ANTIDEPRESSANTS AND THEIR INHIBITORY EFFECTS ON CYTOCHROME P450 HEPATIC ISOENZYMES						
			Cytochrome P450 Inhibited[a]				
Drug	Start Dose (mg)	Max Daily Dose (mg)	1A2	2C	2D6	3A4	
Fluoxetine	20	40	W	M	S	W	
Sertraline	50	200	W	M	S	W	
Paroxetine	20	40	W	W	S	W	
Fluvoxamine	25	300	S	S	W	S	
Mirtazapine	15	45	0	0	W	0	
Bupropion	150	400	0	0	0	0	
Venlafaxine	75	375	0	0	W	0	
Citalopram	20	40	W	0	W	0	
Nefazadone	50–100	600	0	0	W	S	

N, no data; 0, no or negligible inhibitor; W, weak inhibitor; M, moderate inhibitor; S, significant inhibitor.
[a] Examples of drugs metabolized by P450 isoenzymes: 1A2—amitriptyline, theophylline, tacrine; 2C—phenytoin, warfarin, tolbutamide, omeprazole; 2D6—β-blockers, codeine, 1C antiarrythmics; 3A4—carbamazepine, lidocaine, terfenadine, erythromycin, quinidine, astemizole, cisapride.

70%. The choice of antidepressant drug is based on history (previous response by patient or blood relative), side-effect profile, or potential drug–drug interactions. The selective serotonin reuptake inhibitors (SSRIs) are currently the first-line choice for most patients. Patients must be informed that antidepressants are not immediately effective and require daily intake for at least 2 to 3 weeks before symptoms improve. Table 39.2 lists dosage ranges for the newer antidepressants and how they affect the cytochrome P450 isoenzyme system.

For patients who have not responded to maximum dosages after 4 to 6 weeks, treatment alternatives include augmentation with lithium or thyroid hormone, change to a different agent, consultation with a psychiatrist, or electroconvulsive therapy, which remains the most effective treatment for major depression. Once a patient's symptoms have responded to treatment, antidepressants should be continued for 4 to 9 months at the same dose. Maintenance treatment for several years or longer is indicated for patients with age at onset younger than 20 years and a family history of bipolar disease, two previous severe episodes with early recurrence, or three or more previous depressive episodes.

Pharmacologic treatments for bipolar disorder include lithium carbonate, sodium valproate, and carbamazepine. Gabapentin and lamotrigine also have mood-stabilizing properties. Psychiatric consultations are helpful for patients who may need psychiatric hospitalization, who are potentially suicidal, or who are experiencing psychotic symptoms.

ANXIETY DISORDERS

INCIDENCE AND EPIDEMIOLOGY

Anxiety disorders have a high prevalence in medical inpatients (5% to 20%) and outpatients (4% to 14%). Females are two times more likely to suffer from all anxiety disorders except obsessive-compulsive disorder (OCD), for which the risk is the same for men and women. The onset of anxiety disorders, particularly social and simple phobias, is in adolescence, and in those individuals with comorbid depression, it precedes the onset of depression. One-fourth of patients with any anxiety disorder will also have a mood disorder, and 15% will have a substance use disorder. The highest prevalence rates for substance use disorders, however, are among patients with panic disorder (36%) and OCD (33%).

ETIOLOGY AND PATHOGENESIS

Biologic theories postulate excessive or inappropriate autonomic discharges, particularly in the locus coeruleus, a noradrenergic center in the brain. Learning theory explains anxiety disorders as learned through identification and imitation of societal patterns or as a conditioned response to a stressful situation. Family studies have found fivefold higher prevalence rates of anxiety disorders among affected first-degree relatives of patients with panic, generalized anxiety disorder (GAD), and OCD. Twin studies have found 80% to 90% and 10% to 15% concordance for GAD in monozygotic and dizygotic twins, respectively. There are several medical conditions and drugs that can mimic or produce anxiety symptoms, including hyperthyroidism, hypoglycemia, mitral valve prolapse, carcinoid, Cushing's disease, pheochromocytoma, caffeine use, cocaine use, and alcohol withdrawal.

CLINICAL AND LABORATORY FINDINGS

Panic disorder is characterized by the sudden onset of a discrete episode of intense fear that occurs out of the blue. The symptoms peak within 10 minutes of onset and include at least four of the following symptoms: dizziness, tachycardia, dyspnea, sweating, trembling, choking, nausea/abdominal discomfort, depersonalization, paresthesias, flushes or chills, chest pain/discomfort, and fear of dying/going crazy or losing control. The attacks are recurrent, may awaken the person from sleep, and are associated with anticipatory anxiety regarding another attack. Patients frequently go to emergency rooms. Approximately 40% will also experience agoraphobia, an avoidance of situations where escape may be difficult or where help may not be available in case of a panic attack. Travel may be severely restricted to the point of being housebound, or patients may leave home only with a companion. A typical panic attack can be induced in 50% to 75% of panic patients, but not in normal controls, with intravenous infusions of sodium lactate. In the case of social phobia, the person is afraid that he or she will do or say something that will cause humiliation or embarrassment and thus avoids social situations.

GAD is marked by insidious onset of daily, persistent, and excessive worry that is unrealistic. Symptoms fluctuate over the course of years. GAD is associated with motor tension, restlessness, fatigability, autonomic hyperactivity, vague somatic symptoms, irritability, difficulty sleeping/concentrating, exaggerated startle response, and feeling on edge.

Patients with OCD experience recurrent intrusive thoughts (obsessions) and actions (compulsions) that are repetitive, purposeful, and need to be performed according to set rules or in a stereotyped fashion. These thoughts and behaviors cause marked distress, are time-consuming, and significantly interfere with an individual's routine.

Posttraumatic stress disorder results from exposure to an event that is outside the range of usual human experience and is typically life threatening. The event is reexperienced through recurrent dreams, flashbacks, intrusive memories, and so-called anniversary reactions. Thoughts or feelings associated with the trauma or reminders of them are avoided. Patients experience emotional numbing and distancing from relatives and friends and persistent symptoms of arousal, including insomnia, startle response, irritability, and hypervigilance.

OPTIMAL MANAGEMENT

Other psychiatric disorders, such as depression, must be ruled out. Anxiety symptoms that stem from a medical illness often improve when the medical illness is treated. Similarly, eliminating caffeine or making medication adjustments can improve associated anxiety symptoms. Panic disorder responds to SSRIs, tricyclic antidepressants, or monoamine oxidase inhibitors and, for immediate symptom relief, alprazolam. Cognitive-behavioral psychotherapy has been found to be effective, particularly in those panic patients who may not want to take medication. Social phobia responds to antidepressants—chiefly monoamine oxidase inhibitors—and β-blockers. OCD symptoms respond best to a combination of cognitive-behavioral psychotherapy and clomipramine or SSRIs. GAD responds to supportive psychotherapy and relaxation techniques. Short-half-life benzodiazepines are helpful for brief durations, and antidepressants are indicated for comorbid depressive symptoms. Posttraumatic stress disorder may be difficult to treat. A psychiatric consultation is often helpful in defining comorbid conditions, in initiating administration of an appropriate pharmacologic agent, and in providing psychotherapy.

SCHIZOPHRENIA

INCIDENCE AND EPIDEMIOLOGY

Two million Americans suffer from schizophrenia. Higher incidence rates occur in winter and early spring. The prevalence, severity, and morbidity are greater in urban areas and industrialized nations and in lower socioeconomic groups (downward drift). Age at onset is in the teens or early twenties—50% of patients show initial signs before age 25. The odds of these patients having an alcohol or substance abuse disorder is almost five times higher than for the general population. Approximately 47% of schizophrenics will meet criteria for substance abuse/dependence (33.7% alcohol and 27.5% another drug).

ETIOLOGY AND PATHOGENESIS

No etiologic factor has been identified. Genetic studies indicate a ten- to 12-fold higher risk of schizophrenia in first-degree relatives, with monozygotic concordance of 45% to 50%. Many schizophrenic symptoms are associated with excessive dopaminergic activity. High levels of expressed emotion in the families of schizophrenic patients is associated with higher relapse rates.

CLINICAL AND LABORATORY FINDINGS

The prodromal and residual phases of the illness are similar and are marked by social withdrawal, peculiar behavior (such as hoarding), poor personal hygiene, marked lack of initiative, vague/digressive speech, and magical thinking. The active phase consists of grossly impaired functioning with psychotic symptoms (auditory hallucinations and bizarre delusions), incoherent speech, thought disorganization, and flat or grossly inappropriate affect. Schizophrenia may be further categorized by subtype based on predominant symptoms. *Catatonia* is characterized by elective mutism, stupor, negativism, rigidity, or excitability that can lead to exhaustion and death. *Paranoia* has a later onset, the best prognosis, and the highest functioning of the subtypes; delusions are prominent. *Disorganized* schizophrenia is marked by a flat/silly affect, loose associations, and no systematized delusions. The *undifferentiated* type is represented by delusions, hallucinations, and disorganized behavior not meeting the criteria of the other subtypes. Symptoms can be characterized as positive (delusions, hallucinations, hostility) or negative (apathy, inattentiveness, ambivalence, flat affect). Negative symptoms are associated with a poorer prognosis, enlarged lateral ventricles, and cortical atrophy (frontal) on computed tomography scan and with soft neurologic signs, including frontal release and dysdiadochokinesia.

OPTIMAL MANAGEMENT

Owing to the severity of symptoms and impairment that may require psychiatric hospitalization, acute phases of schizophrenia are best managed by psychiatrists. A significant proportion of noncompliant patients will benefit from intramuscular long-acting depot neuroleptics, either haloperidol (50 to 100 mg every 4 weeks) or fluphenazine decanoate (12.5 to 25 mg every 2 to 3 weeks). The new, "atypical" antipsychotics clozapine, risperidone, olanzapine, and quetiapine improve positive and negative symptoms and cause fewer extrapyramidal side effects. Clozapine can cause agranulocytosis in 1% to 2% of patients and requires weekly complete blood counts for the first 6 months and biweekly counts thereafter. Comorbid substance abuse disorders complicate treatment but need to be addressed.

BIBLIOGRAPHY

American Psychiatric Association. *Diagnostic and statistical manual of mental disorders*, fourth ed. Washington, D.C.: American Psychiatric Association, 1994.

Cooper-Patrick L, Crum RM, Ford DE. Identifying suicidal ideation in general medical patients. *JAMA* 1994;272:1757–1762.

Depression Guideline Panel. *Depression in primary care.* Clinical practice guideline, no. 5. AHCPR Publication no. 93-0550. Rockville, Md; US Department of Health and Human Services, Public Health Service, Agency for Health Care Policy and Research, 1993.

DeVane LC. Differential pharmacology of newer antidepressants. *J Clin Psychiatry* 1998;59(supp 20):85–93.

Ford DE, Mead LA, Chang PA, et al. Depression is a risk factor for coronary artery disease in men: the precursors study. *Arch Intern Med* 1998;158(13):1422–1426.

Kessler RC, McGonagle KA, Zhao S, et al. Lifetime and 12-month prevalence of DSM-III-R psychiatric disorders in the United States. *Arch Gen Psychiatry* 1994;51(1):8–19.

Katon WJ, Walker EA. Medically unexplained symptoms in primary care. *J Clin Psychiatry* 1998;59(suppl 20):15–21.

Musselman DL, Evan DL, Nemeroff CB. The relationship of depression to cardiovascular disease: epidemiology, biology and treatment. *Arch Gen Psychiatry* 1998;55(7):580–592.

Pincus HA, Tanielian TL, Marcus SC, et al. Prescribing trends in psychotropic medications: primary care, psychiatry and other medical specialties. *JAMA* 1998;279:526–531.

Regier DA, Rae DS, Narrow WE, et al. Prevalence of anxiety disorder and their comorbidity with mood and addictive disorders. *Br J Psychiatry* 1998;173(suppl):24–28.

Kelley's Textbook of Internal Medicine, fourth edition. Edited by H. David Humes. Lippincott Williams & Wilkins, Philadelphia © 2000.

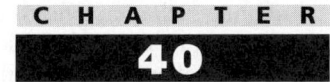

CHAPTER
40

CARE OF THE DYING PATIENT

JOANNE LYNN
BETTY FERRELL

All of us, physician and patient alike, will die. Even with optimal medical care, most of the illnesses described in this text will contribute to patients' deaths. Just a few generations ago, people died rapidly—of infections, accidents, and untreatable illness.

Now, most people will die of heart and lung failure, malignancy, stroke, dementia, or the multifaceted frailty associated with advanced age. These conditions often allow both a full and meaningful life, despite disabilities, and a meaningful closure to life, if patients and families receive competent care and impending death is accepted rather than denied. Indeed, patients, families, and caregivers are all discovering extraordinary opportunities for human growth and activity at the end of life, which are denied to those who experience sudden, unpredicted death, and they are adopting new patterns of practice to encourage comfort and life completion during advanced illness.

■ PROGNOSIS AND THE TIMING OF PALLIATION

Patients, family members, hospice programs, and insurers expect physicians to predict the survival of seriously ill patients. Many people feel that life span is indefinite and that death is largely irrelevant until one becomes a "dying" person, and they look to physicians to declare that status at the right time. Once a person is declared to be dying, social practices allow farewells, attention to spiritual issues, and emphasis on symptom control. Before that designation, these matters are largely avoided.

This view of how physicians can provide prognoses is seriously misleading. Some people, especially those with cancer, do have a distinct terminal phase of decline at the end of life, when they lose weight, restrict food intake, spend most of the time in bed, and predictably die within a few weeks. Similarly, a rapid and obvious decline allows identification and then overt labeling of intensive care patients whose organ systems are going to be overwhelmed within a few hours. Most people with serious chronic illness, however, have a quite ambiguous prognosis until near the very end. Within a week of death, the most accurate statement possible is usually that the patient is likely to live for at least a few months. The most common course is rather rapid death in the context of serious, established chronic disease (Fig. 40.1).

Clinicians would do well to help patients and families prepare for the dying that they are likely to face. Most will not be served

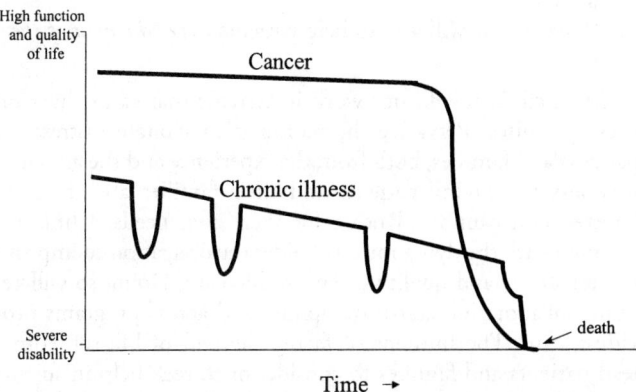

FIGURE 40.1. The time course of the end of life with cancer, in which a "terminal" phase is often evident, and with chronic illness with periodic exacerbations, in which death often seems sudden and its timing unpredictable.

best by a transition model, with a shift from a focus on life prolongation to a focus on living comfortably, which is only declared at the time when the final decline becomes evident. Instead, a combination of palliative measures and life-prolonging measures will best serve most patients. This approach requires thoughtful engagement of a physician and, usually, an interdisciplinary team throughout the course of serious illness. Honest and empathetic communication among all parties concerned allows tailoring of care to the patient's needs and possibilities. One simple way for physicians to identify patients who would benefit from special attention to end-of-life issues is to ask: "Is this patient sick enough that I would not be surprised to find that he or she died in the next few months?" Keeping this question in mind allows earlier identification of patients and families who would benefit from special attention to comfort and to life closure, thereby avoiding the unfortunate tendency to attend to dying only at the brink of death, when little can be done.

■ PROMISES TO PATIENTS

Discontinuity, overwhelming symptoms, confusion about goals, family exhaustion, and mistrust often undermine quality in care at the end of life. Patients and families need skills and reliability in their professional caregivers—enduring commitment, sensitive understanding, and appropriate treatments. The clinician counseling a person who faces an eventually fatal illness will be most effective when he or she is able to promise that the care system serving the patient will reliably deliver the following services.

1. Medical and nursing care will be of the highest quality, in accord with *evidence-based standards*.
2. *Symptoms* of pain and discomfort will be prevented and treated quickly and will never be overwhelming.
3. *No gaps* in care will arise—services will be comprehensive and continuous.
4. Specific *plans will be made* to limit the impact of likely complications.
5. Patient and family can *customize care* to meet their values, dreams, and fears.
6. The use of *patient and family resources* will be decided collaboratively.
7. All caregivers will aim to help patients *make the most of every day*.

Most clinicians do not work in systems that can deliver on these promises. Pervasive shortcomings precipitate distress for patients and families, both from the experience and the anticipatory anxiety. Dying patients and their families are often exhausted and cannot advocate for their own needs. Clinicians working with the dying must shoulder the obligation to improve the reliability and quality of end-of-life care. Doing so will require collaboration across disciplines and across programs providing care. The burdens of facing the end of life sometimes lead patients and families to consider or to seek help in suicide or euthanasia. Practitioners should develop a thoughtful approach to these issues, consistent with the law and the opportunities for care in their localities as well as their own philosophy and beliefs.

■ COMMON PROBLEMS AT THE END OF LIFE

PAIN

Pain is often feared but fortunately can be relieved in most situations. Clinicians should understand the nature, precipitants, responses, and meaning of each patient's pain. The clinical pharmacology of analgesia is treated more fully in Chapter 56. Here we note only that patients near death should be assured of pain relief, even if high doses of opioids are needed or if clouded consciousness or sedation is unavoidable. Respiratory depression is uncommon and can usually be avoided by careful titration of medications. Moreover, once a patient is using opioid drugs for a few days, respiratory depression as a result of their use is quite rare. Usually, cancer pain that is worsening requires escalation of doses to 1.5 times the previous stable dose. Neuropathic pain, however, necessitates anticonvulsants or antidepressant medications in addition to opioids. Patients with difficult pain problems should be referred to palliative care or pain specialists, since a number of new medication regimens and advanced techniques have become available in recent years.

DYSPNEA

Dying from suffocation is a particularly grim passing and should be avoided if at all possible. If a patient faces death from emphysema, ventilator withdrawal, or another condition predisposing to ventilatory failure, the physician and care team must be willing to provide sedation sufficient to assure that the patient does not experience suffocation. This requires using opioids, anesthetic agents, or sedatives. For patients with serious illness who are placed on ventilators, consideration should be given early and often to how to withdraw the ventilator, and protocols for ventilator withdrawal should be clearly understood and rehearsed by staff in those contexts (see Chapter 390). Patients coming to the end of life often experience chronic dyspnea, and oral opioids typically offer enough relief to allow restful sleep or enjoyment of substantial parts of the day (see Chapter 351).

DEPRESSION

Clinicians, patients, and family often discount the patient's sadness and fatigue, attributing such symptoms to the fatal illness. Patients who are seriously withdrawn, anhedonic, uncommunicative, hopeless, or sleepless often benefit greatly from antidepressants (see Chapter 39). Moreover, response comes more quickly and from lower doses than in healthier patients. Amphetamines have rapid onset and elimination, offering advantages when time and therapeutic margins are slim.

INABILITY TO EAT OR DRINK

Patients very near death usually have little appetite. Families can be frightened by this development and feel helpless. They need to understand that reduced intake is natural and does not cause symptoms or distress. Sometimes a small amount of food and drink that has meaning to the patient and family is quite satisfying to all. For some patients, the loss of interest in food or the inability to swallow is part of the eventually fatal condition. This is especially true of dementing illnesses. Tube feeding requires careful consideration. If it is used, plans for discontinuation should be made at initiation and reviewed periodically. Long-term artificial feeding has not been shown to prolong life or improve function in patients with serious chronic illness, including dementia and cancer. The restraints and other complications of nasal routes for tube feeding usually make it necessary to switch to percutaneous gastric routes if artificial feeding is to continue for long. Bowel obstruction in a patient near death usually should not be treated surgically. Ondansetron and other drugs often effectively suppress nausea and emesis, and cramping responds to opioids and other drugs (see Chapters 96 and 98).

DELIRIUM

Metabolic abnormalities, altered sleep, hypoxia, and multiple drugs probably contribute to the commonplace occurrence of delirium in dying persons. Occasionally, a meaningful spiritual experience, such as seeing dead family members or hearing the voice of God, has the features of delirium. The best course is usually to observe for any signs of distress or fear rather than to disrupt a spiritual experience for patient and family. Delirium may have features of terror or bewilderment, or a spiritual experience may become anguished in these ways. Often, in these very sick patients, other measures to relieve delirium must be accompanied by administration of a major tranquilizer, such as haloperidol. Very low doses are often sufficient to restore calm and appropriate behavior.

RESUSCITATION

Any patient who is sick enough that death within a year would not be surprising is a patient who deserves the chance to avoid cardiopulmonary resuscitation (CPR). The care system is primed to respond to any cardiopulmonary collapse with CPR, but persons with serious chronic illnesses are exceedingly unlikely to revive, and even "successful" CPR yields substantial additional disabilities. CPR at the end of life virtually guarantees that death will not be peaceful or supportive to family members. Discussion and decision making about the merits of CPR should begin with the onset of serious and eventually fatal illness and should be repeated as long as needed. CPR or the decision against trying CPR often symbolizes hopefulness or an acceptance of dying, respectively. Clinical teams often need to explore those meanings and possible alternatives.

OTHER PHYSICAL SYMPTOMS

The end of life often entails constipation, skin breakdown, muscle aches, dysphagia, fatigue, fevers, and incontinence. The clinical team must institute routines that prevent most of these complications and treat them early and aggressively. Hospice and palliative care services or consultation are valuable resources.

CAREGIVER SUPPORT AND BEREAVEMENT

Care for a dying loved one is simultaneously one of the most exhausting and most rewarding aspects of life. Clinical teams need to support family caregivers with flexible and thoughtful care plans, opportunities for respite, and emotional support. Grieving starts long before death for most illnesses, and the afflicted family often needs emotional and practical support. After death, many will have unresolved fears and misunderstandings as well as their own grief. Clinical teams should routinely communicate with family shortly after the patient's death and again near the anniversary date, to offer condolences, to answer remaining questions, and to evaluate for complicated grief.

HOSPICE, NURSING FACILITY, HOME CARE, AND OTHER SERVICES

The average duration of disability before death is now more than 3 years. Most people will need the support of services at home or will need to move into a nursing facility. Clinical care teams need to be effective in these settings and know how to utilize the patchwork of community resources. Although hospice programs have dramatically different eligibility requirements, their services are always worth considering, since that is one way to find continuity, comprehensiveness, and skilled symptom management in an affordable package.

QUALITY OF CARE

Patients and families need to be able to choose their care providers on the basis of reliable service quality, and providers need to engage in improvement of quality. The growing array of measurement instruments and experience with quality improvement allows for implementation of improved practices and standards.

ISSUES AT THE TIME OF DEATH

The health care team must ensure prompt pronouncement of death and certification of its cause. Families are often quite unfamiliar with the emotional, religious, and administrative issues that confront them at the time of death, and physicians often must make certain that families have support and guidance. Many patients and families are interested in providing organ or tissue donation, and all suitable patients or families should be offered that opportunity. One particularly important quality measure, especially for home care and nursing facility deaths, is routinely examining a reasonable rate of random autopsies, and clinical teams should ensure that autopsy is available.

◼ PERSPECTIVE

Dying is not primarily a physiological failure of a biochemical system; it is the closing of a human life. Reliable, high-quality health care at the end of life would allow us all to focus on issues of meaningfulness, relationships, and the completion of life's goals rather than being overwhelmed by symptoms and bedeviled by fears. Competent health care is an essential prerequisite to comfortable and meaningful living in the shadow of death.

BIBLIOGRAPHY

Berger A, Portenoy R, Weissman D. *Principles and practice of supportive oncology*. Philadelphia: JB Lippincott, 1998.

Berwick DM. Quality comes home. *Ann Intern Med* 1996;125:839–843.

City of Hope Pain Resource Center, http://mayday.coh.org.

Doyle D, Hanks GWC, MacDonald N, eds. *Oxford textbook of palliative medicine*, second ed. New York: Oxford University Press, 1998.

Field M, Cassell C, eds. *Approaching death: improving care at the end of life*. Washington, D.C.: National Academy Press, 1997.

Jacox A, Carr DB, Payne R, et al. *Management of cancer pain*. Clinical practice guideline no. 9. AHCPR publication no. 94-0592. Rockville, Md.: US Department of Health and Human Services, Public Health Service, Agency for Health Care Policy and Research, 1994.

Jacox A, Carr DB, Payne R, et al. New clinical-practice guidelines for the management of pain in patients with cancer. *N Engl J Med* 1994;330: 651–655.

Lynn J. An 88-year-old woman facing the end of life. *JAMA* 1997;277: 1633–1640.

Lynn J, Harrold JK. *Handbook for mortals: guidance for people facing serious illness*. New York: Oxford University Press, 1999.

Kelley's Textbook of Internal Medicine, fourth edition. Edited by H. David Humes. Lippincott Williams & Wilkins, Philadelphia © 2000.

PRINCIPLES OF CLINICAL EVALUATION

THE CLINICAL APPROACH TO THE PATIENT

JAMES O. WOOLLISCROFT

The patient–physician interaction is the foundation for clinical medicine. For the physician making a diagnosis, monitoring the progression of chronic disease, determining the patient's response to therapy, or assessing and enhancing the patient's health status, the information obtained during the interview and physical examination is often sufficient for an accurate assessment of the patient in the majority of encounters. If needed, it provides the physician direction for subsequent diagnostic and therapeutic interventions. For the patient and physician, it serves as the basis upon which the therapeutic relationship is built and maintained. It also is the forum where treatment plans are discussed and agreed upon and education of the patient is accomplished.

Because accurate information gathering and its interpretation are essential to clinical function, physicians must consider how the clinical interaction is influenced by the patient's expectations for the encounter, by the perceived intrusion of employers and health plans, by cultural norms, and by similar nonmedical issues. Clinicians sometimes forget that the patient's view of this interaction is quite different. Understanding the underpinnings of the clinical encounter and how to optimize the encounter can enhance clinical acumen.

PATIENT'S PERSPECTIVE

For our patients, the language of medicine is often unfamiliar. Consider traditional expressions of risk or outcome in clinical medicine. Physicians tell patients that a procedure has a "low risk" or that the prognosis carries a "75% 10-year survival rate." For the patient, however, the risk or chance of survival is 0% or 100%. Asking the patient his or her understanding of what was said or to repeat instructions or plans provides the opportunity to clarify areas of misunderstanding.

Our increasingly heterogeneous population, with physicians and providers coming from different cultural backgrounds, increases the likelihood of serious miscommunication. Too frequently, physicians assume that their culturally based communication norms are universal, but such is not the case. For example, a distance of 3 to 5 feet between the patient and the physician may be a very comfortable and mutually respectful distance for conversing for many Americans, but patients from different cultural backgrounds may interpret this as aloofness or disinterest. Such unintentional violations of cultural communication norms may inhibit or destroy rapport and prevent the development of a therapeutic relationship.

The expectations of the patient for the physician are in large part culturally determined. Unless specific attention is given to these expectations, the physician may unwittingly try to relate to the patient in a manner that the patient finds unacceptable. For example, some Asian, African, and other peoples view diet as very important when they are ill. If the physician does not address diet in his or her therapeutic instructions, the patient may consider the physician incompetent and not heed the advice. Physicians who do not understand the cultural background of their patients may violate norms for physician behavior, leading to a breakdown in the physician–patient relationship.

The patient's interpretation of symptoms and response to illness is also set in a cultural context. Illness may be viewed as an opportunity to atone for past wrongdoing, and the patient may believe that it is good to suffer. Attempts by the physician to intervene and shorten the suffering may be viewed as contrary to God's will. If the patient is from a different cultural background, the physician should strive to learn about their views of illness and healing and tailor the clinical approach accordingly. The potential for misinterpretation and communication problems increases when patient and physician come from different cultural backgrounds. In all clinical encounters, however, it is important to clarify the patient's understanding and perspective, which will enhance the physician's clinical problem-solving abilities as well as the therapeutic value of the patient–physician interaction.

Patients at different stages of life and illness may ask their physicians to play different roles in their care. Patients who have been very active in their care and decision making may ask their physicians to assume greater responsibility for making important care decisions as an illness progresses. These role changes in an ongoing patient–physician relationship are often signaled in subtle ways. We must be alert and respond to such requests, determine that this is the patient's desire, and then respect the request.

THERAPEUTIC RELATIONSHIP

Patients usually visit physicians for diagnosis of a problem, for continuing care of a known condition, for reassurance, to obtain information, and for disease prevention. Studies of patient–physician interactions show that the patient's satisfaction is enhanced if the physician ascertains the patient's expectations for the interaction and explicitly addresses these expectations. Patients' satisfaction is directly correlated with compliance with recommendations and desirable clinical outcomes, including enhanced control of chronic illnesses. Despite studies documenting the effect of physicians' questioning and communication styles on the interview as an information-gathering tool and as a means to establish rapport and enhance the patient's satisfaction, too frequently clinicians do not use optimal communication techniques. Using a nondirective "patient-centered" approach to establish the patient's reason for seeking care or his or her health status since the last visit allows the patient to establish the agenda for the visit. Once this is accomplished, using a more directed "doctor-centered" approach allows the physician to rapidly concentrate on eliciting the data that are pertinent at that particular interaction. Studies show, however, that physicians often do not allow their patients to complete their opening statements of concerns or symptoms and rapidly apply a directive interview style. This truncates the information elicited from the patient and may prevent the clinician from addressing the patient's concerns.

Of equal importance to verbal communication is nonverbal communication. Through nonverbal communication, the patient is communicating to the physician and the physician to the patient such information as expectations for the encounter, roles to be played by the patient and physician, respect, and the relative power of the participants. It behooves the physician to consider actively the communication that is occurring in the nonverbal realm. Are the patient's words consistent with her or his nonverbal language? Are you conveying a congruent verbal and nonverbal message?

The growth of electronic communication has the potential to change rapidly the dynamic of the patient–physician interaction. Electronic communication with patients has the promise of increased access to care, better education of patients, easy monitoring of chronic disease, and reminders to encourage patient's adherence to therapeutic regimens. Issues of confidentiality, fewer in-person opportunities to assess patients, and erosion of the therapeutic value of the relationship are potential negatives. Choosing the appropriate communication mode for different patients and different situations requires data from studies that are just beginning. While the efficiencies gained through increased reliance on electronic communication are apparent, the costs are often hidden.

The ready availability of medical information on the World Wide Web, ranging from peer-reviewed scientific journals to fallacious claims for therapy, is introducing further complexity into the patient–physician encounter. Increasingly, physicians are asked to comment on information that a patient has found on the Web. This can result in an empowered patient partner, but it can also lead to confusion. Careful explanations are required as to why a given finding or therapy is or is not applicable to the patient bringing you the information.

CLINICIAN'S PERSPECTIVE

From the clinician's perspective, the focus during the clinical encounter is problem solving. Physicians generate hypotheses early during a patient–physician interaction, on the basis of limited information. The physician's problem formulation and the accuracy or quality of the initial set of hypotheses largely determines the accuracy of the final diagnosis. If the clinician frames the problem incorrectly at the outset, it is virtually impossible for him or her to arrive at the right answer.

Although most research has focused on diagnosis, clinicians deal with a wide variety of situations. Healthy persons visit physicians for health maintenance examinations, previously healthy persons come with new signs or symptoms, patients with chronic diseases are seen periodically to monitor disease status and the effect of therapy, and patients with chronic conditions are examined for new signs or symptoms. The expert clinician rapidly switches from one clinical problem to another without consciously recognizing that different issues are addressed and different data are used in the problem-solving process. Patients' data that are potentially important to the physician can be divided into at least three major domains: information required to make a diagnosis, information applied to determine risk of disease, and information to assess the person with the disease.

DIAGNOSIS

When confronted with a patient who has new signs or symptoms, the clinical interaction is designed to elicit information from the patient that facilitates diagnosis and the appropriate diagnostic and therapeutic interventions. Because the clinical approach to diagnosing and treating disease states is the focus for most of this textbook and most teaching and training, I do not consider it further in this chapter.

RISK OF DISEASE

The clinician should consider each patient's risk of disease and whether current diseases, ongoing therapy, or past therapy puts the patient at higher risk of complications or other diseases. The focus for risk determination should be limited to those conditions that it is possible to prevent or those diseases for which early detection methods are available and therapy at an early stage can alter favorably the natural history. The following guidelines provide a framework for risk assessment. The patient's sex and age determine which conditions he or she is most likely to experience. Risks for adolescents are different from risks for the elderly. There are also genetic risks. Are there diseases that run in the patient's family that can be prevented or detected at an early stage? As genetic screening becomes widespread, this will become an increasingly powerful and specific tool. Although environmental risks are usually considered for industrial or work site exposures, they may also be associated with leisure-time activities. Lifestyle and behavioral risks must be assessed. Certain patterns, such as cigarette smoking and alcohol and drug abuse, are independent risk factors that also can magnify environmental risks. Physicians should consider the risk that one disease imposes for the development of other diseases. Is the patient at risk because of current or past therapy? Many therapeutic interventions have side effects that predispose patients to further problems. Appropriate monitoring may reduce this risk.

PERSON WITH THE DISEASE

The third information domain defines the person with the disease. What are the unique attributes of your patient? This question encompasses psychological and social components, including their life experiences, spiritual dimensions, and social support systems. Studies are increasingly emphasizing the importance of this domain to patients. Many physicians, however, infrequently consider this information.

◼ CONCLUSION

A broad knowledge base is insufficient to function as a physician. It is necessary to have the ability to obtain appropriate information from the patient to guide the application of knowledge to each patient's situation. The patient–physician interaction is arguably the most important diagnostic and therapeutic tool clinicians possess, and the approach to the patient can enhance or hinder this tool. Physicians must periodically assess their performances to ensure that the desired outcomes for each patient interaction are being achieved.

BIBLIOGRAPHY

Delbanco TL. Enriching the doctor–patient relationship by inviting the patient's perspective. *Ann Intern Med* 1992;116:414–418.

Kravitz RL, Cope DW, Bhrany V, et al. Internal medicine patients' expectations for care during office visits. *J Gen Intern Med* 1994;9:75–81.

Lipkin M, Putnam SM, Lazare A, eds. *The medical interview: clinical care, education, and research.* New York: Springer-Verlag, 1995.

Mandl KD, Kohane IS, Brandt AM. Electronic patient–physician communication: problems and promise. *Ann Intern Med* 1998;129:495–500.

Mazur DJ, Merz JF. How age, outcome severity, and scale influence general medicine clinic patients' interpretations of verbal probability terms. *J Gen Intern Med* 1994;9:268–271.

Pellegrino E, Mazzarella P, Corsi P. *Transcultural dimensions in medical ethics.* Frederick, Md.: University Publishing Group, 1992.

Rothschild SK. Cross-cultural issues in primary care medicine. *Dis Mon* 1998;44(7):293–319.

Smith RC. *The patient's story: integrated patient–doctor interviewing.* Philadelphia: Lippincott–Raven Publishers, 1996.

Kelley's Textbook of Internal Medicine, fourth edition. Edited by H. David Humes. Lippincott Williams & Wilkins, Philadelphia © 2000.

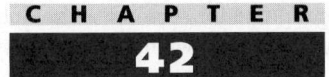

PRINCIPLES OF CLINICAL EPIDEMIOLOGY

JAY M. SOSENKO

This chapter is designed to familiarize the reader with certain aspects of clinical epidemiology. Although the field of clinical epidemiology cannot be fully covered here, selected topics are presented that are relevant to research, clinical practice, and the assessment of the medical literature. The reader who desires a broader discussion of clinical epidemiology or more in-depth information regarding the topics presented is referred to texts on epidemiology and clinical epidemiology in the bibliography.

Clinical epidemiology involves applying epidemiologic methods to the investigation of aspects of clinical medicine. Whereas the overall field of epidemiology commonly studies the general population for factors that affect disease occurrence, research in clinical epidemiology pertains mostly to patients. The clinical epidemiologist may also study disease etiology and prevention, but there is an emphasis on matters concerning the care of patients, including treatment response, cost-effectiveness analysis, and quality of life. Investigations of such patient care outcomes is commonly termed outcomes research. Clinical epidemiology, including outcomes research, uses standard epidemiologic methodology and study designs, which are discussed herein.

◼ TYPES OF STUDIES

CLINICAL TRIALS

In these studies, an intervention—usually a potential treatment or preventive measure—is tested on research participants. Typically, an intervention group (or groups) is compared with a control group that does not receive the intervention, to assess therapeutic benefits and adverse effects. Although the randomization of participants into groups is common to many clinical trials, they may vary greatly in design, including such considerations as placebo use, the number of interventions studied, whether participants and investigators are "blinded" (single-blind vs. double-blind), and whether participants remain on the same arm (parallel design) or are changed to another arm (crossover design) during the course of the study.

OBSERVATIONAL STUDIES

These studies differ from clinical trials in that there are no interventions (treatments) administered to the research participants. Observational studies are particularly useful for examining factors potentially causal to certain diseases, since clinical trials are generally not appropriate for such research. Cohort studies and case–control studies are the two most common types of observational studies.

Cohort studies are based on a design in which the occurrence of a condition is ascertained in a group of individuals exposed to a potential causal factor (exposure) and in a group not exposed to that factor. Prospective (current) cohort studies are those in which the development of the condition occurs after the initiation of the study, while retrospective (historical) cohort studies are those in which the development of the condition occurs before the onset of the study. Prospective cohort studies tend to be performed outside the clinical setting, whereas data for retrospective cohort studies are often derived from clinic and hospital records and also from registries. A study that is designed to follow cigarette smokers and nonsmokers prospectively to compare them for the development of lung cancer is an example of a prospective cohort study, while a study that uses a review of medical records to compare outcomes of different treatments that were administered for lung cancer is an example of a retrospective cohort study.

Case–control studies differ from cohort studies in that the basic design is the measurement of frequencies of exposure in groups with and without a condition. A study that examines the association between lung cancer and cigarette smoking by ascertaining the cigarette smoking history in individuals with (cases) and without (controls) lung cancer is an example of a case–control study. Despite the different designs of cohort and case–control studies, they usually have the same basic purpose—to estimate the association between disease and exposure.

Case–control studies tend to be more applicable to the clinical setting than prospective cohort studies, and they are especially helpful in investigating rare diseases or conditions for which prospective cohort studies would require the long-term follow-up of large numbers of participants. The case–control study design can circumvent this problem, since sufficient numbers of patients with and without a particular condition are often available. For example, a case–control study might be used to examine potential risk factors for rare forms of cancer, such as the case–control study that showed the association between vaginal adenocarcinoma in young women and maternal diethylstilbestrol use.

EPIDEMIOLOGIC MEASURES

The measures discussed here apply to dichotomous outcomes (e.g., the presence or absence of a condition), which are common in observational studies. Clinical trial outcomes may also be dichotomous, but they are often continuous (e.g., cholesterol or blood pressure responses).

INCIDENCE RATE

This is a basic epidemiologic measure that indicates the number of new cases of a condition over the total amount of time that a given population is under observation for the development of that condition. Using a hypothetical example, if 1,000 cigarette smokers are followed for an aggregate duration of 10,000 years for the occurrence of a first myocardial infarction and 20 show signs of that condition, the incidence rate is 20 myocardial infarctions per 10,000 person-years. If 1,000 nonsmokers are followed for the same duration and 10 have myocardial infarctions, the incidence rate is 10 myocardial infarctions per 10,000 person-years.

PREVALENCE RATE

This is the number of existing cases of a condition among a given population at a particular point in time. The prevalence rate is thus a proportion, and it is greater in conditions of either higher incidence or longer duration. If there are 100 individuals with a condition among a population of 100,000, the prevalence rate is 0.001.

RISK

Also termed cumulative incidence, this is the number of new cases of a condition among those who are followed for the development of that condition over a defined period of observation. If 1,000 cigarette smokers are followed for a period of 10 years for the occurrence of a first myocardial infarction and 20 show signs of that condition, the risk is 0.02. If 10 of 1,000 nonsmokers have a first myocardial infarction over 10 years of follow-up, the risk is 0.01. Note that as a proportion, risk has no units; however, it is still a function of the duration of follow-up.

RELATIVE RISK

As discussed earlier, epidemiologic studies are designed to examine the association between a condition and an exposure, such as myocardial infarction and cigarette smoking. Thus, epidemiologic measures have been developed to show the extent of association between a condition and an exposure. The relative risk is a measure used for this purpose. It is the ratio of the risk for those exposed over the risk for those not exposed. The relative risk for the risk data presented above is 2.0. This means that the cigarette smokers had twice the risk of myocardial infarction of nonsmokers. If there had been no difference in the risk between cigarette smokers and nonsmokers, the relative risk would have been 1.0. If those exposed had a lower risk than those not exposed, the relative risk would have been less than 1.0.

RISK DIFFERENCE

Consider a study that assessed the association between another condition and exposure instead of myocardial infarction and cigarette smoking, and the risks for the exposed and nonexposed were 0.2 and 0.1, respectively. The relative risk would be 2.0, the same as that for the myocardial infarction/cigarette smoking example. It is evident, however, that the difference in the risk for the myocardial infarction/cigarette smoking example (0.02 − 0.01 = 0.01) is much lower than the difference in the risk for the other example (0.2 − 0.1 = 0.1). Thus, another measure, the risk difference, provides an added perspective. The magnitude of the risk difference can have public health implications and can be used to make health policy decisions.

TABLE 42.1.	AN EXAMPLE OF THE CALCULATION OF THE ODDS RATIO FROM A CASE–CONTROL STUDY

	Cases	Controls
Exposed	20	10
Not Exposed	180	190
Total	200	200
Odds Ratio	$=\dfrac{\frac{20}{180}}{\frac{10}{190}}$	$=\dfrac{(20)(190)}{(10)(180)}$ $= 2.11$

ODDS RATIO

The relative risk cannot be directly obtained from a case–control study. In that study design, participants are not followed over time, which is necessary to measure risk. Since the purpose of performing case–control studies is to examine the association between a condition and an exposure, a measure of association other than the relative risk must be used. This measure is the odds ratio. It can be calculated as the ratio of the exposure odds in the cases over the exposure odds in the controls (Table 42.1). The odds ratios obtained from case–control studies can closely approximate the relative risk, particularly if a condition is rare. Thus, through the calculation of the odds ratio, case–control studies can also be used to obtain a measure of association between a condition and an exposure.

HYPOTHESIS TESTING

The epidemiologic measures discussed here are not in themselves indicative of statistical significance. Even though a relative risk of 4.0 (a fourfold risk in those exposed) suggests that there is truly an association between a condition and an exposure, one cannot presume that such a result is statistically significant. An observed relative risk can be assessed for statistical significance by first assuming the null hypothesis (no association between a condition and an exposure, a relative risk of 1.0) and then determining the degree of inconsistency (extent of association) between the observed relative risk that was obtained and the null hypothesis. The greater the degree of inconsistency between the relative risk and the null hypothesis, the lower the probability that the null hypothesis is correct (the higher the probability that the condition and exposure are related).

The p value provides a measure of the degree of inconsistency between the null hypothesis and the relative risk. Put more formally, the p value is indicative of the probability that the relative risk is at least as great as that which would have resulted by chance alone, if it is assumed that there is truly no association. If the p value for the relative risk is below a predetermined level, the null hypothesis is rejected, and the result is considered statistically significant. Most studies use a p value of 0.05 as the cutoff for statistical significance. Thus, if a relative risk of 2.0 corresponds to a p value of 0.05, a relative risk that is greater than 2.0 (even further from the 1.0 null value) would be statistically significant at $p < 0.05$. Although the relative risk has been used as an example, this discussion applies to other measures as well.

CONFIDENCE INTERVALS

The confidence interval provides information with regard to both the magnitude of the epidemiologic measures obtained and the significance testing. It is indicative of the range that contains the true magnitude of a measure with a certain level of assurance. For example, if a relative risk of 3.0 has a 95% confidence interval of 1.3–8.5, there is 95% assurance that the true relative risk is somewhere between 1.3 and 8.5. Besides providing information about the range that contains the true relative risk, the confidence interval also indicates whether a measure is statistically significant. In the example cited previously, the relative risk is statistically significant when 0.05 is the designated cutoff for a p value, since the confidence interval does not cover the value of 1.00 (expected, assuming the null hypothesis).

BIAS

In assessing the results of a study, it is insufficient to consider only the epidemiologic measure and its associated p value, since these may have little meaning if a study is biased. Bias occurs when there is a systematic error in the design or conduct of a study that results in a mistaken estimation of the effect of an exposure. Observational studies are generally more subject to bias than are clinical trials, since the latter are undertaken under more controlled conditions. Among observational studies, case–control and retrospective cohort studies may be particularly subject to bias, since they are often dependent on data previously obtained for clinical rather than research purposes. Although prospective cohort studies are still subject to bias, the more standardized manner of data ascertainment for these studies tends to lessen the likelihood. Still, appreciable bias can be found in these studies when there are differences in exposure and outcome between those who remain in the study and those who are lost to follow-up.

Case–control studies may be dependent on the recall of study participants, which can be faulty. Moreover, case–control studies can be biased if the control group is not selected with care. For instance, consider the example of the case–control study presented earlier. If the control group of patients without lung cancer comprises a number of patients with chronic obstructive pulmonary disease (COPD), there may be an underestimation of the actual association between lung cancer and cigarette smoking. This is because cigarette smokers would be overrepresented in the control group. The faulty recall of study participants can lead to recall bias, while the injudicious selection of a control group can lead to selection bias. A number of other kinds of bias (referral, interviewer) can affect studies.

CONFOUNDING

Consider a study examining the relationship between COPD and alcohol intake. One might incorrectly conclude from the data that there is an association between COPD and alcohol intake if there is not an allowance made for cigarette smoking in the analysis of the data. This is because cigarette smoking is a known cause of COPD and it is associated with alcohol use. In this example, cigarette smoking can be viewed as a confounder, since it satisfies two basic conditions: it is a risk factor for a condition under study, independent of the exposure under study, and it is associated with that exposure. Confounding does not always lead to an overestimation of association between a condition and an exposure, in that it can also have the opposite effect and obscure an association which is actually present.

DIAGNOSTIC TEST INTERPRETATION

Diagnostic test interpretation constitutes a field of clinical epidemiology that is applicable to both research and clinical practice. The terms that are commonly used are defined diagrammatically in Table 42.2. The sensitivity of a test indicates the number of those who test positive among those who have the condition. The false negative rate is equivalent to 1 − sensitivity. The specificity of a test indicates the number of those who test negative among those who do not have the condition. The false positive rate is equivalent to 1 − specificity.

In tests with a quantitative result, such as the degree of ST depression in an exercise stress test, the cutoff for test positivity is arbitrary. The values for cutoffs associated with a higher test sensitivity are associated with a lower specificity and a higher false-positive rate. Thus, a less stringent criterion for test positivity is associated with a higher sensitivity and a higher false-positive rate. Receiver–operator curves are used to show graphically how the sensitivity and false-positive rate vary with cutoff values for tests.

The positive predictive value indicates the number of those who have the condition among those who test positive. The negative predictive value indicates the number of those who do not have the condition among those who test negative. Predictive

values vary according to the pretest likelihood that a condition is present in those tested. For a given sensitivity and specificity, a higher pretest likelihood of a condition results in a higher positive predictive value and a lower negative predictive value. Bayes' theorem formulates the relationships of the positive predictive value with test characteristics and the probability of disease. This equation is a useful expression of Bayes' theorem:

$$\text{Positive Predictive Value}$$
$$= \frac{(\text{Sensitivity})(\text{Probability of Disease})}{\begin{array}{c}(\text{Sensitivity})(\text{Probability of Disease}) \ + \\ (\text{False Positive Rate})(\text{Probability of No Disease})\end{array}}$$

BIBLIOGRAPHY

Epstein AM. The outcomes movement: Will it get us where we want to go? *N Engl J Med* 1990;323:266–270.
Feinstein AR. *Clinical epidemiology.* Philadelphia: WB Saunders, 1985.
Friedman LM, Furberg CD, DeMets DL. *Fundamentals of clinical trials.* Littleton: PSG Publishing, 1985.
Griner PF, Mayewski RJ, Mushlin AI, et al. Selection and interpretation of diagnostic tests and procedures. *Ann Intern Med* 1981;94:557–592.
Hennekens CH, Buring JE. *Epidemiology in medicine.* Boston: Little, Brown, 1987.
Herbst AL, Ulfelder H, Poskanzer DC. Adenocarcinoma of the vagina: association of medical stilbestrol therapy with tumor appearance in young women. *N Engl J Med* 1971;284:878–881.
Schlesselman JJ. *Case–control studies.* New York: Oxford University Press, 1982.
Sommer A. Epidemiology and the health care revolution. *Ann Epidemiol* 1997;7:526–529.

Kelley's Textbook of Internal Medicine, fourth edition. Edited by H. David Humes.
Lippincott Williams & Wilkins, Philadelphia © 2000.

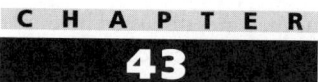

CHAPTER 43

EVIDENCE-BASED MEDICINE

MARK T. O'CONNELL

It is conservatively estimated that over 100,000 people die annually in the United States as a result of negligent or inappropriate medical care. This is equivalent to three 747 airliner crashes every 2 days! Yet, society and the health care system have been slow to respond to this alarming lack of quality control in the world's most expensive health care delivery system. The payers and consumers of health care have predictably, if not belatedly, begun to demand that the policies, systems, and outcomes of health care be continuously measured, analyzed, monitored, and modified so that the quality of care received is explicitly determined and continuously improved. Still, by some current studies as little as less than 30% of medical care is based on valid conclusive evidence that this care is effective or sometimes even necessary.

TABLE 42.2.	DEFINITIONS OF MEASURES USED FOR THE INTERPRETATION OF DIAGNOSTIC TESTS

		Condition	
		+	−
Test	+	TP	FP
	−	FN	TN

Sensitivity = TP/FN + TP
Specificity = TN/FP + TN
FN Rate = FN/TP + FN
FP Rate = FP/FP + TN
Positive Predictive Value = TP/TP + FP
Negative Predictive Value = TN/FN + TN

TP, true-positives; FP, false-positives; FN, false-negatives; TN, true-negatives.

The evidence-based medicine (EBM) paradigm claims that whenever possible, health care decisions should be based primarily on systematically collected data and the valid conclusions that follow from those data. "Best evidence" is being used to justify the rationing of limited resources. Medical evidence is driving the development of clinical pathways and guidelines for care, which are de facto defining "standards of care." Physician behaviors and economic livelihoods are likely to be increasingly affected by the evidence collected and reported about individual and physician group practice patterns, disease-specific outcomes, and resource expenditures.

The nation is calling for accountability from the health care system. At the same time, society is turning to alternative sources of health care, without any significant evidence of effectiveness or value. This paradox reflects a growing general dissatisfaction with our health care system. The tenets of EBM will help to ensure that true quality and value are fundamental characteristics of the American medical care system. Physicians must understand the principles of EBM to efficiently develop valid evidence, accurately interpret this evidence, and optimally apply it to formulating health care policy and providing superior patient care.

Why is this EBM movement gaining momentum and moving to center stage at this time? In part, EBM is an outgrowth of many contemporary factors. As just described, society has recently begun to demand demonstrated value and quality for the expensive health care that it finances and depends on. There is also a relatively new source of evidence in the clinical biomedical literature, in the form of randomized controlled clinical trials. The randomized clinical trial (RCT) is regarded as the optimal study design for determining the effectiveness of treatments and other interventions (Chapter 42). The first RCTs appeared in the medical literature in the 1950s, but 85% of those published have appeared in the literature within the past 5 years. The techniques of meta-analysis have been significantly refined in the past 5 years, bringing vast amounts of previously weak evidence into a more valid context. The computer revolution has delivered this incredibly robust collection of biomedical evidence into the hands of its primary consumers: physicians, patients, and policy makers.

MEDLINE, with its bibliographic citations, and the rapidly growing collections of full-text on-line periodicals, textbooks, and browsable databases of real world clinical data have brought potentially useful medical evidence to those who need it. Just-in-time knowledge servers are becoming part of modern clinical information systems, providing decision makers with context-sensitive previously validated evidence, often in a seamless fashion at the very point of clinical decision making as medical care is being delivered.

EBM has an extremely important personal context for physicians. The EBM paradigm presents a value system that endorses empirical data–driven behavior and moves away from the traditional emphasis on authority and personal opinion and experiences. The EBM paradigm also promotes values, behaviors, and skills that are axiomatic to effective lifelong adult learning. Although EBM includes a set of values and promotes specific attitudes and consequent behaviors, effective practice of EBM requires mastery of an explicit knowledge domain and skills set. EBM, in this sense, can be described as a five-step process: (1)

TABLE 43.1.	EVIDENCE-BASED MEDICINE: A FIVE-STEP PROCESS

1. Identify a gap in knowledge
2. Formulate an explicit, structured question
3. Search for the best evidence to answer the question
4. Critically appraise the evidence for validity and clinical applicability
5. Evaluate the outcomes of evidence-based practices

(From Sackett DL, et al. *Evidence-based medicine: how to practice and teach EMB.* New York: Churchill Livingstone, 1997, with permission.)

---

identify a gap in knowledge; (2) formulate an explicit question to define the information needed; (3) locate the best evidence that answers the question; (4) appraise this evidence for its relevance to clinical practice; and (5) evaluate the outcomes of clinical practice (Table 43.1).

IDENTIFYING A KNOWLEDGE GAP AND FORMULATING A QUESTION

Many studies have shown that physicians frequently encounter gaps in their knowledge while delivering routine care to their patient. In a typical 4-hour clinic session, the busy generalist physician generates over 15 unanswered questions whose answers would have a direct bearing on patient management. Three to four of these questions address significant issues in the diagnostic or therapeutic decisions for these patients. Still, only 20% of these significant questions are ever answered. Physicians continue to practice in the face of missing information, basing decisions on experience and tradition and not on data or evidence.

Yet, many of these clinical questions can be answered, with information contained in the geometrically expanding medical knowledge base. A question that is well stated has a greater likelihood of being well answered. The EBM working group has explicitly stratified clinical questions into eight categories and proposes that a well-formulated question will fit into one of these categories. Understanding the category and structural component of well-formulated questions has been shown to lead to a more efficient strategy in finding the best clinical evidence to answer these questions (Table 43.2).

LOCATING EVIDENCE

In studies of physicians' information needs, physicians usually found the answer to their clinical questions by asking a colleague. Medical journals and textbooks were infrequently used because, for example: "My journals are disorganized," or "I can't get to the library," or "My textbooks are out of date." But information technology has the potential to dramatically alleviate this access-to-evidence problem. Using computers—and more so the internet—to access electronic information sources such as MED-

TABLE 43.2.	TYPES AND STRUCTURES OF WELL-FORMULATED QUESTIONS

Questions About

Identifying and interpreting a clinical finding
Identifying causes of disease
Formulating a differential diagnosis
Selecting and interpreting a diagnostic test
Estimating a prognosis
Selecting a treatment
Screening and preventing a disease
Professional improvement

Elements of Questions

Patient or clinical problem
   what kind of patient or problem?
Questioned intervention
   which test, treatment, exposure?
Comparison intervention
   compared with what test, treatment, or exposure?
Outcome
   what endpoint?

(From Sachett DL, et al. *Evidence-based medicine: how to practice and teach EMB.* New York: Churchill Livingstone, 1997, with permission.)

TABLE 43.3.	EVIDENCE-BASED SEARCHING

Strategies

Explode MeSH terms
Include epidemiologic MeSH terms
Use MeSH subheadings
Use "publication type" field

Example Search

"Should a patient with atrial fibrillation and no other medical problems be treated with warfarin or aspirin to prevent thromboembolic events?"

1. exp Anticoagulants/tu
2. Atrial Fibrillation/dt
3. 1 AND 2
4. exp Research OR exp Clinical Trials
5. 3 AND 4
6. Clinical Trial.pt OR Multi-center Study.pt OR Meta-analysis.pt
7. 3 AND 6
8. 5 OR 7

LINE is a fundamental component of the EBM paradigm. Physicians must develop skills in using computers to access and search the internet (a virtual worldwide CD-ROM), specialized databases, full-text periodicals and textbooks, and other meta-evidence sources such as the Cochrane Collaboration (*www.cochrane.co.uk*) and the Agency for Health Care Policy Research's (*www.ahcpr.gov*) National Clinical Guideline Clearing House (*www.guideline.gov*).

Posing well-designed knowledge gap questions to the search engine interfaces surrounding these knowledge sources is a clinical skill that must be learned and practiced, just as any other skill that is required in clinical care. The EBM working group has established the usefulness of including various evidence-based search terms and strategies in queries of the MEDLINE database (Table 43.3). The value of these strategies in searching other knowledge sources has yet to be established.

CRITICAL APPRAISAL AND APPLICATION OF MEDICAL EVIDENCE

How do we manage the overwhelming quantity of biomedical information? When we are perusing the barrage of periodicals delivered to our doorstep weekly or when we are reviewing the results of one of our electronic searches, how do we efficiently identify the information sources that are most likely to contain valid evidence? How can we "separate the wheat from the chaff?" Pioneers in EBM at McMaster University have established an evolving set of guidelines to help with this problem. By separating sources of clinical information in the biomedical literature into several distinct categories, useful screening questions or "fil-

ters" can be applied. These filters are designed to screen for systematic biases in the methodology used to collect the study data that may adversely affect the validity of the evidence and any reported conclusions. These filters or screening questions are listed in Table 43.4.

To facilitate the understanding and application of scientific evidence, EBM proposes that some aspect of this evidence be

TABLE 43.4.	CRITICAL APPRAISAL OF EVIDENCE FOR VALIDITY AND USEFULNESS: GUIDING QUESTIONS

About a Therapy

" Was the assignment of patients to treatments randomized?"
"Were all of the patients who enterd the trial properly accounted for and attributed at its conclusion?"

About a Diagnostic Test

"Was there an independent, blind comparison with a reference standard?"
"Did the patient sample include an appropriate spectrum of the types of patients to whom the diagnostic test will be applied in clinical practice?"

About a Harmful Exposure

"Were there clearly defined comparison groups that were similar with respect to important determinants of outcome (other than the outcome of interest)?"
"Were outcomes and exposures measured in the same manner in the groups being compared?"

About a Prognosis

"Was there a representative patient sample at a well-defined point in the course of the disease?"
"Was follow-up sufficiently long and complete?"

(From Sachett DL, et al. *Evidence-based medicine: how to practice and teach EBM.* New York: Churchill Livingstone, 1997, with permission.)

TABLE 43.5.	RESULTS, EXAMPLES OF PREFERRED FORMATS

Therapy

Relative risk and confidence intervals (RR, 95% CI)
Relative risk reduction (RRR)
Absolute risk reduction (ARR)
Number needed to treat (NNT)
Number needed to harm (NNH)

Diagnostic Test

Likelihood ratios (LR +, LR −)
Receiver–operator curve (ROC)

reported in standardized formats (Table 43.5). It is suggested that these formats offer the physician and patient a more intuitive and useful description of the meaning and potential impact of clinical information. Specifically, all evaluations of a treatment or other intervention may be reported as the relative risk (RR) along with a 95% confidence interval (95% CI) for the true estimation of the RR. In addition, a description of the absolute risk reduction (ARR) and the derived number needed to treat (NNT) are felt to be of particular importance and usefulness to those involved in clinical decision making. For studies establishing the role and reliability of a diagnostic test, it is suggested that the likelihood ratio (LR) be determined and reported. Similarly, for articles reporting a meta-analysis, a strength-of-effect chart may be included to see the individual effect of contributing studies in the meta-analysis. Several periodicals have already begun to adhere to these recommendations (Chapter 42).

Many factors influence whether valid evidence-based treatment and diagnostic procedures and other clinically important issues actually affect the practice behaviors of individual physicians or the way health care policy evolves. Many of these factors are political, financial, or psychologically grounded. Yet, there are important conceptual factors that all physicians should understand to appropriately interpret the generalizability of any medical evidence (Fig. 43.1). All clinical studies attempt to say something about someone; that is, there is an implied, or specified, reference population. Yet, no clinical study has access to all members of this reference population. The persons actually studied are different from the target population. Studies are conducted in specific places at specific times by specific people. Thus, there are filters that affect the nature of populations who actually participate in clinical studies. Some of these filters are introduced by the study design (e.g., exclusion of all diabetic patients), but other filters are beyond control (e.g., a study conducted at a large inner-city hospital in a poor Southern community with substantial ethnic and cultural diversity). These issues do not affect the validity of a study's result, but it is extremely important for physicians and patients to appreciate the effect that these filters have on the generalizability of any medical evidence (Fig. 43.1).

CRITICAL APPRAISAL OF OUR CLINICAL PRACTICE OUTCOMES

Physicians can no longer practice with the autonomy and minimal scrutiny of previous times. Our practice patterns, our use of resources, and the effectiveness of our interventions will be measured, compared with external standards and with our peers, and reported for all to see. EBM is being cited as the rationale for establishing standards of care, allocating limited resources, and even determining provider reimbursement. Standardized data sets (HEDIS) are used to compare the quality and cost of the care we deliver (Chapter 46). Individual and provider group report cards are becoming a fact of our professional lives. Physicians will be able to apply the tenets of EBM to these data and understand the validity and generalizability of this evidence describing their professional effectiveness. Physician behavior will change in response to this grading and reporting of our clinical activities. EBM provides a framework from which to approach the collection, analysis, and application of this important evidence. The nature of our medical care system and our physician role in this system depends on appropriate management of this information.

HOW CAN PHYSICIANS ASSIMILATE EVIDENCE-BASED MEDICINE INTO THEIR PROFESSIONAL PRACTICES AND VALUES?

Physicians must understand the proper use of clinical evidence to guide the health care delivery system through these dynamic times. EBM has been rapidly adopted by medical educators in the United States. Accrediting agencies expect that the basic tenets of EBM be included in the undergraduate and graduate medical curricula. Physicians in practice are frequently offered opportunities to attend EBM workshops at society meetings and CME (continuing medical education) courses. Many useful websites on the internet provide access to EBM resources and literature. An extremely useful textbook primer, *Teaching and Practic-*

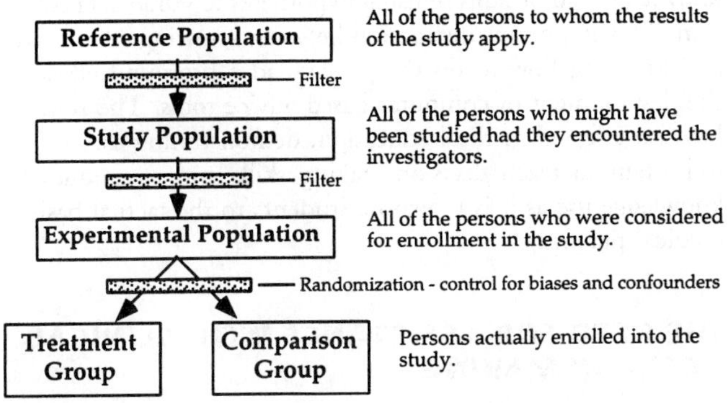

FIGURE 43.1. Generalizability and population filters. Factors that distinguish the reference population from the study and experimental populations act as filters and affect the generalizability and the applicability of a study's results. Factors affecting outcome that are not distributed equally in the experimental groups affect the validity of the study's results.

ing EBM is available. The *Journal of Evidence-Based Medicine* and the *American College of Physicians Journal Club* are two peer-reviewed journals that take an explicit EBM approach to publishing clinical information. It is of paramount importance that physicians understand how EBM is being used to establish definitions of quality, standards of care, and outcomes criteria. Physicians who participate in these decision-making processes assist in protecting the integrity and professionalism of America's medical care. Physicians must expect and demand that clinical decisions be based on the scientific evidence and then also weighed along with the qualitative concerns and values of individual patients, society, and ourselves, the protectors of society's health.

BIBLIOGRAPHY

Chassin MR, Galvin RW. The urgent need to improve health care quality: Institute of Medicine national roundtable discussion on health care quality. *JAMA* 1998;280(11):1000–1005.

Covell DG, Uman GC, Manning PR. Information needs in office practice: are they being met? *Ann Intern Med* 1985;103(4):596–599.

Sackett DL, Richardson WS, Rosenberg W, et al. *Evidence-based medicine: how to practice and teach EBM.* New York: Churchill-Livingstone, 1997.

Weinstein MW. Checking medicine's vital signs. *New York Times Magazine* April 19, 1998; 36–37.

Wennberg DE. Variation in the delivery of health care: the stakes are high. *Ann Intern Med* 1998;128(10):866–868.

Kelley's Textbook of Internal Medicine, fourth edition. Edited by H. David Humes. Lippincott Williams & Wilkins, Philadelphia © 2000.

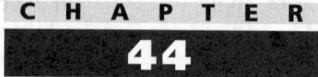

CHAPTER 44

COMPUTERS IN SUPPORT OF CLINICAL DECISION MAKING

EDWARD H. SHORTLIFFE

COMPUTER APPLICATIONS IN MEDICAL CARE

The expanding influence of computers and communications on society is being felt in medicine as well. Essentially all hospitals and clinics depend on computers for administrative and financial functions and for providing access to clinical data. Most physicians have been exposed to the powerful available systems for searching the biomedical literature by computer, either through local networks or from national resources accessed via the Internet. Modern imaging techniques depend on computers for image generation, analytical computers have become mandatory elements in the research laboratory, and information systems and simulation environments are becoming vital topics for medical education. The clinical community has long anticipated the day when computers would be able to assist routinely with diagnosis

and with making decisions about patient management. The pressure for such computer-based innovations is increasing in the era of managed care; both improved clinical productivity and decreased practice variability are often defined as explicit goals. Impressive prototypes and working systems now show that technology increasingly will provide physicians with effective decision-support tools. This chapter describes some of the issues in building such systems and in making them easily available, clinically useful, and broadly acceptable.

ISSUES IN PROVIDING COMPUTER-BASED DECISION SUPPORT

About 30 years ago, the first computer programs for medical diagnosis were shown to be often highly accurate in their diagnostic predictions. Why have such systems resisted widespread implementation and acceptance in the intervening years? The barriers reflect the subtleties and complexities of the medical practice environment and the increasing recognition that good advice from such programs cannot ensure their use and acceptance. Confounding the implementation efforts have been logistical constraints, the sometimes awkward mechanics of computer use, confusion about whether such programs are intended to be tools for clinicians rather than competitors with them, and a pervasive belief that computers do not really "understand" medicine and therefore cannot be expected to reach complex expert decisions. Early successes largely reflect an increased understanding of the importance of such issues and a gradual change in physician attitudes regarding computers and their potential for a beneficial clinical role.

UNDERSTANDING THE NATURE OF MEDICAL KNOWLEDGE

Efforts to construct effective medical decision-support tools are closely tied to research into the nature of medical knowledge and its use for problem solving. Psychological studies have taught us that medical expertise involves the application both of factual knowledge and of skills in using hypotheses to guide data collection. This important distinction between knowing what is true and knowing how to do things has had a profound effect on the development of computer-based advice tools. The research has also affected medical education, demonstrating that it is as important to teach decision-making skills and techniques for knowledge use as it is to expose students to the factual basis of medical practice.

THE NEED FOR ASSISTANCE WITH CLINICAL DECISION MAKING

Knowing how to find the information needed for clinical decision making is as important as trying to memorize it. Innovations such as MEDLINE and its Internet-based implementations such as the National Library of Medicine's PubMed (*http:// www.ncbi.nlm.nih.gov /PubMed /*), are a tribute to the way in which computers can be used to help physicians and others find the information that they need to make good decisions. Computers have superb memories, but until recently they could do little with pieces of text information other than display them. Modern decision-support programs contain detailed clinical information and contain the knowledge to help users determine how that information should be applied. Because computer-based tools offer this kind of expertise, physicians have begun to consult programs to understand clinical guidelines, as well as to obtain reasoned advice about diagnosis and management of specific cases. The ultimate decision-making roles are maintained for provider and patient, but the computer is allowing their decisions to be better informed.

OBSTACLES TO THE EFFECTIVE INTRODUCTION OF DECISION-SUPPORT SYSTEMS

Experience in applying computers in medicine over two decades has shown that logistical issues are the principal causes of system failures, especially for decision-support systems that rely on physician interaction for optimal use. Any medical computing system will fail to be accepted if it is unduly time consuming or if the cost (in time or money) is not clearly justified by the benefit gained. There is also an issue of inertia—the disinclination of busy people to use a computer if it requires an interruption in their normal routine. This implies the need for an integrated model in which computers are used routinely for data-management tasks, perhaps in lieu of traditional pen and paper data-recording techniques, and from which the physician obtains advice or access to guidelines as a by-product of this ongoing interaction. Decision-support tools will thus be more feasible as improved medical record and information systems appear in health systems, hospitals, and offices, supporting the integration of guidelines and reminders into the data-management environment.

Equally important is the design of decision-making tools that are sensitive to the traditional independence and skill of physicians. There is a need for system transparency (an ability for the program to provide explanations of its recommendations, perhaps with supporting links to the original literature sources) and for tactful presentation of advice. Such features make it clear that the unique skills of trained physicians are respected and that the system should be viewed as a knowledge-management tool rather than as the decision maker itself.

Medical informatics researchers have long sought to design interactive techniques that avoid clumsiness, typing, or the need for prolonged training of the intended users. Programs have tended to use a pointing device, such as a light pen or a mouse, as the means for manual selection of items and navigation through a program's features. Options for physician–computer interaction have been greatly expanded by the introduction of hand-held mobile computers, controlled by the use of a pen or stylus and capable of communicating with other computers through wireless networks. Considering the clinical settings in which physicians work, moving from room to room or bed to bed, mobile computing is especially attractive and increasingly affordable.

BRINGING CLINICAL INFORMATION TO THE POINT OF CARE

The introduction of the World Wide Web, the most pervasive application on the evolving Internet (Fig. 44.1), has made it reasonable to expect that physicians will soon use portable devices and wireless communications to access clinically pertinent information and to garner advice from remarkably diverse and distant resources. It is already possible to find a large amount of medical information by searching the Web for topics of interest, although problems with navigation and quality control persist. A wide variety of resources are available, such as MEDLINE search engines, custom-tailored sites for physicians and patients, and libraries of specialized materials such as the compendium of clinical practice guidelines jointly developed by the American Medical Association and the Agency for Healthcare Research and Quality (Fig. 44.2). We will soon see hand-held machines, controlled by the use of a pen and sufficiently portable to be carried like a clipboard, which will provide wireless access to all the information on the Web from the patient's bedside or the clinic examining room.

The use of such network-based information resources will be enhanced if the network serves a wide variety of clinical needs. For this reason, medical computing experts are seeking to ensure that the evolving national network is built with the needs of the health care system in mind. A range of facilities can be provided to practitioners and to patients who seek access to the health care system or to information on disease prevention and health promotion (Fig. 44.3). Serious questions exist regarding management of such a complex range of information resources, including quality control, protection of confidential information, and effective means for finding the best information available for a specific clinical problem. Patients and healthy persons are gaining easy access to many of these resources as well, empowering them in new ways and assisting those who wish to be more actively involved in decision making regarding their own care. At the same time, however, they may be exposed to information of poor quality and without scientific validity, which introduces new responsibilities to physicians as they discuss options and recommendations with patients.

STATUS OF COMPUTERS FOR CLINICAL DECISION SUPPORT

A clinical decision support system is generally viewed as providing patient-specific advice rather than generic information such as that provided by MEDLINE or displayed in text for a clinical practice guideline. Many programs have been developed to address such clinical problems. Since the 1950s, researchers have recognized the relevance of Bayes' rule (Chapter 42) to the task of diagnosis, with computers being used to manipulate the pertinent conditional probabilities. Many bayesian programs are highly accurate in selecting among competing explanations of a patient's disease state. The results of such analyses are probabilities, and their defense is based on Bayes' formula plus the accuracy of the sensitivity, specificity, and prevalence data used. The mathematical orientation of such programs has not always appealed to

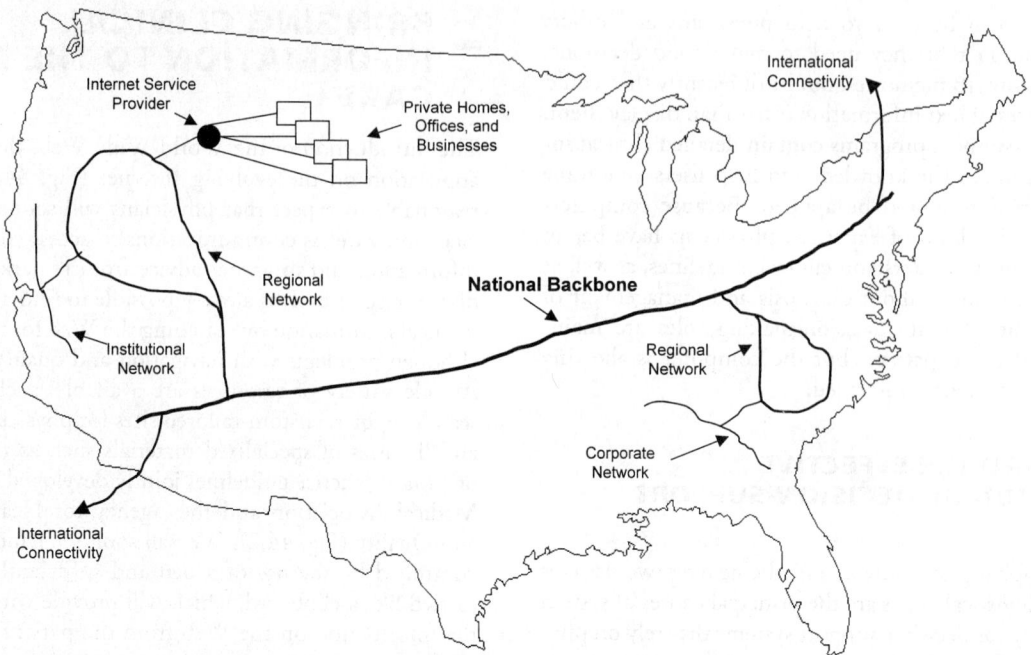

FIGURE 44.1. The Internet allows individual computers in homes and offices to be connected to local Internet Service Providers (ISPs), which are connected in turn to regional networks. High-speed "backbones" connect the regional networks, and international links have made the Internet a global phenomenon. A clinician at a hospital connected to a West Coast regional network can access information from a federal health agency in Washington. The World Wide Web and electronic mail are among the most widely used applications of the Internet, which is the infrastructure on which both are built.

physicians who are used to discussing a more concept-oriented line of reasoning with their consultants.

Many clinical questions deal more with what actions to take in managing a patient than they do with determining the proper disease classification. Researchers have accordingly developed computer-based tools that draw on the methods of decision analysis. One class of programs permits the specification of decision trees, along with associated probabilities and utilities, and then calculates expected utilities and performs sensitivity analyses. A second class has used prespecified decision-analytic models to advise physicians who are not trained in decision analysis; such programs' usefulness is limited to cases that correspond closely to the decision tree provided.

Since the early 1970s, researchers have been applying the techniques of artificial intelligence (AI) to the development of diagnostic and therapy-management consultation programs. AI is the field of computer science that deals with the symbolic (rather than numeric) representation of knowledge and its use in problem solving. The field is closely tied to psychology and to the modeling of logical processes by computer. Of particular relevance is the subfield of AI research known as expert systems. An expert system is a program that uses knowledge derived from experts in a field to provide the kind of problem analysis and advice that the expert may provide.

■ RESEARCH DIRECTIONS

Several barriers continue to limit the effective implementation of decision-support tools in clinical settings. However, rapid technologic progress, especially in the development of powerful but inexpensive single-user computers that provide intuitively pleasing interactive environments, has allowed the introduction of the first commercially available diagnostic programs for physicians. The next major step forward will occur when such programs can be smoothly integrated with the patient's medical record, allowing advice to be generated as a by-product of routine clinical data management.

REPRESENTING MEDICAL KNOWLEDGE

An ongoing research challenge is the need to refine methods for encoding the knowledge used by medical experts. Although powerful techniques exist (e.g., many systems use frames, rules, or belief networks to express relations among medical concepts), several complex challenges remain. For example, physicians use mental models of the three-dimensional associations among body parts and organs when they are interpreting data or planning therapy. Representing such anatomical knowledge and performing spatial reasoning by computer have proved particularly challenging. Similarly, human beings have a remarkable ability to interpret changes in data over time, assessing temporal trends and developing models of disease progression or the response of disease to past therapies. Temporal representation schemes and methods for inferring abstract summaries of temporal trends remain major areas of ongoing research in medical informatics and in computer science in general.

Another kind of expertise is the human skill inherent in knowing how to use what one knows. In medicine, the skill is called *good clinical judgment* to properly differentiate it from the memorization of factual knowledge or of data from the literature. Giving computers factual knowledge does not make them expert unless they also are skilled in the proper application of that

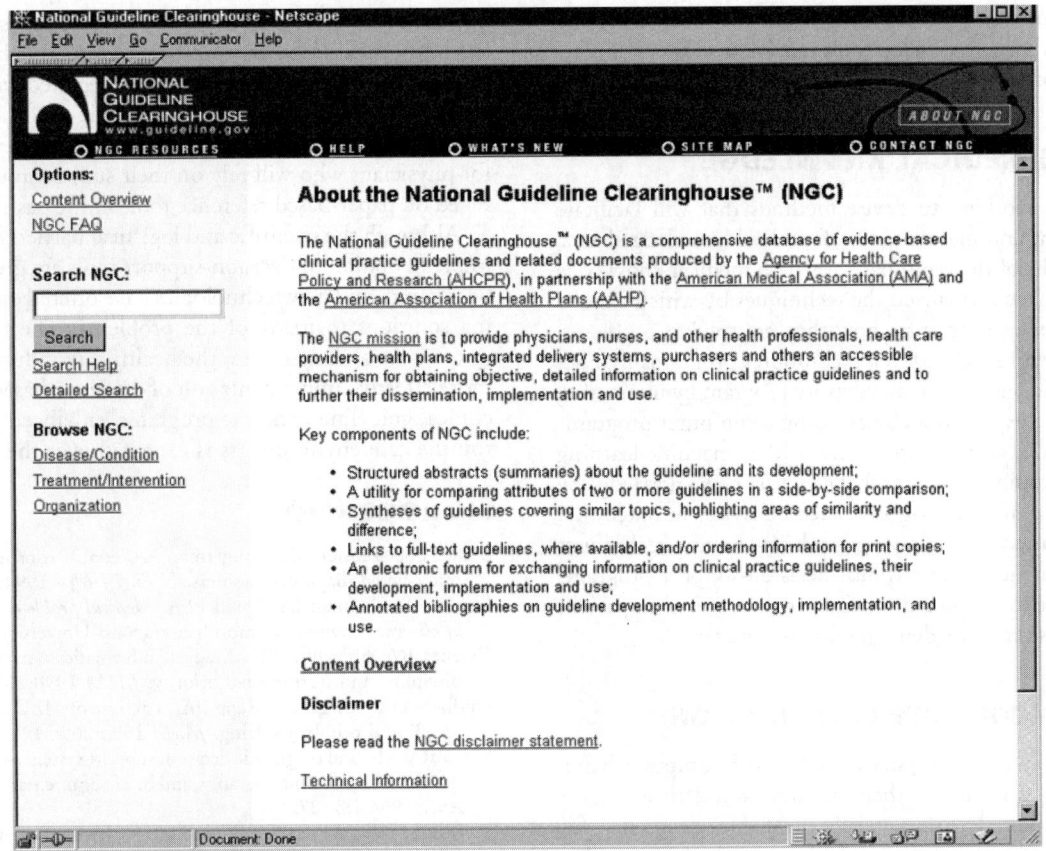

FIGURE 44.2. The Agency for Healthcare Research and Quality, working in collaboration with the American Medical Association, has created a central Internet resource for individuals who wish to find clinical guidelines that have been created and reviewed by authoritative government, academic, or professional groups. Users can search the Web site *http://www.guideline.gov* for guidelines that may be available on any clinical topic.

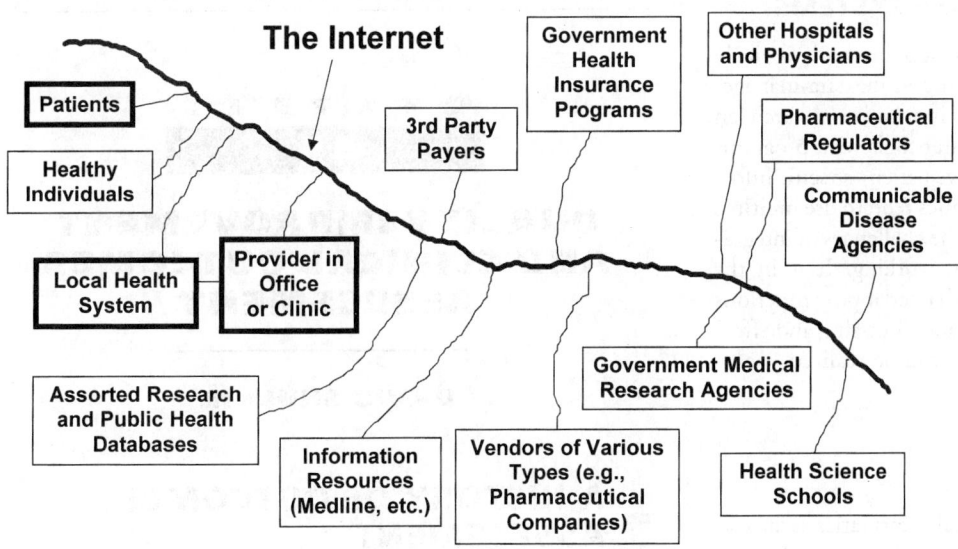

FIGURE 44.3. The evolving national network is increasingly linking persons and computers from a variety of settings that are pertinent to the delivery of health care. Citizens can find health information on the network, and patients are beginning to communicate with their personal physicians by computer and are exploring on-line educational materials regarding their illnesses. Similarly, a wide range of information and communication resources is available to practitioners.

knowledge. Improved understanding of human problem solving is helping researchers to develop tools that more closely simulate the reasoning of expert clinicians.

ACQUIRING MEDICAL KNOWLEDGE

Researchers are working to devise methods that will facilitate the development and maintenance of medical knowledge bases, especially in light of the rapid pace at which medical knowledge evolves. Some have formalized the techniques by which experts should be interviewed to infer how they are solving problems. Efforts have been made to develop computer programs that acquire the knowledge base for an advisory program by interacting directly with the expert, thereby avoiding a computer programmer as intermediary. In addition, the field of machine learning focuses on developing programs that can infer new knowledge by analyzing data from observing associated behaviors or outcomes. There is great interest in applying machine-learning techniques to the development of more robust decision-support programs that are sensitive to regional or institutional variations in patient populations, case mix, or demographic parameters.

PHYSICIAN–COMPUTER INTERACTION

It is often claimed that physicians will resist computer-based tools until they can talk to them as they would to a human consultant. Although commercially available programs for speech understanding by computer are beginning to permit reliable free-form spoken interaction, the resulting dictated material is free text and therefore may be difficult for the computer to interpret and apply properly in a decision-support context. Innovative graphic environments and tools for selecting from menus have demonstrated that computer novices can rapidly learn to use software tools for structured data entry, making the need for speech understanding less of an issue.

INTEGRATION WITH DATABASE SYSTEMS

The successful introduction of decision-support tools is likely to be tied to their effective integration with routine data-management tasks. This suggests the need for innovative research on how best to tie knowledge-based computer tools with programs designed to store, manipulate, and retrieve patient-specific information. Now that health systems and clinics tend to use multiple machines, optimized for different tasks, the challenges of integration are inherently tied to issues of networking. It is in the smooth linkage of multiple machines with overlapping functions that distributed but integrated clinical data processing and effective decision support for busy clinicians will be realized.

■ CONCLUSIONS

With the increasing acceptance of medical informatics as an academic discipline and the training of persons who can work effectively at the interface between medicine and computer science, it is likely that physicians and other health professionals will increas-

ingly be offered clinically useful tools that are sensitive to the realities of the health care environment. Among such systems will be decision-support programs that are integrated with patient data-management systems such as electronic medical records. Such programs will serve as knowledge-access and management tools for physicians who will rely on their support much as they have relied on paper-based reference tools in the past.

Although the scientific and logistical barriers to the successful implementation of decision-support tools are great, progress has been rapid, and new technologies have offered especially promising solutions to many of the problems. The first commercial systems are already in use, the health care industry is calling for more effective implementation of evidence-based advice such as clinical guidelines, and the programs' enhanced integration into routine care environments is expected over the next decade.

BIBLIOGRAPHY

Berner ES, Webster GD, Shugerman AA, et al. Performance of four computer-based diagnostic systems. *N Engl J Med* 1994;330:1792–1796.

Elstein AS, Shulman LS, Sprafka SA. *Medical problem solving: an analysis of clinical reasoning.* Cambridge: Harvard University Press, 1978.

Greenes RA, Shortliffe EH. Medical informatics: an emerging academic discipline and institutional priority. *JAMA* 1990;263:1114–1120.

Lindberg DAB, Siegel ER, Rapp BA, et al. Use of MEDLINE by physicians for clinical problem solving. *JAMA* 1993;269:3124–3129.

Miller RA. Medical diagnostic decision support systems—past, present, and future: a threaded bibliography and brief commentary. *J Am Med Inform Assoc* 1994;1:8–27.

McKinney WP, Barnas GP, Golub RM. The medical applications of the Internet: informational resources for research, education, and patient care. *J Gen Intern Med* 1994;9:627–634.

Shortliffe E. Health care and the Next Generation Internet. *Ann Intern Med* 1998;129:138–140.

Shortliffe EH, Perreault LE, Wiederhold G, Fagan LM, eds. *Medical informatics: computer applications in health care and biomedicine.* New York: Springer-Verlag, 2000.

Sox HC, Blatt MA, Higgins MC, Marton KI. *Medical decision making.* London: Butterworth, 1988.

Kelley's Textbook of Internal Medicine, fourth edition. Edited by H. David Humes. Lippincott Williams & Wilkins, Philadelphia © 2000.

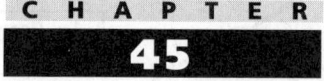

C H A P T E R

45

QUALITY IMPROVEMENT AND CLINICAL OUTCOMES ASSESSMENT

DAVID SHULKIN

■ A HISTORY OF OUTCOMES ASSESSMENT

Although the scrutiny of health outcomes has intensified in recent years, assessing quality of care has a long history in health care. At the turn of the century, Codman, a prominent Boston surgeon, first proposed that physicians evaluate the quality of surgical care by looking at the outcomes of the postoperative patient. In the ensuing decades, state licensure agencies began to inspect for quality of care (1920s). In the 1930s, the Joint Commission of Accreditation of Hospitals (JCAH) was established to evaluate the quality of hospitals, and the federal government initiated its own program for evaluating quality with peer-review standards organizations in the 1950s.

The 1970s witnessed the birth of health services research, and data demonstrated wide variation across small geographic areas for the rates of several common surgical procedures. This finding of wide variations in the use of health care resources prompted questions about the necessity of services being delivered and a corresponding call by payers and policy makers for the development of appropriate standards of care. At the same time came the widespread recognition that medical costs were spiraling out of control. The American business community's response to this cost crisis was the initiation of inspection programs, such as precertification, second-opinion requirements, and intensive use review.

The failure of these efforts to control costs in a fee for service reimbursement model was in part responsible for the rapid dissemination of a managed care approach in the 1980s and 1990s. Increasingly, managed care organizations are tying quality measures to reimbursement, and providers who demonstrate high quality, receive higher levels of compensation than other providers do. Managed care organizations have also been active in disseminating data on quality by issuing "report cards" and other public outcome reports (Chapter 46). This use of quality indicator data has heightened the awareness of the provider community for the need to assess their outcomes in the clinical setting. More recently, the availability of outcomes data through public sources such as the Internet has created a new interest and accessibility for health care data.

Despite the long history of quality improvement in health care, the field has experienced profound transformation in the last decade. The Agency for Health Care Policy and Research (AHCPR), a component of the US Public Health Service, was created to improve the quality, appropriateness, and effectiveness of health care. The agency supports health services research that focuses on understanding the effectiveness of care and the development of clinical practice guidelines. With this resource, the federal government has joined with other agencies, such as the Joint Commission of Accreditation of Healthcare Organizations (JCAHO), the National Committee for Quality Assurance (NCQA), the American Medical Association (AMA), and other organizations to promote use of outcomes data to improve the quality of health care.

APPROACHES TO IMPROVING QUALITY

Historical approaches to quality control in medicine have relied on retrospective case reviews to identify and sanction poor performers. Hospitals were evaluated by looking at structural standards to determine whether they were organized in a way that

was capable of inspecting for quality. These methods focused on the individual provider rather than the health care system in which the practitioners work. Health care providers, payers, and others involved in improving health care quality recognized that these traditional methods of evaluating quality, known as "quality assurance," had become outdated, and they began to seek ways to shift the focus of their quality evaluation programs.

American industry recently discovered the power of continuous quality improvement, a technique originally introduced decades earlier by the American scientist W. Edwards Deming and others, such as Walter A. Shewhart and Joseph M. Juran. Deming believed that only 15% of quality improvement advances could be realized by focusing on an individual's performance and that 85% of quality opportunities could be found in systemic factors. Other quality pioneers soon began to apply and refine these concepts to the field of medicine. In place of chart reviews, continuous quality improvement brings the analysis of trended data that seeks to identify common features or systems among management issues in the patient care delivery process.

A core concept of continuous quality improvement is that the process of delivering patient care should be explicitly designed. In addition to the design component, a continuous quality improvement approach includes an assessment phase in which data are collected to determine how it is being delivered; an analysis phase in which data are interpreted and fed back to clinicians; an intervention phase, in which new ways of delivering care may be initiated; and a reassessment phase, in which the outcome of these interventions are evaluated (Fig. 45.1).

One of the basic tenets of continuous quality improvement is the recognition that outcomes are the result of many factors, such as people, training and supervision, equipment, and the environment in which care is delivered. A multidisciplinary problem-solving approach should be readily evident in the techniques of quality improvement by involving all those who participate in the clinical process, particularly persons who are closest to the work. This means that physicians, nurses, physical therapists, social workers, and unit secretaries often join together to

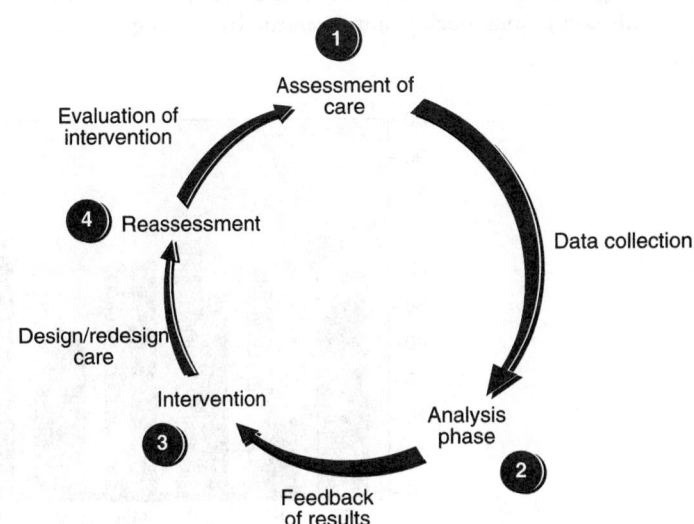

FIGURE 45.1. Approach to continuous quality improvement.

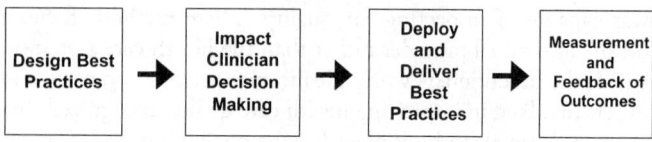

FIGURE 45.2. The model for health care improvement.

understand a problem and identify solutions for improving quality. Improvements often are accomplished by enhanced training, technical advancement, or process changes that can occur through a series of small incremental changes rather than large shifts in practice.

Although the tenets of continuous quality improvement have been embraced in health care for nearly a decade, significant defects in quality still remain. Large deviations for best practice approaches to care are widely documented. Widely publicized cases of drug dosing errors or wrong site amputations are still frequently reported. More advanced work in quality improvement focuses as much on the implementation of new systems for care as on the design of the process. A comprehensive model for health care improvement must include the design of a best practice, changing physician (and other clinicians) decision-making deployment of the best practices, and measurement and feedback of the outcomes (Fig. 45.2).

If any of the latter four steps is not completed, the maximum potential for improvement in quality will probably not be achieved. Further improvement in quality will result from system changes that will reduce clinician reliance on memory and error-proofing processes through standardization and protocol implementation.

OUTCOMES MEASUREMENT AND MANAGEMENT

Quality of care can be most simply defined as doing the right thing for a patient at the right time and with the best outcome. Using this definition, outcomes management is closely aligned with continuous quality improvement by striving to identify

ways to change practice behaviors by correlating variations in patient outcomes with differences in treatment strategies. Outcomes measurements document the impact of a medical intervention on the patient. Traditional outcomes measurements have included mortality, morbidity, and complications of care. For some diagnoses, particularly those involving treatment of high-risk or complex conditions, these measures are adequate in detailing differences in outcomes among groups of patients. However, for most patients, additional and more sensitive measures are needed to document the outcomes of their care. These outcomes measurements may include return to work, the cost of care, patient satisfaction, patient preferences, the functional status before and after treatment for a particular condition, and a measure of appropriateness of care (Fig. 45.3).

TOOLS OF QUALITY ASSESSMENT

Quality improvement tools can help standardize medical treatment and reduce variation, but they are not intended to reduce diagnostic and scientific scrutiny and the clinical reasoning process that is essential to the practice of medicine. The best known of the quality improvement tools is the practice guideline, which documents a standard approach to a clinical problem or use of a technology. Practice guidelines may be developed on the basis of existing scientific evidence or by consensus opinion. Groups within a local clinical setting often develop these guidelines, but they are increasingly being published by professional societies and agencies such as the AHCPR.

Critical pathways are another tool useful in improving quality. Critical pathways detail a clinical plan of care from the start of the clinical intervention, such as admission to the hospital, to a clinical end point, such as discharge from the hospital. The pathway outlines the role of each of the involved health care professionals and provides an overview of the specific aspects of care delivered, such as laboratory tests, pharmaceutical services, and wound care, and the activity level of the patient. These improvement processes aimed at best practice implementation are now being expanded to outpatient areas and systematically

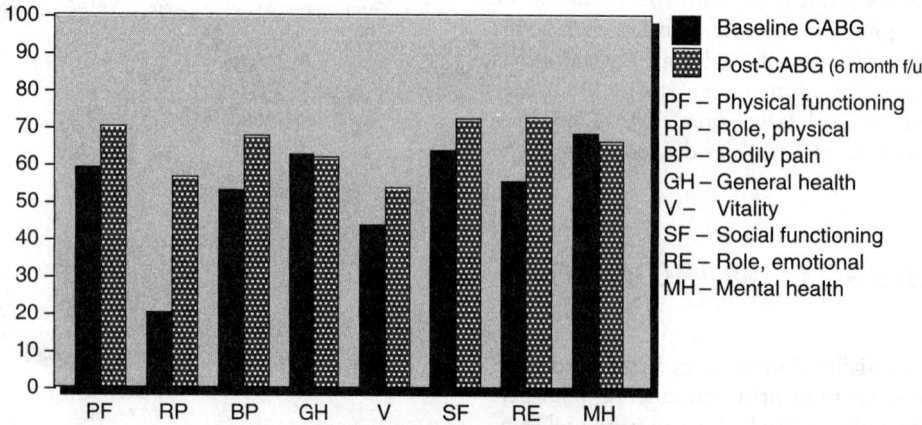

FIGURE 45.3. Functional status measurement before and after a coronary artery bypass graft (CABG).

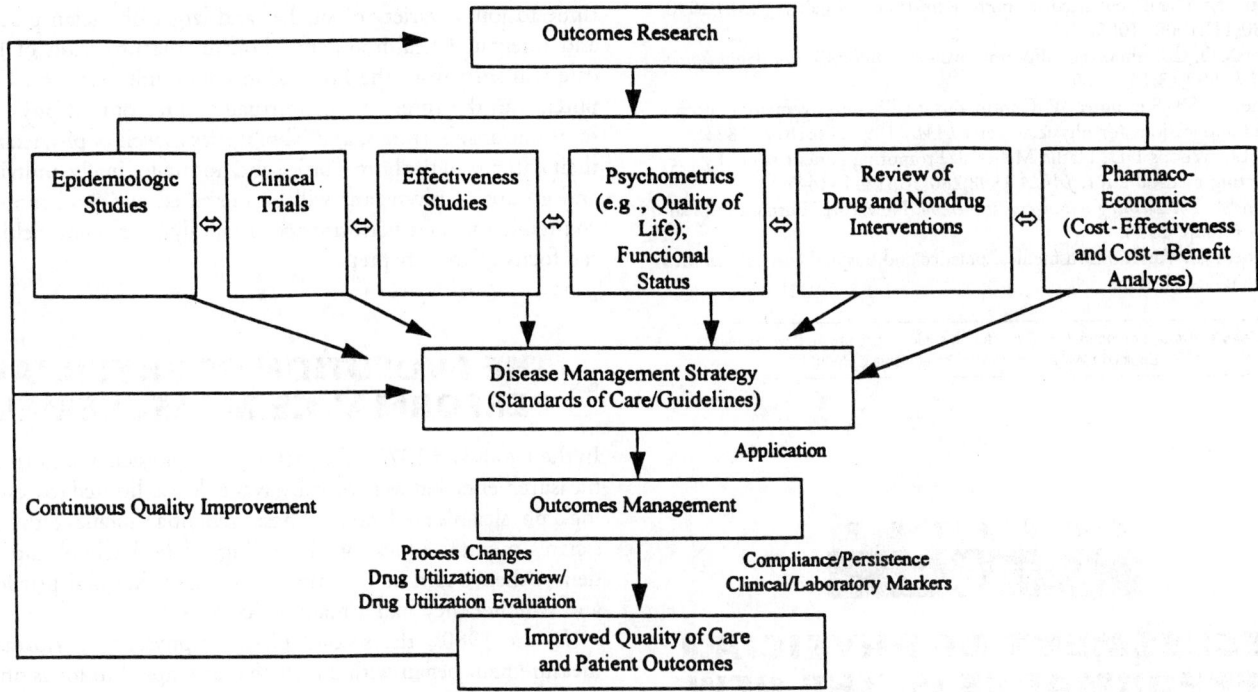

FIGURE 45.4. The science of disease management.

applied over the entire continuum of care—a field now known as *disease management.*

As in clinical trials, studies of patient outcomes must identify confounding factors to appropriately adjust data to allow for a meaningful interpretation. One of the most important of these factors is the severity of the patient's illness. Several commercial severity-of-illness systems are available to clinicians to adjust outcomes. These systems involve abstraction of clinical details from the patients' records and entry of the data into a database that computes expected outcomes that can be compared with the actual outcomes. Many regulatory agencies have begun to mandate use of these severity-of-illness systems for patients treated in hospitals within their jurisdiction.

FUTURE DIRECTIONS IN CLINICAL MANAGEMENT, QUALITY MANAGEMENT, RESOURCE MANAGEMENT, AND DISEASE MANAGEMENT

The burgeoning field of clinical management strategies, although still in their infancy, are likely to take on an even greater importance in health care as we strive for a system that provides appropriate, effective, and cost-efficient care. Future issues in outcomes management include the refinement of comparative databases for clinicians to compare outcomes with one another. Advances in clinical information system technology and electronic medical records will help populate databases to help clinicians understand and improve clinical care delivery. New databases will include details of how care is provided (i.e., process

elements), so the differences in outcomes can be recognized and analyzed. Disease management programs will continue to translate evidence-based findings (Chapter 43) through outcomes research into improvements in the clinical setting (Fig. 45.4).

The concepts of quality improvement and outcomes assessment have begun to be integrated into medical education. Students are increasingly being exposed to these concepts before their introduction to clinical medicine, with reinforcement of these principles after they enter the patient care setting. With the rapid development of integrated delivery systems, implementation of best practice care within an organized model system has provided new opportunities for enhancing quality improvement. New work in health and disease management will coordinate resources of health systems with those of patients, payers, vendors, and other providers to enhance clinical outcomes. These efforts will integrate clinical guidelines, physician and patient education, health risk assessments, care management, and preventive and wellness activities. Most quality improvement efforts have focused on inpatient care or procedures, but quality assessment work will continue to move into the ambulatory setting as more emphasis is being placed on care outside of the hospital. Outcome measurements must gauge the full scope of care with a longitudinal approach that spans inpatient and outpatient care. The continued evolution of quality management will bring about better and more comprehensive measures of care and service that patients face across the entire continuum of care.

BIBLIOGRAPHY

Bowen OR. Shattuck lecture: what is quality care? *N Engl J Med* 1987; 316:1578–1580.

Chassin MR, Galvin RW, and the National Roundtable on Healthcare

Quality. The urgent need to improve health care quality. *JAMA* 1998; 280(11):1000–1005.

Decker MD. Continuous quality improvement. *Infect Control Hosp Epidemiol* 1992;13:165–169.

Kritchevsky SB, Simmons BP. Continuous quality improvement: concepts and applications for physician care. *JAMA* 1991;266:1817–1823.

Leape LL, Woods DD, Hatlie MJ, et al. Promoting patient safety by preventing medical error. *JAMA* 1998;280(16):1444–1447.

Walton M. *The Deming management method.* New York: Putnam Publishing Group, 1986.

Wennberg JE. Variations in medical practice and hospital costs. *Conn Med* 1985;49:444–453.

Kelley's Textbook of Internal Medicine, fourth edition. Edited by H. David Humes.
Lippincott Williams & Wilkins, Philadelphia © 2000.

C H A P T E R

46

ASSESSMENT OF PHYSICIAN PERFORMANCE IN THE NEW CENTURY HEALTH CARE ENVIRONMENT

ROBERTA PARILLO
MARK RIVO
LAURENCE B. GARDNER

Health care delivery and medical practice may be expected to look fundamentally different in the twenty-first century. In his latest book, *The Bleeding Edge: The Business of Health Care in the Next Century,* J.D. Kleinke notes that significant and unprecedented economic pressures on health care providers have compelled health care to change from a cottage industry to a full-scale industrial organization. Several key trends may be expected to shape this new health care marketplace. First, continuing cost-control pressures will likely ensure that capitation (a global payment per individual for a broad range of health services) forever replaces traditional fee-for-individual-service as the dominant form of payment. Purchasers of health care, whether they are individuals, businesses, or the government, will function more as educated, empowered consumers able to assess the value they receive and not merely its cost. Second, integrated health care systems (collaboration of physicians, hospitals and other providers and facilities) competing for these capitated payments will need to provide high-quality, accessible, and affordable care to the covered population of persons along with high user satisfaction. Health care systems that are successful will have collaborative providers, comprehensive information systems, efficient delivery mechanisms and will continuously measure and improve the quality of care and service delivered.

The practice of medicine necessarily will evolve in this new health care marketplace. Third, private, solo physicians will continue to join a variety of smaller and larger physician practices and integrated health systems. Fourth, the provision of most care will shift from the hospital to community settings. Computers and the Internet will "virtually" interconnect physicians to physicians, hospitals, and laboratories as well as physicians to their patients in the home, office and hospital. Finally, individual and groups of physicians will be measured and held more accountable for their performance, a rapidly developing field and the focus of this chapter.

THE EVOLUTION OF PHYSICIAN PERFORMANCE MEASUREMENT

In the 1960s and 1970s, the first phase of physician performance measurements that were broadly available was limited to examining a physician's credentials. These credentials included the physician's medical education, including medical school and residency, their board certification status, their hospital privileges, and whether they had a malpractice history.

In the 1980s, the second phase of physician performance measurement began with efforts that attempted to focus on the outcome of care and to compare physicians against each other (*profiling*) for certain measures. After Medicare's prospective payment system (diagnosis-related groups [DRGs]) put hospitals at financial risk for seniors being admitted, hospitals began to measure and compare physicians based on the length of stay for specific conditions. Quality assurance reviews were also established in which physicians were reviewed whether an individual patient died or suffered a complication that fell outside an established standard of care.

In the 1990s, group/staff model health maintenance organizations (HMOs), such as Kaiser Permanente, and IPA (independent practice association)/Network model HMOs, such as US Health Care, began to measure and compare among physicians their use of health services, the delivery of preventive services to a population of patients, and the satisfaction of their patients with the services delivered. Physician "report cards" were developed, shared with the physician, and used in deciding everything from financial bonuses to termination.

ASSESSING PHYSICIAN PERFORMANCE: THE BASICS

Assessing physician performance, often called *physician profiling,* depends on being able to identify a group of similarly trained physicians (e.g., internists, cardiologists, pulmonologists) who are taking care of a defined population of patients.

A broad spectrum of outcomes may be measured, which reflect the quality of care and service provided. In assessing performance, physicians are often measured against a goal or benchmark. An example of a goal may be that 90% of all adults over age 65 will be immunized against pneumococcus infection and influenza. In this instance, the goal is that all the physicians exceed 90% adult immunization.

The value of physician profiling depends on identifying measurable indicators for that outcome desired and obtaining accurate data easily and without significant cost. Some of the more common data sources used in physician profiling include claims information, office encounter data (e.g., ICD-9 and CPT-4 codes), laboratory results, pharmacy prescriptions, medical records, authorizations (e.g., approved referrals and hospitalizations), and surveys. Great care must be placed on developing a methodology for obtaining the data that is reliable, accurate, and affordable. The resultant data plotted out for each physician typically produces a distribution curve allowing measurement of the overall performance of the group of physicians as well as the variance among physicians using standard statistical methods. A complete discussion of the performance measurement process is beyond the scope of this chapter. Several useful resources are identified at the end of the chapter.

Physician profiling is a fundamental step in the continuous quality improvement (CQI) process that is essential in business today, but it is only recently being adopted by the health care system. The CQI process involves (a) identifying the desired outcome and a measurable indicator, (b) defining the practices or guidelines that must be followed to attain the desired outcome, (c) measuring and providing feedback to those involved, and (d) identifying new ways from the feedback received to attain the desired outcome (Table 46.1).

WHO WILL BE ASSESSING PHYSICIAN PERFORMANCE?

Physician performance measurement is still in its infancy. In September 1998, the National Coalition on Health Care released a report on various quality-of-care initiatives. The report, by Donald Berwick, MD, President of the Institute for Healthcare Quality, argues that case-by-case improvements have not yet brought what is needed to American health care: "a breakthrough example of system-level performance of unprecedented quality at affordable cost, such as the improvements Toyota and other Japanese manufacturers brought to American industry in the 1980s" (Weissenstein).

Yet, it seems certain that the physician performance measurement will become the norm and not the exception in the health care system of the twenty-first century. Today, many health plans and large physician groups have developed sophisticated physician performance measurement standards and systems. In addition, employer coalitions, and three well-known health care organizations are also measuring and reporting on outcomes as part of their mission and goals. These initiatives are briefly summarized in the following sections.

EMPLOYER COALITIONS

In heavily penetrated managed care markets such as California, the Indianapolis and St. Paul areas in the midwest, and Boston, employer coalitions have developed some of their own physician assessment instruments and reports. The Midwest Business Group on Health (MBGH) and the Pacific Business Group

TABLE 46.1.	EXAMPLES OF PHYSICIAN PERFORMANCE MEASURES

Quality of Preventive Services
- Adult immunization rates
- Mammography screening
- Cervical cancer screening
- Smoking cessation effectiveness

Quality of Clinical Care
- β-blocker use after myocardial infarction
- Angiotensin-converting enzyme (ACE)-inhibitor use for congestive heart failure
- hemoglobinA 1C monitoring of diabetics
- Appropriate use of antidepressants
- Rates of hypertensive patients with normal blood pressure
- Documentation of discussing/completing advance directives

Utilization of Care
- Referral rates to specialists
- Pharmacy use
- Emergency room admission rate
- Rates of diagnostic tests ordered
- Office procedure rates
- Hospital admission rates and length of stay

Quality of Physician Office
- Availability of handicapped parking and handicapped-accessible entrances
- Smoke alarms, fire extinguishers, and fire exits available and marked
- Narcotic drugs and prescription pads locked
- Handwashing facilities available and accesible
- General office, waiting, and examining room clean and orderly

Quality of Medical Record
- Legible and signed notes
- Completed problem and medication list
- Documentation of blood pressure and weight at each visit
- Documentation of report received from consultants
- Documentation of inquiry/counseling into smoking, substance abuse, weight

Accessibility of Care
- Is appointment available for physical exam within 30 days?
- Is appointment available within 24 hours for an urgent exam?
- Is there a manual/computerized appointment scheduling system?
- Are no more than 5 adults scheduled per hour?
- Is the office or answering service available at all times?
- Within how many minutes does the physician respond to an emergency call?

Satisfaction with Care
- Are the physician's office manager, receptionist, and nurse friendly and helpful?
- Did the physician adequately listen to the patient's problems?
- Did the physician adequately explain to the patient the diagnosis and treatment?
- Would you recommend this physician to a friend or family member?
- What are patient turnover rates?
- What are physician complaint rates?

on Health (PBGH) have developed measures, gather data, and regularly report their outcomes in all three areas of clinical status, functional status, and member/patient satisfaction. Members use this information to decide what health plan, what physician, and what facility they will select.

JOINT COMMISSION ON ACCREDITATION OF HEALTHCARE ORGANIZATIONS

Founded in 1951 as an independent not-for-profit organization, the Joint Commission on Accreditation of Healthcare Organizations (JCAHO) evaluates and accredits over 18,000 health care organizations and programs, including hospitals, integrated delivery networks, medical groups, and organizations, which provide home care, long-term care, behavioral health care, laboratory, and ambulatory care services.

JCAHO has taken steps to incorporate accountability into its accreditation process through a program called ORYX. Under ORYX, all types of health care organizations, starting with hospitals and other inpatient facilities and soon physician groups, are required to select a performance measurement system and track selected clinical indicators. The plan is to progressively increase the number of reported measures.

NATIONAL COMMITTEE FOR QUALITY ASSURANCE

The National Committee for Quality Assurance (NCQA) is a private not-for-profit organization dedicated to assessing and reporting on the quality of managed care plans. NCQA is governed by a board of directors that includes employers, consumer and labor representatives, health plans, quality experts, policy makers, and physicians.

NCQA began accrediting managed care organizations (MCOs) in 1991 in response to the need for standardized objective information about the quality of these organizations. NCQA has expanded the range of organizations that they accredit or certify to include managed behavioral health care organizations, credentials verification organizations, and physician organizations. Many large employers contract only with NCQA accredited health plans.

NCQA adopted and now manages the evolution of the principal performance measurement tool for managed care, the **H**ealth **P**lan **E**mployer **D**ata and **I**nformation **S**et (HEDIS). HEDIS development had input from large employer leaders and health plan leaders and has quickly became the standardized performance measurement system of choice among managed care plans, many of which report HEDIS data to employer clients. HEDIS 99 includes ten effectiveness-of-care measures that are specific for defined populations. Today, many consumers receive HEDIS data in the form of health plan "report cards" from their individual health plans or through published HEDIS reports in national magazines and local newspapers.

One of the biggest challenges for all accrediting bodies is to obtain standardized information that is comparable across all health plans. This includes specific physician information. NCQA Accreditation 99 requires plans to submit audited HEDIS performance results and evaluates those results against certain performance targets.

AMERICAN MEDICAL ASSOCIATION'S AMERICAN MEDICAL ACCREDITATION PROGRAM

Recently, the American Medical Association (AMA) launched a new program, American Medical Accreditation Program (AMAP). AMAP's accreditation process compares a physician's credentials and practice with written standards, with the intent that meeting or exceeding these standards signifies a physician's commitment to provide high-quality care and to make continual improvements. AMAP's second purpose is to provide a standardized and more efficient way for physicians to meet the requirements of the many organizations that require their credentials and review of their office practice and in the future to accomplish the same objective for the growing array of requirements for clinical measurement, feedback, and improvement.

In September 1998, JCAHO, NCQA, and AMAP formed a joint Performance Measurement Coordinating Council (PMCC). The PMCC convened in January 1999 and set a goal of developing a common measurement agenda to integrate measures development efforts in an attempt to streamline the initiatives, save money, and help speed up and improve the process of producing consistent, broadly applicable measures.

STATE AND FEDERAL GOVERNMENT

In 1998, Wisconsin became the first state to require physicians to turn over medical quality and financial data to a government agency—something 37 other states have required only hospitals to do. Physician performance, particularly as it relates to patient outcomes, is an area of scrutiny that is quickly moving to the forefront of determining health care quality and value.

Legislation was recently passed, authorizing the development of a national uniform data set. Such a uniform set of requirements for collecting and reporting data among physician's offices, medical groups, hospitals, health plans, government, and others will significantly reduce the cost and improve the quality of health care performance reporting.

The Future

Unfortunately for physicians who are being assessed, for purchasers who are trying to buy "value," and for the public who is looking for the best available care, little or no consistency exists in physician performance measures. The public mandate requiring like measures and tools when reporting like outcomes has just started. As we move into the twenty-first century, the existence of so many different assessment measures and performance measurement systems is expensive and confusing and may not always produce accurate and reliable information. However, the impetus to publish accurate performance data is being driven by business, health care organizations, government, and the public. Clearly, a movement toward a uniform, standard system and national database to measure performance and quality accurately and consistently is long overdue, considering how much money is spent on health care every year. Given the new health care marketplace and its premium placed on performance measurement, physicians should take an active role in setting the standards, collecting the data, and reporting the results.

BIBLIOGRAPHY

Ellwood P. Outcomes management: a technology of patient experience. *N Engl J Med* 1988;318:1549–1556.

Kleinke JD. *Bleeding edge: the business of health care in the next century.* Gaithersburg, MD: Aspen Publishers, 1998.

Weissenstein E, Moore JD Jr. Quality under scrutiny. *Modern Healthcare* September 1998:12.

The Informatics Institute
  Contact: Marshall Ruffin, M.D, MPH
  8110 Gathouse Road, suite 401 East
  Falls Church, VA 22042-1210
  Phone: 800 844-0922
  E-mail: marshall@ruffin.com
  Web site: *www.tiinet.com*

The Informatics Institute is a center for education, research, and evaluation of health care information technology. The Institute offers 2-day training sessions in information management in Falls Church, VA, and San Francisco.

Future HealthCare Inc
  Contacts David C. Kibbe, MD, MBA, and Shawn Stockman
  PO Box 9325
  Chapel Hill, NC 27515
  Phone: 800 757-1354 or 919 929-5993
  E-mail: Stockman@interpath.com
  Web site: *www.futurehealthcare*.com

Future HealthCare Inc. is an educational product and consulting firm focused on helping health care organizations use data to improve quality and cost-effectiveness. Future HealthCare offers intensive 2- or 4-day workshops that combine on-site lecture and small group discussion with hands-on, computer-assisted tutorials.

The Institute for Healthcare Improvement
  Contact: Sinead Fitzmaurice
  135 Francis Street
  Boston, MA 02215
  Phone: 617 754-4800
  E-mail: jbert2@ix.netcom.com

The Institute for Healthcare Improvement (IHI) is a nonprofit organization promoting improvement in US and Canadian health systems. IHI offers intensive 2- or 4-day informatics workshops that include hands-on instruction at various locations.

The Managed Care Education Clearinghouse
  Web site: *www.gwumc.edu /mcec /index /htm*

The Managed Care Education Clearinghouse site is designed to be a one-stop shopping center for health professionals learning or teaching about managed care. The site is sponsored and maintained by the George Washington University Medical Center and the Pew Charitable Trusts. Browsers may review and download curricula and other educational materials on managed care, medical informatics, and physician performance measurement.

National Guideline Clearinghouse
  Web site: *www.guideline.gov*

This site is sponsored by the Agency for Healthcare Policy and Research (AHCPR) in partnership with the American Medical Association (AMA) and the American Association of Health Plans (AAHP). Its purpose is to make evidence-based clinical practice guidelines and related abstract, summary, and comparison materials widely available to health care professionals.

Kelley's Textbook of Internal Medicine, fourth edition. Edited by H. David Humes. Lippincott Williams & Wilkins, Philadelphia © 2000.

MEDICAL MALPRACTICE AND RISK MANAGEMENT

KIMBERLY A. COOK
JUAN D. REYES

It is extremely likely that most practicing physicians—especially those practicing in large metropolitan areas—will be involved in a medical negligence case at some time in their careers. Involvement can mean actually being named as a defendant in a lawsuit; it can mean that your conduct is being called into question, but only your employer is actually being sued; it can also mean reviewing material for one side or the other and testifying as an expert witness. What follows is a brief review dealing with medical negligence and risk management, the organization that is devoted to helping physicians avoid malpractice suits and to providing support to physicians during the pendency of a lawsuit, if one is filed.

MEDICAL NEGLIGENCE

Medical negligence is defined as the failure to act as a reasonably prudent physician would act under the circumstances, which causes harm to the patient. This is a two-part equation: the care must be proved to be substandard, and it must have caused the damage or injury that is described in the claim or suit. For example, even if a physician failed to diagnose cancer at a particular point in time, unless the failure affects the patient's prognosis, there is no "causation" and the patient has not proved a case of medical negligence. Similarly, the care may have undoubtedly caused the harm, but if the care was not negligent, there is also no proof of medical negligence. For example, an operation may have resulted in damage to a nerve, but if the nerve damage is a known complication and the surgery was performed correctly, there is no malpractice.

Medical negligence cases can involve matters that have nothing to do with patients, but that can greatly affect the outcome of a case. The most important of these issues is documentation. Documentation is always extremely important. It is critical to record all pertinent findings and *never* add to or change an entry—especially on a later date—without indicating *in the chart* that you are making a change. A jury may well find that negligence was committed based solely on the fact that the chart was altered, because this can call the physician's conduct into question.

It is advisable to note telephone conversations in the chart. Even if the patient is not seen in the office, critical information can be discussed that needs to be documented. Save all phone messages and place them in the chart. If e-mails are generated, retain those as well.

INFORMED CONSENT

One category of medical negligence cases involves informed consent. Informed consent is *not* established by ensuring that the patient signs all the consent forms. Informed consent is a process whereby the patient is counseled as to the risks and benefits of the treatment and also as to the alternative methods of treatment. This discussion should be documented in the chart, particularly the risks of the procedure. The questions asked and responses given should also be recorded, if possible. An office note that reflects that the patient is aware that nerve damage can result from a particular treatment, for example, is extremely helpful in defending a case when that patient sues because he or she suffers that very complication. In some states, if the informed consent is well documented, it creates a presumption in favor of the physician, which can be very difficult for the patient to overcome.

Medical negligence in the context of internal medicine usually comes in one of two forms: (a) failure to perform a particular examination or to make a diagnosis based on an examination that is alleged to be faulty or (b) failure to refer a patient to an appropriate specialist. For example, a 45-year-old male patient in whom a rectal examination is not performed sues when he is diagnosed with rectal carcinoma. A woman diagnosed with breast cancer sues her physician for failure to refer her to a surgical oncologist to investigate the lump the physician believed was benign.

PATIENT EXPECTATIONS

In today's world, in which many people seem to believe that they are entitled to perfect outcomes when treated by a physician and in which an unfortunate number of patients assume that malpractice was committed if the result is anything but perfect, medical negligence claims are all too common. It is unrealistic to assume that if "good medicine" is practiced, a suit will not result. Even if the physician is satisfied with the care, the patient may not be, particularly when there is a personality conflict between doctor and patient.

Because the physician and patient may have very different expectations, it is extremely important for the physician to encourage the patient to speak openly and for the physician to answer all questions asked and, to the extent possible, try to ascertain exactly what the patient expects from the treatment. If the patient anticipates an unreasonable result, it is important for the physician to explain the realistic goals of treatment—and to document these discussions in the chart.

THE ROLE OF RISK MANAGEMENT DEPARTMENT

The scope of the duties of risk management departments vary from institution to institution, but all share one common interest: providing assistance to physicians involved in an actual or potential lawsuit. The risk management department should be kept apprised of all instances in which the physician's involvement in a legal proceeding is sought, even though no formal claim or lawsuit has been filed. Many physicians have allowed themselves to be deposed—usually without being represented by an attorney—in an effort to help a patient (or an attorney) only to find that a lawsuit is then filed against them. It is important to assume that any time sworn testimony is given regarding the care of a patient, a record is being created for a lawyer and perhaps some other physician to review, which might provide the basis for the physician being named as an additional defendant in a lawsuit. The physician should not—and cannot—refuse to cooperate when he has treated a patient who has filed a claim or lawsuit against another physician. However, one should be cautious and inform the risk management department of the fact that sworn testimony has been requested.

The risk management department is dedicated to reducing the risk that a physician will become involved in a malpractice case. This is accomplished by collecting information (and sometimes reporting incidents to the state) to target areas that are particularly problematic in terms of the potential for claims and by conducting "in-services," which try to educate and inform the health care providers.

MALPRACTICE AND MANAGED CARE

With the advent of managed care, malpractice claims—and, therefore, the response of risk management—have changed. Not only can a claim be made when the outcome is unsatisfactory, but the physician can be sued for failing to approve care that is allegedly necessary but not covered by a particular insurance plan. The physician's method of reimbursement can also be called into question. Lawyers for the patient argue that capitated fees suggest that the physician is trying to see too many patients to make up for the reduced charge per patient. They may also claim that there is no incentive for the physician to spend an appropriate amount of time with the patient because the fee per patient, regardless of the amount of time spent or the complexity of the treatment provided, is the same. Although these claims are unfair and focus on issues that have nothing to do with the medical care, they are increasingly allowed by the courts.

Managed care provides different methods whereby unsatisfactory outcomes can be addressed. Some of the new "theories of liability," have been previously discussed. However, the fundamental principles remain the same. The health maintenance organization (HMO) has been an easy target, particularly since the patient has no personal relationship to stand in the way of making a claim. The trend seems to be that the court will hold the HMO responsible for the medical care, because it usually requires the patient to choose from several physicians with whom it has contracted, controls the fees the physicians earn, and can disallow recommended treatment. In many states, the legislatures are also considering passing statutes to ensure that this is the case.

There are instances in which the physician's recommendations for patient care are rejected by the HMO. If this occurs, it is extremely important to document this in the patient's chart or to communicate in writing directly with the managed care entity that denied authorization for the recommended care, setting forth the specific care that has been ordered and the reasons (to the extent that they are known) for the denial.

SETTLEMENT

Another aspect of the process that frustrates many physicians is the evaluation and settlement of claims. It is sometimes hard for the physician to accept that money is paid in a case that he or she feels strongly is medically defensible. However, any physician who has been involved in a trial and who has waited for a jury to deliberate and return a verdict knows very well that medicine sometimes has very little to do with why a case is won or lost. Because the judge and jury are not physicians, each case has to be evaluated by the defense attorneys and by risk management to determine the factors in a particular case that might affect its outcome—even if the case is medically defensible. For example, a record may have been recopied by a doctor after an untoward incident because the paper became soiled; however, the physician makes no reference to the fact that it is being recopied, throws away the first piece of paper, and forgets to record very pertinent information about the patient's condition when the incident occurred. The patient dies and the family files suit. The doctor explains what happened, but in the context of the outcome, the family's lawyer tries to portray the doctor's

actions as a "cover-up." This issue significantly complicates the defense of the case and provides the lay jury with a reason other than the medicine to find in favor of the family.

CONCLUSION

Becoming the target in a medical malpractice case is extremely unpleasant and affects different physicians in varying ways. Some are able to stay removed by viewing the process as an unfortunate complication of practicing medicine. Most, however, are profoundly affected and, understandably, are placed under great stress as a result. Although the lawyer on the other side may view the process as "just business," most physicians interpret a suit as an attack on their ability to practice medicine. It is extremely frustrating to have your training, credibility, and ability as a physician called into question by someone who knows very little about medicine and appears interested only in trying to portray the events in a way to help the patient—frequently a distortion of how things actually occurred.

Medical-legal issues have become increasingly more common and are likely to become even more so. An understanding of the process, however, is hoped to make it less emotionally distressing to the individual physician.

Kelley's Textbook of Internal Medicine, fourth edition. Edited by H. David Humes. Lippincott Williams & Wilkins, Philadelphia © 2000.

RELATED MEDICAL DISCIPLINES

C H A P T E R

48

ADOLESCENT MEDICINE

GAIL B. SLAP

The transition from pediatric to adult health care is often difficult for patients and physicians. Multidisciplinary adolescent clinics have been shown to improve patient satisfaction and compliance but tend to be limited to large academic training centers. In other settings, the internist often assumes care of the adolescent directly from the pediatrician, and because adolescent medicine is outside the core of traditional training in internal medicine, internists frequently are uncomfortable managing their younger patients.

This chapter provides a medical overview of the adolescent population, beginning with a review of the demography and health needs of this age group. The common concerns, such as legality, confidentiality, and rapport, of the physician who cares for adolescents also are discussed. The normal physiologic development and psychosocial development of adolescents are summarized, followed by suggestions for the routine screening examination of the adolescent patient.

DEMOGRAPHIC TRENDS

The World Health Organization defines adolescents as persons between the ages of 10 and 19 years and youths as persons between the ages of 15 and 24 years. Historically, these populations have received little attention in health care policy, because they tend to have fewer traditional medical problems than the very young or the elderly. However, factors have emerged that bring the health needs of youth into the public eye. The 10- to 19-year-old population in the United States has been increasing since 1990 and is expected to reach 43 million by 2020. Compared with the general population, more adolescents will come from minority and impoverished backgrounds, factors that are associated with injury, homicide, unintentional pregnancy, sexually transmitted disease, and inadequate health care.

Two million adolescents (6%) 10 to 18 years of age have chronic conditions that limit their daily function. The leading

cause is mental disorders (32%), followed by chronic respiratory (21%) and musculoskeletal conditions (15%). An estimated 5 million adolescents 12 to 17 years of age have significant emotional or behavioral problems, yet less than one-third receive needed services. Nearly all adolescents with emotional or behavioral conditions and over 85% with chronic medical conditions will survive to require adult medical care.

PUBLIC HEALTH PROBLEMS AMONG YOUTH

INJURY, HOMICIDE, AND SUICIDE

Injury, homicide, and suicide account for over 80% of deaths among 15- to 24-year-old persons in the United States and 55% of youth deaths throughout the world. More years of potential life are lost to injury alone than to cancer and heart disease combined. Motor vehicles account for 75% of adolescent deaths from unintentional injury. One third of adolescents report riding with a driver who has been drinking alcohol, and one quarter report driving after drinking.

Homicide rates among adolescents 15 to 19 years of age are seven times higher for blacks than for whites and six times higher for males than females. The United States ranks first among countries outside Eastern Europe in homicides committed by adolescents under age 18 years.

Suicide is the third leading cause of adolescent death. The rate among adolescents has increased 200% in the past 35 years compared with 17% for the general population. Among those 15 to 19 years of age, white male youths have the highest rate and black female youths have the lowest rate. Known risk factors for youth suicide include a previous attempt, male gender, psychiatric illness, and a family history of suicide. Postulated factors include substance abuse, peer suicide, media reports of suicide, physical abuse, and family dysfunction.

SUBSTANCE ABUSE

The best information on adolescent drug and alcohol use in the United States comes from an annual survey of 50,000 eighth-, tenth-, and twelfth-grade students. In 1998, the rates of use of illicit drugs, alcohol, and tobacco decreased in all three grades for the first time in 6 years. Twenty-two percent of twelfth graders reported daily cigarette smoking, 32% had five or more alcoholic drinks on one occasion within the prior 2 weeks, 23% had used marijuana within the month, and 20% had used another illicit drug. Inhalants were used most by eighth graders, with 12% reporting use within the year.

Risk factors for adolescent substance use include family and peer use; physical and sexual abuse; runaway behavior; family isolation and stress; and emotional and behavioral problems. The signs of use include declining school performance, isolation from family and childhood friends, secrecy, dishonesty, mood swings, and frequent somatic complaints.

SEXUAL AND REPRODUCTIVE HEALTH

The rates of abstinence and condom use among American adolescents increased during the 1990s. Reported use of condoms at last intercourse was 56% in 1997, representing a 22% increase over 7 years. However, the rate of four or more lifetime partners remained high at 16% to 19%. Although pregnancy rates suggest a decline, the United States continues to lead the industrialized world in adolescent pregnancies, deliveries, and abortions.

Of the 12 million cases of sexually transmitted diseases (STDs) reported annually in the United States, 25% occur in adolescents. STD prevalence peaks by age 21 years and then rapidly declines. Biology, as well as behavior, contributes to adolescent risk. The transitional zone from columnar to squamous epithelium is highly susceptible to both infection and dysplasia. This zone recedes into the endocervix from the vaginal canal during adolescence, making it less accessible to infection.

Chlamydia trachomatis is two to three times more prevalent than gonorrhea. It has been isolated in 20% to 60% of adolescents with pelvic inflammatory disease, 40% to 60% of adolescents with cervicitis, 15% of asymptomatic girls, and 8% of asymptomatic boys. The rates of both gonorrhea and chlamydia in adolescents have fallen in the past 10 years, whereas the rates of herpes simplex virus type 2 and human papillomavirus (HPV) have climbed. The association of some types of HPV infection and anogenital cancer has resulted in a declining mean age for cervical intraepithelial neoplasia and invasive cervical cancer.

An estimated 25% of new HIV infections occur in people younger than 22 years of age. The long latency period from HIV infection to the AIDS means that adolescents constitute an asymptomatic and often undiagnosed reservoir for transmission to sexual partners and infants. The risk of HIV infection is increased two- to five-fold by the presence of another STD. Early recognition and treatment of other STDs therefore are central to HIV prevention.

PHYSICIAN–PATIENT RELATIONSHIP

The visit to an internist may be the adolescent's first exposure to the adult health care system. In most cases, the decision to see an internist has been made because the patient feels ready to leave the pediatric setting or wants a more confidential relationship than that previously experienced. Adolescents should be assured of their right to confidentiality, and this should be explained to parents at the time of the first visit. Adolescents and their parents also must understand that confidentiality will not be maintained in life-threatening situations in which parental involvement is essential.

Consent and confidentiality have received increasing attention in state law during the past 10 years. Most states now protect the adolescent's right to medical care, including family planning and substance abuse, without parental consent. The mature minor doctrine states that emancipated minors (i.e., persons younger than 18 years of age who are self-supporting, away at college, in the military, or otherwise independent) can be treated in all states without parental consent. However, adolescent care usually is facilitated by involvement of the parents, and the physician should make every attempt to foster communication within the family about the adolescent's health.

NORMAL DEVELOPMENT DURING ADOLESCENCE

The assessment of growth and development is central to the care of adolescent patients. This holds true for the healthy adolescent who is seen for a periodic screening examination and for the chronically ill adolescent whose pubertal maturation is often delayed.

SOMATIC AND SEXUAL CHANGES OF PUBERTY

The most useful clinical measure of an adolescent's developmental age is the sexual maturity rating or Tanner stage of puberty (Table 48.1). For girls, this is based on breast development and pubic hair growth. For boys, it is based on development of the external genitalia and pubic hair growth. The two components of the pubertal stage of each sex are rated separately on a scale of 1 (prepubertal) to 5 (adult). Puberty in girls normally begins between 8 and 13 years of age with breast development (Fig. 48.1). Puberty in boys typically begins 1 or 2 years later (9.5 to 13.5 years of age) with testicular enlargement (Fig. 48.2). The average duration of puberty is 4 years in girls and 3 years in boys. More than 95% of girls and boys reach a sexual maturity rating of 5 by 16.5 years.

One of the most dramatic changes of puberty is the rapid growth in height. In girls, the height spurt occurs at a mean age of 11.5 years and with a sexual maturity rating of 2 or 3. In boys, it occurs at a later mean chronologic age (13.5 years) and at a later sexual maturity rating (4). Because the timing of the height spurt correlates with the progression through puberty, a child who has grown along a given percentile curve may deviate from that curve in adolescence if puberty is early or late. New height standards include curves that represent children of normal height whose pubertal progression is at the early (+2 SD) or late (−2 SD) limits of normal.

Pubertal growth accounts for 25% of final adult height and 40% of ideal adult weight. The theory that menarche occurs with attainment of a critical body fat is controversial but commonly is used to explain primary and secondary amenorrhea. Menarche occurs at a mean age of 12.8 years in the United States, and 97% of American girls experience menarche by 14.6 years.

Many systemic changes occur during puberty. The slow in-

TABLE 48.1.	STAGES OF PUBERTY		
Stage	**Breast**	**Male Genitalia**	**Pubic Hair**
1 (Preadolescent)	Elevation of papilla only	No enlargement of testes, scrotum, penis	None
2	Breast bud; breast and papilla form small mound and areola widens	Scrotum and testes enlarge; scrotal skin reddens	Sparse, downy hair along labia or base of penis
3	Breast and areola enlarge with no separation of their contours	Penis lengthens, continued growth of scrotum and testes	Darker, coarser hair spreads sparsely over genitalia
4	Areola and papilla project above the level of the breast	Penis broadens, glans develops, testes enlarge, scrotal skin darkens	Hair is adult in type, but area covered is smaller; no spread to medial thighs
5 (Adult)	Areola recedes to breast level; papilla only projects	Adult in size and shape	Adult in type and quantity

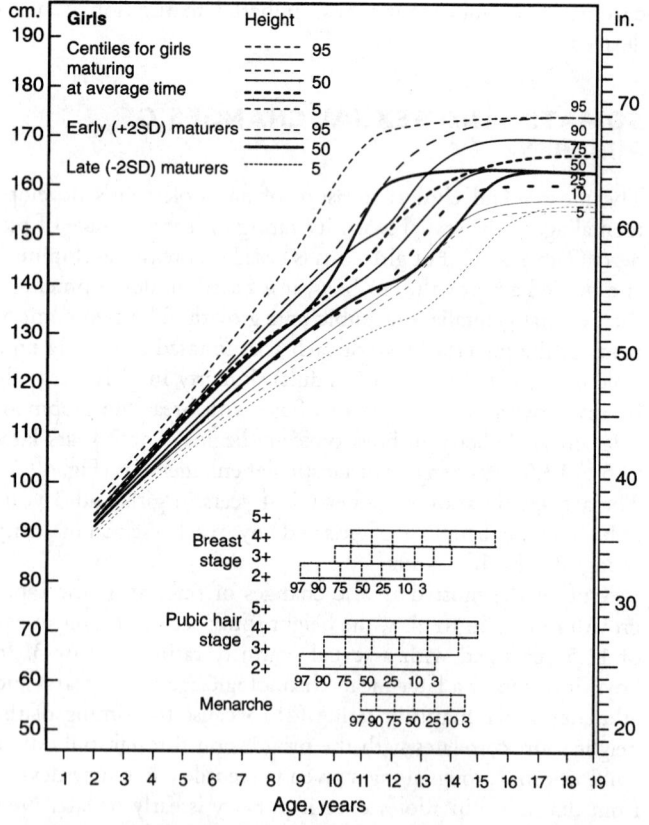

FIGURE 48.1. Percentiles of height for American girls. The heavy solid curves represent girls who are in the 50th percentile for height and 2 standard deviations (SD; 2 years) early or late for puberty. The upper dotted curve represents girls who are in the 95th percentile for height and 2 SD early for puberty. The lower dotted curve represents girls who are in the 5th percentile for height and 2 SD late for puberty. The bottom bars refer to percentile pubertal stage for age (e.g., pubic hair stage 2+ represents stage 2 but not stage 3 pubic hair). (From Tanner JM, Davies PSW. Clinical longitudinal standards for height and weight velocity in North American children. *J Pediatr* 1989;107:317, with permission.)

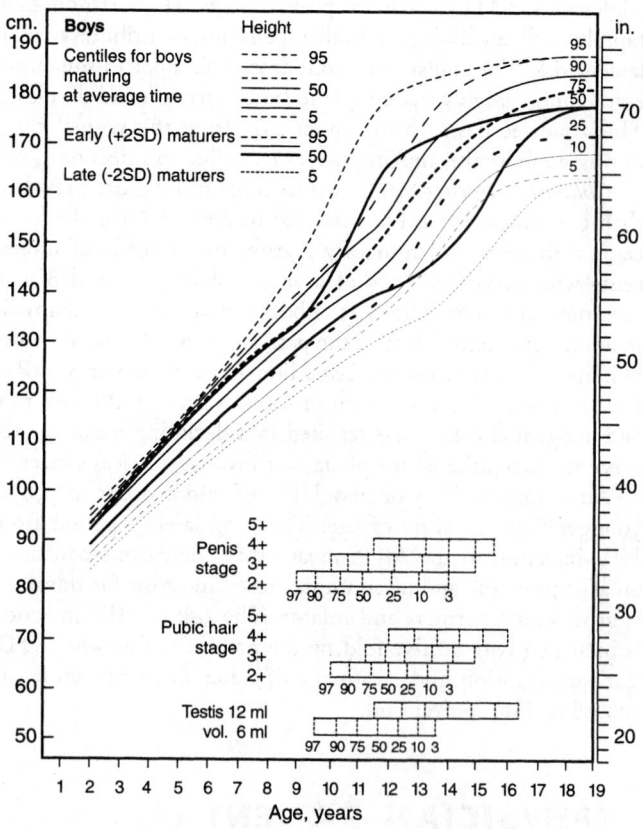

FIGURE 48.2. Percentiles of height for American boys. The heavy solid curves represent boys who are in the 50th percentile for height and 2 standard deviations (SD; 2 years) early or late for puberty. The upper dotted curve represents boys who are in the 95th percentile for height and 2 SD early for puberty. The lower dotted curve represents boys who are in the 5th percentile for height and 2 SD late for puberty. The bottom bars refer to percentile pubertal stage for age (e.g., pubic hair stage 2+ represents stage 2 but not stage 3 pubic hair). (From Tanner JM, Davies PSW. Clinical longitudinal standards for height and weight velocity in North American children. *J Pediatr* 1989;107:317, with permission.)

crease in blood pressure that occurs during late childhood accelerates rapidly during adolescence. The decrease in heart rate that occurs during childhood stabilizes or even increases during adolescence. In boys, heart weight doubles, hemoglobin increases, respiratory rate decreases, and vital capacity increases.

Few detectable gross changes occur in the brain, despite the enormous cognitive change that occurs during adolescence. The brain achieves 95% of final adult weight by the age of 10 years, and electroencephalography does not reveal changes that are specific for puberty.

PSYCHOSOCIAL DEVELOPMENT

The developmental tasks of adolescence fall into three broad categories: the establishment of autonomy, psychosexual development, and future orientation. Young adolescents (11 to 14 years) struggle for independence but retreat to parents during perceived crises. They often are preoccupied with bodily changes and look for reassurance that their development is normal. The capacity for abstract reasoning usually is not fully developed, and the perspective of time tends to be oriented to the present. Middle adolescents (15 to 17 years) usually are near completion of puberty and are more comfortable with their adult bodies. The peer group assumes primary importance, and some family conflict is common. By late adolescence (18 to 21 years), this conflict diminishes as the adolescent establishes an independent identity and begins to work toward realistic adult goals.

■ EVALUATION OF THE ADOLESCENT PATIENT

HISTORY

Most adolescents speak more openly with physicians when interviewed without their parents being present. The parents should be assured that they will join the physician and patient in the office when the physical examination is completed. This gives the physician a chance to obtain additional history from the parents and to discuss the management plan with the patient and parents simultaneously.

Early discussion of the adolescent's family, school performance, social milieu, and interests may guide the remaining history. This also may be the time to discuss sexual activity and the use of cigarettes, alcohol, and drugs. It is essential that these issues be raised at some time during the first visit. The adolescent should understand from the outset that these areas are acceptable for discussion and that confidentiality will be protected whenever possible.

The patient's developmental and immunization histories should be obtained from the parents or the pediatric record. A discussion of nutrition and eating habits is another important part of the adolescent history. Most girls require 2200 to 2500 calories during early adolescence, and most boys require 2500 to 3000 calories. Iron intake is often inadequate in both sexes during adolescence, and girls require three times the amount of iron contained in the average American diet. Obesity, anorexia nervosa, and bulimia are common problems that begin during

adolescence and must be managed in a forthright manner with the adolescent and parents.

PHYSICAL EXAMINATION

Several aspects of the adolescent physical examination differ from the adult examination. Height and weight should be measured annually and plotted on a normative scale to indicate the percentile for chronologic age (Figs. 48.1 and 48.2). The sexual maturity ratings should be performed at each visit (Table 48.1), and progression through the stages should be plotted on a normative scale (Figs. 48.1. and 48.2).

Scoliosis usually becomes clinically apparent during the height spurt and may progress quickly during this time. It is found in 10% of adolescents and is ten times more common in girls. The patient should be examined for asymmetry of the shoulders, scapulae, pelvis, and breasts. When a patient with scoliosis bends forward at the waist, the rib cage protrudes toward the convex side of the curve. If scoliosis is detected, a radiograph of the spine should be obtained to determine the degree, and the patient should be referred for orthopedic evaluation.

Gynecomastia occurs in up to 60% of 14-year-old boys and is most common at genital stage 2. More than 75% of cases are bilateral and resolve within 12 to 18 months. Gynecomastia that persists form more than 2 years requires evaluation.

Fibroadenomas of the breast are common in adolescent girls, accounting for up to 90% of breast lesions in this age group. Conversely, fibrocystic disease is uncommon until late adolescence, and there is usually more tenderness and fluctuation than with fibroadenomas. Although carcinoma of the breast is rare during adolescence, many physicians begin to encourage self-examination during adolescence to establish it as a health habit by adulthood.

Indications for the first pelvic examination include sexual activity, age 18 to 21 years, diethylstilbestrol exposure in utero (now rare among adolescents), and unexplained pelvic pain, menstrual abnormality, or vaginal discharge. Sexually active adolescents should have visits for contraceptive counseling every 3 months, STD screening every 6 months, and a Papanicolaou smear every year.

LABORATORY EVALUATION

The prevalence of iron-deficiency anemia due to rapid growth and nutritional deficiencies warrants a screening hemoglobin or hematocrit in early and late adolescence for boys and girls. Urinalysis should be done in early, middle, and late adolescence. Routine stool check for occult blood, electrolyte analysis, liver function studies, chest radiograph, and electrocardiogram are unnecessary.

The National Cholesterol Education Program does not recommend routine screening for hypercholesterolemia in children and adolescents younger than 20 years of age. Selective screening is recommended for children and adolescents who have one or more of the following: (a) a parent with a blood cholesterol level of 240 mg per deciliter or more; (b) a parent or grandparent who, at or before 55 years of age, was found to have coronary atherosclerosis on coronary arteriography or who had a documented myocardial infarction, angina pectoris, peripheral vascular disease, cerebrovascular disease, or sudden death; (c) an unobtainable biologic family history. Screening should be strongly considered for adolescents with other risk factors for coronary atherosclerosis, such as cigarette smoking, hypertension, obesity, and diabetes mellitus. The recommended test depends on the reason for screening. If done for parental hypercholesterolemia, a random total cholesterol level is recommended first. If the adolescent's level is above 200 mg per deciliter, a 12-hour fasting lipoprotein analysis should be done to measure high-density lipoprotein (HDL) cholesterol and low-density lipoprotein (LDL) cholesterol. If the adolescent's random cholesterol is borderline (170 to 199 mg per deciliter), a second measurement should be obtained and averaged with the first. If the average is borderline or high, a fasting lipoprotein analysis should be obtained. If the initial screen is indicated because of family cardiovascular disease, two separate lipoprotein analyses following 12-hour fasts should be done and the LDL-cholesterol values should be averaged.

Sexually active female adolescents should have testing every 6 months for gonorrhea and chlamydia and a Papanicolaou smear every year. Sexually active male adolescents should have urine leukocyte esterase screening or urine ligase chain-reaction testing for gonorrhea and chlamydia every 6 months. Adolescents with a history of STD or risk factors for HIV infection should have a serologic test for syphilis. HIV screening should be discussed with adolescents who have had multiple sexual partners, a partner at risk for HIV infection, male homosexual intercourse, other STDs, or a history of injection drug use.

IMMUNIZATION

If there is no written documentation of immunization, the primary series for diphtheria–tetanus (dT) and poliovirus should be administered. A dT booster should then be given every 10 years throughout life. The measles–mumps–rubella (MMR) immunization should be administered to all adolescents who have had only one previous MMR inoculation. Hepatitis B immunization is recommended for all adolescents who have not previously received it. The tuberculin skin test should be done for adolescents who are exposed to active tuberculosis, living in homeless shelters or institutions, or working in health care settings.

BIBLIOGRAPHY

American Academy of Pediatrics, Committee on Nutrition. Cholesterol in childhood. *Pediatrics* 101;1998:141–148.
Elster AE, Kuznets NJ. AMA guidelines for adolescent preventive services (GAPS): recommendations and rationale. Baltimore: Williams & Wilkins, 1994.
Emans SJH, Goldstein DP. *Pediatric and adolescent gynecology,* fourth ed. Philadelphia: Lippincott-Raven, 1997.
Friedman SB, Fisher M, Schonberg SK, Alderman EM, eds. *Comprehensive adolescent health care,* second ed. St. Louis: CV Mosby, 1997.
Institute of Medicine. *The hidden epidemic: confronting sexually transmitted diseases.* Washington, DC: National Academy Press, 1997.
Johnston LD, O'Malley PM, Bachman JG. *National survey results on drug use from the monitoring the future study, 1975–1998: Volume 1: Secondary school students.* NIH Pub. No. 99–4660. Washington DC: National Institute on Drug Abuse, U.S. Department of Health and Human Services, Public Health Service, National Institutes of Health. US Government Printing Office, 1999.
Neinstein LS. *Adolescent health care: a practical guide,* third ed. Baltimore: Williams & Wilkins, 1996.
Ozer EM, Brindis CD, Millstein SG, et al. *America's adolescents: are they healthy?* San Francisco, CA: University of California, San Francisco, National Adolescent Health Information Center, 1997.
Strasburger VC, Brown RT. *Adolescent medicine: a practical guide,* second ed. Philadelphia: Lippincott-Raven, 1998.

Kelley's Textbook of Internal Medicine, fourth edition. Edited by H. David Humes.
Lippincott Williams & Wilkins, Philadelphia © 2000.

C H A P T E R
49

PRINCIPLES OF OCCUPATIONAL MEDICINE

MARK R. CULLEN
LINDA ROSENSTOCK

Concomitant with the increasing attention to the adverse health effects of chemical, biological, and physical agents is the challenge to physicians to recognize, diagnose, and treat occupational diseases. To a degree almost unparalleled in any field of clinical medicine, the physician also plays a pivotal role in disease prevention for individual patients and others similarly affected or at risk.

Most men and women in the United States work outside the home; in almost all occupations, they face risks or perceived risks from workplace exposure. Most of these approximately 100 million workers receive medical care from primary care and other first-contact physicians. The goal of this chapter is to define general principles of occupational disease and to describe an approach to incorporating specialized skills and responsibilities of caring for working patients into traditional clinical practice. Although it is not feasible to provide a comprehensive review of occupational diseases here, the final section of this chapter is an overview by organ system of diagnostic categories with known or likely occupational causes.

GENERAL PRINCIPLES OF OCCUPATIONAL DISEASE

ASSESSING CLINICAL MANIFESTATIONS

The clinical and pathologic manifestations of most occupational diseases are indistinguishable from those of other causes. It often is presumed that diseases that arise out of the workplace have such distinctive features that they are readily recognized or that they should be considered only when more common causes have been excluded. Unique clinical and pathologic findings are the exception, however, rather than the rule. For the clinician, the patient usually presents with a disorder such as chronic bronchitis, which may be caused or aggravated by workplace factors (e.g., mineral and grain dusts, irritant gases, plastics constituents) but is explained commonly by another factor, such as cigarette smoking. Other examples include occupationally induced asthma, which may mimic extrinsic or intrinsic asthma, and lung cancer from asbestos exposure or aplastic anemia from benzene exposure, which may be indistinguishable from diseases caused by other agents.

This basic principle does not mean that the occupational origin of these diseases cannot be firmly established by the clinician. It raises the need to maintain an appropriate index of suspicion and to apply other principles and skills in evaluating conditions that are commonly seen or too readily ascribed to nonoccupational or so-called idiopathic origins.

An important temporal relation exists between exposure and disease onset, with long latent intervals for most chronic disease and all occupational cancers. Many occupational diseases of acute onset or episodic occurrence have a predictable temporal pattern between causative exposure and symptoms. For example, for toxins acting as potent respiratory irritants, symptoms may occur within minutes after exposure (as with soluble gases such as chlorine and ammonia) and usually no later than 24 to 48 hours (as with less soluble gases such as phosgene). The link between the outcome and exposure is almost always obvious and readily determined in these settings.

More difficult to diagnose but strongly suggested by characteristic exposure-response patterns, is occupational asthma associated with certain causative agents. For example, asthma due to exposure to Western red cedar dust usually presents as nocturnal asthma (presumably a delayed hypersensitivity reaction), occasionally as an immediate hypersensitivity response shortly after exposure or as both an immediate and a late response. Acute solvent intoxication, characterized by dizziness, disorientation, irritability, headache, and gastrointestinal disturbance, typically occurs within hours of overexposure, abates within hours of leaving exposure, and usually resolves within 24 to 48 hours.

Most chronic disorders occur remote from exposure to the causative factor and may have been unassociated with symptoms at the time of exposure. Most nonmalignant asbestos-related diseases occur at least 20 years after the first exposure, and the average latency is 25 years for asbestos-related lung cancers and 35 years for mesothelioma. However, increased risk occurs years earlier for both of the latter conditions. Knowledge of these latency factors is of crucial importance for the clinician in seeking a history of possible occupational cause and guides an in-depth history of exposures to recent or past employment.

Etiology

Occupational diseases often have multifactorial causation. Occupational factors may act together or in concert with nonoccupational factors in altering risk for disease. The multiplicative risk for lung cancer from asbestos exposure and cigarette smoking is a well-known example. In those heavily exposed to asbestos who do not smoke, the risk is about fivefold, compared with tenfold for smokers without asbestos exposure and 50-fold for those with both exposures. Another example is the increased risk for

compressive mononeuropathies from physical trauma in the setting of diffuse neuropathy, either from toxic or from other causes such as diabetes mellitus. The potentiation of peripheral neurotoxicity from methyl-*n*-butyl ketone in the presence of methyl-ethyl ketone documents the potential interaction of occupational toxins, but the effects of combined exposure remain largely unexplored even when effects of any one agent have been well delineated.

Regardless of whether different factors act synergistically or independently (additively), identification of one or more occupational factors as causative is of major diagnostic and therapeutic importance.

TOXIN EXPOSURE AND DISEASE SEVERITY

For acute and chronic occupational disease, the dose of exposure is a major determinant of risk for or severity of disease. Most occupational exposures to toxins occur by inhalational or dermal routes or both. As with pharmacologic principles of drugs, mechanics of absorption, metabolism, and elimination contribute to cumulative dose. Occupational toxins may be considered to act in one or more of the following ways: as direct cellular toxins, as allergens, and as carcinogens.

Toxins can act as direct cellular toxins, with increasing effect occurring at increasing doses and often no adverse effect observed below a certain threshold dose. Examples include liver and renal toxicity from carbon tetrachloride, central nervous system toxicity in adults exposed to lead, and pulmonary dysfunction from silica dust. In general, increasing doses of exposure to toxins in this group are associated with a greater proportion of exposed persons suffering adverse effects and a greater severity of resultant disease in any given person.

Toxic substances can cause allergic or hypersensitivity reactions, with the exposure dose often affecting the number of exposed persons who become sensitized but even minute exposures capable of precipitating a full-blown response among those sensitized. Examples include the more than 200 agents recognized as causative in occupational asthma, a list that overlaps but is not identical with that associated with occupational dermatitis, and the agents associated with other hypersensitivity pulmonary disorders, such as those caused by cobalt and beryllium.

Toxins are considered carcinogens when increasing risk for tumor occurs with increasing dose and there is no demonstrable safe or threshold level of exposure. Examples are numerous and include asbestos, which acts as a promoter and initiator in carcinogenesis, with lung cancer occurring in as many as 50% of those with heavy exposure who smoke cigarettes and mesothelioma occurring in as many as 10% of those with heavy asbestos exposure independent of smoking status. As with other carcinogens, even small and brief exposures present some theoretical risk, but the risk for these exposures may be unmeasurable and comparable to the increased risk for lung cancer from smoking only a few cigarettes. Understanding a person's risk for cancer after exposure to an occupational carcinogen necessitates extrapolation of risk based on comparability of exposure in epidemiologic studies that define the risk.

TOXICOLOGIC DETERMINATION

Important occupational factors may be difficult to identify and may not have documented clinical significance. An estimated 50,000 chemicals are in widespread industrial use, and about one-third are toxic in doses that may be encountered in the workplace. Identification of these substances often is difficult and made more so by the occurrence of many toxins in mixtures and as contaminants of other products. Hundreds of new substances are introduced annually into the workplace. Toxicologic and human health effects data frequently are inadequate and for some outcomes, such as female reproductive effects, are practically nonexistent.

HOST FACTORS

Host susceptibility factors play a variable role in the occurrence of occupational disease. Although most persons with sufficient exposure to some occupational toxins experience an adverse effect, a significant variation in expression of disease occurs even among those heavily exposed. For example, among those with heavy asbestos exposure, only about 50% develop asbestos-induced pulmonary fibrosis. For some agents that cause occupational asthma, such as platinum, most people who are exposed may become sensitized, but for other agents, such as toluene diisocyanate or Western red cedar, the proportion of those who develop hypersensitivity syndromes is far lower. Atopy has explained the increased risk for some but cannot explain any of the increased risk for sensitization to other agents implicated in occupational asthma and dermatitis.

■ SPECIALIZED SKILLS IN CLINICAL OCCUPATIONAL MEDICINE

OCCUPATIONAL HEALTH HISTORY

The occupational health history is the foundation on which rests any assessment of known or suspected occupational disease. It should become routinely incorporated into the traditional health history, expanded and adapted as demanded by the clinical setting. The occupational history has two main parts: the work and exposure history and the general health history.

Work and Exposure History

In the work and exposure part of the history, information is elicited about the current or most recent job, including job title, type of industry, and nature of work performed. Simply asking the patient to describe a typical day of work can be rewarding and may have benefits beyond the objectives of the history itself, providing the patient an often-welcome opportunity to discuss an important part of his or her life. Information about the job title and industry for all past jobs, including military experience, should be obtained.

Exploration of potentially hazardous exposures is fundamental to this part of the history. Focusing on recent or remote exposures is guided by whether the disorders under evaluation are acute and recurrent or chronic. A checklist approach to general categories of exposure is a good starting point for this inquiry. Additional exposure information beyond that directly obtainable from the patient is often helpful and sometimes necessary. Sources of additional information include environmental monitoring data, specific biologic testing of the patient, product information sheets (material safety data sheets), and data available from the employer, union, and regulatory agencies. Because dose of exposure is important in assessing potential adverse effects, additional queries should address the use of personal protective equipment, the degree of ventilation and general plant hygiene, and the level of technologic safeguards, such as enclosure of hazardous chemicals.

It is important to ask about exposure to nonwork environmental hazards. These are commonly encountered in household and avocational activities and less commonly in the community.

General Health History

In the general health part of the occupational history, the chief complaint and review of systems components of the traditional health history are augmented by exploring the relation between work and symptoms. An important initial question is whether the patient perceives that his or her health problems are work related. Although these perceptions may not be well founded, a patient's suspicion about a workplace problem should be taken seriously. Coworkers with similar complaints provide further evidence that occupational factors may be important; the clustering of even common problems is often the first clue to a work-related disease.

The timing of onset of symptoms and their variation in relation to time at work and association with certain work processes may provide information of particular importance in assessing acute or recurring conditions. It is useful to ask whether symptoms abate when the patient is away from work, such as on weekends and during vacations. The history of such temporal patterns may be of importance in chronic conditions, such as evaluating nonspecific bronchial hyperreactivity resulting from what was initially a specific response to an occupational exposure.

DIAGNOSTIC DECISION MAKING

Determining whether an illness or condition is work related is often important for assigning insurance benefits and making vital decisions about continued work activities. Although the basic principles used to make such decisions are not very different from those used at the bedside in other clinical areas, the decisions often seem more forced and difficult because of the obvious legal and economic ramifications. Moreover, good practice often leads to differing thresholds or standards for making decisions, even in an individual case. For example, if there is any reasonable likelihood that a patient's exposure may be contributing to progression of a lethal or serious disease, removal based on suspicion is appropriate. Workers' Compensation systems typically require a determination based on "more probable than not," a standard defined as a likelihood greater than 50%.

TABLE 49.1.	CRITERIA FOR DETERMINING WORK-RELATED MEDICAL CONDITIONS

The symptoms, signs, and laboratory tests are consistent with the diagnosis.

The temporal pattern of exposure and disease onset is consistent with known time-response characteristics.

The exposure was of sufficient dose given known dose-response characteristics.

Biologic monitoring of exposures or specific end-organ effects is consistent with dose-response characteristics.

Epidemiologic data support effects at a comparable exposure to those experienced by the patient.

No other condition or exposure more readily explains the disease.

Scientific rigor for inclusion in research papers or other reports usually requires a higher degree of certainty about the diagnosis and cause.

The principles for decision making are straightforward. First, there must be clear evidence of exposure to an agent or agents that have toxicologic potential, based on the occupational history, laboratory tests, or outside records. Second, unless there is compelling evidence to cite a single case as a newly described condition, the agent or agents must have been demonstrated or highly suspected from human studies or animal experiments to cause health effects resembling those of the patient. The dose of exposure, to the extent that it can be estimated by history records or tests, should be of a magnitude similar to those levels reported to have such effects. The interval between exposure and onset of effect should be consistent with available evidence. Also important is determining whether other explanations for the disorder are reasonably likely compared with the likelihood that the disorder is work related. In this way, for example, it could be predicted that the rounded opacities seen on the x-ray film of a rock crusher are almost certainly caused by occupational exposure to silica dust (silicosis), because other possible diagnoses presenting radiographically in this way, such as sarcoidosis, are uncommon.

The criteria for determining the work relatedness of a medical condition are summarized in Table 49.1.

■ NOTIFICATION AND FOLLOW-THROUGH

For the physician, the medical treatment of working patients involves special circumstances and evokes special responsibilities that are not usually encountered in traditional practice. Awareness of these is key to the successful practice of clinical occupational medicine.

PHYSICIAN–PATIENT RELATIONSHIP

The physician–patient relationship can be seriously challenged in the diagnosis, treatment, and prevention of occupational dis-

eases, but responses to these challenges can be based on ethical and legal principles derived from general medical practice. One principle addresses the loyalty or allegiance of the physician, which should always remain with the working patient, even when health services are paid for by the employer.

The second principle is maintenance of confidentiality, with the recognition that only in exceptional circumstances should a physician consider violating that fundamental tenet of medical care. In occupational medicine, confidentiality is important for the sake of privacy and because the inappropriate or inadvertent release of information may have serious adverse consequences for the patient, including loss of employment security. After a physician–patient relationship is formed, the same strict rules of confidentiality of the written and verbal release of information should be applied. As in other circumstances, ethical guidelines define two settings in which on a case-by-case basis confidentiality may need to be abandoned: (a) when there are overriding public health consequences, as when other workers may be at significant risk if hazardous conditions or exposures are not disclosed; and (b) when serious harm to the patient will result if information is not revealed. Legal requirements, such as response to subpoena and releasing records for workers' compensation, also may necessitate disclosure. Whether mandated by ethical or legal restraints, the patient should always be informed when an expressed desire for confidentiality cannot be respected.

The third principle of importance is that of informing the patient about medical conditions, including the hazards and potential risks of workplace exposures or diseases, and of discussing decisions that may be anticipated or possible serious consequences such as termination of employment or job relocation. As in other areas of clinical medicine, the physician has an ethical obligation to keep as informed as possible and to recognize when it is in the patient's best interest to seek consultation or referral elsewhere.

REPORTING

In addition to disclosing information to the patient, the physician has broader responsibilities after an occupational disease is diagnosed or suggested. Some of these are legally mandated; some actions not legally required may still have economic or health benefits for the patient. Because occupational diseases are by definition almost all preventable, the potential public health impact of reporting may be significant.

Depending on the medical implications of the problem and considering other factors such as confidentiality, reporting can be accomplished in numerous ways, including notifying the employer, workers and their representatives, public health agencies, and research and regulatory agencies; publishing in scientific journals; and reaching the public through the media. The following summary of potentially important contacts should be considered, recognizing that these same contacts may provide valuable additional information about exposures and therefore may be of assistance at an earlier point in the process of evaluating work-related disease.

Employer

The employer almost always should be notified about identified work hazards or conditions. Many large companies employ professionals who can supply detailed information about the workplace.

Union

Although only about 20% of US workers are members of trade unions, some unions play a key role in workplace health and safety. They may be a source of workplace and exposure information, which may be of assistance in understanding options and implications of job transfer or termination.

Occupational Safety and Health Administration

The state or federal branch of the Occupational Safety and Health Administration (OSHA) serving the physician's region can provide consultation about hazards, including workplace assessments without charge or threat of penalty (through requesting employers). OSHA also serves as the regulatory agency overseeing enforcement of health and safety standards. If necessary, complaints from a patient, the patient's representative, or the patient's physician should prompt an inspection; reports of past inspections also are available and may be an additional source of exposure information.

National Institute for Occupational Safety and Health

The National Institute for Occupational Safety and Health (NIOSH), seated in the Centers for Disease Control and Prevention, is responsible for research and training in occupational health. The many services include supplying information about specific exposures and conducting studies of industries or workplaces with known or suspected health problems.

State and Local Health Departments

Several state and some local health departments are capable of investigating health conditions arising from the workplace. They also may provide information about previously investigated or reported illnesses and injuries and may be the best single referral source for follow-up and intervention for the individual patient and his or her coworkers.

Workers' Compensation

Workers' compensation is a program that covers most US workers, primarily through state programs and for a smaller number through federal programs. Workers' compensation is a no-fault insurance system; in almost all instances, the worker forfeits the right to sue an employer for work-related diseases or injuries in exchange for receiving medical care, rehabilitation, and income replacement.

Because legal duties and responsibilities vary significantly from state to state, the physician needs to become familiar with the major programs that affect his or her patients. This is particularly important in the many jurisdictions in which even a physi-

cian's verbal notification to a patient of the presence of an occupational disease may initiate the beginning of a statute of limitations, the period in which a claim must be filed. The physician plays a key role in the workers' compensation system, with the responsibility to initiate workers' compensation claims, to determine the likelihood of work relatedness of the condition, and to be available for the sometimes onerous and often frustrating task of attendant paperwork.

■ CLASSIFICATION OF OCCUPATIONAL DISEASE BY ORGAN SYSTEM

Classification of major disease groupings with known or strongly suspected occupational causes are presented by organ system in Tables 49.2 through 49.8. Most of these diagnostic categories are associated with multiple occupational factors, but in some, only one agent has been implicated. The information in these tables serves as a useful starting point in considering whether a patient's past or present work is contributing to or causing the diagnosed disorder. For more information about specific diseases, the reader is referred elsewhere in this text and to the bibliography.

TABLE 49.2.	OCCUPATIONAL DISEASES OF THE RESPIRATORY TRACT
Condition	**Examples of Associated Exposures**
Acute or Recurrent Disorders	
Upper respiratory tract inflammation	Fibrous glass, metal dust, welding and plastic fumes
Airway disorders	
Asthma	Western red cedar, toluene diisocyanate
Airway irritation, including nonspecific hyperreactivity	Welding fumes, irritant gases
Byssinosis	Cotton and flax processing
Extrinsic allergic alveolitis	Wood dust, diisocyanates
Toxic pneumonitis	Cadmium, oxides of nitrogen
Pleural effusion	Asbestos
Chronic Disorders	
Interstitial diseases (pneumoconioses)	Silicates, coal dust
Granulomatous disease	Beryllium
Chronic bronchitis	Metal dusts, coal dust
Chronic pleural diseases	
Pleural thickening or rounded atelectasis	Asbestos
Diffuse malignant mesothelioma	Asbestos
Carcinoma	
Upper respiratory tract	Chromium, nickel, hardwood dust
Bronchogenic	Coal tar pitch volatiles, asbestos, arsenic

TABLE 49.3. OCCUPATIONAL HEMATOLOGIC DISORDERS

Condition	Examples of Associated Exposures
Anemia	
Hemolytic	Lead, arsine gas
Hypoproliferative	Benzene
Methemoglobinemia	Nitrites
Stem cell disorders	
Aplastic anemia	Benzene, ionizing radiation
Myeloproliferative disorders	Benzene, ionizing radiation
Acute nonlymphocytic leukemia	Benzene, ionizing radiation
Lymphoproliferative disorders	
Multiple myeloma	Ionizing radiation

TABLE 49.4. OCCUPATIONAL RHEUMATOLOGIC DISORDERS

Condition	Examples of Associated Exposures
Local Disorders	
Raynaud's phenomenon	Vibration, vinyl chloride monomer
Neurovascular compression	Repetitive trauma
Degenerative arthritis	Repetitive trauma
Periarticular disorder	Repetitive trauma
Dupuytren's contracture	Repetitive trauma
Aseptic necrosis	Diving (hypobaric trauma)
Systemic Disorders	
Scleroderma	Coal dust
Acro-osteolysis	Vinyl chloride monomer
Metabolic bone diseases	Fluorine, phosphorus
Diffuse arthralgias, myalgias	Lead
Gout	Lead

TABLE 49.5. OCCUPATIONAL DISORDERS OF THE KIDNEY AND BLADDER

Condition	Examples of Associated Exposures
Acute Renal Disease	
Tubulointerstitial	Carbon tetrachloride
Tubulointerstitial (indirect injury)	Arsine gas, heat
Glomerular	Organic solvents, mercury
Chronic Renal Disease	
Tubulointerstitial	Cadmium, lead
Glomerular	Lead, mercury
Bladder Disease	
Bladder dysfunction (sacral neuropathy)	DMAPM (dimethylaminopropionitrile)
Bladder carcinoma	Benzidine

TABLE 49.6. OCCUPATIONAL GASTROINTESTINAL DISORDERS

Condition	Examples of Associated Exposures
Nonmalignant Liver Disease	
Acute/subacute hepatocellular injury	Carbon tetrachloride, dimethylformamide
Acute cholestatic hepatitis	Methylenedianiline
Chronic persistent hepatitis	Polychlorinated biphenyls
Granulomatous hepatitis	Beryllium
Hepatoportal sclerosis	Arsenic, vinyl chloride monomer
Neoplasms	
Gastric and esophageal	Asbestos
Colon and rectum	Asbestos
Hepatoma	Arsenic, vinyl chloride monomer
Angiosarcoma (liver)	Arsenic, vinyl chloride monomer

TABLE 49.7. OCCUPATIONAL DISORDERS OF THE NERVOUS SYSTEM

Condition	Examples of Associated Exposures
Central Nervous System	
Acute toxic encephalopathy	Organic solvents, manganese
Chronic encephalopathy	Lead, carbon disulfide
Parkinsonian movement disorder	Manganese
Peripheral Nervous System	
Toxic polyneuropathy	N-hexane, lead
Neuromuscular blockade	Organophosphate pesticides
Compression parenchymal mononeuropathy	Repetitive trauma, vibration
Vascular (interstitial) neuropathy	Vibration

TABLE 49.8.	OCCUPATIONAL SKIN DISEASES
Condition	**Examples of Associated Exposures**
Dermatitis	
Irritant contact dermatitis	Detergents, machining fluids
Allergic contact dermatitis	Epoxy resins, nickel
Radiodermatitis	Ionizing radiation
Occupational Acne	
Oil acne and folliculitis	Oil mist, grease
Acne mechanica	Friction, pressure
Chloracne	Polychlorinated biphenyls, dioxins
Disorders Of Pigmentation	
Staining of skin and appendages	Methylenedianiline
Hyperpigmentation	Silver
Hypopigmentation	Quinones
Neoplastic Disorders	
Squamous cell carcinoma	Mineral oils, arsenic
Basal cell carcinoma	Sunlight
Miscellaneous Disorders	
Porphyria cutanea tarda	Polychlorinated biphenyls
Heat-induced lesions	Erythema ab igne
	Miliaria
Cold-induced lesions	Childblains
	Immersion foot
	Frostbite
Lesions induced by ultraviolet radiation	Sunburn
	Delayed actinic changes

BIBLIOGRAPHY

Bernstein IL, Chan-Yeung M, Malo JL, Bernstein DI, eds. *Asthma in the workplace.* New York: Marcel Dekker, 1993.

Cullen MR, Cherniack, MG, Rosenstock L. Medical progress: occupational medicine. *N Engl J Med* 1990;322:594.

Harber P, Schenker MB, Balmes JR. *Occupational and environmental respiratory disease.* St. Louis: CV Mosby, 1996.

Institute of Medicine. *Role of the primary care physician in occupational and environmental medicine.* Washington, DC: National Academy Press, 1988.

Ladou J. *Occupational & Environmental medicine,* second ed. Norwalk, CT: Appleton & Lange, 1998.

Levy BS, Wegman DH. *Occupational health: recognizing and preventing work-related disease,* third ed. Boston: Little, Brown, 1995.

Moore PV. Taking an exposure history. The Agency for Toxic Substances and Disease Registry. *AAOHN J* 1995;43(7):380–394.

Parkes WR. *Occupational lung disorders.* third ed. Oxford: Butterworth-Heinemann, 1994.

Redlich CA, Beckett WS, Sparer J, et al. Liver disease associated with occupational exposure to the solvent dimethylformamide. *Ann Intern Med* 1988;108:680–686.

Rom WN. *Environmental and occupational medicine,* third ed. New York: Lippincott-Raven, 1998.

Rosenstock L, Cullen MR. *Textbook of clinical occupational and environmental medicine.* Philadelphia: WB Saunders, 1994.

Rosenstock L, Hagopian A. Ethical dilemmas in providing health care to workers. *Ann Intern Med* 1987;107:575–580.

Zenz C., Dickerson OB, Horvath EP. *Occupational medicine,* third ed. St Louis: CV Mosby, 1994.

Kelley's Textbook of Internal Medicine, fourth edition. Edited by H. David Humes. Lippincott Williams & Wilkins, Philadelphia © 2000.

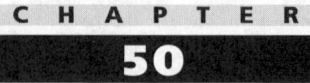

CHAPTER 50

MEDICAL OPHTHALMOLOGY

MICHELE R. PICCONE
STUART L. FINE

INTERPRETATION OF COMMON OCULAR SYMPTOMS

Important ocular symptoms include reduced vision, ocular pain, and redness. Any disturbance of vision requires immediate evaluation. The rapidity of onset, the involvement of one or both eyes, and the determination of whether central or peripheral vision is affected are key historical points. Typically, patients with long-standing poor vision in one eye do not notice any visual impairment until the better eye is occluded.

Acute monocular visual loss may be transient or permanent. *Amaurosis fugax* refers to transient visual loss in one eye that can signify retinal embolic disease from the heart or carotids and can precede central or branch retinal artery occlusion. Giant cell arteritis should be considered in elderly patients with amaurosis fugax. Giant cell arteritis can cause sudden and permanent loss of vision as a result of compromised blood flow to the optic nerve or retina. Prompt treatment with systemic corticosteroids may prevent vision loss in the fellow eye.

Other important ocular symptoms include light flashes (photopsia) and floaters, which may signify a retinal tear, detachment, or vitreous hemorrhage. Distortion of vision (metamorphopsia) can be caused by subretinal fluid or blood from many causes. Binocular diplopia results from eye muscle imbalance caused by neurologic or muscular disorders or by mechanical misalignment of the globes.

The character of ocular pain or irritation can help elucidate the cause. Foreign body sensation results from ocular surface abnormalities such as dry eyes, foreign bodies, conjunctivitis, and herpes simplex keratitis. Burning and itching result from dryness or allergy. Aching or throbbing signifies a deeper process such as intraocular inflammation or elevated intraocular pressure.

Headaches and dizziness rarely have an identifiable ocular basis.

EVALUATION OF THE RED EYE

Redness of one or both eyes is common and can result from mild, superficial disorders with little effect on vision or from

TABLE 50.1.	COMMON SYMPTOMS AND SIGNS OF THE RED EYE			
	Acute Conjunctivitis	Acute Iritis	Acute Keratitis	Acute Angle-Closure Glaucoma
Symptoms				
Incidence	Very common	Common	Common	Uncommon
Vision	Normal	Blurred	Blurred	Markedly blurred
Pain	Mild	Moderate–severe	Moderate–severe	Severe
Photophobia	None–mild	Moderate–severe	Moderate–severe	Moderate
Discharge	Moderate–copious	None	Moderate	None
Halos	None	None	Present	Present
Signs				
Conjunctival hyperemia	Diffusely present	Localized to perilimbal area	Diffusely present	Diffusely present
Pupil abnormalities	None	Small, poorly responsive	Normal	Fixed and moderately dilated
Intraocular pressure	Normal	Low, normal, or high	Normal	High
Corneal epithelial defect	None	None	May be present	None
Corneal opacity	None	None	Local or diffuse	Diffuse
Shallow-anterior chamber	None	None	None	Present
Preauricular lymph node	May be present	None	None	None

severe, deeper problems with profound effect on vision. The redness is nonspecific and results from hyperemia of the conjunctival, episcleral or scleral vessels, which can be caused by inflammatory or infectious processes of the conjunctiva, sclera, cornea, iris, ciliary body, or periocular adnexa (Table 50.1).

Extreme caution should be exercised in prescribing topical corticosteroids for a red eye. Corticosteroids can mask worsening of the disease process, suppress immunity to infectious diseases, raise intraocular pressure, and cause cataracts.

Topical anesthetics should never be dispensed because they are toxic to the cornea, can cause allergic reactions, and can mask the pain of underlying ocular disease.

Contact lens wearers have a higher risk for corneal infections. Thus, a red eye in a contact lens wearer requires special attention.

Any patient who exhibits worsening of symptoms or decreasing visual acuity despite treatment should be referred to an ophthalmologist.

OCULAR TRAUMA

Corneal abrasions can be diagnosed by topical application of fluorescein dye, which stains the denuded corneal epithelial basement membrane. The abrasion appears green when viewed with a cobalt blue light (Fig. 50.1) Corneal abrasions usually are treated with topical antibiotics and cycloplegic agents. In general, small abrasions heal quickly. Large epithelial defects can be patched and monitored daily until healing is complete. Patients generally are more comfortable when the eye is patched, but patching should not be used in corneal abrasions related to contact lens wear or those caused by organic matter (e.g., a thorn or tree branch). The cornea is compromised until the epithelial defect is resolved and should be observed frequently for infection.

The eyelids should be everted and inspected for foreign bodies when foreign body sensation or corneal abrasions are present.

All chemical injuries should be irrigated immediately and copiously with any neutral fluid. Alkali injuries have the worst prognosis because of their rapid corneal penetration.

Hyphema (blood in the anterior chamber) usually results from blunt trauma and frequently coexists with other serious ocular injury (e.g., retinal detachment, lens dislocation, ruptured globe, glaucoma). Hyphema should be treated by an ophthalmologist.

Lacerations of the eyelid margin should be referred to an ophthalmologist for surgical repair. Inaccurate reapproximation of the eyelid margin can result in a permanent eyelid notch with subsequent chronic ocular irritation.

Any ocular injury caused by a sharp object or high-velocity

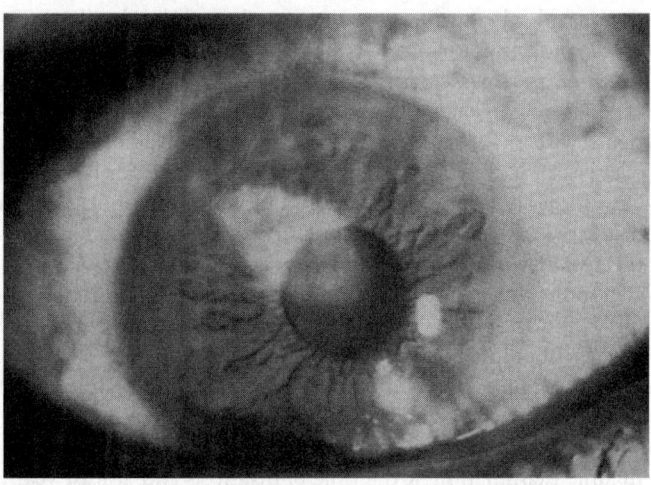

FIGURE 50.1. Neovascularization of the disc and retina.

missile is reason for a high suspicion for a ruptured globe or an intraocular foreign body. Such injuries should be assessed fully and immediately by an ophthalmologist.

OCULAR MANIFESTATIONS OF AIDS

Cytomegalovirus retinopathy causes retinal necrosis. It occurs in 30% of patients with AIDS and is the most common, severe, blinding ocular infection. Intravenous ganciclovir can slow the spread of the infection but does not eradicate the virus; 50% of patients have reactivation despite low-dose maintenance therapy.

Other ocular infections associated with AIDS include herpes simplex retinitis, *Toxoplasma* retinitis, *Pneumocystis carinii* choroiditis, herpes zoster ophthalmicus, and molluscum contagiosum of the eyelids.

Kaposi's sarcoma, a multifocal vascular neoplasm, can affect the conjunctiva, the eyelid margins, and, rarely, the orbit. When Kaposi's sarcoma involves the conjunctiva, it can be mistaken for a subconjunctival hemorrhage. Burkitt's lymphoma can develop in the orbit, causing proptosis with damage to the extraocular muscles and cranial nerves.

Neuro-ophthalmic disturbances, including cranial nerve palsies, papilledema, optic atrophy, and visual field defects, can develop in patients with AIDS. They result from intracranial neoplasms and infectious processes.

DIABETES AND THE EYE

Diabetes can cause retinopathy, glaucoma, an altered refractive state, and cataracts. Diabetic retinopathy is the leading cause of blindness in people younger than 60 years of age in the United States. The likelihood of developing retinopathy increases with the duration of the disease. After 20 years' duration, nearly all patients with type I diabetes have some retinopathy. Patients with type II diabetes may have retinopathy at the time of diagnosis.

Retinopathy can be nonproliferative or proliferative. Nonproliferative retinopathy includes microaneurysms, intraretinal dot and blot hemorrhages, cotton-wool spots, hard yellow exudates, and intraretinal microangiopathy. Proliferative retinopathy refers to neovascularization of the disc and retina (Fig. 50.2), vitreous hemorrhage, and retinal detachment. Vision loss in patients with diabetic retinopathy is most often due to macular edema or vitreous hemorrhage. Macular edema can be treated with focal laser photocoagulation. Proliferative retinopathy can be treated with panretinal laser photocoagulation, which reduces the risk of vitreous hemorrhage from neovascularization.

Proliferative retinopathy typically is asymptomatic until vitreous hemorrhage develops. Because laser treatment can reduce severe visual loss by 50% to 90%, patients with diabetes must undergo regular eye examinations through dilated pupils by an ophthalmologist.

Patients with type II diabetes should have a complete ophthalmic examination at the time of diagnosis and at least yearly thereafter. Patients with type I diabetes should undergo an eye

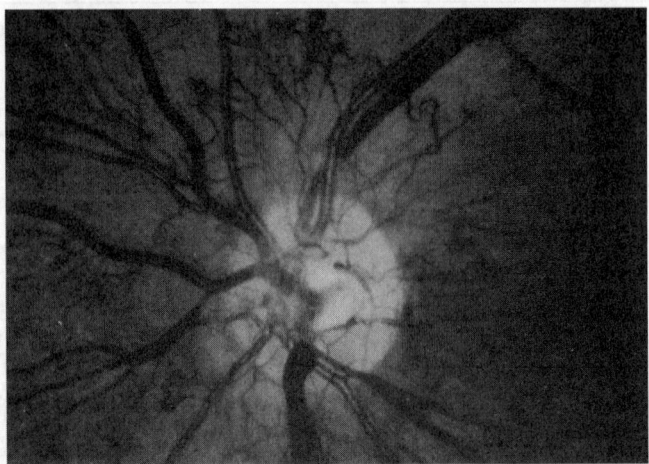

FIGURE 50.2. Corneal abrasion. See color figure 50.2.

examination 5 years after diagnosis and then annually unless and until the severity of retinopathy mandates either more frequent assessment or laser treatment. Forty percent of patients with severe nonproliferative diabetic retinopathy progress to proliferative diabetic retinopathy within 1 year. Pregnant patients with type I diabetes should be examined in the first trimester and every 3 months thereafter because pregnancy can accelerate retinopathy. Ideally, women with diabetes who are planning a pregnancy should undergo a baseline examination before conception. Diabetic blindness is largely preventable.

GLAUCOMA

Glaucoma is a progressive optic neuropathy characterized by cupping of the optic nerve head, irreversible visual field loss, and, usually, elevated abnormal intraocular pressure.

Increased intraocular pressure can result from impaired outflow of aqueous through the anterior chamber angle (open-angle glaucoma) or impaired access of aqueous to the drainage system (closed-angle glaucoma). Treatment is directed toward reducing the intraocular pressure and, when possible, correcting the underlying mechanism.

Chronic open-angle glaucoma accounts for 80% to 85% of all glaucoma. Risk factors are older age, diabetes, family history, myopia, and black race.

Because 25% to 30% of patients with glaucoma have normal intraocular pressures (21.5 mm Hg or lower) on initial presentation, evaluation of the optic nerve and visual field is essential for detection.

AGE-RELATED MACULAR DEGENERATION

Age-related macular degeneration (AMD) is the leading cause of severe vision loss in the Western hemisphere. Age over 65 years, a positive family history, and a history of cardiovascular disease are important risk factors. The condition is rare in blacks.

In the early stage of AMD, characterized by drusen, there typically are no symptoms. *Drusen* are yellow-white deposits behind the retina. Drusen identify an eye at risk for vision loss. Visual symptoms include blurred vision, distortion, and a blank spot in the field of vision. Of those patients with AMD who have visual impairment, 80% have the atrophic or dry form and 20% have the neovascular/exudative or wet form. The neovascular form of AMD results from leakage from abnormal choroidal blood vessels that cause macular detachment. Laser treatment is helpful in selected patients with the neovascular form of AMD.

BIBLIOGRAPHY

American College of Physicians, American Diabetes Association, American Academy of Ophthalmology. Screening guidelines for diabetic retinopathy: clinical guidelines. *Ophthalmology* 1992;99:1626.

Berson FG. *Basic ophthalmology for medical students and primary care residents,* sixth ed. San Francisco: American Academy of Ophthalmology, 1993.

Brown G, ed. *Current concepts in ophthalmology, ocular emergencies,* vol 3. Harrisburg, PA: Pennsylvania Academy of Ophthalmology, 1995.

Diabetic Retinopathy Study Group. Photocoagulation treatment of proliferative diabetic retinopathy study (DRS) findings. *Ophthalmology* 1981; 88:583–600.

Early Treatment Diabetic Retinopathy Study Research Group. Photocoagulation for diabetic macular edema. *Arch Ophthalmol* 1985;103: 1796–1806.

Gold DH, Weingeist TA. *The eye in systemic disease.* Philadelphia: JB Lippincott, 1990.

Jabs DA, Green WR, Fox R, et al. Ocular manifestations of acquired immunodeficiency syndrome. *Ophthalmology* 1989;96:1092–1099.

Spalton DJ, Hitchings RA, Hunter PA. Atlas of clinical ophthalmology. Philadelphia: *JB Lippincott,* 1984.

Kelley's Textbook of Internal Medicine, fourth edition. Edited by H. David Humes. Lippincott Williams & Wilkins, Philadelphia © 2000.

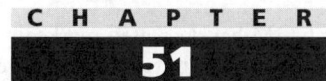

CHAPTER 51

MEDICAL OTOLARYNGOLOGY

ERICA R. THALER
DAVID W. KENNEDY

Although otolaryngology is a surgical subspecialty, much of the field involves nonsurgical treatment of patients. This chapter reviews the medical management of common otolaryngologic disorders, including infections, neoplasms, and emergencies.

■ COMMON OTOLARYNGOLOGIC INFECTIONS

ACUTE OTITIS MEDIA

Definition

Acute otitis media (AOM) is a bacterial or viral infection of the middle ear cleft that occurs with rapid onset and resolves within 1 month. It involves the collection of either purulent or serous fluid in the middle ear.

Incidence and Epidemiology

AOM is most prevalent in the pediatric population, affecting at least 2 million children younger than 3 years of age each year. The incidence peaks in the latter half of the first year of life and falls off dramatically after the first decade. Epidemiologic studies suggest that bottle feeding, smoking in the household, and exposure to large day care facilities increase the incidence of AOM.

Etiology and Pathogenesis

The cause of AOM is multifactorial. Underlying predisposing factors include eustachian tube dysfunction, inadequate aeration of the middle ear cleft, and immunologic immaturity or deficiency. A combination of these and other factors leads to inadequate drainage of fluid from the middle ear space with subsequent viral or bacterial infection. The most common bacteria involved are *Streptococcus pneumoniae, Haemophilus influenzae, Moraxella catarrhalis,* and *Streptococcus pyogenes.* Neonates are more commonly infected by *Staphylococcus aureus* and gram-negative enteric bacilli.

Clinical Findings

Typical clinical findings of AOM are a history of increased irritability, poor oral intake, tugging at the ears, ear pain, and fever. Older children and adults may relate a history of decreased hearing. Generalized symptoms of an upper respiratory tract infection (e.g., rhinorrhea, cough) may be present. A history of imbalance may be elicited. On examination, the auricle and external auditory canal are normal in appearance early in the disease course. The tympanic membrane is thickened, inflamed, bulging, and poorly mobile. Later, perforation may be noted with purulent drainage emanating from the middle ear. Signs and symptoms of complications of AOM include a bulging, doughy, and tender mastoid area, picket-fence fever, mental status changes, and signs of meningeal irritation.

Laboratory Findings

Although laboratory studies are unnecessary in making the diagnosis of AOM, a leukocytosis may be noted. Concern about a possible complication of AOM warrants a contrast-enhanced computed tomographic (CT) scan.

Optimal Management

Evidence suggests that most cases of AOM will resolve spontaneously without antibiotics. However, to treat patients whose AOM will not resolve without intervention and to prevent complications, antibiotic therapy is recommended. First-line therapy for AOM involves a 10-day course of either amoxicillin or trimethoprim-sulfamethoxazole. If these are not successful, broader-spectrum β-lactamase–resistant antibiotics may be necessary. These include amoxicillin-clavulanate, cefaclor, erythromycin-sulfasoxazole, and cefixime. The incidence of β-lactamase–producing pathogens (now 10% to 30%) is rising and may require more aggressive initial antimicrobial regimens. Culture-directed therapy is not necessary for most cases, but may be required for a recalcitrant case or one involving an immunocompromised patient.

OTITIS EXTERNA

Definition

Otitis externa is an infection of the external auditory canal that can be bacterial, fungal, or viral. It typically involves only the skin lining the canal, although cellulitis may extend out onto the auricle. An uncommon variant, malignant otitis externa, is a more severe infection that typically occurs in older patients and involves osteitis of the temporal bone.

Incidence and Epidemiology

Known in the vernacular as "swimmer's ear," otitis externa is more common in warm, humid climates. Maceration of the skin lining the canal from water or trauma to the ear canal predisposes to infection. Malignant otitis externa is more common in elderly, diabetic, and immunosuppressed patients.

Etiology and Pathogenesis

Penetration of the skin lining the canal occurs secondary to a break in the protective cerumen. Edema of the canal and bacterial overgrowth and invasion by virulent organisms then occur. This progression often is assisted by trauma to the canal. The most common bacterial pathogens are *Pseudomonas, S. aureus,* and various anaerobes. The most common fungal pathogen is *Aspergillus.* Malignant otitis externa is caused by *Pseudomonas aeruginosa.*

Clinical Findings

Patients with otitis externa experience a sensation of obstruction. Hearing may be diminished, depending on the degree of inflammation. Pain can be severe, and tragal tenderness is a hallmark sign. The ear canal is edematous and inflamed, often with purulent discharge. The tympanic membrane may not be visible. Cellulitis of the auricle may be present. If the infection is fungal, a white, cottonlike mass may be seen. Malignant otitis externa typically involves granulation tissue, poor response to local therapy, and unremitting pain, particularly at night.

Laboratory Findings

The diagnosis of external otitis is based on the history and physical examination. Occasionally, cultures of purulent discharge help direct antibiotic therapy. If malignant otitis externa is suspected, a CT scan of the temporal bone should be obtained to assess bone destruction. A gallium 67 radionuclide scan will demonstrate osteitis and may be used to follow the course of the disease to determine the duration of antibiotic therapy.

Optimal Management

Treatment of uncomplicated external otitis is directed at drying and acidifying the canal. Many combination topical drops are available, which usually include a topical corticosteroid (dexamethasone or hydrocortisone) and an antimicrobial agent (neomycin, polymyxin, tobramycin, clotrimazole, or nystatin). Placement of a wick into the external auditory canal may be necessary for the drops to penetrate the length of the canal. Excessive debris should be removed. Oral antibiotic therapy is reserved for patients with cellulitis or immunosuppression or for those in whom coexisting otitis media is suspected. When required, ciprofloxacin is a good first-line oral agent because it is effective against both *Pseudomonas* and *Staphylococcus.* Malignant otitis externa should be treated with intravenous antibiotics to cover *Pseudomonas* (aminoglycosides have been used traditionally; fluoroquinolones more recently). Surgery to debride granulation tissue or sequestered cartilage and bone may be necessary.

CHRONIC OTITIS MEDIA

Definition

Chronic otitis media (COM) is defined as inflammation or infection of the middle ear cleft and mastoid air cells of more than 1 months' duration. It may involve simply a persistent serous effusion that will not clear despite antibiotic therapy. COM also may involve cholesteatoma, an epithelial ingrowth into the middle ear that proliferates and invades bone.

Incidence and Epidemiology

The incidence of COM has decreased markedly in the last half-century. This usually is attributed to the advent of multiple broad-spectrum antibiotics used to treat AOM and to the widespread use of pressure-equalization tubes to treat serous otitis media and eustachian tube dysfunction.

Etiology and Pathogenesis

Chronic otitis media can be considered along a continuum of middle ear disease that begins with AOM. Many of the same factors that cause AOM lead to COM (eustachian tube dysfunction, mucosal abnormality of the middle ear, immunologic deficiency). These abnormalities may result in the most mild form of COM, serous otitis media. The normal secretions of the middle ear mucosa are not drained properly and thus fill the middle ear cleft. Alternatively, cholesteatoma may result. Cholesteatoma arises from the ingrowth of epithelial tissue, typically into the middle ear. Retraction of the tympanic membrane secondary to eustachian tube dysfunction or perforation of the tympanic membrane may initiate this process. Secondary infection of the desquamated material then occurs. Organisms involved in COM include staphylococci, *P. aeruginosa, Proteus,* streptococci, and anaerobes. Cholesteatoma causes bony erosion of both ossicles

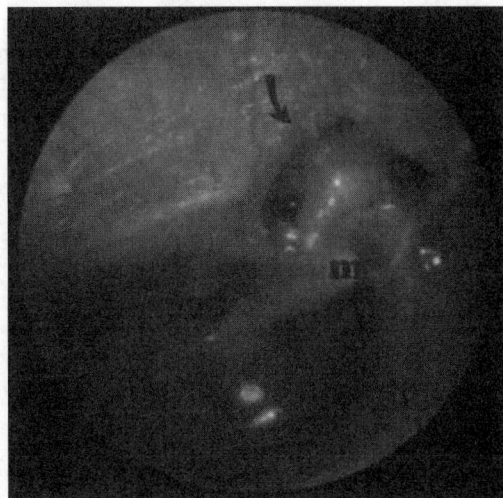

FIGURE 51.1. Otoscopic photograph of right tympanic membrane with large attic retraction pocket causing erosion of the bony external auditory canal. A serous effusion is also present. *m*, malleus short process. See color figure 51.1.

and the temporal bone. This is due to the production of bone-resorbing enzymes or endogenous mediators such as prostaglandin E_2 and interleukin-1.

Clinical Findings

Typical clinical findings of patients with COM range from decreased hearing to purulent and foul-smelling drainage from the ear. Vertigo or unsteadiness may be present, particularly if cholesteatoma has violated the vestibular labyrinth. Otalgia generally is not present and may be a sign of impending intracranial complication. On examination, the normal architecture of the tympanic membrane rarely is found intact. Serous effusion is identified by a retracted tympanic membrane that is poorly mobile and has fluid behind it. Air bubbles may be noted. The presence of unilateral serous otitis media in an adult always should raise the question of a possible nasopharyngeal mass causing eustachian tube dysfunction, and nasopharyngoscopy must be performed. Perforation, retraction pockets, erosion of the ossicles or external auditory canal, purulent discharge, chronic external otitis, and the pearly white cholesteatoma matrix may be visible (Fig. 51.1).

Laboratory Findings

Tuning forks and audiometric testing invariably reveal some degree of conductive loss. Sensorineural loss also may be present. CT scanning may be helpful in determining the extent of bony erosion, particularly invasion of the labyrinth and erosion through to dura.

Optimal Management

Management of COM includes 6 to 8 weeks of antibiotics to prevent recurrent AOM. If, after this time, resolution has not occurred, myringotomy is performed and a pressure-equalization tube may be placed to prevent recurrence. Management of more advanced COM includes systemic antibiotic therapy directed by culture of discharge from the middle ear and topical antibiotic drops. Surgery (some form of tympanomastoidectomy) is necessary to improve aeration of the middle ear, debride infected granulation tissue, and remove cholesteatoma. Intravenous antibiotic therapy may be necessary to treat osteitis of the temporal bone.

SINUSITIS

Definition

Sinusitis is inflammation of the mucous membrane of the paranasal sinuses. Viral sinusitis occurs frequently with upper respiratory tract infections and is self-limiting. Bacterial or fungal sinusitis can be acute or chronic (greater than 12 weeks). Sinusitis frequently is associated with a rhinitis, and to designate this, replacement of both terms with rhinosinusitis is now recommended.

Incidence and Epidemiology

Rhinosinusitis is the most common health care complaint in the United States, affecting more than 31 million people per year. Although typically considered a disease of adult life, rhinosinusitis recently has gained recognition in the pediatric age group.

Etiology and Pathogenesis

The most immediate cause of rhinosinusitis is a disruption of mucociliary drainage of the sinuses. This may be the result of mucosal disease from an upper respiratory tract infection, environmental factors, pollution, or allergies, or it may be due to an underlying anatomical obstruction or narrowing. Pathogens of acute sinusitis include *S. pneumoniae, S. aureus, S. pyogenes,* and *H. influenzae.* Chronic sinusitis frequently is polymicrobial and associated with *Bacteroides* and other anaerobes, *Pseudomonas, Staphylococcus, H. influenzae,* and *Streptococcus viridans.* The incidence of gram-negative chronic sinusitis appears to be increasing significantly. The most common fungus found in sinusitis is *Aspergillus,* but many fungi can be pathogenic.

Clinical Findings

Patients with acute rhinosinusitis complain of pain referred from the involved sinuses, nasal obstruction, purulent nasal discharge, and fever. A history of viral rhinitis, allergic rhinitis, or nasal polyposis may be elicited. The nasal mucosa is edematous and erythematous. If nasal endoscopy is performed, purulent discharge may be seen emanating from the middle meatus along the lateral nasal wall or around the eustachian tube orifice. The presentation of chronic rhinosinusitis is more subtle and difficult to diagnose. Nasal congestion, nasal obstruction, postnasal drip, chronic cough, and headache are among the most common complaints. Nasal endoscopy may reveal abnormal, boggy mucosa and mucopurulent discharge from the middle meatus or spheno-ethmoid recess or the presence of nasal or middle meatal polyps.

Laboratory Findings

The diagnosis of rhinosinusitis is based on the history and physical examination. In acute rhinosinusitis, initial therapy is empiric, but antral puncture and aspiration for culture is a consideration in patients who do not demonstrate early response to therapy or in those who are immunocompromised. In chronic rhinosinusitis, cultures of purulent discharge are helpful as a guide for antibiotic therapy. Traditional sinus radiography is of limited use because it demonstrates the maxillary and frontal sinuses only moderately well and provides poor information with regard to the ethmoid sinuses. A coronal CT scan through the sinuses confirms the presence of mucosal disease and may help to elucidate predisposing anatomical abnormalities.

Optimal Management

Management of rhinosinusitis is predominantly medical. Oral antibiotics and decongestants provide the first-line management of acute rhinosinusitis. Antihistamines are indicated when allergy is a component of the illness. In choosing an antibiotic for the treatment of acute rhinosinusitis, the increasing incidence of resistant *Pseudomonas* and of β-lactamase–producing *H. influenzae* must be borne in mind. A 10- to 14-day course is recommended. In chronic rhinosinusitis, the duration of antibiotic therapy may need to be significantly longer. Topical corticosteroids also are helpful in reducing edema in chronic disease. For refractory chronic rhinosinusitis, a course of oral corticosteroids may help to reduce mucosal edema and shrink nasal polyps (Fig. 51.2). Surgery is reserved for disease that is refractory to medical therapy. Endoscopic sinus surgery involves opening the sinuses,

particularly in the areas surrounding their ostia, and correcting any anatomical abnormalities impairing mucociliary drainage. In occasional cases, long-term intravenous antibiotic therapy may be necessary to eradicate the osteitis that can accompany long-standing sinusitis.

EPIGLOTTITIS AND CROUP
Definition

Both epiglottitis and croup are infections of the upper airway tract, which can rapidly result in respiratory compromise. Epiglottitis is a bacterial infection of the supraglottic airway. Croup is a viral infection predominantly of the subglottic airway, otherwise known as laryngotracheobronchitis.

Incidence and Epidemiology

Croup typically affects children younger than 5 years of age. Until recently, epiglottitis occurred most commonly in children 2 to 4 years of age, but with the advent of the vaccination for *H. influenzae* type B, the incidence is shifting toward the adult population. Both infections occur most commonly during the winter.

Etiology and Pathogenesis

Croup typically is caused by the parainfluenza virus (types 1 and 3). Influenza A virus, rhinovirus, and respiratory syncytial virus also have been implicated. Despite the vaccine, epiglottitis still is caused most often by *H. influenzae* type B.

Clinical Findings

A patient with croup typically has signs and symptoms of an upper respiratory tract infection, including a low-grade fever

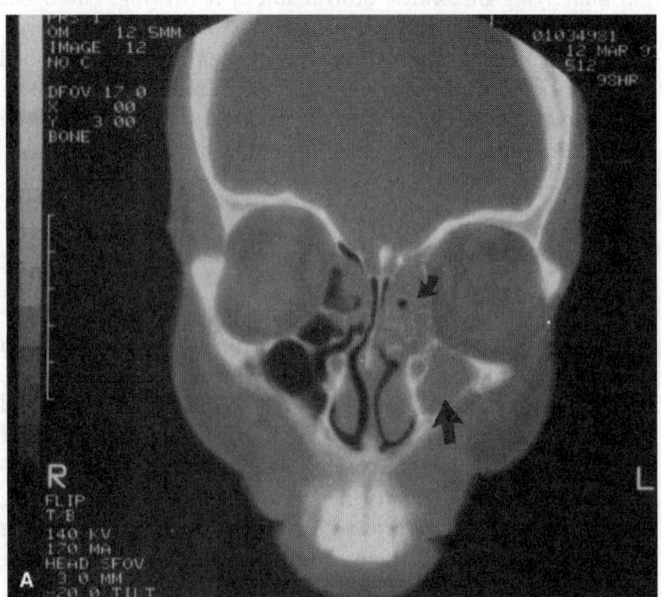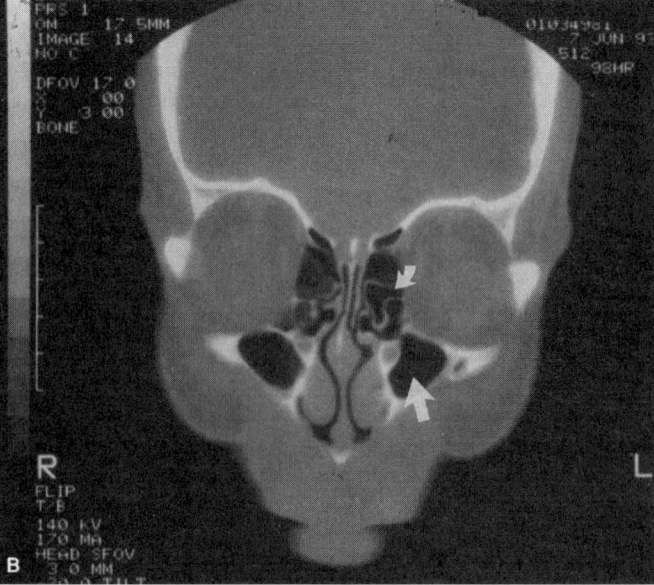

FIGURE 51.2. Before **(A)** and after **(B)** aggressive medical management of chronic left ethmoid (*curved arrow*) and maxillary sinusitis (*large arrow*). (Photographs, courtesy of Donald C. Lanza, MD.)

followed by the gradual onset of a barking, nonproductive cough. Edema of the glottic and subglottic airway leads to stridor, increased work of breathing, and costal retractions. Epiglottitis has a more rapid onset with high spiking fevers and the development of severe odynophagia and dysphagia, often with drooling. "Hot-potato" or muffled speech is present. Stridor develops with the progression of supraglottic edema. Patients have difficulty lying supine secondary to airway obstruction from edematous and inward collapsing aryepiglottic folds. Complete airway obstruction can develop rapidly. Examination of a child with epiglottitis should be extremely limited because agitation can contribute to airway compromise.

Laboratory Findings

In croup, a posteroanterior neck radiograph reveals a "steeple sign" in the subglottic airway with pinpoint narrowing just beneath the glottis. In a patient with recurrent croup, the subglottic area must be evaluated closely for structural abnormalities such as subglottic stenosis, cysts, or hemangiomas. Epiglottitis can be identified on lateral neck radiography by supraglottic edema (hazy, ill-defined structures) or the classic "thumbprint sign" of a swollen epiglottis. Patients with epiglottitis have a greater leukocytosis, and one-third have blood cultures that are positive for *H. influenzae*.

Optimal Management

Assessing the need for and securing the patient's airway are of paramount importance in both epiglottitis and croup. In epiglottitis, some form of airway intervention typically is performed. In croup, however, careful observation and medical therapy may suffice. For a child, airway management may require intubation in the operating room by an anesthesiologist with an otolaryngologist present to perform emergency tracheotomy, if necessary. In an adult, if the patient is cooperative, awake fiberoptic nasal intubation or an awake tracheotomy is the safest means of securing the airway. Croup is treated with racemic epinephrine and corticosteroids to reduce edema and with humidified oxygen to assist in thinning secretions. Epiglottitis is treated with intravenous antibiotics effective against *Haemophilus influenzae*. β-Lactamase–resistant cephalosporins such as cefuroxime or ceftriaxone are excellent first-line agents.

PERIPHERAL VESTIBULAR DISORDERS

Definition

Peripheral vestibular disorders include pathologic condition of the sensory labyrinth or vestibular nerve, leading to a disruption in the patient's sense of balance, which may range in severity from a vague sense of unsteadiness to whirling vertigo. These disorders may be further classified by the cause of the disruption in balance, including trauma, viral or bacterial infection, exposure to ototoxic drugs, autoimmune disorders, and neoplasm.

Incidence and Epidemiology

Dizziness is a common complaint, affecting 90 million Americans each year. It is unknown what percentage of these patients has peripheral vestibular disorders. In general, younger patients are more likely to have peripheral vestibular problems, and older patients are more likely to have central causes to their dizziness.

Etiology and Pathogenesis

There is a myriad of peripheral causes to the subjective sense of imbalance. These include head trauma, resulting in basilar skull fracture or labyrinthine concussion; perilymph fistula, in which there is leakage of the perilymph outside the membranous labyrinth; infection, either viral or bacterial, typically the result of otitis media; ototoxic drugs, including many of the aminoglycosides, and aspirin products; neoplasm, most commonly acoustic neuroma of the vestibular portion of the eighth nerve; and autoimmune disease, including many of the common collagen vascular diseases.

Clinical Findings

A careful history and otoscopic and cranial nerve examinations are critical in determining the cause of balance disorders. The sudden onset of vertigo without change in hearing after a viral infection may suggest viral labyrinthitis. Benign positional vertigo is suggested by a temporary whirling vertigo elicited by certain head positions. Acuity of onset, frequency, duration, and quality are important in identifying the underlying cause. Episodic vertigo associated with episodic hearing loss and tinnitus suggest Menière's syndrome.

A positive positional maneuver such ad Hallpike's test suggest benign paroxysmal positional vertigo. Nystagmus, if present, should be characterized. Fixation-suppressed, horizontal nystagmus is suggestive of an acute-onset peripheral balance disorder. Peripheral cranial nerve deficits, particularly hearing loss (VIII), facial nerve weakness (VII), or sensory loss of the ear canal (V) will help localize the side and site of pathology and may be suggestive of neoplasm.

Laboratory Findings

Routine blood studies may be helpful in determining the etiology of a peripheral balance disorder, but should be ordered judiciously, based on a suggestive history or physical exam. Balance function testing, including electronystagmography, posturography, and rotational chair testing, combine to elucidate whether the balance problem is peripheral or central, the side and even site of the pathology, and whether there has been compensation. An audiometric assessment of the patient's hearing complements these tests. If there is concern about a central etiology, magnetic resonance imaging (MRI) is the radiographic study of choice. Magnetic resonance angiography may be added if there is special concern about vascular compromise.

Optimal Management

Management very much depends on the cause of the peripheral balance disorder. For acute-onset vertigo, meclizine (12.5 to 25 mg three times daily) may be used as an oral vestibulosuppressant. However, this should be tapered as quickly as possible because it may impede the patient's compensation. For many peripheral balance disorders, vestibular rehabilitation or physical therapy aimed at helping the body compensate for the particular vestibular weakness, has proved very effective. This is particularly true for benign paroxysmal positional vertigo, in which a specific positioning maneuver (Epply's maneuver) may be curative. Certain peripheral vestibular disorders have specific treatments, such as diuretics and sodium restriction for Menière's syndrome. Rarely, surgical ablation of some or all of peripheral vestibular neural input may be beneficial when medical therapy or vestibular rehabilitation have failed.

◼ TINNITUS

Definition

Tinnitus is a perceived sound with no external acoustic stimulus. It may be subjective or objective—in the latter case, being audible to the examiner on auscultation. Tinnitus includes a wide variety of noises, ranging from the infrequent high-pitched cricketlike sounds to steady pulsations.

Incidence and Epidemiology

Approximately one-third of the population has at one time or another experienced tinnitus. Only a small percentage of patients have tinnitus that is severe and disabling. Tinnitus almost always accompanies some degree of hearing loss, usually sensorineural.

Etiology and Pathogenesis

Tinnitus that is the product of sensorineural hearing loss may result from cochlear or retrocochlear degeneration. Pulsatile tinnitus may arise from a high-riding jugular bulb, protruding into the middle ear cleft, an arteriovenous malformation, or a glomus tumor. Rapid muscular contractions, of the stapedius muscle, or tensor tympanic and other palatal muscles, may result in a clicklike rapid-fire noise.

Clinical Findings

History and physical examination may elucidate an underlying cause to the tinnitus, for instance, a history of ototoxic drug exposure or head trauma. A glomus tumor or high-riding jugular bulb may be seen on otoscopic examination as a blue mass behind the tympanic membrane. In some cases, pulsatile tinnitus may be objective. The most common physical examination is normal, however, because of the frequent association of tinnitus with sensorineural hearing loss.

Laboratory Findings

Audiometric assessment of a patient with tinnitus is critical. If a hearing loss is unilateral, further investigation of the site of sensorineural hearing loss is warranted to evaluate for retroco-chlear pathology such as tumor. An auditory brain-stem–evoked response (ABR) or MRI are acceptable means of studying this. If a patient's complaints and examination are suggestive of a vascular pathologic condition, magnetic resonance angiography is also important. Serologies are ordered as dictated by a suggestive history. For instance, if the patient has a history of occupational exposure to heavy metals or other industrial pollutants, then screens for these chemicals should be ordered.

Optimal Management

First-line management involves treatment of any underlying cause of tinnitus or sensorineural hearing loss that is reversible, for example, withdrawal of ototoxic drugs such as aspirin. Most often, tinnitus is not treatable. In some circumstances, hearing amplification may help the patient by amplifying external acoustic stimulus out of proportion to the tinnitus. Tinnitus maskers or a variety of other measures may be helpful in enabling the patient contend with tinnitus, including biofeedback, hypnosis, and antidepressant and anxiolytic medications.

◼ HEAD AND NECK CANCER

SQUAMOUS CELL CARCINOMA OF THE UPPER AERODIGESTIVE TRACT

Definition

Epidermoid or squamous cell carcinoma is the most common cancer of the upper aerodigestive tract. It is categorized as keratinizing or nonkeratinizing and arises from squamous mucosa lining the oral cavity, oropharynx, nasopharynx, hypopharynx, and larynx. Even areas of the upper respiratory tract normally covered by pseudostratified columnar epithelium may undergo squamous metaplasia and the subsequent development of squamous cell carcinoma.

Incidence and Epidemiology

Squamous cell carcinoma makes up 90% of oral cavity cancers, 75% of nasopharyngeal cancers, 89% of oropharyngeal and hypopharyngeal cancers, and 71% of laryngeal cancers. These cancers occur more commonly in men, and the average age of onset is 50 to 80 years of age. Synchronous multiple primary tumors occur in about 10% of patients.

Etiology and Pathogenesis

There is a well-known association between the development of squamous cell carcinoma of the upper aerodigestive tract and tobacco and alcohol abuse. Repetitive exposure to these substances is associated with the proliferation of squamous epithelium with premalignant changes, including hyperplasia, keratosis, and dysplasia. Carcinoma in situ develops next in the face of these noxious stimuli. Other known environmental associations include nickel and squamous cell carcinoma of the sinonasal area, eating of betel nuts in squamous cell carcinoma of the oral cavity, and tobacco chewing in squamous cell carcinoma of the gingiva. Metastasis spreads to the cervical nodes first, then to the lungs and liver.

Clinical Findings

Patients have a variety of complaints depending on the location of the lesion. Local pain, persistent hoarseness, foreign body sensation, dysphagia, halitosis, airway compromise, referred otalgia, and trismus are common on presentation. Examination reveals an indurated, tender, often ulcerated lesion. Mobility must be assessed and careful delineation of the submucosal extent of the lesion undertaken. Neck disease may be present on both ipsilateral and contralateral sides. The size of the nodes, skin involvement, and fixation to deep structures should be identified.

Laboratory Findings

A complete set of blood chemistries, blood cell counts, and liver function tests is obtained. Unless otherwise directed by the review of systems or an abnormal blood test result, a chest radiograph is sufficient for metastatic workup before panendoscopy. CT or MRI of the neck should be obtained from the nasopharynx to the clavicles to help define the lesion and identify clinically occult neck disease.

Optimal Management

Management of squamous cell carcinoma of the upper aerodigestive tract is tailored to the site of the lesion and its TNM stage. Surgery and radiation therapy are the primary modalities used, often in combined fashion for advanced tumors. With appropriate multidisciplinary therapy, overall 5-year cure rates are about 65% and can rise to 96% for localized laryngeal tumors. However, oncologic surgery of the head and neck can be functionally and cosmetically debilitating. Careful rehabilitation, psychological support, and close follow-up are critical. Nutritional support is of utmost importance in caring for these patients. Counseling in overcoming alcohol and tobacco addiction also is crucial. Chemotherapeutic protocols are in place for a variety of tumor stages and sites, but are still under investigation.

■ OTOLARYNGOLOGIC EMERGENCIES

IDIOPATHIC SUDDEN SENSORINEURAL HEARING LOSS

Definition

Idiopathic sudden sensorineural hearing loss (ISSNHL) is defined as any sensorineural hearing loss of unknown cause that is instantaneous or occurs within several hours. It is associated with tinnitus in most cases and with vertigo in more than 50% of all cases.

Incidence and Epidemiology

The incidence of ISSNHL is between 5 and 20 per 100,000 population each year. There is no sex predilection. The average age of onset is 46 years. It is most commonly unilateral and occurs most often in the spring.

Etiology and Pathogenesis

Several theories have been proposed to explain ISSNHL. One is that it is the result of a viral infection of the labyrinth. This is supported by evidence of a higher incidence of seroconversion to mumps, rubeola, varicella, cytomegalovirus, and influenza B in patients with ISSNHL compared with control subjects. Another theory is that ISSNHL is of vascular origin. In favor of this theory is the low cochlear tolerance to ischemia. Yamasoba has shown MRI evidence of slow blood flow in the vertebrobasilar system in some patients with ISSNHL. A third theory to explain ISSNHL is the so-called membrane break hypothesis. This suggests that membrane breaks within the inner ear (Reissner's membrane) cause ionic imbalance, allowing admixture of endolymph and perilymph. This imbalance prevents normal transmission of the auditory stimulus. Other diseases that can manifest a sudden hearing loss should be ruled out, including the possibility of acoustic neurinoma or a perilymph fistula.

Clinical Findings

Patients with ISSNHL complain of sudden hearing loss, often on arising in the morning. Tinnitus may be the first sign alerting them to a change. Vertigo is present about half the time. A history of loud noise exposure, scuba diving, flying, or recent head trauma suggests a perilymph fistula. Physical examination reveals a normal external ear and tympanic membrane. Nystagmus may be present. Facial nerve function should be tested carefully, but usually is normal.

Laboratory Findings

Audiographic assessment reveals sensorineural hearing loss. There is no characteristic pattern. Brain-stem audiometry should be obtained if this is unilateral, and an MRI with gadolinium should be performed to evaluate for an acoustic neurinoma if there is any suggestion of retrocochlear pathologic lesion. Blood serology, including an erythrocyte sedimentation rate, a blood glucose level, and a rheumatologic panel, help rule out other causes, particularly of the autoimmune system.

Optimal Management

Many pharmacologic agents have been used unsuccessfully to treat ISSNHL. Bed rest may be helpful, particularly if a membrane rupture has occurred. High-dose corticosteroids have been shown to help patients with moderate hearing loss regain hearing. Inhaled carbogen (95% oxygen and 5% carbon dioxide) has been shown to improve hearing by 1 year after treatment. Fortunately, the natural history of the disease is that 65% of patients recover normal or functional hearing within the first several weeks, regardless of therapy. Causes of sudden hearing loss such as perilymph fistula or acoustic neurinoma usually are treated surgically.

EPISTAXIS

Definition

Epistaxis, or bleeding from the nose, has been categorized as anterior or posterior based on the location of the bleed in the nasal cavity. Anterior epistaxis typically is milder than posterior epistaxis and usually occurs from the region of Kiesselbach's plexus—a capillary network in the mucosa of the cartilaginous nasal septum. Posterior epistaxis typically is arterial, generally from a branch of the sphenopalatine artery.

Incidence and Epidemiology

About one in ten persons has experienced epistaxis. It occurs more commonly in the winter months when drier air diminishes the humidification of the nasal mucosa. The elderly are more affected by the seasonal variation in climate and more often have profuse, posterior bleeds.

Etiology and Pathogenesis

The cause of spontaneous epistaxis is multifactorial. Anatomical abnormalities such as a septal spur may make the mucosa susceptible to drying and crusting, leaving blood vessels more exposed and more susceptible to hemorrhage. Self-inflicted trauma such as repeated nose picking or placement of a foreign body in the nose (more common in children) can lead to epistaxis. Systemic factors such as atherosclerosis and hypertension are associated with an increase in epistaxis. Patients with blood dyscrasias or thrombocytopenia also are more susceptible. Patients who are taking anticoagulants and those who abuse alcohol tend to have profuse, recurrent episodes of epistaxis that are difficult to control. Recurrent epistaxis may also require aspirin therapy to be discontinued.

Clinical Findings

In patients with a mild anterior epistaxis, it often is easy to identify the site of the bleeding. Usually, there are no clinical findings other than the bleed itself. In contrast, in patients with a profuse, posterior epistaxis, many complicating clinical find-

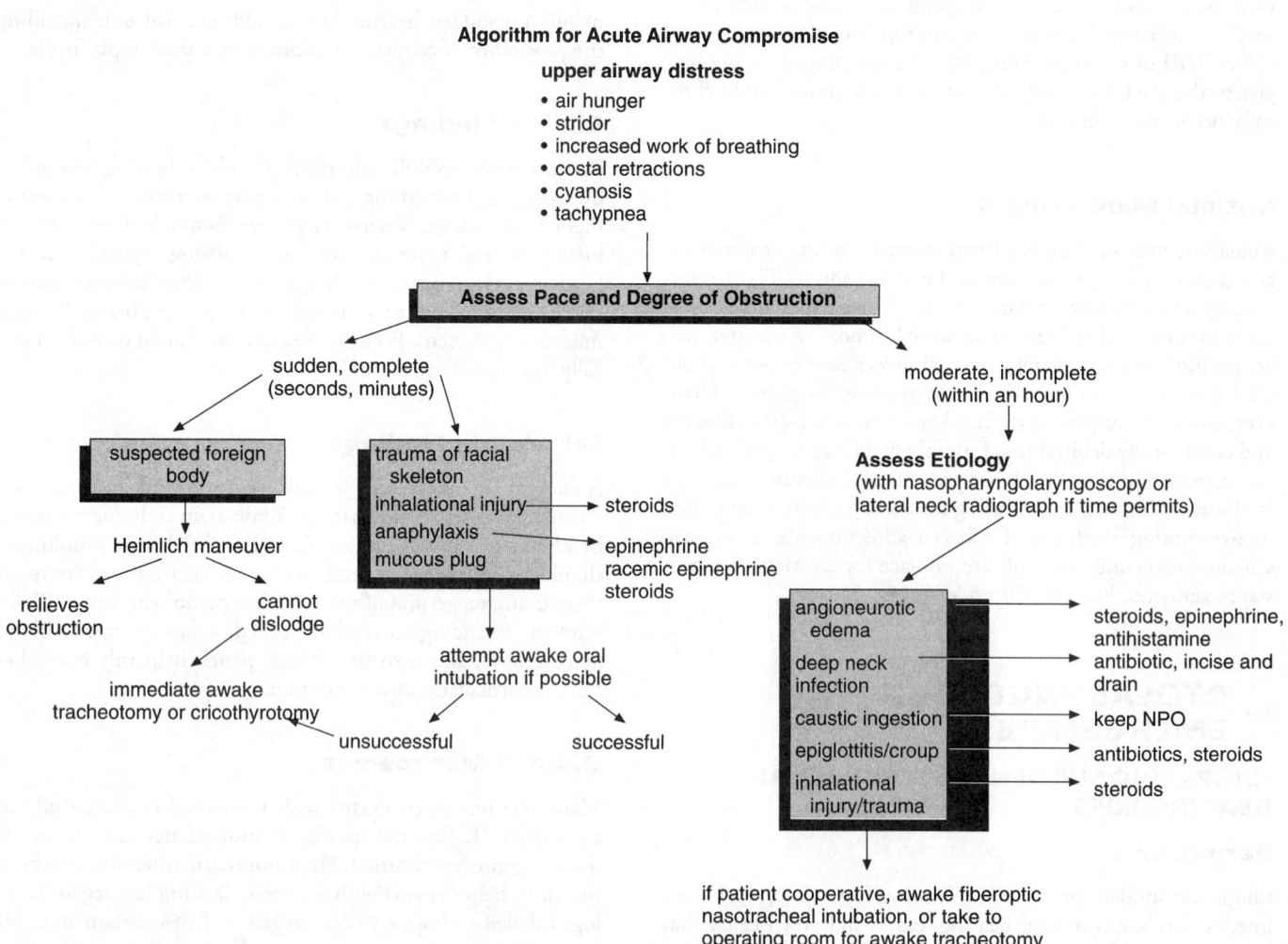

FIGURE 51.3. Algorithmic approach for acute airway compromise.
EVIDENCE LEVEL: C. Expert Opinion.

ings are present. It can be difficult to determine the side and site of the bleeding because blood often emanates rapidly from both nostrils and the mouth. There may be airway compromise and aspiration of blood. Emesis occurs secondary to swallowing of blood. Elevated blood pressure in an anxious patient exacerbates bleeding.

Laboratory Findings

Patients with profuse spontaneous epistaxis of uncertain origin should undergo a hematologic workup to rule out the possibility of an underlying blood dyscrasia. Hemoglobin and hematocrit levels are necessary in deciding to perform a transfusion or to initiate iron supplementation. A carotid arteriogram may be indicated in epistaxis that is recurrent and not controlled with packing. This determines the site of bleeding and allows for concurrent embolization of the bleeding vessel.

Optimal Management

Management of epistaxis first involves a rapid search for the site of bleeding. If found, this can be cauterized with silver nitrate or covered with thrombin-coated Gelfoam or Surgical. If a site is not identified, pressure should be applied to the nares. Control of bleeding that does not respond to pressure held for 10 minutes is achieved by packing the nose. A variety of materials are available. A Merocel sponge coated with antibacterial ointment is one effective method of packing. Ointment-coated gauze in long strips is another. For profuse posterior bleeds, a posterior pack may be necessary. This involves placing a balloon catheter into the nasopharynx, then packing the nasal cavity with gauze. This is secured at the nares. An alternative is the Epistat, which has two balloons, one for the nasopharynx and one for the nasal cavity. Packing is left in place for 48 to 72 hours. If bleeding resumes, embolization or surgical ligation is necessary.

ACUTE AIRWAY COMPROMISE

A discussion of otolaryngologic emergencies would be incomplete without mention of airway compromise. This topic encompasses a wide variety of causes and many subtleties in management that are beyond the scope of this chapter. Instead of a systematic review, an algorithmic approach for the management of acute airway compromise is included in Figure 51.3. This provides a framework for safe airway management by any practitioner involved with patients requiring acute resuscitative measures.

BIBLIOGRAPHY

Fisch U, Nagahara K, Pollak A. Sudden hearing loss: circulatory. *Am J Otol* 1984;5:488–491.

Giebink GS. Preventing otitis media. *Ann Otol Rhinol Laryngol* 1994; 103(Suppl 163):20–23.

Hyams VJ, Batsakis JG, Michaels L. *Tumors of the upper respiratory tract and ear.* Washington, DC: Armed Forces Institute of Pathology, 1988.

Kurihara A, Toshima M, Yuasa R, Takasaka T. Bone destruction mechanisms in chronic otitis media with cholesteatoma: specific production by cholesteatoma tissue in culture of bone-resorbing activity attributable to interleukin-1 alpha. *Ann Otol Rhinol Laryngol* 1991;100:989–998.

Lim DJ, Bluestone CD, eds. Recent advances in otitis media. *Ann Otol Rhinol Laryngol* 1994;(Suppl 164):1–80.

Mattox D, Simmons F. Natural history of sudden sensorineural hearing loss. *Ann Otol* 1977;86:463–480.

Moss AJ. Current estimates from the National Health Interview Survey, United States, 1985. Vital and Health Statistics. Series 10, No. 160. DHHS Pub. No. (PHS) 86-1588. Public Health Service. US Government Printing Office, September 1986.

Wilson W, Byl F, Laird N. The efficacy of steroids in the treatment of idiopathic sudden hearing loss. *Arch Otolaryngol* 1980;106:772–776.

Wilson W, Veltri RW, Laird N, Sprinkle PM. Viral and epidemiologic studies of idiopathic sudden hearing loss. *Otolaryngol Head Neck Surg* 1983;91:653–658.

Yamasoba T, Kikuchi S, Higo R, et al. Sudden sensorineural hearing loss associated with slow blood flow of the vertebrobasilar system. *Ann Otol Rhinol Laryngol* 1993;102:873–877.

Kelley's Textbook of Internal Medicine, fourth edition. Edited by H. David Humes. Lippincott Williams & Wilkins, Philadelphia © 2000.

CHAPTER

52

PRINCIPLES OF WOMEN'S MEDICINE

ERIN N. MARCUS

As women have gained economic and political power in the United States, they have demanded more attention for their unique health problems. Over the past two decades, there has been a proliferation of literature on health issues that affect women primarily, such as breast cancer, as well as research into how ailments such as heart disease differ in women and men.

Because they outlive men and seek out care more frequently, women make up the majority of patients in the United States. A female infant in the United States has a life expectancy of 79 years, 6 more than her male counterpart. The average woman who lives to age 65 can expect to live 19 more years, 3 years longer than a 65-year-old man. Because they live longer, women make up 75% of US nursing home residents.

According to the National Center for Health Statistics (NCHS), women visit doctors' outpatient offices at a rate 1.5 times that of men. Their overall hospitalization rate is higher than men's, and they visit hospital emergency departments slightly more often than men. Women under age 65 are slightly more likely to have health insurance than men, but NCHS surveys indicate they are more likely than men to delay necessary care, regardless of income level.

As with men, cardiovascular disease kills the most women, followed by lung cancer and stroke. Breast cancer, accidents, and chronic obstructive pulmonary disease are the next most common causes of death among women. Certain autoimmune rheumatologic conditions and endocrine conditions are far more common in women than in men.

Multiple cross-sectional surveys indicate that most women in the United States are unaware of the threat of coronary disease and fear breast cancer more than any other condition. A large cross-sectional survey by Legato and associates (1997) found that 58% of women believed they were as likely or more likely to die from breast cancer than from coronary disease. Of those surveyed, 44% considered themselves unlikely to develop heart disease. Perhaps most concerning, 47% of the women at highest risk of coronary disease—those over age 60—said their doctor had never discussed heart disease with them. Yet heart disease is far more prevalent, and deadly, than breast cancer. Phillips and associates (1999) have estimated that of a birth cohort of 1,000 women, 203 will die of cardiovascular causes by the age of 85 years, compared with 33 who will die of breast cancer.

As with the nation as a whole, the ethnic composition of the US female population is changing. Blacks, Hispanics, Asians, Pacific Islanders, and Native Americans make up approximately 28% of women in the United States and overall are growing at a rate faster than that of whites in the population. These women are disproportionately affected by medical issues such as hypertension and diabetes, and many have different assumptions and beliefs about health care and those who provide it. Recent medical decision-making studies have indicated that physicians' own biases may affect how they evaluate women of color with medical problems.

VIOLENCE AGAINST WOMEN

Women are often the target of violence, and all women should be screened for violence in a nonjudgmental, supportive manner. Domestic violence is the leading cause of violent injury to women between the ages of 18 and 44. Sexual assault is common across all age groups. A 1998 Commonwealth Fund survey found that 31% of women reported having experienced domestic violence. Thirty-nine percent reported having experienced some type of abuse or violence in their lifetime. When faced with a victim of abuse or assault, health care workers should carefully document the patient's history and physical findings, assess her immediate safety, and assist her with crisis intervention services.

GYNECOLOGIC ISSUES

Routine gynecologic care is important for all women, because it allows health care providers to detect cancer and sexually transmitted diseases, to provide contraceptive counseling, and to evaluate the patient for conditions with considerable morbidity, such as dysmenorrhea, amenorrhea, sexual dysfunction, menorrhagia, and incontinence.

Over the past two decades, awareness of the need for culturally sensitive and painless pelvic examinations has increased. Young patients may be especially apprehensive about the pelvic examination; similarly, the examination can be uncomfortable for a postmenopausal woman if the examiner fails to use additional lubrication. There are a variety of alternative positions for the disabled patient who cannot lie supine.

GYNECOLOGIC CANCER SCREENING

Since its widespread adoption in the 1970s, Papanicolaou (Pap) screening has drastically reduced the incidence of and mortality from cervical cancer in the United States. Nonetheless, we are experiencing an epidemic of human papilloma virus (HPV), of which several types are associated with cervical cancer, and Pap screening remains extremely important. All young, sexually active women should have an annual gynecologic examination and Pap smear, as should all women older than age 17. Women infected with HIV, who are at an increased risk of invasive cervical cancer, should undergo Pap smear testing every 6 months. Other high-risk women include those who have had first intercourse in their teens when the cervical squamocolumnar junction is believed to be most susceptible to oncogenic change; women with multiple male partners or with men whose previous partners had cervical cancer; women infected with HPV, herpes simplex virus (HSV), or other sexually transmitted diseases; immunosuppressed women; women with a history of substance abuse, including tobacco; and women who have had cervical dysplasia or cancer or endometrial, vaginal, or vulvar cancer.

When to stop annual Pap smear screening remains controversial. No consensus exists among medical groups regarding this issue, but the American College of Obstetricians and Gynecologists now states that low-risk women who have had three consecutive negative annual examinations may, at the discretion of their physician, undergo Pap testing less frequently.

Despite the widespread acceptance of Pap smear testing, many women (particularly those over age 60) have not been adequately screened according to a recent Commonwealth Fund report. Women over age 60 account for 40% of cervical cancer deaths.

There is even less of a consensus regarding screening for ovarian cancer. Manual pelvic examination is insensitive, although a patient with a palpable postmenopausal ovary must be worked up for cancer. Ultrasonography and tumor markers, such as CA 125, are not considered practical screening tests in the general population. However, many physicians use these tests in women at high risk, such as those with a strong family history.

SEXUALLY TRANSMITTED DISEASE SCREENING

In addition to HPV, other sexually transmitted diseases (STDs) such as chlamydia and gonorrhea are very common in the US population, and women are often asymptomatic. All young, sexually active women and women with multiple sexual partners should routinely be screened for chlamydia, the most common bacterial STD in the United States, as well as for gonorrhea. Chlamydia is common throughout all socioeconomic groups in the United States, whereas gonorrhea, syphilis, HSV-2, and HIV are more common in lower-income populations. A recent cross-sectional study of female military recruits by Gaydos and associates found a chlamydia prevalence rate of 9.2%.

Pelvic inflammatory disease accounts for approximately 275,000 hospitalizations annually in the United States, and silent pelvic inflammatory disease may account for many cases of tubal factor infertility.

AIDS, the most deadly STD, is growing faster in women than in any other group. AIDS is the fourth leading cause of death among all US women between the ages of 25 and 44. In certain cities, such as New York, AIDS is the number one cause of death among women in this age group. Most HIV-positive women in the United States are infected through heterosexual sex, and many of these women are in long-term, monogamous relationships at the time they are diagnosed. A study of recently diagnosed women in Rhode Island, for example, found that 70% of those who acquired HIV sexually had been in a long-term stable relationship for at least 2 years.

CONTRACEPTION AND FAMILY PLANNING

Vasectomy remains a relatively underused birth control method in the United States, and most contraception ends up being left up to the female partner. A recent US Centers for Disease Control study of women between the ages of 15 and 44 found that nearly 28% of women who used contraception chose tubal sterilization. Approximately 27% chose oral contraceptives, followed by condom use at 20%. About 11% of the women reported having partners who had had vasectomies. Tubal ligation was highest among black women over age 35, of whom 66% had been sterilized. Women in their 20's most commonly used oral contraceptives. Overall, 5% of the surveyed women said they never used any method of birth control, even though they were sexually active and were not trying to get pregnant.

Given these statistics, it is not surprising that nearly 50% of the 6.3 million pregnancies in the United States annually are unintended. Of these unplanned pregnancies, about 50% occur in women using birth control, whereas 50% occur in women who never practice contraception. The Alan Guttmacher Institute estimates that 43% of unintended pregnancies end in abortion and 13% end in miscarriage.

Nonetheless, access to legal abortion has become more difficult for many women. The number of abortion providers dropped by 14% between 1992 and 1996, and 86% of all US counties lacked an abortion provider in 1996, according to the Guttmacher Institute.

All women at risk of becoming pregnant should be counseled annually on preconception issues, since the fetus' major organs are formed between 17 and 56 days after conception, at a time when many women may not realize they are pregnant. Women should be advised to consume a daily minimum of 400 µg of folic acid to prevent neural tube defects and should be counseled on the avoidance of tobacco, alcohol, and street drugs, as well as herbal supplements, whose safety has not been established in pregnancy. Health care providers should avoid prescribing teratogenic medications to this group and, if this is not possible, should counsel their patients on pregnancy prevention.

MENOPAUSAL ISSUES

Many women seek medical attention during the perimenopause, the transitional years surrounding the last menstrual period,

when hormone levels fluctuate considerably. Health professionals can help perimenopausal women not only by treating hot flashes and other symptoms but also by intervening to prevent osteoporosis and heart disease, which cause considerable morbidity and mortality later on in life.

Menopause is a retrospective diagnosis, made when a woman has not had menses for a year and has a follicle-stimulating hormone (FSH) level greater than 30. Menopause usually occurs between ages 48 and 55. If a woman ceases menstruating before age 40 and is not pregnant, she has premature ovarian failure and must be evaluated for autoimmune and other conditions.

Individual women's responses to menopause vary. In a recent MacArthur Foundation survey of 8,000 adults ages 25 to 74, a majority of postmenopausal women said they felt "only relief" when their menses ceased; 2% of the women reported "only regret." Other surveys have found that major depression is not more common among women at menopause, except among those who had a surgical menopause.

Hot flashes are a true physiologic phenomenon, characterized by a rise in skin temperature, heart rate, and minute ventilation. Between 25% and 75% of women report hot flashes at some point during the perimenopause. Hot flashes are not dangerous but can cause sleep deprivation and diminish quality of life.

Estrogen is the best-established therapy for hot flashes. A dose of 0.625 mg per day of conjugated estrogen is considered the minimum necessary for osteoporosis and coronary artery disease prevention, but some women may need a higher dose to prevent hot flashes. Nonhormonal treatments for hot flashes include clonidine, bellergal, biofeedback, exercise, and avoidance of triggers such as alcohol and caffeine. Many women use herbal supplements such as dong quai and black cohosh, although the efficacy and long-term safety of these supplements are unclear.

The long-term benefits of estrogen use include osteoporosis prevention and treatment, which has been well documented in controlled clinical trials, as well as the primary prevention of coronary artery disease, which has been strongly suggested by many long-term cohort studies. Observational studies also suggest that estrogen may reduce the development of colon cancer and of Alzheimer's dementia. Topical estrogen creams have been found to reduce the risk of recurrent urinary infection and dyspareunia.

There are risks associated with estrogen therapy. Unopposed estrogen markedly increases the risk of endometrial cancer. Therefore, women on estrogen replacement therapy who have not had a hysterectomy must also receive progesterone, which reduces this risk. Estrogen increases the risk of venous thrombosis and of cholelithiasis and increases triglycerides.

The best-publicized and most-feared risk of hormone therapy, breast cancer, remains controversial. The Nurses' Health Study, a cohort study of 121,700 women, found that the relative risk of dying from breast cancer was 1.45 for current hormone users who had used estrogen for 5 years or more, compared with those who had never used it. Other observational studies have yielded conflicting results. The Women's Health Initiative, a 15 year-long US-government–funded study that includes a clinical trial involving 64,500 women, should help elucidate this risk.

Recent data also indicate that estrogen may increase the incidence of new cardiovascular events in women with preexisting heart disease. The Heart and Estrogen/Progestin Replacement Study, a 4-year, controlled clinical trial involving postmenopausal women with documented coronary artery disease, found a statistically significant increase in myocardial infarction and death in the first year of hormone therapy. Over the entire 4-year period, the overall number of coronary events was equal in both the hormone and placebo groups.

Selective estrogen receptor modulators such as raloxifene are a new alternative that may be of benefit in preventing osteoporosis and heart disease. A 2-year controlled trial of raloxifene found that it increased bone mineral density and lowered low-density lipoprotein levels without increasing the rate of endometrial abnormalities. Other studies have found a decrease in breast cancer incidence in women on raloxifene over a 28-month period. However, other literature suggests raloxifene may worsen hot flashes.

BREAST CANCER SCREENING

Mammography is of proven benefit in detecting early cancer and saving lives in women between the ages of 50 and 69. Outside of this age range, however, its use as a screening test is controversial. In a meta-analysis of mammography trial data published in 1995, Kerlikowske and colleagues did not find a statistically significant reduction in breast cancer mortality in women under 50 who were screened. Others have interpreted the individual study results differently, finding a mortality reduction in younger women in five out of the eight major mammography trials.

There is no consensus on screening mammography in women under age 50. As of February 1999, the American Cancer Society recommends screening for all women beginning at 40, whereas the American College of Physicians does not recommend screening of the general population under age 50.

Moreover, there is no clear-cut consensus on when to stop mammography. Women older than 70 have the highest incidence of and mortality from breast cancer, but they have been underrepresented in the major mammography trials. As of 1998, the American Geriatrics Society recommends that women receive mammograms every 2 or 3 years until age 85. Medicare covers annual screening mammograms in all older women.

There may be a high false-positive rate among women who undergo regular mammogram screening. Elmore and colleagues (1998) have estimated that the cumulative risk of a false-positive mammogram result is 49% in women who have ten screening mammograms. Other studies have indicated that false-positive results can cause anxiety, which may interfere with daily life.

OSTEOPOROSIS

Osteoporosis is epidemic in the United States, and its consequences can be deadly. A 50-year-old white woman in the United States has a 50% chance of developing an osteoporotic fracture during the rest of her life. If she breaks her hip, she has a 10% to 20% chance of dying within 1 year. Hip, vertebral, and forearm fractures can also cause significant pain and morbidity.

Osteoporosis prevention must begin early, because bone mass peaks in the third decade of life. All patients should be counseled on the need for adequate calcium and vitamin D intake. Bone mass drops precipitously during perimenopause, and hormone replacement therapy is of benefit in maintaining and augmenting bone mass during this time. There is no consensus on whether initiating hormone therapy after age 65 is of benefit in treating osteoporosis.

All women should have their height measured periodically, because this is an inexpensive means of screening for osteoporosis. Bone mineral density testing should be done periodically in women at increased risk, such as those with a family history of the disease or a personal history of tobacco, phenytoin, steroid, or heparin use or with hyperthyroidism or other endocrinopathies. Women who are undecided about estrogen replacement therapy are also candidates for bone mineral density testing.

Alendronate is effective in preventing and treating osteoporosis, and nasal calcitonin is approved for treating the condition. For more information, see Chapter 465.

HEART DISEASE

Heart disease strikes two out of three women and is a major cause of disability; nearly one in three will die of coronary disease. It is predominantly a disease of older women, largely because of estrogen's protective effects before menopause, and on average strikes women 10 years later than men. As with men, hypertension, obesity, smoking, and hyperlipidemia increase a woman's risk of coronary disease. Diabetic women are at even greater risk than diabetic men.

Women with coronary artery disease most commonly present with angina. Women with angina are more likely to be older and to have hypertension, diabetes, and heart failure than are men with angina. Women are also more likely to have stable angina before their first myocardial infarction.

Women who develop a myocardial infarction are more likely than men to die both in the hospital and within 30 days after infarction, and black women have a particularly high risk of death at this time. Registry reviews by Maynard and associates and others indicate that women with myocardial infarction were not treated as aggressively and were less likely to undergo acute catheterization, angioplasty, thrombolysis, or coronary artery bypass surgery than men. Other reviews have found that women are more likely than men to delay going to the hospital and that women are more likely to present with complicated myocardial infarction at the time they arrive at the hospital. More research is needed on medical and interventional therapies for myocardial infarction and coronary disease in women.

BIBLIOGRAPHY

Barrett-Connor E. Hormone replacement therapy. *Br Med J* 1998;317: 457–461.

Cu-Uvin S, Flanigan TP, Rich JD, et al. Human immunodeficiency virus infection and acquired immunodeficiency syndrome among North American women. *Am J Med* 1996;101:316–322.

Elmore JG, Barton MB, Moceri VM, et al. Ten-year risk of false positive screening mammograms and clinical breast examinations. *N Engl J Med* 1998;338:1089–1096.

Gaydos CA, Howell MR, Pare B, et al. Chlamydia trachomatis infections in female military recruits. *N Engl J Med* 1998;399:739–744.

Hulley S, Grady D, Bush T, et al. Randomized trial of estrogen plus progestin for secondary prevention of coronary heart disease in postmenopausal women. *JAMA* 1998;280:605–613.

Kerlikowske K, Grady D, Rubin SM, et al. Efficacy of screening mammography. A meta-analysis. *JAMA* 1995;273:149–154.

Maynard C, Litwin PE, Martin JS, et al. Gender differences in the treatment and outcome of acute myocardial infarction. Results from the myocardial infarction triage and intervention registry. *Arch Intern Med* 1992;152:972–976.

National Center for Health Statistics. Health, United States, 1998 with Socioeconomic Status and Health Chartbook. Hyattsville, Maryland, 1998.

Phillips KA, Glendon G, Knight JA. Putting the risk of breast cancer in perspective. *N Engl J Med* 1999;340:141–144.

Schulman KA, Berlin JA, Harless W, et al. The effect of race and sex on physicians' recommendations for cardiac catheterization. *N Engl J Med* 1999;340:618–626.

US Public Health Service. *Clinician's handbook of preventive services,* second ed. Washington, DC, 1998.

Wallis L, ed. *Textbook of women's health.* Philadelphia: Lippincott-Raven, 1998.

Wenger NK. Coronary heart disease: an older woman's major health risk. *Br Med J* 1997;315:1085–1090.

Kelley's Textbook of Internal Medicine, fourth edition. Edited by H. David Humes.
Lippincott Williams & Wilkins, Philadelphia © 2000.

CHAPTER
53

PRINCIPLES OF SPORTS MEDICINE

PAUL MCCAFFREY FORD
GORDON O. MATHESON

The optimal care of the physically active patient necessitates an understanding of the physiologic adaptations of exercise training (Table 53.1) and the unique role that exercise plays in promoting health in all patients regardless of the presence of preexisting disease or risk factors for future disease. Comprehensive health care of the exercising population requires a multidisciplinary team to deliver care within the full range of the human performance continuum (Fig. 53.1). Operating within this continuum, the health care disciplines are further integrated by the clinical service programs in which they participate. Clinical activities comprise five major areas:

1. *Human performance and health risk assessment* is aimed at evaluating the performance and health characteristics of a person at any point on the human performance continuum. For the elite athlete, this assessment might include the measurement of human performance capabilities specific to a given sport as well as identification of risk factors that might predict injuries or illnesses unique to that sport. For those

TABLE 53.1.	PHYSIOLOGIC ADAPTATIONS OF EXERCISE TRAINING

Central Adaptations with Training

20–30% increase in cardiac output at maximal exercise
- ⇑ Stroke volume but not maximal heart rate
- ⇑ Contractility
- ⇑ End-diastolic volume
- ⇑ Cardiac mass (hypertrophy with normal myocardial wall thickness)

⇓ Systolic, diastolic, and mean arterial blood pressure at rest and during submaximal exercise
⇓ Peripheral vascular resistance
⇑ Blood volume
- ⇑ Plasma volume
- ⇑ Hemoglobin and red cell mas

Improved ventilatory efficiency (work of breathing)
- ⇑ Maximum V_E
- ⇓ V_E for a given workload
- ⇑ Diffusion capacity

Peripheral Adaptations with Training

⇑ Myoglobin concentration (up to 90%)
⇑ Mitochondrial volume density (up to 120%)
⇑ Capillary density (up to 50%)
⇑ Oxidative enzyme activity (up to 100%)
Muscle fiber hypertrophy (selective fast or slow twitch)
⇑ Muscle glycogen stores
⇑ Fatty acid fuel utilization
⇑ Stores of adenosine triphosphate (20%), P_{Cr} (40%)
Right shift of the lactate threshold

Metabolic Adaptations with Training

⇑ Highly-density cholesterol and ⇓ triglycerides
⇓ Adiposity
Improved insulin-mediated glucose uptake ⇑ and/or retention of bone mineral density

---

P_{Cr}, plasma creatinine; V_E, minute volume, expired.

at the mid range on the human performance continuum, the assessment may use submaximal tests of aerobic capacity, health risk assessment questionnaires, and the assessment of selected risk factors. For people with suboptimal human performance, the assessment focuses on the specific problems resulting from injury or illness, such as deficits in muscular strength and endurance, and on what is required to restore physical competency.

2. *Strength, fitness, and health improvement* is the counseling and education counterpart of "human performance and health

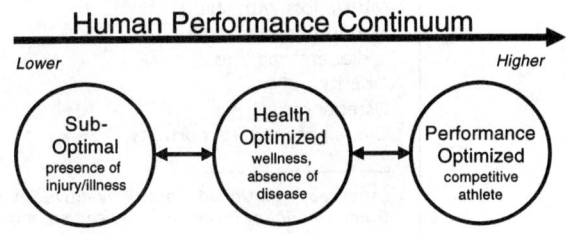

FIGURE 53.1. Human performance continuum.

risk assessment," from which measurements obtained are used to develop a specific program for correcting weaknesses in muscular strength, aerobic capacity, nutritional status, or health risk characteristics.

3. *Exercise medicine* is aimed at the investigation and treatment of medical conditions that can arise or make an impact on participation in exercise. A large segment of work in this field is directed toward prescribing exercise and monitoring the physiologic responses for the purpose of improving physiologic function in chronic diseases. Clinicians providing this care include generalist-based physicians (in the fields of pediatrics, family medicine, and general internal medicine) and specialty-oriented physicians with special interest in exercise (in the fields of cardiology, pulmonary medicine, and exercise physiology).

4. *Musculoskeletal medicine* is concerned with the investigation, diagnosis, and treatment of both surgical and nonoperative musculoskeletal injuries that impair normal exercise capacity. Clinicians providing this care include generalist-based physicians (in the fields of pediatrics, family medicine, and general internal medicine) and specialty-oriented physicians (in the fields of neurosurgery, orthopedics—including specialties of hand, joint replacement, and trauma—and physiatry).

5. *Injury rehabilitation* is a well-developed clinical field that uses a variety of methods and techniques to administer different types of exercise to restore functional capacity after a musculoskeletal injury. Health care professionals in this group include the traditional athletic therapists (athletic trainers, physical and occupational therapists) and complementary medicine approaches (massage and myofascial therapy, chiropractic medicine, and acupuncture)

▆ MEDICAL ASPECTS OF EXERCISE AND SPORTS

BENEFITS OF EXERCISE

Exercise has been demonstrated to have primary, secondary, and tertiary preventive benefits in a wide variety of conditions (Table 53.2). Research has determined that the exercise effect is inde-

pendent of other risk factor modification, requires regular participation, can be effective when started even in middle to late adulthood, and has no clear minimal intensity required, with a linear relation between exercise duration/intensity and health benefits. Adverse effects in the short term are related to the type of exercise performed, previous training and experience, intensity of training and age. Acute cardiac effects, whereas dramatic and of a potential serious nature, are infrequent and can be minimized through application of preexercise screening and optimal selection of exercise type and duration based on coexisting risk conditions. Long-term adverse effects are notable to not include development of or worsening of preexisting osteoarthritis.

SCREENING FOR EXERCISE PARTICIPATION

All physically active patients should be evaluated before participation, using a standard medical history with attention to details of risk factors for cardiac disease and a directed sport-specific musculoskeletal review. The results of this assessment will then direct further cardiovascular risk testing using a standard Bruce protocol exercise treadmill test (Table 53.3) for those asymptomatic patients in an age group (men ≥45, women ≥55 years of age) with two or more risk factors for ischemic cardiovascular disease and for patients with symptomatic cardiac disease. The results of testing, combined with the clinical characteristics, then allow patients to be further categorized into groups that can allow risk stratification and the writing of the appropriate exercise prescription (Table 53.4).

PRINCIPLES OF THE EXERCISE PRESCRIPTION

The current recommendation is for the active patient to accumulate a minimum of 30 minutes of moderate-intensity physical activity in a frequency of 3 to 5 days per week at an intensity to achieve 55% to 90% of maximum heart rate. This activity can include a minimum of 10-minute periods or a single period. Cardiac risk stratification can guide the exercise prescription for those patients with abnormalities found during exercise testing

	Level of Prevention		
Disease	**Primary**	**Secondary**	**Tertiary**
Coronary artery diseases	Y	Y	Y
Depression/anxiety	Y	Y	...
Hypertension	...	Y	Y
Muscle loss with aging	...	...	Y
Non-insulin–dependent diabetes mellitus	...	Y	Y
Obesity	Y	Y	Y
Osteoporosis	Y	Y	Y
Overall premature mortality	Y	...	...

TABLE 53.2. PREVENTION BENEFITS OF EXERCISE

(Adapted from United States Preventive Services Task Force. *Counseling to promote physical activity, Guide to Clinical Preventive Services,* second ed. Baltimore: Williams & Wilkins, 1996:611–625, with permission.)

TABLE 53.3.	PREEXERCISE TESTING RISK STRATIFICATION					
Prescreen Risk Class[a]	**A-1**	**A-2**	**A-3**	**B**	**C**	**D**
	Men ≤45, Women ≤55	Men >45, Women >55	Men >45, Women >55			
Risk factors	None	None	≥2			
Known	No	No	No	Yes	Yes	Yes
Planned exercise intensity						
Intensity <70% maximum heart rate or <60% Vo₂ max	No ETT	No ETT	No ETT	Yes	Yes	Yes
Vigorous ≥ 70% maximum heart rate or ≥60% Vo₂ max	No ETT	Yes	Yes	Yes	Yes	Yes
Postscreen Risk Class	Class A	Class A	Class A	Class B	Class C	Class D
	Apparently healthy	Apparently healthy	Apparently healthy	Low risk	Moderate risk	High risk

[a] (Adapted from Table 5 and text. ACSM, AHA Recommendations for cardiovascular screening, staffing, and emergency policies at health/fitness facilities. *Med Sci Sports Exerc* 1998;30:1009–1018.)

or who have symptomatic cardiac disease (Table 53.4). Physicians counseling patients with regard to exercise will find that most are receptive to counseling. As in all physician-fostered behavioral change, physicians can exert a considerable impact on facilitating behavioral change through developing a therapeutic alliance with the patient, reviewing the relation between exercise and the patient's current and future health, committing the patient to a specific exercise plan, maintaining ongoing support, and using other health care personnel such as health education counselors in an overall supportive environment.

COMMON MEDICAL ISSUES IN THE EXERCISING PATIENT

Fatigue

The differential diagnosis of sustained fatigue in the competitive highly trained or endurance athlete includes those conditions that cause fatigue in the general population and those that occur secondary to training-specific effects alterations in physiologic recovery mechanisms. When the results of the initial examination (including a history, physical examination, and selected testing) are normal, the sustained fatigue is frequently attributed to an exercise-related overtraining syndrome characterized by fatigue, mood changes, perceived or real decrements in athletic performance or recovery from exercise, and frequent infections, usually of the upper respiratory tract. Affecting primarily elite endurance athletes (cyclists, rowers, runners), sustained fatigue has also been reported in activities defined by muscle power training, such as weight lifting. Although current research suggests that this fatigue results from disruption in neuroendocrine

function, whether this set of symptoms truly encompasses a distinct exercise-related syndrome remains unproved, and a consistent diagnostic strategy remains undefined. In addition, the relation between the chronic fatigue syndrome and overtraining in exercise remains unclear. Regardless of this uncertainty, athletes who complain of fatigue benefit from a multidisciplinary evaluation consisting of a thorough medical and psychologic evaluation, review of training history with coaching and athletes, and formulation of long-term training plan that incorporates close attention to the entire training regimen, including influence of competing activities such as schoolwork or other work, amount of sleep and between-exercise rest periods, evaluation of diet, and close attention to training.

Exercised-Induced Asthma

Exercise-induced asthma (EIA) is defined by a drop in FEV₁ (forced expiratory volume in 1 second) of 15% after exercise, occurring in those with or without a prior history of asthma or other atopic illness. Current pathogenic theories suggest a thermal-induced process in which the initial fall in airway temperature during exercise is followed by rapid reheating when ventilation diminishes. The mechanism by which this process results in bronchial narrowing and airway hyperactivity is not well defined. However, clinical observation that the leukotriene modulators can reduce EIA suggests that leukotrienes probably play a major role in this process. Reported in 10% to 25% of athletes in some series, the clinical features of EIA consist of postexercise wheezing or cough, which, in contrast with that which occurs with intrinsic asthma, is not associated with prolonged or intense airway obstruction or a late effect. Other causes

TABLE 53.4.	POSTEXERCISE TESTING RISK STRATIFICATION			
Postscreen Risk Class[a]	**Class A**	**Class B**	**Class C**	**Class D**
Cardiovascular disease features	Apparently healthy	*Clinically stable with:* ■ Coronary artery disease (CAD) ■ Valvular disease ■ Congenital heart disease[b] ■ Cardiomyopathy except hypertrophic or postmyocarditis ■ Exercise treadmill test (ETT) abnormalities that do not meet class C	■ CAD 3-valve CAD or left main disease ■ Acquired valvular heart disease ■ Congenital heart disease ■ Cardiomyopathy except hypertrophic or postmyocarditis ■ ETT abnormalities not related to ischemia ■ Previous ventricular fibrillation or cardiac arrest not related to acute myocardial infarction or cardiac procedure ■ Ejection fraction <30%	■ Unstable angina ■ Uncompensated heart failure ■ Uncontrolled arrhythmias ■ Severe symptomatic aortic stenosis ■ Hypertrophic cardiomyopathy postmyocarditis ■ Severe pulmonary hypertension ■ Other conditions aggravated by exercise (dissecting aortic aneurysm, recent pulmonary embolism)
Clinical characteristics	Apparently healthy	■ NYHA class I or II ■ Exercise capacity >6 metabolic equivalents (METS) ■ No CHF ■ No ischemia or angina at rest or at systolic blood pressure 6 METS ■ Appropriate systolic blood pressure (SBP) rise with exercise ■ Absense of nonsustained or sustained ventricular tachycardia (VT) ■ Ability to self-monitor intensity of exercise	*One or more of the following:* ■ Two or more previous myocardial infarctions ■ NYHA class III or greater ■ Exercise capacity <6 METS ■ Ischemic horizontal or down sloping ST depression ≥1 mm or angina at <6 METS ■ Fall in SBP with exercise ■ Medical problem which physician believes is life-threatening ■ Previous episode of primary cardiac arrest ■ VT at <6 METS	
Exercise risk **Exercise level recommended**	Low 50–90% maximum heart rate or 45–85% maximum oxygen uptake or heart rate reserve[c]	Moderate *Absence of ischemia or significant ETT abnormalities* ■ 50–90% peak heart rate or 45–85% peak measured oxygen uptake or heart rate reserve *Presence of ischemia or significant ETT abnormalities* ■ Upper limit of training heart rate is 10 beats/min less than that associated with abnormality on ETT and/or ischemia		High None recommended for conditioning

[a] Adapted from Table 5 and text. ACSM, AHA Recommendations for cardiovascular screening, staffing, and emergency policies at health/fitness facilities. *Med Sci Sports Exerc* 1998;30:1009–1018.
[b] 26th Bethesda Conference. Recommendations for determining eligibility for competition in athletes with cardiovascular abnormalities. *J Am Coll Cardiol* 1994;24:845–899.
[c] Heart rate reserve is defined as maximum heart rate minus resting heart rate.

of exercise-associated cough such as gastroesophageal reflux, allergic rhinitis, and occult cardiac disease must be excluded. Low ambient temperatures and humidity, exposure to oxidant air pollutants, coexisting respiratory viral infections, and poor physical conditioning worsen severity. Initial treatment with an inhaled β_2-agonist (albuterol) before exercise is the treatment of choice, followed by the addition of inhaled cromolyn sulfate or an oral leukotriene synthesis inhibitor (zileuton) or both, or receptor antagonist (zafirlukast) in selected patients, all of which require daily use. Long-acting β_2-agonists (salmeterol) have had mixed usefulness in clinical use, with some athletes reporting improved control and others having increased symptoms and decreased clinical response to shorter-activity β_2-agonists, a phenomenon attributed to long-term β_2-receptor down-regulation.

Inhaled or oral corticosteroids, the mainstays of intrinsic asthma treatment, play no role in the treatment of EIA.

The Female Athlete Triad

Female athletes training for endurance activities (distance running, cycling, cross-country skiing), those involved in activities in which low body mass provides competitive advantage (gymnastics, ballet, diving, figure skating), and those in sports requiring weight categories for participation (horse racing, rowing) are at risk for the development of exercise-associated amenorrhea, a form of hypogonadotropic hypogonadism in which diminished frequency of luteinizing hormone (LH) pulses results from disturbance of the hypothalamic release of gonadotropin-releasing hormone. The exact mechanism that causes this hypothalamic-pituitary axis disruption is not known, but appears to arise from many interrelated factors including a reduction in critical body fat mass, high caloric expenditures, and inadequate nutritional intake in relation to daily caloric demands of exercise. The subsequent amenorrhea, defined as less than three menstrual periods per 12-month period, results in reduced bone density and subsequent increased stress fractures, primarily of the lower extremity, and decreased fertility; it may also make an impact on athletic performance.

The use of hormone replacement of both estrogen and progesterone is the most common treatment approach, and although a few early reports have demonstrated that such therapy will stabilize and, in some cases, increase vertebral and lower extremity bone density in amenorrheic female athletes, the prevention of stress fractures with hormonal replacement has not been reported in this population.

Whether biphosphonates play a role in this patient population remains to be firmly established. In some female athletes, amenorrhea and osteoporosis are combined with eating disorders to form the so-named "female athlete triad." All female athletes with one component of this triad should be screened for the remaining disorders. In addition to treatment of the hormonal effects of amenorrhea, treatment of these female athletes is optimal when a combination of strategies is provided, including intensive nutritional and psychological counseling and support in addition to standard medical care.

Anemia in the Athlete

The diagnosis and treatment of anemia in the athlete are complicated by both exercise-specific physiologic changes that can interfere with diagnosis and the commonly held but unproven practice of iron supplementation for possible performance enhancement. Athletes may have *pseudoanemia*, in which plasma expansion occurs secondary to intravascular shifts following exercise or to the effects of high-altitude training. *Increased red cell turnover* has also been demonstrated in sports such as running, cycling, and swimming, presumably due to mechanical trauma, increased body temperature, or increased oxidative stress and subsequent increased red cell fragility. The athlete with both low hematocrit and serum ferritin has *iron-deficiency anemia* and should undergo an appropriate clinical evaluation and treatment

with oral iron until the anemia has resolved and the serum ferritin has normalized. Replacement of iron in this group has been demonstrated to reverse performance degradation.

Athletes who have low serum ferritin and a normal hematocrit do not seem to benefit from iron supplementation in terms of performance enhancement. Some clinicians suggest that when the serum ferritin is low and the hemoglobin is in the low-normal range, the differential diagnosis of pseudoanemia, increased red cell turnover, or early iron deficiency may be made and would advocate that a minimum of 2 months of oral iron supplementation be supplied with a repeat of the indices after treatment is completed. Athletes who have subsequent unchanged values presumably have a pseudoanemia or increased red cell turnover while those with increased hemoglobin and or serum ferritin may have had early iron deficiency. Whether treating this group of athletes will enhance performance or forestall performance deterioration before frank anemia develops has not been reported in men or women athletes.

OVERUSE MUSCULOSKELETAL INJURIES

General Principles

Musculoskeletal overuse injuries, because of their subacute to chronic nature, often present a treatment challenge to the clinician. In clinical terms, these injuries occur when the rate of musculoskeletal loading exceeds the rate of adaptation within connective tissue and bone (resulting in the clinical syndrome of tendinosis or stress fracture). All overuse injuries are accompanied by pain that has its onset at some point in the connective tissue remodeling process. Because tissue injury results from the accumulation of repetitive forces applied below the single-cycle failure threshold, treatment requires a fundamental understanding of the factors, often subtle, that contribute to the total load.

It is important to recognize that the onset of pain occurs after substantial accumulation of tissue strain but before complete failure of the tissue. In this sense, even though the onset of pain tends to be a "sudden" event (at least historically), effecting a positive outcome requires attention to the subtle causal factors that led to the accumulated load. With running, for example, the load across the ankle or knee joint can exceed eight times a person's body weight, repeated with each step.

Five factors are commonly associated with overuse injuries. These factors are well recognized for lower-extremity injuries associated with sports such as running, but the general principles may be applied to the upper extremity also. Although these risk factors have not been proved to be causative in clinical trials, either because the studies have not been performed or because the methods used have not permitted definitive conclusions, they remain the time-honored approach used by clinicians treating overuse injuries.

Training errors are factors that create a mismatch between the rate of musculoskeletal loading and the rate of tissue adaptation; these include the total volume of training (number of strain cycles connective tissue and bone are exposed to), the increase of training within a given time frame, and the intensity or pace of training (frequency of strain cycles). Factors that affect *muscular shock absorption* influence the magnitude of the load delivered to the musculoskeletal system. The muscle tendon unit absorbs massive amounts of force over time during physical activity and muscle strength (both concentric and eccentric) and endurance capacity (ability to resist fatigue) are important factors for limiting tissue injury. *Intrinsic biomechanical factors* refers to aspects of lower-extremity alignment that affect the duration, magnitude, and site of the load delivered to the skeleton and include foot type (pes cavus and pes planus), tibial varum, genu valgum, genu varum, the quadriceps angle, femoral neck anteversion, and leg-length discrepancies.

A fourth causative factor consists of *extrinsic biomechanical factors*; these include the contribution to overuse injuries resulting from specific equipment such as shoe type, racquet size, and terrain (rigidity and slope of surface). Finally, *specific tissue pathology* such as osteoporosis or muscle atrophy that may affect the stress:strain relation in a given tissue can affect the onset of overuse injury.

Treatment

The treatment for overuse musculoskeletal injuries relies on elucidating the factors responsible for overload and a detailed, anatomically based physical examination of the injured part. In general, treatment is broken into three phases.

Phase I of the treatment begins when correctable causes of the overuse history are identified, including training errors, intrinsic and extrinsic biomechanical factors, and muscular strength and endurance. The offending activity is stopped, but rarely is there a need for immobilization of a limb because atrophy is a deleterious side effect that can be more incapacitating than the injury, particularly to an athlete. Pain can be managed with local physical therapy modalities, nonsteroidal medication, and ice.

Phase II of the treatment involves the prescription of modified activity to maintain cardiopulmonary fitness. The activity must be non-impact loading (rowing, cycling, swimming, water running). Sports that involve skill maneuvers that do not load the affected part are permissible in this phase. During phase II, there is also the need to provide equipment and technique modifications, including footwear and foot orthoses. Muscular strength and endurance exercises that involve overload are prescribed at this point. The length of phase II depends on the time it takes for the patient to be pain-free on a day-to-day basis. An important aspect of phase II when treating competitive athletes is the clear identification of treatment steps before reintroduction of the sport, a factor that maintains confidence within the doctor–patient relationship.

Phase III begins when this is achieved and involves the reintroduction of impact-loading activities. It is important to note that when activity restarts, the patient commonly has a persistent awareness or discomfort. A written program should be devised using the 10% rule: *no increase in volume or intensity should be greater than 10% more than the last workload increment.* In general, workload increments should allow off days and a rate of progression that ensures that symptoms do not return and relapses are avoided.

BIBLIOGRAPHY

American College of Sports Medicine. American College of Sports Medicine Position Stand and American Heart Association. Recommendations for cardiovascular screening, staffing, and emergency policies at health/fitness facilities. *Med Sci Sports Exerc* 1998;30:1009–1018.

American College of Sports Medicine. American College of Sports Medicine Position Stand. The recommended quantity and quality of exercise for developing and maintaining cardiorespiratory and muscular fitness, and flexibility in health adults. *Med Sci Sports Exerc* 1998;30:975–991.

American College of Sports Medicine. American College of Sports Medicine Position Stand. The female athlete triad. *Med Sci Sports Exerc* 1997;29:1–9.

Andersen RE, Blair SN, Cheskin LJ, Bartlett SJ. Encouraging patients to become more physically active: the physician's role. *Ann Intern Med* 1997;127:395–400.

Blair SN, Koh HW, Carlow CE, et al. Changes in physical fitness and all-cause mortality. *JAMA* 1995;273:1093–1098.

Cumming DC. Exercise-associated amenorrhea, low bone density, and estrogen replacement therapy. *Arch Intern Med* 1996;156:2193–2195.

Garza D, Shrier I, Koh WH, et al. The clinical value of serum ferritin tests in endurance athletes. *Clin J Sport Med* 1997;7:46–53.

Pate RR, Pratt M, Blair SN, et al. Physical activity and public health. *JAMA* 1995;273:402–407.

Regg EW, Cauley JA, Seeley DG, et al. Physical activity and osteoporotic fracture risk in older women. *Ann Intern Med* 1998;129:81–88.

US Preventive Services Task Force. Counseling to promote physical activity. In: *Guide to clinical preventive services*, second ed. Baltimore: Williams & Wilkins, 1996:611–624.

Kelley's Textbook of Internal Medicine, fourth edition. Edited by H. David Humes. Lippincott Williams & Wilkins, Philadelphia © 2000.

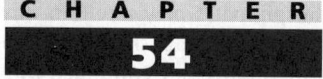

C H A P T E R

54

PRINCIPLES OF REHABILITATION MEDICINE

KRESIMIR BANOVAC
DEBBIE FERTEL
JOSEPH BAUERLEIN

Rehabilitation medicine is integral to the care of patients and should follow most episodes of acute medical and surgical treatment. Passive convalescence after acute or chronic illness or trauma increases the risk for deterioration of a variety of normal and vital functions and for the development of complications. Economically, neglecting rehabilitation in the early stage of convalescence has been shown to be more costly than that of an early aggressive rehabilitation program. The goals of rehabilitation focus on (a) return of function to the baseline level or as close as possible, (b) the adjustment to any residual disability, and (c) the prevention of complications associated with the primary condition and any residual disability.

Optimal therapy requires the skills of a multidisciplinary

TABLE 54.1.	REHABILITATION TEAM
Discipline	**Role**
Physiatrist	Medical care, coordination of rehabilitation
Rehabilitation nurse	Daily care, medication, education, reinforcing patient's independence
Physical therapist	Gross motor skills (sitting, standing, transfers, ambulation)
Occupational therapist	Fine motor skills (hygiene, dressing, feeding)
Recreational therapist	Leisure activity, community reintegration
Psychologist	Psychotherapy to patient and family, assessment of emotional, intellectual and perceptual function
Social worker	Helping family and patient to obtain community resources
Speech therapist	Communication, swallowing, assist in cognitive training
Vocational counselor	Testing of skills and interest, recommend training for alternative occupation
Prosthetist/orthotist	Design and fabrication of prosthesis (artificial limbs) and orthosis (splints and braces)

TABLE 54.2.	GLASGOW COMA SCORE	
Indicator	**Category of Response**	**Grade**
Eye opening	Spontaneous	4
	To voice	3
	To pain	2
	None	1
Verbal response	Oriented	5
	Confused	4
	Inappropriate words	3
	Incomprehensive words	2
	None	1
Motor response	Obeys commands	6
	Localizes pain	5
	Withdraw (pain)	4
	Flexion (pain)	3
	Extension (pain)	2
	None	1

team of rehabilitation specialists. Table 54.1 lists the potential members of a rehabilitation team and their roles. The clinical scenario determines the composition of the team and the setting of the program. The rehabilitation team designs and supervises therapy initially.

The outcome of rehabilitation depends on not only on several patient-related factors, including the motivation and ability of the patient to participate, the interval from the injury to the start of rehabilitation, and the extent of family support, but also on the team. The involvement of family and friends in the rehabilitation process accelerates and facilitates the reintegration of the patient back into the community. As they move back into the community, patients take on more of the responsibility of supervising the continued therapy designed by the rehabilitation team.

■ NEUROREHABILITATION

BRAIN INJURY

In patients with traumatic brain injury (TBI), determination of prognosis after rehabilitation is difficult. Patients with TBI have cognitive deficits as their major disability. Rehabilitation goals can be assessed using the Glasgow Coma Scale (GCS), the most commonly used prognostic indicator (Table 54.2). For patients with mild TBI (GCS score from 13 to 15), the goals are independence in ambulating with or without an assistive device, total independence in activities of daily living (ADL), and reintegration into the community. Many patients demonstrate improve-

ment in problem solving, memory, safety awareness, and recovery of cognitive functions. However, they may initially require supervision at home to ensure safety for several months. Patients with moderate TBI (GCS scores from 9 to 12) may have permanent functional and cognitive deficits, although they may be able to care for themselves and perform some degree of occupational activity. Patients with severe TBI (GCS scores from 3 to 8) are usually dependent on another person for ADL and mobility. They may become ambulatory but are usually not independent owing to impulsive and disinhibited behavior. Often, these patients are left with significant impairments of physical, communicative, and cognitive functions.

SPINAL CORD INJURY

Patients with spinal cord injury (SCI) can be divided into those with complete paralysis and those with incomplete paralysis. Patients with complete SCI have no motor and sensory function below the segment of the traumatized spinal cord. The outcome of the rehabilitation of these patients depends on the degree of reversibility and site of the cord lesion (Table 54.3).

Patients with incomplete SCI may have significant recovery of functional status, although some have permanent disability because of severe spasticity and lack of coordination and proprioception. Furthermore, the process of rehabilitation may be limited owing to additional injuries such as skeletal, thoracic, or abdominal trauma. All patients with brain injury require evaluation of swallowing function and preventive measures to avoid aspiration. Treatments of other complications of SCI are outlined in Table 54.4.

■ ORTHOPEDIC REHABILITATION

The goals of rehabilitation for the patient with orthopedic injury include reduction of pain, return to independence in ADL, and an improvement of strength and endurance. Early mobilization

TABLE 54.3.	PROGNOSTIC EXPECTATIONS AFTER COMPLETE SPINAL CORD INJURY
Cord Injury Level	**Functional Level**
Segments C1–C3	Requires respiratory support ADL dependent on caregivers
Segments C4–C5	Operates a motorized wheelchair Requires assistance with ADL
Segments C6–C8	Operates a manual wheelchair Minimal assistance with ADL
Below T1	Is usually independent in mobility, transfers, ADL, and management of neurogenic bowel/bladder dysfunction

ADL, activities of daily living.

after injury is critical in reducing the incidence of complications associated with extended immobilization. Muscle atrophy, joint contractures, cardiorespiratory deconditioning, deep venous thrombosis, and, less commonly, osteoporosis, orthostatic hypotension, and decubitus ulcers may significantly alter the course of recovery after multiple trauma. Patients with severe injuries and multiple trauma often require 4 to 6 months of rehabilitation.

Some patients with lower-extremity fractures may need adaptive devices (wheelchair, walker, crutches, or cane) until fracture healing and weight bearing allows for their discontinuation. Complication with wound infection or extensive soft-tissue,

TABLE 54.4.	TREATMENT OF COMPLICATIONS OF SPINAL CORD INJURY
Complication	**Treatment**
DVT	Deep venous thrombosis prophylaxis
Brain injury	Seizure prophylaxis
Neurogenic bladder	Intermittent catheterization
Neurogenic bowel	Bowel program (stool softeners, laxatives)
Spasticity	Aggressive range-of-motion exercises Medication may be useful: ▪ GABA (γ-aminobutyric acid) agonist (baclofen) ▪ α_2-adrenergic agonists (clonidine, tizanidine) ▪ Benzodiazepines (clonazepam [klonopin], diazepam) ▪ Calcium release inhibitor (dantrolene [Dantrium])
Agitation	Medication may be useful ▪ β-adrenergic blocking agent (e.g., propranolol) ▪ Neuroleptic (haloperidol)

nerve, or vascular injuries often require more extended rehabilitation to achieve maximal improvement. Patients with limb amputation may require up to 1 year for the wound to heal and the stump to be prepared for a prosthesis, followed by additional time to train the patient in the use of the artificial limb.

CARDIAC REHABILITATION

Cardiac rehabilitation continues its evolution begun 30 years ago. Therapy begins with inpatient treatment after an acute myocardial infarction (phase I). Activities require less than 3 to 4 METs (metabolic equivalents) and include dressing (2 METs), showering (3 METS), and walking upstairs (4 METS). The patient advances to outpatient therapy (phase II) with the degree of structure and monitoring dependent on the risk of recurrent events. Risk is related to the presence and extent of ischemia, the extent of left ventricular dysfunction, and the presence of significant ventricular arrhythmia. Pressure to decrease inpatient length of stay has placed greater emphasis on outpatient therapy. Finally, the maintenance phase (phase III) encourages the patient to maintain lifetime changes that will improve cardiac function and quality of life. Education is critical in all phases and may lead to lifestyle changes that help slow the progression of coronary artery disease. Table 54.5 summarizes the phases of cardiac rehabilitation.

Although cardiac rehabilitation has classically been offered to those patients with coronary artery disease following a myocardial infarction, indications have expanded more recently. Patients with congestive heart failure can obtain significant improvement in their functional capacity and sense of well-being. After cardiac transplantation, recuperation is faster with a rehabilitation program.

PULMONARY REHABILITATION

Pulmonary rehabilitation enhances standard therapy in patients with chronic disabling lung disease. Although pulmonary function measurements do not improve with pulmonary rehabilitation, the functional capacity for ambulation, duration of exercise, and ability to perform ambulatory tasks improves

TABLE 54.5.	CARDIAC REHABILITATION	
Phase	**Duration/Location**	**Goals**
I	Days/inpatient	ADL, less than 3–4 METs Education (weight, diet, stress reduction, smoking cessation)
II	2–3 months/outpatient or home	Progressive activity level Education
III	Lifetime/home	Relieve symptoms Education

TABLE 54.6.	PULMONARY REHABILITATION
Modality	**Goals**
Lower extremity	Treadmills, bicycles, walking, or combination
Upper extremity	Arm ergometer, arm weights to shoulder level
Ventilatory muscles	Hand-held inspiratory resistance devices (especially with chronic obstructive pulmonary disease)
Psychosocial	Diet changes
	Weight control
	Appropriate oxygen therapy
	Exercise
	Smoking cessation

significantly, correlates with improvement in quality of life, and may prolong life expectancy. Historically, pulmonary rehabilitation was indicated primarily in patients with chronic obstructive pulmonary disease (COPD), more recently it has been effective in patients with other disabling chronic lung diseases such as cystic fibrosis, interstitial lung diseases, and neuromuscular disorders. The last decade has seen pulmonary rehabilitation become an integral, vital part of recovery from lung volume reduction and lung transplantation surgery.

A pulmonary rehabilitation program is comprehensive and individualized to allow patients to realistically meet their own goals. Therapy is directed toward maximizing patients' functional capacity within the limits of their pulmonary disease. Ideally, the program includes lower extremity training, upper extremity training, ventilatory muscle muscle training, and psychosocial interventions. All therapy is done while monitoring oxygen saturation, vital signs, and electrocardiograms. Supplemental oxygen in incremental doses needs to be used as indicated. Some patients with severe lung disease have resting hypercapnia, requiring intermittent monitoring of the P_{CO_2} by arterial blood gas or measurement of end-tidal CO_2. Psychosocial intervention is vital to the success of the program (Table 54.6). Patients with chronic lung disease frequently suffer from depression, anxiety, loneliness, low self-esteem, and reduced social support.

BIBLIOGRAPHY

Braddom RL. *Physical medicine & rehabilitation*. Philadelphia: WB Saunders, 1996.

Brotzman SB. *Handbook of orthopaedic rehabilitation*. St. Louis: Mosby-Year Book, 1996.

DeLisa JA, Gans BM. *Rehabilitation medicine*, third ed. Philadelphia-New York: Lippincott-Raven, 1998.

Irwin JS. *Tecklin: cardiopulmonary physical therapy*, third ed. St. Louis: CV Mosby, 1998.

Umphred DA. *Neurological rehabilitation*, third ed. St. Louis: CV Mosby, 1995.

Kelley's Textbook of Internal Medicine, fourth edition. Edited by H. David Humes. Lippincott Williams & Wilkins, Philadelphia © 2000.

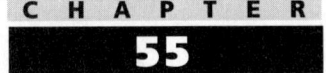

C H A P T E R
55

PRINCIPLES OF CLINICAL PHARMACOLOGY

D. CRAIG BRATER

Many clinicians are repelled by pharmacokinetics because they envision obfuscating mathematical relations that may not seem directly applicable to patient care. Pharmacokinetics need not be intimidating, however, and a physician's ability to design a rational therapeutic regimen can be greatly facilitated by understanding a few simple pharmacokinetic principles. It also is important to realize the limitations of pharmacokinetics. Its practical use represents an attempt to predict in a quantitative fashion how an individual patient will respond to a drug.

Significant variability exists in drug disposition among homogeneous groups of patients, which becomes even greater with such additional influences as disease (Chapter 167), age (Chapter 469), and drug interactions. Hence, clinicians should not be overly rigid in the use of pharmacokinetic values but should view them as best "guestimates" of how an individual patient will handle a drug. These values serve as a starting point of therapy and then must be refined using measures of response in each patient such as blood concentrations of drug and, most important, clinical assessment of response. This is the realm of pharmacodynamics, which describes how an individual patient responds to a dose or concentration of a drug. The pharmacodynamics of drug response also are highly variable among individuals, are influenced, for example, by disease and other drugs, and can be assessed only clinically. Therefore, optimal care of individual patients requires interdigitating of pharmacokinetics with pharmacodynamics.

◼ PHARMACODYNAMICS

In clinical medicine, the term *pharmacodynamics* refers to the response of a patient to a certain dose or serum concentration of a drug; *it is used to define the target concentration of a drug.* Pharmacokinetics then are used to design dosing regimens that allow attainment and maintenance of the desired concentrations, with the overall goal being to obtain the efficacious effects of a drug and avoid the toxic effects.

When drug dose or, more accurately, serum concentration, is related to response, a sigmoid-shaped concentration response curve results (Fig. 55.1*A*). The relation shown in Figure 55.1*A* could be for any response, whether beneficial or toxic. With some drugs, the distinction between concentrations causing desired compared with adverse effects is great (Fig. 55.1*B*). Such drugs are easy to dose, because the objective is to make certain that enough drug is administered to attain benefit with little worry about excessive doses. In this circumstance, recommended

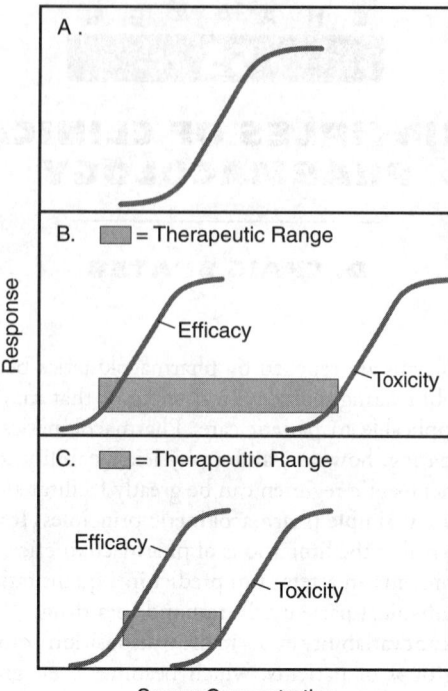

FIGURE 55.1. Schematic curves that relate concentration to response. **A:** A typical sigmoidal concentration response curve. **B:** A drug with a wide therapeutic range. **C:** A drug with a narrow therapeutic range.

doses and concentrations obtained are considerably greater than the minimum necessary. The classic example of this type of drug is penicillin. Clinically used doses are far in excess of those needed to kill bacteria, but, because the dose needed to cause toxicity is massive in comparison (excluding allergic reactions), doses that ensure sufficient drug concentration can be given safely with little, if any, risk of toxicity.

Most cardiovascular drugs have narrower therapeutic indices; that is, the difference between therapeutic and toxic concentrations is small (Fig. 55.1C). With such drugs, as little as a twofold increase in serum concentration can cause toxicity in some patients. Hence, there is little margin for error in dosing, and close attention must be paid to designing a dosing regimen that attains the desired drug concentration without being excessive. Doing so requires knowledge of pharmacokinetic parameters and use of kinetic principles for design of dosing regimens.

Considerable variability in response to a given concentration of a drug occurs among patients. Disease states and patient characteristics also can affect pharmacodynamics, such as the increased sensitivity to central nervous system (CNS) effects of drugs commonly observed in elderly patients (Chapter 469). To compensate for variability in pharmacodynamics, clinicians must be alert to the need to titrate drug doses individually according to clinical response.

PHARMACOKINETICS

The most important pharmacokinetic parameters (bioavailability, volume of distribution [Vd], clearance [Cl], and half-life) and their application are presented in Table 55.1.

TABLE 55.1.	PHARMACOKINETIC PARAMETERS
Parameter (Abbreviation)	**Clinical Application**
Bioavailability (F)	Determines the amount of drug reaching the systemic circulation and therefore the amount at the site of action
Volume of distribution (Vd)	Determines the size of a loading dose
Clearance (Cl)	Determines the maintenance dose
Half-life (T½)	Determines the amount of time needed to reach steady-state serum concentrations (four times the T½)

BIOAVAILABILITY

Bioavailability (F) represents the fraction or percentage of administered drug that reaches the systemic circulation. If the drug is given intravenously, bioavailability is 100% (F = 1.0); if it is given by other routes, bioavailability often is less than 1.0, indicating lack of complete absorption or elimination of the drug before it reaches the systemic circulation. The latter is called either *presystemic elimination* or the *first-pass effect,* and it is important with many drugs. A bioavailability of less than 100% can result from a variety of causes (Table 55.2). The clinical importance of incomplete bioavailability is most readily apparent when a patient is switched from intravenous (IV) to oral therapy. If the bioavailability of a drug is 50%, an oral dose twice that of the IV dose is needed to attain the same amount of drug in the patient. Hence, clinicians must have an awareness of the bioavailability of the drugs they are using so that appropriate IV and oral doses are administered.

Clinicians also should realize that bioavailability can be affected to a substantial degree in many ways. Differences in product formulation can affect the extent of absorption, as can gastrointestinal disorders and drug interactions. For example, inhibition of intestinal wall metabolism and P-glycoprotein secretion of lovastatin or simvastatin can result in increased bioavailability sufficient to increase serum concentrations five- to tenfold with greatly enhanced risk of toxicity. Conversely, ad-

TABLE 55.2.	REASONS FOR INCOMPLETE BIOAVAILABILITY

Incomplete product disintegration
Incomplete dissolution
Physicochemical complex formation (e.g., fluoroquinolone antibiotics and calcium, magnesium, aluminum, or iron)
Intestinal metabolism by CYP3A4
Intestinal secretion from cell back into the gut lumen by P-glycoprotein
Presystemic hepatic metabolism

ministration of most fluoroquinolones in close temporal proximity to many antacids can result in essentially no drug absorption.

The occurrence of such influences and their quantitative importance often are difficult to predict. Consequently, this possibility must be included in the differential diagnosis of vagaries of response to drugs. For example, lack of response of a patient to a loop diuretic should not be ascribed solely to a lack of sensitivity of the patient, but also should include the possibility of incomplete absorption. If a clinician mistakenly assumes only the first possibility, the use of a potentially useful drug may be discontinued. If the drug simply is not being well absorbed, the dose can be increased, or a better and more predictably absorbed preparation can be used. If these possibilities are not considered, they will never be detected, and inappropriate therapeutic behavior may ensue.

VOLUME OF DISTRIBUTION/ LOADING DOSE

The Vd is simply a proportionality factor that describes the concentration of a drug attained by a given dose. If a 100-mg dose of a drug is administered to a patient and results in a serum concentration of 5 mg per liter before any metabolism or excretion has been able to occur, the volume in which the dose has distributed to account for this resultant concentration is 20 L:

$$\text{Initial concentration} = \text{dose}/\text{Vd}$$

Or, in the example cited,

$$5 \text{ mg/L} = 100 \text{ mg}/\text{Vd}$$

Therefore:

$$\text{Vd} = 100 \text{ mg}/5 \text{ mg/L} = 20 \text{ L}$$

This volume does not represent a physiologic space. In general, small Vds usually relate to confinement of the drug in the vascular space or extracellular fluid, whereas very large Vds occur with drugs that distribute extensively into fat (Chapters 167 and 469). Proper use of the Vd is to calculate the loading dose of a drug.

Dosing recommendations for many drugs distinguish between a loading dose and maintenance dosing. The former is used in settings in which an efficacious concentration of drug must be attained quickly in a patient. For example, patients with ventricular ectopy with acute myocardial infarction frequently are given a loading dose of lidocaine to obtain therapeutic concentrations quickly. The dose given is determined by the Vd of lidocaine. For example, the Vd of lidocaine in most patients is 1.1 L per kilogram of body weight, and a typical target concentration is 3 mg per liter. From these values and the patient's weight, a loading dose can be calculated.

If the patient weighs 70 kg:

$$\text{Initial concentration} = \text{loading dose}/\text{Vd}$$

or

$$3 \text{ mg/L} = \text{loading dose}/(1.1 \text{ L/kg}) (70 \text{ kg})$$

Therefore:

$$\text{Loading dose} = (3 \text{ mg/L}) (77 \text{ L}) = 231 \text{ mg}$$

Clinically, such loading doses are commonly administered in increments (e.g., a 100-mg bolus followed by one or two additional 50-mg doses based on the patient's response). So doing allows one to tailor therapy according to response of the individual patient.

Numerous disease states can change drug distribution (Chapters 167 and 469). If such changes are not anticipated, patients may be inappropriately dosed. For example, if a patient has congestive heart failure and needs lidocaine, the loading dose must be modified. By unknown mechanisms, patients with heart failure have a decreased Vd for lidocaine. Consider the potential consequences if such a change is not taken into account; namely, the patient receives the loading dose calculated previously, but the Vd for lidocaine is actually 0.55 L per kilogram (half of its previous value). If 231 mg was administered, the resulting serum concentration would be as follows:

$$\text{Initial concentration} = 231 \text{ mg}/(0.55 \text{ L/kg}) (70 \text{ kg})$$

$$= 231 \text{ mg}/38.5 \text{ L} = 6 \text{ mg/L}$$

Hence, a twofold underestimation of Vd would result in an initial concentration twice that predicted, which could be toxic. If a clinician prospectively considers that a patient's condition (or other concomitantly administered drugs) might affect the Vd of an agent, he or she will be better able to prevent this type of problem. If such a possibility is not considered, a patient's care may be compromised by inappropriate drug dosing. Physicians are accustomed to thinking in terms of doses rather than the pharmacokinetic parameters that dictate those doses. Doing so is not unreasonable, but physicians must avoid the pitfall of assuming that loading doses should be the same for all patients. Generally, if there is any doubt, it is better to administer a dose that is too small rather than one that is too large. If clinical monitoring of the patient reveals insufficient pharmacologic effect, additional drug can be administered. However, if too much drug is given and toxicity ensues, treatment of the adverse effect can be challenging.

Another important consideration when giving a loading dose is the route of administration. Loading doses do not have to be given intravenously and in some instances may be tolerated better if given orally. For example, IV doses of digoxin can cause peripheral vasoconstriction, which may be undesirable. This effect can be avoided with oral dosing. Similarly, phenytoin must be administered cautiously by vein and can precipitate in many IV fluids. Dosing by mouth can prevent such problems. If a loading dose is to be administered by mouth, bioavailability must be taken into account.

The final important point about loading doses concerns the rapidity of administration. Too often, the temptation is to administer a drug as quickly as possible. This causes very high concentrations in serum, which can be associated with adverse effects. Lidocaine is a good example. If the loading dose is given as a rapid-bolus injection, serum concentrations sufficient to cause CNS toxicity frequently occur transiently until distribution into other tissues takes place, lowering the serum concentration to the desired level. However, if the drug is given more slowly, the high serum concentrations can be prevented with less resultant toxicity. For example, when three separate 50-mg bolus doses of lidocaine were given in one study, all patients had CNS toxicity; in contrast, administration of the same dose as a continuous infusion over 18 minutes resulted in toxic effects in less than 10% of patients.

Overall, there is little to gain and a potential for much loss by bolus injection of drugs. Slow, controlled administration is more prudent.

■ CLEARANCE/MAINTENANCE DOSE

Clearance measures the ability to eliminate drug from the body. This value is always given in units of volume divided by time (e.g., milliliters per minute) and sometimes is normalized to body weight or surface area. Because clearance usually is determined by measuring the decline of serum or plasma drug concentrations, the term generally refers to serum or plasma clearance, although whole blood concentrations are measured with some drugs (e.g., cyclosporin A). The value for clearance expresses the volume of serum from which all drug can be removed per unit time. For example, if a drug's clearance is 100 mL per minute, all drug can be removed from 100 mL of serum in 1 minute.

For most drugs, clearance is a constant value. This property is called *first-order,* or *linear,* kinetics. With some drugs, however, elimination pathways can be saturated at higher drug concentrations, in which case, clearance decreases at these higher concentrations. This property is called *zero-order, saturable,* or *Michaelis–Menten* kinetics, and it classically occurs with ethanol, salicylates, and phenytoin. Fortunately, most drugs obey first-order kinetics, which facilitates the design of dosing regimens.

With such drugs, a change in dose results in a proportional change in drug serum concentration, that is, doubling the dose doubles the concentration (Fig. 55.2*A*). Such a relation makes dose adjustments simple. In contrast, for drugs that follow saturable kinetics, a change in dose causes a disproportionate change in drug serum concentration; in other words, doubling the dose may quadruple the serum concentration (Fig. 55.2*B*). Dose adjustments in such circumstances become much less predictable than with drugs that obey first-order kinetics.

The clearance of a drug determines the dose that must be administered to maintain a constant serum concentration. This relation is best illustrated as follows. At steady state, by definition, the rate of drug entry into the body is equal to the rate of exit: rate in equals rate out. In turn, in the simplest case of a constant IV infusion: rate in equals infusion rate.

In all circumstances,

$$\text{Rate out} = (\text{average drug concentration, or } Cp_{average}) \, (Cl)$$

Therefore:

$$\text{Infusion rate} = (Cp_{average}) \, (Cl)$$

or

$$Cp_{average} = \text{infusion rate}/Cl$$

This relation makes intuitive sense in that the higher the infusion rate, the higher the drug concentration; similarly, if the ability to eliminate a drug declines, thereby indicating diminished Cl, as may occur with aging (Chapter 469) or a variety of diseases (Chapter 167), the drug concentration is higher for the same rate of administration.

Lidocaine can be used again as an example. In most patients, the clearance of lidocaine is 9 mL per minute per kilogram. If a steady-state average serum concentration of 3 mg per liter is required in a 70-kg patient, the needed infusion rate can be calculated as follows:

$$Cp_{average} = \text{infusion rate}/Cl$$

$$3 \text{ mg/L} = \text{infusion rate}/(9 \text{ mL/min/kg}) \, (70 \text{ kg})$$

$$\text{Infusion rate} = (3 \text{ mg/L}) \, (630 \text{ mL/min})$$

$$= 1890 \text{ μg/min} = 1.9 \text{ mg/min}$$

Proportionality is a vital factor implied in this relation. For example, if a patient's serum lidocaine concentration is 3 mg per liter at an infusion rate of 1.9 mg per minute and it is deemed necessary to attain a new concentration of 4.5 mg per liter, the infusion rate needed to maintain this new target concentration can be readily calculated as 1.5 times the former infusion rate, namely, 2.85 mg per minute. Expressed in another manner, because of the direct proportionality:

$$\text{Old infusion rate/old serum concentration} = \text{new infusion rate/new serum concentration}$$

In this example,

$$1.9 \text{ mg/min}/ 3 \text{ mg/L} = \text{new infusion rate}/4.5 \text{ mg/L}$$

$$\text{New infusion rate} = (4.5) \, (1.9 \text{ mg/min})/3$$

$$= 1.5 \, (1.9 \text{ mg/min}) = 2.85 \text{ mg/min}$$

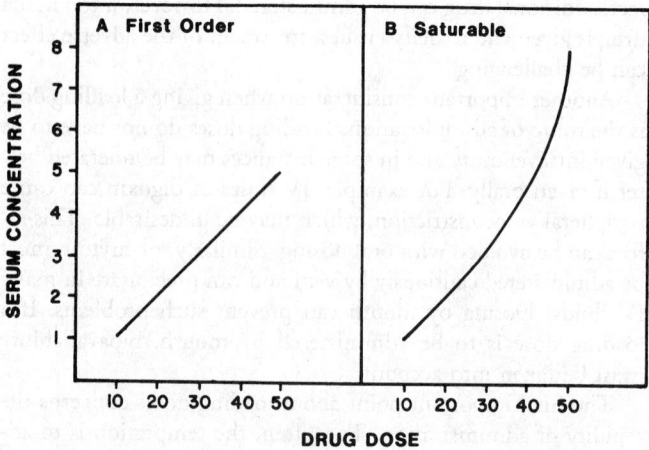

FIGURE 55.2. Relation between the dose of drug administered and the serum concentration that results for a drug that follows first-order kinetics compared with a drug that follows saturable kinetics.

A corollary of this relation is that a difference from normal in the patient's clearance of a drug requires a commensurate change in its administration rate. In the preceding example, if a patient had been administered lidocaine at a rate of 1.9 mg per minute, assuming a normal clearance, but the patient in fact had liver disease or heart failure—both of which diminish the clearance of lidocaine—a potentially toxic serum concentration could develop. If, for example, the patient's clearance of lidocaine was half that of the usual patient (4.5 mL per minute per kilogram), the administration of lidocaine at a rate of 1.9 mg per minute would result in a steady-state serum concentration of 6 mg per liter, which could be toxic.

$$Cp_{average} = 1.9 \text{ mg/min} /(4.5 \text{ mL/min/kg}) (70 \text{ kg})$$

$$= 1.9 \text{ mg/min}/ 315 \text{ mL/min} = 0.006 \text{ mg/mL} = 6 \text{ mg/L}$$

These relations demonstrate that clinicians must be aware of potential influences of patients' diseases and other medications on the ability to eliminate therapeutic agents. Using a standard dose predictably results in some patients having subtherapeutic drug concentrations and others having toxic levels. By recognizing the importance of drug clearance as it dictates the maintenance dose of a drug, clinicians can more reliably design dosing regimens for individual patients.

Administering drugs in the form of a constant IV infusion is less common than intermittent oral dosing. Dosing in this fashion also can be incorporated into the relations presented previously:

$$Cp_{average} = (F) (dose)/(dosing interval) (Cl)$$

where F is the fraction of drug absorbed as defined previously. Note that the combination of these parameters remains an administration rate.

This more comprehensive relation stresses other aspects of maintenance dosing. The effect of incomplete bioavailability should be readily apparent; this must be compensated for by administering larger amounts of drug. In addition, the amount of drug administered can be changed by modifying either the dose itself or the frequency of its administration, or both. Hence, the amount given can be diminished either by decreasing each dose, keeping the dosing interval constant, or keeping each individual dose the same and increasing the interval between doses (Chapter 167). For example, if a patient is receiving 240 mg of a drug every 12 hours, the administration rate is as follows (assuming F = 1.0):

Administration rate = 240 mg/12 h = 20 mg/h

If a clinician wished to halve the administration rate to 10 mg per hour, the dose could be halved to 120 mg, with the frequency of administration maintained at 12 hours,

Administration rate = 120 mg/12 h = 10 mg/h

or the original dose could be maintained at 240 mg and the dosing interval doubled at 24 hours:

Administration rate = 240 mg/24 h = 10 mg/h

Both methods of dose adjustment result in the same average serum concentration of drug. The methods differ, however, in that the more widely spaced dosing interval results in a greater difference between peak and trough drug serum concentrations. With some drugs, too large a magnitude of variation between peak and trough concentrations can be hazardous, with toxicity at the peak and lack of efficacy at the trough. Clinicians must consider this possibility when designing a dosing regimen. If such variations are a problem, they can be prevented by more frequent dosing; alternatively, with many medications, sustained-release preparations have been developed that allow more prolonged dosing intervals and prevent the problem of wide vacillation in serum drug concentrations.

HALF-LIFE/TIME TO REACH STEADY STATE

The concept of half-life often is misused. Traditionally, it has been equated with the capacity for elimination of drug. In reality, it is an indication of the time necessary to reach steady state. Half-life can be affected by changes either in Vd or in clearance. If solely the latter, changes in half-life indeed are a reflection of changes in drug elimination. Such effects would influence the maintenance dose. In contrast, a change in half-life solely on the basis of a change in Vd carries no implications concerning drug elimination and maintenance dose, but rather dictates a need to modify the loading dose. Any change in half-life, however, has the same implications in terms of the time needed to reach steady state.

The half-life of a drug is simply the time necessary for its concentration to decrease by half. This value can be determined easily by measuring the concentrations of a drug as it is eliminated over time. The time needed for a drug to reach steady state is four or five times the half-life. The concept of attainment of a steady state is important when initiating drug therapy but also any time a dosing regimen is changed or the half-life of a drug changes. In both of the latter circumstances, the time needed to reattain a new steady state requires four or five times the half-life. For example, in a patient who is receiving a continuous IV infusion of lidocaine at 2 mg per minute, resulting in a steady-state concentration of 3 mg per liter, it is desired to attain a new concentration of 4.5 mg per liter. As discussed in the previous section, the proportional relation between clearance and $Cp_{average}$ allows easy calculation of the infusion rate needed to attain this new concentration, namely, 3 mg per minute. If the administration rate is increased to this amount, the time needed to reach 4.5 mg per liter is four or five times the half-life of lidocaine.

In most patients, the half-life of lidocaine is about 2 hours; hence, attainment of the new steady-state concentration requires (4 to 5) × 2 = 8 to 10 hours. If the time needed to reach a new steady state is not considered, the clinician might assume that the new concentration of lidocaine would occur quickly. In turn, if the patient does not respond, the clinician might misinterpret this as refractoriness to the drug and thereby change the therapeutic strategy. In reality, the patient may respond to the higher serum concentration of lidocaine once it is reached. In this type of circumstance, if it is deemed necessary for the patient to reach the new steady-state serum concentration quickly, an additional loading dose (calculated from the Vd) must be administered to boost the patient from a concentration of 3 to 4.5 mg per liter. The new infusion rate then would maintain the patient at that concentration.

The alternative scenario also is important. Consider a patient receiving 3 mg per minute of lidocaine with a steady-state serum concentration of 4.5 mg per liter that is causing toxic side effects. If the desire is to decrease the patient's lidocaine concentration to 3 mg per liter, the infusion rate could be switched to 2 mg per minute, and four or five times the half-life, or 8 to 10 hours, would be required to reach the newly defined target concentration. Again, if the time necessary to reach steady state is not considered, the clinician might expect the patient's adverse effects to abate quickly. Such expectations clearly are not realistic.

Another strategy is possible in such a circumstance; namely, lidocaine administration could be stopped completely. If this course of action were followed, it would have to be determined when to recommence administering the lidocaine. Again, knowledge of the half-life is helpful. In this example, the patient's lidocaine serum concentration is 4.5 mg per liter and the half-life is 2 hours. If the lidocaine infusion were stopped, then in 2 hours the concentration would decrease by half to 2.25 mg per liter; similarly, in 1 hour (half a half-life), it would decrease by 1.125 mg per liter to 3.375 mg per liter. Hence, the patient's lidocaine serum concentration would reach the desired new concentration of 3 mg per liter between 1 and 2 hours after the infusion was discontinued. A reasonable strategy would be to discontinue the lidocaine for 75 to 90 minutes and then restart its administration at the new infusion rate.

As noted at the outset of this section, values for half-life per se or changes in half-life in various clinical conditions offer no information about loading or maintenance dosing. This is true because half-life is a function of both Vd and clearance:

$$T\frac{1}{2} = 0.693 Vd/Cl$$

Hence, changes in half-life can occur as a result of changes in Vd, clearance, or both. Knowledge of only the half-life value offers no insight regarding the Vd or clearance of a drug. Therefore, such information is not helpful in determining loading or maintenance doses. Examples with lidocaine and digoxin emphasize these points and are provided in Table 55.3.

In patients with congestive heart failure, the Vd of lidocaine decreases; clearance also decreases, most likely because of congestive hepatopathy. These changes dictate a need to decrease both loading and maintenance doses (to one-half to two-thirds of normal for both) in such patients. Because both parameters decrease in parallel, however, there is no change in lidocaine's half-life; therefore, the time to reach steady state is unchanged. By focusing on half-life, the clinician could be seriously misled in terms of dosing strategy; he or she might conclude that because half-life is unchanged, no adjustment of dosing is necessary. In fact, both loading and maintenance doses need to be modified. Erroneous interpretation of the half-life could thereby result in substantially higher than expected serum concentrations of lidocaine.

In patients with liver disease, a different set of changes occur. In these patients, half-life may be exceedingly prolonged because of the additive effects of an increased Vd (mechanism unknown) and decreased clearance. Hence, the time to reach steady state would be prolonged in such patients, but again the half-life change alone would offer no insight regarding needed modifications of loading and maintenance doses of lidocaine.

The example of digoxin in patients with renal insufficiency also illustrates how overinterpretation of half-life can be misleading. As shown in Table 55.3, both patients with moderate and those with severe renal insufficiency may have half-life values that are similar, despite the fact that the clearance of digoxin in patients with severe renal impairment is considerably less than in patients with moderate renal insufficiency (mandating a much lower maintenance dose in the former). The inability of half-life to discriminate between the two conditions in terms of digoxin elimination occurs because patients with severe renal impairment also have a smaller Vd, which independently affects half-life. Inappropriate interpretation of half-life could lead to potentially disastrous errors in dosing.

DOSING REGIMEN DESIGN

Designing a dosing regimen for an individual patient requires interdigitation of the pharmacokinetic parameters discussed in the preceding sections. Based on data readily available in the

TABLE 55.3.	CHANGES IN LIDOCAINE AND DIGOXIN KINETIC PARAMETERS EMPHASIZING THAT HALF-LIFE IS A FUNCTION OF BOTH VOLUME OF DISTRIBUTION (Vd) AND CLEARANCE (Cl)		
	Vd (Loading Dose)	**Cl (Maintenance Dose)**	**Half-Life (Time to Reach Steady State)**
Lidocaine			
Heart failure	↓	↓	No change
Liver disease	↑	↓	↑↑
Digoxin			
Moderate renal insufficiency	No change	↓	↑
Severe renal insufficiency	↓	↓↓	↑

medical literature, the values for bioavailability, Vd, clearance, and half-life should be estimated for the patient. Such estimates should include consideration of the influence of the patient's age and weight; concomitant disease (e.g., hepatic, renal, and cardiac function); and drug interactions that might influence pharmacokinetic parameters. Clinicians generally are not accustomed to thinking in terms of these parameters. They are facilitated in this regard by the availability of dosing guidelines for individual drugs in readily available reference sources such as the *Physicians' Desk Reference*. However, such guidelines rarely are comprehensive. They usually do not offer sufficient quantitative information about the effects of disease states or drug interactions on the separate pharmacokinetic parameters. Precision of dosing is much improved if regimens are based on pharmacokinetic values. Subsequent chapters provide values for different drugs, which can be used in dosing regimen design.

The approach to designing a dosing regimen can be considered in several steps. First, the need for a loading dose must be determined. This decision is based on the urgency of attaining an efficacious serum concentration combined with knowledge of the drug's half-life and thereby the time required to reach steady-state concentrations if a loading dose is not administered. If a loading dose is elected, the route of administration must be chosen and the dose calculated based on Vd, the desired concentration, and bioavailability (if the drug is not given intravenously):

Loading dose = (desired initial concentration) (Vd)/F

The second step in dosing regimen design is calculation of a maintenance dose that will keep the average serum concentration of the drug at the desired level. This dose is calculated from clearance, the desired concentration, and bioavailability:

Maintenance dose = desired average steady-state concentration (Cl)/F

The route of administration of the maintenance dose also must be selected. If the drug is to be given by mouth, which is the most common situation, a dosing interval must be selected. As a general rule, it is convenient to administer the dose at an interval close to the drug's half-life. When this is done, the difference between peak and trough concentrations at steady state is easily calculated:

Difference between peak and trough = ½dose/Vd

As pointed out, more frequent dosing minimizes the difference between peak and trough concentrations, and widely spaced dosing accentuates the difference. The regimen that is best for an individual patient depends on the drug used and the disease being treated. In some cases (e.g., procainamide), a drug's half-life is short (about 3 hours), precluding its administration every half-life. Conversely, prescribing the drug at more convenient intervals results in excessive vacillation between peak and trough concentrations. To facilitate dosing regimens in such circumstances, sustained-release preparations have been developed that allow wider dosing intervals and minimize drug level fluctuations. With such preparations, the total dose needed is still calculated based on the average steady-state drug serum concentration to be maintained.

The final step in dosing regimen design is using feedback from patient response and measured concentrations of drug in the patient's serum to modify the dosing regimen and tailor therapy to the needs of the individual. If higher serum concentrations are needed, it must be decided whether it is necessary to administer another loading dose or whether it is sufficient simply to increase the maintenance dose and await attainment of a new steady state after a period equal to four or five times the drug's half-life. Conversely, if a lower serum concentration is needed, it must be decided whether simply to switch to a smaller maintenance dose or to discontinue the drug altogether until the desired concentration is reached and then initiate the new maintenance dose. These types of dose adjustments in particular are facilitated by knowledge of the individual pharmacokinetic parameters of a drug in a patient.

Clinicians always should be cognizant of the dynamic nature of drug therapy and the capacity for changes in drug disposition and response. Changes in a patient's primary disease and drug interactions can affect all the pharmacokinetic parameters discussed. The likelihood that handling of and response to a drug will change over time dictates that the clinician be alert for the necessity to change drug dosing regimens. So doing will maximize efficacy and minimize toxicity.

■ THERAPEUTIC DRUG MONITORING

Measuring drug serum concentrations is referred to as therapeutic drug monitoring. This strategy is used to guide therapy for drugs with narrow therapeutic margins for which optimal therapy requires attainment of a drug serum concentration within narrow bounds. Such monitoring allows the highest level of precision in adjusting doses to compensate for variability among individuals.

For example, consider a commonly encountered patient administered lidocaine. As in previous examples, the average Vd of 1.1 L per kilogram and clearance of 9 mL per minute per kilogram can be used to calculate loading and maintenance doses of 231 mg and 1.9 mg per minute, respectively, to attain a target serum concentration of 3 mg per liter in a 70-kg patient. If, however, a patient's pharmacokinetic parameters are at the high end of the range of normal (e.g., 50% higher Vd and clearance), the actually attained lidocaine serum concentration will be 50% lower. If the patient had not responded to the originally derived dosing regimen, the clinician could not distinguish too low a drug concentration from refractoriness to the drug unless a concentration were actually measured. If a low concentration of lidocaine were documented, the preferred strategy would be to increase the dose to attain a desired concentration and then reassess the patient's response.

The converse scenario also is possible, namely, the patient's pharmacokinetic parameters may be at the low end of the normal range. In this case, an actual lidocaine serum concentration as much as 50% higher than expected might occur. If the patient had not responded to lidocaine in this circumstance and it was known that the lidocaine serum concentration was sufficient (if not at the high end of the therapeutic range), the clinician might elect to use another drug rather than give larger doses of lidocaine and risk toxicity.

The actually measured drug concentration is extremely useful in adjusting dosing regimens. The proportionality of the relations between Vd and loading dose and between clearance and maintenance dose makes this possible. Hence, if a steady-state serum concentration of a drug is too low, the desired new target concentration can be defined and the maintenance dose increased proportionately. Such dose adjustments were discussed in detail in the previous section.

Interpretation of measured serum concentrations often is inappropriate (Table 55.4). For example, surveys have shown that as many as half the samples measured for digoxin in a clinical laboratory are useless and potentially misleading. The most common reason for this failing is inattention to simple pharmacokinetic principles. *Proper interpretation requires knowledge of the relation between the time a sample was drawn and the time the dose of drug was administered.* If a value is interpreted based on the belief that it is a trough concentration (obtained immediately before the next dose), whereas it actually is a peak sample or one obtained in the middle of the dosing interval, dose adjustment based on false assumptions may ensue.

Another common error is obtaining a sample during the distribution phase of a drug. This phase is the time necessary for the drug to equilibrate between serum and tissues. Until equilibration occurs, the serum concentration is not reflective of drug concentration at the site of action and, thereby, is not interpretable. For most drugs, equilibration occurs quickly and problems do not occur. For lidocaine and digoxin, however, this potential error must be prevented. After a loading dose of lidocaine has been given, about 30 minutes (and preferably longer) should elapse before a sample is obtained. The distribution phase for digoxin is long, lasting up to 6 hours. Hence, samples for digoxin measurements should never be obtained less than 6 hours after a dose.

A similar error is sampling during the absorption phase when a drug has been administered by other than IV routes. Variability in the time course of drug absorption is immense and is influenced by factors such as drug formulation, disease state, food consumption, and drug interactions. Hence, a drug serum concentration obtained after an oral dose could represent ascent to the peak concentration, the peak itself, or descent from the peak. Which of these possibilities is actually the case cannot be ascertained unless frequent samples are obtained sufficient to define the absorption profile of the drug. Such efforts rarely are indicated.

These three pitfalls in interpretation of drug serum concentrations can be prevented by a simple strategy, namely, obtaining only trough samples. Usually, such values are sufficient to guide therapy and avoid the most common errors that occur in therapeutic drug monitoring.

Proper interpretation of a drug serum concentration during maintenance therapy requires an assessment of whether steady-state concentrations have been reached. So doing requires knowledge of a drug's half-life. If a patient were started on a maintenance regimen and evaluated before steady state was attained, the concentration would increase with continued dosing. If the measured value was interpreted erroneously as the steady-state concentration, inappropriate dosing decisions might ensue. For example, the average half-life for digoxin is about 36 hours. Hence, about a week of dosing is required to reach steady state. If a digoxin serum concentration is obtained after 3 days, found to be less than desired, and in error interpreted as reflective of steady state, a potentially disastrous increase in dose might be prescribed. This type of problem can be prevented by always assessing the patient's drug dosing status with regard to the time needed for steady-state conditions to occur.

Many clinicians tend to overlook lack of compliance with medication regimens as an explanation for measured drug concentrations that differ from those expected. If a person on an outpatient dosing regimen has a drug serum concentration lower than anticipated, the discrepancy could be explained by a greater than expected drug clearance or a lower bioavailability in the specific patient or by poor compliance. All these possibilities must be considered.

A pitfall that must be avoided in therapeutic drug monitoring is using a drug serum concentration itself as a therapeutic goal or definitive diagnostic tool. This is inappropriate because of pharmacodynamic variability among patients; hence, a given drug serum concentration may be subtherapeutic in one patient, ideal in another, and toxic in yet another. A good example of the application of this tenet is digoxin. In a patient with atrial fibrillation in whom digoxin is used to control the ventricular rate, a needed digoxin serum concentration may be high and an average "normal" value of 1.5 ng per milliliter may be subtherapeutic. In contrast, in many patients with congestive heart failure, a concentration of 1.5 ng per milliliter might be ideal. At the other extreme, a patient who is potassium- or magnesium-depleted may experience digoxin toxicity at a serum concentration of 1.5 ng per milliliter.

Proper use of a measured drug concentration in an individual patient requires treatment of the serum concentration value as simply another item of information that must be integrated with other clinical end points to determine how the specific patient is responding to a particular dose and concentration of drug. Once this clinical assessment is made, the concentration value can be used to design or modify the patient's dosing regimen based on pharmacokinetic principles. Optimal therapy is possible only by interdigitating both pharmacokinetic and pharmacodynamic principles.

TABLE 55.4.   REASONS FOR IMPROPER INTERPRETATION OF DRUG SERUM CONCENTRATIONS

Lack of knowledge about the timing of the sample in relation to dosing of the drug
Sampling during the distribution phase
Not realizing the futility of defining a peak concentration after oral dosing
Ignoring the concept of steady state
Ignoring the possibility of noncompliance
Forgetting that there is considerable pharmacodynamic as well as pharmacokinetic variability among patients

CLINICAL TOXICOLOGY

Poisoning is the extreme of pharmacokinetics and pharmacodynamics; its treatment can be considered in terms of the foregoing concepts.

The first principle of clinical toxicology is general support of the patient. Proper ventilation and circulatory support should be the therapeutic focus after which one can consider "detoxification." The pharmacodynamic component of poisoning is consideration of ways to counteract the toxic effect of the poison. The pharmacokinetic component is using methods to either preclude further absorption of the toxin or to enhance its elimination.

Antidotes to some poisons are available. Use of atropine in organophosphate poisoning, *N*-acetylcysteine for acetaminophen overdose, and numerous others are pertinent. See Chapter 57 (Emergency Medicine). Toxicology texts should be accessible for identifying antidotes as well as their mode of administration. In addition, physicians should know how to contact the nearest poison control center, which can provide this information.

All aforementioned pharmacokinetic principles are relevant to poisoning settings. In terms of bioavailability, a number of therapeutic strategies can be used to prevent additional absorption of the poison. Some are as simple as stripping the patient and bathing him or her to remove poisons such as organophosphates, which may be in the clothing and on the skin through which many poisons can be absorbed. With most ingested poisons (except hydrocarbons), emesis can be induced or activated charcoal can be given. With some drugs, activated charcoal actually enhances elimination by interrupting enterohepatic cycling.

Distribution of a drug is also important. Reversing systemic acidemia enhances distribution of salicylate out of the CNS, thereby diminishing its toxicity. Binding of digoxin to Fab fragments actually extracts digoxin out of tissues and back into the plasma where it can be excreted. Distribution of a drug is also significant regarding whether dialytic removal of a poison might be helpful. Drugs with high degrees of protein binding (more than 90%) cannot be removed by dialysis. In addition, drugs with large volumes of distribution (in general more than 1 L per kilogram) are negligibly removed by dialytic procedures including resin hemoperfusion. Most of the body burden of such drugs is in peripheral tissues. As such, even if the dialytic procedure can remove a substantial percentage of poison in the serum, this amount is trivial in proportion to that in the rest of the body.

With some poisons, one can also enhance elimination. The effect of activated charcoal and dialysis has been mentioned. Drugs with renal excretion that is influenced by urinary pH can have their elimination enhanced by adjusting urine pH and enhancing urinary flow. Excretion of organic acids such as salicylate and phenobarbital is increased by an alkaline urine. The converse applies for organic bases.

Some poisons such as methanol and ethylene glycol are metabolized to their toxins. Understanding that this metabolism occurs through alcohol dehydrogenase and knowing that ethanol is the preferred substrate for this enzyme has allowed use of ethanol infusions as therapy for poisoning with these agents.

This example and the principles previously enumerated illustrate how the same principles of clinical pharmacology are logically applied to toxicology.

Refer to Chapter 90, Clinical Pharmacology of Cardiovascular Drugs; Chapter 167, Adjustment of Drug Dosage in Patients with Renal Insufficiency; Chapter 199, Cutaneous Reactions to Drugs; and Chapter 469, Geriatric Clinical Pharmacology.

BIBLIOGRAPHY

Beckmann ML, Brass EP. Advances in managing drug overdoses. *Hosp Formul* 1987;22:432–459.

Gibaldi M, Levy G. Pharmacokinetics in clinical practice. 1. Concepts. *JAMA* 1976;235:1864–1867.

Gibaldi M, Levy G. Pharmacokinetics in clinical practice. 2. Applications. *JAMA* 1976;235:1987–1992.

Holford NHG, Sheiner LB. Understanding the dose-effect relationship: clinical application of pharmacokinetic-pharmacodynamic models. *Clin Pharmacokinet* 1981;6:429–453.

Kulig K. Initial management of ingestions of toxic substances. *N Engl J Med* 1992;326:1677–1681.

Urquhart J. Role of patient compliance in clinical pharmacokinetics. *Clin Pharmacokinet* 1994:202–215.

Wilkinson GR. Clearance approaches in pharmacology. *Pharmacol Rev* 1987;39:1–47.

Williams RL. Dosage regimen design: pharmacodynamic considerations. *J Clin Pharmacol* 1992;32:597–602.

Wood AJJ, Stein CM, Woosley R. Making medicines safer—the need for an independent drug safety board. *N Engl J Med* 1998;339:1851–1854

Kelley's Textbook of Internal Medicine, fourth edition. Edited by H. David Humes. Lippincott Williams & Wilkins, Philadelphia © 2000.

C H A P T E R

56

ALTERNATIVE MEDICINE: PREVALENCE, COST, AND USEFULNESS

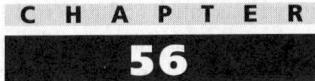

MARK MULTACH

Alternative or complementary medicine is a major growth industry in the United States within the medical, lay, and financial communities. Patients have far outstripped the medical community in their willingness to use these therapies. Americans now make more visits to nontraditional healers than to their family doctors and spend almost as much (out of pocket) on alternative medicine as on unreimbursed physician services ($27 billion versus $29 billion).

Recently, organized medicine has begun to address alternative therapies. Many medical centers have or are developing centers for the study and use of complementary medicine. Research funding, especially at the federal level, is increasing at an unprecedented growth rate.

The allopathic approach to alternative medicine has not been an easy one. Although the traditional medical community deals in epidemiology, biostatistics, randomized placebo-controlled studies, and gold standards, many alternative therapies cannot be studied by this approach. For example, the study of acupuncture has run into difficulties in attempting to carry out double-blind, placebo-controlled studies. The ethical and practical issues have required years of debate to attempt to resolve.

HERBAL MEDICINE AND OTHER NATURAL SUPPLEMENTS

Herbal remedies are used more and more frequently by patients. In the early 1990s, one survey estimated that 54 million Americans used herbal medicines, at a cost of approximately $54 per person per year. Annual sales of botanicals in the United States alone have risen from $1.6 billion in 1994 to $16 billion in sales in 1998, demonstrating the impact since 1994 of Congress's approval of the Dietary Supplement Health and Education Act.

Although more than one-third of the population has tried an herbal remedy within the past few years, more than 60 million Americans used herbal medicines on a more regular basis in 1997. More than 7 million used St. John's wort (in Germany, five times more people use this remedy than Prozac [fluoxetine]), similar to the number using echinacea. Owing in part to release of data recently suggesting a direct effect, ginkgo biloba is used by more than 10 million Americans regularly.

Regulation of this industry is in its infancy. Some manufacturers in the industry have implemented strict quality control measures; however, no such standard is in place across the industry. Contents of "active" (the definition of which is unclear) ingredients may vary by as much as 300% to 1,000% according to manufacturer and even according to batch from a single manufacturer. At the extreme, studies have demonstrated no active ingredient in some products sampled.

Herbal supplements undergo no testing to determine whether they contain what they claim. The Food & Drug Administration (FDA) does not regulate claims of benefit. In fact, the Dietary Supplement Health and Education Act allows that as long as labeling makes no specific claim on the packaging regarding treatment of a disease, companies can sell any supplement. Labeling need only contain promises for improvement of general structure and function. This further complicates the situation for patients. Treatment for specific diseases cannot be listed on the packaging; therefore, no dosages for specific indications can be listed either. Patients are left to their own devices to guess what dosage to use for a specific ailment, which can lead to potential overdoses. Rules regulating advertising for herbal products fall below even the standard set for packaging.

Of equal importance is the potential for adverse reactions or interactions of herbal supplements with prescription drugs or other remedies. Although herbal remedies are advertised as harmless, the problems with many preparations are well documented in both the lay and the medical literature.

Studies of supplements also are the subject of controversy.

In the history of the FDA, regulations have become stricter since the thalidomide scare of the 1960s. Large well-controlled studies are required to look at drug safety and benefit, in addition to ongoing surveillance of drug safety. The literature on supplements falls far short of this level of rigor.

Finally, what constitutes a supplement and what constitutes a drug are unclear. The FDA is responsible for supervision and approval of drugs. The Dietary Supplement Health and Education Act categorized vitamins, minerals herbs, amino acids, some hormones, and other products as *supplements*, which are unregulated by the FDA. Some supplements are chemically similar to prescription drugs but, with the removal of some of the labeling, are distributed as supplements. Cholestin, a popular treatment in China for hypercholesterolemia, contains a yeast and is classified as a supplement. However, a product of the species of yeast, which appears to be the active ingredient, is chemically similar to lovastatin.

Some hope of clearing up the picture is in sight. A presidential commission was appointed 2 years ago and has reviewed the current state of supplements. It has made preliminary recommendations to the FDA on how to regulate supplements. The suggestions included creating a panel, under the auspices of the National Institutes of Health's Office of Alternative Medicine, to review all herbs and to make recommendations regarding claims of current supplements and to recommend that packaging be more extensive in documentation of claims for the patient.

In 1978, in Germany a review panel (referred to as Commission E) was appointed to start an ongoing review process of supplements. The commission included physicians, pharmacists, pharmacologists, toxicologists, representatives of the pharmaceutical industry, and lay persons who reviewed the current literature on herbs then on the market. The commission has produced monographs on more than 300 supplements to date. Based on this ongoing review, approximately 200 supplements have been approved as nonprescription drugs. An English translation of these monographs was made available in August 1998.

In contrast to the paucity of scientific data supporting herbal preparations is the list of current medications that were derived from botanicals. These include aspirin (white willow bark), digitalis (foxglove), paclitaxel (Taxol; from yew tree bark), and oral contraceptives (Mexican yam).

SPECIFIC HERBS

St. John's Wort

Perhaps the best evidence supporting efficacy of a botanical is for St. John's wort (Table 56.1). More than 20 trials to date

---

TABLE 56.1.	**ST. JOHN'S WORT**

- *Production*
  Hypericin (active ingredient) extracted from the stem of the plant *Hypericum perforatum*
- *Dosage*
  Depression: 2–4 g daily (0.2–1 mg of hypericin)
- *Mechanism of Action*—unknown

have been performed following traditional medical literature standards. Trials usually involve a comparison with a placebo or a tricyclic antidepressant. Studies have consistently demonstrated improvement in objective assessments of depression at least equivalent to standard therapy (tricyclic antidepressants) with significantly fewer side effects. Short-term studies showed side effects to be equal to placebo and to be approximately 50% of those of tricyclic antidepressants. Unfortunately, studies were short-term only, lasting less than 6 months at maximum. The most common complaints were photosensitivity (especially in fair-skinned persons), dizziness, gastrointestinal upset, fatigue, and confusion.

Ginkgo Biloba

Ginkgo biloba has been studied in the United States. Its pharmacology and mechanism of action have been reviewed and have shown many unique effects (Table 56.2). Several studies of ginkgo biloba in the United States have shown improvement in objective criteria of neuropsychological functioning in patients with senile dementia, Alzheimer's type. The clinical usefulness of these observations has yet to be demonstrated. The onset of the herb's effect was delayed up to 6 to 8 weeks. Similarly, in studies in the United States and Europe using lower dosages of ginkgo, patients with peripheral vascular disease showed significant improvement.

Echinacea

Echinacea (*Echinacea* angustifolia; purple coneflower) is a genus with a medicinal history going back to Native American medicine (Table 56.3). Although there are many species, the most commonly used medicinally is echinacea purpura. The combination of many species and preparations has made interpretation of the literature very difficult. Many clinical effects have been claimed for echinacea (some infections, chronic fatigue, cancer, and chronic arthritis, to name a few), but it is most frequently used for the common cold. Three studies to date have focused on this application with scientific rigor. In all three studies, cold

TABLE 56.2.	GINKGO BILOBA

- *Production*
  Extracted from the leaves of the plant *Ginkgo biloba*
- *Dosage* (native dried extract, split doses)
  For dementia: 120–240 mg/day
  For peripheral vascular disease: 120–160 mg/day
- *Mechanism of action* (from animal data)
  Improved hypoxic tolerance (especially cerebral tissue)
  Inhibition of cerebral edema in response to trauma/toxin
  Acceleration of regression of cerebral edema
  Inhibition of age-related reduction of muscarinic cholinergic receptors and 1-adrenoreceptors
  Stimulation of choline uptake in the hippocampus
  Inactivation of oxygen radicals
  Improved rheologic properties of the blood
  Increased blood flow (especially microcirculation)

TABLE 56.3.	ECHINACEA

- *Production*
  Derived from the many parts primarily of the plant species *Echinacea purpura* or its extracts
- *Dosage* (native dried extract, split doses)
  Depression: 2–4 g/d (0.2–1 mg of hypericin)
- *Mechanism of action* (many nonspecific effects on the immune system)
  Phagocyte stimulation
  Acute phase reactions
  Monocyte activation (secretion of tumor necrosis factor- α, as well as interleukins 1 and 6)

symptoms were of shorter duration (statistically significant in two of three, the third having a small population limiting its power to detect differences), whereas symptoms were significantly improved in one of three, unchanged in one, and not specifically studied in the third. Some concern has been expressed among both herbalists and allopathic physicians about the immune-enhancing properties of echinacea and potentially harmful immune reactions (severe allergic reactions have been reported). Goldenseal is often found combined with echinaceaz. Studies have demonstrated no benefit from the use of goldenseal.

Kava Kava

Kava kava comes from the dried root of *Piperis methystici G. Forster,* is derived from dried above-ground parts of the plant *Hypericum perforatum* and contains the chemical kavapyrones (kawain). Animal studies have shown significant central nervous system (CNS) depression. As a result of this and observations in humans of drowsiness and slowing of reflexive responses, concern has been expressed over its use, especially in conjunction with other CNS active medications (e.g., alcohol, barbiturates). Adequate studies of kava kava in humans are not available.

Saw Palmetto

Saw palmetto berry is rapidly increasing in use by men for prostate-induced urinary symptoms. Clinical trials (and one meta-analysis) indicate significant decrease in urinary symptoms. The effect is most likely antiandrogenic in nature. Dosages used were 0.5 to 1.0 g per day of the dried berry (0.6 to 1.5 mL of extract).

ACUPUNCTURE

Acupuncture has similarly shown a rapid growth in popularity. Acupuncture includes a number of techniques and tools combined to produce its effects. Various types of needles or other instruments to induce pressure are combined with different types of manipulation of the needle (including twisting, heat [also known as moxibustion], pressure [acupressure], and electricity). In addition to different techniques, a number of historical

TABLE 56.4.	SCHOOLS OR SYSTEMS OF ACUPUNCTURE

- Traditional Chinese medicine
- French energetics
- Korean Hand acupuncture
- Five phases (five elements)
- Auricular
- Myofascial
- Local injection

schools of acupuncture are in existence as well as several newer systems of treatment (Table 56.4).

Approximately 9 to 12 million patients visit acupuncturists yearly, averaging 19 visits per patient. Because this expense is not covered by almost all third-party payers, patients can expect to pay approximately $30 per visit out of pocket. Patients seeking acupuncture care tend to be from a higher socioeconomic group, are younger (25- to 49-year age range on average), and have a higher educational status (college education on average) than the general population. Patients are more likely to be white or of Asian rather than African-American descent. Men and women use acupuncture with about the same frequency. Patients who use acupuncture on a regular basis tend to have chronic medical problems of more than 1 year's duration. Most consult with a traditional physician for the same complaint. However, more than 75% of these patients do not mention acupuncture to their Western-trained physician.

HISTORY OF ACUPUNCTURE

The history of acupuncture dates to 1500 B.C. with the advent of the Taoist philosophy. The first notations of use of acupuncture appear in 500 B.C. with descriptions of the use of stone needles. In 200 B.C., the first definitive description of the principles of health and illness was outlined in the *Yellow Emperor's Internal Classic* in which basic concepts of health and disease were defined. Health was felt to be a balance of *Qi*, the energy flow throughout the body. Illness was a result of some perturbation in this flow. The Internal Classic further defined two systems for describing health and illness: *yin* and *yang*. These systems represented one balanced system of health. Yin represented darkness, passivity, decline, whereas Yang was brightness, excitement, and upwardness. Illnesses and organs were described as either yin (heart, lungs, spleen, liver, kidney, pericardium) or yang (small and large intestines, stomach, gallbladder, bladder). The body balanced these forces in health, whereas in illness there was an imbalance between the two. Treatment was aimed at bringing a healthy balance back by any of a number of modalities including diet and acupuncture.

The second organizing theme of the Internal Classic revolves around *five elements* or natural resources (wood, fire, earth, metal, and water). According to this system, the organs are related to the five elements as well as to each other.

BASICS OF ACUPUNCTURE

The basic principle of acupuncture is modification of body energies focused at specific points along specific lines around the body. Illnesses are felt to be systemic processes in which the energy flow and balance in the body as a whole are disordered. Manipulation of the energy channels along these lines or meridians can realign and rebalance the Qi.

Practitioners use stainless-steel or (more expensive) alloys. Needles may be the single-use type or reusable. The FDA has mandated single use. However, there is still concern about actual adherence to this requirement.

Diseases represent symptoms of a complex dysfunction of the balancing forces just mentioned. Qi flows along a system of *meridians*, imaginary lines running longitudinally in and around the body. Twelve major meridians exist, which communicate by a series of transverse collaterals. In addition, a number of other lines exist, including divergent meridians, 12 muscle meridians, 8 minor meridians, and 12 cutaneous meridians. Each meridian is connected to specific yin and yang organs. Working with the major and minor meridians, 361 acupuncture points are defined. These points are defined in terms related to anatomical structures and easy defined measurements (*Cun*). Each point has a name and serial number description.

The most studied of the acupuncture techniques involves the use of needles and direct manipulation or electrical stimulation. Scientific data relating to other modalities are more scarce. Modern theories and research have attempted to relate the meridians and acupuncture points to anatomical structures and physiologic processes. This approach has had a fair degree of success in defining a scientific basis for acupuncture.

Acupuncture points and major meridians are often associated with underlying nerves. Manipulation of acupuncture points is associated with changes in the release of neurotransmitters, both positive and negative. Some investigators have also found unique electrical properties associated with some acupuncture points and meridians. Many of the effects of acupuncture are clearly associated with nerve function.

In human studies, many observations have begun to elucidate the physiologic processes involved in acupuncture. The effects of acupuncture can be abolished with local pretreatment with procaine, an effect not seen with placebo injections. Acupuncture has been shown to be ineffective in quadriplegics and paraplegics below the level of their neurologic injury. Use of the opiate antagonist, naloxone, eliminates the therapeutic effect of acupuncture, an effect not seen with placebo injections. Alcohol decreases or eliminates the effect of acupuncture, so patients are advised to avoid alcohol before therapy. Finally, corticosteroids are known to inhibit the effect of acupuncture, leading to the recommendation that they be avoided for 6 to 12 weeks before therapy.

In animals, studies have shown a strong association between physiologic processes and efficacy of acupuncture. Use of acupuncture has been shown to induce production of specific messenger RNA sequences and proteins for opiate receptors and endorphins. The effects are blocked with the help of receptor antagonists. Finally, induced hypothalamic lesions (site of β-endorphin release) abolish acupuncture effects.

THERAPY

The acupuncture therapist inserts and immediately knows when the needle was correctly placed. If inserted into an appropriate acupuncture point, the patient describes a sensation of heaviness, fullness, and numbness without pain (*De Qi*). After treatment, the patient usually feels generalized body fatigue; this effect is seen minutes to hours later. As a result, patients are advised to avoid strenuous activity or driving immediately after treatment. A rebound phenomenon may occur 24 to 48 hours later before improvement of symptoms. Note that although there are no studies documenting adverse effects of acupuncture on pregnancy, the lack of such studies on safety has led to naming pregnancy as a relative contraindication to acupuncture.

The most common side effects of acupuncture are warmth, relaxation, a sense of well-being, and an improved energy level. Rarely, patients have a vasovagal episode with the initial needle insertion, nausea, anorexia, and local irritation. Very rare case reports have described pneumothorax, hepatitis B, and pericardial tamponade.

EFFICACY

Acupuncture has been studied in many diseases and ailments, including osteoarthritis, chemotherapy-induced and postoperative nausea, asthma, back pain, fibromyalgia, dysmenorrhea, bladder instability, migraine headaches, chronic pain, substance abuse, and stress.

In patients with pulmonary disease (especially asthma), a small number of studies have been performed. Acupuncture has significant effects on dynamic pulmonary volumes including forced expiratory volume in 1 second (FEV_1), forced vital capacity (FVC), and maximum voluntary ventilation (MVV). Use of acupuncture has been associated with significant reductions (up to 50%) in the cost of caring for these patients, including medication costs, use of laboratory examinations, and need for hospitalizations. Studies have shown that 90% or more of patients with pulmonary disease significantly decrease medication requirements and use. The best-studied example has been methacholine-induced bronchoconstriction. Double-blind studies using sham acupuncture points have shown statistically significant efficacy greater than placebo, although statistically not as effective as bronchodilators.

In patients with chemotherapy-induced or postoperative nausea, single-blind studies have shown statistically significant improvement in symptoms. However, acupuncture is not believed to be as effective as traditional antiemetic medications.

Various pain syndromes have been studied with regard to acupuncture, including postoperative pain, postdental procedure pain, some musculoskeletal conditions (e.g., fibromyalgia, fibromyofascial pain), and low back pain. The argument has been that traditional therapies have such documented toxicity that acupuncture may be an acceptable alternative with at least as much benefit and considerably less potential for toxicity. Studies vary, with little efficacy seen in patients with osteoarthritis but consistent patterns of symptomatic relief in patients with lumbar disk herniation syndromes. In the latter, although in poorly designed studies, improvements have been seen in patients who have failed traditional, conservative therapy.

An area with considerable use for acupuncture therapy is substance abuse (see Chapter 35, Approach to the Problem of Substance Abuse). The quality of the data is similar to other areas of acupuncture treatment. Many studies of varying design and quality have yet to document efficacy beyond placebo thus far.

Other areas of active research include National Institutes of Health (NIH)-funded studies on unipolar depression, osteoarthritis, oral postsurgical pain, and HIV (in combination with Chinese herbal medicine), and even pregnant women with breech presentation to induce version of the baby.

MAGNET THERAPY

Finally, an addition to the armamentarium of some orthopedic surgeons has been the use of magnets in the healing of fractures. Anecdotal reports date back at least two decades. Therapy is applied with local placement of a magnet at the site of the fracture within the cast or stabilizing device. Two well-controlled studies, totaling more than 100 patients, showed statistically significant improvement in symptoms compared with those of controls. However, no data exist as to the benefit in healing. Studies in this area are ongoing.

BIBLIOGRAPHY

Blumenthal M, ed. *The complete German commission E monographs: therapeutic guide to herbal medicines*. Austin, TX: American Botanical Council. 512-926-4900.

NIH Consensus Development Panel on Acupuncture. Acupuncture. *JAMA* 1998;280(17):1518–1524.

NIH Office of Dietary Supplements. *www.usda.gov /fnic /IBID*.

Gruenwald J, Brendler T, Jaenicke C, eds. *Physicians desk reference for herbal medicine*, 1998.

NIH Technology Assessment Workshop on alternative medicine: acupuncture. *J Alternative Comp Med* 1996;2:1–256.

Kelley's Textbook of Internal Medicine, fourth edition. Edited by H. David Humes. Lippincott Williams & Wilkins, Philadelphia © 2000.

C H A P T E R

57

GENERAL PRINCIPLES IN THE APPROACH TO THE PATIENT WITH AN ACUTE EMERGENCY

SHELDON JACOBSON

When a patient presents with an acute, potentially life-threatening complaint or requires immediate resuscitation, an approach must be taken that is different from the traditional practice of internal medicine. To allow rapid assessment and treatment to be carried out simultaneously, the database to initially draw from is usually very limited. There may be no history available other than that given by prehospital personnel. Until the situation becomes less chaotic, care is delivered in a more stereotypical way using resuscitation algorithmic approaches and an analysis of the presenting physical data, especially the vital signs, but also including diagnostic studies and a vectored but thorough comprehensive physical examination. In this overview, we discuss the basic principles in the approach to these situations and the essential issues in the management of a range of presenting problems.

The first and overriding principle is that on arrival, patients are presumed to be unstable or in need of resuscitation until proven otherwise. The ABCDEs (airway, breathing, circulation and cervical spine injury, disrobe, engage) are applied according to the standards of basic cardiac life support (BCLS) promulgated by the American Heart Association. Immediately superimposed on the BCLS algorithms are those of advanced cardiac life support (ACLS), which are also established by the American Heart Association (Fig. 57.1). Note that although these standards were initially focused on the victim of a myocardial infarction who is unstable or sustains a cardiac arrest, the procedures and approaches actually have almost universal applicability to situations involving resuscitation of unstable patients. An overview of the approach to the patient with an acute non-trauma–related emergency has also been developed (Fig. 57.2).

After it has been established that resuscitation is not needed, the next principle is to obtain the presenting complaint and develop the history of the present illness, interpret and treat the abnormal vital signs, or monitor them as the case would require. In addition to the traditional vital signs, namely, respiration rate, pulse, temperature, and blood pressure, the scope of basic vital signs has been enlarged to include the mental status and the determination of the oxygen saturation of arterial blood by pulse oximetry. Given the very short treatment windows for major perturbations of the vital signs, treatment and diagnosis must be carried out at the same time. Thus, immediate management of hypotension, hypoxemia, hypoventilation and malignant hyperthermia can be instituted without a specific primary or underlying diagnosis or a complete understanding of the underlying pathophysiology. Each deviation from the norm of a vital sign suggests a therapeutic option as well as a set of differential diagnostic possibilities.

VENTILATION–RESPIRATION

First, an assessment of the adequacy of the minute ventilation (a proxy for the alveolar ventilation) and cellular respiration (gas exchange as well as cellular oxygen utilization) is needed. The respiratory rate is only one parameter gauging the adequacy of this function. If the respiratory rate is normal (10 to 12 breaths per minute), the patient appears well oxygenated, is alert and oriented, and has a pulse oximetry reading higher than 95%, significant abnormality of alveolar ventilation or cellular respiration is unlikely. Further investigation to monitor the respiratory and ventilatory function may include arterial blood gas determination while the patient is breathing room air, venous or arterial blood lactate, serum creatinine, and electrolytes. This data set will also provide the information needed to determine the patient's alveolar–arterial (A-a) gradient for oxygen, as well as the patient's acid–base status and degree of compensation or inadequate compensation for the acid–base abnormalities. The A-a gradient is a measure of the severity of ventilation/perfusion mismatches. If there is still uncertainty, adequacy of ventilation can also be assessed by bedside pulmonary function testing. These parameters include vital capacity (VC), peak flow, maximal midexpiratory flow rate, the forced expiratory volume in 1 second (FEV_1), and the FEV_1/VC. Normal values for these functions are given in Table 57.1.

In many situations, pulse oximetry is monitored continuously

Universal Algorithm for Adults

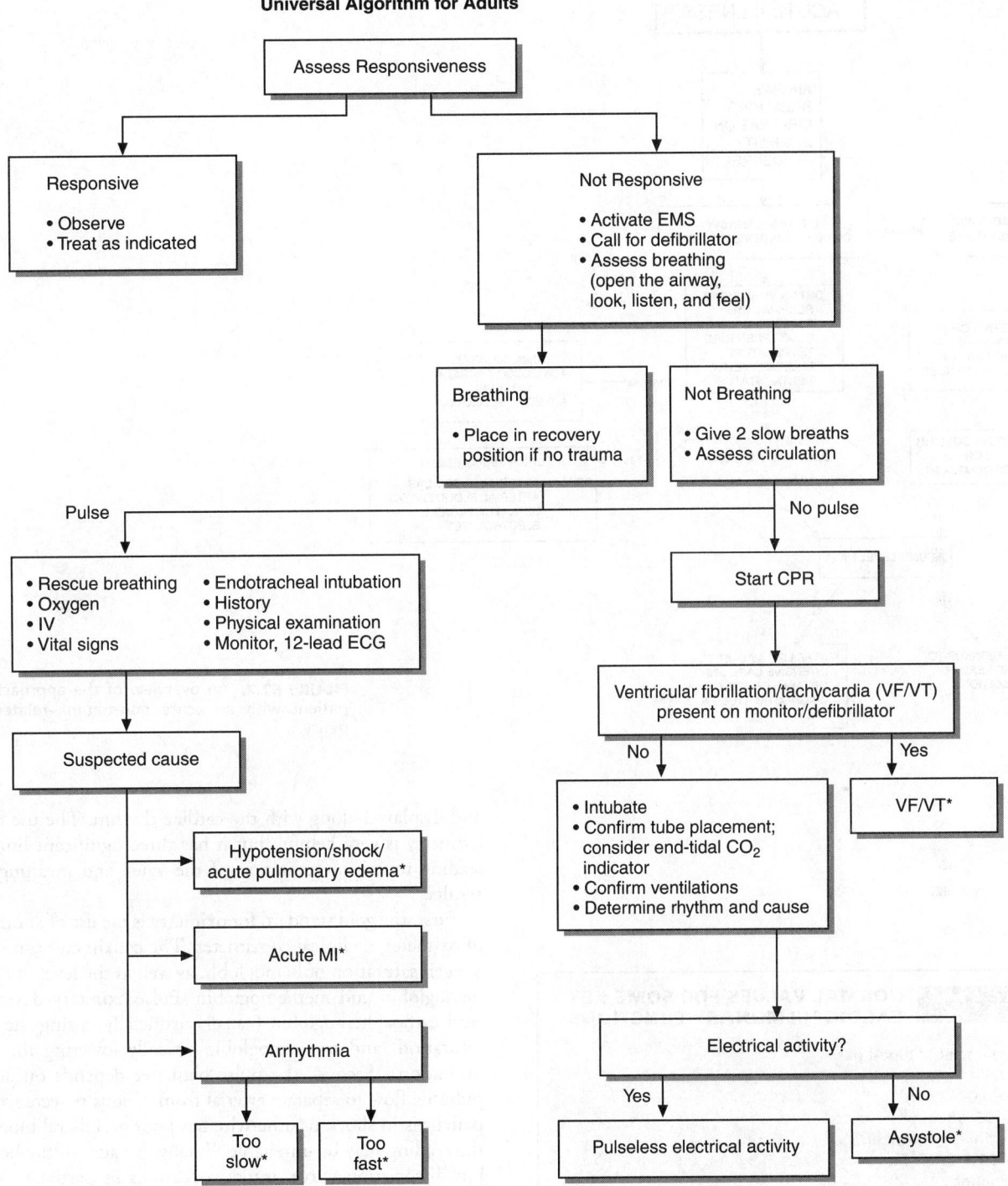

*access specific advance life support protocol

FIGURE 57.1. Standards initially focused on the victim of a myocardial infarction who is unstable or sustains a cardiac arrest; these approaches have almost universal applicability in the resuscitation of unstable patients.

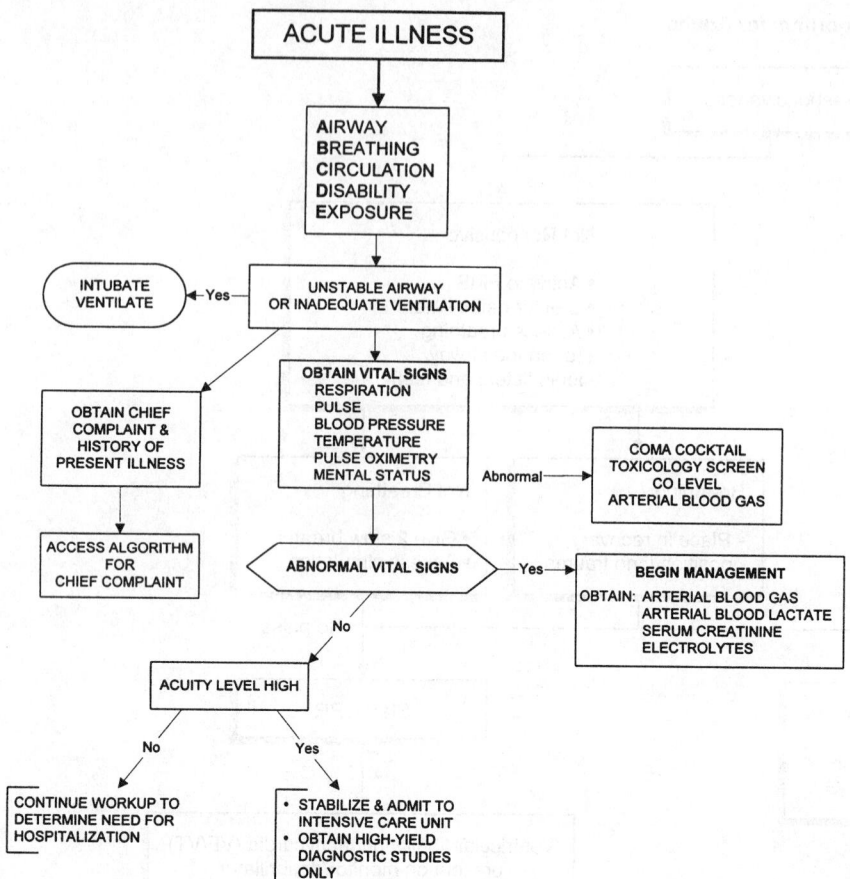

FIGURE 57.2. An overview of the approach to the patient with an acute non-trauma–related emergency.

TABLE 57.1.	NORMAL VALUES FOR SOME KEY CARDIOPULMONARY FUNCTIONS

Room air arterial blood gas
 pH 7.35–7.45
 Paco$_2$ 40–42 min
 Pao$_2$ 95–98 min
Pulse oximetry (room air)
 95–100% saturation
Tidal volume
 6–7 mL/kg
Vital capacity (VC)
 60–70 mL/kg
Forced vital capacity in 1 second = $(FEV_1) - FEV_1/VC = 80$–90%
Peak flow = 400–600 L/sec
Alveolar-arterial oxygen gradient (A-a)
 $A = 150 - Pco_2 \times 0.8$
 $a = Pao_2$
 Normal 10–15 mm Hg (older patients, approximately 1/3 age)
Arterial lactate 0.5–1.5 mmol/L
Venous lactate 0.5–2.2 mmol/L

and displayed along with the cardiac rhythm. The use of pulse oximetry is very helpful, but it has three significant limitations leading to misinterpretation of the value and meaning of the results.

First, the gold standard for oximetry is the use of another type of oximeter, a clinical cooximeter. The cooximeter can measure oxygen saturation of hemoglobin as well as the level of carboxyhemoglobin and methemoglobin. Pulse oximetry devices misread carboxyhemoglobin (usually artificially raising the oxygen saturation) and methemoglobin (usually lowering the oxygen saturation). Second, the pulse oximeter depends on adequate pulsatile flow to separate arterial from venous reflectance. If the patient is in shock or otherwise has poor peripheral blood flow, the reading may be unreliable. Finally, because of the hemoglobin dissociation curve, initial reductions in partial pressure of arterial oxygen (Pao_2) produces minimal decreases in oxygen saturation until the Pao_2 reaches the shoulder of the dissociation curve at a Pao_2 of approximately 60 mm, corresponding to a saturation of approximately 90%. Based on these parameters and the clinical situation, a decision can be made to intervene with endotracheal intubation and ventilatory support of breathing (Table 57.2.). Waveform capnometry, the measurement of the concentration of CO_2 in exhaled air, is very useful because it allows estimation of VC and degree of airway obstruction. In addition, it is very helpful in ascertaining endotracheal tube placement and the adequacy of cardiopulmonary resuscitation.

TABLE 57.2.	**GENERAL INDICATIONS FOR ENDOTRACHEAL INTUBATION AND VENTILATOR MANAGEMENT**

Failure of mechanics of breathing
- Tachypnea >35–40 breaths/min
- Bradypnea <8 breaths/min
- Vital capacity <15 mL/kg (normal 65–75 mL/kg)
- Negative inspiratory force <−25 cm H_2O (normal −65 to −75 cm H_2O)

Failure of oxygenation
- Pao_2 <60 while breathing 50% oxygen via face mask

Failure of ventilation
- $Paco_2$ >60

Unstable airway
- Intermittent obstruction via tongue; not treatable with nasal airway; aspiration of secretions

TABLE 57.3.	**CAUSES OF UNEXPLAINED SINUS TACHYCARDIA**

Pulmonary embolism
Hypoglycemia
Hyperthyroidism
Pheochromacytoma
Occult heart failure
Sinus nodal reentry
Low peripheral vascular resistance
   Vasodilatory medication
   Fistula
   Cirrhosis
   CO_2 narcosis
   Beri-beri heart disease

■ PULSE, RHYTHM, AND CARDIAC MONITORING

The pulse is automatically counted on the cardiac monitor and pulse oximeter. An estimation of the pulse wave by palpation or from the waveform on the pulse oximeter can also be very useful. For example, the patient with critical aortic stenosis has a slow upstroke and a long systolic ejection time, the so-called *pulsus parvus et tardus*, whereas patients with thyrotoxicosis, high fevers, sepsis, arteriovenous fistula, beriberi heart disease, or CO_2 narcosis often have rapid bounding pulses as evidence of their hyperdynamic circulation.

Most acutely ill patients require continuous cardiac monitoring in addition to a baseline standard 12-lead electrocardiogram (ECG) for recognition of characteristic patterns of injury, electrolyte disturbance, infarction, conduction disturbances, or dysrhythmia. The standard 12-lead tracing has been found to be inadequate for diagnosing isolated or predominant right ventricular infarction and true posterior infarction. The former is usually obvious on a V_4R lead, whereas diagnosis of the latter is best served by obtaining a V_8 or V_9 lead. In the future, the standard 12-lead ECG will most likely become a 14-lead study.

Patients with a rapid regular rhythm can have either a sinus tachycardia or a supraventricular or ventricular dysrhythmia. The maximal predicted exercise heart rate in sinus rhythm is approximately 220 beats per minute minus the patient's age with 1 standard deviation (SD) of ten beats. Thus, if a patient has a heart rate greater than this maximal rate at rest, a sinus tachycardia is much less likely. A resting sinus tachycardia can be seen with major physiologic derangements or with an increase in sympathetic tone. Table 57.3 contains a list of differential diagnostic possibilities in patients with unexplained sinus tachycardia. Patients with rapid tachycardias may present with instability of their vital signs due to the rapid rate and decreased diastolic filling time and with heart failure due to the myocardial workload. In some cases of ventricular tachycardia, the loss of the normal sequence of atrioventricular activation and contraction may in and of itself reduce cardiac output. These unstable patients usually require electrical cardioversion as quickly as possible.

Both sinus tachycardia and atrial flutter can present with rates of 140 to 150 beats per minute and thus can be easily confused. Differentiation can be achieved by response to the Valsalva maneuver or carotid massage. With these maneuvers, sinus tachycardia usually slows somewhat and then returns to the prior rate, whereas atrial flutter either shows no change or slows by increases in block (e.g., from 2:1 to 3:1 or 4:1). Atrioventricular (AV) nodal reentry tachycardias either "break" (resolve) with vagal maneuvers or remain constant. Sinus bradycardia, a pulse rate of less than 60, is often due to physical conditioning, increased vagal tone, or sympathetic blockade (Table 57.4). Slow rates are compensated by increasing stroke volume in the normal heart. Patients with heart failure attempt to compensate partially by rate increases, and slow heart rates lead to abrupt declines in cardiac output and progression of heart failure. Sudden slowing of the heart rate can be associated with presyncope or actual loss of consciousness if compensatory increase in the peripheral vascular resistance is inadequate in improving arterial and venous pressure. This is the pathophysiologic mechanism of vasovagal syncope. Occult causes of sinus bradycardia are listed in Table 57.4.

■ BLOOD PRESSURE

In all patients who have potentially life threatening problems, blood pressure monitoring should be instituted as soon as possi-

TABLE 57.4.	**OCCULT CAUSES OF SINUS BRADYCARDIA**

Athletic training
Hypothermia
Sick sinus syndrome
Increased intracranial pressure
Digitalis toxicity
β-blockade
Hypothyroidism
Cardiac ischemia

ble. The bladder of the arm cuff must approximate 60% to 80% of upper arm circumference to reduce artifactual readings. If there is a discrepancy between the indirect measurement and the patient's condition (i.e., low blood pressure measurement without signs of shock, or extraordinarily high readings), measurement of the blood pressure in the forearm or thigh may be helpful. The blood pressure measurements in these sites normally approximate brachial blood pressures. If a significant unresolved discrepancy continues, then direct invasive measurement of the radial blood pressure using a pressure transducer should be carried out. This problem is encountered most frequently in obese patients with pendulous skin folds.

HYPERTENSION

Hypertensive emergencies are defined as an elevated blood pressure with acute end-organ damage. The target organs for this damage are the brain, the heart, and the kidneys. Thus, if a patient presents with a blood pressure of 200/140 and has new focal neurologic signs or symptoms, he or she has, by definition, a hypertensive emergency. The level of hypertension does not correlate with the degree of end-organ damage. In pregnancy, a blood pressure of 140/90 may be the presenting reading in a patient with eclampsia. On the other hand, if during a routine physical examination, an asymptomatic patient is found to have a blood pressure of 200/140 and the only finding on physical examination is some copper wiring and spasm of the retinal arteries, this patient is considered to have a hypertensive urgency. The former patient would be admitted to the intensive care unit and receive parenteral antihypertensive therapy, whereas the latter patient would be started on oral antihypertensive agents and, after some partial response to the inception of treatment with an oral antihypertensive, the patient would be closely monitored in the ambulatory setting while workup is completed. Although many drugs and regimens have been evaluated (including labetalol, other β-blockers, clonidine, captopril, enalopril, nifedipine) the optimal choice or choices for these patients has not been studied. Overly aggressive treatment of the patient with a hypertensive urgency is a common occurrence and can lead to cardiovascular and cerebrovascular events.

HYPOTENSION

Hypotension is defined loosely as a systolic blood pressure of less than 90 mm systolic. However, because very few people walk about with a systolic pressure lower than 100 mm, it is best to consider a systolic blood pressure below 100 mm to be hypotension if the patient cannot assume the upright position and function normally. Even patients with a normal blood pressure may have inadequate systemic perfusion. Because blood pressure equals cardiac output times peripheral vascular resistance, a "normal blood pressure" should not be equated with normal systemic blood flow. In patients with a healthy autonomic nervous system, vasoconstriction can compensate for a blood volume deficit of 15% to 25% before hypotension ensues. During this period of compensated shock, there should be evidence of decreased perfusion of the skin (cold, mottled), a narrow pulse pressure, and decreased urinary output. Sinus tachycardia and orthostatic changes in blood pressure and pulse are not reliable because of the varying response in normal subjects

to positional change and the variable responses of patients to acute hypovolemia. In general, however, a pulse increase of 30 beats per minute or more when the patient stands upright or the development of orthostatic dizziness and hypotension can be viewed as a sign of blood volume loss in the appropriate clinical situation. Smaller changes in orthostatic vital signs may be significant if clinical correlations support the diagnosis.

SHOCK

Hypotension associated with other signs and symptoms of hypovolemia or hypoperfusion (e.g., peripheral cyanosis and mottling, altered mental states) should be considered to place the patient in a state of shock. Although there are various classifications of shock, for practical purposes in the emergency department we can divide them into (a) shock states that can improve—at least to some extent—to volume replacement and (b) cardiogenic shock, which usually does not improve to fluid challenges. Patients with right ventricular infarction and some with very high left ventricular compliance curves (diastolic dysfunction) can respond to volume loading, but most patients with cardiogenic shock decompensate further when given saline rapidly. Patients with so-called distributive shock (e.g., pulmonary embolism, cardiac tamponade, and tension pneumothorax) usually respond to volume loading, at least initially. The patient with cardiogenic shock usually presents with pulmonary and cardiac signs of congestive heart failure; this should be confirmed with a portable chest film. The ECG may reveal extensive damage, often both acute and remote.

All unstable patients should have two large-gauge (no. 18 or larger) intravenous cannulas inserted into a peripheral vein. For the former group of functionally hypovolemic patients, repeated boluses of intravenous saline 200 to 500 mL per challenge dose should be given every 5 minutes while the vital signs, mental state, lung sounds, lactate level, and urinary output are monitored.

TEMPERATURE

Life-threatening problems involving extremes of body temperature present insidiously and are often initially overlooked. Reading via oral or tympanic thermometry should be confirmed by rectal thermometer or a continuous-reading rectal or bladder temperature probe.

HYPOTHERMIA

The differential diagnosis of severe hypothermia is listed in Table 57.5. In general, hypothermia is suspected from the mechanism of injury (e.g., cold water immersion) or the environmental circumstance of the patient. Severe hypothermia with core body temperatures of less than 89° F is associated with depression of cardiac and neuronal function, and the cause of death in such cases at a core temperature of less than 70° F is usually a malignant ventricular rhythm disturbance. Milder degrees of hypothermia may be associated with sepsis, inanition, hepatic or renal failure, electrolyte depletion, drug interaction, or hypoglycemia. Gentle rewarming of frostbitten tissue proceeds *pari passu* (at the same time) with systemic rewarming. Controversy exists as

TABLE 57.5.	CAUSES OF SEVERE HYPOTHERMIA (CORE TEMPERATURE <90° F)

- Exposure/immersion
- Hypoglycemia
- Renal and hepatic failure
- Inanition
- Myxedema coma
- Sepsis

TABLE 57.7.	GLASGOW COMA SCALE

Eye opening	(E)
Spontaneous	4
To Speech	3
To Pain	2
Nil	1
Best Motor Response	(M)
Obeys	6
Localizes	5
Withdraws	4
Abnormal flexion	3
Extensor response	2
Nil	1
Verbal Response	(V)
Oriented	5
Confused conversation	4
Inappropriate words	3
Incomprehensible sounds	2
Nil	1
Coma score (E + M + V) = range 3–15	

(From Jennett B, Teasdale G. *Management of head injuries,* Philadelphia: FA Davis; 1981:78 with permission.)

to the best method of body rewarming in cases of severe hypothermia. We feel it best to simultaneously use both external (radiant heating) and central (e.g., breathing warmed humidified gases) rewarming techniques.

HYPERTHERMIA

Hyperthermia is generally a much more aggressive and destructive disease process than hypothermia. The diagnosis of heatstroke or of another type of critical heat illness should be made when a patient presents with a temperature greater than 104° F and an acute change in mental status. In these situations, time is of the essence and active cooling should be started immediately. The causes of life-threatening hyperthermia are listed in Table 57.6. Active cooling can be achieved by immersion in cold water baths or by evaporative cooling, depending on the ambient humidity and the extent of heat storage and organ damage.

▮ MENTAL STATE

The mental status is the ultimate vital sign because the central nervous system is the most sensitive indicator of the integration of all the physiologic processes of the patient. If the mental status is normal, the other vital signs are unlikely to be significantly abnormal. A number of different indexes and scales are useful in documenting the patient's mental state. These include the Glasgow Coma Scale, which is most useful in head-injured pa-

TABLE 57.6.	LIFE-THREATENING HYPERTHERMIA (TEMPERATURE > 104°F)

- Heatstroke
- Neuroleptic, malignant syndrome
- Malignant catatonia
- Seritonergic crises
- Hypothalamic dysfunction
- Malignant hyperthermia (due to anesthetics and muscle relaxants)
- Adrenergic intoxication (cocaine, hallucinogens)
- Status epilepticus
- Thyroid storm
- Anticholinergic toxidrome

tients (Table 57.7). The Mini-Mental Status Examination is also very helpful in documenting cognitive deficits in patients with dementia (Table 57.8). For the initial evaluation, we are concerned with the patient's position on the continuum from alertness to deep coma. An alert patient is awake and verbal and responds appropriately to questions regarding his or her orientation (person, place, and time). If the patient does not respond to verbal stimulation and appears to be asleep, he or she may be lethargic, stuporous, or comatose.

To differentiate these states, it is necessary to apply a noxious stimulus. This can be achieved by stimulating the extremities with a blunted pin or needle or with a sternal rub. A patient who awakens and is then alert is said to be *lethargic*. A patient who awakens with maximal stimulation and is then cognitively impaired (disoriented and unable to respond appropriately to simple questions) is said to be *stuporous*. Stupor is a very dynamic state, since very few patients remain stuporous for long. Either they awaken or they progress to coma. A number of indexes reflect the depth of coma. Suffice it to say that coma can be either light, in which a patient responds to noxious stimuli, or deep, in which the patient does not respond to stimulation. In the latter situation, the patient has spontaneous cardiopulmonary activity, although with abnormal vital signs, and is functioning on a subcortical or brain-stem level.

COMA

It is important to always be careful to rule out the "locked-in" patient when making the diagnosis of coma. Such patients have either a pontine or lower mid-brain lesion that interrupts the corticospinal and corticobulbar tract. They retain third cranial nerve function but have no voluntary motor function below this level. These patients can blink their answers and have full

TABLE 57.8.	MINI-MENTAL STATE EXAMINATION	Patient's Score	Maximum Score
Orientation (Give 1 point for each correct answer.)			
Time: Ask the patient to identify the current:			
Year		_____	1
Season		_____	1
Date		_____	1
Day		_____	1
Month		_____	1
Place: Ask the patient to identify the:			
State he/she is in		_____	1
Country he/she is in		_____	1
Town or city he/she is in		_____	1
Nature or purpose of building he/she is in		_____	1
Floor of building he/she is in		_____	1
Registration			
Name three objects, taking 1 second to say each. Then, ask the patient to Repeat all three objects. Give 1 point for each correct answer. Then repeat the objects until the patient learns all three. Count trials and record.			
Trials		_____	3
Attention and calculation			
Serial sevens: Ask the patient to count backward from 100 by sevens (93, 86, 79, 72, 65). Stop after five answers. Give 1 point for each correct answer.			
Alternative: Ask the patient to spell "world" backward.		_____	5
Recall (Give 1 point for each correct answer.)			
Ask the patient to name the three objects repeated above.		_____	3
Language (Give 1 point for each correct response.)			
Naming: Point to a pencil and to a watch. Ask the patient to name each as you point		_____	2
Repetition: Ask the patient to repeat, "No ifs, ands, or buts."		_____	1
Three-state command: Ask the patient to follow a three-stage command, such as: "Take this paper in your right hand, Fold the paper in half, Put the paper on the floor."		_____	3
Reading: On a blank piece of paper print the sentence, "Close your eyes," in letters large enough to see clearly. Ask the patient to read and obey the command.		_____	1
Writing: Ask the patient to write a sentence of his or her choice. The sentence should contain a subject, a verb, and an object and should make sense. Ignore spelling errors.		_____	1
Copying: Ask the patient to copy the design shown. Give one point if all sides and angles are preserved and if the intersecting sides form a quadrangle		_____	1
Total		_____	30

The Mini-Mental State Examination (MMSE) is a useful tool for the clinical examination for patients who present with cognitive impairment. The MMSE is simple and easy to administer in the primary care setting and, because it is objectively scored, can be used to document progression of a patient's illness over time. Of a possible 30 points, a total score of 20 to 24 points generally indicates mild impairment, 18 to 19 points indicates moderate impairment, and 15 points or less indicates a severe deficit. Adapted with permission from Folstein MF, Folstein SE, McHugh PR. Mini-mental state. A practical method for grading the cognitive state of patients for the clinician. *J Psychiatr Res* 1975;12:189 [From *Hospital Physician June 1999*]).

comprehension of what is being said unless they also have another defect at the cortical level. Another group of locked-in patients consists of those with very severe and pervasive neuromuscular diseases, such as botulism, myasthenia gravis, periodic paralysis, and amyotrophic lateral sclerosis. This group usually has some residual motor function. Diagnostic signs or laboratory findings help to make the differential diagnosis.

The final group of patients that may present with coma are those who feign coma or feign seizures and postictal states. These patients often have residual motor tone and demonstrate normal opticokinetic nystagmus, indicating that they are awake and are tracking the revolving drum. They also demonstrate normal corneal and blink reflexes. If a definitive answer cannot be obtained, ice water irrigation of their external canals is very useful in confirming the presence of true coma. In the awake patient, ice water causes nystagmus with the rapid component away from the irrigated ear. In true coma with intact brain-stem reflexes, patients respond with tonic deviation of their eyes to the side of the cold water irrigation.

In patients presenting with coma or other acute changes in neurologic functioning, one must exclude either an acute structural lesion, such as a subarachnoid hemorrhage or acute epidural hematoma, or a medical (metabolic or infectious) cause of coma. The central nervous system functioning at 98.6° F has an absolute minute-to-minute requirement for oxygen and glucose. The intervals of hypoxia or hypoglycemia that can be tolerated by the central nervous system without permanent neuronal loss is referred to as the warm ischemia and warm hypoglycemia times, respectively. The warm ischemia time is thought to be 4 to 6 minutes of total absence of perfusion or oxygenation. The warm hypoglycemia time is less readily established and depends on the rate of decline of the blood glucose and the preexisting glucose level. Thus, diabetics who consistently have high blood glucose concentrations may have signs or symptoms of hypoglycemia at a blood glucose level of 80 to 90 mg per deciliter, whereas a previously euglycemic patient may not be symptomatic until a level below 50 mg per deciliter is reached.

These factors have led to the use of the so-called "coma cocktail" in approaching the comatose patient. After a rapid assessment of baseline functioning, including the patients ventilatory and respiratory status, either an accurate bedside glucose is obtained, or a blood glucose is sent to the laboratory and 50 mL of 50% glucose is given intravenously. When a glucose bolus is given, 100 mg of thiamine are also administered to prevent thiamine-deficient patients from developing acute Wernicke's encephalopathy (confusion, ophthalmoplegia, coma). It is far preferable to measure the blood glucose at the bedside than to give a hypertonic bolus of glucose blindly, because the hypertonic bolus can raise the serum potassium to dangerous levels if the patient is already hyperkalemic and hypertonic. In addition, a few patients with cerebral edema may transiently improve owing to the osmatic effect of hypertonic glucose, leading to the wrong diagnostic conclusions.

In most situations, the coma cocktail includes intravenous naloxone to reverse opioid intoxication. The only complication of administering the latter drug is its potential to cause acute narcotic withdrawal in patients who are addicted to narcotics or on methadone maintenance. These patients can be treated using sedation or can be given small incremental doses of morphine, if necessary. There have been a few case reports of false-positive responses to naloxone in patients depressed by sedative hypnotic drugs, but these are few and far between. Because naloxone competes with endogenous opioids for the opioid receptor, the occasional response may be related to this mechanism and not to drug antagonism. At this writing, there appears to be little benefit for the routine use of the benzodiazepine antagonist flumazenil in the coma cocktail. It is most helpful in patients in whom the benzodiazepine effect requires reversal after a procedure has been carried out under conscious sedation with a short-acting benzodiazepine.

OTHER CHANGES

There are two key issues relating to emergencies involving changes in the mental state that are not covered in the definitions given above. These areas are the delirious patient and the patient entering with suicidal or homicidal ideation.

Delirium

Delirium is a condition that can be obvious even to the uninitiated, as in the manifestations of alcohol withdrawal syndrome or delirium tremens. On the other hand, patients with so-called quiet delirium can present with changes in their personality such as paranoid ideation, forgetfulness, or inattention to social and personal relationships. It is useful to think of this state as a reversible, perhaps humoral, alteration of neuronal functioning that is superimposed on the premorbid personality. Delirium is common in intensive care units, especially in patients who already have an underlying dementia.

The management of delirium relates to its secondary nature; that is, the amelioration of the underlying conditions or stressors will lead to reversal of this state. In the interim, consistency of the environment and caregivers and repetition of reassurances and orienting information are very helpful. Because sedation interferes with memory and thus orientation, use of sedative-hypnotic agents in delirious patients is potentially harmful. The exception to this general rule is the patient with an agitated delirium due to the withdrawal of sedative-hypnotic drugs, such as alcohol or benzodiazepines, in whom administration of benzodiazepines are essential.

Suicidal Ideation

Determination of the presence of suicidal or homicidal thoughts or actions must be determined in every responsive patient with an altered mental status. If the patient believes it is safe to confide in the health care provider, this information is usually forthcoming when an inquiry is made. If such a situation is thought to exist, then, while obtaining psychiatric consultation, one should initiate security coverage to safeguard the patient and staff from an immediate acceleration of the thoughts into action. This one-to-one coverage also is important because it prevents the patient from leaving the protected environment of the institution until an appropriate disposition can be made. In the interim, while the psychiatric situation is in flux the practitioner can help defuse the acute situation by supportive measures. The VVV system, **v**alidate, **v**entilate, **v**enture hope of recovery, can be extremely helpful in this context. The provider allows the patient to ventilate his or her thoughts and feelings and then validates the reality of the patient's problems and ventures his or her impression that the problems and situations that precipitated the crisis are amenable to intervention.

The most significant initial problem in these cases is engaging the patient and developing a trusting relationship with him or her. This process is facilitated by using the help system. The provider continuously states that the patient needs help, that help is being provided, and that more help is on the way. By the physician using the word help again and again, the patient, who in reality is frightened and looking for help, will begin to respond positively to the intervention. When all else fails and the patient is displaying accelerating agitation and paranoia, a show of force is necessary. In this procedure, a team approach is used to place the patient into four-point restraints. This team consists of a leader and at least five other persons who can immobilize the patient if he or she does not agree to go into restraints willingly. The time that a patient stays in restraints should be monitored and reassessed frequently because the patient can develop pressure necrosis from the devices used and he or she may aspirate vomitus in the immobilized supine position. Thus, as soon as the patient is secured, a course of chemical restraints is initiated using intravenous short-acting neuroleptic agents, such as haloperidol, and sedation with a short- or intermediate-acting benzodiazepine, such as lorazepam.

PRESENTING COMPLAINT—FOCUSED CARE

There are approximately 30 different presenting complaints or diagnostic categories that encompass almost the entire universe of adult patients seeking care in emergency departments (Fig. 57.3). About 50% of these categories have a high potential for life-threatening disease processes. To arrive at a reasonable number of functional approaches to these subpopulations, we have condensed some major categories and expanded others. Thus, all major trauma patients are grouped together. Our thesis is that understanding the diagnostic entities in each group that are the most critical and prognostically significant allows one to develop a hierarchical approach that is conservative in its use of resources. This approach is also safe in that it will prevent an untoward patient outcome from a missed diagnosis and management opportunity. In the following text, we outline the approach to a number of presenting problems chosen for their high frequency in emergency departments and their responses to appropriate active interventions.

SHORTNESS OF BREATH

The chief complaint of shortness of breath is a common problem and a rather broad diagnostic category, which includes the following potentially life-threatening entities: left ventricular failure; noncardiogenic pulmonary edema; obstructive, restrictive, and neuromuscular diseases of the lung; pneumothorax; pulmonary embolism; metabolic acidosis; salicylate intoxication and severe anemia. Primary hyperventilation syndrome, a psychological entity caused by anxiety or stress, should be seriously considered as the major diagnosis when there is little or no evidence for the presence of the disease categories noted above. However, caution should be taken because hyperventilation may mask the signs and symptoms of the serious underlying condition. The use of bedside pulmonary function testing, arterial blood gas analysis, chest radiography, ECG, and routine complete blood cell count (CBC), blood glucose, and electrolyte testing will narrow the field in most cases to one or two entities, which can usually be isolated on further specific testing.

CHEST DISCOMFORT

A chief complaint of chest pain is almost universally a signal to begin an immediate evaluation of the patient for an acute myocardial infarction or an unstable coronary ischemic syndrome (Chapter 65). In addition, the other disease entities that one must consider in this category are dissecting aneurysm of the aorta, leaking atherosclerotic aortic aneurysm, critical aortic stenosis, pericarditis, acute cor pulmonale, and esophageal rupture. The patient can be evaluated for the relatively benign entities, such as musculoskeletal chest pain and gastroesophageal reflux or spasm, after these other entities are found to be very unlikely. Patients with chest pain can be differentiated by the characteristics of their pain, by the results of the cardiopulmonary examinations, and by the use of the ECG and chest film. After these patients with chest pain have had their initial evaluations, they can be subdivided into three groups or risk categories. These correlate roughly with the pain syndromes of noncardiac pain, atypical chest pain, and ischemic cardiac pain.

- Noncardiac chest pain consists of a pain pattern and supporting data that make diagnosis of an ischemic syndrome unlikely. Noncardiac pain usually begins abruptly or is related to position or breathing. These patients have normal ECGs.
- Atypical chest pain syndromes are present in patients who present with chest discomfort and patterns of discomfort that have features of both ischemic and nonischemic chest pain. The ECGs in this category are either normal or display minor ST segment and I wave abnormalities.
- Cardiac chest pain is actually not strictly a painful sensation as in somatic pain, but it is described as substernal pressure, fullness, or constriction. This is why esophageal disease and myocardial ischemia are so difficult to differentiate; both are visceral stimuli using the same or overlapping autonomic sensory pathways.

In the current medicolegal, professional, and managed care environment, it is crucial for patients with undiagnosed chest discomfort to have their atypical chest pain evaluated acutely over the short term for the presence of cardiac ischemia. Based on a one-time evaluation, approximately 3% of patients with acute cardiac ischemia are missed and discharged from an emergency department. This group of patients has a much higher probability of cardiac arrest than that of similar patients admitted to a hospital. This has led to the concept of chest pain evaluation centers within or in collaboration with emergency departments. In such programs, when all preliminary tests, cardiac enzymes, and serial ECGs are negative over a period of 12 hours or so, these patients can undergo some form of cardiac stress testing. Those patients whose tests show evidence of ischemia or infarction are transferred to the appropriate inpatient locus. Patients who successfully pass these protocols have less than a 1% chance of having active cardiac ischemic disease as the cause of their chest pain.

It is important at this point to touch upon the issue of "silent ischemia," since we tend to become fixated on patients presenting with ischemic chest discomfort while overlooking patients with silent ischemic or variant angina. Silent ischemia is said to be present at some time in over 80% of patients with intermit-

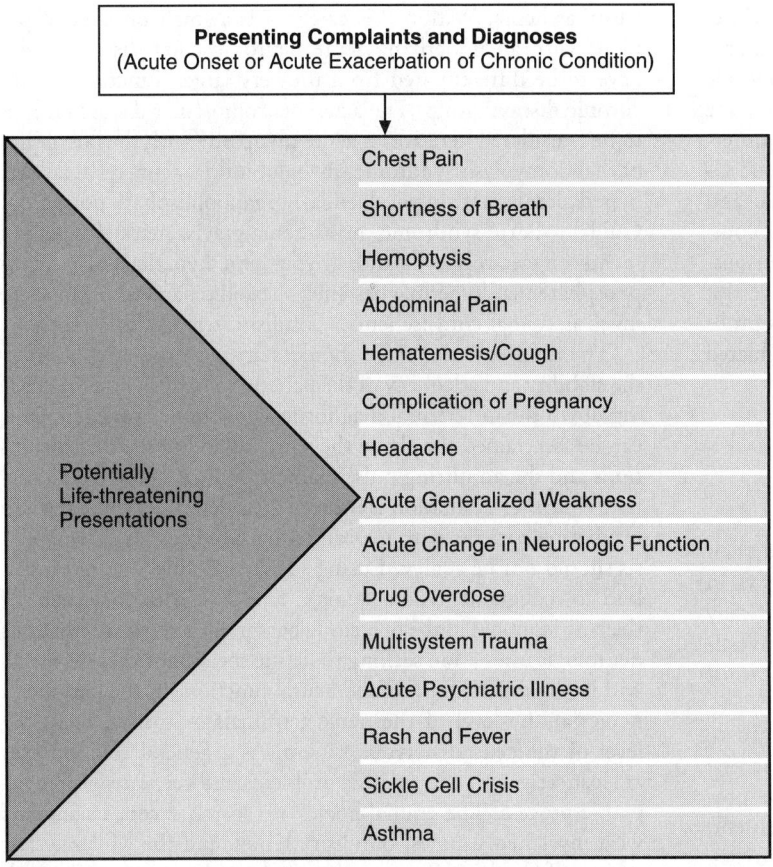

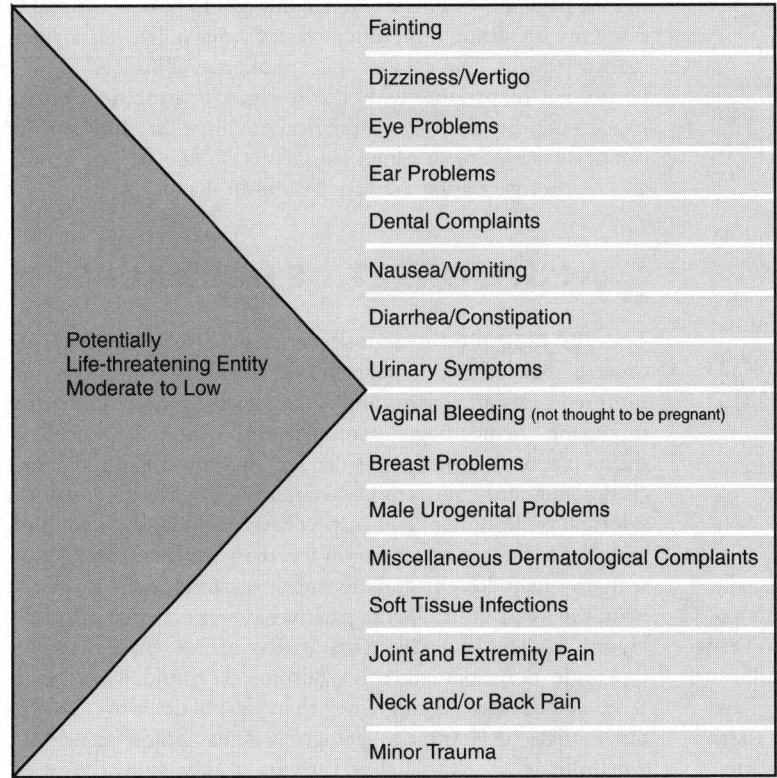

FIGURE 57.3. Presenting complaints or diagnostic categories that encompass almost all adult patients seeking care in emergency departments.

tent or overt ischemia. The lack of chest discomfort occurs either because of a high central pain perception threshold, a small area of myocardium at risk, or some abnormality of the autonomic nerves. Whether the ischemia is truly silent is open to some discussion, because these patients can present with poorly differentiated complaints. These complaints include unexplained fatigue, recent onset of dyspnea on exertion, palpitations, and light-headedness. The undifferentiated nature of these complaints creates significant delays in the recognition of the seriousness of the underlying process. Thus, in patients who have risk factors for coronary artery disease or a past history of this problem, the latter undifferentiated complaints should be evaluated in the context of possible silent ischemia.

ABDOMINAL PAIN

The approach to patients who have abdominal pain as their major complaint also follows the approach developed above in that the immediate life-threatening entities have to be specifically considered initially before the less urgent conditions are investigated. These life-threatening entities include acute myocardial infarction, leaking atherosclerotic aortic aneurysm, and mesenteric ischemia. Leaking aortic aneurysms can be very hard to palpate and can present as renal colic, sciatica, or acute scrotal swellings. In addition, several other acute surgical disease processes require immediate recognition and surgical management. These include gangrenous cholecystitis, ascending cholangitis, and perforation of a hollow viscus with intra-abdominal sepsis (e.g., peptic ulcer, sigmoid diverticulitis, appendicitis). Strangulated closed-loop obstructions, including sigmoid and cecal volvulus and strangulated hernias, are also potentially life-threatening. In women of child-bearing age, the abdominal pain evaluation should include evaluations for possible ectopic pregnancy, ovarian torsion, and extensive pelvic inflammatory disease.

Early surgical consultation and rapid access to an operating room should be the major focus in management for most of these conditions. Fluid resuscitation, treatment for sepsis, and pain control are, of course, key supportive measures. Abdominal computed tomography (CT) imaging with oral and intravenous contrast is extremely useful in delineating most of the processes just noted.

WEAKNESS AND DIZZINESS

A chief complaint of generalized weakness and dizziness usually results in an extended history, physical examination, and laboratory testing often without a resulting satisfactory diagnosis. Perhaps 10% of affected patients have an underlying chronic illness and, as a result of deconditioning or physical disability, have difficulty with their functioning. In a large percentage of these patients, an emotional or psychological illness is a potential source of their symptoms. These psychiatric conditions include anxiety and depression, panic disorder, hypochondriasis, somatization disorders, conversion reactions, and so-called neurocircu-

latory asthenia. Within this category is a small number of patients with an underlying acute neuromuscular disorder, who have to be differentiated from the very large "functional" and chronic disease group. The acute neuromuscular disease entities to be considered here are an acute myopathy with the possibility of rhabdomyolysis syndrome (myoglobinuria, acute renal failure, hyperkalemia, and hypocalcemia), organophosphate poisoning, Guillain–Barré syndrome, myasthenia gravis, marked derangements of electrolyte balance (hypo- and hyperkalemia, hypophosphatemia, hypermagnesemia), periodic paralysis, transverse myelitis, spinal cord ischemia, botulism, tetanus, and rabies.

The differentiation here should start with the evaluation of the stability and adequacy of the patient's airway before proceeding down the differential diagnostic algorithmic approach. This can be ascertained simply by the patient's ability to answer questions and the admitting pulse oximetry values. If there is uncertainty, further evaluation is indicated, as described earlier (when intubating patients with neuromuscular diseases, muscle paralysis should not be achieved using succinylcholine, because it can lead to malignant hyperkalemia). The differentiation, then, of the entities noted in the preceding paragraph requires meticulous neurologic evaluation seeking to define the lesions that may exist within the muscle, at the myoneural junction, in the peripheral nerves at the level of the nerve terminals or trunks, or at the level of the central nervous system. As a general rule, reflexes are lost early with neuropathic problems and very late with myopathic process. The cranial nerves are spared except in patients with myasthenia gravis, botulism, rabies, and the Miller Fisher variant of Guillain–Barré syndrome. In patients presenting with muscle pain and weakness who are thought to have a myopathy, acute myositis should be differentiated from polymyalgia rheumatica (PMR). The creatine phosphokinase (PK) level should be normal in patients with PMR which is associated with a paucity of other findings on physical examination. Both entities can be associated with a high sedimentation rate. Muscle biopsy and electromyography are very helpful in diagnosis.

ACUTE ONSET OF HEADACHE

The most prognostically significant entities associated with acute onset of headache are subarachnoid hemorrhage (SAH) from ruptured berry aneurysms and AV malformations, hypertensive intracranial hemorrhage, meningitis, and hypertensive crisis. If the pain is retro-orbital, consider acute narrow-angle glaucoma, cluster migraine, and temporal arteritis. High-yield historical information leading one to suspect SAH includes sudden onset, with the peak pain appearing in less than 1 minute, association with transient loss of consciousness, occipital location of the pain, the worst headache the patient has ever experienced, meningismus, altered mental status or new neurologic deficits. Although for some patients this syndrome of "thunderclap" headache can be due to migraine, there is no definitive way to differentiate SAH from a "benign" vascular headache without a neuroimaging study. Before carrying out the study, however, one must decide whether the patient is high risk. In most instances, high-risk patients require a lumbar puncture if the imaging study is negative. If the patient has been diagnosed as *mi-*

graineur in the past but has never had a brain imaging study, the diagnosis should be set aside until SAH is ruled out.

Another pitfall is the use of a therapeutic diagnostic test involving the use of antimigraine medications. Patients with a thunderclap headache who have all or most of their pain relieved by these medications should not then be automatically considered to have a benign vascular headache. There are now a number of SAH patients in whom sumatriptan seems to have been effective, although temporarily. Patients with increased intracranial pressure usually have the worst headache pain on arising. Later, they develop nausea and vomiting and become sleepy and cognitively impaired. At that point, there are usually focal localizing signs from the expanding intracranial mass and false localizing signs secondary to the herniation syndromes. The most commonly seen in the latter group are palsies of cranial nerves III and VI.

APPROACH TO MULTISYSTEM-TRAUMA PATIENTS

The internist rather than the surgeon may occasionally treat patients with multisystem trauma. In this circumstance, it is key to recognize the significance of the mechanism of injury as well as to be wary of subtle or hidden diagnoses. In evaluating patients with head or spine injuries, one must be cognizant of the difficulty in discovering other significant injuries of the chest and especially the abdomen. In addition, patients may have what is termed a *distracting injury*. Thus, a patient with a very painful fracture dislocation may not react to a painful injury of the abdomen. Similarly, patients who are intoxicated may have a very high pain threshold, and the extent of their injuries may be grossly underestimated.

Each area of the trunk is divided into zones, each of which has vital structures located within it. In addition, each zone has its own potential for missed injuries and may require special diagnostic studies to "clear" the zone. Thus, the anterior midline zone of the chest has a great potential for these injuries. Many patients will need an ECG and undergo CT scanning of their chest, and many will require an echocardiogram to rule out a myocardial contusion, laceration, or infarction. If the mechanism of injury is sudden acceleration or deceleration, aortic disruption (usually just distal to the left subclavian take-off) should be considered and aortic imaging performed when indicated. Injuries to the upper flank regions can involve the kidneys and great vessels in the retroperitoneum, but also can be associated with injuries to the bases of the lungs.

EMERGENCY EQUIPMENT

Emergency equipment that may be essential in emergency situations outside the hospital, such as in the office setting, is listed in Table 57.9. The use of an automated external defibrillator (AED) is probably the most potentially life-saving piece of equipment. The primary concentration is care within the first 5 minutes because most jurisdictions have prehospital personnel available after that time frame.

TABLE 57.9.	EMERGENCY EQUIPMENT FOR CAR AND OFFICE

1. Cell phone
2. Automatic external defibrillator (probably the most useful piece of equipment)
3. Bag valve mask or valve airway mask device
4. Oral airways
5. Gloves (6 pairs)
6. Sterile saline in bags or pour bottle (4 units)
7. Epinephrine 1/1000 single-dose prefilled syringe for subcutaneous use
8. 50 mL 50% glucose (2 doses) in prefilled syringe
9. Lorazepam 1 mg in prefilled syringes (6–7 doses)
10. IV tubing and cannula
11. 2 blankets
12. Assorted bandages and tape
13. Blood pressure cuff
14. Cold packs
15. Flashlights or lanterns (3 units)
16. Road flares

Kelley's Textbook of Internal Medicine, fourth edition. Edited by H. David Humes. Lippincott Williams & Wilkins, Philadelphia © 2000.

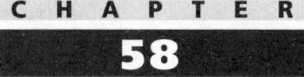

C H A P T E R

58

ANIMAL BITES AND STINGS

FAITH T. FITZGERALD

As travel, pet keeping, and out-of-doors activity increase, so does the risk of animal bites and stings. Injury can result from direct trauma, superinfection, allergy (by far the most morbid), and injected or applied toxins.

INSECTS AND SPIDERS

Although death is rare and due principally to Hymenoptera allergy, the morbidity of arthropod bites in the United States is considerable. Several species infest or attack humans. Nonvenomous but annoying and potentially dangerous arthropods are outlined in Table 58.1.

Stings of *wasps and bees,* which are members of the order Hymenoptera, can be life- threatening to hypersensitive patients (see Chapter 173). Although the venom of Africanized honeybees is no more allergenic or toxic than that of European honeybees, the Africanized bees are more aggressive and multiple stings can lead to death. Local therapy in nonallergic individuals con-

TABLE 58.1.	NONVENOMOUS ARTHROPODS		
Species	**Clinical Picture**	**Diagnosis**	**Therapy**
Mites			
Sarcooptes scabiei (scabies)	Burrow under the skin, causing eczematoid pruritic patches on wrists, elbows, hands, and finger webs. Rarely, cause widespread body rash in immunocompromised hosts (Norwegian scabies).	Microscopic scrapings of lesions show mites or fecal residue.	Launder clothes, bedding; use 1% τ-benzene hexachloride (lindane, Kwell) in nonpregnant victims older than 2 y.
Chiggers	Bite and drop off host. Leave papules or vesicles, some hemorrhagic, on legs and belt line.	History and clinical picture.	Give antipruritics.
Fleas	Allergy to bites results in welts, papules, vesicles, and pruritus.	History and clinical picture.	Pesticide treatment of house and pets.
Lice	Allergy to bites causes welts, pruritus, vesicles, and scratches with superinfection in the pubic area, eyebrows, axillae, and scalp.	Detection of lice or nits by fine combing of hair.	Lindane shampoo and lotion; pyrethrin products; eyelashes: 0.25% physostigmine ophthalmic ointment or thick layer petroleum twice daily. Improve hygiene.
Phthirus pubis (pubic louse)			
Pediculus humanus corporis (body louse)			
Pediculus humanus capitis (head louse)	May be vectors of rickettsial and spirochetal disease.		
Bedbug *Cimex lectularius*	Cause linear pruritic, erythematous papules on hands, face, and neck. May be vectors of hepatitis B.	History, clinical picture, capture of bug.	Hire professional exterminators.
Reduviidae Kissing bug	Found in the southwestern United States and Mexico. Cause papules, urticaria, and hemorrhagic bullae. May transmit *Trypanosoma cruzi*, agent of Chagas' disease.	History, clinical picture, capture of bug.	Hire professional exterminators.
Flies Deerfly, horsefly	Causes painful, nodular hemorrhagic bites, and cutaneous myiasis.	History, clinical picture, extraction of larva in myiasis.	Use topical treatment, surgical for myiasis; avoid exposure.
Mosquitoes	Cause pruritic papules. Greatest danger is as vector for arboviral and parasitic disease.	History, clinical picture.	Use repellents, nets, and exterminators.
Tarantulas	Abdominal hairs may cause dermatitis; painful nonvenomous bites.	History, clinical picture.	Avoidance.

sists of removing the stingers and applying ice. With multiple stings, toxic systemic reactions include faintness, headache, fever, muscle spasms, and gastrointestinal upset. *Fire ants, Solenopsis invicta and S. richteri,* are nonwinged hymenopterans that are endemic in the southeastern United States, where the often multiple bites create painful, burning papules, vesicles, and pustules with potential for necrosis and scarring. Toxic systemic effects include nausea, vomiting, dizziness, and blurred vision. Allergic reactions may also occur.

Hard and soft *ticks* are noted mainly for their carriage of rickettsial, viral, bacterial, spirochetal, and protozoal diseases. Uninfected bites can cause local dermal reactions and, rarely,

a neurotoxic ascending paralysis. Embedded mouth parts can stimulate a granuloma. Ticks should be removed by the application of petrolatum and careful use of blunt forceps. Surgical excision occasionally is required. *Blister beetles* do not bite or sting, but rough contact with their carapace, which contains the vesicant cantharidin, can give painful blisters, which are treated as chemical burns. Several species of caterpillars, including the *saddleback, buck moth,* and *pus caterpillar* of the southern United States, have hairs that penetrate skin and inject venom, causing intense local pain, urticaria, and, rarely, shock. Removal of hairs can be done with cellophane tape or tweezers; antihistamines, corticosteroids, analgesics, and intravenous calcium gluconate help pain and urticaria. The *gypsy moth caterpillar* in the northeastern United States causes an erythematous papular dermatitis.

Of *centipedes,* only the bite of the giant *Scolopendra heros* of the southwestern United States is life threatening, principally to children. It injects hemolytic and cardiotoxic venom, causing local necrosis, severe systemic symptoms, and even rhabdomyolytic renal failure. Treatment is supportive.

Many *spiders* bite, but there are only two major venomous species in the United States: the black widow, *Latrodectus mactans,* and the brown spiders, *Loxosceles.* The female black widow haunts privies, houses, garages, and woodpiles across the United States. It is about 6 mm in diameter and shiny black, with variable red ventral markings sometimes (not always) in an hourglass shape. It is aggressive. About 10% of black widow bites result in envenomation from a neurotoxin, causing an outpouring of various neurotransmitters that produce lactrodectism. A sharp local pain signals the bite. Within a half hour, there is local redness and swelling or a pallid area with a red–blue border. Systemic effects may follow and include muscular rigidity and fibrillations, abdominal pain of such severity as to be misdiagnosed as peritonitis, nausea, vomiting, hypersalivation, swings in blood pressure and pulse, ischemic electrocardiographic changes, cardiac dysrhythmias, hemolysis, rhabdomyolysis, renal failure, hyperglycemia, neutrophilia, coma, and, rarely, death. Muscle relaxants and narcotics treat pain and muscle spasm. An effective antivenin (Lyovac) is a horse serum product, likely to produce hypersensitivity reactions, and is used in severe cases (see Chapter 138).

Loxosceles species, the brown spiders (fiddlebacks), are small, nocturnal, shy creatures with a dark, violin-shaped mark on their backs. They live in homes and clothing, and bite when disturbed. They inject a venom containing necrotizing, hemolytic, and spreading factors. A sudden mild pain at the bite may produce only erythema, induration pain, and pruritus at the site or be followed within hours to days by a characteristic violaceous erythema and necrosis extending to the underlying muscle. Fever, chills, arthralgia, morbilliform rash, malaise, coagulopathy, jaundice, hematuria, renal failure, and, rarely, death may all complicate severe envenomation 24 to 48 hours after the bite. Supportive treatment with splinting and support of the affected part, analgesics, tetanus toxoid, antibiotics for superinfection, and occasional surgical debridement is required. The use of the sulfa drug dapsone, 50 mg orally twice daily for 2 days (increased to 100 mg orally twice daily thereafter if necrosis is progressing), is controversial as benefit is unclear and dapsone can cause agranulocytosis and methemoglobinemia. Intermittent cold packs applied to the site for the first 48 hours also may help.

The two most dangerous species of *scorpions* in the southwestern United States are *Centruroides sculpturatus* and *C. gertschi.* Their venom, delivered by sting from a tail sac, is potent but seldom lethal. Local reactions to many scorpion stings can be severe, but the most venomous southwestern scorpions usually produce little local response. Neurotoxin injection leads within hours to perinasal and oral itching; nystagmus, trismus, numbness, dizziness, agitation, confusion, convulsions; circulatory, renal, and respiratory failure; hemolysis; and death. Therapy is with local ice packs and support. In severe reactions, in very young children, which can be lethal, specific antivenin may be used.

REPTILES

Of *snake bites* in the United States, fewer than 25% are poisonous, and death is rare. Most venomous bites in the United States are caused by rattlesnakes, copperheads, and cottonmouths (all Crotalidae, or pit vipers) or by the coral snake (Elapidae). A few snake bites are by imported exotic species. Confronted by a snake bite victim, the physician must determine the species of snake, which is best done if the reptile is brought in (dead, in a closed container) with the patient. A snake with catlike pupils, a triangular head, and pits between the nostrils and eyes is a pit viper. The coral snake has black bands abutting yellow ("black on yellow, kill a fellow"), and the harmless look-alike snake has red bands adjacent to black ("red on black, venom lack"). Even if the snake is poisonous, not all bites contain venom, and of those that do, the fate of the patient may depend on the size of the snake, the size of the bite, the interval between the bite and the onset of local or systemic signs and symptoms, the field therapy that was given, and the age, size, and general condition of the victim.

Field therapy for snake bite is controversial, but it probably is best to do no more than immobilize the body part, calm the victim, and transport him or her to the hospital as soon as possible. Tourniquets, pressure bands, incision and suction, snake venom extractors, electric shock therapy, and the application of heat or cold to the bite are of no proven benefit and might be harmful. Ingestion of alcohol should absolutely be avoided. Definitive therapy in the hospital depends on the type and severity of envenomation. A severity score for crotalid snake bites has been developed and is useful in predicting the course of events and need for antivenin.

Local effects of pit viper bites include pain, erythema, ecchymosis, local bleeding, and necrosis. Systemic venom produces perioral tingling, a metallic taste, muscle fasciculation, hypotension, disseminated intravascular coagulation, respiratory distress, and renal failure. Large-bore intravenous access should be established and initial blood samples drawn for a complete blood cell count, coagulation studies, renal function tests, and blood for type and cross match. Physical examination should be repeated frequently and laboratory studies repeated after 4 hours in the asymptomatic patient. Electrocardiograms should be obtained on the severely ill and all patients older than 40 years of age. In patients with major systemic symptoms or laboratory derangements, antivenin therapy is given. Because antivenin is horse serum, the patient first should be skin-tested for immediate hypersensitivity. Ten to twenty vials of antivenin, depending on the patient's degree of envenomation, is given intravenously in 500 mg of 5% dextrose and water or normal saline over 1 to 2 hours. Then, based on signs and symptoms, more is given as needed. Local wound care may include debridement, broad-spectrum antibiotics, and tetanus prophylaxis. Should fear of compartment syndrome arise, compartment monitoring and expert surgical consultation are mandated, with fasciotomy only if the pressure is increasing measurably. Extensive debridement is no longer recommended. Serum sickness occurs about 10 days after the receipt of 5 or more vials of antivenin in almost all patients.

Coral snake venom is neurotoxic, and the onset of any neurologic symptoms in a patient with multiple punctures or scratches in the bite (the snake injects venom by chewing) requires specific antivenin (after skin testing), with 3 to 5 vials given intravenously. This may be repeated if symptoms progress. The patient should be observed for at least 48 hours, even in the absence of symptoms, because the onset of toxin effects may be delayed.

Nonvenomous snakes can transmit anaerobic and enteric bacteria, and their bite wounds require careful cleaning and cultures. Antibiotics may be needed if the bites are infected, although rates of infection are low and prophylaxis with antibiotics is not necessary. Tetanus immunization or booster should be considered.

Gila monsters (*Heloderma* species) are the only venomous lizards in the United States and are found in the Southwest. Bites are rare, but the lizard is bulldog-like in the tenacity of its grip. In 70% of bites, a serotonin-containing toxin is injected, causing local edema, tenderness, lymphangitis, and lymphadenitis. Occasionally, the victim experiences weakness, faintness, dizziness, sweating, nausea, vomiting, shock, or coagulopathy. Treatment is supportive.

Information and consultation on venomous bites may be obtained by calling the Antivenom Index in Tucson, Arizona (602-626-6016).

MARINE ANIMALS

The number of sports divers and snorkelers is increasing, and injuries caused by reef and beach creatures are correspondingly more common. Marine injuries and envenomation caused by simple contact are outlined in Table 58.2.

Many species of *fish* and *rays* carry toxic barbs on their tails (e.g., stingray) or fins (e.g., catfish, lionfish, scorpionfish, weaverfish, stonefish, toadfish, ratfish, rabbitfish, leatherback, some sharks). Injury is by deposition of the barb and venom, or the venom alone, leading to local injury or destruction of neural or cardiac tissue, which can be lethal. The local site should be cleaned and soaked in warm [115°F to 120°F (46°C to 48°C)] water for 30 to 60 minutes to inactivate protein toxins. Support and surgical removal of the barb might be required. Antivenins are available for some species. Superinfection with *Vibrio* or *Aeromonas* species can occur.

A bite from the horny beak of the blue-ringed *octopus* of the Pacific, from Australia to Japan, releases a mix of tetrodotoxin, histamine, serotonin, and other poisons into the wound, causing numbness, paralysis, hypotension, and respiratory failure. An-

TABLE 58.2.	**MARINE CONTACT ENVENOMATIONS**	
Species	**Clinical Picture**	**Therapy**
Corals	Cuts, pruritus, urticaria, cellulitis, toxic necrotic lesions, retained mineral fragments in skin, secondary infection.	Irrigation, soap and water, hydrogen peroxide, topical antiseptics. In immunocompromised patients, antibiotic prophylaxis for *Vibrio*, *Alteromonas*.
Sponges	Spicules give irritant dermatitis. Florida fire sponge gives toxic rash, rarely arthritis, erythema multiforme, anaphylaxis.	Remove spicules with adhesive tape, then bathe wound in vinegar. Topical steroids.
Sea urchins	Spines give puncture wounds, granulomas. Some spines toxic (glycosides, acetylcholine, serotonin), giving pain, swelling, hemorrhage locally and systemic paresthesias, paresis, death.	Remove spines. Antibiotics for infection and in immunocompromised.
Cone shell	Radicular tooth causes local injury, systemic neurotoxicity. Mortality may reach 15–20%.	Supportive; neostigmine.
Starfish *Acanthaster planci* (crown-of-thorns)	Poisonous spines give chronic, painful, swollen local lesion.	Supportive, local.
Marine bristleworm	Irritation; some venomous with erythema, swelling, rash at contact site, dysesthesias, paresthesias, pruritus, necrosis.	Remove bristles with adhesive tape. Soak area with dilute ammonia.

Jellyfish
  Portuguese man-of-war (Atlantic)
  Bluebottle (Pacific)
  Box jellyfish (Indopacific, Australia)
	Nematocysts (stinging cells) in tendrils toxic, with potentially severe systemic neurotoxicity (delirium, seizures, paralysis, cardiorespiratory failure, death). Box jelly fish most deadly (15–20% mortality).	Bathe affected sites with seawater, then local 5% acetic acid. Avoid freshwater, alcohol as these cause nematocyst discharge. Provide supportive therapy. Antivenom for box jellyfish only.

Seals, Sea lions (seal finger)	Contact transmits organism (? micrococcus), gives relentless severe pain, erythema, swelling, tenderness.	Tetracycline, 2 g q.i.d. × 1 mo.

other dangerous species, found in the Caribbean, is *Octopus joubini.* Because venomous octopi are small, no octopi less than 6 in. in length should be handled without protective gloves. There is no antivenin.

Numerous species of venomous *sea snakes* live in Indo-Pacific waters. Bites, although rarely lethal, can cause death by rhabdomyolysis and hyperkalemia. Antivenin is available for those associated with extreme toxicity.

MAMMALS

The most common mammal bites are those of dogs, cats, humans, and rats. When *dogs* bite, infection rates reportedly range from 3% to 18%. Cultures may show polymicrobial aerobic and anaerobic organisms, including *Pasteurella canis, P. multocida, Staphylococcus, Streptococcus, Corynebacterium,* and *Capnocytophaga canimorsus* (which in sepsis mimics a Shwartzman reaction), as well as many other. Tetanus, rabies, and mycobacterial disease rarely are transmitted by dog bite in the United States. *Cat* bites become infected 28% to 80% of the time. *Pasteurella multocida* is the major pathogen; it may cause local injury, such as cellulitis, osteomyelitis, septic arthritis, or tenosynovitis, or it may lead to systemic disease with bacteremia, especially in patients with liver disease. Other pathogens include *Erysipelothrix, Streptococcus, Staphylococcus, Moraxella,* and many others. Cat scratches also can carry *P. multocida,* and both bites and scratches can lead to cat-scratch fever (see Chapter 292). *Human* bites typically occur on the knuckles during fistfights, and the potential for both direct injury and infection is high. Organisms implicated in human bite infections include *Streptococcus, Staphylococcus, Corynebacterium, Bacteroides,* and *Eikenella corrodens.* Anaerobes are common. Syphilis, hepatitis B, and, rarely, rabies have been reported from human bites, but no cases of the acquired immunodeficiency syndrome have been reported. *Rat* bites can transmit rat-bite fever and hemorrhagic fever caused by Hantaan virus.

In evaluating bites, initial steps are careful examination for bone or tendon injury, performance of aerobic and anaerobic cultures, meticulous wound irrigation with 1% povidone-iodine (Betadine), and categorization as low or high risk for the development of infection (Table 58.3). In low-risk wounds, antibiotics are unnecessary and suturing may be appropriate. High-risk wounds should be treated with antibiotics but not sutured. Empirical antibiotic therapy for bites should be directed against pasteurellae, streptococci, staphylococci, and anaerobes. A β-lactam antibiotic with β-lactamase inhibitor, and a second-generation cephalosporin with anaerobic activity, or penicillin plus first-generation cephalosporin, or clindamycin and fluoroquinolone, are recommended. In suspected rabies exposure, therapy includes rabies vaccine (1 mL in the deltoid on days 0, 3, 7, 14, and 28) combined with 20 IU rabies immunoglobulin per kilogram of body weight. As much as possible of the immunoglobulin should be infiltrated at the wound site and the residual given intramuscularly at a site distant from the wound. Bite victims should be considered for tetanus and hepatitis B prophylaxis, as well as rabies prophylaxis (see Chapter 318).

BIBLIOGRAPHY

Allen C. Arachnid envenomations. *Emerg Med Clin North Am* 1992;10: 269–298.
Brown CK, Shepherd SM. Marine trauma, envenomations, and intoxications. *Emerg Med Clin North Am* 1992;10:385–408.
Dart RC, Hurlbut KM, Garcia R, et al. Validation of a severity score for the assessment of crotalid snakebite. *Ann Emerg Med* 1996;27:321–326.
Gold BS, Wingert-WA. Snake venom poisoning in the United States: a review of therapeutic practice. *South Med J* 1994;87:579–589.
Reisman RE. Insect stings. *N Engl J Med* 1994;331:523–527.
Talan DA, Citron DM, Abrahamian FM, et al. Bacteriologic analysis of infected dog and cat bites. *N Engl J Med* 1999;340:85–92.
Warrel DA, Fenner PJ. Venomous bites and stings. *Br Med Bull* 1993;49: 423–439.
Human rabies—Texas and New Jersey, 1997. *MMWR* 1998;47:1–5.

Kelley's Textbook of Internal Medicine, fourth edition. Edited by H. David Humes.
Lippincott Williams & Wilkins, Philadelphia © 2000.

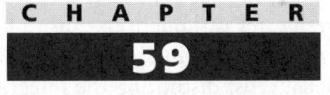

C H A P T E R
59
NEAR DROWNING

LEONARD D. HUDSON
KENNETH P. STEINBERG

Drowning accidents account for an estimated 7,000 to 8,000 deaths in the United States annually; most victims are children and young adults. The incidence of near drowning is unknown, but it has been estimated to be as high as 90,000 cases per year. Conventionally, episodes that result in immediate death are called drowning, and those in which the patient survives, even temporarily, are called near drowning. Although the diagnosis is readily apparent from the clinical setting, there is a broad spectrum of clinical severity determined by factors such as length of submersion, water temperature, volume and type of aspirated liquid, and associated complications or injuries.

Immersion accidents are often classified according to whether they occur in freshwater or saltwater. Differences in serum electrolyte concentrations and blood volume changes between these

TABLE 58.3.	BITE WOUND RISK FOR DEVELOPING INFECTION
High Risk	**Low Risk**
Punctures	Lacerations
Hand and foot wounds	Extremities
Treatment delay over 12 hr	Torso
Immunocompromised host	Face
Human bites	

two forms of drowning were stressed in the early literature. Subsequent experimental studies demonstrated that electrolyte and blood volume changes are usually relatively minor or are so transient as to be clinically inapparent by the time the victim has been transported to a medical facility. The clinical problems associated with drowning in saltwater and freshwater are quite similar and include pulmonary injury, cerebral hypoxia, and hypothermia.

PATHOPHYSIOLOGY

Although most drowning victims inhale a significant quantity of water into the lungs, autopsy studies indicate that little or no fluid enters the lungs in about 10% of cases. This phenomenon has been called dry drowning and is presumably caused by reflex laryngospasm, producing airway obstruction and asphyxiation. When this occurs, resuscitation at the scene of the accident usually results in a rapid return of spontaneous ventilation. Recovery is often dramatic and complete if the anoxic episode has not been prolonged.

The differential diagnosis of the cause of the immersion accident includes diving accidents with head or spinal injury, syncope, cardiac arrhythmia, myocardial infarction, seizure disorders, and scuba diving accidents such as decompression injury and systemic air embolism.

In most cases of near drowning, some degree of lung injury occurs because of the aspiration of water and foreign materials such as organic debris, sand, or vomitus. Seawater is markedly hypertonic compared with plasma and other body fluids. Aspirated saltwater causes alveolar edema by exerting an osmotic effect that draws free water into the lungs and by causing irritant damage to alveolar epithelial cells, increasing their permeability. Aspiration of freshwater is thought to cause a loss of surfactant, leading to alveolar instability, but it also causes damage to epithelial and endothelial cells, disrupting the integrity of the gas exchange barrier. In either situation, even in patients who improve rapidly with resuscitative efforts, the lung injury process may progress, leading to acute respiratory distress syndrome with widespread pulmonary edema and microatelectasis.

Tissue hypoxia related to prolonged submersion accounts for most of the other manifestations of near drowning. These include cerebral hypoxia, metabolic acidosis, depressed cardiac function, and dysrhythmias. Hypothermia, often profound, is seen frequently after near drowning and may contribute to the cardiovascular, metabolic, and central nervous system (CNS) changes.

CLINICAL FEATURES

PULMONARY CHANGES

Approximately 90% of patients admitted to the hospital after near drowning have some evidence of pulmonary aspiration. Gas exchange abnormalities and radiographic changes are extremely common and may progress after the patient reaches the emergency department. The mechanism of hypoxemia appears to be intrapulmonary venoarterial shunting due to alveolar edema and collapse. The chest radiograph often shows patchy, ill-defined infiltrates at the time of admission, with resolution or progression to more widespread involvement occurring over the next 12 to 24 hours. Lung compliance is usually reduced. Pulmonary infection is a common complication and may occur as a result of the lung injury process itself, prolonged intubation with acquisition of nosocomial pathogens, or airway obstruction due to aspirated foreign material.

METABOLIC ABNORMALITIES

Metabolic acidosis with a widened anion gap is extremely common and may persist for several hours, even when resuscitative efforts have been successful. This may reflect delayed lactic acid clearance or persistent tissue hypoxia with ongoing generation of lactic acid.

Experimental observations suggest that significant changes in blood volume or electrolyte concentrations occur only when the quantity of fluid inhaled has been great enough to severely limit survival. Except for life-threatening cardiac dysrhythmias in the period immediately after rescue, such changes are thought to be relatively unimportant determinants of disordered organ physiology after immersion injury.

Aspiration of freshwater leads acutely to hemodilution, a transient increase in blood volume, and dilution of electrolytes, primarily manifested as hyponatremia. These changes may explain the higher incidence of ventricular fibrillation in freshwater near drowning patients.

The aspiration of saltwater causes hemoconcentration, and a reduction in circulating blood volume as free water is drawn from the vasculature into the alveolar space. In those who survive the initial insult, restoration of normal blood volume and electrolyte concentrations is usually complete within 10 to 30 minutes.

Changes in the hematocrit may occur transiently owing to hemodilution or hemoconcentration. Freshwater aspiration may also be associated with mild degrees of hemolysis.

NEUROLOGIC CHANGES

Injury to the CNS is probably the most serious and least reversible clinical event after immersion injury. Cerebral anoxia occurs within minutes after submersion under water and is compounded by circulatory collapse. The resulting cerebral edema leads to further reduction in cerebral perfusion, seizures, and eventually to irreversible brain damage.

Hypoxemia, acidosis, and hypothermia may contribute to neurologic abnormalities at the time of admission. The clinician should also be alert to associated abnormalities that may have predisposed the patient to a serious immersion accident. These include intoxication with alcohol or other drugs and the possibility of CNS trauma (e.g., subdural hematoma, cervical spine fracture associated with a diving injury).

CARDIOVASCULAR ABNORMALITIES

Changes in cardiovascular function after immersion injury result from hypoxemia, acidosis, and hypothermia. The most life-threatening cardiovascular complication of near drowning is the development of ventricular fibrillation, which occurs most commonly in freshwater drowning and in episodes involving massive fluid aspiration. Ventricular fibrillation in hypothermic patients may be extremely refractory to attempts at cardioversion. In such patients, prolonged and aggressive resuscitation efforts are well justified because of the potential for complete recovery.

Bradycardia, hypotension, and myocardial depression are common in the early hours of hospitalization. In addition to ventricular and supraventricular dysrhythmias, the electrocardiogram may show ST-T-wave changes and the presence of J (or Osborn) waves in patients who are hypothermic. J waves represent prolonged depolarization of the ventricle and manifest as a prominent hump at the junction of the QRS complex and ST segment.

Aspiration of a large amount of seawater may result in hypovolemia because of a shift of intravascular fluid to the intraalveolar space. If enough freshwater is aspirated, hypervolemia occurs initially. However, with rapid redistribution of fluid, especially as pulmonary edema develops, hypovolemia may exist by the time the patient reaches the hospital.

HYPOTHERMIA

Hypothermia is a prominent feature of immersion injury and may contribute to many of the physiologic abnormalities seen in near-drowning victims. Hypothermia occurring at the time of the near drowning may also exert a protective effect, particularly in the CNS, by slowing tissue metabolism and minimizing the effects of hypoxia. Ventricular fibrillation is much more common and difficult to treat in patients with a body temperature below 28°C (83°F). When the body temperature is in this range, active core rewarming should be initiated using intravenous solutions warmed to body temperature; warmed electrolyte solutions for gastric, bladder, and peritoneal lavage; and ventilation with warmed, humidified gases. Continuous arteriovenous rewarming or cardiopulmonary bypass should be considered for severe hypothermia. Passive rewarming measures to prevent further heat loss should be undertaken for all hypothermic patients.

■ TREATMENT

The initial treatment should occur at the scene of the immersion accident. The goal of therapy is to restore adequate oxygen delivery as rapidly as possible because tissue hypoxia is the major cause of morbidity and mortality. If the victim cannot be removed from the water quickly, ventilation should be initiated while the victim is still in the water. Attempts to drain water from the lungs are usually ineffective, may delay the initiation of cardiopulmonary resuscitation (CPR), and increase the risk of vomiting and aspiration of gastric contents. An abdominal thrust (Heimlich) maneuver should not be used routinely in submersion victims; it is reserved for cases in which obstruction of the airway with a foreign body is suspected or when the patient does not respond to mouth-to-mouth resuscitation.

Cardiopulmonary resuscitation should be started immediately. After the patient's vital signs have been established, supplemental oxygen should be administered if available and the trachea should be intubated if the patient is comatose and appropriate equipment and personnel are available. After vital signs have been stabilized, the victim should be transported directly to the hospital.

Immediately upon admission to the hospital, electrolytes and arterial blood gases should be checked to assess metabolic and pulmonary function. There is controversy about whether to correct blood gas values for temperature in hypothermic patients. The clinician should be aware of whether or not the laboratory has corrected blood gas values for hypothermia. Intravenous access should be established and electrolyte solutions administered, with careful attention paid to possible electrolyte abnormalities and intravascular volume state. Measures to correct hypothermia should be initiated if indicated. Management of respiratory failure should follow the guidelines for treating the acute respiratory distress syndrome discussed in Chapter 357.

Although occasionally caused by the aspiration of grossly contaminated material, pulmonary infection is most commonly caused by hospital-acquired pathogens. Careful surveillance and institution of directed antibiotic therapy is most important. The use of prophylactic antibiotics is not recommended. When fever and leukocytosis are prolonged despite antibiotic therapy, the clinician should consider the possibility of bronchial obstruction due to aspirated foreign material, infection of the pleural space, or purulent sinusitis.

A variety of pharmacologic and other interventions directed at controlling cerebral edema have been used in victims of near drowning. Elevating the head of the bed, if the patient is hemodynamically stable, may alleviate cerebral swelling. It is also helpful to minimize the risk of further aspiration of gastric contents. Although controlled hyperventilation may be of some benefit in patients with elevated intracranial pressure, there are no data to support the use of corticosteroids or osmotic agents in this setting. Similarly, controlled hypothermia and barbiturate coma have not improved neurologic recovery or survival of patients who are comatose after immersion injury. Uncontrolled intracranial hypertension is associated with a uniformly poor prognosis.

■ SURVIVAL AND PROGNOSIS

Survival depends primarily on the success of initial resuscitative efforts and the recovery of neurologic function. Although respiratory failure can often be severe and prolonged, the prognosis for recovery of lung function is excellent in those who survive. The prognosis for neurologic recovery is influenced by age, duration of submersion, water temperature, and delays in the initiation of adequate CPR. The likelihood of survival is enhanced in children younger than 10 years. The importance of water temperature is emphasized by case reports describing submersion for as long as 40 minutes in extremely cold water with subsequent normal psychometric testing. Such cases are almost entirely limited to children. The immediacy and adequacy of initial CPR is more important than therapy, however sophisticated, after the patient has been taken to the hospital.

Prognosis for neurologic recovery can be assessed on the basis of clinical findings in the first hour of therapy. Spontaneous respiration in the period immediately after CPR is a favorable prognostic factor for neurologic recovery. In one retrospective series, all patients who exhibited spontaneous respirations at the conclusion of CPR survived without significant neurologic sequelae, and those who remained apneic died or survived with severe residual neurologic impairment. In another large series, the level of consciousness on admission to the emergency department was an important predictor. Of those who were alert and fully conscious on arrival or obtunded but arousable, 90% survived without neurologic sequelae. Of those who were comatose on arrival in the emergency department, 55% survived with normal function, 10% survived with persistent brain damage, and 34% died.

BIBLIOGRAPHY

Fields AI. Neardrowning in the pediatric population. *Crit Care Clin* 1992; 8:113–129.

Golden FS, Tipton MJ, Scott RC. Immersion, near-drowning and drowning. *Br J Anaesth* 1997;79:214–225.

Gonzalez Rothi RJ. Near drowning: consensus and controversies in pulmonary and cerebral resuscitation. *Heart Lung* 1987;16:474–482.

Graf WD, Cummings P, Quan L, et al. Predicting outcome in pediatric submersion victims. *Ann Emerg Med* 1995;26:312–319.

Jacobsen WK, Mason LJ, Briggs BA, et al. Correlation of spontaneous respiration and neurologic damage in neardrowning. *Crit Care Med* 1983;11:487–489.

Kyriacou DN, Arcinue EL, Peck C, et al. Effect of immediate resuscitation on children with submersion injury. *Pediatrics* 1994;94:137–142.

Levin DL, Morriss FC, Toro L, et al. Drowning and neardrowning. *Pediatr Clin North Am* 1993;40:321–336.

Modell JH. Current concepts: drowning. *N Engl J Med* 1993;328:253–256.

Modell JH. Biology of drowning. *Annu Rev Med* 1978;29:1–8.

Olshaker JS. Near drowning. *Emerg Med Clin North Am* 1992;10:339–350.

Rosen P, Stoto M, Harley J. The use of the Heimlich maneuver in near drowning: Institute of Medicine report. *J Emerg Med* 1995;13:397–405.

Sachkeva RC. Near drowning. *Crit Care Clin* 1999;15:281–296.

Kelley's Textbook of Internal Medicine, fourth edition. Edited by H. David Humes. Lippincott Williams & Wilkins, Philadelphia © 2000.

CHAPTER

60

TREATMENT OF ANAPHYLAXIS

MARC S. MCMORRIS

Anaphylaxis is an immediate systemic reaction caused by immunoglobulin E (IgE)–mediated release of mediators from mast cells and basophils. An anaphylactoid reaction is a similar reaction independent of IgE. A variety of substances including drugs, foods, latex, insect stings, and other environmental factors have been associated with anaphylactic or anaphylactoid reactions.

The recognition and treatment of anaphylaxis must be insti-

tuted promptly, even if the onset appears mild, because its manifestations can progress rapidly to severe hypotension, as well as shock or acute respiratory obstruction. The differential diagnosis can be broad, including conditions such as vasovagal syncope, adverse drug reactions, seizures, myocardial infarction, arrhythmias, catastrophic asthma, epiglottitis, foreign body aspiration with airway obstruction, mastocytosis, carcinoid, and hereditary angioedema. Vasovagal syncope is generally associated with pallor, diaphoresis and bradycardia in the absence of pruritis or urticaria. Implicit in the diagnosis are risks of airway obstruction, hypotension, tachycardia, gastrointestinal symptoms, and generalized cutaneous reactions alone or in combination. Symptoms generally occur within 5 to 30 minutes of exposure. Urticaria and angioedema are the most common manifestations of anaphylaxis occurring in over 90% of patients. This is followed in frequency by respiratory symptoms, including upper airway obstruction, dyspnea, and wheezing. Gastrointestinal symptoms of nausea, vomiting, or diarrhea are generally less common. Unfortunately, cardiovascular collapse can occur in patients without other antecedent signs or symptoms. One must be aware that anaphylaxis may be biphasic with a recurrence of symptoms 4 to 8 hours after the initial reaction.

Prompt assessment of the clinical symptoms and their severity is essential for appropriate therapy, with attention to the cardiovascular and respiratory systems especially indicated. Aqueous epinephrine is the initial treatment of choice because of its rapid onset of action and favorable effects on target organs; an antiallergic action (i.e., prevents mediator release from mast cells and basophils), bronchodilatation, and a normalizing effect on vascular permeability and systemic hypotension. An H_1 receptor antagonist such as diphenhydramine (Benadryl) should be administered promptly accompanied by monitoring heart rate, cardiac rhythm, and blood pressure. Supplemental oxygen should be given as needed by nasal cannula (Fig. 60.1).

█ HYPOTENSION

Anaphylactic collapse and shock is an ominous manifestation that can result in death if not reversed promptly. A profound drop in blood pressure can be the first sign of an anaphylactic reaction. If there is any evidence of hypotension during the initial evaluation, an intravenous line should be established immediately for fluid replacement, preferably with a large-bore needle or catheter. Hypovolemia primarily reflects massive extravascular loss of fluid, brought on by the increased vascular permeability in anaphylactic reactions. The resultant low filling pressures must be treated specifically with rapid infusions of fluid as the blood pressure is monitored. If repeated doses of aqueous epinephrine and volume expansion are not effective in normalizing blood pressure, other vasoactive drugs may be used. Special consideration must be given to pregnant patients or patients taking β-blocking agents. Refractory patients may respond to glucagon administration or the addition of an H_2 receptor antagonist such as cimetidine or ranitidine. Glucagon has both positive inotropic and chronotropic characteristics. The inotropic effect is not dependent on catecholamines or their receptors and is, therefore, unaffected by β blockade.

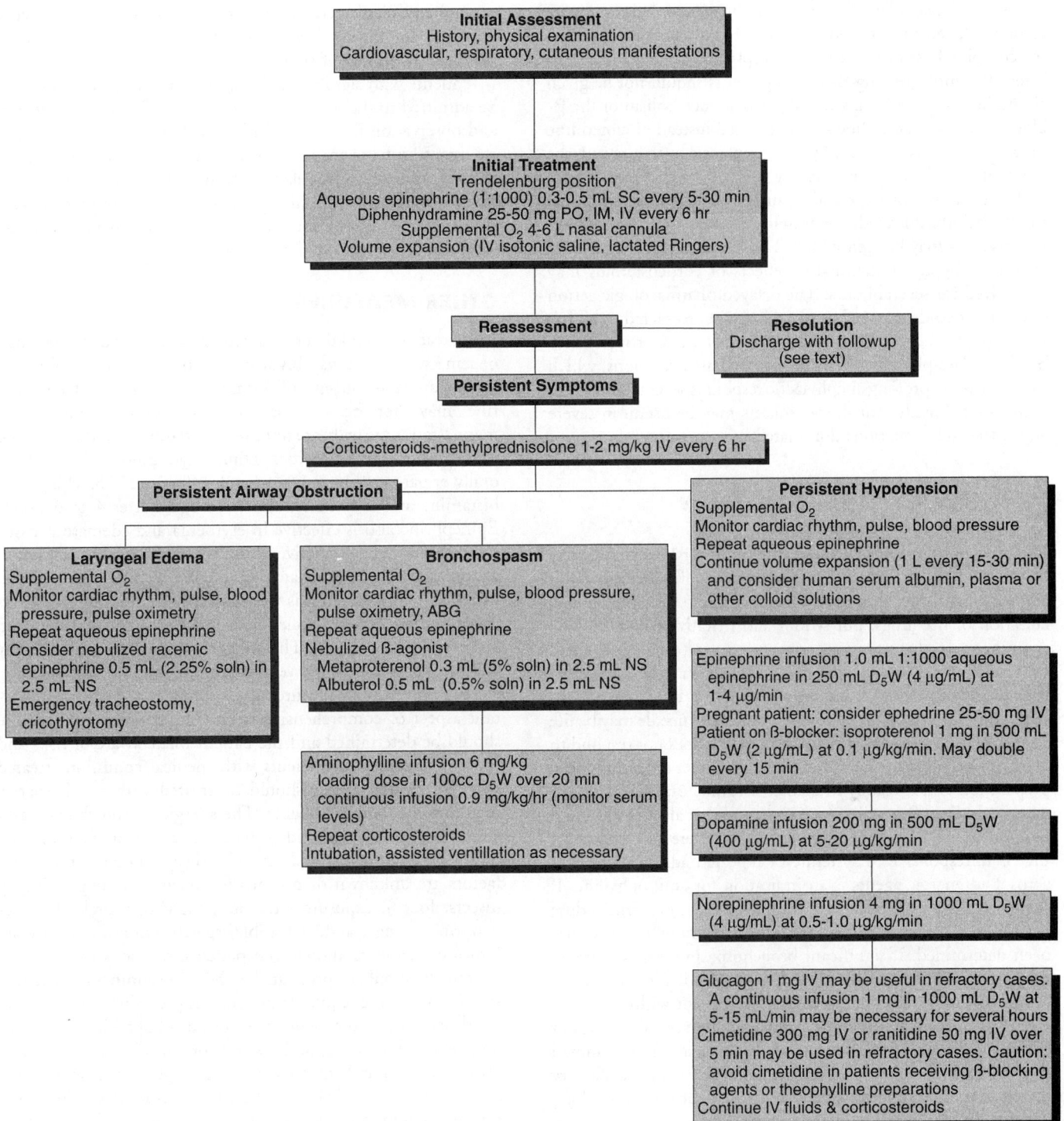

FIGURE 60.1. Treatment of anaphylaxis.

EVIDENCE LEVEL: B. References: Atkinson TP. Anaphylaxis. *Clin Allergy* **1992;76:8. Bechner BS. Anaphylaxis.** *N Engl J Med* **1991;324:1785.**

The cardiovascular effects of histamine in anaphylaxis appear to be mediated through both H_1 and H_2 receptors. Therefore, the combined use of H_1- and H_2-receptor blockers may be indicated. Patients receiving β-blocking agents should not be given cimetidine because it may impair hepatic metabolism of the β-blocking agent. Ranitidine should be used instead of cimetidine in patients receiving theophylline preparations to prevent the possibility of theophylline toxicity.

Intravenous corticosteroids, such as methylprednisolone, should be administered. A resultant increase in adrenergic responsiveness may be seen within 2 hours, although the onset of action of the anti-inflammatory effects of corticosteroids may be delayed for several hours. The delayed pharmacologic action of corticosteroids may be beneficial because protracted or biphasic anaphylactic reactions have been reported. Corticosteroids block the late-phase response of IgE-mediated reactions, which may worsen or prolong anaphylactic responses several hours after their onset. Finally, antishock trousers may be useful in severe and intractable situations dominated by hypotension.

AIRWAY OBSTRUCTION

If airway obstruction is present, the upper or lower tract may be the involved site, with each requiring specific therapy. With angioedema of the larynx, no wheezing may be audible on auscultation of the lungs, but stridor and irritative cough may be prominent. In this situation, aqueous epinephrine is indicated. Endotracheal intubation or a tracheostomy may be imperative if laryngoscopy reveals progression to significant laryngeal obstruction. Tracheal puncture with a large-bore needle may be life saving if rapidly progressive laryngeal edema does not respond to epinephrine and a tracheostomy set with proper operating room preparation is not readily available. If bronchospasm predominates, nebulized β-agonists (metaproterenol or albuterol) should be used in addition to the epinephrine. Severe bronchospasm that is unresponsive to systemic or repeated administration of aerosol adrenergic agents is an indication for aminophylline. If the patient is already receiving theophylline, a lower initial dose is indicated, preferably after the serum theophylline level has been determined. If significant bronchospasm persists, intravenous corticosteroids are indicated, especially if the patient has asthma or has received corticosteroid treatment within the past year. Although corticosteroids may not act for several hours after administration, they should be started as soon as it is determined that other treatment measures are not producing satisfactory results, and they should be delivered at 6-hour intervals. Blood gas determinations and electrocardiographic monitoring is appropriate if significant bronchospasm is present. Supplemental oxygen is indicated if significant respiratory obstruction persists. With $PaCO_2$ elevation denoting respiratory failure, intubation and assistance of ventilation are necessary.

After immediate evaluation and therapy has been instituted, subsequent treatment and follow-up must be individualized to each patient. Patients with mild reactions who respond fully to antihistamine or epinephrine may be sent home when the symptoms subside. However, they should recognize that symptoms may recur several hours later (a possible late-phase re-

sponse) and should return promptly for evaluation if this occurs. Patients also should have oral antihistamines and adrenergic medications to take if symptoms recur.

Patients with significant shock or airway obstruction should be admitted to the hospital for continuous, intensive treatment and observation for at least 24 hours after stabilization, so that resurgent/biphasic anaphylactic reactions can be recognized and treated promptly. The delayed pharmacologic action of corticosteroids may be beneficial in such situations. Complications of shock (cardiac dysrhythmias, hypoxic seizure, metabolic acidosis) should be recognized and treated.

OTHER MEASURES

If the reaction is mild and characterized only by urticaria, angioedema without airway involvement, or gastrointestinal symptoms (nausea, vomiting, colicky abdominal cramping), epinephrine may not be essential or may suffice alone. These manifestations usually are not life threatening, and they respond eventually to antihistamines. Diphenhydramine, 25 to 50 mg orally or parenterally, is a commonly effective H_1-blocking antihistamine and may be administered again after 4 to 6 hours. Epinephrine also is effective in erythema and edematous tissue swelling; its vasoconstrictive action is beneficial, and its onset of action is much faster than that of oral antihistamines. If an injection or insect sting is the cause of the reaction, a venous tourniquet should be applied proximal to the site and loosened at appropriate intervals. The stinger may be removed carefully without compressing the venom sac if it is still in the skin.

The prevention of future anaphylactic episodes is an important aspect of comprehensive treatment. If possible, the cause should be determined and the patient made aware of risks and preventive strategies. Patients with medical conditions treated with β-blocking agents should be treated with an alternative medication if one is available. The allergic person should carry a card or wear a bracelet identifying the allergenic food or drug that poses a health risk and scrupulously avoid that factor. If risk factors are unknown or potentially unavoidable (e.g., stinging insects, foods), exposure reduction, carrying a preloaded epinephrine syringe, and, if feasible, specific immunotherapy are indicated. Patients known to experience reactions to radiocontrast media should be pretreated with antihistamines and corticosteroids before the required radiographic procedures are administered. Patients who experience recurrent idiopathic anaphylaxis may require high doses of daily oral corticosteroids (prednisone, 60 to 100 mg) and must have the appropriate follow-up. Oral aspirin, insulin, penicillin, and cephalosporin "desensitization" can be attempted in patients who are allergic to these medications and who specifically require them for urgent treatment indications. The IgA-deficient patients who require transfusions should receive compatible blood from donors also lacking IgA or carefully washed, cross-matched, red blood cells.

BIBLIOGRAPHY

Atkinson TP, Kaliner MA. Anaphylaxis. *Med Clin North Am* 1992;76(4): 841–855.
Bochner BS, Lichtenstein LM. Anaphylaxis. *N Engl J Med* 1991;324: 1785–1790.

Entman SS, Moise KJ. Anaphylaxis in pregnancy. *South Med J* 1984;77: 402.

Kemp SF, Lockey RF, Wolf BL, Lieberman P. Anaphylaxis. A review of 266 cases. *Arch Intern Med* 1995;155:1749–1754.

Lang DM. Anaphylactoid and anaphylactic reactions, hazards of β-blockers. *Drug Safety* 1995;12:299–304.

Lieberman P. The use of antihistamines in the prevention and treatment of anaphylaxis and anaphylactoid reactions. *J Allergy Clin Immunol* 1990;86:684–686.

Lieberman P. Anaphylaxis and anaphylactoid reactions. In: Middleton E Jr, ed. *Allergy principles and practice*, vol. 2, fifth ed. St. Louis: Mosby, 1998:1079–1092.

Nicklas RA, Bernstein IL, Li JT, et al., eds. The diagnosis and management of anaphylaxis. In: *Supplement to JACI*. St. Louis: Mosby, 1998: S465–S528.

Schwartz LB, Metcalfe DD, Miller JS, et al. Tryptase levels as an indicator of mast-cell activation in systemic anaphylaxis and mastocytosis. *N Engl J Med* 1987;316(26):1622–1626.

Wiggins CA, Dykewicz MS, Patterson R. Idiopathic anaphylaxis: a review. *Ann Allergy* 1989;62:1–4.

Kelley's Textbook of Internal Medicine, fourth edition. Edited by H. David Humes.
Lippincott Williams & Wilkins, Philadelphia © 2000.

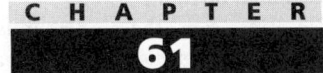

CARDIOPULMONARY RESUSCITATION

KATHLEEN S. SCHRANK

Cardiopulmonary resuscitation (CPR) techniques seek to restore effective cardiovascular and neurologic function following cardiac arrest. These measures are primarily designed for victims of premature sudden cardiac death and are readily used in a variety of medical emergencies; however, they are not intended for reflexive application to those who have truly reached the end of their lives with other severe underlying illnesses. Although the overall death rate from cardiovascular disease has declined, sudden cardiac death still claims over 600 victims each day in the United States. The majority are due to ischemic heart disease, and about two-thirds occur outside the hospital. Until closed-chest CPR and external defibrillation techniques were introduced in the 1960s, death from cardiac arrest was considered inevitable. Since then, widespread public education (on use of CPR, cardiac warning signs, risk reduction, the use of "911"), development of advanced cardiac life support (ACLS) guidelines, and deployment of ACLS treatment to prehospital settings have impacted survival. Today about 20% of victims of primary ventricular fibrillation can survive if the elements of rapid emergency care are in place.

Cardiopulmonary resuscitation techniques include basic life support measures, advanced life support measures, and post-resuscitation stabilization. In cardiopulmonary arrests due to airway obstruction or respiratory failure, CPR alone may restore life. However, resuscitation from cardiac arrhythmias by CPR alone is rare, and the perfusion achieved with CPR declines rapidly with time. Therefore, further rapid interventions are crucial. Ventricular fibrillation (VF) is the most common arrest rhythm; immediate recognition with defibrillation is the most critical action in restoring life to the largest number of arrest victims. Additional interventions are guided by cardiac rhythm and underlying etiologic factors. The ACLS guidelines from the American Heart Association provide an organized framework for cardiac arrest management, and the clinician must consider other causes and actions when a patient fails to respond promptly to them.

■ ADULT BASIC LIFE SUPPORT TECHNIQUES

Basic CPR includes chest compressions and ventilation aimed at maintaining enough perfusion to the brain and heart to preserve cellular viability until effective spontaneous circulation can be restored. Performance is readily learned by health care workers and laypersons; family members of cardiac patients should be encouraged to learn. The rescuer must assess the victim for unresponsiveness; initiate a call for help (generally by telephoning "911"); assess airway, breathing, and circulation status; and begin CPR if arrest is confirmed. The airway is opened by positioning the patient with the head tilted back and chin lifted forward. If cervical spine injury is suspected, then the airway is opened by thrusting the jaw forward, with the neck remaining in a neutral position. The rescuer may then give two slow breaths, watching for chest rise to confirm air flow. If the airway is obstructed, the head and neck should be repositioned. Then a Heimlich maneuver may be done if needed, by placing the heel of the hand between the navel and xiphoid, then thrusting cephalad up to five times. Other methods to relieve obstruction include a finger sweep of the oropharynx, chest compressions, or back blows. Suctioning, laryngoscopy, or cricothyrotomy may be needed if all of the above fail.

Chest compressions are performed with the heel of the hand at a point two-finger breadths above the xiphoid, at a rate of 80 to 100 compressions per minute. Compressions are alternated with breaths (15:2 if one rescuer, 5:1 if two rescuers). The patient must be supine on a hard surface. Compression force determines aortic pressure and should be as vigorous as possible without causing rib fractures. Timing the compression to occupy half of each stroke cycle also improves flow; this tends to occur naturally at the recommended compression rate. The blood flow achieved with CPR drops rapidly with any delay in its initiation and with time. The addition of α-adrenergic drugs augments CPR flow to the heart and brain considerably. Cardiopulmonary resuscitation should be started as soon as arrest is recognized, and continued until a spontaneous pulse is restored or efforts terminated, with brief interruptions for critical interventions such as defibrillation.

The exact means by which CPR provides perfusion remains under debate. Cardiopulmonary resuscitation may directly compress the heart between the sternum and vertebrae, resulting in forward flow because passive closure of the mitral and tricuspid valves prevents backflow (the "cardiac pump" theory). Alternatively, each compression/release cycle produces dramatic changes in intrathoracic pressure, creating a gradient that pulls blood into the chest upon each release, with backflow prevented by competent venous valves; the entire thorax contributes the necessary pressure gradients (the "thoracic pump" theory). Evidence for and against each mechanism exists in various animal models and in humans. In reality, both probably contribute in human CPR, with the thoracic pump mechanism predominating. Trials of alternative methods of CPR based on the latter theory have produced mixed results, with better perfusion but no overall improved survival thus far. Open-chest CPR produces markedly better flow but is not a practical option. Immediate assisted circulation via cardiopulmonary bypass pump is under active investigation.

ADVANCED CARDIAC LIFE SUPPORT GUIDELINES

GENERAL PRINCIPLES

Restarting the heart is the essential first step toward restoration of normal cardiovascular and neurologic function. Cardiac rhythm must be determined initially and again after each intervention or status change, with management shifted accordingly. The patient should be reassessed for the presence of a palpable pulse every few minutes and whenever the rhythm changes. The three major treatment algorithms (ventricular fibrillation, asystole, and pulseless electrical activity) are based on underlying rhythm; each is discussed below. Immediate identification of VF with defibrillation is the highest priority. Common management components include CPR, oxygenation, ventilation, intravenous access, acid–base management, and initial drug therapy with epinephrine.

Optimal ventilation and oxygenation is achieved by early endotracheal intubation with high-flow oxygen. Correct tube placement is critical, and confirmation includes the use of both clinical assessment and bedside devices (end-tidal CO_2 monitors, oximetry, or residual air detection devices). Repeated assessments provide early detection of tube displacement and of pneumothoraces that may occur as a result of the blunt chest trauma of CPR, of procedures, or of positive-pressure ventilation. Vomiting with aspiration frequently complicates emergency intubation; cricoid pressure during intubation plus vigorous suctioning can minimize this risk.

Initial intravenous (IV) access may be rapidly established via the antecubital vein with a large-bore catheter. Central venous access takes more time and expertise, has greater risk, and is less appropriate initially. Drug entry into central circulation is augmented by a fluid bolus given after the drug, plus elevation of the arm. Intraosseous access (tibia, femur, sternum) is an excellent route in children, and sternal devices for adults are now available. Endotracheal administration is effective for several drugs (epinephrine, lidocaine, atropine), especially when intravenous access is delayed. Drugs are absorbed from distal bronchioles, so delivery is improved by using about 10 ml total fluid volume given through a small catheter threaded down the

endotracheal tube. Given by any of these routes, drugs will need 1 to 2 minutes to circulate and begin to act.

Most arrest victims have both metabolic and respiratory acidoses. Hyperventilation provides rapid correction of lethal acidoses and is the primary acid–base intervention. Lowering the CO_2 tension appears to be more beneficial to cellular function than pH correction with base. Excess sodium bicarbonate may produce hypernatremia, hyperosmolality, hypokalemia, or severe alkalosis, so that its use is best guided by arterial blood gas results; if not readily available, then 1 to 2 mEq per kg may be given empirically if the patient does not respond to initial ACLS measures plus hyperventilation. Patients with hyperkalemia and those likely to have had severe metabolic acidosis prior to arrest (drowning, seizures, shock) are most likely to benefit from bicarbonate use combined with hyperventilation.

The initial drug used in arrest management today is epinephrine. It significantly augments central perfusion during arrest via α-adrenergic actions, which constrict only peripheral vessels. The optimal dosage remains controversial, but at least 1 mg is appropriate every 3 to 5 minutes while pulseless. Anecdotal successes with high doses (0.1 to 0.2 mg per kg per dose) have not translated into improved long-range survival in controlled trials, though research is ongoing.

During cardiac arrest care, the rescuer must also look for reversible underlying disorders and situations that merit specific interventions (Table 61.1). Hypovolemia, hypoglycemia, potassium imbalance, or pneumothorax may need prompt correction. Some poisonings have specific antagonists that could be essential. Also, if the patient does not respond to ACLS interventions, everything must be rechecked: intravenous patency, breath sounds, oxygenation, rhythm.

Finally, when efforts are unsuccessful, the clinician must consider termination. The initial situation (presumed downtime), rhythm, duration of effort, transient responsiveness, underlying diseases, and especially the patient's wishes (if known) will all influence this decision. Indeed, in patients with severe illnesses, such decisions are most appropriately made long before cardiac arrest through discussions between the treating physician and the patient or family.

VENTRICULAR FIBRILLATION AND PULSELESS VENTRICULAR TACHYCARDIA

Ventricular fibrillation is the most common arrest rhythm, whereas ventricular tachycardia (VT) is the most survivable; both are managed by the same algorithm (Fig. 61.1). Prompt electrical defibrillation is crucial to survival. Needless delays are common in attempting synchronized cardioversion of pulseless VT, so defibrillation is preferred. The initial trial of defibrillation includes three escalating shocks in rapid succession (assuming that VF/VT persists) to allow better delivery to the heart due to lowered transthoracic resistance. If the rhythm persists, CPR is performed while an endotracheal tube and intravenous line are placed, epinephrine is then given by either route, followed by another defibrillation at 360 J. Next, a series of antiarrhythmic drugs may be alternated with shocks. The drug of choice remains lidocaine. Amiodarone appears to be another excellent choice, although hypotension is a common sequela. Alternatives include

TABLE 61.1.	**SPECIAL SITUATIONS IN CARDIAC ARREST MANAGEMENT**

Situation	Treatment Consideration
Hyperkalemia	Glucose, insulin, bicarbonate, calcium infusions
Hypothermia	No CPR needed if any spontaneous pulse or breathing is present.
	Drugs and electrical therapy may not work prior to rewarming.
	Aggressive rewarming for victims of *rapid-onset* hypothermia.
Intracardiac catheters	Irritation of right ventricle may cause ventricular fibrillation or tachycardia; reposition.
	Catheters may allow massive air embolism, consider aspiration.
Lightning injury	No electrical risk to rescuers. CPR alone may succeed.
	Spontaneous cardiac recovery from asystole may precede return of spontaneous breathing.
Long QT syndromes	Torsades de pointes may occur; magnesium sulfate often effective.
	Identify and remove causative agent in acquired cases.
	After sinus rhythm restored, cautious isoproterenol infusion may prevent recurrence by shortening QT.
Near-drowning	Extreme lactic acidosis is common and needs treatment.
	Consider cervical spine injury.
	Noncardiac pulmonary edema is common (freshwater or saltwater).
Poisonings:	
β-Blockers	Fluid boluses, high-dose pressors/epinephrine, pacing, glucagon
Calcium channel blockers	Same as β-blockers, plus calcium infusion
Cocaine	Benzodiazepines for tachyarrhythmias, α and β blockade
Digoxin	Normalize potassium, consider digoxin Fab antibodies, magnesium
Opiates	Naloxone
Organophosphates	Large doses of atropine, pralidoxime
Tricyclic antidepressants	Alkalinize serum, magnesium sulfate, physostigmine
Pregnancy, viable fetus	Consider open chest CPR, cesarean section unless rapid response to standard advanced cardiac life support

CPR, cardiopulmonary resuscitation.

bretylium, propranolol, magnesium sulfate, phenytoin, or procainamide, although the latter two agents are less useful due to their prolonged loading times. Epinephrine is given every 3 to 5 minutes until pulse is restored. In the case of a known hyperacute myocardial infarction, intravenous thrombolysis may also be considered as an emergency rescue measure after the first few drug–shock–drug–shock trials have failed, since prognosis deteriorates rapidly after each failed defibrillation attempt. After conversion to a safe rhythm, antiarrhythmic drug therapy is continued for 1 to 2 days with whatever drug proved effective (lidocaine if conversion occurred prior to antiarrhythmic drug use), in order to prevent recurrence.

Widespread deployment of automatic external defibrillators for use by the lay public may improve survival from out-of-hospital cardiac arrest. These machines identify VF/VT, advise the rescuer to stand back, and provide shocks if needed. Training is easily added to CPR courses, and these devices are being placed in public venues under local medical oversight. Automatic implanted cardioverter–defibrillators (AICDs) reduce recurrence of cardiac arrest; units deliver a preprogrammed series of shocks internally on recognition of VF/VT. The AICD firing poses no safety risk to hands-on medical personnel, and patient management follows standard ACLS guidelines, with external shocks superimposed for VF/VT if response to or by the AICD is delayed.

ASYSTOLE AND PROFOUND BRADYCARDIAS

Treatment should include CPR, endotracheal intubation, intravenous access, and repetitive doses of epinephrine and atropine (Fig. 61.2). Drug treatment is aimed at stimulating an organized rhythm at an effective rate (primarily through epinephrine's stimulation of cardiac β$_1$ receptors), then adding inotropic support if necessary. Early initiation of external cardiac pacing may also save a small number of patients. Asystole should be confirmed in more than one electrocardiogram (ECG) lead, so that fine VF is not missed. Any correctable problems, such as hyperkalemia, should be addressed early. Aminophylline may prove useful through its competitive inhibition of the binding of endogenous adenosine, which is produced during arrest and acts to suppress automaticity. Overall prognosis is extremely poor, but there are rare survivors with good neurologic function. Most often, asystole is the final rhythm in a prolonged, unwitnessed arrest. Victims with high vagal tone (e.g., hypothermia,

Assess Airway, Breathing, Circulation
Perform CPR until defibrillator attached
VF/VT present

↓

Defibrillate up to 3 times if needed for persistant VF/VT
(200 joules, 200-300 J, 360 J)
Reassess rhythm

↓

Persistent or recurrent VF/VT

↓

Continue CPR
Intubate trachea
Obtain IV access

↓

Epinephrine 1 mg IV push; repeat every 3-5 min until pulse restored

↓

Defibrillate (360 J) within 30-60 sec.

↓

If persistent VF/VT, administer antiarrhythmic medication of probable benefit.
Choices: Lidocaine, amiodarone, bretylium, magnesium sulfate, procainamide, propranolol.
Sodium bicarbonate may be added if hyperkalemia,
bicarbonate-responsive drug overdose or preexisting acidosis.

↓

Defibrillate (360 J) within 30-60 sec after each dose
Pattern should be drug-shock, drug-shock if VF/VT persists.

FIGURE 61.1. Algorithm for ventricular fibrillation and pulseless ventricular tachycardia. (Modified from American Heart Association. *Textbook of advanced cardiac life support,* 1997.)
EVIDENCE LEVEL: A. Reference: *Textbook of Advanced Cardiac Life Support.* **American Heart Association 1997:1–17.**

Assess Airway, Breathing, Circulation.
Perform CPR until monitor / defibrillation attached.
Confirm asystole in more than one lead.
Asystole present

↓

Continue CPR
Intubate trachea
Obtain IV access

↓

Consider and treat possible underlying causes

↓

Consider immediate transcutaneous cardiac pacing

↓

Epinephrine 1 mg IV push;
repeat every 3-5 minutes and consider escalating doses

↓

Atropine, 1 mg IV; repeat every 3-5 minutes to a total of 0.03 - 0.04 mg/kg

↓

Consider termination of resuscitation efforts

FIGURE 61.2. Algorithm for asystole and profound bradycardia. (Modified from American Heart Association. *Textbook of advanced cardiac life support,* 1997.)
EVIDENCE LEVEL: A. Reference: *Textbook of Advanced Cardiac Life Support.* **American Heart Association 1997:1–24.**

drowning) or electrical injury are more likely to have primary asystole with better survival potential.

PULSELESS ELECTRICAL ACTIVITY

The category of pulseless electrical activity (PEA) includes every rhythm that has a reasonable rate but no pulse. Often, the heart muscle is contracting, but without effective output. Therefore, the older term "electromechanical dissociation," which implies absence of muscle contraction, is now used to describe a subset of PEA. Initial management of PEA (Fig. 61.3) includes CPR, endotracheal intubation, intravenous access, and epinephrine. Fluid boluses are recommended early, for correction of potential volume depletion, and pressors may be added once volume is adequate. The clinician must search rapidly for a treatable underlying cause (Table 61.2), particularly profound hypovolemia or tension pneumothorax. Massive myocardial infarction may produce PEA through total pump failure or rupture; survival from full arrest is unlikely. Massive pulmonary embolism may obstruct right heart outflow; if any pulse can be restored, the patient might survive to embolectomy or thrombolysis. Overall survival from PEA is poor because these rhythms are usually the end stage of global heart disease, sepsis, or multi-organ damage.

Assess Airway, Breathing, Circulation
Perform CPR until monitor / defibrillation attached
Assess rhythm
PEA present

↓

Continue CPR
Intubate trachea
Obtain IV access
Assess blood flow using Doppler ultrasound, if available

↓

Consider and treat possible underlying causes

↓

Epinephrine, 1 mg IV push; repeat every 3 - 5 minutes

↓

IV volume infusion

↓

If bradycardia, give atropine 1 mg IV;
repeat every 3 - 5 minutes as needed to a total of 0.03 - 0.04 mg/kg

↓

Consider trial of pressor agent

FIGURE 61.3. Algorithm for pulseless electrical activity. (Modified from American Heart Association. *Textbook of advanced cardiac life support,* 1997.)
EVIDENCE LEVEL: A. Reference: *Textbook of Advanced Cardiac Life Support.* **American Heart Association 1997:1–22.**

TABLE 61.2.	CAUSES OF PULSELESS ELECTRICAL ACTIVITY (PEA)
Acidosis	Hyperkalemia
Air embolism	Hypothermia
Aortic dissection	Hypovolemia
Cardiac valve rupture	Hypoxemia
Drug toxicity:	Myocardial infarction
β-Blockers	Myocardial pump failure
Calcium channel blockers	Myocardial wall rupture
Digoxin/digitalis	Pericardial tamponade
Tricyclic antidepressants	Pulmonary embolism
	Tension pneumothorax

POSTRESUSCITATION MANAGEMENT

Immediate postarrest care includes support of ventilation, oxygenation, and blood pressure. Hypotension is common; evaluation of its hemodynamic significance and cause will guide therapy. Moderate hypertension is not harmful and does not need correction. Electrolytes (especially potassium, magnesium, and phosphorus), glucose, hematocrit, arterial blood gases, chest radiograph, and a 12-lead ECG are needed promptly. Complications of resuscitation efforts (aspiration, rib fractures, liver or spleen lacerations) require prompt recognition. Acute myocardial infarctions cause a large portion of arrests; ECGs, laboratory markers, and echocardiography will assist prompt diagnosis and further interventions. Active ischemia warrants anti-ischemic pharmacotherapy, including nitroglycerin and aspirin. Rhythm monitoring is essential, and antiarrhythmic drugs are needed after VF/VT. Sinus tachycardia is common after arrest and often resolves spontaneously, especially if due to previous epinephrine. Volume depletion, hypoxia, ischemia, congestive heart failure, or agitation may also cause persistent sinus tachycardia.

Brain resuscitation raises several issues distinct from cardiac resuscitation, although rapid restoration of effective circulation is unquestionably the best way to assure brain recovery. The mechanisms of ischemic brain injury remain the focus of intensive research. Neuronal damage begins during cardiac arrest with ischemia and anaerobic metabolism, and a diverse array of processes continue during reperfusion that may produce permanent damage. Contributing factors include local fluxes of potassium and calcium, loss of vasomotor control, endothelial damage, edema, release of tissue mediators, metabolic changes, and induction of apoptosis. Proposed therapies have unfortunately not produced overall improvement. General supportive measures include adequate CPR, oxygenation, and epinephrine during arrest. After arrest, the brain benefits from normal to moderately elevated blood pressure, mild hyperventilation, normalization of glucose, elevation of the head to about 20°, prevention of further insults, and nutritional support. Conditions that increase neuronal metabolic demands (agitation, fever, seizures) must be avoided.

Longer term management and rehabilitation must be tailored to the patient's functional status and underlying disease processes. In the absence of acute infarction, extensive diagnostic studies may be needed to determine etiology, cardiac function, and electrophysiologic stability.

BIBLIOGRAPHY

American Heart Association. *Textbook of advanced cardiac life support.* Dallas, 1997.
American Heart Association, Emergency Cardiac Care Committee and Subcommittees. Guidelines for cardiopulmonary resuscitation and emergency cardiac care. *JAMA* 1992;268:2171–2295.
DeBehnke DJ, Swart GL. Cardiac arrest. *Emerg Med Clin North Am* 1996; 14:57–81.
Halperin HR, Chandra NC, Levin HR, et al. Newer methods of improving blood flow during CPR. *Ann Emerg Med* 1996;27:553–562.
McIntosh TK, Garde E, Saatman KE, et al. Central nervous system resuscitation. *Emerg Med Clin North Am* 1997;15:527–550.
Ornato JP, Peberdy MA. The mystery of bradyasystole during cardiac arrest. *Ann Emerg Med* 1996;27:576–587.
Paradis NA, Halperin HR, Nowak R, eds. *Cardiac arrest: the science and practice of resuscitation medicine.* Baltimore: Williams & Wilkins, 1996.
Shah CP, Thakur RK, Xie B, et al. Implantable cardioverter defibrillators. *Emerg Med Clin North Am* 1998;16:463–489.
Truong JH, Rosen P. Current concepts in electrical defibrillation. *J Emerg Med* 1997;15:331–338.

Kelley's Textbook of Internal Medicine, fourth edition. Edited by H. David Humes.
Lippincott Williams & Wilkins, Philadelphia © 2000.

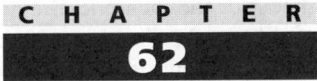

C H A P T E R
62

HYPERTHERMIA AND HYPOTHERMIA

FAITH T. FITZGERALD

Maintenance of body temperature in humans is a balance between heat production and heat loss. The principal source of heat is the oxidation of ingested food. During physical work, including shivering and chilling, muscles generate much additional heat. The loss of body heat occurs through radiation, convection, and evaporation of sweat, with the last of these becoming progressively more important as the surrounding temperature increases. Evaporation of sweat is virtually the sole mode of heat loss at ambient temperatures greater than 35°C (95°F).

Heat sensors through the skin and nervous system send signals to the preoptic nucleus of the anterior hypothalamus, which directs the dissipation of heat by cutaneous vasodilatation (flushing) and sweating, and retention or generation of heat by cutaneous vasoconstriction and muscular activity. Behavioral responses (e.g., seeking shade in the heat or warmth on a cold day) also are important, and impairment of these voluntary actions, as in cognitive dysfunction, can predispose a person to hyperthermia or hypothermia.

Normal body temperatures in healthy adults range from

TABLE 62.1.	HEAT ILLNESS		
Type	**Temperature**	**Symptoms and Signs**	**Therapy**
Heat cramps	Euthermic	Muscle spasms, weakness, fatigue, nausea, vomiting	Remove to cool place, rest and oral fluids
Heat stress	Euthermic to 39°C (102°F)	Tachycardia, hypertension, dizziness, restlessness, mental changes, emotional lability	Remove to cool place, rest and oral fluids
Heat exhaustion	Euthermic to 39°C (102°F)	Nausea, vomiting, irritability, orthostasis, headache, confusion, syncope, weakness, dyspnea, piloerection, profuse sweating	Remove to cool place, intravenous fluids, electrolytes
Heat stroke			
Exertional	>39°C (102°F)	Young people during vigorous exercise: collapse, *sweating,* neurologic changes, lactic acidosis, rhabdomyolysis, renal failure, liver abnormalities	Intravenous fluids, cooling (water spray, fanning, ice packs) support, intensive care; avoid submersion in ice water
Classic	May be >40.5°C (105°F)	Elderly people during heat waves: *no sweating;* neurologic symptoms common; lactic acidosis, rhabdomyolysis, coagulopathy, tachyarrhythmias, hypotension, renal failure, elevated liver enzymes, acute respiratory distress syndrome	

36.1°C to 37.4°C (97°F to 100.2°F), with the highest readings between 4 p.m. and 8 p.m. and the lowest between 4 a.m. and 6 a.m. This diurnal pattern is maintained (although set at a higher level) in most febrile diseases. The average body temperature is lower in the aged, the cachectic, the neurologically impaired, and those with certain disease states such as uremia. In assessing the clinical significance of body temperature, the underlying condition of the patient must be considered: a sustained temperature of 37.7°C (100°F) might be pathologic in an elderly cachectic man and normal in a young and vigorous one.

HYPERTHERMIA

Fever, discussed in Chapter 266, is the complex physiologic response of most vertebrates to immune challenges. Mediated by the hypothalamus, neurologic, endocrine, and behavioral changes are set in motion to achieve a new, higher hypothalamic temperature set point, which appears to have adaptive advantage to the organism. In contract, hyperthermia results when increased body temperature occurs following the breakdown of thermoregulatory homeostasis caused by an uncontrolled rise in heat production, failure of heat dissipation, extreme environmental heat, or, rarely, hypothalamic malfunction. Therefore, fever results from thermoregulation by the body, whereas hyperthermia is a failure of thermoregulation.

Environmental heat illness is caused by increased muscular activity in warm weather, particularly if volume deficiency limits heat dissipation (Table 62.1). Persons with poor conditioning and higher body mass index are at increased risk of exertional heat illness. Elderly patients risk heat stroke because of exposure and neurologic, vascular, or drug-induced predispositions.

Heat stroke, the most severe of environmental heat illnesses, is associated with increased intercellular adhesion molecule–1,

endothelin, and von Willebrand factor antigen, which mediate vascular changes. Mortality can be as high as 10%, even with vigorous treatment. Death occurs from shock, arrhythmia, cardiac ischemia, renal failure, and neurologic dysfunction. Poor prognostic indicators are core temperature higher than 42.2°C (108°F), aspartate aminotransferase level greater than 1,000 during the first 24 hours, and coma of more than 2 hours duration. Although core temperature alone is not prognostic, duration and intensity of hyperthermia are.

Nonexertional causes of dramatic hyperthermia are presented in Table 62.2

Neuroleptic malignant syndrome and familial malignant hyperthermia are discussed in Chapter 266.

TABLE 62.2.	NONEXERTIONAL CAUSES OF DRAMATIC HYPERTHERMIA

Thyrotoxicosis
Pheochromocytoma crisis
Cocaine and amphetamines
Anticholinergics
Alcohol withdrawal
Phencyclidine
Cyclic antidepressants
Monoamine oxidase inhibitors
Lithium
Lysergic acid diethylamide
Phencyclidine
Salicylate toxicity (children)
Serotonin syndrome (meperidine, dextromethorphan, sertraline, selegiline, clomipramine, fenfluramine, imipramine, lithium, phenylzine, amitriptyline, trazodone, and many others in patients taking monoamine oxidase inhibitors)
Hypothalamic injury (rare)

| TABLE 62.3. | FACTORS PREDISPOSING TO HYPOTHERMIA |

Starvation	Autonomic	Burns
Hypothalamic	dysfunction	Paralysis
injury	Sensory receptor	Paresis
Cord injury	dysfunction	Cachexia
Hypoglycemia	Alcohol ingestion	Extremes of age
Thiamine	Phenothiazines	Narcotics
deficiency	Sepsis	Hypopituitarism
Barbiturates	Erythroderma	Hepatic failure
Adrenal	Acute myocardial	
insufficiency	infarction	
Hypothyroidism	Uremia	

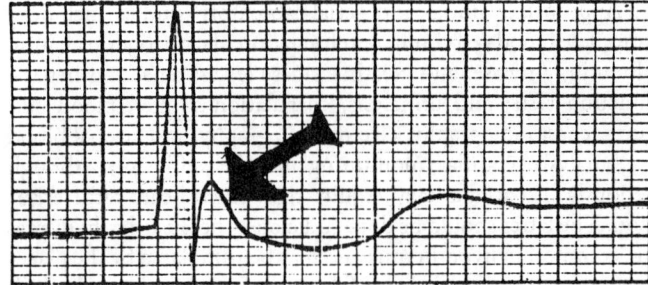

FIGURE 62.1. The camel hump sign, also called the Osborn wave or J wave (*arrow;* 81°F; lead V₅).

HYPOTHERMIA

Human hypothermia has been arbitrarily defined as a rectal temperature of less than 35°C (95°F). Although it occurs mainly in winter and in cold climates, it can happen in any season anywhere the environmental temperature is less than 35°C (95°F). Like hyperthermia, it is generated by exposure plus conditions that compromise thermoregulation (Table 62.3). The body's responses to hypothermia are outlined in Table 62.4.

Below 23.9°C (75°F), all responses are so affected by the cold that the patient loses heat as would a poikilotherm and the victim begins to approach a deathlike state. If a patient appears dead but has a history of hypothermic exposure, he or she should be warmed before being pronounced dead because patients with temperatures as low as 10°C (50°F) have survived.

Physical examination is difficult in a very cold patient. The temperature should be taken with a thermometer designed to read below the standard 34.4°C (94°F) lowest marking. The skin usually is cold, dry, and pale, but may show edema even in the face of intravascular volume depletion. Warm skin on a cold patient suggests that the hypothermia is caused by sepsis, skin disease, or vasodilator drugs. Respiratory compromise ranges from cold-induced bronchorrhea and aspiration pneumonia to noncardiogenic pulmonary edema. Blood gases, warmed by the laboratory to 37°C (98.6°F) as the measurements are made, may show hypoxemia, hypercarbia, and acidemia. Even

if the blood gases show significant hypoxemia, cold protects the patient by decreasing tissue oxygen requirements. Pulse oximeters may not be accurate in patients with hypothermia and vasoconstriction.

Cardiovascular volume is depleted in most patients with chronic hypothermia as a result of the early diuresis described and a later cold-induced renal tubular concentrating defect. Hemoconcentration plus circulatory slowing may lead to intravascular sludging and microvascular occlusion. This, plus myofibrillar enzyme leaks across the cold cell membranes of skeletal and cardiac muscle, can cause dramatic elevations of creatine kinase (including MB) and lactic dehydrogenase. Electrocardiographic changes in hypothermia include increases in the PR interval, QT prolongation, bradycardia, atrial fibrillation with slow ventricular response, nodal rhythm, asystole, and the classic (although not pathognomonic) camel hump sign of Osborn, also called the J wave, a little "hump" on the down slope of the QRS complex, seen at 32.2°C (90°F) and below (Fig. 62.1).

The abdomen may have rigid musculature and decreased bowel sounds. Gastrointestinal submucosal hemorrhage, if present, seldom is of major clinical significance. The amylase level may be increased, the platelet count decreased, and the prothrombin time prolonged. Hepatic and renal clearance of drugs, and their tissue effects, are unpredictable. Renal tubular glycosuria, myoglobinuria, and renal failure may occur.

Consciousness and reflexes are depressed and pupillary reflexes unreliable; the electroencephalogram may be flat below 20°C (68°F), and hypothermia is exclusionary of the diagnosis of brain death by electroencephalography.

Therapy for hypothermia is directed both to discovering and correcting the underlying cause of the hypothermia while rewarming the victim without causing harm. All patients, after blood samples for appropriate laboratory studies have been drawn, should receive 100 mg of thiamine, 50 g of glucose and naloxone (Narcan), 1 to 2 mg intravenously. Other drugs should not be used unless absolutely necessary, given their uncertain effects at the patient's depressed temperature. Because sepsis is hidden in hypothermia, blood cultures and empirical antibiotics may be needed. Stress level corticosteroids are unnecessary unless adrenal insufficiency is a serious possibility. Patients with temperatures less than 32.2°C (90°F) should be admitted to the intensive care unit.

| TABLE 62.4. | THE BODY'S RESPONSE TO COOLING |

Temperature (°C)	Response
37–31.7	Vasoconstriction, shivering, tachycardia, increased blood pressure, diuresis
31.7–23.9	Muscles stiffen, shivering decreases, blood pressure and pulse decrease
23.9 and below	Poikilothermic. Might appear dead.

Appropriate initial and serial laboratory studies include a complete blood cell count; determination of electrolyte, calcium, albumin, amylase, and creatine kinase levels; renal and hepatic function tests; and urinalysis, coagulation studies, blood cultures, chest radiography, electrocardiography, and arterial blood gas analysis. Cardiac monitoring may be sufficient, although seriously ill patients may require right-sided heart catheterization. The latter should be done judiciously because dysrhythmias are common in hypothermia and may be stimulated by the placement of an intracardiac line. Volume replacement should be with normal saline and with dextrose and water. Lactated Ringer's solution should not be used because the hypothermic liver may not be able to metabolize lactate to bicarbonate. The patient should be reassessed continually because physical examination and laboratory studies will change with rewarming.

The great debate in therapy revolves around rewarming therapy itself. Three major methods exist: external active rewarming, central active rewarming, and passive rewarming. External active rewarming includes immersing the patient in hot water or covering him or her with heating blankets. Although this rarely may be necessary in the profoundly cold, asystolic patient, it usually is not required and can be dangerous, leading to more profound hypothermia (the "afterdrop phenomenon"), cutaneous burns, or death. Central active rewarming involves either the use of warmed peritoneal or gastric lavage, which can be complicated by aspiration or infection, or the safer but more difficult to arrange use of warming hemodialysis or inhaled supplemental oxygen delivered as mist, keeping the inspired oxygen at 40°C (104°F) or less to prevent pulmonary burns. All intravenous fluids should be warmed to 37°C (98.6°F).

There is no proven benefit to more rapid rewarming. In all but the most severe cases, passive rewarming (correcting the underlying pathologic process if possible, removing the patient from the cold, and using warm—not hot—blankets) suffices, although airway warming at temperatures less than 32°C (89.6°F) and aggressive central active rewarming at temperatures less than 28°C (82.4°F) may be necessary, especially if the patient is in cardiac arrest.

BIBLIOGRAPHY

Bouchama A, Hammami MM, Haq A, et al. Evidence for endothelial cell activation/injury in heat stroke. *Crit Care Med* 1996;24:1173–1178.

Danzl DF, Dozos RS. Accidental hypothermia. *N Engl J Med* 1994;331: 1756–1760.

Dematte JE, O'Mara K, Buescher J, et al. Near fatal heat stroke during the 1995 heat wave in Chicago. *Ann Intern Med* 1998;129:173–181.

Garners JW, Kark JA, Karnei K, et al. Risk factors predicting exertional heat illness in male marine corps recruits. *Med Sci Sports Exerc* 1996; 28:939.

Mills KC. Serotonin syndrome. A clinical update. *Crit Care Clin* 1997;13: 763–783.

Saper CB, Breder CD. The neurologic basis of fever. *N Engl J Med* 1994; 330:1880–1886.

Simon HB. Hyperthermia. *N Engl J Med* 1993;329:483–487.

Tom PA, Garmel GM, Auerbach PA. Environment-dependent sports emergencies. *Med Clin North Am* 1994;78:305–325.

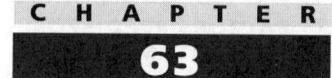

CHAPTER 63

IONIZING RADIATION INJURIES

BRAHM SHAPIRO

PRESENTATION

Accidental radiation injuries are rare and usually involve only a few individuals exposed in a laboratory or industrial accident. There is the extremely unlikely potential for large-scale exposure related to nuclear power and fuel processing. Nuclear war overwhelms meaningful medical response, but terrorism is a potential threat to be planned for.

Patients may have well-defined, acute, whole-body radiation syndromes (Table 63.1) or local radiation burns. Exposures might or might not be associated with radionuclide contamination. Lesser exposures, although causing no acute symptoms, may be carcinogenic and mutagenic. In most instances, radiation exposure is obvious to patient and physician, but rarely unsuspected irradiation can lead to bizarre local burns and myelosuppression.

PATHOPHYSIOLOGY

The ionizing radiations and units of measurement and effect are presented in Tables 63.2 and 63.3. Energy deposited by ionizing radiation results in formation of free radicals and reactive intermediaries, or in direct damage to DNA and other macromolecules. At high doses this leads to acute cell death and swelling. Lower doses cause mitotic arrest of stem cells in marrow, gonads, and gut epithelium. Lymphocytes are highly sensitive, and irradiation causes depletion in marrow, spleen, thymus, and blood. Inflammatory responses are deficient because of leukopenia. Microvascular injury leads to obliterative endarteritis, fibrosis, and atrophy. Delayed effects in survivors of acute injury or individuals with asymptomatic low-dose exposure may lead to carcinogenesis (acute lymphoblastic, myeloblastic, or chronic granulocytic leukemias, or solid tumors of breast, lung, salivary gland, gut, and lymph node) after latent intervals of 3 years to decades. Germ cell irradiation may lead to heritable mutagenesis. Estimated risks of low doses are extrapolated from high doses and depend on the model used. No threshold is assumed, although partial repair of radiation damage to DNA is possible. Effects of radiation exposure are influenced by volume of tissue exposed, dose rate, and modifying factors (e.g., hyperthermia, cytotoxic chemicals). Bone marrow, gut, and gonads are most sensitive, whereas muscle and connective tissue are resistant.

TABLE 63.1.	CHARACTERISTICS OF VARIOUS RADIATION EXPOSURE SYNDROMES

Clinical Syndrome	Absorbed Radiation Dose[a]	Prodrome[b]	Symptoms and Signs	Latent Interval	Prognosis[c]	Duration
Acute Whole-body Radiation Exposure Syndromes						
Asymptomatic	5–50 cGy	None	None (lymphopenia and cytogenetic effects detectable)	—	Complete recovery the rule	Nadir at 4–6 wk
	50–75 cGy	None	None (mild thrombocytopenia and neutropenia)	—	Complete recovery the rule	Recovery by 6–12 wk
	75–100 cGy	Minimal in 15%	Minimal prodrome in 15% (platelets fall to 50% and neutrophils to 75% of baseline)	—	Complete recovery the rule	Prodrome lasts several hours. Recovery by 6–12 weeks
Hematologic						
Mild	100–200 cGy	Mild in 15–25% Lasts <24 hr	Usually asymptomatic, leukopenia and thrombocytopenia	2–4 wk	Complete recovery the rule	Nadir of myelosuppression at 4–6 wk
Moderate	200–400 cGy	Onset with half hr to several hrs. Lasts 6–48 hr. Frequency and severity are dose-dependent	Petechiaae, hemorrhage, infection due to immunosuppression, fever, oropharyngeal lesions, herpes zoster or simplex	2–3 wk	About 50% lethal	Nadir of myelosuppression at 3–5 wk
Severe	400–600 cGy	Severe hemorrhagic phenomena, including fatal cerebral hemorrhage, overwhelming infections (pneumonia, sepsis)		1–2 wk	As dose rises, mortality rate approaches 90%	Nadir of myelosuppression at 2–3 wk. Recovery slow (many weeks) and may be incomplete
Gastrointestinal	600–2000 cGy	Onset in minutes to hrs, lasts from 4 to 48 hr.	Nausea, vomiting, diarrhea, gastrointestinal bleeding, dehydration, shock, hypoproteinemia, gram-negative sepsis	2–7 d	Fatal even if gastrointestinal lesions heal because bone marrow exposure is lethal	Fatal in 3–21 d
Central Nervous System/ Cardiovascular	>2,000 cGy	Onset in minutes, severe, blends with syndrome.	Nausea, vomiting, diarrhea, malaise, drowsiness, tremor, ataxia, convulsions, coma, oliguria, cardiovascular collapse	None, syndrome blends with prodrome	Rapidly and inevitably fatal	Fatal in 3–21 d
Localized Radiation Injuries						
Acute extremity burns (usually caused by handling sealed industrial radiography sources)	>200 cGy	—	No acute changes	2–4 wk	No permanent sequelae	Days to weeks
	200–300 cGy	Erythema, hyperesthesia, paresthesia followed by slowly evolving first-degree burn				

(continued)

TABLE 63.1. (CONTINUED)

Clinical Syndrome	Absorbed Radiation Dose[a]	Prodrome[b]	Symptoms and Signs	Latent Interval	Prognosis[c]	Duration
or	300–600 cGy	—	Erythema; partial epilation; desquamation	2–3 wk	Partial regrowth of hair, residual pigmentation	Days to weeks
Beta radiation burns (usually caused by external contamination by β-emitting radionuclides, i.e., scalp, ears, and shoulders from fallout or legs from walking in contaminated grass)	600–5,000 cGy	—	Erythema, complete epilation followed by slowly evolving second-degree burns.	2–3 wk	Permanent epilation, long-term fibrosis, skin atrophy, finger pulp atrophy, telangiectasia, dermatitis, dysplasia, squamous carcinoma may occur	Healing may take many weeks and long-term sequelae may be present
	>5,000 cGy	—	Injury similar to slowly evolving third-degree thermal burn	10–20 d	Slow healing, tissue loss, scar breakdown. Squamous carcinoma may occur	Healing may take many months. Permanent sequelae are common
Ocular radiation injuries	>200 cGy acute	—	Acute conjunctivitis and anterior uveitis	Occurs within hours	Visual impairment is ususlly progressive. Resolves in days to weeks	May be followed by cataract
	200 cGy cumulative dose	—	Posterior subcapular cataract	Months to many years	Effect on vision varies with severity of cataract, may lead to total blindness	May be cured by surgery. Visual impairment is usually progressive
Reproductive System Effects						
Impaired testicular function	15 cGyt	—	Threshold for transient oligospermia	~6 wk	*Recovery is the rule*	Months
	15–500 cGy	—	Dose-dependent oligospermia/ azoospermia	~6 wk	Recovery possible	Months to 2 yr
	>500 cGy	—	Permanent azoospermia	~6 wk	Permanent azoospermia	Permanent

TABLE 63.1. (CONTINUED)

Clinical Syndrome	Absorbed Radiation Dose[a]	Prodrome[b]	Symptoms and Signs	Latent Interval	Prognosis[c]	Duration
Impaired ovarian function	<100 cGy	—	Usually asymptomatic		Recovery is the rule	—
	100–400 cGy	—	Transient amenorrhea	1–2 mo	Recovery usually occurs within a few to many months	Months to 2 yr
	>400 cGy	—	Permanent amenorrhea and menopausal symptoms	1 mo	Permanent hypogonadism with infertility and hormone deficiency	Permanent
Prenatal intrauterine exposure						
Conception to 2 weeks gestation	Dose-dependent below 10 cGy insufficient risk to terminate pregnancy	Most injuries incompatible with life & fetal loss occurs	Fetal loss may occur before pregnancy evident	—	No effective primary treatment	Permanent
2–6 weeks gestation	''	Major abnormalities of organogenesis (eg, brain, heart, gut, eye).	Evident at prenatal ultrasound or a birth	—	No effective primary treatment	Permanent
6 weeks gestation to term	''	Major malformations rare except for microcephaly & growth retardation.	Evident at prenatal ultrasound, at or after birth to 3 yr	—	No effective primary treatment	Permanent
12 weeks gestation to term	Intrauterine radioiodine	Subsequent bone tumors and leukemogenesis	Years		As for non-radiation-induced disorders	Life-long risk
		Hypothyroidism	Postnatal		Treatable by thyroxine	Life-long deficiencies

[a] Doses given as single acute administrations (fractionation or protraction of dose results in less severe effects).
[b] Prodrome characterized by drowsiness, malaise, fatigue, anorexia, nausea, and vomiting applies to whole-body exposure.
[c] Delayed leukemogenesis may occur 3–10 years or carcinogenesis 10–50 years after recovery from acute exposure (risk low relative to background natural rate).

TABLE 63.2.	CLASSIFICATION OF TYPES OF IONIZING RADIATION	
Radiation Type		**Quality Factor**[a]
High-energy electromagnetic radiation		
γ-Rays (of nuclear origin)		1
x-Rays (of electron origin)		1
Charged particles		
β-Rays		1
Auger and conversion electrons		5
α-Rays		20
Protons		10
Mesons		20
Uncharged particles		
Neurons		20

[a] Quality factor takes into account dose rate, relative biologic effectiveness, and other factors to convert absorbed-radiation dose to dose equivalent. (See Table 63.3)

HISTORY AND PHYSICAL EXAMINATION

Special attention must be paid to the exact nature, timing, and circumstances of exposure, whether radionuclide contamination was possible, and whether radiation dosimeters were worn. Whole-body exposure syndromes evolve through four phases, the duration being inversely related to the dose. A prodrome is followed by a latent interval, the characteristic syndrome, and, if this is survived, recovery. Except for patients with the central nervous system syndrome, most patients with whole-body exposure are seen in the prodromal phase. Subsequent symptoms and signs depend on dose (Table 63.1). Local radiation burns in the early phase manifest only mild paresthesia, pain, and erythema, but over time may evolve to extensive tissue injury and loss. Associated nonradiation injuries also should be noted.

LABORATORY STUDIES AND DIAGNOSTIC TESTS

Appropriate radiation detectors are used to monitor for external and internal radionuclide contamination and to identify the radionuclides. Measurements are also made on the blood, urine, feces, and sputum, or on swabs from the nose, ears, and wounds. Neutron exposure can be deduced from the presence of sodium 24 in blood and from activation of metal objects on the patient. These measurements and those from dosimeters (if worn) are used to calculate absorbed radiation dose. Chromosomal analysis of lymphocytes might also provide estimates of the radiation dose. Serial blood cell counts document initial lymphopenia, which predicts subsequent course, and development of myelosuppression with a nadir at 4 to 6 weeks. Marrow biopsy demonstrates aplasia or hypoplasia. Major electrolyte, fluid, and acid–base disturbances follow loss of gastrointestinal epithelium. Cellular damage may result in the elevation of serum transaminase, lactic dehydrogenase, and uric acid levels. Cultures of blood, urine, and sputum identify infections in these immunocompromised patients. Radiography, arteriography, and three-phase bone scans may be used to evaluate viability of irradiated extremities.

TABLE 63.3.	CLASSIFICATION OF UNITS OF MEASURE FOR IONIZING RADIATION		
Definition	**Traditional Unit**	**Modern SI Unit**	
Absorbed radiation dose: energy deposition per unit volume of tissue	1 rad (100 ergs/g)	= 1 centigray (cGy)	
	100 rad	= 1 gray (Gy)	= J kg^{-1}
Dose equivalent: the biologic effect of a given absorbed radiation dose	rem (radiation equivalent man)	= 1 centisievert (cSv)	
	100 rem	= 1 sievert (Sv)	= J kg^{-1}
Activity: Amount of radioactivity, number of disintegrations per time		becquerel (Bq)	= s^{-1}
	1 curie (Ci)	= 3.7 × 10^{10} Bq	
Exposure: Degree of ionization of air by low energy γ- and x-rays	Roentgen (R)	= 0.000258 coulomb/kg	
LET: Density of ionization and energy deposition per unit path length	Ion pairs/μm	= J m^{-1}	
RBE: Relative effectiveness of a given radiation in producing a given effect compared with a reference radiation (250–400 keV x-rays); RBE is proportional to LET	Ratio or percentage	Ratio or percentage	
Quality factor (Q): Takes into account dose rate, RBE, and other factors to convert absorbed radiation dose to dose equivalent	rad × Q = rem	gray × Q = sievert	

LET, linear energy transfer; RBE, relative biologic effectiveness.

DIFFERENTIAL DIAGNOSIS

Radiation exposure usually is well documented, and there is no differential diagnosis. Rarely, persons exposed to lost industrial radiation sources present with bizarre burnlike lesions or myelosuppression. Failure to consider radiation exposure may result in ongoing exposure.

STRATEGIES FOR OPTIMAL CARE

There is no substitute for prevention. Exposure is minimized by maintaining distance, shielding, and minimizing exposure time. Because radiation accidents are rare and potentially disastrous, detailed and rehearsed response plans by teams, including emergency and nuclear medicine physicians, hematologists, and health physicists, are required. Mass casualties will require triage.

MANAGEMENT

After first aid, patients should be evacuated, with care taken not to spread potential contamination. Hemorrhage, shock, and the airway should be managed in the usual fashion.

External contamination is best managed with soap or nonionic detergent and water. Care should be taken not to abrade skin and cause internal contamination. Contaminated wounds should be irrigated and, if necessary, widely debrided. Contamination of nasopharynx, ears, eyes, and mouth is removed by lavage. Lower respiratory tract contamination resists therapy, but expectorants and bronchoalveolar lavage can be attempted. Ingested contamination can be minimized by reducing absorption (e.g., vomiting, gastric lavage, activated charcoal) or by binding to specific agents (e.g., Prussian blue for cesium, thallium, and rubidium; barium sulfate, alginates, and alumina-containing antacids for strontium and radium; and phytates for calcium, magnesium, zinc, or iron). Once radionuclides are absorbed, isotopic dilution may reduce risk of incorporation. Stable iodide, 300 mg potassium iodide or sodium iodide, administered early reduces thyroid radioiodine uptake (once incorporated into thyroid hormones, this is useless). Radioactive strontium, calcium, phosphate, zinc, and iron can be similarly diluted. Turnover can be accelerated by water diuresis for tritium and by diuretics for radioactive sodium and potassium. Parathyroid hormone may mobilize radioactive strontium, calcium, or phosphate from bone. Chelation enhances renal excretion of radiometals (e.g., calcium or zinc ethylenediaminetetraacetic acid for transuranic and rare earth elements; desferrioxamine for plutonium and iron; penicillamine for copper and cobalt; and dimercaprol for mercury, lead, arsenic, bismuth, chromium, and nickel).

The prodrome of acute whole-body exposure is self-limiting but may require antiemetics and anxiolytics. The central nervous system syndrome is inevitably fatal and only symptomatic management is warranted. In the gastrointestinal syndrome, intravenous fluids, plasma, blood fractions, and broad-spectrum antibiotics benefit some patients. The hematologic syndrome can be self-limiting, and supportive therapy may permit survival until marrow regeneration occurs. This requires reverse isolation, asepsis, and broad-spectrum antibacterial and antifungal therapy with granulocyte levels of less than 800 per L. Activation of latent viral infections necessitates antiviral therapy. Platelet and red blood cell transfusions correct thrombocytopenia and anemia. Recombinant granulocyte colony-stimulating factor may speed recovery. Marrow transplantation also may have a role.

Pain of local injuries is often severe, necessitating narcotics. Local management is similar to that of thermal burns: debridement of nonviable tissue, administration of local and systemic antibiotics, and skin grafting. Severe extremity injuries may require amputation. Healing is slow, and late breakdown of healed lesions is common.

Survivors of acute exposure require education and surveillance for late effects. Management of radiation-induced leukemias and tumors does not differ from that of spontaneous disorders. Visual impairment necessitates cataract removal.

COMPLICATIONS AND PITFALLS

It must be established that a radiation exposure has occurred, as many apparent accidents are false alarms. It is important to allay anxiety associated with radiation exposure; all but the most severely exposed recover completely. Skin decontamination should be gentle to prevent injury and conversion of external to internal contamination. Except for iodides, drugs to reduce incorporation or hasten excretion of radionuclides may cause side effects, and their use should be weighed carefully.

HOSPITALIZATION

Except for trivial exposures and contamination, patients should be hospitalized until radiation exposure has been estimated or the nature of injury is apparent. All patients with hematologic, gastrointestinal, or central nervous system acute exposure syndromes and those requiring chelation therapy, repeated extensive external decontamination, or management of significant local radiation injuries require hospitalization. Major whole-body exposures might be best managed on a hematology or bone marrow transplant service and local injuries in a burn unit.

REFERRAL

Seriously exposures are best treated at institutions with experienced nuclear physicians, hematologists, and facilities for the isolation and treatment of severe hematopoietic suppression. Assistance is available through the Radiation Emergency Assistance Center/Training Sites (REAC/TS) of the Medical and Health Science Division of Oak Ridge Associated Universities (423-481-1000, ext. 1502).

COST EFFECTIVENESS

All hospitals are required to have written radiation accident response plans. Although rarely activated, failure to prepare may lead to dire consequences.

BIBLIOGRAPHY

Mettler FA, Kelsey CA, Ricks RC, eds. *Medical management of radiation accidents.* Boca Raton, FL: CRC Press, 1990:1–405.

Vyas DR, Dick RM, Crawford J. Management of radiation accidents and exposures. *Pediatr Emerg Care* 1994;10:232–237.

Nagataki S, Ashizawa K, Yamashita S. Cause of childhood thyroid cancer after the Chernobyl accident. *Thyroid* 1998;8:115–117.

Pacini F, Vorontsava T, Domidchik EP, et al. Post-Chernobyl thyroid carcinoma in Belarus children and adolescents: comparison with naturally occurring thyroid carcinoma in Italy and France. *J Clin Endocrinol Metab* 1997;82:3563–3569.

Kelley's Textbook of Internal Medicine, fourth edition. Edited by H. David Humes. Lippincott Williams & Wilkins, Philadelphia © 2000.

2

CARDIOLOGY

Elizabeth G. Nabel, Editor

APPROACH TO THE PATIENT WITH CARDIOVASCULAR DISORDERS

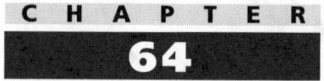

C H A P T E R

64

ESSENTIAL FEATURES OF THE CARDIAC HISTORY AND PHYSICAL EXAMINATION

ELIZABETH G. NABEL

The cardiovascular evaluation consists of the history, the physical examination, and selected laboratory studies. In some situations, the correct diagnosis is based on information from only one of these components. More commonly, it results from the careful integration of information from several or all parts of the evaluation process.

The availability and role of laboratory studies have grown at an impressive rate. Although these specialized studies provide valuable diagnostic information, they do not diminish the central role of the bedside evaluation of patients with suspected cardiovascular disease. The selection of laboratory studies requires a carefully defined differential diagnosis gleaned from the history and physical examination. An accurate and complete clinical assessment allows the physician to more readily detect changes as the patient's course is followed over time (Table 64.1).

TABLE 64.1.	IMPORTANT SYMPTOMS AND SIGNS OF CARDIAC DISEASE	
Symptoms		**Signs**
Dyspnea		Peripheral edema
Fatigue		Pulmonary rales
Chest pain		Heart murmur
Palpitations		Gallop rhythm
Syncope		Irregular pulse

CARDIOVASCULAR HISTORY

Information from the medical history often provides the first clue in the recognition of specific cardiovascular disorders. In some cases, the initial diagnosis is based solely on the history. Many patients with angina pectoris, for example, have entirely normal physical examinations and resting electrocardiograms between episodes of discomfort. Beyond its role in diagnosis, the medical history is central in the determination of the patient's functional capacity or the degree to which the disorder limits his or her activities and lifestyle. This assessment is often used when considering medical, interventional, and/or surgical therapy. When the functional aspect is not concordant with the physical findings and laboratory results, it raises the suspicion that other factors, such as anxiety, depression, or other medical illness, might be contributing to the patient's limitation. Special attention to patients with chronic slowly progressive heart disease is also required because symptoms can develop so insidiously that the patients slowly adjust their lifestyles without recognizing the true extent of disability. It is often helpful to have such patients describe their activities during a typical day.

Through the history, the physician can learn about concurrent disorders or habits, such as diabetes mellitus or cigarette smoking, that can affect cardiovascular function or place it at risk. Careful attention to the patient's medications is similarly important because of their pharmacologic and toxic actions. Several cardiovascular disorders have a heritable tendency, amplifying the importance of a careful family history. This includes inquiry about premature or sudden death.

The major symptoms associated with cardiovascular disease are dyspnea, fatigue, chest pain, palpitations, and syncope. These symptoms are not confined to cardiovascular disorders, and even when they occur in patients with known heart disease, the physician must be alert to possible extracardiac influences.

DYSPNEA

Pulmonary congestion secondary to left ventricular failure or mitral stenosis typically results in dyspnea that is worsened by exertion. Dyspnea is also worsened by the recumbent position (i.e., orthopnea) because the added venous return from the no longer dependent lower extremities contributes to an already engorged pulmonary vascular bed. At times, congestion leads to a nonproductive cough. Patients may awaken after several hours of sleep because of acute respiratory distress (paroxysmal nocturnal dyspnea) that forces them to sit or stand and to seek "fresh air." Wheezing may accompany the dyspnea. Paroxysmal nocturnal dyspnea results from interstitial pulmonary edema. It is more intense and alarming to the patient than is orthopnea, and a longer time is required before the dyspnea improves.

Dyspnea of effort can result from several other causes, including chronic pulmonary disease, poor physical conditioning, and obesity. Differentiating cardiac from pulmonary dyspnea can be particularly difficult. Chronic lung disease can also lead to orthopnea. Anxiety-related dyspnea is usually less predictable than cardiac dyspnea, is often reported as an inability to take a full or deep breath, and is commonly accompanied by other signs of anxiety or by sighing.

Acute pulmonary edema, whether occurring as an initial feature or as a culmination of progressive cardiac failure, is the most severe and dramatic cause of dyspnea in patients with heart disease. The severe breathlessness is typically acute in onset and may be accompanied by cough, at times producing frothy and even blood-tinged sputum. Other causes to be considered in patients with acute, severe dyspnea include pulmonary embolus, pneumonia, and pneumothorax.

FATIGUE

When excessive fatigue results from cardiovascular disease, it is presumed to be a manifestation of inadequate cardiac output and as such is typically related to effort. In evaluating a patient with fatigue, the physician must understand the nature of the fatigue and the intensity of activities that elicit it, and the pattern of development. Fatigue is reported by patients with a wide variety of extracardiac disorders, including anxiety and depression. The use of certain medications can elicit or exacerbate fatigue; examples include excessive diuretic treatment and inordinate lowering of heart rate and blood pressure by antihypertensive or antianginal drugs.

EDEMA

Edema, typically of the lower extremities, is a common complaint of patients with heart failure. Pitting ankle and lower leg edema characteristically involves both lower extremities, increases in magnitude during the day, and decreases overnight because of the enhanced venous return from the legs after assumption of the recumbent position. If the patient is bedridden, edema may be confined to the presacral area. If the elevation of venous pressure is marked and prolonged, fluid accumulates in the liver and abdominal cavity (ascites), prompting the patient to experience an aching or "heavy" discomfort in the right upper quadrant or abdominal distention. Edema can also result when central venous return to the heart is impeded, as in constrictive pericarditis.

Edema occurs in patients with a variety of extracardiac disorders, including local venous insufficiency, lymphatic blockage, and chronic liver or kidney disease. The location of the edema sometimes provides information about its underlying cause. For example, the edema associated with the nephrotic syndrome is often prominent about the face and eyes. Edema limited to the face, neck, and upper arms can result from obstruction of the superior vena cava (e.g., by carcinoma of the lung). Edema confined to one lower extremity is likely to be the result of a local problem (e.g., venous obstruction or inflammation).

CHEST PAIN

Chest pain can be the result of cardiac, vascular, respiratory, musculoskeletal, or gastrointestinal disorders. It can also accompany anxiety. Patients with angina pectoris typically describe pressure-like heaviness or tightness. Many insist that it is not a true pain but rather an uncomfortable sensation. It is characteristically substernal in location and is diffuse rather than focal. Radiation of the discomfort to the left shoulder and arm is common, and it can radiate to the base of the neck and jaw and, less commonly, to the back.

Angina pectoris is typically brought on by physical exertion or emotional stress, lasts a matter of minutes, and is relieved by rest or promptly alleviated by sublingual nitroglycerin. Most patients can describe activities that predictably elicit angina, and some variability in activity tolerance is common. Some patients, for example, report that exertion carried out early in the morning is more likely to precipitate discomfort. Physical activity in cold weather or after meals might also be more likely to provoke angina pectoris. Unfortunately, angina is atypical in one or more of its characteristics in some patients, making its presence more difficult to establish clearly by history. Some patients describe it as sharp or burning. In others, discomfort may be confined to the arms or neck. Some patients experience dyspnea rather than chest discomfort during myocardial ischemia. This angina-equivalent dyspnea resembles angina pectoris in other respects (e.g., duration, relation to stress) and carries the same significance.

Variant angina, also called Prinzmetal's angina, is similar in character to stress-induced angina pectoris but is characteristically unpredictable and nonexertional—features consistent with its cause of coronary artery spasm. Variant angina may occur in the early morning hours, and some patients also report other vasomotor-related symptoms such as migraine headaches or Raynaud's phenomenon.

Angina pectoris that has recently become more frequent or severe or has progressed to occur at rest is considered unstable angina pectoris. Unstable angina also includes angina of recent onset, particularly if it occurs with low levels of activity or at rest. The pain of acute myocardial infarction is characteristically more intense than angina pectoris, lasts longer (30 minutes), radiates more widely, and is not relieved by sublingual nitroglycerin. Nausea and diaphoresis frequently accompany the discomfort. Nonetheless, the intensity of symptoms does vary in patients with acute myocardial infarction, and the physician must remember that as many as 20% of patients with heart attack do not seek medical attention because the symptoms are atypical or mild, or because there are no symptoms. Silent and atypical infarctions appear to be more common in patients with diabetes mellitus and in the elderly.

Although angina pectoris is usually the result of obstructive coronary artery disease, similar discomfort can occur in patients with aortic stenosis, hypertrophic cardiomyopathy, or pulmonary arterial hypertension. One proposed mechanism is ischemia due to the excessive work of the hypertrophied, overloaded ventricle. In patients with pulmonary arterial hypertension, distention of the pulmonary artery may contribute to the discomfort. Acute dissection of the thoracic aorta typically results in excruciating pain that is abrupt in onset and that attains peak intensity almost immediately. Although the distribution of the pain can be similar to that of myocardial pain, the pain of dissection more frequently radiates to the back. A history of hypertension is commonly present. The chest pain from acute pericarditis is sharp and parasternal or precordial. The pain may be referred to the shoulder and ridge of the trapezius muscle. It is aggravated by breathing or twisting of the torso. Patients often report that the pain is diminished by sitting up and leaning forward.

Gastrointestinal disorders such as gastroesophageal reflux, esophageal motor abnormality, and peptic ulcer disease are common causes of substernal and epigastric discomfort. An important part of the evaluation of chest pain is the identification of its relation to food intake, recumbent position, and, at times, the response to antacids. Chest wall injury or inflammation can cause chest pain, but it is typically more focal, often superficial, and may be elicited by local movement and accompanied by chest tenderness. Psychogenic or anxiety-related chest discomfort can have various characteristics. Frequently, it is localized to the cardiac apex, where it may be described as a constant ache lasting for hours or as a brief, sharp, stabbing inframammary pain. This discomfort is not predictably related to exertion. It may be accompanied by other manifestations of anxiety, such as hyperventilation.

PALPITATIONS AND SYNCOPE

Palpitation denotes an awareness of the heartbeat and can be the result of alterations in heart rate, rhythm, or force of contraction. Patients vary remarkably in the degree to which they have symptoms related to such alterations. Some are aware of every premature beat, whereas others are unaware of grossly irregular or potentially serious dysrhythmias. In evaluating a patient with palpitations, it is important to know the type of irregularity he or she experiences, what precipitates it, and whether there are associated symptoms.

Commonly, patients describe a skipped heart beat, which results from the pause and subsequent forceful systole after a premature contraction. Premature heartbeats are occasionally accompanied by a fleeting sharp pain at the cardiac apex. Paroxysms of rapid dysrhythmias are sometimes felt as a beating in the throat or a fluttering in the chest. Dysrhythmias that are sufficiently rapid or slow can interfere with cardiac output and cerebral perfusion, leading to weakness, lightheadedness, or syncope. In patients with coronary artery disease, rapid dysrhythmias can precipitate angina pectoris.

The circumstances associated with palpitations are important. Do they occur after meals or after the drinking of caffeine-containing beverages, with exertion or position change, or during periods of emotional stress? Equally important is the manner of onset and termination of the palpitations. Paroxysmal supraven-

tricular tachycardia, for example, is characteristically abrupt in onset and termination, but sinus tachycardia accompanying anxiety resolves slowly. It can be helpful to have the patient tap out his or her palpitations to assess their rate and regularity.

Dysrhythmias can cause syncope because of excessively slow or rapid heart rates. Syncope resulting from bradycardia secondary to atrioventricular heart block (Stokes–Adams attack) is characteristically abrupt and can occur in any position. Consciousness is usually regained promptly. Syncope caused by rapid dysrhythmias can also be abrupt or can follow a graying-out period of seconds to minutes. The patient may describe palpitations before loss of consciousness, but the absence of palpitations does not exclude a dysrhythmia as the cause of the syncope. In some patients (usually elderly), marked bradycardia with syncope can follow stimulation of a hypersensitive carotid sinus. The stimulation may result from activities such as turning the head abruptly, shaving, or buttoning a tight collar. Aortic stenosis and hypertrophic cardiomyopathy can also cause syncope, typically with or after exertion.

The most common cause of syncope is a vasovagal episode—the common faint. Such episodes usually follow a strong emotional stimulus, such as severe pain or the sight of blood. Orthostatic hypotension is an important cause of syncope, particularly in patients receiving diuretic drugs and in patients with autonomic and peripheral nervous system dysfunction (e.g., from diabetes mellitus). The investigation of syncope should always include inquiry about its relation to position change. Seizure is a potential cause of loss of consciousness in some patients. Information from witnesses with regard to tonic-clonic movements and from the patient about aura, urinary incontinence, and tongue trauma can aid in its recognition.

PHYSICAL EXAMINATION

The cardiac examination is not performed in isolation; it is part of the systematic and complete evaluation of the patient. Extracardiac findings commonly provide key information that points to a specific cardiac diagnosis.

Noncardiac disorders can contribute to or worsen the manifestations of heart disease. To provide optimal treatment, it is essential that these disorders be identified.

The physical examination of a patient with heart disease begins while the patient is providing the medical history. During this time, the physician is listening to and observing the patient.

The examination need not be limited to the resting state. Important information can be obtained in some patients, for example, by evaluation during the Valsalva maneuver after position change or after exercise.

GENERAL INSPECTION

Beyond assessment of the general medical condition, inspection of the patient from head to foot can provide clues to the presence of heritable or acquired systemic disorders that place the patient at risk for specific cardiovascular abnormalities. For example, tall stature, long fingers, and an arm span greater than the patient's height suggests Marfan's syndrome, which can be associated with aortic aneurysm, aortic valve regurgitation, and mitral valve prolapse. Even in the absence of the full features of Marfan's syndrome, a tall, thin stature or sternal abnormalities such as pectus excavatum can be associated with mitral valve prolapse. Recognition of the characteristic appearance of Down's syndrome or Turner's syndrome alerts the physician to possible associated cardiovascular anomalies, such as endocardial cushion defect or coarctation of the aorta, respectively.

The skin, mucous membranes, and nail beds often contain important clues to the diagnosis of cardiovascular disorders. Xanthomas may indicate lipid abnormalities. Thick, taut skin of the face and extremities can result from scleroderma, a condition in which cardiovascular complications can be severe and even life threatening. Cyanosis is most evident in the nail beds and mucous membranes, and its distribution may provide information about its mechanism of development. Central cyanosis due to intracardiac or intrapulmonary shunting of blood may affect the extremities and the oral mucosae. Peripheral cyanosis, which results from localized oxygen desaturation of slowly moving capillary blood (e.g., after cold exposure with peripheral vasospasm), is limited to exposed or distal areas, such as the fingers, toes, and ear lobes. Chronic conditions leading to central cyanosis can result in clubbing of the fingers and toes. Endocarditis and chronic liver disease can also be accompanied by clubbing of the fingers, and clubbing occasionally occurs as an isolated heritable trait.

In patients with infective endocarditis, embolic or immunologic mechanisms can lead to several skin and mucous membrane findings. These include conjunctival petechia and splinter hemorrhage of the nail beds.

BLOOD PRESSURE AND PULSE EVALUATION

Information from the vital signs, particularly the blood pressure and pulse determination, contributes to an assessment of the patient's overall hemodynamic status and in many cases also suggests specific underlying cardiovascular abnormalities.

Arterial Pressure

The accurate determination of blood pressure requires a properly placed sphygmomanometer of appropriate size for the patient (see Chapter 30). The patient must be comfortable and without anxiety during the determination to avoid spurious elevations of the blood pressure. Blood pressure should be measured in the recumbent and standing positions to detect orthostatic hypotension and, during the initial examination, in the left and right arms to recognize certain vascular anomalies, such as some types of aortic coarctation or dissection. If hypertension is suspected, blood pressure should also be measured in the leg.

Attention should be paid to the effects of respiration on the blood pressure. A decline in systolic blood pressure greater than 10 mm Hg during inspiration is called pulsus paradoxus, which is a misnomer because it is not paradoxical but rather an exaggeration of the normally small decline in the pressure during inspiration. Pulsus paradoxus is a cardinal sign of cardiac tamponade, and its detection can lead to identification of a potentially life-threatening situation. However, a paradoxical pulse is not specific for tamponade. Pulmonary insufficiency can result in an exaggerated decrease in blood pressure during inspiration.

Proper analysis of the blood pressure is not limited to isolated consideration of the systolic or diastolic values. The relation of the two, called the *pulse pressure,* is also important. A narrow (reduced) pulse pressure, for example, is commonly present in patients with advanced cardiac failure and in many patients with severe aortic stenosis. In these cases, the systolic pressure is typically limited by the small stroke volume, and the diastolic pressure is increased because of a compensatory rise in systemic vascular resistance. Conversely, situations in which there is a large stroke volume or an abnormal run-off channel from the systemic arterial system lead to a widened (increased) pulse pressure. Examples include aortic regurgitation and large arteriovenous fistula. Fever and bradycardia can also lead to some increase in the pulse pressure.

Pulse Examination

The pulse examination usually begins with palpation of the radial artery to assess heart rate and regularity. Increased heart rate can be an important early sign of a cardiac disorder (e.g., heart failure, pericarditis) as well as a physiologic response to extracardiac factors (e.g., anxiety, hypovolemia, hyperthyroidism). The detection of an unexplained or persistent tachycardia, even when sinus in origin, should always elicit a careful search for its underlying cause. Disorders of pulse rhythm should be characterized by the pattern of their irregularity. The irregularity may occur at regular or repetitive intervals, as in a bigeminal pulse secondary to coupled extrasystoles. In other cases, the irregularity is erratic. Although an electrocardiogram (ECG) is usually required to identify specific dysrhythmias, the pulse rhythm sometimes provides important diagnostic information, particularly when coupled with other physical findings. For example, an "irregularly irregular" radial pulse rate combined with an apical heart rate, as determined by auscultation, that exceeds the radial pulse rate *(pulse deficit)* suggests atrial fibrillation. A rapid, regular pulse rate along with intermittent cannon waves in the jugular venous pulse suggests ventricular tachycardia or, less commonly, junctional tachycardia. In some patients with advanced left ventricular dysfunction, the pulse rate is regular, but the amplitude of every other heart beat is reduced—a phenomenon called pulsus alternans.

The pulse examination includes sequential palpation of the carotid arterial pulses, which is taken as a reflection of the central arterial pulse from left ventricular ejection, and of the major palpable peripheral arteries to detect signs of local vascular disease or certain congenital anomalies (e.g., radial–femoral artery pulse lag due to coarctation). The extent to which the arterial system is surveyed depends in part on the age of the patient and the clinical situation. In adults, the carotid, radial, and femoral arteries and the abdominal aorta are routinely evaluated. In older persons, the popliteal, dorsalis pedis, and posterior tibial vessels are also carefully examined.

The carotid arteries are the primary sites for pulse contour analysis (Fig. 64.1). The artery examination includes assessment of the pulse upstroke, its amplitude, and its duration. All three of these parameters are typically (but not invariably) altered, for

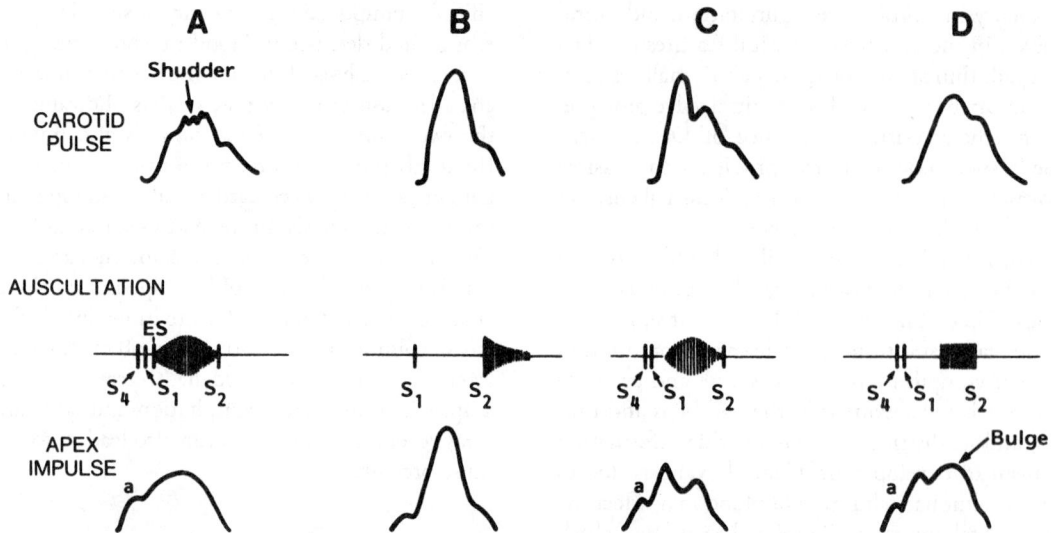

FIGURE 64.1. Examples of carotid pulse, auscultation, and apex impulse findings with aortic stenosis **(A)**, aortic regurgitation **(B)**, hypertrophic cardiomyopathy **(C)**, and myocardial infarction **(D)**. Example D includes mitral regurgitation murmur due to papillary muscle dysfunction and palpable precordial bulge. Apex impulses in A, C, and D also include palpable correlate of the fourth heart sound (a). ES, ejection sound.

example, in patients with severe aortic stenosis. The resultant slow-rising, low-amplitude, and prolonged pulse is called pulsus parvus et tardus. In some patients with severe aortic stenosis, palpation of the carotid artery reveals coarse systolic vibrations or a "shuddering" sensation. The pulse amplitude can be reduced by any disorder that leads to small stroke volume (e.g., advanced cardiac failure). Attention to the upstroke of a low-amplitude pulse can help differentiate primary reduction in stroke volume from that caused by aortic stenosis. Conversely, the carotid pulse is brisk and bounding when significant aortic regurgitation is present. Some patients with aortic regurgitation have a double pulse, in which two discrete systolic peaks can be palpated. Hypertrophic cardiomyopathy with obstruction also can cause a *bisferious pulse.*

The carotid pulse can be altered by local vascular disease, which commonly leads to asymmetry of the pulse amplitudes. Palpation of the carotid vessels must be done with particular caution when local obstructive disease is suspected or when the clinical history suggests the possibility of a hypersensitive carotid sinus. After assessment of the carotid vessels, the other major arteries should be palpated. This is followed by auscultation over the carotid arteries, abdominal aorta, femoral vessels, and other sites where local vascular disease is suspected. The auscultation is performed to detect bruits due to blood flow turbulence that can result from obstructive arterial disease. The intensity of a bruit is also influenced by cardiac output and collateral flow; if an obstruction is very advanced, blood flow may be insufficient to generate audible sound. The duration of the bruit (e.g., extending into diastole) may be more reliably related to the presence of a high-grade obstruction. In patients with hypertension, auscultation in the epigastric area is particularly important because a bruit can indicate renal artery stenosis as a cause for the elevated blood pressure.

Venous Pulse Examination

The jugular venous system is evaluated for its pressure level and wave contour. The former permits an estimation of right-sided cardiac filling pressure, and the latter provides information about the mechanics of right ventricular filling, tricuspid valve function, and the temporal relation of atrial and ventricular systole. For analysis of the jugular venous system, the patient is placed in the position in which the venous blood level and undulations are most visible. Patients with highly elevated jugular venous pressure may have to sit upright. Conversely, persons with low jugular pressure often must be placed fully supine before the individual waves can be identified.

The internal jugular vein is preferred for venous pulse analysis because it is closer and courses in a more direct manner to empty into the right atrium and because it does not have venous valves. Its pressure level and wave contour generally reflect comparable values and events in the right atrium. Pulsations from the external jugular vein are easier to detect but are also more likely to be influenced by the vein's tortuous course and venous valves.

The jugular venous pressure is estimated by measuring the height of the filled jugular vein relative to a reference point, commonly the sternal angle. With normal jugular venous pressure, the top of the column of blood is less than 3 cm above the sternal angle. Elevated pressures can result from right-sided cardiac failure and from conditions that mechanically restrict filling or emptying of the right atrium, such as cardiac tamponade or tricuspid stenosis, respectively. In patients with borderline jugular pressure levels and cardiac failure or tricuspid regurgitation, the application of pressure to the right upper quadrant or periumbilical area may lead to a sustained increase in the jugular pressure level during the maneuver, a response known as *hepato-jugular reflux.*

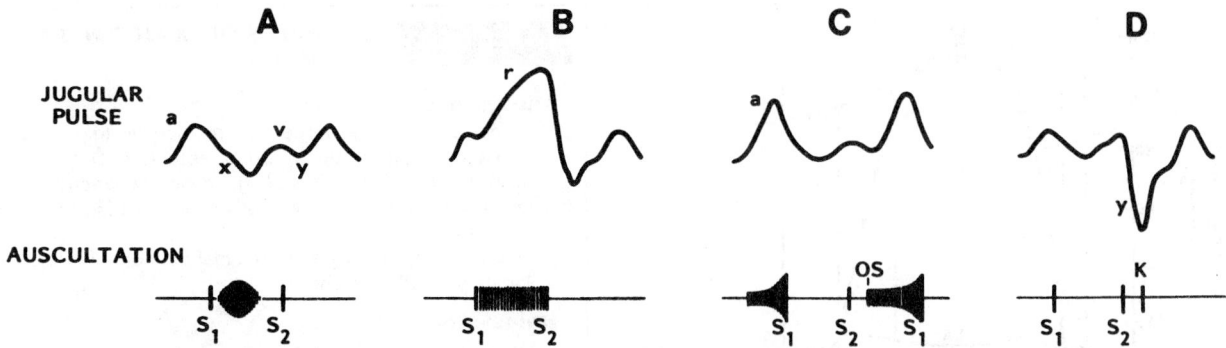

FIGURE 64.2. Examples of jugular pulse and auscultation findings. **(A)** A normal jugular tracing in a patient who has a functional heart murmur. The other tracings are in patients with **(B)** tricuspid regurgitation, **(C)** mitral stenosis with pulmonary hypertension, and **(D)** constrictive pericarditis. r, regurgitant wave; OS, opening snap of mitral valve; K, pericardial knock.

In patients with heart or lung disease, the right-sided filling pressure cannot be taken as an indirect sign of left ventricular filling pressure. The pressure–volume correlations of the two ventricles can be altered to different degrees in individual patients with cardiac disease. An acute disparity in right- and left-sided filling pressures is demonstrated most dramatically in some patients with right ventricular infarction. In this setting, inadequate filling of the left ventricle, to the degree that hypotension results, can occur despite markedly elevated jugular venous and right atrial pressures.

In some patients with obstructive pulmonary disease, an increase in intrathoracic pressure during expiration leads to elevated jugular venous pressure, independent of the right-sided cardiac pressures. In this case, however, the jugular pressure elevation is typically confined to expiration, abating promptly during inspiration. In cardiac failure, the jugular distention persists to some degree throughout the respiratory cycle. Kussmaul's sign represents a paradoxical increase in jugular venous pressure during inspiration. Although not specific, it can indicate restricted cardiac filling secondary to constrictive pericarditis.

The bedside evaluation of the jugular wave contour focuses on the relative magnitude of two outward movements, the *a* and *v* waves, and of two retractions, the X and Y descents (Fig. 64.2A). The *a* wave reflects right atrial contraction, and the resultant emptying and relaxation of the atrium produces the X descent. The subsequent filling of the right atrium against the closed tricuspid valve leads to the *v* wave. The Y descent begins when the tricuspid valve then opens. Identification of the individual venous waves is accomplished by establishing their timing relative to the cardiac cycle, which is best done by simultaneous cardiac auscultation.

In normal persons, the *a* wave is somewhat more prominent than the *v* wave. Abnormally large *a* waves result when atrial contraction occurs against increased resistance to right ventricular filling. The resistance can be at the tricuspid valve level (e.g., tricuspid stenosis) or within the ventricle because of reduced wall compliance, as in pulmonic stenosis or pulmonary arterial hypertension (Fig. 64.2C). Very large *a* waves, called cannon *a* waves, arise when atrial contraction occurs while the tricuspid

valve is closed because of simultaneous ventricular systole. An ectopic ventricular beat can cause a cannon *a* wave. Atrioventricular heart block or ventricular tachycardia with atrioventricular dissociation can lead to sporadic cannon *a* waves, and junctional tachycardia is a potential cause of regularly occurring cannon *a* waves. Because genesis of the *a* wave requires effective atrial contraction, it does not occur in patients with atrial fibrillation.

In patients with tricuspid regurgitation, the usual systolic collapse of the venous pulse wave (X descent) is reduced or replaced by a positive systolic wave. When the tricuspid regurgitation is marked, the regurgitant wave fuses with the usual *v* wave, producing a single, sustained outward wave during systole (Fig. 64.2B). The duration and amplitude of the visible wave are generally related to the severity of the valve regurgitation. If, however, the right atrium is large, the effects of the regurgitant flow on the jugular venous wave may be attenuated.

HEART SOUNDS

The third and fourth heart sounds are low-pitched sounds coincident with the rapid ventricular filling phase of early diastole and with atrial systole, respectively (Fig. 64.3). The third and fourth heart sounds are generated within the ventricle, and either can arise from the left or the right side of the heart. When they result from cardiac disease, they often lead to a characteristic auscultatory cadence that resembles the canter of a horse, explaining their designation as *gallop rhythms*. During rapid heart rates, third and fourth heart sounds can occur almost simultaneously, producing a single prominent summation gallop rhythm.

A left ventricular third heart sound can occur in normal children and young adults. After 35 to 40 years of age, the third heart sound is an abnormal finding whose major clinical implication is cardiac failure secondary to ventricular dysfunction. Ventricular dilatation is often present. A third heart sound is commonly detected in patients with ventricular dilatation caused by volume overload of the ventricle (e.g., from chronic aortic regurgitation).

The fourth heart sound denotes increased resistance to filling of the left or right ventricle because of a reduction in ventricular wall compliance, as occurs with hypertrophy or cardiac ischemia

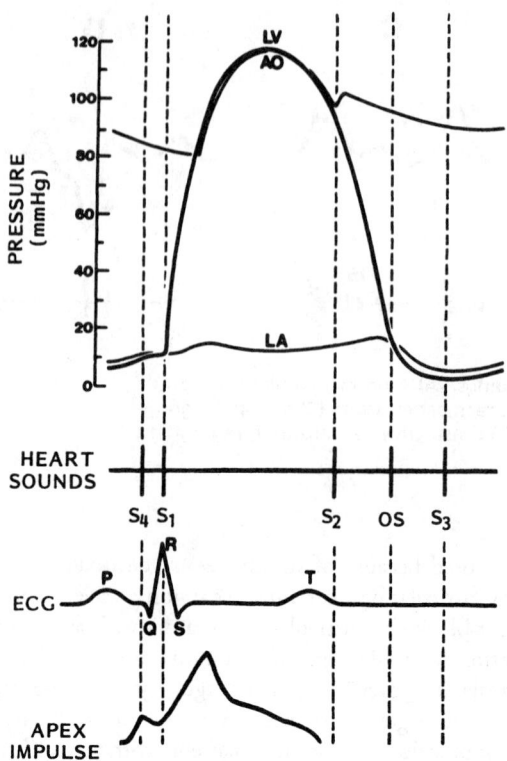

FIGURE 64.3. Diagram of left-sided pressure curves, heart sounds, ECG, and apex impulse. LV, left ventricle; LA, left atrium; Ao, aorta; S$_4$, fourth heart sound; S$_3$, third heart sound; OS, opening snap.

TABLE 64.2.	EXAMPLES OF MAJOR HEART MURMURS

Midsystolic

Increased flow across aortic or pulmonic valve (e.g., secondary to aortic regurgitation or atrial septal defect)
Aortic valve leaflet sclerosis (e.g., in elderly patients)
Aortic or pulmonic outflow obstruction (valvular, subvalvular, supravalvular)
Dilatation of aortic root or proximal pulmonary artery
Papillary muscle dysfunction

Holosystolic

Mitral or tricuspid regurgitation
Ventricular septal defect

Late Systolic

Mitral or tricuspid valve prolapse
Papillary muscle dysfunction

Early Diastolic

Aortic or pulmonic valve insufficiency

Mid-Diastolic

Mitral or tricuspid stenosis
Increased flow across nonstenotic atrioventricular valve (e.g., secondary to mitral regurgitation or atrial septal defect)

Presystolic

Mitral stenosis (with sinus rhythm)

Continuous Murmurs

Patent ductus arteriosus
Cervical venous hum
Ruptured sinus of Valsalva aneurysm
Arteriovenous fistula

(Fig. 64.1A, C, D). The presence of the fourth heart sound does not necessarily imply reduced systolic function of the ventricle or cardiac failure. There is some controversy about the significance of a fourth heart sound in older persons. Some studies have indicated the common presence of a fourth heart sound in healthy persons 50 years of age or older. During the bedside assessment, the clinician must consider the patient's age, the presence or absence of other abnormal signs, and the intensity of the fourth heart sound. The clinical significance of an audible fourth heart sound is greatly strengthened by the presence of its palpable correlate. A prominent audible and palpable fourth heart sound is almost always an abnormal finding. Because vigorous atrial contraction is required for its genesis, a fourth heart sound does not occur in patients with atrial fibrillation.

A left ventricular third or fourth heart sound is best heard at the cardiac apex, with the patient in the left lateral recumbent position. Right ventricular third or fourth heart sounds (e.g., from cor pulmonale) are most prominent at the lower left sternal border or occasionally in the epigastrium.

MURMURS

Murmurs result from turbulence associated with blood flow. Such turbulence within the heart can result from normal flow (e.g., functional murmur) or from increased blood flow across a normal valve (e.g., atrial septal defect). Alternatively, the turbulence can result from a stenotic or incompetent cardiac valve or

directly from an abnormal communication within the heart (Table 64.2). At the bedside, the resultant murmurs should be characterized by their timing, duration, pitch, configuration, intensity, location, and radiation. By convention, a I to VI grading system is used to denote a murmur's intensity; the faintest murmurs are grade I. Murmurs of grade IV or more in intensity have associated thrills (i.e., are palpable). Grade VI murmurs can be heard with the stethoscope removed from the chest surface. Selected murmurs are described in the following paragraphs to illustrate these principles.

The ejection murmur is typically middle- to high-pitched, has a crescendo–decrescendo configuration, and begins shortly after the first heart sound. A common example is the functional ejection murmur occurring in the absence of cardiac disease (Fig. 64.2A). Typically heard best at the left sternal border, it is soft, short in duration, and unaccompanied by other abnormal signs.

The ejection murmur of aortic or pulmonic valve stenosis (particularly if congenital in origin) often begins with a discrete high-frequency ejection sound (Fig. 64.1A). The pulmonic stenosis murmur is most prominent at the left sternal border, but the aortic stenosis murmur is typically heard best at the second right intercostal space, with radiation to the neck. However, the aortic stenosis murmur can be equally or more prominent at the cardiac apex. Although the harsh murmur of severe aortic stenosis is often pronounced enough to result in a thrill, the murmur's intensity is not a consistently reliable guide to the severity of the valve obstruction. The duration of the murmur (particularly the duration to maximal intensity) is more directly related to the degree of stenosis of the aortic or pulmonic valve.

The ejection murmur of hypertrophic cardiomyopathy differs in several respects from that of valvular aortic stenosis. It is typically more midsystolic in onset and may vary in intensity and duration (Fig. 64.1C). It is heard best at the left sternal border, lower than valvular aortic stenosis. Consistent with the subvalvular site of obstruction, it is not accompanied by an ejection sound. Maneuvers that reduce ventricular filling, such as prompt standing or the Valsalva maneuver, increase the duration and intensity of the murmur.

Systolic murmurs from atrioventricular valve regurgitation are also heard best with the diaphragm of the stethoscope but, in contrast to ejection murmurs, are typically plateau in configuration. Some are harsh and can have a honking quality. Although classically holosystolic, regurgitant murmurs can be confined to early, middle, or late systole, depending on the mechanism and amount of the regurgitation. The murmur of mitral valve prolapse, for example, is characteristically late systolic, with its onset after a midsystolic click. On prompt standing or Valsalva maneuver, the click moves toward the first heart sound, and the murmur becomes longer. Regurgitation secondary to papillary muscle dysfunction is often confined to middle or late systole (Fig. 64.1D). The murmur of severe acute mitral regurgitation can be nonholosystolic and can resemble an ejection murmur in quality.

The murmur of mitral valve regurgitation is heard best at the lower left sternal border or cardiac apex, typically with radiation to the axilla. Sometimes the murmur radiates to the back or to the lower left sternal border or even the base of the heart, depending on the direction of the regurgitation jet. The murmur of tricuspid regurgitation is detected at the left sternal border. Like most right-sided murmurs, its intensity is often increased during inspiration, although this characteristic may be lost in the presence of advanced right ventricular failure. Tricuspid regurgitation murmurs are often nonholosystolic.

Uncomplicated ventricular septal defect also results in a holosystolic murmur. It is typically heard best along the left sternal border at the third or fourth interspace. Distinction from mitral regurgitation is based on the murmur's location and radiation, as well as ancillary findings. In the presence of pulmonary arterial hypertension and resultant right-to-left shunting, the murmur associated with a ventricular septal defect becomes shorter and can assume an ejection quality.

The important diastolic murmurs result from aortic or pulmonic insufficiency and from mitral or tricuspid stenosis. The insufficiency murmurs are high-pitched, decrescendo sounds and are most prominent at the left sternal border (Fig. 64.1B). Because pulmonic and aortic insufficiency murmurs are similar in location and quality, they often must be discriminated by associated findings, such as the blood pressure, character of the arterial pulse, and palpation of the ventricles. Faint aortic regurgitation murmurs may be heard only with the patient in the sitting position, leaning forward. Generally, the duration of the

aortic regurgitation murmur is related to the severity of the regurgitation. This association be lost in especially severe regurgitation and with the onset of congestive heart failure. In some patients with severe aortic regurgitation, a low-pitched diastolic murmur (Austin Flint murmur) simulating mitral stenosis can be heard at the cardiac apex.

Mitral or tricuspid stenosis produces a low-pitched rumbling diastolic murmur. The initial component of the murmur occurs in early diastole, during the rapid filling phase of the ventricle. If the patient has sinus rhythm, the murmur recurs or its intensity increases in late diastole as the valvular gradient is increased by atrial contraction (Fig. 64.2C). In some patients, only this presystolic component can be readily detected. The rumble of mitral stenosis is best detected with the patient in the left lateral recumbent position. The rumble of tricuspid stenosis is best heard at the left sternal border.

Murmurs that extend uninterrupted through the second heart sound are called *continuous murmurs*. They can arise in blood vessels (e.g., patent ductus arteriosus, arteriovenous fistula) or, less commonly, in the heart (e.g., ruptured sinus of Valsalva aneurysm). The innocent or cervical venous hum is another continuous murmur, occurring primarily in children but also in older persons during hyperkinetic states such as anemia. Its correct identification is important because it can be confused with patent ductus arteriosus. The hum is heard with the stethoscope bell applied to the right supraclavicular fossa while the patient is in the sitting position. Manual pressure applied to the jugular vein or assumption of the recumbent position attenuates the murmur.

A pericardial friction rub typically has a scratchy, grating quality and is heard best with the stethoscope diaphragm. It consists of a prominent systolic component and one or two diastolic components. At times, only the systolic component can be detected. In a given patient, the number, duration, and intensity of the components can vary considerably over time. The rub is often most prominent at the left sternal border and may be easier to detect with the patient in the sitting position, leaning forward.

BIBLIOGRAPHY

Braunwald E. The history. In: Braunwald E, ed. *Heart disease: a textbook of cardiovascular medicine*, fifth ed. Philadelphia: WB Saunders, 1997.

Constant J. The evolving check list in history-taking. In: *Bedside cardiology*, fourth ed. Boston: Little, Brown and Company, 1993:1.

Dressler W. *Clinical aids in cardiac diagnosis.* New York: Grune and Stratton, 1970.

Fowler NO. The history in cardiac diagnosis. In: Fowler NO, ed. *Cardiac diagnosis and treatment*, third ed. New York: Harper and Row, 1980: 23.

Hurst JW. *Cardiovascular diagnosis: the initial examination.* St. Louis: Mosby, 556.

Kraytman J. Cardiorespiratory system. In: *The complete patient history.* New York: McGraw-Hill, 1979:11.

Kelley's Textbook of Internal Medicine, fourth edition. Edited by H. David Humes. Lippincott Williams & Wilkins, Philadelphia © 2000.

65

APPROACH TO THE PATIENT WITH CHEST PAIN

ELIZABETH G. NABEL

Chest pain is a common symptom that can result from a number of causes (Table 65.1). It may denote serious or even life-threatening disease; on the other hand, it may result from a disorder that is in no way dangerous but is nonetheless disabling because of the patient's concern and anxiety about the discomfort. In either case, identifying the correct etiology requires a thorough understanding of the patient's discomfort and the disorders that can cause chest pain. This includes careful characterization of the chest pain: its manner of onset (sudden or gradual), precipitating factors (e.g., exertion, position, inspiration, food), its character (visceral, pleuritic, superficial), its radiation, any associated symptoms (e.g., dyspnea, nausea), and duration.

Often the diagnosis is strongly suggested by the history and physical findings, but the physician must also appreciate the limitations of the bedside evaluation. Some patients have difficulty describing their symptoms, and some may minimize or exaggerate their discomfort because of denial or secondary gain,

TABLE 65.1.	CAUSES OF CHEST PAIN

Cardiac disease
  Angina pectoris
  Myocardial infarction
  Pulmonary hypertension
  Pericarditis
  Mitral valve prolapse
Dissection of the aorta
Pulmonary disease
  Pulmonary embolism
  Pleuritis
  Pneumothorax
  Pneumonia
  Tumor
Musculoskeletal disease
  Arthritis, bursitis
  Costochondritis
  Intravertebral disk disease
  Muscular spasm
Neural disease
  Intercostal neuritis
  Herpes zoster
Gastrointestinal disorders
  Gastroesophageal reflux
  Esophageal motor disorder (spasm)
  Biliary colic/cholecystitis
  Ulcer disease
Anxiety/hyperventilation

respectively. Moreover, the underlying disorders often do not present in a classic manner but rather are atypical in one or more of their characteristics. With some types of chest pain, such as angina pectoris, the physical examination in the resting state may be entirely normal.

This chapter provides an overview of the disorders that commonly must be considered in a patient with chest pain, along with an approach to the patient with this common symptom. The specific causes and their evaluation and treatment are detailed in other chapters.

CHEST PAIN DUE TO CARDIAC DISEASE

ANGINA PECTORIS

Angina pectoris is typically described as a substernal chest discomfort perceived as a tightness, heaviness, pressure, or burning sensation. It is characteristically nonfocal; that is, the patient does not indicate the location with one finger. The discomfort may radiate to the left shoulder or the arms, or to the neck and jaw. Some patients describe their angina in more atypical terms, such as sharp; a "gas pain"; discomfort in the jaw, teeth, forearms, or back; or discomfort beginning in the epigastric region and radiating up into the chest. Some patients describe it as shortness of breath with no definite discomfort, a symptom called angina-equivalent dyspnea.

Angina results when myocardial oxygen demand is increased to levels that cannot be met through coronary blood flow, usually because of stenotic atherosclerotic lesions in one or more of the epicardial coronary vessels. Accordingly, angina is typically brought on by physical exertion or emotional stress. Most patients with stable angina can identify specific activities or situations that predictably elicit the discomfort; walking up an incline and hurrying are common examples. Some variability in the effort threshold is not uncommon. Activity done in cold weather, after meals, or early in the morning may also be more likely to evoke angina. Some patients report that activity with their arms above their heads is more likely to produce the discomfort. The variable effort threshold for angina in some patients suggests that dynamic alterations in coronary blood flow (e.g., because of an intermittent increase in coronary vasomotor tone) contribute to fixed atherosclerotic stenosis in limiting blood flow. Episodes of stable angina usually begin gradually and last for 2 to 10 minutes. Discomfort is usually relieved promptly by rest or sublingual nitroglycerin.

Stress-induced angina also occurs in some patients with severe aortic valvular stenosis, left ventricular hypertrophy, or pulmonary arterial hypertension in the absence of significant coronary artery stenoses. In these situations, even normal coronary blood flow may be inadequate to meet the heightened myocardial oxygen demand. Angina may also develop in persons with very dilated left ventricles, particularly when accompanied by reduced diastolic coronary perfusion pressure, as in advanced aortic regurgitation.

Angina pectoris that has recently progressed or spontaneously increased in severity, frequency, or duration—particularly if accompanied by rest pain—is considered unstable angina. Patients with the recent onset of angina, particularly if it occurs at low levels of activity or at rest, are also included in this category. Most unstable angina patients have underlying obstructive coronary disease; the unpredictable onset of symptoms or conversion from a stable to an unstable pattern usually results from atherosclerotic plaque fissuring with superimposed platelet- or fibrin-rich thrombi. An unstable pattern can also be precipitated by extracoronary factors (secondary unstable angina). Severe anemia or carbon monoxide exposure, for example, limits blood's capacity to carry or release oxygen and can result in angina under conditions that a patient with coronary disease might otherwise tolerate well. Uncontrolled systemic arterial hypertension, rapid dysrhythmias, or hypoxemia due to pulmonary disease can also provoke angina, as can hyperthyroidism.

Prinzmetal's angina is similar in character and location to stable angina and often responds to nitroglycerin. It characteristically occurs at rest, however, without obvious provocation or a preceding increase in heart rate or blood pressure. These features are explained by its underlying mechanism: transient coronary artery spasm. Often, the episodes occur in the early morning. Some patients with Prinzmetal's angina report other vasomotor-related symptoms such as migraine headache or Raynaud's phenomenon.

ACUTE MYOCARDIAL INFARCTION

Typically, the chest pain of acute myocardial infarction (MI) is severe and prolonged (more than 30 minutes) and is unrelieved by sublingual nitroglycerin. It is often accompanied by nausea and diaphoresis. In some patients, the infarction symptoms are precipitated by vigorous exertion or other stresses that markedly increase myocardial oxygen demand. Commonly, however, acute MI occurs at rest or during normal activities. Some patients, in retrospect, describe crescendo angina before the infarction, but many do not, and MI is often the patient's first clinical feature of coronary heart disease.

The abrupt and unpredictable onset of symptoms arises from underlying acute thrombosis at the site of an ulcerated atherosclerotic plaque. These changes can occur in atherosclerotic lesions that were nonobstructive before the acute event.

Although the features of infarction pain described earlier are characteristic, they are not always present. Indeed, patients vary considerably in the intensity of the acute symptoms. As many as 30% of patients do not seek medical attention, either because the symptoms are atypical or mild or because there are no symptoms (silent infarction). Silent and atypical infarctions appear to be more prevalent in patients with diabetes mellitus and in the elderly.

■ NONISCHEMIC CARDIOVASCULAR CHEST PAIN

The pain of pericarditis is typically sharp and commonly involves the substernal or precordial area, with radiation to the neck, left shoulder, or trapezius ridge. Pericarditis can also result in a steadier, oppressive substernal discomfort that can be difficult to distinguish from that due to myocardial ischemia. Pericardial pain is often worsened by inspiration and by the recumbent position. It is lessened by leaning forward while in the sitting position. The pain of acute aortic dissection is characteristically sudden in onset, intense (reaching peak intensity almost immediately), and prolonged; depending on the site of the dissection, the pain may radiate to the back. It may be "tearing" in quality, and patients often state that it is the worst pain they have ever experienced. A history of hypertension is usually present, unless the patient has Marfan's syndrome or idiopathic cystic medial necrosis.

The atypical discomforts that may occur in patients with mitral valve prolapse have variable characteristics. They may be precordial, fleeting, and unpredictable, without a clear-cut relation to physical effort. The pain is often sharp or like a pin prick, but some patients report substernal discomfort that lasts for hours. In some cases, the autonomic dysfunction that can be associated with mitral valve prolapse may contribute to some of the atypical symptoms.

■ CHEST PAIN DUE TO GASTROINTESTINAL DISORDERS

Gastroesophageal reflux is a particularly common cause of visceral discomfort in the substernal and epigastric areas. It can result in a diffuse burning sensation or the feeling that warm fluid is climbing toward the throat. Some patients report an epigastric pressure sensation. Reflux (as well as primary esophageal motor disorders) can also be associated with frank esophageal spasm with substernal discomfort that is similar in character to that of angina pectoris and that may radiate to the throat and left arm. It may also be relieved by the smooth-muscle relaxant action of sublingual nitroglycerin. Chest pain due to reflux is typically provoked by eating large meals, assuming the recumbent position after eating, bending forward, or straining. However, reflux can be provoked by exercise in some patients. It may be improved by standing upright, drinking water, belching, or taking antacids. Patients with reflux may also experience dysphagia, and some report nocturnal wheezing or coughing due to regurgitation into the bronchi.

Although typically localized in the epigastrium, the pain of peptic ulcer disease may radiate to the back and occasionally to the substernal area. Peptic ulcer discomfort is classically described as gnawing, aching, or dull, and is usually relieved by food or antacids. Discomfort also occurs at night, but early-morning pain before breakfast is unexpected. In some ulcer patients, discomfort is precipitated by eating.

Biliary colic associated with gallstones leads to episodic steady discomfort that usually is sudden, aching, or pressure-like, and is maximal in the epigastrium or right upper quadrant. Radiation to the scapular area is common. Discomfort may persist for 1 hour to several hours before subsiding, and may be followed by a more prolonged uncomfortable sensation or tenderness in the right subcostal area. Nausea and vomiting may accompany the episode.

The discomfort from pancreatitis, although usually localized to the epigastric or periumbilical areas, can radiate to the chest and back, as well as to the flank and lower abdomen. The discomfort is constant and often severe and may be worsened by the supine position. Nausea and vomiting are usually present.

CHEST WALL AND CERVICAL SPINE DISORDERS

The anterior chest discomfort of costochondritis can be either sharp and brief, or a dull ache lasting for hours to days. Localized muscle spasm can contribute to the discomfort. Costochondritis discomfort is usually worsened by chest movement or deep inspiration. Occasionally, the inflammation results in obvious swelling of the tender costochondral junction (Tietze's syndrome). Careful inquiry may reveal recent minor trauma or a new or unusual activity as the cause of chest wall discomfort.

Discomfort from cervical spine disease is usually localized to the neck and back of the head. Because it can radiate to the shoulder and arm, however, it can occasionally be confused with angina pectoris. When cervical radiculitis is present, the patient may report constant aching discomfort in the arm, and there is often a sensory deficit and paresthesias. Weakness may also result. Discomfort may be elicited by movement of the neck, and the neck motion is limited. Bursitis and thoracic outlet syndromes (e.g., neurovascular compression by a cervical rib or scalenus anterior muscle) are additional causes of shoulder pain. Discomfort from these disorders is often elicited by shoulder motion or certain positions rather than exertion itself. Paresthesias may be reported as well.

In its prevesicular phase, herpes zoster involving the left chest can mimic cardiac discomfort. The correct diagnosis is supported by its bandlike dermatome location, its persistence, and the subsequent development of vesicles.

PULMONARY CAUSES OF CHEST PAIN

The discomfort accompanying many pulmonary disorders arises from inflammation of adjacent pleural surfaces. Pleural discomfort usually is sharp or catchlike, and is often unilateral. When the diaphragmatic pleura is involved, the discomfort may radiate to the shoulder. The most important characteristic of pleural pain is its exacerbation by deep inspiration or cough. Movement of the torso may increase its intensity. Associated fever and productive cough suggest pneumonia as the cause. Spontaneous pneumothorax produces an abrupt onset of chest pain with dyspnea. Pulmonary infarction secondary to embolism is another cause of pleuritic pain and may be accompanied by hemoptysis. Massive pulmonary embolism can also lead to central chest pain, similar in character to myocardial ischemia. The combination of chest pain and hemoptysis can also suggest a lung neoplasm.

ANXIETY-RELATED CHEST PAIN

Anxiety-related chest pain can take several forms. Often focal and precordial in location, it may be a constant ache, present for hours or longer. It can also be an unpredictable fleeting or jabbing pain, unrelated to effort. Chest tenderness may accompany the discomfort. Palpitations and somatic complaints are common. Careful inquiry often elicits a relation to emotional stress and other symptoms, such as hyperventilation, characteristic of anxiety states. This chest pain may be partially and variably responsive to several therapeutic measures.

EVALUATION OF THE PATIENT WITH CHEST PAIN

HISTORY AND PHYSICAL EXAMINATION

For the patient with chest pain, the urgency of the evaluation and the decision to perform it in an ambulatory or hospital setting are determined by several factors, including the acuity and severity of the symptoms and findings. When acute chest pain is accompanied by marked dyspnea, hypotension, agitation, or profuse diaphoresis, the diagnostic possibilities may include acute MI, pulmonary embolus, dissecting aneurysm, pericardial tamponade, and pneumothorax; clearly, emergent evaluation is required. Independent of the intensity of the initial symptoms, the physician must also determine if the underlying cause of the chest pain has the potential to progress to a serious or life-threatening state. Discomfort that is not perceived by the patient as severe or that has resolved by the time of presentation can nonetheless represent a serious or unstable condition (e.g., unstable angina). In other cases, particularly when the chest discomfort has occurred episodically over a longer period of time, is not severe, and is not accompanied by acute physical findings or ECG changes, the evaluation may be performed in a more elective manner.

When the characteristics of the chest discomfort are typical, its cause may be strongly suggested by the history. The history, coupled with a careful physical examination, can shorten the list of possible diagnoses or rule out the more serious causes of chest discomfort. The general history and physical examination may also reveal conditions that place the patient at enhanced risk for specific causes of chest discomfort; identification of the classic features of Marfan's syndrome, for example, can suggest the possibility of aortic dissection as a cause of chest pain. The presence of risk factors such as hypertension, cigarette smoking, diabetes mellitus, hypercholesterolemia, or a family history of premature coronary heart disease heightens the risk of coronary heart disease. Risk factors are just that, however; their presence does not prove the diagnosis, nor does their absence exclude it. A patient may also have more than one disorder that can cause chest discomfort. Gastroesophageal reflux and coronary disease often coexist, for example. Also, the stresses associated with one illness (e.g., cholecystitis) may provoke another cause of discomfort, such as angina pectoris in a person with previously unrecognized coronary heart disease.

When chest pain results from musculoskeletal causes, the discomfort may be reproduced by palpation or localized movement. Tenderness on palpation of the epigastrium or right upper quadrant may be present in patients with peptic ulcer or gallbladder disease. Localized chest findings, such as signs of lung consolidation or collapse, pleural rub, or rales, can indicate a pulmonary cause for chest discomfort.

In patients with angina pectoris, the physical examination between episodes of discomfort may be normal. Examination during an episode of angina can help in its recognition. Often, the heart rate and blood pressure are increased during the episode. In some patients, however, the blood pressure may fall, particularly if a large amount of myocardium is rendered ischemic. An audible (and often palpable) fourth heart sound is commonly present, attesting to reduction of ventricular compliance. Some patients develop transient murmurs of mitral regurgitation as a consequence of ischemia-induced papillary muscle dysfunction. The physical examination, of course, is also central in the identification of other disorders, such as aortic stenosis, pulmonary arterial hypertension, or severe systemic arterial hypertension, that can cause or exacerbate anginal chest discomfort.

Physical examination during the early stages of acute MI commonly reveals an obviously distressed patient. The skin may be cool, with diaphoresis. In the absence of a complication, the blood pressure and heart rate are often increased. In patients with acute inferior infarction, bradycardia and hypotension may develop during the early stages due to systemic vagotonia (Bezold–Jarisch reflex). In other patients with acute infarction, the blood pressure may be low because extensive infarction has resulted in cardiac failure. In this case, the heart rate is characteristically increased, unless there is an associated conduction disturbance. Precordial palpation may reveal an apical late systolic bulge, as well as the palpable correlate of a fourth heart sound. An audible fourth heart sound is present in almost all patients with acute infarction, if sinus rhythm is present. An apical systolic murmur, representing mitral regurgitation from papillary muscle dysfunction, is also often evident. In some patients, a friction rub from inflammation of the adjacent pericardium is transiently or intermittently present.

The detection of a new aortic regurgitation murmur in a susceptible patient with severe chest pain can suggest acute proximal aortic dissection. Neurologic defects or asymmetry of the arterial pulses, due to vessel occlusion or compromise, can also occur. Detection of a two- or three-component pericardial friction rub is pathognomonic of pericarditis, although pericarditis can also follow acute MI. Pericardial friction rubs can vary in intensity, and their recognition can be more difficult if only one component is clearly audible. Particularly when the history or physical findings suggest pericarditis, the examination must include a careful search for elevated jugular pressure and paradoxical pulse, which can indicate cardiac tamponade.

LABORATORY STUDIES

For most patients with chest pain, the initial evaluation includes an ECG and chest radiographs. An immediate ECG in any patient with prolonged or severe chest pain is especially important, as it may serve to identify candidates for thrombolytic therapy or emergent angioplasty. The need for and timing of additional laboratory studies are based on the tentative diagnoses derived from the history and physical examination. If, for example, gastroesophageal reflux is suspected, a trial of medical therapy may be chosen, assuming there are no indications or risk factors of advanced disease or complications (e.g., bleeding, dysphagia). If the picture is less clear-cut, if complications are suspected, or if the patient does not respond readily to treatment, then radiographic or endoscopic studies are obtained to confirm the diagnosis and assess its severity. If the diagnostic possibilities include both angina pectoris and a gastrointestinal disorder, the former should be evaluated first before proceeding with procedures such as endoscopy or esophageal studies. If gallstone disease is suspected, the laboratory evaluation initially includes abdominal ultrasonography as well as a blood leukocyte count and standard liver function tests.

Arterial blood gas analysis, ventilation–perfusion scanning, or angiography is required to confirm a tentative diagnosis of pulmonary embolus. If aortic dissection is present, the chest radiograph may demonstrate widening of the mediastinum, but this finding is nonspecific. If the clinical features suggest aortic dissection, an imaging study should be obtained promptly. Emergent transesophageal echocardiography, computed tomography with contrast enhancement, or magnetic resonance imaging can be used. If readily available, transesophageal echocardiography is the study of choice. Aortography may be required to confirm the extent of the arterial disease and to assess coexistent coronary disease.

In a patient with pericarditis, the ECG typically demonstrates a widespread current of injury (ST-segment elevation), and there may be depression of the PR segment. Sinus tachycardia is usually present. An echocardiogram is indicated when pericarditis is suspected; detection of a pericardial effusion supports the diagnosis. Sometimes the echocardiogram can provide information about the underlying cause of the pericarditis and may demonstrate signs (e.g., right ventricular systolic collapse) indicating the hemodynamic effects of the associated effusion. If a diagnosis of pericarditis is made, the laboratory investigation then focuses on the underlying cause. Depending on the clinical situation, this may include skin testing with purified protein derivative, serologic testing for histoplasmosis, analysis of renal function, blood cultures, and blood tests to exclude a systemic inflammatory state, such as lupus erythematosus. Metastatic neoplasm is also included in the list of possible causes in many cases.

EVALUATION OF ISCHEMIC CARDIAC PAIN

Typical chest discomfort that occurs with exercise or emotion and that is relieved by rest or nitroglycerin is presumptive evidence that the patient is experiencing angina. The ECG can aid in its diagnosis and provide information about the myocardial location of the ischemia underlying the angina. Between episodes of discomfort, however, the ECG may be normal, demonstrate nonspecific changes, or show signs of prior infarction. Diagnostically, the ECG is most valuable when it is obtained during an episode of chest discomfort. Typically but not invariably, angina is accompanied by transient ST-segment depression, T-wave inversion, or both. Less commonly, angina may lead to transient normalization of previously depressed ST segments or T waves or to the development of negative U waves. Transient myocardial ischemia also sometimes results in ST-segment elevation, generally indicating substantial (transmural) ischemia. Transient ST-

TABLE 65.2.	STRESS TESTING IN PATIENTS WITH STABLE ANGINA PECTORIS
Test	**Comment**
Exercise electrocardiography	Useful for risk stratification; can aid in selection of treatment regimen
Exercise imaging study (e.g., thallium perfusion or echocardiography)	Particularly valuable if baseline ECG abnormal or hyperventilation-induced ECG changes
Pharmacologic study (e.g., dipyramidole thallium or dobutamine echocardiography)	Particularly helpful for patients who cannot exercise (e.g., due to orthopedic problems)

segment elevation is characteristically present in patients with Prinzmetal's angina.

Exercise testing is usually recommended for patients with suspected angina, provided the symptoms are stable. (Exercise testing is contraindicated in the unstable patient until stabilization has been accomplished.) Beyond providing objective signs of ischemia, the exercise study is helpful in establishing the patient's functional capacity, and it may reveal signs suggesting advanced disease or high-risk state. It may also disclose hypertensive or hyperkinetic responses to exertion, responses that can influence the choice of antianginal medications. The selection of a standard exercise ECG or exercise imaging (e.g., by nuclear medicine or echocardiographic techniques) is based on several factors, including the baseline ECG pattern, concomitant medications, and the estimated pretest likelihood of coronary disease (Table 65.2). Imaging techniques are usually recommended for women (in whom false-positive ECG changes are more common), patients with atypical symptoms (in whom the predictability of exercise testing is reduced because of lower pretest likelihood of disease), and patients with an abnormal resting ECG or hyperventilation-induced ECG changes.

For patients with angina, particularly those with historical or ECG evidence of prior infarction, left ventricular function is a major determinant of prognosis and can influence the selection of bypass surgery. Left ventricular function can be assessed noninvasively by echocardiography or radionuclide ventriculography.

Coronary arteriography is the definitive way to detect the presence and extent of coronary stenosis. Coronary arteriography may be required for diagnosis in patients whose clinical features and noninvasive test results are inconclusive. Cardiac catheterization is recommended for angina patients when revascularization is contemplated because of refractory symptoms, reduced functional capacity, or the presence of signs during exercise testing suggesting advanced disease or high-risk state. The patient's age and left ventricular function also influence this decision. The guidelines for the selection of revascularization are discussed in Chapter 72.

Patients with the presumptive diagnosis of unstable angina are a somewhat heterogeneous group with regard to the extent of coronary disease and prognosis. The evaluation and treatment are influenced in part by an estimation of risk (see Chapter 65). Patients at higher risk include those with prolonged (more than 20 minutes) rest pain, dynamic ECG changes, and associated signs of cardiac failure, hemodynamic instability, or new mitral regurgitation murmur. Up to 20% or so of patients hospitalized with suspected unstable angina may not have obstructive coronary disease.

The ECGs and cardiac enzyme studies, performed serially, help confirm or exclude the diagnosis when acute MI is suspected. As noted previously, an ECG should be obtained immediately to aid in diagnosis and to help identify candidates for thrombolytic therapy. The ECG findings of acute MI are described in Chapters 72 and 84. The initial ECG findings are often nonspecific and may be subtle. Occasionally, the first ECG is normal. A left bundle-branch pattern can obscure the ECG findings of infarction, and in its presence the diagnosis must usually be made by other means.

The most sensitive and specific standard enzyme tests for acute MI are troponin and the MB isoenzyme of creatine kinase. In the first few hours after the onset of pain, the initial troponin and MB values may be normal. Enzyme levels then characteristically rise. Troponin may stay elevated for several days, while the MB isoenzyme falls, usually returning to normal within a few days. Elevated serum levels of troponins may precede elevations of creatine kinase MB and may remain elevated longer. Skeletal muscle injury does not lead to elevated serum troponin levels. Troponin levels are increased in some unstable angina patients and may provide prognostic information.

The blood lactate dehydrogenase level and its isoenzyme pattern may be helpful in the patient who presents several days after suspected infarction. Lactate dehydrogenase activity generally peaks 3 to 6 days after the onset of pain and may remain abnormal for several days after that. Late presentation of acute MI is more commonly detected by persistent elevation of troponin.

Echocardiography is also performed in patients with suspected acute MI. In addition to confirming the presence and location of a segmental wall motion abnormality, the echocardiogram can provide prognostic information by estimating the infarct size and global ventricular function. Some of the complications of acute infarction can also be recognized or confirmed.

◼ TREATMENT

The treatment of the patient with chest pain is determined by its cause.

Patients with reflux are instructed to avoid large meals and postprandial recumbency and to limit ingestion of caffeine and ethanol. Abstinence from smoking is also important. Elevating the head of the bed is often beneficial. Treatment can include antacids and drugs, such as the H_2-receptor blockers that decrease gastric acid secretion.

If recurrent cholecystitis is present, elective surgical therapy is usually recommended. Nonsurgical alternatives are available for some patients with gallstone disease.

For the patient with costochondritis or other chest wall pains, analgesic or nonsteroidal anti-inflammatory drugs and reassurance are usually effective. Occasionally, it is necessary to inject the involved area with local anesthetic.

When pleuritic chest pain is the result of pneumonia, the treatment focuses on the underlying infection. Anti-inflammatory agents such as indomethacin may help control associated pleural discomfort.

When chest pain is due to pulmonary embolus, anticoagulation with heparin is promptly performed. Distinguishing the pleural pain associated with pulmonary embolus from the discomfort of pericarditis is important, as anticoagulation is generally contraindicated in patients with acute pericarditis because of the risk of hemorrhage into the pericardial sac, leading to tamponade. The specific treatment of pericarditis depends on its cause. If tuberculous, fungal, neoplastic, and bacterial causes can be excluded, anti-inflammatory therapy is usually used for presumed idiopathic or postviral pericarditis. Commonly, this begins with salicylates or nonsteroidal anti-inflammatory drugs. Corticosteroid therapy may be required for patients who do not tolerate or respond to the nonsteroidal anti-inflammatory agents.

MANAGEMENT OF CHEST PAIN DUE TO MYOCARDIAL ISCHEMIA

The medical management of the patient with stable angina is not limited to the use of drugs. The patient is instructed to avoid activities that predictably elicit angina and cautioned about exertion after meals or in cold weather. He or she should be encouraged to remain active otherwise, including, if possible, a walking or bicycle exercise program to enhance conditioning. The instruction should include the proper use of sublingual nitroglycerin, including its prophylactic use before necessary activities that the patient thinks might induce discomfort. The patient should also understand the warning signs of progressive angina and the importance of promptly seeking medical evaluation should they occur. This includes angina that is not relieved by two or three nitroglycerin tablets each taken 5 minutes apart. All the preceding should be done compassionately, with appropriate reassurance and care to avoid inducing undue anxiety and incapacitation. Treatment should also include efforts to correct underlying risk factors, such as smoking, systemic arterial hypertension, hypercholesterolemia, and overweight habitus. Aspirin should also be taken daily.

The medicines designed to prevent recurrent episodes of angina fall into three general categories: long-acting nitrates, β-adrenergic blocking drugs, and calcium channel antagonists. There is no universally accepted optimal drug regimen; rather, the choice of regimen is a matter of clinical judgment and is based on several factors, including the pattern and severity of the angina; the pretreatment heart rate, blood pressure, and ventricular function; and the presence or absence of extracardiac disorders that would enhance the likelihood of side effects with a specific agent. The patient's age and occupation can influence the choice. If the angina is mild and infrequent, a single drug, commonly a nitrate or β-blocker, may be chosen. For patients with a significant degree of angina, however, initial therapy often

includes both agents, assuming there is no contraindication to their use.

The antianginal effectiveness of the calcium antagonists appears to be comparable to that of the β-adrenergic blocking drugs. They provide an alternative if the latter are not tolerated or are contraindicated by bronchospastic lung disease. Calcium antagonists also play a front-line role when the clinical characteristics (variable anginal threshold) suggest that vasomotor changes play a prominent role in the angina. This is particularly true for Prinzmetal's angina. Calcium antagonists can also be added to the regimen of patients with exertional angina when symptoms are not effectively controlled by nitrates and β-blockers. The major calcium channel antagonists differ in the degree to which they systematically vasodilate and affect the heart's electrical and contractile functions. Calcium channel drugs are described further in Chapter 90.

Reperfusion therapy with percutaneous angioplasty or coronary bypass surgery is considered for angina patients with refractory symptoms or an unacceptable lifestyle. Surgery is also usually recommended for patients with high-risk angiographic findings, such as obstruction of the left main coronary artery or triple-vessel coronary disease with inducible cardiac ischemia or associated left ventricular dysfunction. In diabetic patients, coronary artery bypass graft is recommended for three-vessel disease and normal left ventricular dysfunction.

Patients with unstable angina and rest pain should be hospitalized in a monitored cardiac unit. In some cases, acute MI must be excluded. Treatment typically includes aspirin and continuous therapeutic heparin infusion, along with antianginal medications as described above. If the episodes prompting admission are severe or prolonged, nitroglycerin is often given initially as an intravenous infusion.

The hospitalized patient with recurrent unstable angina despite medical therapy is at particularly high risk. Cardiac catheterization is indicated for consideration of coronary angioplasty or bypass surgery. Patients with hemodynamic instability and refractory symptoms may benefit from intra-aortic balloon counterpulsation before coronary arteriography.

The symptoms of most hospitalized patients stabilize with medical therapy. If angina recurs as activity is increased or if there are symptoms or signs of ischemia on an exercise study, then coronary arteriography is recommended. Even for patients whose symptoms stabilize in the hospital, coronary arteriography is commonly recommended, if there are no other life-threatening medical illnesses and if the patient's age is not very advanced. The decision to perform revascularization can be influenced by several factors, including the response to medical therapy and the severity of the underlying coronary disease.

The treatment of patients with acute MI and its complications are described in Chapter 73, and several points about the early approach to the patient warrant emphasis here also. The most important step is consideration of reperfusion of the infarct-related artery. Early restoration or maintenance of perfusion of the infarct-related coronary artery is critical. Current approaches include intravenous thrombolytic therapy or immediate (primary) angioplasty. Myocardial necrosis occurs progressively after coronary occlusion; patients must be assessed rapidly as candidates for treatment. This includes excluding patients at prohibitive risk for a thrombolytic complication (e.g., bleeding, stroke). Candidates for thrombolytic treatment generally include patients with ongoing acute infarction who present within 12 hours of symptom onset and have associated ST-segment elevation (current of injury) or new (or presumably new) left bundle-branch pattern along with no contraindications (See Chapter 73 for detailed inclusion and exclusion criteria and a discussion of thrombolytic agent and adjunctive therapy). Aspirin and heparin are also used in the early treatment of patients (e.g., those with non-Q-wave infarction) who do not meet current ECG inclusion criteria for thrombolytic therapy.

For patients in the coronary care unit, the prompt establishment of intravenous access and continuous ECG monitoring are important, as the risk of life-threatening ventricular dysrhythmias is greatest during the first 6 hours of the infarction process. Other immediate measures include oxygen supplementation, along with nitroglycerin and morphine (administered intravenously) for pain relief. Aspirin is administered for its antiplatelet effect. Control of heart rate and blood pressure is important, as they are major determinants of myocardial oxygen demand. Elevated blood pressure may respond to intravenous infusion of nitroglycerin. Nitroglycerin infusion is also often used empirically (e.g., during the first 24 hours); it may aid in pain relief and provide anti-ischemic and some unloading effects. It is important that the drug not lower blood pressure excessively or lead to a reflex increase in heart rate. Particularly when the blood pressure, heart rate, or both are elevated, cautious intravenous use of a β-adrenergic blocking drug (e.g., metoprolol or atenolol) can be beneficial. However, increased heart rate can be a compensatory response to significant left ventricular dysfunction in some patients. β-Adrenergic blocking therapy should not be used in patients with clinically important heart failure or hypotension. If β-blocking action is indicated but there is concern about precipitating left ventricular failure, a short-acting agent (e.g., esmolol) may be useful. Additional cardiac contraindications to β-blocker use include bradycardia and conduction disturbances (complications particularly common during the acute phase of inferior MI). Hypotension can also be especially prominent if there is associated right ventricular infarction. In the absence of overt pulmonary congestion, fluid administration can be performed with caution.

BIBLIOGRAPHY

American Heart Association. *Heart and stroke facts: 1998 statistical supplement.* Dallas, 1998.

Centers for Disease Control and Prevention, National Center for Health Statistics, National Vital Statistics and the United States Bureau of the Census. Health, United States, 1993:31.

Gersh BJ, Braunwald E, Rutherford JD. Chronic coronary artery disease. In: Braunwald E, ed. *Heart disease: a textbook of cardiovascular medicine,* fifth ed. Philadelphia: WB Saunders, 1997: 1289.

Miller AJ. *Diagnosis of chest pain.* New York: Raven Press, 1988:74–76.

Schwartz GG, Karliner JS. Pathophysiology of chronic stable angina. In: Fuster V, Ross R, Topol EJ, eds. *Atherosclerosis and coronary artery disease.* Philadelphia: JB Lippincott, 1996:1389.

Kelley's Textbook of Internal Medicine, fourth edition. Edited by H. David Humes. Lippincott Williams & Wilkins, Philadelphia © 2000.

APPROACH TO THE PATIENT WITH HEART FAILURE

ROBERT J. CODY

EPIDEMIOLOGY AND PRESENTATION

Heart failure (HF) is not a disease. It is a wide-ranging clinical expression of left ventricular (LV) dysfunction, occurring as the result of diverse etiologies. That term is now preferred to congestive heart failure, as not all heart failure patients are "congested," and experts feel that the latter description has limited diagnostic accuracy. Over 500,000 new patients are diagnosed with HF annually in the United States, and this number will likely increase as more patients survive acute myocardial infarction, with progressive LV dysfunction, and as the overall population ages. The goal of therapy is to prevent, or delay, the progression of ventricular dysfunction to advanced stages.

Usually, the clinical manifestations of HF develop in patients with known histories of cardiovascular disease. A history of coronary artery disease or hypertension is common. Heart murmurs also may have been noted in the past. Increasingly, however, the first manifestation of heart disease may be symptoms of HF. In such patients with no history or signs of cardiac involvement, the diagnosis of idiopathic cardiomyopathy often is made. Heart failure is the most common diagnosis leading to hospitalization in patients over age 65. Aging of the myocardium and peripheral vasculature contribute directly to a depression of cardiac performance.

PATHOPHYSIOLOGY OF SYSTOLIC DYSFUNCTION

CARDIAC PUMP FAILURE

Systolic ventricular dysfunction represents failure of the heart as a pump, with loss of systolic power output that subsequently stimulates a cascade of compensatory responses. Systolic ventricular failure can be abrupt in onset, following myocardial infarction, or more insidious in onset, as in idiopathic cardiomyopathy or hypertension. The remodeling process that ensues in response to the inciting myocardial damage involves the contractile proteins, the microvasculature, and the cytoskeletal matrix of collagen, elastin, and other connective tissue elements. Loss of normal ventricular geometry and pumping efficiency further perpetuates the remodeling process but does not predict clinical findings. The presence of a dilated ventricular chamber or a reduced ejection fraction characterizes systolic ventricular dysfunction. The clinical expression of HF can be seen in the presence of normal systolic function. Heart failure with normal systolic function (so-called diastolic HF) is difficult to characterize and is a focus of current studies.

Heart failure is often an insidious process that may remain undetected for many years. To identify the onset and early progression of HF, the best opportunity is within the population of patients with LV dysfunction following acute myocardial infarction. Other processes, such as idiopathic cardiomyopathy or hypertension, do not permit identification of the index event or have a protracted course, so that follow-up of disease progression is difficult. The onset of ventricular dysfunction following acute myocardial infarction is readily linked to its index event. Patients may remain in an asymptomatic state, or rapidly advance to overt congestive HF, by mechanisms that remain obscure. Progression of HF may be secondary to cellular growth factors, abnormal autonomic nervous system activity, activation of hormonal or vasoactive substances, subendocardial ischemia, and mechanical stress factors.

CONDUCTION AND RHYTHM ABNORMALITIES

Conduction abnormalities and cardiac arrhythmias are common in HF. Atrial arrhythmias also occur in the form of premature beats and other atrial arrhythmias. Perhaps the most common atrial arrhythmia in this population is atrial fibrillation. This may occur in acute failure, following an acute myocardial infarction, or at any time during the course of disease progression. Sinus node dysfunction, atrioventricular (AV) junctional block, and intraventricular conduction defects are common and may necessitate permanent pacemaker implantation. Ventricular arrhythmias are common in the HF population. Sudden death accounts for anywhere from 35% to 70% of total mortality. However, not all sudden deaths are due to ventricular tachycardia or fibrillation.

VASCULAR ADAPTATION

A fundamental lesion in HF is the abnormal function of the vasculature. Several mechanisms contribute to vasoconstriction. Clinically relevant information regarding the "myogenic hypothesis," metabolic and local regulating factors, and regional neurogenic control are not well characterized in HF. Intrinsic structural adaptation of the vasculature in HF likely parallels changes observed in hypertension. Preceding long-term structural changes are abnormalities in ventricular vascular coupling, with an increase of characteristic impedance. These rapid changes occur in a time frame that may be too rapid to be explained by structural changes. When "vasoconstrictor mechanisms" are discussed in congestive HF, this concept generally refers to neurohormonal substances that adversely increase vascular tone.

NEUROHORMONAL MECHANISMS

With progressive ventricular dysfunction, the nervous system, particularly the autonomic nervous system, undergoes an adaptive response that favors augmentation of sympathetic nervous system activity and reduction of parasympathetic activity. Early studies demonstrated increased plasma norepinephrine in HF patients, correlated with reduced cardiac performance and increased mortality. Baroreflex and mechanoreflex abnormalities such as the cold pressor test, tilt, and lower body negative pressure were shown to be abnormal. These abnormalities demonstrated partial correction with successful therapeutic interventions.

Activation of the renin–angiotensin system is one of the predominant abnormalities of HF. Studies in milder and asymptomatic HF demonstrate relatively less activation, but values are increased compared to normal. The degree of activity is intensified in the presence of diuretic therapy. In addition to vasoconstriction, angiotensin II stimulates aldosterone secretion by the adrenal gland, producing sodium retention and potassium excretion at the distal nephron. Renin system components have been identified in the myocardium and vasculature, where they adversely affect fibrosis and remodeling, as well as cellular dysfunction.

There are other important factors. Arginine vasopressin is stimulated in the course of congestive HF. It reduces free water clearance and produces vasoconstriction in regional circulations. Natriuretic peptides are produced by cardiac myocytes in response to increased wall stress. When released in the circulation, natriuretic peptides promote sodium and water excretion, as well as vasodilatation. Eventually, activation of opposing vasoconstrictive and sodium-retentive hormonal substances at later stages of HF overwhelms the favorable effects of natriuretic peptides. More recently, the endothelium has been identified as a source of vasoactive substances, such as nitric oxide, which produces vasodilatation, and endothelin, a potent vasoconstrictor.

EDEMA AND SODIUM RETENTION

Sodium and water retention in HF accounts for many of the symptoms that occur in this population. With reduction of glomerular filtration rate, proximal tubular sodium reabsorption is enhanced, with reduction of sodium delivery to the distal nephron. Reduced distal nephron sodium enhances renin secretion from the juxtaglomerular apparatus. Increased renin system activity favors sodium retention and potassium excretion, as well as stimulating vasopressin release, which increase free water retention. A neural environment that is dominated by increased sympathetic nervous system activity and abnormal baroreceptor function produces further renal vasoconstriction. This cascade of events, producing sodium and water retention, accounts for an increase of "classic" HF symptoms and separates symptomatic HF from asymptomatic HF in patients with comparable reduction of ejection fraction.

■ CARDIAC HISTORY

The usual reason for a patient's seeking medical attention is breathlessness or fatigue limiting exercise tolerance. Sometimes the first recognized manifestation of HF is orthopnea or paroxysmal nocturnal dyspnea; in other patients, pedal edema may be the first recognized abnormality. Thus, the secondary manifestations of HF (such as circulatory congestion) bring the patient to medical attention, rather than the primary cardiac contractile abnormality.

PHYSICAL EXAMINATION

GENERAL

Asymptomatic patients may not have distinguishing characteristics on general appearance. Patients with chronic HF will have features of chronic disease, such as pallor and general weakness. In more advanced stages of the disease, wasting of limb-girdle and facial muscles is common, and there may be the appearance of overall cachexia. The abdomen may be distended from hepatomegaly and ascites. Long-standing peripheral edema will be associated with darkened skin due to chronic hemosiderin deposition and scarring from chronic skin lesions. Body weight may be misleading in HF. Accumulation of edema may be insidious and balanced by loss of lean body mass, thereby masking fluid retention. Virtually any weight abnormality may be present, and certainly, the presence of obesity will completely obscure any attempt to characterize weight in relation to the severity of HF.

PULSE AND BLOOD PRESSURE

Tachycardia, in the absence of other known causes, represents chronotropic compensation for the reduced cardiac output of pump failure. A 2:1 ratio of apical to radial pulse may reflect pulses alternans, secondary to the severity of HF. Alternatively, a very slow peripheral pulse may represent sinus node dysfunction (structural or secondary to medications) or heart block. An irregular pulse most typically reflects atrial fibrillation. A narrow pulse pressure is consistent with a low stroke volume or inadequate diastolic filling time. Assessment of the carotids and pulses therefore provides information regarding ventricular contraction and the overall circulatory status.

The measurement of systolic and diastolic blood pressure provides important clues to the etiology of HF. If blood pressure exceeds 140/90 mm Hg on repeated measurements, lowering of the blood pressure is mandatory in HF patients. In contrast, many patients with long- standing HF have hypotension, which is accentuated with upright posture ("orthostatic hypotension"). When documented, this should be correlated with symptoms of dizziness and fatigue. In general, most therapies of HF will produce low blood pressure, and may require adjustment, in the setting of symptomatic orthostatic hypotension.

VENOUS SYSTEM

The magnitude of jugular venous distention provides an estimate of cardiac filling pressure and circulatory volume status. It is most convenient to use the right atrium as the reference point for this measurement by taking the midaxillary point at the nipple level. The simplest stress test is the hepatojugular reflux test performed by exerting constant firm pressure over the right upper quadrant of the abdomen. A positive hepatojugular reflux test may be interpreted as evidence for impaired right ventricular

response to volume load, a dilated heart that can be compressed by a rising diaphragm, and a volume overload state. An alternate approach to stressing the circulation is leg raising or exercise. In evaluating the peripheral venous system, look for varicose veins or prior surgical scars that may increase the tendency for edema, particularly in an asymmetric fashion. Peripheral pitting edema secondary to HF should be distinguished from the heavy ankles of lipedema. The pitting quality of edema distinguishes it from lymphedema.

LUNGS

Tachypnea is a typical finding of HF and may be present under resting conditions during the physical examination. Dyspnea in the course of a patient interview is a finding of inadequate cardiac compensation. The most characteristic finding on pulmonary examination is the presence of rales, indicative of increased pulmonary capillary pressure and transudation of fluid into the alveolar airspace. In general, rales provide an estimate of the severity of LV decompensation, as the height of the rales in the lung fields is proportionate to the severity of the decompensation. Rales will be obscured by the presence of pleural effusion, which is more often a marker of chronic decompensation.

CARDIAC

Precordial palpation provides valuable information in HF, indicating the extent of cardiac enlargement and providing information regarding the degree of contractile impairment and valvular function. Displacement of the apical impulse away from the midsternal line is typical of HF. A diffuse apical impulse is characteristic of ventricular enlargement, and a heaving quality may indicate ventricular dyskinesis or underlying left atrial lift. The palpation of thrills may provide a clue to the presence of valvular disease. Auscultation of the heart should confirm the abnormalities already identified by observation and palpation. In particular, one is interested in the presence of murmurs or diastolic filling sounds. Mitral regurgitation is common in patients with HF and may result in an apical murmur radiating toward the axilla. Tricuspid regurgitation may also be present on auscultation. An accentuated pulmonic closure sound (P_2) suggests pulmonary hypertension, a fourth heart sound (S_4) indicates abnormal atrioventricular filling characteristics, and a third heart sound (S_3) indicates ventricular dysfunction or decompensation.

LABORATORY TESTS

CHEST ROENTGENOGRAPHY

The chest roentgenogram provides an estimate of ventricular chamber size, but it often serves as a screening technique to identify the presence of heart disease. The cardiothoracic ratio measured on a standard posteroanterior chest film provides an estimate of overall heart enlargement. The degree of LV enlargement is better assessed by lateral or oblique views. In the presence of a high pulmonary capillary pressure secondary to LV failure, pulmonary blood volume often is redistributed to the upper lobes in an upright film, producing the cephalization characteristic of left-sided HF. Pulmonary infiltrates and fibrosis occasionally masquerade as HF.

ELECTROCARDIOGRAM

Prior, or acute, myocardial infarction can be identified by Q waves on the electrocardiogram (ECG). Myocardial hypertrophy almost invariably accompanies HF, so that increased voltage or conduction abnormalities are often present. Left ventricular hypertrophy and cardiomyopathy may present with what appears to be localized loss of electrical forces that may be mistaken for a prior myocardial infarction (see Chapter 84). Evidence of atrial conduction delay (i.e., prolongation of the PR interval, QRS duration, and QT interval) is common in HF patients. These changes may predispose to cardiac arrhythmias. Both atrial and ventricular dysrhythmias are a common manifestation of HF, and evidence for their existence may be detected on a random ECG. Longer monitoring periods, especially 24-hour Holter monitoring, are likely to detect these arrhythmias.

BLOOD CHEMISTRY

The most important blood studies in the patient with HF are the serum electrolyte and renal function measurements. A low serum sodium concentration indicates a stimulated renin–angiotensin system as well as increased vasopressin, and will be observed in those patients requiring large doses of loop diuretics. A low serum potassium and contraction alkalosis may be observed with diuretic therapy as well. An elevated blood urea nitrogen or serum creatinine suggests either organic or functional renal impairment, due to vasoconstriction, and decreased cardiac output. Liver function abnormalities may suggest hepatic congestion.

VENTRICULAR PERFORMANCE

Ventricular function can be quantitated by imaging techniques, using either echocardiography or radionuclide gated blood pool scanning. An LV ejection fraction below 45% at rest is considered abnormal. Echocardiography also provides information about valve function and regional wall motion. Doppler flow measurements also identify the functional significance of observed stenotic and regurgitant valve lesions, which provides a better global assessment of the impact of HF on cardiac function, as well as etiologic information.

CARDIAC CATHETERIZATION

Noninvasive methods limit the requirement for contrast determination of LV function at angiography. Coronary angiography is often necessary to clarify etiology. Identification of high-grade coronary artery disease should prompt analysis for revascularization, as ongoing ischemia is a prominent cause for LV dysfunction and HF. Measurement of right heart and pulmonary artery pressures confirms the diagnosis of HF. Right heart catheterization is important when moderate to severe pulmonary hypertension has been suggested by physical examination or noninvasive studies. This procedure is also valuable in the management of complex HF. With quality echocardiography and Doppler studies, right heart catheterization is not required in all patients.

EXERCISE TESTING

Exercise testing can be carried out safely on the patient with HF, and the information obtained from this test is important in diagnostic and therapeutic efforts. An exercise test can be performed either informally in the examining room, by having the patient perform a 6-minute walk test, or formally with the use of a standard stress test using either a bicycle ergometer or a treadmill. The formal test obviously provides more information. Monitoring the ECG during exercise provides additional information that can give a clue to the presence of ischemic heart disease. Performing the stress test while monitoring gas exchange allows more precise assessment of the exercise burden at the point where the patient reaches his or her anaerobic threshold and the peak oxygen consumption that he or she can achieve. Its added value is distinguishing between cardiac, pulmonary, deconditioning, and nonmotivational disability.

■ STRATEGIES FOR MANAGEMENT

MANAGEMENT OVERVIEW

The goals of treatment for congestive HF are several. These include identification of correctable etiologies and cofactors, prevention of disease progression, maintenance of physical activity, reversal of sodium retention, and reduction of the risk of mortality. Of course, some of these factors can only be achieved or optimized through medical therapy of HF, particularly as the disorder reaches advanced stages. The angiotensin-converting enzyme (ACE) inhibitors are recommended for all stages of HF, not only for treatment but to prevent progression of ventricular dysfunction. Spironolactone, an aldosterone antagonist, has recently been shown to significantly reduce mortality when added to standard therapy. Diuretic therapy is used for the symptomatic and clinical relief of edema, but there are no data that identify a primary role for prevention of disease progression. Most clinicians believe that digoxin is safe and effective. More recently, β-adrenergic blockade has emerged as important therapy of HF, dispelling previous misconceptions regarding lack of benefit or even additive risk. It may be necessary to combine drugs with vasodilator properties to achieve desired end points, such as blood pressure reduction or clinical attenuation of mitral regurgitation. Additional issues include control of rhythm disturbances when possible and anticoagulation therapy when indicated. Parenteral therapy is used for decompensation of HF in order to stabilize a patient who has progressive deterioration.

COMORBIDITIES

The first major issue is ongoing myocardial ischemia or infarction. Progressive transmural or endocardial ischemia, or a new myocardial infarction, can produce abrupt decompensation in a previously stable HF patient. The presence of valvular heart disease should be apparent from the physical examination or echocardiographic evaluation. Mitral regurgitation of any origin produces an adverse effect on myocardial function in an otherwise stable HF patient, particularly since the severity of mitral regurgitation is not correlated with the acoustic properties of the accompanying murmur. In addition, the appearance of a new rhythm disorder, most commonly atrial fibrillation, will produce decompensation. Coexistent hypertension may not receive sufficient management in the presence of coexistent HF. In fact, the presence of a systolic arterial pressure of 140 to 150 mm Hg may erroneously be interpreted as evidence of good ventricular function. Quite contrary to this perception, a systolic blood pressure in the 130 to 140 mm Hg range, or a diastolic blood pressure in the 85 to 100 mm Hg range, requires aggressive blood pressure reduction in an individual with ventricular dysfunction and HF. Additional coexisting medical disorders may trigger decompensation. Insulin-dependent diabetes mellitus, progressive renal dysfunction, and pulmonary disease can adversely influence outcome. Pulmonary embolic events and chronic lung disease are not unusual in the HF patient. Pulmonary and upper respiratory infections are common in patients with stable HF, particularly in fall and winter. Likewise, urinary tract infections are not uncommon in the elderly HF population. These disorders are difficult to differentiate from progressive HF yet may trigger decompensation.

PATIENT DIRECTIVES

It is important to emphasize moderate sodium intake to avoid and/or manage advanced congestive HF. This is defined as 2 to 3 g of sodium (80 to 120 mEq), which is defined as the "normal" sodium requirement in humans and is palatable. Replacement of sodium with salt substitutes, which usually provide excess potassium, is often a suitable option. Weight loss in patients who are above ideal body weight is also a goal in the treatment of HF.

Restriction of physical activity produces deconditioning of skeletal muscle and reflex control of the circulation; therefore, it is not recommended. Low-level exercise is tolerated, even in later stages of HF. If necessary, cardiac exercise testing can be used as a means to recommend the level of exercise permitted during chronic follow-up. Dynamic exercise, including swimming and vigorous walking, should be encouraged within the limits of tolerance. The benefits of exercise probably do not extend to isometric forms of exercise, which increase ventricular afterload.

■ CHRONIC PHARMACOLOGIC THERAPY

ANGIOTENSIN-CONVERTING ENZYME INHIBITORS

The hemodynamic benefits of ACE inhibitors in HF and hypertension have been firmly established. The predominant hemodynamic effect of ACE inhibitors is to decrease systemic vascular resistance, associated with a significant increase of cardiac output. In addition, they improve clinical signs and symptoms, as well as improve exercise tolerance in patients with moderate to severe HF treated with diuretics and digoxin. The ACE inhibitors also slow the onset of symptomatic HF and clinical progression in patients with mild HF. The ACE inhibitors have been shown to prolong survival in HF patients, including asymptomatic and symptomatic LV dysfunction in the setting of acute myocardial infarction. As the major etiologic factor for HF in most patients is coronary artery disease or previous myocardial infarction, the observation that limiting LV enlargement and progressive HF after myocardial infarction is beneficial has been a strong factor for the early use of ACE inhibitors.

General guidelines can be identified that are applicable for all ACE inhibitors. First, consider the baseline renal function and extent of diuretic-induced prerenal azotemia, particularly in the elderly patient. Second, initiate ACE inhibitor therapy in relatively small doses. When initiating ACE inhibitors for HF, upward titration from a low starting dose is recommended, followed by progressive increase in ACE inhibitor dosage toward levels utilized in clinical trials that have established long-term benefit. The diuretic dosage should be reduced if hypotension develops. Symptomatic hypotension, or reduction of systolic blood pressure below physiologic lower limits of 80 to 85 mm Hg, would be reason to postpone ACE inhibitor therapy until diuretics are further decreased or until the cause of hypotension has been clarified. However, reduction of blood pressure to the range of 90 to 100 mm Hg should not be considered an adverse effect and is evidence of achieving the therapeutic end point. In patients with HF, renal perfusion and function is typically impaired. With the known underlying renal impairment of HF, transient reduction of renal function may occur but should not discourage continued use of the ACE inhibitor. During longer term use, renal function will return toward baseline in most individuals. Both reducing diuretic dosage and avoiding cyclooxygenase inhibitors, such as indomethacin, and nonsteroidal anti-inflammatory agents is important to minimize the impact of ACE inhibitors on renal function. Other class effects of ACE inhibitors include hyperkalemia, nonproductive cough, skin rash, altered taste, and, rarely, angioedema. Of course, use of ACE inhibitors in pregnant females is contraindicated.

The typical dosage range of ACE inhibitors is supported by clinical trial outcomes. For captopril, initial dosage is 6.25 mg t.i.d., increasing to 50 mg t.i.d. For enalapril, initial dosage is 2.5 mg b.i.d., increasing to 20 mg b.i.d. Lisinopril is initiated at 5 mg daily, increased to 40 mg daily. Quinapril dosage is initiated at 2.5 mg b.i.d. and can be increased to 20 mg b.i.d. Ramapril is initiated at 1.25 mg twice daily, increasing to 20 or 40 mg daily. Fosinopril is initiated at 2.5 mg daily, increasing to 20 mg daily. The final dose chosen for all ACE inhibitors is established according to tolerance, with the realization that the maximal dose might not be achieved.

The specific angiotensin II AT_1 antagonists are beneficial in the treatment of hypertension and demonstrate evidence of benefit in some HF trials. There is currently controversy regarding the role of this class of therapy in HF, and none of these agents has been approved for the treatment of HF. Physicians appear to be using these agents "off label" for the treatment of HF in those individuals suspected of having an ACE inhibitor cough. It is advisable to evaluate the differential diagnosis of cough (including worsening failure) prior to assuming an ACE inhibitor cough.

Another renin system inhibitor is a very old drug, with very recent results in an international trial. Spironolactone is a specific aldosterone antagonist. In high doses, it has weak diuretic properties and has been used for decades, with the adverse potential for gynecomastia in men and hyperkalemia in certain clinical situations. In the recent RALES trial, spironolactone, added to standard therapy of ACE inhibitor, diuretic, and digoxin, produced a highly significant reduction of mortality compared to placebo. The effective target dose in the trial was 25 mg daily, which is much lower then the historical dosage of this drug. At this dose, the risk of hyperkalemia and gynecomastia are low but still present. Evaluation of serum potassium is required at intervals.

OTHER VASODILATORS

In patients who cannot tolerate ACE inhibitors, the combination of hydralazine and isosorbide dinitrate is a very acceptable and proven therapeutic option. In two successive Veterans Administration cooperative trials, this combination has been shown to significantly reduce mortality. In a direct comparison with the ACE inhibitor enalapril, hydralazine/isosorbide dinitrate did not produce as great a mortality reduction as enalapril. However, the combination did produce a greater improvement of exercise duration than enalapril, as well as a small but significantly greater increase in ejection fraction. Hydralazine dosage should be titrated up to 75 or 100 mg 4 times a day, to achieve optimal hemodynamic effect without an undue risk of side effects. Most experience exists with isosorbide dinitrate. This has been administered in doses of 20 to 60 mg 3 or 4 times daily. Nitroglycerin patches may be used, but less information exists regarding their efficacy, compared with isosorbide dinitrate. Tolerance to the hemodynamic benefit of nitrates is well known. It can be minimized by deletion of a daily dose of nitrates (the last dose of the day), or the patch can be removed for several hours each day.

The calcium channel blockers have become popular in cardiovascular medicine. These are pharmacologically diverse compounds. While verapamil was the prototypical agent, diltiazem and the dihydropyridine class of calcium channel blockers are particularly utilized. The prominent vasodilator effect of these agents stimulated the notion that they may be effective for the treatment of HF. However, this has not been substantiated by clinical trials. Therefore, no calcium channel blocker is approved for the treatment of HF, and they should only be used for the treatment of the comorbid conditions of hypertension or active angina.

Vasodilators, such as the α-blockers, and minoxidil failed to demonstrate long-term benefit in HF. Their use should be considered ancillary therapy: to provide intermittent symptomatic relief of HF, for coexistent hypertension, or for symptoms of prostatic hypertrophy (α-blockers).

DIURETICS

By reducing the intravascular volume, these drugs also relieve increased interstitial fluid by allowing its reabsorption into the vascular space. There is no single laboratory test or diagnostic study that provides a simple assessment of volume status in the HF patient. Findings on physical exam remain the most valuable means to assess fluid status. The central venous pressure, particularly its response to abdominal pressure or leg raising, may provide an estimate of venous volume. It is less accurate in the setting of tricuspid regurgitation. Peripheral pitting edema is also a valuable sign of total body volume expansion. The presence of rales also indicates excessive pulmonary fluid. The value of body weight is best determined with serial measurements, where recent fluctuation identifies the need for alteration in diuretic dosage.

The loop diuretics, including furosemide, are the mainstay of diuretic therapy in most patients with HF. Dosage should not exceed known ceiling levels. In mild failure, thiazides may be adequate to attenuate sodium retention. The dosage of loop diuretics must be carefully adjusted and modified when the fluid status changes. Patients should be instructed in sodium intake, the importance of daily weights, and the potential for intermittent adjustment of diuretics.

It is not unusual for a patient with congestive HF to become resistant to diuretics, and several clinical issues can influence such resistance, including renal insufficiency and aging. Edema of the gastrointestinal tract can also reduce drug absorption, thereby limiting efficacy. Different classes of diuretic agents may act at different locations within the nephron, so that combination therapy, as discussed below, may be appropriate in the patient with developing refractory HF. At the very least, a patient should not be considered "refractory to diuretic" if receiving only moderate doses of an oral loop diuretic. There are several approaches to the management of resistance to diuretics that can aid in the optimization of diuretic therapy for the refractory HF patient. A single large bolus of intravenous diuretics may substantially improve urinary flow and natriuresis. Continuous intravenous infusion of a loop diuretic may be efficacious. Perhaps the most versatile and effective approach is the combination of a loop diuretic with a thiazide-type diuretic. Long-standing treatment with a loop diuretic can result in hypertrophy of the distal segment of the nephron, producing enhanced sodium reabsorption. This adverse effect can be overcome by coadministration of a thiazide-type diuretic. If the patient remains resistant to diuretics, additional treatment modalities can be considered. Ultrafiltration, hemofiltration, hemodialysis, or peritoneal dialysis can be utilized for rapid removal of fluid.

Hypokalemia is a common manifestation in patients treated with diuretics and may contribute to dysrhythmias, especially in patients receiving digoxin. Most commonly, diuretic-induced hypokalemia is associated with a metabolic alkalosis and a coexisting chloride deficit. Therefore, chloride is the preferred form of potassium in this setting. Frequent measurement of the serum potassium level is necessary during stages of intense diuresis.

Chronic diuretic therapy also leads to hypomagnesemia. Potassium and magnesium have an interrelationship whereas magnesium is a cofactor in the appropriate function of the

Na^+,K^+-ATPase pump. Therefore, hypokalemia may persist until the magnesium deficiency is corrected. Low serum magnesium levels may contribute to dysrhythmias in patients with HF. Oral magnesium replacement should be considered in all patients with low serum levels and when increased arrhythmias are noted in the setting of intense diuretic therapy.

DIGOXIN

There is a role for digoxin therapy in HF patients in normal sinus rhythm. This was established by multicenter studies demonstrating favorable benefits of digoxin therapy. Furthermore, mechanistic studies have demonstrated beneficial effects of digoxin upon electrophysiologic and neurohormonal abnormalities. Based on most recent clinical trials, use of a standard digoxin dosage of 0.125 or 0.25 mg daily is sufficient. Reduction of the dose to an every-other- day regimen is recommended for patients with significant renal disease (serum creatinine greater than 2.5 to 3.0 mg per dL), the elderly, or patients receiving other drugs that interfere with the metabolism of digoxin. When an individual is receiving digoxin for the first time, a loading dose given either orally or intravenously is required. In patients with atrial fibrillation or advanced HF, the digoxin dosage may be increased to 0.375 mg daily. Routine surveillance of digoxin levels is generally not required when routine doses are utilized. If a patient requires dose reduction for concomitant renal failure, then more routine surveillance of serum levels may be required. Serum levels should be measure at dose nadir, to avoid erroneous determinations.

β-ADRENORECEPTOR BLOCKERS

β-Adrenergic blockade is emerging as the most important "new" breakthrough in the treatment of HF, with at least three major survival analyses demonstrating significant reduction of mortality, with three different drugs. Long considered as "negative inotropes," it is clear that β-blockers exert favorable effects in HF, through reduction of heart rate, suppression of the renin system, and resetting of abnormal sympathetic nervous system and baroreflex abnormalities. The size of the heart decreases, and β-blockers produce a significant increase of ventricular ejection fraction, which would not have been predicted by their putative negative inotropic effects.

A highly significant reduction of mortality with bisoprolol and metoprolol, in their respective trials, prompted early termination of the randomized trials. The target dose of bisoprolol is 10 mg daily; the target dose of metoprolol (in its extended release preparation) is 100 mg b.i.d. A unique "β-blocker" is carvedilol, which also reduced mortality and was associated with dose-dependent clinical improvement. This compound, while predominantly a β-blocker, also has α-blocking and antioxidant properties, with vasodilator effects. The target dose is 25 mg b.i.d. In these trials, the β-blocker was added to standard therapy and therefore should not be considered a substitute for ACE inhibitor therapy.

For all of these drugs, the key to therapy is to begin with the lowest possible dose and gradually advance to the target dose over the course of 1 to 3 months. In complicated patients, up-titration may require close vigilance. At early stages of therapy, observe for signs of increased dyspnea or edema, requiring temporary up-titration of diuretics. Symptomatic hypotension with carvedilol may require a slower rate of up-titration. At all stages, particularly with coadministration of digoxin or amiodarone, monitor for bradycardia or heart block.

ANTIARRHYTHMIC THERAPY AND DEVICES

The absence of synchronized atrial contraction contributes to functional impairment and deterioration in this population. Reasonable attempts should be made to convert a patient to normal sinus rhythm prior to the development of marked left atrial enlargement, which would lessen the likelihood of successful conversion. Pharmacologic or electrical cardioversions in this population are similar to those in other patients with atrial fibrillation. Atrioventricular junctional block and intraventricular conduction defects occur, necessitating permanent pacemaker implantation.

Treatment of ventricular arrhythmias is covered elsewhere in this text. However, electrolyte replacement and optimization of therapy for HF, including effective doses of an ACE inhibitor, should be utilized prior to consideration of specific therapy for ventricular arrhythmia. High-grade ventricular arrhythmias may be noted on routine ambulatory heart rate monitoring in many patients with moderate to severe HF. Sudden death accounts for anywhere from 35% to 70% of total mortality in published studies of the HF population. However, not all sudden death is due to ventricular tachycardia or fibrillation. However, the clinical significance of ventricular premature beats, often in couplets and runs, remains uncertain. Random suppression of these isolated events could expose patients to adverse proarrhythmic actions of many antiarrhythmic drugs, as well as depression of ventricular function. A mortality benefit of amiodarone in HF has been reported but not conclusively established in other HF trials. In HF patients with symptomatic ventricular arrhythmias, implanting a cardiac defibrillator is justified to prevent sudden death.

ANTICOAGULATION

Patients with severe chronic HF are at risk of developing mural thrombi in the dilated left atrium or left ventricle. Patients with chronic atrial fibrillation are particularly at risk of developing atrial thrombi. These thrombi are potential sources of systemic emboli. If clinical symptoms or signs (atrial fibrillation, evidence of thrombi by noninvasive tests such as echocardiography) suggest the presence of intracardiac thrombi, the patient should be treated with warfarin, unless there are specific contraindications. Aspirin may serve as an alternative to warfarin in some individuals.

TREATMENT OF ADVANCED HEART FAILURE

ACUTE MEDICAL MANAGEMENT

The phrase "refractory HF" should be reserved for progressive decompensation despite adequate dosage of digoxin, diuretics, and an ACE inhibitor (or adequate alternate vasodilator regimen). This distinguishes the refractory HF syndrome from forms of acute HF such as cardiogenic shock due to myocardial infarction (see Chapter 71).

In some cases, refractory HF may respond to intravenous diuretic therapy. However, management of refractory HF typically requires short-term hospitalization. Intravenous dobutamine, given in a range of 2.5 to 10 μg per kg per minute over the course of 24 to 96 hours provides clinical and hemodynamic stabilization. The favorable response to short-term dobutamine cannot be extrapolated to continuous or intermittent outpatient therapy. This latter practice remains questionable. Use of intravenous milrinone parallels the use of dobutamine. Milrinone requires an initial bolus dose and has direct vasodilator properties at higher doses of 0.5 and 0.75 μg per kg per minute. The reader should refer to Chapter 71 for additional information.

SURGICAL CONSIDERATIONS

If coronary angiography discloses significant lesions that could be contributing to myocardial dysfunction, coronary bypass surgery or angioplasty should be considered. In the presence of severe LV dysfunction, a myocardial imaging study should be obtained to document reversible ischemia. Ventricular assistance devices are being used as a bridge to transplant in many patients, and studies are in progress to determine their role as primary therapy in patients who are not transplant candidates. Heart transplantation is now a practical clinical approach to the management of severe HF in appropriate patients. The major limiting factor is lack of availability of donor hearts. The reader is referred to Chapter 93 for additional information.

BIBLIOGRAPHY

Cody RJ. Comparing angiotensin-converting enzyme inhibitor trial results in patients with acute myocardial infarction. *Arch Intern Med* 1004; 154:2029–2036.

Cody RJ, Kubo SH, Pickworth KK. Diuretic utilization for the sodium retention of congestive heart failure. *Arch Intern Med* 1994;154: 1905–1914.

Cody RJ. Alteration of hormonal factors in heart failure. In: Hosenpud JD, Greenberg BH, eds. *Congestive heart failure: pathophysiology, diagnosis, and comprehensive approach to management.* New York: Springer-Verlag (in press).

Cohn JN. The management of chronic heart failure. *N Engl J Med* 1996; 335:490–498.

Konstam M, Dracup K, Baker D, et al. *Heart failure: evaluation and care of patients with left ventricular systolic dysfunction.* Clinical Practice Guideline No. 11. AHCPR Publication No. 94-0612. Rockville, MD. US Department of Health and Human Services, June 1994.

Schocken DD, Arrieta MI, Leaverton PE, et al. Prevalence and mortality rate of congestive heart failure in the United States. *J Am Coll Cardiol* 1992;20:301.

Kelley's Textbook of Internal Medicine, fourth edition. Edited by H. David Humes. Lippincott Williams & Wilkins, Philadelphia © 2000.

APPROACH TO THE PATIENT WITH CARDIAC ARRHYTHMIAS

S. ADAM STRICKBERGER
DOUGLAS P. ZIPES
FRED MORADY

Evaluation of the patient with a cardiac arrhythmia begins with the consideration of five questions:

- Does the patient have a cardiac arrhythmia?
- What are the consequences of the arrhythmia?
- Does the patient have associated cardiac problems?
- What is the cause of the arrhythmia?
- What, if anything, should be done?

Does the patient have a cardiac arrhythmia? Obtaining a careful history and performing a thorough physical examination provides the initial clues to the presence of a cardiac arrhythmia. Palpitations, syncope, presyncope, chest pain, or symptoms of congestive heart failure may result from the arrhythmia and are revealed during the history taking. Some patients may be able to tap their fingers in the cadence of a perceived palpitation or recognize the beat tapped out by a physician and, in so doing, establish not only the presence of an arrhythmia but also its rate and rhythm. The patient, or sometimes a close relative, should be instructed in how to determine the pulse rate during the arrhythmia. A rapid, grossly irregular rhythm may suggest atrial fibrillation; a regular rhythm at a rate of 150 beats per minute, atrial flutter with 2:1 conduction; a regular rhythm at a rate of 180 to 200 beats per minute, paroxysmal supraventricular or ventricular tachycardia; or a regular rhythm at a rate of 40 beats per minute, sinus bradycardia or heart block.

The patient's characteristics also help refine the interpretation of data obtained in the history. For example, in a young, otherwise healthy individual with a heart rate of 180 beats per minute, paroxysmal supraventricular tachycardia would be suggested, whereas in an older patient with presyncope, ventricular tachycardia would be more likely. A heart rate of 40 beats per minute in a young person might be a normal sinus bradycardia but signify acquired atrioventricular (AV) block in an elderly individual.

Documenting the arrhythmia by electrocardiogram (ECG) clearly establishes its presence. The electrocardiographic characteristics of the arrhythmia are considered elsewhere in this text. However, physical findings caused by the arrhythmia, in addition to changes in cardiac rate and rhythm, might be helpful. Findings that indicate the presence of AV dissociation, such as a variable peak systolic blood pressure, variable intensity of the first heart sound, and intermittent cannon *a* waves in the jugular venous pulse, suggest arrhythmias like ventricular tachycardia or complete AV block. The second heart sound may be paradoxically split during a QRS complex with a left bundle-branch block contour or widely split without becoming single during expiration caused by right bundle-branch block.

Carotid sinus massage increases vagal tone, which slows the rate of sinus node discharge, and prolongs AV nodal conduction time and refractoriness. These responses can cause (a) a sinus tachycardia to slow gradually or terminate, (b) AV nodal reentry, AV reciprocating tachycardias in the Wolff–Parkinson–White (WPW) syndrome, and some atrial tachycardias to terminate abruptly, and (c) the ventricular response to atrial flutter, atrial fibrillation, and some atrial tachycardias to decrease. Rarely, carotid sinus massage terminates a ventricular tachycardia.

What are the consequences of the arrhythmia? A consideration of the consequences of the arrhythmia in an individual patient is important because arrhythmias are not isolated events and should be managed in the context of the entire clinical situation. When a patient develops a tachyarrhythmia, slowing the ventricular rate is the initial and often most important therapeutic maneuver. Therapy might differ radically for the same arrhythmia in two different patients, however, because the consequences of the tachycardia differ. For example, a supraventricular tachycardia at a rate of 200 beats per minute may produce few or no symptoms in a healthy young adult and therefore might require little or no therapy if it is usually self-limited. The same arrhythmia can precipitate pulmonary edema in a patient with mitral stenosis, syncope in a patient with aortic stenosis, or shock in a patient with acute myocardial infarction. In addition to hemodynamic consequences, the presence of structural heart disease may have other effects. For example, having mitral stenosis may increase the chance of emboli developing in patients with atrial fibrillation. A persistent, uncontrollable tachycardia can result in cardiomegaly and congestive heart failure, often reversible if the tachycardia is stopped. This is called a tachycardia-induced cardiomyopathy. Thus, the presence of heart disease influences the effects of an arrhythmia, but the latter can also cause heart disease.

Does the patient have associated cardiac problems? Whereas the presence of associated cardiac problems influences the consequences of the arrhythmia, certain cardiac lesions are associated with, or predispose to the development of, certain arrhythmias. For example, Ebstein's anomaly is associated with the WPW syndrome. Repair of some congenital cardiac defects such as tetralogy of Fallot can predispose to the subsequent development of cardiac arrhythmias. The presence of a left ventricular aneurysm or a ventricular tumor (usually in infants) can set the stage for ventricular arrhythmias.

What is the cause of the arrhythmia? Information about circumstances that trigger the tachycardia, such as excessive caffeine or alcohol intake, cigarette smoking, or emotionally upsetting events, are important. Nonprescription cold medications can contain sympathomimetic drugs that can produce arrhythmias. Disease states such as ischemia, thyrotoxicosis, hypotension, infection, anemia, or valvular heart disease should be considered.

The cause of the arrhythmia may influence therapy. Electrolyte imbalance, acidosis or alkalosis, hypoxemia, congestive heart failure, and many drugs can produce rhythm disturbances (Table

TABLE 67.1.	**DRUGS ASSOCIATED WITH VENTRICULAR PROARRHYTHMIA**

Antiarrhythmic agents[a]
  Flecainide
  Procainamide
  Propafenone
  Quinidine
  Sotalol
Antibiotics
  Erythromycin
  Pentamidine
  Trimethoprim and sulfamethoxazole
Antifungal agents
  Fluconazole
  Ketoconazole
Antihistamines
  Astemizole
  Terfenadine
Cisapride
Phenothiazine derivatives
Probucol
Tricyclic antidepressants (amitriptyline)

[a] Amiodarone is rarely associated with ventricular proarrhythmia.

67.1), and their identification and treatment can abolish or prevent these arrhythmias. Mild sedation or reassurance may be successful in treating some arrhythmias related to emotional stress. Because therapy always involves some risk, one must be sure, particularly as the therapeutic regimen escalates, that the risks of not treating the arrhythmia continue to outweigh the risks of therapy with potentially hazardous antiarrhythmic measures; correction of precipitating factors is often the simplest and safest form of therapy.

What, if anything, should be done? Therapy of cardiac arrhythmias involves a choice of three modalities: pharmacologic, electrical, and surgical. These are considered in the following sections.

PHARMACOLOGIC THERAPY

Pharmacologic therapy to maintain sinus rhythm is no longer the mainstay of therapy. While drugs still often are used, nonpharmacologic therapy, including catheter ablation and implantable defibrillators, is frequently prescribed for symptomatic paroxysmal supraventricular tachycardia and for the treatment of ventricular tachycardia and fibrillation, respectively. However, pharmacologic therapy is the mainstay of therapy for atrial fibrillation. Many experts believe that ablation therapy for atrial fibrillation will be commonly utilized within 5 to 10 years. A brief discussion regarding ablation therapy follows in this chapter.

The primary objective of pharmacologic therapy is to reach, as rapidly as possible, an effective and well-tolerated serum drug concentration that controls the arrhythmia and to maintain this serum drug concentration for as long as required without producing adverse effects. So-called therapeutic drug concentrations are based on concentrations of drugs that exert therapeutic effects without adverse effects in most patients. The therapeutic serum concentration varies from one patient to another, but for any individual patient, it is the amount of drug required to suppress or terminate the cardiac arrhythmia in that patient without producing adverse effects. Thus, the actual serum concentration of the drug in a specific patient is often of secondary importance. Careful dosing is essential because antiarrhythmic agents have narrow toxic/therapeutic relationships, and important adverse effects can result from amounts of drug that only slightly exceed the amount necessary to produce beneficial effects. An understanding of drug pharmacokinetics—which consists of an understanding of drug absorption, distribution, metabolism, and excretion—is essential.

A complete discussion of the common antiarrhythmic agents can be found in Chapter 90.

ELECTRICAL THERAPY OF CARDIAC ARRHYTHMIAS

CARDIOVERSION AND DEFIBRILLATION

Electrical cardioversion (shock delivered synchronously with the QRS complex) and defibrillation (shock delivered without synchronization to the QRS complex to terminate ventricular fibrillation) appear to terminate most effectively those tachycardias presumed to be due to reentry, including atrial flutter and atrial fibrillation, AV nodal reentry, reciprocating tachycardias associated with the WPW syndrome, most forms of ventricular tachycardia (Fig. 67.1), ventricular flutter, and ventricular fibrillation (Fig. 67.2). The electric shock, by depolarizing all excitable myocardium and prolonging refractoriness, interrupts reentrant circuits and establishes electrical homogeneity that terminates reentry. For elective cardioversion, self-adhesive pads applied in the standard apex–anterior or apex–posterior paddle positions are quite effective. A synchronized shock is used for all cardioversions except for very rapid ventricular tachyarrhythmias, such as ventricular flutter or fibrillation. Shocks generally are titrated when the clinical situation permits. The starting level to termi-

nate atrial fibrillation should probably be 50 to 100 J. For patients with stable ventricular tachycardia, starting levels in the range of 25 to 50 J may be employed. If there is some urgency to terminate the tachyarrhythmia, one can begin with higher energies. To terminate ventricular fibrillation, 200 to 360 J generally is used, although much lower energies terminate ventricular fibrillation when the shock is delivered at the very onset of the arrhythmia. During elective cardioversion, a short-acting barbiturate such as methohexital or an amnesic, such as diazepam, should be used. A physician skilled in airway management should be in attendance, intravenous access should be established, and all equipment necessary for emergency resuscitation should be immediately accessible.

Generally, any tachycardia that produces hypotension, congestive heart failure, or angina and that does not respond quickly and appropriately to medical management should be terminated electrically. Direct current countershock of digitalis-induced tachyarrhythmias is contraindicated because more severe arrhythmias might result from the shock. Electrical cardioversion restores sinus rhythm in 70% to 95% of patients, depending on the type of tachyarrhythmia. If the first shock fails to restore sinus rhythm or does so only transiently, a second shock should be delivered at a higher energy level or after antiarrhythmic drug administration.

Arrhythmias induced by the shock generally are caused by inadequate synchronization, with the shock occurring during the ST segment or T wave. It is important to remember, however, that occasionally even a properly synchronized shock can produce ventricular fibrillation. Postshock arrhythmias usually are transient and do not require therapy. Embolic episodes are reported in 1% to 3% of the patients converted to sinus rhythm from atrial fibrillation. Prior anticoagulation therapy for at least 3 weeks should be considered for patients with atrial fibrillation of more than 48 hours duration. Anticoagulation therapy for at least 3 to 4 weeks after conversion to sinus rhythm appears to be indicated.

Patients with atrial fibrillation who can be considered for electrical cardioversion have new-onset atrial fibrillation or atrial fibrillation of relatively short duration; recurrent emboli or he-

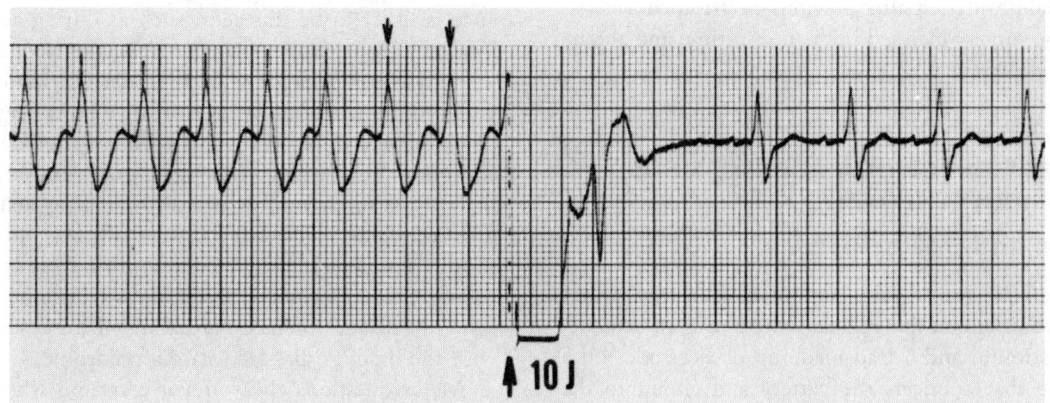

FIGURE 67.1. Electrical cardioversion of ventricular tachycardia. Artifacts indicating synchronization of the external cardioverter to the QRS complex *(inverted arrows)* are seen before delivery of a 10-J shock *(upright arrow)* that is followed by a repetitive ventricular response and the restoration of sinus rhythm.

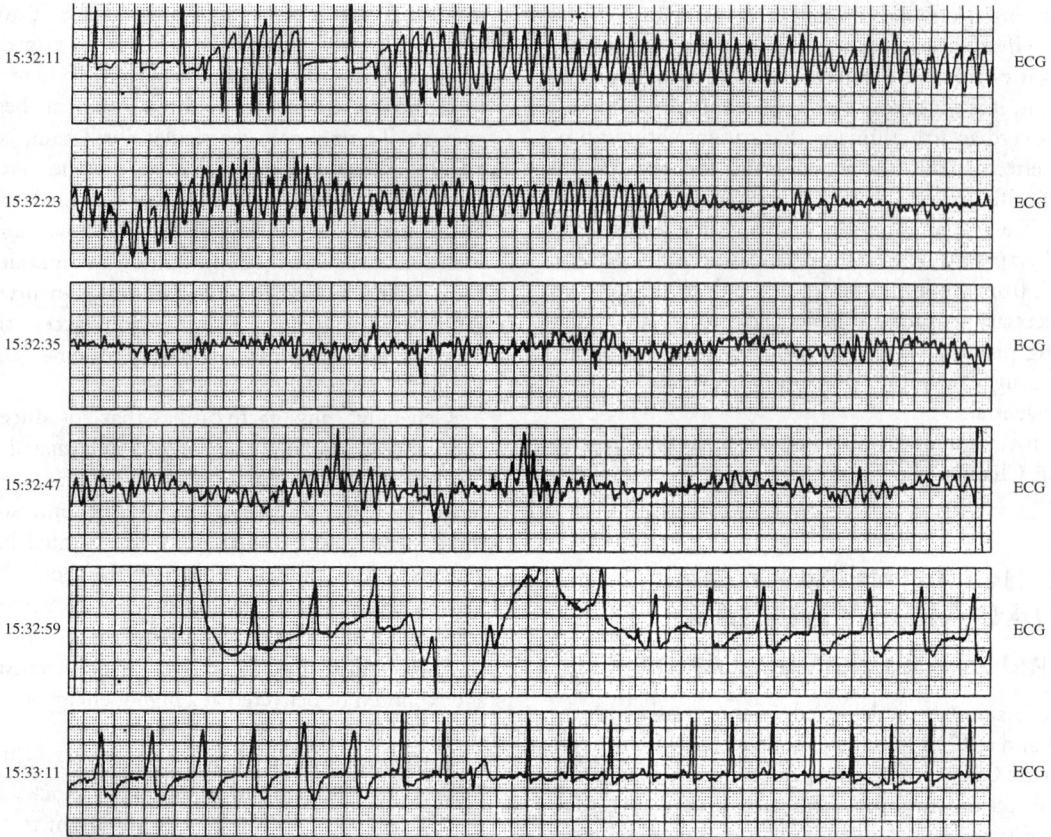

FIGURE 67.2. Direct current defibrillation. Spontaneous onset of ventricular tachycardia occurs in the top strip. It degenerates to ventricular fibrillation, terminated by a transthoracic shock at the end of the fourth strip. Time on left is in hours:minutes:seconds.

modynamic insufficiency during the atrial fibrillation; or a transient precipitating cause removed, such as thyrotoxicosis or correction of mitral stenosis. Patients who are less favorable candidates for electrical cardioversion have atrial fibrillation of long duration, with easily controlled ventricular rates, and no symptoms; sinus node dysfunction; digitalis toxicity; a large left atrium; a history of short-lasting episodes with a high likelihood of spontaneous reversion to sinus rhythm; a history of early reversion to atrial fibrillation after previous electrical conversion attempts; cardiac surgery planned in the near future; and antiarrhythmic drug intolerance.

IMPLANTABLE ELECTRICAL DEVICES FOR TREATING ARRHYTHMIAS

Pacemakers and Defibrillators

A pacemaker is an electronic device composed of a battery power source, an electronic circuit that regulates the timing and characteristics of the stimuli, and a lead made up of electrodes on a catheter or wire that connects the battery and circuit to the heart. Devices called cardioverter–defibrillators are capable of delivering electrical shocks, rather than small-intensity pacing stimuli, directly to the heart to cardiovert or defibrillate.

Treatment of Bradycardia

Drugs generally do not successfully and reliably speed up the heart rate or improve AV conduction for long periods without producing significant side effects in patients who have symptomatic bradycardias. Therefore, regardless of the arrhythmia producing the bradycardia, if the patient is symptomatic with it, pacing is indicated unless the bradycardia is likely to be very brief. Temporary pacing can be used when the rhythm disturbance is likely to be transient, such as during acute myocardial infarction in patients who experience transient AV block.

Permanent pacing for bradycardia is indicated in patients with symptomatic bradycardia of any type as long as it is likely to be permanent or recurrent and is not associated with a transient condition from which the patient may recover, such as acute myocardial infarction, myocarditis, or drug toxicity. Third-degree AV block that is fixed or intermittent and sick sinus syndrome represent the most common indications for permanent pacing. Some patients with sick sinus syndrome also have intermittent episodes of tachycardia and form a subset of patients with the bradycardia–tachycardia syndrome.

Major questions always revolve around who should receive prophylactic pacing. Most agree that the asymptomatic patient with acquired complete AV block or type II second-degree AV block should receive permanent pacing prophylactically because

TABLE 67.2.	FIVE-POSITION PACEMAKER CODE

Chamber-paced
O = none
V = ventricle
A = atrium
D = atrium and ventricle (dual)

Chamber-sensed
O = none
V = ventricle
A = atrium
D = atrium and ventricle (dual)

Mode of response[a]
O = none
I = inhibited
T = triggered
D = atrial triggered and ventricular inhibited (dual)

Programmability, rate modulation
O = none
P = simple programmable
M = multiprogrammable
C = communicating (via telemetry; includes multiprogrammable)
R = rate modulation (via activity sensing, etc.)

Antitachyarrhythmia functions
O = none
P = pacing (antitachyarrhythmia)
S = shock
D = pacing and shock (dual)

---

[a] I indicates that any spontaneous electrical activity sensed by the pacemaker inhibits pacemaker discharge. T indicates that any spontaneous electrical activity sensed by the pacemaker triggers the pacemaker to discharge a pacing stimulus into the refractory period of the chamber where the electrical event was sensed, harmlessly dissipating the ineffective spike. D in this section, in contrast to the D under "chamber-paced" and "chamber-sensed," indicates that atrial and ventricular sensed events inhibit their respective outputs. An atrial paced or sensed event will also trigger ventricular pacing if a ventricular event is not sensed.

these patients commonly develop syncope, presyncope, or sudden cardiac death without pacemaker therapy. More controversial are other groups of patients. For example, it has been suggested that permanent prophylactic pacing reduces sudden death in survivors of acute myocardial infarction complicated by bundle-branch block and transient high-degree AV block. The number of these types of patients who have been carefully studied is small, however, and the data are not conclusive.

Pacemakers can operate in a variety of complex combinations, generally explained by a letter code of five positions (Table 67.2). After a sensed or paced atrial event, the pacemaker delivers a ventricular stimulus after a set AV interval if the P wave does not conduct to the ventricle within that time limit. If the P wave does conduct to the ventricle, then the ventricular spike is inhibited from discharging (Fig. 67.3). In some instances, the pacing mode can change automatically. Generally, mode switching is used in patients who are usually in sinus rhythm but in whom paroxysmal atrial fibrillation occurs. In this instance, the pacemaker will switch from dual-chamber pacing to pacing in the ventricle only.

The various types of pacemakers, the code letters of the first three positions, and their functions are listed in Table 67.3. The nature of the patient's rhythm disturbance determines the type of pacing. By considering the patient's atrial rhythm and capability for AV conduction, one can determine the best mode for pacing (Table 67.4).

All permanent pacemakers have programmable capabilities. That means that the electronically controlled features of the pacemaker can be altered in a noninvasive, reversible fashion using an external programmer. Rate, stimulus output, amplitude or duration, amplifier sensitivity, amplifier refractory period, pacing mode, and other functions are programmable. Thus, pacemaker function can be optimized for specific patient needs, malfunctions can be corrected, and the system can be revised to accommodate changing clinical situations.

Because many patients cannot increase their heart rates with exercise due to sinus node dysfunction or the presence of atrial

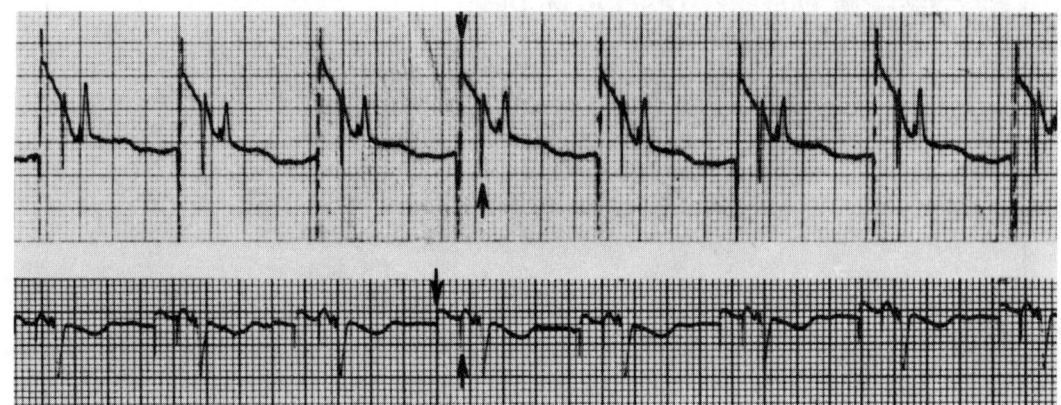

FIGURE 67.3. Dual-chamber pacing. In these two monitor strips from two different patients, two stimuli are apparent. The first *(inverted arrow)* is delivered to the atrium and the second *(upright arrow)* to the ventricle. This is an example of a DDD pacemaker, pacing first the atrium and then the ventricle after a preset atrioventricular interval.

TABLE 67.3.	PACEMAKER SENSING AND PACING

Pacemaker Type	Code	Atrium	Ventricle	Response to Sensed Activity
Atrial asynchronous	AOO	P, S		None
Ventricular asynchronous	VOO	P, S		None
Atrial demand	AAI	P,S		Inhibited by A
	AAT	P, S		Triggered by A
Ventricular demand	VVI		P, S	Inhibited by V
	VVT		P, S	Triggered by V
Atrial synchronous	VAT	S, P	P, S	Triggered by A
Atrial synchronous, ventricular inhibited	VDD	S, P	P, S	Triggered by A, inhibited by V
AV sequential	DVI	P, S	P, S	Inhibited by V
AV sequential	DDI	P, S	P, S	Inhibited by A
				Inhibited by V
AV universal	DDD	P, S	P, S	Inhibited by A
				Inhibited by V
				Triggered by A
Rate-responsive	R			Triggered by physiologic variables such as mechanical vibration, QT, duration, respiration, and others.

P, pacing; S, sensing; A, atrium; V, ventricle.

fibrillation and AV block, several physiologic variables, independent of sinus node function, have been used to alter the pacemaker rate according to physiologic needs. Such approaches for so-called rate-adaptive pacemakers include monitoring changes in the QT interval, respiratory rate, ventricular pressure, and body activity. The activity-sensing pacemaker uses a conventional lead system for sensing cardiac activity and pacing the heart. However, a microphone-like sensor inside the pacemaker pulse generator responds to mechanical vibrations of the body by producing electrical signals proportional to the patient's level of physical activity. As activity increases, the heart is paced more rapidly. Naturally, this pacemaker cannot increase the discharge rate when non-exercise-induced metabolic demands result, such as from mental activity while at rest. A second minor drawback

TABLE 67.4.	PREFERRED PACING MODES[a]

	Atrial Rhythm		
AV Conduction	Normal	Bradycardia	Bradycardia–Tachycardia
Normal	None	AAIR	AAIR
AV block, normal retrograde conduction time	DDD	DDDR	DDIR
AV block, prolonged retrograde conduction time	DDI	DDIR	VVIR, DDIR
AV block without retrograde conduction	DDD	DDDR	DDIR

[a] Depending on the individual patient and clinical circumstances, other modes of pacing may be preferable to those shown here, such as pacemakers with mode switching.
AV, atrioventricular.

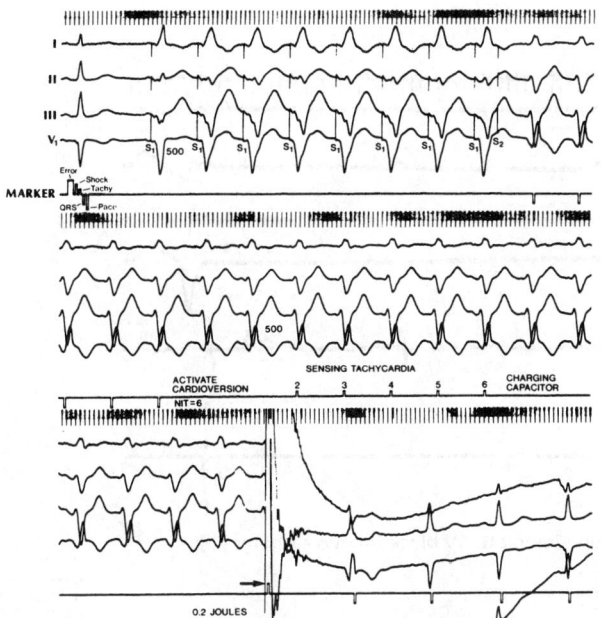

FIGURE 67.4. Implantable transvenous cardioverter. (Top) After a series of eight stimuli (S₁), the S₂ fails to produce a ventricular response. Nevertheless, sustained ventricular tachycardia ensues at a cycle length of 500 milliseconds. The device is activated *(middle)* to cardiovert the ventricular tachycardia if six sequential cycles of the ventricular tachycardia are sensed *(indicated in the marker channel by the small upright square waves)*. The capacitor then charges and at the horizontal arrow in the bottom panel delivers 0.2 J, which terminates the ventricular tachycardia and restores sinus rhythm.

is that the pacemaker produces slight rate increases in the presence of certain environmental noises, such as motion in an airplane. Other pacemakers that measure body temperature or respiratory rate, for example, can respond to metabolic demands. More complex rate-responsive systems incorporate multiple sensors that compensate for the deficits of specific individual sensors.

Treatment of Tachycardia

Pacing to treat patients with tachycardias generally involves three categories of treatment. First, symptomatic bradycardia may result from therapy of a tachycardia. For example, amiodarone results in symptomatic bradycardia in about 2% of patients treated, and these patients may require permanent pacing if they continue to receive amiodarone. Second, pacing can be used to prevent a recurrence of tachycardia. For example, when the tachycardia occurs during the setting of bradycardia, prevention of the latter also may prevent the former. However, this situation does not occur often. By far the most common use of electrical therapy is to terminate the tachycardia already present with an implantable ventricular defibrillator. This can be done with competitive pacing, low-energy synchronous cardioversion (Fig. 67.4), or high-energy defibrillation (Fig. 67.5). These implantable devices monitor the cardiac rate and, when they sense the presence of a tachycardia, deliver competitive pacing stimuli, a synchronized shock, or an asynchronous defibrillation shock. Implantable ventricular defibrillators are the therapy of choice for patients with aborted sudden cardiac death or sustained monomorphic ventricular tachycardia. More recently, implantable

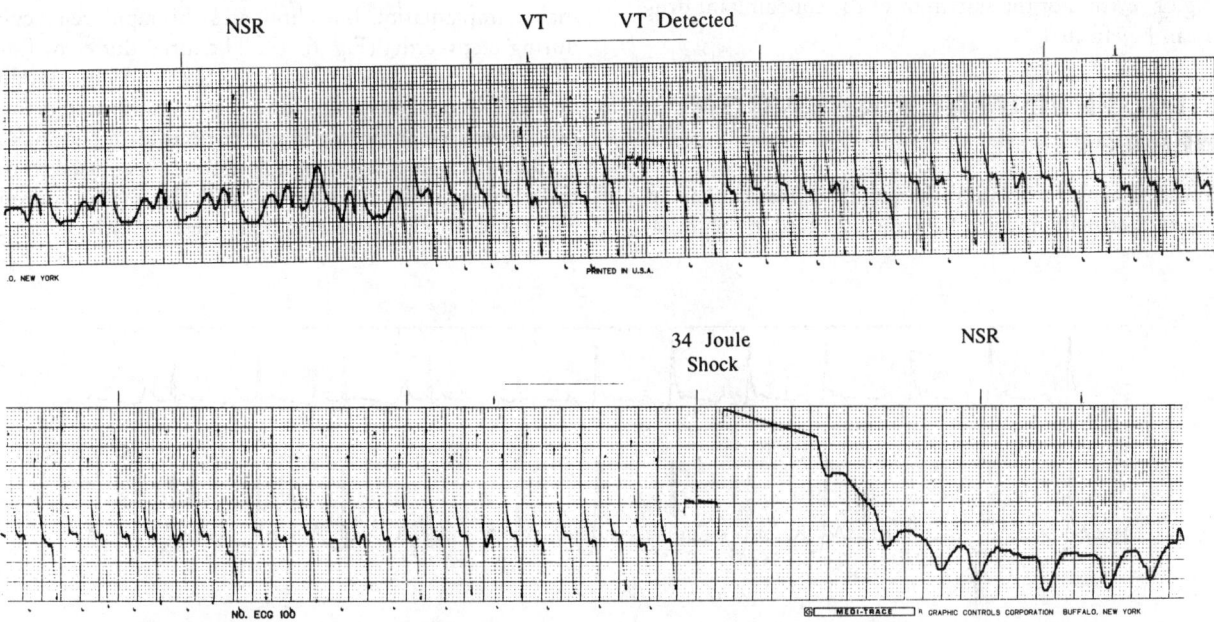

FIGURE 67.5. Cardioversion of ventricular tachycardia. Intracavitary recordings from a cardioverter defibrillator show the transition from sinus rhythm (note negative P waves preceding each ventricular depolarization) to ventricular tachycardia (note change in electrocardiogram and loss of preceding P wave), following a 34-J shock with restoration of sinus rhythm. (From Barold SS, Zipes DP. Cardiac pacemakers and antiarrhythmic devices. In: Braunwald E, ed. *Heart disease: a textbook of cardiovascular medicine*, fifth ed. Philadelphia: WB Saunders, 1996, with permission.)

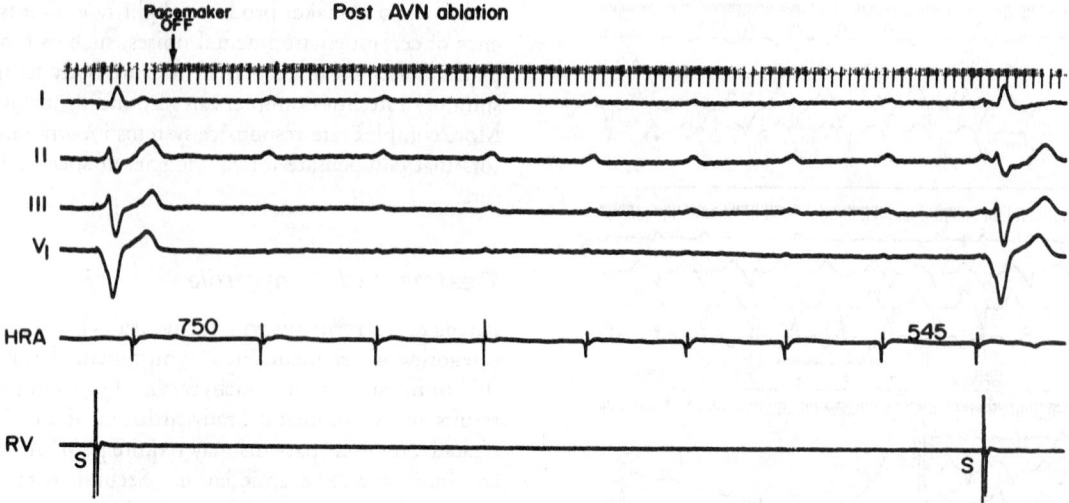

FIGURE 67.6. Ablation of the atrioventricular (AV) junction. Complete AV block follows catheter ablation of the AV junction.

atrial defibrillators designed to treat atrial fibrillation have also been developed. These devices are largely investigational.

General Care

Despite the reliability of modern pacemakers and defibrillators, malfunction can result on occasion, and it is important that the patient be followed closely and regularly in an organized pacemaker/defibrillator clinic. In such a clinic, the electrical function of a system is evaluated to detect malfunction or power depletion. The implant site is checked for erosion or infection, and the patient's overall cardiac status is evaluated so that reprogramming or revision of the system or of the concomitant drug regimen can be effected.

RADIOFREQUENCY ABLATION THERAPY

The purpose of catheter ablation therapy is to treat cardiac arrhythmias by destroying myocardial tissue involved in the initia-

tion or maintenance of the tachyarrhythmia. Ablation is most often accomplished by delivering radiofrequency energy through an electrode catheter placed next to the tissue (usually endocardial) to be destroyed. Other energy sources for cardiac ablation, including laser, microwave, and ultrasound, have also been explored.

Radiofrequency catheter ablation is applied in many different clinical situations. The AV junction can be ablated to produce complete or partial block in patients who have recurrent atrial flutter or fibrillation with a rapid ventricular response that cannot be controlled adequately with drugs. Atrioventricular junction ablation that results in complete AV block requires pacemaker implantation but eliminates the rapid ventricular rates during tachycardia (Fig. 67.6). The atrial flutter or fibrillation still occurs but cannot conduct to the ventricles. Modification of the AV nodal area to produce partial block results in slowing of the ventricular rate without the need for a pacemaker.

Radiofrequency catheter ablation has been used to interrupt the accessory pathway in patients with the WPW syndrome (Fig. 67.7) and to eliminate AV nodal reentry, which is the most

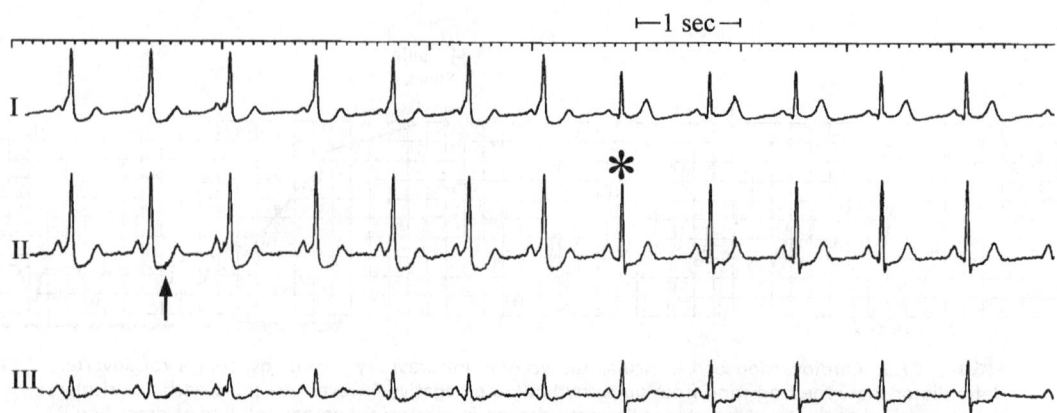

FIGURE 67.7. Successful catheter ablation of an accessory pathway in a patient with the Wolff–Parkinson–White syndrome. The arrow denotes the onset of the application of radiofrequency energy. Accessory pathway function, and the delta wave, is eliminated at the asterisk. Standard ECG leads I, II, and III are shown.

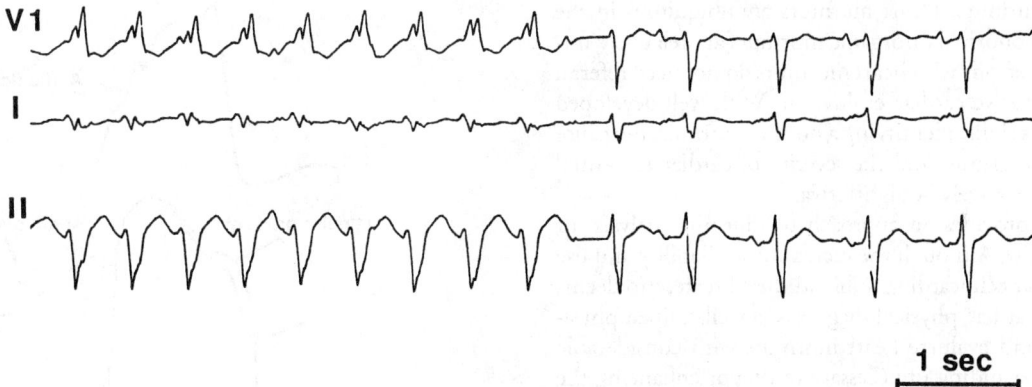

FIGURE 67.8. Successful catheter ablation of sustained hemodynamically tolerated ventricular tachycardia that occurred in a patient with a previous myocardial infarction. The ventricular tachycardia terminated approximately 5 seconds after the onset of radiofrequency energy delivery through an endocardial catheter, restoring sinus rhythm. Standard EKG leads V_1, I, and II are shown.

common mechanism of paroxysmal supraventricular tachycardia. Other supraventricular tachycardias that can be eliminated with ablation include atrial flutter and atrial tachycardia. For patients with ventricular tachycardia, sites of origin or reentrant pathways can be identified electrophysiologically and eliminated with radiofrequency catheter ablation. Success rates are highest in patients with no or minimal structural heart disease and can exceed 95%. In patients with monomorphic ventricular tachycardia due to coronary disease, the ablation success rate is about 80% (Fig. 67.8). Finally, radiofrequency catheter ablation techniques are being developed to treat, and potentially cure, atrial fibrillation.

SURGICAL THERAPY OF TACHYARRHYTHMIAS

The objective of surgery is to excise, isolate, or interrupt tissue in the heart that is critically responsible for the initiation, maintenance, or propagation of the tachycardia while preserving or even improving myocardial function. Indirect approaches have been used to improve cardiac hemodynamics and myocardial blood flow. They may be effective if, for example, ischemia is a cause of the arrhythmia. These include ventricular aneurysmectomy, coronary artery bypass grafting, or relief of valvular insufficiency or stenosis. In the main, however, direct approaches that are focused on myocardial tissue critically involved in the tachycardia are most successful. For instance, the MAZE procedure, in which multiple surgical incisions are made throughout the atria, can be an effective therapy for atrial fibrillation in patients undergoing mitral valve surgery. Other procedures include ventricular endocardial resection in patients with coronary artery disease and ventricular tachycardia. However, implantable ventricular defibrillators have generally replaced surgery for the treatment of ventricular tachycardia. Ablation of monomorphic ventricular tachycardia, when needed, is usually achieved with radiofrequency catheter ablation. Accessory pathway interruption in patients with the WPW syndrome, and AV nodal isolation in patients with AV nodal reentry can also be performed surgically. As with the surgical treatment of ventricular tachycar-

dia, radiofrequency catheter ablation has replaced surgery for most supraventricular arrhythmias. Refer to Chapters 76 and 90.

BIBLIOGRAPHY

Barold SS, Zipes DP. Cardiac pacemakers and antiarrhythmic devices. In: Braunwald E, ed. *Heart disease: a textbook of cardiovascular medicine*, fifth ed. Philadelphia: WB Saunders, 1996.

Zipes DP, Jalife J, eds. *Cardiac electrophysiology: from cell to bedside*, third ed. Philadelphia: WB Saunders, 1999.

Members of the Sicilian Gambit. *Antiarrhythmic therapy: a pathophysiological approach.* Armonk, NY: Futura Publishing, 1994.

Morady F. Radiofrequency catheter ablation. *N Engl J Med* 1999;340: 534–543.

Singh BN, Wellens HJJ, Hiraoka M. *Electropharmacological control of cardiac arrhythmias. To delay conduction or to prolong refractoriness?* Armonk, NY: Futura Publishing, 1994.

Zipes DP. Management of cardiac arrhythmias: pharmacological, electrical and surgical techniques. In: Braunwald E, ed. *Heart disease: a textbook of cardiovascular medicine*, fifth ed. Philadelphia: WB Saunders, 1996.

Kelley's Textbook of Internal Medicine, fourth edition. Edited by H. David Humes. Lippincott Williams & Wilkins, Philadelphia © 2000.

C H A P T E R
68

APPROACH TO THE PATIENT WITH HEART MURMURS

JONATHAN ABRAMS

Evaluation of heart murmurs is one of the most common tasks that an internist or primary care physician must perform in daily practice. It is therefore important that physicians develop basic skills in cardiac physical diagnosis as well as a good understanding of cardiac murmurs. Heart murmurs are ubiquitous in the population, but abnormal or organic murmurs are relatively uncommon. Most persons with heart murmurs do not need referral or further noninvasive cardiac evaluation. With well-developed physical diagnosis skills, identifying a normal murmur, the cause of an abnormal murmur, and the severity of cardiac structural abnormalities is relatively straightforward.

This chapter provides an approach to murmur analysis for the noncardiologist. Although the increasing availability and use of cardiac Doppler echocardiographic studies threatens to deemphasize skills in cardiac physical diagnosis, a well-trained physician can detect and evaluate heart murmurs with considerable proficiency, thus avoiding unnecessary testing or enhancing the value of a Doppler echocardiographic examination by facilitating a complete and accurate synthesis of the underlying cardiac abnormality.

BASIS OF HEART MURMURS

Turbulence of blood within the heart or great vessels is the primary cause of audible cardiac murmurs. Turbulence is directly related to intracardiac sound energy, which produces a murmur when the energy reaches an auditory threshold.

A major factor in the genesis of turbulence and heart murmurs is the velocity of blood flow. Normally, the velocity is maximal in early systole during rapid ejection of blood from the left and right ventricles; innocent or physiologic murmurs and pathologic ejection murmurs tend to be loudest in early systole to midsystole (Fig. 68.1). Because blood velocity is directly related to the pressure difference across a valve, turbulence and murmur intensity usually are greater with increasing degrees of obstruction to blood flow across stenotic valves. Conversely, when cardiac pump function is abnormal or when blood flow is diminished because of other causes, murmurs may become attenuated or even disappear.

The presence of cardiac sound or murmur in diastole is always abnormal because normal diastolic blood flow within the heart is low pressure and low velocity; in the normal heart, there is insufficient intracardiac turbulence to produce audible diastolic vibrations.

Loudness or intensity of cardiac sound is usually roughly proportional to the underlying severity of the cardiac abnormality. Noncardiac factors may also play a role in determining the relative loudness of a murmur. In general, cardiac sound is increased in children and young adults, in thin persons, and in hyperdynamic states such as anxiety, fever, and anemia. Conversely, murmurs may be soft in obese or heavily muscled individuals, women with large breasts, or patients with increased lung volume. The experienced clinician takes these extracardiac factors into account during the assessment of a murmur.

MURMUR IDENTIFICATION

IS A MURMUR ORGANIC?

The most critical question that needs to be answered whenever a murmur is heard is whether the murmur is physiologic and

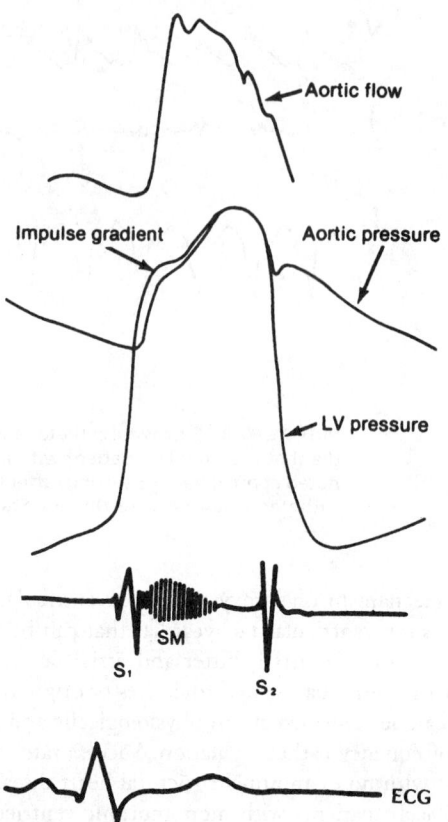

FIGURE 68.1. Pressure–flow relationships of the normal or innocent systolic ejection or flow murmur. In early systole, blood velocity and flow are maximal; the resultant turbulence produces audible cardiac sound vibrations or a heart murmur. The innocent or functional systolic ejection murmur ends within the first 60% to 70% of systole. (From Abrams J. Auscultation of heart murmurs: essentials of cardiac physical diagnosis. *Primary Cardiol* 1981;7:21, reprinted with permission from Primary Cardiology, PW Communications International, Inc.)

normal, or is organic representing intrinsic heart disease. If the murmur is judged to be abnormal, the cause and hemodynamic severity must be assessed. Internists and family practitioners are frequently asked to make determinations about employability, insurability, appropriateness of participation in competitive athletics or recreational sports, the necessity of endocarditis prophylaxis, and the safety of pregnancy and delivery. If a murmur is likely to be pathologic, selection of subsequent cardiovascular testing (e.g., Doppler echocardiography, stress test, cardiac catheterization) and the need to refer the patient to a cardiac specialist are issues that must be confronted by the primary physician. Proficiency in cardiac physical diagnosis is useful because it allows the physician to deal more appropriately with the potential issues raised by detection of a murmur.

The major varieties of cardiac murmurs—systolic, diastolic, and continuous—are diagrammed in Figure 68.2. Most murmurs detected by physicians are systolic, and the odds strongly favor a functional or innocent cause. Diastolic and continuous murmurs are always produced by underlying cardiovascular abnormalities. The most important task of the clinician is to determine if a given systolic murmur is suspiciously or definitely organic; nonsystolic murmurs usually indicate organic heart disease.

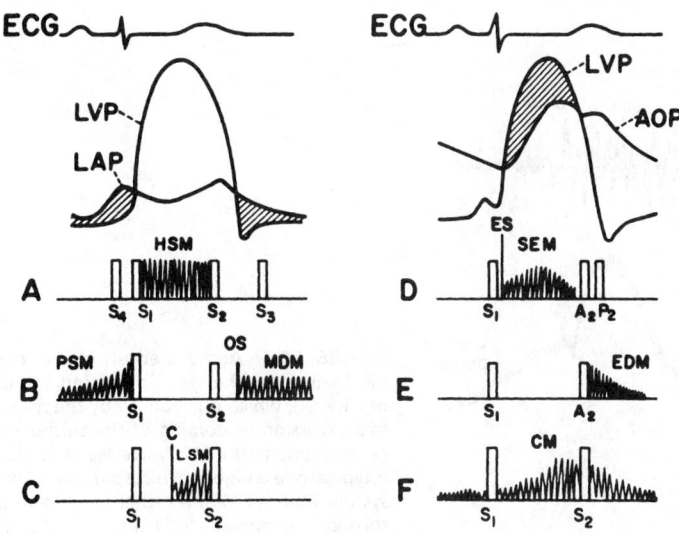

FIGURE 68.2. Intracardiac pressures and heart murmurs in the major cardiac valve abnormalities. **A:** Holosystolic murmur of mitral regurgitation. **B:** Mid-diastolic murmur with late presystolic accentuation of mitral stenosis. **C:** Late systolic murmur of mitral valve prolapse. **D:** Long systolic ejection murmur of aortic stenosis. **E:** Decrescendo diastolic murmur of aortic regurgitation. **F:** A typical continuous murmur, with maximal intensity in late systole spilling over into early diastole. LVP, left ventricular pressure; LAP, left atrial pressure; AOP, aortic pressure; HSM, holosystolic murmur; PSM, presystolic murmur; OS, opening snap; MDM, mid-diastolic murmur; C, midsystolic click; LSM, late systolic murmur; ES, ejection sound; SEM, systolic ejection murmur; EDM, early diastolic murmur; CM, continuous murmur. (From Crawford MH, O'Rourke RA. A systemic approach to the current bedside differentiation of cardiac murmurs and abnormal sounds. *Curr Probl Cardiol* 1979;1:7, with permission.)

EVALUATION OF SYSTOLIC MURMURS

The most critical aspect in auscultation of a systolic murmur is accurate assessment of its length (Fig. 68.3). Because normal ejection dynamics result in markedly reduced blood flow across the aortic and pulmonary valves in late systole (Fig. 68.1), it is abnormal to hear murmur vibrations after the middle third of systole. When there is audible cardiac sound in the last 25% to 30% of systole (a murmur extending up to the second heart sound [S_2]), it almost always indicates underlying abnormality (Figs. 68.2 and 68.3). In the presence of aortic or pulmonic stenosis at the valvular or subvalvular level, the systolic ejection murmur lengthens in relative proportion to the degree of obstruction to outflow (Fig. 68.3). A long systolic ejection murmur that extends into the last third of systole suggests significant outflow obstruction (Fig. 68.4); see Figs. 68.2D and 68.3.

Many systolic murmurs may truly be holosystolic or pansystolic, with the onset of murmur vibrations in early systole (with or just after the first heart sound [S_1]) and continuing to S_2. The most common cause of such a murmur in adults is mitral regurgitation or insufficiency. In mitral or tricuspid valve regurgitation, the sustained systolic pressure difference between the respective ventricle and atrium provides for continuous retrograde blood flow across the atrioventricular (AV) valve into the respective atrium until the end of systole (Fig. 68.2A). Mitral or tricuspid regurgitation can exist without a holosystolic murmur. For instance, the systolic murmur may taper in late systole, ending before S_2, or the murmur may be late in starting, extending up to S_2, as in the classic late systolic murmurs of mitral valve prolapse and papillary muscle dysfunction (Fig. 68.2C).

Doppler echocardiography has revealed that regurgitant flow across the AV valves without an audible murmur is not rare. Although detection of Doppler flow signals suggesting regurgitant flow across the mitral and tricuspid valves without a typical systolic murmur on careful auscultation should raise questions about the physiologic and functional significance of these Doppler "jets," evidence suggests that even the best physical diagnostician occasionally misses organic disease. Whether these flow signals represent Doppler disease rather than true valve abnormality is not always clear. Occasionally, significant AV valve regurgitation can be truly silent to auscultation.

ASSOCIATED CARDIOVASCULAR FINDINGS

Because most pathologic heart murmurs result from hemodynamic perturbations, it follows that evidence of cardiac chamber enlargement, altered carotid arterial pulsations, or abnormalities of the venous pulse commonly are found in patients who have murmurs caused by underlying cardiac disease. Valve opening sounds, normally silent, may be audible when the valvular tissue is thickened, fibrotic, or otherwise abnormal. Table 68.1 lists several associated cardiac abnormalities encountered during physical examination that point to underlying cardiac abnormality; clues to establishing an organic basis of a heart murmur are discussed in a subsequent section. The electrocardiographic or chest radiographic abnormalities may also suggest that a particu-

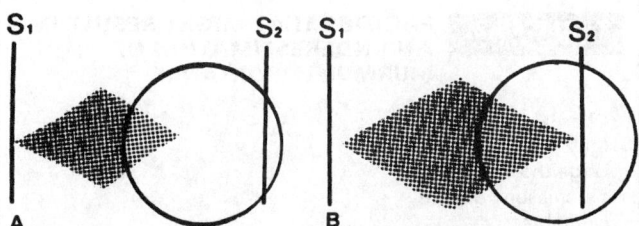

FIGURE 68.3. Importance of assessment of late systole in the evaluation of systolic murmurs. Careful evaluation of the last portion of systole is essential to make a determination as to whether a murmur is ejection in nature or is holosystolic. **A:** An early peaking systolic murmur ends before the last third of systole. This is the usual finding in functional or innocent murmurs, or with mild semilunar valve stenosis. **B:** A long ejection murmur is shown, which peaks late in systole. Sound vibrations extend literally to S_2, suggesting major obstruction to outflow. In severe aortic or pulmonic stenosis, sound vibrations may extend up to and even beyond S_2. (From Abrams J. Auscultation of heart murmurs: essentials of cardiac physical diagnosis. *Primary Cardiol* 1981;7:21; reprinted with permission from Primary Cardiology, PW Communications International, Inc.)

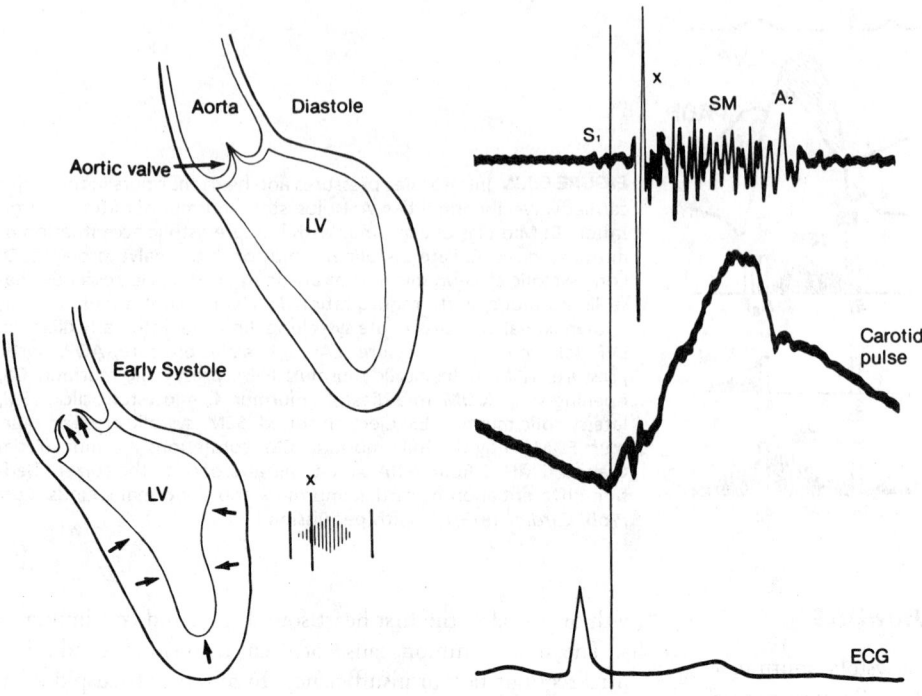

FIGURE 68.4. Aortic stenosis. Note the mechanism for the systolic ejection sound or click (X), which is produced by the maximal excursion or doming of the thickened or noncompliant aortic valve leaflets. This is typical of a congenital bicuspid valve. This systolic murmur (SM) is rather long, lasting throughout systole, indicating significant aortic stenosis. The carotid pulse demonstrates a slowed upstroke with a transmitted murmur or shudder. (From Abrams J. Aortic stenosis. *Primary Cardiol* 1983;9:28; reprinted with permission from Primary Cardiology, PW Communications International, Inc.)

lar heart murmur reflects disease, although the correlation between the murmur and the abnormal test result may be significant or fortuitous.

CAUSES OF A FALSE-NEGATIVE MURMUR

Occasionally, a patient may have serious cardiac structural disease but an unimpressive or no cardiac murmur when a murmur would be expected. Several factors contribute to this phenomenon (Table 68.2). The most likely and most important reason for a false-negative examination result is impaired cardiac function: a low stroke volume or a decreased left ventricular (LV) ejection

---

TABLE 68.1.	FINDINGS ON THE CARDIOVASCULAR EXAMINATION SUGGESTIVE OF ABNORMAL HEART MURMUR

Cardiac rhythm: atrial fibrillation
Carotid arterial pulse
   Small volume
   Slow rising
   Increased amplitude
   Double or bifid
Jugular venous pulse
   Elevated mean pressure
   Very large *a* wave
   Dominant *v* wave
Precordial motion
   Abnormal left ventricular activity: heave, increased forcefulness, palpable *a* wave (S_4), bifid impulse, ectopic location
   Parasternal right ventricular lift or heave
Heart sounds
   Loud S_1
   Wide, fixed, or paradoxical splitting of S_2
   Loud P_2
   Prominent S_4
   S_3 (in adults >age 40)
Abnormal heart sounds
   Midsystolic click
   Ejection click
   Opening snap
   Pericardial knock

TABLE 68.2.	FACTORS THAT MIGHT RESULT IN AN UNDERESTIMATION OF MURMUR IMPORTANCE

Obesity
Muscular chest
Large thorax
Chronic lung disease
Large breasts
Low flow
Low cardiac output or stroke volume
Heart failure
Depressed left ventricular systolic function
Pleural or pericardial fluid or thickening
Pregnancy
Decreased systemic vascular resistance may decrease in regurgitant murmur audibility
Poor stethoscope fit or improper technique (e.g., failure to use the bell and diaphragm appropriately)
Loud ambient noise interference

fraction. If cardiac flow is reduced for any reason, murmur intensity may also be reduced or absent. Heart failure or a low cardiac output can seriously obscure conventional physical findings in cardiac disorders. Factors exogenous to the heart, such as obesity, a large anteroposterior thoracic diameter, pleural or pericardial fluid, or chronic obstructive lung disease, can decrease murmur intensity and audibility.

Intracardiac factors can also decrease murmur intensity. For example, extensive calcification of the mitral valve and chordae is often associated with low flow and can decrease the loudness of the diastolic murmur or opening snap in mitral stenosis. Acoustic factors may play a role in decreasing murmur audibility. Low-pitched sounds or murmurs may not be heard well because the optimal range of hearing for most adults is greater than 1,000 cycles per second. Conversely, many older adults have occult high-frequency hearing deficiency. This can be a problem in murmur detection and identification. The high-pitched "blow" of mild aortic insufficiency is commonly missed, probably because most cardiac events are lower frequency and because persons are not used to listening for cardiac sounds and murmurs with such high frequencies.

It is essential to perform cardiac auscultation in a quiet environment without distractions. The level of noise in hospital rooms, clinics, or physicians' offices can be surprisingly high and usually goes unnoticed. Traffic, construction, and heating and air-conditioning units are common noise pollutants that can subtly interfere with accurate auscultation.

The use of poor-quality or improperly fitted stethoscope ear pieces is a common detriment to good listening. The highest quality stethoscope that a physician can afford is strongly recommended.

CAUSES OF A FALSE-POSITIVE MURMUR

Some murmurs are so prominent that they may result in a diagnosis of a more severe cardiac problem than exists. These can be considered false-positive examination results. Similarly, murmurs that suggest disease despite the absence of an abnormality are false-positive findings.

A common denominator for such murmurs is the presence of a high-flow state, in which the velocity of blood is increased. These individuals often have louder heart sounds and murmurs because of less tissue between the heart and the stethoscope. Children and young adults have prominent murmurs because of the high cardiac outputs in these age groups.

Certain cardiac factors can increase murmur intensity in the presence of organic heart disease and lead to an overestimation of the severity of the valve lesion. A classic example is the enhancement of stenotic murmur audibility in the presence of mixed obstructive and regurgitant lesions of the aortic or mitral valves; the excessive turbulent flow may suggest more serious obstruction than is the case. Even mild degrees of aortic or mitral regurgitation can augment stenotic murmurs.

Pregnancy can produce false-negative and false-positive findings. The enhanced blood volume and cardiac output of middle to late pregnancy typically results in a physiologic ejection murmur or augments the intensity of existing systolic ejection murmurs. Conversely, systemic arterial vasodilatation of pregnancy

can diminish the intensity of mitral or aortic regurgitation murmurs, leading to a false-negative impression of the murmur intensity.

Large-volume flow across the AV valves can produce diastolic filling murmurs without valve obstruction. In severe mitral regurgitation, a mid-diastolic flow rumble may be prominent, suggesting coexisting mitral stenosis though none exists. A similar phenomenon can be heard in cases of major tricuspid regurgitation.

CLUES IN ESTABLISHING AN ORGANIC BASIS OF HEART MURMUR

Alert clinicians can take advantage of careful bedside observations that may aid the diagnosis of an abnormal heart murmur. Any cardiac abnormality detectable on examination in addition to the murmur in question increases the likelihood that the heart murmur has an organic basis (Table 68.1). A systematic assessment of the carotid arterial and venous pulsations, as well as the precordial area, is important in the process of murmur identification.

CAROTID PULSATIONS

Careful attention to the contour and amplitude of the carotid arterial pulse helps to identify an aortic valve abnormality. An increased pulse volume, producing the sensation of a full, briskly rising systolic pulse, should raise the suspicion of aortic regurgitation. A gentle shudder or bifid contour suggests a bisferious pulse, found in pure aortic regurgitation or mixed stenosis and regurgitation. Conversely, a small-volume (hard-to-feel), slow-rising pulse suggests aortic stenosis (Fig. 68.4). In hypertrophic cardiomyopathy, the carotid upstroke is quick and tapping.

JUGULAR VENOUS PULSE

Although less specific than carotid artery findings, alterations in venous pulses may suggest heart disease. An elevated mean venous pressure indicates a high right ventricular (RV) filling pressure, and is consistent with right or biventricular heart failure or with marked pulmonary hypertension. In the latter condition or with a failing right ventricle, the jugular *a* wave is prominent. If there is associated tricuspid regurgitation, which is often acoustically difficult to detect, there is a dominant *V* wave in the venous pulse, often transmitted up the external jugular veins to the ear lobes.

PRECORDIAL MOTION

The presence of an LV or RV lift or heave (a sustained impulse that is palpable into the second half of systole) indicates an abnormality of the respective cardiac chamber. This may be a result of concentric hypertrophy or ventricular dilatation; it suggests that the murmur is likely to have a pathologic basis. Such findings increase the likelihood that an aortic ejection murmur has true hemodynamic importance (LV heave) or that mitral valve disease is severe enough to produce pulmonary hypertension (RV heave). Volume overloading of the heart, as in aortic regurgitation, may produce an apex impulse that is increased in amplitude but normal in contour. When the left ventricle is dilated, the point of maximal impulse of LV apical impulse is displaced leftward and downward from the normal middle left chest fourth and fifth interspaces; RV enlargement produces a parasternal or RV impulse.

ATRIAL FIBRILLATION

Atrial fibrillation is often seen in chronic mitral valve disease, and its presence should increase suspicion of mitral stenosis or insufficiency.

CLICKS AND SNAPS

Audible sounds of valve opening are always abnormal and represent helpful clues to the astute examiner. An opening snap is almost pathognomonic of mitral stenosis. Audible ejection clicks or sounds should focus attention on the aortic valve, usually indicating a bicuspid valve or possibly a dilated aortic root. Aortic ejection clicks are best heard at the apex, not at the aortic area. These sounds are usually loud, occur immediately after S_1, and radiate to the base (Fig. 68.4). Pulmonic ejection sounds are much less common. They should be suggested if the examiner detects an early systolic click at the upper left sternal edge that decreases with inspiration. Pulmonic stenosis (rare in adults) and pulmonary hypertension produce these sounds.

Midsystolic clicks are the hallmark of mitral valve prolapse and may be heard even if there is no systolic murmur. These are high-frequency popping sounds, best heard near the apex in midsystole to late systole. They are frequently accompanied by a late or, less often, holosystolic murmur (Fig. 68.2C), indicating associated mitral insufficiency.

HIGH-FREQUENCY DIASTOLIC MURMUR

The detection of a high-frequency diastolic decrescendo murmur along the left sternal border indicates aortic or pulmonic insufficiency and confirms an abnormality of one of the semilunar valves. A systolic ejection murmur at the base associated with a blowing diastolic murmur beginning with S_2 is probably caused by an aortic valve abnormality. Severe pulmonary hypertension with functional pulmonic insufficiency is virtually identical on auscultation.

Optimal detection of these murmurs, which are often difficult to hear, occurs with the patient sitting up and leaning forward, with the breath held in end expiration. Firm pressure on the diaphragm of the stethoscope is necessary to bring out the high-frequency vibrations of these murmurs.

WHEN TO ORDER A DOPPLER ECHOCARDIOGRAM

CONFIRMATION OF A DIAGNOSIS

If the examiner is not confident about her or his diagnostic skills in cardiac auscultation, obtaining an echocardiogram (with or without Doppler) is an obvious solution to assessing a heart murmur. The tendency to routinely order an echocardiogram is increasing, and this is unfortunate. It is appropriate for experienced physicians to use echocardiography, but this technology should not be used as a "fishing net" that is cast out indiscriminately. The physician should use Doppler echocardiography to confirm an impression or diagnosis of structural heart disease.

ESTIMATION OF SEVERITY

High-quality Doppler echocardiograms may be useful in helping to determine the severity of a known or suggested cardiac lesion. An approximation of the hemodynamic significance of aortic stenosis of mitral stenosis is reliably obtained by noninvasive study. Echocardiograms are somewhat less useful in assessing the precise severity of valvular regurgitant lesions. The size and status of the various cardiac chambers are readily determined by echocardiography, and this is important in the complete assessment of any structural abnormality.

VENTRICULAR FUNCTION

The status of LV function is a critical factor in the assessment of the organic murmurs of aortic stenosis and mitral regurgitation. In pulmonary hypertensive conditions and in cases of tricuspid regurgitation, RV size and performance must be assessed. Two-dimensional echocardiography is useful in evaluating ventricular size and function.

DETECTION OF OCCULT ABNORMALITIES

Doppler echocardiography is often useful in detecting unsuspected problems in patients for whom the physical examination is confusing or misleading. The occasional identification of acoustically silent mitral stenosis in the presence of major aortic stenosis or the diagnosis of significant pulmonary hypertension by Doppler are examples of the utility of this noninvasive procedure. Similarly, documentation of tricuspid regurgitation, often missed at the bedside but commonly present in persons with mitral valve disease or biventricular failure, is an excellent example of the help that a good-quality echocardiogram can provide.

TYPES OF MURMURS

SYSTOLIC MURMURS

Functional or Innocent Murmur

A functional systolic murmur is the most common murmur heard in daily practice. These murmurs are typically not loud, usually of grade 1 to 2 intensity. In high-flow states they may be grade 3, and this degree of loudness can mimic an organic murmur. Characteristically, the murmur is relatively pure in frequency or vibratory. The innocent systolic murmur ends well within the first 60% to 70% of the ejection period. These murmurs are typically best heard at the upper left sternal border. Still's murmur, an innocent murmur in children, is best heard just to the left of the lower sternal edge. If a systolic murmur is clearly maximal at the apex, careful scrutiny is necessary to exclude mitral regurgitation.

Functional murmurs are common in young adults and children. They are frequently found in hyperkinetic states. In older adults with stiffening and thickening of the aortic valve (aortic sclerosis), ejection murmurs are common. In these cases, the murmur tends to be more mixed frequency or harsh, and it radiates to the neck. In isolated aortic stenosis of the elderly, there may be few or no helpful associated cardiac abnormalities. In the aging population, electrocardiogram or chest radiographic abnormalities are common, and the correct diagnosis (i.e., aortic sclerosis versus true aortic stenosis) may require echocardiography.

The assessment of a functional or innocent murmur is in part a diagnosis of exclusion. No other suggestive findings are available, and the murmur meets the criteria presented earlier. Unusual loudness or prominent radiation to the neck or apex, or a particularly long systolic murmur, generally requires Doppler echocardiographic interrogation.

Organic Systolic Murmurs

The major organic murmurs that must be considered in addition to a functional murmur are aortic sclerosis, aortic stenosis, mitral regurgitation, and mitral valve prolapse. A less common systolic murmur is that of hypertrophic cardiomyopathy. These conditions are considered in detail elsewhere in this volume.

In mitral regurgitation or aortic stenosis, a decompensated left ventricle may produce a softer, less impressive systolic murmur, even in the presence of a severe hemodynamic burden. The suggestion of valvular aortic stenosis or mitral regurgitation in a patient with congestive heart failure or a decreased LV ejection fraction mandates a meticulous search for evidence of valve disorder and its severity.

Diastolic Murmurs

The detection of a diastolic murmur virtually always indicates structural heart disease. There are two major variants of diastolic murmurs in the common adult cardiac conditions: the long decrescendo and usually high-frequency murmur of aortic insufficiency (Fig. 68.2E) and the low-pitched rumbling murmur of mitral stenosis (Fig. 68.2B). These murmurs appear at different times in diastole, have markedly different frequency characteristics, and are localized to different areas of the precordium. Occasionally, a mitral stenosis murmur is medium to high frequency and is easily heard close to the sternal border; such a murmur can be readily mistaken for aortic regurgitation.

Nonstenotic Middiastolic Murmurs

Several varieties of *flow rumble* or mid-diastolic flow murmurs are detectable in patients with various cardiac lesions. These murmurs can mimic mitral stenosis, and their presence confirms a significant hemodynamic burden related to the primary valvular abnormality.

TABLE 68.3.	COMMON VARIETIES OF CONTINUOUS MURMURS

Patent ductus arteriosus
Arteriovenous fistula
   Congenital and acquired
   Systemic and pulmonary
Ruptured sinus of Valsalva aneurysm (communication usually into right atrium or right ventricle)
Venous hum (innocent finding in children)
Anomalous origin of coronary artery from pulmonary artery or coronary arteriovenous fistula
"Mammary souffle" of pregnancy
Systemic arterial–pulmonary arterial collaterals or bronchial arterial collaterals in congenital defects
Coarctation of the aorta at coarctation site and collateral vessels
Pseudocontinuous murmur: severe aortic stenosis and regurgitation

In major degrees of mitral or tricuspid regurgitation, when increased blood traverses the respective AV valve during diastolic filling, a mid-diastolic murmur may be audible. These murmurs are relatively short and end well before S_1; they are detected in an apical location, with the patient in a left decubitus position for assessing mitral regurgitation, or located at the lower sternal edge and increasing with inspiration in the case of tricuspid regurgitation. Their presence suggests a big regurgitant leak at the respective valve. A comparable middiastolic murmur can be generated by a large left-to-right shunt at the atrial and ventricular level, when the excessive volume of blood from the shunt returns to the respective ventricle in diastole. A long rumbling diastolic murmur at the apex can simulate mitral stenosis in cases of severe aortic regurgitation. This is the Austin Flint murmur; when diagnosed correctly, the Austin Flint murmur indicates a major degree of regurgitation.

Continuous Murmurs

Continuous murmurs are rare. They indicate blood flow in late systole and early diastole, and result from a communication between a chamber or artery with systemic pressure or resistance with a low-pressure or resistance vessel or chamber, allowing continued blood flow after ventricular ejection has ended. Table 68.3 lists some of the more common continuous murmurs.

■ FURTHER EVALUATION OF PRESUMED ORGANIC MURMURS

Detection of a heart murmur requires confirmation and assessment of severity. Table 68.4 outlines an approach to dealing with presumed organic heart murmurs. Follow-up employs the history, periodic physical examinations, and serial Doppler echocardiography. The health implications of subacute bacterial endocarditis prophylaxis, pregnancy, and athletic and job participation are generally related to the functional impact of the lesion

TABLE 68.4.	APPROACH TO THE PATIENT WITH A MURMUR

Systolic Murmurs

Most common variety of murmur heard in practice
Most are functional or innocent
Consider organic if associated cardiovascular abnormalities are
    present on examination, ECG, or chest roentgenogram
Most common organic murmurs to consider
    Aortic sclerosis of the elderly
    Aortic stenosis
    Mitral regurgitation
    Mitral valve prolapse

Diastolic Murmurs

Always organic
Common
    Aortic regurgitation
    Mitral stenosis
Uncommon
    Flow rumbles in atrioventricular valve regurgitation
    Pulmonic regurgitation
    Continuous murmur

Workup

Echo-Doppler study mandatory if a definite organic murmur is
    diagnosed or suggested
Establish severity of lesion
Careful assessment of ventricular size and function
Ancillary testing to consider
    Radionuclide ventriculogram (resting or with exercise)
    Exercise test for cardiovascular and aerobic function
    Cardiac catheterization

Health Maintenance

Educate patient about endocarditis prophylaxis
Counsel about functional limitation, exercise or job restrictions,
    pregnancy issues

in question, although endocarditis prevention strategies are relevant for even mild or trivial structural abnormalities.

For moderate to severe hemodynamic abnormalities, cardiac catheterization or radionuclide angiography may be required in addition to conventional Doppler echocardiography (see Chap. 77).

BIBLIOGRAPHY

Abrams J. *Synopsis of cardiac physical diagnosis.* Philadelphia: Lea & Febiger, 1984.

Abrams J. *Essentials of cardiac physical diagnosis.* Philadelphia: Lea & Febiger, 1987.

Crawford MH, O'Rourke RA. A systematic approach to bedside differentiation of cardiac murmurs and abnormal sounds. *Curr Probl Cardiol* 1977; 1:1.

Grewe K, Crawford MH, O'Rourke RA. Differentiation of cardiac murmurs by dynamic auscultation. *Curr Probl Cardiol* 1988;13.

Lembo NJ, Dell'Italia LJ, Crawford MH, et al. Bedside diagnosis of systolic murmurs. *N Engl J Med* 1988;318:1572.

Lembo NJ, Dell'Italia LJ, Crawford MH, et al. Diagnosis of left-sided regurgitant murmurs by transient arterial occlusion: a new maneuver using blood pressure cuffs. *Ann Intern Med* 1986;105:368.

Shaver JA, Salerni R, Reddy PS. Normal and abnormal heart sounds in cardiac diagnosis. Part I: systolic sounds. *Curr Probl Cardiol* 1985;10: 1.

Shaver JA, Salerni R, Reddy PS. Normal and abnormal heart sounds in cardiac diagnosis. Part II: diastolic sounds. *Curr Probl Cardiol* 1985; 10:1.

Kelley's Textbook of Internal Medicine, fourth edition. Edited by H. David Humes.
Lippincott Williams & Wilkins, Philadelphia © 2000.

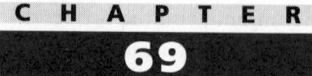

CHAPTER
69

APPROACH TO THE PATIENT WITH SYNCOPE

KRISTIN E. ELLISON
PATRICK T. O'GARA

DEFINITION

The term *syncope* derives from the Greek, *sunkopé,* "to cut short." Syncope is defined clinically as a transient loss of consciousness due to an acute and critical decrease in cerebral blood flow. It is thus distinguished from faintness or dizziness, neither of which is accompanied by true loss of consciousness. Its differential diagnosis is broad, with several benign and a few life-threatening causes. The challenge for the clinician is first to distinguish among the various causes of syncope on the basis of the history, examination, and directed laboratory studies and then to design an effective strategy of treatment and prevention.

EPIDEMIOLOGY

Syncope is a common symptom, accounting for as many as 3% to 5% of all emergency room visits and up to 6% of hospital admissions. By conservative estimates, more than 1 million people in the United States seek evaluation and treatment for syncope each year, at a cost in excess of $1 billion. The prevalence of syncope increases with age; elderly (age greater than 65 years) patients are more likely to have a serious cardiac or neurologic cause. As many as 40% to 50% of patients will have only a single isolated episode and will not require detailed evaluation or complicated treatment. As recently as the 1980s, a cause of syncope was not ascertained in up to 40% of patients. In a tertiary cardiology referral center with emphasis on tilt-table and electrophysiologic testing, the proportion of undiagnosed cases was more recently estimated at only 25%. Diagnosis and treatment remain, in several instances, expensive and not particularly cost-effective, largely because of an overreliance on cardiac and neurovascular testing when the clinical presentation points elsewhere. For the evaluation and management of patients with suspected neurocardiogenic syncope, for example, cost may exceed $16,000 per patient. Attention to the details surrounding the presentation, past medication/drug use, examination (general, cardiac, neurologic), and routine laboratory studies should allow a focused and more cost-effective approach.

PATHOPHYSIOLOGY

The loss of consciousness that defines syncope derives from a critical decrease in cerebral perfusion pressure, leading specifically to a fall in blood flow to the reticular activating system of the brainstem. A fall in mean arterial pressure to 50 mm Hg or below will usually suffice, but preexistent cerebrovascular disease or a rapid fall in mean pressure to a higher minimum level in a patient with chronic hypertension might also precipitate a syncopal event. In most instances, the patient is upright (standing, sitting) and several seconds of premonitory symptoms (lightheadedness, visual disturbance, yawning, diaphoresis, nausea) precedes the loss of consciousness, often allowing time for self-protection. A cardiac cause, such as high-grade atrioventricular (AV) block, termed Stokes–Adams–Morgagni attack, may not be accompanied by such a prodrome. Unconsciousness generally persists for a variable but short period of time (second to minutes), during which the skeletal musculature may relax completely and a few myoclonic jerks or even brief tonic–clonic movements can be seen. The patient will usually regain consciousness without persistent neurologic sequelae. Headache and/or prolonged confusion may point to an alternative diagnosis (e.g., seizure). Alteration in the essential nutrients of the blood necessary for cerebral metabolism, such as with hypoglycemia, hypoxia, or hypercarbia, can cause transient loss of consciousness. However, these disorders are more often associated with somnolence, coma, or another prolonged alteration of mental status.

ETIOLOGIC FACTORS

The major causes of syncope are listed in Table 69.1. The principal cardiovascular causes can be grouped into four general categories that comprise disorders of vasomotor control, cardiopulmonary mechanical lesions, arrhythmias, and cerebrovascular disease. Table 69.2 provides a summary estimate of the relative incidence of the various causes of syncope from among several large and unselected patient populations.

ABNORMALITIES OF VASOMOTOR CONTROL

At least half of all syncopal episodes are related to abnormalities of the autonomic control of the heart and circulation. This category includes postural syncope, neurocardiogenic (vasovagal) syncope, glossopharyngeal syncope, carotid sinus syndrome, and situational syncope (post tussive, micturition, deglutition, defecation, and after other strenuous activities). Receptors in various locations (carotid body, aortic arch, myocardium) are activated by a variety of painful or mechanical stimuli. Afferent nerve

TABLE 69.1. CAUSES OF LOSS OF CONSCIOUSNESS

Syncope
  Abnormalities of vasomotor control
    Orthostatic hypotension
    Vasovagal, vasodepressor, or neurocardiogenic syncope
    Carotid sinus hypersensitivity
    Situational syncope
      Micturition
      Defecation
      Cough
      Deglutition
  Cardiopulmonary mechanical disorders
    Aortic stenosis
    Hypertrophic obstructive cardiomyopathy
    Mechanical valvular malfunction or thrombosis
    Atrial myxoma
    Pulmonary hypertension
    Pulmonary embolus
    Pericardial tamponade
    Pericardial constriction
  Cardiac arrhythmias
    Bradyarrhythmias
      Sinus bradycardia
      Sinoatrial arrest or exit block
      High-degree atrioventricular block
    Tachyarrhythmias
      Supraventricular arrhythmias associated with other cardiovascular abnormalities (e.g., atrial fibrillation in patients with Wolff–Parkinson–White syndrome or aortic stenosis)
      Monomorphic ventricular tachycardia
      Polymorphic ventricular tachycardia in patients with the prolonged QT syndrome
  Cerebrovascular disease
    Vertebrobasilar arterial insufficiency with or without carotid artery disease
    Basilar artery migraine
  Seizures
  Psychiatric illnesses
    Hysterical fainting
    Hyperventilation associated with anxiety
  Metabolic causes
    Hypoglycemia
    Hypoxia
    Hypocapnia
    Alcohol
    Drug effect
  Trauma

impulses then travel to the nucleus tractus solitarius and/or medullary vasodepressor region, stimulating either a release of parasympathetic influences or a withdrawal/inhibition of sympathetic output, resulting in peripheral vasodilatation (vasodepressor component), a fall in blood pressure, and in many instances a concomitant slowing of the heart rate (cardioinhibitory component).

ORTHOSTATIC HYPOTENSION

Orthostatic hypotension (also called postural syncope) is often observed in the elderly and may result in substantial morbidity and mortality from associated falls. It is commonly defined as

TABLE 69.2.	RELATIVE INCIDENCE OF THE VARIOUS CAUSES OF SYNCOPE

Cause	Incidence (%)
Reflex-mediated	
Neurocardiogenic	18
Situational	5
Orthostatic hypotension	8
Cardiac	
Arrhythmias (tachyarrhythmia and bradyarrhythmia)	14
Organic heart disease	4
Neurologic seizures, transient ischemic attacks, migraines	10
Medications	3
Psychiatric	2
Unknown	34

a decrease of 20 mm Hg or more in systolic blood pressure or 10 mm Hg in diastolic blood pressure upon assumption of the upright posture. Such changes can be detected in as many as 20% of medical outpatients older than 65 years of age. Standing results in the pooling of approximately 500 to 700 mL of blood in the lower extremities, splanchnic beds, and pulmonary circulations. The decreased venous return results in a fall in cardiac output and stimulation of cardiopulmonary, aortic, and carotid baroreceptors, which reflexively increase sympathetic, and decrease parasympathetic, tone to maintain the systemic blood pressure. Several conditions, including hypovolemia (hemorrhage, vomiting, diarrhea) and certain drugs (diuretics, nitrates, α-adrenoreceptor blockers, calcium channel) and other agents used in the treatment of hypertension or ischemic heart disease, may contribute to this syndrome.

Patients with autonomic dysfunction not unexpectedly have an increased susceptibility to postural syncope. Autonomic dysfunction may be secondary to systemic disease, such as diabetes mellitus, syphilis, alcoholism, amyloidosis, or adrenal insufficiency. A variety of central and peripheral nervous system disorders, such as Shy–Drager syndrome, Parkinson's disease, Wernicke's encephalopathy, syringomyelia, and inflammatory myelopathies, may also manifest as syncope. These patients often have disturbances of bowel and bladder function and impairment of sweating. They also have chronotropic incompetence, which compounds the hypotension initiated by the inability to increase systemic vascular resistance.

NEUROCARDIOGENIC OR VASOVAGAL SYNCOPE

Neurocardiogenic syncope, also known as neurally mediated, vasovagal, or vasodepressor syncope, is a common disorder of autonomic cardiovascular regulation. Although neurocardiogenic syncope is not life threatening, it can result in significant injury, and failure to recognize this common cause of syncope may result in an unnecessarily costly evaluation. Episodes are often preceded by a prodromal period lasting for a few seconds

to a few minutes. Triggers associated with the development of neurocardiogenic syncope are those that either reduce ventricular filling or increase catecholamine synthesis and release. These include the sight of blood, pain, prolonged standing, a warm environment, hot shower, exercise, or stressful emotional encounters. The individual might be sitting or standing and experiences weakness, nausea, diaphoresis, light-headedness, and, often, a sense of impending darkness. The decreased venous return and fall in cardiac output trigger a paradoxical reflex. The arterial baroreceptors are activated with resultant catecholamine release. When combined with reduced ventricular filling, the sympathetic stimulation leads to vigorous contraction of a volume-depleted ventricle. There is initially tachycardia, decreased blood pressure, and pallor. In susceptible individuals, the mechanoreceptors and vagal afferents (C fibers) in the heart (particularly in the inferior posterior portion of the left ventricular myocardium) are activated . These C fibers project centrally to the dorsal vagal nucleus of the medulla, with the resultant withdrawal of sympathetic influences and increased vagal (parasympathetic) output. This produces cardiac slowing, diaphoresis, pupillary constriction, and, eventually, syncope. The duration of unconsciousness is rarely longer than a few minutes if the conditions that provoke the event can be reversed. Assumption of the supine position or other maneuvers to increase venous return, such as placing the head between the knees when sitting, also help to ameliorate the situation.

Patients with transplanted (denervated) hearts have also experienced cardiovascular responses identical to those observed during neurally mediated syncope. This should not be possible if the response depends solely on the reflex mechanisms described previously. Neurocardiogenic syncope likely results from a variety of mechanisms with various degrees of increased efferent vagal activation and sympathoinhibition. Several neurotransmitters are believed to facilitate neurocardiogenic syncope by inhibiting the release of central sympathetic neurotransmitters. In addition to catecholamines, opioid peptides, arginine vasopressin, nitric oxide, and serotonin are likely to be involved in the modulation of the central nervous system blood pressure and heart rate regulation.

The head-upright tilt-table test is a provocative test for neurocardiogenic syncope. It is generally performed for 30 to 45 minutes at an angle of 60 to 80 degrees. This posture induces the venous pooling that initiates the reflex (Fig. 69.1). Some patients manifest a prominent vasodepressor response, whereas others have a more pronounced cardioinhibitory response. This latter aspect is of importance as only those patients with a significant cardioinhibitory component usually benefit from pacing therapy.

CAROTID SINUS HYPERSENSITIVITY

Carotid sinus hypersensitivity is an uncommon but potentially treatable cause of syncope. Diagnosis is made by performing carotid sinus massage, which should be carried out in the supine position under continuous electrocardiographic monitoring, after listening for bruits. Light massage on alternate sides is then performed for 5 seconds. An abnormal response is defined by

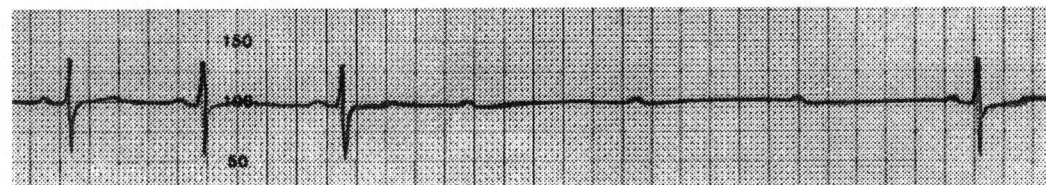

FIGURE 69.1. Surface electrocardiographic lead in a patient who experienced syncope during upright tilt-table testing. Note heart rate slowing followed by high grade atrioventricular block. Loss of consciousness with myoclonic jerks occurred shortly thereafter.

asystole for 3 or more seconds and/or a decrease in systolic blood pressure of 50 mm Hg. A tight collar, shaving, and turning of the head to one side may increase pressure on the carotid sinus. Carotid hypersensitivity occurs predominantly in men, 70% of whom are 50 years of age or older. Activation of carotid sinus baroreceptors, which are located just cephalad to the bifurcation of the common carotid artery, results in inhibition of efferent sympathetic nerve fibers to the heart and blood vessels, activation of cardiac vagal efferent nerve fibers, or both. In susceptible individuals, these responses may result in sinus arrest or AV block (cardioinhibitory response, 34% to 78% of cases), vasodilatation (vasodepressor response, 5% to 10% of cases), or both (mixed response). Certain drugs can cause an abnormal carotid sinus response (digoxin, alpha methyldopa) and should be discontinued if possible. Avoidance of triggers constitutes the primary treatment. Only in severe cases with a clear cardioinhibitory component should a pacemaker be considered.

GLOSSOPHARYNGEAL NEURALGIA

Syncope due to glossopharyngeal neuralgia is preceded by pain in the oropharynx, tonsillar fossa, or tongue, frequently induced by space occupying oropharyngeal tumors. Loss of consciousness is usually associated with asystole rather than with vasodilatation. Afferent impulses in the glossopharyngeal nerve activate efferent cardiac vagal motor neurons in the nucleus ambiguus and the dorsal motor nucleus of the vagus. This results in efferent vagal activation and bradycardia.

SITUATIONAL SYNDROMES

Other less common syndromes that may be caused at least in part by abnormal autonomic cardiovascular control include micturition syncope, defecation syncope, deglutition syncope, and cough syncope. Micturition syncope occurs predominantly in older men, frequently those with prostatic hypertrophy and bladder neck obstruction. Straining (Valsalva) against an obstructed bladder neck and/or activation of bladder mechanoreceptors may contribute to this syndrome. Syncope usually occurs at night during or immediately after voiding. Defecation syncope occurs in both men and women.

Cough syncope typically occurs in men with chronic obstructive lung disease during or immediately after prolonged coughing fits.

Deglutition syncope is rare but may be associated with diseases of the esophagus, particularly esophageal spasm. Activation of esophageal sensory receptors may result in reflex sinus bradycardia or AV block and is triggered by certain foods and liquids.

CARDIOPULMONARY MECHANICAL DISORDERS

Syncope related to cardiopulmonary mechanical disorders often occurs because of an inability to increase cardiac output in the setting of peripheral vasodilatation. The inadequate increase in cardiac output is usually caused by obstruction to ventricular outflow, but it may also result from severe myocardial disease, external cardiac compression, or even severe inflow obstruction. Peripheral vasodilatation may be appropriate (after exercise) or may be caused by activation of mechanoreceptors in the left ventricle, as described previously. In patients with aortic stenosis, syncope is thought to result from mechanical obstruction to LV outflow as well as from the activation of myocardial mechanoreceptors, which impairs the normal vasoconstrictor response in nonexercising vascular beds. Patients with hypertrophic obstructive cardiomyopathy (HOCM) also fail to increase cardiac output normally with exercise and are susceptible to both exertional and postexertional syncope, independent of any rhythm disturbance (such as ventricular tachycardia, or VT), for similar reasons.

Atrial myxoma, a ball-valve thrombus complicating a mechanical prosthesis, and, rarely, severe mitral stenosis may impair left ventricular filling to such an extent that cardiac output becomes significantly reduced and incapable of further augmentation with stress. Underfilling of the left ventricle may result in mechanoreceptor stimulation as described above.

Syncope occurs in as many as 10% of patients with massive (more than 50% obstruction of the pulmonary vascular bed) pulmonary embolism. It may also occur in patients with severe pulmonary hypertension. In these patients, syncope is usually accompanied by other symptoms (e.g., chest pain, dyspnea). In both cases, syncope results from an inability of the right ventricle to maintain or augment cardiac output in the face of pulmonary vascular obstruction. Right ventricular outflow may also be severely restricted in patients with tetralogy of Fallot and infundibular (dynamic) pulmonic stenosis.

Syncope rarely occurs in patients with pericardial tamponade or severe pericardial constriction as a result of decreased ventricular filling and hypotension. Syncope in the setting of acute type

A aortic dissection is more commonly due to pericardial tamponade than to stroke.

CARDIAC ARRHYTHMIAS

Common arrhythmic causes of syncope include bradyarrhythmias due to sinus node dysfunction or AV block, and tachyarrhythmias. Ventricular tachycardia as well as supraventricular tachycardia can result in syncope especially when accompanied by underlying structural heart disease. In normal individuals, cardiac output and systemic arterial pressure usually remain at levels that maintain consciousness at heart rates between 30 and 180 beats per minute. As heart rate decreases, ventricular filling time and stroke volume increase to maintain cardiac output at normal levels. Below 30 beats per minute, stroke volume can no longer increase to compensate for the decrease in heart rate, and syncope may occur. At rates exceeding 180 beats per minute, diastolic filling time is too limited to maintain adequate stroke volume.

Tolerance to an altered heart rate is decreased in association with other comorbidities and selected circumstances such as anemia, cerebrovascular disease, upright posture, cardiopulmonary mechanical disorders, myocardial ischemia, and abnormalities of cardiovascular control. Certain cardiac structural abnormalities are associated with tachyarrhythmias or bradyarrhythmias. For example, hypertrophic cardiomyopathy is associated with VT and sudden death. Patients with cardiac sarcoid are at increased risk for ventricular tachyarrhythmias, cardiac conduction abnormalities, and advanced heart block. Of patients with Ebstein's anomaly of the tricuspid valve, 10% to 25% have AV bypass tracts.

Syncope associated with bradyarrhythmias often occurs with little or no warning. Patients usually regain consciousness and an awareness of their surroundings promptly. Bradyarrhythmias may result from disorders of impulse generation (e.g., sinoatrial arrest) or impulse conduction (e.g., AV block). Bradyarrhythmias are more likely to cause syncope in the elderly or in patients with structural heart disease. Patients with the sick sinus syndrome may have frequent sinus pauses or sinus arrest (more than 3 seconds). Recent pacemaker trials have reported that atrial fibrillation occurs frequently and without symptoms or awareness in this patient population. The need for rate control of rapid atrial fibrillation may exacerbate a tendency to bradycardia among such patients and mandate pacemaker therapy. Atrial fibrillation can be induced by vagal stimulation in some patients.

Patients with syncope associated with paroxysmal atrial fibrillation are predisposed to an abnormal (vagally mediated) neural response such that blood pressure falls at the onset of atrial fibrillation because of the vasodepressor reflex previously described. Although often associated with evidence of cardiac conduction system disease (e.g., prolonged PR interval, bundle-branch block), high-degree AV block may occur episodically in patients with otherwise normal AV conduction. In patients with sinus node dysfunction or AV conduction system abnormalities, attempts should always be made to demonstrate an association between the patient's symptoms and the bradyarrhythmia, so as to target pacemaker therapy.

Syncope due to tachycardia is frequently preceded by rapid palpitations but may occur without warning. In the absence of structural heart disease, supraventricular tachycardia rarely causes syncope in adults. However, in patients with the Wolff–Parkinson–White syndrome and atrial fibrillation, conduction across the accessory AV connection may result in particularly rapid ventricular rates and syncope. Atrial fibrillation may also cause syncope in patients with structural heart disease (e.g., HOCM).

Ventricular tachycardia is a common cause of syncope in patients with structural heart disease. Patients with an acute MI may present with syncope due to ventricular arrhythmias (ventricular tachycardia/ventricular fibrillation; VT/VF). A history of prior MI identifies the substrate for reentrant VT. Certain types of VT may cause syncope in younger individuals without apparent structural heart disease. These include the idiopathic focal VTs, the most common locations of which are the right ventricular outflow tract and the left anterior fascicle. These latter two types of VT are not life threatening but can result in syncope. Patients with abnormalities of ventricular repolarization with long QT syndrome are at risk for polymorphic VT (torsade de pointes). QT prolongation may be congenital and related to the genes encoding for sodium or potassium channels. Many patients with the syndrome have a family history of syncope or early sudden death. In other patients, the disorder is acquired as a result of drug therapy, such as quinidine, procainamide, disopyramide, sotalol, phenothiazines, or electrolyte abnormalities (hypokalemia, hypomagnesemia) that prolong ventricular repolarization. Certain antihistamines (e.g., terfenadine) in combination with drugs (e.g., erythromycin, ketoconazole) or conditions that inhibit hepatic cytochrome P450 metabolism may prolong the QT interval and cause torsade de pointes (Fig. 69.2).

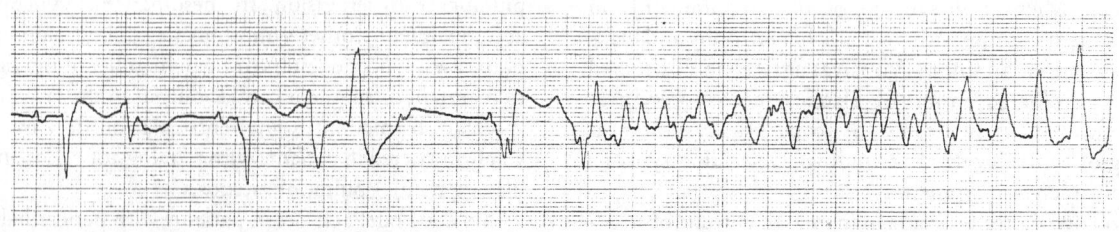

FIGURE 69.2. Acquired long QT syndrome from quinidine therapy with associated bradycardia results in polymorphic ventricular tachycardia (torsade de pointes)

CEREBROVASCULAR DISEASE

It is very unusual for cerebrovascular disease to be the lone cause of syncope. More commonly, cerebrovascular disease lowers the threshold for syncope in patients with other disorders. Syncope as a manifestation of carotid artery disease may occur if the ischemia involves both hemispheres but rarely occurs in the absence of coexistent vertebrobasilar disease. Subclavian steal syndrome can usually be diagnosed on the basis of the history and physical examination. When transient ischemic attacks cause syncope, they are almost always vertebrobasilar in location. Cortical strokes may cause loss of consciousness because of an associated seizure disorder.

Fainting is reported by 12% to 18% of patients with migraine. An uncommon form of migraine may affect the basilar artery in adolescents and cause syncope.

DIFFERENTIAL DIAGNOSIS

SEIZURES

Seizures can mimic syncope and account for loss of consciousness in up to 5% to 10% of patients in reported series. Although profound hypotension associated with bradyarrhythmias or ventricular tachyarrhythmias may result in syncope in supine individuals, loss of consciousness in this position is more often caused by a seizure. Syncope due to cardiac arrhythmia is of rapid onset and brief duration, without preceding aura, and is not followed by a postictal confusional state. Seizure activity is uncommon, as is tongue biting or incontinence, but tonic–clonic movements can occur if the arrhythmia resulting in syncope is prolonged. Epileptic movements within seconds of the onset of syncope are more likely to be indicative of a central nervous system disorder than a cardiac rhythm disturbance. Temporal lobe seizures can be confused with syncope. These seizures may last for several minutes and are characterized by changes in consciousness, confusion, and a variety of autonomic signs, such as flushing and olfactory hallucinations. The clinical picture may be confounded by a syncopal episode that resulted in head trauma and confusion.

Seizure-like activity may occur as a result of syncope when the episode of cerebral anoxia is prolonged. As noted, it is not uncommon for a patient with prolonged episodes of vasovagal syncope to develop myoclonic jerks, particularly if the individual is unable to achieve the supine position. Conspicuous motor activity accompanies syncope due to ventricular arrhythmias in as many as 30% to 40% of cases.

PSYCHIATRIC ILLNESSES

Hysterical fainting is a syncopal disorder felt secondary to a psychiatric condition. It can mimic syncope and be difficult to differentiate from a neurocardiogenic etiology. These episodes usually occur or recur in the presence of observers or in emotionally charged situations, and rarely result in physical injury.

Hyperventilation may cause transient loss of consciousness due to the resultant respiratory alkalosis and cerebral vasocon-

TABLE 69.3. DRUGS CAUSING SYNCOPE
Vasodilators
Nitrates
Calcium channel blockers
Angiotensin-converting enzyme inhibitors
Prazosin (especially first dose)
Hydralazine
Psychoactive drugs
Phenothiazines
Antidepressants (e.g., tricyclic agents, monoamine oxidase inhibitors)
CNS depressants (e.g., barbiturates)
Drugs associated with torsades de pointes
Quinidine
Procainamide
Disopyramide
Flecainide
Sotalol
Terfenadine
Cisapride
Mebefradil
Bepridil
Diuretics
Other mechanisms
Vincristine and other neuropathic drugs
Digitalis
Insulin
Marijuana
Alcohol
Cocaine

striction that may be sufficient to induce cerebral ischemia. Patients usually experience light-headedness, facial pallor, and digital and circumoral numbness and tingling that are not relieved by recumbency.

METABOLIC AND DRUG-RELATED CAUSES

Loss of consciousness associated with drugs or metabolic abnormalities (e.g., hypoglycemia, hypoxia, hypercarbia) is more often prolonged than transient. The onset (and offset) of symptoms associated with these factors is also more gradual than for those associated with true syncope. Common drugs causing syncope are listed in Table 69.3.

TRAUMA

Differentiation of syncope from primary head trauma is important and may be difficult in patients who fall. Younger patients with head trauma may experience retrograde amnesia, complicating the diagnosis of the episode.

HISTORY AND PHYSICAL EXAMINATION

A detailed history of the event from the patient and witnesses is the critical first step in the evaluation of syncope. A diagnosis

TABLE 69.4.   HISTORY AND PHYSICAL EXAMINATION

History

Prior history of syncope; frequency, severity of episodes
Posture before and during the event
Exertional symptoms
Positive family history long QT, syncope, or sudden death
Palpitations, organic heart disease
Premonitory symptoms or sensations
Postictal symptoms, confusion, incontinence, tongue biting
Situational symptoms, coughing, urinating, swallowing, defecating, sensation of pain
Head and neck position before and during event
Time course of onset and recovery from event
Other underlying diseases
Alcohol or drug ingestion
Medications

Physical Examination

Orthostatic blood pressure
Blood pressure in both arms
Skin color and turgor; nail beds
Evidence of trauma or tongue biting
Presence of heart murmurs, rubs, gallops, or bruits
Carotid sinus massage if no bruits
Neurologic examination

may be possible on the basis of the history and examination alone in approximately 30% to 50% of cases. Every effort should be made to obtain information from a witness, when available, who may provide observations of the patient's behavior before, during, and after the event. Such information helps to differentiate syncope from other states of altered consciousness such as dizziness, vertigo, coma, and seizure. Critical issues that should be addressed in the history and physical examination are summarized in Table 69.4.

LABORATORY STUDIES AND DIAGNOSTIC TESTS

After a complete history and examination further information can be derived from the results of carefully selected tests. The relative frequency with which selected test lead to specific diagnosis is listed in Table 69.5.

TABLE 69.5.   RELATIVE FREQUENCY OF DIAGNOSIS PROVIDED BY DIAGNOSTIC TESTS

Test	Percentage
History and physical exam	32
Electrocardiogram	7
Prolonged ECG monitoring	12
Electrophysiologic study	2
Exercise tolerance test	<1

BLOOD TESTS

Routine blood work to help establish the cause of syncope should include serum electrolytes, glucose, and complete blood count. Cardiac arrhythmia may result from hypokalemia. Cardiac enzymes should be evaluated in patients with a history consistent with MI. Blood and urine toxicology screens may reveal the presence of alcohol or other drugs.

ELECTROCARDIOGRAM

The electrocardiogram (ECG) can serve as a useful test and helps to provide a diagnosis in 7% of cases. The ECG may document bradyarrhythmias or tachyarrhythmias. It more commonly provides clues and directs further evaluation. For example, AV block is suggested when bundle-branch block or PR prolongation is present. A prolonged QT interval raises the possibility of polymorphic VT (torsade de pointes) especially in the setting of bradycardia. Q waves consistent with prior MI provide the substrate for reentrant scar–related ventricular arrhythmias as the cause of syncope. Patients hospitalized for syncope should undergo continuous ECG monitoring.

Holter monitoring is appropriate for certain patients evaluated in the ambulatory setting. Prolonged ECG monitoring may establish or confirm the cause of syncope in as many as 12% to 15% of patients. Beyond 24 to 48 hours of ECG monitoring, the diagnostic yield diminishes considerably. Correlation between patients' symptoms and ECG observations is imprecise and occurs in only 25% to 50% of patients. Due to the expense associated with prolonged hospital stays and the imperfect correlation between ECG monitoring and symptoms cited above, there is an increasing reliance on the use of trans-telephonic ECG monitors or event recorders. These monitors are small, portable recorders that are patient-activated to record two ECG channels for up to 30 to 40 seconds. The heart rhythm can be transmitted live or stored for transmission at a later time. The trans-telephonic monitor is particularly useful for patients with palpitations or light-headedness who are at low risk for serious arrhythmia (no structural heart disease) and who have adequate time to activate the recorder during symptoms. For patients with short-lived episodes, continuous recorders with 30 to 45 seconds of activated memory or loop recorders can be provided. These recorders must be worn continuously in order to document events and are typically provided for 2 to 3 weeks. Signal-averaged electrocardiography (SAE) has not been adopted widely in routine practice.

EXERCISE ELECTROCARDIOGRAPHY

Exercise testing is important in those patients with documented or suspected coronary artery disease whose syncope may be due to an arrhythmia triggered by ischemia. Automatic VT and supraventricular tachycardia can also be catecholamine-triggered and exercise-induced. Pharmacologic stress with intravenous dobutamine or adenosine may be useful in patients who cannot exercise. Nuclear or echocardiographic imaging may increase the sensitivity for the detection of myocardial ischemia and is required when pharmacologic stress is necessary. Patients in whom

TABLE 69.6.	FREQUENCY OF DIAGNOSES RESULTING FROM ELECTROPHYSIOLOGIC STUDY FOR UNKNOWN SYNCOPE

Diagnosis	Percentage
Sustained ventricular tachycardia	12
Nonsustained ventricular tachycardia	19
Abnormal sinus node function	7
Prolonged HV interval	3
Abnormal AV node function	2
Supraventricular tachycardia	5
No diagnosis	52

aortic stenosis (AS) or HOCM is the suspected cause of syncope should not undergo exercise testing.

ECHOCARDIOGRAPHY

Echocardiography is indicated in any patient with a suspected cardiac cause (mechanical, arrhythmic) of syncope. In patients in whom adequate acoustic windows can be obtained, transthoracic echocardiography with Doppler interrogation is a highly sensitive and accurate tool for the detection and characterization of valvular (AS), myocardial (HOCM, MI, dilated cardiomyopathy), pericardial (tamponade), and right-sided (pulmonary hypertension) abnormalities associated with syncope. Transesophageal imaging is infrequently required but may be useful when the transthoracic echocardiographic images are technically suboptimal or when a left atrial (myxoma, thrombus) or an aortic (dissection) pathologic process is suspected.

CARDIAC ELECTROPHYSIOLOGIC STUDY

The indications for formal electrophysiologic study in patients with syncope have not been systematically defined. An abnormal

study is more likely to be found in patients with underlying heart disease such as those with prior MI, cardiomyopathy (dilated, hypertrophic, or ischemic) bundle-branch block, preexcitation (Wolff–Parkinson–White syndrome), or for whom documentation of an arrhythmia on ECG or ambulatory monitoring has been obtained. The frequency of diagnoses that result from invasive electrophysiologic testing is shown in Table 69.6. Diagnostic and prognostic information regarding sinus node function, AV nodal and His–Purkinje system conduction, and supraventricular and ventricular arrhythmias can be obtained. Abnormal findings include the induction of sustained monomorphic VT (Fig. 69.3) induction of a supraventricular tachycardia associated with hypotension, prolongation of the HV interval, and prolongation of the sinus node recovery time. Programmed stimulation for induction of ventricular arrhythmias is most sensitive and specific in patients with coronary artery disease. The sensitivity and specificity of the technique are considerably diminished in patients with normal hearts or with structural heart disease due to nonischemic causes.

Prolongation of the HV interval and infrahisian block may indicate that His-Purkinje disease could have been responsible for the syncope. An HV interval longer than 90 milliseconds is abnormal and an indication for pacing in patients with syncope. Some patients with shorter (normal) intervals may still be at risk for AV block.

Prolongation of the sinus node recovery time (more than 1,500 milliseconds) is a specific finding (88% to 100%) but has a low sensitivity for the diagnosis of sinus node dysfunction sensitivity. Continuous ECG monitoring is usually more effective for diagnosis of this abnormality.

Depending on the patient subgroup studied, electrophysiologic testing can establish a cause for syncope in 12% to 70% of subjects. Twenty percent of patients with negative or nondiagnostic study have recurrent syncope; however, the mortality rate is as low as 2%. In contrast, in patients with a possible cardiac cause of syncope, the recurrence rate is approximately 15%, with an associated mortality rate of 7%.

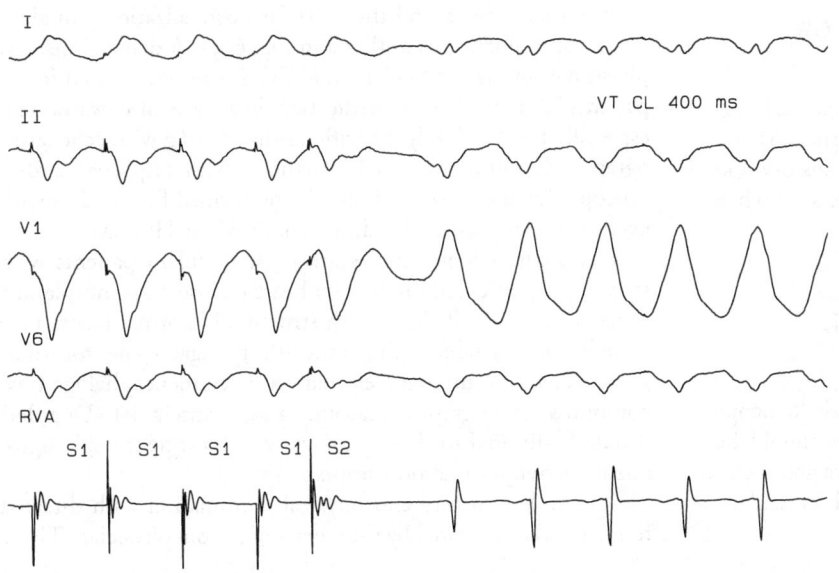

FIGURE 69.3. Surface electrocardiogram leads I, II, V₁, and V₆ and intracardiac electrograms from the right ventricular apex. The figure shows programmed ventricular simulation with administration of a single premature ventricular extra stimulus and the induction of monomorphic ventricular tachycardia with a cycle length of 400 milliseconds. RVA, right ventricular apex; VT, ventricular tachycardia.

Cardiac catheterization and coronary angiography are necessary in some patients to determine the presence and severity of coronary artery disease or the possible anatomical and physiologic basis for an abnormality detected but incompletely characterized by noninvasive means (e.g., tamponade, AS with low cardiac output).

UPRIGHT TILT-TABLE TEST

Upright tilt-table testing at 80° for 60 minutes rarely induces syncope in healthy individuals. However, in patients with neurocardiogenic syncope, this test often induces an event (Fig. 69.1). Upright tilt-table testing for 60 minutes has a sensitivity of 75% and a specificity of 93% for the detection of neurocardiogenic syncope. Addition of intravenous isoproterenol to the tilt protocol increases the sensitivity but decreases the specificity of the test. In severe cases, repeat testing may be considered to evaluate the efficacy of therapeutic intervention.

CAROTID ULTRASONOGRAPHY

Carotid ultrasonography is indicated to define the extent and severity of suspected carotid artery disease, particularly among older patients with audible bruits. Controversy exists as to whether non-invasive carotid testing should be obtained in all patients with syncope at risk for atherosclerotic vascular disease (smoking, hyperlipidemia, audible bruit, claudication, angina). On occasion, magnetic resonance angiography is required for anatomic delineation.

ELECTROENCEPHALOGRAPHY

The diagnostic yield of electroencephalography is very low when seizures are considered unlikely. This test should be reserved for patients in whom the history suggests seizure or in whom comprehensive evaluation has not revealed a cause for loss of consciousness and there remains a suspicion of a neurologic etiology.

CRANIAL COMPUTED TOMOGRAPHY OR MAGNETIC RESONANCE IMAGING

The yield of computed tomography or magnetic resonance imaging, when performed for transient loss of consciousness, is also very low. These studies should be used when the history and physical examination suggest an intracranial process or when head injury is suspected.

■ STRATEGIES FOR OPTIMAL MANAGEMENT

The treatment of syncope depends on the diagnosis. Syncope that is felt to be secondary to a correctable cause should be addressed first. Examples are correction of electrolyte and metabolic abnormalities, removal of offending drugs, and revascularization.

Primary therapy for neurocardiogenic syncope of mild severity includes reassurance and salt loading, when necessary. β-adrenoreceptor antagonists are the next line of treatment and act by decreasing myocardial contractility.

Other pharmacologic agents that have been used to treat this disorder include theophylline, disopyramide, scopolamine, serotonin reuptake inhibitors, and ephedrine. Mineralocorticoids and support stockings may provide additional benefit in patients in whom hypovolemia or venous pooling initiates syncope. Cardiac pacing alone rarely prevents syncope but may be necessary in patients in whom asystole or severe bradycardia is the predominant mechanism. The natural history of neurocardiogenic syncope is variable. Many patients have single or very infrequent episodes, and such patients might not benefit from therapy. There are no known markers that differentiate patients who benefit from therapy from those who do not.

Cardiac arrest survivors, with VT/VF not precipitated by MI, have improved survival with implantable cardiac defibrillators. Anti-arrhythmic therapy may be required for treatment of supraventricular tachycardia. However, for serious episodes or patients who are intolerant of drug therapy, consideration of electrophysiologic study with possible radiofrequency ablation is indicated. Pacemaker therapy is indicated in patients with syncope and conduction system disease not secondary to drug therapy or ischemia.

Hospital admission is required for all patients suspected of cardiac syncope. Patients with cardiac syncope face the highest risk of death in the first 1 to 6 months after presentation. The results of large studies suggest that hospitalization is necessary for patients with evidence of underlying heart disease, a history of chest pain, prior history of arrhythmia, or for those who use medications with proarrhythmic potential. Elderly patients are often hospitalized due to the serious consequences of falling. Motor vehicle driving is regulated by state laws but should be considered on an individual basis. Until it is clear that the syncope has been effectively treated, patients should be instructed to avoid situations such as driving a motor vehicle or operating heavy mechanical equipment.

The cost of an evaluation for syncope will vary depending on the tests ordered and the need for hospitalization. An algorithm for evaluation is outlined in Fig. 69.4. A detailed history, physical examination, and 12-lead ECG is recommended for all patients. A careful drug/medication history is also warranted, especially for the elderly. Specific cardiac testing with echocardiography should be obtained in patients with suspected cardiac syncope. Exercise testing should be performed for patients with exertional symptoms who do not have AS or HOCM.

Electrophysiologic studies are most useful in patients with structural (particularly ischemic) heart disease and unexplained syncope (or VT). Patients with structurally normal hearts may benefit from tilt-table testing if the history suggest a neurocardiogenic cause. Neurologic evaluation (electroencephalography, computed tomography, carotid and transcranial Doppler) should be limited to those patients with focal neurologic signs, seizure activity, or carotid bruits.

A complete history and physical examination with directed tests should be initiated by the emergency room physician. Those

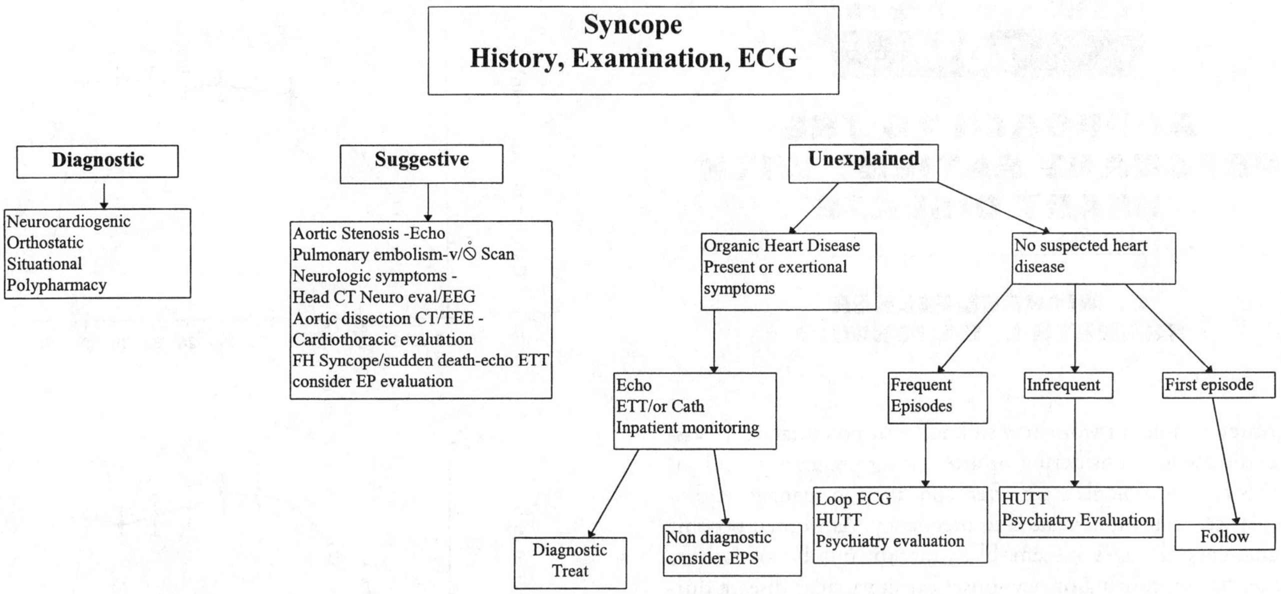

FIGURE 69.4. Flow diagram for the evaluation of syncope. CT, computed tomography; ECG, electrocardiography; EEG, electroencephalogram; EPS, electrophysiology study; ETT, exercise tolerance test; FH, family history; HUTT, head-up tilt test; v/⊚, ventilation perfusion. (Modified from Linzer M, Yang EH, Estes NA III, et al. *Ann Intern Med* 1997;127:76–86.)

patients with ECG abnormalities, history of prior MI, family history of sudden death, or structural heart disease should be referred to a cardiologist/electrophysiologist. Patients with clear seizure activity or focal neurologic deficits warrant cranial computed tomography and additional evaluation. This neurologic workup does not preclude simultaneous cardiac evaluation as 40% of patients with VF will manifest tonic–clonic movements.

PROGNOSIS

Patients with a defined cardiac cause of syncope are at increased risk for sudden and total cardiac death, compared to those with a non-cardiac or unknown cause. Indicators of high risk include significant left ventricular dysfunction, valvular heart disease (AS), hypertrophic cardiomyopathy (with or without obstruction), pulmonary hypertension, known coronary artery disease, long QT syndrome, and preexcitation of the Wolff–Parkinson–White type. Younger patients (under 60 years) without identifiable cardiovascular disease have an excellent prognosis with a low risk of sudden death. However, such patients do experience more frequent recurrences of syncope, though usually without bodily trauma. A normal physical examination and ECG, coupled with the absence of a specific personal or familial cardiac history, usually identifies a low-risk subset.

BIBLIOGRAPHY

Atiga WL, Rowe P, Calkins H. Management of vasovagal syncope. *J Cardiovasc Electrophysiol* 1999;10:874–886.

Brignole M, Gianfranchi L, Menozzi C, et al. Role of autonomic reflexes in syncope associated with paroxysmal atrial fibrillation. *J Am Coll Cardiol* 1993;22:1123–1129.

Coplan NL, Schweitzer P. Carotid sinus hypersensitivity. Case report and review of the literature. *Am J Med* 1984;77:561–565.

Di Girolamo E, Di Iorio C, Sabatini P, et al. Effects of paroxetine hydrochloride, a selective serotonin reuptake inhibitor, on refractory vasovagal syncope: a randomized, double-blind, placebo-controlled study. *J Am Coll Cardiol* 1999;33:1227–1230.

Eagle KA, Black HR, Cook EF, et al. Evaluation of prognostic classifications for patients with syncope. *Am J Med* 1985;79:455–460.

Kapoor WN, Karpf M, Wieand S, et al. A prospective evaluation and follow-up of patients with syncope. *N Engl J Med* 1983;309:197–204.

Kapoor WN, Cha R, Peterson JR, et al. Prolonged electrocardiographic monitoring in patients with syncope. Importance of frequent or repetitive ventricular ectopy. *Am J Med* 1987;82:20–28.

Kapoor WN. Evaluation and management of the patient with syncope. *JAMA* 1992;268:2553–2560.

Linzer M, Varia I, Pontinen M, et al. Medically unexplained syncope: relationship to psychiatric illness. *Am J Med* 1992;92:18S–25S.

Linzer M, Yang EH, Estes NA III, et al. Diagnosing syncope. 1. Value of history, physical examination, and electrocardiography. Clinical Efficacy Assessment Project of the American College of Physicians. *Ann Intern Med* 1997;126:989–996.

Linzer M, Yang EH, Estes NA III, et al. Diagnosing syncope. 2. Unexplained syncope. Clinical Efficacy Assessment Project of the American College of Physicians [comments]. *Ann Intern Med* 1997;127:76–86.

Lipsitz LA. Orthostatic hypotension in the elderly. *N Engl J Med* 1989; 321:952–957.

Mark AL. The Bezold–Jarisch reflex revisited: clinical implications of inhibitory reflexes originating in the heart. *J Am Coll Cardiol* 1983;1:90–102.

Mark AL, Kioschos JM, Abboud FM, et al. Abnormal vascular responses to exercise in patients with aortic stenosis. *J Clin Invest* 1973;52: 1138–1146.

Kelley's Textbook of Internal Medicine, fourth edition. Edited by H. David Humes. Lippincott Williams & Wilkins, Philadelphia © 2000.

C H A P T E R

70

APPROACH TO THE PREGNANT PATIENT WITH HEART DISEASE

G. MICHAEL FELKER
KENNETH L. BAUGHMAN

A greater number of women with known or potential cardiovascular disease are considering or attempting pregnancy, and internists and cardiologists are often consulted to manage cardiovascular complications related to pregnancy. As women become pregnant at older ages, it seems likely that the number of patients with either preexisting or new-onset cardiovascular disease during pregnancy will continue to expand. In this chapter we briefly define the normal physiologic changes that occur during pregnancy, as well as discuss changes in the physical examination and use of noninvasive tests that can complicate the evaluation of these patients. The differential diagnosis of cardiac symptoms appearing during pregnancy is discussed. The diagnosis and treatment of cardiac disorders specific to pregnancy as well as those disorders exacerbated by the physiologic stresses of pregnancy are addressed. Special attention is given to the risks of both diagnostic tests and therapeutic interventions to fetal development and maternal health.

PRESENTATION

The initial signs and symptoms of cardiovascular disease in the context of pregnancy are not significantly different from those in the nonpregnant patient. Evaluation of these signs and symptoms in the pregnant patient, however, is made more difficult by the fact that many symptoms, such as dyspnea on exertion, palpitations, and fatigue, are common during normal pregnancy in women without cardiovascular disease. The unique changes in cardiovascular physiology that occur during pregnancy can mimic other cardiac disorders and are discussed in detail herein.

PATHOPHYSIOLOGY

An appreciation of the normal adaptations of the cardiovascular system to pregnancy is required to understand and treat potential cardiovascular complications associated with pregnancy. Echocardiography has provided substantial insight into the cardiovascular changes that take place during normal pregnancy. The primary changes in cardiovascular physiology are related to increases in cardiac output and circulating blood volume. The time course of changes in cardiac output associated with normal

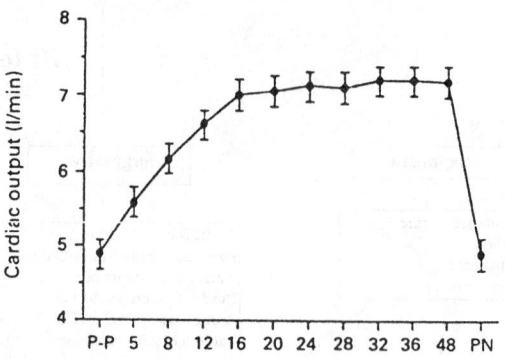

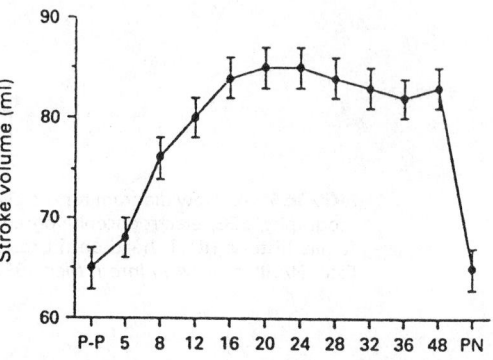

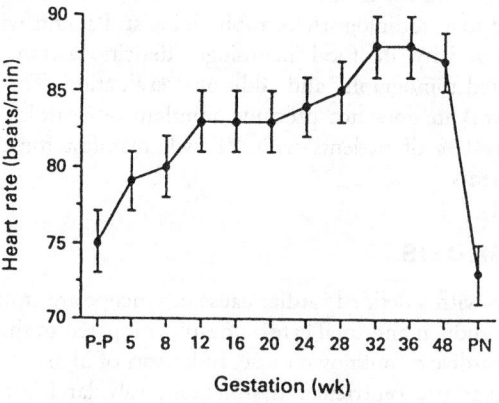

FIGURE 70.1. Changes in cardiac output, stroke volume, and heart rate during pregnancy. P-P, pre-pregnancy; PN, postnatal. (From Hunter S, Robson SC. Adaptation of the maternal heart in pregnancy. *Br Heart J* 1992;68:540–543, with permission.)

pregnancy is shown in Fig. 70.1. Cardiac output in pregnancy begins to increase as early as 5 weeks after the last menstrual period and peaks at 45% over baseline at 24 weeks of gestation. Amplified cardiac output is achieved through rises in both stroke volume and heart rate. During labor, cardiac output increases further, in response to higher demand, primarily accomplished by a rise in stroke volume. Stroke volume is persistently higher in the time period immediately after delivery, possibly owing to relief of venocaval obstruction and a subsequent increase in venous return. These changes in cardiac output may persist into the postpartum period, usually returning to normal within 10 days to 2 weeks after delivery.

In addition to cardiac output, intravascular volume is substantially increased during pregnancy. Plasma volume rises approximately 40% and red cell volume 30% over baseline levels, resulting in mild relative anemia. Multiple changes in neurohumoral activation contribute to this increase in blood volume. Stimulation of the renin–angiotensin axis in response to higher levels of estrogen amplifies circulating aldosterone levels, resulting in enhanced renal tubular absorption of sodium and a subsequent marked increase in total body water, by as much as 8 L by the time of delivery. Mobilization of extracellular fluid and brisk diuresis occur shortly after delivery, resulting in a return to baseline circulating blood volume by 2 weeks postpartum. Systolic blood pressure is relatively unchanged in pregnancy, but diastolic blood pressures are typically 15% lower than in the nonpregnant state, with a concomitant widening of the pulse pressure. These changes are due to a decrease in systemic vascular resistance caused by arteriovenous shunting in the uterus and changes in aortic compliance.

HISTORY AND PHYSICAL EXAMINATION

Cardiac evaluation of the pregnant patient is complicated by the difficulty of differentiating between physiologic and pathologic processes. Many pregnant women have symptoms of palpitations, swelling, dyspnea on exertion, or fatigue despite having no evidence of heart disease. Such symptoms as exertional chest pain or frank syncope are relatively uncommon in pregnancy, however, and require cardiovascular evaluation. Additionally, the significant changes in cardiac physiology that develop during pregnancy can alter substantially the physical examination findings of the pregnant patient. It is crucial for the consulting cardiologist or internist to understand the expected changes in physical findings, to be able to distinguish physiologic from pathologic changes.

Increased total plasma volume results in elevation of jugular venous pressure and lower-extremity edema in more than 80% of normal pregnant women. Growth in uterine size as pregnancy progresses leads to upward movement of the diaphragm and a decrease in lung volumes. Diaphragmatic elevation and higher blood volume may also result in lateral displacement of the left ventricular point of maximal impulse during inspection and palpation of the precordium. Increased stroke volume may produce a rise in the sounds of aortic and pulmonic valve closure as well as a "functional" early systolic murmur over the pulmonic area. In general, diastolic murmurs and gallop rhythms are not normal findings of pregnancy and should suggest underlying structural or functional cardiac abnormalities. In as many as 15% of women, however, a physiologic diastolic murmur is audible at the left sternal border. This murmur is generated by increased blood flow through the internal mammary artery, which stems from enhanced blood flow to the breasts during pregnancy. This mammary souffle may persist in lactating mothers even after delivery. The higher pulse pressure normally seen in pregnancy may also cause Quinke's sign in the peripheral nail beds, leading

to confusion between benign mammary souffle and aortic regurgitation. Echocardiography may be required to distinguish between a physiologic process and underlying valvular heart disease.

LABORATORY STUDIES AND DIAGNOSTIC TESTS

Cardiovascular diagnostic testing in the pregnant patient is complicated by the need to avoid potentially harmful radiation exposure to the developing fetus. Additionally, the interpretation of some diagnostic studies may be made more difficult by the physiologic changes of pregnancy. Diagnostic studies should be selected to minimize risk to the fetus while providing the maximum possible diagnostic information. The potential hazards and benefits of various diagnostic methods are discussed in detail in later sections. Surface electrocardiography and transthoracic echocardiography remain the mainstays of noninvasive cardiac testing in the pregnant patient, providing detailed information on cardiac structure and function without risk to fetal development.

Owing to the elevation of the diaphragm, standard surface electrocardiography may show a leftward shift of the axis of ventricular activation or increased ventricular voltage. These changes are typically within the normal limits of variability, and marked changes from the baseline electrocardiogram should prompt further evaluation for possible cardiac disease. In addition to the changes in stroke volume discussed earlier, echocardiographic studies have shown a mild to moderate increase in left ventricular mass and wall thickness during normal pregnancy. Otherwise, the findings on echocardiography are not substantially different from those of the nonpregnant patient. Visibility of cardiac structures is not impeded by pregnancy, and an adequate echocardiographic window usually can be obtained. The consideration of additional cardiac testing, particularly tests involving radiation exposure—such as with radionuclide studies or coronary angiography—must include careful assessment of the risk to the fetus as well as potential diagnostic or therapeutic benefit to the mother.

RADIATION EXPOSURE AND PREGNANCY

The possibility that radiation exposure will injure the developing fetus is a major concern in evaluating the appropriateness of cardiovascular diagnostic testing in pregnancy. Radiation exposure damages cells both directly and through the generation of ionized water and free radicals. Radiation exposure's potential harmful effects to the developing fetus include growth impairment, structural deformity, gonadal damage, and neoplasia. An increased risk of childhood malignancy associated with in utero radiation exposure has been well documented, as has a dose response with increasing levels of radiation exposure. Exposure during the first trimester is considered more hazardous than later exposure, though there is increased risk associated with exposure during any trimester of pregnancy. There is virtually no data establishing significant fetal damage below 1 rad, though no level of radiation exposure can be considered to carry no risk.

The amount of fetal radiation exposure from a given radiologic procedure varies based on a multitude of factors, including the type of radiation source, size of the patient, distance from the area of investigation, and use of uterine shielding. Consideration of diagnostic testing that uses radiation must include assessment of the dose of radiation to the fetus, fetal age and development, and potential harm to the mother by delaying testing or using alternative means of cardiovascular assessment.

CARDIAC CATHETERIZATION

Standard cardiac catheterization results in an exposure of approximately 500 Gray to a shielded uterus compared with 50 Gray for a standard radiograph. The actual degree of radiation exposure varies, depending on the length and complexity of the procedure. If catheterization is deemed necessary, brachial as opposed to femoral access should be used. Noninvasive studies, such as echocardiography, can generally provide sufficient data regarding left and right ventricular performance to obviate the need for ventriculography during cardiac catheterization. If pulmonary artery catheterization is required for monitoring of hemodynamics in pregnant patients with severe or unstable cardiac disease, it almost always can be performed via an internal jugular approach without the need for fluoroscopically guided catheter placement.

RADIONUCLIDE IMAGING

Radionuclide imaging is frequently used in the nonpregnant patient for noninvasive evaluation of coronary blood flow or ventricular function. Although the degree of fetal radiation exposure is less with these agents than with standard radiologic studies, there is still an increased risk of childhood malignancy associated with the use of these agents in the pregnant patient. In particular, radionuclides eliminated by the kidney may collect in the maternal bladder, resulting in exposure at close proximity to the fetus. In general, these agents should be avoided if possible, especially during the first trimester. If cardiac stress testing is required, stress or dobutamine echocardiography may be used to provide similar information without the potential risks of radiation exposure.

MAGNETIC RESONANCE IMAGING

Magnetic resonance imaging (MRI) is a relatively new technique in the evaluation of cardiovascular disease and holds the promise of a greater degree of noninvasive structural and functional cardiac evaluation than is available with current techniques. There are no data that suggest any untoward effects of this imaging method on either the fetus or the mother, though little long-term data are available. Given this lack of long-term safety data, MRI should be used with caution in the pregnant patient, especially during the first trimester. If this technique proves to be safe, it is hoped that it will allow detailed cardiac evaluation without the fetal radiation exposure inherent in other diagnostic tests.

DIFFERENTIAL DIAGNOSIS

The differential diagnosis of cardiovascular symptoms in the pregnant patient is broad and complicated by the difficulties of distinguishing between physiologic and pathologic processes. Some cardiovascular disorders are specific to the pregnant patient, while others are common in the nonpregnant population but require special consideration during pregnancy. In pregnant patients with complaints of dyspnea, palpitations, or fatigue, interpretation of the history and physical examination may be difficult. In addition to a careful history and physical examination, echocardiography is often a critical aid to establishing a diagnosis in women with undiagnosed cardiovascular disease initially seen in the context of pregnancy. As in the assessment of the nonpregnant patient with heart disease, maintaining a wide differential diagnosis is critical to arriving at appropriate diagnostic conclusions.

In women with known preexisting cardiac disorders, such as valvular or congenital heart disease, the diagnosis is usually straightforward, since an exacerbation of a preexisting condition is more likely than the appearance of a new disorder. In women without known preexisting cardiac disorders, rare but potentially life-threatening cardiovascular disorders, such as peripartum cardiomyopathy or coronary artery dissection, must be prominent among the potential diagnoses if they are not to be overlooked. Hypertensive disorders of pregnancy, including chronic hypertension, gestational hypertension, and preeclampsia, are the most common cardiovascular disorders during pregnancy and are usually apparent on careful evaluation. Optimal management of specific conditions likely to be encountered in the pregnant patient is discussed in detail in the next section.

STRATEGIES FOR OPTIMAL CARE

Optimal treatment of the pregnant woman with cardiac disease must address and balance the well-being of both mother and fetus, requiring an understanding of both maternal pathophysiology and the potential fetal effects of contemplated therapies. Optimal care of the patient with complex cardiac disease in the context of pregnancy often requires close cooperation among members of a multidisciplinary team, including specialists in cardiology, obstetrics, neonatology, and anesthesia. Issues related to the diagnosis and management of specific important cardiovascular disorders in the pregnant patient are discussed herein.

HYPERTENSION IN PREGNANCY

Elevated blood pressure may occur in as many as 10% of pregnancies, and this complication remains a major cause of maternal and fetal morbidity and mortality. Hypertension during pregnancy is associated with higher rates of preterm deliveries, perinatal mortality, and fetal neurologic impairment. Three categories of hypertension in pregnancy are generally recognized: chronic hypertension, gestational hypertension, and preeclampsia. Chronic hypertension is defined as hypertension existing before pregnancy or blood pressure of at least 140/90 mm Hg before 20 weeks' gestation. Owing to the normal physiologic changes of pregnancy, many women with chronic hypertension before pregnancy will be normotensive before 20 weeks' gestation.

Women with severe chronic hypertension (diastolic blood pressure greater than 110 mm Hg) are at higher risk of complications, such as preeclampsia and placental abruption, and pharmacologic treatment in these patients clearly lowers the risk of fetal and maternal morbidity and mortality. In general, fetal and maternal outcomes in patients with mild chronic hypertension (diastolic blood pressure less than 110 mm Hg) are good, and the value of treatment for this degree of hypertension during pregnancy is less clear. Gestational hypertension is defined as asymptomatic elevation of blood pressure after 20 weeks of gestation in a woman with normal blood pressure before pregnancy. Although care must be taken to ensure that gestational hypertension is not an early manifestation of preeclampsia, fetal and maternal outcomes appear to be good with or without treatment in women with simple gestational hypertension. Women with mild, uncomplicated chronic hypertension or gestational hypertension can generally be treated as part of routine obstetrical care. Severe hypertension, especially with evidence of end-organ damage, should prompt inpatient admission and referral to a cardiologist or an obstetrical specialist experienced in dealing with hypertensive disorders of pregnancy.

Pharmacologic treatment of hypertension in pregnancy must be guided by an understanding of both the mechanisms of hypertension and the potential effect of therapy on fetal development. The safety of various antihypertensive medications in pregnancy is outlined in Table 70.1. Methyldopa is a safe and cost-effective antihypertensive agent and traditionally has been the antihypertensive drug of choice in pregnancy. It has an established long-term safety record and substantial evidence of improved fetal outcomes with its use. Despite early concerns about the possibility of fetal growth retardation, β-blockers have now been shown to be relatively safe in pregnancy for the treatment of hypertension. Selective β-blocking agents are preferred over nonselective agents.

Diuretics generally should not be used to treat hypertension in pregnant women, though women with chronic hypertension whose blood pressure has been controlled well by diuretic therapy before pregnancy may continue diuretics during pregnancy. Diuretic therapy should be discontinued if signs of preeclampsia develop. Dihydropyridine calcium-channel blocking agents, such as nifedipine or amlodipine, have not been well studied in pregnancy but have been used safely to treat hypertension in this context. Angiotensin-converting enzyme (ACE) inhibitors have been shown to be teratogenic in both animal and human studies and should be strictly avoided by women who are pregnant or who are contemplating pregnancy.

Preeclampsia is the most severe hypertensive disorder of pregnancy and may progress to eclampsia, a life-threatening seizure disorder. Preeclampsia is defined as the presence of hypertension, edema, and proteinuria after 20 weeks' gestation in a previously normotensive woman. This diagnosis may be difficult to establish in women with preexisting chronic hypertension. The development of proteinuria in a woman with chronic hypertension should strongly suggest the possibility of superimposed pre-

eclampsia. Preeclampsia appears to result from the failure of the normal cardiovascular adaptations of pregnancy, with decreased cardiac output and blood volume and increased systemic vascular resistance. This failure of cardiac adaptation to pregnancy may be the result of failure of the uterine spiral arteries to develop, prohibiting arteriovenous shunting in the uterus and thereby increasing systemic vascular resistance. The precise cause of preeclampsia remains unclear, and many potential etiologic factors, including immunologic phenomena, prostaglandin deficiency, and endothelial dysfunction, have been proposed.

Treatment of preeclampsia depends on the severity of hypertension and proteinuria. Patients with mild preeclampsia may be monitored as outpatients, and the wisdom of aggressive management of hypertension in these patients is unclear. Women with severe preeclampsia or those with progressive symptoms should be treated as inpatients by physicians with experience in the management of this disorder. In women with severe manifestations of preeclampsia or women at term, delivery is the ultimate therapy. Pharmacologic therapy with hydralazine, labetelol, or nifedipine should be used to lower diastolic blood pressure to below 105 mm Hg in women with severe hypertension. Diuretic therapy should be avoided, since volume depletion is common in women with preeclampsia. Women with severe hypertension despite aggressive pharmacologic therapy should undergo delivery regardless of fetal viability. Intravenous magnesium therapy should be given at about the time of delivery to lower the risk of seizure.

VALVULAR HEART DISEASE

Despite a decline in the incidence of rheumatic heart disease, valvular heart disease remains a relatively common concern in both pregnant patients and women contemplating pregnancy. The changes in cardiovascular physiology that accompany pregnancy can unmask previously asymptomatic valvular heart disease or exacerbate a known preexisting condition. Cardiologists and internists can be consulted to assist in the treatment of pregnant patients with native valvular heart disease or prosthetic heart valves or to recommend an appropriate choice of artificial valve for women contemplating future pregnancy.

For patients with disease of native valves, the location and nature of the valvular lesion dictate management. Despite the declining incidence of rheumatic heart disease, the majority of acquired valvular heart disease encountered during pregnancy is rheumatic in origin. Twenty-five percent of women with chronic rheumatic heart disease show initial manifestations during pregnancy, and acute rheumatic fever may recur during pregnancy. Mitral stenosis is by far the most common rheumatic valvular lesion seen in pregnancy and is poorly tolerated, owing to the hemodynamic changes of the pregnant state. The increases in heart rate and blood volume that accompany normal pregnancy may lessen the time for diastolic ventricular filling and greatly amplify the pressure gradient across the stenotic mitral valve. These changes can result in increases in left atrial pressure and a higher incidence of atrial fibrillation, further impairing ventricular filling.

The incidence of symptoms in pregnant women with mitral stenosis increases up to 20 weeks' gestation, by which time the

TABLE 70.1.	MATERNAL AND FETAL CONSIDERATIONS IN THE USE OF CARDIOVASCULAR DRUGS

Drug	Use	Action	Therapeutic Plasma Concentration	Transplacental Passage (Cord/ Maternal Serum Level)	Eliminating Organ
Digoxin	Congestive heart failure, supraventricular tachycardia and tachyarrhythmia	Prolongs refractory period and decreases conduction velocity in atrioventricular node; enhances force and velocity of myocardial contractility	0.5–2 ng/mL	0.6–1	Kidney
Verapamil	Supraventricular tachyarrhythmia involving atrioventricular node	Retards ventricular response to atrial tachyarrhythmia and may cause conversion to sinus rhythm	50–100 ng/mL	0.3–0.4	Liver
β-Adrenergic blocking agents					
Propranolol	Hypertension, hypertrophic obstructive cardiomyopathy, thyrotoxicosis, tachycardia, premature atrial and ventricular contractions, and arrhythmia	Inhibits adrenergic stimulation of cardiac pacemakers, increases threshold of excitability, prolongs refractory period, and delays conduction velocity	50–100 μg/mL	0.1–0.3	Liver
Labetalol	Hypertension	General β- and α-blocking agent	0.7–3 μg/mL	<1	Liver
Metroprolol	Hypertension	β₁-Selective blocking agent	50–100 ng/mL	<1	Liver
Atenolol	Hypertension	β₁-Selective blocking agent	0.2–0.5 μg/mL	<1	Liver
Procainamide	Prevention and treatment of ventricular ectopy, prevention of atrial tachyarrhythmia	Decreases automaticity and conduction velocity in the atrium, atrioventricular node, and conduction system	4–14 μg/mL	0.8–1.3	Kidney
Quinidine	Conversion and prevention of supraventricular and ventricular tachyarrhythmia	Decreases myocardial contractility, automaticity, and conduction velocity and increases refractoriness in conduction system	2–8 μg/mL	0.2–0.9	Liver
Phenytoin	Use limited to acute management of digitalis-induced arrhythmia	Decreases automaticity and potentiates atrioventricular conduction	10–20 μg/mL	~1.0	Kidney
Disopyramide	Ventricular and atrial tachyarrhythmia	Retards conduction in conduction system and ventricle	3–6 μg/mL	0.4	Liver
Lidocaine	Ventricular tachyarrhythmia	Decreases automaticity of Purkinje fibers: increases fibrillation threshold	1.5–4 μg/mL	0.5–0.6	Liver
Diuretics	Chronic hypertension, congestive heart failure, pulmonary edema	Decreases preload	—	Probably 1, but largely unknown	—
Nitrates	Ischemic chest pain, adjunct to management of congestive heart failure and severe pregnancy-induced hypertension	Decreases preload by causing venous dilatation	—	—	—
Nitroprusside	Hypertensive emergencies	Directly effects peripheral vascular smooth muscle to decrease arteriolar resistance and increase venous capacitance	—	Crosses placenta	—

Loading Dose		Maintenance Dose		Drug Interaction	Fetal Complications and Pregnancy Consideration
Oral	i.v.	Oral	i.v.		
1–2.5 mg	0.5–2 mg	0.25–0.75 mg/d	0.25 mg/d	Serum levels may increase when verapamil or quinidine is added	Fetus may tolerate higher levels than adult; because of higher glomerular filtration rate and limited oral absorption, higher doses may be needed in pregnancy
80–120 mg q 6–8 hr	0.15 mg/kg at 0.1 mg/min	20–160 mg q 6–8 hr	0.0025–0.005 mg/kg/min	Do not give with propranolol or to patient with sinus atrioventricular nodal abnormality or severe ventricular dysfunction	Experience is limited; used successfully to treat fetal supraventricular tachyarrhythmia
—	0.5 mg q 5 min to total of 4–10 mg	20–160 mg q 6–8 hr	—	Do not give with verapamil	Fetal brachycardia and growth retardation and neonatal hypoglycemia have been reported; generally absence of significant fetal side effects
—	—	—	—	—	Fetal effects of these drugs are probably slight; experience is limited, and routine use in pregnancy not recommended
—	25 mg/min up to 100 mg and at 10-min intervals to 500 mg	6 mg/kg q 4 hr	1–5 mg/min		The active metabolite *N*-acetylprocainamide may accumulate in the fetus; drug probably safe but should be reserved for patients refractory to quinidine
Do not give	250–500 mg q 6 hr	250–500 q 6 hr	Do not give	May cause digoxin levels to increase; for supraventricular tachyarrhythmia; pretreat with digoxin	Generally considered safe in pregnancy, but neonatal thrombocytopenia and in utero deaths reported
—	100 mg q 5 min to 1 g	300–500 mg/d	—	—	Metabolized slowly; associated with teratogenicity and coagulopathy when given long term; use only for acute management of digitalis toxicity
300 mg	—	100–200 mg q 6–8 hr	—	Does not alter digoxin levels	Pregnancy experience limited to case reports. Do not use routinely in pregnancy
Do not give	1–1.4 mg/kg at 25–30 mg/min	Do not give	1–4 mg/min	—	Preterm newborn has decreased ability to metabolize amides
—	None	Dosages same as in nonpregnant state		Do not use routinely in pregnancy-induced hypertension	Use in pregnancy may decrease plasma volume to point of limiting uteroplacental profusion; use only in situations of clear fluid overload
—	None	—	—	—	Experience limited
—	None	—	3–10 μg/kg/min to a maximum dose of 3.5 mg/kg	—	Cyanide by-product levels higher in fetus than maternal levels, but standard doses do not present a major risk of cyanide toxicity

hemodynamic changes of pregnancy are usually maximal. Management of pregnant women with mitral stenosis should include attempts to decrease circulating blood volume and prevent tachycardia. Diuretic therapy may be indicated in women with pulmonary congestion, but care must be taken to avoid hypovolemia and uterine hypoperfusion. Restriction of physical activity lowers the heart rate and limits cardiac work, and β-blocking agents may be required to further decrease heart rate. Digoxin may be added in patients at high risk of atrial fibrillation, such as those with significant left atrial enlargement.

Vaginal delivery can be accomplished in most women with mitral stenosis, though hemodynamic monitoring may be required during and immediately after delivery. Mitral valvuloplasty or replacement can usually be deferred with careful medical management, but some patients with severe symptomatic mitral stenosis may require correction before delivery. The risks to the mother of open commissurotomy, closed commissurotomy, or valve replacement are similar to those in nonpregnant patients. The risk of fetal loss, however, is higher for both open commissurotomy and valve replacement. Closed commissurotomy is therefore recommended as providing the best chance for satisfactory fetal outcome in centers with experience in this technique. Balloon valvuloplasty has been performed with a low incidence of maternal and fetal complications, but experience with this technique is limited.

Mitral regurgitation and aortic regurgitation are relatively well tolerated in pregnancy, owing to unloading of the left ventricle caused by the decreased systemic vascular resistance accompanying pregnancy. Diuretic therapy and hydralazine for afterload reduction may be safely used in pregnancy for symptomatic patients. Mitral valve prolapse is relatively common in women of childbearing age. Outcomes of pregnancy in the context of this disorder are generally good, even if prolapse is associated with valvular thickening or mitral regurgitation. Isolated rheumatic aortic stenosis rarely occurs, and most patients with aortic valve obstruction have a congenitally bicuspid aortic valve. Moderate aortic stenosis is usually well tolerated, but severe aortic stenosis (aortic valve area less than 1 cm^2) may require termination of pregnancy or surgical intervention.

Evaluation of the safety of pregnancy in women with preexisting prosthetic heart valves must take into account the type of valve, the valve position, and the symptomatic state of the patient. Women with prosthetic heart valves and significant symptoms of heart failure have a substantial risk of both maternal and fetal morbidity and should be strongly discouraged from attempting pregnancy. Even in women without symptoms of heart failure, both bioprostheses and mechanical heart valves present significant difficulties in management. Although bioprosthetic heart valves avoid the necessity for systemic anticoagulation, there is substantial evidence that pregnancy and delivery accelerate the deterioration of such valves. This increased incidence of valve failure appears to be related to the amplified hemodynamic stresses and higher calcium turnover associated with pregnancy.

Alternatively, pregnant patients with mechanical heart valves are at substantially increased risk of thromboembolic complications, and no satisfactory anticoagulation regimen exists for these patients. Mechanical valves in the mitral position are more prone to thromboembolic complications than aortic valves. The optimal regimen for anticoagulation in pregnant patients with mechanical heart valves is not well established. Warfarin must be avoided in the first trimester of pregnancy, owing to its harmful effects on embryonic development; it also may increase the risk of spontaneous abortion or premature delivery. Unfortunately, the use of alternative regimens, such as dose-adjusted subcutaneous heparin, is associated with an increased incidence of potentially severe thromboembolic complications, even when there is an appropriate increase in the activated partial thromboplastin time. Subcutaneous heparin, therefore, does not appear to be sufficient as a sole anticoagulation agent during pregnancy, especially in patients with mechanical mitral valves. Additionally, long-term heparin use is associated with an enhanced risk of severe osteoporosis. Low-molecular-weight forms of heparin may offer an effective and safe alternative to unfractionated heparin or warfarin, but little data are available on their use in pregnancy to date. Most authorities recommend systemic heparin therapy during the first trimester of pregnancy, followed by warfarin therapy from 12 weeks of gestation until 2 to 3 weeks before delivery. Heparin can then be restarted until delivery. Warfarin may be given safely in the postpartum period, even to mothers who are breast-feeding.

PERIPARTUM CARDIOMYOPATHY

Peripartum cardiomyopathy is defined as cardiomyopathy developing during the last month of pregnancy or the first 5 months postpartum, in the absence of preexisting heart disease or other causes of left ventricular dysfunction. Peripartum cardiomyopathy is a rare disorder—it is seen in 1 in 1,300 to 1 in 4,000 deliveries in the United States. Traditional risk factors for this condition include older maternal age, toxemia, twin pregnancies, and multiparity, though new studies have suggested that women without these risk factors may be equally at risk. The source of this condition is unknown. Multiple autoimmune, infectious, toxic, and metabolic factors have been proposed, but none have been verified. Many investigators have found a high incidence of histologic myocarditis in patients with this disorder, but other studies have not reproduced this finding. We have reported the presence of histologic myocarditis in 78% of women with peripartum cardiomyopathy who underwent endomyocardial biopsy early after the diagnosis was clinically established. Most authorities favor an immunologic origin of this disorder, but definitive triggers for autoimmunity have not been identified.

Eighty percent of women with peripartum cardiomyopathy experience symptoms in the first 4 months postpartum, usually symptoms of congestive heart failure, hemoptysis, or embolic phenomena. These symptoms can be confused with those of other disorders, such as toxemia or pulmonary embolism, and some published series on this disorder have created confusion by including patients who did not fit the strict diagnostic criteria outlined here. The diagnosis can be difficult to establish in patients showing initial signs before or immediately after delivery, when symptoms of dyspnea on exertion or orthopnea may be thought to be related to normal pregnancy. In our experience, patients who experience symptoms soon after delivery tend to have a more severe case than patients whose symptoms develop later. The physical examination of patients with peripartum cardiomyopathy shows standard findings of congestive heart failure, including a third heart sound, pulmonary rales, jugular venous distension, and peripheral edema.

Electrocardiography usually shows non-specific ST- and T-wave changes, and echocardiography typically shows severely depressed left ventricular function, with or without left ventricular dilatation. Pulmonary artery catheterization often indicates increased filling pressures and decreased cardiac output, suggesting a diagnosis of cardiomyopathy. Although endomyocardial biopsy can identify patients with histologic myocarditis, the therapeutic benefit of this finding is uncertain, since immunosuppressive therapy is of unclear benefit in these patients. Our practice is to defer endomyocardial biopsy and pulmonary artery catheterization in patients with peripartum cardiomyopathy, except those patients who fail to improve after 2 weeks of standard heart failure therapy. Standard heart failure therapy in patients who experience peripartum cardiomyopathy after delivery is similar to that in nonpregnant patients and should include ACE inhibitors, diuretics, and digoxin. In patients who show signs of peripartum cardiomyopathy during the last month of pregnancy, ACE inhibitor therapy must be avoided, owing to its potential impact on the fetus. Hydralazine may be safely administered as an alternative afterload reduction agent until after delivery in these patients. Thromboembolic complications are common in this disorder, and anticoagulation is recommended after delivery, especially for those patients with persistent left ventricular dysfunction.

The prognosis for patients with peripartum cardiomyopathy varies. Some patients have spontaneous recovery of left ventricular function, and others progress to end-stage dilated cardiomyopathy. The prognosis of patients who recover left ventricular function is excellent, while the prognosis for patients with persistent left ventricular compromise is similar to that for patients with other forms of dilated cardiomyopathy. No features have been identified that predict which patients are likely to make a spontaneous recovery of left ventricular function. Those who recover ventricular function almost always do so within 6 months of their initial symptoms. In patients who progress to dilated cardiomyopathy, cardiac transplantation has been performed, with long-term outcomes similar to those for age-matched controls.

The safety of subsequent pregnancy in women with a history of peripartum cardiomyopathy is the subject of controversy. Women with persistent left ventricular dysfunction are at extremely high risk with subsequent pregnancies and should be advised against conception. In women who have normalized ventricular function, the risk of recurrence with subsequent pregnancy is unknown. Some authors have reported a substantial incidence of recurrence of cardiomyopathy, while other series have indicated no increased risk with subsequent pregnancy and delivery. Stress or dobutamine echocardiography may identify those patients with apparently normal ventricular function at rest who may lack contractile reserve and therefore be at higher risk of recurrence of heart failure under the physiologic stress of pregnancy.

OTHER CARDIOMYOPATHIES AND CARDIAC TRANSPLANTATION

Patients with preexisting left ventricular dysfunction due to dilated cardiomyopathy are at high risk of both maternal and fetal complications during pregnancy. The hemodynamic stresses of pregnancy increase the likelihood of cardiac decompensation in these patients, and ACE inhibitor therapy must be discontinued owing to its teratogenic effects. The hypercoagulable state of pregnancy also raises the risk of thromboembolic complications in this predisposed population. Dilated cardiomyopathy is therefore considered a contraindication to pregnancy.

Hypertrophic cardiomyopathy is usually tolerated well in pregnancy. The changes in hemodynamics that occur with normal pregnancy may serve to diminish obstruction of left ventricular outflow, making severe symptoms during pregnancy less likely. Outflow obstruction can be exacerbated by the acute increases in cardiac contractility and blood loss that occur during delivery, however, and care must be taken to ensure adequate preload and to avoid excessive diuresis. The presence of arrhythmia in women with hypertrophic cardiomyopathy necessitates a thorough evaluation, since sudden death is the most common mode of death in these patients. The β-adrenergic blocking agents are the drugs of choice if pharmacotherapy is required for treatment of arrhythmia. Digoxin should be avoided, because it may enhance the obstruction to ventricular outflow. Patients with hypertrophic cardiomyopathy should be considered for prophylaxis against bacterial endocarditis during delivery.

Pregnancy in women who have undergone cardiac transplantation frequently is complicated by hypertension and hypercholesterolemia and the necessity of immunosuppressive therapy. Women who become pregnant after cardiac transplantation have a higher risk of rejection as well as preterm delivery and other neonatal complications. Routine surveillance for graft rejection via endomyocardial biopsy must be interrupted in light of concerns regarding fetal radiation exposure, leading to potential delays in the recognition of graft rejection until hemodynamic compromise has occurred. Although successful pregnancy and delivery have been reported after cardiac transplantation, pregnancy in this group is generally considered high risk and is discouraged.

PRIMARY PULMONARY HYPERTENSION

Primary pulmonary hypertension (PPH) is a rare disorder of unknown cause, resulting in fixed elevation of pulmonary pressures without evidence of left-sided heart disease, congenital heart disease, or chronic pulmonary emboli. Since this disease disproportionately affects young women, it may be encountered in women who are pregnant or who are considering pregnancy. The prognosis for nonpregnant patients with PPH is grim, and the hemodynamic stresses of pregnancy further exacerbate this condition. Pregnancy in PPH is associated with a maternal mortality rate as high as 50% in the peripartum period; for this reason, pregnancy is contraindicated in the context of PPH. Termination of pregnancy should be recommended to women with this disorder who become pregnant. If delivery is attempted, it should be performed in an intensive care unit with the use of invasive hemodynamic monitoring and subspecialty care in cardiology, maternal–fetal medicine, and anesthesia.

CONGENITAL HEART DISEASE

With improvements in the recognition and treatment of congenital heart disease, more women with these disorders are reaching childbearing age and attempting pregnancy. Although a full discussion of the risks of pregnancy in the various forms of congenital heart disease is beyond the scope of this chapter, several general points can be made. A woman with congenital heart disease who is considering pregnancy should undergo genetic counseling regarding the potential for transmission of congenital heart disease to her children as well as counseling regarding the risks to maternal and fetal health. Children of women with congenital heart disease are at two to tenfold increased risk of having congenital heart disease, depending on the genetics of the specific condition. Treatment of these patients requires a multidisciplinary team approach, including specialists in cardiology, obstetrics, pediatrics, genetics, and anesthesia.

In general, any disorder associated with fixed increases in pulmonary vascular resistance dramatically raises the risk of pregnancy. Eisenmenger syndrome—pulmonary hypertension, right-to-left shunting, and cyanosis—is associated with maternal mortality rates of 40% or more and should be considered an absolute contraindication to pregnancy. As outlined earlier for women with primary pulmonary hypertension, women with pulmonary hypertension stemming from congenital heart disease who attempt delivery should be cared for in an intensive care unit with invasive hemodynamic monitoring. Other forms of uncorrected or partially corrected cyanotic congenital heart disease, such as tetralogy of Fallot, are also associated with poor maternal and fetal outcomes. In general, however, both maternal and fetal outcomes in noncyanotic forms of congenital heart disease are good.

Women with Marfan's syndrome are at risk of aortic dissection during pregnancy, particularly patients with aortic root dilatation, aortic regurgitation, or left ventricular dysfunction. Women with normal aortic root diameters and ventricular function may undertake pregnancy, although cases of aortic dissection in women without aortic root dilatation have been reported. Other forms of inherited connective tissue disease also may predispose to aortic dissection under the increased hemodynamic stresses of pregnancy and delivery. Women with congenital heart disease who wish to become pregnant should undergo careful cardiac evaluation, including echocardiography and stress testing, to evaluate their cardiac reserve and ability to handle the hemodynamic stresses of pregnancy.

PROPHYLAXIS FOR BACTERIAL ENDOCARDITIS

Indications for bacterial endocarditis are generally similar to those in nonpregnant patients. The American Heart Association guidelines do not recommend antibiotic prophylaxis for women with structural heart disease undergoing uncomplicated vaginal delivery, although other authorities do recommend standard antibiotic prophylaxis before delivery for patients with forms of heart disease for which prophylaxis is indicated. Antibiotic prophylaxis is not required for delivery via caesarean section. The standard regimen is 2 g ampicillin administered intravenously or intramuscularly plus gentamicin, 1.5 mg per kilogram, within 30 minutes of delivery, followed by 1 g amoxicillin taken orally or 1 g intravenous or intramuscular ampicillin 6 hours following delivery. Vancomycin may be used in patients with allergy to amoxicillin or ampicillin.

ARRHYTHMIA MANAGEMENT DURING PREGNANCY

The hemodynamic stresses of pregnancy can exacerbate arrhythmia in women with underlying structural heart disease, such as atrial fibrillation in mitral stenosis, or increase the risk of new arrhythmias in women without known cardiac disease. In women with new, unexplained arrhythmias occurring during the final month of pregnancy or in the first 5 months after delivery, the possibility of peripartum cardiomyopathy must be considered. Pharmacologic management of cardiac arrhythmias during pregnancy is complicated by variations in drug absorption and metabolism, resulting in uncertain therapeutic drug levels and necessitating frequent monitoring to avoid toxicity. Moreover, some commonly used antiarrhythmic medications may have adverse affects on fetal development, especially in the first trimester of pregnancy. The safety of many antiarrhythmic medications commonly used during pregnancy is outline in Table 70.1 and is discussed herein.

In general, pharmacologic antiarrhythmic therapy should be avoided in pregnancy if at all possible. Some of the class I agents, such as procainamide, quinidine, and lidocaine, are considered safe for use during pregnancy, though their efficacy in the long-term management of malignant ventricular arrhythmias is questionable in nonpregnant patients. Phenytoin is contraindicated in pregnancy owing to a strong potential for teratogenicity with long-term use. It may be given in acute cases for digoxin toxicity. Although there is some concern about the potential for β-blocking agents to cause growth retardation or fetal bradycardia, these agents are considered to be relatively safe for use during pregnancy. Class III agents, such as sotolol and amiodarone, should be avoided in pregnancy, except in the case of life-threatening ventricular arrhythmias. Calcium channel blocking agents are considered relatively safe in pregnancy, but experience is limited, and they should be used with caution. Digoxin is deemed safe for the treatment of supraventricular arrhythmias, though careful monitoring of drug levels is required to avoid the potential for digoxin toxicity. If possible, nonpharmacologic methods should be used to manage arrhythmias during pregnancy. Electrical cardioversion and cardiac pacing can be performed without untoward effects on the fetus. Electrophysiologic studies or catheter ablation procedures should be deferred until after delivery if possible, to avoid the risk of fetal radiation exposure.

MYOCARDIAL ISCHEMIA AND INFARCTION

Myocardial infarction is a rare complication of pregnancy, but it may become more common with the increasing numbers of older women attempting pregnancy. The mortality rate of myocardial infarction in the context of pregnancy is reported to be as high as 50%. Myocardial ischemia during pregnancy may stem from coronary artery disease, coronary vasospasm, a hypercoagulable state such as the antiphospholipid antibody syndrome, or coronary dissection. Coronary dissection is a rare cause of myocardial ischemia, but it is more common in pregnancy, especially in the immediate postpartum period. Significant fixed coronary artery disease is rare in women of childbearing age, but it could become more common as more women defer childbearing until later in life. In general, women with known coronary artery disease before pregnancy should be discouraged from becoming pregnant, given the increased metabolic demands of the normal changes in cardiovascular physiology, which may worsen symptoms of angina and myocardial ischemia.

Women with coronary artery disease who do become pregnant usually can be treated successfully with medical therapy. If diagnostic testing or risk stratification is required, stress or dobutamine echocardiography should be used, instead of radionuclide techniques. Management of acute coronary syndromes in pregnant patients is complicated by the difficulty in applying the standard therapies used for nonpregnant patients. Thrombolytic therapy should be considered high risk, though little data exist on its use in pregnancy. Heparin may be administered as an antithrombotic agent. Low-dose aspirin, β-blocking agents, and nitrates can be used with caution to treat myocardial ischemia. Calcium channel blocking agents, such as nifedipine, can be administered if coronary vasospasm is suspected.

Coronary angioplasty has been performed during pregnancy, but it should not be done unless absolutely necessary, to avoid fetal radiation exposure. No data exist on the use of primary angioplasty for acute myocardial infarction in pregnant patients. Cardiopulmonary bypass surgery may be attempted during pregnancy if it is required, but it is associated with substantial risk to the fetus from hypothermia and decreased perfusion of the uretroplacental unit. If cardiopulmonary bypass is required, normothermic bypass at high flow volumes is recommended. Patients at more than 20 weeks' gestation should be placed in the left lateral decubitus position to prevent uterine obstruction of venous return. Preparation must be made for emergency caesarean section, in case of severe fetal distress during surgery.

BIBLIOGRAPHY

Dajani AS, Taubert KA, Wilson W, et al. Prevention of bacterial endocarditis: recommendations by the American Heart Association. *JAMA* 1997; 277:1794–1801.

Demakis JG, Rahimtoola SH, Sutton GC, et al. Natural course of peripartum cardiomyopathy. *Circulation* 1971;44:1053–1061.

Hess DB, Hess LW. Management of cardiovascular disease in pregnancy. *Obstet Gynecol Clin North Am* 1992;19:679–695.

Hunter S, Robson SC. Adaptation of the maternal heart in pregnancy. *Br Heart J* 1992;68:540–543.

Kearney P, Singh H, Hutter J, et al. Spontaneous coronary dissection: a report of three cases and review of the literature. *Postgrad Med J* 1993; 69:940–945.

Midei MG, DeMent SH, Feldman AM, et al. Peripartum myocarditis and cardiomyopathy. *Circulation* 1990;81:922–928.

Page RL. Treatment of arrhythmias during pregnancy. *Am Heart J* 1995; 130:871–876.

Pomini F, Mercogliano D, Cavalletti C, et al. Cardiopulmonary bypass in pregnancy. *Ann Thorac Surg* 1996;61:259–268.

Sbarouni E, Oakley CM. Outcome of pregnancy in women with valve prostheses. *Br Heart J* 1994;71:196–201.

Sibai BM. Treatment of hypertension in pregnant women. *N Engl J Med* 1996;335:257–265.

Kelley's Textbook of Internal Medicine, fourth edition. Edited by H. David Humes. Lippincott Williams & Wilkins, Philadelphia © 2000.

CHAPTER 71

APPROACH TO THE PATIENT WITH HYPOTENSION AND SHOCK

TODD M. KOELLING
ROBERT J. CODY

Major advances in the treatment of conditions associated with acute circulatory failure have underscored the importance of early recognition of patients at risk of shock. It is important to draw a distinction between the circulatory derangements of hypotension and shock, because the treatments and outcomes of each differ considerably. Hypotension is the reduction of systemic blood pressure below the usual range of blood pressure for a person. Circulatory shock is a syndrome of inadequate organ and tissue perfusion stemming from extreme circulatory failure. Despite improvements in the treatment of patients with shock, the mortality rates of these patients remain high, in the 30% to 90% range. Hypotension itself is not necessarily associated with circulatory failure and usually is not accompanied by the circulatory shock syndrome. Although hypotension is common in circulatory shock, the actual degree of hypotension need not be striking. Hypotension is often a late sign in the clinical course of shock and generally indicates inadequate compensatory adjustments.

SPECTRUM OF HYPOTENSION

While the thresholds for hypertension and the link between high blood pressure and risk of morbid outcomes has been well established, the same cannot be said for the condition of low blood pressure, or hypotension. Actuarial studies have shown that survival is inversely related to blood pressure at pressures above 110/70 mm Hg; thus, patients who have lower blood pressures (less than 120/80 mm Hg) chronically, in the absence of cardiovascular disease, are protected by the lower readings. Population-based studies of blood pressure have shown that blood pressures lower than 110/60 are associated with increased cardiovascular mortality, suggesting a U-curve relationship between blood pressure and clinical outcome.

Although most physicians and cardiovascular investigators would consider a systemic blood pressure of less than 80/50 mm Hg to be hypotensive, it is not particularly useful to define hypotension by an absolute level of blood pressure because of the wide interindividual and intraindividual variations of systemic blood pressure. For instance, a blood pressure of 90/60 mm Hg is hypotensive for a patient whose usual systemic pressures are 120 to 140/80 to 90 mm Hg but may be normotensive for a young athlete or a woman in her second or third trimester of pregnancy.

Hypotension alone (without symptoms or accompanying cardiovascular abnormalities) is usually not a clinical problem. Continuous blood pressure recordings have demonstrated that a patient's blood pressure may transiently fall below the usual range during the course of a day, particularly while sleeping. Hypotension becomes clinically important when it elicits symptoms of reduced organ perfusion or when it becomes a manifestation of an underlying disease process (e.g., blood loss, myocardial infarction). Symptoms associated with hypotension include light-headedness, weakness, fatigue, syncope, transient ischemic attacks, vision changes, and angina pectoris. The hypotensive event may be positional, transient, or continuous.

ORTHOSTATIC HYPOTENSION

Orthostatic hypotension is defined as a reduction in systolic blood pressure of at least 20 mm Hg or in diastolic blood pressure of at least 10 mm Hg within 3 minutes of standing. Orthostatic hypotension is not a disease, but instead should be considered a physical finding associated with a variety of medical conditions (Table 71.1). Patients who complain of postural symptoms, such as light-headedness, dizziness, blurred vision, or headache, should be evaluated with supine and upright blood pressure readings separated by at least 1 minute after quietly standing.

For most patients, baroreceptor activation with standing increases the heart rate and myocardial contractility to maintain cardiac output, amplifies systemic vasoconstriction to maintain systemic blood pressure (providing adequate cerebral perfusion pressure), and enhances venoconstriction to shift blood volume centrally (bringing ventricular filling pressures and stroke volume back into a physiologic range). These compensatory mechanisms are directed at allowing human beings to shift positions quickly and function in the new position without delay.

A complete medical history may assist in the diagnosis of the source of orthostatic hypotension. The history should focus on previous medical problems as well as medications, alcohol use, and dietary habits. Patients with autonomic dysfunction may also have a history of constipation, urinary difficulties, sexual dysfunction, or night blindness. The physical exam should include supine and upright blood pressures in addition to evaluation of changes in heart rate. Patients with orthostatic hypotension and absence of a rise in pulse with standing may have autonomic dysfunction. Careful attention to the cardiac and neurologic examination findings will also aid in finding a cause for orthostatic hypotension. Cardiac causes of symptomatic orthostatic, intermittent, or continuous hypotension without the

TABLE 71.1.	CAUSES OF ORTHOSTATIC HYPOTENSION

Common
  Dehydration: vomiting, diarrhea, fever, anorexia
  Medications: psychotherapeutic agents (phenothiazines, tricyclic antidepressants), antihypertensive drugs (angiotensin-converting enzyme inhibitors, sympatholytic drugs, vasodilators), diuretics
  Blood loss/anemia
  Hypokalemia
  Deconditioning
  Malnutrition
Neurologic
  Central nervous system diseases: stroke, tumors, Parkinson's disease, multiple sclerosis, spinal cord injuries and diseases, tabes dorsalis, subacute combined sclerosis
  Autonomic nervous system dysfunction
    Primary: Shy–Drager syndrome, Bradbury–Eggleston syndrome, Guillain–Barré syndrome
    Secondary: diabetes mellitus, alcoholism, Wernicke's, amyloidosis, syphilis, myelopathies, neuropathies, various drug groups (sympatholytic agents)
Cardiovascular
  Cardiac: hypertrophic cardiomyopathy
  Vascular: large varicose veins
Endocrine
  Adrenal insufficiency
  Pheochromocytoma
  Hypoaldosteronism/renal salt wasting
  Diabetes insipidus
Other causes
  Idiopathic orthostatic hypotension
  Aging
  Physical deconditioning
  Carcinoid
  Baroreceptor trauma (neck radiation, surgery)

shock syndrome include conduction system disease (sinus node dysfunction, heart block), various tachyarrhythmias, obstructive disorders (valvular stenosis, pulmonary hypertension, atrial myxoma, pulmonary emboli, cardiac tamponade), and ventricular dysfunction (myocardial infarction, cardiomyopathy).

It is not uncommon for an elderly patient to experience orthostatic symptoms (light-headedness, near-syncope) after rising suddenly from a recumbent position. Age alone, however, is not a sufficient explanation for symptomatic orthostatic hypotension. Age-related blunting of autonomic, sinoatrial node, and vascular (arterial and venous) responses does not permit rapid compensation for the shift in central blood volume to more dependent areas (legs, abdomen). Diuretic therapy, malnutrition, hypokalemia, anemia, and deconditioning are also very common factors leading to risk of orthostasis in the elderly. As a result of these varied mechanisms, ventricular filling pressures and volumes drop, leading to a marked reduction in stroke volume.

Patients who have a reversible condition leading to orthostatic hypotension can be successfully treated by removal of the inciting cause. Other patients (particularly the elderly) may have several causes for their symptoms, and treatment can be more difficult. Offending medications should be stopped, lowered in dose, or changed as the initial intervention for orthostatic hypotension. Increasing dietary salt intake may also improve symptoms by providing for intravascular volume expansion. Preventive measures can be helpful, such as educating the patient to rise slowly to a standing position and perform isometric exercises of the upper and lower extremities and abdominal muscles before standing.

If the patient does not respond to these initial measures, medications designed to raise intravascular volume, such as salt tablets and/or fludrocortisone acetate, may be effective. Nonsteroidal antiinflammatory drugs have also been used with the intention of impairing renal salt and water excretion. Patients with supine hypertension and orthostatic hypotension may respond to nonselective β-blockade. Such β-blockers as propanolol, which block both the β$_1$- and β$_2$-adrenoreceptors, can assist in the treatment of orthostatic hypotension by preventing the vasodilatory effect of beta stimulation.

SHOCK

The first known references to the clinical entity of shock came from the eighteenth century in descriptions of dying, war-wounded French soldiers, who were seen to *secousse* (jar) and *ébranlement* (shake). This term was later translated by the English to the expression currently in use (shock). The condition of circulatory shock is a syndrome that occurs when the blood perfusion of the body's organs and tissue is inadequate to meet the ongoing metabolic needs of the cells. If the condition persists, it results in multisystemic derangement of function, organ damage, cell injury, and death.

The initial physiologic response to shock is compensation to the reduction in cardiac output or hypotension. The body responds to the ineffective circulating volume or pressure by recruiting a series of mechanisms of action directed at maintaining adequate perfusion pressure and flow, particularly to vital organs (brain, heart, lungs). Vascular and cardiac baroreceptor reflexes are activated by hypotension, diminished flow, and reduced wall tension (and chemoreceptors by hypoxia) to heighten sympathetic nervous system tone and enhance norepinephrine release at the nerve ending, with eventual spillover into the systemic circulation. The adrenomedullary production and release of epinephrine is enhanced. The renin-angiotensin-aldosterone axis is activated by the heightened sympathetic tone and by a drop in renal blood flow. The elevated angiotensin II levels, along with the augmented sympathetic activity, constrict systemic arterioles to increase systemic blood pressure. The increase in aldosterone and the drop in renal blood flow and glomerular filtration rate lead to salt and water retention by the kidneys. Antidiuretic hormone is released in shock states by a number of nonosmotic stimuli, including angiotensin II, heightened sympathetic tone, and reflex release through volume receptors (e.g., atrial volume-stretch receptors), resulting in water retention.

The retention of salt and water, combined with the constriction of venous capacitance beds by enhanced sympathetic tone, increases central venous and cardiac blood volume, thus augmenting stroke volume and cardiac output. Cardiac output also is increased by baroreceptor reflex–induced tachycardia. The

shock syndrome can be arrested at this point if the underlying cause abates or if the condition is recognized early and is effectively treated. If the condition remains untreated or progresses despite the maximal recruitment of compensatory mechanisms, the patient enters the stage of organ and tissue hypoperfusion and dysfunction, which eventually advances into the final stage of cell injury and death.

CLINICAL MANIFESTATIONS OF SHOCK

Appreciating the spectrum of the clinical manifestations of shock is crucial to making the distinction between hypotension and shock and to monitoring the course and treatment of shock. The initial symptoms and signs of circulatory shock represent the clinical and laboratory test indications of multisystemic hypoperfusion and dysfunction, multiple organ dysfunction and failure, widespread cell injury and death, and the body's responses to this threatening situation. The diagnosis of the shock syndrome is made on the basis of the resulting symptoms and clinical signs (Fig. 71.1).

BLOOD PRESSURE AND PULSE

Although blood pressure and pulse are not the *sine qua non* of shock, they remain central factors and should be checked at frequent intervals. The pulse of a patient in shock may be found to be rapid and faint, or "thready." Reduction of stroke volume in patients in advanced stages of shock may result in blood pressure so low that the usual Korotkoff sounds are not heard with a stethoscope. In this case, a portable Doppler apparatus may aid in the definition of lower systolic pressures. An intra-arterial catheter can be helpful in providing a measurement of the arterial pressure on a continuous basis.

SKIN

Intense vasoconstriction of dermal and subcutaneous arterioles occurs during states of systemic hypoperfusion. The skin, lips, and nail beds appear pale to light blue. The skin becomes cool to the touch, and the palms are frequently moist. In prolonged shock, skin necrosis and ulcers may develop on the digits, particularly when the cutaneous vasoconstriction is complicated by prolonged administration of vasopressor drugs (norepinephrine, dopamine) or the presence of occlusive peripheral vascular disease or coagulopathy. Skin temperature and color may be normal or even warm and pink during the early stages of the venovasodilatory forms of shock (septic shock); the term *warm shock* has been used in this context.

CARDIOVASCULAR SYSTEM

The cardiovascular manifestations of shock generally are a result of inadequate perfusion of organs and tissue. In the hypovolemic and cardiogenic forms of shock, systemic hypoperfusion is related to depressed cardiac output; in the vasodepressor (venovasodilatory) shock states, an abnormality in blood distribution

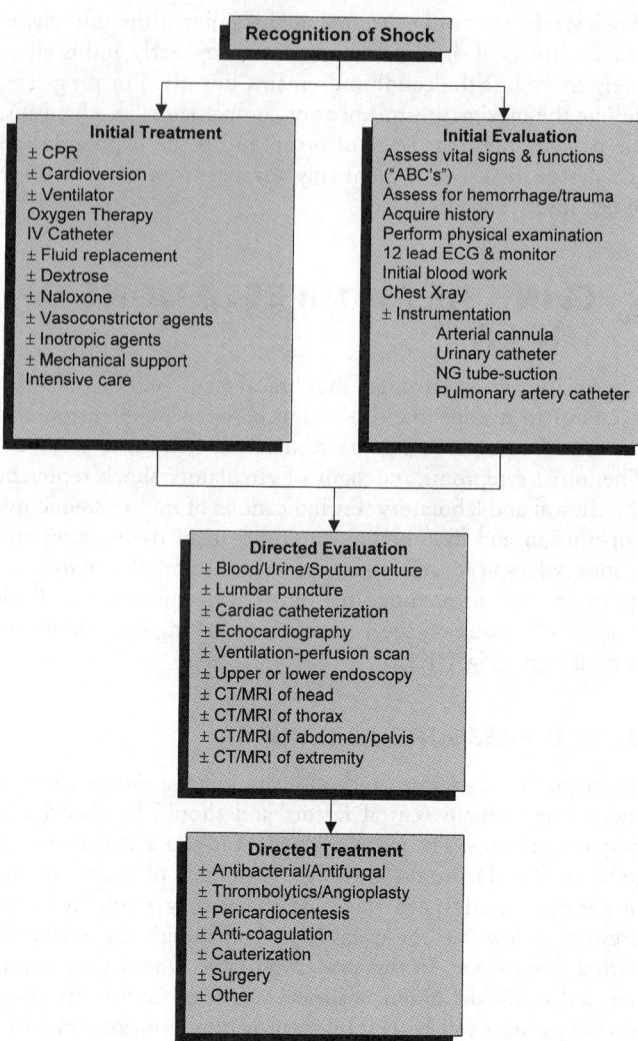

Recognition of Shock

Initial Treatment
± CPR
± Cardioversion
± Ventilator
Oxygen Therapy
IV Catheter
± Fluid replacement
± Dextrose
± Naloxone
± Vasoconstrictor agents
± Inotropic agents
± Mechanical support
Intensive care

Initial Evaluation
Assess vital signs & functions ("ABC's")
Assess for hemorrhage/trauma
Acquire history
Perform physical examination
12 lead ECG & monitor
Initial blood work
Chest Xray
± Instrumentation
    Arterial cannula
    Urinary catheter
    NG tube-suction
    Pulmonary artery catheter

Directed Evaluation
± Blood/Urine/Sputum culture
± Lumbar puncture
± Cardiac catheterization
± Echocardiography
± Ventilation-perfusion scan
± Upper or lower endoscopy
± CT/MRI of head
± CT/MRI of thorax
± CT/MRI of abdomen/pelvis
± CT/MRI of extremity

Directed Treatment
± Antibacterial/Antifungal
± Thrombolytics/Angioplasty
± Pericardiocentesis
± Anti-coagulation
± Cauterization
± Surgery
± Other

FIGURE 71.1. Major steps in the management of circulatory shock. The evaluation and treatment of the shock patient must occur simultaneously and in a proficient manner.

and delivery causes hypoperfusion, despite normal or high cardiac output. A reduction in diastolic arterial pressure to 60 mm Hg or less results in a substantial drop in myocardial perfusion. Myocardial ischemia, particularly of the subendocardial region, is likely to occur in patients with severe untreated shock. During the advanced and terminal stages of shock, certain metabolic factors (e.g., acidosis) also may contribute to myocardial depression.

PULMONARY SYSTEM

Ventilatory defects or ventilation–perfusion mismatch is common in all stages of shock and can account for a significant reduction in the oxygen content of blood. These abnormalities can arise in the context of clear lung fields, as evidenced on physical examination, but often are accompanied by radiographic evidence of atelectasis and diffuse alveolar and interstitial infiltrates. Arterial hypoxemia is markedly exacerbated if adult respiratory distress syndrome (ARDS) develops. The formation

of ARDS lung edema is enhanced by an elevation of pulmonary capillary wedge pressure or a drop in plasma oncotic pressure, but neither is a requirement. Cardiogenic forms of shock can result in pulmonary edema on the basis of high left ventricular filling pressure, which is transmitted to the pulmonary vasculature as high pulmonary venous and pulmonary capillary pressures. ARDS and cardiogenic pulmonary edema may exist together in the same patient (see Chapter 357). The clinical manifestations of bronchoconstriction (wheezing, hypoxemia) may be noted in patients with anaphylactic shock, massive pulmonary embolization, or cardiogenic shock accompanied by high left ventricular filling pressures.

KIDNEYS

Shock with renal hypoperfusion often impairs sodium and water excretion. At this stage, urine output is reduced but generally remains at a level more than 20 mL per hour. The urine sodium concentration drops below 15 mEq per liter, and urine osmolality increases and remains above 400 mOsm. The plasma blood urea nitrogen (BUN)/creatinine ratio increases to more than 10:1; the urine/plasma ratio of BUN remains above 5 and that of creatinine above 30.

Acute renal failure may develop in severe or advanced shock; this threatening condition is often accelerated by underlying renal disease or various drugs (certain antibiotics, nonsteroidal antiinflammatory drugs). In contrast to hypoperfused (but functioning) kidneys, kidneys in failure show signs of dysfunction and anatomic disruption of tubules. Urine sodium concentration usually exceeds 40 mEq per liter, urine osmolality approaches that of plasma (less than 350 mEq per liter), and urine output usually drops to less than 20 mL per hour. Plasma BUN and creatinine values rise, but the plasma BUN/creatinine ratio usually remains at 10:1 or less; the urine/plasma ratio of BUN drops to less than 3 and that of creatinine to less than 20. Coarse granular, renal tubular, or pigmented casts may appear in the urinary sediment. A form of renal failure with high urine output (more than 40 mL per hour) occurs in isolated instances and can occasionally follow a period of oliguric renal failure.

GASTROINTESTINAL SYSTEM

Varying degrees of gastrointestinal hemorrhage that result from gastritis, stress ulcers, and scattered mucosal erosions are common in all stages of shock. Adynamic ileus is not uncommon. Severe shock can cause bowel infarction on the basis of hypoperfusion and intense vasoconstriction, particularly in patients with concomitant mesenteric atherosclerosis. Hepatic hypoperfusion can lead to an elevation of the plasma levels of enzymes, indicating liver cell injury, which may evolve into hepatic necrosis in severe shock. Icterus, a common sign in shock, stems from the liver's inability to conjugate and excrete bilirubin and occasionally to an increased bilirubin load (hemolysis). Hypoglycemia, hypoalbuminemia, depressed clotting factors, and elevated blood lactic acid and ammonia levels may be caused or exacerbated by hepatic hypoperfusion and dysfunction. Plasma amylase may increase as the result of the release of amylase from the pancreas.

NERVOUS SYSTEM

The patient's mental status may range from anxiety in mild shock to confusion, combativeness, lethargy, disorientation, and somnolence in moderate levels of shock and on to obtundation and coma in prolonged or severe stages of shock. Although hypoperfusion is the predominant underlying cause of these symptoms and signs, metabolic factors (hypoglycemia, uremia, hyperammonemia) may contribute to them. Marked cerebral hypoperfusion, ischemia, and edema may elicit decorticate or decerebrate posturing. Advanced stages of shock often are accompanied by dysfunction of vital control centers of the central nervous system, such that abnormal cardiac, vascular, and ventilatory control may ensue. The resulting manifestations include inappropriate heart rate responses, refractory vasodilatation, pooling of intravascular volume in capacitance vascular beds, abnormal ventilatory patterns, inadequate or inappropriate ventilatory responses to acid–base shifts, and profound depression of ventilatory drive.

HEMATOLOGIC SYSTEM

The hematocrit varies widely among patients in shock, depending on the status of extracellular fluid shifts, blood loss, and volume replacement. Varying degrees of coagulopathy stemming from endothelial injury, platelet activation, and hepatic dysfunction are seen in many patients in shock. Disseminated intravascular coagulation (DIC) with diffuse uncontrollable hemorrhage often accompanies terminal stages.

IMMUNE SYSTEM

Although they are not yet well delineated in the context of circulatory shock, immunologic derangements (dysfunction of the reticuloendothelial system, leukocyte dysfunction) may well contribute to the predisposition to infectious complications in the patient with shock. Immune mechanisms play a role in the local release of histamine, cytokines, and other substances in various shock conditions and occupy center stage in the pathophysiologic picture of anaphylactic shock.

MUSCULOSKELETAL SYSTEM

Hypoperfusion of skeletal and muscle structures, in part related to vasoconstriction, can evoke complaints of myalgia, arthralgia, and bone pain. Elevated plasma levels of lactate, creatine phosphokinase (MM type), and other muscle enzymes and myoglobin are manifestations of hypoperfusion of muscle. The release of lactate (lactic acid) from the body's largest organ, skeletal muscle, contributes greatly to the metabolic acidosis present in many shock patients, and the release of myoglobin may contribute to the development of renal failure.

■ CAUSATIVE CLASSIFICATION OF CIRCULATORY SHOCK

A classification of shock according to causative factors is presented in Table 71.2. In the care of critically ill patients, it is

TABLE 71.2.	GENERAL ETIOLOGIC CLASSIFICATION OF CIRCULATORY SHOCK

Hypotensive Shock
 Hypovolemic Shock
  Hemorrhage
   Dehydration
   Vomiting
   Diarrhea
   Diabetic ketoacidosis
   Diabetes insipidus
   Adrenal insufficiency
   High-urine-output renal failure
   Overaggressive diuretic therapy
   Inadequate fluid intake/replacement
  Loss of plasma volume
   Burns
   Desquamated, exudative lesions
   Dumping syndromes
 Increased vascular capacitance
  Septic shock
   Gram-negative organisms
   Gram-positive organisms
   Rickettsia infections
   Viral infections
  Anaphylaxis
  Drugs
   Anesthesia
   Sympatholytics
   Adrenergic blockers
   Vasodilators
   Barbiturates
   Narcotics
  Neurogenic
   Spinal cord injury
   Cerebral damage
   Severe dysautonomia
  Heat stroke
 Cardiogenic shock
  Myocardial infarction
  Myocarditis
  Cardiomyopathy
  Papillary muscle or chordal rupture
  Severe aortic or mitral valve disease
  Ventricular septal or free wall rupture
  Arrhythmia
  Acidosis
  Hypothermia
 Obstruction to flow
  Pulmonary embolism
  Cardiac tamponade
  Tension pneumothorax
  Dissecting aortic aneurysm
  Thrombus or myxoma in heart
  Positive pressure ventilation
Normotensive or hypertensive shock
 Compensated shock
 Overcompensated shock
 Vasoconstrictor administration
 Pheochromocytoma
 Malignant hyperthermia

crucial to understand the causative classification of shock because the most important step in the management of this condition is to recognize and treat the underlying cause.

HYPOVOLEMIC SHOCK

Shock caused by a severe reduction in intravascular volume generally is referred to as hypovolemic shock. This type of shock also has been termed *cold shock* because peripheral hypoperfusion and vasoconstriction result in cold distal extremities. The severity of hypovolemic shock typically is related to the amount and rate of loss of intravascular volume and the responsiveness of the compensatory mechanisms (vasoconstriction, salt and water retention by the kidneys) to the sudden or excessive loss of volume. An acute loss of intravascular volume of 25% or more is required to place a normal person in circulatory shock. Losses in excess of this amount usually overwhelm the compensatory mechanisms and result in severe hypotension and inadequate tissue perfusion. Loss of the same volume over a number of days may not elicit the shock syndrome because, with adequate time, the compensatory responses can reestablish and maintain sufficient intravascular volume and tissue perfusion. Aging and various disease states can reduce the volume loss required to produce circulatory shock and diminish the proficiency of the compensatory responses to avert the development of shock during volume loss.

The most common form of hypovolemic shock is that caused by blood loss, usually through injury. Patients may lose large volumes of blood externally through open lacerations or gastrointestinal lesions or by severe hemoptysis. A source of bleeding may be more difficult to define when the hemorrhage is located in internal body cavities or tissues. For example, each side of the chest cavity can hold 2 to 3 L of blood. Other sites of internal bleeding leading to shock may include the peritoneal space, retroperitoneum, pelvis, and tissues surrounding large bone fractures.

Hypovolemic shock also may occur when plasma volume or extracellular fluid is lost. The patient with major burns can lose large amounts of extracellular fluid into the burn wound, owing to edema and loss of the skin barrier. Similarly, patients with desquamating or exudative skin lesions also may experience hypovolemic shock. A less common source of hypovolemic shock is severe gastrointestinal dumping syndromes due to interference with the normal pyloric mechanism. Contraction of the intravascular space results from hyperosmolar solution in the small intestine. This combines with the release of vasoactive hormones (serotonin, bradykinin, and vasoactive intestinal peptide) to lead to what can be a severe hypotensive condition.

Dehydration can result from a variety of conditions (Table 71.2), which can produce hypovolemic shock. Gastrointestinal losses from vomiting and/or diarrhea are common in infants and in others infected with viruses, bacteria, or parasites. High urine output states, such as diabetic ketoacidosis, diabetes insipidus, renal tubular injury, and overaggressive diuresis, are common sources of hypotension and hypovolemic shock. Lack of fluid intake, inadequate fluid replacement, or excess sweating can also lead to dehydration and hypovolemic shock.

INCREASED VASCULAR CAPACITANCE

Shock precipitated by marked venous dilatation is often referred to as distributive shock, because the central blood volume is redistributed to the peripheral vasculature, particularly to venous capacitance beds. In a broad sense, venovasodilatory shock could be considered a type of hypovolemic shock, since the increased vascular capacitance of these patients causes a reduction of central venous pressure, leading to inadequate diastolic filling of the ventricles. In many cases, venovasodilatory shock can be appropriately termed *warm shock*. In contrast to the vasoconstriction of hypovolemic shock, venovasodilatory shock commonly is associated with hyperthermic or normothermic hands and feet, at least until intense cutaneous vasoconstriction develops during the later stages. Although venovasodilatory shock can be caused by a number of factors (Table 71.2), sepsis and drugs are the most common sources.

Severe sepsis is the most common form of increased vascular capacitance, or venovasodilatory, shock. The study of the sepsis syndrome has elucidated several factors that may contribute to the deterioration to shock. Endotoxin produced by gram-negative bacteria is one of the major factors leading to the fever, systemic hypotension, and tachycardia that characterizes septic shock. Nonetheless, septic shock unrelated to endotoxin may result from infections caused by gram-positive organisms, viruses, *Rickettsieae*, and fungi. Infections also lead to host responses that feed into the syndrome of septic shock. One key element of this response is cytokines. The toxic stimulus (endotoxin) triggers the production of the proinflammatory cytokines tumor necrosis factor and interleukin-1. These compounds promote adhesion of polymorphonuclear cells to the site of the infection, which then produce numerous secondary inflammatory mediators, such as prostaglandins, leukotrienes, bradykinin, and proteases. The hypotensive state created by sepsis mediators may lead to cardiac end-organ damage. Myocardial contractility may also be reduced, owing to circulating myocardial depressant factors and/or DIC.

Anaphylactic shock usually manifests precipitously in response to exposure to an antigen, either in the natural environment or as a result of drug administration. In sensitized persons, the antigen interacts with the IgE-specific antibody on mast cells and other cell surfaces. Mediators liberated from the stimulated cells include histamine, serotonin, kinins, cytokines, and others. Life-threatening anaphylaxis may occur within minutes after exposure to the antigen and is characterized by a varying combination of venovasodilatation, respiratory distress from laryngospasm or bronchospasm, reduction of plasma volume with hemoconcentration, abdominal discomfort, and diarrhea, pruritus, and urticaria.

Shock may also arise from loss of hypotension induced by exogenous vasodilatory agents, such as anesthetics and antihypertensive agents. Patients taking an overdose of prescription or illicit barbiturates, benzodiazepines, or narcotics may experience increased vascular capacitance shock. Hypovolemia, if present, can greatly enhance the tendency to shock in patients taking these medications.

Injury to the spinal cord can produce systemic vasomotor paralysis in the areas caudal to the injury. The loss of peripheral vascular resistance in the involved area can precipitate a drop in central venous pressure, leading to low cardiac output and subsequent organ failure. There is a similar scenario in some patients with cerebral injury and in patients with severe dysautonomia. The drop in systemic blood pressure will usually respond to administration of intravenous fluids or vasoconstrictive medications.

Heat stroke, caused by the inability of the body to dissipate heat fast enough to regulate body temperature, can lead to a form of venovasodilatory shock. In these patients, the body temperature rises to 40°C or higher, with ensuing cutaneous vasodilatation and low peripheral resistance. In this sense, heat stroke is a form of stroke caused by increased vascular capacitance, but it may also be complicated by dehydration, myocardial depression, and DIC.

CARDIOGENIC SHOCK

Shock states associated with cardiac pump failure, generally referred to as cardiogenic shock, are those caused by impaired ventricular systolic performance, inadequate ventricular diastolic filling, cardiac valvular dysfunction, or a combination of these. In cardiogenic shock the impairment of cardiac function leads to compromised oxygen delivery and resultant organ dysfunction and ischemia. Renal responses to depressed cardiac output and systemic pressure (reduced glomerular filtration, increased renin secretion) are often the most sensitive indicator of severe myocardial dysfunction, thus leading to progressive vasoconstriction and salt and water retention. Ventricular filling pressures rise in response to renal factors, leading to a tendency for pulmonary edema and hypoxia and progressive cardiac dysfunction.

Acute myocardial infarction is the most common cause of cardiogenic shock (see Chapter 73). Shock occurs in 5% to 10% of patients hospitalized for acute myocardial infarction and implicates a 40% or higher loss of functioning ventricular myocardium. The Multicenter Investigation of the Limitation of Infarct Size trial determined that older age (more than 65 years), reduced ejection fraction (less than 0.35), infarct size (MB-CPK more than 160 IU per liter), diabetes mellitus, or previous myocardial infarction magnified the probability of cardiogenic shock developing after acute myocardial infarction. Rupture of the ventricular free wall or septum happens in 1% to 2% of patients with acute myocardial infarction and is often heralded by hypotension and shock.

Despite advances in hemodynamic monitoring, pharmacologic intervention, and intra-aortic balloon counterpulsation, the in-hospital mortality rate for postinfarction cardiogenic shock remains higher than 75%. Several studies (uncontrolled) have shown, however, that early reperfusion (within the first 6 to 12 hours) by coronary angioplasty or bypass surgery can reduce in-hospital mortality rates to less than 60%, with probable improvement in long-term survival as well. In-hospital deaths appear to be related directly to age, infarct size, extent of hemodynamic decompensation, and lack of early reperfusion.

Factors other than ischemia can contribute to the development of cardiogenic shock in patients with myocardial infarction. For example, with infarction of the inferior wall, bradycardia and hypotension may be induced by myocardial vagotonic reflexes (Bezold-Jarish reflex); parasympatholytic (atropine) therapy improves this transient, but potentially lethal event in most patients.

Cardiogenic shock may develop in patients with acute myocardial injury from the myocarditides or in patients with severe progressive systolic dysfunction from chronic cardiomyopathy or chronic valvular dysfunction. In these patients, shock is characterized by systemic hypotension (systolic blood pressure less than 90 mm Hg) and depressed cardiac index (less than 2.0 L per minute per square meter) despite an elevated pulmonary capillary wedge pressure (more than 15 mm Hg). Many patients with chronic myocardial weakness may be able to compensate to this level of hemodynamic derangement and remain ambulatory until more critical thresholds are reached.

Acute mitral valvular insufficiency, such as that caused by rupture of the chordae tendineae or papillary muscle, can lead to shock on the basis of inadequate ejection of blood into the aorta. Sudden activation of atrial stretch receptors and reflexes can contribute to hypotension and the hypoperfusion state of massive acute mitral regurgitation. Certain cardiac dysrhythmias, such as ventricular tachycardia or rapid supraventricular tachycardia, often lead to inadequate filling or emptying of the ventricles. The ventricle in fibrillation or asystole does not eject any blood; if this condition is not corrected, shock and death are imminent.

Acidosis can produce myocardial depression in patients who have a pH of less than 7.10 to 7.15. In this context, impaired myocardial function may be associated with the generation of the free radicals O_2^- and OH^-. Severe acidosis also tends to cause arterial vasodilatation, venous vasoconstriction, and a tendency to capillary stasis. Myocardial function may also be depressed in the context of acidosis, owing to the development of DIC and/or pulmonary vasoconstriction. When acidosis alone is the cause of cardiac dysfunction, correction of acidosis by treating the source of the problem (ketoacidosis, uremia, severe diarrhea) will usually result in improved myocardial function.

OBSTRUCTION TO FLOW

Failure of the heart's pumping mechanism also may result from inadequate filling of the ventricles. The prototype for inadequate ventricular filling is pericardial tamponade, in which the pericardial space is filled with fluid or blood under high pressure, preventing adequate filling of the ventricular and atrial chambers. The resultant stroke volume is small, and the heart rate increases in response to the progressive reduction in stroke output. If cardiac output cannot be adequately maintained, blood pressure falls, and shock ensues.

A massive pulmonary embolus may lead to circulatory shock by preventing the emptying of the right ventricle and the filling of the left ventricle. Other causes of shock from obstruction to flow include tension pneumothorax, dissecting aortic aneurysm, and occlusive intracardiac tumors or thrombi. Patients with low central venous pressures may have hypotension and low cardiac output in response to positive pressure ventilation, a form of shock caused by obstruction to flow.

CLINICAL APPROACH AND MANAGEMENT OF SHOCK

Although it is more convenient to discuss the evaluation and treatment of shock separately, the optimal management of shock conditions never allows the separation of these activities. When a patient first shows physiologic signs of shock, a source is not always apparent. The severe hemodynamic derangement and impending organ damage and/or death compel the physician to initiate empirical treatments in an attempt to resuscitate the patient and prevent or minimize long-term consequences. The goal is to stabilize the patient so that definitive diagnosis and treatment are possible.

INITIAL EVALUATION AND TREATMENT

The first step is the recognition of shock, with all subsequent activity directed at stabilizing and treating the shock condition while aggressively and systematically determining the cause. The patient in shock often enters the emergency department with historical evidence (chest pain, recent penicillin injection) or physical signs (trauma, hematemesis) of the cause of shock. In these situations, diagnostic and therapeutic activity is directed toward the suspected problem. Many patients in shock, however, do not have any initially obvious historical or physical clues regarding cause. If the patient is intact mentally, the physician must systematically direct a series of questions to the patient. Many patients in shock enter the emergency department in a lethargic or obtunded state. In this case, the emergency medical technicians, police, family members, or friends accompanying the patient must be questioned. In such cases, an examination of the patient's purse, wallet, and pocket contents for information on medical history, medications, the patient's primary physician, and a friend or relative is usually necessary.

As the patient's clothes are being removed, the physician usually performs a general inspection and palpatory examination, looking for signs of infection, blood loss, trauma, needle marks, and systemic illness. The physical evaluation then must incorporate an examination of the head and neck and major organ systems and regions, including a rectal examination with stool guaiac testing. The physical examination, in concert with the historical information, should at this point provide important clues to the cause and severity of shock and suggest a direction for further diagnostic studies and treatment. Decisions on therapy must parallel all of this activity. With respect to cardiopulmonary resuscitation and life-support measures, the need to initiate these interventions may precede the history, the physical examination, and any laboratory testing. The physician also must be alert to the fact that these life-support measures may have to be instituted, based on established criteria, anywhere along the clinical course.

If the patient appears to ventilate adequately throughout this early course and the initial set of arterial blood gases shows sufficient oxygenation without hypercapnia, a mask oxygen-delivery system would suffice. An arterial blood sample, however, should be drawn, and the blood should be monitored regularly for gases (partial pressures of oxygen [P_{O_2}] and carbon dioxide [P_{CO_2}]),

pH, and lactic acid concentration. If ventilation appears to be inadequate or the arterial blood gas studies indicate hypoxemia or hypercapnia, the patient should be intubated and given assisted ventilation. A catheter should be introduced into an artery, to provide continuous direct recordings of systemic blood pressure and to serve as a convenient conduit for obtaining arterial blood samples. Blood pressure readings using a cuff sphygmomanometer during shock are usually inaccurate or not obtainable, particularly when marked reflex vasoconstriction is present. Conversely, it is imperative not to delay therapy for shock for the sake of placing an arterial catheter.

Twelve-lead electrocardiography is performed early in shock management, particularly for rhythm disturbances or if it is reasonable to suspect that myocardial ischemia–infarction will lead to the patient's demise (because of a history of coronary disease or risk factors). If ischemia or an infarction pattern is present on the electrocardiogram, the physician should consider administering thrombolytic therapy or should call the cardiologist to perform emergency cardiac catheterization/coronary angiography in the patient entering cardiogenic shock, with the intent of achieving early reperfusion via angioplasty or coronary bypass surgery.

The insertion of an intravenous catheter of sufficient size (16 gauge or larger) soon after the patient arrives in the emergency department is important from both a diagnostic and a therapeutic standpoint. As the catheter is inserted, blood samples can be drawn for appropriate laboratory studies (hematocrit, hemoglobin, total white blood cell count with differential cell count, serum electrolytes, glucose, BUN, creatinine, and calcium). About 30 mL of the blood should be refrigerated in the event that a certain analysis is needed on baseline or untreated blood at a later point. In patients with depressed mental status or a history of diabetes mellitus, 50 mL of 50% dextrose solution should be injected into an intravenous line immediately after the withdrawal of blood, to treat the possibility of insulin-induced hypoglycemic shock or shock-induced hypoglycemia. Unless signs of hypervolemia are present, fluid (0.9 N sodium chloride) should be infused as rapidly as possible. Precise recording of fluid input and output and all medications administered begins at this time. Serum electrolytes must be tested on a regular basis throughout the clinical course.

If marked hypotension (systolic pressure less than 70 mm Hg) persists after the rapid infusion of more than 2,000 mL of fluid and in the absence of evidence of hypervolemia, the patient is treated by additional volume administration and low infusion rates of a pressor, such as dopamine (starting at 4 to 5 μg per kilogram per minute). Packed red blood cells should be administered if blood loss was the cause or a major contributor to the shock syndrome. In general, systolic and mean arterial pressures should be brought up to at least 80 mm Hg and at least 65 to 70 mm Hg, respectively, to perfuse the brain and kidneys, and the diastolic pressure should be brought up to at least 60 mm Hg, to perfuse the heart.

The placement of a balloon-tipped, flow-directed pulmonary artery (Swan-Ganz) catheter in the pulmonary artery is one of the early steps in the management of cardiogenic shock. Determination of the left ventricular filling pressure (usually approximated closely by the pulmonary capillary wedge pressure) is crucial in the appropriate and proficient treatment of cardiogenic shock. As many as 20% of patients with acute myocardial infarction and hypotension or shock have inadequate left ventricular filling pressures, some cases caused by volume depletion and others by infarction predominantly involving the right ventricle. Left ventricular filling pressure is poorly estimated by clinical examination, even when it is accompanied by a chest film and central venous pressure recordings.

The Swan-Ganz catheter can greatly assist the physician in the treatment of the shock patient. Placement of this catheter must be considered at this point, particularly if the patient has not yet responded to the previously mentioned therapeutic measures or if a cardiogenic basis for the shock condition is suspected. The pulmonary artery catheter, when interfaced with a pressure-recording system and a thermodilution cardiac output computer, gives an assessment of right and left ventricular filling pressures, cardiac output, stroke volume, and pulmonary arterial pressures. When combined with the data derived from the indwelling systemic arterial catheter, several other hemodynamic parameters can be derived (vascular resistances, stroke work index).

From the directly measured and derived parameters, the physician can rationally direct fluid volume administration and pharmacologic support. For example, a condition of low right and left ventricular filling pressures, low cardiac output and systemic blood pressure, and peripheral hypoperfusion is managed by the additional administration of fluid volume. The same recordings in the context of high cardiac output and low pulmonary and systemic vascular resistances, particularly if marked hypotension or shock persists after more than 3,000 mL of volume administration, suggest a state of profound arteriovenous vasodilatation (sepsis); additional volume administration and vasopressor therapy (dopamine) serve as the primary circulatory support measures in this situation.

The measures used to improve and stabilize cardiovascular status are monitored by the combination of left and right ventricular filling pressures, systemic blood pressure, cardiac output, and clinical status (tissue and organ perfusion, urine output, symptoms). If a patient with infarction-induced cardiogenic shock is found to have a low (less than 12 mm Hg) left ventricular filling pressure, intravenous fluid administration (0.9 N sodium chloride) is begun immediately and continued to bring the left ventricular filling pressure to 15 to 18 mm Hg. If systemic blood pressure, peripheral perfusion, and clinical status improve to a relatively normal level, fluid administration is continued and monitored to keep left ventricular filling pressures at 12 to 18 mm Hg. If the same patient's systemic blood pressure returns to normal (more than 100 mm Hg systolic) but tissue and organ perfusion remains compromised (particularly if cardiac output is less than 2.20 L per minute per square meter), the judicious infusion of a vasodilator is warranted. Nitroglycerin is usually the initial intravenous vasodilator selected. Nitroprusside is a more powerful vasodilator and is chosen when a higher level of afterload reduction is required.

A nasogastric tube should be inserted and the gastric contents visually examined for blood and tested for a guaiac reaction. If the cause of shock is unknown, the gastric specimen should be sent to the special laboratories of the hospital for toxicologic analysis. The nasogastric tube is placed on continuous suction, and the volume withdrawn is recorded. Of course, if gastrointestinal bleeding is suggested earlier as a cause of shock, the nasogastric tube is put in place earlier in the course of treatment.

DIRECTED EVALUATION AND TREATMENT

The management of shock at this point is based on the identification of the type of shock.

Hypovolemic Shock

When hypovolemic shock is recognized, initial management includes elevation of the legs and rapid volume replacement. As the solution is being infused at wide-open rates, a central pressure–monitoring catheter (a flow-directed, balloon-tipped pulmonary artery catheter or, if no cardiopulmonary disease is apparent or suspected, a central venous pressure line) is inserted. Using arterial pressure and systemic perfusion as major end points, the intravascular volume is expanded to raise the central venous pressure to 8 to 12 mm Hg or the pulmonary artery occlusive (pulmonary capillary wedge) pressure to 15 to 18 mm Hg. If the patient remains hypotensive or in shock at these levels, a cardiogenic component must be considered. If the ventricular filling pressures remain low after the infusion of a substantial volume (at least 4 L) and shock persists, continued volume loss or an arteriovenous vasodilatory component must be considered as contributory factors.

There is no single optimal ventricular filling pressure for all patients in shock. A pulmonary capillary wedge pressure of 18 mm Hg may be required to bring cardiac output into an acceptable range in a patient with acute myocardial infarction, whereas a wedge pressure above 15 mm Hg may evoke pulmonary edema in a septic patient with low plasma oncotic pressure. If the plasma oncotic pressure minus the pulmonary capillary wedge pressure exceeds 8 to 10 mm Hg, the risk of pulmonary edema is small. If, however, the wedge pressure approaches or exceeds the plasma oncotic pressure, or if capillary endothelial cell injury has occurred, pulmonary edema is likely to develop. As shock enters a protracted phase and is complicated by pulmonary edema or arterial hypoxemia, the determination of plasma oncotic pressure occasionally may be useful in guiding volume replacement.

Packed red blood cells are given to patients with a depressed hematocrit (30% or less) to expand intravascular volume with little pulmonary extravascular leakage. Local or surgical control of bleeding is obviously important and is initiated early to prevent additional blood loss. Although they are the subject of controversy, large-molecular-weight colloids can be used in an attempt to restrict the administered fluid volume to the intravascular space. The colloids include human serum albumin, plasma substitutes, and glucose polymers (dextrans, hydroxyethyl starch). Human serum albumin, 5 g per deciliter, is an effective but expensive volume expander, particularly in patients whose clinical courses may be adversely affected by low serum albumin and low plasma oncotic pressure. Plasma itself carries the risk of transmitting hepatitis (as does whole blood), and although purified plasma protein derivatives do not transmit hepatitis, they do contain vasoactive contaminants that can cause hypotensive reactions.

The regular use of dextrans (glucose polymers produced by streptococci) has been tempered by their serious side effects, which include anaphylactic reactions, bleeding through interference with platelet function and coagulation, and renal dysfunction. Hydroxyethyl starch (hetastarch), another polysaccharide colloid volume expander, is generally nonallergenic, causes fewer bleeding complications (in doses less than 1,500 mL), and does not lead to renal failure. In contrast to packed red blood cells, a major limitation of the crystalloid and colloid volume expanders is their eventual escape into and equilibration with extravascular spaces, particularly in patients with loss of capillary integrity (ARDS, septic shock).

Increased Vascular Capacitance Shock

A characteristic feature of venovasodilatory shock is its refractoriness to volume-replacement therapy. The acute administration of 4 L or more may have little effect on central filling or systemic pressures or on the clinical manifestations of the shock state. Although intravascular capacity is greatly increased in most of these patients, much of the fluid administered enters extravascular spaces by a drop in the ratio of precapillary to postcapillary sphincter tone and, occasionally, through enhanced capillary permeability. Some patients respond to volume administration alone, but most also require a therapeutic intervention directed at reducing intravascular capacity or effecting a more normal distribution of intravascular volume by augmenting vascular tone.

The patient with marked hypotension (systolic pressures less than 70 to 75 mm Hg) due to venovasodilatory shock is treated initially with vasopressor therapy, such as phenylephrine. Phenylephrine is initiated as a 1 µg per kilogram intravenous loading dose, followed by a drip at 0.5 µg per kilogram per minute; dosing is advanced as needed up to a maximal dose of 5 µg per kilogram per minute (until the mean arterial blood pressure exceeds 65 to 70 mm Hg). Dopamine, given at a starting dose of 5 µg per kilogram per minute and gradually advancing the infusion rate to 10 to 15 µg per kilogram per minute, as needed, may be helpful in patients with severe hypotension and poor renal perfusion. Norepinephrine bitartrate, 0.05 to 0.20 µg per kilogram per minute, may be used in patients who appear to be unresponsive to phenylephrine or dopamine.

As in all forms of shock, the crucial factor for improvement and survival is the prompt recognition and treatment of the underlying cause. It is usually not that difficult to recognize the neurogenic causes of venovasodilatory shock (cerebral or spinal cord injury); diagnosis is based primarily on a good clinical examination. The pharmacologic causes of shock that occur in the hospital or clinic (anesthesia, drug therapy) are readily identifiable and treatable with fluid volume and vasopressors. A similar therapeutic approach can be implemented for unknown drug overdose, with consideration given to the administration of nal-

oxone in certain instances (narcotic overdose). The therapy of anaphylaxis should be initiated immediately on making the diagnosis and includes removing the antigen source or load, if feasible, and administering epinephrine, 0.1 mg intravenously and 0.4 mg subcutaneously. Other support drugs might include bronchodilators, antihistamines, and glucocorticoids.

One of the most difficult forms of venovasodilatory shock to diagnose early is septic or endotoxic shock. The initial manifestation may be only one of the following: hyperventilation, tachycardia, hypotension, reduced tissue perfusion, diminished urine output, altered sensorium (confusion, lethargy), chills, fever, hypothermia, or a change in the white blood cell count. Suspicion should be aroused if one or more of these symptoms is found in a patient who is hospitalized, institutionalized, elderly, subjected to instrumentation (diagnostic tests, indwelling catheters), immunosuppressed, injured (trauma, burns), or chronically ill (chronic renal failure, cirrhosis diabetes mellitus) or who has undergone recent surgery. Early recognition, complete acquisition of cultures, a rational selection and prompt parenteral administration of antibiotics, and circulatory support (volume and vasopressor therapy) are key to survival. The routine use of high-dose parenteral corticosteroids in septic shock is not supported by good clinical trials. A more specific and detailed presentation of the management (e.g., antibiotic selection) of septic shock is presented in Chapter 268.

Cardiogenic Shock

Acute myocardial infarction is the most common cause of cardiogenic shock (see Chapter 73). The continued high mortality rate of this condition has set the stage for a more aggressive diagnostic and therapeutic approach (thrombolytic therapy, catheterization, coronary angioplasty, bypass surgery) in patients with occlusive coronary artery disease.

Unless a patient enters the hospital with symptoms of a myocardial infarction of more than 12 hours' duration, immediate intravenous thrombolytic therapy should be considered. If the patient appears to be advancing to or already shows signs of cardiogenic shock despite early supportive measures (administration of fluid volume or cardiovasculoactive drugs), he or she should undergo urgent cardiac catheterization/coronary angiography in a setting where a catheterization laboratory and cardiologist are readily available and capable of proficiently introducing intra-aortic balloon counterpulsation, performing coronary angioplasty, or directing the patient to emergency coronary bypass surgery. When quickly initiated, this protocol is performed in lieu of thrombolytic therapy in patients who are likely to require invasive studies, considerable instrumentation, or emergency bypass surgery. The overall objective of thrombolytic therapy or catheterization is to pursue the measures necessary to reduce infarct size and minimize the amount of threatened myocardium, thus lessening the patient's chances of progressing to cardiac failure and cardiogenic shock.

After initial hemodynamic stabilization, most patients who have recently experienced myocardial infarction and continued or recurrent circulatory impairment should undergo emergency cardiac catheterization and coronary angiography. The objective is to diagnose and treat definitively a remedial, but otherwise

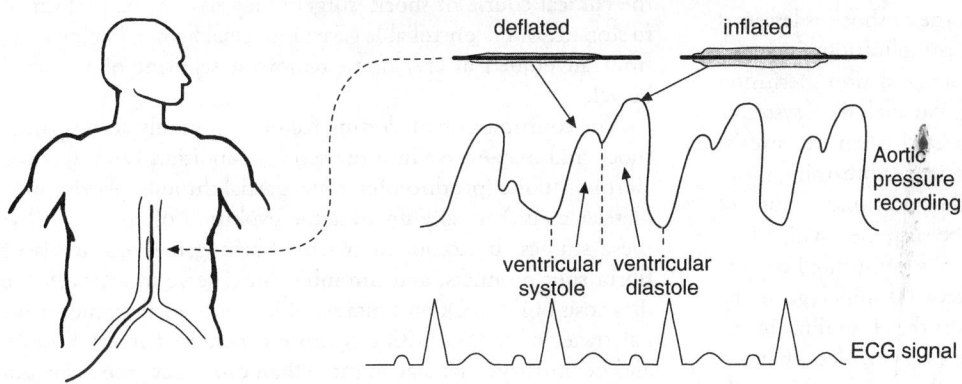

Mechanical support with intraaortic balloon counterpulsation

deflated   inflated

Aortic pressure recording

ventricular systole   ventricular diastole

ECG signal

FIGURE 71.2. Intra-aortic balloon counterpulsation augments central and systemic hemodynamics by balloon inflation within the blood-filled aorta during diastole, thereby increasing coronary myocardial, organ, and peripheral tissue perfusion; diminishing ventricular afterload (resultant increase in stroke volume and cardiac output); and decreasing myocardial oxygen consumption. Balloon inflation and deflation are positioned ("gated") via a continuous electrocardiographic signal.

catastrophic lesion (high-grade left main coronary artery obstruction, high-grade proximal obstruction of two or more coronary arteries, ruptured ventricular septum or wall, massive mitral regurgitation) while the patient is relatively stable. Once the patient has entered a state of clinical shock, the morbidity and mortality rates of cardiac catheterization, coronary angiography, and cardiac surgery rise dramatically. The same general principles apply to the management of noninfarction catastrophic cardiac events (acute severe aortic valvular insufficiency, chordal rupture with severe mitral regurgitation).

Most patients with infarction-induced cardiogenic shock have left ventricular filling pressures higher than 15 mm Hg. Intravenous infusion of nitroglycerin or nitroprusside can be effective in improving cardiac output in patients with preserved arterial pressure, reducing elevated left ventricular filling pressures, and minimizing the degree of mitral regurgitation. The patient with marked hypotension (systolic pressures less than 70 to 75 mm Hg), cardiogenic shock, and left ventricular filling pressure of 18 mm Hg or higher is treated initially with vasopressor therapy, such as phenylephrine. Phenylephrine is initiated as a 1 μg per kilogram intravenous loading dose, followed by a drip at 0.5 μg per kilogram per minute; dosing is advanced as needed up to a maximal dose of 5 μg per kilogram per minute until the mean arterial blood pressure exceeds 65 to 70 mm Hg. The main objective of vasopressor therapy in this context is to elevate systemic blood pressure to achieve and maintain adequate coronary blood flow and perfusion of noninfarcted myocardium. Alternatively, patients with impaired renal blood flow may benefit from intravenous dopamine infusion at a drip rate of 5 to 15 μg per kilogram per minute. Once the mean arterial pressure has increased to more than 70 to 75 mm Hg, dobutamine may be added to augment myocardial contractility if needed.

If peripheral perfusion and systemic blood pressure do not improve to adequate levels with pharmacologic therapies in a patient who otherwise is a reasonable candidate for a major definitive intervention (coronary bypass surgery, heart transplant), mechanical support should be considered (intra-aortic balloon counterpulsation, ventricular assist device). The primary objective of the aforementioned pharmacologic interventions and mechanical support is to stabilize the patient hemodynamically for definitive diagnostic studies (cardiac catheterization and angiography) and a potentially life-saving reparative procedure (coronary angioplasty, bypass surgery, valve replacement). Intra-aortic balloon counterpulsation augments cardiac output by reducing afterload, increases coronary blood flow by enhancing diastolic perfusion pressure and perfusion time, and may decrease myocardial oxygen consumption (Fig. 71.2). Diastolic inflation (30 to 40 mL) and systolic deflation are regulated by electrocardiographic synchronization. Contraindications to balloon counterpulsation include aortic regurgitation and aortic aneurysm.

Obstruction to Flow

Systolic function of the ventricle is directly linked to its state of diastolic filling (preload), as described by the Frank-Starling relation. Diastolic filling of the ventricles can be drastically reduced by several disorders. Pulmonary embolization and cardiac tumors (myxoma) are examples of intracardiac or intravascular obstructions to flow and ventricular filling. Extracardiac or extravascular obstruction of flow by compression occurs during cardiac tamponade, tension pneumothorax, and high positive end-expiratory pressure (PEEP) ventilation. Inadequate ventricular diastolic filling, with resultant reduced stroke volume and cardiac output, is the major mechanism of hypotension and shock in each case.

In the management of cardiogenic shock caused by inadequate filling, it is important to remember that most of the causes are detectable by careful clinical examination and laboratory testing (echocardiography), and most are completely reversible (pericardiocentesis or pericardiectomy for tamponade, chest tube for pneumothorax, resection for myxoma). This group of disorders is among the readily and definitively treatable causes of shock; when any of these conditions is suspected as a cause of hypotension or shock, select diagnostic studies and interventions are initiated as early as possible in the clinical course (e.g., echocardiography and pericardiocentesis for pericardial tamponade).

Complications

The most effective treatment of the complications of shock is prevention. Complications accrue as the severity and duration of shock intensify, and a favorable outcome of shock is lessened greatly as the severity and number of complications increase. Clinically significant ventilatory defects or ventilation–perfusion abnormalities are best detected by the regular analysis of systemic arterial blood gases and should be suspected when the arterial PO_2 falls below 85 mm Hg while the patient is breathing room air. The development of ARDS, the most common cause of death in noncardiogenic shock, should be suspected with a falling arterial PO_2 (particularly as the fraction of inspired oxygen [FIO_2] increases), an arterial PO_2 less than 60 mm Hg, or the finding of diffuse pulmonary infiltrates on the chest film (in the presence of pulmonary capillary wedge pressures less than 15 mm Hg). A systemic arterial PO_2 greater than 60 mm Hg while breathing room air generally can be managed by external oxygen delivery systems (e.g., a mask). A PO_2 less than 60 mm Hg often requires ventilator therapy, occasionally with PEEP, to bring the arterial PO_2 to 60 mm Hg or higher. Ventilator therapy plus PEEP with an FIO_2 of 50% or less is generally preferable to non-PEEP high-FIO_2 delivery (100% oxygen by mask), since a high FIO_2 may lead to toxic changes in the lung within a few hours.

Aspiration pneumonia is not an uncommon complication of shock and can be prevented in most patients by optimal nursing support, proper endotracheal care, and appropriate nasogastric suctioning. Once aspiration pneumonia is suspected and diagnosed, tracheal suction specimens should be submitted for culture. Shortly thereafter, antibiotic therapy is begun.

Renal function is always a major concern in shock states. Once intravascular volume seems adequate or high but urine output remains low (less than 20 mL per hour), a diuretic drug (e.g., intravenous furosemide, starting at 40 to 80 mg) might be administered (see Chapter 140). Failure to respond to incremental doses of the diuretic often heralds the onset of acute renal failure. Select patients with renal dysfunction stemming from renal hypoperfusion may respond favorably to low-dose (1 to 4 μg per kilogram per minute) infusions of dopamine. Drugs with nephrotoxic potential should be avoided or used with caution in shock states because of the marked increase in the susceptibility of the kidneys to injury in this condition. The dosing schedule of drugs cleared by the kidney must be modified once renal dysfunction has developed. Hyperkalemia is a common problem in renal failure of any cause, including shock. Peritoneal or bedside renal dialysis may be required to manage shock-induced renal failure.

Gastrointestinal bleeding is a common complication of shock and is always a threatening event, particularly when coagulation abnormalities develop. Visual inspection and guaiac testing of gastric contents, regular guaiac testing for fecal blood, and monitoring of hematocrit usually allow detection of gastrointestinal bleeding at relatively early stages (before major hemorrhage and the superimposition of hypovolemic shock). Superficial gastric ulceration is the most common source of gastrointestinal bleeding in shock. Gastrointestinal lesions can serve as entry points for infecting organisms and harmful components of luminal contents. Antacids or sucralfate is administered via nasogastric tube and a histamine receptor antagonist (cimetidine, ranitidine) is given intravenously, in an effort to retard and reverse the development of gastrointestinal ulceration. On rare occasions during the clinical course of shock, surgery may have to be performed to stop major uncontrollable gastrointestinal hemorrhaging (e.g., from an eroded artery) or to remove a segment of infarcted bowel.

The consumption of clotting factors commonly accompanies shock and may evolve into the serious condition DIC. Regular clotting studies (prothrombin time, partial thromboplastin time, platelet count) usually uncover the evolution of coagulopathy; these studies, in conjunction with fibrinogen levels, levels of fibrin split products, and thrombin time, serve to establish the diagnosis of DIC. Often a catastrophic event signaling the terminal stages of shock, DIC can cause generalized microthrombi and hemorrhage, damage to more than one organ, renal cortical necrosis, and local (from endotracheal, nasogastric tube, and catheter sites) and diffuse hemorrhage. Fresh-frozen plasma or platelets (if the platelet count is depressed) may be required to stop hemorrhage caused or exacerbated by the consumptive coagulopathy. When more than 2 L of blood is infused in hemorrhagic shock, a unit of fresh-frozen plasma should be administered to avert thrombocytopenia and the dilution of blood clotting factors.

The shock syndrome and its management constitute the ideal situation for iatrogenic complications. Often, diagnostic and monitoring procedures must be performed and major therapies instituted on an emergency basis in settings that are not ideal. Few physicians are optimally trained and experienced in each of the procedures and therapies ultimately required to treat all shock patients. Organizing the management of shock in diagnostic and therapeutic stages, with recruitment of specialists at appropriate times along the clinical course, is an important and effective means of minimizing the complications of shock treatment. A keen awareness of the complications of the diagnostic and therapeutic maneuvers used and vigilance for their occurrence are crucial in the overall treatment of shock. For more information, refer to Chapters 268, 355, 357, and 388.

BIBLIOGRAPHY

Adrogue HJ, Rashad N, Gorin AB, et al. Assessing acid–base status in circulatory failure. *N Engl J Med* 1989;320:1312–1316.

Bates ER, Topol EJ. Limitations of thrombolytic therapy for acute myocardial infarction complicated by congestive heart failure and cardiogenic shock. *J Am Coll Cardiol* 1991;18:1077–1084.

Bengtson JR, Kaplan AJ, Pieper KS, et al. Prognosis in cardiogenic shock after myocardial infarction in the interventional era. *J Am Coll Cardiol* 1992;20:1482–1489.

Califf RM, Bengtson JR. Cardiogenic shock. *N Engl J Med* 1994;330:1724–1730.

Carlson RW, Geheb MA, eds. *Principles and practice of medical intensive care.* Philadelphia: WB Saunders, 1993.

Goldberg RJ, Gore JM, Alpert JS, et al. Cardiogenic shock after acute myocardial infarction: incidence and mortality from a community-wide perspective, 1975 to 1988. *N Engl J Med* 1991;325:1117–1122.

Hands ME, Rutherford JD, Muller JE, et al. The in-hospital development of cardiogenic shock after myocardial infarction: incidence, predictors of occurrence, outcome and prognostic factors. *J Am Coll Cardiol* 1989;14:40–48.

Hardway RM, ed. *Shock: The reversible stage of dying.* Littleton: PSG Publishing.

Kreis DJ Jr, Baue AE, eds. *Clinical management of shock*. Baltimore: University Park Press, 1984.

Leier CV. Acute inotropic support: intravenously administered positive inotropic drugs. In: Leier CV, ed. *Cardiotonic drugs*. New York: Marcel Dekker, 1991.

Moosvi AR, Khaja F, Villanueva L, et al. Early revascularization improves survival in cardiogenic shock complicating acute myocardial infarction. *J Am Coll Cardiol* 1992;19:907–914.

Parillo JE. *Current therapy in critical care medicine*. Philadelphia: BC Dekker, 1991.

Wheeler AP, Bernard GR. Treating patients with severe sepsis. *N Engl J Med* 1999;340:207–214.

Kelley's Textbook of Internal Medicine, fourth edition. Edited by H. David Humes. Lippincott Williams & Wilkins, Philadelphia © 2000.

DISORDERS OF THE CARDIOVASCULAR SYSTEM

CORONARY ARTERY DISEASE

**MIHAI GHEORGHIADE
ROBERT O. BONOW**

In the United States, atherosclerotic coronary heart disease (CAD) is the leading cause of death in both men and women and is a clinically significant disease process in about 11 million persons. The economic toll of CAD is in excess of $60 billion per year. CAD may be asymptomatic; may take the form of stable angina; or, when atherosclerotic plaques rupture and stimulate platelet aggregation and thrombosis, may result in unstable angina, non-Q-wave or Q-wave myocardial infarction (MI), or sudden death. CAD is also the leading cause of left ventricular dysfunction and heart failure in the industrialized world. During the past two decades, the age-adjusted mortality rate from CAD has declined by 50% as a direct result of improved prevention methods and treatment of patients. Despite this progress, cardiovascular disease still accounts for more than 50% of all deaths. The lifetime risk of a CAD-related event (MI or death) at age 40 is 1 in 2 for men and 1 in 3 for women. In less than 1% of patients, CAD is caused by conditions other than atherosclerosis (Table 72.1).

Several factors predispose the coronary arteries to the development and progression of the atherosclerotic process (Table 72.2). Cigarette smoking, hypercholesterolemia, and hypertension can induce changes in endothelial structure and function and promote smooth-muscle-cell proliferation. Diabetes mellitus, genetic factors (family history of premature CAD, ethnic characteristics), male gender, advancing age, and menopause are other strong risk factors that contribute to the progression of coronary atherosclerosis. Additional factors implicated in an increased risk of CAD are physical inactivity, obesity, and psychological factors. Studies indicate that elevated plasma homocysteine levels may also predispose to atherosclerosis, because homocysteine impairs nitric oxide production, stimulates smooth-muscle proliferation, and increases thrombogenicity. Elevated levels of serum lipoprotein(a) appear to correlate with rapid angiographic progression of CAD. Focal inflammation in the coronary arteries in response to reactivation of dormant cytomegalovirus or chlamydia pneumoniae and helicobacter pylori infections may be involved in the pathogenesis of unstable coronary syndromes and could be a risk factor for CAD. Estrogen deficiency, plasma fibrinogen, factor VII, endogenous tissue plasminogen activator, plasminogen activator inhibitor type 1, D-dimer, and C-reactive protein are also emerging cardiovascular risk factors. The importance of genetic factors is underscored by the marked racial differences in the prevalence of coronary risk factors. In the future, genomic analysis will make it possible not only to predict early in life a genetic predisposition for CAD but also to identify the type of pathophysiologic disruption and to develop a rational preventive strategy specific to each person. For example, the Arg3500Gin mutation in the apolipoprotein B gene, which is responsible for familial defective apolipoprotein B-100, causes severe hypercholesterolemia and an increase in the risk of ischemic heart disease.

◼ CHRONIC CORONARY ARTERY DISEASE

Several million persons in the United States suffer from chronic stable angina. Stable angina is characterized by poorly localized chest or left arm discomfort associated with physical exertion or emotional stress and relieved promptly by rest or sublingual nitroglycerin. The discomfort is related to myocardial ischemia that is transient and does not cause myocardial necrosis. It is considered stable if the pattern does not change over a 2-month period.

PATHOPHYSIOLOGY

The most common cause for stable angina pectoris is stenosis of the proximal segments of the left anterior descending, right, or circumflex coronary artery by an atherosclerotic plaque. During an angina attack, myocardial ischemia develops from an imbalance between oxygen demand and oxygen supply, resulting in anaerobic metabolism with formation of lactic acid from glycogen. Causes and effects of myocardial ischemia are illustrated in Fig. 72.1.

TABLE 72.1.	CAUSES FOR CORONARY ARTERY DISEASE OTHER THAN ATHEROSCLEROTIC HEART DISEASE

Congenital anomalies
  Absence of the left circumflex coronary artery
  Coronary artery fistula
  Left coronary artery from pulmonary artery
  Left coronary artery from right coronary sinus
  Right coronary artery from left coronary sinus
  Single coronary artery
Coronary artery aneurysm
  Congenital
  Acquired
Fibromuscular hyperplasia
Trauma
Inflammatory
  Ehlers–Danlos syndrome
  Mycotic aneurysm
  Mucocutaneous lymph node syndrome (Kawasaki)
  Necrotizing arteritis
  Polyarteritis nodosa
  Progressive systemic sclerosis
  Rheumatoid arthritis
  Systemic lupus erythematosus
  Syphilitic arteritis
Coronary dissection
Coronary spasm
Thrombotic/embolic
  Antiphospholipid syndrome
  Atrial fibrillation
  Endocarditis
  Left atrial myxoma
  Marantic endocarditis
  Mitral stenosis
  Mural thrombus
  Paradoxic emboli (PFO)
  Polycythemia vera
  Primary cardiomyopathy
  Primary thrombocytosis
  Prosthetic mitral or aortic valve
  Sickle cell anemia
  Thrombotic thrombocytopenic purpura
Inherited disorder
  Alkaptonuria (atheromatous plaque)
  Fabry's disease (ceramide trihexoside)
  Familial high-density lipoprotein deficiency
  Homocystinuria
  Hunter's syndrome
  Hurler's syndrome
  Primary oxalosis
  Sandhoff's disease
  Takayasu's arteritis
  Tangier disease (cholesterol esters)
Others
  Amyloidosis
  Buerger's disease (thromboangiitis obliterans)
  Fibroelastosis
  Friedreich's ataxia
  Medial calcification
  Obstructive tumors
  Postcardiac transplant
  Progressive muscular dystrophy
  Radiation
  Typhus

PFO, patent foramen ovale.
(Adapted from Wenger NK. Rare causes of coronary artery disease: the heart arteries and veins. In: Hurst JW. *The heart,* 4th ed. New York: McGraw-Hill, with permission.)

Myocardial Oxygen Demand

Most episodes of angina arise from increases in oxygen demand during physical or emotional stress. Myocardial oxygen demand is determined by heart rate, myocardial contractility, and myocardial wall tension. Wall tension, in turn, is related to chamber pressure and volume. An increase in any or all of these variables may develop during exercise or emotional stress and may precipitate myocardial ischemia in patients with compromised oxygen supply.

Myocardial Oxygen Supply

Myocardial oxygen supply is determined by coronary blood flow and the arteriovenous oxygen difference across the coronary bed. Because the arteriovenous oxygen difference is near maximal at rest in most patients, changes in oxygen supply are almost entirely mediated by alterations in blood flow.

Diminished Coronary Vasodilator Reserve

Autoregulation of blood flow occurs primarily at the level of the small coronary arterioles (diameter roughly 200 μm). Coronary vasodilator reserve in the normal coronary circulation allows for a four- to fivefold increase in blood flow to the myocardium in response to physiologic stimuli that promote arteriolar vasodilatation. In contrast, vasodilator reserve is limited or absent in patients with critical atherosclerotic stenoses in the large epicardial arteries. Normal resting flow can be maintained in this context only through compensatory arteriolar dilatation. Thus, coronary vasodilator reserve, which is normally used only during stress, is expended under resting conditions in the patient with CAD to defend resting flow, resulting in diminished reserve during stress. In coronary arteries with severe stenoses that decrease the luminal diameter by 90% to 95%, vasodilator reserve may be completely exhausted under resting conditions.

Thus, the classic understanding of angina pectoris is that myocardial ischemia comes about during stress, when progressive increases in myocardial oxygen demand exceed the ability of the coronary circulation to amplify myocardial blood flow. Although this pathophysiologic mechanism of action does occur and is operative in many patients with CAD, this factor alone is insufficient to explain the full clinical spectrum of chronic stable angina, since it implies that each patient has a stable ischemic threshold—that is, that there is a stable threshold of oxygen demand, determined by heart rate, blood pressure, and contractility, below which ischemia is not present and above which ischemia develops. If this were the case, each patient would have a fixed angina threshold and would experience angina at identical workloads on many different occasions. In clinical practice, this is usually not the case; patients often experience varying thresholds of intensity of exercise at which angina develops.

Endothelial Dysfunction

It is now apparent that patients with coronary atherosclerosis have dynamic fluctuations in the severity of stenosis that may lead to varying angina thresholds. A major component of the

TABLE 72.2.   **CARDIOVASCULAR RISK FACTORS: THE EVIDENCE SUPPORTING THEIR ASSOCIATION WITH DISEASE, THE USEFULNESS OF MEASURING THEM, AND THEIR RESPONSIVENESS TO INTERVENTION**

Risk Factor	Evidence for Association with CVD		Clinical Measurement	Response to Nonpharmacologic Therapy	Response to Pharmacologic Therapy
	Epidemiologic	Clinical Trials	Useful?		
Category I (risk factors for which interventions have been proved to lower CVD risk)					
Cigarette smoking	+++	++	+++	+++	++
LDL cholesterol	+++	+++	+++	++	+++
High fat/cholesterol diet	+++	++	++	++	—
Hypertension	+++	+++ (stroke)	+++	+	+++
Left ventricular hypertrophy	+++	+	++	—	++
Thrombogenic factors	+++ (fibrinogen)	+++ (aspirin, warfarin)	+ (fibrinogen)	+	+++ (aspirin, warfarin)
Category II (risk factors for which interventions are likely to lower CVD risk)					
Diabetes mellitus	+++	+	+++	++	+++
Physical inactivity	+++	++	++	++	—
HDL cholesterol	+++	+	+++	++	+
Triglycerides; small, dense LDL	++	++	+++	++	+++
Obesity	+++	—	+++	++	+
Postmenopausal status (women)	+++	—	+++	—	+++
Category III (risk factors associated with increased CVD risk that, if modified, might lower risk)					
Psychosocial factors	++	+	+++	+	—
Lipoprotein(a)	+	—	+	—	+
Homocysteine	++	—	+	++	++
Oxidative stress	+	—	—	+	++
No alcohol consumption	+++	—	++	++	
Category IV (risk factors associated with increased CVD risk, but which cannot be modified)					
Age	+++	—	+++	—	—
Male gender	+++	—	+++	—	—
Low socioeconomic status	+++	—	+++	—	—
Family history of early-onset CVD	+++	—	+++	—	—

CVD, cardiovascular disease; HDL, high-density lipoprotein; LDL, low-density lipoprotein; +, weak, somewhat consistent evidence; ++, moderately strong, rather consistent evidence; +++, very strong, consistent evidence; —, evidence poor or nonexistent.
(Pearson TA and Fuster V. From Executive summary. 27th Bethesda Conference: Matching the intensity of risk factor management with the hazard for coronary disease events. *J Am Coll Cardiol* 1996;27:957–1047, with permission.)

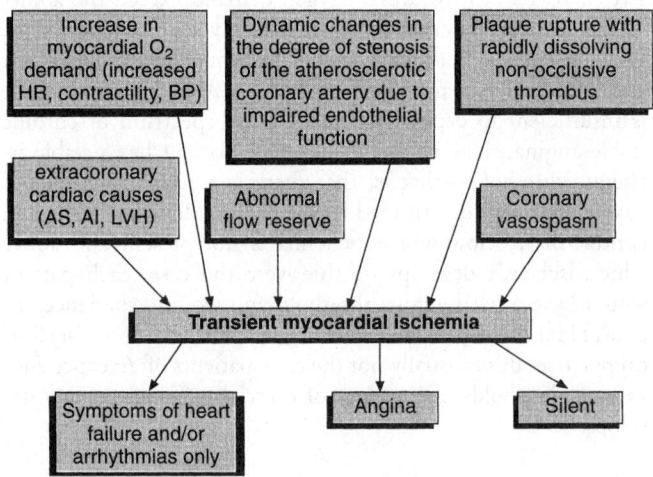

FIGURE 72.1. Causes and effects of transient ischemia. AI, aortic insufficiency; AS, aortic stenosis; BP, systemic blood pressure; HR, heart rate; LVH, left ventricular hypertrophy. (From Maseri A. Role of coronary artery spasm in symptomatic and silent myocardial ischemia. *J Am Coll Cardiol* 1987;9:249–262, with permission.)

pathophysiologic picture of angina is endothelial dysfunction of atherosclerotic arteries, including arteries with plaques that are not themselves flow limiting. Normal arterial endothelial cells produce several vasodilating substances; the most notable of them is endothelial-derived relaxing factor (EDRF), which has been identified as nitric oxide. Nitric oxide is the most potent endogenous vasodilator that is responsible for maintaining normal vascular tone and for inhibiting smooth-muscle growth and proliferation, leukocyte adhesion to the endothelial surface, and platelet aggregation. The release of EDRF by healthy endothelium is continuous and is augmented in response to increases in blood flow. In addition, under normal conditions, both endogenous (acetylcholine, serotonin, thrombin) and exogenous (exercise, mental stress, cold) stimuli promote EDRF production and release, resulting in coronary vasodilatation. In contrast, atherosclerotic coronary artery segments with disrupted endothelium lose the normal ability to dilate in response to these stimuli and manifest a paradoxical vasoconstrictor response that may precipitate an angina attack. Independent of the atherosclerotic process, hypertension, diabetes mellitus, estrogen deficiency, hypercholesterolemia, and cigarette smoking are also associated with abnormal endothelial function.

Circadian Variation

The dynamic alterations in coronary blood flow may follow a circadian pattern. Ischemic episodes become more frequent and occur at lower levels of demand in the early morning hours. This is related to increases in plasma catecholamines and cortisol concentrations that often result in a decrease in coronary blood supply stemming from heightened coronary vascular resistance. In addition, the aggregability of platelets peaks, and fibrinolytic activity declines in the early morning hours.

Pathophysiologic Effects of Myocardial Ischemia

Myocardial ischemia initially causes left ventricular diastolic dysfunction (relaxation failure), since early-stage ischemia impairs the intracellular sequestration of calcium ion in the sarcoplasmic reticulum of the myocyte, allowing persistent tension development during diastole and thus higher left ventricular diastolic pressures. This is followed by regional systolic dysfunction (contraction failure), manifested by diminished systolic thickening and inward systolic wall motion of the ischemic myocardium. These effects of ischemia on left ventricular function usually precede the development of electrocardiographic changes or chest discomfort.

CLINICAL MANIFESTATIONS

Symptoms

Angina pectoris is usually experienced as substernal pressure, heaviness, tightness, burning, or numbness that develops during exercise or emotional stress and is relieved within minutes by resting. The patient often cannot pinpoint the exact location of discomfort. The symptoms often radiate to the left shoulder and the inner surface of the left arm. They may also affect the neck, jaw, and teeth and, less frequently, the left ear, wrist, hand, and the fourth and fifth fingers. Many times, the discomfort is felt only in the neck, shoulder, or arm, without any chest discomfort. In many patients, chest discomfort is associated with dyspnea, and at times it may be perceived only as dyspnea. Patients also may experience diaphoresis, nausea, weakness, or dizziness. The severity is often defined by the grading system developed by the Canadian Cardiovascular Society (Table 72.3).

An angina episode may last a few minutes or up to 15 to 20 minutes. It may occur several times a day or less frequently—once or twice a month. A stable pattern of discomfort may disappear for several months and then reappear at the same or higher intensity and frequency. Patients may have a fixed ischemic threshold, with angina symptoms appearing at a relatively similar level of exertion, or they may describe a varying threshold. If angina develops at different workloads, it suggests that there is an element of vasoconstriction in addition to fixed coronary artery stenosis. Because of the circadian variation of ischemia, angina may be felt only in the morning and with minimal exertion, but later in the day the patient may engage in strenuous activity without chest discomfort. In some patients, the symptoms can be induced by moderate exertion and resolve as the patient progresses to more intense exercise, a phenomenon

TABLE 72.3.	GRADING OF ANGINA PECTORIS BY THE CANADIAN CARDIOVASCULAR SOCIETY CLASSIFICATION SYSTEM
Class	**Description**
I	Ordinary physical activity does not cause angina, such as walking, climbing stairs. Angina [occurs] with strenuous, rapid, or prolonged exertion at work or recreation.
II	Slight limitation of ordinary activity. Angina occurs on walking or climbing stairs rapidly, walking uphill, walking or stair climbing after meals, or in cold, in wind, or under emotional stress, or only during the few hours after awakening. Walking more than two blocks on the level and climbing more than one flight of ordinary stairs at a normal pace and in normal condition.
III	Marked limitations of ordinary physical activity. Angina occurs on walking one or two blocks on the level and climbing one flight of stairs in normal conditions and at a normal pace.
IV	Inability to carry on any physical activity without discomfort—anginal symptoms may be present at rest.

(From Campeau L. Grading of angina pectoris (ltr). *Circulation* 1976;54:522, with permission.)

termed "walk-through angina." On occasion, angina occurs only at night.

Several factors can precipitate an episode of angina. Most notable are any conditions that increase oxygen demand, such as exercise, sexual activity, or emotional distress. The threshold of angina may be decreased by mental stress, excitement, cold temperatures, windy conditions, meals, cigarette smoking, or substance abuse (cocaine or, occasionally, alcohol). Concomitant diseases that strain oxygen demand, such as anemia, hyperthyroidism, or aortic valve disease, also lead to a decrease in the angina threshold. Most ischemic episodes in a patient with stable angina are painless or "silent." The reason for lack of pain or discomfort during some of the ischemic episodes remains unclear. It may be due to a rise in plasma β-endorphin concentration that diminishes pain perception.

Differential Diagnosis

Several conditions can produce an anginal syndrome indistinguishable from that caused by atherosclerotic CAD. These include aortic stenosis, aortic insufficiency, hypertrophic cardiomyopathy, dilated cardiomyopathy, and pulmonary hypertension (either primary or stemming from such conditions as mitral stenosis). Spasm of the large coronary arteries, causing variant (or Prinzmetal's) angina, usually occurs at rest but may be induced by exercise, especially if it develops at the site of a mild atherosclerotic plaque that itself is not flow limiting.

Cocaine also can induce myocardial ischemia that is related to coronary artery vasoconstriction, platelet aggregation, and accelerated atherosclerosis. Chest pain or discomfort is the most common cocaine-related medical problem. Chest pain caused by limited vasodilator reserve of the coronary microvasculature, termed microvascular angina or "syndrome X," can mimic atherosclerotic CAD. This syndrome is more common in women and patients with hypertension and is a typical cause of chest pain with normal coronary arteriograms. Diabetes mellitus may also produce small-vessel disease and myocardial ischemia. In addition, diseases of the coronary arteries other than atherosclerosis may induce angina (see Table 72.1).

Other cardiovascular conditions may cause chest pain unrelated to myocardial ischemia. The pain associated with aortic dissection can mimic a severe angina attack. The chest pain prompted by pulmonary embolism or acute pericarditis usually differs from angina in quality and precipitating factors but occasionally masquerades as myocardial ischemia. Several noncardiac conditions have initial symptoms of chest pain. Usually, they can be distinguished from angina pectoris because of differences in duration, quality, position, and precipitating factors (Table 72.4). In many of these conditions, the discomfort is sharp in nature and well localized and may increase with inspiration.

Physical Examination

Physical examination is a mandatory component of the evaluation of patients with angina, since it is essential to exclude valvu-

lar heart disease or obstructive hypertrophic cardiomyopathy as a noncoronary source of chest pain. In addition, patients who have had an MI may have evidence of left ventricular dysfunction, with a displaced left ventricular impulse, an apical third heart sound, and, from time to time, a murmur of mitral regurgitation. It is also important to probe for signs of hypercholesterolemia, such as arcus senilis, xanthelasma, and tendon xanthomata, which increase the likelihood of atherosclerotic disease. Carotid, abdominal, and femoral bruits and decreased pulses in the legs suggest diffuse atherosclerotic disease. During an angina attack, a fourth or a third heart sound or a mid- to late systolic murmur of mitral regurgitation is often present.

Laboratory Findings

It is important to investigate potential factors that can magnify myocardial oxygen demand and precipitate angina, such as anemia or hyperthyroidism. The development of anemia in the context of a concomitant condition is a common explanation for an increase in angina frequency or intensity in a patient who previously had a stable pattern of angina. The total serum cholesterol level may be elevated, with a decline in high-density lipoproteins (HDLs) or an increase in the low-density lipoprotein (LDL) serum concentration. A normal total serum cholesterol level does not exclude the possibility of severe atherosclerotic CAD.

TABLE 72.4.	DIFFERENTIAL DIAGNOSIS OF EPISODIC CHEST PAIN RESEMBLING ANGINA PECTORIS					
	Duration	**Quality**	**Provocation**	**Relief**	**Location**	**Comment**
Effort angina	5–15 min	Visceral (pressure)	During effort or emotion	Rest, nitroglycerin	Substernal, radiates	1st episode vivid
Rest angina	5–15 min	Visceral (pressure)	Spontaneous (? with exercise)	Nitroglycerin	Substernal, radiates	Often nocturnal
Mitral prolapse	Minutes to hours	Superficial (rarely visceral)	Spontaneous (no pattern)	Time	Left anterior	No pattern, variable character
Esophageal reflux	10 min–1 hr	Visceral	Recumbency, lack of food	Food, antacid	Substernal epigastric	Rarely radiates
Esophageal spasm	5–60 min	Visceral	Spontaneous, cold liquids, exercise	Nitroglycerin	Substernal, radiates	Mimics angina
Peptic ulcer	Hours	Visceral burning	Lack of food, "acid" foods	Foods, antacids	Epigastric substernal	
Biliary disease	Hours	Visceral (wax & wane)	Spontaneous, food	Time, analgesia	Epigastric, may radiate	Colic
Cervical disk	Variable (gradually subsides)	Superficial	Head & neck movement, palpation	Time, analgesia	Arm, neck	Not relieved by rest
Hyperventilation	2–3 min	Visceral	Emotion tachypnea	Stimulus removal	Substernal	Facial paresthesia
Musculoskeletal	Variable	Superficial	Movement palpation	Time, analgesia	Multiple	Tenderness
Pulmonary	30 min +	Visceral (pressure)	Often spontaneous	Rest, time, bronchodilator	Substernal	Dyspnea present

(From Christie LG, Conti CR. Systematic approach to evaluation of angina-like chest pain: pathophysiology and clinical testing with emphasis on objective documentation of myocardial ischemia. *Am Heart J* 1981;102:897.)

It has also been suggested that increased plasma concentrations of fibrinogen, factor VII, plasminogen activator inhibitor type 1, tissue plasminogen activator, and D-dimer enhance blood coagulation and are predictors of MI and sudden death in patients with chronic stable angina. High levels of homocysteine may also be present and have been shown to damage vascular endothelium. Lipoprotein(a) and C-reactive protein, a marker of inflammation and chlamydia pneumoniae and helicobacter pylori infections, are other emerging risk factors for atherosclerosis and acute coronary syndromes. All these measurements, however, should not be obtained routinely in patients with angina or suspected CAD.

Electrocardiography

The electrocardiogram (ECG) may show entirely normal results or nonspecific ST- and T-wave changes or evidence of a previous MI. The patient with Q waves indicative of previous infarction may be unaware of having had an MI, because up to 25% of MIs are unrecognized. Although left or right bundle-branch block, left anterior hemiblock, and atrial or ventricular premature beats may be present, these findings are not specific to CAD.

NONINVASIVE DIAGNOSTIC TESTS

The usefulness of any test in the diagnosis of CAD is its ability to establish the likelihood that atherosclerotic CAD is or is not present. This likelihood, termed the predictive accuracy, is determined by two factors: sensitivity and specificity. Sensitivity measures the percentage of patients with CAD who have a positive test response, and specificity represents the percentage of patients without CAD who have a negative test response. The sensitivity and specificity of common diagnostic tests are noted in Table 72.5.

Another factor that strongly influences the predictive accuracy of any diagnostic test is the prevalence of CAD in the population under study (Bayes theorem), which indicates the likelihood of CAD before testing is performed. The influence of pretest likelihood on the predictive accuracy of a test with high sensitivity and specificity is shown in Fig. 72.2. In patients with a low disease prevalence, such as a general population undergoing routine cardiovascular screening, a test with excellent sensitivity and specificity yields more than three times the number of false-positive as true-positive results. Thus, diagnostic testing is usually reserved for patients with a more moderate pretest likelihood, such as patients with symptoms or several

TABLE 72.5.	NONINVASIVE DIAGNOSTIC TESTS FOR DETECTION OF CORONARY ARTERY DISEASE					
	Sensitivity (%)	Specificity (%)	Criteria for Ischemia Response	Markers of High Risk	Limitations	Relative Cost
Exercise ECG	65	85	ST depression ≥1 mm	ST depression ≥1 mm at low workload and/or lasting >6 mm into recovery Hypotension Poor exercise tolerance	Low sensitivity Low specificity in context of abnormal rest ECG	+
Myocardial perfusion imaging	90	80	Reversible regional perfusion defects	Severe defects Multiple defects Cavity dilatation Increased lung uptake	Attenuation artifacts (breast, diaphragm)	+ + +
Radionuclide angiography	85	80	Reversible regional wall motion abnormality	Resting EF <40% Exercise EF <40% Exercise-induced cavity dilatation	Poor resolution to identify regional wall motion EF responses affected by age, gender, LVH, hypertension	+ + +
Stress echocardiography	80	90	Reversible regional wall motion abnormality	Multiple wall motion abnormalities Wall motion abnormality at low workload	Left ventricular dysfunction Baseline wall motion abnormalities at rest Inadequate image quality in ≈15% of patients	+ +
Ambulatory ECG	?	?	ST depression ≥1 mm lasting >1 min	>60 seconds ST depression/24 h >6 episodes ST depression/24 h	Limited data	+ +

ECG, electrocardiogram; EF, ejection fraction; LVH, left ventricular hypertrophy.

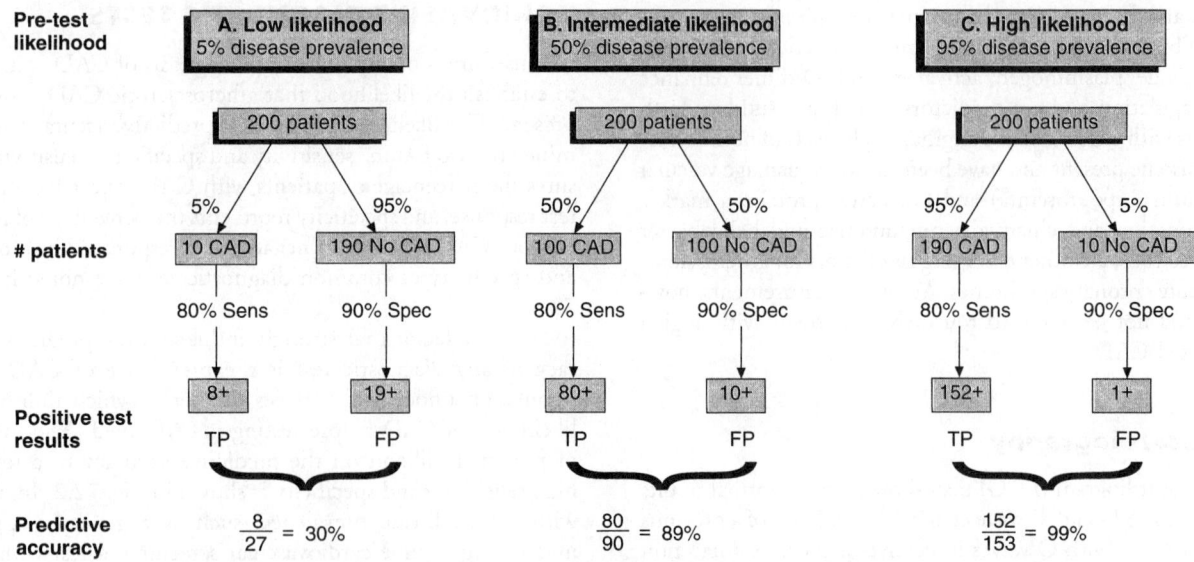

FIGURE 72.2. Effect of disease prevalence, or pretest likelihood, on predictive accuracy of a diagnostic test (Bayes theorem). Three populations of 200 patients undergo a diagnostic test with high sensitivity (Sens) and specificity (Spec), such as tomographic thallium perfusion imaging or stress echocardiography. The sensitivity and specificity determine the number of expected true-positive (TP) and false-positive (FP) responses, from which the predictive accuracy is determined. When applied to patients with low disease prevalence, such as a general population of asymptomatic middle-aged men undergoing routine cardiovascular screening, the test with excellent sensitivity and specificity yields poor predictive accuracy, with over three times the number of false-positive as true-positive test results. The same test achieves higher predictive accuracies in populations with intermediate and high levels of disease prevalence.

coronary risk factors. In patients with a high probability of disease, such as middle-aged men with typical angina and hypercholesterolemia, the diagnosis is usually well established without further testing. Because women have a lower prevalence of CAD than men, the predictive accuracy of any diagnostic test is usually lower in women.

Exercise Electrocardiography

Exercise electrocardiographic testing is usually performed on a motor-driven treadmill that increases in speed and inclination every few minutes according to a preset exercise protocol. Occasionally, exercise electrocardiographic testing is done on a stationary bicycle. Exercise is continued until the patient manifests a cardiac symptom or fatigue or reaches at least 85% of the maximal heart rate predicted for his or her age. The heart rate, blood pressure, and product of heart rate and systolic blood pressure (the rate–pressure product) achieved during exercise are indirect measures of myocardial oxygen demand. The exercise ECG is considered to be indicative of ischemia if at least 1 mm of flat or downsloping ST-segment depression develops during exercise or during the 3- to 5-minute recovery period. ST-segment changes cannot be interpreted in the context of left bundle-branch block, Wolfe-Parkinson-White syndrome, or artificial pacemakers; in these instances, stress testing should be performed with one of the imaging methods discussed later herein. Moreover, exercise-induced ST-segment depression has a lower specificity for CAD in women and in the context of left ventricular hypertrophy, digoxin therapy, mitral valve prolapse, aortic stenosis, supraventricular tachycardia, and anemia.

In addition to ST-segment changes, other variables from the exercise test provide important information regarding the severity of CAD. They include exercise tolerance, exercise-induced symptoms, maximum heart rate and blood pressure, and the heart rate and workload at the onset of ischemia. Exercise-induced hypotension, ST-segment depression of 2 mm or more, ST-segment depression persisting more than 6 minutes during the recovery phase, ischemia at low exercise workloads, and exercise-induced ventricular tachycardia associated with ischemic changes have been linked to extensive CAD.

Myocardial Perfusion Imaging

Thallium 201 (^{201}Tl)

After intravenous administration, thallium is extracted by myocardial cells in proportion to regional myocardial blood flow. Images of the heart soon after thallium administration reflect regional myocardial perfusion. When thallium is administered at peak exercise, regions with exercise-induced ischemia show perfusion defects. Although thallium washes out of the myocardium in proportion to blood flow, it also accumulates in viable myocardium in a manner analogous to potassium ion. Hence, over 2 to 4 hours, thallium defects in previously ischemic myocardium improve or normalize, a phenomenon termed thallium redistribution. Defects related to an infarct do not redistribute and remain irreversible over time. Thallium imaging has a higher sensitivity, specificity, and predictive accuracy than exercise electrocardiographic testing.

In addition to detecting CAD, thallium imaging indicates

the functional severity of CAD. The number, size, and location of stress-induced myocardial perfusion defects reflect the location, extent, and severity of coronary artery stenoses. Lung uptake of ^{201}Tl occurs when left ventricular filling pressures are elevated and is a marker of stress-induced left ventricular dysfunction, usually associated with multivessel CAD. Transient dilatation of the left ventricle after stress is also a marker of severe ischemia and generally indicates multivessel disease. Normal exercise thallium perfusion images are highly predictive of an excellent prognosis, even in patients with known CAD, with a risk of death or MI below 1% per year.

Technetium Tc 99m (^{99m}Tc) Perfusion Agents

Technetium Tc 99m–based agents have a shorter half-life than thallium (6 versus 73 hours), which allows for administration of a higher dose. The higher dose and the higher energy of technetium yield a better image quality and better delineation of perfusion defects than thallium. Sestamibi is the most widely used technetium perfusion agent. Because sestamibi undergoes only a small amount of washout after initial myocardial uptake, the distinction between transient stress-induced perfusion defects and fixed perfusion defects requires two separate injections, one during stress and one at rest. Newer techniques using these agents permit determination of left ventricular function in addition to myocardial perfusion.

Pharmacologic Stress Imaging

In patients who cannot exercise at all or who cannot exercise maximally, perfusion imaging can be done with dipyridamole, adenosine, or dobutamine during pharmacologic stress. This group includes patients with peripheral vascular disease, chronic arthritis, pulmonary disease, and neurologic disorders. In addition, patients receiving β-blockers or rate-lowering calcium channel blockers may not achieve adequate heart rates during exercise and may be candidates for pharmacologic stress imaging.

Radionuclide Angiography

First-pass or gated radionuclide angiography using technetium Tc 99m is useful for the accurate determination of left and right ventricular ejection fractions at rest and during exercise. Although changes in left ventricular function during exercise are sensitive indicators of CAD, the diagnostic accuracy of this test is limited by lack of specificity, since several factors affect the ejection fraction response to exercise. These factors include age, gender, hypertension, left ventricular hypertrophy, and concomitant valvular or myocardial disease. Hence, this test is usually reserved for patients with known CAD, to evaluate left ventricular function as an index of prognosis.

Stress Echocardiography

Stress echocardiography, with imaging either after exercise or during pharmacologic stress, has become another important noninvasive test for CAD. Even though echocardiography cannot quantify the left ventricular ejection fraction as accurately as

radionuclide angiography, its ability to assess regional ventricular function is far superior. Diminished regional systolic wall motion and systolic wall thickening are sensitive markers of regional myocardial ischemia, and the diagnostic accuracy of stress echocardiography is similar to that of myocardial perfusion imaging. The overall sensitivity for detecting the presence and extent of ischemic myocardium, however, appears to be higher with myocardial perfusion imaging.

Cardiac Magnetic Resonance Imaging

Magnetic resonance imaging (MRI) makes visible the heart in any tomographic plane with excellent spatial resolution and precise identification of endocardial and epicardial borders. MRI has a high level of accuracy in determining ventricular volume, ejection fraction, and left ventricular mass, and cine MRI provides accurate assessment of regional wall motion and wall thickening during cardiac cycle. Dobutamine stress testing with cine MRI has been used for CAD detection.

Electron Beam Computed Tomography

Electron beam computed tomography (EBCT) is a widely promoted technique for the detection of calcification within atherosclerotic coronary lesions. Calcification of coronary arteries is a clear indicator that atherosclerosis is present. Nevertheless, calcium detected in coronary arteries by EBCT is a sensitive but perhaps not a specific indicator of angiographically obstructive atherosclerotic lesions. The role of EBCT is primarily to identify patients with early CAD, to establish preventive strategies rather than to identify patients with advanced CAD with coronary artery obstructions. Preliminary evidence has linked calcification to risk of ischemic events, but it is uncertain whether this risk prediction enhances that achieved by assessing more traditional risk factors. The current role of EBCT in clinical practice remains to be determined.

Ambulatory Electrocardiography

Ambulatory electrocardiographic monitoring provides an estimate of the frequency and duration of ischemic episodes that occur during routine daily activities. By quantifying the total duration of ischemia during a 24-hour period, this form of testing has potential value in patients with known CAD, but its sensitivity for detecting CAD is less than that of exercise electrocardiographic testing. Hence, it rarely enters into the diagnostic strategy for CAD diagnosis.

CORONARY ANGIOGRAPHY

In patients with known or suspected CAD, coronary angiography is performed for diagnosis, for risk stratification, and for assessment of the appropriateness and feasibility of myocardial revascularization with coronary artery bypass graft surgery (CABG) or percutaneous coronary revascularization (PCR). Coronary angiography is relatively safe, with a risk of death of less than 0.2% and of a major nonfatal event of less than 0.5%. The most serious nonfatal complications are stroke, MI, and severe bleeding. Coronary angiography is indicated in patients with known or suspected atherosclerotic heart disease, particularly when they are classified by noninvasive testing as being at high risk of experiencing ischemic events. It is also indicated in patients with stable angina who continue to be symptomatic or have signs of ischemia during noninvasive testing, despite adequate medical therapy. Patients who have survived sudden death or who have sustained ventricular tachycardia should also undergo coronary angiography.

At the time of angiography, coronary atherosclerotic lesions are classified as concentric with smooth borders; type 1 eccentric, with smooth borders; type 2 eccentric, with irregularly scalloped borders; or having multiple irregularities. In stable angina, the lesions are usually concentric and smooth. Less frequently, the lesions are eccentric and scalloped, with irregular borders, and may have a hazy appearance. Such complex lesions are thought to represent a ruptured plaque or a partially occlusive thrombus and are more common in unstable angina than in chronic stable angina.

PROGNOSIS AND RISK STRATIFICATION

The prognosis in patients with CAD is related to the extent, severity, and morphologic features of coronary atherosclerotic lesions; left ventricular systolic function; and the severity of myo-

cardial ischemia. Numerous studies indicate that patients with left main coronary artery stenosis or left main equivalent (proximal high-grade stenosis of both the left anterior descending and left circumflex arteries) have the worst prognosis during medical therapy. Coronary anatomy also influences survival in patients without left main disease. In the Coronary Artery Surgery Study registry, in which more than 23,000 patients with suspected or established CAD were evaluated, the 12-year survival was 74% for patients with one-vessel disease, 59% for two-vessel disease, and 40% for three-vessel disease. In patients with preserved systolic function and at least one-vessel disease, 12-year survival was 73%. For moderate left ventricular dysfunction the respective rate was 54%, and for severe left ventricular dysfunction it was 21% (Fig. 72.3). These factors are additive, such that patients with left main disease or three-vessel disease who have left ventricular dysfunction or inducible myocardial ischemia are at greatest risk during medical therapy.

Medically treated women with one- and two-vessel disease and no left main CAD have a survival advantage over men with the same number of diseased vessels. No advantage for women has been observed in the subgroups with three-vessel or left main CAD. In addition to the number of coronary vessels involved, ischemia, and left ventricular function, other factors, such as age, smoking, diabetes, and previous MI, are associated with a poorer prognosis. The smoking history ranks among the most

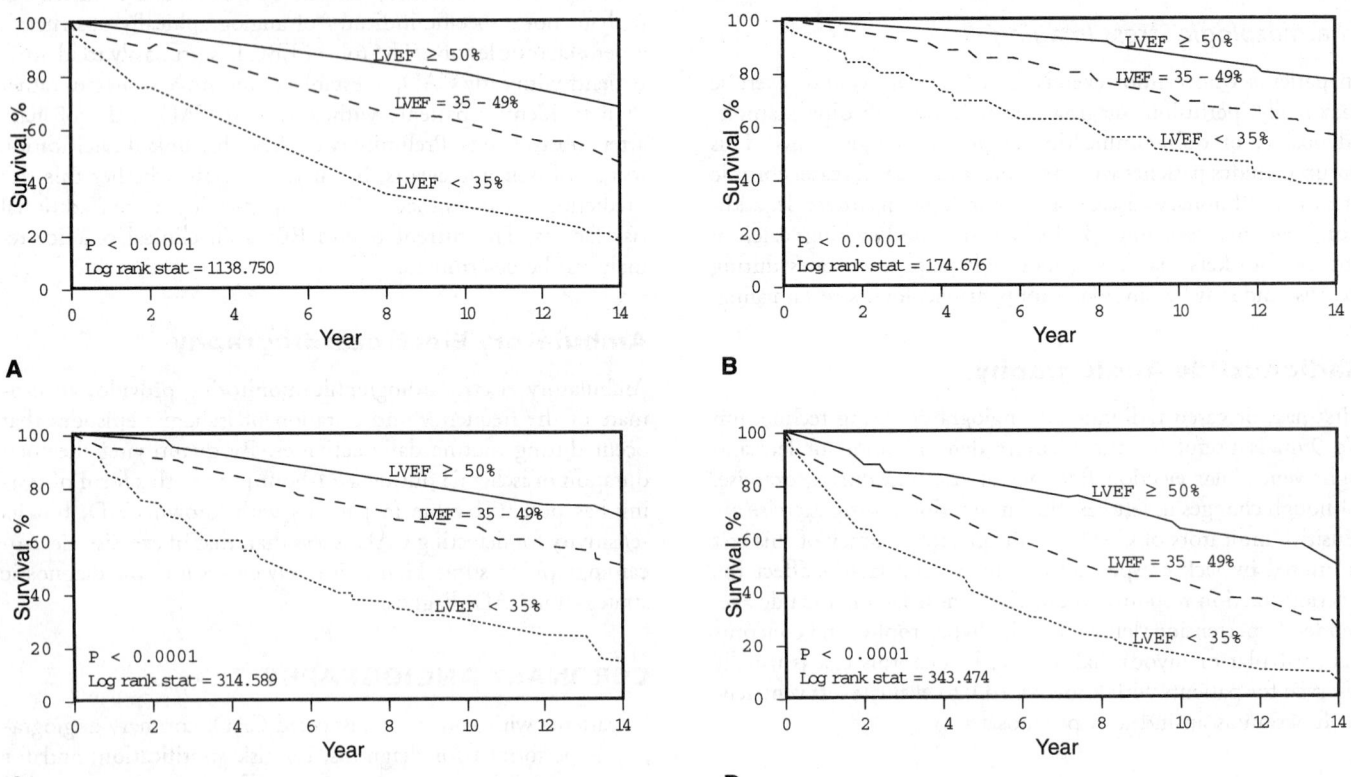

FIGURE 72.3. Graphs showing survival rates for medically treated Coronary Artery Surgery Study (CASS) patients (n = 12,387). **A:** Patients with one-, two-, or three-vessel disease by left ventricular ejection fraction (LVEF). **B:** Patients with one-vessel disease by ejection fraction. **C:** Patients with two-vessel disease by ejection fraction. **D:** Patients with three-vessel disease by ejection fraction. (From Emond M, Mock MB, Davis KB, et al. Long-term survival of medically treated patients in Coronary Artery Surgery Study (CASS). *Circulation* 1994;90:2645, with permission.)

important predictors of survival. Patients on dialysis with a history of MI have a high cardiac mortality (60% at 1 year).

MANAGEMENT

Acute cardiac events, including unstable angina, MI, and sudden cardiac death, are known to result from a disrupted atherosclerotic plaque that leads to occlusive or nonocclusive thrombosis. The atherosclerotic plaque does not need to be stenotic to rupture and cause occlusive thrombosis. Disruption of a nonstenotic plaque may also lead to a mural thrombus, causing growth of the plaque but no acute symptoms. The severity of the stenosis serves as a marker of the extent of the number of nonstenotic plaques in the coronary artery. The likelihood of rupture is related to plaque composition, hemodynamic stress, endothelial factors, and inflammatory causes. Therapy should be aimed at the prevention of plaque disruption and growth, which can lead to both progression and an acute cardiac event. An important decision is whether to treat the patient with medical therapy or to proceed with myocardial revascularization. In either case, risk factors should be addressed and modified appropriately, and general measures should be followed.

Risk Factor Modification

Since modification of risk factors can significantly improve prognosis by slowing plaque progression and disruption, every effort should be made to achieve these goals. Table 72.6 depicts the consensus panel recommendations of the American Heart Association. The major modifiable risk factors are hypertension, hypercholesterolemia, smoking, sedentary lifestyle, obesity, and, possibly, the loss of estrogen effects in postmenopausal women.

Hypertension should be treated aggressively with medications that are likely to lessen left ventricular mass and improve the balance between oxygen supply and oxygen demand, such as β-blockers and angiotensin-converting enzyme (ACE) inhibitors. The use of nisoldipine, a long-acting dihydropyridine calcium channel blocker has been associated with an increased risk of MI in hypertensive patients who have diabetes.

Lowering levels of total cholesterol and LDL cholesterol by diet and drug therapy improves endothelium-dependent coronary vasomotion, thereby contributing to improved myocardial perfusion. In addition, a significant decrease in the serum cholesterol level can prevent atherosclerotic plaque rupture and halt progression (and possibly promote regression) of coronary atherosclerosis. Aggressive management of hypercholesterolemia with diet and a lipid-lowering agent (especially 3-hydroxy-3-methylglutaryl reductase coenzyme A inhibitors or statin) lowers the risk of death and MI and the need for CABG (Table 72.7). Gemfibrozol also reduces cardiovascular events in patients with low HDL. In patients with CAD, total cholesterol should be lowered to below 200 mg per deciliter and LDL cholesterol to below 100 mg per deciliter (2.6 mmol per liter), and HDL cholesterol should be increased to above 35 mg per deciliter (0.9 mmol per liter). Aggressive lipid lowering therapy with statins may be as effective as PCR in stable angina.

Exposure to carbon monoxide and nicotine from tobacco smoke causes immediate constriction of the epicardial coronary arteries and can impair endothelial-mediated endothelial vasodilatation. Cigarette smoking significantly lessens the anti-ischemic effects of nitrates, β-blockers, and calcium channel blockers. Patients who continue to smoke after successful myocardial revascularization procedures are at greater risk of MI and death than nonsmokers. Smoking cessation lessens the risk of MI, which may return to a level similar to that of a person who never smoked. Passive cigarette smoking can also increase the risk of a cardiac event in patients with stable angina.

Weight reduction to an ideal body weight should be achieved. Physical activity is beneficial and may help control hypertension, hypercholesterolemia, and diabetes. A low cholesterol diet lowers serum cholesterol significantly only when combined with high levels of aerobic exercise. Heavy physical exertion, however, can trigger the onset of an acute MI, particularly in sedentary patients.

Hormone replacement therapy in postmenopausal women may be beneficial in limiting cardiovascular events. The use of estrogen combined with a progestational agent is associated with a better lipid profile than the use of estrogen alone, but it is uncertain whether this effect translates into better outcomes. One study has shown that therapy with estrogen and progesterone did not lessen the number of CAD events in postmenopausal women with established CAD. There was a higher rate of thromboembolic events and gallbladder disease early in the course of therapy, which may have offset any long-term beneficial effects from hormone replacement. Given the favorable effects of hormone replacement after several years of therapy, it is appropriate for women already taking these medications to continue.

There is an association between elevated homocysteine and atherosclerosis. Although homocysteine levels can be lowered with folic acid, pyridoxine hydrochloride, and cyanocobalamin, an association between a decrease in homocysteine and improved clinical outcome has not yet been verified. Conditions that lower the threshold for angina, such as anemia, thyrotoxicosis, fever, and hypoxemia, should be corrected. Decongestants (α-antagonists) may aggravate angina and should be avoided if possible. Patients with postprandial symptoms should abstain from large meals. Anxiety should be controlled with medications. Exposure to very low temperatures should be discouraged; however, if they cannot be avoided, the patient should cover the mouth and nose and avoid strenuous exercise. Because sexual intercourse can precipitate angina, nitrates, β-blockers, and calcium channel blockers may be used prophylactically. The use of sildenafil (Viagra) is contraindicated in patients taking nitrates or in patients with severe angina.

Drug regimens, dietary restriction, and the importance of not smoking should be discussed. Patients and family members should be instructed to recognize a change in symptoms that might signal unstable angina or acute MI and to seek medical attention. This is particularly important, because about 50% of patients who have an acute MI experience an increase in the frequency or intensity of angina 1 or 2 weeks before the event. The prognosis of a patient who has an acute MI is related to the time delay in arriving at an emergency department. Although it is important to discuss the prognosis, reassuring the patient and family is also important, since there is an association between anxiety and fatal coronary events, in particular, sudden death.

TABLE 72.6.	GUIDE TO COMPREHENSIVE RISK REDUCTION FOR PATIENTS WITH CORONARY AND OTHER VASCULAR DISEASES
Risk Intervention	**Recommendations**
Smoking Goal: complete cessation	Strongly encourage patient and family to stop smoking. Provide counseling, nicotine replacement, and formal cessation programs, as appropriate.
Lipid management Primary goal: LDL <100 mg/dL Secondary goals: HDL >35 mg/dL; TG <200 mg/dL	Start AHA step II diet in all patients: ≤30% fat, <7% saturated fat, <200 mg/d cholesterol. Assess fasting lipid profile. In post-MI patients, lipid profile may take 4 to 6 weeks to stabilize. Add drug therapy according to the following guide:

LDL <100 mg/dL No drug therapy   LDL 100 to 130 mg/dL Consider adding drug therapy to diet, as follows: ↘   Suggested drug therapy ↗   LDL >130 mg/dL Add drug therapy to diet, as follows: ↘   HDL <35 mg/dL Emphasize weight management and physical activity. Advise smoking cessation.

TG <200 mg/dL Statin Resin Niacin   TG 200–400 mg/dL Statin Niacin   TG >400 mg/dL Consider combined drug therapy (niacin, fibrate, statin).   If needed to achieve LDL goals, consider niacin, statin, fibrate.

	If LDL goal not achieved, consider combination therapy.
Physical activity Minimum goal: 30 minutes 3 or 4 times per week	Assess risk, preferably with exercise test, to guide prescription. Encourage minimum of 30 to 60 minutes of moderate-intensity activity 3 or 4 times weekly (walking, jogging, cycling, or other aerobic activity) supplemented by an increase in daily lifestyle activities (e.g., walking breaks at work, using stairs, gardening, household work). Maximum benefit 5 to 6 hours a week. Advise medically supervised programs for moderate- to high-risk patients.
Weight management	Start intensive diet and appropriate physical activity intervention, as outlined earlier, in patients >120% of ideal weight for height. Particularly emphasize need for weight loss in patients with hypertension, elevated triglycerides, or elevated glucose levels.
Antiplatelet agents/anticoagulants	Start aspirin, 80–325 mg/d, if not contraindicated. Manage warfarin to international normalized ratio = 2 to 3.5 for post-MI patients not able to take aspirin.
ACE inhibitors post-MI	Start early post-MI in stable high-risk patients (anterior MI, previous MI, Killip class II S, gallop, rales, radiographic CHF). Continue indefinitely for all with LV dysfunction (ejection fraction ≤40%) or symptoms of failure. Use as needed to manage blood pressure or symptoms in all other patients.
β-blockers	Start in high-risk post-MI patients (dysrhythmia, LV dysfunction, inducible ischemia) at 5–28 days. Continue 6 months minimum. Observe usual contraindications. Use as needed to manage angina rhythm or blood pressure in all other patients.
Estrogens	Consider estrogen replacement in all postmenopausal women. Individualize recommendation consistent with other health risks.
Blood pressure control Goal: ≤140/90 mm Hg	Initiate lifestyle modification—weight control, physical activity, alcohol moderation, and moderate sodium restriction—in all patients with blood pressure >140 mm Hg systolic or 90 mm Hg diastolic. Add blood-pressure medication, individualized to other patient requirements and characteristics (i.e., age, race, need for drugs with specific benefits) if blood pressure is >140 mm Hg systolic or 90 mm Hg diastolic in 3 months or if *initial* blood pressure is >160 mm Hg systolic or 100 mm Hg diastolic.

AHA, American Heart Association; ACE, angiotensin-converting enzyme; MI, myocardial infarction; TG, triglycerides; LV, left ventricular.
(From Smith SC, Blair SN, Criqui MH, et al. Preventing heart attack and death in patients with coronary disease. AHA, Medical Scientific Statement. Consensus Panel Statement. Circulation 1995;92:2–4, with permission.)

Medical Therapy

Aspirin permanently inhibits platelet cyclooxygenase, resulting in suppression of the biosynthesis of platelet thromboxane A_2, which induces platelet aggregation. Aspirin may also have a beneficial anti-inflammatory effect that results in plaque stabilization. Aspirin, particularly at high doses, may limit the salutary effects of ACE inhibitors in patients with CAD and heart failure. In stable angina, aspirin lowers the risk of MI and sudden death and should be used in all patients at a daily dose of 81 to 324 mg, unless contraindicated.

Clopidogrel, a new thienopyridine, and ticlopidine also block the adenosine diphosphate (ADP) activation of platelets by selectively and irreversibly inhibiting the binding of ADP to its platelet receptor. Both agents can be used instead of aspirin. Clopidogrel may be superior to aspirin in decreasing the combined risk of ischemic stroke, MI, and vascular death. The dose of clopidogrel is 75 mg once a day, and that of ticlopidine is 250 mg twice

| TABLE 72.7. | EFFECT OF STATINS ON CARDIOVASCULAR (CV) EVENT REDUCTION AND LDL-CHOLESTEROL LEVELS |

Clinical Trial	Active Treatment	Dosage (mg/d)	Study Sample Size)	Baseline LDL-C Levels (mmol/L)[a]	% Reduction of LDL-C	On-treatment LDL-C (mmol/L)[a]	CHD Event Reduction (%)[b]
LIPID	Pravastatin	40	9,014	3.89	25	2.92	23
AFCAPS/TexCAPS	Lovastatin	20–40	6,605	3.69	25	2.96	24
PLAC I	Pravastatin	20–40	408	4.24	26	3.13	60
Multinational	Pravastatin	20	1,062	4.71	26	3.47	92
WOSCOPS	Pravastatin	40	6,595	4.97	26	3.67	31
PLAC II	Pravastatin	20–40	151	4.29	27	3.10	60
ACAPS (± warfarin)	Lovastatin	20–40	919	4.06	28	2.92	64 (pooled analysis)
REGRESS	Pravastatin	40	885	4.32	28	3.03	42
CARE	Pravastatin	40	4,159	3.59	28	2.59	24
CCAIT	Lovastatin	40–80	331	4.47	29	3.26	25
KAPS	Pravastatin	40	447	4.89	29	3.39	62
MAAS	Simvastatin	20	381	4.40	31	3.00	24
4S	Simvastatin	20–40	4,444	4.67	34	3.15	34
MARS	Lovastatin	80	270	3.90	38	2.40	24
Post-CABG (± warfarin)	Lovastatin	80	1,351	4.02	60	2.41	12[d]

LDL, low-density lipoprotein; LDL-C, low density lipoprotein cholesterol; LIPID, Long-term Intervention with Pravastatin in Ischemic Disease; AFCAPS/TexCAPS, Air Force/Texas Coronary Atherosclerosis Prevention Study; PLAC I, Pravastatin Limitation of Atherosclerosis in the Coronary Arteries; Multinational, Pravastatin Multinational Study Group for Cardiac Risk Patients; WOSCOPS, West of Scotland Coronary Prevention Study; PLAC II, Pravastatin, Lipids, and Atherosclerosis in the Carotid Arteries; ACAPS, Asymptomatic Carotid Artery Progression Study; REGRESS, Regression Growth Evaluation Statin Study; CARE, Cholesterol and Recurrent Events; CCAIT, Canadian Coronary Atherosclerosis Intervention Trial; KAPS, Kuopio Atherosclerosis Prevention Study; MAAS, Multicentre Anti-atheroma Study; 4S, Scandinavian Simvastatin Survival Study; MARS, Monitored Atherosclerosis Regression Study; Post-CABG, Post Coronary Artery Bypass Graft Trial.
[a] To convert LDL-C values from millimoles per liter to milligrams per deciliter, divide values given by 0.02586.
[b] Coronary heart disease (CHD) events include those coronary outcomes specified in the clinical trial and may include death from CHD, nonfatal myocardial infarction, coronary artery bypass grafting, and percutaneous transluminal coronary angioplasty.
[c] The results are reported for patients randomized to aggressive lovastatin therapy (80 mg) with or without warfarin versus moderate treatment with lovastatin (2.5 mg) with or without warfarin.
[d] Fatal and nonfatal myocardial infarctions.
(From Rosenson RS, Tangney CC. Antiatherothrombotic properties of statins: implications for cardiovascular event reduction. *JAMA* 1998;279:1643–1650, with permission.)

a day. There are no known interactions between these two agents and ACE inhibitors.

Nitrate preparations are potent systemic venous and coronary arterial vasodilators. The paradoxic constriction of atherosclerotic coronary arteries in response to exercise or mental stress, related to endothelial dysfunction and decreased levels of EDRF, can be abolished by nitroglycerin. Nitrates also lower systemic blood pressure and myocardial oxygen demand and inhibit platelet aggregation.

To abort an angina attack, sublingual nitroglycerin or nitroglycerin spray (average dose, 0.4 mg) is the most effective preparation. Nitroglycerin may also be taken prophylactically before activities that typically produce angina. Several long-acting nitrate preparations are available in the form of tablets, topical ointments, and transdermal patches, but these preparations are ineffective in treating an acute angina attack. Tolerance develops rapidly to long-acting nitrate preparations, manifested by the diminished effectiveness of a particular dose and the need for higher doses to maintain efficacy. Intermittent nitroglycerin therapy, consisting of 8- to 12-hour nitrate-free intervals, can be effective in preventing tolerance. Hydralazine, ACE inhibitors, vitamin E, and carvedilol may lessen tolerance to nitrate therapy. Long-acting nitrates may improve exercise tolerance and curb the frequency and severity of angina. There is no evidence, however, that nitrate preparations prevent MI or improve survival.

Nitrate administration is associated with increased production of superoxide anion and the vasopressor hormone endothelin. Intermittent therapy with nitroglycerin may be associated with rebound myocardial ischemia or infarction and heightened sensitivity to endothelin during nitrate-free periods. The most common side effects of nitroglycerin preparations are headaches and dizziness. Dizziness is usually caused by hypotension and can be corrected by assuming a supine position. Patients with critical aortic stenosis or obstructive hypertrophic cardiomyopathy should avoid nitrate preparations. Administration of sildenafil (Viagra) is contraindicated in patients taking nitrates, since the vasodilatory actions are profoundly amplified, resulting in severe hypotension and a potentially fatal event.

The dose of nitrates that prevents angina varies from patient to patient. In general, one should start with a relatively low dose and increase the dose until ischemia is prevented or side effects develop. One of the most common long-acting preparations is isosorbide dinitrate, but 70% to 80% of the oral dose is degraded by its first pass through the liver. In contrast, isosorbide 5-mononitrate, an active metabolite of dinitrate with similar antianginal properties when given orally, is 95% bioavailable because it has a negligible first-pass extraction. Nitroglycerin patches vary in effectiveness among patients, with unpredictable absorption into the systemic circulation.

The β-adrenergic blocking agents are among the most important therapies for CAD. These drugs diminish the frequency of angina attacks and improve exercise tolerance. Although they are well tolerated, such side effects as fatigue and weakness, nightmares, depression, bronchoconstriction, sexual dysfunction, and memory loss can occur. The β-blocking agents differ in their β-receptor selectivity, intrinsic sympathomimetic activity, lipid solubility, and associated β-adrenoreceptor blocking activity. Nonselective β-blockers include propranolol and timolol. Cardioselective β_1-receptor blocking agents (metoprolol) cause less bronchoconstriction and vasoconstriction, but this selectivity is lost when therapeutic doses are used. Some β-blockers (pindolol) have intrinsic sympathomimetic activity, producing low-grade β-simulation at rest and a β-adrenergic blocking effect during exercise. Lipid-insoluble β-blockers (atenolol) are less likely to cross the blood–brain barrier, causing fewer central nervous system side effects. Other β-blockers (labetalol, carvedilol) have vasodilatory properties through a β_2-agonist effect, an α-adrenergic blocking effect, and a direct vasodilatory effect. They are useful in patients with stable angina who have hypertension or are in heart failure.

Although therapy with β-blockers may increase triglyceride and decrease HDL levels, there is no evidence that they cause progression of atherosclerosis; on the contrary, they substantially limit the rate of reinfarction and mortality in patients recovering from acute MI. They are generally well tolerated but are contraindicated in patients with asthma, atrioventricular conduction defects, profound bradycardia, tachy-brady syndrome, severe hypotension, peripheral artery disease, Raynaud's phenomenon, and pheochromocytoma. They should not be used with monoamine oxidase inhibitors, as the unopposed β effect may result in severe hypertension. They should be administered with extreme caution to patients with severe heart failure. Nonetheless, patients with conditions that are often considered contraindications to β-blockade, such as heart failure or pulmonary disease, or older patients, appear to benefit significantly from β-blocker therapy. In particular, post-MI patients with a history of heart failure or left ventricular dysfunction appear to derive the major benefit from β-blockers. Although the potential exists for worsened heart failure in patients with systolic dysfunction, patients receiving ACE inhibitors, diuretics, and digoxin generally tolerate β-blockers well (in particular, extended-release metoprolol, carvedilol, and bisoprolol) when an initially low dose is used (e.g., 12.5 mg extended-release metoprolol once a day, 3.125 mg carvedilol twice a day, or 1 mg bisoprolol per day) followed by a careful, gradual increase in the dose. These agents appear to improve survival substantially in patients with systolic heart failure due to CAD who are already receiving ACE inhibitors.

Because there may be up-regulation of β-receptors during prolonged therapy with β-adrenergic blockers, they should not be discontinued abruptly in patients with ischemic heart disease; this may precipitate unstable angina or MI related to an increase in heart rate and blood pressure. These medications should be weaned gradually over several weeks, if possible. If withdrawal is necessary, strenuous exercise should be avoided, and, if possible, the β-blocker should be replaced with verapamil or diltiazem to decrease heart rate and blood pressure. The β-blockers should be used with caution in patients receiving verapamil and diltiazem, since the combined effect may result in hypotension, bradycardia, and decreased cardiac contractility. ACE inhibitors, in particular ramapril, reduce the rate of death, MI, and stroke in high risk patients for cardiovascular events. This therapy should be strongly considered in patients with stable angina.

Calcium channel blockers (or calcium antagonists) inhibit the entry of calcium ions into the cells via the voltage-dependent L-type calcium channel, which is present in myocytes and vascular smooth-muscle cells. All calcium antagonists cause relaxation of vascular smooth muscle in the arterial and coronary circulation. The net effect on cardiac contractility is a complex interaction between the direct depression of contractility noted with all calcium channel blockers and the reflex sympathetic activation caused by their effect on vascular resistance. Calcium antagonists may lessen the frequency of angina and enhance exercise tolerance. Calcium antagonists are generally well tolerated, but they should be used with extreme caution, if at all, in patients with systolic heart failure, because they may worsen heart failure and increase mortality rates. The use of short-acting calcium antagonists, particularly dihydropyridines, has been associated with a higher risk of MI.

Dihydropyridines (amlodipine, felodipine, isradipine, nifedipine, nicardipine, nimodipine, nitrendipine, nisoldipine) have a predominant effect on the vascular system. Owing to the powerful vasodilatory properties of therapeutic doses, these agents may amplify adrenergic nervous system activity, particularly the short-acting preparations. As a result, these agents usually produce no appreciable slowing of sinoatrial or atrioventricular conduction and may actually increase heart rate and cardiac output. The elevation in heart rate increases myocardial oxygen demand and may also diminish coronary blood flow by shortening the diastolic portion of the cardiac cycle, during which coronary perfusion occurs. Dihydropyridines also may accentuate the circadian variation of adrenergic tone that predisposes to plaque rupture. Thus, short-acting dihydropyridines, alone or in combination with nitrates, may be associated with an increase in anginal attacks or even unstable angina or MI. The intensification of adrenergic nervous system activity may be prevented by a β-blocker; in this context, the negative inotropic effects of the calcium antagonist may predominate. Amlodipine is safe when used for angina, even in patients with systolic dysfunction when it is added to an ACE inhibitor. This may be related to the fact that amlodipine does not enhance neuroendocrine activity (serum norepinephrine concentrations).

Diltiazem and verapamil have balanced myocardial, electrophysiologic, and vascular effects, resulting in a decline in heart rate, atrioventricular conduction, blood pressure, and, particularly with verapamil, cardiac contractility. Bepridil has complex pharmacologic properties, and, in addition to a calcium channel blocking effect, it also inhibits the sodium channel. This may result in prolongation of the QT interval and, occasionally, induction of ventricular tachycardia (torsades de pointes). Bepridil, verapamil, and diltiazem should be avoided by patients with extensive first-degree atrioventricular block (more than 0.24 seconds), second- or third-degree atrioventricular block, tachy-

TABLE 72.8.	**MEDICAL THERAPY FOR STABLE ANGINA ASSOCIATED WITH OTHER MEDICAL CONDITIONS**				
				Calcium Channel Blockers	
Associated Condition	**ASA**	**Nitrates**	**β-Blockers**	**Dihydropyridines**	**Verapamil/Diltiazem**
Systolic heart failure	Yes	Yes	Yes[b]	No[c]	No
Diastolic heart failure	Yes	Yes	Yes	Yes[b]	Yes
Bradyarrhythmias	Yes	Yes	No	Yes	No
Hypertension	Yes	Yes	Yes	Yes	Yes
Aortic insufficiency	Yes	Yes	No	Yes	No
Chronic obstructive pulmonary disease[a]	Yes	Yes	No	Yes	Yes
Peripheral vascular insufficiency	Yes	Yes	Yes[b]	Yes	Yes
Severe mental depression	Yes	Yes	No	Yes	Yes[b]

ASA, aspirin.
[a] Requiring bronchodilators.
[b] Use with caution; may aggravate this condition.
[c] Amlodipine may be used.

brady syndrome, bradycardia, or atrial fibrillation with a slow ventricular response.

Other adverse effects of calcium antagonists include headache, dizziness, hypotension, ankle edema, and nausea. Some of these side effects are limited by the use of long-acting preparations. Constipation is a common complaint in patients receiving verapamil. Verapamil significantly increases the plasma levels of digoxin. Both verapamil and diltiazem raise the level of cyclosporine, and hence they should be used only with extreme caution in patients who have undergone organ transplant and are receiving immunosuppressive therapy. Therapy with β-blockers is preferred over calcium channel blockers in the treatment of stable angina. Patients with stable angina should consume a balanced diet with emphasis on antioxidant-rich fruits and vegetables and whole grains. The need for further supplementation with vitamins E, C, and beta-carotene remains to be determined by the ongoing studies. Medical therapy for stable angina pectoris in patients who have other common medical conditions is shown in Table 72.8.

Myocardial Revascularization

Percutaneous Coronary Revascularization

An estimated 482,000 percutaneous coronary revascularization (PCR) procedures were performed in 1996 in the United States. From 1987 to 1996, the number of procedures increased 211%. In 1996, 67% of PCR procedures were performed on men; 51% were performed on people under age 65. The average cost of PCR in 1995 was $20,370. In many laboratories stents are now used in more than 50% of cases. PCR is the nonsurgical treatment of a stenotic artery that results in dilatation of the coronary lumen by a balloon catheter and/or by another intracoronary device. Balloon angioplasty increases the size of the arterial lumen by disrupting the atherosclerotic plaque and stretching and tearing the media and adventitia. With intracoronary ultrasonographic imaging, arterial dissection is detected in 50% to 80% of patients undergoing this procedure.

Several other devices have been introduced, such as atherectomy catheters, laser catheters, and ablation catheters. Only intracoronary stents with postdeployment inflation and adjunctive therapy with aspirin and ticlopidine or clopidogrel have been proved to decrease angiographic and clinical re-stenosis compared with conventional balloon dilatation. Stenting also can be used for treatment of prolonged total occlusion and coronary vein graft disease. PCR is successful in 90% of patients who undergo this procedure, with success defined as an increase in luminal diameter of at least 20% and a final stenosis severity of less than 50% of the luminal diameter.

Complications develop in less than 5% of patients; they include death (0% to 2%), MI (3% to 5%), and the need for emergency CABG (3% to 7%). Abrupt vessel closure occurs in 2% to 8% of procedures, with an attendant mortality rate of 4% to 10%. Aspirin lowers the rate of abrupt closure when used the day before and the day of angioplasty. Inhibition of the platelet glycoprotein IIb/IIIa receptor, together with low-dose, weight-adjusted heparin, lessens the risk of acute ischemic complications in patients undergoing PCR (Table 72.9). Women and patients with unstable angina have a higher risk of abrupt closure. Angiographic characteristics associated with a high risk of abrupt closure include coronary thrombus, eccentric stenoses, calcified stenoses, stenoses more than 10 mm long, and diffusely diseased arteries. Abrupt closure may require emergency coronary bypass surgery, but now it is successfully managed with percutaneous devices, most notably intracoronary stents.

PCR is indicated in any patient with significant stenosis in a major epicardial artery whose angina does not respond to medical therapy or who has evidence of myocardial ischemia in the territory of the artery to be dilated. This recommendation applies to patients with single or multivessel CAD. PCR should not be performed in arteries with a stenosis of less than 50% and is not indicated in the left main coronary artery.

The main limitation of balloon angioplasty is coronary re-stenosis, which occurs in 30% to 50% of patients within the first 6 months after the procedure. The rate of re-stenosis is

TABLE 72.9.   **CLINICAL TRIALS OF GLYCOPROTEIN IIb/IIIa ANTAGONISTS IN CORONARY INTERVENTION: 30-DAY OUTCOMES**

Trial[b]	N	% All Events[a]		% Death + MI		% MI	
		Placebo	Drug	Placebo	Drug	Placebo	Drug
EPIC	2,099	12.8	8.3	10.3	6.9	8.6	5.2
CAPTURE	1,265	15.9	11.3	9.0	4.8	8.2	4.1
EPILOG	2,792	11.7	5.2	9.1	3.8	8.7	3.7
IMPACT II	4,010	11.6	9.1	8.6	6.9	8.3	6.6
RESTORE	2,141	10.5	8.0	6.4	5.0	5.7	4.2
Pooled	12,307	12.1	8.1	8.7	5.7	8.0	5.0

[a] In each trial, $p \leq 0.05$ (vs. placebo).
[b] EPIC, CAPTURE, and EPILOG data (abciximab) reflect intention-to-treat analyses and represent the primary study end point (all events = death, MI, or urgent/emergency second intervention or coronary bypass surgery). Data from IMPACT II (eptifibatide) and RESTORE (tirofiban) are derived data, calculated on a treated-patient basis and adjusted to reflect the primary end point used for abciximab trials. Both EPILOG and IMPACT II evaluated two treatment strategies against placebo; data for the best treatment comparison are shown. Pooled data are average results for each group weighted for number of patients in each trial.
(From Madan M, Berkowitz SD, Tcheng JE. Glycoprotein IIb/IIIa integrin blockade. *Circulation* 1998;98:2629–2635, with permission.)

much lower after intracoronary stents. Stenting also results in improved outcomes in patients who experience re-stenosis after conventional balloon dilation. Several factors are associated with an increased risk of re-stenosis. Clinical factors include male sex, cigarette smoking, unstable angina, diabetes mellitus, hypertension, hypercholesterolemia, end-stage renal disease, and vasospastic angina. An elevated lipoprotein(a) concentration is also a marker for an increased risk for re-stenosis. Procedural characteristics that predispose to re-stenosis include dilatation of proximal stenoses, saphenous vein grafts, persistently occluded arteries, and stenoses more than 10 mm long. Residual stenosis of more than 30%, a small residual lumen, and the use of an undersized balloon also predispose to re-stenosis. Not all patients who experience re-stenosis after successful balloon angioplasty have recurrent angina. Since re-stenosis is a relatively slow process, it rarely results in MI. The antioxidant agent probucol appears to be effective in lowering the rate of re-stenosis after balloon angioplasty. Stents and platelet glycoprotein IIb/IIIa receptor blocking agents lower the rate of re-stenosis.

Coronary Artery Bypass Graft Surgery

In the United States in 1996 an estimated 598,000 CABGs were performed on 367,000 patients. From 1979 to 1996 the number of procedures increased 424.6%, and the number of patients grew 227.7%. Segments of autologous saphenous vein have been used as conduits, but internal mammary artery grafts are being used more and more, since they have a higher long-term patency rate, particularly when used to bypass the left anterior descending artery. The 10-year patency rate of saphenous vein grafts is 50%; that of an internal mammary graft is about 90%. Endarterectomy is occasionally used in combination with CABG procedures. CABG has been shown to be highly effective in relieving angina and prolonging life. The perioperative mortality rate is usually less than 4%, and the perioperative MI rate has declined from 5% to 8% two decades ago to about 2.5% as methods of myocardial protection during surgery have improved. In patients with chronic CAD, factors associated with an increased risk of

perioperative death are age, female sex, severe left ventricular dysfunction, diabetes, and emergency surgery after failed PCR.

MI is uncommon in the first few years after CABG. The return of angina soon after surgery is related to either incomplete revascularization or early graft closure. Angina occurring very late is related to closure or narrowing of the bypass grafts or progression of atherosclerotic disease in the native vessels. Early use of platelet inhibitor therapy clearly prolongs graft patency. Aspirin should be used in the perioperative period, preferably before but not later than 48 hours after surgery. Usually, 81 to 324 mg of aspirin is an effective dose. Continued cigarette smoking is the most significant risk factor for early graft closure.

The main indication for CABG is relief of symptoms that are not responsive to medical therapy or PCR. Relative contraindications are the complete absence of viable myocardium in the areas supplied by a stenotic artery and coexisting severe noncardiac conditions with a poor prognosis. CABG improves survival in patients with left main disease, three-vessel disease, or two-vessel disease when one of the two vessels involved is a large left anterior descending coronary artery with severe proximal stenosis (Fig. 72.4). This benefit is particularly evident in patients who have left ventricular systolic dysfunction. Some reports suggest that the benefits of CABG on the beating heart, whether through full or limited access (minimally invasive CABG), result in lower mortality and morbidity rates and an earlier return to normal activities.

In selected patients with multivessel CAD, PCR and CABG show similar rates of death or MI and similar improvement in exercise capacity. Patients with diabetes who are on insulin or oral therapy have a significantly lower mortality rate with CABG than with PCR. Patients undergoing PCR are more likely to have persistent angina requiring antianginal medications and a greater need for additional revascularization procedures, including repeated PCR or CABG. For patients with disease of the left main coronary artery, multivessel disease affecting the proximal left anterior descending artery, or three-vessel disease and

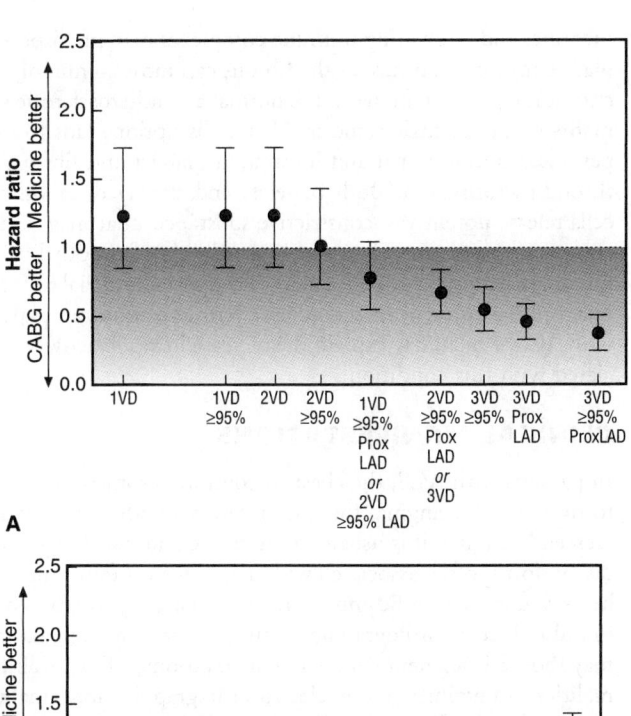

A

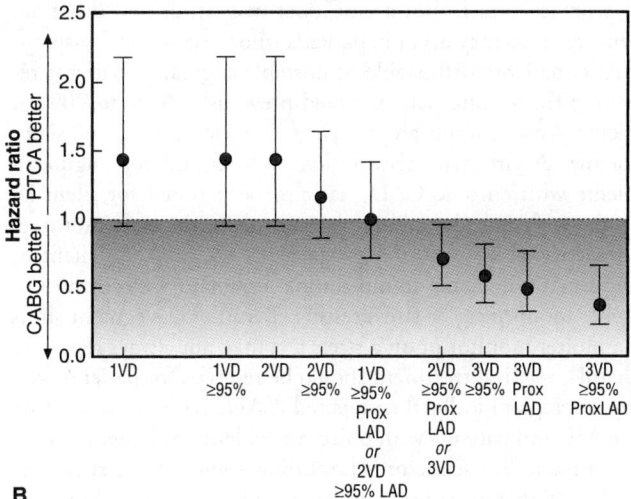

B

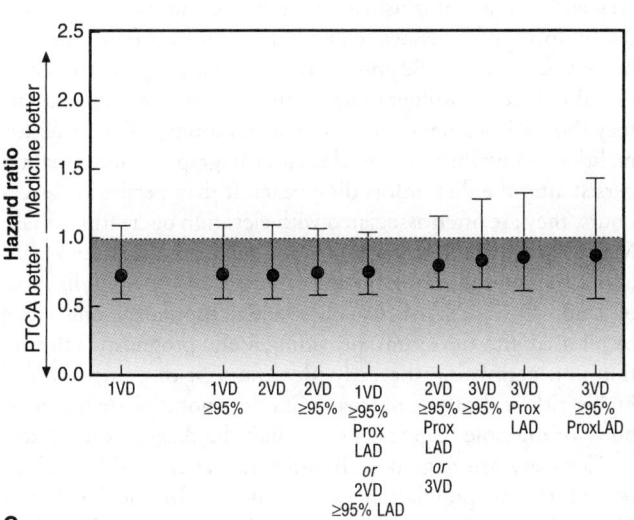

C

FIGURE 72.4. Hazard (mortality) ratios for coronary artery bypass surgery (CABG) versus medicine (**A**), for CABG versus percutaneous transluminal coronary angioplasty (PTCA) (**B**), and for PTCA versus medicine (**C**), calculated from the Cox regression model to evaluate relative survival differences. Points indicate hazard ratios for each level of the coronary artery disease index indicated on the horizontal axis. Bars indicate 99% confidence intervals. The horizontal line at a ratio of 1.0 indicates the point of prognostic equivalence between treatments. Hazard ratios above or below the line favor the treatment indicated. VD, vessel disease; Prox LAD, proximal left anterior descending coronary artery. (From Mark DB, Nelson CL, Califf RM, et al. Continuing evolution of therapy for coronary artery disease: initial results from the era of coronary angioplasty. *Circulation* 1994;89:2015–2025, with permission.)

impaired left ventricular systolic function, CABG is preferred over PCR (see Fig. 72.4).

Angiogenesis

Angiogenesis is an investigational therapy for inducing the growth of new blood vessels. Angiogenic growth factors include vascular endothelial growth factor (VEGF) and fibroblast growth factor. VEGF is a naturally occurring angiogenic peptide that exists in four isoforms. This peptide may stimulate endothelial cell growth, proliferation, and migration. Both recombinant VEGF protein and VEGF gene therapy have produced angiogenesis in animal models. Encouraging results were obtained in patients who were not ideal candidates for coronary revascularization and who received escalating doses of intracoronary recombinant human VEGF. Similar results were obtained with intramuscular injection of the naked DNA coding for VEGF. Although the initial experience with angiogenic growth factors is promising, conclusions are limited by the preliminary nature of the clinical data, including the small number of patients, short follow-up times, and lack of controls.

Transmyocardial Laser Revascularization

Transmyocardial laser revascularization may be used as adjunct therapy for patients with ischemic heart disease who are not suitable candidates for PCR or CABG. This technique uses a carbon dioxide laser to create transmyocardial channels for direct perfusion of the ischemic heart in patients with angina. There is a significant decline in the frequency of angina episodes and the number of hospital admissions for angina after this procedure. The reason for this symptomatic improvement is the subject of uncertainty and controversy, however, since data establishing an improvement after transmyocardial laser revascularization are quite limited.

◼ SILENT ISCHEMIA

Silent ischemia is myocardial ischemia associated with electrocardiographic or hemodynamic abnormalities not accompanied by chest pain or chest discomfort or other anginal symptoms, such as dyspnea. The electrocardiographic and hemodynamic changes during painless episodes are identical to those associated with symptomatic attacks but are of lesser magnitude and duration. Silent ischemia may occur in patients who are completely asymptomatic, patients with stable or unstable angina, or patients recovering from acute MI. As noted previously, 60% to 70% of patients with chronic angina pectoris have episodes of silent ischemia. A circadian distribution, as is found for angina in patients with chronic CAD, has also been noted for silent ischemia, with episodes taking place mostly in the early morning. In patients with CAD, the prognosis is the same for silent or symptomatic ischemia found during ambulatory electrocardiographic monitoring or stress testing. Because ST-segment shifts on a Holter monitor or on a stress test may not always represent ischemia, medical treatment should be reserved for patients who have angiographically documented CAD, patients recovering from MI, and patients with objective evidence of ischemia, such as positive radionuclide or echocardiographic stress test results.

Medical therapy consists of the use of nitrates and β-blockers. If these agents do not suppress or significantly lessen the ischemic episodes, calcium channel blockers should be added. The β-blockers are superior to calcium channel blockers in abolishing silent ischemia, and among the calcium channel blockers, the nondihydropyridines, such as diltiazem, are more effective than the dihydropyridines, such as nifedipine. Revascularization should be considered in patients with silent ischemia who have severe CAD, especially those with left ventricular dysfunction or inducible ischemia on exercise testing.

ACUTE CORONARY SYNDROME

Acute coronary syndrome (ACS) is a clinical syndrome characterized by an increase in the intensity or frequency of angina episodes and is associated with an increased risk of MI and cardiac death. Several scenarios fulfill this broad definition of the syndrome, including a single episode of prolonged rest angina (at least 20 minutes), the new onset of angina (less than 2 months), and acceleration of angina (an angina pattern that becomes more frequent, longer in duration, or lower in threshold). Variant angina, non-Q-wave MI, and postinfarction angina (more than 24 hours) are considered part of the spectrum of ACS. The diagnosis of unstable angina and non-Q-wave MI are usually considered together because they cannot be distinguished clinically or angiographically. In 1990, there were 850,000 new hospitalizations in the United States for this condition, the most common cardiovascular cause for hospital admission.

PATHOPHYSIOLOGY

ACS appearing in the form of prolonged chest pain at rest often results from fissuring or rupturing of the atherosclerotic plaque, leading to thrombus formation. Plaques that are prone to rupture are often insignificant in angiographic features and not flow limiting, and they contain large amounts of extracellular cholesterol covered by a thin cap of fibrotic tissue. The immediate site of plaque rupture is usually marked by an inflammatory process (macrophage-rich areas), suggesting that inflammation plays a role in destabilizing the fibrous cap tissue. Hyperlipidemia, high angiotensin levels, elevated acetoacetic acid levels (as in diabetes),

nicotine, and circulating immune complexes may predispose to plaque rupture. Rupture of the fibrous cap most commonly occurs at the junction between the normal and atherosclerotic segments of an eccentric stenosis. Plaque disruption leads to brief periods of intraluminal and intramural platelet and fibrin-type thrombus formation. Both platelets and damaged endothelial cells release potent vasoconstrictive substances that may lead to coronary vasospasm. There are higher levels of endothelin-1, a potent vasoconstrictor peptide produced by endothelial cells and macrophages present in the atherosclerotic plaques, in patients with ACS, which may explain the increase in vasoreactivity associated with this condition.

CLINICAL MANIFESTATIONS

In patients with ACS, the chest discomfort is somewhat similar to that of stable angina, though in patients with rest angina or crescendo angina, it is usually more severe and lasts longer. The discomfort is often associated with diaphoresis, a fourth or third heart sound, a systolic murmur, and even a dyskinetic apical impulse. Electrocardiographic findings during an angina attack may show ST-segment depression or elevation or T-wave abnormalities; sometimes these electrocardiographic abnormalities persist after the discomfort disappears. If they persist for several hours, they are often associated with elevation of creatine kinase-MB. When there is a typical rise and fall of the creatine kinase-MB level without development of new Q waves, the diagnosis of a non-Q-wave MI is usually made. Troponin T and I may be released into the serum, providing useful prognostic information and permitting the early identification of patients with a higher risk of death. A normal ECG does not exclude the possibility of unstable angina, but it makes the diagnosis less likely.

Coronary arteriographic findings in patients with ACS are related to the population being studied. In the TIMI-IIIB (Thrombosis in Myocardial Ischemia) study, about 5% of patients had left main disease, 15% had three-vessel disease, 30% had two-vessel disease, and 35% had one-vessel disease; 15% had no significant CAD. In contrast, in the Veterans Administration study of unstable angina, 47% had three-vessel, 35% had two-vessel, and 18% had one-vessel disease. Although the extent of coronary stenoses in unstable angina and stable angina appears to be similar, the morphologic features of plaque differ; there are more eccentric lesions with more irregular or hazy borders in patients with unstable angina, suggestive of disrupted atherosclerotic plaques with thrombus formation. Up to 40% of patients studied early after the onset of rest angina have angiographic evidence of coronary thrombi.

NATURAL HISTORY AND PROGNOSIS

Earlier studies reported an infarction rate of 20% to 40% within 3 months of the onset of ACS. In the Veterans Administration studies of unstable angina, the 10-year cumulative mortality was 38% for patients treated medically and 39% for those treated surgically. At present, since patients are initially treated aggressively with β-blockers, nitrates, aspirin, heparin, and glycoprotein IIb/IIIa receptor antagonists and high-risk patients are identified and undergo revascularization, the outcome has improved considerably.

TABLE 72.10.	LIKELIHOOD OF SIGNIFICANT CORONARY ARTERY DISEASE IN PATIENTS WITH SYMPTOMS SUGGESTING UNSTABLE ANGINA		
	High Likelihood	**Intermediate Likelihood**	**Low Likelihood**
	Any of the following features	Absence of high-likelihood features and any of the following	Absence of high- or intermediate-likelihood features but may have
	History of myocardial infarction or sudden death or other known history of coronary heart disease	Definite angina: males <60 or females <70 years of age	Chest pain classified as probably not angina
	Definite angina: males ≥60 or females >70 years of age	Probable angina: males ≥60 or females ≥70 years of age	One risk factor other than diabetes
	Transient hemodynamic or electrocardiographic changes during pain	Chest pain probably not angina in patients with diabetes	T-wave flattening or inversion <1 mm in leads with dominant R waves
	Variant angina (pain with reversible ST-segment elevation)	Chest pain probably not angina and two or three risk factors other than diabetes[a]	Normal electrocardiogram
	ST-segment elevation or depression ≥1 mm	Extracardiac vascular disease	
	Marked symmetric T-wave inversion in multiple precordial leads	ST depression 0.05–1 mm	
		T-wave inversion ≥1 mm in leads with dominant R waves	

[a] Coronary artery disease risk factors include diabetes, smoking, hypertension, and elevated cholesterol.
(From Agency for Health Care Policy and Research Clinical Practice Guidelines. Unstable angina: diagnosis and management. U.S. Department of Health and Human Services Publication no. 94-0602, 1994, with permission.)

EVALUATION AND MANAGEMENT

Patients with suspected ACS should be evaluated initially in a medical facility. The ECG should be obtained during the course of chest discomfort and after its relief. According to the US Agency for Health Care Policy Research, it is important in evaluating patients with chest pain to assess both the likelihood of CAD (Table 72.10) and the likelihood of adverse outcomes (Table 72.11). Elevated troponin I predicts a higher mortality in ACS patients. On the basis of this first evaluation, the patient should be assigned to one of four categories: non-CAD, stable angina, acute MI, or unstable angina. Patients who are judged in the initial evaluation and treatment phase to be at low risk of experiencing adverse outcomes can be evaluated further as outpatients. The follow-up evaluation of these patients should generally occur within 72 hours of their first evaluation. Therapy should consist of aspirin (81 to 324 mg per day), sublingual nitroglycerin as needed, oral β-blockers, and long-acting topical or oral nitrates (Table 72.9). Aspirin lowers the risk of MI by 71%. Ticlopidine and clopidogrel are also acceptable therapy for secondary prevention in patients who cannot tolerate aspirin.

TABLE 72.11.	SHORT-TERM RISK OF DEATH OR NONFATAL MYOCARDIAL INFARCTION IN PATIENTS WITH UNSTABLE ANGINA		
	High Risk	**Intermediate Risk**	**Low Risk**
	At least one of the following features must be present	No high-risk features but must have any of the following	No high- or intermediate-risk features but may have any of the following features
	Prolonged ongoing (>20 min) rest pain	Prolonged (>20 min) rest angina, now resolved, with moderate or high likelihood of CAD	Increased angina frequency, severity, or duration
	Pulmonary edema, most likely related to ischemia	Rest angina (>20 min or relieved with rest or sublingual nitroglycerin)	Angina provoked at a lower threshold
	Angina at rest with dynamic ST changes ≥1 mm	Nocturnal angina	New-onset angina with onset 2 weeks to 2 months before presentation
	Angina with new or worsening MR murmur	Angina with dynamic T-wave changes	Normal or unchanged electrocardiogram
	Angina with S, or new/worstening rales	New-onset CCSC III or IV angina in the past 2 weeks with moderate or high likelihood of CAD	
	Angina with hypotension	Pathologic Q waves or resting ST depression ≤1 mm in multiple lead groups (anterior, inferior, lateral)	
		Age >65 years	

CAD, coronary heart disease; CCSC, Canadian Cardiovascular Society classification.
[a] Estimation of the short-term risks of death and nonfatal MI in unstable angina is a complex and multifaceted problem that cannot be fully specified in a table such as this. Therefore, the table is meant to offer general guidance and illustration rather than rigid algorithms.
(From Agency for Health Care Policy and Research Clinical Practice Guidelines. Unstable angina: diagnosis and management. U.S. Department of Health and Human Services Publication no. 94-0602, 1994, with permission.)

| TABLE 72.12. | CLINICAL TRIALS OF GLYCOPROTEIN IIb/IIIa ANTAGONISTS IN UNSTABLE ANGINA/NQWMI |

Trial	N	% All Events[a]		% Death + Myocardial Infarction (30 days)		% Relative Risk Reduction (30 days)
		Placebo	Drug	Placebo	Drug	
PRISM[b]	3,231	5.9	3.8[f]	7.1	5.8	18
PRISM-PLUS[c]	1,815	17.9	12.9[f]	11.9	8.7[f]	27
PARAGON[d]	2,282	11.7	10.6	11.7	10.6	9
PURSUIT[e]	10,498	15.7	14.2[f]	15.7	14.2[f]	10
Pooled	18,276	13.3	11.4	13.3	11.7	13

PRISM, Platelet Receptor Inhibition for Ischemic Syndrome Management; PRISM-PLUS, Platelet Receptor Inhibition for Ischemic Syndrome Management in Patients Limited by Very Unstable Signs and Symptoms; PARAGON, Platelet IIb/IIIa Antagonism for the Reduction of Acute Coronary Syndrome Events in a Global Organization Network; and PURSUIT, Platelet glycoprotein IIb/IIIa in Unstable angina: Receptor Suppression Using Integrilin Therapy.
[a] "All Events" represents primary end-point comparison in each trial.
[b] Tirofiban monotherapy: 0.6 g/kg/min for 30 min plus 47.5-hr infusion at 0.15 g/kg/min.
[c] Tirofiban (and i.v. heparin): 0.4 g/kg/min for 30 min plus 47.5-hr infusion at 0.1 /kg/min.
[d] Lamifiban: 300-g bolus plus 72-hr infusion at 1.0 g/min.
[e] Eptifibatide: 180-g/kg bolus plus 72-hr infusion at 2.0 g/kg/min.
[f] $p < 0.05$ (vs. placebo).
(From Madan M, Berkowitz SD, Tcheng JE. Glycoprotein IIb/IIIa integrin blockade. *Circulation* 1998;98:2629–2635, with permission.)

Patients at high or intermediate risk of death or nonfatal MI should be admitted to an intensive or intermediate care unit and have serial cardiac enzyme measurements and ECGs to exclude the possibility of acute MI. These patients should be treated with aspirin, intravenous heparin or low-molecular-weight heparin, glycoprotein IIb/IIIa antagonists (Table 72.12), nitrates, and β-blockers (see Table 72.13). Calcium channel blockers should be reserved for patients with hypertension; those with refractory ischemia despite the use of aspirin, heparin, nitrates, and β-blockers; and those with variant angina. Dihydropyridines should not be used as monotherapy. Intravenous thrombolytic therapy is not indicated in patients with ACS unless they have symptoms of prolonged rest pain and elevation of the ST segments in two consecutive leads or a left bundle-branch block.

Patients who continue to have ischemia despite medical therapy and patients whose angina is controlled but who have ischemia on stress testing, left ventricular dysfunction (ejection fraction less than 0.50), or malignant ventricular dysrhythmias should undergo coronary angiography. Patients found to have significant left main stenosis, three-vessel disease, or two-vessel disease with severe stenosis of the proximal left anterior descending artery should undergo CABG, especially if there is associated left ventricular dysfunction. The treatment of the remaining patients with two-vessel disease or one-vessel disease remains the subject of controversy. Patients with inducible ischemia after an episode of unstable angina, especially those with left anterior descending coronary stenosis, are usually candidates for revascularization with PCR or CABG.

▪ VARIANT ANGINA PECTORIS

Variant angina pectoris (or Prinzmetal's angina) is a clinical syndrome of angina that usually occurs at rest and is associated with reversible ST-segment elevation without enzymatic evidence of acute MI. This syndrome is caused by coronary vasospasm, which can be prevented or reversed by nitroglycerin. The spasm may be segmental in nature or involve the entire artery. Although it can develop in patients with normal coronary arteries, most patients have angiographically significant atherosclerotic CAD. Patients with variant angina are at risk of MI and sudden death.

PATHOPHYSIOLOGY

Vasospasm usually happens at the site of, or in close proximity to, an atherosclerotic plaque. Even patients with variant angina who have normal-appearing coronary arteries on angiography have been found to have underlying atherosclerosis at autopsy. It is possible that the loss of endothelial vasodilator function contributes to the coronary vasospasm, in response to stimuli that normally lead to vasodilatation, such as exercise or mental stress, and lowers the threshold for arterial spasm in response to stimuli that promote vasoconstriction. Hyperventilation, exercise, cold exposure, handgrip, histamine, vasopressin, and platelet-mediated vasoactive substances (e.g., thromboxane) may induce vasospasm in patients with variant angina, as may exogenous vasoconstrictors, such as nicotine and cocaine. Hypercholesterolemia has also been implicated in vasospasm, since elevated cholesterol levels impair endothelial function and lower the threshold to ergonovine-induced vasospasm.

CLINICAL MANIFESTATIONS

Chest discomfort usually occurs at rest or during ordinary activities that are not associated with a substantial increase in cardiac work, and most ischemic episodes are not preceded by a rise in heart rate or blood pressure. Vasospasm occasionally can be produced by exercise. The location and radiation are similar to

TABLE 72.13. ACUTE MANAGEMENT OF ACUTE CORONARY SYNDROMES IN RELATION TO RISK OF MYOCARDIAL INFARCTION OR DEATH

	High Risk	Intermediate Risk	Low Risk
Treatment setting	ER → CCU	ER → ICCU, CCU, or ward	ER → Home
Electrocardiographic monitoring	≥48 hr	24–48 hr	ER only
Intravenous	Yes	Yes	No
Analgesic	i.v. narcotic	Usually none unless recurrence	None
Anti-ischemic			
Nitrate	SL; i.v. nitrates	SL; oral or topical	SL; oral or topical
β-blocker	i.v. or oral	Oral	Oral
β-blocker failure	Dihydropyridine added	Dihydropyridine added	Dihydropyridine added
β-blocker contraindicated	Diltiazem or verapamil	Diltiazem or verapamil	Diltiazem or verapamil
Antithrombotic/Antiplatelet			
ASA	Stat to chew, oral daily	Stat to chew, oral daily	Oral daily
ASA intolerance or allergy	Ticlopidine or clopidogrel	Ticlopidine or clopidogrel	Ticlopidine or clopidogrel
Heparin unfractionated	Bolus i.v. ≥48 hr	Bolus i.v., depending on severity/risk, ≥48 hr	No
LWMH	May be an alternative or preferable; use beyond 48–96 hr may increase efficacy	May be an alternative or preferable; use beyond 48–96 hr may increase efficacy	No
IIb/IIIa receptor inhibitors	May add value in medical management and with PCR as an adjunct to heparin and aspirin	Use with PCR	Possible value (oral agents under investigation)
Angiography and revascularization	Should be performed	Reserve for recurrence of ischemia on optimal medical therapy or poor prognosis	Reserve for failure of optimal medical control

ER, emergency room; CCU, coronary care unit; ICCU, intermediate coronary care unit; SL, sublingual; PCR, percutaneous coronary revascularization; LWMH, low-wt molecular-weight heparin; ASA, aspirin.
(Adapted from Cairns J, Theroux P, Armstrong P, et al. Unstable angina: report from a Canadian expert round table. *Can J Cardiol* 1996;12:1279–1292.)

those of stable angina, but the duration is somewhat longer. The discomfort follows a circadian pattern, manifesting predominantly in the early morning. Variant angina is related to heavy cigarette smoking and also has been associated with migraine headaches and Raynaud's phenomenon. There also has been an association with aspirin-induced asthma. Even though variant angina by definition is associated with ST-segment elevation during an ischemic episode, coronary artery spasm can manifest initially as ST-segment depression or T-wave inversion. Ventricular tachycardia is common during prolonged episodes of ST-segment elevation, whether painful or silent.

DIAGNOSIS

The diagnosis is usually based on clinical features and verification of ST-segment elevation during an angina attack that normalizes with sublingual nitroglycerin. Ambulatory electrocardiographic monitoring and exercise testing occasionally can be useful in establishing ST-segment elevation. Because the coronary anatomy in patients with variant angina can vary, all patients with variant angina should undergo coronary arteriography. Intravenous or intracoronary administration of ergonovine is helpful in eliciting spasm in patients with normal coronary arteries or minor atherosclerotic changes. Ergonovine induces coronary vas-

ospasm in more than 90% of patients with variant angina; in contrast, fewer than 1% of patients with atypical chest pain and no CAD have ergonovine-induced vasospasm. A negative ergonovine test effectively rules out coronary spasm as a cause for angina. Ergonovine should be administered only in the cardiac catheterization laboratory.

MANAGEMENT

Medical Therapy

Nitrates and, in particular, calcium channel blockers are extremely effective in preventing coronary artery spasm. Despite an initially positive response, however, patients ultimately may not respond to a single calcium channel blocker. In patients with symptoms refractory to one agent, administration of two calcium channel blockers may be more effective, such as a dihydropyridine combined with diltiazem or verapamil. There may be a rebound of symptoms when therapy with calcium channel blockers or nitrates is abruptly discontinued. β-blockers should not be used in patients with variant angina and normal coronary arteries since blockade of the β2-receptor allows α-receptor-mediated coronary artery vasoconstriction to manifest. In patients with CAD verified by angiography, however, β-blockers can be beneficial. High doses of aspirin should be avoided, since they can increase the severity of vasospasm by decreasing the biosynthesis of prostaglandin I_2.

Myocardial Revascularization

The indications for revascularization in variant angina are the same as in chronic CAD. CABG should be considered for patients with variant angina and significant multivessel atherosclerotic CAD. Bypass surgery is clearly not useful in patients who do not have significant flow-limiting coronary artery stenoses. Patients with single-vessel disease and variant angina refractory to medical management can be successfully treated with PCR, but the re-stenosis rate is higher than in patients with stable angina. Patients should be continued on calcium channel blockers after PCR.

BIBLIOGRAPHY

ACC expert consensus document on coronary artery stents: document of the American College of Cardiology 1. *J Am Coll Cardiol* 1998;32: 1471–1482.

Braunwald E. Shattuck lecture. Cardiovascular medicine at the turn of the millennium: triumphs, concerns, and opportunities. *N Engl J Med* 1997; 337:1360–1369.

Braunwald E, Jones RH, Mark DB, et al. Diagnosing and managing unstable angina. *Circulation* 1994;90:613.

Bypass Angioplasty Revascularization Investigation (BARI) Investigators. Comparison of coronary bypass surgery with angioplasty in patients with multivessel disease. *N Engl J Med* 1996;335:217–225.

Drexler H. Endothelial dysfunction: clinical implications. *Prog Cardiovasc Dis* 1997;4:287–324.

Emond M, Mock MB, Davis KB, et al. Long-term survival of medically treated patients in Coronary Artery Surgery Study. *Circulation* 1994; 90:2645–2657.

Falk E, Shah PK, Fuster V. Coronary plaque disruption. *Circulation* 1995; 92:657–671.

FRagmin and Fast Revascularisation during InStability in Coronary artery disease (FRISC II) Investigators. Invasive compared with non-invasive treatment in unstable coronary-artery disease: FRISC II prospective randomized multicentre study. *Lancet* 1999;354:708–715.

Frazier OH, March RJ, Horvath KA. Transmyocardial revascularization with a carbon dioxide laser in patients with end-stage coronary artery disease. *N Engl J Med* 1999;341:1021–1028.

Gheorghiade M, Bonow RO. Chronic heart failure in the United States: a manifestation of coronary artery disease. *Circulation* 1998;97:282–289.

The Heart Outcomes Prevention Evaluation Study Investigators. Effects of an angiotensin-converting inhibitor, ramipril, on death from cardiovascular causes, myocardial infarction, and stroke in high-risk patients. *N Engl J Med* 2000;342:145–153.

Henry TD. Can we really grow new blood vessels? *Lancet* 1998;351: 1826–1827.

Hollander JE. The management of cocaine-associated myocardial ischemia. *N Engl J Med* 1995;333:1267–1272.

Hulley S, Grady D, Bush T, et al. Randomized trial of estrogen and progestin for secondary prevention of coronary heart disease in postmenopausal women. Heart and Estrogen/Progestin Replacement Study (HERS) Research Group. *JAMA* 1998;280:605–613.

Kullo IJ, Edwards WD, Schwartz RS. Vulnerable plaque: pathobiology and clinical implications. *Ann Intern Med* 1998;129:1050–1060.

Levin GN, Keaney JF, Vita JA. Cholesterol reduction in cardiovascular disease: clinical benefits and possible mechanisms. *N Engl J Med* 1995; 332:512.

Madan M, Berkowitz SD, Tcheng JE. Glycoprotein IIb/IIIa integrin blockade. *Circulation* 1998;98:2629–2635.

Parker JD, Parker JO. Nitrate therapy for stable angina pectoris. *N Engl J Med* 1998;338:520–531.

A Report of the American College of Cardiology/American Heart Association Task Force on Practice Guidelines (Committee on Management of Patients with Chronic Stable Angina). ACC/AHA/ACP-ASIM Guidelines for the management of patients with chronic stable angina. *J Am Coll Cardiol* 1999;33:2092–2190.

Rosenson RS, Tangney CC. Antiatherothrombotic properties of statins: implications for cardiovascular event reduction. *JAMA* 1998;279: 1643–1650.

Ross R. Atherosclerosis: an inflammatory disease. *N Engl J Med* 1999;340: 115–126.

Theroux P, Fuster V. Acute coronary syndromes: unstable angina and non-Q wave myocardial infarction. *Circulation* 1998;97:1195–1206.

Topol EJ, Serruys PW. Frontiers in interventional cardiology. *Circulation* 1998;98:1802–1820.

Weitz JI. Low molecular-weight heparins. *N Engl J Med* 1997;337: 688–698.

Kelley's Textbook of Internal Medicine, fourth edition. Edited by H. David Humes. Lippincott Williams & Wilkins, Philadelphia © 2000.

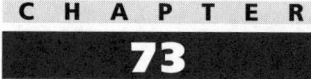

C H A P T E R

73

ACUTE MYOCARDIAL INFARCTION

ROBERT ROBERTS

PATHOGENESIS

Several pivotal observations have significantly altered the diagnosis and treatment of patients with acute myocardial infarction (MI):

1. Acute MI is almost always associated with a thrombus superimposed on significant coronary atherosclerosis.

2. MI is a regional disease limited to the vascular territory of one of the three major vessels or their branches.

3. Q-wave and non-Q-wave infarctions have distinct natural histories. Patients recovering from a Q-wave infarction have a high-risk period of 6 to 12 weeks, followed by a low mortality rate in subsequent years. Patients with Q-wave infarction undergoing early reperfusion (thrombolysis on percutaneous transluminal coronary angioplasty, or PTCA) have the highest risk in the first 24 to 72 hours. In contrast, non-Q-wave infarction has an initially low mortality rate, followed by a prolonged high-risk period of 1 to 2 years; after this interval, the accumulated mortality rate is similar to that of Q-wave infarction.

4. More than half the patients with a first episode of MI (about one-third of the total population) have significant obstructive

atherosclerosis in only one vessel, emphasizing the potential for a second ischemic event.

5. Based on direct experimental and indirect clinical evidence, irreversible injury requires at least 15 to 20 minutes of ischemia.

6. Myocardial necrosis stemming from ischemia begins in the subendocardium and spreads to the epicardium. If the coronary occlusion is complete and sustained, depending on the collateral blood supply, 50% to 90% of the involved myocardium distal to the lesion undergoes ischemia and, subsequently, necrosis, requiring 4 to 6 hours.

7. The evolution of myocardial necrosis is influenced by factors that alter myocardial oxygen supply and demand. Although decreasing demand may limit infarct size, it now appears that increasing supply via coronary perfusion is more effective.

8. Studies indicate that acute MI, at least Q-wave infarction, is more likely to be initiated in the morning (4 a.m. until noon), which corresponds to the time of diminished adrenergic activity, increased plasma fibrinogen levels, and enhanced platelet adhesiveness. The potential causative role of these factors remains to be elucidated.

9. Right ventricular infarction, once considered rare, is now known to occur in conjunction with left ventricular damage in most patients with inferior infarction.

CLASSIFICATION

Traditionally, patients who manifest a Q wave on the electrocardiogram (ECG) have been referred to as having transmural infarction, implying that the pathologic injury extends from the endocardium to the epicardial surface. Subendocardial or nontransmural infarction indicates that injury is restricted to the subendocardium and is associated with electrocardiographic changes limited to the ST-T segments. Because the correlation between electrocardiographic findings and postmortem morphologic findings is often poor, electrocardiographic classification into Q-wave (transmural) and non-Q-wave infarction (subendocardial) is recommended.

CLINICAL FEATURES

The predominant initial symptom is chest discomfort, frequently referred to as discomfort, tightness, or difficulty in breathing rather than pain. Cardiac pain typically radiates to the arm and neck and, less often, to the jaw. Occasionally, the pain starts in the wrist, elbow, or shoulder, or rarely as a toothache, and radiates to the chest. The most consistent feature of chest pain is the retrosternal component. Pain originating or radiating below the rib cage is rare, and pain restricted to the left inframammary region is seldom cardiac in nature. Chest pain associated with infarction is usually not relieved by nitroglycerin. Nausea and vomiting may accompany chest pain, particularly in association with inferior infarction. Esophageal pain is virtually identical to cardiac pain and may also be relieved by nitroglycerin, albeit not immediately, as is often the case with angina.

TABLE 73.1.	PHYSICAL FINDINGS OF ACUTE MYOCARDIAL INFARCTION

Inspection
  Lying with head raised
  Difficulty breathing
  Facial perspiration
  Anxiety
  Ashen look
  Clenched-fist syndrome
  HR ↑–↓
  BP ↑–↓
  Usually PVCs
  a waves in JVP with PVCs
  Kussmaul's sign with inferior acute myocardial infarction
Patient in left lateral position
  Observe dyskinesis
  Palpate prolonged systole
  Palpate dyskinesis
  Palpate atrial contraction
Auscultation
  S_1 and S_2 ↓
  Single S_2
  S_4 usually
  S_3: 10–20%
  Transient systolic murmur
  Pericardial rub

HR, heart rate; BP, blood pressure; JVP, jugular venous pressure; PVC, premature ventricular contractions.

The duration of the pain, its character, and its distribution are extremely unreliable characteristics in differentiating reversible and irreversible injury: fewer than one-third of patients admitted to the coronary care unit are subsequently found to have acute MI.

On physical examination (Table 73.1), one should pay careful attention to the physical appearance, the jugular venous pulses, palpation of the arterial pulses and precordium, and auscultation of the precordium. The patient should be examined in the supine and left lateral decubitus positions. The typical patient is usually anxious, with an ashen or pale face beaded with perspiration, and has the sensation of difficulty in breathing, so that he or she usually lies still with the head propped up on pillows. The patient with severe chest pain may clench the fist and motion toward the sternum, the so-called Levine sign. The patient's appearance, posture, and gestures are in large part dictated by the severity and duration of the chest pain.

The peripheral arterial pulse is often normal, although the rate initially may be slower than normal (60% of patients with inferior infarction in the initial hours) and gradually increase over the next few hours, or it may be faster, as it often is with extensive anterior infarction. Persistent sinus tachycardia beyond the initial 24 hours carries a very high mortality rate. The blood pressure is usually normal, but it may be high as the result of anxiety or low from cardiac failure. Patients with inferior infarction may show signs of bradycardia and hypotension stemming from the so-called von Bejold–Jarisch reflex. Most patients with inferior infarction have concomitant right and left ventricular injury, which can manifest as increased jugular venous pressure, an accentuated A wave, or lack of a decline in venous pressure on inspiration (Kussmaul's sign) owing to the diminished compliance of the right ventricle. The jugular venous pressure may be elevated owing to right ventricular or biventricular failure. About 60% to 70% of patients with inferior infarction in the initial hours show no decrease in jugular venous pulsation on normal inspiration as the result of concomitant right ventricular involvement, despite the absence of right-sided failure.

Depending on the severity, MI may have no discernible effect, may induce an area that is hypokinetic or akinetic, or may actually bulge in the opposite direction during systolic contraction. Within 24 hours of onset of infarction, one can usually palpate an abnormality of the precordial pulsations in patients in the left lateral decubitus position—either lack of a point of maximal impulse or the presence of diffuse contraction. In about 30% to 40% of the patients, atrial contraction is palpable.

The intensity of the first heart sound may be diminished because of decreased contractility. A fourth sound is heard in practically all patients (and, in fact, in many normal persons over age 45). A third heart sound (S_3) is heard in about 20% to 30% of patients, reflecting some degree of left ventricular dysfunction; this may be the only manifestation of cardiac decompensation. In cases of extensive damage, the second heart sound may be single; however, a paradoxical split is rare and reflects severe ventricular decompensation. The presence of a systolic murmur from papillary muscle dysfunction is found at least transiently in most patients in the first 24 hours of acute MI. The pericardial friction rub does not develop as a rule until about 48 to 72 hours. In patients with Q-wave infarction, it is said that if one listens frequently, a transient pericardial rub is heard in most patients; otherwise, it is heard in about 10%.

Patients who have experienced an infarction may show symptoms of worsening cardiac failure. The predominant clinical picture may be one of pulmonary edema, ventricular tachycardia, atrial fibrillation, shock, stroke, pulmonary embolus, heart block, fever, or syncope. Various conditions simulate acute MI, notably acute pulmonary embolus, acute pericarditis, dissecting aortic aneurysm, esophagitis, hiatal hernia, cholecystitis, pancreatitis, and spontaneous pneumothorax.

DIAGNOSIS

ELECTROCARDIOGRAPHIC DIAGNOSIS

The findings on the ECG of acute ischemia or infarction are discussed in Chapter 84. In fewer than half of patients with MI, serial analysis by electrocardiography shows a characteristic profile of ST-segment elevation followed by the development of new Q waves. The rest of the patients may have only minor changes or marked changes consisting of ST-T-segment elevation or depression. When the changes are restricted to the ST-T segment, confirmation by enzymatic and radiographic assessment is essential, since these changes also are associated with ischemia without irreversible injury. In patients with previous MI and residual Q waves or left bundle-branch block, the development of new Q waves may be masked; thus, an electrocardiographic diagnosis becomes more difficult (see Chapter 84).

On the basis of the ECG, patients are divided into those with Q-wave and those with non-Q-wave infarction. In patients with posterior infarction, the more specific manifestation is that of a large R wave in V_1 that is equal to or exceeds that of the S wave, together with new ST changes. In the case of lateral infarction, often the only manifestation is ST-segment depression in the lateral leads; Q waves develop in less than 30% of patients. In patients with inferior infarction who have concomitant right ventricular involvement, one should perform right precordial leads; ST-segment elevation present in these leads is highly suggestive of right ventricular infarction, but otherwise it is difficult to diagnose right ventricular infarction from the ECG. Atrial infarction is suspected if there is an elevation or depression of the PQ segment; changes in the morphologic features of the P wave; or atrial dysrhythmias, such as frequent premature apical beats, atrial flutter, or fibrillation.

DIAGNOSTIC BIOCHEMICAL MARKERS FOR THE EARLY AND LATE DIAGNOSIS OF MYOCARDIAL INFARCTION

More than five million patients with chest pain are seen in emergency clinics throughout the United States annually, but only about 10% of these individuals have suffered acute MI, and about 20% have unstable angina. More than 30% of these individuals have pain of noncardiac origin, and the remainder have pain of cardiac origin with or without ischemia. A major difficulty lies in distinguishing cardiac ischemia from MI, since the history and physical examination are seldom helpful in this regard and the ECG provides a positive specific diagnosis in only about 5% of patients with chest pain (40% of patients with acute MI). This difficulty often results in a large number of patients being admitted unnecessarily to the hospital for exclusion of infarction, such that it is estimated that more than $12 billion is spent in unnecessary admissions. This situation is reflected in the observation that more than 50% of patients admitted with the diagnosis of unstable angina are being discharged within 12 to 24 hours with a noncardiac diagnosis.

The importance of making a diagnosis within hours of arrival in the emergency room is also emphasized by the need for early thrombolytic therapy, which has a mortality of 1% when given immediately compared with 10% when given 6 hours from onset of symptoms. Furthermore, it was shown in the Thrombolysis in Myocardial Infarction (TIMI-III) trial that there was an increased incidence of MI and death among patients with unstable angina who received thrombolytic therapy, compared with the incidence with conventional therapy. The use of glycoprotein IIb/IIIa inhibitors in unstable angina, as opposed to thrombolytic therapy, also emphasizes the need for markers that can differentiate irreversible cardiac injury from the injury of ischemia. Thus, the necessity for early and more appropriate therapy coupled with cost-effective use of resources has underscored the importance of early diagnosis in the emergency room. For the past two decades the diagnostic biochemical marker relied on primarily has been plasma total creatine kinase-MB (CK-MB). While CK-MB has high sensitivity and specificity relative to other conventional markers (lactate dehydrogenase and aspartate aminotransferase), it is not an early marker, since exclusion of infarction may require up to 12 hours from onset of symptoms.

It must be emphasized that in the emergency room a test specific for infarction will be negative 90% of the time, since 90% of patients have not had MIs. The only markers that offer the potential sensitivity and specificity for early diagnosis within the first 6 hours from onset of symptoms are myoglobin and CK-MB subforms. The newly introduced biochemical markers troponin T and troponin I are highly sensitive and specific for MI, but similarly to total CK-MB, they do not increase above normal levels to exclude MI reliably with 90% confidence until about 14 to 16 hours from the onset of symptoms. This delay stems from the fact that only a small amount is released in the early hours. In contrast, myoglobin with a molecular weight of only 17,000 is released rapidly and reaches significant levels above the normal range within 2 to 3 hours. Upon release into the circulation, the tissue isoenzyme CK-MB is acted on by the enzyme carboxypeptidase B, which cleaves the terminal lysine from the MM subunit, resulting in a more negatively charged molecule. This generates two plasma subforms of CK-MB, one referred to as MB-2 (the unmodified tissue form newly released from the tissue) and the other as MB-1 (the modified form being more negative owing to loss of the positively charged terminal lysine), which are normally present in equilibrium in amounts of only one to two units of each subform per liter.

In the initial hours, only minute amounts of CK-MB (MB-2) are released into the circulation of patients with MI, such that exceeding the normal upper limit for total CK-MB in many patients may require 10 to 12 hours. Even the release of one to two units of MB-2, however, will drastically change the ratio from 1:1 to 2:1. Taking advantage of this early change in the ratio provides for a highly specific and early diagnosis of infarction. A prospective, multicenter, double-blind trial was performed in patients with initial symptoms of chest pain. Patients were enrolled consecutively, comparing the sensitivity and specificity of all of the markers for early (less than 6 hours from onset of symptoms) and late diagnosis (more than 6–8 hours) of infarction. The results are summarized in Table 73.2. The CK-MB subforms accurately detected 92% of the patients with infarction within 6 hours of onset and myoglobin detected 79%, with specificity for both markers of 90%. In contrast, total CK-MB and the cardiac troponins had sensitivities of only 75% and 60%, respectively.

Furthermore, it was shown that two samples, one taken on arrival at the emergency room and another 1 hour later, accurately diagnosed 91% of patients with infarction using CK-MB subforms; 78% of patients were diagnosed using myoglobin. Both assays are automated and require about 20 minutes to perform. It is recommended that a sample be obtained on admission and again at 1 hour and every 2 hours thereafter, if necessary, until 6 hours from onset of symptoms. If the plasma ratio of the CK-MB subform remains normal at 6 hours from onset of symptoms, MI can be excluded with a negative predictive value of 99%. Myoglobin analyzed and found to be normal at 6 hours from onset of symptoms has a reliability of 80%. It is also recommended that patients admitted to the hospital with the diagnosis of infarction should be tested every 6 to 8 hours for 24 hours to determine peak activity, to obtain baseline values

TABLE 73.2.	**DIAGNOSTIC SENSITIVITY AND SPECIFICITY OF MARKERS FOR MYOCARDIAL INFARCTION BASED ON A PROSPECTIVE, DOUBLE-BLIND, MULTICENTER TRIAL**						
	Time from Onset of Chest Pain (hr)						
	Early Diagnosis			**Late Diagnosis**			
Marker	**2**	**4**	**6**	**10**	**14**	**18**	**22**
CK-MB subforms							
Sensitivity (%)	21.1	46.4	91.5	96.2	90.6	80.9	53.1
Specificity (%)	90.5	88.9	89.0	90.2	90.0	89.9	92.2
Myoglobin							
Sensitivity (%)	26.3	42.9	78.7	86.5	62.3	57.5	42.9
Specificity (%)	87.3	89.4	89.4	90.2	88.3	88.8	91.3
Troponin T							
Sensitivity (%)	10.5	35.7	61.7	86.5	84.9	78.7	85.7
Specificity (%)	98.4	98.3	96.1	96.4	96.1	95.7	94.6
Troponin I							
Sensitivity (%)	15.8	35.7	57.5	92.3	90.6	95.7	89.8
Specificity (%)	96.8	94.2	94.3	94.6	92.2	93.4	94.2
Total CK-MB activity							
Sensitivity (%)	21.1	40.7	74.5	96.2	98.1	97.9	89.8
Specificity (%)	100.0	98.8	97.5	97.5	96.1	96.9	96.2
Total CK-MB mass							
Sensitivity (%)	15.8	39.3	66.0	90.4	90.5	95.7	95.7
Specificity (%)	99.2	98.8	100.0	99.6	98.9	99.6	99.1

CK-MB, creatine kinase-MB.

for patients undergoing such procedures as cardiac catheterization or PTCA, and to detect early reinfarction. The MB-2 subform returns to normal within about 24 hours and is the most sensitive marker for detection of early reinfarction. The total CK-MB level remains elevated for 72 to 96 hours, and troponin I and T levels remain high, on average, for about 10 days.

The conventional markers, namely, total CK-MB, troponin T, and troponin I, are reliable markers for diagnosis after 12 to 16 hours from onset of symptoms. If CK-MB subforms are used to make an early diagnosis, then the same assay can be used for late diagnosis, since total CK-MB activity can be derived from the subforms. If one chooses to use troponin I or troponin T for late diagnosis, it can be combined with the CK-MB subforms or myoglobin for early diagnosis. There is no advantage to assaying both troponin T and I, since they have a similar plasma temporal profile; troponin I is slightly more specific than troponin T.

The plasma total level of the CK-MB isoenzyme of CK, as assessed by quantitative techniques, is elevated within 6 to 10 hours of onset of infarction and peaks between 12 and 28 hours, with return to normal levels after 72 to 96 hours (Fig. 73.1). Troponin T and troponin I are contractile proteins with a molecular weight of 37,000 and 23,000, respectively. The troponins are released within 6 to 10 hours of onset of infarction, similarly to total CK-MB, and peak at 24 to 36 hours, returning to normal levels within 10 to 12 days. CK has been shown in the conscious canine model to be released only if myocardial necrosis occurs. CK-MB and CK-MB subforms have been shown not to be released in patients with known coronary artery disease (documented on coronary angiograms) during exercise-induced ischemia (documented on thallium scans). It remains to be determined whether troponin T or troponin I is released in the context of myocardial ischemia without necrosis; it is highly unlikely, since these are structural proteins of the sarcomere.

In patients with unstable angina, manifesting as clinical symptoms of pain at rest or increased frequency or severity of angina, total CK-MB activity was elevated in 7%, troponin T

in 13%, myoglobin in 18%, troponin I in 20%, and CK-MB subforms in 27% (Zimmerman et al., 1999). The upper limit of normal for total CK-MB is 7 ng per milliliter, for troponin I is 1.5 ng per milliliter, for troponin T is 0.1 ng per milliliter, and for myoglobin is 85 ng per milliliter. The diagnosis based on CK-MB subforms consists of MB-2 $\geq$2.6 IU per liter, with a ratio of MB-2 to MB-1 of $\geq$1.7 IU per liter. CK-MB and cardiac troponin T levels may be elevated owing to release from skeletal muscle and as the result of musculoskeletal disorders, while cardiac troponin I appears to be highly specific for cardiac injury. False elevations of CK-MB and cardiac troponin T may be observed in patients with renal failure, but these markers will not increase and then decrease, as observed with myocardial injury. Cardiac troponin I is not elevated in patients with renal failure.

MI after noncardiac surgery is also determined reliably from serial analysis of plasma CK-MB, cardiac troponin T, and cardiac troponin I levels every 4 to 6 hours. Levels of other enzymes are markedly elevated as a result of tissue trauma, but these markers are quite specific to myocardial damage. In the context of cardiac surgery, the level of CK-MB, like those of other cardiac enzymes (lactate dehydrogenase, troponin T and I), is almost always elevated, owing to manipulation and involvement of the myocardium; thus, it is not a reliable diagnostic test for infarction.

OTHER LABORATORY FEATURES

The blood glucose may become elevated in the latent diabetic and the electrolytes may be abnormal. Within 24 hours, significant leukocytosis develops, which persists for 7 to 10 days and often reaches levels of 10,000 to 15,000 per milliliter. The sedimentation rate characteristically increases after the first 48 hours.

■ TREATMENT

In the United States in 1997, about 1.5 million persons experienced MI; one-third died, 350,000 of them outside the hospital within 1 to 2 hours of onset of symptoms. Hospitalization of patients in the cardiac care unit has now become routine. Under constant electrocardiographic monitoring and with highly trained medical and nursing personnel, the treatment of dysrhythmias in the cardiac care unit has lowered the mortality rate from MI to 10% to 15%. Most deaths are due to pump failure from destruction of myocardium; thus, the next phase in the approach to therapy was limitation of infarct size, which has been initiated with early reperfusion induced by thrombolytic therapy and, more recently, by primary PTCA. The application of thrombolytic therapy has lowered the in-hospital mortality rate to 6%. The highly vulnerable period for ventricular fibrillation and ventricular tachycardia associated with MI is over after about 36 to 48 hours, so patients are often moved from the cardiac care unit after 2 or 3 days. Patients without complications are generally discharged after about 5 to 8 days.

INITIAL ASSESSMENT

In the initial assessment, the vital signs are checked, and an intravenous infusion is begun. Lidocaine is administered if ven-

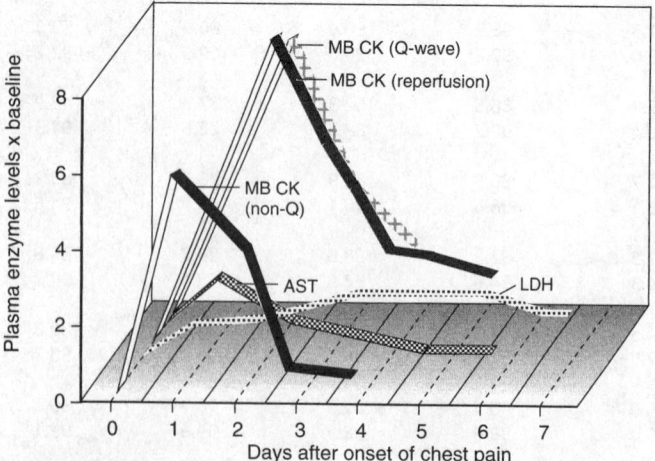

FIGURE 73.1. Typical plasma profiles for the MB isoenzyme of creatine kinase (MB CK), aspartate amino transferase (AST), and lactate dehydrogenase (LDH) activities after onset of acute myocardial infarction.

TABLE 73.3.	INITIAL ASSESSMENT OF ACUTE MYOCARDIAL INFARCTION

Vital signs
Electrocardiograms
Establish I.V. access
Determine if candidate for thrombolytic therapy

TABLE 73.4.	EFFECT OF STREPTOKINASE ON ACUTE MORTALITY

Time from Onset (hr)	Reduction in Mortality (%)	p Value
<1	47	0.0001
<3	23	0.0005
3–6	17	0.03
6–9	11	NS

NS, not significant.

tricular dysrhythmias are present, oxygen is given, and pain is relieved with morphine. An ECG is obtained, and the patient usually is connected to some form of continuous electrocardiographic monitoring (Table 73.3). Aspirin should be given immediately, and the patient should be assessed for thrombolysis and a thrombolytic agent administered within 30 minutes, if there are no contraindications.

ASSURANCE AND PAIN RELIEF

Morphine remains the drug of choice and is extremely effective. It should be given intravenously in small doses (2 to 4 mg), which can be repeated every 5 minutes until relief is obtained. Other analgesics, such as meperidine, may be substituted for morphine, but they tend to be less effective and are just as likely to produce side effects. Intravenous β-blockers are also safe and effective in the relief of pain with acute MI. If the patient is particularly emotionally disturbed, a mild tranquilizer should be given in addition to morphine to allay anxiety.

OXYGEN THERAPY

Hypoxemia often occurs in patients with acute MI, generally as the result of pulmonary edema. Traditionally, oxygen is given routinely via nasal prongs (2 to 4 L). In patients with severe pulmonary edema, it may be necessary to intubate and give oxygen under positive pressure. If the partial pressure of oxygen is normal, oxygen therapy should be discontinued. In patients with uncomplicated infarction, oxygen by nasal prongs is uncomfortable, expensive, and unnecessary.

THROMBOLYTIC THERAPY

Thrombolytic therapy with recombinant tissue-type plasminogen activator (rtPA), streptokinase, acylated plasminogen streptokinase activated complex (APSAC), or recombinant plasminogen activator (rPA) improves ventricular function and diminishes infarct size and mortality rates when administered within the initial 4 to 6 hours. The importance of early administration is shown in Table 73.4: the mortality rate is lessened by almost 50% in patients treated within the first hour, with no significant difference after 6 hours. Studies show some benefit even in patients treated up to 12 hours, but maximal benefit is derived from treatment within the initial 1 to 2 hours. In 60% to 70% of patients, the vessel will recanalize spontaneously after 5 to 10 days. Streptokinase restores coronary patency in about 50% to 60% of patients with acute MI; rtPA or rPA restores patency in about 70% to 80%. Patients undergoing thrombo-

lytic therapy should receive heparin and aspirin. Aspirin lowers mortality and reinfarction rates and is associated with minimal side effects. Heparin, in conjunction with rtPA, has a patency of 80%; with aspirin alone, it is only 52%.

In view of a reocclusion rate of 15% to 20% and a reinfarction rate of 5% to 10% after thrombolysis, there is concern as to whether cardiac catheterization should be performed immediately, followed by angioplasty in patients with appropriate anatomy. The role of conservative versus invasive strategies and immediate versus delayed angioplasty was assessed in several large trials. The TIMI-IIA trial showed that angioplasty performed within 2 hours of receiving rtPA was deleterious compared with angioplasty performed at 18 to 48 hours; similar results were observed in the Thrombolysis in Acute Myocardial Infarction trial and in the European trial. In the second part of the TIMI-II trial, patients were given rtPA within the initial 4 hours of onset of infarction, and half of them underwent cardiac catheterization at 18 to 48 hours, followed by angioplasty if the anatomy was appropriate; the other half were treated conservatively.

The mortality rate at 6 weeks was 4.7% in the conservatively treated group and 5% in the invasively treated group, and at 3 years the mortality rate was 11% in the conservatively treated group and 12% in the invasively treated group. In the conservative group, patients underwent cardiac catheterization for angioplasty or surgery only if there were recurrent ischemic events or if the patient exhibited ischemia on exercise. A similar trial— Should We Intervene Following Thrombolysis? (SWIFT)—in England showed virtually identical results. A newer trial referred to as Partial Angioplasty Combined with Thrombolysis (PACT), however, showed that thrombolysis induced by rtPA followed by angioplasty was associated with minimal bleeding and lower mortality rates than rtPA alone. Further studies are required to confirm these results before PTCA is adopted as routine treatment following thrombolysis.

The role of primary angioplasty has now been assessed in several trials and shown to be associated with a patency of more than 90%, which is consistently better than that of thrombolysis. If primary angioplasty can be performed within 45 minutes of the time the patient arrives at the hospital and if there are skilled surgeons experienced in angioplasty available, PTCA is an acceptable alternative to thrombolysis. In patients with contraindications, such as bleeding disorders, stroke, or hypertension, primary angioplasty is recommended over primary thrombolysis. For patients who have relative contraindications, such as elderly

TABLE 73.5.	INDICATIONS FOR THROMBOLYTIC THERAPY

Chest pain
Electrocardiogram ST ↑ or bundle-branch block
≤12 hr from onset
No contraindications

patients who have had a stroke but have no residual dysfunction, primary angioplasty is recommended. Angioplasty with or without thrombolytic therapy also is used often in patients in cardiogenic shock, but the benefit of this strategy remains to be determined. The long-term effect of angioplasty versus thrombolytic therapy on relief of symptoms and morbidity and mortality rates remains to be determined, particularly since about 30% to 50% of patients experience restenosis within 6 to 8 months after angioplasty. In patients receiving thrombolytic therapy in addition to aspirin and heparin in the TIMI-II trial, a β-blocker (metoprolol) was well tolerated when given on an emergency basis. In patients receiving it within 2 hours of thrombolytic therapy, as opposed to 7 days, there was no difference in ventricular function or mortality rates, but there was a lower incidence of reinfarction and ischemia. These results suggest that β-blockers should be used for immediate rather than delayed treatment.

Patients with chest pain who have ST-T-segment elevation or bundle-branch block and no contraindications are candidates for thrombolytic therapy, but patients with ST-T-segment depression or T-wave inversion are not (Table 73.5). Patients with a bleeding tendency, a previous stroke, hypertension, or peptic ulcer are excluded, as are patients who have undergone surgery in the past 6 weeks (Table 73.6). Age is not a contraindi-

cation. Should patients with non-Q-wave infarction receive thrombolytic therapy, considering that early reperfusion probably occurs spontaneously? In the International Study of Infarct Survival (ISIS)-II trial, a subset of patients with ST-segment depression who received streptokinase showed no benefit compared with placebo. The large prospective TIMI-IIIB trial indicated that patients with unstable angina with ST- or T-wave changes who received rtPA had higher mortality and infarction rates than those who underwent conventional therapy (aspirin and heparin). In patients with non-Q-wave infarction, there was no difference in the incidence of infarction or death compared with placebo.

In this study, thrombolytic therapy was initiated, on average, 9 hours from onset of symptoms. The lack of benefit of thrombolytic therapy in unstable angina is in keeping with the results of several other small trials. It indicates that a nonoccluding thrombus requires an antithrombin to prevent occlusion, whereas a thrombolytic agent increases the levels of plasma thrombin (released from the clot) and has other pro-coagulative effects that induce complete occlusion in some patients. The lack of effect of thrombolysis in patients with non-Q-wave infarction most likely is due to early spontaneous lysis; this precluded any benefit in the TIMI-IIIB trial, since therapy was initiated late (average of 9 hours from onset). Early thrombolytic therapy, such as therapy instituted before hospitalization, may be beneficial, but until such data are available, thrombolytic therapy is contraindicated in patients with chest pain who also have electrocardiographic changes other than ST-segment elevation or bundle-branch block (Fig. 73.2).

Thrombolytic therapy shows maximal benefit when administered in the first 2 to 3 hours after onset of symptoms, but significant benefit occurs when it is given up to 6 hours after onset. Some benefit is documented, particularly for rtPA, up to 12 hours, but there is no benefit after 12 hours. An accelerated dosing regimen of 100 mg rtPA over 90 minutes is recommended. A bolus of 15 mg is followed by an infusion of 50 mg in the next 30 minutes and 35 mg in the remaining 60 minutes. More accelerated dosing regimens are now being evaluated. Streptokinase should be administered as an intravenous infusion of 1.5 million units over 30 to 60 minutes. APSAC is given as

TABLE 73.6.	CONTRAINDICATIONS TO THROMBOLYTIC THERAPY

Absolute contraindications
  Active internal bleeding
  Suspected aortic dissection
  Recent head trauma or known intracranial neoplasm
  Recorded blood pressure >200/120 mm Hg
  Previous allergy to thrombolytic therapy (streptokinase or APSAC only)
  Pregnancy
  Hemorrhagic cerebrovascular accident within 3 mo
  Trauma or surgery within 2 wk
Relative contraindications
  Hemorrhagic retinopathy
  Trauma or surgery >2 wk
  Active peptic ulcer disease
  History of cerebrovascular accident
  Known bleeding diathesis
  Previous treatment with streptokinase/APSAC
  Menstruation
  Prolonged or traumatic CPR

APSAC, acylated plasminogen streptokinase activated complex; CRR, cardiopulmonary resuscitation.

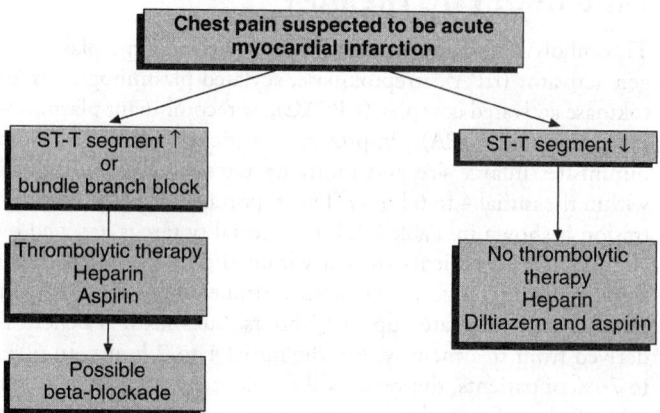

FIGURE 73.2. Algorithm for treatment of chest pain suspected to be acute myocardial infarction.

a bolus of 30 units over 5 minutes; rPA is given as an initial bolus of 15 microunits followed by a second bolus of 15 microunits in 30 minutes. This is followed by full heparinization to maintain the partial thromboplastin time at 1.5 to two times normal for 1 to 3 days. Aspirin also is given throughout this time, at 90 mg per day, followed by 90 to 325 mg per day indefinitely after discontinuation of heparin. Patients with recurrent ischemia or those who exhibit ischemia on stress testing before discharge should undergo cardiac catheterization for possible angioplasty or surgery.

CALCIUM CHANNEL BLOCKERS

Nifedipine and verapamil have been assessed in more than 10,000 patients, and results in unstable angina or acute infarction have shown that these agents are not effective in limiting infarct size or lowering the incidence of reinfarction or death. Diltiazem was shown to limit infarct size in only one study with a small sample size. Thus, the routine use of calcium channel blockers is not indicated for the limitation of infarct size. Nifedipine was shown to be ineffective in preventing reinfarction. Diltiazem was found to be efficacious in preventing reinfarction and death in patients recovering from non-Q-wave infarction and is recommended as a routine prophylactic agent in patients with non-Q-wave infarction (see the section on prophylaxis). Verapamil was shown to be capable of lessening reinfarction and death rates in patients after infarction. In unstable angina, nifedipine should be used only in combination with β-blockers.

NITROGLYCERIN

Studies assessing the effect of intravenous nitroglycerin on the limitation of infarct size are inadequate to derive any definitive conclusions, but all the studies to date have suggested a beneficial effect on infarct size. Two large randomized studies have been performed using nitroprusside: one showed a significant limitation of infarct size, but the other showed opposing results. Nitroprusside is contraindicated in the first 12 hours of acute MI. Neither nitroglycerin nor nitroprusside is recommended for limitation of infarct size; however, in patients with MI and cardiac failure who require a vasodilator, nitroglycerin is recommended over nitroprusside. Three large trials administering nitroglycerin after infarction found no survival benefit.

OTHER ADJUNCTIVE THERAPY

Two large trials recently completed indicate that magnesium was without benefit in the treatment of patients with acute MI. Magnesium was also assessed and found to have no effect on survival. Angiotensin-converting enzyme (ACE) inhibitors have been shown to prolong life in patients with left ventricular dysfunction or cardiac failure. Patients with an ejection fraction of 0.45 or less or those in clinical cardiac failure should routinely receive ACE inhibitors (see Chapter 90).

PHYSICAL ACTIVITY

Patients with uncomplicated infarction should be confined to bed for the first 24 hours, but during this time the patient may use a bedside commode. On the second day, the patient may be permitted out of bed for a total of 1 hour and on the third day for up to 2 hours. It is common practice to transfer the patient out of the cardiac care unit after about 3 days, providing he or she can be moved to a step-down unit or a regular cardiac ward where telemetry or some form of continuous dysrhythmia monitoring is available. By the fifth or sixth day, patients are permitted to ambulate in the room, and by the eighth or ninth day they are usually using the shower by themselves. Early use of a bedside commode often avoids the difficulty of constipation, which may cause straining and precipitate dysrhythmias. Patients are generally discharged at 8 to 10 days and are encouraged to walk daily at home for the next 3 to 6 weeks. They should be followed carefully and frequently by their physicians and typically can return to work in 6 weeks. Many patients engage in submaximal exercise before discharge, which restores confidence and provides information for further stratification. For further discussion of cardiac rehabilitation after MI, see Chapter 89.

DIET

A soft diet is recommended for the first 2 days. The customary suggestion of a diet low in cholesterol, saturated fat, and caffeine during the first 2 to 3 days is probably without scientific basis and should not be routinely applied. Patients are usually given a stool softener to prevent constipation and straining.

TREATMENT OF DYSRHYTHMIAS

For specific examples of the dysrhythmias discussed in this section and discussion of the drugs used, see Chapters 76 and 90.

Ventricular Dysrhythmias

Although the incidence of ventricular tachycardia or fibrillation has been minimized both during transport of the patient and within the hospital, more than 300,000 patients die before reaching the hospital, presumably as the result of dysrhythmias; this is largely because they cannot be reached in time for treatment.

The most effective first-line therapy for the treatment of premature ventricular contractions and prevention of ventricular tachycardia and fibrillation is intravenous lidocaine. In smaller hospitals, where the nursing personnel may be less experienced with MI or where there is no 24-hour coverage by house staff, prophylactic lidocaine may be appropriate. In patients receiving thrombolytic therapy, lidocaine is given consistently as prophylaxis before thrombolytic therapy. In hospitals with a well-trained and experienced cardiac care unit staff, lidocaine should be administered when any of the following types of dysrhythmia appear: five or more isolated ectopic ventricular beats per minute, multifocal ventricular extrasystoles, ventricular beats superimposed on the T wave, or runs of three or more ectopic ventricular beats. Intravenous lidocaine should be given in a bolus of 1 mg per kilogram, followed by an infusion of 2 to 4 mg per minute. Ventricular dysrhythmias, whether they are isolated premature ventricular contractions or runs of ventricular tachycardia, usually subside by 36 to 48 hours. If ventricular ectopy increases with the infusion, an additional bolus of lidocaine can be given.

Patients who experience sustained ventricular tachycardia unresponsive to lidocaine should undergo prompt electrical defibrillation. Patients who have ventricular fibrillation should undergo immediate electroconversion, as should patients with ventricular tachycardia and hemodynamic deterioration. If ventricular fibrillation cannot be immediately cardioverted, it may be necessary to initiate cardiac resuscitation for improved oxygenation before attempting further electroconversion. If ventricular tachycardia or fibrillation persists or recurs despite the use of lidocaine and electrocardioversion, a second antiarrhythmic agent must be added. An effective agent is procainamide, given intravenously in a bolus of 1 to 2 mg per kilogram over 5 to 10 minutes, followed by an intravenous infusion of 20 to 80 mg per kilogram per minute. If this treatment is ineffective, lidocaine is continued, and other agents may be substituted for procainamide (see also Chapter 90). In the case of premature ventricular beats associated with hemodynamic compromise that persists despite lidocaine, procainamide or β-blockade should be considered. In treating dysrhythmias, the physician must also remain cognizant of possible associated hypoxemia, electrolyte imbalance, acidosis, or hypokalemia and hypomagnesemia.

For ventricular fibrillation resistant to repeated electroshock, lidocaine, or other dysrhythmics, bretylium tosylate, 5 mg per kilogram, can be administered intravenously and repeated every 10 to 20 minutes if necessary. If this treatment is effective, an intravenous infusion can be initiated at a rate of 2 mg per minute. If the dysrhythmia continues to recur, electroshock is often more effective after a bretylium bolus. Resistant ventricular fibrillation sometimes can be rendered more susceptible to cardioversion by administering epinephrine, which often converts the fine ventricular fibrillation to a more coarse pattern, which is then more responsive to drugs and electroshock.

Supraventricular Dysrhythmias

The common supraventricular dysrhythmias—sinus tachycardia or bradycardia, atrial ectopic beats, flutter, or fibrillation—seldom require treatment in and of themselves in the acute phase of MI. If sinus tachycardia, which occurs in 20% to 30% of patients, is due to ventricular failure, treatment of the underlying failure is indicated. In patients with persistent sinus tachycardia with minimal myocardial damage and normal hemodynamics, intravenous β-blockade should be initiated. If the tachycardia persists, it may precipitate cardiac failure or more severe dysrhythmias or ischemia. Sinus bradycardia, if it is not associated with hypotension or other symptoms, should not be treated.

Conduction Disturbances

Ischemic injury during MI can induce disturbances in the conduction system at three different levels: the atrioventricular node, the bundle of His, or the right or left bundle branches. The mechanisms of action and treatment are discussed in Chapter 76. First-degree heart block occurs in 5% to 10% of patients with MI and is generally due to disturbances in the conduction

system above the bundle of His. It should be watched carefully but in itself does not require treatment. Second-degree heart block is divided into two types, Mobitz type I (Wenckebach) and Mobitz type II. Of patients with acute MI who show signs of second-degree heart block, 90% have Mobitz type I block. The conduction disturbance is due to ischemia of the atrioventricular node. It is associated with a narrow QRS complex and commonly occurs in patients with inferior MI. It is usually transient and does not persist beyond about 96 hours. It may be intermittent and only rarely progresses to complete atrioventricular block.

Because the conduction disturbance is in the atrioventricular node, there is often a functional escape rhythm with a ventricular response of 60 to 80 beats per minute. If the rate is less than 60 beats per minute or there are symptoms, a transvenous pacemaker is indicated, with the rate set to maintain adequate cardiac output. If complete atrioventricular block develops in this context, it usually progresses from first-degree to Mobitz type I and then to complete heart block in that sequence; it is usually transient and regresses within 5 to 7 days, in a reverse manner to the progression. A pacemaker is indicated in these patients with complete heart block. The mortality rate of complete heart block with inferior infarction is about 25% to 30%, and it remains doubtful whether mortality rates are lowered by a pacemaker. Nonetheless, a pacemaker may relieve the symptoms of cardiac failure. Complete heart block with inferior MI is seldom permanent.

Mobitz type II second-degree heart block is rare, occurring in less than 1% of patients with MI. It is due to a defect below the bundle of His in the fascicles and is almost always associated with anterior infarction and a wide QRS complex. It often progresses to complete atrioventricular block. The mortality rate is 80% to 90% with or without a pacemaker, though a pacemaker is always indicated in the case of Mobitz type II and with complete heart block.

Intraventricular conduction disturbances occur in the right bundle or the anterior or posterior divisions of the left bundle in up to 5% of patients with acute MI. There is no evidence that a pacemaker is helpful for intraventricular conduction defects, but it is generally agreed that patients with existing right bundle-branch block in whom either anterior or posterior fascicular block develops or bilateral bundle-branch block occurs anew (i.e., right bundle-branch block with left anterior or posterior divisional block or alternating right and left bundle-branch block) should have a temporary transvenous pacemaker put in place (see also Chapter 76). The development of concomitant first-degree atrioventricular block adds further risk to these conduction disturbances and should also be considered as an indication for a transvenous pacemaker. It has been suggested that patients surviving acute MI who had bundle-branch block and experienced transient second- or third-degree heart block during infarction should have permanent pacemakers. In one study of such patients, a pacemaker was associated with a decline in the rate of sudden death.

INDICATIONS FOR HEMODYNAMIC MONITORING

Swan-Ganz catheters are probably indicated in less than 10% of patients with MI and remain a somewhat arbitrary choice.

Nevertheless, when there is doubt about the fluid status or if a patient is not responding as expected, one should consider Swan-Ganz catheterization. The following indications serve only as guidelines: cardiogenic shock, hypotension, acute MI during or subsequent to surgery, cardiac failure unresponsive to therapy, persistent sinus tachycardia, vasodilator therapy in patients with systolic blood pressure of less than 120 mm Hg, severe lung disease and suspected left ventricular failure, right ventricular failure from suspected or proven right ventricular infarction, development of mitral regurgitation or ventricular septal defect, or cardiac failure but with unexplained coma, restlessness, hypoxia, acidosis, or oliguria. An intra-arterial catheter for continuous measurement of systemic arterial pressure seldom is used today. The automatic sphygmomanometer devices that periodically estimate blood pressure and transmit the results to a central station often are adequate. In cases of severe hypotension and vasoconstriction, the cuff pressure may be 5% to 10% lower than that of an arterial catheter, but one is primarily interested in the change in pressure, which is correctly reflected by the cuff or automatic devices.

COMPLICATIONS

POSTINFARCTION ANGINA

The complications of acute MI are common and varied (Table 73.7). Chest pain associated with acute MI usually subsides within 12 to 24 hours. Persistent or recurrent pain beyond 24 to 48 hours of onset is an important prognostic symptom reflecting the presence of viable myocardium that is undergoing ischemia, and it indicates that the patient is at increased risk of recurring pain, reinfarction, and death, both immediately and in the long term. Chest pain is much more common after non-Q-wave infarction. In a prospective study of 576 patients with non-Q-wave infarction, the incidence was 43% in the initial 2 weeks, and in two large retrospective studies it was 46% and 50%, respectively. Thus, the incidence of angina after non-Q-wave infarction is 40% to 50% during the 2-week hospital stay, compared with only about 10% to 15% after Q-wave infarction. The incidence of early reinfarction and death in patients with postinfarction angina is three- to fourfold greater than in patients without angina.

Many studies have shown that more than 90% of patients

with postinfarction angina and electrocardiographic changes exhibit multivessel disease on coronary angiography. About 10% have left main disease. Patients should be stabilized with nitrates and diltiazem, after which they may undergo coronary angiography (see the section on postinfarction stratification and investigation). Patients whose condition is refractory to oral nitrates and diltiazem should receive a continuous infusion of nitroglycerin and, if necessary, β-blockers. If their condition remains refractory to medical therapy, coronary angiography should be performed in consideration of surgery or angioplasty. Patients admitted with non-Q-wave infarction without cardiac failure should be treated with diltiazem, 240 to 360 mg per day, in addition to nitrates. Results of a prospective double-blind trial in patients with non-Q-wave infarction showed that diltiazem lowered the incidence of reinfarction and refractory angina by 50%. This salutary effect of diltiazem was in addition to any benefit from nitrates or β-blockers.

EARLY REINFARCTION

The overall incidence of early reinfarction, confirmed by a secondary elevation in plasma CK-MB activity, is 10% to 15% in non-Q-wave infarction. The incidence of reinfarction after thrombolytic therapy is about 5% to 10%. The incidence after Q-wave infarction without thrombolytic therapy is estimated to be less than 5%. Recurrent postinfarction angina, particularly if it is associated with electrocardiographic changes, is highly predictive of reinfarction (see the preceding section on postinfarction angina). Patients recovering from non-Q-wave infarction should undergo routine plasma CK-MB analysis every 12 hours throughout their hospital stay. Patients recovering from Q-wave or non-Q-wave infarction who show signs of postinfarction angina should undergo CK-MB analysis serially every 12 hours for the remainder of the hospital stay. Early reinfarction is an indication for coronary angiography, preferably performed after the patient is stabilized.

An estimated 75% of patients who experience early reinfarction are recovering from non-Q-wave infarction, so early preventive therapy is recommended. In a prospective, double-blind study of 576 patients with non-Q-wave infarction, patients receiving diltiazem (360 mg per day) in combination with conventional therapy exhibited a 50% reduction in early reinfarction and severe angina compared with patients receiving only conventional therapy (80% received nitrates, and 60% were given β-blockers). A new long-term study shows that diltiazem is effective over a 4- to 5-year period in lowering mortality and reinfarction rates in patients with non-Q-wave infarction.

CARDIAC FAILURE

Cardiac failure associated with acute MI develops when 20% or more of the left ventricle is affected. It occurs transiently in 20% to 30% of patients. The decrease in ventricular function is in part reversible: most patients experiencing cardiac failure for the first time recover in 24 to 48 hours. The diminished contractility results in an increase in end-diastolic volume, which, together with decreased compliance from changes in the myocardium or the pericardium, contributes to increased diastolic pressure and

TABLE 73.7.	COMPLICATIONS OF ACUTE MYOCARDIAL INFARCTION

Postinfarction angina
Cardiac failure
Cardiogenic shock
Papillary muscle rupture
Ventricular septal rupture
Cardiac rupture
Pericarditis
Dressler's syndrome
Conduction disturbances
Arrhythmias

pulmonary congestion. In most cases, adrenergic stimulation compensates for the failure; this stimulation increases the heart rate and the force of contraction of the remaining nonischemic myocardium. Heart size remains normal, as does cardiac output (usually).

Because patients are usually normovolemic before the onset of infarction, the sudden development of cardiac failure and loss of fluid into the lungs are associated with decreased vascular volume and relative hypovolemia, which is partly compensated for by increased vascular resistance. Patients in the initial days of cardiac failure associated with acute MI do not retain significant salt and water. Thus, the loss of fluid into the lungs at the expense of vascular volume may precipitate hypotension, which could jeopardize coronary perfusion. Patients with acute MI, due to decreased compliance, are usually operating on the ascending limb of the Starling curve and thus require higher filling pressures to maintain adequate cardiac output. In patients with inferior infarction, particularly with significant right ventricular involvement, the administration of a diuretic may be catastrophic and may produce a condition that simulates cardiogenic shock.

In patients with inferior infarction and pulmonary edema, diuretics should be withheld until the fluid status is assessed. Placement of a Swan-Ganz catheter is indicated, to assess right ventricular function, particularly end-diastolic pressure. If there is hypovolemia, fluids should be administered; if the cardiac output does not rise, dobutamine is indicated. If the jugular venous pressure is elevated, indicating normal fluid states, diuretics and vasodilators should be avoided. If the patient is hypotensive, an intravenous inotropic agent, such as dobutamine (2 to 5 µg per kilogram per minute), should be given, using as an end point the heart rate, which should not be permitted to increase by more than 10%. Patients with mild failure, indicated by a third heart sound with or without basal rales without symptoms of dyspnea, need morphine for pain together with oxygen and the usual supportive measures. In patients with more significant rales who are experiencing hypoxemia or dyspnea, a vasodilator would be appropriate and would achieve the same result as a diuretic without the loss of vascular volume. The preferred vasodilator is intravenous nitroglycerin, initiated at 5 to 10 mg per minute and increased so that there is no more than a 10% decline in blood pressure or heart rate.

In patients whose blood pressure is borderline low and who are in moderate to severe failure, an inotropic agent should be initiated immediately without a vasodilator. Dobutamine is preferred, since it decreases the ventricular filling pressure and induces mild peripheral vasodilatation, which increases coronary flow. In contrast, dopamine does not lower the ventricular filling pressure and, in moderate to high doses, causes vasoconstriction and increased ventricular filling pressure. Dopamine may be combined with a vasodilator or with dobutamine. In patients who are in failure with hypotension or cardiogenic shock, therapy should be initiated with a vasoconstricting agent such as dopamine. If a diuretic is used in the treatment of cardiac failure, a low dose is recommended (e.g., 20 mg furosemide); if this dose is inadequate, a vasodilator or inotropic agent should be added (see Chapter 71).

Digitalis has minimal inotropic effects compared with catecholamines and a long half-life, and it achieves maximal effect after only a loading dose, preferably given over 24 hours. Because most episodes of failure are transient, the initial use of an agent that acts rapidly and has a short half-life is preferred; if failure persists, patients may be started on oral digoxin. Amrinone, another inotropic agent, is given intravenously as a loading dose of 1.5 mg per kilogram, followed by an infusion at 10 to 20 µg per kilogram per minute. Its onset of action is rapid, and its half-life is 1 to 2 hours in patients with cardiac failure. Amrinone, like dobutamine, increases contractility (although less so), lowers left ventricular filling pressure and systemic vascular resistance, and has minimal effect on systemic arterial pressure and heart rate.

CARDIOGENIC SHOCK

Cardiogenic shock occurs in 5% to 10% of inpatients with acute MI and is the most common cause of death. The mortality rate associated with cardiogenic shock is 80% to 100%; the only effective treatment is prevention. Postmortem studies show myocardial necrosis involving 40% or more of the ventricular mass, with areas of old and new infarction indicating previous episodes of infarction. Occasionally, patients with an initial MI may experience shock after an early extension of the infarct. It is rare for patients without histories of ischemic heart disease to experience cardiogenic shock within hours of their first admission. Despite this gloomy prognosis, some patients have reversible injury, and with support they may recover. Every step must be taken to attempt to maintain the systemic circulation until a definitive diagnosis is made and all treatable lesions are excluded.

Cardiogenic shock is a severe form of cardiac failure with manifestations of impaired perfusion of several organs (Table 73.8). Several clinical criteria have been proposed for the diagnosis. These factors are primary cardiac abnormality, a sustained drop in systolic blood pressure to less than 85 mm Hg, a ventricular filling pressure of 16 mm Hg or more, and peripheral organ involvement evidenced by two or more of the following manifestations: oliguria less than 20 mL per hour, impaired mentation or cold and clammy skin, or a cardiac index less than 1.5 L per minute per square meter. The patient is usually drowsy and restless and, in addition to the obvious findings of cardiac failure, has signs of tachycardia, tachypnea, and peripheral vasoconstriction. Hypovolemia, such as may occur with the use of diuretics or vasodilators, dehydration, or sustained ventricular or supraventricular dysrhythmias, must be excluded. Other causes of

TABLE 73.8.	**CRITERIA FOR CARDIOGENIC SHOCK**

Primary cardiac abnormality
BP ≤85 mm Hg
Ventricular filling pressure ≥16 mm Hg
Systemic involvement: oliguria, cold skin, cardiac index ≤1.5 L/
     min/m^2

BP, blood pressure.

shock to be excluded are right ventricular infarction, pulmonary embolus, and tamponade. Now and then, a patient may have hypotension and severe cardiac failure owing to the use of intravenous antiarrhythmic agents, such as procainamide or quinidine, in the context of moderate to severe left ventricular dysfunction.

If adequate oxygen cannot be given by nasal prongs, the patient must be intubated. Every effort must be made to restore the blood pressure. Vasodilators and drugs with a negative inotropic effect are discontinued, pain is relieved, and hemodynamics are monitored. Dopamine should be initiated as an intravenous infusion at a rate of 2 to 5 μg per kilogram per minute and increased as needed by increments of 2 μg per kilogram per minute up to 60 μg per kilogram per minute, if necessary. In monitoring the hemodynamic response, one must assess cardiac output, blood pressure, and overall organ perfusion, as reflected, for example, by urine output. An attempt should be made to improve perfusion with the least possible increase in heart rate. If blood pressure can be maintained at about 90 mm Hg, the use of dobutamine is preferred, since it tends to produce better myocardial perfusion with less of an increase in systemic vascular resistance. Moreover, by lowering pulmonary wedge pressure, it relieves the symptoms of pulmonary congestion. Dobutamine should be initiated as an intravenous infusion of 5 μg per kilogram per minute and increased by 1 to 5 μg per kilogram per minute up to 40 μg per kilogram per minute.

Because the basic defect in cardiogenic shock is impaired contractility, mechanical assist devices should be considered, such as the percutaneous aortic balloon. This device does not improve survival, but in the case of correctable lesions, it helps keep the patient alive until specific therapy for such lesions can be applied. It is particularly useful for patients with ventricular septal or papillary muscle rupture waiting to undergo surgery.

PAPILLARY MUSCLE RUPTURE

Rupture of the papillary muscle occurs now and then within 2 to 7 days after onset of infarction and is characterized by the sudden onset of pulmonary edema stemming from massive pulmonary hypertension and cardiogenic shock. An aggressive surgical approach is indicated, because if the effect of the rupture can be overcome, there is usually enough viable myocardium to allow the patient to survive.

The characteristic finding on auscultation is the new onset of a low-pitched holosystolic decrescendo murmur heard over the precordium with radiation to the axilla. There is often an S_3 as well as an S_4; if there is tachycardia, a summation gallop is present. The arterial pulse may show a brisk, rising upstroke, and, depending on the degree of left ventricular dysfunction, a hyperdynamic apical impulse may be present. Other features can include a giant a wave in the jugular venous pulse as a result of enhanced right atrial contraction from pulmonary hypertension together with a sustained right ventricular impulse along the left parasternal border. There may be wide splitting of S_2 from the shortening of the left ventricular ejection period, as most of the blood is ejected through the mitral valve. Simultaneous palpation with both hands detects the early systolic apical impulse and the late systolic parasternal impulse, which impart a rocking motion to the chest. Diffuse rales are usually evident on auscultation of the lungs.

Prompt recognition is important, and the diagnosis usually can be confirmed by the large v wave in the Swan-Ganz catheter tracing. If it is uncertain whether the patient has a ruptured papillary muscle or a ruptured ventricular septum, analysis of oxygen saturation can be performed with the Swan-Ganz catheter. If no step-up oxygenation from the pulmonary artery to the right atrium is found, this is evidence of a ruptured papillary muscle. In general, an attempt is made to stabilize and maintain the patient on aortic balloon and medical therapy as long as possible before surgery. The mortality rate without surgery is about 90%; early surgery has a mortality rate of about 50%.

VENTRICULAR SEPTAL RUPTURE

Rupture of the ventricular septum is rare after MI; it occurs in less than 1% of patients. It is more common after anterior infarction, and the defect is evident in the apical muscular portion of the septum. If it develops in the context of inferior infarction, the defect is in the basal portion. This complication is more common with the first Q-wave infarction, usually between the first and fifth days of recovery. Ventricular rupture initiates a left-to-right shunt that is always significant, resulting in biventricular failure, pulmonary edema, and cardiogenic shock with rapid deterioration. The predominant feature—over and above the sudden clinical deterioration—is the sudden appearance of a harsh holosystolic murmur that is associated with a thrill felt best at the parasternal area in more than 50% of cases. Rupture of a ventricular septum leads to a hyperdynamic precordium, unless there is severe hypotension; it is always associated with an S_3 and an S_4 and, if tachycardia is present, a summation gallop. Rupture of the ventricular septum is accompanied almost always by massive myocardial damage (in contrast to a ruptured papillary muscle, in which injury may be only moderate). Ventricular septal rupture is more likely to be associated with conduction defects, such as intraventricular or bundle-branch block, than is a ruptured papillary muscle. Right-sided heart failure and elevated jugular venous pressure are more common than with a ruptured mitral papillary muscle.

The diagnosis can be confirmed at the bedside using a Swan-Ganz catheter by finding an oxygen saturation step-up at the right ventricular level. The large v wave observed in the pulmonary occlusive wedge tracing with mitral valve rupture is rare with ventricular septal rupture; when the rupture is massive and associated with significant pulmonary hypertension, it may be present. Patients with this complication almost always require surgery.

CARDIAC RUPTURE

Cardiac rupture after MI is a catastrophe that occurs in less than 1% of patients and is said to be the third most common cause of death in acute MI. Typically, the patient has a Q-wave infarction, and the rupture involves the free wall of the left ventricle. It is more common in women over age 65 and is more likely to occur after the first attack; patients often have preexisting hypertension. Cardiac rupture usually takes place within the first

5 days of an uneventful recovery from acute MI. The event often is heralded by prolonged chest pain, dyspnea, hypotension, neck vein distention, tamponade, and electrocardiographic evidence of electrical mechanical dissociation. Death usually occurs within minutes.

In some cases, the course may be somewhat slowed, and sometimes it may indeed develop into a chronic situation in which the ventricle ruptures into the pericardial cavity. If the pericardium contains the blood, a so-called pseudoaneurysm is formed. The diagnosis of such a false aneurysm can be made by echocardiography or radionuclide ventriculography and confirmed by cardiac catheterization. Treatment of false aneurysm is surgery, which should be performed shortly after the diagnosis because of the danger of rupture of the pericardium. In the more typical urgent cardiac rupture, there is seldom time to initiate therapy. If cardiac rupture is suggested, however, the possibility of taking the patient to the operating room rapidly should be considered; occasionally a patient has been saved.

PERICARDITIS

Pericarditis usually does not develop until at least 48 hours after infarction. It occurs in 5% to 10% of patients with Q-wave infarction and is usually heralded by the appearance of pleural, pericardial pain, as well as pericardial friction rub. The treatment is aspirin. Pericarditis may be the cause of recurring chest pain after the first 48 to 72 hours. It is important to search for pericarditis in patients who have recurrent pain, since it may be inappropriately treated with nitrates or β-blockers or even aggravated by the use of anticoagulants.

DRESSLER'S SYNDROME

Dressler's syndrome is characterized by fever and pleural or pericardial chest pain and usually occurs within 2 to 6 weeks after MI. It is often associated with pain and stiffness of the left shoulder and rarely with a pleural effusion. It is believed to be autoimmune in origin, and the incidence has declined markedly in the past 10 years. Initial treatment consists of salicylates; if the condition does not respond, corticosteroid therapy is instituted.

■ PROGNOSIS OF Q-WAVE AND NON-Q-WAVE INFARCTION

In patients with Q-wave infarction, most deaths occur early. Patients with non-Q-wave infarction do not exhibit the same profile (Fig. 73.3). In patients with non-Q-wave infarction, a highly vulnerable period of reinfarction and death continues throughout most of the first year. Because of this extended period, cumulative survival with non-Q-wave infarction becomes similar to that of Q-wave infarction after about 1 year. The prolonged propensity for reinfarction and ischemia in patients with non-Q-wave infarction is believed to be the major factor accounting for the disparity between the initial and long-term mortality rates (Table 73.9). The hospital mortality rate from non-Q-wave infarction is only 3% to 5%, but the incidence of early reinfarction or extension during the hospital recovery phase in patients with non-Q-wave infarction is about 15%, compared with only 3% to 5% in patients after Q-wave infarction.

Several factors that significantly influence the prognosis of survivors of acute MI are applicable to Q-wave and non-Q-wave

TABLE 73.9.	**COMPARISON OF Q-WAVE VERSUS NON-Q-WAVE MI**	
Characteristics	**Q-Wave MI**	**Non-Q-Wave MI**
Prevalence	47%	53%
Complete coronary obstruction	80–90%	15–25%
Elevated ST-T segment	80%	25%
Depressed ST-T segment	20%	75%
Postinfarction angina	15–25%	30–40%
Early reinfarction	5–8%	15–25%
1-mo mortality rate	10–15%	3–5%
2-yr mortality rate	30%	30%
Infarct size	Moderate to large	Usually small
Residual ischemia	10–20%	40–50%
Acute complication	Common	Uncommon
Therapy		
Thrombolysis	Indicated	Not indicated
β-Adrenergic blockers	Indicated	Retrospective analysis shows ineffective
Calcium channel blockers		
Nifidepine	Possibly detrimental	Not determined
Diltiazem	Not indicated	Recommended
Verapamil	Beneficial	Possibly beneficial but not established

MI, myocardial infarction.

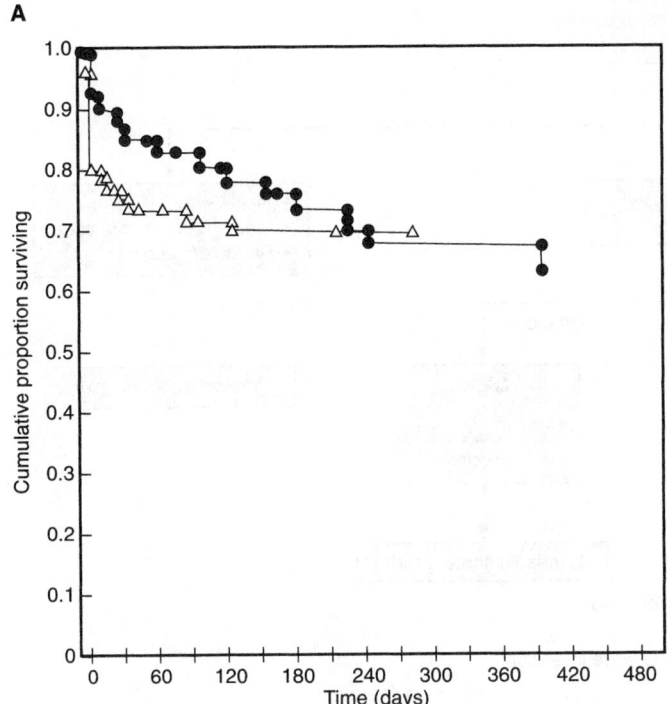

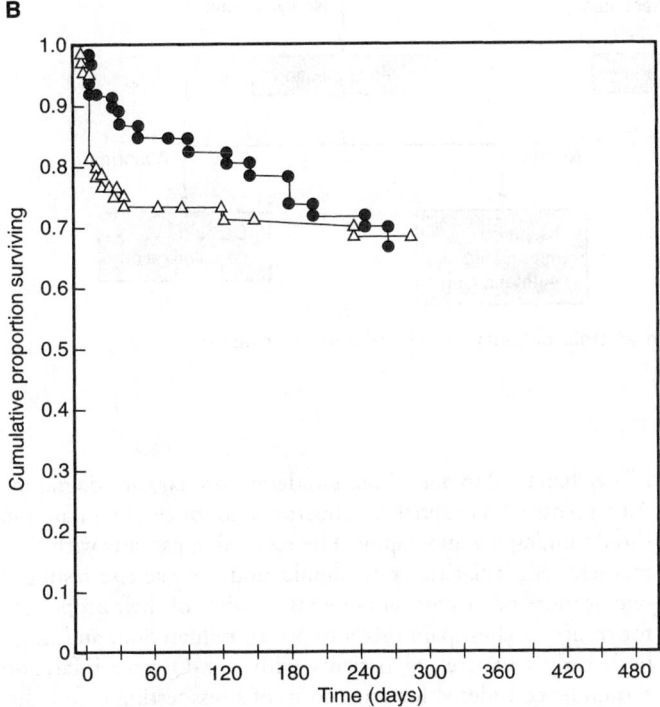

FIGURE 73.3. Survival of patients with Q-wave (*triangles*) and non-Q-wave (*circles*) infarction. **A:** Data from all patients. **B:** Patients without a previous infarction antedating the index infarction. Patients with previous infarction were excluded from the analysis. The cumulative mortality rate is similar in Q-wave and non-Q-wave infarction after about 1 year.

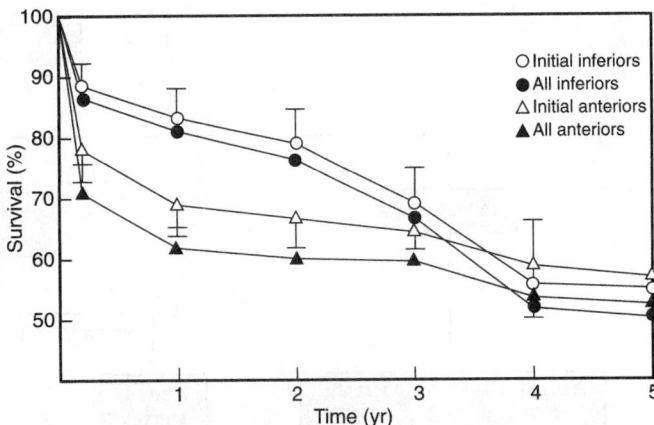

FIGURE 73.4. Survival curves for patients with inferior infarction compared with patients with anterior infarction. Separate curves identify patients with initial infarction as opposed to those who sustained previous infarction. The mortality rate of anterior infarction exceeded the mortality rate of inferior infarction ($p < 0.01$), regardless of initial or previous infarction.

infarction. Predominant among these factors are age, infarct size, the number of vessels with obstructive disease, the site of infarction, residual left ventricular function, and complex dysrhythmias. The most important factors are probably left ventricular function and age. Residual left ventricular function is determined by infarct size, site of infarction, and, to a lesser extent, the number of diseased coronary vessels. The risk of dying with an ejection fraction of less than 0.40 is several times greater than that associated with normal ventricular function. Similarly, the risk of death increases significantly with age and is independent of the other factors. In one series, the 3-year mortality rate of patients under age 50 was 6%, compared with 44% in patients age 70 to 79. The prognosis for survival after infarction is also significantly worse for women than for men, but this may in part reflect the fact that infarction occurs much later in women. Survival for patients after inferior infarction, at least during the first 3 years, is substantially greater than after anterior infarction (Fig. 73.4). In a 15-year study, the proportion surviving after an infarction was 48%, 28%, 18%, and 9% for patients with one-, two-, and three-vessel disease and left main artery disease, respectively.

POSTINFARCTION STRATIFICATION AND INVESTIGATION

Simple, noninvasive testing, together with cardiac catheterization in selected cases, allows for improved management (Fig. 73.5). The physician should consider which of the following treatment plans should be initiated and to what extent: modification of lifestyle; selective pharmacotherapy to relieve symptoms and prolong life; treatment of existing factors, such as smoking, hypertension, or hypercholesterolemia; and revascularization with angioplasty or surgery.

The need for stratification is emphasized by the estimate that

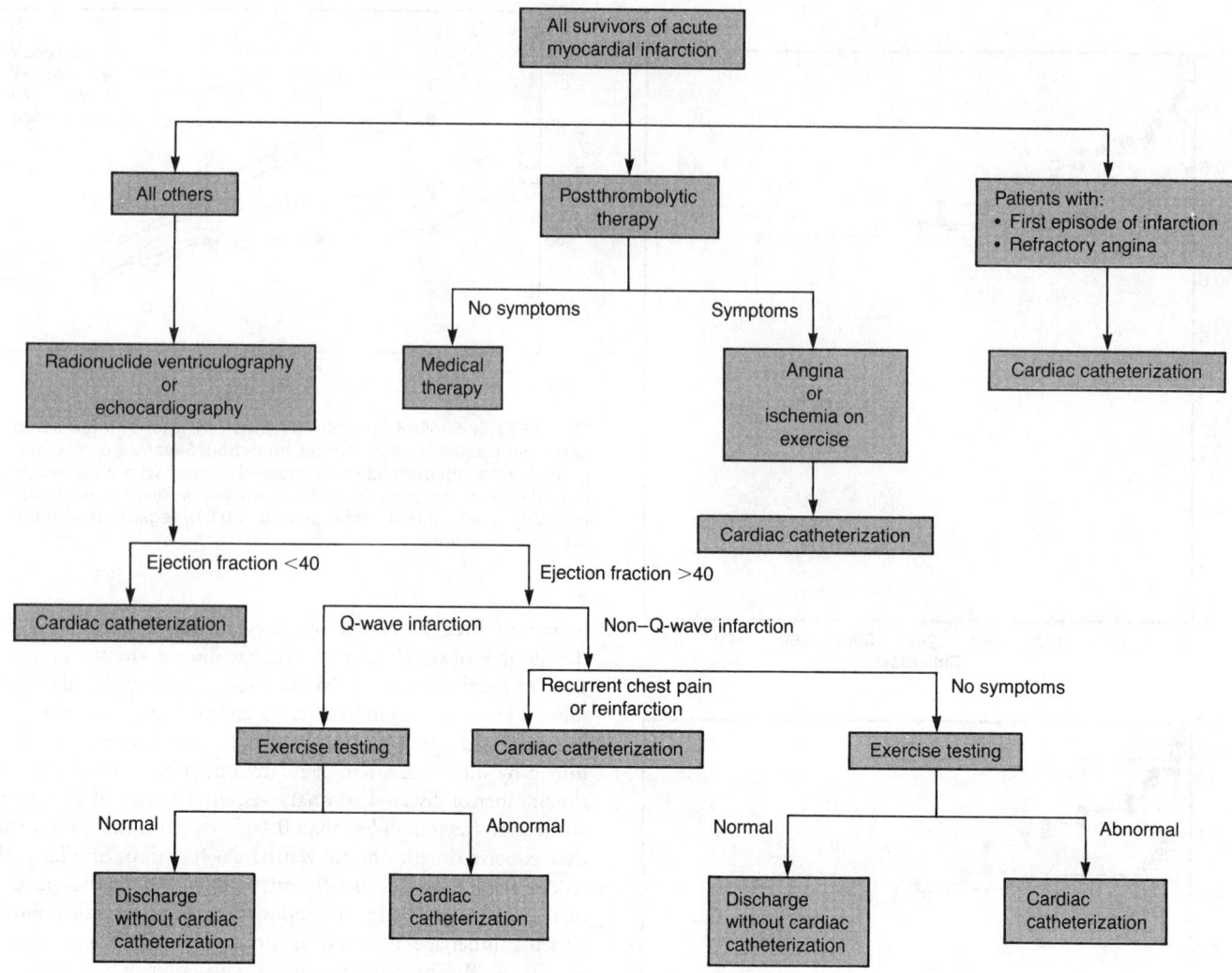

FIGURE 73.5. Protocol to be followed in determining whether patients should undergo noninvasive testing or cardiac catheterization.
EVIDENCE LEVEL: C. Expert Opinion.

only 25% of patients are at high risk after infarction, but they account for about 50% of the deaths. Their symptoms are characterized by an ejection fraction of less than 0.40, electrocardiographic evidence of ischemia on exercise testing, and frequent or complex ventricular dysrhythmias. In contrast, a low-risk group with a 2% mortality rate in the first year make up about 25% of the patients; they have no significant risk factors. This leaves 55% of patients at intermediate risk, with about a 10% chance of dying in the first year. The challenge to the physician is to select those patients in the intermediate group who are likely to have features that, if corrected, would lessen their chance of dying in subsequent years.

All patients surviving MI should undergo an assessment of left ventricular function by radionuclide ventriculography or echocardiography before discharge. Patients treated by thrombolysis probably should have cardiac catheterization only if there is evidence of spontaneous myocardial ischemia or if it is documented on exercise. Patients who have experienced their first episode of infarction should have coronary arteriography and a predischarge stress test. Patients who exhibit an ejection fraction

of less than 0.40 to 0.45 should undergo coronary arteriography. All patients who experience refractory pain or early reinfarction should undergo angiography. The remaining patients with normal left ventricular function should undergo exercise testing if one or more risk factors are present. In view of their propensity for recurrent chest pain (40% to 50%), reinfarction, and death both early and late, all patients with non-Q-wave infarction should be considered for some form of stress testing before discharge, preferably with thallium imaging; those who show significant ischemia should have coronary arteriography.

PROPHYLACTIC THERAPY AFTER INFARCTION

β-BLOCKERS AND CALCIUM CHANNEL BLOCKERS

Four different β-blockers assessed in trials involving more than 30,000 patients have been shown to prolong life in patients after

TABLE 73.10.   INDICATIONS FOR β-BLOCKADE FOR PATIENT

After myocardial infarction
≥60 yr old
Q-wave infarction with ischemia
Ejection <0.45
Concomitant disease (e.g., hypertension)
After cardiac arrest
Ventricular dysrhythmias

infarction: timolol, propranolol, metoprolol, and atenolol. Who should receive β-blockers? About 10% of patients who are at high risk of sudden death or reinfarction and who are likely to benefit from β-blockers have contraindications, such as heart failure, asthma, conduction disturbances, or Prinzmetal's angina. Some patients who have a low annual mortality rate of about 2% also should not receive β-blockers prophylactically. The following are guidelines for the use of β-blockers (Table 73.10) in patients with Q-wave infarction who do not have contraindications to their use:

1. Patients over age 60
2. Patients with Q-wave infarction who exhibit ischemia on exercise
3. Patients with abnormal left ventricular function (ejection fraction less than 0.45)
4. Patients who require β-blockers for concomitant symptoms or disease, such as angina or hypertension
5. Patients who experience an episode of sustained ventricular tachycardia or ventricular fibrillation or have had cardiac arrest during the hospital stay

ANTIPLATELET THERAPY

Most of our therapeutic efforts to date have concentrated on decreasing myocardial demand or attempting to increase flow, but it is now well recognized that coronary thrombosis, partial or complete, has a major role in acute MI, and there is a growing body of evidence that thrombosis plays a part in rest angina. Several studies have shown that aspirin therapy after unstable angina is effective in lowering the incidence of MI and death. The trials assessing aspirin in patients after MI have shown no effect on mortality rates. When coronary events were combined (namely, nonfatal infarction and death), however, a significant beneficial effect was observed. The Food and Drug Administration has approved the use of aspirin once a day in patients after MI; however, there is still little evidence that this treatment is effective. Therefore, the use of aspirin is cautiously recommended in patients at high risk, such as those with a diminished ejection fraction, a previous episode of infarction, or recurring episodes of postinfarction chest pain and those who have been shown to have three-vessel disease or residual ischemia on exercise testing or cardiac catheterization. Patients

who undergo angioplasty are routinely treated on a long-term basis with aspirin.

ANGIOPLASTY AND SURGERY

Patients with left main vessel disease or triple-vessel disease and an ejection fraction below 0.45 are clearly candidates for bypass surgery, using an internal mammary artery if possible. The role of angioplasty is less well defined. It is highly recommended after successful thrombolytic therapy as a means of maintaining patency, despite the fact that 30% of the arteries may re-stenose over the next 6 to 8 months. This therapy is new, and there are no clinical trials assessing medical therapy versus angioplasty. Several trials show comparable results on relief of symptoms with angioplasty or surgery in patients with one- and two-vessel disease. Patients with three-vessel disease in whom an operation would be difficult or in whom the risk of complications could exceed the possible benefit should be considered for angioplasty only in a center experienced with three-vessel angioplasty. Patients with 80% to 90% obstruction of the left anterior descending artery should be considered for angioplasty. About 4% to 5% of the patients who undergo angioplasty require emergency surgery. Only 60% to 70% of patients surviving MI who might otherwise be candidates for angioplasty have the appropriate anatomy for angioplasty. In addition, the high incidence of re-stenosis is a significant factor.

BIBLIOGRAPHY

Bode C, Smalling RW, Berg G, et al. Randomized comparison of coronary thrombolysis achieved with double-bolus releplase (recombinant plasminogen activator) and front-loaded, accelerated alteplase (recombinant tissue plasminogen activator) in patients with acute myocardial infarction. *Circulation* 1996;94:891–898.

Chizner MA. Bedside diagnosis of the AMI and its complications. *Curr Probl Cardiol* 1982;7:1.

Collins R, Peto R, Baigent C, et al. Aspirin, heparin, and fibrinolytic therapy in suspected acute myocardial infarction. *Drug Therapy* 1997;36:847–860.

Gibson RS, Boden WE, Theroux P, et al. Diltiazem and reinfarction in patients with non-Q-wave MI: results of a double-blind, randomized, multicenter trial. *N Engl J Med* 1986;315:423–429.

The Global Use of Strategies to Open Occluded Coronary Arteries in Acute Coronary Syndromes (GUSTO IIb) Angioplasty Substudy Investigators. A clinical trial comparing primary coronary angioplasty with tissue plasminogen activator for acute myocardial infarction. *N Engl J Med* 1997;336:1621–1628.

Ishikawa Y, Saffitz JE, Mealman JE, et al. Reversible myocardial ischemic injury is not associated with increased creatine kinase activity in plasma. *Clin Chem* 1997;43:467–475.

Puleo PR, Meyer D, Wathen C, et al. Use of rapid assay of subforms of creatine kinase MB to diagnose or rule out AMI. *N Engl J Med* 1994;331:561–566.

Thrombosis in Myocardial Ischemia (TIMI) IIIB Investigators. Effects of tissue plasminogen activator and a comparison of early invasive and conservative strategies in unstable angina and non-Q-wave MI. *Circulation* 1994;89:1545–1556.

Zimmerman J, Fromm R, Meyer D, et al. Diagnostic marker cooperative study (DMCS) for the diagnosis of myocardial infarction. *Circulation* 1999;99:1671–1677.

C H A P T E R

74

MYOCARDIAL DISEASES

MICHAEL R. BRISTOW
JOHN B. O'CONNELL
LUISA MESTRONI

Myocardial disease may be defined in several ways. From a clinical standpoint, the term refers to a disorder of heart muscle that leads to demonstrable cardiac dysfunction. Myocardial diseases may be primary—originating in the heart muscle itself—or secondary—that is, resulting from a specific extramyocardial abnormality, such as coronary artery disease, valvular abnormalities, or a systemic process such as hypertension. Many of the primary types of myocardial disease, however, are similar in morphologic and pathophysiologic characteristics to certain secondary cardiomyopathies, and, in fact, they may have common pathogenetic features. The 1995 Task Force on the Definition and Classification of Cardiomyopathies of the WHO/ISFC defined the following types: dilated cardiomyopathy, hypertrophic cardiomyopathy, restrictive cardiomyopathy, arrhythmogenic right ventricular dysplasia, and unclassified forms. The heart muscle diseases associated with specific cardiac or systemic disorders, such as ishemic heart disease, are defined as specific cardiomyopathies. Therefore, the term *cardiomyopathy* denotes any pathologic process that leads to clinically significant myocardial dysfunction. This chapter presents a pathophysiologic, diagnostic, and therapeutic approach to myocardial disease and heart failure.

DILATED CARDIOMYOPATHY

The term *dilated cardiomyopathy* is applied primarily to a form of heart muscle disease characterized by systolic dysfunction and left ventricular dilatation. The most common means of detecting left ventricular dilatation is by echocardiography, in which a left ventricular end-diastolic diameter (LVEDD) of more than 2.7 cm per square meter, coupled with a reduced ejection fraction (less than 0.45), establishes the diagnosis of dilated cardiomyopathy. Although there is usually some degree of cellular hypertrophy in dilated cardiomyopathy on histologic examination, increased wall thickness is not a common feature. The contraction abnormality typically is global, but in diffuse types of heart muscle disease, such as idiopathic dilated cardiomyopathy, there are often areas where segmental contraction is selectively impaired. Similarly, left and right ventricular dysfunction may be disproportionate, with left ventricular dysfunction not uncommonly more prominent. These regional differences in dysfunction tend to disappear as heart failure progresses, such that generalized, globally severe, biventricular dysfunction is the rule at the end stage in most patients with dilated cardiomyopathy.

CAUSES OF DILATED CARDIOMYOPATHY

Table 74.1 lists some of the causes of dilated cardiomyopathy. In the United States, the most common cause of dilated cardiomyopathy is coronary artery disease, listed in Table 74.1 as "postinfarction cardiomyopathy." Depending on the geographic area and other factors, the percentage of cases of heart failure that stem from postinfarction cardiomyopathy ranges from 50% to 90%. In an era in which the treatment of hypertension is aggressive and generally available, the second most common cause of heart failure in our experience is idiopathic dilated cardiomyopathy. A third typical cause is valvular heart disease, partic-

TABLE 74.1. PARTIAL LIST OF INITIAL CAUSES OF DILATED CARDIOMYOPATHY

Direct[a]
  Toxic
    Alcohol
    Anthracyclines
    Catecholamines
    Cobalt
    Phenothiazines
    Radiation
    Uremia
  Infectious
    Protozoan (Chagas' disease)
    Viral (coxsackievirus, other enteroviruses, influenza)
  Metabolic
    Starvation (liquid protein diets, kwashiorkor)
    Thiamine deficiency (beriberi)
  Genetic
  Idiopathic
Indirect[b]
  Ischemic
    Large-vessel coronary disease (postinfarction cardiomyopathy)
    Small-vessel coronary disease
    Global ischemia (cardiac surgery)
    Anemia
    Thromboembolic disorders (thrombotic thrombocytopenic purpura)
  Hypersensitivity
    Idiopathic myocarditis
    Drug reactions (methyldopa, sulfonamides, foreign protein)
    Chagas' disease
  Abnormal loading conditions
    Hypertension
    Valvular heart disease
    Peripartum or postpartum cardiomyopathy
  Endocrine
    Hyperthyroidism
    Acromegaly
    Diabetes
  Infiltration
    Sarcoid
    Hemochromatosis (idiopathic hemochromatosis, hemosiderosis)
    Neoplastic (lymphoma, leukemia)

[a] Mode of action involves direct effect on the heart.
[b] Mode of action involves abnormality of an extramyocardial mechanism followed by secondary myocardial damage.

ularly after several cardiac surgeries for valve replacement. Hypertension remains a leading cause of heart failure in some regions, but it is decidedly unusual as an obvious cause of heart failure in many others. Alcohol cardiomyopathy is relatively common but depends on cultural patterns. These five types of heart muscle disease constitute more than 90% of the cases encountered in most regions of the United States.

There are numerous other types of dilated cardiomyopathy (Table 74.1), and, depending on the region and referral pattern, some of them are relatively common. For example, cardiomyopathy related to chemotherapy with doxorubicin (Adriamycin) may be common in hospitals with large oncologic practices. Peripartum cardiomyopathy may be prevalent where the risk factors for this disorder prevail (e.g., in inner-city hospitals). Myocarditis may become relatively commonplace after epidemics of cardiotropic viruses. A practical approach to finding the source of dilated cardiomyopathy is to construct a differential diagnosis geared toward detecting the types of heart muscle disease that may be reversible (Table 74.2).

Although the initial injury that produces cardiac damage in dilated cardiomyopathy may have several sources, the fact is that the end result is a dilated, poorly contractile ventricle producing a clinical picture that is quite similar across diverse origins. Although some dilated cardiomyopathies do have morphologically unique features, most are indistinguishable on histologic evaluation. Moreover, the clinical signs of biventricular failure are essentially the same regardless of cause.

There are at least two general reasons why diverse causes of dilated cardiomyopathy may have common features. The first is that different types of initial cardiac damage can produce a similar kind of cellular cardiac injury, involving a final common pathway that includes membrane damage, calcium overload, and energy exhaustion. The second reason is that the compensatory mechanisms called into play to cope with pump dysfunction exert powerful influences in their own right, some of which may be harmful. For example, activation of the adrenergic nervous system is an invariable response to pump failure. The physiologic consequences of this activation include peripheral vasoconstriction, which increases systolic wall stress; activation of cardiac adrenergic nerves, leading to amplified cardiac norepinephrine levels and initially to positive chronotropic and inotropic responses, which elevate myocardial oxygen requirements; a contribution to the development of hypertrophy, which increases

TABLE 74.2. POTENTIALLY REVERSIBLE CAUSES OF CARDIOMYOPATHY DETECTABLE BY CATHETERIZATION OR BIOPSY

Myocarditis (idiopathic, drug reactions, collagen vascular disease)
Sarcoidosis
Hemochromatosis
Ischemia ("hibernating" myocardium)
Valvular heart disease (aortic stenosis)
Amyloidosis
Infiltrative neoplastic process (lymphoma)

wall tension and subsequently raises myocardial oxygen demand; and finally, receptor-mediated or non-receptor-mediated cardiotoxicity. Because the adrenergic nervous system invariably is activated after damage to the contractile apparatus, it is not surprising that this powerful compensatory mechanism would contribute to the development of morphologic and dysfunctional features common to diverse etiologic types. The same argument can be put forth for activation of the renin-angiotensin-aldosterone systems and enhanced vasopressin and endothelin secretion, which increase afterload and preload. These multiple harmful signaling pathways produce the aforementioned toxic effects, as well as activating gene programs that lead to progressive remodeling and myocardial dysfunction.

GENETIC BASIS OF CARDIOMYOPATHIES

New studies have confirmed that idiopathic dilated cardiomyopathy is frequently inherited. A defined genetic trait is found in 20% to 35% of cases, but it can be suspected in up to 50%: in these patients, the primary defect lies at the DNA level. At present, the molecular genetics of several systemic diseases that give rise to dilated cardiomyopathy have been defined. Duchenne's muscular dystrophy and myotonic muscular dystrophy result from mutations in the genes encoding dystrophin and MD kinase, respectively. Friedreich's ataxia, a rare cause of cardiomyopathy, has been mapped to chromosome 9 and found to be due to mutations in the frataxin gene. Mutations of the delta-sarcoglycan gene, encoding a cytoskeletal protein of the dystrophin complex, have been identified in the cardiomyopathic Syrian hamster and in human familial cardiomyopathy.

Concerning the adult form of dilated cardiomyopathy, nine different chromosomal loci have been linked to the disease. These map on chromosome 1, 2, 3, 9, 10, 15, X, and a familial dilated cardiomyopathy associated with limb-girdle muscle dystrophy has been mapped on chromosome 6. Two disease genes were identified: cardiac actin, which connects the sarcomere to the cytoskeleton (chromosome 15), and dystrophin (chromosome X), which causes X-linked dilated cardiomyopathy. In this form, with no male-to-male transmission, only the heart is affected in terms of clinical symptoms, and there is no muscle dystrophy. Very recently, the lamin A/C gene has been found to cause an autosomal dominant form of familial dilated cardiomyopathy with conduction defects and variable skeletal muscle involvement. This gene encodes another cytoskeletal protein, an intermediate filament that provides one of the layers of the nuclear envelope, the nuclear lamina. Infantile dilated cardiomyopathy, which can be associated with endocardial fibroelastosis, is caused by the G4.5 gene, which maps on chromosome X and also causes Barth syndrome. The gene function is still unknown.

STRUCTURAL ABNORMALITIES

MORPHOLOGIC CHANGES

With the exception of postinfarction cardiomyopathy, in which the left ventricle has been replaced by scar tissue, the morphologic findings in dilated cardiomyopathy are usually nonspecific.

Increased cell volume and enlarged cardiac nuclear size (both manifestations of hypertrophy) as well as fibrosis are present to a varying degree. In idiopathic dilated cardiomyopathy, however, the amount of fibrosis and hypertrophy does not correlate well with hemodynamic function or with prognosis. Hypertrophy presumably is a response to the increased wall tension and wall stress in the dilated heart as well as to direct effects of hormones and neurotransmitters. The amount of fibrosis in dilated cardiomyopathy is inconsistent, increasing, on average, in control hearts from 4% to 15% to 20% of the total tissue volume on microscopic sections. Some hearts, however, show little or no fibrosis, whereas others have replacement of as much as one-fourth to one-third of the myocardial cell volume. In most cases, the degree of fibrosis does not appear to be extensive enough to cause changes in systolic and diastolic function.

It is relatively common to find a patient with severe heart failure stemming from idiopathic dilated cardiomyopathy with only mild cardiac hypertrophy and little or no fibrosis. The hypertrophy is less advanced than that seen in conditions in which myocardial function can be normal or "supernormal" (e.g., mild hypertension or mild aortic stenosis). Therefore, with the exception of myocardial infarction, anthracycline cardiomyopathy (discussed later in this chapter), and myocarditis, in which dilated cardiomyopathy follows an infectious process, the morphologic abnormalities present in dilated cardiomyopathy appear to be a consequence of the initial myocardial injury and are not responsible for the abnormal cardiac function. These observations indicate that the basic abnormality in most myopathic, noninfarcted, noninfiltrated hearts is functional rather than structural.

DILATED CARDIOMYOPATHIES WITH UNIQUE STRUCTURAL FEATURES

Certain dilated cardiomyopathies have unique structural features that can be recognized in terms of morphologic features and therefore detected in vivo by endomyocardial biopsy. These conditions include anthracycline cardiomyopathy, myocarditis, sarcoidosis, hemochromatosis, Chagas' disease, and amyloidosis. Many of the infiltrative types, such as amyloidosis and hemochromatosis, may have initial symptoms of predominant diastolic dysfunction and restrictive cardiomyopathy, but there is usually some degree of abnormal systolic function. Because some of these conditions may be amenable to medical therapy—such as iron unloading for hemochromatosis, cytotoxic/colchicine therapy for amyloidosis, steroid therapy for sarcoidosis, and various forms of immunosuppression for myocarditis—it behooves the clinician to be acutely aware of these relatively uncommon conditions.

Anthracycline cardiomyopathy is a representative form of dilated cardiomyopathy with unique morphologic and ultrastructural features. Anthracyclines are an extremely valuable class of antitumor agents; the prototype agent, doxorubicin, is the mainstay of the chemotherapeutic treatment of lymphomas, breast cancer, sarcomas, and many other forms of cancer. A unique adverse effect of anthracyclines, however, is a dose-related vacuolation of myocardial cells that ultimately leads to complete loss

of myofibrils. Although there is a direct relationship between the amount of cardiotoxic insult administered (anthracycline dose) and the amount of damage produced, there is substantial individual variability in the dose–response curve. The morphologic abnormality, which can be semiquantitatively graded by examination of endomyocardial biopsy specimens, not surprisingly produces a severity-related adverse effect on systolic pump function. Because the lesion can be graded semiquantitatively and because cardiac function can be studied at the time of endomyocardial biopsy, anthracycline cardiomyopathy creates an opportunity to examine prospectively the structure–function relationship of a diffuse myocardial process in the intact human heart. Figure 74.1 illustrates examples of anthracycline cardiomyopathy, graded as mild (grade 1), moderate (grade 2), or severe (grade 3). The Billingham classification of anthracycline cardiomyopathy also includes grades 1.5 and 2.5. In grade 3, more than 35% of the total number of cells are involved; in grade 2, 16% to 25% of the cells are involved; and in grade 1, fewer than 5% of the cells are affected.

If one examines the development of functional abnormalities relative to the degree of anthracycline change, as judged by the Billingham scale, there appears to be little or no change until a grade 2 abnormality is achieved—that is, until some 20% of the cells are involved. At that point, cardiac dysfunction begins to appear in most patients, and this dysfunction grows rapidly in degree as the anthracycline score rises to 2.5 and 3. Therefore, for anthracycline cardiomyopathy, the structure–function relationship in the intact human heart consists of little change until 20% of the cells are affected and then a rapidly progressive development of cardiac dysfunction as 25% to 35% of the cells become abnormal. The relationship is nonlinear, indicating that small amounts of damage can be tolerated by the heart, either because compensatory changes are invoked or because of an inherent reserve capacity to tolerate myocardial cell loss. Beyond a critical percentage of cellular involvement (about 25%), however, severe heart failure develops rapidly. This fundamental relationship is probably the reason that many patients appear to experience heart failure "suddenly." In most cases, the underlying disease process did not develop suddenly; rather, compensatory mechanisms were supporting cardiac function through the early phases of disease progression.

In most other types of myocardial disease, it is difficult to correlate structure and function, probably because observable structural changes have little to do with what is producing the cardiac dysfunction. This is apparently the case with idiopathic dilated cardiomyopathy with respect to hypertrophy/fibrosis, as described, and also may be the case for some of the infiltrative processes that can lead to cardiac dysfunction, such as myocarditis. In myocarditis and cardiac allograft rejection (which resembles myocarditis in morphologic features), there often is a disparity between the amount of infiltrate observed on histologic examination and the degree of cardiac dysfunction. In both situations, large amounts of lymphocytic infiltrate can be well tolerated in many cases, whereas in other cases a small amount of infiltrate may be associated with marked ventricular dysfunction. For the purely infiltrative processes of cardiac amyloidosis and hemochromatosis, a better correlation between structural abnormality and degree of dysfunction may exist, because the infiltrat-

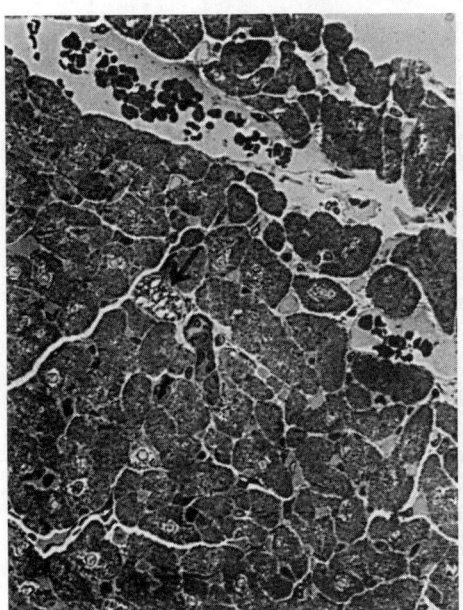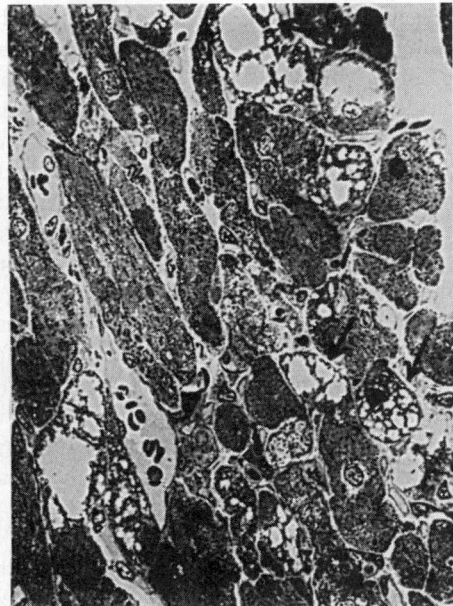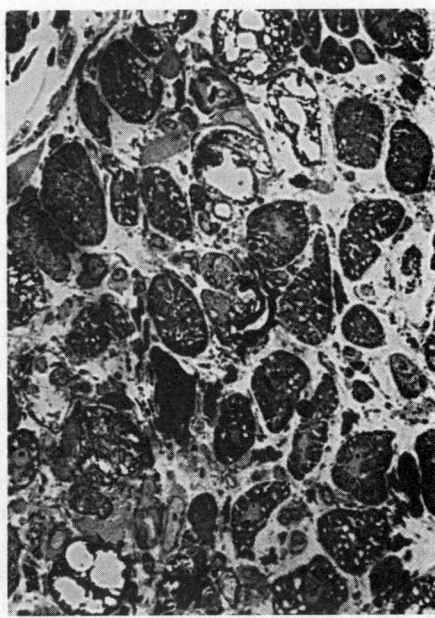

FIGURE 74.1. Examples of anthracycline cardiomyopathy. Left to right: grade 1 (mild), grade 2 (moderate), and grade 3 (severe). Arrows designate vacuolating cells that evidence myofibrillar dropout. (From Bristow MR. Toxic cardiomyopathy due to doxorubicin. *Hosp Pract* 1982;17:106, with permission.)

ing substance causes abnormal function strictly through a replacement process. In the case of infiltration of the heart with T lymphocytes, however, processes other than pure infiltration (e.g., the local production of cytokines) most likely produce the cardiac dysfunction.

In postinfarction cardiomyopathy, it seems obvious that the symptoms are related to myocardial infarction—that is, the replacement of viable myocardium by nonfunctioning scar tissue. The situation is much more complicated than that, however, because postinfarction cardiomyopathy is seen often in patients who survive a myocardial infarct or one or more coronary artery bypass operations and then remain stable for months or years before showing evidence of heart failure. In these patients, it is possible to speculate that the initial insult was a relatively large infarct, involving 10% to 20% of the myocardium, which was initially reasonably well tolerated because of endogenous compensatory mechanisms. In time, however, the noninfarcted myocardium may fall victim to these compensatory changes, to the extent that normally or supernormally contracting viable muscle ultimately becomes myopathic.

Alternatively, a series of silent ischemic events may progressively damage viable myocardium. The fact that biochemical and morphologic changes present in noninfarcted areas of the heart in patients with postinfarction cardiomyopathy are myopathic in nature and similar to those found in idiopathic dilated cardiomyopathy suggests the former explanation in most cases. This scenario typically follows a large anterior infarct in the distribution of the left anterior descending coronary artery, but it may follow occlusion of any large epicardial artery with a large myocardial distribution. Finally, the fact that clinical stability usually ensues in patients who survive infarction but is followed in a certain subset of patients by the later development of heart failure suggests that the responsible progressive myopathic process may

be subject to interventional strategies similar to those currently undergoing trial in the context of idiopathic dilated cardiomyopathy.

PATHOGENESIS

A case can be made for dividing the pathogenesis of myocardial disease into initial and delayed components. By the initial component, we mean the pathogenetic mechanism that accounted for the original impairment of intrinsic contractile function. Various types of initial myocardial injury known to account for dilated cardiomyopathy are shown in Table 74.1. Within this large number of possibilities, however, there may be only a limited number of cellular or molecular mechanisms of action by which injury is effected. Some of them include direct toxic effects, such as those produced by release of cardiac norepinephrine and histamine; free radical formation; direct perturbation of membranes; and release of toxic cytokines.

The most recent advances in molecular genetics suggest that the disease is caused by altered cytoskeletal proteins, at least in a subset of cases. The discovery of mutations of dystrophin and cardiac actin in the human disease and of delta-sarcoglycan in the cardiomyopathic Syrian hamster, causing dilated cardiomyopathy, supports the hypothesis of a defect of force transmission from the sarcomere to the extracellular matrix.

Additionally, myocardial damage may be produced indirectly when myocardial oxygen demand exceeds the ability of the coronary circulation to supply it, leading to exhaustion of energy stores. Factors contributing to this situation are hypertrophy, increased wall stress, and reduced coronary flow. It is conceivable that these conditions lead to relative ischemia, which ultimately damages the highly aerobically dependent myocardium. The best-understood initial, indirect type of damage is from abrupt interruption of coronary flow, which causes myocardial infarction through a metabolic process involving abrupt withdrawal of blood supply. Relative ischemia due to inadequate coronary reserve in dilated cardiomyopathy also would be responsible for delayed cardiac damage. Ultimately, regardless of the type of damage, cardiac cell death probably results from cellular calcium overload, a relatively late-stage phenomenon that produces irreversible cytotoxicity.

Because it may be difficult or impossible to anticipate and prevent most cases of initial myocardial injury, a more likely focus for interventional strategies is in the delayed type of cardiac damage that appears to be responsible for the progressive nature of most forms of myocardial disease. Here the strong suspicion is that neurohumoral factors are playing a harmful role, as discussed earlier. It is highly likely that antagonism or elimination of adrenergic, renin-angiotensin-aldosterone, and vasopressin compensatory mechanisms ultimately afford some degree of protection against progression in myocardial disease and lead to stability or improvement in significant numbers of patients. As discussed later, however, these experimental approaches are still theoretical and have not undergone thorough evaluation. It also is likely that additional harmful compensatory mechanisms of action will continue to be elucidated as heart failure is more thoroughly investigated.

In addition to providing an accessible avenue for intervention, the concept of a delayed type of cardiac damage in myocardial disease is attractive because it is based on factors that are part of well-defined physiologic systems, about which much is known and toward which pharmacologic therapy can be targeted. As the full pathophysiologic picture of heart failure is elucidated in the ensuing decades, secondary prevention strategies in myocardial disease undoubtedly will become increasingly common.

NATURAL HISTORY

The natural history of dilated cardiomyopathy is relatively independent of cause, and the prognosis generally is thought to be poor. Data on prognosis, however, are derived mostly from series of patients from tertiary referral centers, where the patient is usually in an advanced stage of the disease at the time when he or she is first seen. When the population of patients referred to a tertiary referral center is examined, the natural history of dilated cardiomyopathy of unknown cause (idiopathic dilated cardiomyopathy) includes approximately a 30% 1-year mortality rate and a 60% 5-year mortality rate. If postinfarction cardiomyopathy is examined, the survival is perhaps slightly worse, presumably because of the additive adverse effects of the ischemic process. Overall, when one looks at the population of patients referred to tertiary centers, the natural history of dilated cardiomyopathy and heart failure is as bad as or worse than that for many forms of cancer.

Patients with dilated cardiomyopathy die of four general processes. The first two are the most common (more than 80% of patients), whereas the last two are less common. The two most common causes of death are sudden death from arrhythmia and complications related generally to progressive pump dysfunction; in published series, the incidence rates of these two causes of death are usually fairly evenly distributed. Sudden death in the context of cardiomyopathy is particularly frustrating to the clinician, inasmuch as it may occur in a patient who is completely stable and without any antecedent in the form of increased arrhythmic activity. Progressive pump dysfunction can develop either slowly (over years) or rapidly (over weeks to months). The third general category of cause of death in cardiomyopathy covers medical complications related to the underlying disease process, such as embolic stroke, pulmonary embolism, or pneumonia. The fourth category includes deaths unrelated to the underlying disease process.

A number of factors have been shown to correlate with poor prognosis in dilated cardiomyopathy, including a particularly bad ejection fraction or hemodynamics, the presence of high-grade arrhythmia, and the degree of activation of the sympathetic nervous system. With regard to the degree of myocardial dysfunction, it is perhaps surprising that there is not a good overall correlation between hemodynamic indexes and outcome. Arrhythmia quantification correlates even more poorly with outcome; in fact, in some studies there has been no correlation. The best single predictor of outcome in dilated cardiomyopathy or heart failure, in general, is the degree of activation of the sympathetic nervous system, though the correlation is imperfect in this case as well.

RESTRICTIVE CARDIOMYOPATHY

Restrictive cardiomyopathy is defined as severe diastolic dysfunction resulting in altered filling characteristics of the left ventricle, in the context of normal or minimally abnormal systolic function. On echocardiograms, the left ventricular chamber size is normal; however, the walls of the left and right ventricles are thickened, and there is usually associated left atrial enlargement. The hemodynamic abnormalities of restrictive cardiomyopathy are so characteristic that they must be identified before the disease process can be classified as restrictive. The cardiac index is usually normal or slightly low, with a normal or near-normal ejection fraction. The left and right ventricular filling pressures are elevated and may be nearly equal. The ventricular pressure tracings show a dip–plateau configuration that also is found in constrictive pericarditis. In fact, hemodynamic abnormalities in these two states are so similar that it may be difficult to differentiate constrictive pericarditis from restrictive cardiomyopathy. In restrictive cardiomyopathy, however, the left ventricular filling pressures tend to be slightly higher than the right, and that can usually be augmented by rapid volume expansion or exercise. Additional features that can help distinguish restriction from constriction are increased wall thickness on echocardiography in restrictive cardiomyopathy but normal thickness in constrictive pericarditis and thickened pericardium on echocardiography or computed tomography in constrictive pericarditis but normal thickness with restrictive cardiomyopathy. Finally, endomyocardial biopsy is useful in helping discriminate restriction from

TABLE 74.3.	INITIAL CAUSES OF RESTRICTIVE CARDIOMYOPATHY

Direct
  Toxic
    Methysergide
    Anorectic agents
    Radiation
  Infectious: viral myocarditis
  Infiltration: endomyocardial fibrosis
  Genetic
  Idiopathic
Indirect
  Infiltration
    Sarcoid
  Hemochromatosis
  Amyloidosis
  Glycogen storage disease

constriction, because it usually shows more serious interstitial fibrosis or an infiltrative process in restriction.

MORPHOLOGY

Some common causes of restrictive cardiomyopathy are listed in Table 74.3. These pathophysiologic abnormalities result from a multitude of causes, such as infiltration of the myocardium by an abnormal protein (amyloidosis), inflammatory cells (acute viral myocarditis), or heavy metals (hemochromatosis). In these conditions, the myocytes are unable to "relax" or increase in length during diastole; hence, restrictive physiologic features develop. If the endocardium is thickened as a result of fibrosis (endomyocardial fibrosis) or infiltrated (hypereosinophilic syndromes), similar hemodynamic abnormalities may arise. For example, restrictive cardiomyopathy caused by increased endomyocardial fibrosis recently has been reported in association with the anorectic agent fenfluramine. Because the histopathologic abnormalities differ with origin, endomyocardial biopsy is indicated. Recently, patients with nonspecific histologic characteristics showing interstitial myocardial fibrosis have been identified and classified as having idiopathic restrictive cardiomyopathy.

PATHOGENESIS

When a systemic disorder is known, the pathogenesis of the restrictive cardiomyopathy is contingent on the severity of this systemic disease. Early in amyloid heart disease, abnormalities may be confined to conduction disturbances and subtle changes in diastolic function. As abnormal protein is deposited in greater quantities, the conduction disturbance worsens, the electrocardiographic voltage decreases, and diastolic function begins to be compromised. Similarly, in hemochromatosis, the severity of the hemodynamic abnormality is contingent on the degree of iron deposition, and the reversibility is dependent on the degree of secondary fibrosis. In patients in whom no morphologic cause can be identified (idiopathic), the physiologic abnormalities may or may not progress. Forms of genetic transmission of the disease

have been reported. One of them is characterized by desmin deposition; restrictive cardiomyopathy with severe conduction defects, sometimes associated with ventricular wall thickening; and myopathy. The disorder is caused by mutations of desmin or of *CRYAB* genes, which encode a molecular chaperon for desmin. Finally, cardiac amyloidosis can by caused by mutation of transthyretin.

NATURAL HISTORY

In general, the natural history of restrictive cardiomyopathy depends on the cause. Amyloidosis, a disease for which no definitive cure has been established, has a poor prognosis when symptomatic restrictive cardiomyopathy develops. Studies in renal amyloid patients, however, suggest that when a light chain is identified (AL, or primary amyloidosis) the combination of steroids and colchicine at least retards the progression of the disease. Longitudinal studies in patients with cardiac amyloid have not been completed, so the effect on the deposition of amyloid protein in the myocardium is unknown. Hemochromatosis is a potentially reversible process if severe myocardial fibrosis has not developed, and removal of iron by phlebotomy and chelation (desferoxamine) has resulted in substantial hemodynamic improvement. In the hypereosinophilic syndromes, eradication of the source of the eosinophilia may retard the progression of the disease, and, in selected cases, surgery (endocardial resection) has resulted in physiologic improvement. When the restrictive cardiomyopathy is idiopathic, the long-term survival may be quite good (in excess of 10 years).

HYPERTROPHIC CARDIOMYOPATHY

Hypertrophic cardiomyopathy, also known as idiopathic hypertrophic subaortic stenosis, has a prognosis that generally is better than the other two major classes. The definition, as strictly applied, is a hypertrophic left ventricle with disproportionate septal hypertrophy, normal or supernormal systolic function, but varying degrees of diastolic dysfunction. The disproportionate septal hypertrophy may lead to a measurable outflow-tract obstruction, and the mitral valve apparatus may be abnormal as well, leading to mitral regurgitation. Characteristic echocardiographic abnormalities include asymmetric septal hypertrophy and systolic anterior motion of the mitral valve. On catheterization, an outflow-tract gradient may be present at rest or may be provoked by isoproterenol or specialized maneuvers. At a functional level, hypertrophic cardiomyopathy tends to overlap with both restrictive and dilated cardiomyopathy. Systolic function sometimes becomes abnormal in hypertrophic cardiomyopathy, combined with chamber dilatation, and often it is difficult to differentiate a hypertrophic, restricted ventricle from the disproportionately septally hypertrophied ventricle of hypertrophic cardiomyopathy.

MORPHOLOGY

The classic morphologic abnormality in hypertrophic cardiomyopathy is myocardial cellular disarray with disorganization of the

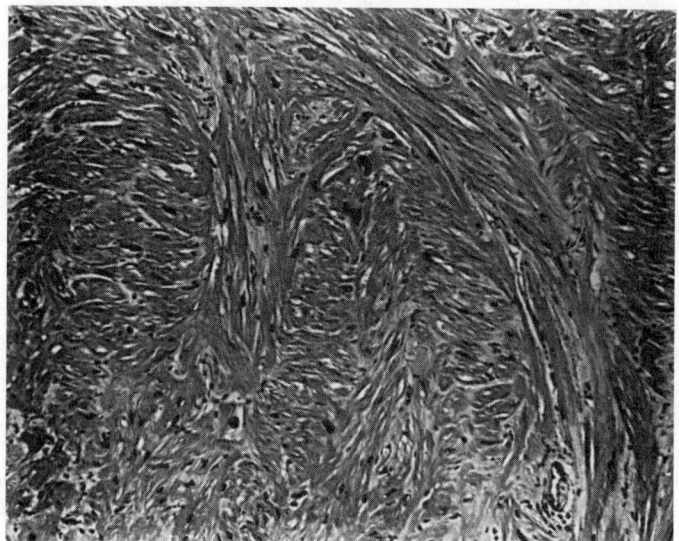

FIGURE 74.2. Myocardial cellular and myofibrillar disarray in hypertrophic cardiomyopathy. (From Tazelaar H, Billingham M. The surgical pathology of hypertrophic cardiomyopathy. *Arch Pathol Lab Med* 1987; 111:257, with permission.)

normally parallel-distributed myocardial cells, and myofibrillar disarray with disorganization of the contractile elements themselves (Fig. 74.2). Myocardial cell and myofibrillar disarray can be found not only in the left ventricle but also in the right ventricle and even in the skeletal muscle.

PATHOGENESIS

Advances in the knowledge of the molecular defects underlying hypertrophic cardiomyopathy indicate that the disease is caused by mutations in genes that encode proteins of the sarcomere. The β-cardiac myosin heavy chain gene (chromosome 14) represents about 35% of cases, α-tropomyosin (chromosome 15) makes up less than 5%, troponin T (chromosome 1) accounts for about 15%, myosin-binding protein C (chromosome 11) comprises 15%, and essential (chromosome 3) and regulatory myosin light chain (chromosome 12) account for less than 1%. Mutations in the cardiac troponin I gene also have been identified (chromosome 19). Finally, a familial form of hypertrophic cardiomyopathy with Wolff-Parkinson-White syndrome has been mapped to chromosome 7, but the specific gene affected has not yet been identified. Mutations in genes encoding β-cardiac myosin heavy chain, α-tropomyosin, and troponin T are associated with myofibrillar disarray and the abnormal mechanical properties that characterize the disease. Despite these findings at the DNA level, it remains to be determined how contractile protein mutations can be transduced into the abnormal structure and function of the heart observed in this disease.

NATURAL HISTORY

The natural history of hypertrophic cardiomyopathy, in general, is better than that of dilated or restrictive cardiomyopathy, with a mortality rate of about 4% per year. Death usually occurs suddenly, presumably because of ventricular arrhythmia. Progression to severe, intractable heart failure based on abnormal diastolic function or progression to systolic dysfunction can and does occur, but this is a less common cause of demise.

Because abnormalities in diastolic function account for most initial symptoms in hypertrophic cardiomyopathy and because arrhythmia is the most common cause of death, it would seem likely that medications designed to improve ventricular compliance or antiarrhythmic agents might favorably influence natural history. Nevertheless, there has been no definitive documentation of any favorable effect on natural history, either by agents that improve diastolic compliance (calcium antagonists) or by antiarrhythmic agents. The genotype appears to modify the risk of heart failure and sudden death. Some myosin mutations are benign, whereas others are associated with premature death. Mutations of cardiac troponin T are also characterized by lowered life expectancy.

RIGHT VENTRICULAR CARDIOMYOPATHY

Right ventricular cardiomyopathy (or arrhythmogenic right ventricular dysplasia) is a heart muscle disease of unknown cause that is characterized by dilatation and/or aneurysmal bulges of the right ventricle in the absence of significant left ventricular involvement. The most common clinical manifestation is the presence of ventricular arrhythmia, ranging from symptomatic ventricular premature beats to ventricular tachycardia. Sudden cardiac death may occur. Right ventricular dysplasia is frequently characterized by inverted T waves in the right precordial leads (beyond V_1 over the age of 12) on electrocardiogram and by ventricular arrhythmia with left bundle-branch block configuration.

MORPHOLOGY

Characteristic of the disease is the fibro-fatty infiltration of the right ventricular myocardium. The left ventricle is usually normal or not severely involved, except in the advanced stages of the disease. The echocardiogram is extremely useful in detecting right ventricular enlargement or wall-motion abnormalities that would confirm the diagnosis of arrhythmogenic right ventricular dysplasia. Right ventricular angiography is also used for the quantification of right ventricular dimensions, contractility, and regional wall motion. Magnetic resonance imaging has the advantage of showing not only right ventricular anatomy but also tissue characterization. This technique can differentiate the fatty infiltration of the right ventricular wall, seen as a white area, compared with the gray color of the normal myocardium.

PATHOLOGY

A definitive (gold standard) diagnosis of right ventricular dysplasia is based on histologic evidence of transmural fibro-fatty re-

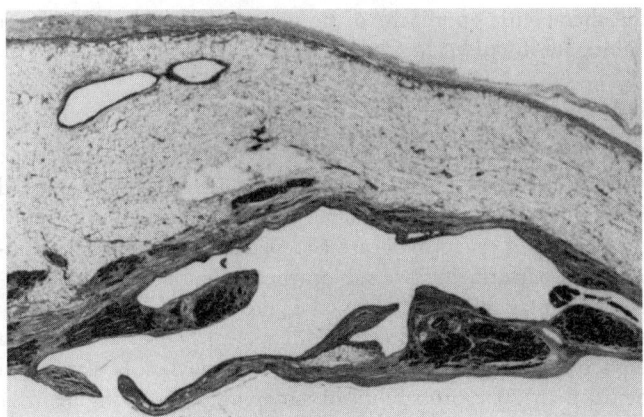

FIGURE 74.3. Histologic section of the right ventricular free wall from a patient with right ventricular dysplasia, showing the replacement of the muscle component by fatty tissue and by a thin layer of subendocardial connective tissue.

placement of right ventricular myocardium (Fig. 74.3). Histologic signs of myocarditis can be present. Nevertheless, endomyocardial biopsy lacks sensitivity, owing to the segmental nature of the disease, and specificity, owing to the normal presence of adipose tissue islands in the right ventricle. The diagnosis relies on the clinical findings of structural, functional, and electrophysiologic abnormalities that are caused by the underlying histologic changes.

PATHOGENESIS

Right ventricular dysplasia has a genetic basis in at least 30% of patients. No gene has been identified so far, but several disease loci have been mapped, on chromosome 1, 2, and 3 and two on chromosome 14. Disease transmission is usually autosomal dominant. In a rare form identified on a Greek island (Naxos syndrome), transmission is autosomal recessive, and heart disease is associated with woolly hair and diffuse nonepidermiolytic palmoplantar keratoderma. This form has been mapped on chromosome 17. It remains unclear whether the genetic background predisposes to a degenerative disease with atrophy and fibro-fatty replacement of the right ventricular myocardium or whether the inflammatory cells found in about 25% of cases indicate an infection or, possibly, genetically determined immune pathogenesis.

NATURAL HISTORY

Right ventricular dysplasia shows a wide variability in clinical expression. The disease can be clinically silent and accidentally discovered at a very advanced age. It has been recognized as a frequent cause of sudden death, particularly in young persons. Finally, the disease can progress to left ventricular involvement, with right and left heart failure mimicking dilated cardiomyopathy.

DIAGNOSTIC WORKUP OF PATIENTS WITH SUSPECTED MYOCARDIAL DISEASE

Regardless of how it is classified, myocardial disease has nonspecific initial symptoms, referable to the heart. These may include signs and symptoms of congestive heart failure (including both congestive and low-output symptoms), chest pain, or arrhythmia. It is important to remember that because of the nonlinear structure–function relationship in dilated cardiomyopathy, overt symptoms and signs appear only after considerable damage has been done, giving the appearance that the damage has developed suddenly. In addition to a history and physical examination with careful elucidation of important factors, such as family history, alcohol or drug intake, recent history of a flulike illness, and history of abnormal physical examination findings or cardiac test results, the routine screening evaluation should include an electrocardiogram and an echocardiogram.

The electrocardiogram may provide clues to myocardial disease, such as conduction delays, an infarct or pseudoinfarct pattern, arrhythmia, or abnormal voltage. An echocardiogram is the easiest way to obtain definitive information about systolic function; it also provides information on the status of the pericardium and the cardiac valves. Also detectable on echocardiography are asymmetric septal hypertrophy and systolic anterior motion of the mitral valve (both signs of hypertrophic cardiomyopathy) as well as certain tissue-signature findings that may suggest an infiltrative process (granular sparkling in amyloid). If a patient is found to have systolic dysfunction and dilated cardiomyopathy, in most cases it is advisable to proceed with definitive invasive cardiac testing, including coronary angiography and endomyocardial biopsy, if these tests are available. In apparent cases of idiopathic dilated cardiomyopathy based strictly on clinical data, some other diagnosis is made by combining these two procedures in 5% to 10% of the cases. That is, myocarditis, some other infiltrative cardiomyopathy, or coronary artery disease may be detected, all of which may change the course of therapy. Consequently, it is important to obtain definitive information on all patients.

Finally, the identification of a genetic form of transmission in a significant proportion of patients with cardiomyopathies suggests the need for family screening. This is justified by the increased risk of disease in the relatives of patients, by the availability of sensitive noninvasive screening methods (in particular echocardiography), by the possibility of early diagnosis and prevention of complications, and by the growing availability of molecular diagnostic techniques. The identification of the molecular basis represents the first step toward a specific therapy for these disorders.

TREATMENT OF MYOCARDIAL DISEASE

Treatment of myocardial disease depends on the specific type of abnormality and its severity. The treatment of most types of myocardial disease, however, can be discussed in terms of general principles, as outlined in the following sections.

SPECIFIC THERAPY

Specific, targeted therapy should be the goal of treatment in all patients with myocardial disease, though, in actuality, this goal is achieved in only a small percentage of patients. The objective is to identify something that potentially can be corrected definitively and then to make that correction. In this category would be forms of myocardial disease and heart failure resulting from valvular heart disease that may respond to correction of the mechanical abnormality, such as aortic stenosis; sarcoidosis, which may improve with steroid therapy; hemochromatosis, which may be remedied by iron unloading; and hypertrophic cardiomyopathy refractory to medical management, which may be corrected by myectomy with or without mitral valve replacement. Patients with moderately severe left ventricular dysfunction and coronary artery lesions amenable to revascularization (in the rare case where the myocardium may be "hibernating" from lack of blood flow) are also possible candidates for specific therapy.

NONSPECIFIC MEDICAL THERAPY

For patients in whom definitive, specific therapy is not possible, nonspecific, symptomatic therapy is the only option. This therapy may consist of no therapy at all, a diuretic for congestive symptoms, the addition of digoxin and afterload reduction for more advanced congestive or low output symptoms, or inhibitors of the renin-angiotensin and adrenergic systems to favorably affect remodeling and lower mortality in dilated cardiomyopathies, or antiarrhythmic therapy for symptomatic arrhythmias. In hypertrophic cardiomyopathy, and possibly in some forms of restrictive cardiomyopathy, therapy to facilitate diastolic function can be attempted. Nonspecific, symptomatic therapy is indicated for patients with myocardial disease who have New York Heart Association class II or III symptoms, with no disability or mild disability, and in whom the prognosis is still relatively good (mortality rate less than 20% per year). Further details of

the therapeutic approach to the patient with congestive heart failure are discussed in Chapter 66.

DEFINITIVE THERAPY

When patients show signs of major disability (New York Heart Association class III or IV) or are at high risk of dying (estimated mortality rate more than 20% per year) for other reasons, definitive therapy in the form of cardiac replacement should be considered and performed if the subject meets eligibility criteria. Cardiac transplantation has emerged as a readily available, relatively straightforward procedure that offers even high-risk patients a high probability (more than 80%) of surviving 1 year and a better than 70% probability of surviving 5 years. Figure 74.4 shows the patient survival rate in the Utah Cardiac Transplant Program compared with the average survival rates calculated from five different natural history studies of dilated cardiomyopathy; it can be seen that survival is dramatically improved with cardiac transplantation. Moreover, after transplantation, patients lead an essentially normal life with excellent functional capacity.

The problem with cardiac transplantation is that the number of donors is limited, probably at an upper limit of 4,000 to 5,000 per year. If 250,000 patients in the United States have myocardial disease (probably an underestimate) and, conservatively speaking, one-fourth of them would benefit from cardiac transplantation, there is a potential donor–recipient mismatch of 1:10. This lifesaving procedure therefore is not available to all patients who could benefit from it. Obviously, medical approaches need to be developed that reverse or stabilize the generally unfavorable natural history of myocardial disease.

▌ RENIN-ANGIOTENSIN SYSTEM INHIBITORS IN DILATED CARDIOMYOPATHIES

Controlled trials with angiotensin-converting enzyme (ACE) inhibitors (enalapril) in dilated cardiomyopathies have confirmed

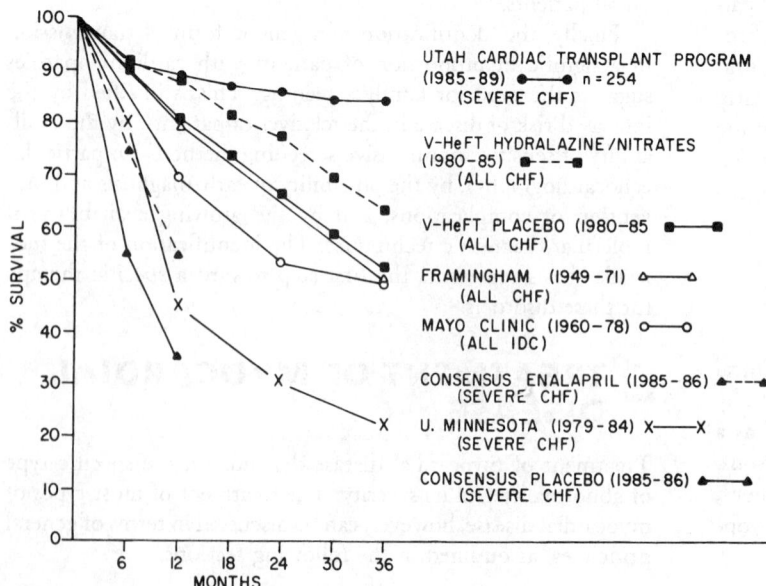

FIGURE 74.4. Survival in a cardiac transplant population (n = 254) with severe, end-stage heart failure due to myocardial disease versus survival in patients with symptomatic treatment or no treatment for heart failure.

a modest decline in mortality rates. The reason behind this decrease in mortality rates and ACE inhibition is not known, although an improvement in the neurohumoral profile and reduction in left ventricular size, leading to an improved myocardial oxygen demand–supply relationship, have been postulated. Recently the addition of the aldosterone antagonist spironolactone has been shown to confer additional survival benefit to subjects with dilated cardiomyopathies (the RALES Trial). Further discussion of the use of renin-angiotensin system inhibitors in subjects with heart failure from primary or secondary cardiomyopathies can be found in Chapter 66.

β-BLOCKING AGENTS IN DILATED CARDIOMYOPATHIES

Because cardiac adrenergic drive is activated in the failing human heart and this sustained activation has multiple potential deleterious effects, it has been postulated that β-blocking agents can favorably affect outcome in dilated cardiomyopathies. Indeed, as observed first in small uncontrolled trials and then later in placebo-controlled medium sized trials, β-blockers consistently improve left ventricular function and attenuate or reverse the remodeling process in subjects with nonischemic or ischemic dilated cardiomyopathies. Recently the β-blocking agents carvedilol, bisoprolol, and metropolol have been shown to substantially reduce mortality in subjects with mild to moderate heart failure from dilated cardiomyopathies. Thus β-blocker therapy in this myocardial disease phenotype has been established. Further discussion of the use of β-blocking agents in subjects with heart failure from primary or secondary cardiomyopathies can be found in Chapter 66.

IMMUNOSUPPRESSION FOR MYOCARDITIS

Uncontrolled trials have demonstrated temporally related improvement in cardiac function after the use of immunosuppressive agents, with concomitant improvement in mononuclear infiltrate on endomyocardial biopsy. Spontaneous improvement also may occur in myocarditis, however, and it is unclear whether immunosuppressive therapy is warranted based on controlled clinical trials. It is clear that immunosuppressive therapy should not be applied generally to patients with idiopathic dilated cardiomyopathy.

CYTOTOXIC/COLCHICINE THERAPY FOR CARDIAC AMYLOID

Evidence suggests that tissue deposition by amyloid may be reversed by using alkylating agents and steroids or colchicine. Although this approach has undergone only limited trials in cardiac amyloid, it is a possible interventional strategy in this relatively common disease that has an otherwise dismal prognosis. Such

an approach should be considered unproved, however, and there is the need for a controlled clinical trial to address the question of efficacy and the risks and benefits.

ANTIARRHYTHMIC THERAPY IN CARDIOMYOPATHIES

Because nearly all antiarrhythmic agents depress cardiac function and because most of them carry a high potential for being proarrhythmic in patients with myocardial disease, routine use of antiarrhythmic agents cannot be recommended in this group of patients. In general, antiarrhythmic therapy should be reserved for patients with a family history of sudden death, those with sustained ventricular tachycardia, or those with symptomatic arrhythmias. In such subjects amiodarone and sotalol are the only agents that have established an adequate safety profile, perhaps because both are Type III antiarrythmics with β-blocking properties. Finally, the use of implantable defibrillators in selected individuals within the above-described clinical settings clearly has efficacy, but is expensive and, as a result, somewhat controversial.

BIBLIOGRAPHY

Bristow MR. β-adrenergic receptor blockade in chronic heart failure. *Circulation* (in press).

Bristow MR. Drug toxicity and the heart: potential molecular mechanisms. In: Symons C, Evans T, Mitchell AG, eds. *Specific heart muscle disease.* Littleton, Mass.: John Wright & Sons, 1983.

Bristow MR. Why does the myocardium fail? New insights from basic science. *Lancet* 1998;352:(Suppl I): 8–14.

Bristow MR, Mason JW, Billingham ME, et al. Dose–effect and structure–function relationships in doxorubicin cardiomyopathy. *Am Heart J* 1981;102:709–718.

CONSENSUS Trial Study Group. Effects of enalapril on mortality in severe congestive heart failure. Results of the Cooperative North Scandinavian Enalapril Survival Study (CONSENSUS). *N Engl J Med* 1987;316: 1429–1435.

Dec GW, Fuster V. Idiopathic dilated cardiomyopathy. *N Engl J Med* 1994; 331:1564–1575.

Eichhorn EJ, Bristow MR. Medical therapy can improve the biologic properties of the chronically failing heart: A new era in the treatment of heart failure. *Circulation* 1996;94:2285–2296.

Fowles RE, Cloward TV, Yowell RL. Endocardial fibrosis associated with fenfluramine-phentermine. *N Engl J Med* 1998;338(18):1316.

Kasper EK, Agema WRP, Hutchins GM, et al. The causes of dilated cardiomyopathy: a clinicopathologic review of 673 consecutive patients. *J Am Coll Cardiol* 1994;23:586–590.

Lange LG, Schreiner GF. Immune mechanisms of cardiac disease. *N Engl J Med* 1994;330:1129–1135.

McKenna WJ, Thiene G, Nava A, et al. Diagnosis of arrhythmogenic right ventricular dysplasia/cardiomyopathy. Task force of the Working Group Myocardial and Pericardial Disease of the European Society of Cardiology and of the Scientific Council on Cardiomyopathies of the International Society and Federation of Cardiology. *Br Heart J* 1994;71: 215–218.

Pitt B, Zannad F, Femme WJ, et al. The effect of spironolactone on morbidity and mortality in patients with severe heart failure. Randomized Aldactone Evaluation Study Investigators. *N Engl J Med* 1999;34(10): 709–717.

Richardson P, McKenna W, Bristow M, et al. Report of the 1995 World Health Organization/International Society and Federation of Cardiology Task Force on the Definition and Classification of Cardiomyopathies. *Circulation* 1996;93:841–842.

Schwartz K, Carrier L, Guicheney P, et al. Molecular basis of familial cardio-myopathies. *Circulation* 1995;91:532–540.

Wigle ED, Rakowski H, Kimball BP, et al. Hypertrophic cardiomyopathy: clinical spectrum and treatment. *Circulation* 1995;92:1680–1692.

Kelley's Textbook of Internal Medicine, fourth edition. Edited by H. David Humes. Lippincott Williams & Wilkins, Philadelphia © 2000.

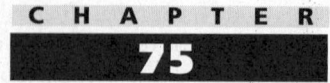

CHAPTER 75

TUMORS OF THE HEART

JOEL S. RAICHLEN
MARTIN G. ST. JOHN SUTTON

Tumors affecting the heart and pericardium are relatively rare, but their identification is extremely important because they may have disastrous clinical consequences that can be prevented or relieved by surgical resection. Unfortunately, most cardiac tumors are clinically silent and those that are not produce a wide variety of nonspecific signs and symptoms. In the past, cardiac tumors were interesting anomalies rarely diagnosed before death. With the introduction of cardiac catheterization, angiographic techniques provided the first means of diagnosing cardiac tumors during life. The development of M-mode echocardiography permitted the noninvasive detection of cardiac masses, but its sensitivity was low; angiography was generally required to assess the size and location of cardiac masses. In the 1980s contrast angiography was largely replaced by two-dimensional echocardiography as the diagnostic method of choice. Today, the diagnosis of cardiac tumors has been enhanced further by the development of transesophageal echocardiography, computed tomography, and magnetic resonance imaging. Guided by this information, elective surgical exploration can be performed for cardiac tumors without the need for invasive studies. The timely removal of cardiac tumors can be curative for most benign tumors and palliative for malignant tumors.

CLINICAL MANIFESTATIONS OF CARDIAC TUMORS

Cardiac tumors are detected in only 5% to 10% of patients because they rarely produce symptoms; when they do so, they are nonspecific and do not suggest the diagnosis. Symptoms, if any, are usually related to the size or the location of the tumor. The clinical manifestations of cardiac tumors result from mass effects, tissue infiltration, embolism, or systemic or immune responses to the tumor or its breakdown products (Table 75.1).

MASS EFFECTS

Clinical signs and symptoms resulting from mass effects occur when tumors protrude into the inflow or outflow tracts of the

---

TABLE 75.1.   CLINICAL PRESENTATIONS OF CARDIAC TUMORS

Specific Manifestations	Clinical Consequences
Mass effects	Mass effects
Obstruction to left-sided heart filling	Pulmonary hypertension
Obstruction of valves	Signs and symptoms of valvular stenosis
Mechanical disruption of valves	Signs and symptoms of valvular regurgitation
Mechanical destruction of cells by tumor	Hemolytic anemia, thrombocytopenia
Inflow- or outflow-tract obstruction	Syncope, dyspnea, ascites, peripheral edema, cor pulmonale, congestive heart failure, paroxysmal nocturnal dyspnea, orthopnea, pulmonary edema
Embolism	Embolism
Coronary emboli	Obstruction, vascular aneurysms
Pulmonary emboli	Chest pain/angina, myocardial infarction
Systemic emboli	Pleuritic chest pain, pulmonary hypertension
	Acute neurologic, abdominal, retroperitoneal, or peripheral ischemic events
Infiltration	Infiltration
Infiltration of ventricular myocardium	Regional dyssynergia, congestive heart failure
Infiltration of atrial or ventricular tissue	Atrial or ventricular tachyarrhythmias
Infiltration of the conduction system	Heart block, sudden death
Pericardial infiltration or constriction	Pleuritic chest pain, constrictive pericarditis, pericardial effusion, cardiac tamponade
Tumor-mediated effects	Tumor-mediated effects
Systemic or immune response to tumor, its breakdown products, or serum proteins mechanically damaged by tumor motion	Constitutional symptoms, rash, polymyositis, hepatic dysfunction, Raynaud's phenomenon, thrombocytosis, leukocytosis, polycythemia, elevated erythrocyte sedimentation rate, hypergammaglobulinemia

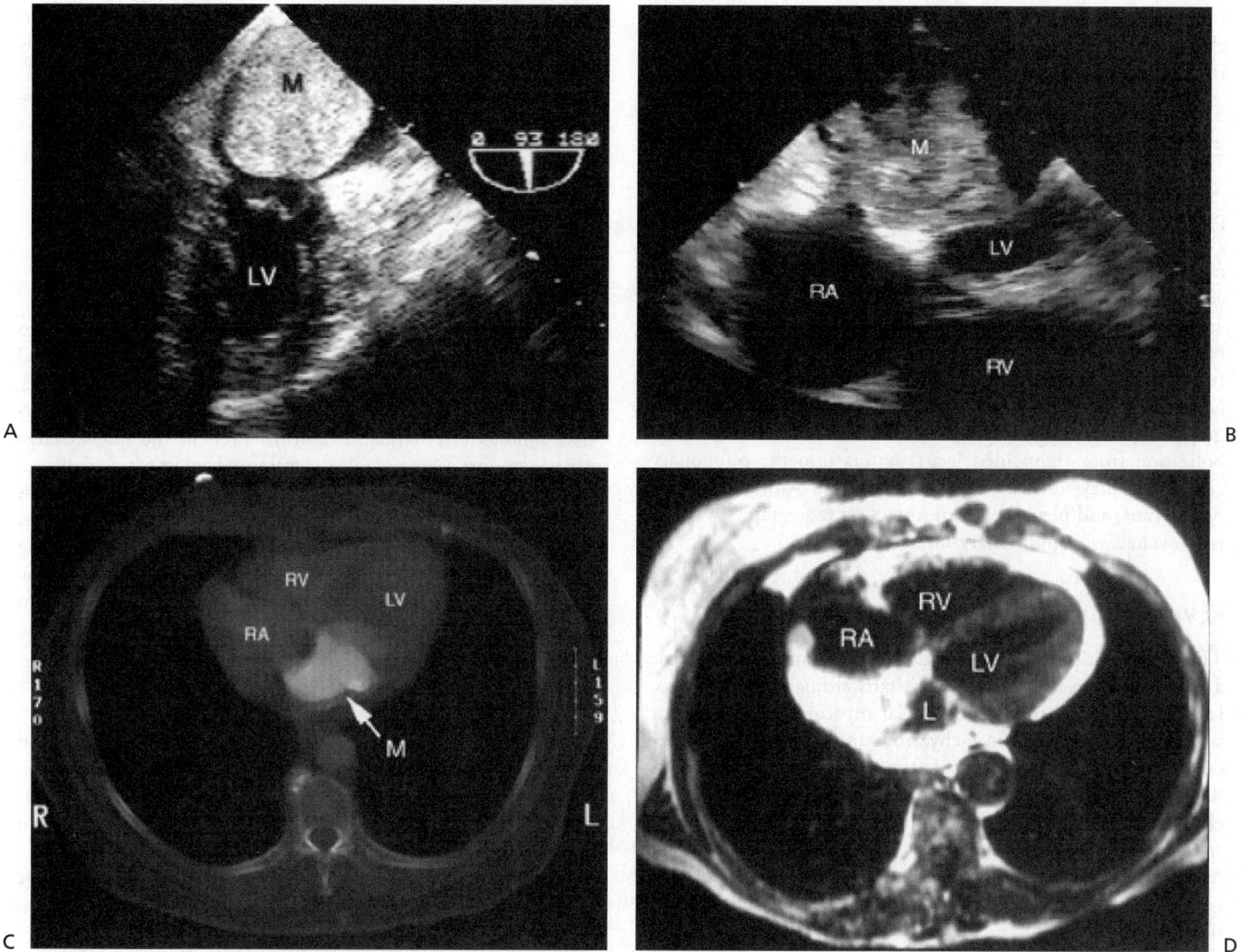

FIGURE 75.1. Imaging of primary tumors. **A:** Transesophageal echocardiogram showing a large myxoma (M) filling the left atrium of the heart. **B:** Transesophageal echocardiogram showing a large left atrial myxoma (M) with a surface made up of irregular projections. **C:** Computed tomographic (CT) scan of the heart showing a densely calcified myxoma (M) filling the left atrium. **D:** T1-weighted electrocardiography-gated magnetic resonance image (MRI) showing lipomatous hypertrophy of the interatrial septum that is contiguous with the epicardial fat surrounding the atria. Note that the tissue intensity is similar to that of the epicardial fat surrounding the ventricles and the subcutaneous fat. L, left atrium; LV, left ventricle; RA, right atrium; RV, right ventricle.

right or left heart chambers, interfering with blood flow (Fig. 75.1A). Minor degrees of obstruction create heart murmurs. As tumors enlarge sufficiently to produce major obstruction to blood flow, they may give rise to frank heart failure. Tumors affecting the right heart chambers can partially or totally obstruct systemic venous return, causing superior vena cava syndrome with facial and upper-extremity edema. Obstruction of drainage from the inferior vena cava or to the egress of blood from the right heart chambers is associated with peripheral edema, hepatomegaly, ascites, and dyspnea on exertion owing to an inability to increase cardiac output. Slowly growing tumors of the left heart chambers may impede diastolic filling, resulting in dyspnea

and pulmonary hypertension mimicking the symptom complex of mitral stenosis.

Cardiac tumors that interfere with atrioventricular or semilunar valve function do so by mass effect or by distortion of the fibrous skeleton of the heart. They cause valvular regurgitation or, less frequently, stenosis, along with their associated murmurs. Severe disruption of mitral valve function can lead to orthopnea, paroxysmal nocturnal dyspnea, or pulmonary edema. Obstruction to aortic outflow can result in chest pain, syncope, or congestive heart failure. Mobile intracardiac tumors—most commonly atrial myxoma—occasionally generate a tumor plop as the forward motion of the tumor is arrested. Depending on the location of mobile tumors, the auscultatory findings may change with body position—murmurs will increase in the upright position and decrease or disappear in the supine position.

EMBOLISM

Many tumors are friable, with irregular, fibrillated surfaces that predispose to in situ thrombus formation and embolization (Fig. 75.1B). Systemic embolization from left-sided heart tumors may occlude local blood flow and become evident as strokes, transient cerebral ischemic attacks, or seizures from emboli to the brain; as acute abdominal pain from infarction of intra-abdominal or retroperitoneal organs; or as sudden onset of extremity ischemia from peripheral emboli. Coronary artery embolism is rare and is associated with the acute onset of chest pain and electrocardiographic findings suggesting myocardial ischemia or necrosis. Embolization from right-sided heart tumors into the pulmonary circulation may also cause acute chest pain, with or without hemoptysis, and pleural effusions on chest radiography when it is associated with pulmonary infarction.

MYOCARDIAL INFILTRATION

Tumor infiltration of the myocardium or pericardium may cause a wide spectrum of clinical and electrocardiographic findings. Infiltration of the atrial or ventricular myocardium or adjacent pericardium may result in tachyarrhythmias as well as nonspecific ST-T wave abnormalities on the resting 12-lead electrocardiogram, indicating altered myocardial repolarization. Other electrocardiographic findings that may be caused by tumor infiltration of the myocardium include reduced QRS voltage, left or right atrial enlargement, and left or right ventricular hypertrophy. Bundle-branch block or varying degrees of heart block may result from infiltration of conduction tissue. Advancing infiltration of the myocardium (Fig. 75.2A) results in regional dyssynergia, followed by clinical evidence of contractile dysfunction and, finally, progressive heart failure. Pericardial infiltration initially may take the form of friction rubs, effusions that can produce cardiac tamponade, or pericardial encasement and clinical signs of constrictive pericarditis.

CONSTITUTIONAL SYMPTOMS

Tumors may be associated with such nonspecific symptoms as fever, malaise, arthralgia, polymyositis, Raynaud's phenomenon, weight loss, and cachexia. Hematologic and hepatic abnormalities include anemia, polycythemia, thrombocytopenia, thrombocytosis, leukocytosis, hypergammaglobulinemia, elevated erythrocyte sedimentation rate, and elevations of hepatic transaminases and alkaline phosphatase levels. These abnormal hematologic and biochemical findings are believed to result from immune responses to the tumor and its breakdown products, to mechanical damage to blood cells and serum proteins by tumor motion, or to tumor secretion products. The combination of these constitutional symptoms, hematologic abnormalities, and cardiac murmurs can mimic bacterial endocarditis. The diagnosis of cardiac tumors from the constellation of nonspecific signs

and symptoms described here depends largely upon the clinician's level of awareness and vigilance. If the presence of a cardiac tumor is even a remote possibility, noninvasive imaging is mandatory to establish the diagnosis and to evaluate the characteristics of the tumor.

■ DIAGNOSTIC IMAGING MODALITIES

CHEST ROENTGENOGRAM

Chest radiography was the first clinical diagnostic technique to suggest the presence of cardiac tumors. Its usefulness was related to its ability to identify intracardiac calcification. Otherwise, chest radiography is of limited diagnostic value, because the cardiac silhouette is frequently normal even in the face of large cardiac tumors. One notable exception is benign pericardial cyst, which frequently appears as a well-defined, round or ovoid mass with sharply circumscribed, smooth borders in the right or, less frequently, the left cardiophrenic angle. Pericardial cysts lie along the cardiac silhouette in all projections, in the cardiophrenic angle in 90% of cases, and adjacent to the left or right atrium in 10% of cases.

ANGIOCARDIOGRAPHY

Tumors appear as filling defects on contrast angiograms and deform or encroach on the lumina of the cardiac chambers or the great vessels entering or leaving the heart. Rarely, arteriography will show evidence of tumor circulation in the form of discrete vessels or as a diffuse blush of dye. Angiography largely has been superseded by the current capabilities of noninvasive imaging techniques and is rarely employed today in the diagnostic evaluation of suspected cardiac tumors.

ECHOCARDIOGRAPHY

Two-dimensional echocardiography was the first diagnostic tool to provide complete images of cardiac tumors. The ability of transthoracic and/or transesophageal echocardiography to make the heart visible in multiple planes allows for determination of the size, location, shape, attachments, and mobility of cardiac masses and their anatomic relationship to surrounding structures. The accuracy with which the specific site of attachment can be determined makes it the only imaging study necessary before surgical excision in the majority of cases. When histologic diagnosis is required, the high-resolution images of the cardiac chambers provided by transesophageal echocardiography can be used to help guide transvascular biopsy. When right atrial tumors are present, imaging of the superior and inferior vena cava must be performed, to ensure that primary tumors do not arise within them and that metastatic tumors do not extend from them into the right atrium (Fig. 75.2B). This is particularly important when surgical resection is contemplated, because such involvement may interfere with the placement of central lines or with caval cannulation for cardiopulmonary bypass.

Echocardiography plays an important role in the evaluation

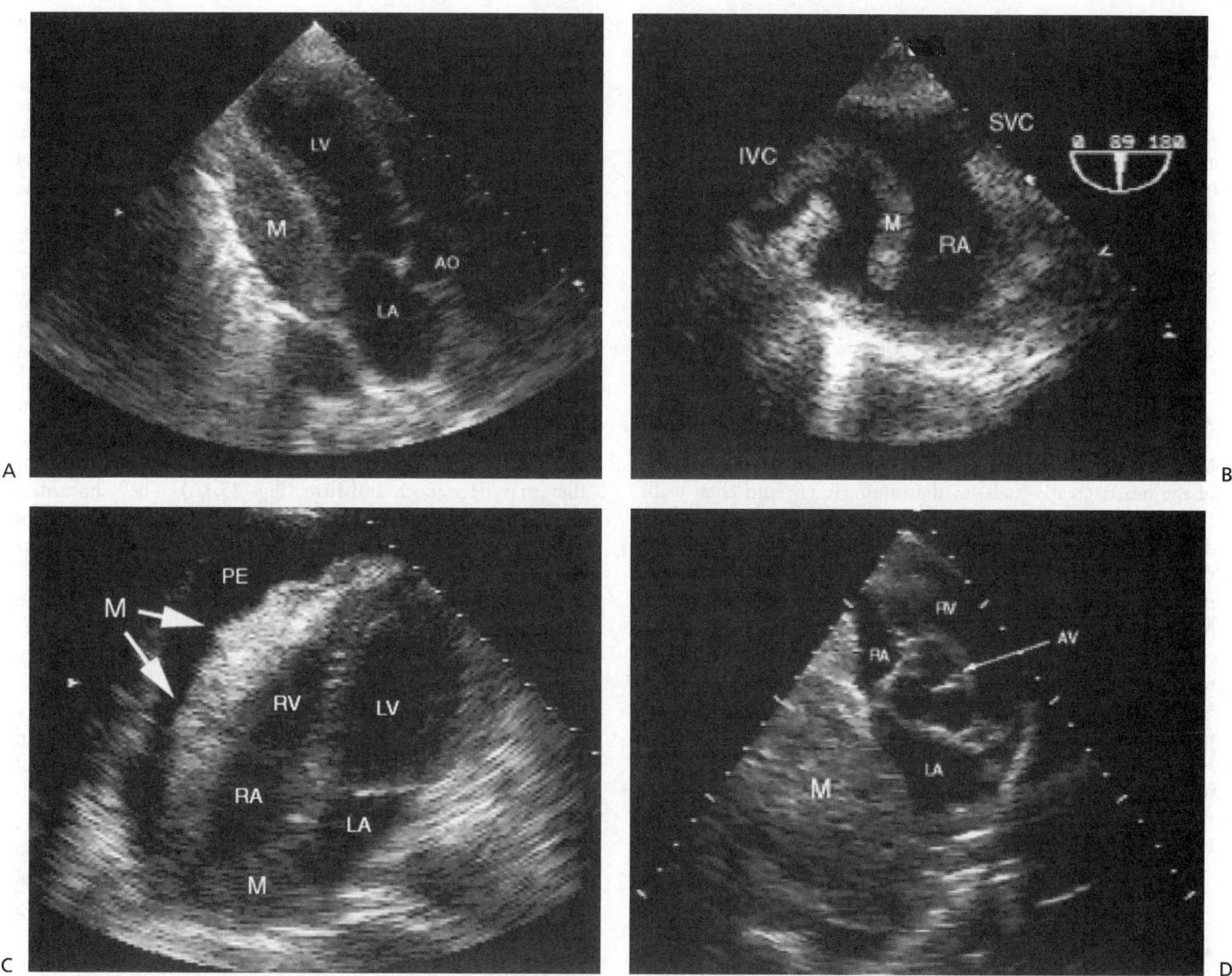

FIGURE 75.2. Metastatic tumors. **A:** Transthoracic echocardiogram showing a metastatic lung carcinoma (M) infiltrating the inferior wall of the left ventricle (LV). **B:** Transesophageal echocardiogram showing tumor mass (M) from a renal cell carcinoma that extends through the inferior vena cava (IVC) and into the right atrium (RA). **C:** Transthoracic echocardiogram showing a pericardial effusion (PE) associated with extensive epicardial metastases (*arrows*) from a metastatic melanoma (M) that also infiltrates the region of the interatrial septum. **D:** Transthoracic echocardiogram showing a large metastatic sarcoma compressing the right atrium (RA) and the left atrium (LA). AO, aorta; AV, aortic valve; RV, right ventricle; SVC, superior vena cava.

of tumors extending from or infiltrating the myocardium. While tumors of moderate size are easily distinguished from adjacent myocardium, small sessile or intramural tumors are more difficult to detect. The presence of a tumor is suggested by differences in echocardiographic intensity compared with the surrounding myocardium and by the identification of areas with asymmetric thickening, especially when they are associated with hypokinetic wall motion.

Echocardiography is the diagnostic study of choice for identifying tumors originating on cardiac valves. When transthoracic echocardiograms do not adequately depict these structures, transesophageal echocardiography should be used, since it provides high-resolution images of the mitral, aortic, and tricuspid

valves. When tumors obstruct cardiac valves or the inflow or outflow regions of cardiac chambers, conventional Doppler echocardiography can provide estimates of the pressure gradients generated as blood passes around the obstructing mass. When tumors disrupt the function of valves, color-flow Doppler echocardiography is useful for assessing the severity of valvular regurgitation.

COMPUTED TOMOGRAPHY

Computed tomographic radiologic imaging techniques are unencumbered by the chest wall, ribs, and lungs that surround the heart. The motion of the heart limits the diagnostic usefulness of conventional computed tomography (CT) imaging of small, mobile, or valvular tumors. Motion artifacts can be limited with more rapid acquisition techniques, such as spiral CT or ultrafast (cine) CT. CT scans are extremely useful in diagnosing cardiac tumors that infiltrate the pericardium, the great vessels, and the tissue surrounding the heart. The relative heterogeneity of the tissue making up the tumors can be characterized, as can its overall radiodensity, which can be compared with that of muscle and subcutaneous fat. CT is also useful in pinpointing the presence of calcifications within tumor masses (Fig. 75.1C). The primary usefulness of CT imaging for cardiac tumors resides in its ability to determine the extent of any myocardial, pericardial, and mediastinal extension of cardiac tumors.

MAGNETIC RESONANCE IMAGING

Magnetic resonance imaging (MRI) provides tomographic views of the heart, great vessels, mediastinum, lungs, and chest wall. By using differences between static tissue and flowing blood and differences in soft-tissue contrast, this technique makes possible the assessment of the extent of tumor invasion into great vessels, the myocardium, the pericardium, and the surrounding tissues. MRI has advantages over CT in the absence of ionizing radiation, the general lack of contrast requirement, and the ability to acquire several orthogonal or oblique projections directly. MRI is also useful for tissue characterization, particularly in differentiating lipomatous tumors with signal intensities similar to subcutaneous fat from thrombi, myxoma, or other soft-tissue tumors (Fig. 75.1D). Although this technique can also suggest the relative homogeneity of a tumor, tissue characterization by MRI cannot distinguish between benign and malignant tumors.

▇ PRIMARY CARDIAC TUMORS

Primary tumors of the heart are rare; their prevalence in autopsy series ranges from 0.0017 to 0.33%. Today, when two-dimensional echocardiography serves as a screening test in the evaluation of many diverse clinical symptom complexes, it is increasingly common for cardiac tumors to be unexpected findings on clinical echocardiograms. When a primary tumor is identified, its classification is aided by knowledge of the distribution and relative incidence of tumors found in the heart (Table 75.2).

BENIGN CARDIAC TUMORS

In large series, roughly 80% of primary cardiac tumors are benign (range, 60% to 90%). The majority of benign cardiac tumors are myxomas, which predominate in adults aged 30 to 60 years, with a 3:1 female predominance. The majority of cases occur sporadically, while about 7% are familial, inherited as an autosomal dominant trait. In a series of 130 myxoma patients, 65% had initial symptoms of valvular heart disease, 36% had embolic phenomena, 5% experienced sudden death, 4% had pericarditis, 3% had myocardial infarction, and 2% had fever of unknown origin. Only 16% of patients were asymptomatic. Myxomas can develop anywhere within the heart, though the

majority are found in the atria. More than 80% are discovered in the left atrium (Fig. 75.1), and most of the remainder are in the right atrium. Less than 2% of myxomas arise in the ventricles; rare cases have been reported in the valve or the inferior vena cava. Occasionally, there can be several myxomas; in this case, biatrial involvement is most common. The findings of several tumors and ventricular involvement are more common in the context of familial myxomas.

For the majority of cardiac myxomas, surgical resection is curative. The size of the tumor and its site of attachment are important in planning the surgical approach. Approximately 90% of myxomas are attached to the interatrial septum in the region of the fossa ovalis. They may be pedunculated or sessile, with a relatively broad base of attachment. They are frequently polypoid and friable, with a gelatinous, mucoid appearance associated with areas of hemorrhage and superficial thrombosis. Their surfaces may have frondlike excrescences (Fig. 75.1B), or they may be smooth and firm (Fig. 75.1A). The echocardiographic appearance of atrial myxomas correlates with the tumor characteristics on surgical inspection. Tumors that appear compliant and deformable are usually gelatinous, papillary, and friable, while those that appear nondeformable are more likely to be firm, smooth, and nonfriable. These differences are important, in that the former group of tumors has a greater frequency of embolization.

The second most common benign cardiac tumor is papillary fibroelastoma. Although these tumors can develop anywhere in the heart, 90% are found on the valves—the aortic and mitral valves more often than the tricuspid and pulmonic valves. Although valvular tumors are usually solitary and asymptomatic, papillary fibroelastomas can sometimes be found several at a time and have been associated with embolization. One study of 56 primary valve tumors found that 93% were benign. Papillary fibroelastomas were the most common histologic type, accounting for 73% of tumors; myxomas were found in 9% and fibromas in 7%. In that study, 53% of mitral valve tumors and 19% of aortic valve tumors produced serious neurologic symptoms or sudden death. In contrast, another study of 42 papillary fibroelastomas found that 93% manifested no symptoms attributable to the tumor.

The remaining benign cardiac tumors are very uncommon. Lipomas are sessile or polypoid tumors that originate in the subepicardium or subendocardium or in an intramuscular location. They are typically encapsulated, they may appear singly or several at a time, and they occur throughout the heart and pericardium. Lipomas are distinguished from lipomatous hypertrophy of the interatrial septum, which represents nonencapsulated adipose tissue that involves the interatrial septum and is in continuity with epicardial fat. In histologic features, both represent homogeneous accumulations of mature fat cells that can be identified by their tissue signature on CT or MR images (Fig. 75.1D).

Fibromas are more common in children than adults, are almost always single, and develop within the ventricular myocardium, most frequently in the septum or the left ventricular free wall. They are firm tumors that may compress surrounding structures. These benign tumors have been resected from the

TABLE 75.2.	DISTRIBUTION OF CARDIAC TUMORS IN ADULTS

Primary benign tumors (2–4% of cardiac tumors)

	Percentage of Benign Tumors (range)	Sites Within the Heart
Myxoma	75 (49–92)	Left interatrial septum > right atrium > ventricles
Papillary fibroelastoma	8 (6–16)	Cardiac valves, left > right
Lipoma	3 (2–7)	Throughout the heart
Fibroma	2 (1–9)	Left ventricle > right ventricle
Hemangioma	2 (≤5)	Throughout the heart
Endodermal heterotopia	1 (≤4)	Atrioventricular node

Primary Malignant Tumors (1–2% of cardiac tumors)

	Percentage of Primary Malignant Tumors (range)	Sites Within the Heart
Angiosarcoma	25 (17–37)	Majority in the right atrium
Rhabdomyosarcoma	13 (3–24)	Throughout the heart
Fibrosarcoma	10 (6–19)	Left atrial predominance
Undifferentiated sarcoma	9 (7–24)	Half in left atrium
Mesothelioma	6 (≤16)	Pericardium
Leiomyosarcoma	6 (≤9)	Majority in left atrium
Malignant fibrous histiocytoma	5 (≤24)	Majority in left atrium
Osteosarcoma	5 (≤9)	Left atrium

Secondary malignant tumors (95–97% of cardiac tumors)

	Percentage of Secondary Malignant Tumors (range)	Routes of Metastasis
Lung carcinoma	30 (26–48)	Direct extension > lymphatic > hematogenous
Breast carcinoma	14 (9–19)	Direct extension, lymphatic
Leukemia	10 (7–14)	Hematogenous
Lymphoma	10 (8–13)	Hematogenous, lymphatic, direct extension
Melanoma	5 (3–8)	Hematogenous
Esophageal carcinoma	4 (3–6)	Direct extension
Renal carcinoma	2 (1–4)	Venous extension, hematogenous

apex or ventricular free wall, but those involving the interventricular septum are frequently inoperable.

Hemangiomas are composed of proliferations of endothelial cells that form blood-filled channels that can create a so-called tumor blush on coronary arteriography. They can arise anywhere in the heart. Endodermal heterotopia (formerly thought to be mesothelioma) involving the conduction tissue is made up of nests of cells that arise in the region of the atrioventricular node. Although these tumors are benign in histologic features, they typically cause complete heart block and have been associated with ventricular fibrillation. They are the most common primary tumor associated with sudden death, followed closely by fibromas.

Rhabdomyomas are the most common tumors among pediatric patients but are exceedingly rare in adults. These tumors usually appear in groups deeply embedded in the right or left ventricular wall. They may regress completely, such that surgery is recommended only for refractory arrhythmias or critical hemodynamic compromise. Rhabdomyomas are found in 58% of children and 18% of adults with tuberous sclerosis, which is a complex of congenital anomalies inherited as an autosomal dominant trait. Teratomas are even more rare adult tumors that

are more frequently found in young patients. They are extracardiac intrapericardial tumors that contain cysts and generally arise from the base of the heart.

PRIMARY MALIGNANT TUMORS

Although primary benign tumors in adults usually develop in the left atrium, primary malignant tumors are more often found in the right atrium. More than 80% of primary malignant neoplasms are sarcomas, making them the second most common type of primary cardiac tumor. The most prevalent primary malignant tumor is angiosarcoma, which is characterized by malignant cells that form vascular channels. These tumors occur throughout adulthood, at mean ages of 40 to 50 years. They are two to three times more common in men. Some 60% to 70% arise in the right atrium. They are aggressive tumors that rapidly expand into the adjacent myocardium and pericardium and frequently metastasize to the lungs and mediastinal lymph nodes.

The malignant cells in rhabdomyosarcoma have features of striated muscle. These tumors have similar incidence rates in all adult age groups and are slightly more prevalent in men. They are found throughout the chambers of the heart and pericardium. Fibrosarcomas, osteosarcomas, and leiomyosarcomas are less common malignant tumors that most frequently develop within the left atrium. Malignant fibrous histiocytoma involves fibroblasts and pleomorphic histiocytoid cells. These tumors have an age at onset similar to that of angiosarcomas, but they exhibit no gender predominance. Over 80% occur in the left atrium, most often on the posterior wall, where they can obstruct pulmonary veins or the mitral valve or cause mitral regurgitation. Malignant mesotheliomas are multicentric tumors that arise from the visceral or parietal pericardium. They may become quite large and compress the great vessels as they enter or leave the heart. In general, these tumors diffusely affect the pericardium and may encase the heart, though they rarely invade the myocardium.

METASTATIC CARDIAC TUMORS

In autopsy series, cardiac metastases have been reported 20 to 40 times more often than primary cardiac tumors; recent estimates suggest that they may occur more than 100 times more frequently. An average of 10% of patients with metastatic malignant disease have myocardial metastases, and another 5% show signs of involvement limited to the pericardium. Cardiac involvement is found in 19% of patients with lung metastases and only 2.7% of patients without lung involvement. Factors suggested to explain this relatively low incidence of cardiac metastasis include mechanical damage of blood-borne metastatic cells as they are deformed by myocardial contraction, metabolic peculiarities of striated muscle, rapid coronary blood flow, and restricted lymphatic connections that are predominantly directed away from the heart, thus requiring metastasis via that route to progress against the direction of lymphatic flow.

Almost all types of malignant tumors have been found to metastasize to the heart; the most common is carcinoma of the lung. In decreasing order, the next most prevalent cancers found to metastasize to the heart are carcinoma of the breast, leukemia, lymphoma, and malignant melanoma. Melanomas are the most likely malignancies to involve the heart; metastases are found in more than 50% of cases in most autopsy series. Cardiac involvement is also found in up to half of all patients with leukemia, one-fourth of patients with bronchogenic carcinoma, and one-fifth of patients with breast carcinoma or lymphoma.

Metastatic tumors of the heart may take the form of intramyocardial masses (Fig. 75.2A), intracavitary masses (Fig. 75.2B), masses extending from the epicardial surface of the heart into pericardial effusions (Fig. 75.2C), or extracardiac masses that surround and/or compress chambers of the heart (Fig. 75.2D). When metastatic tumor involves cardiac chambers, the right side of the heart is more frequently involved than the left. In right atrial metastases, it is important to examine the inferior vena cava, to assess venous extension from the kidney, liver, or other abdominal organ (Fig. 75.2B).

When metastatic disease reaches the heart by direct extension, as in carcinomas of the lung, breast, and esophagus, it usually is associated with diffuse pericardial involvement. Other routes for cardiac metastases include embolic hematogenous spread, as in malignant melanomas and leukemias, and spread via lymphatic channels, as in breast carcinomas and lymphomas. In more than half of patients with cardiac metastasis from lung cancer, the primary tumor is distant from the heart. In these cases, metastasis occurs via lymphatic spread or, less often, by a hematogenous pathway. Lymphatic spread is the most typical route of metastasis in the context of malignant pericardial effusions. Metastases from lung and breast carcinomas may affect the pericardium without obvious cardiac involvement, while melanoma and leukemia usually metastasize to the heart with or without pericardial involvement.

Cardiac metastases to the pericardium may be associated with signs and symptoms of acute pericarditis, constrictive pericarditis, or pericardial effusions that can progress to cardiac tamponade. Pericardial metastases may preclude operative intervention in otherwise resectable noncardiac tumors. Metastatic involvement of the pericardium may take the form of irregularly appearing nodules attached to the visceral or parietal pericardium (Fig. 75.2C). In the context of externally compressing masses, diffuse pericardial thickening may be evident. In a patient with a known primary malignancy, echocardiographic evidence of discrete epicardial masses that move with the cardiac cycle and protrude into a pericardial effusion is highly suggestive of pericardial metastases.

■ TREATMENT AND PROGNOSIS

The recognition of cardiac tumors is important because of the potentially devastating consequences of embolic phenomena and hemodynamic obstruction. Unfortunately, most tumors of the heart metastasize from other organs. Early detection of primary tumors allows for surgical resection, which is frequently curative of benign neoplasms and may prolong survival in patients with malignant ones. Although aggressively debulking primary malignant tumors may retard their dissemination, such operations are only palliative. Postoperative irradiation occasionally is useful in shrinking tumor masses and transiently alleviating symptoms, whereas adjuvant chemotherapy is not often of benefit. Orthotopic cardiac transplantation offers the opportunity of completely removing unresectable tumors. Thus far, it has achieved only limited success in a small number of cases.

In metastatic disease, therapy should be focused on the specific type of tumor and on the clinical manifestations. Cardiac side effects of the malignant growths should be vigorously treated, including medical therapy of heart failure and pacemaker insertion for symptomatic heart block. Hemodynamically significant effusions warrant pericardiocentesis, which may have to be performed repeatedly or require placement of a pericardial–pleural window to obviate life-threatening cardiac tamponade. Reaccumulation of effusions can be prevented by instilling tetracycline, chemotherapeutic agents, or radioisotopes. Excision should be considered for resectable intracavitary tumors causing obstruction or peripheral emboli, particularly when extension and growth of the primary tumor is thought to be under control. Other therapeutic tools should be selected on a tumor-specific basis, such as hormonal and chemotherapy for patients with effusions associated with breast cancer and radiation therapy for pericardial disease in patients with leukemia or lymphoma. With few exceptions, the prognosis remains poor in patients with primary or secondary malignant tumors of the heart.

BIBLIOGRAPHY

Burke A, Virmani R. Tumors of the heart and great vessels. In: xxxxxx, xxxxxxx, eds. *Atlas of tumor pathology*, fascicle 16, third series. Washington, D.C.: Armed Forces Institute of Pathology, 1996.

Casey M, Mah C, Merliss AD, et al. Identification of a novel genetic locus for familial cardiac myxomas and Carney complex. *Circulation* 1998; 98:2560–2566.

Cina SJ, Smialek JE, Burke AP, et al. Primary cardiac tumors causing sudden death: a review of the literature. *Am J Forensic Med Pathol* 1996;17: 271–281.

Edwards FH, Hale D, Cohen A, et al. Primary cardiac valve tumors. *Ann Thorac Surg* 1991;52:1127–1131.

Hehrlein FW, Dapper F. Tumors of the heart. Proceedings of the Third Symposium on Cardiac Surgery. *Thorac Cardiovasc Surg* 1990;38(suppl II):151–210.

McAllister HA, Fenoglio JJ. Tumors of the cardiovascular system. In: xxxxxxxxx, xxxxxxxx, eds. *Atlas of tumor pathology*, fascicle 15, second series. Washington, D.C.: Armed Forces Institute of Pathology, 1978.

Raichlen JS. Cardiac masses, tumors and thrombi. In: St. John Sutton MG, Kotler MN, eds. *Textbook of adult and pediatric echocardiography and Doppler*, second ed. Boston: Blackwell Scientific Publications, 1995.

Salcedo EE, Cohen GI, White RD, et al. Cardiac tumors: diagnosis and management. *Curr Probl Cardiol* 1992;17:75–137.

Siegel MJ, Weber CK. Cardiac and paracardiac masses. In: Gutierrez FR, Brown JJ, Morowitz SA, eds. *Cardiovascular magnetic resonance imaging*. xxxxxxxx: Mosby Year Book, 1992:112–123.

Weiss L. An analysis of the incidence of myocardial metastasis from solid cancers. *Br Heart J* 1992;68:501–504.

Kelley's Textbook of Internal Medicine, fourth edition. Edited by H. David Humes. Lippincott Williams & Wilkins, Philadelphia © 2000.

C H A P T E R

76

CARDIAC ARRHYTHMIAS

BRADLEY P. KNIGHT
DOUGLAS P. ZIPES
FRED MORADY

Cardiac arrhythmias are disorders of the normal heart rhythm. Most frequently, they create palpitations, which consist of an awareness of the heartbeat—usually because of a ventricular contraction that has greater strength than normal, a pause in the normal heart rhythm, extra beats, or combinations of these factors. Less commonly, cardiac rhythm disturbances can produce syncope, near-syncope, angina, congestive heart failure, or death. The ability of patients to perceive palpitations varies greatly. Some patients recognize a slight shortening of the cardiac cycle, whereas others are unaware of episodes of ventricular tachycar-

dia. Some patients complain of palpitations even though they are documented to have sinus rhythm.

Cardiac arrhythmias are caused by a single heartbeat or series of heartbeats that are too slow (bradycardia) or too fast (tachycardia). They can originate in the specialized conduction system, including the sinus and atrioventricular (AV) nodes, His bundle, and Purkinje fibers, or they can originate from atrial or ventricular muscle. In this chapter, cardiac arrhythmias are discussed in relation to their anatomical site of origin. A summary of the pertinent characteristics of arrhythmias is given in Table 76.1.

An arrhythmia feature must be distinguished from an arrhythmia diagnosis. For example, AV dissociation is present when the atria and the ventricles beat independently. It is never a primary disturbance of rhythm, but is the result of an underlying disturbance. When discussing AV dissociation, it must be stated that "AV dissociation is present and is caused by. . ." and then the cause responsible for independent atrial and ventricular discharge must be given.

Artifact deserves early mention in a chapter on arrhythmias. Electrocardiographic artifacts are generated by a variety of sources, including patient movement and electromagnetic interference, and can be confused with arrhythmias. Artifact is best recognized by the presence of a baseline rhythm "buried in" or "marching through" a recording (Fig. 76.1). A high index of suspicion and awareness of the common occurrence of electrocardiographic artifact is required to avoid misdiagnosing artifact as an arrhythmia.

SINUS RHYTHMS

NORMAL SINUS RHYTHM

Sinus discharge at rates of 60 to 100 beat per minute (faster in infants and children) is defined as normal sinus rhythm. The P wave is upright in leads II, III, and aVF and is negative in lead aVR. The P wave can be negative in lead V_1 and sometimes V_2 but is positive in V_3 through V_6. The PR interval exceeds 120 msec. The sinus rate is decreased by vagal stimulation and increased by sympathetic stimulation. Vagal stimulation is dominant at the sinus node; therefore, during simultaneous maximal vagal and sympathetic stimulation, the sinus rate decreases.

SINUS TACHYCARDIA

Sinus tachycardia is present when the sinus rate exceeds 100 beats per minute, usually not exceeding 180 beats per minute in the adult. The maximal sinus rate achieved during strenuous physical activity decreases with age. Sinus tachycardia has a gradual onset and termination, and the P-wave contour can become more peaked and of larger amplitude. It is important to note that carotid sinus massage or other vagal maneuvers result in gradual and transient slowing of sinus tachycardia (Table 76.1).

Although chronic sinus tachycardia has been described in otherwise healthy persons and is called *inappropriate sinus tachycardia,* sinus tachycardia most frequently results from physiologic or pathophysiologic stresses, such as fever, hypotension, congestive heart failure, or thyrotoxicosis. Its presence should

TABLE 76.1. ARRHYTHMIA CHARACTERISTICS

Type of Arrhythmia	P Waves			QRS Complexes		
	Rate	Rhythm	Contour	Rate	Rhythm	Contour
Sinus rhythm	60–100	Regular[a]	Normal	60–100	Regular	Normal
Sinus bradycardia	<60	Regular	Normal	<60	Regular	Normal
Sinus tachycardia	100–180	Regular	May be peaked	100–180	Regular	Normal
AV nodal reentry	150–250	Regular except at onset and termination	Retrograde; difficult to see; lost in QRS complex	150–250	Very regular except at onset and termination	Normal
Atrial flutter	250–350	Regular	Sawtooth	75–175	Generally regular in absence of drugs or disease	Normal
Atrial fibrillation	400–600	Grossly irregular	Baseline undulation, no P waves	100–160	Grossly irregular	Normal
Atrial tachycardia with block	150–250	Regular; may be irregular	Abnormal	75–200	Generally regular in absence of drugs or disease	Normal
AV junctional rhythm	40–100[c]	Regular	Normal	40–60	Fairly regular	Normal; may be abnormal but <0.12 sec
Reciprocating tachycardias using an accessory (WPW) pathway	150–250	Regular except at onset and termination	Retrograde; difficult to see: follow the QRS complex	150–250	Very regular except at onset and termination	Normal
Nonparoxysmal AV junctional tachycardia	60–100[c]	Regular	Normal	70–130	Fairly regular	Normal; may be abnormal but <0.12 sec
Ventricular tachycardia	60–100[c]	Regular	Normal	110–250	Fairly regular; may be irregular	Abnormal, >0.12 sec
Accelerated idioventricular rhythm	60–100[c]	Regular	Normal	50–110	Fairly regular; may be irregular	Abnormal, >0.12 sec
Ventricular flutter	60–100[c]	Regular	Normal; difficult to see	150–300	Regular	Sine wave
Ventricular fibrillation	60–100[c]	Regular	Normal; difficult to see	400–600	Grossly irregular	Baseline undulations; no QRS complexes
First-degree AV block	60–100[e]	Regular	Normal	60–100	Regular	Normal
Type I second-degree AV block	60–100[e]	Regular	Normal	30–100	Irregular[f]	Normal
Type II second-degree AV block	60–100[e]	Regular	Normal	30–100	Irregular[f]	Abnormal, >0.12 sec
Complete AV block Acquired	60–100[b]	Regular	Normal	<40	Fairly regular	Abnormal, >0.12 sec
Congenital	60–100[b]	Regular	Normal	40–60	Fairly regular	Normal, <0.12 sec
Right bundle-branch block	60–100	Regular	Normal	60–100	Regular	Abnormal, >0.12 sec
Left bundle-branch block	60–100	Regular	Normal	60–100	Regular	Abnormal, >0.12 sec

Note: In an effort to summarize these arrhythmias in a tabular form, generalizations have to be made. For example, response to carotid sinus massage may be slightly different from what is listed. Acute therapy to terminate a tachycardia may be different from chronic therapy to prevent a recurrence. Some of the exceptions are indicated in the footnotes; the reader is referred to the text for a more complete discussion. *AV,* atrioventricular; *WPW,* Wolff-Parkinson-White; *DC,* direct-current.
[a] P waves initiated by sinus node discharge may not be precisely regular because of sinus arrhythmia.

TABLE 76.1. *Continued*

Ventricular Response to Carotid Sinus Massage	Physical Examination			Treatment
	Intensity of S_1	Splitting of S_2	*a* Waves	
Gradual slowing and return to former rate	Constant	Normal	Normal	None
Gradual slowing and return to former rate	Constant	Normal	Normal	None unless symptomatic, atropine
Gradual slowing[b] and return to former rate	Constant	Normal	Normal	None unless symptomatic, treat underlying disease
Abrupt slowing caused by termination of tachycardia, or no effect	Constant	Normal	Constant cannon *a* waves	Vagal stimulation, verapamil, digitalis, propranolol, DC shock, pacing
Abrupt slowing and return to former rate; flutter remains	Constant; variable if AV block changing	Normal	Flutter waves	DC shock, digitalis, quinidine, propranolol, verapamil
Slowing, gross irregularity remains	Variable	Normal	No *a* waves	Digitalis, quinidine, DC shock, verapamil
Abrupt slowing and return to former rate; tachycardia remains	Constant; variable if AV block changing	Normal	More *a* waves than *a–c* waves	Stop digitalis if toxic; digitalis if not toxic; possibly verapamil
None; may be slight slowing	Variable[d]	Normal	Intermittent cannon waves[d]	None, unless symptomatic; atropine
Abrupt slowing caused by termination of tachycardia, or no effect	Constant but decreased	Normal	Constant cannon waves	(See AV nodal reentry)
None, may be slight slowing	Variable[d]	Normal	Intermittent cannon waves[d]	None unless symptomatic; stop digitalis if toxic
None	Variable[d]	Abnormal	Intermittent cannon waves[d]	Lidocaine, procainamide, DC shock, quinidine
None	Variable[d]	Abnormal	Intermittent cannon waves[d]	None, unless symptomatic; lidocaine, atropine
None	Soft or absent	Soft or absent	Cannon waves	DC shock
None	None	None	Cannon waves	DC shock
Gradual slowing caused by sinus slowing	Constant, diminished	Normal	Normal	None
Slowing caused by sinus slowing and an increase in AV block	Cyclic decrease then increase after pause	Normal	Normal; increasing *a–c* interval; *a* waves without *c* waves	None unless symptomatic; atropine
Gradual slowing caused by sinus slowing	Constant	Abnormal	Normal; constant *a–c* interval; *a* waves without *c* waves	Pacemaker
None	Variable[d]	Abnormal	Intermittent cannon waves[d]	Pacemaker
May slow slightly	Variable[d]	Normal	Intermittent cannon waves[d]	None, if no symptoms
Gradual slowing and return to former rate	Constant	Wide	Normal	None
Gradual slowing and return to former rate	Constant	Paradoxical	Normal	None

[b] Often, carotid sinus massage fails to slow a rapid sinus tachycardia.

[c] Any independent atrial arrhythmia may exist, or the atria may be captured retrogradely.

[d] Constant if atria are captured retrogradely.

[e] Atrial rhythm and rate may vary, depending on whether sinus bradycardia, tachycardia, and so forth is the atrial mechanism.

[f] Regular or constant if block is unchanging.

Compiled from data in Zipes DP, Maloy LB. *Arrhythmias.* In: Andreoli KG, Zipes DP, Wallace AG, Kinney MR, Fowkes YK, eds. *Comprehensive cardiac care.* 6th ed. St. Louis: CV Mosby, 1987.

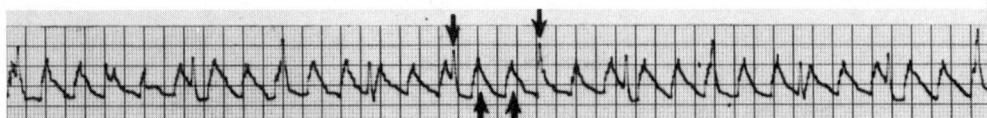

FIGURE 76.1. Artifact mimicking tachycardia. The patient, being monitored on a coronary care unit, brushed his teeth with an electric toothbrush and generated a regular artifact that mimicked a ventricular tachycardia (*upright arrows*). However, the patient's QRS complex (*inverted arrows*) can be seen clearly.

prompt a search for underlying causes. Nonprescription drugs such as decongestants, which contain catecholamines, or alcohol, nicotine, and caffeine can produce sinus tachycardia.

Sinus tachycardia uncommonly is a primary disorder, and therapy focuses on potential causes. The uncommon patient with primary chronic sinus tachycardia may need drug, surgical, or ablative therapy to treat the sinus tachycardia directly.

SINUS BRADYCARDIA

Sinus bradycardia is present when the sinus discharge rate is less than 60 beats per minute. P waves have a normal contour and the PR interval exceeds 120 msec. Excessive vagal or decreased sympathetic tone and anatomical or electrophysiologic abnormalities in the sinus node can cause sinus bradycardia. It is often present in healthy young adults, particularly in athletes, and during sleep. Myxedema, hypothermia, vasovagal reactions, and drugs such as lithium, amiodarone, β-adrenergic blocking agents, and calcium channel blockers can produce sinus bradycardia. Most commonly, it is a benign arrhythmia, and treatment is usually not necessary. Transiently symptomatic sinus bradycardia can be treated with drugs such as atropine or isoproterenol, or with temporary pacing. Chronic symptomatic sinus bradycardia typically requires pacemaker therapy.

SINUS ARRHYTHMIA AND WANDERING PACEMAKER

Sinus arrhythmia is characterized by a phasic variation in sinus cycle length, usually exceeding 120 msec from the maximum to the minimum change in the cycle length. P-wave contour as a rule remains fairly constant, as does the PR interval. Sinus arrhythmia has a respiratory and nonrespiratory form. *Ventriculophasic sinus arrhythmia* occurs when the ventricular rate is slow, such as during complete AV block, and is characterized by shorter PP cycles for the two P waves that flank a QRS complex

and by longer PP cycles for the two P waves that do not include a QRS complex between them. Such changes probably result from the influence of the autonomic nervous system responding to changes produced by the ventricular stroke volume.

Wandering pacemaker is a variant of sinus arrhythmia and is diagnosed when there is a cyclic increase in the RR interval, a PR interval that gradually shortens and may become less than 120 msec, and when a change in the P wave contour that often becomes negative in leads I or II or is lost within the inscription of the QRS complex (Fig. 76.2). As the pacemaker shifts back to the sinus node, these changes may occur in reverse.

Sinus arrhythmia and wandering pacemaker often happen in the very young, particularly in athletes, and probably result from heightened vagal tone. If the patient has no symptoms, treatment is not necessary. For the rare symptomatic patient, the treatment approach is the same as in sinus bradycardia.

SINUS PAUSE OR SINUS ARREST

Sinus pause or sinus arrest is diagnosed when a pause in the sinus rhythm occurs, the duration of which does not equal a multiple of the basic PP interval (Fig. 76.3). Anatomical disruption of the sinus node by ischemia or infarction, degenerative fibrotic changes, the effects of drugs, and excessive vagal tone all can produce a sinus pause or sinus arrest. Sinus pauses can occur after termination of atrial fibrillation in patients with sick sinus syndrome (Fig. 76.4). The arrhythmia may have no clinical significance by itself if latent pacemakers discharge to prevent ventricular asystole. Treatment is as for sinus bradycardia.

SINOATRIAL EXIT BLOCK

Sinoatrial (SA) exit block results when a pause in the PP interval occurs which is equal to a multiple of the basic PP interval. Electrophysiologically, SA exit block results when the sinus node discharges but the impulse is blocked from propagating to the

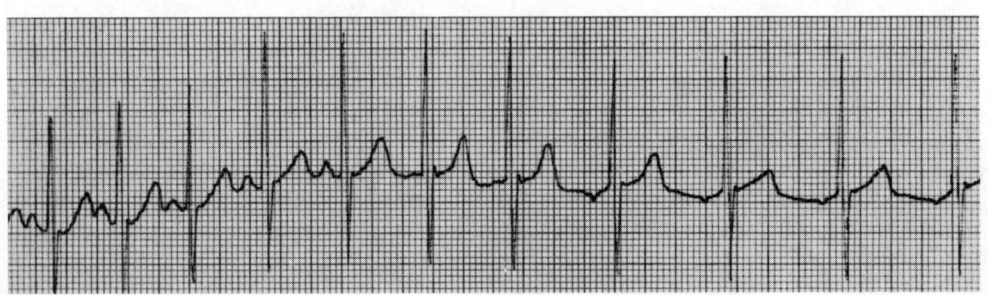

FIGURE 76.2. Wandering pacemaker, monitor lead. Progressive sinus slowing occurs as the P wave becomes isoelectric initially and then negative in the terminal portion of the ECG recording. The P wave once again became positive and varied repetitively in this cyclic manner (not shown).

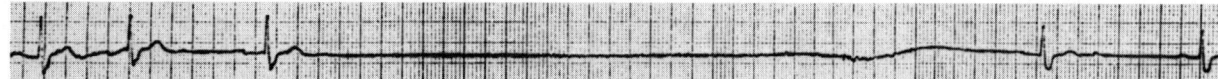

FIGURE 76.3. Sinus pause or sinus arrest, monitor lead. Initial slight sinus slowing is followed by sinus arrest with a junctional escape beat (next to last QRS complex) after almost 8 seconds of asystole. During this time, the patient developed near-syncope. Why other pacemakers did not discharge during that interval is unclear.

atrium. The SA exit block can be type I, during which the PP interval progressively shortens before the pause, and the duration of the pause is less than two PP cycles (see type I Wenckebach second-degree AV heart block), or type II, in which the pause equals two, three, or four normal PP cycles. First-degree SA exit block cannot be recognized electrocardiographically because SA nodal discharge cannot be recorded with the scalar electrocardiogram (ECG). Third-degree SA exit block can present as the complete absence of P waves and mimic sinus arrest. Causes and treatment are the same as for sinus bradycardia.

SINUS NODAL REENTRY

Reentry within the sinus node or involving a part of the sinus node can result in a supraventricular tachycardia with rates of 80 to 200 beats per minute, averaging 130 to 140 beats per minute. During tachycardia, P waves resemble the sinus P wave, and the PR interval is related to the tachycardia rate, usually producing a long RP interval and a shorter PR interval. AV block can occur with persistence of the tachycardia, a hallmark of a tachycardia occurring in the atrium and not requiring participation of the ventricle. Vagal maneuvers can slow and then abruptly terminate the tachycardia. Sinus nodal reentry may account for 1% of cases of symptomatic paroxysmal supraventricular tachycardia. β-Adrenergic blocking agents, calcium channel blockers, or digitalis may be effective therapy.

▇ ATRIAL RHYTHM DISTURBANCES

PREMATURE ATRIAL COMPLEXES

Premature atrial complexes manifest as a premature P wave morphologically different from the sinus P wave. Premature P waves superimposed on the preceding T wave can be difficult to recognize. When such a premature atrial complex blocks in the AV junction before reaching the ventricle, it can be misinterpreted as a sinus pause.

Usually, a premature atrial complex discharges the sinus node

and is followed by a *noncompensatory* pause. On occasion, the premature atrial complex can initiate an aberrantly conducted QRS complex, usually with a right bundle-branch-block contour. Premature atrial complexes can occur in normal persons and can be provoked by drugs, alcohol, caffeine, and tobacco. Premature atrial complexes as a rule do not require therapy, but when they do because of symptoms or precipitation of tachycardias, treatment with digitalis, propranolol, or verapamil may be useful. On occasion, class IA drugs or amiodarone may be tried.

ATRIAL FLUTTER

Atrial flutter is recognized electrocardiographically as sawtooth-shaped atrial complexes, usually at rates of 250 to 350 beats per minute (most often 300 beats per minute), with a 2:1 ventricular response in untreated persons (Fig. 76.5). The flutter waves commonly are negative in leads II, III, aVF, and V_1, and if the AV conduction ratio remains constant, the ventricular rhythm is regular. A varying ratio of conducted beats produces an irregular ventricular rhythm. The classic or type I atrial flutter usually has a rate of 300 beats per minute, whereas type II flutter is faster at 350 to 450 beats per minute. Reentry is the most probable cause of atrial flutter with a counterclockwise macro (large) right atrial circuit due to the impulse traveling cephalad up the right atrial septum and caudad down the right atrial free wall when the flutter waves are negative in II, III, and aVF. When the circuit is in an opposite direction, the flutter waves can be positive or negative. Atrial flutter usually is associated with underlying heart disease, such as rheumatic or ischemic heart disease or cardiomyopathy.

Synchronous direct-current (DC) cardioversion is usually the initial treatment of choice. Rapid atrial pacing can effectively terminate atrial flutter in most patients. Pharmacologic therapy is directed at slowing the ventricular response. If atrial flutter persists, class IA, IC, or III drugs can be tried (Fig. 76.5). Before class I drugs are given, the ventricular rate must be slowed.

Prevention of recurrent atrial flutter is as outlined for prevention of recurrent atrial fibrillation. Radiofrequency catheter ablation can be effective in eliminating typical atrial flutter (Fig.

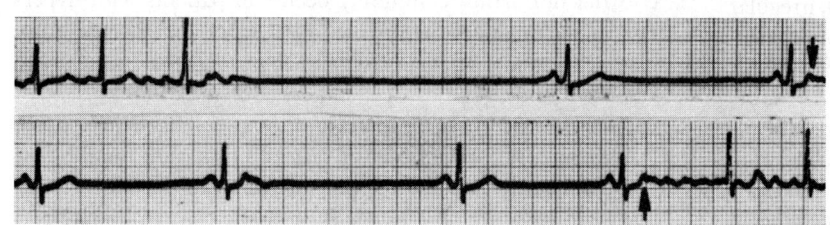

FIGURE 76.4. Sick sinus syndrome, monitor lead. Atrial flutter–fibrillation abruptly terminates and is followed by a slightly irregular sinus bradycardia with intermittent premature atrial complexes (*inverted arrow*). One of these premature atrial complexes (*upright arrow*) reinitiates the atrial flutter–fibrillation.

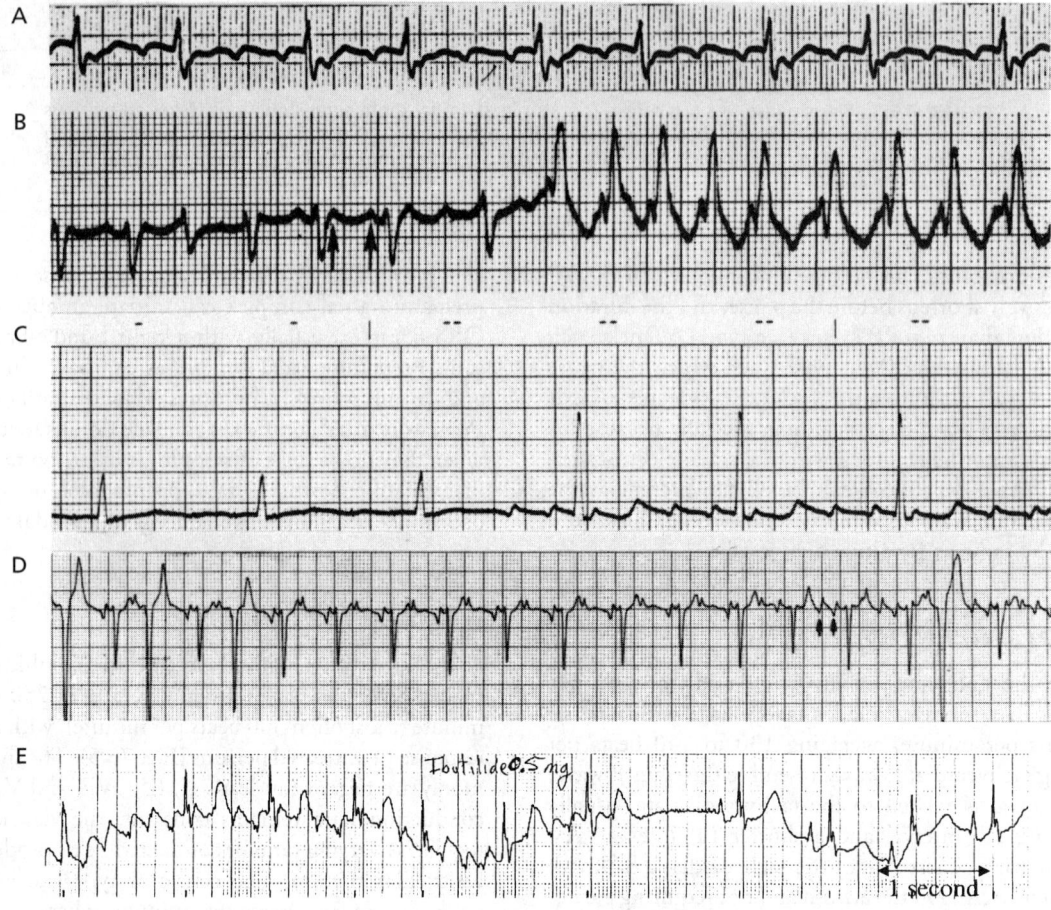

FIGURE 76.5. Atrial flutter. **A:** Relatively slow atrial flutter (200 beats per minute) due to the effects of amiodarone. **B:** Atrial flutter (*arrows*) is difficult to recognize. A long–short cycle sequence initiates functional right bundle-branch block (see section on aberration). **C:** Atrial flutter that is difficult to recognize in lead I (*left*) but obvious when the recording is switched to lead II (*right*). **D:** ECG of a 16-year-old patient with a rapid atrial flutter (*arrows*) induced with physical exertion. Because of an uncontrollable ventricular response, the patient despite his young age, underwent atrioventricular junctional ablation to modify atrioventricular conduction. **E:** Monitor strip showing conversion of atrial flutter to sinus rhythm during an infusion of ibutilide.

76.5). If recurrences cannot be prevented, therapy is directed toward controlling the ventricular rate.

ATRIAL FIBRILLATION

Atrial fibrillation is the most common sustained arrhythmia, and its incidence increases with age. Atrial fibrillation is characterized by totally disorganized atrial depolarization without effective atrial contraction and is most commonly sustained by multiple atrial wavelets of reentry.

Accurate recognition of atrial fibrillation is important because of its high morbidity. Atrial fibrillation appears as small, irregular baseline undulations of varying amplitude and morphology, called F waves, at a rate of 350 to 600 per minute (Fig. 76.6). Many of the fibrillatory impulses are blocked in the AV node, which accounts for the irregular ventricular rhythm. Atrial fibrillation should not be confused with multifocal atrial tachycardia, which is also "irregularly irregular" but has discrete atrial beats separated by isoelectric periods. Regularization and slowing of

the rhythm can occur with heart block and digitalis toxicity. A rapid ventricular response results in less irregularity and can lead to a misdiagnosis of paroxysmal supraventricular tachycardia (Fig. 76.6). In the untreated person with normal AV conduction, the ventricular rate usually is 100 to 160 beats per minute. Conversion of atrial fibrillation to atrial flutter is accompanied by a slowing of the atrial rate, but an increase in the ventricular rate, because fewer impulses block in the AV node. It is easier to slow the ventricular rate during atrial fibrillation than during atrial flutter, because the increased concealed conduction makes it easier to produce AV block.

Atrial fibrillation commonly occurs in patients with hypertension, rheumatic heart disease, atrial septal defect, cardiomyopathy, coronary heart disease, and thyrotoxicosis and in those who have undergone cardiac surgery, but it can be present in patients without structural heart disease, so-called lone atrial fibrillation. The patient who has atrial fibrillation for the first time should be evaluated for precipitating causes.

The therapeutic objective is to slow the ventricular rate and

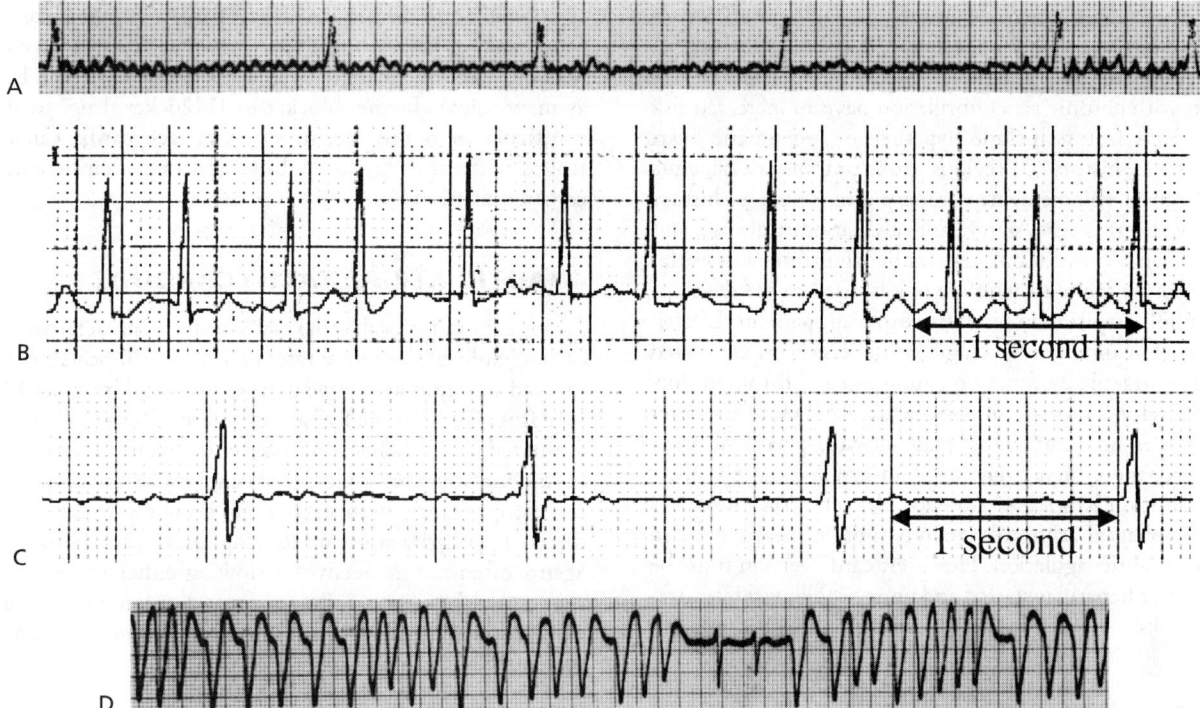

FIGURE 76.6. Atrial fibrillation. **A:** Atrial fibrillation and a slow ventricular response to digitalis therapy are noted. **B:** Monitor strip showing atrial fibrillation with a rapid ventricular response. The irregularity is less obvious when the ventricular rate is rapid but the rhythm is not as regular as paroxysmal supraventricular tachycardia. This patient was unnecessarily treated with adenosine. **C:** Atrial fibrillation with complete atrioventricular block and a wide QRS escape. **D:** Atrial fibrillation in a patient with Wolff–Parkinson–White syndrome. The negative delta wave in lead V$_1$ is consistent with a right-sided accessory pathway. Although atrial activity cannot be seen, the rapid, irregular, wide QRS complexes, with rates exceeding 300 beats per minute at times, interspersed with normal QRS complexes, support the diagnosis of atrial fibrillation with conduction to the ventricle over an accessory pathway.

then to restore atrial systole. If acute cardiovascular decompensation has occurred, electrical cardioversion is the initial treatment of choice. Otherwise, drugs that slow the ventricular response can be used. Sometimes digitalis must be combined with a β-blocker or calcium channel blocker. Digitalis is less effective during exercise. Adequacy of ventricular rate control must be assessed both at rest and with activity. Inadequate rate control can lead to a tachycardia-induced cardiomyopathy. Creation of complete heart block using radiofrequency ablation followed by implantation of a pacemaker is a useful option for patients with medically refractory rapid ventricular rates during atrial fibrillation. This procedure can significantly improve symptoms related to rapid rates but does not restore sinus rhythm. Therefore, continuation of anticoagulation is usually required to prevent thromboembolism.

Conversion to sinus rhythm should be considered in patients with atrial fibrillation when it is likely that sinus rhythm will remain for a relatively long time period, when symptoms are present, or when the ventricular rate cannot be controlled. Electrical cardioversion with a DC shock is the most effective cardioversion technique and can be performed on an outpatient basis. A variety of oral and intravenous drugs are also useful for cardioversion. Pharmacologic cardioversion should be performed while the patient is monitored in the hospital when structural heart disease is present. Intravenous ibutilide is more effective than procainamide. Amiodarone is ineffective at converting atrial fibrillation.

The strongest predictor of recurrent atrial fibrillation is the duration of atrial fibrillation before cardioversion. Atrial fibrillation is more likely to be long-standing in patients with left atrial enlargement. Antiarrhythmic drugs help maintain sinus rhythm. However, sodium channel blockers such as quinidine and flecainide can increase mortality due to proarrhythmia when used chronically in patients with significant underlying structural heart disease. Although not approved by the Food and Drug Administration (FDA) for the treatment of atrial fibrillation, amiodarone effectively prevents recurrences and is relatively safe to use in patients with ventricular dysfunction.

Nonpharmacologic techniques are being developed to manage atrial fibrillation. The Maze and Corridor operations involve open-heart surgery in which surgical incisions are strategically placed in the atria to interrupt atrial fibrillation by preventing reentry. Special catheters are being tested to accomplish this procedure using a transvenous endocardial approach. A subset of patients with apparent atrial fibrillation has a rapidly firing atrial tachycardia arising from the pulmonary veins, resulting in fibrillatory conduction. These patients tend to have frequent uniform premature atrial depolarizations and focal ablation in one of the pulmonary veins can be curative. Implantable transvenous atrial defibrillators permit out-of-hospital conversion for patients who require frequent cardioversion. Multisite atrial pacing may reduce the number of tachycardia episodes in patients with paroxysmal atrial fibrillation.

Patients with chronic atrial fibrillation have an increased risk for stroke. Risk factors include hypertension, rheumatic heart disease, diabetes, history of previous stroke or transient ischemic attack, left atrial enlargement, coronary artery disease, history of congestive heart failure, significant valvular heart disease, and age greater than 65 years. Long-term anticoagulation with warfarin is necessary in patients who are predisposed to the development of emboli. Aspirin can be effective in some patients. Electrical cardioversion and pharmacologic cardioversion are associated with atrial contractile dysfunction (stunning) and thrombus formation. Therefore, short-term anticoagulation before and after cardioversion is necessary in all patients with persistent atrial fibrillation for more than 2 days or of uncertain duration unless a contraindication is present. Absence of a left atrial thrombus by a transesophageal echocardiogram permits safe cardioversion without prior anticoagulation. However, cardioversion must be performed after heparin is started and must be followed by warfarin for 4 weeks.

ATRIAL TACHYCARDIA

Atrial tachycardia can be due to enhanced atrial automaticity, reentry or to triggered activity. In either, AV block can exist without affecting the tachycardia. The atrial rate usually is 150 to 200 beats per minute. The atrial rate can be slightly irregular, and characteristic isoelectric intervals between P waves usually are present (Fig. 76.7). Vagal maneuvers usually do not terminate the tachycardia, even though they may produce transient AV nodal block.

Atrial tachycardia occurs most commonly in patients with structural heart disease such as coronary artery disease or cor pulmonale or in patients after congenital heart surgery or digitalis intoxication. If digitalis is not the cause, it may be given, as may a slow channel blocker or β-blocker drug, to slow the ventricular response. Recurrent atrial tachycardia can be controlled with antiarrhythmic drugs and can often be cured with catheter ablation.

CHAOTIC ATRIAL TACHYCARDIA

Chaotic, or multifocal, atrial tachycardia is characterized electrocardiographically by atrial rates of 100 to 130 beats per minute, marked variation in P-wave morphology, and irregular PP intervals (Fig. 76.8). Usually, at least three P-wave morphologies are noted. This tachycardia occurs frequently in patients with pulmonary disease. Digitalis appears to be an unusual cause, but theophylline administration has been implicated. Therapy is directed primarily at the underlying disease, and antiarrhythmic agents often are ineffective in slowing either the atrial rate or the ventricular response. Potassium and magnesium replacement may suppress the tachycardia. Propranolol should be avoided in patients with bronchospastic disease.

ATRIOVENTRICULAR JUNCTIONAL ESCAPE BEATS

Latent pacemakers are automatic fibers that are prevented from initiating depolarization by a pacemaker, such as the sinus node, that possesses a more rapid rate of firing and keeps them depolarized. Latent pacemakers are found in some parts of the atrium, AV node–His bundle area, and Purkinje system. A latent pacemaker can become the dominant pacemaker by increasing its rate of discharge or by default during bradycardia.

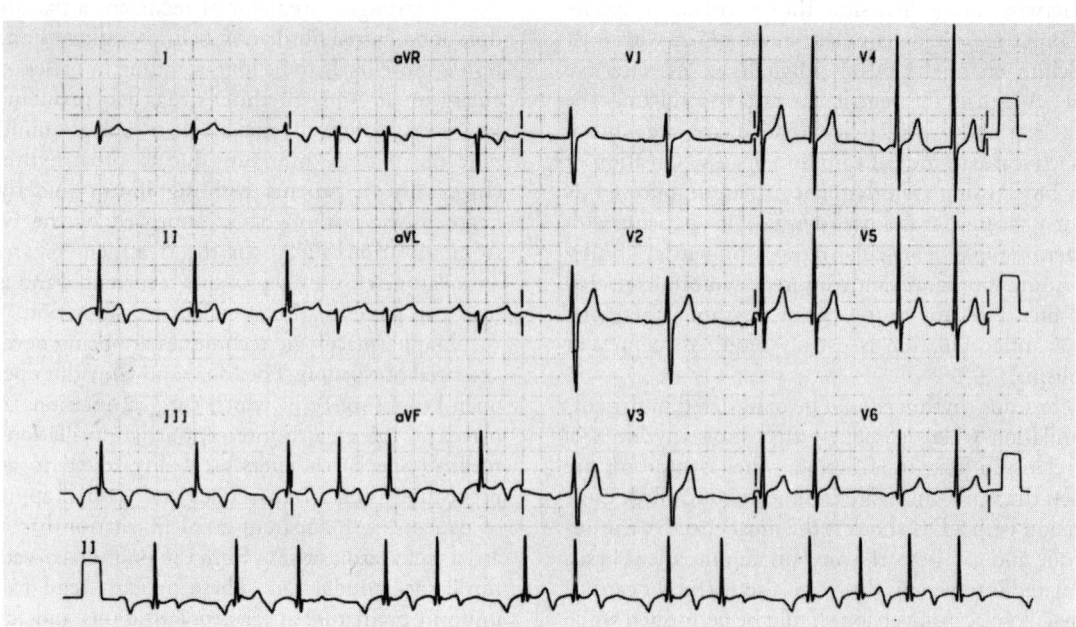

FIGURE 76.7. Atrial tachycardia with varying atrioventricular (AV) nodal block is seen in the 12-lead ECG. Predominantly 2:1, 3:2, and 5:4 AV block is apparent in the lead II rhythm strip (*bottom*).

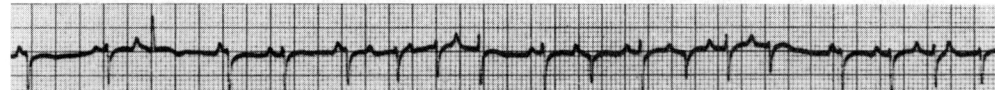

FIGURE 76.8. Chaotic atrial tachycardia. Lead II illustrates frequent premature atrial complexes with multiple morphologies, at times conducting with aberration and often with a prolonged PR interval.

An AV junctional escape beat occurring by default is characterized by a normal QRS complex at a cycle length longer than the normal PP interval with absent, retrograde, fusion, or sinus P waves that do not conduct to the ventricle. This rhythm may be completely normal, and patients most often are asymptomatic.

ATRIOVENTRICULAR JUNCTIONAL RHYTHM

If the AV junctional escape beats continue, the rhythm is called an AV junctional rhythm and is at the inherent rate of the AV junctional tissue of 35 to 60 beats per minute (Fig. 76.9). The ECG displays a normally conducted QRS complex that may conduct retrogradely to the atrium or may occur independently of atrial discharge, producing AV dissociation. Treatment of patients with AV junctional escape beats or AV junctional rhythm usually is not necessary but, if required, can be achieved with drugs that increase the discharge rate of the sinus node and improve AV conduction. Pacing rarely is required.

PREMATURE ATRIOVENTRICULAR JUNCTIONAL COMPLEXES

Premature AV junctional complexes are characterized by a premature supraventricular QRS complex with or without conduction to the atrium. A retrograde P wave can occur before, during, or after the QRS complex, or a nonconducted sinus P wave may occur (Fig. 76.10).

NONPAROXYSMAL ATRIOVENTRICULAR JUNCTIONAL TACHYCARDIA

Nonparoxysmal AV junctional tachycardia usually is characterized by a gradual onset and termination of a supraventricular tachycardia at rates commonly between 70 and 130 beats per minute. Although accepted terminology confers the label of tachycardia to rates exceeding 100 beats per minute, the term nonparoxysmal AV junctional tachycardia has been applied to this rhythm because rates exceeding 60 beats per minute represent, in effect, a tachycardia for the AV junctional tissue.

Nonparoxysmal AV junctional tachycardia occurs most commonly in association with underlying heart disease (inferior myocardial infarction [MI]) or myocarditis, after open-heart surgery, or from excessive digitalis. The last of these can produce the ECG manifestations of junctional exit block, usually of the Wenckebach type. The clinical features vary, depending on the rate of arrhythmia and the underlying cause and severity of the heart disease. Nonparoxysmal AV junctional tachycardia can occur in otherwise healthy persons without symptoms, or it can occur at rapid rates and result in heart failure. It is especially important to recognize slowing and regularization of the ventricular rhythm in patients with atrial fibrillation as being caused by nonparoxysmal AV junctional tachycardia and as a possible early sign of digitalis intoxication.

Generally, monitoring and attention to the underlying heart disease usually are all that are required. The arrhythmia usually abates spontaneously. If the cardiovascular status is compromised, digitalis, slow channel blockers, or β-blockers can be considered. Digitalis may be a cause, and, if so, it should be discontinued. Rarely, catheter ablation is indicated.

ATRIOVENTRICULAR NODAL REENTRANT TACHYCARDIA

AV nodal reentry is characterized by a regular tachycardia with a QRS complex of supraventricular origin, usually at rates between 150 and 250 beats per minute (commonly 180 to 200 beats per minute in adults), sudden onset, and sudden termination. The development of unidirectional block in the AV nodal region is due to the presence of tissues with disparate electrophysiologic properties.

Because anterograde conduction to the ventricle usually occurs over a slowly conducting AV nodal pathway and retrograde conduction occurs over a more rapidly conducting pathway, at the onset of tachycardia the atrial complex blocks in the fast pathway anterogradely, travels to the ventricle over the slow pathway, and returns to the atrium over the previously blocked fast pathway, with the reentry circuit using the two approaches to the AV node (Fig. 76.11). A premature atrial complex that conducts with a long PR interval commonly precipitates AV nodal reentry. The retrograde P wave occurs at the onset or just after the termination of the QRS complex in most cases (Fig. 76.11).

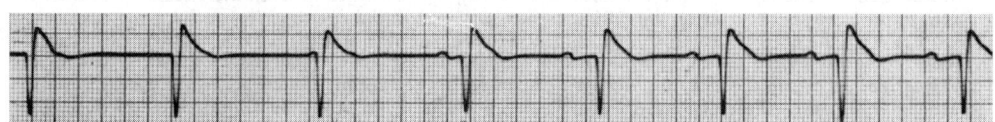

FIGURE 76.9. Atrioventricular (AV) junctional rhythm. Sinus bradycardia permits the escape of an AV junctional rhythm (*left:* 48 beats per minute) until the sinus rate speeds sufficiently to again control the rhythm (*middle*). First-degree AV block is present.

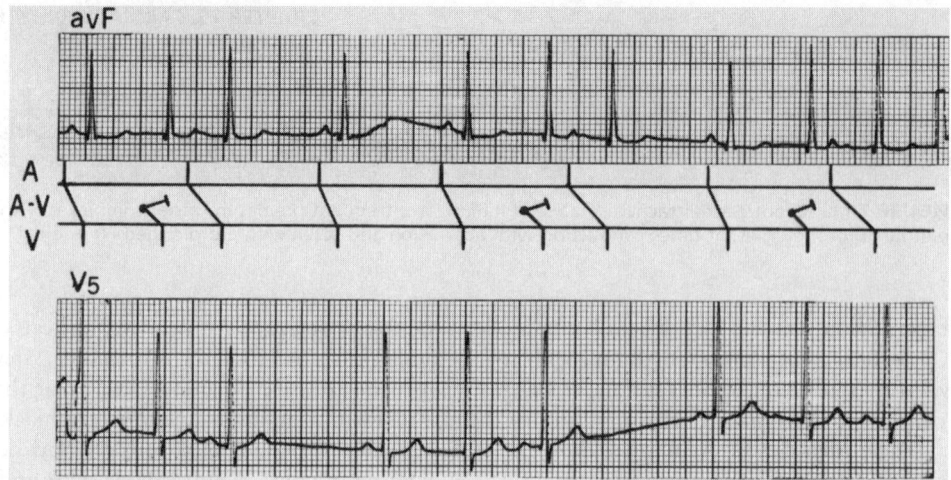

FIGURE 76.10. Premature atrioventricular (AV) junctional complexes are noted in leads aVF and V₅ (onset indicated by dark circles in ladder diagram). They do not block the subsequent sinus impulse, which conducts with a prolonged PR interval. Hence, the premature AV junctional complexes are called interpolated.

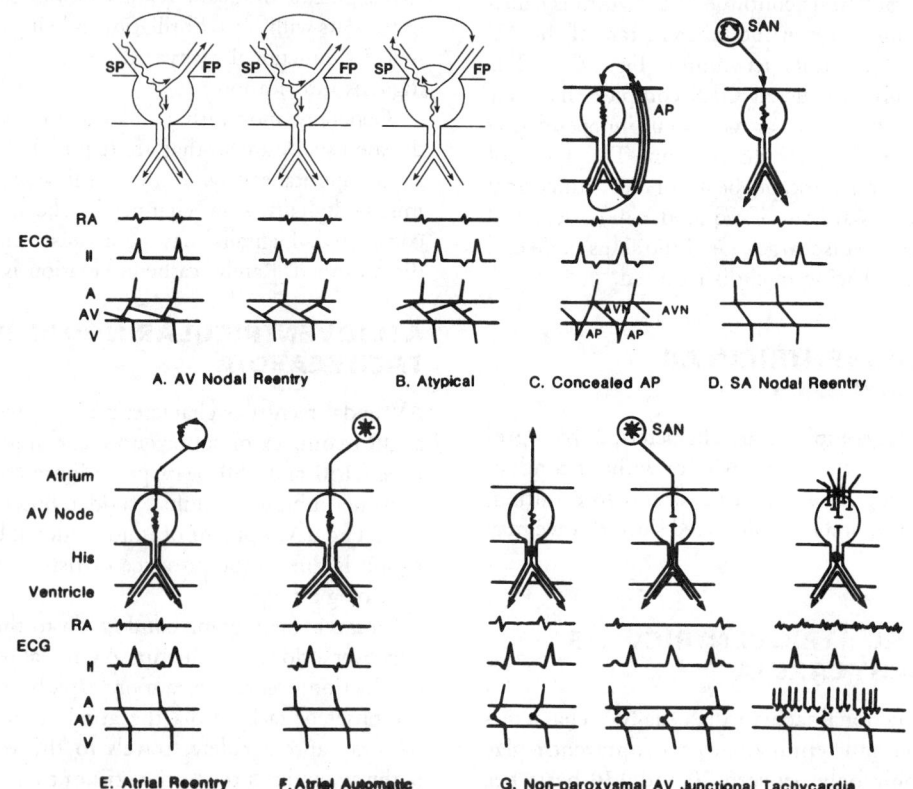

FIGURE 76.11. Diagrammatic representation of various supraventricular tachycardias. In the top portion of each example, a schematic diagram of the presumed anatomical pathways is drawn; in the bottom half, the ECG presentation and the explanatory ladder diagram are depicted. **A:** Atrioventricular (AV) nodal reentry. In the left example, reentrant excitation is drawn with retrograde atrial activity occurring simultaneously with ventricular activity because of anterograde conduction over the slow AV nodal pathway and retrograde conduction over the fast AV nodal pathway. In the right example, atrial activity occurs slightly later than ventricular activity because of retrograde conduction delay. **B:** Atypical AV nodal reentry due to anterograde conduction over a fast AV nodal pathway and retrograde conduction over a slow AV nodal pathway. **C:** Concealed accessory pathway. Reciprocating tachycardia due to anterograde conduction over the AV node and retrograde conduction over the accessory pathway. Retrograde P waves occur after the QRS complex. **D:** Sinus nodal reentry. The tachycardia is due to reentry within the sinus node, which then conducts to the rest of the heart. **E:** Atrial reentry. Tachycardia is due to reentry within the atrium, which then conducts to the rest of the heart. **F:** Automatic atrial tachycardia. Tachycardia is due to automatic discharge in the atrium, which then conducts to the rest of the heart; it is difficult to distinguish from atrial reentry. **G:** Nonparoxysmal AV junctional tachycardia. Various presentations of this tachycardia are depicted with retrograde atrial capture, AV dissociation with the sinus node in control of the atria, and AV dissociation with atrial fibrillation. (From Zipes DP. Specific arrhythmias: diagnosis and treatment. In: Braunwald E, ed. *Heart disease: a textbook of cardiovascular medicine*, third ed. Philadelphia: WB Saunders, 1996, with permission.)

Less frequently, anterograde conduction proceeds over the fast pathway and retrograde conduction over the slow pathway, producing the unusual form of AV nodal reentry. In this instance, the retrograde P wave precedes the following QRS complex at a relatively short AV interval, producing a long ventriculoatrial interval (Fig. 76.11).

AV nodal reentry occurs commonly in patients without structural heart disease and produces a constellation of symptoms ranging from palpitations, nervousness, and anxiety to angina, heart failure, and syncope, depending on the duration and rate of the tachycardia and the presence of structural heart disease. Initial hypotension during tachycardia may evoke a sympathetic response that increases blood pressure and in turn causes a rise in vagal tone that may terminate the tachycardia. The prognosis for patients without heart disease usually is good.

Termination of AV nodal reentrant supraventricular tachycardia initially involves vagal maneuvers, including carotid sinus massage, Valsalva's and Müller's maneuvers, gagging, and, on occasion, exposure of the face to ice water. The drug of first choice is intravenous adenosine (a vagomimetic drug), followed by diltiazem or verapamil or by a short-acting β-blocker such as esmolol. Prevention of recurrences may be more difficult to achieve than termination of the acute episode. Radiofrequency catheter ablation of the slow pathway usually is the initial treatment of choice in symptomatic patients with frequent recurrences because of the high success rate (about 95%), low risk (less than 2%), and effective elimination of future recurrences. AV nodal blocking drugs are most often the initial drugs of choice.

PREEXCITATION SYNDROME

Preexcitation conduction occurs when the atrial impulse activates the whole or some part of the ventricle or when the ventricular impulse activates the whole or some part of the atrium, earlier than would be expected if the impulse traveled through the normal specific conduction system only. In Wolff–Parkinson–White syndrome (preexcitation syndrome), muscular connections composed of working myocardial fibers exist outside the specialized conducting tissue, connecting atrium, and ventricle. They are named *accessory AV pathways* or *connections,* are commonly called *Kent bundles,* and are responsible for the most common variety of preexcitation. When the atrial impulse activates the ventricle over the accessory pathway, three ECG changes result (Fig. 76.12): (a) the PR interval is less than 120 msec during sinus rhythm; (b) the QRS complex duration exceeds 120 msec with a slurred, slowly rising onset of the QRS in some leads (delta wave) and usually a normal terminal QRS portion; and (c) secondary ST-T wave changes occur with T waves that usually are directed opposite to the major delta wave and QRS vectors. The term Wolff–Parkinson–White or preexcitation syndrome is used when the patient has symptoms due to tachyarrhythmias. The anomalous complexes can mask or mimic other cardiac abnormalities such as MI (Chapter 73).

During the electrophysiologic study, a variety of pacing techniques are used to localize the position of the accessory pathway and its role in the tachycardia (Chapter 88). Careful analysis of

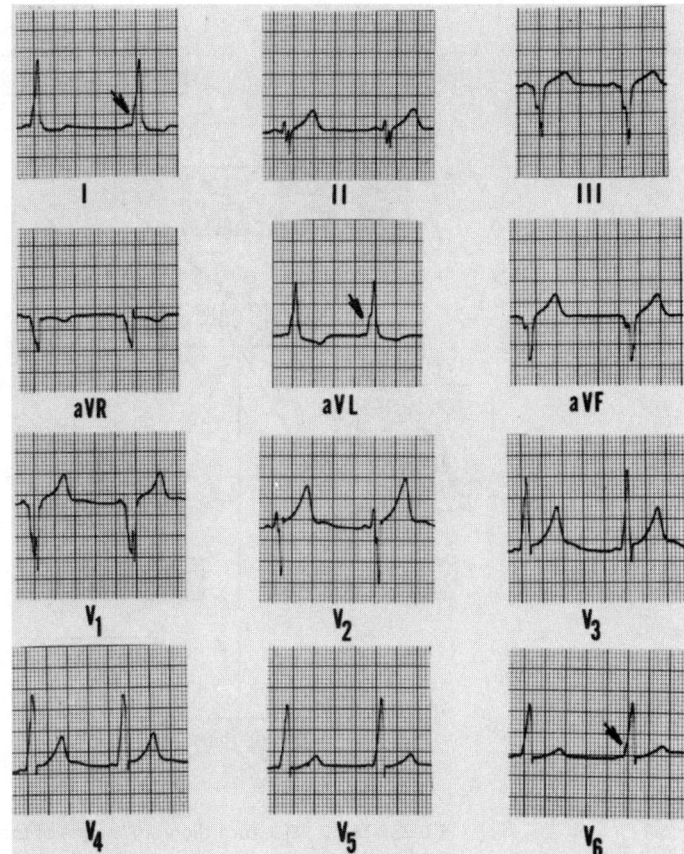

FIGURE 76.12. of a patient with preexcitation and an accessory pathway located in the right posteroseptal region.

the ECG can localize the accessory pathway to one of four major sites (Fig. 76.13).

Because the Kent bundle usually has a longer refractory period during longer cycle lengths than does the AV node, despite the fact that it has more rapid conduction, a premature atrial complex can occur sufficiently early to block anterogradely in the accessory pathway and conduct to the ventricle only over the normal AV node–His bundle pathway. The resultant QRS complex is normal and allows the impulse to return to the atrium over the accessory pathway and initiate the most common type of reciprocating tachycardia, called *orthodromic.* Because the atria may be activated eccentrically (i.e., in a manner other than the normal retrograde activation sequence, starting at the low right atrial septum as in AV nodal reentry), the retrograde P wave may have an unusual contour.

Some accessory pathways are capable only of retrograde conduction. The presence of an accessory pathway that conducts only retrogradely is not apparent by analysis of the scalar ECG during sinus rhythm because the ventricle is not preexcited. Therefore, the ECG manifestations of Wolff–Parkinson–White syndrome are absent, and the accessory pathway is said to be concealed. However, the patient still can have orthodromic reciprocating tachycardia that is identical in appearance to the same tachycardia occurring in a patient who has an accessory pathway capable of bidirectional conduction (Fig. 76.14). The

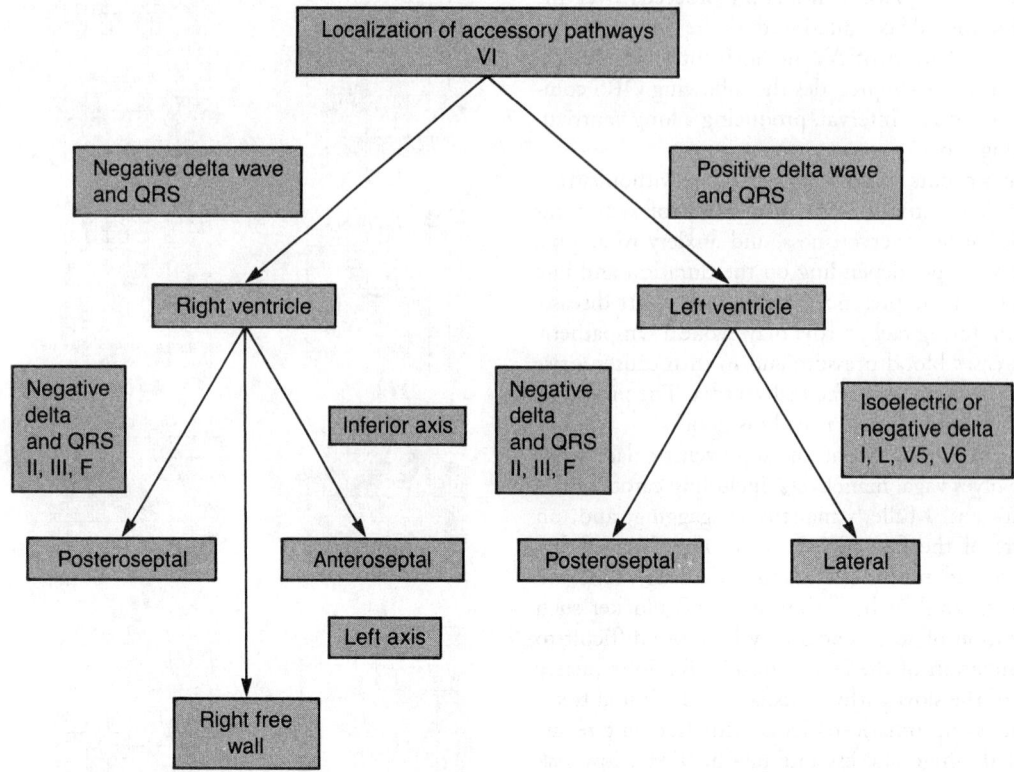

FIGURE 76.13. Electrocardiogram analysis of the sites of accessory pathways in Wolff–Parkinson–White syndrome.

presence of concealed accessory pathways is estimated to account for about 30% of patients with a supraventricular tachycardia referred for electrophysiologic evaluation.

Less commonly, the tachycardia can be antidromic, during which anterograde conduction occurs over the accessory pathway and retrograde conduction occurs over the AV node. The resultant QRS complex is abnormal, owing to total ventricular activation over the accessory pathway (Fig. 76.14). In all patients who have reciprocating tachycardias in which one of the limbs of the tachycardia involves the AV node, vagal maneuvers produce a response similar to that in AV nodal reentry.

About 5% of patients have multiple accessory pathways, and, on occasion, tachycardia can result from anterograde conduction over one accessory pathway and retrograde conduction over the other. An incessant form of orthodromic tachycardia occurs with a long ventriculoatrial interval because of a posteroseptal accessory pathway that conducts very slowly, possibly because it has a long, tortuous route. It is called the *permanent form of junctional tachycardia.* An accessory pathway may also be a "bystander" uninvolved in the mechanism responsible for the tachycardia. SA nodal reentry, AV nodal reentry, atrial tachycardia, atrial flutter or atrial fibrillation that conducts to the ventricle over the accessory pathway does not require the accessory pathway for maintenance of the tachycardia (Fig. 76.14). About 15% to 30% of patients have atrial fibrillation, and 5% have atrial flutter.

The reported prevalence of preexcitation syndrome averages about 1.5 per 1,000 (0.15%), but it is higher in relatives of patients who have Wolff–Parkinson–White syndrome. The acquisition of an accessory pathway is probably congenital. Left-sided pathways are more common than right-sided pathways. Wolff–Parkinson–White syndrome is found in all age groups, with a higher prevalence in men and a decrease in prevalence with age, possibly because of loss of preexcitation. Most adults with preexcitation syndrome have normal hearts, although a variety of acquired and congenital cardiac defects have been reported to be associated with Wolff–Parkinson–White syndrome, most commonly Ebstein's anomaly.

The prognosis for patients with preexcitation syndrome is excellent for those without tachycardia or an associated cardiac abnormality. In most patients with tachycardia, the prognosis is good, but sudden death does occur rarely. Intermittent preexcitation during sinus rhythm or loss of preexcitation after intravenous administration of a class 1 antiarrhythmic agent or with exercise suggests that the refractory period of the accessory pathway is long and the patient is not at risk for the development of a rapid ventricular rate if atrial flutter or fibrillation occurs. Exceptions to these safeguards can be present, however. In the patient without tachycardia, no therapy is indicated. For the patient with recurrent episodes of tachycardia, pharmacologic, electrical, or surgical therapy can be considered. Termination of the acute episode of orthodromic reciprocating tachycardia

RECIPROCATING TACHYCARDIAS

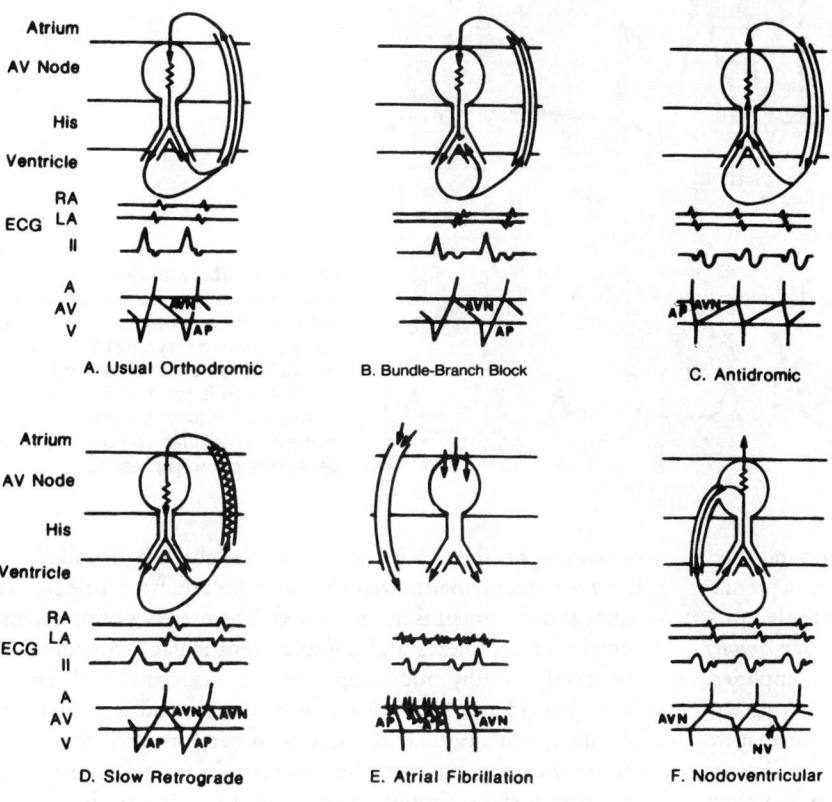

FIGURE 76.14. Schematic diagram of tachycardias associated with accessory pathways. **A:** Orthodromic tachycardia with anterograde conduction over the AV node–His bundle route and retrograde conduction over the accessory pathway (left-sided for this example, as depicted by left atrial activation preceding right atrial activation). **B:** Orthodromic tachycardia and ipsilateral functional bundle-branch block. The impulse must activate the contralateral ventricle, cross the septum, and enter the accessory pathway, making the ventriculoatrial conduction time longer. **C:** Antidromic tachycardia with anterograde conduction over the accessory pathway and retrograde conduction over the AV node–His bundle. **D:** Orthodromic tachycardia with a slowly conducting accessory pathway. **E:** Atrial fibrillation with the accessory pathway as a bystander. **F:** Anterograde conduction over a portion of the AV node and a nodoventricular pathway and retrograde conduction over the AV node. *AVN,* atrioventricular node; *LA,* left atrium; *RA,* right atrium. (From Zipes DP. Specific arrhythmias: diagnosis and treatment. In: Braunwald E, ed. *Heart disease: textbook of cardiovascular medicine,* third ed. Philadelphia: WB Saunders, 1988, with permission.)

characterized by a normal QRS complex should be approached as for AV nodal reentry.

For atrial flutter or atrial fibrillation, drugs that prolong refractoriness in the accessory pathway, often coupled with drugs that prolong AV nodal refractoriness, must be used. In some patients with very rapid ventricular rates, electrical cardioversion should be the initial treatment of choice. Verapamil and lidocaine may increase the ventricular rate during atrial fibrillation in a patient with Wolff–Parkinson–White syndrome, and intravenous verapamil can precipitate ventricular fibrillation. Because verapamil usually is not effective in patients with ventricular tachycardia, a reasonable rule is that intravenous administration of verapamil is contraindicated in any patient with a wide QRS tachycardia. The presence of atrial fibrillation in patients with a concealed accessory pathway should not present a greater therapeutic challenge than it does in patients who do not have an accessory pathway, because anterograde AV conduction occurs only over the AV node.

As in AV nodal reentry, radiofrequency catheter ablation usually is the initial treatment of choice for the symptomatic patient because it eliminates conduction over the accessory pathway (success rate 95%) with minimal complications (less than 2%) and provides a cure of the tachycardia. Surgery rarely is done any longer. Drugs to prevent recurrences are chosen to prolong conduction time or refractoriness in the AV node, the accessory pathway, or both. Digitalis actually can shorten refractoriness in the accessory pathway in some patients and speed the ventricular response during atrial fibrillation.

VENTRICULAR ARRHYTHMIAS

PREMATURE VENTRICULAR COMPLEXES

Premature occurrence of a QRS complex that is bizarre in shape and has a duration usually exceeding the dominant QRS complex (typically greater than 120 msec) characterizes a premature ventricular complex (Fig. 76.15). A large T wave opposite in direction to the major deflection of the QRS complex also is present. A premature P wave does not precede the QRS complex, but a sinus P wave that occurs at its expected time can be present. Because an aberrantly conducted supraventricular complex can mimic the manifestations of a premature ventricular complex, diagnosis of the latter cannot be made unequivocally from the scalar ECG. Most commonly, the premature ventricular complex does not discharge the atria and sinus node because the wave fronts from the anterograde impulse conducted from the sinus node and the retrograde impulse conducted from the premature ventricular complex collide at the AV junction. Therefore, a fully compensatory pause usually follows a premature ventricular complex. That is, the RR interval produced by two sinus-initiated QRS complexes flanking the premature ventricular complex equals twice the normally conducted RR interval. If the premature ventricular complex conducts retrogradely to the atrium and resets the sinus node, a noncompensatory pause occurs. If the sinus impulse is able to conduct to the ventricle despite the premature ventricular complex, the latter is called *interpolated.*

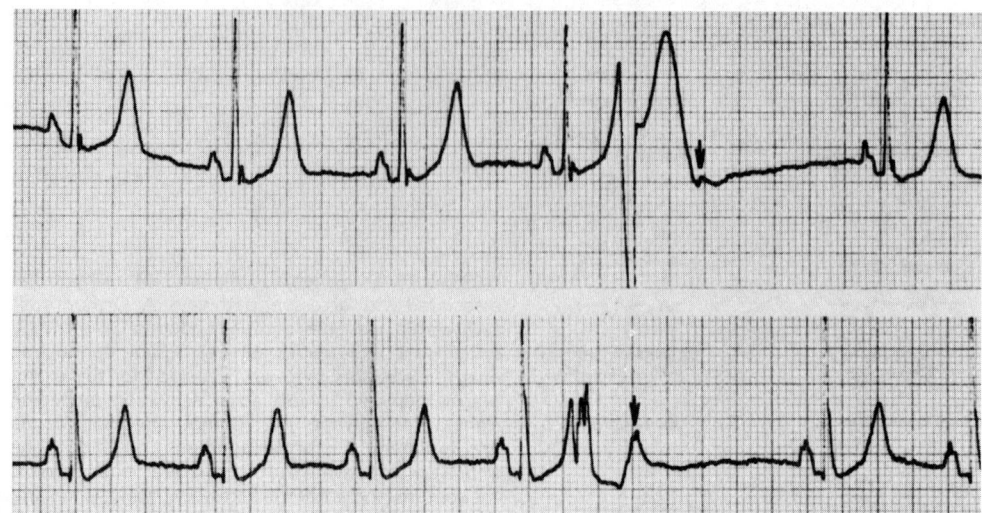

FIGURE 76.15. Multiform premature ventricular complexes. Premature ventricular complexes with different contours occur at a very short coupling interval. The sinus P wave (*arrow*) occurs on time and is blocked because of a refractory AV junction from the premature ventricular complex. A compensatory pause is present.

The term *bigeminy* refers to pairs of complexes and indicates a normal and a premature complex; *trigeminy* indicates a premature complex following two normal beats; *quadrigeminy* is a premature complex following three normal beats. A *pair* or a *couplet* refers to two successive premature ventricular complexes, whereas three successive premature ventricular complexes are called a *triplet*. Arbitrarily, three or more successive premature ventricular complexes are termed *ventricular tachycardia.* Premature ventricular complexes can have different contours and often are called *multifocal.* More properly, they should be called *multiform, polymorphic,* or *pleomorphic,* because it is not known whether multiple foci are discharging or whether conduction of the impulse originating from one site is merely changing.

The prevalence of premature ventricular complexes increases with age. Symptoms may be those of palpitations or discomfort in the neck or chest because of the greater than normal contractile force of the postextrasystolic beat or the feeling that the heart has stopped during the long pause after the premature ventricular complex. Exercise, sleep, or other activities can increase or decrease the number of premature ventricular complexes. Premature ventricular complexes occur in association with a variety of stimuli and can be produced by direct mechanical, electrical, and chemical stimulation of the myocardium. Coronary disease, myocarditis, a variety of medications, electrolyte imbalance, tension states, caffeine, tobacco, alcohol, and autonomic stimulation all can provoke premature ventricular complexes.

The importance of premature ventricular complexes varies, depending on the clinical setting. In the absence of underlying heart disease, premature ventricular complexes have little significance and treatment is not indicated. The presence of premature ventricular complexes and complex ventricular arrhythmias in apparently healthy middle-aged men is associated with an increased incidence of coronary heart disease and a greater risk of subsequent death. It has not been demonstrated that these arrhythmias actually precipitate sudden death in these patients, and they may be simply a marker of heart disease. In a study of patients with asymptomatic ventricular arrhythmias after MI, treatment with flecainide and encainide *increased* mortality 2.5 times compared with the placebo group (Cardiac Arrhythmias Suppression Trial). If ventricular arrhythmias are not associated with structural heart disease, these patients do not have an increased incidence of sudden cardiac death.

Treatment of patients with premature ventricular complexes most often is not indicated, except for the uncommon patient in whom those premature ventricular complexes produce intolerable palpitations. Treatment in general is as for ventricular tachycardia. Premature ventricular complexes in patients with structurally normal hearts often arise from the right ventricular outflow tract and can be treated with radiofrequency ablation.

VENTRICULAR PARASYSTOLE

Parasystole refers to a cardiac arrhythmia characterized electrocardiographically by four basic features: a varying coupling inter-

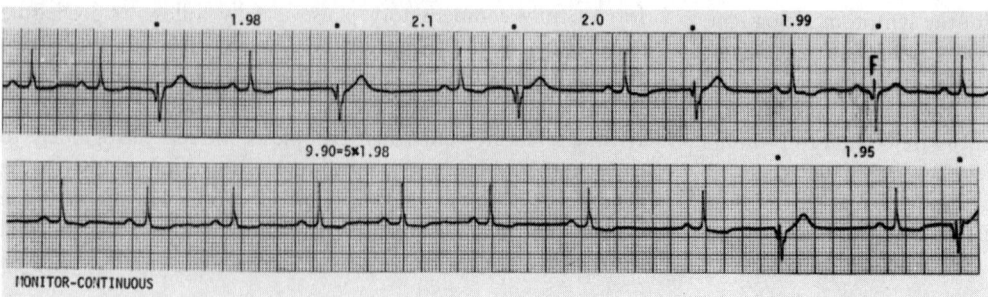

FIGURE 76.16. Ventricular parasystole. Premature ventricular complexes (*dots above tracing*) occur at regular intervals of about 1.98 seconds. The long pause without a premature ventricular complex is 9.9 seconds long, which equals five parasystolic intervals. Note varying intervals and a fusion complex (*F*).

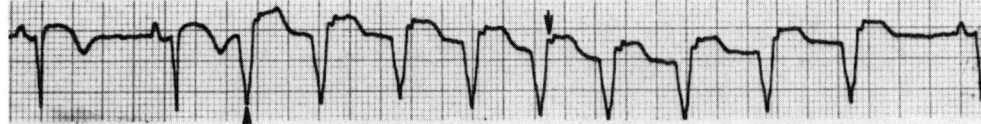

FIGURE 76.17. Ventricular tachycardia with retrograde atrial capture. A late premature ventricular complex (*upright arrow*) initiates a short episode of ventricular tachycardia with retrograde atrial capture (*inverted arrow*).

val between the ectopic or parasystolic complex and the dominant complex, which usually is sinus initiated; a common minimal time interval between manifest interectopic parasystolic intervals, with the longer interectopic intervals being a multiple of this minimal interval; fusion complexes because of the variable intervals between the parasystolic and dominant rhythms; and the presence of the parasystolic impulse whenever the cardiac chamber is excitable (Fig. 76.16). The analogy commonly invoked to represent parasystole is the behavior of a fixed-rate pacemaker. Parasystole can occur in the sinus and AV nodes, atrium and ventricle, and AV junction. Its mechanism presumably is attributable to the regular discharge from an automatic focus that is independent of, and protected from, discharge by the dominant cardiac rhythm.

VENTRICULAR TACHYCARDIA

Ventricular tachycardia arises distal to the bifurcation of the His bundle in the specialized conduction system, the ventricular muscle, or combinations of both tissues. Ventricular tachycardia is diagnosed when three or more premature ventricular complexes occur in a row. Ventricular tachycardia can be sustained, defined arbitrarily in electrophysiologic studies as lasting longer than 30 seconds or requiring termination because of hemodynamic collapse, or nonsustained, in which case it stops spontaneously in less than 30 seconds. AV dissociation may be present, during which atrial activity is independent of the ventricular tachycardia, or the atria may be captured retrogradely by the ventricles, in which case AV dissociation is not present (Fig. 76.17). QRS complexes may exhibit a uniform or monomorphic contour (Fig. 76.18), or they may vary (multiform, polymorphic, pleomorphic; Fig. 76.19).

Ventricular complexes with bizarre configuration or prolonged duration indicate only that conduction through the ventricle is abnormal, and such complexes can occur during supra-

ventricular rhythms as a result of preexisting bundle-branch block, aberrant conduction during incomplete recovery of repolarization (functional; see Fig. 76.5), conduction over accessory pathways (Fig. 76.12), and several other conditions. These complexes do not necessarily indicate the origin of impulse formation or the reason for the abnormal conduction; therefore, the ECG distinction between supraventricular tachycardia with aberration and ventricular tachycardia may be difficult (Table 76.2).

The presence of fusion beats and capture beats provides maximum support for the diagnosis of ventricular tachycardia (Fig. 76.20). Fusion beats indicate activation of the ventricle from two different foci, implying that one of the foci has a ventricular origin. Discharge of the ventricle by the supraventricular rhythm, with a normal configuration of the captured QRS complex at an interval shorter than the wide QRS tachycardia, indicates that the captured beat has a supraventricular origin and suggests that the wide QRS complex tachycardia is of ventricular origin.

Analysis of specific QRS contours can be helpful in the diagnosis of ventricular tachycardia (Table 76.2). During ventricular tachycardia with a right bundle-branch-block appearance, (a) the QRS complex is monophasic or biphasic in V_1, with an initial deflection different from the sinus-initiated QRS complex; (b) the amplitude of the R wave in V_1 exceeds the R'; (c) a small R wave and large S wave or a QS pattern may be present in V_6; and (d) the QRS duration exceeds 140 msec. With a ventricular tachycardia that has a left bundle-branch-block contour, the axis may be rightward, with negative deflections deeper in V_1 than in V_6; a broad, prolonged (greater than 40 msec) R wave may be present in V_1 and V_3; and a small qR or QS pattern may be observed in V_6. A QRS complex that is similar in V_1 through V_6, either all negative or all positive, favors a ventricular origin. An upright QRS complex in V_1 through V_6 may occur, however, because of conduction over a left-sided accessory pathway.

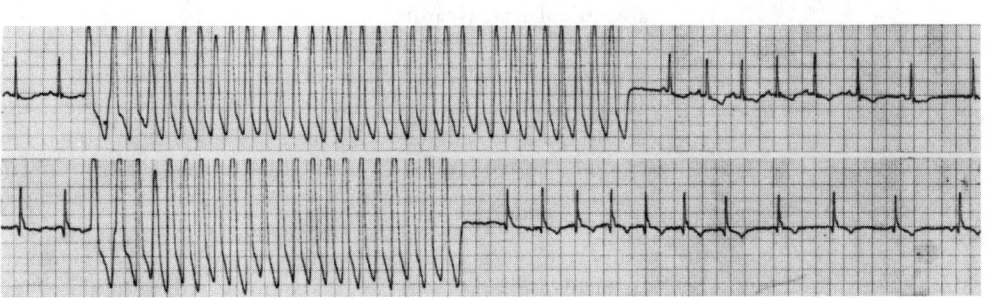

FIGURE 76.18. Monomorphic ventricular tachycardia. A relatively late premature ventricular complex initiates two short episodes of monomorphic ventricular tachycardia. After cessation of the ventricular tachycardia, the atrial rate increases for a short time, probably because of sympathetic discharge provoked by the hypotension resulting from the rapid ventricular tachycardia.

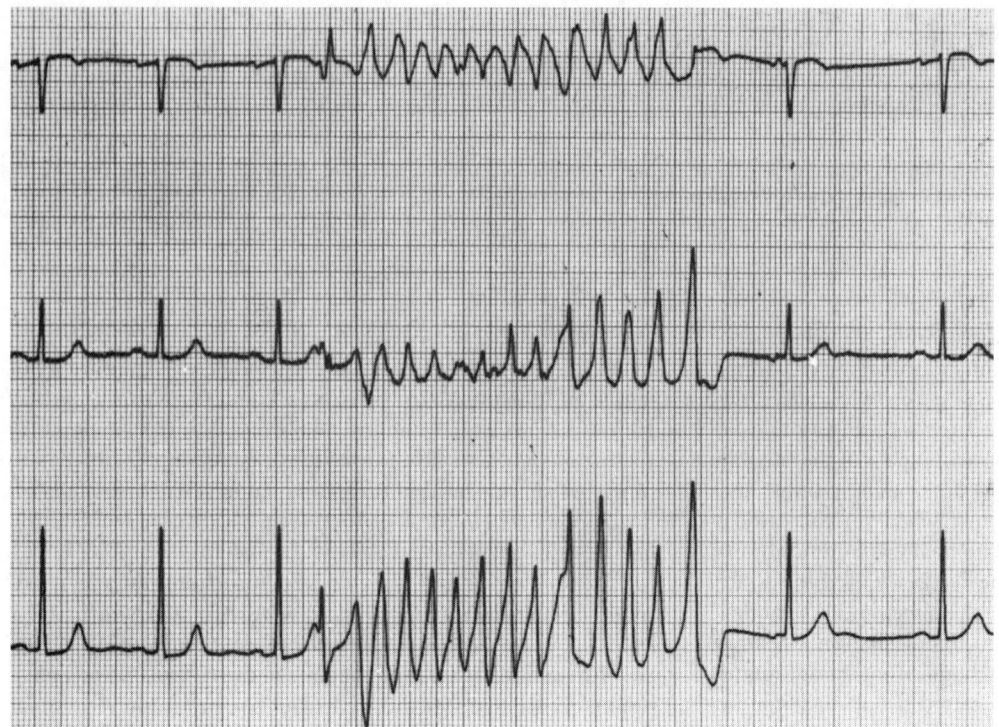

FIGURE 76.19. Polymorphic ventricular tachycardia. A premature ventricular complex occurring in the T wave provokes a short episode of polymorphic ventricular tachycardia. Leads from top to bottom recorded simultaneously are V_1, II, and V_5.

ABERRANCY VERSUS VENTRICULAR TACHYCARDIA

Electrocardiographic features characterizing supraventricular arrhythmia with aberrancy include consistent onset of the tachycardia with a premature P wave; a very short (less than 100 msec) RP interval; a QRS configuration that is the same as that which occurs from known supraventricular conduction at similar rates; linkage of P and QRS rates and rhythms, suggesting that ventricular activation depends on atrial discharge; and slowing or termination of the tachycardia by vagal maneuvers. Uncommonly, vagal maneuvers may terminate a ventricular tachycardia.

Supraventricular beats with aberrancy often have a triphasic pattern in V_1, an initial vector of the abnormal complex similar to that of the normally conducted beats, and a wide QRS complex that terminates a short cycle that follows a long cycle (long-short cycle sequence; Fig. 76.5). During atrial fibrillation, fixed coupling, short coupling intervals, a long pause after the abnormal beat, and runs of bigeminy rather than a consecutive series of abnormal complexes all favor a ventricular origin of the premature complex rather than a supraventricular origin with aberrancy. In the presence of preexisting bundle-branch block, a wide QRS tachycardia with a contour different from that which occurs during sinus rhythm probably is a ventricular tachycardia. A grossly irregular wide QRS tachycardia with ventricular rates faster than 200 beats per minute should raise the possibility of atrial fibrillation with conduction over an accessory pathway (Fig. 76.6). At times, a supraventricular tachycardia can induce a ventricular tachycardia.

When an accurate differential diagnosis between supraventricular tachycardia with aberrancy and ventricular tachycardia cannot be made, one must rely on sound clinical judgment, use of the ECG as only one of several helpful ancillary tests. For example, a wide QRS tachycardia occurring for the first time in a middle-aged man with a history of a previous MI has a greater than 90% chance of being a ventricular tachycardia rather than a supraventricular tachycardia with aberrancy. Rarely, a ventricular tachycardia produces a QRS complex with duration of less

TABLE 76.2.	DIFFERENTIAL DIAGNOSIS OF WIDE QRS TACHYCARDIAS

Supports Supraventricular

Slowing or termination by increased vagal tone
Onset with premature P wave
RP interval ≤100 msec
P and QRS rate and rhythm linked to suggest ventricular activation depends on atrial discharge (eg, 2:1 AV block)
$RSR'V_1$
Long—short cycle sequence
QRS identical to known supraventricular conduction (eg, preexisting bundle-branch block)

Supports Ventricular

Fusion beats
Capture beats
AV dissociation
P and QRS rate and rhythm linked to suggest atrial activation depends on ventricular discharge (eg, 2:1 VA block)
Compensatory pause
Left axis deviation
QRS duration >140 msec
Specific QRS contours

AV, atrioventricular; VA, ventriculoatrial.

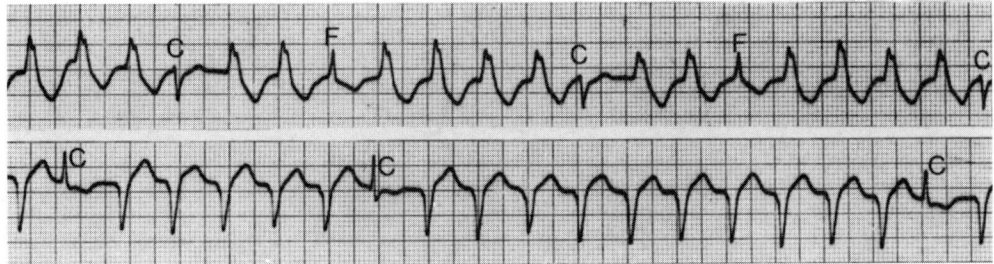

FIGURE 76.20. Ventricular tachycardia with fusion beats (*F*) and capture beats (*C*). Atrial activity is not clearly seen, but atrioventricular dissociation is likely. Note normalization of capture beats and blend of normal beats and ventricular tachycardia to create fusion beats. **Top,** lead V₁; **bottom,** lead II.

than 120 msec, probably when it arises close to the His bundle in the fascicles.

The rate of the ventricular tachycardia, its duration, and the presence of associated heart disease or peripheral vascular disease all help determine the symptoms occurring from the ventricular tachycardia. In addition, the location of impulse formation and, therefore, the way in which the depolarization waves spread across the myocardium may be important. Physical findings vary (Table 76.1).

Ischemic heart disease is the most common cause of ventricular tachycardia, the next being cardiomyopathy, followed by a variety of other causes. Ventricular tachycardia and ventricular fibrillation are responsible for most sudden cardiac deaths. When ventricular tachycardia is recorded in ambulatory patients, it most often starts with a late premature ventricular complex. Short runs of ventricular tachycardia consisting of three or four complexes after MI indicate an increased risk of mortality. Left ventricular dysfunction and ventricular arrhythmias are independently related to mortality risk in the 2 years after MI. Studies are ongoing to identify high-risk patients who might benefit from implantation of a prophylactic cardiac defibrillator.

Termination of the acute episode of ventricular tachycardia depends on the clinical circumstances. Ventricular tachycardia that does not cause hemodynamic decompensation can be treated medically with intravenous lidocaine. Intravenous procainamide or bretylium can be administered next. Intravenous procainamide usually is more effective than intravenous lidocaine. Amiodarone is effective when given intravenously and has recently been approved for this route of administration. Contributing factors such as hypokalemia, ischemia, hypomagnesemia, and extreme bradycardia should be considered and corrected, if present.

If pharmacologic therapy is unsuccessful or if the patient has hemodynamic decompensation with hypotension, shock, angina, congestive heart failure, or symptoms of cerebral hypoperfusion, prompt direct-current electrical cardioversion is indicated. A synchronized shock of 10 to 50 J often is successful. Digitalis-induced ventricular tachycardia is best treated pharmacologically. Striking the patient's chest, sometimes called *thump version,* may terminate ventricular tachycardia by mechanically inducing a premature ventricular complex that presumably interrupts the reentrant pathway. Competitive pacing similarly can terminate ventricular tachycardia. However, these procedures incur the risk of accelerating the tachycardia to ventricular flutter or ventricular fibrillation.

Recurrent episodes usually are treated with class I drugs, sota-

lol, or amiodarone. Propranolol may be useful when fast sinus rates or ischemia contribute to the induction of ventricular tachycardia. Combinations of drugs with different mechanisms of action can be successful when single drugs fail and allow the use of low doses of both agents rather than higher, toxic doses of one drug. Implantable defibrillators have been shown to be more effective in improving survival compared with antiarrhythmic drugs in patients who have experienced a cardiac arrest or sustained ventricular tachycardia. For selected patients, surgery or radiofrequency catheter ablation may be indicated.

Management of ventricular tachycardia with a polymorphic pattern is influenced by whether the QT interval is prolonged. If it is, the ventricular tachycardia may be torsades de pointes, which is treated effectively by accelerating the ventricular rate, usually with pacing. In addition, intravenous magnesium or isoproterenol (used cautiously to increase the rate) successfully has suppressed acquired torsades de pointes. Class IA and possibly classes IC and III antiarrhythmic agents may increase the abnormally prolonged QT interval and worsen the arrhythmia. Class IB drugs may be tried cautiously if the QT interval already is prolonged. When the QT interval is normal, polymorphic ventricular tachycardia is treated as ordinary ventricular tachycardia. For patients with the idiopathic long QT syndrome, β-adrenoreceptor blockade is suggested. For patients who continue to have syncope, left-sided cervicothoracic sympathetic ganglionectomy that interrupts the stellate ganglia and the first three or four thoracic ganglia may be helpful. Implantation of an automatic implantable cardioverter–defibrillator may be advised.

SPECIFIC TYPES OF VENTRICULAR TACHYCARDIA

Fairly specific types of ventricular tachycardia can be identified on the basis of a constellation of distinctive ECG and electrophysiologic features or from a specific set of clinical events.

ACCELERATED IDIOVENTRICULAR RHYTHM

During accelerated idioventricular rhythm, the ventricular rate usually is fairly similar to the sinus rate and ranges between 60 and 110 beats per minute (Fig. 76.21). Fusion beats and capture beats are common as control of the cardiac rhythm passes between the sinus rhythm and the accelerated idioventricular rhythm. The rhythm terminates as the dominant sinus rhythm accelerates or the ectopic ventricular rhythm slows. The ventric-

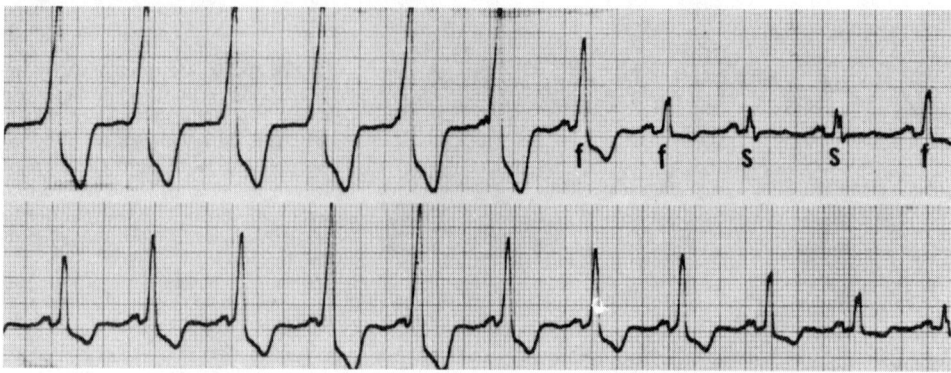

FIGURE 76.21. Accelerated idioventricular rhythm. Gradual speeding of the sinus rate results in fusion beats (*f*) and finally complete sinus capture (*s*), as the idioventricular rhythm focus and sinus node vie for control of the cardiac rhythm.

ular rhythm can be regular or irregular and occasionally shows sudden doubling, suggesting the presence of exit block. Enhanced automaticity is a probable mechanism.

Accelerated idioventricular rhythm primarily occurs in patients with structural heart disease (e.g., acute MI) or digitalis toxicity. Its presence has been used to indicate that coronary reperfusion has been accomplished. Usually, no therapy is required.

TORSADES DE POINTES

The term torsades de pointes refers to a ventricular tachycardia characterized by QRS complexes of changing amplitude that appear to twist about the isoelectric line and occur at rates of 200 to 250 beats per minute (Fig. 76.22). The term connotes a syndrome, not simply an ECG description of the QRS complex, with prolonged QT intervals usually exceeding 500 msec. During the ventricular tachycardia, the peaks of the QRS complexes appear successively on one side and then the other of the isoelectric baseline, giving the typical twisting appearance with continuous and progressive changes in QRS contour and amplitude. Long-short QRS cycle sequences commonly precede the onset of torsades de pointes, which often stops spontaneously with a progressive prolongation of cycle lengths and larger and more distinctly formed QRS complexes, but can degenerate into ventricular fibrillation.

Ventricular tachycardias that are similar morphologically to torsades de pointes but occur in patients without QT interval prolongation should be classified as polymorphic ventricular tachycardias rather than torsades de pointes. The distinction has important therapeutic implications. The most common predisposing factors to the development of torsades de pointes include severe bradycardia, potassium depletion, and class IA and IC antiarrhythmic drugs. Therapy is as described earlier.

LONG QT SYNDROME

The long QT syndrome is characterized by the presence of a prolonged QT interval (usually the corrected QT interval is greater than 500 msec) and often an abnormal U wave (Fig. 76.22). Afterdepolarizations may be important and related to the prolonged, notched, bifid, and sinusoidal T waves that occur. Ventricular tachycardia, commonly of the torsades de pointes variety, occurs.

The syndrome can be divided into a primary or idiopathic group caused by a congenital, often familial, disorder that occasionally is associated with deafness, and an acquired group caused by various drugs (e.g., class IA, IC, and III antiarrhythmic agents, phenothiazines, tricyclic antidepressants, nonsedating antihistamines), metabolic abnormalities (e.g., hypokalemia), the liquid protein diet and starvation, central nervous system lesions, autonomic nervous system dysfunction, coronary artery disease with MI, and other disturbances.

Patients with congenital long QT syndrome who are at increased risk for sudden cardiac death include those who have family members who died suddenly at an early age and those who have experienced syncope. ECGs should be obtained for

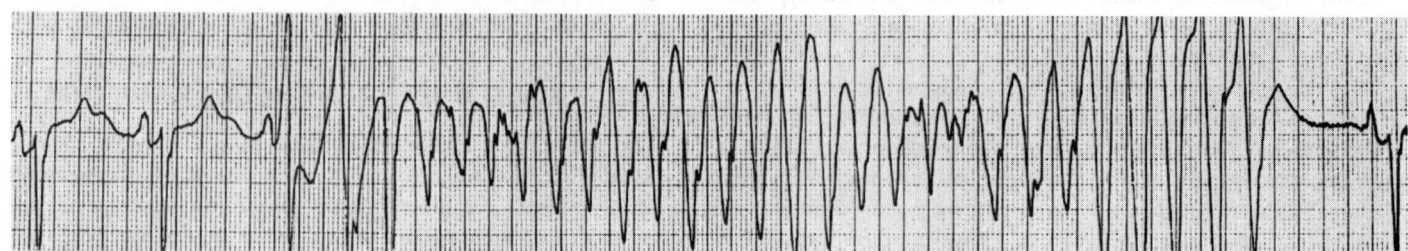

FIGURE 76.22. Long QTU syndrome with torsades de pointes. After two sinus-initiated complexes with obvious QTU prolongation caused by amiodarone, a polymorphic ventricular tachycardia ensues that exhibits the typical contour (not shown) of torsades de pointes.

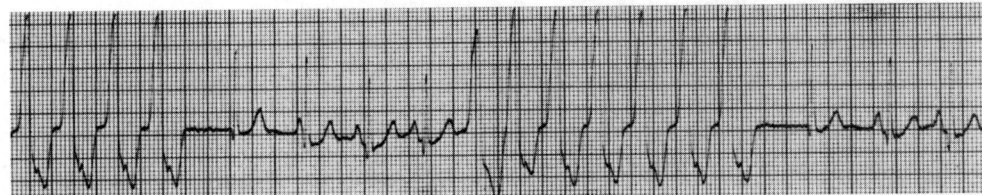

FIGURE 76.23. Repetitive monomorphic ventricular tachycardia. Short bursts of ventricular tachycardia are interrupted by sinus impulses.

all family members when the propositus has symptoms. Genetic abnormalities have been established for this syndrome.

BIDIRECTIONAL VENTRICULAR TACHYCARDIA

Bidirectional ventricular tachycardia is an uncommon ventricular tachycardia characterized by QRS complexes with a right bundle-branch-block pattern, alternating polarity in the frontal plane from −60 degrees to −90 degrees and +120 degrees to +130 degrees, and a regular rhythm. The ventricular rate is between 140 and 200 beats per minute. It occurs commonly, but not exclusively, as a manifestation of digitalis excess, typically in older patients and in patients with severe myocardial disease.

IDIOPATHIC VENTRICULAR TACHYARRHYTHMIAS

Idiopathic ventricular fibrillation may occur in about 1% of all cases of out-of-hospital ventricular fibrillation, affecting mostly men and those in middle age. The cardiovascular evaluation is normal except for the arrhythmia. The natural history is incompletely known, but recurrences are common. Antiarrhythmic drugs and implantable defibrillators are useful therapeutic choices. Some patients have right bundle-branch block and ST-segment elevation. The arrhythmia at times is an early manifestation of a developing cardiomyopathy or arrhythmogenic right ventricular dysplasia, at least in some patients.

Idiopathic ventricular tachycardias with monomorphic contours can be divided into at least three types. Two types, paroxysmal ventricular tachycardia and repetitive monomorphic ventricular tachycardia (Fig. 76.23), appear to originate from the region

of the right ventricular outflow tract. Right ventricular outflow tract ventricular tachycardias have a characteristic ECG appearance of left bundle-branch-block contour in V_1 and an inferior axis in the frontal plane. A third type is left septal ventricular tachycardia that arises in the left posterior septum and sometimes is called a *fascicular tachycardia*. The prognosis for most patients is good. Radiofrequency catheter ablation effectively eliminates these focal tachycardias in symptomatic patients. In others, antiarrhythmic drugs are effective.

BUNDLE-BRANCH REENTRANT VENTRICULAR TACHYCARDIA

Reentry over the bundle branches appears to be responsible for yet another type of ventricular tachycardia. Retrograde conduction over the left bundle-branch system and anterograde conduction over the right bundle branch create a QRS complex with a left bundle-branch-block contour, a frontal plane axis of about +30 degrees, and an HV interval that equals or exceeds that of the normally conducted QRS complex. It is more prevalent in patients with dilated cardiomyopathy. Therapy is as indicated for ventricular tachycardia. Creation of bundle-branch block by catheter ablation can eliminate the tachycardia.

VENTRICULAR FLUTTER AND VENTRICULAR FIBRILLATION

Ventricular flutter and ventricular fibrillation represent severe derangements of the heartbeat that usually lead to death within 3 to 5 minutes unless they are terminated. Ventricular flutter presents as a sine wave in appearance with regular, large oscillations occurring at a rate of 150 to 300 beats per minute (usually

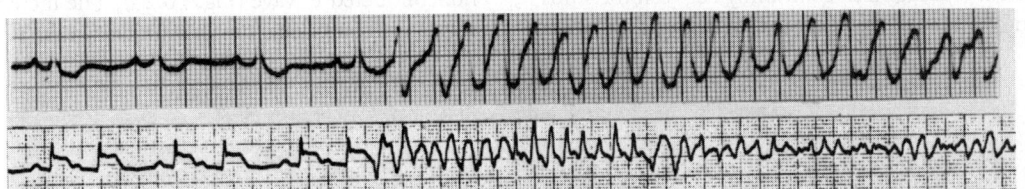

FIGURE 76.24. Ventricular flutter and ventricular fibrillation. In the top electrocardiographic recording, ventricular flutter begins and progresses to ventricular fibrillation (not shown) in this monitor lead. In the bottom recording (lead II), ST-segment elevation indicates the presence of acute inferior myocardial infarction. A 3:2 Wenckebach atrioventricular block is present. A premature ventricular complex initiates ventricular fibrillation.

around 200 beats per minute; Fig. 76.24). The distinction between rapid ventricular tachycardia and ventricular flutter may be difficult and usually is of academic interest only. Ventricular fibrillation is recognized by the presence of irregular undulations of varying contour and amplitude without distinct QRS complexes, ST segments, or T waves (Fig. 76.24). On occasion, the fibrillatory waves are so small as to simulate asystole.

Ventricular flutter or ventricular fibrillation promptly results in faintness followed by loss of consciousness, seizures, apnea, and death. Ventricular fibrillation most commonly occurs in association with coronary artery disease and as a terminal event. It may occur during antiarrhythmic drug administration, hypoxia, ischemia, atrial fibrillation, and rapid ventricular rates in Wolff–Parkinson–White syndrome, after electric shock is administered during cardioversion, or accidentally by improperly grounded equipment.

Ventricular fibrillation probably is responsible for more than 75% of sudden cardiac deaths, with bradycardia and asystole accounting for the remainder. Slow heart rates as a cause of cardiac arrest are associated with a worse prognosis than is ventricular fibrillation. Only 20% to 30% of patients resuscitated from cardiac arrest have acute transmural MIs. Those in whom transmural MIs develop have a recurrence rate of ventricular fibrillation of only 2% at 1 year. Those patients in whom MIs do not evolve have a much higher recurrence rate of ventricular fibrillation. Predictors of death for resuscitated patients include reduced ejection fraction, abnormal wall motion, history of congestive heart failure, history of MI but no acute event, and presence of ventricular arrhythmias.

Immediate nonsynchronized DC electrical shock with 200 to 360 J is mandatory treatment. Cardiopulmonary resuscitation is used only until defibrillator equipment can be applied. *Time should not be wasted with cardiopulmonary resuscitation maneuvers if electrical defibrillation can be done promptly.* After reversion of the arrhythmia to normal sinus rhythm, it is essential to monitor the rhythm continuously and to institute measures to prevent a recurrence. If artificial ventilation is necessary, it is accomplished adequately with a tightly fitting mask and an Ambu bag. Too often, precious time is lost in attempts at intubation by unskilled personnel. A search for conditions contributing to the initiation of the arrhythmia should be made and treated if possible.

◾ HEART BLOCK

Heart block is a disturbance of impulse conduction that can occur at any site, but is recognized commonly between the sinus node and atrium (SA block), between the atrium and ventricle

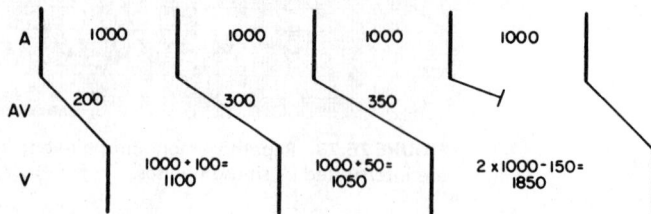

TYPICAL 4:3 WENCKEBACH CYCLE

FIGURE 76.26. Diagrammatic representation of a 4:3 Wenckebach cycle. The sinus cycle length is constant (1,000 msec). The increment in atrioventricular nodal conduction time decreases from 100 to 50 msec, resulting in a shortening of the RR intervals from 1,100 to 1,050 msec. The duration of the RR cycles encompassing the blocked P wave is twice the PP interval minus the increments in the PR intervals.

(AV block), or within the ventricles (intraventricular or bundle-branch block). During AV block, the block can occur in the AV node (between the atrial and His deflections), within the His bundle (producing an H and H′), or distal to the His bundle (between the His bundle and ventricular deflections). Heart block must be distinguished from interference, which is a normal phenomenon characterized by block of an impulse as a result of physiologic refractoriness from a preceding impulse.

FIRST-DEGREE ATRIOVENTRICULAR BLOCK

During first-degree AV block, the PR interval exceeds 200 msec in the adult, but all P waves conduct to the ventricles. The prolonged PR interval can result from conduction delay in the AV node (AH interval), in the His–Purkinje system (HV interval), or at both sites. Occasionally, intra-atrial or intrahisian conduction delay results in PR prolongation. If the QRS complex is normal, the AV delay almost always resides in the AV node, rarely within the His bundle itself. If the QRS complex exhibits a bundle-branch-block pattern, conduction delay can be within the AV node or the His–Purkinje system.

SECOND-DEGREE ATRIOVENTRICULAR BLOCK

Second-degree AV block is divided into type I and type II, as described earlier. In both instances, the AV block is intermittent and usually repetitive. During type I AV block with a regular PP interval, progressive PR interval prolongation precedes the nonconducted P wave (Fig. 76.25). The increment in PR interval conduction delay decreases after the first cycle, resulting in

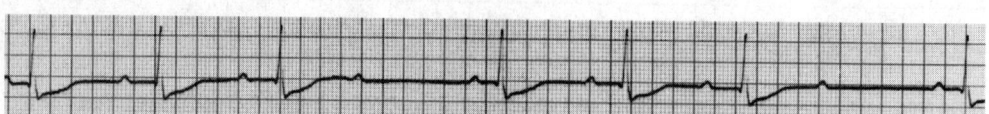

FIGURE 76.25. Type I (Wenckebach) second-degree atrioventricular block. A regular 4:3 conduction ratio is present.

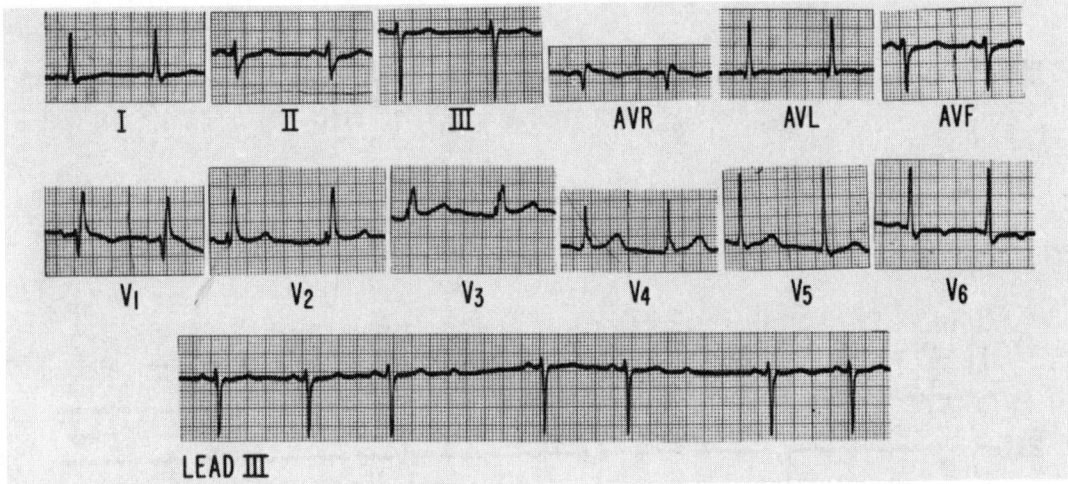

FIGURE 76.27. Type II second-degree atrioventricular (AV) block. Left-axis deviation and right bundle-branch block are present in this patient. Lead II illustrates sudden failure of AV conduction without antecedent PR prolongation.

a PR interval that increases but at a decreasing rate, and an RR interval that progressively decreases (Fig. 76.26). This classic AV Wenckebach structure occurs in less than 50% of the spontaneous clinical examples of type I Wenckebach AV nodal block. During type II AV block, the PR interval remains constant before the nonconducted P wave (Fig. 76.27).

If the QRS complex is normal, the block is more likely to be type I located in the AV node, whereas if a bundle-branch block is present, the block may be located in the AV node or the His–Purkinje system. Almost always, type II AV block occurs in the setting of a bundle-branch block.

As a rule, type I AV block is a more benign conduction disturbance, often not producing symptoms or requiring pacemaker therapy. It almost always occurs in the AV node, but it can occur at other sites. First-degree and type I second-degree AV block can occur in normal healthy persons, such as in well-trained athletes, and during sleep because of the increased vagal tone that occurs during rest (Fig. 76.28). Type II AV block usually is located in the His–Purkinje system and is associated more often with syncope, requiring pacemaker therapy. Type I AV block occurs more commonly during inferior MI, whereas type II AV block occurs more commonly during anterior MI, requiring temporary or permanent pacing, and is associated with a high rate of mortality, usually resulting from pump failure. Type I AV block during inferior MI is transient and does not require temporary pacing.

Two-to-one AV block (Fig. 76.29) and *high-grade AV block* (consecutive block of more than one P wave) can result from type I or type II AV block.

COMPLETE ATRIOVENTRICULAR BLOCK

Complete AV block occurs when no atrial activity conducts to the ventricles, and therefore independent pacemakers control the atria and ventricles. Complete AV block is one type of complete AV dissociation. The ventricular focus usually is located just below the region of block. When complete AV block results from block at the level of the AV node (usually congenital), the QRS complex is normal and the ventricular rate usually is 40 to 60 beats per minute. Atropine and exercise increase the ventricular rate. Acquired complete AV block occurs most commonly distal to the bundle of His because of trifascicular conduction disturbance. The QRS complexes are abnormal, and the ventricular rate usually is less than 40 beats per minute, with no change after atropine or exercise (Fig. 76.30).

A lengthy list of diverse causes can produce AV block, including surgery, electrolyte disturbances, endocarditis, tumors, rheumatoid nodules, calcific aortic stenosis, infiltrative processes, drug toxicity, coronary artery disease, and degenerative processes. In children, the most common cause is congenital, with block occurring at the AV node. Anti-Ro–negative antibodies in the maternal sera of patients with congenital complete AV

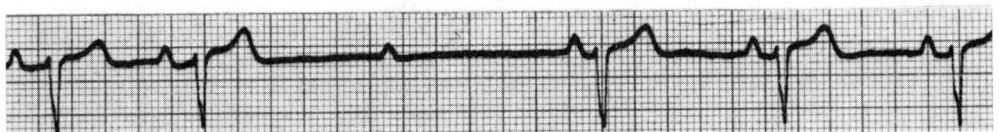

FIGURE 76.28. Vagal-induced type I second-degree atrioventricular block. The rhythm was recorded from a healthy 18-year-old woman during sleep. The PP interval lengthens, and a single P wave is blocked. This is consistent with an increase in vagal tone during sleep and would not be considered abnormal.

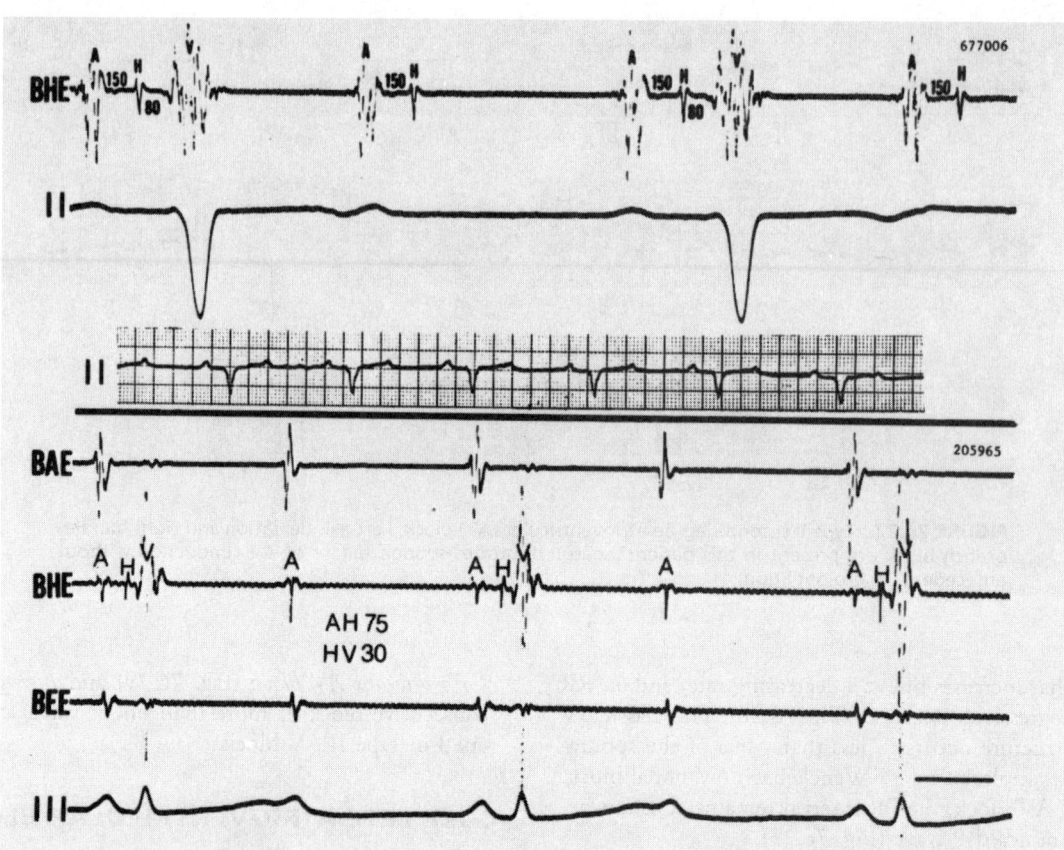

FIGURE 76.29. (Top) The electrocardiographic strip illustrates 2:1 atrioventricular block. From the His bundle recording, it is obvious that the block occurs distal to the His bundle recording site. The bundle of His–ventricular interval is prolonged (80 msec). (Bottom) The 2:1 atrioventricular block evident in lead III is proximal to the His bundle recording site. All intervals are normal. Time line, bottom right, 200 msec. *BAE,* bipolar right atrial electrogram; *BEE,* bipolar esophageal electrogram; *BHE,* bipolar His electrogram. (From Zipes DP. Second degree atrioventricular block. *Circulation* 1979;60:465, with permission of the American Heart Association.)

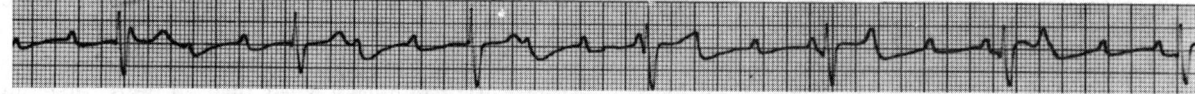

FIGURE 76.30. Acquired complete atrioventricular (AV) block. Tracing recorded in an elderly man with syncope illustrates complete AV block and a ventricular escape rate at about 38 beats per minute. No significant increase in the ventricular escape rate occurred with activity. The patient was treated with permanent pacemaker implantation.

block raise the possibility that placentally transmitted antibodies play a role. Children most often have no symptoms, but those in whom symptoms develop may require pacemaker implantation. For short-term therapy, vagolytic agents such as atropine or sympathomimetic agents such as isoproterenol may be used. Patients with acquired His–Purkinje block usually are symptomatic from Adams–Stokes syncope and require pacemaker implantation.

BIBLIOGRAPHY

Akhtar M, Myerburg RJ, Ruskin JN. *Sudden cardiac death: prevalence, mechanisms and approaches to diagnosis and management.* Baltimore: Williams & Wilkins, 1994.

Knight BP, Morady F. Catheter ablation of accessory pathways. *Cardiol Clin* 1997;15:647–660.

Morady F. Radiofrequency ablation as treatment for cardiac arrhythmias. (Review). *N Engl J Med* 1999;340:534–544.

Olsson SB, Allessie MA, Campbell RWF. *Atrial fibrillation: mechanisms and therapeutic strategies.* Armonk, NY: Futura Publishing Company, 1994.

Podrid PJ, Kowey PR. *Cardiac arrhythmia. Mechanisms, diagnosis and management.* Baltimore: Williams & Wilkins, 1995.

Prystowsky EN, Klein GJ. *Cardiac arrhythmias. An integrated approach for the clinician.* New York: McGraw-Hill, 1994.

Surawicz B. *Electrophysiologic basis of ECG and cardiac arrhythmias.* Baltimore: Williams & Wilkins, 1995.

Zipes DP. Genesis of cardiac arrhythmias: electrophysiological consideration. In: Braunwald E, ed. *Heart disease. A textbook of cardiovascular medicine,* fifth ed. Philadelphia: WB Saunders, 1997.

Zipes DP. Specific arrhythmias: diagnosis and treatment. In: Braunwald E, ed. *Heart disease. A textbook of cardiovascular medicine*, fifth ed. Philadelphia: WB Saunders.

Zipes DP, Jalife J. *Cardiac electrophysiology: from cell to bedside.* 2nd ed. Philadelphia: WB Saunders, 1995.

Kelley's Textbook of Internal Medicine, fourth edition. Edited by H. David Humes. Lippincott Williams & Wilkins, Philadelphia © 2000.

C H A P T E R

77

VALVULAR HEART DISEASE

DAVID S. BACH
KIM A. EAGLE

AORTIC STENOSIS

DEFINITION

Aortic stenosis implies obstruction to left ventricular outflow due to a fixed anatomical abnormality of the aortic valve. Valvular aortic stenosis should be distinguished from nonvalvular forms of left ventricular outflow obstruction, including congenital supravalvular stenosis and subvalvular membrane, ridge or tunnel stenosis, and dynamic subvalvular left ventricular outflow obstruction in hypertrophic obstructive cardiomyopathy.

The normal aortic valve area is 3.0 to 4.0 cm^2. Aortic stenosis is not usually of hemodynamic significance until the valve area is reduced to 25% of normal. It is clinically useful to categorize aortic stenosis as mild, moderate, or severe based on transvalvular gradients and valve area. In general, aortic stenosis is mild when valve area is more than 1.5 to 3.0 cm^2, moderate when valve area is more than 1.0 to 1.5 cm^2, and severe when ≤ 1.0 cm^2. With normal cardiac output, severe aortic stenosis is usually associated with a mean transvalvular pressure gradient ≥ 50 mm Hg. However, there are limitations in the ability to categorize the severity of aortic stenosis based on gradients and estimated valve area. Transvalvular gradients are affected by flow, so patients may have low gradients despite severe aortic stenosis if there is left ventricular systolic dysfunction. Although valve area is independent of flow, there is considerable overlap based on body size; a valve area of 1.0 cm^2 may be adequate in a smaller patient but representative of significant stenosis in a larger patient. Because therapeutic decisions typically are based on the presence of symptoms in the setting of significant aortic stenosis, categorization of disease as mild, moderate, or severe is of lesser clinical importance.

ETIOLOGY, INCIDENCE, AND EPIDEMIOLOGY

In adults, aortic stenosis may be congenital, rheumatic, or senile degenerative (calcific) in origin. Congenital aortic stenosis is

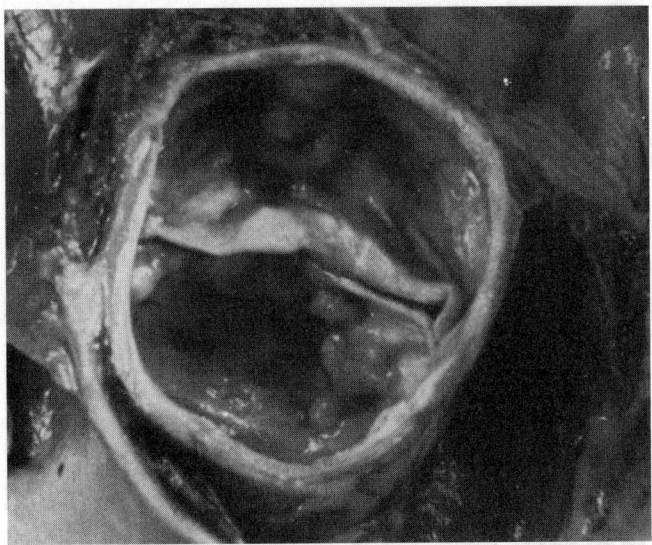

FIGURE 77.1. Bicuspid aortic valve with leaflet calcification. There are two sinuses of Valsalva and two symmetric cusps with no raphe.

much more common in men than women. Although usually associated with a bicuspid aortic valve, other abnormalities such as unicuspid and quadricuspid valves are less commonly present. Bicuspid valves may be true bicuspid valves, with two leaflets and two sinuses of Valsalva or "false" bicuspid valves, with three sinuses of Valsalva and a raphe in one of the valve leaflets, suggesting incomplete commissural development. Rheumatic aortic stenosis may occur in isolation, although it is seen more commonly in conjunction with rheumatic mitral valve disease. Degenerative aortic stenosis occurs exclusively in older adults, with progressive leaflet calcification. Pathology specimens of bicuspid aortic valve and rheumatic aortic stenosis are shown in Figures 77.1 and 77.2, respectively.

PATHOGENESIS

Lesion Pathogenesis

The pathogenesis of the valve lesion in aortic stenosis varies by cause. In congenital aortic stenosis, an abnormal valve is present from birth. However, whereas unicuspid valves can demonstrate significant stenosis from birth, hemodynamically important stenosis associated with most bicuspid valves usually occurs later. Years of mild obstruction and turbulent flow lead to fibrosis, calcification, and rigidity of the valve with subsequent decrease in orifice area. Poststenotic dilation of the ascending aorta is common with congenitally abnormal aortic valves, and associated aortic dissection may occur. In rheumatic disease, aortic stenosis typically manifests years after rheumatic fever. Progressive scarring and adhesion between commissures lead to commissural fusion and a decrease in orifice area. Calcification of the valve may be heavy, especially among older patients. Mild aortic regurgitation is commonly present. Senile calcific aortic stenosis is a gradual, degenerative process, and the progression from a normal aortic valve to stenosis is not fully understood. In general, cusp flexion over years results in calcification and aortic sclerosis,

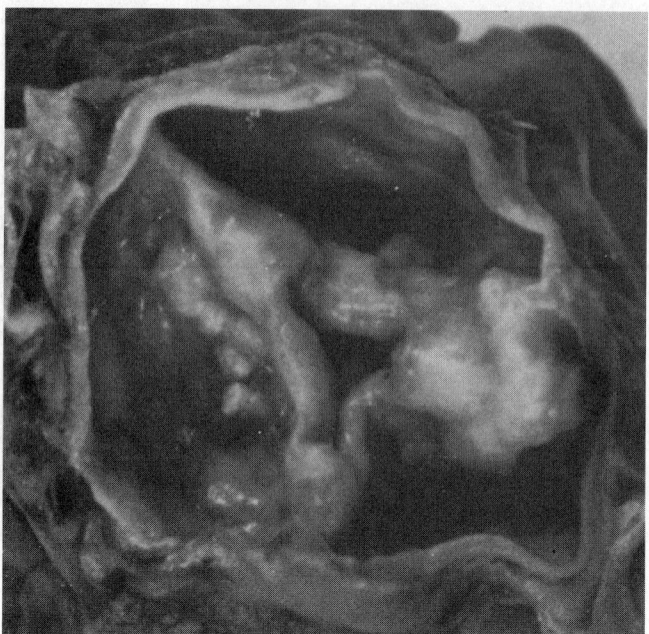

FIGURE 77.2. Rheumatic aortic valve stenosis in an elderly man. Commissural fusion and nodular calcification of the cusps are seen.

which in some patients may be associated with progressive calcification and stenosis. Although calcification occurs in both rheumatic and degenerative aortic stenosis, calcification occurs from the commissures toward the base in rheumatic disease and from the base toward the commissures in degenerative disease. The association between senile calcific aortic stenosis and risk factors for coronary artery and peripheral vascular disease suggests that this may be another form of vascular atherosclerosis.

Hemodynamic Pathogenesis

The common hemodynamic lesion in all forms of aortic stenosis is fixed obstruction to left ventricular outflow. Left ventricular hypertrophy occurs as a compensatory mechanism to maintain left ventricular wall stress in the setting of increased afterload. Left ventricular systolic function at rest is preserved late into the course of disease, although diastolic function may be impaired owing to the increase in left ventricular mass. Cardiac output may fail to increase with exertion in severe disease. Late in the course of aortic stenosis, left ventricular hypertrophy is no longer able to compensate for increased afterload, and the left ventricle dilates with subsequent development of systolic dysfunction.

CLINICAL FINDINGS

History

There is a long latent period before the development of symptoms, during which outflow obstruction and a compensatory increase in left ventricular mass occur. The three classic symptoms associated with aortic stenosis are dyspnea, angina pectoris, and syncope. Dyspnea occurs secondary to increases in left ven-

tricular diastolic, left atrial, and pulmonary venous pressures. Angina pectoris occurs without coronary artery disease resulting from increased oxygen demand from increased left ventricular mass and elevated intracavitary pressures in the setting of a fixed blood supply and from decreased coronary flow due to progressive outflow obstruction. Approximately 50% of patients with senile calcific aortic stenosis and angina pectoris have concomitant coronary artery disease. Syncope may be caused by peripheral vasodilation with exertion, with an increase in peripheral oxygen requirement in the setting of a fixed cardiac output. In addition, syncope at rest or with effort may be due to development of a tachyarrhythmia compromising cardiac output.

Late in the course of disease, a decrease in cardiac output results in congestive heart failure, with symptoms of fatigue, weakness, and peripheral cyanosis. Peripheral edema, hepatomegaly, and ascites may occur as a result of right ventricular failure secondary to pulmonary hypertension. Atrial fibrillation is a late manifestation of pure aortic stenosis, and its presence without other symptoms of advanced disease should suggest the possibility of concomitant mitral valve disease.

During the period in which patients are asymptomatic, mortality is extremely low. However, with the onset of symptoms, prognosis is poor and average survival without intervention is between 2 and 3 years, with the worst prognosis noted among patients with symptoms of congestive heart failure. Sudden death has been reported among patients with severe aortic stenosis and no symptoms of dyspnea, angina, or syncope. However, the incidence is extremely low and the weight of evidence suggests that patients develop typical symptoms of aortic stenosis before a morbid event.

Physical Findings

The classic physical finding of aortic stenosis is pulsus tardus et parvus, a delayed and prolonged arterial pulse of diminished intensity, caused by sustained ejection of blood across the stenotic valve. A prominent anacrotic notch is noted in the ascending limb of the arterial pulse. The pulse contour is typically assessed in the carotid artery. However, rigidity of the carotid arterial wall in older patients may transmit a vigorous pulse that does not accurately reflect central arterial pressure, and assessment of the brachial arterial pulse contour may be more appropriate.

Palpation of the precordium may reveal lateral and inferior displacement of the left ventricular apical impulse because of left ventricular hypertrophy, with a sustained apical impulse and palpable S_4. On auscultation, S_1 is normal. A systolic ejection click may be audible if the valve has not become completely immobile. The aortic component of S_2 is diminished. An S_4 is usually audible and an S_3 may be heard in a patient with congestive heart failure. The classic murmur of aortic stenosis is a harsh, low-pitched, crescendo–decrescendo systolic ejection murmur, which radiates from the base of the heart into the carotids.

Aortic stenosis is distinguished from aortic sclerosis by the abnormal arterial pulse contour and by the murmur peaking in the latter half of systole. Increasing severity of aortic stenosis is associated with the anacrotic notch occurring earlier in systole, progressive delay of the arterial upstroke, and the development of a precordial thrill. On auscultation, there is a progressive decrease in the aortic component of S_2, and the murmur peaks progressively later in systole and encompasses S_2. End-stage aortic stenosis may be associated with a softer murmur owing to decreasing cardiac output.

LABORATORY FINDINGS

Electrocardiogram and Chest Radiograph

The electrocardiogram (ECG) is neither sensitive nor specific for aortic stenosis, but it may show evidence of left atrial enlargement or left ventricular hypertrophy. Similarly, the chest radiograph may remain normal or may show increased size of the cardiac silhouette or evidence of left ventricular hypertrophy. Calcific deposits in the aortic valve can be seen, but their absence on chest radiograph does not preclude calcification of the valve.

Echocardiography and Doppler Imaging

Echocardiography and Doppler imaging are indispensable in the diagnosis and serial assessment of aortic stenosis. These techniques provide an accurate, noninvasive, low-cost, and widely available means to establish the presence, severity, and cause of aortic stenosis; the presence of concomitant valve lesions; and assessment of left ventricular size, mass, and systolic function. Echocardiographic imaging reveals anatomical abnormalities associated with the aortic valve, and a normal aortic valve on echocardiography precludes the presence of aortic stenosis. Left ventricular size, mass, and systolic function can be assessed serially for change. Doppler techniques provide an accurate means for the serial assessment of stenosis severity, with determination of peak instantaneous and mean transvalvular pressure gradients and estimation of valve orifice area based on the continuity equation and orifice planimetry. Transesophageal echocardiography allows additional assessment of valve anatomy for determination of the cause of stenosis. In addition, transesophageal imaging allows assessment of the ascending aorta, including the number of sinuses of Valsalva and the degree and location of poststenotic dilation, both of which impact surgical options for aortic valve replacement.

Cardiac Catheterization

Hemodynamic assessment during cardiac catheterization allows determination of peak-to-peak and mean transvalvular gradients and calculation of the stenotic orifice area using the Gorlin equation. An example of pressure tracings in a patient with aortic stenosis is shown in Figure 77.3. Because the hemodynamic assessment of aortic stenosis can usually be obtained using echocardiography and Doppler, cardiac catheterization for assessment of stenosis severity should be reserved for patients in whom there is a discrepancy between clinical and echocardiographic data. Coronary angiography allows assessment of coronary anatomy among patients with suspicion of coronary artery disease in whom surgical intervention is planned.

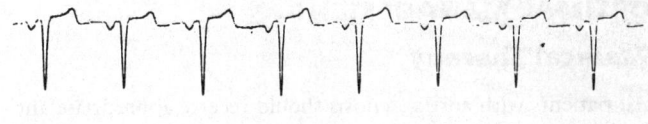

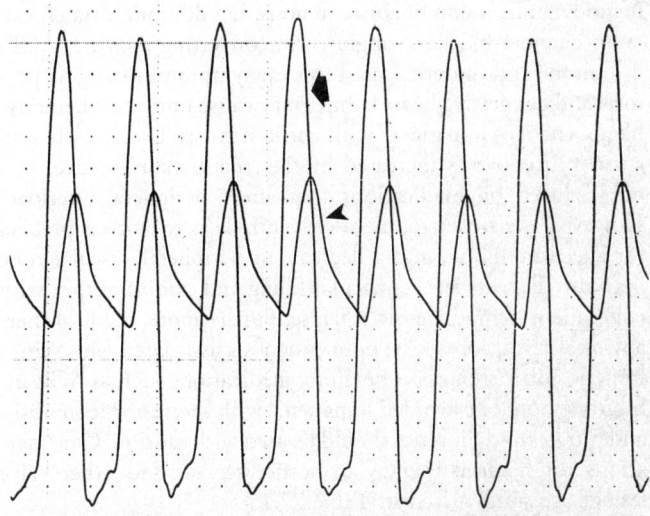

FIGURE 77.3. Simultaneous pressure tracings of left ventricle (*arrow*) and ascending aorta (*smaller arrowhead*) in patient with aortic stenosis. Systolic pressure of ascending aorta (101/59 mm Hg) is diminished and delayed in upstroke compared with that of left ventricle (155/2 mm Hg).

Exercise Testing

Exercise testing has been used with caution, if at all, in patients with significant aortic stenosis because of potential risks, as well as limited diagnostic accuracy for detecting coronary artery disease in the setting of aortic stenosis. Exercise testing is generally not recommended in symptomatic patients with evidence of severe aortic stenosis. However, exercise and pharmacologic stress testing may be useful in some patients. In asymptomatic patients with severe aortic stenosis, exercise testing may identify patients with limited exercise capacity and may provoke symptoms or signs that were not previously reported. In addition, exercise testing may be beneficial in patients with left ventricular systolic dysfunction and evidence of only moderate or mild aortic stenosis. Because gradients are dependent on flow, patients with severe aortic stenosis and low cardiac output have only moderately increased gradients, and it may be difficult to distinguish these patients from others with impaired left ventricular systolic function and only mild or moderate aortic stenosis. Although orifice area is independent of flow, the formulas used to calculate it are known to lose accuracy in low flow states, and calculated orifice area may be low in both groups. Among such patients, it may be useful to assess gradients and orifice area during exercise or dobutamine stress, when cardiac output is increased. When performed, stress testing should be directly supervised by a physician, with careful and frequent assessment of systolic blood pressure. Stress should be terminated for symptoms of angina, dyspnea or light-headedness, or if blood pressure falls.

OPTIMAL MANAGEMENT

Medical Therapy

All patients with aortic stenosis should receive appropriate antibiotic prophylaxis. There is no suitable medical therapy for the hemodynamic lesion of aortic stenosis. In addition, nitrates, calcium channel blockers, angiotensin-converting enzyme (ACE) inhibitors, and diuretics, used to treat symptoms of angina pectoris and congestive heart failure, may cause untoward hemodynamic changes in patients with aortic stenosis. Because left ventricular afterload is increased by the stenotic aortic valve, it is not reduced by medications that affect peripheral afterload. However, the hypertrophied left ventricle is reliant on preload for adequate filling, and a decrease in peripheral vascular tone may also decrease left ventricular filling and cardiac output with consequent hemodynamic collapse. Furthermore, medical therapy does not improve the poor prognosis associated with symptomatic aortic stenosis. Therefore, medications such as ACE inhibitors should be avoided in patients with severe aortic stenosis, and nitrates and diuretics should be used with caution. Considerations for medical therapy in aortic stenosis and other valve lesions are summarized in Table 77.1

Aortic Valve Replacement

Symptomatic patients with significant aortic stenosis should undergo consideration for surgical aortic valve replacement. In patients with aortic stenosis and symptoms of angina pectoris, syncope, or congestive heart failure, aortic valve replacement is associated with symptomatic improvement and increased survival. Left ventricular systolic dysfunction should not preclude consideration for surgical intervention. In the absence of significant comorbid conditions, aortic valve replacement is indicated for virtually all symptomatic patients with aortic stenosis. Aortic valve replacement is also indicated in patients with severe aortic stenosis undergoing coronary artery bypass surgery, surgery on other heart valves, or surgery on the aorta.

Surgical reconstructive procedures for the aortic valve have more limited application than for the mitral valve and are appropriate only for certain congenital aortic valve lesions without significant calcification. Mechanical prostheses have advantages of favorable hemodynamic profile and durability but require long-term anticoagulation because of thrombogenicity. Although stented heterografts do not require anticoagulation, their use is limited by durability and suboptimal hemodynamics associated with smaller prosthesis sizes. Allograft prostheses and the Ross procedure, a "switch" operation in which the normal pulmonic valve is implanted in the aortic position and replaced with a pulmonic allograft, are important alternatives for some younger patients requiring aortic valve replacement, although technical requirements and availability limit their more widespread use. Stentless tissue heterografts offer a new alternative for aortic valve replacement, with advantages of favorable hemodynamics and no requirement for anticoagulation. Considerations for surgical management of aortic stenosis and other valve lesions are summarized in Table 77.2.

Aortic Balloon Valvotomy

In adolescents and young adults, aortic balloon valvotomy plays an important role in delaying or preventing the need for valve replacement surgery. In older adults, balloon valvotomy plays a very limited role in the therapy of aortic stenosis. Although the procedure results in moderate early improvement in transvalvular gradients, the orifice area rarely exceeds 1.0 cm^2 following the procedure. Restenosis of the valve occurs within 6 to 12 months in most patients, and nearly 10% of patients experience periprocedural complications such as stroke and vascular complications. Aortic balloon valvotomy may be useful palliative therapy in selected patients with severe, symptomatic aortic stenosis in whom comorbid diseases preclude surgical intervention, among some patients with severe aortic stenosis who require urgent noncardiac surgery, and as a temporizing measure to im-

TABLE 77.1.	MEDICAL THERAPY IN PATIENTS WITH SEVERE AORTIC AND MITRAL VALVE DISEASE	
Lesion	**Goal of Therapy**[a]	**Medical Intervention**
Aortic stenosis	Avoid decrease in preload, peripheral afterload	Avoid over diuresis, afterload reducing therapy, negative inotropic agents
Aortic regurgitation, acute	Reduce afterload	Nitroprusside or nitroglycerin
	Therapy for pulmonary edema	Diuretics
	Maintain increased heart rate	β-adrenergic agonists or temporary cardiac pacing
Aortic regurgitation, chronic	Decrease systolic blood pressure	Vasodilator therapy with nifedipine, ACE inhibitor
Mitral stenosis	Control heart rate	Negative chronotropy: β-adrenergic or calcium channel antagonists
	Therapy for pulmonary congestion	Salt restriction, diuretics
	Reduce thromboembolic risk	Warfarin if atrial fibrillation or prior embolism
Mitral regurgitation, acute	Reduce afterload and preload	Nitroprusside (with inotropic agent if hypotension), diuretics, intra-aortic balloon counterpulsation
Mitral regurgitation, chronic		Afterload reduction not tested for long-term therapy

ACE, angiotensin-converting enzyme.
[a] General considerations for therapy are prophylaxis against infective endocarditis and prophylaxis against rheumatic fever.

| TABLE 77.2. | SURGICAL AND PERCUTANEOUS INTERVENTION IN PATIENTS WITH SEVERE AORTIC AND MITRAL VALVE DISEASE |

Lesion	Intervention	Indications
Aortic stenosis	Aortic valve replacement	Symptoms of angina pectoris, syncope or heart failure
		Undergoing coronary bypass surgery or surgery on other heart valve or thoracic aorta
	Percutaneous balloon valvotomy	Alternative to valve replacement in selected young patients with congenital aortic stenosis
		Palliative therapy or temporizing measure before aortic valve replacement
Aortic regurgitation	Aortic valve replacement	Symptoms of angina pectoris or congestive heart failure
		Left ventricular systolic dysfunction (ejection fraction <50% at rest) or marked left ventricular dilation (end-diastolic diameter >75 mm or end-systolic diameter >55 mm)
		Undergoing coronary bypass surgery or surgery on other heart valve or thoracic aorta
Mitral stenosis	Mitral valve replacement	Symptoms of heart failure, if not good candidate for percutaneous balloon valvotomy
	Percutaneous balloon valvotomy	If available, with favorable valve morphology and absence of left atrial thrombus or significant mitral regurgitation
Mitral regurgitation	Mitral valve replacement	Symptoms of heart failure
		Left ventricular systolic dysfunction (ejection fraction ≤60% and/or end-systolic diameter ≥45 mm)
	Mitral valve repair	If available with favorable valve morphology and indication for valve replacement
		Some asymptomatic patients with progressive left ventricular dilation, new atrial fibrillation, new severe mitral regurgitation
		Ischemic mitral regurgitation undergoing coronary artery bypass grafting

prove hemodynamics before aortic valve replacement in unstable patients with decompensated congestive heart failure and a prohibitive acute risk of surgery.

Elderly Patients

Because there is no suitable alternative therapy, including aortic balloon valvotomy, aortic valve surgery should be considered in all symptomatic patients with aortic stenosis, regardless of age. Although the operative risk of aortic valve surgery is higher among elderly than younger patients, the surgical procedure is feasible and successful surgery improves survival among elderly patients to that which is normal for their age.

Asymptomatic Patients

Patients with mild aortic stenosis should undergo periodic evaluation including assessment for the development of symptoms and echocardiography with Doppler imaging to evaluate for change in left ventricular size, mass, or function. Asymptomatic patients with moderate or severe aortic stenosis should undergo periodic evaluation more frequently. Patients should be made aware of the importance of angina pectoris, dyspnea, and syncope or presyncope and should promptly report the onset of symptoms.

◼ AORTIC REGURGITATION

DEFINITION

Acute and chronic aortic regurgitation are conditions of left ventricular volume overload caused by incompetence of the aor-

tic valve. As with other forms of valvular heart disease, the severity of aortic regurgitation occurs as a continuum, and the hemodynamic impact of the lesion is affected by factors in addition to regurgitant volume. The severity of aortic regurgitation is defined by its features on Doppler imaging and at cardiac catheterization. However, no gold standard exists against which to judge lesion severity, and overlap occurs between categories. Descriptions of severity are therefore best used in context with other clinical data.

ETIOLOGY, INCIDENCE, AND EPIDEMIOLOGY

In general, aortic regurgitation is caused by congenital or acquired abnormalities of the aortic valve or by acquired abnormalities of the aortic root that affect the competence of the aortic valve. Congenital causes of aortic regurgitation include bicuspid aortic valve and fenestrations of the valve cusps. Acquired abnormalities of the aortic valve can be due to rheumatic disease, hypertensive and atherosclerotic diseases, infective endocarditis, and nonpenetrating trauma. Diseases of the ascending aorta can result in aortic regurgitation, including aortic aneurysm and aneurysm of the sinus of Valsalva, cystic medial necrosis with or without other features of Marfan's syndrome, connective tissue diseases including Reiter's syndrome and ankylosing spondylitis, luetic (syphilitic) aortitis, and aortic dissection. Finally, dysfunction of an aortic valve prosthesis can result in aortic regurgitation.

PATHOGENESIS

Lesion Pathogenesis

The pathogenesis of the lesions responsible for aortic regurgitation varies according to the cause of disease. In congenitally bicuspid aortic valve, turbulent flow due to mild stenosis leads over years to fibrosis and calcification of the cusps, which can result in moderate and rarely severe aortic regurgitation. Bicuspid aortic valve frequently leads to combined aortic stenosis and regurgitation, but severe aortic regurgitation in the setting of bicuspid aortic valve usually implies a secondary process such as infective endocarditis. Aortic valve fenestrations are present at birth and can cause mild or moderate regurgitation.

Rheumatic aortic valve disease occurs years after rheumatic fever. Progressive thickening and retraction of the cusps result in incomplete coaptation and aortic regurgitation. Rheumatic aortic regurgitation typically occurs with some degree of aortic stenosis. Although rheumatic aortic valve disease can occur in isolation, it is more common with concomitant mitral valve disease. Hypertensive and atherosclerotic diseases can cause focal aortic valve calcification and scarring as well as dilation of the aortic root with resultant aortic regurgitation. Although the high prevalence of the underlying diseases makes these causes of aortic regurgitation common, it is usually only mild in severity. Infective endocarditis can cause aortic regurgitation of any severity. Infection of the valve tissue results in a continuum of destructive processes, from leaflet perforation to leaflet flail and leaflet destruction. Rupture of a paravalvular abscess complicating aortic valve endocarditis can lead to a fistula between the ascending aorta and the left ventricle. The degree of valve destruction is influenced by the destructiveness of the organism, chronicity of infection, and host factors. Because the mechanism of regurgitation in infective endocarditis usually relates to destruction of valve tissue, aortic regurgitation usually persists after successful treatment of the infection. Rarely, aortic regurgitation during endocarditis is caused by mechanical interference of a vegetation with normal leaflet coaptation but without significant tissue destruction, and regurgitation may improve or even resolve completely after treatment. Any preexisting congenital or acquired valve lesion can serve as a nidus for infection, and a rapid change in regurgitation severity should raise the possibility of superimposed infective endocarditis. Nonpenetrating trauma can result in avulsion of one or more valve cusps, leading to significant aortic regurgitation.

Diseases of the aortic root can also affect the competence of the aortic valve. Aneurysmal dilation of the aortic root can lead to dilation of the aortic annulus with incomplete leaflet coaptation and aortic regurgitation. Cystic medial necrosis, usually associated with Marfan syndrome, causes characteristic dilation of the sinuses of Valsalva with effacement of the sinotubular junction and aortic regurgitation. Cystic medial necrosis can also occur without other manifestations of Marfan syndrome. Leutic (syphilitic) aortitis is now extremely rare but causes heavy calcification of the aortic root and aortic regurgitation. Aortic dissection can be associated with aortic regurgitation with or without associated aortic aneurysm. Prolapse of the dissection flap through the aortic valve can directly interfere with valve closure and cause aortic regurgitation.

Most mechanical valve prostheses have a small amount of associated regurgitation during normal function, and mild aortic regurgitation is an anticipated finding. Dysfunction of a mechanical prosthesis can result in more significant regurgitation. Bioprosthetic valves typically fail with calcification and fracture of a valve leaflet, resulting in significant regurgitation. Paravalvular regurgitation can occur with both mechanical and tissue prostheses. Severe paravalvular regurgitation suggests partial dehiscence of the prosthesis, caused by either endocarditis or mechanical suture failure.

Hemodynamic Pathogenesis

The initial hemodynamic lesion with both acute and chronic aortic regurgitation is left ventricular volume overload. When chronic, the left ventricle compensates with gradual chamber dilation. Ejection fraction remains normal at rest until late in the disease, and increased left ventricular end diastolic volume permits increased stroke volume and normal forward cardiac output. Systolic hypertension results in a pressure overload component of chronic aortic regurgitation. Increased left ventricular volume causes increased wall tension, and compensatory hypertrophy leads to markedly increased left ventricular mass. The increased left ventricular mass associated with aortic regurgitation occurs with normal or mildly increased wall thickness and significant chamber dilation, whereas hypertrophy in aortic stenosis occurs with markedly increased wall thickness and normal chamber diameter.

Chronic aortic regurgitation is generally tolerated for years without symptoms. Although left ventricular ejection fraction remains normal at rest until late in the course of disease, augmentation with exercise is impaired earlier. Left ventricular end-diastolic pressure is elevated and with severe regurgitation equilibrates with diastolic aortic pressure. Eventually, left ventricular ejection fraction at rest declines as dilation and hypertrophy are unable to compensate for the combined volume and pressure overload, and many patients first note symptoms of dyspnea. Myocardial ischemia occurs in patients with advanced aortic regurgitation because of increased myocardial oxygen demand due to increased left ventricular diameter, stroke volume, and mass and because of decreased oxygen availability due to low perfusion pressure and an eventual decrease in cardiac output.

Acute severe aortic regurgitation results in left ventricular volume overload, but without time for left ventricular dilation, tachycardia is the only compensatory mechanism to maintain forward cardiac output. Left ventricular end-diastolic and left atrial pressures increase rapidly, with pulmonary venous congestion. Unlike chronic aortic regurgitation, acute severe aortic regurgitation is poorly tolerated. Without compensatory chamber dilation, tachycardia alone is usually insufficient to maintain forward cardiac output, and patients frequently present with pulmonary edema and shock.

CLINICAL FINDINGS

History

Patients with chronic aortic regurgitation usually remain asymptomatic for years or decades. Early symptoms include a sensation pounding in the chest, palpitations, or head pounding. Exertional dyspnea may be the first manifestation of left ventricular decompensation, with later development of orthopnea and paroxysmal nocturnal dyspnea. Symptoms of more advanced disease include angina pectoris, which may be nocturnal, and eventually symptoms of right-sided congestive heart failure with ascites and peripheral edema. Asymptomatic patients with severe aortic regurgitation and decreased left ventricular systolic function usually develop symptoms within 3 to 3 years. Sudden death among patients with compensated severe aortic regurgitation has been reported but appears to be rare, occurring with an incidence of less than 0.2% per year. Left ventricular systolic dysfunction and marked left ventricular dilation are associated with a worse prognosis, even if patients remain asymptomatic. Prognosis worsens with the onset of symptoms; mortality rate is estimated to be more than 10% per year among patients with severe aortic regurgitation and angina pectoris and more than 20% per year among patients with symptoms of congestive heart failure.

Acute severe aortic regurgitation usually occurs in the setting of infective endocarditis or acute aortic dissection or, more rarely, after blunt chest trauma. Patients typically exhibit symptoms referable to the underlying disease, including fever with infective endocarditis, and chest or back pain with aortic dissection. Acute severe aortic regurgitation is poorly tolerated and patients frequently present with pulmonary edema or cardiogenic shock.

Physical Findings

Most physical findings associated with severe aortic regurgitation reflect the combination of increased stroke volume and widened pulse pressure. Physical findings can be extensive, and there may be no other single lesion in medicine so rich with associated eponyms. In general appearance, patients can exhibit a bobbing motion of the torso or the head (de Musset's sign) synchronous with the heartbeat. Systolic pulsation of the uvula may be visible (Müller's sign). Arterial pulses are unusually prominent, with exaggerated systolic distention and exaggerated diastolic collapse on palpation (water-hammer or Corrigan's pulse). Palpation of the carotid arteries reveals a bisferiens, or double-peaking pulse. Capillary pulsation is visible in the nail beds when the distal nail is softly compressed (Quincke's pulse). Auscultation of large arteries may reveal a brief, loud systolic (pistol shot) sound. Auscultation of the femoral artery reveals booming systolic and diastolic sounds (Traube's sign); light pressure of the stethoscope proximally reveals a systolic murmur, with a diastolic murmur with pressure distally (Duroziez's sign). The systolic blood pressure is elevated, and the diastolic blood pressure is often very low, revealing a wide pulse pressure.

The left ventricular apical impulse is enlarged and displaced owing to left ventricular enlargement, and may be visible. A systolic thrill may be evident along the base of the heart or in the carotids, caused by the large left ventricular stroke volume. On auscultation, the aortic component of S_2 may be diminished or absent. The murmur of aortic regurgitation is a high-pitched, blowing decrescendo diastolic murmur, loudest at the left or right upper sternal border. Held end-expiration with the patient upright and leaning forward and the stethoscope diaphragm held firmly against the chest aid in the auscultation of soft murmurs of aortic regurgitation. The murmur may radiate to the cardiac apex (Austin Flint murmur), with a low-pitched diastolic rumble that mimics mitral stenosis. A systolic ejection murmur, often louder and more easily heard than the diastolic murmur, is due to large stroke volume and does not necessarily imply aortic stenosis.

Many of the typical physical findings associated with chronic aortic regurgitation are absent in patients with acute aortic regurgitation. Because the left ventricle is not dilated in acute aortic regurgitation, stroke volume is not increased, pulse pressure is not widened, and the associated peripheral arterial manifestations are absent. Although chronic severe aortic regurgitation can usually be diagnosed on physical examination, the detection of acute severe regurgitation is less reliable.

LABORATORY FINDINGS

Electrocardiogram and Chest Radiograph

Neither the ECG nor the chest radiograph is accurate in the detection or estimation of severity of aortic regurgitation. The ECG may reveal evidence of left ventricular hypertrophy or interventricular conduction delay. The chest radiograph may reveal cardiomegaly, dilation of the aortic root, or evidence of pulmonary venous congestion.

Echocardiography and Doppler Imaging

Echocardiography is indicated in patients with suspected aortic regurgitation to confirm the presence and to establish the severity and cause of aortic regurgitation. The dimensions, mass, and systolic function of the left ventricle should be determined, as well as the size and anatomy of the aortic root. Because absolute and subsequent change in left ventricular dimensions directly affect management, accurate quantification is important both at baseline and on subsequent examinations.

Transthoracic imaging allows assessment of aortic valve morphology and may establish the cause of aortic regurgitation with evidence of congenital abnormalities or findings suggestive of infective endocarditis. The proximal 2 to 3 cm of ascending aorta can usually be visualized. Aortic regurgitation is suggested by diastolic fluttering of the mitral valve; acute severe regurgitation is associated with premature closure of the mitral valve. Doppler imaging allows reliable detection and semiquantification of aortic regurgitation. Aortic regurgitation severity is estimated by the size of the regurgitant jet, as well as deceleration characteristics of regurgitant flow. Diastolic flow reversal in the descending aorta suggests severe aortic regurgitation. Transesophageal echocardiographic imaging allows optimal assessment of aortic valve morphology as well as definitive assessment of anatomy of the aorta, including assessment for aortic dissection. An example of bicuspid aortic valve on transesophageal echocardiography is shown in Figure 77.4, and associated aortic dilation and aortic regurgitation are shown in Figure 77.5. Transesophageal imaging is indicated to assess prosthetic valve dysfunction.

Radionuclide Angiography

Radionuclide angiography is a useful noninvasive means for assessment of left ventricular size and function if these data are not

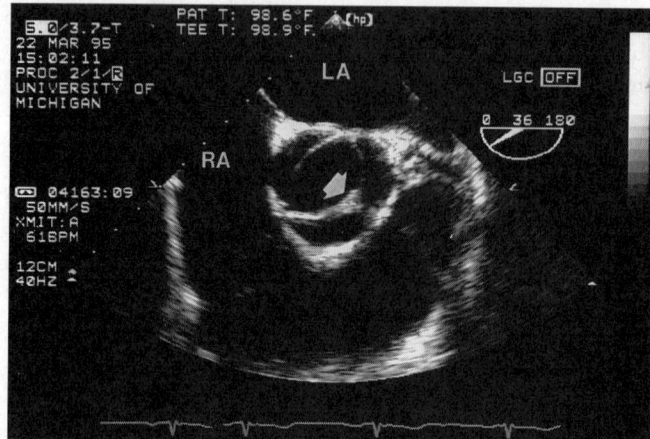

FIGURE 77.4. Transesophageal echocardiogram in patient with bicuspid aortic valve. Three sinuses of Valsalva and leaflet raphe (*arrow*) suggest incomplete commissural development. *LA*, left atrium; *RA*, right atrium.

available on echocardiographic imaging or if there is discordance between clinical data and data from echocardiographic imaging.

Exercise Testing

Exercise testing is useful to assess functional capacity and symptoms in patients with significant aortic regurgitation and equivocal symptoms. Change in left ventricular ejection fraction with exercise has been used as an indication for surgical intervention, although no definitive data support the incremental diagnostic or prognostic value.

Cardiac Catheterization

Cardiac catheterization with coronary angiography allows assessment of coronary anatomy among patients at risk for coronary artery disease in whom surgical intervention is planned. Aortic

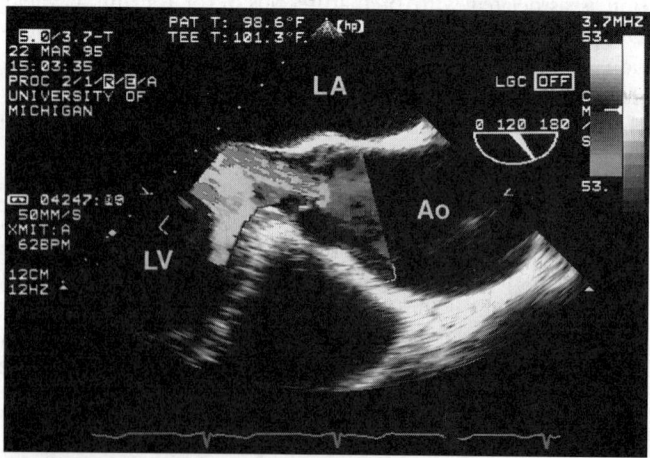

FIGURE 77.5. Transesophageal echocardiogram demonstrating aortic regurgitation in patient with bicuspid aortic valve. Dilation of tubular portion of ascending aorta is present. *Ao*, ascending aorta; *LA*, left atrium; *LV*, left ventricle.

regurgitation severity and aortic root size can be assessed with root angiography, although these data are usually available with noninvasive testing.

OPTIMAL MANAGEMENT

Medical Therapy

Patients with aortic regurgitation should receive appropriate antibiotic prophylaxis. Patients with chronic mild or moderate aortic regurgitation do not benefit from any other form of medical therapy. However, asymptomatic patients with chronic severe aortic regurgitation benefit from long-term vasodilating therapy with nifedipine or possibly ACE inhibitors. Therapy appears to delay the need for aortic valve replacement and results in improved left ventricular size and function after surgery. Therapy should be limited to patients with systolic hypertension, and dose should be titrated upward until systolic blood pressure decreases or side effects develop. Medical therapy is not an alternative to surgery for symptomatic or asymptomatic patients with severe aortic regurgitation and decreased left ventricular systolic function. Asymptomatic patients with moderate or severe aortic regurgitation are able to participate in normal physical activity, including mild intensity exercise, although weight lifting and other isometric exercises should be avoided.

Patients with acute severe aortic regurgitation typically suffer hemodynamic compromise with pulmonary edema and cardiogenic shock. Medical therapy should be directed at aggressive afterload reduction with intravenous nitroprusside or nitroglycerin. Diuretics are useful in the management of pulmonary edema. Because regurgitant volume decreases with a shorter diastolic interval and because diastolic interval decreases with increasing heart rate, maintaining a rapid heart rate using β-agonists or temporary cardiac pacing is useful among patients with acute severe aortic regurgitation and hemodynamic compromise. Intra-aortic balloon counterpulsation is contraindicated.

Serial Testing

Asymptomatic patients with aortic regurgitation and normal left ventricular systolic function should be followed up for evidence of angina or heart failure and for change in left ventricular size and function. Patients with mild aortic regurgitation should be followed up with periodic medical history and physical examination, with additional testing if symptoms develop or if physical examination suggests progression of disease. Patients with moderate or severe aortic regurgitation should undergo serial follow-up, including history, physical examination, and echocardiographic imaging. Patients with chronic, stable aortic regurgitation should be evaluated every 6 to 12 months. Follow-up should be more frequent if there is evidence of left ventricular chamber dilation.

Aortic Valve Replacement

Aortic valve replacement is indicated for patients with severe aortic regurgitation and symptoms of angina or heart failure. In addition, aortic valve replacement is indicated for asymptomatic patients with severe aortic regurgitation and either left ventricular systolic dysfunction (ejection fraction less than 50% at rest) or marked left ventricular dilation (end-diastolic diameter more than 75 mm or end-systolic diameter greater than 55 mm). The risk of surgery increases with progressive left ventricular systolic dysfunction, although functional status and prognosis are improved with aortic valve replacement despite preexisting severe left ventricular systolic dysfunction. Patients with severe aortic regurgitation who require coronary artery bypass grafting or surgery on other heart valves or on the thoracic aorta should also undergo aortic valve replacement.

MITRAL STENOSIS

DEFINITION

Mitral stenosis implies valvular obstruction to left ventricular inflow. Nonvalvular causes of left ventricular inflow obstruction include congenital abnormalities not usually encountered in an adult population, and obstruction due to left atrial tumor or ball thrombus. The normal mitral valve area is 4.0 to 5.0 cm^2. Symptoms occur with exercise or tachycardia when the valve area is approximately 2.0 to 2.5 cm^2; symptoms at rest usually do not occur until the valve area is $\leq$1.5 cm^2. In general, mitral stenosis is considered mild if mean pressure gradient is less than 5 mm Hg and valve area is more than 1.5 cm^2.

ETIOLOGY, INCIDENCE, AND EPIDEMIOLOGY

Mitral stenosis in adults is predominantly of rheumatic origin. Women are affected more often than men. The mitral valve is the most common site of rheumatic valve disease, which may occur in isolation or with concomitant rheumatic involvement of other valves. Heavy mitral annular calcification can extend into the mitral orifice and lead to functional mitral stenosis, most often encountered in elderly persons and in patients with underlying conditions that lead to ectopic calcification. Congenital mitral stenosis is rarely encountered in an adult population and distinguished by "arcade" or "parachute" deformities of the papillary muscles and chordae tendineae.

PATHOGENESIS

Lesion Pathogenesis

Rheumatic mitral stenosis typically manifests years after rheumatic fever, although many patients are unaware of the episode of rheumatic fever. Progressive fibrosis and scarring of the mitral leaflets occur, with the pathologic process extending from the leaflet commissures toward the bases. The chordae tendineae and submitral apparatus are often involved, with scarring and retraction. Calcification of the mitral apparatus is variable, and prominent calcification is more commonly seen in older patients. The anatomy of mitral stenosis forms a continuum, with variable degrees of leaflet and submitral thickening, rigidity, retraction, and calcification. Although mitral stenosis with pliable, noncalcified leaflets is common in developing countries, most patients with mitral stenosis in the United States and other Western countries present late after rheumatic fever with extensive valvular and subvalvular calcification. Nonrheumatic stenosis due to mitral annular calcification occurs with progression from the annulus toward the commissures, whereas rheumatic disease progresses from the commissures to the annulus.

Hemodynamic Pathogenesis

Obstruction to left ventricular inflow causes left atrial dilation and hypertension and resultant pulmonary venous hypertension. Pulmonary arteriolar and capillary vasoconstriction protect against pulmonary edema, although increased pulmonary vascular resistance exacerbates pulmonary arterial and right ventricular hypertension and causes right ventricular hypertrophy. Pulmonary hypertension can be severe late in the course of mitral stenosis, with eventual right ventricular systolic dysfunction. Because the diastolic interval shortens with increased heart rate, left ventricular filling is further compromised in patients with mitral stenosis and tachycardia. Sinus tachycardia, precipitated by physical or emotional stress, results in worsened left atrial hypertension, decreased left ventricular filling, and lower cardiac output. In addition, left atrial dilation predisposes to atrial fibrillation and other supraventricular tachyarrhythmias; the associated rapid ventricular response is poorly tolerated symptomatically and hemodynamically.

The hemodynamics and clinical expression of mitral stenosis are altered by the coincident occurrence of secundum atrial septal defect (Lutembacher's syndrome). The left atrium is decompressed by the atrial septal defect, and left atrial and pulmonary hypertension are attenuated. However, lower driving pressure across the stenotic mitral valve further impairs left ventricular filling. In addition, the presence of mitral stenosis exaggerates volume overload of the right ventricle and pulmonary circulation. In general, low systemic output replaces pulmonary edema among patients with the combination of mitral stenosis and atrial septal defect.

CLINICAL FINDINGS

History

Rheumatic mitral stenosis is a chronic and insidious disease in which the first symptoms typically occur decades after an episode of rheumatic fever that may have been unrecognized or may be no longer recalled. There is usually another long period during which symptoms of mitral stenosis are present but not debilitating. However, once debilitating symptoms occur, usually with associated pulmonary hypertension, prognosis is poor. Whereas 10-year survival rate is more than 80% in patients with mitral stenosis but no symptoms or mild symptoms, it falls to 0% to 15% in patients with debilitating symptoms, and estimated survival is less than 3 years among unoperated patients with advanced mitral stenosis and severe pulmonary hypertension. Among patients with advanced mitral stenosis, mortality is due to progressive heart failure, systemic embolization, pulmonary embolization, and infection.

Early symptoms of mitral stenosis consist of fatigue or dyspnea precipitated by events with associated tachycardia, including strenuous physical exercise, emotional stress, fever, pregnancy, or surgery. Dyspnea may be associated with cough. Later, dyspnea occurs with less strenuous activity and eventually at rest, with eventual development of paroxysmal nocturnal dyspnea and orthopnea that are associated with pulmonary edema and production of frothy, pink sputum. Patients may note palpitations due to atrial or ventricular ectopic beats, paroxysmal atrial tachycardia, or atrial fibrillation. Dyspnea typically worsens with both sinus tachycardia and with tachyarrhythmias owing to the shortened diastolic interval. Hemoptysis is a late symptom, caused by rupture of small bronchial vessels in the setting of significant pulmonary hypertension. Peripheral edema, ascites, and pleural effusion occur late and are caused by right ventricular failure.

The left atrium can become markedly enlarged, and systemic arterial emboli occur secondary to stasis and clotting in the dilated left atrium. Left atrial thrombi may occur in patients in sinus rhythm; the development of atrial fibrillation further increases the risk of thrombus formation. Pulmonary emboli are a late manifestation of mitral stenosis and can be debilitating or fatal.

Physical Findings

Changes in general appearance occur only with advanced mitral stenosis, with evidence of malar flushing due to peripheral cyanosis. Neck vein distention occurs caused by right ventricular failure, and jugular venous *a* waves are prominent in patients in sinus rhythm with tricuspid regurgitation or right ventricular hypertension but are absent with atrial fibrillation. Palpation of the precordium reveals a right ventricular lift or tap at the left sternal border. S_1 may be palpable, whereas the left ventricular apical impulse is diminished or nonpalpable. A diastolic thrill may be appreciable at the left ventricular apex with the patient in the left lateral decubitus position.

Auscultation reveals accentuation of S_1 in patients with pliable mitral leaflets and an increase in the pulmonic component of S_2 in patients with pulmonary hypertension. The classic high-pitched opening snap occurs 50 to 120 msec after the aortic component of S_2 in patients with a noncalcified valve. A low-pitched diastolic rumble occurs after the opening snap, loudest at the left ventricular apex using light application of the stethoscope bell and the patient in the left lateral decubitus position. The murmur intensity increases with simple exercises such as leg lifts or sit-ups. Presystolic accentuation occurs in sinus rhythm. More severe mitral stenosis is associated with longer duration of the diastolic rumble and decrease in the time between the aortic component of S_2 and the opening snap. The murmur of mitral stenosis is differentiated from an Austin Flint murmur of aortic regurgitation by the presence of an opening snap and increased intensity of S_1.

Late signs of mitral stenosis include congestion due to right ventricular failure, with hepatomegaly, ascites, pleural effusion, and peripheral edema. Pulmonary hypertension is associated with the Graham Steell murmur, a blowing diastolic murmur at the right upper sternal border caused by pulmonic insufficiency, and a murmur of tricuspid regurgitation. Murmurs of aortic or mitral regurgitation or both occur with concomitant valve disease.

LABORATORY FINDINGS

Electrocardiogram and Chest Radiograph

Mitral stenosis is associated with "P mitrale" on ECG, with broadened, notched P waves in the inferior leads due to left atrial enlargement. Atrial fibrillation is common. Pulmonary hypertension is associated with right axis deviation and right ventricular hypertrophy. The chest radiograph is associated with classic findings. Left atrial and pulmonary venous hypertension result in apical redistribution and prominent vascularity in the lung parenchyma, with interstitial edema and peribronchial and perivascular cuffing. Edema in the interlobular septa results in Kerley's B lines, horizontal lines at the lung bases extending to the pleural surfaces. With more advanced disease, there may be pulmonary edema and pleural effusions. Fine, diffuse interstitial nodularity may occur due to hemosiderin deposits after recurrent episodes of hemoptysis. The cardiac silhouette reveals prominent pulmonary arteries. Left atrial enlargement results in straightening of the left heart border and splayed bronchi with elevation of the left mainstem bronchus.

Echocardiography and Doppler Imaging

M-mode echocardiography reveals classic findings associated with mitral stenosis, including thickening of the mitral leaflets with decreased excursion, decreased E-F slope, and anterior motion of the posterior leaflet. Two-dimensional imaging reveals variable degrees of thickening and calcification of the mitral leaflets and submitral apparatus. There is a characteristic "doming" or "hockey stick" appearance when the leaflets remain pliable. An example of mitral stenosis with pliable leaflets is shown in Figure 77.6. When thickening and calcification are more advanced, the mitral valve appears as a solid, calcified mass. The left atrium is enlarged and, in the presence of pulmonary hypertension, there is right ventricular enlargement and hypertrophy. The severity of mitral stenosis is established by Doppler-derived transvalvular pressure gradients, and estimation of orifice area using planimetry on two-dimensional imaging or pressure half-time of transmitral Doppler. Tricuspid regurgitation velocity provides an estimate of right ventricular systolic pressure. Color-flow Doppler imaging is useful to assess the presence and severity of associated mitral or aortic regurgitation. Transesophageal imaging is invaluable in the assessment for thrombi within the body or appendage of the left atrium.

Cardiac Catheterization

Invasive techniques usually add little to the anatomical, functional, and hemodynamic information available on echocardiographic and Doppler imaging. Stenosis severity and pulmonary arterial pressures should be assessed at catheterization if right ventricular pressure is elevated out of proportion to stenosis severity on echocardiography or if there is a discrepancy between severity of symptoms and disease on noninvasive imaging. Coro-

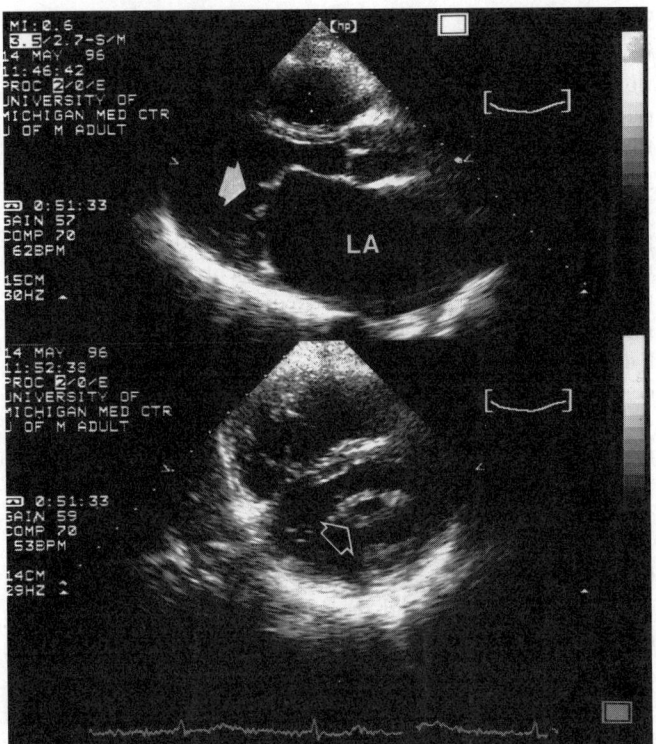

FIGURE 77.6. Transthoracic echocardiogram of patient with rheumatic mitral stenosis. Upper panel shows restricted but pliable leaflets (*arrow*) with doming. Lower panel shows diminished valve orifice *en face* (*open arrow*). *LA,* left atrium.

nary anatomy should be assessed before surgery in patients with risk factors for coronary artery disease.

Exercise Testing

Exercise testing with Doppler imaging is useful among patients with symptoms of dyspnea or fatigue and evidence of only mild or moderate mitral stenosis at rest. Because early symptoms of mitral stenosis are precipitated by tachycardia, exercise may reveal a sharp increase in transvalvular pressure gradients and right ventricular systolic pressure in patients with functionally significant stenosis but only modest abnormalities at rest.

OPTIMAL MANAGEMENT
Medical Therapy

Patients should receive prophylaxis against endocarditis. In addition, patients with a history of rheumatic fever or evidence of rheumatic valve disease should receive secondary prophylaxis against recurrent infection, usually with monthly intramuscular injections of 1.2 million U of benzathine penicillin G. Patients in sinus rhythm with exertional symptoms at rapid heart rate may benefit from rate control using β- or calcium channel blocking agents. Salt restriction and diuretic therapy are useful if there is dyspnea due to pulmonary congestion. Although medical therapy may be useful in patients with mild symptoms of mitral stenosis, surgical or percutaneous intervention is indicated

among patients with severe mitral stenosis and more advanced symptoms or with evidence of significant pulmonary hypertension complicating mitral stenosis.

Patients with mitral stenosis are at risk of systemic embolization. Risk is further increased with advanced age, atrial fibrillation, or history of embolic event. Patients with mitral stenosis and either atrial fibrillation or history of embolization should receive long-term anticoagulation therapy. Long-term anticoagulation is more controversial among patients with mitral stenosis and neither atrial fibrillation nor prior embolic event, but should be considered if mitral stenosis is moderate or severe or if the left atrium is significantly enlarged.

Atrial Fibrillation

Atrial fibrillation is a common complication of mitral stenosis and may exacerbate symptoms owing to both loss of atrial contraction and associated tachycardia. For many patients, the diagnosis of mitral stenosis is first made only after the occurrence of atrial fibrillation. Atrial fibrillation increases the risk of thromboembolism. Acute therapy consists of anticoagulation and rate control. Electrical cardioversion should be performed for hemodynamic instability. Elective cardioversion should be performed weighing the risks of atrial fibrillation, including tolerance of symptoms and risk of thromboembolism, against the likelihood of successful cardioversion and long-term maintenance of sinus rhythm, impacted by the chronicity of atrial fibrillation, and degree of left atrial dilation. Patients should be anticoagulated during and for ≥3 weeks after cardioversion to reduce the risk of systemic embolization, and for ≥3 weeks before cardioversion unless no left atrial thrombus is established on transesophageal echocardiography.

Percutaneous and Surgical Valvotomy

Percutaneous balloon valvotomy results in acute decrease in transvalvular gradient and increase in orifice area in most patients, with good long-term results in some. Echocardiographic imaging identifies patients with favorable valve morphology based on leaflet mobility, absence of leaflet thickening and calcification, and relative sparing of the subvalvular apparatus. In general, the procedure results in a 50% to 60% decrease in pressure gradients and an increase in valve area from about 1.0 to 2.0 cm^2. Event-free survival, with freedom from death, mitral valve replacement, and a another valvotomy, is 50% to 60% at 3 to 7 years and 80% to 90% among patients with the most favorable valve morphology. Acute procedural complications include severe mitral regurgitation in 2% to 10% of patients and persistent, hemodynamically significant atrial septal defect in less than 5% to 12%, with lesser risks of embolic events, myocardial infarction, and left ventricular perforation. Success is greater and procedural risks lower when performed in patients selected for optimal valve morphology and in centers with high procedural volume. Relative contraindications include left atrial thrombus and preexisting moderate or severe mitral regurgitation.

Among appropriately selected patients, there is no difference in hemodynamics, functional improvement, or procedural complications between percutaneous balloon mitral valvotomy and open surgical commissurotomy on either early and later follow-up. Either procedure may delay or avoid mitral valve replacement. Percutaneous balloon mitral valvotomy may be the procedure of choice in appropriate centers with skilled operators for selected patients with favorable valve morphology and absence of both significant mitral regurgitation and left atrial thrombus. Percutaneous balloon valvotomy may be an especially attractive alternative to surgery in young women who wish to bear children, in whom warfarin is contraindicated and tissue prostheses have limited durability.

Mitral Valve Surgery

Intervention is indicated for patients with moderate or severe mitral stenosis and intolerable symptoms, presence of pulmonary hypertension regardless of symptoms, or recurrent thromboembolism despite adequate anticoagulation. Open commissurotomy provides good results in selected patients with mitral stenosis. Patients with significant fibrosis and calcification of the mitral leaflets or with more advanced subvalvular fusion are less likely to have a successful result with either percutaneous balloon valvotomy or open surgical commissurotomy. Mitral valve replacement is indicated for patients who require intervention for mitral stenosis but who are not good candidates for percutaneous valvotomy or open commissurotomy.

The decision of prosthesis type for individual patients begins with an assessment of the relative risks and benefits of each choice. Mechanical prostheses have greater durability but significant thrombogenicity, whereas tissue prostheses have lower thrombogenicity and no independent requirement for anticoagulation but more limited durability. Mechanical prostheses in the mitral position have greater thrombotic risk than those in the aortic position due to the larger orifice area and lower velocity blood flow crossing the prosthesis.

■ MITRAL REGURGITATION

DEFINITION

Mitral regurgitation occurs as an acute or chronic process of left ventricular volume overload due to incompetence of the mitral valve, with blood ejected from the left ventricle into both the low-pressure left atrium and the high-pressure aorta. Trivial amounts of mitral regurgitation are physiologic and normal. Pathologic amounts of mitral regurgitation are typically graded by the size of the regurgitant jet alone or relative to the size of the left atrium. As with aortic regurgitation, semiquantification of mitral regurgitation severity on both noninvasive and invasive testing uses arbitrary criteria, and overlap occurs between categories. Regurgitant volume and regurgitant fraction can be quantified using invasive and noninvasive techniques but are of limited clinical importance.

ETIOLOGY, INCIDENCE, AND EPIDEMIOLOGY

The mitral apparatus is a complex structure comprising the leaflets, annulus, chordae tendineae, papillary muscles, and, in some

respects, the entire left ventricle. Disease or geometric change involving any of these structures can result in mitral regurgitation. Regurgitation caused by abnormal leaflet anatomy can be due to congenital or rheumatic disease, myxomatous degeneration, connective tissue diseases, and infective endocarditis. Congenitally cleft anterior leaflet usually occurs as part of an endocardial cushion defect with associated primum atrial septal defect, paramembranous ventricular septal defect, and abnormalities of the tricuspid valve; regurgitation is present from a young age. Connective tissue diseases associated with mitral regurgitation include systemic lupus erythematosus, rheumatoid arthritis, ankylosing spondylitis, and scleroderma. Valvular involvement in connective tissue diseases is variable; about 50% of patients with systemic lupus erythematosus have detectable mitral regurgitation, and approximately 25% have significant regurgitation. Myxomatous degeneration (mitral valve prolapse) is discussed separately.

Ischemic mitral regurgitation is caused by incomplete mitral leaflet coaptation due to ischemic changes in left ventricular geometry or function and restricted leaflet motion. Sufficient myocardial ischemia can cause transient mitral regurgitation. Any myopathic process that causes left ventricular dilation can cause mitral regurgitation by a similar mechanism, with restricted leaflet motion and incomplete leaflet coaptation. Dysfunction of mechanical and bioprosthetic valves can also lead to regurgitation. Small amounts of paraprosthetic regurgitation are common; larger paravalvular leaks can cause significant regurgitation, often with associated hemolysis. Acute severe mitral regurgitation is caused by infective endocarditis, acute myocardial infarction with papillary muscle rupture or retraction, or prosthetic valve dysfunction.

PATHOGENESIS

Lesion Pathogenesis

Rheumatic disease of the mitral valve usually occurs years after rheumatic fever and may occur with concomitant mitral stenosis or rheumatic involvement of the aortic or tricuspid valve. The leaflets and subvalvular apparatus are typically involved. Mitral annular calcification predominantly occurs in older patients and in patients with conditions associated with ectopic calcification, including patients with end-stage renal failure. Although a common cause of mitral regurgitation, it is not usually severe. Infective endocarditis results in mitral regurgitation caused by destruction of leaflet tissue, submitral structures, or, more rarely, mechanical interference with valve function caused by a vegetation. Coronary artery disease causes mitral regurgitation based on papillary muscle ischemia or infarction with scarring and retraction. Papillary muscle rupture can complicate a small, otherwise hemodynamically well-tolerated myocardial infarction, usually involving the right coronary artery or, less often, the left circumflex artery. Mild mitral regurgitation is a normal finding associated with most mechanical prostheses. Dysfunction of a mechanical prosthetic valve can cause more significant regurgitation, and fracture of a calcified tissue prosthesis results in acute regurgitation. Paravalvular regurgitation of any severity can occur with either mechanical or tissue prostheses owing to annular calcification, infection, or suture failure.

Any myopathic process can be associated with secondary mitral regurgitation caused by left ventricular dilation and incomplete leaflet coaptation. A vicious cycle develops in which the left ventricular volume overload of mitral regurgitation adds to the volume overload of the underlying myopathic process. Progressive left ventricular dilation and progressive mitral regurgitation result in a scenario in which "mitral regurgitation begets mitral regurgitation."

Hemodynamic Pathogenesis

Mitral regurgitation results in left ventricular volume overload with left ventricular ejection into both the high-impedance aorta and the compliant, low-impedance left atrium. In chronic mitral regurgitation, left atrial dilation maintains low left atrial and pulmonary venous pressures. Forward cardiac output is maintained by compensatory left ventricular dilation with increases in left ventricular end-diastolic volume, ejection fraction, and stroke volume. Patients typically remain entirely asymptomatic during this phase of compensated mitral regurgitation, which may last for years. However, prolonged left ventricular volume overload eventually leads to left ventricular systolic dysfunction and pulmonary congestion, with increasing left ventricular end systolic volume and decreasing ejection fraction and forward cardiac output. Because left ventricular emptying does not rely on overcoming high aortic pressure, left ventricular stroke volume remains elevated and ejection fraction remains within the normal range despite progressive systolic dysfunction. Late in the course of disease, left ventricular ejection fraction falls below normal.

In acute severe mitral regurgitation, limited left atrial distensibility leads to acutely increased left atrial and pulmonary venous pressures and pulmonary edema. Although the increased preload associated with acute severe mitral regurgitation results in a modest increase in total left ventricular stroke volume, the absence of compensatory left ventricular dilation results in reduced forward stroke volume and forward cardiac output.

CLINICAL FINDINGS

History

Patients with chronic mitral regurgitation remain asymptomatic for an extended period. Later, patients develop symptoms of fatigue and exertional dyspnea, followed by more overt symptoms of congestive heart failure, including orthopnea and paroxysmal dyspnea. Symptoms are typically insidious at onset, and patients frequently fail to recognize the gradual fatigue and subtle exercise limitations associated with chronic severe mitral regurgitation. In distinction, patients with acute severe mitral regurgitation are almost always symptomatic, with fulminant symptoms of pulmonary edema.

Physical Findings

Patients with chronic severe mitral regurgitation often have a hyperactive precordium and displacement of the left ventricular apical impulse due to left ventricular enlargement. A late systolic left parasternal lift due to left atrial expansion may be present, which, in conjunction with an apical heave, results in a rocking motion of the precordium. An apical systolic thrill may be evident. S_1 is usually normal, although it may be encompassed by the systolic murmur and difficult to appreciate. An S_3 is often present and not necessarily indicative of ventricular failure. The classic murmur of mitral regurgitation is a loud, blowing holosystolic murmur that may obliterate S_1 and S_2. The murmur is usually loudest at the apex with radiation to the axilla or to the back, although it is often audible throughout the precordium. Mitral regurgitation caused by leaflet flail is usually eccentric, and the murmur associated with posterior leaflet flail radiates anteriorly to the left sternal border. The large volume of blood crossing the mitral valve in diastole causes turbulent flow in patients with severe regurgitation, causing a diastolic rumble despite absence of mitral stenosis.

The systolic murmur associated with acute severe mitral regurgitation may be decrescendo rather than holosystolic because of early equilibration of left atrial and left ventricular pressures in the setting of a normal-sized left atrium. The apical left ventricular impulse is not displaced. S_3 and S_4 are common.

LABORATORY FINDINGS

Electrocardiogram and Chest Radiograph

The ECG and chest radiograph may reveal evidence of left atrial or left ventricular enlargement in patients with chronic mitral regurgitation. Later, the ECG may disclose atrial fibrillation.

Echocardiography and Doppler Imaging

Echocardiographic imaging allows assessment of left atrial and left ventricular size and systolic function. Mitral valve anatomy can usually be seen sufficiently to allow assessment of the underlying cause of mitral regurgitation. Examples of incomplete mitral leaflet coaptation and valve perforation due to infective endocarditis are shown in Figures 77.7 and 77.8, respectively. Transesophageal echocardiography provides superb visualization of mitral valve anatomy and almost always allows sufficient visualization to define the cause of regurgitation. Left ventricular wall motion abnormalities associated with coronary artery disease may be evident. However, a small wall motion abnormality accompanying papillary muscle rupture complicating a small myocardial infarction may be obscured by the hyperdynamic left ventricle associated with acute severe mitral regurgitation. Color-flow Doppler imaging allows semiquantitative assessment of mitral regurgitation severity and jet characteristics that may help with determination of cause of regurgitation. Evidence of concomitant valve disease or pulmonary hypertension also may be evident. Among patients with chronic mitral regurgitation, accurate quantitative assessment of left ventricular size and systolic function are important as a baseline with which future studies are compared.

Cardiac Catheterization

Left ventriculography allows assessment of left ventricular ejection fraction and semiquantitative assessment of mitral regurgi-

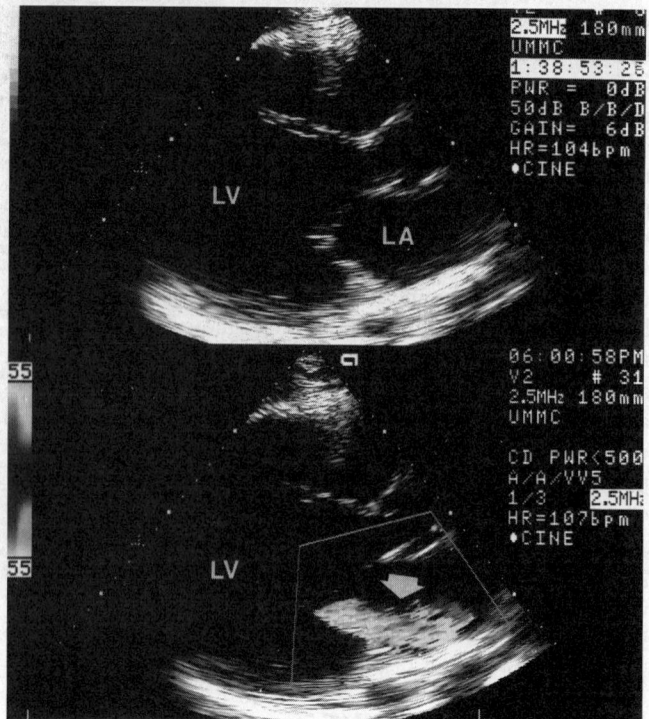

FIGURE 77.7. Transthoracic echocardiogram of patient with dilated cardiomyopathy and mitral regurgitation (*arrow*). There is incomplete mitral leaflet coaptation owing to left ventricular and mitral annular dilation. *LA,* left atrium; *LV,* left ventricle.

tation severity, both of which are usually available using noninvasive imaging. Cardiac catheterization is useful for assessment of coronary anatomy in patients at risk for coronary disease who are undergoing mitral valve surgery and among patients with suspicion for ischemic cause of mitral regurgitation.

Exercise Testing

Mitral regurgitation is a dynamic lesion and, especially in the setting of ischemic mitral regurgitation, severity can worsen with

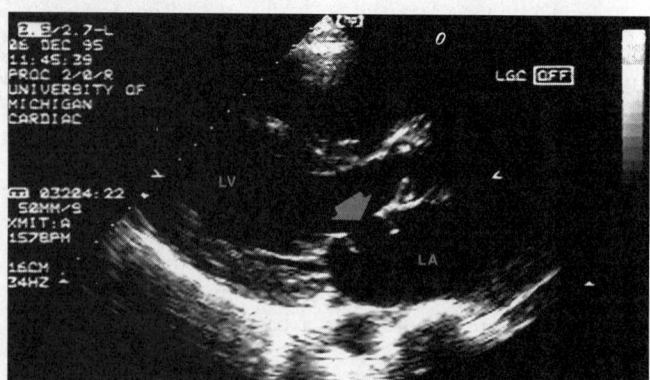

FIGURE 77.8. Transthoracic echocardiogram demonstrating large anterior mitral leaflet perforation (*arrow*) in patient with infective endocarditis. Severe mitral regurgitation was present. *LA,* left atrium; *LV,* left ventricle.

exercise. Although exercise testing is not contributory in most patients, stress testing with Doppler imaging may be useful among patients with exertional symptoms and only mild or moderate mitral regurgitation at rest.

OPTIMAL MANAGEMENT

Medical Therapy

The goal of medical therapy for acute severe mitral regurgitation is to decrease the severity of mitral regurgitation and thereby increase forward cardiac output and minimize pulmonary venous congestion. Nitroprusside decreases afterload and results in lower regurgitant volume and increased forward cardiac output. Nitroprusside is useful alone in normotensive patients with acute severe mitral regurgitation, or in combination with an inotropic agent in patients with hypotension. Intra-aortic balloon counterpulsation is a useful adjunct in patients with acute severe mitral regurgitation and hypotension or pulmonary edema, resulting in decreased afterload, decreased regurgitant volume, and increased forward cardiac output.

As with other patients with valvular heart disease, appropriate antibiotic prophylaxis should be used among patients with chronic mitral regurgitation. Although afterload reducing agents may decrease the severity of mitral regurgitation and are advocated by some for asymptomatic patients with chronic severe mitral regurgitation, the benefits of long-term therapy have not been tested.

Serial Testing

Asymptomatic patients with mild mitral regurgitation and normal left ventricular systolic function should undergo periodic assessment, including history and physical examination on approximately a yearly basis. After the initial documentation of mild mitral regurgitation, echocardiographic imaging should be repeated if there are new symptoms or evidence on physical examination of worsened regurgitation. Patients with moderate mitral regurgitation should undergo yearly assessment, including history, physical examination, and echocardiographic imaging to assess for new symptoms or signs of heart failure and to monitor left ventricular size and function. Asymptomatic patients with severe mitral regurgitation should undergo history, physical examination, and echocardiography every six to 12 months, with more frequent testing if symptoms develop or if there is progressive left ventricular dilation or decreasing left ventricular systolic function on echocardiography. Establishing accurate baseline measures of left ventricular size and ejection fraction are important for future comparison.

Because preoperative left ventricular systolic function is an important predictor of postoperative survival, patients should be referred for surgical intervention before the onset of left ventricular systolic dysfunction. Ejection fraction overestimates left ventricular systolic function in patients with mitral regurgitation because blood is also ejected into the low-impedance left atrium; the ejection fraction remains in the normal range after the onset of systolic dysfunction.

Mitral Valve Surgery

Alternatives for mitral valve surgery include mitral valve repair and mitral valve replacement with or without chordal preservation. Mitral valve replacement without chordal preservation results in loss of ventricular systolic shortening and lower postoperative left ventricular systolic function, functional class, and survival. Mitral valve repair minimizes the use of prosthetic material, thus obviating the need for long-term anticoagulation and reducing the risk of endocarditis. Repair is often associated with more favorable hemodynamics compared with valve replacement, and there is no risk of prosthetic valve failure. However, mitral repair is a more technically demanding procedure requiring substantial surgical skill and expertise, and it may not be feasible for all valves. Intraoperative echocardiography is used to assess the adequacy of repair. Despite a more technically demanding procedure with longer extracorporeal circulation times, mitral valve repair is associated with lower operative and subsequent mortality compared with valve replacement. Mitral valve repair should be considered the surgical procedure of choice if valve morphology is amenable to reconstruction and if appropriate surgical expertise is available.

Mitral valve surgery is indicated for patients with severe mitral regurgitation and either symptoms of heart failure or evidence of left ventricular systolic dysfunction, defined as left ventricular ejection fraction less than 60% or left ventricular end-systolic diameter ≥45 mm. Although severe left ventricular systolic dysfunction before surgery is associated with increased operative and later mortality, symptomatic patients should nonetheless undergo consideration for surgical intervention. Some asymptomatic patients with normal left ventricular systolic function may benefit from early surgical intervention with the goal of preventing the sequelae of chronic mitral regurgitation, if there is a good likelihood of successful valve repair. Asymptomatic patients with severe mitral regurgitation and progressive left ventricular dilation or with atrial fibrillation of recent onset, and patients with new severe mitral regurgitation should be considered for mitral repair.

MITRAL VALVE PROLAPSE

DEFINITION

Mitral valve prolapse is a fairly common syndrome of myxomatous degeneration of the mitral valve leading to redundant leaflets and elongation of chordae tendineae. Patients with mitral valve prolapse syndrome have a propensity to premature valve degeneration with chordal rupture, leaflet flail, and mitral regurgitation. Other features of the syndrome include atypical chest pain, palpitations due to atrial and ventricular arrhythmias, and possibly panic attacks. In distinction, isolated prolapse of a normal mitral valve can be seen on echocardiography in some patients with no propensity to valve degeneration or regurgitation, and mitral valve prolapse may be incorrectly diagnosed. Normal mitral valve leaflets can prolapse into the left atrium in the setting of volume depletion or hyperdynamic left ventricle. On echocardiography, the diagnosis of mitral valve prolapse should be reserved for patients with evidence of prolapse and leaflet thickening or mitral regurgitation, or prolapse with coaptation of the mitral leaflets on the left atrial side of the annulus.

ETIOLOGY, INCIDENCE, AND EPIDEMIOLOGY

Mitral valve prolapse occurs in 2% to 6% of the adult population and is found in more women than men. However, sequelae of mitral valve prolapse, including surgery for mitral regurgitation, appear to be more common in men who carry the diagnosis than in women. Presentation is usually in young adulthood, with evidence of an autosomal dominant inheritance pattern. Mitral valve prolapse is associated with connective tissue diseases, and most patients with Marfan syndrome have mitral valve prolapse. There is an increased incidence of atrial septal aneurysm and secundum atrial septal defect among patients with mitral valve prolapse. Left ventricular dilation can mask the presence of mitral valve prolapse. Patients with Marfan syndrome and chronic severe aortic regurgitation may not have echocardiographic evidence of mitral valve prolapse or mitral regurgitation until after aortic valve replacement and subsequent remodeling of the left ventricle. Increased intravascular volume during the second and third trimesters of pregnancy may similarly minimize prolapse, with fewer associated symptoms and reduced severity of mitral regurgitation.

PATHOGENESIS

Mitral valve prolapse can be diagnosed as an incidental finding on either physical examination or echocardiographic imaging. Myxomatous degeneration of the mitral valve and submitral apparatus can lead to rupture of chordae tendineae. Mitral regurgitation due to mitral valve prolapse may be gradually progressive or may worsen acutely with chordal rupture and leaflet flail.

CLINICAL FINDINGS

History

Patients with mitral valve prolapse can remain asymptomatic and never develop any sequelae of the syndrome. Some patients have symptoms of palpitations or atypical, nonexertional chest pain. Palpitations are due to isolated ectopic beats, supraventricular tachycardia, or, more rarely, ventricular arrhythmias. Sudden cardiac death associated with mitral valve prolapse is rare and presumably related to ventricular arrhythmias. The association between mitral valve prolapse and transient ischemic attacks is controversial, as is the association between mitral valve prolapse and panic attacks. The risk of endocarditis is increased among patients with mitral valve prolapse, especially if there is mitral regurgitation or myxomatous degeneration. Symptoms associated with acute and chronic mitral regurgitation are as previously described.

Physical Findings

Patients with mitral valve prolapse can have a classic appearance of thin body habitus. There is an association between mitral valve prolapse and pectus excavatum and straight back. Auscultation reveals one or more high-pitched mid-to-late systolic nonejection clicks. If there is mitral regurgitation without leaflet flail, the murmur begins in systole after the click. Mitral regurgitation and the associated murmur are holosystolic in patients with flail leaflet. The timing of clicks and intensity of the murmur are affected by left ventricular volume. Maneuvers such as squatting, which increase left ventricular volume, result in clicks later in systole and a murmur of lesser intensity, whereas maneuvers such as standing, which decrease left ventricular volume, result in clicks earlier in systole and a murmur of louder intensity.

LABORATORY FINDINGS

Echocardiography and Doppler imaging are extremely useful in the diagnosis and assessment of mitral valve prolapse. Because of the saddle shape of the mitral annulus, the normal mitral valve can appear to prolapse into the left atrium in some imaging planes, and the diagnosis of mitral valve prolapse should rely on the parasternal long-axis view rather than an apical window. Echocardiographic evidence of myxomatous degeneration includes leaflet thickening, annular dilation, and chordal elongation. Doppler imaging allows detection and semiquantification of mitral regurgitation. To avoid inappropriate diagnosis, caution should be used when there is limited echocardiographic evidence of mitral valve prolapse and absence of leaflet thicken-

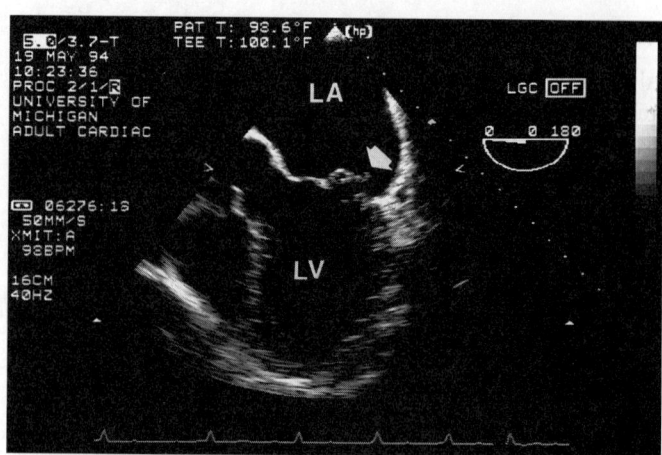

FIGURE 77.10. Transesophageal echocardiogram demonstrating flail anterior mitral valve leaflet (*arrow*) complicating mitral valve prolapse. Severe mitral regurgitation was present. *LA,* left atrium; *LV,* left ventricle.

ing, annular dilation, chordal elongation, or mitral regurgitation. Mitral regurgitation associated with mitral valve prolapse with or without leaflet flail is usually eccentric. Jet eccentricity can lead to suboptimal visualization on transthoracic imaging and underestimation of regurgitation severity. Transesophageal imaging should be used if there is poor visualization of valve anatomy or suspicion of significant mitral regurgitation that is not well demonstrated on transthoracic imaging. Examples of mitral valve prolapse on transthoracic echocardiography and flail mitral leaflet on transesophageal imaging are shown in Figures 77.9 and 77.10, respectively.

OPTIMAL MANAGEMENT

Patients with mitral valve prolapse and either leaflet thickening on echocardiography or mitral regurgitation based on a murmur or on Doppler imaging should receive appropriate antibiotic prophylaxis for prevention of infective endocarditis. Asymptomatic patients require no additional therapy for mitral valve prolapse. Patients should undergo periodic follow-up with history and physical examination, and echocardiographic imaging if there is evidence of mitral regurgitation.

Patients with palpitations usually require no medical therapy other than reassurance. β-adrenergic antagonists are useful for symptomatic relief. Continuous or event-activated ECG monitoring is useful among patients with recurrent or protracted episodes of palpitations. Patients with focal neurologic events who are in sinus rhythm and have no left atrial thrombus should receive antiplatelet therapy with aspirin. Long-term anticoagulation therapy with warfarin is recommended for patients with no contraindication who either have suffered a stroke or have recurrent transient ischemic attacks while receiving aspirin. Timing of surgery for mitral regurgitation follows the same guidelines as described previously. Early surgical intervention should be considered if valve repair is likely.

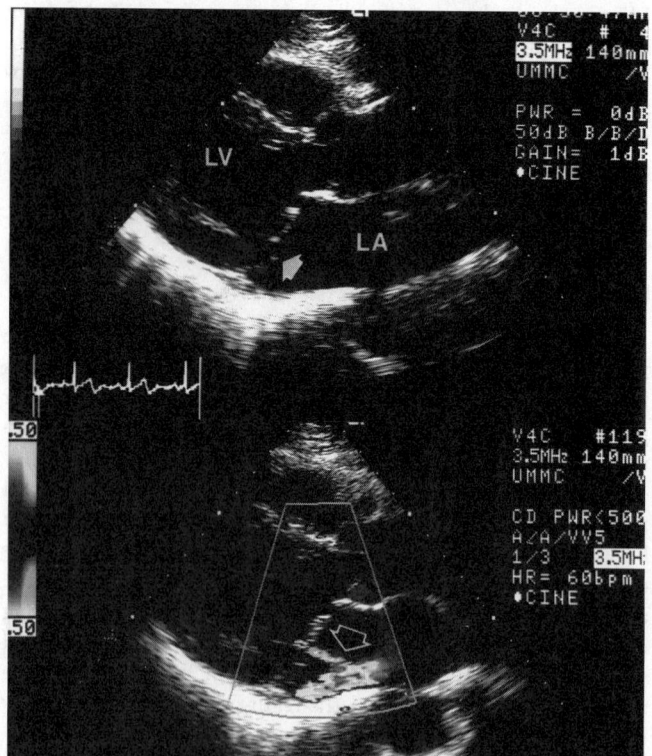

FIGURE 77.9. Transthoracic echocardiogram in patient with mitral valve prolapse. Upper panel demonstrates prolapse of posterior mitral valve leaflet (*arrow*) behind the plane of the mitral annulus. Lower panel demonstrates associated mitral regurgitation (*open arrow*). *LA,* left atrium; *LV,* left ventricle.

TRICUSPID VALVE DISEASE

DEFINITION

Tricuspid stenosis is obstruction to right ventricular inflow due to an anatomical abnormality of the tricuspid valve. Tricuspid regurgitation is incompetence of the tricuspid valve, resulting in ejection of blood from the right ventricle into both the pulmonary artery and the right atrium. Small amounts of tricuspid regurgitation are common and should be considered normal. Semiquantification of tricuspid regurgitation is based on the size of the regurgitant jet relative to the size of the right atrium.

ETIOLOGY, INCIDENCE, AND EPIDEMIOLOGY

Primary abnormalities of the tricuspid valve occur far less often than secondary abnormalities. Primary abnormalities include rheumatic disease, infective endocarditis, carcinoid heart disease, and abnormalities caused by anorectic drugs. Congenital abnormalities of the tricuspid valve include Ebstein's anomaly, tricuspid atresia, involvement in endocardial cushion defect, and other complex congenital lesions and are relatively uncommon in an adult population. Rheumatic disease of the tricuspid valve causes stenosis, regurgitation, or both and is almost always seen in conjunction with involvement of other valves. Approximately 5% of patients with rheumatic mitral valve disease also have involvement of the tricuspid valve. Right-sided endocarditis involving the tricuspid valve, especially common in intravenous drug abusers, causes tissue destruction and significant regurgitation. Carcinoid involvement of the tricuspid valve results in characteristic rigidity of the leaflets. Anorectic drugs are discussed below. Secondary tricuspid regurgitation occurs commonly in association with diseases that cause either right ventricular enlargement or pulmonary artery hypertension.

PATHOGENESIS

Tricuspid stenosis results in increased right atrial pressure, with passive congestion of the systemic venous circulation and hepatomegaly, pleural effusion, ascites. and peripheral edema. Tricuspid regurgitation results in right ventricular volume overload, which, similar to mitral regurgitation, is well tolerated for an extended period.

CLINICAL FINDINGS

Isolated tricuspid valve disease rarely results in significant symptoms. Chronic right ventricular volume overload associated with severe tricuspid regurgitation can eventually cause right ventricular systolic dysfunction. Patients with tricuspid stenosis have jugular venous distension and giant a waves generated by systolic contraction of the right atrium against the stenotic tricuspid valve. Auscultation reveals an opening snap and diastolic murmur similar to mitral stenosis, but distinguished by location at the left sternal border and augmentation with inspiration. Tricuspid regurgitation produces jugular *c-v* waves and a pulsatile liver with hepatojugular reflux. Auscultation reveals a holo-systolic murmur along the left sternal border, increasing in intensity with inspiration. Both tricuspid stenosis and tricuspid regurgitation result in systemic venous congestion with hepatomegaly, pleural effusion, ascites, and peripheral edema.

LABORATORY FINDINGS

In tricuspid stenosis, the ECG may show evidence of right atrial enlargement with peaked P waves in the inferior leads. The right atrium is enlarged on chest radiograph in both tricuspid stenosis and tricuspid regurgitation. Echocardiography reveals thickened, restricted tricuspid leaflets in tricuspid stenosis and may reveal evidence of underlying valvular pathology including rheumatic disease, endocarditis or carcinoid, or the cause of secondary regurgitation. Doppler imaging is useful for quantification of transvalvular gradient in tricuspid stenosis and for semiquantitative assessment of tricuspid regurgitation. Minimal or mild tricuspid regurgitation is common on echocardiography with Doppler imaging and should be considered a normal finding. The presence of tricuspid regurgitation allows estimation of right ventricular systolic pressure from the velocity of the regurgitant jet, which correlates well with pulmonary arterial systolic pressure in the absence of pulmonic stenosis.

OPTIMAL MANAGEMENT

Therapy of secondary tricuspid regurgitation involves treatment of the underlying disease. Systemic venous congestion can be treated with salt restriction and diuretics. Digoxin may be useful if there is right ventricular systolic dysfunction. Surgical alternatives for tricuspid regurgitation include tricuspid valve repair or replacement. Similar to mitral repair, reconstruction is preferable, if feasible. Mechanical prostheses in the tricuspid position have a relatively high rate of thrombosis, and a bioprosthesis is usually preferable.

PULMONIC VALVE DISEASE

DEFINITION

Pulmonic stenosis is valvular obstruction to right ventricular outflow. Pulmonic regurgitation is incompetence of the pulmonic valve with resultant right ventricular volume overload.

ETIOLOGY, INCIDENCE, AND EPIDEMIOLOGY

Isolated pulmonic valve disease is rare. Pulmonic stenosis is nearly always congenital; rare causes include rheumatic disease and involvement in carcinoid syndrome. Small amounts of pulmonic regurgitation are normal. Pathologic pulmonic regurgitation can be caused by rheumatic disease, infective endocarditis, carcinoid disease, or anorectic drugs. Rheumatic involvement of the pulmonic valve is rare and almost exclusively seen in association with rheumatic involvement of other valves. Right-sided endocarditis can involve the pulmonic valve, although isolated pulmonic valve endocarditis is unusual. Significant pulmonic regurgitation is most commonly caused by pulmonary arterial dilation secondary to pulmonary hypertension.

PATHOGENESIS

Pulmonic stenosis results in right ventricular hypertension and right ventricular hypertrophy, although the presence of pulmonic stenosis protects the pulmonary vasculature from increased pressures. Congenital valvular pulmonic stenosis is often accompanied by infundibular right ventricular hypertrophy with secondary subvalvular outflow obstruction. Pulmonic regurgitation is well tolerated for extended periods. Chronic severe pulmonic regurgitation may lead to right ventricular dilation and eventual systolic dysfunction.

CLINICAL FINDINGS

Patients with mild or moderate pulmonic stenosis are usually asymptomatic. Severe pulmonic stenosis is associated with symptoms of fatigue and exertional dyspnea. Patients with pulmonic regurgitation are also typically asymptomatic, although chronic severe regurgitation can eventually lead to right ventricular failure with hepatomegaly, pleural effusion, ascites, and peripheral edema. The murmur associated with pulmonic stenosis is a high-pitched systolic crescendo–decrescendo murmur distinguished from aortic stenosis by location at the left upper sternal border, increase with inspiration, and continuation beyond the aortic component of S_2. The Graham Steell murmur of pulmonic regurgitation is a soft, decrescendo diastolic murmur at the left upper sternal border.

LABORATORY FINDINGS

Echocardiography and Doppler imaging allow accurate assessment of transvalvular pulmonic gradients and semiquantification of pulmonic regurgitation. Minimal or mild pulmonic regurgitation are common findings on echocardiographic imaging and should be considered normal. The anatomy of the pulmonic valve is often visible on transthoracic echocardiography; transesophageal imaging may be useful for additional interrogation.

OPTIMAL MANAGEMENT

Congenital pulmonic stenosis may be amenable to percutaneous balloon valvotomy. Surgical alternatives include commissurotomy and pulmonic valve replacement using mechanical, heterograft, or allograft prostheses. Pulmonic regurgitation usually requires no specific medical therapy. In pulmonic regurgitation due to pulmonary hypertension, therapy is aimed at treatment of the underlying disease.

▪ VALVE DISEASE ASSOCIATED WITH ANORECTIC DRUGS

DEFINITION

An association has been suggested between acquired valvular heart disease and the anorectic drugs dexfenfluramine and fen-

fluramine with or without phentermine, which led to the voluntary withdrawal of both dexfenfluramine and fenfluramine in the United States. The observed lesions include thickening of right-sided heart valves, similar to that observed in carcinoid syndrome, and unusual thickening of left-sided valves with associated regurgitation.

ETIOLOGY, INCIDENCE, AND EPIDEMIOLOGY

The incidence of acquired valve disease associated with anorectic drug use is not known. However, risk appears to be associated with duration of therapy. By some estimates, up to 30% of patients who received dexfenfluramine or fenfluramine and phentermine for 6 to 24 months had echocardiographic evidence of significant aortic or mitral regurgitation. The concentration of valve disease in specific geographic locations raises the possibility that additional factors may have contributed to the development of disease.

PATHOGENESIS

Some of the patients who developed valve disease had echocardiographic and histopathologic findings similar to those observed in patients with carcinoid heart disease. The action of the involved anorectic medications as serotonin-releasing agents raises the possibility that the valve lesions occurred as a result of exposure to increased levels of serotonin, although this hypothesis has not been tested.

CLINICAL FINDINGS

Most patients with echocardiographic evidence of regurgitation were asymptomatic. Some patients presented with murmur on physical examination or with symptoms of fatigue referable to the underlying valve lesions. Because valve lesions associated with anorectic drug use occur in a population of patients with substantial obesity, physical findings may be limited.

LABORATORY FINDINGS

Echocardiographic and Doppler imaging demonstrate thickening of one or more valves with associated regurgitation. As previously noted, in some reports the echocardiographic appearance of affected valves resembles those observed in patients with carcinoid heart disease.

OPTIMAL MANAGEMENT

Screening for valvular heart disease among patients who received anorectic drugs should include history and careful physical examination. Echocardiographic imaging should be used if there is evidence of valve disease based on presence of symptoms, heart murmur, or other clinical findings or if body habitus precludes adequate auscultation. In addition, echocardiographic imaging should be considered for patients who are at risk of cardiac involvement in whom a procedure is anticipated that would require antibiotic prophylaxis in the setting of significant valve disease. The specific regurgitant valve lesions are treated as previously outlined.

BIBLIOGRAPHY

Bach DS. Stress echocardiography for evaluation of hemodynamics: valvular heart disease, prosthetic valve function, and pulmonary hypertension. *Progr Cardiovasc Dis* 1997;39:543–554.

Bonow RO, Carabello B, de Leon AC Jr, et al. Guidelines for the management of patients with valvular heart disease: executive summary. A report of the American College of Cardiology/American Heart Association Task Force on Practice Guidelines (Committee on Management of Patients with Valvular Heart Disease). *Circulation* 1998;98:1949–1984.

Carabello BA, Crawford FA Jr. Valvular heart disease. *N Engl J Med* 1997; 337:32–41.

Connolly HM, Crary JL, McGoon MD, et al. Valvular heart disease associated with fenfluramine-phentermine. *N Engl J Med* 1997;337:581–588.

Enriquez-Sarano M, Schaff HV, Orszulak TA, et al. Valve repair improves the outcome of surgery for mitral regurgitation. A multivariate analysis. *Circulation* 1995;91:1022–1028.

Klodas E, Enriquez-Sarano M, Tajik AJ, et al. Optimizing timing of surgical correction in patients with severe aortic regurgitation: role of symptoms. *J Am Coll Cardiol* 1997;30:746–752.

Lieberman EB, Bashore TM, Hermiller JB, et al. Balloon aortic valvuloplasty in adults: failure of procedure to improve long-term survival. *J Am Coll Cardiol* 1995;26:1522–1528.

Ling LH, Enriquez-Sarano M, Seward JB, et al. Clinical outcome of mitral regurgitation due to flail leaflet. *N Engl J Med* 1996;335:1417–1423.

Scognamiglio R, Rahimtoola SH, Fasoli G, et al. Nifedipine in asymptomatic patients with severe aortic regurgitation and normal left ventricular function. *N Engl J Med* 1994;331:689–694.

Wilkins GT, Weyman AE, Abascal VM, et al. Percutaneous balloon dilatation of the mitral valve: an analysis of echocardiographic variables related to outcome and the mechanism of dilatation. *Br Heart J* 1988;60: 299–308.

Kelley's Textbook of Internal Medicine, fourth edition. Edited by H. David Humes. Lippincott Williams & Wilkins, Philadelphia © 2000.

C H A P T E R

78

CONGENITAL HEART DISEASE IN THE ADULT

THOMAS RYAN
J. KEVIN HARRISON

Congenital heart diseases are those cardiac malformations present at birth. Traditionally, the care of patients with these disorders—even those who survived to adulthood—was provided by pediatricians and pediatric cardiologists. In recent years, it has become increasingly common for internists and "adult" cardiologists to assume the care of these patients as they grow older. Several factors are responsible for this trend.

An estimated more than 500,000 adult patients in the United States have congenital heart disease. Of the 25,000 infants born

with congenital heart disease every year, about 85% are now expected to reach adulthood. As this population continues to grow—in number, complexity, and age—the need for ongoing specialized cardiac care will expand. With aging, the health care requirements of these patients will change as acquired medical problems compound the congenital ones. It is neither feasible nor appropriate to expect the pediatric physician to assume this responsibility throughout the patient's adult life. Training programs and specialized clinics are some examples of recent efforts to address this need.

Various factors have contributed to this growing population of older patients with congenital heart diseases. Perhaps most important are the improvements and innovations in the surgical management of young patients. Over the past several decades, these developments have had a profound impact on survival patterns. The variety and complexity of surgical options have grown so that relatively few lesions remain inaccessible to the surgeon. Despite these often extraordinary advances, few patients can be considered "cured," and most require ongoing cardiac care.

In addition, improvements in cardiac catheterization now allow more accurate diagnoses for patients with congenital heart disease. Percutaneous therapeutic options now exist for some patients who would have previously required surgery.

We can conclude the following: the number of adults with congenital heart disease will continue to grow; most of these patients will undergo palliative or reparative surgery but will require ongoing specialized medical care to provide access to new developments in therapy; and the assessment and management of these patients will become increasingly complex over time.

This chapter focuses on the diagnosis and management of adults with congenital heart disease. Problems unique to older patients, such as those related to pregnancy, are discussed. Only lesions with expected adult survival are covered, and emphasis is placed on the malformations encountered most frequently. Because most adult patients will undergo some form of surgery, postoperative evaluation and management are also stressed. In addition, the final section of the chapter describes some of the newer percutaneous therapeutic options that exist for specific congenital cardiac problems.

■ GENERAL APPROACH TO THE PATIENT

Adults with congenital heart disease may be categorized as having either a natural or an unnatural history. *Natural history* refers to the unoperated condition and includes patients presenting for the first time, those with mild or well-tolerated lesions who have not required intervention, and those who have been considered inoperable or have declined surgical repair. With the increasing availability of accurate diagnostic tools, relatively few patients remain undiagnosed until adulthood. As a result, the population of adult patients with a natural history is shrinking, and most have either mild, simple lesions or very advanced and inoperable defects.

Unnatural history refers to disease whose course has been altered by an intervention, usually surgical. In these patients, a diagnosis has been established and either palliation or repair has been previously performed. In many patients, many procedures have been done over a span of decades, often at different institutions. Unless an up-to-date medical record is available, a major challenge for the physician is to determine the underlying condition and what has been done to alter it. These patients now make up the largest group of patients followed up in most adult congenital heart disease clinics.

The initial evaluation of the adult patient with known or suspected congenital heart disease is greatly facilitated by a thorough review of the medical record. A complete history and physical examination, electrocardiogram (ECG), chest radiograph, and, in most cases, an echocardiogram should be performed. Laboratory studies often include a complete blood count, iron studies, measurement of electrolytes, urea nitrogen, and creatinine, and uric acid and clotting tests. This battery of diagnostic studies provides most of the information needed for a complete initial assessment.

A multidisciplinary approach is recommended for the long-term management of these patients. The involvement of both pediatric and adult cardiologists has several advantages. The array of medical problems encountered in these young patients often includes both congenital and acquired conditions. Input from the different subspecialists is ideal in these situations. The presence of the two cardiologists also facilitates the smooth transfer of care from the pediatric to the adult cardiologist. Other key members of the health care team may include the cardiovascular surgeon, obstetrician, hematologist, geneticist, and nurse specialist.

COMMON AND UNCOMMON CONGENITAL HEART DISEASES: NATURAL SURVIVAL PATTERNS

AORTIC VALVE DISEASE

A congenitally malformed aortic valve that is stenotic at birth is usually either unicuspid or dysplastic. More commonly, the valve is bicuspid and functionally normal at birth but becomes increasingly regurgitant or stenotic in the third of fourth decade. Calcification is rare until later in life. Other forms of left ventricular outflow tract obstruction, including subvalvular and supravalvular aortic stenosis, account for less than 20% of all cases in most series.

Symptoms of aortic stenosis include syncope, exertional dyspnea, and chest pain. Sudden death is uncommon in children. In young patients, the presence of an early systolic ejection sound or "click" is useful to distinguish the valvular from subvalvular and supravalvular forms. The associated systolic ejection murmur, present in almost all patients, is of limited value in assessing severity. In a young patient, evidence of left ventricular hypertrophy on the ECG suggests severe aortic stenosis.

The natural history of congenital aortic valve disease varies. The eventual need for aortic valve replacement is directly related to the severity of stenosis at the time of presentation. In young adults with a nonstenotic bicuspid aortic valve, progression to

significant stenosis is rare. Ongoing surveillance is necessary to detect the development of aortic regurgitation or endocarditis. Echocardiography is a useful adjunct to the physical examination for this purpose. If mild stenosis is present, progression can occur, and about 20% of patients eventually require intervention. If moderate stenosis is present, up to 50% progress to severe stenosis and ultimately need surgery.

Many young adult patients with congenital aortic stenosis have undergone valvotomy in childhood, and the natural history of these patients is especially unpredictable. In one large multicenter registry, about one-third of these patients required aortic valve replacement after 20 years. The indication for surgery was either progressive stenosis, in the majority, or severe regurgitation. Longitudinal follow-up, usually on an annual basis, is recommended in these young patients. To assess the severity of aortic valve disease, echocardiography is most often used for serial evaluation.

PULMONIC STENOSIS

In 80% of cases, obstruction of right ventricular outflow occurs at the level of the pulmonary valve. The valve may be dysplastic, resulting in severe stenosis and often heart failure in infancy, or it may be tricuspid, with thickening and partial fusion of the leaflets, producing a conical or dome-shaped structure. An atrial septal defect (ASD) often accompanies this lesion. Pulmonic stenosis leads to elevated right ventricular pressure and subsequent hypertrophy, which may produce an element of subvalvular obstruction (Fig. 78.1). A systolic, crescendo–decrescendo murmur is generally present from birth, and the diagnosis is rarely overlooked. Symptoms such as fatigue or exertional dyspnea are uncommon until early adulthood and correlate poorly with the gradient. Cyanosis suggests severe stenosis in association with right-to-left shunting through an ASD or patent foramen ovale. Right ventricular failure is a late development. If the stenosis is severe, balloon or surgical valvotomy is undertaken in childhood, usually with excellent results.

The diagnosis of pulmonic stenosis can be confidently made at the bedside. A long and late-peaking systolic ejection murmur heard best at the upper left sternal border indicates significant stenosis. Other indicators of severe stenosis include a soft and very delayed pulmonary closure sound, a right-sided fourth heart sound, and a substernal lift due to right ventricular hypertrophy and dilation.

The adult with pulmonic stenosis has a relatively favorable prognosis. Significant progression is uncommon, so mild to moderate pulmonic stenosis can be managed conservatively. If obstruction is severe or if symptoms accompany moderate pulmonic stenosis, intervention is indicated. In most institutions, percutaneous balloon valvotomy is preferred in both children and adults with valvular stenosis. The procedure is less successful for dysplastic valves. Recurrent stenosis rarely occurs and iatrogenic pulmonic regurgitation is usually mild. Persistent right ventricular dysfunction, probably due to myocardial fibrosis, may occur despite successful repair, especially in older patients. The long-term significance of this requires further study. In most cases, however, adequate valvotomy is associated with relief of symptoms and improved exercise capacity.

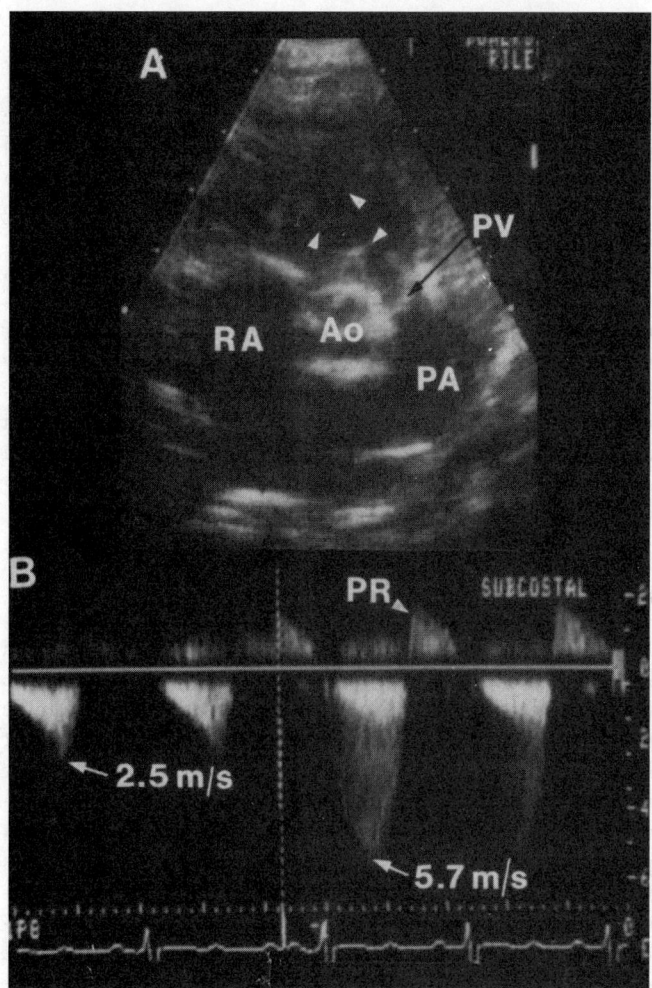

FIGURE 78.1. Two-dimensional echocardiogram (**A**) and Doppler recording (**B**) from a patient with both subvalvular and valvular pulmonic stenosis. In the short-axis view (**A**), right ventricular hypertrophy and infundibular narrowing are apparent (*arrowheads*). The pulmonic valve (*PV*) is thickened. In **B**, Doppler demonstrates both subvalvular and valvular obstruction. A dynamic subvalvular gradient of about 25 mm Hg (*left*) and a maximum gradient at the level of the valve of 130 mm Hg (*right*) are noted. Pulmonic regurgitation (*PR*) is also present. *Ao,* aorta; *RA,* right atrium; *PA,* pulmonary artery. (From Feigenbaum H. *Echocardiography,* fifth ed. Philadelphia: Lea & Febiger, 1994:365, with permission.)

ATRIAL SEPTAL DEFECT

ASDs are classified on the basis of the location of the defect within the septum. The most common type, a secundum ASD, involves the primum portion of the atrial septum and is often encountered in adults. Because of the paucity of symptoms in childhood and the often subtle or unremarkable physical findings, the diagnosis is delayed until adulthood in many patients. With age, the decrease in left ventricular compliance causes elevation of the left atrial pressure and increased left-to-right shunting through the ASD. Thus, for a given ASD size, greater shunting and right ventricular volume overload occurs with age. This increase in the volume load on the right heart may lead to atrial arrhythmias, exercise intolerance, or frank right-sided congestive heart failure, bringing the adult patient with a previ-

ously unrecognized ASD to medical attention. Thus, by the third or fourth decade symptoms are common—usually dyspnea, fatigue, or palpitations. Other presentations in adults include peripheral or central nervous system (CNS) emboli due to paradoxical embolism.

Unrepaired primum ASDs are uncommon in adults. These defects involve the most apical portion of the atrial septum at the insertion of the atrioventricular valve leaflets, which are usually structurally abnormal, most often exhibiting a cleft anterior mitral leaflet. Even after surgical repair, many patients continue to have atrioventricular valve regurgitation. These patients require serial echocardiographic reevaluation. Some eventually require reoperation to prevent ventricular dysfunction and congestive failure.

Venosus ASDs are less common than secundum defects and often lead to symptoms in adulthood. Venosus ASDs involve the superior vena cava–right atrium junction and are truly defects in the floor of the superior vena cava. The right upper pulmonary vein normally travels just posterior to the superior vena cava at this point; the floor of the superior vena cava serves as the "roof" of the right upper lobe pulmonary vein. A venosus defect in the floor of the superior vena cava–right atrium junction "unroofs" the right upper lobe pulmonary vein, which preferentially drains into the lower pressure right atrial chamber. Some speak of this as anomalous pulmonary venous drainage but the right upper lobe pulmonary vein is not anomalously located, and its drainage is correctly rerouted to the left atrium by surgical closure of the venosus defect in the floor of the superior vena cava.

Note that echocardiography, and transesophageal echocardiography in particular, has revolutionized our diagnostic ability to define ASDs in adults. ASDs result in a left-to-right shunt and right ventricular volume overload. Congestive heart failure can develop due to right ventricular failure, manifested by an elevated right ventricular diastolic pressure. Atrial fibrillation is a common late complication, but severe pulmonary vascular disease and pulmonary hypertension are rare. As previously described, symptoms may develop or worsen if left ventricular compliance decreases (e.g., due to hypertension or coronary artery disease), thereby augmenting left-to-right shunting.

Physical findings may be subtle. A fixed and widely split second heart sound is characteristic. The basal systolic ejection murmur is due to increased flow across the pulmonary valve (not due to flow through the defect). Mitral regurgitation may be secondary to mitral valve prolapse in secundum defects or may be due to a cleft mitral leaflet in the case of primum defects. The chest radiograph demonstrates an enlarged right heart and increased pulmonary vascularity (Fig. 78.2). The ECG often reveals incomplete right bundle-branch block. A normal or rightward frontal plane axis suggests a secundum ASD (Fig. 78.3); left axis deviation is characteristic of primum defects (Fig. 78.4). Echocardiography is diagnostic and permits assessment of the location and size of the defect (Fig. 78.5). Associated findings and an estimate of right heart pressure can also be determined noninvasively in most patients.

In adults with symptoms, surgical repair should be recommended unless there is severe pulmonary vascular disease. If surgery is performed in young adults, the outlook is excellent, and long-term survival is better than in older patients who

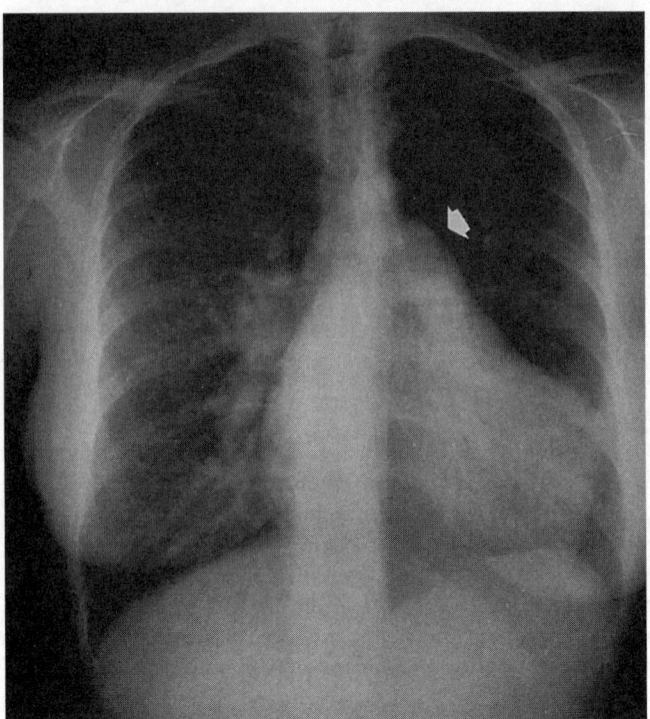

FIGURE 78.2. Chest radiograph from a 28-year-old woman with secundum atrial septal defect. The heart, particularly the right ventricle, is enlarged. The pulmonary artery (*arrow*) is dilated. Pulmonary vascularity is increased.

enlargement in adults include partial anomalous venous connection, either with or without an associated ASD. Abnormal congenital development of the pulmonary veins, allowing part of the pulmonary venous drainage to return to the right heart, physiologically causes left-to-right shunting and right ventricular volume overload. In contrast to that which occurs with ASDs, this shunt is fixed and does not tend to increase with age. These patients are often asymptomatic. Those with large shunt volumes may develop symptoms of palpitations, dyspnea on exertion, and fatigue similar to ASD patients as right ventricular compliance deteriorates. Surgical correction for symptomatic patients is feasible and is most often performed by creating a baffle redirecting the anomalous pulmonary venous return. Such a baffle along the floor of the cava and right atrium can be continued to the atrial septum, where, either through a congenital or surgically created ASD, the pulmonary venous return is redirected properly into the left atrium.

PATENT DUCTUS ARTERIOSUS

Persistent patency of the ductus arteriosus is common in children but uncommon in adults. Risk factors for this condition include female gender, maternal rubella, and birth at high altitude. If the ductus does not close spontaneously within the first 2 months of life, it will probably remain patent. This results in a left-to-right shunt, the magnitude of which depends on the size of the channel and the pressure gradient between the aorta and the main pulmonary artery. Blood pressure measurement typically finds wide pulse pressure, with a low diastolic pressure. A typical continuous machinery-like murmur is present at the upper left sternal border, and often there is evidence of left ventricular volume overload, with cardiomegaly and hyperdynamic pulses. The murmur is often heard best below the left clavicle, but it radiates widely and can be easily heard in the back. With the development of pulmonary vascular disease, the diastolic component shortens and becomes softer.

undergo repair. If surgery is undertaken later in life, the patient may still benefit; this advantage of surgical therapy seems to be maintained even in elderly patients and those with moderate pulmonary hypertension (pulmonary vascular resistance ≤5 Wood units). The management of asymptomatic adults remains controversial. Repair has traditionally been recommended if the left-to-right shunt ratio exceeds 1.5 or 2 to 1. Currently, closure is often recommended in young adults with evidence of right ventricular volume overload based on echocardiography (i.e., right ventricular dilation and paradoxical septal motion). Closure of smaller ASDs, now often detected by transesophageal echocardiography, remains controversial.

Other causes of right heart, right atrium, and right ventricle

The adult who escaped detection and surgical repair as a child is often symptomatic unless the ductus is small and restrictive. If the shunt is large, left heart failure usually develops in adolescence or early adulthood. Pulmonary hypertension and endocarditis are other important complications of this condition. If Eisenmenger's syndrome is present, an important differentiating

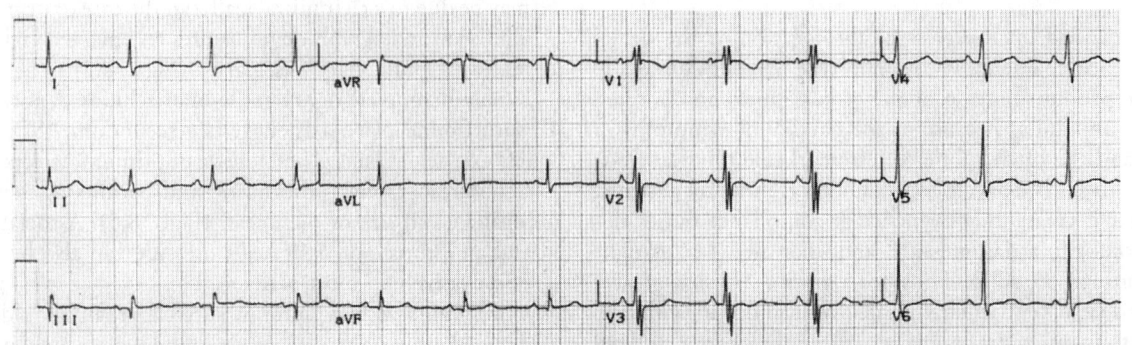

FIGURE 78.3. Electrocardiogram from a patient with secundum atrial septal defect. There is sinus rhythm and incomplete right bundle-branch block. The frontal plane QRS axis is about +30 degrees.

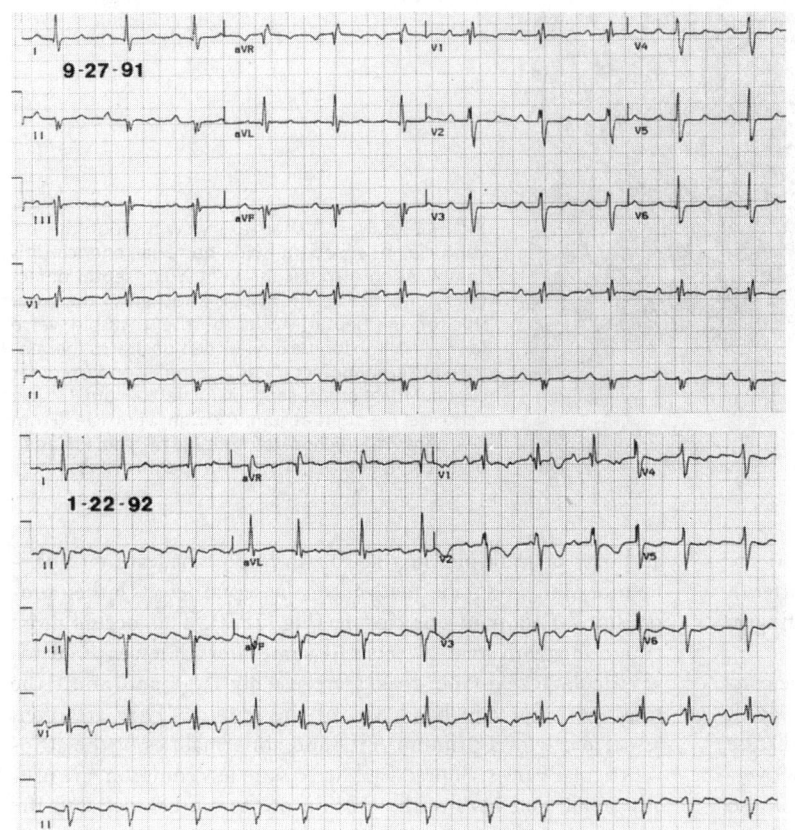

FIGURE 78.4. Serial electrocardiograms from a patient with primum atrial septal defect and mitral regurgitation. The top tracing was recorded before surgical repair. There is sinus rhythm with first-degree atrioventricular block, left-axis deviation, and incomplete right bundle-branch block. The lower tracing was recorded soon after surgical repair. Atrial flutter is noted.

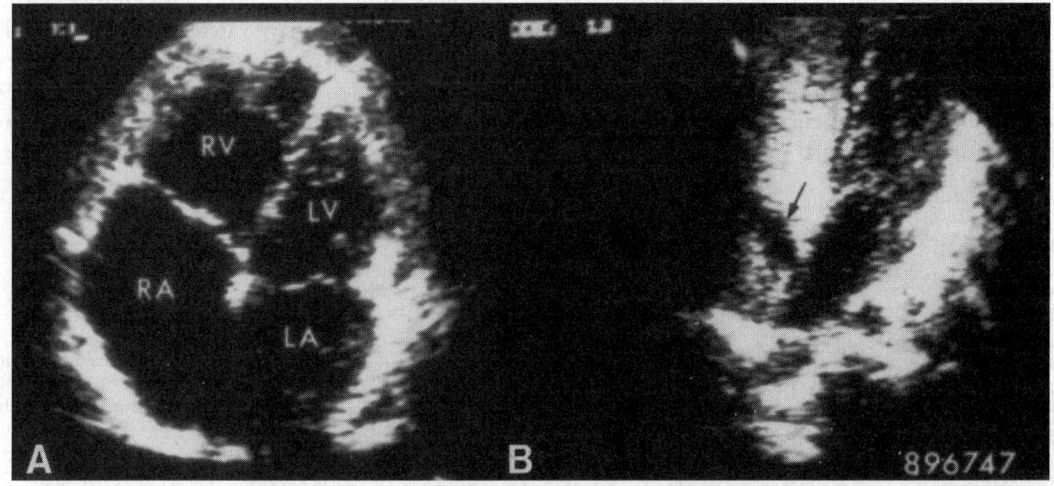

FIGURE 78.5. Two-dimensional echocardiogram from a patient with a large secundum atrial septal defect. **A:** A dilated right atrium (*RA*) and right ventricle (*RV*) are demonstrated, as well as echo dropout in the area of the atrial septum. **B:** Injection of agitated saline through a peripheral vein results in negative contrast effect within the right atrium (*arrow*). This finding is diagnostic of left-to-right shunting through the atrial septal defect. *LA*, left atrium; *LV*, left ventricle. (From Feigenbaum H. *Echocardiography*, fifth ed. Philadelphia: Lea & Febiger, 1994, with permission.)

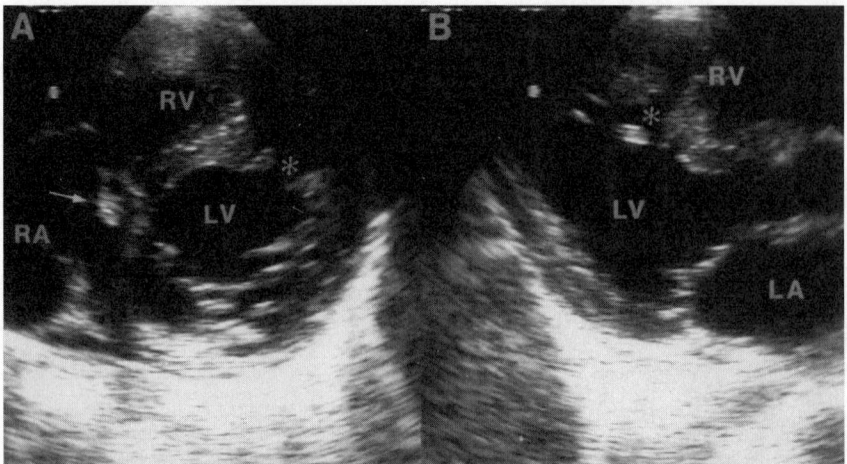

FIGURE 78.6. A: A short-axis view through the left ventricle in a patient with bacterial endocarditis complicating a trabecular ventricular septal defect (*). A large echogenic mass is attached to the atrial side of the septal leaflet of the tricuspid valve (*arrow*). **B:** The long-axis view demonstrates the ventricular septal defect (*) as a complex and irregular channel through the septum. *LA,* left atrium; *LV,* left ventricle; *RA,* right atrium; *RV,* right ventricle. (From Feigenbaum H. *Echocardiography,* fifth ed. Philadelphia: Lea & Febiger, 1994, with permission.)

point is the occurrence of clubbing and cyanosis distal to the site at which the shunt occurs (beyond the left subclavian artery). Thus, the feet and toes are affected, but the hands and fingers are spared.

Surgical closure of the patent ductus in children may be considered curative, but the decision to close a ductus in an adult is more complex. The presence of pulmonary vascular disease and the residual effects of chronic left ventricular volume overload must be taken into account. The procedure itself is also more difficult, primarily because of the calcification of the aortic end of the channel. Transcatheter closure of patent ducti is an alternative for selected adult patients and is discussed in more detail later.

VENTRICULAR SEPTAL DEFECT

Defects of the ventricular septum vary considerably in size and location. All, however, have a left-to-right shunt, the magnitude of which depends on the size of the defect and the pulmonary vascular resistance. The most common type involves the region around the membranous septum. Muscular or trabecular defects can occur anywhere within the muscular portion of the septum

and may be multiple (Fig. 78.6). An important feature of perimembranous and trabecular ventricular septal defects is their propensity for spontaneous closure (Fig. 78.7). This occurs more commonly with small defects and is rare after adolescence. Atrioventricular canal-type defects are usually large and affect the most posterior and basal part of the septum. They are often associated with a primum ASD and abnormalities of the atrioventricular valves. Supracristal defects are less common, are usually small, and involve the portion of the septum between the aortic and pulmonic annuli.

Adults with ventricular septal defect usually have either a small, restrictive defect or a large, unrestrictive defect with elevated pulmonary vascular resistance (Eisenmenger's complex). Patients in the former group are often asymptomatic and present with a loud, harsh holosystolic murmur and associated thrill. Their prognosis is generally favorable, with a cumulative risk of endocarditis (Fig. 78.6) or progressive aortic regurgitation. Obstructive pulmonary vascular disease results in a diminished or reversed shunt and a poor long-term prognosis. This progression is associated with a gradual decrease in the intensity of the murmur. Thus, the disappearance of the murmur in an adult patient generally heralds the development of Eisenmenger's syn-

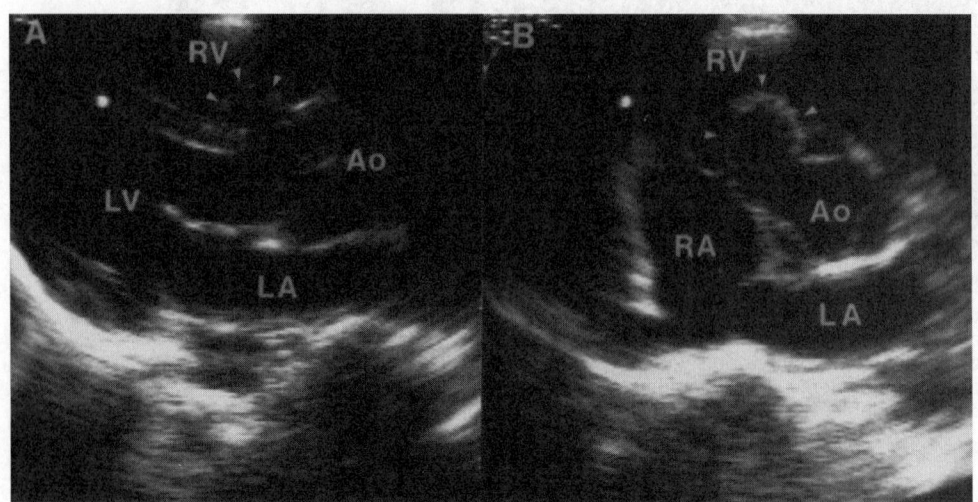

FIGURE 78.7. Two-dimensional echocardiograms from a patient with a perimembranous ventricular septal defect. The defect has closed through formation of a large ventricular septal aneurysm (*arrowheads*). Doppler imaging confirmed a lack of blood flow through the aneurysm. On examination, the patient had no evidence of a residual ventricular septal defect, but significant aortic regurgitation was present. *Ao,* aorta; *LA,* left atrium; *LV,* left ventricle; *RA,* right atrium; *RV,* right ventricle. (From Feigenbaum H. *Echocardiography,* fifth ed. Philadelphia: Lea & Febiger, 1994, with permission.)

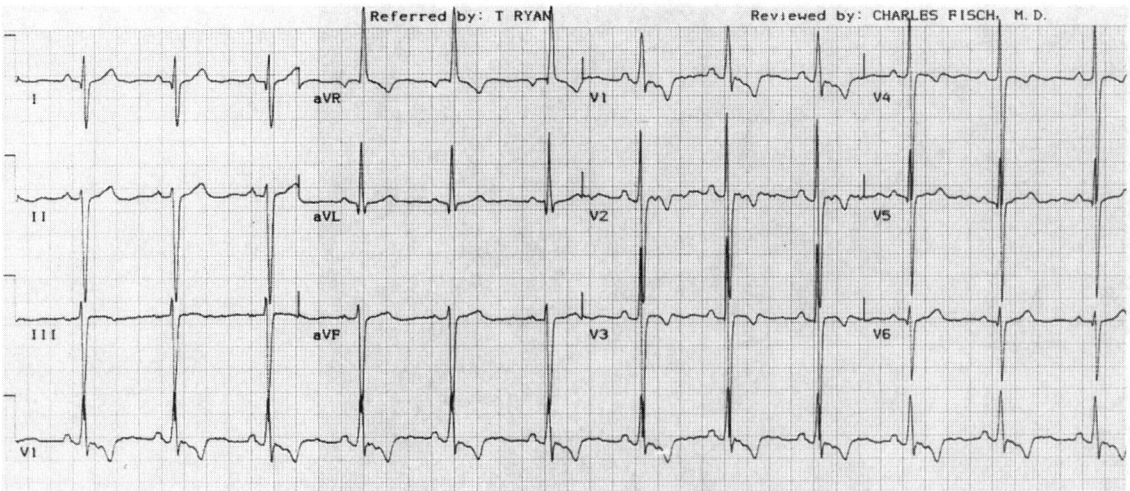

FIGURE 78.8. Electrocardiogram from a patient with complete atrioventricular canal defect and pulmonary hypertension. Sinus rhythm with a right-axis deviation and evidence of right ventricular hypertrophy are found.

drome and should not be misinterpreted as a sign of spontaneous defect closure. In such patients, cyanosis and clubbing develop and exercise tolerance is invariably reduced. Characteristic findings on ECG and chest radiography accompany these changes (Figs. 78.8 and 78.9). The increase in pulmonary vascular resistance is usually fixed, and surgical repair is rarely an option.

Management of the adult patient with a small, isolated ventricular septal defect must take into account the location of the

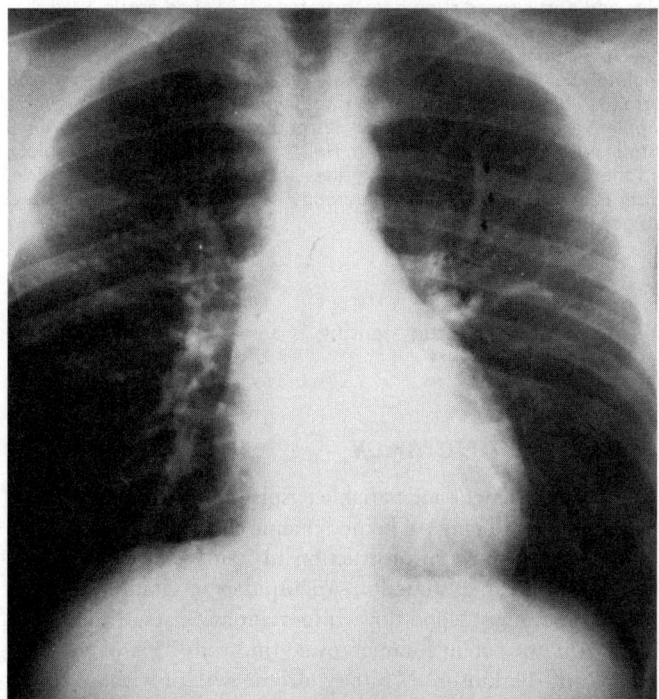

FIGURE 78.9. Chest radiograph from a 23-year-old man with ventricular septal defect. The heart is enlarged. There is evidence of increased pulmonary blood flow, and the pulmonary arteries are dilated (*black arrows*).

defect, the pulmonary vascular resistance, the symptom status, and the presence or absence of associated findings, such as aortic regurgitation. Most patients with a small defect are asymptomatic and have normal pulmonary artery pressure. In the Second Natural History Study of Congenital Heart Defects, the 20-year survival probability for patients with a small ventricular septal defect was over 90%, and 94% of these patients were in the New York Heart Association functional class I. Thus, surgical repair for adults with a small defect and normal pulmonary artery pressure is generally not recommended. The occasional patient with aortic regurgitation in association with a perimembranous or supracristal defect would, in most institutions, be an exception to this rule. In these patients, surgical closure is often recommended to prevent further undermining of the aortic annulus and progressive regurgitation.

AORTIC COARCTATION

Coarctation of the aorta is characterized by a discrete, shelf-like narrowing of the descending aorta just distal to the origin of the left subclavian artery. As in other forms of left ventricular outflow tract obstruction, the elevation in ventricular pressure is proportional to the severity of the obstruction. In coarctation, however, this increase in pressure proximal to the narrowing is transmitted to the head and upper extremities. Hypertension in a young patient should always suggest the possibility of coarctation. Associated findings include a bicuspid aortic valve (in up to 50% of patients) and berry aneurysms of the circle of Willis.

If symptoms do not develop in infancy, most patients remain asymptomatic until adolescence or early adulthood. At that point, however, the outlook deteriorates dramatically if repair is not performed. By age 30, mortality rate approaches 50%. Death may be due to left heart failure, a ruptured cerebral aneurysm, endocarditis, or a dissecting aortic aneurysm. The diagnosis is often made when hypertension is discovered in a young patient. Diminished and delayed pulses in the lower extremities point to the diagnosis. A harsh systolic murmur is usually audible

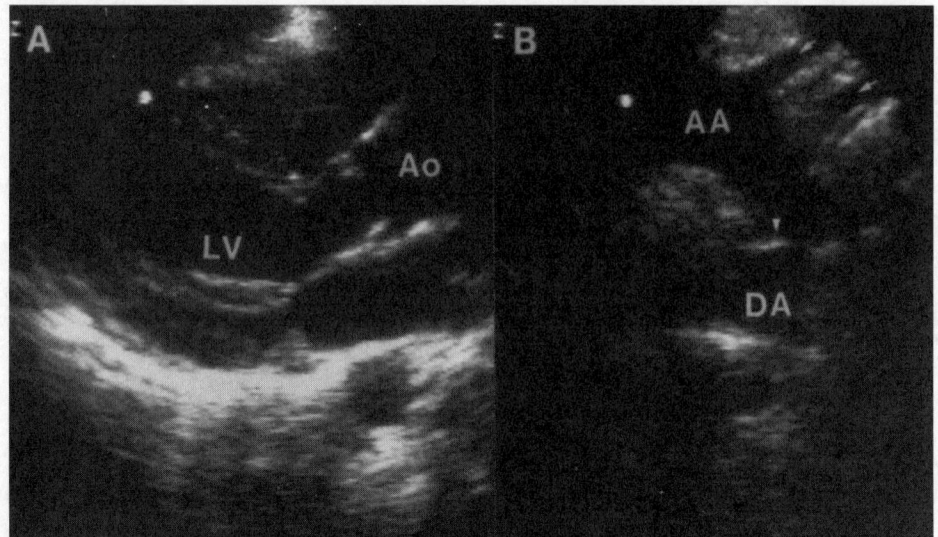

A

B

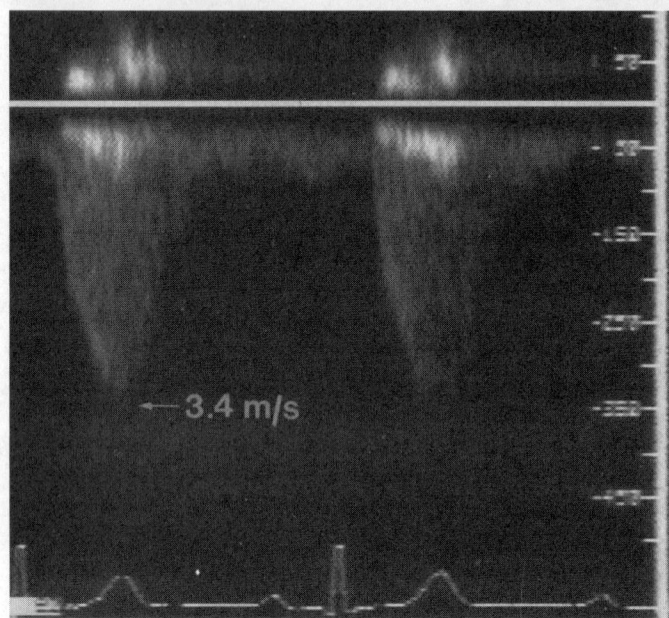

C

FIGURE 78.10. **A:** The long-axis view of a patient with a bicuspid aortic valve and aortic coarctation demonstrates a thickened aortic valve that domes mildly in systole. **B:** A suprasternal long-axis view of the aortic arch (*AA*) demonstrates a discrete, shelf-like narrowing (*arrowhead*) immediately distal to the origin of the arch vessels (*arrows*). The descending aorta (*DA*) beyond the coarctation is well visualized. **C:** Continuous wave Doppler recording of flow in the descending aorta reveals a maximal systolic pressure gradient of 46 mm Hg. The gradient diminishes rapidly, and there is little gradient during diastole. *Ao,* aorta; *LV,* left ventricle. (From Feigenbaum H. *Echocardiography,* fifth ed. Philadelphia: Lea & Febiger, 1994, with permission.)

over the left chest posteriorly. The severity of the coarctation gradient may be estimated by measurement of the systolic blood pressure in the upper extremities compared with that of the lower extremities.

The coarctation can be imaged noninvasively with echocardiography (Fig. 78.10) or magnetic resonance imaging (Fig. 78.11). Echocardiography is useful to measure the pressure gradient across the obstruction and permits simultaneous assessment of associated findings, such as left ventricular hypertrophy or a bicuspid aortic valve.

In most situations, the initial repair of coarctation is performed surgically. Even when the obstruction is eliminated, however, longevity is not returned to normal. Persistent hypertension and the small risk of stroke or aortic dissection adversely affect the long-term prognosis. Deterioration of a bicuspid aortic valve is also a possibility. For restenosis in adults, the procedure

of balloon dilation and stenting is a reasonable alternative to reoperation.

EBSTEIN'S ANOMALY

Apical displacement and variable dysplasia of the tricuspid valve can have a broad range of hemodynamic consequences. Ebstein's anomaly may result in obstruction to right ventricular inflow, right ventricular dysfunction, tricuspid regurgitation, and reduced pulmonary blood flow. Important associated findings include ASD or patent foramen ovale (in up to 75% of patients) and Wolff–Parkinson–White syndrome with or without supraventricular tachyarrhythmias. The clinical course varies, depending on the severity of the deformity and the presence of associated lesions.

Adults with Ebstein's anomaly usually have presenting com-

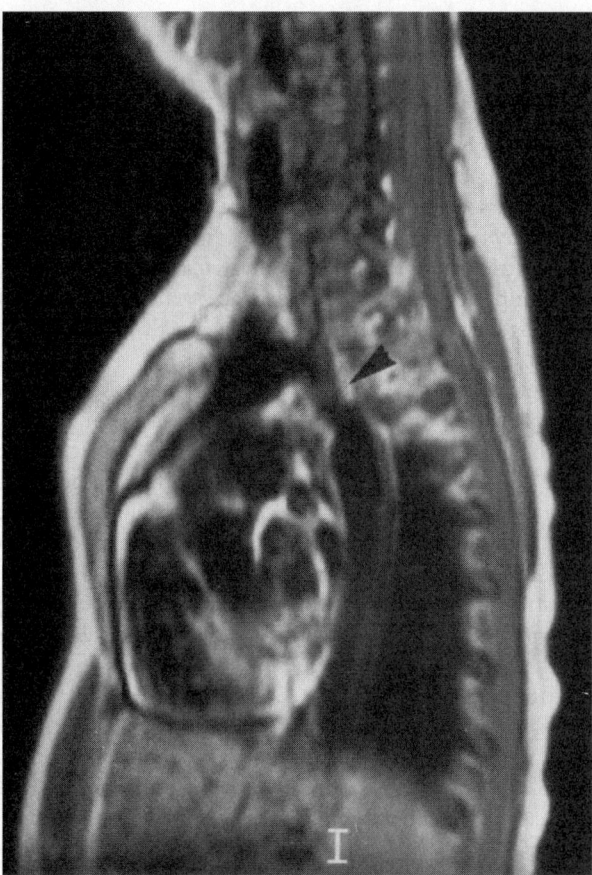

FIGURE 78.11. A magnetic resonance image of the heart in the coronal plane from a patient with aortic coarctation. Narrowing in the descending aorta is indicated by the arrowhead. The distal descending aorta is well visualized. The left ventricular outflow tract is indicated by the asterisk.

plaints of dyspnea and fatigue. Cyanosis is a poor prognostic sign and suggests right-to-left interatrial shunting. Tachyarrhythmias occur in about 25% of patients and may lead to syncope. Management depends on the morphology of the tricuspid valve and the extent of right ventricular hypoplasia. Surgical repair or replacement of the valve is often beneficial to relieve symptoms and eliminate shunting. Selection of the appropriate procedure is primarily made on the basis of echocardiographic findings. The long-term prognosis after repair varies and remains largely uncertain. However, optimal plastic repair is clearly associated with clinical improvement and relief of symptoms.

TETRALOGY OF FALLOT

By far the most common cyanotic congenital cardiac lesion seen in adults, tetralogy of Fallot is encountered in both the unoperated and the surgically repaired state. Although referred to as a "tetralogy" the primary abnormalities are the ventricular septal defect, which is usually large and subaortic, and the right ventricular outflow tract obstruction, which may occur at the valvular, subvalvular, or supravalvular level. Right ventricular hypertrophy and the overriding aorta can be considered secondary. Depending on the severity of the right ventricular outflow obstruc-

tion, effects include variable degrees of right ventricular pressure elevation, reduced pulmonary blood flow, and bidirectional shunting.

The clinical presentation of a patient with tetralogy of Fallot depends primarily on the severity of pulmonic stenosis. If mild, the condition resembles that of a large ventricular septal defect, and cyanosis may not be present. If affected patients do not undergo surgical repair early, their condition progresses to elevated pulmonary resistance, pulmonary artery hypertension, and Eisenmenger's physiology. If severe pulmonic stenosis exists, marked cyanosis and reduced pulmonary blood flow are present early in life. The degree of shunting varies and depends on the balance between pulmonic stenosis and systemic vascular resistance. Cyanotic spells occur during infancy when right-to-left shunting increases. In children, compulsive squatting is classically observed in this condition, presumably an attempt by the child to increase systemic vascular resistance and thereby reduce right-to-left shunting.

The second heart sound is single and loud. A right ventricular heave and palpable systolic thrill are usually present. The ejection murmur is helpful to assess the severity of the pulmonic stenosis. A long, late-peaking murmur suggests severe obstruction. The absence of a murmur may indicate pulmonary atresia. Chest radiography demonstrates right ventricular enlargement and a small main pulmonary artery (Fig. 78.12). The pulmonary vascular markings indicate the magnitude of the decrease in pulmonary blood flow. In about 25% of patients, a right-sided aortic arch is present. Echocardiography is useful and permits assess-

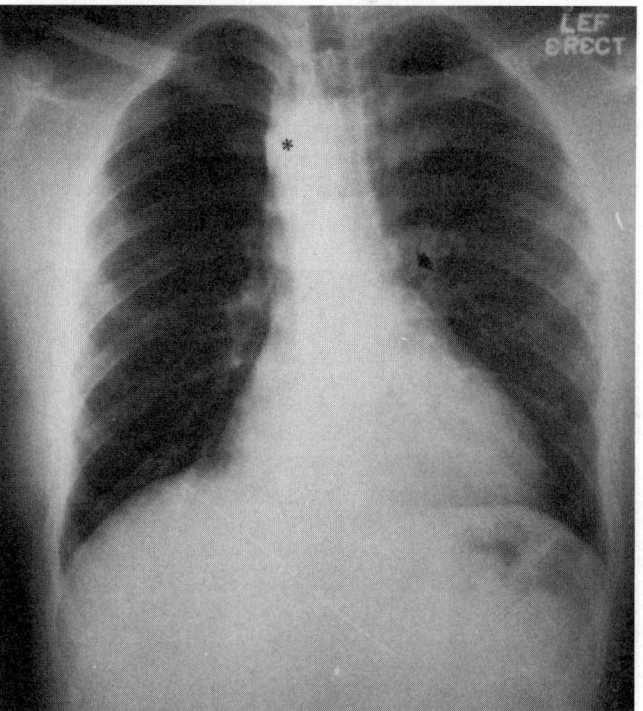

FIGURE 78.12. Chest radiograph from an 18-year-old man with tetralogy of Fallot. The proximal pulmonary artery is small (*black arrowhead*), and the pulmonary vascularity is decreased. The aortic arch is on the right side (*).

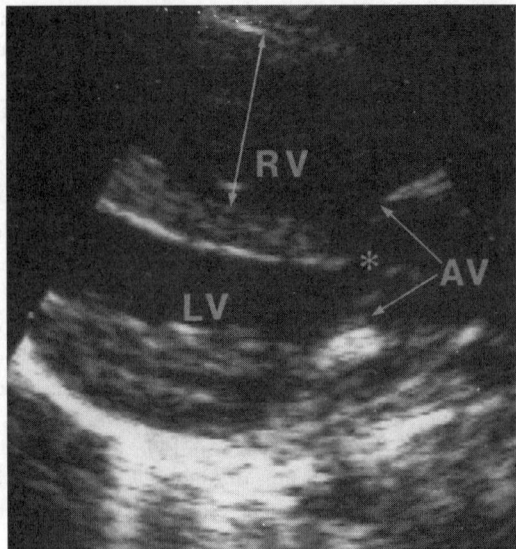

FIGURE 78.13. Long-axis view from a patient with tetralogy of Fallot demonstrates a dilated right ventricle (*RV*), an overriding aorta (*AV*), and a subaortic ventricular septal defect (*). Right ventricular hypertrophy, the other feature of tetralogy of Fallot, is not well illustrated in this image. *LV,* left ventricle. (From Feigenbaum H. *Echocardiography,* fifth ed. Philadelphia: Lea & Febiger, 1994, with permission.)

ment of essentially all the salient features of tetralogy (Fig. 78.13).

LEVOTRANSPOSITION OF THE GREAT ARTERIES

Congenitally corrected, or levo (*l-*), transposition of the great arteries is characterized by ventricular inversion with ventriculoarterial discordance. Thus, the right-sided left ventricle receives the systemic venous blood and pumps it to the pulmonary artery. The left-sided right ventricle receives the pulmonary venous blood and pumps it to the aorta (Fig. 78.14). Circulatory integ-

rity is maintained, but the roles of the two pumping chambers are reversed, forcing the morphologic right ventricle to function as the systemic pumping chamber. Progressive ventricular dysfunction leading to heart failure is a variable and often late event. The clinical consequences of *l*-transposition are primarily the result of the ventricular inversion, as well as the presence or absence of associated anomalies. These include atrioventricular conduction system abnormalities leading to complete heart block, ventricular septal defect, subvalvular pulmonic stenosis, and incompetence of the left-sided atrioventricular valve (the morphologic tricuspid valve resulting in functional mitral regurgitation).

Patients with these associated lesions usually come to the attention of the physician early in life. However, if symptoms do not bring the patient to the physician, the correct diagnosis is often delayed until adulthood. Complete heart block, mitral regurgitation, or left heart failure may lead the patient to seek medical attention. Still, the diagnosis of *l*-transposition is often missed.

Treatment depends on the associated anomalies. Among patients with left heart failure, medical therapy should be instituted. The use of afterload reduction (usually with angiotensin-converting enzyme inhibitors) for treatment of asymptomatic systemic ventricular dysfunction is often used, although the benefit has not been proved. Subvalvular pulmonic stenosis is really a clinical issue unless it is severe, because the morphologic left ventricle ejects to the pulmonary artery. For symptomatic complete heart block, dual-chamber pacing is usually recommended. Surgical treatment of ventricular septal defect or atrioventricular valve regurgitation may also be necessary.

■ POSTOPERATIVE CONGENITAL HEART DISEASE

An increasing proportion of adults with congenital heart disease have undergone some form of surgical repair. Included in this

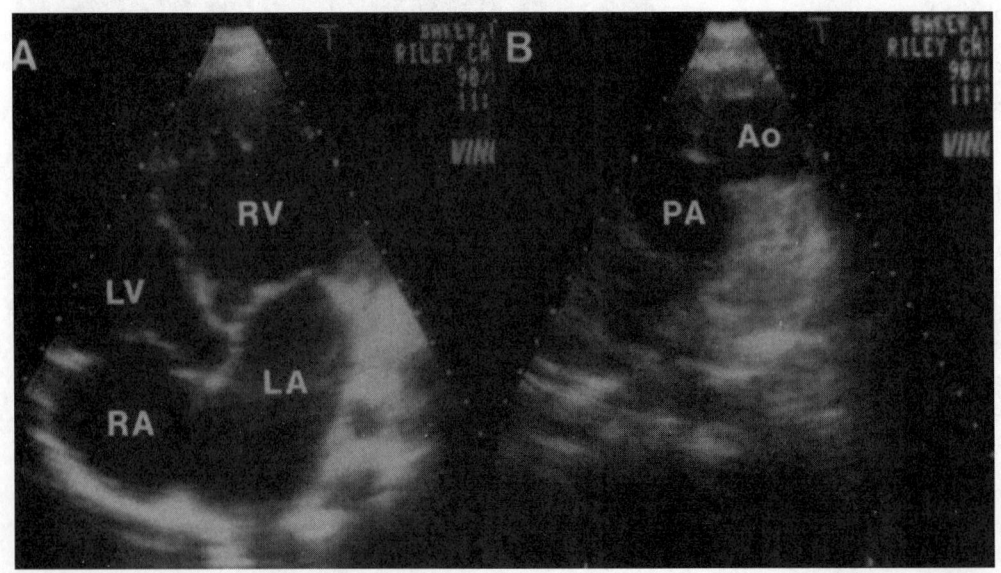

FIGURE 78.14. Apical four-chamber (**A**) and high parasternal short-axis (**B**) views from a patient with l-transposition of the great arteries. **A:** Ventricular inversion is demonstrated. The dilated and trabeculated right ventricle (*RV*) receives blood from the morphologic left atrium (*LA*). The displaced tricuspid valve is apical to the right-sided mitral valve. **B:** The two great arteries arise in parallel, and the aorta (*Ao*) is anterior and to the left of the pulmonary artery (*PA*). *RA,* right atrium; *LV,* left ventricle. (From Feigenbaum H. *Echocardiography,* fifth ed. Philadelphia: Lea & Febiger, 1994, with permission.)

heterogeneous group are those with a simple malformation, such as patent ductus arteriosus (PDA), which was corrected at a young age; those with a more complex lesion, such as tetralogy of Fallot, which was successfully repaired; and those in whom only a palliative procedure, such as a Blalock–Taussig shunt, has been performed. Regardless of the simplicity of the underlying lesion or the degree of surgical success, few patients with congenital heard disease can truly be considered "cured," and most require ongoing surveillance and treatment.

Despite the extraordinary developments over the past few decades in congenital cardiac surgery, most affected young patients are left with residua, anatomical defects left uncorrected or partially corrected by the surgery, or sequelae, abnormalities caused by or resulting from the procedure. Proper diagnosis and management of these patients require a thorough knowledge of the underlying cardiac condition as well as the date and type of intervention. The clinician should also anticipate the potential residua and sequelae that might be encountered and should consider the possible need for further surgical intervention.

SYSTEMIC-TO-PULMONARY ARTERY SHUNTS

Palliation for complex congenital heart disease characterized by inadequate pulmonary blood flow (e.g., tetralogy of Fallot) often involves creation of a vascular connection between the systemic arterial or systemic venosus circulation and the pulmonary arteries. These relatively simple surgical procedures are generally effective, resulting in reduced symptoms and improved oxygenation in most patients. Several variations of this type of shunt have been developed over the years. One of the most effective involves a direct end-to-side anastomosis between the subclavian artery and the ipsilateral pulmonary artery (the Blalock–Taussig shunt). The degree of palliation depends on the magnitude of shunt flow. If the connection is too small, there is no meaningful increase in pulmonary blood flow and thus arterial oxygen content. If the connection is large and nonrestrictive and permits transmission of systemic pressures to the pulmonary circuit, pulmonary vascular obstructive disease may be the late result.

Another form of systemic-to-pulmonary artery connection, the Glenn shunt, creates an end-to-end connection between the superior vena cava and the right pulmonary artery. A late complication of this operation is the development of pulmonary arteriovenous fistulae in the right lower lung. These pulmonary arteriovenous malformations are small and typically diffuse in the right lower lung, and they result in cyanosis. The reason for their development is not known. Often these shunts are disconnected at the time of more definitive surgery. Their anastamotic sites may leave stenosis in the pulmonary arteries, contributing to late obstruction to pulmonary blood flow.

ATRIAL SEPTAL DEFECT

The long-term outlook for the patient with an isolated secundum ASD who underwent patch repair as a child is excellent. Survival is similar to that of age-matched normal subjects; a decrease in right ventricular size occurs in most of the patients, and reoperation is rarely necessary. The risk of endocarditis in these patients is thought to be negligible. The results in patients

operated later in life are slightly less gratifying. In this group, preoperatively pulmonary vascular resistance is a major determinant of outcome. A significant improvement in symptoms is also less likely in the presence of preoperative pulmonary hypertension. The most common late complication in the adult patient is the development of atrial fibrillation. This is estimated to occur in up to 50% of patients who undergo repair beyond age 40 and is an important cause of late morbidity.

TETRALOGY OF FALLOT

Surgical correction of tetralogy of Fallot, when performed early in life, is associated with a markedly improved prognosis; many affected young patients are now reaching adulthood. Residual problems include recurrent right ventricular outflow tract obstruction, right ventricular failure, and severe pulmonic regurgitation. Repair previously included a two-stage process. A palliative systemic-to-pulmonary artery shunt was first created, followed by intracardiac repair at age 1 to 2 years. Definitive surgery involves closure of the ventricular septal defect and relief of the right ventricular outflow obstruction, either by patch enlargement of the outflow tract or repair or replacement of the pulmonary valve. An external right ventricle-to-pulmonary artery conduit or homograft is occasionally required.

Surgical success is the rule in most patients, with the benefits extending through 10 to 20 years of follow-up. Long-term complications include recurrent right ventricular outflow tract obstruction (requiring reoperation in about 15% of patients), severe pulmonic regurgitation, right ventricular failure, advanced heart block, and ventricular dysrhythmias. Left ventricular dysfunction is a late complication that occurs most often in patients who undergo repair later in life. Sudden death, probably secondary to ventricular tachyarrhythmias, also occurs.

D-TRANSPOSITION OF THE GREAT ARTERIES

The surgical management of dextro- or D-transposition of the great arteries has changed in the past decade. Since the early 1960s, an intra-atrial venous switch (the Mustard or Senning operation) was the procedure of choice for transposition. By redirecting venous return at the atrial level, correction of transposition was achieved and 20-year survival rate was about 80% to 85% (Fig. 78.15). With this approach, however, the morphologic right ventricle continued to function as the systemic ventricle. An abnormal response to exercise and a progressive decrease in systolic function were common, thereby accounting for most of the late morbidity and mortality. Atrial dysrhythmias, sinus node dysfunction, atrioventricular block, and sudden death were important late electrophysiologic complications in this type of repair.

In the past decade, intra-atrial repair has gradually been replaced by the arterial switch procedure. This operation is now feasible for infants and children. An important advantage of this approach is the restoration of the normal ventricular arrangement by transferring systemic ventricular function to the morphologic left ventricle.

FONTAN PROCEDURE

The original Fontan operation, used for repair of tricuspid atresia, involved the creation of a direct connection between the

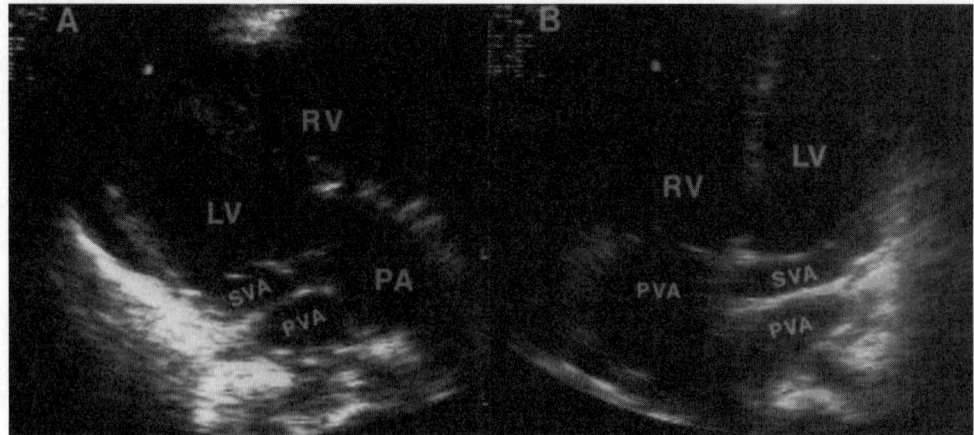

FIGURE 78.15. A: A long-axis view from a patient following an intra-atrial baffle procedure for D transposition of the great arteries. The baffle is easily visualized as a linear structure dividing the atria into a systemic venous atrium (*SVA*) and a pulmonary venous atrium (*PVA*). **B:** The apical four-chamber view again shows the baffle and the orientation of the atria. *LV*, left ventricle; *PA*, pulmonary artery; *RV*, right ventricle. (From Feigenbaum H. *Echocardiography*, fifth ed. Philadelphia: Lea & Febiger, 1994, with permission.)

right atrium and pulmonary artery. In bypassing the rudimentary right ventricle, the procedure maintained separation between the systemic and pulmonary circuits and provided nonpulsatile flow of caval blood to the lungs. Several modifications of the operation have subsequently been developed, and the Fontan surgery is now applied to an increasing number of malformations (e.g., single ventricle with pulmonic stenosis) in which two ventricle repairs are not possible. Recently reported long-term results have been very positive. In properly selected patients, this procedure can result in a marked improvement in symptoms. Survival rate at 5 years approaches 90%, and most patients remain in functional class I or II. Complications include persistent pericardial and pleural effusions, atrial tachyarrhythmias, pulmonary arteriovenous fistulas, and protein-losing enteropathy.

Fontan repair is now being applied to adults, many of whom had undergone previous palliative shunt procedures. Careful selection of candidates for this surgery is critical. The primary predictors of success are adequate systemic ventricular function as defined by left ventricular end-diastolic pressure of less than 10 mm Hg, the presence of sinus rhythm, the absence of atrioventricular valve regurgitation, and the absence of increased pulmonary vascular resistance.

■ MEDICAL MANAGEMENT ISSUES

DYSRHYTHMIAS

The management of dysrhythmias is becoming an increasingly important component in the overall care of adults with congenital heart disease. Certain categories of patients, both before and after surgery, are at particular risk for specific rhythm disturbances. For example, Ebstein's anomaly is frequently associated with Wolff–Parkinson–White syndrome and atrial tachyarrhythmias. In patients with *l*-transposition of the great arteries, atrioventricular block is common, with a 2% annual risk of developing complete heart block.

Postoperative dysrhythmias are common, reflecting both the underlying malformation and the type of surgical repair. The overall risk increases with the patient's age, the complexity of

the lesion, and the severity of ventricular dysfunction. For example, age is an important determinant of likelihood of developing atrial fibrillation or flutter after repair of secundum ASD (Fig. 78.4). Among patients who have undergone a Fontan procedure, decreased ventricular function predisposes to the development of supraventricular dysrhythmias.

Certain types of repair are associated with particular rhythm abnormalities. The Mustard operation for transposition of the great arteries involves the creation of an intra-atrial baffle. Sinus node dysfunction and atrioventricular block are late complications and tend to be progressive. Patients also exhibit an abnormal chronotropic response to exercise. Sudden death occurs in about 5% of patients after Mustard repair. A documented episode of atrial flutter appears to be a marker for increased risk, but the actual mechanism of sudden death is unknown. Both atrial tachyarrhythmias and bradycardia have been implicated, but prevention remains a challenge.

Surgical closure of ventricular septal defect carries a risk of conduction system damage. Right bundle-branch block is a common finding after repair, and transient complete heart block occurs in up to 25% of patients. Persistent complete heart block is present in 1% to 10% of patients, who are at increased risk of sudden death. Pacemaker placement is indicated in most of these patients.

Patients who have undergone repair of tetralogy of Fallot often exhibit right bundle-branch block. More important, however, is risk of sudden death late after repair, which occurs in up to 5% of patients. In most patients, the primary cause is thought to be ventricular tachyarrhythmias. Risk factors include older age at time of surgery, elevated right ventricular systolic pressure (more than 60 mm Hg), and premature ventricular complexes during monitoring. Ventricular arrhythmias in this group are more common in those with significant residual right ventricular outflow tract obstruction with associated severe pulmonary valve insufficiency. These factors taken together suggest that prolonged or severe right ventricular pressure overload is the underlying cause of serious dysrhythmic complications.

CYANOTIC CONGENITAL HEART DISEASE

Tissue hypoxia leads to a rise in erythropoietin production and a resultant increase in red blood cell mass. If this in turn causes an adequate increase in tissue oxygen delivery, erythropoietin release stabilizes and an equilibrium is established at a higher hematocrit level. This condition is called *compensated erythrocytosis.* In some patients, however, an equilibrium state is not achieved and continued expansion of the red cell mass occurs; this has detrimental effects on oxygen delivery, partly because of increased blood viscosity. This condition is referred to as *decompensated erythrocytosis.*

Patients with compensated erythrocytosis have an elevated but stable hematocrit and may be considered iron replete. They exhibit few if any symptoms of hyperviscosity and rarely benefit from phlebotomy. Patients with decompensated erythrocytosis often have significant symptoms of hyperviscosity such as fatigue, headache, visual disturbance, or nightmares. The clinical picture may be complicated by iron deficiency and the creation of microspherocytes (often secondary to phlebotomy). These cells are more rigid than normal erythrocytes, further contributing to the increased blood viscosity.

These conditions are often mismanaged. The risk of thrombotic stroke in adults with cyanotic congenital heart disease is low and is unrelated to the hematocrit level or iron stores. Thus, therapeutic phlebotomy performed to reduce the risk of stroke is unwarranted. Phlebotomy should be considered only after dehydration is excluded and should be reserved for patients with symptomatic hyperviscosity and a hematocrit level above 65%. Withdrawal of 500 mL of blood should be followed by replacement with a similar volume of saline or colloid. As noted previously, repeated phlebotomy may cause iron deficiency and microspherocytes and thereby worsen symptoms. Routine monitoring for iron stores is mandatory, and iron replacement, when indicated, should be done cautiously, usually at a dose of 325 mg per day of ferrous sulfate with biweekly measurements of hematocrits and frequent reevaluation of iron stores.

Many patients with cyanotic congenital heart disease also exhibit defects in hemostasis. In most patients, the bleeding tendency is mild and manifests as easy bruising, epistaxis, or petechiae. Less often, recurrent hemoptysis occurs that may be life threatening. Evaluation of the prothrombin time and activated partial thromboplastin time and deficiencies in the various coagulation factors suggest defects in both the intrinsic and extrinsic coagulation systems. Mild thrombocytopenia and abnormal platelet function also contribute to the bleeding and bruising problems. The use of aspirin, heparin, or nonsteroidal anti-inflammatory agents can aggravate these conditions and should be avoided in these patients. The severity of the bleeding disorder associated with trauma or surgical procedures generally correlates with the hematocrit level. To reduce the operative risk, hemostasis can be temporarily improved by lowering the hematocrit level to 60% to 65%.

INFECTIVE ENDOCARDITIS

The risk of endocarditis in congenital heart disease depends on three factors: the type and severity of the cardiac malformation; whether or not the patient has undergone surgical intervention; and the presence of bacteremia. Lesions that predispose to infection are those associated with a turbulent, high-velocity jet that impacts on an endothelial surface. Thus, a restrictive ventricular

septal defect with a left-to-right jet impinging on the septal leaflet of the tricuspid valve poses a greater risk than a large secundum ASD that is not associated with a jet lesion. Surgical status also influences the relative risk. In some cases, such as ligation of a PDA, surgery substantially lowers the patient's risk. Other surgical devices, such as valved conduit, significantly increase the potential for infection.

Patients can be categorized as having low, intermediate, or high risk based on the underlying lesion and surgical status. Low-risk conditions include secundum ASD, mild pulmonic stenosis, and anomalous pulmonary venous connection. Certain repaired lesions are also considered low risk; these include secundum atrial or ventricular septal defect following patch repair, ligated PDA, repaired tetralogy of Fallot (without a prosthetic valve), and Fontan surgery. Intermediate risk conditions include both unoperated and operated lesions; examples are left-sided valvular regurgitation, bicuspid aortic valve, aortic coarctation, unoperated ventricular septal defect and PDA, and nonvalved conduits (either intracardiac or external). With the highest risk are patients with valved conduits or mechanical prosthetic valves and those with a previous episode of infective endocarditis.

Prevention of endocarditis involves antibiotic prophylaxis and ensuring good personal and dental hygiene. Guidelines developed by the American Heart Association serve as the basis for antibiotic prophylaxis, and these recommendations should be reinforced on a regular basis during clinic visits. The pocket-sized card provided by the association is a convenient and effective way to emphasize the importance of these guidelines. Other measures that help to prevent endocarditis include good general hygiene practices, meticulous skin and dental care, and avoidance of certain female contraceptive devices. All patients with congenital heart disease should be encouraged to undergo twice-yearly dental visits for cleaning and prophylaxis.

PREGNANCY AND CONGENITAL HEART DISEASE

Because of the improvements in medical and surgical management, pregnancy among women with congenital heart disease is becoming increasingly possible. To counsel and manage these patients properly, it is essential to understand the hemodynamic changes associated with normal pregnancy. This condition is often described as a hyperdynamic state with superimposed volume overload. Blood volume and cardiac output increase significantly during pregnancy. The rise in cardiac output is due to increased contractility and heart rate. Despite these alterations, blood pressure changes little, primarily owing to a fall in peripheral vascular resistance. During labor and delivery, fluctuations in intravascular volume, stroke volume, and blood pressure occur. Vaginal delivery is usually associated with a loss of about 500 mL of blood, which partially compensates for the gestational hypervolemia.

Management of women with congenital heart disease ideally begins before conception and focuses on the safety and advisability of pregnancy. If pregnancy is contraindicated (see following text), safe methods of contraception should be presented. The risk of pregnancy to mother and fetus must be covered in detail. This discussion should also include the potential risks of medications and diagnostic procedures. For example, warfarin should not be used during the early stages of pregnancy, and women who are chronically anticoagulated should be switched to heparin before conception. Finally, the risk of heart disease in the offspring should be discussed.

Despite these concerns, there are relatively few congenital malformations in which pregnancy is contraindicated. In general, the most important determinants of outcome are the presence and severity of pulmonary vascular disease and the mother's functional class. Pulmonary hypertension, regardless of the underlying cause, poses a high risk to the mother and a low likelihood of a successful pregnancy. Thus, the presence of Eisenmenger's physiology is widely regarded as a contraindication to pregnancy. Significant heart failure also greatly increases the likelihood of a poor outcome. Mortality in pregnant women with New York Heart Association functional class III or IV is about 7%. Other conditions in which pregnancy should be avoided include severe and symptomatic aortic stenosis, Marfan's syndrome with a dilated aortic root, uncorrected cyanotic heart disease, and unrepaired aortic coarctation. Pregnant women with Marfan's syndrome and an aortic root diameter greater than 40 mm are at risk for aortic rupture. Likewise, coarctation of the aorta during pregnancy has also been associated with rupture, dissection, or stroke. Placental blood flow is also significantly reduced in this condition.

In contrast, most patients with acyanotic congenital heart disease bear the demands of pregnancy with few problems. Those with uncomplicated left-to-right shunts generally do well. If the shunt is large, there is an increased risk of congestive heart failure; if the shunt is reversed, pregnancy should be avoided. In patients with repaired shunt lesions, pregnancy is well tolerated with little additional risk. Isolated ASD is one of the most common conditions and is well tolerated despite the gestational increase in blood volume. With advancing age, however, the possibility of dysrhythmias or paradoxical emboli increases.

Among patients with valvular disease, regurgitant lesions generally fare better than stenotic ones. Severe aortic stenosis often becomes unstable during pregnancy, resulting in heart failure or dysrhythmias. Likewise, severe mitral stenosis is poorly tolerated during pregnancy, often resulting in congestive heart failure, atrial fibrillation, or hemoptysis. In contrast, pulmonic stenosis is better tolerated, even if severe. Because of the decrease in systemic vascular resistance during pregnancy, the severity of left-sided valvular regurgitation rarely worsens and may instead physiologically decrease in severity during pregnancy.

Among the complex forms of disease, unrepaired tetralogy of Fallot is still occasionally encountered in pregnant women. In most, the possibility of clinical deterioration can be anticipated. Because of the hemodynamic changes, right-to-left shunting usually increases, with an associated worsening of cyanosis. Fluctuations during labor and delivery pose an additional risk, occasionally leading to syncope or death. Conversely, in patients who have undergone successful intracardiac repair, the expected risks (with the exception of endocarditis) are substantially less.

EXERCISE AND ACTIVITY RESTRICTIONS

Specific recommendations regarding restriction of activity in adolescents and young adults with congenital heart disease depend on several issues. Although strenuous exercise in certain patients may predispose them to complications or even sudden death, most patients can safely engage in a variety of activities. The overall risk of serious complications is low, and there are few data that demonstrate that a specific activity actually predisposes to sudden death and that avoiding that activity would prolong life. Guidelines take into account the specific cardiac lesion, the type and intensity of exercise, the risk of body collision, and the patient's overall fitness. Certain aspects of the patient's history, such as prior syncope or known dysrhythmias, are also important.

Activities may be categorized as having both a static and a dynamic component. Exercises with a high static component include strenuous isometric activity such as weightlifting or wrestling. Dynamic, or isotonic, activities involve repetitive muscle movements with relatively little developed force (e.g., walking, jogging, low-impact aerobics, cycling). Most activities have an element of both, such as downhill skiing. Recommendations have been published regarding the classification of competitive sports and the relative risks of each to persons with various types of heart disease. For example, athletes with uncomplicated ASD without pulmonary hypertension may participate in all competitive sports. If pulmonary arterial pressure is elevated, only low-dynamic, low-static activities (e.g., golf and bowling) are permitted. In patients with Eisenmenger's physiology, participation in sports is discouraged.

Patients who have undergone repair of complex congenital heart disease constitute a heterogeneous group. For example, after repair of tetralogy of Fallot, patients may be permitted to engage in all forms of sports, provided that the right heart pressure is near normal, that no residual shunting exists, and no significant dysrhythmias have been demonstrated. Patients with right ventricular hypertension or significant right ventricular volume overload should be restricted to low-intensity sports. In addition to the history and physical examination, exercise testing, echocardiography, and ambulatory ECG monitoring are helpful to evaluate these issues.

Adult patients with transposition who have undergone a Mustard or Senning repair usually have limited exercise capacity owing to abnormal systemic ventricular function. The ability of the systemic ventricle to respond to the demands of exercise is blunted, and the risk of exercise-induced dysrhythmias may be increased. For these reasons, patients should be restricted to low- to moderate-intensity exercise of limited duration.

Patients who have undergone Fontan repair for palliation of complex heart disease often experience a marked improvement in functional capacity and a subsequent desire to participate in vigorous exercise. Despite the symptomatic improvement, exercise is usually limited by a reduced cardiac output at rest and during exercise. Most of these patients can safely participate in low-intensity activities if ventricular function is preserved and the presence of significant dysrhythmias has been excluded.

INTERVENTIONAL CARDIAC CATHETERIZATION

Cardiac catheterization has long been a vital diagnostic tool for patients with congenital heart disease. Improvements in digital radiographic imaging, radiographic contrast agents, combined uses of catheterization, cardiac anesthesia, and echocardiography, as well as the direct advances in percutaneous interventional technology, have led to the improved techniques of percutaneous intervention for congenital heart disease. The dream of nonsurgical correction of some of the less complex forms of congenital heart disease has now become a reality for selected individuals.

Percutaneous intervention can also palliate certain congenital heart disorders, thereby postponing the need for surgery. Such interventions can also be combined with surgery in some cases to make the surgery less risky and more effective.

Percutaneous catheter-based intervention to treat patients with congenital heart disease began three decades ago. In 1966, Rashkind described balloon septostomy to treat infants with transposition of the great vessels. This section is an overview of some of these catheter-based interventions for congenital heart disease, which continue to actively evolve.

PERCUTANEOUS TREATMENT OF CONGENITAL VALVULAR DISEASE

One of the most effective and widely accepted percutaneous congenital interventions is that of balloon valvotomy for treatment of persons with pulmonary valvular stenosis. This technique was described in 1982. Indications for the procedure in children and adults include symptomatic valvular pulmonary stenosis, causing chest pain, palpitations, or dyspnea. In addition, asymptomatic persons with severe stenosis, manifested by peak gradients greater than 50 mm Hg, are usually offered balloon valvotomy to prevent late sequelae such as right heart failure.

Classic congenital pulmonary valve stenosis is most easily defined in the lateral radiographic projection during contrast angiography of the right ventricular outflow tract and main pulmonary artery (Fig. 78.16) The systolic doming of the pulmonary valve leaflets and the dilation of the main pulmonary artery just cephalad of the valve defines this disorder. Balloon catheters are selected to dilate the valve to about 1.2 times the size of the measured annulus.

This technique is associated with excellent results and carries a very low complication rate. Immediately after valve dilation, there is usually a dramatic reduction in the transvalvular gradient. Some gradient, between the right ventricle and pulmonary artery, typically about 30 mm Hg, often persists immediately after balloon dilation. This is usually due to right ventricular infundibular narrowing, from the underlying right ventricular hypertrophy, which results in some subvalvular right ventricular outflow tract gradient after relief of the valvular stenosis. This outflow gradient regresses in follow-up, and the long-term echocardiographic and clinical results of the procedure are excellent. Pulmonary valve insufficiency has not been a clinical problem in follow-up and appears to be less severe than that seen previously with surgical pulmonary valvotomy. Less ideal cases of valvular pulmonary stenosis, in patients with dysplastic valves, can still be effectively dilated percutaneously in many persons. These valves, occurring as isolated problems or in association with Noonan's syndrome, consist of thickened fused leaflet tissue. They can be recognized on the lateral angiographic images

of the right ventricular outflow tract as thickened leaflet tissue, lacking the domed appearance in systole and also lacking the supravalvular dilation of the main pulmonary artery. The results of balloon dilation are less ideal and uniform in this group, although many experience effective relief of pulmonary stenosis. Those who are not improved require surgical treatment.

Congenital aortic stenosis in adults is less well suited for percutaneous treatment than is pulmonary valve stenosis. In children with congenital aortic stenosis and in selected young adults with bicuspid aortic stenosis, percutaneous balloon valvotomy has been found to offer effective palliative treatment, postponing the need for valve replacement surgery. In children, balloon valvotomy has been shown to have palliative effects similar to what is seen with surgical valvotomy. In adults, however, the results are less encouraging. Even by the third and fourth decade of life, bicuspid aortic valves are less pliable and are often calcified. These calcified valves are usually not improved significantly by balloon dilation, and restenosis rates are high. Adults with aortic stenosis are usually most effectively treated by valve replacement surgery.

In those suitable for percutaneous balloon aortic valvuloplasty, the procedure is usually performed by way of the femoral artery using retrograde crossing of the stenotic aortic valve. In infants and small children, a venous, prograde approach across the atrial septum may be preferred to avoid femoral artery trauma. After crossing the stenotic aortic valve with a guidewire, a balloon catheter equal in size to the measured diameter of the aortic annulus is positioned. Unlike the pulmonary annulus, overdilation of the aortic annulus is to be avoided in an attempt to avoid aortic annular disruption and aortic valve insufficiency. Complications of the procedure include femoral artery injury or occlusion. Less common but important complications include the creation of severe valvular regurgitation, heart block, myocardial infarction, stroke, and death. In general, although balloon aortic valvuloplasty plays a palliative role in congenital aortic stenosis in children, surgical valve replacement remains the treatment of choice for most adults with congenital aortic stenosis. Congenital mitral valve stenosis is distinctly uncommon and typically responds poorly to balloon dilation. Commissure fusion causing rheumatic mitral valve stenosis in adults responds extremely well to balloon dilation; however, congenital mitral stenosis is usually not improved. Causes of congenital mitral stenosis include supravalvular stricture, a hypoplastic annulus, fibrotic fused leaflet tissue, and abnormal chordal or papillary muscle architecture. These anatomical anomalies respond poorly to balloon dilation, usually not improving the severity of mitral stenosis and often causing leaflet tearing leading to severe mitral regurgitation. Thus, adult patients with congenital mitral valve stenosis, with rare exception, are best treated by surgical valve replacement.

COARCTATION

The treatment of coarctation of the aorta remains controversial. Balloon dilation is effective in reducing the trans-stenotic gradient. Potential complications of the procedure, however, include femoral artery damage and more serious complications such as dissection of the aorta at the dilation site, resulting in

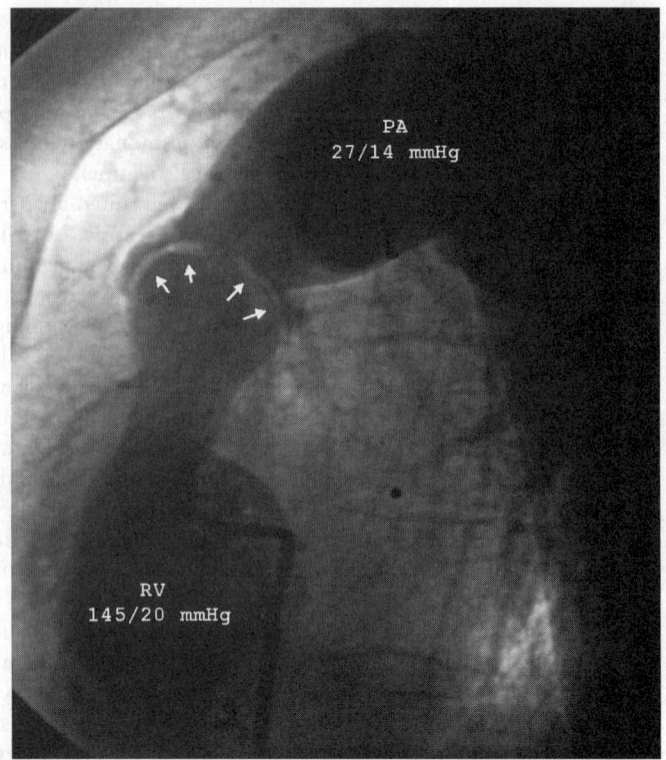

A

PA
27/14 mmHg

RV
145/20 mmHg

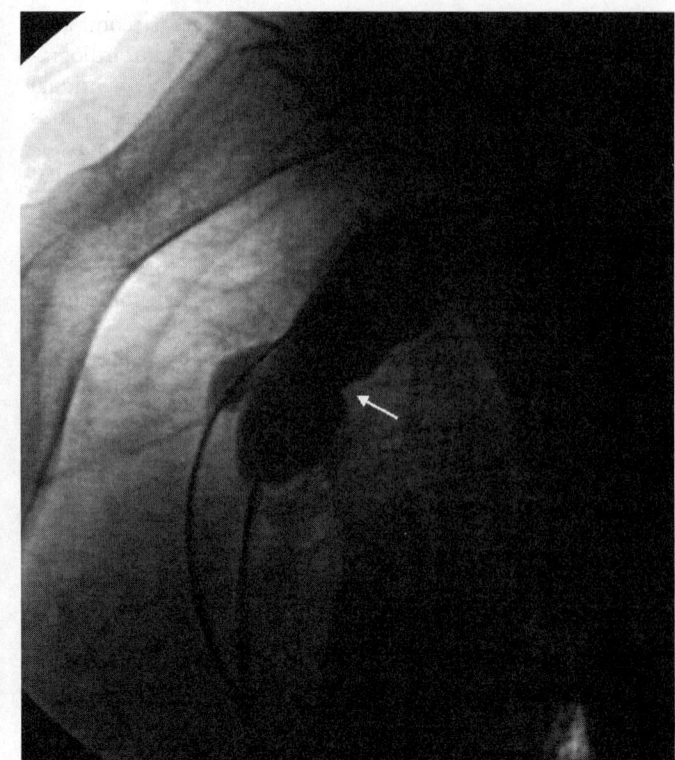

B

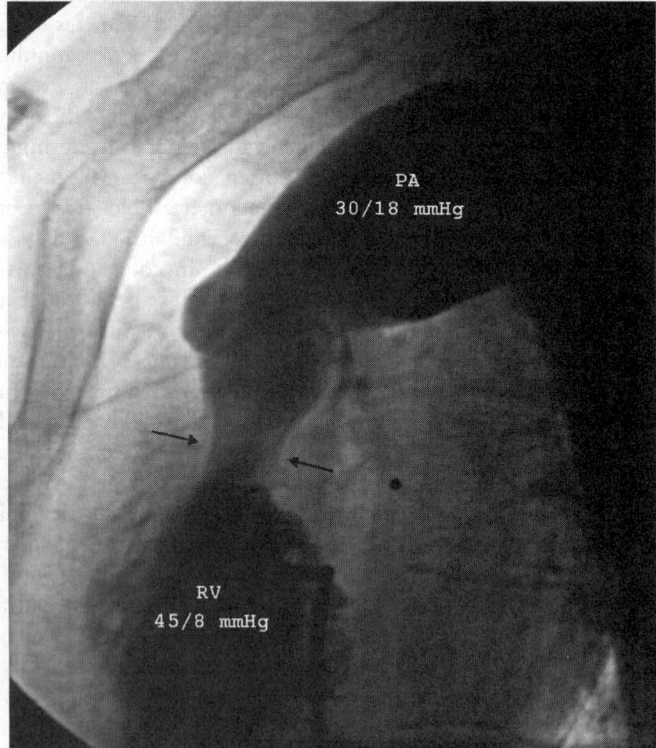

C

PA
30/18 mmHg

RV
45/8 mmHg

FIGURE 78.16. A: Right ventricular angiogram in the lateral projection in a patient with classic congenital pulmonary valvular stenosis. The systolic doming of the stenotic pulmonary valve leaflets is highlighted by the white arrows. Also note the supravalvular dilation of the main pulmonary artery, which is characteristic of this disorder. The peak-to-peak gradient is 118 mm Hg. **B:** Dilation of the valvar pulmonic stenosis using the double-balloon technique. **C:** Lateral angiographic view of the right ventricular outflow tract after balloon dilation of the pulmonary valve stenosis. Note the lack of systolic doming of the valve leaflets and improved leaflet orifice. A small gradient of 15 mm Hg persists immediately after the procedure, which was localized to the mild narrowing of the right ventricular outflow tract (*black arrows*).

acute rupture or late aneurysm formation. Intravascular ultrasonography and stenting of the coarctation site hold promise for limiting these serious complications and improving the hemodynamic results by preventing vascular recoil. Intravascular ultrasonography is important in these procedures in identifying dissections in the wall of the aorta that are often not seen by aortography. Intravascular stenting of the aorta using Palmaz stents has shown excellent early results. Discrete coarctations, especially recurrent coarctation after previous surgery, are ideal indications for percutaneous intervention. Patients who have had previous coarctation surgery have greater risks from repeat surgical intervention. In addition, the periaortic fibrosis in these persons provides an increased margin of safety for percutaneous dilation and stenting.

PULMONARY ARTERY STENOSIS

Balloon dilation of the pulmonary arteries in patients with peripheral pulmonary artery stenosis is the procedure of choice. Peripheral pulmonary artery stenosis may occur as an isolated disorder or may be associated with tetralogy of Fallot, maternal rubella syndrome, or Williams syndrome (Fig. 78.17). Peripheral pulmonary artery stenosis may also occur as a late sequela of previous systemic-to-pulmonary artery shunt surgery. With the exception of the most proximal pulmonary artery lesions, these lesions are not surgically accessible.

Recoil of the dilated pulmonary artery segment is common after balloon angioplasty alone. Stenting of pulmonary artery stenosis has therefore largely replaced balloon dilation. Long delivery sheaths and improved guidewires have made deployment of Palmaz stents to even distal segments of the pulmonary vasculature feasible.

The greatest risks of pulmonary artery stenting are overdila-

tion, dissection, and rupture of the pulmonary artery segment, which are fortunately rare occurrences. Minor dissections often seal and are self-limited, causing small amounts of hemoptysis. This is particularly true in patients who do not have pulmonary hypertension. Life-threatening bleeding may be treated by coil closure of the pulmonary artery branch involved, or they may require surgical intervention.

In addition to pulmonary hemorrhage, a unique and uncommon complication of pulmonary artery stenting is pulmonary edema in the lung distal to the stented segment. This is more likely to occur in patients with severe stenosis and high central pulmonary artery pressure. After relief of the stenosis in these patients, high blood flow rates in the stented segment may cause focal pulmonary edema. This complication, if it occurs, does so within the first 48 hours of the procedure. Supportive care allows resolution of the edema, which usually occurs over the next week.

Stent thrombosis has not been a problem with pulmonary artery stenting owing to the large vessel diameters and high flow rates involved. Aspirin (325 mg per day) is usually prescribed for a period of 3 months.

Procedural success rates have been good, and late clinical and angiographic follow-up has demonstrated excellent long-term results. Follow-up angiography typically reveals some neointimal hyperplasia within the stented segment, but significant restenosis is distinctly uncommon.

PATENT DUCTUS ARTERIOSUS

Percutaneous closure of PDA is now possible for many patients. Closure of PDAs is generally recommended in adults to reduce the risk of endocarditis and left heart failure.

Catheterization-based closure of PDAs was described in the

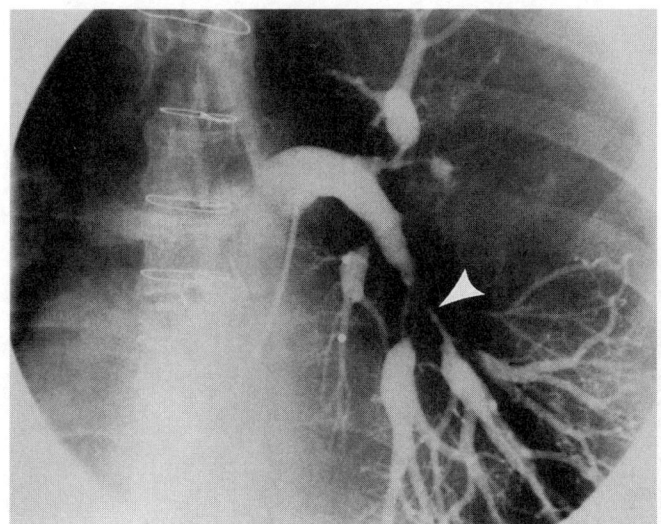
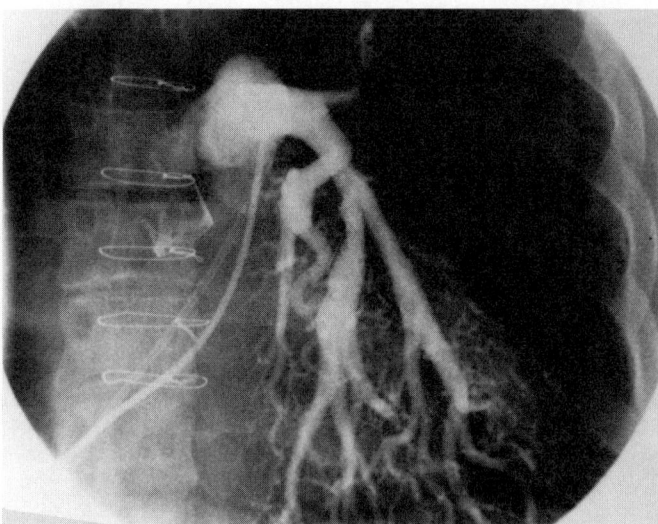

A   B

FIGURE 78.17. A: Left pulmonary arteriogram in the anteroposterior (*AP*) view showing severe peripheral pulmonary artery stenosis, causing severe pulmonary hypertension. **B:** Left pulmonary arteriogram in the AP view 1 year after stenting the left lower lobe pulmonary artery. Three Palmaz stents were used; 2 P308 "kissing" stents in the lower branches and a P188 stent in the more proximal, posteromedial branch. Pulmonary artery systolic pressures improved from 100 mm Hg to 40 mm Hg after stenting of both pulmonary arteries, resulting in marked improvement of exercise tolerance.

1970s. Devices, however, remained suboptimal and percutaneous closure remained limited. In 1991, the use of vascular occlusion coils was described for closure of PDAs. Over the last several years, refinements of this coil occlusion technique have made percutaneous closure more successful. Improvements include the use of detachable coils and coil occlusion bags (Fig. 78.18). The anatomy of the PDA influences the success rate of percutaneous closure. Narrow ducts (less than 4 mm in diameter), with lengths that exceed the diameter, are ideal for coil closure.

Coil embolization is a risk of the procedure. Most embolization is to the pulmonary artery, and most can be percutaneously retrieved using snare techniques and are of no clinical consequence. Percutaneous closure of PDAs is especially advantageous in adult patients for whom surgical closure carries higher risk because of comorbid illnesses and calcified, friable tissue in the region of the ductus.

Coil occlusion techniques are useful in other situations as well. They can be used to occlude systemic-to-pulmonary collateral vessels in patients with Eisenmenger's syndrome and other congenital conditions limiting pulmonary blood flow, when these collaterals are responsible for hemoptysis. This coil occlusion technique can also be used to close coronary–cameral fistulas, as well as other abnormal vascular connections such as anomalous pulmonary venous drainage when dual drainage to the left atrium coexists (Fig. 78.19).

ATRIAL SEPTAL DEFECTS

Perhaps the most exciting area of current investigation is in the area of percutaneous techniques for closure of secundum ASD. Attempts at nonsurgical closure for ASDs is not new. Hufnagel and Gillespie first described such an attempt in 1959. In the 1970s and 1980s, several devices were tested, of which the best known and most widely used was the clamshell device. This

device proved promising but was eventually redesigned because of late wire fractures seen in the radial arms of the device.

Several devices are under active investigation in the United States and Europe. These include the Angel Wings device, the Amplatzer device, the Cardioseal device, the Sideris button occluder, and the AS-DOS device. These devices are designed for catheterization-based closure of secundum ASDs. They are best suited for use in patients with moderate-sized or smaller defects, which have an adequate rim of remaining atrial septal tissue surrounding the defect to which the device may adhere. These devices can also be used to close patent foramen ovales in patients with presumed paradoxical emboli or orthodeoxia.

The Amplatzer, Cardioseal, and Angel Wings devices are perhaps the most encouraging devices currently being studied. Although structurally unique, these devices, share similar delivery and implantation features. They are placed across the atrial septum into the left atrium using a sheathed delivery catheter that is inserted percutaneously into the femoral vein. The left atrial portion of the devices are then deployed, and the catheter is withdrawn slightly to seat this portion of the device against the left side of the atrial septum. Once properly positioned, the right atrial portion of the device is deployed to secure the device in place. The position of the device is confirmed before its final release from the delivery catheter. These procedures are generally performed under general anesthesia. Continuous transesophageal echocardiographic monitoring, as well as fluoroscopy, is vital to ensure optimal device positioning.

Potential risks of percutaneous ASD closure include device embolization, incomplete ASD closure, atrial arrhythmias, thrombus formation on the device with subsequent embolization, and damage to surrounding structures, such as the atrial free walls, atrioventricular valves, and pulmonary veins. These complications have been very uncommon in the recent clinical trials, and procedural success rates have been about 90%.

Two- to three-year follow-up is now available for these de-

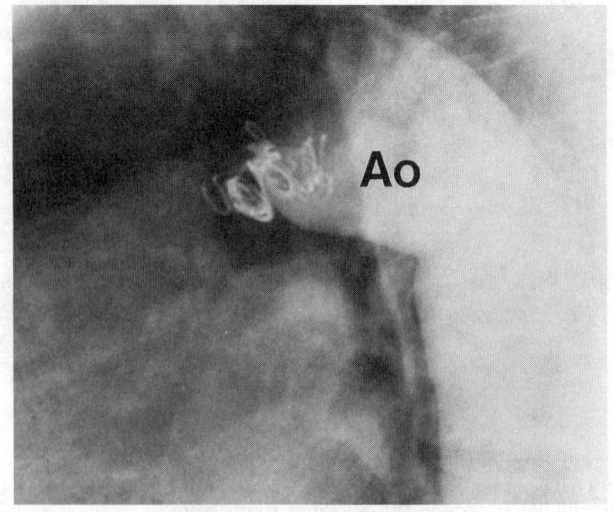
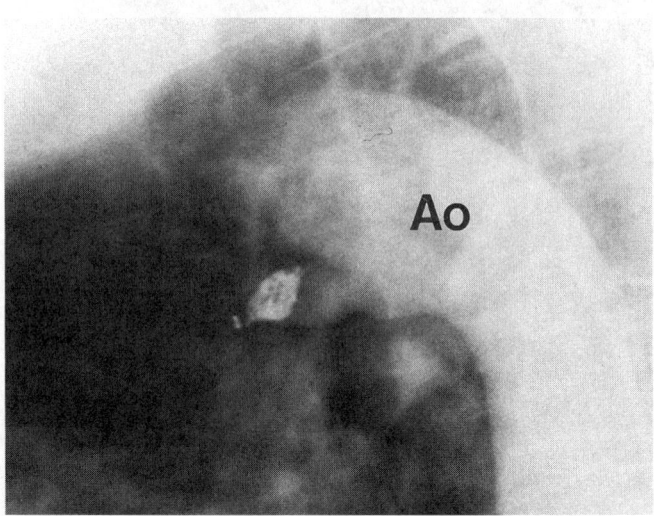

FIGURE 78.18. **A:** Aortography (*Ao*) in the lateral projection after coil closure of a patent ductus arteriosus. **B:** Aortography in the lateral view after closure of a patent ductus using a Gianturco–Griffka vascular occlusion coil bag.

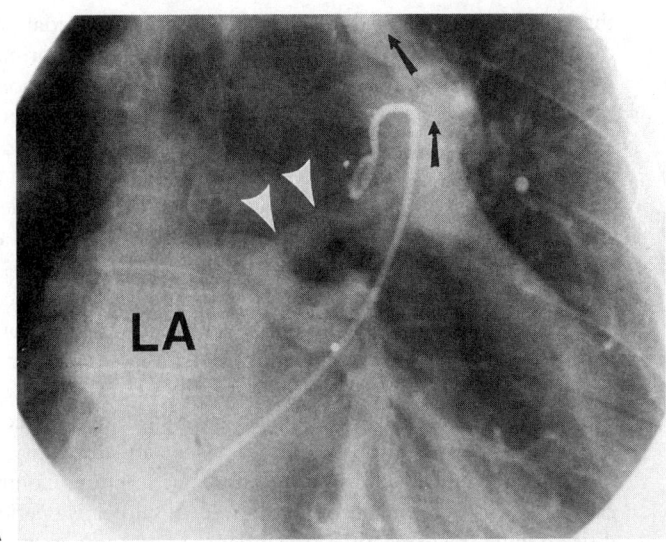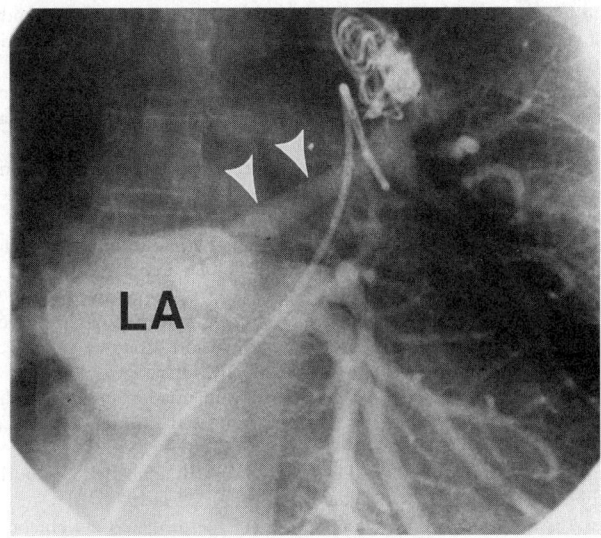

A   B

FIGURE 78.19. **A:** Levophase left pulmonary artery angiogram in the anteroposterior (*AP*) projection demonstrating anomalous pulmonary venous return of the left upper lung draining to the innominate vein (*black arrows*). Dual, normal drainage via a smaller pulmonary vein to the left atrium (*LA*) is also seen (*white arrowheads*). **B:** Levophase left pulmonary arteriogram in the AP projection demonstrating normal left upper lobe pulmonary venous drainage after coil closure of the anomalous pulmonary venous return. A coil matrix is seen, which was deployed to occlude the vertical vein draining the left upper lobe anomalously to the right side of the heart. Note the persistence of the normal left upper lobe pulmonary venous drainage (*white arrowheads*) to the left atrium.

vices, and most patients have been shown to have complete occlusion of the ASD and have had excellent clinical outcomes (Fig. 78.20). Some devices are used with a temporary period of anticoagulation with warfarin, whereas others are used with just aspirin.

In summation, percutaneous treatments for adults with congenital heart disease is in an exciting era of evolution. Improvements in catheterization techniques and new interventional devices have made selected forms of congenital heart defects treatable in the catheterization laboratory, in some cases postponing the need for surgery and in others eliminating the need for surgery altogether.

BIBLIOGRAPHY

Cohen M, Fuster V, Steele PM, et al. Coarctation of the aorta. Long term follow-up and prediction of outcome after surgical correction. *Circulation* 1989;80:840–845.

Das GS, Hijazi ZM, O'Laughlin MP, Mendelsohn AM. Initial results of the US PFO/ASD closure trial. *J Am Coll Cardiol* 1996;27;119A.

Driscoll DJ, Michels VV, Gersony WM, et al. Occurrence risk for congenital heart defects in relatives of patients with aortic stenosis, pulmonary stenosis, or ventricular septal defects. *Circulation* 1993;87(Suppl I):I-114.

Gersony WM, Hayes CJ, Driscoll DJ, et al. Second natural history study of congenital heart defects. Quality of life of patients with aortic stenosis, pulmonary stenosis, or ventricular septal defects. *Circulation* 1993; 87(Suppl I):I-52.

Graham TP. Ventricular performance in congenital heart disease. *Circulation* 1991;84:2259–2274.

Graham TP, Bricker JT, James FW, Strong WB. Task force 1: Congenital heart disease in 26th Bethesda Conference: recommendations for determining eligibility for competition in athletes with cardiovascular abnormalities. *J Am Coll Cardiol* 1994; 24:867–873.

Grifka RG, O'Laughlin MP, Nihill MR, Mullins CE. Double-transseptal, double balloon valvuloplasty for congenital mitral stenosis. *Circulation* 1992;85:123–129.

Kan JS, White RI Jr, Mitchell SE, et al. Percutaneous transluminal balloon valvuloplasty for pulmonary valve stenosis. *Circulation* 1984;69: 554–560.

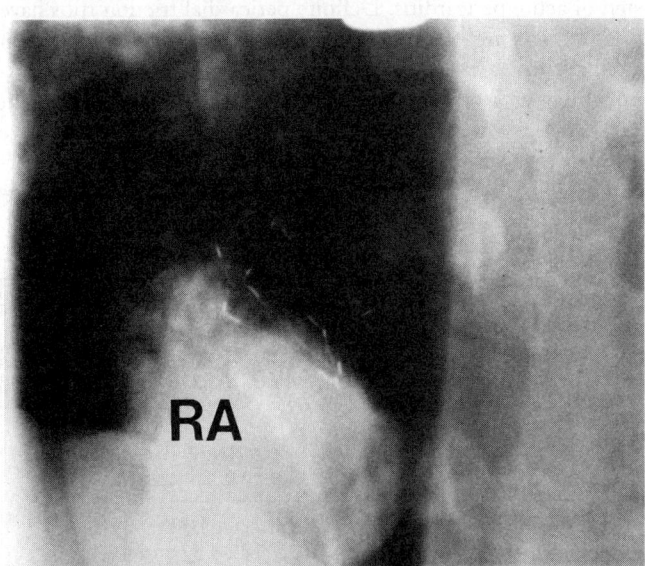

FIGURE 78.20. Right atrial angiogram in the left anterior oblique projection, with cranial angulation, following percutaneous closure of a secundum atrial septal defect using an Angel Wings device. The square wire framework, made of nitinol, is radiographically visible. Each nitinol frame supports a dacron square; the squares are sewn together in the center of the fabric.

Keane JF, Driscoll DJ, Gersony WM, et al. Second natural history study of congenital heart defects. Results of treatment of patients with aortic valvular stenosis. *Circulation* 1993;87(Suppl I):I-16.

Kidd L, Driscoll DJ, Gersony WM, et al. Second natural history study of congenital heart defects. Results of treatment of patients with ventricular septal defects. *Circulation* 1993;87(Suppl I):I-38.

Mullins CE, O'Laughlin MP. Vick GW III, et al. Implantation of balloon-expandable intravascular grafts by catheterization in pulmonary arteries and systemic veins. *Circulation* 1988;77:188–199.

Murphy JG, Gersh BJ, McGoon MD, et al. Long-term outcome after surgical repair of isolated atrial septal defect. Follow-up at 27 to 32 years. *N Engl J Med* 1990;323:1645–1650.

O'Connor BK, Beekman RH, Rocchini AP, et al. Intermediate-term effectiveness of balloon valvuloplasty for congenital aortic stenosis: a prospective follow-up study. *Circulation* 1991;84:732–738.

O'Laughlin MP, Slack MC, Grifka RG, et al. Implantation and intermediate-term follow-up of stents in congenital heart disease. *Circulation* 1993;88:605–614.

Perloff JK, Marelli AJ, Miner PD. Risk of stroke in adults with cyanotic congenital heart disease. *Circulation* 1993;87:1954–1959.

Prieto LR, Foreman CK, Cheatham JP, et al. Intermediate-term outcome of transcatheter secundumatrial septal defect closure using the Bard Clamshell septal umbrella. *Am J Cardiol* 1996;78:1310–1312.

Shah D, Ahzar M, Oakley CM, et al. Natural history of secundum atrial septal defect in adults after medical or surgical treatment: a historical prospective study. *Br Heart J* 1994;71:224–227.

Shim D, Fedderly RT, Beekman RH, et al. Follow-up of coil occlusion of patent ductus arteriosus. *J Am Coll Cardiol* 1996;28:207–211.

Kelley's Textbook of Internal Medicine, fourth edition. Edited by H. David Humes. Lippincott Williams & Wilkins, Philadelphia © 2000.

C H A P T E R

79

PERICARDIAL DISEASES

E. WILLIAM HANCOCK

The diseases that involve the pericardium have many causes, but the pathologic and clinical features of many types of pericardial disease are similar despite the diverse causes. These diseases represent the response of the pericardium to injury. There are three broad pericardial syndromes: acute pericarditis, pericardial effusion, and constrictive pericarditis.

ACUTE PERICARDITIS

ETIOLOGY

Most instances of acute pericarditis are of unknown origin and are assumed to be infections caused by unidentified viral agents. The attribution of idiopathic acute pericarditis to viral infection is based largely on the clinical similarity of idiopathic cases to

the many fewer cases of documented viral cause. Bacterial pericarditis, although relatively rare, occasionally occurs as a primary infection but is more often associated with sepsis, pneumonia, thoracic surgery, trauma, or suppression of a patient's immune responses.

Tuberculous pericarditis is common in many parts of the world and tends to become chronic and to cause tamponade or constriction of the heart. Many other mycobacterial, fungal, and parasitic agents also cause pericarditis.

Many cases of acute pericarditis are noninfective and occur in such conditions as postsurgery (postcardiotomy) syndrome, connective tissue disease, renal failure, radiation, administration of various drugs, or trauma. Many of the noninfective cases probably have a common mechanism related to the nonspecific reaction of the pericardium to injury. The inflammatory response may be mediated by an immunologic reaction. Complicating viral infection may also play a role. Noninfective pericarditis often has relatively little true inflammatory component but consists predominantly of deposits of fibrin on the visceral and parietal surfaces of the pericardium.

CLINICAL FINDINGS

Idiopathic or viral acute pericarditis is often preceded by a low-grade fever, sore throat, and muscular aches. Anterior chest pain, however, is usually the first and most characteristic symptom of the pericarditis itself. The chest pain of pericarditis is classically substernal and pleuritic. It is often sudden in onset and severe and can simulate the chest pain of acute myocardial infarction (MI). The pleuritic component is the most important feature that distinguishes pericardial pain from ischemic chest pain. Other distinguishing features are listed in Table 79.1.

The pericardial friction rub is the most distinctive physical sign of acute pericarditis. Definite pericardial friction rubs have both systolic and diastolic components, and the classic friction rub has three components. The systolic and early diastolic components give a to-and-fro character, and the third component in late diastole due to atrial contraction, adds a highly distinctive element that is virtually pathognomonic of pericarditis. Pericardial friction rubs are best heard with the diaphragm of the stetho-

TABLE 79.1.	DIFFERENCES BETWEEN THE CHARACTERISTIC CHEST PAIN OF ACUTE PERICARDITIS AND THAT OF ACUTE MYOCARDIAL INFARCTION

Acute Pericarditis	Acute Myocardial Infarction
Worse in inspiration	Not affected by breathing
Partially relieved by sitting up	Not affected by position
Radiation, if any, to left shoulder and back	Radiation to jaw, left arm
Not relieved by nitroglycerin	Often relieved by nitroglycerin

scope firmly applied, with the patient in the sitting position, and with breathing suspended in expiration.

LABORATORY FINDINGS

The characteristic abnormalities on electrocardiogram (ECG) in acute pericarditis are ST-segment elevation and PQ-segment depression (Fig. 79.1). These abnormalities reflect subepicardial inflammation of the ventricles and the atria, respectively. ST elevation due to acute pericarditis is usually generalized and present in multiple leads, with the exception of leads aVR and V_1. In some patients, leads III and aVL (when they are cavitary leads) also fail to show ST elevation. The ST-segment elevation of acute pericarditis differs from that of acute MI in its diffuse nature and the lack of reciprocal ST-segment depression in non-cavitary leads. It can be differentiated from the normal variant ST-segment elevation, often termed *early repolarization,* chiefly by the amplitude of the T waves, which tend to be taller compared with the degree of ST-segment elevation, and by absence of PQ segment depression in the normal variant pattern. Depression of the PQ segment is comparable to elevation of the ST segment in its sensitivity and specificity for acute pericarditis.

The serum levels of enzymes, such as creatine kinase, which are used in the diagnosis of acute MI usually remain normal during episodes of acute pericarditis. Moderate rises may occur, however, when a significant degree of myocarditis accompanies the pericarditis. Often, the erythrocyte sedimentation rate and the white blood cell count are elevated.

NATURAL HISTORY

Idiopathic or viral acute pericarditis is a self-limited syndrome in most cases, with a very low probability of permanent adverse effects. A few cases progress to subacute and chronic constrictive pericarditis; usually these patients had a subacute onset of pericarditis initially, were more severely ill during the active phase, and showed pericardial effusion and often pneumonitis and pleuritis with pleural effusion in addition to pericarditis.

A few patients follow a course of relapsing or recurrent acute pericarditis over months or years. The recurrent episodes are usually benign, although the symptoms are distressing. Cardiac tamponade and constrictive pericarditis are unlikely to develop even after numerous relapses of acute pericarditis. These patients are more likely to require treatment with adrenal corticosteroids, which often prevents relapses but also results in hyperadrenocorticism and a liability to corticosteroid withdrawal symptoms.

OPTIMAL MANAGEMENT

The initial diagnostic studies in patients with a clear clinical presentation of acute pericarditis should focus primarily on ruling out a bacterial infection. Cultures of the blood and other sites are indicated when the degree of fever and leukocytosis and the severity of the clinical illness suggest purulent pericarditis as a reasonable possibility. Studies for viral infection are usually not indicated, because the yield is low and the results are usually not useful in management. The tuberculin skin test is usually indicated. When cardiac tamponade is absent, pericardiocentesis done purely for diagnostic studies on the fluid is not indicated unless strong clues point to an infective or neoplastic cause.

After the initial workup, it is usually wise to perform screening tests for rheumatic diseases, such as assays for the rheumatoid factor and the fluorescent antinuclear antibody. A plain chest radiograph usually provides clues to the diagnosis of lung cancer, the most common cause of neoplastic disease presenting as apparently primary pericardial disease.

Treatment of nonspecific acute pericarditis is directed primarily at short-term relief of symptoms. After initial relief of the severe pain with analgesics such as codeine or morphine, it is usually best to prescribe aspirin as an analgesic and anti-inflammatory agent, in doses of 4 to 6 g per day for at least 1 week. Other nonsteroidal anti-inflammatory drugs are more expensive and not necessarily superior to aspirin for the treatment of acute pericarditis. Adrenal corticosteroids, such as prednisone in doses of 60 mg per day rapidly tapering and discontinued after 1 to 2 weeks, are more effective than aspirin and are

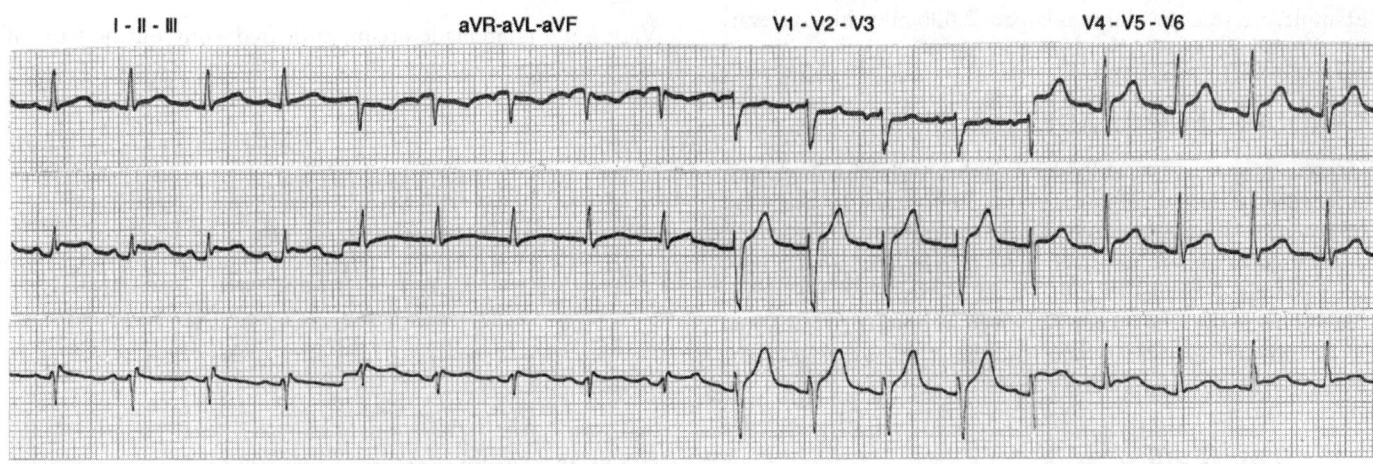

FIGURE 79.1. Electrocardiogram in a patient with acute pericarditis. ST-segment elevation and PQ-segment depression are seen in many leads. The T wave is low compared with the level of ST-segment elevation.

sometimes indicated in severe cases of acute pericarditis. However, corticosteroids should be avoided, if possible, because of the difficulty in withdrawing them later.

The best solution to the problem of corticosteroid dependency is a very gradual tapering of the corticosteroid dose, over as long as 6 to 12 months, accompanied by the use of nonsteroidal anti-inflammatory drugs and other supportive therapy. Colchicine, 1 mg per day given for at least 1 year, is helpful in preventing episodes of recurrent pericarditis in some patients.

▣ PERICARDIAL EFFUSION

The pericardial space normally contains 20 to 30 mL of fluid that is a transudate of plasma. Pericardial effusion is an abnormal increase in the amount of such fluid and may be either a transudate or an exudate. The fluid is often bloody or is virtually equivalent to whole blood, as in trauma, rupture of acute MI, or coagulation defects. Special forms of pericardial effusion occur rarely. One such form is chylous effusion resulting from communication of the thoracic duct with the pericardial space. Another is cholesterol effusion, a form of chronic pericardial effusion in which lipoproteins have become gradually concentrated, probably because of their slower reabsorption.

Pericardial effusion often occurs as a part of a general increase in extracellular fluid volume, as in congestive heart failure and nephrotic syndrome. It also occurs as a feature of virtually any form of pericardial disease; in many of these instances, the pericardial effusion is the essential presenting feature.

The clinical importance of pericardial effusion is primarily related to the degree of compression of the heart that it may produce. The pressure in the pericardial space normally equals the intrapleural pressure, being about equal to the atmospheric pressure but becoming negative with inspiration. When a pericardial effusion develops rapidly, as in traumatic hemopericardium, the pericardium has very little elasticity and the pressure in the pericardial space rises steeply with as little as 200 mL of fluid. The layers of collagen that largely make up the parietal pericardium are wavy, however, and can stretch over time. Thus, a slowly developing pericardial effusion, as in myxedema, for example, can reach a volume as large as 2,000 mL without elevating the intrapericardial fluid pressure significantly.

CARDIAC TAMPONADE

Cardiac tamponade is caused by an abnormally increased pressure within a pericardial effusion that compresses the heart and impedes its filling in diastole. The term "tamponade" is sometimes used in a more restricted sense to refer to a condition of "compromised circulation," that is, hypotension or diminished blood flow to the vital organs. Such a condition is better referred to as *decompensated tamponade*, because it represents only the most severe stage of a graded process.

PATHOGENESIS

As pericardial fluid accumulates, the intrapericardial pressure begins to rise and soon approaches the level of the central venous pressure. From this point, the two pressures rise together, so that in cardiac tamponade of even moderate degree, the central venous pressure (and the jugular venous pressure) can be taken as a close approximation of the intrapericardial pressure. As the intrapericardial pressure rises still further, the right-sided cardiac chambers are compressed. Reduction in volume of the left-sided chambers follows, initially because of reduced output of the right side of the heart secondary to compression, and later as a result of compression of the left-sided chambers. In severe tamponade, all the cardiac chambers are reduced (50% or more) in volume.

Reduction of cardiac filling is followed by reduction in stroke volume. Cardiac output is maintained by tachycardia initially, but becomes reduced later. Arterial pressure is maintained by vasoconstriction in early phases, but it also falls in later stages.

Cardiac tamponade alters the phasic pattern of venous return to the heart during the cardiac cycle. Venous return occurs mainly during systole, when the heart is smallest and least compressed. However, the compression of the heart that exists throughout the cardiac cycle reduces or eliminates the surge of rapid filling in early diastole that occurs both normally and in constrictive pericarditis. This is reflected in the waveform of the venous pulse, which in cardiac tamponade is characterized by a prominent systolic (x) descent and by absence of the normal (y) descent in early diastole. Venous pressure usually varies only slightly with respiration. Kussmaul's sign (increased venous pressure in inspiration) is seen in some cases of constrictive pericarditis but does not occur in uncomplicated cardiac tamponade.

Paradoxical pulse (an abnormal fall in arterial systolic pressure with inspiration) is characteristic of cardiac tamponade (Fig. 79.2). Paradoxical pulse results from an interplay of several factors, including the depth of intrathoracic pressure excursions with breathing. The principal factor, however, is the increased degree of interdependence of the volume of the right and left ventricles. Because both are contained within a relatively fixed overall volume imposed by the tense pericardial effusion, the increase in right ventricular volume with inspiration is accompanied by a greater than normal reduction in the volume of the left ventricle.

CLINICAL FINDINGS

Very acute tamponade occurs most frequently on the basis of acute hemopericardium, caused by such conditions as closed

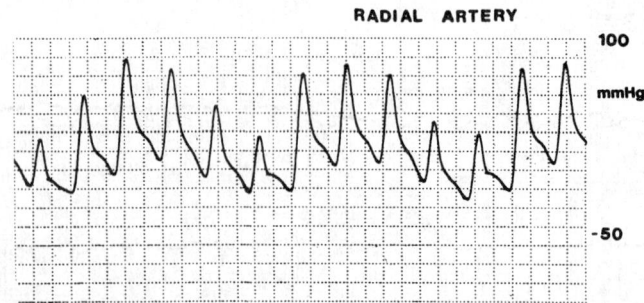

RADIAL ARTERY

FIGURE 79.2. Radial artery pressure recording showing a paradoxical pulse. The systolic pressure falls by 15 to 20 mm Hg with inspiration. The diastolic pressure varies less. The fall in pulse pressure with inspiration reflects a fall in stroke volume.

chest or penetrating trauma, complications of cardiac catheterization, postoperative hemorrhage in cardiac surgical patients, acute dissection of the ascending aorta, or rupture of the heart in acute MI. Sudden hypotension is the hallmark of these cases. Paradoxical pulse is expected but may be undetected because of difficulty in obtaining the blood pressure. Venous pressure elevation is also expected but is often difficult to detect because the relative depletion of intravascular volume is accompanied by constriction of the superficial veins.

Patients with cardiac tamponade associated with medical conditions, such as idiopathic or infective pericarditis, neoplasm, renal failure, or rheumatic diseases, usually present in a less acute manner. The principal symptom is dyspnea, which occurs despite clear lungs. Pleural effusion is often associated and contributes to the dyspnea. Pericardial pain is often absent, and peripheral edema is frequently absent. Jugular venous pressure is nearly always elevated, however, and this is often the key finding in suggesting the diagnosis. The external jugular veins may not be visibly distended because of venoconstriction, but the internal jugular pulsations are seen above the level of the clavicle in the sitting position, usually up to the angle of the jaw.

The other key finding is the paradoxical pulse, which should be sought first by simple palpation and then assessed with the sphygmomanometer. A respiratory variation of 10 mm Hg is a convenient dividing line between normal and abnormal respiratory variation in arterial systolic pressure. Direct arterial pressure recordings are likely to show more variation, usually 15 mm Hg or more in clear instances of cardiac tamponade.

LABORATORY FINDINGS

The ECG in cardiac tamponade often shows low amplitude of the complexes, but this reflects the insulating or short-circuiting effect of the pericardial effusion rather than tamponade itself. Beat-to-beat alternation in the amplitude of the QRS complexes (electrical alternans) occurs in a few cases of cardiac tamponade and is a relatively specific sign. Electrical alternans in pericardial effusion essentially reflects a beat-to-beat change in QRS axis, because the heart swings from one position to another within the pericardial space on successive heartbeats. It is particularly characteristic of neoplastic pericardial effusion, probably because neoplastic effusions are often large effusions with serous fluid and free of adhesions within the pericardial space.

Chest radiographs are expected to show enlargement of the cardiomediastinal silhouette in subacute or chronic pericardial effusion with tamponade, although in very acute cases this may not be evident. The contour of the cardiomediastinal silhouette in pericardial effusion is not sufficiently distinctive for this to be reliable in diagnosis. The plain film may show lucencies, known as *pericardial fat lines*, caused by pericardial fluid adjacent to the epicardial fat, as a sign of pericardial effusion.

Echocardiography is the most valuable diagnostic procedure for the detection of pericardial effusion, demonstrating an echo-free space around the heart (Fig. 79.3; see also Chapter 85). Pericardial effusion can also be demonstrated by other imaging techniques, such as computed tomography (CT) of the chest, magnetic resonance imaging (MRI), radionuclide scans, and contrast angiography, but these methods are more expensive and less convenient than echocardiography. Echocardiographic signs that suggest tamponade include a reduction in the diameter of the right ventricle, an abnormal degree of inward movement (collapse) of the free wall of the right atrium and right ventricle in early diastole, and an abnormal fullness of the inferior vena cava. Echocardiography also shows the exaggerated phasic changes in volume of the right and left ventricle with respiration and Doppler recordings of mitral and tricuspid flow velocity that are related to paradoxical pulse.

OPTIMAL MANAGEMENT

Although the circulation may be supported temporarily by infusion of fluid, with cautious use of dopamine or isoproterenol, the only consistently effective treatment for cardiac tamponade is to remove the pericardial fluid. Removal of the pericardial

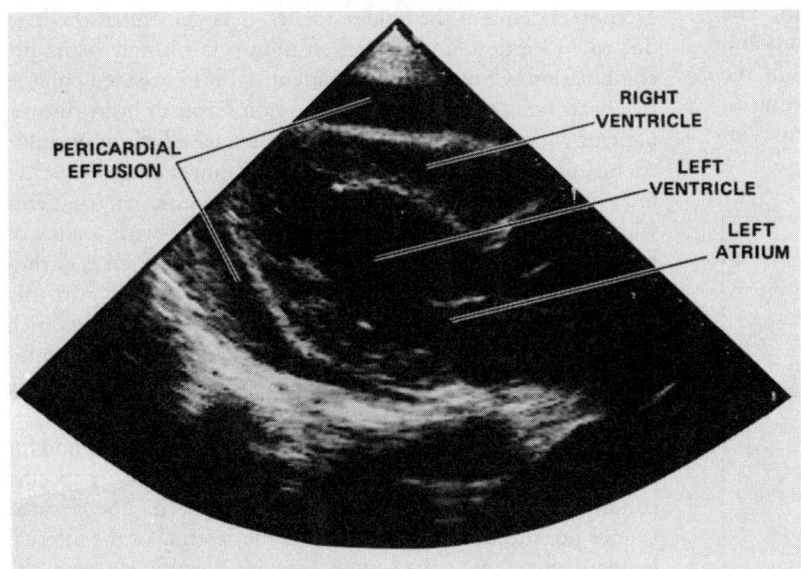

FIGURE 79.3. Two-dimensional echocardiogram showing pericardial effusion in a long-axis parasternal view. A prominent echo-free space is present both anterior to the right ventricle and posterior to the left ventricle. There is little fluid posterior to the left atrium because the space is limited by the attachments of the pulmonary veins.

fluid is indicated if the patient has symptoms or has reduction of arterial pressure, elevation of venous pressure to more than about 10 mm Hg, or a prominent paradoxical pulse. Pericardial fluid can be removed either by needle pericardiocentesis or by one of several surgical procedures. Surgical drainage is more certain to be effective and also provides a biopsy of the pericardium. Pericardiocentesis is less traumatic and is a superior method when physiologic assessment is an important objective of the procedure. Needle pericardiocentesis can be supplemented by balloon pericardiostomy in patients who have recurrent tamponade.

When compression of the heart is due solely to fluid under increased pressure, removal of the fluid leads to an immediate fall in venous pressure, a rise in arterial pressure and cardiac output, and near elimination of the paradoxical pulse. The central venous pressure may remain mildly elevated for 12 to 24 hours until a diuresis allows it to fall further. Occasionally, there is a constricting peel of tissue on the epicardial surface in addition to the pericardial effusion (effusive–constrictive pericarditis). In this case, the central venous pressure remains markedly elevated despite removal of the fluid, and a visceral pericardiectomy is required.

Localized cardiac tamponade occurs occasionally, usually in patients who are recovering from cardiac surgery. Fluid collects in a loculated area and compresses only a portion of the heart. The most common form of localized tamponade is caused by an anterior mediastinal hematoma that compresses the right atrium, simulating superior vena caval obstruction. A loculated pericardial effusion also may compress the left atrium selectively, causing pulmonary edema. Localized tamponade usually requires surgical exploration, both to confirm the diagnosis and to evacuate the fluid.

■ CONSTRICTIVE PERICARDITIS

DEFINITION AND ETIOLOGY

In constrictive pericarditis the heart is compressed, or filling of the heart is limited, by solid tissue surrounding the heart. The solid tissue is usually scar tissue, but malignant solid tumors and organizing blood clot also can constrict the heart. Any of the causes of pericardial disease can produce sufficient scarring to result in constrictive pericarditis (Table 79.2). Most cases in

developed countries are now idiopathic, rather than tuberculous, which was thought to be the most common cause in the past. Previous radiation therapy and cardiac surgery also have become common causes of constrictive pericarditis in the developed countries.

PATHOGENESIS

Because constriction is a subacute or chronic condition, the arterial pressure and cardiac output are usually well maintained by the compensatory control mechanisms of the circulation. Constrictive pericarditis acts more like a rigid shell around the heart than like a continuously imposed positive pressure on the heart. The heart is relatively little compressed at the beginning of diastole when its volume may be less than the volume of the rigid shell; therefore, the early diastolic inflow into the ventricles is not impeded. Filling becomes limited shortly into diastole when the volume of the heart reaches a critical level. Thus, the atrioventricular flow patterns and the associated pressure waveforms are different in constriction than in tamponade. Patients with constrictive pericarditis have a steep early diastolic descent in the venous pressure waveform, followed by a steep rise to a plateau level through the remainder of diastole. The ventricular pressure waveform shows the steep rise particularly well, with a dip-plateau or "square-root" waveform (Fig. 79.4).

Constrictive pericarditis is not always like a rigid shell; it may be more elastic, with a hemodynamic pattern more like that of cardiac tamponade. There is a spectrum of cases between the rigid and elastic forms of constriction; the venous pressure waveform in many of them shows both prominent systolic and diastolic descents, assuming a W or M waveform. In occult constriction of the heart, the elevated filling pressures and abnormal pressure waveforms are seen only after additional intravascular volume has been infused.

CLINICAL FINDINGS

Patients with constrictive pericarditis usually have at least a mild degree of shortness of breath and impaired capacity for physical exertion. Edema of the ankles, ascites, enlargement of the liver due to congestion, and pleural effusion occur, singly or in any combination. Compared with patients with right-sided congestive heart failure caused by the common forms of heart disease, patients with constrictive pericarditis often have little or no ankle edema, probably because they are often younger and have better preserved skin and venous valves in the legs. Thus, many patients with constrictive pericarditis present primarily with ascites or hepatomegaly and are thought to have conditions such as cirrhosis of the liver or abdominal neoplasm. Others present primarily with pleural effusion and are thought to have conditions such as lung cancer or tuberculosis. The key to the differential diagnosis is to recognize the elevated jugular venous pressure during the physical examination.

Elevated jugular venous pressure is virtually a sine qua non for the diagnosis of constrictive pericarditis, unless there are specific conditions that prevent it from being recognized. The elevated venous pressure may be seen in either the external or the internal jugular veins. Unless the venous pressure is extremely high, the

TABLE 79.2.	CONSTRICTIVE PERICARDITIS	
Common Causes		**Rare Causes**
Idiopathic		Bacterial infection
Radiation therapy (in developed countries)		Rheumatic diseases
		Uremia/dialysis
Cardiac surgery (in developed countries)		Neoplasm
		Trauma
Tuberculosis (in less developed countries)		Myocardial infarction

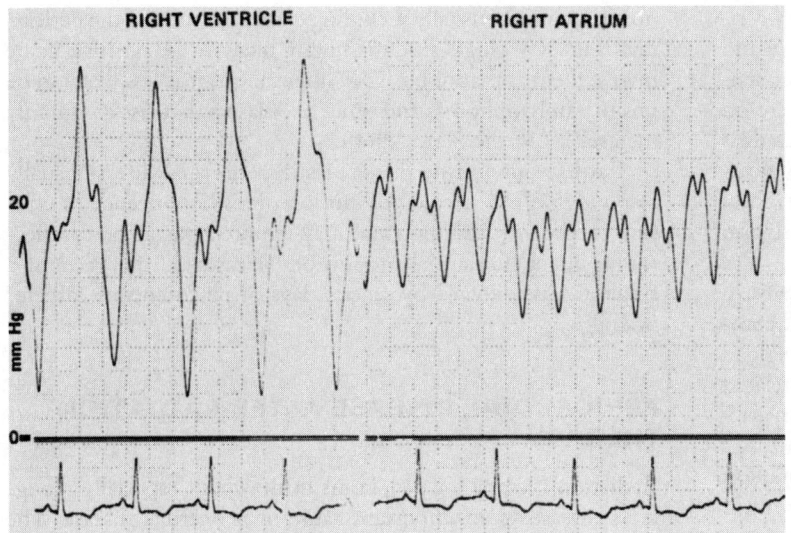

FIGURE 79.4. Pressure recordings in the right ventricle and right atrium in a patient with chronic constrictive pericarditis. Right ventricular pressure falls to a normal nadir in initial diastole but rises quickly to an elevated level for the remainder of diastole, producing a dip–plateau waveform ("square root" sign). Systolic (*x*) and diastolic (*y*) dips are both prominent in the right atrial pressure waveform (*M* or *W* waveform).

venous pulsation is also characteristic, showing a prominent brief dip in early diastole.

The cardiac impulse in constrictive pericarditis sometimes shows a retraction in systole and a prominent outward movement in early diastole. The latter is conspicuous enough in some patients to merit the term *diastolic heartbeat.* There is also an abnormal extra heart sound in early diastole, sometimes termed the *pericardial knock.* The sound is intermediate in both timing and character between a mitral opening snap and a typical third heart sound. Paradoxical pulse is not prominent in most patients with constrictive pericarditis.

LABORATORY FINDINGS

The ECG in patients with constrictive pericarditis is usually abnormal but not distinctive. Atrial fibrillation occurs frequently in long-standing cases, whereas those that are in sinus rhythm often show notched P waves with low amplitude, suggesting disease of the atrial myocardium. Most patients show mild nonspecific abnormalities of the T waves. QRS voltage is often relatively low.

The chest radiograph usually shows normal heart size and clear lungs, with little evidence of redistribution of pulmonary blood flow, in keeping with the level of pulmonary venous pressure, which is usually less than 20 mm Hg even in relatively severe cases. Calcification of the pericardium is seen in a few cases.

Echocardiographic images most often show that the size of the cardiac chambers, the systolic wall motion, and ventricular wall thickness all are normal. The ventricular septum usually shows an abnormal jerky motion in diastole. The pericardium usually appears thickened, but the limited resolution of echocardiography (about 1 mm) makes this a nonspecific finding. However, Doppler studies of the mitral and tricuspid flow velocities, as they vary with respiration, show distinctive exaggerations and are helpful in distinguishing constrictive pericarditis from restrictive cardiomyopathy.

CT and MRI have better resolution than echocardiography and provide more accurate assessment of the thickness of the pericardium. A normal thickness of the pericardium by MRI or CT gives substantial, although not complete, assurance that constriction is not present.

Cardiac catheterization is usually indicated when constrictive pericarditis is diagnosed, both to support the diagnosis and to indicate the severity of the constriction. The classic hemodynamic picture consists of diastolic pressures elevated to the same level in all chambers of the heart, with dip–plateau pressure waveforms in the right ventricle (Fig. 79.3).

Some patients with congestive heart failure, particularly those with amyloidosis or idiopathic restrictive cardiomyopathy, may have findings by cardiac catheterization and angiography that closely simulate those of constrictive pericarditis. Occasionally, a myocardial biopsy or even an exploratory thoracotomy is required for proof.

OPTIMAL MANAGEMENT

Surgical pericardiectomy is usually the only effective treatment and is indicated if the venous pressure is substantially elevated or if significant symptoms are attributable to the constriction. Pericardiectomy for constriction is essentially curative in most uncomplicated cases. However, it is often a difficult operation, with an operative morality risk that is higher than that associated with coronary artery bypass surgery, for example. Constrictive pericarditis is occasionally spontaneously reversible when it develops in the wake of acute pericarditis. In other instances, constriction may be recognizable but may follow a clinically mild course, with the fluid retention controlled by diuretics alone, so that surgery may not be required.

■ SPECIFIC FORMS OF PERICARDIAL DISEASE

UREMIA/DIALYSIS

Pericarditis occurs in advanced renal failure, usually in the form of pericardial effusion with fibrinous deposits on the pericardial surfaces. Tamponade occurs rarely, but with no dialysis the pericarditis reflects an advanced stage of the uremic syndrome and a survival limited to weeks or months. A more important syndrome is the occurrence of pericarditis in patients who are on chronic maintenance dialysis. The genesis of dialysis pericarditis is unknown, because it occurs despite adequate dialysis. Pericardial effusion is usually the predominant manifestation, but chest pain, friction rub, and ECG indications of acute pericarditis also occur frequently.

Cardiac tamponade is difficult to recognize specifically in patients who are on dialysis, because of the hypertension, coronary artery disease, left ventricular failure, and fluid overload that are often associated. Tamponade caused by dialysis-related pericardial effusion often presents as an unexpected drop in arterial pressure during dialysis sessions.

Chest pain and other symptoms of pericardial inflammation may be treated symptomatically, as in idiopathic pericarditis. Corticosteroids may be used in severe cases, and some favor the instillation of triamcinolone, a nonabsorbable corticosteroid, into the pericardial space. Hemodynamic abnormalities severe enough to require intervention are best managed by pericardiocentesis or subxiphoid pericardiostomy, since recurrent tamponade is unusual and progression to constriction is rare.

RHEUMATIC DISEASES

Pericardial involvement in patients with rheumatoid arthritis usually occurs in association with other extra-articular involvement and with a positive serologic test for the rheumatoid factor. The effusive–constrictive pericarditis syndrome is particularly likely to develop in patients with rheumatoid arthritis. Pericarditis occurs eventually in most patients with long-standing systemic lupus erythematosus. It often develops during flare-ups as the syndrome of acute pericarditis. Corticosteroid therapy is more likely to be used in pericardial disease associated with rheumatic diseases than in other forms, but this is because of the indications for corticosteroids in controlling the basic disease process.

NEOPLASM

Neoplasms account for about 50% of the cases of cardiac tamponade among medical patients. Carcinomas of the breast and lung are the most common sources. Neoplastic pericardial disease is prone to cause large pericardial effusions, often with relatively little solid tumor involvement of the pericardium. The neoplasm often spreads from the mediastinal lymph nodes to the heart by way of the lymphatics, and lymphatic obstruction is probably a frequent contributing factor to the effusion.

In general, neoplastic pericardial effusion represents advanced cancer with a short life expectancy, a fact that tends to dictate a conservative approach. Patients with breast cancer that involves the pericardium, however, usually respond to chemotherapy and have a substantial period of survival. Also, pericardial effusion in a patient with neoplasm is not necessarily neoplastic; it may be due to previous radiation therapy, and there is also an increased incidence of idiopathic nonneoplastic pericardial effusion in patients with neoplasms. This tends to dictate an aggressive diagnostic approach, usually including cytologic study of the pericardial fluid. Cytologic study is highly likely to be positive if the involvement is that of breast or lung cancer; it is less likely to be positive in lymphomas and other neoplasms that less commonly metastasize to the pericardium.

Cardiac tamponade in neoplastic pericardial disease usually responds well to needle pericardiocentesis. Recurrence of effusion is relatively common and may require a partial pericardiectomy, but a substantial proportion of cases do not recur if a single tap is followed by several days of percutaneous catheter drainage.

PERICARDIAL DISEASE AFTER RADIATION THERAPY

Radiation therapy for neoplasms in the chest, especially Hodgkin's disease, is an important cause of pericardial disease. The pericardial disease can present as acute or subacute pericarditis, and the onset is months or years, sometimes many years, after the radiation therapy has been completed.

Pericardial disease is usually the most important aspect of the cardiac complications of irradiation, but myocardial fibrosis, coronary artery disease, conduction system disease, and valvular disease also occur in varying combinations in many patients. The differential diagnosis always includes recurrent neoplasm. In addition, radiation disease of the lungs and pleura is often associated and contributes to a complex clinical picture.

Pericardiectomy for radiation-related constrictive pericarditis should only be undertaken for strong indications, because of the added operative risk and often limited long-term results.

TUBERCULOUS PERICARDITIS

Infection of the pericardium by the tubercle bacillus is usually hematogenous and is not necessarily associated with active pulmonary tuberculosis. It may present as acute pericarditis but is more likely to have a subacute course with pericardial effusion. In the developed Western countries, where tuberculous pericarditis has become rare, a negative tuberculin skin test is usually sufficient to effectively exclude this diagnosis. Achieving a positive diagnosis is difficult, because the pericardial fluid is often negative for tubercle bacilli, both on smear and culture. Biopsy of the pericardium gives a higher proportion of positive results.

Antituberculous chemotherapy is often not sufficient to prevent tamponade or constriction in those with active tuberculous pericarditis. Pericardiocentesis is indicated when there is evidence of tamponade, and pericardiectomy is indicated when substantial constriction is demonstrated, regardless of the duration of chemotherapy .

PURULENT PERICARDITIS

Bacterial (purulent) pericarditis usually requires both antibiotic therapy and surgical drainage for a successful outcome. However, purulent pericarditis is likely to progress to constriction within a short time, even when a needle pericardiocentesis or a subxiphoid pericardiostomy has been done. Therefore, a limited pericardial resection is usually indicated at the time the diagnosis is established. Selected cases, particularly those with relatively thin serous effusions, may be managed by antibiotics and catheter drainage alone.

PERICARDIAL DISEASE IN PATIENTS WITH AIDS

Pericardial disease occurs in about 20% of patients with AIDS, and about 25% of these have large pericardial effusions with cardiac tamponade. Many are idiopathic (apparently caused by the HIV itself), but about 50% are caused by bacterial or mycobacterial infection and about 10% by neoplasms such as lymphoma or Kaposi's sarcoma.

POSTCARDIOTOMY SYNDROME

The postcardiotomy syndrome is a syndrome of acute pericarditis that often occurs after cardiac surgery. The mechanism may involve a hypersensitivity reaction to blood, to products of damaged myocardium, to foreign material introduced at the time of surgery, or to viral infection. Pericardial effusion is common and tamponade occurs occasionally. The constrictive pericarditis that occurs after cardiac surgery is probably a late complication of the postcardiotomy syndrome.

PERICARDITIS AFTER MYOCARDIAL INFARCTION

Two types of pericarditis occur after MI. Both are characterized by the syndrome of acute pericarditis, often with some pericardial effusion and rarely with tamponade or constriction. The early form is a direct result of the acute myocardial necrosis and is particularly characteristic of large infarctions. It is seen less often than in the past, probably as a result of the beneficial effect of therapeutic reopening of the infarct-related artery in the early stage of acute MI. The late form of pericarditis after MI, occurring 1 to 2 weeks or more after the acute infarction, is known as *Dressler's syndrome.* It is clinically similar to the postcardiotomy syndrome and probably has a similar pathologic mechanism.

CONGENITAL ABSENCE OF THE PERICARDIUM

Congenital absence of the pericardium occurs occasionally, usually with absence of the left pericardium and rarely a total absence. The condition is generally unimportant, but it may be discovered in chest radiographs because the absence of the pericardium causes unusual prominence of the radiographic shadows of the structures along the left border of the heart shadow, especially the main pulmonary artery. Rarely symptoms and even death result from strangulated herniation of portions of the heart through a partial defect in the pericardium.

PERICARDIAL CYSTS

Pericardial cysts usually present as asymptomatic masses near the right or left pericardiophrenic angle in the chest radiograph. Most are probably congenital. If the differential diagnosis can be resolved noninvasively, surgery is not required.

BIBLIOGRAPHY

Adler Y, Finkelstein Y, Guindo J, et al. Colchicine treatment for recurrent pericarditis. A decade of experience. *Circulation* 1998;97:2183–2185.

Boonyaratavej S, Oh JK, Tajik AJ, et al. Comparison of mitral inflow and superior vena cava Doppler velocities in chronic obstructive pulmonary disease and constrictive pericarditis. *J Am Coll Cardiol* 1998;32:2043–2048.

Correale E, Maggioni AP, Romano S, et al. Pericardial involvement in acute myocardial infarction in the post-thrombolytic era: clinical meaning and value. *Clin Cardiol* 1997;20:327–331.

Dardas P, Tsikaderis D, Ioannides E, et al. Constrictive pericarditis after coronary artery bypass surgery as a cause of unexplained dyspnea: a report of five cases. *Clin Cardiol* 1998;21:691–694.

Estok L, Wallach F. Cardiac tamponade in a patient with AIDS: a review of pericardial disease in patients with HIV infection. *Mt Sinai J Med* 1998;65:33–39.

Guardi LN, Ginsburg RJ, Burt ME. Pericardiocentesis and intrapericardial sclerosis: effective therapy for malignant pericardial effusions. *Ann Thorac Surg* 1997;64:1422–1427.

Merce J, Sagrista-Sauleda J, Permanyer-Miralda G, Soler-Soler J. Should pericardial drainage be performed routinely in patients who have a large pericardial effusion without tamponade? *Am J Med* 1998;105:106–109.

Nataf P, Cacomb P, Regan M, et al. Video-thoracoscopic pericardial window in the diagnosis and treatment of pericardial effusions. *Am J Cardiol* 1998;82:124–126.

Spodick DH. *The pericardium. A comprehensive textbook.* New York: Marcel Dekker, 1997.

Strang JI. Tuberculous pericarditis. *J Infect* 1997;35:215–219.

Kelley's Textbook of Internal Medicine, fourth edition. Edited by H. David Humes. Lippincott Williams & Wilkins, Philadelphia © 2000.

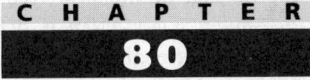

C H A P T E R

80

PULMONARY HYPERTENSION AND COR PULMONALE

LEWIS J. RUBIN

NORMAL PULMONARY CIRCULATION

The pulmonary circulation is normally a high-flow, low-resistance circuit that is capable of accommodating the entire right ventricular output at a pressure that is one-fifth of the level in the systemic circulation. In contrast to the pressure-generator pumping properties of the left ventricle, the thin-walled right ventricle functions primarily as a flow-generator pump. Accordingly, the right ventricle is particularly sensitive to increases in its afterload.

The pulmonary vascular bed has a remarkable capacity to regulate its vascular tone and recruit unused vessels to adapt to physiologic changes. For example, the fourfold or greater increases in cardiac output that occur during maximal exercise are accepted by the normal pulmonary circulation with a minimal increase in pulmonary artery pressure. Similarly, regional decreases in alveolar ventilation and oxygen tension are associated with local vasoconstriction, which redistributes blood flow to adequately ventilated lung units to optimize ventilation–perfusion relations. This phenomenon, known as *hypoxic pulmonary vasoconstriction,* depends on the alveolar and to a lesser degree on the mixed venous oxygen tensions and is potentiated by hypercarbia and acidosis.

The initial phase of the hypoxic pressor response results from inhibition of pulmonary vascular smooth muscle K^+ channel conductance, leading to cellular depolarization and an influx of Ca^{2+} ions through voltage-gated calcium channels. Prolonged or intense pulmonary vasoconstriction leads to a remodeling of the pulmonary circulation, which includes a loss of distal vasculature, extension of smooth muscle into small, nonmuscularized pulmonary arterioles, intimal fibrosis, and, eventually, more severe degrees of vascular obstruction and obliteration. This process, possibly mediated by vascular growth factors, may be responsible for the progression of pulmonary hypertension in chronic hypoxic lung diseases and primary pulmonary hypertension. Evidence suggests that endothelium-derived substances may play an important modulating role in the responses of pulmonary vascular smooth muscle to hypoxia. In conditions such as chronic pulmonary thromboembolism, obstruction of a large component of the vascular surface area is the primary cause of the increased pulmonary artery pressure.

DEFINITIONS

The pressures in the normal pulmonary circulation are shown in Figure 80.1. *Pulmonary hypertension* is defined as a mean pulmonary artery pressure exceeding 25 mm Hg at rest or 30 mm Hg during exercise. Although the term *cor pulmonale* is often equated with overt right-sided heart failure, it is best defined as pulmonary hypertension in the setting of chronic respiratory disease. Right-sided heart failure is a late manifestation of chronic pulmonary hypertension, and its presence should not be required to entertain the diagnosis of cor pulmonale.

TABLE 80.1.	CLASSIFICATION OF PULMONARY HYPERTENSION BASED ON SITE OF PRIMARY INJURY

Postcapillary

Left ventricular failure
Mitral valve disease
Aortic valve disease
Left atrial myxoma or thrombus
Pulmonary venoocclusive disease

Precapillary

Respiratory disorders
   Parenchymal lung disease (obstructive, restrictive, or mixed)
   Restrictive chest wall diseases
   Sleep apnea and hypoventilation syndromes
   High altitude disease
Occlusive pulmonary vascular disease (tumor, air, amniotic fluid, intravenously injected foreign material, schistosomiasis)
Congenital heart disease
   Intracardiac septal defects
   Peripheral pulmonic stenosis
Pulmonary vasculitis
Primary pulmonary hypertension

ETIOLOGY

The causes of pulmonary hypertension can be categorized according to the primary circulatory site of the pathophysiologic insult (Table 80.1). Postcapillary pulmonary hypertension is caused by obstruction of pulmonary venous return, which secondarily produces an increase in precapillary vascular pressure. Precapillary pulmonary hypertension is caused by constriction, obstruction, or obliteration of a substantial component of the pulmonary arterial tree. Although all conditions associated with precapillary pulmonary hypertension share similar hemodynamic profiles, the pathogenesis should be determined, and the approach to therapy should be individualized according to the cause.

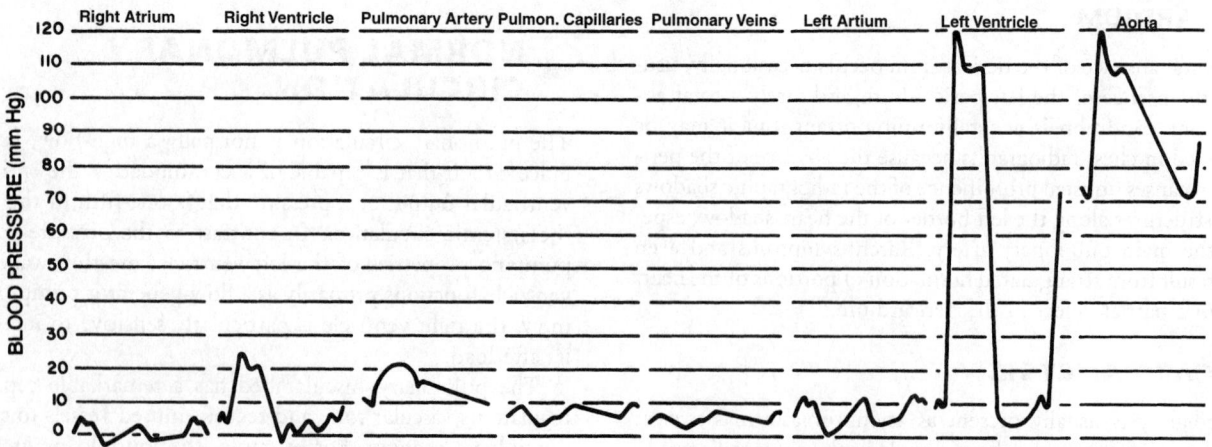

FIGURE 80.1. Pressures in the normal pulmonary circulation contrasted to those in the systemic circulation.

DISTURBANCES OF VENTILATION AND GAS EXCHANGE

The presence and severity of pulmonary hypertension in the setting of chronic respiratory diseases correlate with parameters indicating the degree of impairment in ventilation or gas exchange. For example, the lower the forced expiratory volume in 1 second (FEV_1) in patients with chronic obstructive pulmonary disease, the greater is the likelihood of pulmonary hypertension, particularly when the FEV_1 falls below 1 L. In patients with restrictive lung disease, a vital capacity below 50% of predicted has been correlated with elevations in pulmonary artery pressure.

The strongest correlations have been found with the degree of arterial hypoxemia. Patients with a Pao_2 value less than 55 mm Hg are likely to have pulmonary hypertension, and acidosis or hypercarbia may further contribute to this process.

PULMONARY THROMBOEMBOLISM

Although most patients who experience an acute pulmonary embolism do not have elevations in pulmonary artery pressure, massive embolism can produce vascular obstruction sufficient to raise pressure and cause cardiovascular collapse. Pulmonary hypertension can also be caused by recurrent small-vessel embolism. Most of these patients have never experienced a distinct "embolic event" that necessitated medical attention.

Large-vessel unresolved pulmonary embolism is a potentially treatable cause of chronic pulmonary hypertension. This entity is probably the result of an isolated, often subclinical, embolic event and should be considered in the differential diagnosis of unexplained pulmonary hypertension.

PRIMARY PULMONARY HYPERTENSION

Primary pulmonary hypertension is a rare disease of unknown cause in which substantial and often extreme elevations in pulmonary artery pressure are seen with no known causative factors. This hypertension occurs more often in women, particularly in the childbearing years. A familial association has been found in some patients, which suggests an autosomal dominant mode of genetic transmission with incomplete penetrance, and recent efforts have localized the site of the genes responsible for familial primary pulmonary hypertension. Clinical and pathologic findings consistent with primary pulmonary hypertension have also been found increasingly frequently in patients with portal hypertension and spontaneous or surgically induced portal–systemic shunting. The mechanism responsible is unknown, but one theory suggests that vasotoxins, which are normally metabolized by the liver, reach the pulmonary circulation and induce vascular disease.

Primary pulmonary hypertension is characterized by a spectrum of vascular lesions, from medial hypertrophy of small pulmonary arteries and intimal proliferation of pulmonary arteries and arterioles to more severe destructive vascular abnormalities, such as plexiform lesions and fibrinoid necrosis (Fig. 80.2). Pulmonary veno-occlusive disease is characterized by obliterative changes in the pulmonary venules and secondary changes in the arterial bed.

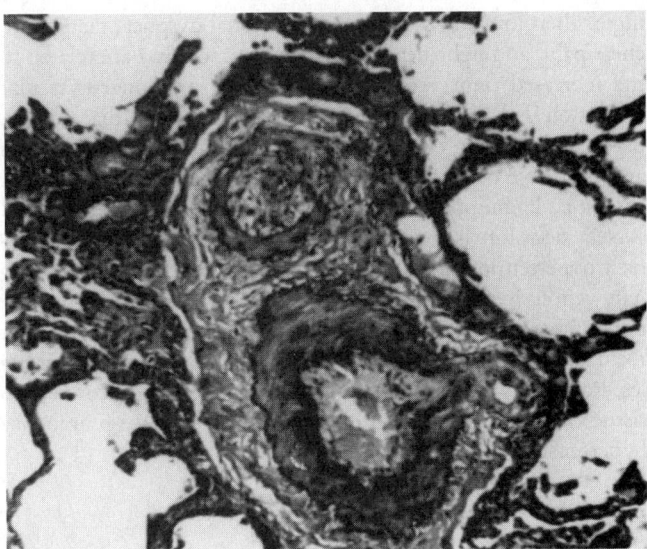

FIGURE 80.2. Pathologic features in the vessels of a patient with primary pulmonary hypertension. Shown are intimal fibrosis and medial hypertrophy in a small pulmonary artery.

PULMONARY HYPERTENSION DUE TO EXOGENOUS SUBSTANCES

A variety of exogenous substances can produce pulmonary hypertension. Drug abusers frequently inject foreign material intravenously, such as cotton fibers and talc, which may obstruct the circulation or induce a granulomatous reaction within the vessel wall and surrounding parenchyma. Inhaled cocaine use has also produced pulmonary vascular disease, presumably because of its potent vasoconstrictor effects. Tea made from the seeds of *Crotalaria fulva* (bush tea) and a herbal remedy from the seeds of *Crotalaria laburnoides* have been implicated in pulmonary vascular disease in several patients, and monocrotaline, an alkaloid derived from *Crotalaria*, has been shown to produce a necrotizing pulmonary arteritis in animal studies.

An epidemic of severe pulmonary hypertension in Europe between 1967 and 1968 coincided with the widespread use of aminorex, a diet suppressant structurally related to amphetamines. More recently, an association between the use of the anorexigens, fenfluramine and dexfenfluramine, which work by inhibiting the reuptake of serotonin in the brain, has been demonstrated in a case-controlled, prospective epidemiologic study. *Infection with HIV has been associated with the development of severe pulmonary hypertension,* which is similar pathologically to primary pulmonary hypertension. The mechanism responsible is uncertain, but the condition appears unrelated to the level of immunocompetence and may be present with no other signs of HIV infection.

■ CLINICAL FEATURES

The symptoms associated with pulmonary hypertension are usually nonspecific, and patients with chronic respiratory disease who develop cor pulmonale may present merely with a worsening of their previous symptoms. Exertional dyspnea, tachypnea, chest pain, and light-headedness are common and are related to the increased right ventricular work. The pulmonary vascular limitation is attributed to the inability to increase cardiac output, particularly during exercise. Syncope, pedal edema, and ascites are indicative of more critical impairments in right ventricular function. Hemoptysis, presumably caused by rupture of small vessels, occasionally occurs in patients with precapillary pulmonary hypertension, but it is more common in those with pulmonary venous hypertension. Hoarseness occurs with severe pulmonary hypertension and is caused by compression of the left recurrent laryngeal nerve by enlarged proximal pulmonary arteries. Raynaud's phenomenon may affect patients with connective tissue diseases or, on occasion, those with primary pulmonary hypertension.

DIAGNOSIS

PHYSICAL EXAMINATION

In addition to findings referable to the underlying diseases, the physical examination can provide important clues to the presence of pulmonary hypertension. Examination of the neck may show jugular venous distention and prominent cv waves, which are indicative of tricuspid insufficiency. Palpation of the precordium may reveal a parasternal lift or, in patients with hyperinflated lungs due to chronic obstructive airways disease, a prominent subxiphoid cardiac impulse. On auscultation, the pulmonic component of the second heart sound is loud, and a pulmonic ejection click may be found. Third and fourth heart sounds heard at the left parasternal region are found in right ventricular failure or severe pulmonary hypertension, respectively. The murmur of tricuspid insufficiency, a holosystolic murmur increasing with inspiration that is best heard along the lower left sternal border, is frequently audible as right ventricular dilation develops. The Graham Steell murmur of pulmonic insufficiency is heard as a diastolic blow at the left second intercostal space.

Examination of the abdomen may disclose tender hepatomegaly due to venous congestion or the pulsatile liver of tricuspid insufficiency. Ascites and edema may indicate overt right-sided heart failure in the absence of other potential causes, such as hypoalbuminemia. Digit clubbing is a common finding in patients with chronic obstructive lung disease, pulmonary fibrosis, cystic fibrosis, and congenital heart disease but is uncommon in other conditions causing pulmonary hypertension, such as primary pulmonary hypertension and thromboembolism.

LABORATORY TESTS

The diagnostic approach consists of two paths: establishing the presence and degree of pulmonary vascular disease and clarifying the cause. Some studies, particularly the more invasive procedures, may be useful for both objectives but are often not undertaken early in the evaluation of patients suspected of having pulmonary hypertension because of the risks entailed.

Pulmonary function testing and arterial blood gas analysis

are useful in detecting unsuspected or deteriorating chronic respiratory disease. Some investigators have suggested performing sleep studies, monitoring oxygen saturation noninvasively in patients with unexplained pulmonary hypertension to exclude sleep apnea or hypoventilation syndromes.

The electrocardiogram (ECG) usually shows evidence of right ventricular hypertrophy, with a frontal plane axis that is generally greater than 100 degrees and an R/S ratio in the right precordial leads (V_1 and V_2) of ≥ 1, and S waves greater than 3 mm in leads V_5 and V_6 (Fig. 80.3). P pulmonale, defined as a P wave greater than 2.5 mm in amplitude in leads II, III, aVF, and V_1 or V_2, is an insensitive marker for pulmonary hypertension, because it can be seen in patients with acute or chronic respiratory diseases in the absence of pulmonary hypertension.

Echocardiography is a useful noninvasive procedure for patients with suspected pulmonary hypertension. Chamber size and wall motion can be assessed, and the presence and severity of tricuspid and pulmonic insufficiency can be evaluated, particularly using Doppler techniques. Echocardiography may provide important information concerning mitral valve disease or left ventricular dysfunction. A right-to-left shunt may be determined using agitated saline or hydrogen peroxide injected intravenously and looking for bubbles traversing to the left side of the heart. Pulmonary artery systolic pressure may also be estimated by Doppler echocardiography, although these measurements are not consistently reliable.

Ventilation–perfusion lung scanning is a critical test in diagnosing the cause of pulmonary hypertension. Patients with recurrent or unresolved thromboembolism have multiple perfusion defects (Fig. 80.4), but the perfusion scan is qualitatively essentially normal for patients with primary pulmonary hypertension. Patients with pulmonary veno-occlusive disease may exhibit a mottled or patchy distribution on perfusion lung scanning. Although there are several anecdotal reports of fatalities during lung scanning of patients with pulmonary hypertension, this test can generally be performed safely and without substantial risk. Scanning of the brain or kidneys after intravenous injection of the tracer may provide evidence of an unsuspected intracardiac or intrapulmonary shunt (Fig. 80.5).

Pulmonary arteriography should be performed for a patient with evidence of pulmonary hypertension who has an abnormal lung scan result to clarify the diagnosis and to determine the extent and site of a clot. Pulmonary arteriography carries increased risk in this setting, but it can be performed safely by using newer contrast materials with less osmotic properties and by performing selective studies with hand injections.

A positive test for antinuclear antibody, usually at a lower titer and in a nonspecific pattern, is obtained for about 25% of patients with primary pulmonary hypertension. An elevated hematocrit level in a patient with pulmonary hypertension should prompt consideration of hypoxemia due to chronic parenchymal lung disease, sleep apnea, or right-to-left shunting. Detailed coagulation studies should be performed for patients with recurrent or major unresolved thromboembolism to exclude antithrombin III, protein C, or protein S deficiencies or the presence of a circulating anticoagulant.

The role of open-lung biopsy in the evaluation of unexplained

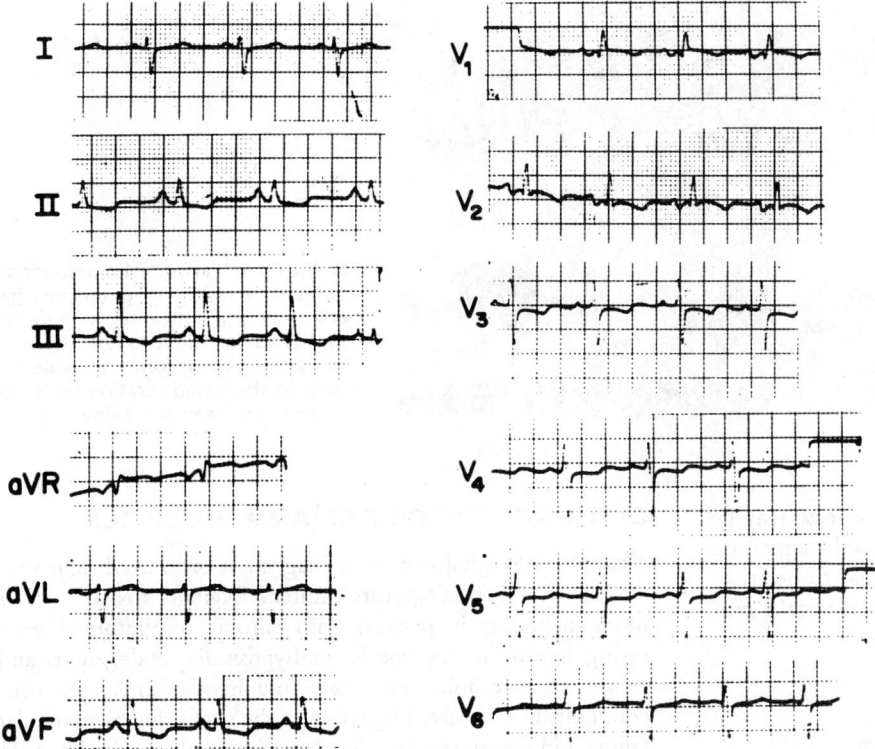

FIGURE 80.3. Electrocardiogram from a patient with primary pulmonary hypertension demonstrating changes of right ventricular hypertrophy.

pulmonary hypertension remains controversial. Although open-lung biopsy can establish the presence of subclinical interstitial lung disease, pulmonary vasculitis, or small-vessel thromboembolism and can clarify the pathologic severity of pulmonary vascular disease, this procedure carries substantial risk in patients with pulmonary vascular disease who are fragile hemodynamically. Open-lung biopsy may be important in guiding appropri-

ate therapy in patients in whom the cause of pulmonary hypertension is not clear on clinical grounds.

A clinical diagnosis of primary pulmonary hypertension can be made when pulmonary artery hypertension (mean pulmonary artery pressure 25 mm Hg at rest) exists in the absence of significant parenchymal lung disease, thromboembolic disease, congenital heart disease, left-sided valvular heart disease, or left ven-

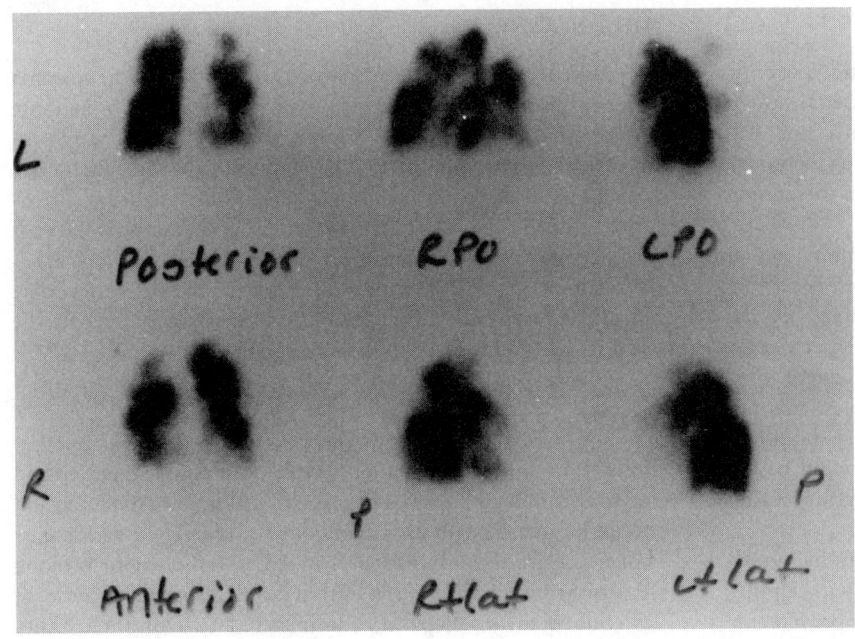

FIGURE 80.4. Perfusion lung scan from a patient with chronic thromboembolic pulmonary hypertension demonstrating multiple perfusion defects.

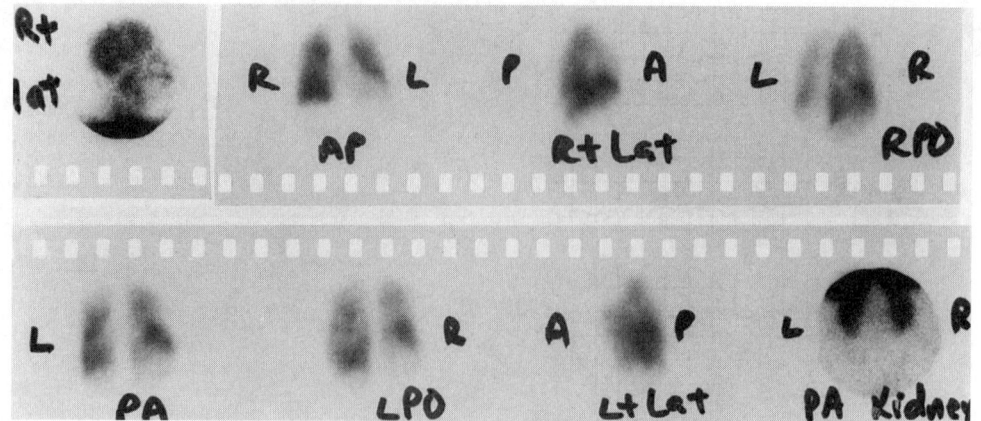

FIGURE 80.5. Perfusion lung scan from a patient with primary pulmonary hypertension demonstrating homogeneous perfusion. Right-to-left shunting through a patent foramen ovale resulted in the demonstration of tracer uptake in the head and kidneys.

tricular dysfunction. Pulmonary veno-occlusive disease may be suspected in a patient who has a chest radiograph suggesting pulmonary edema with Kerley B lines, but cardiac catheterization demonstrates pulmonary hypertension with a normal pulmonary artery wedge pressure.

OPTIMAL MANAGEMENT

TREATMENT OF UNDERLYING DISEASE

Pulmonary hypertension is a manifestation of a variety of disorders affecting the pulmonary circulation. Therapy should address the responsible factors, if possible. Therapeutic measures that improve ventilation and gas exchange, such as bronchodilators, mucolytics, corticosteroids, and respiratory stimulants, may secondarily improve the abnormalities in the pulmonary circulation in patients with parenchymal lung disease. Some bronchodilators, such as the theophylline derivatives and β_2-agonists, also have modest pulmonary vasodilator and inotropic properties that may be beneficial.

Supplemental oxygen therapy can prolong life in hypoxemic patients with chronic obstructive pulmonary disease, although its hemodynamic effects are variable and frequently not dramatic. The maximal effects of oxygen on pulmonary hemodynamics may not be seen for several months after beginning therapy.

The criteria most frequently used for instituting supplemental oxygen therapy are a stable PaO_2 $\leq$55 mm Hg when breathing ambient air or a PaO_2 $\leq$60 mm Hg with P pulmonale on the ECG, a hematocrit greater than 55%, or edema. Patients with documented exercise-induced hypoxemia may also benefit from oxygen therapy. Oxygen should be administered in a manner that raises the PaO_2 to more than 60 mm Hg, and it should be used as continuously as possible. The flow rates should be increased at night for patients who experience desaturation during sleep.

Although most patients with primary pulmonary hypertension do not experience hemodynamic improvement with supplemental oxygen, they may notice symptomatic improvement, which may justify its expense and cumbersome nature.

CARDIAC GLYCOSIDES AND DIURETICS

The value of digitalis in the management of isolated right ventricular dysfunction appears limited. Digitalis toxicity occurs more frequently in patients with chronic respiratory disease, owing in part to the coexistent hypoxemia, endogenous and exogenous catecholamine excess, and hypokalemia with concomitant diuretic use. Digitalis may be useful for biventricular failure and for control of supraventricular tachydysrhythmias in the absence of reversible causes.

Because the right ventricle is sensitive to reductions in preload, diuretics should be used with caution in the setting of cor pulmonale. Small doses of oral furosemide (20 to 40 mg) should be given initially, with the dose increased as needed. In patients with ascites or anasarca that is refractory to furosemide, oral metolazone in initial doses of 2.5 to 5 mg has proved useful. Serum levels of electrolytes, particularly potassium and magnesium, should be monitored periodically when diuretics are administered.

PHLEBOTOMY

Polycythemia is common in patients with chronic hypoxemia and can result in hyperviscosity, which can further contribute to pulmonary hypertension. Supplemental oxygen therapy produces a fall in the hematocrit of patients with chronic obstructive pulmonary disease, although it may take months to occur. Isovolumic phlebotomy is recommended if the hematocrit exceeds 50%, because at this level, the decrease in oxygen carrying capacity produced by phlebotomy is offset by the increases in cardiac output and systemic oxygen delivery, which occur when the viscosity of blood is returned to normal.

ANTICOAGULATION

Unless contraindicated, patients with pulmonary hypertension due to thromboembolism and primary pulmonary hypertension should be treated with anticoagulants for life. The treatment of choice is warfarin, administered in doses sufficient to prolong the prothrombin time to an international normalized ratio of 2:3. Subcutaneous heparin, administered two or three times daily in doses sufficient to prolong the activated partial thromboplastin time to 1.5 times that of the control, may be as effective as warfarin in preventing recurrence and is associated with a lower incidence of bleeding complications.

The use of anticoagulants in other causes of pulmonary hypertension is controversial. The rationale for their use is based on the increased risk of a potentially fatal thromboembolism in patients with a compromised pulmonary vascular bed who are predisposed because they are frequently sedentary and have venous stasis and sluggish pulmonary blood flow. However, the risks of hemorrhagic complications may be increased in patients with the altered hepatic metabolism of warfarin because of right-sided heart failure. Serious adverse effects, including fatal hemoptysis, have been reported in patients with pulmonary hypertension treated with oral anticoagulants.

VASODILATORS

The rationale for the use of vasodilators in some forms of pulmonary hypertension is based on the pathologic findings of medial hypertrophy, implying active vasoconstriction in some forms of pulmonary hypertension, including primary pulmonary hypertension, and on the demonstration that several systemic vasodilators exert similar effects in the pulmonary circulation in experimental models of pulmonary vasoconstriction. Because development of right-sided heart failure results from the increased right ventricular afterload produced by the elevations in pulmonary artery pressure, interventions that reduce afterload could improve right ventricular output.

A variety of vasodilators have been used to treat patients with pulmonary hypertension from diverse causes (Table 80.2). Substantial hemodynamic and symptomatic improvements have been reported for some patients with primary or secondary forms of pulmonary hypertension. Acute deterioration with hypotension, worsening hypoxemia, and death have also been reported. The mixed experience with this approach to therapy emphasizes the need for extreme caution and careful monitoring of cardio-vascular dynamics and gas exchange if vasodilator administration is contemplated.

Because of the risks of protracted adverse effects when a vasodilator is administered to a patient with "fixed" pulmonary vascular disease, some researchers have advocated using potent, short-acting, titratable vasodilators administered intravenously or by inhalation to evaluate the initial responses to this form of therapy. Prostaglandin I_2 (PGI_2), which is now commercially available, has been used in this manner and may be useful in determining whether vasoreactivity exists. Patients who respond to infusion of PGI_2 with increases in cardiac output and decreases in pulmonary artery pressure or pulmonary vascular resistance seem to manifest similar responses when given orally active drugs. Other commercially available intravenous vasodilators such as adenosine, acetylcholine, and prostaglandin E_1 may be useful in a similar fashion, but experience with these drugs in this setting is limited. PGI_2 has also been used as a continuous intravenous infusion for the treatment of severe pulmonary hypertension and may be particularly useful as a bridge to transplantation.

Inhaled nitric oxide (NO), the endothelium-derived relaxing factor, has been used to test vascular reactivity initially and to treat patients with severe pulmonary hypertension for brief periods. Inhaled NO is a fairly selective pulmonary vasodilator, because the molecule readily binds to hemoglobin in the pulmonary capillary bed, rendering it physiologically inactive.

The question about what constitutes a beneficial response to vasodilators is unresolved. Although most investigators agree that a substantial fall in pulmonary artery pressure accompanied by an increase in cardiac output is a beneficial response, this pattern is observed infrequently. More commonly, cardiac output increases while pulmonary artery pressure falls slightly or not at all. Because most patients who manifest an increased cardiac output with vasodilators notice improvement in symptoms, chronic therapy may still be warranted. The generally accepted contraindications to vasodilator therapy are symptomatic

TABLE 80.2.	VASODILATORS USED FOR PULMONARY HYPERTENSION		
Agent	**Trial Dosage**	**Plasma Half-Life**	**Long-Term Therapy**
Nifedipine	10 mg sublingually, repeat once after 15–20 min[a]	3–4 h	10–40 mg PO 3 or 4 times daily or 40–160 mg of extended release preparation once daily[b]
Dilitiazem	30 mg PO[a]	3–5 h	30–90 mg PO 3 times daily or 90–270 mg of extended release preparation once daily[b]
Adenosine	50 μg/kg/min IV, increasing infusion by 50 μg/kg/min every 2 min to a maximum of 300 μg/kg/min	5–10 min	None
Nitric oxide	10–40 ppm in air	2–5 min	None
Prostaglandin I_2 (prostacyclin)	1–12 ng/kg/min IV increasing by 2 ng/kg/min every 10–15 min	3–5 min	2–200 ng/kg/min[b]
Prostaglandin E_1	0.02–0.04 g/kg/min IV	30 min	Under investigation

[a] Not recommended for testing of acute vasoreactivity; doses are for initiation of oral therapy.
[b] Doses of oral therapy should be adjusted based on individual needs and responsiveness.

hypotension, an increase in pulmonary artery pressure, and a deterioration in gas exchange with worsening hypoxemia. This latter event is usually caused by a worsening ventilation–perfusion relation as blood flow increases to poorly ventilated lung units. In patients with right-to-left shunts, vasodilators can increase shunting if systemic vasodilation is greater than pulmonary vasodilation.

TRANSPLANTATION

Combined heart-lung transplantation has been performed successfully in patients with primary pulmonary hypertension or Eisenmenger's syndrome. The major limitations to more widespread application of this approach are the limited availability of suitable organs for transplantation and the limited access to the few centers with the expertise and resources to perform the operation. Additional problems include postsurgical complications, such as transplant rejection, increased susceptibility to opportunistic infections, and adverse effects attributable to immunosuppressant therapy. Bronchiolitis obliterans occurs in as many as 40% of patients after heart-lung transplantation and may be life threatening. Single- or double-lung transplantation has also been performed successfully in patients with pulmonary hypertension in whom right ventricular function was less severely impaired. The greater availability of lungs for transplantation, compared with heart-lung blocs, may make this approach more suitable for widespread applications in the future.

■ PROGNOSIS AND NATURAL HISTORY

Coexistent pulmonary hypertension in the setting of chronic respiratory disease is a poor prognostic sign, with death resulting from respiratory failure or combined cardiopulmonary decompensation commonly occurring within 3 to 5 years.

The median survival from the time of initial diagnosis in primary pulmonary hypertension is 2 to 3 years. Survival is related more to right-sided heart function than to the degree of pulmonary artery pressure elevation. A reduced cardiac output or symptoms indicative of an inability to increase cardiac output with activity, such as syncope, are ominous signs. Spontaneous remissions of primary pulmonary hypertension have been reported but appear to be unusual. Improved survival with oral vasodilator therapy or transplantation has not been evaluated in a prospective, multicenter study fashion, but continuous infusion of PGI_2 has been shown to improve survival in severely affected patients with primary pulmonary hypertension.

BIBLIOGRAPHY

Abenhaim L, Moride Y, Brenot F, et al. Appetite-supressant drugs and the risk of primary pulmonary hypertension. *N Engl J Med* 1996;335: 609–616.

Barst RJ, Rubin LJ, Long WA, et al. A comparison of continuous intravenous epoprostenol (prostacyclin) with conventional therapy for primary pulmonary hypertension. *N Engl J Med* 1996;334:296–301.

Burrows B, Kettel LJ, Niden Ah, et al. Patterns of cardiovascular dysfunction in chronic obstructive lung disease. *N Engl J Med* 1972;286:912–918.

D'Alonzo EG, Barst RJ, Ayres SM, et al. Survival in patients with primary pulmonary hypertension. Results from a national prospective registry. *Ann Intern Med* 1991;115:343–349.

Fuster V, Steele PM, Edwards WD, et al. Primary pulmonary hypertension: natural history and importance of thrombosis. *Circulation* 1984;70: 580–587.

Inbar S, Schrader BJ, Kaufmann E, et al. Effects of adenosine in combination with calcium channel blockers in patients with primary pulmonary hypertension. *J Am Coll Cardiol* 1993;21:413–418.

McMurtry IF, Raffestin B. Potential mechanisms of hypoxic pulmonary vasoconstriction. In: Will JA, Dawson CA, Weir EK, Buckner CK, eds. *The pulmonary circulation in health and disease.* Orlando, FL: Academic Press, 1987:455–468.

Moser KM, Spragg RG, Utley J, Dailey PO. Chronic thrombotic obstruction of major pulmonary arteries. *Ann Intern Med* 1983;99:299–304.

Nocturnal Oxygen Therapy Trial Group. Continuous or nocturnal oxygen therapy in hypoxemic chronic obstructive lung disease: a clinical trial. *Ann Intern Med* 1980;93:391–398.

Pasque MK, Trulock EP, Kaiser LR, Cooper JD. Single-lung transplantation for pulmonary hypertension. Three-month hemodynamic follow-up. *Circulation* 1991;84:2275–2279.

Pepke-Zaba J, Higenbottam T, Dinh-Xuan AT, et al. Inhaled nitric oxide as a cause of selective pulmonary vasodilation in pulmonary hypertension. *Lancet* 1991;338:1173–1174.

Rubin LJ. Current concepts: primary pulmonary hypertension. *N Engl J Med* 1997;336:111–117.

Kelley's Textbook of Internal Medicine, fourth edition. Edited by H. David Humes. Lippincott Williams & Wilkins, Philadelphia © 2000.

CHAPTER 81

VASCULAR MEDICINE

MARK A CREAGER
MARIE GERHARD-HERMAN

Vascular disease constitutes some of the most common causes of disability and death in Western society. Vascular medicine is a subspecialty of medicine that involves the treatment of disorders affecting arteries, veins, and lymphatics. This includes atherosclerosis of the peripheral arteries, arterial aneurysms, vasospastic diseases, venous thromboembolism, venous insufficiency, lymphedema, and the many disorders that predispose to these vascular diseases. In the field of vascular medicine, the vasculature is often thought of as a unique system, since the vessels supplying different organs share many structural and functional features. This concept, along with advances in vascular technology and interventions, has led to the growth of this field.

■ ARTERIAL DISEASE

Arteries are commonly described as large (elastic), medium (elastic and muscular), and small (muscular). Their main function is to deliver oxygenated blood to organs. All arteries are composed of intima, media, and adventitia. The intima, the innermost layer, is normally a thin layer composed of endothelial cells and bounded by the internal elastic lamina. Endothelial cells synthesize vasoactive factors that can relax and constrict blood vessels, as well as factors with anticoagulant and procoagulant activities. The smooth muscle cells of the media are bounded by the internal and external elastic lamina and regulate the tone of the vessels. The outermost layer is the connective tissue matrix of the adventitia, which contains both fibroblasts and smooth muscle cells. Arterial disease results from pathologic narrowing of the lumen, inappropriate vasoconstriction, and structural weakness of the media.

ARTERIAL OCCLUSIVE DISEASE

Symptomatic arterial occlusive disease generally occurs when the luminal diameter is reduced to half of the normal diameter. Acquired arterial stenoses and occlusion may be chronic or acute. Atherosclerosis is the most common cause of peripheral arterial disease. Other causes must be considered in persons without risk factors for atherosclerosis or with an unusual distribution of arterial occlusive disease. These include arteritides such as Takayasu's arteritis and giant cell arteritis, which may cause a localized an inflammatory reaction that results in stenosis of upper and lower extremity vessels, the aorta, or visceral vessels. Other forms of vasculitis (Chapter 181) can also result in symptomatic arterial occlusive disease. Thromboangiitis obliterans, characterized by intimal inflammation and thrombosis, affects the distal arteries of the upper and lower extremities. Arterial occlusion also occurs as a consequence of embolism or thrombosis in situ. Emboli originating in the heart may travel to the aorta and lower extremities. Thrombosis can acutely develop in diseased arteries or occur in normal arteries in patients with some hypercoagulable states or with trauma. Coarctation of the aorta is a congenital cause of arterial narrowing due to hypoplastic growth in a localized area of the thoracic, or more rarely, abdominal, aorta.

PERIPHERAL ARTERIAL DISEASE

Atherosclerosis of the lower extremity causes symptoms in approximately 3% of persons over the age of 50. In contrast, over 25% of persons over age 70 have evidence of peripheral arterial disease by noninvasive testing. The prevalence of peripheral arterial disease is threefold greater when determined by noninvasive testing for arterial stenosis rather than by questionnaires regarding symptoms, consistent with the observation that two-thirds of affected persons are asymptomatic. The risk of peripheral atherosclerosis increases with the presence of known risk factors for atherosclerosis (Table 81.1). Ten percent of symptomatic patients have arterial stenoses limited to the aorta and iliac arteries, and the other 90% have diffuse disease extending to the femoral and tibioperoneal vessels. Patients with only aortoiliac disease tend to be younger and have a high incidence of cigarette smoking. Patients with more extensive disease are likely to be older or have diabetes.

Many patients with mild degrees of peripheral arterial disease remain asymptomatic. Approximately 75% of patients with claudication remain stable with a proper risk factor modification

TABLE 81.1.	ATHEROSCLEROSIS RISK FACTORS FOR PERIPHERAL ARTERY DISEASE
Risk Factor	**Relative Risk**
Diabetes	3.0–4.0
Smoking	2.5–3.0
Hypertension	1.5–2.5
Cholesterol (each 10 mg/dL)	1.1
Age (q 10 yr)	1.6–2.4
Non white	1.3–3.4
Gender	1.0
Homocysteine	1.7–2.6

program and exercise. The remaining 25% have progression of their symptoms. Of those with progressive disease, 1% to 10% eventually require a major amputation. The risk of progression is even greater in patients with diabetes, in whom there is a 17-fold increase in the risk of amputation. Peripheral atherosclerosis is one manifestation of systemic atherosclerosis, and affected persons are likely to have atherosclerosis affecting the coronary, carotid, and renal arteries as well. The risk of a cardiovascular event (myocardial infarction, cardiovascular death, and stroke) is increased six times in those with evidence of peripheral arterial occlusive disease on noninvasive testing. The 5-year survival rate is 44% for patients with severe peripheral atherosclerosis—that is, an ankle brachial index of 0.40.

CLINICAL FINDINGS IN PERIPHERAL ATHEROSCLEROSIS

The inability of blood flow to meet the metabolic demands of exercising muscle results in a symptom called *intermittent claudication*, in which the patient might describe discomfort, pain, cramping, or tiredness of the buttock, thigh, or calf, which occurs with exercise and is relieved with rest. Intermittent claudication should be distinguished from pseudoclaudication, which occurs from lumbar spine disease. In *pseudoclaudication,* leg pain may also occur with standing. Males develop vasculogenic impotence from inadequate pelvic blood flow. Limb-threatening ischemia with forefoot pain at rest, tissue ulceration, or gangrene can occur if the stenoses are so severe that the resting metabolic needs of the tissues are not met.

On physical examination, the patient usually has diminished lower extremity pulses. The femoral, popliteal, posterior tibial and dorsalis pedis pulses should be palpated, because the location of the abnormal pulse may provide an indication of the site of stenosis. For example, a normal femoral pulse but an abnormal popliteal pulse suggests stenosis in the superficial femoral artery. The femoral arteries should be auscultated for bruits providing evidence of stenosis.

With chronic severe disease, the patient may have hair loss, muscle atrophy, cool feet, and nail changes. Pallor occurs with leg elevation because perfusion decreases without the assistance of gravity. Dependent rubor occurs because the capillaries in the distal lower extremity are maximally vasodilated and therefore

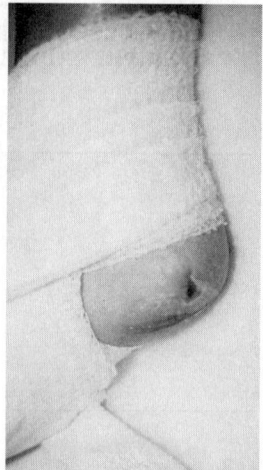

FIGURE 81.1. Arterial ulcer and peripheral arterial disease. Ulcers occur often at sites of pressure from footwear, such as at the heel.

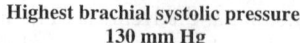
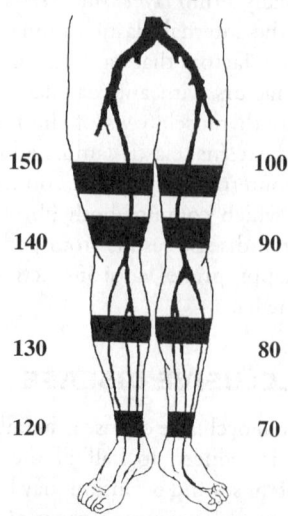

FIGURE 81.2. Segmental systolic blood pressure measurements. Cuffs are placed on the proximal and distal thigh and on the proximal and distal calf. Systolic pressure at each level is given next to the cuff in mm Hg. The systolic pressure of 100 mm Hg in the left proximal thigh indicates more proximal iliofemoral stenosis.

fill rapidly in the dependent position. Ulcers or gangrene can be present on the feet, particularly on the toes and heels, and often at sites of trauma or pressure from footwear when there is severe arterial insufficiency (Fig. 81.1).

TESTING FOR PERIPHERAL ARTERIAL DISEASE

The initial confirmation of peripheral atherosclerotic disease can be acquired noninvasively by determining the systolic blood pressure in the ankle and comparing it with the systolic blood pressure in the arm. Ankle systolic pressure is greater than or equal to arm pressure in the absence of arterial occlusive disease. Conversely, the ankle pressure is usually less than the highest brachial pressure in the presence of peripheral atherosclerosis, with an ankle brachial ratio of ≤0.90 considered abnormal. The ankle:brachial systolic pressure ratio is referred to as the *ankle brachial index.* More extensive information about the location of limb arterial occlusive disease is available through segmental systolic blood pressure measurements performed in the vascular laboratory. Blood pressure cuffs are placed on the proximal thigh, distal thigh, proximal calf, and above the ankle (Fig. 81.2). A Doppler probe is then placed over the dorsalis pedis or posterior tibial artery to determine systolic blood pressures at these cuff locations by listening for the onset of flow when a cuff previously inflated to suprasystolic pressures is deflated. A pressure drop of 20 mm Hg indicates the presence of significant stenosis between the two adjacent levels. Pulse volume recordings (PVR) may also indicate the presence of stenoses. A normal PVR resembles a blood pressure waveform, whereas that distal to a stenosis has a delayed upstroke and diminished amplitude. Doppler waveforms can also be recorded at each level by pulse wave Doppler using duplex ultrasound (Fig. 81.3). When stenosis is present, there is a triphasic waveform proximal to the stenosis to a biphasic or monophasic pattern beyond the stenosis. When pulse wave Doppler waveforms are determined along the length of the artery, an increase in the peak systolic velocity is seen at the site of stenosis. The segmental pressure measurements

may be normal at rest and should be repeated after exercise if the clinical suspicion of peripheral arterial disease is high. A precipitous and sustained drop in ankle pressures occurs after exercise in patients with peripheral arterial disease.

Three-dimensional arterial reconstruction using magnetic resonance imaging (MRI) arteriography and spiral computed tomography (CT) arteriography can provide noninvasive assessment of the distal aorta and iliac vessels, but presently with less clarity than is available with invasive arteriography. Contrast arteriography is necessary to completely evaluate the anatomical extent of disease in the distal aorta and lower extremity arteries.

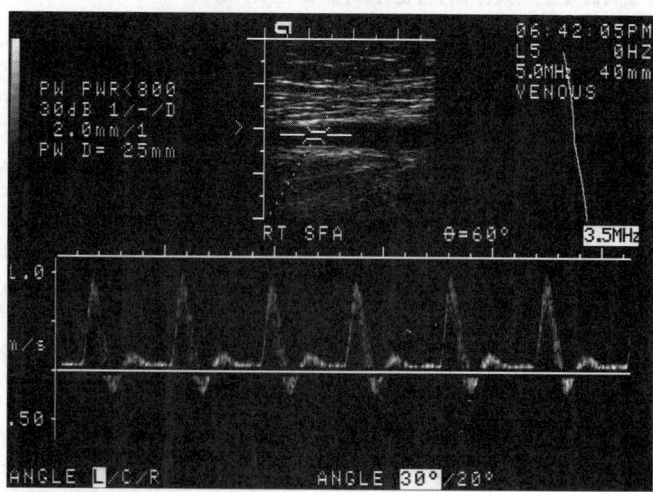

FIGURE 81.3. Pulse-wave Doppler examination. The superficial femoral artery is located with duplex imaging. The Doppler waveform is sampled in the center of the superficial femoral artery. This is a normal triphasic waveform.

It is generally performed only to determine the optimal revascularization procedure. The functional significance of the arterial occlusive disease can be quantified by invasive pressure measurements proximal and distal to the stenosis and can be determined before and after administration of a vasodilator.

MANAGEMENT OF PERIPHERAL ARTERIAL DISEASE

The two goals of treatment in patients with peripheral atherosclerosis are to decrease their considerable cardiovascular risk and to improve symptoms. The identification of peripheral atherosclerosis should prompt evaluation of modifiable risk factors for atherosclerosis such as cigarette smoking, dyslipidemias, hypertension, diabetes, and high homocysteine. Patients should also be evaluated for coexisting cerebrovascular and coronary atherosclerosis. Smoking cessation results in decreased cardiovascular mortality and reduced risk of progression to critical limb ischemia and amputation. Few studies have evaluated the benefits of lipid-lowering therapy on symptom relief in patients with peripheral atherosclerosis. However, in the Scandinavian Simvastatin Survival Study the risk of new or worsening intermittent claudication was reduced by 38% compared with that in the placebo group. Control of diabetes may decrease nephropathy and retinopathy, but it is not known whether this will improve symptoms of claudication or decrease the risk of amputation. Antiplatelet therapy with aspirin and clopidogrel reduces cardiovascular events in patients, including those with peripheral arterial disease. A supervised exercise program can increase pain-free walking time by 50% to 300%. Patients with arterial occlusive disease should be instructed in foot hygiene and told to examine their feet daily to seek urgent treatment for foot ulcers.

Most vasodilators have been ineffective in patients with peripheral atherosclerosis as the resistance vessels of the lower extremity are already vasodilated during exercise to meet the metabolic demands of the tissues. Current pharmacotherapy for peripheral arterial disease includes pentoxifylline and cilostazol. Pentoxifylline is an adenosine diphosphate receptor antagonist that is purported to decrease blood viscosity and improve red cell deformity. Clinical trials with pentoxifylline have reported both favorable and insignificant results compared with placebo. The more severely affected population may be the most responsive.

Cilostazol is a phosphodiesterase inhibitor with vasodilator and platelet-inhibitory properties. Treatment with cilostazol in randomized, controlled trials resulted in improved physical performance, walking ability, and functional status. Cilostazol should not be administered to patients with heart failure because of the potential for increased mortality risk in these patients, which has been described with other phosphodiesterase inhibitors. Carnitine has been evaluated as a therapy for intermittent claudication as patients with peripheral atherosclerosis develop metabolic abnormalities in the skeletal muscle of the lower extremity. Both L-carnitine and propionyl-L-carnitine improved exercise performance in clinical trials. However, carnitine has not been approved for use in the United States. There is ongoing research evaluating the administration of angiogenic growth fac-

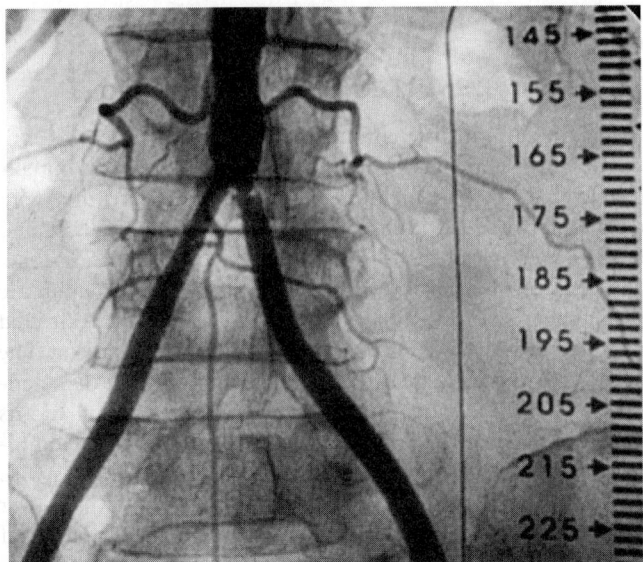

FIGURE 81.4. Contrast arteriography of the distal aorta and iliac bifurcation. A short stenosis is evident at the origin of the left iliac artery.

tors to improve symptoms in patients with claudication and critical limb ischemia.

Percutaneous or surgical intervention is typically reserved for the patient with disabling claudication or limb-threatening ischemia. Percutaneous transluminal angioplasty and stent placement have both high success and high patency rates when used to treat stenoses less than 2 cm in the iliac arteries (Fig. 81.4), but limited success and lower patency rates in the femoral and tibioperoneal arteries. For example, 5-year patency rates after iliac angioplasty are 85% compared with 65% for femoropopliteal angioplasty. The standard operative procedures used for the patient with arterial occlusive disease are bypass procedure around the stenosis or endarterectomy of the diseased segment. More durable results are obtained with bypass grafting procedures. In aortoiliac disease, a bifurcated graft is attached from the distal aorta to the femoral vessels. When one iliac artery is severely diseased and the other is normal, a bypass graft can be placed from one femoral artery to the other femoral artery to improve arterial inflow to the leg beyond the iliac stenosis. The patency rate for both limbs of an aortobifemoral bypass is 85% over 5 years. The patency rates are lower for infrainguinal bypass grafts, varying from 70% over 5 years with femoropopliteal bypass above the knee to 40% over 5 years for femoropopliteal bypass grafts extending below the knee. For prosthetic grafts placed below the knee the patency rate is as low as 20%. When narrowing occurs at the distal anastomosis of a graft, it may be corrected by patching open the anastomosis before it occludes. Patients undergo duplex ultrasound surveillance of their grafts to detect and correct such narrowings before the graft occludes.

Potential complications after peripheral bypass surgery are myocardial infarction, renal failure, bypass graft thrombosis, pseudoaneurysm formation, wound infection, impotence, and death. Preoperative evaluation is recommended to accurately assess the perioperative risk for a cardiovascular event.

SPECIFIC ARTERIAL DISEASES

TAKAYASU'S ARTERITIS

Takayasu's arteritis is a chronic inflammatory disease predominantly in the aorta and its branches. This periarteritis is initially characterized by inflammation of the media and adventitia, with a prominent cellular infiltrate and occasional giant cells at sites of disintegration of the elastic lamina. The inflammation is accompanied by intimal hyperplasia (Fig. 81.5). In the chronic phase, there is fibrosis of the vessel. The pattern of vessels affected varies according to the geographic location of the patient. The aortic arch and its branches are often involved in North American and Japanese patients, whereas the abdominal aorta and its branches are involved in Indian patients. It occurs predominantly in young women. Takayasu's arteritis often begins with fevers, malaise, and myalgias. Occasionally, there is pain over the affected vessels, as in carotodynia. Over time, symptoms of arterial insufficiency such as claudication, cerebrovascular ischemia, or visceral pain occur. These patients may also develop aortic aneurysm or aortic dissection. Bruits are often encountered over the subclavian and carotid vessels. Takayasu's arteritis should be suspected in persons with unequal pulses or blood pressures in their extremities. Takayasu's arteritis is a common cause of renovascular hypertension in India.

There is no diagnostic laboratory test for Takayasu's arteritis. The American College of Rheumatology has listed criteria for reporting this diagnosis, with three of the six criteria resulting in high specificity and sensitivity for the diagnosis (Table 81.2). Angiography can identify the long segmental narrowings that are typical of Takayasu's arteritis. CT and magnetic resonance angiography may demonstrate inflammation in the artery wall. The erythrocyte sedimentation rate has been used to estimate disease activity and may be more reliable when used in combination with systemic complaints or new symptoms of arterial insufficiency.

Medical treatment begins with corticosteroids, which are effective in 60% of the patients. Methotrexate and cyclophosphamide may be added if prednisone alone is ineffective or poorly

TABLE 81.2.	**DIAGNOSTIC CRITERIA FOR TAKAYASU ARTERITIS**[a]

Onset before age 40
Extremity claudication
Decreased brachial pulse
> 10 mm difference in brachial systolic blood pressures
Bruit over subclavian artery or aorta
Angiographic evidence of narrowing or occlusion in the aorta or its proximal branches

[a] Three of six necessary for diagnosis. (Data from Arend WP. The American College of Rheumatology 1990 Criteria for the Classification of Takayasu arteritis. *Arthritis Rheum* 1990;33: 1129–1134, with permission.)

tolerated. These cytotoxic drugs may decrease clinical and angiographic evidence of Takayasu's arteritis. Percutaneous transluminal angioplasty and stenting have been used successfully in short, concentric stenoses. Surgical arterial bypass can be used for patients with symptomatic ischemia; however interventions performed during periods of active disease have dramatically higher restenosis and complication rates.

GIANT CELL ARTERITIS

Giant cell arteritis, also known as *temporal arteritis,* occurs in those over age 50 years. The mean age of onset is 70 years, with the highest prevalence in whites of northern European ancestry. The entity was first described as "thrombotic arteritis of the aged." Giant cell arteritis has been found in the arteries of nearly every organ. The inflammation begins with lymphocyte infiltration, destruction of the elastic lamina, and intimal thickening. The classic findings are focal necrosis and granuloma with multinucleated giant cells in the region of the fragmented elastic lamina. The pattern is one of "skip" lesions, and many sections of the affected artery must be examined before this diagnosis is

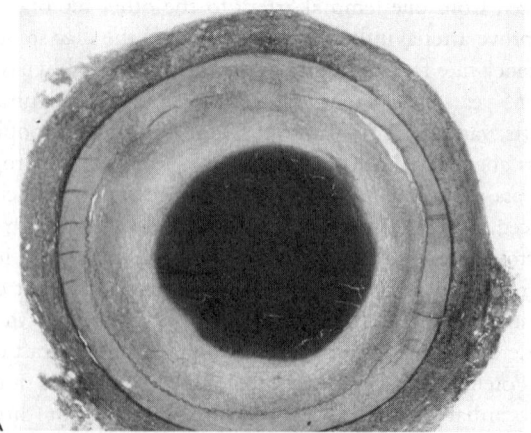
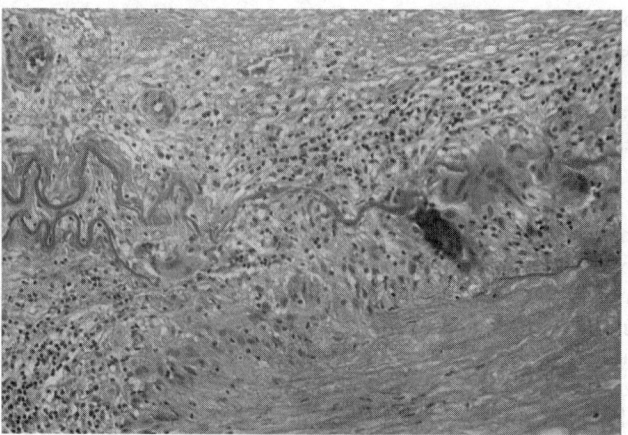

FIGURE 81.5. Arterial histology in Takayasu's arteritis. **A:** Marked intimal hyperplasia is seen in a cross-section of superficial femoral artery. **B:** High-power magnification demonstrates inflammation in the vessel wall.

excluded. The predominant vessels involved include temporal, vertebral, carotid, subclavian, coronary, and brachial arteries, as well as the aorta.

Symptoms at presentation include headache, visual changes, scalp tenderness, weight loss, fever, and malaise. Claudication of the masticatory muscles, tongue, arm, neck, and legs may occur. The presentation can be dramatic with aortic dissection or myocardial infarction. Nearly 50% of the patients have the clinical syndrome of polymyalgia rheumatica. Laboratory findings such as elevated erythrocyte sedimentation rate are common but are not required for the diagnosis. The diagnosis is made from the clinical presentation and confirmed by pathologic examination.

Corticosteroids are the mainstay of treatment for giant cell arteritis, and their use has dramatically decreased the incidence of blindness with temporal arteritis. Death is rare and results from stroke, myocardial infarction, ruptured aortic aneurysms, and aortic dissection. Treatment begins with prednisone, 60 mg per day. The prednisone dose can typically be tapered in 2 to 4 weeks. Remission can occur on occasion after 1 to 2 years of therapy. Surgical intervention may be necessary to achieve limb salvage and to decrease mortality from aortic aneurysm or dissection.

THROMBOANGIITIS OBLITERANS

Thromboangiitis obliterans, also known as Buerger's disease, involves the small and medium arteries in the extremities. The histologic pattern includes extensive intimal inflammation and thickening, thrombosis, and preservation of the media. Migratory superficial thrombophlebitis occurs. The disease mainly affects young male cigarette smokers, but is now reported with increasing frequency in young female cigarette smokers. Patients may present with Raynaud's phenomenon, calf and foot claudication, and gangrene of the digits. Peripheral neuropathy may be present because of severe ischemia. Arteriography reveals segmental occlusions of small and medium arteries, usually those at the distal part of the upper and lower extremities, accompanied by corkscrew collaterals (Fig. 81.6). Treatment must include abstinence from tobacco. New lesions are less likely to develop if the patient stops smoking. Digital ulcers often require debridement. Pharmacologic therapy includes calcium channel blockers and α-adrenergic blockers and possibly vasodilator prostaglandin infusion to decrease vasospasm. The use of pentoxifylline and aspirin has also been advocated, but randomized trials proving benefit of these therapies are lacking.

ACUTE ARTERIAL OCCLUSION

Sudden arterial occlusion may result from embolism or thrombosis. Embolism is the major cause, and the primary source is the heart. Once emboli lodge in an artery, there may be further extension by thrombosis. Sudden arterial occlusion can develop in patients with peripheral arterial disease when thrombosis occurs at the site of atherosclerotic plaque. Arterial thrombosis can also occur in normal arteries in patients with hypercoagulable states and after traumatic injury. The severity and extent of ischemia with sudden arterial occlusion depend on the size of

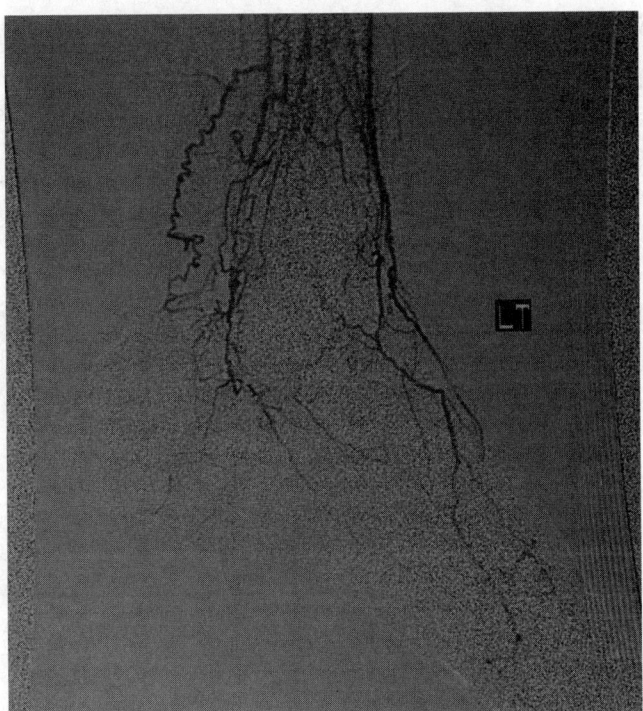

FIGURE 81.6. Distal runoff in lower extremity arteriography. Corkscrew collaterals typical of thromboangiitis obliterans are evident on the left. Segmental arterial occlusions are also noted.

the occluded vessel and the presence or absence of collateral circulation. Pain is present in 80% of patients. Numbness, paresthesias, and weakness may accompany severe ischemia. Pallor and absent pulses distal to the occlusion characterize the physical examination. The presentation is often described as that of the six "p"s: **p**allor, **p**olar (cold), **p**ulselessness, **p**ain, **p**aresthesias, and **p**aralysis. A saddle embolus to the aortoiliac bifurcation can cause such a profound state of leg ischemia that a state of shock ensues (Fig. 81.7).

Assessment of the capillary refill, muscle weakness, sensory loss, and Doppler signals from the vessels can establish the clinical grade of acute limb ischemia (Table 81.3). For limbs that are viable or threatened but not irreversibly ischemic, reestablishing patency of the occluded vessel is achieved through removal or dissolution of the thrombus with thrombolytic therapy, embolectomy, or bypass surgery. Urgent embolectomy is the optimal therapy when a large artery is occluded, and the limb's viability depends on achieving adequate perfusion within hours. The success of thrombolytic therapy depends partly on how soon the agent is administered after the arterial occlusion. This therapy is followed by conventional anticoagulation to prevent recurrent thrombus formation. The hospital course after revascularization may be complicated by the release of potassium, metabolites, and myoglobin from the ischemic tissue into the circulation. If the patient with a viable or threatened limb cannot undergo surgery or thrombolysis, heparin should be administered and the extremity should be kept warm and in a dependent position. The patient must be followed up closely for signs of deterioration at which time the surgical therapy should be reconsidered.

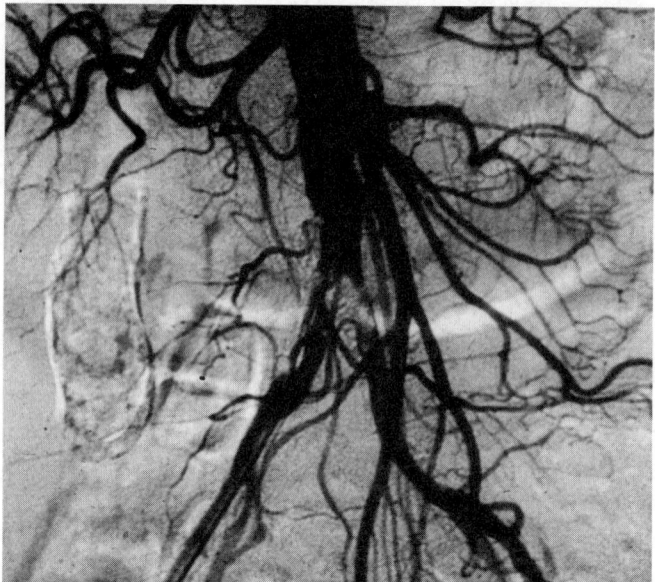

FIGURE 81.7. Angiogram of the distal aorta and iliac bifurcation. A large filling defect consistent with a saddle embolus is seen at the bifurcation.

ATHEROEMBOLISM

Microemboli of lipid and thrombotic atherosclerotic debris commonly originating in the aorta may travel distally resulting in occlusion of small arteries. The clinical presentation is often referred to as *blue toe syndrome*. Affected patients present with pain and cyanosis in their toes and with livedo reticularis and petechiae on their feet and legs. Embolic occlusion of small intramuscular arteries result in calf tenderness. These patients often have fever and eosinophilia. A skin or muscle biopsy demonstrating needle-shaped cholesterol clefts in small arteries is diagnostic of atheroembolism. These lesions can also have significant inflammatory cells and lipid-laden giant cells. Atheroemboli are most often seen after cardiac catheterization but may occur spontaneously from sites of friable atherosclerotic plaque. Antiplatelet therapy may reduce the risk of recurrent atheroem-

bolism. Surgical treatment may be necessary to remove the source of the friable atherosclerotic plaque.

VASOSPASM AND TEMPERATURE-RELATED DISORDERS

Raynaud's Phenomenon

Raynaud's phenomenon is episodic vasospasm resulting in digital ischemia. Episodes of well-demarcated digital pallor or cyanosis follow exposure to cold and emotional distress. The diagnosis is based primarily on the patient's history because simple office maneuvers such as cold water immersion do not reliably induce an episode of digital ischemia in these patients. Raynaud's phenomenon occurs in up to 8% of men and up to 18% of women. The higher prevalence is reported in populations living in colder climates. Unique features of digital arterial circulation contribute to the occurrence of Raynaud's phenomenon. The cutaneous vessels of the fingers and toes are supplied only by sympathetic adrenergic vasoconstrictor fibers. Increased sympathetic efferent activity normally causes vasoconstriction, and may cause profound vasospasm in persons predisposed to Raynaud's phenomenon. Digital arterial narrowing, decreased perfusion, and increased blood viscosity have been postulated as some of the mechanisms that may contribute to Raynaud's phenomenon. Digital blood flow is altered by these changes, and digital ischemia then develops more readily in the presence of vasoconstrictor stimuli.

The classification of Raynaud's phenomenon is separated into primary, not associated with another disease process, or secondary, occurring as a consequence of another disease or treatment. Criteria for the diagnosis of primary Raynaud's phenomenon include history of episodes of bilateral acral pallor or cyanosis, symptoms for more than 2 years, and physical examination with strong, symmetric pulses and no evidence of digital pitting, ulcerations, or gangrene (Table 81.4). In primary Raynaud's phenomenon, nail-fold capillaroscopy, antinuclear antibody, and erythrocyte sedimentation rate are normal. Patients with primary Raynaud's phenomenon have a favorable prognosis.

The presence of asymmetric pulses, or evidence of prolonged

TABLE 81.3.	CLINICAL CATEGORIES OF LIMB ISCHEMIA				
Category of Ischemia	Muscle Weakness	Sensory Loss	Capillary Refill	Arterial Doppler	Venous Doppler
Viable	None	None	Intact	Audible	Audible
Threatened (salvageable with prompt action)	Mild	Mild	Intact	Not audible	Audible
Irreversible (will require major amputation)	Profound	Anesthetic	Absent; marbling pattern present	Not audible	Not audible

(From Ad Hoc Committee on Reporting Standards. Suggested standards for reports dealing with lower extremity ischemia. *J Vasc Surg* 1986;4:80–84, with permission.)

TABLE 81.4.	DIAGNOSTIC CRITERIA FOR PRIMARY RAYNAUD'S PHENOMENON

Bilateral episodes of acral cyanosis or pallor
No digital ulceration, pitting, or gangrene
Strong, symmetric peripheral pulses
Symptoms > 2years
No signs or symptoms of disease associated with secondary Raynaud's phenomenon
Normal erythrocyte sedimentation rate
Normal antinuclear antibody test
Normal nailfold capillaries

(Modified from LeRoy EC, Medsger TA Jr. Raynaud's phenomenon: a proposal for classification. *Clin Exp Rheumatol* 1992;10: 485–488.)

phenomenon are evident before the onset of episodes of digital ischemia. An exception is scleroderma, in which the onset of Raynaud's phenomenon may precede evidence of scleroderma by many years. In cases of secondary Raynaud's phenomenon, the arterial supply to the digits can be assessed by a number of techniques. These include systolic pressure measurements, and blood flow assessment by digital plethysmography or Doppler flow. If abnormal arterial flow is seen, the study can be repeated with warming. If the arterial flow appears normal after warming, vasospasm rather than fixed arterial occlusion is present (Fig. 81.8). Arteriography is not required in most cases and would be indicated only if an obstructive lesion requiring revascularization is sought.

The mainstay of treatment is patient education regarding avoidance of stimuli that precipitate digital ischemic attacks. Patients should be instructed to dress warmly, wearing not only gloves, but sweaters, coats, and hats because reflex sympathetic vasoconstriction occurs in the digits in response to cold exposure elsewhere (e.g., head or trunk). Calcium channel blockers with the exception of verapamil and α-adrenergic blockers have proved to be useful in improving digital blood flow and ameliorating symptoms. Iloprost given intravenously improves healing of ulcers in patients with scleroderma. Selective digital sympathectomy and microarteriolysis may facilitate ulcer healing and

digital ischemia such as digital ulcers, suggests a secondary cause of Raynaud's phenomenon. Secondary causes of Raynaud's phenomenon include connective tissue disease, arterial occlusive disease, thermal or vibration injury, blood dyscrasias, neurologic disorders, drugs, and toxins. Most secondary causes of Raynaud's

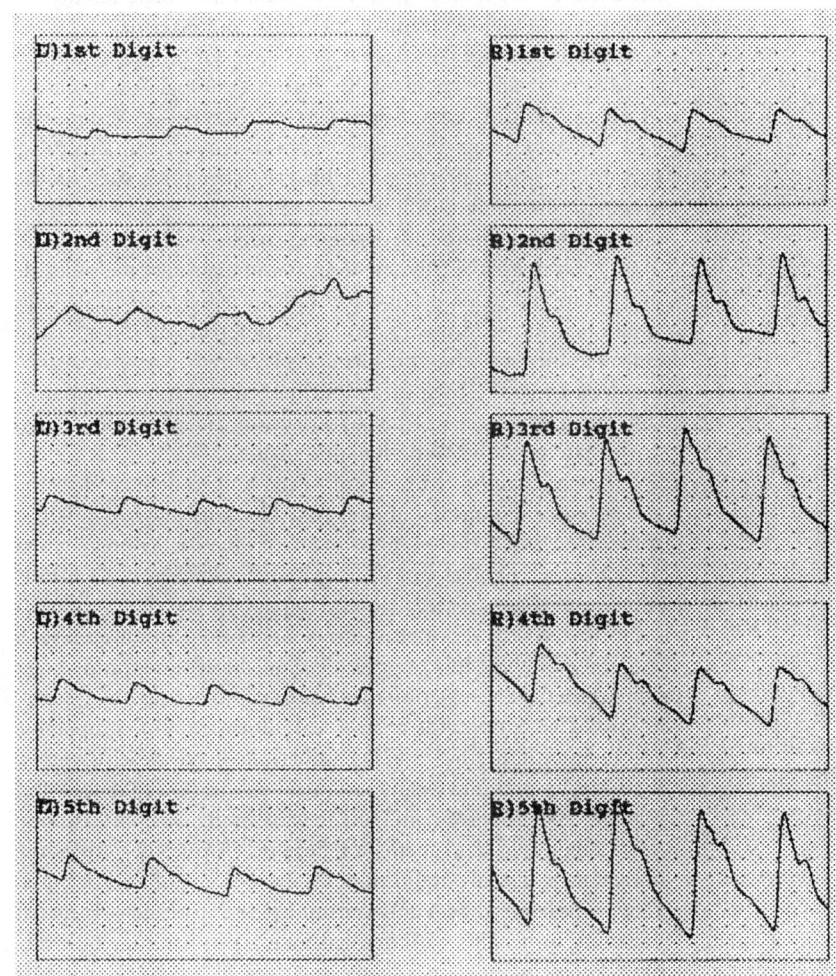

FIGURE 81.8. Photoplethysmography of the digits in the presence and absence of warming. Blunt waveforms consistent with moderate arterial occlusion are evident on the left. The waveforms in the same digits return to normal after warming (*right*).

symptom improvement in severe cases of secondary Raynaud's phenomenon. Cervical and lumbar sympathectomy have also been performed in cases of severe Raynaud's phenomenon, but with limited long-term success.

Acrocyanosis

Acrocyanosis is a rare disorder of the peripheral circulation in the general population but is seen in 20% of patients with anorexia nervosa. Acrocyanosis is seen in adolescents and young women, and patients present with episodes of cyanosis and coldness in the hands and feet. Unlike in Raynaud's phenomenon, the cyanosis extends proximal to the digits. These manifestations are attributed to arteriolar spasm. Cyanosis increases with cold exposure and is relieved by warming. On physical examination, mild edema and excess sweating of the hands and feet may be found. There are no trophic changes or ulceration of the digits. If the patient is examined during an episode, pallor is seen when the extremity is raised above the heart level, ruling against venous obstruction. There should not be physical evidence of central cyanosis. The laboratory evaluation in these patients is normal. The prognosis is excellent, and the disorder is self-limited. In patients with anorexia nervosa, the acrocyanosis generally resolves with weight gain.

Erythromelalgia

Erythromelalgia is an uncommon disorder characterized by erythema, warmth, and burning pain in the extremities. Although there is evidence of arteriolar spasm, this disorder is often thought of as the antithesis of Raynaud's phenomenon. Episodes are precipitated by warmth and relieved by cold. It can be primary, familial, or secondary. There is a striking association between secondary erythromelalgia and myeloproliferative disorders, and the onset of erythromelalgia may precede that of the myeloproliferative disorder by several years. Patients over age 30 should be evaluated with periodic blood counts. Other secondary causes of erythromelalgia include systemic lupus erythematosus, rheumatoid arthritis, spinal cord disease, multiple sclerosis, and drugs such as nifedipine, pergolide, and bromocriptine.

The diagnosis of erythromelalgia is based on clinical history, including erythema, severe burning pain, precipitation by warmth, relief with cooling, and exclusion of disorder such as reflex sympathetic dystrophy and thromboangiitis obliterans. Primary erythromelalgia is not life threatening, but the symptoms can be continuously debilitating. Aspirin is recommended for all patients with erythromelalgia. Sympathectomy has not been effective in treating this disorder. Secondary erythromelalgia requires treatment of the underlying disorders and discontinuation of inciting drugs such as nifedipine and bromocriptine. The prognosis of secondary erythromelalgia is tied to the underlying disease.

ANEURYSMAL DISEASE

An aneurysm is a widening or dilation of a segment of blood vessel and may be defined as an increase in the lumen more than one and a half times that of the nearest normal proximal segment. Aneurysms tend to enlarge over time, since radius relates to wall tension as described by Laplace's law. True aneurysms involve all three layers of the vessel wall; intima, media, and adventitia. They may be fusiform or saccular. Aneurysmal disease is most commonly identified in the thoracic and abdominal aorta, but it may occur in the peripheral and visceral arteries. The incidence, cause, natural history and management vary according on the location. Abdominal aortic aneurysms are described in the following section, since many of these are seen by vascular medicine specialists.

ABDOMINAL AORTIC ANEURYSM

Abdominal aortic aneurysms account for most aortic aneurysmal disease, and most of these occur below the level of the renal arteries. This segment of aorta has decreased elastin lamellae compared with the thoracic aorta. The infrarenal abdominal aorta also lacks vasa vasorum and derives its nutrient supply from the lumen. Abdominal aortic aneurysms occur more often in men than in women. Most abdominal aortic aneurysms are associated with atherosclerosis, whereas cystic medial necrosis accounts for most ascending aortic aneurysms. Important risk factors for the development of abdominal aortic aneurysm in addition to male gender include cigarette smoking, chronic hypertension, and family history of abdominal aortic aneurysm. Other causes include trauma, infection, and arteritis.

Most abdominal aortic aneurysms are asymptomatic. In fact, the diagnosis arises incidentally during radiologic examination in up to 70% of cases. Some patients experience abdominal, back, or flank pain. Expansion of the aneurysm can also cause symptoms by compressing neighboring structures such as the ureter or iliac vein. Embolism of thrombus or atheromatous plaque from within the aneurysm may occlude distal arteries and cause limb ischemia. Physical examination can reveal a pulsatile midabdominal mass, particularly in lean patients or those with large aneurysms. However, 25% are not palpable on physical examination even when the diagnosis is known. Rupture is characterized by severe back or abdominal pain with hemodynamic collapse. Tachycardia, pallor, hypotension, and shock are related to the extent of the hemodynamic insult.

Ultrasonography is the simplest method to detect, measure, and monitor abdominal aneurysms. The sensitivity of this test approaches 100%. However, it may not identify features such as branch vessel involvement or length of the aneurysm. Contrast-enhanced CT is particularly useful in patients with large abdominal girth and is as sensitive as ultrasonography. Techniques such as spiral or helical imaging, faster acquisition times, and three-dimensional reconstruction may further improve CT image resolution. MRI can provide anatomical information of comparable accuracy without the ionizing radiation or contrast. Contrast aortography provides clear anatomical delineation of length and branch vessel involvement, but it is of limited use in assessing the diameter of the aneurysm because thrombus within the lumen may obscure definition of the aortic wall. Abdominal aneurysms larger than 4 cm occur in 1% to 2% of men. Targeted screening in persons with marked increase in risk may be effective. These include first-degree relatives of aneurysm patients

TABLE 81.5.	CLEAR INDICATIONS FOR SURGICAL REPAIR OF ABDOMINAL AORTIC ANEURYSM

Size ≥5 cm
Growth of ≥cm/y
Abdominal aortic aneurysm with symptom of rupture

who are over 50, patients with atherosclerosis, and those with popliteal artery aneurysms because up to 50% have aneurysms elsewhere.

Mortality rates are up to 60% for patients who present to the hospital with rupture of their aneurysms. Therefore, optimal management is focused on elective repair of the aneurysm before rupture (Table 81.5). The timing of surgery depends on symptoms, size of the aneurysm, rate of aneurysm growth, and its potential for rupture. Rupture occurs in 1% to 2% of those with aneurysms less than 5 cm and in 10% to 40% of those with aneurysms greater than 5 cm. However, in a recent study, early elective surgery on abdominal aortic aneurysms of 4 to 5.5 cm did not result in improved mortality at 2, 4, or 6 years compared with a control group with similar aneurysms. The timing of surgery is dependent on the presence of symptoms, aneurysm size, rate of aneurysm growth, and the potential for rupture. Most asymptomatic aneurysms greater than 5 cm should be repaired because of the high likelihood of rupture.

The mortality with elective operative repair is typically less than 5%, and in some reports as low as 1.6%. Risk factors for poor outcome include age, female gender, renal artery involvement, significant blood loss, angina, and renal insufficiency. If surgery is not performed because of size or comorbid conditions, the ultrasonographic assessment should be repeated every 6 to 12 months. Increase in size of aneurysm of more than 1 cm per year or occurrence of any symptoms should prompt reevaluation for surgery, given the threat of rupture. Endovascular repair of abdominal aortic aneurysms is currently under evaluation and holds promise for a less invasive repair for those who are poor operative candidates. However, the first large trials reported with this technique found complication rates up to 20%.

POPLITEAL ARTERY ANEURYSMS

People with a family history of abdominal aortic aneurysm also have an increased likelihood of peripheral aneurysms, including popliteal artery aneurysms. Popliteal artery aneurysms are bilateral in more than 50% of cases. These aneurysms may cause claudication or limb ischemia in cases in which thrombosis of the aneurysm has significantly narrowed the arterial lumen or when there is distal embolization of the thrombus lining the aneurysm. Rupture is an unusual occurrence. Popliteal artery aneurysms also may cause popliteal vein thrombosis because of compression of the companion vein in the confined space of the popliteal fossa. These aneurysms can be diagnosed by duplex ultrasound. Elective resection and bypass grafting constitute the treatment of choice when the distal circulation is adequate. The

risk of limb loss increases after thromboembolic complications have occurred.

ARTERIOVENOUS FISTULA

Arteriovenous fistulas are either congenital or acquired defects in which there is continuity between arteries and veins without intervening capillaries. Small hemangiomas, a spongy texture to the subcutaneous tissue, and dilated superficial veins can be seen on physical examination. A common finding is a palpable thrill or a continuous bruit from turbulence, which results from high-pressure flow entering a low-pressure system. A "machinery" murmur is indicative of a fistula. Venous insufficiency with consequent venous varicosities and edema may be present. Hemodynamically significant shunts can cause high-output heart failure. Evidence of hemodynamic significance includes the development of bradycardia when the fistula is compressed. Comparison between venous oxygen saturation in the involved and noninvolved limbs may be useful in making the diagnosis.

Several syndromes have been described that include arteriovenous fistulas, such as Osler–Weber–Rendu, Parkes–Weber, and Klippel–Trenaunay syndromes. These arteriovenous fistulas may present as late as the second or third decade of life with symptoms of discomfort, heaviness, and increased warmth in the affected region. Hereditary hemorrhagic telangiectasia (HHT) is known as *Osler–Weber–Rendu disease*. This disease affects mucocutaneous and visceral vascular tissue. Patients have family history, telangiectasias, arteriovenous malformations, and epistaxis or gastrointestinal bleeding. Pulmonary arteriovenous malformations are present in up to 20% of affected persons and may be multiple. Hemagiomas and arteriovenous fistulas are noted in Klippel–Trenaunay syndrome, and Parkes–Weber syndrome is associated with arteriovenous malformations. Venous varicosities and limb hypertrophy are present in both.

Most acquired arteriovenous fistulas occur after trauma to the blood vessels. However, infection and malignancy may disrupt vascular walls, and aneurysms can penetrate veins and lead to an arteriovenous fistula. Many acquired arteriovenous fistulas result from percutaneous interventions such as intra-arterial cannulas, cardiac catheterization, intra-aortic balloon pumps, and occasionally percutaneous biopsies. Other causes include penetrating trauma with a knife or bullet.

Diagnosis of arteriovenous fistula is made by noninvasive imaging with duplex ultrasonography or by arteriography. Conservative treatment measures include wearing compressive bandages and pain relief. Cardiac decompensation from high-output state is an indication for repair of the arteriovenous fistula, which amounts to the surgical closure of the fistula and reestablishment of the continuity of the involved artery and vein. This may not be practical in patients with multiple fistulas.

VENOUS DISEASE

Veins are thin-walled tubes with endothelium-lined intima, loosely arranged media, and adventitia. Veins larger than 2 mm in diameter have bicuspid valves located at varying intervals along their length. Valves are common in the extremity veins and absent in the visceral and central nervous system veins. When a person stands, the venous pressure in the feet rises typically from 7 mm Hg up to 90 mm Hg, and as much as 20% of the blood volume is sequestered in the legs within 15 minutes. The calf muscles contract with walking, they squeeze blood into the veins, propelling it toward the heart. The venous valves open when blood is moving centrally and close at other times to prevent blood from flowing back toward the feet. Together, the pumping action of calf muscles and unidirectional action of valves decrease venous pressure in the feet.

The venous system in the lower extremity is composed of superficial, communicating, and deep veins. The superficial veins are those in the skin and subcutaneous tissues down to the level of the muscles. These veins are often visible, in contrast to the deep veins. Veins that supply organs, muscles, and bones constitute the deep venous system. The superficial and deep veins are connected by perforating or communicating veins. Communicating veins are well-developed in the distal lower extremities. One-way valves in the communicating veins allow blood to flow only away from the superficial veins and toward the deep veins.

VENOUS THROMBOSIS

An estimated 500,000 cases of deep venous thrombosis occur in the United States every year. This condition is a major cause of mortality because of pulmonary embolism and morbidity in the form of chronic venous insufficiency. Venous thrombi are composed of fibrin, red cells, platelets, and leukocytes. Venous thrombosis originates in the in valve cusp pockets, in venous sinuses of the calf, and in segments of vein exposed to direct trauma. Deep venous thrombosis occurs in the deep and superficial vessels of the arms and legs as well as in visceral veins. Venous thrombosis can result from any combination of venous stasis, venous endothelial damage, and hypercoagulable state.

Postoperative acute deep venous thrombosis affects up to 70% of orthopedic patients and up to 40% of general surgical patients. Deep venous thrombosis also may complicate other conditions requiring inactivity or prolonged bed rest, such as stroke and congestive heart failure. Deep venous thrombosis may occur during pregnancy and the postpartum period because pregnancy can cause extrinsic venous compression and hypercoagulability. It may result from a hypercoagulable state, including abnormalities of clotting factors, exogenous estrogen administration, and malignancy. Patients at increased risk for deep venous thrombosis should receive prophylaxis with at least one of the measures shown to be effective, such as leg elevation, elastic stockings, low-dose heparin, low-molecular-weight heparin, dextran, and external pneumatic calf compression (Table 81.6).

Clinical Manifestations

Symptoms and signs of venous thrombosis are caused by obstruction to venous outflow, inflammation of venous tissue, or thrombus embolization into the pulmonary circulation. The leg veins are the most common sites of deep venous thrombosis. It

TABLE 81.6.	CONDITIONS INCREASING RISK OF VENOUS THROMBOSIS

Previous venous thrombosis or > two first-degree ralatives with venous thrombosis[a]
Malignancy with recent surgery[a]
Hip or knee surgery[a]
Malignancy
Fracture of pelvis, femur, or tibia
Immobility including bedrest >3 days
Major medical illness such as heart failure or myocardial infarction
General surgery in patient >40 yr

---

[a] Denotes high risk. (Adapted from Hirsh J, Hoak J. AHA Medical/Scientific Statement. Management of deep vein thrombosis and pulmolnary embolism. *Circulation* 1996;93:2212–2245.

occurs in the proximal veins (iliac, common femoral, profunda femoral, superficial femoral, and popliteal veins), the calf veins (tibial, peroneal, soleal, and sural), and the superficial leg veins. Proximal deep venous thrombosis in the lower extremity can manifest as swelling and pain, but may occur without local symptoms. The edema is usually unilateral, occurring only in the affected leg, and may involve the ankle, calf, and thigh. In patients with iliofemoral venous thrombosis, tenderness may be elicited over the femoral veins, and venous collaterals may be evident at the groin. The presentation of lower extremity venous thrombosis is most dramatic in patients with extensive iliofemoral venous thrombosis. Swelling of the entire limb, with pallor and pain is referred to as *phlegmasia alba dolens. Phlegmasia cerulea dolens* is the term applied when the swollen limbs are markedly cyanotic.

Swelling can compromise arterial flow and peripheral pulses may be diminished. There is often thrombosis of nearly all significant deep and superficial leg veins, and there are petechiae and elevated calf compartment pressures. Patients can be in shock given the sequestration of blood and interstitial fluid in the leg. In the most severe cases, there is formation of hemorrhagic bullae, ischemia, and wet gangrene. Calf deep venous thrombosis may present with focal calf discomfort and tenderness. Edema may not occur if only one vein is occluded, since venous return can be accommodated by the other calf veins. Calf vein thrombosis may propagate to the proximal veins in approximately 30% of untreated patients.

Pelvic vein thrombosis can involve the internal iliac veins and the ovarian veins. There are few distinct symptoms when the internal iliac veins alone are involved without extension of thrombus into the common iliac veins. In this case, edema is less likely, since venous return from the leg will not be significantly compromised. The first manifestation in pelvic vein thrombosis is likely to be pulmonary embolism. Patients with prostate cancer and tumor throughout the pelvis may present with pelvic vein thrombosis. One of the most common presentations of pelvic vein thrombosis is ovarian vein thrombosis. Women present with ovarian vein thrombosis most often in the postpartum period and have symptoms of lower quadrant abdominal pain.

Ovarian vein thrombosis can extend to the vena cava, particularly in the presence of malignancy, and can be associated with septic pulmonary emboli. Venous thrombosis of the internal jugular, subclavian, axillary, and brachial veins is becoming more common given the frequent use of central venous catheters.

Neck and arm vein thrombosis may be associated with edema, fever, and local tenderness, These sites are potential sources of pulmonary emboli, with a reported incidence of up to 30%. Very low doses of warfarin may prevent thrombosis with central venous catheters. Paget–Schroetter syndrome or effort thrombosis refers to primary, spontaneous axillary vein thrombosis. It often follows vigorous activity that is unusual for that person or vigorous activity that is unusual for most individuals. Affected patients present with a feeling of tightness and swelling in the dominant arm. Superior vena cava syndrome occurs secondary to obstruction and thrombosis of the superior vena cava as a result of mediastinal spread from a neoplasm, usually carcinoma of the lung. This causes dramatic and painless swelling of the neck and distention of the superficial veins of the upper chest and neck.

Pulmonary embolism and venous thrombosis occur together. In one study, 50% of the patients with proximal vein thrombosis and no suspected pulmonary embolism did indeed have evidence of pulmonary embolism by perfusion lung scanning. Conversely, asymptomatic deep venous thrombosis is found in up to 80% of patients presenting with clinically symptomatic pulmonary embolism. Pulmonary emboli occur more frequently and are larger in patients with proximal vein thrombosis than in patients with calf vein thrombosis. Internal jugular, subclavian, and axillary vein thromboses are potential sources of pulmonary emboli, with a reported incidence of up to 30%. Most clinically significant and fatal emboli arise from thrombi in the proximal veins of the legs.

Diagnosis of Venous Thrombosis

A venous duplex ultrasound scan, combining B-mode imaging and pulse Doppler analysis of venous flow, is the procedure of choice for the initial evaluation of venous disease. Venous ultrasonography is an accurate noninvasive test for confirming the presence of deep venous thrombosis. The sensitivity and specificity exceed 90% in proximal deep venous thrombosis. Two-dimensional real-time images are obtained as the transducer is placed over the common femoral vein and moved distally. Gentle pressure is applied with the probe to determine whether the vein under examination is compressible (Fig. 81.9A). Many thrombi are not visible by ultrasonographic examination; therefore, noncompressibility is the ultrasound criterion for diagnosing deep venous thrombosis (Fig. 81.9B).

Venous flow is evaluated by pulse wave and color Doppler imaging. A lack of respirophasic variation provides additional evidence of venous obstruction. Venous thrombus can be completely lysed with no residual thrombus remaining; however, more often it organizes with narrowing and at times complete occlusion of the lumen. Ultrasonographic findings of thickened walls and valve disorganization indicate previous venous thrombosis. Calf veins are smaller than proximal veins, which makes their evaluation by duplex ultrasonography more difficult. Ve-

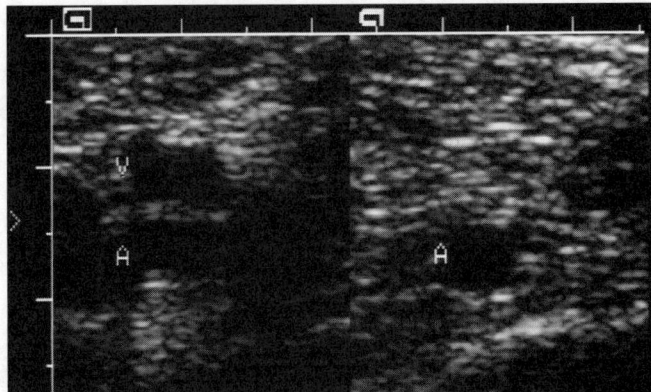

A

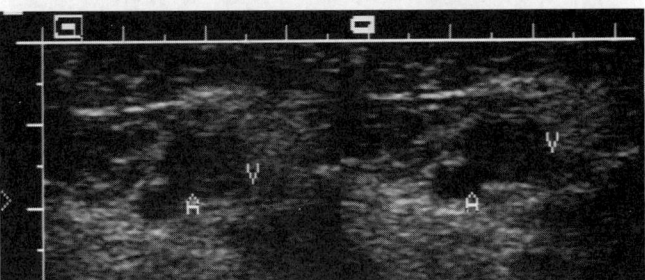

B

FIGURE 81.9. Duplex ultrasonography of the popliteal vein. **A:** The artery and vein are seen on the left, but with gentle compression on the right the vein is completely compressed. **B:** The popliteal vein remains evident with gentle compression, consistent with the presence of venous thrombosis.

nous ultrasonography is used also to diagnosis thrombosis of the internal jugular and arm veins.

Venography is indicated when venous duplex ultrasonography is unavailable or cannot answer the clinical questions. Venography is used to diagnose inferior vena cava and ovarian and iliac vein thrombosis and is used to guide catheter based thrombolytic therapy. Magnetic resonance venography can be used to evaluate the presence of thrombus in veins that are difficult to access by ultrasonography.

Treatment

The objectives of treatment in proximal deep venous thrombosis are to prevent pulmonary embolism and recurrent deep venous thrombosis and to reduce the likelihood of postphlebitic syndrome. Bed rest with leg elevation above the level of the right atrium is indicated for those with edema. Bed rest is usually discontinued after the patient is symptom-free and anticoagulation is therapeutic. Anticoagulation with unfractionated or low-molecular-weight heparin and conversion of the heparin anticoagulant to warfarin for at least 3 to 6 months are prescribed for patients with proximal deep venous thrombosis as described in the following text.

Calf vein thromboses can be treated with standard anticoagulation, or patients can be followed up with sequential ultrasound examination and treatment deferred unless the thrombus extends into the proximal venous system. Extension is estimated to occur in 30% of cases. Compression stockings with a gradient of at least 20 to 30 mm should be prescribed to prevent recurrent edema when patients become ambulatory. Treatment of pelvic vein thrombosis is similar to that for proximal deep venous thrombosis. When pelvic vein thrombosis is associated with pelvic sepsis, any resulting pulmonary emboli can form lung abscesses. Intensive antibiotic therapy is needed, and surgical interruption of the appropriate veins may be required. Treatment of upper extremity venous thrombosis includes anticoagulation with heparin, followed by conversion to warfarin. Elevation with the arm on pillows and the upper body upright is recommended.

Heparin, Low-Molecular-Weight Heparin, and Warfarin Therapy

Heparin therapy, with continuous intravenous infusion of unfractionated heparin or subcutaneous injections of low-molecular-weight heparin, is the initial treatment of choice for deep venous thrombosis. Both can be used in pregnant patients, since heparin does not cross the placenta. Unfractionated heparin is given as an intravenous bolus of 100 U per kilogram (typically 7,500 to 10,000 U) followed by a continuous infusion of 15 U per kilogram per hour (typically 1,000 to 1,500 U per hour). The partial thromboplastin time (PTT) should be checked at 6 hours to confirm that the level is increased to 1.5 to 3.0 times the baseline values. If the PTT is subtherapeutic, the heparin infusion is adjusted and the PTT is determined every 6 hours until therapeutic levels are achieved, then every 24 hours subsequently.

Platelet counts should be checked daily during heparin administration. If potentially life-threatening bleeding (e.g., intracerebral) occurs, the heparin is discontinued and anticoagulation is reversed with protamine sulfate. Hirudin, a direct thrombin inhibitor, may be necessary in patients with heparin-induced thrombocytopenia.

Enoxaparin is the only low-molecular-weight heparin approved for treatment of deep venous thrombosis in the United States. Appropriate patients to consider for therapy are those who do not require prolonged hospitalization, such as those without increased risk of bleeding and without extensive iliofemoral venous thrombosis. The length of hospitalization necessary for patients treated with low-molecular-weight heparin is under evaluation. Patients may require admission to begin therapy with enoxaparin at the dose of 1 mg per kg subcutaneously every 12 hours and to receive education and arrange home services. Dosing with low-molecular-weight heparin is difficult in patients with morbid obesity and those with end-stage renal disease; therefore, heparin levels are determined in these patients 6 hours after the second dose. A level between 0.5 and 1 U per milliliter is therapeutic. Platelet counts should be checked during treatment, since heparin-induced thrombocytopenia can develop. Low-molecular-weight heparin treatment should overlap with warfarin for at least 5 days. Low-molecular-weight heparin should be continued until the international normalization ratio (INR) is therapeutic for 2 consecutive days. Criteria have been proposed for outpatient deep venous thrombosis management (Table 81.7).

Oral anticoagulation with warfarin should begin with a dose of 5 mg daily and may be started on the first or second day of heparin treatment. Lower doses should be considered in the very thin and the elderly, and higher doses in patients who weigh more than 80 kg. Warfarin is contraindicated in pregnant patients because it crosses the placenta and may result in embryopathy. Warfarin achieves its anticoagulant effect by interfering with hepatic production of the vitamin K–dependent clotting factors II, VII, IX, and X. It also interferes with the production of proteins C and S. Warfarin is highly protein-bound in the plasma, and this contributes to a number of drug interactions with other protein-bound drugs. The anticoagulant effect of warfarin is delayed until the preexisting clotting factors are cleared from the circulation.

In the early stages of warfarin administration, a hypercoagulable state can occur owing to the different half-lives of the vitamin K–dependent clotting factors and the vitamin K–dependent coagulation inhibitor, protein C. Therefore, heparin treatment should be continued for 3 to 5 days of warfarin therapy after the prothrombin time indicates adequate oral anticoagulation. The test used to monitor warfarin anticoagulation is the prothrombin time. This test is sensitive to the decrease of factors II, VII, and X. The maintenance dose of warfarin is adjusted to achieve the recommended therapeutic range, which is an INR of 2.0 to 3.0.

TABLE 81.7.	CRITERIA TO CONSIDER FOR OUTPATIENT TREATMENT OF DEEP VENOUS THROMBOSIS	
Inclusion		**Exclusion**
Adult age		Phlegmasia
Hemodynamically stable		Documented pulmonary embolism
Proximal deep venous thrombosis of the leg		Heparin-induced thrombocytopenia
Calf vein thrombosis		Surgery or trauma within 2 weeks
Willing to be treated as an outpatient		Stroke within 2 weeks
		Significant renal dysfunction
		Pregnancy
		Guaiac-positive stool, gastrointestinal bleeding
		Morbid obesity
		Significant comorbid disease
		Potential for poor compliance with regimen

Thrombolysis and Vena Caval Interruption

Catheter-directed thrombolysis with urokinase, streptokinase, and tissue plasminogen activator produces successful clot lysis, but it is also associated with more frequent bleeding complications than heparin therapy is. A potential benefit of thrombolysis is rapid clot lysis, in addition to preservation of venous valves, although this therapy has not been proved to reduce the risk of postphlebitic syndrome. Catheter-directed thrombolysis may be useful in selected patients with deep venous thrombosis in the iliofemoral and axillosubclavian vein, particularly those whose limbs are threatened. Heparin is administered concomitantly at therapeutic doses to decrease the incidence of pericatheter thrombosis. Vena caval interruption should be considered in patients who cannot receive anticoagulation. More controversial indications for vena caval filter are as adjunctive therapy with pulmonary embolectomy and as therapy for patients with deep venous thrombosis and severe underlying lung disease. The initial beneficial effect of vena caval filters for the prevention of pulmonary embolism is subsequently counterbalanced by extension and recurrence of deep venous thrombosis, leading to postphlebitic syndrome.

SUPERFICIAL THROMBOPHLEBITIS

Thrombosis of the greater or lesser saphenous vein or their tributaries is the most common presentation of superficial thrombophlebitis. It is also frequently seen in the cephalic and basilic veins and their tributaries in the upper arm. It may present as tenderness, erythema, and a firm cord along the course of the affected vein. Superficial thrombophlebitis is treated with warm compresses and mild anti-inflammatory analgesic agents. Anticoagulation is not necessary unless superficial thrombosis extends to the saphenofemoral junction, risking propagation into the deep system. Migratory thrombophlebitis is thrombosis that develops in superficial veins at various sites and times. It occurs in the legs, arms, and torso. It is associated with pancreatic cancer and other visceral cancers and is seen in thromboangiitis obliterans or Buerger's disease.

Thrombophlebitis limited to the superficial veins of the anterior chest wall and breast occurs in both men and women and is often referred to as *Mondor's disease.* Patients present with pain, followed by erythema along the course of the thoracoepigastric veins. A firm cord is often palpable by the second day of symptoms. Suppurative thrombophlebitis refers to infection with purulent drainage along the course of a thrombosed vein. It usually results from associated intravenous catheter infection, and is therefore typically in superficial veins. Purulent thrombophlebitis may require drainage in addition to systemic antibiotics. Intravenous drug users are likely to have thrombophlebitis in association with localized abscesses at injection sites. Superficial thrombophlebitis is treated with warm compresses and mild anti-inflammatory analgesic agents. Anticoagulation is not necessary unless superficial thrombosis extends to the saphenofemoral junction, risking propagation into the deep system.

CHRONIC VENOUS INSUFFICIENCY

Chronic venous insufficiency affects many persons under age 60 and is present in up to 3% of the population. The pathophysiology of chronic venous insufficiency includes valve incompetence with associated reflux and venous obstruction. Primary deformities of venous valves and congenital valve rings are rarely the cause of valve incompetence. Incompetency of the venous valves more often follows damage when the cusps are permanently scarred and retracted. Valve incompetence leads to venous hypertension owing to the hydrostatic pressure and the pressure imposed by calf muscle contraction that is not counterbalanced by effective valve closure. Incompetent communicating veins develop as a result of valve damage from prior thrombosis or because increased venous pressure in the deep system overcomes the valve. Flow then refluxes back into the superficial veins and results in the development of varicosities. Lower extremity edema occurs secondary to fluid extravasation into the soft tissues. The elevated venous pressure is transmitted to the subcutaneous tissue and skin, particularly in the distal part of the leg, and forces the extravasation of red cells from the capillaries. This eventually results in brawny hyperpigmentation, induration, skin ulceration, and recurrent bouts of cellulitis. *Lipodermatosclerosis* refers to the hard, tender, thickened subcutaneous tissue that develops in severe cases.

The clinical manifestations of chronic venous insufficiency can be divided into stages according to severity (Table 81.8).

General Management

The goals of management in chronic venous insufficiency are to ameliorate symptoms and reduce the possibility of skin ulceration. This is accomplished by reducing venous hypertension as much as possible. Conservative management includes daily use of graded elastic compression stockings (30 to 50 mm Hg at the ankle), avoidance of prolonged standing, periodic leg elevation during the day, leg elevation throughout the night, and ulcer treatment with medicated compressive dressings. The prototypical antiembolism stockings have a uniform pressure throughout and are used for prophylaxis of deep venous thrombosis in patients at bed rest. They are not effective in reducing edema in ambulatory patients either immediately after diagnosis of deep venous thrombosis or when there is chronic venous insufficiency.

Gradient elastic compression stockings must be prescribed. These have the highest pressure at the ankle and the lowest pressure in the proximal segment of the stocking. Surgical treatment should be considered if these measures fail. Surgical therapy may consist of compression sclerotherapy and ablative surgery for superficial and communicating vein insufficiency. Ablative surgery refers to procedures such as stripping of the greater saphenous vein and division of incompetent communicating veins. Surgical options for valvular incompetence include valvuloplasty for patients with a primary deep vein valve abnormality. Surgical repair of valve incompetence also includes transposing a vein segment with valve incompetence to an adjacent vein segment with a competent valve. Competent valves in a segment of upper extremity vein can be transplanted into a lower extremity vein with incompetent valves. There are venous bypass procedures for patients with chronic venous insufficiency due to obstruction.

TABLE 81.8.	CLINICAL GRADE OF VENOUS INSUFFICIENCY	
Grade of Venous Insufficiency	Physical Examination	Symptoms
1	Dilated superficial veins Normal subcutaneous tissues and skin Ankle edema less than 1 cm	Mild swelling Leg heaviness
2	Many dilated veins Incompetent communicating veins Mild pigmentation changes Mild liposclerosis Lower extremity edema >1 cm	Moderate to severe swelling Heaviness Varicosities Brawny skin changes
3	Many dilated veins Incompetent communicating veins Many venous varicosities Marked skin pigmentation Severe liposclerosis Venous ulcers Edema >2 cm	Severe swelling Calf pain

(Adapted from Reporting standards in venous disease. Prepared by the Subcommittee on Reporting Standards in Venous Disease. *J Vasc Surg* 1988;172–181.)

LYMPHATIC DISEASE

Lymphedema results from excessive accumulation of tissue fluid in the extremities as a result of impaired lymphatic drainage. It can be primary, but is more often secondary or acquired. Lymphedema should be distinguished from the edema of venous insufficiency; however, they do on occasion occur together. Venous edema rarely affects the toes and is characteristically soft and pitting. Lymphedema, in contrast, almost always involves the toes and is usually firm with thickened skin (Fig. 81.10). Primary lymphedema is classified by the age at presentation. Congenital lymphedema results from failure of lymphatic devel-

opment and appears at birth or within the first 2 years of life. There is a familial form of congenital lymphedema with autosomal dominant inheritance called *Nonne–Milroy's disease.* Lymphedema praecox is the most common form of primary lymphedema and occurs between the ages of 2 and 35 years. It is most commonly observed in women and often at the onset of menses or with the first pregnancy. *Meige's disease* refers to a specific form of familial lymphedema with a recessive pattern of inheritance, which manifests at puberty. *Lymphedema tarda* is idiopathic lymphedema occurring after age 35 years. Lymphedema can also occur secondary to malignancy, trauma, infection, burns, surgery, or radiation therapy. Neoplasms are the most common cause of secondary lymphedema and should always be considered when one extremity is lymphedematous. Lymphatic obstruction caused by infections such as filariasis may cause lymphedema in endemic areas.

The characteristic clinical presentation is sufficient to make the diagnosis in many cases of established lymphatic disease. Tests are sometimes necessary to confirm the presence and location of impaired lymphatic flow. MRI and CT can demonstrate thickened skin and a characteristic distribution of edema above the fascial compartment. Lymphoscintigraphy may provide a functional assessment of the lymphatic system. Radiolabeled tracer is injected subdermally between the toes, and transport of the tracer is tracked using the gamma camera. Abnormalities seen include absent or delayed transport, crossover filling with backward flow, and delayed imaging of the lymph nodes. Contrast lymphography is not usually necessary but may be performed before lymphatic reconstructive surgery.

The goal of treatment is to reduce edema and prevent fluid accumulation. Effective therapy includes gradient compression stockings. Local heat application can be useful in decreasing edema. Intermittent external compression pressure machines re-

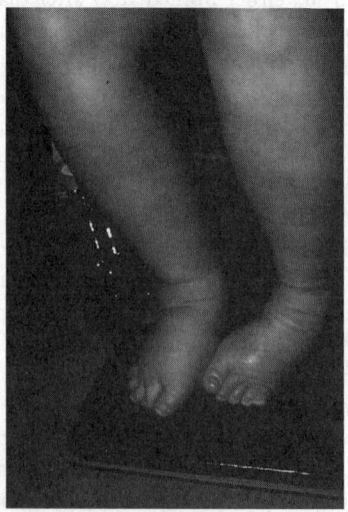

FIGURE 81.10. Lymphedema praecox. Edema is seen throughout the lower extremity and includes the toes.

quire daily use of a minimum of 3 hours. Complex physiotherapy or massage therapy has also been used successfully in lymphedema. Antibiotics are indicated for cellulitis and may be used prophylactically in patients with recurrent episodes of cellulitis. Surgical treatment may be considered in selected cases of severe refractory lymphedema associated with severe extremity disfigurement. Surgical therapy includes excisional procedures and creation of artificial limb channels.

BIBLIOGRAPHY

Ernst CB. Abdominal aortic aneurysm. *N Engl J M* 1993;328:1167–1172.

Hirsh J, Hoak J. AHA Medical/Scientific Statement. Management of deep vein thrombosis and pulmonary embolism. *Circulation* 1996;93:2212–2245.

Hyers TM, Agnelli G, Hull RD, et al. Antithrombotic therapy for venous thromboembolic disease. *Chest* 1998;114:561S–578S.

Kerr GS, Hallahan CW, Giordano J, et al. Takayasu arteritis. *Ann Intern Med* 1994;120:919–929.

Levine M, Gent M, Hirsh J, et al. A comparison of low molecular weight heparin administered primarily at home with unfractionated heparin administered in the hospital for proximal deep vein thrombosis. *N Engl J M* 1996;334:667–681.

Loscalzo J, Creager MA, Dzau VD, eds. *Vascular medicine: a textbook of vascular biology and diseases.* Boston: Little, Brown, 1996.

O'Donnell TF, McEnroe CS, Heggerick P. Chronic venous insufficiency. *Surg Clin North Am* 1990;70:159–180.

Powell JT, for the UK Small Aneurysm Trial Participants. Mortality results for randomized controlled trail of early elective surgery of ultrasonographic surveillance for small abdominal aortic aneurysms. *Lancet* 1998;352;1649–1655.

Prandoni P, Polistena P, Bernardi E, et al. Upper extremity deep vein thrombosis. *Arch Intern Med* 1997;157:57–62.

Szuba A, Rockson SG. Lymphedema: classification, diagnosis, and therapy. *Vasc Med* 1998;3;145–156.

Weitz JI, Byrne J, Clagett GP, et al. Diagnosis and treatment of chronic arterial insufficiency of the lower extremities: a critical review. *Circulation* 1996;94:3026–3049.

Kelley's Textbook of Internal Medicine, fourth edition. Edited by H. David Humes. Lippincott Williams & Wilkins, Philadelphia © 2000.

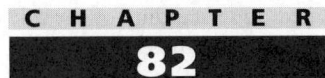

CHAPTER 82

GENETICS OF THE CARDIOVASCULAR SYSTEM

CRAIG T. BASSON
CARL J. VAUGHAN

Recent developments in molecular analysis of cardiovascular disease form the foundation for design of novel diagnostic and therapeutic approaches to patients. Over the last decade, the application of genetic mapping techniques has identified a number of gene defects that cause inherited cardiovascular disorders. Advances have been propelled by the development of a genetic map of highly informative polymorphisms in conjunction with efficient statistical methods for linkage analysis and molecular biologic techniques such as positional cloning. Microsatellite polymorphisms are the most common choice for genetic mapping studies, and the comprehensive genetic maps developed with the support of the Human Genome Project include more than 5,000 microsatellite markers that span the entire genome with an average resolution of 1 centimorgan. These studies have demonstrated a wide variety of defects in structural and contractile proteins, ion channels, transcription factors, signaling molecules, and receptors, which underlie many prominent diseases of the heart and vasculature. Lessons learned in the study of rare monogenic cardiovascular diseases have also provided additional insight into the pathogenesis of more common polygenic disorders such as hypertension and atherosclerosis. While the relative contribution of particular genetic factors to some cardiovascular diseases remains unknown, single- and multiple-gene defects clearly participate in pathogenesis of most cardiovascular disorders. Molecular genetic studies have thus not only defined the mutated disease-causing genes, but have also provided important insights into the cellular and organ physiologic processes whose secrets had remained locked within the genetic code. In this chapter, we describe recent advances in inherited cardiovascular diseases. Although a definitive discussion of all chromosomal loci and genes associated with cardiovascular disease is beyond the scope of this chapter, we will discuss archetypal examples of several categories of cardiovascular disease: (a) dyslipidemias, (b) cardiomyopathies, (c) congenital structural heart disease, (d) arrhythmias, and (e) vascular anomalies.

■ GENERAL APPROACH

As attention increasingly focuses on novel developments in the molecular genetics of cardiovascular disease, a vital, and often overlooked, part of any patient's clinical evaluation is the ascertainment of a family history. A detailed analysis of the family history forms the basis for any subsequent clinical or molecular genetic study. The family pedigree may indicate patterns of heritability (e.g., autosomal versus X-linked or mitochondrial, and dominant versus recessive), provide information on penetrance and expressivity, and focus attention on family members who have not yet been clinically evaluated but who are at risk for a heritable disorder. In the future, genetic testing will become increasingly available in the diagnosis of monogenic cardiovascular disorders, but it currently remains a research tool. As clinicians begin to use DNA-based testing, guidelines need to be developed to indicate when and in whom to conduct such tests. In some cases, DNA-based diagnoses will provide important information to guide diagnosis, surveillance, and therapy. However, genetic testing is not without problems. Used inappropriately, such preclinical testing of asymptomatic individuals may fail to aid management and may be psychologically distressing to patients and their families. Furthermore, establishment of family disease patterns by history, clinical examination, and adjunctive imaging studies is often more than adequate to secure a diagnosis and guide surveillance. Therefore, genetic testing for cardiovascular disease should be applied in a selective manner.

Careful consideration should be given in advance to the likely social, psychological, and economic impact of such testing on a given individual. Patients must be carefully counseled before and after testing by a physician and geneticist with substantial experience in heritable cardiovascular diseases.

GENETICS OF DYSLIPIDEMIAS

Coronary artery disease (CAD) remains the leading cause of morbidity and mortality in the United States. Dyslipidemias, which affect over 140 million adults in the United States, are major risk factors in the development of atherosclerosis and CAD. The term dyslipidemia refers to the abnormal metabolism of plasma lipids and may result from accelerated synthesis or decreased degradation of lipoproteins that transport cholesterol and triglycerides through the plasma. Such abnormal metabolism can be caused by genetic, dietary, or secondary disease factors. Dyslipidemias have been clinically characterized using the Fredrickson classification, which categorizes disorders based on the lipoprotein profile. In this classification, familial hypercholesterolemia (Fredrickson type IIa) and familial combined hyperlipidemia (Fredrickson type IIb or IV) are the most prominent disorders. Other Fredrickson class dyslipidemias are rare; they include type I dyslipidemia, characterized by markedly elevated triglycerides and due to lipoprotein lipase deficiency, and type III hyperlipidemia, in which plasma accumulation of chylomicron remnants and intermediate density lipoprotein occurs.

FAMILIAL HYPERCHOLESTEROLEMIA

Familial hypercholesterolemia (FH) is an autosomal dominant disorder caused by mutation of the low-density lipoprotein receptor *(LDLR)* gene. Familial hypercholesterolemia is common; 1 in 500 individuals is heterozygous for the disorder. Homozygous FH is rare, with a frequency of approximately 1 per million. In addition to elevated serum LDL, affected individuals may exhibit deposition of cholesterol in the cornea (corneal arcus) and in tendons (xanthoma) (Fig. 82.1). In homozygous FH, symptoms of CAD begin in childhood or early adult life. In the heterozygous form, the onset of symptomatic CAD occurs in later life, between ages 40 and 60. Homozygous FH is particularly difficult to treat since the drugs that lower cholesterol depend on a normally functioning LDLR and act primarily by increasing hepatic synthesis of the receptor. Liver-directed *LDLR* gene transfer has been performed in patients with homozygous FH. This approach entails resection of a portion of the liver with harvest of hepatocytes and their infection with a viral vector containing the *LDLR* gene. This technique is not widely available and has only been applied to small numbers of patients. Efforts are ongoing to develop strategies to target the *LDLR* gene to the liver in vivo. This approach has considerable potential and may be a very effective method of lowering LDL in FH. Other strategies that have been employed to lower LDL in patients with homozygous FH include LDL apheresis and hepatic transplantation. Heterozygous FH is treated with a low-cholesterol diet and hydroxymethyl glutaryl–coenzyme A (HMG-CoA) reductase inhibitors (statins), which lower LDL cholesterol by up to 50%.

The *LDLR* locus maps to chromosome 19p13.2-p13.1, and

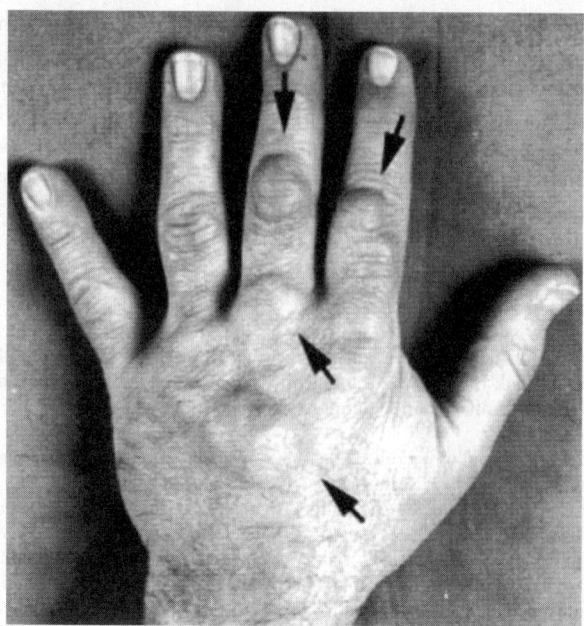

FIGURE 82.1. Tendon xanthoma. Prominent tendon xanthomas *(arrows)* on the hand of a patient affected by homozygous familial hypercholesterolemia. (Courtesy of Dr. Bruce Gordon, Weill Medical College of Cornell University.)

several different mutations in this receptor have been described in FH. Nonsense and frameshift mutations that abrogate translation of the LDLR protein may result in undetectable LDLR levels in the case of homozygous FH or a reduced number of receptors in heterozygous FH. Missense mutations may either hinder intracellular transport and internalization of the receptors (transport-defective alleles) or inhibit receptor binding and endocytosis of LDL. The DNA analysis of FH families is not routinely clinically useful, since diagnosis of specific mutations rarely affects management. A careful family history, with particular attention to the age of onset of myocardial infarction, stroke, and/or peripheral vascular disease, will establish clinical suspicion of FH. The diagnosis can be confirmed by analysis of the lipoprotein profile among family members.

Despite a detailed understanding of the role of the LDLR in FH, our knowledge of the molecular genetic basis for other inherited dyslipidemias remains rudimentary. Familial combined hyperlipidemia (FCH) is the most common dyslipidemia. It occurs with a frequency of 1% in the general population and with a frequency of 10% in patients who have suffered a myocardial infarction. Familial combined hyperlipidemia is characterized by elevated LDL and triglycerides. Although an FCH locus has been described on chromosome 1q21-q23, the specific gene defect responsible for this disorder has not been elucidated.

GENETICS OF CARDIOMYOPATHIES

FAMILIAL HYPERTROPHIC CARDIOMYOPATHY

Familial hypertrophic cardiomyopathy exhibits considerable diversity in terms of its clinical presentation, cardiac morphology, natural history, and molecular genetics. The incidence of the disorder is about 1 in 500. Molecular genetic studies have demonstrated that FHC is genetically heterogeneous and that the defects causing it involve mutations in genes encoding cardiac sarcomere proteins.

The clinical presentation of FHC is highly variable; symptoms may occur at any age and include dyspnea, chest pain, and syncope. Patients may also present with symptoms of overt heart failure. Sudden death may be the initial presentation, most commonly in children and young adults, and often occurs during periods of vigorous physical exertion. Physical findings include a characteristic carotid pulse (pulsus bisferiens), a thrill at the lower sternal border, and a coarse systolic murmur, best heard at the lower left sternal border, that decreases with the patient squatting and is accentuated by the strain phase or phase 2 of the Valsalva maneuver. The electrocardiogram (ECG) is abnormal in most cases of FHC. The most common abnormalities are ST-segment and T-wave abnormalities, followed by increased QRS voltage and evidence of left ventricular hypertrophy. The diagnosis is confirmed with echocardiography (Fig. 82.2), which classically demonstrates asymmetric septal hypertrophy with systolic anterior motion of the anterior mitral valve leaflet and a variable degree of left ventricular outflow tract obstruction. Severity of FHC symptoms may not correlate with the presence or severity of outflow tract obstruction and intracavitary pressure gradient. However, impaired ventricular diastolic filling is generally considered a uniform finding. Because the clinical presentation and spectrum of disease in FHC is so diverse, universally applicable guidelines for management have not been defined. Initial management usually involves therapy with β-blocking drugs or verapamil. Patients with symptoms secondary to outflow tract obstruction that are refractory to pharmacologic therapy may be considered for septal myotomy and myomectomy with or without mitral valve replacement. Septal ablation has also been successfully achieved on an experimental basis through a catheter-based approach by infusion of alcohol

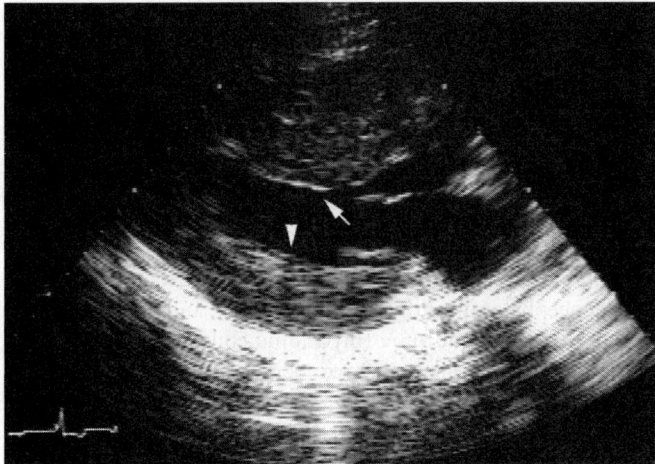

FIGURE 82.2. Hypertrophic cardiomyopathy. Two-dimensional transthoracic echocardiography of a patient with familial hypertrophic cardiomyopathy reveals marked thickening of the left ventricle including the posterior wall *(arrowhead)* and the interventricular septum *(arrow)*. (Courtesy of Dr. Mary Roman, Weill Medical College of Cornell University.)

into the septal perforator branches of the left anterior descending artery. This causes infarction and thinning of the proximal interventricular septum, thus reducing outflow obstruction. Dual-chamber pacemaker therapy has also been used in patients with outflow tract obstruction, but this approach remains controversial. Finally, implantable cardiac defibrillator therapy should be considered in patients at high risk for sudden cardiac death, such as survivors of a cardiac arrest.

Familial hypertrophic cardiomyopathy is inherited as an autosomal dominant trait, although it may also occur in a sporadic manner. Penetrance in familial disease is age-related, with clinical manifestations typically developing by adolescence. Familial hypertrophic cardiomyopathy is a disease of the sarcomere, and mutations in at least eight genes encoding sarcomeric proteins have been described in this disorder. Initial linkage analysis and molecular genetic studies in large families affected by the disorder demonstrated mutations in the cardiac β-myosin heavy chain (β-MHC) gene. To date, molecular genetic studies have revealed mutations in genes encoding the β-MHC (chromosome 14q1), cardiac troponin T (chromosome 1q31), cardiac troponin I (chromosome 19p13.2-q13.2), α-tropomyosin (chromosome 15q2), myosin-binding protein C (chromosome 11p13-q13), ventricular myosin regulatory light chain (chromosome 12q2), ventricular myosin essential light chain (chromosome 3p), and α-cardiac actin (chromosome 15q14). Interestingly, mutation in any of these genes may give rise to a clinically identical phenotype. The numerous *β-MHC* mutations account for 35% to 40% of cases of FHC. Mutations in cardiac troponin T account for disease in approximately 15% of cases, α-tropomyosin 5%, and myosin-binding protein C 10%. The *β-MHC* gene mutations correlate with survival in patients affected by FHC. Several "malignant" mutations have been described that correlate with a poorer prognosis and are associated with a significant risk of sudden death. Conversely, a number of "benign" *β-MHC* mutations are associated with long-term survival. Mutations associated with a worse prognosis are often those that alter the charge in the encoded amino acid residue. Although mutations in cardiac troponin T are often associated with subtle myocardial hypertrophy, survival in these individuals is poor and similar to that of patients with malignant mutation in the *β-MHC* gene. Of note, mutations in myosin-binding protein C are correlated with a benign phenotype and good long-term survival. In addition, cardiac myosin-binding protein C mutations exhibit reduced penetrance until the fifth decade of life, whereas FHC caused by mutations in other genes is almost completely penetrant by the second or third decade. Since left ventricular hypertrophy is relatively common in the elderly and is usually attributed to hypertension, it is possible that mutations in cardiac myosin-binding protein C are more common than expected in the elderly. While rare mutations in α-cardiac actin have been described in patients with dilated cardiomyopathies, recent molecular genetic studies in one family with FHC also have revealed mutations in the α-cardiac actin gene. The cellular mechanisms through which mutated sarcomeric proteins give rise to cardiac hypertrophy in this disorder are unclear. It has been speculated that sarcomeric mutations give rise to abnormal sarcomeric calcium handling, leading to enhanced transcription of cardiac protein genes.

DILATED CARDIOMYOPATHY

Dilated cardiomyopathy is a heterogeneous group of diseases of the myocardium characterized by dilatation and impaired contraction of the left or both ventricles (Fig. 82.3). Dilated cardiomyopathy occurs in approximately 37 per 100,000 individuals, is a frequent cause of heart failure, and is the most common indication for cardiac transplantation in the United States. This disorder usually presents with typical symptoms and signs of congestive heart failure, but it may also present with unexplained fatigue, syncope, and/or sudden death. Metabolic abnormalities (such as vitamin B_1 deficiency), toxins (such as alcohol), and viral infections can cause dilated cardiomyopathy, but there is a growing appreciation that more than 25% of cases are inherited. Familial dilated cardiomyopathy (FDC) has also been described in association with a variety of other cardiac disorders including atrioventricular (AV) block, ventricular tachyarrhythmias, and atrial cardiomyopathy. The application of molecular genetic analysis to this familial disorder has led to the identification of chromosomal locations of several etiologic gene defects.

Autosomal Dominant Cardiomyopathies

Family studies indicate that FDC is transmitted most commonly as an autosomal dominant trait. Less frequently, X-linked and recessive forms are observed. A number of chromosomal loci have been described in autosomal dominant FDC (e.g., chromosome 1p-1q, 1q32, 2q31, 3p25-22, 10q21-23, and 9q13-22). However, the only specific gene implicated thus far is the cardiac actin located on chromosome 15q14. As with FHC, genetic studies of FDC indicate that considerable genetic and clinical heterogeneity exist in this disorder. For example, prominent con-

duction system disease has been described in association with one form of FDC linked to the chromosome 1p-1q locus. Individuals often present in early life with conduction disease and atrial arrhythmias, progressing to congestive heart failure in later life. Missense mutations in the lamin A/C gene have been shown to cause this form of autosomal dominant cardiomyopathy associated with conduction defects. In addition, mutations in desmin, a muscle-specific intermediate filament, as well as cardiac actin have been described in rare families with FDC without conduction defects. Based on observations that mutations in the anchoring portion of cardiac actin cause dilated cardiomyopathy and mutations in cardiac actin that affect actin–myosin binding cause hypertrophic cardiomyopathy, it has been proposed that dilated cardiomyopathy is a consequence of defective transmission of force in cardiomyocytes. The observation that mutations in the nuclear protein lamin A/C cause FDC may suggest that these proteins contribute to force transmission via interaction with cytoskeletal elements. However, the possibility remains that dilated cardiomyopathy may result from nuclear transport dysfunction and cell death.

X-Linked Cardiomyopathy

Two genes related to X-linked cardiomyopathies have been identified: defects in the dystrophin gene are responsible for Duchenne's and Becker's muscular dystrophy, and defects in the tafazzin (G4.5) gene for Barth syndrome. Dystrophin is a member of a large multiprotein complex (the dystrophin-associated glycoprotein complex, or DAG) that links the muscle cytoskeleton to the extracellular matrix, thereby anchoring the cardiomyocytes to the extracellular matrix. In this disorder, characteristic proximal muscle weakness is present, and most patients exhibit a variable degree of cardiac involvement. Heart failure in X-linked Duchenne's muscular dystrophy occurs rapidly after the onset of symptoms in the teens or early 20s. The precise cellular function of tafazzin remains unknown but Barth syndrome secondary to tafazzin mutations is a highly lethal neonatal form of cardiomyopathy associated with other abnormalities including fibroelastosis and neutropenia.

Mitochondrial cardiomyopathies

Mitochondria are maternally inherited, and thus maternal transmission is the hallmark of human mitochondrial disease. Mitochondrial diseases exhibit considerable clinical variability. The development of cardiomyopathy is a common feature of several mitochondrial syndromes such as MELAS syndrome (mitochondrial encephalomyopathy, lactic acidosis, and strokelike episodes); MERFF syndrome (myoclonic epilepsy and ragged red fibers); NADH-coenzyme Q reductase deficiency; Kearn–Sayre syndrome (which also includes a characteristic ocular myopathy and cardiac conduction defects); MIMyCA (maternally inherited myopathy and cardiomyopathy). Mutations in mitochondrial DNA may also occur as secondary genetic abnormalities in other familial and sporadic cardiomyopathies.

Further advances in the genetics of familial cardiomyopathies will not only unravel the molecular pathways that lead to cardiac

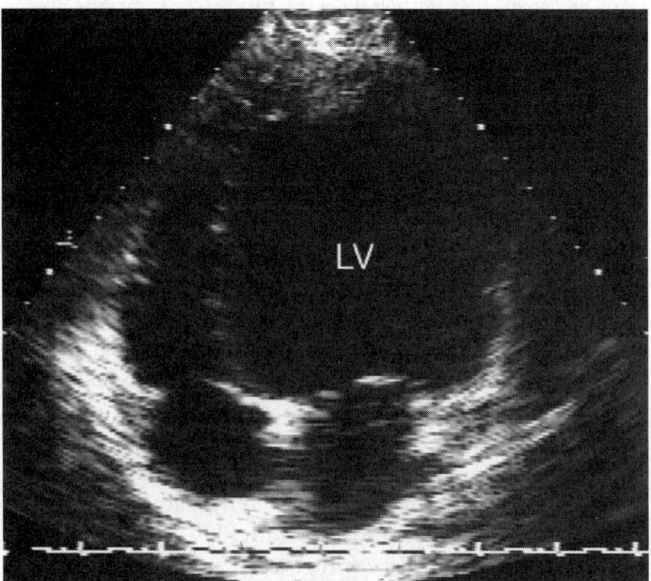

FIGURE 82.3. Dilated cardiomyopathy. Two-dimensional transthoracic echocardiography of a patient with dilated cardiomyopathy reveals marked dilatation of the left ventricular (LV) chamber. (Courtesy of Dr. Mary Roman, Weill Medical College of Cornell University.)

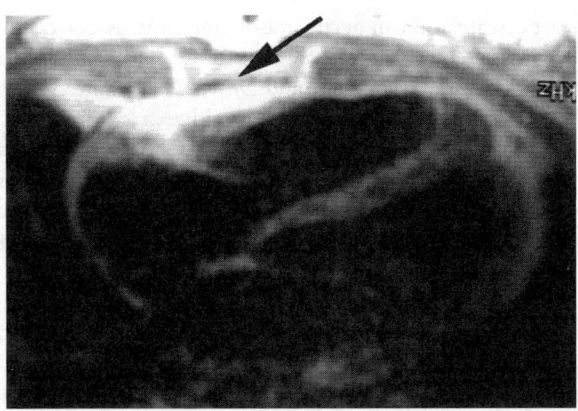

FIGURE 82.4. Arrhythmogenic right ventricular cardiomyopathy. Magnetic resonance imaging of an individual affected by arrhythmogenic right ventricular cardiomyopathy demonstrates extensive fatty infiltration *(bright signal indicated by arrow)* of the anterior wall of the right ventricle. (Courtesy of Dr. Steven Markowitz, Weill Medical College of Cornell University.)

failure but may also direct attention to novel therapeutic targets to prevent or treat these disorders.

ARRHYTHMOGENIC RIGHT VENTRICULAR CARDIOMYOPATHY

Arrhythmogenic right ventricular cardiomyopathy (ARVC) is a recently recognized familial cardiomyopathy characterized by fibrofatty replacement of the right ventricular myocardium. Individuals with ARVC have a propensity to die suddenly from ventricular arrhythmias that originate in the right ventricle and may in fact exhibit left ventricular pathology also. Diagnosis is difficult and may depend on the combined use of electrocardiography, echocardiography, and magnetic resonance imaging (Fig. 82.4). Both autosomal dominant and recessive variants of this disorder have been described and several loci have been reported in the autosomal dominant variant. No specific gene defect has yet been identified. Ultimately, genetic testing in this syndrome will provide an important ancillary diagnostic tool that will assist sudden death risk stratification.

■ GENETICS OF CONGENITAL STRUCTURAL HEART DISEASE

Congenital structural heart disease is estimated to occur in approximately 0.5% of the general population. Early studies of the general population have estimated the risk of recurrent congenital heart disease in a patient with one affected sibling to be 2.3% and in the offspring of an affected mother to be greater than 6.7%. However, the advent and widespread use of diagnostic tools such as color Doppler and transesophageal echocardiography has improved detection of subtle congenital defects, and some studies report an overall neonatal incidence of ventricular septal defects as high as 5%. Bicuspid aortic valve disease and mitral valve prolapse occur in 0.9% and 4% of individuals, respectively. Thus the true incidence of congenital heart defects

has likely been underestimated. Moreover, given that many such defects may be transmitted as autosomal dominant traits, the recurrence risk to an individual with an affected first-degree relative can reach 50%.

SEPTATION DEFECTS

Defects in cardiac septation including atrial septal defect (ASD), ventricular septal defect (VSD), and AV canal septal defects form a major proportion of congenital heart disease. Considerable advances have been made in our understanding of the genetic orchestration of cardiac septation. Mutant genes encoding two transcription factors have been described in families with inherited atrial or ventricular septal defects. Holt–Oram syndrome, also called heart–hand syndrome, is an autosomal dominant condition characterized by upper extremity abnormalities in association with ASDs and VSDs. Mutation of the T-box transcription factor *TBX5* gene causes Holt–Oram syndrome. *TBX5* is expressed in the developing upper limb and heart, and its precise role in cardiogenesis is actively being investigated. Most *TBX5* mutations are truncation mutations (nonsense or frameshift) that result in *TBX5* haploinsufficiency, but missense mutations have been identified. Although *TBX5* haploinsufficiency produces severe malformation of both heart and limbs, the missense mutations thus far identified modify specific DNA binding sites and produce either severe heart or severe limb abnormalities, but not both. Mutations in the homeobox transcription factor gene *NKx2.5* have also been described in families with inherited structural heart disease, in particular ASDs and progressive AV node dysfunction. *NKX* gene family members are homologous to the *Drosophila* tinman gene, which participates in specification of heart muscle progenitors. At least some human *NKx2.5* mutations disrupt the homeobox encoding region of the gene and are predicted to cause disease through *NKx2.5* haploinsufficiency. Mutations in human *NKx2.5* have been described in diverse congenital heart defects, including atrial and ventricular septal defects associated with atrioventricular block, conotruncal defects, and Ebstein's anomaly. The array of anomalies attributable to mutation in *NKx2.5* has led to the suggestion that these anomalies may reflect indirect effects of *NKx2.5* on multiple cardiac structures due to a critical role for *NKx2.5* in early cardiac development and cardiac looping.

CONOTRUNCAL ANOMALIES

Conotruncal defects are cardiac anomalies thought to result from a disturbance of ventricular outflow tract morphogenesis or impairment of branchial arch development. Conotruncal anomalies include truncus arteriosus, tetralogy of Fallot (TOF), interrupted aortic arch, transposition of the great vessels, double-outlet right ventricle, and posterior malalignment VSD (Fig. 82.5). Conotruncal abnormalities account for approximately 15% of congenital heart disease. Conotruncal anomalies have been associated with two overlapping human syndromes: the velocardiofacial syndrome and DiGeorge syndrome. Velocardiofacial syndrome is a syndrome including cleft palate, cardiac anomalies, and a characteristic facial phenotype. DiGeorge syndrome includes absent thymus and parathyroid glands, as well as cardiac outflow

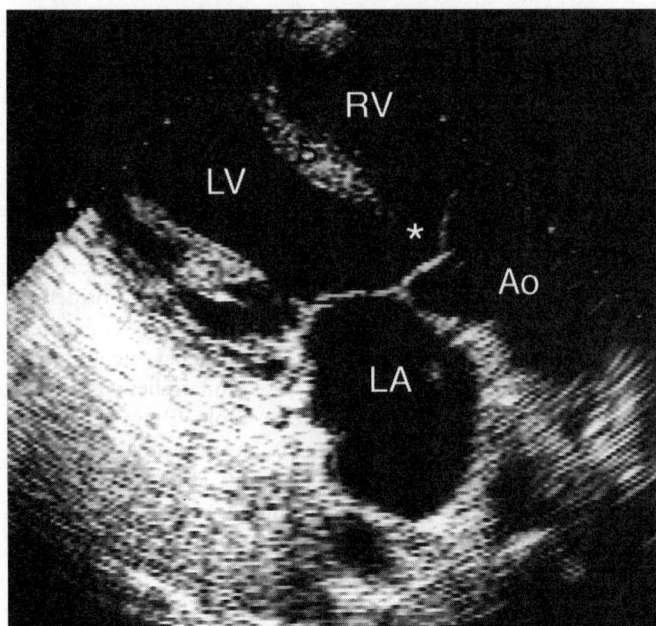

FIGURE 82.5. Double-outlet right ventricle conotruncal defect. Two-dimensional transthoracic echocardiography of a patient with a dou-ble-outlet right ventricle demonstrates typical anatomical features of this and other conotruncal defects such as tetralogy of Fallot. Note the subaortic ventricular septal defect (*) created by the malalignment of the aortic (Ao) outflow tract overriding the interventricular septum dividing the anatomical left ventricle (LV) from the right ventricle. The left atrium (LA) is denoted as well.

tract anomalies with abnormal facies. These syndromes are often aggregated under the acronym CATCH 22 (cardiac anomalies, abnormal facies, thymic hypoplasia, cleft palate, hypocalcemia).

Initial studies described a deletion of chromosome 22q in DiGeorge syndrome, and subsequent analyses showed that deletions in chromosome 22q were present in both isolated cono-truncal abnormalities and the velocardiofacial syndrome. Accordingly, karyotyping and fluorescent in situ hybridization analysis (FISH) with probes specific to the chromosome 22q11 is now a recommended part of the standard evaluation of individuals with conotruncal anomalies. The minimally deleted region of chromosome 22 is currently estimated to be approximately 250 kb of DNA. The CATCH 22 syndrome is thought to result from deletion of contiguous genes and the 22q locus contains a number of genes (e.g., *clathrin heavy chain protein, CDC45L, HIRA,* and *UFDIL*) that are currently under investigation. Further work will define the gene(s) involved and the nature of the aberrant gene product underlying this variable constellation of anomalies.

Tetralogy of Fallot was initially thought to be a multicomponent disorder comprising ventricular septal defect with pulmonic stenosis, overriding aorta, and right ventricular hypertrophy. It is now recognized that TOF is primarily a failure of right ventricular infundibulum development with the accompaning anatomical abnormalities a manifestation of this embryonic field defect. Experimental studies in chick embryos support this concept and indicate that TOF is one form of anomalous conotruncal development. It accounts for approximately 10% of congeni-

tal heart disease and can occur in isolation or in association with ASDs, or AV septal defects, as well as more complex syndromes such as Holt–Oram syndrome and Down's syndrome. Tetralogy of Fallot frequently occurs in patients with extracardiac manifestations that comprise the characteristic CHARGE syndrome (colobomata, heart defects, choanal atresia, retardation, genital hypoplasia, and ear abnormalities). Investigations have revealed that chromosome 22q11 microdeletions are present in 15% of TOF patients as well as in 50% of interrupted aortic arch patients, 35% of truncus arteriosus patients, and 33% of posterior malalignment VSD patients. Microdeletions in chromosome 22q11 have also been described in cases of double-outlet right ventricle. All conotruncal anomalies may reflect de novo genetic events, but they can also be transmitted in an autosomal dominant fashion. Offspring of individuals with conotruncal abnormalities such as CATCH 22 or TOF may have a 50% risk of congenital heart disease. Prenatal diagnosis in families with chromosome 22q11 deletions is clinically available.

GENETICS OF CARDIAC ARRHYTHMIAS

Cardiac arrhythmias are common and lead to considerable morbidity and mortality. It is increasingly recognized that many arrhythmias have a heritable basis including atrial fibrillation, Wolff–Parkinson–White syndrome, and, most notably, the hereditary long QT syndrome (LQTS).

HEREDITARY LONG QT SYNDROME

Long QT syndrome is usually an autosomal dominant genetic disorder characterized (Fig. 82.6) by prolonged ventricular repolarization on the ECG and a predilection for syncope, polymorphic ventricular tachycardia (torsades de pointes), and sudden cardiac death. This syndrome has been clinically characterized in two forms: (a) the Romano–Ward variant and (b) the more rare autosomal recessive Jervell and Lange–Nielsen variant, which is associated with congenital deafness. A number of specific mutations in cardiac sodium and potassium ion channels have been identified in this disorder.

Long QT syndrome is characterized by prolongation of the QT interval and T-wave abnormalities on the ECG (Fig. 82.6). It has been estimated that LQTS is responsible for 3,000 to 4,000 sudden deaths in the United States each year. Symptoms typically begin in teenage years, but they may begin in early childhood or as late as middle age. Syncope occurs in over 50% of gene carriers, and sudden death occurs in 10% to 30% of symptomatic patients, more commonly in those with a history of syncope or resuscitated cardiac arrest. Syncope and sudden death most commonly occur during exercise or emotional stress but may also occur during sleep. Events may be precipitated by drugs that prolong the QT interval or by electrolyte abnormality. Long QT syndrome should be suspected in any case of unexplained syncope, especially when syncope occurs in association with exercise or emotional upset. A corrected QT (QTc) interval of 480 milliseconds in females or 470 milliseconds in males, in the absence of drugs or electrolyte abnormality, corroborates the

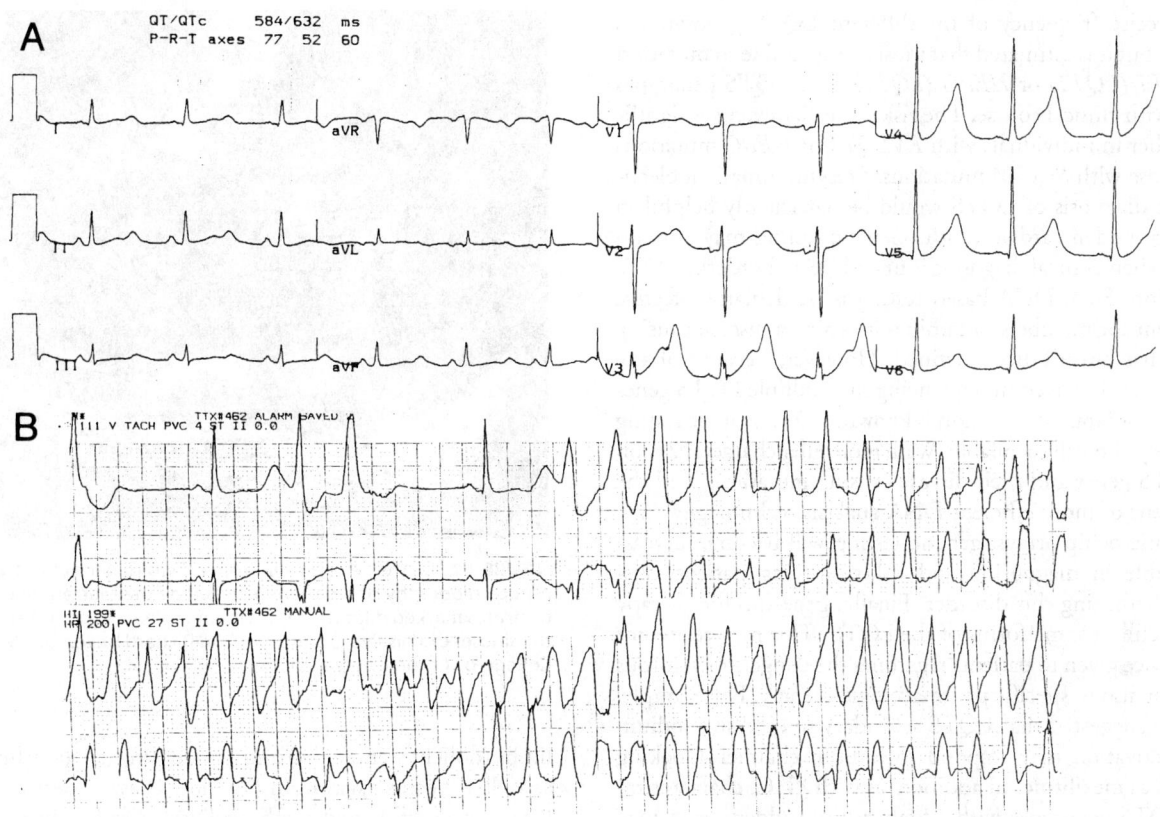

FIGURE 82.6. Hereditary long QT syndrome. **A:** This 12-lead electrocardiogram of a patient who presented with syncope demonstrates marked QTc interval prolongation (632 milliseconds) and bifid T waves consistent with long QT syndrome. **B:** Telemetry recording of the same patient during the onset of polymorphic ventricular tachycardia (torsades de pointes).

diagnosis. In about 10% of patients the QTc will be normal. In addition, T-wave abnormalities are common, especially bifid T waves. There is considerable variability in clinical presentation, at times making diagnosis difficult. To assist diagnosis, diagnostic criteria incorporating electrocardiographic, clinical, and family history have been developed. Therapy is recommended for all symptomatic subjects. Because 30% of LQTS sudden deaths occur as the primary event, some investigators also recommend therapy for all asymptomatic subjects under age 40. Initial therapy for most patients is β-blockade. Other therapies include permanent pacemaker insertion and implantation of cardiac defibrillators, which are increasingly used to prevent sudden death in this disorder.

Molecular genetic studies have revealed that LQTS is genetically and clinically heterogeneous. It results from mutations in genes that encode cardiomyocyte ion channels. Heterozygous mutations in the potassium channel genes *KVLQT1, KCNE1 (minK), KCNE2,* and *HERG,* and the cardiac sodium channel gene *SCN5A,* cause autosomal dominant LQTS. Autosomal recessive LQTS, which is associated with deafness and comprises the Jervell and Lange-Nielsen syndrome, occurs with homozygous mutations in *KVLQT1* and *KCNE1.* Mutation of the *KVLQT1* gene at the *LQT1* locus on chromosome 11 gives rise to an abnormal potassium channel protein (α subunit). Similarly, mutation of the *HERG* gene at the *LQT2* locus on chromo-

some 7 also gives rise to an abnormal potassium channel. Mutations in the *minK* gene have been identified at the *LQT5* locus on chromosome 21. Very recently, a novel potassium channel subunit gene, *KCNE2,* has been cloned and localized to chromosome 21q22.1. *KCNE2* encodes *MiRP1* (Mink-related peptide 1), a small membrane protein that coassembles with *HERG,* and *MiRP1* mutations have been identified in LQTS patients. Mutation of the *SCN5A* gene at the *LQT3* locus on chromosome 3 results in an abnormal sodium channel that fails to inactivate sodium inflow with consequent abnormal myocardial repolarization.

Cardiac potassium channels contribute to the termination of the action potential, and LQTS mutations in these channels have been thought to prolong the cardiac action potential through a "loss-of-function mutation." Sodium channels initiate the myocellular action potential, and then close and remain inactivated. It is generally believed that LQTS mutations in the sodium channel cause it to remain open, thus prolonging the action potential. This concept has been termed a "gain-of-function" mutation. In the case of the HERG channel, it appears that intracellular trafficking of the mutant channel is defective whereby the mutant channel is not translocated from the Golgi apparatus to the cell membrane. Thus, there are a reduced number of normally functioning potassium channels in the cell membrane and consequent abnormal myocellular repolarization.

The precise frequency of the different LQTS genotypes is unknown, but it is estimated that most disease is due to mutation of *KVLQT1 (LQT1)* or *HERG (LQT2)*. The LQTS genotypes correlate with clinical course. The risk of cardiac events is significantly higher in individuals with *KVLQT1* or *HERG* mutations than in those with *SCN5A* mutations. Presymptomatic molecular genetic diagnosis of LQTS would be particularly helpful in preventing sudden cardiac death. Genetic testing may also aid diagnosis when clinical diagnosis is unclear, e.g., borderline QTc prolongation. Such DNA-based testing is particularly effective and efficient for members of families in which a disease-causing mutation has already been defined. However, because of the labor and costs involved in sequencing the multiple LQTS genes when no prior familial mutation is known, LQTS genetic testing is not widely clinically available. With molecular characterization of all LQTS genes and their disease-causing mutations, and the development of more efficient DNA analysis technologies such as DNA microchip arrays, genetic testing will become increasingly feasible in diagnosing and risk-stratifying patients suspected of harboring this disorder. Finally, gene-specific therapy may be useful in some forms of the LQTS. This may relate not only to advice given to patients regarding the dangers of vigorous exercise but also to specific pharmacologic therapy. For example, it has been suggested that LQTS secondary to excessive sodium channel activation may respond to sodium channel–blocking drugs such as mexilitine. In addition, as with FHC, characterization of LQTS genotypes with a high risk of sudden death may prompt consideration of prophylactic implantable defibrillator implantation.

■ GENETICS OF INHERITED VASCULAR DISEASE

There is a wide spectrum of inherited vascular disease. Some disorders reflect disease of large vessels and extracellular matrix assembly, e.g., Marfan's syndrome (fibrillin mutation) and type IV Ehlers–Danlos syndrome (type III procollagen gene mutation). Other inherited disorders reflect disease of the microvasculature, e.g., hereditary hemorrhagic telangiectasia (HHT), also known as Rendu–Osler–Weber syndrome (endoglin or activin receptor–like kinase 1 mutation).

THE MARFAN SYNDROME

Although the Marfan syndrome was recognized as a heritable disorder of connective tissue more than 40 years ago, the precise molecular defect was discovered in 1991. The Marfan syndrome is named after the Parisian pediatrician who in 1896 described severe skeletal abnormalities in a child with the syndrome that now bears his name. The Marfan syndrome is estimated to affect 1 in 20,000 people and exhibits an autosomal dominant pattern of inheritance. In the classic Marfan syndrome, skeletal, ocular, and cardiovascular abnormalities are present. However, there is wide phenotypic variation in the syndrome's expressivity, ranging from mild skeletal involvement and ocular anomalies, to severe neonatal disease with lethal cardiovascular malformations. Skeletal abnormalities comprise a tall thin stature with long thin

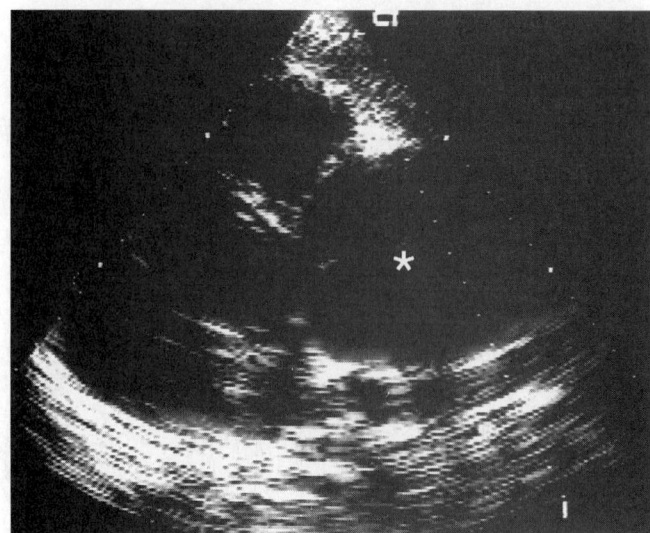

FIGURE 82.7. The Marfan syndrome. Two-dimensional transthoracic echocardiography of a patient affected by the Marfan syndrome demonstrates marked dilatation (6.3 cm) of the aortic root (*) at the level of the sinuses of Valsalva. (Courtesy of Dr. Richard Devereux, Weill Medical College of Cornell University.)

limbs (dolichostenomelia) and "spider fingers" (arachnodactyly) as well as pectus excavatum ("hollow chest"), pectus carinatum ("pigeon chest"), and kyphoscoliosis. Ocular disease includes lens abnormalities with myopia and ectopia lentis as well as a predisposition to retinal detachment. Cardiovascular disease is the most lethal manifestation of the Marfan syndrome and includes dilatation of the ascending aorta (Fig. 82.7), aortic valvular insufficiency, and aortic dissection. The mitral valve is also commonly affected and exhibits thickened nodular leaflets, leaflet fenestration, and disrupted chordal attachments. Mitral valve prolapse with regurgitation and congestive heart failure is a common indication for mitral valve replacement in young children affected by the disorder. Composite aortic valve replacement with ascending aortic conduit surgery (Bental procedure) is usually recommended when moderate aortic insufficiency is present or when the maximal aortic root diameter exceeds 5.5 cm. Clinical studies have shown that pharmacologic therapy with β-blocking drugs may influence both absolute aortic growth rate and aortic growth rate adjusted for age and body size in Marfan patients. Consequently, β-blockade is recommended in most Marfan patients to attenuate aortic dilatation.

The Marfan syndrome is transmitted as an autosomal dominant trait due to mutations in the chromosome 15q fibrillin-1 *(FBN-1)* gene, and approximately 25% of cases represent de novo mutations. Immunohistochemical studies show that the extracellular matrix protein fibrillin, abundant in the aorta and the suspensory ligament of the lens, may be defective or deficient in Marfan patients. Mutations in the related chromosome 5q fibrillin-2 gene cause congenital contractural arachnodactyly, a condition that shares some of the features of the Marfan syndrome but does not include cardiovascular disease. Since the identification of the first mutation in *FBN-1* more than 80 mutations of the gene have been described. Mutations are evenly spaced along the *FBN-1* gene and cause a wide phenotypic spectrum even within families with the same *FBN-1* mutation. Over 60% of the mutations are missense mutations. Cysteine substitutions are particularly common and give rise to instability within the fibrillin molecule. Approximately 30% of mutations result in *FBN-1* haploinsufficiency with resultant defective microfibrillar structure. Most families have unique *FBN-1* mutations, and thus the widespread clinical application of molecular probes to diagnose the Marfan syndrome is limited. Mutational analysis is restricted to families in which a mutation in *FBN-1* has already been described since complete sequence analysis of the large 100-kb *FBN-1* gene is labor-intensive and remains a research tool. In large families, presymptomatic or prenatal screening is possible using haplotype segregation analysis with highly polymorphic markers of *FBN-1*. Recently, *FBN-1* mutations have been described in patients with ascending thoracic aortic aneurysms but without a classic Marfan body habitus. Therefore, *FBN-1* mutations may also contribute to isolated thoracic aortic aneurysmal disease. Genotype/phenotype correlation studies have shown that the clinical criteria used to diagnose the Marfan syndrome are accurate. Therefore, the diagnosis of the Marfan syndrome can be made in most suspected cases through the careful application of these criteria.

SUPRAVALVULAR AORTIC STENOSIS

Supravalvular aortic stenosis (SVAS) is also a disorder of connective tissue matrix assembly that may present as an isolated familial autosomal dominant disorder or as a feature of the autosomal dominant Williams syndrome, which is characterized by SVAS in association with an abnormal "elfin" facies, mental retardation, and hypercalcemia. Rearrangements and deletions in the chromosome 7q11.2 elastin gene are responsible for isolated SVAS, and more complex rearrangements of this chromosomal region are found in Williams syndrome. Studies in mice heterozygous for the elastin gene show an increased number of elastic lamellae and smooth muscle in the arterial wall.

HEREDITARY HEMORRHAGIC TELANGIECTASIA

Hereditary hemorrhagic telangiectasia (HHT), or Osler–Rendu–Weber syndrome, is an autosomal dominant systemic vascular dysplasia with an incidence of 1 in 40,000. The disorder is characterized by mucosal, cutaneous, and visceral telangiectasias that have a predilection for recurrent hemorrhage, especially from mucosal surfaces and within the gastrointestinal tract. In addition, arteriovenous malformations (sometimes with clinically significant shunts) may develop in the pulmonary, cerebral, or hepatic circulations. Pathologic analysis reveals that telangiectasias are lined by a single layer of endothelium attached to a continuous basement membrane. Linkage analysis led to the identification of two loci for HHT, one at chromosome 9q33-q34 *(HHT1)* and the other on chromosome 12q *(HHT2)*. Mutations in the gene encoding endoglin at *HHT1* cause HHT. Endoglin is the most abundant transforming growth factor β (TGF-β) binding protein on the surface of endothelial cells. Mutations in the activin receptor–like kinase *(ALK1)* gene have been described at *HHT2*. It has been suggested that endoglin

binds TGF-β and presents it to the *ALK1* signaling complex, which in turn modulates signal transduction in endothelial cells. This endoglin/*ALK1* cellular pathway is critical for angiogenesis, and although mouse models deficient in endoglin exhibit normal vasculogenesis, they exhibit lethal arrested angiogenesis.

Telangiectasias are components of several other familial syndromes. For example, families with autosomal dominant mucocutaneous venous malformations, such as the "blue rubber-bleb nevus" syndrome, have been shown to have a missense mutation in the endothelial cell specific tyrosine kinase *(TIE2)* gene, which maps to chromosome 9p21.

■ INHERITED CARDIAC TUMORS

Although rare, cardiac tumors may present as components of complex heritable disorders. Cardiac rhabdomyomata and myxomas are the most common tumors of infancy and adulthood, respectively, and both can be heritable traits. Cardiac rhabdomyoma is an important feature of neonatal autosomal dominant tuberous sclerosis. This disorder is characterized by skin lesions and by neurologic and ophthalmologic anomalies. Tuberous sclerosis is most often due to mutations in the *TSCI* gene (chromosome 9q34) or the *TSC2* gene (chromosome 16p13.3). In tuberous sclerosis, rhabdomyomata may be multiple and may occur in more than one cardiac chamber. More than half of all infants with cardiac rhabdomyomata have tuberous sclerosis, and all infants with rhabdomyomata should be evaluated for clinical features of tuberous sclerosis. Importantly, cardiac rhabdomyomata in infants with tuberous sclerosis might not require surgical resection because most spontaneously regress during childhood and patients remain asymptomatic.

Cardiac myxomas are the most common primary cardiac tumor in the general population and occur with a frequency of 7 per 10,000 individuals. Although myxomas are usually sporadic, several autosomal dominant familial syndromes that combine lentiginosis and cardiac myxomas have been described. Previously termed syndromes such as LAMB (lentigines, atrial myxomas, mucocutaneous myxomas, and blue nevi) syndrome and NAME (nevi, atrial myxoma, myxoid neurofibroma, and ephelides) are now grouped under the broader category of Carney complex, which accounts for 7% of all cardiac myxomas. Myxomas in the Carney complex (Fig. 82.8) are often multiple, can occur in any cardiac chamber, and have a predilection to recur after surgical resection. Although usually benign, cardiac myxomas are associated with significant cardiac morbidity due to stroke from tumor embolization and due to heart failure from intracardiac obstruction. Individuals with Carney complex also exhibit spotty pigmentation of the skin, particularly on the face, trunk, lips, and sclera. Extracardiac myxomas may also occur in the breast, testis, thyroid, or adrenal gland. Patients can exhibit a variety of endocrine disorders, including Cushing's syndrome secondary to primary pigmented nodular adrenocortical hyperplasia. The gene defect that produces the cardiovascular and cutaneous disease in Carney complex is unknown. Initial genetic analyses suggested that a gene defect maps to chromosome 2p. More recent linkage analysis in several families affected by the Carney complex has also mapped a disease locus to chromosome

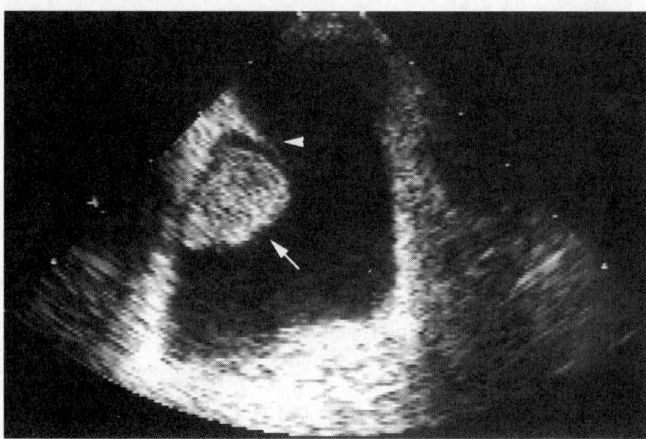

FIGURE 82.8. Right atrial myxoma in the Carney complex. Transesophageal echocardiogram of a woman with autosomal dominant Carney complex. Patient has spotty hyperpigmentation of the skin and had previously undergone cardiac surgery to resect a left atrial myxoma. Echocardiography done after patient presented with constitutional symptoms demonstrated a large pedunculated right atrial myxoma *(arrow)* abutting the eustachian valve *(arrowhead)*.

17q2. Identification of the Carney complex disease gene(s) will enhance our diagnosis and management of patients with cardiac myxomas, and will also provide insights into basic mechanisms that regulate cardiac growth and differentiation.

BIBLIOGRAPHY

Basson CT, Bachinsky DR, Lin RC, et al. Mutations in human TBX5 cause limb and cardiac malformation in Holt–Oram syndrome. *Nat Genet* 1997;15:30–35.

Fatkin D, MacRae C, Sasaki T, et al. Missense mutations in the rod domain of the lamin A/C gene as a cause of dilated cardiomyopathy and conduction-system disease. *N Engl J Med* 1999;341:1715–1724.

Goldmuntz E, Clarke BJ, Mitchell LE, et al. Frequency of 22q11 microdeletions in patients with conotruncal defects. *J Am Coll Cardiol* 1998;32:492–498.

Hobbs HH, Brown MS, Goldstein JL. Molecular genetics of the LDL receptor gene in familial hypercholesterolemia. *Hum Mutat* 1992;1:445–466.

Keating MT. Genetic approaches to cardiovascular disease. Supravalvular aortic stenosis, Williams syndrome, and the long-QT syndrome. *Circulation* 1995;92:142–147.

Kelly DP, Strauss AW. Inherited cardiomyopathies. *N Engl J Med* 1994;330:913–919.

Mah CS, Vaughan CJ, Basson CT. Advances in the molecular genetics of congenital structural heart disease. *Genet Test* 1999;3:157–172.

Maron BJ, Moller JH, Seidman CE, et al. Impact of laboratory molecular diagnosis on contemporary diagnostic criteria for genetically transmitted cardiovascular diseases: hypertrophic cardiomyopathy, long-QT syndrome, and Marfan syndrome. A statement for healthcare professionals from the Councils on Clinical Cardiology, Cardiovascular Disease in the Young, and Basic Science, American Heart Association. *Circulation* 1998;98:1460–1471.

Roden DM, Lazzara R, Rosen M, et al. Multiple mechanisms in the long-QT syndrome: current knowledge, gaps and future directions. The SADS Foundation Task Force on LQTS. *Circulation* 1996;94:1996–2012.

Schott JJ, Benson DW, Basson CT, et al. Congenital heart disease caused by mutations in the transcription factor NKX2-5. *Science* 1998;281:108–111.

Spirito P, Seidman CE, McKenna WJ, Maron BJ. The management of hypertrophic cardiomyopathy. *N Engl J Med* 1997;336:775–785.

Kelley's Textbook of Internal Medicine, fourth edition. Edited by H. David Humes.
Lippincott Williams & Wilkins, Philadelphia © 2000.

DIAGNOSTIC AND THERAPEUTIC MODALITIES IN CARDIOVASCULAR DISEASES

CHAPTER

83

CARDIOVASCULAR RADIOLOGY

ROBERT D. TARVER
DEWEY J. CONCES, JR.
LYNN S. BRODERICK

Despite the development of many sophisticated imaging modalities, the plain chest roentgenogram remains the most commonly used method for the study of the cardiovascular system. Chest roentgenograms make up more than half of all radiographic studies performed. In a significant percentage, the reason for the examination is to help evaluate the cardiovascular status of the patient. Because of the low density of the air-containing lungs, it is possible, without the injection of contrast material, to discern the size and configuration of the heart, the pulmonary arteries and veins, and the aorta. In no other area of the body is detailed anatomy so well shown on plain roentgenograms.

Most chest roentgenograms are performed in the posteroant-erior (PA) projection, with the X-ray tube 6 feet from the plane of the film. Because of the long tube-to-film distance and the fact that the heart is in the anterior portion of the chest, magnification of the heart is minimized to about 10%. Chest roentgenograms are routinely obtained in the upright position in full inspiration. In infants, the anteroposterior (AP) projection, with the patient in the supine position, is used. Portable roentgenograms are almost always performed in the AP position. If possible, the patient is positioned in a sitting position. On occasion, these examinations must be performed with the patient supine, although this is less desirable. Because portable roentgenography is done in the AP projection, there is greater magnification of the heart as compared with PA films performed in the radiology department. The tube-to-film distance is also frequently less on portable roentgenograms than the 6-foot-distance standard for PA films. For these reasons, the apparent cardiac size may be 10% to 20% larger on portable roentgenograms as compared with chest films performed in the radiology department.

The borders of the mediastinum are clearly outlined against the dark, air-containing lung. On the PA view (Fig. 83.1), the upper right margin is usually formed by the superior vena cava. In older or hypertensive patients in whom the aorta is larger, the ascending aorta may become border forming in this segment. The remainder of the right cardiac border is formed by the right atrium. On occasion, if the patient has taken a deep breath, the

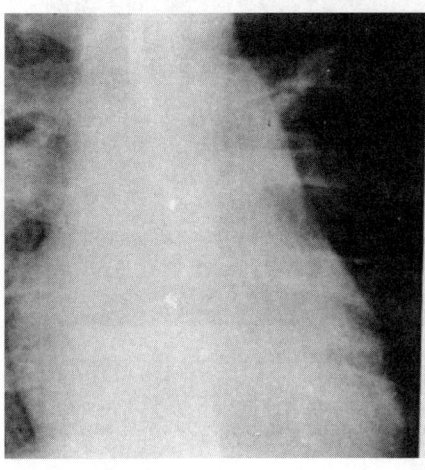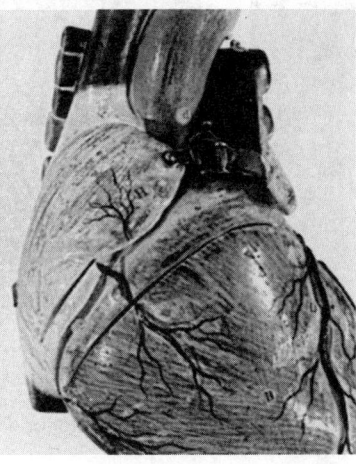

FIGURE 83.1. Comparison of a posteroanterior roentgenogram and anatomical model of the heart, anterior view. The superior right margin is formed by the superior vena cava. The remainder of the right cardiac border is formed by the right atrium. The inferior vena cava joins the right atrium just superiorly to the diaphragm. The left cardiac border comprises the aortic arch, pulmonary artery, left atrial appendage, and left ventricle.

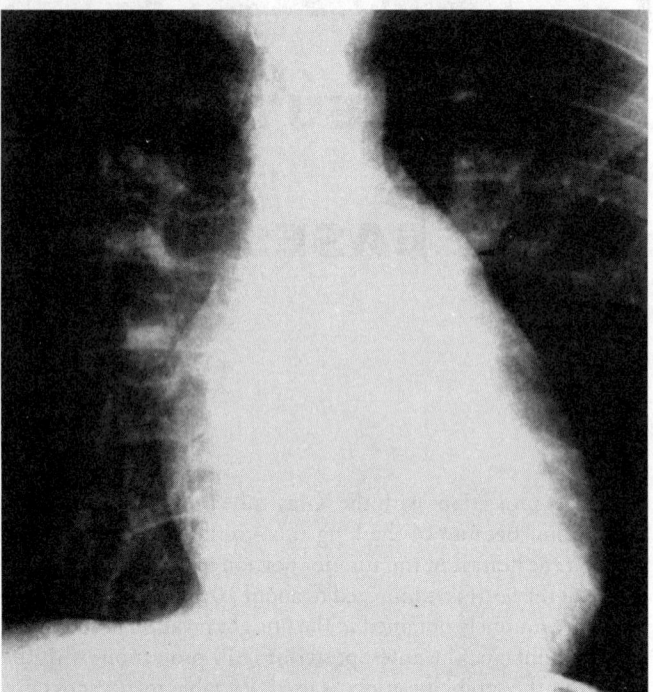

FIGURE 83.2. A 33-year-old woman with atrial septal defect had enlargement of the right atrium and right ventricle. The right cardiac margin is normal in spite of the enlargement of the right atrium. With dilatation of the right ventricle, the heart rotates in a clockwise fashion so that the right ventricular margin may extend to the left cardiac border. This gives the heart a globular shape with some elevation of the apex. Note the enlargement of the pulmonary artery *(arrowhead)*.

inferior vena cava may be discerned as a straight line along the inferolateral aspect of the right cardiac margin. On the left side, the superior margin is made up of the aortic arch. The right margin of the aorta indents the trachea at this level, so that the diameter of the aortic arch may be discerned. Below the aortic arch is a convex bulge comprising the pulmonary trunk and left pulmonary artery. It may vary in size in normal persons and is inclined to be more prominent in young women. Below the pulmonary trunk is the left atrial appendage. This usually cannot be discerned in a normal person; however, with left atrial enlargement, a convex bulge of the left atrial appendage may be apparent below the pulmonary trunk (Fig. 83.2). The remainder of the left cardiac margin and apex is formed by the left ventricle. The right ventricle is not border forming either to the right or to the left. On the lateral view (Fig. 83.3), the superoanterior margin is made up of the ascending aorta. The right ventricle and right atrium make up the inferior aspect of the anterior margin. The posterior margin of the heart superiorly is the left atrium, and more inferiorly it is the left ventricle. The inferior vena cava usually can be seen also as a straight line on the inferior aspect of the posterior cardiac margin. The relationship of cardiac chambers is shown in Figures 83.2 and 83.3.

CARDIOVASCULAR MEASUREMENTS

The size of the heart is related to the size of the patient. Charts are available that compare normal cardiac size with height, weight, and surface areas of patients. From a practical viewpoint, they are rarely used. The most common measurement is the

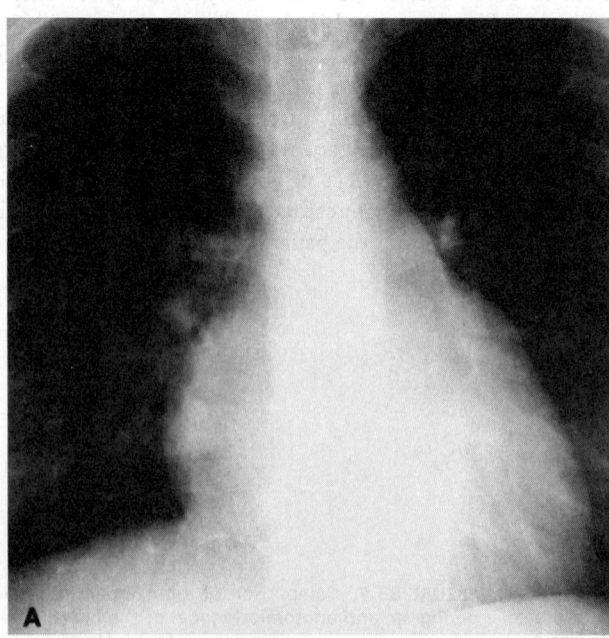

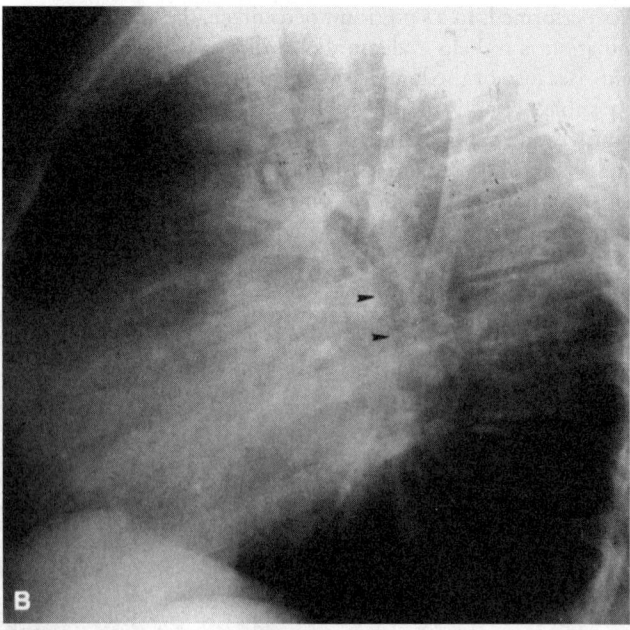

FIGURE 83.3. Mitral stenosis with enlargement of the left atrium and right ventricle. **A:** Posteroanterior view shows the enlarged left atrial appendage forming a convex bulge below the pulmonary artery *(arrowhead)*. **B:** Lateral view shows a dilated right ventricle filling in the retrosternal space. The large left atrium can be seen as a convex bulge posteriorly. Note the posterior displacement of the left lower lobe bronchus by the large left atrium *(arrowheads)*.

cardiothoracic ratio. The greatest distance of the heart to the right of the midline plus the greatest distance of the heart to the left of the midline is divided by the transverse thoracic diameter at the level of the right diaphragm. This ratio is usually between 0.45 and 0.5. The ratio is larger in children and persons of hypersthenic habitus. If serial films are available, the changing cardiac status may best be measured by comparing the transverse cardiac diameter. It must be reemphasized that portable roentgenograms are obtained in the AP projection, which may result in an apparent 10% to 20% increase in the transverse cardiac diameter as a result of differences of magnification. Cardiac size may vary as the result of differences in blood volume as well as cardiac decompensation. Patients who are severely dehydrated may have small cardiac silhouettes that return to normal after hydration. Patients who are overhydrated may have a significant increase in cardiac size despite normal cardiac function. This is commonly seen in a patient receiving intravenous fluids or patients with chronic renal failure on dialysis. A change of transverse cardiac diameter greater than 2 cm on serial roentgenograms performed in the same projection are usually indicative of a change in the physiologic status of the heart.

Aortic size is important in the evaluation of the systemic circuit. Because of changes in the elastic tissue of the aortic media, the aorta gradually dilates throughout life. There is thus a change in aortic configuration with aging. The ascending aorta usually is not discerned in young persons but is readily seen in older persons as well as in those with hypertension or aortic stenosis. A useful measurement is that of the aortic arch, which is made up of the junction of the transverse and descending aorta. The lateral margin is visible on almost all PA roentgenograms. The aorta also has an indentation on the trachea at the same point. In a man in his 40s, the aortic arch diameter is about 3 cm. This can be corrected for age by adding or subtracting 2 mm for each decade of life. A measurement of the aorta in female patients is 2 mm less than that of male patients. Patients with hypertension have significantly larger aortas, usually 4 to 5 mm greater than those of their normotensive counterparts.

ASSESSMENT OF CHAMBER SIZE

The right atrium forms the entire right cardiac border on the PA projection. One might assume, if the right atrium were to enlarge, that the right cardiac margin would extend farther to the right. Although this can occasionally be noted in patients with massive enlargement of the right atrium, the right cardiac margin is rarely changed in patients with right atrial enlargement (Fig. 83.4). When the right atrium enlarges, it frequently does so anteriorly and may be border forming anteriorly, as noted on the lateral projection. This may encroach on the retrosternal space.

With increasing volume, the right ventricle enlarges anteriorly. The heart also rotates in a clockwise fashion (as viewed from below). Normally, the left atrium and left ventricle form the left cardiac border; however, when the right ventricle enlarges as the result of the clockwise rotation, the upper left cardiac border may be formed by the right ventricle. This changes the configuration of the left cardiac border as seen on a PA chest roentgenogram, so that there is straightening or, at times, bulging of the upper left cardiac border, giving the heart a globular shape (Fig. 83.4). There also may be some elevation of the cardiac apex. On the lateral view, the enlarged right ventricle encroaches on the retrosternal space (Fig. 83.2B). Because the retrosternal space may vary depending on the habitus of the patient, this sign has limited value.

The left atrium is a posterior structure. As it enlarges, it forms a convex bulge on the posterosuperior portion of the heart as viewed in the lateral projections. If there is barium in the esophagus, an enlarged left atrium will displace the esophagus posteriorly. The enlarged left atrium also may displace the left lower lobe bronchus posteriorly as viewed on the lateral view (Fig. 83.2B). On the PA projection, an enlarged left atrial appendage may form a convex bulge below the pulmonary artery (Fig. 83.2A). Also, as there is an increase in left atrial size, the enlarged left atrium may be surrounded by air-containing lung, so that its margins are visualized, giving it a double density on the PA roentgenograms.

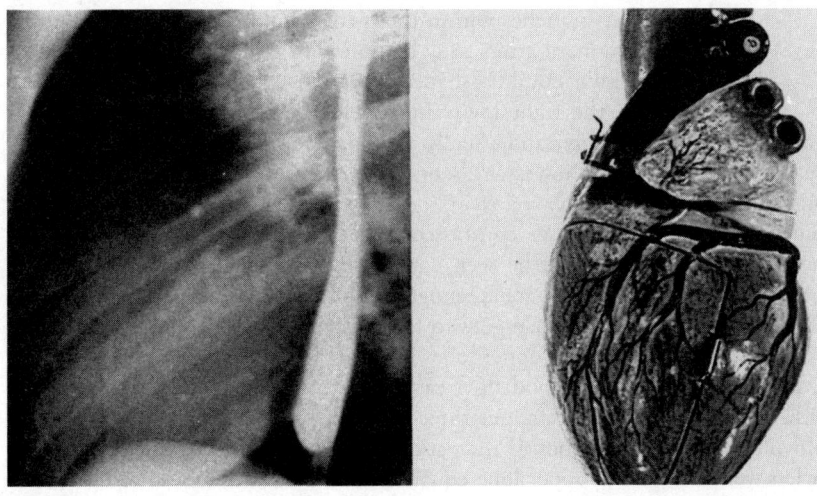

FIGURE 83.4. Lateral view of the chest roentgenogram and cardiac model as viewed from the left side. The anterior margin of the heart is formed by the right ventricle. The right atrium may, on occasion, also form the upper anterior portion of the heart. The posterior margin of the heart is the left atrium superiorly and the left ventricle inferiorly. The inferior vena cava usually can be discerned as a straight line just above the diaphragm.

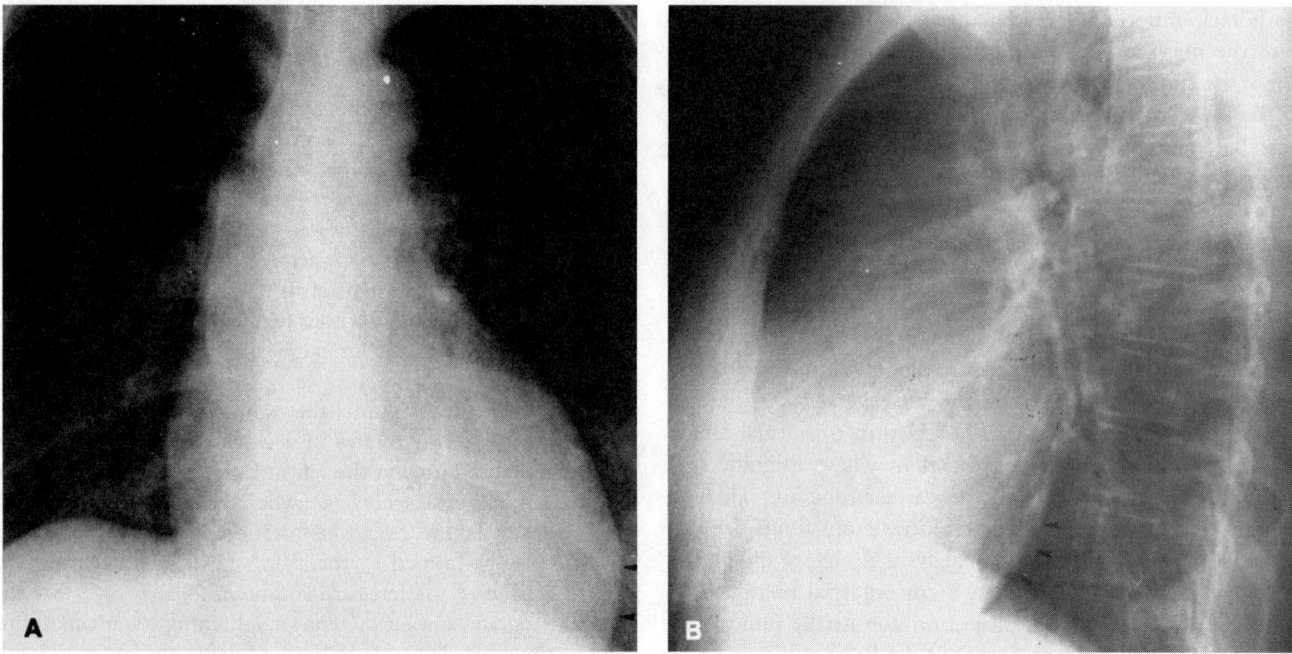

FIGURE 83.5. Aortic insufficiency and dilatation of the left ventricle. **A:** Posteroanterior view shows that the apex of the heart is displaced inferiorly and to the left *(arrowheads).* **B:** Lateral view shows that the dilated left ventricle also extends as a convex bulge along the posteroinferior portion of the heart *(arrowheads).*

The left ventricle forms the left lower lateral aspect of the cardiac silhouette on the PA roentgenogram and the posteroinferior portion on the lateral roentgenogram. As the left ventricle enlarges, it enlarges inferiorly to the left and posteriorly so that the apex moves downward, outward, and posteriorly. This is readily appreciated on both the PA and lateral projections (Fig. 83.5). It must be emphasized that the roentgenogram accurately depicts chamber dilatation; however, there may be thickening of the walls of either the left or the right ventricle without significant cardiac dilatation. When this occurs, there may be little change in the outer configuration of the heart. It is not unusual to have a patient with aortic stenosis and a thickened left ventricle in whom the roentgenographic appearance of the left ventricle appears normal. At times, with left ventricular hypertrophy, there may be an exaggerated rounding of the apex of the heart.

CARDIAC CALCIFICATIONS

The presence of cardiac calcifications may be important clues to the diagnosis of cardiac disease. Calcified coronary arteries usually are associated with significant coronary disease. Calcification of the aortic valve is present in almost 90% of adults with aortic stenosis. On the PA roentgenogram, the aortic valve is superimposed on the spine and a calcified aortic valve frequently may be missed. The mitral valve is located to the left of the spine and slightly more inferiorly, and is more easily seen. Valvular calcification may be better noted on the lateral views. In most radiology departments, chest films are performed with high-kilovoltage settings of 120 to 140 kV. With this high-kilovoltage technique, valvular and coronary artery calcifications are less well

seen. Cardiac fluoroscopy may be helpful in discerning valvular or coronary artery calcifications.

PULMONARY VASCULATURE

ANATOMY

The pulmonary arteries and veins are accurately depicted on a PA roentgenogram. The right lung is better suited for evaluation of the pulmonary vessels than the left. On the left, the heart overlaps a significant portion of the lung. Also on the left, the arteries and veins are parallel and differentiation of these vessels is difficult. On the contrary, the vessels of the right lung are well seen. The right pulmonary artery divides into its upper and lower branches within the mediastinum. The right descending pulmonary artery may be noted on a PA roentgenogram as an inverted comma–shaped structure extending from the hilum into the right lower lung field (Fig. 83.6). The vessels taper smoothly, and usually four or five divisions can be discerned before the vessel disappears in the outer third of the lung. The pulmonary veins in the right lower lung field are horizontal structures as contrasted with the more vertical arteries. They usually can be seen coursing back to the left atrium. On the upright PA roentgenogram, 70% of the blood pumped by the right ventricle goes to the lower lobes. Because of gravitational effects, the upper lobes are relatively underperfused. This difference in blood flow causes the arteries and veins in the lower lobes to be about three times the diameter of the vessels in the upper lobes. If the patient is in the supine position, blood flow to the upper lobe equals that of the lower lobe, and as a result

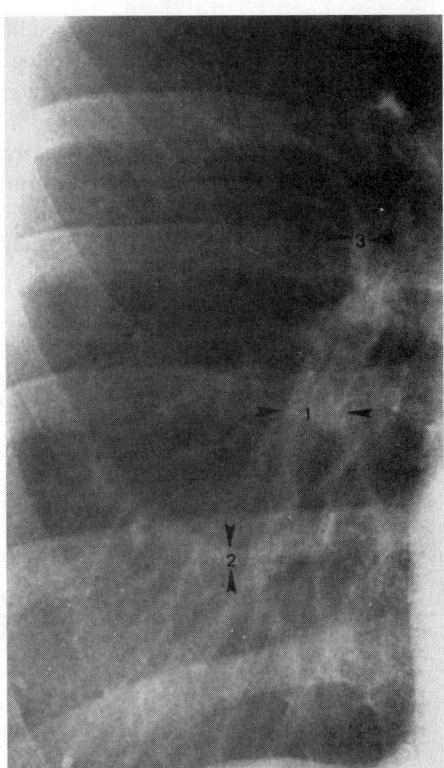

FIGURE 83.6. Right lung of a normal patient. Note the descending branch of the right pulmonary artery (1), which tapers evenly and is shaped like a reversed comma. The pulmonary veins of the right lower lobe are horizontal structures (2) that run almost at right angles to the pulmonary arteries. The vessels in the lower lobes are approximately three times the diameter of the vessels in the upper lobes. The upper lobe pulmonary vein (3) can be seen crossing the right hilum and extending down to the left atrium. The upper lobe pulmonary vein forms the lateral aspect of the right hilum.

there is a significant change in the roentgenographic appearance. This change of perfusion may mimic the changes noted in congestive heart failure. This is one reason that it is always preferable to obtain chest roentgenograms with the patient in an upright position if at all possible. The distal right upper lobe pulmonary arteries and vein are parallel; however, more proximally the artery goes to the higher placed hilum while the veins form one or two vessels that pass laterally, making up the lateral aspect of the hilum, and then descend to enter the left atrium (Fig. 83.6). Because of their differences in course, differentiation of right upper lobe pulmonary arteries and veins is easy.

PULMONARY BLOOD FLOW

Pulmonary vascular size accurately reflects blood flow. If blood flow increases for any reason, the vessels enlarge. If blood flow decreases as a result of pulmonary stenosis or a failing right ventricle, the size of the pulmonary arteries and veins decreases. These lower lobe vessels are larger in a normal person in the upright position because of the increased blood flow to the lower lobes as compared with that to the upper lobes. When there is an increase in pulmonary blood flow, not only does dilatation of the lower lobe vessels occur, but the upper lobe vessels also dilate and there is greater equalization of the size of the upper lobe and lower lobe vessels. It usually takes a doubling of pulmonary blood flow to cause discernible changes on a roentgenogram.

PULMONARY ARTERIAL HYPERTENSION

In patients with significant pulmonary arterial hypertension there is dilatation of the pulmonary arteries in the inner third of the lung. The pulmonary vessels in the middle and outer thirds are normal to decreased in size, and thus there is a marked disproportion in the size of the proximal as compared with the distal vessels. In these patients, pulmonary blood flow is usually decreased; as a result of this, the pulmonary veins are normal to small. This is in contradistinction to the pulmonary vascular changes of increased blood flow in which there is enlargement of both proximal and distal pulmonary arteries and enlargement of pulmonary veins. This disproportionate enlargement of the proximal pulmonary arteries in individuals with pulmonary hypertension is the result of Laplace's law, which states that the tension on the wall is proportional to the radius of the vessel. Larger vessels thus have increased wall tension as compared with medium-sized and smaller vessels, even though the pressure is equal. This causes greater fragmentation of elastic tissue of the arterial wall, and dilatation results. The medium-sized and smaller vessels may actually appear small. This may be secondary to the decreased pulmonary blood flow noted in many of these patients.

PULMONARY VENOUS HYPERTENSION

Pulmonary venous hypertension may be seen in patients with venous stenosis or stenosis of the mitral valve, but most are secondary to left ventricular failure. In a normal person, most blood pumped by the right ventricle goes to the lower lobes. In a patient with pulmonary venous hypertension, there is a reversal of pulmonary perfusion so that most blood flow is to the upper lobes. The relative pulmonary capillary pressure of the lung depends on the position as it relates to the level of the left atrium. It is equal to left atrial pressure at the level of the left atrium. It is less than left atrial pressure above the left atrium, and it is increased above left atrial pressure below the level of the left atrium. In patients with elevated left atrial pressure, pulmonary capillary pressure of the lower lobes may exceed the oncotic pressure of the blood; this is not present in the upper lobes. Thus, there may be interstitial edema limited to the lower lobes that may be roentgenographically manifested by blurring of the margin of the pulmonary vessels and, at times, by increase in linear markings of the lower lobes (Fig. 83.7). This interstitial edema may encircle the bronchi and cause increased density surrounding the bronchi when viewed on end. As a result of the lower lobe interstitial fluid, there may be increased vascular resistance as compared with the upper lobes, which may result in increased upper lobe blood flow and enlarged pulmonary vessels in the upper lobe. This is seen usually as enlargement of the upper lobe veins. These veins course downward, forming the lateral aspect of the hilum, and this may cause enlargement of the hilum of the lung. As interstitial pressure increases, fluid

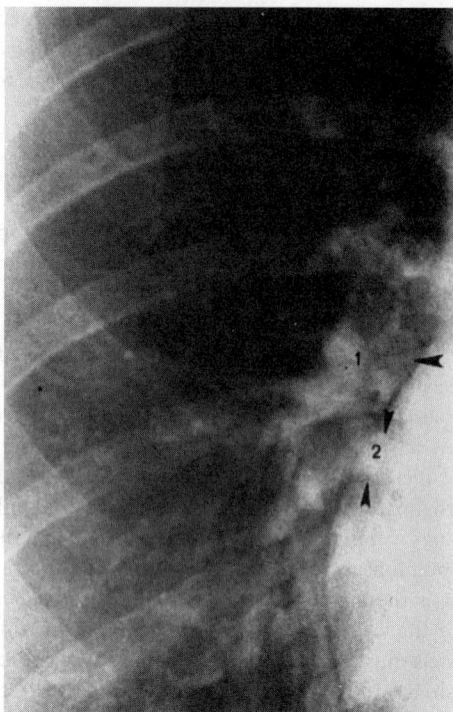

FIGURE 83.7. Severe interstitial pulmonary edema. Note the increased linear markings throughout the right lung. The vessels in both the upper and lower lobes are indistinct because of the interstitial fluid surrounding the vessels. The right upper lobe pulmonary veins are enlarged.

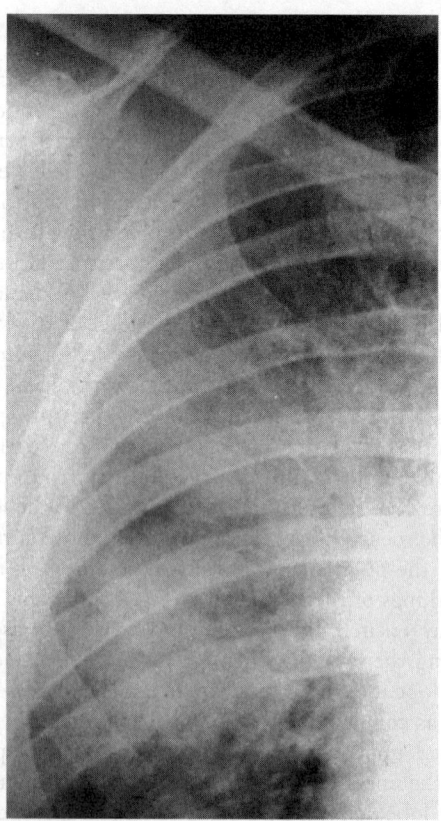

FIGURE 83.8. Pulmonary alveolar edema. The homogeneous perihilar hazy density has been compared to a bat's wing.

may enter the alveoli. This is typically most marked in the perihilar area, giving a so-called bat-wing appearance (Fig. 83.8). No evidence of an air bronchogram exists. The roentgenographic appearance of pulmonary edema secondary to a failing heart should be contrasted to the roentgenographic appearance of pulmonary edema seen with a change in capillary permeability. In the later case, the increased density is more diffuse, involving all segments of both lungs, and air bronchograms may be prominent.

BIBLIOGRAPHY

Braunwald E. *Heart disease: a textbook of cardiovascular medicine,* fifth ed. Philadelphia, WB Saunders, 1996.

Gedgaudas E, Moller JH, Castaneda Zuniga WR, et al. *Cardiovascular radiology.* Philadelphia: WB Saunders, 1985.

Simon M. Physiologic considerations in radiology of the pulmonary vasculature. In: Abrams HL, ed. *Abrams' angiography: vascular and interventional radiology,* fourth ed. Boston: Little, Brown and Company, 1997: 849–867.

Kelley's Textbook of Internal Medicine, fourth edition. Edited by H. David Humes. Lippincott Williams & Wilkins, Philadelphia © 2000.

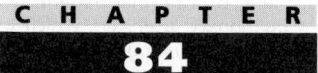

CHAPTER
84

ELECTROCARDIOGRAPHY, EXERCISE STRESS TESTING, AND AMBULATORY MONITORING

CHARLES FISCH

ELECTROCARDIOGRAM

As a noninvasive laboratory procedure for evaluating the heart, electrocardiography is without equal. There is no risk to the patient, the relative cost is minimal, the technique is simple and reproducible, and the record lends itself to serial studies. The procedure may serve as an independent marker of myocardial disease. It often reflects anatomical, metabolic, and hemodynamic alterations. An electrocardiogram (ECG) often is essential for proper diagnosis and therapy. It is without equal for diagnosis of arrhythmias, and it is the procedure of choice in patients presenting with chest pain and syncope, which are the most common presenting symptoms of potential cardiovascular catastrophes.

For proper use of the ECG, its sensitivity and specificity must be understood and considered. The ECG is composed of waveforms, each of which may be influenced differently by a variety of factors and by the sequencing of those factors. The sensitivity and specificity of the test depend to a large extent on the clinical questions asked.

The sensitivity of the ECG for myocardial disorders varies considerably, depending on the cause and on the size and location of the myocardium or specialized tissue involved in a pathologic process. The sensitivity and specificity for arrhythmias are consistently high, and the ECG is the only practical approach to analysis of abnormalities of cardiac rhythm. Because of its major contribution to the care of the patient with cardiac disorders, the ECG has been used continuously and with increasing frequency since it was first introduced in 1903 by Einthoven.

GENERAL CONCEPTS

Depolarization and Repolarization

In the resting state, the outside of the cell or tissue is electrically uniformly positive. Electrodes in contact with the cell membrane record no difference of potential. When the cell is stimulated, sodium enters the cell rapidly and that part of the cell or tissue is said to be depolarized. It is electrically negative with respect to the resting, polarized part of the cell or tissue. Local current is generated, and a potential difference between polarized and depolarized areas can be recorded (Fig. 84.1). The process of depolarization travels rapidly along the length of the cell or tissue, preceded by a positive and followed by a negative field or charge.

Repolarization can be viewed as restitution of the electrical state to that which existed before depolarization. Because repolarization proceeds in the direction of the depolarized or electrically negative part of the cell, repolarization is preceded by a negative and followed by a positive field or charge. When placed in a volume conductor such as the human body, the cell or tissues of the heart impart an electrical field, the voltage difference of which can be recorded from the body surface.

Dipole and Vector

The process of depolarization and repolarization—more specifically, the moving boundary separating the positive and negative fields—can be represented by a single dipole consisting of a positive and a negative charge, representing the respective electrical fields (Fig. 84.1). Such a dipole can also be viewed as a vector that has direction, sense (plus or minus), and magnitude. The arrow of the vector identifies the positive field.

When interpreting an ECG, it is essential to recognize vectors and fields. When depolarization moves toward the recording electrode, also called the exploring electrode, the latter is in the positive field, and the ECG registers an upright positive deflection. Conversely, when depolarization proceeds away from the recording electrode, the electrode is in the negative field, and the ECG registers a downward or negative deflection. The opposite is true for repolarization because repolarization is preceded by a negative field and followed by the positive, repolarized field. The electrode facing the oncoming wave of repolarization is still in the negative field and records a negative deflection. The electrode facing the repolarized area records an upright deflection.

Instantaneous and Mean Vector

At any given moment, the electrical potential can be represented by an instantaneous vector that reflects the net of all electrical forces existing at that particular moment. The sum of all forces generated during total depolarization can be represented by a mean vector. In the case of ventricular depolarization or activation, the resultant vector is referred to as the mean QRS vector.

Activation of the Heart and the Electrocardiographic Waves

The cardiac impulse originates in the sinoatrial node, located in the right atrium at the opening of the great veins (Fig. 84.2), and activates first the right atrium and then the left atrium. The general direction of atrial activation is inferiorly, to the left, and posteriorly, and it is recorded as the P wave. The atrial impulse is delayed in the atrioventricular (AV) node, and the ECG registers an isoelectric PR segment. After the impulse emerges from the AV node, it conducts rapidly along the bundle of His, the right and left bundles, the anterior and posterior divisions (fasci-

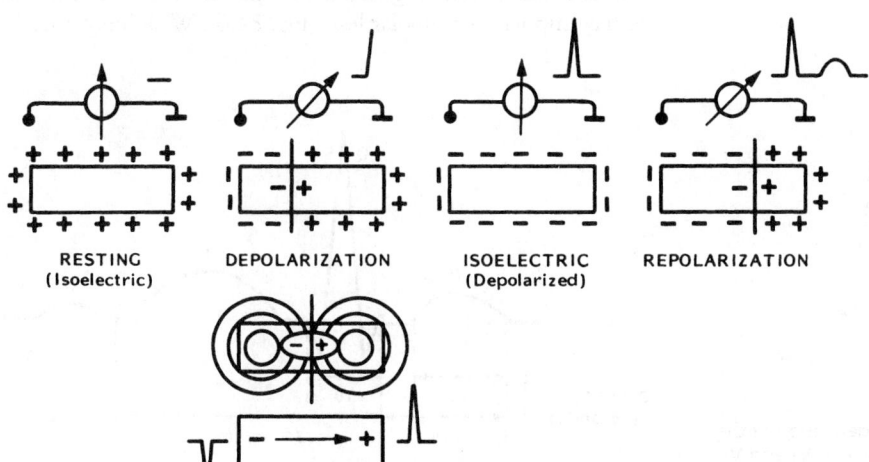

RESTING
(Isoelectric)

DEPOLARIZATION

ISOELECTRIC
(Depolarized)

REPOLARIZATION

FIGURE 84.1. Diagrammatic representation of depolarization and repolarization of the heart. The moving boundary can be represented as a dipole or a vector (see text).

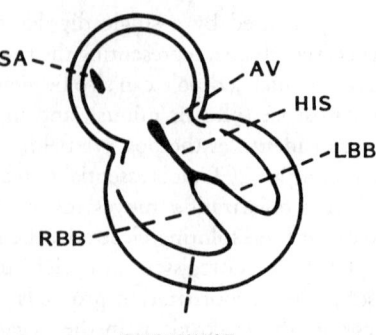

FIGURE 84.2. Specialized tissue. SA, sinoatrial node; AV, atrioventricular node; HIS, bundle of His; RBB and LBB, right and left bundle branches, respectively; PURKINJE, Purkinje fibers.

cles) of the left bundle, and the Purkinje system. The activation (i.e., depolarization) of the ventricles is represented by the QRS complex.

Repolarization follows, with atrial and ventricular repolarization inscribing the Ta and T waves, respectively. The T wave is followed by a U wave, the genesis of which is unclear. There are two prevailing concepts of the generation of the U wave. One suggests that the U wave represents delayed repolarization of Purkinje fibers, and the other states that the U wave is secondary to a diastolic myocardial event.

A more detailed understanding of the order of ventricular activation is essential for proper interpretation of the ECG (Fig. 84.3). The earliest activation of the ventricles occurs in the septum, directed from left to right, anteriorly, inferiorly, and, occasionally, superiorly. This is followed by depolarization of the free ventricular wall, proceeding from the endocardium to the epicardium. The left ventricle, which is considerably thicker than the right, continues to depolarize after depolarization of the right ventricle is completed and generates a strong, unopposed force directed to the left, inferiorly, and posteriorly. In essence, ventricular activation can be represented by two vectors: the early vector reflecting depolarization of the septum directed from left

to right and the second reflecting depolarization of the much larger left ventricle directed to the left, inferiorly, and posteriorly.

NORMAL ELECTROCARDIOGRAM

Normal Values

The magnitude of the electrical potential generated by the heart (Figs. 84.4 and 84.5) is recorded on the ordinate (1 mm = 0.1 mV) of the ECG, and the duration of the event is reflected on the abscissa (1 mm = 0.04 second). The bolder lines on the recording paper identify 0.2-second intervals. Proper standardization of the voltage is indicated by a 10-mm deflection for each 1 mV. To avoid distortion of the ECG pattern due to stylus inertia, it is important that the upstroke be prompt and perpendicular to the baseline.

The maximum duration of a normal P wave is 0.12 second, and its amplitude is 2 mm (0.2 mV). The PR interval varies inversely with the heart rate, but the maximal duration is 0.20 second (perhaps 0.22 second in the presence of sinus bradycardia). The upper limit of the QRS duration is 0.10 second. The QT interval varies from 0.36 to 0.40 second, depending on the patient's heart rate, sex, and age. Because of the influence of a variety of physiologic factors on the duration of the QT interval, mild to moderate deviation from the accepted norm is probably of no clinical significance.

Estimation of Heart Rate

Because there are 300 0.2-second intervals in 1 minute, the heart rate can be determined by dividing 300 by the number of 0.2-second intervals and fractions thereof within one RR cycle. For example, if there are two 0.2-second intervals in an RR cycle, the heart rate equals 300 divided by 2, or 150 beats per minute. Similarly, if there are 2.5 0.2-second intervals in an RR cycle, the heart rate equals 300 divided by 2.5, or 120 beats per minute.

For a more accurate estimate of the heart rate, the number of RR cycles and fractions thereof present in a 3-second period (15 0.2-second intervals equals 3 seconds) is multiplied by 20.

LEADS

The electrical potential generated by the heart can be recorded with a unipolar or a bipolar lead (Fig. 84.6). With bipolar leads,

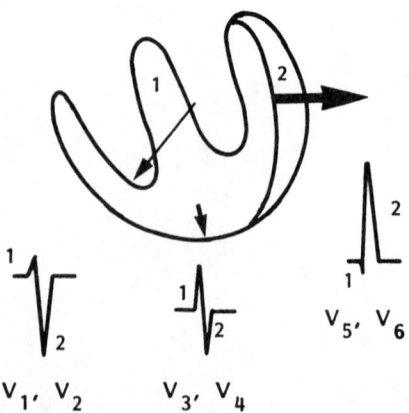

FIGURE 84.3. Sequence of ventricular activation and derivation of the precordial QRS complex. Leads V_1 and V_2, right ventricular; V_3 and V_4, transitional; V_5 and V_6, left ventricular.

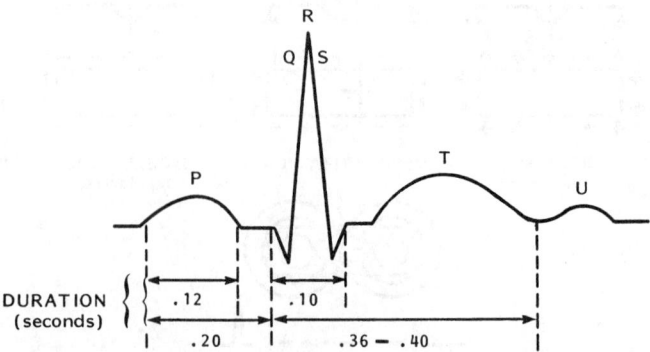

FIGURE 84.4. Electrocardiographic waveforms and normal values.

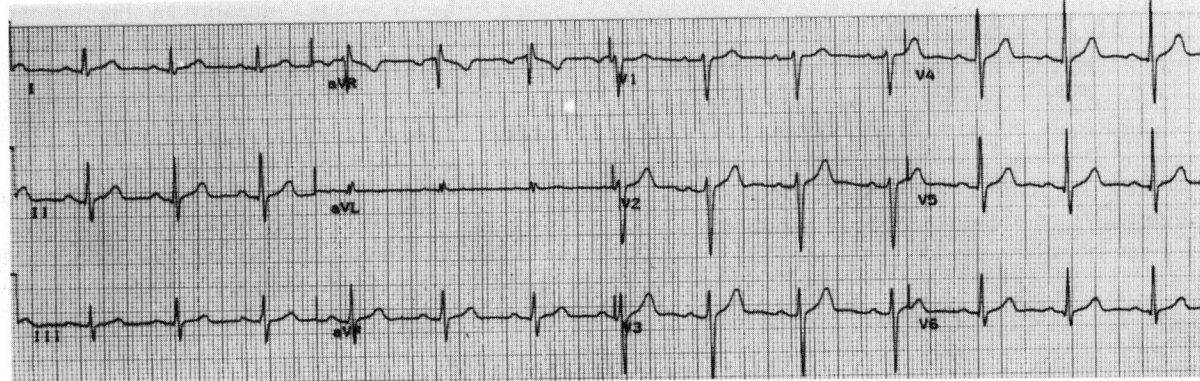

FIGURE 84.5. Normal electrocardiogram.

both electrodes register an electrical potential, and the ECG reflects the difference of potential between the two points. Conversely, the potential of the indifferent electrodes of a unipolar lead is for all practical purposes zero. This zero potential is achieved by connecting the leads from the three extremities into a single common electrode, called the central terminal of Wilson. As a result, unipolar leads record only the potential subtending the exploring electrode rather than a difference between two points, as is the case with a bipolar lead. The exploring electrode determines the polarity of the ECG wave. When the exploring electrode is in the positive field, the ECG records an upright or positive deflection, and when the exploring electrode is in the negative field, the ECG registers a downward or negative deflection.

Bipolar Leads

Lead I is formed by connecting the left and right arms, with the electrode on the left arm designated as the exploring electrode. Lead II is formed by connecting the right arm and the left foot, with the electrode on the left foot designated as the exploring electrode. Lead III is formed by connecting the left arm and the left foot, with the electrode on the left foot designated as the exploring electrode.

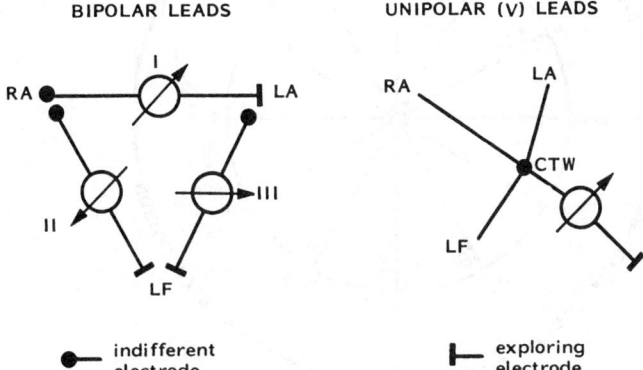

FIGURE 84.6. Bipolar and unipolar leads. RA, right arm; LA, left arm; LF, left foot; CTW, central terminal of Wilson.

Unipolar Leads

The unipolar leads are identified by the letter V. Three unipolar limb leads and six unipolar precordial leads are used.

In leads VR, VL, and VF, the exploring electrode is connected to the right arm, left arm, and left foot, respectively. By disconnecting from the central terminal the limb from which the voltage is being recorded, the amplitude of the wave is augmented by two-thirds, and such leads are identified as augmented leads: aVR, aVL, and aVF, respectively.

The six precordial V leads are recorded from the following points on the thorax: V_1, fourth interspace to the right of the sternum; V_2, fourth interspace to the left of the sternum; V_4, midclavicular line in the fifth interspace; V_3, halfway between V_2 and V_4; V_5, fifth interspace in the anterior axillary line; and V_6, fifth interspace in the midaxillary line. Occasionally, leads V_{3r} and V_{4r} may prove helpful, and these are recorded from the same points as leads V_3 and V_4 but from the right anterior chest wall.

Lead Axis

A line drawn between the two connections of a lead is referred to as the lead axis. The magnitude of deflection of an ECG wave in any lead is greatest if the direction of activation parallels the lead axis and is isoelectric or equiphasic when the direction of activation is perpendicular to the lead axis.

Derivation of the QRS Complex in the Limb Leads

The three bipolar limb leads constitute the Einthoven triangle. The assumptions are that the triangle is equilateral, that the heart is a point source located at the center of this triangle, and that the thorax is a uniform boundary and a uniform volume conductor. Although none of the assumptions are absolutely correct, they are nevertheless useful in analysis of the clinical ECG.

The initial activation of the septum from left to right, inferiorly and anteriorly, and occasionally superiorly projects a negative potential recorded as a Q wave in leads I and aVL. When the initial activation proceeds superiorly, a Q wave is recorded in leads III and aVF (Fig. 84.5). When the initial septal activation is directed inferiorly (a positive potential), an R wave is recorded in leads aVF, II, and III. This usually is followed by activation in a direction from the right shoulder toward the left hip, inscribing a dominant R wave in leads I, II, III, aVL, and aVF. The QRS complex in aVR is negative because of the initial inferior, left-to-right activation of the septum, followed by endocardium-to-epicardium activation of the ventricles. These vectors project a negative potential to the right arm.

PRECORDIAL ELECTROCARDIOGRAM

As the septum depolarizes from left to right, the right ventricular (RV) leads V_1 and V_2 face the positive field and register a small R wave (Figs. 84.3 and 84.5). At the same time, the left ventricular (LV) leads V_5 and V_6 face the negative field and register a small septal Q wave. This is followed by the dominant LV activation from endocardium to epicardium, with the RV leads V_1 and V_2 facing the negative field and registering a deep S wave. Simultaneously, the LV leads V_5 and V_6 face the positive field and register a tall R wave. Leads V_1 and V_2 are considered right and V_5 and V_6 are considered LV leads, leads V_3 and V_4 are septal or transitional and register an equiphasic QRS. The equiphasic configuration is explained by an initial depolarization of the septum from left to right inferiorly and anteriorly inscribing the R wave, followed by depolarization of the LV wall away from leads V_3 and V_4 and inscribing the S wave.

As the electrode is moved from the V_1 to V_6 position, it subtends an increasing myocardial mass, and because the R wave expresses the magnitude of the electrical potential generated by the subtending muscle mass, the amplitude of the R wave increases progressively. The amplitude of the R wave may remain unchanged in leads V_1 and V_2 and occasionally in lead V_3, with a sudden transition of the QRS complex to an LV configuration. With rare exception, after an R wave is recorded in lead V_1, it should neither diminish in amplitude nor disappear in leads

located farther to the left. Ordinarily, an abnormal progression of the R-wave amplitude from V_1 through V_6 suggests a decrease or loss of muscle mass.

In the adult, the precordial T waves are upright, with the exception of those recorded by lead V_1 and rarely by lead V_2, in which the T waves may be inverted (Fig. 84.5). As a rule, a negative T wave from leads other than V_1 should be considered abnormal in adults. Occasionally, the inverted RV T waves present at birth may persist into the teens and rarely into the early 20s and are a normal variant, called the juvenile T waves.

ELECTRICAL POSITION

The frontal axis of the QRS and rotation on the anteroposterior and on the longitudinal (apex to base) axes define the electrical position of the heart.

Axis Deviation

Axis deviation is estimated by plotting the peak values of the R or S wave on two of the three bipolar leads of a hexaxial reference system (Fig. 84.7). From that point, lines perpendicular to the lead axis are drawn. The QRS axis is obtained by connecting the center of the hexaxial lead system and the point where the two perpendicular lines cross (Fig. 84.7).

An axis in the range of -30 degrees to $+90$ degrees is normal. An axis in the range of -30 degrees to -90 degrees is a left axis. A left axis greater than -30 degrees is abnormal, not because of cardiac anatomic position but most likely because of a conduction defect. Left axis deviation of -30 degrees is easily identified by an equiphasic QRS complex in lead II. An axis in the range of $+90$ degrees to $+180$ degrees is right axis deviation. Right axis deviation of $+90$ degrees is recognized by an equiphasic QRS complex in lead I. An axis in the range of -90 degrees to $+180$ degrees is an indeterminate axis.

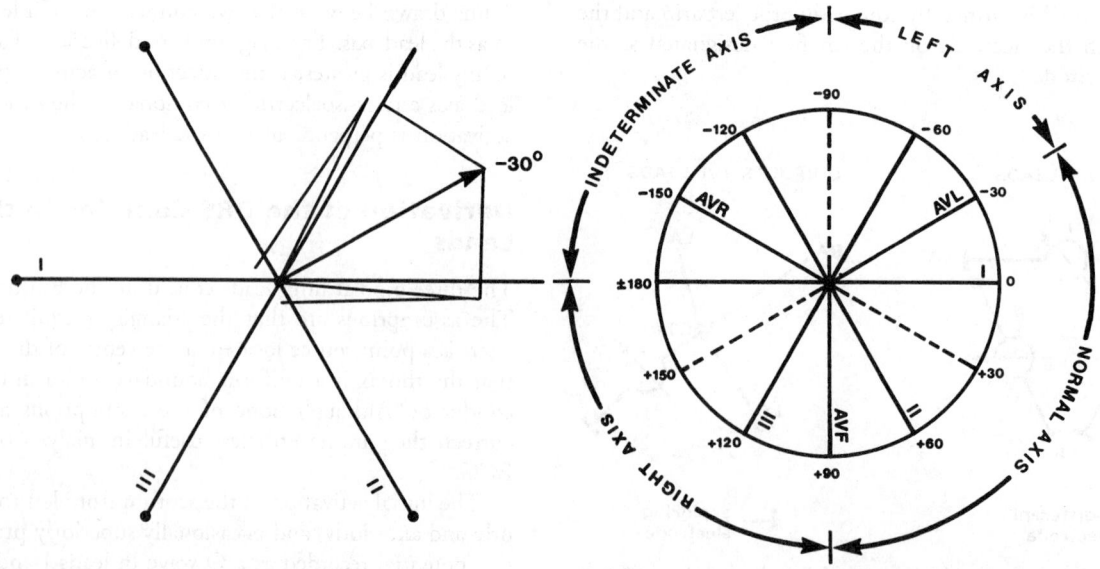

FIGURE 84.7. Plot of QRS axis on hexaxial system *(left)* and range of axis *(right)*.

Rotation on the Anteroposterior Axis

Rotation in the frontal plane on an anteroposterior axis allows the apex of the heart to face the left arm or left foot and points in between. When the apex points in the direction of the left foot, the QRS complex in aVF has the same configuration as the QRS complex in leads V_5 and V_6, and the position is vertical. When the apex points in the direction of the left arm, the QRS complex in lead aVL has the same configuration as the QRS complex in leads V_5 and V_6, and the position is horizontal. When the apex is halfway between the left arm and left foot, the QRS complex is similar in leads aVL and aVF, both resemble the QRS complex in leads V_5 and V_6, and the position is intermediate.

Rotation on the Longitudinal Axis

Rotation on the longitudinal axis (apex to base) is best visualized by viewing the patient in the supine position with the observer facing the diaphragmatic aspect of the heart. Clockwise rotation projects the right ventricle farther to the patient's left, and as a result, the RV QRS complexes (rS) are recorded in leads V_3 and V_4 and occasionally as far to the left as leads V_5 or V_6. Counterclockwise rotation projects the left ventricle to the patient's right, and LV QRS complexes (qR) are recorded in leads V_3 and V_4 and rarely in leads V_1 and V_2.

◼ CONDITIONS PRODUCING ABNORMAL ELECTROCARDIOGRAMS

CHAMBER ENLARGEMENT AND HYPERTROPHY

Atrial Hypertrophy

Right atrial enlargement shifts the P-wave axis to the right. As a result, the P wave in lead I is low or isoelectric; in leads II, III, and aVF, it is increased in amplitude and its configuration *is pointed*. In leads V_1 and V_2, the P wave may be upright and increased in amplitude.

Left atrial enlargement manifests by notching and prolongation of the P wave, encroachment of the P wave on the PR segment, and, not infrequently, left axis deviation of the terminal component of the P wave. In lead V_1, the P wave is negative and prolonged, with an amplitude of 1 mm (0.10 mV) or greater, and its duration is 0.04 second or longer.

P-wave enlargement does not necessarily indicate atrial hypertrophy. Patterns similar to hypertrophy may be caused by chamber dilation, intra-atrial conduction delays, or ectopy.

Ventricular Hypertrophy

Ventricular hypertrophy implies an increase in muscle mass that is manifested by an increased amplitude of the QRS complex. The increased QRS voltage ultimately is associated with changes in the ST segment and T waves.

Left Ventricular Hypertrophy

The QRS voltage criteria for LV hypertrophy include the following:

R wave in lead I plus an S wave in lead III greater than or equal to 2.5 mV

R wave in aVL greater than 1.2 mV

R wave in aVF greater than 2.0 mV

S wave in V_1 greater than or equal to 2.4 mV

R wave in V_5 or V_6 greater than 2.6 mV

R wave in V_5 or V_6 + S wave in V_1 greater than 3.5 mV

The following point system for diagnosing LV hypertrophy has been suggested:

Amplitude of R or S wave in limb leads greater than or equal to 2.0 mV or S wave in lead I or in V_1 or V_2 greater than or equal to 3.0 mV or R wave in V_5 or V_6 greater than 3.0 mV = *3 points*

ST-segment changes with or without digitalis = *1 or 2 points, respectively*

Left atrial enlargement = *3 points*

Left axis deviation of −30 degrees or more = *2 points*

QRS complex duration greater than 0.09 second and intrinsicoid deflection in V_5 and V_6 greater than 0.05 second = *1 point each*

Based on this point system, the diagnosis of LV hypertrophy is probable with 4 points and definite with 5 points. The diagnosis of LV hypertrophy is never secure without associated ST-segment and T-wave changes. Shifts in the ST segment and T wave are directed opposite to the QRS complex; the ST segment is depressed in leads I, aVL, V_5, and V_6, and the T wave is negative and asymmetric, and its ascending limb is steeper, with occasional terminal positive inscription. When the position is vertical, the ST-segment and T-wave changes are recorded in leads II, III, and aVF. The pattern of left atrial preponderance is commonly seen in LV hypertrophy.

Right Ventricular Hypertrophy

Because the right ventricle is about one-third of the thickness of the left ventricle, considerable hypertrophy must take place before the RV mass can generate a voltage that equals or exceeds the voltage generated by the left ventricle. Consequently, the sensitivity of the ECG for RV hypertrophy is low, varying from 40% to 50%.

In general, four patterns indicating RV hypertrophy may be recorded in lead V_1: an rSR', or incomplete right bundle-branch block (RBBB) pattern; a tall R wave with a slurred early upstroke; a qR pattern; and an R/S ratio greater than 1, with an R wave amplitude of 5 mm (0.5 mV) or greater.

If RV hypertrophy exists, correlation of the ECG pattern in lead V_1 with intraventricular pressures suggests the following:

An rSR' pattern indicates an elevated RV pressure, although one that is lower than that of the left ventricle (e.g., atrial septal defect).

A tall R wave with a slur on the upstroke suggests that right and LV pressures are equal (e.g., tetralogy of Fallot).

A qR pattern indicates that the RV pressure exceeds that of the left ventricle (e.g., pulmonary stenosis with an intact septum, primary pulmonary hypertension).

INTRAVENTRICULAR CONDUCTION DEFECTS

Right Bundle-Branch Block

The duration of RBBB is 0.12 second or longer, with a characteristically delayed and slow terminal activation of the right ventricle in a right and anterior direction. In RBBB, the initial septal activation is normal, directed from left to right, and inscribed as an initial small upright R wave in leads V_1 and V_2. Activation of the left ventricle follows, and a notch or an S wave is inscribed in leads V_1 and V_2. Final activation is that of the right ventricle directed to the right and anteriorly, and is inscribed as a prolonged terminal R, the R′ wave.

The R wave in LV leads V_5 and V_6 is tall and narrow, reflecting the normal activation of the left ventricle. A shallow, prolonged S wave reflects the terminal activation of the right ventricle and is recorded simultaneously with the R′ inscribed in leads V_1 and V_2.

Repolarization and the T wave are abnormal in the presence of intraventricular conduction delays. The abnormality is secondary to and obligatory to the abnormal order of depolarization. Such T-wave changes are referred to as secondary T-wave changes. The T-wave change is frequently accompanied by displacement of the ST segment in a direction concordant with the direction of the T wave. A secondary ST-T–wave change does not contribute information other than that inherent in the intraventricular conduction delay. In contrast to the secondary T-wave change, a T-wave change that is independent of QRS alteration and often seen with normal QRS complexes reflects local abnormalities, often prolongation of the excited state (e.g., ischemia). Such T-wave changes are referred to as primary T-wave changes. In RBBB, the T wave is directed opposite to the terminal portion of the QRS, that portion inscribed during the last 0.4 second of the QRS.

Left Bundle-Branch Block

Left bundle-branch block (LBBB) results in late activation of the left ventricle. The initial order of septal activation is reversed, with activation proceeding from right to left, resulting in an initial upright deflection in leads I, aVL, V_5, and V_6. This is followed by activation of the right ventricle, which may be recognized by a notch or a plateau of the R wave in leads I, aVL, V_5, and V_6 . Terminal activation is that of the left ventricle from right to left, inscribing an R′ in leads I, aVL, V_5, and V_6. The pattern in RV leads is that of a QS or rS.

In LBBB, the left intracavitary potential is initially positive, the result of the right-to-left depolarization of the septum. Consequently, the hallmark of myocardial infarction (MI), the Q wave, is not recorded. Only rarely, usually only during the acute phase of infarction, can a diagnosis of MI be made in LBBB.

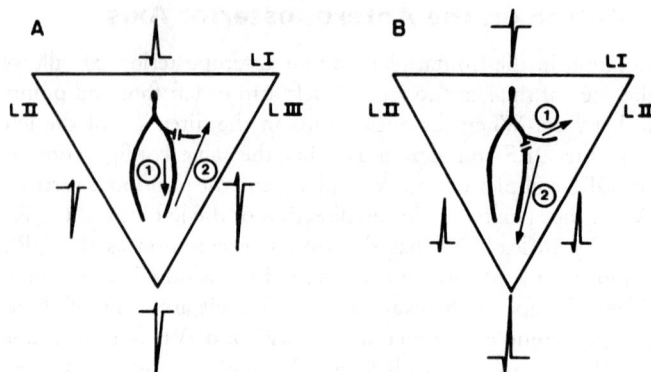

FIGURE 84.8. Left anterior **(A)** and posterior **(B)** divisional (fascicular) block.

Divisional or Fascicular Blocks

The left bundle branch is functionally divided into two fascicles, the anterior and posterior (Fig. 84.8). Block of conduction through either fascicle results in a characteristic ECG pattern.

Left anterior divisional block (LADB) results in initial activation inferiorly, followed by a superiorly directed activation. In leads II, III, and aVF, the initial activation inscribes a small R wave, followed by a dominant, deep S wave. Lead aVL inscribes an initial q wave, and lead I inscribes an initial q or R wave. The QRS duration rarely exceeds 0.10 second and never exceeds 0.12 second. Because of the superiorly oriented mean QRS axis, away from the precordial lead positions, the configuration of the precordial QRS complexes is often that of an RS.

Left posterior divisional block (LPDB) results in initial activation superiorly, followed by an inferiorly directed activation. Leads II, III, and aVF inscribe an initial q wave, followed by a tall R wave. Because this QRS pattern can be recorded in the absence of LPDB, as, for example, in tall, asthenic persons or in patients with chronic obstructive pulmonary disease, a diagnosis of LPDB requires evidence of prior normal intraventricular conduction. The duration of the QRS rarely exceeds 0.10 second and never exceeds 0.12 second.

Although LADB is common, especially in the older persons, LPDB is rare. And while LADB is frequently recorded in patients without evidence of clinical heart disease, LPDB usually is accompanied by clinical evidence of heart disease. As a rule, both are acquired abnormalities.

Incomplete Bundle-Branch Block

Incomplete bundle-branch block is recognized when the QRS complex has the morphology of RBBB or LBBB but the duration is less than 0.12 second.

Nonspecific Intraventricular Conduction Delay

When the QRS duration is 0.12 second or longer but without the configuration of RBBB or LBBB, the intraventricular conduction defect is nonspecific. Such conduction defects are usually due to intramyocardial delays.

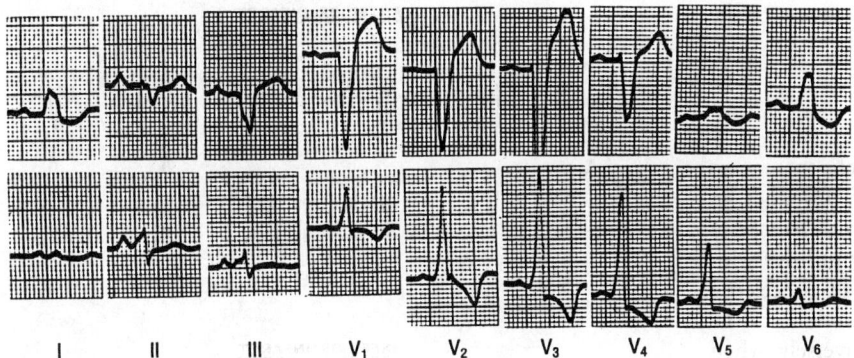

FIGURE 84.9. Left bundle-branch block *(upper)* and Wolff–Parkinson–White syndrome *(lower)*.

WOLFF–PARKINSON–WHITE SYNDROME

The ECG pattern of Wolff–Parkinson–White (WPW) syndrome is characterized by a short PR interval, slur on the upstroke of the R wave or on the downstroke of an S wave (i.e., delta wave), prolonged QRS complex, and often secondary ST-T changes (Fig. 84.9). The WPW pattern results from conduction through an alternative pathway (bundle of Kent), which bypasses the normal AV junction. Conduction through the bypass results in pre-excitation of the ventricle. The abnormal sequence of ventricular activation is responsible for the delta wave and the widening of the QRS complex.

Traditionally, the WPW syndrome has been divided into type A, characterized by a positive delta wave recorded in leads V_1 and V_2, and type B, characterized by a negative delta wave recorded in leads V_1 and V_2. With the introduction of intracardiac electrophysiologic studies, multiple sites of bypass conduction have been identified. The WPW syndrome pattern can be mistaken for intraventricular conduction defects, MI, and RV hypertrophy. Because the ventricular activation through the bypass may result in an initially positive intraventricular potential, WPW syndrome may mask the pattern of MI in a manner similar to that observed with LBBB. About one half of patients with WPW syndrome manifest supraventricular arrhythmias, often with rapid ventricular rates. For additional discussion of WPW syndrome, see Chapter 84.

ABERRATION

Aberration is defined as abnormal intraventricular conduction initiated by a supraventricular impulse originating from the atria or AV junction (Fig. 84.10). Aberration usually is initiated by acceleration of the heart rate, and only rarely is it caused by slowing of the heart rate. In normal and most abnormal hearts, aberration is of the RBBB configuration because the refractory period of the right bundle is normally longer than that of the left bundle. Recognition and differentiation of aberration from ventricular arrhythmias is clinically important because the prognosis and therapy for the two differ significantly.

MYOCARDIAL INFARCTION

The evolution of a classic ECG pattern of MI includes ischemia, injury, and necrosis.

Ischemia

During ischemia, depolarization (i.e., QRS) proceeds normally from endocardium to the epicardium. Conversely, the direction of repolarization (i.e., T wave), which normally proceeds from epicardium to endocardium, is reversed, moving from endocardium to epicardium. The surface leads face the negative field, and a negative T wave is inscribed. The reversal of the order of

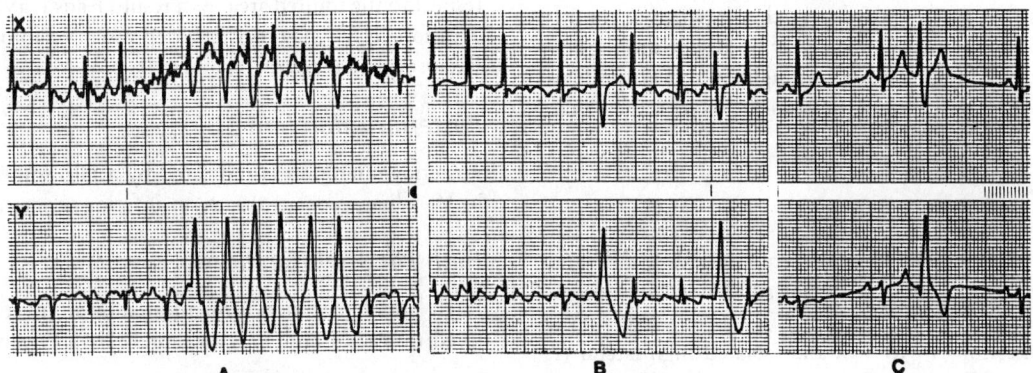

FIGURE 84.10. Ventricular aberration in the presence of atrial fibrillation **(A)**, flutter **(B)**, and sinus rhythm with atrial premature systole **(C)**. The aberration is recognized by the fact that the bizarre QRS complexes follow a relatively prolonged RR cycle, the configuration is that of right bundle-branch block, there is no compensatory pause in panels A and B, and the coupling of the bizarre QRS complex to preceding normal QRS varies. Once initiated, aberration can persist for a number of cycles.

repolarization is most likely caused by delayed recovery of the epicardial layer.

Injury

Normally, during the inscription of the ST segment there is no recordable difference of potential, and the ECG inscribes an isoelectric segment. Injury alters this status, and a difference of potential appears, with the injured area relatively positive with respect to the resting myocardium and the normally isoelectric ST segment displaced. When the exploring electrode faces the current of injury, the ST segment is elevated. Conversely, when the exploring electrode faces the normal muscle, which is relatively negative with respect to the injured myocardium, the ST segment is depressed.

In the intact heart, when the current of injury is subepicardial, the overlying leads record an elevated ST segment, and when the current of injury is subendocardial, the same leads record a depressed ST segment.

Necrosis

Conventionally, the Q wave denotes myocardial necrosis. Normally, the septum depolarizes from left to right, and the left intracavitary potential is negative. Because ventricular depolarization continues from the endocardium to the epicardium, the negativity of the cavity persists. Throughout the inscription of the QRS complex, the potential of the LV cavity is negative, and an intracavitary electrode records a QS pattern. According to the window concept, necrosis of the myocardium results in a window through which the surface electrode records the intracavitary negativity in the form of a Q wave.

Localization of Myocardial Infarction

The general location of MI may be anterior, right ventricular, inferior, or posterior. As a rule, anterior MI results from occlusion of the left anterior descending coronary artery, and occlusion of the right or circumflex coronary arteries results in inferior infarctions. Right ventricular and posterior MIs result from obstruction of the right or circumflex coronary artery, respectively.

A Q wave is frequently recorded in the presence of a nontransmural infarction, and a Q wave may be absent in the presence of a transmural infarction. Accordingly, it appears preferable to refer to MI as Q wave or non-Q wave rather than transmural or nontransmural.

Anterior Infarction

Anterior infarction (Fig. 84.11) is registered in leads I, aVL, and V_1 to V_6. Anterior infarction is further subdivided into septal (V_1, V_2), anterior (V_3, V_4), anteroseptal (V_1 to V_4), lateral (V_5, V_6), extensive anterior (V_1 to V_6), and isolated high lateral (I, aVL). Reciprocal ST-segment changes, namely ST-segment depression, may be recorded in leads II, III, and aVF. This pattern occurs because the distal, reciprocal leads face the normal myocardium, which is relatively negative with respect to the opposite positive field generated by the current of injury.

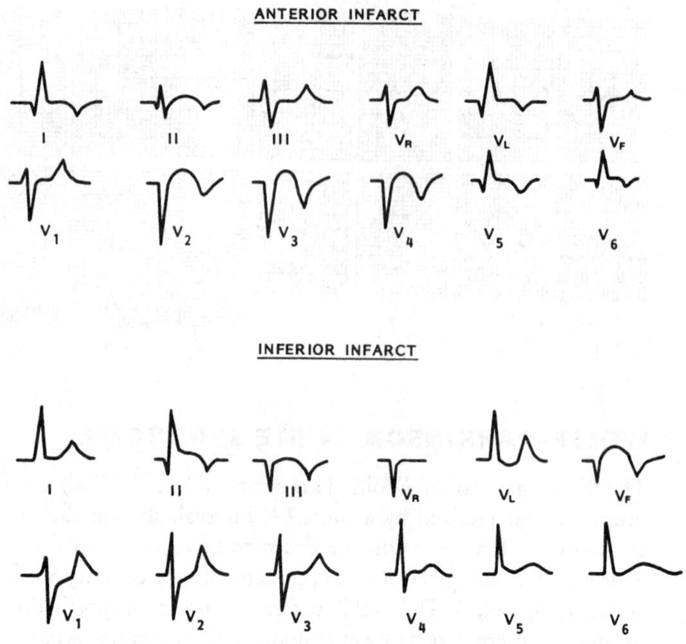

FIGURE 84.11. Diagrammatic presentation of anterior and inferior myocardial infarction.

Right Ventricular Infarction

Right ventricular infarction usually is associated with a diaphragmatic infarct that also involves the inferior part of the septum. It may be recognized by elevation of the ST segment in lead V_1 and occasionally in V_2. Elevation of the ST segment in leads V_{3r} and V_{4r}, however, has the highest sensitivity and specificity for RV infarction.

Inferior or Diaphragmatic Infarction

Inferior or diaphragmatic infarction (Fig. 84.11) is recognized by a Q wave, displacement of the ST segment, and T-wave changes in leads II, III, and aVF. When a positive current of injury is recorded in the inferior leads, the reciprocal leads face the normal myocardium, which at that moment is completely depolarized (isoelectric) and therefore relatively negative with respect to the injured area. As a result, leads I, aVL, V_1 to V_4, and occasionally V_5 may register a depressed, reciprocal ST segment. Reciprocal changes are characteristic of MI.

Posterior Infarction

Posterior infarction is indicated by a tall, somewhat delayed R in V_1 when associated with an inferior or lateral infarction.

High Lateral Infarction

High lateral infarction is manifested by an inverted T wave confined to leads I and aVL and rarely by a Q wave.

Electrocardiographic Diagnosis of Myocardial Infarction

About half of the first ECGs recorded in the course of the evolution of MI are diagnostic of infarction. The remainder may show

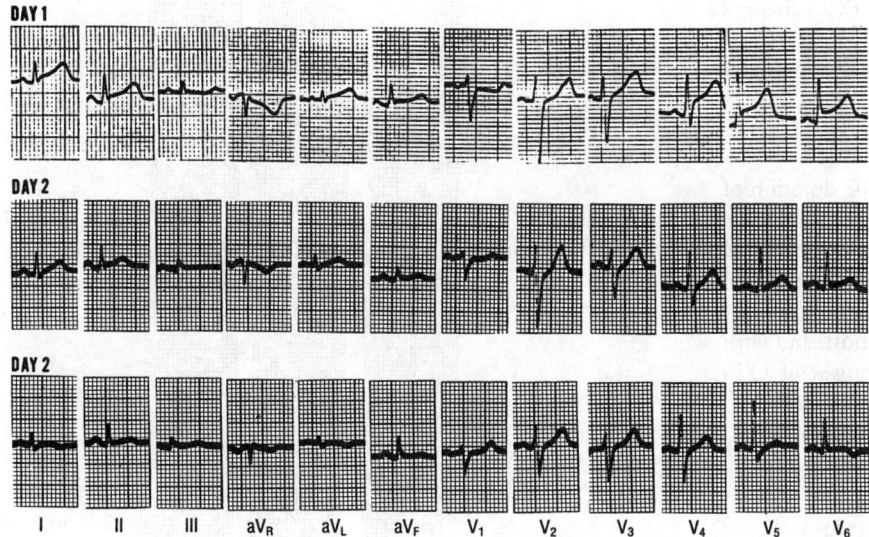

FIGURE 84.12. Acute anterolateral current of injury on day 1 with normalization on day 2. The infarction is manifested by T-wave inversion only *(bottom)*. The latter, if interpreted without serial cardiograms or without correlation with available clinical information, is not diagnostic of infarction.

minimal ST-segment abnormality and often show only T-wave changes. In 10% of patients, the first tracing is normal. The sensitivity of the ECG for MI increases to about 90% with serial tracings and especially when correlated with the clinical and other laboratory findings. In many patients, the infarct is ultimately manifested by T-wave changes only, and because T-wave abnormalities lack specificity, the change must be evaluated in light of all other available data (Figs. 84.12 and 84.13). Comparison with an old ECG, when available, may prove most helpful in the diagnosis of infarctions.

It is frequently difficult or impossible to estimate the age of infarction from a single tracing. With time, the diagnostic feature of infarction, the Q wave, may disappear, leaving only a T-wave abnormality as the residual finding. The ECG may normalize with time, particularly after inferior infarction (Fig. 84.13). Occasionally, the ECG fails to display any evidence of infarction. This is particularly true when the *silent area,* such as the posterior wall, the high lateral segment, or right ventricle, is involved. Similarly, a new infarction may be masked by an old

infarction, intraventricular conduction defects, especially LBBB, and occasionally by WPW syndrome or LADB.

Not all pathologic Q waves indicate infarction. Some are caused by directional changes (e.g., chronic obstructive lung disease, LADB), hypertrophy of the septum (e.g., idiopathic hypertrophic subaortic stenosis, diastolic overload of left ventricle), or myopathies (e.g., congestive cardiomyopathy, progressive muscular dystrophy, amyloidosis). Because most abnormal Q waves are caused by MI, an abnormal Q wave should be considered secondary to infarction until proven otherwise (see Chapter 73).

PERICARDITIS

The current of injury recorded with pericarditis is generated by the involved subjacent myocardium. Characteristically, pericarditis involves the entire heart, and therefore all of the leads, with the exception of aVR, show a current of injury and register an elevated ST segment. Reciprocal ST-segment depression charac-

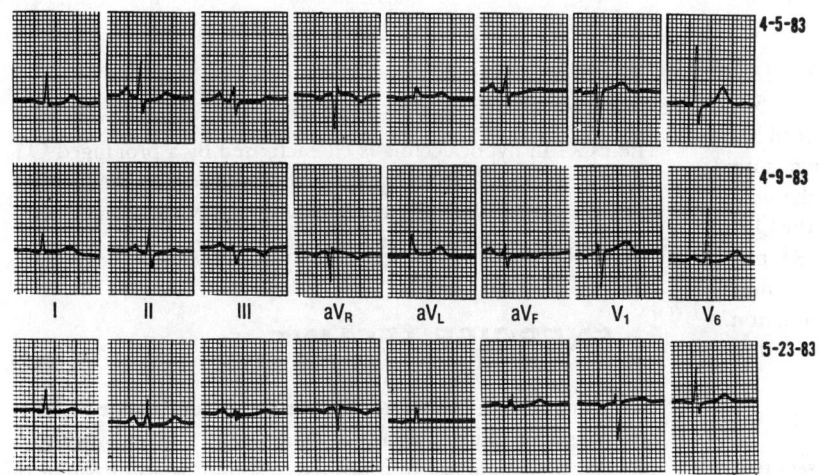

FIGURE 84.13. Acute inferior myocardial infarction manifested by inversion of the T wave in leads III and aVF on April 9, 1983. The electrocardiogram was normal on May 23, 1983.

teristic of MI usually is absent. For more detail of ECG changes with pericarditis (see Chapter 79).

CONDITIONS CAUSING A PROLONGED QT INTERVAL

The QT interval reflects, with some exceptions, the duration of the ventricular recovery time. Prolongation of the QT interval, largely caused by prolongation of phase 2 of the action potential, can be recorded in the presence of hypocalcemia, hypertension, antiarrhythmic drugs, alkalosis, myocardial ischemia, cerebrovascular accident, and bradycardia, after resuscitation, and with other less common conditions. The common causes of QT-interval shortening include hypercalcemia, hyperkalemia, acidosis, and digitalis therapy.

CONDITIONS CAUSING ST-SEGMENT DEPRESSION AND T-WAVE INVERSION

Depression of the ST segment and inversion of the T wave are common findings, which alone rarely indicate a specific cardiac abnormality. As a rule, it is difficult to differentiate between the ST-T changes induced by organic disease, such as coronary heart disease or hypertrophy resulting from hypertension, and other noncardiac causes, such as electrolyte and pH disturbances, endocrine abnormalities, or drug effects. Although the genesis of the ST segment and the T wave differ, these changes, because of their frequent coexistence, are referred to in clinical electrocardiography as ST-T changes.

Determination of the significance of T-wave abnormality is probably the best example of the importance of specificity in interpretation of the ECG. Although the T wave is the most sensitive of all the ECG waveforms because it is altered by a variety of disorders, it lacks the specificity or predictive value that would permit recognition of the cause of the T-wave change. The search for a specific cause of an ST-T change must take into account all available clinical and laboratory information. The information must be evaluated with great care to avoid causing ECG iatrogenic heart disease, with all of its undesirable and often serious sequelae.

ELECTROLYTE ABNORMALITIES

Hyperkalemia

The earliest change of hyperkalemia is peaking or *tenting* of the T wave, usually at a plasma potassium concentration of 5.5 to 7.0 mEq per L (Fig. 84.14). Prolongation of the PR interval and the QRS complex follows. With further rise of plasma potassium concentration, the P-wave amplitude is lowered, and the wave may disappear, the ST segment becomes depressed, and the QRS complex continues to widen. Characteristically, the QRS prolongation is diffuse, involving the initial and terminal components. It may simulate all forms of intraventricular conduction. The terminal event is cardiac standstill or ventricular fibrillation.

Hypokalemia

Hypokalemia is manifested by depression of the ST segment, decrease in amplitude, and inversion of the T wave, which

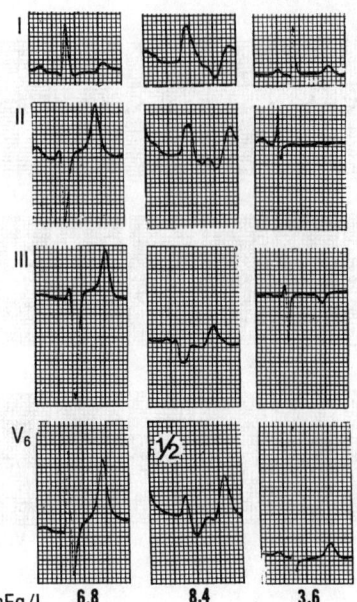

FIGURE 84.14. Electrocardiographic changes of hyperkalemia. After treatment and at a level of 3.6 mEq per L, the PR interval, QRS complex, and T waves are normal. At 6.8 mEq per L, the PR interval and QRS complex are prolonged, with a shift of the QRS axis to the left, and the T waves are symmetric, narrow-based, and tall (so-called tented T waves). At a potassium concentration of 8.4 mEq per L, there is further prolongation of the PR interval, with the P wave becoming difficult to identify, the QRS axis shifted to the right, and the QRS complex prolonged to 0.2 second. The characteristic prolongation of both initial and terminal portions of the QRS is best illustrated in lead V_6. (From Fisch C. Electrolytes and the heart. In: Hurst JW, ed. *The heart*. New York: McGraw-Hill, 1986:1473, with permission.)

merges with a prominent U wave (Fig. 84.15). The changes are best seen in leads V_2 to V_4. The duration of the QT interval is normal; the QU interval is prolonged.

Hypercalcemia

Hypercalcemia is expressed by shortening of the QT interval, largely due to shortening of the ST segment. The ST segment may be absent, with the QRS complex followed by a T wave (Fig. 84.16A). Occasionally, the PR interval is prolonged and the T wave inverted.

Hypocalcemia

The ECG in hypocalcemia is characterized by a prolonged QT interval, primarily resulting from prolongation of the ST segment (Fig. 84.16B). Hypocalcemia with hyperkalemia is a common finding in chronic renal disease (Fig. 84.16C).

■ EXERCISE TESTING

The primary objective of exercise testing is to determine whether the patient exhibits myocardial ischemia at a given workload. The accepted standard of a positive response is a horizontal or downsloping depression of 0.1 mV or greater or, rarely, an eleva-

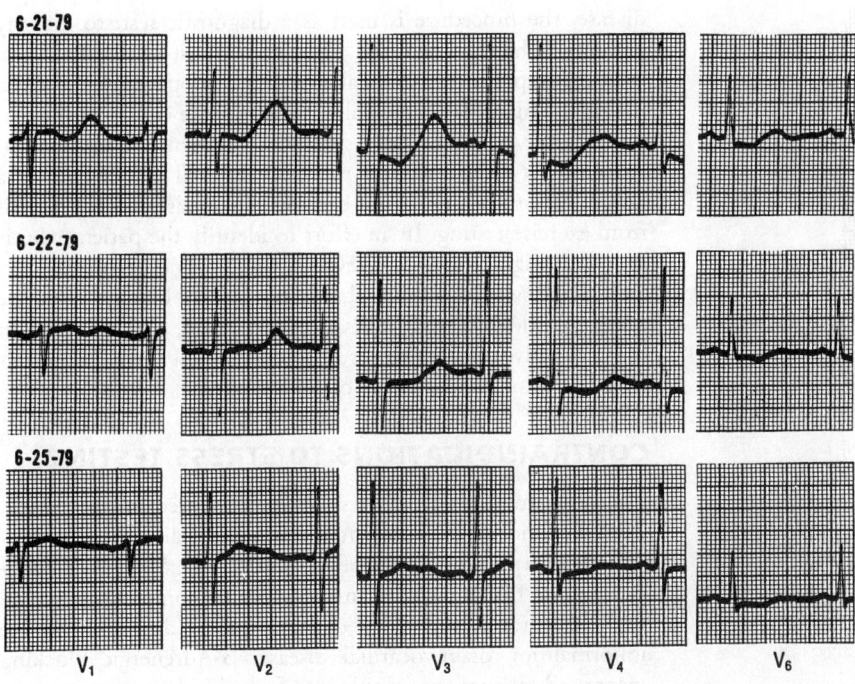

6-21-79

6-22-79

6-25-79

V₁   V₂   V₃   V₄   V₆

FIGURE 84.15. Electrocardiographic changes of hypokalemia. A striking U wave with a marked prolongation of QU interval was recorded on June 21, 1979. The potassium concentration at that time was 1.3 mEq per L. With correction of potassium loss, there was a gradual improvement with a normal QT interval and U wave recorded on June 25, 1979, at a plasma potassium concentration of 3.9 mEq per L. (From Fisch C. Electrolytes and the heart. In: Hurst JW, ed. *The heart.* New York: McGraw-Hill, 1986: 1474, with permission.)

tion of the ST segment, with either of these indications occurring 0.08 second after the QRS, using the TP or PQ segments as the point of reference (Fig. 84.17). The test should be terminated for the following reasons: attainment of the target heart rate, onset of angina or dyspnea, decline in systolic blood pressure, decrease in heart rate, and appearance of three consecutive premature ventricular contractions.

As in any laboratory procedure, the importance of sensitivity and specificity of the test must be recognized. In asymptomatic patients for whom the test is used to detect occult disease, the procedure has a sensitivity of about 50% and a specificity of about 90%. The same values for patients with known three-vessel disease are about 96% and 100%, respectively. The predic-

tive accuracy of the stress test, particularly when applied to coronary artery disease, is in keeping with Bayes' theorem, which indicates that the likelihood that a test is truly positive increases as the prevalence of the disease for which it is being used increases. The test yields maximum benefit when correlated with the history, physical examination, and other laboratory findings.

INDICATIONS FOR EXERCISE TESTING

The primary indication for exercise testing is for symptomatic patients with known or suspected coronary artery disease. Occasionally, the test is used for asymptomatic patients in whom coronary artery disease is likely. For patients with coronary artery

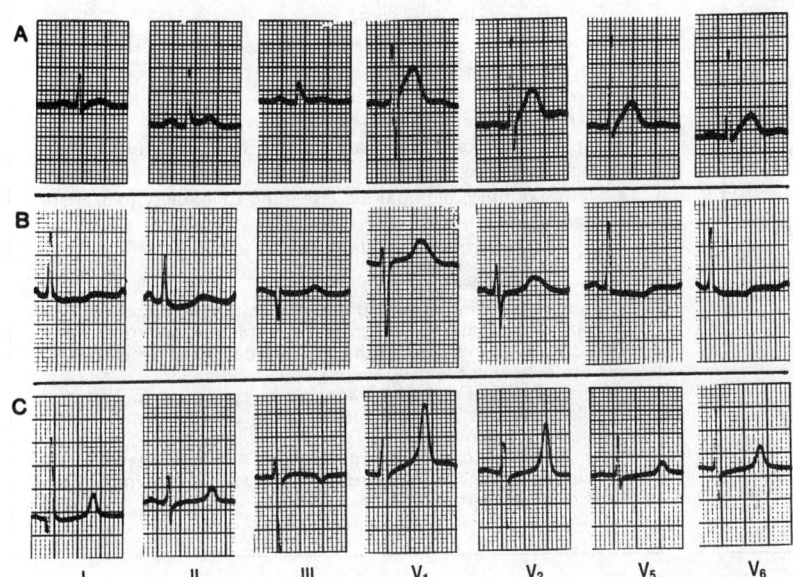

A

B

C

I   II   III   V₁   V₂   V₅   V₆

FIGURE 84.16. **A:** Electrocardiogram (ECG) recorded at a calcium level of 17 mg per dL illustrates the short ST segment characteristic of hypercalcemia. **B:** ECG recorded at a calcium level of 5.9 mg per dL shows prolongation of the ST segment of hypocalcemia. **C:** ECG recorded at a potassium concentration of 6.2 mEq per L, calcium level of 5.3 mg per dL, and phosphorus level of 12.2 mg per dL. The prolongation of the QT interval is due to hypocalcemia, terminated by the tented T of hyperkalemia, and is characteristic of both hypocalcemia and hyperkalemia found in chronic renal disease. (From Fisch C. Electrolytes and the heart. In: Hurst JW, ed. *The heart.* New York: McGraw-Hill, 1986:1475.)

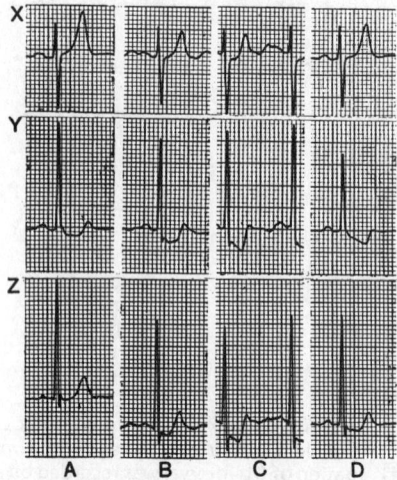

FIGURE 84.17. Simultaneously recorded X, Y, and Z leads illustrate downsloping depression of the ST segment that appears during a stress test: **(A)** resting; **(B)** 7 minutes, stage III; **(C)** 10 minutes, stage III; **(D)** 6 minutes after exercise.

disease, the procedure is used as a diagnostic test; to identify patients at high risk for MI or sudden death (Table 84.1); to evaluate responses to surgical therapy, angioplasty, or medical management; and, occasionally, to follow the course of the disease. In the group without symptoms, patients older than 40 years with two or more of the conventional risk factors or a family history of premature cardiovascular disease may benefit from exercise testing. In an effort to identify the patient who is at low or high risk for new events, the test is used increasingly after acute MI, as a predischarge test 10 to 14 days after the acute episode or 3 to 8 weeks after infarction. The data suggest that a negative test result after MI predicts a less than 2% mortality risk during the first year of follow-up.

CONTRAINDICATIONS TO STRESS TESTING

The contraindications to stress testing are listed in Table 84.2.

ECG abnormalities present at rest make it difficult or impossible to interpret the results of an exercise test. Such abnormalities include LBBB or other intraventricular conduction defects, a WPW pattern, and ST-T changes due to drugs, electrolyte abnormalities, or myocardial disease. β-Adrenergic blocking agents and calcium antagonists interfere with the test by preventing an increase in heart rate and delaying the onset of angina. If possible, these drugs should be discontinued before the test.

TABLE 84.1.	**EXERCISE TEST PARAMETERS ASSOCIATED WITH POOR PROGNOSIS AND INCREASED SEVERITY OF CORONARY ARTERY DISEASE**

Duration of symptom-limiting exercise
  Failure to complete stage II of Bruce protocol or equivalent workload (<6.5 MET) with other protocols
Exercise HR at onset of limiting symptoms
  Failure to attain HR >120 beats/min (off β-blockers)
Time of onset, magnitude, morphology, and postexercise duration of abnormal horizontal or downsloping ST-segment depression
Onset at HR >120 beats/min or <6.5 MET
  Magnitude >2.0 mm
  Postexercise duration >6 min
  Depression in multiple leads
Systolic blood pressure response during or after progressive exercise
  Sustained decrease of >10 mm Hg or flat blood pressure response (<130 mm Hg) during progressive exercise
Other potentially important determinants
  Exercise-induced ST-segment elevation in leads other than a VR
  Angina pectoris during exercise
  Exercise-induced U-wave inversion
  Exercise-induced ventricular tachycardia

Energy expenditure at rest, equivalent to an oxygen uptake of approximately 3.5 mL/kg/min.
HR, heart rate; MET, metabolic equivalent.
(From American College of Cardiology and American Heart Association Guidelines for exercise testing. *J Am Coll Cardiol* 1986; 8:725, with permission.)

TABLE 84.2.	**CONTRAINDICATIONS TO EXERCISE TESTING**

Absolute

- Acute myocardial infarction (within 2 d)
- Unstable angina not previously stabilized by medical therapy[a]
- Uncontrolled cardiac arrhythmias causing symptoms or hemodynamic compromise
- Symptomatic severe aortic stenosis
- Uncontrolled symptomatic heart failure
- Acute pulmonary embolus or pulmonary infarction
- Acute myocarditis or pericarditis
- Acute aortic dissection

Relative[b]

- Left main coronary stenosis
- Moderate stenotic valvular heart disease
- Electrolyte abnormalities
- Severe arterial hypertension[c]
- Tachyarrhythmias or bradyarrhythmias
- Hypertrophic cardiomyopathy and other forms of outflow tract obstruction
- Mental or physical impairment leading to inability to exercise adequately
- High-degree atrioventricular block

---

[a] Appropriate timing of testing depends on level of risk of unstable angina, as defined by AHCPR Unstable Angina Guidelines.
[b] Relative contraindications can be superseded if the benefits of exercise outweigh the risks.
[c] In the absence of definitive evidence, the committee suggests systolic blood pressure >200 mm Hg and/or diastolic blood pressure >110 mm Hg.
(From American College of Cardiology and American Heart Association Guidelines for exercise testing. *J Am Coll Cardiol* 1997; 30(1):265, with permission.)

◼ AMBULATORY MONITORING

A technique for recording the ECG while the patient continues his or her usual daily activities was introduced in 1957 and quickly became a widely used diagnostic tool for the detection of cardiac arrhythmias as correlated with patient symptoms, for the presence of arrhythmias thought to be prognostic and/or of therapeutic importance, and for the evaluation of the efficacy of antiarrhythmic therapy. Ambulatory ECGs (also called Holter or dynamic ECGs) are obtained with a portable tape recorder; later they are scanned and the pertinent data extracted.

Since the early 1960s there have been advances in both recording and playback methodologies. Currently there are two generic forms of ambulatory electrocardiographic recorders: (a) continuous recorders are typically used for 24 to 48 hours to capture arrhythmic events that are common and likely to occur in that time period; and (b) intermittent recorders (loop and event recorders) to detect events that occur less frequently and therefore require longer periods of monitoring (sometimes for weeks or months). Both types have a patient-activated event marker and a time recorder. The most common recording technology to date is the magnetic cassette tape recorder. It allows for playback and interrogation of the entire recording period (full disclosure). Most recorders record two or three leads of the ECG simultaneously. The leads generally used are modified leads V_5 and V_3 and a modified inferior lead. The technique is quite adequate for arrhythmic detection but has limitations for the detection of low-frequency signals such as the ST segment and T waves. Direct recording of the ECG signal in digital format using solid-state recording devices ameliorates these problems. Digital tracings can be analyzed on-line and allow direct transfer to a central analysis facility. The primary limitations in the minds of many clinicians and investigators is, in the case of on-line analysis, the need to "believe" the computer analysis and the inability to verify the computer interpretation because the electrocardiographic data are not recorded and full disclosure is not available. Newer devices are under development to provide for full disclosure by attaching storage devices that can then be interrogated on a separate device. Newer loop recorders may be implanted for longer term monitoring if required.

The characteristics of the patient's symptoms often determine the choice of recording techniques. As the reliability of fully automated systems has not yet been established for clinical use, the technician who scans the results from any of the recording devices plays a vital role in obtaining accurate results. The technician must select pertinent parts of the recordings for printouts that the physician can interpret and must be conscientious and dedicated to the task. Significant portions must not be overlooked. In the case of loss of signal or noise, samples must be printed out for physician decision making. Overreading is essential.

CLINICAL CONSIDERATIONS

There is general agreement that ambulatory electrocardiographic techniques are useful and effective to assess symptoms possibly related to rhythm disturbances such as in patients with otherwise unexplained syncope, episodes of dizziness, or unexplained re-

current palpitations. While other potential uses are numerous and include the evaluation of ischemia in many clinical states, heart rate variability, QT dispersion, T-wave alternans, and signal-averaged analyses, in most instances these analyses are not yet recommended for routine use as the possible sources of inaccuracy are ubiquitous. For research purposes, however, the application of ambulatory electrocardiography may be highly rewarding when performed in laboratories with sophisticated and well-trained physicians and technical professionals.

BIBLIOGRAPHY

American College of Cardiology and American Heart Association. Guidelines for ambulatory monitoring. *Circulation* 1999;100:886–893.

Fisch C. Electrocardiography. In: Braunwald E, ed. *Heart disease,* fifth ed. Philadelphia: WB Saunders, 1997.

Fisch C. Evolution of the clinical electrocardiogram. *J Am Coll Cardiol* 1989; 14:1127–1138.

Friedberg CK, Zager A. "Nonspecific" ST and T-wave changes. *Circulation* 1961;23:655–661.

Gibbons RJ, Balady GJ, Beasly JW, et al. ACC/AHA guidelines for exercise testing. A report of the American College of Cardiology/American Heart Association task force on practice guidelines. *J Am Coll Cardiol* 1997; 30:260–311.

Johnston FD. *Selected papers of Dr. Frank N. Wilson.* Ann Arbor, MI: Edwards Brothers, Inc., 1954.

Lewis T. *The graphic mechanism and graphic registration of the heart beat.* London: Shaw and Sons, Ltd., 1925.

Macfarlane PW, Lawrie VTD. *Comprehensive electrocardiology,* vol. 1. New York: Pergamon Press, 1989.

Pick A, Langendorf R. *Interpretation of complex arrhythmias.* Philadelphia: Lea & Febiger, 1979.

Snellen HA. *Selected papers on electrocardiography of Willem Einthoven.* Leiden University Press, 1977.

Kelley's Textbook of Internal Medicine, fourth edition. Edited by H. David Humes. Lippincott Williams & Wilkins, Philadelphia © 2000.

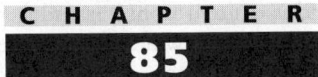

C H A P T E R
85

ECHOCARDIOGRAPHY

WILLIAM F. ARMSTRONG

Echocardiography refers to the use of ultrasound to evaluate cardiac structures and to render clinical diagnoses of heart disease. Initially demonstrated to be feasible in the early 1970s, it has become the single most widely utilized cardiac diagnostic test outside of electrocardiography. This chapter will review the basic principles and clinical utility of echocardiography.

◼ METHODS

ULTRASOUND PRINCIPLES

Clinical echocardiography uses sound waves in the ultrasound frequency range, defined as 1.0 to 10 MHz. For practical imag-

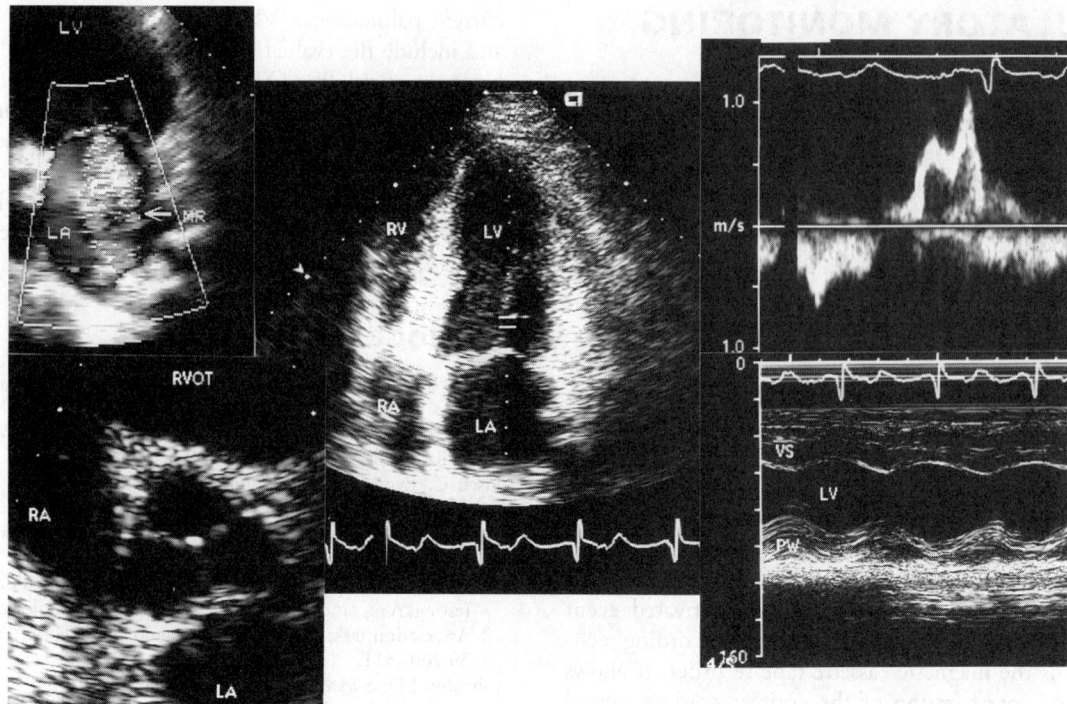

FIGURE 85.1. Composite figure showing the different echocardiographic modalities. The center frame is a four-chamber view from the apex of the left ventricle on which a Doppler cursor line can be seen running through the left ventricle and left atrium. The other four panels illustrate the derived views and modalities that can be obtained from the echocardiogram. The panel in the upper right shows a typical pulsed waved transmitral Doppler recording. Note the biphasic flow above the line, which represents flow from the left atrium to the left ventricle. The bottom right panel is a typical M-mode echocardiogram through the left ventricle. The lower left panel is an expanded, highly detailed view of a normal three-leaflet aortic valve. The upper left panel shows a mitral regurgitation jet recorded in color Doppler flow imaging (here produced in black and white). All four of the smaller images can be derived from the main echocardiographic image. LA, left atrium; LV, left ventricle; VS, ventricular septum; RA, right atrium; RV, right ventricle; RVOT, right ventricular outflow tract; MR, mitral regurgitation.

ing purposes in adult patients, frequencies range from 2.0 to 5.0 MHz. Ultrasound is emitted from a transducer that consists of a series of ultrasound crystals, which also act as receivers. Modern ultrasound equipment sends out a 90-degree array of ultrasound beams, along which there are multiple reflected targets. As the speed of sound in tissue is known (1,450 m per second) the distance of a reflective target can be determined from the round trip transit time of the ultrasound packet from the face of the transducer and back. This series of reflected targets is then converted to an ultrasound image of the heart. Several different ultrasound modes can be utilized for complete cardiovascular evaluation (Fig. 85.1). Repeating this process at frequent intervals creates a series of sequential images that are displayed as a tomographic moving two-dimensional image of the heart (Fig. 85.2). The number of images or frames that can be imaged is limited by the size of the area being interrogated and the speed of sound in tissue. For imaging large sectors of the adult heart, images are acquired at a rate of 30 to 50 frames per second. Newer generation equipment can provide faster imaging frame rates, but only in fairly limited areas.

DOPPLER ULTRASOUND

The Doppler principle states that the frequency of an ultrasound beam reflected from a moving object differs from the transmitted

frequency. If an object is moving toward the transducer, the reflected frequency is higher than the transmitted frequency. Conversely, if the object is moving away from the transducer, the reflected frequency is less than the transmitted frequency. The difference between the transmitted and reflected frequency is the "Doppler shift." The Doppler equation translates this Doppler shift into direction and velocity of motion of the interrogated target.

Doppler ultrasound is used in three basic forms. The first is pulsed Doppler, which effectively is a "steerable stethoscope." It provides an analysis of the direction and velocity of flow at any interrogated site within the imaged frame. A limitation of pulsed Doppler is that the maximum velocity that can be detected is determined by the Nyquist limit and is limited to approximately 2.5 m per second.

Continuous wave Doppler interrogates velocities along a single beam in a continuous fashion and is not limited by any maximum detectable velocity. However, it is limited by "range ambiguity," which implies that it is not possible to determine where along a line of interrogation a velocity originates.

Color flow imaging is a technique in which multiple pulsed Doppler sample volumes are simultaneously interrogated in a region of interest. The Doppler shift is color-encoded to represent both direction and velocity of motion. This effectively

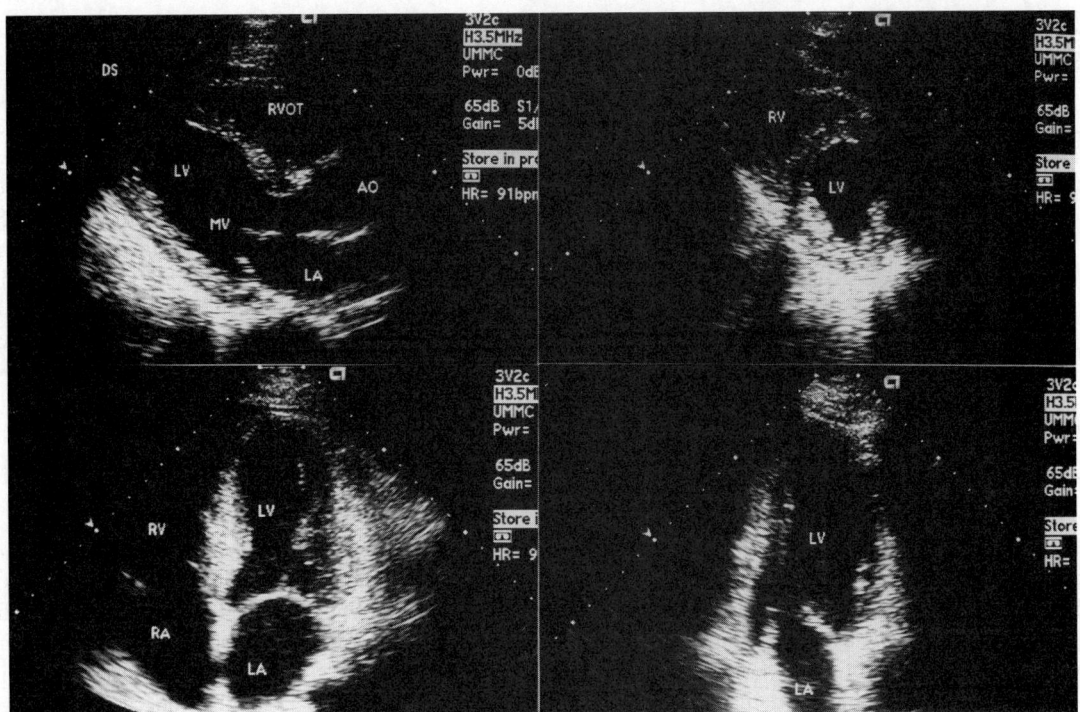

FIGURE 85.2. Four panels illustrating different two-dimensional echocardiographic views. The upper panels were recorded from the parasternal transducer position and the lower two panels were recorded from the apical position. In each case, the orientation of the transducer is rotated 90 degrees to obtain the views on the right after obtaining the view on the left. MV, mitral valve; AO, aorta; other abbreviations per previous figure.

"paints" an image of the velocity of moving blood on top of the two-dimensional image of the heart.

M-MODE ECHOCARDIOGRAPHY

M-Mode echocardiography was the earliest echocardiographic modality utilized clinically. It allowed interrogation of cardiac structures along a single line of interrogation and has been largely supplanted by two-dimensional echocardiography. M-Mode echocardiography has high temporal resolution and still has some value in determining the motion characteristics of rapidly moving structures.

STRESS ECHOCARDIOGRAPHY

Stress echocardiography refers to the utilization of echocardiographic imaging before, during, and/or after cardiovascular stress. By comparing left ventricular wall motion and function at rest and after exercise, the effects of induced ischemia can be detected and hence the diagnosis of coronary artery disease made.

CONTRAST ECHOCARDIOGRAPHY

Gas-filled structures such as microbubbles are intense reflectors of ultrasound. Contrast echocardiography refers to the injection of one of these ultrasound contrast agents into the blood pool. The agent is assumed to parallel the distribution of blood flow

and hence can be used to track flow through the cardiovascular system. Commonly employed ultrasound agents include agitated saline and commercially available perfluorocarbon agents. Saline contrast injections are a valuable means of detecting right-to-left intracardiac shunts, as the bubbles are filtered by the lungs and do not appear in the left heart except in the presence of a shunt such as an atrial septal defect (ASD), patent foramen ovale, etc. Newer commercially available agents are of sufficiently small size to pass through the lungs and fully opacify the left ventricular cavity. In this setting they can be used to enhance endocardial definition and improve wall motion analysis. In addition, they have shown substantial promise for detecting and quantifying myocardial perfusion.

ADVANTAGES AND DISADVANTAGES OF ECHOCARDIOGRAPHY

As with all imaging techniques, echocardiography has a distinct set of advantages and disadvantages. These are outlined in Table 85.1. Perhaps the greatest advantage of echocardiography is that it is an entirely risk-free procedure and confers no known biologic risk to the patients, operators, pregnant women, or fetuses. Standard transthoracic echocardiography is a painless examination that can be accomplished in 15 to 60 minutes, depending on the detail with which the examination must be accomplished.

The major disadvantage of echocardiography is the potential for limited applicability in some patient subsets. Ultrasonography transmits without distortion through fluid and body tissues,

TABLE 85.1. ECHOCARDIOGRAPHY: ADVANTAGES AND DISADVANTAGES

Advantages	Disadvantages
Noninvasive	Limited visualization
Risk-free	in 5–10% of patients
Highly versatile	Potential for overuse
Approaches *all* forms of heart disease	
Rapid	
Portable	
Highly accurate in skilled hands	
High patient acceptance	
High resolution	
Tomographic imaging	

CLINICAL INDICATIONS

The balance of this chapter will deal with individual cardiovascular disease states and the role in which echocardiography can play. It is meant not as an all-encompassing review of echocardiography but only as a brief introduction to basic principles of echocardiography as it relates to specific diseases. Similarly, lines of logical evaluation can be drawn for patients presenting with chest pain, fatigue, arrhythmia, syncope, neurologic diseases, and other complaints for which there are possible cardiovascular etiologies. Table 85.2 outlines many presenting complaints for which echocardiography may be indicated and the preferred echocardiographic methodology for each.

PERICARDIAL DISEASE

Pericardial disease was one of the first forms of organic heart disease diagnosed with echocardiography, and echocardiography remains the imaging modality by which all others are compared for detection of pericardial effusion. Pericardial effusion is manifest as an echo-free space surrounding the heart between the visceral and parietal pericardium. Effusions are typically quantified only as minimal, small, moderate, and large (Fig. 85.3).

but it is not transmitted through bone and it reflects intensively off air-containing structures. As such, obese patients may have poor acoustic windows that limit the ability to visualize the cardiac structures adequately. Additionally, patients with obstructive lung disease represent problematic imaging.

TABLE 85.2. CLINICAL UTILITY OF ECHOCARDIOGRAPHY

	2D	Dop.	CFD	Cont.	TEE	Stress
Pericardial disease	1	2	3	4	4	N/A
Valvular heart disease						
Murmur	1	1	1	3	4	N/A
Mitral stenosis	1	1	1	–	3	3
Mitral regurgitation	1	1	1	–	3	N/A
Aortic stenosis/regurgitation	1	1	1	–	3	3
Prosthetic heart valve dysfunction	1	1	1	–	2	N/A
Coronary artery disease						
Chest pain syndrome	1	3	3	4	4	1
R/O coronary artery disease	1	3	3	4	4	1
Diagnose acute myocardial infarction	1	3	3	4	4	N/A
Complications of infarction						
Aneurysm	1	3	3	4	4	N/A
Thrombus	1	3	3	4	4	N/A
VSD/papillary muscle rupture	1	1	1	3	2	N/A
Assess LV function	1	1	2	4	4	3
Congenital Heart Disease	1	1	1	3	3	3
ASD	1	1	1	2	2	4
Cardiomyopathy						
Dilated	1	1	1	4	4	3
Hypertrophic	1	1	1	4	4	3
Endocarditis	1	1	1	4	2	N/A
Pulmonary hypertension						
Known	1	1	1	2	3	3
Occult	1	1	1	2	3	2
Congestive heart failure	1	1	1	4	4	3
Stroke/source of embolus	1	2	2	1	2	N/A
Aortic dissection	2	2	1	4	1	N/A
Dyspnea evaluation	1	1	1	1	4	1

1, Indicated and essential; 2, often required—may add clinically needed information; 3, necessary in select instances for specific question; 4, rarely necessary. 2D, Two-dimensional echocardiography; R/O, right obstructive; VSD, ventricular septal defect; LV, left ventricle; ASD, atrial septal defect; Cont, contrast echocardiography.

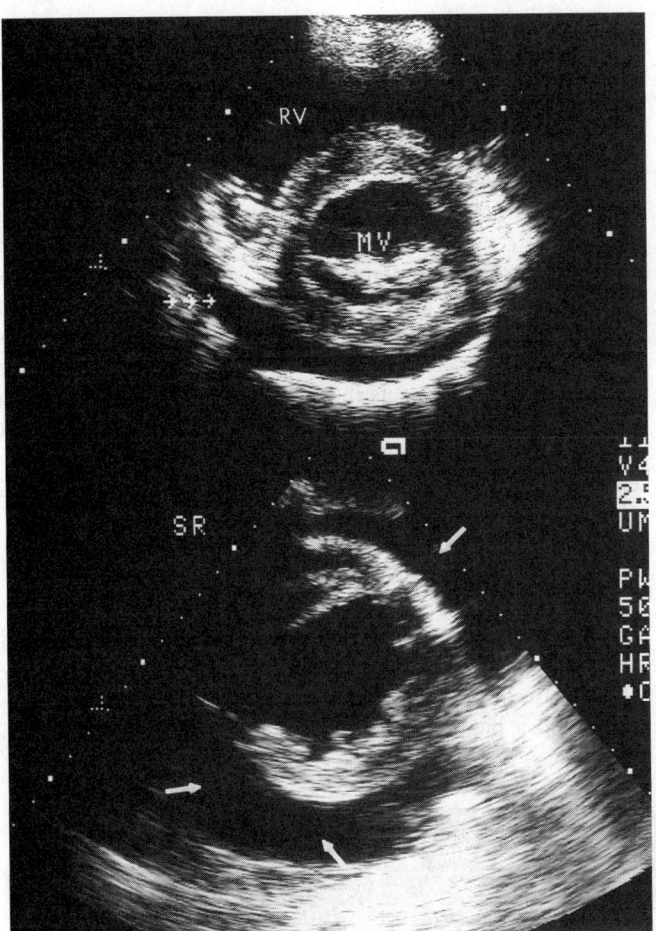

FIGURE 85.3. Short-axis two-dimensional echocardiograms recorded in patients with a small *(upper)* and large *(lower)* pericardial effusion. In the upper panel there is a 1- to 1.5-cm echo-free space posterior to the heart representing pericardial fluid *(arrows)*. In the upper panel there is a larger circumferential effusion *(arrows)* visible both posterior and anterior to the heart in this short-axis view.

Attempts to determine actual fluid volume have met with variable success. In addition to determining the presence of pericardial fluid, echocardiography can play a key role in determining the hemodynamic significance of an effusion. With elevation in intrapericardial pressure, the right atrium and right ventricular outflow tract will show characteristic phasic collapse. This finding is a highly reliable sign of elevated intrapericardial pressure. Echocardiographic evidence of hemodynamic compromise may precede typical clinical evidence of cardiac tamponade.

Constrictive pericarditis remains an elusive diagnosis. Using a combination of M-mode, two-dimensional, and Doppler interrogation, both direct and indirect evidence of constrictive pericarditis can be found with echocardiography. In classic constriction there is an exaggerated interaction between the right and left ventricles during respiration. This is seen as an exaggerated motion of the ventricular septum with the respiratory cycle. This can also be seen on Doppler interrogation of valvular inflows and outflows. Attempts at determining actual pericardial thickness with echocardiography have not met with success. Computed tomography and magnetic resonance imaging remain superior for the determination of pericardial thickness.

VALVULAR HEART DISEASE

Using transthoracic two-dimensional echocardiography, valve morphology can be identified as normal or abnormal, and varying degrees of valve thickening, rigidity, fibrosis, and calcification can be quantified. Doppler ultrasound provides an excellent means for determining the velocity of jets through a stenotic valve, from which both peak instantaneous and mean valvular pressure gradients can be determined. Color flow imaging, supplemented by spectral flow profiles, is an excellent means for determining the severity of regurgitant valvular lesions. In routine clinical practice, regurgitant valvular lesions are characterized qualitatively as absent, minimal, mild, moderate, and severe. Quantitative techniques for determining the severity of valvular insufficiency exist, but they are highly operator-dependent and frequently are not employed in routine clinical practice.

MITRAL STENOSIS

The normal mitral valve consists of two leaflets, the larger of which is the anterior leaflet. When fully opened the leaflets are relatively parallel and the tip of the anterior mitral valve leaflet opens to within 1.0 cm of the anterior ventricular septum. In mitral stenosis there is thickening and fibrosis, predominantly of the tips of the mitral valve leaflets and chordal apparatus (Fig. 85.4). In early mitral stenosis the belly of the leaflet is relatively

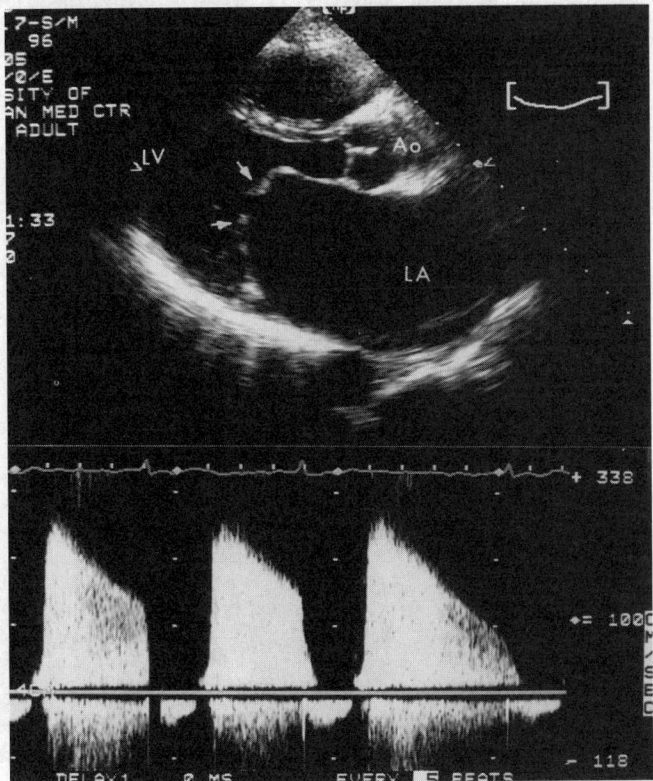

FIGURE 85.4. Mitral stenosis. The upper panel is a parasternal long-axis view recorded in diastole. Note that the left atrium is dilated and that the mitral valve, rather than opening in a straight line, "domes" as the leaflet tips *(arrows)* have restricted mobility. The lower panel is a transmitral continuous wave Doppler recording from which a transmitral pressure gradient can be calculated.

preserved, resulting in a funnel-shaped or domelike opening of the mitral valve. In many instances the actual restrictive orifice can be imaged in its short axis and measured to provide an accurate assessment of the area of the stenotic mitral orifice. Secondary features of rigidity, calcification, and chordal involvement can also be characterized. These features have specific relevance with respect to the feasibility of performing mitral balloon valvuloplasty. Patients with substantial degrees of calcification and rigidity are less likely to have a good result from mitral balloon valvuloplasty.

Quantitation of mitral stenosis relies heavily on Doppler techniques to determine the mean great transmitral gradient. In borderline cases this can be done both at rest and with exercise. Other features of mitral stenosis that can be evaluated using echocardiography include the degree of secondary dilatation of the left atrium, the presence or absence of left atrial thrombus (transesophageal echo required), and the presence of concurrent mitral regurgitation and secondary pulmonary hypertension.

MITRAL REGURGITATION

Both the mechanism and severity of mitral regurgitation can be determined with echocardiography. Mitral valve prolapse with or without leaflet thickening, flail leaflets, concurrent mitral stenosis, and vegetations or other masses can all be reliably identified as the etiologic cause of mitral regurgitation. Transesophageal echocardiography plays an incremental role in determining the mechanism of regurgitation as it relates to potential surgical repair. Mitral regurgitation is quantified as minimal, mild, moderate, and severe. Quantitative techniques for determining its severity exist, including calculation of a regurgitant orifice area and calculation of regurgitant volumes. Most clinical laboratories rely on a qualitative assessment of severity rather than detailed quantitative techniques. The severity of mitral regurgitation is directly proportional to the size of the regurgitant jet within the left atrium (Fig. 85.5). Jets that are eccentric and impinge on a wall will understate the total regurgitant volume, and this must be factored into the clinical assessment. Additionally, highly eccentric jets are more likely to represent the effects of a flail mitral valve leaflet.

AORTIC STENOSIS

As for mitral valve disease, both the anatomical substrate and the severity of stenosis can be determined. In approximately 80% of cases the individual leaflets can be visualized with certainty, and a bicuspid valve be either excluded or diagnosed.

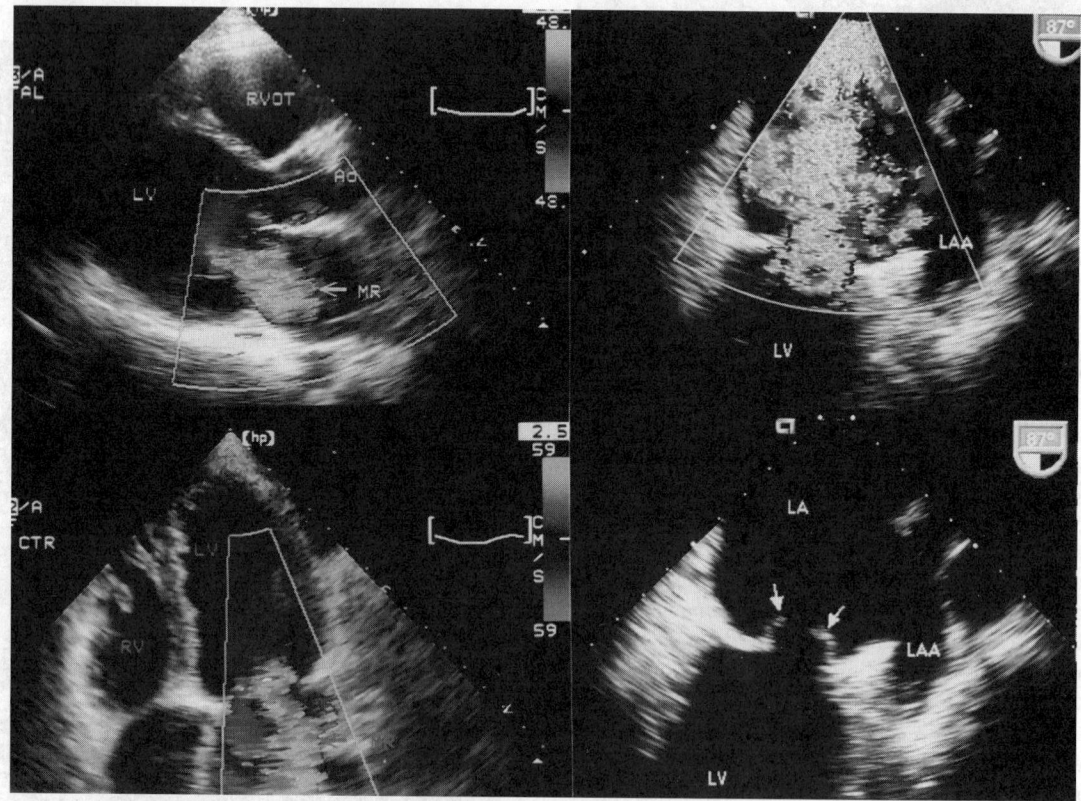

FIGURE 85.5. Four-panel view of patients with mitral regurgitation. The two panels on the left are transthoracic echocardiograms. The upper panel was recorded in a parasternal long-axis view and reveals moderate mitral regurgitation filling approximately 50% of the left atrium. The lower panel reveals a more eccentric mitral regurgitation jet along the lateral wall of the left atrium. The upper right panel is a transesophageal echocardiogram revealing severe mitral regurgitation and the lower panel the same view with the color signal suppressed. In this view, a flail anterior and posterior mitral valve leaflets (arrows) can be visualized as the mechanism for severe mitral regurgitation. LAA, left atrial appendage.

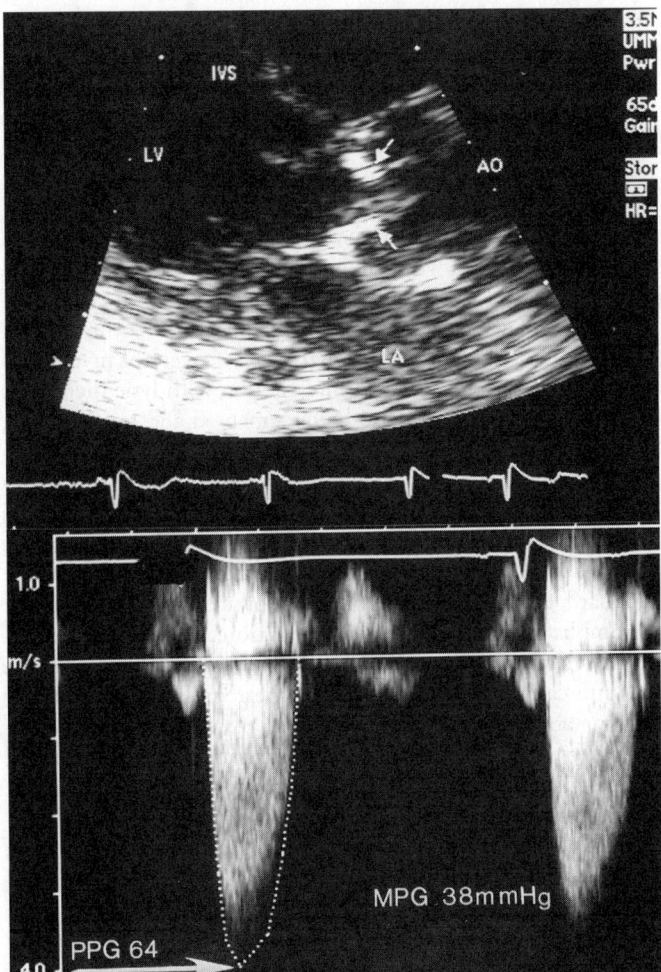

FIGURE 85.6. Two-dimensional echocardiogram and Doppler of a patient with aortic stenosis. The upper panel was recorded in the parasternal long-axis view in systole. Note the thickened aortic valve leaflets with restricted mobility *(arrows)*. The lower panel is a continuous wave Doppler recorded from the apex from which a peak pressure gradient (PPG) of 64 m Hg and a mean pressure gradient (MPG) of 38 m Hg can be calculated.

The degree of leaflet thickening and restriction of motion is easily determined in most patients from the transthoracic echocardiogram (Fig. 85.6). Direct measurement of the stenotic orifice is feasible in only a minority of patients, even with the transesophageal approach. Secondary features of aortic stenosis, including poststenotic dilatation of the aorta and left ventricular hypertrophy, can also be evaluated. Attention should be paid to overall left ventricular function as reduced left ventricular function may result in a reduced gradient in the presence of a severely stenotic valve.

Continuous wave Doppler is essential for determining the peak and mean gradient through a stenotic aortic valve (Fig. 85.6). The gradient determined with transthoracic Doppler ultrasound correlates favorably with simultaneously determined gradients in the catheterization laboratory. The aortic valve gradient may be underestimated in suboptimal quality exams in which the interrogation beam is improperly aligned with the aortic outflow and when compared to nonsimultaneous cardiac catheterization. Doppler ultrasound only rarely overestimates an aortic stenosis gradient. By combining Doppler parameters of flow and a measurement of the left ventricular outflow tract area, aortic valve area can be calculated using the continuity equation.

AORTIC INSUFFICIENCY

Aortic insufficiency is quantified both by color Doppler flow imaging and spectral Doppler. Unlike mitral regurgitation, in which the size of the insufficiency jet correlates well with the severity of regurgitation, the size of an aortic insufficiency jet in general correlates poorly with severity. The actual height or width of a jet, indexed to the left ventricular outflow tract, probably represents the best index of aortic insufficiency severity with color Doppler flow imaging (Fig. 85.7). Additionally, by evaluating the pressure half-time from a spectral display, additional indexes of the severity of aortic insufficiency can be determined.

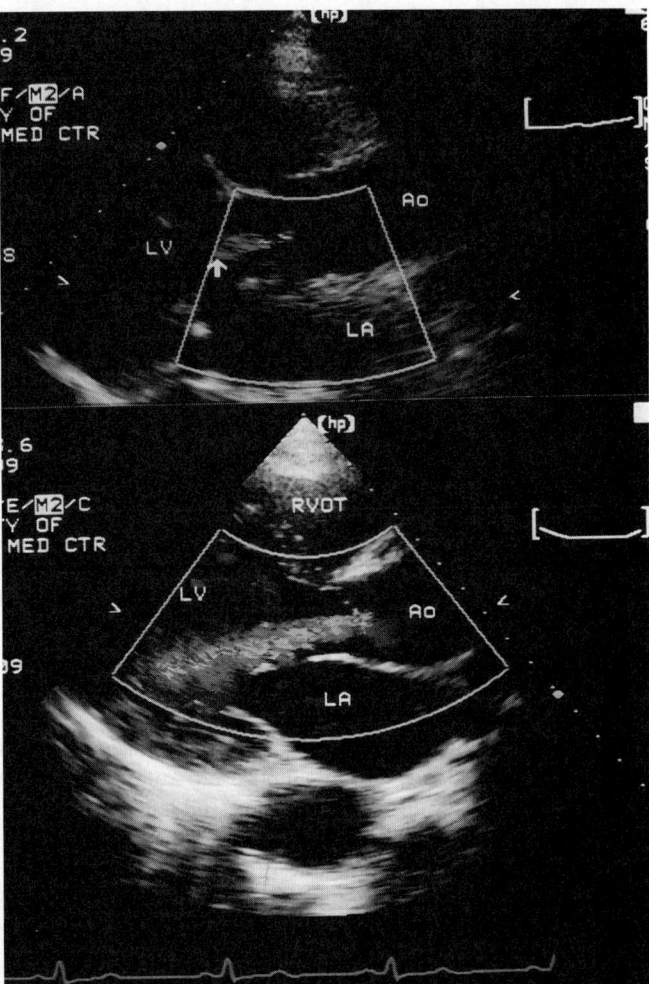

FIGURE 85.7. Parasternal long-axis views of two patients with aortic insufficiency. In each case the images were recorded in diastole. In the upper panel mild aortic insufficiency with a relatively small, narrow jet is seen *(arrow)*. The lower panel demonstrates a greater degree of aortic insufficiency with a wide jet that penetrates down past the tips of the mitral valve leaflets.

TRICUSPID VALVE DISEASE

The majority of tricuspid valve disease encountered is secondary to right heart dilatation and commonly seen in association with pulmonary hypertension. Tricuspid regurgitation is quantified in a manner similar to that for mitral regurgitation. Additionally, right ventricular systolic pressure can be determined from the velocity of a tricuspid regurgitation jet. Primary intrinsic disease of the tricuspid valve is rare. The tricuspid valve may be involved in rheumatic heart disease, in which case mitral involvement virtually always occurs. Isolated tricuspid valve disease can also occur in endocarditis and in the carcinoid syndrome.

PULMONIC VALVE DISEASE

Pulmonic stenosis is largely a disease of childhood. Its quantitation is based on the appearance of the valve as well as on determination of transpulmonic gradients. Mild degrees of pulmonic insufficiency are very common in the normal adult population and do not necessarily represent a pathologic state, unless seen in association with valvular thickening or subsequent chamber enlargement.

CONGENITAL HEART DISEASE

Modern echocardiographic techniques are sufficient for nearly complete characterization of virtually all forms of congenital heart disease in both children and adults. In adults the most common congenital lesion to be detected de novo is the ASD. Its location can be reliably determined as either primum, secundum, or sinus venous. An ASD results in dilatation of the right atrium and ventricle and a relative volume overload of the right ventricle (Fig. 85.8). Additionally, using specialized scanning planes the ASD frequently can be directly visualized with transthoracic echocardiography. Contrast echocardiography with agitated saline is a reliable mechanism for detecting a right-to-left shunt. Transesophageal echocardiography in experienced hands has nearly a 100% accuracy rate for detecting or excluding the presence of an ASD. Transesophageal echocardiography is an excellent method for determining the feasibility of percutaneous ASD closure, based on the ASD size and integrity of the peridefective tissue.

Other congenital lesions that are common in childhood, such as ventricular septal defect (VSD), are infrequently encountered in adult populations as a de novo diagnosis. The combination of two-dimensional imaging and Doppler ultrasound is a reliable mechanism for determining the presence and location of VSDs when suspected. Other than the simpler lesions such as ASDs, the majority of adult congenital heart disease is in a repaired or palliated state. Echocardiography provides virtually all of the information needed to follow patients with repaired tetralogy of Fallot, closed VSD, and previously closed ASD.

▌ CORONARY ARTERY DISEASE

Myocardial ischemia, occurring either during a spontaneous or induced episode of angina or as part of myocardial infarction, results in abnormalities of ventricular wall motion (Fig. 85.9). These abnormalities are detected as a lack of myocardial thickening as well as decreased motion of the endocardium. There is a minimum threshold of involved myocardium required before a wall motion abnormality occurs. However, the majority of Q-wave myocardial infarctions and most non-Q-wave infarcts of substantial size are associated with detectable wall motion abnormalities. Numerous studies have demonstrated that more than 90% of individuals with impending myocardial infarction will have a detectable wall motion abnormality and that the size of this abnormality correlates well with the degree of myocardial necrosis and, similarly, with prognosis. Recovery of myocardial function following successful intervention with lytic therapy or primary angioplasty can also be documented and tracked using echocardiography.

Virtually all mechanical complications of myocardial infarction can be detected with echocardiography. An aneurysm is detected as a distinct bulge in the shape of the left ventricle present both in systole and in diastole. Echocardiography is the standard examination for excluding or diagnosing ventricular thrombus following myocardial infarction. Mechanical complications such as VSD, free-wall rupture, and papillary muscle rupture can be detected. Doppler interrogation is essential for finding abnormal flow associated with a postinfarct VSD and in quantifying the degree of mitral regurgitation. Transesophageal echocardiography plays an incremental role in determining the mechanism and severity of mitral regurgitation. Chronic complications of myocardial infarction such as infarct expansion, chronic left ventricular thrombus (Fig. 85.10), and left ventricular dilatation with reduced left ventricular systolic function can likewise be detected with echocardiography.

Occult coronary artery disease can be detected using stress echocardiography. This technique relies on detection of exercise or pharmacologically induced myocardial ischemia, which is associated with a transient wall motion abnormality. By comparing left ventricular wall motion at rest and with stress, a reliable indicator of the presence of occult coronary artery disease is obtained. In experienced laboratories the accuracy of stress echocardiography for detecting coronary disease is equivalent to radionuclide imaging. Both imaging techniques are superior to routine treadmill ECG alone.

CARDIOMYOPATHIES

Echocardiography is a superb technique for demonstrating the presence of both dilated and hypertrophic cardiomyopathy. Dilated cardiomyopathy of any cause is manifest as dilatation of the left ventricle and is usually secondary to dilatation of the left atrium. Variable degrees of mitral regurgitation are frequently present (Fig. 85.7). Either primary involvement of the right ventricle or secondary involvement due to pulmonary hypertension is not uncommonly seen and is often associated with tricuspid regurgitation. Ejection fraction can be reliably measured by calculation of diastolic and systolic volumes. Complications of ventricular thrombus, secondary mitral and tricuspid regurgitation, and pulmonary hypertension can all be reliably documented. Evaluation of mitral valve inflow may provide valuable

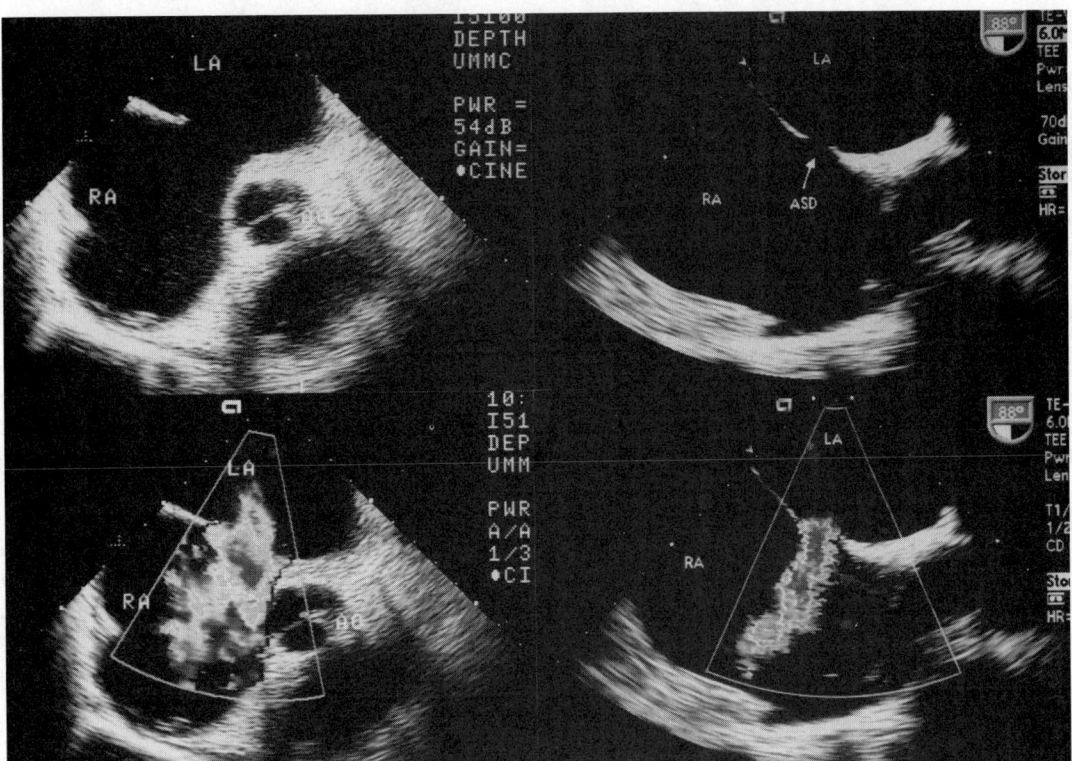

FIGURE 85.8. Transesophageal echocardiograms recorded in two patients with ASDs. On the left is a large ASD seen as echo dropout in the atrial septum on the two-dimensional image. The lower left panel shows the color flow image representing flow from the left atrium to the right atrium. The two right panels represent standard two-dimensional imaging and color flow imaging of a patient with a smaller ASD and predominant left-to-right shunting. ASD, atrial septal defect.

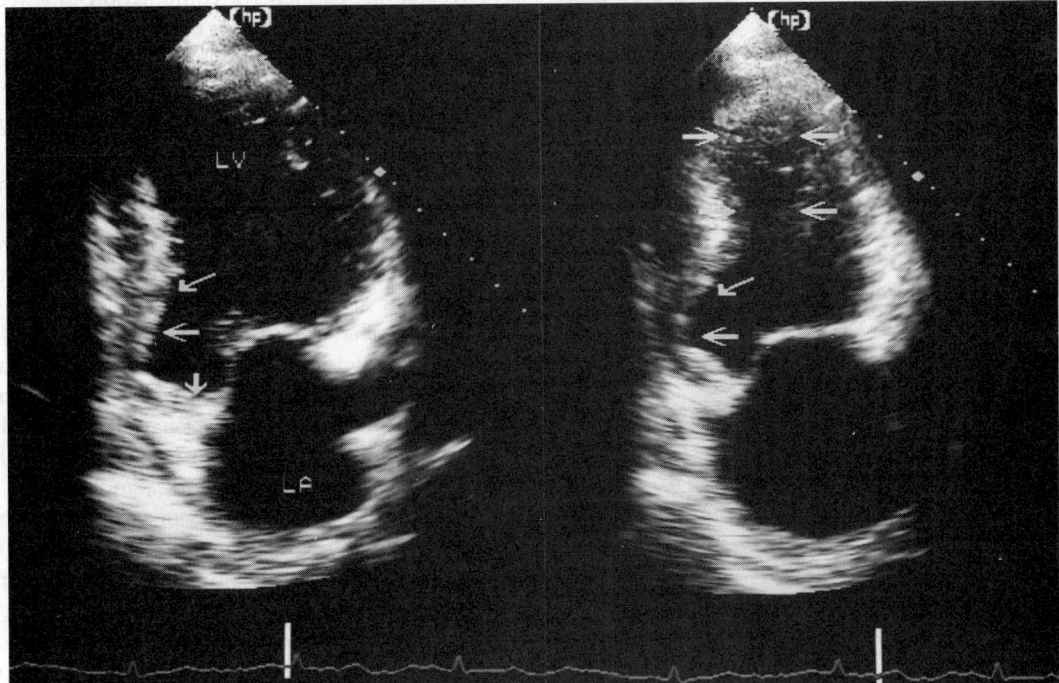

FIGURE 85.9. Apical two-chamber view of a patient with an inferior myocardial infarction. Compare the shape of the left ventricle in diastole and systole to the normal example represented in Figure 85.2. In this example, the left panel is in diastole and the right panel in systole. The proximal inferior wall is dyskinetic and aneurysmal *(arrows).* The remaining walls move normally.

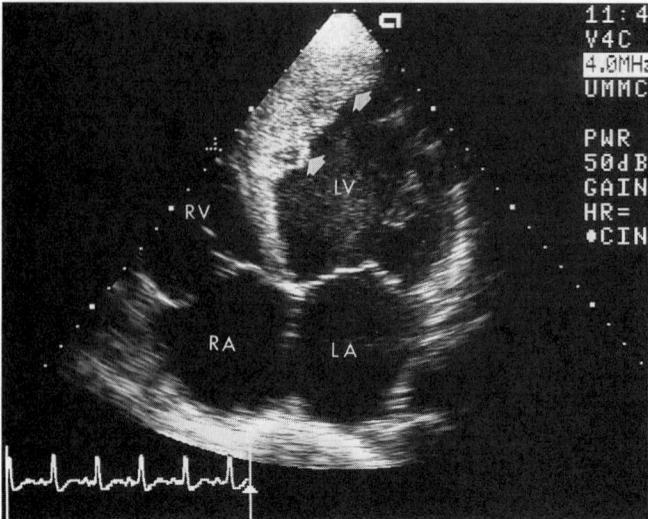

FIGURE 85.10. Apical four-chamber view in a patient with a large anterior apical myocardial infarction and a large mural thrombus. Note the echo-dense mass that fills the apex of the left ventricle. The border of the mass with the blood pool is denoted by white arrows.

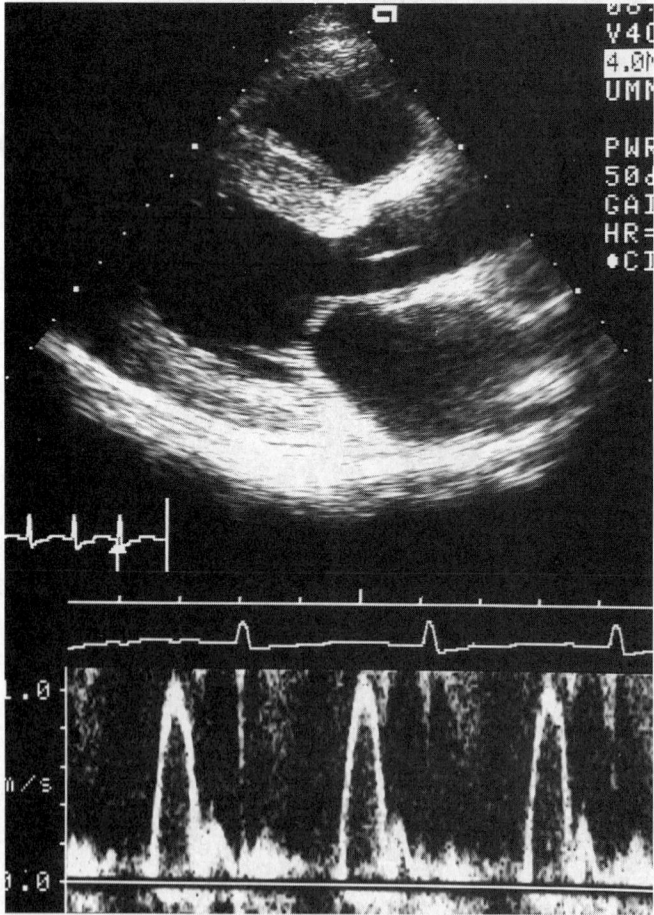

FIGURE 85.11. Parasternal long-axis view of a patient with cardiac amyloidosis. Note the left ventricular hypertrophy and the abnormal texture of the ventricular myocardium, which appears echo-dense and white compared to the normal myocardial texture represented in earlier figures. The lower panel is a transmitral Doppler showing the high E to A ratio, suggestive of a restrictive physiology in this setting.

prognostic information. Patients with end-stage dilated cardiomyopathy reach a "restrictive physiology" phase manifest as a high E-to-A ratio of mitral valve inflow. This finding has been demonstrated to confer an adverse prognosis. Finally, infiltrative cardiomyopathy, such as amyloid, can be reliably diagnosed with echocardiography (Fig. 85.11).

Hypertrophic cardiomyopathy (also called idiopathic hypertrophic subaortic stenosis, or IHSS) is readily diagnosed with two-dimensional echocardiography. In the classic form there is disproportionate and inappropriate hypertrophy of the ventricular septum in association with systolic anterior motion of the mitral valve and dynamic left ventricular outflow tract obstruction. Hypertrophic cardiomyopathy is a very heterogeneous entity, and numerous variations of hypertrophy including diffuse, symmetric left ventricular hypertrophy, isolated apical hypertrophy, and isolated lateral or inferior wall hypertrophy have all been described. The degree of left ventricular outflow tract obstruction can be quantified using continuous wave Doppler, and the degree of associated mitral regurgitation can be quantified with color flow imaging. Two-dimensional echocardiography plays a critical role in the initial diagnosis of hypertrophic cardiomyopathy and in screening of family members once the disease is detected.

OTHER LESIONS

CARDIAC VEGETATIONS AND MASSES

Infectious endocarditis both in acute and chronic forms is associated with valvular abnormalities in well over 95% of patients. A vegetation represents a combination of infected thrombus, inflammatory and infectious material, and platelet fibrin deposition on the valve. Depending on the virulence of the organism, it is variably destructive leading to perforation of the valve leaflets and disruption of the supporting apparatus. Vegetations are detected on two-dimensional echocardiography as mobile, oscillating masses attached to a valvular structure (Fig. 85.12). Varying degrees of valvular insufficiency are present in the vast majority of instances. It is exceptionally uncommon for valvular stenosis to be caused by a vegetation. Typically fresh, active vegetations have a high degree of mobility and oscillatory motion. Their tissue character is rather "soft" and frequently has the same reflective properties as myocardial tissue. Old, healed vegetations take on a far more fibrotic, scarred, and dense appearance. There are several characteristics of vegetations that confer an increased risk of complications, such as progressive valvular destruction, failure to sterilize with antibiotics, and embolic phenomena.

Intracardiac tumors represent a very rare form of organic heart disease. The most common primary benign tumor of the heart is the left atrial myxoma. This typically appears on a stalk arising from the atrial septum. The classic atrial myxoma has a homogeneous texture and is highly mobile. It often results in mitral valve obstruction. The echo appearance of a myxoma is typical enough that confirmatory studies are rarely necessary prior to the recommendation for surgical resection. Other intracardiac tumors including primary malignancies can be easily be

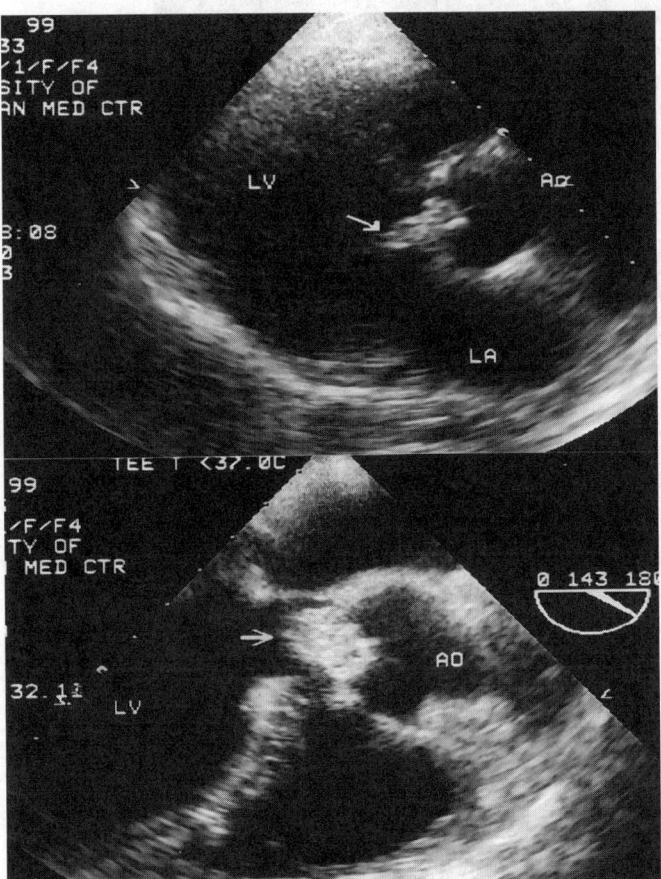

FIGURE 85.12. Parasternal long-axis transthoracic *(upper)* echocardiogram and transesophageal echocardiogram recorded in a longitudinal view *(lower)* in a patient with an aortic valve vegetation *(arrow).* In each case, a large bulky mass is seen nearly replacing the normal aortic valve and prolapsing into the left ventricular outflow tract in diastole.

detected with echocardiography as can metastatic disease. In the majority of instances metastatic disease of the heart is associated with myocardial effusion.

PULMONARY HYPERTENSION

Evidence of both primary and secondary pulmonary hypertension can be demonstrated with echocardiography and Doppler ultrasound techniques. Many causes of secondary pulmonary hypertension, such as congenital heart disease, primary valvular heart disease, and cardiomyopathy, can be easily diagnosed. It is important that the pulmonary artery systolic pressure can be estimated from the tricuspid regurgitation jet (Fig. 85.13). Some degree of tricuspid regurgitation is ubiquitous in patients with pulmonary hypertension. By calculating the transvalvular gradient between the right ventricle and right atrium, and then adding an assumed right atrial pressure, an estimate of right ventricular and hence pulmonary artery systolic pressure can be determined. This correlates favorably over the full physiologic range of pulmonary artery pressures when compared to cardiac catheterization.

DISEASE OF THE AORTA

Disease of the thoracic aorta can be reliably evaluated with transesophageal echocardiography. Transesophageal echocardiography is a highly accurate technique for diagnosing aortic dissection and aortic aneurysm and for documenting the presence of atherosclerotic disease (Fig. 85.14). The accuracy of transesophageal echocardiography for detecting aortic dissection is equal to that of magnetic resonance imaging and computed tomography.

◼ COMMON CLINICAL INDICATIONS

CONGESTIVE HEART FAILURE

Congestive heart failure frequently presents as a combination of dyspnea and fatigue. In many instances the differential diagnosis is between organic heart disease, pulmonary disease, and other major medical illnesses. Two-dimensional echocardiography is a superb tool to quickly screen for the presence of underlying organic heart disease. When present, its nature (valvular heart disease, cardiomyopathy, occult coronary artery disease, pericardial disease, etc.) can be readily ascertained and in the presence of cardiomyopathy the degree of ventricular dysfunction quantified. The American College of Cardiology/American Heart Association position paper on evaluation of patients with congestive heart failure recommends echocardiography as a primary screening tool in virtually all patients with known or suspected congestive heart failure.

CHEST PAIN

In patients with chest pain that could possibly be attributed to organic heart disease, an echocardiogram is an excellent diagnostic tool. A resting wall motion abnormality is frequently detected in patients with acute ischemic syndromes. When ischemic heart disease is suspected, stress echocardiography can reliably identify the presence of underlying coronary artery disease. Other forms of organic heart disease likely to result in chest discomfort include aortic stenosis, chronic and acute disease of the aorta such as dissection (for which transesophageal echocardiography is required), pulmonary hypertension, and valvular and pericardial heart disease. The major consideration in a patient with chest pain is the diagnosis or exclusion of coronary artery disease for which stress echocardiography is frequently necessary. On occasion, the routine resting study demonstrates evidence of occult coronary disease manifested by a previously unrecognized myocardial infarction.

MURMURS

A common indication for performance of an echocardiogram is the elucidation of a cardiac murmur. With careful auscultation a skilled clinician should be able to identify the majority of patients who have a benign flow murmur and likewise identify the origin of a pathologic murmur. Echocardiography is clearly more accurate for determining the severity of valvular stenosis

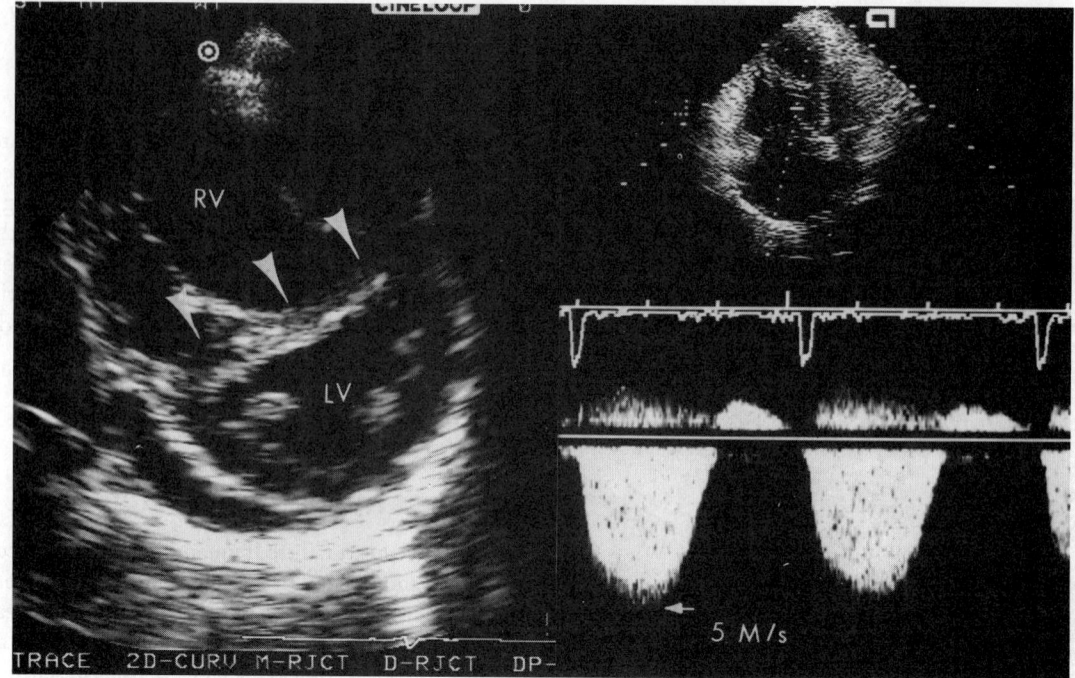

FIGURE 85.13. Two-dimensional echocardiogram and Doppler recorded in a patient with severe pulmonary hypertension. The left panel is a short-axis view at the level of the papillary muscles. Compare the relative size and shape of the right and left ventricles in this patient to the normal example in Figure 85.2. In this case, the left ventricle has assumed a "D"-shaped geometry because of the flattening of the ventricular septum *(arrowheads)*. The right ventricle is dilated and hypertrophied. The right panel is a continuous wave Doppler of a tricuspid regurgitation jet. The peak velocity is 5 m per second, from which a right ventricle to right atrial gradient of 100 m Hg can be calculated. Assuming a right atrial pressure of 14 m Hg, the right ventricular systolic pressure can be estimated to be 114 m Hg.

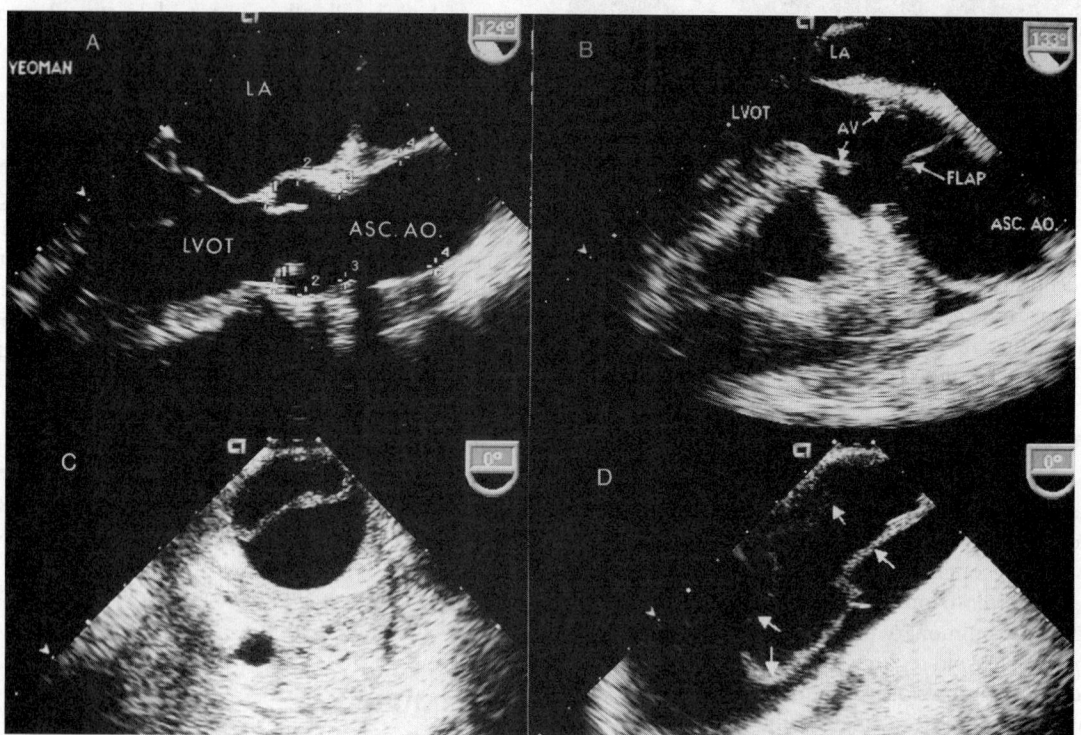

FIGURE 85.14. Four transesophageal echocardiographic images are presented. The upper left panel is a longitudinal view of a normal aorta. Points 1, 2, 3, and 4 represent the anatomical annulus, sinus of Valsalva, sinotubular junction, and ascending aorta, respectively. The upper right panel is a similar long-axis view recorded in a patient with a ascending aortic dissection. A portion of the intimal flap is easily visualized. The lower right panel was recorded in the same patient and shows a larger area of the ascending aorta in which the complex nature of the intimal flap *(arrows)* can be clearly seen. The lower left panel is a transverse view of the descending thoracic aorta in the same patient, demonstrating propagation of the dissection into the descending thoracic aorta.

and regurgitation when compared even to skilled auscultation. Both stenosis and regurgitation of all four cardiac valves as well as determination of intracardiac shunts due to congenital heart disease are reliably determined with echocardiography.

CARDIAC SOURCE OF EMBOLUS

It has been increasingly recognized that many patients with acute neurologic events have underlying cardiac disease that may be a contributing factor. The classic example is a patient with a stroke, subsequently found to have a left atrial thrombus (Fig. 85.15). Other entities that can result in embolization include intracardiac tumors, vegetations, aortic debris, and anatomical defects leading to an intracardiac shunt. The most common entity in the latter category is patent foramen ovale, which can be diagnosed using an intravenous contrast injection, occasionally augmented by either cough or Valsalva. This serves as a reliable mechanism for demonstrating the presence of an occult intracardiac shunt, which can be the source of the cardioembolic phenomena.

The role of echocardiography in determining the source of

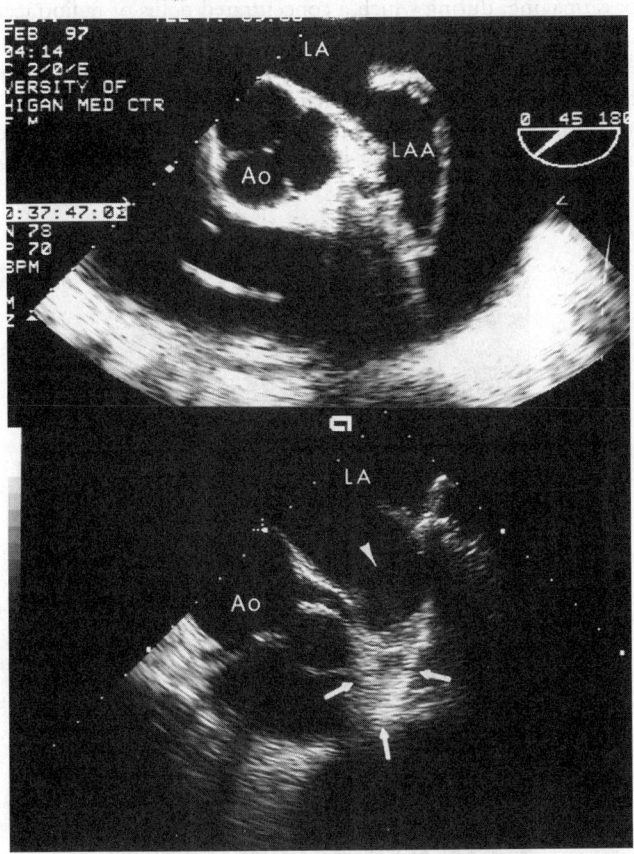

FIGURE 85.15. Transesophageal echocardiograms with specific attention paid to the left atrial appendage. The upper panel shows a normal left atrial appendage without evidence of spontaneous contrast or thrombosis. The lower panel is recorded in a similar view in a different patient. The anatomic boundary of the atrial appendage is noted by the arrows. Note the dense filling defect in the apex of the left atrial appendage and the vaguer, smokelike echoes just superior to the denser thrombosis *(arrows).*

embolus is similar to its role in patients with atrial fibrillation. Patients in atrial fibrillation who undergo conversion have an increased prevalence of embolic events shortly after cardioversion. These embolic events arise from dislodgement of thrombi preexisting in the left atrium, most commonly in the left atrial appendage, or that form due to atrial appendage stunning shortly after cardioversion. Many laboratories have adopted a strategy of transesophageal echocardiography to exclude atrial thrombi prior to cardioversion in patients with atrial fibrillation.

CARDIAC DISEASE IN MAJOR MEDICAL ILLNESSES

Echocardiography serves as a highly accurate screening tool for evaluating the presence of cardiac disease in medical illnesses known to be associated with cardiac abnormalities. This includes evaluation of left ventricular hypertrophy and diastolic dysfunction in patients with recently diagnosed hypertension, evaluation of valvular anatomy in patients with connective tissue diseases such as systemic lupus erythematosus, and screening of patients previously exposed to weight loss drugs. Other roles that echocardiography plays in medical illnesses include documentation of left ventricular function in patients undergoing cancer chemotherapy and detection of secondary right heart involvement in patients with significant lung disease.

█ FUTURE DIRECTIONS

The modern echocardiography laboratory is capable of answering virtually any question regarding the anatomical status of the cardiovascular system. Future developments in echocardiography include new ultrasound platforms that provide higher resolution and higher frame rate images with a greater ability to identify chamber borders. New ultrasound contrast agents, many of which are perfluorocarbon-based, have shown tremendous promise for enhancing the ability of echocardiographic wall motion detection and for determining the status of myocardial perfusion. Equipment advances will provide an intrinsically digital imaging platform, which will obviate the need for videotape and allow instantaneous retrieval of images at remote sites.

BIBLIOGRAPHY

Beattie JR, Cohen DJ, Manning WJ, et al. Role of routine transthoracic echocardiography in evaluation and management of stroke. *J Intern Med* 1998;243:281–291.

Bednarz JE, Krauss D, Lang RM. An echocardiographic approach to the assessment of aortic stenosis. *J Am Soc Echocardiogr* 1996;9:286–294.

Bonow RO, Carabello B, De Leon AC, et al. ACC/AHA Guidelines for the Management of Patients with Valvular Heart Disease. A report of the American College of Cardiology/American Heart Association Task Force on Practice Guidelines (Committee on Management of Patients with Valvular Heart Disease). *Heart Valve Dis* 1998;7:672–707.

Cheitlin MD, Alpert JS, Armstrong WF, et al. ACC/AHA Guidelines for the Clinical Application of Echocardiography. A report of the American College of Cardiology/American Heart Association Task Force on Practice Guidelines (Committee on Clinical Application of Echocardiography). *Circulation* 1997;95:1686–1744.

Pellikka PA. Stress echocardiography in the evaluation of chest pain and accuracy in the diagnosis of coronary artery disease. *Prog Cardiovasc Dis* 1997;39:523–532.

Seward JB, Khandheria BK, Freeman WK, et al. Multiplane transesophageal echocardiography: image orientation, examination technique, anatomic correlations, and clinical applications. *Mayo Clin Proc* 1993;68: 523–551.

Simpson IA, Sahn DJ. Adult congenital heart disease: use of transthoracic echocardiography versus magnetic resonance imaging scanning. *Am J Cardiac Imaging* 1995;9:29–37.

Waggoner AD, Harris KM, Braverman AC, et al. The role of transthoracic echocardiography in the management of patients seen in an outpatient cardiology clinic. *J Am Soc Echocardiogr* 1996;9:761–768.

Kelley's Textbook of Internal Medicine, fourth edition. Edited by H. David Humes.
Lippincott Williams & Wilkins, Philadelphia © 2000.

C H A P T E R
86

RADIONUCLIDE AND MAGNETIC RESONANCE TECHNIQUES

MARK A. LAWSON
GERALD M. POHOST

Both radionuclide and magnetic resonance techniques can be used to evaluate cardiac morphology, function, perfusion, and metabolism. This chapter describes the instrumentation, materials, and methods used with each technique and discusses current and future applications for the diagnosis and management of diseases affecting the cardiovascular system.

◼ RADIONUCLIDE TECHNIQUES

Radionuclide techniques use radionuclides (radioactive isotopes) or agents labeled with radionuclides. Radionuclides used for diagnostic purposes emit photons (γ rays) or positrons (positively charged β particles). Image data are obtained from the interaction of γ photons with the imaging instrument.

INSTRUMENTATION

Single-Photon Planar Imaging

Single-photon planar imaging requires three basic components: (a) a radioactive tracer selected to evaluate specific cardiac pathology or function; (b) a detection device, called a gamma or scintillation camera; and (c) a computer to collect, display, store, and retrieve image data.

In its simplest form, a gamma camera consists of a sodium iodide crystal positioned in front of a tight grouping of photomultiplier tubes. Photons emitted by the radiotracer from within

the heart are detected by the gamma camera through a process of scintillation. As photons strike the crystal, a flash of light, or scintillation, occurs that is detected by the photomultiplier tubes and converted to electrical signals. The position of the scintillation on the crystal is mapped by logic circuits within the camera. The density and distribution of scintillations is recorded by the imaging computer.

Photons emitted by the radiotracer from within the heart can be deflected by surrounding bone and soft tissues before interacting with the gamma camera. This scattering of photons degrades image contrast and spatial resolution. A lead collimator, fastened onto the front of the gamma camera, can improve image quality. A collimator is a lead disk through which a homogeneous distribution of parallel holes is drilled. The lead septa between holes absorb the scattered photons, whereas photons traveling parallel to the holes (mainly nonscattered photons emanating from the field of view) are allowed to pass and interact with the crystal.

Another type of gamma camera contains multiple small crystals, usually arranged in a rectangular array. Each crystal is associated with a photomultiplier tube. These cameras, called multicrystal cameras, detect photons at a faster rate than do single-crystal cameras. Multicrystal cameras are used primarily for first-pass imaging, during which a concentrated bolus of radiotracer is imaged rapidly as it travels through the heart and great vessels. Although multicrystal cameras possess higher count rates, they have lower spatial resolution than do single-crystal cameras.

With the camera positioned over the chest, planar images are acquired in several (usually three) projections (Fig. 86.1). The

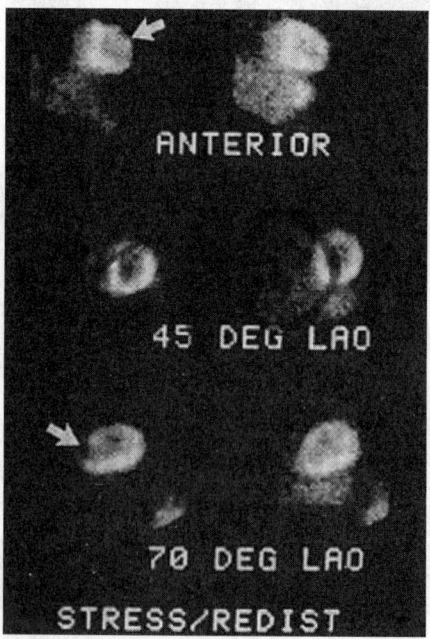

FIGURE 86.1. Planar thallium 201 myocardial imaging study with anterior, 45-degree left anterior oblique (LAO), and 70-degree LAO views obtained immediately after exercise **(left)** and 3 hours later **(right)**. Defects are seen *(arrows)* in the anterolateral and apical walls in the anterior view and in the anterior wall in the 70-degree LAO view. The defects have resolved in the delayed views, demonstrating redistribution with myocardial ischemia.

radioactivity of all structures within the field of view is counted and displayed in the image; photons originating from the heart overlap the activity of structures behind or in front of the heart relative to the orientation of the gamma camera.

Single-Photon Emission Computed Tomography

Single-photon emission computed tomography (SPECT) acquires image data to generate cross-sectional images of the heart in any given orientation. Tomography has the potential to distinguish between structures that overlap one another, and SPECT has been reported to increase the diagnostic accuracy of myocardial perfusion imaging by improving image quality and anatomical localization of defects. Although SPECT may improve accuracy, certain limitations may reduce specificity because of a higher incidence of false-positive results. These limitations include artifacts resulting from attenuation or patient motion, or from reconstruction errors (e.g., center of rotation, orbit, reorientation, and misalignment errors).

Single-proton emission computed tomography acquires image data using a single-crystal camera that rotates about the patient's chest in an arc, stopping momentarily to acquire image data at each stop before rotating to the next stop. From this acquired array of data, a computer reconstructs (using a filtered back-projection algorithm) and displays the desired tomographic images. Cardiac tomographic planes conventionally are displayed in the short, vertical, and horizontal long axes (Color Fig. 86.1). To decrease the image acquisition time, two or three cameras can be mounted on the revolving gantry.

Positron Emission Tomography

Positrons are positively charged β particles generated by certain radionuclides. When a positron encounters an electron, the two annihilate one another and produce two photons with an energy of 511 keV traveling 180 degrees apart. A positron emission tomography (PET) camera consists of a series of detectors arranged in a ring surrounding the body. A computer counts only the photons arriving simultaneously (coincidence detection) on oppositely positioned detectors, and excludes all other photons (i.e., scattered photons) from the image data. These characteristics of PET (less artifact from attenuation and enhanced exclusion of scattered photons) provide images with higher resolution and contrast when compared with single-photon methods.

However, the camera and on-site cyclotron needed to generate the short-lived radionuclides are costly, and their operation requires substantial space and technical expertise. These disadvantages have restricted the widespread application of PET imaging.

RADIONUCLIDES

Technetium 99m

Technetium 99m (^{99m}Tc) is the most commonly used radionuclide in nuclear cardiology laboratories (Table 86.1). It has a single photon peak of 140 keV, which is ideal for detection by

TABLE 86.1.	CHARACTERISTICS OF THALLIUM 201 AND TECHNETIUM 99m	
Characteristic	Thallium 201	Technetium 99m
Photo peak	69–83 keV	140 keV
Half-life	73 hr	6 hr
Activity	2.5–4.0 mCi	25–30 mCi
Excretion	Renal	Hepatobiliary
Myocyte extraction fraction	85%	40%
Viability assessment	Yes	Probably
Attenuation artifact	More	Less
Lung activity uptake	Yes	No
Redistribution	Yes	Minimal
Gated acquisition	No	Yes
Image resolution/ contrast	Lower	Higher
Calculation of left ventricular ejection fraction	No	Yes

imaging equipment. Because of its relatively short half-life of 6 hours, higher activity can be administered. These two characteristics provide images with higher resolution.

Technetium 99m–labeled radiopharmaceuticals are used to evaluate ventricular function as well as myocardial perfusion and infarct size. Agents labeled with ^{99m}Tc can be obtained from a commercial radiopharmacy already prepared for administration. Another source of ^{99m}Tc is a generator kept in the nuclear cardiology department. A ^{99m}Tc generator, about the size of a thermos bottle, contains molybdenum 99 (^{99}Mo), which decays to ^{99m}Tc. By injecting the generator with saline solution, ^{99m}Tc is washed or eluted from the generator and ready to use. The generator can supply ^{99m}Tc-pertechnetate for about a week. However, because ^{99}Mo is a nuclear reactor by-product, it is strictly regulated by the Nuclear Regulatory Commission. It often is more convenient to obtain ^{99m}Tc agents from a commercial radiopharmacy.

Thallium 201

Thallium 201 (^{201}Tl) is a single-photon radionuclide that is the most widely used and best understood agent for assessing myocardial perfusion and viability. Thallium 201 is somewhat less desirable than ^{99m}Tc for gamma camera imaging because ^{201}Tl has a lower photon energy peak (70 to 80 keV) and a longer half-life (73.5 hours). The longer half-life limits the total activity administered to the patient. As a consequence, image quality is somewhat less when compared with that of ^{99m}Tc; however, the difference in image quality does not affect the accuracy of study interpretations. Thallium 201 is produced by a cyclotron and is ordered weekly from a radiopharmacy. It is not regulated by the Nuclear Regulatory Commission.

Positron-Emitting Radionuclides

Positron-emitting radionuclides used in cardiac studies include carbon 11 (^{11}C), nitrogen 13 (^{13}N), oxygen 15 (^{15}O), fluorine 18 (^{18}F), and rubidium 82 (^{82}Rb). Most of these agents are cyclotron-produced, except ^{82}Rb, which is eluted from a generator. These radionuclides have many applications in nuclear cardiology. Carbon 11 is used to label fatty acids (e.g., ^{11}C-palmitate) for evaluation of lipid metabolism and to label carbon monoxide (^{11}CO) for assessment of ventricular function. Labeled ammonia (^{13}NH$_3$) is used as a myocardial perfusion tracer. Other metabolic processes, such as oxygen consumption (^{15}O) and glycolysis (^{18}F-fluorodeoxyglucose), can be evaluated with PET. An important property of PET agents is their short half-lives: 20.4 minutes for ^{11}C, 9.8 minutes for ^{19}N, 2 minutes for ^{15}O, 75 seconds for ^{82}Rb, and 110 minutes for ^{18}F. Because the half-lives are short, repeated injections are possible that can reflect changes in perfusion or metabolism in response to a number of interventions. However, a cyclotron to generate PET agents must be located on site to supply the agents before they decay.

APPLICATIONS

Radionuclide techniques have a number of applications, including assessment of cardiac function, perfusion, viability, and necrosis.

ASSESSMENT OF VENTRICULAR FUNCTION

Radionuclide Ventriculography

Radionuclide ventriculography is used predominantly to assess regional and global ventricular performance (Table 86.2). Three approaches can be used: the gated blood pool method, the first-pass method, and the gated SPECT method. Global ventricular performance can be expressed using the ejection fraction (EF), which is the percentage of blood volume ejected from the ventricle during contraction:

$$EF = (EDV - ESV)/EDV = \text{stroke volume}/EDV$$

where EDV = end-diastolic volume and ESV = end-systolic volume.

Gated Blood Pool Method

By labeling red cells with ^{99m}Tc, radioactivity within the blood pool will be proportional to volume. The counts obtained during end-systole and end-diastole can be substituted in the above equation to calculate the ejection fraction. Technetium 99 pertechnetate binds to red blood cells in the presence of stannous phosphate, allowing ^{99m}Tc to remain in the blood pool; because the heart is the largest blood pool within the chest, it can be imaged with the gamma camera. Gated blood pool ventriculography is performed using a multigated acquisition. It is because of this approach that the study frequently is called MUGA, for "multigated acquisition." That is to say, a series of 16 to 32 equally spaced "snapshots" (or frames) of the cardiac blood pool are acquired during each cardiac cycle, with the first frame being triggered (gated) to the R wave of the patient's electrocardiogram (ECG).

During successive cardiac cycles, the computer assigns incoming image data to frames in sequence. The first MUGA frame is generated by adding together all of the counts acquired during the first temporal segment that follows the R wave. The second frame follows the first, and so on. After a 2- to 10-minute acquisition, sufficient counts accumulate within each frame. The sequence of frames can be viewed repeatedly in a movie (cinegraphic) mode that depicts the events of ventricular contraction and relaxation after the initiating R wave. Global ventricular function is assessed using the ejection fraction calculation and abnormal regional wall motion can be assessed by observing asymmetric contraction of the chamber silhouette in the movie mode (Fig. 86.2). Customarily, studies at rest are acquired in two or three projections, including an anterior and at least one left anterior oblique view. The left ventricular ejection fraction (LVEF) is computed using the projection that best separates the left from the right ventricular cavity, about a 45-degree left anterior oblique view.

TABLE 86.2.	INDICATIONS FOR RADIONUCLIDE VENTRICULOGRAPHY

Rest
- Assessment of global left ventricular function and calculation of left ventricular ejection fraction
- Assessment of regional wall motion
- Identification of ventricular aneurysms and pseudoaneurysms
- Detection of doxorubicin cardiotoxicity
- Evaluation of the status of a cardiac allograft
- Assessment of valvular regurgitation and shunt ratios

Exercise
- Detection of ischemic dysfunction caused by coronary artery disease
- Risk assessment of patients with coronary artery disease
- Determination of optimal timing for valve replacement

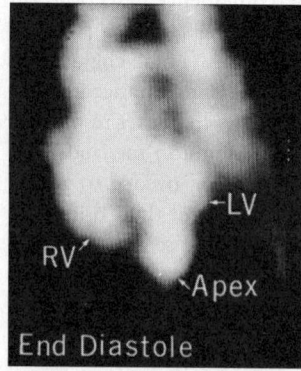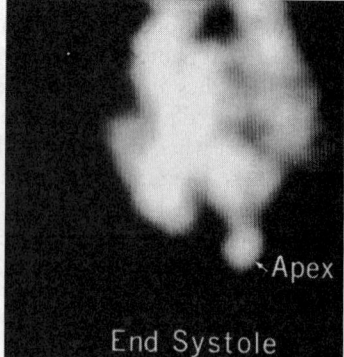

FIGURE 86.2. Equilibrium-gated radionuclide ventriculogram in the left anterior oblique view performed at rest in a patient with an apical aneurysm. The left panel shows end-diastole with the right ventricle (RV) and left ventricle (LV) and its apex. The right panel shows end-systole. In both the end-systolic and end-diastolic frames, a prominent bulge is noted at the apex of the LV, representing an aneurysm of moderate size.

Interpretation of the study begins with a qualitative impression of the movie display by an experienced reviewer to define morphologic abnormalities and evaluate regional and global ventricular function. Computer-aided quantitative analysis of the ventricle determines the ejection fraction. Other indexes of ventricular performance also can be derived, including end-diastolic and end-systolic volumes, and ejection and filling rates.

Gated blood pool studies are performed at rest, or serial studies are combined with exercise to evaluate the response of ventricular performance to stress. The most widely used exercise is performed with the patient semisupine and pedaling a bicycle, which increases the level of stress in a fashion similar to exercise treadmill testing. A 2-minute radionuclide ventriculogram acquisition is obtained at the end of each stage. In general, LVEF should increase with each progressive stage of exercise in patients free of cardiac pathology, reaching a value at least 10% higher than at rest. The development of segmental wall motion abnormalities suggests regional myocardial ischemia caused by coronary artery disease with an overall sensitivity of 86% to 90% and a specificity of 79% to 84%. An abnormal fall or blunting of LVEF is sensitive but not specific for coronary artery disease because untrained normal patients can show an abnormal LVEF response as they achieve their anaerobic threshold.

Gated blood pool studies have been used primarily to evaluate regional and global ventricular function at rest or with stress to diagnose and assess prognosis in patients with ischemic heart disease, valvular heart disease, hypertensive heart disease, congenital heart disease, and cardiomyopathy. In addition, serial studies can be performed over time to monitor left ventricular function in patients who have undergone cardiac transplantation and in those who are receiving cardiotoxic chemotherapeutic drugs (e.g., doxorubicin).

First-Pass Method

The first-pass method acquires images during the initial passage of an intravenously administered bolus of radiotracer through the central circulation and heart. A high-speed or multicrystal gamma camera that acquires images at a rate of 20 frames per second is positioned in the anterior or right anterior oblique projection to optimize separation of the atria from the ventricles. Because there is no background activity at the time of injection, the bolus can be viewed as it passes through the superior vena cava into the right atrium and ventricle, through the pulmonary vasculature, and, finally, into the left atrium and ventricle.

Qualitative analysis consists of visual inspection of sequential frames for abnormalities of morphology and for regional and global ventricular function. Quantitative analysis is performed by outlining the right or left ventricular regions of interest. Time–activity curves reflect radioactivity within the given chamber every 20 to 40 milliseconds, which corresponds to changes in chamber volume.

Gated Single-Proton Emission Computed Tomography Method

Due to the increased count density from ^{99m}Tc, it is clinically feasible to acquire tomographic radionuclide ventriculograms.

Unlike the MUGA and first-pass techniques discussed above, which produce an image of the blood pool, the gated SPECT technique calculates ejection fraction from tomographic perfusion images by comparing the change in ventricular geometry between end-systole and end-diastole.

Tomographic perfusion images are acquired using the procedures discussed later in this chapter. The cardiac cycle is divided into approximately 8 to 16 frames. A computerized automated edge detection algorithm outlines the endomyocardial surface in the end-systolic and end-diastolic frames, and the LVEF is calculated using a modified Simpson's equation (Fig. 86.3).

The added advantages to this technique include the assessment of regional wall thickening and calculation of myocardial mass. Because regional wall motion can be visualized, it is possible to determine myocardial viability (presence of thickening) and evaluate the significance of questionable perfusion defects—most commonly attenuation artifacts whereby seemingly fixed perfusion defects demonstrate normal wall motion. Thus, with gated SPECT techniques, it is possible to simultaneously determine perfusion and function with a single diagnostic study. However, the assessment of ventricular function obtained from this approach is determined during image acquisition, when the

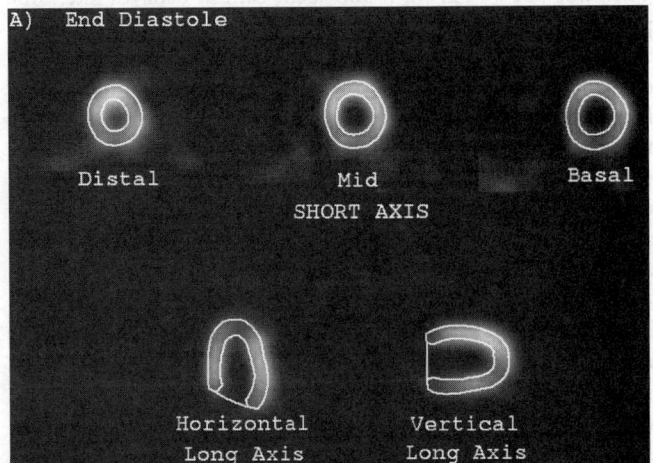

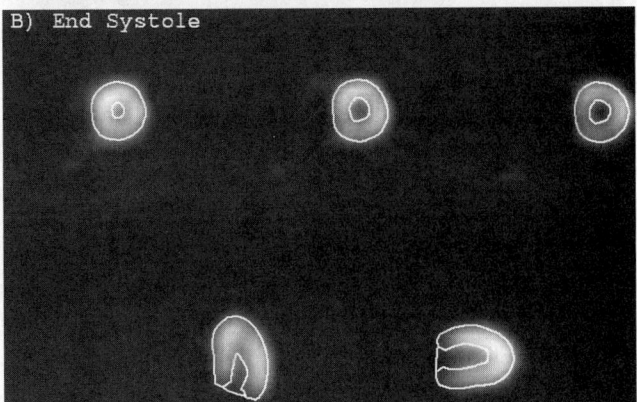

FIGURE 86.3. Gated single-proton emission computed tomography image frames at **(A)** end-diastole and **(B)** end-systole. The endocardial and epicardial surfaces have been outlined by a computerized automated edge detection program.

patient is under the camera in a resting state. If LVEF during exercise is desired, the first-pass technique should be employed.

Positron Emission Tomography

Ventricular function can be evaluated using an equilibrium approach after inhalation of a tracer dose of ^{11}CO. Carbon monoxide labels the red blood cells, allowing blood pool imaging.

ASSESSMENT OF MYOCARDIAL PERFUSION AND VIABILITY

Radionuclide methods to assess myocardial perfusion and viability rely on imaging the distribution of a tracer throughout the myocardium. Myocardium supplied by a stenosed vessel may appear normally perfused under resting conditions. Jeopardized myocardium usually is identified after some cardiovascular provocation accomplished by exercise or pharmacologic manipulation. Perfusion images obtained during stress or coronary vasodilatation are compared with images obtained under resting conditions to identify abnormalities in myocardial perfusion.

Thallium Imaging

Thallium 201 (^{201}Tl), a monovalent cation, behaves like ionic potassium and is actively transported across cell membranes by the Na^+/K^+-ATPase pump. Because it is extracted by myocardial cells with high efficiency (80% to 90%), it is an ideal agent for studying perfusion patterns. Initial extraction of thallium by the myocardium depends on cellular viability and blood flow to myocytes. Thallium 201 is administered at peak exercise or during the peak coronary vasodilative effect of dipyridamole or adenosine (see discussion later in this chapter). Peak myocardial activity distal to a physiologically significant coronary artery stenosis is delayed relative to normally perfused tissue. Regional deficits in myocardial distribution of ^{201}Tl on initial images are related to reduced myocardial blood flow in ischemic viable tissue or nonviable tissue (e.g., acutely infarcted or scarred myocardium). Of all the perfusion agents, thallium uniquely demonstrates the phenomenon of redistribution. Redistribution involves the observation of a defect on initial images resulting from reduced perfusion during stress, following the administration of dipyridamole or adenosine, or even at rest. If the defect is related to underperfused yet viable myocardium, it "fills in" on delayed imaging (Fig. 86.1; Color Fig. 86.1). Redistribution may be better understood by considering myocardial and blood pool activity. Thallium accumulates within viable myocytes over time to a peak and then begins to decrease. Normally perfused myocardium peaks before ischemic myocardium. Clearance or washout of thallium from normal myocardium also is more rapid and parallels blood pool activity. Myocardium that is underperfused during stress achieves equilibrium with blood thallium by extracting thallium as a result of continued bathing by blood containing thallium, albeit at relatively low levels. Over time, the activity levels of normal and underperfused myocardium approach one another. If a sufficient delay (typically 3 to 4 hours) transpires to achieve equilibrium, ischemic but viable myocardium gradually accumulates thallium on serial imaging

studies. The phenomenon of redistribution is the basis for ^{201}Tl imaging in differentiating myocardial ischemia (transient or "reversible" defect) from myocardial infarct or scar (persistent or "fixed" defect).

Exercise

Thallium 201 is administered most commonly during a graded exercise treadmill test. Dynamic changes during exercise include elevation of heart rate, blood pressure, and cardiac output, all of which affect myocardial oxygen consumption (Vo_2). In addition, coronary blood flow increases because of elevation in Vo_2. A mismatch in supply and demand occurs as increases in myocardial metabolic requirements during exercise exceed the ability of the vasculature to supply adequate oxygen and substrate. Myocardial ischemia results in diastolic and systolic left ventricular dysfunction, ischemic ECG changes, and, ultimately, the syndrome of angina pectoris. ^{201}Tl is administered intravenously as a bolus injection during peak exercise, or when the patient develops angina, worrisome ECG changes, or fatigue. Exercise is encouraged for an additional 30 to 60 seconds following injection, and initial imaging (planar or SPECT) should begin within 15 minutes of the termination of exercise. Regional differences in ^{201}Tl distribution are accentuated by exercise-induced regional differences in blood flow, which are proportional to the extent and severity of coronary artery disease. Delayed scans are performed 3 to 4 hours later. The images are evaluated qualitatively and quantitatively for changes in regions with decreased ^{201}Tl uptake between the initial and delayed images.

Additional information regarding ischemic myocardium can be gleaned from thallium imaging. Increased lung uptake of ^{201}Tl during exercise presumably reflects ischemia-induced left ventricular dysfunction. Stress-induced increases in pulmonary capillary wedge pressure and decreases in cardiac output correlate with increases in ^{201}Tl lung accumulation. However, patients with chronic obstructive lung disease also may demonstrate increased ^{201}Tl lung activity, which usually is observed on both the stress and delayed scans. Transient ischemic dilatation of the left ventricular cavity seen on early post-exercise imaging also is a marker of severe, often multivessel, disease. Left ventricular dilatation on early stress images is caused by diffuse subendocardial hypoperfusion, leading to an increase in cavity dimension.

The primary application of exercise–thallium studies is for detection, evaluation, and prognostication of patients with known or suspected coronary artery disease (Table 86.3). When qualitatively interpreted by experienced observers, planar exercise–thallium studies have a sensitivity and specificity of 82% and 88%, respectively, for detecting coronary artery disease. Quantitative planar analysis improves sensitivity to 89%, whereas SPECT acquisitions improve sensitivity to 94% to 95%. In some studies, however, an improved sensitivity with SPECT is offset by a reduction in specificity. Because exercise studies always are performed with ECG monitoring, ECG and radionuclide studies together substantially improve the reliability of either study alone. One of the major roles of exercise–thallium testing is risk stratification of patients for future cardiac events (e.g., myocardial infarction, ischemia-related death). The future cardiac event rate is best predicted by the extent and reversibility

TABLE 86.3. INDICATIONS FOR RADIONUCLIDE-EXERCISE PERFUSION IMAGING

- Diagnosis of coronary artery disease
  As an adjunct to exercise-ECG testing in patients with prior positive stress ECGs having nonanginal or no pain, or in patients with stress-induced angina without ECG changes
- Assessment of prognosis in patients with coronary artery disease
- Assessment of the functional significance of angiographically documented stenoses
- Risk stratification after infarction before hospital discharge
- Assessment of adequacy of therapy or revascularization
- Situations in which the stress ECG alone is unreliable
  Patients with abnormal ST segments and T waves on baseline ECG
  Patients taking digitalis
  Patients with left ventricular hypertrophy
  Patients with ventricular pacemakers
- Evaluation of viability and planning for revascularization

ECG, electrocardiogram.

of perfusion defects. Patients with normal stress thallium perfusion studies are at low risk (0.1% to 0.9% per year) for subsequent events, whereas patients with abnormal thallium scans (with reversible or fixed defects, or both) are at higher risk. A poor prognosis has been reported in patients with a greater number of abnormal segments (especially reversible defects). Finally, exercise–thallium testing is used increasingly as an adjunct to coronary angiography to determine the significance of an angiographically demonstrated coronary stenosis. Whereas coronary angiography only demonstrates coronary arterial morphologic abnormalities, ^{201}Tl distribution relates to the physiologic significance of a stenosis. A radionuclide myocardial perfusion study often is used in concert with coronary angiography to help indicate whether revascularization may be beneficial.

Dipyridamole and Adenosine

Evaluation of coronary artery disease by exercise testing relies on the patient's ability to achieve an adequate level of exercise to produce a technically acceptable study. However, many patients with suspected coronary artery disease cannot achieve a diagnostic level of exercise because of poor physical conditioning, advanced pulmonary disease, peripheral vascular disease, or physical debilitation resulting from arthritic, orthopedic, or neurologic conditions. Pharmacologic agents, such as dipyridamole or adenosine, can be used as an alternative to exercise. Dipyridamole is a coronary artery vasodilator that acts to inhibit adenosine uptake or to stimulate the adenosine receptor located on the coronary endothelium. In normal coronary vessels, dipyridamole and adenosine can cause up to a fivefold increase in myocardial blood flow, whereas in diseased vasculature, blood flow rises to a lesser extent or sometimes even decreases. These vasodilators usually cause only a mild increase in myocardial oxygen demand resulting from a mild increase in heart rate and

a decrease in blood pressure. On occasion, the resulting distribution in blood flow between normal and jeopardized myocardium leads to a decrease in blood flow to the jeopardized myocardium. This situation occurs when the resistance to blood flow becomes substantially lower in the normal vessels, "stealing" blood from the jeopardized myocardium and leading to ischemia. The heterogeneity in ^{201}Tl distribution induced by dipyridamole between normally perfused and jeopardized myocardium is the basis for the detection of stenoses. Adenosine also is a potent coronary vasodilator and has been used in place of dipyridamole in conjunction with myocardial perfusion imaging.

Dipyridamole is administered intravenously over a 4-minute interval (0.14 mg per kg per minute). Blood pressure and heart rate should be measured frequently to ascertain the hemodynamic response to dipyridamole. Two to three minutes after the infusion of dipyridamole is complete, ^{201}Tl is injected intravenously as a bolus. Initial and delayed imaging is performed, and images are interpreted qualitatively and quantitatively in the same manner as exercise studies. A pharmacologic study using adenosine instead of dipyridamole is performed in a similar fashion except that adenosine is administered as a continuous intravenous infusion over 6 minutes (140 µg per kg per minute) and the radionuclide is administered 3 to 4 minutes into the infusion.

The body of literature is greater with dipyridamole than adenosine. The sensitivity and specificity for the detection of coronary artery disease using the dipyridamole-thallium approach is similar to that of exercise thallium studies. Although the ECG results obtained during dipyridamole-thallium studies are not of much clinical importance, the presence of diagnostic ST-segment and T-wave abnormalities in the presence of angina is specific for important coronary artery disease. On the other hand, exercise–ECG testing in conjunction with radionuclide perfusion imaging has the advantage of providing both image and ECG data, enhancing the diagnostic power of the test.

Indications and applications for dipyridamole-thallium testing are similar to those for exercise–thallium testing. However, there are additional situations in which this study appears to be indicated (Table 86.4). Several studies have indicated that patients scheduled to undergo peripheral vascular surgery may benefit substantially from preoperative dipyridamole-thallium testing because these patients have (1) a high prevalence of coexistent coronary artery disease, which often is asymptomatic, and (2) limited exercise capacity because of claudication. Patients with abnormal perfusion scans (especially those demonstrating redistribution) are at increased risk for perioperative cardiac ischemic events and should be considered for perioperative invasive cardiac monitoring or preoperative cardiac catheterization. Exercise–thallium studies performed in patients with left bundle-branch block have been reported to demonstrate perfusion defects (especially in the septal regions) in the absence of coronary artery disease (false-positive results), resulting in lower specificity. These defects are less likely to occur with dipyridamole, and dipyridamole–thallium studies are preferred in patients with left bundle-branch block. Dipyridamole also may be administered safely to patients in the early postinfarction period, who may be unable to perform submaximal exercise–ECG testing before hospital discharge. Although normal perfusion images obtained during dipyridamole–thallium testing identify a low-risk group

TABLE 86.4.	INDICATIONS FOR RADIONUCLIDE-DIPYRIDAMOLE PERFUSION IMAGING

- As a substitute for exercise for patients who are unable to exercise (e.g., those with advanced pulmonary disease, peripheral vascular disease, physical debilitation from arthritic, orthopedic, or neurologic conditions)
- As a substitute for exercise for patients who can exercise but are unlikely to achieve a diagnostic level of exercise (e.g., those who are obese or sedentary, are receiving β-blocker therapy, or are elderly)
- In the presence of left bundle-branch block
- As preoperative risk stratification for patients scheduled to undergo surgery for peripheral vascular disease or aneurysm repair
- In the presence of a fixed-rate ventricular pacemaker

after infarction, redistribution in the infarct zone is reported to be a significant predictor of in-hospital ischemic cardiac events.

Dobutamine

Dobutamine is a positive inotropic agent that stimulates both α- and β-adrenergic receptors. It produces a marked increase in contractility, a modest increase in heart rate, and, consequently, a significant increase in myocardial oxygen consumption leading to ischemia in jeopardized myocardium. Dobutamine–thallium imaging may be an alternative strategy to induce stress in patients with obstructive lung disease in whom dipyridamole is contraindicated. The overall sensitivity (91%) and specificity (79%) of this approach is similar to that reported for the other stress tests.

Study at Rest

Thallium 201 administered at rest is reported to be of value in patients with unstable angina or myocardial infarction for the detection of severe coronary stenoses and evaluation of myocardial viability. The myocardial images often are of lower quality and consequently may be more difficult to evaluate compared with exercise or dipyridamole studies. Segmental contraction abnormalities and ejection fractions have been reported to improve after revascularization in patients who demonstrated resting ^{201}Tl defects that redistributed.

Viability

When a perfusion image defect demonstrates redistribution, it can be said to be viable with a high degree of confidence. On the other hand, up to 50% of defects that persist over a 3- to 4-hour interval have been reported to be viable (confirmed using PET techniques), even though the "fixed" defect should represent nonviable tissue. One reason this occurs is because of a low concentration of blood thallium leading to slower redistribution, which could be incomplete within the 3- to 4-hour period between early and delayed images. Imaging substantially later (e.g., 24 hours) allows adequate time for redistribution to occur to assess viability in defects that appear to be irreversible or fixed on the 4-hour delayed images. Because redistribution of thallium depends on thallium blood levels, a second strategy to promote "fill-in" of fixed defects in viable myocardium is to use a second injection to boost thallium blood pool concentration. A second injection or "reinjection" method has been reported during which a second dose of thallium (usually 1 mCi) is given to augment thallium blood levels after the 3- to 4-hour delayed images have been acquired. Reinjection images are obtained 15 minutes later. If the 3- to 4-hour fixed defect fills in on late or reinjection images, viability has been documented. When the reinjection method is used, the entire study can be completed in a day.

Technetium-Based Agents

Because of the lower photon energy and longer half-life of ^{201}Tl, imaging agents labeled with ^{99m}Tc have been developed and produce images with higher resolution and contrast compared with ^{201}Tl. Two reasons account for this improved image quality. The emitted photon energy of ^{99m}Tc (140 keV) is higher than that of ^{201}Tl, and the half-life (6 hours) is shorter, making the administration of doses with more activity (25 to 35 mCi) feasible.

Technetium ^{99m}Tc Sestamibi

Sestamibi (MIBI) belongs to a family of chemicals known as the isonitriles, which have varying abilities to enter and remain within the myocyte. It is believed that MIBI passively enters myocardial cells (unlike ^{201}Tl) and is sequestered within mitochondria as a result of a large negative transmembrane potential. In contrast to ^{201}Tl, MIBI exhibits minimal redistribution and is believed to be less useful for evaluating viability. However, recent studies have shown that MIBI may play an increasing role in determining viability. Image data obtained from MIBI are similar to those obtained from thallium, and the sensitivity (94%) and specificity (77%) of MIBI for the detection of coronary artery disease or identification of individual coronary artery stenoses are comparable.

Several applications of MIBI are recognized (Table 86.5).

TABLE 86.5.	SITUATIONS IN WHICH TECHNETIUM^{99m} TC SESTAMIBI MIGHT BE THE RADIOTRACER OF CHOICE

- Female patients, especially those with large breasts or small hearts
- Patients with a low likelihood of disease (such patients receive high-dose sestamibi during exercise on the first day of a 2-day protocol)
- Obese patients in whom attenuation might be problematic
- Patients who require a combined perfusion–left ventricular function study
- Patients who require assessment of myocardial perfusion at the time of an acute ischemic episode

Patients in whom soft-tissue attenuation may be problematic, such as obese patients or female patients with large breasts, should be considered for MIBI protocols. MIBI also may be more sensitive for the detection of coronary artery disease in women who have small hearts because of the increased resolution it achieves. Although several of its characteristics make MIBI attractive, it has some potential limitations. MIBI is believed to be less useful than ^{201}Tl for the demonstration of myocardial viability. The fractional extraction of MIBI is lower than that of ^{201}Tl. Because MIBI is excreted through the enterohepatic route, it localizes in splanchnic viscera and can confound the interpretation of inferior and apical myocardial segments when visceral activity is adjacent to the heart.

Because MIBI demonstrates clinically insignificant redistribution, images must be obtained using two separate injections. Two protocols for performing a MIBI perfusion study have been reported: a same-day protocol and a 2-day protocol. For the same-day protocol, a resting study is performed first, after the administration of a low dose of MIBI (8 to 12 mCi). After a delay of 2 to 3 hours, a second, higher dose of MIBI (20 to 30 mCi) is administered during peak exercise or after an infusion of dipyridamole or adenosine. With the 2-day approach, the patient receives a high dose of MIBI at peak stress and undergoes imaging about 30 to 60 minutes later. If the scan is abnormal, the patient returns on another day for resting imaging. However, if the perfusion pattern is normal, the patient need not return on the second day for a resting imaging study.

A so-called hybrid or dual-isotope technique uses ^{201}Tl and MIBI in a convenient, efficient, and practical manner whereby the entire study can be completed within 2 hours. Initially, the patient receives thallium in the resting state and imaging begins about 5 to 10 minutes later. Then, the patient exercises, is injected with MIBI, and undergoes imaging. There is no contamination by ^{201}Tl in MIBI stress images because the gamma camera can discriminate photons of differing energies. Exercise (MIBI) and resting (thallium) images are compared to determine the fate of exercise-induced defects with an overall sensitivity of more than 90% and a specificity of 75% for the diagnosis of coronary artery disease (Color Fig. 86.2).

As a result of high count rates from MIBI, it is possible to assess myocardial perfusion and left ventricular performance using a single radionuclide. The LVEF can be determined using two approaches: gated SPECT and first-pass. Using principles discussed earlier, gated SPECT acquires about eight separate tomograms during a cardiac cycle. Tomograms can be displayed in a continuous loop of ventricular contraction and relaxation.

Other Technetium-Based Agents

Technetium-99m-teboroxime is not a widely used radiotracer, largely because of its elimination and washout characteristics. Like MIBI, it is slowly cleared through the hepatobiliary system, which can interfere with evaluation of the inferior left ventricular wall. Sensitivity decreases if a conventional single-detector gamma camera is used to acquire images. Optimal imaging is accomplished using a multiple-detector gamma camera so that sufficient counts can be obtained before washout (within about 6 minutes). As instrumentation moves toward multiple-detector systems, teboroxime may gain further popularity. However, teboroxime has unique application using a single-detector camera in determining the patency of an infarct-related artery after thrombolysis because its kinetics mimic a pure flow tracer.

Technetium-99m-tetrafosmin is a myocardial perfusion agent with kinetics similar to that of MIBI; however, it offers the advantage of less concentration in splanchnic viscera, thus potentially less interference with left ventricular inferior wall activity. It allows imaging shortly after administration.

Technetium-99m-N-NOET [bis-(N-ethoxy, N-ethyl dithiocarbamato) nitrido] is a new, neutral, lipophilic, myocardial perfusion agent that combines the radiophysical properties of ^{99m}Tc and the redistribution kinetics of ^{201}Tl. These properties are optimal for perfusion assessment by providing high-quality images using a single injection of radionuclide.

Positron Emission Tomography

Regional myocardial blood flow can be evaluated using positron-emitting radiotracers, including ^{13}N-labeled ammonia, ^{15}O-labeled water, and ^{82}Rb. These agents have very short half-lives, on the order of minutes. Multiple injections are used to assess perfusion under various physiologic states (at rest, during exercise, or after the administration of dipyridamole or adenosine). Aside from high-resolution images and the ability to perform multiple studies over a short period, one advantage of PET is the ability to measure myocardial blood flow in milliliters per second per gram of tissue. The PET and SPECT imaging modalities have similar sensitivities and specificities for detecting coronary artery disease. Unfortunately, the equipment and operating costs of PET are substantially more expensive, and it appears that single-photon methods will prevail.

Assessment of Myocardial Metabolism

Myocardial metabolic changes can be visualized using radionuclide methods. During ischemia, myocardial metabolism changes from the oxidation of fatty acids to glycolysis. Labeled fatty acids and glucose analogs have been used to assess changes in myocardial metabolism. The only single-photon method available for the evaluation of fatty acid metabolism uses fatty acids labeled with ^{123}I. PET radiotracers are used more widely to assess the myocardial metabolism. Palmitic acid labeled with ^{11}C can assess transient ischemia and the extent of infarction. An elegant approach to assess myocyte glucose utilization, and therefore viability, uses ^{18}F-fluorodeoxyglucose. ^{18}F-fluorodeoxyglucose accumulates in viable myocardium, which metabolizes glucose. This approach is particularly helpful in assessing viability in regions of asynergic myocardium for which revascularization may be beneficial. If ^{18}F-fluorodeoxyglucose accumulates in a region with a perfusion defect (determined by ^{13}N-ammonia or ^{82}Rb), the region is ischemic but viable. These applications continue to be important primarily for research purposes and are not used widely because of the limited availability and cost of PET instrumentation.

Assessment of Myocardial Necrosis

Technetium-99m-pyrophosphate binds to calcium salts released in regions of acute myocardial necrosis. Usually, adequate deposition of ^{99m}Tc-pyrophosphate for clinical detection occurs between 24 and 72 hours after the onset of infarction. This study is interpreted qualitatively by comparing the degree of uptake of the agent by infarcted myocardium with that of adjacent bony structures. Pyrophosphate imaging is indicated for the detection of myocardial infarction when ECG and cardiac enzyme analyses are nondiagnostic.

Radiolabeled cardiac myosin-specific antibody has been developed and is more specific than pyrophosphate for identification of areas of myocardial necrosis. Uptake occurs within 6 hours of the onset of infarction.

■ MAGNETIC RESONANCE METHODS

Magnetic resonance (MR) is the newest imaging technology. Magnetic resonance imaging (MRI) has excellent temporal and spatial resolution and is ideally suited for visualizing the heart and blood vessels (Table 86.6). Advantages of MRI are its ability to acquire images noninvasively in the absence of ionizing radiation, in any tomographic plane, without interference from surrounding bone or soft tissues. MR spectroscopy (MRS) provides a means of biochemically characterizing tissues by obtaining spectra of metabolites containing MR-sensitive nuclei.

INSTRUMENTATION

The MR instrument (scanner) consists of a large, cylindrical supercooled magnet. The patient is placed in the supine or prone position within the bore of the magnet. This magnet creates a strong magnetic field. Gradient coils are positioned along the length of the magnet and vary the strength of the magnetic field from one point to another. The body coil, acting as an antenna, surrounds the inside of the bore and transmits and receives radiofrequency waves. An operator's console and computer are located in an adjacent room. The computer executes the operator's imaging instructions, sorts out the complex signal received from the patient, and generates the final images.

TABLE 86.6.	**INDICATIONS FOR A CARDIOVASCULAR MAGNETIC RESONANCE IMAGING STUDY**

Assessment of:
- Right and left ventricular function (global and segmental)
- Right and left ventricular volumes
- Aortic disease (e.g., aneurysm, dissection, coarctation)

Central pulmonary arteries
- Complex congenital heart disease
- Cardiac and paracardiac masses
- Pericardial disease
- Valvular regurgitation
- Peripheral and cerebral vasculature

MRI is based on observing the behavior of certain atoms within a magnetic field. Three steps are necessary for imaging. First, with the patient placed in the magnetic field, MR-sensitive nuclei become aligned with the field. Second, radiofrequency energy is applied to perturb the aligned nuclei. Finally, a radiowave signal is received from the perturbed nuclei as they return to their original lower-energy state (i.e., resting orientation).

Atoms and the External Magnetic Field

Atomic nuclei containing odd numbers of protons, neutrons, or the sum of these two possess nuclear spin, that is, they spin about their axis in the same way that the earth spins. The electrical charge associated with each atom also spins, creating a tiny magnetic field. These atoms may be thought of as tiny "bar magnets" that can interact with the magnetic field and radiowaves of the MR scanner. Hydrogen nuclei (or protons) possess this characteristic and are the predominant atomic species in the human body. Hydrogen is the nucleus that is used to generate MR images. Normally, these hydrogen "bar magnets" are oriented randomly within the body. When exposed to an external magnetic field, they align with the magnetic field. As hydrogen nuclei spin, they wobble, or precess, just as a toy top wobbles as it spins. The unique frequency of the wobble (precession) is governed by the Larmor frequency equation: $f = gM$, where f = frequency, g = gyromagnetic ratio, and M = field strength. Each nuclear species has a unique gyromagnetic ratio, and at a field strength of 1.5 T,[1] hydrogen nuclei precess at 64 MHz. By using the gradient coils to produce a graded magnetic field, atoms in different locations precess at slightly different frequencies. For example, if the field strength is less at the head compared with the feet, the precession frequency at the head is slower than at the feet. Hydrogen atoms are localized within the body based in part on this frequency, providing the basis for tomographic MRI.

Radiofrequency Pulse and Relaxation

Image data are obtained by recording the magnitude and rate of relaxation of precessing hydrogen nuclei after the application of radiofrequency energy (radiowaves). Stimulation with radiofrequency energy causes the hydrogen nuclei to "tip over" and become misaligned with the external magnetic field, and to synchronize their precession. The radiofrequency energy is applied as a pulse, and once it is terminated, the perturbed nuclei return or relax back to their original alignment in the magnetic field and their incoherent, random precession. As they relax, energy is released or emitted that is detected by the body coil (antenna). Relaxation is dependent on the interaction of adjacent nuclei, the local chemical and electrical environment, and the external magnetic field. Different tissues relax at different rates, providing contrast between tissues on MR images.

---

[1] Tesla (T) and gauss (G) are units of magnetic strength. One T = 10,000G. For reference, Earth's magnetic field is 50 μT.

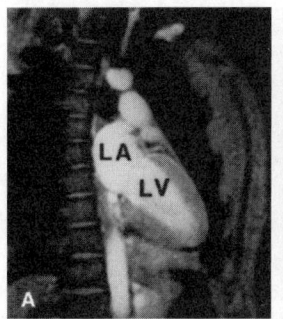 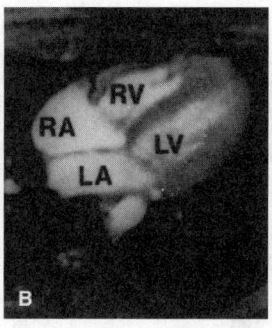 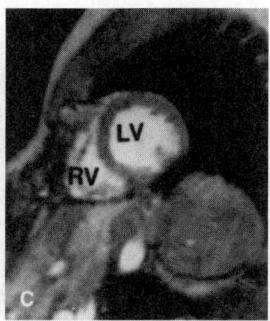

FIGURE 86.4. Midsystolic, gradient-echo magnetic resonance images of the heart in the **(A)** vertical long axis, **(B)** horizontal long axis, and **(C)** midventricular short axis orientations. LA, left atrium; LV, left ventricle; RA, right atrium; RV, right ventricle.

Gating and Pulse Sequences

Cardiovascular MRI applications require gating, or synchronization with the cardiac cycle, because data from repeated cardiac cycles are needed to generate images. Gating enhances image quality and prevents blurring by sampling data during comparable parts of the cardiac cycle. A pulse sequence is a series of gradient and radio-frequency pulses that are generated by the scanner to excite appropriate nuclei to acquire the image data. The two primary sequences used in cardiac imaging are the spin-echo and the gradient-echo pulse sequences. The spin-echo, or "dark blood," sequence provides images with excellent spatial resolution and is used primarily to assess anatomy and morphology. The gradient-echo, or "bright blood," sequence samples multiple data points over a cardiac cycle to improve temporal resolution. Sequential images obtained throughout the cardiac cycle are displayed in movie mode as a continuous loop of ventricular contraction and relaxation, so-called cine MRI. Regional and global ventricular function can be evaluated using this approach. These sequences produce high-quality images with excellent intrinsic contrast between intracavitary blood and the myocardium.

APPLICATIONS

Assessment of Cardiac Anatomy and Morphology

Magnetic resonance imaging (MRI) is unique in its ability to capture an image of the heart in any tomographic plane selected by the operator. Common plane orientations used in cardiac imaging include vertical long axis, horizontal long axis, and short axis (Fig. 86.4). Chamber sizes and wall thickness can be measured and used to determine myocardial mass. The location, extent, and attachment of intracardiac and paracardiac masses and thrombi can be demonstrated by MRI.

Magnetic resonance imaging is invaluable in assessing congenital heart disease. Venoatrial, atrioventricular, and ventriculoarterial connections are readily identified, as are chamber morphology, position, and their relation to the great vessels and other visceral organs. Because MRI is flow-sensitive, atrial and ventricular septal defects can be detected by the presence of turbulent flow using the cine MRI technique (see discussion of turbulent flow later in this chapter). Computer-assisted three-dimensional reconstruction of multi-slice images produces a visual model of complex cardiac anatomy that can be rotated and viewed from any perspective.

Assessment of Ventricular Function

Global and regional right and left ventricular systolic function can be measured from cine MRI. The ejection fraction is calculated from tomographically determined end-systolic and end-diastolic volumes using the area–length method with long-axis images (Fig. 86.5) or Simpson's rule with serial short-axis images. Unlike other imaging modalities, MRI can provide an accurate evaluation of right ventricular function without making geometrical assumptions regarding the shape of the right ventricle. Regional wall motion can be analyzed with cine MRI. Ventricular remodeling and myocardial thinning after myocardial infarction can be readily appreciated.

Valvular Assessment

The received signal from the body (after excitation from the radiofrequency pulse sequence) has both amplitude and phase. Turbulent flow appears as loss of signal (black) in gradient-echo images resulting from randomization of the phases of the blood in the turbulent jet. Accordingly, a regurgitant valve is identified by a jet of signal loss in the respective receiving chamber (Fig. 86.6). The degree of regurgitation can be measured by the size of the jet, the size of the chamber receiving the regurgitant flow, the persistence of the jet during the cardiac cycle, and the size and persistence of the proximal convergence zone.[2]

Turbulent flow also results from stenotic valves. Information similar to that derived from Doppler echocardiography can be obtained by a magnetic resonance technique known as phase velocity mapping. Whereas amplitude data are used to construct anatomical images, phase images (or maps) determine the flow velocity of precessing hydrogen atoms passing through a given plane. Depending on the scanner's specifications, velocities up to 6 to 8 m per second can be measured, making it possible to diagnose severe valvular stenoses.

Assessment of the Pericardium

Because magnetic resonance images can be acquired in any plane, the full extent of pericardial effusions can be defined. Some generalities about fluid composition can be made based on signal

---

[2] The proximal convergence zone is the region of flow acceleration where fluid converges uniformly and radially toward an orifice that is small relative to the proximal chamber.

End-diastolic   **End-systolic**

FIGURE 86.5. End-diastolic and end-systolic gradient echo images of the heart in the **(A)** vertical and **(B)** horizontal long-axis orientations. The left ventricular ejection fraction (LVEF) is determined using the area–length method. Note that the endocardial–blood pool border is outlined to determine changes in cavity size. This patient has had an anterior myocardial infarction with akinesis of the anterolateral wall and dyskinesis of the apex.

intensity. Magnetic resonance imaging can aid in the diagnosis of constrictive pericarditis by measuring the thickness of the pericardium, which normally should be less than 4 mm.

Vascular Imaging and Angiography

Many believe that MRI has become the gold standard for evaluating stable thoracic aortic disease. Intimal flaps, thrombus formation, origin of the tear, involvement of the brachiocephalic vessels, and the presence of aortic regurgitation or pericardial effusion all can be demonstrated during an MRI examination for aortic dissection (Fig. 86.7A). Furthermore, cine MRI can identify flow within the true and false lumina. Three-dimensional reconstruction of the aorta from multislice transaxial images is helpful in planning surgical repair of aortic dissection

and aneurysms (Fig. 86.7B). In coarctation of the aorta, the dimensions of the narrowing and the pressure gradient can be measured. In addition to producing images of the aorta, magnetic resonance angiography of the carotids (Fig. 86.8A) and peripheral vasculature (Fig. 86.8B) can be performed to evaluate the severity of vascular stenoses and the nature of the distal vessel.

FUTURE APPLICATIONS OF CARDIOVASCULAR MAGNETIC RESONANCE IMAGING

Given the rapid development of cardiovascular MRI, continual reference to the literature is necessary to remain current on this powerful diagnostic modality. With these developments, mag-

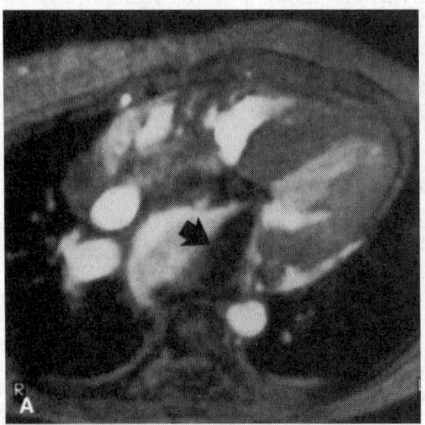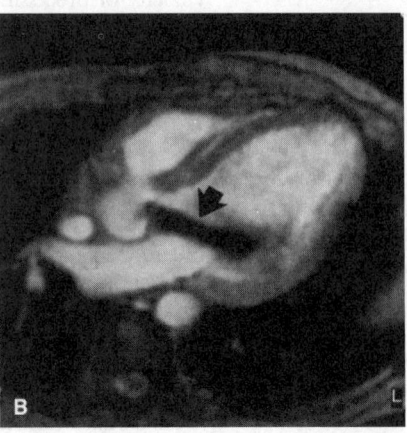

FIGURE 86.6. **A:** Midsystolic, gradient-echo horizontal long axis image of the heart in a patient with severe mitral regurgitation *(arrow)*. **B:** Mid-diastolic, gradient-echo left ventricular outflow tract view of the heart in a patient with severe aortic regurgitation *(arrow)*.

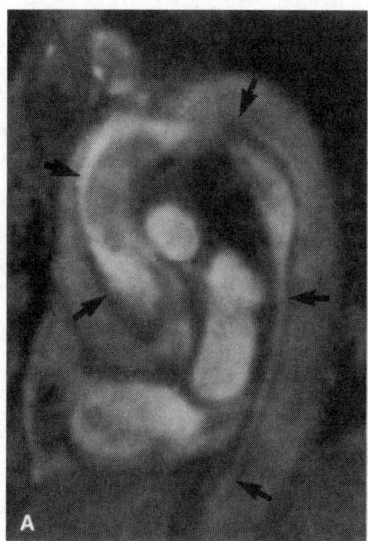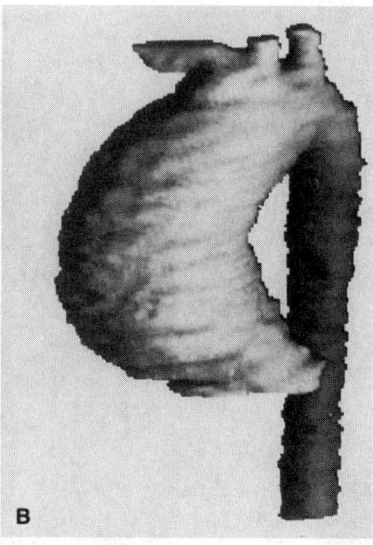

FIGURE 86.7. A: Magnetic resonance angiogram of the aorta in a left anterior oblique projection in a patient with a type I dissection *(arrows)*. **B:** Computer-assisted three-dimensional reconstruction from multiple transaxial magnetic resonance images of an aorta with an aneurysm in the ascending portion.

netic resonance methods should provide an approach to the assessment of many additional aspects of cardiac and vascular pathology.

Coronary Angiography

One of the most important potential MRI applications is magnetic resonance coronary angiography. The coronary arteries can be imaged in-plane or viewed using computer-aided projection

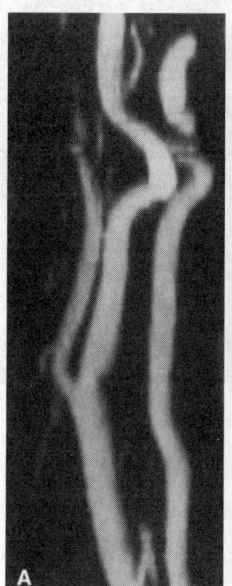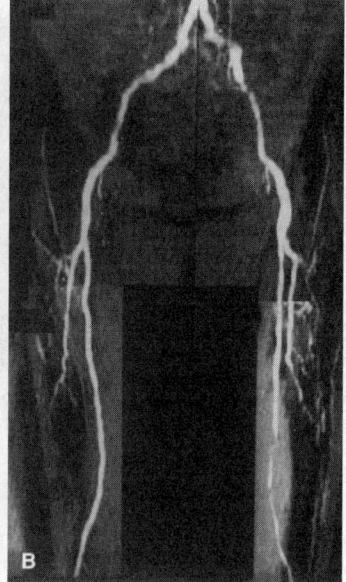

FIGURE 86.8. A: Magnetic resonance angiogram of the carotid and vertebral arteries. There is about a 30% narrowing of the proximal internal carotid artery. **B:** Magnetic resonance angiogram of the lower extremities in a patient with diffuse atherosclerotic disease. Severe disease is noted in the left iliofemoral arteries and bilaterally in the distal anterior tibial arteries. It is important to note that these angiograms are obtained without the administration of contrast agents since intrinsic contrast is provided by flowing blood.

techniques or three-dimensional reconstruction (Fig. 86.9). Coronary magnetic resonance angiography is limited by artifacts and alignment errors resulting from cardiac and respiratory motion, and by interference of high-signal epicardial fat, which reduces artery contrast. As this technique improves, it should be useful in screening for proximal or mid-vessel coronary artery disease in patients who otherwise might be referred for conventional X-ray coronary angiography.

Myocardial Function Assessment with Dobutamine

In a manner similar to stress echocardiography, ischemic wall motion changes can be assessed by cine MRI during an infusion of dobutamine. The relatively longer time required to obtain magnetic resonance images is the disadvantage of this technique. As faster MRI methods become available, this disadvantage probably will disappear.

Myocardial Perfusion Imaging

Contrast-enhanced MRI to evaluate myocardial perfusion uses a first-pass technique during which a bolus of a magnetic resonance contrast agent is injected intravenously and serial magnetic resonance images track the bolus through the cardiac chambers and finally into the myocardium. Paramagnetic resonance contrast agents are chelates of gadolinium. Gadolinium atoms have electrons with unpaired spins. These generate a local magnetic moment that shortens relaxation times in tissues perfused by blood containing gadolinium. In the presence of obstructive coronary stenosis, inhomogeneity in myocardial perfusion is induced after an infusion of dipyridamole. Ischemic myocardium supplied by a stenotic coronary artery has a lower peak signal intensity (which is proportional to the delivery of contrast medium) and a delay in the appearance of contrast.

Spectroscopy

Spectroscopy increasingly is being used to assess myocardial metabolism. Other nuclei besides hydrogen also possess nuclear

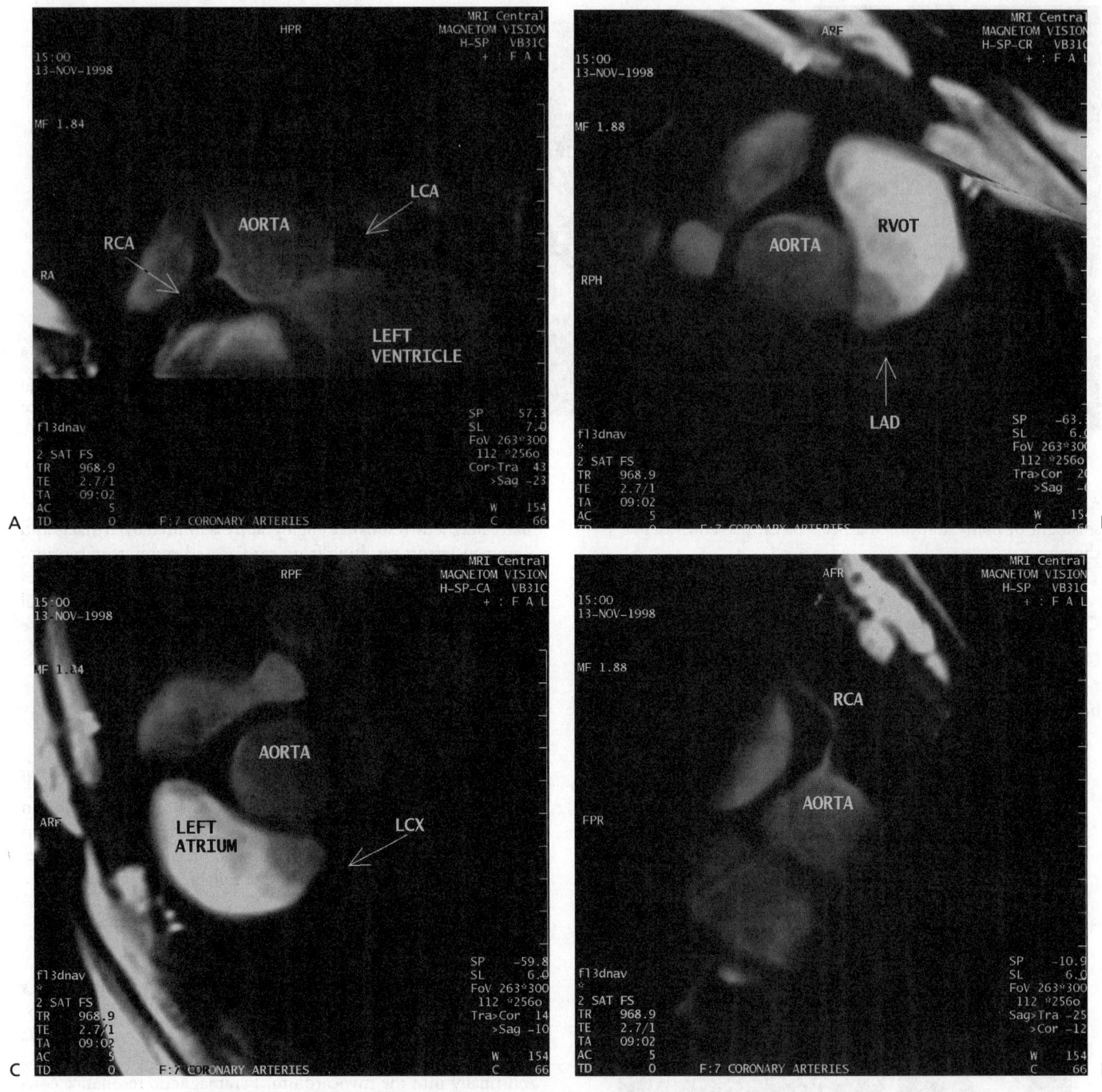

FIGURE 86.9. Coronary magnetic resonance angiograms of the **(A)** right (RCA) and left (LCA) coronary arteries arising from the aortic root, **(B)** left anterior descending (LAD) artery, **(C)** left circumflex (LCx) artery, and **(D)** right coronary artery (RCA).

spin, including ^{31}P, ^{13}C, ^{19}Fl, and ^{23}Na. Magnetic resonance spectroscopy acquires the spectrum of a particular nucleus in a selected region of tissue. For example, the bioenergetic profile of the myocardium can be investigated by acquiring a phosphorus spectrum that demonstrates phosphocreatine, inorganic phosphate, and adenosine triphosphate levels. Spectroscopy has been used to detect ischemia during isometric hand-grip exercise by demonstrating reductions in the phosphocreatine–to–adenosine

triphosphate ratio in jeopardized myocardium in patients with coronary artery disease.

The Comprehensive Magnetic Resonance Cardiovascular Examination

Ultimately, it should be possible for magnetic resonance methods to provide a comprehensive imaging study that includes assessment of cardiac morphology and ventricular function, coronary angiography, and myocardial perfusion imaging. Such an examination would obviate the need for multiple other imaging studies and would make magnetic resonance evaluation for coronary artery disease highly cost-effective.

BIBLIOGRAPHY

Beller GA. *Clinical nuclear cardiology.* Philadelphia: WB Saunders, 1995.

Blackwell GG, Cranney GB, Pohost GM. *MRI: cardiovascular system.* New York: Gower Medical, 1992.

Blackwell GG, Pohost GM. The usefulness of cardiovascular magnetic resonance imaging. *Curr Probl Cardiol* 1994;19:117–175.

Doyle M, Cranney GB, Pohost GM, et al. Magnetic resonance imaging and spectroscopy. In: Pohost GM, O'Rourke RA, eds. *Principles and practice of cardiovascular imaging.* Boston: Little, Brown and Company, 1991:455–552.

Johnson LL, Pohost GM. Nuclear cardiology. In: Schlant RC, Alexander RC, eds. *Hurst's The heart.* Eighth ed. New York: McGraw-Hill, 1993: 2324–2339.

Maddahi J, Rodrigues E, Berman JS. Assessment of myocardial perfusion imaging by single-photon agents. In: Pohost GM, O'Rourke RA, eds. *Principles and practice of cardiovascular imaging.* Boston: Little, Brown and Company, 1991:179–220.

Manning WJ, Atkinson DJ, Grossman W, et al. First pass nuclear magnetic resonance imaging studies using gadolinium–DTPA in patients with coronary artery disease. *J Am Coll Cardiol* 1991;18:959–965.

Manning WJ, Li W, Edelman RR. A preliminary report comparing magnetic resonance coronary angiography with conventional angiography. *N Engl J Med* 1993;328:828–832.

Verani MS. Pharmacologic stress myocardial perfusion imaging. *Curr Probl Cardiol* 1993;18:481–525.

Zaret BL, Wackers FJ. Nuclear cardiology. *N Engl J Med* 1993;329: 775–863.

Kelley's Textbook of Internal Medicine, fourth edition. Edited by H. David Humes.
Lippincott Williams & Wilkins, Philadelphia © 2000.

C H A P T E R

87

DIAGNOSTIC AND THERAPEUTIC CATHETERIZATION

RICHARD A. LANGE
L. DAVID HILLIS

Over the past 40 years, cardiac catheterization has greatly improved our understanding of cardiovascular anatomy, physiology, and pathophysiology. In its early years it was performed sparingly and with substantial risk; however, with increased operator experience and technical improvements, its associated morbidity and mortality have fallen substantially. Today diagnostic catheterization is performed with minimal risk, and therapeutic catheterization (percutaneous coronary revascularization and balloon valvuloplasty) is performed without incident in most patients. Thus, cardiac catheterization plays a pivotal role in the evaluation of patients with suspected or known cardiac disease; in addition, it has become an important therapeutic alternative to cardiac surgery in many patients who require nonmedical therapy.

■ APPLICATION

INDICATIONS

Diagnostic cardiac catheterization is appropriate under several conditions. First, it is often performed to confirm or to exclude the presence of a cardiac condition that is suspected from the patient's history, physical examination, or noninvasive evaluation. In such a circumstance, it allows assessment of the presence and severity of cardiac disease. For example, in a person with progressive angina pectoris or a positive exercise test, coronary angiography allows the physician to visualize the coronary arteries sufficiently to assess the presence and extent of coronary artery disease. Second, catheterization is often helpful in the patient with a confusing or difficult clinical presentation in whom the noninvasive evaluation is inconclusive. For instance, a hemodynamic evaluation or coronary angiography may be useful in the patient with unexplained dyspnea. Third, in a patient being considered for corrective cardiac surgery, catheterization often is performed to assess the suspected abnormality and to exclude associated conditions. For example, catheterization may be performed in the patient with valvular heart disease to evaluate the severity of the valvular abnormality, its influence on overall cardiac function, and the presence of concomitant coronary artery disease that may require revascularization at the time of valvular surgery. Fourth, data obtained at catheterization may provide prognostic information that is helpful in guiding therapy. Such is the case, for example, in the patient with cardiomyopathy, in whom the hemodynamic data obtained at catheterization are used to guide medical therapy and to assess the need for and timing of cardiac transplantation.

Therapeutic catheterization is appropriate in several circumstances. Percutaneous coronary revascularization (angioplasty, atherectomy, or endovascular stenting) may be indicated in the patient with symptomatic atherosclerotic coronary artery disease and suitable coronary anatomy. Because both percutaneous coronary revascularization and coronary artery bypass grafting often are effective in such patients, the factors that influence which procedure is selected include coronary anatomy, the presence of concomitant comorbid medical conditions (which may increase the risk of either procedure), and patient preference. In the patient with symptomatic valvular stenosis, percutaneous balloon valvuloplasty may be performed. With symptomatic, isolated pulmonic stenosis, it is the treatment of choice. With mitral stenosis and favorable valvular anatomy, it is a viable alternative to surgery. In the subject with symptomatic aortic stenosis in whom valve replacement has an unfavorable risk/benefit ratio because of comorbid disease (i.e., chronic obstructive pulmonary disease, hepatic or renal disease, or malignancy), percutaneous aortic balloon valvuloplasty may be considered.

CONTRAINDICATIONS

The only absolute contraindication to catheterization is the refusal of a mentally competent patient to provide informed con-

TABLE 87.1.	RELATIVE CONTRAINDICATIONS TO CARDIAC CATHETERIZATION

- Decompensated heart failure (e.g., pulmonary edema)
- Uncontrolled ventricular irritability
- Uncontrolled systemic arterial hypertension
- Acute or severe renal insufficiency
- Difficulty with vascular access
- Electrolyte imbalance (hypo- or hyperkalemia)
- Digitalis intoxication
- Active infection or febrile illness
- Uncorrected bleeding diathesis
- Severe anemia
- Active bleeding from internal organ
- Severe allergy to radiographic contrast material
- Mental incompetence

sent. Relative contraindications (Table 87.1) mostly involve conditions in which the risks of the procedure are increased or the information obtained from it is potentially unreliable. In these circumstances, the benefits of the data obtained at catheterization must be weighed against the procedure's increased risks. Catheterization usually is not performed in the patient who refuses therapy for the condition for which diagnostic catheterization is recommended.

COMPLICATIONS

Because catheterization is an invasive procedure, its use is associated with certain major and minor risks (Table 87.2). The incidence of complications is higher with therapeutic procedures than with diagnostic ones, but in general either can be performed safely with little morbidity or mortality. Complications are more likely to occur in certain patient groups, including those of advanced (more than 70 years) or very young (less than 1 year) age, marked functional impairment (class IV angina or heart failure), severe left ventricular dysfunction or coronary artery disease (particularly left main disease), severe valvular disease,

TABLE 87.2.	COMPLICATIONS ASSOCIATED WITH DIAGNOSTIC CARDIAC CATHETERIZATION

Complication	Incidence (%)
Major Complications	
Death	0.1
Cerebrovascular accident	0.07
Myocardial infarction	0.07
Arrhythmias (life-threatening)	0.5
Vascular compromise	0.5–1.5
Anaphylaxis (contrast allergy)	0.007
Minor Complications	
Hives	2–3
Nausea/vomiting	5
Vasovagal reactions	3

severe comorbid medical conditions (renal, hepatic, or pulmonary disease), and a history of an allergic reaction to radiographic contrast material. Of those with a known allergy to contrast material, only about 15% have an adverse reaction with its repeat administration, and most of these reactions are minor (e.g., urticaria, nausea, vomiting). In most patients with a previous allergic reaction to radiographic contrast material, angiography can be performed safely, but premedication with glucocorticosteroids and antihistamines and the use of nonionic contrast material are usually recommended.

TECHNIQUES

Cardiac catheterization is generally performed with the patient in the fasting state and mildly sedated. Anticoagulants are discontinued before the procedure (warfarin several days before and heparin 4 to 6 hours before). Antibiotic prophylaxis is not required.

With the *percutaneous femoral approach,* an area 3 to 4 cm below the inguinal ligament is aseptically prepared and locally anesthetized. The femoral vessel is punctured with an 18-gauge (Seldinger) needle, through which a flexible wire is advanced into the vessel's lumen, over which a sheath with a sideport extension is advanced into the vessel. The sideport extension allows continuous monitoring of femoral arterial pressure (through an arterial sheath) or infusion of fluids (through a venous sheath) as catheters are advanced through the sheath to the heart. When the procedure is completed, the catheters and sheaths are removed, local pressure is applied to achieve hemostasis, and the patient remains at bed rest for 8 to 24 hours. Because this approach does not require vascular exposure or repair, it can be performed quickly and repeatedly in the same patient, and it is associated with a low incidence of infection and vascular injury. At the same time, certain conditions make catheterization via the femoral artery difficult, including extensive peripheral vascular disease, morbid obesity, uncontrolled systemic arterial hypertension, bleeding diathesis, and disorders associated with a markedly augmented arterial pulse pressure (e.g., severe aortic regurgitation). Right heart catheterization via the femoral vein may be difficult in the presence of right atrial dilatation.

With the *brachial approach,* an area 1 to 2 cm above the flexor crease of the arm is aseptically prepared and locally anesthetized. A transverse cutdown is performed, and the brachial artery or vein is isolated. Catheters are introduced into the vessel under direct vision, then advanced to the heart. After the procedure has been completed, the catheters are removed, the vein used for right heart catheterization is ligated, and the arteriotomy used for left heart catheterization is sutured. Alternatively, brachial catheterization may be performed percutaneously in a manner similar to the femoral approach.

Catheterization may also be performed percutaneously via the *radial artery.* Since the radial artery is small in caliber, small-diameter catheters must be used, and radial arterial occlusion occurs in 2% to 3% of patients. Catheterization via this approach may be preferred when the patient has a condition that renders the femoral approach difficult or when it is desirable to allow the patient to ambulate soon after catheterization.

If catheterization of the left atrium is desired, the *trans-septal technique* usually is performed. A special catheter is introduced percutaneously in the right femoral vein and advanced to the right atrium. A trans-septal needle is advanced through the catheter and used to puncture the interatrial septum. With the tip of the needle in the left atrium, the catheter is advanced over the needle into the chamber, after which the needle is withdrawn. Through the catheter, the left atrial pressure is measured, and other catheters can be exchanged and positioned for therapeutic procedures, such as mitral valvuloplasty.

Rarely, placement of a catheter in the left ventricle across the aortic (or mitral) valve is not advisable. For example, passage of a catheter across a tilting-disk prosthetic valve may result in the catheter becoming trapped in the prosthetic device. Accordingly, *direct left ventricular puncture* through the chest wall with a needle directed at the cardiac apex is sometimes required. Serious complications, such as cardiac tamponade, hemothorax, pneumothorax, or ventricular fibrillation, occur in about 3% of such procedures.

During routine right heart catheterization, measurements of pressure and oxygen saturation in the vena cavae, right atrium, right ventricle, pulmonary artery, and pulmonary capillary wedge position can be performed, and cardiac output can be quantified (Table 87.3 lists normal values). Measurement of

TABLE 87.3.	NORMAL HEMODYNAMIC VALUES
Measurement	**Value**
Flows	
Cardiac index (L/min/m^2)	2.6–4.2
Stroke volume index (mL/m^2)	35–55
Pressures (mm Hg)	
Aorta/systemic artery	
Peak systolic/end-diastolic	100–140/60–90
Mean	70–105
Left ventricle	
Peak systolic/end-diastolic	100–140/3–12
Left atrium (PCW)	
Mean	1–10
a wave	3–15
v wave	3–15
Pulmonary artery	
Peak systolic/end-diastolic	16–30/4–12
Mean	10–16
Right ventricle	
Peak systolic/end-diastolic	16–30/0–8
Right atrium	
Mean	0–8
a wave	2–10
v wave	2–10
Resistances	
Systemic vascular resistance	
Wood units	10–20
dynes-sec-cm^{-5}	770–1500
Pulmonary vascular resistance	
Wood units	0.25–1.5
dynes-sec-cm^{-5}	20–120
Oxygen consumption (mL/min/m^2)	110–150
AV O$_2$ difference (mL/dL)	3.0–4.5

AV, arteriovenous; PCW, pulmonary capillary wedge.

right-sided pressures helps the physician to evaluate the severity of tricuspid or pulmonic stenosis, to assess the presence and severity of pulmonary hypertension, and to calculate pulmonary vascular resistance. In the absence of pulmonary vein stenosis (a rare condition), the pulmonary capillary wedge pressure accurately reflects the left atrial pressure. The determination of oxygen saturations from the various right heart chambers is used to assess the presence, location, and magnitude of intracardiac left-to-right shunting, such as occurs with atrial or ventricular septal defect or patent ductus arteriosus. Occasionally, angiography is performed to define right-sided anatomical abnormalities or to evaluate the severity of right-sided valvular regurgitation.

For optimal measurement of right heart pressures, a relatively stiff, large-lumen, nonflotation catheter is used. It is advanced until it "wedges" in a small pulmonary artery. The catheter's position in the pulmonary capillary wedge location is confirmed by obtaining blood with an oxygen saturation of above 95%. Alternatively, a softer, balloon-tipped, flotation catheter can be used. With this catheter, the acquisition of a blood sample to confirm the pulmonary capillary wedge position is often difficult, and the fidelity of the pressure recordings is not as good as those obtained with a stiffer, large-lumen catheter; however, its ease of passage and paucity of complications make it more suitable for use by operators with limited experience. Furthermore, because it is flow-directed, it often can be advanced through the right heart without fluoroscopic guidance. Finally, adding a thermistor to the flotation catheter's distal portion allows measurement of cardiac output by thermodilution.

With left heart catheterization, mitral and aortic valvular function, left ventricular pressures and function, systemic vascular resistance, and coronary artery anatomy can be assessed. To perform angiography or to measure the pressure in the left ventricle, a catheter is usually advanced retrograde across the aortic valve. In rare circumstances in which this is impossible (e.g., severe aortic stenosis or a tilting-disk prosthetic valve in the aortic position), transseptal catheterization is performed, and the catheter is advanced to the left ventricle antegrade across the mitral valve.

HEMODYNAMIC MEASUREMENTS

CARDIAC OUTPUT

The blood flow measurement most often performed during catheterization is the quantitation of cardiac output. This variable allows assessment of overall cardiovascular function, vascular resistances, valve orifice areas, and valvular regurgitation. In the catheterization laboratory, the three common methods of measuring cardiac output are the Fick principle, the indicator dilution technique, and angiography.

Fick Technique

The Fick principle, introduced by Adolph Fick in 1870, is based on the fact that when a substance is consumed by an organ, its concentration is the product of blood flow to the organ and the substance's arteriovenous difference across the organ. Using the lung as the organ of interest and oxygen as the substance, one can calculate pulmonary blood flow using the formula:

Cardiac output (L/minute)

= oxygen consumption (mL/minute)/arteriovenous oxygen difference (mL/L)

In the absence of intracardiac shunting, pulmonary and systemic blood flows are similar, so that the Fick method provides a measurement of systemic blood flow. The results of the Fick method are most reliable when the arteriovenous oxygen difference is wide (e.g., a low cardiac output) and least reliable when it is narrow (e.g., a high cardiac output; Table 87.4).

The oxygen consumption is determined by collecting a timed sample (usually for 3 to 4 minutes) of expired air in a receptacle called a Douglas bag. From the volume of air collected and the difference in oxygen content between inspired and expired air, the amount of oxygen consumed per minute can be determined. Alternatively, oxygen consumption can be estimated with a metabolic rate meter. With this device, a plastic hood is placed over the patient's head and the oxygen content of expired air is monitored continuously as it is withdrawn from the hood with a blower motor.

In some catheterization laboratories, an assumed value for oxygen consumption is derived from a formula or nomogram. The average oxygen consumption for adults is 125 (range 65 to 250) mL per minute per square meter of body surface area. Because oxygen consumption varies greatly from one patient to another, the use of an assumed value is potentially unreliable. In general, oxygen consumption is higher in men than in women and decreases gradually with age. It increases with hyperthyroidism, hyperthermia, and exercise, and it decreases with hypothyroidism and hypothermia.

The determination of the arteriovenous oxygen difference across the lungs requires that blood be obtained from the vessels entering the lungs (pulmonary artery) and draining the lungs (pulmonary vein). In the absence of right-to-left shunting, the oxygen content of pulmonary venous blood is similar to that of systemic arterial blood. Therefore, in practice, a systemic arterial (rather than a pulmonary venous) blood sample is procured. The oxygen contents of systemic arterial and pulmonary arterial blood are measured directly or calculated from the oxygen saturation using the formula:

$$O_2 \text{ content (mL/dL)} = \text{saturation} \times \text{Hgb (g/dL)} \times 1.34 \text{ (mL } O_2/\text{g Hgb)}$$

where 1.34 is the oxygen-carrying capacity of 1 g of hemoglobin (Hgb). The normal arteriovenous oxygen difference is 3.0 to 4.5 mL/dL.

The following is an example of the calculation of cardiac output using the Fick principle:

Oxygen consumption = 250 mL per minute
Hemoglobin = 15 g per dL
Oxygen saturation of systemic arterial blood = 95%
Oxygen saturation of pulmonary arterial blood = 70%
Conversion factor = 10 (number of deciliters per liter)

$$\text{Cardiac output (L per minute)} = 250 \text{ mL per minute}/(0.95 - 0.70)(15 \text{ g per dL})(1.34 \text{ mL } O_2/\text{g})(10 \text{ dL/L})$$
$$= 5.0 \text{ L/minute}$$

Indicator Dilution Method

With indicator dilution, a known amount of indicator is injected as a bolus into the circulation and allowed to mix completely in the blood, after which its concentration is measured. A time–concentration curve is generated (Fig. 87.1), and a minicomputer calculates the cardiac output from the area of the inscribed curve.

Thermodilution

The most widely used indicator to measure cardiac output is cold solution. A balloon-tipped, flow-directed, polyvinyl chloride catheter with a thermistor at its tip and an opening 25 to 30 cm proximal to the tip is inserted into a vein and advanced to the pulmonary artery, so that the proximal opening is located in the vena cavae or right atrium and the thermistor is in the pulmonary artery. A known amount of cold fluid is injected through the proximal port; it mixes completely in the right ventricle and causes a change in blood temperature, which is detected by the thermistor. The thermodilution method is relatively inexpensive and easy to perform, and does not require arterial sampling or blood withdrawal. In most patients, it accurately determines pulmonary blood flow, which (in the absence

TABLE 87.4.	METHODS FOR DETERMINING CARDIAC OUTPUT AND CONDITIONS IN WHICH THEY ARE MOST (OR LEAST) RELIABLE

Method	Most Reliable	Least Reliable
Fick	Low cardiac output	High cardiac output
Thermodilution	High cardiac output	Pulmonic regurgitation
		Tricuspid regurgitation
		Intracardiac shunting
Indocyanine green	High cardiac output	Aortic regurgitation
		Mitral regurgitation
		Low cardiac output
		Intracardiac shunting
Angiographic	Normal-shaped ventricle	Extensive segmental wall motion abnormalities
		Dilated ventricle
		Aortic regurgitation[a]
		Mitral regurgitation[a]

[a] In these circumstances, angiographic output is greater than forward cardiac output (see text).

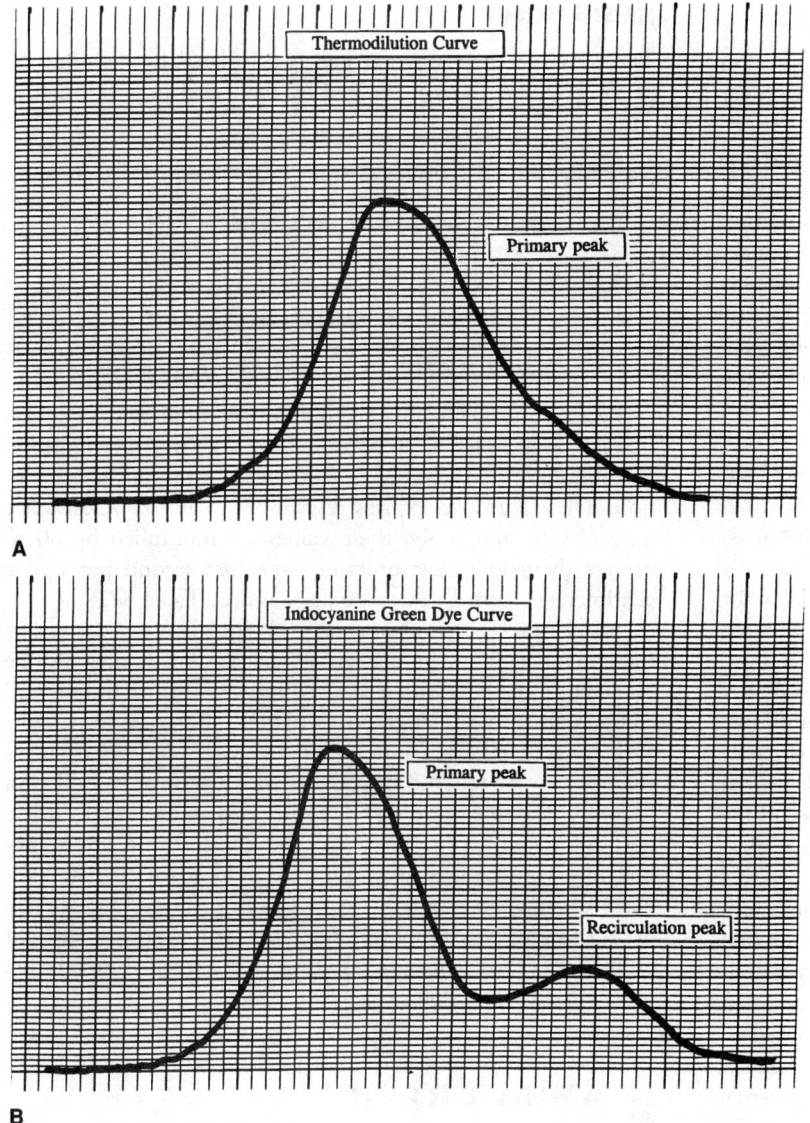

FIGURE 87.1. Time–activity curves for the indicator dilution technique of determining cardiac output: thermodilution **(A)** and indocyanine green **(B)**. With indocyanine green, there is a primary peak and a recirculation peak; with thermodilution, only a primary peak is observed.

of intracardiac shunting) is similar to systemic blood flow. However, certain conditions may render the results of the thermodilution technique unreliable, including tricuspid or pulmonic regurgitation and intracardiac shunting (Table 87.4).

Indocyanine Green

The second most widely used indicator to measure cardiac output is indocyanine green. This water-soluble, nontoxic substance is usually introduced through a catheter positioned in a right heart chamber, and its concentration is sampled in arterial blood withdrawn at a constant rate through an optical densitometer. The lungs and left heart serve as sites of complete mixing, and there is no degradation of indocyanine green between the site of injection and sampling. As with thermodilution, a time–activity curve is inscribed, and the cardiac output is determined from the area of the curve, excluding the recirculation peak (Fig. 87.1). The results obtained with this method compare favorably with those of other techniques for measuring cardiac output, but it

may provide inaccurate results if the recirculation peak cannot be easily separated from the primary peak (e.g., low cardiac output) or if one of the valves between the site of injection and sampling (mitral or aortic) is regurgitant (Table 87.4).

Angiographic Method

From the left ventriculogram, the volume of blood ejected with each heartbeat (stroke volume) can be determined. It is then multiplied by the heart rate, yielding the angiographic cardiac output. In patients with mitral or aortic regurgitation, a portion of the blood ejected from the left ventricle regurgitates into the left atrium or ventricle and does not enter the systemic circulation. In these patients, the angiographic cardiac output is higher than the forward output. The measurement of cardiac output by the angiographic method is potentially erroneous in patients with extensive segmental wall motion abnormalities or misshapen ventricles, in whom the determination of stroke volume may be inaccurate (Table 87.4).

PRESSURES

One of the most important functions of cardiac catheterization is to measure and record intracardiac pressures. Once a catheter is positioned in a cardiac chamber, it is connected through fluid-filled, stiff, plastic tubing to a pressure transducer, which transforms the pressure signal into an electrical signal that is recorded. The accurate measurement of pressure requires close attention to the details of the catheter system, including proper transducer balancing, removal of air bubbles and blood from the catheters and connections, and avoidance of an excessive length of plastic tubing. All transducers should be referenced to the same zero level and their position adjusted if the patient's position changes. Pressure transducers should be calibrated frequently against a mercury manometer to ensure proper function.

During catheterization, pressures are usually measured directly from each of the cardiac chambers—right atrium, right ventricle, pulmonary artery, ascending aorta, and left ventricle. In contrast, a left atrial pressure is seldom measured directly unless a trans-septal catheterization is performed. Because the left atrial pressure is transmitted to the pulmonary capillaries, it is recorded "indirectly" as the pulmonary capillary "wedge" pressure. To measure the wedge pressure, an endhole catheter is placed in the main pulmonary artery and advanced until it is wedged in a small pulmonary artery. If the catheter is adequately wedged, the tracing observed is that of a transmitted left atrial pressure, and the blood aspirated through the catheter is fully saturated (oxygen saturation ≥95%). Normal values for intracardiac pressures are shown in Table 87.3.

In addition to measuring pressures from each cardiac chamber, pressures from certain chambers are examined simultaneously to identify or exclude a gradient between them that is indicative of valvular stenosis. Thus, left ventricular and left atrial (or pulmonary capillary wedge) pressures are recorded simultaneously to identify the diastolic gradient of mitral stenosis (Fig. 87.2A). Likewise, left ventricular and aortic (or systemic arterial) pressures are recorded simultaneously to determine if there is a systolic gradient indicative of left ventricular outflow tract obstruction (Fig. 87.2B).

RESISTANCES

The resistance of a vascular bed is calculated by dividing the pressure gradient across the bed by the blood flow through it. Thus:

Systemic vascular resistance = mean systemic arterial pressure

— mean right atrial pressure/systemic blood flow

Pulmonary vascular resistance

= mean pulmonary artery pressure

— mean left atrial pressure/pulmonary blood flow

Because a properly obtained pulmonary capillary wedge pressure is similar to left atrial pressure (except in the rare condition of pulmonary vein stenosis), it can replace it in the above equation. These formulas express resistances in arbitrary resistance units. More commonly, these values are multiplied by 80 to express them in metric units of dynes per second per square centimeter. Normal values are displayed in Table 87.3.

An elevated systemic vascular resistance is often present in the patient with systemic arterial hypertension. It may also be observed in patients with a reduced forward cardiac output and compensatory arteriolar vasoconstriction (often seen in patients with congestive heart failure). Conversely, systemic vascular resistance may be reduced in patients with arteriolar vasodilation (due, for example, to sepsis) or those with an increased cardiac output (due, for example, to an arteriovenous fistula, severe anemia, fever, or thyrotoxicosis). Elevated pulmonary vascular resistance often is observed in patients with primary lung disease or Eisenmenger's physiology and those with a greatly elevated pulmonary venous pressure resulting from left-sided myocardial or valvular dysfunction.

◼ ANGIOGRAPHY

During angiography, radiographic contrast material is injected into the cardiovascular structure of interest as cineangiography

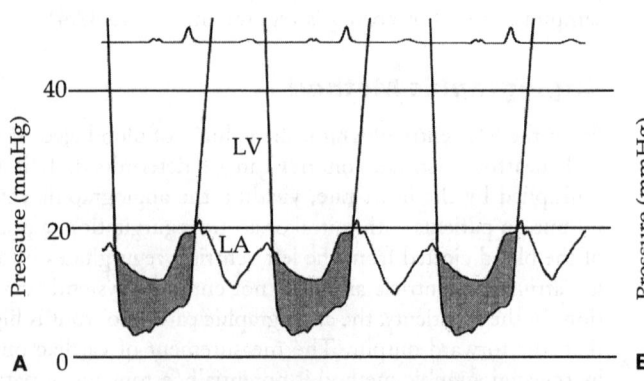
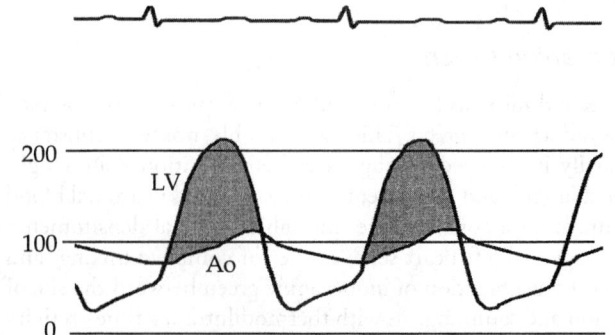

FIGURE 87.2. A: Simultaneous pressure recordings from the left atrium and left ventricle, demonstrating a diastolic gradient in a patient with mitral stenosis. **B:** Simultaneous pressure recordings from the left ventricle and aorta, demonstrating a systolic gradient in a patient with aortic stenosis. Gradients are indicated with shading.

is performed on 35-mm film at 30 to 60 frames per second. The resultant cineangiogram permits the study of cardiac structures in real time, in slow motion, or by single frame. Alternatively, angiographic images can be projected onto a high-resolution screen and converted with computer processing from an analog to a digital form. Digital angiography allows image enhancement, computer processing, and quantitative analysis, features that are not available with routine cineangiography. With computer digitization, less radiographic contrast material is required, and the angiographic images can be stored on a central computer or computer-accessible medium (optical disk, magnetic tape, or compact disk) and recalled later for processing and analysis.

LEFT VENTRICULOGRAPHY

With cineangiography of the left ventricle, global and segmental left ventricular function, left ventricular volumes and ejection fraction, and the presence and severity of mitral regurgitation can be assessed. Typically, a power injector is used to deliver 30 to 60 mL of contrast material over 3 to 4 seconds through a catheter in the left ventricular cavity, and the silhouette is filmed in one (single-plane) or two (biplane) projections (Fig. 87.3).

Using a standard area–length formula, left ventricular volumes and ejection fraction are determined. Specifically, end-diastolic and end-systolic volumes are measured, from which stroke volume is derived (the difference between end-diastolic and end-systolic volumes) and the ejection fraction is calculated (the quotient of stroke volume and end-diastolic volume). The angiographic cardiac output is the product of stroke volume and heart rate.

In addition to providing information about volumes and global systolic function, left ventriculography allows assessment of segmental wall motion. A segment of the left ventricular wall with reduced systolic motion is said to be hypokinetic; a segment that does not move is akinetic; and a segment that moves paradoxically during systole is dyskinetic.

CORONARY ANGIOGRAPHY

Selective coronary angiography is usually performed to determine the presence and severity of fixed, atherosclerotic coronary artery disease and to guide subsequent percutaneous (e.g., angioplasty) or surgical (e.g., bypass grafting) therapy. It is sometimes used to evaluate the presence of dynamic alterations in coronary

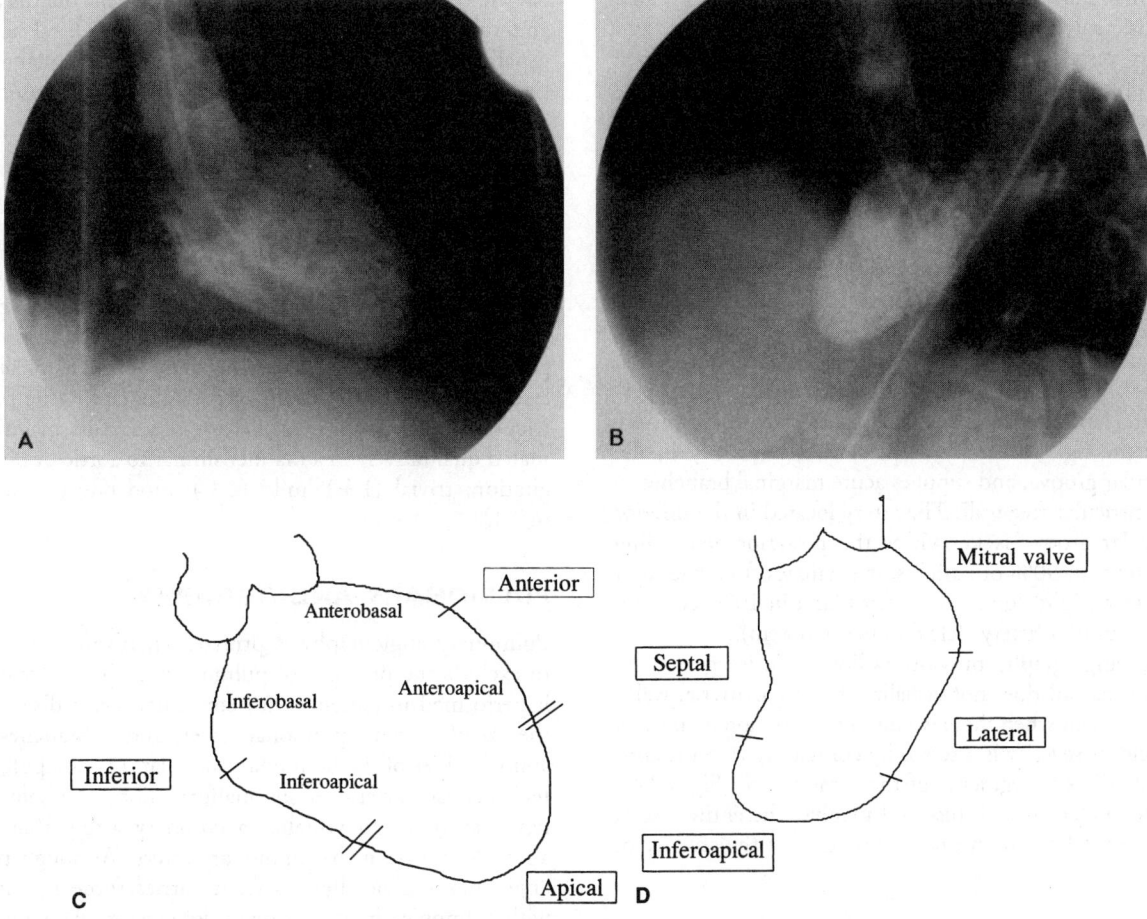

FIGURE 87.3. With biplane ventriculography, two projections 90 degrees apart in obliquity are performed: 30E right anterior oblique **(A)** and 60 degrees left anterior oblique **(B)**. The segments of the left ventricle that are visualized with each obliquity are labeled **(C, D)**. With typical single-plane ventriculography, only the right anterior oblique view is obtained.

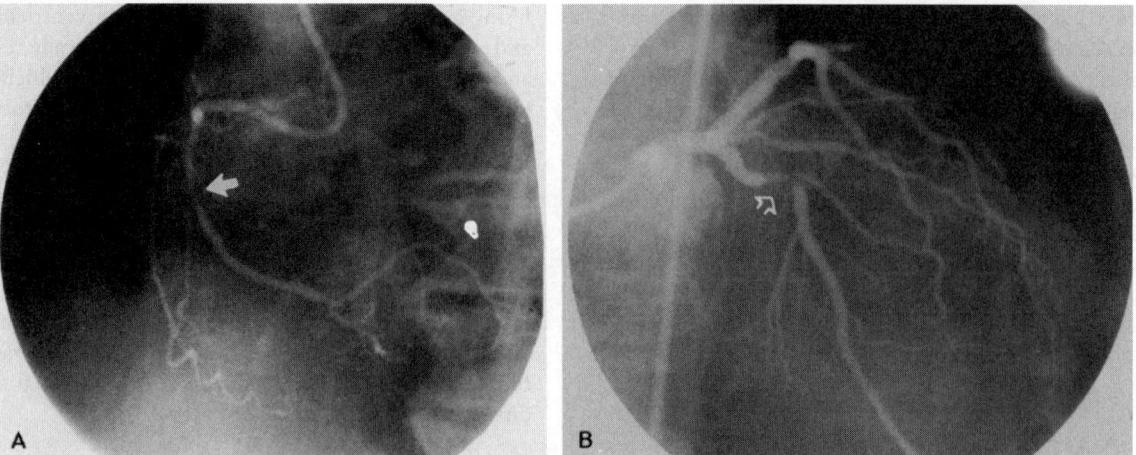

FIGURE 87.4. Coronary angiograms from a patient with an 80% stenosis in the right coronary artery (**A,** *arrow*) and a 90% stenosis in the left anterior descending coronary artery (**B,** *arrow*).

arterial tone (coronary arterial spasm), to define congenital abnormalities of the coronary arteries, and to establish the patency of bypass grafts. Under fluoroscopic guidance, the ostia of the native right and left coronary arteries or bypass grafts are engaged selectively with a catheter, and radiographic contrast material is injected manually as cineangiography is performed. Because atherosclerotic coronary arterial stenoses are often eccentric and the coronary vessels overlap one another, images are obtained in multiple obliquities to procure a complete angiographic assessment of each arterial segment.

The left main coronary artery arises from the left coronary cusp and divides into the left anterior descending and left circumflex arteries. The left anterior descending courses in the anterior interventricular groove and provides a variable number of septal perforators, which perfuse the interventricular septum, and diagonal branches, which perfuse the high lateral left ventricular wall. The left circumflex artery is located in the posterior atrioventricular groove and provides obtuse marginal branches—also called circumflex marginal branches—that perfuse the lateral left ventricular free wall. The right coronary artery arises from the right coronary cusp, courses anteriorly in the atrioventricular groove, and supplies acute marginal branches to the right ventricular free wall. The artery located in the inferior interventricular groove is known as the posterior descending coronary artery. In 90% of patients, it emanates from the right coronary artery (right-dominant system), and in 10% its origin is the left circumflex artery (left-dominant system).

Coronary angiography provides radiographic images of the coronary lumina but does not visualize the actual arterial walls. A stenosis is present when there is a discrete reduction in luminal diameter, and its severity is assessed by comparing it to presumably normal adjacent segments of the same artery (Fig. 87.4). Thus, if atherosclerosis is diffuse and involves the entire artery, angiography may lead to an underestimation of the severity of disease.

AORTOGRAPHY

Aortography is accomplished with the rapid injection of a large amount (50 to 60 mL over 2 seconds) of radiographic contrast material into the aorta. With proximal aortography, the severity of aortic valve regurgitation, the location of saphenous vein bypass grafts, and the anatomy of the proximal aorta and its branches can be assessed. Examples of anatomical abnormalities of the aorta that can be visualized by aortography include annuloaortic ectasia, dissection, coarctation, patent ductus arteriosus, and ruptured sinus of Valsalva aneurysm. Distal aortography usually is performed to assess the presence of vascular abnormalities, such as aneurysml dissection, intraluminal thrombus, coarctation, or branch vessel stenosis.

RIGHT VENTRICULOGRAPHY

Cinenangiography of the right ventricle allows assessment of global right ventricular function and possible anatomical abnormalities of the right ventricle, including its outflow tract. Because the right ventricle is asymmetric, there are no reliable ventriculographic methods for quantifying right ventricular volumes and ejection fraction. With right ventriculography, the presence of tricuspid regurgitation can be assessed and its magnitude estimated qualitatively in a manner similar to aortic or mitral regurgitation: trivial (1+), mild (2+), moderate (3+), or severe (4+).

PULMONARY ANGIOGRAPHY

Pulmonary angiography is primarily performed to confirm or to exclude the presence of pulmonary emboli. Occasionally, it is performed in patients with congenital heart disease to assess the size of the main pulmonary artery and its branches, to detect abnormalities of the pulmonary vasculature (e.g., pulmonary artery stenosis, arteriovenous malformation, anomalous pulmonary veins), or to visualize a coronary artery that originates anomalously from the pulmonary artery. Although pulmonary angiography generally is safe, it carries some risk in patients with pulmonary hypertension or right ventricular failure. In such patients it should be performed only when noninvasive techniques fail to assess the suspected condition adequately or when the potential benefits outweigh the risks.

ASSESSMENT OF VALVULAR HEART DISEASE

VALVULAR STENOSIS

In patients with valvular stenosis, the effective valve orifice area can be calculated with data obtained during catheterization using principles of standard fluid dynamics. The pressures on either side of a stenotic valve are recorded simultaneously (Fig. 87.2) and the flow across it is measured, after which the valve area is calculated with the equation of Gorlin and Gorlin:

Valve orifice area (cm^2) = flow across the valve/constant

$$\times \text{ mean pressure gradient}$$

The mean pressure gradient is the average gradient during systole (for aortic or pulmonic valves) or diastole (for mitral or tricuspid valves). The cardiac output is the flow across the valve.

Although the normal mitral valve orifice is 4 to 6 cm^2, substantial stenosis may occur before a pressure gradient (Fig. 87.2A) or clinical symptoms appear. A mitral valve with an effective area of 1 cm^2 or less is considered severely stenotic; 1.1 to 1.5 cm^2, moderately stenotic; and 1.6 to 2 cm^2, mildly stenotic.

The normal aortic valve has a cross-sectional area of 3 to 4 cm^2, but hemodynamically important aortic stenosis (Fig. 87.2B) does not develop until the valve orifice area falls below 1 cm^2. An aortic valve area of 0.7 cm^2 or less is severely stenotic; 0.8 to 1 cm^2, moderately stenotic; and 1.1 to 1.3 cm^2, mildly stenotic. The term "critical" aortic stenosis is reserved for an aortic valve area of 0.5 cm^2 or less.

The normal pulmonic valve has a cross-sectional area similar to that of the aortic valve. By convention, the severity of pulmonic stenosis is estimated solely according to the peak right ventricular pressure rather than the Gorlin-derived valve area. Pulmonic stenosis with a peak right ventricular pressure of 30 to 50 mm Hg is considered mild; 50 to 100 mm Hg, moderate; and above 100 mm Hg, severe.

The tricuspid valve is normally large, with an orifice area of 6 to 10 cm^2. The patient with a tricuspid valve area of less than 3 cm^2 and right-sided heart failure is said to have significant tricuspid stenosis and is considered a candidate for valvuloplasty, commissurotomy, or valve replacement.

VALVULAR REGURGITATION

The presence and severity of mitral regurgitation may be evaluated qualitatively by observing the amount of radiographic contrast material that regurgitates into the left atrium during left ventricular systole on a standard left ventriculogram. The magnitude of regurgitation is estimated as trivial (1+), mild (2+), moderate (3+), or severe (4+). To obtain a quantitative assessment of the severity of mitral regurgitation, the volume of blood that regurgitates from the left ventricle into the left atrium per minute (regurgitant volume) can be calculated by measuring the difference between the angiographic cardiac output (determined by left ventriculography) and the forward cardiac output (determined by the Fick or thermodilution method). The regurgitant fraction is the percentage of the total angiographic output that regurgitates into the left atrium: it is the quotient of the regurgitant volume and the angiographic output. Typically, valvular regurgitation with a regurgitant fraction of 0.6 or more is severe; 0.40 to 0.59, moderate; 0.20 to 0.39, mild; and below 0.20, trivial.

The presence and severity of aortic regurgitation may be evaluated qualitatively by observing the amount of radiographic contrast material that regurgitates into the left ventricle during ventricular diastole by aortography; it is also graded as trivial (1+), mild (2+), moderate (3+), or severe (4+). As with mitral regurgitation, a quantitative assessment of the severity of aortic regurgitation can be obtained by calculating the regurgitant volume and fraction.

INTRACARDIAC SHUNTING

LEFT-TO-RIGHT SHUNT

In patients with known or suspected congenital heart disease or unexplained heart failure, cardiac catheterization may be performed to assess the presence, location, and magnitude of intracardiac shunting. Several techniques may be used (Table 87.5).

Oximetric Assessment

Oximetric detection and localization of intracardiac left-to-right shunting are based on the principle that oxygenated blood shunted from the left side of the heart to the right side causes an abnormal increase ("step-up") in the oxygen content or saturation of blood in the chamber into which shunting occurs. To detect the presence and site of the left-to-right shunt, blood samples are obtained from the pulmonary artery, right ventricle,

TABLE 87.5. COMPARISON OF METHODS TO DETECT, LOCALIZE, AND QUANTIFY INTRACARDIAC LEFT-TO-RIGHT SHUNTING

Method	Able to Localize?	Able to Quantify?	Minimal Q$_p$/Q$_s$ Reliably Detected
Oximetry	Yes	Yes	1.5–1.9 at level of atrium 1.3–1.5 at level of ventricle 1.3 at level of great vessels
Indocyanine green	No	Yes	1.35
Angiography	Yes	No	Unknown

Q$_p$, pulmonic blood flow; Q$_s$, systemic blood flow.

TABLE 87.6.	OXIMETRIC ASSESSMENT OF THE PRESENCE, SITE, AND SIZE OF LEFT-TO-RIGHT INTRACARDIAC SHUNTING IN A PATIENT WITH A VENTRICULAR SEPTAL DEFECT[a]		
Chamber	O_2 Saturation (%)	O_2 Content (mL/dL)	O_2 Content Difference (mL/dL)
Vena cavae	65	13.1	0.4
Right atrium	67	13.5	2.2
Right ventricle	78	15.7	0.2
Pulmonary artery	79	15.9	0
Systemic artery	97		

Site of O_2 "step-up" = right ventricle   Mixed venous chamber = right atrium

Q_p = 250 mL/min/(0.97 − 0.79)(15 g/dL)(1.34 mL O_2/g hemoglobin)(10 dL/L) = 6.91 L/min

Q_s = 250 mL/min/(0.97 − 0.67)(15 g/dL) (1.34 mL O_2/g hemoglobin)(10 dL/L) = 4.14 L/min

Q_p/Q_s ratio = 6.91/4.14 = 1.7

[a] Measured oxygen consumption = 250 mL/min; Hemoglobin = 15 g/dL.

right atrium, and vena cavae, and the oxygen content or saturation of each sample is evaluated for evidence of such a step-up. An abnormal step-up is present when the right atrial oxygen content is more than 1.9 mL per dL higher than that of the vena cavae, the right ventricular oxygen content is more than 0.9 mL per dL higher than that of the right atrium, or the pulmonary arterial oxygen content is more than 0.5 mL per dL higher than that of the right ventricle. The oxygen content of blood can be measured directly or calculated from the saturation [saturation × hemoglobin (g per dL) × 1.34 mL O_2 per g hemoglobin].

The oximetric quantitation of shunting is accomplished by calculating pulmonic (Qp) and systemic (Qs) blood flows according to the Fick principle, where

Qp (L per minute) = oxygen consumption (mL per minute)

/arteriovenous oxygen content difference across the lungs

(mL per L)

and

Qs (L per minute) = oxygen consumption (mL per minute)

/arteriovenous oxygen content difference across the body

(mL per L)

The arteriovenous oxygen content difference across the lungs is the difference in oxygen contents between pulmonary arterial and venous blood. The arteriovenous oxygen content across the body is the difference in oxygen contents between systemic arterial and mixed venous blood, with the latter obtained from the chamber immediately before (proximal to) the site of the shunt. For example, if a ventricular septal defect is present, the mixed venous chamber is the right atrium; if a patent ductus arteriosus is present, the mixed venous chamber is the right ventricle. An example of the calculations for a patient with an intracardiac left-to-right shunt is presented in Table 87.6.

The oximetric determination of intracardiac left-to-right shunting is highly specific but relatively insensitive, in that an oximetric assessment reliably demonstrates the presence of a moderate or large shunt but may fail to detect a small shunt (Table 87.5).

Indocyanine Green Assessment

As described previously, when a bolus of indocyanine green is introduced into a right heart chamber and its concentration is measured in systemic arterial blood, a concentration–time curve is inscribed, which is characterized by a primary peak and a recirculation peak. In the patient with left-to-right intracardiac shunting, the inscribed curve demonstrates prominent early recirculation (Fig. 87.5) due to indocyanine green's rapid recirculation to the systemic arterial system through the intracardiac shunt. Because the area of the inscribed recirculation curve is proportional to shunt flow, the magnitude of shunting can be calculated with this technique. Although this method cannot identify the site of left-to-right shunting, it can detect shunts with a Qp/Qs as small as 1.35; thus, it is somewhat more sensitive than oximetry.

Angiographic Assessment

When radiographic contrast material is introduced into a left-sided chamber during angiography in a subject with left-to-right intracardiac shunting, its movement into a right-sided chamber may be visualized. The reliability of any angiographic technique for detecting or localizing intracardiac left-to-right shunting depends on the location of the defect and the obliquity in which the angiogram is performed. Left-sided angiography may be used to detect and localize certain kinds of intracardiac left-to-right shunts. For example, the interventricular septum may be visualized by performing left ventriculography in a 40-degree to 50-

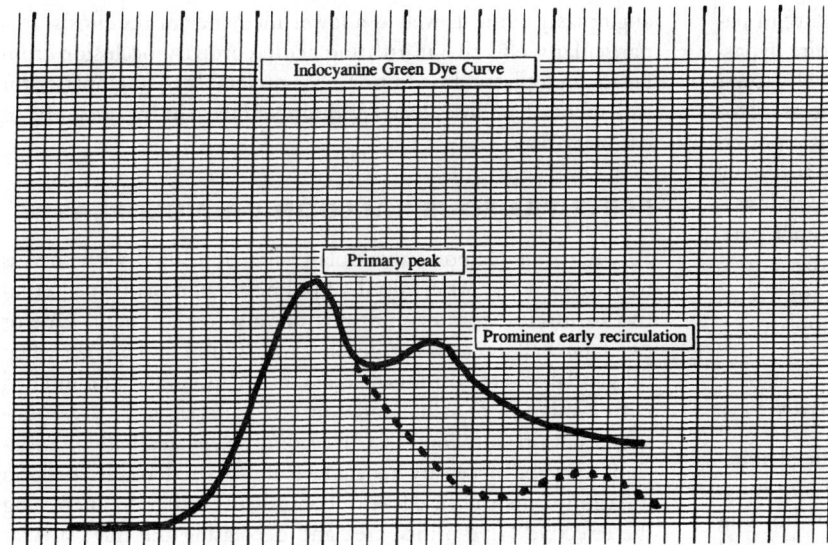

FIGURE 87.5. An indocyanine green curve from one patient with *(solid line)* and one patient without *(dotted line)* left-to-right intracardiac shunting. With the shunt, there is prominent early recirculation.

degree left anterior oblique projection, allowing the diagnosis of a ventricular septal defect. A communication between the thoracic aorta and the pulmonary artery (i.e., patent ductus arteriosus or aortopulmonary window) may be identified by performing aortography in the left anterior oblique or left lateral projection.

Atrial septal defects and anomalous pulmonary venous drainage are difficult to visualize angiographically. Although angiography can detect and localize certain intracardiac left-to-right shunts, it cannot measure the magnitude of shunting.

RIGHT-TO-LEFT SHUNT

In the patient with right-to-left intracardiac shunting, the passage of unoxygenated blood from the venous circulation to the systemic circulation results in arterial desaturation (less than 95%). When desaturation is due to other conditions (i.e., ventilation–perfusion mismatch or hypoventilation), it is corrected when 100% oxygen is administered; this does not happen when the arterial desaturation is due to right-to-left shunting. Thus, demonstration of a systemic arterial oxygen saturation below 95% that does not correct with the administration of 100% oxygen (via face mask) is consistent with right-to-left intracardiac shunting.

■ INTERVENTIONAL CATHETERIZATION

PERCUTANEOUS TRANSLUMINAL CORONARY ANGIOPLASTY

For many patients with atherosclerotic coronary artery disease, percutaneous transluminal coronary angioplasty (PTCA) is the treatment of choice. With PTCA, a distensible balloon is inflated under high pressure within the coronary stenosis, with resultant disruption of the plaque and aneurysmal dilatation of the vessel. These alterations provide new pathways for blood flow in the diseased coronary artery, leading to increased luminal size. Angioplasty is performed percutaneously, with local anesthesia;

compared with bypass surgery, it usually involves a shorter hospitalization, and its procedure-related mortality (1%) is similar.

Percutaneous transluminal coronary angioplasty is performed with special equipment consisting of a large-lumen guide catheter, a flexible wire, and a balloon catheter. The guide catheter is positioned in the coronary ostium, and angiography of the diseased coronary artery is performed to visualize the stenosis. The flexible wire is advanced through the guide catheter, navigated across the stenosis, and positioned in the distal arterial segment. The deflated balloon catheter is then advanced over the wire and positioned at the stenosis, after which it is inflated for 1 to 5 minutes at 3 to 15 atmospheres of pressure with a mixture of saline and radiographic contrast material. If the stenosis is adequately dilated, the balloon catheter and wire are removed. If the dilatation is considered inadequate, additional inflations at higher pressure or for a longer time may be performed, or the initial balloon may be replaced with a larger one. When a satisfactory result is obtained, a final angiogram is performed.

Percutaneous transluminal coronary angioplasty has been widely used in several clinical circumstances (Table 87.7). In

TABLE 87.7.	ACCEPTED INDICATIONS FOR PERCUTANEOUS CORONARY REVASCULARIZATION

- Stable angina pectoris not adequately responsive to medical therapy
- Objective evidence of significant ischemia in a moderate area of myocardium while receiving medical therapy
- Unstable angina pectoris
- Acute myocardial infarction ("primary angioplasty")
- Provocable or spontaneous ischemia after myocardial infarction (with or without antecedent treatment with a thrombolytic agent)
- Significant coronary artery stenosis in a survivor of cardiac arrest or sustained ventricular tachycardia in the absence of myocardial infarction

experienced hands, it is an effective therapeutic modality in patients with limiting angina who would otherwise require bypass surgery for symptomatic relief. Overall, PTCA's initial success averages about 90%. Acute coronary occlusion—due to coronary arterial dissection, thrombosis, or vasospasm—is reported in 3% to 7% of patients undergoing angioplasty. It is usually corrected with additional dilatations, placement of an endovascular stent, or urgent bypass surgery, so that the overall peri-procedural mortality is only 0.5% to 1%. During the 4 to 6 months after successful PTCA, 35% to 50% of stenoses recur, but this restenosis is usually amenable to repeat angioplasty.

DIRECTIONAL CORONARY ATHERECTOMY

The atherectomy device consists of a rigid cylindrical metal housing with a cut-out section ("cutting window") 5 to 9 mm long. Opposite the cutting window is a balloon fixed to the housing unit. The atherectomy device is advanced over a wire positioned across the stenosis and positioned with its cutting window facing the atheromatous plaque. When the balloon is inflated, the cutting window is pushed against the atheromatous plaque. A cup-shaped rotating cutter is slowly advanced through the metal housing, shaving portions of the plaque and depositing the shaved debris in the catheter tip. Enlargement of the coronary artery lumen is achieved by removal of atherosclerotic material and dilatation due to balloon inflation. Accordingly, the increase in luminal diameter achieved with atherectomy is substantially greater than that of balloon angioplasty alone. With atherectomy, the rates of initial success, abrupt closure, and restenosis are similar to those of balloon angioplasty. However, the incidence of local vascular complications and periprocedural myocardial infarction is higher with atherectomy, and its size and relative rigidity make it poorly suited for use in small, tortuous, or angulated coronary arteries.

ROTATIONAL CORONARY ATHERECTOMY

High-speed rotational atherectomy ("rotablation") uses a diamond-coated elliptical metal drill, or "burr," to debulk atherosclerotic plaque. The burr, which rotates at speeds up to 200,000 rpm, is passed over a guidewire that has been advanced through the coronary stenosis. The rotablator selectively ablates the most fibrous, calcific plaque, whereas the normally elastic arterial wall deflects away from the rotating burr. This technique is used primarily for coronary stenoses that are long, calcified, or ostial in location.

ENDOVASCULAR STENTS

Intracoronary stents consist of metal coils or metallic mesh cylinders wrapped tightly around a deflated angioplasty balloon. The balloon catheter is advanced over an angioplasty guidewire into the coronary artery and, once properly positioned, is inflated to expand the stent. After balloon deflation, the stent retains its expanded cylindrical configuration, forcing intraluminal irregularities against the vessel wall. Stenting results in a much greater increase in luminal diameter than that achieved with balloon

angioplasty alone as well as a lower incidence of restenosis. It is particularly effective in treating acute coronary occlusion from failed angioplasty. In addition, it is preferable to angioplasty for treatment of stenoses located in saphenous vein bypass grafts or coronary ostia.

PERCUTANEOUS BALLOON VALVULOPLASTY

Percutaneous balloon valvuloplasty has been used with success in patients with aortic, mitral, or pulmonic stenosis as an alternative to surgical commissurotomy or valve replacement. One or two large balloon catheters (each 15 to 20 mm in diameter when fully inflated) are positioned across the stenotic valve and inflated with a mixture of saline and contrast material at 3 to 5 atmospheres of pressure for 15 to 30 seconds. Repeated balloon inflations may be necessary to achieve the desired result. Balloon inflation splits the fused valve commissures, thereby increasing the effective valve orifice area and decreasing the transvalvular pressure gradient. Percutaneous balloon valvuloplasty is associated with a mortality of 1% to 2%.

Percutaneous mitral balloon valvuloplasty is usually successful in patients with symptomatic mitral stenosis and suitable valve anatomy. It is ineffective when the mitral leaflets are markedly thickened, immobile, or heavily calcified, or if subvalvular fibrosis is extensive. In the average patient, percutaneous balloon mitral valvuloplasty increases the effective orifice area from 1 to 2 cm^2. Because it is performed through a transseptal approach, it should not be attempted in the patient with a left atrial thrombus or recent cerebrovascular event.

In the adult patient with aortic stenosis, percutaneous balloon valvuloplasty is only modestly successful in that the transvalvular pressure gradient is reduced by about 50% and the valve area is increased to only 0.7 to 1.0 cm^2. Stenosis recurs in most patients within 6 to 12 months. Hence, aortic balloon valvuloplasty is a short-term palliative procedure to be used only in severely ill patients who are poor surgical candidates.

Pulmonic balloon valvuloplasty is used primarily in infants and children, but its use in adults with pulmonic stenosis is well described. It is the treatment of choice for isolated, noncalcific pulmonic stenosis.

ENDOMYOCARDIAL BIOPSY

Through a long sheath positioned across the tricuspid valve, a routine bioptome can be advanced to obtain small pieces (1 to 2 mm^2) of myocardial tissue from the right ventricular side of the interventricular septum. Endomyocardial biopsy is used most often to detect transplant rejection and to monitor immunosuppressive therapy in survivors of cardiac transplantation. Less commonly, it is undertaken in the patient with suspected infiltrative cardiomyopathy (sarcoidosis, amyloidosis, hemochromatosis, carcinoid). In experienced hands, complications are uncommon; cardiac perforation occurs in only 0.3% to 0.5%, and the procedure-related mortality is roughly 0.05%.

BIBLIOGRAPHY

Bittl JA. Advances in coronary angioplasty. *N Engl J Med* 1996;335:1290–1302.

Boehrer JD, Lange RA, Willard JE, et al. Advantages and limitations of methods to detect, localize, and quantitate intracardiac left-to-right shunting. *Am Heart J* 1992;124:448–455.

Glazier JJ, Turi ZG. Percutaneous balloon mitral valvuloplasty. *Prog Cardiovasc Dis* 1997;40:5–26.

Landau C, Lange RA, Hillis LD. Percutaneous transluminal coronary angioplasty. *N Engl J Med* 1994;330:981–993.

Mueller HS, Chatterjee K, Davis KB, et al. ACC expert consensus document. Present use of bedside right heart catheterization in patients with cardiac disease. *J Am Coll Cardiol* 1998;32:840–864.

Pepine CJ, Allen HD, Bashore TM, et al. ACC/AHA guidelines for cardiac catheterization and cardiac catheterization laboratories. American College of Cardiology/American Heart Association Ad Hoc Task Force on Cardiac Catheterization. *Circulation* 1991;84:2213–2247.

Reifart N, Vandormael M, Krajcar M, et al. Randomized comparison of angioplasty of complex coronary lesions at a single center. Excimer Laser, Rotational Atherectomy, and Balloon Angioplasty Comparison (ERBAC) Study. *Circulation* 1997;96:91–98.

Ryan TJ, Bauman WB, Kennedy JW, et al. Guidelines for percutaneous transluminal coronary angioplasty. A report of the American Heart Association/American College of Cardiology Task Force on Assessment of Diagnostic and Therapeutic Cardiovascular Procedures (Committee on Percutaneous Transluminal Coronary Angioplasty). *Circulation* 1993;88:2987–3007.

Serruys PW, van Hout B, Bonnier H, et al. Randomised comparison of implantation of heparin-coated stents with balloon angioplasty in selected patients with coronary artery disease (Benestent II). *Lancet* 1998; 352:673–681.

Topol EJ, Serruys PW. Frontiers in interventional cardiology. *Circulation* 1998;1802–1820.

Kelley's Textbook of Internal Medicine, fourth edition. Edited by H. David Humes. Lippincott Williams & Wilkins, Philadelphia © 2000.

CHAPTER
88

ELECTROPHYSIOLOGIC TESTING

FRED MORADY

Electrophysiologic testing plays an important role in the management of patients who have serious arrhythmias. Invasive electrophysiologic studies often are important in guiding the management of patients who have had ventricular tachycardia, the aborted sudden death syndrome, paroxysmal supraventricular tachycardia, Wolff–Parkinson–White (WPW) syndrome, unexplained wide-QRS complex tachycardias, and unexplained syncope. Electrophysiologic testing also may be helpful in the management of patients in whom abnormalities of sinus node function or atrioventricular (AV) conduction are suspected.

This chapter describes the diagnostic information that can be obtained through electrophysiologic testing and reviews the clinical situations in which an electrophysiologic test is appropriate. The field of interventional electrophysiology, consisting of several types of catheter ablation techniques, is described in Chapter 76.

TECHNICAL ASPECTS AND RISKS

Electrophysiologic studies are performed in a catheterization laboratory or procedure room in which fluoroscopy is available. Depending on the clinical indication for the study, two to four electrode catheters are inserted percutaneously, with local anesthesia, into a femoral, brachial, subclavian, or internal jugular vein and positioned in the right atrium, across the tricuspid valve for recording the His bundle electrogram, in the coronary sinus for recording left atrial depolarizations, or within the right ventricle.

The use of multipolar electrode catheters that have four or more electrodes allows use of the distal pair of electrodes for pacing and the proximal electrodes for recording intracardiac electrograms. Pacing is performed with a programmable stimulator capable of introducing premature stimuli, referred to as extrastimuli, in a synchronized fashion. Electrophysiologic testing usually requires both overdrive pacing and the scanning of early diastole with one or more extrastimuli. Pacing generally is performed with stimuli that are 1 to 2 milliseconds in duration and that have a current intensity twice the late diastolic threshold. If necessary, the arterial pressure can be continuously monitored with a short cannula inserted into a femoral, brachial, or radial artery. When left atrial or ventricular mapping is required, either a trans-septal approach is used to enter the left atrium or left ventricle, or an electrode catheter is introduced into a femoral or brachial artery and passed across the aortic valve into the left ventricle.

When performed competently by appropriately trained personnel, the mortality rate of electrophysiologic testing is less than 0.1%, and the risk of nonlethal complications also is low. A potentially lethal complication is perforation of a cardiac chamber by an electrode catheter, which may result in cardiac tamponade requiring needle pericardiocentesis or an emergency thoracotomy. The risk of thromboembolic complications can be minimized by the use of heparin during the electrophysiologic study. The most common complications are thrombophlebitis or hematoma formation at the site of catheter insertion, and the incidence of these complications is about 1% to 2%.

Hemodynamically unstable, sustained ventricular tachycardia or ventricular fibrillation may be induced in the course of electrophysiologic testing. Because this usually is intentional, it is not considered to be a complication. Sustained, monomorphic ventricular tachycardia often can be terminated by rapid pacing. Ventricular fibrillation and sustained ventricular tachycardias that cannot be terminated by pacing and that result in severe hypotension are terminated by direct-current countershock as soon as the patient loses consciousness.

Rarely, ventricular tachycardia or ventricular fibrillation either cannot be terminated by direct-current countershock or recurs repeatedly shortly after conversion to sinus rhythm. Electromechanical dissociation after termination of ventricular tachycardia or ventricular fibrillation is another rare complication of electrophysiologic testing. Immediate cardiopulmonary resuscitation is required if one of these complications occurs. Because these complications are most likely to occur in patients with unstable coronary syndromes or severe congestive heart failure, such patients should not undergo electrophysiologic testing.

EVALUATION OF SINUS NODE FUNCTION

Sinus node function is evaluated primarily by determination of the sinus node recovery time. The right atrium is paced at several rates between 100 and 200 beats per minute for 30 to 60 seconds at each rate. The interval between the last paced atrial depolarization and the first spontaneous sinus depolarization is the sinus node recovery time (Fig. 88.1). The sinus node recovery time is adjusted for heart rate by subtraction of the baseline sinus cycle length, which yields the corrected sinus node recovery time. The upper limit of normal of the corrected sinus node recovery time is 550 milliseconds.

A prolonged sinus node recovery time indicates an abnormal-

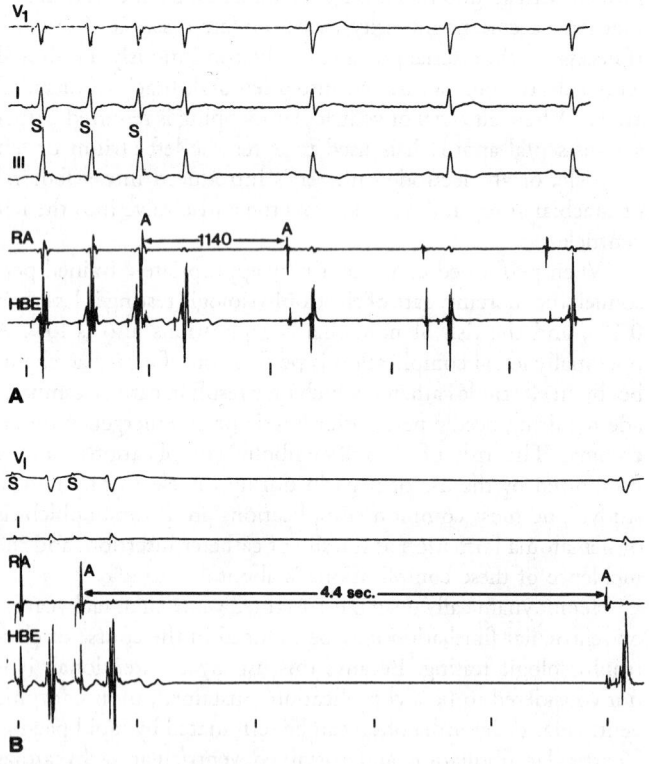

FIGURE 88.1. Examples of normal and abnormal sinus node recovery times. Shown are leads V₁, I, and III; the intracardiac electrogram recorded in the right atrium (RA); and the His bundle electrogram. The last two or three stimuli (S) of a 45-second pacing train at a rate of 120 to 150 beats per minute are seen. The sinus node recovery time is the interval between the last paced atrial depolarization and the first spontaneous atrial depolarization originating in the sinus node. It is corrected for heart rate by subtracting the baseline sinus cycle length. The time lines in this and all subsequent figures represent 1-second intervals. **A:** The sinus node recovery time is 1,140 milliseconds and the corrected sinus node recovery time is 140 milliseconds (upper limits of normal are 500 to 550 milliseconds). **B:** The sinus node recovery time is 4.4 seconds. The sinus cycle length was 840 milliseconds, and therefore the corrected sinus node recovery time is 3.56 seconds, which is markedly prolonged. A, atrial electrogram.

ity of sinus node automaticity, although not necessarily a clinically significant degree of sinus node dysfunction. The sensitivity of the sinus node recovery time for the sick sinus syndrome is about 75% to 80%, with a specificity in the range of 90%. Another indicator of sinus node function is the sinoatrial conduction time, which can be measured directly by recording a sinus node depolarization or indirectly by an overdrive pacing or an extrastimulus technique. Although this test provides a measure of conduction of impulses through the sinoatrial junction, it has little or no clinical value.

In patients who have the sick sinus syndrome and a documented bradyarrhythmia associated with symptoms, there is no need for electrophysiologic testing to assess sinus node function; if the symptoms and bradyarrhythmia are severe enough to warrant a permanent pacemaker, a pacemaker should be implanted if a correctable reason for the sinus node dysfunction cannot be identified. If there is uncertainty about whether a permanent pacemaker is necessary, an electrophysiologic test may be helpful in guiding management of these cases. For example, a patient who complains of dizzy spells or light-headedness may have a resting sinus bradycardia of 40 to 50 beats per minute or sinus pauses of less than 3 seconds in duration; these abnormalities are suggestive of sinus node dysfunction but are not in themselves severe enough to justify pacemaker implantation. If this patient is found to have a markedly abnormal sinus node recovery time (corrected sinus node recovery time more than 1 to 1.5 seconds), this degree of sinus node dysfunction may justify implantation of a permanent pacemaker. However, if the sinus node recovery time is normal or only slightly prolonged, it may be appropriate to follow the patient clinically and to defer pacemaker implantation.

EVALUATION OF ATRIOVENTRICULAR CONDUCTION

The status of the AV conduction system is assessed during an electrophysiologic study by recording the His bundle electrogram and by determining the response to atrial pacing at incremental rates. The His bundle electrogram is recorded by positioning an electrode catheter across the tricuspid valve, which allows division of the PR interval into two components: the atrial His (AH) interval, which reflects AV nodal conduction, and the His ventricular (HV) interval, which reflects conduction in the His–Purkinje system (Fig. 88.2). The normal ranges of the AH and the HV intervals are 70 to 145 milliseconds and 35 to 55 milliseconds, respectively. When there is AV block during sinus rhythm or atrial pacing, the level of block within the AV conduction system can be localized to the AV node or to the His–Purkinje system by determining if the block occurs proximal or distal to the His bundle depolarization.

Prolongation of the AH interval and mild prolongation of the HV interval are rarely of clinical significance. However, marked prolongation of the HV interval (100 milliseconds) in patients with a bundle-branch block is associated with about a 25% risk of progression to high-degree AV block over 3 years and may be an appropriate indication for a permanent pacemaker in pa-

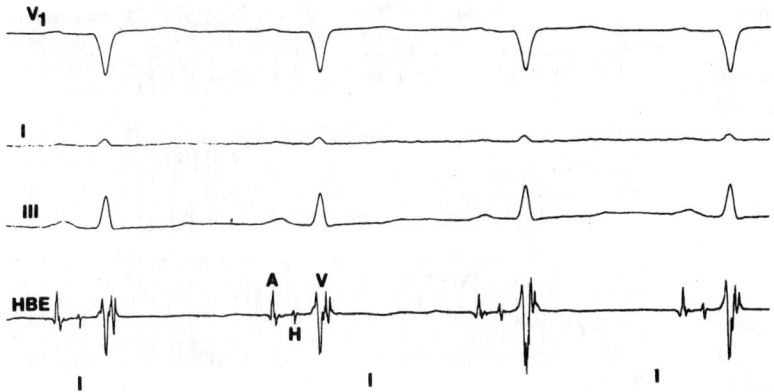

FIGURE 88.2. The His bundle electrogram. Also shown are leads V_1, I, and III. The atrial depolarization (A) corresponds to the P wave on the ECG, and the ventricular depolarization (V) corresponds to the QRS. The His bundle deflection (H) occurs between the A and the V and cannot be seen on the ECG. The AH interval reflects AV nodal conduction, whereas the HV interval reflects infranodal conduction.

tients who have otherwise unexplained syncope or who require treatment with antiarrhythmic drugs that may further depress infranodal conduction.

During incremental atrial pacing, physiologic block occurs within the AV node when the rate approaches 140 to 170 beats per minute (Fig. 88.3A). Block distal to the His bundle depolarization may be physiologic under certain circumstances, as during

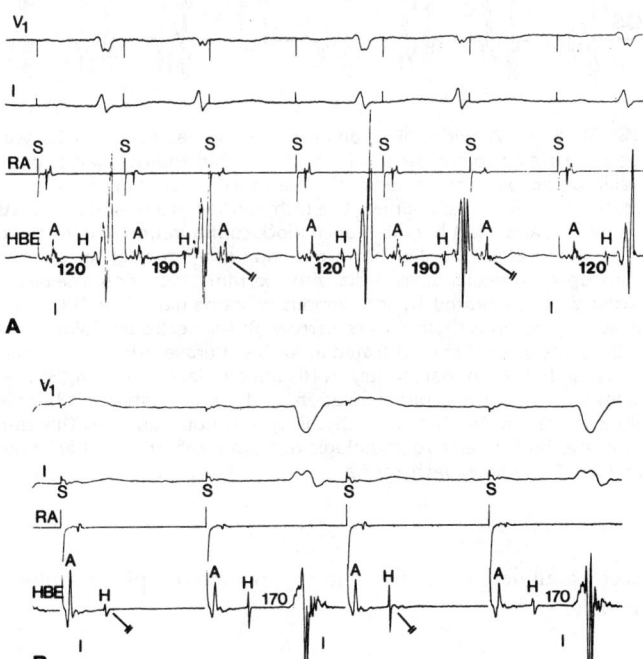

A

B

FIGURE 88.3. Atrioventricular (AV) block during atrial pacing. Shown are leads V_1 and I, the right atrial electrogram (RA), and the His bundle electrogram. **A:** Physiologic AV block within the AV node. The AV nodal Wenckebach block occurs during atrial pacing at a rate of 170 beats per minute. There is progressive prolongation of the AH interval, then block between the atrium and His bundle. A His bundle depolarization is not present when the block occurs, indicating that the block was within the AV node. **B:** Pathologic infranodal AV block. This patient had a left bundle-branch block and a prolonged baseline HV interval of 170 milliseconds (upper limits of normal, 55 milliseconds). During atrial pacing at a rate of 100 beats per minute, the AH interval was constant at 150 milliseconds but there was 2:1 infranodal block. This type of block is abnormal. A, atrial depolarization; H, His bundle deflection; S, pacing stimuli.

rapid atrial pacing (more than 200 beats per minute) when there is 1:1 conduction through the AV node. Infranodal AV block is pathologic when it occurs during relatively slow rates (less than 150 beats per minute; Fig. 88.3B). Pathologic block distal to the His bundle depolarization indicates tenuous conduction in the His–Purkinje system, is associated with an increased risk of high-degree AV block, and usually is an indication for implantation of a permanent pacemaker.

Spontaneous AV block that occurs within the AV node is rarely an indication for a pacemaker, but AV block that occurs below the AV node usually is. Because the level of AV block can often be determined on a clinical basis, electrophysiologic testing usually is not necessary to evaluate whether a patient with second- or third-degree AV block requires a permanent pacemaker. An electrophysiologic study is indicated to evaluate AV conduction if the results of clinical evaluation are inconclusive. An HV interval of 100 milliseconds or longer, spontaneous block distal to the His bundle electrogram, or pathologic infranodal block during atrial pacing usually indicates the need for a permanent pacemaker.

■ EVALUATION OF PAROXYSMAL SUPRAVENTRICULAR TACHYCARDIA

MECHANISMS OF TACHYCARDIA

Paroxysmal supraventricular tachycardia (PSVT) that is caused by reentry usually can be induced by atrial or ventricular pacing during an electrophysiologic test. Because the most common mechanisms of recurrent PSVT are AV nodal reentry, orthodromic tachycardia (in which the AV node is the anterograde limb of a reentry circuit and an accessory pathway is the retrograde limb), and intra-atrial reentry, a patient's PSVT usually can be reproduced in the electrophysiology laboratory. By observing several features of the tachycardia, including the method of initiation, the sequence of atrial activation, and the responses to atrial and ventricular pacing, the precise mechanism of tachycardia can be determined.

In AV nodal reentrant tachycardia, which is the most common type of PSVT, there are two pathways for conduction of impulses through the AV node; these two pathways have different conduction properties and degrees of refractoriness. In the typical AV nodal reentrant tachycardia, a reentry circuit incorporates the more slowly conducting pathway as its anterograde limb and the more rapidly conducting pathway as its retrograde limb.

INDICATIONS FOR TESTING PATIENTS WITH PAROXYSMAL SUPRAVENTRICULAR TACHYCARDIA

In patients with documented episodes of PSVT, management on purely a clinical basis is often appropriate. However, several clinical situations may indicate electrophysiologic studies, and these are described in the following sections.

Unexplained Wide-QRS Complex Tachycardia

The 12-lead electrocardiogram (ECG) often provides clues to determining whether a wide QRS complex tachycardia represents PSVT with a bundle-branch block or ventricular tachycardia. In some cases, it may not be possible to discern the mechanism of a wide QRS complex tachycardia from the ECG or even from analysis of recordings obtained with an esophageal lead. An electrophysiologic study helps in these cases by establishing the mechanism of the tachycardia, thereby allowing appropriate therapy (Fig. 88.4).

Paroxysmal Supraventricular Tachycardia Associated With Severe Symptoms

Some patients with PSVT may have serious symptoms, such as syncope, severe chest pain, or pulmonary edema. Instead of treating these patients purely on a clinical basis, it often is appropriate to perform an electrophysiologic test to establish the mechanism of the PSVT and to guide management. In most cases, it is possible to eliminate the PSVT by catheter ablation using radiofrequency energy. If pharmacologic therapy is chosen for the patient, the efficacy of the therapy can be determined by electropharmacologic testing. The end point of electropharmacologic testing is inability to induce the tachycardia or slowing of the tachycardia to the point where it is no longer associated with severe symptoms.

Recurrent Paroxysmal Supraventricular Tachycardia Not Responding to Pharmacologic Therapy

An electrophysiologic test is performed to determine the mechanism of the PSVT and to eliminate the tachycardia using a radiofrequency catheter ablation technique. For most patients, the diagnosis and cure of PSVT can be accomplished during a single electrophysiology procedure.

Because of the favorable risk/benefit profile of radiofrequency ablation, electrophysiologic testing with a view toward catheter ablation is appropriate for patients with recurrent PSVT who

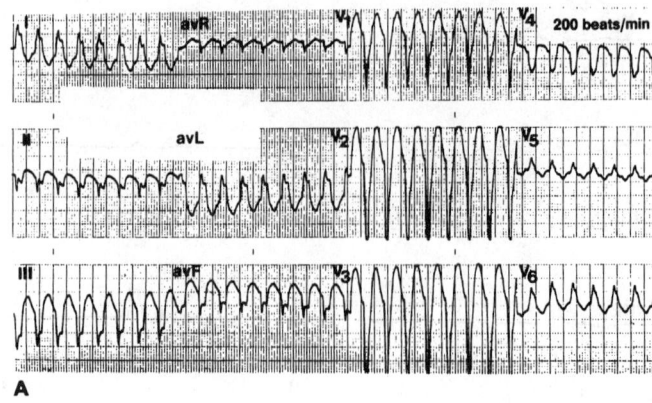

A

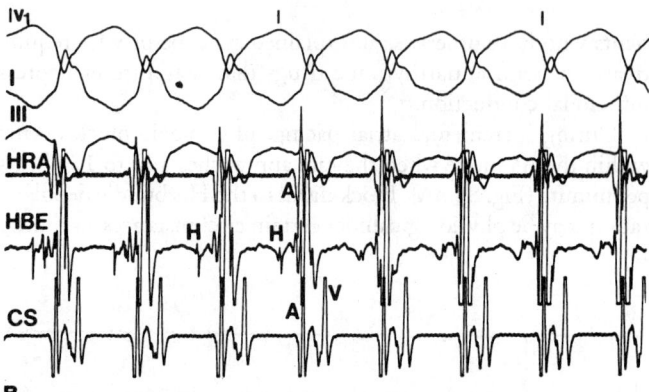

B

FIGURE 88.4. A wide QRS complex tachycardia. **A:** This ECG was recorded in a 60-year-old man with a history of an anterior wall myocardial infarction who presented to the hospital complaining of rapid palpitations and light-headedness. The tachycardia has a rate of 200 beats per minute and a left bundle-branch block configuration. There are no clues on the ECG that allow differentiation of ventricular tachycardia from supraventricular tachycardia with aberrant conduction. The tachycardia was terminated by intravenous procainamide. The QRS complexes during sinus rhythm were narrow. **B:** An electrophysiologic test in the same patient demonstrated inducible supraventricular tachycardia caused by AV nodal reentry. A His bundle depolarization (H) precedes each ventricular depolarization, and a rate-related left bundle block is present. Ventricular tachycardia was not inducible. This case illustrates how an electrophysiologic test can clarify the mechanism of a wide QRS complex tachycardia.

elect to undergo curative therapy instead of pharmacologic therapy.

Recurrent Paroxysmal Palpitations of Uncertain Cause

Using trans-telephonic electrocardiographic monitoring and continuous loop ambulatory electrocardiographic monitoring, it should be possible to document the cardiac rhythm in most patients who have recurrent palpitations. But at times it may be impossible to document the cause of symptoms in a patient who has recurrent episodes of paroxysmal palpitations compatible with PSVT. An electrophysiologic study may be indicated in a patient who has recurrent symptoms of paroxysmal tachycardia in whom documentation of the cause of symptoms cannot be obtained by monitoring (see Chapter 76).

EVALUATION OF WOLFF–PARKINSON–WHITE SYNDROME

In addition to orthodromic tachycardia, another type of tachycardia that may be associated with WPW syndrome is atrial fibrillation or flutter with a rapid ventricular response. Because accessory pathways may have rapid conduction properties and a short refractory period, atrial fibrillation or flutter may result in extremely rapid ventricular rates in patients with the WPW syndrome. The ventricular rate may exceed 250 to 300 beats per minute, resulting in severe hemodynamic compromise and a risk of degeneration into ventricular fibrillation.

Another type of tachycardia that may occur in patients who have WPW syndrome is antidromic tachycardia. This is a reentrant tachycardia that is much less common than the orthodromic variety. In this type of tachycardia, the accessory pathway is the anterograde limb of the reentry circuit, and the AV node is the retrograde limb. Ventricular activation therefore occurs in an eccentric fashion through the accessory pathway, resulting in a wide QRS complex tachycardia that has the appearance of ventricular tachycardia on the ECG.

The goals of electrophysiologic testing in patients with WPW syndrome are to define the refractoriness and conduction properties of the accessory pathway, to induce and establish the mechanism or mechanisms of tachycardia that the patient has had, to determine the number of accessory pathways and their locations, and to ablate the pathways using radiofrequency energy. Programmed atrial stimulation and ventricular stimulation are used to define the refractory periods and to induce tachycardias. Localization of accessory pathways (mapping) is accomplished by searching either for the earliest site of atrial activation along the tricuspid and mitral annulus during orthodromic tachycardia, or for the earliest site of ventricular activation during pre-excited QRS complexes. The sites of earliest atrial and ventricular activation indicate the atrial and ventricular insertion sites of the accessory pathway, respectively. Sometimes rapid atrial pacing may be used to induce atrial fibrillation, allowing determination of the ventricular rate and the shortest interval between two consecutive, pre-excited QRS complexes. If the shortest interval is less than 250 milliseconds, then the risk of cardiac arrest resulting from atrial fibrillation is increased.

Because electrophysiologic studies are performed in patients who are supine and inactive, the results of testing in the baseline state may not accurately reflect conditions present during states of sympathetic activation, such as exercise or emotional stress. Accessory pathways usually are responsive to sympathetic stimulation, and it often is appropriate to induce sympathetic activation to obtain a more accurate assessment of the tachycardia that a patient may experience spontaneously. This is done by infusing isoproterenol, usually at a rate of 1 to 2 μg per minute, during the electrophysiologic test.

In the past, an electrophysiologic study was performed in patients with WPW syndrome to identify high-risk patients who

were appropriate candidates for surgical ablation of the accessory pathway, either for the purpose of electropharmacologic testing or to identify the number and locations of accessory pathways as a prelude to surgery. After radiofrequency catheter ablation of accessory pathways was demonstrated to be highly effective and relatively safe, almost all electrophysiology procedures in patients with WPW syndrome have been performed for the purpose of ablating the accessory pathways. Appropriate candidates for an electrophysiologic test and catheter ablation include patients with WPW syndrome who have experienced potentially dangerous arrhythmias, who have been refractory or intolerant to pharmacologic therapy, or who prefer definitive therapy over long-term pharmacologic therapy (Fig. 88.5).

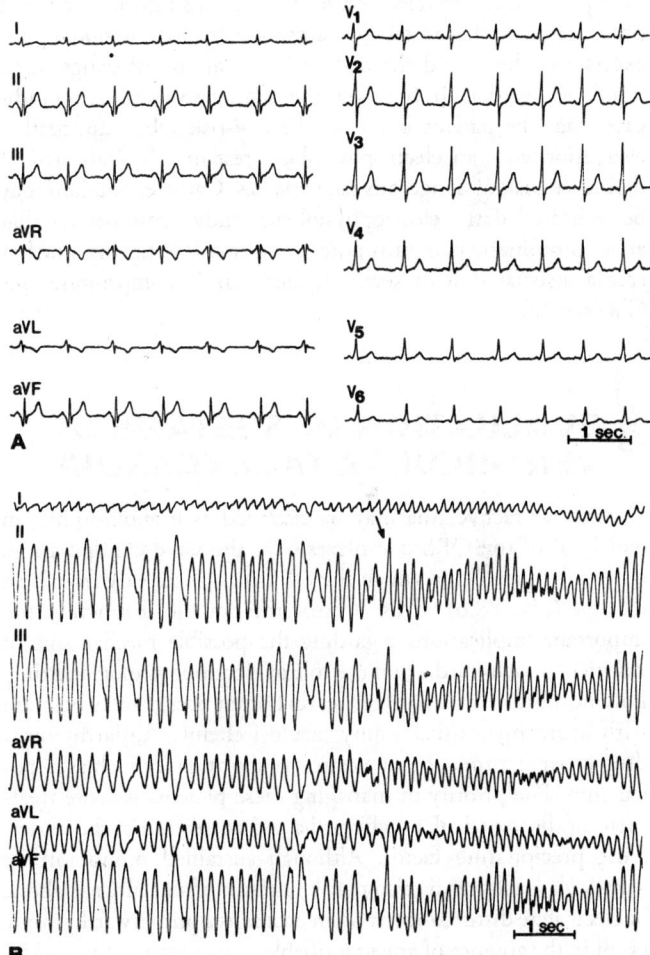

FIGURE 88.5. Life-threatening atrial fibrillation induced during an electrophysiologic test in a patient with Wolff–Parkinson–White syndrome and recurring severe palpitations. **A:** The electroencephalogram during sinus rhythm demonstrated a short PR interval and delta waves characteristic of Wolff–Parkinson–White syndrome. Mapping demonstrated the presence of a right free wall accessory pathway. **B:** Atrial fibrillation was induced by rapid atrial pacing. The frontal plane leads are shown. There was rapid conduction through the accessory pathway and an average ventricular rate of 330 beats per minute. The arrow in lead II marks the point at which the atrial fibrillation degenerated into ventricular fibrillation, which was terminated by a direct-current countershock. The electrophysiologic test demonstrated the life-threatening potential of atrial fibrillation in this patient.

An asymptomatic patient may have delta waves and a short PR interval on an ECG, and there is usually no role for electrophysiologic testing in this situation. The WPW pattern on the ECG does not necessarily imply that symptomatic arrhythmias will occur, and it is usually appropriate to postpone evaluation and treatment until the time at which symptomatic arrhythmias arise. However, thorough evaluation of an asymptomatic patient who has a WPW pattern on the ECG may be appropriate if, for example, there is concern about the possible consequences of the first episode of tachycardia occurring during strenuous athletics or affecting those who have potentially high-risk occupations, such as airline pilots or school bus drivers. Noninvasive evaluation may be helpful in screening these patients. If the electrocardiographic manifestations of ventricular pre-excitation disappear during exercise or after intravenous infusion of 1 g of procainamide, the accessory pathway refractory period is not excessively short, and the patient is not at risk of dangerously rapid tachycardias. If, however, the noninvasive evaluation indicates that the patient is not in the low-risk subgroup, further evaluation with an electrophysiologic test may be indicated to define the risk of dangerous tachycardias. Catheter ablation may be indicated if the electrophysiologic study demonstrates that an asymptomatic patient is potentially at risk of having a tachycardia associated with severe hemodynamic compromise (see Chapter 76).

EVALUATION OF SUSTAINED VENTRICULAR TACHYCARDIA

Ventricular tachycardia may be classified as monomorphic, in which all of the QRS complexes have the same configuration, or as polymorphic, in which the QRS complexes vary from beat to beat (Fig. 88.6). This electrocardiographic distinction has important implications regarding the possible mechanisms of ventricular tachycardia and the role of electrophysiologic testing. Polymorphic ventricular tachycardia often occurs in association with acute myocardial injury, acute ischemia, antiarrhythmic drug proarrhythmia, or an electrolyte abnormality such as hypokalemia. The priority in managing these patients is acute treatment of the ventricular tachycardia and correction of the underlying precipitating factor. Although sustained monomorphic ventricular tachycardia also may be a result of an acute metabolic or electrolyte disturbance; it often occurs as a primary arrhythmic event in the absence of any identifiable acute precipitating factor. Electrophysiologic testing plays an important role in the long-term management of patients with this type of ventricular tachycardia.

MECHANISMS OF VENTRICULAR TACHYCARDIA

The underlying mechanisms of sustained monomorphic ventricular tachycardia include reentry, abnormal automaticity, and triggered activity. The most common mechanism of ventricular tachycardia is reentry, and this type of ventricular tachycardia

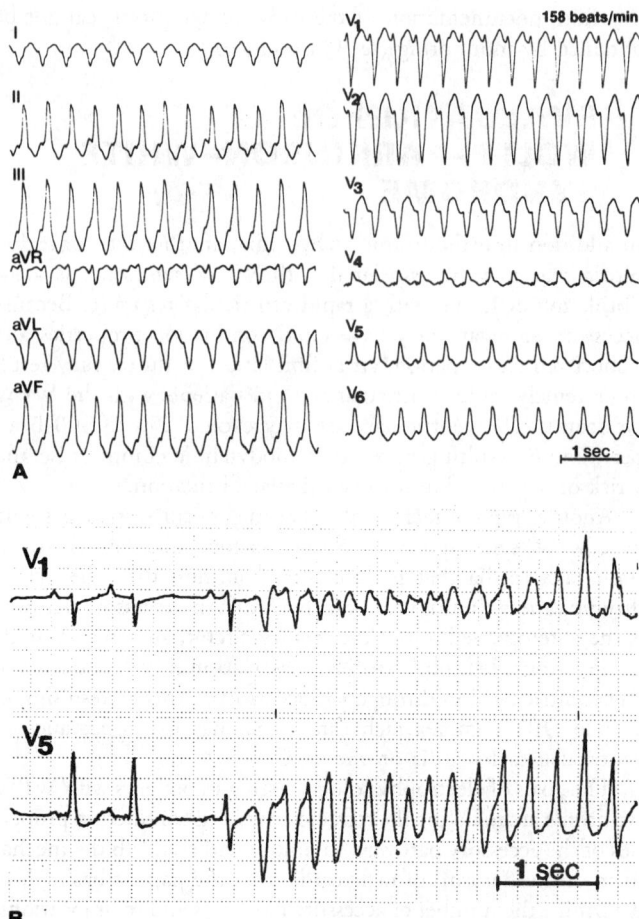

FIGURE 88.6. Examples of monomorphic and polymorphic ventricular tachycardia (VT). **A:** Sustained monomorphic VT, at a rate of 158 beats per minute, in a patient with coronary artery disease and a history of an anterior myocardial infarction. All of the QRS complexes in each lead have the same configuration. This type of VT often is a primary dysrhythmia, which is not caused by an identifiable precipitant (such as ischemia) or by a metabolic abnormality, and which often can be reproduced during electrophysiologic testing. **B:** An example of polymorphic VT at an average rate of 300 beats per minute. The QRS complexes vary from beat to beat in leads V$_1$ and V$_5$, which were recorded simultaneously. This episode of polymorphic VT occurred in a patient who was hypokalemic and did not recur after the hypokalemia was corrected. If the cause of this type of VT can be identified and corrected, there is usually no role for electrophysiologic testing.

usually is inducible by programmed ventricular stimulation. Automatic ventricular tachycardias are not inducible by pacing but may be induced by an infusion of isoproterenol, and ventricular tachycardia caused by triggered activity may be provoked with atrial and ventricular pacing at critical rates.

Many types of therapy directed toward ventricular tachycardia are nonspecific and do not depend on the specific mechanism of ventricular tachycardia. Some forms of therapy, however, are mechanism-specific, and electrophysiologic testing allows identification of patients who are appropriate candidates for these mechanism-specific therapies. These therapies include the use of β-blocking agents for catecholamine-sensitive ventricular tachycardia; the use of calcium channel blockers for ventricular tachycardia caused by triggered activity; catheter ablation of the right bundle for bundle-branch reentry tachycardia; and catheter ablation of a critical zone of slow conduction in the ventricular tachycardia reentry circuit of patients with a prior myocardial infarction.

SENSITIVITY AND SPECIFICITY OF PROGRAMMED VENTRICULAR STIMULATION

The most common mechanism of sustained monomorphic ventricular tachycardia in patients with coronary artery disease (CAD) is reentry, and the sensitivity of electrophysiologic testing in reproducing a spontaneous episode of ventricular tachycardia is high (greater than 90%) for patients with CAD. In patients with other types of heart disease, such as dilated or hypertrophic cardiomyopathy or valvular heart disease, automatic types of ventricular tachycardia may be more common, and the sensitivity of electrophysiologic testing in inducing sustained monomorphic ventricular tachycardia is lower (65% to 75%) than in patients with CAD.

A standard stimulation protocol for inducing ventricular tachycardia has not been as universally accepted. Typical stimulation protocols incorporate the sequential use of one, two, and three extrastimuli introduced during sinus rhythm or after eight-beat pacing trains at rates of 100 to 150 beats per minute. The yield of monomorphic ventricular tachycardia increases as the number of extrastimuli increases, and about 25% of clinically significant monomorphic ventricular tachycardias require three extrastimuli for induction (Fig. 88.7A).

It also is possible to induce polymorphic ventricular tachycardia or ventricular fibrillation, which often are nonspecific arrhythmias and which do not have clinical significance; the yield of these nonspecific dysrhythmias also increases as the number of extrastimuli increases (Fig. 88.7B). Because nonspecific polymorphic ventricular tachycardia and ventricular fibrillation may require direct-current countershock to terminate, programmed ventricular stimulation protocols should be designed to minimize the induction of these arrhythmias. For example, limitation of coupling intervals to 200 milliseconds improves the specificity of programmed stimulation without compromising the yield of clinically important forms of ventricular tachycardia.

ELECTROPHARMACOLOGIC TESTING

In patients who have frequent episodes of sustained ventricular tachycardia, the efficacy of antiarrhythmic drugs usually can be assessed by noting the clinical response to treatment. Because sustained monomorphic ventricular tachycardia often occurs in a sporadic and unpredictable fashion, it often is not possible to assess antiarrhythmic drug efficacy on a clinical basis.

The ability to induce ventricular tachycardia in the electrophysiology laboratory allows the use of electropharmacologic testing to assess antiarrhythmic drug efficacy. After a baseline study in which ventricular tachycardia is shown to be inducible, antiarrhythmic drug therapy is instituted, and the effects of the drug on inducibility and other characteristics of the ventricular tachycardia are observed. Initial drug testing can be performed

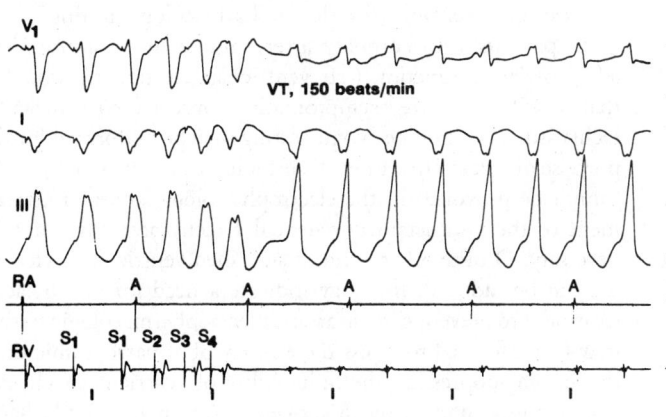

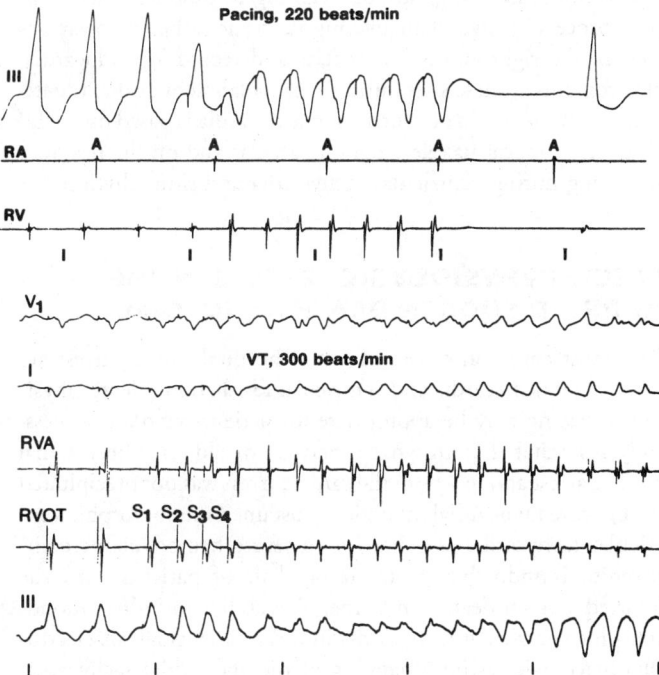

FIGURE 88.7. Induction of monomorphic and polymorphic ventricular tachycardia by programmed stimulation. **A:** Monomorphic ventricular tachycardia (VT), 150 beats per minute, was induced by programmed stimulation with three extrastimuli (S_2, S_3, S_4) introduced at the right ventricular outflow tract (RV). The VT had a right bundle branch block configuration that was identical to a previously documented spontaneous episode of VT. Atrioventricular dissociation is seen in the right atrial recording. **B:** Monomorphic VT often can be terminated by rapid ventricular pacing, as shown here. Right ventricular pacing at a rate of 220 beats per minute terminated the VT. **C:** Polymorphic VT, 300 beats per minute, also induced by programmed stimulation with three extrastimuli (S_2, S_3, S_4). The QRS morphologies in leads V_1, I, and III vary from beat to beat. The VT required direct-current countershock to terminate. This type of polymorphic VT induced by programmed stimulation often is a nonspecific finding.

at the time of the first electrophysiologic study with drugs that can be administered intravenously, such as procainamide or propranolol. With most antiarrhythmic drugs, however, electropharmacologic testing requires a second electrophysiologic test after a steady-state plasma drug concentration has been achieved with oral therapy. Electropharmacologic testing usually is performed after four or five doses of an antiarrhythmic drug have been administered. In the case of amiodarone, which has unusual pharmacokinetic properties, electropharmacologic testing usually is delayed until 10 to 14 days of an oral loading dose has been administered.

The most desirable end point of electropharmacologic testing is the complete suppression of ventricular tachycardia induction. The inability to induce ventricular tachycardia after initiation of drug therapy generally predicts that the antiarrhythmic drug will have long-term effectiveness in preventing spontaneous episodes of ventricular tachycardia. However, it is often not possible to completely suppress the induction of ventricular tachycardia with antiarrhythmic drugs, and in some instances this may not be necessary. It may be appropriate to implement long-term treatment with a drug that has been demonstrated to be effective in markedly slowing ventricular tachycardia to the point that it is hemodynamically stable and not associated with severe symptoms. This type of response to electropharmacologic testing predicts a low risk of arrhythmia-related death.

MAPPING OF VENTRICULAR TACHYCARDIA

Patients who have recurrent sustained ventricular tachycardia unresponsive to antiarrhythmic drug therapy may be appropriate candidates for definitive therapy aimed at eliminating the site or sites of origin of ventricular tachycardia by various surgical or catheter ablation techniques. In these patients, electrophysiologic testing is performed to identify the sites of origin of ventricular tachycardia using various mapping techniques. The mapping process involves maneuvering electrode catheters to various sites in the right and left ventricles and recording endocardial electrograms at these sites during ventricular tachycardia. Identification of the origin of ventricular tachycardia is based on analysis of the endocardial electrogram patterns and on the response to pacing during ventricular tachycardia and sinus rhythm.

ELECTROPHYSIOLOGIC TESTING IN THE ABORTED SUDDEN DEATH SYNDROME

The most common causes of out-of-hospital cardiac arrest are ventricular tachycardia and ventricular fibrillation. Electrophysiologic testing may be appropriate for patients who are successfully resuscitated from what otherwise would have been lethal cardiac arrest and in whom the cardiac arrest was not precipitated by an acute myocardial infarction. Sustained monomorphic ventricular tachycardia associated with severe hemodynamic compromise is inducible in about one-half of patients with the aborted sudden death syndrome. The ability to induce monomorphic ventricular tachycardia in these patients allows electropharmacologic testing, mapping of the ventricular tachycardia

in patients who may be candidates for catheter or surgical ablation, and selection of the appropriate detection criteria in patients who are candidates for devices such as the automatic internal cardioverter–defibrillator. However, because a large-scale multicenter study (Antiarrhythmics Versus Implantable Defibrillators; AVID) demonstrated that the implantable cardioverter–defibrillator is superior to antiarrhythmic drug therapy for increasing survival after ventricular fibrillation or sustained ventricular tachycardia associated with severe symptoms, the role of electropharmacologic testing in survivors of cardiac arrest has rapidly waned. In addition, because the sensitivity of programmed ventricular stimulation is lower in patients with cardiomyopathy and other types of heart disease than in patients with CAD, a negative electrophysiologic test for a patient with the aborted sudden death syndrome who does not have CAD does not rule out the possibility that the cardiac arrest was caused by a primary episode of ventricular tachycardia or ventricular fibrillation. In light of these considerations, and to improve cost-effectiveness, an implantable cardioverter–defibrillator now often is implanted without a prior electrophysiologic test in patients who have survived a cardiac arrest and in whom a correctable cause for the cardiac arrest cannot be identified.

NONSUSTAINED VENTRICULAR TACHYCARDIA

For patients with symptomatic nonsustained ventricular tachycardia, electrophysiologic testing may be used to guide therapy of those who have infrequent arrhythmia episodes and in whom assessment of drug efficacy is not clinically possible. If ventricular tachycardia is inducible by programmed stimulation, drug efficacy can be determined by electropharmacologic testing.

In patients with coronary artery disease and compromised left ventricular function (left ventricular ejection fraction less than 0.35) who have asymptomatic, nonsustained ventricular tachycardia, electrophysiologic testing may be performed for the purpose of risk stratification. If sustained ventricular tachycardia cannot be provoked in the electrophysiology laboratory, treatment of the nonsustained ventricular tachycardia may not be necessary. On the other hand, if sustained ventricular tachycardia can be induced, this may indicate a need for prophylactic treatment to prevent cardiac arrest. Electropharmacologic testing may be performed to assess the efficacy of antiarrhythmic drug therapy in suppressing the inducibility of ventricular tachycardia. A multicenter study (Multicenter Automatic Defibrillator Implantation Trial; MADIT) demonstrated that an implantable cardioverter–defibrillator improves survival compared to conventional medical therapy in patients in whom the inducible ventricular tachycardia is not suppressed by an antiarrhythmic drug. Therefore, electrophysiologic testing is useful in identifying patients with coronary artery disease and nonsustained ventricular tachycardia who are appropriate candidates for antiarrhythmic drug therapy or an implantable cardioverter–defibrillator.

In patients with nonsustained ventricular tachycardia who do not have coronary artery disease, electrophysiologic testing generally is not useful for the purpose of risk stratification. In such patients, the decision to institute prophylactic antiarrhythmic therapy to prevent cardiac arrest must be made on a clinical basis.

LIMITATIONS OF TESTING PATIENTS WITH VENTRICULAR TACHYCARDIA

Electrophysiologic testing has several limitations when performed in patients with ventricular tachycardia. First, because the ventricular tachycardia is not caused by reentry or because of an unknown reason, some patients with documented sustained ventricular tachycardia may not have inducible ventricular tachycardia, especially patients without CAD. Second, patients who have had a spontaneous episode of sustained monomorphic ventricular tachycardia often have more than one type of monomorphic ventricular tachycardia inducible during electrophysiologic testing, and the clinical importance of these additional configurations may be unclear. Third, although polymorphic ventricular tachycardia or fibrillation is usually a laboratory artifact in patients who have never had a cardiac arrest, the clinical significance of this type of induced arrhythmia is often unclear in patients who have been resuscitated from a cardiac arrest and for whom there is no documentation of the precipitating arrhythmia.

EVALUATION OF UNEXPLAINED SYNCOPE

Electrophysiologic testing may be helpful in uncovering an arrhythmic cause of syncope in patients whose syncope remains unexplained after a complete clinical, neurologic, and noninvasive cardiac evaluation. Electrophysiologic findings indicating abnormalities likely to be related to syncope consist of inducible monomorphic ventricular tachycardia; inducible paroxysmal supraventricular tachycardia associated with significant hypotension; a markedly prolonged sinus node recovery time (corrected sinus node recovery time more than 1 to 1.5 seconds); a markedly prolonged HV interval of 100 milliseconds or more; and pathologic infranodal block during atrial pacing. Some abnormalities may be nonspecific or not severe enough to be considered a likely cause of syncope, including inducible polymorphic ventricular tachycardia or ventricular fibrillation; inducible paroxysmal supraventricular tachycardia not associated with hypotension; mild prolongation of the sinus node recovery time; mild prolongation of the HV interval; and slow conduction or prolonged refractoriness in the AV node.

The diagnostic yield of electrophysiologic testing because of unexplained syncope is in the range of 30% to 60% for patients who have underlying heart disease and 5% or less for those who do not have structural heart disease. The threshold for performing an electrophysiologic test should be high for patients with syncope who are free of heart disease. For these patients, electrophysiologic testing often is reserved for cases of syncope associated with serious injury or that has proven to be recurrent and problematic.

The arrhythmia that most commonly causes syncope in patients who have heart disease is ventricular tachycardia, and it is always important to thoroughly investigate an episode of syncope in this type of patient. Even one episode of unexplained syncope is an appropriate indication for electrophysiologic testing of patients who have significant structural heart disease to rule out a serious or potentially lethal arrhythmia as the cause of syncope.

An electrophysiologic test that does not demonstrate any diagnostic abnormalities in patients with unexplained syncope generally predicts a benign prognosis and a low risk of sudden death. This suggests that electrophysiologic testing is effective in ruling out potentially lethal arrhythmias as the cause of syncope. Although the reasons are unclear, 70% to 80% of patients may have no further recurrences of syncope after undergoing an electrophysiologic test that does not reveal any diagnostic abnormalities. However, about 20% of patients with unexplained syncope and a negative electrophysiologic test result may have had a falsely negative electrophysiologic test result during follow-up, and the most commonly missed abnormalities are symptomatic bradycardias related to sinus node dysfunction or AV block. The absence of abnormalities during electrophysiologic testing in these patients suggests that these symptomatic bradycardias may be related to transient fluctuations in autonomic tone instead of an intrinsic sinus node or AV conduction system abnormality. For additional discussion of syncope, see Chapter 69.

BIBLIOGRAPHY

Antiarrhythmics Versus Implantable Defibrillators (AVID) Investigators. A comparison of antiarrhythmic drug therapy with implantable defibrillators in patients resuscitated from near-fatal ventricular arrhythmias. *N Engl J Med* 1997;337:1576–1583.

Calkins H, El-Atassi R, deButleir M, et al. Diagnosis and cure of Wolff–Parkinson–White syndrome or paroxysmal supraventricular tachycardias during a single electrophysiologic test. *N Engl J Med* 1991;324:1612–1618.

Guidelines for clinical intracardiac electrophysiological and catheter ablation procedures: a report of the American College of Cardiology/American Heart Association Task Force on Practice Guidelines (Committee on Clinical Intracardiac Electrophysiologic and Catheter Ablation Procedures). *J Am Coll Cardiol* 1995;26:555–573.

Kim SG. Management of survivors of cardiac arrest: is electrophysiologic testing obsolete in the era of implantable defibrillators? *J Am Coll Cardiol* 1990;3:756–762.

Link MS, Costeas XF, Griffith JL, et al. High incidence of implantable cardioverter–defibrillator therapy in patients with syncope of unknown etiology and inducible arrhythmias. *J Am Coll Cardiol* 1997;29:370–375.

Marinchak RA, Rials SJ, Filart RA, et al. The top ten fallacies of nonsustained ventricular tachycardia. *Pacing Clin Electrophysiol* 1997;20:2825–2847.

Mason JW. A comparison of electrophysiologic testing with Holter monitoring to predict antiarrhythmic-drug efficacy for ventricular tachyarrhythmias. *N Engl J Med* 1993;329:445–451.

Moss AJ, Hall J, Cannom DS, et al. Improved survival with an implanted defibrillator in patients with coronary disease at high risk for ventricular arrhythmia. *N Engl J Med* 1996;335:1933–1940.

Wilber DJ, Kopp D, Olshansky B, et al. Nonsustained ventricular tachycardia and other high-risk predictors following myocardial infarction: implications for prophylactic automatic implantable cardioverter–defibrillator use. *Prog Cardiovasc Dis* 1993;36:179–194.

C H A P T E R

89

PRINCIPLES OF CARDIAC CONDITIONING AND REHABILITATION

VICTOR F. FROELICHER
JONATHAN N. MYERS

Cardiac rehabilitation was conceived in the 1960s as a treatment for patients who had suffered a myocardial infarction (MI). Before the 1970s, the patient who suffered an MI was almost completely immobilized for 6 weeks or more and was even washed, shaved, and fed to keep the work of the heart to a minimum. This approach was thought to provide the heart with the opportunity to form a firm scar. Also, the patient was told not to expect to be able to return to a normal life. These were incorrect beliefs, particularly in the situation of an uncomplicated MI. Prolonged immobilization not only did not speed healing but exposed the patient to the additional risks of venous thrombosis, pulmonary embolism, muscle atrophy, lung infections, and deconditioning. Equally serious was the psychological result of such an approach, often leading to psychological impairment. Thus, the old approach to rehabilitation was an attempt to correct iatrogenic impairment.

Today, the physician's approach to the acute MI has completely changed. A relatively brief period of time monitored by the high technology in the coronary care unit is followed by early mobilization, sitting at the bedside, graduated exercise, and, in the uncomplicated patient, discharge from the hospital in less than 1 week. This policy has been shown by randomized trials to be safe from the point of view of cardiac complications. Inpatient rehabilitation is brief, but educational videos and pamphlets can begin the patient's education. Iatrogenic deconditioning is not a problem because a walking program can begin very early. Psychological rehabilitation takes place in the doctor's office along with prescribing exercise and education. Certainly, all patients do not need all rehabilitative interventions, but exercise programs, educational sessions, group therapy, and psychological and vocational counseling are available in most communities for those who need them. The approach to exercise has also changed; the current emphasis is on physical activity rather than fitness.

■ BASIC EXERCISE PHYSIOLOGY

The cardiorespiratory response to exercise depends on the type of exercise, the environmental conditions, and the physiologic status of the patient. Changes that occur with a single bout of acute exercise are called responses and are temporary. Adaptations are long-lasting changes in structure or function that occur with training (regular exercise) and improve the body's response to subsequent exercise.

Dynamic exercise (bicycling, walking, running, swimming) involves the movement of large muscle masses. Because this movement is rhythmic, a drop in total peripheral resistance and a "pumping" action in the skeletal muscle that returns blood to the heart occur. Dynamic exercise evokes a series of cardiovascular adjustments, which supply the active muscles with sufficient blood, dissipate the heat generated, and maintain blood supply to the heart and brain. Local increases in metabolites cause dilation of the arteries and arterioles in active muscles, resulting in a decrease in systemic vascular resistance proportional to the muscle mass involved. To maintain arterial blood pressure, sympathetic activity increases, which causes constriction of the resistance vessels in the splanchnic bed, kidneys, and nonworking muscles. The generalized vasoconstriction in inactive tissues and the increased venous return result in maintenance of the heart's filling volume and pressure. The increase in pulmonary blood flow causes a moderate increase in mean pulmonary artery pressure. The extent to which basic hemodynamic and metabolic variables change from rest to a moderately high level of exercise is illustrated in Figure 89.1.

Isometric exercise (lifting a weight, forceful squeezing or pressing) involves a constant muscular contraction, which limits blood flow. Instead of an increase in cardiac output and blood flow, blood pressure must be increased to force blood into the active, contracting muscles. Dynamic exercise can be graded to increase myocardial oxygen demand gradually, whereas isometric exercise is more difficult to grade and increases myocardial oxygen demand quickly without as great an increase in cardiac output. Although isometric exercise can enhance peripheral muscle tone and function, it does not result in the same beneficial cardiac and hemodynamic effects as does dynamic exercise.

■ RESPONSE TO ACUTE EXERCISE

HEART RATE

The body's initial hemodynamic response to dynamic exercise is an increase in heart rate. The elicited heart rate response is proportional to the workload and depends on the person's age and physical condition. Maximal heart rate is an important determinant of maximal cardiac output (because cardiac output = heart rate × stroke volume) and, therefore, also of exercise capacity.

BLOOD PRESSURE

The systolic and diastolic blood-pressure response to exercise varies with the type and intensity of the exercise and the age of the person. In dynamic exercise of moderate to heavy intensity, there is a gradual linear increase in systolic pressure of about 40 mm Hg at maximum, whereas diastolic pressure stays about the same or decreases. The increase in cardiac output during exercise is balanced by a reduction in peripheral resistance, such that mean arterial pressure increases only modestly.

BLOOD FLOW

At rest, a large portion of the cardiac output is directed to the spleen, liver, kidneys, brain, and heart, with only about 20%

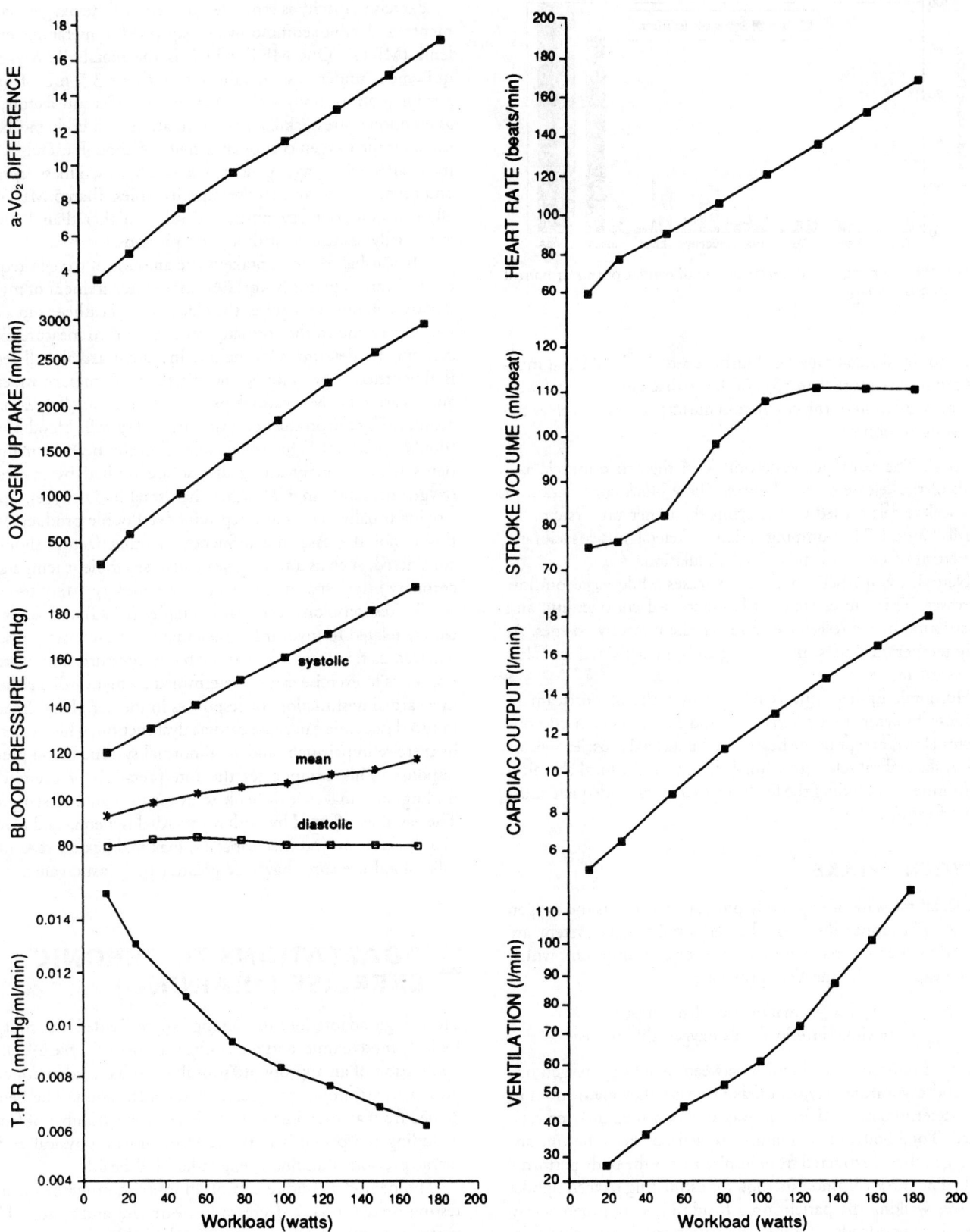

FIGURE 89.1. Basic hemodynamic and metabolic variables and the magnitude of the response from rest to a moderately high level of exercise. Units for a–$\dot{V}O_2$ difference are milliliters of O_2 per 100 mL of blood. *TPR*, total peripheral resistance. (From Myers JN. The physiology behind exercise testing. *Prim Care* 1994;21:415, with permission.)

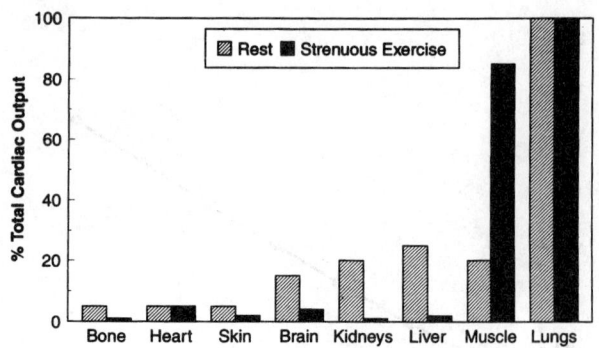

FIGURE 89.2. Changes in the distribution of cardiac output from rest to strenuous work.

going to the skeletal muscles. During exercise, the skeletal muscles can receive more than 85% of the cardiac output (Fig. 89.2).

The regulation of the circulation during exercise involves the following responses:

Local. The resistance vessels dilate in the active muscle as a result of the release of metabolites. These block constriction in the local vessels caused by the sympathetic nervous system.

Mechanical. The pumping action of skeletal muscle facilitates the return of blood to the central circulation.

Neural. Sympathetic outflow increases while vagal outflow decreases. This causes tachycardia, increased contractility, and constriction of the resistance vessels in the nonactive tissues. As body temperature rises, the sweat glands are activated and skin vessels dilate.

Humoral. Epinephrine is released into the bloodstream in response to sympathetic activation and has a generalized constrictor effect, except in the heart and the skeletal muscle. Sensors within skeletal muscle detect small changes in the local chemical environment, providing the feedback to maintain adequate muscle perfusion.

OXYGEN UPTAKE

The usual measure of total body physiologic work is the oxygen uptake. The upper limits of the cardiopulmonary system are defined by the maximal oxygen uptake (or consumption), which can be expressed by the Fick principle:

$$\dot{V}O_2max = \text{maximal cardiac output} \\ \times \text{maximal arteriovenous oxygen difference}$$

It is important to distinguish between total body oxygen uptake and myocardial oxygen uptake because they are distinct in their determinants and in the way they are measured or estimated. Total body, or ventilatory, oxygen uptake is the amount of oxygen that is extracted from inspired air as the body performs work. The most common method for estimating oxygen uptake involves walking the patient on a treadmill using progressively increasing workloads. If direct measurement is not available, oxygen uptake is best estimated by the peak work rate performed rather than by the total exercise time, because the latter depends on the protocol used and the patient's endurance and muscular strength.

Exercise capacity is estimated in terms of the oxygen requirements, and values commonly are expressed in metabolic equivalents (METs). One MET, which is the metabolic oxygen requirement under basal conditions, is about 3.5 mL of oxygen per kilogram of body weight per minute. Certain factors, such as emotional stress, skill and coordination, and body mechanics, can alter the oxygen cost of an activity. Although exercise capacity is affected by age, gender, exercise status, illness, genetics, and other factors, an exercise capacity of less than 5 METs usually carries a poor prognosis, and values higher than 10 METs are usually associated with a good prognosis.

Myocardial oxygen uptake is the amount of oxygen required by the heart to perform work. Accurate measurement of myocardial oxygen uptake requires the placement of catheters in a coronary artery and in the coronary venous sinus to measure oxygen content. Its determinants include intramyocardial wall tension (left ventricular pressure × end-diastolic volume), contractility, and heart rate. Myocardial oxygen uptake can be reasonably estimated by the product of heart rate and systolic blood pressure (double product). This is valuable clinically because many patients with coronary artery disease are limited by myocardial oxygen demand (angina) rather than total body oxygen uptake. Angina usually occurs at a reproducible double product. When this is not the case, the influence of other factors should be considered, such as a recent meal, adverse ambient temperature, coronary artery spasm, or changes in coronary artery tone.

The response on electrocardiography (ECG) and angina are closely related to myocardial ischemia (coronary artery disease), whereas exercise capacity, systolic blood pressure, and heart rate responses to exercise can be determined by myocardial ischemia, myocardial dysfunction, or responses in the periphery. Exercise-induced ischemia can cause cardiac dysfunction, which can result in exercise impairment and an abnormal systolic blood pressure response. This complicates the interpretation of exercise test findings and makes it difficult to assess the cause of symptoms. The variables affected by both myocardial ischemia and myocardial dysfunction (exercise capacity, maximal heart rate, and systolic blood pressure) have the greatest prognostic value.

ADAPTATIONS TO CHRONIC EXERCISE (TRAINING)

Physiologic adaptations to training can be divided into morphologic, hemodynamic, and metabolic categories (Table 89.1). The application of an appropriate stimulus results in adaptation; the greater the stimulus, the greater is the adaptation. The benefits gained from an exercise program depend on a number of factors, including the patient's initial level of fitness, physical endowment, previous training, age, gender, and health.

The hemodynamic results of an exercise program include a resting bradycardia, a decrease in heart rate and systolic blood pressure at any matched submaximal workload, an increase in maximal oxygen uptake and maximal cardiac output, an increase in total blood volume, and a more rapid return toward baseline in recovery. These hemodynamic adaptations not only improve exercise capacity but also make the heart more efficient, such

TABLE 89.1.	PHYSIOLOGIC ADAPTATIONS TO PHYSICAL TRAINING IN HUMANS

Morphologic Adaptations

Myocardial hypertrophy

Hemodynamic Adaptations

Increased blood volume
Increased end-diastolic volume
Increased stroke volume
Increased cardiac output
Reduced heart rate for any submaximal work load

Metabolic Adaptations

Increased mitochondrial volume and number
Greater muscle glycogen stores
Enhanced fat utilization
Enhanced lactate removal
Increased enzymes for aerobic metabolism
Increased maximal oxygen uptake

that any submaximal workload can be performed with less demand on the heart muscle.

SCIENTIFIC BASIS FOR EXERCISE PROGRAMS IN PATIENTS WITH CORONARY HEART DISEASE

In terms of prognosis, exercise training has been definitively shown to improve morbidity and mortality. Although few of the randomized trials in cardiac rehabilitation individually have shown significant reductions in mortality, taken together, these trials demonstrate a substantial 20% to 25% reduction in the rate of mortality from cardiovascular causes.

Although some studies of exercise training have demonstrated cardiac changes (enhanced contractility, decrease of exercise-induced ST-segment depression), these studies have used high-intensity training among highly selected patients. Larger, randomized trials using standard training programs in unselected patients have shown modest improvements in thallium perfusion images. Several randomized trials have demonstrated that intensive dietary and lipid-lowering therapy along with exercise may retard or reverse the progression of atherosclerotic lesions in some patients. Certainly, however, the statin drugs are much more effective in this regard.

Advances in the treatment of cardiovascular disease and data supporting the value of secondary prevention have increased greatly the spectrum of patients who may benefit from cardiac rehabilitation. In addition to patients who have sustained MIs, this group now includes patients with chronic heart failure and patients who have undergone coronary artery bypass grafting, cardiac transplantation, catheter interventions, and pacemaker implantation. Of the roughly 1 million persons in the United States who survive acute MIs annually, only 10% to 15% undergo formal outpatient rehabilitation. Not all patients need a formal exercise program, but directing these services to the patients who need them the most remains one of the important challenges for the field.

PHASES OF CARDIAC REHABILITATION AFTER MYOCARDIAL INFARCTION

The typical phases in cardiac rehabilitation are coronary care unit and inpatient care (phase I), convalescence in an outpatient or home program (phase II), and recovery in a long-term community-based or home program (phase III). Phase I has been greatly shortened by thrombolysis and catheter interventions. Most education comes in quick bursts of information, but fortunately the public is much better informed. Reimbursement agencies have greatly decreased funding for Phase III, which usually is supported for only 1 year. Monitored programs usually are reimbursed for only a small proportion of high-risk patients.

SEVERITY OF THE MYOCARDIAL INFARCTION

Electrocardiography

The ECG pattern predicts the clinical course and outcome surprisingly well. The greater the number of areas with Q waves and the greater R-wave loss, the larger is the MI. Non–Q-wave MIs are associated less commonly with congestive heart failure or shock, but they can be complicated. It once was thought that non–Q-wave MIs were unstable and needed intermediate intervention, but this has been shown not to be the case. Also, calcium antagonists are not indicated for non–Q-wave MIs, but they should receive β-blockers just like patients with Q-wave MIs.

Inferior infarctions usually are smaller than anterior infarctions, result in less of a decline in ejection fraction, and are less likely to be associated with shock or congestive heart failure. Anterior infarctions are more likely to cause aneurysms and a greater decrease in ejection fraction.

Size of the Myocardial Infarction

The size of an MI can be judged by the creatine phosphokinase level, mostly by the muscle–brain fraction (CK-MB) released. In general, the higher the amount of MB released and the longer the creatine phosphokinase level remains elevated, the larger is the MI. Troponin now is available as a cardiac enzyme, reflecting damage.

Complicated and Uncomplicated Myocardial Infarction

Morbidity and mortality are much higher in patients with complicated MIs than in those with uncomplicated MIs. The criteria for a complicated MI are presented in Table 89.2. The most important clinical predictors are previous MI and the presence of congestive heart failure or cardiogenic shock. The progressive ambulation program should be delayed until patients with complications reach an uncomplicated status and then should proceed at a slower than normal pace.

EARLY AMBULATION

The program should begin with range-of-motion exercises and sitting with legs dangling and should progress to ambulation

TABLE 89.2.   CRITERIA FOR CLASSIFYING A MYOCARDIAL INFARCTION AS COMPLICATED

Continued cardiac ischemia (pain, late enzyme rise)
Left ventricular failure (congestive heart failure, new murmurs, roentgenographic changes)
Shock (blood pressure drop, pallor, oliguria)
Important cardiac dysrhythmia (more than six premature ventricular contractions per minute, atrial fibrillation, ventricular tachycardia)
Conductions disturbances (bundle-branch block, atrioventricular block, hemiblock)
Severe pleurisy or pericarditis
Complicating illnesses
Marked creatine phosphokinase rise without a noncardiac explanation or after thrombolysis

and calisthenics. After the patient has been transferred from the intensive care unit, self-care activities can begin and an upright posture should be encouraged as much as can be tolerated. Before exercise is allowed, the patient's condition must be medically stable. There should be no evidence of congestive heart failure, dangerous dysrhythmias, or unstable angina. The blood pressure should remain within 20 mm Hg of the resting level. The heart rate usually should remain within 20 beats per minute of the resting level, and the rating of perceived exertion should not exceed 14. If complications arise, the activity should be discontinued and restarted later at a lower level. The patient should be able to walk up stairs before hospital discharge and should be able to perform activities of daily living independently by the time of hospital discharge (3- to 4-MET level).

EXERCISE TESTING BEFORE HOSPITAL DISCHARGE

Exercise testing after acute MI has been shown to be safe. When performed before hospital discharge, it should be submaximal ($\leq$5 METs). This test has many benefits, including clarification of the response to exercise, determination of an exercise prescription, and recognition of the need for medications or interventions. It can have a beneficial psychological effect on recovery and begins the outpatient rehabilitation process.

RETURN TO WORK AND RECREATIONAL ACTIVITIES

Historically, decisions regarding the patient's return to work, driving, and sexual and recreational activities have been based on clinical judgments rather than physiologic assessments. These decisions should be based on the consequences of the coronary event (ischemia, symptoms of congestive failure or dysrhythmias), the nature of the patient's occupational or recreational activities, and the patient's response to the predischarge exercise test. In general, if the patient does not exhibit any untoward response to submaximal exercise testing and achieves 5 or more METs, it is unlikely that he or she will encounter difficulties during activities of daily living. More strenuous job or recrea-

tional requirements should not be undertaken until a symptom-limited exercise test can be performed, and exercise capacity can be determined and related to the desired physical activities. Factors influencing return to work include age, work history, severity of cardiac damage, financial compensation for illness, employer ignorance, termination of employment, and, most important, the patient's perception of his or her health status.

The transition from an outpatient to a home-based maintenance program occurs more rapidly. Randomized trials have demonstrated that patients can return to work quickly and safely during rehabilitation and that participation in a rehabilitation program facilitates this process. Researchers at Stanford University have advocated home exercise that is unmonitored or monitored by telephone or microprocessor. The safety and efficacy of these home programs have been shown to be similar to those of more conventional programs.

MEDICAL EVALUATION FOR THE EXERCISE COMPONENT

The following is one approach to assessing patients, placing them in a "niche" so the clinician knows how to react to their symptoms and test results. The tools for assessment begin with the history and physical examination. The first step in evaluating patients for outpatient cardiac rehabilitation is to determine whether their coronary heart disease is stable. "Stability" is determined primarily by the presence or absence of myocardial ischemia, congestive heart failure, and dysrhythmias. The hallmark symptom of ischemia is chest pain. Most patients have chest pain of some type and the pain commonly is ignored. After patients are told about heart disease, these routine pains may become frightening. It is important to separate nonischemic from ischemic chest pain. All chest pain should not be called angina pectoris. Angina becomes unstable when it changes its pattern (i.e., occurs more frequently, at rest, or at lower workloads). Increasing symptoms of congestive heart failure include sudden weight gain, edema in the lower extremities, dyspnea on exertion, and paroxysmal nocturnal dyspnea. Although there was early concern that thrombolytic agents could leave patients more likely to experience ischemia, their benefits have been shown to extend over 10 years. In addition, β-blockers are a must drug because they reduce mortality after MI by 25%. Statins appear to reduce cardiovascular events by up to 50%.

In patients who are stable, further assessment can proceed. Initially, the ischemic threshold should be determined by the onset of angina pectoris or ST-segment depression at a particular heart rate, double product, or workload. Once this is clarified, myocardial function should be determined. Clinical clues that suggest the possibility of myocardial dysfunction include a history of congestive heart failure, cardiogenic shock, a previous MI, a large anterior MI, cardiomegaly, a large creatine phosphokinase elevation, multiple Q waves, and underlying problems such as cardiomyopathy or valvular heart disease. These patients must be watched for signs and symptoms of congestive heart failure. They are usually limited by their maximal cardiac output, which leads to early fatigue and pulmonary symptoms, rather than to chest pain. A strong effort should be made to explain the symptoms related to congestive heart failure. In patients who have sustained MIs, the symptoms could be caused by mitral valve insufficiency, resulting from papillary muscle dysfunction or rupture, or from a dilated mitral annulus.

In addition to myocardial ischemia and dysfunction, the other key features of heart disease are arrhythmias, valvular function, and exercise capacity. These five features are important because they usually explain the patient's symptoms and help to establish the prognosis. Evaluation of these features is necessary for optimal management, including individualization of the rehabilitation program. The ECG, chest radiograph, and exercise test are next in importance after a careful history and physical examination. The exercise test is the key to prescribing exercise. Specialized tests such as echocardiography, nuclear imaging, and cardiac catheterization can be used to confirm impressions, clarify incongruous clinical situations, or identify coronary pathologic or anatomical patterns requiring revascularization.

EXERCISE PRESCRIPTION

The major ingredients of the exercise prescription are the frequency, intensity, duration, mode, and rate of progression. Based on numerous studies performed over the last several decades, it usually is accepted that increases in maximal oxygen uptake are achieved if a person exercises dynamically for a period ranging from 15 to 60 minutes, three to five times per week, at an intensity equivalent to 50% to 80% of the person's maximum capacity. Short periods for warm-up and cool-down are strongly encouraged for participants in cardiac rehabilitation programs.

Remember, however, that the prescription is for fitness and increasing aerobic capacity. Increasing physical activity through simple activities such as brisk walking appears to provide the same health benefits with less risk and to be more convenient.

CONTRAINDICATIONS TO EXERCISE TRAINING AND SAFETY

Absolute contraindications to exercise training include unstable angina, dissecting aortic aneurysm, complete heart block, uncontrolled hypertension, uncontrolled congestive heart failure, dysrhythmias, thrombophlebitis, and other complicating illnesses. Relative contraindications include frequent premature ventricular contractions, controlled arrhythmias, intermittent claudication, metabolic disorders, and moderate anemia or pulmonary disease. If these contraindications are observed, the incidence of exertion-related cardiac arrest in cardiac rehabilitation programs is extremely low, and, because of the availability of rapid defibrillation, death rarely occurs. A survey evaluating more than 51,000 participants over a 5-year period demonstrated that only one to three fatalities occurred per million hours of participation in a cardiac rehabilitation program.

MONITORING OF THE EXERCISE COMPONENT

It now is recognized that only a small percentage of patients referred for cardiac rehabilitation require supervised continuous

TABLE 89.3.	**CRITERIA FOR ELECTROCARDIOGRAPHIC MONITORING DURING CARDIAC REHABILITATION**

Severely depressed left ventricular function (ejection fraction <30%)
Resting complex ventricular arrhythmia (Lown type 4 or 5)
Ventricular arrhythmia appearing or increasing with exercise
Decrease in systolic blood pressure with exercise
Survival of sudden cardiac death
Myocardial infarction complicated by congestive heart failure, cardiogenic shock, or serious ventricular arrhythmia
Severe coronary artery disease and marked exercise-induced ischemia
Inability to self-monitor intensity because of physical or intellectual impairment

Criteria advocated by the American College of Cardiology and the American Heart Association Subcommittee on Cardiac Rehabilitation.

ECG monitoring during exercise. Table 89.3 presents a list of criteria for ECG monitoring outlined by the American College of Cardiology.

PHASE III (MAINTENANCE PROGRAM)

Progression to an out-of-hospital maintenance program is desirable after patients have participated in a phase II program for a suitable period. The time required before patients move to a maintenance program can vary considerably, but rarely exceeds 12 weeks. The purpose of phase III is to maintain training adaptations, prevent recurrence of events or symptoms, and maintain progress. It is important that patients understand how to monitor their own exercise intensity and recognize symptoms and that they have a basic knowledge of their particular disease and medications. This maintenance program should most often be a self-monitored walking program, although physicians can play an important part in this process by encouraging patients.

Performing an exercise test before the maintenance program is useful to provide an outgoing exercise prescription, confirm the safety of exercise for a given patient, and assess the risk for future cardiac events.

FUTURE DIRECTIONS IN THE UNITED STATES

As suggested by Ribisl and colleagues, a new era requires a new model. The old model of a standard, fixed 36-session program in which every patient receives the same intervention regardless of specific needs or characteristics, is outmoded and a disservice to patients. Part of the reason for adhering to the old model was failure to interact with third-party payers in the design of appropriate programs that met patient needs. The security of a safe and reliable means of obtaining reimbursement was the driving force behind this approach, and programs have been reluctant to make any change because of a fear that revenues would be lost. Some observations and suggestions follow and then recommendations are provided of several models for consideration. These models are based on impressions of trends and opportunities that exist today. With cardiac rehabilitation care serving approximately 15% to 20% of eligible patients, utilization is low.

The treatment plan for patients with cardiovascular disease is rarely limited to a single diagnosis. It is unusual to find an older patient who is free of other diagnoses of chronic disease. Many patients with cardiac disease are likely to have one or more additional conditions, such as obesity, diabetes, chronic obstructive pulmonary disease (COPD), arthritis, or other complications that must be taken into account in the intervention plan.

There is a clear lack of awareness among those in the medical profession who are responsible for making decisions regarding the treatment options available to their patients in the community. Because training in preventive strategies has never been an integral part of medical education, efforts must be made to convince current practitioners and medical students about the benefits to patients.

Cardiac rehabilitation needs to be restructured by adding newer cost-effective techniques to survive the current reformation of health care. Traditional rehabilitation will be best delivered at centers in the community rather than by following the current fragmented approach in which each hospital has a competitive program. Newer models involve the use of other medical and paramedical professionals, volunteers, and communication with patients by telephone, internet and the postal service.

TREATMENT MODELS

Four specific models are presented, with research documenting their efficacy.

Center-Based Model

Physician referral could be improved as general practitioners become more responsible for triage and have the option of directing patients to a center with multidisciplinary specialists available. Health care managers must be convinced that cardiac rehabilitation is effective. The necessary components of this triaging approach include initial assessment by a team of specialists, risk stratification, exercise prescription (often just a walking program with indirect supervision, when medically appropriate), dietary instruction, lipid abnormality classification and treatment, psychological and vocational counseling, education, and a discharge plan.

The Center-Based Model is the classic model that was the prototype for most programs in recent history. Its major shortcomings are lack of adequate referral. Physician referral could be improved if general practitioners become more responsible for triage and have the option of directing patients to a center with multidisciplinary specialists available.

Home-Based Model

The Home-Based Model has been in place for over a decade, and numerous studies in the literature have documented its effectiveness. This model has been validated at Stanford University

in a 1-year randomized clinical trial including 160 women and 197 men 50 to 65 years who were sedentary and free of cardiovascular disease. It included physician referral, assessment, prescription, and multiple interventions. Regular feedback and home visits were carried out to prevent relapses. Home-based exercise was as effective as group exercise in producing these changes. Lower-intensity exercise training was as effective as higher-intensity exercise training in the home setting.

Volunteer Community Model

The Volunteer Community Model is a unique approach that was developed by Lorig and colleagues in patients with arthritis. These investigators trained nonmedical lay volunteers (who themselves had arthritis) to direct educational programs of self-management in the community to help patients with arthritis deal with their disease outside the medical setting. Lorig and colleagues have since expanded this model to include four chronic disorders (coronary heart disease, COPD, stroke, and arthritis).

Health Risk Appraisal Model

A randomized 12-month trial comparing claims data was performed in a large insured population. After assessment with a Health Risk Appraisal (HRA) instrument accomplished by mail, feedback on risk factors and recommendations for change were provided again by mail using an educational packet of self-management materials. This study demonstrated a considerable cost-trend reduction from a simple mail-based health promotion program. The insurance company was so pleased with the reduction in claims that the program has been continued.

CONCLUSION

Much of what began under the label of cardiac rehabilitation now has been assimilated into routine care. Hospital accreditation guidelines specify a multidisciplinary approach that includes progressive ambulation for the cardiac patient. Cardiac rehabilitation has redirected interest to humanistic concerns, providing a balance to the emphasis on high technology. The average patient does not require all components of cardiac rehabilitation, but usually can benefit from some of them. Analyses of controlled trials reveal a decrease in mortality among patients with MIs who have participated in exercise programs. Physiologic studies support the occurrence of beneficial hemodynamic and metabolic changes in a wide range of cardiac patients. Therefore, the physician should consider an exercise program as part of the routine therapeutic regimen.

BIBLIOGRAPHY

American College of Sports Medicine. *Guidelines for exercise testing and exercise prescription,* fourth ed. Philadelphia: Lea & Febiger, 1991.
Dennis C, Houston-Miller N, Schwartz RG, et al. Early return to work after uncomplicated myocardial infarction. Results of a randomized trial. *JAMA* 1988;260:214.

Fletcher GF, Balady G, Blair SN, et al. Statement on exercise: benefits and recommendations for physical activity programs for all Americans. A statement for health professionals by the Committee on Exercise and Cardiac Rehabilitation of the Council on Clinical Cardiology. *Circulation* 1996;94(4):857–862.

Fries R, Long M, Forsythe D. Randomized controlled trial of cost reductions from a health education program. *Am J Health Promotion* 1994;8:216.

Froelicher VF, Herbert W, Myers J, Ribisl P. How cardiac rehabilitation is being influenced by changes in health-care delivery. *J Cardiopulm Rehabil* 1996;16(3):151–159.

Froelicher VF, Myers J, Follansbee WP, Labovitz AJ. *Exercise and the heart*, third ed. St Louis: CV Mosby, 1993.

Greenland P, Chu JS. Efficacy of cardiac rehabilitation services with emphasis on patients after myocardial infarction. *Ann Intern Med* 1988;109:650.

King AC, Haskell WL, Taylor CB, et al. Group versus home-based exercise training in healthy older men and women: a community-based clinical trial. *JAMA* 1991;266:1535–1542.

Lorig K, Holman H, Sobel D, et al. *Living a healthy life with chronic conditions: self-management of heart disease, arthritis, stroke, diabetes, asthma, bronchitis, emphysema.* Palo Alto, CA: Bull Publishing, 1994.

Oldridge NB, Guyatt GH, Fischer ME, Rimm AA. Cardiac rehabilitation after myocardial infarction: combined experience of random clinical trials. *JAMA* 1988;260:945.

Ries AL, Kaplan RM, Limberg TM, Prewitt LM. Effects of pulmonary rehabilitation on physiologic and psychosocial outcomes in patients with chronic obstructive pulmonary disease. *Ann Intern Med* 1995;122:823–832.

Ryan TJ, Anderson JL, Antman EM, et al. ACC/AHA guidelines for the management of patients with acute myocardial infarction: executive summary. A report of the American College of Cardiology/American Heart Association Task Force on Practice Guidelines (Committee on Management of Acute Myocardial Infarction). *Circulation* 1996;1:94(9):2341–2350.

Kelley's Textbook of Internal Medicine, fourth edition. Edited by H. David Humes.
Lippincott Williams & Wilkins, Philadelphia © 2000.

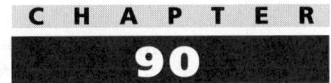

CHAPTER 90

CLINICAL PHARMACOLOGY OF CARDIOVASCULAR DRUGS

D. CRAIG BRATER

This chapter presents some general concepts of clinical pharmacology as applied to specific cardiovascular drugs. The material in this chapter should be combined with that of other chapters in the text dealing with the same drugs and the diseases for which they are used. A general discussion of clinical pharmacology, with definitions of terms and concepts, is presented in Chapter 55. A discussion of specific aspects of clinical pharmacology in the aged appears in Chapter 469 and Chapter 167 covers the adjustment of drug dosages in patients with renal insufficiency.

DRUGS USED FOR CONGESTIVE HEART FAILURE

For a general discussion of the approach to patients with heart failure, see Chapter 66.

ANGIOTENSIN-CONVERTING ENZYME INHIBITORS AND OTHER PRELOAD- AND AFTERLOAD-REDUCING AGENTS

Vasodilators and, particularly, angiotensin-converting enzyme (ACE) inhibitors have revolutionized the treatment of congestive heart failure (CHF). As a result of disappointing results with inotropic agents and particularly because ACE inhibitors are the only class of pharmacologic agent that has proved to have a salutary impact on survival in patients with heart failure, these drugs are indicated in all patients with left ventricular dysfunction, including those who are asymptomatic. A few patients (perhaps 10%) are not able to tolerate ACE inhibitors, primarily owing to persistent cough or hypotension. For the former, angiotensin antagonists are a logical choice. Despite compelling evidence of efficacy, surveys show that the number of patients receiving ACE inhibitors is disappointingly low, even when patients are cared for by a cardiologist. A goal should be that 90% of patients with left ventricular systolic dysfunction receive an ACE inhibitor.

Disposition and Effect

Initial work demonstrating the feasibility of using vasodilators in CHF was performed with nitroprusside. Because nitroprusside has a short duration of action and must be given intravenously, its use was limited to acute studies in intensive care settings.

Nitrate preparations cause venodilation and thereby decrease preload. They are most effective in patients with elevated cardiac filling pressures. In patients whose filling pressures are not increased, nitrates should be avoided or used with caution because profound hypotension can occur. The numerous nitrate preparations available for clinical use have identical pharmacologic effects but differ in their times of onset and durations of action (Table 90.1). Transdermal delivery systems provide remarkably stable blood concentrations of nitroglycerin, but tolerance to the patches or sustained intravenous infusions of nitroglycerin develops within about 8 hours. The cyclic variation in nitroglycerin serum concentrations that occurs with all other preparations allows the vascular endothelium to remain responsive to the nitrate. As such, patches should be removed at night to allow responsiveness to be restored by morning.

Hydralazine and some dihydropyridine calcium antagonists (e.g., amlodipine) have been used to reduce afterload in patients with CHF. Such an effect is particularly useful in patients with increased peripheral vascular resistance and with normal or slightly elevated cardiac filling pressures. In hypotensive patients, afterload reducing agents must be used cautiously if at all because they occasionally cause profound hypotension. If the patient also has increased filling pressure, combining afterload reduction

| TABLE 90.1. | Nitrate Preparations Used for Preload Reduction in Heart Failure and for Angina |

Preparation	Dose Range (mg)	Frequency of Dosing (hr)	Onset of Effect (min)	Duration of Effect (hr)
Glyceryl trinitrate (nitroglycerin)				
Aerosol	1–2 sprays	As needed	8	0.3–0.5
Sublingual	0.15–0.6	0.5	4–8	0.3–0.5
Oral (slow-release)	6.5–19.5	4–6	45–120	4–6
Buccal	1–3	3–4	4–10	6–8
Ointment (2%)	7.5–60 (1/2–4″)	4–6	30–120	3–8
Patches[a]	10–20	12–24	60–180	24
Isosorbide dinitrate				
Sublingual	2.5–15	2–4	15–60	1–3
Oral				
Timed-release	5–80	4–6	45–120	4–6
Chewable	5–10	2–4	60–90	2–3
Isosorbide mononitrate (oral)	20	12	30–60	12
Erythrityl tetranitrate				
Sublingual	5–15	6–8	2	0.2–0.7
Oral	5–30	6–8	60–90	3–6
Pentaerythritol tetranitrate (slow-release)	20–80	4–6	60–90	3–4

[a] For information about patches, see text.

with nitrates is helpful; alternatively, agents with mixed effects are useful.

After oral administration, hydralazine reaches peak concentrations within 30 to 120 minutes. Clinically observed effects occur within 20 to 30 minutes of dosing. Hydralazine has an elimination half-life of 2 to 4 hours, but the biologic effect in both CHF and hypertension appears to be longer. As a result, when used for afterload reduction, dosing every 6 hours is sufficient; when used to treat hypertension, hydralazine can be given every 12 hours. As an antihypertensive, daily doses of hydralazine greater than 200 mg seldom are needed. In contrast, it is unusual for patients with CHF to respond to 200 mg per day, and typical doses in this disorder are 300 to 400 mg per day. The reason for the different dose requirements is unknown but may simply represent the higher degree of peripheral vasoconstriction in severe CHF compared with hypertension. Hydralazine commonly induces sympathetically mediated reflex tachycardia in hypertensive patients, whereas in CHF the improved cardiac function decreases sympathetic tone so that tachycardia is infrequent.

Dihydropyridine calcium channel antagonists decrease arteriolar resistance. Although effective in afterload reduction, they are used more frequently as antianginal or antihypertensive agents. Calcium channel antagonists are discussed in the section on antianginal agents.

ACE inhibitors have relegated all other afterload-reducing regimens to secondary alternatives. A number of these drugs are available. The main distinguishing feature is duration of action and degree of dose adjustment needed in patients with renal insufficiency (Table 90.2). As noted previously, ACE inhibitors extend the life of CHF patients, and they also have documented benefit in patients with asymptomatic left ventricular dysfunction. In the few patients who do not tolerate these drugs, angiotensin antagonists are logical second choices, although they have

not yet been proved to decrease mortality. If neither group of drugs is effective, the combination of nitrates and hydralazine should be considered.

Effects of Disease

Because the usual strategy for use of nitrates is to start with low doses and titrate upward based on clinical response, minor changes in their disposition that might occur are moot. Hydralazine shows no substantial changes in its disposition in various disease states. Dihydropyridine calcium antagonists are discussed in later sections.

The pharmacokinetics of nitroprusside have not been well studied. It is metabolized to thiocyanate, which is eliminated by the kidney over a half-life of 2 or 3 days. As such, the metabolite accumulates in patients with renal insufficiency. The adverse effects of nitroprusside, other than hypotension, are due to thiocyanate. Its accumulation can cause central nervous system (CNS) side effects, such as restlessness, agitation, and toxic psychoses. Because the compound is excreted so slowly, it is important to monitor all patients clinically and with measurements of circulating thiocyanate. Particular caution is needed in patients with renal impairment. If thiocyanate concentrations reach 10 mg per deciliter, caution is paramount and nitroprusside administration should be discontinued. If severe toxicity develops, thiocyanate can be removed by hemodialysis.

Because all ACE inhibitors depend to some degree on the kidney for excretion, their pharmacokinetics are altered in renal impairment (Table 90.2). Dosing needs modification, depending on the level of renal function. In patients with severe renal insufficiency, doses of one-fifth to one-sixth of the normal dose of some of these drugs should be used. The half-lives of ACE inhibitors are prolonged in renal insufficiency, so the time to

TABLE 90.2.	Pharmacokinetic Features of ACE Inhibitors and Angiotensin Antagonists			
		Half-Life (Hours)		
Drug	**Bioavailability (%)**	**Normal Renal Function**	**Severe Renal Insufficiency**	**Dose in Patients with Severe Renal Insufficiency (Fraction of Normal)**
ACE Inhibitors				
Benazepril	28–37	11–20		1/4
Captopril	60–70	2	20	1/6
Cilazapril	45–75	36–49		1/4
Delapril		1.2	2.3	1/2
Enalapril	36–44	5	15	1/3
Fosinopril	25–29	11–15	17–32	1/2
Imidapril	40	8–14	35	1/2
Lisinopril	25–50	30	54	1/2
Moexipril	22			1/4
Pentopril		4		Avoid
Perindopril	17–20	1.2–5	27	1/10
Quinapril	46–60	2	32	1/4
Ramipril	28	7–11	16	2/3
Spirapril	50	2		1/3
Temocapril		7–15	8–20	1/2
Trandolapril	40–60	16–242		1/3
Angiotensin Antagonists				
Candesartan	42	9–13	13	1/2
Eposartan	6–29	5–7		2/3
Irbesartan	60–80	12–20		No change
Losartan	33–36	2–3		No change
Telmisartan	43	24		Unknown
Valsartan	23–39	5–10		Unknown

ACE, angiotensin-converting enzyme.

reach steady state is greater (four times the half-life). The frequency of dose increments should be such that steady state is attained at one dose before a change is made. In other clinical conditions such as CHF and in the elderly, no additional changes in disposition appear to occur, except those caused by the patient's renal function. Similar considerations apply to angiotensin antagonists (Table 90.2).

Drug Interactions

Pharmacokinetic drug interactions have not been described with these preload- and afterload-reducing agents. Various pharmacodynamic interactions can occur with other drugs affecting cardiovascular hemodynamics. These are predictable based on the additive pharmacology of the drugs; a good example is the combined effect of nitrates and hydralazine.

DIURETICS

Disposition and Effect

All diuretics except spironolactone must reach the urine to be effective, because their active sites are on the luminal surface of renal tubular cells. As such, patients with renal insufficiency may have very high serum concentrations of a diuretic but negligible

response because no drug can reach the urinary site of action. Hence, therapeutic strategies with diuretics are based on attaining sufficient amounts of drug in the urine.

The carbonic anhydrase inhibitor acetazolamide has a half-life of 13 hours, which extrapolates to a time needed to reach steady state of 2 to 3 days.

Mannitol inhibits sodium reabsorption throughout the nephron, with predominant effects at the proximal tubule and the thick ascending limb of the loop of Henle. In patients with severe renal disease, the half-life of mannitol increases from about 1 to 36 hours. Its administration in such patients can result in retention of mannitol with potentially disastrous consequences as the osmotic effect draws water into the vascular space, resulting in volume expansion, which can be sufficient to precipitate heart failure. Mannitol should be used with caution (if at all) in patients with renal insufficiency.

Unlike mannitol, which is filtered at the glomerulus, loop diuretics enter the tubular lumen by being actively secreted by the organic acid transport pathway of the proximal tubule. Negligible amounts of these drugs are filtered because they are highly bound to serum proteins, as reflected by their small volumes of distribution. The renal elimination of bumetanide and furosemide is fast, accounting for their short half-lives (1 hour). Ethacrynic acid probably has similar pharmacokinetic characteristics.

Torsemide is a longer-acting agent, with a half-life of about 4 hours.

The efficacy of the loop diuretics, combined with the short half-life, extrapolates to an intense, short-lived diuresis. In patients with normal renal function, peak diuretic effect occurs within 30 minutes after intravenous dosing and within 1 to 2 hours after oral administration. The diuresis then lasts for 2 to 3 hours (4 to 6 hours for torsemide), after which the kidney's reabsorptive capacities for sodium return. In fact, in this postdiuretic recovery period, the nephron avidly reabsorbs sodium; if dietary intake is too high, the sodium loss caused by the drug can be completely nullified by sodium retention. Therefore, dietary sodium restriction is an important adjunct to therapy with these agents.

Response to all the loop diuretics appears similar. The maximal response in terms of the fractional excretion rate of sodium is about 20%. This compares with a value of about 5% for thiazide diuretics. The loop diuretics differ in terms of potency; that is, different amounts are used to elicit the same response. As such, 1 mg of bumetanide equals 20 mg of torsemide, 40 mg of furosemide, and 50 mg of ethacrynic acid. Because ethacrynic acid has been reported to be more likely to cause ototoxicity, it is less commonly used. Torsemide use has recently been shown to decrease hospitalization rates and improve quality of life compared with furosemide in patients with CHF. This is presumably due to its complete and predictable absorption and longer duration of effect.

Thiazide diuretics also reach the urine by active secretion at the proximal tubule. They have a minor effect to inhibit sodium reabsorption in the proximal nephron and cause most of their effect by blocking sodium reabsorption at the distal tubule. Many different thiazide compounds are marketed, with limited or no data available concerning their pharmacokinetics. The maximal natriuretic response obtainable with each is the same, but they differ in potency (i.e., different milligram amounts are used). The only clinically relevant difference is the duration of action: short (1 to 5 hours; bendroflumethiazide and trichloromethiazide), intermediate (5 to 15 hours; hydrochlorothiazide, hydroflumethiazide, and indapamide), and long-acting (15 to 50 hours; the remainder plus metolazone). The choice of drug should depend on the desired duration of action. Unwanted potassium loss appears to be greatest with the long-acting thiazides, and in most settings short- or intermediate-acting agents are preferable. The choice is probably best determined by which is least expensive.

Although the efficacy of thiazides is modest and as single agents they are not effective in most patients with CHF, thiazides can be particularly effective when combined with loop diuretics. Chronic dosing with loop diuretics can result in diminished efficacy over time owing to hypertrophy of distal nephron segments wherein they avidly retain sodium. These nephron sites are blocked by thiazide diuretics so that their combination with a loop diuretic results in a synergistic response. The combination also results in substantial potassium loss so that patients must be monitored for development of hypokalemia. In addition, the overall diuretic response in some patients can be substantial and actually result in severe volume depletion. Thus, patients should

be monitored frequently at the outset of such combination therapy.

Distally acting agents act at portions of the nephron where potassium is secreted. Hence, in addition to inducing sodium excretion, they block potassium excretion and are commonly referred to as potassium-retaining or potassium-sparing diuretics. All other diuretics cause potassium loss concomitant with natriuresis. Amiloride and triamterene differ from spironolactone in acting independently of aldosterone, in reaching their sites of action from the lumen rather than the peritubular side of the nephron, and in being secreted into the lumen by the organic base transport pathway of the proximal tubule. Amiloride (7 to 11 hours) and triamterene (2 to 5 hours) have relatively short elimination half-lives, so their onset of action is quick and they reach steady state within about 1 day. Triamterene's activity resides in a sulfate ester conjugate. Clinically, the effects of both drugs are similar. The natriuretic effects of all distally acting diuretics are small, so they are used more frequently for their potassium-retaining properties than as natriuretic agents.

Spironolactone is a competitive antagonist of aldosterone and acts by eliminating the effects of this mineralocorticoid. The disposition of spironolactone is complex and poorly understood. The drug is a long-acting agent and requires 3 or 4 days to reach maximum effect, so nothing is gained by changing doses more frequently. Because of these kinetic characteristics and the dependence on aldosterone for efficacy, when used as a diuretic spironolactone is best reserved for settings of primary or secondary (e.g., hepatic cirrhosis) hyperaldosteronism.

Effects of Disease

As renal function declines either because of primary renal disease or as a secondary manifestation of other conditions like CHF, the access of diuretics into the urine decreases in parallel. As such, in patients with creatinine clearance values less than about 40 mL per minute, all diuretics except those affecting the loop of Henle have negligible effects as single agents. In addition, distally acting diuretics carry an unacceptable risk of producing hyperkalemia in patients with renal impairment and are contraindicated. Hence, the mainstay of diuretic therapy in patients with diminished renal function of any cause is loop diuretics. These agents retain their efficacy in patients with renal insufficiency if adequate amounts of the diuretic reach the site of action. The therapeutic strategy in such patients is to administer a large enough dose to allow delivery of adequate amounts of diuretic into the urine. This can be accomplished with the doses suggested in Table 90.3.

Diuretics are mainstays of therapy in patients with heart failure, although no formal efficacy trials have been conducted. If renal function is normal in these patients, loop diuretics are delivered to the site of action as efficiently as in normal subjects. It is reasonable to presume that the same is true for other diuretics. Because many patients with heart failure have mild decrements in renal function, they most likely need doses two or three times greater than normal. Such a strategy ensures sufficient access of diuretic into the urine with negligible risks. Even when sufficient drug reaches the nephron in such patients, the tubular response is subnormal and the maximal sodium excre-

TABLE 90.3. Maximum Single Doses of Loop Diuretics in Various Clinical Conditions

Clinical Condition	Dose of Loop Diuretic (mg)					
	Bumetanide		Furosemide		Torsemide	
	IV	Oral	IV	Oral	IV	Oral
Renal insufficiency						
$Cl_{Cr} < 50$	2–3	2–3	80–120	160–240	20–50	20–50
$Cl_{Cr} < 20$	6–8	6–8	160–200	320–400	50–100	50–100
Nephrotic syndrome	2–4	2–4	80–160	160–320	50–100	50–100
Cirrhosis	1	1	40	80	10	10
Congestive heart failure	2–3	2–3	40–80	80–160	50–100	50–100

Cl_{Cr}, creatinine clearance; IV, intravenous.

tion rate attainable is diminished (e.g., to about 10% of filtered sodium). Clinically, this phenomenon means that the patient will never have the intensity of diuretic response that occurs normally. Yet, larger single doses of diuretic are not useful in overcoming this effect; instead, effective doses should be administered more frequently, such as three or four times a day rather than once or twice.

Patients with hepatic cirrhosis commonly develop secondary hyperaldosteronism; as a result, the drug of choice is spironolactone. The dose must be titrated to a level sufficient to block the effects of endogenous aldosterone, realizing that dosage changes require 3 or 4 days to reach a steady state. Because renal function is relatively normal in patients with cirrhosis, the diuretics that must reach the urine to be active retain their efficacy, but response is subnormal. Because of this change in the pharmacodynamics of response, effective doses often must be administered more frequently to obtain the needed overall response.

Patients with nephrotic syndrome and normal glomerular filtration rates deliver normal amounts of diuretic into the urine. Much of this drug can bind to the albumin in the urine, which is the hallmark of this condition. As such, doses two to four times normal are needed to result in adequate amounts of unbound, pharmacologically active drug at the site of action.

In the edematous disorders, one might speculate that the absorption of drugs would be altered; edema of the gut wall, altered intestinal perfusion, or changed gastrointestinal motility all might affect absorption. Studies in patients with nephrotic syndrome, cirrhosis, and heart failure have shown normal bioavailability of loop diuretics, although the time course of absorption is slowed. Oral doses do not have to be increased in those with the edematous disorders to compensate for malabsorption.

Drug Interactions

Nonsteroidal anti-inflammatory drugs (including aspirin) decrease the effects of probably all diuretics. This most likely occurs by an independent effect of these drugs to stimulate sodium reabsorption at the thick ascending limb, thus diminishing the overall response to the diuretic. Clinically, the effect is often minor or negligible, but it is sometimes sufficient to require

discontinuing the nonsteroidal drug, increasing the diuretic dose, or switching to a more effective diuretic.

Diuretic agents lower blood pressure and are often used as antihypertensives. Their effects are predictably additive to other antihypertensives. In addition, with many nondiuretic antihypertensives, reflex fluid retention occurs, expanding intravascular volume and nullifying the blood pressure-lowering effect. This phenomenon is called *pseudotolerance,* because it does not represent true tolerance to the drug. Use of a diuretic in this setting often causes a synergistic antihypertensive effect.

CARDIAC GLYCOSIDES

The positive inotropic effect of digitalis glycosides has been believed to be particularly beneficial for heart failure, and their electrophysiologic effect—slowing conduction through the atrioventricular node—has been useful for controlling the rate of ventricular response in patients with atrial fibrillation. However, until recently, a definitive trial assessing the efficacy of digoxin had not been conducted. The Digitalis Investigation Group (DIG) trial has now shown that digoxin does not affect mortality but that in patients with left ventricular ejection fractions less than 0.45 it improves symptoms and decreases morbidity. Thus, digoxin is a logical choice in such patients who have not responded adequately to ACE inhibitors and diuretics.

Questions have also been raised about the efficacy of digitalis glycosides in patients with atrial fibrillation. In this setting, these drugs have been used both to convert patients to sinus rhythm and to control the rate of ventricular response in patients with persistent atrial fibrillation. One study found that digoxin was no different from placebo in converting to sinus rhythm in patients who had been in atrial fibrillation for 7 days or less. Other drugs may be more efficacious in this setting, although direct comparative trials have not been performed. Digitalis glycosides clearly are effective in maintaining the rate of ventricular response in patients with atrial fibrillation. However, these drugs often do not satisfactorily control the ventricular response during exercise, particularly in younger patients. Other drugs, such as verapamil and diltiazem, are effective both at rest and during exercise and may be preferable in many patients.

TABLE 90.4.	Pharmacokinetic Properties of Digoxin
Bioavailability (%)	75
Renal excretion (%)	70
Volume of distribution (L/kg)	3.12 Cl_{Cr} + 3.84
Clearance (mL/min/kg)	
No heart failure	1.02 Cl_{Cr} + 0.81
Heart failure	0.88 Cl_{Cr} + 0.33
Half-life (hr)	40
Therapeutic range (ng/mL)	0.8–2.0

Disposition and Effect

Although other preparations of cardiac glycosides are available, digoxin and digitoxin are those used clinically. Digoxin's use is so dominant that it alone is discussed here. Digoxin is eliminated predominantly by the kidney and thus requires dosage adjustment in patients with diminished renal function.

Parameters for digoxin pharmacokinetics are listed in Table 90.4. Both the volume of distribution and the clearance of digoxin depend on renal function. Therapy often is initiated with a loading dose, although this strategy results in a higher incidence of toxicity than if a maintenance dose is used and steady-state serum concentrations are gradually attained. Hence, a loading dose should not be used unless therapeutic effects are truly needed quickly.

If a loading dose of digoxin is to be given, it can be calculated (as discussed in Chapter 56) based on the patient's weight and renal function from the values in Table 90.4. It can be given intravenously, intramuscularly, or orally (preferred, except in the emergency setting). Intravenous administration results in transient arteriolar constriction with increased peripheral vascular resistance, an undesirable effect in patients with heart failure. Intramuscular administration often can result in erratic absorption. Although decreases in splanchnic blood flow or edema of the gut in cardiac disease might be predicted to cause malabsorption of cardiac glycosides, there is no evidence that this occurs. Lastly, if a loading dose is given, spreading the dose over a 24-hour period in four divided doses is sufficient and prevents the high serum concentrations that occur with a large single dose. Because of the long half-life of digoxin, dosing can be limited to once a day, which facilitates compliance. Maintenance doses must be based on renal function.

The therapeutic range for digoxin serum concentrations is listed in Table 90.4. Values must be interpreted relative to each patient because there is considerable overlap between therapeutic and toxic concentrations. For example, patients with atrial fibrillation often require serum concentrations considerably higher than normal to control the rate of ventricular response, and they do not suffer adverse effects. In contrast, numerous conditions increase the sensitivity to the toxic effects of digitalis glycosides, such as potassium and magnesium depletion and hypercalcemia. In these settings, normal glycoside serum concentrations can be associated with toxicity. Hence, serum concentration measurements should be interpreted in the context of clinically evaluated end points of drug efficacy and toxicity.

Digitalis toxicity occurs frequently, with most surveys finding an incidence in hospitalized patients of about 15%. Toxicity can be fatal, particularly if it goes unrecognized, emphasizing the importance of maintaining a high index of suspicion. Although classic symptoms of digitalis intoxication occasionally occur, symptoms are more commonly absent or are nonspecific (e.g., nausea) and could be caused by the primary disease. Similarly, although some cardiac dysrhythmias are classically associated with digitalis toxicity, ventricular premature beats are most common, and toxicity can cause virtually any dysrhythmia. Digitalis toxicity is often difficult to diagnose because many of its manifestations may be attributable to exacerbation of the primary disease. Obtaining glycoside serum concentrations can sometimes be helpful. If these concentrations are high, a clinical diagnosis of toxicity is supported but not confirmed. If the concentrations are normal, however, toxicity still cannot be excluded, because many conditions (e.g., hypokalemia) increase sensitivity to the toxic effects of digitalis. A very low concentration is evidence against a diagnosis of toxicity, but exclusion of digitalis as the culprit occurs only if the concentration is zero. A definitive diagnosis is established only when the signs or symptoms revert with cessation of digitalis administration.

If digitalis toxicity is diagnosed, the drug should be stopped while factors are assessed that may have increased the sensitivity to the effects of the glycoside. If found, such factors should be treated (e.g., with administration of potassium or magnesium supplements). Treatment of life-threatening ventricular dysrhythmias should avoid quinidine-like agents and focus on lidocaine-like drugs or phenytoin. The latter may be particularly effective for digitalis toxic dysrhythmias. If toxicity is severe, antigen-binding fragments (Fab) can be used to bind digitalis glycosides and remove them from sites of activity.

If glycoside serum concentrations are measured, the cautions noted in Chapter 55 must be followed. The largest source of error that renders laboratory values uninterpretable is sampling during the long distribution phase (up to 6 hours) of digitalis glycosides. This pitfall can be avoided by obtaining samples just before the patient is to receive the next dose (a trough concentration)

Effects of Disease

Digoxin has been studied extensively in various disease states. As indicated in Table 90.4, both the volume of distribution and the clearance depend on renal function. Digoxin excretion by the kidney occurs by filtration at the glomerulus and secretion into the urine at the distal nephron. Secretion occurs via the same P-glycoprotein that accounts for multidrug resistance to many chemotherapeutic agents. As discussed in the following section on drug interaction, this secretory component is subject to inhibition by other drugs. It also appears that reabsorption of filtered drug can occur in the renal proximal tubule. This reabsorptive component is enhanced in settings of prerenal azotemia in which overall proximal tubular reabsorption is increased. As a result, in patients with volume depletion or with exacerbated heart failure in which prerenal effects occur, the reabsorption of digoxin increases, thereby decreasing renal elimination over and above the effects of decreased glomerular filtration itself. Clinically, patients with prerenal azotemia may need even greater reductions in digoxin maintenance doses than dictated by their creatinine clearance. Caution should be used in such patients. Otherwise, maintenance doses of digoxin can be calculated from the values in Table 90.4.

Elderly patients need dosage adjustment based on renal function; in other words, there is no change in clearance due to age itself.

Thyroid disease has an independent effect on digoxin clearance. Hyperthyroidism results in increased clearance, with the converse in hypothyroidism. By unclear mechanisms, the same directional relations occur with the volume of distribution. Hence, in patients with thyroid disease, both loading and maintenance doses of digoxin should be adjusted. As thyroid function normalizes, so do the kinetic parameters of digoxin, which will require changes in dosing.

Drug Interactions

Because of the narrow therapeutic range of digitalis glycosides, drug interactions have been assiduously sought. Several drugs can affect the absorption of cardiac glycosides. The bile acid sequestrants cholestyramine and colestipol bind digoxin and digitoxin in the gut and can prevent or diminish their absorption (i.e., decrease bioavailability). If patients are receiving a cardiac glycoside and one of these agents, the interaction probably can be avoided if the glycoside is taken either 1 hour before or at least 4 hours after the sequestrant.

Interactions to decrease the absorption of digoxin have been reported with various other drugs, including antacids, kaolin-pectin, neomycin, and sulfasalazine. Their occurrence is less predictable than with the bile acid sequestrants, but their potential should be kept in mind. To avoid such interactions, doses of glycosides can be separated from those of potential interactants.

About 10% of patients harbor colonic bacteria that can degrade digoxin. This may be the case in a patient who needs large doses of digoxin to attain normal serum concentrations of the drug. If these bacteria are killed by broad-spectrum antibiotics, degradation diminishes, allowing more drug to be absorbed. In such patients, if a broad-spectrum antibiotic is started, digoxin serum concentrations should be observed closely so that appropriate dosage reduction can be instituted before toxicity ensues.

A unique approach to treating digoxin toxicity (particularly overdoses) uses Fab to change the distribution of digoxin, effectively extracting it into the circulation from tissue sites of action (e.g., cardiac muscle). Digoxin serum concentrations increase considerably when Fab fragments are administered, but the pharmacologic effect of the glycoside is diminished because the measured amounts in serum are bound to the Fab fragments and are therefore inactive. These drug–Fab complexes then can be excreted by the kidney.

Several drugs, especially quinidine, decrease the secretory component of the renal excretion of digoxin by blocking P-glycoprotein. An interaction occurs in at least 90% of patients who are administered both quinidine and digoxin, with a doubling of the digoxin serum concentration. Hence, maintenance of a constant serum concentration requires halving the dose. There is some debate as to whether the increased serum concentration during this interaction extrapolates to increased cardiac

effects and risk of toxicity. Most authorities recommend adjusting the digoxin dose to attain the same concentration as would be sought when using digoxin alone. Because the interaction with quinidine is so predictable, the digoxin dose should be halved if concomitant quinidine therapy is begun. The similar interaction that occurs with amiodarone, spironolactone, verapamil, flecainide, and diltiazem is less predictable in terms of magnitude of effect, so with these interactants, the dose of digoxin should be adjusted based on measured serum concentrations.

Numerous pharmacodynamic interactions occur with cardiac glycosides, predominantly by increasing sensitivity to their toxic effects. Drugs causing potassium or magnesium depletion or hypercalcemia increase the risk of toxicity. In these settings, the physician must rely on clinical end points of therapeutic response rather than on measured concentrations.

NONGLYCOSIDE INOTROPIC AGENTS

Because of disappointments with the overall efficacy of digitalis glycosides, other inotropic agents have been and are still being explored. These include sympathomimetic agents and drugs that inhibit cardiac phosphodiesterase. The phosphodiesterase inhibitors have generally been disappointing, particularly because of their early promise. The first of these agents, amrinone, showed short-term efficacy but caused thrombocytopenia with long-term use. Milrinone and similar agents appeared to be promising initially, but long-term efficacy trials showed increases in mortality. Milrinone is now available for intravenous infusion for short-term use. There are no promising agents of this type on the horizon.

Disposition and Effect

Dopamine is an endogenous catecholamine. Its clinical usefulness relates to its activation of cardiac β_1-receptors to increase inotropism, its activation of renal dopaminergic receptors to increase renal blood flow, and its activation at higher doses of peripheral α-adrenergic receptors to cause vasoconstriction. The last effect is often unwanted, and dosing is usually aimed at maintaining infusion rates low enough to avoid increases in peripheral vascular resistance. Because dopamine is eliminated rapidly, it must be administered as a continuous intravenous infusion, with titration of the rate according to monitored end points of its cardiovascular effects. Typical infusion rates are 10 to 30 μg per kilogram per minute; α-mediated vasoconstriction becomes more prevalent at greater doses.

Dobutamine has for the most part supplanted dopamine as an inotropic agent. It does not increase peripheral vascular resistance. Dobutamine has a short half-life (about 2.5 minutes) with a large clearance (60 mL per kilogram per minute) and a small volume of distribution (0.2 L per kilogram). It is administered as a continuous intravenous infusion; the short half-life means that steady state is attained within about 10 minutes. Hence, the dose can readily be titrated according to cardiovascular end points, with usual infusion rates of 2.5 to 10 μg per kilogram per minute.

Milrinone is available for intravenous administration in patients refractory to other agents. It causes peripheral vasodilation and positive inotropic effects. Its salutary effect most likely occurs by both mechanisms. A loading dose of 50 mg per kilogram is administered based on a volume of distribution of about 0.45 L per kilogram. Maintenance doses are usually 0.375 to 0.75 μg per kilogram per minute, with rates titrated according to response. When the dosing rate is changed, however, the physician must remember that about 5 hours is required to reach new steady-state concentrations. Clearance is about 5 mL per kilogram per minute and depends on renal function. The half-life may increase from 1 to about 3 hours in patients with renal insufficiency. Patients with severe renal insufficiency should receive doses that are one-third of those of patients with preserved renal function.

Effects of Disease

No studies have assessed the influence of diseases on the disposition of and response to sympathomimetic agents. Because the infusion rates of these drugs can be so readily titrated against clinical response, there is little need for such data. The pharmacokinetics of milrinone differ in patients with renal insufficiency compared with normal volunteers, mandating dose adjustment as previously indicated.

Drug Interactions

Dopamine is metabolized by monoamine oxidase. Hence, inhibitors of this enzyme can greatly impair the clearance of dopamine, and caution should be used if they are given together. In contrast, dobutamine is metabolized by catechol O-methyltransferase, so the same considerations do not apply. Drug interactions have not been described with milrinone.

β-ADRENERGIC ANTAGONISTS

Disposition, effects of disease, and drug interactions with β-adrenergic antagonists will be discussed in the section on antianginal agents. Historically, these drugs were thought to be contraindicated in patients with CHF owing to their negative inotropic effects and potential ability to precipitate CHF itself. More recent studies have shown that the elevated sympathetic tone in patients with CHF has long-term deleterious effects; as such, β-antagonists can be efficacious. Short-term studies with a variety of agents (metoprolol, bisoprolol, practolol, alprenolol, acebutolol, bucindolol, labetalol, and carvedilol) showed that they could be used safely and that they improved cardiac function and alleviated symptoms. More recently, larger long-term trials, particularly with carvedilol and metoprolol have indicated decreases in mortality. β-Adrenergic antagonists clearly are helpful in patients with symptomatic systolic dysfunction. Whether all β-antagonists have the same efficacy is not known, so it is prudent to use those with proven benefit.

ANTIARRHYTHMIC AGENTS

Disposition and Effect

Antiarrhythmic agents can be broadly grouped according to their electrophysiologic effects on the heart, as discussed in Chapter 76, but these classifications are less than optimal because they do not precisely take into account all mechanisms of action. Pharmacokinetic parameters are presented in Table 90.5 for the strictly antiarrhythmic drugs. β-Adrenergic antagonists and calcium channel antagonists are discussed with antianginal agents.

Therapy with all the quinidine-like drugs is complicated because all are converted to active metabolites and because the short half-lives mandate either frequent dosing or use of a sustained-release preparation. The contribution of quinidine's metabolite to overall pharmacologic effect is debated; in contrast, it is clear that N-acetylprocainamide (NAPA) and mono-N-desisopropyldisopyramide (MND) are active. With NAPA, the rate of formation depends on whether a patient is a fast or slow acetylator of procainamide. Its elimination depends on the level of renal function. On average, a patient with normal renal function has higher serum concentrations of procainamide than of NAPA, and therapy can be based on measurements of procainamide serum concentrations and clinical evaluation. With decreased renal function, however, NAPA preferentially accumulates and may greatly exceed procainamide concentrations. Because the two compounds have different cardiac effects, interpreting serum concentrations becomes impossible. Instead, emphasis should be placed on clinical end points of response. Alternatively, procainamide can be avoided in patients with renal disease.

The metabolite of disopyramide (i.e., MND) has only about one-fourth the efficacy of the parent drug as an antiarrhythmic, but its effects are 20 times greater as an anticholinergic agent. Its accumulation in patients with renal disease increases the risks of adverse effects from disopyramide, so, if possible, this drug should be avoided in such patients.

Use of the quinidine-like drugs sometimes requires a loading dose, which can be given orally or intravenously (except disopyramide). The latter route must be used with caution because profound hypotension can occur if the rate is too rapid (particularly with quinidine). Infusion rates of 10 to 20 mg per minute should be used, with careful monitoring of the patient.

Lidocaine is the agent of choice for ventricular tachyarrhythmias in most patients, particularly those with an acute myocardial infarction. It has poor bioavailability because of a large first-pass effect, so its use has been restricted to parenteral administration. Mexiletine and tocainide were developed as lidocaine-like agents that could be given orally. Lidocaine is converted in the liver to monoethylglycinexylidide (MEGX) and other metabolites. MEGX does not contribute to the beneficial effects of lidocaine but instead is thought by some to contribute to the CNS toxicity associated with lidocaine (agitation, restlessness, and, in its worst form, seizures).

Lidocaine therapy usually is instituted with a loading dose calculated from the volume of distribution (Table 90.5), which is affected by different disease states. Several methods are used for loading, the most common of which is repeated bolus administration of 50- to 100-mg doses every 10 to 15 minutes. Rapid-bolus administration results in very high serum lidocaine concentrations for a short time, which are sufficient to cause CNS side effects. A better method for attaining desired concentrations is to calculate the total loading dose needed and then to administer half the amount as a bolus injection over 2 to 3 minutes.

TABLE 90.5.	PHARMACOKINETIC PARAMETERS OF SOME ANTIARRHYTHMIC DRUGS						
Drug	Bioavailability (%)	Renal Excretion (%)	Active Metabolites	Vd (L/kg)	Cl (mL/min/kg)	Half-Life (hr)	Effect of Disease
Amiodarone	22–86	0	Desethylamiodarone	70	2	25–50 days	Renal disease: presumably no change
Bretylium	25	100	None	5.0	10	6–11	Renal disease: 1/5 normal Cl
Cibenzoline	85–100	50–60	None	4.0–7.3	9–15	6–15	Renal disease: 1/3 normal Cl CHF: 2/3 normal Vd; normal Cl Elderly; 1/2 normal Vd; 1/2 normal Cl
Disopyramide	65–85	40–60	Mono-N-desisopropyl disopyramide (MND)	0.6	1.5–2.1	4–10	Renal disease: ↓ Cl of parent and MND Cirrhosis: 3/4 normal Cl CHF: 1/2 normal Cl
Dofetilide	>90	70	None	3.3	5.8	7	Renal disease: 1/4 normal Cl
Flecainide	90–95	40	Meta-O-desalkyl-flecainide	5.5–7.3	9–16	7–12	Cirrhosis: 1/5 normal Cl
Ibutilide		<5	Negligible effects	11–15	24–31	6–9	Renal disease: no change Elderly: no change CHF: no change
Lidocaine	30	5	Monoethylglycine-xylidide (MEGX)	1.6	10	1.5–2	Renal disease: No change Cirrhosis: 1 1/2 normal Vd; 1/2 normal Cl; bioavailability 90% CHF: 1/2 normal Vd; 1/2 normal Cl
Mexiletine	90	30–55	None	5.9–10.1	6.3–8.3	8–12	Renal disease: no change AMI: no change Cirrhosis: 1/4 to 1/3 normal Cl
N-acetylprocainamide (NAPA)	80–90	60–85	None	1.2–1.7	2–3.3	6–10	Renal disease: 1/4 normal Cl
Phenytoin	100	2	None	0.6	$V_{max} = 8.4$ mg/kg/d $K_m = 8.5$ mg/L	24	Renal disease: ↓ protein binding Cirrhosis: ↓ binding
Procainamide	75–85	50–70	NAPA	2.4	8.5–10	2.5–3.5	Renal disease: accumulation of parent and NAPA CHF: no change
Propafenone	5–12	<1	5-OH-propafenone	2.5–4.4	11–14	3–17	Renal disease: no change Cirrhosis: ↓ Cl
Quinidine	70–80	15–40	3-OH-quinidine (contribution to effect unknown)	2–3.5	2.5–5	5–12	Renal disease: no change Elderly: 1/2 normal Cl CHF: 1/2 normal Vd and 1/2 normal Cl
Sotalol	100	75–90	None	0.7–2.4	1.5–2.1	5–8	Renal disease: 1/5 normal Cl
Tocainide	90–100	40	None	2.2	2–2.5	12–14	Renal disease: 1/2–1/4 normal Cl CHF: no change

AMI, acute myocardial infarction; CHF, congestive heart failure; Cl, clearance; Vd, volume of distribution.

The rest of the bolus is then given as a continuous infusion over 20 minutes, followed by the maintenance infusion rate calculated from the clearance of lidocaine and the target steady-state serum concentration.

In some patients, the serum concentration of lidocaine increases after maintenance on the same dose for 24 hours or more. With time, the protein binding of lidocaine increases because the concentration of the binding protein, α_1-acid glycoprotein (an acute-phase reactant), increases. The unbound, pharmacologically active concentration of lidocaine remains unchanged, and hence no dose adjustment is necessary. Because conventional clinical laboratories measure only total serum concentrations of drugs, as opposed to unbound, free concentrations, it is impossible for the clinician to know whether an increased lidocaine concentration in this setting is due to a change in elimination or to the protein-binding phenomenon described. As a result, it is important to correlate clinical assessment with the laboratory measurement and with other indexes of response.

Mexiletine and tocainide are well absorbed and have half-lives that allow dosing two or three times a day. Both drugs are rapidly absorbed, so that sufficiently high peak concentrations occur to cause adverse effects (CNS effects, nausea, vomiting) in many patients. The rate of absorption can be slowed without affecting the extent of absorption (bioavailability) by simply taking the medication with a meal. Because the extent of absorption is not affected, the average steady-state concentration is not altered by this maneuver; instead, the magnitude of difference between peak and trough concentrations is minimized.

Flecainide, encainide (now discontinued), and propafenone modify fast sodium channels. It was thought originally that these drugs would have wide application for the treatment of ventricular dysrhythmias. However, the use of encainide and flecainide was found to increase mortality in patients with ventricular ectopy after a myocardial infarction due to proarrhythmic effects. Propafenone has a complicated pharmacology. It is administered as a racemic mixture; one stereoisomer is a sodium channel blocker; the other, a β-adrenergic antagonist. In addition, propafenone is converted to an active metabolite by CYP2D6. This isoenzyme is polymorphically distributed, such that about 10% of whites are poor metabolizers and cannot form the active metabolite.

Phenytoin is most often used as an anticonvulsant but can be of benefit in some dysrhythmias, particularly those caused by digitalis. Its pharmacokinetics are complex because at clinically used doses it obeys Michaelis–Menten (saturable) kinetics. As such, an increase in dose may result in a disproportionate increase in the serum concentration. For example, if a dosage of phenytoin of 150 mg per day results in a serum concentration of 7.5 mg per liter, a doubling of the dose to 300 mg per day may result in a doubled serum concentration of 15 mg per liter. A further increase in dose to 400 mg per day, however, may not result in a proportional increase in serum concentration to 20 mg per liter, but rather cause the concentration to increase to 30 mg per liter, with a risk of toxicity. When increasing doses of phenytoin, small increments should be used. Because the half-life of phenytoin is at least 1 day, when doses are changed about 1 week must elapse before a new steady state is reached. The half-life is long enough to allow once-a-day dosing.

It is occasionally necessary to administer a loading dose of phenytoin (usually about 1 g in adults). Loading doses can be given intravenously or, preferably, orally. Phenytoin precipitates in many intravenous solutions, and it is best given as a slow bolus dose directly into an accessible port as proximal to the patient as possible. The total loading dose should be divided into 200- to 300-mg doses, which can be administered every 30 to 60 minutes orally or intravenously.

Bretylium, amiodarone, N-acetylprocainamide, sotalol, ibutilide, and dofetilide are antiarrhythmic agents that prolong repolarization. Bretylium and sotalol were developed first as antihypertensives. The efficacy of both was poor compared with that of the other agents, so they have not been used to treat hypertension. Bretylium, used for refractory ventricular tachyarrhythmias, is administered almost exclusively in intensive care unit settings as intermittent intravenous doses or as a constant intravenous infusion. Loading doses of bretylium can be given as two or three single intravenous boluses of 5 to 10 mg per kilogram every 5 to 10 minutes; alternatively, 5 to 10 mg per kilogram can be infused over 15 minutes and repeated twice if needed. With initial administration, bretylium causes catecholamine release from peripheral nerve endings, which increases blood pressure. The catecholamine depletion that follows can cause hypotension.

Amiodarone is effective in many patients with dysrhythmias refractory to other agents. The disposition of amiodarone also makes it difficult to use. Its exceedingly long half-life—usually 25 to 50 days but sometimes 100 days or more—means that a change in dosage does not result in a new steady state for 6 months or more. Similarly, if the patient develops adverse effects, considerable time is required for the drug to dissipate. Because of the length of time needed to reach steady state, a loading dose is usually given. Although numerous dosing schedules have been proposed, a reasonable approach would be 1,200 mg per day for 2 weeks; the usual maintenance dose of 400 mg per day alternating with 600 mg per day then is instituted.

NAPA, the active metabolite of procainamide, has been developed as an antiarrhythmic agent itself. NAPA has different electrophysiologic effects than procainamide, and its use prevents one of the most common adverse effects of procainamide—drug-induced systemic lupus erythematosus. NAPA has good bioavailability and is eliminated predominantly by renal routes; its relatively short half-life requires frequent dosing.

Sotalol, ibutilide, and dofetilide prolong the QT interval and thereby are unequivocally associated with risk of torsades de pointes. Use of these drugs should be by cardiologists who are expert in arrhythmias and their treatment. Adenosine has proved extremely useful in converting supraventricular tachyarrhythmias to sinus rhythm. It is given as a 6-mg bolus dose, repeated in 10 minutes, if necessary. Many patients have a sensation of shortness of breath with its administration.

Effects of Disease

The influence of disease on the disposition of antiarrhythmics can be anticipated by the data in Table 90.5 that specify the routes of excretion of the individual drugs. For agents with predominant excretion by renal routes, renal disease (including the moderate renal decline of the elderly) decreases clearance and requires modification of maintenance doses. In contrast, if hepatic elimination predominates, primary liver disease and congestive hepatopathy affect clearance. Although studies have assessed the influence of various clinical conditions on the disposition of antiarrhythmic agents, many gaps in our knowledge remain and caution should be used if a potential elimination pathway is affected by the patient's disease.

Quinidine is primarily eliminated by hepatic routes, and renal insufficiency does not appreciably affect its pharmacokinetics. Elderly patients and patients with CHF have clearances of quinidine that are about half of normal, so maintenance doses should be about half those normally used. The dose then can be increased if needed, based on measured quinidine serum concentrations and clinical response. By mechanisms that are not understood, patients with CHF also have a diminished volume of distribution for quinidine; in such patients, if a loading dose is given, it should be half that normally used.

The disposition of procainamide is complex because of its conversion to NAPA. In patients with renal impairment, both parent drug and NAPA accumulate, the latter preferentially because it is more dependent on renal routes of elimination than is procainamide. If procainamide must be used in such patients, caution is mandatory. In patients with CHF, the disposition of procainamide is unchanged.

Disopyramide and its metabolite accumulate in patients with renal disease. Because the metabolite has greater potency in terms of adverse anticholinergic side effects, its accumulation in such patients would be expected to result in considerable toxicity. Hence, disopyramide should be avoided in patients with decreased renal function. Patients with liver disease or CHF also have diminished clearances of disopyramide. If used in such patients, maintenance doses should be 50% to 75% of normal doses.

Lidocaine, for all practical purposes, depends exclusively on hepatic metabolism for its elimination, so its disposition is unaffected by renal disease. In patients with liver disease or CHF, however, the clearance of lidocaine is about 50% of normal. Maintenance infusion rates must be decreased. Changes in the volume of distribution of lidocaine also occur in these settings by mechanisms that are not understood. In patients with cirrhosis, the volume of distribution is increased and a loading dose up to 1.5 times normal may be needed. It is probably best to administer a normal loading dose and then use a supplemental dose that is 50% of normal, if clinically indicated. The converse occurs in patients with CHF: the volume of distribution is half the normal value, and loading doses in such patients should be half of those usually used.

Although mexiletine and tocainide are similar with respect to the relative contribution of the kidney (40%) and the liver (60%) for elimination, they appear to differ with respect to effects of disease. In patients with renal disease, the disposition of mexiletine is unchanged, but for tocainide clearance is 50% to 75% of normal and maintenance doses should be proportionally decreased. Patients with acute myocardial infarction eliminate mexiletine normally, although those with CHF have not been studied. CHF does not affect the disposition of tocainide. Patients with cirrhosis have considerably impaired elimination of

mexiletine and should receive maintenance doses one-fourth to one-third of normal. The effects of liver disease on the disposition of tocainide have not been studied.

In both renal and hepatic disease, the protein binding of phenytoin is decreased. This does not, however, result in an increase in the unbound, pharmacologically active concentration. Hence, dosing does not have to be altered. Total phenytoin serum concentrations decrease in this setting, so the target serum concentration is less. For example, in patients with severe renal insufficiency, the desired total drug serum concentration is 7 to 12 mg per liter instead of 10 to 20 mg per liter in patients with normal renal function. In both cases, the unbound drug concentration is about 1 to 2 mg per liter.

Bretylium depends exclusively on the kidney for excretion, so its use should be avoided in patients with renal disease. If it must be given, maintenance doses as low as 20% of normal should be used. Alternatively, a normal loading dose should be given with no further dosing.

Because amiodarone depends entirely on the liver for its elimination, one would predict no influence of renal disease on its disposition. Similarly, hepatic impairment may decrease its elimination, and amiodarone should be used with extreme caution in such patients (although no studies have addressed this question).

N-Acetylprocainamide is excreted by renal routes, and patients with severe renal insufficiency need reductions in maintenance doses to one-fourth those normally used.

Both sotalol and dofetilide are highly dependent upon the kidney for elimination. They should be avoided in patients with severe renal insufficiency. Patients with mild to moderate decreases in renal function should receive lower doses and should be monitored closely clinically.

Adenosine is eliminated from plasma by cellular uptake. There is no appreciable change in patients with renal or hepatic disease.

Drug Interactions

Antiarrhythmic drugs are frequently used in combination, and their effects in concert represent a pharmacodynamic drug interaction. Similar interactions occur with other drugs; for example, the quinidine-like effect of phenothiazines is additive to that of quinidine itself, procainamide, and disopyramide. By understanding the pharmacology of the antiarrhythmics, adverse pharmacodynamic interactions can be avoided.

Numerous pharmacokinetic drug interactions occur with antiarrhythmic agents, both with the antiarrhythmic itself being affected and with the antiarrhythmic affecting the handling of other drugs. Drug interactions should be anticipated, using the general patterns of effect shown in Table 90.6. For example, cimetidine clearly inhibits the metabolism of several drugs, and it should be expected to do so with other drugs for which hepatic elimination is a major pathway of elimination. Amiodarone also has a spectrum of effects like cimetidine. In contrast, rifampin and phenytoin increase the metabolic elimination of numerous drugs, and they would be expected to have a similar effect on other metabolized agents. Adenosine's effects are blocked by xanthines, including theophylline and caffeine. In contrast, dipyrid-

TABLE 90.6.	DRUG INTERACTIONS WITH SOME ANTIARRHYTHMIC AGENTS
Drug	**Interaction**
Adenosine	Theophylline and caffeine block effects
	Dipyridamole enchances effects
Amiodarone	Decreases clearance of digoxin, flecainide, quinidine, phenytoin, procainamide, and warfarin
Disopyramide	Decreases clearance of warfarin
	Clearance increased by phenytoin, phenobarbital, and rifampin
Dofetilide	Clearance decreased by cimetidine (renal secretion) but not ranitidine
	Clearance decreased by ketoconazole (decreased metabolism and renal secretion)
Flecainide	Decreases clearance of digoxin and propranolol
	Clearance decreased by cimetidine, amiodarone, and allopurinol
Lidocaine	Clearance decreased by cimetidine, metoprolol, and propranolol
Mexiletine	Clearance increased by phenobarbital, phenytoin, and rifampin
N-acetylprocainamide	Clearance decreased by trimethoprim (renal secretion)
Phenytoin	Increases clearance of carbamazepine, clonazepam, cyclosporine, diazepam, digitoxin, doxycyline, glucocorticoids, methadone, warfarin, quinidine, theophylline, valproate, and disopyramide
	Clearance increased by carbamazepine, phenobarbital, and rifampin
	Clearance decreased by amiodarone, chloramphenicol, chlorpromazine, cimetidine, disulfiram, isoniazid, methylphenidate, and propoxyphene
Procainamide	Clearance decreased by amiodarone (metabolic effect) and by cimetidine, ranitidine, and trimethoprim (renal secretion)
Propafenone	Decreases clearance of digoxin in a dose-related fashion, causing increases in digoxin serum concentrations of 35–85%
	Decreases clearance of warfarin and increases its effects by about 25%
Quinidine	Decreases clearance of digoxin (renal secretion), which causes a doubling of digoxin serum concentration
	Clearance increased by rifampin and phenytoin
	Clearance decreased by amiodarone, cimetidine, and verapamil
Tocainide	Clearance decreased by cimetidine

amole blocks adenosine uptake, thereby prolonging and enhancing adenosine's effects.

Propafenone increases serum digoxin concentrations 35% to 85% and increases the prothrombin time by about 25% in patients taking warfarin. Propafenone is converted to its active metabolite by CYP2D6, so inhibitors of this isoenzyme, such as quinidine, decrease formation of the metabolite.

Understanding the pathways of elimination of antiarrhythmic agents and the pharmacology of potential interactants allows anticipation of drug interactions and appropriate modification of dosing strategies.

ANTIANGINAL AGENTS

Disposition and Effect

Nitrates, β-blockers, and calcium channel antagonists are the mainstays of therapy for angina. Numerous nitrate preparations are available, as previously discussed (Table 90.1). Their use in patients with angina follows the same pharmacologic principles as for treatment of those with CHF.

β-Adrenergic antagonists decrease myocardial oxygen demands primarily by decreasing heart rate and particularly by blocking exercise- or stress-induced increases in rate. β-Blockers can be conveniently grouped according to their pharmacologic characteristics: nonselective, cardioselective, or with intrinsic sympathomimetic activity (ISA). Nonselectivity implies the ability to block all β-receptors. Cardioselectivity means that at low doses the agent has a relative selectivity to block β_1-receptors, which mediate chronotropy and renin release; at higher doses, selectivity disappears. ISA indicates that the drug has partial agonist activity; at low levels of endogenous sympathetic activity, these drugs have agonist properties; when endogenous activity increases, these β-blockers become antagonists. Clinically, these agents do not diminish (and in fact may increase) resting heart rate, but they block exercise- or stress-induced increases in heart rate.

Clinically, the most useful means for discriminating among these agents, other than selectivity and ISA, is the primary route of elimination. Some obey primary renal excretion (nadolol, atenolol, acebutolol), and others are eliminated predominantly by the liver (propranolol, timolol, metoprolol). Pindolol is eliminated by both routes. The importance of this characteristic is in predicting the need for dose modification in patients with disease. For example, patients with renal insufficiency require decreased doses of nadolol, and patients with liver disease require dose modification of propranolol. Alternatively, if a patient has renal disease, a β-blocker eliminated by the liver can be used.

Pharmacokinetic data for β-adrenergic antagonists are pre-

TABLE 90.7.   Pharmacokinetic Parameters of Some β-Adrenergic Antatonists

Drug	Bioavailability (%)	Renal Excretion (%)	Active Metabolites	Vd (L/kg)	Cl (mL/min/kg)	Half-Life (hr)	Effect of Disease
Nonselective							
Esmolol	0	0	None	2–3.5	200–300	8–10 min	Renal disease: no change Cirrhosis: no change
Propranolol	36	0	4-OH-propranolol	4–4.5	12	2.5–5	Cirrhosis: bioavailability doubles; 1/2 normal Cl Hyperthyroidism: 2 × normal Vd and Cl
Timolol	50–60	15	None	1.7	7.7	2.7	?
Nadolol	30–50	60–75	None	1.5	1–3	14–24	Renal disease; 1/4–1/2 normal Cl
Cardioselective							
Metoprolol	50	5–10	α-OH-metoprolol	4.9	10–20	2.5–5	Cirrhosis: bioavailability ↑ to 85%; 1/2 normal Cl Hyperthyroidism: 2 × normal Vd and Cl
Atenolol	45–55	75–85	Hydroxyatenolol	0.7–1.2	1.3–2.1	6–9	Renal disease; 1/4–1/2 normal Cl Hyperthyrodism: no change Cirrhosis: no change
Betaxolol	80–90	15	None	5–10	4.7	14–22	Renal disease: 1/2 normal Cl Elderly: 1/2 normal Cl
Bisoprolol	80–90	50	None	2.9	1.8–3.4	9–12	Renal disease: 1/3–1/2 normal Cl
Intrinsic Sympathomimetic Activity							
Nonselective							
Pindolol	75	35–40	None	2.1	7–7.7	3–4	Renal disease: no change Elderly: no change Cirrhosis: no change
Cardioselective							
Acebutolol	20–60	15–30	Diacetolol	1.2	8.8	3–4	Renal disease: 1/3–1/2 normal Cl of metabolite
Combined β and α Antagonism							
Carvedilol	25	<2	Negligible effects	1.5–2	8.7	2–8	Renal disease: no change Cirrhosis: bioavailability triples; 1/2 normal Cl
Labetalol	11–86	<5	None	5.6–9	21–31	3–8	Renal disease: no change Elderly: bioavilability doubles Cirrhosis: bioavailability doubles

Cl, clearnace; Vd, volume of distribution.

sented in Table 90.7. Propranolol, metoprolol, and atenolol have active metabolites, but they probably contribute negligibly to the overall pharmacologic effect. In contrast, the metabolite of acebutolol, which is also cardioselective and has ISA, contributes substantially to the activity of this agent; in fact, the dosage modification required in patients with renal disease is due to changed handling of the metabolite rather than of the parent drug. Similarly, the long half-life of the metabolite allows less frequent dosing than would be necessary with the parent compound alone.

One of the convenient features of the β-blockers is that response can be easily evaluated clinically. Whether a dose has been administered sufficiently to cause β-blockade can be determined simply by assessing whether the heart rate increases with exercise. In a formal evaluation, exercise on a treadmill can be used. However, testing also can be accomplished easily in an office setting by having the patient walk up and down stairs or by determining whether the transient increase in heart rate with standing is blocked. If any of these tests show that increases in heart rate are not blocked, the patient can be given larger doses of the β-blocker. It is important to note that β-blockade usually cannot be documented reliably by assessing effects on resting heart rate because in most patients, the contribution of β-adrenergic tone to resting heart rate is negligible. Proper assessment, therefore, entails evaluation of the effects on exercise-induced increases in heart rate.

Calcium channel antagonists have proved useful in treating patients with angina, not only to block a coronary vasospastic component of the syndrome but also to reduce afterload and thus diminish myocardial oxygen demands. Although verapamil, diltiazem, and the various dihydropyridines share the feature of calcium channel blockade, these drugs also manifest a spectrum of pharmacologic effects. Simplistically, verapamil is at one end of the spectrum, having the greatest slowing of atrioventricular nodal conduction and the least effect of lowering peripheral vascular resistance. The dihydropyridines are at the opposite end, being the most potent in terms of decreasing resistance and having negligible effects on cardiac conduction. Diltiazem is intermediate in both regards.

Pharmacokinetic parameters for the calcium antagonists are presented in Table 90.8. All depend on hepatic elimination, and verapamil and diltiazem are converted to active metabolites. The contribution of norverapamil to the overall pharmacologic effect is unknown. Desacetyldiltiazem appears to contribute substantially to the overall effects of diltiazem; it reaches serum concentrations of about half that of the parent drug, and it is about one-third as potent.

In addition to formation of an active metabolite, the pharmacology of verapamil is made more complex by the fact that it exists as two stereoisomers, of which the 1-form is active. When given orally, stereoselective first-pass metabolism of the active isomer occurs, so that relatively more of the inactive form reaches the systemic circulation. This phenomenon accounts for the finding that after oral dosing, greater total serum concentrations of verapamil are required to produce the same effect as with intravenous dosing. After intravenous dosing, the total concentration represents half-active and half-inactive drug. In contrast, after oral dosing, the total verapamil concentration is predominantly inactive drug. The relation between the active 1-isomer and response is the same for both routes of administration. A corollary of this stereoselective pharmacology is that measurement of total serum concentrations of verapamil is not helpful and is likely to be misleading.

Effects of Disease

Clear patterns are evident when assessing the impact of different diseases on the disposition of β-blockers. Those with predominant elimination by the liver show striking changes in disposition in patients with cirrhosis. For example, with propranolol and metoprolol, clearance is about half normal in such patients. Presystemic elimination also is decreased, which increases the bioavailability of both drugs. These two changes have a multiplier effect on serum drug concentrations: thus, if the bioavailability doubles together with a decrease in clearance to half normal, the average serum concentration quadruples (Chapter 55). Sub-

TABLE 90.8. Pharmacokinetic Parameters for Calcium Channel Antagonists

Drug	Bioavailability (%)	Renal Excretion (%)	Active Metabolites	Vd (L/kg)	Cl (mL/min/kg)	Half-Life (hr)	Effect of Disease
Amlodipine	52–88	<10	None	21.4	7–13.5	34–50	Cirrhosis: 1/2 normal Cl Renal disease: no change Elderly: 1/2 normal Cl
Diltiazem	30–40	<4	Desacetyldiltiazem	2.2–7.8	14–20	3.5–5	Renal disease: no change
Felodipine	4–36	0	None	8–12	12–24	10–25	Elderly: 1/2 normal Cl Renal disease: no change CHF: 1/2 normal Cl; bioavailability doubles
Isradipine	15–20	0	None	1.6–4	10.5	2–8	Cirrhosis: bioavailability doubles; 1/4–1/2 normal Cl Elderly: 1/3–1/2 normal Cl
Nicardipine	6.5–30	<1	None	0.6–0.9	7–17	4–12	Renal disease: no change Cirrhosis: 1/5 normal Cl Elderly: no change
Nifedipine	40–50	<1	None	0.8–1.3	6–15	3.5–4	Cirrhosis: bioavailability ↑ to 90%; 1/3–1/2 normal Cl Elderly: 1/2 normal Cl Renal disease: no change
Nimodipine	5–13		None	0.9–2.3	14–19	1–6	Cirrhosis: AUC quadruples
Nisoldipine	4–8	0	None	1.6–7.1	8–16	7–15	Renal disease: no change Cirrhosis: bioavailability doubles: 1/4 normal Cl Elderly: AUC triples
Nitrendipine	5–30	<0.1	None	2–6	19–21	8–12	Cirrhosis: AUC quadruples Renal disease: no change
Verapamil	12–33	3–4	Norverapamil	2–6	14–20	2–5	Cirrhosis: bioavailability ↑ to 70%; 1/2 normal Vd; 1/4–1/3 normal Cl Elderly: 1/2 normal Cl Renal disease: no change

AUC, area under the serum concentration versus time curve; Cl, clearance; CHF, congestive heart failure; Vd, volume of distribution.

stantial decreases in dose must be made to compensate for these effects. If the dose is given intravenously so that bioavailability is not a factor, the magnitude of dose adjustment needed depends solely on changes in clearance. Although timolol has not been studied in patients with cirrhosis, its disposition is so similar to that of propranolol and metoprolol that one would expect similar qualitative changes.

Hyperthyroidism affects the disposition of propranolol and metoprolol, and one would predict similar effects with other hepatically eliminated β-blockers. Both the volume of distribution and the clearance double in hyperthyroid patients, so the loading dose should be twice the usual amount. In addition, on average such patients require a maintenance dose twice normal. As the hyperthyroidism is treated and the patient returns to the euthyroid state, disposition parameters regress toward normal, and doses of these β-blockers should be diminished. The disposition of atenolol is not affected by hyperthyroidism, making it a desirable β-blocker in such patients. Effects of thyroid dysfunction on disposition of other β-blockers is unknown.

The β-blockers eliminated predominantly by the kidney require decreased maintenance doses in patients with renal insufficiency. On average, patients with severe renal impairment require maintenance doses 25% to 50% of normal. In such patients, the half-life is prolonged (e.g., up to 40 hours for atenolol), so that the time needed to reach steady state may be lengthy. Alternatively, in patients with renal disease, a β-blocker eliminated by hepatic routes can be used so that no dose adjustment is needed.

Pindolol has substantial elimination by both renal and hepatic routes, so neither renal nor hepatic disease affects its overall disposition. One would predict that patients with combined renal and hepatic disease will need dosage modification of this drug.

Because the calcium channel antagonists are eliminated by hepatic metabolism, it can be predicted that renal dysfunction will not affect their elimination. Conversely, liver disease has

been shown to affect the disposition of a number of these drugs (Table 90.8). With cirrhosis, the bioavailability of a number of these agents roughly doubles, similar to the effects observed with β-blockers eliminated by hepatic metabolism. Clearance of these drugs is also reduced in patients with hepatic disease. Because of the multiplier effect, patients with cirrhosis should receive substantially decreased maintenance doses. By mechanisms that are not understood, the volume of distribution of verapamil is decreased to about half normal in patients with cirrhosis, so they should receive proportionally lower loading doses.

Drug Interactions

Drug interactions described with β-blockers and calcium antagonists are listed in Table 90.9. Propranolol and metoprolol are affected by other drugs that influence hepatic metabolism. These drugs are metabolized by CYP2D6, and their metabolism is predictably decreased by drugs such as quinidine, which inhibit this isoenzyme. Although timolol has not been studied, one would expect it to be subject to similar interactions because it is also metabolized by this isoenzyme. Interactions have not been described for those β-blockers eliminated by the kidney.

Calcium antagonists are metabolized by CYP3A4; verapamil and diltiazem also inhibit this isoenzyme. Thus, these two drugs inhibit other substrates for this isoenzyme, such as cyclosporine. Of particular note is the effect of verapamil and diltiazem on the metabolism of lovastatin and simvastatin. Both calcium antagonists can dramatically increase serum concentrations of these two hydroxymethyl glutaryl-coenzyme A (HMG-CoA) reductase inhibitors (also called statins) sufficient to cause rhabdomyolysis. Other HMG-CoA reductase inhibitors are not subject to this interaction and should be used instead.

Antianginal agents are an excellent example of the ability to use predictable pharmacodynamic interactions to the patient's advantage by combining them. The effects of antianginal drugs on the determinants of myocardial oxygen demand are presented

TABLE 90.9.	Drug Interactions with β-Adrenergic Antagonists and Calcium Channel Antagonists
Drug	**Interaction**
β-Adrenergic Antagonists	
Propranolol	Decreases clearance of diazepam and lidocaine
	Absorption decreased by antacids and cholestyramine
	Clearance decreased by chlorpromazine, cimetidine, diltiazem, and quinidine
Metoprolol	Decreases clearance of lidocaine
	Clearance increased by rifampin
	Clearance decreased by cimetidine, oral contraceptives, propafenone, and diltiazem
Calcium Channel Antagonists	
Verapamil	Decreases clearance of substrates for cytochrome P4503A4, including carbamazepine, quinidine, cyclosporine, lovastatin and simvastatin; decreases renal secretion of substrates for P-glycoprotein such as digoxin
Diltiazem	Similar to verapamil
Dihydropyridine calcium antagonists	Clearance decreased by inhibitors of cytochrome P4503A4 including ketoconazole, itraconazole, erythromycin, amiodarone, and others

TABLE 90.10.	**Effects of Antianginal Agents on Determinants of Myocardial Oxygen Demands**				
Determinant	Nitrates	β-Blockers	Verapamil	Diltiazem	Dihydropyridine Calcium Antagonists
Heart rate	↑	↓	—	—	↑
Contractility	↑	↓	↓	↓	—
Wall tension					
Preload	↓↓	—	—	—	—
Afterload	↓	a	↓	↓	↓↓

—, no effect.
a Modest ↑ with nonselective, no effect with cardioselective, modest ↓ with agents having intrinsic sympathomimetic activity.

in Table 90.10. Logical combinations of these drugs can be used for additive efficacy; for example, reflex tachycardia caused by nitrates or dihydropyridines can be blocked by β-adrenergic antagonists. Similar additional pharmacodynamic interactions that occur with these drugs are predictable, based on the known pharmacology of the interactants.

ANTIHYPERTENSIVE AGENTS

Disposition and Effect

Previous sections have discussed nitroprusside, hydralazine, ACE inhibitors, angiotensin antagonists and β-adrenergic and calcium channel antagonists, all of which are effective antihypertensives (Tables 90.2, 90.7, and 90-8). Pharmacokinetic parameters for additional antihypertensive drugs are presented in Table 90.11.

The central α_2-adrenergic agonists decrease blood pressure by suppressing the concentration of circulating catecholamines, thereby decreasing peripheral vascular resistance. Methyldopa, clonidine, and moxonidine have a substantial component of renal elimination; in contrast, guanabenz and guanfacine depend exclusively on hepatic function. Despite the short half-lives of guanabenz and methyldopa, their duration of effect is long enough to allow dosing twice a day.

Doxazosin, prazosin, terazosin, trimazosin, and urapadil block α_1-adrenergic receptors in the periphery. The selectivity of this effect still allows catecholamines to activate α_2-receptors, suppressing their release. Hence, in contrast to nonselective peripheral adrenergic antagonists such as phentolamine and phenoxybenzamine, administration of these drugs is not associated with increases in circulating catecholamine concentrations. This effect may account, at least in part, for the usual absence of reflex tachycardia in association with their use. Prazosin is metabolized to two compounds that are active. They are eliminated by secretion into the bile and do not attain sufficient systemic concentrations to exert an effect. Although the half-lives of prazosin and trimazosin are short, they can be administered twice a day for the treatment of hypertension. Doxazosin and terazosin usually can be given once a day.

Diazoxide can be administered orally, but it is usually given intravenously for hypertensive emergencies. An early hypothesis was that diazoxide was so avidly bound to serum proteins that large, rapid intravenous bolus doses were required to attain enough unbound drug at the arteriolar site of action to be effective. As such, early guidelines suggested initial doses of 300 mg, with repeated administration as needed. Subsequent studies proved the initial postulate to be false and also noted that the large doses that had been recommended too often resulted in hypotension. Doses of 1 mg per kilogram should be given; they can be repeated every 10 to 15 minutes until desired blood pressures have been reached.

Two interesting aspects of the pharmacology of diazoxide are its propensities to cause hyperglycemia and to cause sodium retention. These effects are somewhat paradoxical, because diazoxide is derived from a sulfonamide structure, just as are oral sulfonylureas and thiazide diuretics. Patients with non–insulin-dependent diabetes are particularly susceptible to the hyperglycemic effects of diazoxide and should be monitored closely. Sodium retention is usually not problematic and does not occur unless sodium is given to the patient. If it does occur, diuretics may be needed.

Minoxidil, an extremely potent vasodilator, is reserved for patients with refractory hypertension. It is not used in mild or moderate hypertension because its potent vasodilating effects predictably cause reflex tachycardia, requiring concomitant use of β-blockers, and fluid retention sufficient to mandate use of diuretics. Hence, multidrug therapy is always needed. In addition, minoxidil causes hair growth, and the hirsutism can be a particularly worrisome cosmetic problem in women. When used as an ointment to stimulate hair growth, less than 5% of a dose is absorbed. Although minoxidil has a short half-life, it can be administered twice a day.

Labetalol has both nonselective β- and α-adrenergic antagonist effects (Table 90.7). The ratio of these separate pharmacologic activities is about 7:1. Labetalol has two asymmetric carbon atoms in its structure. It is administered as a racemate, which therefore contains four structurally distinct stereoisomers (RR, RS, SR, and SS). The RR isomer accounts for the β-blocking activity, the SR isomer is responsible for the α-blockade, and the other two configurations are inactive. As a result, the pharmacology of labetalol is little different from separate but concomitant administration of two drugs with the same pharmacologic activity of the active stereoisomers of labetalol.

Treatment of Malignant Hypertension

The choice of antihypertensives differs, depending on whether the patient has mild hypertension or accelerated or malignant

TABLE 90.11. **Pharmacokinetics of Antihypertensive Agents**

Drug	Bioavailability (%)	Renal Excretion (%)	Active Metabolites	Vd (L/ kg)	Cl (mL/min/ kg)	Half- Life (hr)	Effect of Disease
Central α₂-Adrenergic Antagonists							
Clonidine	75–95	40–70	None	2.0–4.0	3–5	7–18	Renal disease: 1/3–1/2 normal Cl
Guanabenz		0		5		4	Cirrhosis: 1/3 normal Vd; 1/5 normal Cl
Guanfacine	60–100	25–35	None	3.9–6.5	2.6–5.2	12–23	Renal disease: no change
Methyldopa	25–30	50–65	Methyldopamine	0.5–0.6	3.3–5.7	1.3–1.8	Renal disease ↑ effect; ? accumulation of metabolite; give 1/2 normal dose
Moxonidine	90	60–60	None	1.8–3.0	12–15.3	1.5–3	Renal disease: 1/3–1/2 normal Cl
Peripheral α₁-Adrenergic Antagonists							
Doxazosin	60–70	1	None	1.0	1.2–2.2	18–20	Renal disease: no change
Prazosin	50–70	<10	6- and 7–0 demethylated prazosin	0.6–0.8	2.4–3.3	2.5–4.5	Elderly: 1 1/2 normal Vd CHF 1/2–2/3 normal Cl Renal disease; no change
Terazosin	80–90	10–15		0.25–0.43	1.1	10–18	Elderly: 1/2 normal Cl CHF: no change
Trimazoson	63		1-Hydroxytrimazosin		0.9	2.9	
Urapadil	63–80	10–15	N-Demethyl urapadil	0.4–0.8	1.8–3.8	1.8–4.8	Renal disease: no change Cirrhosis: 1/4 normal Cl Elderly: 1/2 normal Cl
Direct Vasodilators							
Cardralazine		70–80	None	0.7		2.5	
Diazoxide	85–90	20	None	0.18	0.1	15–30	Renal disease: ↓ binding and possible ↑ response; give 1/ 2–2/3 normal dose
Fenoldopam	5–7	<1		0.2–0.7	25–38	0.2	
Hydralazine	10–35	<10	None	6–8	75–140	0.7–1.0	CHF: 1/2 normal CL Renal disease: no change
Minoxidil	95	12–20	Minoxidil sulfate	2.6–5.0	20–24	3–4	Renal disease; ↑ effect—mechanism unknown; 1/2 normal Cl
Miscellaneous							
Guanadrel		40		10	41	4	Renal disease: 1/5 normal Cl
Ketansirin	50	<4	None	5–10	6–10	6–14	Cirrhosis: 1/2 normal Cl

CHF, congestive heart failure; Vd, volume of distribution; Cl, clearance.

hypertension. The approach in the former case is discussed in Chapter 30; the latter represents a special use of these agents.

Nitroprusside is the gold standard for hypertensive emergencies because of its potency and short duration of action. It is effective in virtually all patients, and the short duration of effect allows precise control of the degree of lowering of the blood pressure. This drug is particularly useful in patients with hypertensive encephalopathy or in those with cerebrovascular disease in whom the goal is to lower the diastolic blood pressure quickly to about 110 mm Hg, with subsequent gradual lowering to

normal. Rapid attainment of normal blood pressures in such patients can result in cerebrovascular compromise. Although nitroprusside is the ideal agent for treating these patients, it requires an infusion pump and intra-arterial monitoring of blood pressure.

Other drugs used for hypertensive emergencies include intravenous diazoxide and labetalol and oral clonidine. Labetalol can be administered as either intermittent bolus injections or as a continuous intravenous infusion. With the former method, an initial dose of 20 mg is administered as a bolus dose over 2 to

5 minutes. Ten to 15 minutes later, 40 mg can be administered, with additional 80-mg doses every 10 to 15 minutes until the goal blood pressure or a total dose of 300 mg is reached. This dosing strategy is aimed at using small doses initially to prevent a too-pronounced fall in blood pressure, thus allowing gradual titration of the pressure to desired levels. If an infusion pump is available, labetalol can be administered at a rate of 2 mg per minute, with end points the same as with intermittent dosing. This method also results in controlled titration of blood pressure.

Although the use of labetalol and repeated small doses of diazoxide allows controlled pressure lowering in most patients, the longer duration of action of these drugs is undesirable if an adverse effect occurs or if the antihypertensive effect is greater than desired. Hence, these drugs do not supplant nitroprusside in patients at greatest risk, but they are useful alternatives when nitroprusside cannot be used or if the precise degree of titration that occurs with nitroprusside is not needed.

Clonidine offers the advantage of oral administration, thus avoiding the expense of intravenous dosing, but it is not appropriate for all patients. The use of clonidine entails the administration of 0.2 mg initially, followed by 0.1 mg every hour until a total dose of 0.8 mg or the desired blood pressure is reached. This oral titration allows gradual lowering of the blood pressure. Such doses of clonidine frequently cause patients to be sleepy, however, and the drug therefore should not be used in patients in whom one is closely monitoring end points of cerebral perfusion, such as alertness.

The efficacy of oral nifedipine has been described in patients with severe hypertension. Administration of a 10-mg capsule orally or sublingually can cause prompt lowering of blood pressure in 15 to 30 minutes. Although this regimen is attractive in its simplicity, too many adverse effects occur and this therapy should be abandoned.

Effects of Disease

The effects of disease on the disposition of a number of the antihypertensives were discussed in prior sections, and the effects on additional agents are presented in Table 90.11. Of the centrally acting α_2-adrenergic agonists, clonidine, moxonidine, and methyldopa have substantial renal elimination. Patients with severe renal insufficiency require maintenance doses of clonidine and moxonidine one-third to one-half of those normally used. Studies with methyldopa have been equivocal in terms of demonstrating clinically relevant changes in clearance related to renal disease; on the other hand, patients with renal disease have greater blood pressure lowering from methyldopa than do those with normal renal function. The mechanism by which an increased effect occurs is not understood, but such patients should receive lower doses of methyldopa.

Guanabenz and guanfacine are eliminated exclusively by the liver, and disposition is predictably altered in patients with cirrhosis. Pronounced declines in the clearance of guanabenz to 20% of normal occur, mandating decreased maintenance doses. By unknown mechanisms, the volume of distribution is also about one-third of normal in patients with cirrhosis. Because loading doses of guanabenz are rarely if ever administered, this change has little clinical relevance. With the pronounced altera-

tions in the disposition of guanabenz that occur in cirrhosis, clonidine, methyldopa, or moxonidine should be used in such patients if a centrally acting α_2-agonist is to be given.

Prazosin clearance is decreased in patients with CHF to one-half to two-thirds of normal. Elderly patients appear to eliminate prazosin normally but have an increased volume of distribution. Because a loading dose strategy is not used with this drug, no change in dosing is needed. Conversely, the clearance of doxazosin, terazosin, and urapidil is reduced in elderly patients, and they should receive half the usual dose.

Although both diazoxide and minoxidil are primarily eliminated by the liver, the response to both drugs is increased in patients with renal disease. Changed protein binding is a postulated mechanism for the effect with diazoxide, but no data support (or refute) this hypothesis. Initial doses of both drugs should be decreased in patients with renal insufficiency, with subsequent increases dictated by clinical endpoints. One would expect liver disease to affect the disposition of diazoxide and minoxidil; although studies have not been published that address this question, it would seem reasonable to exercise cautious dosing in such patients.

Drug Interactions

Drug interactions with β-adrenergic antagonists and calcium channel antagonists were presented previously (Table 90.9). Of the remaining antihypertensive agents, clinically important drug interactions are pharmacodynamic. These drugs frequently are used in combination for their additive effects. For example, potent vasodilators such as hydralazine, dihydropyridine calcium antagonists, and minoxidil frequently cause reflex tachycardia and fluid retention, which can be sufficient to negate their pressure-lowering effect (pseudotolerance). In this setting, the addition of β-blockers or diuretics restores antihypertensive efficacy. Understanding the pharmacology of the various antihypertensives allows rational combination of these agents to achieve a beneficial drug interaction.

Adverse pharmacodynamic drug interactions also occur with these agents. For example, nonsteroidal anti-inflammatory drugs can blunt the natriuretic effect of most diuretics and the antihypertensive effect of β-blockers and ACE inhibitors.

ANTICOAGULANT, THROMBOLYTIC, AND ANTIPLATELET AGENTS

Disposition and Effect

Drugs that affect hemostasis are among the most exciting drugs for cardiovascular disorders. New drugs are being developed at a rapid pace, many of which are biologic agents. These, in turn, spawn frenzied development of nonbiologic agents with the same pharmacologic effects. For example, the first available agent that blocks platelet glycoprotein IIb/IIIa receptors is a hybridized monoclonal antibody. Its efficacy has resulted in intense efforts to develop nonpeptide inhibitors of this receptor that provide more flexibility in terms of route of administration, ability to

| TABLE 90.12. | Pharmacokinetics of Anticoagulants, Fibrinolytics, and Inhibitors of Platelet Function |

Drug	Bioavailability (%)	Renal Excretion (%)	Active Metabolites	Vd (L/kg)	Cl (mL/min/kg)	Half-Life (hr)	Effect of Disease
Anticoagulants							
Desirudin		50–60		0.27	2.2	2–3	Renal disease: 1/6 normal Cl
Heparin (low-molecular-weight)	65–99 Subcutaneous	80–90		0.06–0.19	0.2–1.0	1.8–4.5	Renal disease: 1/2 normal Cl Cirrhosis: no change
Hirudin				0.53	2.3	2.8	
Tirofiban		80		0.3–0.6	3.4–5.0	1.2–1.6	Renal disease: 1/2 normal Cl Cirrhosis: no change Elderly: 3/4 normal Cl
Warfarin	100	0		0.11–0.20	0.02–0.08	35–45	Renal disease: no change Cirrhosis: ↑ effect CHF: ↑ effect Elderly: no change
Fibrinolytics							
Alteplase		0		0.10–0.13	5.4–9.8	0.5–1.2	
Anistreplace		0		0.08	0.9	1.2	
Reteplase		0		0.8	4.4–5.3	0.3	
Streptokinase		0		0.02–0.08	1.7	0.6	
Antiplatelet Agents							
Dipyridamole	45			2.4	2–4	12	
Iloprost	15–20	0		0.7–0.8	16–20	0.3–0.5	Renal disease: 1/2 normal Cl Cirrhosis: 1/2 normal Cl Elderly: no change
Sulotroban		52–62			10	0.7–3.0	Renal disease: 1/5 normal Cl
Ticlopidine	80–90	2	2-Keto-ticlopidine			24–33	Renal disease: no change Elderly: 1/3 normal Cl
Vapiprost		<1		0.8–0.9	7.3–10.3	1.1–1.4	

CHF, congestive heart failure; Cl, clearance.

dose chronically, and so on. The pharmacokinetics of anticoagulants, thrombolytics, and platelet inhibitors are listed in Table 90.12.

The pharmacokinetics of heparin are difficult to evaluate because of imprecision of assays for heparin. Heparin consists of many different polymeric constituents, it follows saturable elimination kinetics, and there is great variability in its effect among patients. As a result, reported values for heparin disposition parameters vary over a tenfold range. This variability has been the stimulus for developing low-molecular-weight heparins, which are far less variable in their kinetic profile. This lower variability accounts for their equal and sometimes superior efficacy with less toxicity compared with conventional heparin. Conventional heparin has an average molecular weight of 15,000 (range, 3,000 to 30,000), whereas that for low-molecular-weight heparins is 4,000 to 5,000. This low molecular weight allows these heparins to be filtered by the glomerulus, causing them to depend on the kidney for elimination in contrast to conventional heparin.

Excluding the use of low doses of subcutaneously administered heparin for prophylaxis, the usual goal of therapy is to maintain an activated partial thromboplastin time (aPTT) 1.5 to 2.5 times the control value. To do so, conventional heparin can be given in several ways. If a continuous intravenous infusion is used, a loading dose of 70 to 75 U per kilogram should be given, followed by an infusion rate of 1,000 U per hour. The anticoagulant effect should be measured in about 6 hours, at which time most patients will have reached steady state. If the aPTT is not in the desired range, the infusion rate can be adjusted by increments (or decrements) of 100 to 200 U per hour, with assessment of anticoagulant effect 6 hours after the change in regimen. When the desired anticoagulant effect is obtained, follow-up monitoring should occur on a daily basis.

A less preferable mode of administration is intermittent intravenous injections of heparin. With this method, a dose of 70 to 100 U per kilogram is administered every 4 hours. Doses are adjusted based on aPTT measurements obtained about 30 minutes before a dose. This method is inferior to continuous intravenous infusion of heparin because the level of anticoagulation vacillates within the dosing interval, and the time at which peak effects occur is associated with greater-than-needed anticoagulation. This probably accounts for the greater incidence of side effects that occurs with intermittent intravenous administration.

Heparin also can be administered subcutaneously as 7,000

to 10,000 U every 8 hours or 10,000 to 15,000 U every 12 hours. With this route, doses should be adjusted to maintain an aPTT 2 to 2.5 times control 6 hours after a dose. This method is preferred only when intravenous access is problematic or impossible.

Unfractionated heparin is highly heterogeneous, making its clinical pharmacology complex. Low-molecular-weight heparins (enoxaparin, dalteparin, and ardeparin) have been developed, which have more predictable pharmacokinetics. These preparations do not require monitoring of aPTT; rather, they are administered subcutaneously in fixed doses. Because they are primarily eliminated by the kidney, doses need to be decreased in patients with diminished renal function. These preparations have been shown to be effective for prevention and treatment of deep venous thrombosis and in pulmonary embolism. In the former condition, they allow treating some patients on an ambulatory basis, avoiding hospitalization. Recently, enoxaparin was also approved for use in patients with acute coronary syndromes.

A variety of thrombin inhibitors have been and are still being tested. Most of these agents are either hirudin itself or modifications thereof. Hirudin is the anticoagulant in leech saliva. Early trials with hirudin and its analogs were disappointing, but in retrospect the reason therein was because they were designed ignoring fundamental principles of clinical pharmacology. As a consequence, wrong doses were used. These drugs may eventually prove to live up to their previous expectations. Currently, lepirudin is approved for anticoagulation in patients who have had heparin-induced thrombocytopenia. Its dose is based on a desired aPTT 1.5 to 2.5 times normal. Since lepirudin depends on the kidney for elimination, lower doses are needed in patients with decreased renal function.

Warfarin depends exclusively on hepatic metabolism for elimination. Warfarin obeys stereoselective metabolism in that the clearance of the active S($-$) isomer is about 1.5 times as great as that of the inactive isomer. Because the volume of distribution is the same for each stereoisomer, the half-life for the active isomer is shorter (24 to 33 hours) than that for the inactive isomer (35 to 58 hours). The goal of therapy with warfarin is to maintain a prothrombin time 1.5 times control, using the international normalized ratio (INR). A loading dose is usually administered as 10 mg per day for 2 or 3 days. A large single loading dose should not be given because it can cause precipitous falls in clotting factor VII, with risk of bleeding. Maintenance doses average 5 mg per day, but because there is considerable variability among patients, the dose should be titrated to obtain the desired INR. Because of the half-life of the active isomer of warfarin, attaining a steady state requires about 1 week of dosing.

Streptokinase and urokinase are thrombolytic agents used to lyse clots in peripheral and pulmonary veins, in peripheral and coronary arteries, and in shunts. Although the two agents have different mechanisms of action, their ultimate effect is to initiate fibrinolysis. Streptokinase differs from urokinase in being a foreign protein; thus, it is antigenic, and an initial loading dose must be administered that is sufficient to overwhelm circulating antibodies that are present in anyone who has had a previous streptococcal infection (i.e., virtually everyone). In addition, the antigenicity requires a 6- to 12-month lapse of time between exposures to streptokinase. With these drawbacks, urokinase

would seem to be a preferable agent. Unfortunately, it is more expensive, rendering it the usual second choice.

For systemic intravenous administration, both streptokinase and urokinase initially require loading doses to attain a therapeutic effect (streptokinase, 250,000 U in 20 to 30 minutes; urokinase, 4,400 U per kliogram over 10 minutes). This streptokinase dose is sufficient to overcome endogenous antibodies in 85% to 90% of patients. Maintenance doses are streptokinase, 100,000 U per hour for 24 to 72 hours, and urokinase, 4,400 U per kilogram per hour for 12 to 24 hours, with the duration of infusion, depending on the entity being treated.

Various regimens have been used for regional infusion. Some use a loading dose (10,000 to 20,000 U of streptokinase) and others do not. Infusion rates have ranged from 1,000 to 5,000 U per minute, with durations of infusion usually of up to 1.5 hours.

With systemic and even with regional administration, streptokinase and urokinase result in a systemic thrombolytic state and the risk of bleeding. A thrombolytic agent specifically directed to a thrombus therefore would be desirable and would offer a theoretical therapeutic advantage. As such, attention has focused on modifying streptokinase to make it more clot-specific (e.g., anisoylated plasminogen streptokinase activator complex, anistreplase) and using tissue plasminogen activator ([tPA] and similar agents). Both restore patency in thrombotically occluded coronary arteries but unfortunately do not obviate the risk of bleeding.

Several types and dosing regimens of tPA are available, with considerable debate as to advantages and disadvantages. All tPA agents are pharmacologically the same. Differences are in their pharmacokinetics and, hence, their dosing regimens. Alteplase is approved for use in acute myocardial infarction, acute stroke, and massive pulmonary embolus. Studies are ongoing to assess its benefit in acute coronary syndromes. For myocardial infarction, accelerated dosing is preferred wherein an initial intravenous bolus of 15 mg is administered. Subsequent infusion rates are based on body weight. For patients weighing more than 67 kg, 50 mg is administered over 30 minutes followed by another 35 mg over 60 minutes. For patients ≤67 kg, 0.75 mg per kilogram is infused over 30 minutes followed by another 0.5 mg per kilogram over 60 minutes. For treatment of stroke, 0.9 mg per kilogram (maximum dose = 90 mg) is administered over 60 minutes, with 10% of the dose given as an initial bolus. Reteplase is administered as two separate 10-U bolus doses 30 minutes apart. The bolus doses are administered over 2 minutes.

Choice of these thrombolytics is largely driven by cost, a component of which is convenience of dosing.

Low-dose aspirin, ticlopidine, clopidogrel, dipyridamole, inhibitors of the glycoprotein IIb-IIIa receptor, and drugs in development that are either prostaglandin analogs or block thromboxane receptors are used to inhibit platelet aggregation. The activity of aspirin (acetylsalicylic acid) depends on the acetyl moiety; hence, nonacetyl salicylate derivatives are ineffective. Once aspirin is absorbed across the gastrointestinal epithelium, the acetyl group is cleaved and irreversibly binds to platelet cyclooxygenase, thus preventing thromboxane A_2 synthesis and inhibiting platelet aggregation. The dose required for this effect is minuscule. At very low doses, platelets are most likely acetylated in the portal circulation rather than systemically. Low doses of aspirin are sufficient to inhibit platelet aggregation, and if aspirin is used for this purpose, doses of one adult aspirin per day should not be exceeded. This admonition particularly applies to the use of aspirin for prophylaxis against myocardial infarction. Ticlopidine is as efficacious as aspirin, but because it is more expensive and causes more adverse effects, it is reserved for patients who cannot take aspirin. Clopidogrel is similar in effects to ticlopidine but does not have the same risk of neutropenia. Thus, its therapeutic margin seems greater.

Dipyridamole is used more frequently than compelling data would indicate. It causes increased concentrations of cyclic adenosine monophosphate in the platelet and thus inhibits aggregation. Because this mechanism differs from that of aspirin, it has been postulated that the combination would have a synergistic, or at least additive, effect. Efficacy has been demonstrated in some conditions. The half-life of dipyridamole is long enough to allow twice-daily dosing.

Prostaglandin I_2 inhibits platelet aggregation, whereas thromboxane is a potent aggregant and vasocontrictor. Iloprost is a PGI_2 analog and sulotroban and vapiprost are thromboxane inhibitors that are under development.

The final common pathway in platelet aggregation involves activation of the platelet glycoprotein IIb/IIIa receptor. The first inhibitor of this receptor to be approved for use is a humanized monoclonal antibody, abciximab. It has been studied in the setting of angioplasty, where it prevents the rethrombosis that occurs in many patients, particularly those at high risk. Because this agent is a protein, it must be given intravenously. Intense efforts have focused on developing other IIb/IIIa antagonists, in particular seeking nonpeptide, orally available agents. To this end, tirofiban and eptifibatide have recently become available. Abciximab and eptifibatide are approved for use in high-risk patients with percutaneous transluminal coronary angioplasty (PTCA) plus patients undergoing acute coronary syndromes. Tirofiban is approved for the latter. All are used in combination with aspirin and heparin and are being actively studied for broader indications.

Effects of Disease

Several attempts to assess the influence of hepatic and renal disease on the disposition of heparin have been reported, with conflicting results. Such patients may have disease-induced alterations in hemostasis that make them more susceptible to bleeding with heparin. It does not appear, however, that changes in pharmacokinetics are of concern. Because low-molecular-weight heparins are primarily excreted by the kidney, doses need adjustment in patients with renal insufficiency.

Warfarin is eliminated exclusively by hepatic metabolism and would be expected to be subject to altered disposition in patients with hepatic dysfunction. Neither patients with liver disease nor those with viral hepatitis, however, have been shown to have altered pharmacokinetics. Patients with liver disease are more sensitive to the anticoagulant effects of warfarin, however, probably because of decreased synthesis of vitamin K. A similar phenomenon occurs in patients with CHF, in whom warfarin disposition is normal but the congestive hepatopathy causes decreased

synthesis of clotting factors. In hyperthyroid patients, the degradation of clotting factors increases, similarly increasing sensitivity to warfarin but via a different mechanism. Hence, several clinical conditions affect the sensitivity to warfarin, but none is associated with pharmacokinetic changes.

Patients with renal disease have diminished protein binding of warfarin because of accumulation of endogenous organic acids that displace the anticoagulant from binding sites on albumin. The unbound pharmacologically active concentration, however, remains the same. Therefore, any increased sensitivity to warfarin in patients with renal disease is due to the bleeding diathesis that occurs in such patients.

Disease-induced effects on the disposition of streptokinase, urokinase, tPA, and dipyridamole have not been described. Increased sensitivity to their effects is predictable in diseases associated with clotting abnormalities.

Doses of iloprost need adjustment in patients with hepatic or renal disease. Sulotroban doses need to be substantially lower in patients with renal disease, whereas with ticlopidine, elderly patients require lower doses.

Drug Interactions

No definitive pharmacokinetic drug interactions have been described with heparin. The antiplatelet effects of large doses of penicillins and the hypoprothrombinemic effects of cephalosporins containing the methylthiotetrazole side chain (cefamandole, moxalactam, cefoperazone, and others) increase the risk of bleeding during heparin administration.

Numerous drug interactions have been described with warfarin, not only because of the frequency of their occurrence but also because of their potential severity (Table 90.13). The effect of cholestyramine on absorption can be obviated by administering warfarin 1 hour before a dose of this resin. The protein-binding interactions are transient. After displacement from albumin, the free concentration of warfarin reaches a new steady-state concentration the same as before the interaction; as such, no change in dose is required. Numerous drugs induce hepatic

---

TABLE 90.13. **Drug Interactions With Warfarin**

Absorption

Decreased absorption caused by cholestyramine and presumably colestipol

Protein Binding

Decreased binding caused by chloral hydrate, clofibrate, diazoxide, ethacrynic acid, mefenamic acid, phenybutazone, phenytoin, and salicylates

Metabolism

Increased metabolic degradation caused by carbamazepine, chronic ethanol intake, glutethimide, griseofulvin, phenobarbital, phenytoin, and rifampin

Decreased metabolism caused by amiodarone, chloramphenicol, cimetidine, clofibrate, disulfiram, acute ethanol intake, oral contraceptives, propafenone, and sulfinpyrazone

metabolism of warfarin, thus requiring increased doses of the anticoagulant. This interaction requires about 2 weeks to reach its full effect and dissipates slowly. Dosing adjustments should be based on the measured INR. Several drugs also inhibit the metabolism of warfarin. In contrast to the slow onset of induction, these inhibitory effects occur quickly. As a consequence, if any of the inhibiting drugs listed in Table 90.13 are added to a stable regimen, the warfarin dose should be halved in anticipation of the effect, with further adjustments based on INR. The dissipation of the inhibitory effect depends on the rate of elimination of the inhibiting drug. For example, owing to the prolonged half-life of amiodarone, its effects persist for months. Conversely, the effects of cimetidine dissipate within 2 or 3 days.

LIPID-LOWERING DRUGS

DISPOSITION AND EFFECT

The binding resins cholestyramine and colestipol are not absorbed. By binding bile acids, they decrease the absorption of cholesterol. An indirect effect—increasing low-density lipoprotein receptor numbers (up-regulation)—also serves to lower serum cholesterol concentrations. The binding properties of these resins are nonspecific, and they can interact with many drugs. To avoid such interactions, dosing with other agents should precede administration of the resin by at least 1 hour or should be delayed until at least 4 hours afterward.

Little is known about the disposition of most lipid-lowering drugs. Clofibrate is the most studied. It is not active but is rapidly metabolized to *p*-chlorophenoxyisobutyric acid (CPIB), the active moiety, which in turn is either excreted in the urine or conjugated in the liver, with renal excretion of the conjugates. This metabolite can cause a severe myopathy, so considerable caution must be exercised with its use in patients in whom CPIB may accumulate.

The development of gemfibrozil, another derivative of fibric acid, was motivated by the adverse effects of clofibrate. Its half-life (7.5 hours) allows twice-daily administration. Gemfibrozil disposition is normal in patients with renal disease, and it should be used in preference to clofibrate in such patients.

Doses of nicotinic acid (niacin) must be titrated gradually upward in patients to minimize the common side effects related to cutaneous vasodilation. Beginning doses are usually 50 to 100 mg three times a day, with gradual increases to 1 to 3 g three times daily. Because the adverse effects seem to be related to rapidly increasing serum concentrations, they can be minimized by taking the nicotinic acid with food, which slows its rate of absorption without affecting bioavailability.

Probucol is eliminated slowly, with a half-life of 20 to 50 days. With this long half-life, once-daily dosing is sufficient.

Lovastatin and similar agents (simvastatin, pravastatin, fluvastatin, cerivastatin, and atorvastatin) are the most effective lipid-lowering agents. Lovastatin and simvastatin are converted to numerous active metabolites, which probably account for their effectiveness. The others are primarily active as the parent compounds. By inhibiting HMG-CoA reductase, these drugs increase the number of low-density lipoprotein (LDL) receptors,

thereby lowering LDL 30% to 40%. The statins are particularly effective when combined with bile acid–binding resins. Atorvastatin has greater efficacy than the other statins in that at maximally effective (and tolerated) doses it lowers LDL more than the other drugs in the class.

It has recently been discovered that the isoenzyme responsible for metabolism of lovastatin and simvastatin is cytochrome P4503A4 (CYP3A4). In turn, inhibitors of CYP3A4 such as verapamil, diltiazem, ketoconazole, and others cause substantial increases in concentration of parent drug with risk of myopathy. Alternative statins should be used if substrates or known inhibitors of CYP3A4 are to be coadministered.

Effects of Disease

The disposition of clofibrate is considerably affected by both renal and hepatic disease. In renal insufficiency, CPIB accumulates in a disproportionate fashion because excretion of the metabolite itself is decreased; the conjugates of CPIB also accumulate and then are hydrolyzed back to CPIB in vivo. Because of the severe myopathy that can occur from clofibrate, it is best to avoid it in this setting; gemfibrozil is a better alternative. Patients with cirrhosis also have diminished clearance of clofibrate. If its use cannot be avoided, maintenance doses in such patients should be about half of normal doses.

For the remaining lipid-lowering drugs, the paucity of data makes their use in patients with hepatic or renal disease potentially hazardous. Nicotinic acid is eliminated by hepatic routes, and its disposition is thereby unchanged in patients with renal disease. Although no data are available concerning its handling in patients with liver disease, nicotinic acid can cause elevated liver function tests in such patients and should be avoided. Because of the slow elimination of probucol, which depends on hepatic metabolism, this drug is best avoided in patients with liver disease.

Atorvastatin serum concentrations are markedly increased in patients with cirrhosis (up to 15-fold). This drug should be avoided in patients with liver disease. Fluvastatin also accumulates in such patients but to less degree. If used in patients with liver disease, doses should be one-third to one-half normal. Both lovastatin and simvastatin accumulate in elderly patients, who should receive doses that are half those of younger patients.

Drug Interactions

Cholestyramine and colestipol can bind many drugs in the gastrointestinal tract and thus decrease their bioavailability. Physicians should have a high index of suspicion that the binding resins will affect the absorption of any drug. Some drugs undergo biliary secretion followed by reabsorption, a process called *enterohepatic circulation*. With such agents, the resins can interrupt this recycling and sequester drug in the gut. The overall effect is increased elimination of the drug. This process occurs with cardiac glycosides, and the binding resins have been advocated as potential therapeutic agents in overdoses of digoxin and digitoxin. Similar effects would be expected with other drugs that undergo enterohepatic cycling.

Clofibrate is avidly bound to serum albumin and can displace warfarin from binding sites. Because this interaction is transient, no change in warfarin dosing is needed due to this effect alone. In contrast, clofibrate also inhibits the hepatic metabolism of warfarin, decreasing clearance and mandating a decrease in the maintenance dose to about half of normal. This inhibition is stereoselective. As discussed previously, warfarin is administered as a racemate, whereas only the S(−) isomer is active. Clofibrate selectively decreases the metabolism of the active isomer.

Gemfibrozil and probucol do not interact with oral hypoglycemics and warfarin. Whether they affect disposition and response to other drugs is unknown.

Lovastatin and simvastatin are metabolized by CYP3A4. Inhibition of this isoenzyme by drugs such as ketoconazole, erythromycin, verapamil, and diltiazem can cause substantial increases in concentration of both the parent drugs and their active metabolites. This effect enhances the risk of myopathy and rhabdomyolysis. If potential inhibitors of CYP3A4 are a necessary part of therapy, then alternative HMG-CoA reductase inhibitors should be used.

BIBLIOGRAPHY

Alexander JH, Harrington RA. Recent antiplatelet drug trials in the acute coronary syndromes. *Drugs* 1998;56:965–976.

The Digitalis Investigation Group. The effect of digoxin on mortality and morbidity in patients with heart failure. *N Engl J Med* 1997;336:525–533.

Frishman WH. Carvedilol. *N Engl J Med* 1998;339:1759–1765.

Goodfriend TL, Elliott ME, Catt KJ. Angiotensin receptors and their antagonists. *N Engl J Med* 1996;334:1649–1654.

Lefkovits J, Plow EF, Topol EJ. Platelet glycoprotein IIb/IIIa receptors in cardiovascular medicine. *N Engl J Med* 1995;332:1553–1559.

Riaz K, Forker AD. Digoxin use in congestive heart failure. *Drugs* 1998;55:747–758.

Roden DM. Risks and benefits of antiarrhythmic therapy. *N Engl J Med* 1994;331:785–791.

The SOLVD Investigators. Effect of enalapril on mortality and the development of heart failure in asymptomatic patients with reduced left ventricular ejection fractions. *N Engl J Med* 1992;327:685–691.

Stevenson LW. Inotropic therapy for heart failure. *N Engl J Med* 1998;339:1848–1850.

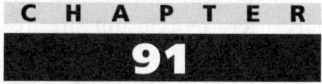

CHAPTER 91

USE OF ANTICOAGULANT DRUGS

MICHAEL D. EZEKOWITZ

Parenteral anticoagulation is usually achieved with heparin, which was first identified in 1916 by McLean, a medical student. Warfarin was first used in humans in 1953. Chronic anticoagula-tion requires the oral administration of warfarin. It acts by directly competing with vitamin K, thereby inhibiting synthesis of vitamin K–dependent coagulation factors.

HEPARIN

STRUCTURE AND COMPOSITION

Heparin is made up of a heterogeneous group of highly sulfated glycosaminoglycan molecules of different sizes and structures that are highly negatively charged. Heparin molecules vary according to (a) size, depending on the number of disaccharide residues; (b) constituents, depending on whether glycuronic or iduronic acid is present; and (c) sulfation and charge, depending on the extent and positioning of sulfate residues. All these factors contribute to functional heterogeneity between heparin molecules. Commercial preparations of heparin are heterogeneous. Their components have molecular weights ranging from 3,000 to 30,000 (mean, 15,000). Only about one-third of the heparin molecules have the specific pentasaccharide sequence required for binding with antithrombin III (ATIII). This fraction is responsible for most of its anticoagulant effect. Commercial heparin is most commonly obtained from the lungs or intestinal mucosa of cows or pigs, from which it is extracted as either the sodium or calcium salt.

MECHANISMS OF ACTION

The anticoagulant effect of heparin is mediated largely through its ability to bind to and catalyze ATIII. At high concentrations, heparin also catalyzes the inhibition of factor IIa. At concentrations at which heparin is used clinically, this interaction is thought to be of little importance. More important, the heparin–ATIII complex inhibits the activated coagulation enzymes X, XI, XII and IX (Xa, XIa, XIIa, and IXa). Thrombin and Xa are the coagulation factors that are most sensitive to inactivation; on average, inhibition of thrombin is about ten times greater than the inhibition of Xa, but relative sensitivities vary.

ACTIONS

The synthesis of heparin by mast cells, which are present in the perivascular tissues, suggests that heparin is not involved in maintaining blood fluidity. However, vascular endothelial cells synthesize heparin-like heparan sulfate molecules, suggesting that the heparin–antithrombin system plays an important physiologic role in the prevention of intravascular thrombosis.

Congenital deficiency states for heparin have not been described. Congenital deficiency of ATIII does occur and is associated with a hypercoagulability state. ATIII deficiency is inherited as an autosomal dominant disorder in which carriers have ATIII levels between 40% and 60% of normal. Affected persons have a high prevalence (30%–80%) of thromboses, which often occur before the fifth decade, are recurrent, may occur in unusual locations, and are associated with a positive family history of thrombosis.

Heparin may increase vessel wall permeability and activation of lipoprotein lipase. It may inhibit platelet function, reduce proliferation of vascular smooth muscle cells, inhibit delayed hypersensitivity reactions, and suppress aldosterone secretion and angiogenesis.

All heparin fractions can interfere with platelet function. There is evidence that large heparin molecules that have no or low affinity for ATIII are particularly potent inhibitors of platelets. Platelet inhibition, combined with increases in vascular permeability, probably accounts for dissociations between the antithrombotic and hemorrhagic effects of heparin.

PHARMACOKINETICS

Heparin is not absorbed after oral administration and therefore must be given by injection. The preferred routes of administration are intravenous and subcutaneous. Intramuscular injection may produce large hematomas by accidental puncture of an intramuscular vein. There is evidence that heparin administration by intermittent intravenous injection is associated with more bleeding than is administration by continuous intravenous infusion.

The efficacy and safety of heparin administered by either continuous infusions or subcutaneously are comparable, provided that the dosages used are adequate. However, if the subcutaneous route is selected, the initial dose must be sufficiently high to counteract the reduced bioavailability associated with this method of administration. If an immediate anticoagulant effect is required, the initial subcutaneous dose should be accompanied by an intravenous bolus injection to avoid the 1- to 2-hour delay in anticoagulant effect that occurs with subcutaneous heparin alone.

After its injection and passage into the bloodstream, heparin binds to a number of plasma proteins that can reversibly neutralize its anticoagulant activity and so reduce its bioavailability. Heparin also binds to endothelial cells and macrophages, further complicating its pharmacokinetics. Differences between individuals in protein- and cell-binding capacity for heparin contribute to the variability of the anticoagulant response commonly seen in patients with thromboembolic disorders and to the laboratory phenomenon of heparin resistance (see discussion later in this chapter).

Neither liver nor renal disease appears to influence heparin pharmacokinetics at standard therapeutic concentrations. Similarly, there is no convincing evidence that heparin pharmacokinetics is influenced by concomitant use of other medications. Heparin elimination is, however, increased in patients with acute pulmonary embolism by a mechanism that is poorly understood. Bleeding while on heparin therapy is increased by any process that additionally impairs hemostatic mechanisms. Such a process may include reduction in platelet numbers (e.g., lymphoproliferative disorders, therapeutic agents) or function (e.g., polycythemia rubra vera, aspirin) or reduction in the concentration of coagulation proteins (e.g., hepatic disease, oral anticoagulants). Pregnancy, malignancy, acute thrombosis, and major surgery may be associated with heparin resistance owing to an increase in procoagulant activity.

There appears to be no clinically important difference in the bioavailability of sodium or calcium heparin. When the two salts

have been directly compared in clinical trials assessing subcutaneous heparin prophylaxis for deep venous thrombosis, antithrombotic efficacy and hemorrhagic side effects have been similar.

After administration of an intravenous bolus of heparin, activity falls rapidly as equilibration occurs with binding to plasma proteins and cellular constituents, particularly endothelial cells. This is followed by a more gradual clearance that can best be explained by a combination of a saturable and a nonsaturable mechanism. The saturable phase of heparin clearance appears to be due to uptake by endothelial cells and macrophages, with depolymerization and metabolism to smaller less sulfated derivatives. The nonsaturable mechanism obeys first-order kinetics—the rate of clearance is linearly related to dose and can be accounted for by renal elimination.

The relative contribution of each of these mechanisms to clearance of heparin depends on the dose and size of the heparin fractions administered. Low doses of standard heparin are eliminated predominantly by the highly efficient but low-capacity saturable mechanism. With larger doses of heparin, capacity of the saturable mechanism is exceeded, so that at high doses renal clearance predominates. Larger heparin molecules are preferentially cleared by the saturable mechanism; this has important implications for dose-response relations and for differences between the pharmacokinetic properties of standard and low-molecular-weight heparins.

MONITORING HEPARIN THERAPY

Because there is no suitable chemical assay for heparin, the investigation of its kinetics has depended on measurements of its biologic activity. Currently used methods for measuring heparin activity are summarized in Table 91.1.

CLINICAL USE OF HEPARIN

The results of randomized controlled trials confirm that a relation exists between the clinical effectiveness of heparin and its ex vivo effect on the activated partial thromboplastin time (aPTT) for the following conditions; prevention of recurrent thrombosis in patients with proximal vein thrombosis; prevention of mural thrombus in patients with acute myocardial infarction; prevention of recurrent ischemia in patients who have had streptokinase therapy for acute myocardial infarction; and prevention of coronary artery reocclusion after tissue plasminogen activator.

Maintaining the aPTT ratio above 1.5 is associated with protection against thrombosis, but bleeding complications may occur within the therapeutic range. The risk of bleeding is increased by a number of factors, which include both the heparin dose and the degree of prolongation of the aPTT. A satisfactory approach is to give an initial bolus of 5,000 U intravenously unless contraindicated (e.g., surgery within 24 hours) followed by an infusion of 32,000 U over 24 hours. This is the average infusion rate required to achieve optimal anticoagulation. Because of the short half-life of heparin at therapeutic doses, infusion rates should be adjusted on the basis of aPTTs performed as closely as 6 hours apart, with the first performed 6 hours after

TABLE 91.1.   MEASUREMENT OF HEPARIN ACTIVITY

Method	Procedure	Therapeutic Range
Heparin assay	Thrombin or factor Xa is added to plasma sample; measure time to clotting	0.3–0.7 U/mL
Protamine titration of thrombin time	Protamine is added to thrombin-treated plasma sample; measure amount needed to inhibit clot formation	0.2–0.4 U/mL
Activated partial thromboplastin time (aPTT)	Kaolin and cephalin are added to a decalcified plasma sample; measure clotting time on recalcification	1.5–2.5

heparin is initiated. A heparin dose adjustment nomogram has been developed for aPTT reagents for which the therapeutic range is 1.9 to 2.7 times control (based on a protamine titration heparin level of 0.2 to 0.4 U). With this protocol, an aPTT above the lower limit of the therapeutic range was reached in 82% of patients after 24 hours and in 91% after 48 hours. This nomogram is not applicable to all aPTT reagents and should be adapted to the heparin responsiveness of the local thromboplastin in use.

In postmyocardial infarction patients who have received thrombolytic therapy, particularly streptokinase, a systemic lytic state may be observed with prolongation of clotting parameters. When intravenous heparin is given in this situation, the same 5,000-U intravenous bolus may be given, followed by 24,000 U over a 24-hour period (for the first 24 hours only adjusted upward if aPTT values are below the therapeutic range).

When the subcutaneous route is used for therapeutic anticoagulation, a suitable initial heparin dosage is 17,500 U every 12 hours. The dosage should be reduced to 12,500 U every 12 hours after thrombolytic therapy; at this lower dose, the heparin level does not exceed 0.1 anti-Xa U per milliliter and therefore coagulation monitoring is not required. For patients at particularly high risk, three studies have demonstrated that the efficacy of low-dose heparin is improved without compromising safety by adjusting the dose to achieve a minimal heparin effect. One of these studies, which aimed for an aPTT at the upper limit of normal, used a mean daily dose of 15,000 U of heparin; the other two prolonged the aPTT ratio to 1.1 to 1.2 with a mean daily dose in excess of 18,000 U. The adjusted dose regimen has limitations for routine use because it requires careful monitoring and the use of a responsive aPTT system.

SIDE EFFECTS

Bleeding

Four variables have been reported to influence bleeding during heparin treatment: (a) the dose of heparin; (b) the method of heparin administration; and patient factors such as (c) concur-

rent illness and (d) concurrent medication (Table 91.2). Pooled analysis of randomized trials comparing different methods of heparin administration yields an average incidence of major bleeding of 6.8% in the continuous-infusion group and 14.2% in the intermittent intravenous group (odds ratio 0.42; p .01). However, the comparison is confounded by the difference in the 24-hour heparin dose, which was greater in the intermittent intravenous group in five of the six studies. Thus, the observed increase in bleeding could be contributed to by the higher dose of heparin in the intermittent intravenous group.

For studies comparing continuous intravenous heparin with subcutaneous heparin, there was a similar bleeding incidence of 5.2% and 4.1%, respectively (odds ratio 1.1). Other factors that predispose to anticoagulant-induced bleeding are a serious concurrent illness, chronic heavy alcohol consumption, and a reduced functional capacity.

The concomitant use of aspirin has long been identified as a risk factor for heparin-induced bleeding. This observation bears close examination because the combination of heparin and aspirin is used often in the initial treatment of acute coronary artery syndromes. Aspirin increases operative and postoperative bleeding in patients who receive the very high doses of heparin required during open heart surgery. However, the risk of adding aspirin to a short course of regular therapeutic doses of heparin does not appear to be excessive.

Renal failure and patient age and gender also have been implicated as risk factors for heparin-induced bleeding. The reported association with female gender has not been consistent among studies and remains in question. The influence of patient-related factors on heparin-associated bleeding is illustrated by a recent

TABLE 91.2.   FACTORS INFLUENCING BLEEDING RISKS OF HEPARIN

Doses of heparin
Concurrent illness and medication
Method of heparin administration
Interindividual differences in protein and cell binding

study of patients with proximal vein thrombosis. Patients received an initial intravenous bolus of 5,000 U of heparin followed by a continuous infusion of 30,000 U per 24 hours for patients with clinical risk factors for bleeding and of 40,000 U per 24 hours in patients free of risk factors for bleeding. The incidence of major bleeding was 11% in the high-risk group (who received the lower starting dose) and 1% in the low-risk group (who received the higher starting dose).

Bleeding during an intravenous infusion usually can be managed with supportive measures and by stopping the infusion, because the half-life for heparin therapeutic levels is approximately 60 minutes, and heparin effect is rapidly lost. It may be necessary to reverse heparin effect more rapidly if bleeding is life threatening (e.g., massive gastrointestinal or intracranial bleeding) or if a heparin overdose has occurred when heparin elimination will be markedly delayed. The anticoagulant effects of heparin can be reversed with protamine sulfate, which binds firmly with heparin. The dose of protamine sulfate is determined by the amount of circulating heparin, which in turn depends on the amount of heparin that was administered and the time elapsed since the last heparin dose. The full neutralizing dose is 1 mg of protamine sulfate for 100 U heparin; this must be reduced to half of this at 1 hour and to one-fourth of this at 2 hours. Protamine should be infused over 10 minutes to avoid hypotension and may need to be repeated because of its rapid clearance. Smaller repeated doses of protamine will be required to reverse therapeutic doses of heparin that have been given subcutaneously.

Thrombocytopenia

The reported incidence of heparin-associated thrombocytopenia varies widely. Thrombocytopenia is more common with heparin derived from bovine lung than that derived from porcine gut. Pooled analysis of recent prospective studies of full-dose intravenous heparin (thrombocytopenia defined as a platelet count less than 100×10^9 per liter) yielded a prevalence of thrombocytopenia of 5.4% for bovine and 1.3% for porcine heparin. The prevalence of thrombocytopenia in association with low-dose subcutaneous heparin appears to be lower than with full-dose intravenous therapy. Arterial thrombosis as a complication of heparin-induced thrombocytopenia (HIT) is also rare (0.18%). Arterial thrombosis occurs as a consequence of platelet aggregation in vivo, but venous thrombosis could result from heparin resistance caused by the neutralizing effect of heparin-induced release of platelet factor 4.

Thrombocytopenia usually begins between 3 and 15 days after the commencement of heparin therapy (median 10 days), but it has been reported within hours of commencing heparin in patients who have been exposed to heparin previously. The platelet count usually returns to baseline levels within 4 days after stopping heparin. Heparin-associated thrombocytopenia is thought to be caused by an IgG–heparin immune complex involving both the Fab and Fc portions of the IgG molecule. If the platelet count falls progressively or precipitously to less than 100,000 per milliliter, heparin should be stopped and an alternative management strategy instituted. If warfarin treatment has already been started and the international normalized ratio

---

TABLE 91.3.	**POTENTIAL PROBLEMS WITH THE INTERNATIONAL NORMALIZATION RATIO**

Lack of reliability at the onset of warfarin therapy
Loss of accuracy and precision when thromboplastins with high ISI values are used.
Loss of accuracy with automatic clot detectors
Lack of reliability of the ISI result provided by the manufacturer
Incorrect calculation of the INR because an inappropriate normal control plasma is used to calculate the patient's prothrombin time ratio

INR, international normalized ratio; ISI, international sensitivity index.

(INR) is approaching or in the therapeutic range, warfarin can be continued without the addition of alternative treatment (Table 91.3). If warfarin has not been started and heparin is being used to treat venous thromboembolism, a caval filter can be inserted or an alternative antithrombotic agent used. Two alternative antithrombotic agents have been evaluated in descriptive studies. These are the snake venom ancrod and the heparinoid Lomoparin (Organon).

The diagnosis of suspected HIT can be confirmed by laboratory tests. A test based on ^{14}C serotonin release of washed donor platelets plus heat-treated patient serum in the presence of therapeutic (0.1 U and high 100 U per milliliter) heparin concentrations has been shown to be both sensitive and specific.

Osteoporosis

The incidence of osteoporosis occurs as a complication of heparin therapy has been difficult to determine, because the need for long-term heparin treatment is rare. When it occurs, randomization to heparin or alternative therapy is usually not clinically justifiable. In one randomized trial that did address this question, 1 of the 20 women allocated to long-term antenatal heparin prophylaxis (10,000 U twice daily) developed clinical osteoporosis, whereas no patients in the control group did. A number of other descriptive series and case-controlled studies have also evaluated clinical or radiologic end points. Taken in combination, these studies suggest that heparin-induced osteoporosis is largely confined to patients who receive moderately high doses ($\geq$20,000 U per 24 hours) for more than 5 months.

OTHER SIDE EFFECTS

Heparin has been reported to produce two distinct types of skin lesions—urticarial lesions and skin necrosis. *Urticarial lesions* occur at the site of subcutaneous injection and may be caused by a contaminant in heparin. Changing to a different preparation (i.e., a different salt or different animal origin) may resolve this problem. *Skin necrosis* usually occurs as a complication of subcutaneous heparin but has also been observed in association with the intravenous route of administration. The mechanism of skin necrosis is uncertain; it is inconsistently associated with thrombocytopenia but may be caused by a heparin-associated immune reaction. Histologic studies have found hemorrhagic infarction of skin and subcutaneous fat with acute necrotizing angiitis, in keeping with a hypersensitivity reaction. Skin necrosis seems to be unrelated to the source of the heparin, and, consequently, a different preparation of standard heparin is unlikely to be tolerated. The heparinoid Lomoparin, which has minimal cross-reactivity with standard heparin, may be a safe alternative in these patients, but this has yet to be demonstrated equivocally. Generalized hypersensitivity reactions may also occur as a result of heparin. Symptoms include urticaria, conjunctivitis, rhinitis, bronchospasm, angioneurotic edema, and anaphylactic shock.

Selective hypoaldosteronism is a rare but probably real side effect of heparin administration, which appears to be caused by inhibition of 18-hydroxycorticosterone synthesis from corticosterone. It is usually of no clinical importance, although significant metabolic derangements and death have been reported in a few cases.

LOW-MOLECULAR-WEIGHT HEPARINS

Smaller heparin molecules bind less to plasma proteins and endothelial cells, are cleared predominantly by nonsaturable renal mechanisms rather than by the rapid saturable cellular route, inhibit platelet function to a lesser extent, have little affect on vascular permeability, and have a higher anti-Xa to anti IIa ratio than larger heparin molecules. A number of low-molecular-weight heparins (LMWHs) have been approved for use in North America.

Biochemistry and Anticoagulant Effects of LMWHs

LMWHs are fragments of heparin produced by either chemical or enzymic depolymerization. LMWHs are approximately one-third of the size of heparin with a molecular weight distribution of 1,000 to 10,000 and a mean molecular weight of 4,000 to 5,000. Depolymerization of heparin results in a change in the anticoagulant profile of the resulting low-molecular-weight fractions, with a progressive loss of their ability to catalyze thrombin inhibition. In addition to LMWHs produced by depolymerization, two other glycosaminoglycans have been developed for clinical use. These are dermatan sulfate and the heparinoid Lomoparin, which is a mixture of heparan sulfate (80% of the mixture), dermatan sulfate, and chondroitin sulfate.

LMWHs produce their anticoagulant effect by binding to ATIII through the same unique pentasaccharide sequence as standard heparin, which is present on less than one-third of LMWH molecules. Because a minimum chain length of 18 saccharides (including the pentasaccharide sequence) is required for ternary complex formation (heparin–ATIII–thrombin), only the larger molecules in each preparation are able to inactivate thrombin. In contrast, all LMWH fragments that contain the high-affinity pentasaccharide sequence catalyze the inactivation of factor Xa. Almost all standard heparin molecules contain at least 18 saccharide units, whereas only 25% to 50% of different LMWHs contain fragments of this or greater length.

Pharmacokinetics of LMWHs

The pharmacokinetics of LMWHs differs from standard heparin largely because of the reduced binding and clearance by plasma proteins, macrophages, and endothelial cells. These differences likely account for their longer plasma half-life, which is approximately two- to fourfold longer than standard heparin. Minimal protein binding contributes to excellent bioavailability of LMWHs at low doses and a predictable anticoagulant dose response. Because they are cleared principally by the kidneys, the half-life of LMWHs is largely independent of the dose administered, and, unlike standard heparin, it is prolonged with renal failure.

Antithrombotic and Hemorrhagic Effects of LMWHs

When compared with standard heparin in experimental models of thrombosis and hemorrhage, LMWHs are slightly less effective as antithrombotic agents but produce much less bleeding. The improved antithrombotic to bleeding ratio with LMWHs is thought to be the result of less impairment of platelet function, reduced binding of von Willebrand's factor, and reduced effects on vascular permeability. LMWHs have been compared with standard heparin and have been shown to be more effective in preventing venous thrombosis in high-risk patients and to be more effective and safer for the treatment of venous thrombosis. Together with more uniform bioavailability and predictable dose-response relations, these properties open the way for therapeutic anticoagulation with LMWHs without the need for frequent monitoring. This could make it feasible to treat some acute thrombotic disorders on an outpatient basis, an advance that would reduce cost and improve patient convenience.

Unresolved Issues with LMWHs

Like standard heparin, LMWHs do not cross the placental barrier, and descriptive studies suggest they are safe and effective in pregnancy, but experience is limited. As previously noted, the long-term use of standard heparin may be complicated with osteoporosis. It is not known if the risk of osteoporosis is reduced or eliminated by LMWHs.

There is an impression that the incidence of thrombocytopenia is lower with LMWHs than with standard heparin, but this has never been confirmed in a properly designed clinical study. There are reports that LMWH can be associated with thrombocytopenia, both in previously unexposed individuals and in those with a history of HIT, and that LMWH preparations cross-react with plasma from patients with recent HIT. In contrast to the LMWHs, the heparinoid Lomoparin, which is essentially free of contaminating heparin, has minimal cross-reactivity in in vitro assays for HIT and has been used successfully in patients with a history of HIT. Prospective studies of large numbers of patients treated with LMWH are required to resolve these issues.

WARFARIN

MECHANISM OF ACTION

Oral anticoagulants produce their anticoagulant effect by interfering with the cyclic interconversion of vitamin K and its 2,3 epoxide (vitamin K epoxide). Vitamin K is a cofactor for the post-translational carboxylation of glutamate residues to γ-carboxyglutamates (Gla) on the N-terminal regions of vitamin K–dependent proteins.

PHARMACOKINETICS AND PHARMACODYNAMICS OF WARFARIN

Warfarin is rapidly absorbed from the gastrointestinal tract and reaches maximal blood concentrations in healthy volunteers in 90 minutes. The dose-response relation of warfarin differs among healthy subjects and can vary to a much greater extent among sick patients. Because of the variations in dose response in individual patients during the course of anticoagulant therapy, their anticoagulant dosage must be monitored closely.

Drugs can influence the pharmacokinetics of warfarin by reducing its absorption from the intestine or by altering its metabolic clearance (Table 91.4). The anticoagulant effect of warfarin is reduced by cholestyramine, which impairs its absorption. It can be potentiated by drugs that inhibit the metabolic clearance of warfarin either through stereoselective or nonselective pathways. Stereoselective interactions can affect the oxidative metabolism of the S-isomer or R-isomer of warfarin. Inhibition of metabolism of S-warfarin is more important clinically because this isomer is five times more potent as a vitamin K antagonist than the R-form. Therefore, drugs that inhibit clearance of the S-isomer prolong the prothrombin time (PT) to a much greater degree than drugs that inhibit the metabolic clearance of the R-isomer. The clearance of S-warfarin is inhibited by phenylbutazone, sulfinpyrazone, disulfiram, metronidazole, and trimethoprim-sulfamethoxazole, all of which have been documented to potentiate the effect of warfarin on the PT. In contrast, drugs such as cimetidine and omeprazole inhibit only the metabolic clearance of the R-isomer. They have only moderate potentiating effects on the PT in patients treated with oral anticoagulants. Amiodarone inhibits the metabolic clearance of both the S- and R-isomers and has an important potentiating effect on the anticoagulant effect of warfarin. The anticoagulant effect of warfarin is inhibited by drugs such as barbiturates, rifampicin, and carbamazepine, which increase its metabolic clearance by inducing activity of hepatic mixed oxidases. Chronic alcohol use has the potential to increase the clearance of warfarin by hepatic enzyme induction.

TABLE 91.4.	INTERACTIONS WITH WARFARIN		
Level of Evidence	Potentiation	Inhibition	No Effect
I	Alcohol (if concomitant liver disease), amiodarone, anabolic steroids, cimetidine, clofibrate, cotrimoxazole, erythromycin, fluconazole, isoniazid (600 mg daily), metronidazole, miconazole, omeprazole, **phenylbutazone**[a], piroxicam, propafenone, propranolol[b], **sulfinpyrazone, (biphasic with later inhibition)**	Barbiturates, carbamazepine, chlordiazepoxide, cholestyramine, **griseofulvin**, nafcillin, rifampin, sucralfate, high vitamin K content foods/enteral feeds, large amounts of avocado	Alcohol, antacids, atenolol, bumetadine, enoxacin, famotidine, fluoxetine, ketorolac, metoprolol, naproxen, nizatidine, psyllium, ranitidine[c]
II	Acetaminophen, chloral hydrate, ciprofloxacin, dextropropoxyphene, disulfiram, itraconazole, quinidine, phenytoin (biphasic with later inhibition), tamoxifen, tetracycline, flu vaccine	Dicloxacillin	Ibuprofen, ketoconazole
III	Acetylsalicylic acid, disopyramide, fluorouracil, ifosphamide, ketoprofen, lovastatin, metozalone, moricizine, nalidixic acid, norfloxacin, ofloxacin, propoxyphene, sulindac, tolmetin, topical salicylates	Azathioprine, cyclosporine, etretinate, trazodone	
IV	Cefamandole, cefazolin, gemfibrozil, heparin, indomethacin, sulfisoxazole		Diltiazem, tobacco, vantomycin

[a] In a small number of volunteer subjects, an inhibitory drug interaction occurred.
[b] Drugs outlined in **bold** are those that have supporting level I evidence from both patients and volunteers.
[c] Level II evidence of potentiation in patients.

Hereditary resistance to warfarin has been described. The affected persons require warfarin in doses 5 to 20 times higher than average to achieve an anticoagulant effect. This disorder is thought to be caused by an altered affinity of the receptor for warfarin because the plasma warfarin levels required to achieve an anticoagulant effect are much higher than average.

Subjects receiving long-term warfarin therapy are sensitive to fluctuating levels of dietary vitamin K, which is obtained predominantly from phylloquinone in plant material. Important fluctuations in vitamin K intake occur in both apparently healthy and sick subjects. Increased intake of dietary vitamin K sufficient to reduce the anticoagulant response to warfarin occurs in patients on weight reduction diets (rich in green vegetables) and those treated with intravenous nutritional fluid supplements rich in vitamin K. The effects of warfarin can be potentiated in sick patients with poor vitamin K intake (particularly if they are treated with antibiotics and intravenous fluids without vitamin K supplementation) and in those in states of fat malabsorption. Hepatic dysfunction also potentiates the response to warfarin through impaired synthesis of coagulation factors. Hypermetabolic states produced by fever or hyperthyroidism increase responsiveness to warfarin, probably by increasing the catabolism of vitamin K–dependent coagulation factors. Drugs can influence the pharmacodynamics of warfarin by inhibiting the synthesis of vitamin K–dependent coagulation factors, by increasing the metabolic clearance of vitamin K–dependent coagulation factors, and by interfering with other pathways of hemostasis. The anticoagulant effect of warfarin is augmented (a) by the second- and third-generation cephalosporins because these antibiotics inhibit the cyclic interconversion of vitamin K, (b) by thyroxine because this hormone increases the rate of metabolism of coagulation factors, and (c) by clofibrate through an unknown mechanism. Although heparin increases the anticoagulant effect of warfarin, it causes only a slight prolongation of the PT at therapeutic levels.

Drugs such as aspirin in high doses, other nonsteroidal anti-inflammatory drugs, high doses of penicillins, and moxalactam can increase the risk of warfarin-associated bleeding by inhibiting platelet function. Aspirin in high doses can also produce gastric erosions, which increase the risk of serious upper gastrointestinal bleeding. The risk of clinically important bleeding is increased when high doses of aspirin are used in combination with high-intensity warfarin therapy (INR 3.0 to 4.5). In contrast, a recent study has reported that low doses of aspirin (100 mg per day), which retain their antithrombotic efficacy and have only minimal gastric side effects, increase the efficacy of warfarin without significantly increasing the risk of major bleeding.

Sulfonamides and many broad-spectrum antibiotics may augment the anticoagulant effect of warfarin by eliminating bacterial flora and thereby producing vitamin K deficiency. However, these agents potentiate the anticoagulant effect of warfarin only in patients on a vitamin K–deficient diet. It is prudent to take special care when treatment with any new drug is necessary in patients who are being treated with oral anticoagulants and to monitor the INR time more frequently during the initial stages of combined drug therapy, with dose adjustments made when appropriate.

MONITORING ORAL ANTICOAGULANT THERAPY

The PT test is the most common method for monitoring oral anticoagulant therapy. The PT is responsive to depressions of three of the four vitamin K–dependent procoagulant clotting factors (factors II, VII, and X). These are reduced by warfarin at a rate proportional to their respective half-lives. The PT is performed by adding calcium and thromboplastin to citrated plasma. The term "thromboplastin" refers to a phospholipid–protein extract of tissues, usually lung, brain, or placenta, which contains both the tissue factor and the phospholipid necessary to promote the activation of factor X by factor VII. During the first few days of warfarin therapy, the PT reflects primarily the depression of factor VII, which has a half-life of approximately 6 hours. Subsequently, the test is prolonged also by depression of factors II and X. The responsiveness of a given thromboplastin to warfarin-induced changes in clotting factors mirrors the strength of the activation of factor X by factor VII as the levels of both of the clotting factors decrease. An unresponsive thromboplastin produces accelerated stimulation of factor X, resulting in a lesser prolongation of the PT for a given reduction in clotting factors than that caused by a less responsive thromboplastin.

A calibration model adopted in 1982 is used to standardize the reporting of the PT by converting the PT ratio observed with the local thromboplastin into an INR, calculated as follows:

$$INR = observed\ ratio_c\ Patient\ Pt_c/\ Control\ PT$$

where C is the power value that represents the international sensitivity index (ISI). The ISI is a measure of the responsiveness of a given thromboplastin to reduction of the vitamin K–dependent coagulation factors compared with the international reference preparation; the lower the ISI, the more responsive is the reagent. The INR system loses accuracy and precision when thromboplastins with high ISI values are used (Table 91.3).

PRACTICAL DOSING

After administration of coumarin, an observable anticoagulant effect is delayed until newly synthesized dysfunctional vitamin K–dependent clotting factors replace the normal clotting factors as the latter are cleared from the circulation. Depending on the dose administered, the delay may range from 2 to 7 days. An approach to warfarin dosing and monitoring is as follows: if a rapid anticoagulant effect is required, an initial dose is administered in combination with heparin, which is then discontinued when the INR has been in the therapeutic range for at least 2 days. If treatment is not urgent (e.g., chronic stable atrial fibrillation) and the patient is under the age of 70 years, treatment can be commenced with an anticipated maintenance dose of 4 to 5 mg per day, which achieves a steady-state anticoagulant effect in 5 to 7 days. PT (INR) monitoring is usually performed after 5 to 7 days after institution of therapy, then weekly for 1 to 2 weeks, and then less often, depending on the stability of INR results. If the INR response remains stable, testing can be drawn out to intervals as long as every 4 to 6 weeks. If adjustments to the dose are required or clinical situations or drug changes occur, then the cycle of more frequent monitoring is repeated until a stable dose response is again achieved.

Some patients on long-term coumarin therapy are difficult to manage because they have unexpected fluctuations in dose response. The unexpected fluctuations in dose response could be due to changes in diet, inaccuracy in PT testing, undisclosed drug use, poor patient compliance, surreptitious self-medication, or intermittent alcohol consumption. We recommend an initial dose of 3 mg daily for patients over 70 years of age. For these patients particularly, concomitant monitoring of blood pressure is essential to reduce the incidence of intracranial bleeding.

MANAGEMENT OF PATIENTS WITH HIGH INR VALUES

An approach to managing patients with high INR values has been developed. The following guidelines are suggested:

1. If the INR is above the therapeutic range but below 6.0, if the patient is not bleeding, and if rapid reversal is not indicated for reasons of surgical intervention, the next few doses can be omitted and warfarin therapy can be resumed at a lower dose when the INR is in the therapeutic range.
2. If the INR is above 6.0 but below 10.0 and the patient is not bleeding or when rapid reversal is required because the patient requires elective surgery, vitamin K_1 can be given subcutaneously in a dose of 0.5 mg to 1 mg with the expectation that a demonstrable reduction of the INR will occur at 8 hours and that in many patients the INR will be in the therapeutic range of 2.0 to 3.0 within 24 hours. If the INR remains high at 24 hours, an additional dose of 0.5 mg vitamin K_1 can be given. Warfarin treatment can then be resumed at a lower dose.
3. If the INR is above 10.0 but below 20.0 and the patient is not bleeding, a higher dose of vitamin K (3 mg to 5 mg) should be given subcutaneously with the expectation that the INR will be reduced substantially at 6 hours. The INR should be checked in 6 hours and vitamin K can then be repeated, if necessary. Subcutaneous injection of vitamin K is preferred over intravenous injection in these circumstances because rapid intravenous infusion of vitamin K can produce anaphylactoid reactions.
4. If a very rapid reversal of an anticoagulant effect is required because of serious bleeding or major warfarin overdose (e.g., INR more than 20.0), vitamin K in a dose of 10 mg should be given by slow intravenous infusion (e.g., over 20 to 30 minutes) and the INR checked every 6 hours. It may be necessary to repeat vitamin K at 12-hour intervals and supplement with plasma transfusion or prothrombin complex concentrate, depending on the urgency of the situation.
5. In case of life-threatening bleeding or serious warfarin overdose, replacement with prothrombin complex concentrate is indicated, supplemented with intravenous vitamin K (10 mg), which should be repeated as necessary, depending on the INR.
6. If continued warfarin therapy is indicated after high doses of

vitamin K administration, heparin can be given until the effects of vitamin K have been reversed and the patient becomes responsive to warfarin.

CLINICAL INDICATIONS

PREVENTION OF VENOUS THROMBOEMBOLISM

Oral anticoagulants are effective in preventing venous thrombosis after hip surgery and major gynecologic surgery when used at a targeted INR of 2.0 to 3.0 (Table 91.5). Benefit has been demonstrated when treatment is commenced a number of days before surgery, the evening before surgery, or on the first postoperative day. The risk of clinically important bleeding with the less intense regimen is small, but because warfarin prophylaxis is more complicated to use than fixed low-dose heparin, warfarin is generally reserved for very-high-risk patients such as those with previous venous thrombosis or those having major orthopedic procedures. For patients undergoing elective hip replacement or major knee surgery, low-molecular-weight heparins have been shown to be more effective than warfarin commenced postoperatively or the night before surgery.

Very low fixed doses of warfarin (1 mg daily) have been reported to be effective in one small study in patients having gynecologic surgery and in a larger study in which 1 mg of warfarin per day was effective in preventing subclavian vein thrombosis in cancer patients with indwelling subclavian catheters. It is surprising that the very-low-dose warfarin was associated with an increase in fibrinolysis in the gynecologic patients. One recent randomized study demonstrated that warfarin in a fixed dose of 1 mg is ineffective in preventing postoperative venographically proven venous thrombosis in patients having hip and knee surgery. The other studies in hip surgery—one uncontrolled and another based on fibrinogen uptake studies—produced similar findings. Although it is attractive because of its safety and simplicity, the 1-mg dose is now clearly ineffective in patients having hip and knee replacements and should not be used for those with these high-risk conditions. Levine and associates reported that low-dose warfarin with a targeted INR of 1.5 is effective in preventing thrombosis in patients with stage IV breast cancer.

TREATMENT OF DEEP VENOUS THROMBOSIS

Initial therapy is with heparin or low-molecular-weight heparin. Caution is advised in patients having spinal or epidural anesthesia because of the risk of bleeding and paraplegia. Antithrombotic therapy should be commenced only when the needle has been removed and contraindicated if bleeding has occurred. Oral anticoagulant therapy is indicated for up to 3 months in patients with proximal vein thrombosis and in patients with symptomatic calf vein thrombosis. A less intense regimen (INR 2.0 to 2.5) is as effective as the more intense regimen (INR 3.0 to 4.5) but is associated with a much lower incidence of bleeding. More recently, studies in patients with proximal vein thrombosis evaluating short-course compared with long-course heparin treatment

TABLE 91.5.	**ANTITHROMBOTIC REGIMENTS TO PREVENT VENOUS THROMBOEMBOLISM**
Method	**Description**
LDUH	5,000 U heparin given q8–12 hr, starting 1–2 hr before operation
Adjusted-dose subcutaneous heparin (ADH)	3,500 U heparin given q8h with postoperative dose adjustments by ± 500 U to maintain aPTT at high-normal value

LMWH and heparinoids[a]	**General surgery**
	Moderate risk
	  Dalteparin, 2,500 U 1–2 hr before surgery and once daily after surgery
	  Enoxaparin, 2,000 U 1–2 hr before surgery and once daily after surgery
	  Nadroparin, 3,100 U 2 hr before surgery and once daily after surgery
	  Tinzaparin, 3,500 U 2 hr before surgery and once daily after surgery
	High risk
	  Dalteparin, 5,000 U 10–12 hr before surgery and once daily aftery surgery
	  Daparoid, 750 U 1–2 hr before surgery and twice daily after surgery
	  Enoxaparin, 4,000 U 10–12 hr before surgery and once daily after surgery
	  Enoxaparin, 3,000 U twice daily starting 12–24 hr after surgery
	Orthopedic surgery
	  Ardeparin, 50 U/kg twice daily starting 12–24 hr after surgery
	  Dalteparin, 5,000 8–12 hr before surgery and once daily starting 12 h after surgery
	  Danaparoid, 750 U 1–2 hr before surgery and twice daily after surgery
	  Enoxaparin, 3,000 U twice daily starting 12–24 hr after surgery or 4,000 U once daily starting 10–12 hr before surgery
	  Nadroparin, 40 U/kg starting 2 h before surgery and once daily after surgery or 4,000 U once daily after surgery for 3 d: the dose is then decreased to 60 U/kg once daily
	  Tinzaparin, 50 U/kg 2 hr before surgery and once daily after surgery or 75 U/kg once daily starting 12–24 hr after surgery
	Acute spinal injury
	  Enoxaparin, 3,000 U twice daily
	Multiple trauma
	  Enoxaparin, 3,000 U twice daily starting 12–36 hr after injury
	Medical conditions
	  Dalteparin, 2,500 U once daily
	  Danaparoid, 750 U twice daily
	  Enoxaparin, 3,000 U once daily

Adjusted-dose perioperative warfarin	Start daily dose (5 mg) the day of or the day after operation; adjust dose for INR 2–3 by day 5
Preoperative and postoperative two-step warfarin	Start 1–2.5 mg/d 5–14 d before operation, aiming for 2- to 3-sec increase in prothrombin time at time of operation; give 2.5–5 mg/d, aiming for an INR 2–3 in postoperative period
Minidose warfarin	Start 1 mg/d 10–14 d before operation, aiming for INR 1.5 after operation
IPC/ES	Start immediately before operation, and continue until fully ambulatory

[a] Dosage expressed in anti-Xa units; use with caution in patients having spinal or epidural anesthesia/analgesia. Ardeparin, enoxaparin, dalteparin, and danaparoid are approved by the Food and Drug Administration.
aPTT, activated partial thromboplastin time; INR, international normalized ratio.

have confirmed the initial observation that moderate-dose warfarin is associated with a low rate of recurrent venous thromboembolism and a low incidence of bleeding.

ACUTE MYOCARDIAL INFARCTION

Intravenous heparin or low-molecular-weight heparin is indicated in the acute phase of myocardial infarction. There is evidence that less intense warfarin therapy (INR 2.0 to 3.0) is effective in preventing stroke and venous thromboembolism in patients with acute myocardial infarction and that a higher intensity (INR 3.0 to 4.5) is effective in reducing recurrent infarction, stroke, and death.

The early evidence that oral anticoagulants are effective for the early treatment of acute myocardial infarction comes from studies performed in the 1960s and 1970s, which reported that a low-intensity warfarin regimen (presumptive INR 1.5 to 2.5) is effective for preventing stroke and pulmonary embolism. Three randomized trials evaluated the effectiveness of oral anticoagulants in patients with acute myocardial infarction. Two of these, the MRC study and the Veterans Affairs Cooperative Study, showed a significant reduction in stroke; the third, the Bronx

Municipal Study, reported a nonsignificant trend. The Bronx Municipal Study showed a significant reduction in mortality, whereas the other two showed no effect on mortality. All three studies showed a reduction in the incidence of clinically diagnosed pulmonary embolism.

The early evidence that oral anticoagulants are effective in the long-term management of acute myocardial infarction comes from analysis of pooled data from seven randomized trials published between 1964 and 1980, which showed that oral anticoagulant therapy during a 1- to 6-year treatment period reduced the combined end points of mortality and nonfatal reinfarction by approximately 20%.

The question of the value of oral anticoagulants has been reopened by the results of three more recent studies. The study by the Sixty-Plus Reinfarction Study Group was limited to patients over the age of 60 who had been treated with oral anticoagulants for at least 6 months. Although there was a significant reduction in reinfarction and in stroke in patients randomized to receive continuing anticoagulant therapy, the findings were limited by its lack of generalizability as a "stopping trial" in a select age group. The study by Smith and associates had no age restriction and showed a 50% reduction in the incidence of the combined outcomes of recurrent infarction, stroke, and mortality. The most recent study, Anticoagulants in the Secondary Prevention of Events in Coronary Thrombosis (ASPECT) trial, also had no age restriction and reported a higher than 50% reduction in reinfarction and a 40% reduction in stroke.

All three contemporary studies used high-intensity regimens (INR of 2.7 to 4.5 in the first; 2.8 to 4.8 in the other two), and all reported an increased incidence of bleeding with anticoagulants. Indirect support for the efficacy of oral anticoagulants in patients with coronary artery disease comes from a randomized trial of patients with peripheral arterial disease. Compared with an untreated control group, a relatively high-intensity oral anticoagulant regimen (INR 2.6 to 4.5) produced a significant (50%) reduction in mortality (6.8% to 3.3% per year). Studies are ongoing, evaluating the role of warfarin and aspirin in combination among survivors of myocardial infarction.

PROSTHETIC HEART VALVES

There have been no clinical trials comparing oral anticoagulants with an untreated control group in patients with prosthetic heart valves (for ethical reasons); however, a trial with aspirin as the comparator found that the bleeding in the warfarin group was significantly less than in those who received antiplatelet drugs (relative risk reduction 60% to 79%). The incidence of bleeding was highest in the warfarin group. The minimum effective intensity of anticoagulant therapy has been evaluated in three studies that compared the efficacy and safety of two levels of intensity of warfarin therapy. The first included only patients with tissue heart valves and showed that the less intense regimen (INR 2.0 to 2.25) was as effective but produced less bleeding than the more intense regimen (INR 2.5 to 4.0). The second study, which included patients with mechanical prosthetic heart valves, compared a very-high-intensity regimen prothrombin ratio (INR 7.4 to 10.8) with a lower-intensity regimen (INR 1.9 to 3.6). There was no difference in effectiveness between the two regimens, but the higher-intensity regimen produced significantly more

bleeding. A third study, which included patients with mechanical prosthetic valves, all of whom received aspirin and dipyridamole, compared the efficacy and safety of a low-intensity regimen (INR 2.0 to 3.0) with a high-intensity regimen (INR 3.0 to 4.5). No difference in efficacy was found between those in the two regimens, but, as in the previous studies, the high-intensity regimen was associated with a statistically significant increase in bleeding.

Thus, two studies have now demonstrated that moderate-intensity warfarin treatment is as effective as a high-dose regimen, although in one, all patients also received aspirin and dipyridamole. A recently completed randomized trial has shown that the addition of aspirin in a dose of 100 mg per day to warfarin (INR 3.0 to 4.5) results in a marked improvement in efficacy when compared with warfarin (INR 3.0 to 4.5) plus placebo. The combined low-dose aspirin and high-intensity warfarin regimen produced a significant and clinically impressive reduction in general mortality, in cardiovascular mortality, and in stroke, without a significant increase in major bleeding or cerebral hemorrhage.

ATRIAL FIBRILLATION

Five primary prevention trials, all with relatively similar study designs, were performed. Three were carried out in the United States—the Stroke Prevention in Atrial Fibrillation trial (SPAF), the Boston Area Anticoagulation Trial for Atrial Fibrillation (BAATAF), and the Stroke Prevention in Atrial Fibrillation trial (SPINAF). One trial was carried out in Denmark—the Copenhagen Atrial Fibrillation, Aspirin, Anticoagulation study (AFASAK); and the other was performed in Canada—the Canadian Atrial Fibrillation Anticoagulation study (CAFA). In two of the trials (AFASAK and SPAF), a third group of subjects was randomized to aspirin therapy. To be eligible for enrollment in these studies, patients were required to be good candidates for anticoagulant therapy. All five trials reached consistent conclusions, with a pooled 68% risk reduction on intention-to-treat analysis. All trials reached a statistically significant difference ($p < 0.05$) except for the Canadian study, which was stopped prematurely after the results of other trials became available. In patients who remained on treatment with warfarin, the reduction of stroke risk was greater than 80%. The rates of hemorrhagic complications were low, with little difference between the rate of major or intracranial hemorrhage in the warfarin, aspirin, or control groups. Minor hemorrhage was increased by approximately 3% per year in the warfarin group. Results from the aspirin treatment arms of the two original studies that randomized patients to aspirin therapy were consistent with a small benefit. In the AFASAK study, which used a 75-mg daily dose of aspirin, the 14% reduction in stroke was not statistically significant, whereas in the SPAF trial a 325-mg daily dose of aspirin was associated with a 44% reduction of risk of stroke.

The European Atrial Fibrillation Trial (EAFT) study compared anticoagulant therapy, aspirin, and placebo in patients with atrial fibrillation who had sustained a stroke or transient ischemic attack within the preceding 3 months. There was a 68% reduction in stroke risk with anticoagulant therapy and a 16% stroke risk reduction in the aspirin group. Of interest, the reduction in stroke risk with an aspirin dose of 300 mg per day was comparable to the reduction observed in the AFASAK study, which used an aspirin dose of 75 mg per day. None of the patients in the anticoagulant group of the EAFT suffered an intracranial hemorrhage.

In the second phase of the Stroke Prevention in Atrial Fibrillation (SPAF II) trial using an intention-to-treat analysis, warfarin was slightly more effective than aspirin for preventing ischemic stroke. This difference was almost entirely offset, however, by a higher rate of intracranial hemorrhage in the warfarin group, in patients over 75 years of age who had a rate of intracranial hemorrhage 1.8% per year compared with approximately 0.3% in the other trials. The intensity of anticoagulant therapy was higher in the SPAF II trial than in the primary prevention studies. In addition, most patients who suffered an intracranial hemorrhage during any of the trials had relatively high levels of anticoagulation, with estimated INRs greater than 3.0 at the time of the hemorrhage. Therefore, the high rate of cerebral hemorrhage observed in the anticoagulant group in the SPAF 2 study was possibly related to the high intensity of anticoagulation in the elderly patients who may be at particularly high risk for intracranial hemorrhage when INR values are greater than 3.0. In addition, when an on-treatment analysis was performed, the benefit of warfarin over aspirin in both the under- and over-75-year group was about 50%.

In a pooled analysis of the primary prevention trials, it was determined that increasing age, history of hypertension, history of diabetes mellitus, and a previous transient ischemia attack or stroke are independent predictors of a higher risk of stroke in patients with atrial fibrillation. Accordingly, in patients under the age of 65 without risk factors, anticoagulation does not seem to be of benefit. However, in patients under the age of 65 with risk factors and over the age of 65 with or without risk factors, anticoagulation significantly reduces the risk of stroke, particularly in women.

EVALUATION OF WARFARIN AND ASPIRIN IN COMBINATION

The SPAF III study evaluated 1,044 patients with atrial fibrillation who also had at least one prespecified risk factor for thromboembolic disease. The prespecified risk factors increased were congestive heart failure or left ventricular fractional shortening less than 25%, previous thromboembolism, systolic pressure greater than 160 mm Hg, or being a woman over 75 years of age. Patients were randomly assigned either to a combination of low-intensity, fixed-dose warfarin adjusted to an INR of 1.2 to 1.5 for initial dose adjustment and aspirin 325 mg per day or to adjusted-dose warfarin for an INR of 2.0 to 3.0. The mean INR in the combination group was 1.3 compared with 2.4 for those taking adjusted-dose warfarin. The trial was terminated after a mean follow-up of 1.1 years when the rate of ischemic stroke and systemic embolization in the combination therapy group was 7.9% per year, compared with 1.9% per year in the dose-adjusted group (RR 74%; $p < 0.0001$). The rates of major bleeding were similar in both treatment groups. Thus, following the regimen of low-intensity, fixed-dose warfarin plus aspirin was not sufficient for stroke prevention in patients with nonvalvular atrial fibrillation who were considered to be at high risk for thromboembolic complications. This study further confirmed the benefit of therapeutic dose warfarin over aspirin; the dose of warfarin was below the therapeutic level.

PATIENTS CONSIDERED AT LOW RISK ON ASPIRIN

A separate component of the SPAF III study identified patients with atrial fibrillation considered at low risk because of the absence of four prespecified thromboembolic risk factors (recent congestive heart failure or left ventricular fractional shortening less than 25%, previous thromboembolism, systolic blood pressure higher than 160 mm Hg at study enrollment, or being a woman over 75 years of age). It is noteworthy that a history of diabetes mellitus was not used as a risk factor. All were given aspirin at 325 mg per day with an ischemic stroke rate of 1.4% per year. For such patients, treatment with warfarin was (1.1% per year) and may not justify the risk, expense, and inconvenience of life-long anticoagulation. Thus, it appears that these patients would be protected with either aspirin or warfarin.

STROKE PREVENTION IN PATIENTS WITH ATRIAL FIBRILLATION: SUMMARY

Patients without risk factors for hypertension, diabetes, previous transient ischemic episodes, or stroke who are under the age of 65 do not require either warfarin or aspirin prophylaxis. Patients between the ages of 65 or 75 without risk factors can be treated with aspirin or warfarin. All patients over 75 or those of any age with risk factors would benefit from warfarin. Any patient with poor ventricular function and atrial fibrillation would benefit from warfarin.

IDEAL THERAPEUTIC RANGE FOR ANTICOAGULATION

From the results of several studies, it appears that anticoagulation therapy with warfarin should be monitored carefully, and an INR between 2.0 and 3.5 is the optimum range for most indications. Among elderly patients, however, an upper limit to the INR of approximately 3.0 is appropriate.

SILENT CEREBRAL INFARCTION

Cerebral infarction in patients with atrial fibrillation may vary from being clinically silent to catastrophic. The prevalence of silent cerebral infarction and its effect as a risk factor for symptomatic stroke are important considerations for the evaluation of patients with atrial fibrillation.

The Veterans Affairs Cooperative Study was a double-blind, controlled trial designed primarily to determine the efficacy of warfarin for the prevention of stroke in neurologically normal patients with nonrheumatic atrial fibrillation. It also was designed to evaluate patients with silent cerebral infarction. Computed tomography scans of the head were performed at entry, at the time of any subsequent stroke, and at termination of follow-up on all patients who completed the study without a neurologic event. Of 516 evaluable scans performed at entry, 76 (14.7%) had evidence of one or more silent infarcts. Age (p 0.011), a history of hypertension (p 0.003), active angina (p 0.012), and elevated mean systolic blood pressure ($p < 0.001$) were associated with the presence of this finding. Silent cerebral infarction occurred during the study at rates of 1.01% and 1.57% per year for the placebo and warfarin treatment groups, respectively (RR, 1.55, 95% CI 0.40 to 6.11 NS). Silent cerebral infarction at entry was not an independent predictor of later symptomatic stroke, but active angina was a significant predictor; 15% of the placebo-assigned patients with angina developed a stroke compared with 5% of the placebo-assigned patients without angina.

ADVERSE EFFECTS OF ANTICOAGULATION

Bleeding is the main complication of oral anticoagulant therapy. The risk of bleeding is influenced by the intensity of anticoagulant therapy, by the patient's underlying clinical disorder, presence of hypertension and by the concomitant use of high doses of aspirin, which both impair platelet function and produce gastric erosions.

Four randomized studies have demonstrated that the risk of clinically important bleeding is reduced by lowering the therapeutic range from 3.0–4.5 to 2.0–3.0. Although this difference in anticoagulant intensity is associated with a reduction of the dose of warfarin of only approximately 1 mg, the effect on bleeding is profound.

The risk of major bleeding has been reported to be increased by age over 65 years, a history of stroke or gastrointestinal bleeding, atrial fibrillation, and the presence of serious comorbid conditions such as renal insufficiency or anemia. Bleeding that occurs when the INR is less than 3.0 is often associated with an obvious underlying cause or an occult gastrointestinal or renal lesion.

The most important nonhemorrhagic side effect of warfarin is skin necrosis. This uncommon complication, usually observed on the third to eighth day of therapy, is caused by extensive thrombosis of the venules and capillaries within the subcutaneous fat. An association has been reported between warfarin-induced skin necrosis and protein C deficiency and, less commonly, protein S deficiency, but this complication can also occur in nondeficient persons.

The pathogenesis of this striking complication is unknown. A role for protein C deficiency seems probable and is supported by the similarity of the lesions to those seen in neonatal purpura fulminans, which complicates homozygous protein C deficiency. The reason for the unusual localization of the lesions remains a mystery. The treatment of patients with coumarin-induced skin necrosis who require lifelong anticoagulant therapy is problematic. Warfarin is relatively contraindicated, and long-term heparin is inconvenient and associated with osteoporosis. A reasonable approach in such patients is to restart warfarin at a low dose, such as 2 mg, under the coverage of therapeutic doses of heparin and to increase the warfarin gradually over several weeks. This approach should prevent an abrupt fall in protein C levels before

a reduction in the levels of factors II, IX, and X and has been shown to be free of recurrence of skin necrosis in a number of recent case reports.

Oral anticoagulants cross the placenta and can produce a characteristic embryopathy, central nervous system abnormalities, or fetal bleeding. Warfarin should not be used in the first trimester of pregnancy and should, if possible, be avoided throughout the entire pregnancy. Heparin is preferred when anticoagulants are indicated in pregnancy. There is convincing evidence that warfarin does not induce an anticoagulant effect in the breast-fed infant when the drug is administered to a nursing mother.

BIBLIOGRAPHY

Atrial Fibrillation Investigators. Risk factors for stroke and efficacy of antithrombotic therapy in atrial fibrillation: analysis of pooled data from five randomized controlled trials. *Arch Intern Med* 1994;154:1449–1457.

Cairns JA, Hirsh J, Lewis HD Jr, et al. Antithrombotic agents in coronary artery disease. *Chest* 1992;102:456S–481S.

Cruickshank MK, Levine MN, Hirsh J, et al. A standard heparin nomogram for the management of heparin therapy. *Arch Intern Med* 1991;151: 333–337.

Fennerty AG, Levine MN, Hirsh J. Hemorrhagic complications of thrombolytic therapy in the treatment of myocardial infarction and venous thromboembolism. *Chest* 1989;95:88S–97S.

Hirsh J. Heparin. *N Engl J Med* 1991;324:1565–1574.

Hirsh J, Levine MN. Review: low molecular weight heparin. *Blood* 1992; 79:1–17.

Hull R, Raskob G, Pineo G, et al. A comparison of subcutaneous low-molecular-weight heparin with warfarin sodium for prophylaxis against deep-vein thrombosis after hip or knee implantation. *N Engl J Med* 1993;19:1370–1376.

Hull RD, Raskob GE, Pineo GF, et al. Subcutaneous low-molecular-weight heparin compared with continuous intravenous heparin in the treatment of proximal-vein thrombosis. *N Engl J Med* 1992;326:975–982.

Poller L. A simple nomogram for the derivation of International Normalised Ratios for the standardisation of prothrombin time. *Thromb Haemost* 1988;60:18–20.

Sutcliff FA, MacNicholl AD, Gibson GG. Aspects of anticoagulant action: a review of the pharmacology, metabolism and toxicology of warfarin and congeners. *Q Rev Drugs Met Drug Interact* 1987;5:225.

Kelley's Textbook of Internal Medicine, fourth edition. Edited by H. David Humes. Lippincott Williams & Wilkins, Philadelphia © 2000.

CHAPTER
92

PRINCIPLES AND APPLICATIONS OF CARDIAC SURGERY

JOHN G. BYRNE
RAYMOND H. CHEN
DAVID H. ADAMS

Surgical intervention for cardiovascular disorders is indicated when the outcome of the planned operation is expected to be superior to medical treatment. Cardiac surgery is usually indicated when symptoms are refractory to medical management but may also be indicated to provide survival benefit.

The modern era of cardiac surgery can be summarized by the events of recent decades. The 1950s were notable for the development of cardiopulmonary bypass and early attempts at correction of congenital abnormalities. During the 1960s, the surgical treatment of congenital abnormalities and valve replacement surgery became commonplace. The 1970s were characterized by the widespread growth of coronary artery bypass graft (CABG) procedures for the treatment of coronary artery disease. During the 1980s, cardiac transplantation and valve reparative procedures became accepted treatment options. The 1990s have been notable for the development of minimally invasive and video-assisted techniques for cardiac surgery, and the new millennium may bring the development of "robotic" computer-assisted cardiac surgery.

INDICATIONS FOR CARDIAC SURGERY

ISCHEMIC HEART DISEASE

Elective or Urgent Surgery

The inability to medically control severe anginal symptoms is the most common indication for elective or urgent cardiac surgery in ischemic heart disease. Transarterial catheter dilatation techniques, with or without intra-arterial stents, are now widely used as first-line invasive therapy for patients with disabling angina and relatively limited coronary obstructions who fail to improve with medical therapy. Early recurrent obstructions after balloon dilatation, or stent restenosis, however, are relatively common, and many patients ultimately require CABG for symptomatic relief.

An important factor to measure, when considering CABG, is the magnitude of inducible myocardial ischemia, as reflected both by the patient's symptoms and by the response to exercise stress testing. Other important considerations include the nature and condition of the coronary arteries, as well as the many patient-related factors that determine the patient's risk profile for surgery. Patients with several comorbidities, such as generalized atherosclerosis, diabetes mellitus, respiratory insufficiency, and renal failure, have a much higher risk for surgery. For obvious reasons, it is inappropriate to recommend CABG in patients whose life expectancy is limited due to coexisting major medical illnesses or terminal cancer.

Patients with multivessel disease and good ventricular function have similar survival when managed by percutaneous transluminal coronary angioplasty (PTCA) or CABG, but freedom from reintervention and return of angina is much better with CABG (Fig. 92.1). Patients with multivessel coronary artery disease or significant left main coronary artery disease or both in the setting of depressed left ventricular function have improved long-term survival with CABG over medical management (Figs. 92.2 and 92.3). This may be especially true for diabetics, as documented in the Bypass Angioplasty Revascularization Investigation (BARI) trial. Long proximal left coronary artery obstruction also generally precludes safe and effective

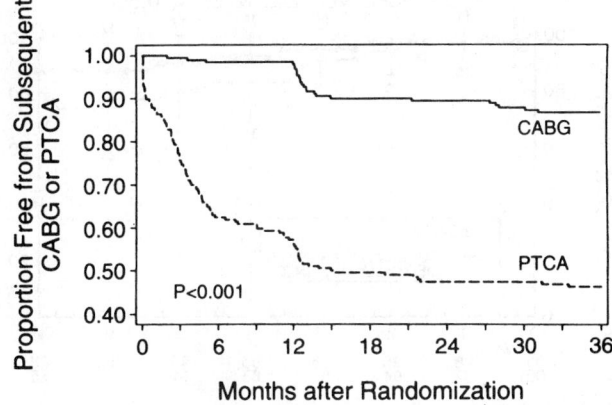

FIGURE 92.1. Proportion of patients remaining free from subsequent intervention (CABG or PTCA) after the initial revascularization procedure. (From King SB III, Lembo NJ, Weintraub WS, et al. A randomized trial comparing coronary angioplasty with coronary bypass surgery. *N Engl J Med* 1994;331:1044.)

PTCA/stent procedures, and patients with diabetes are best managed with surgical revascularization.

Emergency Surgery

Patients who develop mechanical complications of acute myocardial infarction (MI) are candidates for emergency cardiac surgery. These include patients with (a) ruptured ventricular free wall resulting in tamponade, (b) ruptured ventricular septum resulting in a ventricular septal defect, (c) ruptured papillary muscle resulting in severe mitral regurgitation, and (d) severe pump impairment resulting in cardiogenic shock. Needless to

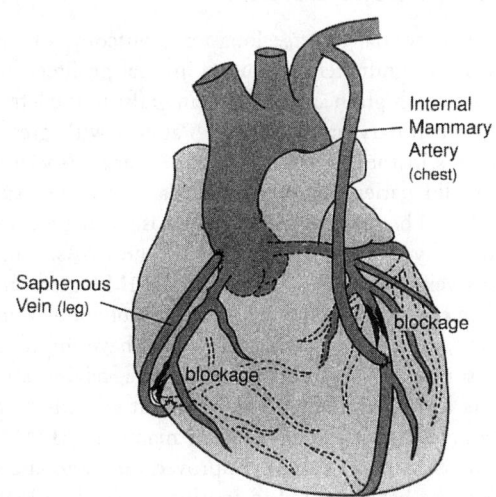

FIGURE 92.2. Anatomical depiction of two-vessel bypass operation, using the LIMA graft to the left anterior descending artery and aortocoronary saphenous vein graft to the posterior descending artery. (From Burrows SG, Gassert CA. *Moving right along after open heart surgery.* Atlanta: Pritchett & Hull Associates, 1990:43.)

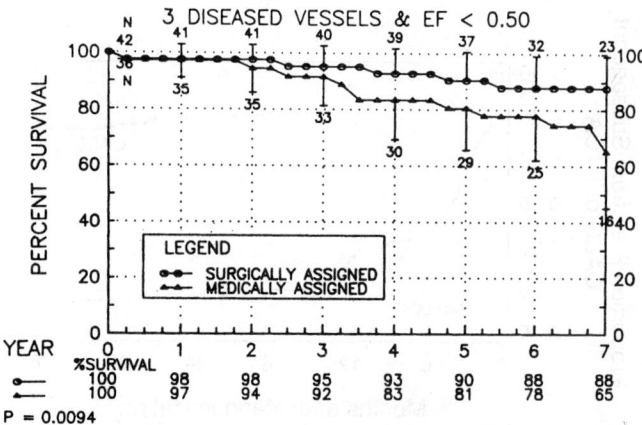

FIGURE 92.3. Survival in the CASS randomized trial of patients with three-vessel disease and ejection fractions less than 0.50. After seven years of follow-up, 88% of patients assigned to surgical treatment versus 65% of those assigned to medical treatment are alive (p = 0.0094). (From Killip T, Passamani E, Davis K, et al. Coronary Artery Surgery Study: a randomized trial of coronary bypass surgery: eight years follow-up and survival in patients with reduced ejection fraction. *Circulation* 1985;72:102.)

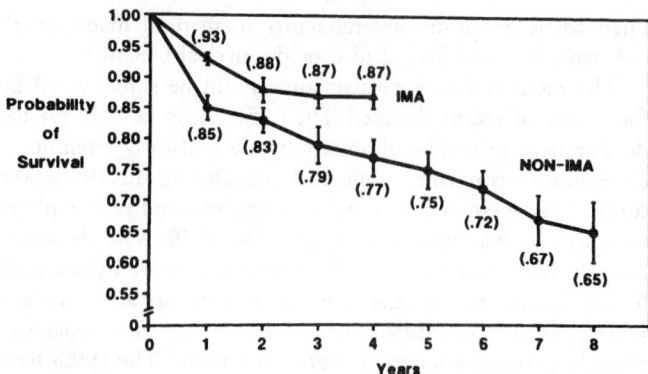

FIGURE 92.4. Actuarial Kaplan–Meier survival estimates for cornary artery bypass patients 70 years of age and older. The NON-IMA group had only vein grafts, whereas the IMA group included patients who had one internal mammary artery graft and at least one vein graft. The projected survival for up to 4 years was statistically significant (p < 0.001). (From Gardner TJ, Greene PS, Rykiel MF, et al. Routine use of the left internal mammary graft in the elderly. *Ann Thorac Surg* 1990; 49:188.)

say, the operative risk in these patients is very high, but in general their only chance for survival involves surgical therapy. An acute MI without cardiogenic shock is not usually an indication for undertaking CABG. However, patients who develop postinfarct angina have an increased risk for reinfarction, either in the original infarct zone or in another portion of the heart supplied by a second coronary artery with severe obstruction, and are generally best served by transcatheter or surgical intervention. Patients who require emergency CABG are usually best served by all-vein bypass grafting, because of the concerns regarding early decreased flow in the internal mammary artery (IMA) in the setting of potential high inotropic requirement.

Long-Term Considerations

The major potential adverse long-term outcome of CABG is saphenous vein graft stenosis due to intimal proliferation. This risk is especially high in saphenous vein grafts to the left anterior descending coronary artery (LAD). Patients with greater than 50% stenosis in these grafts had worse 7- and 10-year survival rates than did patients with greater than 50% stenosis of the native LAD. The problem of late stenosis can be avoided to some extent by grafting one or both of the IMAs, rather than saphenous veins, to the LAD (Fig. 92.4). IMA grafts have improved late graft patency compared with saphenous vein grafts. In addition, patients receiving IMA grafts have improved early and late survival compared with patients receiving saphenous vein grafts alone. The late survival benefit extends to patients older than age 70 for the left internal mammary (LIMA) graft. The improved patency and the improved early and late survival for IMA grafts have resulted in routine use of the LIMA graft, making it the gold standard for elective CABG operations, and have ameliorated somewhat the long-term risk of saphenous vein graft stenosis in CABG. Furthermore, "all-arterial" reconstruction, by use not only of both IMA, but also of free radial arteries,

has gained favor because of presumed improved patency of the arterial conduits. Use of bilateral IMA grafts in diabetics, however, increases the risk of deep sternal wound infection.

VALVULAR HEART DISEASE

Deformities of the cardiac valves, resulting in valvular stenosis or regurgitation generally culminate in chronic and progressive cardiac functional deterioration. Pressure or volume overloading of the heart results, with cardiac enlargement and progressive deterioration of contractile function. Although congenital bicuspid aortic valve and rheumatic mitral valve disease were once the most common indication for valve surgery, the most common indication for valvular heart surgery is degenerative calcific aortic stenosis and degenerative mitral regurgitation.

Aortic Valve Disease

Patients with critical aortic stenosis often benefit dramatically from aortic valve replacement (AVR). The indication for valve replacement is based primarily on symptoms, but occasionally patients with asymptomatic high-grade aortic stenosis (systolic gradient more than 100 mm Hg) are also candidates for surgery (Fig. 92.5). In fact, most patients in this subgroup have symptoms with forced exertion. In aortic regurgitation, symptoms usually direct surgical therapy, but asymptomatic patients with echocardiographic documentation of severe cardiac dilatation (end-systolic dimension greater than 55 mm Hg) or dysfunction (ejection fraction less than 0.30) are also appropriately referred for AVR.

Mitral Valve Disease

Another common condition for which cardiac valve surgery is indicated is chronic progressive mitral regurgitation. Many such patients need valve surgery to prevent clinical heart failure. The

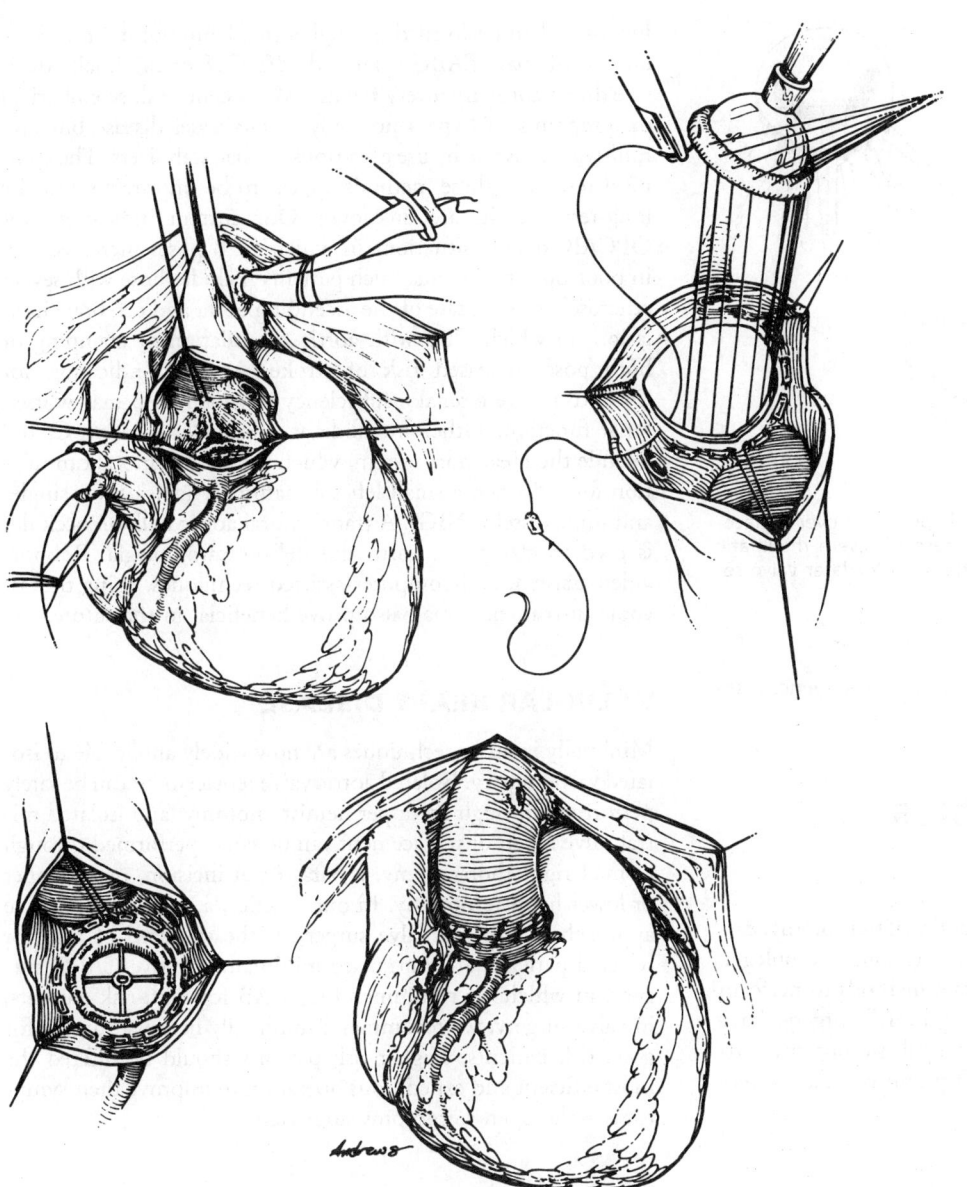

FIGURE 92.5. Aortic valve replacement. The sclerotic leaflets are excised, and the new valve is secured to the native annulus with the interrupted sutures. (From Cooley DA. *Techniques in cardiac surgery, second edition.* Philadelphia: W.B. Saunders, 1984:179.)

indication for surgery in most patients is also related to symptoms, but asymptomatic patients with echocardiographic documentation of cardiac dysfunction are also appropriately referred. If these patients develop significant cardiac dilatation, cardiac functional recovery may not occur after valve replacement or repair. Mitral valve repair is generally preferred over replacement and is usually possible except in the case of severe rheumatic mitral disease (Fig. 92.6). Successful repair obviates the need for later valve re-replacement owing to bioprosthetic structural valve degeneration and the need for life-long anticoagulation in the case of mechanical valves.

HEART FAILURE

Patients with severe heart failure refractory to medical management may be candidates for surgical therapy. Heart transplantation is reserved for patients without other major medical comor-

bidities. Ventricular assist devices (VADs) may be used as "bridge to transplant," "bridge to recovery," or possibly as permanent devices (Fig. 92.7). Given the limited number of available donor hearts, nontransplantation procedures such as high-risk CABG or mitral valve repair with VAD backup may be the only suitable option. Ventricular volume reduction surgery has also been suggested as an option for end-stage dilated cardiomyopathy but remains highly controversial.

OTHER INDICATIONS FOR CARDIAC SURGERY

The many other possible indications for open heart surgery include congenital deformities of the heart, such as ASDs and aneurysmal disease of the thoracic aorta resulting in dilatation, dissection, or rupture. Primary cardiac tumors, although rare, almost always require surgical removal and reconstruction of the affected portion of the heart. Surgical treatment of atrial

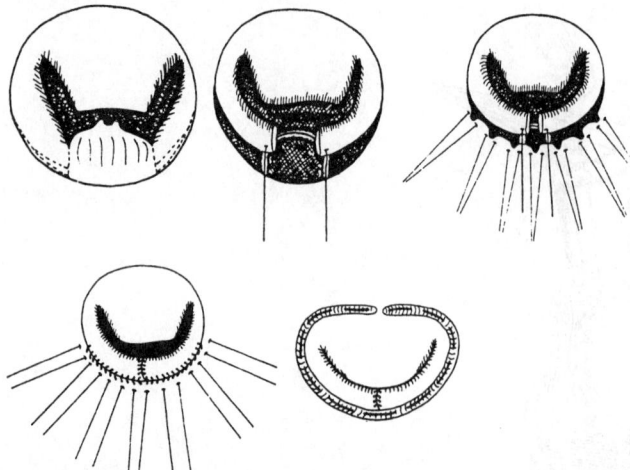

FIGURE 92.6. Mitral valve repair is generally preferred over replacement and is usually possible except in the case of severe rheumatic mitral disease. Successful repair obviates the need for later valve rereplacement.

fibrillation by the Cox–Maze procedure may also benefit selected patients.

■ SURGICAL STRATEGIES

ISCHEMIC HEART DISEASE

Most CABGs are performed using conventional sternotomy, cardiopulmonary bypass (CPB), aortic clamping, and cardioplegia. Recently, however, efforts to develop safe methods to perform surgery without CPB, so-called "beating heart" surgery, have evolved. When performed by means of a full sternotomy, off-bypass CABG is termed *OPCAB* or **o**ff-**p**ump **c**oronary **a**rtery

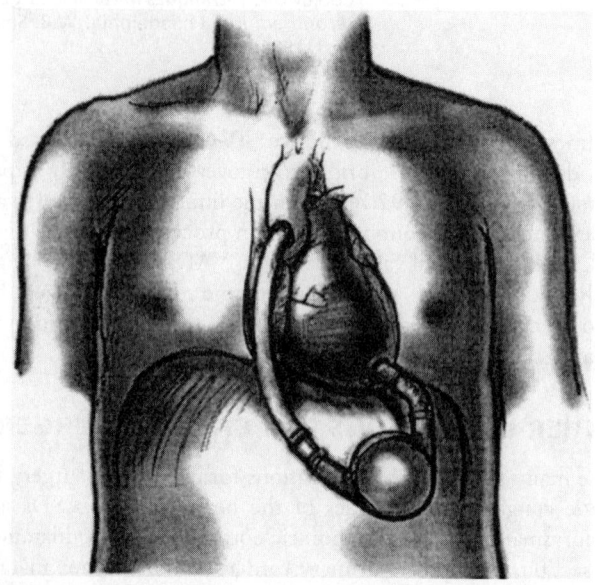

FIGURE 92.7. Ventricular assist devices (VADs) may be used as "bridge to transplant," "bridge to recovery," or possibly as permanent devices.

bypass. When performed through a small anterior left thoracotomy, off-bypass CABG is termed *MIDCAB* or **m**inimally **i**nvasive **d**irect **c**oronary **a**rtery **b**ypass. Many centers have embarked on programs to bypass not only single-vessel disease but also multivessel disease by use of various cardiac stabilizers. The technical results of these methods appear to be improving, but the long-term results are unknown. Our current indications for OPCAB include situations in which CPB poses increased risk in poor-option patients. Such patients include those with severe atherosclerotic disease of the ascending aorta and cerebral circulation, in which CPB with aortic cannulation or clamping or both pose increased risk of stroke. Another indication for OPCAB is severe renal insufficiency in which CPB may worsen renal function. Other methods at minimally invasive CABG include the Heartport system, which uses transfemoral cannulation for CPB and a small left submammary incision for single- and multivessel CABGs. A transfemoral aortic balloon occluder is used to clamp the aorta and deliver cardioplegia. Robotic, video-assisted, and computer-assisted techniques, using thorascopic instruments, may also prove beneficial in the future.

VALVULAR HEART DISEASE

Minimally invasive techniques are now widely applicable to isolated valve surgery. Isolated aortic valve replacement can be safely performed through an upper hemisternotomy, and isolated mitral valve repair or replacement can be safely performed through a small right thoracotomy, a parasternal incision, or an upper or lower hemisternotomy. In our practice, a minimally invasive approach to isolated valve surgery is the standard of care for selected patients. In contrast to minimally invasive CABG surgery, in which we recommend OPCAB for high-risk patients, in valve surgery, we recommend minimally invasive surgery for good-risk patients. Higher-risk patients should be offered the most efficient and expeditious operation to improve their symptoms—the open sternotomy approach.

HEART FAILURE

Transplantation

The classic Shumway technique of left and right atrial cuff anastomoses is still used today but is limited because it fails to effectively transplant the atria and because it essentially represents a ventricular transplant with a loss of atrioventricular (AV) synchrony. Many transplantation surgeons today favor the bicaval technique, in which a complete heart transplantation is performed by excising the recipient atria and performing separate left atrial and bicaval anastomoses so that the complete donor heart is transplanted, not just the ventricles. This preserves AV synchrony and long-term function (Fig. 92.8).

Ventricular Assist

VADs fall into two categories: short-term postcardiotomy failure assist devices and more long-term devices. We currently use the ABIOMED system for short-term support and the HeartMate,

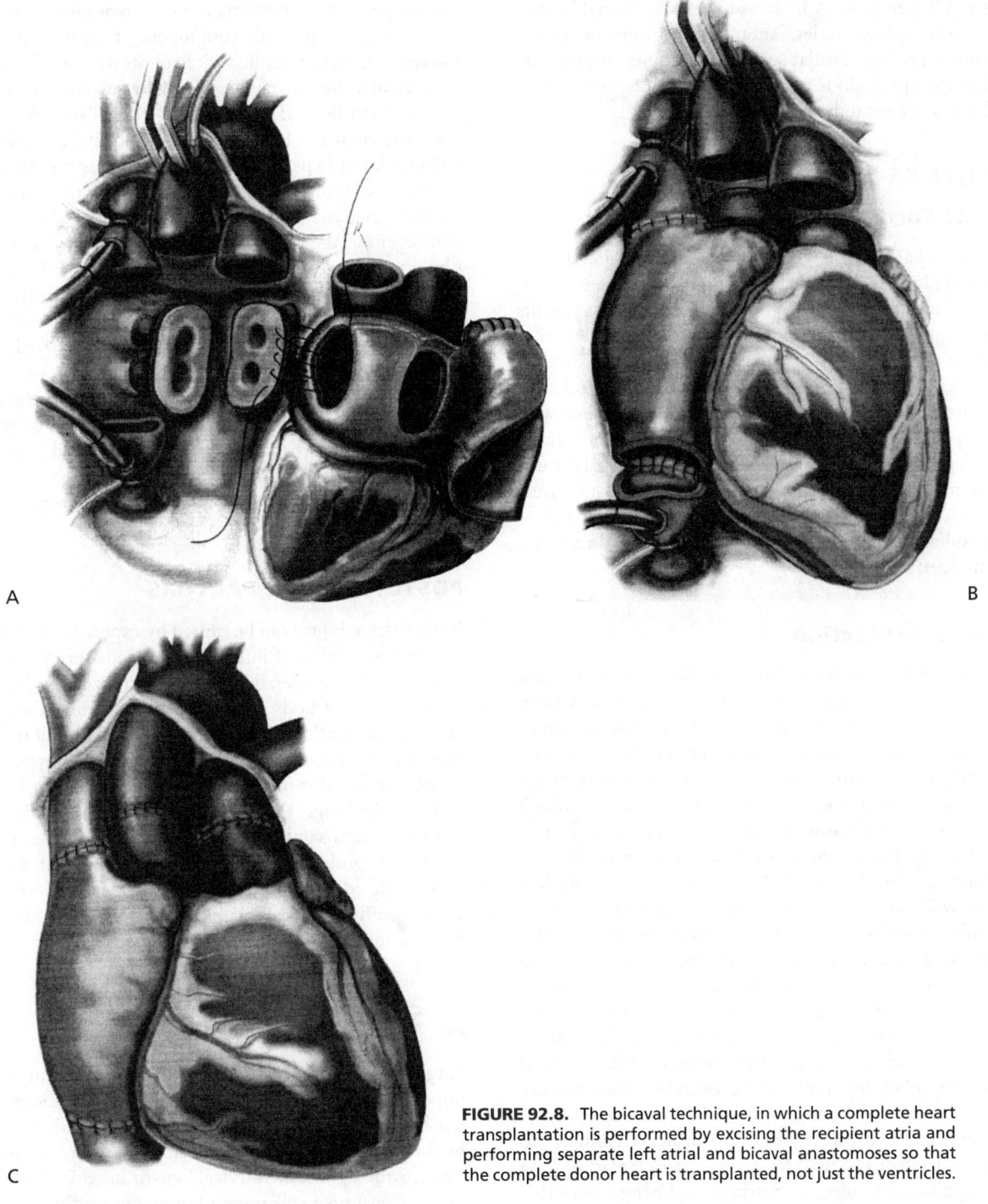

FIGURE 92.8. The bicaval technique, in which a complete heart transplantation is performed by excising the recipient atria and performing separate left atrial and bicaval anastomoses so that the complete donor heart is transplanted, not just the ventricles.

TCI, for long-term support. Both can be used for bridge to recovery and bridge to transplant, but most frequently the short-term devices are used for bridge to recovery and the long-term devices are used for bridge to transplant. The ABIOMED system can be used for both left (LVAD) and right (RVAD) support and requires systemic anticoagulation. The HeartMate system is an LVAD only and is generally implanted on a semielective basis. It does not require systemic anticoagulation. Current trials are evaluating VADs for use as permanent devices.

ESTIMATING THE RISKS OF CARDIAC SURGERY

PATIENT-RELATED FACTORS

The presence of diabetes mellitus, renal insufficiency, intrinsic lung disease, and neuropsychiatries factors may influence the decision for cardiac surgical intervention. Patient characteristics that influence the risk of surgery include the patient's age, with elderly patients having higher surgical risks for all types of cardiac procedures. Women have an increased operative mortality after CABG in most reported series. Another factor influencing risk and outcome is previous cardiac surgery. Outcomes are generally worse when the operation is performed as an emergency procedure or because of hemodynamic instability.

OPERATIVE FACTORS

Effects of Cardiopulmonary Bypass

Exposure of the patient's blood to an extracorporeal circuit initiates a cascade of inflammatory changes and complement activation. Experimentally, this type of inflammatory response results in end-organ injury to the lungs, liver, and kidneys. Another consideration when a patient is placed on CPB is the need to prime the circuit with up to 2 L of fluid and to provide anticoagulation to avoid clotting when the blood comes in contact with the extracorporeal system. Use of relatively large doses of heparin prevents microthrombosis but may result in a protracted disruption of the patient's coagulation function, even after the usual attempts to reverse the heparinization effect with drugs such as protamine sulfate. Thus, bleeding complications remain a major threat with open heart surgery.

Myocardial Protection

The most significant challenge, however, with cardiac surgical procedures that involve total bypass of the heart results from the need to interrupt blood flow to the heart and to induce complete ischemia while the surgery is performed. Although rare, inadequate myocardial protection can lead to surgical mortalities owing to cardiac pump failure, or to cardiogenic shock, which develops immediately after the operation as a result of the heart's intolerance to the protracted anoxic interval required for performing the procedure. Various techniques have evolved to allow surgeons to work in and on a still and bloodless environment by developing solutions and administration techniques that allow both induced arrest and metabolic support of the arrested heart during protracted periods of cardiac anoxia. These cardioplegic techniques, as well as a host of later refinements and additions, have become a mainstay for protecting the heart from ischemic injury during long and complicated cardiac surgical operations. The other important development in reducing injury to the heart during cardiac surgery began with the experimental work of Shumway and others, who investigated techniques to protect donor hearts to be used for cardiac transplantation. The benefit of significant cooling, by markedly reducing myocardial metabolic demands especially in the arrested heart, was clearly demonstrated and has become an accepted adjunct to myocardial protection.

Avoidance of Intraoperative Cerebrovascular Accidents

Patients with peripheral vascular disease, especially those with significant intracranial cerebrovascular disease, may have inadequate brain perfusion on CPB with focal or generalized central nervous system injury as a result. Although extracorporeal bypass circuits generally approximate the normal mean perfusion pressure, the phasic pulsatile component of normal circulatory hemodynamics is not duplicated. Patients with significant obstructive vascular disease may be especially susceptible to the loss of phasic blood flow. If the patient is cooled systematically, however, the body's tolerance to less adequate perfusion may be enhanced, but bypass perfusion flow support may still be inadequate. In addition, there may be embolization of aortic atherosclerotic material from perfusion cannulas, which injure such end organs as the brain. Intraoperative epiaortic echocardiography is one way to identify potential mobile debris. Avoidance of manipulation of an aorta with mobile debris or heavily calcified aorta may also help reduce the incidence of intraoperative CVA. When a "porcelain aorta" is encountered, circulatory arrest without aortic cannulation may be the only option to ensure that no atheroma forms an embolism to the brain.

Extracorporeal perfusion technology and its physiologic foundations have become highly sophisticated, but many patients, especially elderly ones with generalized atherosclerosis, continue to sustain complications as a result of the need for extracorporeal CPB during surgery.

POSTOPERATIVE FACTORS

Primary lung injury can be caused by exposure to CPB, with the resultant activation of inflammatory mediators and with edema formation. Long operations are characterized by the significant accumulation of body fluid, with weight gains often exceeding 10% of a patient's normal body weight as a result of hemodilution and the circulatory support provided by bypass. Furthermore, embolization of atheromatous material can affect the brain and also the lungs, gut, kidneys, and liver. In addition to these factors, there is significant risk of systemic or wound infections because of prolonged intraoperative exposure of the mediastinum, pericardium, and pleura. Patients with an immune or vascular insufficiency, especially those with severe diabetes, may have an increased risk of surgery-related infection.

■ SUMMARY

Surgical therapy for cardiovascular disease continues to be an important adjunct to medical treatment. In patients who have not benefited from medical management, cardiac surgery may be the only option for symptomatic relief. In addition, surgery can provide significant survival benefit in selected groups of patients. Continued collaboration between cardiologists and their surgical counterparts will result in further refinement in referral strategies for patients with significant cardiovascular disease.

BIBLIOGRAPHY

Aklog L, Adams DH, Couper GS, et al. Techniques and results of direct-access minimally invasive mitral valve surgery: a paradigm for the future. *J Thorac Cardiovasc Surg* 1998;116:705–715.

The Bypass Angioplasty Revascularization Investigation (BARI) investigators. Influence of diabetes on 5-year mortality and morbidity in a randomized trial comparing CABG and PTCA in patients with multivessel disease. *Circulation* 1997;96:1761–1769.

Calafiore AM, Di Gammarco G, Teodori G, et al. Midterm results after minimally invasive coronary surgery (LAST operation). *J Thorac Cardiovasc Surg* 1998;115:763–771.

Caracciolo EA, Davis KB, Sopka G, et al. Comparison of surgical and medical group survival in patients with left main equivalent coronary artery disease. Long-term CASS experience. *Circulation* 1995;91:2335–2344.

Carpentier AF, Lessana A, Relland JY, et al. The "physio-ring": an advanced concept in mitral valve annuloplasty. *Ann Thorac Surg* 1995;60:1177–1186.

Chen RH, Kadner A, Adams DH. Surgical techniques in heart transplantation. *Graft* 1999;2:119.

Killip T, Passamani E, Davis K. Coronary artery surgery study (CASS): a randomized trial of coronary bypass surgery. Eight years follow-up and survival in patients with reduced ejection fraction. *Circulation* 1985;72:V102–V109.

King SB III, Lembo NJ, Weintraub WS, et al. A randomized trial comparing coronary angioplasty with coronary bypass surgery. Emory angioplasty versus Surgery Trial (EAST). *N Engl J Med* 1994;331:1044–1050.

Loulmet D, Carpentier A, d'Attellis N, et al. Endoscopic coronary artery bypass grafting with the aid of robotic assisted instruments. *J Thorac Cardiovasc Surg* 1999;118:4–10.

Shumway NE. Forty years of thoracic transplantation at Stanford. *Transplant Proc* 1999;31:46.

Kelley's Textbook of Internal Medicine, fourth edition. Edited by H. David Humes. Lippincott Williams & Wilkins, Philadelphia © 2000.

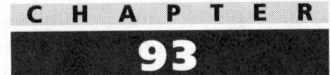

CHAPTER 93

MEDICAL MANAGEMENT OF THE CARDIAC TRANSPLANT PATIENT

KEITH AARONSON
ROBERT CODY

Cardiac transplantation is the most successful treatment available for patients with truly end-stage heart disease. Nearly 85% of patients survive the first postoperative year, with a subsequent mortality rate of only 4% per year. Compared with larger centers, survival is worse at low-volume transplantation centers (less than nine transplantations per year). For patients who meet the strict selection criteria, survival is much greater than would be expected for the natural history of their disease. Severe heart failure is the reason for undergoing transplantation for nearly all recipients. For ambulatory patients, disease severity is commonly documented by a severe reduction in oxygen consumption during exercise testing, but other indicators of severity of illness should also be considered. Implantable defibrillators and improved surgical and catheter-based techniques have substantially reduced the need for transplantation as a treatment for refractory angina or recurrent malignant ventricular arrhythmias. Despite the growing number of patients placed on the transplant waiting list, the restricted availability of donor hearts has limited the

annual number of transplantations to approximately 2,400 in the United States and 3,500 worldwide. Given this severe organ shortage, every effort is made to ensure that patients accepted for the transplant waiting list are free of comorbid conditions (including advanced age) that would further limit post-transplant survival.

Periodic follow-up of the transplant recipient should be performed by an experienced cardiac transplantation team. However, the frequency and intensity of routine follow-up with the transplant center are reduced as the time from transplantation increases. As the number of transplantation survivors grows, an increasing number of internists will encounter these patients in their daily practice. Therefore, a basic knowledge of cardiac transplantation and immunosuppression and its complications is important for the practicing internist, who will often be the initial point of contact for patients who have returned to their communities. With the appropriate knowledge of the altered physiology of the transplanted heart, and of immunosuppressant drug interactions, many of the common problems encountered by these patients (e.g., colds, hypertension, hyperlipidemia, diabetes) can be well treated by an internist. In some managed care settings, internists have been increasingly called on to evaluate all recipient problems before the patient may be seen at the transplant center. The threshold for contacting the transplantation team must be low, and access to specialized care for this small but fragile population should be readily available. For their part, the transplantation cardiologist, coordinator, and surgeon must be highly accessible and should attempt to coordinate their care with the internist, whenever possible.

The post-transplantation management of the heart transplant recipient reflects the constant tensions inherent in the use of immunosuppressant therapies: inadequate immunosuppression risks organ rejection, whereas overvigorous immunosuppression increases the risk of infection, malignancies, and other drug complications (discussed in the following text). Optimal management attempts to balance these conflicting risks by individualizing immunosuppressant therapy to each recipient's needs.

■ IMMUNOSUPPRESSANTS AND THEIR COMPLICATIONS

Most heart transplant recipients initially receive a three-drug regimen for chronic maintenance immunosuppression: cyclosporine (or, less commonly, tacrolimus), azathioprine or mycophenolate mofetil, and prednisone.

CYCLOSPORINE AND TACROLIMUS

By inhibiting the enzymatic action of calcineurin, cyclosporine reduces the transcription of inflammatory cytokines, most notably interleukin-2, thereby inhibiting T-cell activation and proliferation. Cyclosporine dosing is guided by trough blood levels, with higher targeted levels early after transplantation or when rejection is present or frequent (Table 93.1). Cyclosporine is metabolized by the liver through the cytochrome P4503A4 system. Because many other drugs either compete for use of this enzyme system or increase its activity, their coadministration

TABLE 93.1. TARGET THERAPEUTIC CYCLOSPORINE LEVELS

Time After Transplantation (mo)	MC-TDx Level (ng/mL)	HPLC Level (ng/mL)
0–3	300–400	250–300
3–6	250–350	200–250
6–12	200–250	150–200
>12	150–200[a]	100–150[a]

HPLC, high-pressure liquid chromatography; MC-TDx, monoclonal fluorescence polarization immunoassay.
[a] Possibly lower in long-term recipients with low risk of rejection.

with cyclosporine markedly affects its blood levels (Table 93.2). Physicians must be aware of these potential drug interactions, and blood levels should be closely monitored whenever a change in cyclosporine levels is anticipated.

Cyclosporine use is associated with numerous unwanted side effects, most of which appear to result from calcineurin inhibition. The most serious adverse drug effects include renal dysfunction (decreased glomerular filtration rate, hyperkalemia, hypermagnesemia), hypertension, hyperlipidemia, diabetes, gout, osteoporosis, and cholelithiasis. Common neurotoxicities include tremulousness and peripheral neuropathy; seizures generally occur only when cyclosporine levels are high or when patients predisposed to them. Hirsutism is common and may be a troubling side effect for women. Gum hyperplasia may require periodontal attention to prevent oral infections. Hepatotoxicity is infrequent. As transplant physicians have gained greater familiarity with cyclosporine, targeted drug levels and dose-related toxicities have decreased.

Although structurally different, tacrolimus (previously called FK-506) also inhibits calcineurin activity. It is routinely used in preference to cyclosporine at some centers. Increased doses of tacrolimus alone (without increased corticosteroids) have been successfully used to treat cellular rejection. Neurotoxicity and nephrotoxicity appear to be more common with tacrolimus than with cyclosporine, but this may in part reflect less familiarity with the drug and more aggressive immunosuppression. However, hypertension appears to be less common, whereas diabetes may be more common. Hirsutism does not occur with tacrolimus and generally resolves when patients are switched to it from cyclosporine.

AZATHIOPRINE AND MYCOPHENOLATE MOFETIL

Both azathioprine and mycophenolate mofetil (MMF) reduce DNA synthesis. MMF selectively inhibits inosine monophosphate dehydrogenase, a critical enzyme in the de novo purine synthesis pathway, on which T- and B-lymphocyte biosynthesis depend. Azathioprine blocks numerous enzymes required for DNA synthesis and so less selectively inhibits immune cell proliferation than does MMF. MMF also inhibits growth factors that may be important in the development of coronary allograft vasculopathy. In studies of both heart and kidney transplant recipients, patients on MMF tend to have fewer serious rejection episodes but more infections. Both drugs may cause leukopenia, and dose adjustments may be required to prevent this. Because both azathioprine and allopurinol are metabolized by xanthine oxidase, azathioprine doses must be reduced by one-third to one-half when allopurinol is given. Other potential adverse effects of azathioprine include hepatitis and pancreatitis. Abdominal discomfort, vomiting, diarrhea, and gastrointestinal hemorrhage may occur with MMF use.

TABLE 93.2. EFFECTS OF COMMONLY USED DRUGS ON CYCLOSPORINE AND TACROLIMUS LEVELS

Increased Cyclosporine and Tacrolimus Levels	Decreased Cyclosporine and Tacrolimus Levels
Calcium channel blockers	Anticonvulsants
Diltiazem	Phenobarbital
Nicardipine	Carbamazepine
Verapamil	Phenytoin
Antibiotics	Antituberculars
Clarithromycin	Rifabutin
Erythromycin	Rifampin
Antifungals	Neuroleptics
Clotrimazole[a]	Phenothiazines
Fluconazole	
Itraconazole	
Ketoconazole	
Hormonal therapies	
Estrogen	
Danazol	
Methyltestosterone	
Oral contraceptives	
Other drugs	
Allopurinol	
Bromocriptine	
Metaclopramide	
Methylprednisolone (high-dose)	
Isoniazid	

[a] Decreases tacrolimus only (not cyclosporine).

CORTICOSTEROIDS

Corticosteroids inhibit the production of T-cell lymphokines, which amplify macrophage and lymphocyte responses and cause lymphocytolysis. Corticosteroid side effects are legion. High doses are used early after transplantation, with prednisone doses commonly reduced to 0.3 mg per kilogram at 1 month and 0.1 mg per kilogram by 3 months after transplantation in patients not experiencing frequent rejection. Many patients ultimately can be weaned from corticosteroids and successfully maintained on a two-drug regimen.

REJECTION

Rejection is the most common cause of death in the first year after heart transplantation. Hyperacute rejection manifests within hours of transplantation as a result of preformed recipient antibodies directed against the donor graft. Fortunately, the use of ABO blood group–compatible donors and prospective donor-specific cross-matching for recipients with preformed anti-HLA (human leukocyte antigen) antibodies has made this a rare, though usually fatal, event.

Acute cellular rejection occurs far more commonly. About two-thirds of patients experience at least one rejection episode in the first post-transplant year, with the greatest risk occurring in the early post-transplant months. The risk is substantially lower after the sixth month and is very low after 1 year. Rejection is more common in younger patients and in multiparous women, in recipients of female donors, in those who develop anti-HLA antibodies or experience a cytomegalovirus infection or a previous rejection episode, and when immunosuppression is decreased either by the physician or by a poorly compliant patient. Perioperative treatment with either polyclonal (antithymocyte or antilymphocyte globulins) or monoclonal (OKT3) antibodies reduces early rejection but increases infections and may increase future development of post-transplant lymphoproliferative disorder (see Malignancies). Newer monoclonal antibodies directed against the interleukin-2 receptor are under study for this indication.

Rejection may present as episodes of undo fatigue or malaise, palpitations, a mild reduction in exercise capacity, or even frank heart failure, but most episodes are asymptomatic. Noninvasive methods of detecting rejection are still neither sensitive nor specific enough to supplant endomyocardial biopsy, which remains the standard approach (although limited experience with serial monitoring of intramyocardial electrograms from pacemakers implanted at the time of transplantation is encouraging). Therefore, surveillance right ventricular endomyocardial biopsies are performed routinely on all patients regardless of symptoms, with extra biopsies performed whenever rejection is suspected clinically. A typical schedule would be to perform weekly biopsies for the first month, biweekly biopsies for the next 2 months, monthly biopsies for the 4th to 6th months, and bimonthly biopsies for the 7th through 12th months. Biopsy frequency subsequently decreases to every 3 to 12 months as the time from transplantation lengthens. If any biopsy shows rejection, the frequency of subsequent biopsies increases until the rejection is no longer present. Because the decision to institute antirejection treatment reflects not just the histologic grade of rejection but the effect of rejection on cardiac function, some measure of cardiac function (either echocardiography or measurement of right heart and pulmonary wedge pressures and cardiac output by pulmonary artery catheterization) is performed with each biopsy.

Rejection is graded by the International Society of Heart and Lung Transplantation (ISHLT) scale from grade 0 (none) to 4 (severe). Experts differ on the threshold for treating asymptomatic rejection. Patients with milder grades of asymptomatic rejection may be treated by increasing the level of background immunosuppression; or, when they occur late in the post-transplantation period, they may not require specific treatment. Those with higher grades of rejection, with rejection associated with a reduction in ventricular function or poor hemodynamics, and with rejection occurring closer to the time of transplantation are treated more aggressively. Treatment, when indicated, generally includes high-dose glucocorticoids. More severe rejection episodes and corticosteroid-refractory episodes are treated with either antithymocyte/antilymphocyte globulins or OKT3. A follow-up biopsy is required 1 to 2 weeks after a course of treatment to ensure that the rejection has resolved. Treatment of right or left ventricular dysfunction, when present, is the same as for the nontransplant recipient.

Humoral rejection is an antibody-mediated process directed against HLA class II antigens present on the donor vascular endothelium. The diagnosis is suspected when a recipient has ventricular dysfunction without cellular rejection, which is confirmed by immunofluorescence staining of biopsy specimens showing deposition of IgG, C3, and C4 on coronary endothelium. Humoral rejection generally occurs in the first 3 months after transplantation, appears to be more common when antilymphocyte antibodies are used for rejection prophylaxis and is associated with an increased fatality rate and a higher incidence of cardiac allograft vasculopathy. Affected persons are treated with high-dose intravenous glucocorticoids, antithymocyte globulin, cytoxan, plasmapheresis, and heparin.

INFECTION

Infections are a constant risk for the post-transplant patient. The lungs are the most common site of infection, followed by the blood, urine, gastrointestinal tract, and operative wounds. Corticosteroids may make the signs of infection subtle. Prompt clinical evaluation of the recipient with low-grade fever, malaise, or a nonproductive cough is essential. A careful history and physical is often supplemented with a chest radiograph and a low threshold for pursuing other diagnostic testing as appropriate. As immunosuppressive medications are reduced over time, the overall risk of infection decreases.

Common pathogens and sites differ by post-transplantation period. In the first few months after transplantation, bacterial infections predominate, with the usual nosocomial pathogens resulting in intravascular catheter-induced bacteremias, urinary tract infections, pneumonias, and mediastinitis. Prophylactic treatment with oral nystatin or clotrimazole troches is required to prevent oral and esophageal candidiasis, but candidemia may also occur. Without prophylaxis, herpes simplex virus is common from 2 to 4 weeks after transplantation, but routine use of acyclovir can eliminate this risk. In the second and third months after transplantation, aspergillosis may cause pneumonia with frequent hematogenous dissemination.

The most important pathogen in the third through sixth months cytomegalovirus (CMV). CMV-negative recipients of a CMV-positive donor have the highest risk and progress to the most severe illness (primary infection), but CMV-positive recipients are also at risk for clinical illness. CMV may cause a mononucleosis-like febrile illness (CMV syndrome) or tissue-invasive disease (pneumonia, hepatitis, esophagitis, or colitis). CMV infection is associated with the development of allograft vasculopathy, and persistent CMV replication is associated with severe coronary disease. CMV infection up-regulates major histocompatibility antigens and is associated with an increased risk of subsequent rejection. Patients at risk are given ganciclovir either prophylactically or preemptively (after detection of CMV by antigen assay or polymerase chain reaction [PCR] but before clinically manifested illness) to prevent CMV illness and as treatment for established disease. Oral valacylovir effectively prevents CMV disease in renal transplant recipients and may be an attractive alternative to ganciclovir, but it has not yet been approved by the Food and Drug Administration for this indication.

Although far less common, toxoplasmosis also may occur during this period, with encephalitis, hepatitis, and myocarditis the typical presentations. Toxoplasmosis only occurs in toxoplasmosis-negative recipients of a positive donor and can be completely prevented by prophylaxis with pyrimethamine for the first 6 weeks after transplantation. *Pneumocystis carinii* pneumonia previously occurred in about 20% of recipients, with the peak incidence in the third through sixth months, but prophylaxis with trimethoprim-sulfamethoxazole for the first year after transplantation has made this illness uncommon. *Legionella* (pneumonia) and *Listeria* (meningitis and bacteremia) should be considered in the appropriate settings.

After the first 6 months, recipients remain at risk for the usual community-acquired bacterial infections, but parasitic and fungal infections and herpes zoster are also encountered. A nodular pulmonary infiltrate should prompt consideration of nocardiasis.

CORONARY ALLOGRAFT VASCULOPATHY

Development of coronary artery disease in the transplanted heart is the single most common cause of death in patients who survive the first post-transplantation year. Although classically described as a diffuse, concentric process, focal lesions may occur as well. Complete obliteration of secondary and tertiary epicardial vessels may occur, and the development of collaterals is unusual. Angiographic evidence of coronary allograft vasculopathy (CAV) is present in 50% of patients by 5 years after transplantation, but the more sensitive intravascular ultrasonography (IVUS) technique detects CAV in 80% to 100% of patients at 5 years. That CAV is limited to the transplanted heart attests to its immunologic nature, but hypercholesterolemia, hypertriglyceridemia, obesity, glucose intolerance, possibly smoking, and CMV infection all play a role. Denervation renders most patients incapable of experiencing angina (although partial reinnervation with atypical presentations of angina may occur), so CAV presents most commonly as heart failure, ventricular arrhythmias, or sudden death, if not first detected by annual surveillance coronary angiography or IVUS.

Coronary artery bypass surgery or catheter-based interventions may be performed with good short-term success if the anatomy is suitable, but this is often not the case, and progression of disease may be rapid. In one study, the 1-year survival rate after the demonstration of any 40% proximal or mid-vessel lesion was only 63%, with only 23% of heart failure patients surviving 1-year. Treatment and prevention of CAV are based on attention to the reversible risk factors just noted.

HMG-CoA reductase inhibitors (statins) reduce the incidence of both CAV and fatal rejection and should therefore be pursued in all patients, with a goal low-density lipoprotein (LDL) level of less than 100 mg per deciliter. However, myositis is more common in patients receiving statins with cyclosporine, so careful monitoring is warranted. Lovastatin, in particular, should be avoided. Diltiazem was shown to reduce the incidence of angiographically detectable CAV in a randomized trial and many centers use this routinely, with appropriate decreases in cyclosporine dosing. Some centers substitute MMF for azathioprine in patients with established CAV, based on limited clinical data suggesting that mycophenolate may decrease the incidence of CAV in new transplant recipients. Retransplantation is the most successful treatment for this condition, but it is controversial, considering the poorer survival for second-transplant recipients and the persistent shortage of donor organs. Those centers that perform retransplantation (about 50% of US centers) do so in only young and otherwise ideal candidates.

MALIGNANCIES

Nearly 12% of all deaths after heart transplantation result from malignancy. Most of the common malignancies (e.g., those of the lung, breast, colon, prostate, and cervix) are not appreciably increased in solid organ transplant recipients. When present, these cancers respond to therapy as would be expected in nonimmunosuppressed patients.

Two types of malignancies occur with particular frequency in heart and other solid organ transplant recipients. Post-transplant lymphoproliferative disorder (PTLD) occurs in nearly 2% of transplant recipients. Lymphotropic effects of the Epstein–Barr virus are thought to underlie this condition. Its development is related to the aggressiveness of immunosuppression and particularly to the prolonged use of prophylactic OKT3. Tumors are frequently present in extranodal sites, particularly in the gastrointestinal tract, lung, and central nervous system. The spectrum of disease runs from localized, benign lesions that respond to a reduction in immunosuppression to much more aggressive tumors that may be fatal despite lesion excision (when feasible), chemotherapy, and radiation.

The incidence of skin cancers is increased about 20-fold in cardiac transplant recipients. Locally invasive cancers may be fatal. An increased incidence is seen with all immunosuppressive regimens, but azathioprine may especially enhance this risk. Patients must be encouraged to use effective techniques to reduce sun exposure. All suspicious lesions should be biopsied, and yearly dermatologic screening is advisable.

The cardiac transplant recipient trades one set of problems for another. Post-transplant success requires frequent monitoring and constant vigilance on the part of both the patient and the treatment team. In most cases, these efforts are rewarded with good recipient survival and a substantially improved quality of life.

BIBLIOGRAPHY

Aaronson KD, Schwartz JS, Chen T-M, Mancini D. Development and prospective validation of a clinical index to predict survival in ambulatory patients referred for cardiac transplant evaluation. *Circulation* 1997; 95:2660–2667.

Costanzo MR, Augustine S, Bourge R, et al. Selection and treatment of candidates for heart transplantation. A statement for health professionals from the Committee on Heart Failure and Cardiac Transplantation of the Council on Clinical Cardiology, American Heart Association. *Circulation* 1995;92:3593–3612.

Halle AA, DiSciascio G, Massin EK. Coronary angioplasty, atherectomy, and bypass surgery in cardiac transplant recipients. *J Am Coll Cardiol* 1995;26:120–128.

Hosenpud JD, Bennet LE, Keck BM, et al. The Registry of the International Society of Heart and Lung Transplantation: Sixteenth Official Report—1999. *J Heart Lung Transplant* 1999;18:611–626.

Hunt SA. Twenty-fourth Bethesda Conference: Cardiac Transplantation. *J Am Coll Cardiol* 1993;22:1.

Kobashigawa J, Miller L, Renlund D, et al. A randomized active-controlled trial of mycophenolate mofetil in heart transplant recipients. Mycophenolate Mofetil Investigators. *Transplantation* 1998;66;507–515.

Kobashigawa JA, Katznelson S, Laks H, et al. Effect of pravastatin on outcomes after cardiac transplantation. *N Engl J Med* 1995;333:621–627.

Mancini DM, Eisen H, Kussmaul W, et al. Value of peak exercise oxygen consumption for optimal timing of cardiac transplantation in ambulatory patients with heart failure. *Circulation* 1991;83:778–786.

Merrigan TC, Renlund DG, Keay S, et al. A controlled trial of ganciclovir to prevent cytomegalovirus disease after heart transplantation. *N Engl J Med* 1992;326:1182.

Shroeder JS, Gao SZ, Alderman, et al. A preliminary study of diltiazem in the prevention of coronary artery disease in heart transplant recipients. *N Engl J Med* 1993;328:164.

Kelley's Textbook of Internal Medicine, fourth edition. Edited by H. David Humes. Lippincott Williams & Wilkins, Philadelphia © 2000.

3

GASTROENTEROLOGY

Peter G. Traber

APPROACH TO THE PATIENT WITH DIGESTIVE AND HEPATOBILIARY DISORDERS

APPROACH TO THE PATIENT WITH DYSPHAGIA

JOEL E. RICHTER

Dysphagia, from the Greek roots *dys* (with difficulty) and *phagia* (to eat), means either difficulty initiating a swallow (oropharyngeal dysphagia) or the sensation that foods, liquids, or both are hindered in their passage from mouth to stomach (esophageal dysphagia). It is important to differentiate dysphagia from odynophagia (pain with swallowing), although it is often difficult to separate the two clearly.

Dysphagia is common in all age groups, increasing in prevalence with advancing years. It is a significant cause of disability and a contributor to health care costs. Studies in nursing homes show that 30% to 40% of patients have swallowing disorders, resulting in a high incidence of aspiration pneumonia. Dysphagia also affects social well-being; the fear or reluctance to eat with others can lead to social isolation, malnutrition, and depression.

Table 94.1 outlines the common causes of dysphagia; however, many disorders overlap, producing both oropharyngeal and esophageal dysphagia. A thorough history, including medication use, can lead to an accurate diagnosis of the cause of dysphagia in 80% to 85% of patients with swallowing disorders.

■ INTEGRATED FUNCTION OF SWALLOWING

Swallowing, or deglutition, has been divided into three stages—oral, pharyngeal, esophageal—all regulated and coordinated by the swallowing center in the medulla.

The oral stage is largely voluntary and highly variable, depending on taste, environment, degree of hunger, and motiva-

tion. The preparatory stage entails the chewing of food and the forming of it into an oral bolus. Aided by adequate dentition, food is broken down to a size and a consistency appropriate for swallowing and mixed with saliva. Fine tongue movement is critical for confining the food bolus to the midline and pushing it up and back toward the palate while propelling the bolus into the pharynx. This process requires proper function of the striated muscles of the tongue and pharynx, and is the stage of swallowing most likely to be abnormal in patients with neurologic or skeletal muscle disease.

The pharyngeal stage requires the fine-tuned, coordinated sequence of contractions and relaxations resulting in the transfer of the bolus material from the pharynx to the esophagus. Food in the pharynx stimulates sensory receptors, sending impulses to the swallowing center in the brain stem. The central nervous system then initiates a series of involuntary responses occurring over a 1-second period. The soft palate is elevated and retracted with complete closure of the nasal pharynx, preventing swallowed material from entering the nasal cavity. The vocal cords are closed, and the epiglottis swings back and down to close the larynx. The larynx is pulled up and forward by the muscles attached to the hyoid bone, stretching the opening of the esophagus and the upper esophageal sphincter (UES). The UES relaxes during elevation of the larynx. Contractions of the pharyngeal constrictor muscles propel the bolus into the open mouth of the esophagus. Respiration is suspended during the swallow. The pharyngeal swallowing response is complex. Sensory information is carried along cranial nerves V, VII, IX, and X; the motor responses are carried along cranial nerves V, VII, X, and XII.

In the esophageal stage, digested material from the mouth is transported to the stomach. This active process requires contraction of both longitudinal and circular muscles of the tubular esophagus and coordinated relaxation of the sphincters. Swallowing shortens the longitudinal muscles, providing a structural base where the circular muscle contraction forms the peristaltic wave. This primary wave moves from the striated muscle of the upper esophagus through the esophageal body at 2 to 4 cm per second. Primary peristalsis is initiated by a swallow; secondary peristalsis can be initiated at any level of the esophagus in response to local luminal distention. This type of peristalsis clears

TABLE 94.1	COMMON CAUSES OF DYSPHAGIA

Oropharyngeal dysphagia
Neuromuscular diseases
  Cerebrovascular accidents
  Parkinson's disease
  Brain stem tumors
  Multiple sclerosis
  Amyotrophic lateral sclerosis
  Peripheral neuropathies (diphtheria, diabetes, polio)
Skeletal muscle disorders
  Polymyositis/dermatomyositis
  Muscular dystrophies (myotonic dystrophy, oculopharyngeal dystrophy)
  Myasthenia gravis
  Metabolic myopathies
Mechanical obstruction
  Inflammatory status
  Extrinsic compression (thyromegaly, cervical osteophyte)
  Postsurgical changes
  Zenker's diverticulum
  Cricopharyngeal bar
Miscellaneous
  Decreased saliva (medications, radiation, Sjögren's syndrome)
  Alzheimer's disease
  Depression
Esophageal dysphagia
Mechanical obstruction
  Benign strictures (peptic, corrosive, radiation)
  Webs and rings (Schatzki's)
  Neoplasm
  External compression (vascular, thyroid, mediastinal mass)
  Diverticulum
Motility disorders
  Achalasia
  Spastic motility disorders
  Scleroderma
  Miscellaneous (diabetes, alcohol, gastroesophageal reflux disease)

ingested material incompletely transported by a primary peristaltic wave and material regurgitated from the stomach.

OROPHARYNGEAL DYSPHAGIA

PRESENTATION

Patients with oropharyngeal dysphagia have trouble initiating swallowing, with symptoms occurring within 1 second of swallowing. They identify the cervical esophagus as the problem area. Associated complaints may include nasal regurgitation, coughing, choking, dysarthria, and nasal speech (Fig. 94.1). Laryngeal penetration and aspiration may occur in these patients without concurrent choking or coughing. The cough reflex may be diminished from altered sensation relating to an underlying neurologic disease or from desensitization due to chronic aspiration.

The physical examination usually reveals a neurologic or neuromuscular condition contributing to the symptoms. Hemiparesis secondary to a previous cerebrovascular accident, palpebral ptosis and end-of-the-day weakness indicative of myasthenia

gravis, or a fenestrating gait and paucity of movement characteristic of Parkinson's disease can lead to a precise diagnosis. Specific deficits of the cranial nerves involved in swallowing may also aid in the evaluation.

Oropharyngeal dysphagia should not be confused with globus, a sensation of a lump or tightness in the throat. It is a more constant symptom that usually does not interfere with swallowing and actually may be relieved during deglutition. It can be associated with or aggravated by stress and gastroesophageal reflux.

COMMON CAUSES

Neuromuscular diseases are responsible for about 80% of cases of oropharyngeal dysphagia. Strokes are the most common neurologic condition in the elderly. Symptoms are typically abrupt in onset and are usually associated with other neurologic deficits, particularly those of the cranial nerves. However, small lacunar infarcts, deep in the brain, may produce dysphagia as a sole primary symptom. Cerebral and brain stem cerebrovascular accidents can produce oropharyngeal dysphagia. The mechanism producing the former is probably brain stem distortion secondary to cerebral edema; the latter results from direct brain stem injury caused by vertebrobasilar artery disease. Bilateral brain stem involvement is more severe and less likely to show recovery than unilateral involvement. If recovery occurs, it usually does so within the first 6 to 9 months after the stroke.

Some degree of oropharyngeal dysphagia is present in up to 50% of patients with Parkinson's disease; 95% show abnormalities on video-esophagography. Clinically significant dysphagia may appear early in the course of Parkinson's disease, but it usually is a late manifestation. Tongue tremor and hesitancy in initiating a swallow are well-recognized features of this disease.

Inflammatory myopathies (polymyositis and dermatomyositis) present with oropharyngeal dysphagia in 60% to 70% of patients. These patients may show dramatic improvement with steroid therapy. Two forms of muscular dystrophy involve the striated muscles of the pharyngoesophageal region. Myotonic dystrophy is a familial disease characterized by myopathic facies, myotonia, swan-neck deformity, muscle wasting, frontal baldness, testicular atrophy, and cataracts. Oculopharyngeal dystrophy is an autosomal dominant disorder occurring after age 60 in patients of French–Canadian ancestry. Dysphagia followed by ptosis is a common presentation.

Myasthenia gravis is characterized by weakness on repetitive use of voluntary muscles. Typically, muscle strength tends to worsen toward the end of the day, partially returns with rest, and improves dramatically with administration of anticholinesterase drugs. Myasthenia gravis has a peak incidence in the third decade for women and the seventh decade for men. Dysphagia occurs in nearly two-thirds of patients; the first manifestation is often nasal regurgitation of fluids and weakness in chewing. Other common symptoms include generalized weakness, ptosis, diplopia, and dysarthria characterized by a fading voice that becomes more nasal after sustained conversation or when the patient is challenged with repetitive phrases.

Oropharyngeal dysphagia can also occur with a steroid myopathy and hyper- or hypothyroidism.

Dysphagia

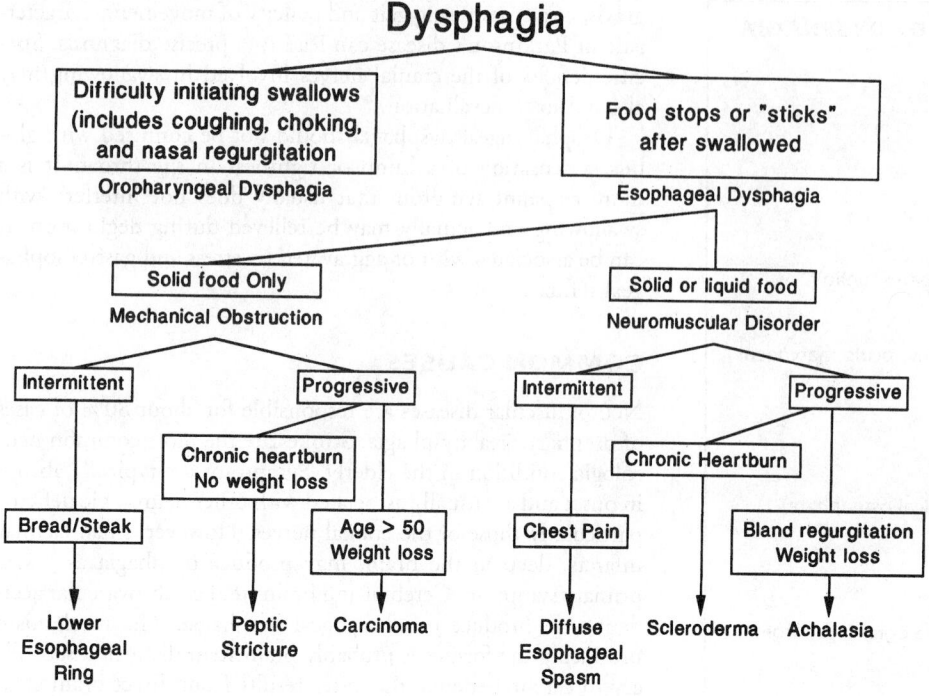

FIGURE 94.1. Diagnostic algorithm for the symptomatic assessment of the patient with dysphagia. (Modified from Castell DO, Donner MW. Evaluation of dysphagia: a careful history is crucial. *Dysphagia* 1987;2:65–71.)
EVIDENCE LEVEL: B. Reference: AGA Medical Position Statement on Management of Oropharyngeal Dysphagia. *Gastroenterology* 1999;116:452–478.

Anatomical abnormalities causing mechanical obstruction and oropharyngeal dysphagia include neoplasms, infections (e.g., retroperitoneal abscesses), thyromegaly, lymphadenopathy, and, rarely, cervical osteophytes. UES dysfunction may be associated with a Zenker's diverticulum or cricopharyngeal bar. Once thought to be related to discoordination of UES relaxation (cricopharyngeal achalasia), recent studies show that the UES relaxes appropriately but opens incompletely because of reduced muscle compliance resulting from myositis and fibrosis. To compensate for this decrease in cross-sectional area, intrabolus pressure and

hypopharyngeal pressure increase, leading to dysphagia and diverticula formation. Patients usually present after age 50 with variable symptoms, including regurgitation of previously eaten foods, solid and liquid dysphagia, cough, and halitosis. Cricopharyngeal myotomy is the treatment of choice.

DIAGNOSTIC STUDIES

Barium examination of the oropharynx and esophagus during swallowing is the most useful test (Fig. 94.2). The extremely

Dysphagia

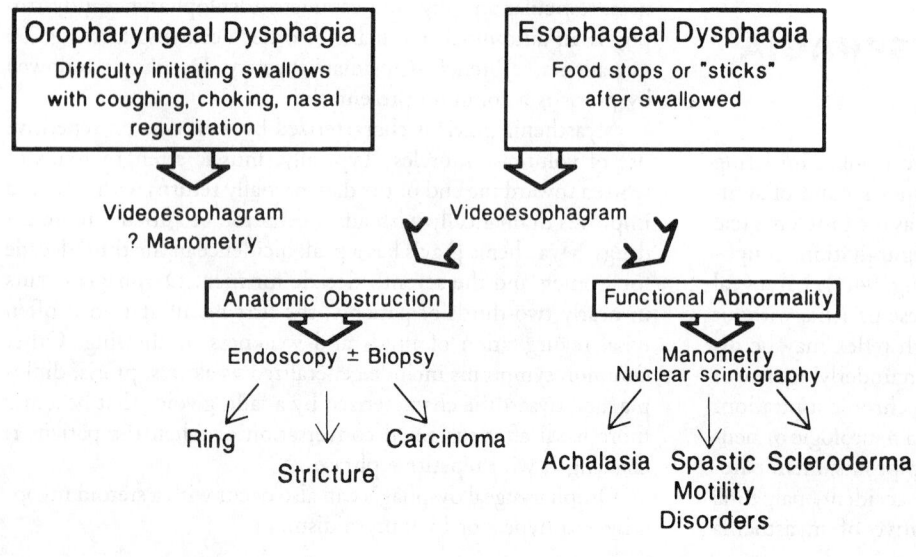

FIGURE 94.2. Algorithm for the appropriate use of diagnostic tests in evaluating the patient with dysphagia. The barium esophagogram, preferably using the video technique, is the initial diagnostic test for patients presenting with either oropharyngeal or esophageal dysphagia.
EVIDENCE LEVEL: B. Reference: AGA Medical Position Statement on Management of Oropharyngeal Dysphagia. *Gastroenterology* 1999;116:452–478.

rapid sequence of events in this area cannot be evaluated adequately by standard barium techniques. Examination of the oropharyngeal area should include videotaping and the use of both liquids and different consistencies of semisolid and solid boluses. Playback of the videotape allows careful evaluation of the swallowing mechanism and identification of subtle abnormalities resulting from neurologic or muscular diseases. The administration of various consistencies of barium and food products helps identify patients who can swallow safely without aspiration and assists in the formulation of therapeutic interventions. Conventional esophageal manometry is less helpful. Appropriate evaluation of the oropharyngeal region requires self-contained intraluminal transducer systems and on-line computer analysis to assess UES and pharyngeal dynamics accurately. These techniques require special facilities and expertise and are not routinely done. Endoscopic visualization of vocal cord movement and ultrasound are useful for imaging tongue movements and laryngeal transport.

ESOPHAGEAL DYSPHAGIA

PRESENTATION

Esophageal dysphagia is caused by various mechanical or neuromuscular (motility) defects that prohibit the passage of food down the esophagus. The patient often describes this problem as food "hanging up" somewhere behind the sternum. Localized to the lower sternum or the epigastric area, the lesion is most likely in the distal esophagus. Localization to the lower part of the neck may indicate dysfunction in this area, but often the symptoms are referred from a more distal blockage.

Figure 94.1 shows a simple algorithm for the evaluation of patients with dysphagia. After obtaining a general medical history, including medication use, a detailed history of swallowing should emphasize the duration of the symptoms and the types of food and liquids that cause them. Patients reporting dysphagia that occurs with both solids and liquids are most likely to have an esophageal motility disorder. If the dysphagia occurs only after swallowing a solid bolus, such as a large piece of meat, but never when the patient initially drinks a beverage, the physician should consider the possibility of a mechanical obstruction. Intermittent solid food dysphagia, particularly for bread or steak in an otherwise healthy person, should suggest a lower esophageal (Schatzki's) ring. Dysphagia is the rule if the luminal diameter is less than 13 mm but is unlikely if the diameter is larger than 20 mm. Progressive solid food dysphagia may be associated with a peptic stricture or carcinoma. Patients with peptic strictures usually have a long history of heartburn and regurgitation and no weight loss. Although the esophagus may be markedly narrowed, these patients have a good appetite and will modify their diet to maintain their weight. On the other hand, patients with cancer of the esophagus tend to be older men with marked weight loss, as much from anorexia as from esophageal luminal narrowing.

Intermittent dysphagia for solids and liquids associated with chest pain should suggest spastic motility disorders. Progressive solid and liquid food dysphagia may be associated with sclero-derma or achalasia. Scleroderma of the esophagus generally is seen in women giving a long history of heartburn. On the other hand, patients with achalasia are equally distributed between men and women, and they complain of bland regurgitation, choking, coughing, and weight loss. All of these disorders are discussed in further detail in Chapter 106.

The physical examination is usually of limited value. Patients with esophageal cancer may have cervical and supraclavicular lymphadenopathy and marked weight loss. Patients with scleroderma may present with the CREST syndrome: digital calcinosis, Raynaud's disease, esophageal dysmotility, sclerodactyly, and telangiectasia.

DIAGNOSTIC STUDIES

A barium esophagogram should be the initial test performed (Fig. 94.2; Chapter 106). Barium outlines irregularities in the esophageal lumen, defines sites of anatomical obstruction, and assesses liquid transit through the body of the esophagus. In patients with dysphagia for liquids and solids, this test accurately defines achalasia and diffuse esophageal spasm. In patients with solid food dysphagia, a barium swallow performed with tablets of various sizes (6, 8, 12.5 mm), marshmallows, or food products may help identify anatomical abnormalities such as subtle rings, strictures, or segmental regions of poor motility. An upper gastrointestinal series is not a suitable substitute for a barium esophagogram when esophageal disease is suspected because this study focuses on the stomach, with only spot films of the pharynx and limited full-column examination of the esophagus.

There is a good correlation between radiographic findings and subsequent endoscopic examination. If the barium studies reveal an obstructing lesion, endoscopy with biopsy and brush cytology can establish the diagnosis. Immediate therapeutic intervention can be accomplished with the use of dilators over a wire or blunt bougie dilators. Endoscopy should not be the initial test for patients presenting with dysphagia. The use of a narrow endoscope and light sedation tends to miss rings and strictures, particularly if the luminal diameter is greater than 13 mm, as a result of poor esophageal insufflation and distention.

If the barium studies are normal or suggest a motility disorder, esophageal manometry is the next step (Chapter 106). Motor abnormalities of the esophagus can be intermittent, and manometry allows more prolonged evaluation of the esophagus than barium studies. Manometric studies are diagnostic of achalasia and spastic motility disorders and may suggest the presence of a scleroderma esophagus.

BIBLIOGRAPHY

Baron TH, Richter JE. The use of esophageal function tests. *Adv Intern Med* 1993;38:361–386.

Castell DO, Donner MW. Evaluation of dysphagia: the careful history is crucial. *Dysphagia* 1987;2:65–71.

Logenmann JA. Swallowing physiology and pathophysiology. *Otolaryngol Clin North Am* 1988;21:613–623.

Kelley's Textbook of Internal Medicine, fourth edition. Edited by H. David Humes.
Lippincott Williams & Wilkins, Philadelphia © 2000.

C H A P T E R
95

APPROACH TO THE PATIENT WITH NONCARDIAC CHEST PAIN

HENRY P. PARKMAN

Chest pain is a common clinical problem. The symptom of chest pain is frightening for patients due to the possibility of cardiac disease and its mortality. However, of the 750,000 patients with chest pain undergoing cardiac catheterization each year, normal coronary arteries are demonstrated in 20% to 30%. These patients have noncardiac, or unexplained, chest pain (NCCP). It is estimated that 4% of the population have frequent episodes of NCCP.

Patients with NCCP may be seen by a variety of physicians including internists, family practitioners, cardiologists, and gastroenterologists. Evaluation and treatment of patients with NCCP is a major clinical challenge, since the cause of the chest pain can often be elusive and the patients can remain extremely symptomatic with resultant poor functional status and repeated visits to physicians and emergency rooms. A significant proportion of patients (44%) with NCCP actually continue to believe that they have heart disease. Patients with NCCP have a good prognosis with mortality rate similar to that of the general population. Several studies have suggested that a definitive diagnosis of the cause of the patient's NCCP helps to reassure the patient, improve quality of life, and reduce the number of urgent office and emergency room visits.

TABLE 95.1.	CAUSES OF CHEST PAIN

Cardiovascular
  Coronary artery atherosclerosis
  Coronary artery spasm
  Valvular heart disease
    Aortic valvular disease
    Mitral valve prolapse
  Pericarditis
  Microvascular angina
  Dissecting thoracic aortic aneurysm
Noncardiac
  Gastrointestinal
    Esophageal
      Gastroesophageal reflux disease
      Esophageal dysmotility (e.g., diffuse esophageal spasm)
      Esophageal hyperalgesia
    Gastric
      Gastric ulcer, especially in the fundus
  Pulmonary
    Mediastinitis
    Pneumonia
    Lung cancer
    Pulmonary embolism
    Pneumothorax
    Pulmonary hypertension
  Musculoskeletal
    Costochondritis/Tietze's syndrome
    Arthritis of shoulder/spine
    Rib fracture
    Fibromyalgia
  Psychiatric/psychogenic
    Hyperventilation syndrome
    Anxiety
    Panic disorder
    Somatization disorder
    Depression
  Miscellaneous
    Herpes zoster

◼ DIFFERENTIAL DIAGNOSIS (TABLE 95.1)

CARDIAC DISORDERS

Coronary artery disease is the most important cause of chest pain due to the risk of myocardial infarction and death. Patients with recurrent chest pains should be evaluated for coronary artery disease first, often entailing exercise stress with thallium testing and/or coronary arteriography. If these suggest underlying coronary artery disease, the patients are then treated appropriately. However, patients with underlying coronary artery disease may also have NCCP. Up to 36% of patients with recurrent chest pains and known coronary artery disease may have gastroesophageal reflux disease (GERD) precipitating their symptoms. Ischemic heart disease and GERD can coexist in the same patient and may produce identical symptoms. Acid suppression can lead to marked improvement in the chest pain in some patients.

Chest pain is commonly associated with mitral valve prolapse and usually described as a brief sharp or sticking pain, but it may be a dull ache over the chest that may last for hours. Breathlessness, palpitations, faintness, and fatigue may be associated

symptoms. Esophageal motor abnormalities, primarily diffuse esophageal spasm (DES), and panic disorder have been described in many patients with mitral valve prolapse, which may also cause chest pains.

Microvascular angina refers to abnormalities in the small endocardial vessels without lesions in the larger epicardial vessels. These patients have chest pain despite normal coronary arteriograms. Diagnosis requires sophisticated cardiac catheterization. Increased microvascular resistance is the hallmark of the disease. The prevalence of this disorder among patients with recurrent chest pain and normal coronary arteries in the general population is unknown, since evaluation for this disorder is not usually performed. It has been suggested that stress thallium or exercise gated blood pool scintigraphy might be used as a screening test for this disorder. The diagnosis would be suggested by ischemic ST segment response and/or abnormal left ventricular ejection fraction in response to exercise associated with the patient's typical chest pain in the absence of coronary artery disease. Patients with microvascular angina have also been found to have coexistent esophageal motility abnormalities, making it unclear as to whether the chest pain symptoms are from the esophagus or heart. The long-term prognosis for these patients appears to be excellent, with little evidence of heart attacks or cardiac deaths.

ESOPHAGEAL DISORDERS

Esophageal disorders are probably the most common cause of NCCP, accounting for 20% to 60% of cases. The common causes of esophageal chest pain are esophageal motility disorders and GERD. Esophageal hyperalgesia (hypersensitivity) has been suggested as a third mechanism.

Esophageal Motor Abnormalities

Diffuse esophageal spasm is an esophageal motor disorder that is clinically manifested by substernal chest pain and/or dysphagia (see Chapter 94). Chest pain, usually the most prominent symptom, is generally retrosternal and may have radiation pattern similar to that of angina. Symptoms are intermittent and nonprogressive. Esophageal manometric findings are high-amplitude, nonperistaltic contractions that are interspersed with normal peristaltic contractions. Although this disorder is occasionally thought to be synonymous with esophageal chest pain, DES actually accounts for less than 5% of patients with NCCP.

The "nutcracker" esophagus describes manometric findings of high-amplitude peristaltic esophageal contractions (see Chapter 106). In contrast to DES, the esophageal contractions are always peristaltic. This finding is present in 12% of patients with NCCP. It is unclear as to whether this entity has true clinical or pathophysiologic significance, since often the high-pressure contractions correlate poorly with the occurrence of chest pain. When these patients are treated with the calcium channel blocker nifedipine, to reduce the amplitude of esophageal contractions, there is little symptomatic improvement in the chest pain. Moreover, the patient's symptoms may improve on low-dose trazodone, an antidepressant, without a change in the manometric abnormalities. Nutcracker esophagus may also be associated with GERD and symptoms of chest pain may improve with antireflux treatment.

Gastroesophageal Reflux Disease

Although heartburn is the classic symptom, GERD may cause atypical symptoms such as chest pain (see Chapter 106). Prolonged esophageal pH monitoring has allowed better recognition of GERD as one of the most common identifiable causes of NCCP. It is possible that in some patients acid-sensitive receptors in the esophagus interpret the reflux as chest pain. Occasionally, the reflux of acid into the esophagus may precipitate esophageal spasm.

Esophageal Hyperalgesia

Esophageal hyperalgesia has recently been suggested as a cause of unexplained chest pain. Graded distention of an intraesophageal balloon in patients with NCCP has been used to show that they are more sensitive to esophageal distention, with patients reporting an exaggerated perception of pain compared to controls. Esophageal balloon distention can produce chest pain in approximately 50% of patients with NCCP compared to only 10% to 20% of normal subjects. Furthermore, the volumes used to elicit chest pain in patients are relatively low compared to the higher volumes needed in normal subjects. The chest pain may be related to lower pain threshold to balloon distention, suggesting that there is enhanced sensitivity to distention (hyperalgesia) as a result of a lower visceral pain threshold. In some patients with NCCP, intraesophageal balloon distention produces nonperistaltic esophageal contractions consistent with spasm distal to the balloon simultaneously with reproduction of patients' chest pain.

MUSCULOSKELETAL DISORDERS

Musculoskeletal causes may account for 10% to 30% of patients with NCCP. The pain is often a dull, aching, or nagging pain with variable intensity and duration. Alternatively, it may be a sharp pain that is accentuated by movement especially on arising in the morning. The diagnosis of musculoskeletal chest pain involves eliciting tenderness on palpation of trigger points on the chest wall, which is similar to the spontaneously occurring pain.

Tietze's syndrome is characterized by pain, tenderness, and swelling of a costal cartilage usually involving the second, left costosternal or sternoclavicular joints. Trauma to the cartilage from repeated coughing or sudden movements is proposed as mechanisms for this disorder. Costochondritis is similar to Tietze's syndrome, although it more commonly affects multiple junctions with frequent symmetry, especially of the lower ribs.

PSYCHIATRIC/PSYCHOGENIC DISORDERS

Patients with NCCP have a high prevalence of depression, anxiety disorders, and somatization disorders. Panic disorder is the most common anxiety-related disorder in NCCP. Up to one-third of patients with chest pain and normal coronary arteries have panic disorder. Panic disorder is characterized by frequent (at least three attacks in 3 weeks) periods of intense fear or discomfort accompanied by shortness of breath, palpitations, chest pain or discomfort, sweating, faintness, choking, and fear of losing control, "going crazy," or dying. Chest pain in panic disorder may be an important factor in the health care seeking of these patients. It is an important disorder to recognize since some patients may have depression and suicidal ideation.

■ HISTORY AND PHYSICAL EXAMINATION

Information obtained during the history and physical examination, carefully selected diagnostic tests, and therapeutic trials of medications are used to evaluate the patient for the different

TABLE 95.2. EVALUATION OF NONCARDIAC CHEST PAIN

History and physical examination
Initial baseline testing
  Chest radiography
  Electrocardiography
Evaluate for cardiac cause
  Stress thallium test
  Coronary arteriography
Reevaluate for musculoskeletal causes
  Physical examination
  Therapeutic trial with nonsteroidal anti-inflammatory drug
Evaluate for esophageal disorders
  Diagnostic testing
    Esophageal manometry
    Esophageal pH monitoring
  Therapeutic trial
    Proton pump inhibitors
Evaluate for psychological causes

the detection of a musculoskeletal cause. Cutaneous signs of scleroderma may suggest GERD as a cause of chest pain.

DIAGNOSTIC TESTS

The initial diagnostic phase of the evaluation involves ruling out the possibility of cardiac disease. Most patients with chest pain should have initial evaluation for a cardiac source because the presence or absence of coronary disease cannot be reliably established from symptoms alone. Depending on the patient's age and gender, the cardiac evaluation may involve an electrocardiogram, exercise stress testing with thallium imaging, and coronary arteriography. Once coronary artery disease is excluded, evaluation proceeds for other, more benign causes of chest pain. Evaluation of NCCP is often tailored to the individual patient. The evaluation may include upper gastrointestinal radiologic examination or upper endoscopy, esophageal manometry, and 24-hour esophageal pH monitoring.

ENDOSCOPY OR X-RAYS

The upper gastrointestinal tract (esophagus and stomach) is evaluated for mucosal disorders (esophagitis, ulcer, mass lesions) with either barium studies or upper gastrointestinal endoscopy (esophagogastroduodenoscopy). Although these tests are frequently normal, important therapeutic information is obtained if they are positive. It should be remembered that a normal study does not rule out an esophageal cause for chest pain.

If dysphagia is an associated symptom, a barium esophagram is the procedure of choice to detect structural lesions of the esophagus such as strictures, achalasia, or even esophageal cancer. Careful observation of esophageal function during fluoroscopy is important, since esophageal aperistalsis, spasm, or GERD may be demonstrated. A hiatal hernia on barium swallow has been found to correlate poorly with GERD.

Upper endoscopy can also identify a significant number of patients with NCCP with acid-peptic disorders (esophagitis, gastritis, duodenitis, or ulcer disease). In one study of 100 patients with NCCP, esophagitis was present in 24 patients and gastroduodenal ulcer in 6. However, other studies have suggested that endoscopic evidence of esophagitis is seen in fewer than 10% of patients with NCCP. The advantage of endoscopy over radiology is the better mucosal detail that endoscopy provides and the ability to perform biopsies directly. Endoscopy is more reliable in detecting reflux esophagitis, pill-induced esophagitis, and Barrett's esophagus, a complication of long-standing GERD. Endoscopy is thus generally preferable over barium studies in evaluation of patients with NCCP. However, upper endoscopy gives little information about the physiologic function of the esophagus.

ESOPHAGEAL MANOMETRY AND PROVOCATIVE TESTING

Esophageal manometry is used to evaluate patients with NCCP primarily for spastic motility disorders of the esophagus (see

cardiac, esophageal, musculoskeletal, and psychiatric causes of chest pain (Table 95.2).

A detailed description of the chest pain, including aggravating and alleviating factors, is important. Esophageal disorders giving rise to chest pain can be perceived as chest pain similar to that of angina. In many cases, it is not possible from the history to distinguish between cardiac and esophageal causes of chest pain. This is not surprising in view of the close proximity of these two organs and the fact that both organs are innervated by similar distribution of the vagus nerve (parasympathetic) and sympathetic nervous system. Associated symptoms of dysphagia (difficulty swallowing), odynophagia (pain on swallowing), and heartburn may be helpful to direct the etiology of chest pain to the esophagus. However, these associated symptoms are not always present in patients with esophageal chest pain; furthermore, they can be present to some degree by chance occurrence in patients with cardiac pain. Esophageal discomfort is usually not brought on by exertion or relieved by rest. At times, however, GERD can be triggered by exercise, as angina can. Features suggesting an esophageal origin include pain that continues for hours, pain related to meals, and pain relieved with antacids. Chest pain due to esophageal spasm can be associated with deglutition, especially with foods that are cold or hot. Similar to patients with angina, patients with esophageal spasm may also obtain relief with sublingual nitroglycerin and calcium channel blockers.

Besides inquiring about the common risk factors for coronary artery disease, one needs to inquire about the use of cocaine. Cocaine use may also induce myocardial ischemia.

Patients with atypical chest pain should be screened for generalized anxiety states, panic disorder, and depression. Chest pain associated with intense fear or discomfort and the sense of impending doom or dying should raise the suspicion of panic attacks. These patients often have other somatic complaints.

The physical examination is occasionally helpful to detect cardiac valvular disease, such as aortic stenosis and mitral valve prolapse. Eliciting tenderness on palpation of the chest wall, as well as reproduction of the patient's typical pain, is helpful in

Chapter 106). Esophageal manometry is useful to specifically diagnose achalasia and DES. However, most of the time esophageal manometry will be normal or show nonspecific findings. The two major esophageal motor abnormalities, DES and achalasia, are found in only 3% and 1%, respectively, of patients undergoing esophageal manometry for NCCP. Other manometric diagnoses, such as nutcracker esophagus and nonspecific esophageal motor disorders, are present more frequently in patients with chest pain; however, the relationship of these nonspecific findings to chest pain has been questioned. Occasionally, evidence of low LES pressure or low-amplitude esophageal contractions may suggest GERD, which can be verified by subsequent esophageal pH monitoring. Due to the high prevalence of normal or nonspecific findings on esophageal manometry in patients with NCCP, it has been suggested that esophageal manometry not be used as one of the initial tests in patients with unexplained chest pain.

Acid perfusion of the esophagus (Bernstein's test), intravenous infusion of edrophonium, and esophageal balloon distention are provocative tests that have been used during esophageal manometry to correlate abnormal findings (such as acid in the esophagus or esophageal dysmotility) with the clinical symptoms of chest pain. If positive, they may help to reassure the patient that there is an esophageal and not a cardiac cause of the chest pain. These provocative tests do not determine cause and effect, and they might not help to direct therapy confidently.

AMBULATORY ESOPHAGEAL pH MONITORING

Ambulatory 24-hour monitoring of esophageal pH is helpful in determining the presence of GERD (see Chapter 106). This is the best test for quantifying abnormal amounts of acid reflux and/or demonstrating a causal relationship between the acid reflux and chest pain. During the study, diary cards and event markers are used to time the patient's symptoms and can be used to correlate atypical symptoms of reflux, such as chest pain, to episodes of acid reflux. The symptom index is calculated as the percentage of chest pain episodes that occurred when the esophageal pH was less than 4. The higher the symptom index, the more likely the chest pain is secondary to reflux. Often a symptom index of greater than 50% is used to demonstrate a correlation of symptoms to acid reflux. The value of the symptom index is that it directly associates the chest pain events with acid reflux. Furthermore, it can be positive even when the esophageal acid exposure is normal. Patients with a positive symptom index but normal acid exposure represent a group that may be hypersensitive to physiologic amounts of acid reflux. The symptom index can also be useful when the test is being performed on gastric acid suppressant medications or if a patient has several different types of symptoms.

THERAPEUTIC TRIAL

An alternative approach to esophageal pH monitoring in the evaluation of a patient for GERD as a cause of chest pain is with a therapeutic trial of a gastric acid suppressant medication. This has been gaining popularity, especially with the availability of effective gastric acid suppression with the proton pump inhibitors and for physicians without easy access to esophageal pH monitoring testing. With this approach, one places a patient on an acid suppressant treatment for 2 to 4 weeks and monitors the frequency of chest pain episodes. A reduction in the number of chest pain episodes suggests that GERD was the cause. Usually proton pump inhibitors, such as omeprazole 20 mg PO b.i.d. or lansoprazole 30 mg PO b.i.d., are used to ensure that gastric acid secretion is suppressed and that elimination of acid reflux has occurred. If there is response to the therapeutic trial, the patient may be placed on the medication that helped his or her symptoms. If there is not a response, esophageal and gastric pH monitoring on medication is often used to determine if gastric acid secretion was suppressed.

◼ STRATEGIES FOR OPTIMAL CARE

ESOPHAGEAL CHEST PAIN

Gastroesophageal Reflux Disease–induced Chest Pain

Treatment of GERD initially includes nonsystemic therapy with dietary modifications and postural measures (see Chapter 106). Antacids may be useful to acutely relieve the symptoms. Stopping drugs that reduce LES pressures may be helpful. These include anticholinergics, nitrates, calcium channel blockers, β-adrenergic agents, and certain tranquilizers. Fatty foods, chocolate, and alcohol also reduce LES pressure and may contribute to GERD.

Antisecretory agents are the main treatment for NCCP caused by GERD. These include H_2-receptor antagonists (cimetidine, ranitidine, famotidine, and nizatidine) and proton pump inhibitors (omeprazole and lansoprazole). Chest pain resulting from GERD appears to be harder to treat than conventional symptoms of GERD, such as heartburn. Patients often need intensive therapy with t.i.d./q.i.d. or double-dose b.i.d. H_2 receptor agonists, or up to b.i.d. dosing of proton pump inhibitors.

Prokinetic agents, such as cisapride and metoclopramide, increase LES pressure and increase gastric emptying, both of which may improve symptoms of reflux. Although prokinetic agents are useful in mild symptoms of GERD, they have not been studied in NCCP resulting from GERD. Usually for NCCP, they are used as adjunctive therapy to gastric acid suppressants.

The final type of antireflux treatment is surgery (see Chapter 106). The most common antireflux operation is the Nissen fundoplication, which involves wrapping the fundus around the gastroesophageal junction to augment LES pressure. With the introduction of potent antisecretory agents, surgical treatment is required in only a minority of patients (less than 3% of patients). Surgery should be attempted in patients with NCCP only with objective evidence of reflux as a cause of symptoms, preferably by both esophageal pH monitoring and some response to gastric acid–suppressive therapy.

Spastic Esophageal Motor Disorders

Treatment of spastic esophageal motility disorders has not been as successful as that for GERD (see Chapter 106). Treatment for esophageal motility disorders such as DES and nutcracker esophagus centers on smooth muscle relaxants to reduce the high-amplitude esophageal contractions. If dysphagia is also a problem, reduction of LES pressure may also improve the chest pain. Medications used for spastic esophageal motility disorders include nitrates, calcium channel antagonists, and anticholinergic agents. Oral or sublingual nitrates, such as isosorbide dinitrate (Isordil), has been shown to reduce the frequency of symptoms and lower the high-amplitude contractions in the esophageal body. The frequency of side effects, most notably headache and hypotension, usually precludes increasing the dosage of nitrates to effectively relieve the chest pain. The calcium channel antagonists nifedipine and diltiazem both reduce esophageal contraction amplitude, but demonstrations of symptomatic improvement have been inconsistent. Anticholinergic agents, such as hyoscyamine (Levsin) or dicyclomine (Bentyl), reduce the amplitude of esophageal contractions; however, their effectiveness in treating esophageal motility disorders is unknown. In patients with recalcitrant DES, pneumatic dilatation of the lower esophageal sphincter may be tried. Surgical therapy, such as long esophageal myotomy, although tried in the past, is best avoided.

INCREASED VISCERAL NOCICEPTION

Treatments for functional gastrointestinal disorders, including NCCP, have often included psychotropic medications. It is likely these therapies are mediated through visceral analgesic action that alters abnormal nociception (visceral hypersensitivity). Often tricyclic antidepressants are used at doses lower than those for treatment of depression. Imipramine 25 to 100 mg taken at bedtime has been reported to result in significant improvement in patients with NCCP who do not have reflux disease. The antidepressant trazadone 25 to 100 mg per day (at night) has been shown to be beneficial in decreasing symptoms associated with abnormal esophageal motility. The conventional antidepressant amitriptyline (Elavil) may also be useful but has anticholinergic side effects.

MUSCULOSKELETAL DISORDERS

Treatment of patients with musculoskeletal chest pain includes local therapy, nonsteroidal anti-inflammatory drugs, and, occasionally, corticosteroid–lidocaine injections.

PANIC DISORDER

Panic disorder can be approached with cognitive behavior therapy and pharmacologic therapy. The tricyclic antidepressants are often considered first-line therapy. Imipramine administration is beneficial; however, it may take up to 24 weeks for response. Benzodiazepines, such as alprazolam, may be used for initial control and have been used for this disorder. Serotonin uptake inhibitors, such as fluoxetine, have shown promising results.

■ COMPLICATIONS AND PITFALLS

A pitfall in the approach to patients with NCCP is a failure to recognize that GERD and panic disorder may cause chest pain. Today there is specific treatment available for chest pain due to GERD. Furthermore, patients with known underlying coronary artery disease can have noncardiac causes, especially GERD, accounting for some of their chest pain. GERD as a cause of chest pain in patients with coronary artery disease is also important to recognize because medications used to treat ischemic heart disease, especially nitrates and calcium channel blockers, can decrease the LES pressure and predispose patients to more reflux. If chest pain symptoms are chronic (more than 5 to 10 years duration) and due to GERD, the patient may be at risk for Barrett's metaplasia, which is best evaluated with endoscopy.

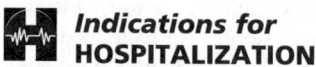 *Indications for* **HOSPITALIZATION**

Usually hospitalization in patients with NCCP occurs when there is still the concern that the pain is from cardiac ischemia. This occurs in patients who have not been adequately evaluated for cardiac disease or patients with a change in their typical pain episodes.

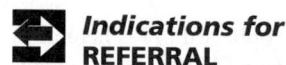 *Indications for* **REFERRAL**

Patients may be referred to gastroenterologists for several reasons, including (a) upper endoscopy procedure; (b) esophageal pH monitoring and/or esophageal manometry; (c) consultation to determine if the chest pain is of gastroenterologic origin; (d) aggressive treatment for GERD and spastic esophageal motor disorders. Patients may be referred to a psychiatrist or a psychologist for psychological disorders. Generally speaking, panic attacks are best treated by a specialist.

■ CONCLUSION

Through appropriate evaluation, many patients with NCCP may be found to have a reason for their symptoms. Esophageal disorders, musculoskeletal disorders, and panic disorders can often be diagnosed. With esophageal manometry and esophageal pH monitoring, an esophageal etiology can be demonstrated in 50% of patients with NCCP, with GERD being more prevalent than esophageal motor disorders. Occasionally, empiric treatment, especially for GERD, is undertaken both for therapeutic and diagnostic reasons. Patients with esophageal hyperalgesia (altered sensory perception) or panic disorder may respond to psychotropic medication.

BIBLIOGRAPHY

Achem SR, Kolts BE, MacMath T, et al. Effects of omeprazole versus placebo in treatment of noncardiac chest pain and gastroesophgeal reflux. *Dis Dis Sci* 1997;42:2138–2145.

Beitman BD, Mukerji V, Lamberti JW, et al. Panic disorder in patients with chest pain and angiographically normal coronary arteries. *Am J Cardiol* 1989;63:1399–1403.

Cannon RO III, Quyyumi AA, Mincemoyer R, et al. Imipramine in patients with chest pain despite normal coronary angiograms. *N Engl J Med* 1994;330:1411–1417.

Fass R, Fennerty MB, Ofman JJ, et al. The clinical and economic value of a short course of omeprazone in patients with noncardiac chest pain. *Gastroenterology* 1998;115:42–49.

Goyall RK. Changing focus on unexplained esophgeal chest pain. *Ann Intern Med* 1996;124:1008–1010.

Hewson EG, Sinclair JW, Dalton CB, et al. Twenty-four-hour esophgeal pH monitoring: the most useful test for evaluating noncardiac chest pain. *Am J Med* 1991;90:576–583.

Katerndahl DA, Trammell C. Prevalence and recognition of panic states in patients presenting with chest pain. *J Fam Pract* 1997;45:54–63.

Richter JE. Practical approach to the diagnosis of unexplained chest pain. *Med Clin North Am* 1991;75:1203–1207.

Singh S, Richter JE, Hewson EG, et al. The contribution of gastroesophageal reflux to chest pain in patients with coronary artery disease. *Ann Intern Med* 1992;117:824–830.

Voskuil J-H, Cramer MJ, Breunelhof R, et al. Prevalence of esophageal disorders in patients with chest pain newly referred to the cardiologist. *Chest* 1996;109:1210–1214.

Kelley's Textbook of Internal Medicine, fourth edition. Edited by H. David Humes. Lippincott Williams & Wilkins, Philadelphia © 2000.

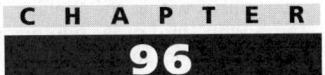

CHAPTER 96

APPROACH TO THE PATIENT WITH ABDOMINAL PAIN

ROBERT B. STEIN
GARY R. LICHTENSTEIN

The approach to the patient with abdominal pain is one of a physician's greatest challenges. Abdominal pain is a common symptom that involves the patients' subjective reaction to a stimulus. It is essential that treating physicians have an understanding of the pathophysiologic basis of abdominal pain so that they may be better able to determine its cause and prescribe appropriate therapy. This chapter reviews the physiologic aspects of abdominal pain, as well as the methods most suitable for evaluation and management of acute and chronic abdominal pain.

ANATOMICAL BASIS OF ABDOMINAL PAIN

The perception of pain (nociception) most commonly begins at the level of the pain neuroceptors (nociceptors). The free periph-

eral ends of these fibers are ubiquitous and may respond to a variety of stimuli, such as stretch, spasm, inflammation, or ischemia. Two types of fibers transmit painful impulses: A δ fibers and C fibers. Type A δ fibers are found predominantly in skin and muscle. They are myelinated, rapidly conducting, and yield sharp, well-localized pain. Type C fibers are unmyelinated and are distributed in muscle, mesentery, abdominal viscera, and peritoneum. Compared to type A δ fibers, type C fibers conduct stimuli slowly and produce a poorly localized, dull or burning pain. Acute injury often leads to sharp pain transmitted by type A δ fibers, followed by a dull ache or discomfort transmitted by type C fibers.

The majority of nociceptors in the abdominal viscera are type C fibers. Thus, it is common for patients with abdominal pain to present with a dull, poorly localized pain. Nociceptors within the abdominal viscera are less sensitive and fewer than those within the skin. The fact that endoscopic biopsies and polypectomies can be performed without causing any discomfort to the patient supports this fact. However, mucosa that is inflamed or interrupted may cause significant pain, likely resulting from the release of a variety of chemical substances (e.g., bradykinin).

Visceral afferent (sensory) fibers penetrate the serosa of hollow abdominal organs to enter the submucosa and muscularis layers. This is in contrast to solid organs such as the liver, which only have nociceptors on their surfaces and capsules. This explains why large hepatomas may not elicit abdominal pain until they involve or stretch the liver capsule.

There are three orders of neurons that transmit pain signals from the abdominal organs to the brain. Viscera afferent neurons leave the abdominal organs and travel via splanchnic nerves to regional ganglia (e.g., celiac, superior mesenteric). The cell bodies of the visceral afferent fibers are located in the dorsal root ganglia of spinal afferent nerves (Fig. 96.1). Fibers then carry impulses to the dorsal horn of the spinal cord where they synapse with the second-order neurons. These neurons then cross the anterior commissure and ascend the spinal cord via the contralateral lateral spinothalamic tract. Upon entering the brain stem, synapse occurs with the third-order neurons, which carry painful impulses to the somatosensory cortex of the cerebrum via the thalamus, and to the limbic system and frontal cortex. The somatosensory cortex makes possible the discrimination of painful stimuli, whereas the limbic system and frontal cortex provide the emotional aspects of pain.

Inhibitory fibers descend from the cerebral cortex and connect to the dorsal horn via the thalamus and brain stem. These inhibitory fibers allow modulation of painful stimuli and release important neurotransmitters, which effect the interpretation of pain.

STIMULANTS OF ABDOMINAL PAIN

Sensory receptors are generally of two distinct types: mechanoreceptors and chemoreceptors. Mechanoreceptors are primarily located in the walls of the hollow organs, within the muscle layers, and between the muscularis mucosa and submucosa. Visceral

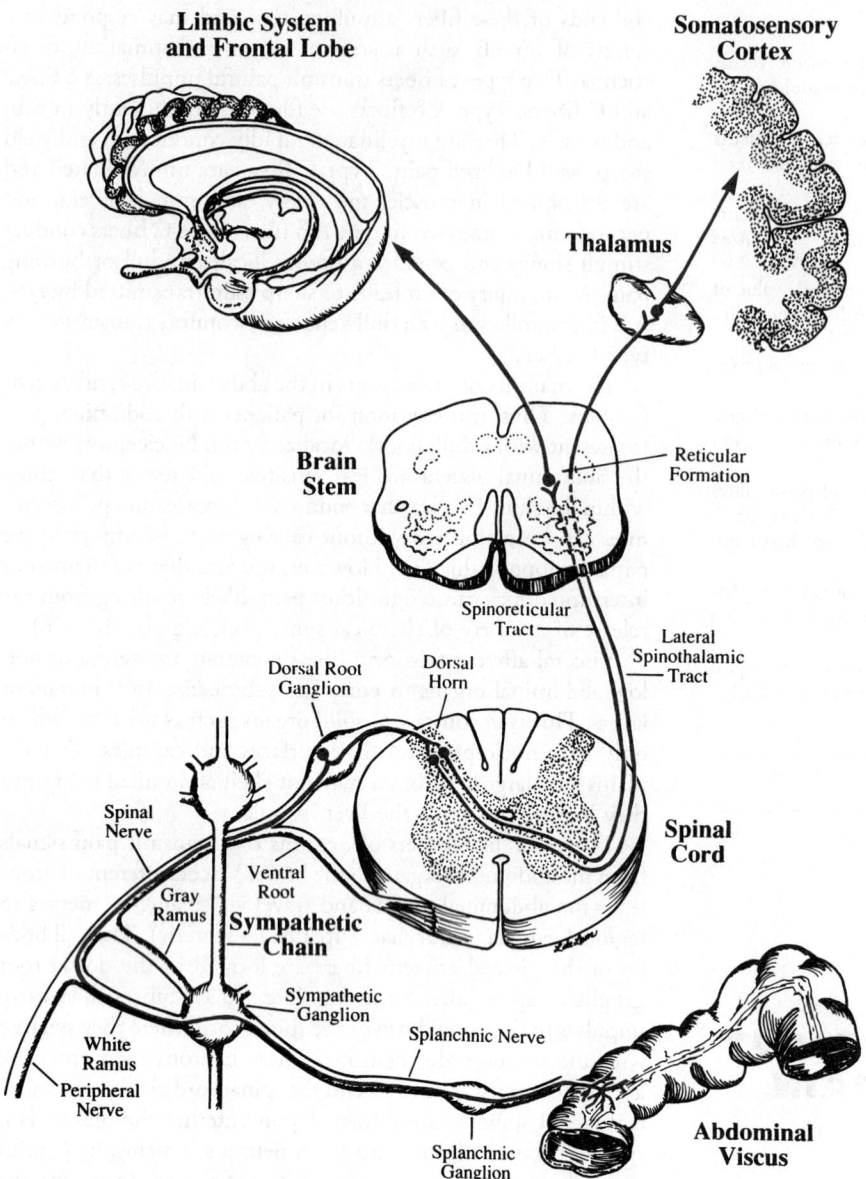

FIGURE 96.1. Neuronal pathways mediating abdominal visceral pain sensation. Three orders of neurons carry pain signals from the abdominal organ to the brain. The first-order neuron travels from the abdominal organ to the regional splanchnic ganglion along the corresponding splanchnic nerve, through a ganglion of the sympathetic chain, and then by way of the white ramus communicans to the spinal nerve. From there, it traverses the dorsal root (its cell body lies in the dorsal root ganglion) to enter the dorsal horn of the spinal cord, where it synapses predominantly within laminae I and V. The second-order neurons leave the dorsal horn, cross the midline, and ascend primarily in two tracts. The spinothalamic tract neurons travel through the brain stem to various nuclei within the thalamus, where they synapse with third-order neurons that go predominantly to the somatosensory cortex. This area mediates the sensory and discriminative aspects of pain. Spinoreticular tract neurons synapse within reticular formation nuclei located primarily in the pons and medulla. From there, third-order neurons travel predominantly to the limbic system and frontal cortex, mediating aspects of pain that have to do with feelings and actions. (Yamada T, ed. *Textbook of Gastroenterology.* 2nd ed. Philadelphia: JB Lippincott 1995:752).

mechanoreceptors are most sensitive to stretch (e.g., as occurs during bowel obstruction) and are not responsive to cutting or crushing. This is in sharp contrast to somatoparietal receptors, which are exquisitely sensitive to the latter. Visceral mechanoreceptors are also located on the surfaces of solid abdominal organs and within the mesentery. Stretching or torsion of the mesentery, as occurs during sigmoid volvulus, usually leads to marked abdominal pain. Pathologic processes within solid organs such as the liver or spleen may not cause any pain until the process causes stretching of the capsule.

Abdominal visceral receptors also respond to a variety of chemicals and neurotransmitters. Inflammation, ischemia, mechanical injury, and tissue necrosis are some of the conditions that result in the release of substances such as bradykinin, substance P, histamine, prostaglandins, and serotonin. Accumulation of these chemicals activates nociceptors and has other direct and indirect effects on the circulation and tissues adjacent to

the involved area. Additionally, the endorphins that usually are released are important stimulants of inhibitory pathways.

TYPES OF ABDOMINAL PAIN

There are three major types of abdominal pain: visceral, parietal, and referred. Visceral pain is perceived as dull, gnawing, or burning pain that is poorly localized. It is often described as an "uncomfortable" feeling rather than pain. Visceral pain may be elicited by numerous stimuli such as muscle contractions or spasm, mural distention, ischemia, or necrosis. Visceral pain is often accompanied by autonomic disturbances, including nausea, vomiting, pallor, and diaphoresis. Patients often feel restless and attempt to move about to relieve the discomfort.

In contrast to visceral pain, parietal pain is sharp, well localized, and more intense. Parietal pain often indicates the anatomi-

TABLE 96.1.	SEGMENTAL DISTRIBUTIONS OF CUTANEOUS HYPERALGESIA RESULTING FROM PAIN IN ABDOMINAL VISCERA

Abdominal Viscera	Segmental Distribution of Cutaneous Hyperalgesia
Esophagus (lower)	T4–T7
Stomach	T5–T10
Liver, gallbladder	T5–T10
Pancreas	T6–T9
Small intestine	T5–T10
Colon, rectum	T8–L1, S1–S4
Kidney, ureter	T8–L2
Urinary bladder	T10–L2, S2–S4
Ovary, fallopian tube	T9–L1
Uterus	T9–L2, S1–S4
Cervix	T10–T12, S2–S4
Testicle, epididymis	T9–T12

(From Cevero F, Morrison JFB, eds. *Visceral sensation.* Amsterdam: Elsevier, 1986:87, with permission.)

cal site of the stimulus (e.g., right upper quadrant pain in a patient with acute cholecystitis). Parietal pain is not usually associated with autonomic disturbances. Patients experiencing parietal pain attempt to lie still as even small movements often exacerbate the pain.

Referred pain combines features of both visceral and parietal pain and is felt at sites distant to the involved organ, usually along cutaneous dermatomes whose afferent nerve roots enter the same levels of the spinal cord as the affected organ (Table 96.1). Referred pain is usually well localized, and it increases in intensity as organ damage progresses.

HISTORY

MODE OF ONSET

Often the key to the correct diagnosis of abdominal pain is found in the patient's historical account of his or her symptoms. The mode of onset of the pain is one such piece of the history that may be of paramount importance. Acute abdominal pain is commonly predated by prodromal symptoms, which may be helpful in determining the diagnosis of more acute pain. For example, a patient may report several months of biliary colic prior to the development of acute right upper quadrant pain of gangrenous cholecystitis. Conversely, the sudden onset of severe abdominal pain without prior symptoms may be more difficult to diagnose and often is the result of an intra-abdominal catastrophe, such as mesenteric infarction or perforated viscus.

Abdominal pain may begin after an injury (e.g., acute pancreatitis after blunt abdominal trauma), and it is useful to ask what the patient was doing when the pain began. Obtaining a menstrual history in women is also important, as acute lower abdominal pain may be the result of intrauterine or ectopic pregnancy.

LOCATION

The location of abdominal pain is often helpful in constructing a differential diagnosis to determine its cause (Table 96.2). However, it must be remembered that abdominal pain can be diffuse or localized. In addition, the pain may be referred to a dermatomal distribution distant from the involved organ. Pain from gastric or duodenal ulcers is usually localized to the epigastrium, whereas peri-umbilical pain is often small intestinal in origin. Pain below the umbilicus may be related to a colonic process, such as diverticulitis, or tubal or ovarian disorders. Gallbladder and biliary pain is often localized to the right upper quadrant but may be referred to the right shoulder or right scapula.

It is also important to realize that abdominal pain may migrate over time. One well-described example is pain that occurs during the course of acute appendicitis. Initially, the pain begins in the mid-abdomen, but over time the pain moves toward the right lower quadrant and McBurney's point. This should be distinguished from referred pain, where pain is felt at locations remote from the involved organ (e.g., phrenic irritation referred to the shoulder region).

RELIEVING OR AGGRAVATING FACTORS

An important part of the history is determining which factors improve or aggravate the pain. The patient's position often provides a clue to the diagnosis. Peritonitis often results in the patient's lying still, as even small movements may exacerbate the pain. Alternatively, the visceral pain that accompanies mesenteric ischemia often leads the patient to writhe around in an attempt to find a comfortable position. Pancreatitis is associated with worsening pain when the patient lies supine, leading these patients to sit upright or lean forward to relieve pressure and irritation on the posterior peritoneum. Psoas muscle irritation, as may occur in Crohn's disease complicated by a psoas abscess, often results in the patient's lying supine with the right leg flexed at the hip and knee. Diaphragmatic irritation from a subphrenic abscess or hepatic congestion may result in avoidance of deep breathing or coughing.

The relationship of abdominal pain to food is also important. Uncomplicated duodenal ulcer pain is often relieved by the ingestion of food, whereas gastric ulcers are aggravated during meals. Patients with small intestinal obstruction usually complain of postprandial pain. More proximal obstruction leads to symptoms shortly after meals, whereas terminal ileal disease may lead to pain that occurs hours after food ingestion. Patients with mesenteric ischemia classically complain of periumbilical pain after meals, resulting in anorexia and weight loss. Patients with pancreatitis avoid eating, as ingestion of any food or liquid may exacerbate their pain. Acute cholecystitis is also commonly associated with right upper quadrant pain shortly after a meal. Patients with irritable bowel syndrome often complain of lower abdominal cramping following meals, although a detailed account of the types of foods that seem to provoke symptoms is usually unrewarding. The patient's use of medications may also be helpful in diagnosing certain disorders. Patients who take large doses of antacids or histamine-2 receptor antagonists for relief of symptoms may have esophagitis, hiatal hernia, or peptic

TABLE 96.2.	COMMON CAUSES AND CHARACTERISTICS OF ACUTE ABDOMINAL PAIN

Disorder	Location	Character	Onset	Relieving/ Worsening Factors	Radiation	Intensity	Pattern
Appendicitis	Periumbilical then RLQ	Diffuse initially; localized later	Progressive	Motion increases pain	RLQ	Moderate	Constant
Cholecystitis	RUQ	Localized	Acute	Biliary colic	Back and right scapula	Moderate	Waxing and waning
Diverticulitis	LLQ	Localized	Progressive	Motion and bowel movement increase pain	LLQ and left lower back	Moderate or mild	Constant
Small-bowel obstruction	Periumbilical	Diffuse	Progressive	Nasoenteric suction lessens pain; food ingestion increases pain	None	Moderate	Waxing and waning
Mesenteric ischemia/ infarction	Periumbilical	Diffuse	Acute	Worsening of pain with eating	None	Severe	Episodic
Renal colic	Unilateral flank pain	Localized	Acute	Movement lessens pain	Flank or back	Severe	Colicky with crescendo/ decrescendo pattern
Ruptured ectopic pregnancy	Suprapubic, LLQ or RLQ	Localized	Acute	Movement decreases pain	None	Moderate	Constant
Perforated peptic ulcer	Midepigastric, RUQ or LUQ	Localized initially; diffuse later	Acute	Pain changes with ingestion of food	None	Severe	Constant
Gastroenteritis	Periumbilical	Diffuse	Progressive	Bowel movement changes pain	None	Moderate or mild	Waxing and waning
Acute pancreatitis	Hypogastric, back or LUQ	Localized	Acute	Leaning forward lessens pain	Middle of back	Moderate or severe	Constant

LUQ, left upper quadrant; LLQ, left lower quadrant; RUQ, right upper quadrant.
(Adapted from Glasgow RE, Mulvihill SJ. Abdominal pain, including the acute abdomen. In: Feldman M, ed. *Sleisenger and Fordtran's gastrointestinal and liver disease: pathophysiology/diagnosis/management,* fifth ed. Philadelphia: WB Saunders, 1998:80.)

ulcer disease. Alternatively, patients with gastritis or peptic ulcer disease who attempt self-medication for analgesia may exacerbate their pain by taking high doses of nonsteroidal anti-inflammatory drugs (NSAIDs).

TEMPORAL RELATIONSHIP OF ABDOMINAL PAIN

The timing and duration of abdominal pain are also important in determining its cause. Pain that is acute in onset and well localized may point to a more severe process such as ruptured appendix or ectopic pregnancy, whereas dull, intermittent pain is more characteristic of mesenteric ischemia. Colicky pain, or pain that comes and goes over time, classically is reported by patients with cholelithiasis or nephrolithiasis. Pain from gallstones may occur following meals but commonly develops in the evening hours, lasts from minutes to hours, and occurs inter-mittently in an unpredictable manner. Determining the progression of the pain is also helpful, as pancreatitis or appendicitis may take hours to reach peak intensity, whereas patients with intra-abdominal catastrophes, such as a ruptured abdominal aortic aneurysm, present with immediate onset of severe pain.

Determining the duration of abdominal pain is also important. Patients who present within hours of the onset of pain are more likely to have an acute process such as mesenteric infarction. Conversely, those who seek attention after weeks of pain are less likely to have a life-threatening process, and more likely to have a more chronic process, such as inflammatory bowel disease or irritable bowel syndrome.

QUALITY/CHARACTER

Determining the character or quality of the perceived pain is also helpful in delineating its source. Dull pain is more characteristic of visceral irritation, whereas somatoparietal pain usually leads to more severe, well-localized pain. Oftentimes, patients use a variety of terms to help depict their pain, such as burning, stabbing, gnawing, cramping, or aching. Depth of the pain may also be reported. A patient with pancreatic cancer may present with a feeling of deep aching in the midepigastrium and back, whereas acute appendicitis presents as a relatively superficial anterior pain that is more easily reproducible on physical examination. Cramping pain may be associated with distention of a hollow viscus secondary to obstruction, whereas burning midepigastric pain is classically reported by patients with peptic ulcer disease.

INTENSITY

The intensity of the pain is often characterized as mild, moderate, or severe. However, pain is a subjective experience and depends on a variety of factors, including perception of pain, personality, and prior painful experiences. What one person describes as severe pain another may describe as trivial. Close visual evaluation of a patient in pain is often very helpful, as a patient sitting comfortably likely has less intense pain that one writhing in distress. Grading pain on a scale (e.g., scale from 1 to 10) has limited value at one point in time but may be useful in measuring the intensity of pain over time.

OTHER SIGNS AND SYMPTOMS

Many conditions causing abdominal pain are associated with other systemic signs and symptoms. Nausea and vomiting are commonly associated with abdominal pain, and their temporal relationship to the onset of the pain should be noted. Acute viral gastroenteritis is usually associated with nausea and vomiting early in its course. Alternatively, patients with small-bowel obstruction often develop abdominal pain that precedes the onset of vomiting. Colonic obstruction usually leads to later vomiting; however, reflex vomiting may occur as a result of conditions such as cecal volvulus. Anorexia commonly occurs as an early symptom of appendicitis, and patients with mesenteric ischemia often have persistent anorexia and subsequent weight loss.

Diarrhea and constipation also commonly are associated with abdominal pain. Gastroenteritis and colitis often are accompanied by diarrhea. Bloody diarrhea usually suggests more severe colitis secondary to infection, ischemia, NSAIDs, or inflammatory bowel disease. Frank rectal bleeding accompanying abdominal pain may suggest more severe ischemia or bowel infarction. Alternating diarrhea and constipation is a classic presentation of irritable bowel syndrome. Lower abdominal pain and constipation may be a sign of colonic neoplasm, although these patients may develop a paradoxical diarrhea.

Pyrexia accompanying abdominal pain presents a broad differential diagnosis. Patients with gastroenteritis may develop fevers early in the course of illness, whereas patients with walled-off abscesses may develop late, intermittent fevers. High fevers and rigors combined with right upper quadrant pain are suggestive of cholangitis, whereas left lower quadrant pain and a fever is characteristic of diverticulitis.

Acute onset of jaundice, abdominal pain, vomiting, dark

urine, and clay-colored stools suggests biliary tract disease or hepatitis. Pancreatic carcinoma involving the head of the pancreas typically presents with painless jaundice. Abdominal pain in association with neurologic disturbances and photosensitivity suggests porphyria. Inflammatory bowel disease, lupus, and vasculitis may all cause abdominal pain and associated skin disorders.

Abdominal pain may also be associated with urogenital signs or symptoms. Colicky flank pain radiating to the groin is likely to be secondary to renal calculi and is often accompanied by hematuria. Abdominal pain and pneumaturia suggests an enterovesicular fistula complicating diverticulosis or Crohn's disease. A careful menstrual history should always be obtained, as lower abdominal pain may be the result of ectopic pregnancy, ovarian cyst, or ovulation.

PAST MEDICAL HISTORY

Evaluation of the patient's past medical and surgical history may provide additional information as to the etiologic factors involved in their abdominal pain. Patients who have had prior abdominal surgeries are likely to develop adhesions, which may be the cause of small-bowel obstruction. Abdominal aortic aneurysm repair often results in compromise of the arterial supply to the left colon, resulting in ischemic colitis. A patient with cholelithiasis who presents with distal small-bowel obstruction may have a gallstone ileus.

Patients with concomitant coronary artery disease or arrhythmias are prone to develop small intestinal ischemia. Additionally, congestive heart failure may lead to hepatic congestion and subsequent diaphragmatic irritation. In patients with a history of cirrhosis, the onset of diffuse abdominal pain should raise the concern for spontaneous bacterial peritonitis. Furthermore, abdominal pain may be a result of medications taken to treat underlying illnesses, as gastric or duodenal ulcers should be suspected in patients with chronic arthritis taking large doses of NSAIDs.

FAMILY AND SOCIAL HISTORY

A detailed review of the patient's family and social history may reveal other important clues to the cause of their symptoms. The diagnosis of inflammatory bowel disease is more likely in an individual with one or more affected family members. Excessive use of alcohol is a common cause of pancreatitis, hepatitis, and gastritis. Cocaine abuse may lead to vascular compromise, resulting in mesenteric ischemia. Recent foreign travel or camping trips raise the possibility of intestinal parasite infection.

■ PHYSICAL EXAMINATION

The general appearance of a patient in abdominal distress may reveal obvious or subtle clues to their diagnosis. A patient's expressions, position, breathing pattern, and gestures are often as important as the abdominal exam itself. Following a review of their general appearance, vital signs should be checked. The presence of fever or tachycardia may point to an acute process, such as cholangitis or diverticulitis. Acute onset of pain and hypotension often is a clue to an abdominal catastrophe, such as ruptured aortic aneurysm. Elderly patients or those on high-dose steroids mask fevers and require even closer attention. Atrial fibrillation may predispose patients to mesenteric ischemia as a result of left atrial emboli. Patients with hepatitis or common bile duct obstruction often are icteric or jaundiced. Spider angiomas suggest chronic liver disease. Patients with vascular disease may have weak distal pulses resulting from poor peripheral perfusion.

ABDOMINAL EXAMINATION

Prior to palpation it is important to inspect the abdomen for the presence of surgical scars, distention, hernias, or abnormalities of the overlying skin such as ecchymoses or engorged veins. Following inspection, auscultation should be performed, allowing for sufficient time to determine the quality and character of the bowel sounds. Diffuse peritonitis usually leads to absent bowel sounds, whereas early intestinal obstruction results in "tinkling," high-pitched sounds. A succussion splash, which can be elicited by placing the stethoscope on the abdomen and moving the patient from side to side, may be detectable in a patient with gastric outlet obstruction. A bruit may be audible over the mid-abdomen in a patient with an aortic aneurysm, whereas auscultation over the liver may reveal a hepatic bruit in a patient with a large hepatoma.

Palpation of the abdomen should begin with light palpation at an area distant from the region of greatest pain. This allows the patient to "get comfortable" with the examination rather than be fearful that the examiner will cause more pain. Percussion is useful to detect fluid or gas within the abdomen. Shifting dullness suggests the presence of ascites or blood within the abdominal cavity. Percussion is also used to determine the size of the liver and spleen. Once palpation is begun, it is important to slowly increase pressure rather than use sudden or abrupt movements. Rebound tenderness suggests peritoneal irritation, as does guarding, which can be localized or generalized. It is also often useful to gently shake the bed from side to side, which may be a more subtle way to detect peritonitis.

GENITAL, RECTAL, AND PELVIC EXAMINATIONS

Rectal, genital, and pelvic examination should be part of every physical examination in patients with acute abdominal pain. Intra-abdominal disorders may not initially involve the anterior abdominal wall and may first be detected during rectal examination (e.g., appendicitis). Stool should be tested for occult blood. External genital examination is useful and may lead to a diagnosis of an inguinal hernia—a common cause of small-bowel obstruction. In women, a pelvic examination is essential as it may lead to discovery of disorders of the fallopian tubes or ovaries, whereas the presence of cervical motion tenderness suggests pelvic inflammatory disease.

LABORATORY STUDIES AND DIAGNOSTIC TESTS

BLOOD AND OTHER LABORATORY TESTS

A complete blood count with differential should be obtained from every patient with acute onset of abdominal pain. Anemia often points to gastrointestinal bleeding, which may be occult. Microcytic anemia suggests a more chronic process, such as colonic polyps or neoplasm. Leukocytosis and bandemia may suggest an ominous process, such as gangrenous cholecystitis, whereas more minor elevations in the white blood cell count are often present in patients with less serious disorders, such as viral gastroenteritis. Conversely, severe leukopenia may indicate overwhelming infection and sepsis syndrome. Eosinophilia may point to an allergic reaction or parasitic infection, whereas lymphopenia may be the result of a viral infection (e.g., cytomegalovirus). Thrombocytopenia, secondary to splenic sequestration, is often seen in patients with cirrhosis and may lead to bleeding diatheses.

Urinalysis should always be performed in patients complaining of abdominal pain. The urine specimen can be examined for glucose, bile, blood, protein, and ketones. Microscopic examination for white and red blood cells, bacteria, and crystals may lead to a diagnosis of pyelonephritis or renal calculi. A urine pregnancy test should also be performed in all women of childbearing age who present with acute abdominal pain.

Serum electrolytes and glucose should be obtained, as well as blood urea nitrogen (BUN) and creatinine. An elevated BUN-to-creatinine ratio suggests dehydration but may be seen in patients with upper gastrointestinal bleeding or renal insufficiency. Elevated serum amylase and lipase are suggestive of pancreatitis. Measurement of liver-associated enzymes is often helpful and should be evaluated in all patients who present with upper abdominal pain or jaundice. Obstructive jaundice usually results in hyperbilirubinemia and elevations of alkaline phosphatase and γ-glutamyltranspeptidase. The presence of abdominal pain accompanied by elevations of alanine aminotransferase and aspartate aminotransferase indicates hepatocellular injury, perhaps secondary to viral or alcoholic hepatitis. Mild abnormalities are common, however, and minor elevations may be a result of a variety of causes such as minor infections, congestive heart failure, or drug reactions. An elevated prothrombin time (PT, international normalized ratio) is commonly found in patients with cirrhosis. Hypoalbuminemia may also be a manifestation of cirrhosis, but it can also be the result of other chronic abdominal processes such as inflammatory bowel disease or neoplasm. Patients with ascites who develop abdominal pain should undergo diagnostic paracentesis to rule out spontaneous bacterial peritonitis.

RADIOGRAPHIC EXAMINATION

Determination of the type of radiologic evaluation to be performed should be guided by the historical presentation, physical examination, and laboratory results. A plain abdominal series, including upright and supine views of the abdomen, is essential in all patients who present with acute onset of abdominal pain. In patients who cannot stand, a later left decubitus film may supplant the upright view. These radiographs can detect free intraperitoneal air secondary to perforated viscus and are sensitive in the detection of abnormal gas patterns (e.g., small-bowel obstruction). Pneumobilia, although rarely identified, suggests the presence of a fistula between the small bowel and the biliary tree. A "ground glass" appearance suggests the presence of ascites. Gallstones are usually not visualized on plain abdominal radiographs, whereas up to 70% of renal calculi are opaque and can be seen on the plain abdominal series. A chest radiograph may detect pneumonia or effusion, accounting for abdominal or flank pain in some patients. Furthermore, an upright chest radiograph can usually rule out the presence of even small amounts of free intraperitoneal air.

In addition to plain radiographs, ultrasonography and computed tomography (CT) examinations should be performed when appropriate and may even be the tests of first choice in certain situations. Ultrasonography is particularly advantageous for detection of cholelithiasis or biliary ductal dilatation. Ultrasound examination is also beneficial in diagnosing pelvic disorders such as ovarian cysts and ectopic pregnancy. Abdominal CT scan is significantly more expensive than ultrasonography but is the best method of detecting many intra-abdominal processes (e.g., appendicitis). CT is particularly sensitive for evaluation of retroperitoneal abnormalities, such as pancreatic neoplasm or retroperitoneal hemorrhage/abscess, and can often detect changes that occur within the mesentery (e.g., fat stranding secondary to diverticulitis) or intestinal wall (e.g., ischemia). CT is useful for evaluation of vascular structures as well, and can diagnose such problems as dissecting aortic aneurysm and portal or splenic vein thromboses. CT is beneficial following abdominal trauma, as lesions such as splenic rupture and liver laceration may be detected and managed quickly.

ENDOSCOPY

The use of endoscopy to evaluate abdominal pain depends on the timing and nature of the pain, in combination with the patient's other comorbidities. For example, a patient who develops acute abdominal pain may be suffering from a perforated duodenal ulcer, in which case endoscopy is contraindicated. Alternatively, it would be appropriate to perform upper endoscopy in a patient with more chronic epigastric pain suggestive of an uncomplicated gastric ulcer. Flexible sigmoidoscopy and/or colonoscopy are often indicated in patients with lower abdominal pain accompanied by rectal bleeding to rule out the presence of colitis secondary to ischemia, infection, NSAIDs, or inflammatory bowel disease. Colonoscopy may also be required to decompress a sigmoid volvulus. Cholangitis secondary to an obstructing gallstone or mass is characterized by fever, chills, and acute right upper quadrant pain, and may best be treated by emergency endoscopic retrograde cholangiopancreatography (ERCP) with stone extraction or biliary stenting.

LAPAROSCOPY

Diagnostic laparoscopy is an invasive procedure that may be useful in a subset of patients who have abdominal pain of uncer-

tain origin. Laparoscopy may be performed on an emergency basis in an extremely ill patient, or on an elective basis in patients with more chronic abdominal pain where the diagnosis remains elusive despite all other noninvasive tests. Additionally, laparoscopy can be therapeutic, as a patient diagnosed with appendicitis during laparoscopy can often undergo a laparoscopic appendectomy rather than the more invasive open procedure.

MODIFIERS OF CLINICAL PRESENTATION OF ABDOMINAL PAIN

An individual presenting with abdominal pain may under special circumstances have specific factors, which modify the approach that the health care deliverer takes to diagnose the problem. In particular, individuals who are very young or very old, who are pregnant, or who are immunocompromised present a special challenge in the diagnosis of abdominal pain.

AGE

The diagnosis of abdominal pain in individuals who are either very young or very old is often challenging since the clinical history may be difficult to ascertain or may be unreliable. Despite having significant abdominal pathology, laboratory parameters can be misleadingly normal.

Several etiologies of acute abdominal pain need to be considered in infants and children. In infancy, the development of the abdominal wall has not occurred, and splinting of the recti musculature in response to peritoneal irritation does not readily occur. In infants who present with abdominal pain, the following etiologies should be strongly suspected in the differential diagnosis: small intestinal intussusception, pyelonephritis, Meckel's diverticulitis, gastroesophageal reflux disease, acute appendicitis, and infectious intestinal enteritides. Slightly older children presenting with acute abdominal pain may have bacterial cystitis, mesenteric lymphadenitis, Meckel's diverticulitis, acute appendicitis, or inflammatory bowel disease, whereas in adolescents pelvic inflammatory disease, inflammatory bowel disease, acute appendicitis, and other disorders that are commonly encountered in the adult population should be considered. In children of all ages the presence of abdominal pain as a sequel of abuse is common and must be included among the differential diagnostic possibilities. In the elderly adult population with acute abdominal pain, the differential diagnostic spectrum encompasses other specific causal factors, such as biliary tract disease, malignancy, bowel obstruction, complications of peptic ulcer disease, and hernia-related pain.

In light of the lack of standard clinical and laboratory findings in this patient population, astute clinical judgment with aggressive intervention is imperative to help reduce the often-late diagnoses that occur in these patients at extremes of age, with resultant increased morbidity.

PREGNANCY

Pregnancy increases the challenge for the diagnostician who is attempting to uncover the cause of acute abdominal pain. Abdominal discomfort may arise from the presence of uterine enlargement and its sequelae. Additionally, attempts to perform radiographic examinations are typically avoided (especially early on in pregnancy) due to potential teratogenic fetal effects. Furthermore, pregnancy abrogates the body's ability to ward off infection. Finally, the abdominal examination itself is more difficult during pregnancy. The specific causes of abdominal pain in the pregnant patient are similar to those in age-matched nonpregnant controls. During pregnancy, common causes for abdominal pain include acute appendicitis, pyelonephritis, cholecystitis, ovarian (such as torsion or cyst rupture) and adnexal disease.

Anatomical variations due to displacement of abdominal viscera from the gravid uterus require knowledge of typical pregnancy-associated presentations of these common disorders. The position of the appendix after the fifth month of gestation is positioned superior to the right iliac crest with its tip positioned more medially subsequent to displacement by the enlarged uterus. As pregnancy progresses, the appendiceal tip becomes displaced more superiorly, such that at 8 months of gestation its position approximates the right subcostal margin. During pregnancy the presence of fever is less commonly seen despite the presence of significant abdominal pathologic processes. Additionally, leukocytosis is frequently encountered during pregnancy, thus making its interpretation in the presence of abdominal pain more difficult. This becomes important when evaluating the patient for the presence of appendicitis, since rapid diagnosis with early surgical intervention has been demonstrated to reduce morbidity and rate of fetal loss.

IMMUNOCOMPROMISED HOST

The presence of an immunocompromised host is certainly a potential modifier of disease presentation. Immunocompromised patients comprise those individuals with congenital immunodeficiency syndromes (e.g., common variable immunodeficiency) or those with acquired immunodeficiency syndromes [such as medication-induced states (e.g., corticosteroids or other immunosuppressants, or chemotherapeutic agents), or disease-related states (e.g., AIDS)]. In general, these individuals are susceptible to diseases that may occur commonly in the general population (e.g., appendicitis, cholecystitis, and diverticulitis), or disease states that occur specifically in the immunocompromised population (such as graft-versus-host disease, cytomegalovirus infection, or neutropenic enterocolitis). Regardless of the cause of the immune compromised status, the typical signs and symptoms of peritonitis (fever, guarding, rebound, and abdominal pain) may be minimal or absent. Patients may not appear acutely ill and white blood counts may not be elevated; however, a left shift to immature forms is commonplace and should be sought. The primary methods for detection of abnormalities that may develop are frequently endoscopic and/or radiographic. Radiographic assessment might include CT scans or plain abdominal radiographs. In general, these examinations should be performed more frequently in this patient population than in nonimmunocompromised hosts.

ACUTE ABDOMINAL PAIN

The term *acute abdominal pain* refers to a disorder of less than 24 hours' duration presenting with signs and symptoms of pain localized to the abdominal region. Regardless of the acuity of the situation, it is critical to provide an early, efficient, and accurate diagnosis so that appropriate specific therapeutic intervention can occur. If the pain is chronic, the diagnostician should ascertain if there has been an acute worsening of a chronic condition requiring urgent intervention. An astute clinician may also detect signs that the patient being evaluated has a psychological basis of abdominal pain. If discovered, this may prevent the need for unnecessary, sometimes costly, and possibly risky procedures.

Whatever the acuity of the situation, the history and physical examination remain the most important elements extracted in the determination of an accurate early diagnosis. A precise evaluation of the location, severity, character, chronology, exacerbating and relieving factors, other associated symptoms, and associated other medical history is essential. A complete and thorough physical examination enables the diagnostician to verify diagnostic suspicion raised while taking the history. Subsequently, by using specific laboratory and imaging modalities, the establishment of a precise diagnosis frequently is successful.

Several areas of particular importance that often help the physician to determine the urgency of the situation include the vital signs (especially the presence of hypotension, orthostatic hypotension, fever, tachycardia, bradycardia, tachypnea, or hypopnea). Additionally, diaphoresis, pallor, clamminess, mental confusion, and restlessness serve as indicators of a possible pending catastrophe. At the other end of the spectrum, less subtle findings include respiratory arrest, coma, shock, and cardiovascular arrest. In assessing patients with acute abdominal pain, detailed laboratory evaluation may signify the presence of acute pathology and help to establish its cause. Several tests, including liver enzymes, bilirubin, amylase, lipase, white blood cell count with differential, hemoglobin, and urinalysis with microscopic evaluation, should be done. Leukocytosis with the presence of polymorphonuclear leukocytes or bands is an important finding, but its presence does not necessarily indicate the need for surgical intervention (e.g., acute cholecystitis). Additionally, individuals with acute clinical deterioration, such as a perforated appendix, requiring emergency surgical intervention may present with a normal white blood cell count.

In evaluating patients with acute abdominal pain there are several commonly encountered diagnoses that should be considered, including acute appendicitis, diverticulitis, acute cholecystitis, acute pancreatitis, perforated gastric or duodenal ulcer, small-bowel obstruction, acute mesenteric ischemia, endometriosis, acute salpingitis, abdominal aortic aneurysm ectopic pregnancy, tubo-ovarian abscess, gastroenteritis, viral hepatitis, inflammatory bowel disease, nonulcer dyspepsia, gastroesophageal reflux disease, and ovarian cysts or torsion. Characteristics of some of these disorders are listed in Tables 96.2 and 96.3.

CHRONIC ABDOMINAL PAIN

Clinicians in nearly all specialties and subspecialties are commonly faced with treating a patient who acknowledges the pres-

TABLE 96.3.	INTRA-ABDOMINAL AND EXTRA-ABDOMINAL CAUSES OF ACUTE AND CHRONIC ABDOMINAL PAIN

Luminal

Small-bowel obstruction
   Abdominal wall hernia
   Neoplasm
   Adhesion
Colonic neoplasm
Colonic volvulus
Small intestinal intussusception
Crohn's disease
Mesenteric ischemia
Ulcerative colitis
Vasculitis with bowel involvement
   Systemic Lupus Erythematosis
   Henoch–Schönlein purpura
Peptic ulcer disease
Gastroesophageal reflux disease

Hepatobiliary

Biliary obstruction
   Gallstone
      Choledocholithiasis
      Cholecystitis
   Stricture
   Tumor
   Parasite
   Hemobilia

Genitourinary

Endometriosis
Ovulation ("Mittelschmertz")
Ovarian cyst
Renal capsule distension
Nephrolithiasis with recurrent ureteral obstruction
Recurrent pyelonephritis
Bladder outlet obstruction
   Benign prostatic hypertrophy
   Prostatitis
   Prostate cancer
   Urethral stricture or neoplasm
Uterine fibroid necrosis

Neurologic

Neuropathy
Abdominal epilepsy
Abdominal migraine
Cutaneous neuropathy
Radiculopathy
Vertebral collapse with nerve root compression
Amyloidosis
Slipped-rib syndrome

Other

Familial Mediterranean fever
Porphyrias
   Acute intermittent porphyria
   Variegate porphyria
   Protoporphyria
Heavy-metal poisoning
Torsion
   Spleen
   Testicle
   Omentum
Abdominal aortic aneurysm dissection or rupture
Pancreatitis
C1q esterase deficiency

ence of chronic abdominal pain (Table 96.3). The majority of incidents are short-lived and minor in nature, and in some estimates occur in up to 15% of individuals. Individuals afflicted with chronic abdominal pain due to any specific cause may experience significant disruption of their lives (e.g., work, family function, and other social interactions), a higher rate of narcotic/analgesic use and dependency, and lowered self-esteem.

Chronic Intermittent Abdominal Pain

Individuals afflicted with chronic intermittent abdominal pain are not infrequently erroneously regarded as having "functional abdominal pain." The pain may be present for several hours to several days at a time with intervening periods of complete relief. The critical solution to discerning the particular etiology of patients with chronic intermittent abdominal pain is extracting a careful medical history.

The cause of chronic abdominal pain can be established by ascertaining the factors that trigger its onset. Onset of pain in terms of proximity to meals is often helpful. Patients with mesenteric ischemia, gastroesophageal reflux disease, peptic ulcer disease, and chronic pancreatitis often complain of pain after meals. Individuals who note the onset of abdominal pain occurring at monthly intervals might include patients with endometriosis or ovulation-related pain. Pain that has its onset in specific positions is suggestive of the presence of a nerve root irritation by a neoplasm, vertebral pathologic process, or compression or entrapment of a nerve. If jaundice is present in the presence of intermittent abdominal pain, the presence of a gallstone occluding the common bile duct or recurrent pancreatitis due to gallstone disease should be considered. In a person with perineal disease, such as severe hemorrhoids, fissures, or fistulas, the consideration of Crohn's disease should be entertained. The presence of an "abdominal mass" that comes and goes should raise the suspicion of intestinal intussusception or an abdominal hernia. If an individual has a distended abdomen with visible peristalsis, bowel obstruction should be considered. The presence of a rash such as palpable purpura should suggest the presence of a vasculitis, which can be seen in disorders such as systemic lupus erythematosus, polyarteritis nodosa, or Henoch–Schönlein purpura. These disorders may affect the bowel by causing a small-vessel vasculitis with subsequent abdominal pain.

Pain relieved by defecation may signify the presence of colonic obstruction secondary to a colonic neoplasm or may occur in persons with irritable bowel syndrome. Intermittent lower abdominal pain radiating to the back or flank area associated with hematuria may signify the presence of nephrolithiasis. The presence of suprapubic pain relieved by urination may signify bladder outlet symptoms resulting from prostatitis, benign prostatic hypertrophy, or use of medications such as anticholinergics.

Upper abdominal pain worsened by the ingestion of food and relieved by vomiting suggests the presence of a partial functional or organic obstruction of the upper luminal digestive tract and may result from peptic ulcer disease, duodenal carcinoma, gastroparesis, duodenal Crohn's disease with stricturing, surgical stricture of the proximal small bowel, and other similar obstructive factors.

There exist several disorders that are difficult to differentiate from underlying intestinal pathology. A common source of such confusion is from the "slipped-rib syndrome," a disorder in which the intercostal nerve, and not the abdominal viscera, is the source of pain. In this disorder the patient is noted to experience recurrent left upper quadrant or right upper quadrant pain that may or may not radiate to the back. On physical examination, superior retraction of the inferior portion of the lowest rib will frequently reproduce the pain. In addition, the patient may relate that certain positions relieve or exacerbate the pain. The performance of an intercostal nerve block relieves the pain temporarily and serves as a diagnostic test. Similarly, it is sometimes difficult to differentiate abdominal wall pain from that of an intra-abdominal cause. To help differentiate these specific factors, Carnett's test can be performed. This test is performed by first asking the patient to fold his or her arms. The examiner then determines the site of maximal discomfort when abdominal palpation is performed. The patient is asked to attempt to sit up partially—a maneuver that places tension on the abdominal wall. The patient is then asked to attempt to sit up once again while the examiner palpates in the same area as previously. If the palpation in this region elicits more pain than the initial examination, then this is felt to be consistent with abdominal wall–related pathology as the source of pain. Several specific diagnoses may cause the Carnett's test to be positive including cutaneous nerve entrapment, hernias of the abdominal wall, and rectus sheath hematomas. A similar source of commonly overlooked pain is the presence of abdominal pain at sites of previous surgery (e.g., scars or trocar sites). These sites require special attention during the performance of a physical examination. Hernias may become obvious when an increase in abdominal pressure occurs with careful examination of the local areas of pain. Local nerve blocks may be successful in elimination of pain at former surgical sites if hernias are not present.

In the evaluation of patients who have chronic abdominal pain of unknown cause it is important to pay attention to details. Simple laboratory tests may reveal the source of pain in some patients with an unrevealing physical examination. The presence of abnormal liver tests suggests the need to image the hepatobiliary system via transabdominal ultrasound, abdominal CT, abdominal magnetic resonance imaging (MRI), endoscopic ultrasound, or ERCP. If iron-deficient anemia is present, disorders such as Crohn's disease, ulcerative colitis, peptic ulcer disease, gastric or duodenal neoplasms, colonic or small-bowel neoplasm, or ischemic bowel disease might be considered. In evaluation for the presence of such disorders, endoscopic evaluation of the luminal gastrointestinal tract (e.g., esophagogastroduodenoscopy, sigmoidoscopy, colonoscopy, enteroscopy), small-bowel radiography (e.g., enteroclysis or small-bowel meal), or imaging of the mesenteric vasculature (e.g., mesenteric angiography or magnetic resonance angiography) might be considered for diagnostic evaluation. If the patient reports intermittent abdominal distention and a change in bowel habit, an obstruction series or CT evaluation when symptoms are present might diagnose the presence of intermittent small-bowel obstruction, intussusception, or an intermittent obstructing internal hernia. Hematuria or urinary tract infection detected on urinalysis should be followed by appropriate imaging or evaluation of the genitourinary system in selected patients (e.g., cystoscopy, intravenous pyelo-

gram, transcutaneous ultrasonography, or CT). The use of abdominal and pelvic ultrasonography and CT imaging is helpful for the evaluation of lower abdominal or pelvic pathology. If these are unsuccessful in establishing a specific diagnosis, hormonal therapy and laparoscopy are sometimes required.

Chronic Persistent Abdominal Pain of Known Cause

Individuals afflicted with incurable, chronic, persistent abdominal pain of known cause often present great challenges to health care providers. Patients with abdominal cancers (e.g., colon cancer, gastric cancer, pancreatic cancer, lymphoma) or cancers that are metastatic to abdominal organs or lymph nodes (e.g., pancreatic cancer with lymph node or hepatic metastases) frequently suffer from chronic abdominal pain. In individuals with chronic pancreatitis, chronic abdominal pain often plagues their ability to perform their activities of daily living. Furthermore, patients with mesenteric ischemia frequently complain of postprandial abdominal pain.

Therapy of these disorders is focused on treatment of the underlying pathologic process and relief of the abdominal pain. The relief of pain may require drug treatment, nerve blocks or destruction, or nerve stimulation. The use of NSAIDs may help with musculoskeletal pain syndromes but is less effective for chronic abdominal pain. Anxiolytics are not effective for the treatment of chronic abdominal pain but rather function to lessen the anxiety associated with the pain. Dependency may be problematic if long-term anxiolytic use is attempted. Antidepressants (e.g., nortriptyline, amitriptyline, and doxepin) have also been used successfully in individuals who have chronic pain states and have analgesic efficacy independent of their antidepressant effects. Opioids have also been used for the treatment of chronic abdominal pain; however, the potential for dependency must be realized when initiating therapy. In addition, techniques have been used for chemical and surgical nerve destruction. For example, the use of a celiac plexus block may be performed by injecting a nerve-destroying substance (e.g., ethanol) into the celiac nerve ganglia in individuals with pancreatic adenocarcinoma, often with encouraging results. In individuals with short life spans (typically less than 6 months) it is similarly appropriate to consider surgical techniques such as rhizotomy or cordotomy for pain relief; however, the clinician needs to be cognizant of the possible complications that can occur as a result of this technique (such as bowel and bladder dysfunction or worsening of pain). In addition, transcutaneous electrical nerve stimulation and dorsal column stimulation are relatively safe and simple procedures that may provide moderate pain relief to some individuals.

Chronic Functional Abdominal Pain

Chronic intractable abdominal pain or chronic undiagnosed (functional) abdominal pain is defined as abdominal pain that has been present for at least 6 months without any identifiable cause despite appropriate diagnostic evaluation. This disorder occurs more commonly in women than men and is frequently associated with a history of sexual or physical abuse. Functional abdominal pain needs to be differentiated from other similar common disorders (e.g., nonulcer dyspepsia) that may require quite different therapies. Patients with functional abdominal pain often have pain elsewhere (not only abdominal pain). Despite repeated histories and physical examinations, there is no evidence for another cause that would explain the symptom complex. Typically the pain does not change in intensity, location, or character in response to physiologic states (such as eating or defecation), or, if it does vary, it does so in an unpredictable fashion. The pain is often worse during times of stress and is often associated with many other somatic complaints. The pain responds poorly to standard therapies; thus, patients may undergo many unnecessary procedures.

In general, individuals afflicted with functional abdominal pain may have many psychological impairments, including depression, sleep alterations, anxiety, diminished activity, loss of sexual desire, and preoccupation with the abdominal pain. Depression is especially common and can be quite debilitating in certain individuals with functional abdominal pain.

Unless there are specific indications for performing more involved and perhaps more invasive diagnostic procedures than those that have already been performed for individuals with chronic abdominal pain of more than 6 months' duration, the testing is unlikely to be fruitful. Frequently, abnormalities identified are of little or no importance in terms of their relationship to the patient's complaints. Certainly, if a patient has not had an adequate etiologic evaluation, the appropriate workup should be performed.

Similar to many other chronic disorders, there is presently no cure for functional abdominal pain. Thus, it is important to discuss this with the patient and to help establish realistic therapeutic expectations. In caring for the patient with functional abdominal pain, frequent contact is important with continued reassurance. The goal should be to improve the quality of life of the patient by discussing improvement in patient functioning, not necessarily elimination of pain (since such a goal is in all likelihood unachievable). Patients should also be encouraged to take an active role in their care. A multidisciplinary approach is recommended, incorporating the fields of psychiatry or psychology, neurology, pain management, physical therapy, relaxation therapy, and other similar ancillary treatments (such as biofeedback and hypnosis).

■ STRATEGIES FOR OPTIMAL CARE

COMPLICATIONS AND PITFALLS

Establishment of an accurate diagnosis as quickly and efficiently as possible helps to minimize the patient's suffering and may avoid complications. The rapidity with which the diagnosis must be established varies with the presentation. Few conditions require immediate operative intervention to the extent that an orderly procedure cannot be followed in the workup and evaluation of patients with abdominal pain. Some exceptions to this are exsanguinating hemorrhage, vascular catastrophe, and perforated viscus, which require urgent evaluation and diagnosis. Thus, the clinician should approach nearly all patients in a logical fashion, with particular attention to the history and physical examination. All individuals who present with abdominal pain should have rectal and pelvic examinations performed because significant pathology can be uncovered by these examinations.

In evaluating individuals with abdominal pain there are several points that should be emphasized: (a) Disorders of the chest can mimic abdominal disorders and need to be considered in the evaluation of patients. (b) Acute mesenteric ischemia and infarction may be difficult to diagnose since there are typically nonspecific abdominal findings. (c) Don't assume that the location of the pain is of no consequence. Upper abdominal pain is a common complaint in individuals with cholecystitis, pancreatitis, or peptic ulcer disease. Midabdominal pain may represent appendicitis, intestinal obstruction, or mesenteric vascular occlusion, whereas lower abdominal pain may represent appendicitis, diverticulitis, ureteral colic, ectopic pregnancy, or ovarian cyst torsion. (d) Don't assume that observing the patient's actions is not helpful. As a rule of thumb, if a patient prefers to lie still in bed, parietal pain (e.g., peritonitis) may be present, whereas a patient moving about restlessly likely has visceral pain (e.g., intestinal or ureteral obstruction, biliary colic). (e) Physical examination must include a thorough evaluation of all hernias, especially in obese patients because small hernias are especially difficult to palpate in such individuals.

Indications for HOSPITALIZATION

Although there are established guidelines for determining when an individual needs to be admitted to the hospital, there have been very few randomized controlled trials to determine when this is necessary in patients with abdominal pain. When dealing with the very young, the elderly, or immunocompromised patients with acute abdominal pain, admission should be considered even in the presence of normal vital signs and normal laboratory parameters. These patients may not mount the same response to severe insult (e.g., bowel perforation, mesenteric ischemia) that is commonly seen in other individuals. Patients with chronic recurrent abdominal pain presenting with similar symptoms to their baseline pain often can be managed as outpatients. If, on the other hand, a patient with chronic abdominal pain has a sudden onset of severe acute abdominal pain on top of his or her chronic abdominal pain, admission should be contemplated to rule out more serious diagnoses. Patients who have abdominal pain in association with fever, vomiting, orthostatic hypotension, tachycardia, abdominal guarding, abdominal rebound, leukocytosis, a new finding of hyperbilirubinemia, or mental confusion should be strongly considered for admission to firmly establish a quick diagnosis and to closely observe their response to treatment.

BIBLIOGRAPHY

Bender J. Approach to the acute abdomen. *Med Clin North Am* 1989;73: 1413–1422.

Gershon MD, Kirchgessner AL, Wade PR. Functional anatomy of the enteric nervous system. In: Johnson LR, ed. *Physiology of the gastrointestinal tract*, Vol 1. New York: Raven Press, 1994:381–390.

Glasgow RE, Mulvihill SJ. Abdominal pain, including the acute abdomen. In: Feldman M, eds. *Sleisenger and Fordtran's Gastrointestinal and liver disease: pathophysiology, diagnosis, management*, fifth ed. Philadelphia: WB Saunders, 1998:80–89.

Haubrich WS. Abdominal pain. In: Haubrich, ed. *Bockus Gastroenterology*, fifth ed. Philadelphia: WB Saunders, 1995:11–29.

Klein KB. Approach to the patient with abdominal pain. In: Yamada T, ed. *Textbook of gastroenterology*, second ed. Philadelphia: JB Lippincott, 1995:750–771.

Levitt MD. Approach to the patient with abdominal pain. In: Kelley, ed. *Kelley's Textbook of internal medicine*, third ed. Philadelphia: Lippincott-Raven Publishers, 1997:593–599.

Silen W. Abdominal pain. In: Fauci, eds. *Harrison's Internal medicine*, fourteenth ed. New York: McGraw-Hill, 1998:65–68.

Silen W. *Cope's Early diagnosis of the acute abdomen*. New York: Oxford University Press, 1991.

Vitello JM, Nyhus LM. The patient's complaints and what they mean. In: Nyhus LM, ed. *Abdominal pain: a guide to rapid diagnosis*. Norwalk: Appleton & Lange, 1995:1–11.

Kelley's Textbook of Internal Medicine, fourth edition. Edited by H. David Humes. Lippincott Williams & Wilkins, Philadelphia © 2000.

CHAPTER
97

APPROACH TO THE PATIENT WITH ACUTE ABDOMEN

STEWART C. WANG
MICHAEL W. MULHOLLAND

The term *acute abdomen* denotes a clinical disorder of sudden onset that manifests with signs and symptoms focused in the abdominal region. Pain is usually the predominant symptom and is most often caused by a progressive underlying abdominal disorder. Surgical management often is needed and must be undertaken without inordinate delay. Sometimes, however, the acute abdomen is neither an intra-abdominal disorder nor a condition that necessitates operative intervention. The physician needs to consider the many causes of acute abdominal pain and to be vigilant for the need for an emergency operation, because delay invites a cascade of complications or death. The most common causes of the acute abdomen are listed in Tables 97.1 and 97.2.

PRESENTATION

ABDOMINAL PAIN

Pain usually is the first symptom. The pain may develop acutely de novo or may represent exacerbation of existing chronic pain.

TABLE 97.1. COMMON ABDOMINAL CAUSES OF ACUTE ABDOMEN

Gastrointestinal tract
- Appendicitis
- Peptic ulcer disease
- Small- and large-intestinal obstruction
- Gastric and intestinal perforation
- Intestinal ischemia
- Meckel's diverticulitis
- Colonic diverticulitis
- Chronic inflammatory bowel disease
- Gastroenteritis

Pancreas, biliary tract, liver, and spleen
- Acute pancreatitis
- Acute calculous cholecystitis
- Acalculous cholecystitis
- Acute cholangitis
- Hepatic abscess
- Ruptured hepatic tumor
- Acute hepatitis
- Splenic rupture
- Spontaneous bacterial peritonitis

Urinary tract
- Renal or ureteral stone
- Acute pyelonephritis

Reproductive organs of women
- Ruptured ovarian cyst or follicle
- Torsion of ovary
- Tubal (ectopic) pregnancy
- Acute salpingitis
- Pyosalpinx
- Endometritis
- Rupture of uterus

Abdominal wall
- Rectus muscle hematoma

Retroperitoneum
- Aortic aneurysm
- Retroperitoneal hemorrhage

In general, only stimulation of the visceral and parietal peritoneum produces pain. The stimuli for visceral pain are distention of the gastrointestinal (GI) tract or other hollow abdominal organs, traction on the intestinal mesentery, or inflammation or ischemia. Chapter 96 discusses the causes and mechanisms of abdominal pain. When pain fibers of the visceral peritoneum are activated, pain is sensed in a pattern generally corresponding to the embryologic origin of the diseased organ—foregut, midgut, or hindgut. The distribution of visceral pain from different abdominal organs is illustrated in Fig. 97.1.

Visceral pain usually is sensed as intense midline discomfort, is vaguely characterized, and is poorly described by the patient. The small intestine from the second part of the duodenum to the ileocecal valve, the appendix, the ascending colon, and the right half of the transverse colon all derive from the midgut of the embryo. Visceral pain of midgut origin is sensed in the periumbilical region of the abdomen. Obstruction in any portion of the intestine that derives from the midgut, including the appendix, causes pain that is felt in the periumbilical region. Only when transmural inflammation or ischemia develops is the adjacent parietal peritoneum stimulated. When painful parietal stimulation occurs, the location of pain shifts to the part of the

TABLE 97.2.	EXTRA-ABDOMINAL CAUSES OF ACUTE ABDOMEN

Supradiaphragmatic
  Myocardial infarction
  Acute pericarditis
  Lower lobe pneumonia
  Pneumothorax
  Pulmonary infarction
Endocrine
  Diabetic ketoacidosis
  Addisonian crisis
Hematologic
  Sickle cell crisis
  Acute leukemia
Drug-induced
  Lead toxicity
  Narcotic withdrawal
Metabolic
  Acute porphyria
  Familial Mediterranean fever
  Hyperlipidemia
Central and peripheral nervous system
  Herpes zoster
  Tabes dorsalis
  Nerve root compression

abdomen over the inflamed or ischemic organ, and the pain becomes somatic. In the case of the appendix, the shift is to the right lower quadrant. When an obstructed loop of small intestine becomes gangrenous, the location of the pain shifts to correspond to the location of involved overlying parietal peritoneum.

Parietal pain is more sharply felt than visceral pain, usually is well localized, and is easily described. Parietal irritation is characteristically associated with splinting of the overlying anterior abdominal musculature, a phenomenon called *guarding*. Any motion of the parietal peritoneum, as by percussion or depression and release of the abdominal wall, elicits the sharp

pain known as *rebound tenderness*. If the process is progressive, bowel sounds become hypoactive and disappear. The cardinal signs of peritoneal irritation—pain, guarding, rebound tenderness, and absent bowel sounds—thus become established.

In addition to pain sensed in the abdomen, visceral disease often is associated with characteristic patterns of pain sensed in areas anatomically distinct from the abdomen. The patterns of radiation of pain often can provide a useful clue to the organ involved (Fig. 97.1). In gallbladder disease, the radiation is to the right scapular region. In pancreatitis, the radiation is to the middle of the back in the region of L1 and to the left of this vertebra when the body or tail of the pancreas is involved. When a duodenal ulcer penetrates posteriorly, the radiation is straight through to the back to the area of L1. Diaphragmatic irritation is referred to the shoulder region in the distribution of dermatomes C3, C4, and C5. Renal colic radiates from the flank to the groin or testicle.

ASSOCIATED GASTROINTESTINAL SYMPTOMS

Anorexia

Anorexia is a nonspecific symptom that accompanies many acute abdominal disorders. It is almost invariably present in acute appendicitis, and the diagnosis should be questioned if the patient does not have anorexia. Anorexia is less prominent for the gynecologic or urologic causes of the acute abdomen.

Vomiting

Vomiting usually develops in the course of acute abdomen as a reflex consequence of activation of visceral afferent fibers to the medullary vomiting center. Such reflex vomiting usually is not progressive, nor are unpleasant symptoms ameliorated by vomiting. In contrast, vomiting due to mechanical obstruction of the

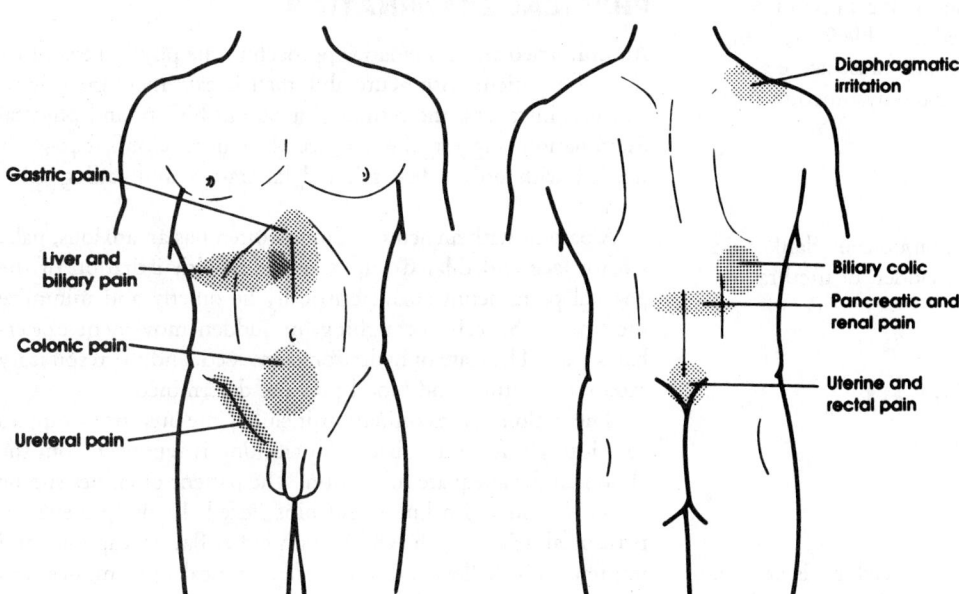

FIGURE 97.1. Common patterns of referred pain among patients with acute visceral pain.

GI tract is progressive. Vomiting caused by obstruction may lead to intravascular fluid depletion. Electrolyte imbalance characterized by hypochloremic, hypokalemic alkalosis occurs when the obstruction is proximal in the small intestine. More distal intestinal obstruction causes delayed vomiting and distention and may lead to hypovolemia but rarely to electrolyte imbalance.

Abdominal Distention

Abdominal distention is caused by accumulation of swallowed air, the gas of bacterial metabolism, and fluids secreted from the GI tract above the level of obstruction. Distention denotes mechanical intestinal obstruction or paralytic ileus. When distention is caused by ileus, bowel sounds are absent on auscultation of the abdomen. Distention caused by mechanical obstruction is accompanied by hyperactive, high-pitched bowel sounds except in the late stages, when vascular compromise of the GI tract and peritonitis develop.

Constipation

Constipation may be present as a symptom of an underlying disease, such as cancer of the sigmoid colon, that has produced a complication such as perforation. Constipation also may be caused by paralytic ileus. An important indication of mechanical intestinal obstruction is obstipation, the absence of bowel movements or flatus.

Diarrhea

Copious watery diarrhea suggests gastroenteritis. GI ischemia caused by mesenteric venous thrombosis is associated with dark, bloody diarrhea. Bloody diarrhea also may be associated with chronic inflammatory bowel disease.

Jaundice

The presence of jaundice in patients with acute abdominal pain usually indicates a hepatobiliary disorder as the cause of acute abdomen (see Chapter 103). As indicated in Table 97.1, prehepatic causes of jaundice also can occasionally cause acute abdomen. Jaundice also can be caused by hepatic dysfunction from abdominal sepsis.

Urologic Symptoms

Frequency, dysuria, hematuria, and suprapubic or flank pain indicate a lesion in the kidneys, ureter, bladder, or urethra and necessitate investigation and treatment.

▋ HISTORY AND PHYSICAL EXAMINATION

HISTORY

Past Illness

A complete record of all previous surgical procedures is crucial. A history of previous appendectomy or cholecystectomy allows one confidently to exclude disorders of the appendix or gallbladder as causes of symptoms. A history of peptic ulcer may be an important clue in the diagnosis of a perforated peptic ulcer. A history of previous attacks of renal calculi, inflammatory bowel disease, or abdominal aortic aneurysm is important.

Family History

Family history is particularly important in ruling out medical causes of acute abdomen such as familial Mediterranean fever and sickle cell anemia.

Drug Therapy

The cause of acute abdomen may be directly related to the use of drugs. Use of estrogen-containing oral contraceptives may lead to development of hepatic adenoma, which can bleed and precipitate acute abdominal pain. Patients taking anticoagulant drugs are susceptible to intramural hematoma of the intestine and to retroperitoneal hemorrhage. Corticosteroids may be important in two ways. First, sudden withdrawal of corticosteroids after long-term therapy may precipitate an Addisonian crisis, which may be manifest as abdominal pain. Second, the presence of corticosteroids masks development of the typical signs and symptoms of acute abdomen.

Menstrual History

The correct and expeditious diagnosis of the cause of acute abdominal pain is most difficult among women of childbearing age. For this reason, an accurate and detailed history of menstrual function and sexual activity is critical in the care of young women. Particular attention must be paid to timing of symptoms relative to anticipated menstrual periods, previous episodes of pelvic inflammatory disease, and the possibility of pregnancy.

PHYSICAL EXAMINATION

An unhurried and systematic approach to the physical examination of a patient with acute abdomen is extremely important. In most instances, the results of a careful history and physical examination suggest the correct diagnosis. Confirmation is needed with only a few selected laboratory and radiographic tests.

A patient with an acute abdomen often has an anxious, pale, sweaty face and dilated pupils. Patients with irritation of the parietal peritoneum characteristically lie quietly and minimize movement. Sneezing, coughing, or sudden movement exacerbates pain. The state of hydration is assessed, and the respiratory rate, temperature, and blood pressure determined.

The abdominal examination includes the area from nipples to midthigh, front and back. All clothing is removed from the abdomen for adequate inspection. The patient often lies supine or on the side with knees and hips flexed. In the presence of peritoneal irritation, the abdomen is either flat or scaphoid, and respiration is shallow and intercostal. Surgical scars, masses, and potential sites of hernias are evaluated.

After inspection, auscultation is performed before palpation. All four quadrants are auscultated, and the presence and character of bowel sounds are assessed. Bowel sounds are considered absent if no tones are audible over at least a 2-minute period of auscultation. A silent abdomen, if associated with pain and tenderness, is an ominous finding. If hyperactive bowel sounds are present, pitch and association with waves of abdominal pain are evaluated. Vascular bruits are assessed.

After auscultation, gentle percussion is performed to elicit rebound tenderness. Percussion starts in the quadrant farthest from the site of pain; percussion of the painful quadrant is performed last. Gentle palpation to assess the tone of the abdominal wall ensues. Deep palpation is performed last. Intentional attempts to elicit rebound tenderness by means of rapid release of the abdominal wall after deep palpation usually are not helpful and eliminate the possibility of sequential examinations. The sine qua non of an inflammatory process such as appendicitis is localized or *point tenderness,* best elicited by means of gentle, one-finger palpation. If the inflamed appendix is deep in the pelvis, point tenderness may be elicited only by means of rectal or vaginal examination.

Digital rectal examination is performed on all patients. The stool on the examining finger is tested for guaiac positivity. Pelvic examination is performed on all female patients. Any external ostomies or fistulas are examined digitally.

MODIFIERS OF CLINICAL PRESENTATION

Several factors modify the appreciation of pain and the development of signs of peritoneal irritation in an acute abdomen (Table 97.3). The two extremes of age, infancy and old age, inhibit the full expression of peritoneal irritation, particularly the development of guarding. Patients undergoing corticosteroid therapy and those with Cushing's syndrome may have deceptively few signs of peritoneal irritation even though they have well-devel-

TABLE 97.3.	FACTORS THAT MAY LIMIT THE EXPRESSION OF THE SIGNS AND SYMPTOMS OF THE ACUTE ABDOMEN

Endocrine or metabolic factors
   Corticosteroid therapy
   Cushing's syndrome
   Diabetes
Extremes of age
   Infancy (<2 y)
   Old age (>70 y)
Retroperitoneal abnormality
Vascular compromise of the intestine
Postoperative status
Central nervous system disorder
   Coma
   Paraplegia
Pregnancy
Neutropenia

oped peritonitis. Diabetes mellitus inhibits expression of the signs and symptoms of acute abdomen to a lesser degree. Patients with diabetes, however, may rapidly experience gangrenous cholecystitis and may have relatively less pain and tenderness than patients without diabetes who have a similarly advanced abnormality. Abdominal signs are less well developed when the abnormality is retroperitoneal. Retroperitoneal perforation of the duodenum often is not diagnosed promptly because of the lack of explicit abdominal signs. Patients with severe acute pancreatitis also may have severe pain and abdominal tenderness but relatively less guarding or rebound tenderness. For reasons that are not well understood, patients with vascular compromise of the intestine and even intestinal infarction have pain out of proportion to the abdominal signs of guarding and tenderness.

Acute abdominal abnormality is difficult to diagnose immediately after operations performed for another abdominal condition. Pain, abdominal tenderness, and fever are common and are expected after any abdominal operation, thus the presence of these signs and symptoms delays the diagnosis of acute abdominal disease. Patients in a coma or who have paraplegia do not have abdominal signs or symptoms. In both conditions, systemic signs (fever, hypotension, leukocytosis) are the usual, and often late, indicators of abdominal disease. Among patients with paraplegia, abdominal pain may be limited to diaphragmatic irritation that causes shoulder pain in the distribution of C3, C4, and C5.

AGE

The diagnosis of acute abdominal conditions can be difficult in the two extremes of age. In infancy, the abdominal wall is not well developed, and splinting of the rectus muscles in response to an intra-abdominal inflammatory process does not occur. Infants are unable to communicate well, and the cardinal signs of peritoneal irritation may be difficult to elicit. Systemic signs of fever and dehydration, although they tend to occur early, are not helpful because they are common among children. Elderly patients may not have systemic manifestations even in the presence of well-developed generalized peritonitis. Leukocytosis may not be apparent, and abdominal signs may be misleading. In the two extremes of life, the management of acute abdominal pain calls for the best clinical judgment and the judicious use of early laparotomy.

CORTICOSTEROID THERAPY

Patients taking corticosteroids who have acute abdominal disorders of any cause often do not have full expression of the usual manifestations of acute abdomen. It is common, for example, for findings at physical examination of the abdomen to be relatively normal among patients with toxic megacolon and multiple colonic perforations if the patient is taking corticosteroids. The findings at examination also are relatively normal among corticosteroid-treated patients with acute perforation of a duodenal ulcer. The signs of peritonitis (pain, guarding, and rebound tenderness) may be poorly developed, and fever is suppressed. The patient may not appear acutely ill despite rapid progression of infection. The white blood cell (WBC) count may not be elevated, but usually a marked shift to immature forms is present. Radiologic examination, either plain radiography of the abdomen or computed tomography (CT), is performed more frequently than it is for other patients.

PREGNANCY

Diagnosis of the cause of acute abdomen during pregnancy is complicated. The pain may originate from the pregnant uterus, and uterine enlargement displaces organs from their normal positions. Abdominal examination is difficult, and radiologic evaluation is avoided. Acute appendicitis, acute cholecystitis, and acute pyelonephritis are the most common causes of the acute abdomen among pregnant women. The point tenderness of appendicitis in pregnancy often is shifted away from McBurney's point to a more lateral position in the right upper quadrant of the abdomen. Two specific causes of acute abdomen that occur frequently during pregnancy are rupture of splenic artery aneurysm and rupture of subcapsular hematoma of the liver. The former becomes manifest as severe epigastric pain associated with hypotension and without tenderness of the uterus. Immediate surgical exploration is life saving. Subcapsular hematoma of the liver typically occurs among multiparous woman in the third trimester of pregnancy and is associated with toxemia and disseminated intravascular coagulation. In both disorders hemoperitoneum and shock often are followed by death of the fetus. In the evaluation of acute abdominal abnormalities among pregnant patients, a useful rule is to examine and treat the patient as aggressively as and for the same conditions as nonpregnant patients. The best guarantee of a healthy infant is a well mother.

NEUTROPENIA

Acute abdominal pain is frequent among patients with severe neutropenia (fewer than 100 cells per microliter). Patients with acute leukemia or aplastic anemia and those undergoing bone marrow transplantation before engraftment or aggressive systemic chemotherapy are are particular risk. Among these patients, a syndrome of fever, diffuse abdominal pain, and watery diarrhea may mimic an abdominal disorder. These symptoms often are caused by neutropenic colitis, a pathologic entity characterized by mucosal ulceration, invasive bacterial infection, and sepsis. The terminal ileum and ascending colon are most commonly affected. Cecal edema may occur among many such patients. Laparotomy is indicated if the presence of perforation or full-thickness necrosis is suggested.

■ LABORATORY STUDIES AND DIAGNOSTIC TESTS

A careful history interview and physical examination suggest the correct diagnosis in most cases of acute abdomen. Laboratory and radiologic or ultrasonographic examinations have to be se-

lective and are directed at confirming the diagnosis suggested by the history and physical findings (Fig. 97.2).

All patients with acute abdomen need a complete blood cell count, including hemoglobin, hematocrit, and WBC count with differential. Leukocytosis with a shift to the left indicates acute inflammation, usually a bacterial infection. Leukopenia suggests a viral infection. A low WBC count with severe shift to the left (increase in immature forms or in cells with toxic granulation) occurs among elderly persons or in the presence of an abscess, but elderly patients may show little change in the number or shift of the WBC count.

All patients with acute abdomen need urinalysis. The results rapidly rule out diabetic ketoacidosis and urinary tract infection. The presence of gross or microscopic blood in the urine suggests renal or ureteral calculi and is an indication for intravenous pyelography. A urine pregnancy test rules out pregnancy as a confounding factor. Serum amylase is measured if pancreatitis is suggested. Liver enzyme tests are performed if cholecystitis, cholangitis, or hepatitis is included in the differential diagnosis. Serum electrolytes, urea, and creatinine are measured for elderly patients, when a patient has vomiting or diarrhea, and when the pathologic process has existed for a prolonged period.

Plain radiographs of the abdomen are obtained when generalized peritoneal irritation is present or when the presence of intestinal obstruction or infarction or renal calculi is suggested. When a perforated viscus is a possibility, three views of the abdomen are obtained—supine, upright, and right or left decubitus. The views include both sides of the diaphragm and the pelvis so that the presence of free air and free peritoneal fluid can be detected. About 75% of patients with perforated peptic ulcer have free air under the diaphragm or evidence of free air on decubitus radiographs. The extent of pneumoperitoneum, however, usually is much more pronounced in colonic perforation. The presence of gas in the biliary tree is ascertained. The presence of gas indicates abnormal communication between the GI tract and the biliary system. Pneumatosis, the presence of gas within the intestinal wall or in the portal vein, usually is a grave sign in the context of acute abdominal pain; it indicates intestinal infarction.

Specialized tests include ultrasonography, radionuclide scanning, CT of the abdomen, GI contrast studies, endoscopic examination of the upper or lower GI tract, and laparoscopy. Ultrasonography is the preferred primary method for examination of the gallbladder and biliary tract. Radionuclide scanning is quite sensitive for confirming the presence of acute cholecystitis. Ultrasonography is preferred as a first method for examination of the liver, the reproductive organs, and retroperitoneal structures such as the aorta. CT is preferred for examination of the pancreas and for detection of localized intra-abdominal or retroperitoneal inflammatory processes. An increase in the availability of abdominal CT has reduced the number of abdominal explorations for pancreatitis. CT also has become the preferred examination to evaluate complications of acute diverticulitis.

Not all patients need all of the listed tests. A young man with typical signs and symptoms of appendicitis and normal findings of urinalysis usually needs no additional testing and needs an emergency operation. Many patients, however, need more involved investigations than those listed earlier. Laparoscopy has

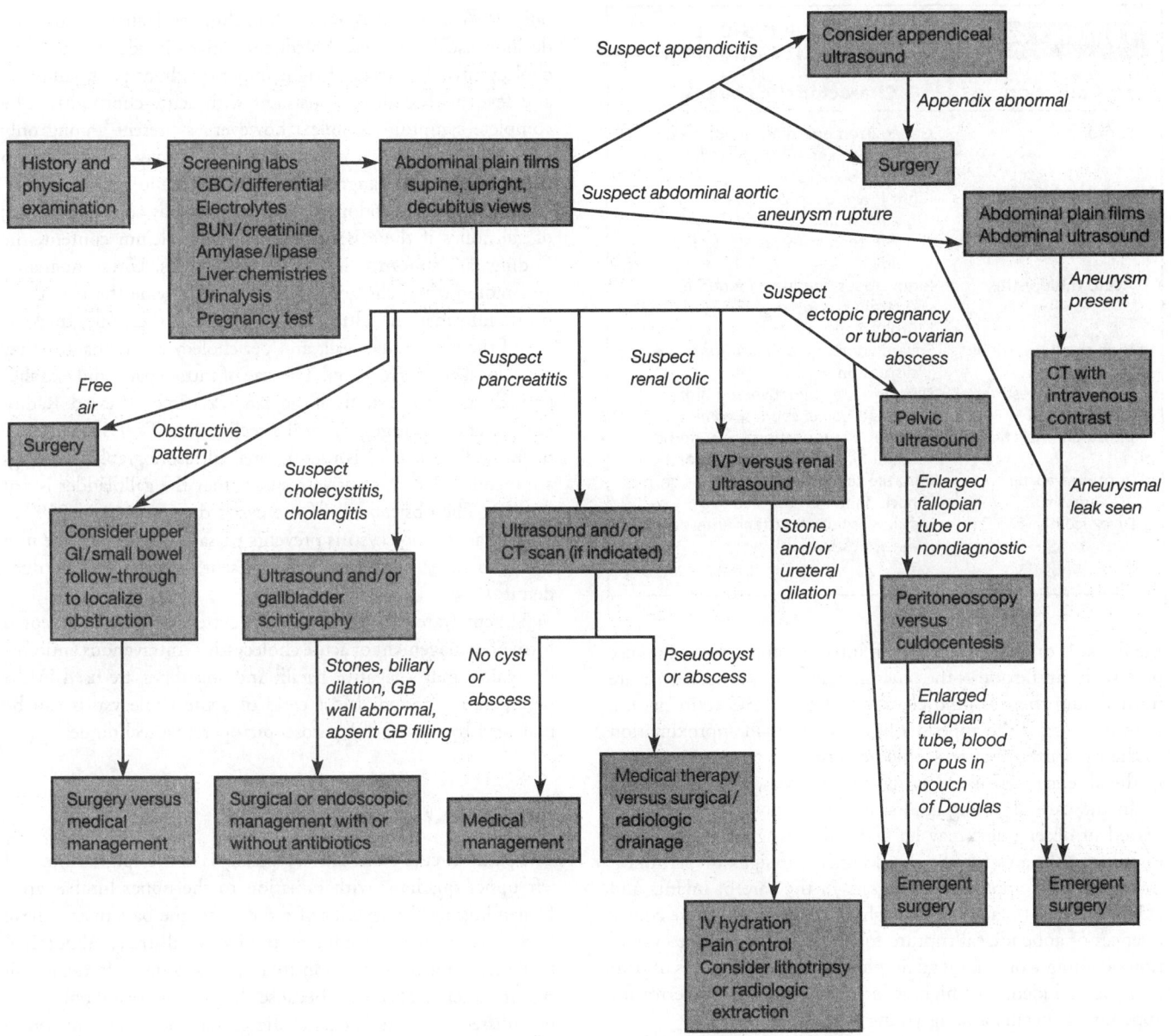

FIGURE 97.2. Evaluation of acute abdomen.
EVIDENCE LEVEL: C. Expert Opinion.

a rapidly developing role in the diagnosis of acute inflammatory abdominal conditions. In many instances it allows minimally invasive surgical treatment. For example, laparoscopy is a valuable procedure for young women because a gynecologic condition cannot be easily distinguished from appendicitis or right upper quadrant pain may be caused by the Fitz-Hugh–Curtis syndrome, in which perihepatic inflammation is a complication of salpingitis.

■ DIFFERENTIAL DIAGNOSIS

The characteristic physical findings associated with acute abdominal abnormalities are summarized in Table 97.4.

ACUTE APPENDICITIS

Acute appendicitis always is included in the differential diagnosis of abdominal pain. The patient typically has periumbilical pain and anorexia with or without nausea and vomiting. After a variable time, usually hours, the pain moves to the right lower quadrant as the parietal peritoneum becomes involved in the inflammatory process. Low-grade fever is usual. The most characteristic sign is point tenderness at McBurney's point, which is located one-third of the distance from the anterior superior iliac spine to the umbilicus. The exact point of maximal tenderness, however, depends on the anatomic location of the appendix. When the appendix is in a pelvic location, the point of maximal tenderness may be elicited best by means of rectal examination. In retrocecal appendicitis, tenderness often is higher and more lateral, toward

TABLE 97.4.	CHARACTERISTIC PHYSICAL FINDINGS OF ACUTE ABDOMEN
Condition	**Characteristic Features**
Peritonitis	Generalized guarding, tenderness, rebound tenderness, hypoactive or absent bowel sounds
Appendicitis	Right lower quadrant tenderness, guarding and rebound
	Discrete tenderness at McBurney's point
Acute cholecystitis	Right upper quadrant tenderness and guarding, positive
	Murphy signs
High small-intestinal obstruction	Severe vomiting, dehydration, no distention
Low small-intestinal obstruction	Distention, hyperactive and high-pitched bowel sounds, vomiting
Intestinal infarction	Pain out of proportion to tenderness, rectal bleeding if venous infarction
Ruptured aortic aneurysm	Pulsatile tender mass, hypotension, back pain
Diverticulitis	Left lower quadrant tenderness and mass, obstipation

the flank. If oriented medially, an inflamed appendix may cause pain with hip flexion—the *psoas sign*. Findings at urinalysis are normal, and there is mild elevation of the WBC count with a leftward shift. If the appendix lies posteriorly in approximation to the right ureter, microscopic hematuria or pyuria may occur in the absence of primary urinary tract disease.

In the care of young adults, if the diagnosis is in doubt, a period of observation may be planned during which the same examiner evaluates for the development of signs of peritoneal irritation. This approach is less safe in the care of infants and elderly persons because of the higher incidence and grave consequences of appendiceal rupture for these groups. In the evaluation of young women, pregnancy and other pelvic causes of pain must be excluded. The highest incidence of diagnostic error for appendicitis occurs among young women.

ACUTE CHOLECYSTITIS

The pain of acute cholecystitis occurs almost invariably in the right upper quadrant. Radiation to the right scapular region or the right shoulder is common. The pain frequently occurs 1 or 2 hours after a meal, quickly reaches maximum intensity, and may persist for a prolonged time. Pain relief usually necessitates narcotic analgesia. A history of intolerance of fatty foods or biliary colic often is elicited. Fever usually is low grade. The classic findings are guarding and tenderness in the right upper quadrant with or without a palpable, tender mass. Sudden arrest of inspiration occurs when the patient inspires deeply while the right upper quadrant is being palpated—*Murphy's sign*. The inspiratory arrest is caused by stimulation of parietal peritoneum by the inflamed gallbladder fundus.

Results of liver tests may be normal, and leukocytosis often is low grade. A mild rise in serum transaminase and bilirubin values may be present, although clinical jaundice is present in

only 10% of cases. A serum bilirubin level above 5 mg per deciliter usually implies choledocholithiasis in addition to acute cholecystitis. The triad of right upper quadrant pain, jaundice, and fever with chills is consistent with acute cholangitis. The complete symptom complex, however, is present among only 60% of patients with cholangitis, and it may be difficult to differentiate acute gangrenous cholecystitis and cholangitis.

Although plain abdominal radiographs may contain evidence of gallstones if there is sufficiently high calcium content, the findings are abnormal in only 10% of cases. Ultrasonography and radionuclide cholangioscintigraphy provide the best diagnostic information. Ultrasonography shows the stone, thickening of the gallbladder wall, and pericholecystic edema and may show localized perforation. The size of intrahepatic and extrahepatic ducts and the status of the pancreas can be assessed. Radionuclide cholescintigraphy with a technetium Tc 99m derivative of iminodiacetic acid is useful when ultrasonographic findings are inconclusive. A positive result is that the gallbladder is not imaged. The obstruction of the cystic duct present in 95% of cases of acute cholecystitis prevents passage of radionuclide into the gallbladder. Radioactivity is present, however, in the duodenum.

Urgent (rarely emergency) cholecystectomy is the accepted form of management of acute cholecystitis. Intravenous antibiotics against gram-negative bacilli and anaerobes are used in the perioperative period. Most cases of acute cholecystitis can be managed by means of laparoscopic operative techniques.

ACUTE PANCREATITIS

The pain of acute pancreatitis typically is in the epigastrium and left upper quadrant with radiation to the upper lumbar area. Depending on the severity of the disease, the patient may have hypovolemia, hypotension, or respiratory distress. Abdominal tenderness out of proportion to accompanying abdominal wall rigidity often is observed. Because the peripancreatic phlegmon may dissect down either paracolic gutter, the clinical presentation may sometimes be confused with that of acute appendicitis or acute diverticulitis. Leukocytosis (15,000 cells per microliter) with a left shift often is present in acute pancreatitis. An elevated serum amylase level is present in more than 75% of cases. Plain abdominal radiographs may show dilatation of the stomach, air in the duodenum, an isolated dilated loop of proximal small intestine (sentinel loop), or dilatation of the transverse colon caused by ileus in intestinal segments that abut the inflamed pancreas.

The amount of air in the GI tract often militates against adequate evaluation of the pancreas by means of ultrasonography, and CT has become the most informative method of examining the pancreas for inflammation (Fig. 97.3). The availability of abdominal CT has markedly reduced the number of exploratory laparotomies performed on patients with pancreatitis. Other reliable diagnostic techniques include paracentesis with determination of amylase concentration in the peritoneal fluid when ascites is present.

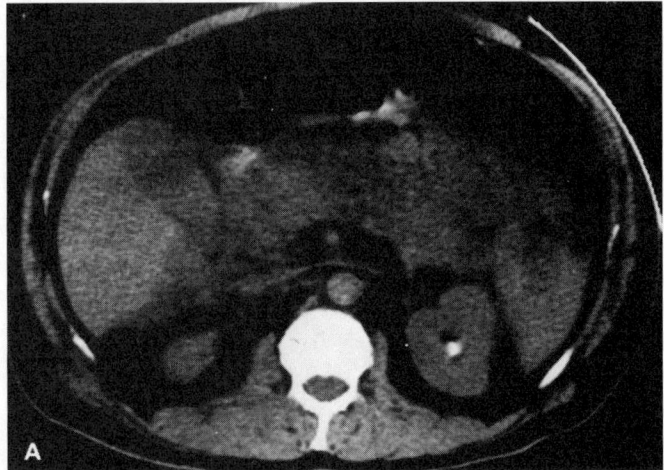
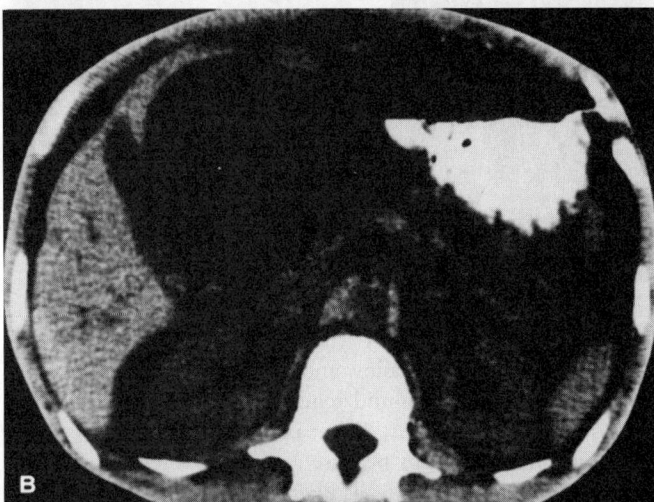
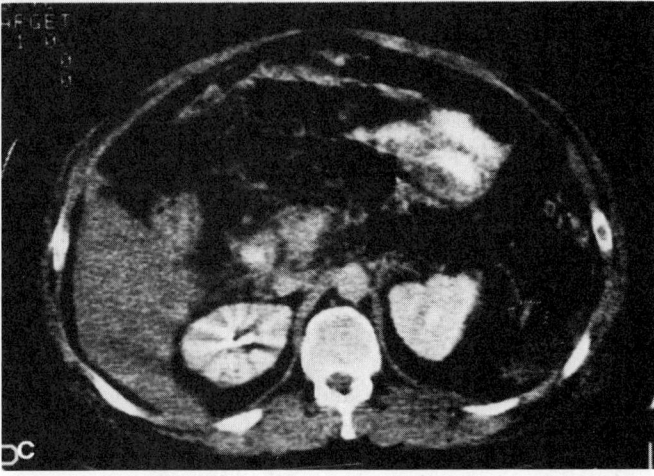

FIGURE 97.3. Computed tomographic scan of the upper abdomen shows pancreatic phlegmon associated with acute pancreatitis **(A)**, pancreatic pseudocyst and associated dilatation of the pancreatic duct **(B)**, and peripancreatic gas in the presence of pancreatic abscess **(C)**.

ACUTE OBSTRUCTION OF THE SMALL INTESTINE

The most common causes of small-intestinal obstruction are adhesive bands from previous operations and hernias (inguinal, femoral, umbilical, incisional). The onset of complete small-intestinal obstruction is heralded by the development of visceral pain in the distribution of the midgut. Pain usually is felt in the midline around the umbilicus. The discomfort occurs intermittently in concert with periods of increased peristaltic activity. Soon after the onset of obstruction, patients may be nearly free of pain between periods of peristalsis. With the development of intestinal distention, however, residual discomfort remains between the episodes of intense colic. The pain of small-intestinal obstruction is severe and gnawing and yet vague and difficult to describe. If pain is not the first symptom, the diagnosis of small-intestinal obstruction should be questioned.

Abdominal distention, obstipation, and vomiting occur after the pain begins. Physical examination is directed at assessment of the completeness of obstruction and at detection of accompanying intraperitoneal inflammation. Information from plain abdominal radiographs is confirmatory in most instances. The loops of the small intestine usually are distended with fluid and swallowed air (Fig. 97.4). Upright radiographs contain air-fluid levels. In classic cases, the colon and rectum have a paucity of gas. A precise knowledge of the site of obstruction in the small intestine is not necessary in most cases of complete obstruction. *Barium contrast studies should not be performed* to obtain such information preoperatively.

Two challenges confront surgeons treating patients with adhesive small-intestinal obstruction: differentiating simple and strangulated obstruction and differentiating partial and complete obstruction. With modern operative techniques and perioperative support, the perioperative mortality for simple mechanical obstruction is about 1%. The presence of intestinal infarction increases this risk to 5% to 10%. A delay in diagnosis or operative therapy of 12 hours, during which time strangulation may occur, increases mortality 50%. It follows, therefore, that impending strangulation should be sought strenuously and managed promptly. There are, however, no definite clinical criteria to differentiate simple and strangulated mechanical small-intestinal obstruction. Even experienced clinicians have difficulty detecting intestinal infarction. The classically taught clinical signs of strangulated obstruction, continuous abdominal pain, signs of peritonitis, abdominal mass, tachycardia, leukocytosis, and acidosis do not reliably confirm the presence of intestinal strangulation. The presence of erythema of the overlying skin of an incarcerated hernia is an advanced sign, but its absence does not rule out strangulation. Because of the difficulty in differentiating simple from complicated obstruction and the serious consequences of strangulation, prompt surgical treatment is considered when complete obstruction has been diagnosed.

It sometimes is difficult to determine whether obstruction is partial or complete. The finding of stool or gas in the colon at radiography or the passage of flatus after the onset of obstructive symptoms does not eliminate complete obstruction from consideration. Colonic gas and stool may already have been present at the time of obstruction. Symptomatic improvement that accom-

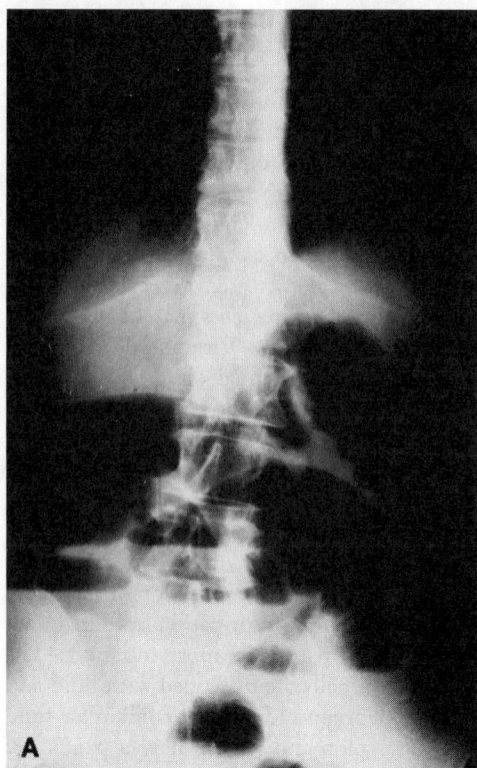
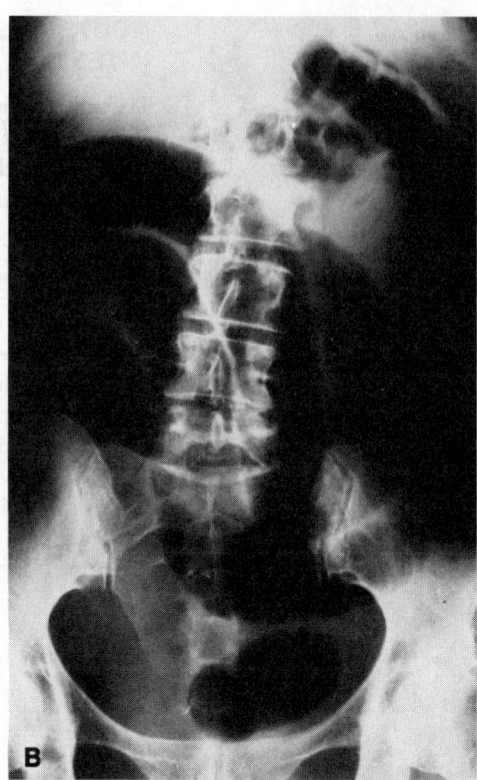

FIGURE 97.4. Plain supine (A) and upright (B) radiographs of the abdomen of a patient with complete intestinal obstruction show dilated loops of small intestine and air-fluid levels.

panies nasogastric decompression of the upper GI tract and restoration of intravascular volume also may be misinterpreted, because temporary relief may occur even if obstruction is complete.

Nonoperative treatment is indicated only if the obstruction is believed to be incomplete. Marked improvement of partial obstruction is expected within 1 or 2 days if nonoperative treatment is chosen. Serial radiographs should document distal passage of gas from the small intestine into the colon. Repeated clinical examinations should show clear and progressive improvement. Most important, a disciplined plan must be established. If patients do not meet criteria for improvement with nonoperative therapy, prompt surgical exploration should be undertaken.

PERFORATED PEPTIC ULCER

Patients with perforated peptic ulcer commonly have sudden onset of severe upper abdominal pain with or without radiation to the shoulders. The pain tends to diminish for 15 to 30 minutes, only to recur as constant, severe pain. A history of known peptic ulcer disease or dyspepsia is present among two-thirds of patients. The patient is anxious and appears acutely ill at examination. Tachycardia and fever are present, but hypotension rarely occurs early. If a patient with an acute abdomen has hypotension, other diagnoses, such as perforated colon, gangrene of the intestine, pancreatitis, cholangitis, or ruptured aortic aneurysm should be suspected.

Physical examination shows a flat or scaphoid, rigid abdomen. The patient lies immobile. With the abdominal wall splinted, respiration is shallow and intercostal. Abdominal rigidity, tenderness, and rebound tenderness are prominent. Bowel sounds usually are absent, and at percussion liver dullness may be diminished or absent because air is interposed between the liver and the abdominal wall. Plain abdominal radiographs are obtained with multiple views—supine, upright, and right decubitus (Fig. 97.5). Free air, however, is present in only about 75% of cases. Leukocytosis may be moderate, but anemia usually is absent. Serum amylase levels usually are within normal limits. If the serum amylase level is elevated, the value rarely exceeds three times the upper limit of normal. The accepted treatment is surgical. If the perforated ulcer is in the duodenum, closure of the perforation is accomplished with a direct suture technique or by means of suture closure over a buttressing piece of omentum (the Graham patch technique).

If the patient has a history of peptic ulcer or if perforation occurs during medical therapy, a definitive ulcer operation is undertaken if the patient has no other serious illness, the perforation is less than 48 hours old, and the patient has not experienced preoperative shock. When a decision is made to perform a definitive ulcer operation, proximal gastric (highly selective) vagotomy is the preferred procedure. When the perforated ulcer is gastric, the treatment of choice is antrectomy or excision of the ulcer and closure. Omental patch closure occasionally is performed for gastric perforation if the patient's condition is precarious.

COLONIC PERFORATION

Colonic perforation occurs as a complication of closed-loop obstruction, diverticulitis, or carcinoma. Impressive pneumoperi-

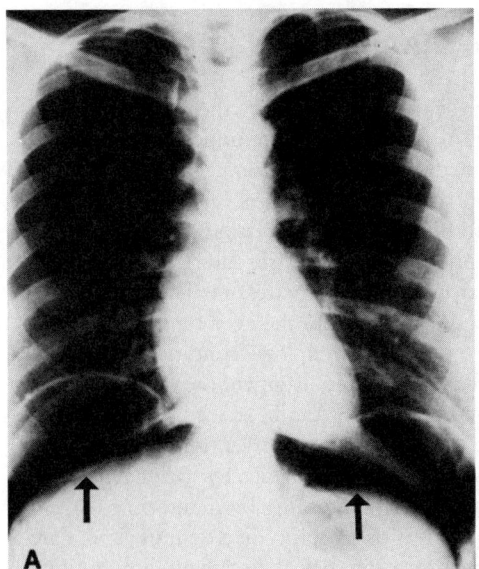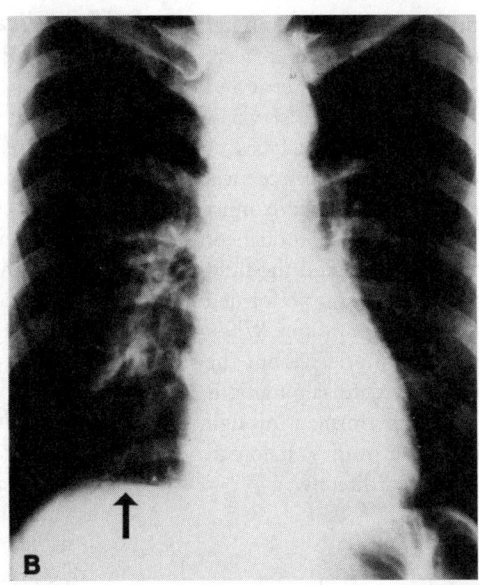

FIGURE 97.5. Upright chest radiographs of two patients with perforated peptic ulcer show massive **(A)** and minimal **(B)** amounts of free intraperitoneal air.

toneum often occurs, and septic shock develops quickly. In diverticular disease, perforation may occur as a primary event in the inflamed diverticulum or as a secondary event when a contained pericolic abscess from a previously inflamed diverticulum ruptures freely into the peritoneal cavity. A history of left lower quadrant pain and physical findings of a left-sided pelvic inflammatory mass are common.

Rapid resuscitation and broad-spectrum antibiotic coverage for the mixed aerobic and anaerobic colonic flora are instituted, and an operation is performed without delay. The goal of surgery is to resect the diseased colonic segment, to perform lavage of the peritoneum, and to construct a totally diverting colostomy. Primary colonic anastomosis under these conditions is unwise.

ACUTE DIVERTICULITIS

True colonic diverticula are uncommon. True diverticula are congenital, contain all the layers of the intestinal wall, and involve the right colon, usually as single lesions. Although true diverticula can be obstructed and become inflamed, they are rarely perforated. In most instances, the term *diverticulosis* refers to the presence of multiple pseudodiverticula in the colon. Pseudodiverticula contain only mucosa and submucosa as they penetrate the muscular layers of the colonic wall. Diverticulosis typically involves the sigmoid colon (95% of cases), but it can involve the descending colon or even the entire colon. The diverticula represent outpouchings of the mucosa and submucosa at points of weakness in the muscular wall at the site of perforating vessels. Most diverticula are adjacent to the longitudinal smooth-muscle bands of the taeniae coli, because these are the sites at which colonic vessels perforate the intestinal wall. The mucosal herniation is caused by an increase in intraluminal pressure.

Diverticulosis is common in western countries. It is a frequent problem among the elderly. In the absence of complications, diverticulosis does not necessitate specific treatment aside from common-sense admonitions to maintain appropriate fiber con-

tent in the diet. Diverticulosis occasionally has been associated with massive colonic bleeding caused by erosion of colonic arterioles subjacent to the mucosa of a diverticulum.

Diverticulitis is believed to occur when the ostium of one or more diverticula is obstructed with fecal material. Because the diverticula are outpouchings of the colon, obstruction and inflammation in effect constitute pericolonic inflammation. An inflamed diverticulum can rupture either freely into the peritoneal cavity, causing generalized peritonitis, or, more commonly, intramesenterically with walling off by surrounding tissue, resulting in a pericolic abscess. Such a contained abscess can perforate and cause diffuse peritonitis. Colonic obstruction can be caused by a pericolic abscess as the result of mechanical obstruction or spasm. Colonic obstruction usually occurs when many diverticula in the same segment of intestine are inflamed. A peridiverticular abscess can rupture into an adjacent viscus, usually the bladder, to cause a colovesical fistula, which allows air into the urine and causes chronic urinary tract infection. Diverticulitis causes acute abdomen when free or localized perforation or colonic obstruction occurs.

When generalized peritonitis has occurred, emergency surgery is needed to remove the diseased segment of intestine. An end-colostomy is constructed, and the rectal stump is closed or exteriorized as a mucous fistula. A second operation, usually months later, is performed to close the colostomy. When perforation produces a localized abscess, the situation is less urgent. A period of nasogastric decompression and therapy with systemic antibiotics, sometimes combined with percutaneous abscess drainage, may allow elective surgical therapy—resection and primary anastomosis—under optimal circumstances. Most patients with colonic obstruction caused by diverticulitis can be treated conservatively, and the need for an operation can be determined on the basis of clinical response within 7 to 10 days.

GYNECOLOGIC DISEASES

Gynecologic causes of acute abdomen, such as ruptured or twisted ovarian cyst, ectopic pregnancy, and acute salpingitis, often must be differentiated from acute appendicitis or another surgical condition. Menstrual and sexual histories are crucial. At pelvic examination, inflammatory disease of the uterus and fallopian tubes is indicated by tenderness when the cervix is moved, iliac fossa tenderness, or the finding of an adnexal mass at bimanual examination. Microscopic examination of any cervical discharge is mandatory, and any secretions from the cervix must be subjected to aerobic and anaerobic culture. The pouch of Douglas can be aspirated by means of colposcopy and the fluid examined for blood and bacteria. A pregnancy test is performed for all patients of childbearing age who have symptoms. When the findings on abdominal examination are impressive but the distinction between acute appendicitis and acute salpingitis is uncertain, laparoscopic examination may be performed through a small, subumbilical midline incision. The ovaries, fallopian tubes, uterus, and appendix can be visualized directly.

RUPTURED ECTOPIC PREGNANCY

An acute intra-abdominal crisis occurs when a tubal pregnancy ruptures into the peritoneal cavity. Sudden lower abdominal pain develops and is rapidly followed by generalized peritonitis and hypovolemic shock caused by intra-abdominal bleeding. At pelvic examination the cervix may look blue, and blood may be present at the cervical os. The uterus may be slightly enlarged, and a hematoma may be appreciated in the cul de sac. Laboratory studies show anemia and moderate leukocytosis. A pregnancy test result is positive. When necessary, peritoneoscopy or culdocentesis confirms the diagnosis. Emergency surgical intervention is needed to control hemorrhage.

RUPTURED ABDOMINAL AORTIC ANEURYSM

When abdominal aneurysms rupture, they do so most commonly posteriorly into the retroperitoneum. An initially contained retroperitoneal perforation may then rupture into the free peritoneum with sudden exsanguination. Ruptured aortic aneurysm must be kept high on the list of differential diagnoses, particularly when acute abdomen is associated with back pain and hypovolemic shock. The most important physical finding is a palpable, pulsatile mass in the abdomen. Plain abdominal radiographs in anteroposterior, lateral, and oblique projections, especially cross-table lateral, show aneurysmal calcification of the vessel wall. Ultrasonography is the most useful study for the diagnosis of aneurysm. When ruptured aortic aneurysm is suggested, any complex radiologic investigation needed, such as intravenous pyelography or aortography if a suprarenal aneurysm is suggested, is conducted in the operating room. An emergency operation is mandatory to control bleeding and to replace the aneurysmal segment with a synthetic graft.

■ STRATEGIES FOR OPTIMAL CARE

The essential questions to answer in the care of a patient with acute abdomen include the following: What is the nature of the pathologic process? Is hospitalization necessary for supportive care, observation, or further diagnostic testing? Is surgical evaluation indicated?

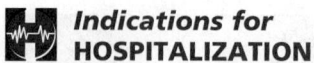

Indications for HOSPITALIZATION

For patients with acute abdominal pain, the need for hospitalization is related to the nature of the underlying pathologic condition found during the evaluation. If the underlying pathophysiologic condition necessitates surgical intervention, the timing of hospitalization is best determined in conjunction with the surgical consultant (see later). When medical therapy is indicated as the primary treatment, as for gastroenteritis, hepatitis, or endometritis, the need for hospitalization is dictated by the patient's physiologic condition when he or she comes to medical attention. Many of the potential causes of acute abdomen preclude or can be exacerbated by continued oral intake even if surgical intervention is not needed. The need to provide adequate analgesia, hydration, and nutrition while the patient takes nothing by mouth in situations such as acute pancreatitis, colonic diverticulitis, and flare-ups of chronic inflammatory bowel disease often necessitates hospitalization for supportive care. The need to monitor responses to medical therapy such as administration of antibiotics and electrolyte replacement also may dictate hospitalization.

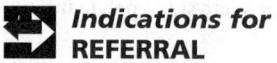

Indications for REFERRAL

Indications for referral are related to the nature of the pathologic condition found during the primary evaluation. When critical intra-abdominal disorders such as ruptured abdominal aortic aneurysm, ectopic pregnancy, perforated viscus, or acute cholangitis are high on the list of possible diagnoses, immediate surgical consultation is indicated before extensive laboratory or diagnostic tests are initiated to prevent the considerable morbidity or mortality associated with any delay in definitive treatment. In less urgent situations, the history and physical examination and laboratory and diagnostic evaluations proceed to determine the cause of the underlying pathologic condition. If pathophysiologic processes that may necessitate surgical intervention remain on the list of diagnostic possibilities after this evaluation, surgical consultation is indicated. Most patients with acute abdominal pain need surgical evaluation.

SURGICAL MANAGEMENT

Once a referral has been made for surgical evaluation, the surgical consultant needs to answer the following questions: Is an operation needed immediately? If so, what amount of preoperative investigation is necessary? If an immediate operation is not indicated, what follow-up plan should be adopted, and what changes in the patient's condition indicate the need for an operation? The most common causes of acute abdomen are pathologic processes contained in the abdomen. Extra-abdominal causes are uncommon but must always be considered and excluded. Not all pathologic processes within the abdomen that cause acute abdomen are surgical conditions; examples include acute pancreatitis and acute salpingitis.

Immediate Operation

Rarely is an operation indicated so immediately that time cannot be devoted to performing necessary laboratory or radiographic tests. The most striking example of such an abdominal emergency is that of a patient with back or abdominal pain and a pulsatile abdominal mass. The single most important consideration in the differential diagnosis in such a case is leaking aortic aneurysm. Sending the patient to the radiology department for abdominal radiographs or intravenous pyelography can cause fatal delay. The patient is taken to the operating room immediately. If radiologic examination is considered critical, the examination can be performed in the operating room. Similarly, a young woman with a positive pregnancy test, peritonitis, and hemorrhagic shock needs immediate laparotomy to control bleeding from a ruptured ectopic pregnancy. Another, less urgent example is a patient with a perforated viscus and intestinal obstruction associated with septic shock (Table 97.5).

TABLE 97.5.	DIFFERENTIAL DIAGNOSIS OF ACUTE ABDOMEN THAT MAY NECESSITATE SURGICAL INTERVENTION

Gastrointestinal tract
  Appendicitis
  Perforated peptic ulcer
  Mechanical intestinal obstruction
  Intestinal perforation
  Intestinal ischemia
  Colonic diverticulitis
  Inflammatory bowel disease
  Meckel's diverticulitis
Pancreas, biliary tract, liver, spleen
  Acute pancreatitis
  Acute calculous cholecystitis
  Acalculous cholecystitis
  Acute cholangitis
  Hepatic abscess
  Ruptured hepatic tumor
  Splenic rupture
Urinary tract
  Renal or ureteral stone
Reproductive organs of women
  Ectopic pregnancy
  Tubo-ovarian abscess
  Ovarian torsion
  Uterine rupture
  Ruptured ovarian cyst or follicle
Retroperitoneum
  Abdominal aortic aneurysm rupture
Supradiaphragmatic region
  Pneumothorax
  Pulmonary embolus
  Acute pericarditis
  Empyema

Immediate Operation Not Needed

For many patients with acute abdominal pain, the need for immediate surgical intervention is not evident. In such cases, it is imperative that a management plan be developed early. The plan must set prospective goals for clinical improvement that if not met prompt surgical exploration. The management plan includes repeated examination of the abdomen by the same observer at intervals determined by the severity of the signs and symptoms. In this way, the development of signs of peritoneal irritation can be detected early and a decision to operate made appropriately. If the patient's condition continues to improve, surgical intervention becomes unnecessary. Follow-up care can include repeated blood tests or abdominal ultrasonography or radiography. There are times, however, when no method of investigation provides enough information for a confident diagnosis, and exploratory laparotomy is needed. The importance of laparotomy for diagnosis must not be overlooked, but the decision to operate must be judicious.

BIBLIOGRAPHY

Ambrosetti P, Grossholz M, Becker C, et al. Computed tomography in acute left colonic diverticulitis. *Br J Surg* 1997;84:532–534.

Grossman SJ, Joyce JM. Hepatobiliary imaging. *Emerg Med Clin North Am* 1991;9:853–874.

Irish MS, Pearl RH, Caty MG, et al. The approach to common abdominal diagnosis in infants and children. *Pediatr Clin North Am* 1998;45: 729–772.

Johnson GL, Johnson PT, Fishman EK. CT evaluation of the acute abdomen: bowel pathology spectrum of disease. *Crit Rev Diagn Imaging* 1996;37:163–190.

Levine JS, Jacobson ED. Intestinal ischemic disorders. *Dig Dis* 1995;13: 3–24.

Navez B, d'Udekem Y, Cambier E, et al. Laparoscopy for management of nontraumatic acute abdomen. *World J Surg* 1995;19:382–387.

Neff CC, vanSonnenberg E. CT of diverticulitis: diagnosis and treatment. *Radiol Clin North Am* 1989;27:743–752.

Salky BA, Edye MB. The role of laparoscopy in the diagnosis and treatment of abdominal pain syndromes. *Surg Endosc* 1998;12:911–914.

Silen W. *Cope's early diagnosis of the acute abdomen,* 16th ed. New York: Oxford University Press, 1983.

Tarraza HM, Moore RD. Gynecologic causes of the acute abdomen and the acute abdomen in pregnancy. *Surg Clin North Am* 1997;77:1371–1394.

Kelley's Textbook of Internal Medicine, fourth edition. Edited by H. David Humes.
Lippincott Williams & Wilkins, Philadelphia © 2000.

C H A P T E R

98

APPROACH TO THE PATIENT WITH NAUSEA AND VOMITING

WILLIAM L. HASLER

Nausea and vomiting are nonspecific symptomatic responses to a variety of conditions. *Nausea* is the subjective sensation of an impending urge to vomit, usually perceived in the throat or epigastrium. *Vomiting* is the forceful ejection of gastroesophageal contents from the mouth. Although usually preceded by nausea, vomiting may occur without nausea. *Retching* may precede vomiting but involves no discharge of gastric contents from the mouth.

Nausea and vomiting should be differentiated from other symptoms. *Regurgitation* is the effortless return of gastroesophageal contents into the mouth without nausea or somatic muscle contraction. *Rumination* is regurgitation with rechewing and re-swallowing of food, often multiple times after a meal. *Anorexia* is loss of appetite, which may or may not be associated with nausea. *Early satiety* is a sensation of gastric fullness before completion of a meal. Nausea may be part of the general feeling of *indigestion,* which includes discomfort, heartburn, anorexia, and bloating.

Nausea and vomiting have socioeconomic effects on patients' lives. Most patients with nausea due to enteric infection restrict their activities. Pregnant women with first-trimester nausea report fatigue, sleep disturbances, and irritability. Nausea and vomiting after cancer chemotherapy or in the postoperative period reduce time spent on leisure activities, household tasks, and socializing. Employee productivity is markedly impaired by acute enteric infection, nausea of pregnancy, and cancer chemotherapy. Postoperative nausea and vomiting greatly increase the costs of the operation of outpatient surgical centers.

PATHOPHYSIOLOGY

Vomiting is caused by coordinated interaction of neural, humoral, somatic muscular, and gastrointestinal myoelectric and muscular phenomena. What is known about the pathways that mediate vomiting comes from studies involving ablation of neural structures in experimental animals. The mechanisms that result in nausea are less well understood. Whereas vomiting may be generated in decerebrate animals, nausea requires activation of selected cerebrocortical sites.

ACTIVATION OF THE EMETIC RESPONSE

Vomiting is initiated by stimulation of structures in the central (CNS) and peripheral nervous systems (Fig. 98.1). The area postrema in the dorsal medulla of the brainstem represents the chemoreceptor trigger zone in response to a number of neurochemical activators. Other CNS and peripheral afferent sites mediate emesis after other stimuli. Because of its location and lack of a tight blood-brain barrier, the area postrema is an interface to receive neural input and to sample chemical activators in the bloodstream and cerebrospinal fluid. The area postrema stimulant apomorphine, a dopamine D_2 receptor agonist, induces emesis when applied to the structure, and ablation of the area postrema prevents apomorphine-evoked emesis. Drugs (digoxin, opiates, nicotine, ergot alkaloids, some cancer chemotherapies), metabolic disorders (uremia, diabetic ketoacidosis, hypoxemia, hypercalcemia), radiation therapy, and exposure to bacterial toxins induce vomiting through activation of the area postrema. In addition to D_2 receptors, the area postrema is rich in muscarinic M_1, histaminic H_1, and serotonergic 5-HT$_3$ receptors; there are therapeutic roles for antagonists of these receptor subtypes.

Other CNS sites may provide stimuli for emesis. Cerebral pathways mediate vomiting caused by exposure to noxious

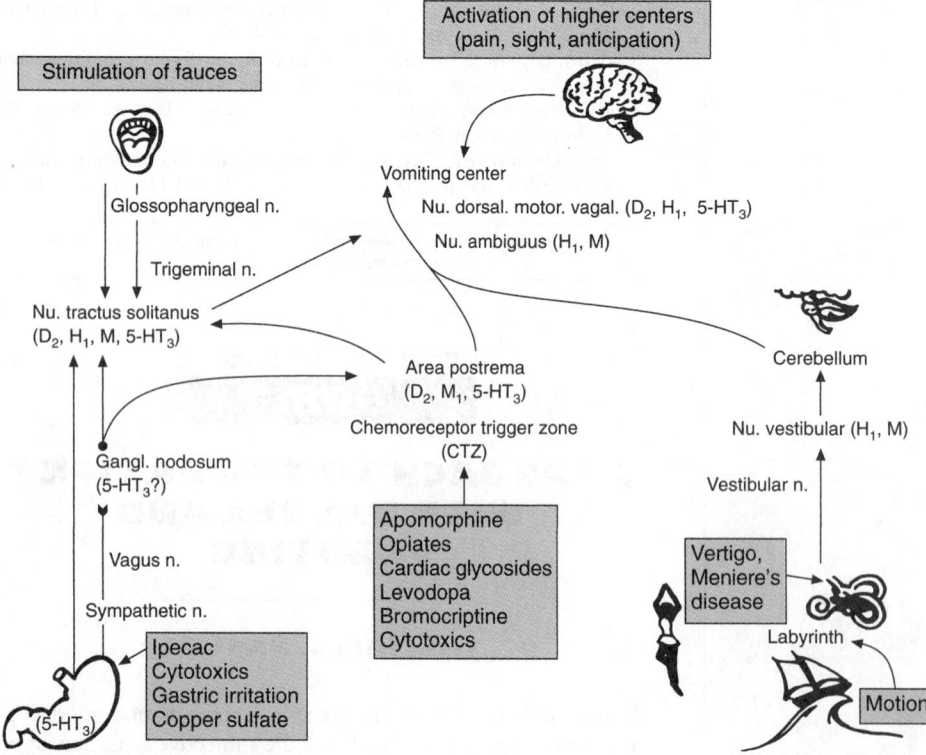

FIGURE 98.1. Afferent neural pathways and receptor populations involved in vomiting as determined by means of experimental studies with animals. Selected brainstem nuclei coordinate vomiting after activation of cortical, oral, vestibular, or peripheral afferents or the area postrema. (Mitchelson F. Pharmacological agents affecting emesis. *Drugs* 1992; 43(3):295–315, with permission.)

odors, visual stimulation, somatic pain, and unpleasant tastes. Activated brainstem vestibular nuclei mediate emesis caused by motion sickness, labyrinthine infections or tumors, or Meniere's disease through pathways independent of the area postrema. Muscarinic M_1 and histaminergic H_1 but not dopaminergic or serotonergic pathways have important roles in motion sickness. Therefore use of antimuscarinic and antihistaminergic agents to manage this condition brings about an antiemetic response.

Gastric irritants such as copper sulfate, salicylate, and antral distention activate afferent nerves that project from the stomach. Nongastric intraperitoneal afferent stimuli that evoke emesis include distention of the colon, small intestine, and bile ducts, peritoneal inflammation, and mesenteric vascular occlusion. Stimuli also may originate from the heart and pharynx. These findings explain emesis induced by peritonitis, mesenteric ischemia, and myocardial infarction. Emetic responses to many peripheral stimuli are mediated by vagal pathways. Vagotomy prevents emesis after intragastric exposure to copper sulfate and reduces vomiting provoked by the chemotherapeutic agent cisplatinum and by abdominal irradiation. Area postrema ablation, however, has little effect on copper sulfate–evoked vomiting. Serotonergic 5-HT_3 (and possibly 5-HT_4) receptors mediate the effects of many peripherally active emetic agents. Thus serotonin receptor antagonists are effective in controlling vomiting caused by selected peripheral exposure to stimuli such as cisplatinum.

CENTRAL NERVOUS SYSTEM COORDINATION OF THE ACT OF VOMITING

Multiple brainstem sites mediate the act of vomiting in response to emetic stimuli from the activator sites. These include the nucleus tractus solitarius, the dorsal vagal and phrenic nuclei, medullary nuclei involved in respiration, the nucleus ambiguus, which supplies the laryngeal and pharyngeal musculature, and the trigeminal, facial, and hypoglossal nuclei, which serve the facial and tongue muscles. Once activated, these structures provide somatic stimulation to the diaphragm along cervical spinal pathways and to the external muscles through the thoracolumbar spinal nerves. Neurotransmitters involved in these processes are poorly understood.

PERIPHERAL RESPONSES TO INITIATION OF VOMITING

Somatic Muscular Events Associated with Vomiting

Emesis is caused by a stereotypical series of somatic muscle actions. During retching, inspiratory thoracic, diaphragmatic, and abdominal muscles contract concurrently against a closed glottis. The resulting high positive intra-abdominal pressure forces gastric contents into the esophagus and herniates the gastric cardia into the thorax. High negative intrathoracic pressure prevents expulsion of luminal contents into the mouth. In contrast, both intra-abdominal and intrathoracic pressures are positive during vomiting because of a lack of diaphragmatic contraction in the crural region that allows transmission of the high positive abdominal pressure into the thorax. With vomiting, the high positive intrathoracic pressure is the force for expulsion of luminal contents into the mouth. Oral propulsion of the vomitus is facilitated by movement of the hyoid bone and larynx up and forward. Glottic closure prevents pulmonary aspiration of gastroesophageal contents. Elevation of the soft palate prevents passage of the vomitus into the nasal cavities.

Gastrointestinal Myoelectric and Motor Events Associated with Nausea and Vomiting

Gastrointestinal motility is regulated by oscillatory electrical activity known as the *slow wave,* which controls the maximal frequency and the direction of contractions (see Chapter 129). In the stomach, a pacemaker in the gastric body generates slow waves at three cycles per minute that propagate to the pylorus. Small-intestinal slow waves originate in the proximal duodenum at 11 to 12 cycles per minute. Patients with nausea from pregnancy, gastroparesis, nonulcer dyspepsia, and motion sickness have abnormalities of gastric slow-wave frequency, including accelerated (tachygastria) or decelerated (bradygastria) cycling. Because slow-wave amplitudes are very low with tachygastria, this condition causes gastric atony. Bradygastria produces chaotic but infrequent slow waves that produce uncoordinated and ineffective gastric contractions. The causative relation between gastric dysrhythmias and the sensation of nausea is unclear.

With vomiting, gastrointestinal myoelectric and motor events are more pronounced. Before emesis, intestinal slow waves are abolished and followed by bursts of electrical spikes that propagate orally. A retroperistaltic contractile complex begins in the middle small intestine and propagates into the stomach, causing enterogastric reflux. Pyloric closure, antral contraction, and lower esophageal sphincter relaxation facilitate evacuation of the intragastric contents. Blockade of these motor events by atropine does not prevent emesis, indicating that they are not strictly needed for vomiting to occur but enhance evacuation of luminal contents.

Endocrinologic and Autonomic Responses to Induction of Nausea and Vomiting

Levels of circulating hormones and neurotransmitters are altered with nausea and vomiting. Vasopressin levels increase during motion sickness and after administration of apomorphine and cisplatinum. Among monkeys, vasopressin V_1 antagonists prevent motion-induced emesis. This finding suggests a possible pathogenic role of vasopressin. Levels of other transmitters such as epinephrine, β-endorphin, and cortisol change during nausea and vomiting, but the pathogenic importance of these alterations is uncertain. Autonomic neural disturbances are caused by the proximity of brainstem nuclei that mediate vomiting to those that control respiratory, vasomotor, cardiac, and salivary activity. Pallor, diaphoresis, hypersalivation, defecation, tachycardia, and hypotension may occur with nausea. Bradycardia, blood pressure variations, and respiratory interruption may occur with retching or vomiting.

DIFFERENTIAL DIAGNOSIS OF NAUSEA AND VOMITING

The differential diagnosis of nausea and vomiting is extensive. It includes a broad range of pathologic and physiologic conditions that affect the gastrointestinal tract, peritoneal cavity, central nervous system, and endocrine and metabolic functions (Table 98.1).

MEDICATIONS

Drug reactions are among the most common causes of nausea and vomiting and usually occur soon after initiation of therapy. The most extensively studied medications that evoke emesis are cancer chemotherapeutic agents. Emesis from chemotherapy may be acute, delayed, and anticipatory. Potent agents that induce acute vomiting within hours of administration include cis-

---

TABLE 98.1.   DIFFERENTIAL DIAGNOSIS OF NAUSEA AND VOMITING

Medications

Cancer chemotherapy
 Severe—cisplatinum, dacarbazine, nitrogen mustard
 Moderate—etoposide, methotrexate, cytarabine
 Mild—fluorouracil, vinblastine, tamoxifen
Analgesics
 Aspirin
 Nonsteroidal anti-inflammatory drugs
 Auranofin
 Anti-gout drugs
Cardiovascular medications
 Digoxin
 Antiarrhythmics
 Antihypertensives
 β-Blockers
 Calcium channel antagonists
Diuretics
Hormonal preparations
 Oral antidiabetic agents
 Oral contraceptives
Antibiotics
 Erythromycin
 Clarithromycin
 Tetracycline
 Sulfonamides
 Antituberculous drugs
 Acyclovir
Gastrointestinal medications
 Sulfasalazine
 Azathioprine
Central nervous system active
 Narcotics
 Anti-parkinsonian drugs
 Anticonvulsants
Antiasthmatic agents
 Theophylline

Disorders of the Gastrointestinal Tract and Peritoneal Cavity

Mechanical obstruction
 Gastric outlet obstruction
 Small-intestinal obstruction
 Superior mesenteric artery syndrome
Functional gastrointestinal disorders
 Gastroparesis
 Chronic intestinal pseudoobstruction
 Nonulcer dyspepsia
 Irritable bowel syndrome
 Pancreatic adenocarcinoma
Radiation therapy
Intraperitoneal inflammatory disease
 Ulcer disease

Cholecystitis
Pancreatitis
Hepatitis
Crohn's disease

Central Nervous System Causes

Increased intracranial pressure
 Malignant tumor
 Infarction
 Hemorrhage
 Abscess
 Meningitis
 Congenital malformation
Emotional responses
Psychiatric disease
 Psychogenic vomiting
 Anxiety disorders
 Depression
 Anorexia nervosa
 Bulimia
Labyrinthine disorders
 Motion sickness
 Labyrinthitis
 Tumors
 Meniere's disease

Endocrinologic and Metabolic Causes

Pregnancy
 Uremia
 Diabetic ketoacidosis
 Hyperparathyroidism
 Hypoparathyroidism
 Hyperthyroidism
 Addison's disease

Infectious Causes

Gastroenteritis
 Viral
 Bacterial
Nongastrointestinal infection
 Otitis media

Miscellaneous Causes

Postoperative nausea and vomiting
Cyclic vomiting syndrome
Cardiac disease
 Myocardial infarction
 Congestive heart failure
Ethanol abuse
Jamaican vomiting sickness
Hypervitaminosis
Starvation

platinum, nitrogen mustard, and dacarbazine, which act by activating 5-HT$_3$ receptors on vagal afferent fibers and the area postrema. In contrast, acute vomiting from less emetogenic agents such as cyclophosphamide and delayed and anticipatory nausea are mediated by serotonin-independent pathways. Analgesics such as aspirin or nonsteroidal anti-inflammatory drugs induce nausea through direct irritation of mucosal afferent fibers. Other drugs with emetic properties include cardiac antiarrhythmics, antihypertensive agents, diuretics, antidiabetic drugs, contraceptives, antibiotics such as erythromycin, and gastrointestinal medications such as sulfasalazine.

INFECTIOUS AND TOXIC CAUSES

Infectious illness produces nausea and vomiting that usually is of acute onset. Acute enteric infection is most prevalent among children younger than 3 years and often occurs in the autumn and winter. Viral gastroenteritis may be caused by rotaviruses, reoviruses, adenoviruses, and the Hawaii, Snow Mountain, and Norwalk agents. Bacterial infection with *Staphylococcus aureus*, *Salmonella* organisms, *Bacillus cereus*, and *Clostridium perfringens* also produces nausea and vomiting, in many cases through the action of toxins on the area postrema. Nausea among immunosuppressed patients is caused by gastrointestinal infection with cytomegalovirus or herpes simplex virus. Nongastrointestinal infections that produce nausea include otitis media, meningitis, and hepatitis.

DISORDERS OF THE GASTROINTESTINAL TRACT AND PERITONEAL CAVITY

Gastrointestinal and peritoneal disorders represent prevalent causes of nausea and vomiting. Gastric or small-intestinal obstruction produces prominent nausea that may be relieved by vomiting. Gastric outlet obstruction often is intermittent, whereas small-intestinal obstruction usually is acute and associated with abdominal pain. Superior mesenteric artery syndrome is a rare condition in which the duodenum is compressed by the overlying superior mesenteric artery as it originates from the aorta, producing anatomic obstruction. This syndrome occurs among patients who have had profound weight loss, a recent surgical procedure, or prolonged bed rest.

Motility disorders such as gastroparesis or chronic intestinal pseudoobstruction produce nausea due to an inability to clear retained food. Gastroparesis is caused by diabetes, scleroderma, systemic lupus erythematosus, amyloidosis, or pancreatic adenocarcinoma. It also can develop after vagotomy or in the absence of other diseases. Idiopathic gastroparesis may be preceded by a viral prodrome of diarrhea, fever, headache, or myalgia. Chronic intestinal pseudoobstruction may be hereditary or caused by a systemic disease that produces gastroparesis. Paraneoplastic pseudoobstruction occurs with some malignant tumors such as small-cell carcinoma of the lung. Nausea may be prominent among patients with nonulcer dyspepsia who also may have delayed gastric emptying.

Abdominal radiation therapy produces emesis among as many as 80% of patients by means of effects on the structure and function of the gastrointestinal tract. Involvement of seroto-

nergic pathways is indicated by the ability of 5-HT$_3$ receptor antagonists to reduce emesis evoked by abdominal irradiation.

Abdominal disorders that do not involve the gastrointestinal lumen may produce nausea and vomiting. Inflammatory conditions such as pancreatitis, appendicitis, and cholecystitis activate afferent pathways from the peritoneum. Biliary colic in the absence of inflammation produces nausea through activation of afferent fibers from distention of the biliary tree. Fulminant hepatic failure results in nausea, presumably because of retention of unknown emetic toxins and increased intracranial pressure.

CENTRAL NERVOUS SYSTEM CAUSES

Many emetic stimuli produce symptoms through action on the cerebrum or brainstem. Increased intracranial pressure from malignant tumors, infarction, hemorrhage, or infection may produce emesis with or without nausea. Emotional responses to unpleasant smells, tastes, or memories may induce vomiting. Psychogenic vomiting occurs most commonly among young women, often with a history of psychiatric illness or social difficulties. Other psychiatric conditions accompanied by nausea include anxiety disorders, depression, anorexia nervosa, and bulimia.

Labyrinthine disorders such as labyrinthitis, tumors, and Meniere's disease produce nausea and vomiting, often with vertigo. Motion sickness is evoked by repetitive movements that activate the vestibular nuclei and is associated with extensive autonomic activation that produces pallor, diaphoresis, and salivation. Space sickness, experienced by most astronauts in zero gravity, is related to motion sickness but may not have the associated autonomic phenomena.

ENDOCRINOLOGIC AND METABOLIC CONDITIONS

Endocrinologic and metabolic causes of nausea include uremia, diabetic ketoacidosis, hyper- and hypoparathyroidism, hyperthyroidism, and Addison's disease. Pregnancy is the most common endocrinologic cause of emesis, which occurs among about 70% of pregnant women. The condition peaks in the ninth week of gestation and is not deleterious to either mother or fetus. Hyperemesis gravidarum, however, a condition of intractable vomiting that complicates 1% to 5% of pregnancies, may produce dangerous fluid and electrolyte abnormalities. The cause of nausea of pregnancy is unknown but is believed to be hormone-related. Acute fatty liver of pregnancy, a condition distinct from first trimester nausea, produces third-trimester emesis and can be complicated by liver failure, disseminated intravascular coagulation, and fetal or maternal death.

MISCELLANEOUS CONDITIONS

Nausea and vomiting complicate 17% to 37% of operations, more commonly among women. Postoperative nausea and vomiting occur more frequently after general anesthesia and abdominal and orthopedic procedures, rather than after laparoscopic and extra-abdominal procedures other than orthopedic operations. Cyclic vomiting syndrome produces discrete attacks of intractable vomiting. The mean age at onset is 5 years; the syndrome occurs very rarely among adults. Children with this syndrome typically have eight attacks per year that last an average of 20 hours. The pathogenesis is likely multifactorial, but a strong association with migraine headaches has been reported and some patients respond to antimigraine therapy. Posterior myocardial infarction produces nausea due to diaphragmatic irritation. Nausea may occur in congestive heart failure from passive congestion of the liver and gastrointestinal tract. Excess ethanol induces vomiting through local action on the gastrointestinal tract and through action on the brainstem. Jamaican vomiting sickness occurs after one eats unripe akee fruit. Excess vitamin intake and extended fasting or starvation also may cause nausea.

HISTORY AND PHYSICAL EXAMINATION

HISTORICAL FEATURES

A detailed history provides useful diagnostic information about the cause of unexplained nausea and emesis. Acute vomiting (1 to 2 days) most often is caused by infection, a medication or toxin, or accumulation of endogenous toxins, as in uremia or diabetic ketoacidosis. Chronic vomiting (more than 1 week) usually is caused by a long-standing medical or psychiatric condition.

Timing of Nausea and Vomiting

The timing of symptoms provides clues to the underlying disease. Vomiting soon after a meal occurs with gastric obstruction from ulcer disease or a malignant tumor. Psychogenic vomiting also occurs soon after eating, but most patients control the act of emesis until a convenient receptacle is available. Patients with gastroparesis may report nausea within 5 minutes of eating, but most have symptoms more than 1 hour after a meal. Nausea and vomiting from inflammatory conditions such as cholecystitis and pancreatitis may occur in the first postprandial hour. With some cases of esophagitis or ulcer disease, nausea may abate with eating. Vomiting early in the morning is characteristic of first-trimester pregnancy, uremia, and chronic alcoholism.

Character of the Vomitus

The characteristics of the vomitus can assist in diagnosis. Return of undigested food suggests achalasia or Zenker's diverticulum. Vomiting of partly digested food hours or days after ingestion suggests gastric obstruction or gastroparesis. Bile in the vomitus excludes obstruction proximal to the ampulla of Vater, whereas blood or coffee-ground material suggests a process with mucosal damage such as an ulcer or malignant tumor. However, retching and vomiting can induce hematemesis from Mallory–Weiss tears across the gastroesophageal junction. Voluminous, clear, acidic vomitus suggests gastric hypersecretion from Zollinger–Ellison syndrome. Feculent emesis occurs with distal intestinal or colonic obstruction, intestinal bacterial overgrowth, and gastro-

colic fistula. Odorless emesis may be found with gastric achlorhydria.

Symptoms Associated with Nausea and Vomiting

Abdominal pain occurs with ulcer disease, intestinal obstruction, and inflammatory disorders such as cholecystitis and pancreatitis. Vomiting may relieve nausea and pain in ulcer disease and intestinal obstruction but has no effect in inflammatory conditions. The presence of diarrhea, fever, or myalgia suggests enteric infection. Weight loss and malnutrition occur with chronic illness, but psychogenic vomiting rarely produces weight loss. Meningitis or CNS lesions are suggested by headaches, visual changes, altered mentation, and neck stiffness. In these disorders, emesis may be effortless, there may be no nausea, or emesis may be projectile. Labyrinthine diseases become manifest with tinnitus or vertigo. Chest pain, dysphagia, or jaundice suggests pregnancy or cardiac, esophageal, or hepatobiliary disease. Associated symptoms also indicate the severity of the underlying condition and help to direct treatment. Prolonged vomiting may produce substantial fluid and electrolyte loss, which may be manifested as postural light-headedness, rapid heart rate, and mouth dryness.

Complications of Nausea and Vomiting

Gastrointestinal hemorrhage may be caused by retch-induced mucosal tears across the gastroesophageal junction, known as Mallory–Weiss tears. A more severe complication, Boerhaave's syndrome, occurs when retching or vomiting produces complete esophageal rupture with mediastinitis or peritonitis. Among patients with impaired consciousness, emesis may be complicated by pulmonary aspiration of acidic material that leads to severe chemical pneumonitis.

PHYSICAL EXAMINATION FINDINGS

The physical examination assists in the diagnosis and management of nausea and vomiting. Fever suggests infection or inflammation. Tachycardia or orthostatic hypotension indicates dehydration, which is supported by finding a loss of skin turgor or dry mucous membranes. Skin examination may show sclerodactyly in scleroderma or jaundice with hepatobiliary disease. Oral examination may reveal loss of dental enamel, common in bulimia. Adenopathy raises the possibility of a neoplasm. Hepatomegaly also is found in malignant disease, as is benign hepatic disease. An absence of bowel sounds indicates ileus, whereas high-pitched hyperactive bowel sounds with a distended abdomen are a sign of intestinal obstruction. A succession splash on side-to-side movement occurs in gastric obstruction or gastroparesis. If abdominal tenderness or guarding is found, inflammation or infection such as an ulcer, cholecystitis, pancreatitis, or peritonitis is considered. The finding of gross or occult fecal blood at rectal examination prompts evaluation for an ulcer or neoplasm. At neurologic examination, focal signs, papilledema, and impaired mentation suggest a CNS process, whereas nuchal rigidity is consistent with meningitis. Asterixis is present in metabolic diseases such as uremia or hepatic failure. Patients with gastrointestinal motility disturbances may have peripheral or autonomic neuropathy.

LABORATORY STUDIES AND DIAGNOSTIC TESTING

A thorough history interview and examination provide the information necessary for a diagnosis and for treatment of most patients with nausea and vomiting. However, some patients require blood studies, structural evaluations, or assessment of gastrointestinal function for diagnosis and treatment (Fig. 98.2).

LABORATORY TESTING

Laboratory tests are ordered on the basis of findings in the history and physical examination. With long-standing symptoms or dehydration, serum electrolyte measurements can show hypokalemia or an elevated blood urea nitrogen level relative to creatinine level. Metabolic alkalosis may be caused by loss of hydrogen ions in the acidic vomitus and contraction of the extracellular space from dehydration. A complete blood cell count can be used to rule out anemia from inflammation or blood loss, leukocytosis from an inflammatory source, or leukopenia from a viral infection. Chronic blood loss also may be suggested by a low serum iron level and iron saturation of transferrin. Hypoalbuminemia

occurs with some chronic diseases and in conditions with gastrointestinal protein loss. Amylase, lipase, and liver chemical analyses are performed when pancreatic or hepatobiliary disease is suspected. Endocrinologic and metabolic causes can be assessed through serum pregnancy testing, thyroid function testing, and measurement of blood urea nitrogen, creatinine, glucose, ketones, calcium, and plasma cortisol. Specific serologic markers can be obtained for presumed collagen vascular diseases such as lupus erythematosus, whereas antineuronal nuclear antibodies are present with paraneoplastic intestinal pseudoobstruction (usually from small-cell carcinoma of the lung). The presence of meningitis is confirmed by means of lumbar puncture.

STRUCTURAL EVALUATION

Structural investigation may be needed to exclude organic disease as a cause of emesis. Flat and upright abdominal radiographs are obtained as a screening examination. Air-fluid levels in the small intestine with an absence of colonic air suggests intestinal obstruction, whereas diffuse luminal distention with absent bowel sounds indicates ileus or chronic pseudoobstruction. Subdiaphragmatic free air indicates visceral perforation. Small-intestinal barium radiography may help confirm suspected partial intestinal obstruction. If symptoms are intermittent and intermittent obstruction is highly likely, enteroclysis may provide a more detailed assessment of the small-intestinal lumen. If colonic obstruction is a consideration, colonoscopy or barium enema radiography are performed before small-intestinal contrast studies. Upper gastrointestinal endoscopy or contrast radiography may be performed in cases of suspected ulcer disease or outlet narrowing. Endoscopy affords the advantage of allowing biopsy of abnormal mucosa. Endoscopy also may suggest gastroparesis, demonstrating retained food in the absence of outlet obstruction. For suspected pancreaticobiliary disease, ultrasonography or computed tomography may be useful. Biliary scintigraphy may provide findings that suggest acute cholecystitis. Computed tomography or magnetic resonance imaging of the head is indicated if the signs and symptoms indicate a CNS cause. If intestinal ischemia is a consideration, mesenteric angiography or magnetic resonance imaging of mesenteric flow may provide enough information for a diagnosis.

STUDIES OF GASTROINTESTINAL MOTOR AND MYOELECTRIC ACTIVITY

When luminal obstruction has been excluded, functional causes of nausea such as gastroparesis and pseudoobstruction are entertained. The clinician may treat the patient empirically with medication designed to stimulate gastrointestinal motility. An alternative is to test gastrointestinal motor and myoelectric activity to characterize the functional defects (see Chapter 129).

Quantification of Gastric Emptying

Gastroparesis is diagnosed through the demonstration of delayed gastric emptying of an ingested meal. Scintigraphic measures of the emptying rates of solid (such as technetium Tc 99m sulfur colloid in scrambled eggs) or liquid (such as indium In 111

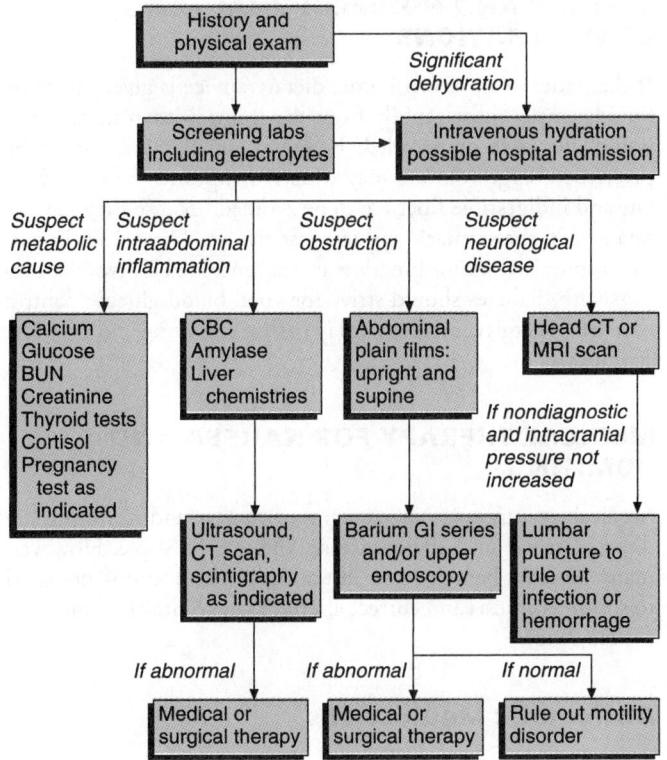

FIGURE 98.2. Evaluation of nausea and vomiting.
EVIDENCE LEVEL: C. Expert Opinion.

diethylenetriamine pentaacetic acid [DTPA] in water) radionuclides are the most commonly used tests of gastric emptying. Gastroparesis affects solid-phase emptying to a greater extent than does liquid-phase emptying. Thus solid-phase scintiscans are more sensitive for diagnosis. Other means of quantifying gastric emptying are under investigation including magnetic resonance imaging and ultrasonography. A promising new technology is the carbon C 13 octanoate breath test. Because this test involves ingestion of a nonradioactive ligand, it may be used in examinations of children and pregnant women, for whom scintigraphy is relatively contraindicated.

Gastrointestinal Manometry

When scintigraphy does not provide enough information for a diagnosis of the cause of nausea, gastrointestinal manometry can be performed. Because of the discomfort involved and the personnel required, this test is performed only in specialized centers. Under fasting conditions, the stomach and small intestine exhibit a pattern known as the migrating motor complex, which consists of three phases that repeat every 90 to 120 minutes. The most propulsive phase, phase III, clears undigested debris from the upper gastrointestinal tract. Absence of gastric phase III, found in some cases of gastroparesis, is a predisposing factor for bezoar formation. Loss of intestinal phase III may lead to bacterial overgrowth. The postprandial period exhibits irregular, continuous contractions. The absence of this fed pattern in the stomach correlates with delayed solid-phase gastric emptying.

In addition to defining gastric dysmotility, manometry also is used to characterize small-intestinal motor disturbances. In intestinal pseudoobstruction, barium radiography may show intestinal dilatation and delayed transit. Manometry of the small intestine provides more specific information regarding the neuropathic or myopathic nature of the condition. Pseudoobstruction resulting from enteric nerve dysfunction, as with the familial visceral neuropathies or early scleroderma, produces intense, uncoordinated bursts of motor activity, whereas smooth-muscle dysfunction in familial visceral myopathy or late scleroderma produces contractions of very low amplitude. These patterns can be nonspecific, thus surgical full-thickness intestinal biopsy may be needed to document degeneration of nerve or muscle layers.

Electrogastrography

Gastric myoelectric disturbances are diagnosed in referral centers by means of electrogastrography, a technique with which slow waves are measured using cutaneous electrodes over the stomach. Recordings for healthy persons show a rhythm of three cycles per minute that increases in amplitude after eating. Patients with nausea may have symptoms that correlate with abnormally rapid (tachygastria) or slow (bradygastria) rhythms or with an absence of the postprandial signal increase. Because many patients with delayed gastric emptying have altered slow-wave activity, electrogastrography has been proposed as a nonradioactive means of diagnosing gastroparesis. Electrogastrographic findings also may be abnormal among some patients with nausea who have normal gastric emptying. The suggestion is that this test may help define patient populations with primary slow-wave dysrhythmia.

■ STRATEGIES FOR OPTIMAL CARE

Care of a patient with nausea and vomiting involves assessment of the cause and the severity of the condition and initiation of therapy to prevent complications.

🏥 Indications for HOSPITALIZATION

The first decision in treating a patient with vomiting is to determine whether intravenous resuscitation is needed. Poor skin turgor or orthostatic pulse or blood pressure changes indicate that more than 10% of body fluids have been lost, mandating intravenous infusion of saline solution (0.45% or 0.9%). Potassium supplements may be started for hypokalemia if urine output is adequate. Intravenous fluids can be given in the emergency department or outpatient clinic if the patient is expected to resume adequate oral intake at home. If prospects for oral replenishment are uncertain, hospitalization should be considered. Patients with mechanical obstruction or ileus may benefit from nasogastric suction. The threshold for hospitalization should be lowered for patients with diabetes, patients with concurrent diarrhea, persons with another chronic debilitating disease, and very young or very old patients; these persons become rapidly dehydrated.

DIETARY AND NONMEDICINAL CONSIDERATIONS

If the patient can return home, dietary advice is given. Because liquids empty more rapidly from the stomach than do solids, a liquid diet is recommended. Frequent, small meals should be prescribed; large volumes may worsen symptoms. Foods rich in fats and indigestible fiber are to be avoided because they may be retained in the stomach and increase nausea. Drugs that impair gastrointestinal motor function are discontinued if possible. Persons with diabetes should strive for good blood glucose control because hyperglycemia may delay gastric emptying and promote symptoms.

MEDICAL THERAPY FOR NAUSEA AND VOMITING

Medical or surgical management of nausea and vomiting are directed at the underlying disease whenever possible. However, many patients benefit from initiation of medications designed to suppress emesis and correct aberrant gastrointestinal function (Table 98.2).

Antiemetic Medications

Antiemetic drugs that act on CNS muscarinic, cholinergic, histamine, or dopamine receptors reduce symptoms in many cases. Use of these agents is tailored to the underlying emetic stimulus.

TABLE 98.2. ANTIEMETIC AGENTS FOR SPECIFIC CLINICAL INDICATIONS

Clinical Indication	Mechanism of Antiemetic Action
Motion Sickness Treatment and Prophylaxis	
Meclizine, dimenhydrinate	Vestibular histamine receptor antagonism
Scopolamine	Vestibular muscarinic receptor antagonism
Antiemetic Control of Area Postrema Stimulation	
Phenothiazines	CNS dopamine receptor antagonism
Butyrophenones	CNS dopamine receptor antagonism
Prokinetic Stimulation of Gastrointestinal Motility	
Cisapride	$5\text{-}HT_4$ receptor facilitation of enteric cholinergic nerve function
	$5\text{-}HT_3$ receptor antagonism (weak)
	Direct smooth muscle stimulation
Metoclopramide	$5\text{-}HT_4$ receptor facilitation of enteric cholinergic nerve function
	CNS and gastric dopamine receptor antagonism
	$5\text{-}HT_3$ receptor antagonism (weak)
Domperidone	Area postrema and gastric dopamine receptor antagonism
Erythromycin	Enteric motilin receptor agonism
Bethanechol	Smooth muscle muscarinic agonism
Octreotide	Somatostatin analog
Leuprolide	Gonadotropin-releasing hormone analog
Prophylaxis of Cancer Chemotherapy Emesis	
Ondansetron, granisetron	CNS and peripheral $5\text{-}HT_3$ receptor antagonism
Metoclopramide	Dopamine receptor antagonism; $5\text{-}HT_3$ receptor antagonism
Phenothiazines	Dopamine receptor antagonism
Corticosteroids	?Inhibition of prostaglandin synthesis
Benzodiazepines	Prevention of anticipatory nausea by means of sedation; ?Action on CNS GABA receptors
Cannabinoids	?Inhibition of prostaglandin synthesis; ?Stimulation of production of endogenous endorphins

CNS, central nervous system; 5-HT, serotonin; GABA, γ-aminobutyric acid.

and urinary retention impair the usefulness of these drugs for some persons.

Dopamine antagonists, including phenothiazines (prochlorperazine, chlorpromazine) and butyrophenones (droperidol, haloperidol), are the most commonly prescribed antiemetics. These agents act on area postrema D_2 receptors and are effective against emesis caused by gastroenteritis, medications, and toxins and by some chemotherapeutic agents, abdominal irradiation, and surgery. Antidopaminergic agents produce many CNS side effects, including drowsiness, insomnia, anxiety, mood changes, confusion, dystonic reactions, parkinsonian symptoms, and irreversible tardive dyskinesia. Through effects on the pituitary gland, antidopaminergic agents may induce hyperprolactinemia that leads to breast engorgement, galactorrhea, and sexual dysfunction. Other side effects include blood dyscrasia and jaundice. Many antidopaminergic drugs have effects on other receptor subtypes and provoke antihistaminic and antimuscarinic side effects.

Prokinetic Agents for Gastroparesis and Intestinal Dysmotility

Gastrointestinal motility disorders may respond to drugs that stimulate gastric emptying and intestinal transit. These agents often are given before meals to enhance gastric emptying with a dose at bedtime to effect gastrointestinal clearance of undigested residue during sleep. Cisapride has become the initial drug of choice in the care of selected patients with gastroparesis and pseudoobstruction. Cisapride acts by means of $5\text{-}HT_4$ receptor facilitation of gastrointestinal cholinergic transmission and potently stimulates gastric emptying. Rare side effects include headache, abdominal cramps, and diarrhea due to colonic stimulation. Cisapride should be prescribed judiciously because of reports of potentially fatal cardiac arrhythmias among patients with cardiac disease or taking other medications.

Like cisapride, metoclopramide acts by means of $5\text{-}HT_4$ receptor facilitation of gastric cholinergic function, but the drug also acts as a dopamine D_2 antagonist in the stomach and brainstem. The prokinetic properties of metoclopramide are limited to the proximal gastrointestinal tract, thus the drug is useful for gastroparesis but not for small-intestinal or colonic dysmotility. Because of central antidopaminergic side effects, metoclopramide is poorly tolerated by as many as 20% of patients.

Domperidone is a dopamine D_2 antagonist with prokinetic properties. It crosses only into CNS regions with porous blood-brain barriers such as the area postrema and thus exhibits a superior side-effect profile to that of metoclopramide. The drug is prescribed throughout much of the world but is not available in the United States. Because of a lack of enteric cholinergic stimulation, domperidone is a weaker prokinetic agent than are metoclopramide and cisapride, but the drug still has marked symptomatic efficacy in the treatment of patients with gastroparesis. Although dystonic reactions do not occur with domperidone, hyperprolactinemia is a problem because of the incomplete blood-brain barrier of the anterior pituitary gland.

Other prokinetic agents can be used to manage gastrointestinal motor dysfunction. The macrolide antibiotic erythromycin induces upper gastrointestinal contractions and promotes gastric

Antihistamines such as meclizine and dimenhydrinate are useful for vomiting with labyrinthine disorders, such as motion sickness or labyrinthitis. They also are effective in controlling nausea caused by uremia or the postoperative state. Antihistamines are safe, although sedation and dryness of the mouth may limit their use. Newer, less sedating antihistamines such as astemizole have limited antiemetic activity.

Drugs such as scopolamine that antagonize muscarinic receptors in vestibular pathways also are effective in controlling motion sickness when given orally or transdermally. Side effects from antimuscarinic agents such as dryness of the mouth and eyes, sedation, impaired concentration, headache, constipation,

emptying through action on receptors for the hormone motilin, the physiologic regulator of the migrating motor complex. Some patients with gastroparesis and pseudoobstruction respond to erythromycin, but this agent has a narrow dose range of efficacy that limits its utility: low doses have no effect and high doses induce abdominal pain, nausea, and diarrhea. Macrolide derivatives with no antimicrobial activity but with prokinetic properties are being developed. The direct muscarinic stimulant bethanechol has motor stimulatory properties in the upper gastrointestinal tract and on rare occasions is used to manage gastroparesis. However, because it induces spastic rather than propagative motility and because it produces side effects such as diaphoresis, abdominal pain, nausea, and chest pain, bethanechol is rarely prescribed for dysmotility syndromes. The somatostatin analog octreotide, which evokes small-intestinal complexes that resemble the migrating motor complex, may reduce nausea and vomiting among patients with scleroderma who have pseudoobstruction and bacterial overgrowth. The gonadotropin-releasing hormone analog leuprolide evokes propagative gastrointestinal motor complexes and reduces nausea and bloating among patients with small-intestinal dysmotility syndromes.

Management of Emesis Resulting from Cancer Chemotherapy

Extensive investigation has focused on antiemetic regimens to prevent or control nausea and vomiting that complicate cancer chemotherapy. Most programs include multiple drugs that act on distinct receptor sites. For highly emetogenic agents such as cisplatinum, prophylactic regimens usually include 5-HT$_3$ antagonists such as ondansetron and granisetron. These agents also are effective against emesis induced by radiation therapy and the postoperative state. Side effects of 5-HT$_3$ antagonists include headache, constipation, and rare elevations in liver enzyme levels. Metoclopramide in high doses is useful for prophylaxis of chemotherapy-induced emesis, possibly stemming from weak 5-HT$_3$ antagonism. Other antidopaminergic agents such as prochlorperazine and domperidone are used with efficacy with some forms of chemotherapy. Corticosteroids have potent antiemetic effects against chemotherapeutic agents through unknown mechanisms. Intravenous benzodiazepines such as lorazepam are included in antiemetic regimens because they produce sedation and reduce anticipatory nausea. In prophylaxis against chemotherapy-induced emesis, cannabinoids such as tetrahydrocannabinol and nabilone are as efficacious as or slightly better than antidopaminergics. Cannaboids, however, produce severe side effects such as somnolence, ataxia, syncope, seizures, and hallucinations, which are prominent in the elderly. The mechanisms of the antiemetic effects of cannabinoids are unknown.

Miscellaneous Antiemetic Therapies

Other medications are efficacious in selected instances. Tricyclic antidepressants are used to manage nausea associated with depression and have been shown to be effective in the treatment of patients with unexplained functional nausea. Patients with nausea due to opiate withdrawal have responded to opiate antagonists such as naloxone.

SURGICAL AND OTHER NONMEDICATION MANAGEMENT OF NAUSEA AND VOMITING

Nonmedication therapies have been proposed for some conditions of chronic emesis. Acupuncture and acustimulation have been used to control nausea of pregnancy, motion sickness, and postoperative nausea. Among patients with diabetes and gastroparesis, enteral feedings through a jejunostomy can reduce symptoms and decrease the number of hospitalizations. Intravenous hyperalimentation may be needed for severe pseudoobstruction. Patients with gastroparesis after vagotomy may improve after surgical removal of the stomach. Electrical pacing of the stomach has been reported to benefit some patients with severe gastroparesis, but this technology is unproved.

BIBLIOGRAPHY

Borison HL, Wang SC. Physiology and pharmacology of vomiting. *Pharmacol Rev* 1953;5:193.

Camilleri M, Hasler WL, Parkman HP, et al. Measurement of gastrointestinal motility in the GI laboratory. *Gastroenterology* 1998;115:747–762.

Eckhauser FE, Conrad M, Knol JA, et al. Safety and long-term durability of completion gastrectomy in 81 patients with postsurgical gastroparesis syndrome. *Am Surg* 1998;64:711–717.

Jantunen IT, Kataja VV, Muhonen TT. An overview of randomised studies comparing 5-HT$_3$ receptor antagonists to conventional anti-emetics in the prophylaxis of acute chemotherapy-induced vomiting. *Eur J Cancer* 1997;33:66–74.

Lin HC, Hasler WL. Disorders of gastric emptying. In: Yamada T, ed. *Textbook of gastroenterology,* 2nd ed. Philadelphia: JB Lippincott, 1995: 1318.

Mitchelson F. Pharmacological agents affecting emesis: a review, I, II. *Drugs* 1992;43(4):443–463.

Parkman HP, Harris AD, Krevsky B, et al. Gastroduodenal motility and dysmotility: an update on techniques available for evaluation. *Am J Gastroenterol* 1995;90:869–892.

Reynolds JC, Putnam PE. Prokinetic agents. *Gastroenterol Clin North Am* 1992;21:567–596.

Kelley's Textbook of Internal Medicine, fourth edition. Edited by H. David Humes. Lippincott Williams & Wilkins, Philadelphia © 2000.

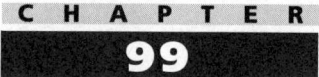

C H A P T E R

99

APPROACH TO THE PATIENT WITH DIARRHEA

CAROL E. SEMRAD
EUGENE B. CHANG

▌ PRESENTATION

Diarrhea is a symptom that is extremely common and bothersome. It is one of the most common problems encountered by physicians in outpatient and inpatient settings and is a major cause of work absenteeism and medical expense. In developing countries, infectious diarrhea is a major cause of morbidity and mortality, predominantly among children, accounting for about 3 million deaths per year. In the United States, acute infectious diarrhea alone accounts for 2.2 million physician visits per year. The elderly have the highest mortality followed by adults who are immunocompromised or have cardiovascular disease. In the pediatric population, each child has an average of 7 to 15 episodes of diarrhea before the age of 5 years. In this age group, diarrhea accounts for 9% of all hospitalizations and causes 300 to 500 deaths a year. The morbidity and mortality from diarrheal disease in the United States could be reduced if inexpensive oral rehydration solutions were used earlier in the course of illness.

Although most cases of diarrhea are transient and benign, some are chronic and debilitating, and often associated with underlying disease. Diarrhea may be described as an increase in frequency, size or loosening of bowel movements. Because individual persons have different definitions of diarrhea, it is important to differentiate true diarrhea from conditions, such as fecal incontinence or functional bowel disease, associated with increased frequency or loose consistency of stool but a normal stool weight. Most adults who consume an average, low-residue western diet have less than 200 g of stool per day. Those with stool weights more than 200 g per day most likely have diarrhea. The average daily stool weight among infants is far less than that among adults; an output of 200 g per day represents diarrhea. Some patients with severe diarrhea have dehydration and metabolic disturbances, particularly if they are unable to take fluids orally. Findings such as fever, weight loss, and abdominal pain may be important clues to the cause of diarrhea. The context in which diarrhea occurs is an important factor in evaluation and management. The causes of diarrhea among hospitalized or intensive care patients differ from those among outpatients. The causes of diarrhea among immunocompromised hosts differ from those among normal hosts.

PATHOPHYSIOLOGY

Every day about 8 to 10 L of fluid enters the small intestine of an adult. About 2 L are from dietary intake, the rest are from salivary, gastric, pancreatic, biliary, and intestinal secretions. About 80% of this fluid is reabsorbed in the small intestine, and all but approximately 100 mL of the remaining fluid is absorbed in the colon. Water and electrolytes are absorbed in the intestine by a number of processes. Sodium is transported into absorptive (villous) small-intestinal epithelial cells predominantly by nutrient-dependent cotransporters. This results in the paracellular flow of Cl^-, K^+, and water. In addition, water may be transported transcellularly in the small intestine by the sodium-glucose cotransporter. There also are nutrient-independent Na^+ transporters on the luminal surface of absorptive epithelial cells in the small intestine and colon. These include Na^+–H^+ exchange in the jejunum, coupled Na^+–H^+ and Cl^-–HCO_3^- exchange in the ileum and proximal colon, and Na^+ channels in the distal colon. Short-chain fatty acids (SCFAs) generated

by bacterial degradation of unabsorbed carbohydrate and soluble fiber are absorbed with sodium in the colon, further promoting fluid absorption.

The intestine (small intestine and colon) also secretes water and electrolytes into the lumen. Apical chloride channels in crypt epithelial cells open when intracellular levels of cyclic nucleotides or calcium are increased in response to exposure to toxins, hormones, neurotransmitters, and immune mediators. When the apical chloride channels open, Na^+ and water are drawn paracellularly into the lumen. Bicarbonate is secreted in the ileum through a less well understood mechanism. The balance between absorptive and secretory processes in the intestine must be tightly regulated to avoid diarrhea. Net absorption of fluid and electrolytes normally far outweighs net secretion. Diarrhea occurs when the amount of fluid delivered to or secreted by the colon cannot be completely reabsorbed and stool output is more than 200 g per day.

Diarrhea arises from two basic pathophysiologic mechanisms—increased active anion secretion and decreased absorption of water and electrolytes (Table 99.1). In most diarrheal diseases, both processes are affected, resulting in net secretion, luminal fluid accumulation, and increased stool weight. Increased active anion secretion may have a number of different causes, including exposure to enterotoxins, hormones, neuropeptides, inflammatory mediators, bile salts, laxatives, medications, and insecticides. Examples include excessive stimulation of anion secretion by prosecretory agents such as vasoactive intestinal polypeptide (VIP), 5-hydroxytryptamine (serotonin; 5-HT), tachykinins, and prostaglandins. Prostaglandins are produced by inflammatory cells and stimulate sustained increases in levels of cyclic adenosine monophosphate (cAMP) in intestinal epithelial cells. As a result, anion secretion is stimulated and Na^+ and Cl^- absorption is inhibited, which leads to development of profuse watery diarrhea. Active secretion also is a component of diarrhea associated with celiac disease. In this disease, rapid epithelial cell turnover in the proximal small intestine causes crypt hyperplasia. Because crypt cells are believed to be the main sites of active anion secretion, these events give the celiac mucosa a secretory phenotype that is constantly active because of constant stimulation by inflammatory mediators.

Decreased absorption of water and electrolytes is an equally important cause of diarrhea. It can be caused by several different mechanisms. Besides their effect on active anion secretion, bacte-

TABLE 99.1.	**PATHOPHYSIOLOGIC MECHANISMS OF DIARRHEA**

Decreased absorption of water and electrolytes
    Inhibited or defective absorption of water and electrolytes
    Luminal presence of osmotically active agents
    Increased propulsive motor activity that causes decreased contact time
    Increased intestinal permeability
Increased secretion of water and electrolytes
    Stimulated anion secretion
    Secretion from hyperplastic crypts

rial enterotoxins, such as cholera toxin and *Escherichia coli* heat-stable toxin, and prosecretory agents, such as VIP and 5-HT, activate specific signaling pathways in villous epithelial cells that lead to functional inhibition of Na^+ and Cl^- absorption. Clinical studies with healthy human subjects suggest that secretagogues such as VIP appear to inhibit Na^+ and Cl^- absorption more so than they stimulate active anion secretion. Other mechanisms of decreased absorption of water and electrolytes in the intestine include (a) ingestion of a poorly absorbed, osmotically active solute such as magnesium or lactose by persons with lactase deficiency, (b) decreased absorptive surface area, as caused by mucosal damage, intestinal resection, or enteroenteric fistula, (c) hypermotility that causes decreased contact time between luminal fluid and absorptive mucosal surface area, and (d) impairment of mucosal barrier function (increased permeability) that causes back flux of water and electrolytes into the intestinal lumen.

MECHANISMS OF DIARRHEA

Mechanisms That Cause Specific Diarrheal Diseases

General Mechanisms of Inflammation-induced Diarrhea

Diarrhea is one of the cardinal manifestations of diseases that cause inflammation of the intestinal mucosa, including infection, celiac disease, or inflammatory bowel disease (IBD). Loss of surface area for water and electrolyte absorption due to mucosal damage is the main mechanism. However, diarrhea also occurs when the intestinal epithelium and mucosal architecture are intact but the lamina propria is expanded by infiltration of inflammatory cells. Inflammatory mediators such as prostaglandins, leukotrienes, platelet-activating factor, histamine, and hydrogen peroxide have been postulated on the basis of the results of in vitro studies to cause active intestinal secretion. However, studies performed on chronically inflamed intestine show selective decreases in secretory, absorptive, and barrier functions and increases in antigen-presenting surface molecules. These responses may represent a physiologic adaptation of the epithelium to down-regulate metabolic processes or undergo a phenotypic shift aimed at augmenting intestinal mucosal defense functions. Inflammatory mediators also may induce, directly or through neural activation, hypermotility that causes rapid intestinal transit and reduced contact time between luminal fluid and the absorptive surface area. Changes in splanchnic and mesenteric capillary blood flow and lymphatic drainage also may be contributing factors.

Diarrhea Due to Inflammatory Bowel Disease

Diarrhea associated with IBD is proportional to the extent and degree of mucosal inflammation and can have numerous causes (Table 99.2). In ulcerative colitis, inflammation and ulceration of the colonic mucosa can cause exudation of protein, blood, and pus into the intestinal lumen that results in bloody diarrhea. If diarrhea is voluminous, however, it is usually caused by de-

TABLE 99.2.	**PATHOPHYSIOLOGIC MECHANISMS OF DIARRHEA IN INFLAMMATORY BOWEL DISEASE**

Mucosal injury and loss of digestive and absorptive functions
  Loss of absorptive surface area
  Increased mucosal permeability
  Ulceration with plasma-like exudate
  Impaired or down-regulated enterocyte transport functions
  Decreased mucosal digestive functions
Increased net secretion
  Anion secretion stimulated by inflammatory mediators
  Inhibited absorption by inflammatory mediators
  Increased epithelial turnover and immaturity of villous function
  Anion secretion stimulated in the colon by unabsorbed bile salts and fatty acids
Intestinal dysmotility
  Rapid transit
  Decreased luminal fluid–mucosa contact time
Anatomic alterations
  Short bowel from surgical resection
  Enteroenteric fistula
  Paradoxic diarrhea caused by partial intestinal obstruction
  Bacterial overgrowth caused by strictures or an incompetent ileocecal valve
  Pouchitis
Other potential mechanisms
  Mucosal atrophy from prolonged parenteral hyperalimentation
  Antibiotic-associated colitis (*Clostridium difficile*)
  Medication

creased absorption of fluid and electrolytes across the diseased mucosa and stimulation of fluid secretion by inflammatory mediators in both the colon and small intestine.

Along with the inflammation-induced effects on mucosal function and integrity described earlier, persons with Crohn's disease and small-intestinal involvement may have impaired mucosal digestive function caused by increased cellular turnover and a greater proportion of immature villous cells along the crypt-villus axis. Thus the expression of brush border hydrolases such as lactase, sucrase–isomaltase, and aminopeptidases can be markedly decreased, reducing the overall mucosal capability to digest oligosaccharides and oligopeptides. Chronic inflammation also is associated with decreased expression or function of critical nutrient-transporting proteins, such as sodium glucose transporter 1 (SGLT1). The net effect of the presence of incompletely digested and nonabsorbed nutrients is to increase the osmolar load of the colon. When the capacity of the colon to reabsorb water and electrolytes is overwhelmed, diarrhea occurs.

Among persons with Crohn's disease who have inflammation of or have undergone resection of the terminal ileum, malabsorption of bile salts or fat may cause diarrhea. If less than 100 cm of ileum is involved, bile salts but not fats are malabsorbed. Malabsorption of α-hydroxy bile acids, in particular, stimulates colonic secretion and increases mucosal permeability. This results in watery diarrhea, which can be alleviated with the binding resin cholestyramine. When more than 100 cm of ileum is involved, fat malabsorption frequently develops. In this case, the extent of bile-salt wasting exceeds the synthetic capacity of the liver, resulting in negative bile salt balance and depletion of the body's total bile-salt pool. As a result, there are insufficient bile salts in the intestinal lumen for proper micelle formation, which is necessary for fat digestion and absorption. Unabsorbed long-chain fatty acids reach the colon and are hydroxylated by bacteria. In this form they stimulate net fluid secretion, increase mucosal permeability, and induce colonic hypermotility. This results in diarrhea, which may be lessened by a low-fat diet. Administration of cholestyramine in this case may make diarrhea worse by further increasing bile-salt losses and fat malabsorption.

Other causes of diarrhea in Crohn's disease include bacterial overgrowth due to stricture-related stasis or an incompetent ileocecal valve, paradoxical diarrhea from partial intestinal obstruction, and intestinal hypermotility with rapid transit. Some patients with Crohn's disease have diarrhea from complications of altered intestinal anatomy. An enteroenteric fistula may bypass large amounts of small intestine. Extensive resection of the small intestine may cause short-bowel syndrome. In both cases diarrhea is caused mainly by an insufficiency of absorptive surface area. Immediately following resection some patients have hypersecretion of acid caused by hypergastrinemia that may exceed the absorptive capacity of the remaining intestine and cause diarrhea.

Disturbances in SCFA acid metabolism and absorption in the colon of patients with IBD also may contribute to diarrhea. SCFAs have several important functions in the colon. They promote vectorial Na^+ and water absorption, are a leading source of energy for colonocytes, and have trophic effects on the mucosa. Decreased availability of SCFAs has been associated with the development of diversion colitis and may aggravate ulcerative colitis. Both the availability and absorption of SCFAs may be markedly impaired in ulcerative colitis. For example, the bacterial flora can be altered by medications such as antibiotics, steroids, and immunomodulatory agents that adversely affect the production of SCFAs. This may decrease colonic Na^+ absorption, make the mucosa unable to withstand injury and heal itself, further compromise fluid absorption, and cause diarrhea.

In some patients with continent reservoir ileostomies, ileorrhea may develop from partial obstruction and overgrowth of anaerobic bacteria caused by fecal stasis. Patients with an ileoanal anastomosis after colectomy and mucosal proctectomy may have diarrhea caused by intestinal spasms and diminished absorptive capacity. This usually resolves 6 to 12 months later, after ileal adaptation (villous hyperplasia and increased nutrient transporters) and enlargement of the ileal reservoir. These patients also can have pouchitis (inflammation of the ileal reservoir) that causes bleeding and diarrhea. Net fluid secretion in this instance is thought to be caused by a decrease in absorptive function related to partial villous atrophy, bacterial overgrowth, and increased mucosal permeability of the pouch. Iatrogenic causes should be considered when a patient with IBD has diarrhea. Antibiotic-associated and medication-induced diarrhea can occur but are often overlooked.

Diarrhea Caused by Transmissible Agents

In most instances of infectious diarrhea, pathogens are acquired through the fecal-oral route. Enteric pathogens (Table 99.3) fall

---

TABLE 99.3. PATHOGENS THAT CAUSE INFECTIOUS DIARRHEA

Watery diarrhea
  Enterotoxigenic (*Escherichia coli* toxins, *Vibrio cholerae* toxin)
  Enteroadherent (enteroadherent *E. coli*, cryptosporidia, giardia)
  Food-borne toxins[a] (*Bacillus cereus, Clostridium perfringens* and *C. botulinum, Staphylococcus aureus, V. parahaemolyticus*,[b] ciguatoxin, scromboid toxin)
  Invasive (rotavirus, Norwalk agent, *Salmonella* species,[c] enteroinvasive *E. coli*[c])
  Organisms of the immunocompromised (*Mycobacterium avium-intracellular complex, cryptosporidia, Isospora belli, microsporidia, cyclospora,* HIV enteropathy)

Bloody diarrhea
  Invasive (*Campylobacter jejuni*,[c] *Aeromonas* organisms,[c] *Yersinia enterocolitica, Vibrio parahaemolyticus*,[c] *Vibrio fulnificus*[c])
  Destructive (*Shigella* organisms,[c] enterophemorrhagic *E. coli*, *C. difficile*,[b] *Entamoeba histolytica schistosomiasis*[b])
  Organisms of the immunocompromised host (cytomegalovirus)

---

[a] Symptoms usually occur several hours after the ingestion of contaminated food. Vomiting is common.
[b] Diarrhea may be watery or bloody.
[c] Some strains both produce an enterotoxin and invade; may initially manifest as watery diarrhea, which then turns bloody.

---

into three groups—bacterial, viral, and parasitic (see Chapter 113).

Bacterial Pathogens

Several mechanisms are responsible for diarrhea caused by bacterial pathogens. *Vibrio cholerae* and *E. coli* (enterotoxigenic *E. coli* [ETEC]) colonize the intestine and produce enterotoxins that disturb water and electrolyte transport in the absence of mucosal damage. Cholera toxin and the heat-labile enterotoxin of *E. coli* bind to the Gm1 ganglioside of the luminal surface of enterocytes, gain entry into the cell, activate adenylate cyclase, and increase intracellular cAMP levels. This results in direct stimulation of active Cl^- secretion and inhibition of nutrient-independent Na^+ and Cl^- absorption in epithelial cells. These enterotoxins also indirectly stimulate secretion by binding to receptors on enterochromaffin cells that release hormones that activate the enteric nervous system. Heat-stable *E. coli* toxin (STa) also causes secretory diarrhea and is a frequent cause of traveler's diarrhea. This agent binds to intestinal guanylate cyclase (GCC) (the receptor for the gastrointestinal hormone guanylin) present in the brush border membrane of enterocytes. Activation by STa increases intracellular cyclic guanosine monophosphate (cGMP), which like cAMP stimulates anion secretion and inhibits Na^+ and Cl^- absorption.

These enterotoxins cause high-volume diarrhea without fecal leukocytes or blood. Loss of fluid and electrolytes into the intestinal lumen may cause hypovolemia, acidosis, and decreased perfusion to vital organs—the main cause of morbidity and mortality. Because nutrient-dependent sodium cotransporters are not affected by these toxins, oral rehydration solutions containing

Na^+ and glucose or glucose polymers are very effective in promoting intestinal fluid absorption and preventing death.

Oral rehydration solutions that contain glucose polymers, such as rice-based solutions, lessen diarrhea. For the same osmotic load, glucose polymers are digested by amylase and hydrolases at the brush border membrane into many more glucose monomers than are present in standard glucose-containing solutions. Because absorption of glucose monomers occurs immediately upon digestion, this results in absorption of both the fluid ingested and some of the enteric secretions. The small-intestinal epithelium must be relatively intact for polymeric solutions to be beneficial. If not, the polymers are digested in the lumen but not absorbed; the result is an increase in luminal osmols and worsening diarrhea.

Campylobacter, Salmonella, Shigella, and enteroinvasive *E. coli* (EIEC) are invasive organisms that injure the intestinal mucosa and cause diarrhea with fecal leukocytes and often blood. *Campylobacter* is the most common species of these organisms on a worldwide basis. The degree of mucosal injury, inflammation, and exudate depends on the virulence of the pathogen and on host susceptibility. Although most of these diseases are self-limited, relapses can occur among patients with *Campylobacter* infection. Enterohemorrhagic *E. coli* (EHEC) infection, as with *E. coli* O157:H7, is associated with ingestion of undercooked meats and raw milk. The organism elaborates Shiga-like cytotoxins that cause bloody, but noninflammatory diarrhea (absence of fecal leukocytes). In a small number of cases, EHEC and *Shigella* organisms can cause hemolytic-uremic syndrome and thrombotic thrombocytopenic purpura.

Enteroadherent *E. coli* (EAEC) organisms cause diarrhea through a mechanism that is not fully understood. As implied by the name, these organisms are not invasive and do not stimulate appreciable mucosal inflammation. They adhere to the luminal surface of enterocytes and disrupt the glycocalyx and cause effacement of the microvillous membrane, disorganization of the terminal web, crypt hyperplasia, and villous atrophy. These changes decrease brush border hydrolase activity, and the decrease may cause substantial nutrient malabsorption and osmotic diarrhea. EAEC infection is a cause of diarrhea in infancy.

A number of bacterial pathogens contaminate foods and elaborate toxins. *Staphylococcus aureus* infection is one of the most common causes of food poisoning. The organisms elaborate several toxins that cause profuse vomiting and stimulate net intestinal fluid secretion. Symptoms may occur within several hours of ingestion of preformed toxin. Some strains of *Bacillus cereus* that contaminate fried rice produce an illness characterized by nausea and vomiting. Other *Bacillus* species that contaminate meats, baked goods, and salads cause abdominal cramps and diarrhea. *Clostridium perfringens* multiplies in unrefrigerated foods and when ingested binds to the intestinal mucosa and elaborates an enterotoxin that stimulates net fluid secretion and causes motility abnormalities. Crampy abdominal pain is therefore a prominent feature that differentiates this illness from diarrhea caused by other enterotoxigenic bacteria. *Vibrio parahaemolyticus* infection is associated with food poisoning from raw or spoiled shellfish. It produces several enterotoxins, some of which stimulate net intestinal fluid secretion and others that are cytotoxic and proinflammatory. Persons with this disorder have watery diarrhea or dysentery.

Viral Pathogens

Infection with rotaviruses and Norwalk virus causes acute, self-limited diarrhea. Rotavirus infection is a leading cause of diarrhea among children younger than 2 years. Norwalk virus primarily infects older children and adults. These viruses injure the small-intestinal mucosa and cause villous blunting, shortening of microvilli, and mononuclear infiltration of the mucosa. Decreased brush border hydrolase activity is common and may seriously impair nutrient absorption. Diarrhea is caused by decreased fluid absorption related to loss of villous surface area and an increase in luminal osmols. A rotavirus enterotoxin NSP4 has been identified that stimulates intestinal fluid secretion by a calcium-dependent signaling pathway and may contribute to the development of diarrhea. Rotavirus also stimulates intestinal fluid secretion by activation of the enteric nervous system.

Parasitic Pathogens

Chronic diarrheal diseases occasionally are caused by intestinal parasites such as helminths (cestodes, nematodes, trematodes) and protozoa, particularly among persons from areas where these organisms may be endemic or public sanitation is poor. Diarrhea is not always a manifestation of helminthic infection. Most cestodes, for example, cause few gastrointestinal symptoms even when worm loads are large. Helminthic organisms that colonize the small intestine are more likely to produce diarrhea and nutrient malabsorption and usually cause eosinophilia. Of the intestinal nematodes, *Capillaria philippinensis, Ascaris lumbricoides, Trichinella spiralis, Ancylostoma* (hookworms), and *Strongyloides stercoralis* may cause diarrhea. Trematodes such as *Schistosoma* species deposit eggs in the intestinal mesenteric venules and incite a host inflammatory response that may cause diarrhea.

Protozoa that cause diarrhea include *Giardia lamblia, Cryptosporidium* species, and *Amoeba* species. *Giardia lamblia* is a major cause of waterborne outbreaks of diarrhea and traveler's diarrhea. Person-to-person transmission also occurs, particularly in day care centers, in guardian institutions, and among homosexuals. After ingestion of cysts, trophozoites develop and multiply in the small intestine, where they adhere to the mucosal surface and cause effacement of the brush border microvillous membrane, partial villous atrophy, and reduction of brush border hydrolase activity. Diarrhea is caused by impaired fluid absorption. Malabsorption of carbohydrate and peptides can contribute to the development of diarrhea.

Cryptosporidium infection is an important cause of waterborne diarrheal illness among humans and domestic animals. Transmission also can occur by the fecal-oral route from infected animals and persons. *Cryptosporidium* infection usually produces acute, often severe, crampy, watery diarrhea that is self-limited and lasts several days to weeks. The organisms attach to small-intestinal epithelial cells, but the mechanism by which they cause diarrhea is not well understood.

Entamoeba histolytica is transmitted in contaminated water and by the fecal-oral route. *E. histolytica* cysts multiply in the small intestine and mature into trophozoites, which penetrate the mucosa of the large intestine. Severe mucosal inflammation and ulceration develop from the acute inflammatory response of the host and the innate cytotoxic properties of the organisms. The histologic lesion of amebic infection is characteristically a flask-shaped ulcer that features a small mucosal ulcer and a large submucosal area of tissue necrosis. Chronic complications of amebic infection involve most commonly the liver and lung. A hepatic abscess (typically single and in the posterior aspect of the right lobe) when aspirated yields a dark, odorless, and thick necrotic material that resembles anchovy paste. Pulmonary amebic abscesses or bronchopleural fistulas develop in some patients with hepatic amebiasis; they are caused by amebic emboli or contiguous spread.

Diarrhea Caused by Opportunistic Pathogens or Developing in a Susceptible Host

Antibiotic-associated Colitis

Antibiotic-associated colitis is caused by *Clostridium difficile*, a common nosocomial pathogen in health care and long-term care facilities. The disease is caused by poor hand washing by health care workers who spread the organism and alteration of intestinal flora by antibiotics to favor growth of *C. difficile*. Although any antibiotic can cause antibiotic-associated colitis, clindamycin, cephalosporins, and ampicillin are most commonly involved. Diarrhea is caused by two exotoxins. Toxin A is a potent stimulator of intestinal fluid secretion, increases intestinal permeability, and activates a profound inflammatory response in the lamina propria. Toxin B is cytotoxic and causes epithelial and mesenchymal cell destruction.

Diarrheal Pathogens in Immunocompromised Hosts

Immunocompromised hosts are vulnerable to common diarrheal pathogens as well as opportunistic pathogens. *Giardia lamblia* infection is an important cause of diarrhea among persons with AIDS and common variable hypogammaglobulinemia. Unusual pathogens such as *Legionella* organisms and *Candida albicans* also can cause diarrhea among immunocompromised hosts. Opportunistic pathogens including *Cryptosporidium* species, *Isospora belli*, *Mycobacterium avium-intracellulare* complex, Microsporida, and cytomegalovirus (CMV) are important causes of diarrhea among patients with AIDS. CMV infection can cause profuse watery diarrhea or bloody diarrhea due to mucosal inflammation and ulceration. *Cryptosporidium* infection causes intractable watery diarrhea among persons with AIDS. There is no effective treatment.

Other Diseases

Tropical sprue and Whipple's disease cause intestinal inflammation, villous blunting, and crypt hyperplasia similar to celiac disease. The process causes decreased fluid absorption and diarrhea. Tropical sprue occurs among persons who live in or travel to the tropics. It is associated with overgrowth of predominantly coliform bacteria in the small intestine. Whipple's disease is an infectious disease of the small intestine caused by the organism *Tropheryma whippelii*. Those with the *HLA B27* genotype may be more susceptible to this disease.

Noninfectious Diarrheal Diseases Associated with an Abnormal Mucosa

Diseases of the intestine such as IBD, celiac disease, microscopic colitis, eosinophilic and allergic gastroenteritis, and acute radiation enteritis are associated with inflammation of and usually injury to the intestinal mucosa. These diseases cause diarrhea by several different mechanisms, including loss of surface area, nutrient malabsorption, increased intestinal permeability, and stimulation of secretion by inflammatory mediators.

In microscopic colitis (collagenous and lymphocytic) the endoscopic appearance of the colon is normal (see Chapter 114). Diagnosis can be made only by means of colonic biopsy, which characteristically shows normal crypt architecture but increased numbers of intraepithelial lymphocytes and of lymphocytes and plasma cells in the lamina propria. Collagenous colitis is differentiated from lymphocytic colitis by the additional presence of a thickened subepithelial collagen layer. Microscopic colitis causes watery and sometimes high-volume diarrhea. It occurs predominantly among older women and is associated with celiac disease, autoimmune disease, and arthritis. In most cases, mucosal inflammation is diffuse, causing pancolitis. The diagnosis is made from multiple biopsy specimens obtained at flexible colonoscopy.

Diarrhea is a frequent complication of bone marrow transplantation. Soon after transplantation diarrhea usually is caused by the toxic effects of cytoreductive therapy on rapidly dividing cells in the intestinal epithelium. Graft versus host disease (GVHD) is another cause of diarrhea among these patients. In mild cases, the intestinal mucosa appears endoscopically normal, but biopsy specimens obtained from the stomach, small intestine, colon, or rectum contain apoptosis of crypt or gastric gland cells. In more severe cases, exploding crypts (crypts filled with cell debris), chronic inflammation, and villous flattening are found, and they account for watery diarrhea. In the most severe cases, the intestinal epithelium is denuded with exudation of protein, pus, and blood; the result is bloody diarrhea. Chronic GVHD occurs more than 3 months after transplantation and has clinical and radiologic features similar to those of visceral scleroderma. These patients often have diarrhea and nutrient malabsorption.

Noninfectious Diarrheal Diseases Associated with a Normal Mucosa

Diarrhea associated with a normal intestinal mucosa is most likely functional. Functional diarrhea can be caused by (a) the presence of osmotically active substances in the lumen, (b) a decrease in contact time for fluid absorption, as in rapid intestinal transit, (c) defects in specific ion or nutrient transporters, or (d) defects in the regulation of intestinal water and electrolytes.

Osmotic Diarrhea

The presence of poorly absorbed solute in the intestinal lumen can cause diarrhea and limit the ability of the intestine to effi-

TABLE 99.4.	**MEDICATIONS AND DIETARY PRODUCTS ASSOCIATED WITH DIARRHEA**

Agents that cause osmotic diarrhea
  Mg^{2+} containing antacids
  Mg^{2+} containing laxatives (milk of magnesia, magnesium citrate, Epsom salts)
  PO_4^- containing laxatives (Fleets Phospho-Soda, neutral phosphate)
  Polyethylene glycol (bowel preparation)
  Lactulose
  Sorbitol (chewing gum, dietetic foods and candies, elixirs)
  Mannitol (drug additive, elixirs)
  Fructose (pears, prunes)
Agents that cause secretory diarrhea
  Antibiotics
  Phenolphthalein laxatives
  Ricinoleic acid (castor oil)
  Anthraquinones, senna, bisacodyl, dicotyl laxatives
  Methylxanthines (theophyline, caffeine)
  Furosemide
  Cholinergic agents (bethanechol, organophosphates)
  Mesalamine
  Prostaglandins (misoprostol)
  Prokinetic agents (cisapride, metoclopramide)
  H_2 blockers, proton-pump inhibitors
  Protease inhibitors
  Cardiovascular medications (quinidine, quinine, angiotensin-converting enzyme inhibitors)
  Ethanol
  Heavy metals
Agents that cause malabsorption and diarrhea
  Orlistat (inhibits lipase)
  Cholestyramine (binds bile salts)
  Colchicine (villous blunting)
  Methotrexate (villous blunting)
  Metformin, acarbose (inhibits intestinal α-glucosidases)
Chemotherapeutic agents commonly associated with diarrhea
  5-Fluorouracil[a]
  Interleukin-2
  Irinotecan, topotecan
  Methotrexate[a]
  Cyclophosphamide (high-dose with bone marrow transplant)[b]
  Docetaxel
  Thiotepa (high-dose with bone marrow transplant)[b]
  Daunorubicin, doxorubicin
  Cytosine arabinoside
  Azacitidine

---

[a] Cytotoxicity enhanced with leucovorin.
[b] Causes severe mucositis with malabsorption and diarrhea.

ciently absorb water and electrolytes. Both exogenous (Table 99.4) and endogenous factors can cause osmotic diarrhea. Magnesium-containing antacids, bowel lavage solutions (polyethylene glycol), and sorbitol (chewing gum, elixir preparations) represent exogenous sources of luminal osmolytes. Endogenous causes include small-intestinal conditions in which nutrient digestive or absorptive capability is impaired and nutrient, water, and electrolyte malabsorption and diarrhea occur; examples are primary or acquired lactase deficiency and rare defects in sugar transport proteins. Lactose intolerance due to acquired lactase deficiency is the most common endogenous cause of osmotic diarrhea. Its prevalence is highest among Asians, Native Americans, and African Americans. Symptoms due to lactose malabsorption depend on the amount ingested. Unabsorbed lactose is metabolized by colonic bacteria to CO_2, H_2, and SCFAs. Ingestion of a small amount of lactose may cause gas and bloating but not diarrhea. Diarrhea does not occur because SCFAs are absorbed along with sodium and water in the colon. However, ingestion of larger amounts of lactose overwhelms the capacity of the colon to absorb SCFAs and results in acidic osmotic diarrhea.

Decreased Contact Time for Fluid Absorption

Rapid intestinal transit occurs in most cases of diarrhea. It is caused by reflexive propulsive activity in response to an increase in luminal volume or the effect of the disease on intestinal smooth muscle. In only rare instances is a primary motility disorder thought to cause diarrhea. Some children with toddler's diarrhea and adults with painless diarrhea (irritable bowel syndrome [IBS] variant) may have continuous propulsive migrating motor complexes that are not halted with eating. This causes rapid intestinal transit, wasting of carbohydrates in the colon, and an osmotic diarrhea. Persons with IBS may have diarrhea of other causes. such as microscopic colitis, celiac disease, or laxative abuse. Many persons with IBS do not have true diarrhea but rather frequent, loose stools of normal weight.

Congenital Diarrhea

Infants with rare congenital ion transport disorders have watery diarrhea at birth. Congenital chloride diarrhea is associated with metabolic alkalosis and chloride-rich, acidic stools. The genetic defect resides in the down-regulated in adenoma (*DRA*) gene, which codes for an anion exchanger normally expressed in the ileum and colon. The defect impairs $Cl^- - HCO_3^-$ or $Cl^- - OH^-$ exchange in the intestine. Congenital sodium diarrhea is associated with metabolic acidosis and sodium-rich, alkaline stools. These infants appear to have defective $Na^+ - H^-$ exchange in jejunal brush border membranes. The genetic defect has not yet been identified. In both diseases, patients need aggressive oral fluid replacement therapy for life. In microvillous inclusion disease, brush border membranes do not reach the luminal surface (or are invaginated from the apical surface) of villous epithelial cells and are found intracellularly or misplaced in the basolateral membrane. The result is a devastating loss of surface area for nutrient and fluid absorption and the need for lifelong parenteral nutrition.

Defective Regulation of Intestinal Water and Electrolytes

The intestine normally is maintained in a net absorptive state by the sympathetic nervous system. However, when extrinsic adrenergic nerves are cut, as occurs during transplantation of the small intestine, diarrhea develops but resolves. This phenomenon suggests local factors in the intestine also regulate water and electrolyte absorption. Enteric nerves, endocrine cells, immune cells, and mesenchymal cells in the intestine all are capable of releasing proabsorptive and prosecretory substances that may influence water and electrolyte transport. In rare instances, tumors produce one or more of these prosecretory substances and cause secretory diarrhea. These patients usually have high-volume, watery diarrhea that does not resolve with fasting. Examples include tumors that produce VIP (VIPoma, watery diarrhea, hypokalemia, achlorhydria syndrome or pancreatic cholera), 5-HT, and bradykinin (carcinoid syndrome), gastrin (gastrinoma or Zollinger–Ellison syndrome), and calcitonin (medullary carcinoma of the thyroid). Nutrient malabsorption also may occur among persons with gastrinoma due to denaturation of pancreatic enzymes and precipitation of bile salts by the large acid load presented to the duodenum.

Defective regulation of intestinal water and electrolyte transport also occurs in diabetic diarrhea. Persons with diabetes often have severe watery diarrhea (more than 500 g per day), dehydration, and nocturnal incontinence. Among a subset of persons with diabetes, autonomic neuropathy appears to be a contributing factor because treatment with the α_2-adrenergic agonist clonidine lessens the diarrhea. This diagnosis requires clinical signs of autonomic neuropathy and the exclusion of fecal incontinence and other causes of diarrhea, such as bacterial overgrowth.

Other Diarrheal Diseases

Nosocomial diarrheal diseases are caused by iatrogenic factors such as medication (e.g., antibiotics or sorbitol-containing elixirs), tube feeding, and *C. difficile* infection related to poor hand washing. They most commonly occur in hospitals, nursing homes, and guardian institutions. Persons who reside in institutions and nursing homes also are susceptible to food poisoning and infectious diseases that are transmitted by the fecal-oral route.

Factitious chronic diarrhea is caused by the secretive use of laxatives or diuretics that either stimulate anion secretion or cause osmotic diarrhea (Table 99.4). In some cases of chronic diarrhea, no cause can be found despite an extensive evaluation. When referred to tertiary care centers, some patients are found to have fecal incontinence, microscopic colitis, and bile-acid induced diarrhea. For other patients no cause of diarrhea is found (chronic idiopathic diarrhea). These persons should be treated symptomatically. For many, the diarrhea resolves spontaneously.

■ HISTORY

The following questions should be answered when any patient comes to medical attention with diarrhea: Is it truly diarrhea? Is the diarrhea acute (less than 2 to 3 weeks' duration) or chronic (more than 4 weeks' duration)? What are the other symptoms? What are the circumstances? Routine questions should be asked about stool texture and frequency, blood in the stool, fever, vomiting, abdominal pain, weight loss, travel, diet, drug use, alcohol, abdominal operations, chemotherapy, radiation therapy, incontinence, immune status, and underlying disease.

To determine whether a patient truly has diarrhea, questions should be asked about consistency and frequency of stools relative to baseline bowel habits. Persons with IBS or fecal incontinence often have frequent, small stools of normal weight rather than diarrhea. Diarrhea that is of new onset, occurs daily or at night, or is associated with metabolic disturbances usually is caused by organic disease.

Acute diarrhea usually is infectious or related to use of new medications. Chronic diarrhea can be caused by a vast number of different diseases. Associated symptoms provide clues to the cause of diarrhea. Low-grade fever occurs with viral or toxigenic diarrhea, whereas high fever occurs with invasive bacterial infections, amebiasis, CMV colitis, or IBD. Fainting, dizziness on standing, or weakness suggests high-volume diarrhea. Weight loss with acute diarrhea indicates fluid loss, whereas with chronic diarrhea it usually indicates nutrient malabsorption. Nausea and vomiting are most often found with viral infections or food poisoning. Abdominal cramps may be caused by infection but can be caused by carbohydrate malabsorption. Severe abdominal pain occurs with invasive or cytopathic bacterial infection and intestinal ischemia. Blood in the stool indicates an infectious, inflammatory, or ischemic process. Associated neurologic symptoms occur with botulism and exposure to marine toxins (scromboid, ciguatera). Diarrhea sometimes occurs with a systemic illness such as hepatitis, legionnaires' disease, Rocky Mountain spotted fever, and toxic shock syndrome.

The setting in which diarrhea occurs provides important clues as to causation. Recent travel, restaurant dining, or ingestion of foods that were imported, poorly cooked, or left out at room temperature may point to an infectious cause of diarrhea. Diarrhea may occur with new use of medications, over-the-counter drugs, or herbal products or with changes in diet. Diarrhea due to *C. difficile* infection is common among patients in hospitals and nursing homes and those with a history of antibiotic use. Immunocompromised persons may have diarrhea caused by common organisms or those unique to the impaired host. Among the elderly and those predisposed to thrombosis, diarrhea with pain out of proportion to physical findings suggests intestinal ischemia.

■ PHYSICAL EXAMINATION

Attention is paid to vital signs, volume status in particular, and the findings of the abdominal and rectal examinations. High fever suggests the presence of invasive organisms. Hyperventilation may be a sign of metabolic acidosis caused by bicarbonate loss in the stool. Orthostatic vital signs (a drop in blood pressure greater than 10 mm Hg and a rise in pulse of more than 20 beats/min on standing) are reliable indicators of volume depletion except among persons taking cardiac medications, such as β-blockers or calcium channel blockers, and elderly persons with vascular disease. Skin tenting, dry mucous membranes, resting tachycardia, hypotension, sunken eyeballs, and a scaphoid abdomen are all signs of severe dehydration due to voluminous diarrhea.

Patients with chronic diarrhea are evaluated for signs of malnutrition and vitamin and mineral deficiency caused by malabsorption. These signs include weight loss, muscle wasting, tetany, oral and skin lesions, peripheral neuropathy, ataxia, and edema. Edema may indicate protein-losing enteropathy.

The abdomen is examined for distention, bowel sounds, tenderness, and masses. A stool swab for culture, when necessary, is obtained before the rectal examination because lubricants contain bacteriostatic agents that can interfere with bacterial growth. The rectum is examined for stool texture, masses, and sphincter tone. Rectal villous adenoma and carcinoid tumor may be detected during the examination. Most persons with diarrhea do not have solid stool in the rectum except for those with diarrhea associated with fecal impaction. Stool should be tested for occult blood. Persons with high-volume diarrhea are often incontinent of stool. Among those with cholera, fluid with mucous flecks (rice-water stools) pours out of the rectum.

LABORATORY STUDIES AND DIAGNOSTIC TESTS

STOOL TESTS

Stool Tests for Intestinal Inflammation

Stool studies for the presence of intestinal inflammation are readily performed but lack specificity. Fecal lactoferrin (an iron-binding glycoprotein released from leukocytes during an inflammatory reaction) is the most sensitive (about 90%) but least specific test in supporting a diagnosis of invasive bacterial enteritis. Microscopic examination for fecal leukocytes is the least sensitive test (about 50%) but has the greatest specificity. A negative result of a fecal occult blood test has the same negative predictive value for an invasive bacterial enteritis as does a negative fecal lactoferrin test.

Stool Culture

Stool culture results are positive in only 40% to 60% of cases of dysentery. Special culture techniques are needed for the diagnosis of *Yersinia, Campylobacter,* and *V. cholerae* infections. Growth of colonies on sorbitol–MacConkey agar indicates EHEC infection, but confirmation by means of vero cell toxin testing or strain-specific serotyping is critical for diagnosis.

Stool for Ova and Parasites

Microscopic analysis of stool for parasites is performed before any barium studies, because barium interferes with depiction of parasites for weeks. In ideal circumstances, one stool test for *Giardia* antigen should be performed in cases of chronic diarrhea because with chronic infection *Giardia* organisms adhere to the small-intestinal mucosa and few are found in the stool. *Cryptosporidium* organisms are not detected by means of routine microscopic examination of the stool. Special staining is needed for detection.

Stool for *Clostridium difficile* Toxin

The test for toxin B (cytotoxin) is performed by means of adding a sterile stool filtrate to human fibroblasts grown in culture and observing for cell death within 2 to 3 days. A more rapid test that has about the same sensitivity is an enzyme immunoassay

to detect toxin A. The sensitivity is about 90% when three stool samples are tested.

Stool Sudan Stain for Fat

Sudan staining is a qualitative test for fat in the stool that is valid only if the patient is eating a high-fat diet. The test is 90% sensitive with fat malabsorption of more than 10 g per day. The result sometimes is positive in the presence of high-volume secretory diarrhea, in which as much as 14 g per day of fat can be passed in the stool.

Stool Alkalinization and Cathartic Screen

Addition of NaOH or KOH turns stool pink when phenolpthalein-containing laxatives are present. The test is easy to perform, and a positive result leads to an inexpensive and rapid diagnosis. If the result is negative and laxative abuse is highly likely, stool and urine are tested for anthraquinones, docusate salts, magnesium, SO_4, PO_4, and diuretics. Although stool magnesium output can increase to 50 mmol per liter with diarrhea, levels higher than this suggest laxative abuse.

Stool Electrolytes

Stool electrolyte measurements are useful in differentiating secretory diarrhea from osmotic diarrhea (Table 99.5). Secretory diarrhea is characterized by high stool sodium and bicarbonate concentrations and the absence of a stool osmotic gap. Osmotic diarrhea is characterized by a low stool sodium concentration and the presence of a stool osmotic gap more than 100 mOsm per kilogram H_2O. Direct measurement of stool osmolality may be falsely elevated when stool specimens are not processed immediately; the delay allows colonic bacteria to generate large amounts of SCFAs from unabsorbed carbohydrates and soluble fibers. This occurs even in stool samples that are refrigerated. To avoid this problem, plasma osmolality rather than stool osmolality is used in the following calculation:

$$\text{Stool osmotic gap} = 290 \text{ mOsm/kg} - 2 \times (\text{stool } [Na] + [K])$$

The normal gap is usually less than 50 mOsm/kg H_2O, and plasma osmolality equals stool osmolality. When stool electrolyte concentrations are far less than those in plasma, surreptitious addition of water to the specimen must be considered.

Stool pH

A low stool pH (less than 7.0) can indicate carbohydrate malabsorption, due to the presence of SCFAs, or gastrinoma, due to hypersecretion of acid. This test is most helpful in the care of infants and children.

Fasting Stool Volume

A 24- to 48-hour measurement of stool volume while the patient is fasting provides useful information about whether diarrhea is functional (less than 250 mL per day), osmotic (low volume),

TABLE 99.5.	**STOOL OSMOTIC GAP AS A GUIDE TO THE PATHOPHYSIOLOGIC PROCESS AND DIAGNOSIS OF DIARRHEA**
Plasma osmolality or 290 mOsm/kg H_2O − 2 [Na + K] mmol/L	= Stool osmotic gap
Stool [Na] >90 mmol/L and Osmotic gap <50 mOsm/kg H_2O	= Secretory diarrhea or osmotic diarrhea caused by Na_2SO_4 or Na_2PO_4 ingestion[a]
Stool [Na] <60 mmol/L and Osmotic gap >100 mOsm/kg H_2O	= Osmotic diarrhea; if stool volume does not return to normal with fasting, suspect surreptitious Mg ingestion[b]
Stool [Na] >150 mmol/L and Stool osmolality >375–400 mOsm/kg H_2O	= Suspect contamination of specimen with concentrated urine
Stool osmolality <200–250 mOsm/kg H_2O	= Suspect contamination of specimen with dilute urine or water

[a] Normal stool SO_4 and PO_4 are usually <10 mmol; exact values not established. In Na_2SO_4- or Na_2PO_4-induced diarrhea, stool Cl^- concentrations are <20 mmol/L.
[b] Normal stool Mg on regular diet is 10–45 mmol/L; during fasting, the concentration should be <10 mmol/L. In Mg-induced diarrhea, stool Mg^{2+} concentration is usually >50 and often >100 mmol/L.
Source: Powell DW. Approach to the patient with diarrhea. In Yamada T, ed. *Textbook of gastroenterology,* 2nd ed. Philadelphia: JB Lippincott, 1995, with permission.

or secretory (high volume more than 1 L per day). Intravenous fluids are administered during the fast.

Quantitative Stool Fat Test

A 72-hour stool collection for fat while the patient consumes a high-fat diet (70 to 100 g fat per day) is performed when (a) malabsorption is highly likely and the qualitative test result for stool fat is negative, (b) a qualitative test result for stool fat is positive and it is believed the positive result is caused by high-volume diarrhea, and (c) diarrhea is of undetermined origin. If the test result is positive, specific diagnostic tests are performed on the basis of the likelihood of pancreatic disease, bacterial overgrowth, mucosal disease, or lymphatic obstruction.

FLEXIBLE SIGMOIDOSCOPY

Examination with a flexible sigmoidoscope performed without intestinal preparation is useful in the detection of pseudomembranes, mucosal inflammation, and melanosis coli. Even if the mucosa appears normal, biopsy specimens are obtained to look for microscopic colitis, infiltrative disease, certain infectious diseases, and laxative abuse.

BLOOD HORMONE LEVELS

For patients with high-volume secretory diarrhea of undetermined origin, measurement of serum levels of gastrin, VIP, somatostatin, cortisol, neurokinins, and calcitonin may be considered. When carcinoid syndrome is suspected, serotonin and urine 5-hydroxyindoleacetic acid are measured.

ACUTE DIARRHEA

DIFFERENTIAL DIAGNOSIS

Normal Hosts

Acute diarrhea (less than 2 to 3 weeks' duration) may be caused by infection or ingested toxins, drugs, or dietary products. The most common cause is infection caused by viruses and food-borne toxins (Table 99.3). Viral diarrhea usually occurs among children, their family members, and day care workers. Diarrhea caused by food poisoning usually occurs within several hours of the meal. Associated symptoms include low-grade fever, vomiting, and abdominal cramps.

Pathogens that cause traveler's diarrhea usually are acquired through the fecal-oral route. They include enterotoxigenic bacteria (*E. coli, V. cholerae*), which cause high-volume watery diarrhea without blood or pus, and other organisms such as *Campylobacter, Shigella, Salmonella,* viruses, and parasites. Giardiasis is the most common parasitic infection in the United States. It is contracted though ingestion of contaminated water. Sporadic waterborne outbreaks of cryptosporidiosis also have occurred on farms and in cities.

Most acute infectious diarrheal diseases are self-limited, but some may persist for more than 3 or 4 weeks. In some instances the long duration may be caused by secondary lactase deficiency, and diarrhea improves with a lactose-free diet. Outbreaks of diarrhea lasting as long as a year occurred in Brainerd, Minnesota, and other rural areas. They were associated with ingestion of raw milk. No organism has yet been identified.

Bloody stool has a limited differential diagnosis that includes invasive bacterial enteritis (*Campylobacter, Shigella, Yersinia*), *E. histolytica,* cytopathic toxins (*C. difficile, E. coli,* or Shiga toxin), IBD, and intestinal ischemia. Persons with infection by invasive or cytopathic organisms often have severe abdominal pain and fever. Systemic manifestations of enteric bacterial infection include arthritis, urethritis and conjunctivitis (*Salmonella, Shigella, Campylobacter, Yersinia*), and hemolytic-uremic syndrome (EHEC, *Shigella*).

A number of drugs and dietary products cause acute diarrhea (Table 99.4). Antibiotics are the most common cause. About 25% of antibiotic-associated diarrhea is caused by *C. difficile* toxin. *C. difficile* infection can cause watery or bloody diarrhea with fever and abdominal pain. In other cases of antibiotic-associated diarrhea the cause is unknown. Other drugs that commonly cause diarrhea include antacids, prokinetic agents (cisapride, metoclopramide), prostaglandins, and drug elixirs that contain sorbitol. Diarrhea caused by drugs usually is watery and without associated symptoms. Cholinergic poisoning with organophosphate insecticides may occur among migrant farmers, landscapers, or those who ingest medicinal teas. The classic presentation is diarrhea, severe abdominal cramps, copious salivation, and pulmonary edema. Dietary substances that cause diarrhea include lactose (among those with lactase deficiency), sorbitol (elixirs, dietetic candies, gum), fructose (pears, prunes, apple juice), and Olestra (a nondigestible fat substitute).

Immunocompromised Hosts

Although many new anti-retroviral drugs, especially protease inhibitors, cause diarrhea, the development of these compounds has resulted in a marked decrease in infectious diarrhea among persons with HIV infection in developed countries (see Chapter 114). Nevertheless, persons with HIV disease and a CD4 cell count less than 150 cells per cubic millimeter and other immunocompromised hosts are still at risk of diarrhea caused by common infectious organisms and by CMV, *M. avium-intracellulare* complex, *Cryptosporidium* organisms, *I. belli*, Microspora, and *Cyclospora* organisms.

Diarrhea is common among recipients of bone marrow and intestinal transplants. Soon after bone marrow transplantation, diarrhea usually is caused by cytoreductive therapy (Table 99.4). Twenty to 80 days after transplantation, diarrhea usually is caused by GVHD or infection. Persons with GVHD also may have a skin rash, jaundice, buccal mucositis, and abdominal pain, which help secure the diagnosis. Endoscopic intestinal biopsy, however, often is necessary to differentiate GVHD from infection. Immediately after small-intestinal transplantation, diarrhea appears to be caused by disruption of adrenergic neurons. Later it is caused by rejection, GVHD, or infection. A patient with neutropenia who has a fever, diarrhea, and abdominal pain may have neutropenic colitis (typhlitis), which can be fatal unless colonic resection is performed.

Patients with Cancer

Diarrhea is common among patients who undergo chemotherapy (Table 99.4) or radiation therapy to the abdomen. It usually is caused by the toxic effects of chemotherapy or radiation therapy on the gastrointestinal tract. Interleukin-2, 5-fluorouracil

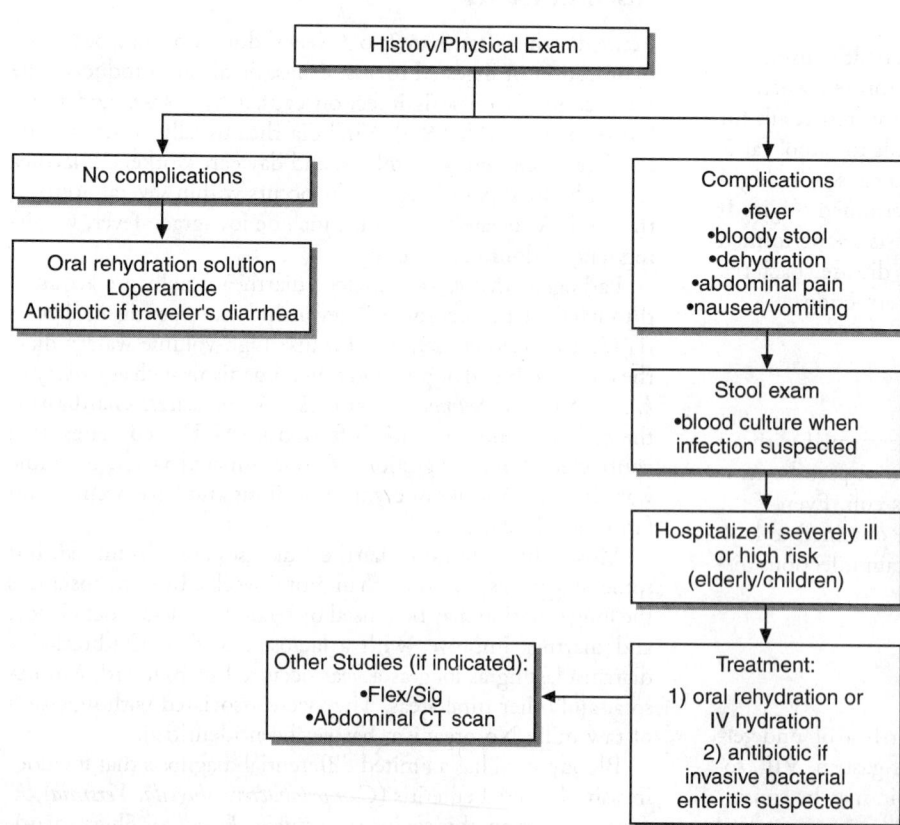

FIGURE 99.1. Approach to normal hosts with acute diarrhea.

plus leucovorin, and irinotecan (CPT-11) are the chemotherapeutic agents that most commonly cause diarrhea. Almost all patients have more frequent bowel movements after abdominal or pelvic radiation. Diarrhea also can occur many years after radiation therapy as the result of ischemia, enteroenteric fistula, or bacterial overgrowth. Radiation enteritis proctitis also can cause bloody diarrhea owing to ischemia.

Persons in Hospitals, Mental Health Facilities, or Nursing Homes

Diarrhea occurs among 30% to 50% of patients in intensive care units and can be caused by antibiotics, other drugs, fecal impaction, the underlying disease, or tube feeding. Among hospitalized patients *C. difficile* infection is the most common cause of diarrhea, whereas *Salmonella, Shigella,* or parasitic infection is extremely rare, especially in tertiary care hospitals. Among critically ill persons, increased mucosal permeability, low serum albumin levels, and dysmotility contribute to decreased intestinal fluid absorption. Tube feeding with formulas low in sodium content may contribute to diarrhea in this setting. Among nursing home residents, viral infections are the most common cause of diarrhea. About one-fourth of residents have *C. difficile* toxin in their stool. Sporadic outbreaks of *Salmonella* and EHEC infection also occur. In guardian institutions, patients are at increased risk for diarrhea caused by infection by *Shigella* species, *Giardia* species, *E. histolytica* and helminths.

EVALUATION

In cases of uncomplicated acute diarrhea among normal hosts (Fig. 99.1), no evaluation is necessary. Stool specimens are obtained for examination for ova and parasites only when the history suggests exposure to parasites or when diarrhea does not resolve. When diarrhea is associated with fever, a screening stool test (see earlier) is performed to differentiate inflammatory from noninflammatory diarrhea. A stool occult blood test is the easiest to perform, and the results are immediately available. If invasive bacterial enteritis is highly likely, stool culture is performed even if stool screening results are negative. If a patient has bloody diarrhea, a stool culture is performed; the microbiology laboratory should be notified about suspicious organisms for best diagnostic yield. If the culture result is negative, colonoscopy and biopsy are performed. IBD sometimes can be differentiated histologically from infectious enteritis and intestinal ischemia on the basis of the presence of irregular, branching crypts, a feature associated with chronic inflammation.

Among immunocompromised hosts with diarrhea, stool is obtained for culture, examination for parasites, and detection of *C. difficile* toxin (Fig. 99.2). If fever is present, blood cultures

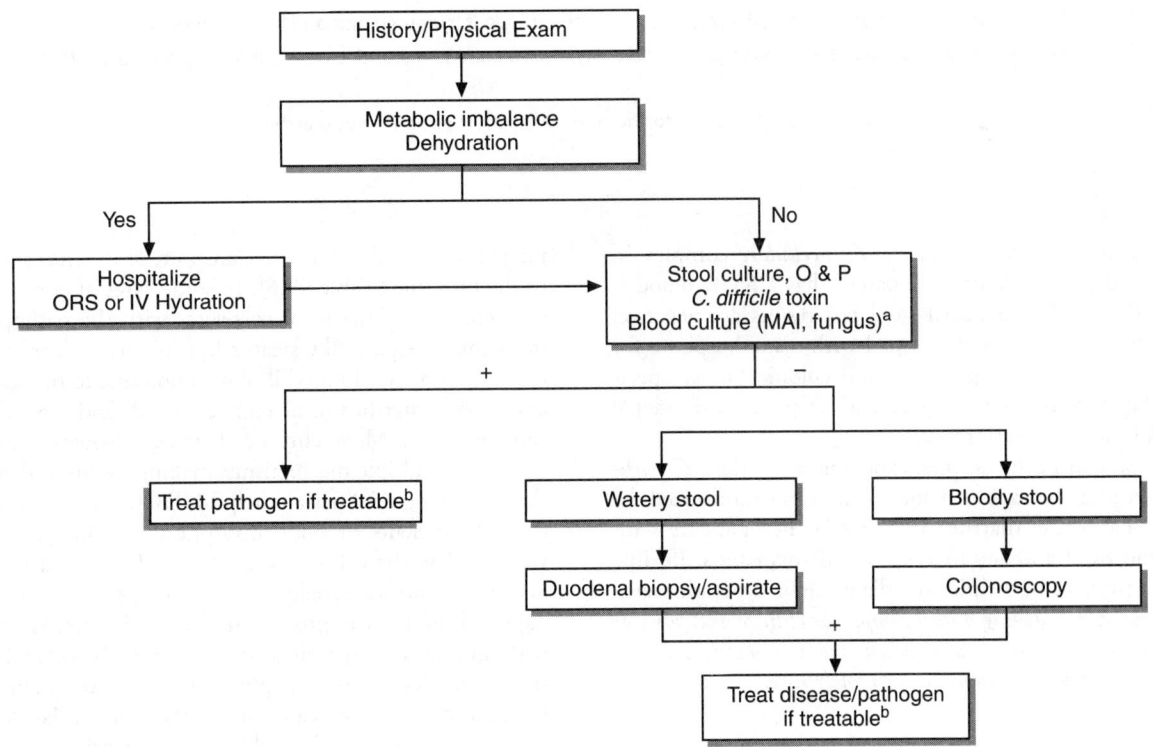

a Obtain if patient has fever.

b If disease can not be treated, aim therapy at reducing diarrheal output (antimotility agent, octreotide, ORS) and providing nutrition support.

FIGURE 99.2. Approach to the immunocompromised host with diarrhea.

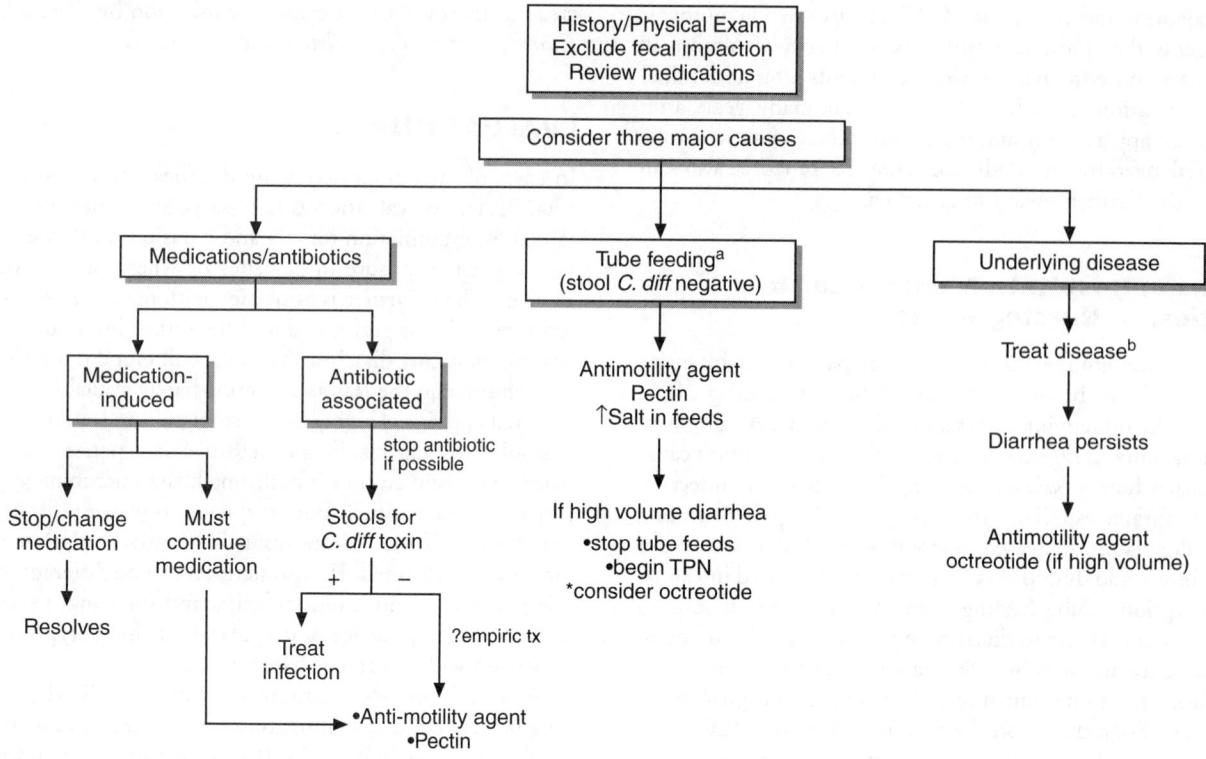

ª Rarely the cause of diarrhea. ?Infected formula. Try diluting formula if hyperosmolar and jejunal feeding.

ᵇ Underlying disease may cause increased gut permeability, hypoalbuminemia or dysmotility that may not be treatable.

FIGURE 99.3. Approach to the hospitalized/ICU patient with diarrhea.

are obtained for bacteria, *M. avium-intracellulare* complex in particular, and fungus. When the patient has a fever, blood is present in the stool, and initial stool test results are negative, full colonoscopy should be performed with a stool aspirate for culture, *C. difficile* toxin, parasites, and colonic biopsy specimens. If the stool is watery, upper endoscopy with duodenal aspirate and biopsy is performed.

When a patient in the hospital experiences diarrhea, *C. difficile* infection must be excluded and medications scrutinized for those that may cause diarrhea (Fig. 99.3). For patients with blood in the stool and negative results of toxin tests, flexible sigmoidoscopy may be helpful for diagnosis if a pseudomembrane is present. *Obtaining a stool sample for culture and parasite examination is not recommended when diarrhea develops in the hospital because these infections are extremely rare.*

CHRONIC DIARRHEA

DIFFERENTIAL DIAGNOSIS

Chronic diarrhea (more than 4 weeks' duration) may be caused by malabsorption of nutrients or poorly absorbable solute, de-

ranged water and electrolyte transport, or inflammatory diseases of the intestine (Table 99.6). In some cases of chronic diarrhea, the character of the stool correlates with the pathophysiologic mechanism (e.g., bulky steatorrhea in chronic pancreatitis, watery diarrhea after limited ileal resection due to bile salt wasting, and bloody diarrhea in ulcerative colitis), and a rapid diagnosis can be made. Most chronic diarrheal diseases, however, are caused by multiple mechanisms, making a clinical diagnosis difficult. A few guidelines are helpful. Diarrhea due to malabsorption of nutrients or poor absorption of solute usually is low volume (less than 1 L per day) and diminishes with fasting. Secretory diarrhea usually is high volume (more than 1 L per day) and does not improve with fasting. Inflammatory diarrhea with mucosal destruction is associated with blood and pus in the stool and edema. History, physical examination, and screening blood and stool tests can narrow the differential diagnosis so that the cause is found quickly and efficiently.

Malabsorption

Malabsorption can be caused by a number of diseases, drugs, or dietary products that impair intraluminal digestion, mucosal absorption, or nutrient delivery. Impairment of intraluminal

TABLE 99.6.	CAUSES OF CHRONIC DIARRHEA

Inflammatory disease
   Inflammatory bowel disease
   Microscopic colitis
   Eosinophilic and allergic gastroenteritis
Malabsorptive disease
   Impaired digestion (pancreatic insufficiency, bacterial overgrowth, extensive ileal resection)
   Impaired mucosal absorption (chronic infection, celiac disease, tropical sprue, radiation enteritis, lymphoma, Whipple's disease, amyloidosis)
   Lymphatic obstruction (lymphoma, Kaposi's sarcoma, severe congestive heart failure, constrictive pericarditis)
Irritable bowel syndrome
Medications (see Table 99.4)
Radiation
Abdominal surgery
   Cholecystectomy
   Truncal vagotomy
   Short-bowel syndrome
Ischemic bowel
Laxative abuse (see Table 99.4)
Endocrine (hyperthyroidism, adrenal insufficiency)
Villous adenoma
Systemic mastocytosis
Hormone-producing tumors (gastrinoma, carcinoid syndrome, VIPoma, medullary thyroid carcinoma)
Heavy metals

digestion can be caused by pancreatic insufficiency, bacterial overgrowth, ileal resection, drugs (orlistat, cholestyramine), or hypersecretion of acid. Impairment in mucosal absorption can be caused by diseases associated with a normal intestinal mucosa (acquired lactase deficiency, abetalipoproteinemia) or with an abnormal intestinal mucosa (chronic intestinal infection, celiac disease, Crohn's disease, tropical sprue, Whipple's disease, radiation enteritis, lymphoma). Some drugs (colchicine, methotrexate, neomycin) also impair mucosal absorption. In short-bowel syndrome, the intestinal mucosa is normal, but the surface area for absorption is markedly decreased. Impairment in nutrient delivery usually is caused by diseases that cause lymphatic obstruction (lymphoma, tumor, tuberculosis, constrictive pericarditis, severe congestive heart failure). Hypoproteinemic edema is characteristic in these conditions.

Symptoms of nutrient malabsorption are predominantly related to impaired absorption of fat and carbohydrate. Steatorrhea (greasy, foul smelling stools that are difficult to flush) is the hallmark of malabsorption. Stools may be bulky or watery depending on whether triglycerides or fatty acids are malabsorbed. Watery steatorrhea is caused by fatty acid–induced stimulation of fluid secretion in the colon. Malabsorption of carbohydrate causes osmotic watery diarrhea, abdominal bloating, and cramps. Weight loss may be caused by nutrient malabsorption or decreased oral intake to avoid diarrhea. Poor absorption of carbohydrates, cations, or anions also causes osmotic watery diarrhea.

Poorly absorbed sugars include lactulose (used in therapy for hepatic encephalopathy), sorbitol (present in elixirs, dietetic candy, and chewing gum), and fructose (present in pears, prune juice, and apple juice). Magnesium, phosphate, and sulfate are present in laxatives. These poorly absorbed solutes exert an osmotic force in the lumen; they draw fluid and electrolytes from plasma to the lumen. An increased stool osmotic gap is found in all cases of osmotic diarrhea except for those caused by laxatives containing phosphate and sulfate. In the latter case, the stool osmotic gap is normal but stool Cl^- concentration is low because SO_4 and PO_4 anions displace Cl^- to maintain stool osmolality equal to plasma.

Deranged Water and Electrolyte Transport

A number of different diseases cause watery diarrhea by altering water and electrolyte transport. In some of these diseases (bile acid diarrhea, diabetic diarrhea, microscopic colitis, laxative abuse, villous adenoma, hormone-secreting tumors, congenital transport disorders), diarrhea is caused by decreased absorption or stimulation of fluid secretion in the intestine. In others (IBS, toddler's diarrhea), dysmotility with rapid intestinal transit may play a role. In many of these diseases, the pathophysiologic mechanisms underlying the disorders are not well understood (postvagotomy syndrome, postcholecystectomy syndrome, binge drinking, idiopathic diarrhea).

Bile acid diarrhea may be caused by ileal disease or resection, primary malabsorption of bile salts, or postcholecystectomy or postvagotomy syndrome. Primary malabsorption of bile salts has been reported among infants and adults; it presumably is caused by defective intestinal bile acid transport proteins. Diarrhea due to primary bile salt malabsorption generally improves with fasting and cholestyramine treatment.

Diarrhea due to the presence of hormone-secreting tumors and congenital diarrhea are rare and are characteristically high volume and unresponsive to fasting. In VIPoma, VIP and other peptides are secreted from a pancreatic adenoma or neural crest tumor (in children) that causes watery diarrhea, hypokalemia, and achlorhydria. In the carcinoid syndrome, serotonin, bradykinin, prostaglandins, and other substances are secreted from metastatic tumors and cause diarrhea, flushing, abdominal cramps, bronchospasm, and right-sided heart valve lesions. Skin flushing and diarrhea also may be manifestations of systemic mastocytosis. Patients with the Zollinger–Ellison syndrome (gastrinoma) often experience diarrhea, in part because of the large gastric acid load presented to the small intestine.

There are two conditions in which high-volume diarrhea is associated with metabolic alkalosis—congenital chloride diarrhea and large villous adenoma of the intestine. The mechanism by which the latter causes diarrhea is unclear, although prostaglandins may play a role.

Diabetic diarrhea is associated with severe autonomic neuropathy, which perturbs water and electrolyte transport and motility. The incidence of celiac disease and pancreatic insufficiency also is reported to be higher among these patients. Thus the diagnosis of diabetic diarrhea rests on the exclusion of other identifiable causes.

In IBS, stools are more liquid and frequent, but the volume usually does not increase, and patients rarely lose weight. Dysmotility leading to carbohydrate wasting in the colon and food sensitivities may have a role in this disorder. Lactose intolerance, microscopic colitis, and celiac disease are considered in the differential diagnosis.

Laxative abuse is found in about 25% of patients evaluated for chronic diarrhea. It occurs most often among young women with eating disorders and among middle-aged women (often health care workers) who obtain secondary gain from ongoing medical attention. These patients often appear to have diarrhea while fasting, either self-induced surreptitiously or caused by manipulation of their stool collections. Over-the-counter laxatives containing phenolphthalein can be detected by means of alkalinization of the stool. Other laxatives (anthraquinones, docusate salts, Mg^{2+}, SO_4, Na_2PO_4, Na_2SO_4, diuretics) are detected only by means of laboratory stool and urine analysis. A room search, although complicated by ethical and legal issues, often is helpful in the diagnosis. This disorder is difficult to diagnose, and the patients are difficult to treat because they go to great lengths to hide their abuse. They often leave the care of physicians when they are confronted with the diagnosis.

Inflammatory Disease

Inflammatory diarrhea can be watery or bloody depending on whether there is destruction of the intestinal epithelium. Fever, abdominal pain, blood in the stool, and hypoproteinemia are characteristic signs of inflammatory destruction of the intestinal epithelium. The pattern of abdominal pain, the clinical situation, and the character of bloody stools provide clues to causation. Left-sided abdominal pain and frequent passage of small, bloody stools suggests left-sided colitis due to IBD. Among the elderly, this must be differentiated from ischemic colitis. Right-sided abdominal pain and bloody stool may be caused by Crohn's disease or chronic infection of the terminal ileum (tuberculosis, *Yersinia* infection, or histoplasmosis). Microscopic colitis causes watery diarrhea predominantly among middle-aged women. Some have associated celiac disease.

Patients with rectal inflammation, as in ulcerative and infectious proctitis, may have normal stool weight but experience tenesmus, incontinence, and increased stool frequency. These symptoms are caused by reduction in the capacity of the rectal vault from muscular irritation and decreased absorptive and barrier properties of the mucosa, making it difficult to form solid stool. Infectious proctitis due to gonorrhea, herpes, syphilis, chlamydiosis, or amebiasis is possible if there is a history of anal intercourse.

Eosinophilic gastroenteritis is caused by infiltration of the gastrointestinal tract with eosinophils. The cause is unknown.

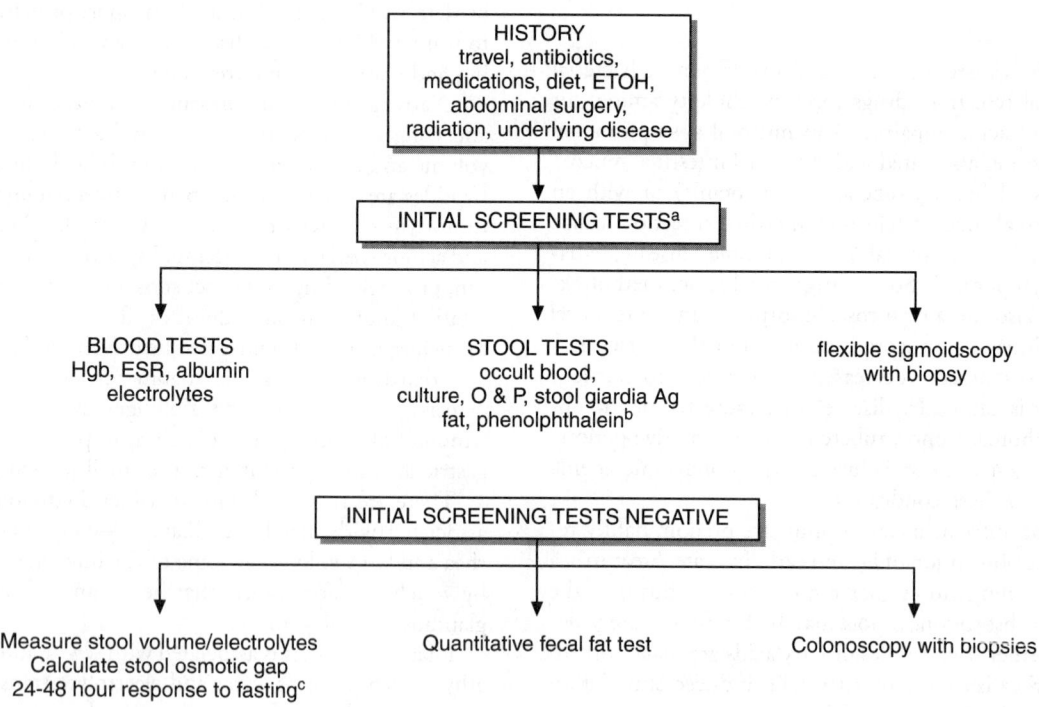

a If initial screening test positive, treat disease or obtain further tests for specific diagnosis as indicated.

b If laxative abuse suspected, send stool and urine for cathartic screen.

c If secretory diarrhea send thyroid function tests, blood levels for VIP, gastrin, calcitonin, cortisol and urine for 5-HIAA and heavy metals.

FIGURE 99.4. Evaluation of chronic diarrhea.

Some of these patients have allergic eosinophilic gastroenteritis. Any area of the gastrointestinal tract (esophagus to anus) can be involved, but the most common location is the stomach and small intestine. When the small-intestinal mucosa is involved, patients may have watery or bloody diarrhea. Allergic gastroenteritis is caused by specific food antigens that when ingested cause vomiting, abdominal cramps, and diarrhea. It most commonly occurs among infants and children.

EVALUATION

In most cases of chronic diarrhea, diagnostic evaluation is performed in the outpatient setting. Patients with dehydration, metabolic disturbances, or malnutrition may need admission to the hospital for a more expeditious evaluation. Before any tests are performed, a careful history must be obtained to ascertain the use of prescription drugs, over-the-counter drugs, or herbal preparations, dietary habits, and the presence of fecal incontinence. If lactose intolerance is likely or the patient has begun to use a new medication or dietary product, a lactose-free diet is tried or a change in medication is made before further evaluation.

An informative history can streamline tests that can establish a specific diagnosis. However, when this is not the case, initial screening tests (blood and stool) and flexible sigmoidoscopy are performed to differentiate organic disease from functional disease (dysmotility, laxative abuse) (Fig. 99.4). Initial screening tests include blood tests to look for electrolyte abnormalities, anemia, a low serum albumin level, and an elevated sedimentation rate—all signs of organic disease. Stool is tested first for occult blood, ova and parasites, *Giardia* antigen, fat, and phenolphthalein, and a stool culture is performed. Detection of *Giardia* antigen by means of enzyme-linked immunosorbent assay is as sensitive as examination of duodenal aspirate or biopsy in ascertaining the presence of chronic *Giardia* infection and is less

invasive. Flexible sigmoidoscopy with biopsy can be useful in detecting inflammatory (IBD, microscopic colitis), infectious (shistosomiasis), infiltrative (amyloidosis), and cathartic (use of anthracene laxatives) lesions.

A careful history, screening blood and stool tests, and flexible sigmoidoscopy provide specific diagnostic clues in about 80% of cases. The other 20% of persons with chronic diarrhea may need inpatient evaluation. Measurement of stool volume in response to a 24- to 48-hour fast, quantitative fecal fat test, and colonoscopy with biopsy provide a specific diagnosis in many of these cases. The response of diarrhea to fasting, measurement of stool electrolytes, and calculation of the stool osmotic gap helps differentiate osmotic diarrhea from secretory diarrhea (Table 99.5). If the fecal fat test result is positive, specific tests for malabsorption are performed. Colonoscopy allows visualization of the right colon and terminal ileum, sometimes revealing Crohn's disease, collagenous colitis, or villous adenoma. If no diagnosis is made after these tests and diarrhea is secretory, blood is obtained for measurement of thyroid function and hormone levels.

■ STRATEGIES FOR OPTIMAL CARE

MANAGEMENT

Fluid therapy is most important in the management of diarrhea, especially for infants and the elderly, because morbidity and mortality are caused by intravascular volume depletion. Persons with moderate to severe diarrhea lose large amounts of Na^+, Cl^-, K^+, HCO_3^-, and water in the stool; the result is hypokalemia, non–anion gap metabolic acidosis, and prerenal azotemia. When large diarrheal losses are replaced with water or oral solutions low in sodium content (juice, soda, sports drinks), hyponatremia results. Oral rehydration solutions (Table 99.7), in partic-

TABLE 99.7.	**COMPOSITION OF ORAL SOLUTIONS**					
Solution	**Na[a]**	**K[a]**	**Cl[a]**	**Base[a]**	**Carbohydrate[a,b]**	**Osmolality[c]**
WHO-ORS	90	20	80	10[d]	111 (20)	310
Rice-based[e]	90	20	60	10	— (40)	260
Sports drink	20	2.5	11	0	111 (20)	145
Ginger ale	3	1	2	4[f]	500 (90)	540
Apple juice	3	28	30	0	690 (124)	730
Chicken broth	250	8	250	0	0	450
Tea	0	0	0	0	0	5

WHO-ORS, World Health Organization oral rehydration solution.
[a] Millimoles per liter.
[b] Grams per liter in parentheses. All solutions contain glucose except the rice-based formula.
[c] Milliosmoles per kilogram.
[d] Citrate.
[e] Lessens diarrhea; 70 and 50 mmol Na solutions are more palatable and can be used to control less severe diarrhea.
[f] Bicarbonate.
Source: Modified from Avery ME, Snyder JD. *N Engl J Med* 1990;323:891.

ular the rice-based solutions, are designed for maximal intestinal fluid absorption and must be started early in the course of moderate to severe diarrhea for optimal results. For patients with hypotension or who are unable to drink, an intravenous solution containing potassium and a base (Ringer's lactate) is started.

Patients with chronic, high-volume diarrhea lose zinc and magnesium in the stool. Failure to replace zinc losses may result in zinc deficiency, which may then worsen diarrhea. Because magnesium is poorly absorbed and can make diarrhea worse, intramuscular or intravenous replacement of magnesium often is necessary. Serum electrolytes, blood urea nitrogen, creatinine, and magnesium are monitored to guide therapy. Food can be taken as tolerated except perhaps for lactose by patients with secondary lactase deficiency.

Patients with acute infectious diarrhea should not be treated with antibiotics except those with traveler's diarrhea and those likely to have invasive bacterial enteritis. Antibiotic therapy for EHEC infection is controversial. For travelers, antibiotic treatment to prevent diarrhea is not generally recommended. A single oral dose of a quinilone and an antimotility agent at the onset of symptoms relieves traveler's diarrhea within 24 hours in most instances. For patients with severe diarrhea, high fever, or bloody stools, a quinilone taken orally twice a day for three days is recommended for adults. *Antimotility agents should not be used* because of concern about promoting bacterial invasion or prolonging intestinal infection. Persons with diarrhea caused by *C. difficile* toxin should stop taking the offending antibiotic (if possible) and be treated with metronidazole. Treatment with oral vancomycin is reserved for patients with severe or refractory infection. For hospitalized patients with persistent diarrhea and negative results of stool tests for *C. difficile* toxin, empirical antibiotic treatment can be tried. The use of *Saccharomyces boulardi* (*S. cerevisiae*) to prevent or control *C. difficile* infection has not been shown to be effective.

Management of chronic diarrhea consists of fluid repletion and specific therapy for the underlying condition. Lactase deficiency is managed with a lactose-free diet or Lactaid. Pancreatic insufficiency is managed with exogenous pancreatic enzymes. Celiac disease is managed with a gluten-free diet. Tropical sprue and bacterial overgrowth are managed with antibiotics. Patients with limited ileal resection are treated with cholestyramine, and those with extensive ileal resection are treated with a low-fat diet and an antimotility agent. Severe diarrhea due to GVHD is controlled with steroids and antithymocyte globulin or mycophenolate mofetil (CellCept) combined with parenteral nutritional support. When the underlying condition cannot be controlled or does not respond to available treatments, as in the case of chronic intestinal infections, cancer-related diarrhea, and GVHD, management is aimed at lessening diarrhea and maintaining adequate nutrition. Antimotility agents can be tried, but octreotide (often at high doses) often is more effective in lessening diarrhea. Anti-inflammatory agents are used in the treatment of patients with IBD and to maintain remission.

Antidiarrheal agents can be grouped into four categories: bismuth subsalicylate, antimotility agents, antisecretory agents, and anti-inflammatory agents. Bismuth subsalicylate has both anti-microbial and antisecretory properties and is used most often in the prevention or control of traveler's diarrhea. Antimotility agents (opiates) slow intestinal transit and increase contact time for fluid reabsorption. Loperamide does not cross the blood-brain barrier, and therefore use of this agent is associated with fewer side effects. Tincture of opium is the most potent drug, but it can cause sedation and induce drug dependence. Antimotility agents usually are reserved for those with mild to moderate diarrhea who do not have fever or blood in the stool. Antimotility agents should not be used or are used with caution to treat patients with high-volume diarrhea (use may cause underestimation of fluid losses), invasive bacterial enteritis (may enhance bacterial invasion and delay clearance), or ulcerative colitis (may precipitate toxic megacolon).

No specific agent inhibits intestinal fluid secretion. Octreotide, the long-acting somatostatin analog, inhibits all gastrointestinal secretions and is effective in decreasing secretory diarrhea from any cause. It is most often used to treat patients with severe diarrhea due to HIV disease, GVHD, or chemotherapy and those who have undergone extensive intestinal resection with an end jejunostomy. Octreotide or long-acting octretoide also are useful in the management of diarrhea due to hormone-producing tumors. It acts by inhibiting formation and secretion of these hormones. Undesirable side effects of octreotide include increased risk of gallstones, malabsorption (at doses higher than 300 μg per day), and pseudoobstruction. Patients with diabetes who have diarrhea have been reported to respond to treatment with α_2-adrenergic agents (clonidine and lidamidine) and to treatment with octreotide. Proton-pump inhibitors are effective in decreasing diarrhea among patients with gastrinoma, short-bowel syndrome with acid hypersecretion, and congenital chloride diarrhea.

Steroids and 5-aminosalicylic acid decrease prostaglandin and leukotriene production, and the decrease results in decreased intestinal fluid secretion. Steroids also promote sodium and chloride absorption. These agents are effective in the management of IBD and microscopic colitis. Indomethacin inhibits production of prostaglandins but not of leukotrienes. It may decrease diarrhea in cases of radiation enteritis and villous adenoma but exacerbates diarrhea due to IBD.

COMPLICATIONS AND PITFALLS

Failure to recognize large diarrheal fluid losses contributes to morbidity and mortality, especially among infants and the elderly. Small diarrheal losses among infants rapidly lead to dehydration. Oral administration of rehydration solutions must be started early in the course of diarrhea. Solutions that contain glucose do not lessen diarrhea but keep up with fluid losses. Parents need to be instructed to continue giving oral solutions despite continued diarrhea. Oral solutions that contain glucose polymers (rice-based) do lessen diarrhea. Adults are told to monitor urine output as a gauge of adequate hydration. Standard oral solutions (Table 99.7) are appropriate only in mild cases of diarrhea.

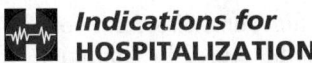

Indications for
HOSPITALIZATION

Any person with diarrhea accompanied by severe dehydration, inability to drink, metabolic disarray, severe abdominal pain, high fever, or a toxic appearance needs admission to a hospital for supportive care and diagnostic evaluation. There should be a lower threshold to admit patients with compromised immune function, elderly persons, or very young persons. These groups have the highest morbidity and mortality from diarrheal diseases.

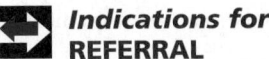

Indications for
REFERRAL

Severe diarrhea necessitates a more streamlined evaluation, which often includes endoscopic studies. Patients may need early referral to a specialist. Persons with chronic diarrhea of undetermined causation (idiopathic) are referred to a tertiary center that can perform specialized tests, such as tests for bile salt malabsorption and permeability studies.

▪ COST-EFFECTIVENESS

The cost of a single positive result of a stool culture performed indiscriminately for patients with diarrhea is about $1,200. The cost of a positive result of a stool culture can be drastically decreased if cultures are limited to patients with a positive result of a screening test for inflammation or when suspicion of invasive bacterial enteritis is high. Maximal diagnostic yield from a stool culture is obtained when the laboratory is notified to culture for specific organisms such as *Yersinia, Cholera,* or EHEC when these are suspected. Stool culture and examinations for parasites should not be performed when diarrhea develops while a patient is in the hospital unless there is reason to suspect an outbreak of *Salmonella* or *Campylobacter* infection. For patients with chronic diarrhea and no etiologic clues, a careful history and physical examination, limited blood and stool screening tests, and flexible sigmoidoscopy are performed before more expensive and invasive tests.

BIBLIOGRAPHY

Avery ME, Synder JD. Oral therapy for acute diarrhea. *N Engl J Med* 1990: 323:891–894.

Chang EB, Sitrin M, Black D, eds. *Gastrointestinal, hepatobiliary and nutritional physiology.* Philadelphia: JB Lippincott, 1996:91–118.

Donowitz M, Kokke FT, Saidi R. Evaluation of patients with chronic diarrhea. *N Engl J Med* 1995;332:725–729.

Field M, Semrad CE. Toxigenic diarrheas, congenital diarrhea and cystic fibrosis: disorders of intestinal ion transport. *Annu Rev Physiol* 1993; 55:631–655.

Fine KD. Diarrhea. In: Sleisenger MH, Fordtran JS, eds. Gastrointestinal

and liver disease: pathophysiology/diagnosis/management, 6th ed., vol 2. Philadelphia: WB Saunders, 1998:128–152.

Montrose MH, Keely SJ, Barrett KE. Electrolyte secretion and absorption: small intestine and colon. In: Yamada T, ed. *Textbook of gastroenterology,* 3rd ed., vol 1. Philadelphia: JB Lippincott, 1999:320–355.

Powell DW. Approach to the patient with diarrhea. In: Yamada T, ed. *Textbook of gastroenterology,* 3rd ed., vol 1. Philadelphia: JB Lippincott, 1999:858–909.

Schiller LR. Review article: anti-diarrhoeal pharmacology and therapeutics. *Aliment Pharmacol Ther* 1995;9:87–106.

Kelley's Textbook of Internal Medicine, fourth edition. Edited by H. David Humes.
Lippincott Williams & Wilkins, Philadelphia © 2000.

C H A P T E R
100

APPROACH TO THE PATIENT WITH CONSTIPATION, FECAL INCONTINENCE, AND GAS

JEFFREY L. BARNETT

Constipation implies difficulty extruding stool; fecal incontinence implies difficulty withholding it. At first glance, these symptoms appear completely unrelated, if not opposite. However, they share a common pathophysiologic mechanism and can even coexist in the same person. For example, long-standing constipation with straining predisposes to fecal incontinence later in life. Chronic fecal impaction among children or the elderly may manifest as overflow fecal incontinence. Irritable bowel syndrome (IBS) and various neuromuscular diseases may produce both constipation and fecal incontinence. Structural anorectal disorders such as rectal prolapse and hemorrhoids may be associated with both of these symptoms. Gaseousness, particularly bloating and flatulence, may accompany constipation and fecal incontinence or occur as an independent problem. Although belching and flatus production are universal, when taken to excess, these are particularly disturbing symptoms for many patients.

▪ CONSTIPATION

Constipation can be defined as a symptomatic decrease in the frequency of bowel movements. Misconceptions persist about the need for daily evacuation. Normal stool frequency varies, but most persons pass at least two or three stools per week. Women and blacks are more likely to report infrequent defecation than are men and whites. To a patient, constipation may mean not only decreased stool frequency but also passage of dry stools, excessive straining, lower abdominal fullness, and a sense of incomplete evacuation. Although these symptoms are more difficult to assess objectively than is bowel movement infrequency, they deserve serious attention by the physician.

PATHOPHYSIOLOGY

Constipation is caused by one of two mechanisms—obstruction of the movement of luminal contents or poor colonic propulsive activity (Table 100.1). Obstruction of colonic flow may be

TABLE 100.1.	DIFFERENTIAL DIAGNOSIS OF CONSTIPATION

Obstruction
Poor colonic propulsion
Structural disorders
  Colon cancer
  Benign stricture
  Extraluminal tumors
  Anorectal lesions
    Rectocele
    Anal stricture
    Hemorrhoids
    Fissure
Functional disorders
  Hirschsprung's disease
  Anal spasm
  Irritable bowel syndrome
  Defecation disorders
    Paradoxic puborectalis contraction (anismus)
    Rectal prolapse
Medication
  Anticholinergics
  Antidepressants
  Calcium channel blockers
  Diuretics
  Calcium supplements
  Iron pills
  Aluminum antacids
  Opiates
  Bismuth compounds
  Barium
Metabolic conditions
  Hypothyroidism
  Uremia
  Hypercalcemia
  Hypokalemia
  Pregnancy
  Pheochromocytoma
  Porphyria
Neuromuscular disorders
  Diabetes mellitus
  Scleroderma
  Amyloidosis
  Myotonic dystrophy
  Central nervous system lesions
  Multiple sclerosis
  Parkinson's disease
  Chagas' disease
  Ganglioneuromatosis
  Intestinal pseudoobstruction
Psychogenic disorders
  Depression
  Anorexia nervosa
Idiopathic disorders
  Colonic hypersegmentation
  Colonic hypoactivity

caused by luminal narrowing or a functional disorder. Poor propulsive activity in the colon may be caused by inhibition of motility (drugs, electrolyte disturbances, metabolic diseases) or diffuse nerve and muscle diseases (multiple sclerosis, familial visceral myopathy).

Several obstructing lesions cause constipation, the most important of which is carcinoma of the colon. Although carcinoma of the colon often becomes manifest with gross or occult blood in the stool, changes in bowel habit, ranging from a subtle decrease in stool frequency to constipation, also may occur. These symptoms usually occur over weeks or months but in rare instances are present for more than 1 year. Benign causes of colonic obstruction such as strictures caused by diverticular disease, colonic ischemia, or inflammatory bowel disease can produce similar symptoms. Anal strictures, foreign bodies, or sphincter spasm due to painful fissures or hemorrhoids may interrupt normal stool passage.

In the absence of an anatomic lesion, a disturbance in motility can produce functional colonic obstruction. A classic example of this is Hirschsprung's disease, or aganglionosis. This disorder is characterized by an absence of myenteric neurons in a segment of distal colon proximal to the sphincter. The aganglionic segment remains contracted, causing proximal obstruction and dilatation. This congenital condition occurs most often among infants with obstipation soon after birth, but in rare instances a short segment of aganglionosis can cause constipation among older children and adults. A more diffuse form of functional colonic obstruction may occur among patients with constipation associated with IBS. Hypersegmenting contractions of colonic circular muscle impede the forward movement of luminal contents in these patients. This spastic type of constipation may be associated with crampy abdominal pain and passage of scybalous (hard, dry) stools.

Constipation may be caused by drugs, metabolic abnormalities, and systemic diseases. Patients may suffer unknowingly if a physician fails to warn them about the constipating effects of such commonly prescribed medications as codeine, aluminum- or calcium-containing antacids, and iron compounds. Depressed patients often report constipation, a condition that may be exacerbated by the anticholinergic properties of antidepressants. Such metabolic disturbances as hypercalcemia and hypokalemia cause constipation by decreasing colonic smooth-muscle contractility. Constipation is a common gastrointestinal (GI) symptom among patients with diabetes mellitus, particularly those with autonomic neuropathy. Patients with progressive systemic sclerosis also may report constipation, but slow transit is caused by atrophy and fibrosis of colonic smooth muscle in this disease.

Neurogenic causes of constipation highlight the importance of both the extrinsic and intrinsic enteric nervous systems to normal colonic function. Central lesions due to Parkinson's disease, multiple sclerosis, or cerebrovascular accidents may cause constipation, although the symptoms may be caused in part by debilitation, inactivity, and poor bowel habits. Damage to the parasympathetic sacral nerves can lead to paralysis of the distal colon and rectum, making defecation an especially difficult problem for persons with spinal cord injuries. Chagas' disease, a parasitic infection, is an example of constipation caused by damage to the intrinsic enteric nervous system. The trypanosome organism infiltrates the GI tract and causes inflammation and degeneration of the myenteric plexus ganglion cells. Constipation associated with esophageal involvement suggests this infection among patients who have lived in or traveled to South America.

Changes in hormone levels have been associated with constipation. High levels of circulating catecholamines and low levels of thyroid hormone can depress GI motility and cause severe constipation among patients with pheochromocytoma and hypothyroidism, respectively. Elevated progesterone levels have been associated with increased intestinal transit time and reduced in vitro contractility of GI smooth muscle. Constipation during pregnancy and during the luteal phase of the menstrual cycle may be caused by increasing levels of this hormone.

Chronic idiopathic intestinal pseudoobstruction is a rare disorder characterized by recurrent episodes of intestinal obstruction without mechanical blockage. In addition to the small intestine, any other portion of the GI tract and occasionally the bladder can be involved. Although familial cases have been described, the underlying defect is unknown. Morphologic evidence of both neuropathy and myopathy has been reported.

Often no underlying cause of chronic constipation can be identified. Idiopathic constipation, a disorder more common among women, can be divided into two types: slow colonic transit (colonic inertia) and defecatory disorders (outlet obstruction). Colonic inertia involves poor transit of colonic contents throughout the colon and is demonstrated by delayed movement of radiopaque markers. Defecation disorders are a heterogeneous group of conditions characterized by poor evacuation of contents from the rectosigmoid colon. These mechanisms overlap and may coexist in the same patient, but the division is useful in conceptualizing and treating patients with chronic symptoms. Slow transit of luminal contents can be caused by a weakly propulsive or a spastic hypersegmenting colon. These disorders may be caused by abnormalities of the colonic smooth muscle or the myenteric plexus. Colonic inertia typically underlies severe constipation among young to middle-aged women who describe little pain but annoying bloating and marked stool infrequency. On the other hand, constipation among the elderly typically manifests as straining or evacuation difficulty rather than infrequency of stools.

Patients with long-standing constipation often have a disorder of the defecatory mechanism. Straining is common, and passage of even a large barium balloon or plastic sphere often is difficult. During attempted defecation, paradoxic contraction of the puborectalis and external sphincter muscles may produce functional outlet obstruction (anismus or rectosphincteric dyssynergia). Chronic straining itself is associated with increased descent of the perineal floor, which leads to a mechanically inefficient bulging motion of the anorectum. Abnormal perineal descent may cause chronic stretch injury to the pudendal nerve, which innervates the puborectalis muscle and external anal sphincter. This damage may cause incompetence of the anal sphincter and fecal incontinence. Occult and complete rectal prolapse may cause both partially obstructed defecation from rectal intussusception and, like perineal descent, chronic pudendal nerve injury. A large rectocele (anterior rectal herniation) may interfere with defecation because during straining, stool preferentially fills this sac and is therefore poorly expelled.

DIAGNOSTIC EVALUATION

The diagnostic evaluation of patients with constipation begins with a detailed history and physical examination. Important historical points include symptom duration and progression, a description of stool characteristics, and the presence of anorectal pain or bleeding. A directed history may uncover subtle symptoms suggesting hypothyroidism, collagen vascular disease, or esophageal or bladder dysfunction. A careful drug history must include such over-the-counter medications as antacids, vitamins, and bismuth compounds. The physical examination includes a thorough anorectal examination for tumors, hemorrhoids, and fissures. Anorectal neurogenic function is assessed by means of perianal cutaneous sensation, the anal wink reflex, and adequacy of anal canal tone. Examination during squeeze and straining maneuvers may uncover evidence of rectal prolapse, rectocele, and anismus. Appropriate laboratory studies can confirm suspected electrolyte or metabolic disturbances.

If the initial evaluation suggests the possibility of colonic obstruction, a structural study of the colon, such as barium radiography or endoscopy, is performed to exclude luminal narrowing. Flexible sigmoidoscopy or colonoscopy allows excellent visualization of the mucosa and tissue biopsy, which allow definitive diagnosis of anatomic lesions. A barium examination allows better evaluation of mild strictures or complicated diverticular disease, but the barium may be difficult to remove from a partially obstructed colon.

Once anatomic obstruction is ruled out, an attempt at treatment is made for patients with simple constipation. Most patients improve and no further diagnostic evaluation is necessary. However, a few patients with chronic refractory symptoms need further evaluation (Fig. 100.1).

The transit of stool through different segments of the colon is evaluated by means of following the progression of swallowed radiopaque markers over several days. Colonic inertia (slow transit throughout) can be differentiated from normal transit with functional outlet obstruction. Inertia in localized regions of the colon also can be identified. Marker studies are particularly useful for objective documentation of decreased stool frequency. A surprisingly large number of patients, albeit still a minority, have completely normal colorectal transit times. Some even deny stool output, although abdominal radiographs clearly show disappearance of markers. Many of these patients have psychologic factors that influence their symptoms. The approach to further evaluation and treatment is quite different from that of patients with abnormal colorectal transit.

Anal manometry is used to assess the function of the internal and external anal sphincters. Rectal distention normally initiates a reflex that relaxes the internal anal sphincter and contracts the external anal sphincter. Loss of this reflex suggests Hirschsprung's disease, a diagnosis that must be confirmed by means of rectal biopsy. Unexplained poor relaxation of the internal sphincter and paradoxic contraction of the external sphincter during defecation have been described as causes of constipation. Severe idiopathic constipation is associated with impaired rectal

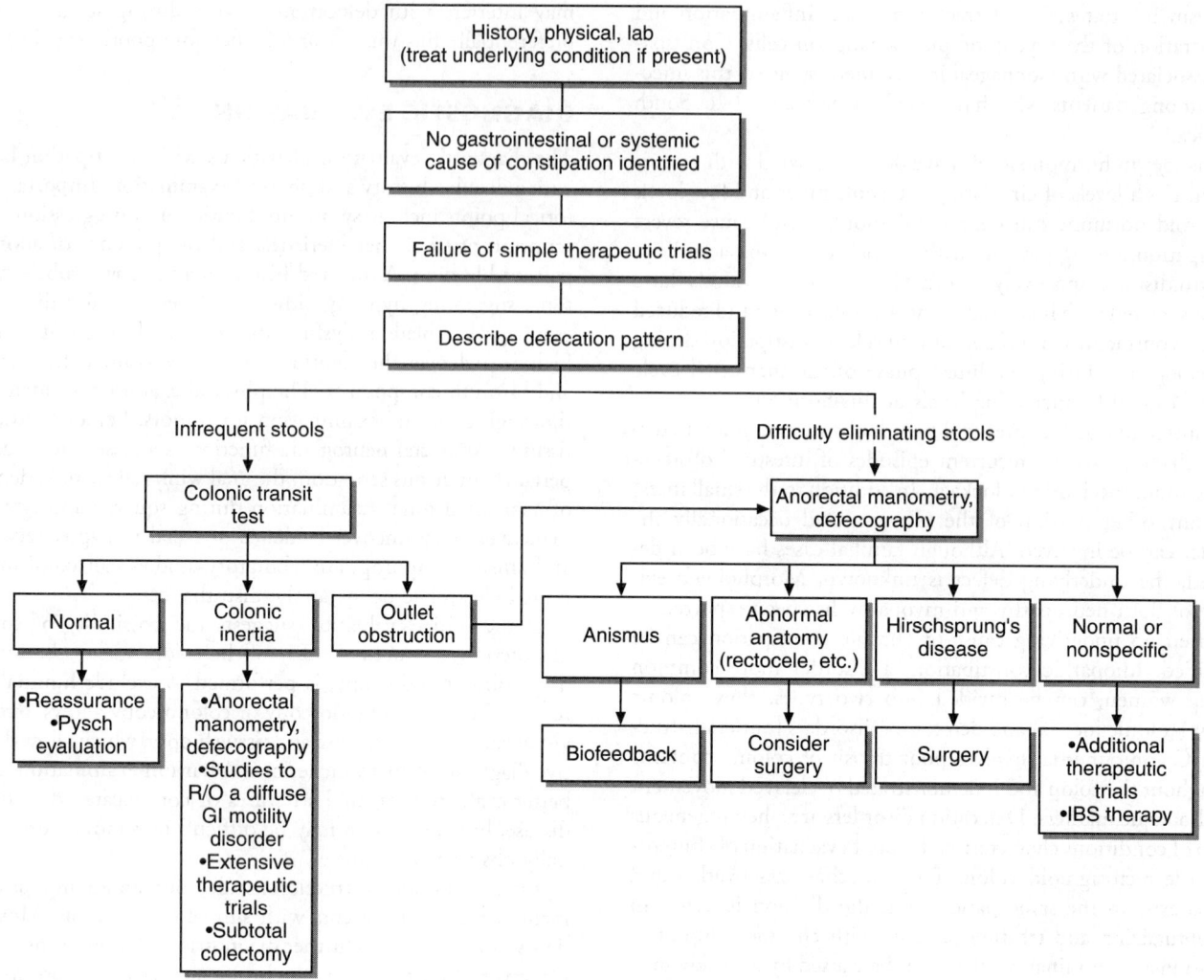

FIGURE 100.1. Algorithm for the approach to the patient with constipation.
EVIDENCE LEVEL: C. Expert Opinion.

sensation to balloon distention. An overly compliant rectum combined with a sensory loss may interfere with the normal urge to evacuate among these patients.

Defecography and serial specialized radiographs allow dynamic evaluation of the defecation process. The anorectal angle helps maintain fecal continence. Squatting in preparation for defecation straightens this angle to allow normal stool passage. Straining relaxes the puborectalis sling muscle to further straighten the anorectal angle. Failure to relax this muscle causes constipation among some patients. Abnormal perineal descent, obstructing enteroceles, rectoceles, and rectal prolapse also can be identified with defecography.

STRATEGIES FOR OPTIMAL CARE

Metabolic abnormalities must be corrected and constipating medications changed if possible. Daily exercise such as walking or running is encouraged. Adequate hydration and dietary fiber intake (20 to 30 g) is emphasized. The patient is encouraged to

allocate a limited time for defecation after a chosen meal. This approach takes advantage of the gastrocolonic reflex and helps establish a bowel routine.

Simple constipation often responds to daily fiber supplementation. Dietary fiber and hydrophilic colloid laxatives consist of poorly absorbed plant polysaccharides. Fiber products increase fecal volume and shorten colonic transit time by increasing the colonic bacterial mass and retaining luminal water. Greater fecal bulk enlarges the colonic diameter, which decreases intraluminal pressure. This may ease the straining associated with passage of small, scybalous stools. Fiber supplements such as psyllium, methylcellulose, and polycarbophil are available in various forms. These products are taken on a daily basis as a dietary supplement, not "as needed" in the manner of a laxative. Coadministration of at least 8 ounces (240 mL) of fluid is recommended, because GI obstruction can occur with use of these agents. Fiber supplementation merits at least a 2- to 3-week trial. The patient must be warned that symptoms of flatus and bloating may transiently worsen. Fiber products must be used cautiously by patients with a dilated, atonic colon or a severe defecation disorder because of risk of fecal impaction.

If fiber supplementation alone is unsuccessful, short-term or intermittent use of laxatives may be necessary. Saline (magnesium hydroxide, magnesium citrate), lubricant (mineral oil), and hyperosmotic (lactulose, polyethylene glycol) laxatives are best suited for this use. Emollient laxatives or stool softeners are of marginal benefit. Stimulant laxatives should be used for only brief periods because they can damage myenteric neurons and cause dependency. Chronic use of stimulant laxatives is a predisposing factor for a dilated, featureless colon recognized at barium enema examination as cathartic colon. Anthraquinone laxatives often cause benign hyperpigmentation of the colorectal mucosa (melanosis coli). The changes of cathartic colon and melanosis coli may be reversible on withdrawal of the laxative.

The spastic constipation of IBS occasionally responds to smooth muscle relaxants such as nitrates, anticholinergics, and calcium channel blockers, but these medications are of unproven benefit and cause constipation among many patients. Patients with hypoperistalsis need medication to stimulate smooth-muscle activity. Although many stimulants have been tried, none has yet proved efficacious in the management of constipation.

Nonpharmacologic therapies occasionally are beneficial to certain constipated patients. Psychotherapy and relaxation techniques help some patients with depression or IBS. A specific biofeedback technique has successfully retrained persons with constipation caused by anismus.

Surgery is rarely needed and is considered only to manage long-standing intractable symptoms or serious complications. A marker transit study combined with a defecation study allows a rational physiologic approach to surgical therapy. The procedure of choice for slow transit ascertained at marker study is colectomy with ileorectal anastomosis. Although colectomy is beneficial to some patients, chronic postoperative symptoms of diarrhea, persistent constipation, and acute small-intestinal obstruction are not unusual. The possibility of a diffuse motility disorder of the GI tract must be considered before this operation is performed. Lesser resections have a lower success rate and a high incidence of anastomotic leaks but can be considered if regional motility disorders or localized segments of dilatation can be identified. Some patients with prominent rectocele who have improved defecation dynamics when digital pressure is exerted on the posterior vaginal wall may benefit from surgical repair of this lesion. Rectopexy and operations to support the pelvic floor may improve defecation for patients with rectal prolapse or abnormal perineal descent.

COMPLICATIONS

Chronic constipation may have a role in the development of rectal prolapse, hemorrhoids, and anal fissure. Severe and even life-threatening complications (Table 100.2) are most common among elderly or debilitated patients. Fecal impaction, or fecaloma, may produce local mechanical problems such as urinary tract obstruction. Stercoral ulcers due to pressure necrosis from the fecal mass can bleed or perforate. Fecal impaction and less commonly perineal nerve damage may lead to incontinence. Fecal incontinence in turn can contribute to urinary tract infec-

TABLE 100.2.	**COMPLICATIONS OF CONSTIPATION**

Hemorrhoids
Anal fissures
Rectal prolapse
Cecal perforation
Volvulus
Ischemic colitis
Fecal impaction
   Colonic obstruction
   Urinary tract obstruction
   Stercoral ulceration
Fecal incontinence
   Decubitus ulcers
   Urinary tract infection
Laxative use
   Cathartic colon
   Melanosis coli

tion and decubitus ulcers, both common causes of sepsis among the elderly.

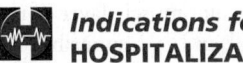

Indications for HOSPITALIZATION

Hospitalization rarely is needed even for severe constipation.

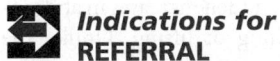

Indications for REFERRAL

Referral is appropriate if an underlying metabolic, neurologic, or anorectal cause of constipation is identified that requires the expertise of a specialist or a colorectal surgeon. Refractory symptoms despite fiber and laxative trials among women with idiopathic constipation and persistent constipation or recurrent fecal impaction in the elderly are indications for referral to a gastroenterologist with expertise in physiologic testing and medication regimens.

FECAL INCONTINENCE

The unintended release of fecal contents is a socially disabling and embarrassing symptom. Direct questioning may be needed to ascertain that a patient with "loose stools" or "bowel problems" has fecal incontinence, because the presence of this symptom is not always volunteered readily. The prevalence of fecal incontinence is highest among women, the elderly, and persons in long-term care facilities. About 10% of elderly persons living in residential facilities are incontinent of stool at least once a week.

PATHOPHYSIOLOGY

Rectum and Its Contents

The contents, motility, compliance, and sensation of the rectum are important determinants of fecal continence. Nearly everyone has experienced fecal urgency during an acute diarrheal illness. Large volumes of liquid stool delivered to the rectum challenge the continence mechanisms of even healthy persons. In general, bulky solid stools are easiest to control. The ability of a normally compliant rectum to accommodate and sense material presented to it is an important determinant of continence and defecation. Neuropathic damage from long-standing diabetes and poor distensibility caused by radiation proctitis may interfere with normal rectal reservoir function and predispose to fecal incontinence.

Anal Canal and Sphincters

The anal canal is a slit 3 to 4 cm long and slightly anteroposterior that is the final barrier to fecal flow. It is normally closed by tonic contractions of the surrounding sphincter musculature. Spongy vascular anal cushions help fine-tune this closure. Prolapsing tissue or previous hemorrhoidectomy may interfere with this seal to allow minor seepage. The internal sphincter muscle is the thickened distal portion of the circular muscle layer of the rectum. It is under involuntary control and is responsible for most of the resting sphincter tone. The external sphincter is a surrounding sleeve of striated muscle that extends a small distance below the caudal margin of the internal sphincter. It helps to maintain a degree of resting tone but is predominantly responsible for the augmented tone needed to maintain continence during periods of rectal distention or sudden increases in abdominal pressure, such as during coughing or lifting. Unlike the rectum, which is sensitive only to distention, the mucosa of the anal canal can detect touch, pain, and temperature.

When material enters the distal rectum, anal sampling may occur to differentiate flatus from liquid or solid stool and allow selective passage of these materials. Traumatic childbirth injuries and damage to the sphincter muscles during operations for anal fissure or hemorrhoids may be a predisposing factor to incontinence. Neuropathic damage to the sphincters be caused by various conditions such as diabetes, spinal cord injury, or more commonly chronic constipation with straining (stretch injury to the pudendal nerve) and degenerative changes associated with aging.

Puborectalis Muscle and Defecation

The puborectalis muscle attaches to the symphysis pubis and wraps around the posterior aspect of the anorectal junction to form a sling. Tonic contraction of this muscle produces an approximate right angle between the axes of the anus and rectum to act as a barrier to passage of rectal contents. The origin and innervation (sacral branches) of the puborectalis muscle and external sphincter are similar, so these muscles act in concert. Stool entering the rectum causes reflex relaxation of the internal sphincter so that anal sampling can occur. External sphincter contraction maintains continence during rectal accommodation to the bolus. The act of voluntary withholding increases the anterior pull of the puborectalis muscle and accentuates the acuteness of the angle to better maintain continence. When the decision is made to defecate, sitting or squatting increases (straightens) the anorectal angle to facilitate stool passage. If the person is resisting strongly the call to stool, simply relaxing conscious control allows defecation. Otherwise, a Valsalva maneuver is performed to increase intra-abdominal pressure, and pushing relaxes the puborectalis muscle to further straighten the angle. The pelvic floor descends, the rectum contracts, the sphincter relaxes, and the bolus is expelled. Traumatic or neuropathic injury to this muscle may cause major fecal incontinence.

DIAGNOSTIC EVALUATION

Symptoms of fecal incontinence range from minor soiling or poor control of flatus to complete loss of control of even solid stools. Important characteristics to consider include the severity and chronicity of symptoms, the patient's age and sex, predisposing anorectal trauma, and the presence of diarrhea or constipation, associated sensory abnormalities, and underlying neuromuscular disease (Table 100.3). Incontinence associated with toilet-training difficulties among children or with acute episodes of constipation among the elderly suggests fecal impaction. Incontinence associated with hematochezia may suggest ulcerative or radiation proctitis. Nocturnal incontinence is typical of diabetic autonomic neuropathy. New-onset incontinence associated with pelvic or lower extremity sensorimotor loss suggests spinal cord disease. Symptoms immediately after childbirth suggest traumatic disruption of the sphincter.

The social context and circumstances surrounding fecal incontinence must be considered. Incontinence associated with anxiety and urgency in IBS may reflect lack of an available toilet facility. Fecal soiling among demented or mentally disabled persons may be caused by a communication or recognition problem. Physical disabilities may prevent timely defecation among persons without access to physical assistance.

A directed physical examination offers clues to the cause of fecal incontinence. Anal sphincter deformities, perianal infection, tumors, fistulas, and prolapsing hemorrhoids may be apparent at simple inspection. Absence of the anal wink in response to a pinstroke suggests neuropathic damage. Digital examination allows evaluation of sphincter tone at rest and during squeeze and may help detect fecal impaction or a low-lying tumor.

The diagnostic evaluation is specifically tailored to the clinical presentation. Soiling associated with an acute diarrheal illness or fecal impaction may necessitate no specific anorectal evaluation other than that of the underlying bowel problem. Likewise, identification of a rectal mass or fourth-degree laceration after childbirth necessitates no further anorectal studies, and the appropriate surgical procedure may be performed.

The extent of evaluation of less obvious causes of fecal incontinence depends in part on the availability of tools and local expertise. Inspection of the distal colon either endoscopically or radiographically is necessary in most cases to rule out proctitis, tumor, or impaction. Anorectal manometry with perfused cathe-

TABLE 100.3.	**CAUSES OF FECAL INCONTINENCE**

Diarrhea
Fecal impaction
Irritable bowel syndrome
Anal abnormality
  Anal carcinoma
  Congenital abnormalities
  Protruding internal hemorrhoids
  Rectal prolapse
  Perianal infections
  Fistula
  Injury
    Surgical (e.g., hemorrhoidectomy, fistulotomy)
    Obstetric
    Accidental trauma
Rectal abnormality
  Rectal carcinoma
  Rectal ischemia
  Proctitis
    Inflammatory bowel disease
    Radiation-induced lesion
    Infectious disease
Neurologic diseases
  Central nervous system
    Stroke, dementia
    Toxic/metabolic
    Cord injury, tumors
    Multiple sclerosis, tabes dorsalis
  Peripheral nervous system
    Diabetes, others
    Cauda equina lesions
  "Idiopathic" (primary neurogenic)
    Childbirth injury
    Chronic constipation
    Descending perineum
    Old age

Source: Barnett JL. Anorectal disease. In: Yamada T, ed. *Textbook of gastroenterology,* 3rd ed. Philadelphia: JB Lippincott, 1999: 2083–2106, with permission.

ters, balloons, or transducers allows measurement of resting and maximal squeeze sphincter function (see Chapter 129). The rectoanal inhibitory reflex can be measured by means of inflating a rectal balloon and detecting diminution of baseline tone. Simple balloon inflation also allows estimation of rectal sensation, and more sophisticated techniques with pressure-volume relations can estimate rectal compliance. Defecography is a radiographic study that allows dynamic assessment of the function of the sphincter and the puborectalis muscle during expulsion of a simulated barium paste stool (see Chapter 129). It also can help detect internal rectal prolapse and exaggerated perineal descent. Needle electromyography may be indicated under special circumstances for direct assessment of the symmetry and degree of denervation and reinnervation of the external sphincter muscle fibers. Anal endosonography is a particularly sensitive means of detecting subtle sphincter muscle defects. Standardized tests to measure leakage of rectally infused saline solution or resistance to passage of solid spheres can be used to test the integrated continence mechanisms.

STRATEGIES FOR OPTIMAL CARE

Underlying causes of fecal incontinence such as proctitis or a spinal cord tumor are managed specifically. Even if the underlying etiologic factor is not easily corrected, symptoms often respond to relatively simple measures. Fecal impaction is cleared with enemas, and a treatment plan for constipation is instituted. Loose or frequent stools are controlled with fiber agents or antidiarrheal drugs. Debilitated patients or those with neurologic disease or injury may respond best to a bowel program of regular, timed defecation. Fiber agents and anticholinergics may help to control incontinence among patients with IBS who have postprandial urgency symptoms by solidifying stools and blunting the gastrocolonic response. Sphincter exercises may be an adjunct to the foregoing measures by improving tone and awareness of the pelvic floor.

Persistent fecal incontinence is managed with a trial of biofeedback therapy. This simple technique of operant conditioning attempts to improve sphincter contractility and rectal sensitivity to distention through use of visual or auditory cues. Among motivated patients, success rates of about 70% are achieved after only two or three sessions when combined with medical therapy and a bowel program. Severe neurogenic lesions causing marked sphincter dysfunction or poor rectal sensation, trauma, surgically induced sphincter deformities, and refractory IBS respond poorly to anal biofeedback therapy.

Fecal leakage in association with third-degree hemorrhoids or persistent rectal prolapse may respond to surgical repair of these conditions. Incontinence caused by obstetric injury or previous anal surgery may be cured after simple repair of the external anal sphincter. Other causes of fecal incontinence unresponsive to medical therapy may improve after a variety of operations, including postanal repair, anterior reefing procedure, gracilis muscle transposition, and even placement of an artificial sling. Surgical expertise and careful patient selection are critical, because results vary and the procedures are not without complications. Placement of a colostomy is considered for patients with persistent fecal incontinence who have not had successful medical therapy and are not candidates for a more specialized surgical procedure. Diversion of the fecal stream in this manner may improve quality of life for selected patients and may even be life saving for debilitated patients or those in long-term care who are at risk of sepsis caused by urinary tract or decubitus ulcer infections.

▬ GAS

PRESENTATION AND PATHOPHYSIOLOGY

Eructation, or belching, is the retrograde passage of upper GI gas from the mouth. Involuntary belching is a normal process after a meal and is caused by release of swallowed air after gastric distention with food. Medications or foods such as mints and tomatoes that decrease lower esophageal sphincter tone may facilitate the process. Air swallowing, or aerophagia, is responsible for most upper GI gas, so symptoms may occur with any process that causes hypersalivation such as gum chewing, smoking, and oropharyngeal irritation. Chronic habitual eructation usually is caused by voluntary aerophagia. These often anxious patients have been shown to swallow before each belch; air is released from the esophagus before it even reaches the stomach. Many patients have chronic symptoms of gastroesophageal reflux or functional dyspepsia, which they believe are temporarily relieved by belching.

Flatulence, the frequent passage of gas through the rectum, like belching, rarely suggests serious organic disease in the absence of other worrisome symptoms or signs. Although the intestine at any given time usually contains less than 200 mL of gas, several times that amount may be excreted per day. Healthy young men pass gas an average of 14 times per day, and up to 25 expulsions is considered normal. Although flatus is composed in part of swallowed air (nitrogen and oxygen), in the absence of aerophagia the composition is determined primarily by the activity of the colonic flora and the ingestion of carbohydrates. Nonabsorbable dietary carbohydrates (legumes, beans) and portions of ingested sugars (fructose, sorbitol in fruits and candies) and starches that escape small-intestinal absorption reach the colon and are metabolized by bacterial fermentation into hydrogen, carbon dioxide, and sometimes methane. The volume and composition of flatus therefore is affected by diet, intestinal transit, and alterations of colonic flora produced by antibiotics or bowel cleansing.

HISTORY AND PHYSICAL EXAMINATION

Patients with gaseousness may describe bad breath, belching, chest pain, dyspepsia, excessive bloating, abdominal discomfort, loud bowel sounds, or flatulence. These symptoms often reflect a functional disorder such as aerophagia, nonulcer dyspepsia, and IBS. Symptoms among these patients typically are not nocturnal or progressive and have been present at least intermittently for months or years. The possibility of a severe organic disorder must be considered, however, especially if vomiting, weight loss, fever, bleeding, or steatorrhea is present. A careful dietary history may relate symptoms to ingestion of legumes, beans, wheat products, fruit, candy, and carbonated beverages. The consumption of milk products must be specifically addressed, because lactose intolerance can develop even later in life. Medications, especially those that slow GI motility, such as anticholinergics, antidiarrheal agents, and narcotics may cause bloating and other symptoms.

DIFFERENTIAL DIAGNOSIS

Important disorders to consider when a patient has gaseousness include obstruction, GI dysmotility, and malabsorption or maldigestion. Partial obstruction at the pylorus or duodenal bulb may be caused by peptic ulcer disease. Hernia, Crohn's disease, or adhesions from abdominal operations may produce intestinal obstruction that if subtle, may masquerade as unexplained bloating or gaseousness. Tumors of the GI tract, particularly ovarian cancer among women, can manifest as bloating without weight loss or frank obstruction. Autonomic neuropathy from diabetes or neuromuscular dysfunction as a result of systemic sclerosis may produce bloating, early satiety, and nausea. Stasis from these

or other GI motility disorders predispose a patient to bacterial overgrowth. When the normally sterile upper GI tract becomes overgrown with anaerobic bacteria, these organisms metabolize ingested foodstuffs into gas and organic acids and cause diarrhea, bloating, and flatulence. Similar symptoms may be caused by giardiasis and malabsorption (celiac sprue) or maldigestion (pancreatic insufficiency).

LABORATORY STUDIES AND DIAGNOSTIC TESTS

Extensive testing is not necessary if a patient with gaseousness has no worrisome symptoms to suggest a specific organic disorder. Simple laboratory tests, including a blood cell count, chemical screen, and stool studies, and abdominal radiography help rule out specific disorders and relevant systemic diseases. Barium examination or endoscopy may be indicated if intestinal obstruction, peptic ulcer disease, or malabsorption is an important concern. Hydrogen breath tests can be used to diagnose bacterial overgrowth, lactase insufficiency, and carbohydrate intolerance, especially if ingestion of the test food reproduces the patient's typical symptoms.

STRATEGIES FOR OPTIMAL CARE

In the absence of a specifically identified disorder, therapy for gaseousness consists of reducing swallowed air and dietary restrictions to reduce colonic production of bacterial gas. Aerophagia is reduced by means of elimination of gum chewing, eating hard candies, smoking, and chewing tobacco. For chronic belching, simply identifying the process of air swallowing for the patient might relieve symptoms. If not, anxiolytics or behavioral modification may be considered. A patient with flatus may benefit from a low-flatus diet, which restricts beans, onions, legumes, fruits, wheat products, starches, and milk. Simethicone and activated charcoal are used with occasional success, although the mechanism is uncertain and efficacy is not clearly shown. Lactase enzymes can be tried for gaseousness produced by milk products and bacterial α-galactosidase for that produced by nondigestible oligosaccharides (beans, legumes).

BIBLIOGRAPHY

Barnett JL. Anorectal diseases. In: Yamada T, ed. *Textbook of gastroenterology*, 3rd ed. Philadelphia: JB Lippincott, 1999:2083–2106.

Camilleri M, Thompson G, Fleshman JW, et al. Clinical management of intractable constipation. *Ann Intern Med* 1994;121:520–528.

Levitt MD. Follow-up of a flatulent patient. *Dig Dis Sci* 1979;24:652–654.

Levitt MD, Lasser RB, Schwartz JS, et al. Studies of a flatulent patient. *N Engl J Med* 1976;295:260–262.

Mavrantonis C, Wexner SD. A clinical approach to fecal incontinence. *J Clin Gastroenterol* 1998;27:108–121.

Perman JA, Boatwright DN. Approach to the patient with gas and bloating. In: Yamada T, ed. *Textbook of gastroenterology*, 3rd ed. Philadelphia: JB Lippincott, 1999:815–826.

Sultan AH, Kamm MA, Hudson CN, et al. Anal-sphincter disruption during vaginal delivery. *N Engl J Med* 1993;329:1905–1911.

Wald A. Approach to the patient with constipation. In: Yamada T, ed.

Textbook of gastroenterology, 3rd ed. Philadelphia: JB Lippincott, 1999: 910–926.

Kelley's Textbook of Internal Medicine, fourth edition. Edited by H. David Humes. Lippincott Williams & Wilkins, Philadelphia © 2000.

C H A P T E R
101

APPROACH TO THE PATIENT WITH AN ABDOMINAL OR RECTAL MASS

**ILIAS SCOTINIOTIS
MICHAEL L. KOCHMAN**

PRESENTATION

The signs and symptoms of an intra-abdominal or pelvic mass can be caused by the effects of the mass on surrounding structures or by the indirect, systemic effects of the underlying process, which is usually neoplastic or inflammatory. The diagnostic approach is in large part determined by the clinical presentation. With the increasing use of cross-sectional imaging, a mass may be detected incidentally in a patient, posing a different set of diagnostic questions and issues.

Pain is frequently the presenting symptom of an abdominal mass. The location of the pain often is determined by the developmental origin of the organ involved (see Chapter 96). Gastrointestinal or genitourinary bleeding, whether macroscopic or microscopic, is an important finding and always must be sought when a mass is suspected. Through disruption of mucosal integrity, blood in the stool or urine directs the investigation toward the mucosa of the respective system. If bleeding is not present, the lesion is more likely to be extrinsic to the gastrointestinal or genitourinary epithelium and may not be accessible to endoscopic investigation.

Luminal obstruction is a frequent presentation of masses that originate in the organs of the digestive tract. The nature of this presentation is related to luminal diameter and the relation of the mass to surrounding structures. Masses in the head of the pancreas frequently cause obstruction of the common bile duct, which courses through the pancreatic head, and less commonly obstruction of the duodenum, which courses adjacent to the pancreatic head. In the colon, the progressively smaller size of the lumen makes a distal mass much more likely to cause obstruction than a proximal mass. Masses arising in the small intestine are relatively rare, and do not account for most episodes of small-intestinal obstruction, which is more commonly attributable to adhesions that are sequelae of earlier surgery (often gynecologic, intestinal, or colonic, less commonly biliary or gastric), intra-abdominal infection (peritonitis), or irradiation. Impinge-

ment of a mass on surrounding blood vessels that leads to syndromes of vascular insufficiency, such as lower extremity edema or intestinal ischemia, may denote the presence of a large lesion. The presence of ascites in the setting of an abdominal mass suggests the presence of peritoneal metastasis.

The systemic constitutional effects of an abdominal mass often may be the only presentation. High fever points toward an intra-abdominal abscess. Unexpected loss of more than 5% to 10% of body weight suggests the presence of malignant disease. Paraneoplastic syndromes are a rare presentation of abdominal tumors. Cases of pseudoachalasia related to hepatoma and of dermatomyositis or polymyositis related to malignant gastrointestinal disease have been described. Gastric cancer may cause microangiopathic hemolytic anemia, chronic disseminated intravascular coagulation, membranous nephropathy, sudden appearance of seborrheic keratosis (Leser–Trélat sign), or filiform pigmented lesions in skin folds (acanthosis nigricans). Unexplained deep venous thrombosis in an elderly patient raises the possibility of an underlying adenocarcinoma (Trousseau's syndrome).

Discovery of abdominal masses among adults without symptoms is increasing in frequency as cancer screening recommendations put forth by professional societies become widely adopted. This is true of colorectal cancer, for which screening with fecal occult blood testing and sigmoidoscopy is recommended. In this era of increased availability of cross-sectional imaging techniques, it is not uncommon to find an abdominal mass during investigations for unrelated problems. More than 20% of adults have benign liver cysts or tumors, such as hemangioma or focal nodular hyperplasia, and 30% of adults older than 50 years have cystic renal lesions. Among patients with incidental masses, careful radiologic description coupled with evaluation of the clinical situation determines the need for further testing.

PATHOPHYSIOLOGY

The clinical consequences of an abdominal mass depend on its location and the underlying etiologic factors. A pancreatic mass can compromise the exocrine function of the gland. The profound weight loss associated with pancreatic cancer is initially caused by fat malabsorption due to reduced pancreatic secretion from tumor obstruction of the pancreatic duct. Lesions in the head of the pancreas obstruct a greater length of the main pancreatic duct and therefore cause a greater degree of malabsorption.

In the liver, unaffected parenchyma has great capacity to compensate functionally for the injury caused by a mass lesion. Even very large liver lesions do not manifest with hepatic failure. Because the hepatic parenchyma is enclosed within Glisson's capsule, an expanding mass frequently causes pain. If there is diffuse underlying injury due to cirrhosis, the development of a mass lesion can unmask hepatic failure; deterioration causes jaundice, coagulopathy, ascites, or encephalopathy. The same is true of the kidneys, where development of renal failure is a rare complication of a mass lesion in the absence of severe underlying renal disease.

In most hollow abdominal organs, such as the stomach, small intestine, colon, and rectum, the capacity of the organs is such that a mass can grow to great size before intestinal function is affected. Given the great surface area of these organs, a discrete mass is unlikely to manifest with maldigestion or malabsorption. The absence of afferent pain fibers from the wall of the digestive tract also renders growth of these lesions painless until local invasion into the peritoneum or adjacent structures occurs. Mass lesions in the hollow organs therefore can be clinically inapparent until they reach an advanced stage.

HISTORY AND PHYSICAL EXAMINATION

The nature of any pain symptoms must be defined carefully with respect to duration, food ingestion, and defecation. Pain that closely follows a meal suggests a lesion in the gastrointestinal tract. The location and radiation of pain can help localize the lesion, and the temporal relation to meals can help localize a proximal or distal lesion. Defecatory pain points to the anal canal as the source and suggests a rectal abscess, fissure, or anal canal tumor. Decreased frequency of defecation (constipation) or decreased caliber of the stool point to a lesion in the distal colon. Fecal incontinence, urgency, or a sensation of incomplete evacuation suggests a rectal lesion, especially if blood coats the stool. Blood also may be mixed with stool, suggesting a source in the colon. Melena generally indicates a proximal source in the stomach, small intestine, or right colon. Other causes of black stool, such as iron or bismuth ingestion, must be ruled out. The term *hematochezia*, denoting the passage of bright red blood per rectum, is an ineffective descriptor because it has been used in different contexts. It is more valuable to describe precisely the appearance of the blood-containing stool. Dysuria or hematuria may indicate that the mass either originated in or extends into the urinary tract. The latter can occur in the setting of an inflammatory mass, such as that caused by Crohn's disease, which also can cause pneumaturia if an enterovesicular fistula is present.

Important aspects of the social history include the use of alcohol, which predisposes to hepatic or pancreatic lesions, or risk factors for viral hepatitis. A family history of neoplasia, such as colorectal polyps or cancer, may suggest a genetic predilection. A history of blunt abdominal trauma is sought, because that can lead to formation of a duodenal hematoma or pancreatic pseudocyst.

Fever greater than 38°C (100.4°F) in a patient with an abdominal mass suggests an intra-abdominal abscess. Neoplasms that commonly cause fever, such as renal cell carcinoma and hepatocellular carcinoma, are not associated with such severe temperature elevations.

The characteristics of an abdominal mass at palpation can be revealing. Tenderness with rebound suggests that the mass is inflammatory and associated with localized or generalized peritonitis. A firm, nontender, nonpulsatile mass is likely to be neoplastic. In most instances of intra-abdominal neoplasia, however, the mass is not detectable at physical examination before it extends regionally. Ability to palpate a neoplasm therefore usually indicates a poor prognosis. Evidence of lymphadenopathy at examination suggests metastatic disease. Gastric cancer, for ex-

ample, may spread to intra-abdominal lymph nodes and supraclavicular nodes (Virchow's node) or may involve a periumbilical nodule (Sister Mary Joseph's node). Digital rectal examination allows palpation of approximately half of all rectal neoplasms. It is an important component of the physical examination because it also allows stool testing for occult blood by means of a guaiac-based test. A positive test result has a positive predictive value between 10% and 20% for colorectal cancer among persons who have no symptoms and undergo screening, but that value is substantially higher if a patient has a known abdominal mass.

LABORATORY STUDIES AND DIAGNOSTIC TESTS

Laboratory testing plays a minor role in the evaluation of a suspected abdominal or rectal mass, although a complete blood cell count is an important initial test. The leukocyte count is important if an infectious cause of the mass is being considered. The hemoglobin and red blood cell count indices allow assessment of the chronicity of gastrointestinal bleeding. In the setting of a hepatic mass, abnormalities in measurements of hepatic function, such as conjugated bilirubin, albumin, and international normalized ratio, suggest underlying cirrhosis. Use of immunologic tests for serum tumor markers has been controversial in the diagnosis of malignant abdominal tumors. Neuroendocrine tumors express synaptophysin and chromogranin A. Measurement of mucin-related carbohydrate antigens CA 19-9 and CA 242 has approximately 75% sensitivity for pancreatic adenocarcinoma but is fairly nonspecific. The test result can be positive for other cancers of the gastrointestinal tract, such as hepatobiliary or gastric cancer, among many patients with chronic pancreatitis, and among healthy persons. Measurement of carcinoembryonic antigen also is nonspecific for colorectal cancer; levels are elevated in the presence of benign liver and pancreatic disease. Carcinoembryonic antigen testing has limited use in the followup care of patients who have undergone surgical resection of colorectal cancer for the detection of recurrence. α-Fetoprotein, another oncofetal protein, is secreted by most but not all hepatocellular carcinomas. Overall, serum tumor markers are unreliable for diagnosis but may corroborate the diagnosis of a malignant disease under the appropriate clinical circumstances.

If a patient with an abdominal mass has ascites, it is important to perform diagnostic paracentesis for evaluation of the serumascites albumin gradient. A difference in serum-to-ascites albumin concentrations lower than 1.1 suggests that the ascites is not related to portal hypertension and is likely to indicate peritoneal metastasis. Cytologic examination of ascitic fluid has a sensitivity of about 50% for peritoneal carcinomatosis if adequate volume is aspirated but is highly specific. Increased levels of triglycerides in ascitic fluid (chylous ascites) strongly suggest underlying lymphoma.

In the case of masses of the stomach, small intestine, colon, or rectum, the most important diagnostic test is endoscopy coupled with endoscopic biopsy, which can be performed under sedation. A conventional upper gastrointestinal endoscope can reach lesions as far as the third portion of the duodenum. An enteroscope is needed to see jejunal lesions, and a side-viewing duodenoscope is used for better visualization of a mass in the region of the ampulla of Vater. In the lower gastrointestinal tract, anoscopy and rigid proctoscopy have limited diagnostic value when flexible fiberoptic endoscopy can be performed instead. Flexible sigmoidoscopy allows examination of the distal 60 cm of colon, which usually translates to an area around the mid descending colon. The examination can be undertaken after easy preparation with two cleansing enemas. The 180-cm colonoscope allows inspection of the entire colon and rectum (see Chapter 127).

The diagnostic use of endoscopic retrograde cholangiopancreatography (ERCP) is limited to masses of the pancreatic head or biliary tract. High-grade, abrupt obstruction of both the pancreatic duct and common bile duct (double duct sign) has high specificity for cancer of the pancreatic head. Cytologic brushings obtained at ERCP have less than 50% sensitivity for cancer of the bile duct or pancreas. A development in imaging of the biliary tree is magnetic resonance cholangiography, the clinical utility of which as an alternative, noninvasive modality remains to be fully elucidated.

Despite the great utility of endoscopic procedures in the diagnosis of an abdominal mass, these examinations should not always be undertaken if the mass is believed to be inflammatory or infectious. Inflammation of the wall may increase the risk of perforation during endoscopy, and endoscopic biopsy is not always definitive in identifying the cause of inflammation. Radiologic evaluation of the mass is a reasonable alternative.

Many cross-sectional imaging techniques are of use in evaluating abdominal masses. Ultrasonography is effective in imaging the hepatic parenchyma and the biliary system but is otherwise limited for use in the abdomen by gas in overlying intestine. In the kidneys, ultrasonography can be used reliably to diagnose most benign simple cysts. Computed tomography has emerged as the preferred technique for abdominal imaging because it allows a comprehensive evaluation of the viscera (see Chapter 128). Magnetic resonance imaging (MRI) can help define difficult to characterize lesions such as focal nodular hyperplasia and focal fatty infiltration.

CT is the standard for evaluation of renal and adrenal masses. MRI currently carries no appreciable advantage over CT in the evaluation of renal masses. CT also is widely used for imaging of the pancreas, in which contrast enhancement can be used reliably to detect masses more than 2 cm in diameter. In evaluation of pancreatic masses, however, CT is limited in defining involvement of peripancreatic vessels and peritoneal metastases, both of which are important indicators that the tumor is unresectable. These challenges have been addressed by the development of endoscopic ultrasonography (EUS), which can give greater detail about the pancreatic parenchyma and surrounding blood vessels and lymph nodes. With an endoscope fitted with an ultrasound probe, images of the pancreatic parenchyma can be obtained through adjoining parts of the stomach and duodenum. EUS is superior to other imaging modalities in the detection of small pancreatic masses. It is the most accurate method of local staging of pancreatic masses and of rectal masses. Because it also allows detailed visualization of the intestinal wall, EUS also is useful in evaluating submucosal lesions throughout the

digestive tract, including the esophagus, stomach, small intestine, and rectosigmoid colon.

DIFFERENTIAL DIAGNOSIS

The differential diagnosis of an abdominal mass is broad. It includes infectious, inflammatory, vascular, traumatic, and neoplastic lesions. These can be difficult to differentiate on the basis of history and physical findings alone given the nonspecific presentation. Careful radiologic characterization of the lesion is important because both the prognosis and the management decisions depend on the cause of the mass.

The importance of radiologic characterization is nowhere more important than in the liver (Fig. 101.1). With advanced imaging techniques, it is possible to diagnose most liver lesions, such as cysts, hemangioma, adenoma, focal nodular hyperplasia, focal fatty infiltration, and hepatocellular carcinoma. The presence of multiple lesions always prompts a search for an extrahepatic primary malignant tumor, usually carcinoma of the breast, colon, rectum, or lung. Even with the most advanced radiologic means, however, differentiating a liver tumor from an abscess may be difficult. Pyogenic (bacterial) liver abscesses may be single or solitary and mimic metastatic disease. They may arise from hematogenous spread of bacteria or from local spread from contiguous infections, often cholangitis. The diagnosis is considered even when patients have nonspecific symptoms such as low-grade fever and malaise, because 50% of patients with a liver abscess lack signs or symptoms referable to the right upper quadrant. Amebic abscess is a rare entity in the United States and is preceded in 90% of cases by a history of bloody diarrhea (dysentery) within the previous year. Abscess formation with an indolent presentation also can occur in the subphrenic space, arbitrarily defined as the space between the diaphragm and the transverse colon. In 90% of cases, this is a delayed complication of operations on the biliary tract, stomach, or duodenum.

In the evaluation of a suspected upper abdominal mass, the malignant potential of the mass is determined by its location, best defined with CT (Fig. 101.2). A mass arising in the stomach is adenocarcinoma until proved otherwise, because benign tumors of the stomach rarely grow to considerable size. Adenocarcinoma accounts for 95% of all cancers of the stomach and may defy endoscopic biopsy diagnosis if it presents in its infiltrating form, linitis plastica. Lymphoma is the second most common malignant tumor of the stomach, but it often manifests as an infiltrating, submucosal lesion rather than a single, ulcerating mass. A mass in the small intestine is less likely to be malignant than is a mass in the stomach. Benign small-intestinal tumors include adenoma, leiomyoma, lipoma, and less commonly hamartoma, fibroma, and angioma. The most common malignant tumors of the small intestine are adenocarcinoma (40% to 45%), carcinoid tumor (30%), leiomyosarcoma (10%), and lymphoma (15%). Throughout the gastrointestinal tract, the diagnosis of lymphoma is considered in the evaluation of patients with AIDS or profound immunosuppression.

A solid mass in the pancreas, as in the stomach, is caused by cancer until proved otherwise (Fig. 101.3). Pancreatic cancer usually arises from the epithelium of the pancreatic duct (ductal

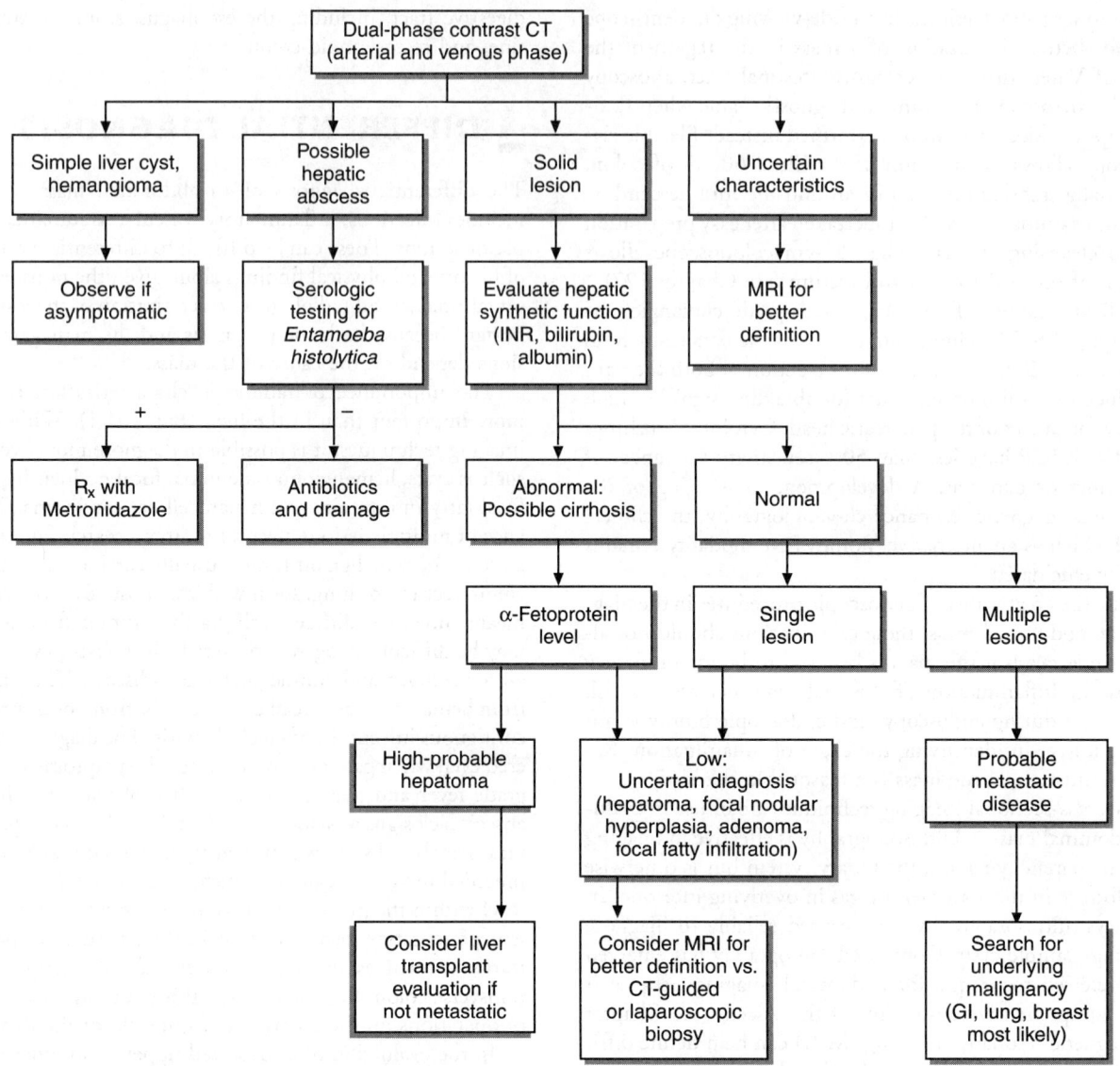

FIGURE 101.1. Evaluation of a liver mass.
EVIDENCE LEVEL: B. Reference: Saim S. Imaging of the hepatobiliary tract. *N Engl J Med* 1997; 336:1889–1894.

adenocarcinoma). Other types of solid pancreatic masses are functional neuroendocrine tumors (insulinoma, gastrinoma, and VIPoma) and pancreatic lymphoma. When a pancreatic mass contains cystic components, the differential diagnosis includes inflammatory lesions such as pancreatic pseudocyst. The challenge lies in differentiating this benign lesion from a cystic pancreatic neoplasm, such as mucinous cystadenoma or cystadenocarcinoma. Mucinous cystic neoplasms occur more commonly among women (6:1 female-to-male ratio) between the ages of 40 and 60 years. Patients often have large, complex cysts that harbor foci of adenocarcinoma, which are difficult to visualize with any imaging modality. Because of that possibility, any large cystic lesion of the pancreas that is not clearly a pseudocyst complicating pancreatitis is evaluated for possible resection.

Neuroendocrine tumors of the gastrointestinal tract (carcinoids) arise most commonly in the appendix, followed by the ileum, rectum, and stomach. They are usually indolent with low rates of growth and therefore often have metastasized to mesenteric lymph nodes, liver, or lung by the time they come to medical attention. The symptoms of neuroendocrine tumors usually are caused by local effects of tumor growth, including obstruction and intussusception. Small-intestinal carcinoids in particular can cause obstruction due to an associated severe desmoplastic reaction in the mesentery, which is nearly pathognomonic at CT. Carcinoid syndrome, which comprises flushing, diarrhea, and valvular lesions and is attributed to secretion of serotonin, is experienced by less than 5% of all patients with carcinoids. It occurs only in the setting of hepatic metastases except for a few cases of foregut-derived carcinoids the venous drainage of which bypasses the liver.

Tumors arising from smooth muscle (leiomyoma or leiomyosarcoma) or submucosal or mesenteric fat (lipoma or liposarcoma) can occur throughout the digestive tract. Leiomyoma can arise from the muscularis mucosa or from the muscularis propria.

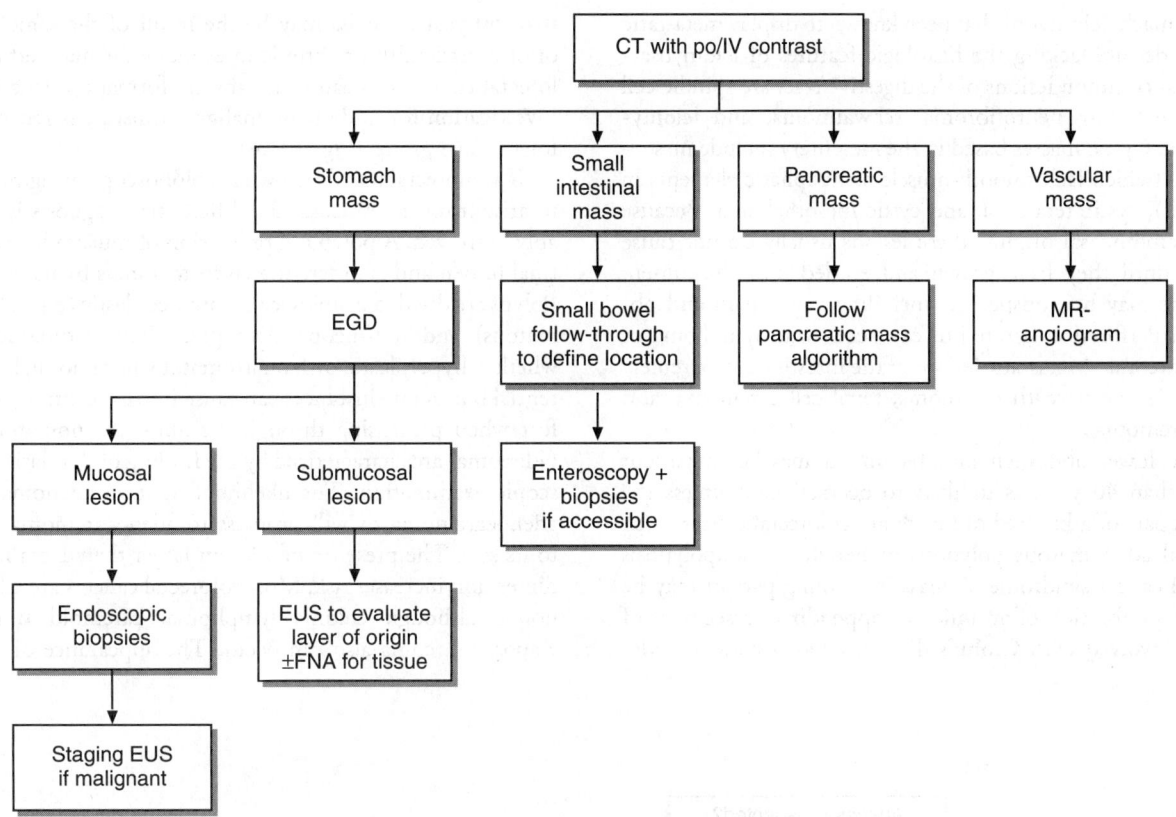

FIGURE 101.2. Evaluation of a suspected upper abdominal mass.
EVIDENCE LEVEL: C. Expert Opinion.

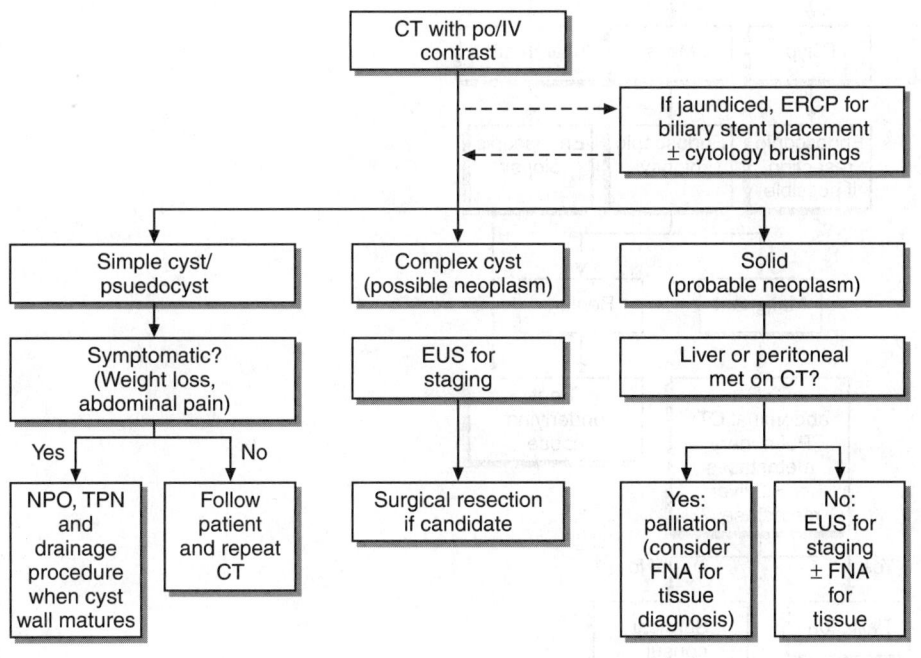

FIGURE 101.3. Evaluation of a pancreatic mass.
EVIDENCE LEVEL: C. Expert Opinion.

In the stomach, leiomyoma has been known to display metastatic potential despite lacking the histologic features of leiomyosarcoma. Less common lesions of the digestive tract are spindle cell tumors, including neurofibroma, schwannoma, and leiomyoblastoma. Cystic masses based in the mesentery include mesenteric cysts (which lack smooth-muscle or lymphatic elements in their walls), cystic teratoma, and cystic mesothelioma. Because of their submucosal origins, these lesions usually do not cause bleeding until they have grown and eroded into the lumen. Symptoms may be nonspecific, including vague pain and obstruction. Perforation is rare but can occur with lymphoma or leiomyosarcoma. Metastatic lesions of the intestine are extremely rare, but can occur with melanoma, renal cell carcinoma, and breast carcinoma.

In the lower abdomen and rectum, a mass in a patient younger than 40 years is unlikely to be malignant unless the patient is part of a kindred of hereditary colorectal cancer, such as familial adenomatous polyposis or hereditary nonpolyposis colorectal cancer syndrome. A mass in a young patient may be caused by perforation of an inflamed appendix or a segment of intestine involved with Crohn's disease. Among patients older than 50 years, a mass may be the result of the same processes or of diverticulitis or chronic intestinal ischemia. Perforated colorectal cancer also can cause abscess formation, so a thorough investigation for underlying malignant disease is recommended for this age group (Fig. 101.4).

If a colorectal mass is shown at colonoscopy or sigmoidoscopy to arise from the mucosa, the differential diagnosis is considerably narrowed. A polyp is a protrusion of mucosa into the intestinal lumen and is differentiated from a mass by its smaller size. Polyps are divided histologically into neoplastic (typically adenomatous) and non-neoplastic types. Nonadenomatous polyps whether hyperplastic or hamartomatous have no malignant potential but in rare instances can cause intussusception or discomfort when prolapsing through the anus. Adenomatous polyps (adenoma) are characterized by the finding of dysplasia at microscopic examination. The likelihood that an adenoma contains adenocarcinoma or will progress to adenocarcinoma is related to its size. The presence of a lesion larger than 1 cm in greatest dimension increases risk. Most colorectal cancers are adenocarcinoma, although colonic lymphoma, carcinoid tumor, and Kaposi's sarcoma also can occur. The appearance of colorectal

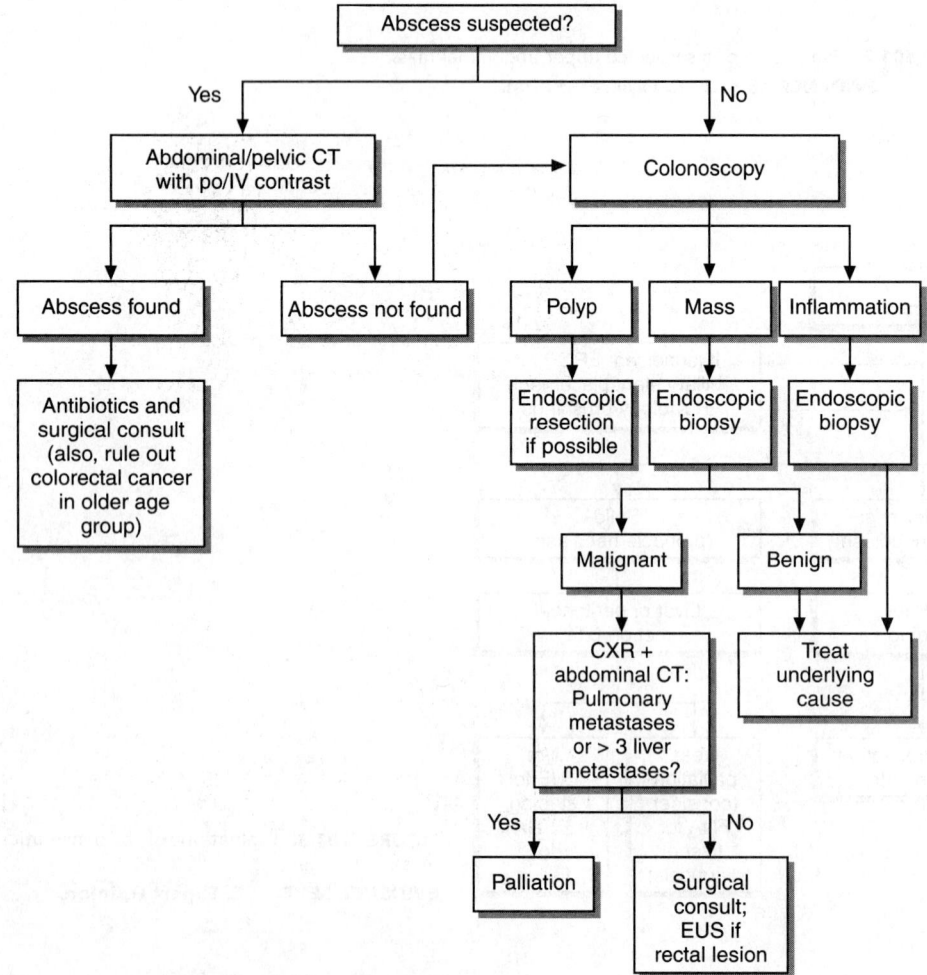

FIGURE 101.4. Evaluation of colorectal abnormality.

cancer can be mimicked by colitis cystica profunda, a rare, benign disease characterized by large, submucosal, mucus-filled cysts that is most common in the rectum. Because these distinctions can be difficult to make at endoscopy, a biopsy is performed on any polypoid or mass lesion.

A renal mass can be infectious, neoplastic, or congenital. Perinephric abscess, a complication of acute pyelonephritis, can be differentiated from a tumor at CT. Any solid renal mass that becomes enhanced with intravenous administration of contrast material during CT is presumed malignant. The most common malignant tumor is renal cell carcinoma, which often has systemic manifestations. The differential diagnosis of a solid renal mass also includes transitional cell carcinoma of the renal pelvis with parenchymal invasion, renal lymphoma, and a renal oncocytoma. Cystic renal masses most often are simple cysts, which are found at CT among 30% of patients older than 50 years. However, renal cysts also can harbor cancer. This is especially true among patients with von Hippel–Lindau disease or tuberous sclerosis (who also have renal angiomyolipoma), or among the 90% of patients undergoing long-term dialysis (more than 5 years) who have renal cysts. About 1% to 2% of these patients eventually have renal cell carcinoma.

A mass with a history of blunt trauma to the abdomen suggests the possibility of hematoma. The abdominal organs most susceptible to this type of injury are the spleen, the kidneys, and the retroperitoneal duodenum. A pulsatile mass found with abdominal palpation suggests an aortic aneurysm, although transmitted pulsation to a solid mass can be deceptive and confusing.

■ STRATEGIES FOR OPTIMAL CARE

MANAGEMENT

The discovery of an abdominal mass is a cause of great anxiety to a patient, so a physician is bound to feel urgency to arrive rapidly at a diagnosis. However, abdominal masses rarely constitute a medical emergency. It is important, therefore, to formulate a stepwise, logical approach that utilizes the strengths of the diagnostic modalities available in a cost-efficient and logical way.

The initial step is always an effort to define the characteristics and location of the mass. The information gleaned from physical examination must be complemented by appropriate radiologic evaluation. In the hepatobiliary system, CT has emerged as the optimal diagnostic test, except when gallstone disease (cholelithiasis or choledocholithiasis) is the presumptive diagnosis. Contrast-enhanced CT can be used to classify most focal liver lesions, such as a cyst, hemangioma, or metastasis. MRI is the state-of-the-art modality used in atypical cases and has largely supplanted liver biopsy in the diagnosis of liver lesions such as focal nodular hyperplasia, focal fatty infiltration, and some cases of adenoma. If the nature of a focal lesion is unclear, a directed biopsy can be undertaken under laparoscopic guidance. Patients with focal

hepatocellular cancer or a solitary metastatic lesion are referred to a surgeon specialized in treatment of diseases of the hepatobiliary tract for possible resection. Resection of multifocal hepatocellular carcinoma or multiple metastatic lesions usually is not possible. The finding of metastatic liver lesions prompts a thorough, directed search for a primary source. Hepatic adenoma is resected when possible because of the risk of rupture or hemorrhage and the rare occurrence of malignant transformation. Focal nodular hyperplasia, which is more common than adenoma but less frequently symptomatic, can be followed, because it imparts no malignant risk. A patient with adenoma or focal nodular hyperplasia should stop taking oral contraceptives.

Outside the liver, CT again is an important early diagnostic tool. It offers a comprehensive analysis of the abdomen and pelvis, which includes the presence of enlarged lymph nodes. When malignant growth is suspected, CT is a diagnostic and staging study.

The need to obtain tissue for histologic diagnosis of an abdominal mass depends on the index of suspicion of malignancy and on the accessibility of the mass to biopsy techniques. For a mass in the stomach, colon, or rectum, endoscopic biopsy is easy if the mass involves the mucosa. For a mass in the pancreas, obtaining tissue for diagnosis is difficult unless the mass involves the ampulla; further evaluation with cholangiopancreatography or MRI often is necessary. In the evaluation of renal masses, percutaneous needle sampling to define the nature of a mass is not recommended. In the case of a cystic renal mass, malignancy cannot be reliably ruled out with fine-needle aspiration cytologic examination, and the therapeutic benefit of aspiration is limited, because the recurrence rate of benign cysts exceeds 90% unless sclerosis is performed. In the evaluation of solid renal masses, percutaneous biopsy is not recommended unless a diagnosis of lymphoma is suspected, because of the risk of needle track seeding.

The management of nonmalignant abdominal masses depends on the underlying cause, the presence of symptoms, and the risk of malignant transformation. Intra-abdominal abscesses are drained, and therapy is directed at the underlying disease, whether it is inflammatory bowel disease, urinary or biliary obstruction, pancreatitis, or vascular insufficiency. Pancreatic pseudocysts can be drained percutaneously, endoscopically, or surgically. Indications for drainage include symptoms (abdominal pain, nausea, continuing weight loss) or suspicion of infection. The staging and management of malignant abdominal tumors are discussed in Chapters 115, 116, 118, and 126.

COMPLICATIONS AND PITFALLS

A pitfall in the management of a mass lesion is a missed malignant tumor. A tumor can be missed because biopsy material from the lesion gave false-negative results for malignancy or the biopsy missed the target lesion. For that reason, if a biopsy result does not confirm a diagnosis or does not agree with the clinical or endoscopic impression, it is important to repeat the biopsy or proceed with an alternative sampling technique. If an abdominal mass lies outside the intestinal lumen and is therefore not accessible to endoscopic biopsy, laparoscopy is considered.

The evaluation of an abdominal mass involves procedures that in rare instances lead to serious complications. Intravenous administration of contrast material for CT exposes patients to the risk of anaphylactic reaction or acute renal failure. Endoscopic procedures are associated with a risk of hemorrhage or perforation, although these complications are rare (less than one in 500 procedures). The risk increases in the presence of active intestinal inflammation or other systemic disease. ERCP causes pancreatitis in 5% of cases. The risks of each diagnostic procedure and the comorbidity must be considered in determining how to proceed in the care of each patient.

 ### Indications for
HOSPITALIZATION

Most abdominal or rectal mass lesions can be evaluated on an outpatient basis. Endoscopic and radiologic tests are routinely performed as outpatient procedures. Patients with intestinal obstruction, intractable pain or vomiting, suggestion of an intra-abdominal abscess, or active gastrointestinal bleeding are evaluated in the hospital.

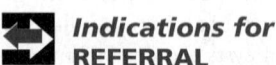 ### Indications for
REFERRAL

If ERCP or EUS is indicated, it is preferable to refer the patient to a gastroenterologist with experience in advanced endoscopic procedures. The diagnostic accuracy of EUS in particular depends on the level of experience of the examiner. Early consultation with a surgical colleague is desirable even if surgery is not imminent to allow timely investigation of comorbid factors and discussion with the patient of the indications for surgery and its attendant risks and the alternatives. For malignant lesions, a multimodality approach with the collaboration of medical specialists, surgical specialists, oncologists, and radiation therapists is optimal management.

BIBLIOGRAPHY

Akriviadis EA, Llovet JM, Efremidis SC, et al. Hepatocellular carcinoma. *Br J Surg* 1998;85:1319–1331.

Fuchs CS, Mayer RJ. Gastric carcinoma. *N Engl J Med* 1995;333:32–41.

Kulke MH, Mayer RJ. Carcinoid tumors. *N Engl J Med* 1999;340:858–868.

Rosewicz S, Wiedenmann B. Pancreatic carcinoma. *Lancet* 1997;349:485–489.

Saini S. Imaging of the hepatobiliary tract. *N Engl J Med* 1997;336:1889–1894.

Wolf JS Jr. Evaluation and management of solid and cystic renal masses. *J Urol* 1998;159:1120–1133.

Kelley's Textbook of Internal Medicine, fourth edition. Edited by H. David Humes. Lippincott Williams & Wilkins, Philadelphia © 2000.

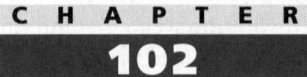

APPROACH TO THE PATIENT WITH GASTROINTESTINAL BLEEDING

GRACE H. ELTA

Gastrointestinal (GI) bleeding is a common clinical problem that varies in severity from life-threatening hemorrhage to slow, insidious bleeding that produces only iron deficiency. The annual rate of hospitalization for upper GI bleeding has been estimated to be 36 to 102 patients per 100,000 members of the general population, and the rate is twice as common among men as among women. Lower GI bleeding is less common, requiring approximately 20 hospitalizations per 100,000 persons. The rate of both acute upper GI and acute lower GI bleeding is higher among patients who take aspirin than among those who do not, and the risk appears to be dose related. Most bleeding episodes from both upper GI and lower GI sources resolve spontaneously. However, patients with severe and persistent bleeding have high mortality rates and may need invasive interventional techniques. Early and accurate diagnosis among patients with severe bleeding facilitates therapeutic maneuvers that lower mortality. The foundation of management of GI bleeding is rapid assessment and appropriate resuscitation.

PRESENTATION

The presentation of GI bleeding depends on its acuity and the source. Chronic GI blood loss may manifest with unsuspected iron deficiency anemia or the finding of occult blood in routine screening stool examinations. More severe cases of chronic or unrecognized GI bleeding may manifest with symptoms of anemia, such as pallor, dizziness, angina, or dyspnea. Acute GI bleeding usually has a much more obvious presentation. Bleeding from the upper GI tract often manifests with hematemesis, or bloody vomitus. This may be from recent bleeding, which causes bright red vomitus, or previous bleeding, which gives vomitus a coffee grounds appearance. Melena is black, tarry, loose, malodorous stool caused by the presence of degraded blood in the intestine and generally indicates an upper GI source, although the bleeding may originate in the proximal colon or small intestine. Other causes of black stool, such as iron or bismuth ingestion, must be ruled out. Hematochezia, or bright red blood from the rectum that may be mixed with stool, generally indicates a lower GI lesion.

ASSESSMENT AND RESUSCITATION

The first step in assessment of GI bleeding is to determine the urgency of the situation. Agitation, pallor, hypotension, and tachycardia may indicate shock, which necessitates immediate volume replacement. Shock occurs when blood loss approaches 40% of blood volume. If there is no evidence of hypotension and tachycardia, the presence of orthostatic vital signs helps establish the diagnosis of lesser degrees of intravascular volume depletion. Postural hypotension of 10 mm Hg or greater usually indicates 20% or greater reduction in blood volume. If the patient has acute bleeding, intravenous access must be established. If the patient has signs of shock or continued bleeding, a large-bore central intravenous line is useful. Blood samples are obtained immediately for assessment of hematocrit, platelets, and coagulation factors and blood typing and cross-matching.

The initial hematocrit of a patient with acute bleeding poorly reflects the degree of blood loss. Because hematocrit is expressed in terms of red blood cell volume as a percentage of total blood volume, it does not drop until blood volume has been restored. This repletion of blood volume from extravascular fluid begins immediately but takes 24 to 48 hours to equilibrate completely. Therefore a patient with acute bleeding needs close attention to blood pressure and heart rate. Gross evidence of ongoing bleeding is better for evaluating blood loss than are laboratory tests. In contrast, hematocrit is an accurate reflection of the degree of anemia among patients with chronic blood loss. However, the severity of iron deficiency, reflected by microcytic indices and low serum ferritin, is a better indicator of the duration of bleeding.

Patients with severe acute GI bleeding need admission to an intensive care unit. Intravascular volume is repleted with normal saline solution to prevent the consequences of shock while blood is being cross-matched for transfusion. The specific criteria that define when a patient needs transfusions vary with the age of the patient, the presence of concomitant cardiopulmonary disease, and the presence of continued bleeding. In general, the hematocrit is maintained above 30% for elderly patients and above 20% for young, healthy patients. With continued evidence of bleeding, the decision to transfuse cannot be based on hematocrit alone. Plasma volume after acute GI bleeding also often is overexpanded by intravenous fluids; thus the hematocrit immediately after transfusion may be an underestimate of final value. In general, packed red blood cells are the primary source of blood. Transfusion of whole blood is reserved for the unusual circumstances of massive blood loss and need for coagulation factor replacement. If results of coagulation tests are abnormal, as is the case among many patients with cirrhosis, fresh frozen plasma and platelets may have to be administered. Even patients with an initially normal prothrombin time and platelet count eventually need plasma and platelet transfusions when repeated transfusions are performed. In rare instances patients who undergo massive transfusions need calcium supplementation to counter the effects of calcium-binding agents in banked blood.

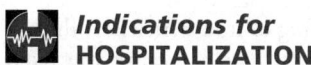

Indications for HOSPITALIZATION

Patients with ongoing bleeding, a need for transfusion, or endoscopic findings that put them at risk of recurrent bleeding need to be admitted to the hospital. Changes in practice over the last 10 years show that hospitalization days have decreased considerably and that more than 90% of patients with upper GI bleeding undergo endoscopy within 24 hours of admission. Twenty-five percent of these endoscopic examinations include endoscopic hemostatic therapy. An important change in the management of nonvariceal upper GI bleeding has been the use of upper GI endoscopy to assess the risk of rebleeding and allow outpatient care of selected patients, which has led to considerable cost savings. Because most of the hospital cost of providing care for patients with upper GI hemorrhage is the hospital bed cost, shortening the length of stay or eliminating the need for hospitalization can greatly lower costs.

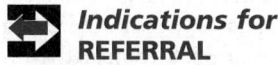

Indications for REFERRAL

Patients with GI bleeding need early referral for endoscopy because in most instances this examination is necessary for diagnosis. Early endoscopy also allows an accurate prognosis for the bleeding episode and allows endoscopic therapy.

LOCATION OF BLEEDING

In the case of obvious upper GI bleeding that manifests with hematemesis, a nasogastric tube is placed to further assess the rate of ongoing blood loss. When upper GI bleeding is only suspected, as when a patient has melena or a history of epigastric symptoms or disease, the presence of blood in a nasogastric tube confirms the upper GI tract as the source. Not infrequently, however, duodenal bleeding with melena may not produce blood in the nasogastric aspirate because the pylorus is competent and there is little duodenogastric reflux. Therefore a normal nasogastric aspirate does not preclude the upper GI tract as the bleeding source. Testing for occult blood in nasogastric aspirates rarely is necessary because the blood often is obvious. A simple positive test result for occult blood may merely indicate nasogastric tube trauma. The one occasion on which occult blood testing is helpful is when a coffee grounds aspirate appearance is produced by food. When occult testing of a gastric aspirate is performed, it is important not to rely on standard stool kits, which give false-negative results in acidic solutions.

Hematochezia usually indicates a lower GI source. However, a patient with rapid bleeding from an upper GI source may pass bright red blood through the rectum because of rapid GI transit. Therefore placement of a nasogastric tube and even performance of an upper endoscopic examination are considered if there is any clinical question about the bleeding location in a patient with hematochezia.

For patients with occult bleeding or iron deficiency, the history and physical examination often help localize the likely source of blood loss. However, patients may have more than one GI lesion, so a lesion in the upper GI tract may accompany a problem in the intestine. Therefore many of these patients need diagnostic evaluation of the entire GI tract.

ACUTE UPPER GASTROINTESTINAL BLEEDING

Approximately 80% of episodes of upper GI bleeding are self-limited and necessitate only supportive therapy. Recent mortality rates for upper GI hemorrhage vary from 3.5% to 7% in the United States, although a large study in the United Kingdom showed a mortality rate of 14%. Patients with continued or recurrent bleeding have mortality rates of 25% to 30%. Factors predictive of a poor prognosis for upper GI bleeding include the age of the patient (over 60), severity of the initial bleeding, concomitant illnesses, the cause of bleeding, and signs of recent hemorrhage. The most important prognostic indicator is the cause of bleeding. Variceal hemorrhage has much higher rebleeding and mortality rates than other diagnoses. Onset of bleeding during hospitalization has a mortality of 33% compared with only 7% among patients who start to bleed before admission. Patients who need emergency surgical treatment have a surgical mortality as high as 30%; those undergoing elective operations have a surgical mortality of 10%.

Endoscopic visualization of signs of recent bleeding, such as active arterial spurting, oozing of blood, visible vessel, or fresh or old blood clot, is an important predictor of outcome among patients with peptic ulcer bleeding (Table 102.1). The rebleeding rate among patients with arterial spurting from an ulcer is higher than 70%; for patients with a visible vessel, which may be hidden by an adherent clot, it is 50%. This contrasts to other less common signs such as black eschar, oozing, or clot, which are associated with rebleeding rates of 6% to 8% compared with no rebleeding of ulcers without stigmata.

ETIOLOGY

The three major causes of upper GI bleeding are peptic ulcer disease, gastropathy (or gastric erosions), and varices (Table 102.2). The distribution of causes varies with the patient population studied. In all endoscopic series, 10% to 15% of patients have no diagnosis confirmed, and as many as 20% to 30% have more than one diagnosis. The patients with no endoscopic diagnosis have an excellent prognosis.

Peptic Ulcer

Duodenal, gastric, or stomal ulcers account for 40% to 50% of upper GI bleeding. Continued bleeding or recurrent bleeding is an indication for endoscopic therapy. Multipolar electrocoagulation, heater probe, neodymium: yttrium-aluminum-garnet (Nd:YAG) laser therapy, and injection therapies all are therapeutic options through flexible endoscopy. These therapeutic endoscopic methods are accepted for cessation of bleeding. They are also used for prevention of rebleeding among patients at high risk with signs of bleeding identified at endoscopy. Early surgical therapy is considered for persistent or recurrent bleeding from ulcers not controlled with endoscopic techniques. Only when a patient has an inoperable condition would alternative treatment such as angiographic embolization with gelatin foam or autologous clot be reasonable. Intra-arterial infusion of vasopressin is

TABLE 102.2.	FINAL DIAGNOSES OF CAUSE OF UPPER GASTROINTESTINAL BLEEDING AMONG 2,225 PATIENTS
Diagnosis	**Percentage of All Diagnoses**
Duodenal ulcer	24.3
Gastric erosions	23.4
Gastric ulcer	21.3
Varices	10.3
Mallory/Weiss tear	7.2
Esophagitis	6.3
Erosive duodenitis	5.8
Neoplasm	2.9
Stomal ulcer	1.8
Esophageal ulcer	1.7
Miscellaneous	6.8

Source: Modified from Silverstein FE, Gilbert DA, Tedesco FJ, et al. The national ASGE prognosis in upper gastrointestinal bleeding. II. Clinical prognosis factors. *Gastrointest Endosc* 1981;27:80–93, with permission.

TABLE 102.1.	SIGNS OF HEMORRHAGE AND RISK OF REBLEEDING	
Sign	**Incidence (%)**	**Risk of Rebleeding (%)**
Spurting arterial bleeding	8	85–100
Nonbleeding visible vessel	17–50	18–55 (mean, 43)
Adherent clot (no visible vessel)	18–26	24–41
Older signs	12–18	5–9
No signs	10–36	0

Source: Modified from Johnston JH. Endoscopic risk factors for bleeding peptic ulcer. *Gastrointest Endosc* 1990;36:S16–S20, with permission.

relatively ineffective in the control of ulcer bleeding, presumably because the vessels that bleed tend to be large.

Gastric Erosions or Gastropathy

The term *gastritis* should be reserved for pathologists; it is defined histologically and may have no endoscopic or clinical correlate. Gastropathy can be divided into several etiologic categories. Drug-induced gastropathy due to use of aspirin or other nonsteroidal anti-inflammatory drugs (NSAIDs) is generally a self-limited disease that heals rapidly after discontinuation of the offending agent. The GI hemorrhage caused by drug-induced gastropathy is common because of the widespread use of these medications but is usually minor and transient.

Alcohol is also a gastric mucosal irritant, although it is uncertain whether alcohol in the doses usually consumed causes gastropathy or whether some of the damage that occurs among persons with alcoholism is related to underlying portal hypertension. Gastropathy associated with portal hypertension frequently is present in patients with cirrhosis. The GI hemorrhage from this lesion can be recurrent and difficult to manage but rarely is massive. In the unusual case of profuse chronic blood loss from portal gastropathy, portosystemic shunting and propranolol are reported to be effective.

Stress gastritis is an important type of gastropathy that causes serious hemorrhaging. It occurs among patients in intensive care units who have risk factors such as respiratory failure, hypotension, sepsis, renal failure, thermal burns, peritonitis, jaundice, and neurologic trauma. Risk of bleeding for an individual patient varies with the number of risk factors. Endoscopic evidence of stress gastropathy is found among almost all patients in intensive care units, although only 2% to 10% of these patients have serious bleeding. All therapeutic modalities for clinically significant bleeding are associated with high failure rates and high morbidity.

Endoscopic therapy usually is the first and safest choice for treatment although it has not been studied for this specific indication. The presence of multiple bleeding sites precludes use of endoscopic therapy in the care of some patients. In contrast to therapy for bleeding ulcers, angiographic control of bleeding due to stress gastropathy by means of intra-arterial administration of vasopressin reportedly has a good success rate because of the small vessel size in these superficial lesions. Operative mortality is extremely high for stress gastropathy, and rebleeding after surgery is common, so surgery is the last alternative. The main emphasis in the management of stress gastropathy is prophylaxis. Routine use of high-dose antacids, H_2 blockers, or sucralfate for patients at risk has been shown to decrease the incidence of bleeding. Use of agents that improve mucosal defense without altering intragastric pH, such as sucralfate, may lower the rate of nosocomial pneumonia among patients breathing with respirators, although these data are controversial.

Varices

Hemorrhage from esophageal varices often is massive and has a high mortality rate. The highly specialized therapy for variceal bleeding necessitates an early and accurate diagnosis. The presence of cirrhosis does not assure that varices are the bleeding source because 30% to 60% of patients with cirrhosis who have upper GI bleeding have a nonvariceal source. In addition to standard resuscitation measures, patients with variceal hemorrhage are treated with intravenous octreotide or vasopressin plus nitroglycerin, sclerotherapy or band ligation, and occasionally balloon tamponade. When sclerotherapy or band ligation fails the patient eventually may need portosystemic shunting. This traditionally has necessitated a surgical procedure, which carries high risk among patients with advanced cirrhosis. As an alternative, transjugular intrahepatic portosystemic shunting (TIPS) achieves portal decompression and allows time for consideration of liver transplantation (see Chapter 105).

Other Causes of Upper Gastrointestinal Bleeding

Mallory–Weiss tears are retching-induced superficial tears in the gastric or esophageal mucosa close to the gastroesophageal junction. Many patients with this lesion give a history of vomiting foodstuffs before vomiting blood. However, the presence of blood with the first emesis does not rule out this diagnosis. Patients often have a history of alcohol intake. Mallory–Weiss tear usually responds to conservative management but may necessitate therapy with endoscopic hemostatic techniques or even intra-arterial vasopressin.

Gastric varices usually accompany esophageal varices and are caused by underlying liver disease. It is important, however, to consider splenic venous thrombosis as the cause of the increased venous pressure when gastric varices are associated with minimal to absent esophageal varices. This may occur as a complication of pancreatitis owing to contiguous inflammation from the body and tail of the pancreas. These patients are best treated with simple splenectomy and have an excellent prognosis because of the lack of underlying liver disease.

Esophagitis and esophageal ulcers account for approximately 8% of instances of upper GI hemorrhage. The primary cause of these lesions is peptic reflux. Other etiologic factors are irradiation, infectious esophagitis caused by pathogens such as *Candida* organisms or herpesvirus, pill-induced damage, and sclerotherapy-induced ulcers. Persistent or recurrent bleeding is managed aggressively with therapeutic endoscopic or angiographic techniques because esophageal lesions are less amenable to surgery than is peptic ulcer disease.

Hemorrhage from erosive duodenitis is closely related to duodenal ulcer bleeding but usually is less severe because the lesions are shallower and involve smaller vessels. It accounts for approximately 5% of cases of upper GI hemorrhages.

Neoplasms are an uncommon source of upper GI bleeding but do cause persistent or recurrent bleeding. Surgical removal of the neoplasm often is indicated. However, for patients at poor risk who have known metastatic disease, other means of hemostasis such as endoscopic therapy or angiographic embolization of tumor vessels is quite successful.

Vascular ectasia, or angiodysplasia, which occurs less commonly in the stomach or duodenum than in the colon, cause 5% to 7% of cases of upper GI bleeding. The lesions may be associated with hereditary hemorrhagic telangiectasia (Osler–Weber–Rendu disease), chronic renal failure, aortic valve disease, or radiation therapy. They also occur sporadically among elderly persons. Therapeutic endoscopic methods of ablation have been successful in some instances, although when the lesions are multiple, recurrences are common. Because it improves platelet function, estrogen therapy is effective in decreasing blood loss from vascular ectasia among patients with renal disease. Estrogen-progesterone therapy has been shown to decrease transfusion requirements among patients with normal kidney function who have chronic bleeding from vascular ectasia. An unusual variant of gastric vascular ectasia is watermelon stomach. The endoscopic appearance is a column of vessels that run along the top of longitudinal rugal folds that traverse the antrum and resemble the stripes on a watermelon.

Aortoenteric fistula is a rare cause of bleeding, but it must be diagnosed promptly. This fistula occurs primarily among patients who have undergone insertion of a Dacron graft because of an aortic aneurysm and in whom the graft has eroded into the duodenum, usually the third portion. Most patients with aortoenteric fistulas have relatively minor bleeding one or two times (herald bleeds) before fatal exsanguinating hemorrhage occurs. A high index of suspicion in the evaluation of patients who have undergone operations on the aorta may allow early surgical intervention.

Hematobilia and hemosuccus pancreaticus, or bleeding into the GI tract through the ampulla of Vater, is rare. Causes include liver trauma or liver biopsy, cancer, hepatic arterial aneurysm, hepatic abscess, gallstones, and pancreatic pseudocyst. The diagnosis may be made endoscopically but requires angiographic confirmation. The lesions may be managed with angiographic embolization or surgery.

Dieulafoy's syndrome is protrusion of a ruptured artery into the proximal portion of the stomach with essentially no surrounding ulceration. The cause of bleeding is thought to be not a primary ulcerative process but pressure erosion of the overlying epithelium by the ectatic vessel. These lesions often respond to electrocoagulation, although surgical ligation may be needed.

DIAGNOSTIC APPROACH

Whether all patients with upper GI bleeding should undergo a diagnostic examination is controversial. Those with self-limited minor bleeding and other more serious medical problems may not need an examination, because endoscopic diagnosis has not been shown to alter prognosis. However, for most patients, even those with relatively little bleeding, an accurate diagnosis is desirable to direct further care (Fig. 102.1). For some patients with profuse bleeding, the diagnostic examination or endoscopy can be used for therapeutic maneuvers.

History and Physical Examination

While initial resuscitation measures are being implemented, a history interview is conducted and a physical examination performed. The history often raises specific diagnostic possibilities. A history of peptic disease or dyspeptic symptoms suggests ulcer bleeding. Recent use of aspirin or NSAIDs must always be ascertained. A history of ingestion of alcohol or a caustic substance

is important. A history of cirrhosis, or symptoms of cirrhosis such as ascites, may suggest the need for urgent endoscopy to diagnose variceal bleeding. Other medical conditions, such as having undergone aortic graft surgery, coagulopathy, cancer, or a recent nosebleed, may suggest diagnoses.

Physical examination of the skin may provide diagnostic clues. Signs of cirrhosis or evidence of underlying malignant disease, such as Kaposi's sarcoma, may be present. Findings of lymphadenopathy or abdominal masses may suggest malignant disease. Abdominal tenderness in the epigastrium is a common sign of peptic disease. Hepatic or splenic enlargement may occur with liver disease or some malignant disorders. When a patient has upper GI bleeding, results of a rectal examination may indicate the magnitude of blood loss by demonstrating maroon or melenic stools in patients with severe bleeding.

Endoscopy

Barium contrast studies have been replaced by endoscopy in the diagnosis of upper GI bleeding. The much greater accuracy and therapeutic potential of endoscopy generally makes it the diagnostic procedure of choice. Diagnostic endoscopy is viewed as a safe and simple procedure by both patient and physician, although morbidity and mortality rates of 1.0% and 0.1%, respectively, have been reported. Endoscopy is contraindicated when the patient is uncooperative or is likely to have a perforated viscus. Endoscopy can be used for precise location of the bleeding when there is continued bleeding or when signs of bleeding persist. For some patients with massive hemorrhage, the source of bleeding cannot be discerned at endoscopy. For patients whose bleeding has stopped and no signs of bleeding remain, a lesion seen at endoscopy, such as a clean ulcer base, is the presumed source. Sometimes more than one lesion or no lesions are identified. Under these circumstances, no definitive diagnosis can be made, and these patients need to undergo another examination if they bleed again.

The timing of the diagnostic endoscopy depends on the severity and suspected cause of the hemorrhage. Patients who do not stop bleeding with simple supportive care need urgent endoscopy to guide further therapeutic techniques. For patients with underlying cirrhosis, endoscopy is performed as soon as possible after the bleeding episode because these patients often have more than one site of potential hemorrhage, and the diagnosis of bleeding varices alters future approaches to treatment. In most instance, when bleeding ceases, diagnostic endoscopy can be postponed for 24 hours without seriously altering diagnostic accuracy. When there are no complications and both patient and physician are comfortable without a specific diagnosis, an empiric trial of treatment may be indicated. Barium radiography may be used in this situation to rule out more serious lesions and avoid endoscopy altogether.

Radionuclide Scanning

Localization of the site of GI bleeding can be accomplished by means of scanning for extravasation of intravascular radiolabeled

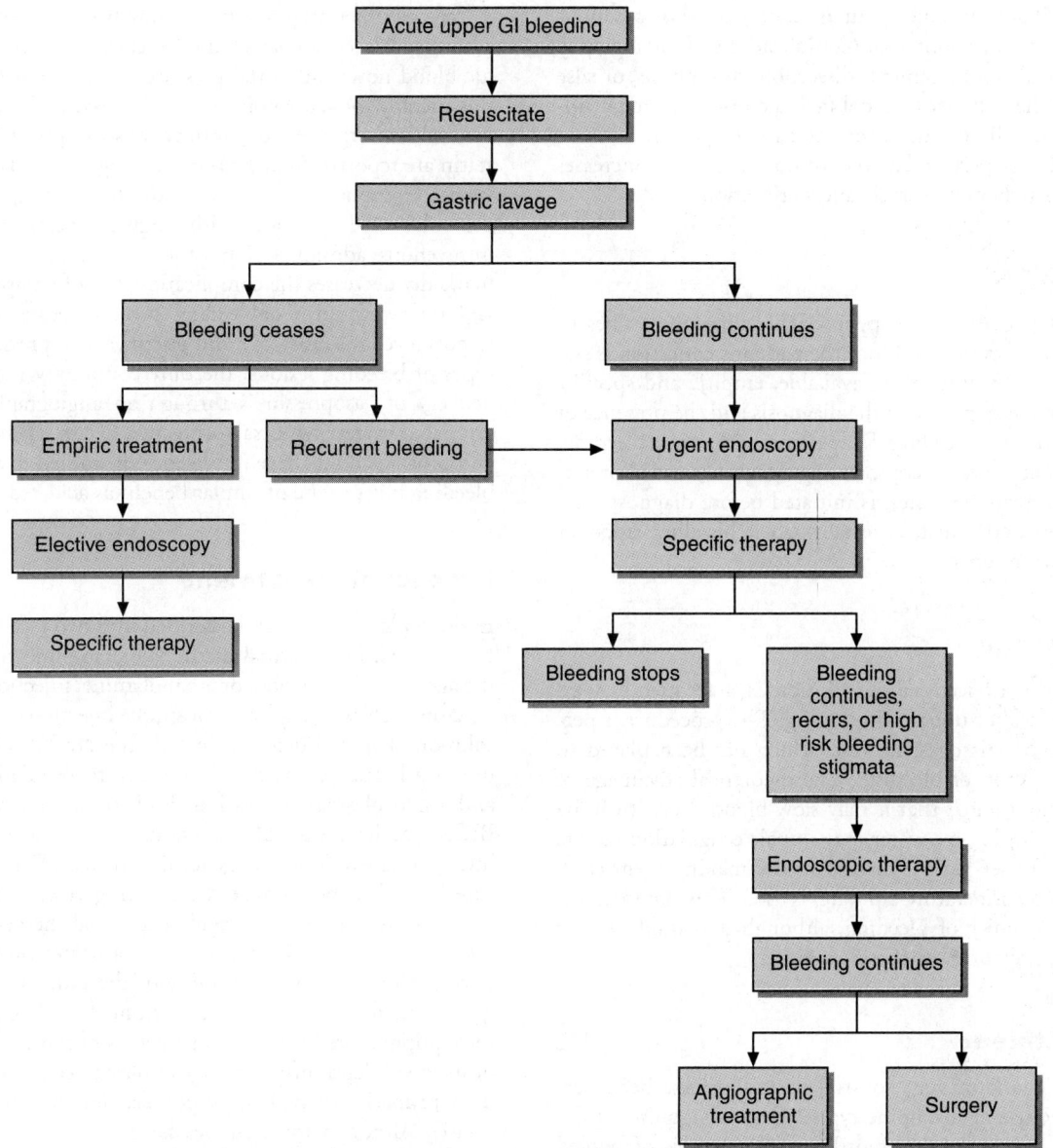

FIGURE 102.1. Evaluation of nonvariceal upper gastrointestinal bleeding.
EVIDENCE LEVEL: C. Expert Opinion.

material. In one method technetium Tc 99m sulfur colloid is used, and scans are obtained soon after injection. Another method with technetium Tc 99m pertechnetate–labeled red blood cells allows repetition of scans for 24 to 36 hours after injection to detect intermittent bleeding. These techniques can reveal bleeding when the rate of blood loss is as low as 0.5 mL per minute and have no associated morbidity. The disadvantage of radionuclide scanning is that the bleeding merely is localized to an area of abdomen; the scans do not show the specific location or the responsible lesion. For this reason, radionuclide studies often are used as a screening tool to determine whether a patient has sufficient bleeding to warrant angiography. The value as an angiography screen has been questioned, but the scans may allow more selective angiographic studies and thereby decrease the load of contrast material.

Angiography

Angiography is used as a diagnostic examination in acute upper GI bleeding only when endoscopy has not provided enough information to establish a diagnosis. The source of blood loss must be arterial and flowing at a rate of 0.5 to 0.6 mL per minute to detect extravasation. Angiography may be chosen as a therapeutic alternative for delivery of intra-arterial vasopressin to patients with stress gastropathy or for embolization of inoperable bleeding ulcers or neoplasms. Angiography also can be used to diagnose difficult cases of recurrent GI bleeding from an unknown source. Angiographic demonstration of vascular ectasia may suggest the source of bleeding, although for patients who are not actively bleeding, the diagnosis is uncertain since these are frequent lesions. Angiography provides an accurate diagnosis in 50% to 75% of instances but is associated with a serious complication rate of about 2%. Complications of angiography are related to catheter placement (dissection, thrombosis, or false aneurysm) or the contrast material (allergic reactions, renal failure). When embolic occlusion of vessels with gelatin foam or autologous clot is performed, the complication rate increases with potential ischemic necrosis and perforation.

MANAGEMENT

Treatment of patients with upper GI bleeding always begins with resuscitation measures. Once the patient's condition is stable, two types of treatment are available, empiric and specific. Specific treatment depends on the diagnosis and the presence or absence of continued bleeding. For patients with severe bleeding, specific treatment is endoscopic or angiographic control or surgery. Empiric treatment often is initiated before diagnostic examinations are performed, especially when bleeding stops, as occurs in most instances.

Gastric Lavage

Gastric lavage with iced saline solution is a frequently used method of control of upper GI bleeding. The procedure is performed through a nasogastric tube, which has been placed to identify the location of bleeding. The theoretical advantage of use of a cold solution is that it may slow blood flow. It can be argued, however, that ice water may impair coagulation factors and that it increases patient discomfort by making them cold. Therefore room temperature tap water is used. This allows monitoring of the rapidity of bleeding, although it is unlikely that appreciable therapeutic benefit is obtained.

Drug Treatment

More than 25 randomized, controlled studies have been performed on the use of histamine type 2 (H_2) antagonists in the management of upper GI hemorrhage. An analysis of pooled results from treatment of more than 2,500 patients suggested that treatment may reduce the rate of surgical intervention 20% and of death 30%, although these reductions were only marginally significant. Because even a moderate reduction in mortality is desirable and because H_2-blockers are without great toxicity, these agents are commonly administered to patients with ulcer bleeding despite the lack of proven efficacy. Although it has been suggested that more potent acid suppression with continuous intravenous administration of H_2-antagonists or with high doses of omeprazole may be more effective than standard doses of H_2-antagonists, this effect had been difficult to demonstrate. In a comparison of omeprazole and placebo in the treatment of ulcer patients at high risk with bleeding signs at endoscopy who were not treated by means of endoscopy, it was found that high-dose omeprazole (40 mg twice a day) significantly lowered the rates of further bleeding and surgical intervention. Although potent acid suppression is unlikely to replace endoscopic therapy, it appears to be the medical treatment of choice, perhaps because clotting activity is stabilized.

Several other drug treatments have been studied. Intravenous administration of somatostatin decreases acid secretion, splanchnic blood flow, and portal pressure. Evidence of the efficacy of this therapy for acute nonvariceal GI bleeding is not strong. For variceal hemorrhage, both intravenous vasopressin and somatostatin are reported to be helpful, although these data are controversial. Complications of vasopressin therapy are primarily cardiovascular and increase with higher doses. Sublingual or intravenous administration of nitroglycerin with vasopressin markedly decreases the complication rate of vasopressin therapy and improves control of bleeding, perhaps because of a reduction in portal venous resistance and portal venous pressure. For other types of bleeding lesions, the only commonly used method of delivery of vasopressin is through an angiographically placed arterial catheter. Mucosal protective agents such as sucralfate and prostaglandins have not been well studied in the control of bleeding but may be of similar benefit as acid-reducing therapy.

Endoscopic Treatment

Endoscopic methods can be divided into two types, thermal and nonthermal. Nonthermal methods include injection of sclerosing agents such as alcohol or ethanolamine, injection of vasoconstrictors such as epinephrine, or simple injection of normal saline solution. Thermal methods include the Nd:YAG laser therapy, use of a heater probe, multipolar electrocoagulation (BICAP), and argon plasma coagulation. Both the heater probe and the BICAP device are small, mobile units that can be used in the intensive care unit or emergency department. Direct probe pressure is used to tamponade the bleeding vessel, then the tissue temperature is raised to coagulate and seal the vessel. Nd:YAG laser therapy is as effective as use of a heater probe or BICAP device. However, the immobility or the Nd:YAG laser, the requirement for trained support personnel, and the high cost of the equipment reduce the attractiveness of this therapy. Because of its lower depth of injury, argon plasma coagulation has been used primarily to manage superficial lesions such as vascular ectasia. Although most studies have not shown improvement in mortality rates with endoscopic therapy, a meta-analysis of numerous trials suggested that mortality is improved, although the results reached statistical significance only for laser therapy. It is now widely accepted that in addition to controlling upper GI bleeding, therapeutic endoscopic methods can prevent rebleeding of high-risk ulcers when signs of bleeding are found. However, a lack of standardized definitions of the various signs of recent hemorrhage and sufficient knowledge of the course of development of each sign continue to be problems in deciding when this preventive therapy is warranted.

Angiographic Treatment

Intra-arterial delivery of vasopressin through angiographically placed catheters is successful in the management of upper GI bleeding when the bleeding vessel is of small caliber, as in stress gastropathy. Embolization is an effective alternative when the bleeding vessel is large, as in hemobilia or in inoperable cancer or ulcer bleeding.

Surgical Treatment

The indications for urgent surgical therapy for GI bleeding have remained essentially the same over the last 50 years except that now endoscopic therapy may be tried as a first approach. Patients who continue to bleed for more than 24 hours, need more than six to eight transfusions, or have recurrent bleeding despite endoscopic treatment need surgery. This decision may be delayed for patients who are at poor operative risk and can undergo angiographic treatment or when a specific diagnosis has a known high surgical mortality rate, such as stress gastropathy or acute variceal hemorrhage. If the patient requires surgery, decisions must be made quickly, before the patient's condition deteriorates.

ACUTE LOWER GASTROINTESTINAL BLEEDING

Lower GI bleeding is defined as bleeding that originates below the ligament of Treitz. The average patient is older than the average patient with upper GI bleeding. The mortality rate for lower GI bleeding is reported to be 3.6%, similar to that for upper GI bleeding. The mortality is markedly higher when bleeding begins after hospitalization. A decrease in mortality from acute lower GI bleeding has been witnessed in the past three decades. This decrease has been attributed to better localization and diagnosis of bleeding by means of colonoscopy and angiography, which allow more selective surgical and angiographic treatment. It also may be attributed to better resuscitation care and medical and surgical management.

ETIOLOGY

The two major causes of acute lower GI bleeding are diverticulosis and angiodysplasia (Table 102.3). As in the case of upper GI bleeding, 80% of bleeding episodes resolve spontaneously, and 20% are associated with persistent blood loss. Among patients whose bleeding ceases, about 25% have recurrent bleeding. Un-

TABLE 102.3.	FINAL DIAGNOSES OF MAJOR LOWER GASTROINTESTINAL BLEEDING
Diagnosis	**Percentage of all Diagnoses**
Diverticulosis	43
Angiodysplasia	20
Undetermined	12
Neoplasia	9
Colitis	
Radiation	6
Ischemic	2
Ulcerative	1
Other	7

Source: Boley SJ, DiBiase A, Brandt LJ, et al. Lower intestinal bleeding in the elderly. *Am J Surg* 1979;137:57–64, with permission.

like upper GI bleeding, most lower GI bleeding is slow and intermittent and does not necessitate hospitalization. The most common causes of chronic lower GI bleeding are hemorrhoids and colonic neoplasia.

Diverticulosis

Diverticular bleeding occurs among only about 3% of patients with diverticulosis. However, it is the most common cause of lower GI hemorrhage because of its high prevalence in the Western world. Despite the left-sided preponderance of diverticula, angiographic studies have demonstrated that 70% of bleeding diverticula occur in the right colon. In contrast, colonoscopic studies have suggested a higher incidence of bleeding diverticula in the left colon. Regardless of the most common location, better localization of the bleeding source with either angiography or colonoscopy allows directed surgical therapy and is associated with lower postsurgical rebleeding rates. When diverticular bleeding ceases spontaneously, no further therapy is indicated because most patients do not have recurrences. Approximately 20% of patients have recurrent diverticular bleeding, and they need elective surgical excision of the portion of the colon bearing the bleeding site. In the event of failure to localize the bleeding area, right hemicolectomy or subtotal colectomy is indicated when the patient's general medical condition and anticipated life span warrant such aggressive therapy. Among the 20% of patients with persistent hemorrhage from diverticulosis, angiography can be used for both diagnosis and treatment.

Bleeding from diverticula is presumed to be caused by penetration of a colonic artery into the dome of the diverticulum. The artery ruptures into the diverticular sac and causes copious bleeding, but clinical evidence of diverticulitis or inflammation usually is not present. Diverticulosis is thought not to produce occult heme-positive stool or slow bleeding.

Angiodysplasia

Vascular ectasia, or angiodysplasia, is a common cause of both lower GI hemorrhage and slow, intermittent blood loss. Most of the lesions are degenerative and are associated with aging, unlike the congenital vascular lesions that occur throughout the GI tract among various age groups. Two-thirds of patients with colonic angiodysplasia are older than 70 years. Angiodysplastic lesions usually are multiple, less than 5 mm in diameter, and primarily involve the cecum and right colon. There appears to be some clinical association with aortic value stenosis. The diagnosis of vascular ectasia can be made with colonoscopy or angiography. Both diagnostic modalities frequently depict the lesions without demonstrating active bleeding. Despite this limitation, if no other source of GI bleeding is identified, the presence of angiodysplasia in a patient with recurrent or persistent GI bleeding is an indication for treatment. Intra-arterial administration of vasopressin has been successful for control of continued hemorrhage. When bleeding has ceased, endoscopic techniques of hemostasis may be tried. When there are too many lesions or when bleeding reoccurs despite therapeutic colonoscopy, right hemicolectomy or subtotal colectomy is indicated depending on the location of the lesions. Medical therapy with estrogen and progesterone has decreased transfusion requirements among patients with inoperable lesions or those with presumed small-intestinal angiodysplasia, which cannot be reached with colonoscopy or enteroscopy.

Neoplasms

Benign and malignant neoplasms of the colon are common lesions that like diverticulosis and angiodysplasia occur predominantly among the elderly. Neoplasms rarely cause hemorrhage but usually manifest with intermittent episodes of a small amount of bleeding or occult blood in the stools. The diagnosis is made by means of colonoscopy or barium enema radiographic examination. Treatment is by means of surgical or colonoscopic excision. Tumors of the small intestine are rare but may be diagnosed by radiography of the small intestine or enteroclysis.

Other

Hemorrhoids are probably the most common cause of minor intermittent lower GI bleeding. The characteristic clinical history is bright red blood on the toilet tissue or around the stool but not mixed in the stool. Bleeding often occurs with straining or passage of hard stool. A similar history is common among patients with anal fissures, although fissures tend to be more painful. However, rectal polyps and carcinoma may have a similar history, so patients always are evaluated with flexible sigmoidoscopy. Perianal disease is managed with sitz baths, stool softeners, avoidance of straining, and ointments or suppositories. It is unknown whether actual therapeutic benefit is obtained with local application of medications containing lubricants and hydrocortisone, but many patients report symptomatic relief. When bleeding or other symptoms continue to be troublesome, hemorrhoidal banding or surgery may be indicated.

The amount of bleeding from inflammatory bowel disease and ischemic, infectious, or radiation-induced colitis usually is small to moderate; it rarely is massive. The blood is mixed with the stool, and often there are other symptoms of the disease, such as diarrhea, pain, and tenesmus. Diagnosis and management of these entities must be individualized according to diagnosis.

Meckel's diverticulum is the most frequent congenital anomaly of the intestinal tract. It is caused by incomplete obliteration of the vitelline duct, which leaves an ileal diverticulum that may contain gastric mucosa capable of acid secretion. Most Meckel's diverticula remain asymptomatic. The most common complication, bleeding, usually occurs in childhood, although in rare instances it occurs among adults. The diagnosis can be made by means of radiolabeled technetium scanning, but false-negative findings are not uncommon. Barium filling of the diverticulum may occur, especially with enteroclysis. Mesenteric angiography may show the site of bleeding. Surgical excision is the treatment of choice.

Intussusception may become manifest with maroon stools and is almost always accompanied by crampy abdominal pain. Uncommon among adults, intussusception usually has a leading point such as a polyp or malignant tumor. The diagnosis may be suggested by plain abdominal radiographs and the findings of a sausage-shaped mass at physical exam. Barium enema radio-graphic examination may be useful for diagnosis and, among children, for therapeutic reduction. Treatment of adults for intussusception usually is surgical.

Ileal or colonic varices, which have a predilection to occur around ostomies, may cause massive lower GI bleeding. The diagnosis often is made by means of angiography, and treatment is portosystemic shunting with surgery or TIPS. Multiple lesions of colonic vascular ectasia among patients with portal hypertension, called portal colopathy, can cause hematochezia or Hemoccult-positive stools. Solitary rectal ulcer, which may be caused by internal prolapse of the rectal mucosa, also causes lower GI bleeding, although bleeding rarely is massive. Colonic ulcers, especially in the cecum, may be related to use of NSAIDs. Aortoenteric fistulas not associated with prosthetic grafts have been found in the ileum and colon. The diagnosis usually is made at angiography, the treatment is surgical.

DIAGNOSTIC APPROACH

All patients with lower GI bleeding need a diagnostic examination unless the overall prognosis is too poor to warrant further testing (Fig. 102.2). For most patients whose bleeding ceases spontaneously, elective colonoscopy after routine preparation is indicated. Patients with continued bleeding need an urgent diagnosis. If a perianal or rectal source is suspected, simple proctoscopy can be performed quickly and may provide the diagnosis. For most colonic bleeding, a more thorough examination is needed. If the bleeding is slow to moderate, rapid intestinal lavage by means of nasogastric intubation allows adequate preparation for urgent colonoscopy. In the presence of rapid bleeding, the colonoscopic view may be obscured, so immediate angiography must be performed. Before angiography, upper GI endoscopy is considered to rule out an upper GI source of bleeding.

History and Physical Examination

A thorough history and physical examination often point to the correct diagnosis. For example, a prior diagnosis of hemorrhoids or inflammatory bowel disease is important. Symptoms that occur in association with bleeding, such as abdominal pain or diarrhea, suggest specific diagnoses. A recent history of anorexia or weight loss may indicate malignant disease. The finding of an abdominal mass at physical examination also suggests cancer.

Colonoscopy

Colonoscopy has generally replaced barium enema radiographic examination for diagnostic evaluation of lower GI bleeding. Several series have demonstrated the superior diagnostic sensitivity of colonoscopy even over that of double-contrast barium enema examination. Ten percent to 20% of patients with lower GI bleeding and normal results of barium enema examinations have abnormal colonoscopic findings. When lower GI bleeding is the clinical indication for colonoscopy, the diagnostic yield is high (40% to 50%). If results of a barium enema examination are abnormal, colonoscopy usually is still indicated for biopsy or therapeutic maneuvers. For these reasons, most clinicians favor

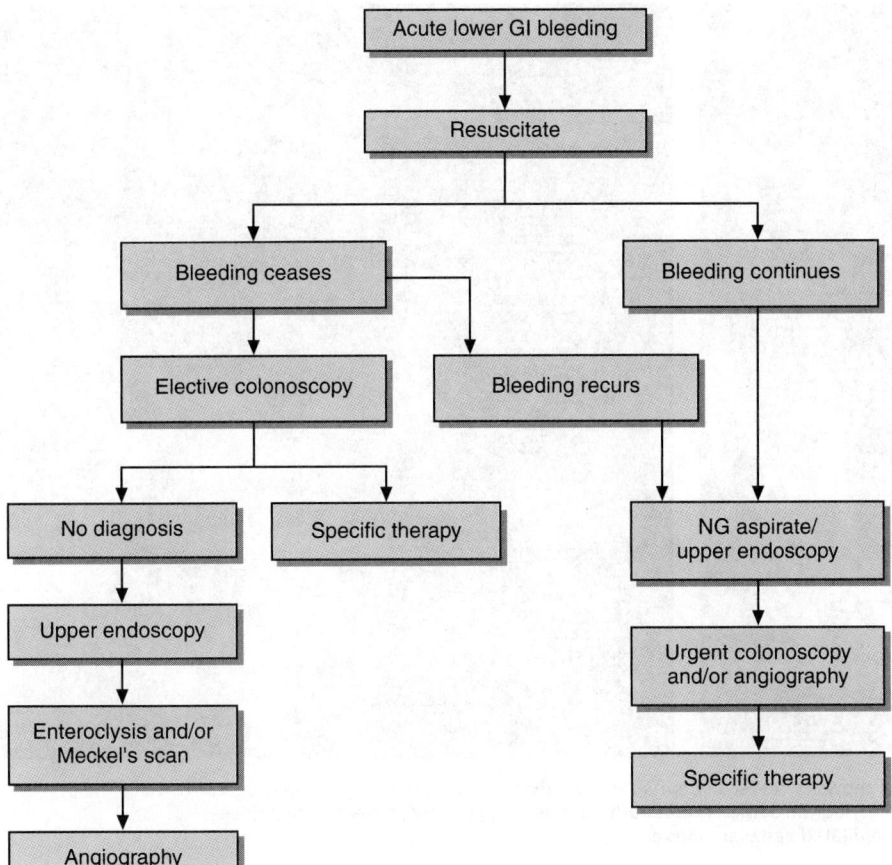

FIGURE 102.2. Evaluation of lower gastrointestinal bleeding.
EVIDENCE LEVEL: C. Expert Opinion.

colonoscopy as the primary examination. In the rare instances in which full colonoscopy is not technically feasible or when the colonoscopic findings do not provide enough information for a diagnosis, a barium enema examination is helpful. Patients with rapid, ongoing blood loss need diagnostic angiography or urgent colonoscopy after purging.

Angiography

For a patient with rapid bleeding, angiography offers accurate diagnosis and therapy. Most angiographers prefer that radionuclide scans be obtained first to demonstrate active bleeding and direct the angiographic examination. When dye extravasation does not occur, angiography can lead to a presumptive diagnosis, such as angiodysplasia (Fig. 102.3). Rare small-intestinal lesions, such as arteriovenous malformations or neoplasms, may be demonstrated. Despite the diagnostic accuracy of both colonoscopy and angiography, the source of bleeding in many patients with a presumed lower GI source is not found. Most of these patients undergo repeated studies.

TREATMENT

Resuscitation must be the initial step in patient care. Most patients whose bleeding stops need elective treatment of the source of bleeding depending on the diagnosis. Urgent therapeutic ma-

neuvers are indicated when a patient needs transfusion of more than three units of red blood cells.

Intra-arterial Administration of Vasopressin

For patients with extensive bleeding, vasopressin is infused at a rate of 0.2 units per minute after selective catheterization of the bleeding vessels. Contrast injection is repeated in 30 minutes to confirm cessation of hemorrhage. If hemorrhage is controlled, the vasopressin dose is reduced to 0.1 unit per minute and maintained for about 12 hours. If the hemorrhage persists, the dose may be increased to 0.3 unit per minute. If vasopressin therapy fails, the patient needs surgery. Embolization techniques are used as a last resort in the care of patients who cannot withstand surgical treatment.

Therapeutic Colonoscopy

When bleeding has ceased or is slow, electrocoagulation techniques may be used to manage angiodysplasia. There are a few reports of this type of therapy for bleeding diverticula, although the success and complication rates are not yet known.

Surgery

Accurate localization of bleeding sites with angiography and colonoscopy has led to improved mortality and rebleeding rates

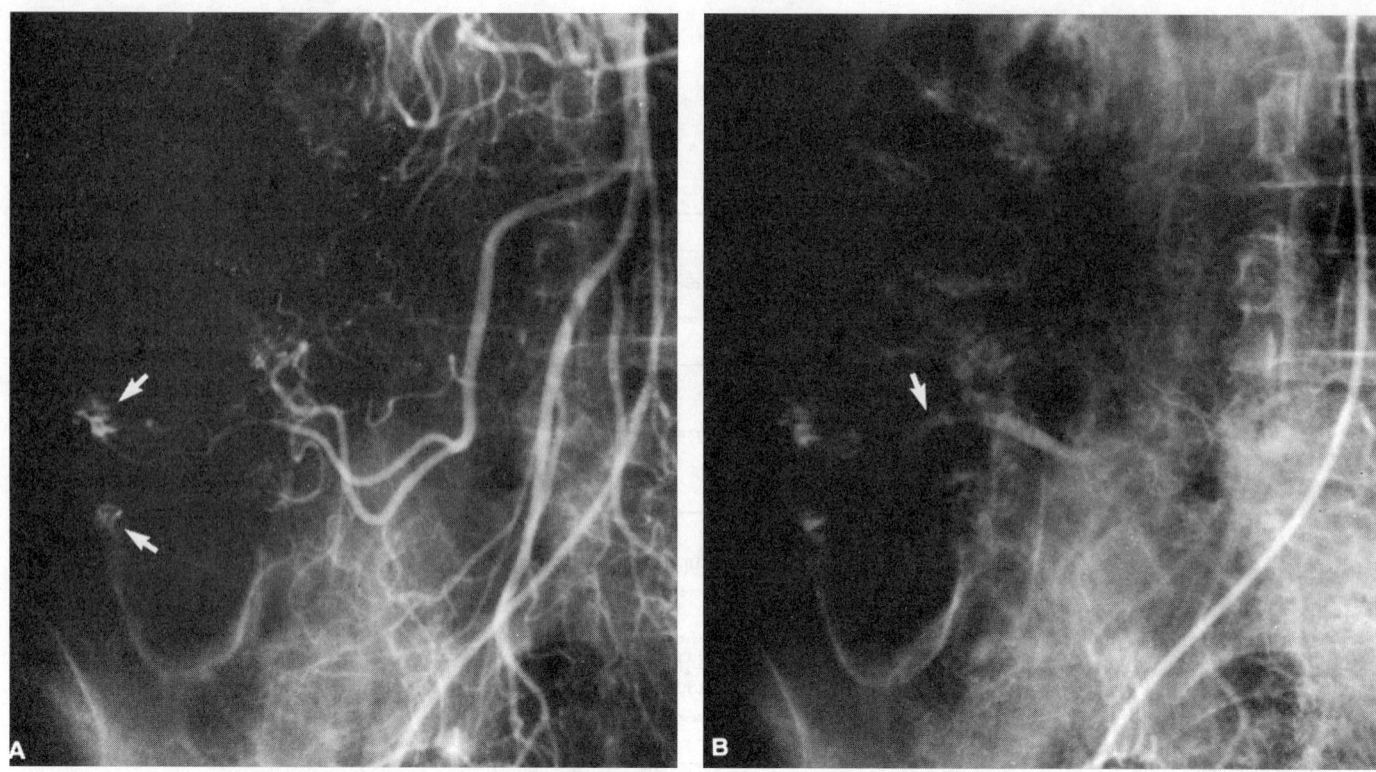

FIGURE 102.3. A: Angiogram shows two vascular tufts (*arrows*) that suggest cecal angiodysplasia. **B:** Venous image from the same arteriogram demonstrates early venous filling (*arrow*), reflecting arteriovenous communication through a dilated vascular ectasia.

among patients with lower GI bleeding. For the difficult situation of recurrent bleeding without demonstration of bleeding site, a subtotal colectomy may be indicated when the patient's overall prognosis is good.

OCCULT GI BLEEDING

Occult GI bleeding is defined as bleeding of which the patient is unaware and which is manifested by guaiac-positive stools or iron deficiency anemia. Absorption of dietary iron (average, 1 to 2 mg a day) equals or just exceeds iron loss through normal daily occult GI bleeding (average, 1 mg a day). Large amounts of blood may be lost in the GI lumen and yet remain occult. Ingestion of more than 200 mL of blood is required to produce melena, and a bolus of more than 150 mL of blood into the cecum is required to produce melena or hematochezia.

Hemoglobin components in stool depend on the bleeding site. Bleeding from the upper GI tract allows degradation of hemoglobin and conversion of heme to porphyrins, which are not detectable with conventional guaiac-based tests (can be negative with losses of 30 mL of blood per day). The hydration of stools also affects guaiac positivity; liquid or soft stools are much more likely to be positive. In addition the presence of fruits and vegetables that have peroxidase activity or of red meat can cause false-positive results. In general blood loss must exceed 10 mL a day for a Hemoccult test result to be positive half the time. Hemoquant, which is a quantitative measurement of stool heme-

derived porphyrin, is much more accurate in measuring GI blood loss. However, the high cost of the Hemoquant test and the requirement of collection of a stool specimen (possibly leading to decreased compliance) has hampered widespread use.

The best discriminant of iron deficiency is serum ferritin level, which correlates better with iron stores than do either serum iron and transferrin saturation or hypochromic microcytic indices. Iron deficiency presents primarily with fatigue, which is multifactorial and not caused by anemia alone. Pica, or compulsive eating behavior for ice or soil, is associated with iron deficiency. Physical findings include koilonychia, glossitis, cheilitis, and esophageal webs.

Most of the lesions that cause gross GI bleeding can also cause chronic oozing and occult bleeding. In Western countries acid-peptic disease accounts for 30% to 70% of instances of occult bleeding. In tropical countries, hookworm infestation is the most common cause. A few specific causes of occult bleeding that were not mentioned in the discussion of gross bleeding deserve comment. Large hiatal hernias are associated with iron-deficiency anemia thought to be caused by longitudinal erosions (Cameron's erosions) in the gastric mucosa at the level of the diaphragmatic hiatus. Long distance runners may have iron deficiency caused by occult bleeding due to mesenteric ischemia or repetitive jarring. A common cause of occult GI bleeding is gastroduodenal and small-intestinal damage due to use of aspirin and other NSAIDs. If the occult bleeding is caused by use of NSAIDs and the patient needs to continue use of these drugs, switching to enteric-coated aspirin, nonacetylated salicylates, or a less damaging NSAID may decrease mucosal irritation. Another alternative is cotreatment with prostaglandins or proton pump inhibitors (PPIs), which has been shown to be effective in the prevention of gastropathy and ulcers due to NSAIDs. Prophylactic treatment with H_2-blockers appears effective against duodenal disease but not gastric disease. It remains unclear who should receive prophylaxis because most patients taking NSAIDs do not have appreciable upper GI bleeding, and routine prophylaxis with prostaglandins or PPIs is expensive and has side effects. It seems reasonable to recommend cotreatment with prostaglandins or PPIs in the care of patients who have marked upper GI bleeding but need to continue NSAID intake.

Current health care maintenance recommendations include yearly testing of three stool specimens for the presence of blood after the age of 40 to 50 years. This may allow for early detection and better cure rates for colonic carcinoma, the second most common cause of cancer deaths in the United States (see Chapter 116). Unfortunately, patients with asymptomatic colorectal cancer often have fecal blood levels below the threshold of guaiac tests and within the normal range of quantitative tests. Several studies have shown Hemoccult detection rates for asymptomatic colon cancer of 20% to 30% with compliance rates for screening programs in the range of 30% to 60%. Therefore it is not surprising that fecal blood screening confers only marginal reductions in cancer mortality.

The amount of diagnostic evaluation indicated for patients with occult bleeding depends on the severity of blood loss, age of the patient, and clinical history (Fig. 102.4). All patients who have anemia due to GI blood loss warrant evaluation. Depending on drug history, symptoms, and age, this may consist of endoscopic examination of either the upper or the lower GI tract. Many patients need study of both potential sites of blood loss, because concurrent lesions are common. In the absence of anemia or GI symptoms in a patient older than 40 years, colonoscopy or air-contrast barium enema examination plus sigmoidoscopy is adequate. For young patients without GI symptoms or anemia, simple follow-up hematocrit readings and examinations of stool samples may be sufficient because diagnostic studies are both expensive and uncomfortable.

GASTROINTESTINAL BLEEDING FROM AN UNKNOWN SOURCE

A few instances of chronic bleeding or recurrent acute bleeding elude diagnosis despite upper and lower GI radiography and upper GI and lower GI endoscopy. It has been estimated that as many as 5% of patients do not have an identifiable source of bleeding despite extensive examination. The cause of most instances of GI bleeding of obscure origin is thought to be vascular ectasia.

For young patients a radionuclide scan for Meckel's diverticu-

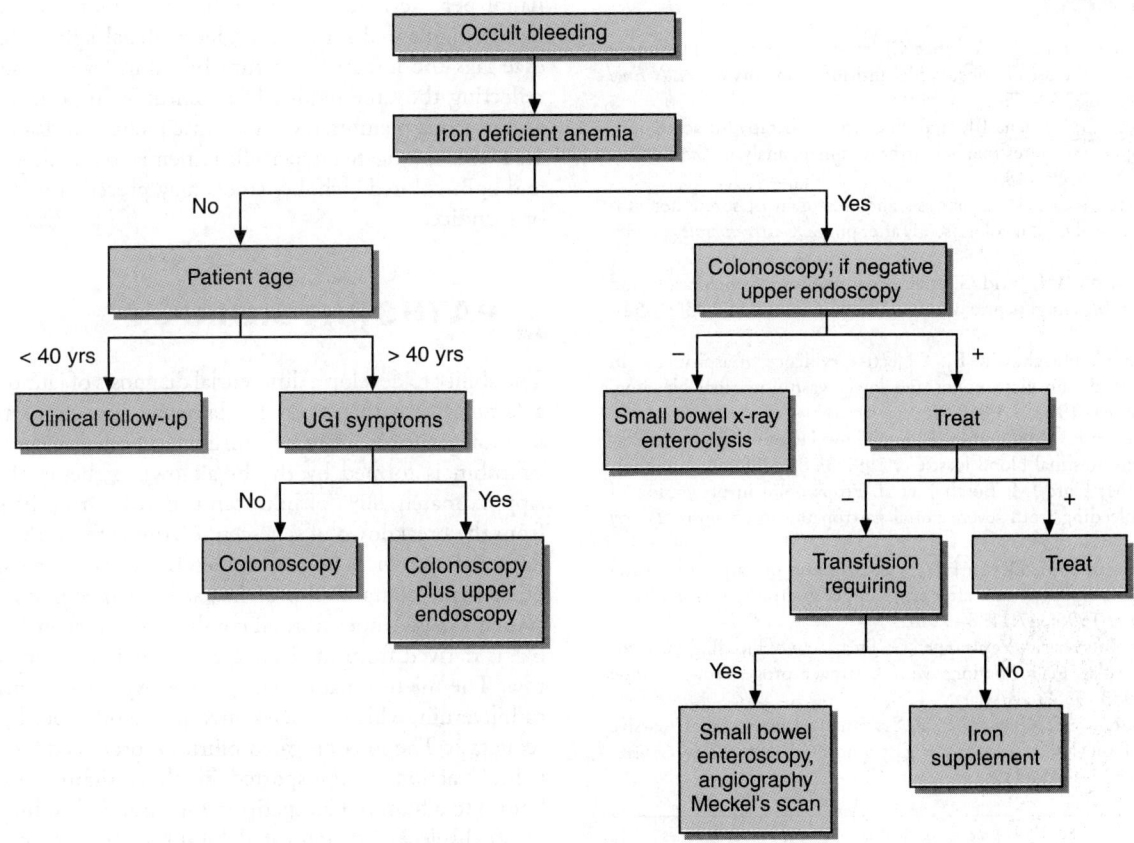

FIGURE 102.4. Evaluation of occult gastrointestinal bleeding.
EVIDENCE LEVEL: C. Expert Opinion.

lum is valuable. A useful approach toward identifying small-intestinal sources of bleeding is enteroclysis or small-intestinal infusion radiography. This necessitates oral intubation and fluoroscopic positioning of the tip of the tube at the duodenojejunal junction. Barium is then rapidly injected with methylcellulose and water to achieve a double contrast effect. If the results of the small-intestinal studies are negative among patients bleeding from an unknown source and the blood loss can be offset with iron supplementation, no further evaluation may be necessary. If transfusions are needed, however, visceral angiography or small-intestinal enteroscopy is indicated. Angiography for patients who are not actively bleeding may reveal vascular anomalies or small-intestinal tumors not identified with other studies. Small-intestinal enteroscopy has been reported successful in making a diagnosis for 30% of patients with bleeding of obscure origin that has eluded all other diagnostic tests. Intraoperative transluminal endoscopy has been useful in locating small-intestinal angiodysplastic lesions. Endoscopic thermal ablation of angiodysplasia is recommended when the lesions are accessible. If ablation is unsuccessful or not feasible because of the presence of multiple lesions, surgical resection of the involved segments may be necessary. A therapeutic trial of estrogen-progesterone therapy for the possible underlying diagnosis of vascular ectasia may be worthwhile even if there is not a definite diagnosis. Rare instances of bleeding from an unknown source defy diagnosis, or the patient is too ill for surgery and must undergo transfusions as needed.

BIBLIOGRAPHY

Allison MC, Howatson AG, Torrance CJ, et al. Gastrointestinal damage associated with the use of nonsteroidal anti-inflammatory drugs. *N Engl J Med* 1992;327:749–754.

Cook DJ, Guyatt GH, Salena BJ, et al. Endoscopic therapy for acute nonvariceal upper gastrointestinal hemorrhage: a meta-analysis. *Gastroenterology* 1992;102:139–148.

Jensen DM, Machicado GA. Diagnosis and treatment of severe hematochezia: the role of urgent colonoscopy after purge. *Gastroenterology* 1988; 95:1569–1574.

Khuroo MS, Yattoo GN, Javid G, et al. A comparison of omeprazole and placebo for bleeding peptic ulcer. *N Engl J Med* 1997;336:1054–1058.

Lanas A, Sekar C, Hirschowitz BJ. Objective evidence of aspirin use in both ulcer and non-ulcer upper and lower gastrointestinal bleeding. *Gastroenterology* 1992;103:862–869.

Morris AJ, Wasson LA, MacKenzie JF. Small bowel enteroscopy in undiagnosed gastrointestinal blood loss. *Gut* 1992;33:887–889.

Perez-Ayuso RM, Pigre JM, Bosch J, et al. Propranolol in prevention of recurrent bleeding from severe portal gastropathy in cirrhosis. *Lancet* 1991;337:1431–1434.

Rockall TA, Logan RFA, Devlin HB, et al. Selection of patients for early discharge or outpatient care after acute upper gastrointestinal haemorrhage. *Lancet* 1996;347:1138–1140.

van Cutsem E, Rutgeerts P, Vantrappen G. Treatment of bleeding gastrointestinal vascular malformations with oestrogen-progesterone. *Lancet* 1990;335:953–955.

Wagner HE, Stain SC, Gilg M, et al. Systematic assessment of massive bleeding of the lower part of the gastrointestinal tract. *Surg Gynecol Obstet* 1992;175:445–449.

CHAPTER

103

APPROACH TO THE PATIENT WITH JAUNDICE

RICHARD H. MOSELEY

Jaundice, or icterus, is yellow pigmentation of the skin, mucous membranes, sclerae, and body fluids. It is caused by excess accumulation in tissue of bilirubin, a distinctively colored degradative product of heme. It is a dramatic sign of liver disease or, less commonly, hemolysis, and has been recognized for centuries.

PRESENTATION

Jaundice is the clinical manifestation of hyperbilirubinemia. Yellow discoloration of the skin caused by chronic ingestion of large amounts of foods rich in carotene or lycopene, such as carrots or tomatoes, respectively, or of drugs such as quinacrine and busulfan is readily differentiated from jaundice with the documentation of normal serum bilirubin levels and the absence of scleral icterus. Jaundice usually is detectable when serum bilirubin levels are greater than 2.5 to 3 mg per deciliter (43 to 51 μmol per liter). It is more difficult to appreciate jaundice of darkly pigmented skin and under artificial light. Clinical jaundice lags the increase in serum bilirubin level by several days, reflecting the time required for bilirubin to permeate the skin and mucous membranes. As a consequence, in disorders associated with conjugated hyperbilirubinemia, darkening of the urine and light-colored (acholic) stools may precede the development of jaundice.

PATHOPHYSIOLOGY

The ability to develop a differential diagnosis of jaundice requires a familiarity with certain fundamental aspects of the normal physiologic mechanism of bilirubin production and excretion. Bilirubin is formed by the breakdown of heme (Fig. 103.1). Approximately 80% of bilirubin is derived from heme released from the breakdown of senescent erythrocytes in the reticuloendothelial system. The rest comes from the heme moieties of other heme-containing proteins, such as myoglobin and tissue cytochromes. Under normal conditions, less than 1% of bilirubin is derived from ineffective erythropoiesis in the bone marrow. The microsomal enzyme, heme oxygenase, converts heme to biliverdin, which is then converted to bilirubin by biliverdin reductase. The unconjugated bilirubin produced by these enzymatic reactions is transported in blood tightly but reversibly bound to albumin. Competition for albumin binding by certain drugs displaces unconjugated bilirubin. In neonates this may result in diffusion of bilirubin across the blood-brain barrier

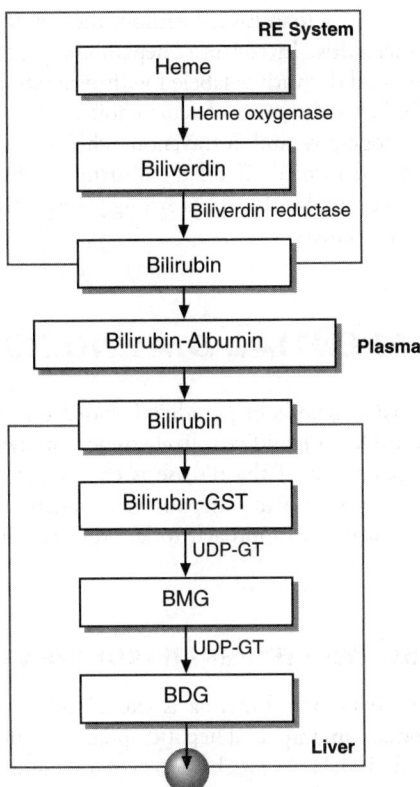

FIGURE 103.1. Bilirubin metabolism. The conversion of heme to biliverdin by microsomal heme oxygenase occurs predominantly in the reticuloendothelial cells of the spleen. Biliverdin undergoes further oxidation by cytosolic biliverdin reductase to form bilirubin. Unconjugated bilirubin circulates in plasma largely bound to albumin. After dissociation from albumin, bilirubin is taken up by the liver, where it is bound to the cytosolic proteins, glutathione S-transferases (GST). Glucuronidation of bilirubin is catalyzed by microsomal uridine diphosphoglucuronyl transferase (UDPGT), and the reaction results in formation of bilirubin monoglucuronide (BMG) and bilirubin diglucuronide (BDG). Conjugated bilirubin is then excreted into bile.

and bilirubin encephalopathy or kernicterus. Because of its tight albumin binding and hydrophobicity, unconjugated bilirubin is not filtered or secreted by the kidney. Instead, unconjugated bilirubin is avidly taken up by the liver.

Hepatic uptake of bilirubin across the sinusoidal membrane is mediated, in part, by a protein termed *organic anion transporting polypeptide* (OATP). Other proteins, yet to be cloned, such as bilitranslocase, also mediate the sinusoidal uptake of unconjugated bilirubin. In the hepatocyte, bilirubin is bound to cytosolic binding proteins and transported to the endoplasmic reticulum, where it is converted to a water-soluble form by means of conjugation as a diglucuronide. This process facilitates its excretion into bile and is mediated by the microsomal enzyme, bilirubin uridine diphosphoglucuronyl transferase (UDPGT).

Hepatic bilirubin uptake and conjugating activity are preserved in most forms of liver disease. Biliary excretion represents the rate-limiting step in overall bilirubin metabolism. This step is mediated by a canalicular multispecific organic anion transporter (cMOAT) that has been identified as an adenosine triphosphate (ATP)–binding cassette transporter that belongs to the family of multidrug resistance proteins (MRP2).

Jaundice can be classified pathophysiologically as the result of unconjugated or of conjugated hyperbilirubinemia. Unconjugated hyperbilirubinemia occurs when there is a defect in bilirubin metabolism before hepatic uptake. Conjugated hyperbilirubinemia results when the defect occurs after hepatic uptake. This classification scheme is artificial: even in pure hemolytic states, serum conjugated bilirubin levels are elevated somewhat, albeit to a lesser extent than the rise in unconjugated bilirubin. Likewise, liver disease, in which predominantly conjugated hyperbilirubinemia occurs, also may raise levels of serum unconjugated bilirubin. Hemolysis may accompany certain forms of liver disease, such as Wilson's disease, and intrahepatic cholestasis may be associated with hemolytic disorders, such as the jaundice associated with sickle cell anemia. Hemolytic disorders also are associated with pigment gallstone formation, which may lead to obstructive jaundice.

HISTORY AND PHYSICAL EXAMINATION

Many clues to the cause of jaundice and the presence of liver disease can be obtained from a carefully performed history interview and physical examination. These clues include the following:

- History of exposure to infectious agents, such as the hepatitis viruses, drugs, organic solvents, alcohol, or other hepatotoxins
- History of gallstones, previous operations on the biliary tract, and previous episodes of jaundice or inflammatory bowel disease
- Family history of jaundice or liver disease
- The presence of pruritus, fever, or abdominal pain
- Signs of chronic liver disease, including palmar erythema, spider angiomas, parotid gland enlargement, gynecomastia, Dupuytren's contracture, and testicular atrophy
- Physical findings of chronic cholestasis, including excoriation, xanthelasma, and xanthoma
- Physical signs of inflammation or malignant disease, including hepatomegaly, splenomegaly, palpable gallbladder, tenderness with palpation, mass lesions, and cachexia

Age and sex are important clues. Viral hepatitis occurs more commonly among younger adults; choledocholithiasis and malignant disease occur among older patients. Primary biliary cirrhosis and choledocholithiasis are more common among women; pancreatic cancer and primary sclerosing cholangitis are more common among men.

LABORATORY STUDIES AND DIAGNOSTIC TESTS

Serum levels of total, conjugated, and unconjugated bilirubin confirm the clinical diagnosis of jaundice and direct further evaluation. A complete blood cell count, reticulocyte count, and microscopic examination of a peripheral blood smear are useful in identifying hemolysis as the predominant cause of jaundice. Serum bilirubin levels typically do not exceed 5 mg per deciliter with hemolysis. Routine liver function tests (serum albumin and prothrombin time [PT]) and liver chemical analysis (serum alanine aminotransferase [ALT], aspartate aminotransferase [AST], and alkaline phosphatase) should be performed. In the absence of hemolysis, the finding of isolated hyperbilirubinemia indicates Gilbert's syndrome or familial hyperbilirubinemia as the cause of jaundice.

Elevation of the serum alkaline phosphatase and transaminase activities of a patient with jaundice points to the presence of hepatobiliary disease. As more fully discussed in Chapter 104, the pattern of liver chemistry abnormalities is helpful in differentiating hepatocellular from cholestatic liver injury. Hepatocellular injury invariably causes an increase in serum aminotransferase activity, but marked (fourfold or greater) elevations of serum alkaline phosphatase activity are typically seen among patients with cholestatic disorders. If serum alkaline phosphatase level is normal, extrahepatic obstruction is unlikely.

Imaging of the biliary tree is an early and important step in the evaluation of patients with jaundice who are thought to have cholestatic jaundice. The role of these studies is to determine whether bile duct dilatation is present and, if it is present, the site and cause of the obstruction. Ultrasonography (US) and computed tomography (CT) are the primary imaging modalities used. US is less expensive than CT and obviates use of contrast agents and ionizing radiation. Although US can readily depict cholelithiasis, it is more limited than CT in detecting the level and type of obstruction. US evaluation of the pancreas and distal common bile duct may be obscured by overlying intestinal gas. Obesity also may limit the technical quality of US. CT may be indicated as the first-line imaging study if malignant disease is suspected because it provides information about pancreatic abnormality, retroperitoneal lymph node involvement, and ability to resect the tumor.

If bile duct dilatation is found, or if bile duct dilatation is absent but clinical suspicion for bile duct obstruction is high, direct visualization of the biliary tree with either endoscopic retrograde cholangiopancreatography (ERCP) or percutaneous cholangiography (PTC) is warranted. In certain cases, such as that of a patient who has undergone cholecystectomy and is likely to have choledocholithiasis, direct visualization of the bile duct as the initial diagnostic study may be the most appropriate and cost-effective approach. The choice between ERCP and PTC, two invasive studies, is governed by the availability of skilled personnel, the patient's clotting function, the anticipated need for therapeutic intervention (sphincterotomy, placement of biliary stents or drains), earlier operations, such as Roux-en-Y gastrojejunostomy, and the anticipated level of obstruction. ERCP is favored over PTC for distal lesions; PTC is favored over ERCP for proximal lesions.

Magnetic resonance cholangiopancreatography (MRCP) is a relatively new technique of noninvasive visualization of the bile ducts and pancreatic ducts without the use of contrast material. Early trials suggest it may be useful in the evaluation of jaundice. Endoscopic ultrasonography (EUS) is another imaging modality that has demonstrated utility and accuracy in the diagnosis of choledocholithiasis. For patients with a low to moderate likelihood of having choledocholithiasis, EUS may be a more cost-effective strategy than ERCP without the potential complication of pancreatitis. In contrast, hepatobiliary imaging with iminodiacetic acid derivatives labeled with technetium 99m, although useful in the diagnosis of acute cholecystitis, has no role. Oral cholecystography and intravenous cholangiography also should not be performed. If biliary obstruction has been excluded or hepatocellular disease is strongly suspected, liver biopsy may be warranted.

◾ DIFFERENTIAL DIAGNOSIS

The differential diagnosis of jaundice is based on whether the disease responsible for jaundice is likely to be hemolytic, hepatocellular, or cholestatic. If the disease is cholestatic, it depends on whether the process is intrahepatic or extrahepatic. An algorithm for the diagnostic approach to jaundice is shown in Fig. 103.2.

UNCONJUGATED HYPERBILIRUBINEMIA

Unconjugated hyperbilirubinemia is caused by an increase in bilirubin production, impaired hepatic uptake, or impaired conjugation (Table 103.1). As much as 85% of total serum bilirubin is the unconjugated form in these disease states. Increased red blood cell destruction in disorders associated with ineffective erythropoiesis and in hemolytic disorders increases bilirubin production. Examples include ineffective erythropoiesis associated with pernicious anemia, sideroblastic anemia, thalassemia, and lead poisoning and congenital and acquired hemolytic conditions, including hereditary spherocytosis, hemoglobinopathy, autoimmune hemolysis, and hemolysis associated with drug use or sepsis. Reductions in hepatic blood flow due to congestive heart failure or portosystemic shunting impair the delivery and uptake of bilirubin to hepatocytes. Impaired hepatic uptake at the sinusoidal membrane occurs in Gilbert's syndrome and after administration of certain drugs, such as sulfonamides, penicillin, salicylates, and rifampin. The hyperbilirubinemia of Gilbert's syndrome is mild (2 to 4 mg per deciliter) and is exacerbated by fasting and intercurrent viral infection. Reduced activity of UDPGT leads to impaired bilirubin conjugation and occurs among neonates and patients with Gilbert's and Crigler–Najjar type I and II syndromes. UDPGT activity can be induced by phenobarbital, effectively reducing the jaundice in Crigler–Najjar type II syndrome.

CONJUGATED HYPERBILIRUBINEMIA

Conjugated hyperbilirubinemia can occur in a wide spectrum of hepatobiliary diseases, including disorders associated with acute or chronic liver injury, extrahepatic biliary obstruction, and the familial abnormalities of bilirubin excretion—Dubin–Johnson and Rotor's syndromes. Cholestasis, or impaired bile formation, is the most common cause of jaundice. Cholestasis can be categorized further as a functional defect in bile formation at the level of the hepatocyte (intrahepatic chole-

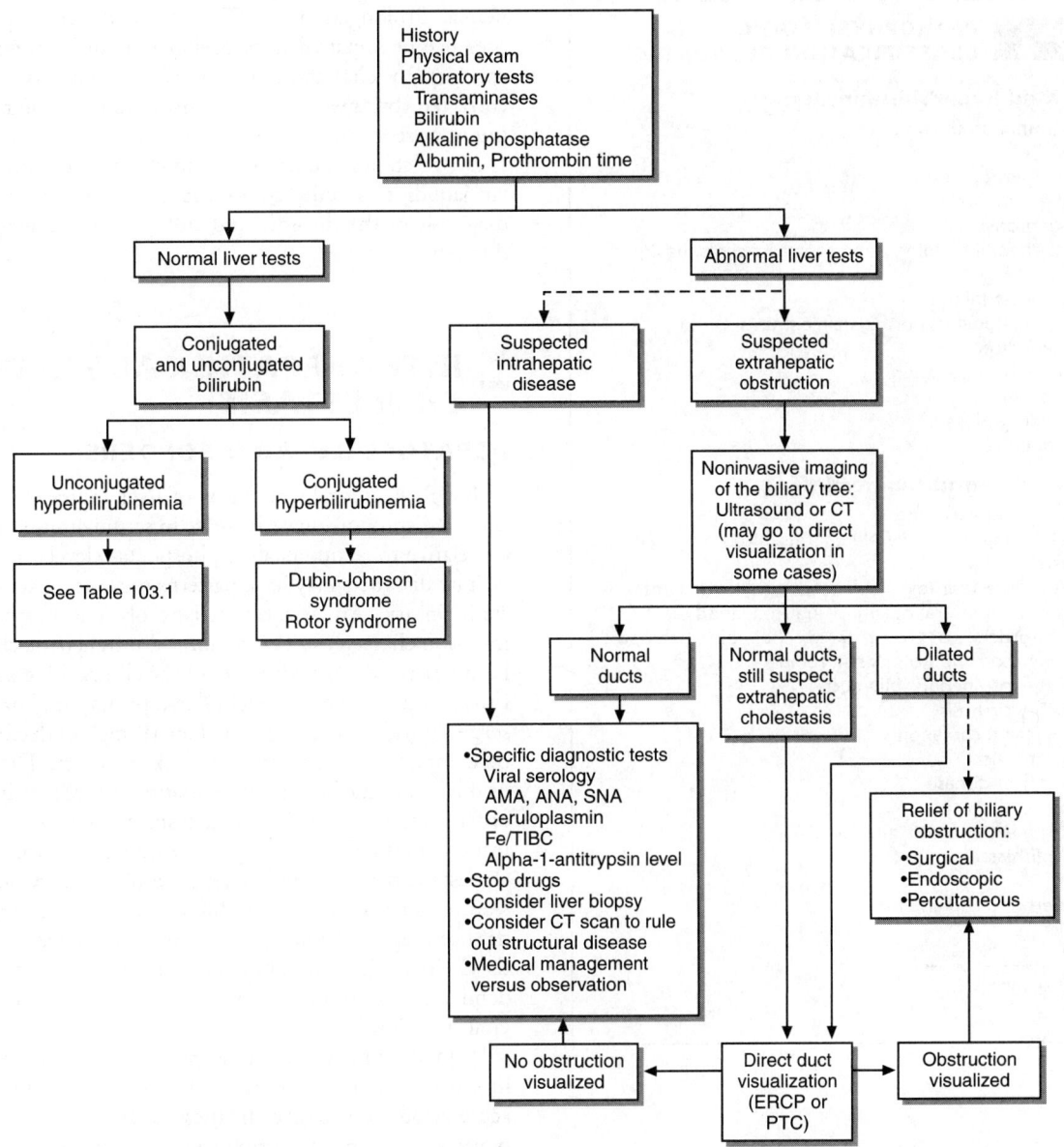

FIGURE 103.2. Evaluation for jaundice. *Dotted line,* alternative approach for certain patients. *AMA,* antimitochondrial antibody; *ANA,* antinuclear antibody; *SMA,* smooth-muscle antibody; *Fe/TIBC,* iron/ total iron binding capacity.

EVIDENCE LEVEL: C. Expert Opinion.

stasis) or obstruction of bile flow within the biliary tract (extrahepatic cholestasis). The most common causes of intrahepatic and extrahepatic cholestasis are listed in Table 103.2. Hepatobiliary disorders associated with a cholestatic pattern of jaundice often are accompanied by pruritus. Extrahepatic biliary obstruction may manifest with signs of cholangitis, such as fever, right upper quadrant abdominal pain, leukocytosis, and hypotension. Serum alkaline phosphatase levels are disproportionately elevated relative to serum aminotransferase levels, and serum cholesterol levels may be elevated. A prolonged PT, reflecting malabsorption of fat-soluble vitamin K, is corrected by means of parenteral administration of vitamin K.

Jaundice produced by disorders associated predominantly

with hepatocyte necrosis or dysfunction has a hepatocellular pattern. Examples of such disorders include acute viral hepatitis, autoimmune hepatitis, and most forms of drug-induced hepatotoxicity. Malaise, anorexia, nausea, and vomiting may dominate the clinical signs and symptoms of these disorders. Disproportionate elevations in serum aminotransferase levels relative to serum alkaline phosphatase levels reflect the underlying hepatocellular damage and necrosis. In complete biliary obstruction, serum bilirubin level tends to plateau over time between 10 and 30 mg per deciliter. Levels greater than 30 mg per deciliter are more likely to occur among patients with hepatocellular disease. Additional factors, such as renal failure, excessive hemolysis, and sepsis, are present among patients with severe hyperbilirubi-

TABLE 103.1. PATHOPHYSIOLOGIC CLASSIFICATION OF JAUNDICE

Unconjugated Hyperbilirubinemia

Increased bilirubin production
  Hemolysis
  Ineffective erythropoiesis
Impaired bilirubin uptake
  Gilbert's syndrome
  Drugs (e.g., rifampin, radiographic contrast agents, flavispidic acid)
  Congestive heart failure
  Surgical or spontaneous portosystemic shunts
  Neonatal jaundice
Impaired bilirubin conjugation
  Gilbert syndrome
  Crigler–Najjar syndrome
  Neonatal jaundice

Conjugated Hyperbilirubinemia[a]

Impaired canalicular excretion
  Hepatocellular injury (e.g., viral hepatitis, alcoholic hepatitis, cirrhosis)
  Intrahepatic cholestasis (e.g., intrahepatic cholestasis of pregnancy, total parenteral nutrition–induced jaundice)
  Familial disorders of conjugated bilirubin transport (Dubin–Johnson and Rotor's syndromes)
Disorders of the intrahepatic bile ducts
  Primary biliary cirrhosis
  Primary sclerosing cholangitis
  Liver allograft rejection
  Graft versus host disease
  Neoplasms
Disorders of the extrahepatic bile ducts
  Choledocholithiasis
  Neoplasms
  Primary sclerosing cholangitis
  Biliary strictures

[a] See also Table 103.2.

TABLE 103.2. DIFFERENTIAL DIAGNOSIS OF CHOLESTATIC SYNDROMES

Intrahepatic	Extrahepatic
Acute hepatocellular disorders	Choledocholithiasis
Viral hepatitis	Biliary strictures
Alcoholic hepatitis	Cholangiocarcinoma
Drugs	Pancreatic carcinoma
Chronic hepatocellular injury	Pancreatitis
Primary biliary cirrhosis	Periampullary carcinoma
Sclerosing cholangitis	Biliary atresia
Chronic active hepatitis	Choledochal cysts
Drugs	Miscellaneous disorders
Total parenteral nutrition	
Systemic infection	
Postoperative state	
Benign recurrent causes	
Miscellaneous conditions	

nemia. Prolongation of PT in these disorders points to the presence of impaired hepatocellular synthetic function and, in contrast to cholestatic forms of jaundice, is typically not corrected by means of administration of vitamin K. The importance of differentiating intrahepatic from extrahepatic causes of cholestatic jaundice and cholestatic from hepatocellular jaundice is reflected in the divergent approaches to the diagnosis of the disorder and treatment of patients with these different processes.

INTRAHEPATIC CAUSES OF CHOLESTASIS

HEPATOCELLULAR DISORDERS

Although hepatocellular forms of liver injury characteristically cause a disproportionate increase in serum aminotransferase levels relative to serum alkaline phosphatase levels, several hepatocellular disorders may have patterns more consistent with cholestatic injury. An atypical variant of acute hepatitis A viral infection characterized by prolonged intrahepatic cholestasis has been described. Usual features of the clinical illness include pruritus, fever, diarrhea, weight loss, pronounced jaundice, and serum bilirubin levels greater than 10 mg per deciliter followed by complete recovery after 12 weeks or more. The importance of this syndrome lies in differentiating this relatively benign disorder from extrahepatic obstruction. Acute hepatitis B virus infection, particularly among the elderly, may manifest with a cholestatic pattern. Cholestatic hepatitis with atypical histologic features, such as ductular proliferation and acute pericholangitis, has been reported among liver transplant recipients with hepatitis C virus infection. Cholestasis also is a characteristic of epidemic, or waterborne, non-A, non-B hepatitis, or hepatitis E viral infection.

A predominant cholestatic picture, with striking elevations in serum alkaline phosphatase levels, occasionally occurs with acute alcoholic hepatitis. In these cases, liver biopsy specimens typically contain signs of cholangitis that involves intralobular bile ducts in the absence of extrahepatic obstruction. The degree of cholestasis found at liver biopsy is a highly significant indicator of poor outcome among patients with alcoholic hepatitis.

PRIMARY BILIARY CIRRHOSIS

Chronic nonsuppurative destructive cholangitis, commonly known as primary biliary cirrhosis (PBC), is a chronic, progressive cholestatic syndrome of unknown causation that is most common among women in the sixth or seventh decade of life. The most common symptoms of PBC are pruritus and fatigue of insidious onset. Jaundice is present among about one-fourth of patients when they come to medical attention. Physical findings among patients with PBC can be variable. For patients with symptoms, examination is more likely to reveal hepatomegaly, splenomegaly, hyperpigmentation, excoriation, and signs of chronic liver disease, such as spider angioma and palmar erythema. The physical finding of xanthelasma correlates with moderate elevations in serum lipid levels, whereas xanthoma usually are a reflection of severe hyperlipemia.

More than 80% of patients with PBC have at least one associated autoimmune disease and nearly 50% have two or more such disorders, often manifesting themselves after the diagnosis is made. Keratoconjunctivitis sicca is the most commonly reported association.

The triad of an elevated serum alkaline phosphatase level (corroborated by similar elevations in 5′-nucleotidase, γ-glutamyl transpeptidase [GGTP], or leucine aminopeptidase level), detectable titers of antimitochondrial antibody, and an elevated serum IgM level is of considerable discriminatory value in the diagnosis of PBC. Percutaneous liver biopsy with special stains for copper is critical in the diagnostic approach when PBC is suspected.

PRIMARY SCLEROSING CHOLANGITIS

Primary sclerosing cholangitis (PSC) is a chronic, progressive inflammatory disorder that primarily affects the extrahepatic and intrahepatic bile ducts and leads to fibrosis and stricture of the biliary tract (see Chapter 125). Obstruction of the biliary tree is manifested as chronic cholestasis that results in secondary biliary cirrhosis, portal hypertension, and hepatic failure.

Physical findings of PSC may include jaundice, hepatomegaly, and splenomegaly. Early in the development of PSC, however, the physical findings may be entirely normal. Later stages of the disease are characterized by the signs of chronic liver disease and of portal hypertension common to other forms of cirrhosis. The development of cholangiocarcinoma is another late complication of PSC. The hallmark of PSC is the presence of multiple areas of stenosis of bile ducts (see Chapter 125).

Biliary tract abnormalities resembling PSC have been described as a complication of AIDS. Clinical manifestations include fever, right upper quadrant pain, nausea, and vomiting. Marked elevations of serum alkaline phosphatase levels and lesser changes in serum aminotransferase and bilirubin levels are found. Cholangiography reveals intrahepatic and extrahepatic ductal dilatation with focal stricture formation or beading and decreased arborization and terminal pruning of secondary and tertiary intrahepatic biliary radicles. Endoscopic sphincterotomy results in symptomatic and biochemical improvement among some patients with concomitant stenosis of the papilla of Vater. Opportunistic infection of the biliary tract with cytomegalovirus or *Cryptosporidium* species and resultant cholangitis have been proposed as a pathogenic mechanism for this cholestatic syndrome.

Histiocytosis X, cystic fibrosis, and hepatic metastases from adenocarcinoma of the pancreas and colon may manifest with cholangiographic findings identical to those of PSC. A caustic form of sclerosing cholangitis has been found after injection of a scolicidal solution for the management of hepatic *Echinococcus* cysts. This form of sclerosing cholangitis affected only the parts of the biliary tract that came in contact with this agent. Progressive cholestasis associated with diffuse intrahepatic duct involve-

TABLE 103.3.	DRUGS ASSOCIATED WITH INTRAHEPATIC CHOLESTASIS
Amoxicillin[a]	Ketoconazole
Amoxicillin/clavulanic acid	Methimazole
Atenolol	Methyltestosterone
Azathioprine	Nitrofurantoin[b]
Captopril	Phenylbutazone
Chlorpromazine[a]	Procainamide
Chlorpropamide	Prochlorperazine
Cyclosporine	Propafenone
Danazol	Sulfonamides
Erythromycin	Sulindac
Estrogens	Thiabendazole
Floxuridine	Tolazamide
Flurazepam	Tolbutamide
Flutamide	Trazodone
Gold salts	Trimethoprim-sulfamethoxazole
Griseofulvin	Valproic acid[b]
Haloperidol	Warfarin
Imipramine	

[a] Reports of vanishing bile duct syndrome have been described.
[b] Typically cause hepatocellular injury, although cholestasis has been described.

ment that mimics PSC has been found after bone marrow transplantation.

DRUG-INDUCED INTRAHEPATIC CHOLESTASIS

Cholestasis is a common feature of drug-induced liver injury and typically is manifested as bland cholestasis (e.g., estrogenic steroids) with minimal biochemical or histologic evidence of hepatic inflammation or as an inflammatory cholestasis (e.g., phenothiazines), which often is accompanied by systemic features of a hypersensitivity reaction, such as fever, rash, arthralgia, and eosinophilia, and histologic features of hepatocellular necrosis. A wide spectrum of drugs have been implicated (Table 103.3).

CHOLESTASIS ASSOCIATED WITH TOTAL PARENTERAL NUTRITION

Several different biochemical and histologic patterns of hepatic dysfunction have been recognized during administration of total parenteral nutrition (TPN). Steatosis appears to be related to TPN formulas containing large amounts of carbohydrates as the only caloric source. Intrahepatic cholestasis, although more common among newborn premature infants, also occurs among adults during hyperalimentation, particularly patients with inflammatory bowel disease. Twofold elevations in serum alkaline phosphatase and total bilirubin levels are encountered and abnormalities in ALT levels characteristically are more pronounced than elevation in AST levels. GGTP level appears to be the most sensitive indicator of TPN cholestasis in the pediatric population. Several mechanisms have been proposed, including direct effects of constituents of TPN solutions and intraluminal effects resulting from the interruption of oral intake or loss of intestinal surface area. Elevated biliary levels of the cholestatic bile acid lithocholate, which normally is formed by bacterial degradation of chenodeoxycholate, have been described among patients with abnormalities in liver chemical values during TPN. Antibiotic suppression of putative intestinal bacterial overgrowth among patients receiving TPN may be effective in preventing cholestasis.

Extrahepatic forms of cholestasis must be considered in the differential diagnosis of jaundice among patients receiving long-term hyperalimentation. Several factors that work in concert to promote bile stasis during TPN are thought to be responsible for the increased incidence of gallbladder sludge, cholelithiasis, and acalculous cholecystitis among these patients.

JAUNDICE IN BACTERIAL INFECTIONS

Cholestatic jaundice among patients with bacterial infections is a well-recognized clinical syndrome. The pathogenic mechanism is thought to involve circulating bacterial endotoxin, because cholestasis is associated with infection with a variety of gram-negative bacteria and is found in the absence of documented bacteremia. Sepsis-associated cholestasis is not restricted to gram-negative bacteria. Clinical hepatic dysfunction usually is overshadowed by the symptoms and signs of the underlying disease, although the sudden appearance of jaundice with a high fever may herald the systemic infection. Conjugated hyperbilirubinemia occurs and levels typically are within the range of 5 to 10 mg per deciliter. Twofold to threefold elevations in serum alkaline phosphatase levels occur among about one-half of all patients, but serum aminotransferase levels usually are normal.

POSTOPERATIVE JAUNDICE

Postoperative jaundice is a commonly encountered cholestatic syndrome. The importance lies in determining the cause among the various etiologic or contributory factors. Increased bilirubin production may be the result of transfusions, particularly of stored blood; resorption of blood from hematomas and other extravascular spaces; or hemolysis, which is encountered often among patients undergoing cardiac surgery. Careful review of the anesthesia record may point to hepatocellular dysfunction from anesthetics, such as halothane and other haloalkanes, and to periods of relative hypotension or hypoxemia. The perioperative use of potentially hepatotoxic drugs and the presence of occult infection should be considered. The transfusion requirement should be documented; as many as 90% of cases of transfusion-transmitted hepatitis occur within 5 to 12 weeks after transfusion. Concurrent renal impairment may decrease the clearance of conjugated bilirubin. After biliary tract surgery, biliary strictures or retained common bile duct stones may be present. When all causative factors have been addressed and excluded, the impairment in bile secretion that leads to the development of jaundice by the second or third postoperative day is referred to as *benign postoperative intrahepatic cholestasis*. Early postoperative jaundice among patients undergoing cardiopulmonary bypass surgery (so-called *pump jaundice*) may have poor prognostic im-

plications independent of the underlying mechanism of hyperbilirubinemia.

BENIGN RECURRENT INTRAHEPATIC CHOLESTASIS

The clinical features of benign recurrent intrahepatic cholestasis, a relatively uncommon familial syndrome, are characterized by recurrent episodes, lasting an average of 3 to 4 months, of pruritus, anorexia, weight loss, and jaundice. During attacks, serum bilirubin levels range from 10 to 20 mg per deciliter with a predominant increase in the conjugated fraction; serum alkaline phosphatase levels are increased; and liver biopsy samples exhibit striking central-zone bile stasis and a mild portal inflammatory infiltrate. Findings at ERCP performed to rule out extrahepatic obstruction in such patients routinely are normal. Liver chemistries and histologic features return to normal between episodes, and progression to chronic liver disease does not occur.

INTRAHEPATIC CHOLESTASIS OF PREGNANCY

Intrahepatic cholestasis of pregnancy is differentiated from other liver diseases occasionally encountered during pregnancy by its relative benignity. Familial studies support an autosomal dominant mode of inheritance with variable expression. Epidemiologic studies have shown a high frequency of this disorder among Scandinavians and Chilean Indians. Although the pathogenesis is not completely understood, abnormal sensitivity to endogenous estrogens appears to play a primary role. Women with a history of intrahepatic cholestasis of pregnancy have clinical and laboratory abnormalities of the syndrome when challenged with oral contraceptives when they are not pregnant.

Pruritus is the principal symptom of intrahepatic cholestasis of pregnancy. The onset most often occurs during the third trimester. Jaundice, reflecting underlying conjugated hyperbilirubinemia, typically is mild. Twofold to fivefold elevations of AST and ALT levels may occur, and serum alkaline phosphatase and cholesterol levels are increased. Percutaneous liver biopsy, rarely necessary in the diagnosis, reveals varying degrees of cholestasis with minimal or no inflammatory reaction. Pruritus and laboratory abnormalities resolve promptly after delivery, underscoring the self-limited nature of this disorder. However, increased risk of fetal distress, prematurity, and stillbirths has been demonstrated.

FAMILIAL FORMS OF INTRAHEPATIC CHOLESTASIS

Arteriohepatic dysplasia (Allagille's syndrome) is an autosomal dominant form of infantile cholestasis characterized by survival into adulthood. Well-defined clinical features include hepatic ductular hypoplasia, abnormal facies, peripheral pulmonic stenosis, and vertebral anomalies. A nonsyndromic form of paucity of interlobular bile ducts resembling that described among infants and children has been reported among adults. This disorder, possibly familial, may progress rapidly to end-stage biliary cirrhosis.

MISCELLANEOUS DISORDERS

A syndrome of chronic intrahepatic cholestasis resembling PBC has been described among patients with sarcoidosis. Clinical and biochemical features include insidious onset of pruritus, jaundice, hepatomegaly, marked elevations in serum alkaline phosphatase level, and hypercholesterolemia. Mitochondrial antibodies typically are absent. The pathogenesis of this disorder is thought to involve progressive destruction of bile ducts by portal and periportal granulomas that leads to a biliary form of cirrhosis.

Hepatic involvement is common among patients with both the primary and secondary forms of amyloidosis. Mild hepatic dysfunction occurs even with extensive hepatic infiltration, manifesting primarily as hepatomegaly and moderate elevations in serum alkaline phosphatase levels. Severe intrahepatic cholestasis, however, has been reported among a small percentage of patients with systemic amyloidosis. Hepatomegaly, ascites, and pruritus often are present, and striking elevations in serum bilirubin, alkaline phosphatase, and cholesterol levels occur. Liver biopsy demonstrates prominent amyloid deposition in periportal regions with relative sparing of central-zone hepatocytes. Interference of the movement of bile into septal bile ducts by amyloid deposits is thought to be the mechanism of cholestasis.

The cause and pathophysiologic mechanism of intrahepatic cholestasis associated with extrabiliary Hodgkin's disease and other lymphomas are poorly understood. Attempts to relate the cholestasis to abnormal hormones elaborated by the tumor have been unsuccessful. Intrahepatic cholestasis may occur with thyrotoxicosis, even in the absence of congestive heart failure.

∎ EXTRAHEPATIC CHOLESTASIS

Structural or mechanical obstruction of the bile ducts most often is caused by choledocholithiasis, pancreatic and periampullary cancer, or biliary strictures. Biochemical features are similar to those of intrahepatic cholestasis; they include striking elevations in serum bilirubin and alkaline phosphatase levels. Symptoms such as abdominal pain, fever, and chills may assist in the diagnosis, but extrahepatic obstruction can occur in the absence of such symptoms. Initial evaluation may be aided by abdominal US and, in certain clinical settings, such as suspected retained common bile duct stones, by direct visualization of the biliary tree and anatomic definition of the level of obstruction with ERCP or PTC.

CHOLEDOCHOLITHIASIS

Stones in the bile ducts figure prominently in the differential diagnosis of cholestasis and are classified as primary (arising de novo), secondary (originating and migrating from the gallbladder), recurrent (re-forming after biliary tract surgery), or retained (overlooked at surgery). Primary bile duct stones often are associated with biliary infections and intrahepatic stones. Among Asians they may be part of the syndrome referred to as *recurrent pyogenic cholangitis*. Differentiation between retained and recurrent stones is hampered by the absence of reliable information regarding the time required for a ductal stone to re-form. Recurrent stones are more likely to be composed of bile pigments, whereas retained stones contain primarily cholesterol.

Clinical features include epigastric pain that radiates to either right or left upper quadrant, nausea, vomiting, and jaundice due to ductal obstruction. Acute pancreatitis or angina pectoris caused by a reflex decrease in coronary blood flow also may be a part of the presentation. Fever and rigor signify the development of obstructive cholangitis.

BILIARY STRICTURES

The cause of more than 90% of all benign strictures involving the major bile ducts is iatrogenic injury, which occurs mainly during operations on the biliary tract. An ischemic basis of this type of stricture has been postulated. Postoperative pain, fever, jaundice, and excessive discharge through drains or the abdominal incision should alert the physician to the possibility of bile duct injury. The critical aspect of the management of biliary strictures is prevention.

CHOLANGIOCARCINOMA

Biliary cancer, despite its relative rarity, should be considered in the differential diagnosis of extrahepatic cholestasis. Sixty percent of patients are men, in contrast to the female preponderance for primary carcinoma of the gallbladder, and the presentation typically is in the sixth or seventh decade of life. Infestation with liver flukes (*Clonorchis sinensis, Opisthorchis felineus*, and *O. viverrini*), ulcerative colitis, and congenital choledochal cysts all appear to be associated with bile duct carcinoma. The clinical features are similar to those of other forms of extrahepatic obstruction, and the disorder commonly mimics benign biliary stricture or sclerosing cholangitis.

PANCREATIC CAUSES

Pancreatic carcinoma and periampullary carcinoma often have features of extrahepatic obstruction. Benign disorders occur less often, but stenosis of the distal segment of the common bile duct has been recognized increasingly as a common complication of chronic alcoholic pancreatitis. Partial obstruction may be manifested as anicteric elevation in serum alkaline phosphatase level; episodic or persistent jaundice; secondary biliary cirrhosis; and less commonly, suppurative cholangitis with microabscesses or macroabscesses in the liver. Histologic findings of alcohol-induced liver injury are notably absent among such patients. Surgical biliary decompression is recommended in the treatment of patients with persistent stenosis of the intrapancreatic portion of the common bile duct. Strictures of the distal common bile duct also have been described among patients with cystic fibrosis.

MISCELLANEOUS DISORDERS

Although choledochal cysts are congenital malformations, as many as one-half of patients with cysts do not come to medical attention until adulthood. Symptoms at presentation are those of acute cholangitis: right upper quadrant abdominal pain, fever, and jaundice. Diagnosis is accomplished best with abdominal US and ERCP. Surgical therapy consists of resection of the abnormal duct in view of the malignant potential of congenital choledochal cysts. Caroli's disease is an intrahepatic variant of cystic disease of the biliary tract. Periampullary duodenal diverticula, usually incidental findings at endoscopy or barium radiographic studies, rarely may cause structural extrahepatic obstruction.

Hemobilia caused by hepatic trauma, rupture of an aneurysm of the hepatic artery, biliary ascariasis, hepatobiliary neoplasms, choledocholithiasis, or a ruptured liver abscess may cause extrahepatic obstruction and gross or occult gastrointestinal blood loss. Extrahepatic biliary obstruction also can be caused by metastatic disease, most commonly tumors of gastrointestinal origin. Patients often are assumed to have hepatic metastasis, and response to chemotherapy differentiates certain neoplasms, notably lymphoma and small-cell lung cancer. Nonneoplastic disease, specifically tuberculous adenitis, has been reported to cause extrinsic extrahepatic obstruction in rare instances. Other unusual infectious causes of bile duct obstruction are ascariasis and candidiasis.

▬ STRATEGIES FOR OPTIMAL CARE

Management of most of the diseases that cause jaundice is discussed in the disease-specific chapters. Management of extrahepatic biliary obstruction is discussed briefly here. The two goals of such management are, first, to drain bile above the obstruction, thereby relieving pruritus and reducing the risks of secondary biliary cirrhosis, cholangitis, and hepatic abscesses and, second, to remove or bypass the cause of obstruction.

Temporary drainage of obstructed ducts can be achieved for almost all patients by means of placement of percutaneous or nasobiliary catheters above the level of obstruction at the time of diagnostic PTC or ERCP, respectively. In cases of inoperable malignant obstruction, internal biliary stents are preferred over percutaneous transhepatic stenting or surgical bypass because of lower short-term morbidity and cost. Plastic biliary stents offer the advantage of low cost and ease of placement, but a short patency period necessitates replacement. Self-expanding metallic stents, on the other hand, remain patent for longer periods but are expensive and cannot be exchanged. Membrane-covered stents that have the combined attributes of metal and plastic stents are under development.

Although patients with jaundice and biliary obstruction have increased postoperative morbidity and mortality, principally because of sepsis and renal failure, elective preoperative percutaneous biliary drainage does not appear to reduce operative risk but increases hospital stay and cost.

The management of choledocholithiasis has been dramatically altered by the advent of laparoscopic cholecystectomy. The main indication for ERCP and endoscopic sphincterotomy (ES) once was choledocholithiasis among patients who had undergone cholecystectomy or patients with choledocholithiasis and an intact gallbladder considered to be at high surgical risk or those suffering from complications, such as cholangitis or severe acute pancreatitis, which carry a high surgical mortality rate. Four strategies currently are followed in the care of a patient scheduled to undergo laparoscopic cholecystectomy: (a) preoperative ERCP and ES if common bile duct stones are present; (b) intraoperative cholangiography with postoperative ERCP and ES if common bile duct stones are present; (c) intraoperative cholangiography with laparoscopic common bile duct exploration if common bile duct stones are present; and (d) postoperative ERCP only for patients with recurrent symptoms that suggest biliary obstruction from retained common bile duct stones. The optimal strategy has not been defined but requires that the likelihood of a common bile duct stone be balanced against the the rate of technical failure and the risk of complications from any given intervention. The risk of pancreatitis from ERCP is approximately 5% and is nearly doubled if ES is performed. Laparoscopic common bile duct exploration is technically difficult, is not performed at most centers, and frequently necessitates postoperative ERCP. Nevertheless, there is a growing trend away from preoperative ERCP with greater experience in laparoscopic common bile duct exploration.

Despite advances in the endoscopic management of choledocholithiasis, 2% to 5% of stones are resistant to conventional endoscopic techniques. Extracorporeal shock wave lithotripsy may be effective but is limited by availability and cost. Intracorporeal laser-induced shock wave lithotripsy involves positioning with a conventional duodenoscope and use of a laser fiber close to the stone in the common bile duct for the delivery of laser pulses. This may become, in combination with conventional endoscopic extraction, the preferred management of complicated common bile duct stones.

COMPLICATIONS AND PITFALLS

Although bile duct dilatation found at US or CT has a high predictive value for obstruction, this finding may be absent in certain settings in which extrahepatic obstruction is present. Intermittent or partial obstruction, as is the case among as many as one-third of patients with choledocholithiasis, may not cause detectable bile duct dilatation. Encasement of the bile ducts by cholangiocarcinoma or diffuse fibrosis from PSC may prevent dilatation even if a dominant stricture is present. For the same reason, intrahepatic ductal dilatation may be limited in the presence of cirrhosis. Therefore, if on the basis of clinical evaluation, extrahepatic obstruction is suspected, direct visualization of the bile ducts with either PTC or ERCP should be pursued.

Acute biliary obstruction may cause serum transaminase elevations disproportionate to serum bilirubin and alkaline phosphatase elevations, often more than 2,000 U per liter. The levels rapidly decline to near normal within 72 hours, unlike serum transaminase levels in disorders associated with hepatocellular jaundice, which typically remain elevated for longer periods (ischemic hepatitis is a notable exception).

Indications for HOSPITALIZATION

Symptoms and signs of cholangitis (abdominal pain, fever, leukocytosis, and hypotension) necessitate immediate hospitalization. Among elderly patients with suspected biliary obstruction, hospitalization may be warranted, even in the absence of these symptoms and signs. For disorders associated with hepatocellular jaundice, a decision regarding hospitalization is based on factors other than the mere finding of jaundice, including the presence of coagulopathy, the need for intravenous therapy and parenteral nutrition, and the need for inpatient therapy for the underlying disorder.

Indications for REFERRAL

Acute viral hepatitis is the most common cause of jaundice among young adults. If uncomplicated, it may not necessitate referral. For other disorders associated with hepatocellular jaundice or intrahepatic cholestasis a likely diagnosis may be rendered by the referring physician, and the need to refer depends substantially on the clinical setting and the degree of reassurance needed by the patient. The need for liver biopsy among such patients may lead to a referral. Biliary obstruction from either choledocholithiasis or a malignant tumor is more likely among older patients, and in most cases the expertise of a gastroenterologist is needed.

BIBLIOGRAPHY

Bass NM. An integrated approach to the diagnosis of jaundice. In: Kaplowitz N, ed. *Liver and biliary diseases,* 2nd ed. Baltimore: Williams & Wilkins, 1996:653–672.

Bearcroft PW, Lomas DJ. Magnetic resonance cholangiopancreatography. *Gut* 1997;41:135–137.

Berg CL, Crawford JM, Gollan JL. Bilirubin metabolism and the pathophysiology of jaundice. In: Schiff ER, Sorrell MF, Maddrey WC, eds. *Schiff's diseases of the liver,* 8th ed. Philadelphia: Lippincott-Raven, 1999: 147–192.

Frank BB. Clinical evaluation of jaundice. A guideline of the Patient Care Committee of the American Gastroenterological Association. *JAMA* 1989;262:3031–3034.

Roy-Chowdhury J, Jansen PLM. Bilirubin metabolism and its disorders. In: Zakim D, Boyer T, eds. *Hepatology: a textbook of liver disease,* 3rd ed. New York: Raven Press, 1996:323–361.

Scharschmidt BF, Goldberg HI, Schmid R. Current concepts in diagnosis. Approach to the patient with cholestatic jaundice. *N Engl J Med* 1983; 308:1515–1519.

Turgeon DK, Moseley RH. Jaundice and abnormal liver chemistries. In: Henderson JM, ed. *Gastrointestinal pathophysiology.* Philadelphia: Lippincott-Raven, 1996:153–183.

Woodley MC, Peters MG. Approach to the patient with jaundice. In: Yamada T, ed. *Textbook of gastroenterology,* 2nd ed. Philadelphia: JB Lippincott, 1996:893–908.

Kelley's Textbook of Internal Medicine, fourth edition. Edited by H. David Humes.
Lippincott Williams & Wilkins, Philadelphia © 2000.

CHAPTER 104

APPROACH TO THE PATIENT WITH ABNORMAL LIVER CHEMISTRIES

RICHARD H. MOSELEY

The approach to the patient with abnormal liver chemistries is not governed by any well-defined diagnostic algorithms. Instead, a systematic approach to patients with suspected liver disease involves, first, an understanding of the diverse panel of available measurements of liver function and serum markers of hepatobiliary disease. From this panel, a group of indices most appropriate to the particular clinical problem is selected. A single test is rarely sufficient in the analysis of most clinical problems, but the selection process is facilitated by several distinct patterns of liver injury.

HISTORY AND PHYSICAL EXAMINATION

As in most disease states, an accurate history is critical. Systemic symptoms of liver disease (e.g., anorexia, weight loss, chills and fever, nausea, and vomiting) are nonspecific and typically of little help in the differential diagnosis. Valuable information can be elicited by questions regarding family history, drug use (prescription and over-the-counter medications), alcohol consumption, illicit substance use/abuse, exposure history, sexual and menstrual history, occupational or environmental history, travel history, past surgery (including anesthesia records, if available), and transfusion history.

Familial forms of intrahepatic cholestasis such as arteriohepatic dysplasia (Alagille's syndrome) are well described. Hemochromatosis, Wilson's disease, and α_1-antitrypsin deficiency are examples of liver diseases transmitted by an autosomal recessive mode of inheritance, and genetic factors may play a role in other hepatobiliary disorders, such as primary sclerosing cholangitis and autoimmune hepatitis.

Given the relatively nonspecific presentation of drug-induced liver disease, drug-related hepatic injury may not be suspected initially in a patient with abnormal liver chemistries. Difficulties in diagnosis are compounded by the unknown hepatotoxicity of newly introduced agents. Nevertheless, the possibility of drug-induced liver injury should be considered in all patients with a seemingly nonspecific change or worsening in liver chemistries; such considerations are aided by a complete drug history. Alcohol and nonprescription medication use is an important part of this inquiry. Alcoholic patients should always be questioned about acetaminophen use because of its propensity to cause hepatotoxicity at even therapeutic doses.

Viral hepatitis should be investigated in patients with abnormal liver chemistries and a history of exposure to or contact with jaundiced persons, syringes or needles (including tattoo paraphernalia), or blood and blood products. A history of recent ingestion of raw oysters or steamed clams should suggest hepatitis A infection. Additional risk factors associated with hepatitis A in the United States include homosexual contact and contact with children attending day care centers. The patient's source of water is occasionally relevant, because private water supplies are often implicated in hepatitis A outbreaks. The development of abnormal liver chemistries in the "healthy" hepatitis B carrier warrants strong consideration of hepatitis D virus superinfection. Recent travel to areas endemic for viral hepatitis should be noted; water-borne outbreaks of hepatitis E most commonly occur in Southeast Asia and the Indian subcontinent. Abnormalities in smell (dysosmia) and taste (dysgeusia) may be noted by patients with viral hepatitis. Arthritis, abrupt in onset, with a strong predilection for proximal interphalangeal joints and often accompanied by an interstitial rash, occurs during the prodromal phase in 20% of patients with hepatitis B.

Sexually transmitted diseases are an important cause of abnormal liver chemistries; therefore, a sexual history should be included in the evaluation. The number of sexual partners that the patient has had in the preceding 6 months should be determined, considering that the average incubation period of hepatitis B is from 6 to 12 weeks. A sexual history in the female patient should always include information on contraceptive use. A menstrual history may reveal the presence of secondary amenorrhea, a common complication of chronic liver disease.

Although the use of hepatotoxins such as carbon tetrachloride, chloroform, and trinitrotoluene has diminished, liver injury associated with accidental or occupational exposure to workplace chemicals remains a significant problem. Although an itemized list is beyond the scope of this chapter, exposure to industrial and environmental hepatotoxins should be elicited by a thorough occupational history.

The nature of and indications for previous abdominal surgery should be ascertained. Information concerning the gross appearance of the liver at the time of surgery may prove valuable. In the postoperative patient, surgical and anesthesia records should be reviewed for the inhalational agent administered, the presence and duration of intraoperative hypotension, and the amount of blood product support required. Chronic liver disease is a late complication of jejunoileal bypass surgery; biliary strictures, retained and recurrent stones, or papillary stenosis should be considered in the postcholecystectomy patient with abnormal liver chemistries.

Generalized pruritus may be a presenting symptom in patients with liver disease, particularly cholestatic syndromes. Pruritus in the jaundiced patient is frequently nocturnal and is most pronounced on the palms and soles. The presence or absence and character of abdominal pain may provide some clues toward establishing a cause of abnormal liver chemistries. In contrast to the intense and rapidly developing right upper quadrant abdominal pain of acute extrahepatic obstruction as in choledocholithiasis, the pain associated with acute viral hepatitis is a heavy or dragging sensation. Pain from primary and metastatic tumors of the liver may be distinguished by its dull or boring character, although hemorrhage into the tumor may result in the sudden appearance of severe pain.

Physical findings of some discriminative value in the patient with abnormal liver chemistries include stigmata of chronic liver disease (e.g., spider angiomata, palmar erythema, parotid gland enlargement, gynecomastia, Dupuytren's contracture, and testicular atrophy), hepatomegaly and liver consistency, splenomegaly, gallbladder distention, and abdominal tenderness. Although the degree of hepatomegaly can vary in all forms of hepatobiliary disease, a liver span of more than 15 cm is more often associated with passive congestion from right-sided heart failure or neoplastic and infiltrative processes (e.g., amyloidosis, myeloproliferative disorders, and glycogen and lipid storage disorders). A pulsatile liver may be encountered in tricuspid insufficiency. A hepatic bruit or friction rub should alert the examiner to the possibility of an underlying hepatocellular carcinoma. Murphy's sign (inspiratory arrest during deep palpation of the right upper quadrant) can be elicited in those with acute cholecystitis. Punch or fist tenderness may help to differentiate hepatobiliary from pleural-based pain. Jaundice manifested by yellow pigmentation of the skin, mucous membranes, and sclerae typically requires a serum bilirubin concentration higher than 3 mg per deciliter for detection; artificial light makes detection at low levels more difficult. Sunflower cataracts and Kayser–Fleischer rings are highly suggestive of Wilson's disease.

LABORATORY STUDIES AND DIAGNOSTIC TESTS

TESTS OF LIVER FUNCTION

Laboratory determinations that reflect hepatic disease are often called liver function tests, although only some are true measurements of hepatic function. Therefore, the use of this term should be discouraged. Tests that examine the liver's ability to excrete substances into bile, particularly organic anions, fall within this strict definition, as do laboratory assessments of the liver's synthetic and metabolic capacity.

BILIRUBIN

Tests of bilirubin metabolism are important in the assessment of hepatic function because bilirubin is an endogenous organic anion, derived primarily from the degradation of hemoglobin from senescent erythroid cells. Total serum bilirubin is separated into two fractions, a water-soluble, direct-reacting conjugated form and a lipid-soluble, indirect-reacting form representing unconjugated bilirubin. Almost all the bilirubin normally present in serum is the unconjugated fraction. Hyperbilirubinemia, clinically manifested as jaundice, is accordingly classified as either predominantly unconjugated or predominantly conjugated, simply by subtracting direct from total serum bilirubin to estimate the indirect, or unconjugated, bilirubin. Increased production of bilirubin, impaired transport into hepatocytes, or defective bilirubin conjugation within the hepatocyte are disorders associated with unconjugated hyperbilirubinemia. Up to 85% of total serum bilirubin is the unconjugated form in these disease states.

Besides the rate of hemolysis, the liver's ability to conjugate bilirubin determines the degree of unconjugated hyperbilirubinemia observed. Even in severe hemolytic disorders, total serum bilirubin rarely exceeds 5 mg per deciliter in the presence of normal hepatic function. In contrast, in hepatocellular disorders with impaired intrahepatic excretion of bilirubin and in extrahepatic obstruction, a conjugated hyperbilirubinemia is observed. In these settings, typically more than 50% of the serum bilirubin is in the direct-reacting form.

Urine bilirubin is invariably conjugated bilirubin and thus is encountered only in conditions in which serum levels of direct or conjugated bilirubin are elevated. The tea-colored appearance of urine caused by the presence of bilirubin must be differentiated from similar discoloration by hemoglobinuria and myoglobinuria. Bilirubinuria may precede the clinical appearance of jaundice, largely because of the low (less than 1 mg per deciliter) renal threshold for excretion of conjugated bilirubin.

SERUM BILE ACIDS

Two primary bile acids (cholic and chenodeoxycholic acid) are synthesized in the liver from cholesterol and converted by intestinal bacteria to the secondary bile acids (deoxycholic, ursodeoxycholic, and lithocholic acid). Although serum bile acids are almost always elevated in moderate to severe liver disease, poor diagnostic sensitivity in patients with mild liver disease has prevented the widespread application of serum bile acid determination. The finding of normal fasting levels of cholic acid conjugates, however, may be helpful in supporting a diagnosis of Gilbert's syndrome in patients with unconjugated hyperbilirubinemia.

CLOTTING FACTORS

Liver disease is a common cause of impaired coagulation. Normal serum activities of the vitamin K-dependent coagulation factor proenzymes (factors II, VII, IX, and X), as assessed by the one-stage prothrombin time (PT), require intact hepatic synthesis and adequate intestinal absorption of lipid-soluble vitamin K. A prolonged PT can therefore be seen in patients with hepatocellular disorders that impair hepatic synthetic function (e.g., hepatitis, cirrhosis) and in those with cholestatic syndromes that interfere with lipid absorption. Hepatocellular injury can be differentiated from cholestatic causes of PT prolongation by the parenteral administration of vitamin K; intact hepatic function is established by an improvement in the PT of more than 30% within 24 hours. A prolonged PT in acute viral hepatitis signifies severe hepatocellular necrosis, may antedate other manifestations of hepatic failure, and is associated with a worse prognosis. Plasma concentrations of individual proteins may be useful clinical guides; in view of its short half-life, factor VII is the best index of the severity of liver disease and of prognosis.

ALBUMIN

Albumin is quantitatively the most important of several plasma proteins formed in the liver. Accordingly, the measurement of total concentration of serum albumin is a useful test of hepatic synthetic function. The relatively long half-life of serum albumin (20 days) makes the serum albumin level a better index of severity and prognosis in patients with chronic liver disease than in patients with acute hepatic injury in whom levels are usually normal or only minimally depressed. Nutritional factors (i.e., the availability of amino acids) are critical determinants of the rate of albumin synthesis. Moreover, alterations in serum albumin levels may reflect disturbances in synthesis and changes in the rate of catabolism, dilution by expanded plasma volume (as seen in cirrhosis), or enhanced loss through the gastrointestinal tract or kidneys.

IMMUNOGLOBULINS

Although measurement of serum globulins does not fulfill the operational definition of a liver function test, the hypergammaglobulinemia commonly observed in patients with liver disease indirectly represents functional impairment of the reticuloendothelial cells of the hepatic sinusoids. Hypergammaglobulinemia higher than 3.0 g per deciliter in a patient with chronic hepatitis is more consistent with autoimmune liver disease than viral hepatitis. A predominant rise in the immunoglobulin A (IgA) fraction is observed in hypergammaglobulinemia associated with alcoholic cirrhosis. A disproportionate elevation of IgM is a feature that differentiates primary biliary cirrhosis from other liver diseases, specifically autoimmune hepatitis, which are associated with prominent hypergammaglobulinemia. A specific diagnosis, however, is rarely established by quantitative determinations of immunoglobulins. Instead, hyperglobulinemia demonstrated on serum protein electrophoresis is a clue to the presence of chronic liver disease.

TESTS OF HEPATIC METABOLISM

Drug metabolism is another critical hepatic function, and liver disease is often associated with impaired drug metabolism. The most widely performed tests of hepatic metabolic capacity are the antipyrine clearance determination and the aminopyrine demethylation breath test. Although these quantitative tests may be noninvasive predictors of hepatic histology, difficulties with interindividual differences in the metabolism of a single drug and intraindividual differences in the metabolism of different drugs make interpretation difficult.

■ SERUM MARKERS OF HEPATOBILIARY DYSFUNCTION

Routine biochemical laboratory tests are not true indices of hepatic function. Instead, they serve as markers of hepatobiliary dysfunction—specifically, hepatocellular necrosis, cholestasis, or infiltrative processes.

AMINOTRANSFERASES (TRANSAMINASES)

Aspartate aminotransferase (AST; serum glutamic-oxaloacetic transaminase [SGOT]) and alanine aminotransferase (ALT;

serum glutamic-pyruvic transaminase [SGPT]) are important markers of hepatocellular injury. AST is found in various tissues (notably cardiac and skeletal muscle, kidney, and brain), but ALT is limited primarily to the liver. Given the tissue distribution of the two enzymes, elevations of serum ALT are a more specific reflection of hepatocellular disease than serum AST levels. Within the liver cell, AST is present in mitochondria and the cytosol, and ALT is localized to the cytosol. The highest serum elevation of both enzymes is seen in patients with viral, toxin-induced, and ischemic hepatitis; smaller elevations (less than 300 units) relative to the degree of histologic necrosis are usually seen in cases of alcoholic hepatitis. The AST/ALT ratio in serum is a useful indicator of alcoholic liver disease: a ratio above 2 is highly suggestive of alcohol-induced hepatic injury. In contrast, in patients with acute and chronic viral hepatitis (and extrahepatic biliary obstruction), an AST/ALT ratio of less than 1 is typical, although an AST/ALT ratio above 1 has been associated with cirrhosis in patients with chronic hepatitis B infection. Thus, an AST/ALT ratio above 1 in the setting of nonalcoholic chronic liver disease may signify underlying cirrhosis. In the presence of cirrhosis, however, this ratio may be less useful in differentiating alcoholic from nonalcoholic forms of liver disease.

Although these indices of hepatocellular injury do not predict histologic findings, serial determinations of serum AST and ALT levels may reflect the extent of hepatocellular injury and are useful in following the progression of liver disease. Decreases in AST and ALT levels in serum, however, may be either a sign of recovery from an acute injury or, particularly in the case of fulminant hepatic failure, an indication of limited hepatic reserve after overwhelming hepatocyte necrosis.

ALKALINE PHOSPHATASE

In the liver, alkaline phosphatase appears to be an integral enzyme of the exterior surface of the bile canalicular membrane. Hepatocellular injury invariably results in increases in serum aminotransferase activity, but significant (fourfold or greater) elevations of serum alkaline phosphatase activity are typically seen in patients with cholestatic syndromes. Lesser increases in levels lack specificity and may be present in all forms of liver disease. Alkaline phosphatase activity can also be demonstrated in bone, placenta, intestine, kidney, and leukocytes. Liver and bone are the predominant sources of serum alkaline phosphatase activity in normal persons, with less than 20% derived from the intestine. In pregnancy, a substantial fraction may be derived from the placenta. Ectopic production of an alkaline phosphatase isoenzyme occurs in patients with cancer, and elevations may therefore be observed in the absence of bony or hepatic metastases. Low levels of serum alkaline phosphatase have been reported in acute hemolytic anemia complicating Wilson's disease, hypothyroidism, pernicious anemia, zinc deficiency, and congenital hypophosphatasia.

OTHER ENZYME MARKERS OF CHOLESTASIS

Although the alkaline phosphatase isoenzymes can be separated electrophoretically, alternative approaches are used in clinical practice. Serum γ-glutamyl transferase or transpeptidase (GGTP) determination establishes the hepatic origin of an elevated alkaline phosphatase by virtue of its localization within the hepatobiliary tree. Alcohol consumption, presumably through enzyme induction, raises serum enzyme levels, and this finding has been invoked as a sensitive marker of chronic alcohol consumption that occurs independently of any liver damage. Serum GGTP levels are also elevated in patients with pancreatic disorders, myocardial infarction, uremia, chronic obstructive pulmonary disease, rheumatoid arthritis, and diabetes mellitus and in those using microsomal enzyme-inducing drugs such as anticonvulsants and warfarin.

Determination of serum 5'-nucleotidase (5'-NT) or serum leucine aminopeptidase (SLAP) levels plays a role similar to that of serum GGTP determination. Despite their presence in a wide variety of other body tissues, elevated enzyme levels in the nongravid patient are specific for hepatobiliary disease and correlate well with elevated alkaline phosphatase levels of hepatic origin. SLAP levels are elevated in pregnancy, and conflicting data exist concerning 5'-NT levels in pregnancy. In patients with cancer, elevated 5'-NT levels are a sensitive marker in the diagnosis of metastatic disease to the liver. A normal 5'-NT level does not necessarily exclude liver disease in the setting of an elevated alkaline phosphatase, because these markers may not increase parallel with early or mild hepatic injury.

LACTATE DEHYDROGENASE

Although commonly available, measurement of total serum lactate dehydrogenase (LDH) has limited diagnostic specificity for hepatocellular disease, and fractionation of LDH to determine levels of the isoenzyme of hepatic origin (LDH-5) is rarely indicated. Moderate elevations of LDH are often seen in hepatocellular disorders such as viral hepatitis and cirrhosis and are less common in cholestatic disorders.

◼ DISEASE-SPECIFIC MARKERS

The laboratory tests previously outlined alert the physician to the presence of hepatobiliary disease. Additional markers of specific disorders are discussed in the following section.

VIRAL SEROLOGY

Diagnosis of acute hepatitis A is based on the serologic detection of hepatitis A virus-specific IgM antibody (IgM anti-HAV; Chapter 119) (Table 104.1). Seropositivity first becomes detectable at the onset of clinical illness and is invariably present at the onset of jaundice. This serologic marker typically persists for 120 days, far exceeding both clinical and biochemical resolution of illness. Prolonged periods of seropositivity of more than 200 days have been observed. Nevertheless, it is best regarded as a marker of acute or recent hepatitis A viral infection. In contrast, IgG anti-HAV is present primarily in convalescent sera and persists for long periods after infection, perhaps for life.

Several serologic tests are available to establish hepatitis B viral

TABLE 104.1.	SEROLOGIC DIAGNOSIS OF ACUTE VIRAL HEPATITIS
Disease	**Serologic Test**
Hepatitis A	IgM anti-HAV
Hepatitis B	HBsAg, IgM anti-HBc
Hepatitis C	Anti-HCV, HCV RNA
Hepatitis D	HBsAg, anti-HDV

HBc, hepatitis B core; HBsAg, hepatitis B surface antigen.

infection (Chapter 119). Hepatitis B surface antigen (HBsAg) is the first marker detectable in serum, preceding elevations in serum aminotransferases and the onset of symptoms. HBs antigenemia typically lasts for 1 to 2 months in self-limited infections. Antibody to core antigen (anti-HBc) is detected in serum about 2 weeks after the appearance of HBsAg; typically, a window or lag period then occurs before specific antibody to HBsAg (anti-HBs) appears. During this period and in the 10% of patients who do not manifest detectable levels of HBsAg, anti-HBc may be the only detectable serologic marker of recent infection with hepatitis B virus. HBeAg is considered to be a marker of hepatitis B virus (HBV) replication and infectivity. During the recovery phase of acute HBV infection, HBeAg-to-anti-HBe seroconversion precedes HBsAg-to-anti-HBs seroconversion. In patients with chronic hepatitis B, seroconversion from HBeAg to anti-HBe is usually associated with loss of HBV DNA in serum and remission of liver disease. Tests for HBV DNA should be reserved for patients with chronic HBV infection to assess HBV replication and candidacy and response to antiviral therapy.

Infection with the hepatitis C virus (HCV) is identified using an enzyme-linked immunosorbent assay (ELISA) to detect circulating antiviral antibodies (Chapter 119). Because increased serum γ-globulins or other serum components may produce false-positive results by ELISA, a recombinant immunoblot has been used to supplement the ELISA in the diagnosis of HCV. Nevertheless, determining whether viremia underlies the finding of antibody to HCV by any method requires the demonstration of HCV RNA by the polymerase chain reaction. The appearance of antibody to HCV may be delayed up to 6 months after acute infection.

Infection with hepatitis D virus should be considered in any HBsAg-positive patient with acute or chronic hepatitis, especially if the disease is severe or the patient is in a high-risk group. Serologic confirmation of hepatitis D coinfection or superinfection is accomplished by testing for hepatitis D antigen and anti-hepatitis D antibodies. At least one acute and one convalescent serum sample should be assayed for anti-hepatitis D, because this antibody can be transient, at low titer, and appear late in infection. Total (predominantly IgG) antibodies to hepatitis D virus are usually detectable in high titer in superinfections. Persistence of IgM anti-hepatitis D typically predicts progression to chronic hepatitis D infection.

IMMUNOLOGIC TESTS

Immunologic abnormalities occur in a wide spectrum of liver diseases. The antinuclear antibody reaction in autoimmune hepatitis is of the homogeneous pattern by immunofluorescence, and a titer of 1:160 or more is usually required. Antimitochondrial antibodies are present in over 90% of patients with primary biliary cirrhosis and in about 25% of patients with autoimmune hepatitis and drug-induced liver injury. In fact, an antimitochondrial antibody titer higher than 1:40, even in the absence of serum alkaline phosphatase elevation, strongly suggests primary biliary cirrhosis. Smooth muscle antibodies, reactive to S actin, may be detected in up to 70% of patients with autoimmune hepatitis, in about 50% of patients with primary biliary cirrhosis, and in occasional patients with acute viral hepatitis. A circulating antineutrophil cytoplasmic antibody (ANCA) has been reported in up to 87% of patients with primary sclerosing cholangitis.

Human leukocyte antigens (HLA) have also been associated with a wide spectrum of liver diseases; specifically, HLA-B8 and -DRw3 have been associated with autoimmune hepatitis, and HLA-A3 and -B14 have been linked to hemochromatosis. The increased incidences of these HLA haplotypes, however, are neither absolute nor diagnostic. Thus, although HLA typing provides information on gene frequencies, it is not routinely recommended.

CERULOPLASMIN

Determination of the serum concentration of ceruloplasmin, a copper transport protein in plasma, is particularly useful in the diagnosis of Wilson's disease. Although not directly involved in the pathogenesis of this autosomal recessive copper storage disorder, low levels of ceruloplasmin (less than 20 mg per deciliter) are found in about 90% of homozygotes and about 10% of heterozygotes. In contrast to Wilson's disease, serum ceruloplasmin is typically elevated in primary biliary cirrhosis, another disorder associated with increased hepatic copper concentrations. Increased serum levels in this disorder and other forms of liver disease reflect the role of ceruloplasmin as a nonspecific acute-phase reactant. Accordingly, normal values are sometimes seen during the chronic active hepatitis phase of Wilson's disease. Pregnancy and exogenous estrogen administration may also lead to elevated values for this protein. Likewise, hypoceruloplasminemia may result from the drop in hepatic synthetic function observed in non-wilsonian fulminant hepatic injury, and less commonly in severe malnutrition, other protein-losing states, and Menkes' syndrome.

IRON STORAGE PARAMETERS

Measurements of serum iron level and total iron-binding capacity (or transferrin) are useful in the diagnosis of the hepatic iron overload state, hemochromatosis (Chapter 123). Transferrin is normally 20% to 45% saturated, and the serum iron level and percent saturation of transferrin are elevated early in the course of this disorder. However, these tests have a relatively low degree of specificity in patients with liver disease; increased serum iron levels, with normal transferrin saturation, are common in pa-

TABLE 104.2. COMPARISON OF MARKERS IN HEMOCHROMATOSIS AND ALCOHOLIC LIVER DISEASE

Marker	Normal Range	Alcoholic Liver Disease	Hemochromatosis
Transferrin-iron saturation (%)	20–50	50–60	>62
Serum ferritin (ng/mL)	15–300	300–1,000	500–6,000
Hepatic iron concentration (μg/g dry weight)	300–1,800	1,800–5,000	10,000–30,000
Iron index (liver iron in μg/g dry weight divided by [patient's age × 55.8])	<1.1	<1.6	>1.9

tients with alcohol-induced liver injury. Acute elevations in serum iron levels have also been observed in acute viral hepatitis. Assays of serum ferritin may more closely estimate total body iron stores, and elevated serum ferritin levels are common early in the course of hemochromatosis before any histologic evidence of liver injury. Other forms of hepatocellular necrosis and systemic infection are associated with elevated serum ferritin levels disproportionate to body iron stores. For this reason, quantitative determination of tissue iron concentration on liver biopsy remains the definitive test for the diagnosis of hemochromatosis. Representative iron storage parameters in symptomatic hemochromatosis are shown in Table 104.2, compared with parameters encountered in alcoholic liver disease.

A genetic test for hemochromatosis is now available. Approximately 85% of patients with hemochromatosis are homozygous for a C282Y mutation in a gene referred to as *HFE*. A second mutation, H63D, is associated with hemochromatosis when it occurs in C282Y/H63D compound heterozygotes. At present, the cost of this molecular diagnostic test limits its use as a screening tool, although it has great applicability in studies of family members. Genetic testing should be performed in all first-degree relatives of the affected patient, known as the *proband,* and in the spouse of the proband. If the spouse does not carry one of the mutations, the biologic children would not need to be tested because they would be heterozygotes. Because cirrhosis is rarely observed in patients with hemochromatosis who are younger than 40 years old, treatment most likely can be started and liver biopsy avoided in C282Y homozygotes, unless patients are 40 years and older or unless they exhibit abnormal serum aminotransferases.

α-FETOPROTEIN

A sensitive radioimmunoassay for α-fetoprotein, a major serum protein during fetal life, has been used to screen for primary hepatocellular carcinoma. Whereas 70% to 90% of patients with hepatocellular carcinoma have elevated serum α-fetoprotein, significant elevations also occur in patients with germ cell tumors, other gastrointestinal malignancies, and such nonneoplastic hepatic disorders as autoimmune hepatitis, viral and alcoholic hepatitis, and primary biliary cirrhosis. To enhance the specificity of this test in the diagnosis of hepatocellular carcinoma, concentrations exceeding 400 ng per milliliter have been generally cited, although this arbitrary cutoff may exclude up to one-third of

patients with biopsy-proven hepatocellular carcinoma. A monoclonal radioimmunoassay may improve the specificity of α-fetoprotein screening.

α1-ANTITRYPSIN

α_1-Antitrypsin is a 52-kd glycoprotein synthesized in the liver (and to a lesser extent in monocytes and macrophages) that migrates in the α_1-globulin fraction on serum protein electrophoresis. Normal serum levels (150 to 350 mg per deciliter) may increase postoperatively and in association with inflammation, malignancy, pregnancy, and estrogen therapy. Persons homozygous for the electrophoretically slowest of the genetic variants of this protein (Pi ZZ [Pi, protease inhibitor]) have markedly decreased serum α_1-antitrypsin levels and are predisposed to the early onset of chronic active hepatitis and cryptogenic cirrhosis and hepatocellular carcinoma. Heterozygotes (Pi MZ) have serum levels 50% to 60% of normal. The inability of the hepatocyte to process and secrete the Z protein, which differs from the normal M protein by a single amino acid substitution, results in the characteristic presence of periodic acid–Schiff (PAS)–positive, diastase-resistant globules in periportal hepatocytes on percutaneous liver biopsy. The diagnosis of α_1-antitrypsin deficiency should be entertained in a patient with liver chemistry abnormalities showing a hepatocellular injury pattern when an absent α_1-globulin peak is observed on serum electrophoresis. It should be confirmed by serum α_1-antitrypsin activity determination and genetic Pi typing.

SERUM AMMONIA

Urea formation in the liver via the Krebs–Henseleit cycle is required for the disposal of ammonia, the toxic product of nitrogen metabolism. Thus, elevated serum ammonia levels are common in acute and chronic forms of liver disease. Striking elevations in fulminant hepatic failure result from the impaired conversion of ammonia to urea in the setting of severe hepatocellular necrosis, whereas the hyperammonemia present in patients with cirrhosis and portal hypertension primarily reflects the portosystemic shunting of ammonia derived from colonic bacteria. The serum ammonia determination, most accurately measured on arterial blood, is best regarded merely as an aid in the differential diagnosis of encephalopathy; serial determinations have little role in clinical practice.

PERCUTANEOUS LIVER BIOPSY

Unlike most of the laboratory tests previously discussed, no predictive value can be assigned to a specific morphologic feature observed with a percutaneous liver biopsy. For proper biopsy interpretation, all clinical, biochemical, immunologic, and radiographic data should be correlated with the histologic features. The positive predictive value of a prebiopsy diagnosis ranges from 88% for alcoholic liver disease to 56% for fatty liver. Elevations of serum transaminases more than three times normal also correlate positively with enhanced prebiopsy diagnostic accuracy. Other major applications of liver biopsy include determining the indication for antiviral therapy in chronic viral hepatitis and establishing the diagnosis in patients with unexplained hepatomegaly, suspected systemic disease (e.g., tuberculosis, sarcoidosis, or fever of unknown origin), and suspected primary or metastatic carcinoma.

DIFFERENTIAL DIAGNOSIS

Initially, nonhepatic causes must be considered (Table 104.3). Then, a proper diagnostic approach must be selected for the patient with suspected liver disease. Liver disease can be classified into four major types: cholestatic, hepatocellular, infiltrative, and immunologic. Depending on the target of the immune response, immunologic injury results in either a cholestatic picture (when the bile ducts are involved preferentially, as in primary biliary cirrhosis) or a hepatocellular form of injury (when the primary insult is to the hepatocyte membrane, as in viral and autoimmune hepatitis). Cholestasis can be categorized further as either a functional defect in bile formation at the level of the hepatocyte (intrahepatic cholestasis) or a structural impairment in bile secretion and flow (extrahepatic cholestasis). Evaluation is aided by the presence of these relatively discrete patterns of liver injury and tests of discriminative value in the detection of these patterns. Routinely, serum aminotransferase activity, serum alkaline phosphatase, serum total and direct bilirubin, serum total protein, with albumin and globulin fractionation, and PT should be determined in all patients with suspected liver disease before disease-specific markers are sought.

A pattern of typical abnormalities seen in the various forms of hepatobiliary injury emerges from this battery of tests (Table 104.4). Additional diagnostic information may be provided by testing for disease-specific markers (Table 104.5). Further laboratory evaluation of any patient with evidence of chronic (greater than 6 months) hepatitis should include, at the minimum, serum protein electrophoresis, serum ferritin, antinuclear antibody, serum ceruloplasmin, hepatitis B viral serology, and antibody to HCV.

CHOLESTATIC INJURY

The differential diagnosis of a patient with abnormal liver chemistries consistent with cholestatic injury (elevated serum alkaline phosphatase and bilirubin levels with or without moderately elevated serum aminotransferase levels) is a formidable clinical challenge. Although no symptoms or signs are pathognomonic for intrahepatic or extrahepatic forms of cholestasis, a history of previous biliary tract surgery, the presence of abdominal pain or significant weight loss, palpable gallbladder or abdominal mass, fever or other signs of cholangitis, and an elevated serum

---

TABLE 104.3.	**NONHEPATIC CAUSES FOR ABNORMAL LIVER CHEMISTRIES**	
Test	**Nonhepatic Causes**	**Discriminating Tests**
Albumin	Protein-losing enteropathy	Serum globulins, α_1-antitrypsin clearance
	Nephrotic syndrome	Urinalysis, 24-hr urinary protein
	Malnutrition	Clinical setting
	Congestive heart failure	Clinical setting
Alkaline phosphatase (AP)	Bone disease	GGTP, SLAP, 5'-NT
	Pregnancy	GGTP, 5'-NT
	Malignancy	AP electrophoresis
Serum AST	Myocardial infarction	MB-CPK
	Muscle disorders	Creatine kinase
Bilirubin	Hemolysis	Reticulocyte count, peripheral smear, urine bilirubin
	Sepsis	Clinical setting, cultures
	Ineffective erythropoiesis	Peripheral smear, urine bilirubin, Hgb electrophoresis, bone marrow examination
	"Shunt" hyperbilirubinemia	Clinical setting
GGTP	Alcohol, drugs	History
Ferritin	Systemic disease, chronic inflammation	Clinical setting
Prothrombin time	Dietary deficiency of vitamin K, antibiotic and anticoagulant use, steatorrhea	Response to vitamin K, clinical setting

GGTP, γ-glutamyl transpeptidase; Hgb, hemoglobin; MB-CPK, creatine phosphokinase isoenzyme; 5'-NT, 5'-nucleotidase; SLAP, serum leucine aminopeptidase.

TABLE 104.4. ROUTINE BIOCHEMICAL TESTS IN THE PATIENT WITH IDEALIZED HEPATOBILIARY DISEASE

Test	Hepatocellular Necrosis	Cholestasis	Infiltrative Process
Aminotransferase	+ + to + + +	0 to +	0 to +
Alkaline phosphatase	0 to +	+ + to + + +	+ + to + + +
Total/direct bilirubin	0 to + + +	0 to + + +	0 to +
Prothrombin time	Prolonged	Prolonged; responsive to vitamin K	Normal
Albumin	Decreased in chronic disorders	Normal	Normal

0, normal; + to + + +, increasing degrees of abnormality.

amylase should point to an extrahepatic cause (e.g., choledocholithiasis, pancreatitis, cholangiocarcinoma, or carcinoma of the pancreas). Fever and right upper quadrant abdominal pain, however, may occur in drug-induced cholestasis. Moreover, in this common cause of intrahepatic cholestasis, discontinuing the offending drug may not lead to immediate resolution of the cholestatic picture. Hyperbilirubinemia resulting from extrahepatic biliary obstruction, in contrast to that observed in acute and chronic forms of hepatocellular injury, over time tends to level off and rarely exceeds 35 mg per deciliter. In addition, a daily increase of 1.5 mg per deciliter in total serum bilirubin is characteristic of extrahepatic obstruction. Partial obstruction or obstruction involving only a portion of the intrahepatic biliary tree may result in an elevated serum alkaline phosphatase level in the absence of hyperbilirubinemia.

Conversely, a normal alkaline phosphatase level in a jaundiced patient strongly rules against the presence of extrahepatic obstruction. Nevertheless, none of the routine biochemical laboratory tests can distinguish reliably between intrahepatic cholestasis and extrahepatic biliary obstruction. Furthermore, within 24 to 48 hours after acute extrahepatic obstruction, profound elevations in serum AST and ALT levels may be observed, followed by a rapid decline. For an approach to the differential diagnosis of cholestasis, see Chapter 103.

TABLE 104.5. DIAGNOSIS OF SELECTED HEPATOBILIARY DISORDERS

Form of Liver Injury	Supporting Data
Hepatocellular	
Viral hepatitis	Viral serology
Alcoholic hepatitis	AST <300 and AST/ALT >2
Drug-induced hepatitis	Eosinophil count
Autoimmune hepatitis	Immunoelectrophoresis
	Antinuclear antibody
	Anti–smooth muscle antibody
Wilson's disease	Serum ceruloplasmin
Hemochromatosis	Serum iron/total iron-binding capacity
	Serum ferritin
	Liver biopsy (hepatic iron index)
α₁-Antitrypsin (AAT) deficiency	Protein electrophoresis
	Serum AAT level
	Pi typing
Cholestatic	
Primary biliary cirrhosis	Antimitochondrial antibody
	Immunoelectrophoresis
Primary sclerosing cholangitis	Endoscopic retrograde cholongiopancreatography
Infiltrative	
Hepatocellular carcinoma	α-Fetoprotein
Hepatic granulomas	Liver biopsy

ALT, alanine aminotransferase; AST, aspartate aminotransferase.

HEPATOCELLULAR INJURY

Although other features, such as serum bilirubin levels and PT, may vary and correlate with the severity of the injury, elevated serum aminotransferases are characteristically associated with hepatocellular forms of injury and reflect the release of intracellular enzymes from necrotic hepatocytes. As a rule, aminotransferase levels higher than 400 units indicate hepatocellular injury. In contrast, milder degrees of serum aminotransferase elevation (less than 300 units) are of little diagnostic benefit, since they are observed in cholestatic disorders as often as in acute and chronic hepatocellular disease. Establishing the cause of hepatocellular necrosis usually requires more information than routine laboratory results provide. However, the nature and degree of aminotransferase elevation may help in distinguishing between alcoholic hepatitis and ischemic, viral-, or drug-induced hepatitis. Ischemic liver injury is sometimes indistinguishable from acute viral hepatitis. A disproportionate and marked elevation in serum transaminases in the setting of generalized malaise, anorexia, jaundice, and tender hepatomegaly characterizes both disorders. Measures to improve hepatic blood flow (e.g., correction of hypotension or congestive heart failure), however, are accompanied by a more rapid fall in serum aminotransferase levels than is seen in the course of acute viral hepatitis. Normal values are occasionally found within 48 to 72 hours in cases of ischemic hepatitis. Suggestive features of drug-related hepatotoxicity include a history of recent institution of therapy and indirect evidence of a hypersensitivity reaction, such as rash, arthralgia, and eosinophilia. Profoundly abnormal AST and ALT levels, with preservation of an elevated AST/ALT ratio, are seen in alcoholic patients with acetaminophen hepatotoxicity, and measurement of acetaminophen blood levels should be considered strongly in the proper setting.

Endocrine disorders are rare but recognized causes to consider. Hyperthyroidism, independent of congestive heart failure or concomitant unrelated liver disease, can result in jaundice and a prolonged PT; serum aminotransferases and alkaline phosphatase are typically less than 250 units per liter and less than threefold elevated, respectively. Moderate elevations in serum aminotransferases and vague constitutional symptoms may suggest the diagnosis of Addison's disease.

A high index of suspicion is required in the diagnosis of Wilson's disease. Ceruloplasmin levels should be determined routinely in patients younger than age 35 with a pattern of abnormalities suggesting HBsAg- and HCV-negative chronic hepatitis, autoimmune hepatitis, or cryptogenic cirrhosis. Ingestion of nutritional supplements (e.g., vitamin A) and herbal products and the use of unconventional forms of therapy should also be considered in the setting of hepatocellular injury of unknown origin.

INFILTRATIVE DISORDERS

Isolated elevation of serum alkaline phosphatase, confirmed by SLAP, 5'-NT, or GGTP to be of hepatic origin, strongly suggests an infiltrative process, whether a localized (primary biliary cirrhosis) or systemic granulomatous disease, such as sarcoidosis, miliary tuberculosis, coccidiomycosis, histoplasmosis, brucellosis, Q fever, or a drug reaction (e.g., allopurinol, quinidine), or, alternatively, the first indication of metastatic carcinoma to the liver. Serum alkaline phosphatase levels elevated more than three times in patients with cirrhosis should raise concern of the development of hepatocellular carcinoma. The triad of an elevated serum alkaline phosphatase level, detectable titers of antimitochondrial antibody, and an elevated serum IgM level in a middle-aged woman is of considerable discriminative value in the diagnosis of primary biliary cirrhosis. Alternatively, in a patient with a history of malignancy, the presence of an elevated serum alkaline phosphatase warrants an evaluation for metastases.

The absence of diagnostic findings on abdominal ultrasonography, computed tomography of the abdomen, technetium sulfur colloid nuclear imaging, and invasive tests such as endoscopic retrograde cholangiopancreatography (ERCP) is a major indication for performing a percutaneous or laparoscopic liver biopsy. A decision tree that can be used in the approach to the patient with an elevated alkaline phosphatase is shown in Figure 104.1.

THE LIVER IN SYSTEMIC DISORDERS

The liver may be a target organ in a vast array of systemic disorders. In particular, but by no means exclusively, the presence of coexistent cardiac, pancreatic, and inflammatory bowel disease should be considered in the approach to any patient with abnormal liver chemistries. A prolonged PT, often disproportionate to other signs of liver dysfunction, is the most common abnormality in patients with congestive heart failure. Patients with clinically inapparent left-sided heart failure may present with a picture like that of acute or chronic hepatitis. Hemochromatosis, in turn, may present as a congestive cardiomyopathy. Distal common bile duct stenosis is a well-described complication of chronic alcoholic pancreatitis to be considered in the setting of persistent anicteric alkaline phosphatase elevations. Hepatobiliary manifestations of clinical importance occur in up to 10% of patients with inflammatory bowel disease. Membranoproliferative glomerulonephritis and essential mixed cryoglobulinemia have been associated with chronic HCV infection. Hematologic disorders, such as polycythemia rubra vera, myeloproliferative disorders, and paroxysmal nocturnal hemoglobinuria may predispose to hepatic vein thrombosis. Patients with renal cell carcinoma may present with liver chemistry abnormalities, primarily elevated alkaline phosphatase levels, in the absence of of hepatic metastases. Bacteremia, particularly with gram-negative organisms, should be considered in any ill person with disproportionate elevations of serum bilirubin compared with levels of alkaline phosphatase and aminotransferases.

Liver diseases peculiar to the gravid female include intrahepatic cholestasis of pregnancy, toxemia, and acute fatty liver of pregnancy, although viral hepatitis is the most common cause of jaundice during pregnancy. Fatty liver should be considered in the obese patient presenting with mildly elevated levels of serum transaminases and alkaline phosphatase. A form of nonalcoholic liver disease resembling alcoholic hepatitis and cirrhosis has been described. Previously considered to be a disorder predominantly seen in middle-aged, obese women with hyperglycemia or hyperlipidemia, nonalcoholic steatohepatitis (NASH) is now recognized to exhibit a broader clinical profile. Diagnosis relies on the presence of macrovesicular steatosis and parenchymal inflammation with or without Mallory bodies, fibrosis, and cirrhosis in liver biopsy specimens in the absence of a history of excessive alcohol consumption. Abnormal serum aminotransferases are the most common biochemical abnormality in this disorder, although there is a lack of association between biochemical abnormalities and the degree of steatosis. In general, serum aminotransferases are only mildly to moderately elevated; less than one-third of patients have serum AST or ALT levels more than threefold elevated. Weight reduction in obese patients may lead to improvement in serum aminotransferase abnormalities.

Multitransfused hemophiliacs have a high incidence of asymptomatic abnormalities in liver chemistries, and liver biopsies demonstrate a wide histologic spectrum of liver disease, ranging from mild chronic persistent hepatitis to chronic active hepatitis and cirrhosis. The prevalence of HCV seropositivity in these patients is very high.

In AIDS patients, mild to moderate increases in serum aminotransferase activities are common. Increases in alkaline phosphatase levels and jaundice are less common. Macrosteatosis and nonspecific portal inflammation are the most common histologic abnormalities on liver biopsy; in the past, information provided by liver biopsy had little effect on therapy or survival. Liver biopsy is more sensitive than bone marrow aspiration and biopsy at detecting mycobacterial infection.

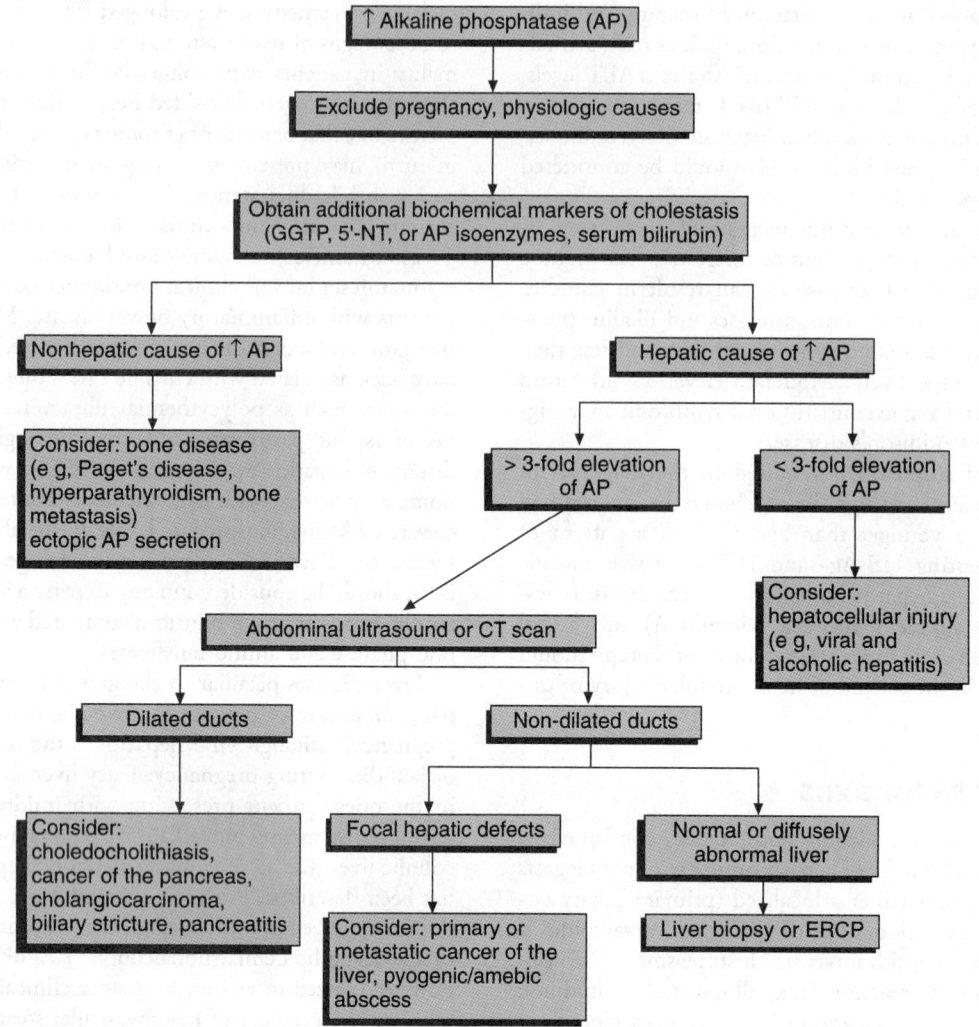

FIGURE 104.1. Diagnosing the patient with elevated serum alkaline phosphatase levels. *CT,* computed tomography; *ERCP,* endoscopic retrograde cholangiopancreatography; *GGTP,* serum γ-glutamyl transpeptidase; *5'-NT,* 5'-nucleotidase.
EVIDENCE LEVEL: C. Expert Opinion.

ELEVATED AMINOTRANSFERASES IN ASYMPTOMATIC PERSONS

Several studies, performed before HCV antibody testing, addressed the issue of evaluating asymptomatic patients with moderately elevated serum aminotransferase levels. Apart from determinations of ferritin, ceruloplasmin, α_1-antitrypsin, and markers for hepatitis B virus, blood tests have little discriminative value. A high incidence of obesity and regular alcohol use has been demonstrated in these patients. Fatty infiltration consequently is the most common finding on liver biopsy; however, histologic findings of chronic persistent or active hepatitis in many patients support the use of percutaneous liver biopsy in the diagnostic approach to patients with persistently elevated levels of serum aminotransferases. In studies performed since the advent of serologic tests for HCV, some patients with asymptomatic elevations in serum ALT have evidence of HCV infection. Therefore, antibody to HCV should be routinely determined. Asymptomatic anti–HCV-positive patients often are found to have chronic liver disease on liver biopsy even with no serum ALT elevations. This has led some authors to recommend that all anti–HCV-positive patients (confirmed by recombinant immunoblot) should undergo liver biopsy, regardless of serum ALT levels. However, liver biopsy may be avoided in anti–HCV-positive patients with normal ALT levels whose serum HCV-RNA is also negative.

Indications for HOSPITALIZATION AND REFERRAL

Because abnormalities in liver chemistries are merely markers of hepatocellular injury, decisions regarding hospitalization should not be made on the basis of the degree of abnormality. Even tests of liver function, serum albumin, serum bilirubin, and PT cannot be used as the sole criteria for admission, with the exception of a prolonged PT in acute viral hepatitis.

The diagnostic tests previously discussed suggest but rarely provide a specific diagnosis in a patient with suspected liver disease. Nevertheless, information obtained from these tests should facilitate the efficient use of other noninvasive and invasive tests such as ultrasonography, computed tomography, radionuclide hepatobiliary scanning, percutaneous transhepatic cholangiography, endoscopic retrograde cholangiopancreatography, and laparoscopy. Liver biopsy has a key role in the evaluation of patients with abnormal liver chemistries, and referral is usually on this basis. However, a likely diagnosis can be rendered by the referring physician, and the need to refer may depend substantially on the clinical setting and the degree of reassurance required by the patient.

BIBLIOGRAPHY

Baker AL. Liver chemistry. In: Kaplowitz N, ed. *Liver and biliary diseases,* second ed. Baltimore: Williams & Wilkins, 1996:207–220.

Craxi A, Almasio P. Diagnostic approach to liver enzyme elevation. *J Hepatol* 1996;25(suppl 1):47–51.

Freidman LS, Martin P, Munoz SJ. Liver function tests and the objective evaluation of the patient with liver disease. In: Zakim D, Boyer TD, eds. *Hepatology: a textbook of liver disease,* third ed. Philadelphia: WB Saunders, 1996:791–833.

Kamath PS. Clinical approach to the patient with abnormal liver test results. *Mayo Clin Proc* 1996;71:1089–1095.

Moseley RH. Approach to the patient with abnormal liver chemistries. In: Yamada T, ed. *Textbook of gastroenterology,* second ed. Philadelphia: JB Lippincott, 1995:909–927.

Moseley RH. The evaluation of abnormal liver function tests. *Med Clin North Am* 1996;80:887–906.

Pratt DS, Kaplan MM. Evaluation of the liver: laboratory tests. In: Schiff ER, Sorrell MF, Maddrey WC. *Schiff's diseases of the liver.* Philadelphia: Lippincott-Raven, 1999:205–244.

Kelley's Textbook of Internal Medicine, fourth edition. Edited by H. David Humes.
Lippincott Williams & Wilkins, Philadelphia © 2000.

CHAPTER
105

APPROACH TO THE PATIENT WITH CHRONIC LIVER DISEASE AND FULMINANT HEPATIC FAILURE

CHARMAINE A. STEWART
MICHAEL R. LUCEY

Cirrhosis is a diffuse pathologic process in which the normal structure of the liver is replaced by regenerative nodules of hepatocytes separated by bands of fibrosis. Cirrhosis may result from

TABLE 105.1.	CAUSES OF CIRRHOSIS

Chronic Toxic Insults
Alcohol

Chronic Viral Infection
Hepatitis B ± hepatitis D
Hepatitis C

Inherited Metabolic Disease
Wilson's disease
Hemochromatosis
α_1-Antitrypsin deficiency

Secondary Metabolic Disease
Secondary hemosiderosis

Autoimmune Disorders
Chronic autoimmune hepatitis (autoimmune chronic active hepatitis)

Chronic Biliary Disorders
Primary biliary cirrhosis
Secondary biliary cirrhosis
Primary sclerosing cholangitis
Biliary atresia
Alagille's syndrome
Caroli's syndrome
Cystic fibrosis

No Apparent Cause/Miscellaneous
Cryptogenic cirrhosis
Congenital hepatic fibrosis

various forms of chronic hepatic insult (Table 105.1). It is often associated with three sets of clinical phenomena: hepatocellular insufficiency, portal hypertension, and cholestasis. Although these syndromes usually coexist in a cirrhotic patient, they are separated here for purposes of description.

PORTAL HYPERTENSION

PATHOPHYSIOLOGY

The portal vasculature is normally a high-flow, low-pressure, low-resistance system. The normal portal pressure is 5 to 10 mm Hg (7 to 14 cm H_2O). Portal hypertension occurs when resistance to flow causes an increase in blood pressure within the portal vein. *Portal hypertension* is defined as a portal blood pressure of 5 mm Hg greater than the pressure in the inferior vena cava (IVC) or as a direct measurement of a portal pressure of 30 cm H_2O or more. Although cirrhosis is the most common cause in the developed world of an increase in resistance to portal flow, not all portal hypertension is due to cirrhosis. The origin of portal hypertension may be subdivided into presinusoidal, sinusoidal, and postsinusoidal causes (Fig. 105.1). Portal hypertension is usually a feature of chronic liver injury, but it may be seen clinically in some acute circumstances, including the more protracted forms of acute hepatic failure, such as submassive hepatic failure and acute forms of Budd–Chiari syndrome or veno-occlusive disease of the liver.

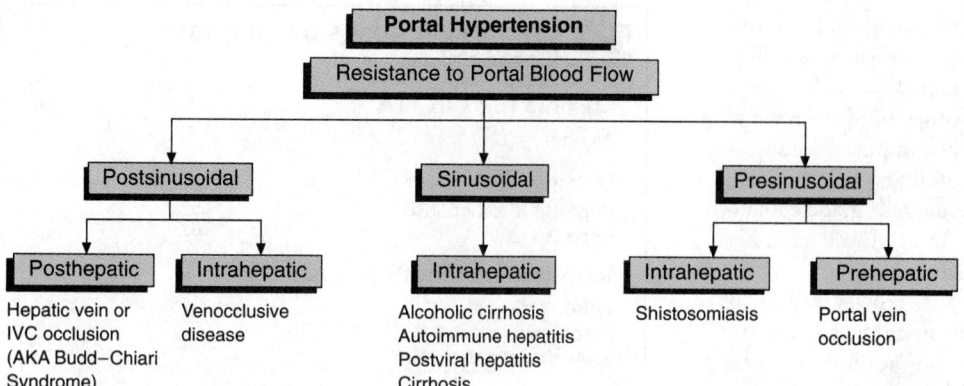

FIGURE 105.1. Theoretical subclassification of portal hypertension according to the locus of obstruction to portosystemic communication.

Portal pressure may be measured by direct placement of a catheter in the portal vein, either by a puncture from the skin through the liver (percutaneous transhepatic portal pressure) or by a transjugular route. Today, the latter is often a prelude to placing a transjugular intrahepatic portosystemic shunt (TIPS). This approach also allows measurement of the IVC or free hepatic vein pressure and calculation of the transsinusoidal pressure gradient. A transjugular approach can be used to measure the wedged hepatic vein pressure, an indirect measure of the portal vein pressure when a transhepatic incursion into the portal vein is ill advised. Wedged hepatic venous pressures have been validated as an estimate of portal pressure in alcoholic cirrhosis only.

CLINICAL FEATURES OF PORTAL HYPERTENSION

PORTOSYSTEMIC COLLATERALS

The portal and systemic systems are connected through many collateral vessels. When portal pressure is increased, these collaterals dilate and are called *varices*. The most common site of variceal development is the lower esophagus, followed by the stomach and rectum. Mesenteric varices or stomal varices are less common. When the portal pressure rises higher than 12 mm Hg, esophageal varices are likely to bleed. Endoscopic studies have shown that variceal size, the presence of red marks on the variceal surface (red wale marks), and decompensated cirrhosis (Child–Pugh class C) are predictors of future hemorrhage (Table 105.2). Varices at other sites such as the stomach may also bleed.

Portal hypertensive gastropathy, another important clinical manifestation of portal hypertension, is present in at least 50% of patients with cirrhosis who have varices that have bled. Endoscopically, "lizard skin" mosaic pattern with diffuse erythema with or without cherry-red spots (submucosal hemorrhage) or a hemorrhagic appearance. Histology reveals diffusely dilated, tortuous mucosal and submucosal arteries, capillaries, and veins. Portal gastropathy leads to oozing, which can become a source of significant blood loss, even requiring transfusion.

SPLENOMEGALY

Portal hypertension commonly results in splenomegaly, although the correlation between splenic size and portal pressure

measurements is poor. Splenomegaly leads to hypersplenism, which causes consumption and sequestration of white cells and platelets and results in leukopenia and thrombocytopenia, respectively. Another cause of thrombocytopenia in affected patients is relatively low levels of thrombopoietin, a growth factor that is produced by the liver and stimulates platelet production.

ASCITES

Ascites is the accumulation of serous fluid in the peritoneal cavity. It is often associated with fluid collection in a hemithorax, termed *cirrhotic hydrothorax*. Cirrhotic hydrothorax usually occurs on the right side and occasionally is found without overt ascites. The mechanisms underlying ascites formation in portal hypertension include altered Starling forces in the portal circulation as a result of increased portal pressure and reduced portal venous oncotic pressure as a result of hypoalbuminemia, altered renal sodium handling, increased hepatic, and possibly splanchnic lymph formation. Peripheral arterial vasodilatation theory was recently proposed as the initial defect, resulting in increased vascular capacity and relative hypovolemia. Transient sodium and water retention occurs as a compensatory mechanism to refill the intravascular circulation. These mechanisms eventually fail, and, in conjunction with hypoalbuminemia, from liver failure, ascites develop. This is further contributed to by the inabil-

TABLE 105.2.	**CHILD–TURCOTTE–PUGH SCORE**		
	Points		
Factor	**1**	**2**	**3**
Encephalopathy	None	1, 2	3, 4
Ascites	Absent	Slight	Moderate
Bilirubin (mg/dL)	1–2	2–3	>3
Albumin (g/dL)	>3.5	2.8–3.5	<2.8
Prothrombin time (seconds prolonged)	1–4	4–6	>6
Bilirubin (mg/dL)	1–4	4–10	>10

Grading (total score): 1–6, class A; 7–9, class B; 10–15, class C.

ity of the kidneys to handle sodium and water loads, followed by sodium retention and increased peripheral blood volume with a concomitant reduction in central blood volume.

Increasing abdominal girth and rapid weight gain are the most common symptoms associated with new-onset ascites. Ascites is detected clinically by dullness on percussion of the abdominal flanks that moves as the patient changes position ("shifting dullness") and by a fluid wave. Small volumes of ascites (less than 1500 mL) are often clinically undetectable and require an imaging study such as computed tomography (CT) scanning or sonography for confirmation.

Investigation of new-onset ascites that is unexplained by standard clinical investigations should always include diagnostic paracentesis. In addition to examination of the fluid for culture and cytology, diagnostic paracentesis allows calculation of the serum/ascites albumin gradient (serum albumin [grams per deciliter] minus ascites albumin [per deciliter]). This is the most reliable method of distinguishing ascites due to portal hypertension from all other forms of ascites and has replaced the use of the exudate–transudate paradigm (Table 105.3). Portal hypertensive ascites has a serum/ascites albumin gradient of 1.1 g per deciliter or more; ascites not associated with portal hypertension has a value of less than 1.1 g per deciliter. Similarly, analysis of portal hypertension-induced hydrothorax yields the same results.

Patients with ascites are best managed with a combination of loop diuretic, such as furosemide, and a distal-acting aldosterone-inhibiting diuretic, such as spironolactone. Both drugs achieve synergy in producing diuresis and saluresis.

Refractory ascites is ascites that does not respond to maximal diuretic therapy or results in diuretic-related side effect, such as renal insufficiency or hyponatremia. At the end of the spectrum of refractory ascites is hepatorenal syndrome (HRS).

TABLE 105.3.	CLASSIFICATIONS OF ASCITES BY SERUM/ASCITES ALBUMIN CONCENTRATION GRADIENT

High Gradient (>1.1 g/dL)

Cirrhosis
Alcoholic hepatitis
Congestive/restrictive heart failure
Massive hepatic metastases
Fulminant hepatic failure
Budd–Chiari syndrome
Veno–occlusive disease
Portal vein occlusion
Acute fatty liver of pregnancy
Myxedema

Low Gradient (<1.1 g/dL)

Peritoneal carcinomatosis
Tuberculous peritonitis (without cirrhosis)
Pancreatic ascites (without cirrhosis)
Bile leak
Nephrotic syndrome
Systemic lupus erythematosus
Bowel obstruction or infarction

HEPATORENAL SYNDROME

Hepatorenal syndrome is defined as renal insufficiency in the presence of liver failure and the absence of parenchymal or obstructive renal disease that does not respond to volume expansion. In HRS, the kidney responds to reduced effective circulating volume with intense vasoconstriction of the renal circulation. Reduced renal blood flow and glomerular filtration rate ensue.

All cirrhotic patients who develop new-onset renal failure should undergo renal sonography to exclude intrarenal and postrenal structural lesions. Doppler sonograms allow assessment of renal vasoconstriction. The diagnosis of HRS should be suspected in any patient with advanced hepatic failure and portal hypertension who has developed renal insufficiency without response to plasma volume expansion. Renal insufficiency is progressive over weeks or days in the presence of severe liver disease without intrinsic renal disease, ongoing infection, hypovolemia, or nephrotoxic agents such as nonsteroidal anti-inflammatory agents.

Laboratory evidence of HRS includes low glomerular filtration rate, as indicated by serum creatinine greater than 1.5 or 24-hour creatinine clearance less than 40 mL per minute, absence of proteinuria, and lack of ultrasonographic evidence of obstructive uropathy or parenchymal kidney disease. Other laboratory evidence that supports this diagnosis is urine volume less than 500 mL per day; urine sodium less than 10 mEq per liter; urine osmolality greater than plasma osmolality; urine red blood cell count less than 50 per high-power field; and serum sodium less than 130 mEq per liter. There are two forms of HRS. Type I is rapidly progressive and associated with early mortality, whereas type II is more chronic and lasts from weeks to months.

HRS often overlaps other forms of acute renal insufficiency, particularly prerenal uremia and acute tubular necrosis. The patient often has a history of one or more precipitating factors, including hypovolemia from blood loss, diuretics, paracentesis, or lactulose; use of cyclooxygenase inhibitors, which precipitate HRS on account of the role of intrarenal prostaglandins in the maintenance of renovascular tone; or exposure to other hepatotoxins, including intravenous dye or aminoglycosides. The serum creatinine level underestimates glomerular filtration in patients with cirrhosis and ascites.

The prognosis of patients with HRS is grave. Renal failure is an independent poor prognostic indicator of survival from liver transplantation. The role of liver transplantation, with or without renal grafting, in patients with HRS remains controversial.

HEPATIC ENCEPHALOPATHY

The principal mechanism for the development of hepatic encephalopathy in cirrhotic patients is the transmission of portal blood to the right heart through intrahepatic or extrahepatic shunts, thereby bypassing the hepatic mass. This tendency is exacerbated by surgically created portosystemic shunts or TIPS. Although chronic hepatic encephalopathy is caused by nitrogenous substances arising from the gut, it is still uncertain which substances are the actual mediators of the syndrome. Candidates

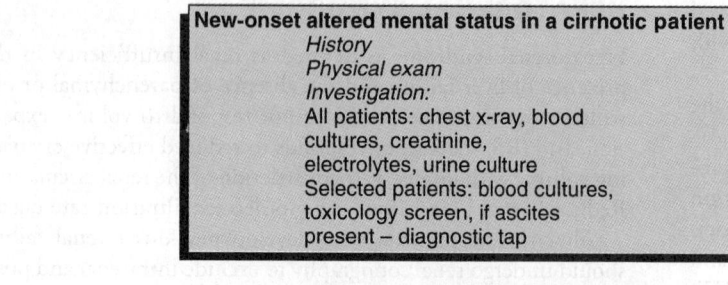

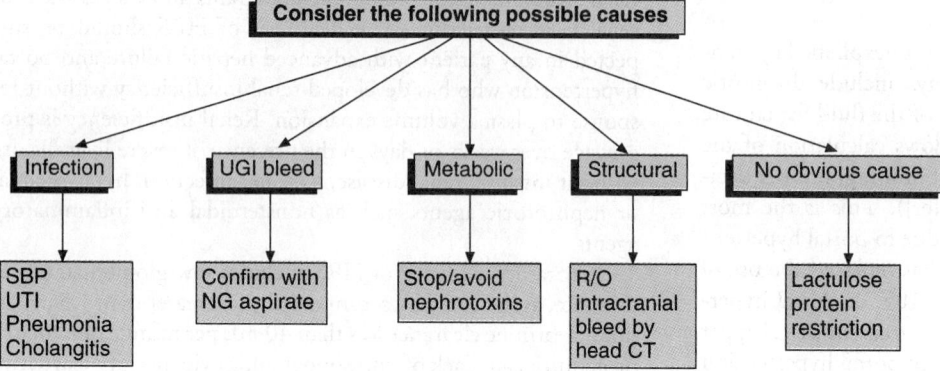

FIGURE 105.2. New-onset altered mental status in a cirrhotic patient.

include ammonia, either directly or through a disturbance in the balance of excitatory/inhibitory neurotransmitters; aromatic amino acids enhancing either "false neurotransmitters" or synergistic neurotoxins including mercaptans, fatty acids, and phenols; γ-aminobutyric acid (GABA); and endogenous or exogenous benzodiazepine ligands.

Clinically, chronic hepatic encephalopathy varies from a subtle alteration in higher cerebral function detectable only on neuropsychometric testing to a broad range of neuropsychological syndromes up to and including coma. Among its characteristic features are variability in severity with rapid reversibility, especially in patients using lactulose.

As shown in Figure 105.2, the new onset of a change in mental status in a patient with cirrhosis can have a bewildering variety of precipitating causes. It may be the mode of presentation of infections, electrolyte abnormalities or covert gastrointestinal bleeding that might otherwise go unnoticed. If, despite a thorough investigation, no precipitating cause is found for apparent hepatic encephalopathy that fails to resolve with standard measures, one should consider other progressive neurologic disorders. Wilson's disease is an important diagnosis not to miss. Occasionally, patients with portosystemic shunts develop an idiopathic syndrome of cerebrospinal demyelination.

PULMONARY MANIFESTATIONS OF CHRONIC LIVER DISEASE

Two distinct pulmonary disorders are associated with portal hypertension and result from right-to-left intrapulmonary shunting. The first is called the *hepatopulmonary syndrome,* characterized by pulmonary capillary vasodilatation and hypoxemia without associated pulmonary hypertension. This phenomenon is mediated by nitric oxide. The other disorder is the *portopulmo-*

nary syndrome, characterized by portopulmonary hypertension as the primary feature, which may preclude liver transplantation.

CHOLESTASIS

PATHOPHYSIOLOGY

Cholestasis is characterized by pruritus, jaundice, and elevated alkaline phosphatase; it results from impairment of bile secretion and specific defects in the secretion of anions (Chapter 103). Jaundice often is a feature of cholestasis, but it may precede the onset of pruritus and elevated alkaline phosphatase by several weeks to years. Approximately 20% to 50% of jaundiced patients experience pruritus. The cause of this symptom is unknown but has been attributed to the poor excretion of pruritogenic agents in bile. Cholestyramine, a bile acid chelating agent, may be used as first-line therapy. In refractory cases, the opiate antagonist, naltrexone, which works by inhibiting endogenous opiatelike agents has proved effective. Also, rifampin, which inhibits bile acid uptake into hepatocytes, may also be used. Phenobarbital and ursodeoxycholic acid are also efficacious in the management of pruritus.

CLINICAL FEATURES OF CHOLESTASIS

Hyperlipidemia occurs in patients with chronic cholestasis owing to impaired excretion of cholesterol and phospholipids into bile. It has been traditionally thought that the hyperlipidemia of cholestasis does not lead to atherosclerotic disease, but this is controversial.

Fat malabsorption and steatorrhea may result from impaired bile acid delivery and poor micelle formation. Reduced absorption of the fat-soluble vitamins, A, D, E, and K is a consequence of fat malabsorption; therefore, replacement of these vitamins is recommended. Also, calcium–fatty acid complexes may form, and this impairs calcium absorption. The bone disease that is prevalent in chronic cholestasis is osteoporosis, although osteomalacia may also be found. These patients are best evaluated with bone densitometric studies. If osteopenia is diagnosed, an oral diphosphonate is indicated.

HEPATOCELLULAR INSUFFICIENCY

PATHOPHYSIOLOGY

Hepatocellular insufficiency is a pathologic deficiency of one or more of the paradigmatic hepatocellular activities: protein synthesis, metabolism and excretion of bilirubin and bile salts, and metabolism of endogenous proteins and xenobiotics. When hepatocellular insufficiency is life-threatening, with or without portal hypertension, it is called *end-stage liver failure*. Because estimates of prognosis in chronic liver failure are inaccurate, end-stage liver failure remains an imprecise concept. Hepatocellular insufficiency may arise acutely in response to a sudden massive destruction of liver, but it more commonly occurs in patients with chronically diseased livers, in whom much of the functioning hepatic mass has been lost because of cirrhosis. Liver failure resulting from cirrhosis is usually more gradual in onset and less uniform in presentation than that in acute liver injury. Coagulopathy and hypoproteinemia may predominate in one patient, whereas encephalopathy may be more prominent in another. In addition, other factors such as vitamin K deficiency or the presence of a portosystemic stent may affect the clinical features at a particular time.

CLINICAL FEATURES OF HEPATOCELLULAR INSUFFICIENCY

Coagulopathy

The liver is the site of synthesis of many protein factors involved in the regulation of hemostasis, including factor I (fibrinogen), factor II (prothrombin), and factors V, VII, IX, X, XII, and XIII, high-molecular-weight kallikrein, protein S, protein C, and antithrombin III.

Inadequate hemostasis accompanies liver failure both because of impaired synthesis of clotting factors as a result of a substantial reduction in functioning hepatic mass and because of vitamin K deficiency in cholestatic disorders. Hepatic synthesis of clotting factors II, VII, IX, and X requires vitamin K. Occasionally, patients with liver failure and autoanticoagulation develop clinical evidence of a hypercoagulable state, such as deep venous thrombosis or pulmonary embolus. This is explained, presumably, by a relatively greater perturbation to the synthesis of anticoagulant factors, such as protein S, protein C, and antithrombin III, than to the procoagulant factors.

The clinical manifestations of coagulopathy include easy bruising, bleeding from the gums and nose, and minor degrees of anorectal bleeding. Hemorrhage from varices is multifactorial

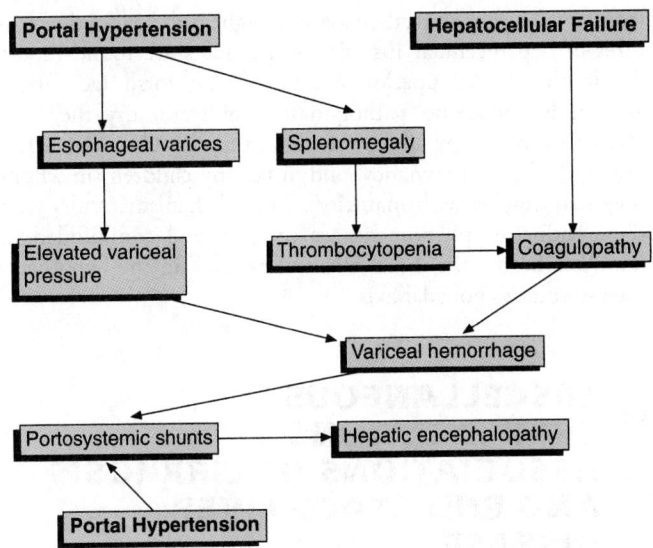

FIGURE 105.3. Interaction of portal hypertension and hepatocellular failure, leading to variceal hemorrhage and hepatic encephalopathy.

in origin, and coagulopathy is one contributing factor (Fig. 105.3).

Hypoalbuminemia

Hypoalbuminemia in chronic liver disease has a complex pathogenesis. In some patients with cirrhosis and ascites, a reduced serum albumin concentration is the result of dilution rather than reduced synthesis. Indeed, given that its half-life in serum is 20 days, albumin is a poor indicator of "acute" hepatic injury. The reduction in serum albumin in many cirrhotics also depends on nutritional status.

Endocrine Effects

Male patients with cirrhosis display a combination of androgenic failure and feminization, whereas cirrhosis in females is complicated by amenorrhea and anovulation (Table 105.4). Spider an-

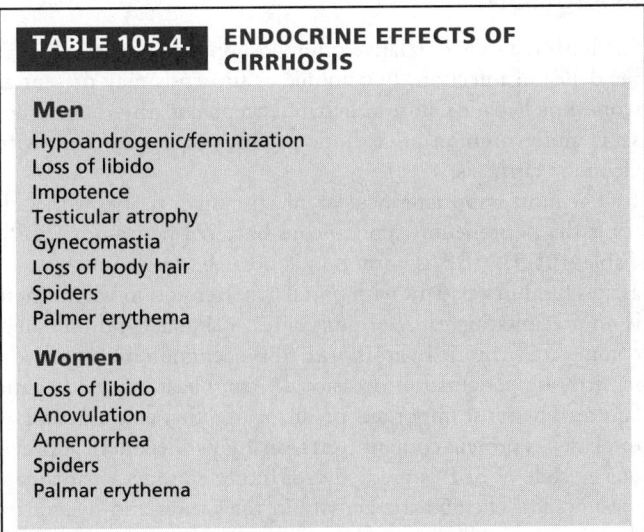

TABLE 105.4.	ENDOCRINE EFFECTS OF CIRRHOSIS

Men
Hypoandrogenic/feminization
Loss of libido
Impotence
Testicular atrophy
Gynecomastia
Loss of body hair
Spiders
Palmer erythema

Women
Loss of libido
Anovulation
Amenorrhea
Spiders
Palmar erythema

giomata and palmar erythema are thought to be endocrine features of hepatocellular insufficiency. Spiders are found in the distribution of the superior vena cava (upper torso, face, arms, and hands) and are not pathognomonic of liver injury: they may also occur in healthy adults (in whom they usually number less than six), during pregnancy, and in healthy children (in whom they may resolve with maturity). The mechanisms underlying these endocrine phenomena are complex and confounded in many studies by the direct effect of alcohol on the hypothalamus–pituitary–gonadal axis.

MISCELLANEOUS COMPLICATIONS/ ASSOCIATIONS OF CIRRHOSIS AND END-STAGE LIVER DISEASE

ENDOCRINE DISORDERS

The presence of diabetes mellitus accompanying cirrhosis should prompt investigation for hereditary hemochromatosis. Disorders of thyroid function, particularly hypothyroidism, are common in primary biliary cirrhosis and to a lesser extent in chronic autoimmune hepatitis. Unrecognized hypothyroidism may be the cause of clinical deterioration in a previously stable cirrhotic.

BONE DISEASE

Many forms of chronic liver disease are complicated by disorders of bone metabolism (hepatic osteopenia). The causes are multifactorial, including immobility leading to lack of sunlight, disordered hepatic metabolism of vitamin D, and the effect of ethanol on bone. Hepatic osteodystrophy is particularly common in chronic cholestatic disorders, especially primary biliary cirrhosis. Clinically, it produces vertebral collapse and pathologic fractures of the long bones.

INFECTION

Cirrhosis is a state of relative immunosuppression, with a higher incidence of infection. Pneumonia or urosepsis may present as worsening hepatic failure or hepatic encephalopathy. Tuberculosis is more common in cirrhotic patients, especially those with alcoholic cirrhosis.

The most important locus of infection in cirrhotics with ascites is the peritoneum (spontaneous bacterial peritonitis [SBP]; Table 105.5). SBP is a monomicrobial bacterial infection of ascites fluid in a patient with portal hypertension in whom there is no precipitating cause of peritonitis. A similar syndrome may complicate cirrhotic hydrothorax. SPB occurs almost exclusively in cirrhotic patients but occasionally complicates acute hepatic failure. The most important predictor of a first episode is a low total ascites protein content (less than 1 g per deciliter). A previous episode of SBP is predictive of future episodes. Inadequate opsonic and chemotactic activity in the ascites and overall reduced systemic clearance of bacteria are the putative mechanisms

TABLE 105.5.	SPONTANEOUS BACTERIAL PERITONITIS (SBP): KEY CHARACTERISTICS

Occurs with cirrhosis and ascites
Total ascites protein <1 g/dL
Previous episodes of SBP are predictive
Low ascitic opsonic activity
Presentation protean, subtle: requires high index of suspicion
Diagnosis by paracentesis: >250 polymorphonuclear leukocytes/mm³ diagnostic
No organism found in 30–50% of cases
Escherichia coli, Klebsiella pneumoniae, Streptococcus pneumoniae found rarely anaerobes
3–5 days intravenous cephalosporin may be sufficient; oral quinolones, or co-trimoxazole reduces incidence of recurrence

in the pathogenesis of SBP. Gram-negative aerobes such as *Escherichia coli* and *Klebsiella pneumoniae* or gram-positive aerobes such as *Streptococcus pneumoniae*, and rarely anaerobes, are most commonly responsible for SBP.

SBP often has a subtle presentation lacking characteristic signs or symptoms of peritonitis. Consequently, SBP must be suspected whenever a cirrhotic patient with ascites develops a sudden deterioration in hepatic or renal function, worsening malaise, encephalopathy, or an unexplained leukocytosis. SPB should also be sought when a cirrhotic patient develops fever and abdominal pain more typical of acute peritonitis. Small pockets of infected ascites may be present that are detectable only by sonography or CT scanning and are hazardous to aspirate. In such cases, it is often wise to presume SBP and institute appropriate antibiotics rather than to attempt a difficult aspiration.

The key to recognizing SBP is diagnostic paracentesis. The diagnosis of SBP is made by finding more than 250 polymorphonuclear cells (PMN)/mm³. A very elevated PMN count in ascites (e.g., more than 5,000/mm³) suggests an intra-abdominal abscess or a secondary cause of peritonitis. Demonstration of an organism is not required for the diagnosis; in fact, no organism is identified in 30% to 50% of cases of SBP. A culture of multiple organisms from ascites suggests a perforated viscus.

All patients in whom SBP is suspected should receive blood cultures, a chest radiograph, and urine microscopy and culture in pursuit of blood-borne sepsis and other sites of infection.

MALIGNANCY

Hepatoma may manifest as right upper quadrant pain, weight loss, and deteriorating hepatic function. Alternatively, hepatoma is increasingly being recognized as an asymptomatic phenomenon in at-risk persons, especially during evaluation for liver transplantation. Maleness, cirrhosis, chronic hepatitis B (HBV) infection, or chronic hepatitis C (HCV) infection, and hemochromatosis are risk factors for hepatoma. A very high incidence of hepatoma occurs in children with tyrosinemia. Serum α-fetoprotein and either liver ultrasonography or magnetic resonance imaging (MRI) of the abdomen are appropriate screening tools for patients who are at risk for hepatoma.

Cholangiocarcinoma may arise de novo, or it may complicate primary sclerosing cholangitis and occasionally other cystic dis-

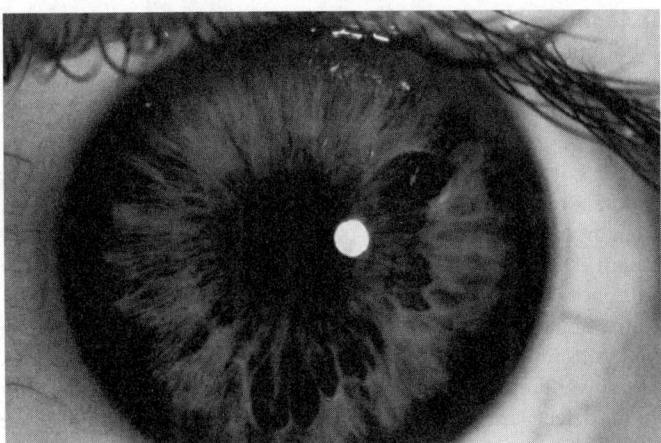

FIGURE 105.4. Kayser–Fleischer ring. See color figure 105.4.

TABLE 105.6.	IMPORTANT DATA IN ANY PATIENT PRESENTING WITH PUTATIVE LIVER DISEASE

Duration of symptoms
?Previous similar episodes
Current or past history of jaundice, pruritus, ascites, hemorrhage, confusion or altered mental state; men: impotence, painful gynecomastia; women: amenorrhea
Past medical history: operations, blood transfusions, hepatitis, hemorrhage
Review of symptoms: alcoholism (CAGE questions), hypothyroidism, diabetes mellitus heart failure, psychiatric disease, emphysema, sexual/lifestyle history
Social history: IV drug use, occupation, marital/social status
Family history: liver disease, death from cirrhosis, gastrointestinal hemorrhage, alcoholism
Current medications

Important Observations on Clinical Exam

Neurologic: mental status, asterixis, gait
Hands: palmar erythema, spider nevi, Dupuytren's contracture, finger clubbing, muscle wasting
Eyes: scleral icterus, xanthomata, Kayser–Fleischer rings
Skin: spider nevi, jaundice, excoriations, easy bruising, purpura
Head/neck: muscle wasting
Abdomen: distended vessels, ascites, hepatomegaly, splenomegaly, rectal examination

CAGE, questionnaire for alcoholism evaluation.

orders such as Caroli's disease. It is often difficult to make a definitive diagnosis of cholangiocarcinoma (Fig. 105.4).

APPROACH TO THE PATIENT WITH LIVER DISEASE

When a physician encounters a patient with newly recognized liver disease for the first time, he or she should consider whether it represents an acute injury to a previously healthy liver or the first presentation of a previously unrecognized chronic liver disease. Many of the clinical features of liver injury, such as jaundice and encephalopathy, are common to the acute or chronic state. A careful history and physical examination are of fundamental importance in distinguishing acute and chronic liver disease (Table 105.6). For example, a history of subtle features of chronic liver injury, such as pruritus or amenorrhea, which predate the presentation of overt liver disease may provide important clues. Patients may not recognize the significance of previous illnesses such as jaundice or hepatitis unless asked specifically. Similarly, careful attention should be paid to a history of exposure to sources of liver injury, such as alcohol, blood transfusions, intravenous drug use, and sexual history. The history and physical examination allow the formulation of a differential diagnosis and selection of investigations.

The same approach applies to new-onset deterioration in a patient with established cirrhosis. Usually, acute deterioration occurs because of a precipitating event, which may be ameliorated even when the underlying liver disease is intractable other than by liver transplantation. The precipitating events include infection, variceal hemorrhage, and the ill-advised use of toxins such as intravenous dye or medicines.

INVESTIGATION OF PATIENTS WITH CIRRHOSIS

LIVER TESTS

Profiles of serum transaminases, bilirubin, albumin, and alkaline phosphatase are not specific for diagnosis of cirrhosis but indicate broader categories of liver injury such as hepatocellular injury or cholestasis, which often coexist in an individual patient (Chapter 104). The best measures of hepatic synthetic function are the prothrombin time and the serum albumin level. The long half-life of albumin makes it a suitable measure of synthesis in chronic liver injury only. The measurement of specific clotting factors is of little practical usefulness, although factor V has the theoretical advantage of being vitamin K-independent and synthesized exclusively in the liver.

The totals of these measures of synthetic and excretory function are included in the empirically derived global measure of hepatic function, the Child–Pugh score (Table 105.2).

NONSPECIFIC TESTS

Many commonly measured laboratory parameters may be deranged in end-stage liver disease. For example, the impact of cirrhosis and ascites on renal function was described in the section on HRS. Cirrhosis and ascites are often accompanied by hyponatremia. This is dilutional in origin and is contributed to by marked hyperaldosteronism and exacerbated by diuretics. It is a grave prognostic sign when hyponatremia persists despite withholding diuretics and restricting intake of fluids and salt. Hematologic abnormalities common in end-stage liver disease include leukopenia and thrombocytopenia due to hypersplenism, iron-deficiency anemia, and macrocytosis due to target cells. Disease-specific noninvasive tests are discussed in detail in Chapter 104.

LIVER IMAGING STUDIES

Liver imaging studies include sonography with Doppler imaging, CT scanning, MRI, angiography, and CT angiography. All patients with putative chronic liver disease who are undergoing investigation should have at least one baseline structural imaging study, the choice of which depends on local expertise and resources. Many patients with chronic cholestatic liver disease receive a cholangiogram, either endoscopic retrograde cholangiopancreatography, percutaneous transhepatic cholangiography, or more recently, magnetic resonance cholangiography. Endoscopic retrograde cholangiopancreatography remains the method of choice for distinguishing primary sclerosing cholangitis from other chronic cholestatic processes.

LIVER BIOPSY

Histopathologic examination of liver tissue may be helpful in confirming the presence of cirrhosis or in estimating the degree of activity of chronic hepatitis. It may assist making the diagnosis of specific conditions including hemochromatosis, Wilson's disease, α_1-antitrypsin deficiency, autoimmune chronic hepatitis, chronic cholestatic disorders such as primary biliary cirrhosis, and congenital hepatic fibrosis, among others. Liver biopsy is the only unequivocal way of diagnosing acute cellular rejection in a liver allograft. Guided biopsies may be useful for diagnosing hepatic malignancy. Liver biopsy is sometimes eschewed in patients with hepatic masses who are being considered for liver transplantation, to avoid spreading malignant cells outside the hepatic capsule. On the other hand, liver biopsy has little clinical usefulness in diagnosis or management of acute hepatic injury and often yields relatively nonspecific findings in chronic liver diseases.

Percutaneous liver biopsy is the most common method of obtaining liver tissue. It is usually carried out as a day-case outpatient procedure. Outpatient liver biopsy should be limited to patients with preserved hematology and coagulation parameters: hemoglobin greater than 10 g, platelet counts $\geq$70,000 and prothrombin time $\leq$15 seconds or international normalized ratio up to 1.3. Patients with renal failure may have platelet dysfunction, and a platelet count of 100,000 is required for an outpatient procedure. Patients whose measures fall outside these parameters may still be suitable for percutaneous liver biopsy after replenishment of platelets, clotting factors, or fresh frozen plasma. However, our policy is to observe for at least 16 hours all patients who require blood products to have a percutaneous liver biopsy. Transjugular liver biopsy is an alternative for these patients. It is often wise to have had an imaging procedure (CT, sonogram, or MRI) before proceeding to biopsy to identify mass lesions or unusual structural anomalies, such as atrophic right hepatic lobe.

Minor complications of percutaneous liver biopsy include vasovagal reaction with hypotension, bradycardia, and nausea; pain at the site of insertion; or shoulder tip pain. Pain usually resolves within 2 to 4 hours upon administration of simple analgesia. Percutaneous liver biopsy may be followed by a dull ache in the right upper quadrant for 24 hours. More significant complications include perforation of a viscus, pneumothorax, or

hemorrhage. Puncture of the gallbladder is followed by intense abdominal pain and is not likely to go unrecognized. Similarly, pneumothorax, leading to pain and difficulty in breathing, is readily diagnosed. Significant hemorrhage may manifest as a subtle onset of hypotension and dizziness hours after the procedure. For this reason, our policy is to keep outpatients for 4 hours after the procedure while their blood pressure and heart rate are monitored. Patients are advised to go to an emergency room if they experience severe pain, difficulty in breathing, or dizziness after discharge home. Significant hemorrhage may require ablation of a bleeding vessel by angiography or ultimately laparotomy. Hemorrhage is the cause of occasional mortalities after liver biopsy. The presence of cancer in the liver and coagulation defects are the principal risk factors for postprocedure bleeding.

Alternatives to percutaneous liver biopsy include transjugular biopsy, laparoscopic guided biopsy, and open liver biopsy. The main advantage of transjugular biopsy is that bleeding from the liver should remain within the vascular space. Laparoscopic liver biopsy has its devotees, but, except for occasional patients with anomalous atrophy of the right hepatic lobe, it has no advantages over percutaneous liver biopsy. There are few indications if any for open liver biopsy.

WHY DO PATIENTS WITH END-STAGE LIVER DISEASE DIE?

Acute gastrointestinal hemorrhage, bacterial infection, and multisystem failure, particularly the combination of hepatic and renal failure, are the most common modes of death in patients with cirrhosis. Bacterial infection may present as SBP, pneumonia, urinary tract infection, cholangitis, or occasionally meningitis. A few patients, less than 5% in the United States, die of hepatocellular carcinoma, although this percentage is higher in areas of greater prevalence for hepatitis B and C. As shown in Figures 105.2 and 105.3, hemorrhage, infection, and multisystem failure often interact in the same patient and carry a high mortality. Thus, 20% to 25% of patients with cirrhosis die during hospitalization for their initial variceal bleed. Similarly, in one large series, 50% of cirrhotic patients died within 1 year of their initial episode of SBP. Ninety percent of patients who develop renal failure in addition to acute alcoholic hepatitis (usually an event within chronic alcoholic liver disease) die in the same hospital admission.

END-STAGE LIVER FAILURE

Although therapy may control the initial decompensating event (e.g., acute sclerotherapy for bleeding esophageal varices or antibiotics for SBP), these measures do not change the long-term mortality unless liver failure is corrected. Therapies that reverse liver failure include abstinence from alcohol in patients with end-stage alcoholic cirrhosis, corticosteroids for autoimmune chronic hepatitis, specific therapies for metabolic disorders such as hemochromatosis and Wilson's disease, and liver transplantation for many forms of cirrhosis. Patients with alcoholic liver disease, especially acute alcoholic hepatitis, can make substantial recoveries after withdrawal from alcohol.

Liver transplantation has become the treatment of choice in the developed world for end-stage liver disease (Chapter 132). Its wider application is limited by an inadequate supply of donor organs and its cost.

MANAGING THE COMPLICATIONS OF CIRRHOSIS, PORTAL HYPERTENSION, AND HEPATOCELLULAR FAILURE

BLEEDING ESOPHAGEAL VARICES

A minority of esophageal varices bleed. Variceal hemorrhage is most likely in patients with large varices, varices with longitudinal red marks on their surface, and decompensated cirrhosis as shown by Child–Pugh class (Table 105.2). Elevation of portal pressure higher than a threshold of 12 mm Hg is critical to the initiation of variceal bleeding. Prophylactic therapy with non-cardioselective β-blockade such as propranolol reduces the portal pressure and the incidence of first or recurrent variceal bleeding in high-risk patients, but it remains controversial whether this translates into a survival benefit. Patients with cirrhosis and features of portal hypertension should undergo endoscopy to assess the presence, size, and surface markings of esophageal varices to determine whether prophylactic β-blockade is appropriate. Prophylactic variceal injection sclerotherapy is not recommended in cirrhotic patients with varices who are found to have a high risk for an initial bleed.

Variceal hemorrhage—whether a first or a subsequent bleed—is always an emergency. Once an upper gastrointestinal bleeding source has been confirmed, either by presentation of hematemesis or by gastric aspiration in those who present with melena or subtle signs of decompensation, the patient should be managed with supportive and specific therapy (Chapter 107). Upper gastrointestinal endoscopy rarely reveals blood issuing from an esophageal varix; more commonly, blood is present in the esophagus and stomach in the presence of esophageal varices. Unless another source of bleeding is identified, such as an actively bleeding gastric varix or a gastric or duodenal ulcer, the esophageal varices are the presumed source of hemorrhage and should be treated accordingly. It is often impossible to get an adequate view of all the stomach owing to adherent clot, and this must be reviewed at a later date to rule out gastric varices or other pathology. Injection sclerotherapy direct into the varix using sodium tetradecyl sulfate, ethanolamine, or 5% morrhuate sodium is the standard approach for varices that have recently bled. Ligation banding per endoscopy is an alternative to sclerotherapy but can be technically difficult during vigorous hemorrhage.

Balloon compression using a Sengstaken–Blakemore tube is a complementary approach often used to control persistent bleeding. Endotracheal intubation and mechanical ventilation to protect the airway are standard procedures in the United States before placing the tube. Balloon tamponade is effective in controlling bleeding in 80% of cases, but rebleeding occurs in the same hospital admission in at least 50% of these cases. Prolonged use (more than 12 hours) of the inflated esophageal balloon increases the risk of esophageal perforation, especially if the patient has received extensive recent sclerotherapy.

Intravenous octreotide (50 μg bolus followed by 50 μg per hour for 48 hours) appears to be as effective as vasopressin and has considerably fewer side effects. It acts by producing splanchnic vasoconstriction. Intravenous vasopressin (0.2 to 0.4 units per minute) is the longest-established pharmacologic agent for controlling variceal hemorrhage, although studies of its efficacy are equivocal. Vasopressin is usually administered with glyceryl trinitrate to limit cardiac side effects. Terlipressin, an analogue of vasopressin without cardiac effects, has been promoted as an alternative. If bleeding persists or recurs, TIPS is the treatment of choice. When performed by an experienced interventional radiologist, TIPS is a very effective method for controlling acute or recent variceal bleeding. It is also the best method to control bleeding gastric varices. Emergency operative portosystemic shunting carries a high mortality and has been replaced by TIPS.

Serial sclerotherapy or band ligation until variceal obliteration is the standard of care for longer-term management. Patients should also receive β-adrenergic blockade using a nonselective adrenergic β-antagonist.

Late recurrent bleeding is common despite sclerotherapy or banding. Each episode should be managed as for an initial bleed. When Child–Pugh class A patients rebleed despite appropriate sclerotherapy or banding, an operative portosystemic shunt can be considered. Child–Pugh class B and C patients need evaluation for liver transplantation.

ASCITES

Management of ascites due to portal hypertension is directed at controlling fluid overload, avoiding precipitating renal failure, and, in selected patients, providing prophylaxis against SBP. The key to ascites control is dietary restriction of sodium and judicious use of diuretics. Limiting sodium chloride intake to 2 g per day is not excessive and is compatible with a palatable diet. Furosemide and spironolactone are the most widely used diuretics; careful monitoring of serum sodium and potassium levels is required when these agents are used. Painful gynecomastia is a common and troublesome side effect of spironolactone in men with cirrhosis who have ascites. In these patients, amiloride should be substituted for spironolactone. Whenever the serum creatinine level exceeds 2.0 mg per deciliter (an arbitrary figure) or the serum sodium level is below 125 mEq per liter, the diuretic regimen must be reviewed. Hyponatremia of $\leq$125 mEq per liter demands withholding all diuretics and restricting fluid intake to initially 1.5 L per day in addition to sodium restriction. There is no need to restrict fluid when the serum sodium concentration exceeds 125 mEq per liter.

In patients with advanced disease, in those whose sodium restriction and diuretics are inadequate, or in those whose complications such as renal failure or electrolyte imbalance limit their use, ascites can become very difficult to control (intractable ascites). Intractable ascites is managed by intermittent large-volume paracentesis, usually performed as an outpatient procedure. Ten or more liters of ascitic fluid can be removed at one time.

The role of albumin replacement (12.5 g of albumin for each liter of ascites removed) is controversial. Limiting removal to 2 L and using intravenous albumin is a reasonable, although unproven, precaution in patients with an elevated serum creatinine level. Recently, it has been shown that a functioning TIPS improves ascites control, reducing or eliminating the need for diuretics in some patients with large-volume ascites. A functioning TIPS increases urinary sodium clearance while correcting the increased serum levels of renin, aldosterone, and norepinephrine. TIPS should be considered for any patient who requires paracentesis on a weekly basis.

Cirrhotic hydrothorax, occurring with ascites or as an isolated phenomenon, is sometimes a difficult clinical problem causing dyspnea. It is managed using the same approach as for ascites alone. However, cirrhotic patients with hydrothorax are especially suitable for TIPS. Any patient with intractable ascites or troublesome cirrhotic hydrothorax should be considered for liver transplantation.

Prophylactic therapy against SBP has been studied with quinolones or trimethoprim-sulfamethoxazole, which significantly reduces the incidence of SBP in patients who are at risk. A reasonable plan is to limit prophylaxis to patients who are awaiting liver transplantation, who are considered to be at high risk for a first episode of SBP, or who have had a previous episode of SBP.

CHRONIC HEPATIC ENCEPHALOPATHY

Acute exacerbations of hepatic encephalopathy in cirrhotic patients should always prompt a search for a precipitating cause: gastrointestinal bleeding, new-onset renal failure or electrolyte disturbance, infection (especially SBP), or intracranial hemorrhage (Fig. 105.3). Medication should be reviewed, particularly among hospital inpatients, to check for inadvertent administration of benzodiazepines or other central nervous system depressants.

Lactulose is the mainstay of management of chronic hepatic encephalopathy. The dosage should be titrated to produce two or three soft bowel movements daily. The value of antibiotics in the management of chronic hepatic encephalopathy is less certain. The theoretical risk of ototoxicity, particularly if the patient develops renal failure, has led some experts to eschew the use of neomycin. Metronidazole is a safer alternative if lactulose is insufficient. Restriction of dietary protein intake is a time-hallowed response to chronic hepatic encephalopathy. Recent studies suggest that modest protein replenishment is safe in most cirrhotic patients. Protein restriction should be reserved for acute management of episodes of severe encephalopathy and for patients with disabling chronic encephalopathy.

HEPATOMA

Small localized unilocular hepatomas, discovered when screening with α-fetoprotein measurements or imaging studies, may be resectable, even from a cirrhotic liver. Alternatively, it is appropriate to consider these patients for liver transplantation. A full discussion of hepatoma can be found in Chapter 126.

FULMINANT HEPATIC FAILURE

Acute hepatic injury presents as a sudden increase in previously normal liver transaminases. Fulminant hepatic failure refers to a specific subgroup of patients with severe acute hepatic injury, defined as the development of acute hepatic encephalopathy within 8 weeks of the onset of symptomatic hepatocellular disease in a previously healthy person. Submassive hepatic necrosis is similar to fulminant hepatic failure except that it is slower in onset. Submassive hepatic necrosis (synonyms: subfulminant hepatic failure, subacute hepatic failure) is defined by the development of acute hepatic encephalopathy within 9 to 24 weeks of onset of symptomatic hepatocellular disease in a previously healthy person.

CLINICAL FEATURES

Acute hepatic injury with no hepatic encephalopathy always resolves, except when it is due to other ongoing systemic disease or when the elevated transaminases represent the first recognition of previously covert chronic liver disease. The incidence of acute hepatic injury is unknown. An estimated 2,000 cases of fulminant hepatic failure and subacute hepatic necrosis occur in the United States annually and 80% of these patients die. Outcome is determined by the course of encephalopathy, which is measured on a four-grade scale (Table 105.7). Cerebral edema, leading to increased intracranial pressure (ICP), is a common feature of severe fulminant hepatic failure and may cause permanent cerebral injury and death. Fulminant hepatic failure and submassive hepatic necrosis are always accompanied by severe coagulopathy.

The causes of fulminant hepatic failure are shown in Table 105.8. Wilson's disease is usually included among the causes of fulminant hepatic failure despite the fact that it is a covert chronic disorder. A history of heavy alcohol use also suggests chronic injury, even though alcoholics are at particular risk for acetaminophen-induced hepatic failure. When presented with an apparent case of acute hepatic injury, the physician must always answer two questions. Is this really an acute illness or is it the first presentation of a previously unrecognized chronic disorder? Are single or multiple factors contributing to acute hepatic injury?

PREDICTING OUTCOME IN FULMINANT HEPATIC FAILURE AND SUBACUTE HEPATIC NECROSIS

In general, the deeper the coma, the worse the outcome. For example, patients who develop grade III or IV coma have a higher mortality rate than hepatic failure patients in whom encephalopathy never progresses beyond grade II. Paradoxically, rapid onset of encephalopathy is a favorable prognostic sign. Consequently, most acetaminophen-induced fulminant hepatic failure patients who experience grade III coma recover spontaneously. Delay in the onset of encephalopathy after the onset of jaundice indicates a lack of spontaneous recovery and is unfavorable prognostic factor. For this reason, submassive hepatic necrosis has a particularly poor outcome.

Criteria for determining the prognosis of fulminant hepatic failure are shown in Table 105.9. It distinguishes between acet-

TABLE 105.7.	CLINICAL GRADES OF ACUTE HEPATIC ENCEPHALOPATHY		
Grade	**Mental State**	**Asterixis**	**Electroencephalogram Result**
I	Altered affect, subtle loss of mental acuity, slurred speech	Slight or none	Normal
II	Accentuation of stage I, confusion, drowsiness, inappropriate behavior, loss of sphincter control	Easily elicited	Abnormal, generalized slowing
III	Sleepy but arousable, marked confusion, can answer simple questions only	Present when patient can cooperate	Always abnormal
IV	Coma IVa—responds to pain IVb—no response to pain	Cannot cooperate	Always abnormal

aminophen-induced fulminant hepatic failure and that due to all other causes. Drug-induced hepatic failure, other than that caused by acetaminophen, has a poor prognosis. Examples include hepatic failure due to phenytoin or halothane. HBV- and HAV-induced hepatic failure has a better outcome than idiopathic (presumed viral) fulminant hepatic failure. It is unclear whether HCV causes hepatic failure. Patients younger than 2 years or older than 40 years have a poor prognosis. Renal failure is also a poor prognostic factor. As mentioned, coagulopathy is

always present. Some have recommended serum factor V levels as an indicator of when to proceed to transplantation. A factor V level of less than 20% is a poor prognostic indicator. Acidosis is a poor prognostic factor, particularly in acetaminophen-induced fulminant hepatic failure.

MANAGEMENT

Patients with uncomplicated acute hepatic injury can be treated in their local hospitals, but their physicians may alert a transplantation center so that expeditious transfer can be arranged if encephalopathy develops. All patients with fulminant hepatic failure should be transferred to an intensive care unit at a liver transplantation center. Anti-HBc (hepatitis B core antibody)

TABLE 105.8.	CAUSES OF FULMINANT HEPATIC FAILURE

Viral Infection

Hepatitis A
Hepatitis B
Hepatitis D
Other viruses (less common)
Cytomegalovirus
Epstein–Barr virus
Varicella
Herpes

Poisons, Chemicals, and Drugs

Amanita phalloides
Acetaminophen
Tetracycline
Phosphorus
Halogenated volatile anesthetics (especially halothane)
Isomazid
Methyldopa
Valproate
Monoamine oxidase inhibitors

Ischemia and Hypoxia

Hepatic vascular occlusion
Acute circulatory stroke
Heat stroke
Gram-negative sepsis

Miscellaneous

Acute fatty liver of pregnancy
Reye's syndrome
Wilson's disease
Hodgkin's disease and other lymphomas
Hereditary fructose intolerance
Galactosemia, tyrosinemia
Idiopathic (also called non-A non-B)

TABLE 105.9.	PROGNOSTIC CRITERIA FOR PREDICTING REQUIRED LIVER TRANSPLANTATION IN PATIENTS WITH FULMINANT HEPATIC FAILURE

Acetaminophen Toxicity

pH <7.3 (regardless of grade of encephalopathy)
  or
Prothrombin time[a] >50 s and serum creatinine >3.4 mg/dL (300 μmol/L) in patients with grade III or IV encephalopathy

All Other Causes

Prothrombin time[a] >50 s (regardless of grade of encephalopathy)
  or
Any three of the following variables (regardless of grade of encephalopathy):
  Age <10 years or >40 years
  Liver failure due to halothane or other drug idiosyncrasy or idiopathic hepatitis
  Duration of jaundice prior to encephalopathy >7 d
  Prothrombin time[a] >25 s
  Serum bilirubin >17.5 mg/dL (300 μmol/L)

The prothrombin time thresholds have been reduced for application in the United States because of differences in laboratory methods to assay prothrombin time between United States and Europe. In Europe, prothrombin time thresholds in this table should be multiplied by 2.
Adapted from O'Grady JG, Alexander GJM, Hayllar KM, Williams R. Early indicators of prognosis in fulminant hepatic failure. *Gastroenterology* 1989;97:439.

IgM, HBsAg, and anti-HAV IgM should be checked to identify patients with acute HBV and HAV. Antibodies to cytomegalovirus, Epstein–Barr virus, herpes simplex virus, and varicella should also be checked. Serum ceruloplasmin levels should be determined, and the patient's eyes should be examined by slit-lamp for corneal rings. An unusually low serum alkaline phosphatase level (lower than 80 units) or high serum and urinary copper levels may also indicate underlying Wilson's disease. The physician should look for toxic insults (e.g., *Amanita* mushrooms, drugs) and consider acute onset of chronic disease.

Hepatic failure patients who have ingested acetaminophen should receive a full course of *N*-acetylcysteine. There is unconfirmed evidence that *N*-acetylcysteine may be beneficial even in non–acetaminophen-related hepatic failure. Although considerable data support a role for circulating benzodiazepines in the development of acute (and chronic) hepatic encephalopathy, there is no place for flumazenil in treating fulminant hepatic failure unless it is within a defined research protocol.

Aminoglycosides, radiographic dye, and other potentially nephrotoxic agents should be used cautiously to avoid renal toxic effects. Some practitioners advocate early introduction of dialysis for better management of fluid balance. Hepatic failure may be complicated by hypoglycemia and coma, which could be misinterpreted as being caused by cerebral edema. Correcting hypoglycemia in hepatic failure may require large amounts of dextrose. Hypokalemia and acidosis may also complicate hepatic failure. Coagulopathy should be corrected by fresh frozen plasma before invasive procedures (placement of central lines, placement of ICP monitor) or whenever there is evidence of hemorrhage (intracranial hemorrhage, gastrointestinal bleeding). In most circumstances, it is not necessary to give fresh frozen plasma simply to correct a prolonged prothrombin time of up to 30 seconds.

Hypotension is common in fulminant hepatic failure, despite high cardiac output, because of associated low systemic vascular resistance. Hypotension may exacerbate low cerebral perfusion pressure (CPP) consequent to raised ICP. Assisted ventilation should be undertaken in patients with grade IV coma or in patients with evidence of hypoxia or respiratory distress, because pulmonary edema and adult respiratory distress syndrome are features of deteriorating hepatic failure. Ventilation also maintains hypocapnea as an adjunct to controlling elevated ICP.

Patients with fulminant hepatic failure or subacute hepatic necrosis have a high risk for sepsis. Daily cultures of blood, urine, and other body fluids are advisable. This is particularly important because sepsis may prevent liver transplantation. The syndrome of high-output hypotension mimics septicemia. Unexplained fever despite broad-spectrum antibiotic coverage warrants consideration of an antifungal prophylaxis.

Cerebral edema is the single most dangerous complication of fulminant hepatic failure. Patients with hepatic failure may have rapid and extreme changes in cerebral perfusion pressure precipitated by positional changes and movement. Acute elevation in ICP may manifest as seizures, changes in pupillary responses, and cerebral posturing. The immediate response to clinical signs of increased ICP should also exclude hypoglycemia, because it may mimic acute changes in mental status. Hypoglycemia is a particular risk for patients with acetaminophen-related

fulminant hepatic failure or patients with the microvesicular fat deposition disorders (e.g., Reye's syndrome, acute fatty liver of pregnancy, valproate poisoning). Only mannitol has been shown to offer a therapeutic benefit to the elevated ICP/reduced CCP syndrome of hepatic failure. Dexamethasone is of no value. The ability of barbiturate coma and ventilator-driven hypocapnea to reverse ICP elevations associated with hepatic failure is unknown, but often tried on an empiric basis.

Because ICP is subject to rapid changes, ICP monitoring in the treatment of severely ill patients with fulminant hepatic failure has received much attention. However, it is associated with side effects and uncertain clinical usefulness.

Liver transplantation is a life-saving procedure for patients with hepatic failure or submassive hepatic necrosis that does not respond to medical management. The most important indicators of the need for liver transplantation are the level of encephalopathy and the trend of change in encephalopathy. Unfortunately, because acute hepatic encephalopathy can vary between grades II and III in a matter of minutes, making a decision based on these factors remains difficult. Even when listed as a highest emergency status, it is not unusual for a patient in North America to wait 72 hours or longer for a suitable donor. During this time, further deterioration, especially worsening cerebral edema, may make transplantation impossible. For this reason, human heterotopic auxiliary transplants, live-donor segmental liver transplantation, extracorporeal perfusion through human or pig livers or artificial hepatocyte perfusion devices, and xenografts have been attempted to sustain the patient until spontaneous recovery develops or a suitable organ is found. The outcome of liver transplantation in patients with fulminant hepatic failure is somewhat worse than that for transplantation performed for other causes. One-year survival rates of 50% to 60% are common.

BIBLIOGRAPHY

Arroyo V, Gines P, Gerbes A, et al. Definition and diagnostic criteria of refractory ascites and hepatorenal syndrome in cirrhosis. *Hepatology* 1996;23:164–176.

Basile AS, Jones EA, Skolnick P. The pathogenesis and treatment of hepatic encephalopathy: evidence for the involvement of benzodiazepine receptor ligands. *Pharmacol Rev* 1991;43:27–71.

Blei AT, Olafsson S, Webster S, et al. Complications of intracranial pressure monitoring in fulminant hepatic failure. *Lancet* 1993;341:157–158.

Bornman PC, Krige JEJ, Terblanche J. Management of esophageal varices. *Lancet* 1994;343:1079–1084.

Gines P, Quintero E, Arroyo V, et al. Compensated cirrhosis: natural history and prognostic factors. *Hepatology* 1987;7:122–128.

Harrison PM, Keays R, Bray GP, et al. Improved outcome of paracetamol-induced fulminant hepatic failure by late administration of acetylcysteine. *Lancet* 1990;335:1572–1573.

Lee WM. Acute liver failure. *N Engl J Med* 1993;329:1862–1872.

O'Grady JG, Alexander GJM, Hayllar KM, et al. Early indicators of prognosis in fulminant hepatic failure. *Gastroenterology* 1989;97:439–445.

Perrault J, McGill DB, Ott BJ, et al. Liver biopsy: complications in 1000 inpatients and outpatients. *Gastroenterology* 1978;74:103–106.

Runyon BA. Care of patients with ascites. *N Engl J Med* 1994;330:337–342.

Schrier RW, Arroyo V, Bernardi M, et al. Peripheral arterial vasodilation hypothesis: a proposal for the initiation of renal sodium and water retention in cirrhosis. *Hepatology* 1988;8:1151–1157.

Kelley's Textbook of Internal Medicine, fourth edition. Edited by H. David Humes. Lippincott Williams & Wilkins, Philadelphia © 2000.

DISORDERS OF THE ALIMENTARY TRACT

C H A P T E R

106

DISEASES OF THE ESOPHAGUS

JOEL E. RICHTER

The esophagus is a relatively simple tubular organ connecting the oropharynx to the stomach. The pleasures of eating and maintaining adequate nutrition require a normal, healthy esophagus. The three major functions of the esophagus are to transport ingested material from the oropharynx to the stomach, to prevent regurgitation of food and gastric contents from the stomach into the esophagus, and to allow venting of ingested air to reduce abdominal bloating.

ANATOMY AND PHYSIOLOGY

The esophagus can be divided functionally into three regions: the upper esophageal sphincter (UES), the esophageal body, and the lower esophageal sphincter (LES).

UPPER ESOPHAGEAL SPHINCTER

The UES consists of striated muscle formed primarily by the horizontal fibers of the cricopharyngeus muscle, located at the level of the C5-6 vertebrae. The UES, like the striated muscles of the oropharynx and upper portion of the esophagus, is innervated like skeletal muscle, receiving motor input directly from the brain stem (nucleus ambiguus) to the motor end plates in the muscle. The UES is tonically closed and opens momentarily in response to a swallow. The UES also serves as a secondary barrier preventing aspiration of gastroesophageal contents.

BODY OF THE ESOPHAGUS

The esophageal body consists of an empty tube lined by squamous mucosa. It has a submucosal layer and two layers of mus-

cles: inner circular and outer longitudinal muscles. No serosa overlies the muscle layers. The upper portion of the esophagus is primarily striated muscle; the lower two-thirds is predominantly smooth muscle. The nerve network for the esophageal body lies between the muscle layers. Meissner's (submucosa) plexus is between the muscularis mucosa and the circular muscle layer. Auerbach's (myenteric) plexus is between the circular and longitudinal muscle. Similar to the LES, innervation of the smooth muscle portion of the esophageal body is primarily through the vagus nerve from neurons arising in the dorsal motor nucleus of the brain stem and nerve endings in the myenteric plexus.

At rest, the esophageal body is quiet without motor activity. Normal esophageal motor activity is characterized by the orderly progression (peristalsis) of a contraction along the esophagus in coordination with relaxation and contraction of the UES and LES (Fig. 106.1). These activities are initiated by the voluntary act of swallowing, but perpetuation through the distal esophagus is under the control of the enteric nervous system.

LOWER ESOPHAGEAL SPHINCTER

The LES is a high-pressure zone of smooth muscle that straddles the diaphragm and is the major component of the antireflux barrier. At rest, the sphincter is tonically contracted, preventing the reflux of gastric contents. On swallowing, the LES relaxes and stays relaxed until the peristaltic wave reaches the end of the esophagus and produces sphincter closure. LES relaxation is vagally mediated by preganglionic cholinergic nerves and postganglionic noncholinergic, nonadrenergic nerves. The candidates for inhibitory neurotransmitters include vasoactive intestinal polypeptide (VIP) or nitric oxide.

The tonic contractions of the LES are predominantly due to intrinsic muscle activity. LES pressure fluctuates greatly over time, even from minute to minute. Much of this is due to various extraesophageal factors that modulate LES pressure, including the foods ingested (proteins increase and fats decrease LES pressure) and other factors such as cigarette smoking and gastric distention, both of which decrease LES pressure. The latter factor is a critical trigger for transient LES relaxation, which is important in the venting of ingested gases. In response to transient increases in intra-abdominal pressure, LES pressure increases to a greater degree than the pressure increases in the abdomen below, thus preventing gastroesophageal reflux (GER). In addition, many hormones and peptides affect LES pressure.

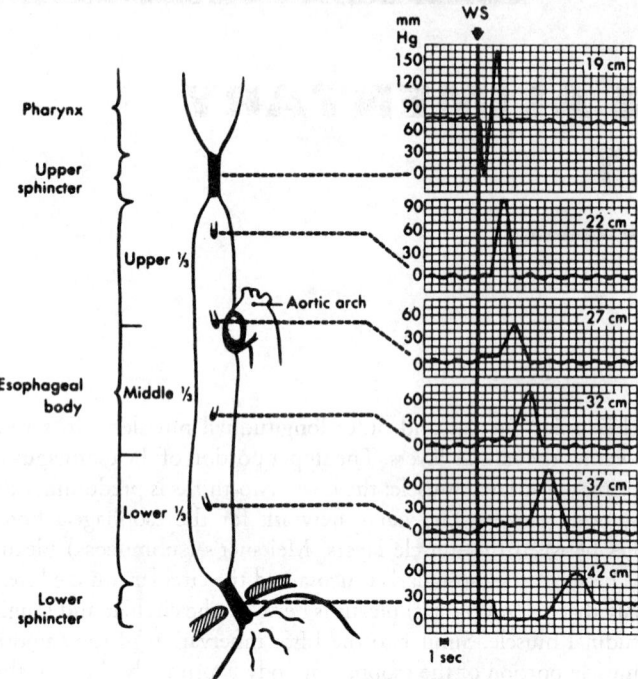

FIGURE 106.1. Manometric pressure changes with a swallow of an 8-mL bolus (*WS*). Distance (cm) from nares is shown on tracings. Proximal and distal tracings are from the upper (UES) and lower (LES) esophageal sphincters, respectively. Immediately after a swallow, UES pressure falls transiently. Shortly thereafter, LES pressure falls and remains low until the peristaltic contraction passing aborally through the UES and then through the esophageal body closes the LES. (From Dodds WJ. Examination of the Esophagus. In: Margulis AR, Burhenne HJ, eds. *Alimentary tract radiology,* fourth ed. St. Louis: CV Mosby, 1989:529, with permission.)

For example, gastrin, motilin, substance P, and pancreatic polypeptide increase LES pressure, whereas secretin, cholecystokinin, glucagon, and VIP decrease LES pressure.

DIAGNOSTIC PROCEDURES

A thorough history and physical examination are critical in evaluating patients with esophageal disorders and often identify the diagnosis and direct further testing. The barium esophagogram is the most important test for the diagnosis of structural and motor abnormalities of the esophagus (Chapter 94). A proper examination should include videotaping of the oropharyngeal and esophagus portions of swallowing, as well as full-column and air-contrast views of the distended esophagus to identify mucosal irregularities, masses, and regions of lumenal narrowing. Endoscopic ultrasonography is useful in diagnosing and staging benign and malignant esophageal neoplasms (Chapter 127). Endoscopic ultrasonography is superior to computed tomography in evaluating the depth of tumor infiltration and assessing regional lymph node metastases. Manometry is the definitive test for diagnosing esophageal motility disorders because it allows accurate measurements of sphincter pressures and esophageal pressure waves and more completely evaluates abnormalities of esophageal peristalsis (Chapter 129). Fiberoptic endoscopy with

biopsy and brush cytology is the best way to identify mucosal abnormalities of the esophagus (Chapter 127). Prolonged ambulatory monitoring of the esophagus (up to 24 hours) is the most reliable way to diagnose GER disease (Chapter 129).

GASTROESOPHAGEAL REFLUX DISEASE

Gastroesophageal reflux disease (GERD), with its major symptom heartburn, is the most common disorder of the esophagus. It is the major indication for antacid consumption and probably the most prevalent condition originating from the gastrointestinal tract. In a recent Gallup survey, 44% of adult Americans experienced heartburn at least once every month, and 10% complained of weekly symptoms. Over 40% of the subjects took antacids for their heartburn, but only one in four discussed this complaint with a physician. Pregnant women have the highest prevalence of heartburn: at least 25% have daily symptoms, usually in the third trimester.

GERD is defined as the sequelae, both clinical and histopathologic, of the movement of gastroduodenal contents into the esophagus. GERD, however, represents a spectrum of disease and occurs in many healthy persons without adverse consequences. Episodes of "physiologic reflux" are typically postprandial, short-lived, and asymptomatic and almost never occur at night. Pathologic reflux leads to inflammatory changes and mucosal injury (reflux esophagitis) and usually symptoms.

PATHOPHYSIOLOGY

The pathophysiology of GERD results from the complex interplay of multiple factors (Fig. 106.2). The common denominator for acid reflux is the creation of a common cavity representing equilibration of intragastric and intraesophageal pressures. The

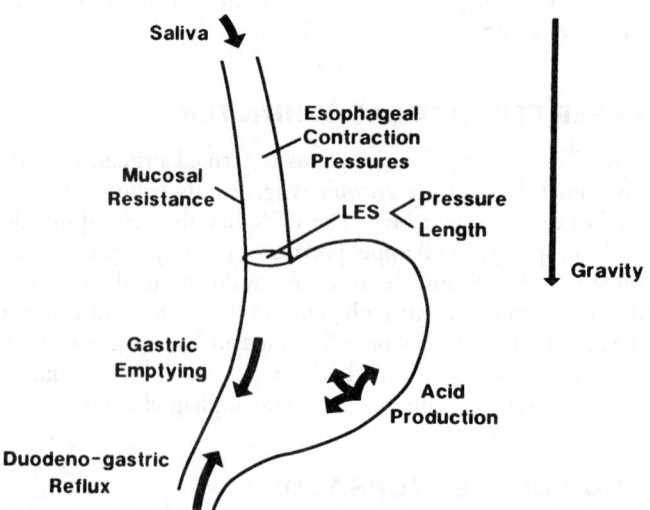

FIGURE 106.2. Major factors in the pathophysiology of gastroesophageal reflux disease.

LES is the major barrier against GER, with a secondary component from the crural diaphragm during inspiration, but the measurement of a single LES pressure is not very discriminatory. Rather, transient LES relaxation, occurring with either normal or low LES pressure, is the major mechanism that promotes free reflux of gastric contents. Transient relaxation accounts for nearly all episodes of reflux in normal subjects and 65% of episodes in patients with GERD. Other patients have reflux because of very low baseline LES pressures with either transient increases in intra-abdominal pressure (stress reflux) or spontaneous reflux across an atonic sphincter.

Esophageal acid clearance normally occurs as a two-step process. First, swallow-induced peristaltic esophageal contractions rapidly clear fluid volume from the esophagus. Next, the small amount of residual acid is neutralized by saliva, which has a pH of 6.4 to 7.8. Dysfunction of the esophageal clearance mechanisms contributes to esophagitis, particularly in patients with severe motility disorders such as scleroderma or in patients with sicca complex.

The nature and volume of gastric contents are important. The primary role of acid is indisputable, but its mechanism of mucosal damage involves the action of coexisting pepsin more than direct damage from acid alone. In animal models, bile salts and pancreatic enzymes can produce esophagitis, but their importance in human disease is unknown. Acid hypersecretory states, such as the Zollinger–Ellison syndrome, are associated with a high prevalence of esophagitis. Delayed gastric emptying promotes GER, but this is an important factor in only 10% to 15% of patients with GERD.

The same degree of acid exposure may lead to variable degrees of mucosal damage, probably related to individual variations in esophageal mucosal resistance. Factors contributing to mucosal resistance include mucus, bicarbonate ions secreted by submucosal glands, stratified squamous cells and their tight junctions, and mucosal blood flow.

The relation between a sliding hiatal hernia and the development of GERD remains controversial. Most patients with esophagitis have a sliding hiatal hernia, but many persons with hiatal hernias do not have GERD. A large irreducible hernia may interfere with normal esophageal clearance by acting as a fluid trap, promoting acid reflux during swallow-induced LES relaxation, particularly in the supine position.

CLINICAL PRESENTATIONS

Heartburn is the classic symptom of GERD, but associated symptoms include dysphagia, odynophagia, regurgitation, water brash, and belching. Patients describe their heartburn as a retrosternal burning pain that also may be noted in the epigastrium, neck, throat, and occasionally the back. It often occurs postprandially and is exacerbated by recumbency or bending over. In the patient with heartburn, dysphagia should suggest the presence of a peptic stricture. Alternative diagnoses include severe inflammation without stricture, peristaltic dysfunction, and an esophageal cancer arising in Barrett's esophagus. The presence of odynophagia usually represents ulcerative esophagitis. The effortless regurgitation of acid fluid, especially postprandially and at night, is highly suggestive of GERD. Water brash is the sudden appearance in the mouth of a slightly sour or salty fluid from the salivary glands in response to intraesophageal acid exposure.

Patients with GERD may present with extraesophageal symptoms, including chest pain (Chapter 94) and respiratory and ear, nose, and throat problems. In these patients, the clinical symptoms of heartburn or regurgitation may be mild or even absent. Chronic cough, recurrent aspiration pneumonia, and pulmonary fibrosis may be related to GERD. Some studies suggest a close association between asthma and GERD: up to 80% of asthmatics have evidence of excessive acid reflux by pH testing. Hoarseness, sore throat, halitosis, vocal cord granuloma, and even laryngeal cancer may be caused by intermittent aspiration of gastric contents.

DIAGNOSIS

In most patients with classic symptoms of heartburn or regurgitation, the history is sufficiently typical to permit a trial of therapy without the need for diagnostic tests. The following situations should lead to early investigation: esophageal symptoms not responding to medical therapy, dysphagia and atypical presentations of suspected GERD, possible complications of reflux disease, and before consideration of antireflux surgery. Tests for GERD evaluate different variables in the disease spectrum (Table 106.1). There is no single best selection of tests; these tests must be applied selectively based on the information desired.

All patients with persistent reflux symptoms or frequent relapses after histamine receptor antagonist therapy should have endoscopy to identify the possible presence of esophagitis or other complications of GERD. Patients with esophagitis and complications need biopsies to exclude associated malignancies and Barrett's esophagus. However, most patients with GERD have no evidence of esophagitis at the time of endoscopy.

The barium esophagogram should be the first diagnostic procedure in most patients with dysphagia. An optimal double-contrast barium esophagogram detects erosive and ulcerative esophagitis in about 90% of cases. However, the radiologic detection of mild (nonerosive) esophagitis is unreliable. The barium esophagogram is also the preferred method for identifying a hiatal hernia and is good for identifying GER fluoroscopically, particularly with provocative maneuvers.

Prolonged esophageal pH monitoring is helpful in patients

TABLE 106.1.	CATEGORIES OF DIAGNOSTIC TESTS FOR GASTROESOPHAGEAL REFLUX DISEASE
Potential for Reflux	**Acid Sensitivity**
Hiatal hernia	Acid perfusion Bernstein test
Manometry	24-h pH test with symptom correlation
Esophageal Damage	**Presence of Abnormal Reflux**
Barium esophagogram	Barium esophagogram
Endoscopy	24-h pH test
Mucosal biopsies	

with atypical presentations or difficult management problems. It has essentially replaced the acid perfusion Bernstein test. The most common indications include noncardiac chest pain, suspected pulmonary or ear, nose, and throat presentations of GERD, and intractable reflux symptoms associated with a negative workup. Prolonged pH monitoring also should be conducted before antireflux surgery if there is any question about the diagnosis. It is the best test for diagnosing GERD, with a sensitivity of 85% and a specificity above 95%.

Manometry of LES pressure is not a sensitive diagnostic test: less than 25% to 50% of patients with GERD have a low resting LES pressure (less than 10 mm Hg). Manometry is reserved for patients in whom another diagnosis is suspected (e.g., achalasia), and it is mandatory before antireflux surgery to ensure adequate esophageal pump function.

STRATEGIES FOR OPTIMAL CARE MANAGEMENT

The rationale for GERD therapy depends on a careful definition of specific aims (Table 106.2). In patients without esophagitis, the therapeutic goal is simply to relieve the acid-related symptoms. In patients with esophagitis, the ultimate goal also is to heal esophagitis while attempting to prevent further complications such as strictures and Barrett's metaplasia. These goals are set against a complex background, since GERD is a chronic condition and patients with esophagitis generally experience relapse when medical therapy is stopped.

Lifestyle Modifications

Lifestyle changes, which form the cornerstone of effective reflux treatment for all patients, are summarized in Table 106.3.

Antacids and Alginic Acid

Antacids and alginic acid are useful for treating mild, infrequent reflux symptoms, especially those brought on by lifestyle indiscretions. They are ineffective in healing esophagitis. Antacids work primarily by neutralizing acid, although for relatively short periods. Therefore, patients need to take these agents frequently, usually 20 to 30 minutes after meals and at bedtime. Aluminum hydroxide antacids containing alginic acid form a highly viscous solution that floats on the surface of the gastric pool and acts as a mechanical barrier. Alginic acid tablets (Gaviscon) effectively prevent episodes of upright acid reflux.

Prokinetic Drugs

Bethanechol and metoclopramide are prokinetic drugs that effectively relieve heartburn symptoms, but their efficacy in treating esophagitis is equivocal. Bethanechol (25 mg) and metoclopramide (10 mg) are given 30 minutes before meals and at bedtime. Side effects are common in both young and elderly patients. The prokinetic drug cisapride is more effective than placebo and equal to H_2 antagonists in controlling reflux symptoms and healing mild esophagitis. Cisapride promotes the release of acetylcholine at the myenteric plexus, thereby increasing LES pressure, improving peristalsis amplitude, and accelerating gastric emptying. At a dose of 10 mg 30 minutes before meals and bedtime, cisapride has minimal side effects; the most common are abdominal cramps, borborygmi, and diarrhea. However, recent concerns have been raised about serious cardiac arrhythmias (ventricular fibrillation, torsades de pointes, QT prolongation) and death associated with drug interactions with cisapride. These drugs include common antibiotics (e.g., clarithromycin, erythromycin), antifungal agents (e.g., fluconazide, ketoconazole), and antiviral agents (e.g., indinavir, ritonavir). When taken with cisapride, these drugs inhibit the cytochrome P450 enzyme that metabolizes cisapride, thereby potentially increasing cisapride blood level to dangerous levels. Cisapride also may be useful in maintenance therapy of patients with reflux symptoms and mild esophagitis.

H_2 Antagonists

H_2 antagonists is a family of drugs that achieved the first real breakthrough in the treatment of GERD and continues to be

TABLE 106.2.	GENERAL APPROACH TO THE MANAGEMENT OF GASTROESOPHAGEAL REFLUX DISEASE		
	Symptoms without Esophagitis	**Mild Esophagitis**	**Severe Esophagitis or Intractable Symptoms**
Acute	Lifestyle changes	Lifestyle changes	Lifestyle changes
	PRN medication	Daily medications	Daily medications
	H_2-antagonists	H_2-antagonists	Proton pump inhibitor
	Antacids	Cisapride	
	Alginic acid		
	Prokinetics		
Maintenance	PRN medications as above	H_2-antagonists	Proton pump inhibitor
		Cisapride	Antireflux surgery
PRN, as need arises.			

TABLE 106.3.	LIFESTYLE MODIFICATIONS FOR GASTROESOPHAGEAL REFLUX DISEASE AND THEIR MECHANISMS OF ACTION		
Decreases LES Pressure	**Improves Acid Clearance**	**Direct Esophageal Irritants**	**Decreases Gastric Distention**
Avoid certain foods (fats, chocolate, coffee, carminatives) Avoid certain medications (theophylline, progesterone, antidepressants, nitrates, calcium channel blockers)	Elevate head of bed Upright position after meals	Avoid citrus, spicy, or tomato-based products Avoid medications causing pill-induced esophagitis	Avoid large meals Take evening meals several hours before retiring Lose weight

LES, lower esophageal sphincter.

the backbone of therapy for mild reflux esophagitis. Despite advertising to the contrary, all H$_2$ antagonists (cimetidine, ranitidine, famotidine, nizatidine) are equally effective in improving reflux symptoms and healing mild to moderate esophagitis, when properly dosed. H$_2$ antagonists are usually given once or preferably twice a day. Recent data on patterns of acid exposure show that the bulk of acid reflux occurs during the early evening hours after dinner and decreases markedly during the sleeping hours. Therefore, it may be preferable to take an H$_2$ antagonist 30 minutes after dinner rather than at bedtime. Heartburn can be decreased significantly by H$_2$ antagonists, and esophagitis is healed in about 60% of patients after up to 12 weeks of treatment. Healing rates differ, depending primarily on the degree of esophagitis before therapy. Mild esophagitis heals in 75% to 90% of patients; moderate and severe esophagitis heals in only 40% to 50% of patients. H$_2$ antagonists may also be effective in preventing the relapse of GERD in patients with reflux symptoms and mild esophagitis. Recently, these drugs at lower doses are available over the counter for intermittent relief of heartburn and the prevention of episodic heartburn events.

Proton Pump Inhibitors

Omeprazole and lansoprazole are potent, long-acting inhibitors of both basal and stimulated acid secretion. They act by selective, noncompetitive inhibition of the H$^+$/K$^+$-ATPase pump on the parietal cell. Proton pump inhibitors completely abolish reflux symptoms in most patients with severe GERD, usually within 1 to 2 weeks. Complete healing of esophagitis occurs after 8 weeks in 80% of patients. Omeprazole and lansoprazole are superior to H$_2$ blockers in relieving symptoms and healing esophagitis, particularly in patients with severe reflux symptoms and severe esophagitis, as well as maintenance therapy to prevent relapse of esophagitis for up to a year.

Side effects are minimal with both short- and long-term use. One concern with long-term use of proton pump inhibitors is that profound hypoacidity stimulates gastrin release, promoting the proliferation of enterochromaffin-like cells in the gastric fundus. In the rat model, prolonged use of omeprazole causes gastric

carcinoids. However, in extensive human studies in which patients on continuous omeprazole were followed for up to 7 years, no cases of gastric carcinoids or even dysplasia were observed.

Antireflux Surgery

Antireflux surgery, done openly or by laparoscopic techniques, attempts to maintain a segment of the tubular esophagus below the diaphragm and usually includes wrapping the stomach around the distal esophagus to produce increased LES pressure. Long-term relief of symptoms occurs in about 80% of patients followed up for up to 20 years. Critical for successful antireflux surgery are the preservation of esophageal function, confirmed by esophageal testing before surgery, and an experienced surgeon. Indications for antireflux surgery include younger patients with severe GERD who otherwise would require lifelong medical therapy, recurrent difficult-to-dilate strictures, nonhealing ulcers, severe bleeding from esophagitis, and aspiration symptoms from related reflux disease.

COMPLICATIONS

Peptic strictures represent the end stage of ongoing reflux, mucosal damage, healing, and secondary fibrosis. Patients with strictures present with slowly progressive dysphagia for solids, usually without much weight loss. Radiographically, peptic strictures are commonly found in the lower esophagus and are characterized by smooth-walled, tapered, circumferential narrowings. The benign nature of the stricture must be confirmed by endoscopy and biopsies. Therapy of peptic strictures consist of a careful review of dietary and medication habits, aggressive antireflux therapy, and bougienage. Patients should chew their food well while taking fluids liberally and avoid potentially damaging pills, such as aspirin, nonsteroidal anti-inflammatory drugs, or potassium chloride. Aggressive acid suppression, particularly with proton pump inhibitors, may reduce the need for subsequent dilations. Dilating (stretching) the narrowed distal esophagus with blunt bougies, either passed freely or over a guide wire, can markedly relieve the symptoms of dysphagia.

Barrett's esophagus is secondary to severe esophagitis and produces a unique reparative process in which the original squamous epithelium lining is replaced by metaplastic columnar epithelium. The prevalence of Barrett's esophagus varies, depending on the population being studied. Patients with symptomatic GERD have a prevalence rate of 5% to 12%; those with esophagitis, scleroderma, and peptic strictures can have higher rates (11% to 44%). The diagnosis of Barrett's esophagus is best made by endoscopy and confirmed by biopsy. Although Barrett's epithelium may comprise three types of mucosa, only the specialized columnar epithelium has malignant potential.

Therapy for Barrett's esophagus is no different from that for any other form of esophagitis. The major concern is the increased prevalence and incidence of adenocarcinoma of the esophagus. The prevalence is an estimated 10%, a 30- to 40-fold increase over the general population, whereas incidence varies, ranging from 1 case in 46 to 441 patient-years of follow-up. The columnar lining of the esophagus may evolve over time through increasing degrees of dysplasia to cancer. For this reason, endoscopic surveillance is recommended in patients with Barrett's esophagus to detect high-grade dysplasia or early cancer, thereby permitting curative surgical resection.

OTHER INFLAMMATORY DISORDERS OF THE ESOPHAGUS

Inflammatory disorders of the esophagus are usually acute in onset and characterized clinically by odynophagia and dysphagia. An algorithm for evaluating patients with odynophagia is shown in Figure 106.3.

INFECTIOUS ESOPHAGITIS

Infections of the esophagus are rare in the general population, but, when present, should prompt a search for an immunodeficiency. Esophageal infection is seen primarily in three groups of immunocompromised patients: HIV-positive patients, cancer patients with granulocytopenia after chemotherapy, and organ transplant recipients receiving immunosuppressive therapy. Other predisposing conditions include malignancy, alcoholism, diabetes mellitus, and therapy with corticosteroids or other immunosuppressive agents.

The most common causes of infectious esophagitis are *Candida*, herpes simplex virus, and cytomegalovirus. Candidal esophagitis is most common in HIV-infected patients and in granulocytopenic cancer patients; viral esophagitis predominates in bone marrow transplant recipients. Both candidal esophagitis and viral esophagitis are seen after solid organ transplantation. Less common causes of infectious esophagitis include histoplasmosis, *Mycobacterium tuberculosis, Mycobacterium avium* complex, *Cryptosporidium, Pneumocystis carinii,* Epstein–Barr virus, HIV, and gram-negative and gram-positive bacteria. Mixed infections are present in about 30% of patients.

Esophageal infections should be suspected in the immunocompromised patient presenting with odynophagia, dysphagia, or chest pain. Oral thrush is commonly sought, but its presence does not preclude the possibility of infections with other organisms besides *Candida*, and its absence does not exclude the presence of *Candida*. Endoscopy with brush cytology, biopsy, and culture is the best initial diagnostic test.

Patients with candidiasis present with discrete, 3- to 5-mm,

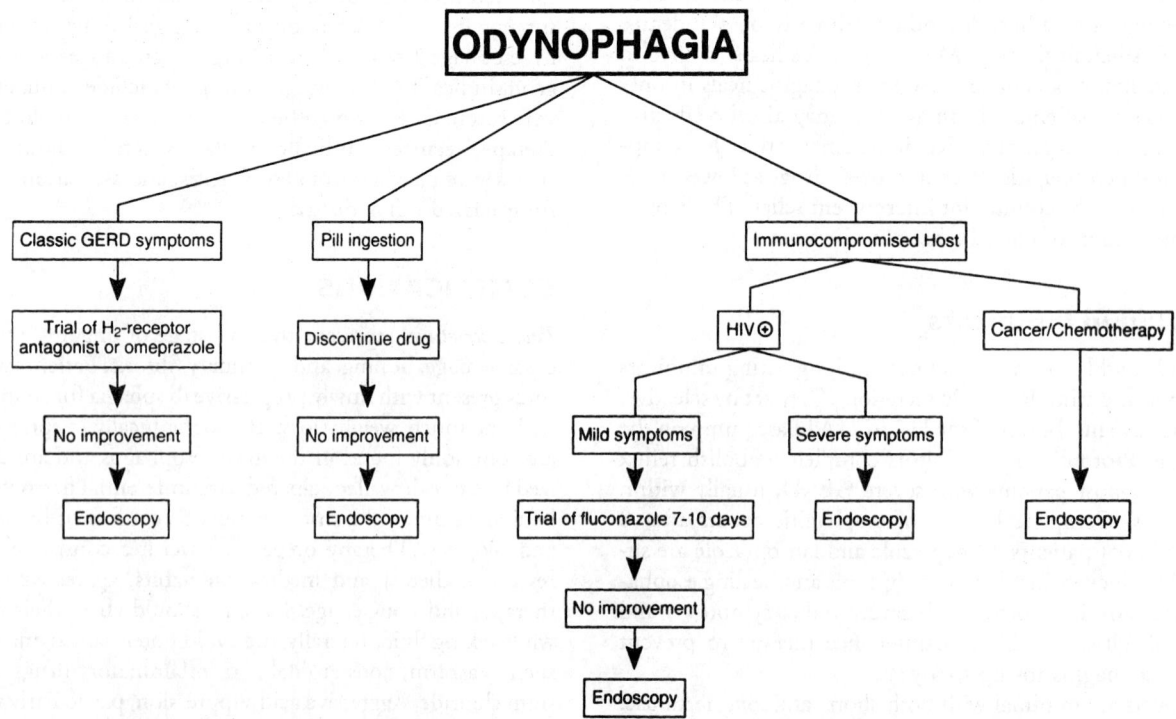

FIGURE 106.3. Approach to the patient with odynophagia. (Modified from Wilcox CM. Esophageal disease in the acquired immunodeficiency syndrome: etiology, diagnosis and management. *Am J Med* 1992;92:412–421.)

EVIDENCE LEVEL: B. Reference: Speckler SJ. AGA Technical review of treatments of patients with dysphagia. Gastroenterology 1999;117:233–254.

TABLE 106.4.   TREATMENT REGIMENS FOR COMMON ESOPHAGEAL INFECTIONS

	Infection	Treatment
Candida	Minimal compromise (i.e., diabetes, steroids)	Nystatin 1–3 million U q.i.d. Clotrimazole 100 mg t.i.d.
	AIDS patients	Ketoconazole 200–400 mg/d Fluconazole 100 mg/d
	Failure of above	Amphotericin B 0.3 mg/kg/d
Herpes simplex virus	Immunocompetent patient	Supportive care Analgesics Topical anesthetics
	Immunocompromised patients	
	Mild cases	Acyclovir 200–400 mg 5×/d orally
	More severe cases	Acyclovir 15 mg/kg/d IV
Cytomegalovirus		Ganciclovir 5 mg/kg IV q 12 hr Foscarnet 60 mg/kg/d IV q 8 hr
HIV		Prednisone 40 mg/d

Modified from Wilcox CM, Karowe NW. Esophageal infection: etiology, diagnosis, and management. *Gastroenterologist* 1994;2:188.

raised yellowish plaques or confluent cheeselike exudates. The diagnosis is most easily established by brushing the plaques and smearing the material on a clear glass slide, allowing it to dry, applying 10% potassium hydroxide, and examining the slide for the appearance of typical branch hyphae and budding yeast. Fungal cultures and histologic examination of biopsy specimens are also helpful. Treatment for candidal esophagitis depends on the severity of the infection and the nature of the underlying immune defect (Table 106.4).

Herpetic esophagitis is characterized early in its course by clear vesicles. Because the vesicles are short-lived, the usual finding is that of discrete, small, superficial ulcers with a punched-out appearance and raised yellow edges. The intervening mucosa often appears normal. Brushing and biopsies show cytologic changes that may suggest herpetic infection (Cowdry type A inclusions).

Cytomegalovirus esophagitis appears as an extensive area of mucosal injury with inflammatory exudate and ulcerations. The ulcers are deep, progress in size, and occasionally perforate. Biopsy specimens, brush cytology, or viral cultures may show evidence of this virus.

Esophageal ulcerations have been described in patients with seroconversion to HIV. These patients present with a syndrome characterized by fever, myalgia, maculopapular rash, and odynophagia. Endoscopy shows multiple discrete esophageal ulcerations; electron microscopic examination of tissue shows retroviral organisms, indicating HIV as the direct cause.

Treatment of these viral esophagitides is summarized in Table 106.4.

PILL-INDUCED ESOPHAGITIS

More than 50% of the cases of pill-induced esophagitis result from tetracycline and its derivatives, particularly doxycycline. Other commonly prescribed medications causing esophageal injury include slow-release potassium chloride, iron sulfate, quinidine, corticosteroids, and nonsteroidal anti-inflammatory drugs.

A common factor is a history of improper ingestion. Nearly 50% of the reported patients took little or no fluid while swallowing the pills or took them just before bedtime. Patients with pill-induced esophageal injury generally complain of odynophagia and retrosternal burning; only a few report that the pills get stuck in their chest. Endoscopy, the first investigative study, usually reveals discrete ulcers at the level of the aortic arch or distal esophagus. Patients with pill-induced esophagitis improve with withdrawal of the offending medication. Symptomatic resolution and endoscopic healing is usually evident in 3 days to 6 weeks. In addition to drug discontinuation, other therapies include palliation of odynophagia with viscous lidocaine, prevention of acid reflux, and assurance of adequate nutrition. Rarely, patients develop strictures requiring dilation. To prevent further pill-induced esophageal injuries, patients should be encouraged to ingest all pills with 8 ounces of water while standing or sitting upright and should be discouraged from taking pills just before bedtime.

ESOPHAGEAL MOTILITY DISORDERS

Functional disturbances of the esophagus, from either neurologic or muscular disorders, may involve the striated or smooth muscle segments of the esophagus. The skeletal muscle causes of oropharyngeal dysphagia are discussed in Chapter 94; the common smooth muscle esophageal disorders are discussed in the text that follows.

ACHALASIA

Achalasia is characterized by a double defect in esophageal function. The LES does not appropriately relax, offering resistance to the flow of liquids and solids from the esophagus into the stomach. In addition, there is loss of peristalsis in the lower two-thirds (smooth muscle portion) of the esophagus. Achalasia usually manifests between the ages of 25 and 60 years; men and women are affected equally. Its cause is unknown. The two most popular theories suggest that achalasia is secondary to a viral infection or a degenerative disease of the neurons. In South America, infection with the protozoan *Trypanosoma cruzi* produces ganglion damage and an achalasia-like syndrome with megaesophagus.

Pathophysiology

Abnormalities in muscle and nerves can be detected in achalasia, although a neural lesion is thought to be of primary importance. Three major neural anatomical changes are described: loss of ganglion cells within Auerbach's plexus, degeneration of the vagus nerve, and qualitative and quantitative changes in the dorsal motor nucleus of the vagus. There is selective damage to inhibitory neurons with marked reduction of VIP and nitric oxide receptors, which may account for the observed motility disturbances. Further evidence of denervation is the exaggerated contractions in the LES and esophageal body observed when these patients are given methacholine. This response indicates denervation hypersensitivity.

Clinical Presentation

Nearly all patients with achalasia have dysphagia for solids; most also have dysphagia for liquids. The onset is gradual, and most patients have symptoms for an average of 2 years before the diagnosis is made. Postural changes, such as throwing the shoulders back, lifting the neck, and performing a rapid Valsalva maneuver, help improve esophageal emptying. Fullness in the chest and regurgitation of undigested nonacidic food are seen in many patients. Undigested food may be regurgitated postprandially or at night, causing choking, cough, and aspiration pneumonia. Chest pain occurs in some patients and is more common in younger patients with earlier disease. It is surprising that heartburn is described by some achalasia patients, presumably because of the fermentation of intraesophageal contents. Weight loss is very common and usually progresses with the duration of the disease.

Diagnosis

With suspected achalasia, the first test is a barium esophagogram. Early in the course, the esophagus may appear normal in diameter but with a loss of normal peristalsis. As the disease progresses, the esophagus becomes more dilated and tortuous with retained food and air–fluid levels (Fig. 106.4*A*). The distal esophagus is characterized by a smooth, symmetric, tapering "bird beak" appearance. Clues to the diagnosis may also be found on chest radiographs, which demonstrate a widened mediastinum, thoracic air–fluid level, and absence of the gastric air bubble. Diagnosis of achalasia is confirmed by esophageal manometry, which reveals such characteristic features as absence of peristalsis in the distal smooth muscle esophagus, incomplete or abnormal LES relaxation, elevated LES pressures, and elevated intraesophageal pressures relative to gastric pressures (Table 106.5). All achalasia patients should undergo upper gastrointestinal endoscopy to differentiate primary achalasia from pseudoachalasia, usually secondary to an adenocarcinoma.

Strategies for Optimal Care Management

The goal of therapy in achalasia is to diminish the high residual LES pressure after swallowing. If esophageal emptying is improved, esophagus stasis and its consequences are reduced. Although peristalsis rarely returns, the patient feels as if swallowing is nearly normal. Three treatments are available: pharmacologic therapy, pneumatic dilation, and surgical myotomy.

Smooth muscle relaxants, including sublingual isosorbide dinitrate or calcium antagonists such as nifedipine, can be used prophylactically with meals or as necessary for pain or dysphagia. These medications provide variable relief of symptoms, and their effectiveness tends to decrease with time.

TABLE 106.5.	MANOMETRIC CHARACTERISTICS OF THE ESOPHAGEAL MOTILITY DISORDERS				
		Spastic Motor Disorders			
	Achalasia	**DES**	**Nutcracker**	**Hypertensive LES**	**Scleroderma**
Striated muscle/UES	Normal	Normal	Normal	Normal	Normal
Smooth muscle	Aperistalsis	Intermittent peristalsis Simultaneous, repetitive High amplitude Long duration Spontaneous	Normal peristalsis High amplitude	Normal peristalsis	Low-amplitude peristalsis *or* Aperistalsis
LES	Incomplete relaxation High pressure	Occasional LES dysfunction	Normal	High pressure Normal relaxation	Low or no pressure

DES, diffuse esophageal spasm; LES, lower esophageal sphincter; UES, upper esophageal sphincter.

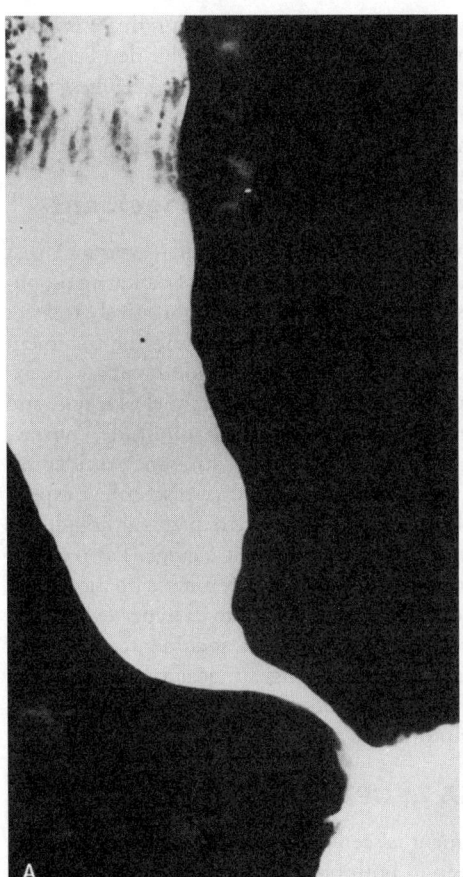
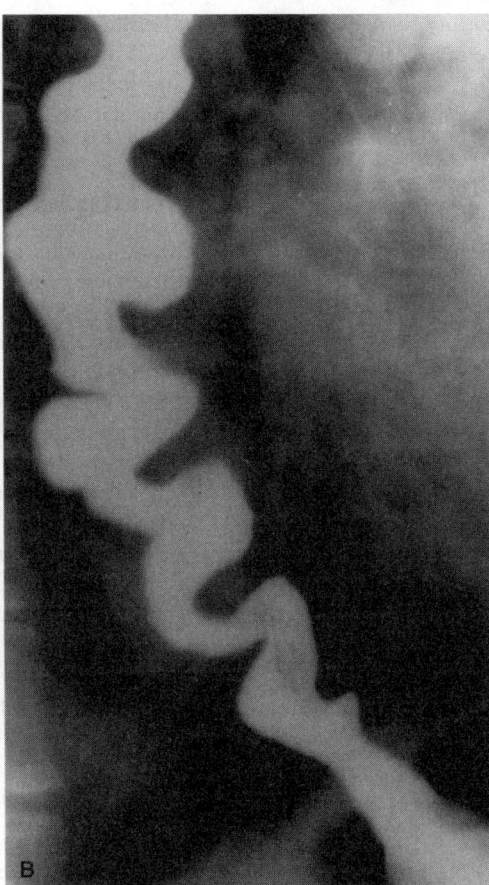

FIGURE 106.4. A: Achalasia characterized by a moderately dilated esophagus with lack of peristalsis and retention of barium and secretions, forming an air–fluid level in the proximal esophagus. Spastic LES relaxes incompletely, causing a bird-beak appearance of the distal esophagus with poor emptying. **B**: Diffuse esophageal spasm characterized by a nondilated esophagus and multiple spastic contractions, causing the barium to move to and fro and the esophageal lumen to have a segmented appearance.

Recent studies suggest that botulinum toxin injections via endoscopy directly into the lower sphincter may relieve symptoms for 3 to 12 months. The toxin inhibits the release of acetylcholine, which overcomes the unopposed excitation of the smooth muscle esophagus resulting from selective loss of inhibitory neurons in the myenteric plexus.

Pneumatic dilation involves placing a balloon across the LES; it is then inflated to a pressure adequate to tear the muscle fibers of the sphincter. Good to excellent results occur in 50% to 90% of patients. The procedure can be done on an outpatient basis, recovery is rapid, and discomfort is short-lived. About 30% of patients require subsequent dilations. Perforation, a major complication, is reported in about 5% of patients and usually requires surgical repair.

Heller myotomy involves incising the circular muscle of the LES and more distal esophagus down to the mucosa and allowing the muscle to protrude through. Myotomy produces good to excellent results in 60% to 90% of cases, and the operative mortality is low. Disadvantages of surgery are the morbidity associated with the operation, a long hospital stay, increased costs compared with pneumatic dilation, and an increased risk of postoperative GER. To prevent the latter problem, many surgeons now add a loose antireflux operation to the myotomy. Laparoscopic and thorascopic techniques for esophageal myotomy are under investigation (Chapter 131).

SPASTIC MOTILITY DISORDERS

Spastic motility disorders produce manometric patterns different from those of achalasia. They are characterized by normal peristalsis intermittently interrupted by simultaneous contractions, high-amplitude or long-duration waves, or dysfunction of the LES. Confusion has arisen as to whether these manometric abnormalities are separate, distinct entities or are variations of diffuse esophageal spasm (Table 106.5). However, the similarities among these disorders in presentation, natural history, and treatment suggest that they often overlap and should be best designated as spastic motility disorders of the esophagus.

Pathophysiology

The cause of spastic motility disorders is unknown, and no specific characteristic pathologic lesion is present. Spastic motility abnormalities are commonly associated with other medical conditions, particularly GER. Central nervous system processing could produce some of these manometric abnormalities. Psychologically stressful interviews, loud noises, or difficult mental tasks can produce simultaneous waves and increase contraction amplitudes in the distal esophagus of normal persons and patients with spastic motility disorders. These patients also appear to have both a motor and sensory component to their spastic disorder. Acid instillation may stimulate sensitive neural receptors, producing discomfort independent of motility changes. Esophageal balloon distention can reproduce esophageal pain at low distending volumes without noticeable motor changes.

Clinical Presentation

Spastic disorders of the esophagus generally present during middle age and are more common in women. Dysphagia and chest pain are the cardinal symptoms, and most patients present with both. Dysphagia for liquids and solids is present in 30% to 60% of patients. This symptom is intermittent and varies daily from mild to very severe, but usually it is not progressive or severe enough to interfere with eating or to cause weight loss. Intermittent anterior chest pain, sometimes mimicking angina pectoris, is reported by most patients. Pain episodes last from minutes to hours and may require narcotics or nitroglycerin, further confusing the distinction between esophageal and cardiac pain. Many patients also have symptoms compatible with the irritable bowel syndrome, as well as urinary and sexual dysfunction in women.

Diagnosis

Spastic motility disorders are best defined by esophageal manometry (Table 106.5). The patient's chief symptom is an important factor in the prevalence and type of motility disorder identified (Fig. 106.5). In patients with diffuse esophageal spasm, the barium esophagogram may reveal severe lumen-obliterating tertiary contractions that trap barium and delay transit, producing a to-and-fro movement of the bolus (Fig. 106.4*B*). Patients with other spastic motility disorders often have a normal barium esophagogram. Endoscopy may be done, but its major role is to

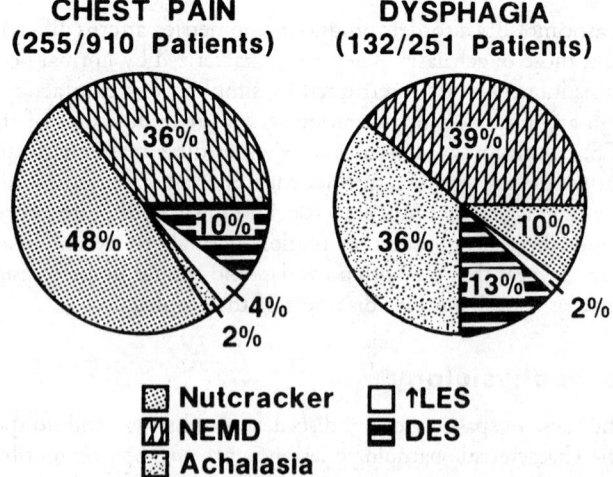

CHEST PAIN (255/910 Patients)   **DYSPHAGIA** (132/251 Patients)

- ▨ Nutcracker   □ ↑LES
- ▧ NEMD   ▬ DES
- ▦ Achalasia

FIGURE 106.5. Incidence of esophageal motility disorders in patients with noncardiac chest pain (*left*) and dysphagia (*right*) in a 3-year experience with nearly 1,200 consecutive patients undergoing esophageal manometry. The chief complaint is an important factor in the prevalence and type of motility disorders identified. *NEMD*, nonspecific esophageal motor disorder; *↑LES*, hypertensive lower esophageal sphincter; *DES*, diffuse esophageal spasm. (From Katz PO, Dalton CB, Richter JE, et al. Esophageal testing of patients with noncardiac chest pain or dysphagia. *Ann Intern Med* 1987;106:593–597, with permission.)

identify possible structural lesions or to rule out reflux esophagitis. Provocative tests, such as edrophonium chloride (Tensilon) and balloon distention, may be able to provoke the chest pain. Ambulatory 24-hour pH monitoring is useful to identify associated GERD, which is present in 20% to 50% of these patients.

Strategies for Optimal Care Management

Many patients respond favorably to confident reassurance that their chest pain is not coming from their heart and has an esophageal origin. GER should be identified and aggressively treated. Otherwise, no single drug has proven efficacy in the treatment of spastic esophageal motility disorders. Smooth muscle relaxants, such as long-acting nitrates, calcium channel blockers, and anticholinergic agents, may decrease high-amplitude contractions but have not relieved chest pain consistently. Antidepressant medications may reduce the amount of discomfort experienced as well as the patient's reaction to pain, although the esophageal motility abnormality does not change. Passive dilation of the esophagus is of no value, but pneumatic dilation helps some patients with diffuse esophageal spasm or hypertensive LES who complain of severe dysphagia with documented delays in esophageal emptying. Rarely, a long surgical myotomy helps some patients, but aggressive interventions must be used cautiously because symptoms may not be relieved.

SCLERODERMA ESOPHAGUS

Esophageal involvement is seen in 70% to 80% of patients with scleroderma. It is seen in both progressive systemic sclerosis and the CREST syndrome (calcinosis, Raynaud's, esophageal involvement, sclerodactyly, and telangiectasias). The pathophysiology involves an abnormality in muscle excitation and responsiveness owing to muscle atrophy and decreased cholinergic excitation. The classic manometric features of advanced scleroderma include low LES pressure, peristaltic dysfunction of the smooth muscle portion of the esophagus characterized by low-amplitude contractions or aperistalsis, and preserved function of the striated esophagus and oropharynx (Table 106.5). As a result of these manometric abnormalities, patients may have dysphagia and severe GERD. It is surprising that dysphagia for solids and liquids is reported by less than 50% of patients with scleroderma. More severe dysphagia suggests esophagitis, often with an associated stricture. Esophagitis is present in most patients.

Management of scleroderma centers on the treatment of GER and its complications. Patients should chew their food well and drink plenty of fluids. GERD should be identified and aggressively treated using H_2 antagonists or proton pump inhibitors. Strictures respond to frequent dilations. In severe cases, antireflux surgery may be warranted.

Benign and malignant tumors of the esophagus are discussed in Chapter 115.

■ MISCELLANEOUS ESOPHAGEAL DISORDERS

ESOPHAGEAL DIVERTICULA

Esophageal diverticula are outpouchings of one or more layers of the esophageal wall. They occur in three main areas: immediately

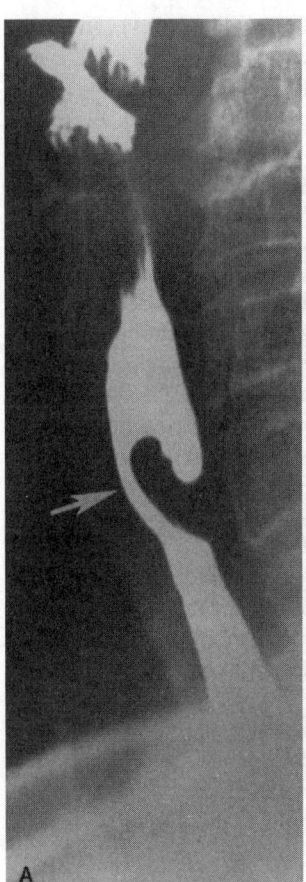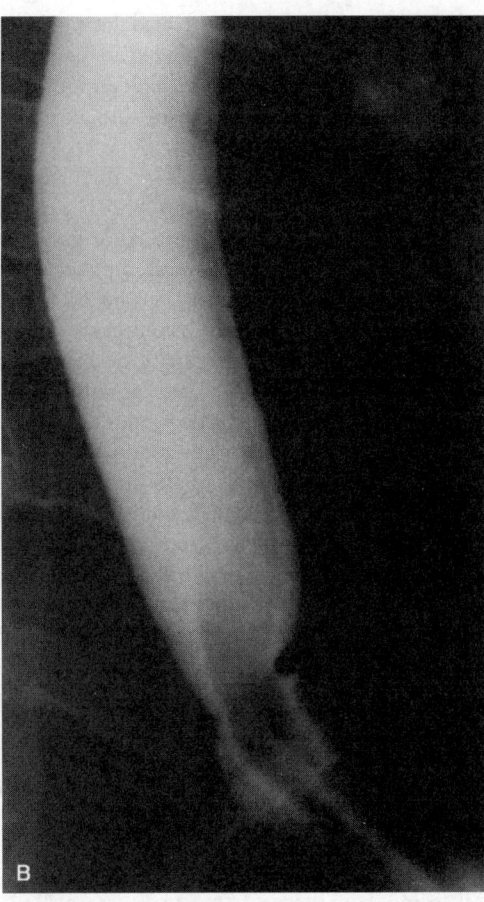

FIGURE 106.6. A: Small Zenker's diverticulum, representing an outpouching immediately above the incompletely opened and noncompliant upper esophageal sphincter (*arrow*). **B**: Lower esophageal (Schatzki's) ring characterized by a smooth, thin (less than 4 mm) symmetric narrowing at the level of the squamocolumnar junction above a small hiatal hernia.

above the UES (Zenker's diverticulum), near the midpoint of the esophagus (traction diverticulum), and immediately above the LES (epiphrenic diverticulum). Zenker's diverticulum is seen in older patients, who complain of cervical dysphagia, gurgling in the throat, halitosis, regurgitation of foul food, and sometimes a neck mass (Fig. 106.6*A*). It was originally thought to be related to discoordination of UES relaxation, but recent studies show that the sphincter opens incompletely because of reduced muscle compliance. To compensate for this decreased cross-sectional area, the hypopharyngeal bolus pressure increases, leading to dysphagia and diverticula formation. Traction diverticula are usually asymptomatic. They are thought to be secondary to external inflammatory processes such as tuberculosis or to a localized segmental motility disorder. Epiphrenic diverticula are invariably associated with esophageal motility disorders, especially achalasia. Diverticula are best diagnosed by a barium esophagogram; endoscopy is rarely required. Symptomatic diverticula require surgery.

RINGS AND WEBS

The lower esophageal (Schatzki's) ring at the squamocolumnar junction is the most common cause of intermittent dysphagia for solids (Fig. 106.6*B*). Rings are usually found in patients over age 50 and are rarely seen before age 30. The origin of the lower esophageal ring is unknown, but it may be a complication of GERD. The diagnosis is made with the barium swallow using the prone position, having the patient perform the Valsalva maneuver, or having the patient swallow a marshmallow or tablet to bring out the ring. Treatment includes reassurance, adjustments in eating habits, dilation of the ring with a blunt bougie, and treatment of associated GERD.

Webs are membranous narrowings covered entirely by squamous mucosa, which can occur anywhere along the esophagus but are found primarily in the upper 2 to 4 cm of the esophagus. Some webs are congenital; others are associated with iron-deficiency anemia (Paterson–Kelly or Plummer–Vinson syndrome). Most webs are asymptomatic and are incidental radiologic findings. Symptomatic patients are usually women who report dysphagia for solids rather than liquids. Diagnosis is made by the lateral view on the barium esophagogram. Treatment with bougienage is often successful.

BIBLIOGRAPHY

Baehr PH, McDonald GB. Esophageal infections: risk factors, presentation, diagnosis and treatment. *Gastroenterology* 1994;106:509–532.

Baron TH, Richter JE. The use of esophageal function tests. *Adv Intern Med* 1993;38:361–386.

Biot WJ, Devesa SS, Kneller RW, et al. Rising incidence of adenocarcinoma of the esophagus and gastric cardia. *JAMA* 1991;265:1287–1289.

Clouse RE. Spastic disorders of the esophagus. *Gastroenterologist* 1997;5:112–127.

Richter JE. Extraesophageal presentations of gastroesophageal reflux disease. *Semin Gastrointest Dis* 1997;8:75–89.

Sloan S, Rademaker AW, Kahrilas PJ. Determinants of gastroesophageal junction incompetence: hiatal hernia, liver esophageal sphincter, or both? *Ann Intern Med* 1992;117:977–982.

Sontag SJ. The medical management of reflux esophagitis. Role of antacids and acid inhibition. *Gastroenterol Clin North Am* 1990;19:683–712.

Spechler SJ. Comparison of medical and surgical therapy for complicated gastroesophageal reflux disease. Department of Veterans Affairs gastroesophageal reflux disease study group. *N Engl J Med* 1992;326:786–792.

Vaezi MF, Richter JE. Current therapies for achalasia: comparison and efficacy. *J Clin Gastroenterol* 1998;27:21–35.

Kelley's Textbook of Internal Medicine, fourth edition. Edited by H. David Humes. Lippincott Williams & Wilkins, Philadelphia © 2000.

CHAPTER 107

GASTRODUODENAL ULCER DISEASE AND GASTRITIS

DAVID C. METZ
JOHN H. WALSH

Peptic ulcers are defects in the gastrointestinal mucosal lining that extend through the submucosa into the muscle layer. They require the presence of aggressive noxious substances including acid and pepsin for their formation and therefore are classified as an acid-peptic disorder. Peptic ulcers are rarely due simply to excessive secretion of acid. Most cases represent an imbalance between aggressive factors and factors that undermine mucosal integrity, especially the presence of gastric inflammation (gastritis). Chronic gastric infection with the gram-negative bacterium, *Helicobacter pylori* (*H. pylori*), is the most important factor that predisposes to peptic ulceration. *H. pylori* gastritis causes peptic ulceration by having an indirect effect on gastric acid secretion (especially with regard to duodenal ulcers) and by causing gastritis, thereby undermining gastric mucosal integrity (especially with regard to gastric ulcers). Gastropathy due to the ingestion of nonsteroidal anti-inflammatory drugs (NSAIDs) is the second most common cause of ulcers. Although NSAIDs do not cause gastritis per se, they undermine mucosal integrity by depleting gastric mucosal prostaglandins. Rarer causes of gastritis are not generally associated with the presence of peptic ulceration.

■ EPIDEMIOLOGY OF PEPTIC ULCER DISEASE

Duodenal ulcers are common. Although their incidence and prevalence appear to be decreasing, approximately one in ten persons are affected during their lifetime (Fig. 107.1). The illness is often considered to be a disease of young and middle-aged adults, but the incidence of first-time ulcers peaks after age 50. The incidence of duodenal ulcer in men has been decreasing during the past 30 years, but no decrease has been found in women. Therefore, the male-to-female ratio has dropped from 4 to 1 to almost 1 to 1 in the United States.

Hospitalizations for gastric ulcer have not decreased during the past 20 years. In the United States and Western Europe, however, there has been a large drop in duodenal ulcer disease hospital admissions in men during the latter part of this century. The most dramatic decrease has been in elective hospitalizations, but ulcer-related mortality also has decreased. The age-adjusted mortality rates for duodenal ulcer have decreased during the past 20 years from about 4 in 100,000 in men and 0.8 in 100,000 in women to about 1 in 100,000 in men and 0.5 in 100,000 in women. Age-adjusted mortality rates for gastric ulcer in men have fallen from about 4 per 100,000 to 1.5 per 100,000; in women they have remained between 1.1 and 1.2 per 100,000. On the other hand, rates of ulcer complications such as bleeding, perforation, gastric outlet obstruction, and penetration into the pancreas have shown much less change (Fig. 107.2).

Bleeding is the most common complication and is the most common cause of death from peptic ulcer. Mortality from bleeding occurs almost exclusively in older patients who have at least one additional major disease. Some evidence suggests that the rates of duodenal ulcer are beginning to stabilize in the United States (Fig. 107.1).

Major factors associated with ulcers are chronic *H. pylori* infection, smoking, and the use of NSAIDs (Fig. 107.3). About 15% to 20% of *H. pylori*–infected subjects develop ulcers during their lifetime. Eradication of this infection markedly decreases the recurrence of peptic ulcers. Much of the decrease in ulcer incidence observed in recent years may be due to the decrease in *H. pylori* gastritis in developed countries such as the United States. The overall association between cigarette smoking and duodenal ulcer is strong. Smokers have a higher incidence of duodenal ulcer, and after treatment their ulcers heal more slowly and recur more rapidly than do ulcers of nonsmokers. Death rates from ulcer in smokers also are higher; however, this finding may reflect a higher frequency of other smoking-related diseases. NSAIDs are implicated in the formation of gastric and duodenal ulcers, and bleeding from gastric and duodenal ulcers is increased in patients taking aspirin or other nonsteroidal agents.

DISEASES WITH INCREASED ULCER RISK

Two conditions have a clear association with peptic ulceration. *H. pylori* gastritis is associated with both duodenal and gastric ulcers. Multiple endocrine neoplasia syndrome type I (MEN-I) is a rare, dominantly inherited disorder characterized by enteropancreatic neuroendocrine tumors (especially nonfunctional tumors, gastrinomas, and insulinomas), parathyroid hyperplasia, and pituitary tumors (especially prolactinomas and adrenocorticotropic hormone [ACTH]-secreting tumors). Zollinger–Ellison syndrome characterized by the triad of an enteropancreatic neuroendocrine tumor, gastric acid hypersecretion, and peptic

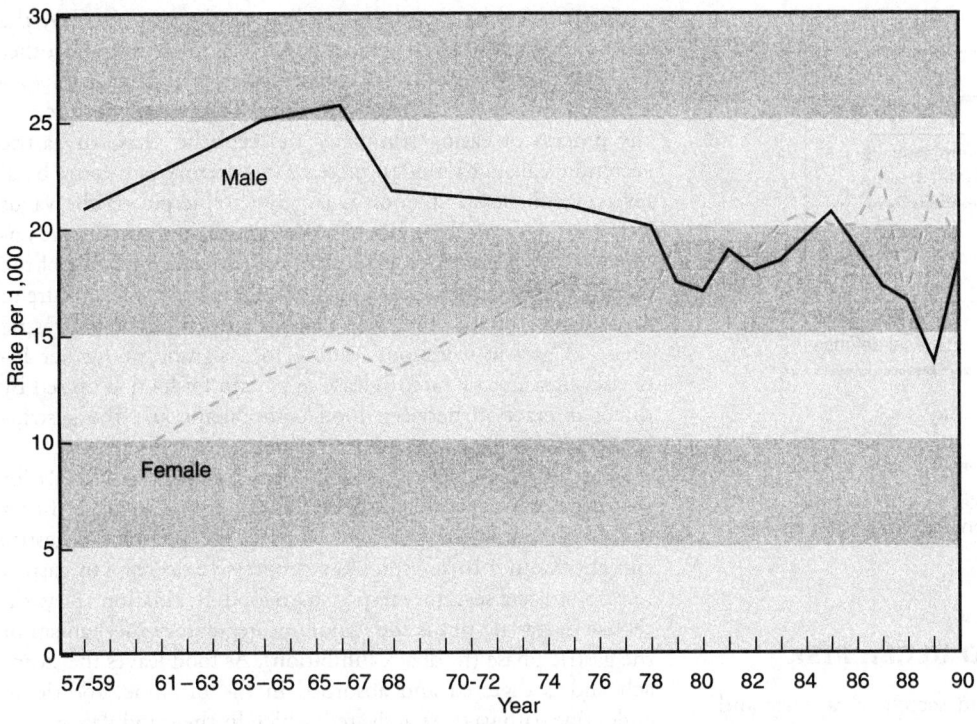

FIGURE 107.1. One-year period prevalence by sex for peptic ulcer disease. Data from the National Center for Health Statistics. (From Kurata JH. Epidemiology: peptic ulcer risk factors. *Semin Gastroenterol Dis* 1993;4:2–12, updated since 1990 by personal communication, with permission.)

ulceration (almost exclusively of the duodenum) develops in more than 50% of MEN-I patients. This accounts for about 25% of all patients with gastrinoma—itself a rare disorder with an annual incidence of approximately 0.5 per million. Familial hyperpepsinogenemia, C1-esterase deficiency, and Neuhauser's syndrome are rare disorders associated with peptic ulcer.

Peptic ulcer is common in patients with chronic obstructive pulmonary disease. The risk is not explained simply by the association of both diseases with smoking. Duodenal ulcers are common in cirrhosis, regardless of the underlying cause. Several series have found that patients with cirrhosis and esophageal varices

are as likely or more likely to bleed from duodenal ulcer as from the varices. Alcohol abuse without cirrhosis is not associated with an increased ulcer risk. Some patients with renal failure have unexplained acid hypersecretion, which frequently is associated with duodenal ulcer. A larger percentage of these patients experience decreased acid secretion associated with hypergastrinemia but no ulcer disease. After renal transplantation, complications of peptic ulcer disease are common. Weak associations with duodenal ulcer have been found in coronary heart disease, polycythemia vera, Crohn's disease, the carcinoid syndrome, and myasthenia gravis.

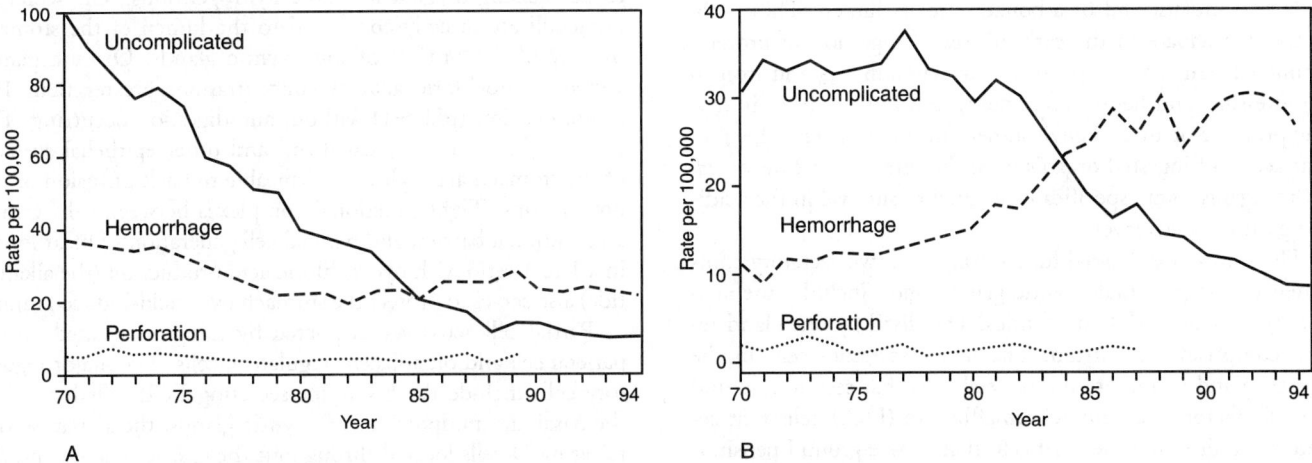

FIGURE 107.2. Hospitalization rates for uncomplicated or bleeding duodenal (**A**) and gastric ulcers (**B**). Data from the National Center for Health Statistics. (From Kurata JH. Epidemiology: peptic ulcer risk factors. *Semin Gastroenterol Dis* 1993;4:2–12, updated since 1990 by personal communication.)

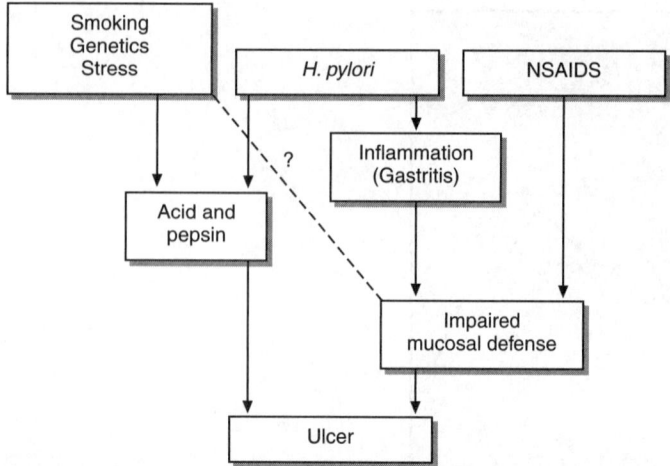

FIGURE 107.3. Pathogenesis of peptic ulcer. (Modified from Soll AH. Pathogenesis of peptic ulcer and implications for therapy. *N Engl J Med* 1990; 322:909–916.)

DISEASES WITH DECREASED ULCER RISK

Gastric atrophy leads to decreased acid secretory capacity and decreases the risk of duodenal ulcer. The most extreme example is pernicious anemia in which achlorhydria results from autoimmune destruction of parietal cells (type A gastritis). Many persons with chronic *H. pylori* infection have pangastritis (type B gastritis) in which progressively lower acid secretory capacity develops with time. The risk of duodenal ulcer decreases in proportion to acid secretion, but the risk for gastric ulcer is maintained in these patients until acid secretion is quite low.

■ NORMAL PHYSIOLOGY OF GASTRIC SECRETION

The epithelial lining of the stomach secretes acid, pepsin, intrinsic factor, mucus, and bicarbonate into its lumen. These substances participate in the early phases of digestion of protein, permit efficient absorption of dietary vitamin B_{12} and iron in the intestine, and help protect the gastric mucosa from injury. The presence of an acid environment in the stomach helps prevent access of ingested organisms to the intestine. However, *H. pylori* organisms are specifically adapted to survival in the acidified gastric mucus layer.

The stomach is divided functionally into two secretory components. The proximal oxyntic gland region includes the anatomical corpus (body) and fundus. The distal pyloric gland region comprises the antrum. The major secretory cells in the oxyntic gland region are the parietal cells that secrete acid and intrinsic factor, the enterochromaffin-like (ECL) cells that secrete histamine, and the chief cells that secrete group I pepsinogen. The G and D cells in the pyloric gland region secrete the hormones gastrin and somatostatin, respectively. Throughout the stomach, mucous neck cells and surface epithelial cells secrete group II pepsinogen, mucus, and bicarbonate.

Gastric secretion varies according to the time of day, the time and types of food intake, psychological states, and other metabolic activities of the body. Secretion is highest in the evening and lowest in the early morning. The thought of food or the process of eating stimulates the cephalic phase of gastric secretion, causing a modest increase in secretory rate above basal levels. Cephalic stimulation is largely cholinergic via the vagus nerve and is strongly antagonized by muscarinic cholinergic antagonists, such as atropine. Gastrin is the major mediator of the gastric phase of acid secretion. Antral distention and exposure to protein and certain other food constituents stimulate the gastric phase of gastric secretion, leading to a significant further increases in secretory rate. Release of gastrin by food is caused by direct interaction between food components and the gastrin-secreting G cells that line antral glands.

Gastrin release also is mediated by receptors on G cells for gastrin-releasing peptide, a neuropeptide found in nerve fibers that innervate antral glands. Lowering the pH of the gastric contents from 4 to 1 results in a progressive decrease in gastrin release and acid secretory responses to food. Regulation of gastrin release by gastric pH is the major autoregulatory mechanism of the gastric phase (feedback inhibition). As food leaves the stomach and is digested and absorbed in the intestine, additional endocrine pathways are activated, which further modulate gastric secretion (the intestinal phase of gastric acid secretion).

Parietal cells are located in the middle and lower parts of oxyntic glands. In the unstimulated basal state, tubulovesicles are present in the cytoplasm. When the parietal cell is stimulated, the tubulovesicles fuse with one another and with the apical membrane to form the secretory canalicular complex. Secretory canaliculi are lined with proton pumps (H^+,K^+-ATPase enzymes), which traverse the apical cellular membrane and are responsible for acid secretion. Energy derived from the hydrolysis of adenosine triphosphate (ATP) is used to pump hydrogen ions into the secretory canaliculi in exchange for potassium ions. Equimolar amounts of chloride enter the canaliculi through nearby chloride channels, producing hydrochloric acid. Other channels permit efflux of potassium ions, making them available to be exchanged again for more hydrogen ions. The secretory canaliculi are directly connected to the lumen of the stomach by way of the orifices of the oxyntic glands. Oxyntic glands secrete hydrochloric acid at concentrations greater than 100 mmol per liter (pH ~1) without autodigestion occurring. The linings of the secretory canaliculi and other epithelial surfaces of the stomach are highly impermeable to back-diffusion of hydrogen ions. Tight junctional complexes between cells creates an additional barrier, and parietal cell generation of bicarbonate in a 1 to 1 ratio with hydrochloric acid production (the alkaline tide) also serves to protect the stomach from acid-induced injury.

Partial cell activity is regulated by receptors located on the parietal cell and on adjacent regulatory cells. The major regulatory cells include the histamine-secreting ECL cells located in the basal and midportions of oxyntic glands, the somatostatin-releasing D cells located throughout the gastric mucosa and the gastrin-releasing G cells located primarily in the antrum. The three principal parietal cell receptors are the histamine H_2 receptor, which responds to histamine released from ECL cells; the muscarinic cholinergic receptor, which responds to acetylcholine released from vagal nerve fibers; and the cholecystokinin (CCK)-B/gastrin receptor, which responds to circulating gastrin released from antral G cells. CCK/gastrin receptors are also found on ECL cells, where activation leads to the release of histamine and D cells that release somatostatin. Somatostatin acts as a master feedback regulator that inhibits ECL and G cells by binding to type 2 somatostatin receptors on these cells. Mucosal nerves contain other inhibitory peptides such as galanin and neuropeptide Y, which may mediate neural inhibition of ECL and G cells as well.

ACID SECRETORY CAPACITY

The ability to secrete acid is determined by the number of functional parietal cells. Basal acid output rates in normal subjects after an overnight fast are 0 to 10 mmol per hour in men and 0 to 8 mmol per hour in women. The rate of acid secretion at any given time is the fraction of the maximal acid secretory capacity that is stimulated by endogenous regulators of parietal cell activity. Parietal cell mass is estimated by measurement of acid secretion rates during maximal stimulation with histamine, gastrin, or a synthetic analogue of one of these agents such as pentagastrin. The normal rate of maximal acid output (MAO) ranges from 10 to 48 mmol per hour in men. Normal MAO levels are about 25% lower in women. Peak acid output is somewhat higher than MAO. Basal acid output averages about 10% of MAO and rarely exceeds 20%.

Increased MAO is often found in duodenal ulcer patients, especially patients with Zollinger–Ellison syndrome. About 25% of idiopathic duodenal ulcer patients have MAO rates higher than the upper limit of normal. Parietal cell hyperplasia in these patients is probably explained by the trophic effect of gastrin on the acid-secreting gastric mucosa. Decreased MAO (hypochlorhydria) is found in many patients with chronic gastritis. Total absence of gastric acid secretion during maximal stimulation is known as achlorhydria. Patients with pernicious anemia have achlorhydria combined with insufficient intrinsic factor secretion. Many other patients with chronic atrophic gastritis have achlorhydria but retain the ability to secrete enough intrinsic factor to permit intestinal absorption of cobalamin sufficient to prevent development of pernicious anemia.

Operations used to treat peptic ulcer disease also decrease MAO. Vagotomy decreases gastric responsiveness to stimuli but has little effect on parietal cell mass. Subtotal gastric resection, surgical removal of part of the parietal cell region along with antrectomy, decreases acid secretion out of proportion to the number of parietal cells removed. Resection strictly limited to the antrum also leads to decreased acid secretion, possibly by removing the trophic effect of gastrin. Antisecretory drugs cause temporary, reversible decreases in MAO.

MUCOSAL CYTOPROTECTION

Mucosal cytoprotection depends primarily on adequate mucosal blood flow, which permits normal secretion of mucus and bicarbonate (HCO_3^-) as well as the delivery of protective factors, especially prostaglandins. The process of mucus secretion involves extrusion of the apical portions of the mucus-secreting gastric surface cells and mucous neck cells. The mucus contained within the cells streams out through the apical defects to form the gastric mucus layer, consisting of an adherent semisolid glycoprotein gel overlaid by soluble mucus. Bicarbonate secretion by surface mucus cells under and within the mucus layer may permit neutralization of the pH near the gastric surface mucosa. Thus, the combination of mucus and bicarbonate secretion, by providing a less acidified environment near the cell surface than in the lumen, helps the gastroduodenal mucosa defend itself from damage.

Stimuli of mucus and bicarbonate secretion in vivo include reflexes induced by gastric mucosal irritation, cholinergic stimulation, and acid secretion. Prostaglandins are the major stimulants of bicarbonate and mucus secretion and are thus the primary underlying mediators of mucosal cytoprotection. Pepsin can partially digest the mucus gel, suggesting that increased peptic activity may decrease the thickness of the mucus layer predisposing to ulceration. However, dissolving gastric mucus with mucolytic agents has had no apparent adverse effects in animal models of peptic ulcer. In contrast, studies have shown that both gastric and duodenal ulcer patients secrete less bicarbonate than do control subjects, and pH levels at the mucosal cell surfaces of peptic ulcer patients are lower than in normal subjects.

Growth factors including fibroblast growth factor, transforming growth factor-α, heparin-binding growth factor, and hepatocyte growth factor contribute to mucosal integrity by promoting normal proliferation of mucosal cells and promoting healing of mucosal lesions.

GASTRITIS

Patients with either gastric or duodenal ulcer usually also have gastritis. Gastritis is best defined as chronic inflammation of the gastric mucosa and therefore is a histologic diagnosis. Acute gastritis (or gastropathy) is typically a consequence of gastric mucosal irritation by noxious substances such as NSAIDs (including aspirin), alcohol, or bile, but the histologic findings are typically quite bland. An exception to this rule is the marked inflammation that occurs with acute *H. pylori* infection, although this syndrome is rarely recognized clinically. Chronic gastritis is almost always caused by *H. pylori* infection, and it resolves after cure of the infection. In chronic *H. pylori* gastritis, the antral mucosa is infiltrated with inflammatory cells. Patients with *H. pylori*-induced duodenal ulcers also have histologic evidence of duodenal inflammation associated with gastric metaplasia of the duodenal bulb that may be colonized by *H. pylori* organisms. Patients with *H. pylori*-induced gastric ulcers often have chronic gastritis in association with intestinal metaplasia of the gastric mucosa with varying degrees of gastric atrophy (loss of glands). Other specific causes of chronic gastritis are rare and tend not to be associated with peptic ulcer disease.

HELICOBACTER PYLORI GASTRITIS

Helicobacter pylori is a gram-negative spiral bacterium 1.5 to 3.5 μm in size. Its appearance is characterized by its helical shape

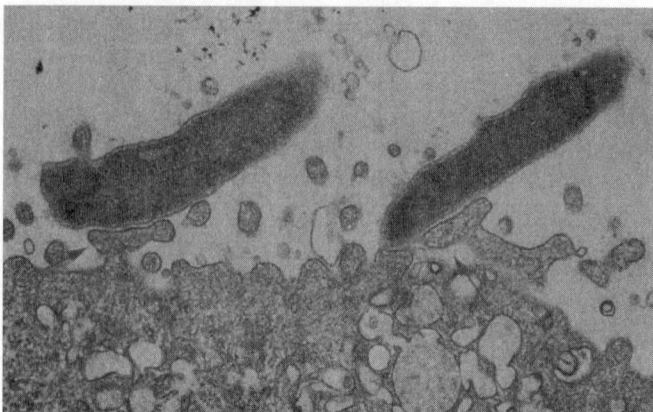

FIGURE 107.4. Electron micrograph of adherence. *Helicobacter pylori* has a unique habitat: it lives only in gastric epithelium, including metaplastic gastric epithelium, wherever it occurs. Only gastric epithelium expresses specific adherence receptors in vivo that can be recognized by the organism. Note the organism adhering to gastric epithelium. (From American Gastroenterological Association. Digestive health initiative: *Helicobacter pylori:* the new factor in management of ulcer disease. Bethesda, MD, 1995, with permission.)

as well as by six sheathed unipolar flagella that provide motility (Fig. 107.4). The organism produces urease, which appears to be important in colonization of the gastric mucosa. Although difficult to culture, organisms are detectable with standard histologic stains (hematoxylin and eosin) but are best seen if special silver-based stains such as Giemsa, Warthin Starry, or Genta stains are used. *H. pylori* appears to be pathogenic for humans exclusively, but a number of other members of the *Helicobacter* genus that infect other mammalian species have been discovered. For example, *H. felis* infects cats, *H. mustelae* infects ferrets, and *H. acinonyx* infects cheetahs. *H. heilmannii* (formerly *Gastrospirillum hominis*) is another human *Helicobacter* species, which is not felt to be pathogenic.

Epidemiology of *Helicobacter pylori* Infection

Helicobacter pylori gastritis is one of the most common human infections, with over 2 billion people infected worldwide. In developing countries with low standards of hygiene, the prevalence of *H. pylori* infection increases dramatically in early childhood (Fig. 107.5). In certain countries, up to 90% of the population is infected by age 10. Spontaneous clearance of the organism is extremely uncommon, resulting in chronic life-long infection in untreated persons. In developed countries such as the United States, the prevalence of *H. pylori* infection is lower, with approximately 30% of the adult population infected. The age-specific prevalence of *H. pylori* increases by roughly 1% per annum until late middle age when it increases sharply (Fig. 107.5). This increase is likely due to the poorer living standards prevalent in the United States when this cohort of people were young. The risk of acquiring *H. pylori* infection in adulthood in the developed world is low, roughly 0.5% per annum.

Overcrowding and low socioeconomic status appear to be important factors in the development of *H. pylori* infection.

Members of large families tend to have a higher prevalence of infection, and the last in a series of siblings is more likely to be infected than first-borns. Institutional outbreaks of the infection have also demonstrated a higher prevalence in overcrowded conditions.

Some racial and ethnic groups have an increased risk for harboring *H. pylori* infection, although this may reflect socioeconomic status in childhood (when the infection is acquired) rather than ethnicity per se. African Americans have a higher prevalence of infection than Hispanics, and whites have the lowest prevalence. *H. pylori* infection appears to occur equally in both sexes.

Because *H. pylori* infects only humans, it must be transmitted directly from one person to another. The method of transmission is not well understood, but epidemiologic studies support fecal–oral spread and the organism has been isolated from human feces. Iatrogenic transmission has been documented through contaminated endoscopes, pH probes, biopsy forceps, and nasogastric tubes. These data suggest that exposure to gastric secretions may be required for oral–oral spread. The organism can survive in milk for up to 6 days and in water for up to 14 days. There is no evidence of sexual transmission.

Pathophysiology of *Helicobacter pylori* Infection

Although most persons infected with *H. pylori* are asymptomatic, approximately 15% develop peptic ulcer disease (both gastric and duodenal ulcers) and about 0.05% develop gastric cancer or lymphoma. The World Health Organization has categorized *H. pylori* as a class 1 carcinogen.

H. pylori infection can be divided into an early stage, characterized by colonization of the host stomach, and a late stage, characterized by clinical disease. Colonization requires that the

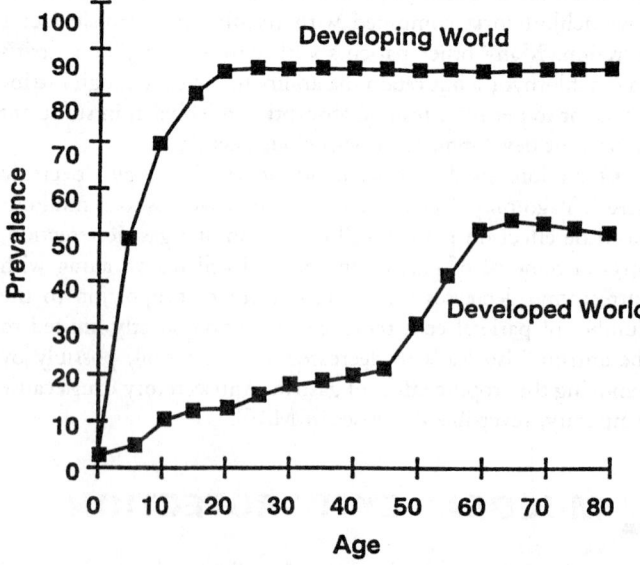

FIGURE 107.5. Age-specific prevalence of *Helicobacter pylori* infection in developing and developed countries of the world. (Modified from Marshall BJ. *Helicobacter pylori* gastritis. *Am J Gastroenterol* 1994; 89(suppl):S116–S128.)

organism overcome normal host defenses. Urease may be important in early colonization by creating a protective nonacidic microenvironment shielding the organism from gastric juice. Urease-negative *H. pylori* mutants are unable to colonize the stomachs of experimental animals. Motility is another important colonization factor. Amotile mutant organisms without flagella are poor colonizers, presumably because these organisms cannot penetrate the mucus layer overlying the gastric epithelium. Adherence to the gastric epithelial layer is another essential factor enabling *H. pylori* to colonize the human stomach, because without this ability, organisms would be washed out with normal gastric emptying.

Various bacterial adhesion molecules that bind specifically to receptors on the gastric surface of mucus cells have been described. Thus, although organisms can be seen swimming freely in the gastric lumen, it appears that most are located within the unstirred mucous layer lining the gastric epithelium where ideal growth conditions prevail (i.e., low oxygen and high carbon dioxide tensions). Colonization also occurs in areas of gastric metaplasia containing surface mucus cells outside the stomach. The organism is noninvasive, and its subsequent effects are due to its products or possibly due to phagocytosis by mucosal immune cells.

Virulence factors associated with *H. pylori* infection can be divided into those that lead to gastritis (occurring in all infected persons) and those that lead to additional clinical disease entities (occurring only in some persons). Urease and various other enzyme products of *H. pylori* organisms are important in undermining mucosal integrity, thereby leading to gastritis. These effects all lead to an undermining of mucosal integrity, which predisposes to acid-peptic disease by decreasing mucosal cytoprotection. The Vac A gene, which encodes for a toxin that causes vacuolization of infected culture cells, is present in all *H. pylori* isolates, but only 50% of them express the toxin. Vac A cytotoxin has been associated with the development of peptic ulcer disease. Cag A is also a marker for pathogenicity. The precise function of the Cag A protein has not yet been elucidated, but expression of Cag A is associated with peptic ulcer disease as well as gastric cancer and lymphoma. Two other virulence genes have been described: the Pic B gene, which may act as an amplifier of Cag A, and the Ice A gene, which appears to be important in bacterial adherence.

One of the unique features of *H. pylori* infection is the organism's ability to survive symbiotically within its human host despite inducing a robust immune response. Because the organism itself is not invasive, the host response must be due to bacterial products that diffuse across the basement membrane into the gastric mucosa or are taken up by M cells in Peyer's patches of the intestine. The immune response is probably ineffective because the organism stimulates a predominantly TH2 (antibody) response, which is unable to eradicate the infection even though secretory immunoglobulin (IgA) is produced. Tissue injury is probably mediated by the organism's ability to induce host production of interleukin-8 and other cytokines from cells within the gastric mucosa. This results in chemotaxis of activated polymorphonuclear leukocytes, which release various secondary substances that induce an inflammatory response. A lymphoproliferative response is also characteristic of chronic *H. pylori* infection.

The host inflammatory response is probably important in altering membrane permeability, permitting "off shore" organisms to obtain nutrition from the colonized host. For the development of disease processes other than gastritis, additional host factors may be required. In support of this theory, gastric metaplasia of the duodenal bulb and gastric acid hypersecretion appear to be important for the development of duodenal ulceration, whereas gastric atrophy (and relative hypochlorhydria) may be important for the development of gastric ulceration or gastric carcinoma. Patients with an excessive lymphoproliferative response may be predisposed to the development of gastric lymphoma.

OTHER SPECIFIC CAUSES OF GASTRITIS

Specific infiltrative diseases of the stomach may cause gastritis associated with pain. Ménétrier's disease (hypertrophic gastritis associated with protein-losing enteropathy), tuberculosis, syphilis, sarcoidosis, and eosinophilic granuloma of the stomach are rare gastric diseases that may be symptomatic. Chronic autoimmune gastritis (with or without pernicious anemia) is characterized by infiltration of the gastric mucosa by chronic inflammatory cells early on leading to loss of gastric glands and intestinal metaplasia as it progresses. The condition is generally asymptomatic and is associated with achlorhydria due to autoimmune-mediated loss of parietal cells. *Helicobacter heilmannii* (formerly *Gastrospirillum hominus*) is another spiral bacterium that occasionally infects humans. It is far more rare than *H. pylori* infection, tends to cause a less exuberant inflammation, and is believed to be nonpathogenic. Peptic ulceration is rare with all these other specific causes of gastritis.

■ EFFECTS OF *HELICOBACTER PYLORI* GASTRITIS ON NORMAL GASTRIC PHYSIOLOGY

In acute *H. pylori* infection, hypochlorhydria may accompany the acute gastritis, which is mediated by bacterial proteins. Epidemic achlorhydria has been described in institutional outbreaks as well as in studies in which the organism has been iatrogenically transmitted through nasogastric tubes. The inhibition of acid output in these patients continues for weeks to months but recovers in most individuals within about 9 months. It is unclear whether persons with persistent hypochlorhydria are especially predisposed to ultimately developing gastric atrophy.

The effects of chronic *H. pylori* infection on gastric acid secretion results in a spectrum of effects from hypergastrinemia and gastric acid hypersecretion on one extreme to hypo- or even achlorhydria on the other extreme. In antral predominant gastritis, a major effect appears to be exerted on somatostatin-secreting D cells, such that the feedback inhibition of luminal acid on antral gastrin release is altered. Consequently, hypergastrinemia leads to excessive stimulation of ECL and parietal cells and mild acid hypersecretion. Meal-stimulated gastrin release is also excessive in patients with chronic *H. pylori* infection. Thus, chronic antral predominant infection leads to antral G-cell hyperfunction, inappropriate hypergastrinemia, hypersecretion of acid, and the potential for duodenal ulcer disease. Progressively lesser degrees of hypergastrinemia and hypersecretion have been noted in patients with *H. pylori*-positive nonulcer dyspepsia and asymptomatic infections.

In pangastritis or corpus-predominant infection, parietal cell function is altered by local *H. pylori*-induced inflammation, and secretory responses are inhibited. Tumor necrosis factor-α is felt to be one of the more important mediators of this effect. Thus, chronic *H. pylori* infection involving the acid secretory component of the stomach ultimately leads to hypo- or achlorhydria and gastric atrophy. Gastric ulceration may develop in affected patients owing to a loss of mucosal cytoprotection as long as the environment is not totally anacidic. Hypergastrinemia in these patients may result from both a physiologic response to a decrease in acid output and antral D-cell dysfunction leading to G-cell hyperfunction. Long-standing gastric atrophy may ultimately progress to intestinal metaplasia and possibly gastric carcinoma. *H. pylori* is also associated with gastric lymphomas, which sometimes occur in mucosa-associated lymphoid tissue, called *maltomas*. Maltomas may regress after *H. pylori* eradication. Figure 107.6 summarizes the disease states associated with *H. pylori* infection.

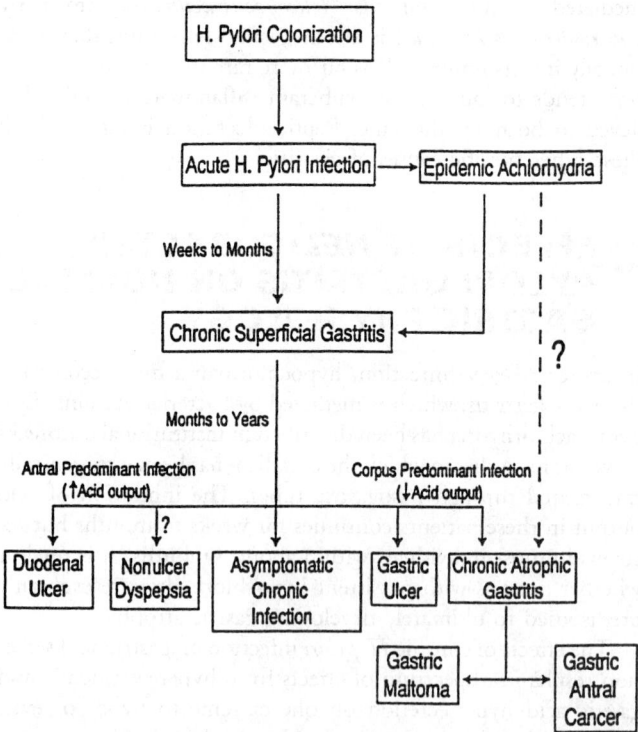

FIGURE 107.6. Algorithm describing the potential outcomes of *Helicobacter pylori* infection in susceptible persons. Acute gastritis (sometimes with epidemic achlorhydria) develops in virtually all colonized persons and progresses to chronic superficial gastritis. Patients with antral-predominant infection develop relative gastric hypersecretion and become predisposed to duodenal ulceration (and possibly nonulcer dyspepsia). Patients with corpus-predominant pangastritis develop relative gastric hyposecretion and become predisposed to gastric ulceration (and possibly gastric carcinoma or maltoma). Most patients with chronic infection remain asymptomatic throughout life.

ULCER PATHOPHYSIOLOGY

Ulcers are formed when the mucosa of the stomach or duodenum cannot resist the corrosive effects of acid on its surface. Exogenous factors, primarily *H. pylori* infection and NSAID usage, contribute to the formation of most peptic ulcers. Peptic ulceration occurs in about one in six patients with *H. pylori* infection. Conversely, approximately 70% of all gastric ulcers and about 90% of all duodenal ulcers are a consequence of *H. pylori* infection. Most non–*H. pylori*-associated peptic ulcers are due to NSAIDs. Hypersecretory states such as Zollinger–Ellison syndrome account for a minority of cases of peptic ulcer. In approximately 20% of patients with duodenal ulcers, none of these predisposing factors can be identified.

Gastric ulcer is not associated with any consistent abnormality in acid secretion, although some acid is needed for gastric ulcer formation. Gastric ulcer in the setting of achlorhydria, therefore, usually indicates gastric cancer. Ulcers of the gastric body are associated with altered mucosal defenses (due to *H. pylori* infection or NSAID use) with sufficient acid secretion to account for pepsin activation and autodigestion of the gastric mucosa. However, patients with distal antral ulcers, pyloric channel ulcers, or gastric ulcers associated with duodenal ulcers have mild gastric acid hypersecretion, similar to those found in idiopathic duodenal ulcer disease wild.

After *H. pylori* gastritis, prostaglandin deficiency is the next most important cause of altered mucosal defense leading to peptic ulceration in the presence of activated pepsin. Prostaglandins are produced by cyclooxygenases in the gastric mucosa. Inhibition of cyclooxygenase by aspirin or other NSAIDs is associated with acute gastropathy and peptic ulcers. Elderly patients taking high doses or combinations of NSAIDs, especially those with a history of peptic ulcer disease, have a particular risk for peptic ulceration (Table 107.1). The pathophysiologic mechanism for ulcer formation is presumed to be decreased mucosal production by cyclooxygenase of prostaglandin E_1 and E_2. These prostaglandins normally inhibit acid secretion, stimulate bicarbonate secretion, and mucous secretion, and maintain mucosal blood flow. Two forms of cyclooxygenase are in the stomach. The constitutively expressed cyclooxygenase-1 (COX-1) appears to be more important in maintaining mucosal integrity than the inducible

TABLE 107.1.	ESTABLISHED RISK FACTORS FOR NSAID-RELATED DAMAGE

Ulcer history
Older age
High-dose NSAID therapy
Combinations of NSAIDs
Recent use of NSAIDs
Corticosteroid use

NSAIDs, nonsteroidal anti-inflammatory drugs.
The role of alcohol consumption, tobacco use and low socioeconomic status in promoting NSAID damage remains unproven. There is no evidence for synergy between NSAIDs and *Helicobacter pylori* infection.

TABLE 107.2.	RELATIVE ULCEROGENIC RISK OF NSAIDS AND ASPIRIN
Very low	COX II inhibitors[a]
Low	Diflunisal (Dolobid)
	Diclofenac (Voltaren)
	Ibuprofen (Motrin)
	Salsalate (Disalcid)
Medium	Fenoprofen (Nalfon)
	Ketoprofen (Orudis)
	Naproxen (Naprosyn)
	Sulindac (Clinoril)
	Aspirin
High	Azapropazone
	Meclofenamate (Meclomen)
	Indomethacin (Indocin)
	Piroxicam (Feldene)
	Tolmetin (Tolectin)

COX, cyclooxygenase.
[a] COX II inhibitors may delay healing of active ulcers.

COX-2. NSAIDs that inhibit COX-2 more than COX-1 may produce fewer ulcers than those that are very active against COX-1 (Table 107.2).

As mentioned previously, bicarbonate secretion into the unstirred mucous layer adjacent to the gastric mucosa maintains local pH close to 7 until the pH of the gastric contents falls below 2. Decreased local secretion of bicarbonate in both gastric and duodenal ulcer patients undermines this protective pH gradient. The decreased bicarbonate release typical of idiopathic duodenal ulcer disease can be reversed by cure of *H. pylori* infection, suggesting that it is a secondary phenomenon. On the other hand, pancreatic bicarbonate secretion is normal or increased in patients with ordinary duodenal ulcer disease.

Most patients with idiopathic duodenal ulcer disease have normal to slightly elevated rates of basal acid secretion. The average maximal acid secretion rate in duodenal ulcer patients is 50% to 100% higher than that in the normal population, and the average basal acid secretion rates also are higher than those in the normal population to about the same extent. The mild acid hypersecretion in idiopathic peptic ulcer disease is most likely due to antral-predominant *H. pylori* infection, which accounts for most cases.

Rarely, peptic ulceration does occur exclusively from excessive acid hypersecretion. Zollinger–Ellison syndrome is the prototypical example of such a condition. The continuously high rate of acid secretion accounts for the especially severe duodenal ulcers seen in patients with this syndrome. In addition, delivery of large acid loads to the small intestine results in an osmotic diarrhea, inactivation of pancreatic lipase with resultant fat malabsorption, and proximal small intestinal dilatation. Acid hypersecretion is the only important pathophysiologic factor in Zollinger–Ellison syndrome, and control of the acid hypersecretion with antisecretory drugs abolishes all the symptoms of gastrinoma. Hyperhistaminemia is another rare cause of basal acid hypersecretion. Patients with systemic mastocytosis or basophilic leukemia may have a clinical syndrome that resembles Zollinger–Ellison syndrome with acid hypersecretion due to excessive histamine stimulation of parietal cells but without hypergastrinemia. Idiopathic hypersecretion, defined as a basal acid output of more than 10 mmol per hour without hypergastrinemia or other obvious explanation, is much more common than Zollinger–Ellison syndrome. Most, if not all, of these persons have antral-predominant *H. pylori* infection. Vagal hyperactivity is an alternative cause of the hypersecretion in these patients.

Increased psychological stress has often been associated with gastrointestinal symptoms suggestive of peptic ulcer. It has been difficult to demonstrate any consistent pattern of environmental stress associated with new ulcer craters in patients on ulcer maintenance trials receiving either antiulcer drugs or placebos. It is likely that some subpopulations of ulcer patients have psychological trigger mechanisms that favor recurrence of ulcers. However, no mechanism for the psychological induction of ulcers has been defined. Symptoms of nonulcer dyspepsia, a form of functional bowel disease, often are worsened by stress and may be confused with stress-induced ulcer symptoms.

Stress ulcer is the term given to gastric mucosal lesions that arise in the setting of trauma, shock, hemorrhage, sepsis, burns, or other severe medical illness. The lesions may be diffuse or solitary ulcers or erosions. The body of the stomach rather than the antrum is involved most often. These lesions often bleed. The incidence of stress ulcer has decreased markedly in recent years. This improvement may be due to better management of hypovolemia and sepsis, but it also may reflect increased prophylactic use of antacids and antisecretory agents in patients at risk in intensive care settings. Gastric acid is required for stress ulcers to form, but patients rarely have acid hypersecretion. The formation of these lesions probably can be explained best by a combination of mucosal ischemia and systemic acidosis. Lesions do not form if the pH in the gastric lumen is kept above 3.5 to 4. Lesions appear to form only when mucosal blood flow is diminished. Acidosis increases the severity of the lesions, and correction of acidosis decreases their formation. The presence of bile acids, alcohol, or NSAIDs in the gastric lumen may accentuate the lesions. Also, cancer chemotherapeutic agents can enhance formation of such lesions.

◼ PEPTIC ULCER

NATURAL HISTORY

Initial Healing

About 80% of cases of duodenal ulcer treated with H_2-receptor antagonists, H^+,K^+-ATPase inhibitors, antacids, sucralfate, or bismuth compounds heal within 4 weeks, and more than 90% heal within 12 weeks. Untreated patients with duodenal ulcer often have no symptoms within 2 weeks of diagnosis, but only 20% to 50% of untreated duodenal ulcers heal within 4 weeks. Treated patients become asymptomatic more rapidly than the ulcer heals. Patients with gastric ulcer take longer to heal than those with duodenal ulcer. Large ulcers take longer to heal than small ulcers, and smoking is the major environmental factor associated with slow ulcer healing. Young women and patients with NSAID-induced gastric ulcers exhibit especially rapid healing.

About 15% to 20% of duodenal ulcers and about 30% of gastric ulcers fail to heal after 4 to 6 weeks of treatment with H_2-receptor antagonists. Proton pump inhibitors produce somewhat better initial healing rates. About 50% of the unhealed ulcers heal after the treatment period is doubled. Less than 5% of patients are extremely resistant to treatment with standard medical therapy. Patients with Zollinger–Ellison syndrome fall into this category. Such patients often respond to more complete inhibition of acid secretion with higher doses of proton pump inhibitors. Occasionally, they may require surgery. Patients with a gastric ulcer that does not heal after 12 weeks should receive special consideration for surgery because of the possibility of an undiagnosed cancer.

Recurrence

Peptic ulcer disease is characterized by recurrent episodes of ulceration. About 75% of patients with a single prior episode of gastric or duodenal ulcer experience a second ulceration if *H. pylori* is not eradicated. The usual site of recurrence is close to the initial crater. Recurrences occur in about one-third, one-half, and two-thirds of patients within 3, 6, and 12 months of ulcer healing, respectively. Most of these recurrences are symptomatic, but about one-fourth are painless.

Factors that decrease the likelihood of ulcer relapse include first episode of ulcer, youth, female sex, discrete use of NSAIDs that are subsequently avoided, and not smoking. Maintenance therapy with nocturnal H_2-receptor antagonists reduce the recurrence rate from over two-thirds at 1 year to approximately one-fourth, although cure of *H. pylori* infection is the most important factor in preventing recurrence. Older studies showed that cure of *H. pylori* infection reduces the recurrence rate to less than 10%, although more recent studies in the United States have uncovered a curious form of peptic ulcer that recurs after effective cure of *H. pylori* infection in up to 25% of patients. Patients with a history of chronic, recurrent ulcer disease, smokers who continue to smoke, NSAID users who continue to use NSAIDs, and patients with endoscopic or radiographic evidence of a scarred duodenal bulb are more likely to have early recurrences.

Complications

Gastrointestinal hemorrhage is the most common complication of peptic ulcer disease and is the leading cause of death associated with ulcers. The incidence of bleeding in patients with peptic ulcer may be as high as 10% to 20%. This figure is difficult to establish because many ulcers are discovered only because of bleeding (i.e., patients present with bleeding de novo). Patients who have one episode of bleeding are more likely to have bleeding from recurrent ulcers than are patients who have experienced peptic ulcers without bleeding. In patients with recurrent symptomatic ulcer disease, the incidence of bleeding probably is less than 2% over 10 years. In contrast, up to one-third of patients with a single episode of bleeding have more bleeding within 1 or 2 years.

Ulcer bleeding is caused by erosion of the ulcer (diameter ≥ 0.5 mm) into an artery. About 80% of bleeding ulcers stop without specific treatment; the rest require either endoscopic hemostasis or surgery. There is some evidence that high doses of proton pump inhibitors decrease persistent or recurrent bleeding, but the usual antisecretory therapy has little or no effect. Twenty percent of patients with a bleeding ulcer that stops have recurrent bleeding within 2 weeks. The most useful endoscopic sign that predicts recurrent bleeding is the visible vessel, a segment of artery that protrudes into the base of the ulcer crater. Patients with this sign may benefit especially from prophylactic endoscopic hemostasis.

The mortality rate from bleeding peptic ulcers (for many years, about 8% to 10%) may now be starting to decline as a consequence of aggressive endoscopic management in recent years. The cause of death has also changed. Otherwise healthy patients rarely die of ulcer hemorrhage. Death most often occurs in older patients with one or more associated serious illnesses, such as cardiorespiratory failure, malignancy, or burns.

Recurrence of bleeding after healing of an actively bleeding ulcer also is common. This type of rebleeding may occur at any time but is most common in the first 2 years after an initial bleeding episode. Each episode of bleeding carries about a 30% to 40% risk of another bleeding episode in the patient's lifetime. Continued use of NSAIDs increases the chance of rebleeding. Recurrent bleeding can be decreased by diminishing acid secretion surgically or by long-term treatment with antisecretory drugs. *H. pylori* eradication also decreases the risk of recurrent bleeding.

Delayed gastric emptying can be caused either by mechanical obstruction to gastric outflow or by functional disturbances of gastroduodenal motility. In peptic ulcer disease, mechanical obstruction results from scarring or edema of the duodenal bulb or pyloric canal. Duodenal ulcer is the most common cause, but gastric ulcer, especially in the pyloric channel, may also cause obstruction. Acute antisecretory therapy may reduce edema and restore normal gastric emptying in some patients. Patients who do not respond rapidly and who do not develop normal gastric emptying within 2 or 3 days of continuous nasogastric suction and acid inhibition usually require surgical treatment.

Gastric outlet obstruction is a relatively rare complication of peptic ulcer disease in the United States, occurring in less than 2% of patients with duodenal or gastric ulcer. Recurrent obstruction is common in patients with a previous episode of obstruction managed by medical treatment. Many of these patients require surgical treatment.

Perforation, a dramatic complication of peptic ulcer disease, is relatively rare, affecting less than 2% of peptic ulcer patients. Although patients may develop de novo perforation, a history of ulcer symptoms is common. The average duration of symptoms before perforation is 5 years. Patients with Zollinger–Ellison syndrome are more likely to present initially with an ulcer complication such as perforation than are patients with idiopathic peptic ulcer disease. Penetration of ulcers into the pancreas may cause pancreatitis or pain that mimics pancreatitis. Leakage into the lesser sac can lead to the formation of an inflammatory mass or abscess.

Penetration or perforation can also lead to the formation of fistulae between the stomach or duodenum and nearby organs. Gastrocolic fistula may be secondary to gastric ulcer, but this complication is far more commonly due to malignant tumors. Fistulae may develop between the duodenum and the bile duct in patients with duodenal ulcer. Perforation almost always is treated surgically, but penetration may be treated medically unless a specific complication develops that requires surgical therapy.

CLINICAL PRESENTATION OF PEPTIC ULCER DISEASE

Peptic ulcer is a major consideration in the differential diagnosis of epigastric pain or discomfort. Although the characteristic pain is a dull ache in the epigastrium relieved by food or antacids, there are many variations. For example, duodenal ulcer pain is midepigastric in only about 80% of patients. About 15% of patients have right upper quadrant pain, and 5% have left upper quadrant pain. In addition, about 25% of duodenal ulcer patients have pain that sometimes radiates into the back, and up to 50% have heartburn in association with epigastric pain. Bleeding ulcers may be painless and manifest as hematemesis, melena, anemia, or even hematochezia. Patients with perforated ulcers typically present with severe generalized abdominal pain associated with signs of peritonitis (the acute abdomen). Patients with ulcer-induced gastric outlet obstruction may present with repeated episodes of vomiting, leading to dehydration and chloride depletion.

It is usually impossible to distinguish between duodenal ulcer and gastric ulcer by symptoms alone. The pain of both gastric and duodenal ulceration is typically located in the epigastrium and is episodic. Other features common to both gastric and duodenal ulcers include the intensity and quality of the pain, its radiation to the back (in about 25%), the high frequency of symptom relief with antacids and association with other symptoms such as bloating or belching (in about 50%).

However, the occurrence of certain features of peptic ulcer disease differs between duodenal and gastric ulcer patients. Duodenal ulcer pain typically occurs at night, especially within the first few hours of reclining. It is less common on arising. Food ingestion does not tend to induce duodenal ulcer pain and often relieves it. One-fourth to one-third of patients cannot relate their pain to any variable such as diet or time of day. About 50% of duodenal ulcer patients complain of intense pain at some time, but less than 20% describe the pain as "gnawing." Duodenal ulcer pain characteristically occurs in clusters, interspersed with relatively symptom-free intervals but about 30% of patients with duodenal ulcer have pain almost every day. Anorexia, nausea, vomiting, and weight loss are not typically considered symptoms of uncomplicated duodenal ulcer, but surveys of duodenal ulcer patients find that between 25% and 50% of patients report these symptoms in various combinations. About 20% of patients with duodenal ulcer have increased appetite, possibly because food relieves their symptoms.

Symptoms that may suggest gastric ulcer are pain that occurs within 30 minutes after eating, continuous rather than episodic pain, anorexia, nausea, vomiting, and weight loss. These symptoms also are more common in gastric cancer. Heartburn is somewhat less common in gastric ulcer than in duodenal ulcer. Ulcers that lie in the pyloric channel are a subtype of gastric ulcer that are especially likely to produce food-induced symptoms, including pain, nausea, and vomiting. A history of NSAID ingestion is more common in patients with gastric ulcer than in those with duodenal ulcer, but nonspecific epigastric symptoms commonly occur with no ulceration at all in patients who take these agents.

The physical examination is not useful in establishing the diagnosis of uncomplicated peptic ulcer. Midepigastric tenderness is a common but nonspecific finding. The physical examination is useful to exclude other potential causes of epigastric pain, such as musculoskeletal tenderness, neuropathy, and abdominal masses. The succussion splash, a sign that the stomach contains excessive air and fluid, is suggestive of gastric outlet obstruction. Patients with free perforation of ulcers usually have abdominal rigidity and signs of generalized peritonitis. Patients with localized ulcer perforations may have more subtle and localized physical findings.

DIFFERENTIAL DIAGNOSIS OF PEPTIC ULCER

Because of the significant variation in presentation of patients with duodenal or gastric ulcer, no rigid set of symptoms and signs can be considered typical of an ulcer. The only reliable method of definitively diagnosing a gastric or duodenal ulcer, nonulcer dyspepsia, or gastric cancer is endoscopic or radiographic examination (see "Diagnosis of Peptic Ulcer Disease"). The differential diagnosis of peptic ulceration is thus an important consideration in all patients presenting with epigastric pain (Table 107.3).

Nonulcer Dyspepsia

Ulcerlike symptoms without evidence of an ulcer crater is known as nonulcer dyspepsia (NUD). This condition is at least as common as peptic ulcer and cannot be distinguished by history. The cause of NUD is unknown. Up to 50% of affected patients have delayed gastric emptying. However, there is a very poor correlation between changes in symptoms and changes in gastric emptying rates after administration of agents that accelerate gastric emptying; this suggests that motility disturbances may be an effect rather than a cause of the syndrome. Patients with NUD often are hypersensitive to balloon distention of the stomach, suggesting an important neural role in the pathogenesis of

TABLE 107.3.	DIFFERENTIAL DIAGNOSIS OF DYSPEPSIA

Peptic ulcer disease (gastric and duodenal)
Nonulcer (functional) dyspepsia
Gastroesophageal reflux disease
Drug-induced dyspepsia and gastropathy
Gastric or duodenal tumors (benign, malignant)
Crohn's disease of the stomach and duodenum
Pancreatic disease (benign, malignant)
Hepatobiliary disease
Neuromuscular pain

this condition. The diagnosis of NUD usually is applied to patients who have epigastric symptoms lasting for more than 4 weeks and in whom appropriate diagnostic evaluation, including upper gastrointestinal endoscopy, reveals no obvious cause for the pain. There are no definite clinicopathologic correlates for patients with NUD. Features that suggest NUD rather than peptic ulcer are onset at an earlier age, female sex, precipitation by food, daily occurrence, impaired sleep pattern, relative rarity of gnawing pain, and worsening of symptoms during periods of stress.

Attempted *H. pylori* eradication often is the initial approach to management of dyspeptic patients with positive *H. pylori* serology without further diagnostic workup. This treatment effectively prevents recurrent peptic ulcer but produces long-term benefit in only a minority of patients with *H. pylori*-positive NUD. Patients with NUD often respond to antacids or H_2-receptor antagonists in about the same way as patients with peptic ulcer. This therapeutic approach may suffice for symptomatic treatment, but it does not provide useful diagnostic information or guidance for treatment if the pain recurs. Other drugs that may be useful are prokinetic drugs to increase gastric emptying and low doses of tricyclic antidepressants to reduce the pain threshold.

Gastroesophageal Reflux Disease

The cardinal symptom of reflux esophagitis is heartburn (also called pyrosis). Reflux pain may arise in the epigastrium, but it typically radiates into the chest. It is generally burning in nature, but it may also be felt as a constriction. Associated symptoms include regurgitation of food and acid into the mouth, difficulty swallowing (dysphagia), laryngeal or pulmonary symptoms (e.g., wheezing, coughing, hoarseness), and bleeding. Heartburn is typically caused by reflux of gastric juice (containing acid and activated pepsin) into the lower esophagus, but it may also be caused by reflux of bile or by local fermentation of ingested foodstuffs (as can occur in achalasia). Symptoms of heartburn are increased under conditions of increased abdominal pressure (e.g., during pregnancy, when bending over or straining), during food ingestion (food increases acid secretion and certain foodstuffs such as garlic, fat, and chocolate decrease lower esophageal sphincter tone), or when the person is supine rather than upright. Thus, heartburn commonly occurs at night, and it may awaken the person from sleep.

Distinguishing typical heartburn from the abdominal symptoms of peptic ulcer is generally not difficult because typical ulcer pain does not have a retrosternal radiation. However, up to 50% of ulcer patients (especially those with duodenal ulcer) also have heartburn. These patients are likely to have both esophageal reflux and peptic ulcer. Therefore, the presence of heartburn should not sway the physician away from considering a peptic ulcer.

Gastritis and Drug-Induced Dyspepsia

Except for the typical endoscopic findings that occur with erosive gastropathy due to NSAID ingestion, gastritis is a histologic diagnosis that requires tissue biopsy. Erythema found on endoscopic examination is insufficient for a diagnosis of gastritis, whether it occurs with or without abdominal pain. Moreover, a clinical diagnosis of gastritis cannot be made based on the presence of epigastric pain with or without a history of ingestion of noxious agents, such as alcohol or NSAIDs.

There appears to be a poor correlation between the amounts of NSAIDs ingested and the subsequent development of pain or mucosal disease. Endoscopic studies have shown that NSAID-induced mucosal disease occurs in up to 50% of patients, but most often the lesions are asymptomatic and of unclear clinical significance. Furthermore, NSAID-associated pain may or may not be associated with mucosal disease. The ulcerogenic potential of aspirin is less than that of certain NSAIDs (e.g., indomethacin and piroxicam) but is greater than that of ibuprofen (Table 107.2). Thus, the only sure way of determining whether NSAID use is the cause of epigastric pain in a particular individual is to discontinue the agent.

Many other drugs cause epigastric distress, nausea, and sometimes vomiting, often in the absence of endoscopic findings. Nausea and vomiting are symptoms that typically occur with digitalis or theophylline toxicity or after chemotherapy for various malignancies. Certain chemotherapeutic agents (e.g., 5-fluorouracil) typically cause mucositis, which may occur anywhere along the gastrointestinal tract. Acute epigastric pain may also result from acute gastric inflammation (gastropathy) after ingestion of other noxious agents such as alcohol. However, there also is no way of clinically distinguishing the pain of acute gastropathy from that of peptic ulceration without an endoscopy. It is important to obtain a complete recent drug history in all patients with epigastric pain.

H. pylori gastritis is associated with abdominal pain when there is either gastric or duodenal ulceration. However, the association between *H. pylori* gastritis and NUD is controversial, with the prevailing view that pain is generally not a typical feature of the chronic gastritis of *H. pylori* infection but that a small subgroup of patients with NUD may have *H. pylori* gastritis–induced symptoms.

Epigastric pain indistinguishable from that of peptic ulceration is a feature of certain specific infiltrative diseases of the stomach, including Ménétrier's disease (hypertrophic gastritis associated with protein-losing enteropathy), tuberculosis, syphilis, sarcoidosis, and eosinophilic granuloma of the stomach. These conditions all are diagnosed by endoscopic or surgical biopsy.

Gastroduodenal Neoplasia

Upper gastrointestinal cancer (especially gastric carcinoma) is found in less than 2% of patients with epigastric pain. Symptoms especially suggestive of gastric cancer include continuous pain, early satiety, a persistent sensation of a full stomach, pain increased by food, nausea, vomiting, and weight loss. Age is not useful in distinguishing the pain of benign from malignant gastric disease because both are most common in the elderly. Most gastric carcinomas are seen as infiltrative lesions that are easily recognized endoscopically or by barium radiography. A small proportion of patients present with gastric ulceration that can be difficult to distinguish from a benign gastric ulcer. Patients known to be achlorhydric almost never develop benign gastric ulcers. On the other hand, most patients with gastric carcinoma produce some gastric acid. Therefore, achlorhydria is a useful finding in patients presenting with gastric ulceration, indicating probable malignancy, but the presence of acid is not helpful in distinguishing benign from malignant disease. Malignant ulcers commonly have heaped-up irregular margins, but this also may occur with benign ulcers. Failure of a gastric ulcer to heal with standard ulcer treatment is believed to be relatively specific for malignant ulcer. Therefore, histologic examination of biopsies taken from the ulcer base and margins and endoscopic confirmation of complete healing is recommended to rule out malignancy for gastric ulcers that occur in a setting of chronic *H. pylori* gastritis. In contrast, duodenal ulcers are almost never malignant.

Gastric lymphoma also may cause ulcerlike symptoms or may present with symptoms of gastric outlet obstruction, including vomiting and electrolyte depletion. Some gastric lymphomas (maltomas or other gastric non-Hodgkin's lymphomas) appear to be related to *H. pylori* infection and may regress after the organism is eradicated. Other malignant lesions that cause gastric outlet obstruction include pancreatic carcinoma and primary carcinoma of the duodenum, which is exceedingly uncommon.

Crohn's Disease

Crohn's disease may involve any portion of the alimentary tract from lips to anus. However, gastroduodenal Crohn's disease is uncommon; when it does occur, antecedent disease is commonly elsewhere in the gastrointestinal tract. Rarely, patients with primary gastroduodenal Crohn's disease present with epigastric symptoms indistinguishable from peptic ulceration. Radiologic studies may be useful in distinguishing gastroduodenal Crohn's disease from typical peptic ulcer disease in patients with established Crohn's disease elsewhere. However, duodenal involvement may produce a radiographic appearance resembling chronic duodenal ulcer disease so that endoscopic biopsy is generally more helpful. Duodenal or gastric biopsies may reveal inflammation with granulomas.

Pancreatic Disease

Acute or chronic pancreatitis, pancreatic pseudocyst, and pancreatic carcinoma all may produce upper abdominal pain. Pancreatic pain usually radiates into the back, but it may be primarily epigastric. Alternatively, peptic ulcer pain also sometimes radiates to the back. For example, penetration of a duodenal ulcer into the pancreas may lead to back pain and even cause pancreatitis. Pancreatic disease always should be considered in the differential diagnosis of epigastric pain, especially before making the diagnosis of NUD.

Hepatobiliary Disease

Symptoms of cholecystitis, biliary colic, or hepatitis can usually be distinguished readily from those of peptic ulceration. However, the pain of peptic ulceration is occasionally located in the right upper quadrant pain. Furthermore, nausea and vomiting may accompany hepatobiliary disease in addition to peptic ulceration.

Neurologic Syndromes

Acute or chronic pain arising from diseases of the lower thoracic spine may refer to the anterior abdomen. Nerve entrapment at the border of the rectus abdominis sheath or in surgical scars can also cause chronic abdominal pain. Epigastric pain should be distinguished from pain in the ribs or costochondral cartilage. Neuritis from herpes zoster or diabetic mononeuritis multiplex may involve the epigastric region. Careful examination including attention to the thoracic cage and vertebrae usually reveals the nature of the pain in these situations.

DIAGNOSIS OF PEPTIC ULCER DISEASE

Routine laboratory studies are not generally useful in establishing a primary diagnosis of peptic ulcer disease, but they may be useful in defining the specific cause of an ulcer or in classifying genetic subtypes of ulcer. *H. pylori* testing is essential in all patients with documented ulceration because cure of the infection significantly reduces the likelihood of a subsequent recurrence. Fasting serum gastrin and acid secretory measurements are the major methods for identifying or excluding a gastrinoma or other hypersecretory state. Serum calcium measurement is a good screening test for the presence of MEN-I–associated hyperparathyroidism. Hemoglobin and hematocrit measurements are useful for monitoring chronic or recurrent ulcer bleeding. Ultimately, however, peptic ulceration can be diagnosed only by endoscopy or by a barium radiographic study.

Diagnosis of *Helicobacter pylori* Gastritis

The diagnosis of *H. pylori* gastritis may be made using either invasive or noninvasive methods (Table 107.4). Invasive diagnostic methods detect organisms either directly (e.g., by histo-

TABLE 107.4.	DIAGNOSTIC TESTS FOR *HELICOBACTER PYLORI* INFECTION[a]	
Test	**Sensitivity (%)**	**Specificity (%)**
Invasive		
Histology	95	<100[b]
Culture	~60	100
Biopsy urease test	90–95	98–100
Noninvasive		
Serology[c]	95	95
Urea breath test	95–98	95–98
Stool antigen	95	95

[a] Published values in clinical trials may be somewhat higher than those encountered in clinical practice.
[b] Limited by observer error and histologic stains used.
[c] Not useful for post-therapy cure determination.

logic identification with appropriate stains or bacterial culture) or indirectly (e.g., by rapid urease testing of biopsy specimens). Noninvasive methods detect organisms indirectly either by identifying a humoral immune response to the infection (e.g., by serum antibody testing) or by detecting metabolites of the bacterial enzyme urease (e.g., by urea breath testing). Recently, a direct noninvasive stool antigen test that identifies bacterial antigens in stool has also become available.

The gold standard for the diagnosis of *H. pylori* infection is identification of organisms on endoscopic biopsy (at least two antral specimens taken 3 to 5 cm from the pyloris). Gastritis is readily apparent on standard histologic slides stained with hematoxylin and eosin, but it may be difficult to identify organisms with certainty using standard stains. Special silver-based stains including Giemsa, Warthin Starry, and Genta stains provide adequate sensitivity and specificity for diagnosing the infection histologically. Studies evaluating these special staining techniques have shown an accuracy of almost 100%, although certain investigators believe that inter- and intraobserver variability may confound the detection of organisms histologically.

The most specific method of diagnosing *H. pylori* infection is culture of antral biopsy specimens. However, this method has not become routine in clinical practice because the organism is fastidious and false-negative results are common. Cultures may become more important in future clinical practice because the likelihood of encountering a resistant organism increases (at present, metronidazole resistance can be as high as 60% in certain populations and clarithromycin resistance as high as 10% or more).

Rapid urease testing of biopsy specimens is a highly effective method of detecting *H. pylori* infection that is independent of pathologic interpretation bias. These tests all contain urea-impregnated agar and a pH indicator leading to a change in color if urease is present in the biopsy specimen. The sensitivity and specificity of rapid urease testing are more than 90%.

Antral biopsies should always be obtained if an ulcer is identified during upper endoscopy. However, noninvasive testing should be the primary diagnostic approach in patients who do not need endoscopy. Serologic testing is simple and widely available. The major factor determining the accuracy of antibody testing is the specificity of the antigen used. Early *H. pylori* antibody assays using sonicated extract of *H. pylori* organisms suffered from cross-reactivity with other *Helicobacter*-like organisms. The HMCAP antigen has been shown to be highly specific and is used in a number of commercially available antibody tests. Serologic tests are highly sensitive and specific, but they cannot distinguish between a previously treated *H. pylori* infection and a currently active one. However, with no prior course of therapy specifically directed against *H. pylori* infection, a positive antibody test implies active infection, because spontaneous bacterial clearance is extremely rare and monotherapy with antibiotics given for other reasons generally fails to cure the infection. Quantitative serologic tests are available as laboratory-based enzyme-linked immunosorbent assays (ELISAs), but rapid qualitative office-based immunoprecipitation serologic tests are almost as accurate.

Office-based qualitative testing kits either use serum that re-

quires centrifuged blood specimens or whole blood that requires only a fingerstick to provide a capillary tube of blood. These testing kits are potentially the diagnostic antibody tests of choice because of low cost and ease of performance, but they may not be as accurate as the serum tests. A potential limitation of all methods of antibody testing is the occasional patient who fails to generate a normal humoral immune response (less than 5% of patients).

The principle of urea breath testing relies on the fact that *H. pylori* organisms produce large amounts of urease. In the presence of *H. pylori* infection, ingested urea is acted on by bacterial urease releasing labeled carbon, which is absorbed, circulates as bicarbonate, and is exhaled as carbon dioxide. With no *H. pylori* infection, the ingested urea passes through the stomach, is absorbed in the small bowel, and is excreted unchanged in the urine. However, a fraction enters the colon and is metabolized to ammonia and carbon dioxide, so that urea breath testing is most accurate during the first hour after urea ingestion. Breath testing is especially useful for documenting cure of *H. pylori* gastritis after antibiotic therapy in addition to confirming active infection in patients who have negative antibodies.

Urea breath testing can be performed using two types of carbon labeling, the carbon-13 (^{13}C) urea breath test and the ^{14}C urea breath test. The ^{13}C test is nonradioactive, but the ^{14}C test available in the United States uses only 1 μCi of C^{14} providing a radiation exposure that is equivalent to $\frac{1}{30}$ of a chest x-ray per test. C^{13} breath analysis requires a mass spectrometry unit that is expensive and not generally available although breath samples can be mailed to an off-site laboratory for analysis. ^{14}C breath analysis is performed using a standard scintillation counter, which is available in most medical centers.

Stool antigen testing for *H. pylori* gastritis has also received approval by the Food and Drug Administration (FDA). Trials have shown this test to be extremely accurate for initial diagnosis and for confirming cure of *H. pylori* infection after antibiotics. The test identifies bacterial antigens in stool with an immunoprecipitation assay. Its cost is highly competitive, and it may become the noninvasive diagnostic modality of choice if patients demonstrate willingness to provide stool (instead of breath) for diagnosis.

H. pylori testing must be done without confounding factors that may cause false-negative results. For determination of cure, testing should not be performed any earlier than 4 weeks after completion of the antibiotic regimen. Testing earlier than 4 weeks cannot distinguish between antibiotic-induced suppression of infection and true cure. Furthermore, exposure to proton pump inhibitor medications, monotherapeutic antibiotic regimens, sucralfate, or bismuth compounds may also suppress an infection sufficiently to cause a false-negative test. These caveats apply similarly to biopsy and breath testing methods.

Fasting Serum Gastrin Measurements

Radioimmunoassay measurement of serum or plasma gastrin should be made in patients in whom gastrinoma is suspected on clinical or genetic grounds. Examples include duodenal ulcer patients with hypercalcemia or a family history of MEN-I, with

TABLE 107.5.	DIFFERENTIAL DIAGNOSIS OF HYPERGASTRINEMIA

Appropriate Hypergastrinemia

Antisecretory therapy (H_2-receptor antagonists or proton pump inhibitors)
Atrophic gastritis (with or without pernicious anemia)
Vagotomy
Chronic renal failure
Chronic *Helicobacter pylori* infection (pangastritis)

Inappropriate Hypergastrinemia

Zollinger–Ellison syndrome (gastrinoma)
Chronic *H. pylori* infection (antral predominant)
Retained antrum syndrome (after Billroth II gastrectomy)
Massive intestinal resection (transient)
Gastric outlet obstruction (reversible)

suspected or documented gastric acid hypersecretion (unexplained diarrhea or enlarged gastric folds), with ulcers refractory to ordinary medical management and any patient in whom ulcer surgery is planned.

Normal fasting serum gastrin concentrations are less than 100 pg per milliliter in most laboratories. Values are much higher in most patients with gastrinoma, but some gastrinoma patients have only a modest elevation of serum gastrin levels. Hypergastrinemia may be appropriate (i.e., a physiologic response to absent gastric acid secretion) or inappropriate (i.e., in the presence of gastric acid secretion; Table 107.5). Prolonged neutralization of gastric contents interrupts the normal inhibition of gastrin release by luminal acid and leads to increased serum gastrin and eventually to hyperplasia of G cells. Potent antisecretory drugs, including H_2-receptor antagonists and H^+,K^+-ATPase inhibitors, are the major causes of appropriate hypergastrinemia. H_2-receptor antagonists typically cause only mild elevations that do not persist for more than 24 hours.

The most common natural cause of appropriate hypergastrinemia is atrophic gastritis, especially the type associated with pernicious anemia. Other common causes of appropriate hypergastrinemia are surgical vagotomy, chronic renal failure, and the chronic pangastritis sometimes associated with *H. pylori* infection. Gastrinoma is the prototypical cause of inappropriate hypergastrinemia, but other causes exist as well. The most important of these is chronic antral-predominant *H. pylori* infection in which prolonged low-grade hypergastrinemia leads to antral G-cell hyperfunction. The retained antrum syndrome should also be considered in patients who previously have undergone ulcer surgery (specifically a Billroth II resection).

Most gastrinoma patients have an abnormal serum gastrin response to intravenous secretin injection. After a bolus injection of 2 units per kilogram of secretin, a prompt increase in serum gastrin of more than 200 pg per milliliter occurs in 87% of patients with gastrinoma. Similar increases are rarely obtained in patients with hypergastrinemia from other causes including achlorhydria, which highlights the fact that gastrinoma is best diagnosed by measuring serum gastrin and acid secretory mea-

surements at the same time to confirm inappropriate hypergastrinemia.

Acid Secretory Studies

Measurements of basal and stimulated gastric acid output can be made directly by nasogastric intubation and pentagastrin stimulation. Absence of acid after stimulation virtually excludes the diagnosis of peptic ulcer because it signifies true achlorhydria. MAO of less than 10 mmol per hour after pentagastrin stimulation is rare in patients with duodenal ulcer, but it does not rule out gastric ulcer in which the primary defect is due to a loss of mucosal cytoprotection. Increased acid output levels occur in about one-third of patients with duodenal ulcer. Increased basal acid output to above 10 mEq per hour is found in almost all patients with gastrinoma. However, most patients with basal acid output levels of more than 10 mEq per hour have idiopathic hypersecretion. Idiopathic hypersecretion is generally distinguished from gastrinoma by a normal serum gastrin level. Increasing the diagnostic threshold for gastrinoma to a basal acid output of 15 mEq per hour improves the diagnostic specificity but reduces the sensitivity of acid secretory testing.

Endoscopy

Upper gastrointestinal endoscopy permits direct visual examination of the esophageal, gastric, and proximal duodenal mucosa. Ulcers are seen as depressions with white or yellow bases surrounded by normal gastric or duodenal mucosa, often with erythematous or edematous edges. The sensitivity and specificity of endoscopic examination for the diagnosis of gastric and duodenal ulcers are over 90% in the hands of experienced endoscopists. Endoscopic criteria distinguishing ulcers from erosions include the appearance of depth and a size over 5 mm. Upper gastrointestinal endoscopy provides an opportunity to rule out other structural disease that may cause abdominal pain (e.g., erosive esophagitis and gastric cancer) and permits access for endoscopic biopsy of the gastrointestinal mucosa (i.e., to identify malignancy, Barrett's metaplasia, infiltrative gastropathies, Crohn's disease, or *H. pylori* infection). Material can also be obtained for culture.

Radiographic Examination

Most gastric and duodenal ulcers can be diagnosed by ordinary barium radiographic examinations. The greatest precision can be achieved by optimizing the radiographic technique and by using double-contrast radiography. Radiographic examination is somewhat less accurate than endoscopy for the diagnosis of small ulcers, especially those in scarred duodenal bulbs. Radiography is especially useful for identifying infiltrative diseases, such as lymphoma or linitis plastica and extrinsic compression of the stomach and duodenum by mass lesions.

TREATMENT OF PEPTIC ULCER DISEASE

Nonspecific Measures

Dietary manipulations are not of proven benefit in peptic ulcer disease. Milk and cream diets used in the past may have been harmful, because milk is a strong stimulant for acid secretion and cream can cause hyperlipidemia. High-fiber diets may be of modest benefit. Bland diets have no rationale or effectiveness and should not be prescribed for ulcer treatment. Because smoking is associated with poor healing and increased ulcer recurrence rates, discontinuation of smoking is a reasonable adjunct to ulcer treatment. However, no study has yet demonstrated a specific benefit in this approach. The role of alcohol restriction in patients with documented peptic ulcer is controversial. Patients with alcoholic cirrhosis have a higher rate of duodenal ulcer than does the general population, but ingestion of 1 to 2 ounces of alcohol per day by noncirrhotic persons does not adversely affect healing. However, heavy alcohol intake may increase the rate of ulcer recurrence after initial healing.

Discontinuation of aspirin or NSAIDs is important both for ulcer healing and for reducing recurrence rates. They should be replaced by acetaminophen, if possible. If they cannot be discontinued, an NSAID with relatively low ulcerogenic potential, such as ibuprofen, should be used. Studies are currently underway regarding specific COX-2 inhibitor NSAIDs that are likely to have a lower risk for peptic ulcer complications. Other measures that may decrease ulcer formation in NSAID-dependent patients are *H. pylori* eradication and chronic treatment with misoprostol or acid-inhibiting drugs.

Cure of *Helicobacter pylori* Infection

Cure of *H. pylori* gastritis accelerates the healing of *H. pylori*-associated duodenal and gastric ulcers, greatly diminishes the likelihood of ulcer relapse and may also decrease the likelihood of ulcer complications. Thus, effective antibiotic therapy in patients with active or remote peptic ulcers cures the disease as opposed to the use of maintenance antisecretory therapy which only limits ulcer diatheses by controlling acid output (Fig. 107.7). Recent studies in the United States have found that peptic ulcers may recur after effective cure of *H. pylori* infection in up to one-fourth of patients.

Evidence in support of anti-*H. pylori* therapy for other *H. pylori*-associated conditions also exists. For example, effective antibacterial therapy in patients with gastric lymphoma (90% of whom are infected with *H. pylori*) causes tumor regression in about 50% without the need for chemotherapy. In addition, many authorities recommend therapy for young *H. pylori*-positive undifferentiated dyspeptic patients without significant risk factors for serious underlying disease (i.e., no bleeding, dysphagia, weight loss, or anemia). The rationale for this approach is that it definitely benefits the 15% who have ulcers, and it may benefit some of the remainder who likely have functional pain, thus avoiding upper endoscopy in those who respond. The downside of this approach is that the precise cause of the pain

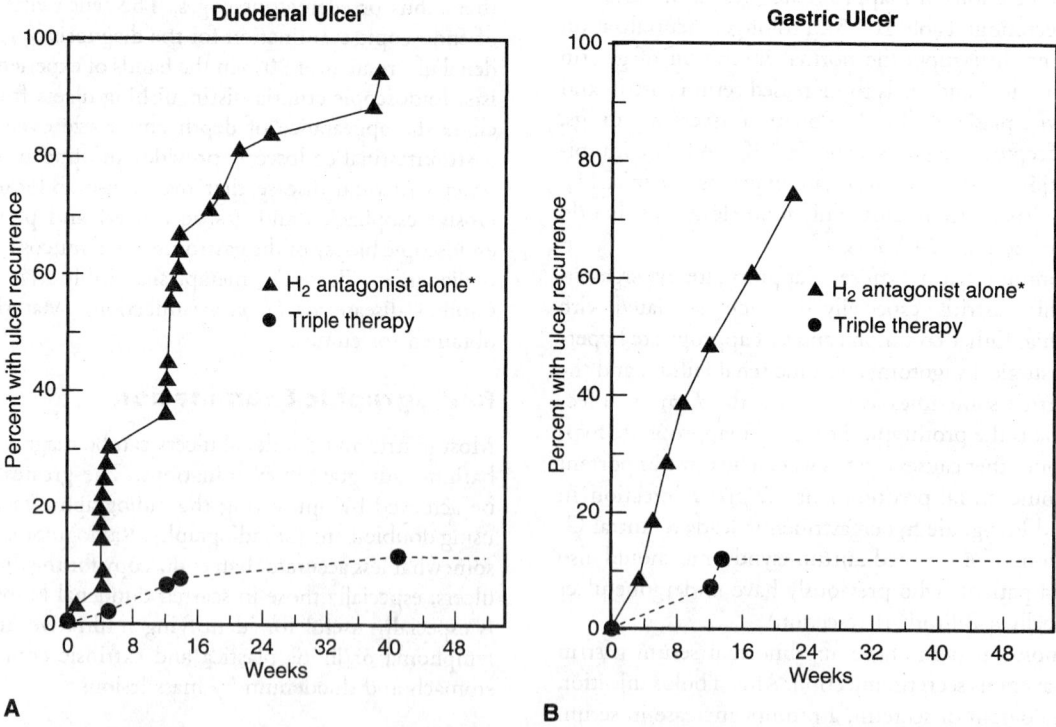

FIGURE 107.7. A: Life-table recurrence of duodenal ulcers for the year after successful healing with H₂-antagonist alone or triple therapy plus H₂-antagonist. **B:** Life-table recurrence of gastric ulcers for the year after successful healing with H₂-antagonist alone or triple therapy plus H₂-antagonist. (From Graham DY, Lew GM, Klein PD, et al. Effect of treatment of *Helicobacter pylori* infection on the long-term recurrence of gastric or duodenal ulcer: a randomized, controlled study. *Ann Intern Med* 1992; 116:705–708, with permission.) Recent US data have suggested that the recurrence rate after cure of *H. pylori* infection may be somewhat higher (approaching 20%).

may not be elucidated, that other non–*H. pylori*-associated conditions (e.g., Barrett's esophagus) may be missed, that antibiotic resistance may become a problem, and that this approach may not be cost-effective in the long term because patients may ultimately need endoscopy anyway. Because a relation between NUD and *H. pylori* is not generally accepted, most authorities would not favor treating nonulcer dyspeptics with antibiotics until all other possible causes for their dyspepsia have been excluded.

Further indications for anti-*H. pylori* therapy are somewhat controversial. These include elderly infected patients who require NSAIDs for long-term arthritic complaints and persons at significant risk for gastric antral cancer (e.g., persons with a strong family history of gastric cancer, persons from high-risk areas, or persons with previously recognized premalignant conditions diagnosed on endoscopic evaluation for some other indication). The prevailing thought is that there is insufficient evidence to recommend therapy for esophageal reflux patients who require maintenance proton pump inhibitor therapy (both conditions may predispose to atrophy but whether this is of any concern or not has not yet been shown). Despite these areas of controversy, there is clear agreement that one should test for *H. pylori* infection only if one is planning on treating a patient with a positive result.

The optimal therapeutic regimen for curing *H. pylori* infection is not yet established, but consensus is emerging that triple-therapy combinations should be used to ensure adequate cure rates. In addition to having a cure rate of over 90%, the ideal regimen should be simple and easily tolerated and have a low likelihood of inducing bacterial resistance. Standard triple therapy with metronidazole (250 mg t.i.d.), a bismuth compound (e.g., two chewable Pepto-Bismol tablets q.i.d), and tetracycline (500 mg q.i.d.) with meals (with standard doses of antisecretory therapy to heal ulcers as well) provides excellent results. The cure rate after completion of 14 full days of triple therapy was as high as 95% in controlled trials. In clinical practice, however, the true cure rate is lower because this regimen is poorly tolerated and patient compliance is a significant problem. Tetracycline can be replaced with amoxycillin (2 g per day in divided doses) for an improved side-effect profile, although efficacy is sacrificed slightly by making this substitution. Substituting clarithromycin instead (500 mg t.i.d.) may improve the side-effect profile without reducing overall efficacy. The FDA has approved a blister pack containing all the drug components of standard triple therapy (including the antisecretory agent for ulcer healing) under one label, called Helidac (Proctor & Gamble) with eradication rates of 77% to 82%, as detailed in the product labeling. Whether this packaging results in improved compliance is unknown.

An important component of standard triple therapy is bismuth. Bismuth has no efficacy as monotherapy for *H. pylori*, but it is extremely useful in combination regimens. Resistance to bismuth preparations has not been reported. Thus, by reducing the overall *H. pylori* burden significantly, this highly effective luminally active agent may limit the likelihood of resistance developing to other regimen components during therapy. Triple-therapy regimens consisting of 400 mg b.i.d. of ranitidine bismuth citrate (Tritec) with clarithromycin (500 mg q.i.d.) and

a second antibiotic (metronidazole or amoxicillin) also have excellent cure rates and are better tolerated than standard triple therapy.

Proton pump inhibitor–based triple therapy regimens are arguably the current regimens of choice for *H. pylori* therapy. The rationale for combining antibiotics with proton pump inhibitors such as omeprazole or lansoprazole is that the proton pump inhibitors appear to have independent activity against *H. pylori* organisms in vitro, possibly secondary to increasing gastric pH. Proton pump inhibitor therapy alone does not cure *H. pylori* gastritis. The FDA has approved proton pump inhibitor–based triple-therapy regimens consisting of lansoprazole (30 mg b.i.d.) or omeprazole (20 mg b.i.d.) combined with two antibacterial agents; amoxicillin (1 g b.i.d.); clarithromycin (500 mg b.i.d.); or metronidazole (500 mg b.i.d.). For example, 14 days of lansoprazole (30 mg b.i.d.) with amoxicillin (1 g b.i.d.) and clarithromycin (500 mg b.i.d.) was approved based on a cure rate of 86% to 92%. The MOC regimen, consisting of metronidazole (500 mg b.i.d.), omeprazole (20 mg b.i.d.), and clarithromycin (250–500 mg b.i.d.) also appears to be effective (over 90% cure rate) and well tolerated. A 7-day course of treatment may be sufficient.

Metronidazole should be avoided in patients who previously received metronidazole monotherapy for other indications (e.g., for vaginitis), because pretreatment resistance may be important in limiting efficacy. Metronidazole-containing regimens should also be avoided in patients who drink alcohol and who are unlikely to stop alcohol intake during treatment to avoid the possibility of a disulfuram effect from therapy. Little is known about the possible effect of clarithromycin resistance on the efficacy of second-generation triple-therapy regimens. Clarithromycin resistance is relatively uncommon at present but in time, with widespread use of clarithromycin monotherapy for other indications (e.g., respiratory tract infections), resistance may become more of a problem. In this situation, clarithromycin could be replaced with amoxicillin, although overall efficacy may be reduced. Amoxicillin resistance has been described but is extremely rare. An anti-*H. pylori* regimen for patients who have failed therapy with other regimens has been described by European investigators to include standard triple therapy plus omeprazole (so-called quadruple therapy). There is little experience with this regimen in the United States.

Monotherapy or dual therapy for *H. pylori* infection should be avoided (even though certain proton pump inhibitor dual therapy regimens with clarithromycin have been approved by the FDA). The most effective single agent appears to be clarithromycin with an efficacy of less than 50% (in doses of 500 mg q.i.d.). In addition to being relatively ineffective, these regimens run the risk of inducing organism resistance.

There is no evidence yet that widespread treatment of all patients with documented *H. pylori* infection leads to the elimination of, or even a significant reduction in, the worldwide prevalence of this ubiquitous infection. For worldwide eradication of *H. pylori* infection to occur, vaccine development will need to be successful. Currently, there are many problems involved in developing effective vaccines for *H. pylori*; nevertheless, ongoing work is promising.

TABLE 107.6.	ANTIULCER THERAPY

Histamine$_2$-receptor antagonists (cimetidine, ranitidine, famotidine, nizatidine)
Proton pump inhibitors (omeprazole, lansoprazole)
Antacids
Prostaglandins (misoprostil)
Anticholinergics
Sucralfate
Bismuth formulations

Medical Management of Peptic Ulcer Disease

Several drugs are effective for healing active peptic ulcers. Some may also decrease the rate of ulcer recurrence if given on a continuous basis after healing. Drugs that are effective fall into three major categories: those that inhibit acid secretion, those that neutralize acid secretion, and those that improve cytoprotection resulting in a local environment that permits healing to occur (Table 107.6).

H$_2$-Receptor Antagonists

Antagonism of the H$_2$-receptor on the gastric parietal cell markedly inhibits basal and stimulated gastric acid secretion. H$_2$-receptor antagonists including cimetidine, ranitidine, famotidine, and nizatidine all have similar activities but vary in potency. However, they are nearly equipotent in prescribed dosage formulations. A single dose of a H$_2$-receptor antagonist can inhibit acid secretion for 6 to 12 hours. H$_2$-receptor antagonists can produce prolonged inhibition if given as continuous intravenous infusions.

Oral H$_2$-receptor antagonist regimens for duodenal ulcer disease have evolved from multiple daily doses to a single nocturnal administration. A single nocturnal dose of drug produces the same healing response as do multiple doses. The most frequently recommended nocturnal doses that produce equivalent healing rates are 800 mg cimetidine (Tagamet), 300 mg ranitidine (Zantac) or nizatidine (Axid), and 40 mg famotidine (Pepcid). Nighttime administration inhibits nocturnal acid secretion but has no effect on secretion during the subsequent day. Experience with treatment of duodenal ulcer has indicated that nocturnal acid has a special role in duodenal ulcer pathogenesis.

After 4 weeks of treatment, about 80% of duodenal ulcer patients treated with H$_2$-receptor antagonists have complete healing of their ulcers, compared with about 40% healing in patients treated with placebo. About 50% of the remaining patients who have not healed at 4 weeks heal after another 2 to 4 weeks of treatment. Regardless of healing, most patients become asymptomatic within 2 weeks of treatment with active drug or placebo. The optimal H$_2$-receptor antagonist dosage schedule for treating gastric ulcers has not been established with certainty. Gastric ulcers heal more slowly than duodenal ulcers do, and most authorities recommend 6 to 8 weeks of therapy. With gastric ulcer, the healing rate is related to the size of the ulcer. Patients with a gastric ulcer larger than 1 cm may require 3

months or more for complete healing. The effectiveness of H$_2$-receptor antagonists for the management of acutely bleeding ulcers has not been shown conclusively. There is little, if any, effect on the percentage of patients with acute bleeding who stop bleeding spontaneously, even with high doses of drugs given by continuous intravenous infusion.

Maintenance therapy for recurrent ulcer prevention is also usually given as a single nocturnal dose. However, the dose itself is generally reduced by 50% (i.e., 400 mg cimetidine, 150 mg ranitidine or nizatidine, and 20 mg famotidine). Prophylactic H$_2$-receptor antagonists reduce the recurrence rate at 1 year from over two thirds to about one fourth of patients (Fig. 107.8). The effects of maintenance therapy on the occurrence of complications have not been established fully, but decreased incidence of recurrent bleeding from ulcers has been reported. Certain hypersecretory states, including Zollinger–Ellison syndrome (see text that follows), require more frequent administration of high-dose H$_2$-receptor antagonists (up to 7 g per day in divided doses up to every 4 hours). Patients with severe reflux esophagitis may also require multiple daily doses for good symptomatic responses. These patients and patients with Zollinger–Ellison syndrome may be managed more effectively with omeprazole or lansoprazole, longer-acting H$^+$,K$^+$-ATPase inhibitors.

The side effects of single nocturnal doses of H$_2$-receptor antagonists are minimal. Used in larger doses, such as for treatment of Zollinger–Ellison syndrome, cimetidine has some side effects not usually associated with the other agents. These include alterations in drug metabolism resulting from inhibition of hepatic production of cytochrome P-450 enzymes, gynecomastia due to a direct antiandrogen effect of the drug, and possibly increased confusion in older patients or metabolic encephalopathy in hospitalized patients with serious liver or kidney disease. All H$_2$-receptor antagonists can elicit allergic reactions, such as drug

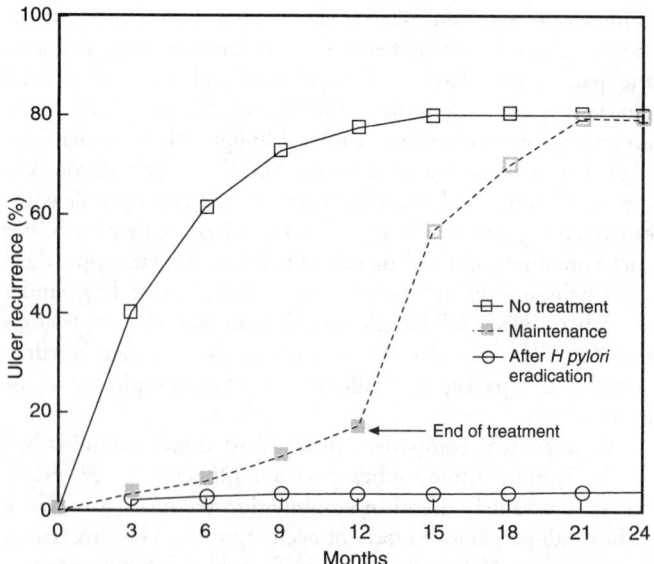

FIGURE 107.8. Recurrence rates for patients with healed duodenal ulcer are high during the first year after healing, but recurrences can be suppressed by nightly H$_2$-receptor blocker treatment. As soon as the H$_2$-blocker treatment is stopped, ulcers recur at their previous rapid rate.

rash and hepatitis, but these are rare. Thrombocytopenia has been reported as well, but its clinical significance is small.

H^+,K^+-ATPase (Proton Pump) Inhibitors

Omeprazole (Prilosec) and lansoprazole (Prevacid) are two H^+,K^+-ATPase inhibitors that are FDA-approved for use in patients with peptic ulcer disease in the United States. Additional H^+,K^+-ATPase inhibitors that may soon become available for general use are rabeprazole and pantoprazole. H^+,K^+-ATPase inhibitors have been used extensively in hypersecretory forms of peptic ulcer disease (in addition to gastroesophageal reflux disease). H^+,K^+-ATPase inhibitors are substituted benzimidazoles, which bind covalently to luminally active proton pumps via disulfide bonds at one of three essential transmembrane cysteines in the fifth or sixth transmembrane portion of the α subunit of the enzyme. This inactivates the parietal cell acid pump irreversibly with inhibition of all types of acid stimulation (Fig. 107.9). H^+,K^+-ATPase inhibitors have a prolonged half-life approximately equal to the time taken to regenerate intracellular H^+,K^+-ATPase, about 48 to 72 hours.

Proton pump inhibitors cause more rapid healing of duodenal and gastric ulcers than H_2-receptor antagonists and are now more commonly used than H_2-receptor antagonists for primary ulcer treatment. For example, ulcer healing rates after 2 weeks of therapy with proton pump inhibitors (omeprazole 20 mg or lansoprazole 30 mg once daily in the morning before breakfast) are roughly equal to the 4-week healing rates produced by H_2-receptor antagonists. Their efficacy in H_2-receptor antagonist–refractory duodenal ulcers has also been shown. The long-lasting profound inhibition of acid by omeprazole or lansoprazole has made these agents the drugs of choice for the treatment of Zollinger–Ellison syndrome. The therapeutic goal is to reduce acid secretion rates at less than 10 mEq per hour in patients with intact stomachs (less than 5 mEq per hour in those with prior gastric surgery). This generally requires twice-daily dosing. Proton pump inhibitors are also more effective than H_2-receptor antagonists for the treatment of erosive esophagitis.

Proton pump inhibitors have a better side-effect profile than do H_2-receptor antagonists. Hypochlorhydria-induced hypergastrinemia is more pronounced with proton pump inhibitors than with H_2-receptor antagonists because of a more profound and longer inhibition of gastric acid output. Achlorhydria causes hypergastrinemia as a consequence of loss of feedback inhibition of gastric mucosal G cells. In rats, high-dose H^+,K^+-ATPase inhibitor therapy given for 2 years produces severe ECL cell hyperplasia associated in some instances with carcinoid tumors of the stomach. In humans treated for up to 11 years, changes in ECL cells are minimal. ECL cell carcinoids occur in humans under only two hypergastrinemic conditions: MEN-I syndrome with Zollinger–Ellison syndrome and pernicious anemia. Other side effects of proton pump inhibitor used for brief periods to heal peptic ulcers are not significant.

Antacids

Antacids were the first agents proved to be more effective than placebo for acute duodenal ulcer healing. They have been used for centuries to treat dyspepsia. Development of H_2-receptor antagonists led to some loss of enthusiasm for antacids. A major objection to antacids was the high incidence of diarrhea caused by the large doses considered necessary for adequate neutralization of acid. Low-dose antacids have been found to heal ulcers effectively, a finding that could lead to an increased use of antacids as single agents for ulcer treatment because of the low cost and acceptable side effects of lower doses.

Most antacids are combinations of magnesium and aluminum hydroxides. The most prominent side effect of magnesium is diarrhea. The most obvious side effect of aluminum is constipation, but other metabolic effects may be more important. Aluminum hydroxide can lead to phosphate depletion and may cause metabolic bone disease in patients with renal failure. Calcium carbonate is an effective antacid, but it may cause hypercalcemia and acid rebound due to stimulation of gastrin release if large doses are used.

When antacids are given during fasting, neutralization of gastric pH is brief, lasting less than 30 minutes. On the other hand, antacids given 1 hour after meals can produce gastric neutralization for the next 2 hours. An additional dose 3 hours after a meal can add another hour of neutralization. Small doses of antacid, such as two antacid tablets four times a day, are as effective as higher doses. This dose of antacid does not neutralize gastric acidity well, despite its efficacy for healing. Since all low-dose antacid regimens shown to heal ulcers have contained aluminum, the aluminum rather than the neutralization may be the important therapeutic factor. Low-dose antacid therapy is effective for duodenal or gastric ulcers. Tablets are as effective as liquids.

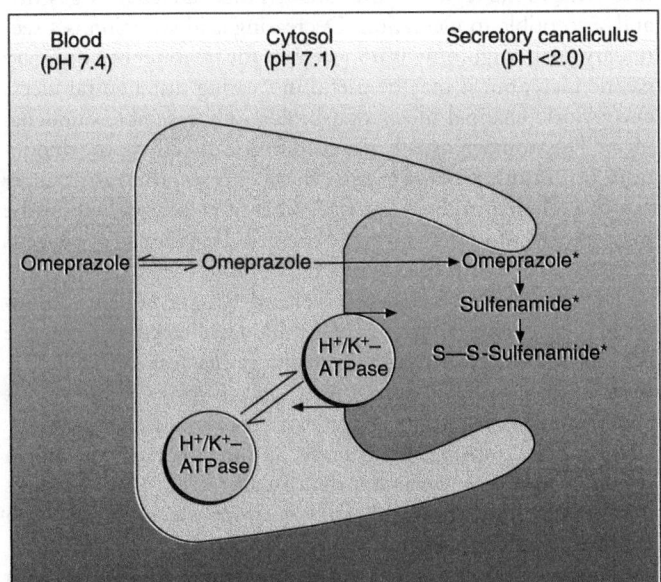

FIGURE 107.9. Action of omeprazole on a gastric parietal cell. With the appropriate stimulus, the H^+,K^+-ATPase can move from cytoplasmic vesicles (where it is inactive) to the secretory canalicular membrane (where it is active). Omeprazole enters the cytoplasm freely. In the canaliculus, it is protonated and converted to a sulfenamide, which then is bound covalently by disulfide bonds to H^+,K^+-ATPase and inhibits secretion. (From Maton PN. Omeprazole. *N Engl J Med* 1991;324: 965–975, with permission.)

Prostaglandins

Prostaglandins are best known for their cytoprotective properties, but they may act primarily as acid inhibitors. Misoprostol, a prostaglandin E_1 analogue, inhibits acid secretion by activating the adenylate cyclase inhibitory guanosine triphosphate–binding protein, G_i. Prostaglandins inhibit direct mucosal damage produced by aspirin or alcohol in rats. The major beneficial effect may be to maintain mucosal blood flow rather than to prevent damage to the surface epithelial cells. However, prostaglandins may have a special protective action on damage produced by NSAIDs. The healing rates of peptic ulcer produced by prostaglandins and by doses of H_2-receptor antagonists that inhibit acid secretion to a similar extent are about equal, but these doses of prostaglandins produce abdominal cramps and diarrhea in many patients. Another potential effect that arouses concern is the ability to cause uterine contraction and thus induce abortion.

Anticholinergic Agents

Anticholinergic drugs that inhibit acid secretion have been available for many years. The maximal inhibition of acid secretion produced by these drugs is only about 30% to 40%. These agents also have side effects that reduce their acceptability to patients, the most common being dryness of the mouth because of inhibition of salivary secretion. Used alone, ordinary anticholinergic agents are not recommended for ulcer treatment. They have been used as adjuncts to other agents, especially H_2-blockers, in patients with gastric acid hypersecretion that is difficult to control with a single agent. This situation used to occur commonly in patients with Zollinger–Ellison syndrome but is now managed more effectively with proton pump inhibitors.

Sucralfate

Sucralfate is an aluminum sulfate disaccharide that has minimal acid-neutralizing capacity, does not alter acid or pepsin secretion, but is effective for ulcer treatment. Its mechanism of action is unknown, but it is presumed to act locally on the gastric and duodenal mucosa. Possible mechanisms include binding to the ulcer base, local neutralization of pepsin, stimulation of mucosal prostaglandin synthesis, and local effects of the aluminum component. No specific side effects have been noted. Sucralfate and H_2-receptor antagonists produce similar rates of ulcer healing. The only apparent disadvantages to sucralfate are the need to give it at least twice a day, the large size of the tablet, and the lack of *H. pylori* eradication regimens that include sucralfate.

Bismuth Formulations

Colloidal bismuth, formulated as tripotassium dicitratobismuthate, can produce ulcer healing rates as high as those of other ulcer treatments. Periods of remission after ulcer healing may be longer after bismuth treatment than after H_2-blockers. The mechanisms for ulcer healing by bismuth are unclear but may include its known antibacterial effect against *H. pylori*. Other bismuth compounds, including bismuth subsalicylate, share this antibacterial effect. Regimens that include bismuth plus one or more antibiotics have been effective in eradicating *H. pylori* infections, although bismuth compounds alone rarely produce true eradication. Bismuth compounds also appear to have mucosal protective effects that are independent of antibacterial effects. Bismuth compounds do not inhibit acid secretion. One major side effect of bismuth is blackening of the tongue and stool. More serious side effects could result from absorption of bismuth into the circulation. Colloidal bismuth compounds are absorbed poorly, and blood levels rarely approach toxic concentrations; however, bismuth is excreted into the urine and stool for several weeks after treatment is stopped.

Surgical Management of Peptic Ulcer Disease

Some of the complications arising from ulcer disease require surgical treatment. The most definite indications for surgery are hemorrhage not responsive to medical management (including endoscopic hemostasis), gastric outlet obstruction not reversed by medical management, perforation, and malignancy. Other potential indications for surgery include recurrent episodes of self-limited hemorrhage, potentially resectable gastrinoma (unresponsiveness to medical therapy is extremely uncommon in the proton pump inhibitor era), and symptomatic ulcers in patients who are unwilling to take or are refractory to medical therapy (especially smokers).

Partial or Total Gastrectomy

The most effective operation for treatment of gastric ulcer is simple antrectomy. The major goal of surgery for gastric ulcer is to remove the region of the stomach most affected by gastritis and susceptible to ulceration. Decreasing acid secretion is a secondary goal. Vagotomy is unnecessary for treatment of ordinary gastric ulcer, but it may be useful in treating distal antral ulcers and pyloric channel ulcers that biologically resemble duodenal ulcer. The stomach usually is anastomosed directly to the duodenum (a Billroth I anastomosis). In most cases, the gastric ulcer can be included in the resection. When it is located high in the stomach, the ulcer may need to be resected separately, or a bleeding site may need to be oversewn.

Partial gastric resection also is effective for treatment of duodenal ulcer. The goal of surgery for duodenal ulcer is to decrease the amount of acid emptied from the stomach into the duodenum or jejunum. The rate of recurrence is lower if resection is combined with vagotomy. The amount of stomach resected usually is more than the antrum alone, and the operation is known as a *subtotal gastrectomy* rather than an antrectomy. Anastomosis may be performed with a Billroth I (gastroduodenal) or a Billroth II (gastrojejunal) anastomosis.

Total gastrectomy is the treatment of choice for patients with Zollinger–Ellison syndrome unresponsive to medical management, but this is rarely required in the proton pump inhibitor era. A better surgical option for carefully selected gastrinoma patients (non–MEN-I patients with unifocal, nonmetastatic primary tumors) is local tumor resection. This nongastric approach to gastric acid hypersecretion has low morbidity and can lead to cure, defined as normalization of serum gastrin levels, negative secretin testing, and negative imaging in up to 50% of patients. Total gastrectomy is also used for some patients with more than one recurrent ulcer despite a prior subtotal gastrectomy. However, postoperative symptoms and complications tend to be greater for total than for subtotal gastrectomy.

Vagotomy

Vagotomy removes the cephalic phase of gastric secretion and is one of the oldest forms of surgical treatment for ulcer. It may be performed as the only operation for treatment of duodenal ulcer, or it may be combined with a subtotal gastrectomy. Truncal vagotomy involves cutting both major trunks of the vagus nerve, either in the abdomen just below the diaphragm or in the chest. This operation impairs normal gastric emptying and must be combined with a second procedure to enhance emptying, either pyloroplasty or gastrojejunostomy. Highly selective vagotomy minimizes the side effects of vagotomy caused by the need for an emptying procedure and by gastric and intestinal vagal denervation. This type of vagotomy is also known as a proximal gastric vagotomy or a parietal cell vagotomy. Individual branches of the vagus nerve that innervate the stomach proximal to the antrum are dissected along the blood vessels and cut. If performed properly, this operation causes a decrease in acid secretion similar to that achieved with truncal vagotomy and does not require a separate procedure to enhance gastric emptying.

Closure of Perforation

Perforated ulcers often require only simple closure with an omental patch. Sometimes closure is combined with a more definitive operation, such as vagotomy. Bleeding ulcers not included in resections can be oversewn to achieve hemostasis in the operating room.

Complications of Ulcer Surgery

Recurrent ulceration after ulcer surgery is of major concern. The operation associated with the lowest rate of symptomatic ulcer recurrence, other than total gastrectomy, is subtotal gastrectomy combined with vagotomy. Recurrences occur in less than 5% of such patients. They tend to occur early and are rare more than 2 years after surgery. The trade-off for lower recurrence rates is the higher morbidity associated with motility disorders because of the more extensive resection. Truncal vagotomy with pyloroplasty and highly selective vagotomy are associated with higher recurrence rates than is resection plus vagotomy. Recurrences occur at a relatively steady rate of about 1% per year. Unless the surgeon is especially experienced with the operation, highly selective vagotomy tends to produce higher recurrence rates than truncal vagotomy.

The rate of recurrence of bleeding in patients who undergo surgery for bleeding ulcers is higher than the rate of recurrence of symptomatic ulcer in patients operated on for other reasons. It is difficult to obtain an accurate estimate of postoperative bleeding rates from ulcer, but they probably are at least 10% in patients treated with subtotal gastrectomy and vagotomy and considerably higher in patients treated with vagotomy alone. It is unknown whether surgical treatment is more effective than medical maintenance treatment for prevention of recurrent ulcer bleeding. The effects of combining surgery with *H. pylori* eradication have not been determined.

Mortality rate in patients requiring emergency surgery for bleeding ulcers may be as high as 20% to 25%, depending on other medical conditions associated with the bleeding. Mortality rate of those having elective operations for ulcer is only about 1%. The perioperative mortality and morbidity are greatest for subtotal gastrectomy, intermediate for vagotomy with pyloroplasty, and lowest for highly selective vagotomy without pyloroplasty.

Diarrhea and dumping syndromes are relatively common in patients who have had gastric resections or pyloroplasty. They are relatively uncommon in patients with highly selective vagotomy without pyloroplasty.

Ulcer operations routinely lead to early postoperative weight loss. This weight loss is due chiefly to decreased food intake rather than to malabsorption of nutrients. Malabsorption of calcium and iron leads to metabolic bone disease and iron-deficiency anemia in many patients with subtotal gastrectomy and in fewer patients with vagotomy alone. These late complications develop slowly and may not be appreciated for several years.

Reflux of bile into the stomach produces an endoscopic picture often known as *bile gastritis*, which is characterized by edema and erythema. It is unclear whether this endoscopic picture is associated with any specific symptoms.

Marginal or anastomotic ulcers, also known as *stomal ulcers,* are ulcers that develop at a gastroenteric stoma after an operation that includes gastroenteric anastomosis. Usually, these ulcers form on the intestinal side of the anastomosis. They result from exposure of the intestinal mucosa to acid. The jejunal mucosa is less resistant to acid than is the duodenal bulb, probably because the duodenal bulb mucosa can secrete bicarbonate. The highest rates of marginal ulcers occur in patients treated with gastrojejunostomy without gastric resection or vagotomy. After partial gastrectomy and vagotomy, the rate of marginal ulceration is only 1% to 2%. The major causes of anastomotic ulcers are incomplete vagotomy or ingestion of NSAIDs. Treatment in the past always included reoperation to complete the vagotomy, to resect more stomach, or both. However, most patients with anastomotic ulcer can now be managed suitably with H^+,K^+-ATPase antagonists.

Cancer in the residual stomach is a potential late complication of subtotal gastrectomy. Several recent surveys have indicated that the risk of this complication is low, and some have questioned whether it is a significant risk. If it occurs, the interval from operation to carcinoma is almost always more than 15 years and often more than 20 years. Untreated *H. pylori* infection may play a role in the development of postgastrectomy gastric carcinomas.

BIBLIOGRAPHY

Graham DY, Lew GM, Klein PD, et al. Effect of treatment of *Helicobacter pylori* infection on the long-term recurrence of gastric or duodenal ulcer: a randomized, controlled study. *Ann Intern Med* 1992;116:705–708.

Graham DY, Malaty HM, Evans DG, et al. Epidemiology of *Helicobacter pylori* in an asymptomatic population in the United States: effect of age, race, and socioeconomic status. *Gastroenterology* 1991;100:1495–1501.

Hentschel E, Brandstatter G, Dragosics B, et al. Effect of ranitidine and amoxicillin plus metronidazole on the eradication of *Helicobacter pylori* and the recurrence of duodenal ulcer. *N Engl J Med* 1993;328:308–312.

Hopkins RJ, Girardi LS, Turney EA. Relationship between *Helicobacter pylori* eradication and reduced duodenal and gastric ulcer recurrence: a review. *Gastroenterology* 1996;110:1244–1252.

Isenberg JI, Thompson JC. Medical progress and ulcer disease: three key observations that changed the compass. *Gastroenterology* 1997;113:1031–1033.

Langman MJS, Weil J, Wainwright P, et al. Risks of bleeding peptic ulcer associated with individual nonsteroidal antiinflammatory drugs. *Lancet* 1994;343:1075–1078.

Lee J, O'Morain C. Who should be treated for *Helicobacter pylori* infection? A review of consensus conferences and guidelines. *Gastroenterology* 1997; 113(suppl 6):S99–S106.

Metz DC. Peptic ulcer disease: diagnosis and treatment. In: Dimarino AJ, Benjamin SB, eds. *Gastrointestinal disease: an endoscopic approach*, vol. 1. Cambridge, MA: Blackwell Science, 1997:285–304.

NIH Consensus Conference. *Helicobacter pylori* in peptic ulcer disease. NIH Consensus Development Panel on *Helicobater pylori* in Peptic Ulcer Disease. *JAMA* 1994;272:65–69.

Walsh JH, Peterson WL. The treatment of *Helicobacter pylori* infection in the management of peptic ulcer disease. *N Engl J Med* 1995;333:984–991.

Kelley's Textbook of Internal Medicine, fourth edition. Edited by H. David Humes. Lippincott Williams & Wilkins, Philadelphia © 2000.

C H A P T E R

108

MOTOR DISORDERS OF THE GASTROINTESTINAL TRACT

CHUNG OWYANG

Disorders of gastric and intestinal motility are associated with a number of common gastrointestinal complaints, including heartburn, nausea, vomiting, chest and abdominal pain, diarrhea, and constipation. Historically, inadequate methods to record gut motor activity made it difficult to establish a connection between the patient's symptoms and dysfunctional motility. Interest in gastrointestinal motility problems has increased largely because of advances in monitoring techniques that have led to improved understanding of the normal patterns of motor activity in the gastrointestinal tract.

Gastrointestinal motor function is regulated by a complex hierarchy of interdependent pathways, including the inherent properties of the longitudinal and circular muscle layers, extraintestinal and enteric neural elements, and substances that act in endocrine and paracrine capacities. The enteric nervous system is the repository of the motor "programs" that result in luminal transit. Dysfunction can occur at all levels of this hierarchy, resulting in altered gastrointestinal transit and thereby disrup-

tion of the secretory and absorptive events that complete the intraluminal digestive process.

Classification of clinical disorders associated with altered gastrointestinal motility has been hampered by inadequate knowledge of the normal motility patterns in the gut and the mechanisms of their regulation. One approach to classifying these clinical syndromes (Table 108.1) is based on whether transit in the involved region of the gastrointestinal tract is delayed, accelerated, or reversed (retrograde). This approach is useful because the practical consequence of disordered motility is abnormal transit of the luminal contents, though the relationship between transit and the patterns of muscle contractions that determine transit remains unclear. Other classifications of gastrointestinal motility disorders are based on descriptions of abnormal contractile patterns. To understand motor dysfunction by these criteria, it is necessary to have some knowledge of the normal myoelectrical and motor activities of the gastrointestinal tract.

Gastric electrical pacemaker activity originates on the greater curvature at the junction between the proximal and distal stomach. Rhythmic depolarizations generated by the pacemaker, known as slow waves, cycle at a frequency of 3 cycles per minute (cpm) in humans. Under quiescent conditions, slow waves partially depolarize gastric smooth muscle but do not cause contraction. Additional depolarizations provided by neurohumoral stimulation (action potentials) are the triggers for phasic gastric contractions, which follow the spread of the slow waves and are peristaltic. Thus, gastric slow waves control the maximal frequency and the direction of contractions in the distal stomach, whereas action potentials determine the amplitude and duration of contractions.

In the fasting state, the stomach and small intestine have a rhythmic, periodic contractile activity that is divided into three phases: phase I is defined by the absence of motor activity, phase II by irregular contractions, and phase III by a brief burst of regular contractions lasting about 5 minutes, which begins at a pacemaker site along the greater curvature of the gastric body and migrates down the intestine—hence the name *interdigestive migratory motor complex* (IMMC). Occasionally, phase III activity begins in the duodenum and not at the gastric pacemaker. Gastric phase III activity appears to be initiated by the gastrointestinal peptide motilin. The entire cycle repeats about every 90 to 120 minutes, until the pattern is interrupted by the ingestion of food. The IMMC has been referred to as the "intestinal housekeeper" because of its action of sweeping the stomach and small intestine of debris in the fasting state. Loss of phase III activity is associated with gastric bezoar and bacterial overgrowth in the small intestine and subsequent malabsorption. The postprandial motor pattern features persistent irregular contractions that are thought to be necessary for proper mixing and absorption of the intraluminal contents. The periodicity, propagation, and duration of the IMMC are functions of the enteric nervous system. Interruption of the fasting pattern by eating requires an intact vagovagal axis and probably intact enteroenteric reflexes as well. The duration of phases I and II is affected by whether the person is awake or asleep; phase II activity is more prominent during the waking state.

These motor patterns are altered during abnormal circum-

TABLE 108.1.	CLINICAL SYNDROMES OF DISORDERED GASTROINTESTINAL MOTILITY

Transit delayed due to obstruction
  Primary
    Achalasia and related disorders
    Pyloric stenosis, congenital or due to duodenal ulcer, pyloric channel ulcer, tumor of the distal stomach, gastric bezoar
    Aganglionosis coli (Hirschsprung's disease)
  Secondary
    Intestinal obstruction (acute and subacute)
Transit delayed due to defective propulsion
  Primary
    Postvagotomy gastroparesis
    Aberrant gastric pacemaker (extachygastria)
    Chronic idiopathic intestinal pseudo-obstruction
      Visceral myopathies (sporadic or familial)
      Visceral neuropathies (sporadic or familial)
    Diverticular disease of the colon
    Idiopathic constipation
      Functional
      Neuropathy due to laxative abuse
  Secondary
    Oropharyngeal dysphagia
    Ileus
      Acute abdomen
      Abdominal operations
      Electrolyte disturbances—hypokalemia, hypocalcemia, hypomagnesemia
      Drug toxicity—anticholinergics, adrenergic agonists, calcium channel blockers, opiates, cytostatic drugs, dopamine agonists
    Diabetic gastroenteropathy
    Progressive systemic sclerosis, dermatomyositis
    Dysautonomia (Shy–Drager syndrome)
    Chagas' disease
    Myxedema ileus, hypoparathyroidism, pregnancy
    Paraneoplastic syndrome
    Infiltrative diseases—amyloidosis, pernicious anemia malignancy
    Infectious—viral gastroenteritis, Guillain-Barré syndrome, botulism
Accelerated transit
  Primary
    Gastric incontinence (dumping syndrome)
    Postvagotomy diarrhea
    Intestinal hurry (irritable bowel syndrome)
    Rectosphincteric incontinence
  Secondary
    Carcinoid syndrome
    Infective and postinfective diarrhea
    Purgative abuse
Retrograde transit
  Primary
    Rumination
    Vomiting
  Secondary
    Gastroesophageal reflux
    Duodenogastric reflux (biliary gastritis)
    Vomiting (metabolic)
    Bacterial overgrowth in small intestine

(From Wingate DL. Synopsis of clinical syndromes. In: Christensen J, Wingate DL, eds. *A guide to gastrointestinal motility*. Bristol, England: Wright-PSG, 1983:230, with permission.)

stances in different ways, depending on the location of the abnormality. For example, as with the heart, ectopic pacemakers in other gastric regions will cause tachygastria resulting in the dissociation of electro-mechanical activities and gastric atonia. Alterations in CNS modulation of gut motor function are associated with abnormal clusters of contractions and loss of IMMC activity. This type of abnormality has been reported in patients with irritable bowel syndrome. Disorders of extrinsic innervation, such as truncal vagotomy and diabetic neuropathy, can be associated with an altered response to food. Diseases that cause an enteric neuropathy (eg, visceral aganglionosis) are associated with disturbed IMMC activity, which can take the form of abnormal periodicity, propagation, or duration of phase III activity. Finally, intestinal myopathic disorders, such as hollow visceral myopathy and progressive systemic sclerosis, are associated with abnormalities in electrical slow-wave activity, resulting in infrequent, weak contractions and leading to poor intestinal propulsion but normal contractile patterns.

Diagnosis of gut motor disorders generally relies on evidence of abnormalities in gastrointestinal transit or in the contractile patterns that are typical of each region of the gastrointestinal tract. Tests commonly used to assess gastrointestinal transit include barium transit and radioscintigraphy. Both techniques require exposing the patient to ionizing radiation. Barium transit studies generally provide only qualitative information because of the wide variation in results noted in normal subjects. In addition, these studies are diagnostic only if marked delay or acceleration of transit is observed. Radioscintigraphy requires isotopic labeling of standardized solid or liquid meals and following with a gamma camera. This test is considered more sensitive than the use of barium and is the test of choice for measuring gastric emptying.

Evaluation of contractile activity requires the placement of pressure-sensitive sensors within the lumen of the gut, typically in the form of a multilumen, perfused tube attached to pneumohydraulic pumps and external pressure transducers. This technique allows continuous recording of changes in intraluminal pressure and thus provides an indirect measurement of contractile activity. Recent improvements in monitoring techniques using advanced, solid-state devices permit prolonged (up to several days), ambulatory recordings of upper gastrointestinal motility. It is also possible to record electrical slow waves emanating from gastrointestinal smooth muscle using electrodes attached to the skin overlying the stomach (electrogastrography). The electrical slow waves establish the frequency with which muscle contractions occur, which varies depending on the region of the gastrointestinal tract examined. Tachydysrhythmias and bradydysrhythmias can develop in the gastrointestinal tract and may result in delayed gastric emptying.

GASTRIC DYSMOTILITY

The stomach plays an important role in the early stages of digestion because of its ability to store, triturate, and deliver nutrients to the duodenum. Normal gastric emptying is the result of a well-coordinated interplay of hormonal, secretory, and neuromuscular events. The emptying of liquids and solids is controlled by different regions of the stomach. The proximal stomach acts as a reservoir that allows food to be accommodated without a significant change in intragastric pressure; this is referred to as *receptive relaxation*. In addition, this region of the stomach evidences sustained or tonic contractions that exert a steady pressure on the proximal gastric contents, regulate the pressure gradient between the stomach and duodenum, and control gastric emptying of liquids. Loss of receptive relaxation in the proximal stomach can result in rapid emptying of liquids and symptoms of "dumping." Emptying of solids is regulated by the phasic motor activity of the distal stomach. The churning action of this region triturates the solid food particles until they are about 1 mm in diameter and can pass through the pylorus. Abnormalities of motor function of the distal stomach may result in retention of solid food particles.

DELAYED GASTRIC EMPTYING

ETIOLOGY

Disorders of delayed gastric emptying are more common than those associated with rapid emptying. Mechanical or outlet obstruction as well as functional obstruction can cause delayed gastric emptying. In adults, mechanical obstruction is typically a complication of peptic ulcer disease, though tumors of the distal stomach and gastric bezoars should be considered when making the diagnosis. Bezoars, which are concretions of food or foreign matter formed as a result of functional and mechanical gastric obstruction, can produce gastric ulceration, bleeding, and, in rare cases, perforation.

Functional obstruction, or gastroparesis, is associated with several clinical situations; the common denominator is the presence of ineffective electromechanical activity. Gastric atonia may be a result of tachygastria, which develops when a rival ectopic pacemaker, usually in the antrum, generates an oscillatory pattern at an abnormally high frequency (more than 4 cpm) that overdrives the rest of the stomach. During tachygastria, the stomach is atonic, because the electrical activity is of insufficient amplitude to induce contraction. Clinical conditions associated with the development of gastric slow-wave dysrhythmias are listed in Table 108.2. Reversible causes of gastroparesis include medications, such as opiates, anticholinergics, calcium channel

TABLE 108.2.	CLINICAL CONDITIONS ASSOCIATED WITH THE DEVELOPMENT OF GASTRIC SLOW-WAVE DYSRHYTHMIAS

Anorexia nervosa
Diabetic gastroparesis
Idiopathic gastroparesis
Functional dyspepsia
Gastric ischemia
Gastroparesis associated with abdominal malignancy
Unexplained nausea and vomiting
Nausea of the first trimester of pregnancy
Motion sickness
Renal failure

blockers, β-adrenergic agonists, and dopaminergic agonists. Altered metabolism from diabetes mellitus, hypothyroidism, hypoparathyroidism, and pregnancy may delay gastric emptying, as can electrolyte disturbances, including hypokalemia, hypocalcemia, and hypomagnesemia.

Postvagotomy gastroparesis is occasionally a complication of peptic ulcer surgery. Gastroparesis is also found in the context of neuromuscular disorders, such as chronic idiopathic pseudo-obstruction and myotonic dystrophy. Patients with diabetes mellitus can experience gastric stasis as a result of autonomic neuropathy or poorly controlled blood glucose in the absence of neuropathy, a condition that frequently is associated with tachygastria. Occasionally, infiltrative disorders, such as amyloidosis, and collagen vascular diseases, such as progressive systemic sclerosis and dermatomyositis, are associated with delayed gastric emptying. Many patients have idiopathic gastroparesis, which may be the result of a viral or other insult leading to temporary or permanent gastric neural or muscular damage.

CLINICAL FEATURES

Delayed gastric emptying should be suspected in patients who complain of nausea, vomiting, postprandial abdominal pain, early satiety, or bloating. It can be accompanied by reflux of acidic gastric contents into the esophagus, resulting in heartburn or chest pain. The vomitus in gastroparesis may be foul smelling or contain bits of food ingested more than 12 hours previously. The medical history should be reviewed carefully for evidence of previous gastric surgery, peptic ulcer disease, diabetes mellitus, thyroid disease, or psychiatric illness. Physical examination is generally not helpful unless the symptoms are severe, resulting in dehydration or malnutrition. Abdominal distention may be present, and occasionally a succussion splash is present several hours after a meal.

Peptic ulcer disease and mechanical gastric outlet obstruction should be ruled out before the diagnosis of gastroparesis is made. This is typically accomplished with an upper barium study or endoscopic examination. Abdominal radiographs in the supine and upright positions can be useful, particularly if a perforation is suspected. Other tests to consider include serum glucose to rule out diabetes; serum calcium, potassium, and magnesium to rule out electrolyte disturbances; and thyroid function tests if they are clinically indicated.

Delayed gastric emptying is best diagnosed using radioscintigraphy methods. Incorporation of a radioisotope into a test meal allows for quantitative, noninvasive measurement of solid- and liquid-phase gastric emptying (Fig. 108.1). Solid-phase gastric emptying provides a more accurate gauge of clinical disease than liquid-phase emptying. Generally, gastric emptying is considered to be delayed if the time for emptying half the gastric contents exceeds normal values by two standard deviations. If gastric scintigraphy is equivocal, manometry of the stomach and duodenum may confirm the diagnosis. Patients with gastroparesis may have less frequent, lower-amplitude contractions and loss of antral phase III activity (Fig. 108.2). They may also evidence a reduced contractile response to a meal during gastrointestinal manometry. Patients with gastric neuropathy may show irregularity of the IMMC, whereas those with gastric myopathy may have a low amplitude of antral contractions but normal frequency of antral phase III activity. In questionable cases, electrogastrography studies may indicate that some forms of gastroparesis are related to electrical dysrhythmia. The normal frequency of electrical slow waves in the antrum is 3 cpm. Some patients with gastroparesis have a frequency in excess of 6 cpm—hence the designation *tachygastria* (Fig. 108.3). These diagnostic tests are complementary and may help identify specific causes of gastroparesis, thereby helping to individualize treatment.

TREATMENT

Management of gastroparesis initially should be directed toward correcting reversible causes, such as electrolyte imbalances, re-

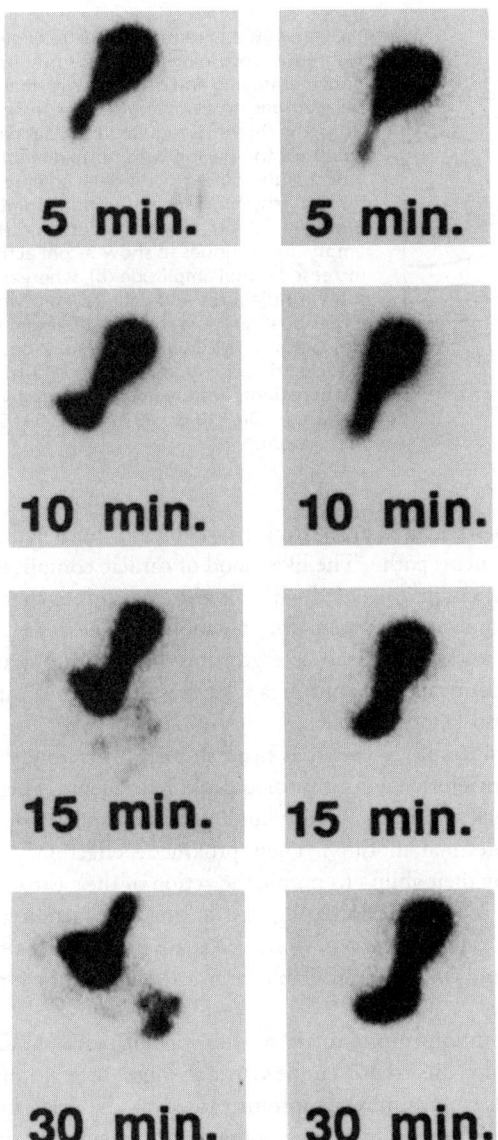

FIGURE 108.1. Solid-phase gastric emptying study: films taken 5, 10, 15, and 30 minutes after ingestion of Tc-99m sulfur colloid–labeled scrambled eggs with toast. Early movement of the meal from the proximal to the distal stomach is apparent. The sequence on the left shows normal gastric emptying. Tracer is present in the small bowel after 30 minutes. On the right, no gastric emptying is apparent after 30 minutes. Subsequent scans can be obtained after 60 and 120 minutes.

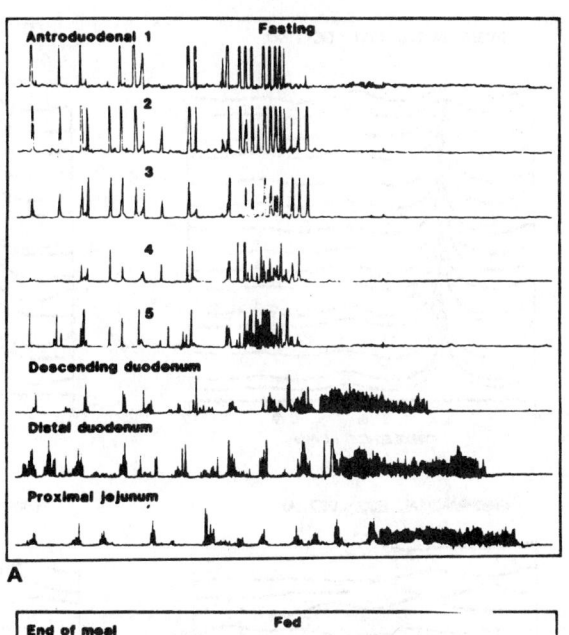

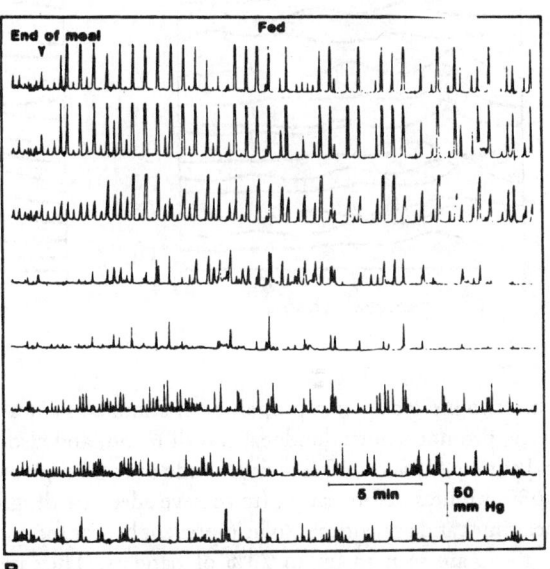

FIGURE 108.2. Normal gastrointestinal motility. **A:** Normal interdigestive migrating motor complex (fasting). Phase III activity is visible in the antrum, pressure activity is gradually moving into the duodenum, and gradual change is occurring in the configuration of the waves as they move through the antroduodenal junction. **B:** Normal fed activity. Irregular, but persistent phasic pressure activity is seen in the distal antrum and proximal small bowel. (From Malagelada JR, Camilleri M, Stanghellini V. *Manometric diagnosis of gastrointestinal motility disorders.* New York: Thieme, 1986:45, with permission of the Mayo Foundation.)

moving causative medications, and optimizing care of underlying medical illnesses, such as diabetes mellitus. Correction of hyperglycemia may improve gastric motor function in diabetic patients, since an elevated blood glucose level has been shown to evoke gastric dysrhythmias and impair gastric contractions. Prokinetic drugs that stimulate gastric emptying are effective in many patients. Cholinomimetic drugs, such as bethanechol, increase the amplitude of contractions in gastrointestinal smooth muscle, but the contractions are often not coordinated and therefore are rarely used for the treatment of gastroparesis.

Metoclopramide, the prototypical dopamine receptor antago-

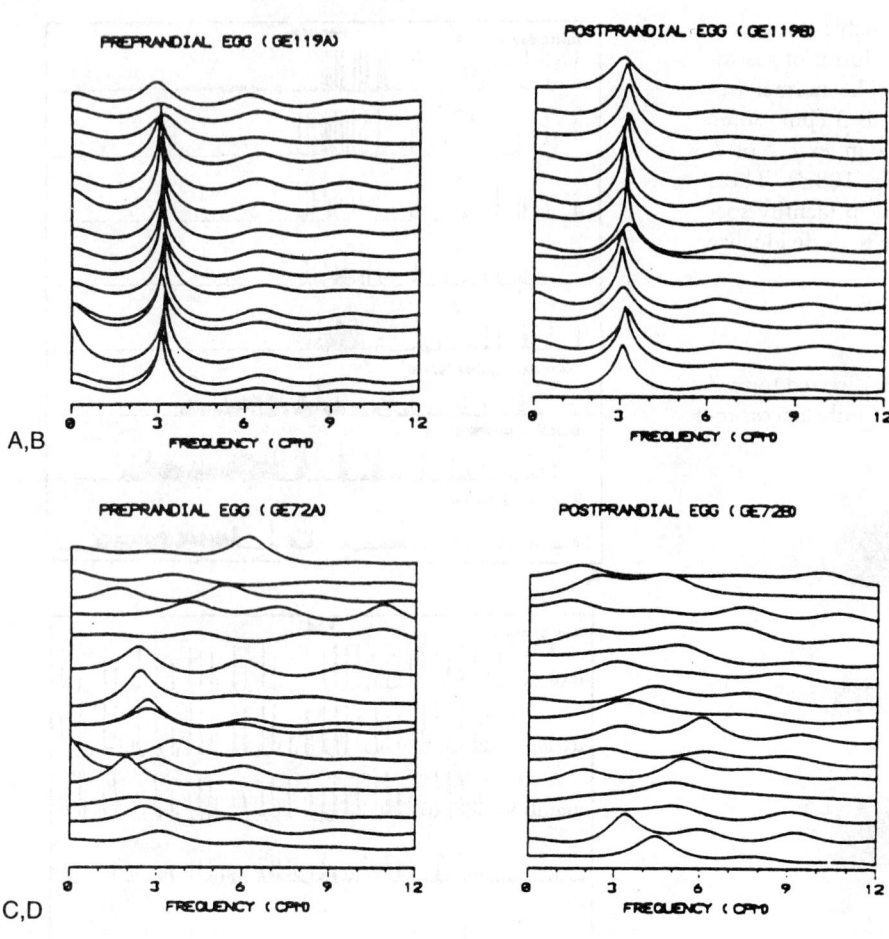

FIGURE 108.3. Frequency spectra of electrogastrographic recordings of a person with normal gastric emptying and a patient with diabetes and delayed gastric emptying. Under fasting conditions, the rhythm is regular at 3 cycles per minute (cpm) for the person with normal emptying (**A**), whereas the patient with delayed emptying exhibits dysrhythmic activity without dominant frequency (**C**). After eating, the person with normal emptying continues to show 3-cpm activity with increased signal amplitude (**B**), whereas the person with diabetes and delayed emptying shows a chaotic slow-wave rhythm (**D**). (From Chen JD, Lin Z, Pan J, McCallum RW. Abnormal gastric myoelectric activity and delayed gastric emptying in patients with symptoms suggestive of gastroparesis. *Dig Dis Sci* 1996;41:1538–1545, with permission).

nist, has cholinergic agonist properties. It stimulates antral contractility, promotes antroduodenal coordination, and also has a central antiemetic action. Metoclopramide (5 to 30 mg) is taken about 30 minutes before eating (to achieve adequate drug levels by mealtime) and at bedtime (to help prevent bezoar formation). Side effects are seen in up to 20% of patients. They include agitation; irritability; drowsiness; extrapyramidal signs, such as restlessness and dystonic reactions; menstrual disorders; and galactorrhea. Parkinsonism and tardive dyskinesia have been reported in the elderly. Tachyphylaxis may develop after prolonged use.

Domperidone is a second-generation prokinetic drug with antidopaminergic properties that crosses the blood–brain barrier poorly and therefore has fewer side effects than metoclopramide. Unlike metoclopramide, domperidone has no cholinomimetic effects. Antiemetic properties are maintained because of its effect on the chemoreceptor trigger zone. The usual dose is 10 to 30 mg, 30 minutes before meals and at bedtime. At present, domperidone is an investigational drug in the United States.

Cisapride is effective for treating gastroparesis and other motility disorders. It appears to act in part by stimulating acetylcholine release by myenteric plexus fibers. Cisapride has no known antidopaminergic properties and does not cross the blood–brain barrier. The usual dose is 10 to 20 mg, 30 minutes before meals and at bedtime. The most common reported side effect is mild diarrhea. Cisapride may cause cardiac arrythmias, especially in

patients who have preexisting heart disease, renal failure, and diabetic neuropathy. The likelihood of cardiac complication increases if cisapride is used with certain medications that use the cytochrome P450 system for metabolism. These medications include antibiotics, such as erythromycin, clarithromycin, and troleandomycin, and antifungals, such as fluconazole, intracomazole, and ketoconazole.

Considerable interest has been shown in macrolide analogs of the antibiotic erythromycin as prokinetic agents. These drugs have weak antibiotic activity but a potent stimulatory effect on gastrointestinal motility. Their prokinetic effect may be mediated by their ability to mimic the action of the gastrointestinal peptide motilin by initiating gastric phase III activity; hence, they are called *motilides*. These drugs are in the latter phases of testing and will not be available for routine clinical use for several years.

In addition to prokinetic medications, patients should eat a low-residue diet to prevent bezoars and ingest several small, low-fat meals to minimize symptoms caused by the delay in gastric emptying. Some studies suggest that gastric pacing may improve symptoms and gastroparesis and accelerate gastric emptying in patients with gastroparesis. More controlled studies are necessary to further investigate the role of gastric pacing in clinical practice. Surgery is seldom indicated for the treatment of nonmechanical gastroparesis and should be considered only after other options have failed and a thorough evaluation suggests that normal motility exists in other regions of the digestive tract.

RAPID GASTRIC EMPTYING

ETIOLOGY

Dumping syndrome is a complication of vagotomy and drainage procedures for peptic ulcer disease or malignancy. All standard anti-ulcer procedures cause dumping syndrome, but superselective vagotomy appears to have a lower incidence than truncal vagotomy. Persistent dumping syndrome generally occurs in 8% to 15% of patients after gastric surgery.

CLINICAL FEATURES

Symptoms may develop in both the early and late postprandial periods. Early symptoms typically occur within 15 to 30 minutes after starting a meal and include nausea, nonproductive vomiting, anxiety, dizziness, sweating, flushing, abdominal cramping, and diarrhea. The pathophysiologic basis for these symptoms appears to be related to disruption of the normal neuromuscular pathways that regulate gastric emptying. Truncal vagotomy disrupts receptive relaxation in the proximal stomach and thereby diminishes gastric reservoir capacity. Furthermore, resection of the pyloric sphincter results in decreased resistance to the flow of liquids and altered processing of solid particulates. This combination culminates in the dumping of hypertonic solutions into the jejunum. The early vasomotor symptoms associated with dumping probably are caused by rapid blood volume contraction due to rapid secretion of fluid into the bowel caused by the presence of a hypertonic solution. This is associated with reflex splanchnic vasodilatation stemming from jejunal distention, plasma hyperosmolarity, and acute release of vasoactive gut peptides.

The late symptoms associated with the dumping syndrome generally occur about 2 hours after a meal and include hypoglycemic symptoms, such as diaphoresis, hunger, tremulousness, weakness, and confusion. The pathophysiologic basis for these symptoms appears to be related to the rapid delivery and absorption of simple sugars from the jejunum, causing a sudden rise in serum glucose and an exaggerated insulin response, resulting in hypoglycemia. Rapid caloric delivery to the intestine also releases numerous vasoactive hormones, which may further increase lightheadedness or even lead to syncope and shock. The diagnosis of dumping syndrome is based on a clinical constellation of symptoms and signs in patients who have undergone vagotomy. Evidence of a postprandial increase in hematocrit or plasma osmolarity, indicating hemoconcentration, is consistent with the diagnosis. Gastric scintigraphy confirms rapid emptying of a liquid meal in most cases.

TREATMENT

Treatment of the dumping syndrome focuses on slowing gastric emptying and lessening the volume and hypertonicity of the liquid boluses entering the small intestine. Eating six to eight small, low-carbohydrate meals per day, avoiding large amounts of liquids (especially hypertonic fluids), and separating ingestion of the liquid and solid components of the meal are effective strategies for many patients. Some patients report that assuming a recumbent posture after a meal has benefit, possibly by helping maintain intravascular volume and slowing gastric emptying. Late dumping symptoms are managed by avoiding simple carbohydrates at mealtime. Medications that delay gastric emptying, such as opiates and anticholinergics, and gel-forming fiber products, such as pectin, that slow gastrointestinal transit and postpone carbohydrate absorption may be useful in selected patients. In some studies, the somatostatin analog octreotide has been found to be effective in difficult cases, since it not only delays gastric emptying but also has inhibitory effects on meal-stimulated release of vasoactive hormones, which may be important pathogenetic factors.

INTESTINAL DYSMOTILITY

Disorders of intestinal motility have symptoms of nausea, bloating, and abdominal pain in addition to malabsorption and diarrhea, owing to bacterial overgrowth from intestinal stasis. Many conditions lead to acute intestinal dysmotility, but the most common is acute intestinal pseudo-obstruction in the postoperative period or accompanying severe illness. As with gastroparesis, severe localized or generalized neuromuscular disease can lead to chronic intestinal dysmotility, such as advanced diabetic visceral neuropathy or chronic intestinal pseudo-obstruction.

ACUTE INTESTINAL PSEUDO-OBSTRUCTION

ETIOLOGY

Acute intestinal pseudo-obstruction was first described by Ogilvie in 1948 and is also referred to as Ogilvie's syndrome. Typically, it involves the small and large intestines and develops in older patients who have undergone surgery or suffer from a severe systemic illness or infection that inhibits intestinal neuromuscular function. It may be associated with or exacerbated by electrolyte disturbances (hypokalemia, hypocalcemia, hypomagnesemia) or medications, such as antidepressants, anticholinergics, calcium channel antagonists, or opiates.

CLINICAL FEATURES

Patients with acute intestinal pseudo-obstruction show signs of abdominal distention with or without nausea during an acute illness or after surgery. The abdomen is tympanitic on examination, and bowel sounds are often minimal or absent. Serum electrolytes should be obtained to rule out metabolic abnormalities, and abdominal radiographs should be examined to exclude perforation and to assess the magnitude of luminal distention. Most patients have a moderately dilated colon without air-fluid levels. The cecum is usually dilated to larger than 10 cm in diameter. If obstruction is suspected, a Gastrografin enema or gentle sigmoidoscopy without air insufflation is performed. Barium should be avoided, because it may form an impaction or induce a peritoneal reaction if perforation has occurred.

TREATMENT

Initial management should be conservative. Oral intake should be discontinued, and decompression through nasogastric and rectal tubes should be initiated. Metabolic and electrolyte disturbances should be corrected and medications that slow bowel motility discontinued. Contrast studies should be avoided, but a Gastrografin or equivalent enema sometimes is required to rule out mechanical obstruction. If the cecal diameter exceeds 12 cm, colonoscopic decompression may be attempted to lower the risk of perforation. If the condition persists, tube cecostomy has been used with some success. Occasionally, in the presence of necrosis or perforation, a right hemicolectomy may be required. Perforation occurs in about 15% of patients.

One double-blind, placebo-controlled trial confirmed rapid and dramatic improvement of acute colonic pseudo-obstruction in patients treated with intravenous neostigmine (2 mg). All treated patients had prompt evaluation of flatus and/or stool, with reduction of abdominal distention and only minimal side effects. This treatment should be considered before colonoscopic or surgical intervention in patients whose conditions do not improve with conservative management.

CHRONIC INTESTINAL PSEUDO-OBSTRUCTION

ETIOLOGY

Chronic intestinal pseudo-obstruction may be idiopathic and familial, or it may be due to systemic disease or medications that inhibit intestinal motility. Familial and idiopathic cases often develop in childhood or adolescence and result from damage to the myenteric plexus (visceral neuropathy) or smooth-muscle layers, with replacement of myocytes by fibrosis (visceral myopathy). There may be dysfunction of smooth muscle in other organs, such as the ureters, bladder, and urethra; fibrosis of the ocular lens; and periportal fibrosis of the liver. Scleroderma is the most common systemic disease leading to chronic intestinal pseudo-obstruction, but other conditions include rheumatologic diseases; infiltrative diseases, such as amyloidosis; and neuromuscular diseases, such as myotonic dystrophy, muscular dystrophy, Chagas' disease, and Parkinson's disease. The abrupt onset of chronic pseudo-obstruction in an older patient should raise the suspicion of a paraneoplastic reaction, most often due to small-cell lung carcinoma. Many commonly used drugs can affect gastrointestinal motility. Phenothiazines and antiparkinsonian drugs can inhibit colonic and small-bowel motility and thus cause colonic pseudo-obstruction and adynamic ileus. Other agents, such as anticholinergics, calcium channel antagonists, and smooth-muscle relaxants, also can diminish intestinal tone as well as the amplitude and frequency of peristaltic contractions. Chronic intestinal pseudo-obstruction may affect the entire gut, including the esophagus, stomach, small intestine, and colon.

CLINICAL FEATURES

At one end of the spectrum of intestinal pseudo-obstruction, patients may be asymptomatic; at the other end, they may show recurrent symptoms and signs of small-intestinal obstruction. Symptomatic patients usually have varying amounts of abdominal pain, distention, and vomiting. As a rule, the symptoms are related to eating. Chronic intestinal pseudo-obstruction often leads to intestinal bacterial overgrowth, which may cause diarrhea and steatorrhea. Patients with predominantly colonic involvement have initial symptoms of constipation. When both the small bowel and colon are affected, diarrhea may alternate with constipation, depending on the severity of steatorrhea and the relative involvement of the small intestine and colon. Many patients with small-intestinal pseudo-obstruction have esophageal symptoms, including dysphagia, chest pain, heartburn, and regurgitation. Gastric involvement may further aggravate the symptoms of vomiting and bloating. This limits food intake, and weight loss and malnutrition can be profound. On physical examination there is evidence of malnutrition, with pallor, cheilosis, and edema. The abdomen may be distended and tympanic, with varying bowel sounds.

Laboratory studies show evidence of malnutrition with hypoalbuminemia, anemia, and vitamin B_{12} deficiency. Electrolyte abnormalities and acid–base disturbances result from diarrhea or vomiting. There may be excessive fecal fat. Abdominal radiographs with or without barium often show diffuse dilatation of the stomach, small intestine, and colon with or without air-fluid levels, though selective gastric and duodenal dilatation is noted in some cases. Scleroderma or infiltrative diseases may cause thickened small-intestinal folds. Diverticular disease or pneumatosis intestinalis may be present. Absent fasting IMMC activity and failure to convert to the fed motor pattern with meal ingestion are seen with gastrointestinal manometry. Intravenous pyelography may show a dilated bladder or ureters. Patients with bacterial overgrowth are diagnosed by hydrogen breath testing or jejunal cultures. In patients with known systemic diseases, the clinical scenario coupled with judicious use of radiographic and functional tests can provide an accurate diagnosis. Diagnosis of idiopathic and familial cases, however, may require a full-thickness intestinal biopsy taken at laparotomy to examine for destruction of the muscle layers or myenteric plexus.

TREATMENT

Nutrition supports are key to the treatment of patients whose abdominal symptoms frequently are worsened by eating. Adult patients should consume 1,500 to 1,800 calories/day, divided into four equal feedings. At least half of the calories should come from supplemental formulas, such as Ensure, Isocal, or Vivonex, because liquid empties faster from the stomach and moves more easily through the small bowel. In severe cases, long-term parenteral nutrition is needed. Broad-spectrum antibiotics are useful in treating the bacterial overgrowth syndrome: a 10-day course often results in weight gain and cessation of diarrhea, a remission that may last weeks to months. Metabolic or electrolyte disturbances should be corrected, and medications that inhibit motility should be discontinued. Prokinetic medications are used with varying degrees of success. Cisapride may be more effective than metoclopramide for treating intestinal motor dysfunction. The somatostatin analog octreotide decreases bacterial overgrowth and minimizes symptoms in scleroderma patients with intestinal pseudo-obstruction.

INTESTINAL DYSMOTILITY IN DIABETES

ETIOLOGY

Up to 20% of patients with long-standing diabetes have diarrhea or constipation. There are many potential causes of diarrhea, including bacterial overgrowth from intestinal stasis, bile acid delivery to the colon, or impaired autonomic neural regulation of intestinal absorption leading to active secretion. Constipation probably is due to impaired colonic neural function. A defect in the colonic motor response to a meal is noted in some diabetics.

CLINICAL FEATURES

Diabetic diarrhea is watery and nonbloody and may be associated with tenesmus. The diarrhea may awaken the patient at night. Constipation and diarrhea can be intermittent or alternating. The physical examination typically shows peripheral or autonomic neuropathy. Patients with diabetic diarrhea should undergo stool analysis for total volume and fecal fat content. Most patients have a near-normal daily volume, but some excrete 500 to 1,000 mL/day, suggesting a secretory process. The presence of steatorrhea warrants evaluation for small-intestinal bacterial overgrowth with a culture of a jejunal aspirate or with a hydrogen breath test after ingestion of glucose. In a healthy patient, ingested glucose is absorbed by intestinal enterocytes and metabolized without production of hydrogen. In the patient with bacterial overgrowth, the glucose is metabolized by luminal bacteria, which produce hydrogen that is absorbed, transported to the lungs, and exhaled in the breath. Bacterial overgrowth usually occurs only in the presence of abnormal small-intestinal motility in diabetics. This may be confirmed with gastrointestinal manometry showing the absence of IMMC activity in the small intestine during the fasting state. Secretory diarrhea in diabetics can be documented by intestinal perfusion studies using the nonabsorbable marker polyethylene glycol to determine whether active secretion is taking place in the small intestine.

TREATMENT

Intestinal complications of diabetes are markers of advanced disease. Once intestinal symptoms begin, they are likely to recur. Bacterial overgrowth is treated with oral antibiotics. Recurrent episodes of bacterial overgrowth can be treated with prokinetic agents, but they are less effective in the context of intestinal dysmotility than in cases of gastroparesis. A trial of cholestyramine may be useful to rule out bile acid diarrhea. For mild diarrhea, antidiarrheal opiates, such as loperamide, are useful. The α-adrenoceptor agonist clonidine is effective in some dia-

betics with secretory diarrhea that is presumed to stem from impaired mucosal adrenergic innervation. In patients with constipation with or without alternating diarrhea, fiber supplementation is the simplest and most reliable therapy.

BIBLIOGRAPHY

Camilleri M, Annras S. Dysmotility of the small intestine. In: Yamada T, ed. *Textbook of gastroenterology*, third ed. Philadelphia: JB Lippincott, 1999:1584–1610.

Chen JD, McCallum RW. Clinical applications of electrogastrography. *Am J Gastroenterol* 1993;88:1324–1336.

Hasler WL. Disorders of gastric emptying. In: Yamada T, ed. *Textbook of gastroenterology*, third ed. Philadelphia: JB Lippincott, 1999: 1341–1369.

Hasler WL. Physiology of gastric emptying and gastric motility. In: Yamada T, ed. *Textbook of gastroenterology*, 3rd ed. Philadelphia: JB Lippincott, 1999:188–215.

Hasler WL, Soudah HC, Owyang C. Mechanisms by which octreotide ameliorates symptoms in the dumping syndrome. *J Pharmacol Exp Ther* 1996;277:1359–1365.

Horowitz M, Fraser R. Disordered gastric motor function in diabetes mellitus. *Diabetologia* 1994;37:543–551.

Krishnamurthy S, Schuffler MD. Pathology of neuromuscular disorders of the small intestine and colon. *Gastroenterology* 1987;93:610–639.

Malagelada JR, Camilleri M, Stanghellini V. *Manometric diagnosis of gastrointestinal motility disorders*. New York: Thieme, 1986.

McCallum RW, Chen JDZ, Lin Z, et al. Gastric pacing improves emptying and symptoms in patients with gastroparesis. *Gastroenterology* 1998;114: 456–461.

Reynolds JC, Putnam PE. Prokinetic agents. *Gastroenterol Clin North Am* 1992;21:567–596.

Sarna SK, Otterson MF. Small intestinal physiology and pathophysiology. *Gastroenterol Clin North Am* 1989;18:375–404.

Sawyers JL. Management of postgastrectomy syndromes. *Am J Surg* 1990; 159:8–14.

Kelley's Textbook of Internal Medicine, fourth edition. Edited by H. David Humes. Lippincott Williams & Wilkins, Philadelphia © 2000.

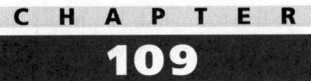

CHAPTER
109

IRRITABLE BOWEL SYNDROME

YEHUDA RINGEL
DOUGLAS A. DROSSMAN

IRRITABLE BOWEL SYNDROME AS A FUNCTIONAL GASTROINTESTINAL DISORDER

Functional gastrointestinal disorders (FGIDs) are the clinical conditions seen most frequently in gastroenterology practice, and they account for a major portion of primary care. FGIDs are defined as a "variable combination of chronic or recurrent

TABLE 109.1.	FUNCTIONAL GASTROINTESTINAL DISORDERS

Esophageal disorders
  Globus
  Rumination syndrome
  Functional chest pain of presumed esophageal origin
  Functional heartburn
  Functional dysphagia
  Unspecified functional esophageal disorder
Gastroduodenal disorders
  Functional dyspepsia
  Aerophagia
  Functional vomiting
Bowel disorders
  Irritable bowel syndrome
  Functional abdominal bloating
  Functional constipation
  Functional diarrhea
  Unspecified functional bowel disorder
Functional abdominal pain
  Functional abdominal pain syndrome
  Unspecified functional abdominal pain
Functional biliary disorders
  Gallbladder dysfunction
  Oddi's sphincter dysfunction
Anorectal disorders
  Functional incontinence
  Functional anorectal pain
  Pelvic floor dyssynergia

TABLE 109.2.	DIAGNOSTIC CRITERIA FOR IRRITABLE BOWEL SYNDROME

Twelve weeks or more in the past 12 months of abdominal discomfort or pain that has two of three features[b]
  Relieved with defecation
  Onset associated with a change in frequency of stool
  Onset associated with a change in form (appearance) of stool

The following symptoms are not essential for the diagnosis, but when/if present they increase confidence in the diagnosis and may be used to identify subgroups of IBS

  Abnormal stool frequency (>3/day or <3/week)
  Abnormal stool form (lumpy/hard or loose/watery stool) more than one-fourth of defecations
  Abnormal stool passage (straining, urgency, or feeling of incomplete evacuation) more than one-fourth of defecations
  Passage of mucus more than one-fourth of defecations
  Bloating or feeling of abdominal distension more than one-fourth of days

[a] In the absence of structural or metabolic abnormalities to explain the symptoms.
[b] The 12 weeks need not be consecutive.

gastrointestinal (GI) symptoms not explained by structural or biochemical abnormalities." In the absence of any obvious, specific morphologic or physiologic marker for the disorder, the diagnosis is mainly based on the clinical signs and symptoms. Symptom-based criteria for defining and diagnosing FGIDs, later known as "Rome criteria," were first developed by a multinational working team in 1990. The Rome criteria subclassified FGIDs into five groups according to the anatomical region (esophageal, gastroduodenal, bowel, biliary, and anorectal) and a separate category, functional abdominal pain (Table 109.1).

Although many hypotheses have been proposed to explain the pathogenesis of the various symptoms experienced by patients with FGIDs, their pathophysiologic basis is still unclear. At present, the evolving theory suggests that the symptoms result from dysregulation of intestinal motor, sensory, and central nervous system (CNS) function. Irritable bowel syndrome (IBS) is the most common and best-studied disorder among the group of FGIDs. It is characterized by symptoms of abdominal pain, bloating, and disturbed defecation (diarrhea or constipation). Many of the physiologic aspects of IBD as well as our biopsychosocial understanding of the disease and general approach to diagnosis and treatment also may be relevant to other FGIDs.

DEFINITION

IBS is a group of functional bowel disorders in which abdominal discomfort or pain is associated with defecation or change in bowel habit and with features of disordered defecation (Rome

II). Since there are no markers for IBS, the disorder is defined by a cluster of clinical symptoms. The first symptom-based criteria for the diagnosis of IBS were developed by Manning in 1978. The Manning criteria include abdominal distention, relief of pain with bowel movement, more frequent stools with onset of pain or looser stools with onset of pain, the passage of mucus, and the sensation of incomplete evacuation. These criteria have been used widely in epidemiologic and clinical studies. A consensus and more comprehensive criteria for the definition of patients with IBS and other functional GI disorders were developed by the Rome multinational working team in 1990. The revised Rome criteria for IBS are shown in Table 109.2.

EPIDEMIOLOGY

IBS affects about 10% to 20% of adolescents and adults in Western countries (14% to 24% of women and 5% to 19% of men). There are no reported ethnic differences, and the rate appears to decline among older subjects. Although only 30% of IBS patients seek medical attention, IBS is still one of the most commonly seen disorders in the general population and in medical settings. It accounts for 12% of primary care visits and 28% of cases seen in gastroenterology practice. Whether a patient seeks health care is influenced by social and cultural factors, the presence and severity of pain, and psychosocial disturbances.

Patients most often report going to the doctor because of severe pain, bloating, bowel symptoms, and associated psychological distress. Women see physicians for symptoms of IBS more often in Western countries, whereas in India and Sri Lanka it is primarily men. The disorder poses a considerable socioeconomic burden. On average, IBS patients take off three times more workdays in a year, pay significantly more average annual visits to physicians, and spend 42% more on health care than people without bowel symptoms.

ETIOLOGY AND PATHOGENESIS

Although no unique pathophysiologic mechanism of action has been identified, IBS can be understood in terms of several contributing features. Motility disorders traditionally have been implicated in the etiologic picture of IBS. Patients with IBS have exaggerated intestinal motor activity in response to intrinsic stimuli (meals, intraluminal balloon distention) or environmental stimuli (psychological stress). Specific motility patterns are associated with different subtypes of IBS: slowed or delayed intestinal transit occurs in constipation-predominant IBS, and accelerated transit is present in diarrhea-predominant IBS. These findings are not unique to IBS, however, and there is little correlation between pain and motor abnormalities.

Visceral hypersensitivity and altered pain perception have been suggested as another major factor in the pathophysiologic origin of IBS. Several studies have shown that patients with IBS experience the urge to defecate at lower rectal volume and have lower pain thresholds to rectal distention. The pathophysiologic mechanisms by which visceral hypersensitivity and pain are generated and modulated are still poorly understood. This may involve dysregulation of the gut control mechanism at different levels between the enteric nerve system and the brain.

The CNS has a major role in conducting and processing afferent visceral information, including pain signals. Studies using functional brain imaging (positron emission tomography, functional magnetic resonance imaging) have shown differences in regional brain activity between patients with IBS and normal controls in response to rectal distention. These findings emphasize the role of the CNS in modulating the conscious sensory experience of visceral sensation and pain in IBS. Symptoms of IBS and other FGIDs can be produced not only by peripheral dysfunction at the level of the gut (abnormal intestinal motor or sensory function) but also by dysfunction at any level of the gut control mechanism, including the autonomic nervous system, spinal pathways, and CNS.

The gut is physiologically responsive to stressful stimuli and emotions. A variety of studies have shown that psychological distress can cause prolonged motor abnormalities as well as a reduction in the threshold at which people experience afferent GI sensations. Moreover, psychological factors, through their effects on the CNS, also can influence patients' symptom perception (sensation intensity/severity)—via affective and cognitive centers in the brain—and illness behavior.

Patients with IBS have a higher prevalence of comorbid affective disorders, personality disturbances, and psychiatric illnesses compared with normal populations, all of which up-regulates symptom experience and behavior. Therefore, more frequent and severe psychological difficulties are found among patients who frequently seek medical care for more severe symptoms. Psychological tests fail to identify a specific pattern of psychological symptoms or traits that are unique to any of the FGIDs, including IBS.

One explanation of the link between psychological stress and symptom experience and behavior relates to the high incidence of abuse history (up to 50%) among women in GI referral practices, particularly for those with functional diagnoses. Abuse history is associated with more severe symptoms, poorer daily func-

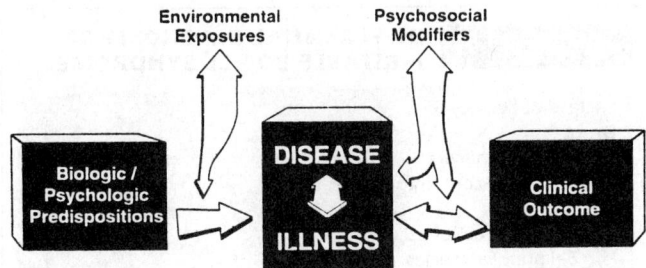

FIGURE 109.1. Schematic representation of the biopsychosocial model (see text for details.) (From Drossman DA. Gastrointestinal illness and the biopsychosocial model [Presidential Address]. *Psychosom Med* 1998; 60:258–267, with permission.)

tion, greater psychological distress, and poorer health outcome. This may be mediated through CNS pathways that amplify the pain experience or the patient's perceived ability to cope with it.

Since both physiologic and psychological factors contribute to symptoms and illness, a biopsychosocial model of illness and disease is helpful in explaining patients' clinical symptoms and behavior (Fig. 109.1). Environmental stress, thoughts, and emotions can have various influences on aspects of gut physiologic mechanisms of action, the symptom experience, health behavior, and outcome. A biopsychosocial approach addressing all of these factors is necessary for establishing more comprehensive and effective diagnosis and treatment of patients with IBS.

DIAGNOSIS

CLINICAL SYMPTOMS

Abdominal pain associated with a change in the consistency or frequency of stools and relieved with defecation is the hallmark of IBS. The abdominal pain often is poorly localized and may be migratory and varying in nature. It often occurs after a meal, during psychological stress, or at the time of menses. Associated symptoms can include bloating or a sensation of distention, presence of mucus in the stool, urgency, and a feeling of incomplete evacuation. IBS can be diarrhea predominant, constipation predominant, or a combination of both at varying times. Symptoms that awaken the patient from sleep, the onset of symptoms at an older age, or the presence of GI bleeding, weight loss, or fever suggest a diagnosis other than IBS and may require further evaluation. It should be noted that IBS can coexist with other GI diseases (inflammatory bowel disease). A positive diagnosis of IBS is based on identifying unequivocal symptoms suggestive of the disorder using symptom-based criteria (Rome, Manning) and a modest effort to exclude other diseases.

DIAGNOSTIC STRATEGY

The initial evaluation involves limited diagnostic screening tests, including blood tests, stool tests, and sigmoidoscopy. Additional studies depend on the patients' history and dominant symptom. Examples of testing include the lactose hydrogen breath test in

TABLE 109.3.	DIFFERENTIAL DIAGNOSIS OF IRRITABLE BOWEL SYNDROME

Lactase deficiency
Drugs
   Laxative/cathartics
   Magnesium-containing antacids
Infection
   Bacterial infection
      Salmonella species
      Campylobacter jejuni
      Yersinia enterocolitica
      Clostridium difficile
   Parasitic infection
      Giardia lamblia
      Entameba histolytica
   Opportunistic infections in immunocompromised host
Inflammatory bowel disease
   Crohn's disease
   Ulcerative colitis
Malabsorbtion
   Chronic pancreatitis
   Celiac sprue
Metabolic disorders
   Diabetes mellitus
   Thyrotoxicosis
Endocrine-producing tumors
   Gastrinoma
   Carcinoid
   VIPoma
Psychiatric disorders
   Depression
   Somatization disorders
Intestinal pseudo-obstruction
   Primary visceral myopathy/neuropathy
   Secondary myopathy/neuropathy (scleroderma, diabetes)
Other colonic diseases
   Microscopic/collagenous colitis
   Villous adenoma

a patient with diarrhea-predominant symptoms or plain abdominal radiography during an acute episode for a patient with pain, gas, or bloating as the primary symptom. If the initial screening evaluation gives normal results, the physician should withhold further diagnostic studies and begin treatment with a follow-up visit within 4 to 6 weeks. Other factors must be considered in planning a diagnostic strategy, including the duration and severity of symptoms, age at onset, family history of colon cancer, change over time (getting worse or better), previous diagnostic evaluations, and psychosocial status. Good clinical judgment based on a thorough history and physical examination can help minimize unneeded investigative studies.

SPECIFIC DIAGNOSTIC TESTING

The initial evaluation should include a complete blood count, sedimentation rate, serum chemistries, evaluation of the stool for ova, parasites and blood, and sigmoidoscopy. Colonoscopy or barium enema with sigmoidoscopy is recommended if the patient is older than 50 years. The presence of the following signs should raise the suspicion of other diagnosis (Table 109.3) and may lead to further studies: history of weight loss, onset of symptoms in an older patient, nocturnal awakening, family history of carcinoma or inflammatory bowel disease, fever, abnormal physical finding (abdominal mass, hepatomegaly), abnormal laboratory result (occult blood in stool, anemia, leukocytosis, elevated sedimentation rate, abnormal chemistries).

If any of the initial tests show abnormal results or if a first therapeutic trial fails, further investigative studies may be necessary. Those patients with constipation as their predominant symptom should undergo colonic function tests, such as colonic transit time and anorectal manometry (see Chapter 100). Patients with mainly diarrhea may require stool tests (volume, electrolytes, fat, white count), small-bowel evaluation (small-bowel follow-through radiography and endoscopy with duodenal aspirate and biopsy), breath tests to exclude bacterial overgrowth, and colonic biopsies to exclude collagenous/lymphocytic colitis (see Chapter 111). Additional small-bowel radiographic studies should be considered for patients with bloating and pain, to exclude partial obstruction.

◼ TREATMENT STRATEGY

PHYSICIAN–PATIENT RELATIONSHIP

Once a diagnosis of IBS has been established, the physician's confidence in the diagnosis should be conveyed to the patient along with reassurance and education about the condition and its consequences. An effective physician–patient relationship is the basis for any treatment program. This relationship is achieved through adhering to the following recommended guidelines. First, the physician must conduct a nonjudgmental, patient-centered interview to identify his or her symptoms, fears, and concerns; exacerbating factors; and psychosocial contributions. Second, the physician should clearly explain the disorder, including its pathophysiologic characteristics, natural history, chronic nature, and the role of environmental stress and psychosocial factors on the symptoms. Third, attention must be paid to the patient's beliefs and expectations, making efforts to integrate them realistically into a plan of care that helps the patient better control symptoms. This plan includes developing strategies that address symptoms, cognition, and modes of behavior. Finally, it is essential to provide continuity of care while setting limits on the frequency of clinical visits and the extent of additional testing. A specific treatment strategy is based on the nature (diarrhea, constipation, pain/bloating) and severity (mild, moderate, severe) of the symptoms.

TREATMENT APPROACH BASED ON SEVERITY

The severity of IBS is determined by the intensity and constancy of the symptoms, the nature of the physiologic disturbances (diarrhea or constipation), the degree of psychosocial difficulties, and the frequency of health care use. Most patients with IBS do not see physicians for their symptoms. The majority (about 70%) of the patients who do see physicians have mild and infrequent symptoms associated with little disability and no overt psychological difficulties. These patients often are seen in primary care and usually require only reassurance, education, and dietary or lifestyle changes. Patients with moderate symptoms (about 25% of those who see physicians) experience more intense and frequent symptoms that occasionally interfere with daily activities (missing work) and may be associated with psychological distress. These patients may require pharmacologic and/or behavioral treatments. Only a small proportion of IBS patients (about 5%) have severe symptoms. They experience more constant abdominal pain, often in the context of psychological difficulties (depression) that chronically interfere with daily functioning. They frequently use health care services and may undergo extensive testing. These patients usually are referred to tertiary centers and often need psychopharmacologic (antidepressants) and/or psychological (cognitive-behavioral) treatment. Patients with the most refractory symptoms should be referred to specialized functional GI disorders or pain treatment centers.

SPECIAL TREATMENTS
Dietary Modifications

Identifying offending dietary substances and making dietary modifications can be helpful with some patients. Food items that may be associated with IBS symptom exacerbation include lactose (in lactose intolerant individuals), caffeine, fatty foods, alcohol, gas producing foods (e.g., cabbage, beans), sorbitol (>10 gm/day) and other offending food items that aggravate GI motility. Recommendations for dietary changes should usually also involve life style changes and encouragement for health promoting behaviors.

Pharmacotherapy

Most patients with IBS require no prescribed medications. Medications are best used intermittently or for short-term periods, mainly during exacerbations, and only as part of a complete management plan. Placebo effects may occur in as many as 70% of patients and should be considered when assessing the benefit of any drug treatment. Nevertheless, individual symptoms may respond to specific agents. The use of medication directed at the gut depends on the dominant symptom (pain, diarrhea, or constipation). When pain and bloating are the main symptoms, such anticholinergic agents as dicyclomine hydrochloride or hyoscyamine sulfate can be used, preferably before meals for postprandial pain. Other antispasmodics, such as octylonium, cimetropine, mebeverine, or peppermint oil, are not available in the United States. There are a few new medications, currently in clinical trials, that are directed at minimizing gut sensitivity. They include serotonin receptor antagonists and the kappa opioid antagonist fedotozine. In more severe or refractory cases, low doses of antidepressants should be considered. They often are used for their neuromodulatory and analgesic properties as well as for their psychotrophic effects. Tricyclic agents, such as desipramine (50 to 150 mg) or amitriptyline (25 to 100 mg), have been studied best and appear to be effective. However, serotonin re-uptake inhibitors, such as fluoxetine or paroxetine, may be preferred for older patients or those with associated constipation because of their less prominent anticholinergic effects.

When diarrhea is the primary symptom, antidiarrhea agents, such as loperamide (4 to 8 mg per day), may help diminish urgency, stool frequency, and soiling and increase stool consistency. For patients with constipation, increasing dietary fiber (25 g per day) may be effective. If this solution is not sufficient, osmotic laxatives, such as milk of magnesia, sorbitol, or lactose, may be added. Stimulant laxatives (senna phenolphthalein) should be avoided on a long-term basis. The use of promotility agents, such as cisapride, also has been suggested for patients with colonic inertia but may be helpful only for those with milder symptoms.

Psychological Treatments

Referral for psychological treatment usually is recommended for patients with disabling symptoms or associated psychiatric disorders (major depression). Several psychological treatments have been used in patients with IBS, including cognitive-behavioral therapy, dynamic psychotherapy, hypnotherapy, and relaxation training (arousal reduction). There are several well-designed studies that suggest their beneficial effect. Psychological treatments appear to be superior to conventional medical treatment in minimizing psychological distress, improving coping, and reducing bowel symptoms. No one specific treatment was found to be superior. The most important aspect of treatment is the patient's acceptance of the need for treatment and the motivation to engage in it. A physician's willingness to address both biologic and psychological aspects of the illness and to develop an effective therapeutic relationship (adopting a biopsychosocial approach) with patients can contribute significantly to the success of treatment.

BIBLIOGRAPHY

Drossman DA. Psychosocial sound bites: exercises in the patient–doctor relationship. *Am J Gastroenterol* 1997;92:1418–1423.
Drossman DA. Gastrointestinal illness and the biopsychosocial model [Presidential Address]. *Psychosom Med* 1998;60:258–267.
Drossman DA. An integrated approach to the irritable bowel syndrome [Review]. *Aliment Pharmacol Ther* 1999;13(suppl 2):3–14.
Drossman DA, Corazzione E, et al. *Rome II. The functional gastrointestinal disorders. Diagnosis, pathophysiology, and treatment.* 2nd ed. McLean, VA: Degnon Associates, 2000.
Drossman DA, Li Z, Andruzzi E, et al. U.S. householder survey of functional GI disorders: prevalence, sociodemography and health impact. *Dig Dis Sci* 1993;38:1569–1580.
Drossman DA, Talley NJ, Olden KW, et al. Sexual and physical abuse and gastrointestinal illness: review and recommendations. *Ann Intern Med* 1995;123:782–794.
Drossman DA, Whitehead WE, Camilleri M. Irritable bowel syndrome: a technical review for practice guideline development. *Gastroenterology* 1997;112:2120–2137.
Gaynes B, Drossman DA. The role of psychosocial factors in irritable bowel syndrome. In: Whorwell PJ, Houghton LA, eds. *Bailliere's clinical gastroenterology* 1999; 13(3):437–452.
Patrick DL, Drossman DA, Frederick IO, et al. Quality of life in persons with irritable bowel syndrome: development of a new measure. *Dig Dis Sci* 1998;43:400–411.
Thompson WG, Longstreth GF, Drossman DA, et al. Functional bowel disorders and functional abdominal pain. *Gut* 1999; 45(Suppl 2); II43–II47.

Kelley's Textbook of Internal Medicine, fourth edition. Edited by H. David Humes. Lippincott Williams & Wilkins, Philadelphia © 2000.

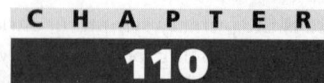

DISORDERS OF DIGESTION AND ABSORPTION

DENNIS J. AHNEN

The human gastrointestinal tract is extraordinarily well adapted for efficient digestion and absorption of nutrients; more than 90% of ingested and endogenously secreted fat, protein, and carbohydrate is digested and absorbed. Disorders at any level of this process, however, can cause nutritional deficiency.

■ NORMAL NUTRIENT ASSIMILATION

Normal nutrient digestion and absorption is a highly coordinated process. For the major nutrients, digestion, absorption, and metabolism can be considered to occur in four phases: hydrolysis in the intestinal lumen, hydrolysis at the enterocyte brush border, transport from the lumen into the enterocyte, and intracellular processing and secretion from the enterocyte into the portal or lymphatic circulation.

FAT ASSIMILATION

Dietary fat consists predominantly of triglycerides, phospholipids, and cholesterol. Although fat intake varies widely worldwide (15% to 50% of total caloric intake), the average American diet consists of roughly 42% fat, containing about 100 g of triglycerides, 2 to 8 g of phospholipids, and 0.2 to 0.5 g of cholesterol per day. In addition to ingested fats, about 9 g per day of phospholipid and 1 to 2 g per day of cholesterol are secreted into the intestinal lumen each day (mostly from bile). Overall, more than 95% of ingested and secreted lipid is digested and absorbed, predominantly in the proximal jejunum.

Triglycerides are composed of three fatty acids linked by ester bonds to glycerol. Considerable variability exists in the relative amounts of the saturated fatty acids (palmitic and steric) versus the unsaturated fatty acids (oleic and linoleic) in the diet. Certain essential fatty acids cannot be adequately synthesized by humans and must be ingested and absorbed. Phospholipid structure is similar to that of triglycerides, with one of the hydroxyl groups of glycerol linked to one of several polar head groups (choline, serine, ethanolamine) instead of a fatty acid. Cholesterol has a multiringed sterol nucleus; it is the most abundant sterol in human tissue and is the precursor of other steroid hormones and bile acids.

Dietary fats are not soluble in water and spontaneously form lipid aggregates. Triglycerides tend to aggregate into lipid droplets. Phospholipids are amphipathic molecules that have a propensity to aggregate into phospholipid bilayers, with their polar head groups on the outside and their hydrophobic fatty acids in the interior. These aggregates form the structural bridges between water-soluble proteins and nonpolar lipids, such as in the phospholipid bilayer of biologic membranes. Other water-insoluble nutrients, such as cholesterol and fat-soluble vitamins, are sequestered in the hydrophobic interior of triglyceride and phospholipid aggregates.

Triglyceride Digestion and Absorption

The overall process of triglyceride digestion and absorption is depicted in Fig. 110.1. Lipolysis of ingested triglycerides is initiated in the stomach by the action of gastric lipase, an acidic lipase (pH optimum of 3 to 6) that preferentially hydrolyzes medium-chain triglycerides. Gastric lipase may be particularly important for neonatal digestion of milk fat, which is rich in medium-chain triglycerides. The bulk of intraluminal lipolysis in the adult is mediated by pancreatic lipase. Bile acids can displace pancreatic lipase from the lipid droplet, and another pancreatic protein, colipase, is required to restore lipase activity in the presence of bile acids. The lipase–colipase complex acts on the first and third positions of triglycerides, yielding β-monoglyceride and two free fatty acids (Fig. 110.1).

The products of triglyceride hydrolysis (fatty acids and β-monoglyceride) are solubilized within the intestinal lumen in combination with secreted bile acids to form mixed micelles. Bile acids are amphipathic, with their hydrophobic and hydrophilic regions clustered at different ends of the molecule. As a result, they can form aggregates, with their hydrophilic domains (solid circles in Fig. 110.1) oriented on the external surface and their hydrophobic domains on the interior surface. Fatty acids and β-monoglycerides are also amphipathic and become oriented within the micelle with their hydrophobic regions clustered in the interior of the mixed micelle. The bile acid micelle increases the solubility of fatty acids and β-monoglycerides by a factor of 100 to 1,000, thus increasing the delivery of the lipolytic products through the aqueous environment of the intestinal lumen to the enterocyte brush border.

At the enterocyte brush border, fatty acids and β-monoglycerides are released from the micelle to diffuse through the adjacent microvillar membrane. Transport through the microvillar lipid bilayer traditionally has been thought to be by passive diffusion, but more recent data suggest that it also may be facilitated by a fatty acid–binding protein in the microvillar membrane. Once taken up by the enterocyte, fatty acid and β-monoglyceride transport to the endoplasmic reticulum is mediated by the intestinal fatty acid–binding protein. The mechanism for transport of other glycerides and lipids is not certain, but it may require a separate fatty acid–binding protein. Within the cytosol, fatty acids are acylated to fatty acid acyl coenzyme A (CoA). Re-esterification of β-monoglycerides with fatty acid acyl-CoA to form triglycerides is mediated by acyltransferases on the inner surface of the endoplasmic reticulum.

The re-esterified triglycerides become incorporated into another type of lipid aggregate, the chylomicron (Fig. 110.1), which consists of a central lipid droplet composed predominantly of triglycerides plus small amounts of cholesterol esters and free cholesterol. The droplet is coated with a monolayer of

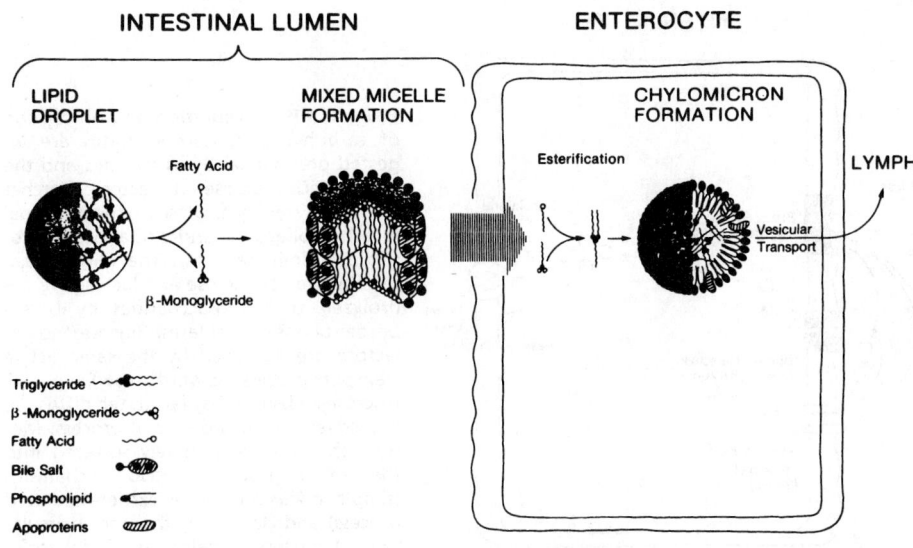

INTESTINAL LUMEN   ENTEROCYTE

LIPID DROPLET   MIXED MICELLE FORMATION   CHYLOMICRON FORMATION

Fatty Acid   Esterification   LYMPH

β-Monoglyceride   Vesicular Transport

Triglyceride
β-Monoglyceride
Fatty Acid
Bile Salt
Phospholipid
Apoproteins

FIGURE 110.1. Digestion and absorption of triglycerides. Triglycerides are ingested as lipid droplets (shown in partial cross section) and hydrolyzed by lipase in the intestinal lumen to fatty acids and β-monoglycerides. Fatty acids and β-monoglycerides are solubilized by bile acid micelles (shown in partial cross section) and absorbed from micellar solution by passive and carrier-mediated transport systems. In the enterocyte, they are re-esterified to triglycerides; incorporated into chylomicrons (shown in partial cross section), which are secreted by exocytosis; and cleared by the intestinal lymphatics.

phospholipids that are oriented with their polar head groups to the exterior and their hydrophobic domains to the interior. Several apoproteins (apoA-I, apoA-IV, and apoB-48) also are incorporated into the phospholipid monolayer. These amphipathic apoproteins are synthesized by the enterocyte and become associated with the chylomicron surface within the endoplasmic reticulum and Golgi apparatus. Apoprotein function is not fully understood, but apoA-I is a cofactor for the plasma cholesterol esterification enzyme lecithin–cholesterol acyltransferase, apoA-IV has been shown to be a satiety factor in rats, and apoB-48 appears to be required for coordinated intestinal triglyceride transport. Chylomicrons are packaged into membrane-bound transport vesicles in the Golgi apparatus, transported to the basolateral membrane, secreted by exocytosis into the lamina propria, and selectively taken up into lymphatics.

Phospholipid Digestion and Absorption

Phospholipid digestion and absorption is similar to those of triglycerides. Within the intestinal lumen, phospholipids are hydrolyzed by phospholipase A_2, a 14-kd enzyme secreted by the pancreas as a proenzyme. Trypsin-mediated cleavage of seven N-terminal amino acids results in enzyme activation. Phospholipase A_2 requires both bile salts and calcium for activity. Phospholipase A_2 hydrolyzes the fatty acid at position 2 of phospholipids to form lysophospholipids, which are then solubilized in mixed micelles and taken up into the enterocyte by both passive diffusion and facilitated transport. Intracellularly, lysophospholipids can be re-esterified to phospholipids or degraded by lysolecithinase. Phospholipid assimilation, like that of triglycerides, is more than 90% efficient in the proximal small bowel.

Cholesterol Digestion and Absorption

Cholesterol plays an important role as a component of biologic membranes (modulates fluidity) and as a substrate for steroid hormone and bile acid synthesis. Free cholesterol is the predominant sterol in the diet and in biliary secretions. The small amount of cholesterol ester in the intestinal lumen is hydrolyzed to free cholesterol by pancreatic cholesterol esterase. This enzyme has an absolute requirement for trihydroxy bile acids and is capable of hydrolyzing triglycerides, phospholipids, and esters of vitamins A, D_3, and E. Free cholesterol is solubilized in bile acid micelles; then cholesterol is transported across the jejunal brush border by an energy-requiring process that, in all likelihood, is facilitated by a specific carrier protein. Most of the absorbed cholesterol is re-esterified in the endoplasmic reticulum. Both free cholesterol and cholesterol esters are incorporated into chylomicrons for secretion. Only about half of dietary cholesterol is absorbed into the enterocyte, and its absorption depends critically on the presence of bile acids.

Fat-Soluble Vitamin Assimilation

The fat-soluble vitamins (A, D, E, K) are hydrophobic molecules that are absorbed in a manner similar to that of lipids. Their absorption depends critically on bile acid solubilization. Vitamin A (retinol) is ingested primarily as the provitamin beta carotene, which is solubilized in mixed micelles and passively absorbed from micellar solution. Beta carotene is cleaved intracellularly to two molecules of retinol. Retinol is esterified, incorporated into chylomicrons, secreted, and cleared by the lymphatics. Vitamin A is stored exclusively in hepatic lipocytes as retinol ester.

Most vitamin D is synthesized endogenously in the skin, but it undergoes significant enterohepatic circulation. As a result, substantial vitamin D deficiency can occur in the context of fat malabsorption. Vitamin D is stored in the liver and in peripheral tissues. A portion of vitamin E (alpha tocopherol) is ingested as an ester. The ester is mostly hydrolyzed to alpha tocopherol in the intestinal lumen by nonspecific pancreatic lipase. Absorption of vitamin E is similar to that of vitamin D, with little re-esterification before secretion in chylomicrons.

Vitamin K_1 (phylloquinone) is ingested with food, and vitamin K_2 (menadione) is derived from bacterial sources. Vitamin K_1 appears to be absorbed by active transport, whereas vitamin K_2 is absorbed passively. Both vitamins are secreted largely un-

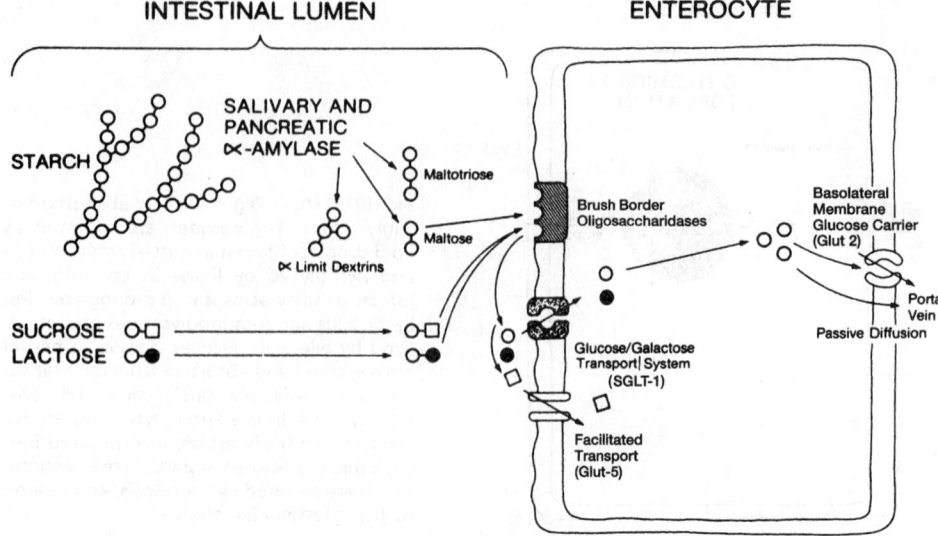

FIGURE 110.2. Digestion and absorption of carbohydrates. Carbohydrates are ingested predominantly as starches and the disaccharides sucrose and lactose. Starches are hydrolyzed by amylases in the intestinal lumen to oligosaccharides (maltose, maltotriose, α-limit dextrins). The oligosaccharides as well as sucrose and lactose are hydrolyzed to monosaccharides by brush-border oligosaccharidases. Glucose and galactose are absorbed by the same active transport process (upward arrow), whereas fructose is absorbed by facilitated diffusion, a passive (downward arrow) process. Monosaccharides are passively secreted into the lamina propria by two mechanisms (simple diffusion and a carrier-mediated process) and cleared by the portal circulation. ○, glucose; ■, galactose; □, fructose.

changed into chylomicrons. There is little tissue storage and rapid turnover of the total body pool of vitamin K.

CARBOHYDRATE DIGESTION AND ABSORPTION

The average American diet contains about 250 g of carbohydrates, which accounts for about 45% of daily caloric intake. About half of ingested carbohydrate consists of starch. Two-thirds of ingested starch is amylopectin, a large (10^6 kd) glucose polymer containing both α_{1-4}- and α_{1-6}-linked glucose molecules, and one-third is amylose, a smaller (100 kd) α_{1-4}-linked glucose polymer. The disaccharides sucrose and lactose constitute about 15% of ingested carbohydrates, and the mushroom disaccharide trehalose is a small component of the diet. Monosaccharides (glucose, galactose, fructose, sorbitol, maltodextrins) are being ingested in increasing amounts in processed and dietetic foods and in soft drinks and now compose up to 10% of ingested carbohydrate. The remainder of dietary carbohydrate (about 10 gm per day) consists of undigestable fiber (cellulose, hemicellulose, gums, and pectins). Although these fibers are not digested in the small intestine, they can be fermented by colonic bacteria. The overall process of carbohydrate digestion and absorption is depicted in Fig. 110.2.

Both salivary and pancreatic amylase enzymes are capable of cleaving the internal α_{1-4}-linked glucose bonds of starch. Salivary amylase activity ordinarily is short-lived, because it is not active at the acidic pH of the stomach. The bulk of ingested starch is hydrolyzed by pancreatic amylase to oligosaccharides. The end products of amylase action are α_{1-4}-linked glucose polymers (maltose and maltotriose) as well as a series of α-limit dextrins containing both α_{1-4} and α_{1-6} linkages (Fig. 110.2 and Table 110.1). Sucrose, lactose, and the oligosaccharide products of intraluminal starch hydrolysis are further hydrolyzed to their component monosaccharides by a series of oligosaccharidases of the jejunal brush border (Fig. 110.2 and Table 110.1). Through the combined action of these enzymes, luminal oligosaccharides are hydrolyzed to glucose and smaller amounts of galactose and fructose.

Monosaccharides are transported across the enterocyte by members of two distinct families of transporters, the secondary active sodium/glucose co-transporter SGLT-1 and the facilitated glucose transporters Glut-5 and Glut-2. Glucose and galactose entry across the microvillar membrane is mediated by SGLT-1 and driven by the Na^+,K^+,-ATPase-generated sodium gradient across the apical cell membrane (Fig. 110.3). Fructose enters the cells by facilitated transport that is probably mediated by the Glut-5 transporter. Ingestion of large amounts of fructose found

TABLE 110.1.	OLIGOSACCHARIDASES OF THE INTESTINAL BRUSH BORDER	
Substrate	**Enzyme**	**Products**
Maltose, Maltotriose, α_{1-4}-linked glucose oligosaccharides	Maltase	Glucose
Sucrose	Sucrase-α-dextrinase	Glucose and fructose
α-limit dextrins (α_{1-6} links)	Sucrase-α-dextrinase	Glucose
α-limit dextrins (α_{1-4} links)	Sucrase-α-dextrinase	Glucose
Lactose	Lactase	Glucose and galactose
Trehalose	Trehalase	Glucose

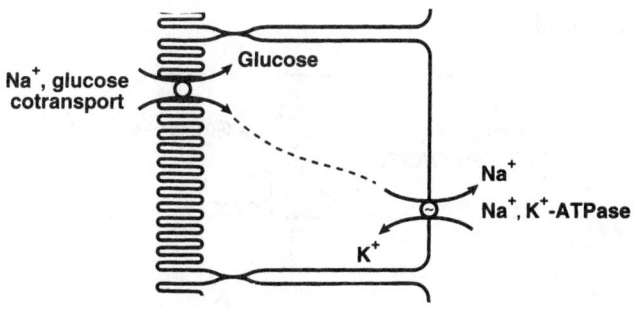

FIGURE 110.3. Glucose and galactose transport across the enterocyte. Glucose and galactose are actively cotransported with sodium across the enterocyte brush border by the transport protein SGLT-1. A homotetramer of four SGLT-1 subunits of protein forms the functional cotransporter. Sodium passes down the concentration gradient generated by the sodium–potassium ATPase pump located on the basolateral membrane of the enterocyte and glucose or galactose is cotransported on a 1:1 molar ratio with sodium.

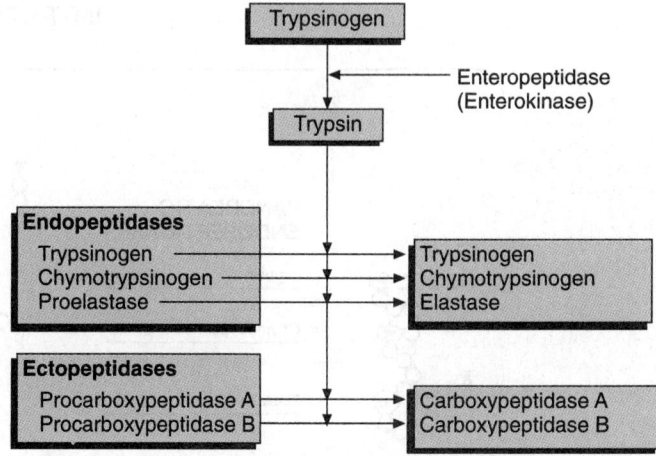

FIGURE 110.4. Activation of the pancreatic protease proenzymes in the intestinal lumen. Trypsinogen is cleaved to the active protease trypsin by the microvillar membrane enteropeptidase. Trypsin can then mediate the proteolytic activation of additional trypsinogen as well as the other proenzymes.

in some soft drinks can overwhelm this transport system and result in osmotic diarrhea. Similarly, sorbitol, which is widely used in dietetic foods, is poorly absorbed by the normal intestinal tract and also can induce osmotic diarrhea. Once inside the cell, the sugars can be used by the enterocyte as an energy source, but most are secreted across the basolateral membrane into the interstitial space. The bulk of the secreted glucose exits by a sodium-independent facilitated transport system (Glut-2), and a smaller fraction (up to 25%) diffuses passively down its concentration gradient through the basolateral membrane. Glucose passes to the portal circulation by passive diffusion. The intestinal assimilation of dietary starch and sucrose is efficient, with nearly 100% assimilation within the jejunum. The efficiency of lactose assimilation varies considerably among different populations (see "Lactase Deficiency").

PROTEIN DIGESTION AND ABSORPTION

The average American diet consists of 70 to 100 g per day of protein (about 10% of total caloric intake). In addition, 20 to 30 g per day of endogenous protein is secreted into the intestinal lumen through biliary, pancreatic, and intestinal secretions. Proteins are composed of α-amino acids linked by peptide bonds. There are 20 common amino acids found in protein. Of these, eight essential amino acids (Table 110.2) must come from dietary sources, because they cannot be synthesized by human

cells. The overall scheme of protein digestion is shown in Figs. 110.4 through 110.6.

Protein digestion is initiated in the stomach by the action of a group of enzymes, the pepsinogens, that are secreted by chief cells as inactive precursors. At acidic pH, pepsinogens are converted to pepsins by autocatalytic cleavage. The extent of gastric proteolysis depends on many factors, including the rate of gastric emptying, the gastric pH, and the type of protein digested. Gastric proteolysis undoubtedly increases the efficiency of protein digestion, but gastric function is not essential for normal protein digestion.

The bulk of intraluminal proteolysis is mediated by pancreatic proteases through a highly ordered series of events. The pancreas secretes both endopeptidases (trypsin, chymotrypsin, elastase), which are capable of cleaving internal peptide bonds, and carboxypeptidases (carboxypeptidase A and B), which in turn are capable of cleaving the carboxy-terminal amino acid from peptides. All these pancreatic proteases are synthesized and secreted as inactive precursors. Within the small-bowel lumen, trypsinogen is hydrolyzed (by removal of the N-terminal hexapeptide) to the active protease trypsin by enteropeptidase (enterokinase). Enterokinase is a protease that is released from the intestinal brush border by bile acids. Trypsin is then capable of cleaving additional molecules of trypsinogen to trypsin, as well as the other inactive enzymes to their active counterparts (Fig. 110.4). Dietary proteins are initially cleaved by the pancreatic endopeptidases, each of which has a different substrate specificity (Fig. 110.5). The resultant peptides are the preferred substrates for the pancreatic carboxypeptidases. The end products of this ordered sequence of intraluminal proteolysis are basic and neutral amino acids (40%) and a series of oligopeptides (60%).

The oligopeptide products of pancreatic proteases are hydrolyzed further by a series of brush-border oligopeptidases (Fig. 110.5), which remove the amino-terminal amino acid from oligopeptides. A comparable series of brush-border carboxypeptidases can cleave the carboxy-terminal amino acid from oligopep-

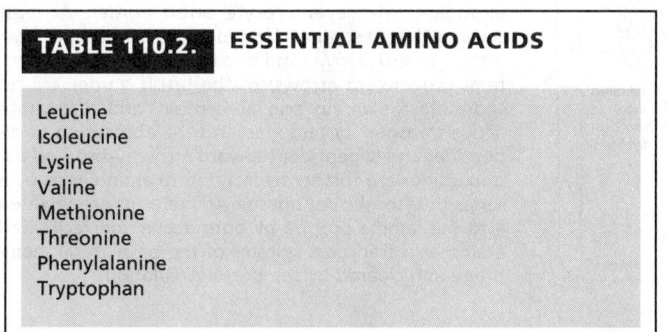

TABLE 110.2.	**ESSENTIAL AMINO ACIDS**
Leucine	
Isoleucine	
Lysine	
Valine	
Methionine	
Threonine	
Phenylalanine	
Tryptophan	

INTESTINAL LUMEN

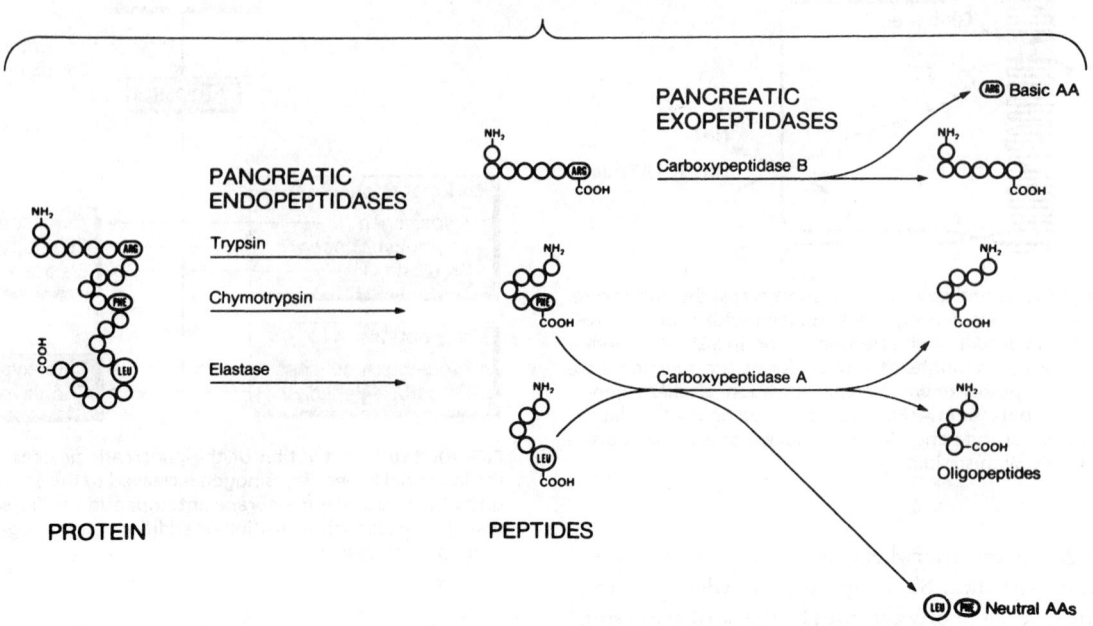

FIGURE 110.5. Intraluminal digestion of proteins by pancreatic proteases. Although protein digestion is initiated in the stomach, most proteolysis is mediated by the sequential action of pancreatic endopeptidases (trypsin, chymotrypsin, elastase) and exopeptidases (carboxypeptidases A and B). The endopeptidases cleave internal peptide bonds. Each of the pancreatic endopeptidases has a different specificity; thus, a series of oligopeptides results from their action. The carboxypeptidases can then cleave the carboxy-terminal amino acid from the oligopeptides. Trypsin preferentially cleaves peptide bonds on the carboxyl side of basic amino acids, resulting in small peptides with basic carboxy-terminal amino acids. These peptides serve as substrates for carboxypeptidase B, which cleaves the basic carboxy-terminal amino acid from the peptide. Chymotrypsin preferentially cleaves peptide bonds adjacent to aromatic neutral amino acids, and elastase preferentially cleaves bonds adjacent to aliphatic neutral amino acids. The peptides created by chymotrypsin and elastase are then subject to cleavage by carboxypeptidase A, to release the neutral carboxy-terminal amino acid. The products of pancreatic proteolysis therefore are free amino acids and oligopeptides.

ENTEROCYTE

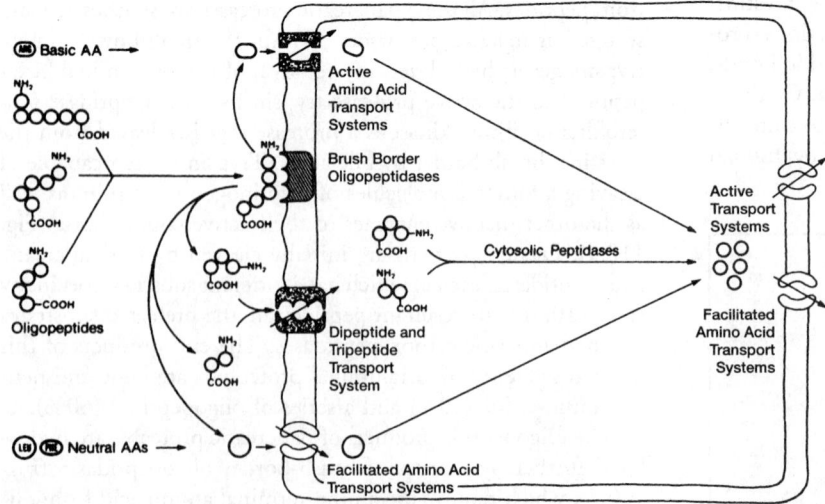

FIGURE 110.6. Brush-border digestion and absorption of proteins. The oligopeptides that are produced by pancreatic protease digestion are further hydrolyzed to free amino acids, dipeptides, and tripeptides by oligopeptidases of the enterocyte brush border. At least seven different sodium-dependent active transport systems (upward arrows) and two facilitated transport systems (downward arrows) of the brush border are responsible for amino acid absorption, and a separate active transport system mediates the absorption of dipeptides and tripeptides (upward arrow). Absorbed oligopeptides are further hydrolyzed to amino acids by a series of cytosolic peptidases. Amino acids are secreted into the lamina propria by both active and facilitated amino acid transport systems of the basolateral membrane and cleared by the portal circulation.

TABLE 110.3.	AMINO ACID TRANSPORTERS OF THE ENTEROCYTE APICAL AND BASOLATERAL MEMBRANE		
Transport System	Location (Apical/Basolateral)	Substrates	Sodium Dependence
B	Apical	Neutral amino acids	Yes
$B^{0,+}$	Apical	Neutral and basic amino acids	Yes
Imino	Apical	Imino acids (proline, hydroxyproline)	Yes
β	Apical	β-amino acid (taurine)	Yes
X^-_{AG}	Apical	Acidic amino acids	Yes
$b^{0,+}$	Apical	Neutral and basic amino acids	No
L	Both	Large hydrophobic neutral amino acids	No
y^+	Both	Basic amino acids	No
A	Basolateral	Neutral amino acids	Yes
ASC	Basolateral	Three and four-carbon neutral amino acids (alanine, serine, cysteine)	Yes
asc	Basolateral	Three and four-carbon neutral amino acids	No

tides, and a family of endopeptidases are capable of cleaving internal peptide bonds of oligopeptides. The final products of the brush-border oligopeptidases are free amino acids, dipeptides, and tripeptides.

The jejunal brush border contains a series of amino acid transporters with different or overlapping specificities. At least six sodium-dependent secondary active transporters for α-amino acids, one active transporter for taurine (a β-amino acid), and three sodium-independent facilitated transporters can mediate amino acid uptake across the microvillar membrane (Table 110.3). System B is thought to be the major apical transport system for neutral amino acids, whereas the X^-_{AG} and imino systems are thought to be critical for acidic and proline-containing amino acid transport, respectively. The relative importance of the other transport systems for neutral and basic amino acids is not yet known.

Many amino acids are more efficiently absorbed as constituents of di- and tripeptides than as single amino acids. One active transport system thus far has been characterized for dipeptides and tripeptides. Dipeptides and tripeptides containing compact amino acids (proline, hydroxyproline, glycine) are the optimal substrates for this sodium-dependent active transport process. Undoubtedly, additional transport systems for amino acids and oligopeptides will be identified.

Absorbed di- and tripeptides are hydrolyzed almost completely to amino acids by a series of cytosolic oligopeptidases that are entirely different from those in the brush border. The three best characterized of these enzymes are cytoplasmic dipeptidase, which hydrolyzes neutral dipeptides; cytosolic prolidase, which specifically hydrolyzes dipeptides containing proline or hydroxyproline; and cytosolic tripeptidase, which has strong affinity for tripeptides containing an amino-terminal proline.

About 10% of absorbed amino acids are used by the enterocyte for protein synthesis, with glutamine being preferentially used as a source of energy. The remainder of absorbed amino acids are transported across the basolateral membrane by several amino acid transport systems (three facilitated and two active transport systems have been described; see Table 110.3). Overall protein assimilation is efficient. More than 95% of dietary and endogenous proteins within the intestinal lumen are absorbed by the proximal and middle small bowel.

ASSIMILATION OF FOLATE AND OTHER WATER-SOLUBLE VITAMINS

Most dietary folates are polyglutamic acid conjugates of folic acid. Hydrolysis of the polyglutaminated folate probably is mediated by a specific brush-border hydrolase that deconjugates the polyglutamate to monoglutaminated folate. The monoglutamyl product is absorbed by an energy-dependent transport process. Relatively little is known about the absorption of the other water-soluble vitamins. Animal studies suggest that there are active transport mechanisms for ascorbic acid, biotin, inositol, nicotinic acid, and thiamine. Para-aminobenzoic acid and pyridoxine appear to enter the cell by simple diffusion, whereas choline and riboflavin are absorbed by carrier-mediated facilitated diffusion.

IRON ABSORPTION

Normally, 1 or 2 mg of iron is absorbed daily. Heme iron, which is found in animal protein, is about six times more efficiently absorbed than the non-heme iron of grains and cereals. Most heme iron is absorbed as an intact metalloporphyrin by gastric and intestinal epithelial cells. The iron is released from heme after absorption by oxidative cleavage mediated by heme oxygenase. In contrast, absorption of nonheme iron depends on several intraluminal factors. Iron is poorly absorbed from ferric salts unless it is reduced, because ferric iron is insoluble in aqueous solution above pH 3. In addition, a number of dietary factors can either increase or decrease nonheme iron solubility in the gut. Organic anions, such as phosphate, phytate, and phosphoproteins, can bind iron and render it insoluble, whereas some amino acids, such as histidine and lysine, complex with iron and make it more soluble. Nonheme iron is absorbed most efficiently in the duodenum, where it is taken up by a carrier-mediated transport process. Once in the cell, iron is either bound to ferritin or transferred to plasma bound to transferrin. The iron–transferrin complex is taken up by the hepatocyte by receptor-mediated endocytosis. The efficiency of iron absorption is enhanced when body iron stores are depleted and diminished when body iron stores rise. The mechanism of regulation is not known, but when the efficiency of iron absorption improves, the absorption of other metals, such as zinc, nickel, manganese, cobalt, and lead, also improves.

SPECIALIZED ILEAL ABSORPTIVE MECHANISMS

Cobalamin (Vitamin B₁₂)

Cobalamin is produced by bacteria and absorbed by animals after ingestion of contaminated foods or after production by the intestinal microflora in ruminants. In humans most dietary cobalamin comes from meat, milk, egg products, and dietary supplements. Cobalamin always is bound tightly to proteins and undergoes a series of protein transfers during its absorption. In ingested tissues it is bound to intracellular enzymes (methylmalonyl-CoA mutase and methyltetrahydrafolate-homocysteine transferase). It is released from these enzymes by gastric proteases and transferred to a family of glycoproteins called R proteins. Both intrinsic factor and R proteins are secreted into gastric juice. Pancreatic proteases subsequently hydrolyze the R protein, freeing cobalamin to bind to intrinsic factor. The cobalamin–intrinsic factor complex is not absorbed in the proximal small bowel but binds to specific receptors on the brush border of the distal ileum. This binding is calcium dependent and requires a neutral pH. The mechanism of uptake and transcellular transport of cobalamin is not clear, but intrinsic factor does not appear to be transported across the enterocyte. Before secretion into the lamina propria, cobalamin is transferred to yet another carrier protein, transcobalamin II. Intestinal malabsorption of cobalamin thus can result from gastric disease that interferes with intrinsic factor secretion, pancreatic insufficiency with failure to release intrinsic factor from R proteins, ileal disease or dysfunction (Crohn's disease, radiation injury, tropical sprue), or bacterial overgrowth (see "Bacterial Overgrowth").

Bile Acids

About 10% of bile acids are absorbed by passive diffusion in the proximal small intestine. The remainder reaches the terminal ileum, where it is absorbed by the sequential action of two secondary active transport systems (conjugated bile acid–anion cotransport across the brush border and bile acid–anion countertransport across the basolateral membrane). Ileal bile acid absorption normally is very efficient—more than 90% of secreted bile acids are reabsorbed into the portal circulation to be extracted by the liver and resecreted into the bile. If bile acids are not absorbed at the terminal ileum, they may enter the colon, where they induce electrolyte and water secretion. Severe bile acid malabsorption, which cannot be compensated for by increased hepatic bile acid synthesis, leads to a decrease in biliary bile acid secretion below the critical concentration necessary to produce mixed micelles, with resultant malabsorption of lipids and fat-soluble vitamins.

Bile acid malabsorption can be assessed by direct measurement of fecal bile acids or fecal excretion of radiolabeled conjugated bile acids, but these assays are cumbersome and not commonly available. Measurements of selenium-75-homocholic acid taurine (^{75}SHCAT) or [^{14}C]glycocholate or [^{14}C]taurocholate are more widely used to detect bile acid malabsorption. Plasma levels of 7α-hydroxy-4-cholestene-3-one and lathosterol plasma levels have been shown to reflect bile acid production rate in the liver. Since hepatic synthesis is highly correlated with intestinal loss of bile acids, these plasma sterol measurements may become more convenient ways to measure bile acid malabsorption.

DISORDERS OF DIGESTION AND ABSORPTION

CLINICAL FEATURES OF MALABSORPTION

The dominant symptoms of malabsorption depend on whether there is a generalized defect in nutrient assimilation or a defect in the assimilation of a specific nutrient, such as lactose. A simplified approach to patients suspected of having generalized malabsorption is shown in Fig. 110.7. In generalized malabsorption, the major symptoms result from the loss of calories into the stool (weight loss), an increase in stool volume (diarrhea), colonic fermentation of unabsorbed carbohydrates (abdominal bloating, distention, and flatulence), and deficiency of dietary nutrients (malnutrition). Patients with generalized malabsorption may experience weight loss despite a good and sometimes increasing appetite. They also may have anorexia and lessen their dietary intake because of such symptoms as bloating, cramping, and diarrhea after meals. Abdominal discomfort is common, but significant abdominal pain is unusual and should suggest alternative or additional diagnoses. Nongastrointestinal symptoms, such as short stature or infertility, can be the initial manifestations of chronic subclinical malabsorption.

If diarrhea is defined strictly as increased stool volume (>200 mL), almost all patients with generalized malabsorption have diarrhea. The diarrhea results from a combination of osmotic and secretory factors (see Chapter 99). The increased stool volume may or may not be associated with liquid stools, however. Some patients with significant steatorrhea continue to have formed, albeit bulky, stools. Oil or undigested food particles may be seen in the stool. Usually, the stool is pale, yellow, spongelike and difficult to flush down the toilet.

Carbohydrates that are not absorbed in the small bowel can be fermented by colonic bacteria. The resultant gases (predominantly hydrogen and carbon dioxide) contribute to the symptoms of abdominal distention, bloating, and flatulence. The short-chain acids produced by carbohydrate fermentation also can contribute to the osmotic load in the colon and inhibit colonic water absorption.

Deficiency of specific dietary nutrients may be superimposed on the symptoms of generalized malabsorption or may be the initial abnormality. Weakness and lethargy are among the most typical early symptoms of generalized malabsorption and usually are caused by anemia, dehydration, hypokalemia, and hypomagnesemia. Deficiency of iron, folate, or cobalamin can result in

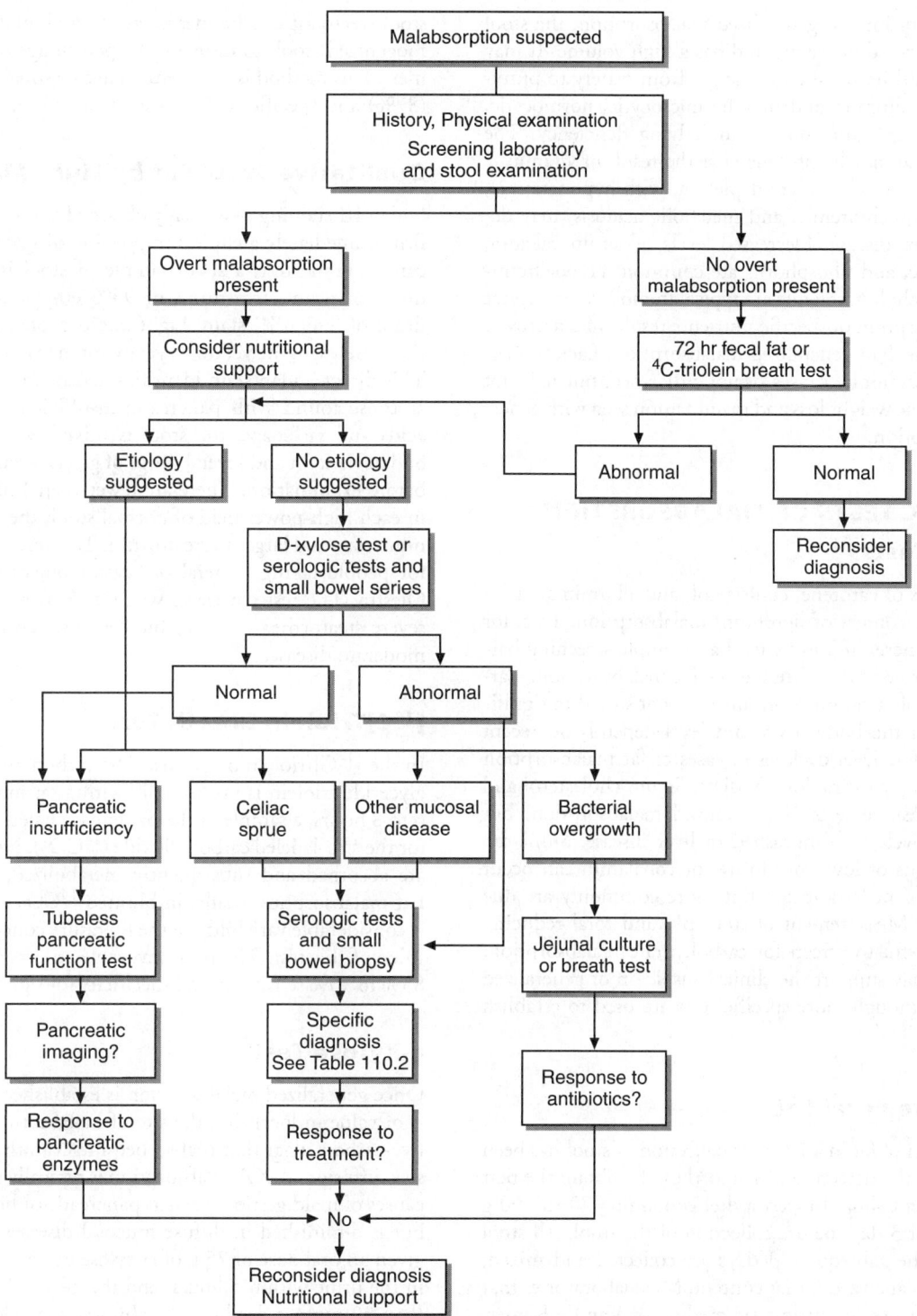

FIGURE 110.7. Approach to the patient with suspected generalized malabsorption. See text for details of specific diagnostic tests and treatment.

anemia. Excessive bruising or bleeding (vitamin K deficiency), paresthesia or tetany (hypocalcemia or hypomagnesemia), and pathologic fractures due to osteoporosis or osteomalacia (calcium and protein deficiency) are the common initial manifestations of specific dietary deficiencies. On clinical examination, pallor, muscle wasting, and hair loss often are present. Follicular hyper-

keratosis, chelosis, and glossitis are common signs of nutritional deficits. The abdomen may have a doughy consistency, because of dilated, fluid-filled loops of small intestine. Peripheral edema develops as the result of hypoalbuminemia, and there may be clubbing of the nails or evidence of peripheral neuropathy.

Laboratory test results vary depending on the severity and

type of malabsorption. In generalized malabsorption, the stool is usually semiformed or watery and has a high volume. It may appear greasy, and its consistency ranges from watery to putty-like. Anemia is common and may be microcytic, normocytic, or macrocytic, depending on the underlying deficiency. The prothrombin time may be prolonged as the result of vitamin K deficiency. Profound electrolyte depletion, with hyponatremia, hypokalemia, hypochloremia, and metabolic acidosis, may develop with severe disease. Decreased levels of serum calcium, magnesium, zinc, and phosphorus are common. Hypoalbuminemia and hypocholesterolemia are typical in moderate to severe disease. Malabsorption of specific nutrients results in a narrower clinical spectrum than generalized malabsorption. Lactose malabsorption, for example, causes osmotic diarrhea, but it is not associated with the weight loss and malnutrition seen with generalized malabsorption.

DIAGNOSTIC TESTS OF MALABSORPTION

Screening Tests

The serum levels of carotene, cholesterol, and albumin are routinely low in the context of significant malabsorption. Tests for these nutrients therefore can be used as a simple screening battery; however, none of them are specific for malabsorption. Carotene, a fat-soluble vitamin A precursor, is not stored in significant quantity in the body; its serum level depends on recent dietary intake. The level declines in cases of fat malabsorption and is low in people eating low-fat diets. Serum cholesterol and albumin are sensitive tests of generalized malabsorption, but both nutrient levels are diminished in liver disease. Similarly, anemia with signs of low iron, folate, or cobalamin can occur in the context of malabsorption but more commonly are due to other causes. Measurement of stool pH and total reducing substances is useful to screen for carbohydrate malabsorption. All these tests may support the clinical suspicion of generalized malabsorption, though more specific tests are used to establish the diagnosis.

Quantitative Fecal Fat

The quantitation of fat in a 72-hour collection of stool has been the standard for the detection of steatorrhea. To obtain the best results, the patient should ingest a diet containing 70 to 100 g of fat for at least 3 days before collection of the stool. All stool specimens for the subsequent 3 days are collected and mixed, and an aliquot is analyzed for fat content. Most laboratories that measure fecal fat use the titrimetric method of Van de Kamer, but near infrared reflectance analysis may have better reproducibility. Normally, more than 95% of the dietary fat intake is absorbed. Stool fat in excess of 6 g per day is considered abnormal. Falsely elevated results can be obtained from patients taking mineral oil, castor oil, or the fat substitute Olestra.

Quantitative fecal fat determinations are difficult to complete, and collections of stool are unpleasant for both the patient and the staff. Usually, the samples are sent to outside laboratories for analysis, delaying the availability of results. As a result, many other diagnostic tests for steatorrhea have been developed. The stool steatocrit can be measured in an aliquot of acidified, homogenized stool, to estimate the percentage of fat in the specimen. This method is reported to have reasonably high sensitivity (87%) and specificity (97%) for steatorrhea.

Qualitative Stool Fat by Light Microscopy

Sudan III staining of a freshly obtained stool specimen can confirm immediately a clinical impression of severe steatorrhea. To carry out the test, a small sample of stool is mixed with two drops of water, two drops of 95% ethyl alcohol, and several drops of Sudan III stain. Light microscopic examination shows the presence of the yellow to yellow-orange refractile fat globules. This direct Sudan stain identifies neutral fats in the stool, such as those found with pancreatic insufficiency. To detect fatty acids and fat soaps, the stool is mixed with several drops of Sudan III stain and several drops of glacial acetic acid and heated before examination. There are fewer than 100 tiny fat globules in each high-power field of normal stool; the globules are more numerous and larger in steatorrhea. Test results are false-positive for people taking mineral oil, castor oil, or the fat substitute Olestra. The test correlates well (>85%) with the presence of severe steatorrhea (>15 g) but has low sensitivity for mild to moderate disease.

[^{14}C]Triolein Breath Test

In the [^{14}C]triolein breath test, the carbon 14–radiolabeled triglyceride triolein is taken orally with a fat meal. Each hour for 6 to 8 hours, a sample of the patient's exhaled breath is analyzed for the ^{14}C-labeled carbon dioxide ($^{14}CO_2$). Normally, the lipids are absorbed and subsequently metabolized, releasing $^{14}CO_2$. Fat malabsorption results in blunted $^{14}CO_2$ production. There is considerable variability in the literature concerning the clinical value of this test. The most favorable reports suggest that it has 85% to 90% sensitivity and specificity for significant steatorrhea.

D-Xylose Test

Once generalized malabsorption is established, the D-xylose test is of value in localizing the site of malabsorption. D-Xylose is a five-carbon sugar that is absorbed intact in the jejunum by passive diffusion. D-Xylose absorption is typically normal in luminal causes of maldigestion, such as pancreatic or bile acid deficiency, but is diminished in diffuse mucosal diseases. Normal subjects given an oral dose of 25 g of D-xylose excrete 4.5 g of the xylose in the urine within 5 hours, and the 2-hour blood level is more than 30 mg per deciliter. An abnormal D-xylose test has about 80% sensitivity and specificity for detecting mucosal dysfunction. False-positive test results may occur with renal disease, delayed gastric emptying, ascites (increased volume of distribution of xylose), and bacterial overgrowth (intraluminal bacterial use of xylose).

Small-intestinal Radiographs

Radiologic evaluation of the small intestine sometimes is useful in distinguishing between luminal and mucosal causes of generalized malabsorption. The presence of pancreatic calcifications suggests the possibility of pancreatic insufficiency. The small-intestinal mucosal pattern is usually normal in pancreatic or biliary causes of malabsorption, whereas it is frequently abnormal in mucosal diseases. The pattern of mucosal abnormality also can suggest the type of mucosal disease. Dilated small intestine (>3 cm in caliber) with variable mucosal fold thickening (>3 mm) typically is seen in celiac and tropical sprue, short bowel syndrome, and bacterial overgrowth. Markedly thickened mucosal folds with or without dilatation are seen in malabsorptive disorders associated with infiltration of the intestinal wall with fluid (blood, lymph, edema) or cells (tumor, inflammation). The thickened folds may be straight and regular, as in lymphangiectasia, abetalipoproteinemia, or amyloidosis, or irregular and distorted, as in Whipple's disease, lymphoma, or Crohn's disease.

Small-intestinal Biopsy

In mucosal causes of malabsorption, small-intestinal biopsy may establish a specific diagnosis or show a pattern that is seen in several disorders (villous atrophy). Biopsy specimens may be obtained either with a suction instrument or at the time of endoscopy. The endoscopic appearance of scalloped duodenal folds or loss of duodenal folds suggests the diagnosis of villous atrophy. Once the biopsy specimens are obtained, they should be oriented before fixation, to ensure optimal interpretation (Fig. 110.8).

Tests for Intestinal Bacterial Overgrowth and Specific Nutrient Malabsorption

Although other tests for intestinal bacterial overgrowth are simpler, jejunal cultures remain a standard for documenting small-intestinal bacterial overgrowth. In this test, a nasogastric tube is passed into the proximal jejunum. Several samples of jejunal secretions should be obtained for aerobic and anaerobic cultures. A culture result showing more than 10^5 aerobic organisms per milliliter or any anaerobic growth is considered abnormal (10^3 to 10^5 organisms per milliliter is suggestive of abnormality).

The D-[^{14}C]xylose test measures the release of $^{14}CO_2$ after ingestion of 1 g of D-xylose containing a trace amount of D-[^{14}C]xylose (see Chapter 129). Bacterial fermentation of D-[^{14}C]xylose in the small intestine results in a prompt increase in $^{14}CO_2$ in the breath. The test has 90% to 95% sensitivity and specificity for small-intestinal bacterial overgrowth.

Several breath hydrogen tests have been developed on the principle that most hydrogen in the breath comes from fermentation of undigested carbohydrates by intestinal bacteria (see Chapter 100). The bile acid breath test measures $^{14}CO_2$ in the breath after oral administration of cholyl-L-[^{14}C]glycine and can be used to detect either bile acid malabsorption or bacterial overgrowth. If the radiolabeled bile acid is not absorbed normally in the ileum or is deconjugated by bacteria in the small intestine, the [^{14}C]glycine is fermented to $^{14}CO_2$, which is measured in the exhaled breath. All breath hydrogen tests have the limitation that 10% and 25% of normal subjects do not have enough hydrogen-producing bacteria in the intestine to cause fermentation. Cobalamin absorption classically is measured with a dual-labeled Schilling test. Increased serum homocysteine and/or methylmalonic acid levels are a relatively sensitive screening test for cobalamin deficiency.

MALDIGESTIVE SYNDROMES

Exocrine Pancreatic Insufficiency

The two most common causes of exocrine pancreatic insufficiency in adults are chronic pancreatitis (see Chapter 117) and pancreatic carcinoma (see Chapter 118); in children, the most common cause is cystic fibrosis. Regardless of the source, pan-

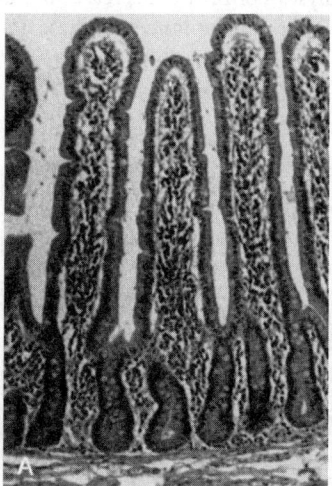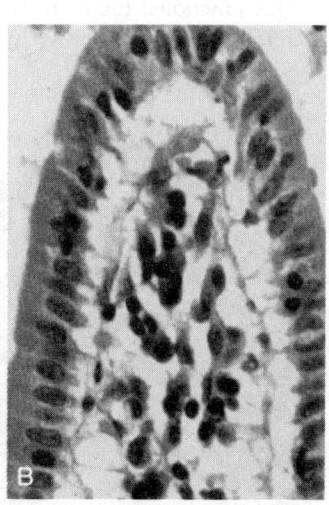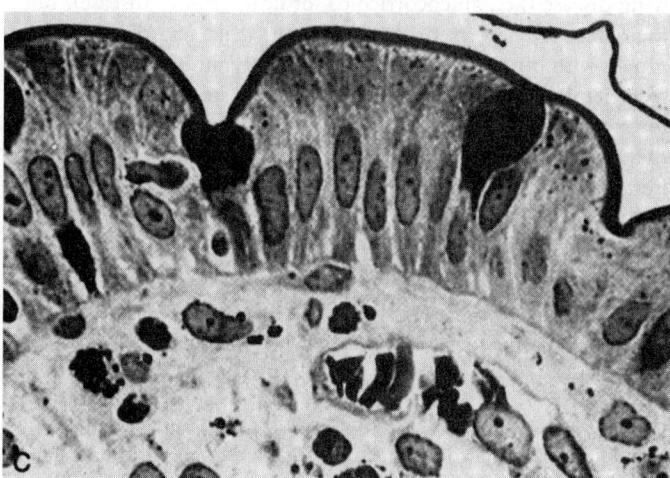

FIGURE 110.8. Histologic appearance of normal jejunum. **A:** The villi are long and slender, and the villus/crypt length ratio is 4:1. Scattered cells are present in the lamina propria. **B:** The enterocytes are columnar with basal nuclei. A few intraepithelial lymphocytes (dark round nuclei) are present. **C:** Electron microscopy of columnar enterocytes with scattered goblet cells (black-stained mucus) and a uniform microvillus surface. (From Misiewicz JJ, Bartram CI, Cotton PB, et al., eds. *Slide atlas of gastroenterology.* London: Gower Medical Publishing, 1985, with permission.)

creatic insufficiency can result in severe malabsorption, with fecal fat excretion of more than 35 g per day.

The diagnosis of exocrine pancreatic insufficiency is suggested by the presence of significant steatorrhea together with normal D-xylose absorption or normal small-intestinal radiographs. The diagnosis is supported by radiologic evidence of pancreatic disease (calcification) and endocrine pancreatic insufficiency. Pancreatic secretory testing is the best means of directly evaluating pancreatic function (see Chapter 117). In clinical practice, the diagnosis of exocrine pancreatic insufficiency often rests on indirect tests, such as the bentiromide test (PABA) and the pancreolauril tests, which measure urine, plasma, or breath levels of the pancreatic hydrolytic products of orally administered substrates. Fecal levels of chymotrypsin or elastase levels also are diminished in patients with pancreatic insufficiency. Often the diagnosis is established by clear improvement in malabsorption in response to a trial of pancreatic enzyme replacement.

Bile Acid Deficiency

Solubilization of fatty acids requires bile acids; thus, moderate steatorrhea can develop in disorders that cause deficient bile acid delivery to the intestinal lumen (bile duct obstruction, intrahepatic cholestasis). In ileal disease or resection, failure of bile acid reabsorption leads to depletion of the bile acid pool. Inherited defects in ileal bile acid transport have been identified, and ileal bile acid absorption is particularly sensitive to the effects of radiation. These partial defects in bile acid absorption more commonly cause diarrhea, as a result of the effects of unabsorbed bile acids on colonic fluid secretion, than frank malabsorption. In states of bile acid deficiency, the symptoms of malabsorption often are overshadowed by other symptoms of the underlying disease (obstructive jaundice, active Crohn's disease of the ileum). Specific defects in ileal bile acid uptake can be measured with a bile acid breath test.

Bile acid depletion can improve with treatment of the underlying disease (i.e., glucocorticoids for ileal Crohn's disease), but the defect often is fixed (ileal resection). Bile acid diarrhea improves with binding resins, such as cholestyramine, but they can worsen bile acid depletion and its associated steatorrhea. Therapy for steatorrhea is directed at improving fat absorption, supplementing fat-soluble vitamins, and minimizing symptoms. Vitamin B_{12} and bile acid malabsorption typically co-exist with ileal disease.

MALABSORPTIVE SYNDROMES

Celiac Sprue

Until recently celiac sprue (gluten-sensitive enteropathy, nontropical sprue) was thought to be a relatively uncommon disorder characterized by chronic diarrhea and overt generalized malabsorption. Recognition of cases with milder clinical expression, wider use of endoscopic biopsy of the duodenum, and, in particular, immunologic screening methods have changed that view dramatically. Screening studies have suggested that celiac sprue may be very common, affecting as many as one in 200 individuals. The prevalence of celiac sprue is higher in patients with

selective IgA deficiency (up to 10%) and Down's syndrome (up to 16%).

Celiac sprue is thought to be an immune disorder in genetically predisposed individuals that produces injury to the small-intestinal mucosa and is triggered by the gliadin fraction of gluten. Gliadin is a protein constituent of wheat, barley, rye, and perhaps oats. Genetic factors are important in the pathogenesis of celiac sprue. About 10% of first-degree relatives of patients with celiac sprue also have the disease, and concordance of disease in identical twins has been reported. Genetic susceptibility to celiac disease is likely multigenic. Linkage with the HLA-DQ2 and/or -DQ8 gene loci account for part of the genetic predisposition, but a non-HLA locus on the short arm of chromosome 6 and other loci also appear to be involved.

An autoimmune response to gliadin-related peptides is suggested as a mechanism of injury in celiac disease by both histologic and immunologic features of the disease. The small-intestinal lamina propria is infiltrated heavily with lymphocytes and plasma cells, some of which have been shown to be capable of producing antigliadin antibodies, and there is an increased number of γ/δ T-cell receptor–positive intraepithelial lymphocytes. The presence of circulating antibodies to gliadin and a variety of autoantibodies (antireticulin, anti-endomysial, anti-tissue transglutaminase) suggests that humoral immunity also plays a part in the response.

Celiac sprue causes varying degrees of diffuse injury to enterocytes, resulting in sloughing of cells from the villi and compensatory crypt hyperplasia. On histologic examination, the total thickness of the mucosa is normal (Fig. 110.9); the villi are atrophic, however, and the crypts are elongated. The surface epithelium, which is normally columnar, appears cuboidal, and there is a loss of the normal basal polarity of the enterocyte nuclei. The crypts are hyperplastic and hyperproliferative. The lamina propria has higher than normal numbers of plasma cells and lymphocytes and more intraepithelial lymphocytes. Electron microscopy shows shortened and sparse microvilli and loss of tight junctions. Enzymatic analyses confirm a decrease in the concentration of digestive hydrolases in the mucosa. These ab-

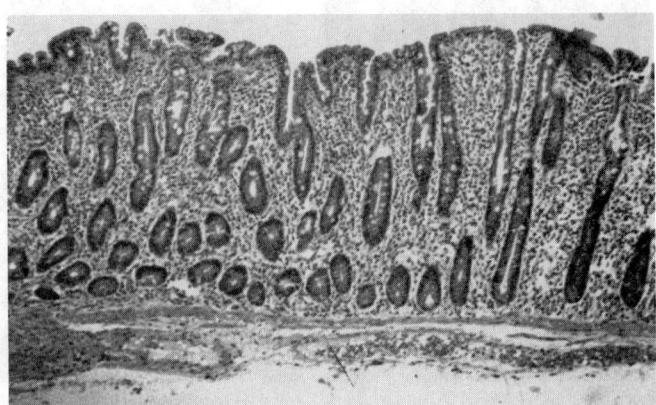

FIGURE 110.9. Histologic appearance of the jejunum in a patient with celiac sprue. Villi are absent (total villous atrophy). The crypts are hyperplastic. The lamina propria is infiltrated with mononuclear cells. (From Misiewicz JJ, Bartram CI, Cotton PB, et al., eds. *Slide atlas of gastroenterology*. London: Gower Medical Publishing, 1985, with permission.)

normalities result in both fewer numbers and impaired functional capacity of absorptive cells.

The length of intestine affected in celiac sprue varies and correlates with the severity of symptoms, but the degree of involvement diminishes from proximal to distal sites. Thus, malabsorption of nutrients that normally are absorbed in the proximal small intestine (fat, protein, carbohydrate, iron, calcium, vitamin D) is more common than malabsorption of bile acids or cobalamin.

Clinical Findings and Diagnosis

The clinical features of celiac sprue vary widely, and spontaneous exacerbations and remissions of symptoms occur. Celiac sprue that manifests during childhood may go into remission during adolescence, only to recur in adulthood. The symptoms, signs, and laboratory data in celiac sprue span the entire spectrum described earlier for generalized malabsorption. The clinical manifestations of celiac sprue may be as subtle as short stature or as severe as malabsorption with dehydration, emaciation, and adrenocortical insufficiency. Nongastrointestinal symptoms may predominate (Table 110.4).

Several clinical features suggest the diagnosis of celiac sprue. A family history of the disorder is helpful. The spontaneous remission seen in adolescence is not observed in other causes of malabsorption. Dermatitis herpetiformis, a pruritic, papulovesicular rash typically present over the elbows, knees, and buttocks, develops in 10% to 25% of patients with celiac sprue. Almost all (85% to 90%) patients with dermatitis herpetiformis have abnormal small-bowel biopsy results, but the intestinal involvement can be patchy, and the disease is often mild and asymptomatic.

The diagnosis of classic celiac sprue rests on findings of mucosal malabsorption, small-intestinal biopsy results showing villous atrophy, and resolution of the disorder after gluten withdrawal. The malabsorption may be generalized, with steatorrhea, or more selective (iron, folate, vitamin D deficiency). The D-xylose test shows abnormal results in about 70% of patients, and a small-intestinal series typically shows dilatation of the small intestine and various degrees of thickening of the mucosal folds.

TABLE 110.4.	EXTRAINTESTINAL MANIFESTATIONS OF CELIAC DISEASE
Short stature	
Delayed puberty	
Oligomenorrhea	
Infertility	
Iron-deficiency anemia	
Osteomalacia or osteoporosis	
Hypoalbuminemia	
Depression	
Ataxia	
Arthritis	

Villous atrophy is seen in other diseases (Table 110.5), but celiac sprue is the most common cause of total villous atrophy. The presence of circulating antigliadin, anti-endomysial, or anti-transglutaminase antibodies supports but does not establish the diagnosis. Evidence of a prompt clinical response and histologic signs of improvement in the small bowel with institution of a strict gluten-free diet confirm the diagnosis.

Serologic studies increasingly are being used to aid in the diagnosis of celiac sprue. The relative sensitivity and specificity of these tests from one laboratory are shown in Table 110.6, but these results vary among laboratories. For screening of low-risk populations, the anti-endomysial antibody test has slightly better performance characteristics but is more expensive than the IgA antigliadin test. A negative result on either test suggests an alternative diagnosis. In subjects with a high or moderate probability of having the disease, the anti-endomysial test is preferred because of its higher specificity. The IgG anti-gliadin test is used only in subjects with selective IgA deficiency. Serologic screening of asymptomatic subjects is not recommended at present, because clinical benefit has not been established and any potential benefit requires adherence to a difficult dietary regimen.

Some patients with celiac disease in childhood experience remission of disease later in life and can have normal jejunal mucosa and few or no symptoms while on a gluten-containing diet. Such individuals are said to have latent celiac disease and are at risk of recurrent symptoms. Patients who have never had a biopsy result suggestive of celiac disease but who have characteristic immunologic abnormalities are said to have potential celiac disease.

Optimal Management

The therapy for celiac sprue includes nutritional repletion and strict gluten withdrawal. Gluten withdrawal may not be simple to achieve, because gluten-containing grains are ubiquitous in processed foods. The patient must be both well informed and highly motivated to achieve strict gluten withdrawal. The clinical response to gluten avoidance correlates with the length of intestine involved. Improvement in symptoms usually takes place within 1 to 2 weeks of initiation of therapy, but the histologic features may take several months to normalize. Less than 10% of patients with the diagnosis of celiac sprue fail to respond to a gluten-free diet (so-called refractory sprue). Some of these patients respond to a trial of prednisone. Relapse of symptoms after adequate gluten withdrawal is common and usually is caused by failure to maintain a strict gluten-free diet. If symptomatic recurrence persists despite adequate dietary control, the possibility of a secondary complication, such as intestinal lymphoma, should be considered.

Tropical Sprue

Tropical sprue is a syndrome of uncertain origin that results in progressive mucosal injury to the entire small intestine and probably represents more than a single entity. It should be suspected in residents of tropical regions with chronic diarrhea and malabsorption of at least two unrelated nutrients (xylose and

TABLE 110.5.	HISTOLOGIC CHARACTERISTICS OF THE SMALL INTESTINE

Normal	Villus-to-crypt ratio 3–4:1, columnar epithelial cells, scattered mononuclear cells in the lamina propria (Fig. 110.8)
Disorders in which small-intestinal biopsy is diagnostic	
Whipple's disease	Blunting of villi, PAS-positive macrophages in the lamina propria, bacteria on electron microscopy (Fig. 110.11).
Hypogammaglobulinemia	Partial villous atrophy, lack of plasma cells and lymphocytic infiltrate in lamina propria, sometimes nodular lymphoid hyperplasia
Abetalipoproteinemia	Enterocytes filled with lipid droplets (Fig. 110.12)
Amyloidosis	Amyloid deposition in the mucosa and submucosa
Disorders in which small-intestinal biopsy may be diagnostic	
Celiac sprue	Most common cause of total villous atrophy, crypt hyperplasia, lymphocytic infiltration of lamina propria (Fig. 110.9)
Intestinal lymphangiectasia	Dilated lymphatics in the lamina propria
Intestinal lymphoma	Infiltration of lamina propria and displacement of crypts with malignant lymphocytes
Crohn's disease	Fissuring ulcerations, noncaseating granulomas
Parasitic infestations	*Giardia* or cryptosporidic trophozoites attached to epithelial cells, invasive *Isospora*
Radiation enteritis	Acute: partial villous atrophy, no crypt hyperplasia, decreased mitosis in crypts
	Chronic: mucosal ulceration or atrophy, obliterative endarteritis in submucosa
Disorders in which the small-intestinal biopsy result is abnormal but not diagnostic	
Tropical sprue	Partial villous atrophy, lymphocytic infiltration of lamina propria (Fig. 110.10)
Small intestinal bacterial overgrowth	Partial villous atrophy and lymphocytic infiltration of lamina propria in a patchy distribution

PAS, periodic acid–Schiff.

vitamin B$_{12}$). The disorder may manifest within months of arriving in the tropics, after many years of tropical residence, or after return to a temperate climate from the tropics. Tropical sprue is not uniformly prevalent in the tropics; it is common in Haiti, the Dominican Republic, India, Indonesia, and Southeast Asia but rare in Jamaica, the Bahamas, and Africa.

One form of tropical sprue probably results from bacterial infection of the gastrointestinal tract. The data suggesting that tropical sprue is an infectious disease are the geographic distribution of its occurrence; the seasonal appearance of disease, peaking between April and June; the appearance of epidemics and focal outbreaks of the disease; the apparent declining incidence of the disease; the relatively rapid appearance of the disease in visitors to endemic areas; and the response of affected patients to antibiotic therapy. Enterotoxigenic coliform bacteria have been isolated in the proximal small intestine of patients with tropical sprue, but no specific strains have been found consistently. Chronic protozoal infection (*Cryptosporidium parvus, Isospora belli, Cyclospora cayetanensis*) also has been suggested as a cause of the syndrome. Nutritional factors are important in tropical sprue. There is a much lower incidence of the disease in tropical countries whose populations are generally well nourished (Puerto Rico). The rapid and often dramatic response to folate therapy highlights the importance of this nutritional element.

Pathogenesis

Tropical sprue can affect any or all regions of the small intestine, often in a patchy distribution. The small-intestinal mucosa shows partial to subtotal villous atrophy and infiltration of the lamina propria with a mixture of lymphocytes and plasma cells (Fig. 110.10). No histologic features completely distinguish

TABLE 110.6.	RELATIVE PERFORMANCE CHARACTERISTICS OF SEROLOGIC TESTS FOR CELIAC SPRUE IN A GENERAL POPULATION

Antibody	Prev	Sens	Spec	PPV
IgA antiendomysial	<1%	85–95%	97–100%	95–100%
IgA antigliadin	<1%	80–90%	85–95%	12%
IgG antigliadin	7%	75–85%	75–90%	2%

Prev, prevalence in the general population; Sens, sensitivity; Spec, specificity; PPV, positive predictive value in a general population at low risk for celiac disease.
Kelley CP. Use of serum antibodies to diagnose celiac disease. In Rose BD, ed. *Up to Date in Medicine*. Up to Date in Medicine, Inc., 1999.

tropical from celiac sprue, but total villous atrophy is much less common in tropical sprue.

Clinical Findings and Diagnosis

Patients with tropical sprue usually suffer a progressive course that begins with fatigue and diarrhea and leads to abdominal distention and watery diarrhea. Late in the course of the disease, severe anemia (combinations of B_{12}, folate, and/or iron deficiency) and progressive malnutrition are noted. Although most of the features of tropical sprue are similar to those of celiac sprue, there are several distinctions. Megaloblastic anemia due to vitamin B_{12} deficiency is much more common in tropical sprue, because the entire small intestine is affected. Abdominal pain also is more typical of tropical sprue (90%) than celiac sprue (30% to 50%). A pellagroid or eczematous rash over the ankles and wrists is characteristic of tropical sprue, but it is distinct from the dermatitis herpetiformis seen in celiac sprue.

The diagnosis of tropical sprue is based on the clinical syndrome of progressive malabsorption and malnutrition, an appropriate residence or travel history, evidence of malabsorption caused by mucosal disease; a typical small-intestinal biopsy result showing partial villous atrophy (Fig. 110.10); and an appropriate response to specific therapy. Because this disease occurs in the tropics, the differential diagnosis includes parasitic and tuberculous enteritis as well as inflammatory bowel disease, gluten-sensitive enteropathy, and the other causes of mucosal malabsorption (Table 110.5).

Optimal Management

Patients with early symptoms of tropical sprue respond within a few days to folate therapy. Patients with signs of disease lasting longer than 4 months should be treated with tetracycline, 500 mg four times daily for the first month and then 500 mg twice daily for 5 to 11 months, and folate, 0.5 mg per day for 6 to

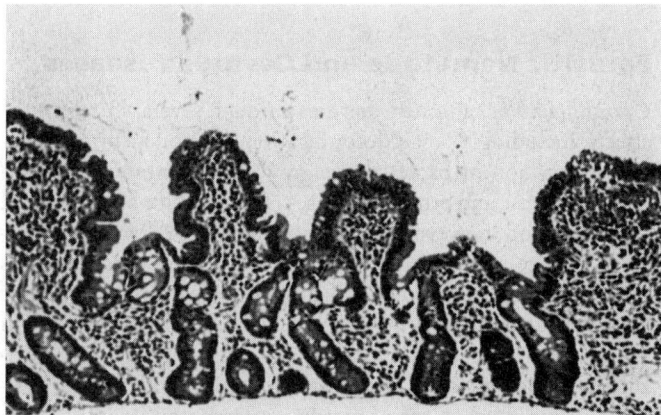

FIGURE 110.10. Histologic appearance of the jejunum in a patient with tropical sprue. The villi are shortened (partial villous atrophy). The crypts are mildly hyperplastic. (The villus/crypt ratio is 1:1.) The lamina propria is infiltrated with mononuclear cells. (From Misiewicz JJ, Bartram CI, Cotton PB, et al., eds. *Slide atlas of gastroenterology*. London: Gower Medical Publishing, 1985, with permission.)

12 months. Failure to improve progressively on this therapy should prompt reevaluation of the diagnosis.

Whipple's Disease

Whipple's disease is a rare, chronic systemic bacterial infection that appears to strike predominantly white men. Many organs can be affected in Whipple's disease, but gastrointestinal involvement with generalized malabsorption is the most common clinical picture. A bacterial cause for Whipple's disease had long been suspected because of evidence of numerous, weakly gram-positive bacilli in many tissues, including enterocytes and macrophages of the intestinal lamina propria (Fig. 110.11) and by the clinical response to antibiotics. The organism responsible for Whipple's disease (*Tropheryma whipellii*) was originally identified by a polymerase chain reaction–based assay and later cultured in human phagocytes in vitro.

The intestinal features of Whipple's disease may be patchy, but they are typically most severe in the proximal small intestine. Clubbing of the villi and periodic acid–Schiff (PAS)–positive macrophages in the lamina propria are seen in intestinal biopsy specimens (Fig. 110.11). Similar PAS-positive macrophages may infiltrate other organs, including the remainder of the gastrointestinal tract, mesenteric and peripheral lymph nodes, heart, brain, lung, spleen, liver, and pancreas.

Clinical Findings and Diagnosis

Although involvement of the small intestine with resultant progressive malabsorption is the usual reason that patients with Whipple's disease seek medical attention, it is the extraintestinal symptoms that suggest the specific diagnosis. The most common extraintestinal features of Whipple's disease are arthritis and arthralgia. The joint symptoms may predate the development of diarrhea and malabsorption by many years. Low-grade fever and lymphadenopathy are typical, and murmurs of aortic or mitral insufficiency are found in about 25% of patients. Central nervous system involvement can cause a host of neurologic abnormalities (personality changes, dementia, visual disturbances, hypothalamic symptoms, meningoencephalitis, spastic paresis, encephalopathy, posterior column disease).

The diagnosis of Whipple's disease is based on the clinical picture of generalized malabsorption with prominent extraintestinal manifestations and positive results of small-intestinal biopsy. Steatorrhea occurs in more than 90% of patients, and decreased D-xylose absorption is found in 75%. Because the disease primarily involves the proximal small intestine, vitamin B_{12} or bile acid malabsorption is uncommon. Radiographic studies show irregular thickening of the duodenal and jejunal folds with dilatation of the jejunal loops. Small-intestinal biopsy specimens show blunting of the villi and PAS-positive macrophages in the lamina propria (Fig. 110.11). The diagnosis is confirmed by microscopic evidence of characteristic bacteria within enterocytes or macrophages.

Optimal Management

A typical regimen for treatment of Whipple's disease is 1.2 million units procaine penicillin and 1 g streptomycin daily for 10

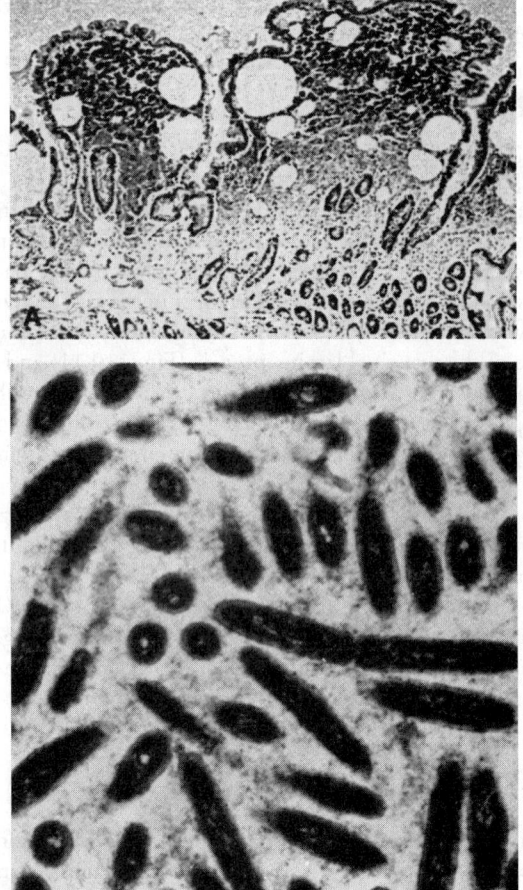

FIGURE 110.11. Histologic appearance of the small intestine in a patient with Whipple's disease. **A:** The villi are widened by the infiltration of periodic acid–Schiff–positive macrophages. **B:** Electron microscopic appearance of the bacteria (*Tropheryma whipellii*) seen in Whipple's disease. (From Misiewicz JJ, Bartram CI, Cotton PB, et al., eds. *Slide atlas of gastroenterology*. London: Gower Medical Publishing, 1985, with permission.)

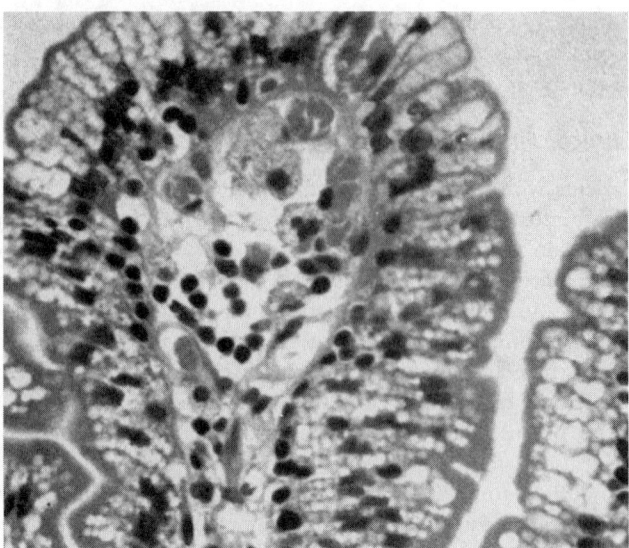

FIGURE 110.12. Histologic appearance of small intestine in a patient with abetalipoproteinemia. The villous architecture is normal. The enterocytes are columnar, but they are filled with lipid droplets. (From Misiewicz JJ, Bartram CI, Cotton PB, et al., eds. *Slide atlas of gastroenterology*. London: Gower Medical Publishing, 1985, with permission.)

days, followed by trimethoprim–sulfamethoxazole, one double-strength tablet twice daily, or tetracycline, 1 g per day for 1 year. With treatment, a sense of well-being and improved appetite usually return within a few weeks, and the malabsorption is corrected within the first few months. A second biopsy of the small intestine shows clearing of the bacteria from the enterocytes, but the PAS-positive macrophages may persist for several years. Whipple's disease may relapse after therapy, without significant gastrointestinal involvement. Neurologic symptoms are the most difficult to treat; they may or may not respond to antibiotic therapy.

Abetalipoproteinemia

Abetalipoproteinemia results from a genetic defect in triglyceride transport and secretion. It is a rare autosomal recessive disorder that has a high prevalence among Mediterranean Jews. In at least some families, the disease appears to be caused by a mutation in a microsomal triglyceride transport protein. The disease results

in a failure of β-lipoprotein (chylomicrons and very low density lipoprotein) assembly. The resultant impairment in chylomicron secretion from the enterocyte leads to triglyceride accumulation within the enterocyte and mild fat and fat-soluble vitamin malabsorption in infancy. Characteristically, small-intestinal biopsy shows normal villous architecture, but the enterocytes are filled with lipid droplets (Fig. 111.12). Neurologic symptoms develop late in the course of the disease, and the typical acanthocytic red blood cells appear later still. Markedly low serum triglyceride (<10 mg per deciliter) and cholesterol (<50 mg per deciliter) levels are noted frequently. No effective therapy exists for the extraintestinal manifestations; however, nutrition may be improved with the use of a low-fat diet supplemented with fat-soluble vitamins and medium-chain triglycerides.

Parasitic Nematode and Cestode Diseases

Giardia lamblia can cause diarrhea through several intraluminal effects, including bile salt deconjugation and uptake by the parasite, promotion of bacterial overgrowth, and inhibition of enterocyte lactase and other hydrolases. The presence of generalized malabsorption, however, is closely related to the organism's ability to induce enteropathy. Giardial enteropathy occasionally is seen in immunocompetent subjects, but it is a common source of villous atrophy and mild to moderate fat malabsorption in immunodeficient subjects, particularly those with common variable immunodeficiency or the acquired immunodeficiency syndrome. The mechanism of giardial enteropathy is not known. The diagnosis of giardiasis can be made by examination of the stool or duodenal aspirate by wet preparation.

Infestation with *Cryptosporidium* protozoa or *Isospora belli* usually leads to an acute diarrheal illness (see Chapter 321) that sometimes is associated with generalized malabsorption. As with giardiasis, immunodeficient subjects are at higher risk of primary, persistent, and recurrent coccidiosis. The protozoa may be seen on stool examination, but the diagnosis usually is made by small-intestinal biopsy. Small-intestinal biopsy in these cases shows evidence of partial villous atrophy with a mixed eosinophilic, lymphocytic, and polymorphonuclear infiltrate in the lamina propria. Cryptosporidia may take the form of basophilic bodies along the microvillus border. Various forms of *Isospora* may be evident within epithelial cells. Strongyloidiasis and capillariasis also can cause generalized malabsorption. *Diphyllobothrium latum* can provoke vitamin B_{12} malabsorption, and *Ascaris lumbricoides* can bring about vitamin A malabsorption.

Immunodeficiency States and Malabsorption

About 10% of patients with selective IgA deficiency or common variable immunodeficiency syndrome have diarrhea and steatorrhea. The latter patients often have long histories of recurrent sinopulmonary infections before the onset of diarrhea and malabsorption. Often, malabsorption is caused by giardiasis, but other chronic infections can elicit similar symptoms. The diagnosis of malabsorption is established in the usual manner, but stool cultures and examination for ova and parasites establish the correct diagnosis. Small-intestinal radiographs may show nodular lymphoid hyperplasia (Fig. 110.13). The small-intestinal biopsy sample is characterized by villous atrophy and cellular infiltration of the lamina propria, but the appearance is distinguished from those of other conditions by the absence of plasma cells in the lamina propria and the presence of *Giardia lamblia* trophozoites adherent to the luminal mucosa. Nodular lymphoid

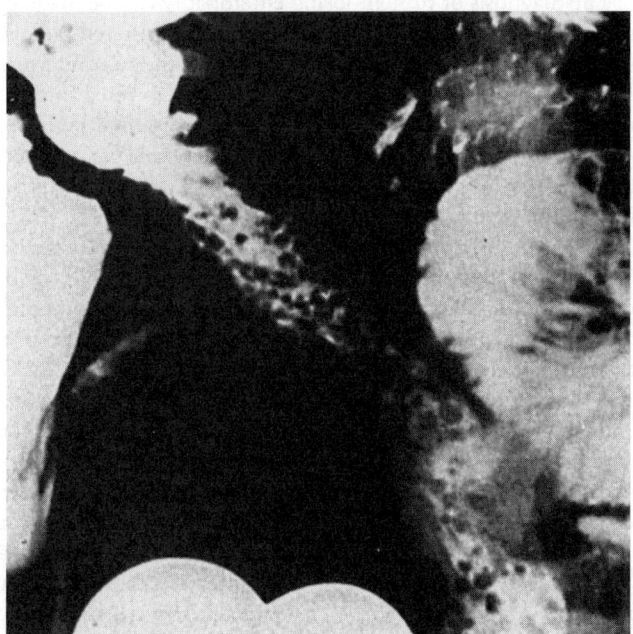

FIGURE 110.13. Loop of small intestine showing nodular lymphoid hyperplasia in a patient with hypogammaglobulinemia and generalized malabsorption. (From Misiewicz JJ, Bartram CI, Cotton PB, et al., eds. *Slide atlas of gastroenterology*. London: Gower Medical Publishing, 1985, with permission.)

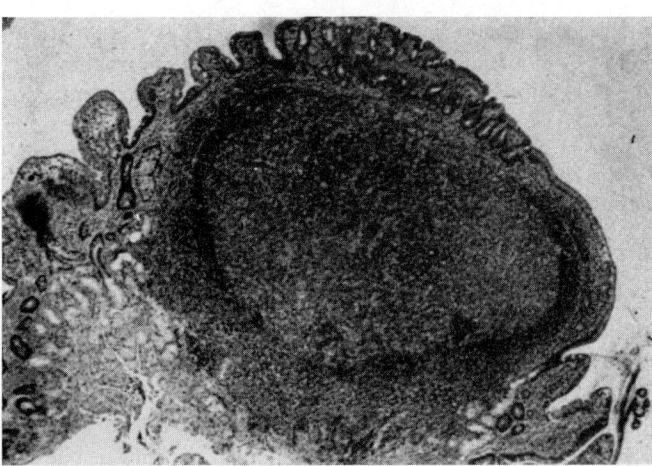

FIGURE 110.14. Histologic appearance of nodular lymphoid hyperplasia of the small intestine. The mucosa overlying the lymphoid nodule is flattened. (From Misiewicz JJ, Bartram CI, Cotton PB, et al., eds. *Slide atlas of gastroenterology*. London: Gower Medical Publishing, 1985, with permission.)

hyperplasia also may be found on histologic examination (Fig. 110.14). Diarrhea and malabsorption usually resolve with therapy of the enteric infection.

Diarrhea with or without malabsorption occurs frequently in the context of the acquired immunodeficiency syndrome and contributes to the progressive weight loss and cachexia seen in this disease. A specific treatable infectious agent should be sought—the most common are *Cryptosporidium* species, *G. lamblia*, *I. belli*, *Mycobacterium avium-intracellulare*, and cytomegalovirus. Often, however, a specific agent that accounts for the diarrhea is not found. Secondary lactase deficiency and bile acid and cobalamin malabsorption are particularly common in this context and can respond to specific therapy. Symptomatic antidiarrheal therapy also can be effective.

Small-intestinal Resection

The end result of a small-intestinal resection on nutrient assimilation depends on the length and site of the resection and the functional capacity of the remaining bowel. In general, resections that leave more than half of the jejunum intact do not result in significant malabsorption, but larger resections are associated with varying degrees of malabsorption. Even small resections of critical sites within the small intestine can provoke specific deficiencies, however. Patients with resections that include the duodenum and proximal jejunum have a high incidence of iron and calcium deficiency, whereas resections of the distal ileum are associated with vitamin B_{12} and bile acid malabsorption. Any resection that includes the ileocecal valve is associated with a greater risk of postoperative diarrhea, because it shortens the duration of nutrient retention in the small intestine and may allow bacterial overgrowth due to the retrograde spread of colonic bacteria. Not surprisingly, the capacity of the residual small intestine to absorb nutrients is an important factor in the clinical consequences of small-intestinal resection. Resection is followed by adaptation of the small-intestinal remnant, which may lead to diminishment of the severity of malabsorption over time. The mechanism of adaptation is unknown, though trophic hormones, luminal nutrients, and neural factors have been proposed as important elements. Adaptation appears to occur more readily in children than adults.

Clinical Findings and Diagnosis

Usually, it is not difficult to make the diagnosis of malabsorption stemming from small-intestinal resection, because the symptoms begin immediately after surgery. The clinical picture ranges from isolated nutrient deficiencies to generalized malabsorption and malnutrition. Resections of less than 100 cm of ileum typically are associated with modest (20% to 50%) declines in bile salt absorption. Although these declines lead to increased loss of bile salts into the colon, enhanced hepatic synthesis of bile salts is capable of maintaining the bile acid pool size, thereby preventing fat malabsorption. The presence of excessive amounts of bile salts in the colon, however, produces increased colonic water secretion and diarrhea. With larger resections of the ileum (>100 cm), more extensive bile salt malabsorption can provoke bile salt depletion and steatorrhea.

Optimal Management

Parenteral nutrition should be instituted routinely after major small-intestinal resections. Enteral feeding can be resumed quickly if the length of resection is moderate. If the resection is extensive, however, it is prudent to initiate enteral feeding slowly, with several small feedings containing little fat. The amount of fat in the diet should be increased progressively to tolerance. Once the diet is stabilized, the severity of malabsorption can be assessed and nutritional therapy instituted as outlined in the section on nutritional management of generalized malabsorption.

Moderate bile acid malabsorption (small ileal resection) and the diarrhea it produces can be treated effectively with cholestyramine, though such treatment can make the diarrhea associated with fat malabsorption (large ileal resection) worse. After a large small-intestinal resection, some patients have marked gastric or intestinal hypersecretion, which can cause both diarrhea and malabsorption. Treatment with an H_2 receptor antagonist or a proton pump inhibitor may result in prompt improvements in some patients, and the somatostatin analog octreotide has been effective in others. Bacterial overgrowth can complicate small-intestinal resection, particularly if the ileocecal valve is resected; this problem can be improved substantially by administering courses of broad-spectrum antibiotics. If adequate nutrition cannot be maintained orally, long-term home parenteral nutrition must be considered.

Protein-Losing Enteropathy

Protein-losing enteropathy is a syndrome characterized by loss of protein with or without loss of lipids and lymphocytes

TABLE 110.7.	DISORDERS CAUSING PROTEIN-LOSING ENTEROPATHY
Mechanism of Action	**Diseases**
Lymphatic obstruction	
Mechanical	Lymphangiectasia, retroperitoneal fibrosis, lymphoma, Whipple's disease
Elevated lymphatic pressure	Constrictive pericarditis, pulmonic stenosis, superior vena caval obstruction
Exudative protein loss	
Neoplastic	Gastric, colonic, esophageal, and small-intestinal cancer; familial polyposis; Gardner's syndrome; juvenile polyposis
Ulcerative	Inflammatory bowel disease, gastritis, infectious enteritis, radiation enteritis
Nonmalignant, nonulcerative	Hypertrophic gastropathy, allergic gastroenteropathy, celiac sprue, tropical sprue

(lymph) into the gastrointestinal tract (Table 110.7). The syndrome can be caused by a variety of disorders, including mesenteric lymphatic obstruction, with loss of lymph into the gut lumen, and mucosal disorders that result in the exudation of protein-rich secretions into the lumen. Increased fecal protein loss often occurs in patients with HIV-related conditions, regardless of the presence opportunistic infections. Protein loss into the gut can cause hypoproteinemia, which can lead to edema, and the lymph loss may provoke immunodeficiency.

The diagnosis of protein-losing enteropathy can be made by measuring the appearance of parenterally administered radiolabeled albumin in the stool or, more simply, by the α_1-antitrypsin clearance test. Normally, α_1-antitrypsin is not secreted into the small intestine, but it is present if there is substantial intestinal protein loss. Because α_1-antitrypsin is degraded in the stomach, this test is not useful for the diagnosis of hypertrophic gastropathy or other gastric conditions causing protein loss.

Lymphangiectasia can stem from a primary developmental abnormality or from obstruction of the enteric lymphatics by retroperitoneal fibrosis, pancreatitis, lymphoma, or Whipple's disease. The syndrome is characterized by loss of lipid and protein-rich lymph into the intestinal lumen, with resultant hypocholesterolemia, hypoalbuminemia, edema, chylous effusions, and diarrhea. In addition to nutrients, immunoglobulins and lymphocytes are also lost into the gut; this results in lymphocytopenia, decreased serum immunoglobulins, and, in many cases, cutaneous anergy. The diagnosis is supported by documentation of protein loss into the gut and small-intestinal biopsy results showing evidence of broad villi with dilatation of the mucosal and submucosal lymphatics (Fig. 110.15). Severe right-sided congestive heart failure, particularly that caused by constrictive pericarditis, can resemble lymphangiectasia in its clinical manifestations. Dilated lymphatics may be present on small-intestinal biopsy but the two disorders are distinguishable by the cardiac findings.

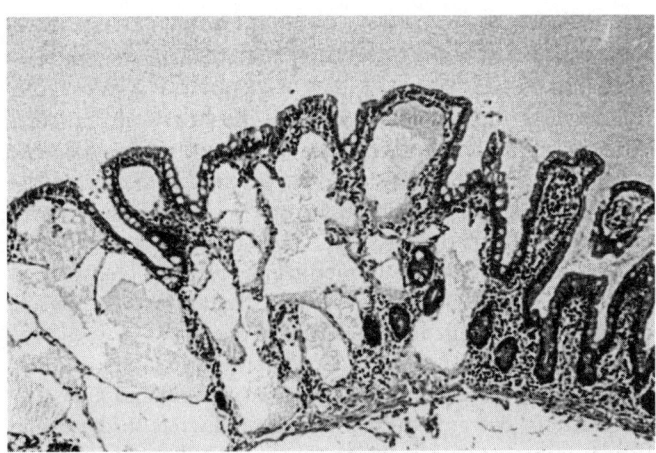

FIGURE 110.15. Lymphangiectasia of the small intestine. Markedly dilated lymphatics are present in the lamina propria, causing widening of the villi. The patchy nature of the lesion can be seen. (The villi at right are normal.) (From Misiewicz JJ, Bartram CI, Cotton PB, et al., eds. *Slide atlas of gastroenterology.* London: Gower Medical Publishing, 1985, with permission.)

Neoplastic and ulcerative diseases of the gut can provoke exudative protein loss into the small intestine (Table 110.7). Occasionally, hypoalbuminemia and edema are the dominant abnormalities in these disorders. Hypertrophic gastritis is the most common gastric cause of protein-losing enteropathy. Allergic gastroenteropathy is discussed in Chapter 114.

Optimal Management

Therapy for protein-losing enteropathy depends on the causative disorder. If the underlying cause is not correctable, dietary therapy is useful. With lymphatic obstruction, the combination of low-fat diet and medium-chain triglycerides results in a decrease in lymphatic flow and may moderately lessen the protein loss.

Small-intestinal Lymphoma and α Heavy Chain Disease

Lymphoma of the small intestine can cause malabsorption by diffuse infiltration of the lamina propria and submucosa. The normal mucosa is replaced progressively, and mucosal ulceration as well as lymphatic obstruction may occur. The association of malabsorption and intestinal lymphoma is particularly common in α heavy chain disease, an unusual disorder of B lymphocytes that initially appears to be infectious but subsequently progresses to intestinal lymphoma. These disorders are characterized by progressive symptoms of diarrhea and malabsorption with prominent abdominal pain. Small-intestinal radiographs show nodular, irregular thickening of the mucosa in advanced disease. The small-intestinal biopsy result differs from that of celiac or tropical sprue in that there is no crypt hyperplasia and the lamina propria is infiltrated with a monomorphic population of lymphocytes. The malignant nature of the lymphocytic infiltrate may not be obvious at first. Thus, a full-thickness biopsy is sometimes necessary to make the diagnosis. Specific therapy for lymphomas and α heavy chain disease is discussed in detail in Chapters 233

through 235, but nutritional support is occasionally necessary for the associated malabsorption.

DISORDERS WITH COMBINED MALDIGESTIVE AND MALABSORPTIVE FEATURES

Bacterial Overgrowth

Relatively few ($<10^3$ organisms per milliliter) bacteria can be found within the lumen of the normal small intestine. Bacterial growth is prevented by the hostile acid environment of the stomach as well as by the rapid transit of intestinal contents. Furthermore, colonic bacteria are prevented from refluxing into the small intestine by the ileocecal valve. Accordingly, achlorhydria, small-intestinal strictures, blind loops, large fistulas, ileal resections, and motility disorders can result in the proliferation of bacteria within the small intestine.

Intestinal bacterial overgrowth can cause diarrhea and malabsorption through a combination of intraluminal and mucosal effects. Anaerobic bacteria produce folate but consume both vitamin B_{12} and D-xylose (bacterial overgrowth is one nonmucosal source of an abnormal D-xylose test result). Certain bacteria have the capacity to deconjugate bile salts, and anaerobic bacteria can ferment carbohydrates with the resultant production of gas (carbon dioxide and hydrogen) and short-chain organic acids. In addition to their effects on intraluminal nutrient digestion and solubilization, bacteria can have a direct toxic effect on the enterocyte. Small-intestinal biopsies in patients with bacterial overgrowth may uncover partial villous atrophy in a patchy distribution.

Clinical Findings and Diagnosis

The clinical features of bacterial overgrowth are those seen with any disorder of generalized malabsorption. Weight loss, diarrhea, anemia, and fat-soluble vitamin deficiency are the most common clinical findings. The anemia seen in bacterial overgrowth usually stems from vitamin B_{12} deficiency (bacterial utilization); folate deficiency is uncommon, because bacteria can produce folate. The malabsorptive symptoms often are overshadowed by the underlying cause of the bacterial overgrowth. Bacterial overgrowth should be considered in patients with diarrhea or malabsorption in the context of possible intestinal stasis, such as postoperative partial intestinal obstruction, Crohn's disease, intestinal pseudo-obstruction, or autonomic neuropathy. The diagnosis of bacterial overgrowth can be made by small-intestinal culture or by the D-[^{14}C]xylose breath test.

Optimal Management

Anatomic causes of bacterial overgrowth usually must be treated surgically. If surgical correction is not feasible, antibiotic therapy is appropriate. If jejunal cultures have been taken, the choice of antibiotics is dictated by the results of the cultures. Broad-spectrum, nonabsorbable antibiotics are appealing, but they have not been tested widely for this disorder (rifaximin has been shown to be effective in European trials). An absorbable broad-spectrum antibiotic, such as tetracycline or chloramphenicol, is also a reasonable first choice. Because of the importance of anaerobic bacteria, metronidazole is a useful alternative. Antibiotics typically are taken for a period of 7 to 10 days (250 to 500 mg tetracycline four times a day, 50 mg chloramphenicol per kilogram per day in four divided doses, or 250 mg metronidazole three times a day). Frequently, a single 7- to 10-day course of therapy can result in several months of improvement. Some patients may experience a shorter duration of response, requiring longer or cyclic therapy for improvement, and some patients may not respond or may become resistant to the effects of antibiotics over time. If malabsorption cannot be corrected, nutritional supplementation may be required.

Zollinger–Ellison Syndrome

Diarrhea is a prominent symptom in about 30% of patients with gastrinoma (see Chapter 107). Steatorrhea is less common (5%), but it can result from inactivation of pancreatic lipase and protonation of fatty acids, making them less soluble in bile salt micelles (below pH 6); precipitation of bile acids (below pH 5); and injury to the small-intestinal mucosa. Symptoms respond promptly to successful acid suppression.

Crohn's Disease

Crohn's disease of the small intestine (regional enteritis) is a common cause of malnutrition, owing to inadequate oral intake, increased gastrointestinal losses, and malabsorption. Crohn's disease can provoke malabsorption by direct mucosal inflammation and injury, enteric fistulas, bacterial overgrowth, and loss of functional absorptive surface due to disease and/or intestinal resection. The terminal ileum is the most common site of disease, and, for this reason, selective bile acid or vitamin B_{12} malabsorption may be evident (see Chapter 111).

Radiation Enteritis

Radiation therapy to the small intestine can cause generalized malabsorption through direct injury to the mucosa and bacterial overgrowth of the small intestine. The risk of radiation enteritis increases with the dose of radiation (>50 Gy) and with the concomitant presence of atherosclerotic vascular disease or fixation of the intestine (previous laparotomy).

Acute radiation injury results in suppression of cell proliferation in the intestinal crypts, which can lead to ulceration of the mucosa. Months to years after completion of radiation therapy, progressive obliterative endarteritis may appear, causing a progressive ischemic injury that can lead to generalized malabsorption. The terminal ileum is particularly prone to direct radiation injury; thus, bile acid and cobalamin malabsorption is typical. Ischemic injury also can result in fibrosis, strictures, and fistulas that predispose to bacterial overgrowth of the small intestine.

Malabsorption induced by radiation injury may take the form of specific lactose, bile acid, or cobalamin malabsorption with resultant diarrhea and/or anemia or severe generalized malabsorption and malnutrition. The diagnosis can be missed because symptoms of weight loss and diarrhea may be attributed to the disease for which the radiation was given. An abnormal D-xylose test or a small-intestinal radiograph establishes the mucosal nature of the disease. The small-intestinal series may show irregular thickening of the mucosal folds, particularly of the ileum. With more severe injury, there may be strictures and enteroenteric fistulas. These radiologic features can be difficult to differentiate from those found in Crohn's disease or invasion of the intestine by cancer. Often, the coexistence of radiation proctitis helps clarify the cause of the small-intestinal disease. Ileal biopsy specimens obtained at colonoscopy may be diagnostic. Occasionally, laparotomy is required to establish the diagnosis.

No specific therapy for radiation enteritis exists, though there have been reports of benefit from glucocorticoids and sulfasalazine. Bacterial overgrowth stemming from discrete strictures and fistulas improves with resection, but intestinal resection is hazardous in this context because anastomotic leaks may result from ischemia. Treatment with broad-spectrum antibiotics may be useful for associated bacterial overgrowth. Lactose cobalamin and bile acid malabsorption respond to specific therapy. Nutritional management is critical in severe disease.

Amyloidosis

Significant small-intestinal involvement develops in about 70% of patients with systemic amyloidosis (see Chapter 235). The involvement is diffuse, with initial perivascular deposition of amyloid followed by muscular, neural, and submucosal infiltration. Malabsorption may result from ischemic injury and bacterial overgrowth. The diagnosis is established by rectal or small-intestinal biopsy. There is no specific therapy for amyloidosis of the small intestine. Antibiotics for documented bacterial overgrowth and nutritional support are the cornerstones of management.

Ischemia of the Small Intestine

Malabsorption is an uncommon complication of chronic ischemia of the small intestine, but it can result from either direct injury to the intestinal wall or bacterial overgrowth originating from an ischemic stricture.

MISCELLANEOUS DISORDERS

Generalized malabsorption may develop in diabetes mellitus either because of pancreatic insufficiency or because of bacterial overgrowth deriving from autonomic insufficiency and intestinal stasis. Thyrotoxicosis can cause a shortened gastrointestinal transit time and mild malabsorption, usually without significant malnutrition. Partial villous atrophy is evident on small-intestinal biopsy in both hypothyroidism and hypoparathyroidism. Some malignancies that do not directly involve the gastrointestinal tract have been associated with unexplained partial villous atrophy and malabsorption.

A variety of drugs can cause defects in nutrient absorption. Neomycin given orally in doses higher than 2 g per day can precipitate bile salts, resulting in poor micellar solubilization of fat. Sulfasalazine interferes with folate absorption. Cholestyramine binds bile salts in a dose-dependent manner, resulting in impaired micellar solubilization and modest malabsorption of fat. Colchicine can produce generalized malabsorption characterized by partial villous atrophy and infiltration of the lamina propria with lymphocytes. These features are reversible with discontinuation of the drug. Somatostatin and its analogs have provoked modest steatorrhea as the dose-limiting toxicity. Ethanol occasionally can lead to mild generalized malabsorption.

DISORDERS OF SPECIFIC NUTRIENT ASSIMILATION

Disorders of specific nutrient assimilation are caused by an isolated defect in an enzyme or transport system and are not associated with generalized malabsorption or malnutrition. The clinical features depend on the specific nutrient affected.

Lactase Deficiency

Lactase deficiency is the most common defect of nutrient assimilation in the world. Normally, lactase levels peak in the infant intestine just before delivery. In most populations, excluding those from northern Europe, lactase mRNA and protein levels fall significantly between the ages of 2 and 15 years (constitutional lactase deficiency). Transient secondary lactase deficiency typically develops after enteric infections, and a rare autosomal recessive form of hereditary lactase deficiency is associated with low levels of lactase even in the neonate.

Lactase deficiency results in a failure of lactose hydrolysis, with resultant malabsorption of the disaccharide. Unabsorbed lactose may cause osmotic diarrhea; furthermore, when it reaches the colon, it is fermented by colonic bacteria to form carbon dioxide, hydrogen, and short-chain fatty acids, producing abdominal bloating and flatulence. Typically, these symptoms begin within 1 to 2 hours after the ingestion of lactose. Because this disorder is so common, a trial of lactose withdrawal is used early in the workup of postprandial bloating, flatulence, and diarrhea. A specific diagnosis can be made with either a lactose tolerance test or a lactose hydrogen breath test. Although lactase levels can be measured directly in peroral jejunal mucosal biopsy specimens, this is not usually necessary.

Secondary lactase deficiency is seen routinely in diffuse mucosal disease of the small intestine, such as celiac or tropical sprue, or in acute enteritis caused by viral, bacterial, or parasitic infestation. Such deficiency may persist after the acute form of enteritis has resolved and should be suspected when diarrheal symptoms do not resolve after an episode of acute enteritis. Secondary lactase deficiency is very common (up to 70%) in HIV-infected patients and is particularly severe in those with advanced disease.

Therapy for primary and secondary lactase deficiency includes lactose withdrawal or replacement. High concentrations of lactose are present in milk, ice cream, cheese, and many desserts, sauces, and stuffings. Withdrawal of these foods alone may reduce dietary lactose below the level at which symptoms develop. Low-lactose milk is now widely available. In addition, lactase may be added to milk or ingested with meals.

Hereditary Sucrase-α-Dextrinase Deficiency

Congenital defects of sucrase-α-dextrinase are unusual; only about 100 cases have been well studied, but the incidence is particularly high among natives of Alaska and Greenland. One type of the disorder (about 20% of the total) results from a defect in synthesis of both sucrase and α-dextrinase, but the more common type is associated with selective absence of sucrase activity. The symptoms of sucrase-α-dextrinase deficiency begin in childhood, when sucrose-containing formulas or foods are ingested. The resultant osmotic diarrhea may lead to severe dehydration and malnutrition. Sucrase-α-dextrinase deficiency can be confirmed by an abnormal sucrose tolerance test result, an abnormal sucrose hydrogen breath test result, or a decreased enzyme level in a jejunal biopsy specimen. Patients with sucrase-α-dextrinase deficiency can be treated by simple withdrawal of sucrose-containing foods.

Glucose–Galactose Malabsorption

Glucose–galactose malabsorption is a rare autosomal recessive disorder caused by mutations in the sodium-dependent glucose and galactose cotransporter of the enterocyte brush border (SGLT-1). The failure of glucose and galactose uptake into the enterocyte results in osmotic diarrhea after ingestion of glucose or starch. The onset of diarrhea occurs when oral feeding is started, and diarrhea may lead to severe dehydration and even death if the cause is not recognized. A specific diagnosis can be established by an abnormal oral glucose tolerance test result combined with a normal D-xylose test result.

Fructose Malabsorption

A rare congenital form of fructose malabsorption has been described, but the biochemical basis of the disease is not yet known. It does not appear to be due to mutations in the Glut-5 fructose transporter of the intestinal brush border.

Genetic Amino Acid Transport Disorders

Hartnup's disease and cystinuria are genetic defects in amino acid transport (neutral amino acids and basic amino acids plus cystine, respectively) in the small intestine and proximal renal tubule. Lysinuric protein intolerance is a genetic defect in basic amino acid transport in all tissues. This defect causes postprandial hyperammonemia due to ornithine deficiency, which impairs the urea cycle. These disorders do not cause nutritional defects because the affected amino acids can be absorbed by other amino acid and peptide transporters.

Selective Bile Acid Malabsorption

Mutations in the ileal cobalamin receptor can cause a rare form of selective cobalamin malabsorption. This autosomal recessive disease typically appears in children (0 to 5 years of age); the symptoms are failure to thrive, infections, megaloblastic anemia, neuropathy, and mild generalized malabsorption. Similarly, mutations in the ileal bile salt transporter can cause leaks in the enterohepatic circulation, leading to severe chronic diarrhea and malabsorption in adults.

BIBLIOGRAPHY

Bia JC. Malabsorption syndromes. *Digestion* 1998;59:530–546.

Brasitus TA, Sitrin MD. Intestinal malabsorption syndromes. *Ann Rev Med* 1990;41:339–347.

Bruno MJ, Haverkort EB, Tytgat GN, et al. Maldigestion associated with exocrine pancreatic insufficiency: implications of gastrointestinal physiology and properties of enzyme preparations for a cause-related and patient-tailored treatment. *Am J Gastroenterol* 1995;90:1383–1393.

Davidson NO. Intestinal lipid absorption. In: Yamada T, ed. *Textbook of gastroenterology*, third ed. Philadelphia: Lippincott Williams and Wilkins, 1999:428–456.

Ganapathy V, Leibach FH. Protein digestion and assimilation. In: Yamada T, ed. *Textbook of gastroenterology*, third ed. Philadelphia: Lippincott Williams and Wilkins, 1999:456–488.

Grant JP, Chapman G, Russell MK. Malabsorption associated with surgical procedures and its treatment. *Nutr Clin Pract* 1996;11:43–52.

Gudmand-Hoyer E, Skovbjerg H. Disaccharide digestion and maldigestion. *Scand J Gastroenterol* 1996;216:111–121.

Haghighi P, Wolf PL. Tropical sprue and subclinical enteropathy: A vision for the nineties. *Crit Rev Clin Lab Sci* 1997;34:313–314.

Kagnoff MF. Celiac disease: a gastrointestinal disease with environmental, genetic, and immunologic components. *Gastroenterol Clin North Am* 1992;21:405–425.

Marousis CG, Cerda JJ. Malabsorption: a clinical update. *Compr Ther* 1997;23:672–678.

Saltzman JR, Russell RM. Nutritional consequences of intestinal bacterial overgrowth. *Compr Ther* 1994;20:523–530.

Traber PG. Carbohydrate assimilation. In: Yamada T, ed. *Textbook of gastroenterology*, second ed. Philadelphia: Lippincott Williams and Wilkins, 1995:405–427.

Kelley's Textbook of Internal Medicine, fourth edition. Edited by H. David Humes. Lippincott Williams & Wilkins, Philadelphia © 2000.

CHAPTER

111

INFLAMMATORY BOWEL DISEASE

LAWRENCE S. FRIEDMAN
DANIEL K. PODOLSKY

Inflammatory bowel disease (IBD) encompasses at least two forms of idiopathic intestinal inflammation: ulcerative colitis (UC) and Crohn's disease (CD). The latter is also called regional enteritis, regional ileitis, Crohn's ileitis, and granulomatous colitis. Although many other inflammatory disorders affect the gastrointestinal (GI) tract, they can be distinguished from UC and CD by the presence of a specific underlying etiologic agent or by the character and manifestations of the inflammatory activity. In contrast, the causes of the major forms of IBD are unknown.

In the absence of identifiable causative agents, UC and CD are defined empirically by their typical clinical, pathologic, endoscopic, radiologic, and laboratory features. Although these features usually allow the clinician to distinguish between UC and CD, the validity of this diagnostic distinction remains uncertain. UC and CD are at least partly distinct in their initial pathogenetic events, but they have many key pathophysiologic processes in common. Moreover, UC and CD each may encompass several variants, which are at least partially distinct. For example, patients with CD may manifest different complications (fistulas) and may express different inflammatory mediators, perhaps owing to underlying genetic differences between the two groups. Thus, patient subgroups defined by disease location, specific pathologic findings (the presence or absence of granulomas in patients with CD), or disease complications may reflect a multiplicity of diseases with some shared features.

Regardless of this uncertainty, the broad classification of IBD into UC and CD that has emerged from extensive clinical experience and investigation over more than 60 years serves as a useful framework for the evaluation and treatment of these patients. Nonetheless, in some patients it is impossible to distinguish with confidence UC from CD affecting the colon using any of the conventional diagnostic criteria; such cases are often labeled "indeterminate colitis."

EPIDEMIOLOGY

The incidence and prevalence of the major forms of IBD have been studied extensively in many populations (Table 111.1). These studies document a wide variation in incidence and prevalence rates and support the conclusion that both environmental and genetic factors contribute to the pathogenesis of UC and CD. The rates of UC and CD in men and women are essentially equivalent, but significant differences are found among different racial and ethnic groups. The highest prevalence rates are reported in non-Hispanic whites, with significantly lower rates in American black and Hispanic populations. Ashkenazi Jews have higher rates of IBD than do other populations in the same coun-

TABLE 111.1. EPIDEMIOLOGIC FEATURES OF INFLAMMATORY BOWEL DISEASE

Incidence (per 100,000)	1–10 (CD), 2–18 (UC)
Prevalence (per 100,000)	20–100 (CD), 40–100 (UC)
Race	White > black > Hispanic
Sex	M ≈ F
Age at onset	Peak 15–25, second peak 50–80 (CD)
Ethnic	Jewish > non-Jewish
Smoking	Associated with CD, inversely associated with UC
Relapse association	Nonsteroidal anti-inflammatory drugs, oral contraceptives (CD), refined sugar?

CD, Crohn's disease; UC, ulcerative colitis.

try, supporting the notion that genetic factors contribute to some of the epidemiologic variation.

Higher rates of both UC and CD among first-degree relatives of patients have been observed consistently in different populations. In general, there appears to be a substantially greater probability that IBD will develop among siblings than among unrelated controls. In parents or children, the relative risk may be fivefold or greater. Enhanced risk in first-degree family members seems to be due to genetic rather than environmental factors. However, the increased risk does not conform to any simple mendelian pattern of inheritance, and even among first-degree relatives, the overall prevalence of IBD is generally below 10%.

Incidence and prevalence rates of IBD among inhabitants of different countries typically vary in proportion to socioeconomic development. A North–South gradient in rates has been noted, with especially high rates in Scandinavian and other northern European countries. In general, the incidence and prevalence rates of UC and CD vary in parallel among populations, but there are exceptions—for instance, UC is relatively common in Japan, but CD is rare. The prevalence of CD increased steadily (as much as sixfold) from the early 1960s through the 1980s in Western Europe and the United States, but the rates for UC remained essentially unchanged during this interval. The overall incidence and prevalence rates of the two disorders are roughly equivalent in these populations, with incidence rates for each ranging from 3 to 10 per 100,000 and prevalence rates ranging from 30 to 50 per 100,000.

Other epidemiologic associations may provide clues to pathogenesis. The incidence of UC is inversely associated with smoking, and clinical relapses have been related to cessation of smoking. Nonetheless, attempts to use nicotine for therapeutic intervention have provided equivocal results at best. In contrast, the incidence of CD parallels smoking. Oral contraceptive use may be associated with a higher risk of CD, and increased consumption of acetaminophen and other non-narcotic analgesics (nonsteroidal anti-inflammatory drugs), as well as simple sugars, may play a part in flare-ups of CD. Both UC and CD may manifest at virtually any age, from early childhood to the ninth decade. The onset is usually in the second and third decades, however, with a smaller increase in incidence in the fifth and sixth decades.

PATHOGENESIS

The precise cause or causes of UC and CD are unknown. Considerable evidence suggests that they result from an interaction between genetically determined host susceptibility and acquired environmental influences. Observations supporting the inference that genetically determined factors contribute to the development of IBD in humans include variations in the prevalence rates of the diseases among different populations, cosegregation of IBD with disorders thought to be genetically determined in some kindreds, and the higher risk of disease in first-degree relatives of a patient with UC or CD. The high degree of concordance of disease in monozygotic twin pairs in Sweden (as high as 67% when the proband has CD and 20% when the proband has UC, compared with 8% for nonidentical twins) provides especially compelling support for the central role of genetic factors.

Although genetic factors may predispose to UC and CD, the development of disease requires either cooperative interaction among more than one genetic locus or initiating "environmental" (most likely intestinal luminal) factors or both. The rate of disease in first-degree relatives of patients with IBD (generally 5% to 10%) is too low simply to reflect recessive inheritance of a single mendelian "disease gene," even with variable penetrance. Furthermore, the fact that the identical twin of a patient does not uniformly show signs of IBD clearly implies that disease development does not solely reflect genetically defined host susceptibility.

Identification of disease-associated genes has not yet been confirmed, but several candidate genetic loci have been studied. Genome-wide screens using anonymous DNA markers scattered throughout all chromosomes have been carried out in members of kindreds multiply affected with IBD. Such screens permit identification of a region of the genome linked to a disease without previous bias as to the likely location of the genes. Application of these techniques has identified a putative susceptibility locus for CD, *IBD1*, in the pericentromeric region of chromosome 16 in some families from northwestern Europe and America, particularly Ashkenazi Jews. The locus is not linked with UC. Other loci on chromosomes 3, 7, and 12 have been linked to both UC and CD, suggesting that UC and CD share some, but not all, susceptibility genes; however, these associations require confirmation. Intensive efforts will be needed to identify the specific gene responsible for the linkage with CD on chromosome 16 and to determine whether the gene or genes identified in the multiply affected kindreds are similarly important in the great majority of patients with CD who have no family history of IBD.

Extensive attempts have been undertaken to find associations with major histocompatibility complex loci. A higher incidence of HLA-DR2 (and lower rate of DR4 and DRw6) among patients with UC and a higher incidence of haplotypes DR1 and DQw5 in patients with CD have been reported but require confirmation. The possibility of a genetically encoded aberration in immune response is also supported indirectly by the frequent finding of a distinctive form of antineutrophil cytoplasmic antibodies (ANCAs) in the serum of patients with UC and 70% of their first-degree relatives and of anti–*Saccharomyces cerevisiae* antibodies (ASCAs) in the serum of 70% of patients with CD and some of their first-degree relatives. Although it is unlikely that ANCAs have a direct role in the pathogenesis of UC, they may reflect genetically defined dysregulation of immunoglobulin production, as further indicated by the disproportionate infiltration of IgG-producing B lymphocytes in IBD tissue. In contrast, the finding of ASCAs in patients with CD may reflect an increase in intestinal permeability to luminal antigens, as is typical of this disorder.

Genes responsible for the expression of colonic mucin glycoproteins are also candidates for genetic contributors to IBD. Alterations in colonic mucin glycoproteins have been found consistently in patients with UC and unaffected identical twins of patients with UC, but not in patients with CD. It is unclear which structural genes are responsible for the altered glycoprotein profile (apoprotein genes or those responsible for glycosylation). Finally, altered levels of expression or biological activity of cytokines and other regulatory peptides in patients with IBD (see "Pathophysiology") may be the result of genetic variation (e.g., relative expression and activity of interleukin [IL]-1 and IL-1 receptor antagonist, alterations in the production of IL-2 by mucosal lymphocytes, and variations in the expression of IL-4 and IL-10).

Recently developed animal models of IBD support the notion that chronic intestinal inflammation can derive from the interaction of several genetic factors. Specifically, in various mouse models, alteration of several different murine genes has resulted in a form of IBD. For example, colitis has been found in mice made deficient in T lymphocytes bearing the α/β class of receptors as well as those made deficient in IL-2, the major histocompatibility complex class II molecules, the G protein $G_{i\alpha}$, mdr1, and intestinal trefoil factor, among others, by gene deletion techniques. In addition, generalized inflammation of the GI tract has been noted in IL-10-deficient mice and transforming growth factor β (TGF-β)–deficient mice as well as in HLA-B27 transgenic rats. These findings suggest that IBD in humans could be the consequence of alterations in one of a number of genes controlling the immune response. Alternatively, IBD could reflect a spectrum of disorders resulting from alterations of various genes, in each case leading to similar manifestations owing to shared common pathways of inflammation and tissue injury.

Several observations suggest that CD4$^+$ lymphocytes are essential for the development of IBD. These observations include the direct demonstration of activated CD4$^+$ lymphocytes in patients with IBD, the ability of therapeutic agents that modulate lymphocyte activation to ameliorate disease activity, and the apparent requirement for CD4$^+$ T cells in murine models. Indeed, adoptive transfer of a subpopulation of CD4$^+$ lymphocytes (CD45RB^{hi}CD4$^+$) to SCID mice results in an IBD-like colitis in recipient mice. Moreover, prolonged remission of CD has been noted in a series of patients who underwent allogeneic bone marrow transplantation for treatment of coincidental leukemia. Genes encoding products that play a role in lymphocyte activation or down-regulation might contribute to a chronic immune response in IBD. Candidate genes are those that encode for aberrant antigen-presenting molecules, elements of the T-cell-receptor complex and its secondary signaling pathways, or cytokines that attenuate immune activation. Regardless of whether there is an intrinsic genetic alteration of the immune system, there is increasing evidence that CD is associated with a so-called TH1 response, in which CD4$^+$ lymphocytes of this subtype predominate (see "Pathophysiology"). In contrast, UC may be characterized by a predominance of the TH2 T-lymphocyte subset.

Gene products necessary for sustaining epithelial integrity also may play a role in the pathogenesis of IBD. Genes whose products could control mucosal barrier function include structural elements of the epithelial cells themselves, epithelial products that form the overlying continuous viscoelastic mucous coat (mucin glycoproteins or trefoil factors), or cytokines/growth factors.

Much effort has been directed toward the identification of environmental factors that may play a causative role in IBD.

The role of environmental factors is suggested by clinical improvement when patients with IBD are placed on bowel rest or an elemental diet and by experimental germ-free animal models. Several transmissible agents—including atypical mycobacteria, cell wall–deficient bacteria, and the measles virus—have been suggested as specific etiologic agents, but associations have been inconsistent. Bacterial products, rather than a specific species of bacteria, may be critical to the development of IBD. The bacterial flora produce a complex mixture of proinflammatory and chemotactic substances (e.g., formylated peptides), and injection of bacterial cell wall products into genetically susceptible animals can result in granulomatous enteritis with features similar to those of CD. Furthermore, the development of colitis in genetically altered mice (IL-2-deficient mice) appears to depend on the presence of intestinal flora, even if the flora do not contain bacteria that are pathogenetic by conventional mechanisms of action. The therapeutic benefit of oral antibiotics and elemental diets in some patients with IBD may be due to reductions in luminal bacterial populations that contribute to intestinal inflammation. Bacterial flora, epithelial cell barrier function, and mucosal immune responses also may be modulated by other environmental agents. These include some medications (nonsteroidal anti-inflammatory agents may impair the mucosal barrier), smoking, and diet.

PATHOPHYSIOLOGY

Although the hypothesis previously outlined provides a framework for understanding the initiation of IBD, its major clinical manifestations depend on a series of immunologic and inflammatory events. Immunoregulatory molecules, cytokines in particular, play a major role in the up-regulation of lymphocytes, macrophages, and neutrophils and facilitate amplification of immune responses by enhancing the recruitment and activation of inflammatory cells. They are produced by and also may activate epithelial cells, endothelial cells, smooth-muscle cells, and fibroblasts. Indeed, the recognition of the close integration of the epithelium with the mucosal immune system has been an important recent development. The proinflammatory cytokines also mediate systemic manifestations of inflammation, such as fever and hepatic production of acute-phase reactants. Other important effects include the enhanced production of collagen and other extracellular matrix components by smooth muscle, thereby leading to fibrosis and stricture formation in CD.

Alterations in many cytokines have been found in association with IBD, including proinflammatory cytokines (synthesis and secretion of tumor necrosis factor [TNF-α], IL-1, and IL-6 in involved tissue), regulatory cytokines (IL-2 and interferon-γ), and a hematopoietic cytokine (granulocyte–macrophage colony-stimulating factor). Patients with IBD also may have a relative deficiency of down-regulatory cytokines, including IL-1 receptor antagonist (IL-1RA), a natural inhibitor of the cytokine IL-1, and IL-10, as well as relative insensitivity to IL-4. As noted earlier, there is increasing evidence that patients with CD have a predominance of TH1 lymphocytes in affected bowel. These CD4$^+$ lymphocytes produce IL-2 and interferon-α, which activate macrophages to generate proinflammatory cytokines (TNF-α, IL-1, IL-6) and cytokines, which reinforce further T-lymphocyte activation, particularly IL-12 and IL-18. To date, there is less compelling evidence that in UC the cytokines produced by TH2 lymphocytes predominate (e.g., IL-5).

Among their many effects, cytokines facilitate the recruitment of acute inflammatory cells to sites of disease. Indeed, in recent years there has been increasing recognition of a family of cytokines, designated chemokines, that may be especially important in cell recruitment. Chemokines include IL-8 and related peptides that contribute to neutrophil recruitment and activation as well as monocyte chemoattractant protein 1, which may play a role in macrophage activation. Chemokine activities are augmented by other inflammatory mediators, both cytokines and noncytokines (TGF-β, leukotrienes, formylated peptides, and complement fragment C5a, in addition to IL-8, all of which attract and activate neutrophils). Redundancy in the effects of immune and inflammatory mediators has been found as a common feature of inflammation within the mucosa.

In addition to cytokines, neuropeptides may play an important role in regulating many of these same inflammatory responses and modulating the functional effects of cytokines and other mediators. Increased concentrations of some neuropeptides, such as substance P, somatostatin, and vasoactive intestinal polypeptide, are present in IBD tissues, and their receptors may be found on many cell populations. These peptides may substantially modulate lymphocyte activation and other mucosal inflammatory responses.

Collectively, chemotactic molecules and cytokines recruit neutrophils and other leukocytes to IBD-affected tissues through various mechanisms of action, including sequential events in which circulating leukocytes roll on the vascular endothelial surface, attach, and then migrate into the tissue. Several cytokines and other inflammatory mediators induce the expression of adhesion molecules on local endothelium and stimulate leukocyte activation, thereby enhancing these processes. Key vascular adhesion molecules (e.g., E-selectin, which is necessary for neutrophil adhesion to endothelium) are expressed on intestinal endothelium in association with active IBD.

Recruitment of acute inflammatory cells leads to the production of additional key mediators of inflammation, with resulting amplification of these processes. These products include additional cytokines and chemokines as well as "nonspecific" mediators of inflammation. Among the latter, arachidonic acid metabolites (leukotrienes and prostaglandins) seem to be especially important. Leukotrienes are chemotactic; prostaglandins, along with other metabolites and some cytokines, promote intestinal electrolyte and fluid secretion, thereby contributing to diarrhea. Activation of inflammatory cells results in the production of reactive oxygen metabolites that may serve as the final common pathway of actual tissue damage. Although reactive oxygen metabolites may be produced by many cell populations, neutrophils and macrophages appear to be the major source.

In addition to their proinflammatory role, it seems as though cytokines and other regulatory peptides have a key role in the down-regulation of inflammation and the reestablishment of mucosal integrity and healing. Several cytokines appear to have potent anti-inflammatory effects that counterbalance the proinflammatory peptides. In addition to IL-1RA, which seems to act as a competitive inhibitor of IL-1, peptides with direct down-regulating properties include IL-10, IL-4, and TGF-β (though in some contexts the latter may augment inflammatory responses). Cytokines, especially TGF-β, and trefoil peptides may facilitate mucosal healing after ulceration. Insulin-like growth factors and some cytokines may promote healing through fibrosis, though these processes may lead to the formation of strictures.

PATHOLOGY

ULCERATIVE COLITIS

The inflammatory process in UC is confined to the mucosa and superficial submucosa of the colon and rectum. UC rarely spares the rectum, and the inflammatory process typically extends in a continuous manner proximally from the rectum. The length of proximal extension varies among patients, involving the entire colon (pancolitis or universal colitis) at onset in approximately one-third of patients.

The histopathologic features are characteristic but nonspecific and may be seen in other intestinal inflammatory conditions (Fig. 111.1A). They include the presence of significant numbers of neutrophils within the lamina propria and the crypts, where they form microabscesses. Depletion of goblet cell mucin is also common. In addition to neutrophil infiltration, many lymphocytes and other leukocyte populations are present. This mixed population of inflammatory and immune cells reflects the constituents of both an acute and a chronic inflammatory response. The presence of the features of chronic inflammation distinguish UC (and CD) from many other forms of intestinal inflammation, including most forms of infectious colitis. The absence of inflammation in the deeper layers of the bowel (except in the most severe form of the disease, designated fulminant colitis) is characteristic. In conjunction with severe inflammation and the coincident production of a complex mixture of inflammatory mediators (see earlier discussion), extensive superficial mucosal ulceration develops.

On the macroscopic level, as seen through the sigmoidoscope or colonoscope, mild inflammation is evidenced by mucosal edema and mild granularity, which contrasts with the smooth, glistening appearance of the normal mucosa. With more severe inflammation, diffuse friability (bleeding on contact) is apparent and may progress to become areas of broad superficial ulceration, frequently covered with a mucopurulent exudate (Fig. 111.1*B*). Areas of regenerative or residual inflammatory tissue may be apparent as pseudopolyps. In parallel with histopathologic findings, macroscopic involvement is diffuse, extending proximally to a varying degree, though the most severely affected mucosa is almost always present most distally. In especially severe disease, complete destruction of the mucosa is apparent; it may be accompanied by marked thinning of the deeper muscular layers in patients with fulminant colitis, when the colon is examined after colectomy.

CROHN'S DISEASE

CD is much more varied in its pathologic and clinical manifestations. Active disease is characterized by an infiltrate in which

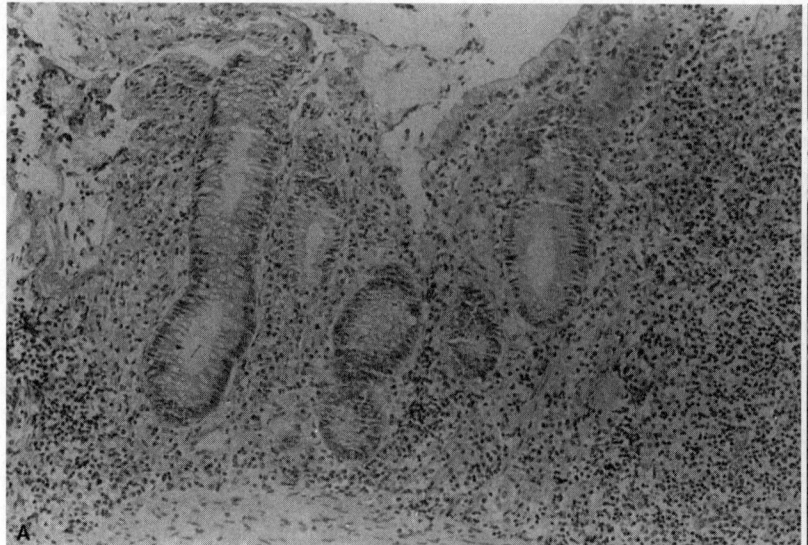
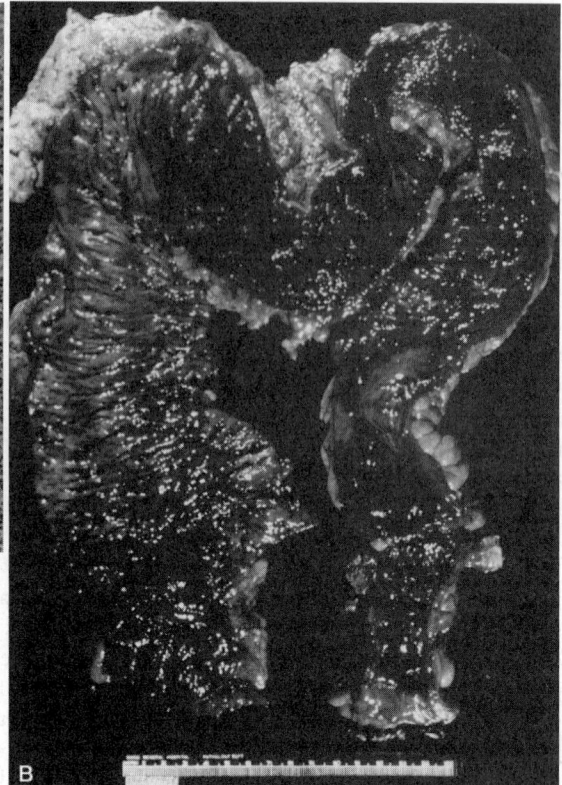

FIGURE 111.1. A: Histopathologic picture of acute ulcerative colitis. This photomicrograph shows some of the typical features of acute ulcerative colitis. Note the presence of microabscesses formed by collections of neutrophils within the lumen of the crypt. Also note the epithelial destruction and the intense, diffuse acute and chronic inflammatory infiltrate in the lamina propria. **B:** This surgical specimen exhibits the characteristic features of severe ulcerative colitis, with diffuse destruction of the mucosal surface and overlying mucopurulent exudate.

macrophages and lymphocytes predominate. The aggregation of macrophages into noncaseating granulomas is found in most patients, but this is not an invariable feature of the disease. In contrast to the continuous and diffuse inflammatory process found in UC, inflammation in CD can be patchy, and segmental involvement of different areas is typical.

Although the acute and chronic inflammatory infiltrate in the mucosa can resemble that found in UC, extension of the inflammatory process into the deeper layers of the bowel wall is a distinguishing feature, and transmural involvement is typical (Fig. 111.2A). Mucosal ulceration occurs frequently. The earliest mucosal lesions of CD are aphthoid ulcerations overlying Peyer's patches and areas of dense lymphoid infiltration. Perhaps as a further consequence of the transmural nature of the inflammatory process, more advanced ulcers are typically deep and linear, often serpiginous or fissure-like, in contrast to the broad superficial ulcers found in UC. Linear ulceration with intervening areas of intact mucosa, often heaped up due to infiltration with large numbers of immune and inflammatory cells, leads to a cobblestone appearance. Inflammation actually may extend through the serosa, frequently leading to adherence to adjacent intraabdominal and pelvic structures. Pathologic anatomic connections, designated fistulas, may develop within these areas of inflammation, leading to various clinical syndromes depending on the involved sites. Thus, fistulas may communicate between different segments of the luminal GI tract (small intestine and colon, colon and stomach) or between the bowel and other organs (bladder and vagina). Fistulas also typically extend from the terminal ileum or distal colon to the skin, particularly in the perianal region. Microperforation or blind tracts (sinuses)

stretching from the bowel lumen may become occluded, leading to abscess formation. Collagen deposition within the bowel wall is also common and may lead to stricture formation, which usually is not found in UC. Macroscopically, the bowel wall may be substantially thickened, though narrowed areas of fibrosis and stricture are also found (Fig. 111.2B). At surgery, mesenteric fat is often seen creeping over the bowel.

Although CD may affect any region of the GI tract, involvement of the terminal ileum or colon is most common. In about 30% of patients, disease is present only in the small intestine (usually the terminal ileum). In approximately 30% of cases, only the large bowel is affected, and in 40% the large bowel and small intestine are affected. In contrast to UC, CD involvement of the colon is usually segmental, and in many patients the rectum is spared. "Skip areas" are often present between regions of disease. In a few patients, however, Crohn's colitis may be diffuse, with rectal involvement, making its distinction from UC more difficult. Although it is less common, CD may involve more proximal areas of the GI tract entirely, including the mouth, esophagus, and stomach. Moreover, a distinctive form of focal microscopic gastritis has been found in a substantial proportion of patients with CD of the small intestine or colon or both. This type of gastritis is frequently asymptomatic.

■ CLINICAL FEATURES

ULCERATIVE COLITIS

The cardinal symptom of UC is bloody diarrhea. Because of irritability of the inflamed rectum, bowel movements are fre-

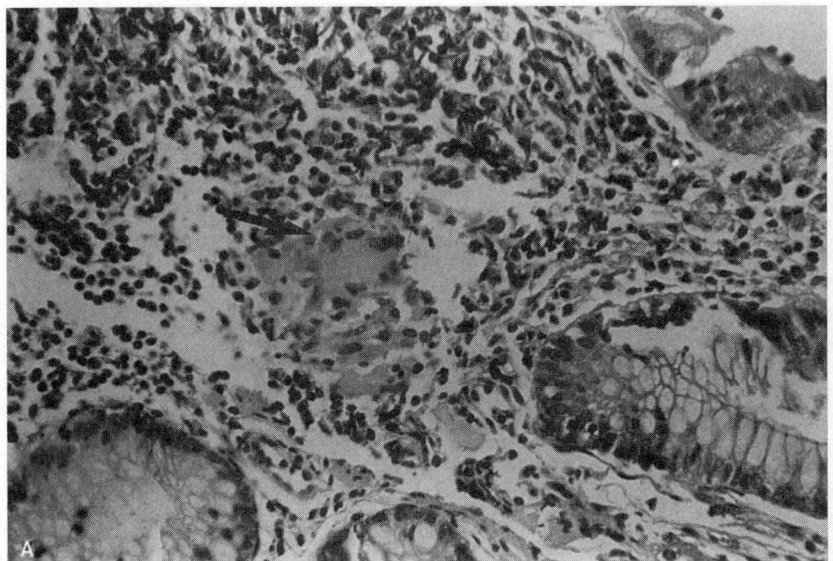
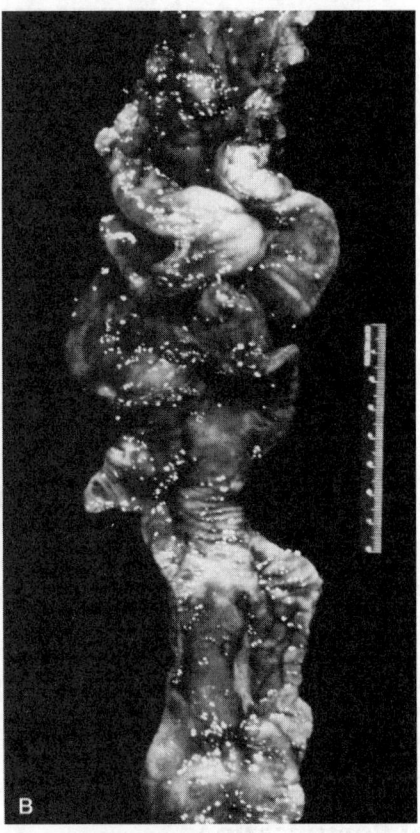

FIGURE 111.2. A: Histopathologic features of Crohn's disease. This photomicrograph exhibits some of the typical features of Crohn's disease, including a complex chronic inflammatory infiltrate in the lamina propria that extends to deeper layers. Poorly formed noncaseating granulomas can be seen, though they are not uniformly present. (From Friedman LS, Graeme-Cook F, Schapiro RH. Inflammatory colitides. In: Boland CR, ed. *Colon, rectum, and anus.* Philadelphia: Current Medicine, 1996. [Feldman M, ed. *Gastroenterology image collection*, vol. 4.], with permission.) **B:** Surgical specimen of Crohn's ileitis shows some of the features typical of Crohn's disease, including marked thickening of the intestinal wall due to transmural inflammation and resulting luminal compromise. The mucosal surface itself has linear ulcerations, in contrast to the diffuse mucosal ulcerations typical of ulcerative colitis.

quent but often small in volume. Symptoms can include fever, crampy lower abdominal pain, rectal pain, tenesmus, and rectal urgency. The severity of the inflammation and the resulting symptoms varies in part with the extent of colonic inflammation. When inflammation is confined to the rectum or rectosigmoid, blood is occasionally present only on the surface of the stool, and systemic symptoms are usually absent. With more extensive colonic inflammation, blood is typically mixed with the stool, and fatigue, fever, and weight loss are common.

Of patients with UC, approximately one-third have pancolonic disease at onset, slightly less than half have disease limited to the distal colon (proctosigmoiditis), and the rest have disease of intermediate extent (generally left-sided disease). Over time, left-sided disease develops in as many as 70% of patients, and 35% of those with proctosigmoiditis experience proximal extension of the disease process.

The activity of UC often is classified as mild, moderate, or severe on the basis of symptoms, physical findings, and laboratory abnormalities (Table 111.2). Disease activity during a first attack of UC is mild in more than 50% of patients. In most such cases, the disease is limited to the rectum or rectosigmoid and is characterized by mild diarrhea, often with rectal bleeding.

Approximately 25% of patients have a moderately severe first attack of UC, characterized by up to six bloody bowel movements a day, abdominal pain, fatigue, and low-grade fever. In many cases, the onset of the attack is mild, and symptoms worsen gradually over days or weeks. Approximately 20% of patients experience more severe disease, characterized by frequent bouts of bloody diarrhea, profound fatigue, fever, tachycardia, weight loss, abdominal pain and tenderness (occasionally with rebound), anemia, and hypoalbuminemia. The outcome of an initial attack of UC usually correlates with the extent of disease and the severity of symptoms. More than 90% of patients with a mild initial attack achieve clinical remission with medical therapy (confirmed on sigmoidoscopy), whereas up to 25% of patients with a severe initial attack prove unresponsive to medication and may require colectomy.

Typically, UC follows a chronic relapsing course characterized by intermittent acute attacks interspersed with periods of remission. Some patients (<5%), however, have no recurrence after an initial acute attack. In an even smaller percentage of cases, symptoms are chronic and continuous. Neither the severity of the first attack nor the extent of colonic inflammation at the time of diagnosis predicts the frequency of relapses. For

TABLE 111.2.	SPECTRUM OF SEVERITY OF ULCERATIVE COLITIS		
Feature	Mild	Moderate	Severe or Fulminant
Bowel frequency per day	<4	4–6	>6
Rectal bleeding	Intermittent	Usual	Continuous and severe
Fever	No	Possibly	Yes
Pulse	Normal	May be >90/min	Often >90/min
Abdominal tenderness	Absent	Often present	Present with distention
Hematocrit (%)	Normal	>30	≤25–30
Albumin	Normal	Normal	Reduced
Erythrocyte sedimentation rate (mm/hr)	<30	May be >30	>30

patients younger than 50, the median time until relapse after resolution of the first attack is approximately 2 to 3 years; for older patients the median time to relapse is longer (see "Inflammatory Bowel Disease in the Elderly"). The severity of the first attack does correlate with the subsequent overall rate of colectomy, which may be as high as 50% within 2 years after a severe first attack of UC, compared with 10% or less during this interval for patients with initial signs of mild disease or proctitis. Overall, approximately 25% of patients ultimately require colectomy.

Local Complications

Patients with an initial severe acute attack of UC can experience various complications. Colonic perforation is more likely during the initial attack of UC than with subsequent attacks, because of the lack of colonic fibrosis and scarring at the outset. Perforation occurs most often in the sigmoid colon. Over time, strictures of the colon occasionally develop as a consequence of hypertrophy and thickening of the muscularis mucosa, particularly in patients with extensive colitis and continuous symptoms. Strictures may result in exacerbation of diarrhea and fecal incontinence or in symptoms of colonic obstruction. Distinguishing benign stricture formation from malignant stricture can be especially difficult.

The most serious complication of acute UC is toxic megacolon, in which the inflammatory process extends beyond the submucosa into the muscularis, leading to the inability of the colon to contract and subsequent colonic distention. Fever, tachycardia, anemia, and leukocytosis usually are present. Additional signs of toxicity often include dehydration, altered mental status, electrolyte disturbances, and hypotension. On physical examination, the abdomen is distended as a result of colonic dilatation, and there is often rebound tenderness over the colon; bowel sounds are hypoactive or absent. Although it is associated with pancolitis in most cases, toxic megacolon now and then also develops in the context of more limited disease and colitis stemming from other causes, including infectious colitis and Crohn's colitis. Risk factors for toxic megacolon in patients with severe colitis include the use of antimotility agents, such as anticholinergic drugs and narcotic analgesics; barium enema examination; colonoscopy; and hypokalemia. Plain radiographs of the abdomen are useful in establishing the diagnosis of toxic megacolon

and in following the course of the disease. Colonic dilatation is usually maximal in the transverse colon or whichever segment of the colon is highest in the abdominal cavity when the patient is supine; the luminal diameter exceeds 6 cm. Colonoscopy and barium enema should be avoided when toxic megacolon is suspected on the basis of physical examination and plain abdominal radiographs.

Once toxic megacolon is recognized, aggressive medical therapy should be initiated. The patient should be given nothing by mouth, and a nasogastric tube should be put in place. Fluids and electrolytes, parenteral glucocorticoids, and, in many cases, intravenous broad-spectrum antibiotics are administered. Intravenous cyclosporine has been found to be beneficial in some patients with severe or fulminant UC (see "Immunosuppressive Agents"). If the patient's clinical symptoms do not improve and radiography shows no change in 24 to 48 hours, surgical intervention, generally a subtotal or total colectomy, is necessary. Patients with severe UC or toxic megacolon unresponsive to intravenous glucocorticoids sometimes have cytomegalovirus inclusion bodies on colonic mucosal biopsy specimens and respond to the withdrawal of glucocorticoids and treatment with intravenous ganciclovir. Surgery is mandatory after colonic perforation, which is associated with a mortality rate above 40%, compared with a mortality rate of 2% for patients with toxic megacolon operated on before perforation.

Ulcerative Colitis and Colon Cancer

Patients with long-standing UC have a markedly higher risk of colon cancer compared with the general population. The risk of colon cancer correlates with the extent of colitis and begins to rise in patients who have had pancolitis for 8 to 10 years and in those who have had left-sided colitis (not beyond the splenic flexure) for 15 years—and possibly sooner. The magnitude of the risk of colon cancer in patients with UC appears to vary, with average incidence rates of 0.5% to 1.0% per year for patients with pancolitis of at least 10 years' duration. The risk of cancer is greatest in patients who have UC early in life, because of the long period they are at risk. The average age at onset of colon cancer in patients with UC is in the fourth decade, compared with later middle age and old age in the general population.

Compared with colon cancer in the general population, colon cancer in patients with UC is more likely to be multicentric and submucosal. Methods used to screen the general population for colorectal cancer, such as examination of the stool for occult blood, do not apply to patients with UC, because of the high incidence of bleeding due to colitis. Therefore, surveillance colonoscopy is used to screen at-risk patients for colon cancer or dysplasia, a histologic lesion in which mucosal cells are marked by nuclear stratification, loss of nuclear polarity, and nuclear and cellular pleomorphism. Dysplasia may be classified as low grade, high grade, or indefinite, depending on the degree of cellular atypia. Dysplasia often precedes the development of invasive colon cancer and may be used as a marker to identify patients at high risk of harboring invasive cancer or experiencing it in the future. Indeed, up to 88% of colons resected for malignancy in UC are found to have associated dysplasia elsewhere in the specimen.

Invasive cancer is particularly likely when dysplasia arises in the vicinity of a suspicious lesion or mass (so-called dysplasia-associated lesion or mass); in such cases, there is at least a 40% chance that the lesion is a carcinoma. Similarly, there is a 40% chance that carcinoma is present in the colon when surveillance colonoscopy detects high-grade dysplasia. In addition, there is as much as a 20% chance that a colon contains carcinoma when surveillance colonoscopy shows low-grade dysplasia.

Although the association between dysplasia and UC is well established, the benefits of surveillance colonoscopy to detect dysplasia are still debated. The benefits of surveillance colonoscopy may be limited: 20% of cases of colon cancer develop in patients not found to have dysplasia on previous routine surveillance colonoscopy, interpretation of mild dysplasia is difficult in the context of active inflammatory disease, and a reduction in cancer mortality rate attributable to surveillance has been difficult to establish. Additional genetic markers of colon cancer, such as mutations of the p53 and *ras* genes, have been identified in some patients with UC and colonic dysplasia or cancer, but their role in the development of cancer in UC and their value in screening require more study.

The usual approach to surveillance is to perform colonoscopy every 1 to 2 years in patients with ulcerative pancolitis of at least 8 to 10 years' duration or of at least 15 years' duration in those with left-sided colitis. Generally four biopsy specimens are taken every 10 cm throughout the colon. Noninflamed areas, masses, strictures, and flat lesions, in particular, should be biopsied. High-grade dysplasia is an indication for colectomy, and experience suggests that low-grade dysplasia, if confirmed by a second pathologist, should also be an indication for colectomy. In a patient who is unwilling or unable to undergo repeated surveillance colonoscopy, prophylactic colectomy is an option in terms of lowering the risk of colon cancer.

CROHN'S DISEASE

Compared with UC, CD is more varied in its initial clinical symptoms and course, in part because of the diversity of anatomic involvement and in part because of the transmural nature of the inflammatory process. At first, approximately 40% of patients have disease involving the ileum and cecum, 30% have

TABLE 111.3.	PATHOGENESIS OF DIARRHEA IN CROHN'S DISEASE

Intestinal inflammation (prostaglandin E_2, cytokines)
Bacterial overgrowth
Bile salt malabsorption
Lactose intolerance
Fistulas
Short bowel syndrome (previous intestinal resection)

disease confined to the small intestine, and 30% have disease confined to the colon, with pancolitis in 30% of the latter patients and segmental or left-sided (distal to the splenic flexure) disease in 70%. Less often, CD involves the oral cavity, esophagus, stomach, or duodenum, though there is increasing appreciation of the frequent presence of asymptomatic gastric inflammation.

Patients with CD most often initially experience the triad of diarrhea, abdominal pain, and weight loss. The onset of disease can be insidious, and the mean duration of symptoms is more than 12 months before patients seek medical evaluation. In patients with colonic disease, diarrhea is often small in volume and associated with rectal urgency and tenesmus. In patients with disease confined to the small intestine, stool volume is larger (Table 111.3). In patients with severe terminal ileal inflammation or those who have undergone surgical resection of the terminal ileum, watery diarrhea may develop from stimulation of colonic fluid and electrolyte secretion by bile salts unabsorbed in the terminal ileum; steatorrhea ultimately may result from frank bile salt deficiency. Steatorrhea also may result from bacterial overgrowth, with deconjugation of bile salts as a consequence of strictures in the small intestine. Additionally, diarrhea may stem from fistulas between intestinal segments.

Patients with ileocolonic CD often have crampy right-lower quadrant pain after eating, an effect of partial intermittent obstruction of the ileum. Associated symptoms include abdominal distention, nausea, and vomiting. Weight loss may result from diffuse intestinal inflammation, malabsorption, or decreased intake of food because of anorexia or abdominal pain. Colonic CD is associated with rectal bleeding and perianal involvement more often than small-intestinal CD. Patients with gastroduodenal CD may have early symptoms of epigastric pain suggestive of a duodenal ulcer or postprandial vomiting due to duodenal stenosis.

On physical examination, patients with active or long-standing CD will often appear pale and ill, sometimes with evidence of weight loss and muscle wasting. The abdomen is often tender, with evidence of thickened bowel loops, a thickened mesentery, or an abscess on palpation, most often in the right-lower quadrant. Perianal involvement is characterized by inflammation, induration, and fistulous openings. Laboratory findings may include anemia resulting from chronic disease, blood loss, or deficiencies in iron, folate, or vitamin B_{12}. The white blood cell count often is mildly elevated and may be markedly elevated in patients with an intra-abdominal abscess. Thrombocytosis also may develop in the context of active disease. It is more likely that the erythrocyte sedimentation rate will be high in colonic

TABLE 111.4.   CROHN'S DISEASE ACTIVITY INDEX (CDAI) FORMULATED BY THE NATIONAL COOPERATIVE CROHN'S DISEASE STUDY GROUP[a]

Variables	Weighting Factor
Number of liquid or soft stools in past 7 days	2
Abdominal pain (0 = none; 1 = mild; 2 = moderate; 3 = severe)	5
General well-being (0 = well; 1 = slightly unwell; 2 = poor; 3 = very poor; 4 = terrible)	7
Number of complications (arthritis, iritis, uveitis, fever >100°F, aphthous stomatitis, erythema nodosum, pyoderma gangrenosum, fissure, fistula, abscess)	20
Taking opiates/Lomotil for diarrhea (0 = no; 1 = yes)	30
Abdominal mass (0 = none; 2 = questionable; 5 = definite)	10
Decrease in hematocrit from normal	6
Percentage below standard weight	1

[a] The total is obtained by summing the products of the grade of each variable and its weighting factor. A score <150 signifies remission; a score >450 signifies severe disease.

disease than in ileal disease, but it also can be normal. Hypoalbuminemia reflects severe disease and malnutrition.

Because of the varied clinical features of CD, no single parameter reflects disease activity in every case. For clinical studies, several numeric systems have been devised for assessing disease severity and response to therapy (Table 111.4). Ancillary measures of intestinal inflammatory activity include the erythrocyte sedimentation rate and acute-phase reactants in serum, such as C-reactive protein or orosomucoid levels.

Complications

Patients with CD can experience a variety of intestinal complications; depending on the predominant complication, the pattern of disease in an individual case is designated as *inflammatory*, *fistulizing*, or *stricturing*. A mixed clinical picture of these types also is relatively common. Fistulas develop in 20% to 40% of patients with CD. Fistulas are usually enteroenteric or enterocutaneous and occasionally enterovesical or enterovaginal, resulting from extension of the inflammatory process through the intestinal wall into an adjacent organ or the skin. The terminal ileum is involved most often and may be associated with fistulas extending to other loops of small intestine or to the sigmoid colon. Most enteroenteric fistulas in patients with CD are small in diameter and may represent incidental findings on barium contrast studies, but occasionally fistulas are large enough to cause diarrhea, malabsorption, or weight loss. Abdominal pain typically stems from active Crohn's inflammation rather than the presence of a fistula. Enterocutaneous fistulas may cause particular problems and frequently are the result of anastomotic leaks

after surgical resection for active disease. Rectovaginal fistulas usually develop in the context of active rectal CD and may lead to a foul vaginal discharge or, now and then, the passage of gas or stool through the vagina. Enterovesical fistulas from diseased ileum or sigmoid to the bladder may produce pneumaturia and recurrent polymicrobial urinary tract infections.

From time to time, free intestinal perforation can occur in CD, but it is less common than in UC because of the characteristic thickening of the bowel wall due to transmural inflammation. Abscesses, which develop in up to 20% of patients with CD, often arise from the terminal ileum and may form between loops of intestine, in the mesentery, or between the intestine and peritoneum. They may also extend into the iliopsoas and retroperitoneal regions, resulting in hip or back pain. Rarely, hepatic or splenic abscesses develop, and, in the postoperative period, anastomotic leaks can lead to intra-abdominal abscesses. Patients with intra-abdominal abscess show signs of fever and abdominal pain and may have a tender abdominal mass on examination as well as leukocytosis with a "shift to the left".

Intestinal obstruction may complicate the course of CD, particularly of the small intestine, in up to 30% of cases; it results from thickening of the intestinal wall by the inflammatory infiltrate, muscular hyperplasia, fibrosis from previous inflammation, or adhesions. Symptoms include crampy midabdominal pain and diarrhea that worsens after meals and improves with fasting. Occasionally, prolonged episodes of severe pain are accompanied by nausea and vomiting.

Perianal disease, seen in approximately 25% of patients with CD, stems from ulceration of the anal canal, with subsequent formation of perirectal abscesses or fistulas. Fistulous openings are usually in the perianal skin, but they also can be in the scrotum, vulva, or groin. Initial symptoms include drainage of serous or mucoid material, redness, induration, and pain that is typically worsened by defecation, sitting, or walking. Sometimes deep perirectal abscesses are evidenced by fever in the absence of localizing symptoms.

Several complications in patients with CD result from intestinal malabsorption due to ileal inflammation or previous ileal resection. Cholesterol gallstones form with increased frequency because of a decrease in the size of the bile salt pool as a result of malabsorption of bile salts. The frequency of calcium oxalate kidney stones is also higher in patients with CD compared with the general population. Calcium oxalate stones are thought to form when fatty acids, normally absorbed in the terminal ileum, reach the colon owing to small-intestinal disease or resection and bind calcium, permitting oxalate, bound to sodium as sodium oxalate, to be absorbed in the colon. Hydronephrosis may develop in patients with CD as a consequence of obstruction of the right ureter by an inflammatory mass surrounding the terminal ileum.

As in UC, the incidence of colon cancer is higher in patients with Crohn's colitis than in the general population. The risk increases with the duration and extent of disease—in patients with extensive Crohn's colitis it is 20 times that of the general population. Surveillance colonoscopy has been recommended for patients with extensive Crohn's colitis, but it has not been evaluated in prospective trials. The risk of adenocarcinoma of the small intestine is also higher in patients with CD of the small intestine. Cancers usually arise in areas of active inflammation, but as many as a third may develop in noninflamed segments. Surgically bypassed loops of small intestine once were thought to be particularly susceptible to developing cancer, but this apparent association reflects the long duration of CD in patients who underwent intestinal bypass many years ago, when that operation was a standard surgical approach to small-intestinal CD.

SPECIAL PATIENT GROUPS

INFLAMMATORY BOWEL DISEASE IN THE ELDERLY

Although IBD affects young adults primarily, epidemiologic studies have shown consistently that nearly 16% of patients with CD and 12% of those with UC are older than 60 at the time of diagnosis. Older patients with UC tend to have less extensive disease: most have proctitis or limited left-sided colonic inflammation. In contrast, ischemic colitis, a major diagnostic consideration in an elderly patient with acute colitis, almost always spares the rectum. Bloody diarrhea is the typical first symptom, but constipation is a more common initial symptom in older patients than in younger patients. On average, the first attack of UC tends to be more severe in older than in younger patients and is more likely to lead to toxic megacolon and higher mortality rates. Nonetheless, after the initial attack, in most older patients UC follows a mild course with no impact on survival, presumably because the extent of colonic inflammation is limited. Although the risk of colon cancer increases with age in the general population, there is no additional risk in patients with late-onset UC, owing to the limited extent and short duration of disease.

Like younger patients, older patients with CD usually have abdominal pain, diarrhea, rectal bleeding, and weight loss. Older patients are more likely to have left-sided colonic or rectal involvement without associated small-intestinal disease. In fact, two-thirds of patients with isolated anorectal or distal colonic CD are older than 50 at the time of diagnosis. In the older age group, women are affected twice as often as men, and there is less likely to be a family history of IBD. The prognosis of CD in the elderly is also good; the disease generally has a mild course. Colonic CD tends to be more responsive to medical treatment than small-intestinal CD. Moreover, postoperative recurrence is less common in elderly patients than in younger patients. Relative mortality rates from CD or colon cancer related to CD among elderly patients do not exceed those of the general population, in contrast to younger patients, in whom the relative mortality rate is markedly higher.

INFLAMMATORY BOWEL DISEASE IN CHILDREN

In 15% of patients with UC and approximately 30% of patients with CD, the onset of illness is before age 20. In general, the clinical picture of UC in childhood resembles that of UC in adulthood. Although GI symptoms of CD are similar in children and adults, extraintestinal manifestations are more often found on initial examination in children than in adults. In addition, growth failure is a major initial complaint in 30% of children with CD. In children with long-standing disease, linear growth, bone development, and sexual maturation may be delayed markedly; such delays can antedate the onset of intestinal symptoms. Factors contributing to growth retardation include malnutrition due to poor oral intake as a result of anorexia and the avoidance of food, as well as malabsorption and increased caloric requirements stemming from extensive intestinal inflammation. Glucocorticoid therapy also can contribute to growth retardation.

PREGNANCY AND INFLAMMATORY BOWEL DISEASE

IBD often occurs in young adults in the peak of reproductive life. Fertility in women with UC appears to be normal, but some studies have suggested that fertility is impaired in women with CD. A decline in the birthrate among women with CD may relate to avoidance of sexual activity or pregnancy, emotional or cosmetic factors, or early menopause rather than a decreased rate of fertility per se. Among men with IBD, infertility sometimes results from reversible abnormalities in sperm number and function caused by the drug sulfasalazine. Most pregnancies in women with IBD lead to the delivery of healthy infants, and the incidence of spontaneous abortions, stillbirths, prematurity, and congenital abnormalities is similar to that of the general population. Some studies have indicated that the incidence of fetal complications is slightly higher when the mother's disease is active during pregnancy.

The best predictor of the activity of IBD during pregnancy is the activity of disease at the onset of pregnancy. Patients in remission at the time of conception are likely to remain in remission during the course of pregnancy, and the relapse rate during the course of pregnancy is no greater than that in nonpregnant patients followed over the same time period. On the other hand, when the disease is active at the time of conception, it remains so throughout pregnancy in two-thirds of patients. Onset of IBD during pregnancy is no more severe than in nonpregnant women. When UC occurs for the first time or recurs during pregnancy, attacks are most likely to manifest during the first trimester or in the postpartum period. Diagnostic radiographic studies or endoscopy with sedation may be required for a pregnant patient with active IBD but are best avoided during the first trimester. The 5-aminosalicylates and glucocorticoids appear to be safe for use during pregnancy, but immunosuppressants and metronidazole, in general, should not be administered.

DIAGNOSIS

In most cases, the diagnosis of IBD can be strongly suspected on the basis of clinical symptoms of diarrhea, bloody diarrhea, abdominal pain, or perianal abscess. In some cases, fever, growth retardation, or an extraintestinal manifestation may be the first problem. In patients with diarrhea, stool cultures for enteric pathogens and examinations for ova and parasites should be carried out and may be repeated during an exacerbation of IBD, to exclude infectious enterocolitis. Various nonspecific markers of inflammation have been used to monitor disease activity, including the erythrocyte sedimentation rate, serum albumin level, serum C-reactive protein or orosomucoid levels, and presence of α_1-antitrypsin in stool. In some patients with small-intestinal CD, features of malabsorption may require evaluation. Anemia can be caused by iron deficiency as a result of blood loss or, occasionally, duodenal inflammation and malabsorption of iron. Macrocytic anemia may stem from folate or, rarely, vitamin B_{12} deficiency due to duodenal or terminal ileal inflammation, respectively. Other features of malabsorption include hypocalcemia and vitamin D deficiency, hypoalbuminemia, and frank steatorrhea due to bile salt deficiency. ANCAs are found in the serum of approximately 70% of patients with UC, and ASCAs are found in the serum of approximately 70% of patients with CD. These tests are not recommended for routine clinical practice, however, and are seldom needed to make a diagnosis. Liver function tests may be indicated to screen for primary sclerosing cholangitis and other liver diseases associated with IBD.

The principal techniques used to confirm the diagnosis of IBD are endoscopy (sigmoidoscopy and colonoscopy) and contrast radiography. They often are used in a complementary fashion, depending on the clinical question being addressed (Table 111.5). Endoscopy is useful in defining the extent of mucosal inflammation and detecting mild inflammation, and air-contrast

radiography is appropriate for assessing colonic distensibility, detecting strictures, and defining fistulas. Barium enema, in particular, is contraindicated in patients with moderate or severe UC or Crohn's colitis because of the possibility of precipitating toxic megacolon.

In patients with colitis, colonoscopy is superior to barium enema in providing direct assessment of the extent and severity of inflammation. In addition, colonoscopy permits histologic examination of mucosal biopsy specimens. In UC, inflammation almost invariably begins in the rectum and extends proximally to a varying degree, without skip areas. Mild UC is characterized by loss of the fine vascular pattern seen in the normal colonic mucosa. Additional findings may include erythema, edema, and granularity, resulting from the uneven reflection of light from the irregular mucosal surface. Exudate or mucopus may be observed with more active disease, and the mucosa may exhibit friability (bleeding on contact). In more severe disease, mucosal bleeding is spontaneous, and ulcerations are evident. Colonoscopy should be avoided in patients with severe colitis or deep ulceration, because of the risk of toxic megacolon or colonic perforation.

The earliest manifestation of CD is aphthous ulcer with intervening areas of normal mucosa. In more severe disease, ulcers may be large and stellate or linear and, in some cases, long and serpiginous. Often a characteristic cobblestone appearance

TABLE 111.5. CLINICAL, ENDOSCOPIC, AND RADIOLOGIC FEATURES OF ULCERATIVE COLITIS AND CROHN'S DISEASE		
Feature	**Ulcerative Colitis**	**Crohn's Disease**
Clinical		
Fever	Only in severe cases	Common
Abdominal pain	Uncommon	Common
Diarrhea	Common	May be absent
Rectal bleeding	Very common	Occasional
Weight loss	Uncommon	Common
Signs of malnutrition	Uncommon	Common in small-bowel Crohn's disease
Perianal disease	Rare	Common
Abdominal mass	No	Common
Intestinal complications		
Stricture	Rare	Common
Fistulas	Rare	Common
Toxic megacolon	Occasional	Rare
Perforation	Uncommon	Uncommon
Risk of malignancy	Increased	Increased
Endoscopic		
Friability	Characteristic	May occur
Aphthous and linear ulcers	Rare	Common
Cobblestone appearance	Never	Common
Pseudopolyps	Common	May occur
Rectal involvement	Usual	Half of cases of Crohn's colitis
Distribution	Continuous	Discontinuous (skip lesions)
Radiologic		
Distribution	Continuous or symmetric	Discontinuous, often asymmetric
Ulceration	Fine, superficial	Deep, with submucosal extension
Fissures	Never	Often
Strictures or fistulas	Rare	Common
Ileal involvement	Dilated ("backwash ileitis")	Narrowed, nodular

is noted. In contrast to UC, the rectum may or may not be involved in CD. Colonoscopy is particularly useful for evaluating strictures and mass lesions (permitting biopsy for diagnosis) and for conducting surveillance examinations for dysplasia. Benign strictures are usually concentric and smooth, and malignant strictures are more likely to be rigid, nodular, or eccentric. Occasionally, benign strictures can be dilated with a balloon passed through the colonoscope. Polypectomy may be performed through the colonoscope, but pseudopolyps are not premalignant and do not require excision.

In general, radiographic findings do not correlate with the activity of disease; some patients with markedly abnormal radiographic studies may be asymptomatic, and improvement in radiographic findings may lag behind clinical improvement. The diffuse ulceration of UC is seen clearly on air-contrast barium enema or the postevacuation film of a single-contrast barium enema. In early UC, the results of barium enema may be normal or show only limited distensibility, narrowing of the lumen, and shortening of the colon. The mucosa may appear slightly irregular or granular. In more severe UC, the mucosa may evidence coarse granularity and nodularity. "Collar button" ulcers that penetrate the mucosa and inflammatory polyps (pseudopolyps) may be present.

Severe rectal inflammation can result in enlargement of the presacral space. In approximately 15% to 20% of patients with pancolitis, inflammation extends into the terminal ileum as backwash ileitis, marked by mucosal irregularity, dilatation of the terminal ileum, and a deformed ileocecal valve. In chronic UC, the colon is shortened and has a tubular appearance owing to a loss of haustral markings (Fig. 111.3). A mass protruding

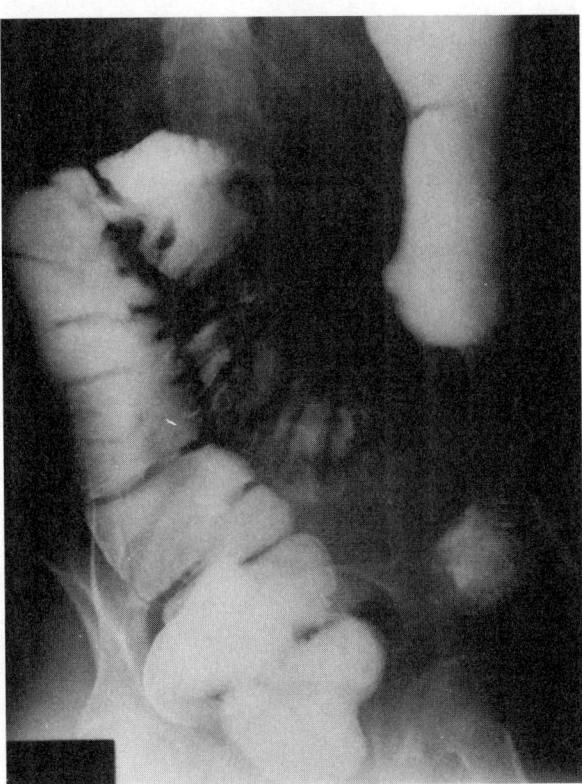

FIGURE 111.4. Barium enema showing features of Crohn's colitis. In contrast to ulcerative colitis, which affects the colon diffusely, Crohn's disease typically spares the rectum and exhibits segmental involvement.

into the lumen; a flattened, rigid area; or a stricture suggests the possibility of colon cancer, but radiologic methods fail to detect cancer in patients with UC in up to 15% of cases.

Early CD is identified on air-contrast barium enema as small, discrete (aphthous) ulcers. Aphthous ulcers also may be seen in various other conditions, including shigellosis, amebiasis, and Behçet's syndrome. In more severe CD, barium enema or small-bowel radiographs may show ulcers that are larger and deeper and often stellate or linear with nodularity of the intervening mucosa (cobblestone appearance; Fig. 111.4). As a result of transmural inflammation and fibrosis, the bowel wall may lack distensibility, the lumen may be narrow, and frank strictures may be noted. Long segments of luminal narrowing stemming from circumferential inflammation and fibrosis may produce a characteristic string sign. Fistulas are studied better by radiography than by endoscopy (Fig. 111.5). Involvement of the stomach and duodenum, almost always seen in association with involvement of the jejunum or ileum, is marked by mucosal infiltration and stiffening, in some cases suggesting tumor.

Computed tomography is particularly useful in the evaluation of patients with CD because of its ability to identify thickening of the bowel wall and abscesses (Fig. 111.6). This technique also may be used to direct percutaneous drainage of abscesses. In some centers, scanning with white blood cells labeled with indium In 111 is used to assess the extent and activity of disease on the basis of the homing of neutrophils to sites of active inflammation. Disease activity also can be estimated by quantitating radiolabeled neutrophils in stool. Although these techniques are

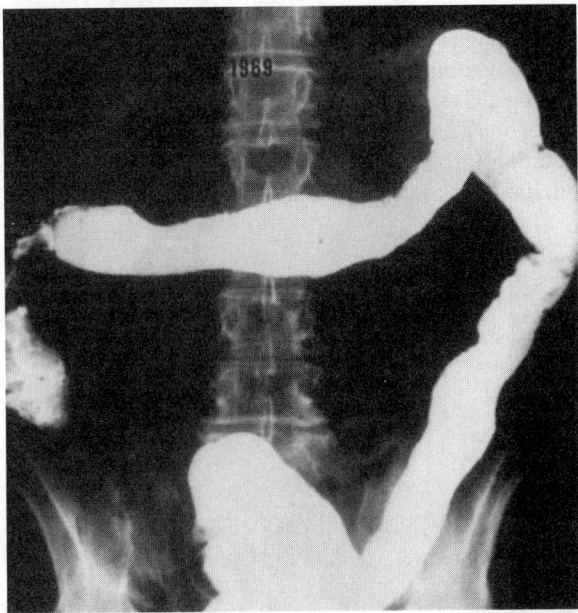

FIGURE 111.3. Barium enema of chronic ulcerative colitis. As a result of long-standing inflammatory disease, the colon becomes foreshortened with a loss of the characteristic haustral markings, leading to a tubular appearance of the colon. (From Friedman LS, Graeme-Cook F, Schapiro RH. Inflammatory colitides. In: Boland CR, ed. *Colon, rectum, and anus.* Philadelphia: Current Medicine, 1996. [Feldman M, ed. *Gastroenterology image collection*, vol. 4.], with permission.)

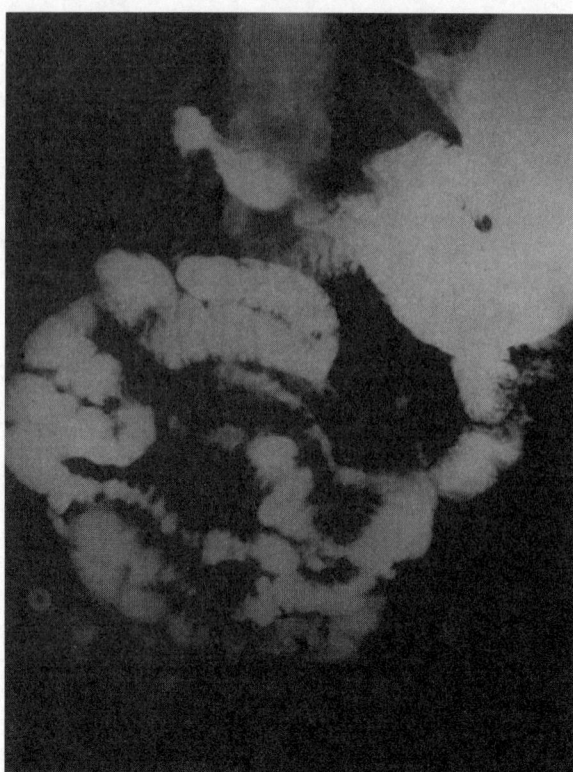

FIGURE 111.5. Upper gastrointestinal and small-bowel follow-through barium study in Crohn's disease, showing extensive involvement of the small intestine by Crohn's disease and obvious impairment of the lumen by inflammatory disease.

TABLE 111.6.	DIFFERENTIAL DIAGNOSIS OF INFLAMMATORY BOWEL DISEASE

Infectious colitis
   Campylobacter
   Shigella
   Salmonella
   Clostridium difficile
   E. coli O157:H7
   Amebiasis
   Herpes simplex
   Gonorrhea
   Chlamydia
   Lymphogranuloma venereum
   Yersinia enterocolitica
   Plesiomonas
   Aeromonas
Ischemic colitis
Diverticulosis
Carcinoma
Lymphoma
Radiation enteritis
Carcinoid syndrome
Eosinophilic enteritis
Vasculitis
Behçet's syndrome
Drugs (e.g., nonsteroidal anti-inflammatory drugs, oral contraceptives)
Endometriosis

E. coli, Escherichia coli.

sensitive for detecting intestinal inflammation, they are not specific for IBD, and white blood cell scanning is limited by relatively poor resolution.

DIFFERENTIAL DIAGNOSIS

In the patient with onset or flare-up of IBD, the most challenging problem often is to distinguish IBD from acute infectious colitis caused by various enteric pathogens (Table 111.6). *Yersinia* ileitis can mimic acute appendicitis or Crohn's ileitis but is cured readily by antibiotic therapy. Many bacterial pathogens, most notably campylobacter and salmonella, can provoke illness resembling UC. Diarrhea caused by infectious agents rarely continues beyond a few weeks, and stool cultures for bacterial pathogens, testing for *Clostridium difficile* toxin, and, in some cases, examination for ova and parasites as well as serologic tests for

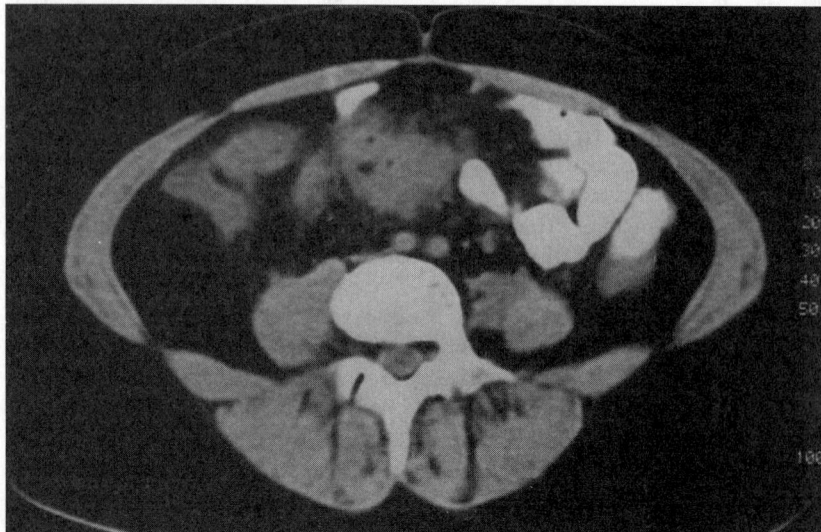

FIGURE 111.6. Computed tomography scan in Crohn's disease shows a right-lower-quadrant inflammatory mass, which must be distinguished from frank abscess formation.

amebiasis identify most cases of acute infectious colitis. Occasionally, the onset of IBD actually follows a bacterial illness or viral gastroenteritis. Histologic examination of rectal biopsy specimens obtained by sigmoidoscopy on initial evaluation helps distinguish acute self-limited colitis from idiopathic IBD; only the latter is associated with abnormal crypt architecture.

In patients with prolonged diarrhea, the diagnosis of giardiasis must be considered. Intestinal tuberculosis, which usually involves the cecum and ileum, must be distinguished from CD in patients from endemic areas; pulmonary tuberculosis may be absent. Intestinal stenosis and draining fistulas sometimes can be caused by chronic fungal infections, such as blastomycosis, as well as actinomycosis. In homosexual men who practice anal intercourse, several pathogens can cause proctitis that resembles ulcerative proctitis, including chlamydia, lymphogranuloma, herpesvirus, cytomegalovirus, syphilis, and gonorrhea. In human immunodeficiency virus–infected patients, diarrhea and abdominal pain may be prompted by various opportunistic infections, including those caused by cytomegalovirus, *Mycobacterium avium* complex, *Cryptosporidium*, *Microsporidium*, and *Isospora*.

Additional diagnostic considerations vary with the patient's age and the clinical picture. In the elderly, ischemic colitis must be considered. In contrast to UC, ischemic colitis spares the rectum because of extensive collateral circulation and usually resolves spontaneously within days to weeks. Distinguishing Crohn's colitis from diverticulitis may be challenging. Both diseases can be accompanied by abdominal pain, fever, diarrhea, and rectal bleeding. In general, attacks of diverticulitis are acute, in contrast to the chronic course of IBD. In elderly patients, a syndrome of segmental colitis, characterized by patchy mucosal erythema and hemorrhage involving a segment of colon containing diverticula, may be confused with IBD. Diversion colitis in a segment of colon that has been bypassed surgically can mimic CD (the condition for which the bypass may have been performed originally) and can be triggered by a deficiency of intraluminal short-chain fatty acids as a result of interruption of the fecal stream. Microscopic colitis, either lymphocytic or collagenous colitis, typically takes the form of chronic watery diarrhea in middle-aged women. In contrast to IBD, the colonic mucosa looks normal on endoscopy, and histologic features are diagnostic. Radiation proctitis usually results from pelvic irradiation and is marked by mucosal friability, ulcerations, atrophy, and telangiectases. Colitis caused by a variety of drugs, such as nonsteroidal anti-inflammatory drugs, gold, estrogen, and allopurinol, sometimes mimics or exacerbates IBD. Ulcerative jejunoileitis is a rare complication of celiac disease that can lead to abdominal pain, diarrhea, and malabsorption and may mimic CD.

Hemorrhoids or anal fissures are a possibility in patients with mild UC and initial symptoms of rectal bleeding. Irritable bowel syndrome, characterized by crampy lower abdominal pain, diarrhea, constipation, or alternating diarrhea and constipation, may be considered in a young person with mild CD, but bleeding and signs of inflammation are absent, and radiographic and endoscopic studies are invariably normal in this condition. Occasionally, intestinal lymphoma can produce symptoms similar to those of CD, including fever, abdominal pain, diarrhea, and weight loss. Radiographic and endoscopic features are also similar, and, in such cases, definitive diagnosis depends on intestinal biopsy.

VARIANT FORMS OF INFLAMMATORY BOWEL DISEASE

LYMPHOCYTIC AND COLLAGENOUS COLITIS (MICROSCOPIC COLITIS)

In addition to the major forms of IBD, over the past two decades other forms of nonspecific inflammatory disorders affecting the intestinal tract have been recognized. The pathogenetic relationship of these disorders to UC and CD remains unclear. In general, the inflammatory processes and resulting symptoms are of modest severity in these variant forms of IBD. They include lymphocytic colitis (also called microscopic and minimal change colitis) and collagenous colitis. Although these initially were described as distinct inflammatory conditions on the basis of pathologic changes on mucosal biopsies, their differences probably reflect a spectrum of findings that can be present in the context of a single disease.

Patients with lymphocytic or collagenous colitis experience mild, often watery diarrhea. Blood is found only rarely in the stools. Both entities are characterized by microscopic inflammatory changes in the absence of macroscopic abnormalities on endoscopic or radiologic examination. Some patients with microscopic colitis have crypt abscesses on mucosal biopsy, but more typically a modest increase in lamina propria lymphocyte populations is the dominant histopathologic finding. The mucosa of patients with collagenous colitis exhibits marked expansion (to 10 μ or more) of the basement membrane beneath the colonic surface epithelium, presumably composed predominantly of collagen. The inflammation or the deposition of collagen may be continuous through the colon or patchy. Whether the deposition of collagen is a secondary consequence of mild lymphocytic inflammation or a primary alteration is unknown. Similarly, the role of the collagen in the pathogenesis of diarrhea is uncertain. Changes usually occur within the right colon, so colonoscopic examination for mucosal biopsy may be necessary to document the disease.

These subtle forms of colonic inflammation sometimes respond to symptomatic treatment with an antidiarrheal agent (loperamide or diphenoxylate) or to sulfasalazine or other 5-aminosalicylic acid (5-ASA) compounds. The therapeutic responses suggest that these disorders share at least some pathophysiologic properties with the major forms of IBD, especially UC. This impression is reinforced by the observation that these patients exhibit some of the same immune-associated markers present in patients with UC, such as circulating ANCAs. Preliminary observations suggest that patients with lymphocytic or collagenous colitis respond to treatment with bismuth subsalicylate, two tablets by mouth four times a day for 8 weeks. In most cases, lymphocytic colitis resolves spontaneously within 3 years. In severe refractory cases, diversion of the fecal stream has resulted in cessation of diarrhea and reversion of the collagen layer.

DIVERSION COLITIS AND POUCHITIS

Two distinctive forms of intestinal inflammation can develop after certain surgical procedures. Diversion colitis is found in the defunctionalized segments of the bowel after exclusion from the path of flow of luminal contents. The mucosa in these bypassed segments can appear quite friable and even ulcerated, owing to broad, typically superficial inflammation. Patients may void small-volume, possibly bloody stools frequently. Diarrhea can be accompanied by abdominal pain and systemic signs of inflammation, including anorexia and fever. This lesion can result from depriving the surface epithelial cells within the affected segment of their primary metabolic fuel (glutamine for the small-intestinal epithelium and short-chain fatty acids for the colonic epithelium), which they normally derive directly from the lumen. Compromise of the mucosal barrier can lead to penetration of luminal proinflammatory substances and result in mucosal inflammation. Efforts to treat diversion colitis with short-chain fatty acids have yielded mixed results. Occasionally, patients respond to nonspecific anti-inflammatory agents, such as glucocorticoids, though reestablishing continuity of the colon or resecting the affected segments are the most effective approaches, when feasible.

With the increasing use of procedures in which a neorectum is created from the ileum after total colectomy (ileal pouch–anal anastomosis or ileoanal pull-through) in patients with UC or familial polyposis, the development of idiopathic inflammation in the pouch has become a well-recognized complication. Pouchitis is more common in patients with a history of UC than in those with a history of polyposis, suggesting that a predisposition to intestinal inflammation also contributes to this disorder. In these patients, biopsy of the pouch mucosa is essential to exclude the possibility of underlying CD, which can be mistaken for UC before colectomy. The mucosa is typically friable and exhibits diffuse, nonspecific inflammation on biopsy; the presence of granulomas indicates CD. Patients experience rectal urgency and frequent bowel movements. Fever and other constitutional symptoms may accompany local manifestations. Treatment is empiric. Some patients respond to the antibiotics metronidazole or ciprofloxacin. Alternatively, patients can be treated with topical or oral 5-ASA or glucocorticoids. In the most refractory cases, takedown of the pouch and conversion to conventional ileostomy may be necessary.

■ EXTRAINTESTINAL MANIFESTATIONS

Both UC and CD are associated with various extraintestinal manifestations. The most common extraintestinal manifestation of IBD, occurring in 25% of cases, is arthritis, usually in the form of migratory pain or painful swelling involving the knees, hips, ankles, elbows, and wrists. Symptoms involving fewer than five joints (pauciarticular) tend to be acute and self-limited and correlate with relapses of IBD and the presence of other extraintestinal manifestations. Control of bowel inflammation generally results in dramatic improvement in arthritis. A second pattern of peripheral arthritis is characterized by involvement of five or more joints (polyarticular), persistence of symptoms for months to years independent of the activity of IBD, and an association with uveitis. Deformity of joints is uncommon. A similar type of arthritis is seen in association with various enteric infections.

A less common type of arthritis seen in patients with IBD is sacroiliitis with or without ankylosing spondylitis; the incidence of this condition is 30-fold higher in patients with UC than in the general population. In 80% of patients, the human leukocyte antigen HLA-B27 is present. Ankylosing spondylitis tends to pursue a relentlessly progressive course; the activity of arthritis does not parallel that of bowel disease. Patients experience lower back pain, morning stiffness, and a stooped posture. Characteristic radiographic changes include squaring of the vertebrae, straightening of the spine (resulting in the so-called "bamboo spine"), and blurring and patchy sclerosis of the margins of the sacroiliac joints. Frank ankylosing spondylitis is uncommon; a more limited process affecting the sacroiliac joints is often evident.

Hepatic complications of IBD include fatty liver, primary sclerosing cholangitis, chronic hepatitis, and cirrhosis. Fatty liver develops in approximately 50% of hospitalized patients with IBD and may relate to weight loss and malnutrition. Up to 20% of patients with IBD have asymptomatic elevations of the serum alkaline phosphatase level, and frank primary sclerosing cholangitis is found in 1% to 4% of patients with UC (but a much smaller percentage of those with CD). Early biliary ductal changes may be confined to intrahepatic bile ducts (formerly termed pericholangitis) and can be confirmed only by liver biopsy. Ultimately, progressive periductal fibrosis develops. In more advanced cases, the serum bilirubin level may be elevated, and gross changes may be seen on endoscopic retrograde cholangiopancreatography. Findings include strictures and focal dilatations of the intrahepatic and extrahepatic biliary tree, suggestive of sclerosing cholangitis. Approximately 75% of patients with primary sclerosing cholangitis have associated IBD. Primary sclerosing cholangitis pursues a course independent of the activity of colitis and may even have its onset after colectomy for UC. Patients may have symptoms of fever, right-upper-quadrant pain, and jaundice stemming from episodes of bacterial cholangitis. Dominant strictures may be seen at the bifurcation of the common bile duct, and cholangiocarcinoma develops at this site in up to 10% of cases. In advanced cases, there may be secondary biliary cirrhosis and portal hypertension.

Dermal complications of IBD, seen in approximately 15% of patients, include erythema nodosum, pyoderma gangrenosum, and, in rare instances, Sweet's syndrome (neutrophilic dermatosis). Erythema nodosum, most common in children with CD, is characterized by raised, tender nodules, usually over the anterior surface of the tibia. The course of erythema nodosum parallels that of bowel disease and improves with resolution of bowel disease. Approximately one-third to one-half of patients with pyoderma gangrenosum have IBD (more often UC than CD), but pyoderma gangrenosum occurs in fewer than 5% of patients with IBD. The typical lesion is an expanding discrete ulcer on the leg with a necrotic base. The ulcer may become large and deep, resulting in destruction of surrounding soft tissue. Lesions usually develop during an attack of acute colitis, but their subsequent activity can be independent of that of bowel disease. Pyoderma gangrenosum usually improves with control of bowel disease.

The principal ocular complications of IBD, seen in less than 5% of cases, are episcleritis and uveitis. Episcleritis takes the form of scleral injection and burning and generally responds to treatment with topical glucocorticoids. Uveitis, or iritis, is an inflammatory lesion of the anterior chamber of the eye, with initial symptoms of eye pain, photophobia, blurred vision, and conjunctival injection. Because vision can be impaired, it is important to make an immediate diagnosis by slit-lamp examination, so that therapy with topical glucocorticoids and atropine can be initiated.

The risk of thromboembolic events, including deep venous thrombosis and pulmonary embolism, is higher in patients with UC and CD. In as many as 50% of patients with IBD and venous thrombosis, activated protein C resistance, due to factor V Leiden mutation, can be detected. Other factors that contribute to a thromboembolic tendency include activation of clotting factors, such as factor VIII and fibrinogen; decreased levels of antithrombin III; and thrombocytosis. The risk of amyloidosis, particularly involving the kidney, is higher in patients with CD and may result in renal insufficiency. Low bone mineral density is common at diagnosis in patients with CD but not UC, and long-term therapy with corticosteroids also may contribute to osteopenia. Rare pulmonary complications of IBD include pulmonary infiltrates with eosinophilia, bronchiolitis obliterans with organizing pneumonia, necrobiotic pulmonary nodules, serositis, glomerulonephritis, and myelodysplastic syndromes. Aphthous stomatitis is common in both UC and CD.

MEDICAL THERAPY

SUPPORTIVE MEASURES

Antidiarrheal agents, such as loperamide or diphenoxylate, may be used in patients with mild symptoms of IBD to reduce the frequency of bowel movements and to relieve rectal urgency. In patients with moderate or severe colitis, antidiarrheal agents must be used with particular caution because they predispose to the development of toxic megacolon. Anticholinergic agents, such as tincture of belladonna, dicyclomine hydrochloride, or propantheline bromide, may minimize abdominal cramps and rectal urgency, particularly when administered before meals to lessen peristalsis. These drugs are contraindicated in patients with severe colitis. Narcotics are best avoided because of the risk of dependency.

In patients with severe IBD requiring hospitalization, repletion of fluids and electrolytes is essential, and blood transfusions may be required for patients with profound anemia. Some patients with refractory chronic anemia respond to treatment with recombinant human erythropoietin. Those patients with anorexia or malnutrition may benefit from supplementation of oral intake with defined-formula diets. Parenteral nutrition may be required, for instance, for patients with chronic small-intestinal obstruction not amenable to surgical resection, a previous massive small-bowel resection and insufficient remaining small intestine, or severe, uncontrollable diarrhea.

Specific deficiencies of iron, calcium, magnesium, zinc, vitamin D, vitamin K, and vitamin B_{12} may require correction. Specific therapy may be indicated for extraintestinal manifestations of IBD, as discussed in the chapters describing those entities. If possible, nonsteroidal anti-inflammatory drugs, which can exacerbate IBD, should be avoided. The value of elemental diets consisting of amino acids, monosaccharides, essential fatty acids, vitamins, and minerals as primary therapy for IBD is the subject of controversy. Experience suggests that such elemental diets limit the activity of CD and achieve remission nearly as often as glucocorticoids but that remission is unlikely to be sustained. Moreover, most patients find these diets unpalatable and monotonous.

As for any chronic illness, particularly one that manifests in the prime of life, education and emotional support are crucial to successful management. Patients should be encouraged to learn about their illness and to participate fully in therapeutic decision making. Stress and psychosomatic factors do not cause IBD but may exacerbate it. A sympathetic physician committed to long-term care is vital. In the United States, the Crohn's and Colitis Foundation of America is an excellent source of information and support for patients. There is no specific curative drug treatment for IBD. Because of the multiplicity of drugs (each with limitations) as well as the variability of disease among patients with IBD, therapy must be individualized (Table 111.7).

5-AMINOSALICYLATES

The original 5-aminosalicylate, sulfasalazine (Azulfidine), remains a useful first-line drug in the treatment of UC and Crohn's colitis of mild to moderate severity. Sulfasalazine consists of 5-ASA (or mesalamine) linked by an azo bond to sulfapyridine. The 5-ASA is the active (therapeutic) component of the drug; sulfapyridine prevents proximal absorption and ensures delivery of 5-ASA to the colon. In the colon, bacteria split the azo bond to release 5-ASA, which exerts a topical action on inflamed colonic mucosa, presumably by inhibiting prostaglandin and leukotriene synthesis, inhibiting granulocyte chemotaxis and activation, and scavenging reactive oxygen metabolites. Much of the freed sulfapyridine is absorbed systemically, accounting for most of the toxicity of sulfasalazine.

Sulfasalazine (up to 1.5 g orally four times daily) induces remission of acute attacks of UC in up to 80% of cases. Once remission is achieved, continued maintenance therapy with doses of 500 mg four times daily or 1 g twice daily lowers the subsequent relapse rate by 50%. Sulfasalazine is also beneficial for active Crohn's colitis, but its efficacy in small intestinal, ileocecal, and perianal CD is less predictable. The role of sulfasalazine in maintaining remission in CD is uncertain; total daily doses as high as 3 to 4 g may prevent relapses or postsurgical recurrences of CD.

Up to half of patients taking sulfasalazine experience side effects; the most common are anorexia, nausea, vomiting, epigastric discomfort, and headache. These effects are dose related and are most likely to occur in patients who are slow acetylators of sulfapyridine on a genetic basis. Reversible decreases in sperm number and function are common in men taking sulfasalazine

TABLE 111.7.	APPROACH TO THE TREATMENT OF INFLAMMATORY BOWEL DISEASE
Clinical Problem	**Options**
Proctitis and distal colitis	Topical 5-aminosalicylic acid Topical hydrocortisone
Ulcerative colitis	
Mild to moderate	Oral sulfasalazine Oral 5-aminosalicylic acid Oral prednisone
Severe	Oral Prednisone or i.v. hydrocortisone (or equivalent) i.v. cyclosporine
Refractory disease or high corticosteroid requirement	Addition of 6-mercaptopurine or azathioprine to standard therapy
Maintenance of remission	Oral sulfasalazine Oral 5-aminosalicylic acid
Crohn's disease	
Mild to moderate	Oral sulfasalazine Oral 5-aminosalicylic acid Oral prednisone Oral metronidazole
Severe	Oral prednisone or i.v. hydrocortisone (or equivalent) Methotrexate?
Perianal disease	Oral metronidazole or ciprofloxacin Oral prednisone Addition of 6-mercaptopurine or azathioprine to standard therapy
Refractory disease, high corticosteroid requirement, or fistulas	Addition of 6-mercaptopurine or azathioprine to standard therapy Infliximab (anti–tumor necrosis factor α antibody)
Maintenance of remission	Oral 5-aminosalicylic acid (especially after surgery and for ileitis) 6-Mercaptopurine or azathioprine

and, on isolated occasions, may result in infertility. Rare, idiosyncratic reactions to sulfasalazine include fever, rash, neutropenia, agranulocytosis, pancreatitis, hepatitis, pneumonitis, polyarteritis, pulmonary fibrosis, and lupus erythematosus. Most such side effects can be attributed to the sulfapyridine component of sulfasalazine, which, in general, should not be reinstituted after an idiosyncratic reaction. Folic acid (1 g per day taken orally) is often prescribed with sulfasalazine, which may limit the intestinal absorption of folate.

Because 5-ASA is the active component of sulfasalazine and because sulfapyridine accounts for most of the drug's toxicity, several alternative formulations of 5-ASA have been developed. Formulations of 5-ASA effective in the treatment of colonic IBD, and in some cases distal small-intestinal IBD, include enemas, suppositories, and various encapsulated and slow-release preparations (Table 111.8). Enemas or suppositories containing 5-ASA (or a related compound, 4-ASA) are beneficial in the treatment of distal UC confined to the rectum or rectosigmoid colon. Oral delayed-release preparations of 5-ASA (mesalamine) include Asacol, in which 5-ASA is coated with an acrylic resin that dissolves at an intraluminal pH greater than 6, and Pentasa,

in which 5-ASA in the form of microgranules is coated with a semipermeable membrane of ethyl cellulose, permitting slow release of 5-ASA throughout the small intestine and colon. In another formulation, olsalazine (Dipentum), 5-ASA is linked to a second 5-ASA molecule instead of sulfapyridine, creating a dimer and permitting delivery of 5-ASA to the distal small intestine and colon.

The various oral formulations of 5-ASA are associated with fewer side effects than sulfasalazine, though olsalazine may cause diarrhea in up to 20% of patients. Rare cases of acute pancreatitis and pericarditis as well as nephrotoxicity have been associated with the use of oral 5-ASA. In general, the 5-ASA compounds appear to be as effective as sulfasalazine in the treatment of ulcerative and Crohn's colitis and in the maintenance of remission of UC, and they are probably more effective than sulfasalazine in preventing relapses of CD, though they are more expensive. Because it is released in the small intestine, Pentasa may be useful in the treatment of small-intestinal CD, but other 5-ASA compounds, such as Asacol, can be administered to maintain remission in patients with ileitis at doses larger than 3 g per day. Because 5-ASA compounds are potentially nephrotoxic, renal function should be monitored in patients treated with these drugs.

GLUCOCORTICOIDS

Glucocorticoids are the most widely used agents in the treatment of moderate to severe UC or CD. These compounds can affect many factors contributing to inflammatory activity in IBD. Glucocorticoids are potent inhibitors of the release of arachidonic acid from cell membranes and of the inflammatory response. In addition, they inhibit the release of IL-1 and IL-2 from immune cells. They are available in oral, intravenous, and rectal formulations of varying potency and duration of action. Despite their effectiveness in suppressing severe IBD, there is no evidence that continued use of glucocorticoids after remission is achieved helps prevent relapse of the disease.

In patients with severe UC or CD, initial therapy consists of intravenous hydrocortisone (300 mg per day), solumedrol (60 mg per day), or the equivalent. Continuous infusion may be preferable to intermittent dosing. Once clinical remission is achieved, a tapering regimen of oral prednisone is instituted. Corticotropin (ACTH; 120 U per day) is as effective as 300 mg per day of intravenous hydrocortisone for the treatment of CD and UC and may be more effective than hydrocortisone in the few patients with a first attack or relapse of UC not previously treated with glucocorticoids. For patients with moderately severe disease, treatment can be initiated on an outpatient basis with oral prednisone (40 to 60 mg per day); once remission is achieved, the drug is tapered over 2 to 3 months. Although the ultimate goal is to discontinue glucocorticoids, some patients require long-term treatment with low-dose prednisone (10 to 15 mg per day) because of continued smoldering disease activity.

Numerous side effects complicate the use of glucocorticoids, including fluid retention, acne, glucose intolerance, adrenal suppression, a predisposition to severe infections, glaucoma, cataracts, peptic ulcer disease, hypertension, osteoporosis, emotional lability or frank psychiatric disorders, and Cushing's syn-

TABLE 111.8.	5-AMINOSALICYLATES				
Drug	Brand Name	Formulation	Initial Dose	Maintenance Dose	Comments
Mesalamine enemas	Rowasa enemas	4-g 5-ASA in 100 mL diluent	1 enema PR q.h.s.	1 enema PR q 2–3 days	May need to taper
Sulfasalazine	Azulfidine	5-ASA linked to sulfapyridine, split by bacterial azoreductases in colon	500 mg p.o. b.i.d., increase over 1 week to 1–1.5 g q.i.d.	500 mg p.o. q.i.d. or 1 g b.i.d.	Numerous side effects (20% of patients; see text); often given with folic acid 1 mg p.o. q.d.
Olsalazine	Dipentum	5-ASA linked to 5-ASA, split like sulfasalazine in colon	500–1,000 mg p.o. b.i.d.	500 mg p.o. b.i.d.	Causes diarrhea in 20% of cases; may improve with dose reduction and administration with meals
Mesalamine	Asacol	5-ASA coated with acrylic resin, released in alkaline pH (terminal ileum, colon)	400–800 mg p.o. t.i.d., can increase to 1,600 mg t.i.d.	800–1,600 mg t.i.d.	Effective in terminal ileitis as well as colitis
Mesalamine	Pentasa	5-ASA microspheres coated with ethyl cellulose, slowly released throughout distal stomach, small bowel, and colon	1 g p.o. q.i.d.	500 mg-1 g p.o. q.i.d.	Some efficacy in small-bowel CD and UC

5-ASA, 5-aminosalicylic acid; CD, Crohn's disease; UC, ulcerative colitis.

drome. Every attempt should be made to avoid prolonged use of glucocorticoids. In some cases, long-term alternate-day glucocorticoid therapy may be useful in suppressing disease activity with fewer side effects.

Topical hydrocortisone (hydrocortisone enemas or foam) commonly is used in the treatment of distal colitis. As the dose increases, however, so do systemic absorption and the frequency of adverse systemic side effects. Therefore, several topical glucocorticoid preparations with enhanced potency and diminished systemic bioavailability, such as budesonide, have been developed and are undergoing clinical trials. Although not yet generally available in the United States, budesonide undergoes extensive first-pass metabolism and has fewer systemic side effects than conventional glucocorticoids. Oral formulations of budesonide are also being studied.

IMMUNOSUPPRESSIVE AGENTS

The immunosuppressant azathioprine and its metabolite 6-mercaptopurine are used most often in conjunction with glucocorticoids in the treatment of CD and UC unresponsive to standard therapy alone (glucocorticoids, sulfasalazine). Their precise mechanism of action in IBD is uncertain, but they may have an inhibitory effect on T-cell production. Immunosuppressants are particularly useful in treating Crohn's fistulas, limiting or eliminating glucocorticoid requirements or preventing prompt relapse after a course of standard medical therapy or surgical resection. Although azathioprine and 6-mercaptopurine appear to prevent relapses of CD or UC in remission, long-term maintenance therapy with these drugs must be balanced against concerns about a possible higher risk of malignancy. As yet unconfirmed evidence suggests that there is no benefit to continuing these drugs if a patient taking one of them has been in remission for more than 4 years.

Azathioprine or 6-mercaptopurine is generally administered in an oral dose of 50 mg per day. The dose is increased gradually to a maximum of 1.5 mg per kilogram per day for 6-mercaptopurine or 2.0 mg per kilogram per day for azathioprine, as tolerated. There is usually a latent period of about 2 months and sometimes up to 6 months before a therapeutic effect is observed. Because of this delayed onset of benefit, these medications are not helpful in controlling acute disease activity and generally should not be used unless therapy for a year or more is contemplated. Adverse effects of both drugs include acute pancreatitis in approximately 3% and fever and rash in 2% of patients. Nausea is common, and diarrhea develops in some patients. Bone marrow suppression is uncommon with a standard dose of 50 mg per day but may be a problem at higher doses; peripheral blood counts should be monitored during therapy. Rare patients experience profound leukopenia within 7 to 14 days of starting these drugs because of a deficiency of the enzyme thiopurine methyltransferase, which results in increased intracellular accumulation of 6-thioguanine. Both drugs should be administered with great caution to patients receiving allopurinol, owing to competitive inhibition of the pathways responsible for their metabolism.

Cyclosporine, an immunosuppressant used to prevent rejection of transplanted organs, has been used with success in the treatment of refractory IBD. Cyclosporine has a more rapid onset of action than azathioprine or 6-mercaptopurine, and clinical benefit is often seen within 1 to 2 weeks. The most encouraging results have been reported in severe UC—intravenous cyclosporine (4 mg per kilogram per day) given by continuous infusion may result in a dramatic response, thereby preventing or at least delaying the urgent need for surgery. On the other hand, cyclosporine is unlikely to be useful for long-term management of IBD because of its expense and many side effects, including hypertension and renal dysfunction. Tacrolimus, a newer immunosuppressant with properties similar to those of cyclosporine, is also undergoing clinical evaluation in patients with IBD, but preliminary studies have not established its superiority to cyclosporine.

Methotrexate, a folic acid antagonist that interferes with the action of IL-1, has shown promise in the management of both UC and CD unresponsive to standard therapy. The most widely used regimen consists of intramuscular injections of 25 mg once a week for 12 weeks. Potential side effects include acute alveolitis in up to 10% of patients and hepatic fibrosis. In general, the use of such agents as cyclosporine and methotrexate should be confined to centers performing controlled trials of novel agents to treat IBD.

Infliximab, an anti-TNF-α chimeric monoclonal antibody, was recently approved by the U.S. Food and Drug Administration for the treatment of moderate to severely active CD unresponsive to conventional therapy. The drug is given as a single infusion of 5 mg per kilogram over at least 2 hours. Additional doses at 2 and 6 weeks are recommended for patients with fistulizing disease, but reports of anaphylactoid reactions and lymphomas in rare patients treated with infliximab suggest that caution is required in using the drug, despite clinical remission rates of approximately 70%. In addition, a serum sickness–like illness has been reported in up to 25% of patients treated again after a prolonged interval following initial infusion. The drug is not recommended for use in children. Limited experience suggests that thalidomide, which also inhibits TNF, has beneficial effects in CD, but its use is closely restricted.

ANTIBIOTICS

Metronidazole is useful in the treatment of perineal CD, Crohn's colitis, and pouchitis. Its mechanism of action in IBD is unclear. The standard dose is 10 to 20 mg per kilogram per day (750 to 1,500 mg per day) in divided doses. Occasionally, there may be dramatic healing of perianal disease, rectovaginal fistulas, and complex perineal abscesses. Metronidazole may be especially effective in controlling Crohn's colitis, despite a lack of effect in UC. However, the use of metronidazole is limited by a high rate of often intolerable side effects, which are dose related; these include a metallic taste, furry tongue, GI upset, and disabling paresthesias. Moreover, there is a high relapse rate when the drug is discontinued, and the safety of long-term therapy with metronidazole, which may have carcinogenic potential, is uncertain. Other orally administered antibiotics, such as ciprofloxacin, may be helpful in the treatment of perineal CD and possibly Crohn's ileitis or UC. Broad-spectrum intravenous antibiotics often are administered to patients with severe or fulminant UC or toxic megacolon, but they are of unproven therapeutic benefit.

OTHER DRUGS UNDER INVESTIGATION

Numerous other agents have been reported to be effective in the treatment of IBD, at least anecdotally. Some have undergone limited clinical trials, but none is used routinely. Fish oil contains eicosapentanoic acid, which diverts the metabolism of arachidonic acid from leukotriene B_4 to leukotriene B_5 and has been reported to have a glucocorticoid-sparing effect in IBD. Specific inhibitors of 5-lipoxygenase, which catalyzes the formation of leukotriene B_4, have shown limited promise in preliminary studies, particularly in patients not taking sulfasalazine. Agents that bind to the leukotriene B_4 receptor have shown some benefit in IBD. A variety of agents that inhibit specific inflammatory mediators and cytokines are under study, including IL-10 and IL-11. An antisense oligonucleotide that inhibits expression of the intracellular adhesion molecule ICAM-1 has shown promise in a highly preliminary trial. Mycophenilate mofetil, a newer immunosuppressant, has had an effect in patients with CD who cannot tolerate azathioprine. Enemas containing sodium cromoglycate, a stabilizer of mast cell membranes, have been efficacious in distal UC. Hydroxychloroquine, which is thought to act by correcting a defect in the ability of antigen-bearing epithelial cells to stimulate suppressor T cells, occasionally results in remissions in UC. Superoxide dismutase, a scavenger of reactive oxygen metabolites, has shown some benefit in limited clinical trials. Nicorette gum and transdermal nicotine, evaluated because of an association between the cessation of tobacco use and the development of UC, have been of limited clinical benefit in patients with UC. In unresponsive perineal CD, hyperbaric oxygen has been reported to have efficacy.

■ STRATEGIES FOR OPTIMAL CARE

ULCERATIVE COLITIS

In patients with ulcerative proctitis or distal colitis, initial therapy with hydrocortisone or 5-ASA enemas is often effective. Alternatively, oral sulfasalazine, or another oral 5-aminosalicylate, may be administered in gradually increasing doses. Once clinical remission is achieved, the frequency of enemas can be decreased to every other day or every third day, or a lower (maintenance) dose of an oral 5-aminosalicylate can be given. Patients who do not respond to enemas or oral 5-aminosalicylates may require a trial of oral prednisone beginning at a dose of 40 mg per day.

For patients with more extensive colitis that is mild in activity, oral sulfasalazine (or another oral 5-aminosalicylate) can be tried, starting at a dose of 500 mg twice a day and increasing to 1 to 1.5 g four times a day over a week. Patients unresponsive to oral aminosalicylate may need a trial of oral prednisone at an initial dose of 20 to 60 mg per day. Patients with moderately severe disease probably should be given oral prednisone at the outset. Once clinical remission is achieved, the dose of oral prednisone can be tapered at a rate of 2.5 to 5 mg per day per week to 20 mg per day, at which point the rate of tapering may be slowed to 2.5 to 5 mg per day every other week. At some point, it is reasonable to start an oral aminosalicylate, which can be continued as maintenance therapy once the oral prednisone is discontinued.

Patients with severe UC require hospitalization and parenteral glucocorticoids. Dehydration and hypokalemia should be corrected, and the patient should be monitored for the development of toxic megacolon. Malnourished patients may need parenteral nutrition. Intravenous hydrocortisone (300 mg per day) or its equivalent should be administered. The value of intravenous broad-spectrum antibiotics in severe colitis is uncertain, but they should be considered for patients with clinical signs suggesting sepsis. Once the patient's clinical condition improves, intravenous glucocorticoids can be discontinued and oral prednisone begun.

In patients with UC that does not respond to oral aminosalicylates or glucocorticoids, therapy with immunosuppressive agents may be considered. For patients with mild to moderately severe disease, azathioprine or 6-mercaptopurine can be tried, but these agents may require several months for a response. In patients with severe UC, a trial of intravenous cyclosporine can be considered; if it is effective, clinical improvement should occur within a week. Patients unresponsive to aggressive medical therapy can be considered for colectomy (see "Ulcerative Colitis" below).

CROHN'S DISEASE

In patients with Crohn's colitis or ileocolitis of mild to moderate severity, oral sulfasalazine or an alternative 5-aminosalicylate should be tried, as described for UC. Patients unresponsive to an oral aminosalicylate or those with more severe disease should be started on oral prednisone (40 mg per day). If an intraabdominal abscess is present, broad-spectrum antibiotics should be administered, and the abscess should be drained. Because abdominal pain is often the predominant symptom in patients with CD, efforts should be undertaken to identify the basis of the pain; specifically, the possibility of intestinal obstruction caused by a fibrotic stricture should be explored and, if necessary, treated surgically or, if it is accessible, endoscopically. If diarrhea is the predominant symptom, additional explanations, such as a fistula or bacterial overgrowth, may need to be investigated. Antibiotics (metronidazole or ciprofloxacin) also may be effective as primary treatment for patients with disease of the large bowel and possibly the ileum.

Patients with severe CD often require hospitalization, intravenous hydration, and parenteral glucocorticoids. Patients unresponsive to corticosteroids alone may need immunosuppressive drugs as well. Surgical intervention should be considered when prolonged courses of high-dose glucocorticoids are needed or when a specific complication requiring surgical intervention is identified (see next section). For patients with perianal disease, a course of oral metronidazole or ciprofloxacin may be worthwhile. Treatment with infliximab can be considered for patients with refractory symptomatic fistulas. Nutritional repletion and supplementation may be necessary for the malnourished patient. In the patient with terminal ileal disease or a previous ileal resection, supplemental vitamin B_{12} is often mandatory.

■ SURGICAL THERAPY

ULCERATIVE COLITIS

Up to 25% of patients with extensive UC ultimately require colectomy. The most common indication for surgery is the fail-

ure of medical therapy to control colonic inflammation. In most cases, intractability manifests as chronic diarrhea severe enough to impair the patient's quality of life. In some cases, surgery is considered when it is not possible to wean the patient from high-dose glucocorticoids. In children, intractability manifests primarily as growth failure. Additional indications include the failure of extraintestinal manifestations of colitis to respond to medical management and the finding of dysplasia or carcinoma on colonoscopy. Emergency colectomy may be necessary for toxic megacolon or severe fulminant colitis. Rarely, severe hemorrhage is an indication for emergency colectomy.

The standard operation for UC is proctocolectomy with a Brooke ileostomy, which may be performed in one or two stages. A two-stage procedure is generally favored for patients who are severely ill (e.g., those with toxic megacolon). Advantages of proctocolectomy and ileostomy are that the procedure is curative and associated with excellent technical and functional results. Disadvantages are the need for an ostomy with an appliance and the risk of impaired sexual function in men.

An alternative to standard proctocolectomy and ileostomy is ileal pouch–anal anastomosis, in which the colon is removed, but the muscularis of the rectum is left in place after dissection of the rectal mucosa and submucosa. A pouch constructed from the terminal ileum is sewn to the dentate line at the anorectal junction. A temporary diverting loop ileostomy is commonly created to protect the ileal pouch–anal anastomosis until it heals. The major advantage of the ileal pouch–anal anastomosis is that it maintains bowel continuity. Initially, patients have numerous bowel movements and frequent fecal incontinence, which improves gradually over 12 months. Additional potential complications include the formation of an abscess in the ileal pouch and pouchitis, a syndrome characterized by diarrhea, rectal bleeding, malaise, and both endoscopic and histologic evidence of inflammation of the pouch. In some cases, pouchitis is responsive to oral antibiotics, such as metronidazole (250 to 500 mg three times a day for 7 to 10 days). Approximately 2% of patients require excision of the ileal reservoir and placement of a permanent ileostomy.

CROHN'S DISEASE

Ultimately, most patients with CD undergo surgery for the disease. Although surgical resection is not curative, intractability and failure of medical therapy often result in the need for surgery in CD. Additional indications are intestinal obstruction, symptomatic fistulas, abscesses, toxic dilatation, perforation, and cancer.

In patients with small-intestinal CD, the most common surgical procedure is segmental resection for intestinal obstruction or fistula. Only grossly involved bowel is resected, because resection of intestine that is macroscopically normal but microscopically abnormal does not lessen the frequency of recurrence. In fact, the frequency of ileal recurrence after resection for ileitis or ileocolitis is approximately 50% after 10 years. The site of recurrent disease is almost invariably proximal to the anastomosis. In a patient operated on for acute appendicitis but found instead to have acute ileitis, ileal resection should not be performed, because of the likelihood that acute ileitis will be self-limited; however, appendectomy should be performed so that diagnostic confusion is avoided in the future.

To preserve bowel length and lower the chance that short bowel syndrome will result from repeated intestinal resections, strictureplasty is often carried out for patients with an intestinal obstruction caused by a fibrotic stricture in the absence of substantial inflammation. The technique involves making a longitudinal incision of the stricture, followed by transverse closure. Segmental or total resection of the colon is ultimately required in 50% of patients with Crohn's colitis. However, recurrence rates are as high as 75% 10 years after segmental resection. The rate of recurrence of the disease in the small intestine after total colectomy is approximately 25%. For patients with extensive rectal CD, total proctocolectomy with a Brooke ileostomy may be considered. An ileal pouch–anal anastomosis is inappropriate in the context of Crohn's colitis, because of the invariable recurrence of CD in the pouch.

PROGNOSIS

Both UC and CD are generally chronic, relapsing diseases, but in an individual case the course is unpredictable. For patients with a first attack of UC, the risk of relapse approaches 90% after 25 years of follow-up. However, at any point in time, half of all patients with UC are in remission. Colectomy is ultimately required in 25% of patients. The mortality rate is slightly higher than that of the general population after the initial attack, reflecting patients with severe acute pancolitis. After that, the mortality rate is not increased, and more than 90% of patients lead full, productive lives.

At least 50% of patients with CD require surgery, and most of them experience a subsequent symptomatic recurrence; another surgical procedure is required in at least a third of the patients who undergo surgery. Intestinal obstruction is most likely to occur in patients with small-intestinal CD, and fistulas and abscesses are most likely in those with ileocolonic disease; the latter group has a higher risk of postsurgical recurrence than the former. Compared with the general population, life expectancy is slightly lower in patients with CD. Death rates are highest in the immediate postoperative period, and death tends to occur during the first 5 years after diagnosis. Although most patients lead active lives, the disease may be continually active and debilitating in 15% to 20% of cases.

BIBLIOGRAPHY

Feldman M, Scharschmidt BF, Sleisenger MH, eds. *Sleisenger and Fordtran's gastrointestinal disease,* sixth ed. Philadelphia: WB Saunders,1998.

Fiocchi C. Inflammatory bowel disease: etiology and pathogenesis. *Gastroenterology* 1998;115:182–205.

Hanauer SB, Meyers S. Management of Crohn's disease in adults. *Am J Gastroenterol* 1997;92:559–566.

Kirsner JB, ed. *Inflammatory bowel disease,* fifth ed. Philadelphia: Saunders, 2000.

Kornbluth A, Sachar DB. Ulcerative colitis practice guidelines in adults. *Am J Gastroenterol* 1997;92:204–211.

O'Sullivan MA, O'Morain CA. Nutritional therapy in Crohn's disease. *Inflamm Bowel Dis* 1998;4:45–53.

Podolsky DK. Inflammatory bowel disease, parts I and II. *N Engl J Med* 1991;325:928–937, 1008–1016.

Sands BE. Biologic therapy for inflammatory bowel disease. *Inflamm Bowel Dis* 1997;3:95–113.

Snapper SB, Syngal S, Friedman LS. Ulcerative colitis and colon cancer: more controversy than clarity. *Dig Dis* 1998;16:81–87.

Targan SR, Shanahan F, eds. *Inflammatory bowel disease: from bench to bedside.* Baltimore: Williams & Wilkins, 1994.

Yamada T, ed. *Textbook of gastroenterology,* third ed. Philadelphia: JB Lippincott, 1999.

Kelley's Textbook of Internal Medicine, fourth edition. Edited by H. David Humes.
Lippincott Williams & Wilkins, Philadelphia © 2000.

CHAPTER

112

MESENTERIC VASCULAR DISEASES

JAMES C. STANLEY

Mesenteric vascular diseases are a heterogeneous group of clinically significant illnesses that have become recognized with increasing frequency due to the more common imaging of the intestinal circulation during study of vascular and nonvascular diseases of the abdomen. Considerable information exists regarding some of these diseases, whereas knowledge about others is anecdotal. It is important to recognize differences among the common ischemic diseases (Table 112.1) and common splanchnic aneurysms (Table 112.2).

MESENTERIC MACROVASCULAR CIRCULATION

Mesenteric blood flow is derived from the celiac, superior mesenteric, and inferior mesenteric arteries. The celiac artery arises from the aorta between the crura of the diaphragm. This vessel courses ventrally for nearly 2 cm, then divides into the common hepatic, left gastric, and splenic arteries. The superior mesenteric artery arises from the aorta behind the pancreas. Superior mesenteric artery blood flow averages 600 mL per minute, accounting for approximately 15% of the cardiac output. Blood flow increases by about 100% in the superior mesenteric artery after a solid meal. Clearly, the range of normal blood flow to the small intestine is great.

The first two branches of the superior mesenteric artery are the inferior pancreaticoduodenal and middle colic arteries. These vessels are the source for important collateral flow between the superior mesenteric artery and the celiac artery, as well as the inferior mesenteric artery. The inferior mesenteric artery arises from the aorta approximately 5 cm above its bifurcation. This

TABLE 112.1.	MESENTERIC ISCHEMIC DISEASE		
	Acute Embolic Occlusion	**Low-Flow States**	**Chronic Arteriosclerotic Occlusive Disease**
Usual pathology	Embolic occlusion of SMA beyond collaterals from CA and IMA, from dislodged atrial thrombus (due to atrial fibrillation)	Cardiac failure	Aortic spillover arteriosclerosis causing critical stenoses of at least two of the three major splanchnic arteries. Usually involves orificial stenoses of CA and SMA
Gender ratio (M/F)	2:1	1.5:1	1:2
Clinical manifestation	Marked disparity between acute excruciating midabdominal pain and a paucity of early physical findings	3- to 4-day history of vague abdominal pain, distention	Gradual but progressive development of postprandial pain, lasting 3–4 h. Associated "small-meal syndrome" and weight loss
Diagnostic studies	Emergent arteriography, operative diagnosis	Arteriography, occasional barium enema in subacute cases reveals colon "thumb printing"	Lateral aortography
Treatment	Emergent SMA embolectomy, chronic anticoagulation	Improve cardiac function, vasodilators (glucagon) and fluids	Bypass or endarterectomy of CA and SMA
Mortality	Operative mortality 60% without intestinal infarction, 95% with intestinal infarction	Low, but 60% with intestinal infarction	Operative mortality less than 10%

SMA, superior mesenteric artery; CA, celiac artery; IMA, inferior mesenteric artery.

vessel branches into the left colic artery and the superior rectal arteries.

MESENTERIC MICROCIRCULATION

The stomach's mucosa constitutes more than half of the gastric wall mass, has the most active metabolism, and receives about 75% of the resting gastric blood flow. The stomach's muscularis layer constitutes over one-third of the gastric wall mass but receives less than 25% of the resting gastric blood flow. Capillaries of the muscularis externa and muscularis mucosa exist in parallel, whereas capillaries of the submucosa and mucosa are arranged in series, so that blood must first pass through the submucosal plexus before entering the juxtaposed mucosal plexus.

The small intestine's three anatomical layers are dominated by the villi and microvilli of the mucosa. The villi's high capillary density facilitates exchange of large quantities of fluid between the blood and transporting surface. The mucosa of the small intestine receives over 50% of this organ's resting blood flow, whereas the muscularis externa, constituting half of the small intestine's mass, receives only 10% to 15% of the total blood flow. Serosal blood vessels must first pierce the muscularis externa before forming an extensive submucosal plexus. From this plexus, one group of arteries pierces the muscularis mucosa at the base of the villi to form a capillary network about the glands lining the mucosal crypts. A second group of arteries enters the base of the villi and provides extensive branches to the tip of the villi. The colon has a similar microcirculation, with more than 75% of its blood flow perfusing the mucosa.

Intramural collateral blood vessels are derived mostly from precapillary microvascular channels. Two-thirds of these collateral vessels originate from extramural marginal vessels; the rest arise from intramural vessels. The primary hemodynamic determinant of collateral flow is passive; modest vasodilatation in an ischemic bowel segment is the only active component. It is unlikely that consistent reflex vasoconstriction or vasodilatation occurs in the vessels of adjacent nonischemic bowel, as was thought for some time.

SPLANCHNIC ISCHEMIA

MICROCIRCULATORY CONSEQUENCES OF INTESTINAL ISCHEMIA

Severe reductions in intestinal blood flow cause cellular hypoxia, accumulation of oxygen free radicals, elevation of portal venous pressure, adverse effects of digestive enzymes on the gut tissues themselves, and intraluminal bacterial proliferation. The entire cellular coverage of the villus may be destroyed before reperfusion takes place. Non–neutrophil-derived reactive oxygen metabolites cause further injury, with reperfusion of ischemic intestinal tissues. An early susceptibility to ischemic injury and invasion of the microcirculation by intestinal bacteria, evident by the presence of portal venous gas (Fig. 112.1), causes intestinal ischemia to be much more damaging than that affecting other tissues, such as skeletal or cardiac muscle.

The small intestine can sustain modest reductions in blood flow without ischemic injury, as long as there is no more than a 50% decrease in oxygen consumption. Drugs that influence

TABLE 112.2.   SPLANCHNIC ARTERY ANEURYSMS

Aneurysm Location	Frequency in Splanchnic Circulation	Male/Female Ratio	Contributing Factors	Frequency of Reported Rupture	Site of Rupture	Mortality with Rupture
Splenic artery	60%	1:4	Medial degeneration; arterial fibrodysplasia; multiple pregnancies; portal hypertension; trauma; chronic pancreatitis with arterial erosion by pseudocysts	2% bland aneurysms, 95% with pregnancy	Intraperitoneal within lesser sac; intragastric with pancreatitis-related aneurysms	25% bland and unassociated with pregnancy; during pregnancy 70% maternal, 75% fetal
Hepatic artery	20%	2:1	Medial degeneration; blunt and penetrating liver trauma; infection related to intravenous substance abuse	20%	Intraperitoneal and biliary tract with equal frequency	35%
Superior mesenteric artery	5.5%	1:1	Medial degeneration; infection related to bacterial endocarditis, often associated with nonhemolytic streptococci and more recently with bacteremia from intravenous substance abuse	Uncommon, thrombosis more common	Intraperitoneal and retroperitoneal	50%
Celiac artery Gastric and gastroepiploic arteries	4% 4%	1:1 3:1	Medial degeneration Periarterial inflammation; medial degeneration	13% 90%	Intraperitoneal 70% intestinal tract; 30% intraperitoneal	50% 70%
Pancreaticoduodenal, pancreatic, and gastroduodenal arteries	3.5%	4:1	Pancreatitis-related arterial necrosis and arterial erosion by pseudocysts in 60% of gastroduodenal and 30% of pancreaticoduodenal artery aneurysms; medial degeneration	75% inflammatory, 50% noninflammatory	85% intestinal tract; 15% intraperitoneal	50%
Jejunal, ileal, and colic arteries	3%	1:1	Medial degeneration; connective tissue diseases	30%	Intraperitoneal and intestinal tract	20%

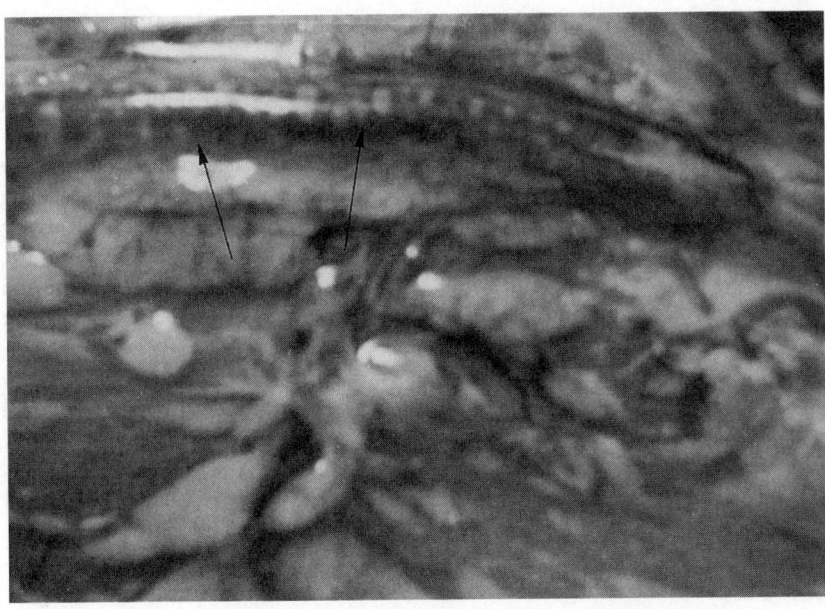

FIGURE 112.1. Portal venous air bubbles *(arrows)* associated with the invasion of a profoundly ischemic bowel wall by gas-forming bacteria. (From Wakefield TW, Stanley JC. The intestine. In: Zelenock GB, ed. *Clinical ischemic syndromes: mechanisms and consequences of tissue injury.* St. Louis: CV Mosby, 1990, with permission.)

mesenteric blood flow, such as glucagon, have major effects on intestinal motility. Agents that decrease intestinal motility may lessen oxygen needs of the gut and increase its tolerance to subcritical ischemia. Perhaps most important in this effect is the relaxation of the intestine's muscularis mucosa, with subsequent decreases in the resistance to blood flow from submucosal vessels to mucosal and villous vessels.

ACUTE EMBOLIC MESENTERIC VASCULAR OCCLUSION (TABLE 112.1)

The most catastrophic form of treatable intestinal ischemia is macroembolism involving the superior mesenteric artery. Such emboli have a cardiac origin in nearly 95% of patients. Most originate from atrial thrombi associated with arteriosclerotic heart disease and atrial fibrillation or from ventricular thrombi following myocardial infarction. Men are affected twice as often as women. Nearly 5% of all peripheral emboli involve the superior mesenteric artery. Half of these patients have had prior episodes of embolism of extraintestinal vessels, most often involving the femoral or popliteal arteries. Superior mesenteric artery emboli usually lodge beyond the origin of the inferior pancreaticoduodenal and middle colic arteries (Fig. 112.2). This effectively isolates the distal superior mesenteric arterial circulation and causes critical ischemia of the distal jejunum, entire ileum, and right colon.

Patients experiencing acute superior mesenteric artery embolic occlusions usually present with intense unremitting midabdominal pain with nausea and vomiting. This may be accompanied by explosive diarrhea. Early physical examination is usually normal, without evidence of abdominal tenderness, rigidity, or mass lesions. The diagnosis should be suspected in the face of such a disparity in the severity of symptoms and the absence of physical findings.

Leukocytosis, hemoconcentration, and systemic acidosis often accompany embolic occlusion of the superior mesenteric

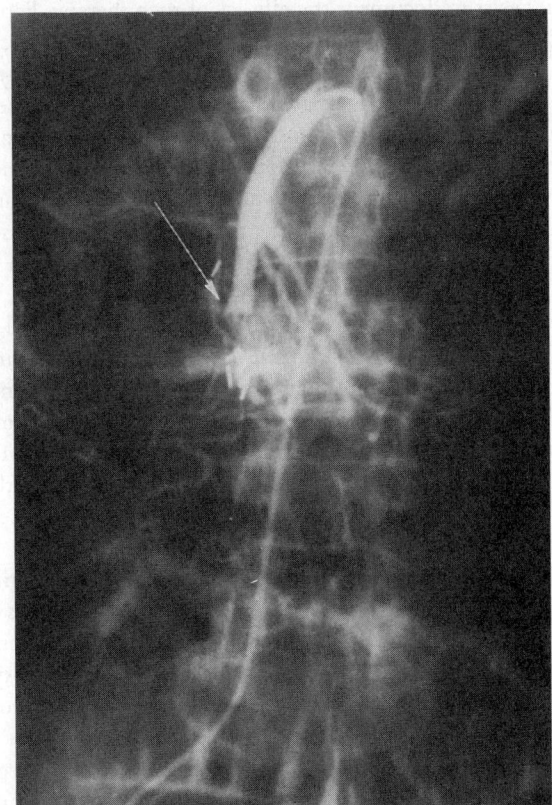

FIGURE 112.2. Superior mesenteric artery embolus *(arrow)* of cardiac origin, causing occlusion of this vessel beyond the inferior pancreaticoduodenal and middle colic arterial branches. (From Wakefield TW, Stanley JC. The intestine. In: Zelenock GB, ed. *Clinical ischemic syndromes: mechanisms and consequences of tissue injury.* St. Louis: CV Mosby, 1990, with permission.)

artery. Bowel infarction may be accompanied by elevated levels of serum amylase, inorganic phosphates, creatinine phosphokinase, and alkaline phosphatase, but none of these are reliable biochemical markers of intestinal ischemia.

Early radiographic features of superior mesenteric artery embolism are usually minimal. Tissue invasion by gas-forming organisms, with evidence of mesenteric or portal venous gas on abdominal films, implies a grave prognosis. Computed tomography may document intravascular gas, as well as intestinal wall thickening accompanying gut infarction.

Patients suspected of acute superior mesenteric artery embolism should undergo emergency arteriographic study and operation. Arteriographic studies usually reveal a characteristic meniscus sign at the site of acute embolic occlusion. Revascularization of ischemic intestine is best performed by superior mesenteric artery embolectomy. Intestines appearing marginally viable at initial operation should be allowed to remain, with the intent of undertaking a second-look operation 24 to 36 hours later. Reperfusion of the intestine after embolectomy may cause sloughing of ischemic mucosa and massive gastrointestinal hemorrhage, a serious problem in patients who require anticoagulants to lessen further peripheral embolization.

Vasodilators have been advocated as a logical means of improving flow to noninfarcted, marginally viable intestine associated with acute mesenteric embolic occlusion, but no controlled studies exist to document the efficacy of such therapy. Papaverine requires intra-arterial administration and may be associated with tachyphylaxis if administered over prolonged periods of time. Glucagon is not associated with autoregulatory escape and when administered intravenously has the same effect as superior mesenteric artery catheter infusion. The usefulness of low molecular weight dextran has not been documented in clinical studies.

Aggressive diagnosis and prompt surgical therapy has lessened the mortality of superior mesenteric artery embolism from 95% with intestinal infarction to 60% without infarction.

Microembolization from aortic atherosclerotic material, diseased heart valves, prosthetic valves, or infective endocarditis may also cause acute intestinal ischemia. These minute emboli usually produce segmental intestinal infarctions. Clinical manifestations of microemboli are those of an acute abdomen and frequently lead to operations without suspicion of the underlying disease. Limited bowel resections are appropriate in these settings.

Other causes of acute mesenteric ischemia deserve mention. In particular, acute superior mesenteric artery thrombosis may present in a manner similar to that of embolic occlusion. In most instances of thrombosis, the underlying arteriosclerosis affects the proximal superior mesenteric artery, and the prodromata of intestinal angina may precede the thrombotic event. The entire midgut, including the proximal jejunum, becomes ischemic. Acute mesenteric thrombosis necessitates an urgent endarterectomy or bypass procedure; outcomes are less salutary than with operative interventions for embolism. Unfortunately, thrombolytic therapy and balloon angioplasty has little value in this setting because of attending hemorrhage from the reperfused intestine.

LOW-FLOW NONOCCLUSIVE MESENTERIC ISCHEMIA (TABLE 112.1)

The second most common lethal form of intestinal ischemia follows nonmechanical reductions in mesenteric blood flow. Patients at particular risk are those in cardiac failure. Men are affected 50% more often than women. Digitalis in this setting causes an increase in mesenteric vascular resistance, as will many vasopressors used for the management of acute cardiac failure. Elderly patients who become hypovolemic from various illnesses, ranging from simple dehydration to sepsis, are also at high risk for nonocclusive mesenteric ischemia.

The most vulnerable portion of the intestine to low-flow ischemia is the colon's splenic flexure because of its watershed blood supply. However, the entire intestine may be affected by low flow. The incidence of nonocclusive intestinal ischemia remains ill defined, mainly because many patients have self-limited unreported sequelae, such as mild ischemic colitis.

Nonocclusive mesenteric ischemia is often manifest by a 3- or 4-day history of vague lower or midabdominal discomfort with distention, accompanied later by nausea and vomiting. The severity often becomes intense with transmural bowel infarction and peritoneal irritation. The latter is usually accompanied by leukocytosis. Biochemical evidence of intestinal infarction is an unreliable diagnostic finding. Plain radiographic studies may reveal bowel wall edema, and barium enema studies often reveal a "thumb-printing" pattern in the colon, indicative of submucosal hemorrhage and edema. Arteriographic studies in low-flow intestinal ischemia usually exhibit delayed arterial emptying and delayed venous filling, with a segmental or diffuse appearance of vasoconstriction. The latter is reversible with intra-arterial administration of papaverine or another vasodilator.

Treatment of low-flow nonocclusive mesenteric ischemia requires restoration of a normal hemodynamic state by appropriate administration of blood, colloids, and electrolyte fluids in conjunction with management of the patient's compromised cardiac status. Cardiac function may deteriorate further with additional intestinal ischemia, an event that may be lessened by the administration of various vasoactive drugs. Theoretically glucagon, which has inotropic and chronotropic actions, has the potential to improve cardiac function at the same time it produces splanchnic vasodilatation and reduces intestinal motor activity. Papaverine, administered directly into the superior mesenteric artery by a percutaneously inserted catheter, may also be used in these patients. The efficacy of these pharmacologic therapies has not been documented in controlled studies. Nevertheless, patients with low-flow nonocclusive intestinal ischemia appear to benefit when treated aggressively by these means. Operation should be undertaken only when transmural infarction is suspected and resection of the bowel appears necessary. The mortality of low-flow nonocclusive intestinal ischemia when intestinal infarction has occurred is 60%.

CHRONIC ARTERIOSCLEROTIC MESENTERIC VASCULAR OCCLUSIVE DISEASE (TABLE 112.1)

The most common form of chronic intestinal ischemia is due to splanchnic arteriosclerosis. The incidence in women is nearly twice that in men. Smoking is a prominent risk factor in these women, but lipid disorders, hypertension, diabetes mellitus, or premature menopause do not appear with frequencies great enough to explain this gender difference.

Arteriosclerotic stenoses typically affect the origins and proximal few centimeters of the three major intestinal arteries. Most of these stenoses represent coexisting spillover aortic arteriosclerosis. Total occlusion or a narrowing of more than 90% in both the celiac and superior mesenteric arteries affects more than 95% of patients with symptomatic splanchnic arteriosclerosis (Fig. 112.3). The inferior mesenteric artery, although involved with hemodynamically significant stenotic disease in nearly 50% of cases, tends to be the least likely of the three major splanchnic arteries to become occluded. Because of the usual efficiency of the collateral circulation, chronic single-vessel intestinal occlusive disease rarely causes gut ischemia.

Clinical manifestations of splanchnic arteriosclerotic occlusive disease depend on the adequacy of the mesenteric collateral circulation. When the collateral blood supply is inadequate, intestinal angina occurs, manifest by midabdominal pain within 10 to 15 minutes of eating. This usually persists for 3 to 4 hours until the ingested food has completed its transit through the small intestine. The severity of intestinal angina usually pro-

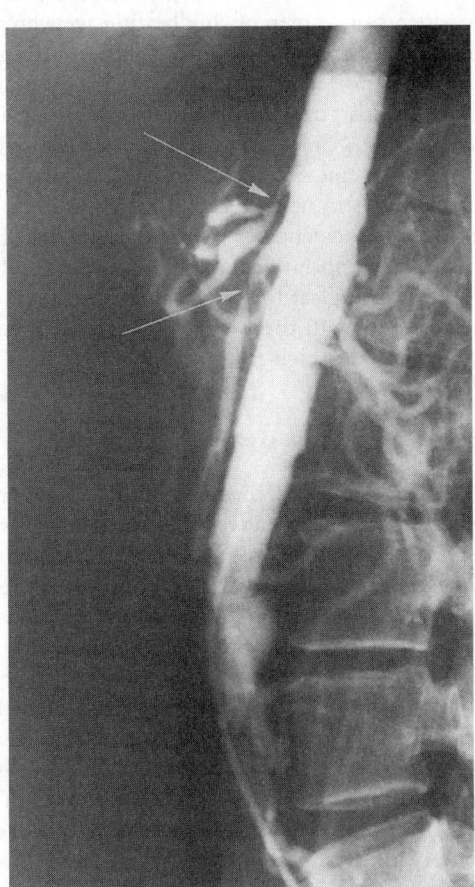

FIGURE 112.3. Arteriosclerotic stenoses *(arrows)* of the proximal celiac and superior mesenteric arteries. (From Wakefield TW, Stanley JC. The intestine. In: Zelenock GB, ed. *Clinical ischemic syndromes: mechanisms and consequences of tissue injury.* St. Louis: CV Mosby, 1990, with permission.)

gresses and is often associated with a 10- to 15-kg weight loss by the time it is diagnosed. Eating less food causes less pain, and weight loss occurs because of the reduced food intake, often referred to as "small-meal syndrome."

Transabdominal ultrasonography of the proximal intestinal arteries offers a noninvasive means of screening patients suspected of having chronic arteriosclerotic splanchnic artery occlusive disease. However, lateral aortography is necessary to confirm the presence of ostial obstructions of the major mesenteric arteries. There are no pathognomonic tests for chronic mesenteric ischemia.

Treatment of chronic intestinal ischemia due to arteriosclerotic disease necessitates revascularization of the intestines. Endarterectomy of the celiac and superior mesenteric arteries or bypass procedures involving these vessels are the most successful means of restoring normal blood flow to the intestines. The mortality of such surgery is less than 10%, and amelioration of symptoms occurs in over 90% of survivors. Experience with percutaneous balloon angioplasty has been limited; the procedure carries the risk of acute embolic infarction of the intestines.

SPLANCHNIC ARTERY ANEURYSMS (TABLE 112.2)

Splanchnic artery aneurysms are an unusual but important group of diseases. Nearly 22% of these aneurysms present as emergencies, including 8.5% that are fatal. The most commonly involved vessels, in decreasing order of frequency, include the splenic, hepatic, superior mesenteric, celiac, gastric–gastroepiploic, jejunal–ileal–colonic, pancreaticoduodenal–pancreatic, and gastroduodenal arteries (Fig. 112.4).

SPLENIC ARTERY ANEURYSMS

Aneurysms of the splenic artery account for more than 60% of splanchnic artery aneurysms. Their incidental recognition in 0.78% of abdominal arteriographic studies probably reflects their prevalence in the general population. Splenic artery aneurysms are usually saccular, occur at bifurcations, and are multiple in 20% of patients (Fig. 112.5).

Women are affected four times more often than men. Three distinct conditions are associated with these aneurysms: (a) arterial fibrodysplasia, (b) portal hypertension with splenomegaly, and (c) multiple pregnancies with 40% of the women exhibiting these lesions having completed six or more pregnancies. These aneurysms often exhibit arteriosclerotic changes; but arteriosclerosis is considered a secondary event, not a primary cause of these aneurysms. Trauma and inflammatory disease, such as chronic pancreatitis with pseudocyst erosion of the splenic artery, are less common but important causes of some aneurysms. Microaneurysms of the splenic artery, usually associated with connective tissue disorders, are of less clinical importance.

Most splenic artery aneurysms are asymptomatic. These aneurysms may be suspected with signet ring calcifications in the left upper quadrant on plain abdominal radiographs. However, diagnosis is usually the result of arteriography performed for some other disease. Ultrasonography, computed tomography,

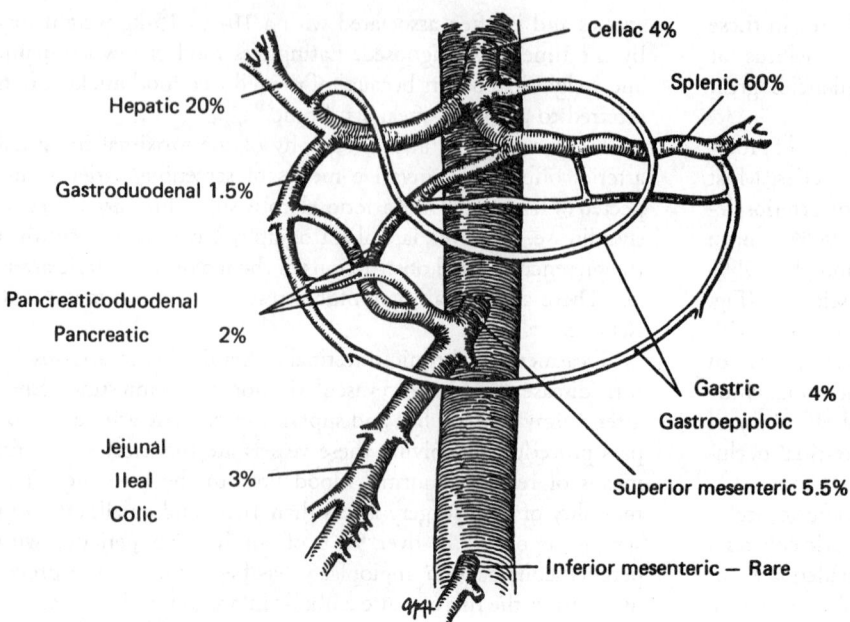

FIGURE 112.4. Distribution of splanchnic artery aneurysms. (From Stanley JC, Zelenock GB. Splanchnic artery aneurysms. In: Rutherford RB, ed. *Vascular surgery*, fourth ed. Philadelphia: WB Saunders, 1995, with permission.)

or magnetic resonance imaging may prove useful in the initial recognition of splenic artery aneurysms, but arteriography is usually necessary to confirm their presence.

Life-threatening rupture affects less than 2% of bland splenic artery aneurysms in nonpregnant women. Symptoms of a "double rupture" occur in 25% of such cases, with bleeding into the retrogastric area occurring first and frank intraperitoneal hemorrhage and shock developing later when the lesser space tamponade is lost. The contention that rupture is less likely to occur in calcified aneurysms, normotensive patients, or patients older than 60 years is not supported by clinical experience. Rupture has affected nearly 95% of aneurysms recognized during pregnancy; maternal mortality is 70% and fetal mortality 75% in this setting.

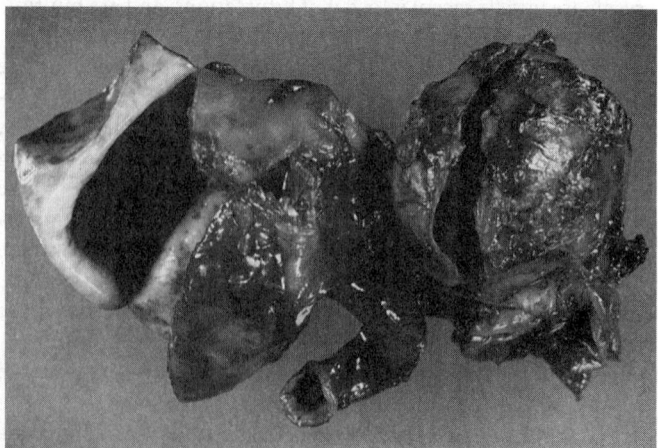

FIGURE 112.5. Splenic artery aneurysms are usually saccular and occur at branchings. (From Stanley JC, Zelenock GB. Splanchnic artery aneurysms. In: Rutherford RB, ed. *Vascular surgery*, fourth ed. Philadelphia: WB Saunders, 1995, with permission.)

Operative intervention is easily justified for aneurysms in pregnant patients or women of childbearing age who might become pregnant, and for symptomatic aneurysms. Aneurysm size greater than 2.5 cm is a relative indication for surgical therapy.

Treatment consists of aneurysmectomy or ligation and exclusion of the aneurysm. Splenectomy may be necessary if the aneurysm is within the splenic parenchyma. The mortality rate for ruptured aneurysms in nonpregnant patients is 25%. Thus, on the basis of a 2% incidence of rupture with an accompanying 25% mortality rate, operative mortality must be less than 0.5% to justify elective surgical therapy. Catheter-directed occlusion of these aneurysms with thrombogenic material is an available alternative therapy for high-risk patients.

HEPATIC ARTERY ANEURYSMS

Hepatic artery aneurysms account for 20% of all splanchnic artery aneurysms. Men are affected twice as often as women. These aneurysms are usually recognized during the sixth decade of life. Causes include atherosclerosis (32%), acquired medial degeneration (24%), trauma (22%), and infection associated with illicit drug use (10%). Traumatic pseudoaneurysms are increasingly recognized in contemporary times with the greater use of computed tomography to evaluate the injured patient. Periarteritis nodosa, cystic medial necrosis, and other arteriopathies are uncommon causes of these aneurysms. Most aneurysms of the hepatic artery are solitary, being fusiform when less than 2 cm in diameter and saccular when more than 2 cm in diameter. Hepatic artery aneurysms are extrahepatic in 80% of cases and intrahepatic 20% of the time.

Most hepatic artery aneurysms are asymptomatic. Symptoms, if present, characteristically include right upper quadrant and epigastric pain, which when severe is similar to that of pancreatitis. Large aneurysms uncommonly obstruct the biliary tract. Hepatic artery aneurysms are discovered most often during arteriographic evaluations of other gastrointestinal or abdominal diseases.

Rupture of a hepatic artery aneurysm causes bleeding into the peritoneal cavity and biliary tract with equal frequency. The latter results in hematobilia with acute gastrointestinal bleeding and fever from cholangitis. Melena and chronic anemia are uncommon with this complication. Hepatic artery aneurysms rupture in less than 20% of cases. The mortality with rupture approaches 35%.

Aneurysms of the common hepatic artery are treated by aneurysmectomy or exclusion, often without arterial reconstruction. If the aneurysm is in the proper hepatic artery, blood flow to the liver should be restored after aneurysmectomy, preferably with an autologous vein graft. Simple ligation or percutaneous transcatheter obliteration of a hepatic artery aneurysm may also be appropriate in selected patients. Partial hepatectomy is rarely required but may be necessary to successfully treat hematobilia due to intraparenchymal aneurysms.

SUPERIOR MESENTERIC ARTERY ANEURYSMS

Aneurysms of the superior mesenteric artery account for 5.5% of all splanchnic artery aneurysms. Men and women are affected equally. Infection accounts for nearly 50% of cases, occurring most often as a result of nonhemolytic streptococcal infection originating from left-sided bacterial endocarditis. Infection associated with illicit intravenous drug abuse is a second cause, increasing in frequency. Medial degeneration, atherosclerosis, and trauma are less common causes. Aneurysms in young patients are usually mycotic, whereas those in patients older than 50 years are most often noninfectious in origin.

Superior mesenteric artery aneurysms are usually recognized when vascular calcifications are identified on radiographs of the abdomen or arteriograms performed for unrelated diseases. Epigastric pain is not uncommon. Symptoms of intestinal angina may accompany nonmycotic lesions, in which aneurysmal dissection or thrombus has compromised intestinal blood flow. The reported frequency of rupture is low, but thromboembolic complications of these aneurysms is relatively high, and most lesions should be treated operatively. Mortality is 50% with rupture. Aneurysmectomy with formal arterial reconstruction is preferred in most cases. However, simple ligation of vessels entering and exiting the aneurysm has been successful in about 30% of reported cases. The operative mortality rate in treating superior mesenteric artery aneurysms is less than 15%.

CELIAC ARTERY ANEURYSMS

Celiac artery aneurysms represent 4% of splanchnic artery aneurysms. Most exhibit medial degeneration. There is no gender predilection. Celiac artery aneurysms are usually asymptomatic or cause vague abdominal discomfort. The rupture rate approaches 13%, with a mortality of 50%. Treatment usually consists of aneurysmectomy and arterial reconstruction. Celiac artery ligation may be done in selected cases if circulation to the liver is adequately maintained through collateral vessels. More than 90% of operations for celiac artery aneurysms are successful.

GASTRIC AND GASTROEPIPLOIC ARTERY ANEURYSMS

Aneurysms of the gastric and gastroepiploic arteries account for 4% of all splanchnic artery aneurysms. Gastric artery aneurysms are ten times more common than gastroepiploic artery aneurysms. Men are three times more likely to be affected than women. These aneurysms are usually acquired, most as a result of medial degeneration or as a consequence of periarterial inflammation. They often present as vascular emergencies without prior symptoms. Rupture occurred in more than 90% of reported cases, with 70% causing serious gastrointestinal bleeding and the rest caused life-threatening intraperitoneal hemorrhage. Nearly 70% of patients with rupture die from this complication.

Ligation of aneurysmal vessels with or without aneurysm excision is appropriate for extragastric lesions. Intramural lesions should be excised with the involved portion of the stomach.

JEJUNAL, ILEAL, AND COLONIC ARTERY ANEURYSMS

Aneurysms affecting the intestinal branches of the superior and inferior mesenteric arteries account for 3% of all splanchnic artery aneurysms. Men and women are affected equally. These aneurysms are recognized most often in the seventh decade of life. Ninety percent of these aneurysms are solitary, except for microvascular aneurysms associated with connective tissue disorders. Congenital or acquired medial defects cause most of these lesions. Certain aneurysms represent the sequelae of an endarteritis from septic cardiac emboli.

Most mesenteric artery branch aneurysms are incidental findings during exploratory surgery for intestinal or intraperitoneal bleeding. Seventy percent of these aneurysms cause abdominal pain or bleeding, and some may represent as a tender abdominal mass. Arteriography is necessary to establish a preoperative diagnosis.

The risk of rupture is 30% and the reported mortality with rupture is 20%. Treatment of these small aneurysms usually consists of ligation or aneurysmectomy for extraintestinal aneurysms, and bowel resection for intramural aneurysms.

PANCREATICODUODENAL, PANCREATIC, AND GASTRODUODENAL ARTERY ANEURYSMS

Pancreatic and pancreaticoduodenal artery aneurysms account for 2% of all splanchnic artery aneurysms. Gastroduodenal artery aneurysms represent an additional 1.5% of these lesions. These aneurysms are among the most hazardous of all splanchnic artery aneurysms. Men are affected four times more often than women. The most common cause is periarterial inflammation, which usually occurs as a consequence of pancreatitis with vascular necrosis or vessel erosion by an adjacent pseudocyst (Fig. 112.6). Most patients with these aneurysms have epigastric pain and

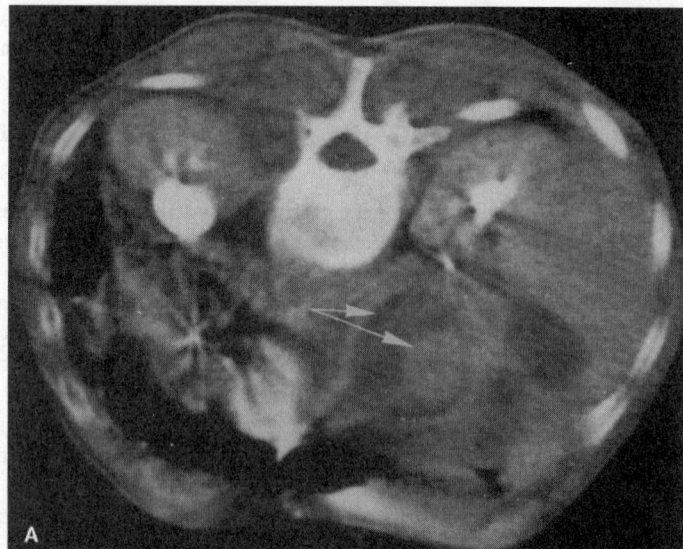

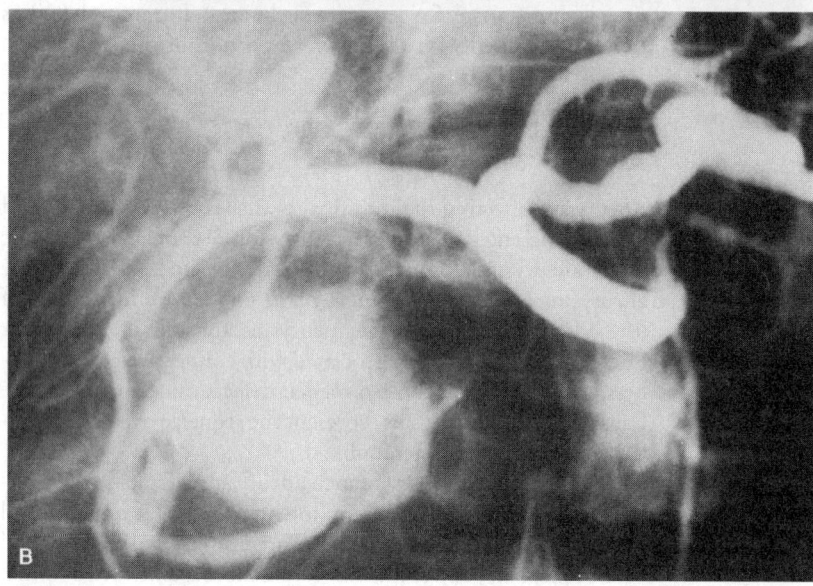

FIGURE 112.6. Gastroduodenal artery aneurysm in a patient with alcoholic-related pancreatitis and pseudocyst erosion of the artery. **A:** CT scan. **B:** Arteriography. (From Eckhauser FE, Stanley JC, Zelenock GB, et al. Gastroduodenal and pancreaticoduodenal artery aneurysms: a complication of pancreatitis causing spontaneous gastrointestinal hemorrhage. *Surgery* 1980;88:335–344, with permission.)

discomfort. This may reflect the fact that about 60% of gastroduodenal and 30% of pancreaticoduodenal artery aneurysms are complications of pancreatitis. Asymptomatic aneurysms of these vessels are unusual.

Aneurysmal rupture of gastroduodenal and pancreaticoduodenal aneurysms occurs in 75% of inflammatory lesions and 50% of noninflammatory lesions. Bleeding into the biliary or pancreatic ductal system may also occur. Endoscopy, ultrasonography, computed tomography, and magnetic resonance imaging often contribute to the diagnosis, but arteriography is essential to confirm the presence of these lesions. Mortality with rupture approaches 50%.

Operative intervention with aneurysmectomy is justified in all reasonable-risk patients. Aneurysms embedded within the pancreas are best treated by suture–ligation of entering and exiting vessels from within the aneurysm. Eventual extirpation of the diseased pancreas may be necessary. Transcatheter embolization may temporarily control acute bleeding from some of these aneurysms but is associated with a high rate of rebleeding and abscess formation.

BIBLIOGRAPHY

Harward TRS, Smith S, Seeger JM. Detection of celiac axis and superior mesenteric artery occlusive disease using abdominal duplex scanning. *J Vasc Surg* 1993;17:738–745.

Jarvinen O, Laurikka J, Salenius JP, et al. Acute intestinal ischaemia—a review of 214 cases. *Ann Chir Gynaecol* 1993;83:22–25.

Kaleya RN, Boley S. Acute mesenteric ischemia. *Crit Care Clin* 1995;11:479–512.

Kurland B, Brandt LJ, Delany HM. Diagnostic tests for intestinal ischemia. *Surg Clin North Am* 1992;72:85–105.

McAfee MK, Cherry KJ Jr, Naessens JM, et al. Influence of complete revascularization on chronic mesenteric ischemia. *Am J Surg* 1992;164:220–224.

Simpson R, Alon R, Kobzik L, et al. Neutrophil- and non-neutrophil-mediated injury in intestinal ischemia reperfusion. *Ann Surg* 1993;218:444–453.

Stanley JC, Fry WJ. Pathogenesis and clinical significance of splenic artery aneurysms. *Surgery* 1974;76:898–909.

Stanley JC, Zelenock GB. Splanchnic artery aneurysms. In: Rutherford RB, ed. *Vascular surgery*, fourth ed. Philadelphia: WB Saunders, 1995:1124–1139.

Wakefield TW, Stanley JC. The intestine. In: Zelenock GB, D'Alecy LG, Fantone JC III, et al., eds. *Clinical ischemic syndromes: mechanisms and consequences of tissue injury.* St. Louis: CV Mosby, 1990:439–456.

Wolf EL, Sprayregan S, Bakal CW. Radiology in intestinal ischemia. Plain film, contrast, and other imaging studies. *Surg Clin North Am* 1992;72:107–124.

Kelley's Textbook of Internal Medicine, fourth edition. Edited by H. David Humes. Lippincott Williams & Wilkins, Philadelphia © 2000.

CHAPTER 113

GASTROINTESTINAL INFECTIONS

C. M. THORPE
ANDREW G. PLAUT

From ancient times to today, infections of the gastrointestinal (GI) tract occur throughout the world. GI infections are more common and have a higher impact in developing countries, among children, and in persons with protein-calorie malnutrition or immunodeficiency. These illnesses are clinically challenging because they are caused by a variety of microbes that have many mechanisms for causing disease, and the severity of infection can range from trivial discomfort to severe or even fatal illness. The care of patients with GI infections calls for careful attention to supportive measures, such as fluid and electrolyte replacement, as well as an informed decision regarding the risks and benefits of specific antimicrobial therapies.

Our understanding of how to prevent and treat GI infections is well advanced, but the causative organisms are highly persistent, and outbreaks and sporadic incidents remain among the most common events seen in medical practice. Although GI infections are usually associated with diarrhea, recent clinical observations and research have identified newer agents that are important in causing nondiarrheal illness. One example is *Helicobacter pylori,* a gram-negative spiral rod that can colonize the gastric mucosa and is associated with peptic ulcer disease and possibly gastric malignancy. Furthermore, the clinical spectrum of some diarrhea-causing agents has been redefined in the era of immunosuppression due to HIV infection or due to drugs used in organ transplantation.

This chapter provides a guide for evaluating patients with GI infection, reviews some of the pathogenic mechanisms of these organisms, and highlights some specific infectious agents that cause predominantly diarrheal disease. The distinction between *colonization* and *infection* is important, as a normal, abundant, and varied GI microflora is found in everyone. Many of these microorganisms harmlessly colonize mucosal sites, but only a few species, under circumstances not always clear, cause clinically apparent illnesses that we refer to as infections.

WORKUP AND LABORATORY EVALUATION OF PATIENTS WITH ACUTE DIARRHEA

In patients with infectious diarrhea the primary objectives are to relieve symptoms and limit fluid loss from diarrhea and vomiting (see also Chapter 99). Many patients treated with supportive measures alone will recover spontaneously. The identification and drug eradication of the causative agent may be secondary objectives. In general, extensive efforts to identify the cause of illness are justified only when the infection is severe or protracted, if it affects many individuals in an obvious outbreak, or if specific antimicrobial therapy is being planned for a given patient. An aggressive diagnostic approach may, however, be justified if the host is very young, debilitated, or immunocompromised.

Evaluation begins with a careful history to clearly establish the context of the illness. Where has the patient been working and traveling? Are others ill? Were foods possibly contaminated? Is the patient malnourished, aged, very young, immunocompromised, or less likely to spontaneously clear an infection than would a normal person? Have there been social practices such as receptive anal intercourse that may encourage acquisition of unusual infections? Is the infected person already on antimicrobial therapy for other reasons (suggesting antibiotic-associated diarrhea)?

Once the setting of the infection is established, the clinician should determine which intestinal organ is most involved. GI infections dominated by vomiting suggest the presence of preformed toxins, although any invasive bacterium or virus can trigger central vomiting centers. Pain has much localizing value: if periumbilical, infection or distention of the small intestine with fluid or gas is likely, while infraumbilical pain on either side suggests colonic involvement. Painful evacuation (tenesmus) occurs with anorectal inflammation that causes high-frequency but low-volume bowel movements containing mainly mucus, sometimes blood, but little stool. High-volume diarrhea suggests that the infection is interrupting the normal balance of gut secretion and absorption, which is typical for infections caused by the protozoan *Giardia lamblia,* certain toxin-producing bacteria such as *Vibrio cholerae,* and certain strains of *Escherichia coli.* Despite their severity, secretory diarrheas are not typically associated with stool blood or mucus because enterotoxins usually do not induce inflammation or tissue destruction. In contrast, stools containing blood and mucus are more likely with enteroinvasive agents such as *Shigella* species or *Entamoeba histolytica,* and these are also more likely to cause fever and generalized symptoms. Common microbial causes of acute diarrhea and common clinical presentations are summarized in Table 113.1.

Efforts to identify the specific cause of a gut infection are most productive in the inflammatory-type diarrheas. Laboratory evaluation should begin with an examination for gross or occult

TABLE 113.1.	MICROBIAL CAUSES OF ACUTE DIARRHEA

Secretory: High-volume watery diarrhea, noninflammatory, dehydrating, few fecal leukocytes
  Vibrio cholerae
  Toxigenic *E. coli* (ETEC strains)
  Giardia lamblia
  Viruses
Inflammatory: Low-volume diarrhea, mucus and blood, many fecal leukocytes
  Shigella species
  Certain *E. coli* (EIEC and STEC strains)
  Entamoeba histolytica (not many leukocytes)
  Clostridium difficile
  Campylobacter jejuni
  Salmonella species
Mixed or variable type
  Yersinia enterocolitica
  Cryptosporidium
Food poisoning
  Clostridium perfringens
  Bacillus cereus
  Staphylococcus aureus
Traveler's diarrhea
  Toxigenic *E. coli* (ETEC strains)
  Invasive *E. coli* (EIEC strains)
  Shigella species
  Salmonella species
  Giardia lamblia
  Viruses

TABLE 113.2.	PRACTICAL CONSIDERATIONS IN THE CARE OF PATIENTS WITH ACUTE DIARRHEA

Stool volume is more important than frequency; replace solutes and water.
Use antidiarrheal drugs sparingly in management of inflammatory diarrheas.
Amebiasis, *Campylobacter,* and *Escherichia coli* diarrheas may mimic ulcerative colitis.
Ask patients of both sexes about specific sexual practices.
Location of abdominal pain often identifies the major organ involved.
Sigmoidoscopy can injure or perforate the inflamed colon.
Barium x-ray examinations of the inflamed colon may worsen the illness.
Some protozoan parasites (amebae, giardia) do not cause peripheral eosinophilia.
Counsel travelers about diarrhea before departure.
Bacterial overgrowth syndromes are easily overlooked.
Older people get colon cancer. Gross or occult fecal blood persisting after gut infections requires careful follow-up.

fecal blood and fecal neutrophils, which suggest invasive infection. Stool cultures should be obtained for outpatients and for those inpatients admitted to the hospital with a community-acquired diarrhea, and specimens should be tested for *Salmonella* species, *Shigella* species, *Campylobacter* species, and Shiga toxin–producing *E. coli* (STEC). However, culture yields for these pathogens are too low to warrant such culture studies on patients who develop diarrhea after 3 days in the hospital. GI infections beginning in hospital are much more likely to be due to nosocomial causes, e.g., *Clostridium difficile*. In the United States, routine culture for *Yersinia* species, *Aeromonas* species, and other less common bacterial pathogens is not recommended except in selected cases. Culture for *Neisseria gonorrhoeae* or specific testing for *Chlamydia trachomatis* are appropriate in those patients with diarrhea who engage in receptive anal intercourse. If there is a history of anal intercourse, and rectal pain or mucoid discharge is a clinical feature, culture for herpes simplex virus may also be helpful. Prior antibiotic use should prompt a search for *C. difficile* toxin in the stool. Parasites can also cause diarrhea, of which the three most common are *G. lamblia, E. histolytica,* and *Cryptosporidium parvum.* Stool examination for ova and parasites should be done when diarrhea occurs in the following epidemiologic and clinical situations: (a) patients who engage in anal intercourse, (b) patients who have recently traveled to parasite-endemic areas; and (c) patients with rectal pain or itching, severe tenesmus, persistent diarrhea, or chronic diarrhea with weight loss.

Sigmoidoscopy can be valuable in patients with bloody stools; features of acute proctitis such as rectal pain, tenesmus, and bloody discharge; a history of anal surgery or insertive anal intercourse; or recent antibiotic use (to exclude pseudomembranous colitis). The examination should be conducted without preliminary bowel cleansing or laxatives, and with limited insufflation of air to reduce the risk of perforation. Cultures and smears from specific lesions can be of great value in identifying the cause of the infection and guiding therapy. Practical considerations in the evaluation of acute diarrhea are summarized in Table 113.2.

PATHOGENESIS OF ACUTE ENTERIC INFECTIONS

Entry of microorganisms into the gut has one of three outcomes: immediate expulsion, colonization, or clinically apparent infection. Expulsion is most likely and occurs when microbes cannot withstand natural barriers. Gastric acidity, bile acids, intestinal motility, competition from established microbes, and the secretory immune system of the small and large bowel all promote rapid removal of gut microbes. Colonization occurs when organisms multiply after first binding to specific host cells; by definition, colonizing organisms do not provoke a significant inflammatory response. These bacteria constitute the normal gut flora but can cause infection if they become enteroinvasive or if they are translocated to other tissues, such as the peritoneal cavity, biliary tree, and urinary tract.

Despite their clinical importance, true enteric infections are the least likely outcome of bacterial or parasite entry into the gut. The risk of infection can be enhanced in patients whose gut defensive systems are compromised or those on drugs that modify the normal gut microflora. When infection occurs, microbes or microbial products can produce direct tissue injury or stimulate host inflammatory and/or metabolic events, resulting in clinical illness. The depth of tissue penetration of enteric

TABLE 113.3.	DEPTH OF TISSUE PENETRATION OF ENTERIC PATHOGENS

No entry strictly necessary (preformed toxin)
  Staphylococcus aureus
  Bacillus cereus
Enterocyte binding, trivial cell injury
  Vibrio cholerae
  Toxigenic *E. coli*
Mild injury to intestinal epithelium
  Giardia lamblia
  Cryptosporidium
Invasion of intestinal epithelium with cell injury or death
  Shigella species
  Most *Salmonella* species
  Campylobacter jejuni
  Yersinia enterocolitica
  Enteroinvasive *E. coli*
  Clostridium difficile
  Entamoeba histolytica
  Probably most viral agents
Passage through superficial epithelial cells to deeper tissues
  Rotavirus (via M cells to lymphoid follicles)
  Salmonella typhi (to regional lymphoid tissue and blood)
  Mycobacterium avium complex (to lamina propria macrophages)

pathogens is summarized in Table 113.3. It should be noted, however, that some pathogens do not fit neatly into a single category. For example, STEC can cause tissue damage without invading. During the infectious process, the microorganism can undergo changes that allow enhancement of virulence, illustrating how well infectious agents have adapted to their hosts. These findings also indicate that the study of infectious bacteria in a laboratory setting may not identify critical virulence attributes that are induced during infections in a natural host, although such information is essential for understanding pathogenesis and for vaccine development.

Enteric pathogens have developed many strategies to disrupt normal functioning of the GI tract. Some pathogens are capable of binding to and damaging enterocytes without invasion. Some produce toxins that affect host cells. Some pathogens are capable of invading through intestinal epithelium to deeper tissues of the intestine or regional lymph nodes. Examples of pathogens that are known to enter and multiply within intestinal epithelial cells include *Salmonella, Shigella, Yersinia,* and *Campylobacter.* In contrast, *Vibrio cholera* is an infectious agent that binds noninvasively to the enterocyte and produces potent enterotoxins without causing significant tissue destruction but markedly altering intestinal function.

Bacterial toxins are a heterogeneous group of proteins that can be encoded by bacterial chromosomal DNA, plasmids, or chromosomally integrated bacteriophage. Toxin production is carefully regulated by the pathogen. Some known regulators of bacterial toxin synthesis include environmental pH, osmolality, and temperature, but often more subtle and less understood environmental features also may change toxin synthesis. Toxin synthesis is often coordinated with other virulence determinants in the same organism. For example, in *V. cholerae,* synthesis of cholera toxin is coregulated with formation of an essential intestinal colonization factor, the toxin-coregulated pilus. Simultaneous expression of multiple virulence determinants in bacteria is thought to reflect a coordinated response to host factors.

Enterotoxins cause intestinal secretion and diarrhea by stimulating adenylate cyclase–cyclic adenosine monophosphate (cAMP), the guanylate cyclase–cyclic guanosine monophosphate (GMP) system, or other less well-defined signaling pathways. For example, *V. cholerae* enterotoxin is a protein that initiates several intracellular biochemical steps leading to an increase in cyclic AMP, which in turn inhibits the coupled influx of Na^+ and Cl^- across the brush border of the enterocyte in the small intestine. Cholera toxin also stimulates Cl^- secretion by gut crypt cells. This combined oversecretion and underabsorption by the small intestine results in volume accumulation in the gut, with high-volume diarrhea that characterizes this disease. In its most severe form known, as cholera gravis, patients can pass liters of "rice water" stool in a day, resulting in severe dehydration. Thus clinical cholera, a profound and sometimes fatal illness, is the result of a toxin that does not directly kill intestinal cells.

Some bacterial products are cytotoxins that damage the intestinal mucosa by inducing disturbances in cell protein synthesis or by igniting acute inflammation that leads to necrosis and ulceration. For instance, when injected into rodent intestine, *C. difficile* enters cells and toxin A disrupts the actin cytoskeleton, leading to fluid secretion, mucosal damage, and intestinal inflammation. Although some toxins are shown to cause damage in vitro, proof that they mediate disease in vivo has been verified for only certain well-studied pathogens. Therefore, many details of how cytotoxins injure gut tissue remain uncertain.

Finally, some GI pathogens do not invade host cells or produce pathogenic toxins, but they clearly cause diarrhea. Examples of such infectious agents are *G. lamblia* and enteropathogenic *E. coli.*

COMMON ACUTE BOWEL INFECTIONS

In the industrialized world, one-third of carefully evaluated cases of acute diarrhea can be ascribed to known bacterial agents, and the number of such identifiable agents is increasing. In developing countries and warm climates, bacterial agents are responsible for more than half of diarrhea cases. In all countries combined, enteroinvasive agents such as *Shigella, Salmonella,* and *Campylobacter jejuni* are responsible for diarrhea in about 15% of patients, but other microbial agents can dominate in particular seasons of the year, or in outbreaks and other special circumstances. These agents include *Yersinia enterocolitica, Aeromonas* species, *Plesiomonas shigelloides,* STEC, *V. cholerae,* and noncholera vibrios.

The three protozoan parasites most commonly associated with diarrheal disease are *G. lamblia, E. histolytica,* and *Cryptosporidium parvum.* Other parasitic agents are also important in certain settings and include *Blastocystis hominis, Dientamoeba fragilis,* and *Strongyloides stercoralis.* A newly recognized coccidian organism, *Cyclospora cayetanensis,* may also be associated with diarrhea in both immunocompetent and immunocompromised patients.

Viral pathogens are important causes of diarrhea in the United States in all ages. Rotavirus, a double-stranded RNA virus, is one of the most important causes of sporadic and epidemic gastroenteritis in children under 2 years old. Calciviruses, a group of single-stranded RNA viruses usually named for the location where first isolated, are an important cause of epidemic outbreaks among older children and adults. Norwalk virus is the best known example of the calcivirus family and is thought to be responsible for 40% of viral gastroenteritis outbreaks in the United States. Less commonly, enteric adenoviruses and astroviruses have been associated with gastroenteritis. At least a third of viral gastroenteritis cases in the United States are thought to be caused by as-yet-undescribed agents.

SALMONELLOSIS

Salmonella species are major causes of enteric infection worldwide. In the United States, they account for 5% to 10% of acute infectious diarrheas, and more than 40,000 cases of nontyphoidal salmonellosis are reported annually. Only 1% to 5% of cases are actually reported, indicating that the number of *Salmonella* infections is likely to be 800,000 to 4 million per year. About 500 persons die annually from conditions related to acute salmonellosis in the United States. Salmonella taxonomy has changed in the past several decades, primarily due to new information about molecular genetic relationships. There are two species of *Salmonella: S. enterica* (whose multiple subspecies and serovars are distinguished by somatic and flagellar antigen serology) and *S. bongori*. Most human pathogens are included in the subspecies of *S. enterica* subsp. *enterica* and more than 2,000 named serotypes of *Salmonella* can cause human disease. The nomenclature of the species *S. enterica* is confusing because the serotypes that constitute this species are referred to by serotype designation. For example, *S. enterica* subsp. *enterica* serovar *heidelberg* is referred to as simply *S. heidelberg. S. enterica* subsp. *enterica* serovar *typhi*, or *S. typhi*, is the cause of typhoid fever, a systemic illness of great importance worldwide but uncommon in the United States. *S. typhi* affects about 500 individuals annually in the United States, and even in these cases the majority are imported by travelers from areas where this organism is endemic. Nontyphoidal *S. enterica* serovars are of greater importance in the United States; approximately half of all isolates identified are either *Salmonella typhimurium* or *Salmonella enteriditis*.

Salmonella enterica strains have a reservoir in domestic and farm animals including poultry, cattle, and pigs, and thus find their way into human foods. Poultry and eggs are particularly troublesome, and in the United States, an estimated 0.01% of eggs with intact shells contain salmonellae, and many chickens sold are contaminated. Outbreaks of *Salmonella* infection from contaminated food continue to occur as in a recent U.S. outbreak of *S. enteritidis* traced to a commercial ice cream manufacturer. About 1 in 1,000 Americans and 15 in 1,000 persons in developing countries are asymptomatic carriers of *Salmonella* species.

Nontyphoidal *Salmonella* gastroenteritis begins with chills, headache, nausea, and vomiting 6 to 48 hours after exposure, soon followed by abdominal pain and diarrhea. Occasionally,

respiratory symptoms such as cough will prompt patients to describe their illness as an "intestinal flu." This tissue-invasive pathogen causes fever in about half of patients. Although salmonellosis involves the ileum and colon only in its early phases, a severe, prolonged colitis may develop that can only be distinguished from shigellosis, *campylobacter* infection, and other nonbacterial colitides by stool culture. The ability of *S. typhimurium* and *Salmonella choleraesuis* to bind to and invade mammalian cells *in vitro* requires the synthesis of several bacterial proteins, and genetically engineered mutants having deletions of any one of these proteins cannot invade. These proteins appear to be induced by carbohydrate or protein components on host epithelial cells, suggesting that *Salmonella* species are able to sense and respond to the *in vivo* environment. Once they enter the blood, salmonellae can reach and invade any tissue, and thus may cause a variety of infections including endocarditis, cholecystitis, splenic abscess, meningitis, and septic arthritis.

Conditions predisposing to salmonellosis include the postgastrectomy state, hypochlorhydria, altered intestinal motility, prior antibiotic administration, sickle cell anemia, chronic liver disease, and immunodeficiency that accompanies neoplastic diseases and AIDS. Thus, already in 1987, recurrent *Salmonella* bacteremia was included in the U.S. Centers for Disease Control and Prevention (CDC) case definition of AIDS. Diagnosis of nontyphoidal salmonellosis is made by finding this easily cultured pathogen in stool or blood. Uncomplicated disease in adults usually resolves spontaneously and warrants only symptomatic and supportive therapy (Table 113.4).

In immunocompetent patients, antimicrobial treatment of *Salmonella* gastroenteritis does not substantially improve the symptoms or outcome, and it may prolong the excretion of the organisms. This can contribute to the maintenance and extent of the environmental reservoir of antibiotic-resistant salmonel-

---

TABLE 113.4.   ANTIMICROBIAL TREATMENT FOR ENTERIC INFECTIONS[a]

Salmonella, Shigella, Campylobacter
  Ciprofloxacin 500 mg PO q 12h × 3 d or *norfloxacin* 400 mg PO q12h × 3 d
Traveler's diarrhea, unknown organism
  Ciprofloxacin 500 mg PO q12h × 3 d or *norfloxacin* 400 mg PO q12h × 3 d
Entamoeba histolytica (asymptomatic cyst passer)
  Paromomycin 500 mg PO t.i.d. × 7 d or *iodoquinol* 650 mg PO t.i.d. × 20 d or *diloxanide furoate* 500 mg PO t.i.d. × 10 d or *metronidazole* 750 mg PO t.i.d. × 10 d
Entamoeba histolytica (acute, dysenteric)
  Metronidazole 750 mg PO t.i.d. × 10 d or *tinidazole* 1 g PO q12h × 3 d or *ornidazole* 500 mg PO q12h × 5 d, each followed by either *iodoquinol* 650 mg PO t.i.d. × 20 d or *paromomycin* 500 mg PO t.i.d. × 7 d
Giardia
  Metronidazole 250 mg PO t.i.d. × 5 d or tinidazole 2 g PO × 1 dose
Clostridium difficile
  Metronidazole 250 mg PO q.i.d. (or 500 mg PO t.i.d.) × 7–10 d or vancomycin 125 mg PO q.i.d. × 7–10 d

---

[a] Specific antibiotic regimens are revised frequently.

lae. In contrast, antimicrobial therapy in the immunocompromised or debilitated host can be of critical importance. AIDS patients often have high relapse rates after treatment of *Salmonella* bacteremia. Consequently, aggressive therapy (several weeks of parenteral antibiotics followed by oral therapy totalling 6 to 8 weeks) is recommended. Prophylaxis with antimicrobial therapy should be considered following treatment because even after aggressive therapy, relapses can occur in patients with AIDS. *Salmonella* strains that are resistant to quinolones have recently been identified, possibly due to the use of antimicrobial therapy and feed supplementation in food animals. Because of multidrug resistance of nontyphoidal salmonellae, seriously ill patients or those with complex infections such as endocarditis may require treatment with a third-generation cephalosporin even before antimicrobial susceptibilities are determined. Fecal excretion of salmonellae may occur for 6 to 8 weeks after the patient recovers, but some patients become chronic carriers. Control of human salmonellosis will eventually require reduction of salmonellae in foods from animal sources.

S. typhi causes typhoid fever and is not strictly an intestinal diarrheal disease. Humans are the only natural hosts and acquire the illness by fecal–oral contamination, often from a chronic carrier. Since there is no known animal reservoir, typhoid fever occurs under conditions of poor sanitation, and the marked decline in cases in the United States can be attributed to public health measures, not specific eradication of the agent by antimicrobials. Typhoid fever consists of fever, chills, sweats, headache, and abdominal pain beginning about 5 to 14 days after exposure, and it may last for weeks if untreated. Constipation, not diarrhea, typifies the early stage of the disease. A characteristic rash ("rose spots") may be found, predominantly on the trunk. In the second week there is a threat of GI hemorrhage and perforation due to infection of lymphoid follicles throughout the lower bowel. Diarrhea at this stage is common. Although the gut is the site of entry, the illness quickly involves other organs. The case fatality rate is about 2% in the United States and much higher (12% to 30%) in developing countries, where typhoid fever is made more severe by compromised host defenses and poor nutrition. Diagnosis is by culture of *S. typhi* or *S. paratyphi* from blood, bone marrow, or stool.

Chloramphenicol resistance and a high relapse rate have prompted the use of amoxicillin and trimethoprim–sulfamethoxazole as alternative oral therapies, although multidrug resistance of *S. typhi* has emerged as a problem in many endemic areas, such as the Indian subcontinent, Southeast Asia, and Africa. For critically ill patients or patients from areas where multidrug resistance is a problem, initiating therapy with agents active against potentially multidrug-resistant *S. typhi* should be considered while sensitivity testing is undertaken. The best choices are ciprofloxacin or ceftriaxone. Chronic colonization of the biliary system by salmonellae is a source of infection for others and occurs in about 1% of patients recovering from typhoid fever.

Safe and immunogenic vaccines to prevent typhoid fever are available, but efficacy is not 100%. Immunity requires both cell-mediated and humoral responses. Several commercial vaccines are currently available for travelers to endemic areas, including a live attenuated oral vaccine and a parenteral polysaccharide vaccine. These vaccines are ineffective against infections by nontyphoid salmonellae.

SHIGELLOSIS

Shigella species account for 2% to 3% of acute diarrheal diseases in the United States and are most prevalent in children and the poor. There is no animal reservoir; humans are the only known host. Illness is usually acquired by direct fecal–oral contact or fecal contamination of food, accounting for the disease's association with poor sanitation and crowding, and the recognition that shigellosis could be easily transmitted by anal–oral sex. One factor that favors transmission and explains the occasional food- or water-borne outbreaks is the low number of organisms needed for infection.

The genus *Shigella* consists of four species: *S. dysenteriae, S. flexneri, S. boydii,* and *S. sonnei.* The first three have various serotypes. *S. sonnei* causes the mildest illness and is the commonest species infecting otherwise healthy people in the United States, but an increase in *S. flexneri* infections among adult U.S. males has been linked to anal–oral transmission in homosexuals. *S. flexneri* is predominant in Mexico, South America, and most other tropical countries. In the past 30 years, major pandemics of *S. dysenteriae* have occurred on multiple subcontinents, including Central America, Southeast Asia, and Central and East Africa. Shigellosis is a common cause of dysentery, the general term describing diarrhea consisting of low-volume stools containing blood, mucus, and fecal leukocytes. Fever is found in about half of patients, and febrile seizures in children are possible. Shigellae have their principal effects on the colon. The mucosal inflammatory response is intense as the shigellae penetrate, divide in, and lyse epithelial cells. Tenesmus is common and may lead to rectal prolapse in severely ill children who have many painful evacuations. On sigmoidoscopy the colorectum is very red, edematous, typically ulcerated, and coated with patchy mucus, and the degree of inflammation leaves little doubt as to why crampy pain and low-volume diarrhea, often with bloody stools, are the typical manifestations. However, in some patients shigellosis results in watery, nonbloody diarrhea. Though more commonly seen with infections by other agents, these milder symptoms may occur in shigellosis. Hemolytic-uremic syndrome and postinfectious arthritis have been described. Definitive diagnosis is made by culture of stool or fecal mucus, and swabs of rectal mucosa can also give positive results. Culture of fresh samples or immediate inoculation of plates or transport media is necessary, as shigellae do not survive well at room temperature.

Shigella dysenteriae produces a potent polypeptide toxin (Shiga toxin) that has cytotoxic and enterotoxic properties *in vitro.* Shiga toxin, which is closely related in structure to enterotoxins of *E. coli,* probably participates in the cell lysis typical of this infection, and its enterotoxic properties also contribute to the secretory component of the illness.

Shigellosis is usually self-limited, but antibiotics may shorten both the course of diarrhea and the duration of pathogen excretion in stool. Although resolving cases do not require antimicrobial drugs, these agents may be lifesaving in severe cases, and treatment may interrupt person-to-person transmission. The fluoroquinolones are the treatment of choice for adults. Vaccine development for shigellosis has not yet been successful, but the use of recombinant microbiologic techniques to identify the most antigenic or virulent attributes of shigella may in time lead to successful vaccines.

CAMPYLOBACTER INFECTION

Infections due to *Campylobacter* species were long thought to be uncommon, but through improved methods of stool culture they are now recognized as the cause of 10% to 15% of cases of acute diarrhea in the United States. Groups at high risk for infection include infants and young adults. *Campylobacter,* like *Salmonella,* has a large animal reservoir and can be cultured from healthy cattle, sheep, swine, poultry, and domestic animals. Human infection is typically acquired by the eating of contaminated poultry, reminiscent of the transmission of *Salmonella,* but outbreaks have also been traced to consumption of raw milk or untreated river or stream water. Two species—*C. jejuni* and *C. coli*—account for almost all clinical isolates in most series. A third species, *C. fetus,* tends to be associated with chronic infections in gay men or immunocompromised hosts.

The typical illness begins with abdominal cramps and diarrhea 2 to 4 days after exposure. Anorexia and malaise are also typical, and some patients have bloody diarrhea. As with nearly all bacterial pathogens, not every encounter with *Campylobacter* causes illness. In one volunteer challenge study, only 18% of healthy subjects became ill, usually within 3 days, but 70% of all subjects excreted large numbers of the organism in the stool. The incidence of clinical illness was higher with larger oral inocula (although as few as 500 to 800 organisms can cause illness), and attack rates rose when organisms were given with food or drugs that reduce gastric acidity.

Campylobacter enteritis has many systemic features, and the early phases of the illness have an influenza-like character. Fever occurs in about half of patients and may precede diarrhea, attesting to the tissue-invasive and inflammatory nature of this infection. The pain of *Campylobacter* enteritis may be intense and easily confused with a surgical abdomen. The jejunum and ileum are the main sites of infection, but the colon is involved in some patients. Fecal leukocytes and blood in the diarrheal stool are common. A reactive arthritis 10 to 14 days after the onset of illness has been described, a cause of Reiter's syndrome. An association between *Campylobacter* infection and the Guillain–Barré syndrome, an acute inflammatory demyelinating polyradiculoneuropathy, has now been clearly documented. This serious sequel of otherwise typical *Campylobacter* enteritis is thought to occur due to molecular mimicry of host antigens by the infecting microorganism.

Campylobacter enteritis is among the forms of infectious gastroenteritis most easily confused with idiopathic ulcerative colitis, and corticosteroids may aggravate symptoms of *Campylobacter* infection and promote tissue injury. *Campylobacter* enteritis also mimics ulcerative colitis by its slow resolution, as diarrhea sometimes lasts 2 weeks. In most patients, systemic symptoms are usually much relieved before diarrhea stops. Diagnosis is made by stool culture, but *Campylobacter* species are relatively fastidious organisms requiring specialized media and other conditions for growth. Despite such technical obstacles, this organism should be sought routinely in patients with recent onset of bloody stools to avoid confusion with other forms of colitis. Properly collected and cultured specimens should yield the organism in 90% of typical cases but less common *Campylobacter* species may be overlooked using these methods. A specific search for major *Campylobacter* species is now the practice in most large laboratories.

Therapy involves the usual attention to fluid and electrolyte replacement and supportive measures. Antimicrobial agents shorten clinical illness and decrease the duration of fecal excretion, but since their routine use may encourage the emergence of resistant organisms, only severe, prolonged, or complicated illness should be treated with antibiotic therapy. Resistance to fluoroquinolones requires a single mutation in the DNA gyrase gene, and there has been a dramatic worldwide increase in resistance to fluoroquinolones. The organism is usually susceptible to the macrolide family to which resistance emerges less rapidly. For these reasons, macrolide antibiotics are the preferred agents for *Campylobacter* infections.

AMEBIASIS

Entoamoeba histolytica is the protozoan parasite that causes amebiasis. In the subtopics and tropics, asymptomatic carriage of *E. histolytica* cysts is common (up to 80% in some populations), but asymptomatic carriage in the United States is relatively uncommon. The majority of cases of symptomatic amebiasis in the United States are imported by travelers from endemic areas, with less than 5% of cases occurring through fecal contamination in nursing homes, day care centers, and through anal–oral sexual encounters. Humans can harbor nonpathogenic amebae that are morphologically indistinguishable from *E. histolytica;* these nonpathogenic amebae, termed *Entamoeba dispar,* do not invade tissue and do not need treatment. *E. histolytica* and *E. dispar* can be distinguished by techniques such as polymerase chain reaction (PCR) and isoenzyme analysis, but these methods are not presently available for routine diagnostic use.

E. histolytica infection is acquired by fecal–oral transmission of cysts or trophozoites excreted by patients who are ill with the disease. Cysts can survive outside the human host for up to 10 days; once ingested, they excyst to become trophozoites, a poorly understood process essential for disease to occur. *E. histolytica* trophozoites are invasive and preferentially attack the colonic mucosa to cause focal necrosis and ulcerations. Lesions are more abundant in the cecum and ascending colon than elsewhere. Although it is uncertain as to how this organism lyses cells and causes the necrotizing ulcerations responsible for the clinical illness, increased expression and secretion of cysteine-type proteinases correlate with the virulence of different strains of *E. histolytica.* Although pathogenic strains can activate the alternative complement pathway, their trophozoites are resistant to killing by complement and can survive in the bloodstream to subsequently invade the liver. The ability of this parasite to cause tissue damage is a complex interaction of host and microbial factors.

Amebiasis has several clinical patterns of infection, including acute amebic dysentery, nondysenteric amebiasis, and the asymptomatic carrier state. Amebae can also disseminate from the bowel to produce extraintestinal infection, including liver and brain abscess as well as infection of serosal surfaces such as pleura, peritoneum, and pericardium. Acute amebic dysentery is characterized by severe abdominal cramps, chills, fever, and liquid bowel movements containing bloody mucus. Fecal leukocytes are present, but numbers are less than in the invasive bacterial diarrheas. The disease can be fulminant and extensive, involving the entire colon with widespread hemorrhagic ulceration. Perforation may occur in severe disease.

Sigmoidoscopy, which should always be performed with great caution and without cleansing of the colon, shows intense inflammation. The classically described oval ulcers with undermined edges and intervening normal mucosa are only seen in some patients. Mucosal ulcers in amebiasis contain numerous trophozoites, and microscopic examination of fresh scrapings held near 37°C is useful. Amebic trophozoites are about four times the diameter of an erythrocyte and when kept warm have slow, unidirectional movement along pseudopods.

Stool examination for trophozoites of *E. histolytica* is an art acquired with practice and patience; overdiagnosis is common because coexistent nonpathogenic amebae, erythrocytes, and cell debris can be confusing. Searching for trophozoites in stool mucus is often fruitful, as they originate in colonic ulcers teeming with organisms. Immunologic diagnostic tests are now being developed; for example, the Enzymeba test is based on stool examination for histolysin, the major cysteine proteinase of *E. histolytica*. This test has 87.5% sensitivity and 100% specificity for infection. Another assay based on the use of monoclonal antibodies to detect galactose-specific adhesin (present only on pathogenic strains of *E. histolytica*) has 97% sensitivity and 100% specificity. These tests are not widely available.

As with *Campylobacter* enteritis, it is important to differentiate acute amebic colitis from idiopathic ulcerative colitis, as corticosteroids can greatly aggravate amebiasis and convert it to a fulminant illness. Severe amebiasis may be indistinguishable from the acute toxic dilatation that complicates inflammatory bowel disease, so proper diagnosis may avoid the disaster of an unwarranted emergency colectomy. Nondysenteric intestinal amebiasis is a milder illness characterized by frequent watery or soft stools. Chronic amebic infection creates amebomas, lesions that must be differentiated from other chronic inflammatory and neoplastic diseases of the colon. Amebic liver abscess is characterized by fever, right upper quadrant pain, and the presence of spherical cavities in the liver that can be detected by various hepatic imaging techniques. These are not true abscesses but rather pockets of necrotic debris from which thick brown fluid can be aspirated. Diagnosis is confirmed by serologic testing, which is generally available in large medical centers or in public health laboratories.

Treatment of amebiasis varies with the clinical syndrome. Acute amebic dysentery should be treated with an antitrophozoite agent, such as metronidazole, tinidazole, or ornidazole, followed by diloxanide furoate, iodoquinol, or paromomycin (compounds active against cysts). Treatment of asymptomatic cysts is optional for patients who live in endemic areas. For those in nonendemic areas, cyst treatment with diloxanide furoate, paromomycin, or iodoquinol is recommended. Invasive disease, such as liver abscess, is treated with metronidazole followed by a luminal agent.

GIARDIASIS

Giardia lamblia is the most common protozoal infection of the intestinal tract worldwide. Prevalence varies from 2% to 5% in industrialized countries to 20% to 30% in the developing world. Giardiasis is endemic in the United States as either acute diarrhea or a chronic illness, usually acquired by consuming water contaminated with the feces of humans or domestic or wild animals. Drinking apparently clear water from streams or wells in mountainous areas is a common source of this microbe, and patients should be asked about recent hiking or camping trips. Transmission of giardiasis is common in day care centers and institutions for the mentally ill and retarded, and among homosexual men. The major clinical importance is in young children and the immunocompromised, but healthy persons may have severe illness caused by this protozoan parasite.

Patterns of clinical giardiasis are diverse, ranging from asymptomatic carriage to severe chronic diarrhea, malabsorption, and growth retardation in children. The acute illness, which often is falsely attributed to a number of bacterial causes, is characterized by periumbilical abdominal cramps, nausea and vomiting, and watery diarrhea that may lead to significant fluid depletion. The means by which *G. lamblia* causes high-volume diarrhea is unknown. Diarrhea is very occasionally absent in the acute infection. Many cases are short-lived and spontaneously clear without therapy. However, giardiasis often becomes a chronic intestinal infection and then can present in several ways: a nonspecific chronic diarrheal syndrome not associated with other significant symptoms, or a postinfectious malabsorptive syndrome characterized by abdominal distress, gas, bloating, and general malaise, without much diarrhea. As many as 50% of asymptomatic patients have biochemical evidence of carbohydrate, fat, and micronutrient malabsorption, and giardiasis has been reported as one of the causes of protein-losing enteropathy. Allergic and inflammatory phenomena, including urticaria and arthralgias, have also been described in association with giardiasis.

Diagnosis is made by finding trophozoites or cysts in stool or in intestinal fluid or tissue. However, stool examination for trophozoites or cysts is positive in only one-third to one-half of confirmed cases. Because *Giardia* organisms have a predilection for the proximal small intestine, the agent can also be recovered from duodenal or proximal jejunal aspirates. This is accomplished by tube or at endoscopy, or by a novel string test in which the free end of a thread is taped to the patient's cheek while the remainder is coiled into a swallowed gelatin capsule; when retrieved and examined microscopically, it may contain many adherent trophozoites. Alternatively, a small intestinal biopsy with examination of both the adherent mucus and the mucosal tissue may reveal the trophozoites.

Several drugs are effective in the treatment of giardiasis, including metronidazole, tinidazole, and quinacrine, but only metronidazole is readily available in the United States. Other less effective options include furazolidine (used in metronidazole failures) and paromomycin (for use in pregnancy).

VIRAL DIARRHEA

Viral diarrhea is a common cause of acute infectious diarrhea in the United States in both children and adults. The typical illness is characterized by fever, nausea, vomiting, cramps, and watery diarrhea. Although technically an invasive diarrheal disorder, the diarrhea is not inflammatory, so polymorphonuclear leukocytes and blood are often not found in stool. Frank bloody diarrhea should direct attention to bacterial or protozoan agents. The two most common and well-documented viral agents causing diarrhea are the rotaviruses and the calciviruses. Other less commonly identified viruses include enteric adenoviruses, astroviruses, and non–group A rotaviruses. Although there are few comprehensive community surveys, the incidence of rotavirus diarrhea alone is an estimated 3.5 million cases per year in the United States. Nearly everyone in the United States has had either symptomatic or asymptomatic rotavirus exposure during childhood.

Rotaviruses (named for their wheel-like appearance on electron microscopy) are among the RNA–reovirus group and cause enteric illness in children up to 2 years of age. In North America, rotavirus disease is most common in the winter, whereas infections in the tropics occur throughout the year. Symptomatic infection has an incubation period of 1 to 3 days, after which there is a sudden onset of vomiting lasting for 3 days and watery diarrhea lasting for 3 to 8 days. Fever and abdominal pain are common. Rotavirus can cause a delay in gastric emptying, making vomiting worse. While there are few sequelae of infection, inadequate fluid replacement in young children can result in severe dehydration and even death. Presumptive diagnosis can be confirmed serologically by finding viral antigens in the stool with a solid-phase ELISA assay. An effective live oral vaccine has been licensed in the United States and is administered in three doses with other childhood vaccines. The use of the vaccine has been restricted recently because of a high incidence of interssuception.

Norwalk and Norwalk-like diarrhea are caused by a heterogeneous group of viruses classified as calciviruses. They have been named for the location of recognized outbreaks (e.g., Snow Mountain virus or Montgomery County virus). These agents have not been cultured, but Norwalk and several other related Norwalk-like virus illnesses can be confirmed by a rise in serum antibody titer or by the detection of viral antigen in stool specimens. Oral vaccines for Norwalk virus are in early development.

Spread of Norwalk viruses may occur by person-to-person transmission, but more often through the ingestion of contaminated water or foods such as shellfish and salads. Infections occur at all ages, although adults typically have a milder illness than do children. This may be the result of partial immunity (most children have detectable antibody by age 10), which can attenuate the degree of disability from these ubiquitous viruses. Diarrhea in Norwalk disease is accompanied by abdominal pain, nausea, poor appetite, myalgias, and low fever lasting 1 to 4 days. There are no significant long-term sequelae.

Treatment of viral diarrhea requires adequate fluid and electrolyte replacement and supportive care. No specific drug therapy is known to be of benefit.

ESCHERICHIA COLI INFECTIONS

Escherichia coli is a normal component of the intestinal microflora in all normal people. Pathogenic *E. coli* organisms have acquired the potential to cause disease by uptake of DNA that encodes for virulence factors, and in this way differ from nonpathogenic strains. Currently, six categories of *E. coli* can be distinguished by epidemiologic, clinical, and pathogenic mechanisms: enterotoxigenic (ETEC), enteropathogenic (EPEC), enteroinvasive (EIEC), Shiga toxin–producing *E. coli* (STEC), enteroaggregative (EAggEC), and diffuse adherent (DAEC).

ETEC strains cause infant diarrhea in tropical and developing countries and diarrhea among travelers but are relatively uncommon in the United States. These organisms have fimbriae by which they attach to enterocytes of the small intestine. They cause diarrhea by liberating a heat-stable or heat-labile toxin, or both. Labile toxin is closely related in structure and biologic effects to the toxin of *V. cholerae*.

EPEC strains cause diarrhea in humans, but they have not been shown to be toxigenic or capable of invading epithelial cells. Unlike most other diarrheogenic *E. coli*, EPEC strains have a characteristic interaction with epithelial cells that can be demonstrated by electron microscopy. EPEC organisms adhere very closely to the surface of enterocytes and alter the cell by destroying the microvilli and causing rearrangement of the cell's cytoskeleton. These cell changes are called *attaching and effacing lesions*. The ability of EPEC to cause these lesions is encoded by plasmid-associated genes as well as a 35-kb chromosomal DNA insertion known as a pathogenicity island. Illness due to EPEC occurs in infants but can sporadically affect adults in outbreaks. Diarrhea is watery with little blood.

EIEC strains cause enteroinvasive intestinal infection similar to that of *Shigella* species. Both *Shigella* and EIEC organisms have 120- to 140-Md plasmids that encode genes that allow these bacteria to invade and spread intercellularly. The illness caused by EIEC organisms is centered in the colon and can be similar to *Shigella* dysentery, with fever, cramps, and low-volume, bloody, frequent stools. As is the case with *Shigella*, however, diarrhea can be watery.

STECs, also called "enterohemorrhagic *E. coli*" or "EHECs," are important pathogens in the developed world. STEC organisms can asymptomatically colonize the gut, cause a mild watery diarrhea, or cause severe hemorrhagic colitis. Although STEC organisms are noninvasive, they have acquired the ability to synthesize Shiga toxins structurally related to that elaborated by *Shigella dysenteriae*. The genes encoding these toxins are carried on lysogenic bacteriophage in STEC organisms. Like EPEC, most STEC strains can also form attaching and effacing lesions. Infection has been food-borne in several large outbreaks in the United States, and this illness has major clinical and commercial importance. In one outbreak in the United States, more than 500 children and adults were stricken with STEC infection by eating contaminated hamburger meat in fast-food restaurants. An outbreak in Georgia was traced to a children's pool in a water park. STEC organisms have often been isolated from diarrheal outbreaks in day care centers, nursing homes, and schools. Of great clinical importance, STEC strains have been implicated in 63% to 92% of patients with the hemolytic-uremic syndrome, a serious sequela of STEC infection due to the systemic effects of Shiga toxins. While the appearance of these agents in outbreaks rather than individual cases is a distinguishing feature, the illness can be confused with idiopathic ulcerative colitis. One of the STEC serotypes, O157:H7, does not ferment sorbitol and can be readily distinguished from other *E. coli* strains on sorbitol-enriched MacConkey plates as colorless colonies. Laboratories that use this single criterion for STEC screening will identify only this serotype. However, it has been recognized that many other serotypes can also cause infection, so the best screening tests for STEC infection are not based on sorbitol fermentation but rely on identification of Shiga toxins in the stool by enzyme-linked immunosorbent assay.

DAEC and EAggEC are distinguished by their patterns of adherence to epithelial cells. DAEC are recovered more frequently from stools of children with diarrhea than those without, but data implicating these agents in diarrheal disease are inconclusive. EAggEC organisms are pathogenic, and at least some strains can secrete a heat-stable enterotoxin (East1) and a heat-labile protein that is immunologically similar to hemolysin. EaggEC have recently been shown to be associated with diarrhea in patients with HIV.

PSEUDOMEMBRANOUS ENTEROCOLITIS

Pseudomembranous enterocolitis is an inflammatory lesion of the colon that usually occurs in a setting of oral or parenteral antibiotic use, but it may also be seen during cancer chemotherapy, in patients infected with HIV, and occasionally in the absence of other risk factors. The illness can range from a mild to intense inflammation of the colon caused by one or more toxins of the responsible agent, *Clostridium difficile*, a strictly anaerobic, gram-positive bacterium.

Uncomplicated diarrhea is a common side effect of antibiotics themselves; for example, ampicillin and clindamycin cause self-limited diarrhea in up to 25% of patients. These drug side effects are relieved when drugs are stopped, distinguishing them from the disease caused by *C. difficile*. Pseudomembranous colitis begins during the period of antibiotic use or may start up to 4 weeks after the drug has been discontinued. The illness is characterized by diarrhea, fever, abdominal pain, and fecal leukocytosis; frank bleeding is unusual. Adults are more susceptible than children, and the occasional patient with *C. difficile* colitis will develop severe or fulminant disease. When fulminant, *C. difficile* colitis can be complicated by hypotension, very elevated peripheral leukocytosis, abdominal distention, toxic megacolon (Fig. 113.1) and even colonic perforation, but diarrhea may be minor or even absent. Sigmoidoscopy shows scattered or confluent pale yellow plaques extending proximally from the most distal rectum on an edematous and erythematous mucosa (Figure 113.2). An adherent pseudomembrane consisting of large amounts of mucus and cellular debris may obscure the underlying plaques. Often there is a poor correlation between the sigmoidoscopic and clinical findings, both of which are highly variable. Contrast radiography can aggravate the inflammation and should be avoided if the clinical setting and sigmoidoscopy are consistent with the diagnosis. These patients do not need colonoscopy for diagnosis, and this more invasive procedure is best avoided.

The clinical terms pseudomembranous colitis, antibiotic-associated colitis, and *C. difficile* colitis are interchangable. Antimicrobials probably trigger the illness by changing the enteric flora to allow entry or overgrowth of *C. difficile*. This organism is absent from stools of normal individuals in North America but appears in about 20% of patients who have diarrhea while receiving antimicrobial therapy, and in 95% of patients with pseudomembranous colitis. All antimicrobial drugs—particularly ones with activity against enteric bacteria—have been implicated in pseudomembranous colitis, but broad-spectrum penicillins and

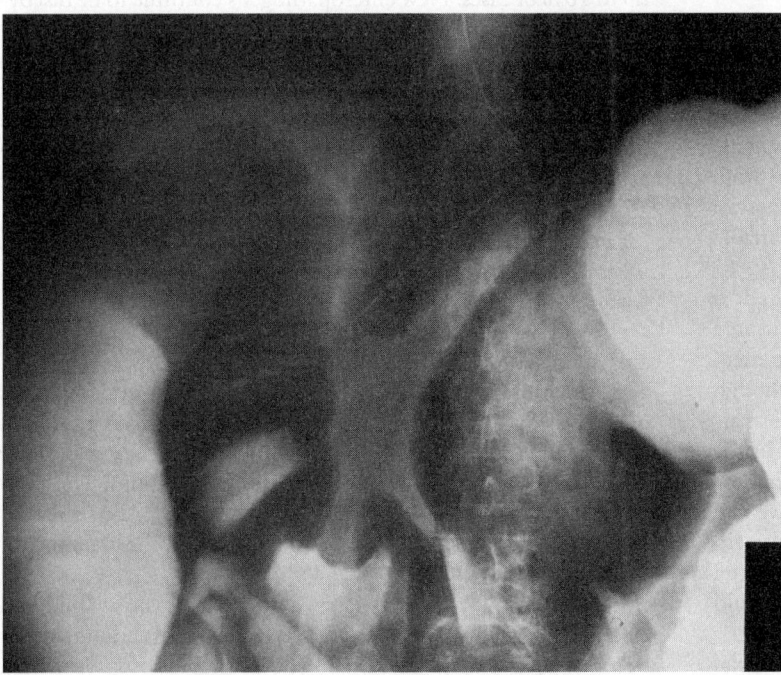

FIGURE 113.1. Toxic megalocolon in a patient with *C. difficile* colitis. (Courtesy of Dr. Robert R. Paul.)

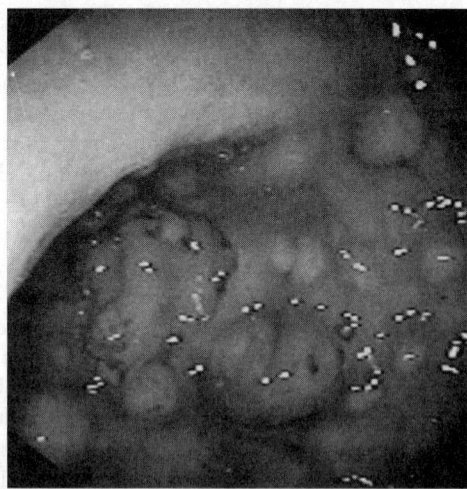

FIGURE 113.2. Sigmoidoscopic appearance of pseudomembranes in a patient with *C. difficile* colitis. (Courtesy of Dr. Sharon B. Turissini.)

cephalosporins are most commonly implicated. Tetracycline and metronidazole are rarely involved.

People colonized by *C. difficile* may pass heat-resistant spores that represent a risk for patient-to-patient transmission by personnel in the hospital setting; these may be extremely difficult to control. For this reason, enteric precautions are essential in managing hospitalized patients with *C. difficile.* These precautions include private rooms, dedicated toilet facilities, and careful attention to handwashing by hospital personnel.

C. difficile produces two high molecular weight cytotoxins, A and B. Toxin A causes mucosal damage, intestinal inflammation, and fluid secretion in animal models and is a neutrophil chemoattractant in humans. Toxin B is not known to be enteropathogenic *in vivo.* The toxic effects of toxin A are mediated through damage to the cellular cytoskeleton after binding to an enterocyte receptor.

The A toxin causes actinomorphic (sunlike) rounding in cell culture and is blocked by specific antitoxin. This test is time consuming but has a sensitivity of 94% to 100% and a specificity of 99%. Alternatively, *C. difficile* infection can be confirmed by demonstrating toxin B in stool filtrate. Several rapid immunoassays for *C. difficile* antigens or toxins are available. The stool cytotoxin test remains the gold standard, but the commercial immunoassays are faster and cheaper and provide reasonable sensitivity and specificity.

Prompt cessation of antimicrobials should be considered, if possible. Patients with mild diarrhea may require no additional treatment, but oral metronidazole and oral vancomycin are effective in treating more severe or persistent infections. Although the pharmacokinetics of oral vancomycin make it an ideal treatment of *C. difficile* colitis, its clinical overuse has resulted in the development of resistance in other organisms, e.g., the enterococci. Thus, metronidazole, which is much less expensive but usually effective, is the initial treatment of choice. Oral bacitracin is also active against *C. difficile,* but it is expensive and has been associated with a high relapse rate. Antiperistaltic agents should be avoided because they worsen the clinical disease.

Up to 20% of patients relapse within 3 weeks after an initial course of therapy. Management of relapse with metronidazole or vancomycin may be unnecessary if the relapse is not clinically severe, but a second course is advised for more severe or persistent diarrhea. Additional relapses are notoriously treatment-resistant. To treat persistent relapsing infection, rifampin, cholestyramine to bind toxins, treatments with the yeast *Saccharomyces boulardii,* and even fecal enema bacteriotherapy have been tried, but no generally acceptable therapy for recurrent infection has been described.

TRAVELER'S DIARRHEA

Traveler's diarrhea is a category of acute diarrheal illnesses typically contracted within a week of travel to a foreign country. These ailments are caused by bacterial, viral, or protozoal pathogens. Visitors to Latin America, Asia, the Middle East, and Africa are most often affected. More than 30 million people travel annually from an industrialized to a developing country, and of these 50% can expect to experience an episode of acute diarrhea. This illness is usually self-limited but often modifies the traveler's agenda.

Traveler's diarrhea usually begins 3 to 6 days after arrival in a foreign country and is accompanied by nausea, malaise, and vomiting. Fever occurs in about half of patients. About 20% of patients have fever or bloody stools, suggesting infection with an invasive organism. Patients are usually much improved in 72 hours, although symptoms may persist in some patients for more than a month.

The vast majority of these cases are infectious, and the specific agent involved is highly dependent on the country visited, the nature of the travel, and the foods consumed. Toxigenic *E. coli* (ETEC strains) cause up to 40% of cases, and *Shigella, Salmonella,* viruses, and *G. lamblia* are each implicated in about 5% to 10% of cases. *E. histolytica, C. jejuni, Cryptosporidium,* and *Aeromonas* are responsible in certain countries. Viruses such as rotavirus and the Norwalk family of viruses are responsible for up to 10% of cases. New enteropathogens continue to be discovered, and sometimes one need not travel at all to become exposed; that is, it is sufficient that one's food has traveled. An example of this phenomenon is the coccidian parasite *Cyclospora cayatenensis,* first described as a disease of travelers in the 1980s but now recognized as a pathogen that can be acquired by the eating of fresh fruits and vegetables imported from endemic areas.

Travelers become ill by eating leafy vegetables, poorly stored meat and seafood, dairy products, and water (or ice) that is fecally contaminated. Foods cooked at high temperature, beverages made with boiled water, and soda in tightly capped bottles are usually safe. The consumption of eggs, custard, mayonnaise, and milk- or cream-based sauces while traveling in many parts of the world should be avoided, and hot foods cooked in a cloud of steam at roadside may be the safest to eat. Contrary to popular belief, the grand and majestic hotels in the developing world do not have uniformly high standards of sanitation, but they do provide comfortable accommodations for the short period of recovery.

Treatment of traveler's diarrhea primarily involves fluid and electrolyte replacement. Even in the tropics most adults do not become rapidly dehydrated, so hypotonic solutions containing glucose taken with salted crackers, or salty soups combined with fruit juices and complex carbohydrates such as rice, potatoes, or bread (which promote active glucose–sodium cotransport), can usually meet fluid and salt requirements. Oral rehydration therapy with standardized, prepackaged mixtures of salts and carbohydrates in water is recommended for children with mild or moderate dehydration, and can be purchased at almost any pharmacy in the world. Many patients require no therapy beyond compounds that reduce stool frequency. Oral bismuth subsalicylate may reduce stool frequency by 50%, and loperamide by 80%, although such drugs should not be used in patients with fever or dysentery (bloody stools) because they may exacerbate invasive bacterial infections. Antimicrobial therapy is recommended for illness that is moderate or severe, including abdominal pain or cramps, fever or dysentery, or prolonged symptoms. Fluoroquinolones are the antibiotics of choice for adults, and usually a short course (3 days or less) is sufficient. Antibiotic therapy reduces the duration of diarrhea from an average of 3 days to less than 1 day. The combination of loperamide and an antimicrobial drug is particularly effective, reducing symptoms while eradicating the organism.

The role of chemoprophylaxis in preventing traveler's diarrhea remains controversial. The primary prophylaxis for traveler's diarrhea should be avoidance of food that may be fecally contaminated. For most travelers, chemoprophylaxis is unnecessary, expensive, and carries the risk of side effects. Furthermore, in this era of increasingly resistant microbes, widespread use of prophylactic antimicrobials must also be weighed against concerns about increasing antimicrobial resistance in enteric pathogens abroad. For travelers to high-risk areas who have underlying illness or cannot use food and water precautions, prophylaxis with bismuth subsalicylate, fluoroquinolones, trimethoprim–sulfamethoxazole, or doxycycline may be considered. Prophylaxis should begin on the first day in the country and should continue for 2 days after returning. Prophylaxis longer than 3 weeks is not advisable because of the cost, potential drug toxicity, and interference with the development of natural defense mechanisms against these infections.

INFECTIOUS PROCTITIS AND PROCTOCOLITIS

Infectious causes of proctitis should be considered in any patient with a history of anal intercourse. Proctitis implies sigmoidoscopic evidence of inflammation limited to the rectum and is often associated with constipation, tenesmus, rectal bleeding, and perirectal pain. Sexually transmitted microorganisms causing this illness include *N. gonorrhoeae, C. trachomatis,* herpes simplex virus, and *Treponema pallidum.* Proctocolitis suggests inflammation extending beyond the rectum, and in those patients diarrhea may accompany symptoms of proctitis. The most common infectious agents causing proctocolitis extending above the rectum are *S. flexneri, C. difficile, C. jejuni, C. trachomatis,* and *E. histolytica.*

AIDS

Gastrointestinal pathogens are common in HIV-infected patients and may affect any organ. Patients may have no symptoms, or they may be quite ill or sometimes debilitated from these infections. Diarrhea is common in those infected with HIV: it occurs in 30% to 60% of North American and European patients with clinical AIDS and in 90% of patients in developing countries. Many microorganisms cause acute, treatable illness, only some of which are classified as opportunistic pathogens, and they are acquired by anal–oral sexual practices. Homosexuals or bisexuals who have AIDS are more likely to have diarrhea with an enteric pathogen than are heterosexuals or intravenous drug users with HIV. The finding of an enteric pathogen, however, does not necessarily imply that symptoms can be ascribed to that particular organism, since similar enteric pathogens can be identified in up to half of asymptomatic patients. Multiple coinfections are common in AIDS patients.

As always, evaluation should begin with a careful history to help focus diagnostic efforts. Stools should be cultured for bacterial pathogens, assayed for *C. difficile* toxin, and examined for parasites. More extensive workup by endoscopy and biopsy is often required. Empirical treatment may be justified; for example, patients with symptoms of esophagitis, particularly if accompanied by oral thrush, may receive treatment with fluconazole for presumptive candidiasis, reserving more invasive investigation for refractory cases. The subject of AIDS is also covered in Chapters 98, 114, and 343.

FOOD POISONING SYNDROMES

The term *food poisoning* describes the nausea, vomiting, abdominal cramps, chills, fever, and diarrhea that quickly follow consumption of food contaminated with bacteria or their toxins, or with toxic chemicals. Food poisoning should be considered when the illness starts within hours after ingestion of a meal, and if others eating the same foods or in the same locale are also affected. A specific diagnosis in the individual patient is usually not made, nor is a search justified, as uneventful recovery is the rule. In large outbreaks, public health authorities may deem it necessary to identify a source.

The pathogenic mechanism of microbial food poisoning involves ingestion of preformed bacterial toxin or the ingestion of an organism that then rapidly produces toxin *in vivo. Staphylococcus aureus* and *Bacillus cereus* are examples of organisms that can grow in food and make such toxins. Symptoms typically begin 1 to 6 hours after food ingestion. Vomiting and diarrhea are the hallmarks of staphylococcal food poisoning, whereas nausea and vomiting alone characterize *B. cereus* toxin ingestion. However, *B. cereus* also can cause long-acting food poisoning 8 to 16 hours after food ingestion, this form characterized by diarrhea and cramping abdominal pain. Another common cause of the 8- to 16-hour food poisoning syndrome is *Clostridium perfringens* type A, an organism that elaborates a potent enterotoxin capable of changing small intestinal solute and water transport. The abdominal cramps and diarrhea of *C. perfringens* disease usually is impossible to distinguish from other gut infections.

In all but extremely ill, elderly, or debilitated patients, treatment of microbial food poisoning syndromes is best limited to symptomatic treatment because these illnesses are usually relieved within 24 hours. Dominant vomiting in these diseases may result in hypochloremic alkalosis and consequent hypokalemia, both of which are of clinical importance.

MISCELLANEOUS INTESTINAL INFECTIONS

SMALL INTESTINAL BACTERIAL OVERGROWTH SYNDROME (BLIND-LOOP SYNDROME)

The normal proximal small intestine is sparsely populated by bacteria (usually less than 10^3 per milliliter), consisting of a mixture of aerobes and anaerobes. However, these numbers may soar to 10^7 per milliliter to 10^9 per milliliter if intestinal motility or other gut clearance mechanisms are abnormal. This condition, known as bacterial overgrowth syndrome, stasis syndrome, blind-loop syndrome, or stagnant-loop syndrome, leads to malabsorption of dietary fat and fat-soluble vitamins and can result in weight loss, steatorrhea, macrocytic anemia, vitamin deficiency syndromes, and chronic diarrhea. Recognition of this group of disorders is important because treatment to correct the stasis or eradicate the responsible microorganisms is highly effective; however, these syndromes are commonly overlooked.

Clinical malnutrition due to bacterial overgrowth was first recognized in elderly patients with jejunal diverticula, but since then it has been found in any condition involving stasis in the small intestine. Such stasis occurs behind strictures or adjacent to fistulae due to inflammation such as Crohn's enteritis, in postirradiation states, and in neoplasms such as ovarian malignancies that secondarily involve the gut mesentery. Bacterial overgrowth is also found in postsurgical patients with inadequate emptying of reconstructed loops (such as the afferent loop of the Billroth II gastrectomy), in gastric achlorhydria, or in intrinsic motility disorders such as scleroderma of the small intestine, diabetes mellitus, and chronic pseudo-obstruction. Malabsorption is directly attributable to the type and number of bacteria in the upper gut, and these are largely anaerobes. Bacteria interfere by competing directly for nutrients such as vitamin B_{12}, which they can remove from intrinsic factor or other cobalamin binders en route from the stomach to the receptor sites in the terminal ileum. Perhaps of more direct importance, bacteria in the upper gut can modify or partially degrade bile acids, which renders them ineffective for the absorption of dietary triglycerides and fat-soluble vitamins. Bacterial deconjugation or dehydroxylation of bile acids changes their solubility and micelle-forming properties, which are needed for the absorption of dietary lipids. Bacterial overgrowth can also cause focal damage to the enteric mucosa, perhaps contributing to the malabsorption problem.

The main nutritional consequences are weight loss and macrocytic anemia, and the patient may have chronic diarrhea. However, diarrhea is often absent despite flagrant bacterial overgrowth, perhaps explaining why these disorders are clinically overlooked. Workup of patients suspected of having bacterial overgrowth or stagnant-loop syndromes should include contrast roentgenography of the small intestine to define the abnormal anatomy and to assess motility and clearance of gut contents. The diagnosis is firmly established by finding large numbers of bacteria in aspirated jejunal contents of the malnourished patient. Specific arrangements should be made with the bacteriology laboratory for quantitation and anaerobic growth of the aspirated sample. Diagnostic breath tests have also been developed; these include hydrogen breath analysis after ingestion of lactulose or glucose, or measurement of expired $^{14}CO_2$ after ingestion of ^{14}C-xylose or ^{14}C–bile acids. These tests have significant false-positive and false-negative results. The breath hydrogen or $^{14}CO_2$ response after antibiotic therapy may be used to judge the efficacy of treatment. Vitamin B_{12} deficiency can be documented by measuring the serum vitamin B_{12} level and by doing a Schilling test. In the blind-loop syndrome, serum vitamin B_{12} is abnormal in both stage I (oral vitamin B_{12} alone) and stage II (oral vitamin B_{12} with intrinsic factor) tests.

Experienced clinicians often treat stasis syndromes without documenting bacterial overgrowth if the clinical circumstances strongly suggest the diagnosis. The basis of treatment is eradication of the overgrowing bacteria and caloric and vitamin replacement if nutritional depletion is severe. Specific therapy should include broad-spectrum antibiotic therapy with metronidazole, ampicillin, tetracycline, or clindamycin. The diet may be augmented by medium-chain triglycerides whose absorption is not dependent on bile acids. A gratifying weight gain of 5 to 15 kg is not unusual with proper treatment of a severely malnourished patient. A single course of antibiotic therapy often results in a prolonged remission, although repeated courses of antibiotics may be required. Correction of the anatomical disorder leading to overgrowth is not usually necessary but should be considered in the appropriate patient if antibiotic and other forms of therapy are ineffective.

TROPICAL SPRUE

Tropical sprue is a malabsorptive disorder of unknown cause that is endemic in the tropics, particularly southern India, Southeast Asia, and the Caribbean; it is rare in Africa. It occurs both in the indigenous population and in visitors from temperate climates. Tropical sprue can develop in visitors as soon as 2 weeks after their arrival, although a lengthy stay of months to years is more the rule. Occasionally, the illness appears several months after the visitor has been home. This illness should not be confused with nontropical sprue (celiac disease), a sensitivity to ingested gluten for which treatment is entirely different.

Chronic illness is usually preceded by an episode of acute infectious diarrhea that never fully resolves. The epidemiologic and clinical features, coupled with the response to antibiotic therapy, support the view that tropical sprue is one of several postinfectious malabsorption states whose full range of causes has not been identified. The differential diagnosis includes chronic bacterial or parasitic infections (chronic giardiasis, cryptosporidiosis, S. stercoralis infection) and neoplasms (mainly primary intestinal lymphoma). HIV should be in the differential diagnosis until serologically excluded.

The full tropical sprue syndrome is characterized by chronic diarrhea, folic acid deficiency, vitamin B_{12} deficiency, malabsorption of various nutrients, megaloblastic anemia, edema, and hypoalbuminemia. Tropical sprue should be suspected in any person who has lived in the tropics, complains of diarrhea and weight loss, and has evidence of folic acid deficiency. Jejunal biopsy shows blunting (not usually absence) of the villi and infiltration of the lamina propria with lymphocytes and plasma cells.

Treatment consists of folic acid, vitamin B_{12} replacement, and tetracycline. The prognosis is good, although therapy for several months may be necessary.

WHIPPLE'S DISEASE

This rare intestinal illness, largely confined to white males of European ancestry, is characterized by malabsorption and systemic illness. Bacteria in gut tissues were observed by electron microscopy many years ago but only recently were identified by polymerase chain reaction amplification of the microbial 16S ribosomal RNA in patient tissues. This revealed a gram-positive actinomycete unrelated to any known genus, now named *Tropheryma whippelii*. Details on the clinical manifestations of Whipple's disease are found in Chapter 110.

BIBLIOGRAPHY

Belongia EA, Osterholm MT, Soler JT, et al. Transmission of *Escherichia coli* 0157:H7 infection in Minnesota child day-care facilities. *JAMA* 1993;269:883–888.

Diarrheal disease: current concepts and future challenges. Proceedings of a symposium organized by the Royal Society of Tropical Medicine and Hygiene, United States Naval Medical Research Unit No. 3 and the Pathological Society of Great Britain. *Trans R Soc Trop Med Hyg* 1993; 87(Suppl 3):31–34.

Dupont HL, Ericsson CD. Prevention and treatment of traveler's diarrhea. *N Engl J Med* 1993;328:1821–1827.

Gaunt PN, Piddock LJ. Ciprofloxacin resistant *Campylobacter* spp. in humans: an epidemiological and laboratory study. *J Antimicrob Chemother* 1996;37:747–757.

Herwaldt BL, Ackers ML. An outbreak in 1996 of cyclosporiasis associated with imported raspberries. *N Engl J Med* 1997;336:1548–1556.

Kelly CP, Pothoulakis C, LaMont JT. *Clostridium difficile* colitis. *N Engl J Med* 1994;330:257–262.

LaMont JT, ed.: *Gastrointestinal infections: diagnosis and management.* New York: Marcel Dekker, 1997.

Kelley's Textbook of Internal Medicine, fourth edition. Edited by H. David Humes. Lippincott Williams & Wilkins, Philadelphia © 2000.

C H A P T E R

114

GASTROINTESTINAL DISEASES WITH AN IMMUNE BASIS

CHARLES O. ELSON

Lymphoid cells comprise approximately 25% of the cells in the intestinal mucosa, thus representing a major component of the immune system. The intestinal immune system is organized in three interconnecting cellular compartments: Peyer's patches and lymphoid follicles, lamina propria lymphoid cells, and intraepithelial lymphoid cells (Fig. 114.1). The cell compartments are segregated by differences in physical location and structure and by the types and functions of the cells within them. The antigenic challenge to the mucosal immune system is enormous. Intestinal lymphoid cells are in a constant state of response to these antigens, as evidenced by the large numbers of plasma cells present continuously in the mucosa and by studies of germ-free animals in which the intestinal immune system is poorly developed.

PEYER'S PATCHES AND LYMPHOID FOLLICLES

Peyer's patches are organized lymphoid aggregates with follicles that extend from the epithelial layer down into the lamina propria and sometimes to the submucosa. Similar, smaller structures, many with but a single follicle, are dispersed throughout the human intestine. Peyer's patches and related lymphoid follicles lack afferent lymphatics. Instead, they have a specialized epithelium containing M cells that actively phagocytose and pinocytose antigenic materials in the intestinal lumen and deliver them to lymphoid cells below. Peyer's patches serve as sites of induction of immune responses, containing B-cell and T-cell precursors as well as antigen-presenting cells, but they are deficient in mature effector cells such as plasma cells or cytotoxic T cells, probably because differentiating B and T cells leave Peyer's patches after being stimulated there. The route of antigen exposure is critical. Peyer's patch cells respond almost exclusively to antigens delivered from the intestinal lumen. Peyer's patches and related follicles are a preferential site for the induction of IgA responses, which is the major immunoglobulin at mucosal surfaces.

Lymphocytes induced in the Peyer's patch and intestinal follicles leave these structures through efferent lymphatics that drain into mesenteric lymph nodes, where further division and maturation occur. From there, they travel by the thoracic duct into the circulation and are dispersed widely in the body. However, they tend to selectively accumulate or "home" to the intestine and other mucosal sites through the interaction of integrin receptors on lymphocytes that bind to ligands on the endothelial cells in the mucosa.

LAMINA PROPRIA LYMPHOCYTES

The intestinal lamina propria contains an abundance of B cells, plasma cells, T cells, and macrophages, as well as a lesser number of other cells, such as eosinophils and mast cells. Approximately 70% to 90% of the plasma cells in the intestine produce IgA, 5% to 15% produce IgM, and only 3% to 5% produce IgG, with IgE and IgD plasma cells occurring infrequently. Plasma cells are terminally differentiated, end-stage cells whose estimated half-life is about 5 days, indicating that their repopulation must be dynamic and continuous. Approximately two-thirds of

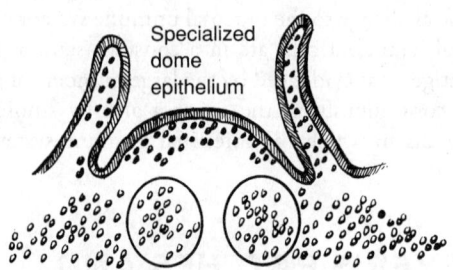

Specialized dome epithelium

Peyer's patch/lymphoid follicles

Inductive site
Antigen-sampling M cells
Precursor B and T cells
Preferential IgA responses

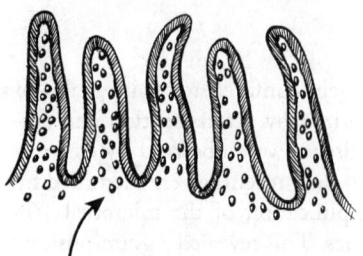

Intraepithelial lymphocytes (IEL)

Effector site
Mostly CD8+ T cells, both $T\alpha\beta$ and $T\delta$
Thymic-independent T cell subset
Cytotoxic activity in vitro
Produce cytokines that modulate epithelial function

Lamina propria lymphocytes (LPL)

Effector site
Large number plasma/B cells: IgA > IgM > IgG
Activated/memory T cells; mainly CD4+
Predominance of helper T cell activity
Macrophages, eosinophils present

FIGURE 114.1. Important features of the major compartments of the intestinal immune system.

lamina propria T cells have the CD4$^+$ helper or inducer phenotype, and one-third have the CD8$^+$ suppressor or cytotoxic phenotype, similar to that found in peripheral blood. Macrophages make up about 10% of lamina propria isolates, and mast cells constitute 1% to 3%. Mast cells are abundant in the lamina propria of the intestine and are present in the deeper layers of the bowel wall. At least two types of mast cells exist: the mucosal mast cell, which predominates in the lamina propria, and the connective tissue mast cell, which predominates in the deeper intestinal wall. The two types respond differently to various agonists and inhibitors—an observation of potential clinical importance. For example, mucosal mast cells are not inhibited by disodium cromoglycate. Eosinophils are a normal constituent in humans, but neutrophils are not. Natural killer cells and function seem to be deficient in the intestinal lamina propria, although precursors of lymphokine-activated killer cells are well represented. Lamina propria T cells differ from peripheral T cells in activation requirements and intracellular signaling pathways. They have surface markers of activated memory cells but proliferate poorly when stimulated in culture. They do produce cytokines *in vitro* but do not actively produce cytokines *in situ,* perhaps due to the influence of regulatory cells. The mechanism of this paradox of activated but hyporesponsive cells has yet to be elucidated.

INTRAEPITHELIAL LYMPHOCYTES

The third compartment of the intestinal immune system is represented by lymphocytes that are physically located within the epithelial layer, averaging 1 lymphocyte per 6 to 20 epithelial cells. The cellular composition of this compartment is quite different from that of the Peyer's patch or the lamina propria.

The predominant cell type is the T cell, most of which bear the CD8 marker.

A variety of T-cell types are represented, including both αβ and γδ T-cell receptor–bearing cells. The latter is a major population in some species but represents only 5% to 7% of intraepithelial lymphocytes (IELs) in humans. These and some other IEL T cells appear to be generated directly in the gut epithelium rather than in the thymus, as are conventional T cells. The role of such thymic-independent IELs in health or disease is unclear. Unlike lamina propria cells, IELs have full cytotoxic capabilities, including natural killer, antibody-dependent cellular cytotoxicity, and T-cell cytotoxicity, but the exact role of such cells in mucosal defense is unknown. Because IELs increase in number after roundworm infestations, one hypothesis is that they may have a cytotoxic function directed primarily at parasites. IELs are increased in experimental graft-versus-host disease, prompting the suggestion that an increase in IELs may be a marker for cell-mediated immune responses in the intestine. There is some evidence that IELs may defend the epithelium against viral infections by secreting interferon or other cytokines, or perhaps by direct cytotoxicity for virally infected epithelial cells. Although we know very little about their precise function in gut-associated lymphoid tissue, IELs are in a site that would expose them to a great variety of antigenic stimuli and have the potential to participate in host defense and possibly mediate diseases. IELs are increased in number in some intestinal diseases, including celiac disease, dermatitis herpetiformis, and tropical sprue, but their role in these diseases is unknown.

ROLE OF THE EPITHELIUM

The epithelium is being increasingly recognized as an active participant in mucosal immune responses. Epithelial cells are in direct contact with IELs and in close apposition to lamina propria lymphocytes. Important interactions, or "cross-talk," between epithelial cells and mucosal lymphocytes appear to occur through the secretion and response to various cytokines. The barrier function of the epithelial layer is mediated in large part by tight junctions between enterocytes. Exposure of epithelium to interferon-γ (IFN-γ), a cytokine known to be produced by IEL, diminishes tight-junction resistance and reduces barrier function. At the same time, IFN-γ up-regulates class II major histocompatibility complex (MHC) molecules on enterocytes. Increased class II MHC expression on intestinal epithelium is common at sites of chronic intestinal inflammation in humans. The role of epithelial cell class II MHC molecules *in vivo* is unclear, but epithelial cells can present foreign antigen to primed T cells in vitro; such presentation has stimulated suppressor rather than helper cells. Epithelial cells actively produce many cytokines, some of which influence immune responses. These include interleukin-8 (IL-8), a chemokine for neutrophils and lymphocytes, which is secreted rapidly during invasion of epithelial cells by bacteria. Epithelial cells produce transforming growth factor–β (TGF-β) and IL-6, both cytokines that promote IgA responses. TGF-β is also a potent inhibitor of many lymphocyte functions; its local secretion may be an important mechanism limiting inflammation in the normal gut.

SECRETORY IgA AND ITS TRANSPORT SYSTEM

The epithelium plays a crucial role in the transport of IgA into the gut lumen. Most plasma cells at mucosal sites produce IgA. IgA is produced as a monomer of 150-kd plus a dimer of 320 kd. IgA dimer is covalently coupled to a 15-kd protein known as J chain before secretion from plasma cells. Dimeric IgA, but not monomeric IgA, is able to bind to the polymeric immunoglobulin receptor (pIgR, also known as secretory component), a 70-kd receptor molecule produced by and present on the surface membrane of gut epithelial cells. J chain appears to be required for this binding to occur. After binding, the dimeric IgA–pIgR complex is endocytosed in a coated pit type of vesicle, transported to the apical membrane by a microtubule-dependent process, and released into the lumen (Fig. 114.2). Polymeric IgM is transported in a similar manner. In addition to transporting IgA into the lumen, pIgR confers to IgA a resistance to proteolysis. Once released into the lumen, secretory IgA has antiviral, antitoxin, and antibacterial functions, primarily by decreasing the ability of such cells or substances to bind or adhere to mucosa.

The liver can actively transport IgA into bile; this transport also is mediated by pIgR. In some species, particularly rodents, pIgR is present on hepatocytes, and most IgA enters the intestine by this route. In humans, pIgR is present on bile ductular cells but not on hepatocytes, and this is not a major pathway of IgA transport. Because the same mechanism can transport immune complexes of IgA bound to antigen, this system may serve as an excretory route for the clearance of intestinal antigens out of the body. In humans, bile ductular cells, in addition to expressing pIgR on their surface membrane, express HLA-DR antigens.

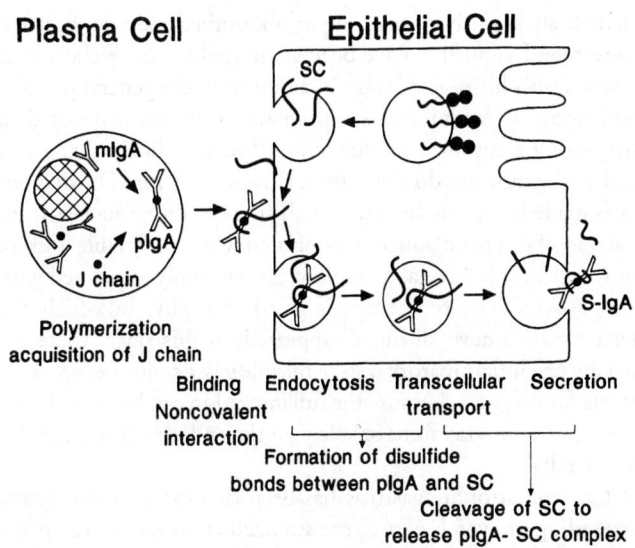

FIGURE 114.2. Model of the selective transport of J-chain-containing polymeric IgA (pIgA) through an epithelial cell. mIgA, monomeric IgA; SC, secretory component. (From Mestecky J, McGhee JR, Elson CO. Intestinal IgA system. *Immunol Allergy Clin North Am* 1988;3:356, with permission.)

The transport of immune complexes and the expression of HLA-DR antigens by these ductular cells may be important in certain diseases, such as primary biliary cirrhosis and chronic graft-versus-host disease, in which there is a progressive destruction of bile ductular cells of apparent immune origin.

REGULATION OF THE RESPONSE TO ANTIGENS IN THE INTESTINE

Development of immunity to an antigen after an intestinal exposure is a well-known phenomenon that has been documented repeatedly after natural infections in humans and oral immunization regimens in experimental animals. "Natural" antibodies, such as the hemagglutinins, are examples of immunization at an intestinal surface. However, such exposure can also result in a state of specific systemic unresponsiveness, called *oral tolerance*. The factors that determine which result predominates are not understood, but presumably the answer lies in complex regulatory cell interactions within the intestinal immune system. Oral tolerance has been demonstrated in animals after feeding them a variety of different antigens, and it has also been demonstrated in humans. Feeding of autoantigens to experimental animals to induce oral tolerance ameliorates autoimmune diseases, and trials are under way to determine whether this may be an effective and nontoxic form of therapy for humans with autoimmune disorders.

CHRONIC ATROPHIC GASTRITIS

Chronic atrophic gastritis is a nonerosive inflammation of the gastric mucosa. Although a variety of upper abdominal complaints, such as dyspepsia, upper abdominal pain or fullness, nausea, and vomiting, have been attributed to chronic atrophic gastritis, this histologic lesion is common in the general population, most of whom are asymptomatic. Care must be used in attributing symptoms to this lesion, but it is likely that some patients' symptoms do result from chronic gastritis. The diagnosis is made by gastric biopsy, which shows a mononuclear infiltrate in the gastric mucosa associated with a variable loss of gastric glands; intestinal metaplasia is commonly associated with the gastritis. The final stage is gastric atrophy, in which the gastric glands have all but disappeared; at this stage, there are usually few inflammatory cells. Multiple gastric biopsies are preferable for diagnosis because the inflammation can be focal. Diagnosis based on x-ray films or solely on the endoscopic appearance is not reliable.

Chronic atrophic gastritis has been divided into two types, depending on which part of the stomach is involved and on the presence or absence of antibodies to parietal cells. In type A gastritis, inflammation affects the body and fundus of the stomach, but the antrum is spared. Serum anti–parietal cell antibodies and hypergastrinemia are common. Gastric acid secretion is usually low or absent. Patients with type A gastritis have an increased incidence of concomitant autoimmune disorders such as Hashimoto's thyroiditis, hypothyroidism, Graves' disease, insulin-dependent diabetes mellitus, Addison's disease, hypoparathyroidism, and vitiligo. The cause of the gastric lesion appears to be autoimmune damage to gastric parietal cells in the body and fundus of the stomach. The major autoantigens recognized by parietal cell antibodies are the α and β subunits of H^+, K^+-ATPase, the gastric proton pump responsible for acid secretion, which is localized on the cannicular (luminal) surface of the parietal cell. A subset of patients with type A gastritis develop *pernicious anemia* with absolute achlorhydria, an absence of intrinsic factor, and vitamin B_{12} malabsorption. The clinical features of these patients are those of vitamin B_{12} deficiency, including anemia, glossitis, neuropathy, memory impairment, and depression. There are usually few or no gastrointestinal symptoms. In addition to serum anti–parietal cell antibodies, antiintrinsic factor antibodies are common. The diagnosis is made by establishing the presence of achlorhydria, a low vitamin B_{12} level, an abnormal Schilling test result, and serum antibodies to intrinsic factor. Treatment consists of monthly vitamin B_{12} injections, 100 μg IM or daily cobalamin 1 mg PO.

In type B gastritis, inflammation affects the antrum and the body of the stomach; antibodies to parietal cells are not found. Serum gastrin levels are generally normal, although gastric acid secretion is often reduced. There is no association with autoimmune disorders, as is seen in type A gastritis. Instead, most cases are due to infections of the gastric mucosa with *Helicobacter pylori* (see Chapter 107). Gastrointestinal symptoms are more common than in type A gastritis. The incidence of chronic type B gastritis increases with age and is also is strongly associated with duodenal ulcer, gastric ulcer, gastric polyps, and gastric cancer. Because type B gastritis is much more prevalent than type A gastritis, it is numerically more important as a precursor lesion for gastric ulcer and cancer.

CELIAC SPRUE

Celiac sprue is a disease characterized by an abnormal small-bowel mucosa and malabsorption due to a reaction to dietary gluten proteins, which responds to a withdrawal of wheat and other gluten-containing grains from the diet. This disorder has a variety of names, including celiac disease, nontropical sprue, idiopathic steatorrhea, adult celiac disease, and gluten-sensitive enteropathy, all of which describe the same disorder. The prevalence of this disorder in the population is unknown because individuals may have the lesion without any symptoms. The pathology, clinical features, and treatment are discussed in Chapter 110.

When normal-appearing jejunal mucosa of celiac patients is exposed to gliadin, there ensues a rapid infiltration with inflammatory cells, damage and shedding of mature epithelial cells, compensatory proliferation of crypt cells, and an increased turnover of the epithelium. Crypt cells have poorly developed microvillus membranes, and they secrete rather than absorb fluids and electrolytes. The preponderance of crypt cells and deficiency of villus cells in the mucosa accounts for the deficient microvillus enzymes, poor nutrient absorption, net fluid secretion, and diarrhea of these patients. The exact pathogenesis of this abnormal response to gliadin is unknown. One theory postulates a missing intestinal peptidase and toxic damage by inadequately digested gliadin peptides, but there is little support for this idea. An immunologic pathogenesis is best supported by the evidence. An increase in IELs, particularly of $\gamma\delta$ T cells, is a characteristic feature of active celiac sprue. There is also an increase in lymphocytes, particularly $CD4^+$ T cells, and plasma cells in the lamina propria. Several immunologic abnormalities occur in celiac patients, including increased serum and mucosal antibodies to gliadin and increased serum antibodies to nongliadin antigens. Antibodies to certain autoantigens, such as connective tissue reticulin (endomysium), nuclear antigens, thyroid and parietal cells, also occur in these patients (Table 114.1). Although serum IgG antigliadin is more frequently elevated than IgA antigliadin, serum IgA antigliadin appears to be disease-specific and has been used as a screening test for celiac sprue. Serum antibodies to gliadin and to endomysium can be useful adjuncts for the diagnosis and follow-up of celiac sprue and are now available through commercial laboratories. Gliadin exposure has been shown to stimulate the release of cytokines by intestinal T cells of patients, indicating the presence of sensitized T cells in situ. The smallest gliadin peptide able to trigger the disease (ten amino acids long) is also the smallest size able to trigger sensitized T cells in vitro

TABLE 114.1.	SERUM ANTIBODIES USEFUL IN SCREENING FOR CELIAC DISEASE	
Antibody	**Sensitivity (%)**	**Specificity (%)**
IgG antigliadin	90–100	60–90
IgA antigliadin	50–90	90–100
IgA antireticulin	25–50	98–100
IgA antiendomysium	91–100	92–100

when presented in association with class II MHC antigens such as HLA-DR. The autoantigen recognized by antiendomysium has been identified as tissue transglutaminase. This enzyme may form a complex with glutamine-rich gliadin peptides, and the resulting complex may be the actual target of immune attack. Celiac sprue is strongly associated with class II HLA DR genes; 95% of patients carry two alleles (DQBI*0201 and DQAI*0501) that encode a specific DQ2 glycoprotein. This association implies that interactions between this HLA-DQ2 product and CD4$^+$ T cells are important in disease pathogenesis. Both B cells and T cells probably play a role in disease pathogenesis, in concert with a genetically determined susceptibility encoded at least in part by genes in the MHC.

The prognosis for most patients who are correctly diagnosed and appropriately treated is excellent. However, there are some serious complications that can develop in a minority of patients. Adult patients with celiac sprue have a higher incidence of primary small-bowel lymphoma and carcinoma than the population at large. Unexplained worsening of symptoms with abdominal pain, bleeding, or weight loss suggests this complication. It is unclear as to whether malignancy is less common in those adhering to a strict gluten-free diet, but it would seem best for the physician to assume so.

Ulcerative ileojejunitis may complicate celiac sprue; the major symptoms are abdominal pain, diarrhea, and intestinal bleeding. Intestinal obstruction or perforation not uncommonly complicates the course. Treatment with corticosteroids and immunosuppressives has been unsuccessful.

Refractory sprue is a rare occurrence in which patients no longer respond to gluten withdrawal, even though they did initially. Some of these patients may respond to treatment with corticosteroids or immunosuppressive drugs, such as azathioprine, but others pursue a relentlessly downhill course.

Collagenous sprue may represent a subset of refractory sprue; in this condition, collagen is deposited in the lamina propria beneath the epithelium, but the lesion otherwise is typical of celiac sprue. However, patients generally do not respond to gluten withdrawal or to other treatments, and their prognosis is poor.

Dermatitis herpetiformis is a skin disease that is closely linked to celiac sprue. It is an intensely itchy, chronic, usually papulovesicular eruption that occurs twice as often in males as in females and has a peak incidence in the second to fourth decades. Skin lesions tend to occur suddenly and are usually symmetrically distributed on the extensor surfaces, such as the knees and elbows, but also at other sites such as the scapula, sacrum, face, and scalp. It may occur in clusters, which explains its name but nongrouped lesions are also common. Mucous membrane lesions are uncommon. Healed lesions are often hyperpigmented and scarred. Intestinal biopsy reveals that most patients with dermatitis herpetiformis have a partial villus atrophy, similar to that seen in celiac patients, although the lesions tend to be patchy and less severe, and there are rarely any intestinal symptoms associated. Patients have an equally high incidence of the HLA-B8 DR3 haplotype, as do patients with celiac sprue. The intestinal and skin lesions respond to withdrawal of gluten from the diet.

The diagnosis is achieved by the characteristic clinical appearance and by biopsy. Histologically, the lesion is characterized by subepidermal vesicles due to neutrophil and eosinophil infiltration. Direct immunofluorescence reveals granular pockets of IgA1 at dermal papillary tips of involved and uninvolved skin. Complement components such as C3 are frequently found in the same areas as the IgA. These IgA1 deposits are possibly involved in the immunopathogenesis of the skin lesions, but the exact mechanism is unknown. The disease runs a long course, with spontaneous exacerbations and remissions. Rapid symptomatic relief of acute flares can be achieved with treatment with dapsone or sulfapyridine. The optimal long-term treatment is a gluten-free diet, which has been shown to greatly or completely alleviate the skin lesions and decrease the IgA deposits in the skin, although the response can be delayed for 6 months or longer. The gluten-free diet also improves the intestinal lesions and theoretically reduces the risk of intestinal lymphoma, an occurrence that has been reported in patients with dermatitis herpetiformis.

INFLAMMATORY BOWEL DISEASE

Ulcerative colitis and Crohn's disease are discussed in Chapter 111.

COLLAGENOUS COLITIS/ LYMPHOCYTIC COLITIS

Collagenous colitis is a clinicopathologic syndrome characterized by watery diarrhea and crampy abdominal pain, with a distinctive pathologic lesion consisting of a subepithelial collagen band, prominent chronic inflammatory cells in the lamina propria and epithelium, and damage of surface epithelium (Fig. 114.3). It

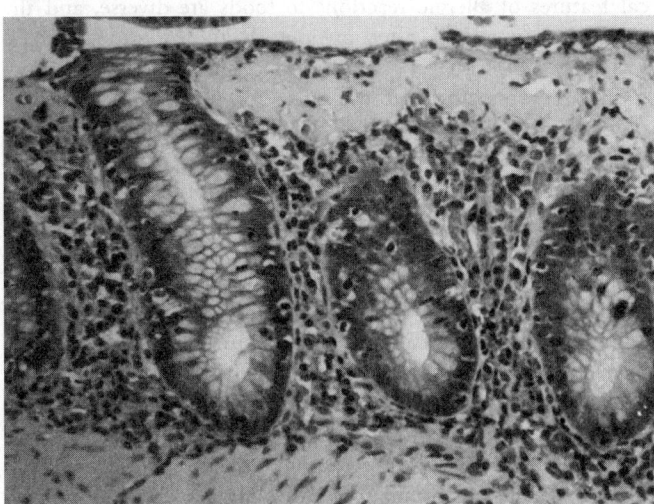

FIGURE 114.3. Features of collagenous colitis illustrated here include marked damage of surface epithelium (flattening), prominent subepithelial collagen band, numerous intraepithelial lymphocytes, and increased chronic inflammatory cells in the lamina propria. H&E, original mag ×3,200. (From Lazenby AJ, Giardello FM. Collagenous and lymphocytic colitis. *Semin Colon Rectal Surg* 1993;4:84, with permission.)

afflicts middle-aged to elderly women predominantly, but it occurs sporadically in younger women and in men. Its pathogenesis is unknown but presumably represents an autoimmune process. There are significant associations with autoimmune thyroid disease and with enteropathic arthritis as well as sporadic associations with a variety of immune-mediated disorders. The colon mucosa appears normal to the endoscopist. Diagnosis requires colon biopsy; multiple biopsies should be taken proximal to the rectosigmoid regardless of endoscopic appearance because the lesion can be patchy. In some patients, a similar lesion can occur in the small bowel as well. A related condition, *lymphocytic colitis,* has only the increased chronic inflammation in lamina propria and epithelium but similar symptoms. Treatment is with antidiarrheal medications and a trial of sulfasalazine. Some cases may require a course of prednisone. A 2-month course of bismuth has been reported to benefit some patients.

INTESTINAL ALLERGY

Adverse reactions to foods are commonly reported by patients. There are multiple possible mechanisms for such reactions, only one of which is allergy. Food allergy or hypersensitivity has been defined as an immunologic reaction, usually IgE-mediated, resulting from the ingestion of food or a food additive. Allergic reactions to food are most common in infancy and early childhood, occur only in certain individuals, may be triggered by the ingestion of a small amount of the food, and are unrelated to any physiologic effect of the food or food additive. Symptoms tend to resolve with age despite continued exposure or reexposure to the offending food antigen and despite continued IgE reactivity to it, as evidenced by positive immediate skin test responses. The mechanisms for the remission of symptoms with age is unknown, but they probably account for the relative infrequency of allergic reactions to food antigens in adults. The clinical features of allergic reactions to foods are diverse, and the major manifestations often are outside the intestine, such as urticaria, tinnitus, serous otitis, asthma, and anaphylaxis. However, symptoms limited to the intestine, such as nausea, vomiting, diarrhea, and intestinal cramping, can also occur within a few hours of food ingestion. The pathogenesis of IgE-mediated food reactions is the same as that for other forms of allergy. The cross-linking of IgE molecules on the surface of mast cells by the allergen stimulates the release of potent mast cell mediators that cause vasodilatation and vasopermeability, stimulation of mucus production, smooth-muscle contraction, stimulation of pain fibers, and attraction of inflammatory cells. Patients may have noticed an association between the ingestion of a particular food and the acute onset of their symptoms, in which case the diagnosis is obvious. If the patient has not made any such association and particularly if the symptoms are chronic, the diagnosis relies on dietary manipulations in which various foods or food groups are removed from the diet. If the patient improves, the relevant foods are added back to the diet to determine whether the symptoms are reliably reproduced. If so, this indicates only that the patient is having an adverse reaction to food and not that the reaction is necessarily IgE-mediated. Demonstration of the latter requires some measure of the presence of IgE antibody specific for the food antigen by skin testing *in vivo* or by a number of *in vitro* assays. In selected instances, double-blind food challenges may be necessary to establish the diagnosis; this is the most rigorous but also the most cumbersome and least practical method of diagnosis. Biopsy of the intestine is only useful to exclude other diseases as a cause of symptoms. Pathologic analysis shows only edema of the mucosa, or the result is normal. When an adverse reaction to food is established, the differential diagnosis includes other forms of immunologic reaction (non–IgE-mediated), food poisoning, food idiosyncrasy, and pharmacologic and metabolic food reactions. Treatment consists mainly of avoidance of the food allergen.

EOSINOPHILIC GASTROENTERITIS

Eosinophilic gastroenteritis is an illness characterized by peripheral eosinophilia, infiltration of some part of the intestine with eosinophils, and gastrointestinal symptoms. Three clinical patterns have been identified, depending on which layer of the bowel wall is predominantly affected. The most common is mucosal involvement with variable degrees of malabsorption, intestinal blood loss, iron deficiency anemia, and hypoproteinemia secondary to protein-losing enteropathy. Symptoms are usually intermittent and include nausea, vomiting, diarrhea, and abdominal pain. A history of atopy and food intolerance is often obtained. Stools frequently contain occult blood and Charcot–Leyden crystals, a distinctive-appearing breakdown product of eosinophils. Eosinophilic infiltration is found readily on endoscopic biopsies. The diagnosis is based on the biopsy, the clinical history, and the eosinophilia. The differential diagnosis includes intestinal lymphoma, polyarteritis nodosa, regional enteritis, hypereosinophilic syndrome, and intestinal parasites; other causes of malabsorption and of protein-losing enteropathy may need to be considered in selected cases.

The second type of clinical presentation is one in which the deeper muscle layers are predominantly involved. The resulting thickening and rigidity of stomach or small bowel results in symptoms of gastric or small-bowel obstruction, such as nausea, vomiting, and crampy abdominal pain. In most patients, the process is limited to the antrum and pylorus. An allergic history and a history of food intolerance is common. The differential diagnosis includes infiltrating gastric carcinoma or lymphoma, Crohn's disease, polyarteritis, and eosinophilic granuloma. The diagnosis usually requires a full-thickness biopsy.

The third and least common presentation is predominant serosal involvement and eosinophilic ascites. The diagnosis is made by laparotomy by demonstration of a thickened serosa with eosinophilic infiltration. Although this and the other clinical patterns of the disease can occur alone, they not uncommonly overlap.

The pathogenesis of eosinophilic gastroenteritis is not well understood. Immunologic reactions to foods are postulated to account for about one-half of these patients. The treatment proceeds as for any allergic reaction to foods: identification and avoidance of the food responsible. The cause of the disease in the other one-half is unclear, but corticosteroid therapy seems beneficial for most patients.

IMMUNODEFICIENCY DISEASES

SEVERE COMBINED IMMUNODEFICIENCY

Severe combined immunodeficiency is a disease of infancy, and patients usually do not survive past 2 years of age unless they receive a bone marrow transplant or are given replacement therapy. They can have chronic diarrhea and malabsorption, which are usually of infectious origin, and candidiasis. These patients are extremely prone to infections, including enteric infections with *Salmonella, Shigella,* or enteropathogenic *Escherichia coli.* However, respiratory infections are always the greater clinical problem and the one to which the patient ultimately succumbs. Small bowel biopsy shows the absence of plasma cells, edema, blunted villi, crypt hyperplasia, a mononuclear infiltrate of the lamina propria, and periodic acid–Schill (PAS)–positive macrophages reminiscent of those seen in Whipple's disease. The defect is thought to be at the level of the bone marrow stem cell (Table 114.2), and the treatment usually is bone marrow transplantation.

X-LINKED AGAMMAGLOBULINEMIA (BRUTON'S)

Individuals with X-linked agammaglobulinemia show the early onset of recurrent bacterial infections associated with low or absent serum and secretory immunoglobulins, an absence of circulating B cells, and an absence of plasma cells in the gut or lymphoid tissues. Although the patients have recurrent respiratory infections with bacteria such as staphylococci, streptococci, and *Haemophilus influenzae,* these patients generally do not have clinically apparent gastrointestinal tract disease. They may rarely have chronic diarrhea, malabsorption, or bacterial overgrowth

TABLE 114.2.	GENE MUTATIONS CAUSING SELECTED IMMUNODEFICIENCIES	
Disease	Chromosome Site	Gene Product Encoded
X-linked agammaglobulinemia	Xq21.2–22	Btk, B-cell tyrosine kinase
Severe combined immunodeficiency		
X-linked	Xq13	Interleukin-2 receptor γ chain
Autosomal recessive	—	Adenosine deaminase, nucleoside phosphorylase
Hyper-IgM syndrome, X-linked	Xq26	CD40 ligand
Wiskott–Aldrich syndrome	Xp11, 23	Wiskott–Aldrich protein

of the small intestine, and they occasionally may have infection with *Giardia* or rotavirus. The reasons for the relative absence of intestinal problems in this group are unclear.

COMMON VARIABLE HYPOGAMMAGLOBULINEMIA

Common variable hypogammaglobulinemia (CVH) is a heterogeneous group of disorders characterized by hypogammaglobulinemia, impaired ability to produce antibodies after challenge, and an increased incidence of infections. The age at onset, the clinical symptoms, and the pattern of immunologic deficiency are variable. The diagnosis requires an abnormally low level of two or more immunoglobulin isotypes. The T-cell defects may or may not be associated. Most patients have recurrent infections of the upper and lower respiratory tract with highly virulent encapsulated bacterial pathogens. Patients with CVH have a very high incidence of gastrointestinal abnormalities, including diarrhea in 60% and malabsorption in approximately 10% to 20%. Disaccharidase deficiency and protein-losing enteropathy also occur. Small-bowel biopsy shows markedly reduced numbers of plasma cells, and a variable number of patients have partial or complete villus atrophy which does not respond to gluten-free diet. Chronic infection with *Giardia lamblia* can occur in these patients and may be associated with a striking nodular lymphoid hyperplasia, which is evident on barium x-ray studies or endoscopy. CVH is frequently associated with atrophic gastritis, achlorhydria, and, in some cases, pernicious anemia. The latter is differentiated from classic pernicious anemia by an earlier age of onset, the absence of plasma cells from the gastric lamina propria, and the absence of antibodies to parietal cells or to intrinsic factor. Patients also have increased incidence of collagen vascular diseases and malignancy, especially reticuloendothelial neoplasms, although there is no increased incidence of primary lymphoma of the intestine. A subset of patients, perhaps 4% to 8%, can develop a segmental colitis resembling inflammatory bowel disease. Therapy is directed at treating various infections as they occur and employs chronic administration of intravenous γ-globulins.

SELECTIVE IgA DEFICIENCY

Selective IgA deficiency is the most common immunodeficiency state of humans; it affects 1 of 500 to 3,000 persons in the general population. It is characterized by a deficient serum IgA level (<0.05 mg per milliliter) with normal or even elevated IgG or IgM levels. The continued production of secretory IgA in some patients and a compensatory increase in secretory IgM in others may explain why most patients with selective IgA deficiency remain well. The clinical syndrome is that of recurrent bronchosinopulmonary infection. Some of these symptomatic patients have a concomitant IgG subclass deficiency. Chronic infection with *G. lamblia* and nodular lymphoid hyperplasia are uncommon. There is an association of IgA deficiency with celiac sprue; such patients are clinically indistinguishable from other patients with celiac sprue and respond well to a gluten-free diet. This association may reflect a common genetic background; both conditions are associated with an increased frequency of

HLA-B8. There is also an association between selective IgA deficiency and atrophic gastritis, pernicious anemia, and with other autoimmune diseases.

THYMIC APLASIA

Thymic aplasia (DiGeorge's syndrome) is a rare, congenital disorder with multiple abnormalities of structures derived from the embryonic third and fourth pharyngeal pouches, including facial abnormalities, congenital heart disease, and hypoplasia of the parathyroid and the thymus. The clinical features are dominated by hypocalcemia, congenital heart disease, and in those who survive the neonatal period, an increased susceptibility to infection. Gastrointestinal problems include chronic candidiasis, diarrhea, and malabsorption. Histologic examination of a small-bowel biopsy frequently yields abnormal results, revealing partial villus atrophy, crypt hyperplasia, and abnormal PAS-positive macrophages. The T-cell functions are markedly impaired; B-cell function is frequently normal, perhaps because of some residual helper T-cell activity. Treatment is largely supportive, but transplantation of a normal thymus can be helpful.

INTESTINAL LYMPHANGIECTASIA

Abnormalities of intestinal lymphatics in these patients result in protein-losing enteropathy, hypoalbuminemia, hypogammaglobulinemia, and lymphopenia. The major clinical symptoms are diarrhea and edema, which begin in the first to third decades. Severe diarrhea with steatorrhea occurs in approximately 20% of patients. Chylous effusions occur in approximately 50%. A small intestinal biopsy shows dilated intestinal lymphatics, although these may occur only in a patchy fashion. The patients have reduced levels of serum immunoglobulins and reduced cellular immune responses, both of which result from excessive loss of immunoglobulin and lymphocytes into the intestinal lumen. The cause of the lymphatic abnormality is unknown. Similar intestinal lymphangiectasia can occur secondary to other diseases such as Whipple's disease, lymphomas, inflammatory states, congestive heart failure, and constrictive pericarditis. Patients have an increased incidence of tuberculosis but otherwise fare remarkably well against other types of pathogens. Treatment of the secondary lymphangiectasia is directed to the primary disease. A low-fat diet improves serum protein and lymphocyte levels in approximately half of patients.

AIDS

CD4$^+$ helper T cells, the major target of HIV, are markedly depleted in the gut epithelium and lamina propria, as they are in other lymphoid tissues. This mucosal CD4 cell depletion is likely to have as profound an effect on mucosal immunity as it has on systemic immunity and to be a major factor in the large number of intestinal infections that occur in these patients. The damage done to the intestinal mucosa by the infections can result in malabsorption and malnutrition, which further reduce immune function, leading to chronic wasting and death.

Gastrointestinal symptoms are common in AIDS. The initial

infection with HIV may be associated with a viral-like syndrome, including anorexia, nausea, vomiting, and diarrhea. Diarrhea is often prominent in patients after the disease is well established and may represent the major clinical problem. The diarrhea is frequently caused by infection with any of a variety of opportunistic protozoal, viral, bacterial, or fungal pathogens. The diagnosis of such infections is accomplished by stool culture, examination of the stools for ova and parasites, and gastrointestinal biopsy. The most common agents are *Entamoeba histolytica*, *G. lamblia*, cytomegalovirus, herpes simplex, *Candida*, *Salmonella typhimurium*, *Mycobacterium avium complex*, and *Cryptosporidium*.

Although diarrhea usually results from infection with one or more of the pathogens previously described, diarrhea occurs in some patients in the absence of any identifiable infection. This diarrhea is frequently accompanied by steatorrhea, weight loss, and malnutrition. Intestinal biopsies are abnormal; jejunal biopsies show partial villus atrophy, crypt hyperplasia, and increased numbers of IELs. Rectal biopsies indicate focal crypt epithelial cell degeneration (i.e., apoptosis) and frequently show viral inclusions. The cause of this AIDS-associated enteropathy is unknown, but viral infection and local autoimmune reactions have been proposed. Treatment is supportive, with particular attention paid to correction of nutritional deficits.

AIDS patients can develop Kaposi's sarcoma, an angioproliferative disorder thought to be of endothelial cell origin. The gastrointestinal tract is involved in about one-half of patients, almost always in association with oral or skin lesions. The flat to nodular vascular lesions are usually submucosal but sometimes extend into the mucosa and become ulcerated. Intestinal bleeding may occur. Most patients succumb to infection rather than to the tumor itself. Treatment with chemotherapy can relieve symptoms but has not been shown to enhance survival.

BIBLIOGRAPHY

Ferguson A, Arranz E, O'Mahony S. Clinical and pathological spectrum of coeliac disease—active, silent, latent, potential. *Gut* 1993;34:150–151.
Lazenby AJ, Giardello FM. Collagenous and lymphocytic colitis. *Semin Colon Rectal Surg* 1993;4:84–92.
MacDermott RP, Elson CO. Mucosal immunology I: basic principles. *Gastroenterol Clin North Am* 1992;20:397–634.
Marsh MN. Gluten, major histocompatibility complex, and the small intestine. A molecular and immunobiologic approach to the spectrum of gluten sensitivity ("celiac sprue"). *Gastroenterology* 1992;102:330–354.
Shearer WT, Buckley RH, Engler RJ, et al. Practice parameters for the diagnosis and management of immunodeficiency. The Clinical and Laboratory Immunology Committee of the American Academy of Allergy, Asthma, and Immunology (CLIC-AAAAI) [published erratum appears in *Ann. Allergy Asthma Immunol.* 1991;77:262]. *Ann Allergy Asthma Immunol* 1996;76:282–294.
Smith PD, Mai UEH. Immunopathophysiology of gastrointestinal disease in HIV infection. *Gastroenterol Clin North Am* 1992;21:331–345.
Ten RM. Primary immunodeficiencies. *Mayo Clin Proc* 1998;73:865–872.
Toh BH, van Driel IR, Gleeson PA. Pernicious anemia. *N Engl J Med* 1997;337:1441–1448.
Wershil BK, Walker WA. The mucosal barrier, IgE-mediated gastrointestinal events and eosinophilic gastroenteritis. *Gastroenterol Clin North Am* 1992;21:387–404.
Wilcox CM, Rabeneck L, Friedman S. AGA technical review: malnutrition and cachexia, chronic diarrhea, and hepatobiliary disease in patients with human immunodeficiency virus infection. *Gastroenterology* 1996;111:1724–1752.

Zins BJ, Sandborn WJ, Tremaine WJ. Collagenous and lymphocytic colitis: subject review and therapeutic alternatives. *Am J Gastroenterol* 1995;90: 1394–1400.

Kelley's Textbook of Internal Medicine, fourth edition. Edited by H. David Humes. Lippincott Williams & Wilkins, Philadelphia © 2000.

CHAPTER
115

UPPER GASTROINTESTINAL NEOPLASMS

ANIL K. RUSTGI

This chapter encompasses the salient features of the common benign and malignant esophageal, gastric, and small intestinal neoplasms. Upper gastrointestinal (GI) neoplasms are common in the United States but are even more so worldwide.

CANCER OF THE ESOPHAGUS

SQUAMOUS CELL CARCINOMA

Esophageal squamous cell carcinoma is the most common esophageal malignancy worldwide, although there is great geographic variation. Worldwide incidence is 2.5 to 5.0 for men and 1.5 to 2.5 for women per 100,000 population. However, high incidence areas, which include China, India, Iran, regions around the Caspian Sea, and South Africa, have rates exceeding 100 per 100,000 population. In the United States, African Americans have a four- to fivefold increased risk compared to white Americans. There is also an increase with each decade of life after age 40. It is a cancer that is more common in men than women regardless of ethnicity and age.

ETIOLOGIC FACTORS AND PREDISPOSING CONDITIONS

The geographic variation in esophageal squamous cell carcinoma strongly hints at the contribution of environmental factors or the interplay of environmental and acquired genetic factors. Tobacco and alcohol are the greatest risk factors for esophageal squamous cell carcinoma in North America and Western Europe. While often patients may have excessive intake of tobacco and alcohol together, studies have established that tobacco and alcohol act independently as risk factors. At the same time, there is a large increase in risk with patients who consume both tobacco and alcohol, with the amount and duration of use as critical parameters.

Vitamin and trace mineral deficiencies are crucial as risk factors. Vitamins A, C, and E demonstrate antioxidant effects. Cer-

tain trace elements, such as selenium, molybdenum, and zinc, show an inverse association with mortality from esophageal cancer mortality in high-incidence areas. Achalasia is a predisposing risk factor as there is a 5% prevalence of patients with achalasia of long-standing duration that ultimately develop esophageal squamous cell carcinoma. The interval from symptomatic achalasia to esophageal cancer is about 20 years, although the relative risk is unclear.

Patients with head and neck squamous cell carcinoma are at an increased risk for the development of esophageal cancer, which probably reflects the fact that patients with both cancers use tobacco and alcohol. Synchronous or metachronous esophageal cancers may develop at an annual rate of approximately 5% in patients with head and neck squamous cell cancer. A genetic predisposition to esophageal cancer is rare but is noteworthy in the condition of tylosis palmaris, an autosomal dominant disorder that involves hyperkeratosis of palms and soles. Such patients are predisposed to esophageal squamous cell carcinoma and oropharyngeal leukoplakia, especially by age 45. Other factors implicated in the pathogenesis of esophageal squamous cell cancer include chronic lye ingestion, exposure to ionizing radiation, celiac sprue, human papillomavirus infection, Plummer–Vinson syndrome, esophageal diverticula, and hot maté drinking.

PATHOLOGIC FACTORS

Early esophageal cancer, while not usual in the United States, may be superficial and manifest as an ulcer, plaque, or small polypoid lesion. Discrimination between early cancer and contiguous normal squamous mucosa may be enhanced by employing vital staining dyes such as toluidine blue or Lugol's iodine solution, which stain normal mucosa only. Advanced esophageal squamous cell cancers are invariably fungating, ulcerated, and sometimes annular. Submucosal invasion may produce nodules that are friable and may cause strictures. The vast majority of squamous cell cancers are found in the proximal to mid-esophagus.

PATHOGENESIS

The progression from normal squamous mucosa to epithelial dysplasia and eventually to cancer is the hallmark of esophageal squamous cell cancer. However, dysplasia may or may not be present at the time of pathologic analysis. Tobacco tars and cigarette smoke contain various chemical carcinogens, such as aromatic amines, *N*-nitroso compounds, and polycyclic aromatic hydrocarbons. In addition, alcohol may contain constituents that are directly or indirectly carcinogenic. Ethanol itself may facilitate the absorption of other carcinogens. Exposure of the squamous mucosa to high concentrations of combinations of carcinogens over a long period of time likely results in mucosal injury. Genetic alterations may accrue as a result, predisposing to malignant transformation. Frequent genetic alterations include cyclin D_1 oncogene amplification and *p53* tumor suppressor gene mutation. Animal models have been helpful to elucidate underlying molecular mechanisms. In this context, rats that are administered nitrosoamines can develop esophageal papillomas and squamous cancer. Transgenic mice with overexpression of the cyclin D_1 oncogene targeted specifically to the oral–esophageal epithelium develop severe dysplasia, a precursor to cancer.

CLINICAL FEATURES AND NATURAL HISTORY

Early esophageal squamous cell carcinoma may or may not be associated with symptoms. Growth of cancer is manifest by dysphagia as well as odynophagia. Nausea, vomiting, and hematemesis may result. Anorexia and weight loss may ensue from malnourishment. Mediastinal involvement by the cancer is suggested by retrosternal pain or radiation of pain to the back. Other symptoms may include cough, hoarseness, and bone pain. Cough may be the result of aspiration pneumonia or, rarely, tracheoesophageal fistula. Hoarseness is due to recurrent laryngeal nerve involvement. Skeletal metastases may cause bone pain. Esophageal cancer usually presents in an advanced stage. Unfortunately, about 75% of untreated patients succumb to disease within a year. The average survival of untreated patients with advanced cancer is approximately 9.5 months.

DIAGNOSIS

Evaluation involves by establishment of tissue diagnosis followed by staging and therapeutic planning. Initial diagnostic tests usually entail barium swallow supplemented with a tablet and flexible fiberoptic endoscopy. Staging involves computed tomography (CT) scan, endoscopic ultrasonography, and radionuclide bone scan. Bronchoscopy should be considered if tracheal invasion is suspected.

Barium swallow x-rays are useful in the evaluation of dysphagia. The radiologic appearance of early esophageal cancer may consist of a granular mucosal appearance with ulcerations. A polypoid, infiltrative, or ulcerative appearance can be the distinguishing features of advanced esophageal cancer. However, ultimately the accurate diagnosis of esophageal cancer requires endoscopy with biopsy/cytology. Multiple biopsies will increase the diagnostic yield in up to 96% of cases.

High-incidence areas, such as northern China, merit endoscopic screening in the general population. Screening in high-risk areas of China has been effective; 5-year survival was nearly 90% after operative resection for cancer cases detected. However, general screening in the United States is not feasible for esophageal squamous cell carcinoma given the lack of cost-effectiveness. Screening should be undertaken in patients with tylosis, achalasia, and head and neck cancer, perhaps every 1 to 2 years.

After diagnosis is established, staging of the cancer is necessary in order to optimize treatment options and management (Table 115.1). CT of the chest and abdomen is useful for lymph node, pulmonary and hepatic involvement. Endoscopic ultrasonography is particularly helpful in assessing depth of esophageal invasion and local lymph node involvement. Bone scan may be necessary to rule out bone metastasis.

TREATMENT

Advanced esophageal cancer makes curative surgical resection difficult, if not impossible. Although nearly 60% of patients may

TABLE 115.1.	TNM STAGING SYSTEM FOR CANCER OF THE ESOPHAGUS
Primary Tumor (T)	
TX	Primary tumor cannot be assessed
T0	No evidence of primary tumor
Tis	Carcinoma in situ
T1	Tumor invades lamina propria or submucosa
T2	Tumor invades mucularis propria
T3	Tumor invades adventitia
T4	Tumor invades adjacent structures
Lymph Node (N)	
NX	Regional lymph nodes cannot be assessed
N0	No regional lymph node metastasis
N1	Regional lymph node metastasis
Distant Metastasis (M)	
MX	Presence of distant metastasis cannot be assessed
M0	No distant metastasis
M1	Distant metastasis

be surgically explored, only two-thirds of such patients undergo resection. Thus, a total of 40% of patients will require palliative therapy. Overall, 1- and 5-year survival rates are approximately 18% and 5%, respectively.

Curative surgical resection remains the key for esophageal cancer. Surgical approaches include transthoracic esophagectomy, transhiatal esophagectomy, and, to a lesser extent, en-bloc resection for cancers of the distal esophagus and the cardia. An additional consideration is selection of esophageal replacement with stomach, colon, or jejunum.

Surgery alone may be curative in more than 60% of diseases in patients with T1 or T2 (N0 M0) lesions. For patients with locally advanced disease and good performance status, many expert centers recommend neoadjuvant chemotherapy and radiation therapy followed by surgical resection. Neoadjuvant chemotherapy or radiation therapy alone does not appear to yield any survival advantages, and combination neoadjuvant therapy requires further evaluation.

Advanced disease often dictates palliative approaches with simultaneous meticulous attention to nutrition and analgesia support. Palliative measures include external-beam radiation therapy, brachytherapy, endoscopic dilatation with insertion of expandable metal stents, endoscopic laser treatment, and photodynamic therapy.

Key prognostic factors include performance status, presence or absence of aneuploidy, and cyclin D_1 oncogene amplification; aneuploidy and cyclin D_1 gene amplification are poor prognostic parameters. Ultimately, selection of patients for neoadjuvant therapy will be influenced by identification of key clinical and biologic parameters.

ESOPHAGEAL ADENOCARCINOMA

Barrett's esophagus is an important precursor to esophageal adenocarcinoma In addition, many adenocarcinomas of the gastric cardia may arise in short segments of Barrett's metaplasia. The incidence of esophageal adenocarcinoma, as well as adenocarcinoma of the gastric cardia, has increased at a rate of 4% to 10% annually over the past decade.

EPIDEMIOLOGIC FACTORS

The annual age-adjusted incidence rates of adenocarcinoma of the esophagus and gastric cardia in white men is 1.3 and 2.8 per 100,000, respectively, and is more common than in women. The incidence increases with each decade after age 40. The incidence of adenocarcinoma arising in Barrett's esophagus varies but may approach 500 cases per 100,000. This figure corresponds to nearly a 125-fold increased risk when compared to the general population in the United States. The prevalence of adenocarcinoma at the time of initial diagnosis of Barrett's esophagus is approximately 8%. The reason for the rapid increase in incidence of these two cancers is unknown but may be attributable to the rise in Barrett's esophagus and gastroesophageal reflux disease, and possible increasing eradication of *Helicobacter pylori* infection.

ETIOLOGIC FACTORS AND PREDISPOSING CONDITIONS

Barrett's esophagus encompasses metaplastic change from normal esophageal squamous epithelium to intestinalized columnar epithelium. As a premalignant condition, it is the most important risk factor for esophageal adenocarcinoma. It is conceivable that cigarette smoking and alcohol may be important once Barrett's esophagus has developed, but this is not established. Patients with Barrett's esophagus are identified at an average age of 55 years. It typically affects whites, a feature shared with esophageal adenocarcinoma. Chronic gastroesophageal reflux disease plays a role in the development and progression of Barrett's esophagus, but clearly other factors are important. Patients with cystic fibrosis and scleroderma may be at increased risk for Barrett's esophagus.

PATHOLOGIC FACTORS

Barrett's esophagus is distinguished by an intestinal columnar epithelium. A salient feature is the presence of goblet cells that can be histologically confirmed with Alcian blue stain. Various intestinal markers, such as villin and sucrase–isomaltase, among others, have been found to be increased in Barrett's esophagus. Barrett's metaplasia can progress to dysplasia, either low grade or high grade, which is the immediate precursor to carcinoma in situ and carcinoma. Esophageal adenocarcinoma is more likely to arise in long-segment Barrett's esophagus (more than 3 cm above the gastroesophageal junction) than in short-segment Barrett's esophagus (less than 3 cm), although the latter is definitely documented. Esophageal adenocarcinoma may have different stages of differentiation and grow longitudinally to the proximal esophagus and/or the proximal esophagus, thereby making classification of this cancer and gastroesophageal junctional adenocarcinoma difficult.

PATHOGENESIS

The transition of Barrett's metaplasia to adenocarcinoma involves progression through low-grade dysplasia, high-grade dysplasia, and carcinoma in situ. While gastroesophageal reflux may play a role, suppression of acid secretion does not ameliorate the progression of disease. Some investigators advocate the notion that bile reflux may be contributory, as demonstrated in a rodent model of esophagojejunostomy. The molecular mechanisms underlying the sequence of changes in Barrett's esophagus are being elucidated. Seminal studies have demonstrated that abnormal DNA content, as reflected by aneuploidy measured through flow cytometry, is associated with dysplasia and adenocarcinoma. Additionally, *p53* tumor suppressor gene mutations, *p16* tumor suppressor gene alterations by virtue of mutation or promoter hypermethylation, and microsatellite DNA instability are all important genetic alterations.

CLINICAL MANIFESTATIONS AND NATURAL HISTORY

Early esophageal adenocarcinoma may be silent or a consequence of gastroesophageal acid reflux disease and its complications, such as ulcers and stricture. Symptoms attributable to advanced esophageal adenocarcinoma include dysphagia, odynophagia, weight loss, chest pain, nausea, vomiting, cough, and GI bleeding.

Only a subset of Barrett's patients develop adenocarcinoma. Most esophageal adenocarcinomas have high-grade dysplasia in the surrounding mucosa. Patients with low-grade dysplasia may progress or regress at follow-up. However, patients with high-grade dysplasia who undergo esophagectomy may have foci of adenocarcinoma in nearly one-third of resected specimens. Esophageal adenocarcinoma can spread through the esophageal wall or metastasize to lymph nodes, lungs, or liver, among other structures. The prognosis is poor without treatment in a manner reminiscent of that for esophageal squamous cell cancer.

DIAGNOSIS

The squamocolumnar junction is displaced proximally in Barrett's esophagus and encompasses the junction between the stratified squamous epithelium and specialized metaplasia. The mainstay of diagnosis is endoscopy with confirmation of Barrett's esophagus by histopathologic examination demonstrating the intestinal columnar epithelium with goblet cells. Barium swallow x-ray may be useful in assessing esophageal motility, but more importantly, if there is mucosal irregularity or stricture present. Also, since scleroderma may be complicated by Barrett's esophagus, barium swallow x-rays may be helpful. The development of early esophageal cancer may be manifest by superficial erosions, nodules, or plaques superimposed on Barrett's esophagus, and therefore the index of suspicion must be high to warrant directed biopsies. Progression of cancer is associated with polypoid mass, ulcerated mass, as well as stricture formation. The approaches to staging of esophageal adenocarcinoma are the same as that for esophageal squamous cell cancer with endoscopic ultrasonography and CT scan.

In contrast to screening for esophageal squamous cell cancer in the United States, screening for Barrett's esophagus is of paramount importance. While there remains controversy as to the appropriate frequency of endoscopic screening, certain principles nonetheless prevail. Barrett's metaplasia likely requires endoscopy every 3 years; Barrett's esophagus with low-grade dysplasia merits endoscopy every 6 months for a year and, if stable, annually thereafter; and finally, the finding of high-grade dysplasia requires repeat endoscopy in a month. If high-grade dysplasia is reconfirmed, then esophagectomy should be recommended when appropriate.

THERAPY

Since the 5-year survival for esophageal adenocarcinoma is less than 10%, early diagnosis is imperative; moreover, detection of dysplasia in Barrett's esophagus carries even greater importance. Adenocarcinoma necessitates surgical resection, assuming that the patient is an appropriate candidate and there is no distant metastatic disease. The entire Barrett's segment should also be removed, given the propensity for contiguous dysplastic lesions and synchronous cancers. Recently, the potential of multimodal therapy has been investigated. Neoadjuvant or preoperative therapy may have a beneficial role. For instance, when patients were randomized to receive 5-fluorouracil and cisplatin chemotherapy before surgery, median survival improved from 11 to 16 months compared to surgery alone. Significantly, 3-year survival was 32% in the chemotherapy and surgery arm versus surgery alone, where it was less than 10%. Radiation therapy alone, in the neoadjuvant or adjuvant setting, has not been demonstrated to be efficacious as of yet. Patients who cannot undergo surgical resection due to poor performance status or the coexistence of mitigating comorbid illnesses are candidates for palliative approaches as outlined for esophageal squamous cell cancer.

◼ BENIGN ESOPHAGEAL TUMORS

Leiomyomas are the most common benign esophageal tumors. Men are affected more commonly than women. Typically solitary, leiomyomas are submucosal with smooth overlying mucosa and higher occurrence in the distal esophagus. Squamous cell papillomas are usually discovered incidentally. They are typically small, sessile, and polypoid. Histologically, they are characterized by a papillated appearance. Other benign tumors include granular cell tumor, fibrovascular polyps, hemangiomas, lymphangiomas, lipomas, and fibromas.

GASTRIC CANCER

The most common gastric cancer is adenocarcinoma, with lymphomas and leimyosarcomas as less common types. Benign neoplasms are rare.

Epidemiologic Factors

While there is geographic variation in the incidence of gastric cancer worldwide, there is a greater incidence in developing na-

tions. Individuals who emigrate from high-risk areas to low-risk or low-incidence areas keep the risk of their original country. This has been observed in people emigrating from South Americas to the United States or from Japan to Hawaii. The annual incidence of gastric cancer in the United States is 10.9 per 100,000 among men and 5.0 per 100,000 among women. This has been decreasing steadily from the 1930s when gastric cancer was more common, although gastroesophageal junctional cancers have been increasing recently.

Etiologic Factors and Predisposing Conditions

For decades the focus has been on the role of dietary factors. Diets rich in salt—especially fish, meats, and pickled foods—as well as carbohydrates appear to predispose to gastric cancer. *N*-Nitroso compounds can form in the stomach by nitrosation of ingested nitrates, which are common in diet. It is felt that salt is a cocarcinogen.

Apart from dietary factors, there are a number of conditions that predispose to gastric cancer (Table 115.2). These include pernicious anemia, the stomach remnant S/P subtotal gastrectomy for benign disease, Ménétrier's hypertrophic gastropathy, chronic atrophic gastritis with intestinal metaplasia, gastric adenomatous polyp, and chronic gastric ulcer. In particular, the intestinal type of gastric cancer is often associated with chronic atrophic gastritis and intestinal metaplasia. It has also been demonstrated that in high-incidence areas of gastric cancer, superficial gastritis occurs early in childhood, and this likely progresses to chronic atrophic gastritis with intestinal metaplasia by adulthood. The discovery that *H. pylori* causes gastritis led to the supposition that *H. pylori* was related to gastric carcinogenesis. This was substantiated by studies in which individuals who were seropositive for *H. pylori* infection had a much higher incidence of gastric cancer than seronegative individuals. This risk was determined to be a three- to sixfold increase for patients with *H. pylori* infection. It also was found that families from developing nations who were of low socioeconomic status and lived under crowded conditions had higher *H. pylori* infection rates, especially during childhood.

TABLE 115.2.	CONDITIONS THAT PREDISPOSE TO GASTRIC ADENOCARCINOMA
Nonfamilial:	
Chronic gastrititis, especially chronic atrophic gastritis	
Intestinal metaplasia	
Gastric adenomatous polyp	
Postgastrectomy stump	
Gastric epithelial dysplasia	
Ménétrier's disease	
Chronic peptic ulcer	
Familial:	
Family history of gastric cancer	
Hereditary nonpolyposis colorectal cancer type II	
Blood group A	

Pathologic Factors

Adenocarcinoma accounts for nearly 95% of all gastric cancers; the remainder are lymphomas (see later section) and sarcomas. Depth of invasion is a key prognostic factor for gastric adenocarcinoma. In this context, when limited to mucosa or submucosa, there is a favorable prognosis. Grossly, gastric adenocarcinomas may be either fungating or polypoid masses or, alternatively, ulcerating. Importantly, these tumors may infiltrate adjacent structures. Other types of gastric adenocarcinomas requiring attention are linitis plastica and the superficial type. The linitis plastica lesion, found in up to 10% of gastric adenocarcinomas, is due to an infiltrating tumor comprising anaplastic cells that evoke a desmoplastic response. Since spread is throughout the stomach, the result is a nondistensible stomach that can be appreciated radiographically and endoscopically. Unfortunately, metastasis is common. In contrast, superficial tumors are limited to the mucosa and spread laterally, thereby making resection more plausible.

While there are several histologic classifications of gastric adenocarcinoma, the Lauren classification is the most commonly accepted. It divides gastric adenocarcinoma into the following: (a) an *intestinal* (because it resembles intestinal carcinoma), well-differentiated type; and (b) a *diffuse,* infiltrating, poorly differentiated type that carries a worse prognosis. The intestinal type was noted to be more prevalent among male individuals, among older individuals, and in the setting of intestinal metaplasia, whereas the diffuse type occurred more commonly in younger individuals. The most common type in populations with a high incidence of gastric cancer, such as that seen in developing countries, was intestinal. In addition, the intestinal type is typically a fungating or polypoid mass, and is associated with *H. pylori* infection. The worldwide decline in gastric cancer suggests that the intestinal type of gastric cancer, which accounts for the majority of gastric tumors, results mainly from environmental causes. In contrast, diffuse-type gastric cancer, with its proclivity for younger individuals, its association with blood group A, and its similar incidence in high- and low-risk areas, most likely is controlled to a larger extent by genetic factors than by environmental factors. Nearly 50% of gastric adenocarcinomas are in the gastric antrum or pylorus, and the remainder are found more proximally. Recently, there has been a dramatic increase in these cancers in the cardia and the gastroesophageal junction, although not in association with *H. pylori* infection.

Pathogenesis

The mechanism by which *H. pylori* predisposes to gastric cancer has not yet been elucidated. However, several mechanisms have been postulated. *H. pylori* bacteria harbor several virulence factors, especially urease, which produces ammonia. These factors damage the gastric mucosa that is exacerbated by the host immune response to the infection. Prolonged infection with *H. pylori* results in insidious destruction of the gastric mucosa leading to atrophic gastritis, with the subsequent development of intestinal metaplasia. It is likely that ingested nitrites that are converted to nitrates augment abnormal cellular proliferation. Independently, *H. pylori* infection may also contribute to abnormal cell proliferation, thereby leading to DNA damage. Among the key genetic alterations in gastric carcinogenesis are abnormalities in growth factors (e.g., transforming growth factor α, K-sam), the *p53* tumor suppressor gene, and the phenomenon of microsatellite DNA instability.

Animal models have proved to be useful in recapitulating gastric cancer. A high rate of induction of gastric adenocarcinoma was first accomplished in rats with the nitrosamine *N*-methyl-*N*-nitro-*N'*-nitrosoguanidine (MNNG). Since then, *N*-methyl-*N*-nitrosourea (MNU) has been infused into the mouse glandular stomach and yielded gastric adenocarcinoma. Recently, transgenic mouse models have been developed in which transforming growth factor–overexpressing transgenic mice develop a hypertrophic gastropathy resembling Ménétrier's disease. Additionally, with *Helicobacter* inoculation into *p53-* deficient mice, there is acceleration of gastritis.

Clinical Features and Natural History

Gastric cancer in its earliest stages is usually not accompanied by symptoms. However, more typically, the cancer is either locally advanced or metastatic. The most common symptoms are weight loss, abdominal pain, nausea, anorexia, dysphagia, melena, early satiety, and ulcer-type pain. Gastric cancer has a poor prognosis if left untreated, and even intervention occurs when the disease is advanced. It can spread transmurally to local lymph nodes, and distantly to lungs, liver, and bone. Specialized instances include palpable supraclavicular lymph node (Virchow's node) and spread to ovaries (Krukenberg's tumor).

Diagnosis

The diagnosis of a luminal mass by upper GI radiography or fiberoptic endoscopy is straightforward. All suspicious lesions require biopsies for histopathologic analysis. Areas of abnormalities in the setting of intestinal metaplasia merit close scrutiny to detect early gastric cancer. Generally speaking, gastric ulcers should be biopsied as well. If benign, there will be chronic inflammation; however, atypia may be due to inflammation. The presence of malignant cells underscores the diagnosis of gastric cancer. Repeat biopsies may be necessary to resolve ambiguity. Benign gastric ulcers are much more common than gastric cancer arising in the ulcer. Ulcers may also arise from other causes, such as ethanol- or nonsteroidal anti-inflammatory drug–mediated injury.

It is important to distinguish masses or ulcers from submucosal lesions, such as leiomyomas or carcinoids, as biopsy may not be capable of diagnosing the submucosal lesions. Upon diagnosis of gastric cancer, other modalities should be employed to gauge penetration and extent of disease (Table 115.3). In this context, endoscopic ultrasonography can assess depth of invasion and CT scan can allow for determination for local and distant metastases. Apart from spread to lymph nodes, lungs, and liver, gastric adenocarcinoma can also metastasize to bone, thereby warranting bone scan under certain circumstances.

A controversial topic in the United States is the use of screening for gastric cancer in patients with chronic atrophic gastritis or intestinal metaplasia. It is generally not done given the low

TABLE 115.3.	STAGING OF GASTRIC CARCINOMA		
Stage	**Stage Grouping**		
IA	T1	N0	M0
IB	T1	N1	M0
	T2	N0	M0
II	T1	N2	M0
	T2	N1	M0
	T3	N0	M0
IIIA	T2	N2	M0
	T3	N1	M0
	T4	N0	M0
	T4	N0	M0
IIIB	T3	N2	M0
	T4	N1	M0
IV	T4	N2	M0
	Any T	Any N	M1

incidence of disease in this population. However, patients who have under undergone gastric cancer surgery or who have dysplasia should be enrolled in screening and surveillance endoscopy. Since patients who have had a subtotal gastrectomy for benign ulcer disease are at increased risk for gastric cancer, they should be subjected to screening for gastric cancer, but only after 15 to 20 years has passed since the initial surgery. In contrast, screening endoscopy for gastric cancer in Japan is prevalent.

Treatment

The only chance for cure of gastric adenocarcinoma is surgical resection, but this is in the setting of disease being limited to the stomach. The vast majority of patients present with extension to lymph nodes and adjacent organs or spread to distant organs, thereby obviating the need for curative surgical resection. It should be noted that surgery for early gastric cancer carries a very favorable prognosis, approaching a 5-year survival of 80% to 90%. Recently, endoscopic mucosal resection has gained attention, especially in Japan.

The surgical approach for distal gastric adenocarcinoma involves subtotal gastrectomy and may be accompanied by extensive lymphadenectomy (the latter recommended by Japanese surgeons). If the gastric adenocarcinoma has invaded adjacent organs, removal of those organs may be required. Proximal tumors require total gastrectomy with distal pancreatectomy and splenectomy. Limited gastric surgery is pursued for excessive hemorrhage or obstruction. The 5-year survival rate in the United States is about 15% for all gastric cancers.

While GI tumors in general are not responsive to chemotherapy, gastric cancer may be sensitive. Partial response rates approaching 20% to 30% may be evident with single agents, such as doxorubicin, mitomycin C, and 5-fluorouracil. This may be increased with combinations of chemotherapeutic agents, without necessarily prolonging survival. Radiation therapy is largely ineffective and palliative. The results of combination chemotherapy and radiation require long-term study. Terminally ill patients may benefit from palliative measures such as laser treat-

ment or prosthesis placement with the intent of maintaining lumen patency.

BENIGN GASTRIC NEOPLASMS

Recognition of benign gastric neoplasms is important to avoid unnecessary therapeutic interventions. Chief among this category are submucosal leiomyomas, which are typically in the middle to distal stomach. They may grow into the lumen with ulceration and bleeding. They can also grow into the serosa, leading to compression. On upper GI series radiographs, leiomyomas are smooth with an intramural filling defect. Endoscopic examination reveals overlying mucosa, and biopsies may not be diagnostic. Bleeding leiomyomas should be surgically removed.

Gastric polyps may be predominantly either adenomatous or hyperplastic. Adenomas are usually found in middle-aged to elderly patients. They carry a low likelihood of becoming gastric cancer but can nonetheless progress to that stage through the intermediate dysplastic state. Gastric adenomas may be associated with familial adenomatous polyposis, an inherited syndrome with autosomal dominant mode of inheritance. In general, gastric adenomas are benign, but they may ulcerate and bleed. They may be suspected or inferred on upper GI radiography, but confirmation requires endoscopy. Whether sessile or pendunculated, polypectomy is predicated by size and bleeding.

Other benign gastric neoplasms include lipoma, carcinoid, neurofibroma, lymphangioma, and hamartoma.

GASTRIC LYMPHOMA

The stomach is the most common extranodal site for lymphoma and represents over half of all GI lymphomas (Table 115.4), typically non-Hodgkin's lymphoma. Gastric lymphoma may be associated with chronic atrophic gastritis and intestinal metaplasia. Although symptoms and signs are reminiscent of gastric adenocarcinoma, diagnosis of lymphoma is imperative because 5-year survival is much better, approaching 50%.

Gastric lymphoma may present as an ulcer or ulcers, or as a submucosal lesion; endoscopic biopsy is critical. Apart from conventional histopathologic examination, immunoperoxidase staining of lymphoid markers is helpful. Treatment involves surgical resection, the extent of which is predicated on location of

TABLE 115.4.	GASTROINTESTINAL LYMPHOMAS
B-cell	
Low grade of mucosa-associated lymphoid tissue	
Mediterranean lymphoma	
Malignant lymphoma, centrocytic	
Burkitt-like lymphoma	
T-cell	
EATL	
Non-EATL	

EATL, enteropathy-associated T-cell lymphoma.

disease. Radiation therapy and chemotherapy are necessary (4,000 cGy to the upper abdomen and 2,000 cGy to the liver). Long-term survival approaches 80% when disease is limited to the stomach. Lymph node involvement requires combination chemotherapy and radiation therapy with careful attention to perforation and tumor lysis. However, disseminated disease merits particular focus on chemotherapy, with radiation therapy reserved for debulking large lesions.

An important gastric lymphoma subtype is mucosa-associated lymphoid tissue (MALT) lymphoma. MALT lymphoma is a low-grade B-cell lymphoma that is associated with chronic *H. pylori* infection. There have been reports of regression of MALT lymphoma with eradication of *H. pylori* infection, however, this should not supplant careful deliberation about radiation therapy and chemotherapy.

SMALL INTESTINAL CANCER

Malignancies in the small intestine are rare but primarily include adenocarcinomas, lymphomas, leiomyosarcomas, and carcinoids.

Adenocarcinoma

Nearly 50% of small intestinal malignancies are adenocarcinomas and predominantly occur in the duodenum and proximal jejunum. Predisposing conditions include familial adenomatous polyposis (especially around the ampulla of Vater in up to 12% of patients), hereditary nonpolyposis colorectal cancer type II, Crohn's disease, and celiac sprue. In familial adenomatous polyposis, small intestinal adenomas are usually proximal and, as indicated, in or around the ampulla of Vater, perhaps reflecting the potential synergy between a hyperproliferative mucosa and exposure to bile. Distal polyps in the jejunum and terminal ileum are unusual. Hereditary nonpolyposis colorectal cancer, another inherited form of colon cancer, can be associated with extracolonic cancers, especially endometrial, ovarian, gastric, renal, bladder, and pancreatic; recently, small intestinal adenocarcinoma as a manifestation has also been acknowledged. Adenocarcinoma complicating Crohn's disease can be difficult to diagnose due to underlying inflammation but should be suspected if stricture or obstruction is present. Nonetheless, it may be found incidentally. Celiac sprue can be complicated by malignancy, especially adenocarcinoma or lymphoma, apart from jejunal ulceration and stricture. For both Crohn's disease and celiac sprue, it is likely that adenocarcinoma of the small intestine could develop with long duration of disease.

If a patient is discovered to have small intestinal adenocarcinoma, it should be surgically resected. Unfortunately, chemotherapy and radiation therapy offer little promise. After resection, it would be prudent to survey with small-bowel follow-through x-ray film series or enteroclysis to monitor for potential recurrence. Small-bowel endoscopy, while advisable for any suspicious lesions or areas, is not necessarily feasible if the lesion is inaccessible to this approach.

Lymphoma

The small intestine is the second most common site (after stomach) for GI lymphomas, most of which are non-Hodgkin's type.

Of these, nearly 60% are diffuse histiocytic lymphomas. The disease may be focal or diffuse. Typical symptoms are diarrhea, steatorrhea, and/or abdominal pain or obstruction. Lymphomas complicating celiac sprue are generally of the T-cell type. A variant of small intestinal lymphomas is Mediterranean lymphoma, which comprises malabsorption in association with α-chain protein in the serum. One should also be wary of small intestinal lymphomas in patients with AIDS.

When localized to the small intestine, lymphoma should be treated with radiation therapy at a dose of 3,500 to 4,000 cGy. The response is often excellent, with cure possible in up to 75% of patients. However, lymph node involvement decreases the response rate to radiation. Therefore, combination chemotherapy should be added involving such agents as cyclophosphamide, doxorubicin, vincristine, and prednisone. Surgical resection is helpful for obstructing or bleeding lesions. Undifferentiated as well as Burkitt's lymphomas require more aggressive combination therapy. The overall response of small intestinal lymphoma is contingent on histologic profile and stage, but survival ranges from 40% to 60% at 2 years.

Carcinoid Tumor

Carcinoid tumors may occur in the small intestine, especially in the terminal ileum and appendix. The syndrome is present in the face of liver metastasis. The details of carcinoid tumor and syndrome are discussed in Chapter 118.

Other Neoplasms

Rare malignant small intestinal neoplasms include leiomyosarcomas and neurofibrosarcomas. Benign lesions include leiomyoma, lipoma, lymphoid hyperplasia, neurofibroma, and lymphangioma.

■ SUMMARY AND FUTURE DIRECTIONS

Esophageal, gastric, and small intestinal neoplasms, both benign and malignant, are important in the United States and worldwide from epidemiologic, diagnostic, and therapeutic perspectives. In particular, the progression from Barrett's esophagus to esophageal adenocarcinoma has received much attention in the United States. Advances are being made through an understanding of underlying molecular mechanisms, through the employment of cell culture techniques and animal models, and through correlation of genetic and biochemical alterations with stage of disease. Ultimately, these will translate into improvements in chemoprevention with the focus on premalignant lesions, such as esophageal squamous dysplasia, Barrett's esophagus, and intestinal neoplasia. In addition, earlier diagnosis through molecular tools will lead to more meaningful therapeutic and survival outcomes for malignant esophageal and gastric neoplasms. Experimental therapeutics, notably the advent of gene therapy and the potential application of *H. pylori* immunization therapy, also offer hope.

REFERENCES

Forman D. *Helicobacter pylori* infection and cancer. *Br Med Bull* 1998;54: 71–78.

Fuchs CS, Mayer RJ. Gastric carcinoma. *N Engl J Med* 1995;333:32–41.

Gammon MD, Schoenerg JB, Ahsan H, et al. Tobacco, alcohol, and socioeconomic status and adenocarcinoma of the esophagus and gastric cardia. *JNCI* 1997;89:1277–1284.

Parsonnet J, Friedman GD, Vandersteen DP, et al. *Helicobacter pylori* infection and the risk of gastric carcinoma. *N Engl J Med* 1991;325: 1127–1131.

Walsh T, Noonan N, Hollywood D. A comparison of mutimodal therapy and surgery for esophageal adenocarcinoma. *N Engl J Med* 1996;335: 462–467.

Kelley's Textbook of Internal Medicine, fourth edition. Edited by H. David Humes. Lippincott Williams & Wilkins, Philadelphia © 2000.

C H A P T E R
116

COLORECTAL NEOPLASIA

C. RICHARD BOLAND

The epithelium of the colon and rectum is one of the most rapidly proliferating tissues in the body. The rapid cell turnover permits the large intestine to renew itself on a continuing basis to provide an effective interface between the host and the fecal stream. The regulation of epithelial cell proliferation, migration, and cell death is critical to the maintenance of the proper number of cells in each epithelial crypt. Cell division occurs at the bases of the crypts, and the daughter cells destined for maturation migrate up the crypt toward the surface, where they undergo apoptosis and are shed after 2 to 3 days. Neoplasia occurs as a result of clonal expansion of a cell that has undergone a genetic alteration that results in loss of normal growth control, which permits an inappropriate accumulation of cells. Benign neoplasia (in the colon and rectum this constitutes an adenoma) can grow larger, but it is incapable of invasion and metastasis. Malignant neoplasia—cancer—evolves from benign neoplasia through the stepwise acquisition of additional genetic alterations that ultimately permit malignant cellular behavior.

In this chapter, the term "colon" will be used to refer to the colorectum; issues of clinical significance to rectal lesions will be specified.

■ COLORECTAL POLYPS

DEFINITION

Colorectal polyps are any excrescences found in the colon or rectum, which does not imply any specific pathologic variety. However, the pathogenesis and natural history are dependent on the pathologic characteristics of the polyp. Adenomatous polyps and hyperplastic polyps make up the vast majority of what is found in the colorectum. Adenomas are the most common and important of these, as they are the precursors of cancer. There is a longer list of much less prevalent hamartomatous polyps, such as juvenile polyps. Submucosal lesions may have a polypoid appearance, but the behavior of these depends on what is beneath the colonic epithelium.

INCIDENCE AND EPIDEMIOLOGIC FACTORS

Adenomatous polyps increase in prevalence with advancing age and can be found in at least 40% of the population. Not every adenomatous polyp will necessarily increase in size, and only a small fraction of them progress to cancer. The tendency to develop adenomas has a strong familial component that probably reflects both genetic and environmental influences. The significance of adenomas is that they serve as markers of an increased risk of colorectal cancer, and their removal is associated with a significant reduction in that risk.

Hyperplastic polyps make up about 15% to 20% of colorectal polyps, and their incidence increases with age. Only rarely do they grow more than 1 cm in diameter, and they are not premalignant lesions. They occur predominantly in the distal colon and rectum; unlike adenomas, they are uncommon in the proximal colon.

Juvenile polyps are the principal variety in children, may occur in 1% to 2% of young children (under 10 years), and are quite rare in adults. Peutz–Jeghers polyps are a unique pathologic variety of hamartoma that is pathognomonic of the eponymous syndrome.

Other polypoid lesions of the colorectum include inflammatory polyps (which are a consequence of inflammation and repair, but are not neoplastic) and any submucosal lesion that elevates the normal overlying mucosa. The submucosal lesions include lipomas, lymphoid nodules, carcinoids, metastatic tumors from other organs, and many others.

ETIOLOGIC FACTORS AND PATHOGENESIS

An adenomatous polyp develops when both alleles of the adenomatous polyposis coli gene *(APC)* are inactivated in a colorectal epithelial cell. The first allele is usually lost by a point mutation that creates a premature stop codon in one allele, also called a "nonsense mutation," which results in the synthesis of a truncated protein. The second allele is typically deleted from the nucleus by a poorly understood process that results in a loss of heterozygosity (LOH). The normal, or "wild-type," APC protein regulates the intracellular concentration of β-catenin, which plays a role in mediating proliferation, migration up the crypt, and adhesion of the epithelial cell to other epithelial cells (Fig. 116.1). As the colorectal epithelial cell leaves the zone of proliferation and moves toward the surface of the epithelium, the APC protein expression is triggered, which leads to a fall in intracellular β-catenin, cessation of proliferation, initiation of the cell death program, and weakening of the intercellular adhesion apparatus. Loss of the two APC alleles permits β-catenin to remain at a high level, which provides a substantial growth advantage

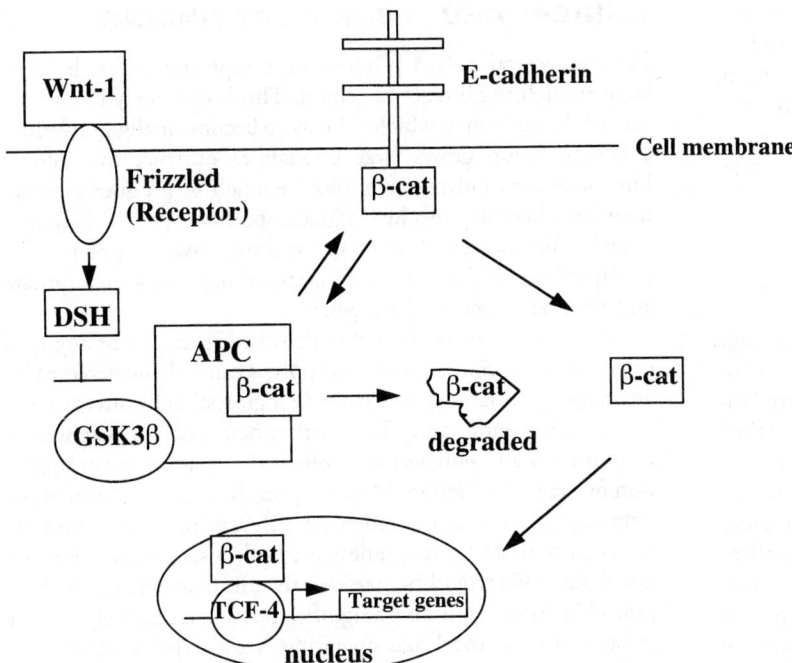

FIGURE 116.1. Regulation of β-catenin by the adenomatous polyposis coli gene *(APC)* in the colonic epithelial cell. Cellular proliferation and intercellular adhesion are controlled in part by β-catenin, which is regulated by *APC*. Not all of the members of this signaling pathway have been identified in the colon; it is likely similar to the WNT pathway of lower organisms, as indicated here. When β-catenin is present at a critical concentration in the cell, it binds to TCF-4, moves to the nucleus, and promotes the expression of proliferation-associated "target genes," including c-*myc* and cyclin D. β-Catenin is also part of the intercellular adhesion complex, as indicated by E-cadherin in the figure. *Wnt-1* signaling through the "frizzled" receptor activates DSH, which then inhibits GSK3β, which is required for activation of *APC* and the subsequent degradation of β-catenin. Thus, Wnt signaling leads to cellular proliferation. When the epithelial cell matures and migrates to the top of the colonic crypt, this signaling pathway is turned off. The APC protein is expressed and phosphorylated by GSK3β and binds to β-catenin, leading to its degradation. Expression of the proliferation-associated target genes falls, mitosis is inhibited, and degradation of the E-cadherin complex permits the dying cell to detach from the crypt and fall into the colonic lumen. The absence of APC from the colonic epithelial cell permits unrestrained growth, and the intact intercellular adhesion promotes the formation of a tumor mass.

for that cell's progeny. This permits a clone of cells to grow at the top of the crypt that have intact intercellular adhesion characteristics; senescence and detachment of the cell do not occur. An adenomatous polyp is the result.

Some adenomas grow larger, some regress, and others do not change in size. At least one explanation for this variable behavior is that half of all adenomas acquire a mutation in codons 12 or 13 of the K-*ras*-2 proto-oncogene, which further facilitates polyp growth. The *ras* gene mutations are most common in large, tubulovillous adenomas. Hyperplastic polyps have been much less extensively studied, but one model suggests that they are the result of *ras* mutations without concomitant *APC* mutations; these are not considered to be neoplasms or to be premalignant. A few colorectal polyps have features that are both adenomatous and hyperplastic, and these should be expected to act like adenomas.

A critical event in the evolution of adenoma-to-carcinoma progression is the loss of both alleles of the *p53* tumor suppressor gene. This typically occurs first by the acquisition of a point mutation in an evolutionarily conserved portion of the *p53* gene, which alters the amino acid encoded (a missense mutation) and alters the function of the protein. As described previously for the *APC* gene, the genomic instability of the adenoma may eventually lead to loss (LOH) of the other, wild-type copy of *p53*. Loss of both *p53* alleles frequently mediates the transition from the benign adenoma to cancer. The tumor progression sequence and the putative genetic lesions that occur with each step are outlined schematically in Fig. 116.2.

The pathogenesis of the juvenile polyp is unknown, but the identification of two tumor suppressor genes that are associated with juvenile polyposis coli (JPC; see below) suggests that this polyp represents a low-grade, poorly understood neoplasm. In-

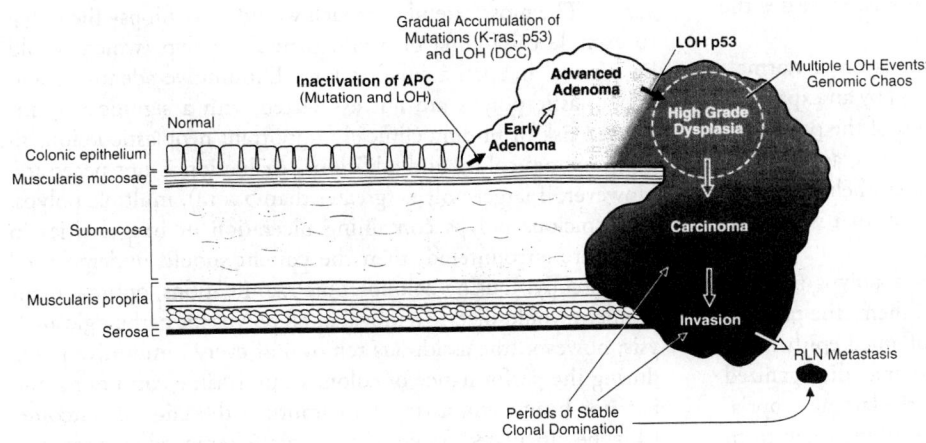

FIGURE 116.2. Tumor progression and genetic alterations in colorectal cancer development. This is a proposed model of the genetic events by which normal colorectal epithelium first enters into a neoplastic growth pathway (biallelic inactivation of the *APC* gene), undergoes additional growth in a variety of directions depending on the accumulated genetic events that might include K-*ras* mutations, *p53* mutations, or LOH at tumor suppressor gene loci), and the adenoma-to-carcinoma transition that occurs upon the inactivation of the *p53* gene (which will involve processes that inhibit the products of both *p53* alleles). (From Boland CR, Sato J, Appelman HD et al. Microallelotyping defines the sequence and tempo of allelic losses at tumour suppressor gene loci during colorectal cancer progression. *Nature Medicine* 1995;1:902–909, with permission.)

flammatory polyps are made up of non-neoplastic but disorganized tissue that results from cycles of epithelial damage and repair. These are seen in the setting of chronic inflammation, usually inflammatory bowel disease. Their principal importance is that inflammatory polyps are found in colons with increased malignant risk, and these polyps may grossly resemble an adenoma or cancer.

PATHOLOGIC FACTORS

Adenomatous polyps are defined by their size, their morphologic configuration, and their histopathologic features. The most important clinical issue is size. Polyps smaller than 6 mm are "diminutive," polyps 6 to 9 mm are "small," and those greater than 10 mm are considered large and clinically important. Polyps on a distinguishable stalk are considered pedunculated, which facilitates their complete removal colonoscopically, and those without a stalk are considered sessile. The histopathologic features of a polyp correlate generally with size and the accumulation of genetic abnormalities. Most small adenomatous polyps are tubular adenomas, characterized by a complex network of branching adenomatous glands. Larger adenomas are more likely to acquire a "villous" component, in which the adenomatous glands extend straight down from the surface to the center of the polyp, microscopically creating fingerlike projections. Tubulovillous (or villoglandular) adenomas have a combination of both.

Some polyps will develop a focus carcinoma completely surrounded by adenoma. If the malignant lesion does not invade the *muscularis mucosae,* it is not considered invasive, and is usually termed carcinoma in situ or, simply, high-grade dysplasia. As a clinical issue, noninvasive cancer in the head of a polyp virtually never metastasizes.

Every adenoma is at least mildly dysplastic. All parts of the spectrum from mild dysplasia to carcinoma may be found in adenomatous polyps. The likelihood of encountering carcinoma increases directly in proportion to the size of the adenoma. The likelihood of finding carcinoma in diminutive or small adenomas is 1.3%. In adenomas 1 to 2 cm in size, 9.5% contain carcinoma; in adenomas greater than 2 cm, 46% have cancer. Villous features are more commonly seen in larger adenomas, and the presence of villous features, even in a small adenoma, increases the likelihood that cancer will be present.

Juvenile polyps are made up of a surface layer of normal-appearing colonic epithelium, which is elevated by an expansion of the underlying lamina propria. The interior of the polyp also is filled with dilated, mucous-filled glands, edema, and inflammatory cells. The coexistence of adenomatous epithelium should be carefully sought within juvenile polyps, since that is thought to be the source of the malignant potential.

Inflammatory polyps are also called pseudopolyps (really a misnomer because their morphology renders them true polyps). These lesions are covered with normal or inflamed epithelium, and are filled with inflammatory cells, edema, disorganized glands, vascular engorgement, and fibrosis of the lamina propria. The significance of these lesions is in distinguishing them from true neoplasms, which commonly occur in inflamed colons.

CLINICAL AND LABORATORY FINDINGS

Most colorectal polyps produce no symptoms. A few become large enough to obstruct the colon. This is extremely rare in the case of the adenoma, which is likely to become malignant before a benign lesion grows large enough to obstruct the colonic lumen. Benign polyps rarely bleed enough to produce anemia; however, they may produce a guaiac-positive stool if the polyp is large and located close to the rectum. Juvenile polyps may prolapse beyond the anus in children, or they may autoamputate and thus be passed in the stool.

There are no blood tests that detect the presence of any type of polyp in the colon. Colorectal polyps can only be detected by an imaging procedure (such as a radiologic test) or by direct visualization using endoscopy. The current best mode of diagnosis is colonoscopy and polypectomy followed by pathologic examination of the excised lesion. Novel approaches, such as "virtual colonoscopy," are in development, which may provide a noninvasive, computerized tomographic method to screen for colorectal neoplasia. This would be particularly advantageous when the a priori likelihood of finding a significant lesion is relatively low. At present, this approach has operating characteristics similar to a barium enema, but is less sensitive than colonoscopy.

OPTIMAL MANAGEMENT

Adenomatous polyps are common and are often found in the course of routine screening in asymptomatic patients (see next section on colorectal cancer). When encountered, they should be completely removed colonoscopically. A partial biopsy is not adequate management, as it can lead to an underestimation of the pathologic processes. Polyps can be removed by electrocautery using either biopsy forceps as a monopolar electrode ("hot biopsy") or by snare cautery, which is most often employed to completely excise pedunculated lesions. Polyps containing only adenomatous tissue (with any grade of dysplasia) are adequately treated by total polypectomy. Even cancer in the head of a polyp is adequately treated if the margin of resection shows unambiguous excision of the cancer with an uninvolved excision margin. Surgical resection is not necessary in this case.

Many adenomatous polyps are discovered during flexible sigmoidoscopy. If a diminutive (less than 6 mm) polyp is encountered during sigmoidoscopy, the optimal management is controversial. The most careful approach would be to biopsy the polyp to exclude carcinoma or a villoglandular polyp (which would be unusual in such a small lesion). Diminutive adenomas and hyperplastic polyps are not associated with a significantly increased risk of finding clinically important neoplastic lesions in the proximal colon, and additional evaluation is not necessary. However, if larger polyps (greater than 5 mm), multiple polyps, or suspicious polyps containing ulceration or irregularities in shape are encountered, then the patient should undergo total colonoscopy. During colonoscopic examinations, optimal management would dictate removal of all polyps for pathologic analysis; however, the assiduous removal of every diminutive polyp during the performance of colonoscopy is time consuming and has not been demonstrated to improve the clinical outcome. Most pedunculated polyps can be totally removed colonoscopically. However, large (greater than 9 mm) sessile polyps should either be removed by an endoscopist with interventional expertise or may require surgery. Large polyps that are not removed should undergo multiple biopsies to assist in making a decision about the need for surgical removal.

COLORECTAL CANCER

DEFINITION

Colorectal cancer is a malignant neoplasm of the colon that has developed through the multistep accumulation of critical mutations in growth-regulatory genes that permit invasion and metastasis to occur. Colorectal cancers usually (and probably always) evolve from pre-existing adenomas, although not necessarily from a polyp. The initial adenomatous lesion may have been small and flat. By the time a cancer is found clinically, the progenitor adenomatous tissue may no longer be present due to different rates of proliferation and the relative growth advantage of the malignant tissue.

INCIDENCE AND EPIDEMIOLOGIC FACTORS

Cancer of the large bowel (colon and rectum) is the most common neoplasm of the gastrointestinal (GI) tract and is the second most common cause of cancer-related mortality in the United States. Colorectal cancer occurs at some time in the lives of 5% to 6% of the population of the United States. The clinical importance of this disease is based both on the incidence of this disease and on the fact that early detection leads to a substantial improvement in outcome.

The incidence of colorectal cancer varies widely among nations. It is highest in industrialized countries, such as the United States, Western Europe, and Australia, and is much lower in developing countries. The principal exception to this rule is Japan, an industrialized nation with an incidence of colorectal cancer less than one-fourth that in the United States. It is of considerable interest that the incidence of colorectal cancer is increasing rapidly in Japan at the same time that other sweeping cultural changes have taken place. Within the high-risk regions, cancers of the colon and rectum are slightly more common in men than women, and the incidence rates are equal between blacks and whites. The most important risk factor in the United States is age. The incidence is very low before age 40, and the relative risk increases as an exponential function of age thereafter. The rates of colorectal cancer have been slowly increasing in the United States over the past four decades, although the mortality rate has fallen slightly, presumably due to earlier detection and improved management.

Frequent aspirin users have a relative risk of 0.6 (aspirin is protective) for colorectal cancer mortality, compared with nonusers. A similar degree of protection is conferred by other anti-inflammatory drugs, and this is thought to be accomplished by the inhibition of cyclooxygenase 2 (Cox-2) activity.

The age-adjusted relative risk for colorectal cancer among patients with one affected first-degree relative is 1.72. More than one affected first-degree relative increases the risk to 2.75, and the presence of an affected relative under the age of 45 increases the relative risk to 5.37. The existence of relatives with colorectal cancers occurring after age 60 do not add substantially to the familial risk. A similar degree of incremental risk is associated with first-degree relatives with adenomatous polyps, with additive risks when there are multiple or young relatives affected.

ETIOLOGIC FACTORS AND PATHOGENESIS

Although diets rich in fat and total calories have been implicated as a factor in the high incidence of colorectal cancer in the Western world, there are undoubtedly multiple factors that contribute to the pathogenesis of this disease. Per-capita ingestion of meat correlates with increased risk, whereas dietary fiber, the nondigested residue of complex plant carbohydrates, appears to protect against colorectal cancer. People in geographic locations with low levels of selenium in the soil have higher incidences of colorectal cancer, and selenium supplements may reduce mortality. However, excessive dietary selenium can be toxic, and routine supplementation is not recommended. Interventional trials that modify diets in patients who have already developed one or more adenomatous polyps have failed to reduce the recurrence rates of small adenomas, even when followed for up to 4 years. It may require decades of significant dietary modification to reduce the rates of new neoplasms.

The international differences observed in colorectal cancer incidence appear to be mediated in part by environmental, probably dietary, factors. Groups that migrate from low- to high-incidence regions experience a change in cancer incidence that gradually matches that in the new region.

Colorectal cancer develops through the multistep accumulation of genetic alterations—including point mutations and genetic deletions—as described above in the section on polyps. Whereas adenomas represent benign clonal expansions of colonic epithelium that have lost one level of growth control, carcinomas are clonal expansions that emerge from adenomas, in which there have been additional genetic modifications that permit invasion and metastasis. One genetic accident that can mediate adenoma-to-carcinoma conversion is biallelic inactivation of the *p53* gene. The likelihood of accumulating the critical combination of genes required for the malignant phenotype is low, and in spite of the underlying genomic instability in neoplastic tissue, this process requires many years (or even decades) and occurs in only a small proportion of all adenomas.

Although all cancers evolve through the accumulation of genetic alterations, not all cancers use the same pathway. All colorectal neoplasms are driven by genomic instability, which increases the mutational rate in the tissue. However, there are many ways to mutate the genome. About 85% of colorectal cancers have a type of genomic instability called *chromosomal instability*, which results in chromosomal deletion and numerous LOH events. These tumors are aneuploid, and have only one copy of both *APC* and *p53*; the single, remaining copies of these two genes in the tumors are mutated and inactive.

The 15% of colorectal cancers without chromosomal instability are diploid and have a form of hypermutability known as *microsatellite instability (MSI)*. MSI results from loss of the DNA mismatch repair (MMR) system, and short, repetitive DNA sequences are very prone to mutation during new DNA strand synthesis. There are about 10^5 of these simple repetitive "microsatellite" sequences in our genome, and most are in noncoding regions; those mutations are not thought to be biologically important. However, there are some microsatellite sequences in the coding regions of critical genes, such as the transforming growth factor (TGF) β_1 type II receptor ($TGF\beta_1 RII$), which is critical for inhibiting epithelial proliferation in the colon. Most tumors with MSI have a mutation in this sequence, which inactivates the gene and promotes growth. Several other genes with coding microsatellites are mutated in such tumors, including the insulin-like growth factor type 2 receptor (which is a component of the TGF-β signaling pathway), the apoptotic gene *BAX*, two of the DNA MMR genes themselves, *hMSH6* and *hMSH3*, the *E2F4* gene, and even *APC*.

The DNA MMR system consists of a complex of several proteins, as described below (see the section on hereditary non-polyposis colorectal cancer). In about 80% to 90% of sporadic cancers with MSI, one of the DNA MMR genes, *hMLH1*, has undergone hypermethylation of its promoter, which silences the expression of the gene, resulting in loss of DNA MMR function and MSI. Abnormalities of gene methylation can be found throughout the non-neoplastic tissue in these colons, but the mechanism responsible is unknown.

CLINICAL FINDINGS

Early colorectal cancers, the ones that clinicians are most interested in finding, produce no symptoms whatsoever. Symptomatic colorectal neoplasia has two characteristic modes of presentation. The first of these is lower intestinal obstruction, which occurs when tumors (usually in the sigmoid colon or rectum) become large enough to obstruct the lumen. Second, tumor bleeding may result in hematochezia (most often with distal tumors) or iron deficiency anemia (more often noted with cancers in the cecum or ascending colon). The tendency for intestinal neoplasms to ooze blood has been exploited in the effort to detect asymptomatic cancers at an early stage. On physical examination, an abdominal mass or enlarged liver is found only in advanced disease. Occult bleeding can be detected by rectal examination. Rarely, colon cancers perforate spontaneously and present with an acute abdomen.

PATHOLOGIC FACTORS

Adenocarcinoma accounts for over 95% of malignancies of the colon and rectum. The prognosis in colorectal cancer is directly related to the penetration depth of the malignancy rather than to the total tumor bulk. Dukes initially categorized staging for rectal cancer, but this system has undergone repeated modification and adaptation to include colonic cancers as well. An internationally accepted classification and the historical precursors of colorectal cancer staging are outlined in Table 116.1.

Cancers of the colon spread by direct extension through the wall of the bowel into the pericolic fat and mesentery, to the mesenteric lymph nodes, and via the portal vein to the liver. Additional spread may occasionally be evident throughout the peritoneal cavity, to the lungs, and less commonly to other distant sites. Rectal carcinoma spreads by direct extension into the

TABLE 116.1	**STAGING OF COLORECTAL CANCER**[a]

Dukes (Rectal Cancer)

A. First-stage. Growth limited to bowel. No extension to perirectal adipose tissue or nodes. (85% 5-year survival).

B. Second-stage. Extension of growth into perirectal adipose tissue. No nodal metastases. (64% 5-year survival).

C. Third-stage. Nodal metastases regardless of depth of penetration.

D. Fourth-stage. Distant spread such as liver. Termed "D" by Turnbull.

Astler and Coller (Colorectal Cancer)

A. Growths limited to mucosa (100%).

B_1. Growths extending into muscularis propria but not perimural adipose tissue. No nodal metastases (67%).

B_2. Growths extending into perimural adipose tissue. No nodal metastases (54%).

C_1. Growths not extending into perimural adipose tissue. Nodal metastases present (43%).

C_2. Growths extending into perimural adipose tissue. Nodal metastases present (22%).

TNM Staging (Colorectal Cancer)

0. Tis, N0, M0 (100%)

I. T1, N0, M0 (100%): T2, N0, M0 (85%)

II. T3, N0, M0 (70%): T4, N0, M0 (30%)

III. Any T, N1, M0 (60%): Any T, N2, N3, M0 (30%)

IV. Any T, any N, M1 (3%)

---

[a] Staging of rectal and colon carcinoma and predicted outcomes, based on the modified Dukes' staging, the Astler and Coller modifications, the American Joint Commission of Cancer (AJCC), and the Union Internationale Contra le Cancer (UICC), with 5-year survival.
Tis, in situ; T1, invades submucosa; T2, invades muscularis propria; T3, invades through muscularis into subserosa or perimural tissues; T4, invades through serosa or into other organs or tissues. N0, no nodal metastases; N1, 1–3 regional nodal metastases; N2, 4 or more regional nodal metastases; N3, metastasis, in any node along course of major named blood vessel. M0, no distant metastases; M1, presence distant metastases.
(Modified from Fisher ER, et al. Dukes' Classification revisited. *Cancer* 1989;64:2354; and Cooper HS, Slemmer JR. Surgical pathology of carcinoma of the colon and rectum. *Semin Oncol* 1991;18:367.)

perirectal fat (since the rectum is below the peritoneal reflection and has no serosa) and to the regional lymph nodes. Rectal cancers metastasize to the liver or other distant sites somewhat less frequently and are more likely to be associated with progressive local disease in the pelvis after an initial resection (which can be very difficult to manage). This tends not to occur after proximal resections. Anastomotic recurrences are relatively uncommon with current surgical management and are most often seen after resections of high rectal lesions in which tumor was inadvertently left behind in an attempt to preserve the rectum.

LABORATORY FINDINGS

Most early colorectal cancers are not associated with any laboratory abnormalities. Screening for early colorectal cancers can be performed by looking for occult colonic bleeding by means of a barium enema or a colonoscopic exam.

The amount of blood lost from a colorectal neoplasm is related to the size of the lesion. The ability to detect an occult neoplasm with a fecal occult blood test (FOBT) is a function of both the amount of blood in the stool and its dispersion throughout the stool. As a practical matter, more distally located lesions are more likely to be associated with a positive FOBT since blood will be distributed on the surface of the stool, where it will be sampled. Small (2 cm) colorectal cancers—the targets of screening—will typically add only 1 to 2 mL of blood to the physiologic loss of about 0.7 mL of blood per day. Guaiac-based FOBTs detect the peroxidase activity associated with blood. Therefore, maneuvers that make the FOBT more sensitive may lead to falsely positive tests, as the test detects ordinary blood losses or the peroxidase activity from red meat, or fresh fruits and vegetables, in the diet.

Advanced colorectal cancers, especially those from the cecum or proximal colon, may present with anemia since the lesions may become large (greater than 3 to 4 cm) and hemorrhagic before they cause obstruction. Adenocarcinomas may produce elevations of the plasma carcinoembryonic antigen (CEA), an oncofetal glycoprotein. When found, this may be helpful to determine residual or recurrent tumor burden, but the CEA is not an effective screening test because it is neither sensitive nor specific for colorectal cancer. CEA levels may be spuriously elevated in the presence of severe liver disease.

OPTIMAL SCREENING AND MANAGEMENT

Screening with Fecal Occult Blood Tests

In asymptomatic patients, colon cancer may be found by screening the stools for occult fecal blood. When found by screening an asymptomatic individual, colorectal cancer is more likely to be detected at a pathologic stage that is associated with favorable patient survival. Nevertheless, controversy surrounds the selection of patients to be screened and the methods employed to detect occult fecal bleeding. Guaiac-based FOBTs, such as Hemoccult cards and other similar products, are positive in only about half of persons with colon cancer, and the sensitivity will vary depending on how the screening is performed. The test can be made more sensitive, for example, by rehydrating the cards with a drop of water before development; however, nearly 10% of patients will test positive. In one large study using this maneuver, annual screening for occult fecal bleeding reduced colorectal cancer mortality by 33%, principally by detecting tumors at an earlier, more curable stage. However, the increased sensitivity achieved by rehydration reduced the specificity of a positive test from about 5%–10% down to 2.2%. When conventional (non-rehydrated) FOBTs are used and the screening frequency is reduced to every other year, the reduction in mortality falls to 15% to 18%. More intensive screening increases the diagnosis of early cancers but requires more resources.

To screen efficiently for asymptomatic colorectal cancer, the number of false-positive fecal occult blood tests must be limited. This can be accomplished by restricting the ingestion of rare beef during the period preceding and during testing. As alluded to above, guaiac-based slide tests should not be rehydrated prior to their development, since this tends to increase false-positive

results, particularly when the diet is high in peroxidase-containing foods, such as beef and certain fruits and vegetables. Large doses of vitamin C may mask fecal bleeding by inhibiting the peroxidase reaction. When properly performed, less than 2% of asymptomatic patients over age 50 will have positive tests. When evaluated with colonoscopy (or, as an alternative, sigmoidoscopy plus air contrast barium enema), a bleeding colonic lesion is found in approximately half of the group with a positive screening test, and 10% of the group will have colorectal cancer. Stage I or II cancers are found in 65% to 90% of asymptomatic patients whose tumor has been detected by screening with an FOBT.

Screening with Sigmoidoscopy

A second, complementary approach to screening is flexible sigmoidoscopy, which is very sensitive and, when coupled with biopsy, specific for neoplasia; however, it screens only the distal half of the colon. This has been recommended beginning at age 50, to be repeated every 4 years. Sigmoidoscopy has been shown to reduce the incidence of fatal cancer in the distal colorectum by 70% to 79% for a period of 10 years in two case-control studies.

The finding of one or more adenomatous polyps larger than 5 mm at sigmoidoscopy indicates the need for a full colonoscopy, at which time all polyps should be removed. Follow-up examinations may be safely deferred for at least 3 years (and perhaps as much as 5 years) after all lesions have been completely removed. The finding of hyperplastic polyps or diminutive (less than 6 mm) adenomas is more controversial, but the best evidence suggests that patients with these findings are not at significantly greater risk to have clinically important lesions in the proximal colon than those who have no lesions in the distal colon. The appropriate follow-up may require modification based on other factors, such as a prior history of colorectal lesions or a family history of neoplasia.

The management of patients with a positive family history of "sporadic" colon cancer (one or more relatives with cancers or polyps but without a familial cancer syndrome) is a challenge at this time. Annual or frequent colonoscopy in such patients, particularly those with a single affected relative, has a low yield, and the cost of surveillance per neoplastic lesion is high. For unknown reasons, familial risk is relatively less important in rectal cancer.

Surveillance of High-risk Patients

Surveillance (follow-up after treatment of the initial lesion) of patients who have had adenomatous polyps removed is more controversial. It is more important to initiate a follow-up program in patients who have had larger (greater than 1 cm), multiple, or more dysplastic lesions removed. In these higher risk patients, the recommendations for follow-up examination are similar to those for patients who have had cancers resected. For patients who have had a single, small (less than 1 cm) adenomatous polyp removed, a single follow-up examination is recommended after 3 years. If this examination reveals no recurrent neoplasia, patients may be screened in a manner similar to those in the general population. Patients with intermediate degrees of risk (those with a single adenomatous polyp 1 to 2 cm in diameter, or those with multiple diminutive polyps ranging from 1 to 5 mm in diameter) require a less well-defined surveillance schedule. Assuming that all lesions have been completely removed from the colon, the first follow-up examination may be deferred for 3 years. If this reveals additional neoplasia, which will occur in about 40% of cases, the test should be repeated again in 3 years. It is not known as to whether longer screening intervals, such as 5 to 10 years, will be sufficient to prevent cancer. Longer intervals are appropriate for most patients, but this approach is not perfect, and some patients will develop interval cancers. Colonoscopic surveillance can produce a dramatic reduction in subsequent cancer incidence (perhaps on the order of 75% to 90%), but this program requires a considerable investment of resources.

Symptomatic Disease

If there are symptoms or signs suggestive of large intestinal disease, diagnostic colonoscopy (not just sigmoidoscopy) should be undertaken, regardless of the presence or absence of occult blood in the stool, since an FOBT is not sufficiently sensitive to exclude neoplasia. Flexible sigmoidoscopy is recommended as a screening test of the distal colon and rectum for asymptomatic individuals over age 50. Only two-thirds of colorectal neoplasms occur within the reach of this instrument, so it is inadequate as a solitary means to evaluate a patient with symptoms suggesting a neoplasm, with anemia, or with a positive FOBT.

Treatment of Colon Cancer

Some colorectal cancers, particularly those found in adenomatous polyps, can be excised colonoscopically. Most cancers require surgical resections. Principles of surgical therapy are based on the blood supply and lymphatic drainage of the colon. For most cancers, surgical excision with a 5-cm margin is the optimal therapy; however, this is based more on tradition than on data. Cancers of the cecum, ascending colon, and hepatic flexure are best treated with a right hemicolectomy and ileocolonic anastomosis. Cancers of the distal transverse colon, splenic flexure, or proximal descending colon may be treated by extended right hemicolectomies or segmental resections. Distal descending colon or sigmoid colon cancers are treated by a segmental resection ("low anterior resection") and primary colonic anastomosis. The treatment of colon cancers (above the level of the rectum) does not require a colostomy.

Treatment of Rectal Cancer

The treatment of rectal cancer is more complex than that of colorectal cancers and depends on its location in the rectum, the depth of invasion, and size. Rectal cancers in the proximal third of the rectum (more than 12 cm from the anus) can usually be resected with an operation that preserves the lower rectum and anus. Cancers in the mid-lower rectum (in the lowest 7 to 8 cm) may require a proctocolectomy, which necessitates ab-

dominoperineal resection and a sigmoid colostomy. In order to avoid such radical surgery, local resection may be undertaken for rectal cancers when the tumor is small (less than 3 cm), polypoid, not fixed to submucosal tissues, and involves less than 25% of the circumference of the rectum. This approach may be chosen for patients with more advanced tumors who are at greater risk for surgical complications or who adamantly refuse to accept a colostomy.

Cancer in Adenomatous Polyps

Cancers that are confined to the head of a polyp and do not invade the stalk can be removed by colonoscopic polypectomy. When there is a clear margin of benign tissue between the cancer and the cut edge of the polyp, the incidence of recurrent disease is very low and the patient may be safely managed without a colonic resection. When a clear margin of benign tissue is not evident or when invasion occurs in a sessile lesion, colonic resection is indicated. In the rare instance when a poorly differentiated carcinoma occurs in a colonoscopically removed polyp, the outcome is less certain, and a formal cancer operation should be considered, depending on the clinical circumstances of the patient.

Follow-up of Colon Cancer

Patients who have had a cancer removed have a 5% likelihood of developing a metachronous tumor during the subsequent 10 years. The chance of recurrent neoplasia is twice as high in patients who have multiple synchronous lesions, either adenocarcinomas or adenomatous polyps. Patients who have had cancers removed should be reexamined with colonoscopy 6 to 12 months after the initial surgery. If new neoplastic lesions are encountered, these should be removed and the patients examined again in 1 year. If no new neoplastic lesions are encountered, the surveillance interval may be increased to 3 years indefinitely, except in cases where hereditary nonpolyposis colorectal cancer is suspected, as these require more frequent surveillance.

Adjuvant Postoperative Chemotherapy for Colon Cancer

Approximately 50% of all patients with large intestinal cancers undergo resection and have a long-term disease-free survival. The development of metastatic cancer remains a substantial threat in patients who have been told that their surgery was successful in terms of removing the primary tumor. Adjuvant therapy is the treatment of patients who have undergone successful resections with the intent of preventing tumor recurrences. Adjuvant therapy is not indicated in patients with stage I or II colon cancers [i.e., cancer limited to the wall of the colon (Dukes A or B1)] and is not associated with lymph node metastasis because the cancer-free survival rate after removal of these tumors is already better than 80% and chemotherapy does not significantly improve survival in this combined group. A modest but statistically insignificant improvement in 7-year disease-free survival from 71% to 79% has been reported for patients with stage II cancers.

Stage III cancer (i.e., with regional lymph node involvement) should be treated with adjuvant chemotherapy. The use of combined 5-fluorouracil (5-FU) and levamisole in patients with stage III cancers improves the 3.5-year disease-free survival from 47% to 63% and delays the time to recurrence. Adjuvant therapy requires the weekly administration of intravenous 5-FU for 1 year and a 3-day course of oral levamisole every 2 weeks. The toxicity may be unacceptable in some patients, and 30% are unable to complete the full year of treatment. Currently, the use of 5-FU and leucovorin has emerged as an alternative to 5-FU/levamisole, and a variety of regimens have been tested, all meeting similar results. No superiority in survival for either levamisole, leucovorin, or other drug in combination with 5-FU has been established; however, some of the leucovorin-containing regimens are of equal benefit but may be completed in only 6 months. Attempts have been made to improve outcome by portal venous infusion of chemotherapeutic agents to increase delivery to the liver, but this has not been shown to significantly decrease liver metastases to date. Modified forms of 5-FU are currently being tested to reduce toxicity.

Adjunctive Radiation Therapy for Rectal Cancer

Radiation therapy has a role as an adjunct to surgery for rectal cancer. Combined postoperative adjuvant therapy using 4,500 to 5,040 cGy plus a 5-FU–based chemotherapy regimen reduces recurrence rates in stage T3 and T4 (deeply invasive or regionally metastatic rectal cancer) by 34%. Many patients will find this regimen difficult to complete, but the benefits may be lifesaving. Chemoradiation may be used preoperatively to convert an apparently nonresectable tumor to one that can be surgically removed in some instances, and is increasingly being used in all rectal cancers.

Metastatic Colorectal Cancer

Intensive postoperative surveillance programs may detect an isolated focus of metastatic disease in the liver. Patients in whom additional metastases can be excluded should be offered surgical resection since medical therapies do not cure this disease. There are no successful modalities for treatment of widespread metastatic disease at this time. Chemotherapy (5-FU and other drugs) may produce partial tumor shrinkage in 15% to 25% of patients with advanced metastatic disease; however, no chemotherapeutic regimen has been proven to significantly prolong life in this disease. Chemotherapeutic regimens have played a palliative rather than curative role in metastatic disease. Hepatic artery infusions of chemotherapeutic agents have been used in numerous trials, but evidence from randomized controlled trials has yet to show a significant survival advantage for this therapy. Radiation therapy may provide symptomatic relief for some patients with localized metastatic lesions and may be used as a palliative measure.

■ FAMILIAL COLORECTAL CANCER SYNDROMES
FAMILIAL ADENOMATOUS POLYPOSIS

Familiality is a major issue in colorectal cancer, but only a small proportion of such cancers reflect inherited syndromes. The most easily recognized of these is familial adenomatous polyposis (FAP), which is an autosomal dominant disease characterized by the development of multiple adenomatous polyps, beginning in adolescence, followed by the appearance of carcinoma at a median age of about 40 to 45 years. This disease occurs in about 1 in 10,000 births, and it may occur as a "new mutation" in perhaps 25% to 30% of cases. Gardner's syndrome, most of Turcot's syndrome, and other eponymous variations of FAP are all attributable to germ line mutations in the same gene and highlight the phenotypic variation characteristic of this disease.

Etiologic Factors, Pathogenesis, and Disease Manifestations

Familial adenomatous polyposis is caused by a germ line mutation in the *APC* gene, located on chromosome 5q, as described above. Virtually all of the disease-causing mutations described create a prematurely truncated protein product of the *APC* gene. Every cell in the body carries this germ line mutation in FAP, and these cells are phenotypically normal. When the second, wild-type allele is mutated or lost from an individual colonic epithelial cell, it undergoes clonal expansion and evolves into an adenomatous polyp. This same process of biallelic inactivation occurs during the evolution of a sporadic adenoma as discussed above. However, in FAP, the likelihood is greater that many adenomas will develop early in life because the germ line lesion is present in every colonic cell from birth. Patients with FAP are at risk to develop small intestinal adenomas, fundic gland hyperplasia in the stomach, and extraintestinal manifestations including mandibular and cranial osteomas, dental abnormalities, fibromas, lipomas, epidermoid and sebaceous cysts, desmoid tumors, and pigmented lesions in the ocular fundus. FAP patients are at risk for periampullary adenomas and carcinoma. The phenotypic manifestations of the disease can, in part, be predicted based on the location of the mutation in the *APC* gene. Of particular interest, certain mutations occurring at the beginning (5′ end) of the *APC* gene can produce a mild form of FAP called attenuated adenomatous polyposis coli (AAPC), or attenuated FAP, in which only a few polyps may develop, and the onset of adenomas and cancer is delayed by a decade or more compared with the classic forms of the disease. This is still FAP, but it is a mild form that is likely to be underdiagnosed.

One mutation in the *APC* gene does not inactivate the gene but creates a microsatellite tract, which is intrinsically unstable and is predisposed to developing another, inactivating mutation. This sequence variation, I1307K, is present in 6% of Ashkenazi Jews but is relatively weak in its expression as a cancer-predisposing gene. Individuals carrying I1307K may develop multiple colorectal adenomas, may have as much as a two- to threefold increase in cancer risk, and develop cancers approximately a decade earlier than usual.

Optimal Management of Fap

In FAP, screening sigmoidoscopy should be performed annually beginning in adolescence. The median age for first polyp is about age 16; the polyps occur diffusely, but the onset will be later in the attenuated forms of the disease. Considerable variation in phenotype may occur within families, presumably because of the presence of independently inherited "modifier" genes. A diagnostic blood test, the truncated protein test, is available for FAP based on the fact that the *APC* gene is mutated in a way that produces a prematurely truncated gene product in most cases. Each family will have its own unique mutation; unfortunately, only 60% to 70% of mutations will be detected with this test. If the test is positive in an index family member, it is extremely sensitive and specific to definitively rule the disease in or out in the relatives.

Treatment of FAP calls for either a total proctocolectomy or a subtotal colectomy with ileorectal or ileo-anal anastomosis in certain circumstances. Complete removal of all colorectal tissue is the most effective means of preventing the cancer; however, if the rectum is relatively free of polyps, a rectum-sparing operation in conjunction with an intensive program of proctoscopic follow-up may be elected as alternative, although less certain, management. The advantages of sparing the rectum are unfortunately associated with a 10% risk for the development of rectal cancer in spite of vigorous follow-up. Sulindac 300 to 400 mg per day can reduce the number of polyps in the colons and rectums of patients with FAP, but cancers have developed in spite of this treatment regimen. Patients who have undergone colectomies are still at risk for the development of malignant neoplasms in the periampullary region (10% to 15% of patients) and abdominal desmoid tumors (5% to 10% of patients). Patients with the I1307K permutation may not require surgery, and may be managed with frequent colonoscopy.

HEREDITARY NONPOLYPOSIS COLORECTAL CANCER (OR LYNCH SYNDROME)

Hereditary nonpolyposis colorectal cancer (HNPCC) refers to familial colorectal cancer that is not FAP. In those instances in which a germ line mutation in one of the DNA MMR genes is linked to the disease, the term Lynch syndrome may be used. The clinical diagnosis of HNPCC can be confidently made (using the "Amsterdam criteria") when there are three affected family members, one of whom is a first-degree relative of the other two, when one member has been affected by cancer prior to age 50. Some true Lynch syndrome kindreds fail to meet these criteria because of small family size or incomplete penetrance of

the disease. The incidence of this disease is uncertain, but it accounts for about 3% to 4% of all colon cancers, and perhaps 1 in 500 births, making it a relatively common genetic disease. The key feature of the disease is an increased risk to develop cancer of specific organs—especially the colon and endometrium—at uncharacteristically early ages (Table 116.2).

Etiologic Factors, Pathogenesis, and Disease Manifestations

Lynch syndrome is an autosomal dominant disease caused by a germ line mutation in one of the DNA MMR genes (Fig. 116.3). Mutations in any one of these genes cause the same syndrome (Table 116.3). Development of cancer occurs along a different pathway than occurs in most sporadic cancers or in FAP. Every cell in the body carries the germ line mutation in one allele of one DNA MMR gene. A genetic accident occurs in the matching allele in one cell, which then develops MSI. Neoplasia evolves as genes controlling growth accumulate inactivating mutations at microsatellite sequences.

Now that the disease can be confidently diagnosed, it is known that penetrance of the disease is incomplete; 91% of men and 69% of women with Lynch syndrome develop cancer during their lifetimes, and colon cancer develops in only 74% and 30% of men and women, respectively. Women have a 20% to 42%

TABLE 116.3. INCIDENCE OF GERM LINE MUTATIONS IN LYNCH SYNDROME

HNPCC Gene	Incidence/Proportion of Families
hMSH2	31%
hMLH1	33%
hPMS1	Rare (one family)
hPMS2	4%
hMSH6	Rare (a few families)
Undetermined loci	32%

HNPCC, hereditary nonpolyposis colorectal cancer.

TABLE 116.2. ESTIMATES OF CANCER RISK BY ORGAN SITE IN LYNCH SYNDROME

Cancer Site	Lifetime Cancer Risk	Relative Risk	Median Age (y)
Any cancer by age 70	91% (men), 69% (women)	—	—
Colon or rectum	74% (men), 30% (women)	—	46
Endometrium	20–42% (by age 70)		46
Stomach	—	4.1	54
Ovaries	—	3.5	40
Small intestine	—	25	53
Hepatobiliary system	—	4.9	66
Kidney	—	3.2	66
Ureter	—	22	56
Kidney/ureter	—	75.3	—

Single base mispairs   **Insertion or deletion loops**

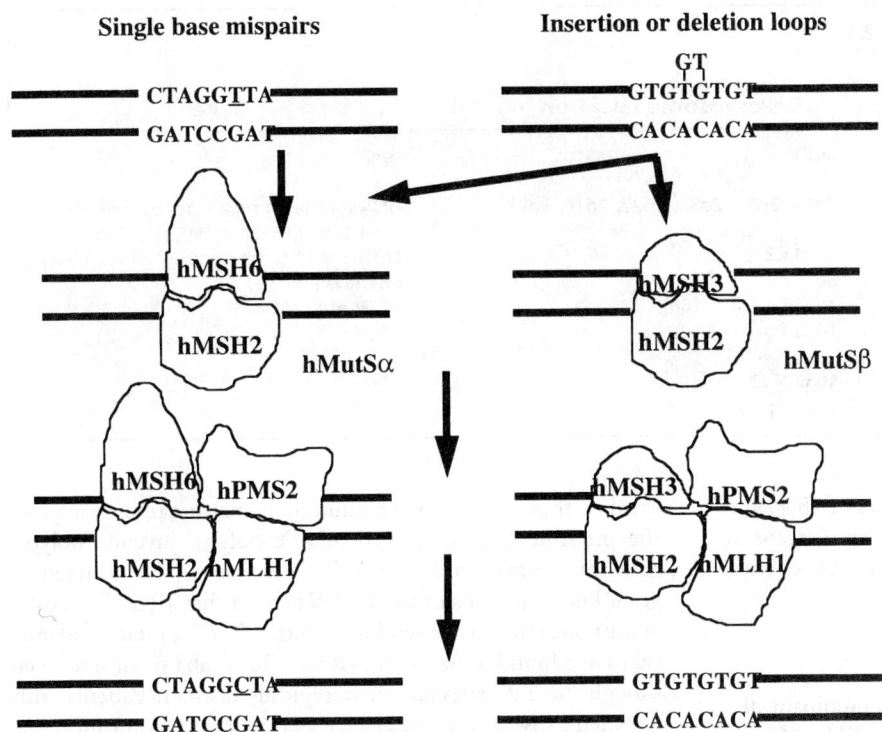

FIGURE 116.3. The DNA mismatch repair (MMR) system. The DNA MMR proteins work as a multimeric complex to repair base pair mismatches and heteroduplex loops that develop during new DNA synthesis. The hMSH2/hMSH6 protein complex binds to single-base mispairs, whereas the hMSH2/hMSH3 complex also can mediate the repair of insertion/deletion loops that sometimes form during the replication of a microsatellite sequence. The hMLH1/hPMS2 protein complex distinguishes the newly synthesized strand from the template strand and targets the mutant one for repair. Loss of any of these proteins results in loss of the DNA MMR function.

risk for endometrial cancer, depending on the registry, which is similar to the risk for colon cancer. In three separate registries, the incidence of colon cancer has been linear, and 1.6% per year from ages 25 to 75. In HNPCC, there are no phenotypic markers of disease; diffuse polyposis does not occur. Solitary adenomatous polyps may develop as early as the second decade, and the adenomas are unusually aggressive, rapidly evolving into villous adenomas or cancers. Colon cancer in this setting has an early onset (mean age 40 to 45 years, the same as in FAP), more than two-thirds of the cancers occur in the proximal colon, and multiple primary malignancies are common. There are additional risks for the early development of cancer in the stomach, small intestine, ureter, renal pelvis, brain, and other sites. Interestingly, there is no increased incidence of breast or lung cancers in HNPCC kindreds.

When the disease is suspected, the tumor can be assayed for MSI, which can be detected in paraffin-embedded, archival tumors that were removed decades earlier. The fact that 15% of sporadic tumors have MSI (most due to epigenetic silencing of the *hMLH1* gene) is a confounding factor. Immunohistochemistry may be useful to identify the mutant gene once MSI is found, and the germ line mutation in a DNA MMR gene may be found in blood samples by a variety of genetic tests. Currently, the mutant DNA MMR gene can be found in about half of HNPCC families. Some (less than 10%) of HNPCC tumors do not have MSI, which suggests that additional mechanisms for this disease remain to be discovered.

Optimal Management of Lynch Syndrome

In HNPCC, a full colonoscopic exam is required beginning at about age 25 (depending on the pattern of tumor development in the family), and this should be repeated every 1 to 2 years because of the aggressive pattern of tumor evolution in this disease. Diagnostic blood tests are being developed for HNPCC, but this is a more complex problem, since there are multiple genes that produce this syndrome. As in FAP, once the mutation is found in an individual family, it may be applied with confidence in those relatives. Patients with HNPCC are best treated with a subtotal colectomy and ileorectal anastomosis in order to limit the amount of residual colon at risk for cancer. Proctectomy is usually not necessary in the management of this syndrome, but annual proctoscopic surveillance is required after surgery. The endometrium represents a substantial cancer risk, and removal is recommended when childbearing is no longer an issue. The ovaries are at increased risk for cancer, and oophorectomy may be a reasonable step at the time of hysterectomy. The risk of cancer in the other organs is relatively low, and specific screening measures have not been recommended.

OTHER FAMILIAL POLYPOSES AND COLORECTAL CANCER (TABLE 116.4)

PEUTZ–JEGHERS SYNDROME

Peutz–Jeghers syndrome (PJS) is a rare, autosomal dominant disease inherited by a germ line mutation in a serine/threonine kinase located on chromosome 19p called SKT11 or LKB1. The diagnosis can be made because of the dark pigmented macules around the mouth, digits, and elsewhere. Affected patients get characteristic PJ polyps throughout the GI tract that can cause obstruction or intussusception. The polyps, which themselves are benign hamartomas, have a diagnostic branching smooth-muscle component to them. Despite traditional opinions to the

TABLE 116.4.	POLYPOSIS SYNDROMES	

Polyposis Syndrome	Chromosome Location	Gene
Familial adenomatous polyposis, Gardner's syndrome, Turcot's syndrome	5q21	*APC*
Hereditary nonpolyposis colorectal cancer, or Lynch syndrome	2p16, 3p21, 2q32, 7p22, 2p16, 3p22	DNA mismatch repair genes: *hMSH2, hMLH1, hPMS1, hPMS2, hMSH6*
Peutz–Jeghers syndrome	19p13.3	*LKB1/STK11* (a serine/threonine kinase)
Hereditary mixed polyposis syndrome	6q	unknown
Juvenile polyposis coli	10q22.3–24.1, 18q21.1	*PTEN* or *SMAD4*
Bannayan–Riley–Ruvalcaba syndrome, a variant of JPC	10q23	*PTEN*
Cowden's disease	10q22–23	*PTEN*

contrary, PJS patients have a lifetime risk of cancer of 48%, and these occur earlier than in the general population. Organs at risk for cancer include the GI tract, pancreas, breast, ovaries, and testes.

JUVENILE POLYPOSIS COLI

Juvenile polyposis coli (JPC) is a rare, autosomal dominant disease caused by a germ line mutation in either the *SMAD4* gene on chromosome 18q or the *PTEN* gene on chromosome 10q. The diagnosis is made by finding ten or more juvenile polyps in an individual, followed by family analysis and testing for germ line mutations in *SMAD4* or *PTEN*. In JPC, the polyps are limited to the colon, but in some instances, generalized GI involvement with juvenile polyps may occur. In some cases, the polyps can be removed by repetitive endoscopic polypectomy; however, in other cases, polyp formation may be more extensive, complications such as chronic blood loss or protein-losing enteropathy may be present, and resection of segments of the large or small bowel may be required. Patients with JPC are at increased risk for cancer of the colon at an early age, presumably due to the evolution of adenomatous epithelium in the polyps.

A syndrome known as Bannayan–Riley–Ruvalcaba syndrome (and by several other names) is a rare variant of JPC, associated with characteristic macular pigmented lesions, macrocephaly, and other congenital anomalies, and linked to germ line mutations only in the *PTEN* gene.

COWDEN'S SYNDROME

Cowden's syndrome is a rare, autosomal dominant disease characterized by pathognomonic skin and tongue papules. About a third of these patients have multiple hamartomatous polyps of the intestine (including hyperplastic polyps, juvenile polyps, ganglioneuromas, and others). This disease has been linked to germ line mutations of the *PTEN* gene, as has JPC. Curiously, at least one family has been found with a *PTEN* mutation identical to one found in Bannayan–Riley–Ruvalcaba syndrome, even though these diseases are phenotypically distinct. Patients with Cowden's disease are not at increased risk for colon cancer, although the nature of the *PTEN* gene as a tumor suppressor gene is manifested in a risk for early-onset breast and thyroid cancers in affected patients.

BIBLIOGRAPHY

Boland CR. Malignant tumors of the colon. In: Yamada T., ed. *Textbook of gastroenterology*, third ed. Philadelphia: JB Lippincott, 1999: 2023–2082.

Boland CR. Hereditary non-polyposis colorectal cancer. In Vogelstein B, Kinzler KW, eds., *The genetic basis of human cancer*. New York: McGraw-Hill, 1998:333–346.

Boland CR, Sinicrope FA, Brenner DE, et al. Gastrointestinal cancer prevention and treatment. *Gastroenterology* 2000; 118:S115–S128.

Cohen AM, Minsky BD, Schilsky RL. Cancer of the colon. In: DeVita VT, Hellman S, Rosenberg SA, eds. *Cancer: principles and practice of oncology*, fifth ed. Philadelphia: JB Lippincott, 1997:1144–1197.

Cohen AM, Minsky BD, Schilsky RL. Cancer of the rectum. In: DeVita VT, Hellman S, Rosenberg SA, eds. *Cancer: principles and practice of oncology*. Philadelphia: JB Lippincott, 1997:1197–1234.

Winawer SJ, Fletcher RH, Miller L, et al. Colorectal cancer screening: clinical guidelines and rationale. *Gastroenterology* 1997;112:594–642.

Kelley's Textbook of Internal Medicine, fourth edition. Edited by H. David Humes. Lippincott Williams & Wilkins, Philadelphia © 2000.

DISORDERS OF THE PANCREAS, LIVER, AND BILIARY TRACT

CHAPTER

117

PANCREATITIS

JAMES H. GRENDELL

■ PANCREATIC EXOCRINE FUNCTION

The exocrine pancreas is the master digestive gland of the body, secreting about 1 L of bicarbonate-rich, clear fluid into the small intestine every day. This fluid, pancreatic juice, contains the digestive enzymes necessary for the intraluminal hydrolysis of dietary macronutrients (protein, starch, fat, nucleic acids) and fat-soluble vitamin esters into smaller molecules that can either (a) be absorbed directly by enterocytes or (b) be acted upon further by constituents of bile or intestinal brush-border enzymes to permit absorption by the small intestine.

FUNCTIONAL ANATOMY

The pancreas lies deep within the abdominal cavity. In the adult, it is about 12 to 20 cm long and weighs 70 to 120 g. The head of the gland is apposed to the curvature of the duodenum, with the body and tail extending obliquely posterior to the stomach toward the gastric surface of the hilum of the spleen (Fig. 117.1A). Posteriorly the distal common bile duct enters the head of the pancreas and passes through the pancreatic parenchyma to reach the duodenal ampulla (Fig. 117.1B).

The pancreas has a rich arterial blood supply derived from interconnected branches of both the celiac and superior mesenteric arteries (supplying the head and part of the body) and the splenic artery (supplying the rest of the body and tail). The venous drainage of the pancreas enters the hepatic portal venous system, emptying either directly into the portal vein or into the splenic vein.

Pancreatic lymphatics generally follow the course of the arteries and veins, with most lymphatic drainage entering the pancreaticosplenic lymph nodes and some the pancreaticoduodenal and pre-aortic nodes. Pancreatic lymphatics interconnect exten-

sively with those of other nearby organs and retroperitoneal tissues.

The sympathetic and parasympathetic efferent innervation of the pancreas is supplied by the vagus and splanchnic nerves by way of the hepatic and celiac plexuses. The vagal (parasympathetic) efferent fibers pass through these plexuses but do not synapse until they reach the parasympathetic ganglia in the interlobular septa of the pancreas. The postganglionic fibers then

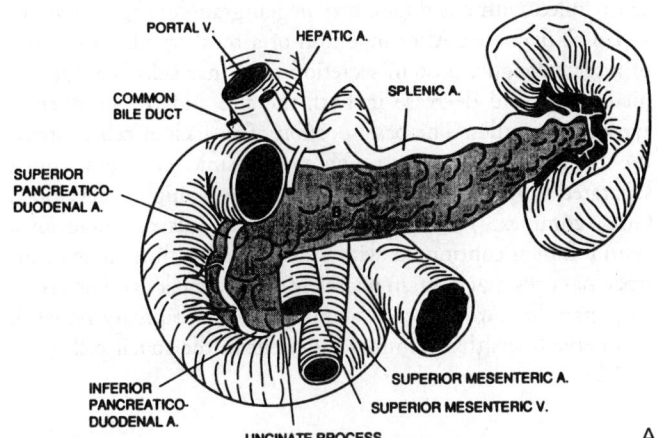

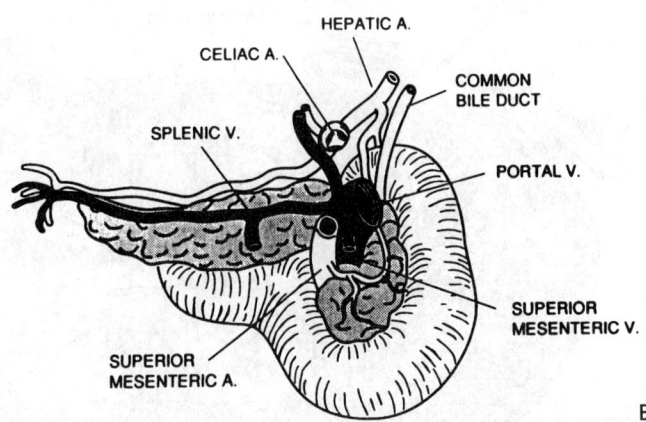

FIGURE 117.1. (A) Anterior and **(B)** posterior views of the pancreas and some surrounding structures. A, artery; B, body; H, head; T, tail; V, vein. (From Grendell JH. Embryology, anatomy, and anomalies of the pancreas. In: Haubrich WS, Schaffner, F, Berk JE, eds. *Bockus Gastroenterology,* fifth ed. Philadelphia: WB Saunders, 1995; 2815, with permission.)

supply the acini, ducts, and islets of Langerhans. Sympathetic nerves arise from the lateral gray matter of the thoracic spinal cord and pass through the greater splanchnic nerves to synapse in the celiac ganglia. The postganglionic fibers follow the distribution of the hepatic, splenic, and superior mesenteric arteries to innervate pancreatic blood vessels. Visceral afferent fibers (which appear to mediate pain) travel through the vagus nerves to the celiac ganglia and splanchnic nerves to reach the thoracic sympathetic chain and the spinal root ganglia.

HISTOLOGIC FACTORS

The pancreas is divided into lobules surrounded by connective tissue septa containing blood vessels, lymphatics, nerves, and exocrine secretory ducts. On microscopic examination, the parenchyma of the lobules consists mainly of the acini involved in exocrine secretion (more than 80% of the gland). Scattered among the acini are the islets of Langerhans (1% to 2% of the gland), which are responsible for pancreatic endocrine secretion.

Acinar cells are tall and pyramidal, situated on a basal lamina. They are highly specialized for the synthesis, storage, and secretion of large amounts of protein, mainly in the form of digestive enzymes. In the resting state, the apical portion of the acinar cell is filled with eosinophilic zymogen granules that are about 1 μm in diameter. After ingestion of a meal or administration of a secretagogue, protein secretion by acinar cells is accompanied by a rapid decrease in both the size and the number of zymogen granules. The basal portion of the acinar cell contains the nucleus and extensive rough endoplasmic reticulum, and is separated from the zymogen granules by a highly developed Golgi complex. The apices of the acinar cells converge on a central lumen continuous with a duct lined with flattened centroacinar cells that contain relatively few organelles and no secretory granules. Around each acinus lie a rich capillary network and nerve fibers that terminate adjacent to the acinar cells (Fig. 117.2).

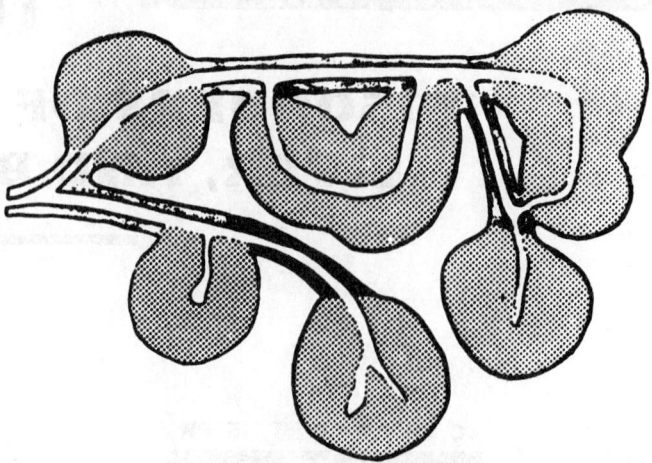

FIGURE 117.3. The complex relationship between pancreatic ducts (*heavily shaded*) and acini *(stippled)*. Acini may exist as terminal structures of ducts or form anastomotic loops that connect to ducts at both ends. (From Bockman DE. Anatomy of the pancreas. In: Go VLW, Gardner JD, Brooks FP, et al. eds. *The exocrine pancreas: biology, pathobiology, and diseases.* New York: Raven Press, 1986:1, with permission.)

The acini empty into intralobular ducts lined by cuboidal epithelium. These then join to form interlobular ducts that empty into the main pancreatic duct. These larger ducts, lined primarily by tall columnar cells, with occasional goblet and argentaffin cells, are accompanied by arterial and venous blood vessels and nerves, and are surrounded by extensive connective tissue.

Casts of the pancreatic duct system formed by retrograde injection of the duct with silicon demonstrate that the organization of ducts and acini is complex. Acini are not merely spherical units at the ends of the duct system, similar to a bunch of grapes. Rather, acini are commonly curved, branching tubules that anastomose, occasionally loop, and ultimately end blindly (Fig. 117.3).

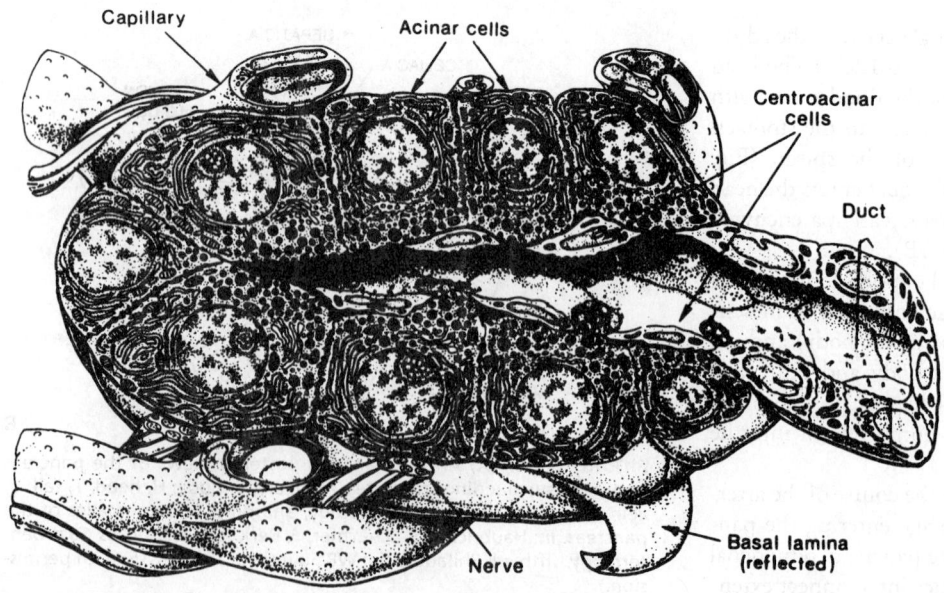

FIGURE 117.2. The organization of the pancreatic acinus and surrounding capillaries and nerves. (From Fawcett DW. *Bloom and Fawcett: a textbook of histology,* eleventh ed. New York: Chapman & Hall, 1986: 718, with permission.)

Recently, stellate cells have been identified in the pancreas that appear to be very similar to the extensively studied stellate cells of the liver (where they have also been called lipocytes and fat storage, or Ito, cells). When activated, these cells undergo a marked morphologic change to resemble myofibroblasts and express genes for collagen synthesis. In the liver these cells are the major cell type responsible for the synthesis of extracellular collagen and are believed to be the critical factor in the development of fibrosis in response to liver injury. It is likely that stellate cells play a similar role in the pancreas.

The endocrine pancreas consists of about 1 million islets of Langerhans that are about 0.2 mm in diameter, typically round or oval, and separated from the surrounding exocrine tissue by fine fibers of connective tissue. The most common types of islet cells are the insulin-secreting β cell (in the center of the islet) and the glucagon-secreting α cell (in the periphery). The other major cell types are the somatostatin-secreting δ cell and the pancreatic polypeptide–secreting cell.

Each islet is surrounded by an extensive network of capillaries lined by fenestrated endothelium. Afferent arterioles bring blood into the capillary glomerulus. This blood then travels from the islets in efferent capillaries, bathing the surrounding exocrine tissue and creating an insuloacinar portal system. Other arterioles supply blood directly to acinar tissue without passing through islets. The result of the insuloacinar portal system is that acini surrounding islets (peri-insular acini) are exposed to much higher concentrations of islet hormones (e.g., insulin, glucagon) than acini located away from islets. This may explain the observation that peri-insular acini have larger cells and nuclei and more zymogen granules (with different enzyme composition) than other acini.

COMPONENTS OF PANCREATIC JUICE

Water and Electrolytes

Pancreatic juice is isosmotic with extracellular fluid, with water entering passively along osmotic gradients. The major cations are Na^+ and K^+, which are secreted at concentrations similar to plasma concentrations and independent of secretory rates. Although the total anion concentration does not vary with secre-

tory rate, the amounts of the major cations, HCO_3^- and Cl^-, do. At low secretory rates the concentration of HCO_3^- is only 30 to 60 mmol per liter, but it rises to about 135 mmol per liter at high secretory rates, with a corresponding decrease in Cl^- concentration.

This flow-related reciprocal relation of HCO_3^- and Cl^- concentrations in pancreatic juice appears to involve two components. Firstly, acinar cells secrete a plasma-like fluid with a low HCO_3^- concentration, whereas centroacinar and duct cells secrete bicarbonate-rich fluid. Because the fluid secretory capacity of the centroacinar and duct cells is much greater than that of the acinar cells, the bicarbonate-rich fluid predominates at higher rates of stimulated secretion. Secondly, HCO_3^- in pancreatic juice is exchanged for Cl^- in the pancreatic duct in a time-dependent diffusional process. At high secretory flow rates, more of the HCO_3^- escapes this exchange process.

In addition to the four main cations and anions, pancreatic juice also contains Ca^{2+} (1 to 2 mEq per liter) and minute amounts of Mg^{2+}, Zn^{2+}, HPO_4^{2-}, and SO_4^{2-}.

Proteins

In humans, pancreatic juice has a protein concentration ranging from about 1% to about 10%. Most of these proteins are digestive enzymes or cofactors, which include 20 isozymes of 12 different enzymes. The remainder are pancreatic secretory trypsin inhibitor, several trypsin-like enzymes that do not serve primarily as digestive enzymes, plasma proteins, and glycoproteins.

The four major categories of digestive enzymes are proteases (digesting proteins and peptides), amylase (digesting starch), lipases (digesting triglycerides and phospholipids), and nucleases (digesting nucleic acids) (Table 117.1). In addition, pancreatic juice contains colipase, a peptide cofactor that contributes to lipolysis by binding to bile salt–lipid surfaces, enhancing the ability of lipase to digest triglycerides. All the proteases, as well as phospholipase and colipase, are secreted by the pancreas as inactive proenzymes (zymogens). After entering the intestinal lumen, trypsinogen is converted to trypsin by enterokinase (enteropeptidase), an intestinal brush-border enzyme. Trypsin then can activate the other proenzymes as well as trypsinogen mole-

TABLE 117.1.	SITES OF ACTION OF PANCREATIC DIGESTIVE ENZYMES		
Enzyme	**Substrate**	**Site of Action**	**Products**
Amylase	Carbohydrates (amylase, amylopectin, glycogen)	α-1,4 Linkage between hexoses (but not at branch points or end points)	Maltose, maltotriose, α-limit dextrins
Endopeptidases (trypsin, chymotrypsin, elastase)	Peptides, proteins	Internal peptide bonds	Smaller peptides
Exopeptidases (carboxypeptidase A and B)	Peptides, proteins	Peptide bonds at carboxyl terminal	Smaller peptides
Lipase	Triglycerides	Ester linkage of fatty acid in position 1	Fatty acids, monoglycerides
Phospholipase	Phospholipids (e.g., lecithin)	Ester linkage in position 2	Fatty acid, 1,1-diglyceride (e.g., lysolecithin)

cules. Unlike the other digestive enzymes, amylase, lipase, and ribonuclease are secreted in active form.

The acinar cell synthesizes and secretes in low concentration a trypsin inhibitor capable of inhibiting trypsin and, to some extent, chymotrypsin. The presence of pancreatic secretory trypsin inhibitor appears to be a protective mechanism against damage to the pancreas due to premature activation of trypsin in pancreatic tissue or juice. However, once pancreatic juice enters the intestine, trypsinogen is activated by enterokinase so rapidly and to such an extent that the relatively small amount of trypsin inhibitor present does not interfere with the normal digestive process. An additional protective mechanism against the potential harmful effects of premature trypsin activation within the pancreas is the ability of several trypsin-like molecules synthesized by the acinar cell and of trypsin itself to destroy trypsin and trypsinogen molecules.

CELLULAR MECHANISMS OF SECRETION

Water and Electrolytes

Most of the stimulated secretion of water and electrolytes by the pancreas appears to come from centroacinar cells and the epithelial cells lining the intralobular and small interlobular ducts. The peptide hormone secretin is the most potent stimulus for water and bicarbonate secretion, binding to receptors on the basolateral surface of the duct cells, producing an increase in intracellular cyclic AMP (cAMP) concentration resulting in activation of protein kinase A. However, the peptide hormone cholecystokinin (CCK) and, particularly, cholinergic neural stimulation also appear to contribute to the observed postprandial increase in water and bicarbonate secretion by potentiating the effects of secretin. Bicarbonate is secreted by pancreatic centroacinar and duct cells against large concentration and electrochemical gradients. Most of the HCO_3^- is derived from CO_2 in blood, which is converted to HCO_3^- by the action of the enzyme carbonic anhydrase. The HCO_3^- is exchanged for Cl^- at the apical (luminal) cell surface by an active process that appears at least in part driven by the active secretion of H^+ across the basolateral cell surface into the interstitial space mediated by an Na^+, H^+ pump (in turn driven by Na^+, K^+-ATPase) and other active proton transport mechanisms. Secretion of Cl^- across the apical cell surface is an important step in water and electrolyte secretion, and it takes place through a Cl^- channel that is the cystic fibrosis transmembrane conductance regulator (CFTR). The primary cations, Na^+ and K^+, reach the pancreatic duct by paracellular routes.

Proteins

The secreted proteins of the exocrine pancreas, primarily digestive enzymes, are synthesized on ribosomes of the rough endoplasmic reticulum in acinar cells. Newly synthesized proteins enter the cisternal space of the endoplasmic reticulum through insertion into the membrane of a lipophilic "signal" or "leader" sequence of amino acids at the amino-terminal end of each protein. Once inside the cisternal space, the signal peptide is cleaved by peptidases, resulting in the secretory protein that will remain membrane-bound until secreted into the acinar lumen. The secretory proteins are transported as a mixture to the Golgi complex in transition vesicles that bud from the endoplasmic reticulum. Additional post-translational processing (e.g., glycosylation, peptide cleavage) occurs in the Golgi complex. The final mixture of secretory proteins buds from the Golgi complex to form condensing vacuoles that ultimately become zymogen granules, the storage compartment for digestive enzymes and other secretory proteins immediately before secretion. In zymogen granules, secreted proteins appear to be arranged in a tightly packed, crystalline-like state. Zymogen granules move toward the apices of acinar cells by a process involving microtubules. When the acinar cell is stimulated to secrete, the zymogen granule membrane and plasma membrane fuse, and a fusion pore forms, opening the zymogen granule and leading to release of digestive enzymes and other secreted proteins into the fluid component of the acinar lumen (exocytosis).

Stimulation of protein secretion by pancreatic acinar cells is due to specific binding to receptors on the basolateral cell surface by the cholinergic neurotransmitter acetylcholine and, at least in some species, by CCK. This begins an intracellular cascade by which phospholipase C is activated by a G-protein–mediated mechanism.

Phospholipase C in turns cleaves phosphatidylinositol to inositol 1,4,5-triphosphate (1,4,5-IP_3) and 1,2-diacylglycerol (DAG). The 1,4,5-IP_3 causes an increase in cytosolic calcium concentration due to the release of calcium from intracytoplasmic stores. Protein kinase C is activated by DAG, and calcium activates several additional protein kinases and a protein phosphatase by binding to calmodulin. These protein kinases and phosphatases are believed to bring about digestive enzyme secretion by altering the phosphorylation of a number of proteins, producing specific effects yet to be fully identified.

REGULATION OF PANCREATIC SECRETION

Basal

During the basal or fasting state, the volume of pancreatic juice secreted into the duodenum is low, with enzyme secretion about 10% of maximal levels and bicarbonate secretion only 2% of maximal. However, brief periods of increased pancreatic enzyme and bicarbonate secretion occur about every 60 to 120 minutes in temporal association with the increased motor activity of phase III of interdigestive migrating motor complexes (see Chapter 108). Cholinergic neural input is the primary regulator of the increase in both motor and secretory activity, and secretion of the peptide motilin from duodenal endocrine cells into the blood appears to play a role in the initiation of phase III. α-Adrenergic tone acts as an inhibitor of pancreatic secretion in the fasting state.

Postprandial

After ingestion of a meal, the exocrine pancreas secretes bicarbonate and enzymes at about 60% to 75% of the levels attained after intravenous infusions of maximally effective doses of secretagogues such as secretin and CCK. The meal-related regulation of secretion is usually divided into cephalic, gastric, and intestinal phases, although considerable overlap occurs.

The cephalic phase is stimulated by the thought, sight, taste, or smell of food. It can produce a secretory response 25% to 50% of maximal and is regulated primarily by vagal cholinergic innervation. The gastric phase has not been studied extensively. However, gastric distention produces a small increase in pancreatic secretion that appears to be mediated by vagal cholinergic reflexes. Current data do not support a significant role for gastrin in this process. By determining the rate of entry of acid and nutrients into the duodenum, gastric emptying strongly influences the intestinal phase, which is the predominant phase in the pancreatic response to a meal.

During the intestinal phase secretin is released into the blood from the duodenum in response to duodenal acidification. Fatty acids and bile may also help stimulate the secretion of secretin. The rise in plasma secretin concentration after a meal (potentiated by vagal cholinergic stimulation and circulating CCK) is responsible for the increase in pancreatic water and bicarbonate output.

Increased enzyme secretion is stimulated by fatty acids, oligopeptides, amino acids, and Ca^{2+} entering the intestine. This leads to release of CCK from the duodenum into the circulation and activation of cholinergic enteropancreatic reflexes, both of which stimulate pancreatic enzyme secretion. As is the case with secretin-stimulated water and bicarbonate secretion, cholinergic neural input appears to be essential for the full effect of physiologic levels of CCK to be exerted on pancreatic secretion, particularly in humans. Because studies examining human pancreatic tissue have thus far failed to demonstrate conclusively the presence of high-affinity (secretion-stimulating) CCK receptors on pancreatic acinar cells, it is possible that CCK may regulate pancreatic secretion in humans by binding to afferent or efferent vagal neurons rather than to acinar cells themselves.

FEEDBACK REGULATION

Feedback inhibition of pancreatic enzyme secretion by intraduodenal pancreatic proteases such as trypsin, chymotrypsin, and elastase has been clearly demonstrated in the rat. Several studies suggest that bile acids may also participate in feedback inhibition in some species. More limited data in humans support the existence of feedback inhibition of enzyme secretion by intraduodenal proteases, mediated by cholinergic nerves. The relative importance of this in either normal physiology or disease remains to be determined.

INHIBITORS OF EXOCRINE SECRETION

Postprandial exocrine secretion by the pancreas reaches only 60% to 75% of the maximal levels attained when pharmacologic concentrations of secretagogues are administered. This suggests the existence of physiologic inhibitory mechanisms. The islet cell peptides glucagon, pancreatic polypeptide, and somatostatin (also released from the small intestine) have all been suggested as possible mediators of such inhibitory processes.

Another potential candidate is peptide YY (PYY), found in intestinal endocrine cells in the ileum and colon and released in response to intraluminal lipid. PYY and perhaps other factors may act as the "ileal brake" to reduce pancreatic secretion after digestion of a meal has been largely completed. It is likely that inhibitors of pancreatic exocrine secretion act primarily by altering cholinergic neural transmission.

PANCREATIC BLOOD FLOW

Although ingestion of a meal increases overall splanchnic and portal blood flow, postprandial changes in pancreatic blood flow have not been extensively evaluated. The pancreas has a rich arterial blood supply; and physiologic levels of stimulation (due to CCK, secretin, or duodenal acidification) do not appear to increase total pancreatic perfusion. This indicates that, under physiologic conditions, pancreatic secretion is not limited by blood flow.

ACUTE PANCREATITIS

Acute pancreatitis is an inflammatory process arising in the exocrine pancreas, with variable involvement of peripancreatic tissues or remote organ systems. It ranges in severity from a mild, self-limited disease to a catastrophic one with multiple potentially severe complications and the risk of death. However, if the patient survives and the primary cause of pancreatitis can be identified and eliminated, the pancreas usually returns to normal clinically, biochemically, and morphologically (at least insofar as these aspects are routinely assessed).

Various studies report an incidence of acute pancreatitis from about 10 to as high as 50 per 100,000 per year. Although some series suggest a substantial increase in incidence over approximately the last 30 years, it is unclear to what extent this reflects improvements in our ability to make the diagnosis.

ETIOLOGIC FACTORS

Gallstone disease and excessive alcohol use account for about 70% to 80% of cases of acute pancreatitis in industrialized countries (Table 117.2). Other definable etiologic factors account for about 10% of cases, including genetic hyperlipidemia (with serum triglycerides typically higher than 1,000 mg per deciliter on presentation with acute pancreatitis), chronic hypercalcemia, surgery (particularly upper abdominal surgery and thoracic procedures involving cardiopulmonary bypass), solid organ transplantation (liver, heart, kidney), abdominal trauma (blunt or penetrating), endoscopic retrograde cholangiopancreatography (ERCP; incidence of 1% to 10%), sphincter of Oddi manometry (incidence of 10% to 20%), and infections (e.g., ascariasis, clonorchiasis, mumps, cytomegalovirus infection). Pancreatic cancers and ampullary tumors infrequently present as acute pancreatitis, as do, even more rarely, cancers metastatic to the pancreas. Benign anatomic abnormalities interfering with emptying of the pancreatic duct, such as choledochal cysts or duodenal diverticula, are also uncommon causes of acute pancreatitis.

Nearly 90 drugs have been implicated as potential causes of acute pancreatitis, although strong confirmatory evidence is

---

TABLE 117.2. **MAJOR CAUSES OF ACUTE PANCREATITIS**

Gallstone disease

Chronic excessive alcohol use

Drugs (e.g., azathioprine, 6-mercaptopurine, didanosine, pentamadine, sulfonamides, valproic acid, lisinopril, enalapril, furosemide, methyldopa, estrogens, tetracycline, metronidazole, erythromycin, nitrofurantoin, isoniazid, rifampicin, cimetidine, ranitidine, acetaminophen, salicylates, some nonsteroidal anti-inflammatory drugs)

Infections (e.g., ascariasis, clonorchiasis, mumps, coxsackievirus, cytomegalovirus, tuberculosis, *Mycobacterium avium* complex)

Blunt or penetrating abdominal trauma

Surgery

Endoscopic retrograde cholangiopancreatography, sphincter of Oddi manometry

Genetic hypertriglyceridemia

Chronic hypercalcemia

Pancreatic or ampullary tumors

Sphincter of Oddi dysfunction

Duodenal disease (e.g., peptic ulcer, Crohn's disease, periampullary diverticulum)

Choledochal cyst

Toxins (organophosphate insecticides, scorpion venom)

Pancreas divisum

Vasculitis (e.g., polyarteritis nodosum, systemic lupus erythematosus, thrombotic thrombocytopenic purpura, Henoch–Schönlein purpura)

Cystic fibrosis

Hereditary disease (e.g., mutation in cationic trypsinogen gene)

Idiopathic disease

---

available for only about 20 (Table 117.2). Some of these drugs typically produce acute pancreatitis within a month of starting treatment, presumably by a hypersensitivity reaction. These include azathioprine, mercaptopurine, sulfonamides, metronidazole, lisinopril, enalapril, and aminosalicylates. Other drugs (e.g., didanosine, pentamidine, and valproic acid) may produce pancreatitis after months of administration, suggesting perhaps the cumulative effects of the drug or toxic metabolites,

A still debated potential cause of acute pancreatitis is pancreas divisum, a variant of pancreatic ductal anatomy that involves 5% to 7% of the general population. In these persons, the duct of Santorini, draining the larger portion of the gland (arising from the embryologic dorsal pancreas) through the accessory papilla, does not fuse with the duct of Wirsung, draining the smaller embryologic ventral pancreas through the major papilla. In persons with pancreas divisum, the accessory papilla may be inadequate to accommodate the volume of pancreatic secretions under some circumstances, leading to relative obstruction to flow and recurrent acute pancreatitis. This appears to be the case for some patients; but given the prevalence of pancreas divisum, it is important to evaluate for other potential etiologic factors before ascribing pancreatitis to this common anatomical variant.

Another controversial proposed cause is sphincter of Oddi dysfunction. This has been diagnosed on the basis of finding, by endoscopic sphincter of Oddi manometry, a transient or fixed elevation of basal sphincter pressure of more than 40 mm Hg.

Patients with AIDS have an incidence of acute pancreatitis of as high as 4% to 20% in some series. This is due in part to infections involving pancreatic tissue (cytomegalovirus infection, cryptosporidiosis, cryptococcosis, toxoplasmosis, or infection with *Mycobacterium tuberculosis* or *Mycobacterium avium* complex) and in part to drug toxicity (e.g., didanosine, pentamidine, trimethoprim–sulfamethoxazole). Patients with AIDS also frequently have an elevated serum amylase concentration in the absence of pancreatitis either by clinical evaluation or by pancreatic imaging studies. It is unclear as to whether this hyperamylasemia is due to abnormalities in renal tubular function, increases in the salivary isoamylase fraction of total serum amylase, or subclinical pancreatic inflammation below the threshold for detection by imaging studies.

About 10% of adult patients are categorized as having idiopathic acute pancreatitis, although some series quote figures as high as 20% to 30%, depending on the criteria used to classify patients etiologically. Several studies have suggested that occult gallstone disease (biliary microlithiasis or gallbladder sludge) can be demonstrated in 50% to 75% of these patients by microscopic examination of bile or duodenal juice for cholesterol and bilirubinate crystals or by repeated abdominal ultrasonographic examinations. Treatments directed at gallstone disease (e.g., cholecystectomy, endoscopic sphincterotomy, or ursodeoxycholic acid therapy) significantly reduce the likelihood of recurrent acute pancreatitis in these patients. Other work has suggested that sphincter of Oddi dysfunction may account for 15% of cases of acute pancreatitis otherwise considered idiopathic. In addition, studies are under way to determine whether some less common mutations of CFTR may result in otherwise unexplained episodes of recurrent acute pancreatitis in adults.

Acute pancreatitis complicates anywhere from 1 in 100 to 1 in 4,000 pregnancies, generally due to gallstone disease and occurring in the third trimester. Acute pancreatitis in childhood is uncommon; the leading causes are trauma, biliary tract disease, drugs, and infections. Other causes in children include genetic hyperlipidemia (chylomicron disease), congenital malformations (pancreas divisum; choledochal, pancreatic ductal, or duodenal duplication cysts), cystic fibrosis, Reye's syndrome, and glycogen storage disease type I.

Recently, the genetic defect has been identified in some kindreds with hereditary pancreatitis, which is inherited as an autosomal dominant trait and may present in childhood or adolescence as recurrent acute pancreatitis.

These patients have a point mutation in the gene coding for cationic trypsinogen on chromosome 7, which impairs a mechanism in the acinar cell that protects the pancreas against the premature activation of trypsinogen to trypsin. About 20% of cases of acute pancreatitis in children are ultimately classified as idiopathic, although some of these may turn out to be related to less common mutations in CFTR.

PATHOGENESIS

Acute pancreatitis is believed to begin as an autodigestive process within the gland resulting from premature activation of zymogens (digestive enzyme precursors) within the acinar cell, duct system, or interstitial space. As trypsinogen activation to trypsin can lead to activation of all other zymogens, this appears to be an essential early step, a concept supported by the finding that a mutation in the trypsinogen gene results in hereditary pancreatitis. Whether trypsinogen is autoactivated or whether this process is mediated by other molecules such as lysosomal enzymes remains undetermined. Premature digestive enzyme activation can then result in acinar cell damage and necrosis and pancreatic edema and inflammation. In addition to digestive enzyme activation, oxidative stress, impaired microcirculation of blood in the pancreas, and release of cytokines (in particular interleukin-1 (IL-1), tumor necrosis factor, platelet-activating factor, and nitric oxide) also appear to contribute to both pancreatic injury and extrapancreatic complications (Fig. 117.4).

Extension of this inflammatory process beyond the pancreas frequently leads to localized complications and can result in various systemic complications (Table 117.3). For reasons that remain unknown, in about 75% to 85% of cases the inflammatory process is self-limited, involving only the pancreas and peripancreatic tissues and resolving spontaneously in a few days to a week. In the other 15% to 25%, a severe course ensues, with multiple local and systemic complications, prolonged hospitalization, and risk of death.

The overall mortality rate for hospitalized patients with acute pancreatitis is about 3% to 5%. Many of the systemic complications of acute pancreatitis appear to result from the development of a cytokine-mediated systemic inflammatory response syndrome.

Gallstone disease initiates the autodigestive process resulting in acute pancreatitis when a stone, usually only a few millimeters in diameter, migrates down the common bile duct and reaches the duodenal papilla (Fig. 117.5). Impaction of a stone at the papilla may then lead either to a sudden increase in pressure in the pancreatic duct, resulting in a "secretory block" of digestive enzymes at the level of the acinar cell, or to reflux of bile or duodenal juice into the pancreatic duct. Other etiologic factors involving obstruction of the bile or pancreatic duct may function in a similar way, although it is unclear why conditions such as pancreatic and ampullary tumors or pancreas divisum only infrequently produce acute pancreatitis.

The mechanisms by which acute pancreatitis is induced by causative factors other than gallstones, pancreatic infections, or direct trauma to the gland remain unknown. However, experimental studies and some clinical observations suggest that development of a secretory block in the acinar cell may be a common feature of acute pancreatitis due to a number of causes.

Although acute pancreatitis that develops after a single binge involving excessive alcohol (ethanol) use has been occasionally reported, it is unclear if alcohol was the primary or sole cause in these cases. Typically, alcoholic acute pancreatitis occurs in persons with long-standing heavy ethanol use. Although chronic alcoholics have been reported to have about a 15-fold increased risk of developing acute pancreatitis compared to nonalcoholic controls, only about 5% of chronic heavy-alcohol users develop

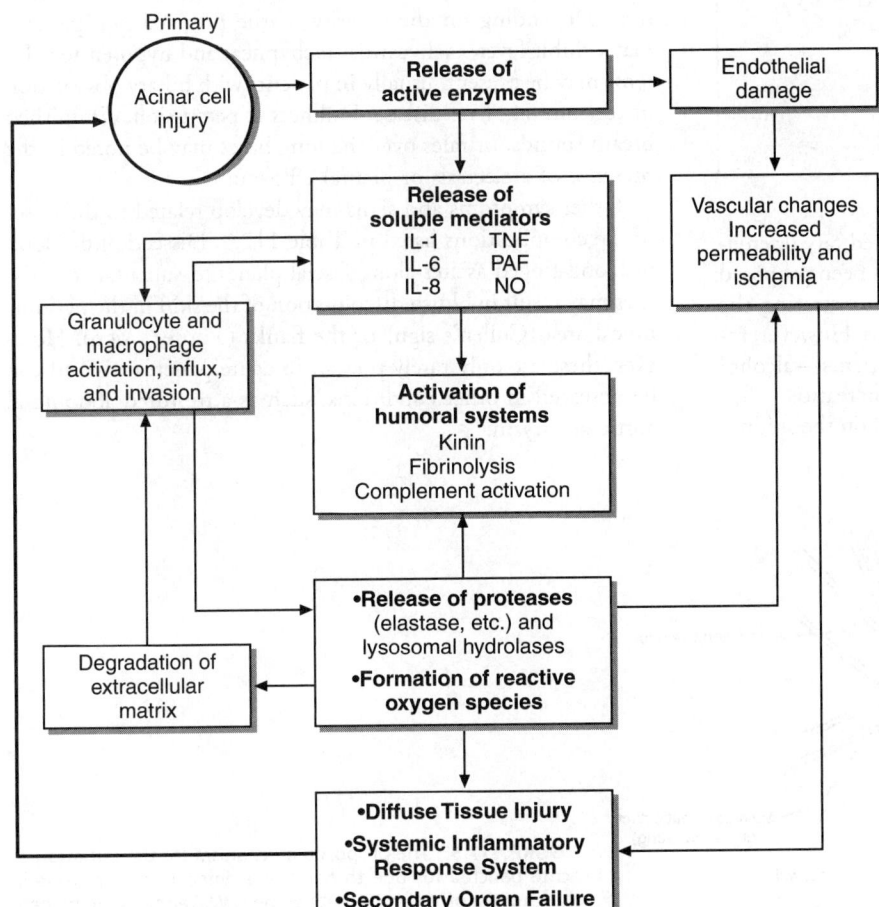

FIGURE 117.4. Proposed mechanisms involved in the pathophysiology of acute pancreatitis. IL, interleukin; TNF, tumor necrosis factor; PAF, platelet-activating factor; NO, nitric oxide. (Modified from Gorelick FS. Acute pancreatitis. In Yamada TA, Alpers DH, Owyang C, et al. eds. *Textbook of gastroenterology,* second ed. Philadelphia: JB Lippincott, 1995: 2064.)

TABLE 117.3.	COMPLICATIONS OF ACUTE PANCREATITIS

Local
Pancreatic
  Inflammatory mass ("phlegmon")
  Peripancreatic effusion
  Infected necrosis or abscess
Nonpancreatic
  Ileus and functional gastric outlet obstruction
  Ascites or pleural effusion
  Bile duct obstruction
Systemic
Cardiovascular
  Hypovolemia
  Hypotension and shock
Pulmonary
  Hypoxemia
  Atelectasis
  Pleural effusion
  Respiratory failure (adult respiratory distress syndrome)
Renal
  Oliguria
  Azotemia and acute renal failure
Metabolic
  Hypoalbuminemia
  Hypercalcemia
  Hyperglycemia
  Hypertriglyceridemia
  Metabolic acidosis
Hematologic
  Vascular thrombosis
  Disseminated intravascular coagulation
Hemorrhagic
  Stress gastritis and ulcers
  Pseudoaneurysm
  Gastric varices
Other
  Peripheral fat necrosis
  Encephalopathy

pancreatitis, indicating a major role for other hereditary or environmental risk factors. Alcoholic pancreatitis has been proposed to develop only in a gland that is already demonstrating the morphologic abnormalities of chronic pancreatitis. However, recent reports suggest that—at least for some patients—alcohol can produce acute and potentially reversible pancreatitis.

A variety of possible adverse effects of ethanol on the sphinc-ter of Oddi and the pancreas have been described both in humans and in experimental animals. These have included an increase in pressure or spasm of the sphincter of Oddi, protein plug formation in the pancreatic ducts, increased fragility of lysosomes and zymogen granules in acinar cells, and various alterations in pancreatic juice, including an increase in protein concentration and in the ratio of trypsin to trypsin inhibitor. Alcohol-related abnormalities in acinar cell signaling or in defense mechanisms against oxidative stress have been proposed. Whether or how these factors may be involved in the development of alcoholic acute pancreatitis remains to be established.

CLINICAL FEATURES

Abdominal pain, the primary manifestation of acute pancreatitis, is present in about 95% of patients. Pain is epigastric and radiates to the back in one-half to two-thirds of patients and is typically worsened by ingesting food or alcohol or by vomiting. Cessation of eating and drinking, leaning forward (doubling up), or assuming a knee-to-chest position may provide some relief of pain. Nausea, vomiting, and abdominal distention are also common symptoms. Hematemesis, melena, or diarrhea infrequently occur.

On examination, abdominal tenderness is usually present. It may be mild and limited to the epigastrium or marked, diffuse, and accompanied by abdominal rigidity and rebound tenderness. Depending on the severity of the presentation, patients may exhibit fever, tachycardia, tachypnea, and hypotension. Icterus may be present, usually in patients with biliary obstruction or concomitant liver disease. Dullness to percussion, diminished breath sounds, or rales over the lung bases may be noted in the presence of atelectasis or pleural effusion.

Other symptoms and signs may develop related to the onset of the complications listed in Table 117.3. Dissection of blood or blood-tinged ascites along fascial planes to subcutaneous tissues may result in bluish discoloration of the skin in the periumbilical area (Cullen's sign) or the flanks (Turner's sign). However, these are only rarely present in acute pancreatitis and can be observed in other conditions, such as a ruptured abdominal aortic aneurysm.

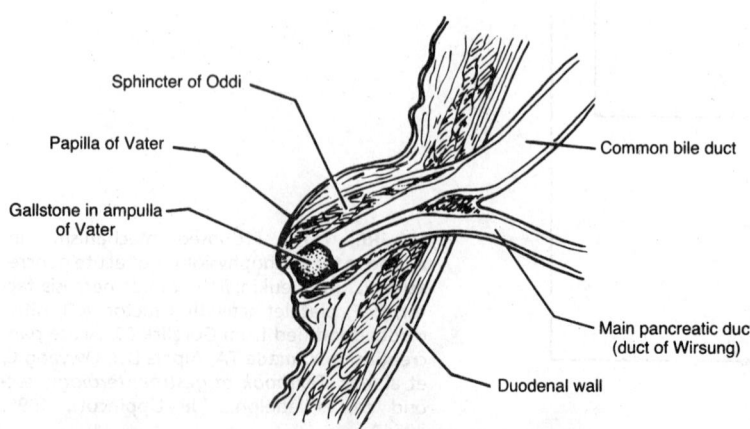

FIGURE 117.5. The proposed mechanism for the initiation of acute pancreatitis due to gallstones: impaction of a stone in the ampulla of Vater. (From Steinberg W, Tenner S. Acute pancreatitis. *N Engl J Med* 1994;330:1198, with permission.)

DIAGNOSIS

Although the diagnosis of acute pancreatitis may be strongly suggested by the history and physical examination, a number of other diseases may present in a very similar way. Therefore, laboratory testing or abdominal imaging is necessary to confirm the diagnosis.

Laboratory Testing

During the development of acute pancreatitis, digestive enzymes leak from damaged acinar cells or ducts and eventually reach the systemic circulation, raising the circulating levels of these enzymes above normal. Measurement of the serum amylase concentration has been used for the diagnosis of acute pancreatitis for over 70 years; if measured within the first hours from the onset of symptoms, the level appears to be elevated in 80% to 85% of all patients with acute pancreatitis but in only 65% to 70% with acute pancreatitis due to alcohol abuse. Serum amylase levels may also be elevated in several conditions that can closely mimic acute pancreatitis (e.g., cholangitis, gastrointestinal (GI) perforation or ischemia, ruptured ectopic pregnancy) as well as in diseases of the salivary glands and in acute or chronic renal failure (due to diminished renal excretion of amylase). Determination of serum lipase concentration, at least by some methods, is as sensitive as or more sensitive than amylase (perhaps because lipase levels remain elevated in serum longer than amylase levels) and has greater specificity. This is so despite the fact that lipase levels may also be elevated in other diseases (such as GI perforation or ischemia) or due to acute or chronic renal failure. However, all of the current methods of measuring lipase (especially some of the autoanalyzer methods) may not perform equally well, particularly in terms of specificity. Clinical studies indicate that elevations in serum amylase or lipase due to impaired renal function should not exceed three times the upper limit of normal.

Measurement of urinary amylase excretion, serum amylase isozymes, or serum concentrations of other pancreatic enzymes (e.g., trypsin, elastase, phospholipase, procarboxypeptidase) has not proven to be more useful than standard serum amylase or lipase determinations. Although measurement of serum alanine aminotransferase (ALT) or aspartate aminotransferase (AST) is not useful in making the diagnosis of acute pancreatitis, a three-fold or greater increase above the upper limit of normal of ALT or AST in a patient with acute pancreatitis suggests gallstones as the cause.

Abdominal Imaging

Abdominal imaging, particularly computed tomography (CT), has made the greatest contribution to the rapid and accurate diagnosis of acute pancreatitis and many of its complications. Abdominal ultrasonography may be useful in determining whether gallstones are the cause of an episode of acute pancreatitis; however, the sensitivity of ultrasonography in diagnosing acute pancreatitis is low, and examinations are often technically inadequate in patients with significant ileus. The CT scan may be normal in 15% to 30% of patients with mild acute pancreati-

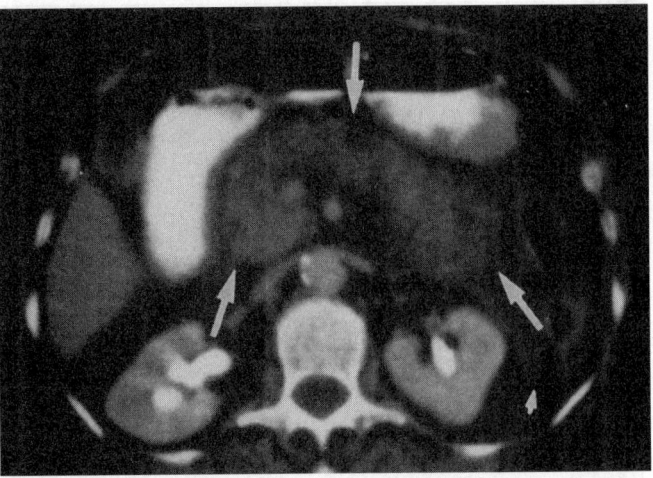

FIGURE 117.6. Typical findings on computed tomography in acute pancreatitis. The pancreas is edematous and inhomogeneous *(large arrows)*, and inflammation has resulted in an increase in the density of the tissue surrounding loops of intestine near the tail of the pancreas *(small arrow)*. (From Grendell JH. Acute pancreatitis. In: Grendell JH, McQauid KR, Friedman SL, eds. *Current diagnosis and treatment in gastroenterology.* Stamford, CT: Appleton & Lange, 1996:435, with permission.)

tis, although the gold standard for establishing the diagnosis in these patients is often uncertain. CT is virtually always abnormal in moderate to severe disease (Fig. 117.6). Thus, CT is the most useful means—short of laparotomy—for differentiating severe acute pancreatitis from other catastrophic intra-abdominal processes that can mimic pancreatitis.

Thus far, magnetic resonance imaging (MRI) has not improved on CT as a technique for diagnosing acute pancreatitis or its complications. However, it may be a useful substitute for evaluating patients who cannot receive intravenous contrast agents for CT or if detailed, noninvasive imaging of the bile or pancreatic ducts is also desired (magnetic resonance cholangiopancreatography).

Estimation of Severity

Extensive efforts have been devoted to establishing methods for predicting the severity of acute pancreatitis, so that the 75% to 85% of patients who will have a relatively mild course can be differentiated from those patients destined for more serious illness and possible death.

Assessment of Ranson's criteria (based mainly on patient age and various laboratory values) has been the most commonly used prognostic indicator in the United States, whereas the modified Glasgow (Imrie) criteria, similar to Ranson's criteria, have been used in the United Kingdom (Table 117.4). For both sets of criteria, the more risk factors a patient accrues, the greater the probability of a prolonged, complicated course and death. However, neither the Ranson nor the Glasgow score can be computed until the patient has been hospitalized for 48 hours, and neither can be recomputed to follow the patient's course. A more useful but complex scoring system is the Acute Physiologic and Chronic Health Evaluation (APACHE) II score, which can be

TABLE 117.4.	**RANSON'S AND MODIFIED GLASGOW CRITERIA OF SEVERITY**

RANSON'S

GALLSTONE PANCREATITIS

On admission to hospital:
   Age >70 y
   WBC >18,000/µL
   Glucose >220 mg/dL
   Lactate dehydrogenase >400 U/L
   AST >250 U/L
Within 48 h of hospital admission:
   Decrease in hematocrit >10 points
   Increase in BUN >2 mg/dL
   Serum calcium <8 mg/dL
   Base deficity >5 mmol/L
   Fluid deficit >4 L

PANCREATITIS DUE TO CAUSES OTHER THAN GALLSTONES

On admission to hospital:
   Age >55 y
   WBC >16,000/µL
   Glucose >200 mg/dL
   Lactate dehydrogenase >350 U/L
   Aspartate aminotransferase >250 U/L
Within 48 h of hospital admission:
   Decrease in hematocrit >10 points
   Increase in BUN >5 mg/dL
   Serum calcium <8 mg/dL
   PaO_2 <60 mg Hg
   Base deficit >4 mmol/L
   Fluid deficity >6 L

MODIFIED GLASGOW

Highest value observed during initial 48 h after admission:
   Age >55 y
   WBC <15,000/µL
   Gluose >180 mg/dL
   BUN >45 mg/dL
   PaO_2 <60 mm Hg
   Serum calcium <8 mg/dL
   Serum albumin <3.3 g/dL
   Lactate dehydrogenase >600 U/L

BUN, blood urea nitrogen; WBC, white blood cell count.

calculated at the time of admission and then recalculated throughout the course of hospitalization to measure improvement or worsening. However, the APACHE II score has been criticized for assigning too heavy a weighting to age.

In addition, because a number of studies have suggested that obesity is a risk factor for morbidity and mortality in acute pancreatitis, it has been proposed that the use of APACHE II for estimating the severity of acute pancreatitis could be improved by adding a factor to account for body mass index. When values obtained at 48 hours after admission are compared, the Ranson, Glasgow, and APACHE II scores perform similarly in predicting the severity of disease.

Dynamic (bolus contrast-enhanced) CT has been used as a predictor of severity, but the criteria have not been well standardized, the optimal timing of the examination is uncertain, and the technique is costly. In addition, there is a risk of nephrotoxi-

city from intravenous contrast agents; and concern has been raised, based on work in experimental models of pancreatitis, that pancreatitis could be worsened due to contrast-induced alterations in the pancreatic microcirculation. So far there has been no convincing evidence for the latter from clinical observation.

MRI and various laboratory tests are being evaluated as potential indicators of severity. The laboratory tests have the advantage of being relatively simple and inexpensive, and include measurement in blood of C-reactive protein, IL-6 and IL-8, leukocyte elastase, and, in urine or blood, trypsinogen activation peptide. Some initial reports are promising, but these tests require more extensive validation in general clinical practice.

Although a number of predictors (especially APACHE II) effectively define or stratify groups of patients for clinical research, none so far is clearly superior to close observation and careful judgment by an experienced physician as a basis for making therapeutic decisions.

DIFFERENTIAL DIAGNOSIS

Various relatively common intra-abdominal processes may present similarly to acute pancreatitis, and some may even elevate serum amylase or lipase levels. These include penetrating duodenal ulcer, perforated gastric or duodenal ulcer, cholangitis, intestinal ischemia or infarction, and ruptured ectopic pregnancy. A ruptured abdominal aortic aneurysm may present with similar symptoms and signs as well as such uncommon entities as acute intermittent porphyria, familial Mediterranean fever, and lead poisoning.

MANAGEMENT

The goals of therapy of acute pancreatitis are to provide supportive care, to decrease pancreatic inflammation and its consequences, and to prevent or to identify and treat complications.

Mild Acute Pancreatitis

Most patients have a mild, self-limited course requiring only bed rest, no oral intake, intravenous hydration and electrolytes, and analgesia. Traditionally, meperidine has been the analgesic of choice because of reports that it is less likely than other opiates to raise sphincter of Oddi pressure. However, the clinical importance of this is uncertain, and other narcotics can be substituted if needed. Nasogastric suction does not shorten the course of the disease but is useful in relieving symptoms of nausea, vomiting, or abdominal distention. Patients may be cautiously fed once abdominal pain and tenderness have abated and serum amylase or lipase values have begun to approach normal.

Severe Acute Pancreatitis

The care of the patient with severe acute pancreatitis poses a much greater challenge. In the earliest stages, vigorous resuscitation with intravenous hydration and electrolytes is critical to prevent or treat hypovolemia and shock. Volume requirements may be remarkably large; and these patients often need an intensive care unit with careful attention to monitoring of hemodynamics (including mean arterial pressure, cardiac index, and pulmonary capillary wedge pressure), urine output, and respiratory and renal function. Patients should initially be kept at bed rest with no oral intake, and large amounts of intravenous narcotic analgesics are typically needed for pain relief as well as nasogastric suction for treatment of severe ileus, nausea, and vomiting.

Several pharmacologic agents have been tried to inactivate trypsin and other serine proteases (e.g., aprotinin, gabexate), decrease pancreatic secretion (atropine, somatostatin and the somatostatin analog octreotide), or reduce inflammation (corticosteroids, indomethacin). None of these approaches has been shown to be beneficial in good clinical studies. In addition, the efficacy of early peritoneal lavage or operative approaches ("necrosectomy," debridement and drainage) in the absence of documented pancreatic infection remains to be demonstrated.

The recognition that cytokines and other mediators of inflammation are major contributors to both pancreatic injury and the later development of systemic complications in severe acute pancreatitis has engendered optimism that pharmacologic therapy directed either at inhibiting proinflammatory cytokines (e.g., IL-1, tumor necrosis factor, platelet-activating factor) or augmenting anti-inflammatory ones (e.g, IL-10) may prove to be effective in reducing the severity of acute pancreatitis. Unlike the activation of trypsin and other zymogens within the pancreas that may be largely completed by the time a patient is first seen by a physician, production of cytokines and development of distant organ dysfunction develop later, providing a possible "interventional window" during which drugs which specifically block the effects of inflammatory mediators could prevent or mitigate some of the life-threatening complications of severe pancreatitis (Fig. 117.4). However, the first such agent tested in a large, prospective, randomized, placebo-controlled trial, a potent antagonist of platelet-activating factor, failed to show any benefit. Nevertheless, a variety of other experimental drugs are at various stages of evaluation for this purpose.

In addition to organ failure, septic complications of acute pancreatitis are a major cause of morbidity and mortality. Earlier attempts to prevent this by prophylactic administration of antibiotics failed to show a benefit. However, the patients studied were on the milder end of the spectrum of severity (and thus less likely to develop septic complications) and the antibiotic used, ampicillin, was later shown not to penetrate inflamed pancreatic tissue well. Renewed interest in the use of prophylactic antibiotics has resulted from recent small studies suggesting a benefit from administration of either imipenem or a quinolone (e.g., ciprofloxacin) and metronidazole to patients with predicted severe pancreatitis. However, the currently available studies have limitations; and there is concern that prolonged use of prophylactic antibiotics, particularly imipenem, may increase the frequency of fungal infections. Until results of larger and more definitive studies are available, if prophylactic antibiotics are to be given, their use should be restricted to patients with predicted severe pancreatitis or suspected cholangitis. The combination of ciprofloxacin and metronidazole is the best choice to reduce the risk both of fungal infection for the patient and of development of imipenem-resistant organisms in the hospital.

Four randomized controlled studies have examined the value of ERCP with sphincterotomy and stone extraction, if indicated, in diminishing the severity of presumed gallstone pancreatitis. Gallstones should be suspected as the most likely cause in high-incidence areas (e.g., Hong Kong) and among patients who abstain from or moderately use alcohol, in women, in persons older than age 60, in those with a serum ALT elevated above the upper limits of normal by a factor of at least 3, in those with a history of gallstones, or in those with a dilated common duct visualized on abdominal ultrasonography or CT. If associated cholangitis is suspected due to the presence of right upper quadrant abdominal pain and tenderness, fever higher than 39°C, leukocyte count greater than 20,000 per milliliter, or bilirubin greater than 5 mg per deciliter, then urgent ERCP should be performed. However, in Western societies cholangitis is associated with acute gallstone pancreatitis in fewer than 10% of cases. Currently available studies yield conflicting results concerning whether ERCP performed within 24 to 72 hours of hospital admission reduces the severity of the disease for patients with presumed gallstone pancreatitis of moderate to severe degree who do not have cholangitis.

Oral feedings should not be resumed too soon for patients with severe acute pancreatitis or major complications (e.g., organ failure or infected pancreatic necrosis or abscess), as this may lead to exacerbation of the disease and further complications. Such patients should receive either enteral tube feedings (preferably of an elemental diet delivered to the more distal jejunum to reduce pancreatic stimulation) or total parenteral nutrition (TPN). Enteral feeding has the advantages of fewer complications and lower cost, and it may promote maintenance of intestinal mucosal integrity, thus reducing the risk of septic complications resulting from bacterial translocation from the gut. Lipid emulsions can be safely used as a component of TPN if care is taken to maintain the serum triglyceride concentration below 500 mg per deciliter. Oral feedings should not be started until any major complications have been effectively treated and the patient is free of pain and nausea and has near-normal serum amylase or lipase concentrations. If operative debridement and drainage is performed for infected necrosis or abscess (or if used for sterile necrosis), surgical placement of a tube jejunostomy greatly facilitates subsequent nutritional management.

COMPLICATIONS

In the initial 24 to 48 hours after admission, shock is the most lethal potential complication. Shock results from a combination of factors: marked hypovolemia due to transudation and exudation of fluid into the retroperitoneum and peritoneum, third-spacing of fluid into the dilated stomach and intestine, and (in some patients) a "leaky capillary" syndrome, as well as from myocardial depression due to unidentified factors presumably released as a consequence of the inflammatory process. Treatment is vigorous rehydration guided by hemodynamic monitoring in an intensive care unit, supplemented by vasopressor administration, if needed.

Although hypocalcemia is common and one of the adverse prognostic factors in the Ranson and Glasgow criteria for severity, clinically significant reductions of circulating ionized calcium are uncommon. Calcium administration is required only for patients with clinical findings related to hypocalcemia. If hypomagnesemia is also present, magnesium correction is required. The mechanisms by which hypocalcemia occurs are uncertain, but the disorder is probably multifactorial and may involve sequestration of calcium in saponified fat in the retroperitoneum and peritoneum, a decrease in the serum albumin concentration, and an impaired mobilization of calcium by parathyroid hormone.

Elevations in serum transaminases, alkaline phosphatase, and bilirubin are common in acute pancreatitis. However, they are usually mild and of no clinical significance, except as a possible indicator of gallstones as an etiologic factor (e.g., ALT more than three times the upper limit of normal). Jaundice is present in about 15% to 20% of patients, with total serum bilirubin usually below 4 mg per deciliter. A higher level or protracted elevation indicates coexisting parenchymal liver disease (e.g., alcoholic hepatitis or cirrhosis, chronic viral hepatitis) or obstruction of the common bile duct by a gallstone, tumor, pancreatic inflammatory mass, or pseudocyst. Surgical or endoscopic intervention may be required for treatment of bile duct obstruction.

Pulmonary abnormalities are common in patients with acute pancreatitis. About 60% of patients demonstrate hypoxemia on room air arterial blood gas determination; and 30% to 60% have abnormal chest film findings, ranging from atelectasis and pleural effusions (usually left-sided) to diffuse bilateral infiltrates indicative of adult respiratory distress syndrome. At about 3 to 7 days after admission, respiratory failure develops in about 5% to 10% of patients, requiring mechanical ventilation. Acute renal failure may also develop during the first week in the hospital, necessitating dialysis. The presence of respiratory or renal failure is associated with a markedly increased mortality rate approaching 50% in some series, but both complications are reversible if the underlying pancreatic inflammation abates and other complications (e.g., sepsis) do not supervene.

Patients with moderate to severe acute pancreatitis are at risk for septic complications resulting from infected pancreatic necrosis or abscess. This usually presents a week or more after admission as clinical deterioration (e.g., worsening pain or nausea and vomiting), fever (especially if higher than 39.5°C), or leukocytosis (especially if greater than 20,000 per milliliter). Over the past 20 years, earlier diagnosis and aggressive treatment of infected pancreatic necrosis and abscess have led to a reduction in mortality rates for septic complications from 70% to 80% to 10% to 20%. This has resulted from the widespread use of CT scanning and needle aspiration in the early evaluation of patients with suspected infected necrosis or abscess. Suspicious (low-density) areas in the pancreas or of fluid collections adjacent to it should be aspirated, sent for culture, and, most importantly, immediately Gram-stained. The presence of both bacterial organisms and polymorphonuclear leukocytes on the Gram-stained smear strongly indicates infected necrosis or abscess. Patients with these findings generally should undergo emergency surgery with extensive debridement and drainage. Several recent reports have proposed that some patients can be adequately treated with endoscopic or percutaneous catheter drainage or even antibiotics alone. However, the selection criteria have yet to be established in terms of which patients may do well with nonoperative approaches because the viscous nature of the infected material and the frequent presence of loculations make catheter drainage difficult and antibiotic penetration uncertain. Patients who develop signs of recurrent sepsis after initial operative treatment for infected necrosis or abscess should be carefully evaluated for possible fungal (usually *Candida*) sepsis.

Operative debridement and drainage has been proposed to benefit patients with severe acute pancreatitis who have sterile necrosis (CT-guided aspirates negative for bacterial or fungal organisms), particularly if it is complicated by respiratory or renal failure. However, it has not been established that this group of patients does better after surgery than similar patients treated only with aggressive nonoperative care.

Two-thirds to three-fourths of patients with acute pancreatitis have fluid collections (peripancreatic effusions) demonstrated early in their illness by abdominal ultrasonography or CT. Only about 10% to 15% of patients with acute pancreatitis develop an encapsulated collection of inflammatory fluid and pancreatic juice—a pseudocyst. If pseudocysts are asymptomatic or only mildly symptomatic (e.g., mild pain), acute pseudocysts should be followed by ultrasonography or CT for at least 6 weeks to determine if they will resolve (about half will) or decrease in size without treatment. Asymptomatic acute pseudocysts less than 6 cm in diameter or those diminishing in size can be watched without treatment indefinitely.

Symptomatic acute pseudocysts, expanding pseudocysts, and those larger than 6 cm in diameter (particularly if larger than 10 cm) should be considered for therapy if they persist for more than 6 weeks after an episode of acute pancreatitis. In the past the standard definitive treatment was open internal drainage of the pseudocyst into the stomach, duodenum, or a Roux loop of jejunum. More recently in selected patients, newer approaches, including minimally invasive (laparoscopic) surgical techniques, percutaneous catheter drainage, and endoscopic internal drainage, have been successfully employed. The treatment decision should be based on the specific circumstances for a given patient and the local expertise. For clinically infected pseudocysts (patients who typically have fever, leukocytosis, and pseudocyst aspirates demonstrating both polymorphonuclear leukocytes and bacterial organisms on Gram-stained smear), percutaneous catheter drainage is as effective as the previous operative approach (open external drainage), with a lower rate of pseudocyst recurrence and fistula formation.

Significant hemorrhage (requiring blood transfusion) is a rare complication of acute pancreatitis. Potential causes include stress gastritis, Mallory–Weiss tear, development of a pseudoaneurysm in the peripancreatic arterial circulation, bleeding from small vessels in the wall of a pseudocyst into the cyst contents, or gastric varices due to splenic vein thrombosis. Bleeding from stress gastritis, a Mallory–Weiss tear, or gastric varices usually presents with hematemesis, melena, and a falling blood hemoglobin concentration, and is best diagnosed by upper GI endoscopy. Bleeding from a pseudoaneurysm or into a pseudocyst from the cyst wall may not communicate with the GI tract (in which case it is best diagnosed by CT); or it may result in bleeding via the pancreatic duct (hemosuccus pancreaticus), with melena and blood or clot at endoscopy in the region of the duodenal papilla without any mucosal lesion that could account for it. Angiography is of great value in identifying the site of bleeding from a pseudoaneurysm. Frequently, pseudoaneurysms can be definitively treated by angiographic embolization, but some require direct operative control.

MANAGEMENT AFTER RECOVERY FROM ACUTE PANCREATITIS

Once a patient has recovered from an attack of acute pancreatitis, the most likely cause should be identified and treated, if possible, to prevent a recurrence. Patients with gallstone disease should generally undergo cholecystectomy. However, if the gallbladder has already been resected or if the patient is not a good operative candidate, endoscopic sphincterotomy is also highly effective. For the occasional patient with a gallbladder in place and cholesterol gallstones who, for whatever reason, cannot undergo surgery or ERCP, bile acid dissolution therapy can be considered. If alcohol is the cause, patients should be strongly advised to abstain. Genetic hyperlipidemia requires treatment with diet, avoidance of contributing factors (e.g., alcohol, estrogens, thiazides), good control of diabetes mellitus if present, and, in some cases, lipid-lowering drugs. If a specific drug is believed to be the causative factor, it should not be restarted.

In a relatively small number of patients, no etiologic process is established after the initial history and physical examination, determination of serum triglyceride and calcium concentrations, and abdominal ultrasonography. Several reports have suggested that at least half of these patients have occult gallstone disease (e.g., microlithiasis, biliary sludge); this is best identified by stimulating the gallbladder to contract with cholecystokinin and examining the bile or duodenal juice for cholesterol and bilirubinate crystals or by performing repeated abdominal ultrasonographic examinations for sludge in the gallbladder. Other studies have proposed that about 15% of these patients may have sphincter of Oddi dysfunction. Genetic hyperlipidemia is often missed because serum triglycerides are not measured until after the patient has been fasting for several days, by which time triglyceride levels may have fallen substantially. The more common causes of "idiopathic" acute pancreatitis and the means of diagnosing them are given in Table 117.5.

CHRONIC PANCREATITIS

Chronic pancreatitis is an inflammatory process involving the pancreas that results in irreversible fibrosis of the gland and atrophy of both exocrine and endocrine tissue. The pancreatic ducts are often involved, with the formation of intraductal protein plugs (which may calcify), ductal strictures, and dilatation of ducts upstream from strictures. Individual episodes of acute pancreatitis do not appear to lead to chronic pancreatitis in the absence of a significant stricture of the main pancreatic duct or its outflow. There are few reliable data on the prevalence or incidence of chronic pancreatitis. Estimates of prevalence from autopsy data range from 0.04% to 5%. One prospective study from Denmark in 1978–1979 estimated a prevalence of 26 cases per 100,000 population, whereas data from Germany covering the period 1988–1995 suggested an incidence of 6.6 cases per 100,000 population per year, resulting in a prevalence of about 132 cases per 100,000 population.

ETIOLOGIC FACTORS

In industrialized countries, alcohol consumption accounts for about 70% of cases (Table 117.6). Typically patients give a history of at least 6 to 12 years of consumption of 150 to 175 g of ethanol per day. However, there does not appear to be a

---

TABLE 117.5.	POSSIBLE CAUSES OF OCCULT ("IDIOPATHIC") ACUTE PANCREATITIS
Cause	**Useful Diagnostic Tests**
Occult gallstone disease (ultrasound-negative)	Biliary drainage for crystal analysis; repeated abdominal ultrasound exams (ERCP)
Undiagnosed hypertriglyceridemia	Previous serum triglyceride values, if available; serum triglyceride determination *after* patient resumes regular diet and medications
Abnormalities of the ampulla, bile duct, or pancreatic duct	ERCP
Sphincter of Oddi dysfunction	ERCP with sphincter of Oddi manometry
Pancreatic cancer; ampullary or other tumors	CT-guided fine-needle aspiration biopsy ERCP; serial determination of serum CA 19–9 levels
Cystic fibrosis	Measurement of sweat chloride; molecular genetic testing

ERCP, endoscopic retrograde cholangiopancreatography; CT, computed tomography.

TABLE 117.6.	MAJOR CAUSES OF CHRONIC PANCREATITIS

Chronic excessive alcohol use (70% of cases in industrialized countries)
Tropical chronic pancreatitis (primarily in India, Indonesia, Africa)
Chronic obstruction of the pancreatic duct
　Ampullary stenosis or neoplasm
　Pancreatic tumors
　Pseudocysts
　Pancreatic duct stents
　Traumatic or inflammatory strictures
　Pancreas divisum (uncertain)
Pancreatic trauma
Genetic hypertriglyceridemia
Hyperparathyroidism
Cystic fibrosis (including *CFTR* mutations that do not produce pulmonary disease)
Hereditary disease (e.g., mutation in the cationic trypsinogen gene)
Idiopathic disease (10–30% in industrialized countries)

statistical threshold for alcohol consumption because consumers of 1 to 20 g of ethanol per day have a small but statistically significant increase in the risk of developing chronic pancreatitis compared with abstainers. The form in which alcohol is consumed does not appear to affect the risk. A diet high in protein and either very high or very low in fat may predispose to chronic pancreatic injury from alcohol. Genetic, dietary, and other environmental predisposing factors probably have a significant influence on the risk of chronic pancreatitis because only 10% to 15% of individuals with the highest levels of alcohol use develop this disease.

The tropical or nutritional form of chronic pancreatitis is observed primarily in areas of India, Indonesia, and Africa. Patients typically present in childhood with abdominal pain and diffuse pancreatic calcifications, malnutrition, and diabetes mellitus, and they often die in early adulthood of complications of the disease. Although malnutrition appears to be a major factor, with patients consuming a low-protein and very-low-fat diet, it is not the only one; regions of India with comparable degrees of childhood malnutrition do not always have comparable prevalences for tropical chronic pancreatitis.

Long-standing obstruction of the main pancreatic duct or outflow from it may lead to obstructive chronic pancreatitis. This type of obstruction can result from papillary stenosis or ampullary neoplasms, pancreatic tumors, endoscopically placed pancreatic duct stents, pseudocysts, and strictures of the pancreatic duct as a consequence of trauma or, rarely, a severe episode of acute pancreatitis. Whether pancreas divisum can result in chronic pancreatitis (in addition to producing episodes of recurrent acute pancreatitis) remains a matter of dispute, with different clinical studies yielding conflicting results. Obstructive chronic pancreatitis, which appears to be a distinct type of chronic pancreatitis, is characterized by dilatation of the main pancreatic duct and acinar atrophy and fibrosis. However, unlike the case of alcoholic chronic pancreatitis, protein plugs or stones in the pancreatic duct are very uncommon; and morphologic and functional abnormalities may regress substantially once the obstruction is relieved.

Chronic pancreatitis may also develop in association with pancreatic trauma, genetic hyperlipidemia, hyperparathyroidism, and cystic fibrosis. A hereditary form presents with symptoms usually beginning in childhood and an autosomal pattern of inheritance with about 80% penetrance. The genetic defect is a point mutation on the gene on chromosome 7 coding for the pancreatic zymogen cationic trypsinogen, which renders the molecule less susceptible to intracellular mechanisms that protect the acinar cell against the premature activation of trypsinogen to trypsin. Other familial clusterings of what may be hereditary chronic pancreatitis have been described, with the onset of disease in the third or fourth decade.

About 10% to 30% of patients with chronic pancreatitis in industrialized countries have no apparent definable etiologic factor and are classified as having an idiopathic form. These patients seem to cluster in two age groups: a younger one (approximately age 15 to 30 years), in whom abdominal pain predominates, and an older group (approximately age 50 to 70 years), with pancreatic exocrine insufficiency and diabetes mellitus, often in the absence of pain. Recent studies have suggested that patients with idiopathic chronic pancreatitis have an increased incidence of a variety of defects in the *CFTR* gene that do not produce the pulmonary abnormalities typical of classic cystic fibrosis but that may alter pancreatic secretion in a way predisposing to development of chronic pancreatic injury. A possible autoimmune cause for some cases of idiopathic chronic pancreatitis has also been proposed.

PATHOGENESIS

The pathogenesis of chronic pancreatitis remains uncertain. For alcohol-related disease, current theories can be broadly divided into two main types. The first is that alcohol-related alterations in the physicochemical properties of pancreatic juice or in the function of the sphinchter of Oddi lead to duct obstruction as the principal cause of pancreatic damage (duct obstruction theories). The second is that repeated or continuous injury to pancreatic acinar cells produces inflammation, necrosis, and fibrosis, with duct obstruction, when present, as a secondary event (toxic–metabolic theories).

The leading variant of the duct obstruction theories proposes that protein plugs (some of which may calcify) initially precipitate in intralobular and small interlobular ducts due to one or more changes in pancreatic juice, such as an increase in protein and calcium concentration and viscosity, a decrease in citrate concentration, and alterations in solubility and the function of specific proteins (e.g., lithostathine, glycoprotein 2). Obstruction to smaller ducts produced by these plugs could trigger the inflammatory process, leading to fibrosis, atrophy, and ultimately involvement of the main pancreatic duct. Consistent with this theory is the finding that protein plugs are often found in pancreatic juice from patients with alcoholic chronic pancreatitis; a clinical natural history study involving serially performed ERCP suggested that in most patients branch ducts are deformed early in the course of the disease, before the main duct suffers increasing damage. Conversely, however, protein plugs can be found in the pancreatic juice from alcoholics without chronic pancreatitis and even in normal controls. This theory also fails to explain why protein plugging would occur early in chronic pancreatitis, before any reduction in pancreatic juice flow, and how the plugging of small ducts would initiate such a severe inflammatory response.

The toxic–metabolic theories propose that chronic pancreatitis results from chronic or repetitive injury to pancreatic acinar cells, leading to inflammation, atrophy, and fibrosis. Ductal plugging and stricturing could occur as a secondary event, perhaps related to decreased secretion and periductal fibrosis. In these theories, alcohol could act primarily by producing a direct toxic injury to acinar cells or by causing low-grade recurrent or persisting "acute" pancreatitis, which could be analogous to the role proposed for alcoholic hepatitis in the pathogenesis of cirrhosis of the liver.

There is insufficient evidence to consider any theory concerning the pathogenesis of alcoholic chronic pancreatitis (or of any other cause of chronic pancreatitis) as established. Probably more than one mechanism is involved, and it is likely that different mechanisms may predominate in different patients or even at different stages of the disease in the same patient.

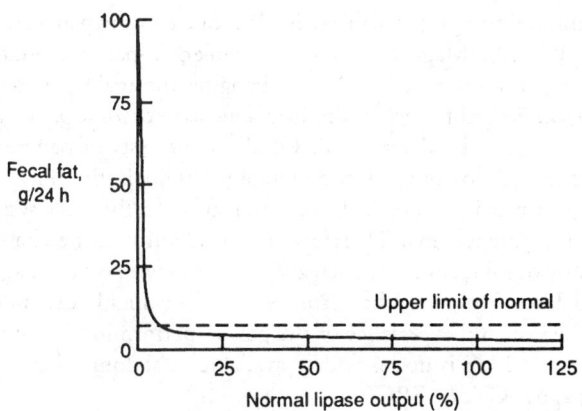

FIGURE 117.7. The relation of fecal fat excretion to secretion of pancreatic lipase into the duodenum in patients with chronic pancreatitis. Steatorrhea is not observed until lipase secretion is reduced to less than 10% of normal. (Adapted from DiMagno EP, Go VLW, Summerskill WHJ. Relations between pancreatic enzyme outputs and malabsorption in severe pancreatic insufficiency. *N Engl J Med* 1973;288:813.)

CLINICAL FEATURES

Pain is the most common presenting symptom. It is usually epigastric, dull, and constant in character, radiating to the back, to both upper quadrants, and even (occasionally) to the lower quadrants, particularly the left. The pain may be partially relieved by sitting bent forward or lying prone. In about half of patients, episodes of pain last for several days, with intervening pain-free intervals; the other half have near-constant pain. Pain is typically worsened by ingesting food or alcohol and may be accompanied by nausea and vomiting. For some patients, the pain diminishes or resolves completely over long periods of time (5 to 15 years), coincident with the appearance of pancreatic calcifications, steatorrhea, and diabetes ("burnout" of the gland). About 10% to 20% of patients with chronic pancreatitis have little or no pain, particularly the older age group of patients with idiopathic disease.

Patients with chronic pancreatitis typically lose weight due to pain and nausea, malabsorption due to pancreatic exocrine insufficiency, and poorly controlled diabetes mellitus. Overt steatorrhea occurs in about 30% to 50% of patients after the pancreas's capacity to secrete lipase and other digestive enzymes has been reduced to less than 10% of normal (Fig. 117.7). The quantity of fat in the stool in pancreatic insufficiency generally exceeds that found in other diseases producing steatorrhea. In the absence of ingestion of exogenous lipid oils (e.g., mineral oil), a history of oil leakage from the anus or an "oil slick" in the toilet is highly suggestive of pancreatic insufficiency. Although body stores of fat-soluble vitamins (A, D, E, and K) may be diminished, clinical deficiencies are rarely observed. Hypoproteinemia is also uncommon.

Clinically evident diabetes mellitus occurs in about 50% of patients, usually after the diagnosis has been well established. However, patients with little or no pain may present initially with diabetes, as may patients with tropical chronic pancreatitis. For similar durations of diabetes, retinopathy and neuropathy appear to occur as often as in primary forms of diabetes; however, ketoacidosis and nephropathy are uncommon.

During episodes of pain, patients with chronic pancreatitis usually have demonstrated mild to moderate epigastric tenderness without guarding or rebound tenderness. Generally, the abdominal tenderness is less impressive than the degree of pain reported. A rounded, palpable abdominal mass suggests the presence of a pseudocyst, although most are not palpable. Bulging flanks and shifting dullness indicate the possible presence of pancreatic ascites, and dullness to percussion or diminished breath sounds at the lung bases may be signs of a pancreatic pleural effusion.

DIAGNOSIS

Chronic pancreatitis should be suspected when a patient presents with the typical pattern and character of abdominal pain, particularly if accompanied by symptoms suggestive of steatorrhea or diabetes mellitus. The finding on plain abdominal film of calcifications in the region of the pancreas (Fig. 117.8) is present

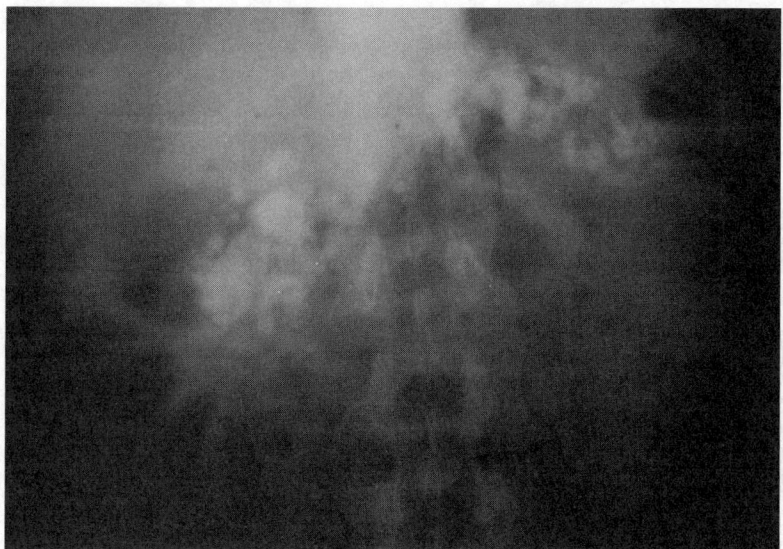

FIGURE 117.8. Abdominal plain film demonstrating calcifications throughout the pancreas in a patient with chronic pancreatitis.

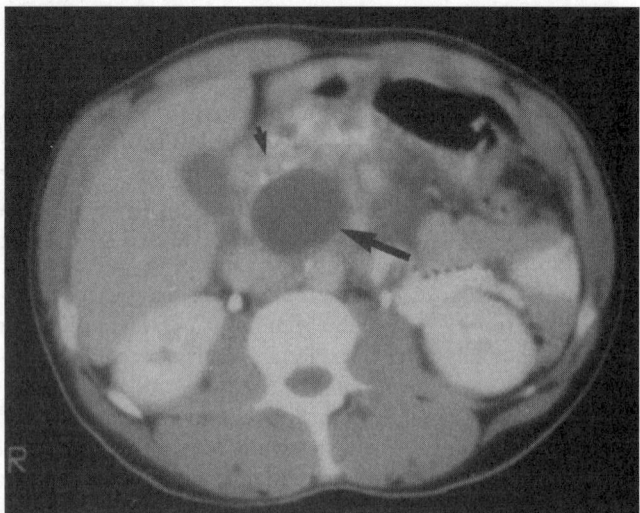

FIGURE 117.9. Typical findings on computed tomography in chronic pancreatitis. There is an area *(small arrow)* containing multiple bright-appearing calcifications and a pseudocyst *(large arrow)* in the head of the pancreas. (From Forsmark CE. Chronic pancreatitis and pancreatic insufficiency. In: Grendell JH, McQuaid KR, Friedman SL, eds. *Current diagnosis and treatment in gastroenterology*. Stamford, CT: Appleton & Lange, 1996:441, with permission.)

in about one-third of patients and establishes the diagnosis with a high degree of reliability; no further diagnostic testing is necessary. In increasing order of sensitivity, cost, and invasiveness, abdominal ultrasonography, CT, and ERCP can be used to confirm the diagnosis in patients without calcification on plain film. On ultrasonography and CT scanning (Fig. 117.9), typical findings are calcifications (which can be below the resolution of plain film), dilatation of the pancreatic duct, and pancreatic pseudocysts. ERCP provides exquisitely detailed views of the pancreatic duct system, demonstrating strictures and ectatic changes in the pancreatic duct and its main branches (which are

common findings, particularly in alcoholic chronic pancreatitis; Fig. 117.10). Magnetic resonance cholangio-pancreatography provides a noninvasive means of imaging the main pancreatic duct, but its utility and role in the diagnosis of chronic pancreatitis remains to be determined. Of all of the tests of pancreatic structure, endoscopic ultrasonography (EUS) is the only one that can provide a detailed evaluation of both the duct system and the parenchyma. Therefore, it can identify subtle changes in early or mild chronic pancreatitis not seen with other imaging modalities. However, the accuracy of EUS is highly dependent on the skill and experience of the person performing the procedure, and EUS is not as widely available as abdominal ultrasonography, CT, or ERCP.

An alternative approach to the diagnosis of chronic pancreatitis is the testing of pancreatic exocrine function. The most sensitive and reliable tests involve collection of either duodenal or "pure" pancreatic juice (by cannulation of the pancreatic duct at ERCP) and measuring either the concentration of bicarbonate after administration of secretin or the concentration of one or more of the pancreatic digestive enzymes after administration of a test meal or CCK (or its analog cerulein). These direct tests of function are most useful in suspected mild or early chronic pancreatitis, particularly if idiopathic or due to causes other than alcohol, a situation in which calcifications or abnormalities in the pancreatic duct are frequently not present on imaging studies. However, direct test of pancreatic function are technically cumbersome, expensive, and not widely available. Indirect or "tubeless" tests of pancreatic function include measurement of fecal concentrations of the pancreatic enzymes chymotrypsin or elastase, and the bentiromide and pancrealauryl tests. These latter two tests involve oral administration of a test substance that is cleaved by pancreatic enzymes in the small intestine, releasing a marker that can be measured in urine or blood. Unfortunately, these inexpensive and relatively convenient indirect tests are reliable only in patients with advanced disease (e.g., those with steator-

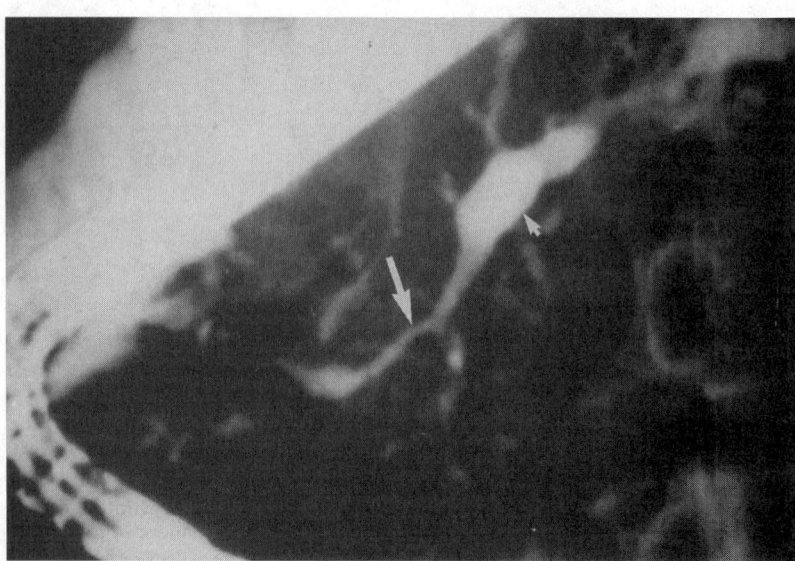

FIGURE 117.10. Typical findings on endoscopic retrograde pancreatography in chronic pancreatitis. Throughout the pancreatic duct, there are multiple alternating areas of stricture *(large arrow)* and duct dilatation *(small arrow)*, creating a "chain of lakes" appearance.

rhea), for whom the diagnosis is generally not difficult to establish by plain film or other abdominal imaging.

The most sensitive imaging studies, EUS and ERCP, and the direct tests of pancreatic function (e.g., secretin stimulation test for measurement of bicarbonate concentration) are abnormal in most patients with chronic pancreatitis and correlate well in those with moderate to severe disease. However, in patients suspected of having mild or early chronic pancreatitis, any two of these three tests yield conflicting results in 15% to 30% of cases, creating diagnostic uncertainty that is difficult to resolve in the absence of pancreatic histologic examination, which is rarely available.

The hallmark of pancreatic insufficiency is the presence of steatorrhea which is defined as fecal fat excretion of more than 7 g per 24 hours on a diet of 100 g of fat per day. Qualitative stool fat determinations (Sudan staining) generally become positive when steatorrhea results in a stool fat excretion of 12 to 15 g per day or more.

DIFFERENTIAL DIAGNOSIS

The differential diagnosis in patients with upper abdominal pain includes peptic ulcer disease, gastric or pancreatic cancer, chronic partial obstruction of the small intestine, and functional abdominal pain syndromes. Steatorrhea from pancreatic insufficiency must be distinguished from that due to diseases of the small intestine.

MANAGEMENT

Pain

For patients with alcoholic chronic pancreatitis, abstinence from alcohol may result in improvement in pain, particularly for patients with early or mild disease (before the development of extensive calcifications and steatorrhea). Oral analgesics, including potent narcotics, are often needed for pain relief. For patients disabled either by pain or by the amount of narcotics required to control pain, a trial of high doses of a nonenteric-coated pancreatic enzyme supplement (e.g., Viokase or Ku-Zyme HP, 8 with meals and at bedtime along with a gastric proton pump inhibitor) can be instituted in the hope of ameliorating pain by enhancing feedback inhibition of pancreatic enzyme secretion. This approach appears to have the greatest prospects for success in patients with idiopathic chronic pancreatitis without steatorrhea. Results of celiac plexus and splanchnic nerve blocks have generally been disappointing; even if some pain relief is achieved, it is usually short-lived.

Thoracoscopic splanchnicectomy performed in the mediastinum is being evaluated to determine if it will result in a more effective and durable form of pain relief.

Patients whose pain is not adequately managed by oral analgesics and who have not responded to a trial of pancreatic enzymes should be considered for operative treatment. Preoperative evaluation by CT and, frequently, ERCP is essential in determining the type of operation to be performed and in identifying complications (e.g., pseudocysts or pancreatic cancer). Patients with alcoholic chronic pancreatitis often have alternating areas of stricture and dilatation of the pancreatic duct ("chain of lakes" appearance). For these patients a lateral pancreaticojejunostomy (modified Puestow procedure) produces resolution or significant improvement in pain in 70% to 80% of patients when pain is assessed at 6 months after surgery. However, when pain is assessed 3 to 5 years after surgery, successful outcomes decrease to about 50%.

Patients with dominant strictures in the body or tail of the pancreas should undergo distal pancreatectomy. Patients with inflammatory masses of the head of the pancreas or nondilated ducts generally benefit most from resection of the head of the pancreas, either by a modified Whipple procedure or by one of several duodenum-sparing techniques. Carefully selected patients have been reported to have good results in 80% to 85% of cases, and these good results have tended to persist over time. However, pancreatic resection carries the risk of precipitating or worsening diabetes and insulin dependence.

Rarely patients who continue to have incapacitating pain after previous unsuccessful attempts at surgical relief undergo total pancreatectomy. However, this should be considered an extreme measure because of the extent of the operation and the difficult-to-manage diabetes that results. In this setting, autotransplantation of the pancreas or of pancreatic islets has been attempted to try to prevent or mitigate diabetes.

A number of approaches have been tried to reduce the need for surgery in patients with chronic pancreatitis and poorly controlled pain. A combination of antioxidants has been administered to prevent or reduce oxidative injury to the pancreas, and the inhibitory somatostatin analog octreotide has been given to reduce the metabolic workload of the gland; but neither of these is of proven efficacy.

Currently, there is considerable interest in endoscopic dilatation and stenting of strictures and removal of stones from the pancreatic duct and in destruction of pancreatic duct stones with extracorporeal shock wave lithotripsy. Uncontrolled studies in highly selected groups of patients report symptom improvement in 60% to 70% of patients over several years of follow-up. Prospective randomized, controlled trials are needed to assess the benefits and risks of these approaches in comparison with those of surgery and symptomatic medical care.

Malabsorption

Patients with significant degrees of steatorrhea should receive pancreatic enzyme supplements with meals and snacks. Generally, a total of at least 30,000 units of lipase taken before and during each meal substantially reduces (but usually does not completely correct) steatorrhea, and permits stabilization of body weight and amelioration of diarrhea and bloating. As pancreatic enzymes are degraded by gastric acid, the effectiveness of enzyme supplementation can be enhanced by acid suppression, neutralization of acid by bicarbonate, or the use of enteric-coated preparations. For the rare patient unable to tolerate a fat intake sufficient to maintain an adequate body weight despite pancreatic enzyme supplementation, medium-chain triglycerides can be added to the diet, which do not require intraluminal lipolytic activity for their absorption.

COMPLICATIONS

Pseudocyst

About 10% of patients with chronic pancreatitis develop pseudocysts, usually in the body or tail of the gland. Pseudocysts less than 6 cm in diameter are usually asymptomatic, but larger ones can produce pain and relatively infrequently become infected, bleed, rupture, or obstruct the bile duct or GI tract. Pseudocysts are easily diagnosed by abdominal ultrasonography or CT. Asymptomatic pseudocysts in patients with chronic pancreatitis do not require treatment and may resolve spontaneously. Symptomatic pseudocysts and pseudocysts greater than 6 cm in diameter that are expanding should be treated. Open operative internal drainage has been the standard treatment; however, percutaneous catheter drainage and endoscopic internal drainage are being increasingly employed, and laparoscopic operative techniques have been developed. Clinically infected pseudocysts should be drained using percutaneous catheters.

Pancreatic Ascites and Pleural Effusion

Leakage of pancreatic juice from a pseudocyst or disrupted duct may result in collections of fluid with high protein and amylase concentrations in the peritoneum or in the pleural space, usually on the left. In about half of these patients, conservative treatment with no oral intake, TPN or jejunal feeding of an elemental diet, octreotide administration to decrease pancreatic secretion, and repeated aspiration of ascites or pleural effusions leads to resolution in 2 to 3 weeks. The remaining patients should undergo ERCP to identify the site of leakage and to plan therapy. Selected patients can be successfully treated by endoscopic stenting of the pancreatic duct. Others, depending on the location of the leak, will require distal pancreatectomy or internal drainage of a pseudocysts or damaged duct to a Roux limb of jejunum.

Bile Duct or Duodenal Obstruction

Bile duct or duodenal obstruction occurs in 5% to 10% of patients with chronic pancreatitis. Bile duct obstruction typically develops due to fibrosis in the head of the pancreas that produces a long, tapered stricture of the common bile duct. This is usually diagnosed by a combination of liver tests (elevated serum levels of alkaline phosphatase and bilirubin), abdominal ultrasonography, and ERCP. Biliary bypass surgery is warranted only in patients who develop cholangitis or whose liver tests or liver biopsy findings show evidence of progressive damage attributable to chronic bile duct obstruction. Endoscopic stenting of the common bile duct is an option in patients who are poor operative candidates. Duodenal obstruction can result from a large pseudocyst or an inflammatory mass in the head of the pancreas. If clinically significant, drainage of the pseudocyst or gastrojejunostomy is required.

Splenic Vein Thrombosis

Inflammation or compression of the splenic vein due to chronic pancreatitis can produce splenic vein thrombosis with spleno-megaly, gastric varices, and upper GI bleeding. This should be suspected in any patient with known pancreatic disease or a history of chronic heavy alcohol use who presents with upper GI bleeding and is found at endoscopy to have gastric varices in the absence of significant esophageal varices. Splenectomy is highly effective in treating this condition.

Pancreatic Cancer

Patients with chronic pancreatitis of any etiology appear to have an increased risk of developing pancreatic cancer. This increase appears to be modest for most etiologic factors but may be substantially higher for patients with tropical or hereditary chronic pancreatitis. The diagnosis of pancreatic cancer in patients with chronic pancreatitis is often very difficult to make because the symptoms, signs, and CT, ERCP, or EUS findings can be very similar. A progressive rise in the serum level of the tumor marker CA 19-9 suggests a cancer. Cytologic examination of aspirates of pancreatic juice or brushings from the pancreatic duct has a sensitivity of only 25% to 50% for the diagnosis of pancreatic cancer; CT-guided fine-needle aspiration biopsies have a sensitivity of 80% to 85%. Although K-ras mutations are found in pancreatic juice or aspiration biopsies of most patients with pancreatic cancer, its specificity is not known because K-ras mutations have also been reported in specimens from patients with chronic pancreatitis without apparent pancreatic cancer. Thus, no recommendations for screening patients with chronic pancreatitis for pancreatic cancer can be made at this time. Unfortunately, at the time of diagnosis, pancreatic cancer in patients with chronic pancreatitis is only very rarely curable by surgery.

BIBLIOGRAPHY

Adler G, Nelson DK, Katschinski M, et al. Neurohormonal control of human pancreatic exocrine secretion. *Pancreas* 1995;10:1–13.

Baron TH, Morgan DE. Acute necrotizing pancreatitis. *N Engl J Med* 1999; 340:1412–1417.

Bradley EL III. A clinically based classification system for acute pancreatitis. *Arch Surg* 1993;128:586–590.

Forsmark CE, Grendell JH. Complications of pancreatitis. *Semin Gastroint-est Dis* 1991;2:165.

Grendell JH. Nonsurgical therapy of acute pseudocysts. In: Bradley EL III, ed. *Acute pancreatitis: diagnosis and therapy*. New York: Raven Press, 1994.

Ho HS, Frey CF. Current approach to the surgical management of chronic pancreatitis. *Gastroenterologist* 1997;5:128–136.

Layer P, Keller J. Pancreatic enzymes: secretion and luminal nutrient digestion in health and disease. *J Clin Gastroenterol* 1999;28:3–10.

Mengener K, Baillie J. Chronic pancreatitis. *Lancet* 1997; 350:1379–1385.

Norman J. The role of cytokines in the pathogenesis of acute pancreatitis. *Am J Surg* 1998;175:76–83.

Steer ML, Waxman I, Freedman S. Chronic pancreatitis. *N Engl J Med* 1995;332:1482–1490.

Steinberg W, Tenner S. Acute pancreatitis. *N Engl J Med* 1994; 330:1198–1210.

Kelley's Textbook of Internal Medicine, fourth edition. Edited by H. David Humes. Lippincott Williams & Wilkins, Philadelphia © 2000.

PANCREATIC CANCER AND GUT NEUROENDOCRINE TUMORS

DANIEL G. HALLER

▌ PANCREATIC CANCER

Adenocarcinoma of the pancreas is one of the most enigmatic malignancies of the gastrointestinal (GI) tract in terms of etiologic factors, diagnosis, and therapy. As one of the leading causes of cancer death, this tumor represents one of the greatest challenges for patients and physicians alike. Unlike esophageal and gastric cancer, there are no clear epidemiologic risks for this cancer. Although there are minor geographic and gender differences, these are less strong than for other common tumors. The most consistently documented environmental risk is cigarette smoking, documented by case-control and case-cohort studies. Dietary factors similar to those observed in colorectal cancer, such as diets high in animal fat and low in fiber and antioxidant vitamins, have also been implicated in the development of pancreatic cancer. Although a number of medical factors, such as chronic pancreatitis and diabetes, are variably associated with a higher risk of developing pancreatic cancer, causative links have not been definitively established. Recently, a familial pancreatic cancer has been described, although studies would suggest that such genetic causes account for a relatively small proportion (less than 5%) of cases. However, the ability to screen a known high-risk patient population could allow for earlier diagnosis and therapy.

NATURAL HISTORY AND DIAGNOSIS

The biology of pancreatic cancer has begun to impact on the understanding of pancreatic carcinogenesis and prognostication. Specific point mutations in the K-*ras* and *p53* oncogene have been described in most pancreatic cancer specimens. K-*ras,* in particular, has been thought to be one of the earlier genetic events in the development of pancreatic cancer. Locoregional extension of tumor is an early and common event, and provides both an explanation for poor outcome and the rationale for combined-modality treatment programs. Because of the location of the pancreas and the propensity for locoregional spread, preoperative staging is of primary importance in selecting optimal patients for surgical resection. The majority of patients present with unresectable or metastatic disease, and diagnostic techniques to spare such patients unnecessary surgery are of chief importance. For the small number of patients who do undergo surgical resection, the expected 5-year survival ranges from 5% to 25%. Preoperative staging studies include either computed tomography (CT) or magnetic resonance imaging (MRI) (see

Chapter 128) and endoscopic ultrasound (see Chapter 127). In many institutions, magnetic resonance angiography has replaced standard angiograms as the diagnostic study of choice to assess vascular involvement; such involvement typically represents a relative contraindication to surgical resection with curative intent. Endoscopic retrograde cholangiopancreatography may also be useful in some patients to define the nature of a pancreatic mass, to obtain cytologic specimens for definitive diagnosis, and to distinguish tumors of the pancreas from those of the ampulla of Vater or the duodenum. Endoscopic ultrasonography is now being used in many institutions both to assess resectability based on vascular involvement and for transduodenal biopsies to obtain histologic diagnosis. Although adenocarcinoma is the most common malignancy of the pancreas, other tumors—with widely divergent natural histories and treatments—may also develop in the pancreas and surrounding structures, such as islet cell tumors, lymphomas, germ cell tumors, and low-grade pancreatic neoplasms. For this reason, histologic or cytologic confirmation of malignancy is imperative, particularly when therapeutic decisions, such as neoadjuvant treatment, are under consideration. Fine-needle aspiration of the pancreas is generally considered safe, although it is anecdotally associated with tracking of tumor cells in the path of the biopsy needle. The decision to perform a major surgical resection or combined-modality chemotherapy and radiation therapy without a preoperative or intraoperative biopsy is controversial.

TREATMENT

For patients with pancreatic cancer that appears resectable by preoperative staging, surgery remains the standard curative treatment option. The pancreaticoduodenectomy (Whipple's procedure) is the procedure of choice for most patients with tumors of the head or body of the pancreas, with operative mortality as low as 2% in centers that perform large numbers of cases. For tumors in the tail of the pancreas, distal pancreatectomy may be considered, although few patients with tumor in this location present in a localized manner to allow curative resection. Conversely, patients who present with painless jaundice alone (attributable to a small tumor strategically placed in the head of the pancreas) are most likely to be cured with surgery. Late postoperative complications include the development of pancreatic exocrine insufficiency, which may complicate the interpretation of weight loss in a patient with a history of pancreatic cancer. This condition is easily remedied by administration of exogenous enzymes. Only a small proportion of patients who undergo Whipple's procedure develop insulin dependence.

There are many patients with pancreatic cancer who have localized but unresectable disease. Some local problems can be dealt with by nonsurgical techniques, including biliary stenting by endoscopy for obstructive jaundice (see Chapter 127). In some patients whose survival is thought to be good (better than 6 to 9 months), optimal therapy for biliary and duodenal obstruction may include surgery to bypass the tumor. For patients with pain, either with localized tumor or with metastases, celiac axis nerve bloc may help to minimize dependence on narcotics.

Active antitumor therapy for patients with unresectable pancreatic cancer has traditionally consisted of radiation, typically given in conjunction with 5-fluorouracil (5-FU)–based chemotherapy. The initial trials of such therapy were carried out by the Mayo Clinic and confirmed by the Gastrointestinal Tumor Study Group (GITSG). The GITSG trial established that, when radiation is given, 4,000 cGy with 5-FU was superior to 6,000 cGy alone and equivalent to 6,000 cGy with 5-FU, in terms of median survival (10 versus 6 months). Although considered by most to be standard practice, few other studies have confirmed or addressed the potential superiority of combined-modality chemoradiation to radiation alone. In selected centers with appropriate equipment, intraoperative radiation, given before standard external-beam radiation, is the preferred treatment, with higher intraoperative doses of radiation allowing for the possibility of better local control of the primary tumor. Although retrospective studies have suggested benefit from intraoperative radiation in local control and overall survival, there are no data from large, randomized controlled trials to confirm this conclusion.

In some institutions, preoperative (neoadjuvant) chemoradiation has been used in two groups of patients: those with tumors thought initially to be resectable and those with tumors considered initially to be of borderline resectability. There is a clear downstaging effect from such treatment, but the proportion of patients whose tumors are rendered resectable for cure, despite their initially having been thought to be unresectable, is unclear. Nonrandomized comparisons of preoperative chemoradiation to surgery followed by chemoradiation have not demonstrated a survival advantage to the neoadjuvant approach, likely because improvements in local control of the primary tumors may not limit the development of life-threatening metastatic disease. However, many investigators still prefer neoadjuvant therapy for patients with resectable pancreatic cancer because of improved tolerability when such treatment is given preoperatively.

For patients who undergo curative resection of pancreatic cancer, the 5-year survival rate in most series is poor, ranging from 5% to 25%, supporting the need for effective adjuvant therapy to control micrometastases remaining after surgery. In spite of the number of patients who could benefit from such treatment, there have been few prospective trials addressing the role of postoperative adjuvant treatment. The most widely accepted, yet controversial, study is from the GITSG. In 1973, this group began a randomized trial comparing surgery alone to postoperative radiation with both concurrent and sequential chemotherapy with 5-FU. Accrual to the trial was extraordinarily slow, in part due to fear of complications of postoperative treatment. For the 43 patients who were randomized, the median survival for the combined-modality treatment was 20 months, compared to 11 months for the surgery-alone group. The 5-year survival was 14% and 5%, respectively. When the trial closed to randomized accrual, the group subsequently entered more patients into the combined-modality treatment, with similar results. Nonrandomized, retrospective studies of postoperative combined-modality therapy support the results from the GITSG trial, but there are no large, contemporaneous controlled trials to fully confirm the level of benefit of this widely accepted treatment. It is nonetheless the standard of care in most large institutions in which pancreatic resections are performed, making it difficult to perform prospective randomized trials in which surgery alone is the standard arm. A new adjuvant therapy trial is comparing two schemes of postoperative combined-modality therapy for resected patients, one using 5-FU and the other gemcitabine, with either drug given sequentially with radiation and concurrent continuous infusion 5-FU.

ADVANCED DISEASE

Many patients with pancreatic cancer present with metastatic disease and most develop it during the course of their illness, resulting in poor survival and mandating the development of successful systemic treatment and supportive care strategies. Although early trials of biologics, such as K-ras vaccines and antisense compounds, are currently under way, the mainstay of systemic therapy for pancreatic cancer remains cytotoxic chemotherapy. Broad phase II trials of new agents have typically shown that pancreatic cancer is generally considered to be a relatively chemotherapy-resistant disease. Until recently, only a few drugs showed any measurable antitumor activity by standard drug screening and clinical trials techniques, including 5-FU, mitomycin, and streptozocin. Combination therapy with these drugs has not yielded significantly improved benefits, and standard practice until recently has been to administer 5-FU for palliation. Measurable response rates with this drug are typically less than 10%, and palliative benefits have been difficult to quantify.

Recently, a new drug, gemcitabine, has entered clinical practice for the management of advanced pancreatic cancer. Noted to have some activity in early clinical testing, phase II trials were similarly encouraging. A phase III trial of gemcitabine compared to weekly 5-FU alone has been completed, in which gemcitabine was considered to be superior to 5-FU in clinical benefit (palliation). Using a scale of clinical benefit response, which combines measures of pain control and performance status, 24% of the gemcitabine-treated patients were responders, compared to 5% for 5-FU. Few patients in either group exhibited clear tumor response by conventional measures, but median survival for gemcitabine was superior (5.7 versus 4.4 months, $p = 0.0024$). At 1 year, survival was also superior for gemcitabine. In a separate study, some objective responders were seen when patients who had previously failed on 5-FU were given gemcitabine. Currently, both 5-FU and gemcitabine represent legitimate treatment options for patients with advanced pancreatic cancer. In addition, early reports of activity of docetaxel, topotecan, and cisplatin combined with gemcitabine have led to new treatment regimens that are presently under clinical investigations.

■ GUT NEUROENDOCRINE TUMORS

Gastrointestinal hormones coordinate in a highly integrated fashion the intake, processing, absorption, and distribution of essential nutrients. Like other endocrine transmitters, gut hormones are secreted from endocrine cells into the blood, where they circulate to reach target tissues. However, unlike classic endocrine tissues in which homogeneous cells are concentrated in glands, endocrine cells of the gut are scattered along the GI mucosa as isolated cells. In the intestine, endocrine cells originate

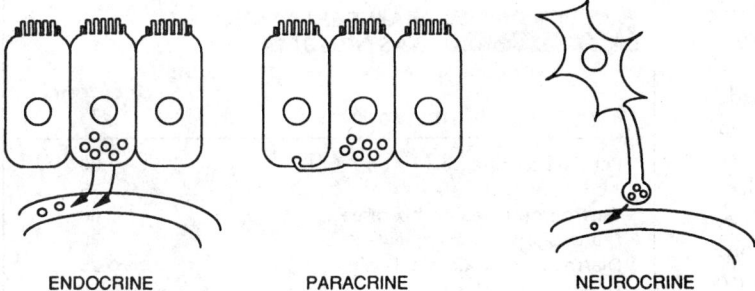

ENDOCRINE   PARACRINE   NEUROCRINE

FIGURE 118.1. Transmitters of the gastrointestinal tract. The mechanisms of secretion for hormones, paracrine transmitters, and neurocrine agents of the gastrointestinal tract are represented schematically.

from stem cells within the crypts. Electron-dense, hormone-containing, secretory granules are located toward the bases of the cells, which lie in proximity to capillaries. Exposure of endocrine cells to stimuli such as food, changes in lumen pH, or other intestinal secretions within the gut lumen initiates the intracellular events resulting in secretion of hormone into adjacent capillaries. On reaching the systemic circulation, these transmitters bind to specific hormone receptors on respective target tissues to exert their physiologic effects.

Endocrine cells of the gut have been identified cytochemically by their ability to reduce silver solutions (argentaffinity) and to take up silver ions from solution (argyrophilia) or to form isoquinolones and fluoresce after hot-formaldehyde treatment. This latter method uses the acronym APUD (*a*mine *p*recursor *u*ptake and *d*ecarboxylation) to identify amine-containing cells. Specific hormone-containing cells can be distinguished by their electron microscopic appearance and immunohistochemical properties.

Peptide transmitters of the GI tract also have been identified in pancreatic islets and in neurons of the brain and gut. Peptides of neural origin may function as typical neurotransmitters acting directly through synapses on target cells, or they may be secreted from nerve endings into the bloodstream to reach distant targets (neurocrine action; Fig. 118.1).

GASTROINTESTINAL HORMONES

Many GI hormones are similar in amino acid sequence. This evidence is taken to imply a common ancestry and evolution through gene duplication and divergence. Six groups of peptides have been identified in the GI tract. These include the gastrin–cholecystokinin family, the secretin family, the pancreatic polypeptide (PP) group, the opioids, the tachykinins, and the bombesin-like peptides. Several GI peptides share no structural homologic features with other mammalian peptides. These so-called "orphan peptides" include somatostatin, motilin, and neurotensin. Bioactive GI peptides that have been extracted from the GI tract are listed in Table 118.1.

CHARACTERISTICS OF ENDOCRINE TUMORS OF THE GASTROINTESTINAL TRACT

Endocrine tumors of the pancreas often present as fascinating and bizarre diagnostic puzzles. The specific manifestations of

these tumors depend on the release of biologically active substances. The released mediators include the hormones gastrin, insulin, vasoactive intestinal peptide (VIP), glucagon, and somatostatin, and biologically active amines such as serotonin and its metabolites. Discrete syndromes result from the overproduction and secretion of each of these potential transmitters and provide an intriguing array of clinical findings for the physician. Endocrine tumors of the pancreas share many similarities in location, histologic features, growth rate, manner of spread, association with multiple endocrine neoplasia type I (MEN I) syndrome, and response to hormonal treatment and chemotherapy. In the management of gut neuroendocrine tumors, clinicians must always keep in mind that individual patients may have signs or symptoms of hormone-related disorders, or of tumor bulk, or both. In some diseases, such as gastrinomas, there has

TABLE 118.1.	PEPTIDES OF GASTROINTESTINAL TRACT

Hormones
  Gastrin
  Cholecystokinin
  Secretin
  Glucose-dependent insulinotropic peptide
  Pancreatic polypeptide
  Motilin
  Insulin
  Glucagon
  Enteroglucagon
  Peptide YY
  Somatostatin
Neurotransmitters or neuromodulators
  Cholecystokinin
  Somatostatin
  Gastrin-releasing peptide
  Neuropeptide Y
  Vasoactive intestinal polypeptide
  Neurotensin
  Calcitonin gene–related peptide
  Galanin
  Peptide HI
  Pancreastatin
  Substance P
  Substance K
  Enkephalin
  Dynorphin
Paracrine transmitters
  Somatostatin
  Peptide YY

been a paradigm shift for morbidity and mortality away from the complications of gastrinemia toward the more typical tumor-related complication of metastatic disease.

Histologically, endocrine tumors of the pancreas are made up of small, uniform cells with little mitotic activity. On electron microscopic examination, these cells contain abundant secretory granules. Hormone-secreting tumors stain positively with selective markers, such as chromogranin A, neuron-specific enolase, or antisera against specific hormones. Because of their innocuous histologic appearance, endocrine tumors of the pancreas once were thought to be benign, and some were given the name carcinoid ("cancer-like") tumor. Despite their appearance, most GI hormone–secreting tumors behave in a malignant manner. Within the GI tract, most endocrine tumors are found in the pancreas, where they are believed to be of islet cell origin. Glucagon-secreting tumors (glucagonomas) almost invariably are confined to the pancreas. Most gastrin-secreting tumors (gastrinomas) also are found in the pancreas, despite the fact that there are no gastrin cells in the adult pancreas. Some gastrinomas may also be found in the gut and in paraintestinal lymph nodes. Carcinoid tumors, which demonstrate uniform serotonin production, may originate in any organ derived from the primitive endoderm, although the most common sites are the appendix, rectum, and small intestine.

Gut neuroendocrine tumors are typically slow growing and often are diagnosed only because of their elaboration of bioactive transmitters. These tumors usually metastasize to the liver but may spread to lymph nodes, bone, and lung.

Many endocrine tumors of the pancreas are associated with MEN I and are accompanied by tumors of the pituitary and parathyroid. The pancreatic tumors usually secrete GI hormones, including gastrin, insulin, glucagon, PP, and, rarely, VIP. MEN I is inherited as an autosomal dominant disorder and affects 1 in 20,000 individuals. Genetic mutations responsible for the disorder (the *MEN1* gene) have been localized to a specific area on the long arm of chromosome 11 (11q13), and recently the gene has been identified and named menin. The function of the gene is currently not well defined. Hyperparathyroidism with accompanying hypercalcemia is the most common clinical manifestation of MEN I. Pancreatic tumors occur in 50% to 65% of patients with this syndrome, and gastrinoma is the most common functioning islet cell tumor. Patients with endocrine tumors associated with MEN I seem to have longer life expectancies than do those with sporadic endocrine tumors of the pancreas, implying that MEN I–associated pancreatic tumors have a less malignant course than sporadic pancreatic tumors.

GASTRINOMAS

Gastrin-secreting tumors are the most common endocrine tumors of the GI tract, with an incidence of 0.5 to 1.0 per million population. Zollinger and Ellison originally reported the syndrome in 1955, when they described two patients with atypical peptic ulceration, gastric hypersecretion, and non–β-cell islet tumors. The compilation of symptoms and physical findings caused by a gastrin-secreting tumor is referred to as Zollinger–Ellison syndrome (ZES; see also Chapter 107). Before

TABLE 118.2.	MANIFESTATIONS OF GASTRINOMA	
Manifestation		**Incidence (%)**
Peptic ulcer disease		80
Abdominal pain		75
Gastroesophageal reflux disease		60
Diarrhea		30
Diarrhea and abdominal pain		25
Upper gastrointestinal tract bleeding		10
Perforated ulcer		7

the availability of radioimmunoassays for measuring blood levels of gastrin, patients had severe complications of gastric acid hypersecretion. Typical manifestations of the disease included intractable or complicated peptic ulcer disease with abdominal pain and multiple ulcers or ulceration in unusual locations, such as the jejunum. More recently, it has become difficult to distinguish patients with gastrinoma from those with common peptic ulcer disease; this is likely the result of common and effective therapies for reducing gastric acid secretion.

The clinical manifestations of gastrinoma are listed in Table 118.2. Abdominal pain remains the most prominent symptom, occurring in about 75% of patients. Pain usually is caused by peptic ulceration of the stomach, duodenum, or jejunum. Diarrhea is also common, and results from the destruction of mucosal integrity by gastric acid hypersecretion, excessive fluid secretion, and the deleterious effects of gastric acid on pancreatic enzymes and bile acids leading to malabsorption. Gastrinoma accounts for 0.1% of all patients with peptic ulcer disease.

Because peptic ulcer disease is common, a high index of suspicion is needed to make the diagnosis of a gastrin-secreting tumor (Table 118.3). Gastrinoma should be suspected in individuals with peptic ulcer disease who have diarrhea or multiple ulcers, or ulcers in unusual locations such as the jejunum. Suspicion should be high in patients with a family history of peptic ulcer disease, pancreatic tumor, MEN I, or manifestations of MEN I such as hyperparathyroidism or hypercalcemia. Anyone considered for surgery for peptic ulcer disease should be evaluated for

TABLE 118.3.	PATIENTS IN WHOM TO SUSPECT GASTRINOMA

Duodenal or gastric ulcer associated with
   Diarrhea
   Family history of peptic ulcer disease
   Hypercalcemia
   Nephrolithiasis
   Multiple endocrine neoplasia type I
Ulcers in the distal duodenum or jejunum
Recurrent peptic ulcer after ulcer surgery
Ulcer disease refractory to medical therapy or ulcer surgery
Evidence of gastric rugal hypertrophy
Unexplained secretory diarrhea
Refractory gastroesophageal reflux disease

gastrinoma because its existence may alter the surgical approach or the need for surgery.

The single best test for gastrinoma is measurement of serum gastrin (see also Chapter 107). In general, the higher the serum gastrin level, the more probable is the diagnosis of gastrinoma, particularly in the setting of low gastric pH. A serum gastrin level of more than 1,000 pg per milliliter in the presence of a gastric pH of less than 3 is virtually diagnostic of gastrinoma. Other causes of hypergastrinemia include antisecretory therapy, such as H_2 blockers and H^+,K^+-ATPase inhibitors, renal failure, retained gastric antrum, extensive small-bowel resection, gastric outlet obstruction, G-cell hyperfunction, and achlorhydria, which accompanies diseases such as pernicious anemia and atrophic gastritis.

When serum gastrin levels are only mildly elevated, several provocative tests can be used to make the diagnosis of gastrinoma. The most useful of these is the secretin stimulation test, in which 2 units per kilogram of secretin is infused and serial serum gastrin levels are measured over 30 minutes. If gastrin levels increase by more than 200 pg per milliliter and if basal acid hypersecretion is present, then the diagnosis of gastrinoma is confirmed.

After the diagnosis of gastrinoma is confirmed, it is important to localize the tumor because many gastrinomas may be cured by surgical resection. Imaging studies used to localize the primary tumor and identify metastases include ultrasonography (including endoscopic ultrasonography), CT, MRI, angiography, and nuclear medicine scanning, including radiolabeled somatostatin scans. Angiography or MRI may be useful in determining whether an identified tumor appears resectable. Intraoperative ultrasonography may help localize tumors that were not identified before surgery. Patients who have not had a primary tumor localized before laparotomy may have an excellent prognosis, primarily because of low tumor burden.

Before the availability of effective gastric acid antisecretory therapy, the leading causes of death in gastrinoma were complications arising from gastric acid hypersecretion. With the development of H_2 receptor antagonists and H^+,K^+-ATPase inhibitors, gastric acid secretion can be controlled; death now results from the malignant nature of the tumor itself. Therefore, the treatment of gastrinoma is aimed at controlling acid secretion while localizing the tumor to effect a surgical cure. In a recent series of 212 patients with gastrinoma followed at the U.S. National Institutes of Health for a mean of nearly 14 years, one-third of the patients died. However, none of them died from acid-related causes. Gastrinoma tumor growth was responsible for half of the deaths, and the other half died of non-ZES-related causes. Tumors localized to the lymph nodes or duodenal wall often are cured by surgical resection, with subsequent normalization of serum gastrin levels. Tumors of the pancreas fare less well because they often have metastasized by the time of diagnosis. In patients with gastrinomas and MEN I, parathyroidectomy usually reduces serum gastrin levels and may improve symptoms, and should be indicated as an initial surgical approach to this syndrome. Gastrinomas associated with MEN I often are multiple, lowering the likelihood of surgical resection being curative. If curative surgery is not possible, medical treatment can be combined with tumor-debulking procedures. Standard medical management consists of the administration of high doses of H_2 receptor antagonists or an H^+,K^+-ATPase inhibitor to control acid secretion and symptoms, with or without surgery. Control of symptoms can be achieved in nearly all patients using an H^+,K^+-ATPase inhibitor, such as omeprazole.

For patients who have metastatic disease at the time of diagnosis, several chemotherapeutic approaches have been adopted. However, because of the low incidence of gastrinoma, many treatment protocols have incorporated all patients with islet cell tumors. Most protocols include streptozocin, alone or in combination with 5-FU or doxorubicin. The overall success of chemotherapy in islet cell tumors, while not extensively tested, has shown objective response rates in excess of 50% in patients treated with doxorubicin and streptozocin, with some complete responses in both tumor size and excess hormone secretion. Chemotherapy may be the only option for patients suffering from the bulk effects of metastatic disease. The synthetic analog of somatostatin, octreotide, has been shown to reduce gastric acid secretion and serum gastrin levels, and may improve symptoms. However, because there are more effective therapies for controlling gastric acid, octreotide usually is not recommended as initial therapy.

INSULINOMAS

Insulinomas, which arise from β cells of the pancreas, usually are solitary, benign neoplasms that secrete large amounts of insulin. The disease has an incidence of 8 per 10 million population, occurs primarily in the fifth to seventh decade of life, and is associated with MEN I in 10% of cases. The hallmark of insulinoma is uncontrolled insulin release from an autonomously functioning neoplasm that causes profound and life-threatening hypoglycemia. Symptoms range from mild confusion to coma, and associated with hypoglycemia is a compensatory adrenergic surge that is responsible for tachycardia, palpitations, and diaphoresis. Rarely, the presentation of an insulinoma results from the mass of the tumor itself, with complications such as pancreatic or biliary duct obstruction, or abdominal or back pain that may resemble adenocarcinoma of the pancreas.

The first step in the evaluation of suspected hypoglycemia is measurement of the fasting blood glucose level. Whipple's triad describes features associated with clinical hypoglycemia: a fasting glucose level of less than 2.5 mmol per liter, signs and symptoms of hypoglycemia during prolonged fasting, and prompt reversal of symptoms after the administration of glucose.

Measurement of fasting glucose and insulin levels is critical for determining the cause of fasting hypoglycemia (Table 118.4). Normally, proinsulin undergoes cleavage of a connecting peptide (C peptide) to yield the active insulin molecule. Excess production of endogenous insulin is accompanied by high circulating levels of C peptide. Hypoglycemia caused by insulinoma can be distinguished from that caused by the surreptitious injection of insulin. This is attributable to the fact that in the latter condition C-peptide levels are low because the production of endogenous insulin is suppressed when insulin is injected. However, the effect of ingestion of oral hypoglycemics, such as sulfonylureas (which release endogenous insulin), can be distinguished from the effects of insulinoma only by a careful history or by detection

TABLE 118.4.	CAUSES OF HYPOGLYCEMIA AND DIAGNOSTIC TESTS		
	Serum Insulin Levels	C-Peptide Levels	Other
Excess Insulin			
Insulinoma	Increased	Increased	
Insulin administration	Increased	Decreased	Insulin antibodies
Oral hypoglycemic drugs	Increased	Increased	Positive drug test
Autoimmune hypoglycemia	Decreased	Decreased	Antibodies to insulin or insulin receptor
Decreased Glucose Production			
Liver disease/ethanol ingestion	Decreased	Decreased	Diagnosed by history, abnormal liver function tests
Akee fruit ingestion	Decreased	Decreased	Diagnosed by history

of hypoglycemic agents in the blood or urine. Hypoglycemia resulting from decreased glucose production is accompanied by low insulin levels and is easily distinguished from insulinoma.

Within 24 hours of fasting, 70% to 80% of patients with insulinoma have elevated insulin levels and hypoglycemia. In the absence of surreptitious drug use, this test is diagnostic of insulinoma. Measurement of proinsulin levels increases the sensitivity of testing to 90%. If insulin levels are not elevated with this test, prolonging the fast from 24 to 72 hours will reveal an additional 10% to 15% of patients with the disease. Fasting as a provocative test should be conducted in the hospital, where patients can be monitored carefully so that complications of hypoglycemia do not develop. Additional provocative tests include stimulation with the hypoglycemic agent tolbutamide, calcium infusion, or glucagon administration. A rapid increase in circulating insulin levels in response to one of these agents is a strong indication of insulinoma.

Up to 80% of insulinomas are single, benign lesions that are small at the time of diagnosis, presumably because they present with symptoms of hypoglycemia early in their course. Once the diagnosis of insulinoma has been established, an attempt should be made to localize the tumor, since the only curative therapy is surgical resection. Ultrasonography of the pancreas, abdominal CT, MRI, or nuclear medicine scanning should be performed, but many insulinomas escape detection by these modalities. Insulinomas are not rich in somatostatin receptors, thus making radiolabeled somatostatin scans less sensitive. Angiography produces positive results in about 60% of patients; with the simultaneous infusion of calcium, the sensitivity increases to 85%. Depending on experience, endoscopic or intraoperative ultrasonography may have a high sensitivity, complementing other techniques. Metastases are much less common with insulinomas than with other endocrine tumors of the pancreas. The presence of MEN I should not preclude localization of the tumor and attempted curative surgery, even though it is more probable that multiple tumors exist.

Once the diagnosis of insulinoma has been made, it is important that subsequent hypoglycemia be prevented. This can be achieved by monitoring hypoglycemic symptoms and giving small, frequent meals while attempts are made to localize the tumor. The antihypertensive agent diazoxide suppresses insulin release and controls the symptoms of hypoglycemia in about

50% of patients with insulinomas. Octreotide also may reduce insulin secretion and raise blood glucose levels, but its long-term use in these patients remains unclear. For insulinomas that cannot be removed surgically, chemoembolization of liver metastases or systemic chemotherapy may reduce tumor size and insulin secretion.

GLUCAGONOMAS

Glucagon-secreting tumors are rare neoplasms that arise from α cells of pancreatic islets. Most glucagonomas are malignant and 50% are metastatic at the time of diagnosis. The manifestations of the tumor result from the increased secretion of glucagon, the primary physiologic actions of which are to cause gluconeogenesis, glycogenolysis, and decreased GI motility. A triad of a characteristic rash, anemia, and diabetes associated with an α-cell pancreatic neoplasm typifies the glucagonoma syndrome. The disease often occurs in the fifth decade and can be associated with the MEN I syndrome.

The most common manifestation of glucagonoma is mild diabetes or glucose intolerance, which is directly attributable to the excess secretion of glucagon (Table 118.5). Accelerated gluconeogenesis leads indirectly to decreased levels of circulating amino acids. The rash, *migratory necrolytic erythema,* occurs in more than 70% of patients and typically develops only after the tumor has metastasized. Up to one-third of patients experience thromboembolic phenomena, although the cause of the clotting tendency is unknown. Weight loss, mucositis, stomatitis, and neuropsychiatric manifestations also may be associated with glucagonoma.

TABLE 118.5.	CLINICAL MANIFESTATIONS OF GLUCAGONOMA

Glucose intolerance or diabetes mellitus
Necrolytic migratory erythema
Anemia
Weight loss
Thromboembolic disease
Low circulating amino acid levels
Psychoneurologic manifestations

Chronic dermatitis in conjunction with diabetes or glucose intolerance is highly suggestive of glucagonoma. However, only measuring fasting levels of glucagon can make the diagnosis. In this syndrome, glucagon levels often exceed 1,000 pg per milliliter (normal levels are less than 150 pg per milliliter). Renal failure, liver disease, or stress can cause less extreme elevations of glucagon, which usually are easily distinguishable from glucagonoma. Because patients usually are seen late in the disease course, glucagonomas often are larger than 5 cm in diameter, and are found most often in the body or tail of the pancreas. Radiolabeled somatostatin receptor scans may be used to localize these tumors and to identify metastases.

Surgical resection is the preferred therapy for glucagonoma and offers the only hope for cure. Although many patients have large tumors or metastatic disease at the time of diagnosis, debulking the tumor may reduce serum glucagon levels, ameliorate symptoms, and provide long-term palliation. Chemotherapeutic regimens, such as doxorubicin and streptozocin, may reduce tumor burden, which may result in improvement of symptoms. Octreotide may normalize serum glucagon levels and improve symptoms, including neuropsychiatric manifestations, but has had no reproducible effect on tumor growth. Interferon, alone or in combination with chemotherapy or octreotide, has been shown to improve the rash, decrease glucagon levels, and reduce tumor size in glucagonoma and other islet cell tumors.

VASOACTIVE INTESTINAL POLYPEPTIDE–SECRETING TUMORS

Tumors that secrete VIP are rare, occurring in 1 in 10 million individuals. These tumors differ from other endocrine tumors of the pancreas in that they usually are not associated with MEN I. Their clinical manifestations are directly attributable to the effects of elevated serum VIP levels. The syndrome is characterized by profuse watery diarrhea, hypokalemia, and achlorhydria, and is referred to as the WDHA syndrome, pancreatic cholera, or Verner–Morrison syndrome. The major manifestation of VIP-secreting tumors is profound intestinal secretion, with large volumes of fluid that overwhelm the absorptive capacity of the colon, resulting in watery diarrhea. Virtually all patients have stool volumes of more than 700 mL per day, and 70% excrete more than 3 L per day, even during imposed fasting. With excessive stool losses, hypokalemia and dehydration often occur. Because of the gastric inhibitory effects of VIP, achlorhydria is common.

VIP-secreting tumors should be considered during the evaluation of secretory diarrhea. Elevated circulating VIP is the hallmark of this disease, and levels exceeding 60 pmol per liter are diagnostic. Seventy-five percent of these tumors are confined to the pancreas, 20% are ganglioneuromas, and a few involve the lung, colon, or liver. VIP-secreting tumors often are large, and 75% can be localized by CT.

The initial goal in the treatment of VIP-secreting tumors is to control the diarrhea and replace fluid and electrolyte losses. Intravenous fluid administration often is necessary during the early course of the illness until the diarrhea can be reduced. Octreotide is extremely useful in reducing diarrhea in this disease. As with other endocrine tumors, surgical resection is the only curative approach, and once the tumor has been localized it should be removed. About one-half of these tumors are metastatic at the time of diagnosis. However, surgical debulking or hepatic artery embolization and systemic chemotherapy in selected patients have led to improvement of symptoms related to hormone secretion or bulky tumors.

SOMATOSTATINOMAS

Somatostatin has profound inhibitory actions on the GI tract. As a regulatory hormone, it reduces gastric and pancreatic secretion, gallbladder motility, and the secretion of many other hormones. As a result, somatostatin may reduce both the secretion and the target tissue response of hormones. Tumors that elaborate somatostatin are rare, usually arise in the pancreas (rarely from the intestine), and often are large tumors with hepatic or lymph node metastases at the time of diagnosis.

The clinical manifestations of somatostatinomas include diabetes mellitus, steatorrhea, and gallstones. These findings result from the inhibitory effects of somatostatin on insulin secretion, pancreatic exocrine secretion, and gallbladder contraction, respectively. Almost all patients have reduced gastric acid secretion or achlorhydria.

The diagnosis of somatostatinoma can be confirmed by documenting elevated somatostatin levels in serum. The radiographic diagnosis and treatment of these tumors is similar to that of other pancreatic islet cell tumors.

OTHER HORMONE-SECRETING TUMORS

Rarely, islet cell tumors produce other hormones. About 10% of islet cell tumors secrete adrenocorticotropic hormone (ACTH), and about 10% of all ectopic ACTH production is from endocrine tumors of the pancreas, making these lesions an uncommon cause of Cushing's syndrome. Even less common are tumors that produce neurotensin. PP-producing tumors may present as a pancreatic mass, yet despite high circulating levels of PP, this disease does not have prominent clinical manifestations. Nonfunctioning endocrine tumors may also occur, and a high index of suspicion for these lesions is important in the diagnosis of a patient with a pancreatic mass, poorly differentiated histology on biopsy, and a clinical course that seems more benign than typical adenocarcinoma of the pancreas. Histopathologic examination, with immunohistochemical stains, frequently resolves this diagnostic problem.

CARCINOID TUMORS

Carcinoid tumors differ from other hormone-secreting tumors of the GI tract because they secrete nonpeptide transmitters. Because these tumors originate from cells of the peripheral neuroendocrine system, they can occur anywhere in the GI tract, lungs, or other tissues. Carcinoid tumors are the most common neuroendocrine tumors of the GI tract, with 1 to 2 new cases per 100,000 in the United States each year.

Carcinoid tumors are made up of small, round, uniform cells that stain for argentaffin. The cells contain numerous

TABLE 118.6.	CARCINOID TUMORS		
	Foregut	**Midgut**	**Hindgut**
Anatomical distribution	Bronchi, stomach, duodenum, pancreas	Small bowel, cecum, ascending colon	Transverse and descending colon, rectum
Argyrophilic	+++	+	Usually absent
Argentaffin staining	+	+++	+
Secretory products	5-HTP histamine, serotonin	Serotonin	Rare
Clinical symptoms	Flushing rare	Flushing, diarrhea	Rare
Metastases	Bone	Liver	Bone

5-HTP, 5-hydroxytryptophan.

neurosecretory granules in which silver particles are accumulated, accounting for their argyrophilia. In addition, these granules contain chromogranins, neuron-specific enolase, and synaptophysin.

Pathophysiologically, carcinoids can be divided into those that originate from the foregut, midgut, or hindgut (Table 118.6). Foregut carcinoids arise from the respiratory tree, pancreas, stomach, or proximal duodenum and can produce any of several potential transmitters, including 5-hydroxytryptophan (5-HTP), serotonin, histamine, and ACTH. Flushing may occur with foregut carcinoids, although it is less common than with midgut carcinoids. This symptom probably results from the production of histamine, as it responds to treatment with antihistamine medications.

Carcinoids of the midgut arise in the duodenum, jejunum, ileum, or right side of the colon. These tumors usually contain large amounts of serotonin and are argentaffin-positive. Midgut carcinoids are primarily responsible for carcinoid syndrome, which invariably occurs only once they have metastasized to the liver. Tumors that have not metastasized rarely produce this syndrome, presumably because the transmitters are metabolized and inactivated in the liver before reaching the systemic circulation. The appendix is the most common site of carcinoids, representing one-third of all newly diagnosed cases. Carcinoids of the hindgut, although less common, are being discovered more often with the routine use of sigmoidoscopy. These tumors may produce serotonin, but they often contain other mediators, such as neuropeptides or catecholamines.

The classic symptoms of carcinoid syndrome are flushing, diarrhea, and asthma, although other findings include facial telangiectasia and valvular heart disease. Flushing typically is of the face and upper body, and although initial attacks are transient, they become longer lasting as the disease progresses. Episodes of flushing may be accompanied by diarrhea. Elevated plasma serotonin levels are found in most patients with carcinoid syndrome, and this is believed to be the most probable cause of symptoms, including diarrhea. However, a few patients do not have elevated serotonin levels, and some patients are asymptomatic despite high levels of circulating serotonin. Treatment with serotonin antagonists does not affect flushing, making it likely that other mediators contribute to different manifestations of carcinoid syndrome. Cardiac fibrosis involving the tricuspid and

pulmonic valves may be the result of growth factors elaborated by these tumors. In the GI tract, carcinoids often cause a desmoplastic reaction that can result in kinking or obstruction of the bowel (Fig. 118.2).

In a patient suspected of having a carcinoid tumor, measurement of serotonin or serotonin metabolites is critical for the diagnosis. The major metabolite of serotonin is 5-hydroxyindoleacetic acid (5-HIAA), which is excreted primarily in the urine. Normally, urinary 5-HIAA levels range from 2 to 8 mg per day. Elevated urinary 5-HIAA levels are suggestive of carcinoid tumors; however, many foods that are rich in serotonin, including certain fruits and nuts, particularly bananas, pineapples, walnuts, and pecans, can cause false-positive results. Measurement of platelet serotonin levels is not affected by the ingestion of serotonin-rich foods and may complement urinary 5-HIAA levels. Serial plasma or urinary serotonin measurement is not useful because of wide variations during the day. Provocative testing with the infusion of pentagastrin releases serotonin in 75% and

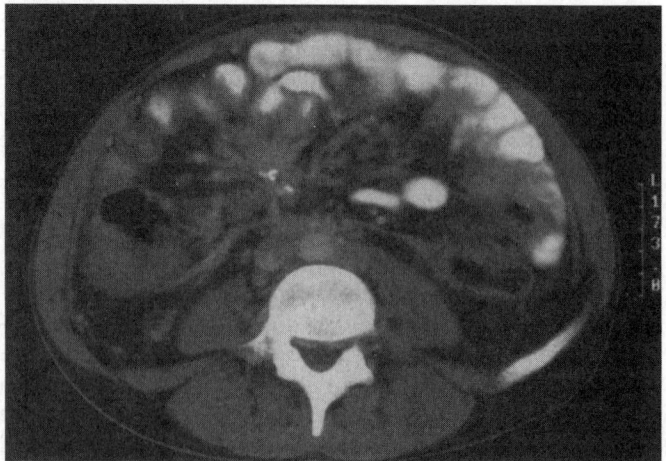

FIGURE 118.2. An abdominal computed tomographic scan with intravenous and oral contrast media shows a spiculated, calcified mesenteric mass in a 34-year-old man with a carcinoid tumor of the small bowel. In the mesentery, these tumors classically induce a desmoplastic reaction, which results in radiating strands of tissue that fix and separate small-bowel loops. The scan also shows para-aortic and aortocaval lymphadenopathy. (Courtesy of Dr. Erik Paulson, Duke University Medical Center, Durham, NC.)

causes flushing in nearly 100% of patients with carcinoid syndrome. This test can be used when the diagnosis remains unclear, even after the measurement of urinary 5-HIAA or platelet serotonin levels. Plasma chromogranin A levels may also be monitored, and levels of greater than 5,000 µg per milliliter have been shown to be an independent predictor of poor prognosis.

Up to 50% of patients with carcinoid tumors do not have symptoms of carcinoid syndrome. The diagnosis is difficult in these cases and usually is made only after the tumors produce abdominal pain or evidence of metastatic disease.

Once the diagnosis of carcinoid syndrome has been made, the tumor should be localized. Many carcinoid tumors occur outside the GI tract. Most bronchial carcinoids can be detected by chest radiography. Tumors of the stomach, duodenum, or colon can be detected by endoscopy, but those of the small bowel beyond the reach of the endoscope are difficult to detect by any modality. Small-bowel barium radiography or CT may show thickening or fixation of small-bowel loops suggestive of carcinoid tumor. Ultrasonography, CT, or MRI can detect liver metastases. Localization with radiolabeled molecules, such as the catecholamine [131I]MIBG (*m*-iodobenzylguanidine), and radiolabeled somatostatin analogs has been used to identify APUD tumors. Comparisons of conventional CT scans and radiolabeled somatostatin analogs have suggested that these techniques are complementary. Positron emission tomography performed with 11C-labeled 5-HTP, which is taken up by carcinoids, has been used for the identification of metastases.

The treatment of carcinoid tumors depends on their size, location, and, perhaps, somatostatin receptor status. Surgery usually is recommended for appropriate candidates. However, anesthesia must be undertaken cautiously because severe hypotension can occur during its induction. Premedication with octreotide has been advocated to prevent or treat crises (Fig. 118.3). The size of the primary tumor correlates well with the presence of metastases to lymph nodes and liver.

Appendiceal and rectal carcinoids smaller than 1 cm rarely metastasize, whereas those larger than 2 cm may be associated with local and distant metastases. For tumors smaller than 1 cm, excision alone is sufficient therapy. For larger tumors, more extensive cancer surgery should be undertaken to achieve more

accurate staging and potentially curative resection of locoregional disease. For incidentally found appendiceal carcinoids larger than 2 cm, a right hemicolectomy usually is performed after initial appendectomy. When local lymph nodes are involved in resection specimens from GI carcinoids, patients may live for extended periods without apparent recurrence, but long-term follow-up usually demonstrates continuing relapse over many years.

In addition to primary surgery, cytoreductive surgery for palliation or cure should be considered for neuroendocrine tumors of the GI tract. Surgical palliation of bowel obstruction from tumor masses or mesenteric fibrosis may improve the quality of life significantly in patients with carcinoid tumors. Hepatic surgery for liver metastases may render some patients free of disease for prolonged periods, and cytoreduction of large liver metastases also may reduce or eliminate symptoms caused by hormone release. The most aggressive form of liver-directed surgery liver transplantation also has been performed in highly selected patients with metastatic neuroendocrine tumors. As with all such surgery, patient selection is paramount, with ideal candidates having a long disease-free interval since initial diagnosis and a demonstrably long period of indolent disease confined to the liver, as well as exhaustive sequential staging studies demonstrating no evidence of extrahepatic tumor.

Other forms of liver-directed therapy can be considered for patients who have liver-only or liver-dominant disease but who are not ideal candidates for transplantation or extensive surgical resection. In some cases, less morbid surgical techniques, such as cryosurgery or radiofrequency ablation, provide acceptable cytoreduction. Nonsurgical techniques also are being investigated, such as hepatic arterial embolization and chemoembolization. Early studies have suggested a role for surgical hepatic arterial ligation in the treatment of typically hypervascular neuroendocrine liver metastases. Ligation of the hepatic artery may provide brief, but profound, regression of tumor masses and clinical syndromes resulting from hormone release, but this technique has largely been replaced by selective arteriographic embolization. These techniques, performed by interventional radiologists, may provide equivalent tumor control with less morbidity. Retrospective studies of patients treated with these procedures have demonstrated that more than half of all patients with carcinoid and islet cell tumors experience an objective regression, the duration of which may be prolonged with the addition of systemic chemotherapy, particularly in the more chemosensitive islet cell tumors.

In addition to surgery and liver-directed therapies, another local treatment option is radiation therapy. As with other malignant tumors, radiation to bone metastases or bulky tumors may provide substantial relief of symptoms. Hepatic radiation also may be beneficial in selected patients with hormone-producing or painful liver metastases.

For many patients with metastatic gut neuroendocrine tumors, local therapy alone is insufficient for the palliation of symptoms caused by hormone release or tumor bulk. For patients in whom hormone-related syndromes cause the most problems, somatostatin analog often provides the most effective control, without significant toxicity. This drug usually should not be used for trivial symptoms that can be controlled with

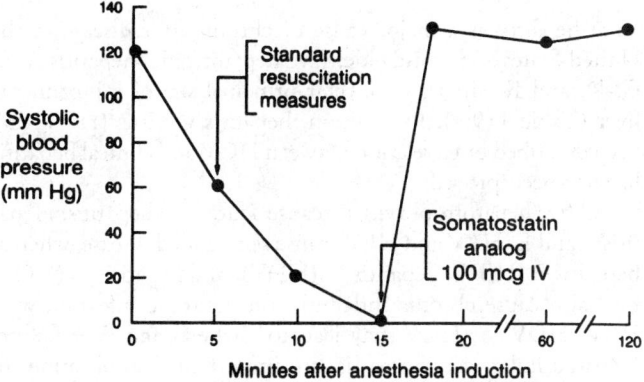

FIGURE 118.3. Response of carcinoid crisis to somatostatin analog therapy. (From Moertel CG. An odyssey in the land of small tumors. *J Clin Oncol* 1987;5:1502, with permission.)

other medications, and the cost and need for frequent subcutaneous injections has made somatostatin analog an unattractive option for some patients. However, for patients whose symptoms from islet cell or carcinoid tumor syndromes are severe or life threatening, somatostatin analog is standard therapy. There is emerging evidence that response to somatostatin analog may be predicted by the presence of somatostatin receptors in tissue specimens; this observation also appears to be true for somatostatin radionuclide imaging. A long-acting octreotide acetate formulation has largely supplanted the use of frequent subcutaneous dosing.

For patients who are unresponsive to somatostatin analog, or who have ceased to respond, additional systemic treatments are required, particularly when tumor bulk is the chief clinical problem. For more than a decade, interferon-α has been used in investigational protocols for the treatment of patients with carcinoid and islet cell tumors. In carcinoid tumors, occasional tumor regression is observed with interferon, with a higher proportion of patients achieving reductions of 5-HIAA, with relatively brief symptom control. Higher response rates, with more prolonged duration, have been observed in patients with islet cell tumors who are treated with interferon. Studies are under way to evaluate the use of interferon combined with somatostatin analog and with systemic chemotherapy.

Systemic chemotherapy has not been evaluated extensively and systematically in patients with gut neuroendocrine tumors, in part because of the indolent natural history of many of these malignancies and in part because there are a variety of nonchemotherapeutic options. For selected patients, however, systemic chemotherapy is a valid option, particularly for islet cell tumors and for poorly differentiated gut neuroendocrine tumors with aggressive biologic potential.

In carcinoid tumors, drugs that have been studied most often include 5-FU, streptozocin, doxorubicin, and dimethyltriazenoimidazole carboxamide. Objective remissions for each of these drugs used as a single agent occur in less than 20% of patients. Combinations of these drugs have been investigated prospectively in large-scale cooperative group trials. Overall, the combination of 5-FU and streptozocin has been the most consistently active and tolerable regimen, with a suggestion of a survival advantage compared with other regimens in phase III trials. Systemic chemotherapy for islet cell tumors typically has been much more successful and represents a legitimate treatment option for patients with bulky tumors or poorly controlled syndromes. In early trials, the combination of 5-FU and streptozocin was found to produce objective responses in most patients with islet cell tumors. With the identification of doxorubicin as an active agent in islet cell tumors, combination chemotherapy with this drug also has been investigated. A trial comparing streptozocin and doxorubicin with streptozocin and 5-FU demonstrated that the doxorubicin-containing regimen was superior, with a 69% objective remission rate and a significantly superior median survival. Long-term, durable responses were seen in some patients. This regimen should be considered standard therapy for patients with islet cell tumors who are considered candidates for systemic chemotherapy. For patients with poorly differentiated gut neuroendocrine tumors, the selection of chemotherapy is similar to that for small-cell carcinomas of the lung.

BIBLIOGRAPHY

Burris HA, Moore MJ, Anderson J, et al. Improvements in survival and clinical benefit for gemcitabine as first-line therapy for patients with advanced pancreas cancer: a randomized trial. *J Clin Oncol* 1997:15; 2403–2413.

Glimelius B, Hoffman K, Sjoden PO, et al. Chemotherapy improves survival and quality of life in advanced pancreatic and biliary cancer. *Ann Oncol* 1996;7:593–600.

Janson ET, Holmberg L, Stridsberg M, et al. Carcinoid tumors: analysis of prognostic factors and survival in 301 patients from a referral center. *Ann Oncol* 1997;8:685–690.

Kulke MH, Mayer RJ. Carcinoid tumors. *N Engl J Med* 1999;340: 858–868.

Lynch HT, Smyrk T, Kern SE, et al. Familial pancreatic cancer: a review. *Semin Oncol* 1996;23:251–275.

Marx S. Multiple endocrine neoplasia type I: clinical and genetic topics. *Ann Intern Med* 1998;129:484–494.

Oberg K. Neuroendocrine gastrointestinal tumors: a condensed overview of diagnosis and treatment. *Ann Oncol* 1999;10:S3–S8.

Rubin J, Ajani J, Schirmer W, et al. Octrotide acetate long-acting formulation versus open label subcutaneous octreotide in malignant carcinoid syndrome. *J Clin Oncol* 1999;17:600–606.

Whittington R, Neuberg D, Tester WJ, et al. Protracted fluorouracil and concurrent radiation in the management of locally unresectable pancreaticobiliary carcinoma. *J Clin Oncol* 1995;113:227–232.

Yeo CJ, Cameron JL, Lillemoe KD, et al. Pancreaticoduodenectomy for cancer of the head of the pancreas. 201 patients. *Ann Surg* 1995; 221: 721–733.

Yu F, Venzon DJ, Serrano J, et al. Prospective study of the clinical course, prognostic factors, causes of death and survival in patients with long-standing Zollinger–Ellison syndrome. *J Clin Oncol* 1999;17:615–630.

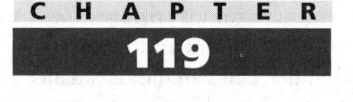

CHAPTER 119

VIRAL HEPATITIS

FREDERICK NUNES

Viral hepatitis is a major cause of chronic liver disease in the United States and worldwide. Five hepatotropic (hepatitis A, B, C, D, and E) viruses have their principal site of injury in the liver (Table 119.1). In addition, hepatitis G virus (HGV) has been described but a relation between HGV and clinical hepatitis has not been proved.

All five hepatotropic viruses cause acute viral hepatitis. Hepatitis A and E (HAV and HEV) cause self-limited disease, whereas hepatitis B (HBV), hepatitis D (HDV), and hepatitis C (HCV) may also cause chronic inflammation. Chronic infection with HBV, HDV, or HCV may lead to cirrhosis and liver failure. Hepatocellular carcinoma is an important complication of chronic viral hepatitis and cirrhosis. This chapter discusses the diagnosis and therapy of the five well-characterized hepatotropic hepatitis viruses (Table 119.1). Other viruses, such as cytomega-

					Prevalence of Chronic Infections (US)
Virus	**Genome**	**Transmission**	**Can Cause Chronic Disease**	**Prevention of Transmission**	
A	RNA	Oral/fecal	No	Pre- and postexposure immunization	0
B	DNA	Percutaneous Permucosal	Yes	Pre- and postexposure immunization	1–1.25 million
C	RNA	Percutaneous Permucosal	Yes	Blood donor screening and risk behavior modification	3.9 million
D	RNA	Percutaneous Permucosal	Yes	Pre- and postexposure immunization	70,000
E	RNA	Oral/fecal	No	Safe drinking water	0

TABLE 119.1. **HEPATOTROPIC VIRUSES**

lovirus (CMV), Epstein–Barr Virus (EBV), adenovirus, or members of Flaviviridae—all of which can affect the liver as part of a systemic disturbance—are not considered here.

The clinical presentation of patients with acute viral hepatitis is similar, regardless of the causative virus. Many cases are subclinical or present as a flulike illness that would not be recognized as being due to viral hepatitis unless liver chemistry blood tests are performed. Serum transaminase levels are often greater than 20 times the normal limit. A minority of patients present with the classic pattern of a viral prodrome, followed by overt jaundice. Specific serologic tests usually identify the offending viral agent (Chapter 104).

The development of chronic viral infection depends on host and virus factors. Treatment of chronic viral hepatitis is therefore aimed at both host immune modulation and direct antiviral treatment. Host immune modulation, particularly with interferon-α, has been the major approach to date. Interferons have a number of toxicities. Interferon-treated patients often develop a flulike syndrome, with fever, chills, nausea, and myalgia. Neurologic or psychological effects such as sleep disturbance, depression, or agitation may limit long-term use of interferon. Hematologic (white blood cells and platelet decreases) and endocrine (thyroid dysfunction) effects necessitate laboratory monitoring while a patient is on therapy.

HEPATITIS A

INCIDENCE AND EPIDEMIOLOGY

HAV has a worldwide distribution and is almost universally prevalent during childhood in developing countries because of poor sanitary conditions and overcrowding. Hepatitis A is transmitted almost exclusively through the fecal–oral route. HAV infections frequently occur in small outbreaks caused by fecal contamination of drinking water or food. Travel to endemic areas is a common source of infection for persons from nonendemic areas. In the United States, 125,000 to 200,000 acute infections occur per year, with highest attack rates in late childhood (ages 5 to 14).

ETIOLOGY

HAV is an RNA-containing virus. Although HAV isolates may vary in nucleotide sequence, they all belong to one serotype.

PATHOGENESIS

HAV is not cytopathic, and the mechanisms by which it leads to cellular injury have not been defined.

CLINICAL FINDINGS

HAV causes a self-limited infection. Hepatitis A is most often a subclinical disorder in children, but adults are usually symptomatic. Cholestasis may be a prominent feature of type A infection but is unusual with the other well-described hepatitis viruses. The viral incubation period ranges from 15 to 45 days. Most cases are self-limited, and many are unrecognized by the host. When acute HAV infection results in jaundice, patients continue to shed virions for up to 14 days after the onset of jaundice. In rare instances, HAV causes fulminant hepatitis that may lead to death (Chapter 105). Persons with underlying chronic liver disease, such as chronic hepatitis B and C, have an increased risk for severe HAV infection.

LABORATORY FINDINGS

The diagnosis of acute HAV is made by serology (Fig. 119.1). Anti-HAV IgM antibody is positive in acute infections. It occurs early and lasts generally 3 to 6 months after the onset of clinical disease. As the IgM antibody decreases, IgG anti-HAV rises and persists probably for life. Tests for total (IgG and IgM) anti-HAV are helpful in determining immunity to HAV reinfection, but are not helpful in making a diagnosis of acute HAV.

OPTIMAL MANAGEMENT

The treatment of patients with HAV infection is supportive. In rare cases of HAV infection that result in fulminant hepatic failure, orthotopic liver transplantation may be indicated.

HAV vaccine is an attenuated strain of HAV grown on tissue

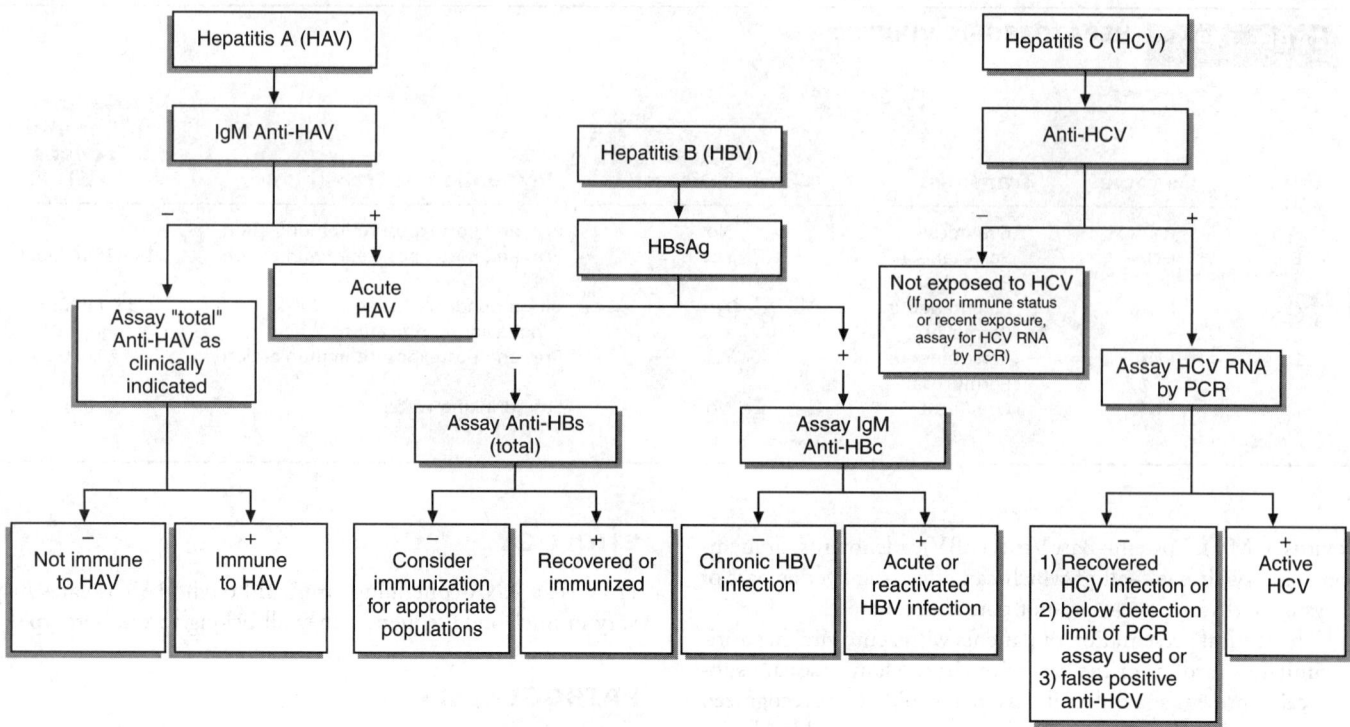

FIGURE 119.1. Approcah to diagnosis of Hepatitis A infection.
EVIDENCE LEVEL: C. Expert Opinion.

culture cells and chemically inactivated. The HAV vaccine confers immunity in 80% to 90% of those treated and is effective for *preexposure* prophylaxis (Table 119.2). Its use is recommended for persons traveling to endemic areas. Other possible candidates include children in communities with high rates of

HAV infection, day care center staff, staff of custodial institutions, sewage workers, homosexual men, intravenous drug abusers, and residents in communities experiencing hepatitis A outbreaks. Immune globulin is effective as postexposure prophylaxis for HAV. Postexposure prophylaxis is recommended within 2 weeks of exposure for household and sexual contacts of patients with HAV infection.

TABLE 119.2.	HEPATITIS A PREEXPOSURE AND POSTEXPOSURE PROPHYLAXIS

Preexposure

Populations at increased risk for HAV infection or the adverse consequences of infection

    Travel or work in countries with intermediate or high endemicity of infection

    Children in communities with high rates of HAV and periodic HAV outbreaks

    Homosexual men

    Intravenous drug users

    Persons who have chronic liver disease

    Persons who have clotting-factor disorders

    Food handlers

    Sewage workers

Vaccination in outbreak settings

Routine examination of children 2 years of age and accelerated vaccination of older children

Postexposure (non vaccinated)

Close personal contact

Day care centers

Common source exposure

HAV, hepatitis A virus.

HEPATITIS B

INCIDENCE AND EPIDEMIOLOGY

Worldwide, there are approximately 300 to 350 million HBV carriers. The prevalence of HBV infection varies greatly throughout the world. Endemic areas with a high prevalence of infection include certain parts of Africa, Asia, and the Mediterranean basin. Approximately 40,000 to 320,000 acute HBV infections occur per year in the United States, with a prevalence of chronically infected persons of approximately 1 to 1.25 million. The virus is primarily transmitted by percutaneous exposure or by inapparent skin or mucosal exposure. HBV has been found in almost every body fluid obtained from an infected person. Intimate (sexual) contact and perinatal transmission are important nonpercutaneous means of HBV transmission. The incidence of chronic disease depends on the person's age and immunologic status at the time of infection. The proportion of patients who become chronically infected declines with age, ranging from 90% for infants infected at birth to 70% for those infected in childhood and less than 5% for healthy adults.

| TABLE 119.3. | DIAGNOSIS OF HEPATITIS B |

| | HBsAg | Core Antibody | | HBsAb | HBeAg | HBeAb | HBV DNA | Comments | Antiviral Treatment |
		IgM	Total						
Not exposed	−	−	−	−	−	−	−	Immunize susceptible children, high-risk persons, health care workers	No treatment
Acute	+	+	−	−	+	−	+		Supportive care
Chronic high-replicative form	+	−	+	−	+	−	+		Treatment considered
Chronic non- or low-replicative form	+	−	+	−	−	+	−		No treatment
Mutant HBV	+	−	+	−	−	− or +	+	Pre–core mutation interrupts synthesis of HBeAg	Treatment considered
Recovered	−	−	+	+	−	−	−	HBsAb may be undetectable in patients with remote infection	No treatment
Immune	−	−	−	+	−	−	−	Titers >10 IU/mL considered immune	No treatment

HBsAg, hepatitis B surface antigen—protein that forms the outer envelope of the virus; HBcAb, hepatitis B core antibody—antibody formed against core protein surrounding the viral DNA; HBeAg, hepatitis B e antigen—structural portion of core protein indicative of active replication of HBV; HBeAb, hepatitis B e antibody—antibody formed against a structural portion of core protein indicative of active replication of HBV; HBsAb-antibody directed against the surface antigen; HBV DNA, hepatitis B DNA—presence of DNA may be assayed by a variety of methods.

ETIOLOGY

HBV is a DNA-containing virus that replicates in the liver via an RNA intermediate, using reverse transcriptase activity. A number of virally encoded proteins are produced and secreted into the serum. These proteins and the immune response they induce form the basis for the diagnosis of HBV (Fig. 119.1; Table 119.3).

PATHOGENESIS

HBV is not cytopathic, except perhaps when the expression of the virus is greatly enhanced such as in immunosuppressed persons. The damaging effects of infection are thought to result from the immune response of the host to virally encoded proteins. Portions of the DNA genome may integrate into the host's genome.

CLINICAL FINDINGS

Most patients with acute HBV infection are asymptomatic or present with mild flulike symptoms. Jaundice occurs in less than one-third of cases. The incubation period varies from a few weeks to 6 months. A prodrome of fever, arthralgias or arthritis, and rash may occur in 10% to 20% of cases of acute HBV infection. This prodrome is due to circulating hepatitis B surface antigen (HBsAg)/antibody to HBV surface antigen (anti-HBs) com-plexes that activate complement after depositing in the synovium and walls of cutaneous blood vessels. These symptoms generally resolve early in the illness, before the symptoms of liver disease become apparent.

LABORATORY FINDINGS

Detection of HBsAg in serum establishes the diagnosis of HBV infection. HBsAg appears in the blood about 6 weeks after infection and is usually cleared within 3 months in patients with transient disease. Persistence of HBsAg after 6 months from the onset of the infection implies chronic infection. The presence of IgM antibody to HBV core antigen (anti-HBc IgM) signifies an acute or reactivated chronic infection. Polyclonal anti-HBs is generally detectable 3 months after infection and implies recovery and immunity to HBV. However, in a subset of individuals with chronic HBV infection, both HBsAg and anti-HBs are detectable.

HBV DNA is a sensitive measure of viral replication. HBe antigen (HBeAg) is a secreted product that is produced as a result of intracellular modification of the protein product of the gene, which encodes precore and core protein. The presence of HBeAg in the bloodstream correlates with HBV viral DNA synthesis and thereby correlates with viral replication and infectivity. Antibody to HBV e antigen (anti-HBe) is usually an indicator of lower infectivity. Occasionally, HBV DNA is positive in the setting of a negative HBeAg. This finding is due to the

TABLE 119.4	TREATMENT OF CHRONIC VIRAL HEPATITIS		
Virus	**Approved Treatments**	**Variations of Standard Treatment**	**Experimental Treatments**
Hepatitis A	Supportive		
Hepatitis B	1. Interferon alfa-2b 5 mIU subcutaneously daily for 16 weeks. 2. Lamivudine 100 mg daily	Interval of treatment Duration of treatment	Nucleoside analogues Therapeutic vaccine
Hepatitis C	1. Intron A combined with ribavirin 1,000–1,200 mg/d for 6–12 mos 2. Interferon alfa-3 mIU subcutaneously 3×/wk for 12 months	Higher dose Daily administration Longer duration of treatment	Longer-acting interferons
Hepatitis D	Interferon alfa-2b 9 mIU subcutaneously 3×/wk		
Hepatitis E	Supportive		

expression of a mutant form of HBV, referred to as the "non-e-antigen–secreting, precore mutant virus." In patients with chronic HBV infection, a liver biopsy can assist in assessment of the degree of inflammation, in evaluation for presence of scar tissue, and in detection of viral antigens.

OPTIMAL MANAGEMENT

Serologic and molecular tests assist in determining prognosis and stratifying patients for treatment. The various forms of HBV infection are outlined in Table 119.3. Treatment is indicated for patients with a replicative form of infection (HBeAg or HBV DNA–positive or both). Interferon alfa-2b (Intron A) is an approved treatment for HBV infection. The standard dose of interferon alfa-2b for patients with well-compensated chronic HBV is 5 million units subcutaneously daily or 10 million units subcutaneously three times per week for 4 to 6 months (Table 119.4). Interferon therapy is associated with approximately 40% con-

version from a replicative form to a nonreplicative form of HBV infection recognized serologically by HBV e Ag becoming undetectable. Clearance of HBV DNA and remission of disease can be obtained in approximately one-third of treated persons. Patients with higher serum aminotransferases and lower HBV-DNA levels are more likely to respond (Table 119.5). Patients with normal serum aminotransferases or patients with decompensated cirrhosis are generally not candidates for interferon therapy.

Lamivudine, an agent that inhibits reverse transcriptase enzymes is an approved therapy for chronic hepatitis B associated with viral replication and active inflammation. Treatment with this type of antiviral medication is restricted to HBV, because the other known hepatitis viruses do not require a reverse transcriptase enzyme for replication. HIV testing should be offered to all patients before initiating lamivudine therapy because a lower dose is administered to treat HBV than HIV. If a patient is HIV-positive, combination therapy with a higher dose of lami-

TABLE 119.5.	INDICATION FOR TREATMENT
Indications for Treatment	**Positive Predictive Factors for Treatment**
HBV	
Persistent elevation of serum aminotransferases	High serum aminotransferease
HBsAg+, HBeAg+, HBV DNA+	Low serum HBV DNA
Chronic hepatitis on liver biopsy	Short duration of illness before treatment
Compensated liver disease	Active histologic hepatitis
	Fibrosis on liver biopsy
	No major current illnesses
	Absence of immunosuppression, including HIV
HCV	
Persistent elevations of serum aminotransferase	HCV genotypes 2 or 3
	Age <45 yr
Serum HCV RNA+, anti-HCV+	Duration of disease <5 yr
Chronic hepatitis on liver biopsy	Absence of cirrhosis
Compensated liver disease	Low levels of HCV RNA before treatment

HBV, hepatitis B virus; HBeAg, hepatitis B e antibody; HBsAg, hepatitis B surface antibody; HCV, hepatitis C virus.

TABLE 119.6.	PASSIVE AND ACTIVE IMMUNIZATION FOR PREVENTION OF HEPATITIS B		
Population Exposure	**Immunoglobulin Administered**	**Vaccine Administered**	**Comments**
Newborn of an HBV-infected mother	Yes	Yes	
All newborns	No	Yes	Recommended
Children 11–12 who have not been vaccinated	No	Yes	Recommended
High risk	No	Yes	Includes health care workers

vudine combined with other antiviral agents is desired to lower the probability of HIV drug resistance. Lamivudine is administered orally and is rarely associated with serious side effects at the standard HBV dose of 100 mg per day. Dose adjustment is necessary for impaired renal function. Lamivudine therapy is approved for 1 year; however, the optimal duration of therapy is not known. Relapse after discontinuation of lamivudine treatment is common. Lamivudine-resistant mutants arise in approximately 25% of patients treated for 1 year, but the long-term significance of these mutants is not known.

Newer approaches under investigation include therapeutic vaccines and multiple nucleoside analogues in combination.

Orthotopic liver transplantation is an accepted treatment for end-stage liver disease due to chronic HBV (Chapter 132). Although initial results were poor owing to aggressive recurrent HBV infection, long-term survival has been achieved by treatment with HBV immunoglobulin to block graft infection.

The primary strategy for the prevention of HBV is immunization. Transmission of HBV can be prevented by preexposure prophylaxis with HBV vaccine or, after exposure, by the combination of vaccination and HBV immune globulin (HBIG). Postexposure prophylaxis is recommended for exposed persons, including babies born to infected mothers. Preexposure prophylaxis with HBV vaccine is recommended for all babies at birth, children ages 11 to 12 if not previously vaccinated, and high-risk persons of any age including health care workers (Table 119.6).

HEPATITIS C

INCIDENCE AND EPIDEMIOLOGY

Hepatitis C is widely prevalent throughout the world. Hepatitis C is a common cause of chronic liver disease, and in the United States it affects approximately 3.9 million people. The incidence of acute HCV infection in the United States has declined since its peak in 1989. Currently, there are approximately 35,000 acute new infections of HCV in the United States each year. Most infected persons (greater than 75%) develop a chronic infection. Hepatitis C is transmitted through percutaneous and permucosal routes. The major identified risk factors are listed in Table 119.7. Transmission of HCV is most efficient via percutaneous exposure, such as the sharing of contaminated needles among intravenous drug users or the transfusion of infectious blood products. Screening tests to exclude infectious donors has markedly decreased the risk of transfusion-associated HCV now

estimated between 0.01% and 0.001% per unit transfused. The incidence of HCV among intravenous drug users has declined because of changing drug use practices. Intravenous drug users account for approximately 50% of all new acute infections and 50% or more of chronic infections. It may be difficult to obtain a history of injection drug use because many patients have stopped intravenous drug exposure many years before the recognition of HCV.

The incidence of sexual transmission of HCV is not certain, but it probably occurs, although rarely. At present, no specific recommendations are made to change sexual practices in monogamous relationships, in which one partner is anti-HCV–positive. Sexually active patients who are anti-HCV–positive, but who are not in a long-term monogamous relationship, should be advised to use "safe sex" barrier precautions. Maternal–fetal transmission occurs occasionally (<5%) at the time of birth. Coinfection of the mother with HIV appears to facilitate transmission of HCV to the neonate. Infection of the neonate after birth occurs rarely, and at present breast-feeding is not discouraged for mothers chronically infected with HCV. Household contact is not considered a risk factor for HCV infection; however, anti-HCV–positive persons should not share personal items such as toothbrushes and razors.

There is a high prevalence of anti-HCV antibody among alcoholic patients with liver disease. Alcohol use appears to increase HCV replication, progression to fibrosis and cirrhosis, and risk of hepatocellular carcinoma. Whether this potential synergistic relation between alcohol and HCV occurs with more modest alcohol intake is not yet clear. It seems prudent, however, to counsel HCV-infected persons to abstain or minimize alcohol intake.

TABLE 119.7.	RISK FACTORS FOR THE ACQUISITION OF HEPATITIS C VIRUS (HCV)

- Blood transfusions before 1992
- Intravenous drug use
- Body piercing and tattooing
- Infants born to infected mothers
- Frequent exposure to blood products (chronic renal failure, organ transplantation, hemophilia)
- Infants born to HCV-infected mothers
- Intranasal cocaine use
- Hemodialysis
- Occupational exposure to blood and blood products

ETIOLOGY

HCV is an RNA-containing virus of the family Flaviviridae, identified in 1989 by molecular biologic techniques. HCV is a genetically heterogeneous family of viruses with at least six distinct genotypes and many subtypes identified worldwide. Genotype 1 is the most common in the United States present, found in approximately 75% of infected patients. The frequency of the various genotypes varies among geographic regions.

CLINICAL FINDINGS

Most acute and chronic HCV infections are clinically asymptomatic. The incubation period after exposure to HCV ranges from 2 weeks to 2 months. If symptoms or jaundice occur as a result of acute HCV infection, symptoms generally last 2 to 12 weeks. A small number of persons with chronic HCV have signs and symptoms of liver disease. The major manifestation of chronic HCV infection may be chronic fatigue, but it may be difficult to determine whether symptoms are attributable to chronic HCV or to another cause. Other symptoms may include mild right upper quadrant discomfort, nausea, anorexia, myalgias, and arthralgias.

Clinically apparent extrahepatic manifestations of HCV develop in 1% to 2% of chronically infected people. The most significant of these are essential mixed cryoglobulinemia and membranoproliferative glomerulonephritis. Cryoglobulinemia may present as skin rashes, myalgias and arthralgias, glomerulonephritis, and the presence of serum cryoglobulins. Porphyria cutanea tarda is associated with chronic HCV and excessive hepatic levels of iron. The possible association between HCV and diabetes mellitus is under active clinical and laboratory investigation.

There is a spectrum of HCV disease outcomes; thus, estimating prognosis in individual patients is difficult. However, longitudinal studies suggest that cirrhosis develops in at least 20% of patients over a 10- to 20-year period. Those who have had chronic HCV for an extended period of time and have developed moderate to severe hepatitis are at risk for progression to cirrhosis, hepatic failure, and hepatocellular carcinoma. In the United States, an estimated 8,000 to 10,000 persons die annually as a result of HCV-associated liver disease, and chronic HCV infection is the most common reason for performing liver transplantation in many liver transplantation centers (Chapter 132). The number of deaths attributed to HCV is expected to triple over the next 10 to 20 years based on a cohort effect of persons infected with HCV in the 1970s and 1980s.

LABORATORY FINDINGS

Serum alanine aminotransferase (ALT) is usually less than five times the upper limit of normal. The incidence of persistently normal ALT levels among carriers is not well known but may be as high as 15%. Occasional normal ALT levels occur in many infected individuals. Alkaline phosphatase, albumin, prothrombin time, serum bilirubin, and platelet count are normal until the development of advanced liver disease. Iron and ferritin levels may be slightly elevated.

The diagnosis of HCV infection is based on serologic tests to detect anti-HCV antibody and molecular tests to identify viral RNA (Fig. 119.1; Table 119.8). Initial testing to detect HCV antibody (anti-HCV) is performed with second- or third-generation enzyme immunoassay (EIA). False-positive HCV EIA tests occur particularly when screening low-prevalence populations such as blood donors. Confirmation of HCV exposure requires a supplemental test such as the second-generation recombinant immunoblot assay. Anti-HCV antibody titers are present in almost all patients 1 month after onset of acute HCV, but may never become detectable in immunosuppressed or immunocompromised persons. The anti-HCV antibody is not neutralizing, and it does not confer immunity (Fig. 119.1).

Testing for the presence of HCV RNA in serum or liver tissue is the gold standard for diagnosing active HCV infection. This may be required in patients with acute HCV and patients on dialysis, patients who are taking corticosteroids or immunosuppressive mediations, and patients who have hypogammaglobulinemia.

The presence of HCV RNA in the serum is detectable by the reverse transcription–polymerase chain reaction (RT-PCR) assay. This assay can be very sensitive (100 or less viral genomes per milliliter of serum). However, RT-PCR is not standardized and is subject to variability as a result of specimen handling, serum storage conditions, and PCR technique. Controversy exists as to the value in a clinical, rather than a research, setting of quantifying the HCV viral load. HCV viral load does not correlate with severity of hepatitis nor does it portend a poor

TABLE 119.8.	DIAGNOSTIC TESTS FOR HEPATITIS C VIRUS (HCV)	
Method	**Test**	**Purpose**
Serologic	Detect Anti-HCV Antibodies	
	Enzyme immunoassay (EIA)[a]	Screening for HCV
	Second-generation recombinant immunoblot assay (RIBA-2)	Used as supplemental antibody test
Molecular	Detect and characterize HCV RNA	
	Qualitative reverse transcriptase polymerase chain reaction (RT-PCR)	Confirm active HCV infection
	Quantitative test for HCV RNA level	Determine viral RNA levels and may correlate response to treatment
	Genotype determination	Correlates with response to therapy

[a] Not all patients with active HCV infection are detected with EIA screening.

prognosis. In many studies, a low level of viremia correlates with probability of response to antiviral therapy.

Genotype 1 is the most common in the United States, and affected patients are less likely to respond to antiviral therapy compared with those with genotypes 2 and 3.

A liver biopsy is not necessary for diagnosis but assists in determining the degree of inflammation and presence of scar tissue. In general, there is a poor correlation between serum ALT level and liver disease activity determined by histology. A liver biopsy is also helpful in excluding other causes of liver disease, including iron overload, autoimmune liver disease, and alcoholism.

OPTIMAL MANAGEMENT

No effective vaccine is available for HCV, perhaps as a result of the great deal of variability of the hepatitis C viral envelope. Postexposure prophylaxis with immunoglobulin is not effective in blocking HCV infection and is not recommended.

Interferon-α monotherapy and the combination of interferon-α and ribavirin are two regimens approved for the treatment of HCV in the United States. Three recombinant alfa interferons have been approved for treatment of chronic HCV in the United States (interferon alfa-2a, alfa-2b, and alfacon-1). The optimal dose, interval of administration, and duration of treatment with interferon-α is not known. The standard therapy for chronic HCV with these interferons in a patient with well-compensated liver disease, is 3 million units three times per week, or in the case of alfacon-1 interferon, 9 μg three times per week for 12 months administered by subcutaneous injection (Table 119.4). Long-term response to therapy for hepatitis C is defined as persistently negative serum HCV RNA by PCR for at least 6 months after completion of treatment. A long-term response is observed in approximately 10% to 15% of patients treated with interferon-α monotherapy for 6 to 12 months. The presence of HCV genotype 1, cirrhosis, a high viral load as measured by quantitative PCR, or a long duration of infection (greater that 15 years of probable infection), are negative predictors for a long-term response to interferon monotherapy (Table 119.5).

Flulike side effects of fever, malaise, headache, chills, arthralgias, and myalgias occur within 8 hours of interferon-α administration. These side effects can be ameliorated by acetaminophen. Later side effects include fatigue and malaise. Severe depression may occur and limit treatment with interferon-α. Thyroid dysfunction has been reported in 2.55% to 20% of patients. Interferon-α is generally contraindicated in patients with severe depression, autoimmune hepatitis, uncontrolled hyperthyroidism, coronary heart disease, or decompensated cirrhosis.

The combination of interferon and ribavirin is associated with higher sustained response rates compared with the three interferon-α monotherapies now available. Ribavirin is an oral nucleoside analogue with activity against a wide spectrum of viruses. The mechanism by which it improves the sustained response to interferon therapy is not known. Ribavirin causes a dose-related hemolytic anemia necessitating frequent hemoglobin monitoring. Because ribavirin is teratogenic, patients must use a medically accepted form of birth control while on therapy and for 6 months after discontinuation of therapy.

Combination therapy with interferon and ribavirin leads to a sustained response (loss of HCV RNA from the serum for at least 6 months after completion of treatment) in approximately 30% to 40% of previously untreated patients.

Orthotopic liver transplantation is an accepted treatment for end-stage liver disease secondary to HCV. HCV is the most common indication for orthotopic liver transplantation in the United States (Chapter 132). Response rates may be higher or lower depending on the HCV genotype.

Future research will aim to optimize combination treatment regimes. Alternative forms of interferon may require less frequent administration and improved sustained response rates. Future therapies may include anti-inflammatory agents, anti-fibrotic agents, immune modulators, and compounds that directly inhibit HCV encoded enzymes.

■ HEPATITIS D

INCIDENCE AND EPIDEMIOLOGY

HDV is transmitted by blood and blood products. HDV infection has a worldwide distribution, but the areas of highest endemic rate are the Mediterranean countries, the Middle East, and certain parts of South America. It is found infrequently in Asia, Western Europe, and North America. In nonendemic areas such as North America, HDV occurs most commonly among intravenous drug users and multiply transfused patients.

ETIOLOGY

HDV is a small circular RNA-containing virus. HDV is a defective virus that can infect only in the presence of HBV infection. Acute HDV infection may occur coincident with acute HBV infection or as a superinfection in a person chronically infected with HBV.

PATHOGENESIS

The delta agent may be cytopathic, but the precise mechanism of hepatic injury is not known.

CLINICAL FINDINGS

HDV coinfection with HBV causes severe acute disease, but a low risk of chronic infection. Superinfection with HDV of a chronic HBV-infected person generally results in chronic HDV infection and a higher risk for severe chronic liver disease.

Typically, acute HDV is accompanied by a biphasic aminotransferase pattern, with one peak level resulting from HBV-induced liver cell injury and the other from the delta agent. The serologic response to acute HDV infection as measured by commercial immunoassays is often undetectable or represented by transient appearance of IgM antibody. By methods confined to research laboratories, delta antigen and HDV RNA can be detected transiently in liver tissue and serum during acute infection.

LABORATORY FINDINGS

Acute and chronic HDV is diagnosed by the presence of HDV antibody (anti-HD). IgM anti-HD and delta antigen, although helpful in diagnosing acute HDV infection, are not routinely available in the United States.

OPTIMAL MANAGEMENT

An HDV vaccine is not available. Prevention is best obtained by immunizing against HBV and education to reduce high-risk behaviors. HDV may also be treated with interferon alfa-2b (Table 119.4). In one randomized controlled trial, there was a 50% response rate to 9 million units of interferon alfa-2b administered three times per week subcutaneously for 48 weeks. However, relapse at the end of treatment was common.

▍ HEPATITIS E

INCIDENCE AND EPIDEMIOLOGY

HEV is transmitted through the oral–fecal route. The incubation period is 40 days on average, with a range of 15 to 60 days. Large outbreaks of HEV have been identified in India, Bangladesh, and Central and South America. The case fatality rate is reported as 1% to 3% overall and 15% to 25% in pregnant women. Sporadic cases can occur in developed countries after travelers return from an endemic area.

ETIOLOGY

HEV is a RNA-containing virus. Blood-borne transmission has not been demonstrated, and a carrier state has not been observed. Antibody to HEV is detectable at disease presentation.

PATHOGENESIS

There is no chronic hepatitis or carrier state resulting from this agent.

LABORATORY FINDINGS

Serologic testing for HEV is not routinely available but may be obtained through a research laboratory.

OPTIMAL MANAGEMENT

Therapy is supportive.

BIBLIOGRAPHY

Alter M, Gallagher M, Morris T, et al. Acute non A-E hepatitis in the United States and the role of hepatitis G virus infection. *N Engl J Med* 1997;336:741–746.

Alter M, Mast E. The epidemiology of viral hepatitis in the United States. *Gastroenterol Clin North Am* 1994;23:437–455.

Centers for Disease Control. Hepatitis B virus: a comprehensive strategy for eliminating transmission in the United States through universal childhood vaccination: recommendations of the Immunization Practices Advisory Committee (ACIP). *MMWR* 1991;40:1–19.

Centers for Disease Control. Prevention of hepatitis A through active and passive immunization: recommendations of the Advisory Committee on Immunization Practices (ACIP). *MMWR* 1996;45:1–30.

Davis GL, Esteban-Mur R, Rustgi V, et al. Interferon alfa-2b alone or in combination with ribavirin for the treatment of relapse of chronic hepatitis C. International Hepatitis Interventional Therapy Group [comments]. *N Engl J Med* 1998;339:1493–1499.

Hoofnagle J, DiBiscegli A. The treatment of chronic viral hepatitis. *N Engl J Med* 1997;336:347–356.

Lai C, Chien R, Leung N, et al. A one-year trial of lamivudine for chronic hepatitis B. Asia Hepatitis Lamivudine Study Group. *N Engl J Med* 1998;339:61–68.

Lindsay K, Davis G, Schiff E, et al. Response to higher doses of interferon alfa-2b in patients with chronic hepatitis C: a randomized multicenter trial. *Hepatology* 1996;24:1034–1040.

McHutchinson JG, Gordon SC, Schiff ER, et al. Interferon alfa-2b alone or in combination with ribavirin as initial treatment for chronic hepatitis C. Hepatitis Interventional Therapy Group [comments]. *N Engl J Med* 1998;339:1485–1492.

Poynard T, Leroy V, Cohard M, et al. Meta-analysis of interferon randomized trials in the treatment of viral hepatitis C: effects of dose and duration. *Hepatology* 1996;24:778–789.

Takahashi M, Yamada G, Miyamoto R, et al. Natural course of chronic hepatitis C. *Am J Gastroenterol* 1993;88:240–243.

Kelley's Textbook of Internal Medicine, fourth edition. Edited by H. David Humes. Lippincott Williams & Wilkins, Philadelphia © 2000.

AUTOIMMUNE HEPATITIS AND PRIMARY BILIARY CIRRHOSIS

GILLIAN ANN ZELDIN
ALBERT J. CZAJA

Autoimmune hepatitis (AH) is a disorder of unknown cause that is characterized by progressive destruction of hepatic parenchyma, which often results in cirrhosis and a high mortality if untreated. This diagnosis is made after exclusion of toxic, metabolic, and viral causes of chronic liver injury and differentiated from the cholangiopathies of primary biliary cirrhosis and primary sclerosing cholangitis. It is uncommon, with a female predominance (70%) and onset in the third to fifth decade (onset before age 30 in 50%). It is often associated with other autoimmune disorders. Histologically, AH is characterized by periportal hepatitis (also referred to as piecemeal necrosis or interface hepatitis). Hypergammaglobulinemia and liver-associated autoantibodies are found in the serum.

Diagnostic criteria were established by the International Autoimmune Hepatitis Group in 1992 (Table 120.1). Notably, there is no diagnostic requirement for 6 months of disease activity, since patients with AH may present acutely. If antibodies against nuclear, smooth muscle and liver–kidney–microsomal antigens are absent, then the less common asialoglycoprotein receptor (anti-ASGPR), soluble liver antigen, liver cytosol, and

TABLE 120.1.	**CRITERIA OF THE INTERNATIONAL AUTOIMMUNE HEPATITIS GROUP OF THE DIAGNOSIS OF AUTOIMMUNE HEPATITIS**		
Criterion		**Probable**	**Definite**
Risk factors			
Exposure to blood			
Yes, but unrelated to disease		x	
No			x
Alcohol use			
<25 g/d (for women) or <35 g/d (for men)			x
<40 g/d (for women) or <50 g/d (for men)		x	
Use of hepatotoxic drugs			
No			x
Yes, but unrelated to disease		x	
Laboratory findings			
Abnormal AST or ALT levels		x	x
Serum alkaline phosphatase < 3× normal			x
Total globulin, γ-globulin, or IgG levels			
>1.5 × the upper limit of normal			x
>1.0–1.5 × the upper limit of normal		x	
Titer of antibodies to nucleus, smooth muscle, or liver/kidney microsome type 1			
> 1:80 (for adults)			x
Low titers or presence of other autoantibodies		x	
Viral markers			
Negative for IgM antibodies to hepatitis A virus, hepatitis B surface antigen. IgM antibodies to hepatitis B core antigen, antibodies to hepatitis C virus, antibodies to cytomegalovirus, and Epstein–Barr virus		x	x
False-positive for antibodies to hepatitis C		x	
Histologic findings			
Interface hepatitis or piecemeal necrosis		x	x
Concurrent lobular hepatitis		x	x
No biliary lesions or other changes		x	x

ALT, alanine transaminase; AST, aspartate transaminase.

liver-pancrease autoantibodies suggest the probable diagnosis of AH. Although no subtypes of AH are formally recognized, types 1, 2, and 3 are used clinically, and several overlap and outlier variants are characterized (Table 120.2)

INCIDENCE AND EPIDEMIOLOGY

The incidence of AH in Western Europe is less than 1 per 100,000 persons per year, but AH accounts for about 20% of chronic liver disease among patients of North America. The prevalence of AH is highest among the white populations of Northern Europe, North America, and Australia with a high incidence of human leukocyte antigen (HLA) DR3 and DR4 alleles. The Japanese population has a low incidence of HLA-DR3, and AH in Japan is HLA-DR4–associated.

PATHOGENESIS

Although the pathogenesis of AH is unknown, two theories prevail: autoantigen-mediated injury and antibody-dependent cell-mediated cytotoxicity in a genetically sensitive host. Evidence for antibody-dependent cell-mediated injury would require antigen–antibody complexes on the hepatocyte surface targeted by

natural killer cells with Fc receptors, aberrant display of HLA class II antigens on the hepatocyte surface to facilitate presentation of normal cell material to other antigen-processing cells, and intrinsic suppressor T-lymphocyte defects that would facilitate unmodulated B-cell production of immunoglobulins against hepatocytes. Thus far, none of the autoantibodies associated with AH have been established as pathogenic, and only non-antigen–specific suppressor T-cell defects have been demonstrated and may not be disease-specific.

AUTOIMMUNE HEPATITIS SUBTYPES AND VARIANT SYNDROMES

Autoimmune hepatitis type 1 is characterized by antibodies to smooth muscle or nuclear antigens, may present at any age, and has a strong female predominance. Almost 50% of patients also have an extrahepatic immunologic disease. The presence of anti-ASGPR is specific for AH type 1, and persistence during immunosuppressive therapies is associated with relapse. Specific HLA allelic risk factors have been identified, and type 1 is steroid-responsive. Type 2 affects mainly children (95%) and can present in a chronic or fulminant manner. Female-to-male ratio is 10:1, and it is commonly associated with concurrent immune disorders including vitiligo, autoimmune thyroiditis, and insu-

TABLE 120.2.	VARIANT FORMS OF AUTOIMMUNE HEPATITIS
Syndrome	**Distinguishing Features**
Overlap variants	
Autoimmune hepatitis an biliary cirrhosis	Mitochondrial antibodies Histologic cholangitis Hepatic copper deposition Cholestatic laboratory changes Responsiveness to corticosteroid therapy
Autoimmune hepatitis and primary sclerosing cholangitis	Chronic ulcerative colitis Histologic cholangitis Cholestatic laboratory changes Abnormal cholangiogram Recalcitrance to corticosteroids
Autoimmune hepatitis and chronic viral infection	
Autoimmune dominant	Titer of smooth muscle or antinuclear antibodies >1:160 Titer of smooth muscle and antinuclear >1:40 Piecemeal necrosis (interface hepatitis), lobular hepatitis, and portal plasma cell infiltrates
Viral dominant	Titer of smooth muscle or antinuclear antibodies <1:320 Antibodies to liver/kidney microsome type 1 and hepatitis C viremia Portal lymphoid aggregates, steatosis, or bile duct injury
Outlier variants	
Autoimmune cholangitis	Absence of mitochondrial antibodies Antinuclear antibodies Smooth muscle antibodies common Histologic features of bile duct injury Concurrent cholestatic laboratory changes Antibodies to carbonic anhydrase Normal cholangiogram Unpredictable response to corticosteroids and ursodeoxycholic acid
Cryptogenic chronic hepatitis	Absence of smooth muscle, antinuclear, or liver/kidney microsome type 1 antibodies at presentation Histologic finding identical with those of autoimmune hepatitis HLA-B8, HLA-DR3, or HLA-AI-B8-DR3 common Possible antibodies to soluble liver antigen or liver-pancreas Possible late appearance of conventional autoantibodies Responsiveness to corticosteroid therapy

HLA, human leukocyte antigen.

lin-dependent diabetes. Frequently there are autoantibodies to parietal cells, islets of Langerhans, or thyroid antigens. The type 2a variant occurs in young women, and type 2b in older men, and it is often associated with hepatitis C and rarely with concurrent autoimmune disorders. Type 3 is not established as a distinct subgroup but is characterized by the presence of antibodies to soluble liver antigen, mitochondrial, liver membrane and smooth muscle antigens and the absence of nuclear, liver–kidney–microsomal and rheumatoid factor autoantibodies.

Several atypical forms of autoimmune hepatitis exist, but they lack firm diagnostic features or established treatment strategies. Overlap syndromes have features associated with autoimmune hepatitis and another type of chronic liver disease, whereas outlier syndromes have findings that are incompatible with autoimmune hepatitis according to the criteria codified by the international panels (Table 120.2). Autoimmune cholangitis is a chronic hepatocellular inflammation with bile duct injury seen on histologic examination, but affected patients have a normal cholangiogram. It has features of both autoimmune hepatitis and primary biliary cirrhosis, but lacks antimitochondrial antibodies.

Disease-specific antibodies to carbonic anhydrase are commonly present. Antinuclear and anti–smooth muscle antibodies are present in autoimmune cholangitis and are seen in conjunction with elevated serum alkaline phosphatase or bilirubin. Affected patients have variable clinical responsiveness to corticosteroids and ursodeoxycholic acid, and histologic improvement is not common.

 ## CLINICAL FEATURES

The presentation of AH is diverse, ranging from asymptomatic transaminase elevations to subfulminant hepatitis. The most common symptom is fatigue, anorexia and weight loss, and the presence of pruritus or pain argues against this diagnosis. Occasionally, patients present with cirrhosis, and the complications of portal hypertension. Women may develop primary or secondary amenorrhea as the initial manifestation. Before treatment most patients have elevated serum transaminase levels, bilirubin, and alkaline phosphatase. The hypergammaglobulinemia of AH is

TABLE 120.3.	**EXTRAHEPATIC IMMUNOLOGIC DISORDERS ASSOCIATED WITH AUTOIMMUNE HEPATITIS**
Autoimmune thyroiditis	Nephritis
Graves' disease	Coombs'-positive hemolytic anemia
Chronic ulcerative colitis	
Systemic sclerosis	Idiopathic thrombocytopenic purpura
Pernicious anemia	
Rheumatoid arthritis	Erythema nodosum
Leukocytoclastic vasculitis	Fibrosing alveolitis

polyclonal but predominantly of the immunoglobulin G fraction. Cryoglobulins may be present, but are rarely clinically significant. Extrahepatic immunologic disorders are often associated with AH (Table 120.3)

Liver biopsy is necessary for diagnosis of AH to assess the severity and stage of inflammation and assist with the determination of prognosis. AH is characterized by periportal mononuclear infiltrates extending into the lobule (piecemeal necrosis), but some patients may have a predominantly plasma cell infiltrate. Patients with severe cases have necrosis from portal tracts to the central vein or nonspecific cirrhotic histology at the time of biopsy. Histologically, AH may occasionally be difficult to distinguish from viral chronic viral hepatitis, primary biliary cirrhosis, or primary sclerosing cholangitis. Periportal hepatitis on biopsy predicts cirrhosis for 17% of patients but 5-year survival is normal. Survival rate drops to 58% at 5 years if cirrhosis is established on biopsy. Bridging necrosis or multilobular necrosis is intermediate with 45% 5-year mortality rate, and 82% develop cirrhosis within 5 years. Rarely, hepatocellular carcinoma can occur in cirrhosis.

MANAGEMENT

Without immunosuppressive therapy, patients with autoimmune hepatitis usually progress to liver failure, with a mean survival of 5 years. The indications for treatment are based on symptoms, clinical progression, and manifestations of inflammation by laboratory or histologic evaluation. Cirrhotic patients with inflammatory activity on histology may still respond to corticosteroids, and a trial should be initiated. Prednisone alone or a lower dose of prednisone in combination with azathioprine is effective. The combination is preferred because of a lower risk of corticosteroid-related side effects such as osteopenic bone disease, obesity, cushingoid features, brittle diabetes, hypertension, or emotional lability. Initial treatments are either prednisone 30 mg per day and azathioprine 50 mg per day or 60 mg of prednisone per day with a weekly tapering of prednisone to 10 mg per day (combination therapy) and 20 mg per day (single-drug regimen).

Patients with multilobular necrosis on histologic examination who have no normalization of at least one laboratory parameter or whose pretreatment hyperbilirubinemia does not improve during a 2-week treatment period have a high rate of immediate mortality. These patients should be evaluated for liver transplantation if there are features of decompensation.

Remission is defined as an absence of symptoms, serum aspartate aminotransferase less than two times normal, and other serum markers normal and inactive or very minimally active biopsy. Sixty-five percent of patients experience remission within 2 years of therapy. When remission is achieved, corticosteroids should be tapered to the lowest possible maintenance dose. Liver biopsy examination before drug withdrawal is necessary to establish remission. More than 50% of patients have inflammatory activity on liver tissue examination. Histologic remission can lag behind biochemical evidence of remission by several months, and therapy should be extended for this duration. Relapse occurs in 50% of patients within 6 months of discontinuation of therapy.

Progressive symptoms, increasing aspartate transaminase and bilirubin levels, or worsening inflammation of liver biopsy defines treatment failure, which occurs in 9% of treated patients. High-dose prednisone alone (60 mg daily) or prednisone (30 mg daily) in conjunction with azathioprine (150 mg daily) induces clinical remission in 70% of failures within 2 years of the increased therapy. No remission after 3 years of continuous therapy (incomplete response, 13%) requires long-term maintenance with low dose ($\leq$10 mg) prednisone. Ten-year survival rates for treated patients with and without cirrhosis at presentation are 89% and 90%, respectively, and are comparable to a healthy age- and sex-matched cohort (94% at 10 years).

LIVER TRANSPLANTATION

Liver transplantation is effective therapy for decompensated disease in patients who have failed therapy or have advanced disease at presentation. Five-year survival rate after transplantation is 92%. Recurrence of autoimmune hepatitis in the graft is a common event (20% to 30%) with an incidence that increases over time as immunosuppressive therapy is reduced. Although response to treatment is poor, patient and graft survival do not appear to be decreased. Transplant recipients with AH should not undergo complete withdrawal of corticosteroid, and azathioprine should probably be part of the immunosuppressive regimen.

PRIMARY BILIARY CIRRHOSIS

DIAGNOSIS AND EPIDEMIOLOGY

Primary biliary cirrhosis (PBC) is a chronic cholestatic liver disease characterized by progressive inflammatory destruction of smaller intrahepatic bile ducts. The diagnosis should be considered in the setting of elevated serum alkaline phosphatase, hypercholesterolemia, and antimitochondrial antibodies. The natural history of PBC is that of a slowly progressive cholestasis marked by fatigue, pruritus, and the development of cirrhosis with its concomitant complications. PBC usually affects middle-aged women, and presentation is rare in those younger than 30 years or over 80 years. PBC is diagnosed in all races, but is more frequently seen in whites. PBC accounts for up to 2% of deaths from cirrhosis worldwide. It is diagnosed more frequently in developed countries, but whether this represents improved access to health care or a true difference in disease incidence is not known.

ETIOLOGY AND PATHOGENESIS

Although the cause of PBC is unclear, immunologic and genetic factors appear to play a role. For example, antimitochondrial antibodies are present in 95% of patients with PBC. In general, this family of antibodies are non-species—and non-organ—specific, and their presence or titer does not affect the course or severity of the disease. However, one of the antimitochondrial antibodies, anti-M2, appears specific for PBC. It is directed against the pyruvate dehydrogenase complex on the inner membrane of the mitochondrion. Additional immunologic abnormalities associated with PBC include IgM hypergammaglobulinemia, circulating immune complexes, and decreased populations and function of suppressor T cells. Other (extrahepatic) autoimmune diseases associated with PBC include systemic scleroderma, CREST syndrome (calcinosis, Raynaud's disease, esophageal dysmotility, sclerodactyly, and telangiectasia), autoimmune thyroiditis, rheumatoid arthritis, psoriatic arthritis, and Sjögren's syndrome. A genetic component to the pathogenesis of PBC is suggested by its link to the HLA-DRw8 antigen. However, the lack of concordance of disease in identical twins suggests that some triggering event is required to initiate PBC in a genetically susceptible person.

The pathogenesis of PBC appears to be due to two related processes that culminate in hepatic damage and the clinical features of the disease. Activated lymphocytes may be the mediators of the chronic small bile duct destruction that is the hallmark of this disease. In contrast to that which occurs in healthy persons, patients with PBC express increased amounts of class I (HLA-A, HLA-B, and HLA-C) and class II (HLA-DR) histocompatibility antigens on bile duct cells. These may provide a better target for activated cytotoxic T lymphocytes. Histologically, the bile duct lesions resemble those that are known to be mediated by cytotoxic T lymphocytes, such as graft-versus-host disease and rejection of transplanted organs.

CLINICAL FEATURES

Many of the clinical manifestations of PBC are caused by the gradual destruction of small intrahepatic bile ducts (Table 120.4). The resulting diminution in the number of such ducts

TABLE 120.4.	PRESENTATION OF PRIMARY BILIARY CIRRHOSIS	
Feature	**Percent**
Asymptomatic	25
Fatigue	65
Pruritus	50
Hepatomegaly	25
Splenomegaly	15
Xanthelasma	10

results in retention of bile acids, bilirubin, copper, and other substances that are normally secreted or excreted into bile, causing further damage to the liver cells. Other substances concentrate in the blood and soft tissues, causing symptoms such as itching. The pruritus is not due to the naturally occurring primary or secondary bile acids but to some other substance that is secreted into bile and bound by cholestyramine, a nonabsorbed, quaternary ammonium resin. In addition, serum levels of endogenous opioids are increased in those with PBC, and opioid antagonists relieve itching in some patients.

Hyperlipidemia and xanthoma formation are also consequences of long-standing cholestasis. Approximately 10% of patients eventually develop xanthelasmas that correlate with the degree of hypercholesterolemia. These lesions can be found on the palms of the hands, on the soles of the feet, over the extensor surfaces of the elbow and knees, on the eyelids or buttocks, and in the tendons of the ankles and wrists. The impaired secretion of bile causes a diminished concentration of bile acids in the intestinal lumen. If bile acids fall below the critical micellar concentration, complete digestion and absorption of neutral triglycerides in the diet may become inadequate. This accounts for the fat malabsorption seen in some patients and can be accompanied by malabsorption of the fat-soluble vitamins A, D, E, and K and by calcium malabsorption.

Some PBC patients with sicca syndrome may also suffer from pancreatic insufficiency. The pathogenesis of the osteopenic bone disease that occurs in at least 25% of PBC patients is likely to be multifactorial in nature and can lead to vertebral compression and long bone fractures. In patients whose osteoporosis is due to PBC, liver transplantation eventually leads to increased bone mineral density. Copper retention can rarely result in the finding of Kayser—Fleischer rings on eye examination or renal tubular acidosis because of excessive deposition of copper in the distal renal tubule.

Natural history studies have identified several variables associated with decreased survival in patients with PBC, such as bilirubin level greater than 10 mg per deciliter. The course of the disease has been described as being divided into three periods: a lengthy presymptomatic phase of up to 20 years, a symptomatic phase of pruritus, fatigue, and mild jaundice that may span 10 years, and a preterminal phase accompanied by marked jaundice and the complications of cirrhosis. The preterminal phase may be approximately 2 years, unless transplantation intervenes. Statistical models to predict survival have been validated and are valuable in management of medical care and the timing of liver transplantation. The most powerful predictor is the serum bilirubin level. Patients with bilirubin levels higher than 10 mg per deciliter usually survive less than 2 years; such a finding should prompt evaluation for liver transplantation. Other indications for liver transplantation include hepatorenal or hepatopulmonary syndromes, complications of portal hypertension, severe osteoporosis, evidence of malnutrition, and hepatocellular carcinoma (rare).

Many patients are asymptomatic at the time of diagnosis, but the signs and symptoms of cholestasis develop as the disease progresses. Once symptoms appear, and fatigue, pruritus, muscle wasting, progressive jaundice, and hepatic dysfunction develop. These can culminate in the complications of cirrhosis and portal hypertension and the need for liver transplantation. The diagnosis of PBC should be considered in patients with unexplained cholestasis or elevation of serum alkaline phosphatase. A percutaneous biopsy is necessary to confirm the diagnosis and determine prognosis. The pathognomonic lesion is characterized by patchy destruction of interlobular bile ducts with a mononuclear inflammatory infiltrate. Granulomas may be present but are not required for the diagnosis of PBC.

The severity of histologic damage can be classified into stages I to IV. Procedures to exclude other causes of cholestasis may include ultrasonography (which demonstrates normal-sized bile ducts), and computed tomography helps exclude ductal dilatation and may reveal portosystemic collaterals suggestive of portal hypertension. Endoscopic retrograde cholangiopancreatography may be used in patients lacking appropriate markers. The PBC patient has normal large bile ducts, but may have irregularities of smaller bile ducts. In end-stage PBC the physical signs of cirrhosis will be present and can include spider angiomata, temporal and extremity wasting, ascites, and signs and symptoms of hepatic encephalopathy.

TREATMENT

There is no proven medical treatment for the underlying disease of PBC, although drugs such as ursodeoxycholic acid, colchicine, and methotrexate are promising, and their use is associated with improvement in histology in some patients. Ursodeoxycholic acid (12 to 15 mg per kilogram body weight per day) improves serum bilirubin, alkaline phosphatase, aminotransferases, and IgM levels in several trials. It has also been reported to decrease pruritus in up to 50% of patients. Note that it has been shown to improve survival and to delay time to transplantation. Recently, pretransplantation treatment with ursodeoxycholic acid has been shown not to have an adverse impact on post-transplantation survival. Several small trials have demonstrated that methotrexate can effect a reduction in serum alkaline phosphatase and cholesterol and improve histology in some patients with PBC. However, other trials have not shown efficacy. A National Institutes of Health–sponsored double-blind, randomized controlled trial of methotrexate for treatment of PBC is currently underway. Corticosteroids, D-penicillamine, and azathioprine do not alter the course of the disease or improve survival and have no role in treatment of PBC.

Transplantation is the treatment of choice for PBC patients with complications of portal hypertension, severe symptomatic osteopenic bone disease, intolerable symptoms of pruritus, or a predicated survival of less than 2 years (Table 120.5). In properly selected candidates, liver transplantation is highly successful in treating PBC, and 5-year survival rates exceed 75%. Under adequate immunosuppression, recurrent PBC in the graft is rare.

The pruritus that accompanies cholestasis may limit normal activity, lead to sleep deprivation, and prompt suicidal ideation. It is often the earliest specific compliant and is characteristically worse at bedtime. Pruritus may occur during the third trimester of pregnancy and persists after delivery in some patients. Currently, treatment options for pruritus may not completely relieve symptoms in all patients. Therefore, transplantation may be considered in patients whose quality of life is greatly diminished by the pruritus, regardless of evidence of hepatic decompensation. Cholestryamine, a nonabsorbed resin relieves pruritus in many patients, with a usual dosage of 4 g in divided doses per day. The onset of action may be delayed by several weeks. Colestipol is as effective as cholestyramine. Antihistamines may be helpful in the early phases of PBC, when pruritus is not severe, and may primarily induce sleep.

Fat malabsorption can lead to complaints of nocturnal diarrhea, bulky stools, weight loss despite good appetite, increased caloric intake, and malabsorption of vitamins A, D, E, and K associated with clinical syndromes of deficiency. Steatorrhea can be treated with a low-fat diet supplemented by medium-chain triglycerides. If sicca syndrome accompanies PBC, then pancreatic insufficiency may be present and can be evaluated by the bentiromide test. If present, it can be treated with pancreatic enzyme replacement. Fat-soluble vitamin levels should be measured and specific supplements provided. Cholestyramine can bind these supplements and should be administered in separately timed doses.

Osteopenic bone disease is a nearly universal finding in women with PBC. Testing for vitamin D deficiency is essential, and supplementation is appropriate to prevent osteomalacia. Patients may require high-dose calcium supplementation and bisphosphonates and estrogen therapy if the patient is postmenopausal. Advanced osteoporosis with bone fracture is an indication for hepatic transplantation.

Hypercholesterolemia as a complication of chronic liver disease is unique to the cholestatic liver disorders and to PBC in particular. Some patients with PBC are initially diagnosed during evaluation for hypercholesterolemia. Serum cholesterol can exceed 300 mg per deciliter, but it is predominantly composed of high-density lipoprotein. Despite the elevation in cholesterol, a Mayo Clinic case-matched controlled retrospective study has demonstrated that PBC patients do not have an increased risk for coronary artery disease. As patients develop advanced cirrhosis, serum cholesterol may fall dramatically.

TABLE 120.5.	COMPLICATIONS OF PRIMARY BILIARY CIRRHOSIS	
Complication		**Percent**
Hypercholesterolemia		85
Osteopenia		75
Pruritus		70
Fat-soluble vitamin deficiency		20

BIBLIOGRAPHY

Czaja AJ. Autoimmune hepatitis. Evolving concepts and treatment strategies. *Dig Dis Sci* 1995;40:435–456.

James SP, Hoofnagle J, Strober W, et al. Primary biliary cirrhosis: a model autoimmune disease. *Ann Intern Med* 1983;99:500–512.

Johnson PJ, McFarlane I. Meeting report: International Autoimmune Hepatitis Group. *Hepatology* 1993;18:998–1005.

Jones EA, Bergasa NV. The pruritus of cholestasis. *Hepatology* 1999;29:1003–1006.

Kaplan MM. Primary biliary cirrhosis. *N Engl J Med* 1996;335:1570–1580.

Lindor KD, Dickson ER, Baldus WP. Ursodeoxycholic acid in the treatment of primary biliary cirrhosis. *Gastroenterology* 1994;106: 1284–1290.

Neuberger J. Transplantation for primary biliary cirrhosis. *Semin Liver Dis* 1997;17:137–146.

Pasha TM, Dickson ER. Survival algorithms and outcome analysis in primary biliary cirrhosis. *Semin Liver Dis* 1997;17:147–158.

Ratziu V, Samuel D, Sebagh M, et al. Long term follow up after liver transplantation for autoimmune hepatitis: evidence of recurrence of primary disease. *J Hepatol* 1999;30:131–141.

Roberts SK, Therneau T, Czaja AJ. Prognosis of histologic cirrhosis in type 1 autoimmune hepatitis. *Gastroenterology* 1996;110:848–857.

Kelley's Textbook of Internal Medicine, fourth edition. Edited by H. David Humes. Lippincott Williams & Wilkins, Philadelphia © 2000.

TABLE 121.1.	MINOR TYPES OF ALCOHOLIC LIVER DISEASE

Alcoholic fatty liver with perivenular fibrosis
Alcoholic foamy degeneration (alcoholic microvesicular steatosis)
Sclerosing hyaline necrosis
Alcoholic cirrhosis with chronic hepatitis[a]
Cholestasis
Iron overload

---

[a] A significant percentage of these patients may have concomitant hepatitis B or hepatitis C infection.

CHAPTER 121

ALCOHOLIC LIVER DISEASES

DAVID W. CRABB
LAWRENCE LUMENG

INCIDENCE AND EPIDEMIOLOGY

In the United States, at least 18 million people are problem drinkers and alcoholics, and alcohol abuse with or without alcohol dependence is one of the most important causes of chronic liver disease. Cirrhosis accounts for 75% of all medical deaths among alcoholics. The peak incidence of alcoholic liver disease (ALD) occurs in the age range of 40 to 55 years, and the male-to-female ratio is about 3:1. ALD includes three major histologic stages: fatty liver (or steatosis), hepatitis, and cirrhosis. Two or more of these histologic stages of ALD often coincide, as they represent a spectrum of the liver's response to injury from alcohol. A common concurrence is alcoholic steatosis and hepatitis, called *alcoholic steatohepatitis;* it should be distinguished from nonalcoholic steatohepatitis (NASH). Alcoholic hepatitis also frequently coexists with cirrhosis. Simple alcoholic fatty liver is the most benign and reversible form of ALD. By comparison, alcoholic hepatitis is much more serious and is the most important precursor of (although not an absolute requisite for) cirrhosis. Before the discovery of hepatitis C virus, it was noted that cirrhosis often developed in alcoholic patients without being preceded by alcoholic hepatitis. This puzzle is now partly solved because we know that roughly 20% to 40% of alcoholics with cirrhosis are infected with hepatitis C virus and that hepatitis C virus acts at least additively, if not synergistically, with alcohol to produce cirrhosis. In addition to the major types of ALD just listed, Table 121.1 summarizes several minor types. Among the minor types, alcoholic fatty liver with perivenular fibrosis is also a known precursor of alcoholic cirrhosis.

ETIOLOGY

The cause of ALD is multifactorial. In the past, it was attributed to malnutrition (e.g., "Laennec's nutritional cirrhosis"). However, alcoholic cirrhosis occurs in well-nourished persons, and cirrhosis does not occur in patients with simple malnutrition. Epidemiologic studies have shown a direct correlation between national per capita consumption of alcohol and prevalence of ALD and between individual alcohol consumption and the risk of alcoholic hepatitis or cirrhosis. Historically, a dramatic decrease in ALD was associated with diminished alcohol intake during war rationing and prohibition. Both the amount of ethanol ingested and the duration of intake are important factors in the induction of ALD. A daily intake of ethanol as low as 40 g in men or 20 g in women over more than 10 years results in a significant increase in the incidence of cirrhosis. Note that 1 ounce of 80-proof spirits, a 12-ounce bottle of 4% beer, or a 4-ounce glass of wine each contains approximately 10 to 12 g of ethanol.

Other studies have suggested that alcoholic hepatitis or cirrhosis is unlikely in persons who consume less than 80 g of alcohol per day for 10 to 20 years. The amount of ethanol that can be safely consumed is uncertain, but it is probably less than 20 g per day for men and less than 10 g for women. Neither the pattern of drinking nor the type of alcoholic beverage plays an important role in the development of liver disease. In comparison with agents such as carbon tetrachloride, ethanol is a weaker hepatotoxin, and studies suggest that a threshold cumulative dose must be consumed, amounting to 600 kg for men and 150 to 300 kg for women to produce liver injury. To achieve a cumulative dose of 600 kg of ethanol, one has to consume 72 ounces of beer, 1 liter of wine, or 8 ounces of distilled spirits per day for 20 years.

The notion that ethanol itself can cause ALD is supported by animal experiments. Rats and baboons chronically given large amounts of ethanol in a nutritionally balanced diet developed fatty liver and increased hepatic collagen. About 30% of the baboons, but not the rats, developed cirrhosis after 1 to 5 years. Rats fed by constant intragastric infusion of a nutritionally adequate liquid diet containing ethanol and comprising 50% of total calories developed fatty liver, necrosis, and fibrosis. However, a secondary role of dietary imbalance or malnutrition can-

CHAPTER 121: ALCOHOLIC LIVER DISEASES

TABLE 121.2.	EVIDENCE FOR NUTRITIONAL FACTORS IN ALCOHOLIC LIVER DISEASE

- Hepatitis (nonalcoholic steatohepatitis) and cirrhosis similar to those seen in alcoholics are seen in some obese patients, especially those who have diabetes, or hyperlipidemia or have undergone bypass surgery.
- Nutritional deficiencies caused by decreased dietary intake, impaired absorption, altered metabolism, diminished utilization, decreased storage, and increased excretion are common among alcoholics.
- Intravenous amino acids have led to significant improvement of ascites, serum bilirubin, and plasma albumin in patients with alcoholic hepatitis in several controlled trials.
- The degree of liver injury produced in alcohol-fed rats can be modulated by carbohydrate content or by the amount and type of protein and fat (fats that worsen ethanol-induced injury are fish oil (containing ω-3 polyunsaturated fatty acids) and polyunsaturated fat; fats that tend to decrease ethanol-induced injury are medium-chain triglycerides or saturated fats) in the diet.
- As the fat content in the Japanese diet has increased, there has been an increase in the incidence of alcoholic hepatitis.
- Epidemiologic studies suggest that alcoholic liver disease is more common in populations that consume more polyunsaturated fats and in alcoholics who are obese.
- Polyunsaturated lecithin (particularly dilinoleoyl phosphatidylcholine) can reduce the severity of fibrosis in the baboon model of alcoholic liver injury.

not be dismissed. Arguments in favor of nutritional contributions to ALD are shown in Table 121.2.

Genetic, hormonal (gender-related), immunologic, and environmental factors are also important in modulating the individual variation in susceptibility to the toxicity of ethanol. In the baboon model, only a small proportion of the animals developed cirrhosis. In humans, no more than 35% of heavy drinkers develop alcoholic hepatitis, and only 20% develop cirrhosis. Alcoholic hepatitis and cirrhosis develop with shorter duration of alcohol abuse and after lower cumulative alcohol intake in women than men. This gender-related differential susceptibility may be due to a lower volume of distribution for ethanol and

decreased first-pass (gastric or hepatic or both) metabolism of ethanol in women and other sex hormone-related factors that lead to increased alcohol metabolism, altered cytokine release, inadequate induction of hepatic fatty acid–binding capacity, and insufficient compensatory increases in ω-hydroxylation in females. Postulated immunologic mechanisms are complex and involve the effects of ethanol, acetaldehyde, and endotoxin on an array of cytokine interactions that include activation of Kupffer cells, hepatic stellate cells, and sinusoidal endothelial cells. Further details of these interactions are discussed in a later section. Finally, there is a high prevalence of hepatitis B and C infections in alcoholics with cirrhosis, suggesting an interaction between viral infections and ethanol.

■ METABOLISM OF ETHANOL

Ethanol is rapidly absorbed from the gastrointestinal tract, and most of it is metabolized in the liver. When moderate amounts of ethanol (e.g., 10 to 30 g) are consumed by normal adult males in the "fed" state, a sizable first-pass metabolism of ethanol can be easily detected, but whether the stomach or liver or both is responsible for this phenomenon is debated. In favor of gastric metabolism are the facts that gastric mucosa contains alcohol dehydrogenase (ADH) and that peak blood alcohol levels are higher in those with decreased gastric ADH activity, such as women and patients who have a gastrectomy or chronic gastritis or who are taking cimetidine. However, the total ethanol oxidizing capacity of the stomach is low, suggesting a hepatic contribution.

After absorption, ethanol is distributed in the body water space. In the liver, it is metabolized to acetaldehyde by ADH in the cytosol and the cytochrome P450IIE1 (CYP2E1) in microsomes (Table 121.3 and Fig. 121.1). The role of catalase is very minor. Because there is no way to store ethanol and no feedback control of the rate of ethanol oxidation, its metabolism dominates other oxidative pathways, producing dramatic metabolic changes described in the following text.

ADH is responsible for the bulk of ethanol oxidation. The ADH reaction rate is controlled by the amount of ADH, the

| TABLE 121.3. | ETHANOL-METABOLIZING ENZYMES IN HUMANS |

Enzymes	Intracellular Location	Polymorphisms
Alcohol-Metabolizing Enzymes		
Alcohol dehydrogenase	Cytosolic	*ADH2*1, 2*2, 2*3* *ADH3*1, 3*2*
Cytochrome P45OIIE1	Microsomal	Promoter variants
Catalase	Peroxisomes	None known
Acetaldehyde-Metabolizing Enzymes		
Aldehyde dehydrogenase-2	Mitochondrial	*ALDH2*1,* *ALDH2*2*
Aldehyde dehydrogenase-1	Cytosolic	None known

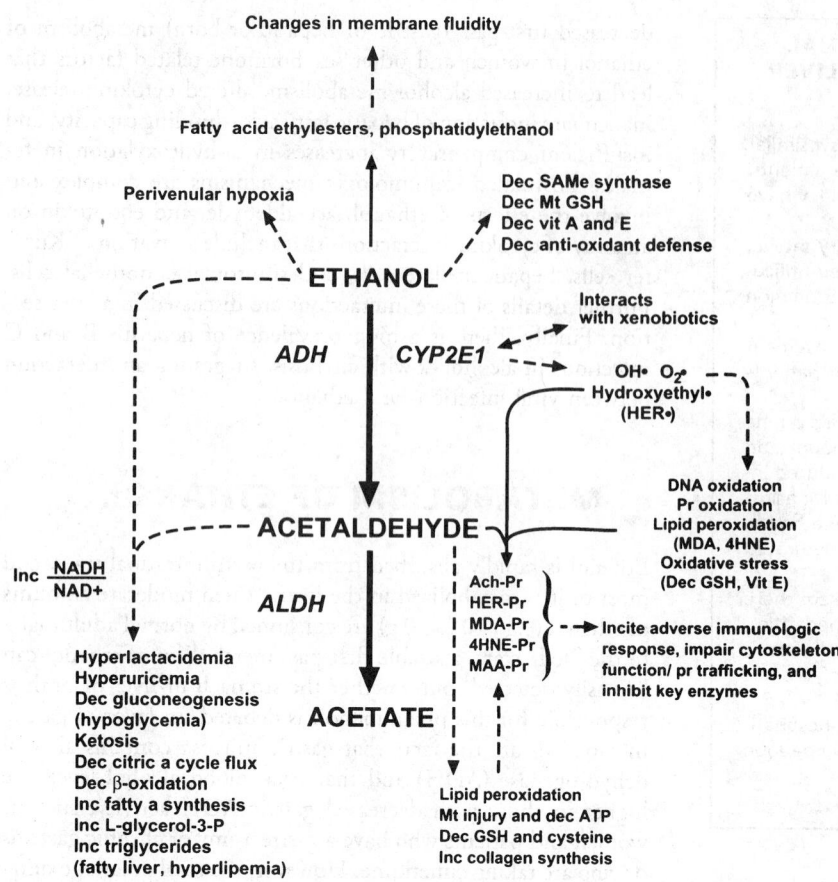

FIGURE 121.1. Pathways of ethanol metabolism and metabolic effects of ethanol, acetaldehyde, and acetate. *Dec,* decreased; *Inc,* increased; *Mt,* mitochondrial; *SAMe, S-*adenosyl-methionine; *GSH,* glutathione; *ADH,* alcohol dehydrogenase; *CYP2E1,* cytochrome P450 IIE1; *ALDH,* aldehyde dehydrogenase; *vit,* vitamin; *Pr,* protein; *Ach,* acetaldehyde; *HER,* hydroxyethyl radical; *MDA,* malondialdehyde; *4-HNE,* 4-hydroxynonenal; *MAA,* malondialdehyde-acetaldehyde.

acetaldehyde level, and the free $NADH/NAD^+$ ratio in the cytosol. The latter is ultimately determined by the rate of mitochondrial electron transfer. ADH is not inducible with chronic alcohol exposure; rather, its content and the ethanol elimination rate are decreased with fasting, protein deficiency, and liver disease. In humans, there are seven ADH gene loci, two of which are polymorphic. Different people, especially of different racial groups, inherit different sets of ADH isoenzymes. The kinetic properties of the various ADH isoenzymes differ widely in vitro. Although the *ADH2*2* allele appears to be protective against alcoholism, no specific ADH polymorphism has been firmly identified as a factor that predisposes to the development of ALD.

CYP2E1 is associated with NADPH–cytochrome P450 reductase in the microsomal membrane and reduces molecular oxygen to water as ethanol is oxidized to acetaldehyde. Although CYP2E1 normally oxidizes only a small fraction of alcohol, it is inducible by chronic alcohol use, especially in the perivenular zone, and it may contribute to the increased rates of alcohol elimination in heavy drinkers. CYP2E1 can also be induced by starvation and by a diet high in fat. CYP2E1 has a high K_m for ethanol and may be more important in ethanol metabolism at high blood levels. CYP2E1 and other P450 isoenzymes that can oxidize ethanol also metabolize certain drugs. Alcoholics, when sober, exhibit increased metabolism of these drugs (Table 121.4); however, since ethanol competes with these drugs for metabolism, there is a decreased rate of drug elimination when

the patient drinks. Acute alcohol ingestion also increases the pharmacodynamic action of several drugs (Table 121.4). The interaction between induction of CYP2E1 in alcoholics and acetaminophen-induced hepatitis is clinically very important. Although therapeutic doses of acetaminophen are harmless when consumed by alcohol-naive persons, in alcoholics such doses can produce serious and sometimes fatal liver disease with extremely high aminotransferase levels, massive perivenular hepatic necrosis, pancreatitis, and renal failure. This disorder is sometimes called the "acetaminophen–alcohol syndrome." Thus, heavy drinkers should be warned to avoid acetaminophen entirely.

Acetaldehyde is further oxidized by aldehyde dehydrogenases (ALDHs; Table 121.3) to acetate, which is released from the liver and metabolized by heart and muscle. The enzymes are inhibited by disulfiram (Antabuse). Consumption of alcohol while taking disulfiram or several other drugs results in the accumulation of acetaldehyde, producing vasodilation, cutaneous flushing, tachycardia, nausea, and vomiting (Table 121.4). This reaction is also observed in about 50% of Asians who are deficient in ALDH2. These individuals drink less and have a low prevalence of alcoholism. High blood acetaldehyde levels are also observed in alcoholics when they drink. This is probably due to the adaptive increase in ethanol oxidation and reduction in the ability of mitochondria to oxidize acetaldehyde. The increased acetaldehyde level in alcoholics perpetuates alcoholic liver injury because acetaldehyde is much more toxic than ethanol.

TABLE 121.4.	INTERACTIONS BETWEEN CHRONIC ALCOHOL ABUSE AND DRUG ACTIONS AND METABOLISM	

Increased Drug Metabolism	Increased Drug/Chemical Toxicity	Increased Drug Tolerance
Pentobarbital	Acetaminophen	Anesthetics
Meprobamate	Vitamin A	Barbiturates
Warfarin	Isoniazid	Meprobamate
Tolbutamide (and other sulfonylureas)	Phenylbutazone	Benzodiazepines
	Halothane	
Phenytoin	Enflurane	
Cocaine	Carbon tetrachloride	
Rifampin	Benzene	
Aminopyrine	Nitrosamines	
Methadone	Cocaine	

Increased Pharmacodynamic Effect	Antabuse-like Reactions
H_1 antihistamines	Tolbutamide
Barbiturates	Metronidazole
Benzodiazepines	Griseofulvin
Chloral hydrate	Quinacrine
Meprobamate	Pargyline
Narcotics	Reserpine
Phenothiazines	Phenylbutazone
Phenytoin	Moxalactam and several other second- and third-generation cephalosporins

METABOLIC EFFECTS OF ETHANOL OXIDATION

Oxidation of ethanol is coupled to the production of NADH. As shown in Figure 121.1, the high NADH concentration shifts the equilibria of several enzymatic reactions toward the formation of reduced metabolites (e.g., conversion of pyruvate to lactate and of dihydroxyacetonephosphate to L-glycerol-3-phosphate). Increased lactate formation results in mild hyperlacticemia and contributes to hyperuricemia owing to impaired renal excretion of urate. The reduction in pyruvate and dihydroxyacetone phosphate concentrations inhibits gluconeogenesis and may result in hypoglycemia. Alcoholic hypoglycemia occurs during fasting, when blood glucose levels are maintained by gluconeogenesis. Alcoholic ketoacidosis also occurs in alcoholics who are fasting while drinking heavily. They exhibit very high free fatty acid levels, low insulin levels, and high levels of glucagon and catecholamines.

The concentration of β-hydroxybutyrate (not detected by urine dipsticks) characteristically exceeds that of acetoacetate. Increased NADH concentration in the mitochondria inhibits other NAD^+-linked pathways, such as the citric acid cycle, amino acid oxidation, and fatty acid oxidation. Fatty acid synthesis is also accelerated with chronic alcohol exposure. Increased levels of L-glycerol-3-phosphate and fatty acids result in accelerated synthesis of triglycerides. The liver secretes some of this fat as very low density lipoprotein (VLDL), increasing plasma VLDL. The secretion of VLDL does not keep pace with the increased synthesis of triglycerides, so the liver cells become filled with fat.

Ethanol oxidation by way of CYP2E1 produces an array of metabolic effects. In addition to being inducible by chronic alcohol use and high fat intake, this enzyme is unusually "leaky" and generates reactive oxygen species (ROS) including hydroxyl radical ($OH^{\cdot-}$), superoxide anion ($O_2^{\cdot-}$), and hydrogen peroxide (H_2O_2). Thus, CYP2E1 is a major source of oxidative stress. This P450 enzyme also has unusual capacity to activate many xenobiotics to toxic metabolites and thereby contributes to a wide spectrum of alcohol-related pathology.

PATHOGENESIS OF ALCOHOLIC LIVER DISEASE

ALCOHOL-INDUCED FATTY LIVER OR STEATOSIS

The altered hepatic $NADH/NAD^+$ ratio produced by ethanol and the inhibition of fatty acid oxidation are largely responsible for the development of alcoholic fatty liver. Because the high periportal to low perivenous oxygen gradient normally present within the liver acinus is made steeper by chronic alcohol ingestion, perivenous hepatocytes become much more hypoxic. As a result, the effect of alcohol metabolism on the redox state and on fat accumulation is most severe in perivenous cells. Fat accumulation does not continue indefinitely because the redox state changes are attenuated with continuing chronic alcohol use. The fat that accumulates in alcoholic fatty liver can come from different sources: diet, adipose tissue, and de novo hepatic synthesis from carbohydrates, depending on the diet.

ALCOHOL-INDUCED CELL DEATH AND FIBROSIS

The mechanisms by which chronic alcohol consumption leads to irreversible liver damage are also summarized in Figure 121.1. The accumulation of fat is accompanied by induction of microsomal proteins and fatty acid–binding protein and by retention of secretory proteins (due to impaired cytoskeleton function and protein trafficking pathways caused by formation of acetaldehyde–protein adducts) and water. This causes the hepatocytes to swell and is called *ballooning* or *hydropic degeneration*. This swelling interferes with blood flow to the perivenous zone. There is also increased oxygen consumption in the liver of rats after prolonged alcohol consumption. Increased oxygen consumption coupled with decreased blood flow may induce perivenular hypoxia and thus pericentral apoptosis/necrosis and fibrosis.

Other mechanisms of ethanol hepatotoxicity include the induction of physical alterations in cell membranes. Acute exposure to ethanol increases membrane fluidity, whereas chronic alcohol consumption usually results in compensatory decreases in the fluidity of plasma and subcellular membranes, which may affect activities of membrane-bound receptors and enzymes involved in signal transduction. Changes in membrane fluidity can be mediated by the formation of abnormal lipids such as fatty acid ethyl esters and phosphatidyl ethanol. Alcohol use also adversely affects antioxidant defense in hepatocytes by decreasing the activity of *S*-adenosylmethionine synthase, diminishing mitochondrial glutathione contents, and depleting the stores of vitamins A and E. In addition, alcohol use promotes the oxidation of DNA, proteins, and lipids as a result of increased production of ROS.

Lipid peroxidation is a well-known deleterious chain reaction of lipid radical formation that is initiated by ROS attack on unsaturated lipids in cell membranes. Lipid peroxidation has been demonstrated in experimental animals exposed to alcohol and in patients with ALD. Lipid peroxidation leads to production of reactive aldehydes such as malondialdehyde (MDA) and 4-hydroxynonenal (4-HNE). ROS are generated principally by CYP2E1 in hepatocytes and Kupffer cells, but debate exists about their relative quantitative importance. CYP2E1 is more active in perivenular hepatocytes where glutathione levels are normally lowest; therefore, high levels of ROS and other radicals such as hydroxyethyl radicals (HER derived from $OH^{·-}$-radical attack on ethanol) are generated in the perivenular zone of the liver where alcohol-induced injury is most pronounced. In addition to tissue damage, lipid peroxidation may also promote collagen production by transformed hepatic stellate cells. Iron overload, which accompanies chronic alcohol abuse, accelerates ROS production, accentuates lipid peroxidation, and is likely to contribute to liver injury. Induction of microsomal enzymes also increases the hepatotoxicity of a number of agents (Table 121.4). For instance, hepatic vitamin A is metabolized more rapidly in alcohol-fed animals, depleting vitamin A stores and causing increased toxicity of vitamin A when it is given as a supplement. Acetaldehyde is an important factor in hepatic injury because it injures mitochondria, thereby depleting cellular adenosine triphosphate. It chemically reacts with glutathione and cysteine and modifies proteins, phospholipids, and components of the cytoskeleton by forming adducts.

In addition to acetaldehyde, a number of reactive aldehydes derived from lipid peroxidation and HER have been shown to react with proteins. As shown in Figure 121.1, these adducts include acetaldehyde-, HER-, MDA-, 4-HNE- and mixed malondialdehyde–acetaldehyde–protein adducts. Antibodies directed against membrane and soluble proteins of the hepatocyte modified by acetaldehyde and by HER are detected in alcoholics and constitute a possible immune component to liver injury. Acetaldehyde damages the cytoskeleton, and this inhibits protein secretion. Abnormal transport of proteins through the Golgi apparatus may also alter the properties and function of surface proteins. A major acetaldehyde-modified protein in alcohol-fed rats was recently identified to be an enzyme in the bile salt synthetic pathway (Δ^4-3-ketosteroid 5β-reductase). In addition, Mallory bodies are formed from cytokeratin intermediate filaments. Injury to the intermediate filaments may contribute to ballooning degeneration.

Recent research has implicated a complex cascade of autocrine and paracrine cytokine pathways that involves increased intestinal permeability and increased absorption of endotoxin (lipopolysaccharides [LPS]), oxidative stress and activation of Kupffer cells, proliferation and transformation of hepatic stellate cells, and stimulation of sinusoidal endothelial cells (Fig. 121.2). Cytokines are a diverse group of mediators that exhibit inflammatory, cytotoxic, fibrogenic, and growth-promoting properties. Patients with alcoholic hepatitis frequently have elevated levels of endotoxin, tumor necrosis factor (TNF)-α, interleukin (IL)-1, and IL-8 in circulation. IL-8 and TNF-α levels in particular correlate inversely with survival from alcoholic hepatitis.

The mechanisms whereby alcohol or acetaldehyde activates Kupffer cells are not completely known. Recent studies point to injured hepatocytes, endotoxin, and perhaps ethanol per se as important factors. Hepatocytes injured by ethanol release chemotactic factors to attract monocytes and neutrophils. Injured hepatocytes also release factors that activate Kupffer cells. Chronic alcohol ingestion is thought to allow the increased absorption of endotoxin by increasing intestinal permeability. Endotoxin can activate Kupffer cells by binding first to a LPS-binding protein and then to a surface glycoprotein called CD14. Kupffer cells can also be activated by ethanol oxidation by CYP2E1. Oxidative stress from endotoxin and CYP2E1 activates an oxidative stress-sensitive nuclear transcription factor, NF-κB, which coordinately increases the expression of a wide range of genes. Activated Kupffer cells secrete TNF-α, transforming growth factor TGF-β1, platelet-derived growth factor (PDGF), IL-8, IL-6, and IL-1, as well as ROS, nitric oxide, proinflammatory/vasoactive eicosanoids, and proteolytic enzymes. TNF-α exhibits a sensitizing effect on hepatocytes, making ethanol much more toxic. IL-8 functions as a major neutrophil chemotactic agent and activates neutrophils. IL-6 is an acute-phase reactant and also serves as a hepatocyte-stimulating factor. PDGF promotes proliferation of stellate cells, whereas TGF-β1 induces stellate cells to transform into myofibroblasts; the latter secrete collagen, metalloproteinases, proteoglycans, and other matrix material. Stellate cells are also important in regulating portal pressure and in modulating inflammatory responses,

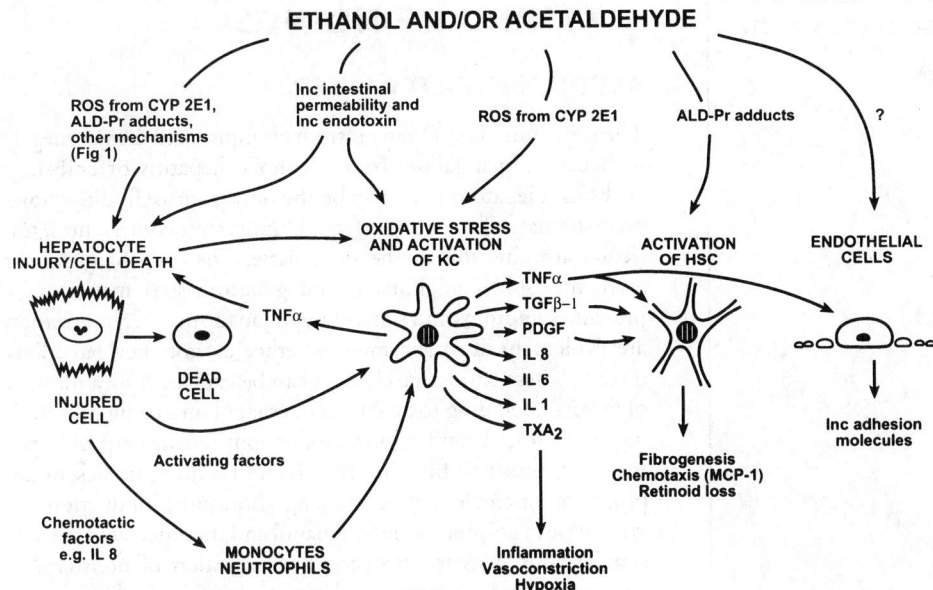

FIGURE 121.2. Effects of ethanol and acetaldehyde on hepatocytes, Kupffer's cells, stellate cells, and endothelial cells. This figure summarizes the toxicity of ethanol on the liver cells, the mechanisms of activation of Kupffer's (*KC*) and hepatic stellate cells (*HSC*), and the roles played by various cytokines in alcoholic liver disease. *ROS,* reactive oxygen species; *ALD-Pr,* aldehyde-protein; *TXA₂,* thromboxane A₂. The other cytokines are defined in the text.

as in the expression of monocyte chemoattractant protein-1 (MCP-1), a monocyte-specific chemokine.

In addition to cytokines, acetaldehyde, malondialdehyde (MDA), and 4-HNE can induce stellate cells to express collagen genes. In alcoholic hepatitis and cirrhosis, sinusoidal endothelial cells are known to express important adhesion molecules that include E-selectin, vascular cell adhesion molecule (VCAM-1), and intracellular adhesion molecule (ICAM)-1. Selectins and ICAM-1 are required for neutrophils to tether to the sinusoidal wall, whereas other molecules, notably VCAM-1, mediate lymphocyte tethering. These adhesion molecules bind neutrophils and lymphocytes by way of β_1 and β_2 integrins.

PATHOLOGY

ALCOHOLIC FATTY LIVER

The fatty liver is enlarged and firm and may be pale yellow. Microscopically, there is great variation in the number of fat droplets found and the number of cells affected, with a distinct tendency for fat accumulation in the perivenous and midzones of the liver lobule. Occasionally, hepatocytes rupture to form a fatty cyst, and then a lipogranuloma. Generally, there is sparse cell necrosis or inflammation. Fatty liver may be complicated by intrahepatic cholestasis and mild cholangiolitis in the absence of extrahepatic biliary obstruction. Perivenular fibrosis may be present and has been shown to be a precursor of cirrhosis. Another variant known as *alcoholic foamy degeneration* is characterized by pericentral hepatocytes filled with foamy, microvesicular fat, focal cell necrosis, but no inflammation.

ALCOHOLIC HEPATITIS

In alcoholic hepatitis, ballooning degeneration, focal hepatocyte necrosis, and a neutrophilic inflammatory infiltrate occur. About

30% of patients develop alcoholic hyaline (i.e., aggregates of perinuclear, eosinophilic, amorphous material). Although highly suggestive of ALD, hyaline is also seen in other diseases (Table 121.5). Hepatocellular necrosis and neutrophilic infiltration of the liver are considered absolute criteria for the diagnosis of alcoholic hepatitis. Other pathologic findings in alcoholic hepatitis include steatosis and fibrosis (steatohepatitis) and cirrhosis. On a case-by-case basis, it is difficult to distinguish histologically alcoholic hepatitis from NASH (see Chapter 123). However, statistically, periportal fibrosis, bile duct proliferation, and cirrhosis are more frequently seen in alcoholic steatohepatitis, and nuclear vacuolation is much less prevalent. Pericellular and perisinusoidal fibrosis seen in both alcoholic steatohepatitis and NASH give rise to a characteristic "chicken wire" appearance,

TABLE 121.5.	DIFFERENTIAL DIAGNOSIS OF LIVER DISEASES EXHIBITING MALLORY'S HYALINE

Steatohepatitis
  Alcoholic steatohepatitis
  Nonalcoholic steatohepatitis (see Table 121.6)
Chronic hepatitis C
Drug-induced hepatitis (e.g., griseofulvin or amiodarone)
Chronic cholestatic disorders
  Primary biliary cirrhosis
  Primary sclerosing cholangitis
  Chronic biliary obstruction
Wilson's disease
Hepatocellular neoplasms/masses
  Hepatocellular carcinoma
  Hepatic adenoma
  Dysplastic hepatocellular nodule
  Focal nodular hyperplasia
Indian childhood cirrhosis
Weber–Christian disease
Abetalipoproteinemia

TABLE 121.6.	**CONDITIONS ASSOCIATED WITH NONALCOHOLIC STEATOHEPATITIS**

Nutritional/metabolic
  Obesity
  Diabetes mellitus and hyperglycemia
  Hyperlipidemia
  Accelerated weight loss
  Acute starvation
  Total parenteral nutrition
Gastrointestinal
  Jejunoileal or jejunocolonic bypass
  Extensive small-bowel resection
  Gastroplasty
Drugs
  Amiodarone
  Synthetic estrogens
  Tamoxifen
  Nifedipine
  Corticosteroids
Miscellaneous
  Limb lipodystrophy
  Weber–Christian disease
  Abetalipoproteinemia
Idiopathic

and perivenular sclerosis leads to deposition of a collar of collagen in the wall of the central vein. Conditions known to be associated with NASH are listed in Table 121.6. In a few cases of alcoholic hepatitis, there is sclerosing hyaline necrosis, that is, severe, irregular, confluent, centrilobular necrosis with obliteration of the central vein by collagen.

ALCOHOLIC CIRRHOSIS

The end stage of ALD is cirrhosis, characterized by fibrous bands connecting portal triads with central veins and by regenerative nodules. The nodules are typically small (1 to 3 mm) and uniform in size. Although fibrosis may be reversible, regression is impossible when significant nodular regeneration occurs. Over time and with abstinence from alcohol, nodular regeneration becomes more vigorous and forms large nodules; hence, mixed micro-/macronodular or macronodular cirrhosis develops. There is commonly superimposed fatty change and alcoholic hepatitis. There may also be increased stainable iron in biopsy samples. Iron overload in alcoholic cirrhosis can be differentiated from genetic hemochromatosis by gene analysis of HFE mutations or by quantitative iron analysis. In genetic hemochromatosis, the hepatic iron index (hepatic iron content expressed as μmol per gram dry weight divided by the patient's age) in the cirrhotic liver is greater than 1.9, whereas that in the cirrhotic liver of alcoholics is invariably less than 1.9. In some patients with alcoholic cirrhosis, there is portal inflammation with piecemeal necrosis. This feature may reflect an autoimmune component of ALD, unsuspected Wilson's disease (particularly in young patients), or most commonly, coexistent chronic viral hepatitis (particularly hepatitis C virus infection).

CLINICAL FINDINGS

ALCOHOLIC FATTY LIVER

The spectrum of ALD ranges from asymptomatic hepatomegaly to hepatocellular failure from alcoholic hepatitis or end-stage cirrhosis. Hepatomegaly may be the only positive finding; however, stigmata of alcoholism (e.g., Dupuytren's contractures, testicular atrophy, loss of the male pattern of body hair, palmar erythema, spider angiomata, and gynecomastia) may also be present. Symptoms and signs of hypogonadism and feminization are evident in alcoholic men, whether or not they have liver disease. These endocrine changes can be explained by a number of factors, including toxic effects of ethanol on Leydig cells leading to decreased testosterone production; impairment of hypothalamic–pituitary function by ethanol resulting in lack of appropriate increase in luteinizing hormone; induction of aromatase in adipose tissue by ethanol and thus increased conversion of androgens to estrogens; and ingestion of nonsteroidal estrogens found in plants called *phytoestrogens* in alcoholic beverages that then can lead to increased estrogenic effect.

More advanced disease may cause weakness, cachexia, fever, anorexia, nausea, vomiting, jaundice, hepatic tenderness, splenomegaly, or ascites. Most likely, such cases represent a combination of fatty liver and alcoholic hepatitis, since the classic lesions of alcoholic hepatitis are difficult to find in livers massively infiltrated with fat. Rarely, alcoholic fatty liver is complicated by cholestasis and produces a picture that mimics both alcoholic hepatitis and extrahepatic biliary obstruction. Patients with alcoholic fatty liver may suffer fat embolism, alcohol withdrawal symptoms, or hypoglycemia.

ALCOHOLIC HEPATITIS

Patients with alcoholic hepatitis usually complain of anorexia, nausea, malaise, weakness, abdominal pain, icterus, weight loss, and fever; however, a few are totally free of symptoms. At the opposite end of the clinical spectrum, many patients present with severe jaundice, ascites, azotemia, and hepatic encephalopathy and may progress rapidly to death. Such patients commonly deteriorate early in the hospital stay, despite stopping drinking. Physical examination reveals the findings summarized in Table 121.7.

ALCOHOLIC CIRRHOSIS

Patients with alcoholic cirrhosis may be asymptomatic in 10% to 20%, but commonly present with the complications of chronic liver disease and the usual stigmata. Among male patients with cirrhosis from a variety of causes, hypogonadism and feminization are most prominent in patients with ALD and are comparable to those with genetic hemochromatosis. Complications of alcoholic cirrhosis include cachexia, coagulopathy, ascites, spontaneous bacterial peritonitis, hepatorenal syndrome, hepatic encephalopathy, hepatocellular carcinoma, and gastrointestinal bleeding from esophageal and gastric varices (Chapter 105). Other less common causes of bleeding are ectopic varices and portal hypertensive gastropathy.

TABLE 121.7.	CLINICAL FINDINGS IN ALCOHOLIC HEPATITIS

Finding	Incidence (%)
Hepatomegaly	95
Hepatic tenderness	50–70
Signs of portal hypertension (splenomegaly, prominent abdominal veins, and ascites)	40–70
Stigmata of chronic parenchymal liver disease and alcoholism (bruising, leukonychia, palmar erythema, spider angiomata, edema, parotid gland enlargement, and testicular atrophy)	30–60
Jaundice	55
Fever	50
Upper gastrointestinal bleeding	30
Hepatic encephalopathy	20

LABORATORY FINDINGS

Macrocytosis is common in alcoholics, and its presence in an otherwise healthy person suggests occult alcohol abuse. Some cases are characterized by the presence of thick macrocytes caused by folate deficiency or a toxic effect of alcohol on the bone marrow. In most cirrhosis, regardless of the cause, the macrocytes are thin target cells resulting from changes in the lipid composition of the red cell membrane. Thin target macrocytes disappear very slowly with improvement in liver function.

ALCOHOLIC FATTY LIVER

In alcoholic fatty liver, hyperbilirubinemia (usually less than 5 mg per deciliter) is observed in about 25% of cases. In almost all types of ALD, serum aspartate aminotransferase (AST) and alanine aminotransferase (ALT) are usually less than 300 IU per liter. In contrast to viral and toxic hepatitis and NASH in which serum ALT is equal to or higher than serum AST, the serum AST is usually higher than serum ALT (with the AST/ALT ratio ≥ 2 in 80% of the cases) in ALD. In the absence of cholestasis, alkaline phosphatase is only modestly elevated (less than 300 IU per deciliter). In patients with ALD, a γ-glutamyltranspeptidase to alkaline phosphatase ratio of more than 5 is characteristic. Serum albumin and globulin levels are abnormal in less than 25% of patients with alcoholic fatty liver, and the serum globulin level rarely exceeds 4 g per deciliter.

ALCOHOLIC HEPATITIS

Laboratory abnormalities are more severe in alcoholic hepatitis. Anemia occurs in 50% to 70% of patients, secondary to toxic effects of ethanol on the bone marrow, impaired vitamin B_6 metabolism, folic acid deficiency, iron deficiency from blood loss, or hypersplenism. Leukocytosis is observed in 25% to 75% of cases. Leukopenia and thrombocytopenia are present in 10% to 15% and may reflect folate deficiency, alcohol-induced marrow suppression, or hypersplenism. Serum AST and ALT are elevated in all cases of alcoholic hepatitis, and alkaline phosphatase is elevated in 80% of cases. Peak AST levels rarely exceed 300 IU per liter except in patients with sclerosing hyaline necrosis or acetaminophen overdose, in which case AST levels may be much higher. Serum bilirubin is increased in 90% of the cases. Serum albumin is usually decreased and prothrombin time is often prolonged. Electrolyte abnormalities are common in alcoholic hepatitis and include hyponatremia, hyperchloremia due to partial renal tubular acidosis, hypokalemia from poor dietary intake, vomiting, or diarrhea, hypomagnesemia from increased urinary loss, and respiratory alkalosis.

ALCOHOLIC CIRRHOSIS

The liver test abnormalities in alcoholic cirrhosis are less pronounced than those in alcoholic hepatitis. In fact, in compensated cirrhosis, many of the liver tests are nearly normal. Laboratory abnormalities may include mild increases in AST, ALT, and alkaline phosphatase, depression of serum albumin, elevation of serum globulins (greater than 4 g per liter), prolongation of prothrombin time, leukopenia, thrombocytopenia, and anemia. Hypersplenism by itself rarely leads to platelet counts lower than 40,000/μL, and splenectomy is almost never indicated.

DIAGNOSIS AND MANAGEMENT

There are two pitfalls in the diagnosis of ALD: (1) failing to consider ALD in patients not fitting the stereotype of the skid-row alcoholic and (2) assuming that abnormal liver tests in an alcoholic patient are due to ALD. Alcoholism should be considered in any patient with liver disease, and a careful drinking history should be obtained from the patient and a reliable third party. The history should include either the most commonly used simple questionnaire called the CAGE test or the more detailed screening instrument, the MAST test. The MAST test has a shortened version of 12 questions rather than the long version of 25 questions. The CAGE test uses the following questions: Have you felt the need to CUT DOWN on drinking? Are you ANNOYED by references to your drinking? Do you feel GUILTY about your drinking? Do you ever need an EYE-OPENER (i.e., an alcoholic drink in the morning)? A positive response to two or more of these questions strongly suggests the possibility of alcohol abuse and should prompt a more thorough history. The sensitivity of the CAGE test for alcohol abuse is 70% to 96%, and the specificity is 91% to 99%. The diagnostic accuracy of the CAGE test is about 80%, whereas that of the MAST test is 90%. However, the CAGE test is easier to use than the MAST.

The history should also include an estimate of the number of grams of ethanol consumed daily and the duration of drinking. As pointed out earlier, up to 40% of patients with presumed alcoholic liver disease are infected with hepatitis C virus, and testing for hepatitis C virus antibody is mandatory.

A liver biopsy is necessary to differentiate fatty liver, alcoholic hepatitis, and cirrhosis reliably. Before the discovery of hepatitis C virus, it was reported that up to 20% of liver biopsies done on alcoholic patients showed nonalcoholic (and sometimes treatable) liver diseases. Appropriate blood tests and biopsy should be performed to exclude nonalcoholic causes of liver disease and to define the severity of disease. However, tense ascites, severe thrombocytopenia (less than 80,000/μL), or prolonged prothrombin time (international normalized ratio [INR] greater than 1.4) may preclude percutaneous needle biopsy. If a percutaneous biopsy cannot be performed, a safer but more expensive alternative is a transjugular liver biopsy.

DIFFERENTIAL DIAGNOSIS

Alcoholic Fatty Liver

As outlined in Table 121.8, fatty liver can result from many processes. Several series of focal fatty changes, either focal fat or focal fat sparing, found by ultrasonography or computed tomography (CT) have been reported. This lesion should not be confused with space-occupying lesions such as tumor or abscess. ^{99m}Tc-sulfur colloid scanning or magnetic resonance imaging (MRI) is useful in distinguishing focal fatty change from space-occupying lesions because the scan is normal in the former. However, ultimately a liver biopsy may be necessary to make the diagnosis. When one encounters massive hepatomegaly (the liver span exceeds 15 cm in the midclavicular line), the differential diagnosis includes fatty liver, right heart failure, constrictive pericarditis, Budd–Chiari syndrome, infiltrative processes (e.g., amyloidosis, myeloproliferative disorders, reticuloendotheliosis, and lipid storage diseases), and neoplasms. In evaluating the cause of hepatomegaly, a helical CT scan with dual contrast and arterial/venous phases should be performed to exclude neoplasms, because this is more sensitive in detecting focal hepatic masses than either ultrasonography or sulfur colloid scan.

TABLE 121.8.	**DIFFERENTIAL DIAGNOSIS OF FATTY LIVER**

Macrovesicular Fat (Large Droplets)

Alcoholic steatohepatitis
Nonalcoholic steatohepatitis (see Table 121.6)
Hepatitis C
Toxic causes: methotrexate, halogenated hydrocarbons, and so on
Wilson's disease

Microvesicular Fat (Small Droplets)^a

Reye's syndrome
Parenteral alimentation
Intravenous tetracycline
Toxic shock syndrome
Jamaican vomiting disease
Acute fatty liver of pregnancy
Salicylate overdosage in children
Valproic acid
Yellow fever
Certain metabolic diseases: cholesterol ester storage disease, galactosemia, and Wolman's disease

---

^{a} Microvesicular fatty liver is usually the result of mitochondrial damage and metabolic defects.

Alcoholic Hepatitis

The distinctive histologic appearance of alcoholic hepatitis usually establishes the diagnosis. However, it is mimicked by nonalcoholic steatohepatitis (NASH). Clinically, patients with alcoholic steatohepatitis are usually much sicker than those with NASH. Since fever, leukocytosis, right upper quadrant pain, jaundice, and cholestasis can occur in those with alcoholic hepatitis, imaging of the liver and biliary tree by US or CT may be necessary to exclude extrahepatic cholestasis. Since these noninvasive tests are more specific (86% to 100%) than sensitive (50% to 95%) in detecting extrahepatic biliary obstruction, endoscopic retrograde cholangiopancreatography or percutaneous transhepatic cholangiography may be required to exclude obstruction.

Alcoholic Cirrhosis

Alcoholic cirrhosis is usually micronodular but may be macronodular. Thus, the differential diagnosis of alcoholic cirrhosis includes posthepatitic cirrhosis (whether due to chronic viral infection, drugs, metabolic disorders, or autoimmune hepatitis), the cirrhotic stage of primary biliary cirrhosis, secondary biliary cirrhosis, Wilson's disease, hemochromatosis, and cirrhosis caused by NASH. These diagnoses require a careful history of drug use and exposure to hepatitis viruses, tests for hepatitis B surface antigen, hepatitis C antibody, autoantibodies (antinuclear, anti-DNA, antimitochondrial, and anti–smooth muscle antibodies), serum ceruloplasmin, α_1-antitrypsin level, copper and iron studies, and the measurement of the metal content of the liver biopsy. Alcoholic cirrhosis with features of chronic active hepatitis may reflect superimposed hepatitis B or C or an autoimmune process incited by alcoholic injury. Disease processes that mimic cirrhosis (e.g., constrictive pericarditis, Budd–Chiari syndrome, veno-occlusive disease, idiopathic portal hypertension, portal vein thrombosis, and myeloid metaplasia) should be considered.

PROGNOSIS AND TREATMENT

Alcoholic Fatty Liver

Alcoholic fatty liver is benign unless accompanied by perivenular fibrosis or foamy degeneration. Patients with these conditions have a high risk for developing hepatic failure or cirrhosis. Treatment includes abstinence from alcohol and correction of nutritional deficits. Bedrest has no proven value. Under this regimen, fatty liver regresses in 3 to 6 weeks.

Alcoholic Hepatitis

The early mortality rates for alcoholic hepatitis vary from 19% to 78% (mean 49%). In the subset of patients with severe disease and spontaneous hepatic encephalopathy, the early mortality rate was higher (59%). It is not surprising that the worst prognosis was observed in patients with severe jaundice, encephalopathy, renal failure, ascites, and variceal bleeding. Several laboratory tests are prognostic indicators: prothrombin time of more than 4 seconds above control despite vitamin K treatment, total bilirubin greater than 5 mg per deciliter, and serum creatinine that increases more than 0.6 mg per deciliter during the first 10 days of hospitalization. The severity of fibrosis or cirrhosis found on liver biopsy is also a prognostic indicator. That is, with little fibrosis, the 5-year survival rate was 72%, but with severe fibrosis, it was 48%. In a series with 6-year follow-up, no patients with alcoholic hepatitis who continued to drink reverted to a healthy liver, 58% had persistence of alcoholic hepatitis, and 42% progressed to cirrhosis. In other series, up to 80% ultimately developed cirrhosis. In patients who abstained or reduced drinking, 70% reverted to normal, 15% continued to have alcoholic hepatitis, and 15% developed cirrhosis. A 50% mortality rate over 7 years was found in patients with alcoholic hepatitis who continued heavy drinking. This mortality rate decreased to 24% in those who reduced drinking or abstained.

In a Veterans' Affairs Cooperative Study that involved 280 patients with severe alcoholic liver injury, more than two-thirds of those with alcoholic hepatitis and cirrhosis had died within 2 years of follow-up. One study evaluated the predictive power of Child's–Turcott–Pugh scoring system, the combined clinical laboratory index of the University of Toronto, and Maddrey's discriminant function to predict 30-day mortality of patients with alcoholic hepatitis who participated in the VA Cooperative Study. All three scoring systems correlated with survival, but Maddrey's discriminant function exhibited the highest predictive value.

Maddrey's discriminant function

$$= 4.6 \times [\text{PT (seconds)} - \text{control}] + \text{bilirubin (mg/dL)}$$

where PT = prothrombin time.

A discriminant function higher than 32 predicts a 50% mortality within 1 month. Other studies indicate that the presence of hepatic encephalopathy is as predictive as the discriminant function.

Cessation of alcohol drinking is paramount in the treatment of alcoholic hepatitis and is best accomplished by detoxification, followed by referral to an intensive outpatient alcohol treatment program and then to Alcoholics Anonymous or to an outpatient follow-up counseling program. Other supportive therapy includes a nutritious diet.

Protein calorie malnutrition is common finding in patients with ALD. In the VA Cooperative Study on Alcoholic Hepatitis, more than 75% of patients with severe liver disease exhibited signs of kwashiorkor, marasmus, or both, and malnutrition worsened prognosis of alcoholic hepatitis. Several small controlled trials have tested the effect of parenteral amino acid therapy or enteral amino acid/protein therapy in alcoholic hepatitis. Uniformly, these trials have shown faster improvement in serum bilirubin, serum albumin, and ascites and no deterioration in hepatic encephalopathy. Amino acid mixtures enriched in branched-chain amino acids are not superior to standard mixtures. Only one of the controlled trials has demonstrated an improved mortality rate. Certainly, most patients with alcoholic hepatitis are malnourished, and this should be addressed either enterally or parenterally.

Corticosteroids modulate the immune system and inhibit fibrogenesis. The use of corticosteroids (prednisone, prednisolone, or 5-methylprednisolone in the dosage range of 35 to 80 mg per day for 4 to 6 weeks) in the treatment of alcoholic hepatitis has been extensively studied by at least 12 randomized controlled trials. Five studies showed decreased mortality with corticosteroids, and seven showed no difference. These studies have been subjected to meta-analyses and demonstrated the following: (1) Only patients with hepatic encephalopathy or Maddrey's score higher than 32 should be treated with corticosteroids. (2) Treatment with corticosteroids should exclude patients with gastrointestinal bleeding, active infection, renal failure, and acute pancreatitis. (3) Corticosteroids reduces mortality risk by 25%. (4) One has to treat seven patients to avoid one death. In all, we believe that corticosteroid therapy benefits some patients with severe alcoholic hepatitis who have no contraindications.

Anabolic–androgenic corticosteroids such as oxandrolone have been tested in an attempt to enhance recovery, that is, to increase the removal of hepatic fat, to stimulate protein synthesis, and to accelerate cell repair and hepatic regeneration. Oxandrolone was tested in a VA Cooperative Study in a 30-day trial in patients with moderate to severe alcoholic hepatitis and compared with prednisolone or placebo. Oxandrolone did not improve survival in the short term, but surprisingly, it improved long-term outcomes in patients who ingested sufficient calories during the trial. Oxandrolone cannot be recommended for clinical use until more data are available.

Propylthiouracil has been used to treat alcoholic hepatitis, possibly by decreasing the hypermetabolic state induced by alcohol and protecting perivenous cells from hypoxic injury. It also inhibits neutrophil myeloperoxidase. In one study, propylthiouracil improved symptoms and laboratory tests, but in another series of more severely ill patients, it was not effective. In the largest controlled trial, 310 patients with ALD were randomized to either propylthiouracil or placebo and followed up for up to 2 years. Propylthiouracil therapy resulted in a cumulative mortality rate half of that in the placebo group among moderately ill patients and in a subgroup of severely ill patients. Thus, propylthiouracil therapy may benefit patients with moderate to severe alcoholic hepatitis. However, since these earlier studies, there has been little subsequent interest in the use of propylthiouracil. It should not be used routinely pending further studies.

Several other agents including polyunsaturated lecithin and S-adenosylmethionine are being tested in multicenter trials. The potential actions of polyunsaturated lecithin may include phospholipid replacement for liver cell membranes, attenuation of activation of Ito cells, and stimulation of collagenase activity. S-adenosylmethionine administration has been shown to be useful in experimental animals by replenishing this transmethylating agent, enhancing the synthesis of polyamines, and providing cysteine for glutathione synthesis.

Alcoholic Cirrhosis

The prognosis of alcoholic cirrhosis depends on whether the patient continues to drink, the coexistence of alcoholic hepatitis, and the severity of the disease. The Copenhagen Study Group for Liver Disease indicated that the 5-year survival rate was nearly 85% for abstainers without jaundice, ascites, or gastrointestinal bleeding. Continued drinking lowered survival to 60%. The presence of jaundice or ascites reduced the survival rate to 50%

in abstainers and to 30% in drinkers. Gastrointestinal bleeding carried the worst prognosis, with a 5-year survival rate of 35% in abstainers and 20% in drinkers. It is prudent to urge complete abstinence for patients with any form of ALD.

Alcoholic cirrhosis has been treated with corticosteroids without effect on survival. Prophylactic nonselective portocaval shunting also does not improve survival; it merely shifts the cause of death from gastrointestinal bleeding to hepatic coma. Colchicine (1 mg per day, 5 days per week) improved survival in one study with a 14-year follow-up and is being studied further in an ongoing VA Cooperative Study.

Advanced (Child's B or C) alcoholic cirrhosis can be treated by liver transplantation provided that patients (1) do not have other alcohol-related comorbid disorders, (2) have undergone intensive outpatient treatment and rehabilitation, and (3) have at least a 6-month period of documented abstinence (Chapter 132). Guidelines for treatment for alcoholism before transplantation vary from center to center, but the 2-year survival of these carefully selected patients compares well with those undergoing transplantation for other indications. In addition, the quality of life of these transplant recipients is excellent with many of them returning to part-time or full-time employment. The rates of recidivism vary between 10% and 30%, depending on the candidate selection process and the criteria in defining recidivism. End-stage ALD now accounts for approximately 25% of adult liver transplantations in the United States.

A PRACTICAL CLINICAL APPROACH TO AN ALCOHOLIC PATIENT WITH LIVER DISEASE: MEDICAL EVALUATION OF SICK ALCOHOLIC PATIENTS

It is common for alcoholic patients to be admitted to the hospital seriously ill. These patients must be cared for on an emergency basis before their liver disease or alcoholism can be directly addressed. Four categories of medical emergencies are encountered: metabolic disorders, infections, altered neurologic status, and abnormal renal function.

METABOLIC DISORDERS

Two problems unique to alcoholic patients are alcoholic ketoacidosis and hypoglycemia. These conditions may be confused with intoxication. They are readily reversible by administration of fluids and glucose. Most patients are phosphate- and magnesium-deficient as well and need to have these electrolytes replaced.

INFECTIONS

Alcoholics are very prone to infections as a result of malnutrition, immunosuppression by alcohol, and liver disease. The most severe infections may be heralded only by a deterioration in mental status, hypotension, or nonspecific symptoms and frequently are not accompanied by fever. Bacteremia and spontaneous bacterial peritonitis are common in patients with cirrhosis who are unwell and require hospitalization (Chapter 105). Other infections include pneumonia and lung abscess, bacterial meningitis, and urinary tract infections. Patients with possible infections should have a chest x-ray, urinalysis, blood cultures, and perhaps lumbar puncture. A sample of ascites, if present, should be analyzed for serum ascites albumin gradient, cell count, differential, and culture in blood culture bottles at bedside. An absolute neutrophil count over 250/μL indicates infection. Direct inoculation of ascitic fluid into blood culture bottles at the bedside substantially improves the chances of culturing an organism, since the concentration of bacteria in the fluid is low. The presence of *Bacteroides* species or multiple organisms strongly suggests the possibility of a perforated viscus. Many studies now support the prophylactic use of antibiotics active against gram-negative rods for all cirrhosis patients with gastrointestinal bleeding—variceal or not.

If examination of the ascites suggests infection, the patient should be started on a third-generation cephalosporin to treat the most likely organisms, streptococci and enteric gram-negative rods. The use of aminoglycosides should be avoided because of a high risk for renal impairment. A repeat paracentesis should be done 48 hours after initiation of therapy. If the neutrophil count has not decreased, secondary bacterial peritonitis or a resistant organism should be suspected. Many trials support the use of quinolones as secondary prophylaxis for recurrent spontaneous bacterial peritonitis and primary prophylaxis in cirrhosis patients who have a high risk for developing spontaneous bacterial peritonitis, which may be particularly useful for patients awaiting transplantation.

ALTERED NEUROLOGIC STATUS

It is difficult to evaluate sick, intoxicated alcoholic patients. The major differential diagnoses are stroke; head trauma; chronic or acute subdural hematoma; meningitis; hypoglycemia; hyponatremia; postictal state; drug, ethylene glycol, or methanol ingestion; Wernicke–Korsakoff syndrome; hepatic encephalopathy; and alcohol or drug withdrawal syndromes. If trauma is a serious consideration, an urgent head CT scan is mandatory. CT scans are highly desirable before performing lumbar puncture on almost any patient, unless the clinical suspicion of meningitis is high, in which case lumbar puncture should be done promptly and antibacterial therapy initiated. Alcoholic patients often abuse drugs other than alcohol, and they may ingest toxic substances by mistake. Depressant drugs, narcotics, and phenothiazines can be detected by rapid blood and urine tests. Methanol or ethylene glycol poisoning is suggested by unexplained metabolic acidosis. Because the requirement for thiamine is increased by carbohydrate, alcoholic patients should be given thiamine on admission to the hospital before receiving dextrose solutions. Supplementation of other water-soluble vitamins, especially pyridoxine and folate, is advisable. Vitamin K should be given if the prothrombin time is prolonged.

Hepatic encephalopathy may be difficult to diagnose (see also Chapter 105). Generally, there is physical evidence of chronic liver disease. The presence of fetor hepaticus (the odor of methionine catabolites) is distinctive. Arterial blood levels of ammonia are usually elevated. Asterixis is an indicator of metabolic encephalopathy but is not specific or sensitive, and it disappears with deep coma. An electroencephalogram may help to distinguish hepatic encephalopathy from alcohol withdrawal. When hepatic encephalopathy is diagnosed, a careful search must be made for the factors that precipitated it (e.g, gastrointestinal bleeding; electrolyte and acid–base imbalance; high protein intake; severe constipation; noncompliance with medications; drug use, including acetaminophen, sedatives, and narcotic analgesics; infection; renal failure; and hepatoma). Alcohol withdrawal syndromes and their treatment are described in Chapter 440. Drug therapy of patients with liver disease must take into consideration alterations of pharmacodynamics and pharmacokinetics, as outlined in Table 121.4.

RENAL DYSFUNCTION

Patients with ALD may have renal dysfunction at the time of admission, or it may develop during hospitalization. If the patient has advanced, chronic liver disease with tense ascites or has been treated vigorously with diuretics, the hepatorenal syndrome should be considered (Chapter 105), but other causes of renal failure should be excluded. The urine sodium is low (less than 10 mEq per liter) initially, and the urine osmolarity is high, with no proteinuria and an acellular urinary sediment. Potentially reversible renal disease must be considered (e.g., a drug side effect, radiocontrast-induced nephropathy, urinary tract obstruction, sepsis, rhabdomyolysis, and acute tubular necrosis). Intravascular volume depletion must be excluded by measuring the central venous pressure or pulmonary artery wedge pressures and performing a fluid challenge. The therapy for hepatorenal syndrome should include paracentesis and careful crystalloid and colloid administration; fresh frozen plasma may be superior to albumin. Peritoneovenous shunts have not been shown to improve survival in hepatorenal syndrome. A potential role of placement of a transjugular intrahepatic portal-systemic shunt in the treatment of hepatorenal syndrome is being assessed, but preliminary data indicate that it is also ineffective.

EVALUATION OF ALCOHOLIC PATIENTS WITH SUSPECTED OR WORSENING LIVER DISEASE

Alcoholic patients may have historical or physical findings that suggest liver disease or that previously diagnosed liver disease has worsened. Of course, it cannot be assumed that the abnormalities all are due to alcohol abuse. The patient may have nonalcoholic liver disease or may have ALD with superimposed viral hepatitis, drug hepatitis, hepatoma, or biliary obstruction. Up to 30% of patients with ALD may have gallstones, usually bilirubin pigment stones. Therefore, a systematic approach should be taken to delineate the liver disease or diseases present. The patient should be closely questioned about ingestion of drugs or toxins. Exposure to viruses (e.g., by sexual contact, blood and blood product transfusions, or intravenous or nasal drug use) must be investigated. The physical examination should be directed toward finding stigmata of chronic liver disease, organomegaly, abnormal masses, visible or palpable gallbladder, abdominal tenderness, Murphy's sign, and so on. The finding of stigmata requires further investigation and often mandates liver biopsy. The liver tests may help to decide which diagnostic (and often invasive) tests to perform next, but they do not help in the differential diagnosis of intrahepatic versus extrahepatic causes of cholestasis. Hepatomegaly suggests fat, tumor, mass, or infiltrative lesions.

Ultrasonography or CT scan should be performed before biopsy so that mass lesions can be biopsied under radiologic guidance. Jaundice raises many possibilities, including biliary tract obstruction. Radiologic imaging should be performed to look for dilated ducts. If the ducts are dilated, obstruction is present, and a cholangiogram should be obtained. If the patient has symptoms suggestive of intermittent obstruction (attacks of pain or symptoms of biliary infection) but no dilation of the ducts, a cholangiogram should also be performed. If neither biliary obstruction nor masses are present, the appropriate blood tests should be obtained and the liver should be biopsied. In particular, serum iron saturation, ferritin, ceruloplasmin, and urine copper studies should be done before the biopsy so that liver metal content can be analyzed if these measurements suggest hemochromatosis or Wilson's disease.

PREVENTION

The prevention of ALD depends on the development of effective treatment of alcoholism. The success of therapies for alcohol abuse varies from 30% to 90%. Improved results await programs for the detection of alcohol abuse in an early stage when the patient still has support from family and employers; methods for monitoring alcohol consumption in patients who are under treatment; and the development of pharmacologic agents that reduce the urge to drink. There is evidence from animal and clinical studies that serotonin uptake inhibitors and opioid antagonists can improve the results of alcoholism treatment, and naltrexone was recently approved for use in treatment of alcoholism in conjunction with behavioral or psychological therapy. Additional medications to reduce craving, such as acamprosate, are expected to be approved in the coming years.

BIBLIOGRAPHY

Beresford TP. Predictive factors for alcoholic relapse in the selection of alcohol-dependent persons for hepatic transplant. *Liver Transpl* Surg 1997;3:280–291.
Crabb DW. Ethanol oxidizing enzymes: roles in alcohol metabolism and alcoholic liver disease. *Prog Liver Dis* 1995;13:151–172.
Hoofnagle JH, Kresina T, Fuller RK, et al. Liver transplantation for alcoholic liver disease: executive statement and recommendations. Summary of a National Institutes of Health workshop held December 6-7, 1996, Bethesda, Maryland. *Liver Transpl* Surg 1997;3:347–350.
Ishii H, Ku Rose I, Kato S. Pathogenesis of alcoholic liver disease with particular emphasis on oxidative stress. *J Gastroenterol Hepatol* 1997;12(suppl):S272–S282.
Lieber CS. Hepatic and other medical disorders of alcoholism: from pathogenesis to treatment. *J Stud Alcohol* 1998;59:9–25.
Lieber CS, Leo MA. Metabolism of ethanol and some associated adverse effects on the liver and the stomach. *Recent Dev Alcohol* 1998;14:7–40.
Lin HZ, Yang SQ, Zeldin G, et al. Chronic ethanol consumption induces the production of tumor necrosis factor-alpha and related cytokines in liver and adipose tissue. *Alcohol Clin Exp* Res 1998;22(suppl):231S–237S.

Marsano LS, Pena LR. The interaction of alcoholic liver disease and hepatitis C. *Hepatogastroenterology* 1998;45:331–339.

Mezey E. Dietary fat and alcoholic liver disease. *Hepatology* 1998;28:901–905.

Ramond MJ, Poynard T, Rueff B, et al. A randomized trial of prednisolone in patients with severe alcoholic hepatitis. *N Engl J Med* 1992;20:326:507–512.

Schenker S, Bay MK. Medical problems associated with alcoholism. *Adv Intern Med* 1998;43:27–78.

Thurman RG, Bradford BU, Iimuro Y, et al. The role of gut-derived bacterial toxins and free radicals in alcohol-induced liver injury. *J Gastroenterol Hepatol* 1998;13(suppl):S39–S50.

Yoshihara H, Noda K, Kamada T. Interrelationship between alcohol intake, hepatitis C, liver cirrhosis, and hepatocellular carcinoma. *Recent Dev Alcohol* 1998;14:457—469.

C H A P T E R

122

DRUG-INDUCED HEPATIC INJURY

SHELLY C. LU
LAWRENCE S. MALDONADO

Drug-induced hepatic injury is associated with more than 800 different drugs, accounting for 4% to 7% of adverse drug reactions. Although adverse drug reactions comprise only 2% to 3% of hospital admissions for jaundice, they cause up to 25% of cases of fulminant hepatic failure and 40% of acute hepatitis cases in persons older than 50 years. Furthermore, drugs cause chronic liver diseases such as chronic active hepatitis, cirrhosis, and liver tumors. Drugs cause disproportionately more of the serious forms of liver disease. The clinician evaluating a patient with abnormal liver test results must be aware that drug-induced hepatic injury can mimic almost any liver disorder.

Most drugs and xenobiotics (chemicals taken up by the body but not incorporated into the normal cellular metabolic economy) enter the body as lipophilic compounds through the gastrointestinal tract and hepatocyte membranes. Hepatic biotransformation converts endogenous substances and exogenous chemicals to more polar compounds that can be excreted in the bile or urine. The process of hepatic excretion involves three important steps: membrane transport of organic substances, biotransformation, and bile secretion. *Membrane transport* refers to specific mechanisms by which charged and uncharged molecules enter hepatocytes at their sinusoidal poles and leave at their sinusoidal or canalicular poles. Although many of these mechanisms are poorly characterized, specific transport mechanisms have been identified for bile acids, organic anions, organic cations, and neutral organic compounds. In addition, many lipo-

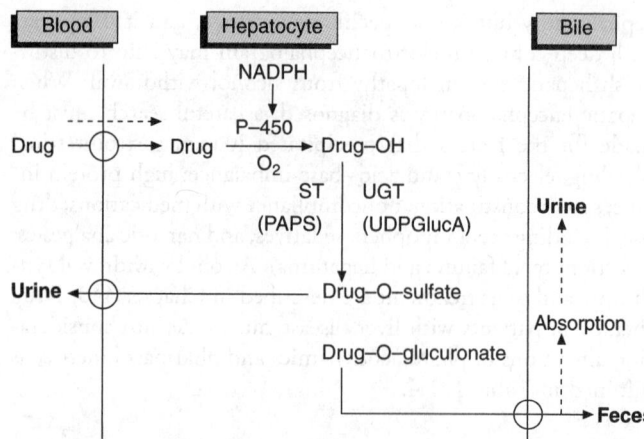

FIGURE 122.1. Scheme of hepatic biotransformation. Drugs may enter the hepatocyte by specific membrane transport processes shared with endogenous substances or by simple diffusion through the plasma membrane based on lipophilia. Once inside the cell, the drug may access sites of biotransformation by lateral diffusion through intracellular membranes or by binding to nonspecific sites on cytosolic proteins (e.g., ligandin). In this typical example, biotransformation then proceeds by P-450–catalyzed hydroxylation (phase 1) and subsequent sulfation or glucuronidation (phase 2) of the hydroxyl group. If the drug already contains an appropriate acceptor group, phase 2 can proceed directly. The highly polar metabolites are then exported by carrier-mediated transport processes. GSH and glucuronide conjugates are probably transferred preferentially to bile, whereas sulfate conjugates are transferred to plasma and then eliminated in urine. Polar metabolites excreted in bile may be absorbed from the intestine and appear in urine. *ST,* sulfotransferase; *UGT,* UDP-glucuronosyltransferases, *PAPS,* 3'-phosphoadenosine-5'-phosphosulfate; *UDPGlucA,* UDP-glucuronic acid.

philic substances bound to plasma proteins diffuse passively into hepatocytes. These substances are processed or metabolized in hepatocytes and appear mainly in bile. Excretion in bile is not the fate of all compounds metabolized in the liver, however. Some polar products of biotransformation are transported into plasma and eliminated in urine (Fig. 122.1).

■ BIOTRANSFORMATION

The processes of hepatic biotransformation usually are equated with drug metabolism. The hepatocyte contains a wide variety of enzymes that can process drugs. These enzymes are found in the endoplasmic reticulum, the cytosol, and, to a lesser extent, other organelles. Table 122.1 lists the key families of enzymes involved in hepatic biotransformation. Each enzyme represents a large family of distinct gene products, all of which share a common cofactor or endogenous cosubstrate. Different xenobiotics induce specific gene products. The substrate specificity of individual components of any enzyme family is tremendously redundant. Nevertheless, subject to genetic control, individual forms of any family may exhibit some unique substrate specificity. Although biotransformation usually detoxifies xenobiotics, the products of these reactions sometimes are more toxic than the parent compounds.

Most drugs are metabolized by the liver in two sequential

TABLE 122.1.	CONSTITUENTS OF HEPATIC BIOTRANSFORMATION	
Enzyme Family	**Cofactor**	**Subcellular Location**
Cytochrome P-450	NADPH, O_2	Endoplasmic reticulum
Glucuronosyltransferases	UDP-glucuronic acid	Endoplasmic reticulum
Sulfotransferases	PAPS	Cytosol
GSH S, transferases	GSH	Cytosol and endoplasmic reticulum

GSH, reduced glutathione; *NADPH,* nicotinamide adenine dinucleotide phosphate; *PAPS,* 3′-phosphoadenosine-5′-phosphosulfate; *UDP,* uridine diphosphate.

processes, known as phase 1 and phase 2 reactions. In phase 1, a series of reactions involving oxidoreductases, hydrolases, and transferases transforms solutes into more polar substances. Most oxidations are performed by the mixed-function oxidase system. In phase 2, these metabolites are conjugated with glucuronic acid; glycine, sulfates, glutathione (GSH); and other substances, yielding more polar products for subsequent excretion. Some drugs are metabolized primarily by phase 2 reactions. Knowledge of the sequence and relative importance of these reactions in handling drug metabolism is critical in understanding the hepatotoxicity of certain drugs. For example, acetaminophen is metabolized predominantly by phase 2 reactions, resulting in polar, nontoxic metabolites. However, about 5% of an ingested dose is oxidized by cytochrome P-450, producing a reactive, toxic intermediate (see Acetaminophen-Induced Hepatotoxicity).

Advanced liver disease impairs phase 1 reactions, but leaves phase 2 reactions relatively preserved. For example, cirrhosis severely impairs cytochrome P-450 metabolism of diazepam but does not affect glucuronosyltransferase metabolism of another benzodiazepine, oxazepam. Awareness of such considerations helps in managing drug therapy in patients with advanced liver disease.

Another important feature of hepatic biotransformation is the zonation or lobular heterogeneity of enzymes, cofactors, cofactor synthesis, and induction. In rodents, phenobarbital induces cytochrome P-450 selectively in zone III of the hepatic acinus (centrilobular). Hepatotoxins activated by cytochrome P-450 and detoxified by GSH tend to produce zone III necrosis, possibly because of the larger content of cytochrome P-450 and smaller content of GSH in this location.

In addition to genetics and liver disease, other factors that affect biotransformation include age, gender, nutrition, cofactor availability, pregnancy, and the concomitant use of other drugs. Different enzymes have different developmental patterns, even within the same supergene family. Although severe malnutrition has major effects on the metabolism and pharmacokinetics of drugs, moderate undernutrition has little effect. Exceptions include GSH S-transferase–mediated reactions and glucuronidation. Fasting decreases levels of GSH and enhances the toxicity of drugs detoxified by GSH, such as acetaminophen. Fasting also may affect glucuronidation by limiting the availability of its cosubstrate, uridine diphosphate-glucuronic acid (UDP-GlucA). In animal studies, various phase 1 and 2 activities decrease late in pregnancy. Similar studies in humans are lacking.

CYTOCHROME P-450

Cytochrome P-450, phospholipids, and nicotinamide adenine dinucleotide phosphate (NADPH)-cytochrome P-450 reductase are the main components of the mixed-function oxidase system. Only one form of NADPH-cytochrome P-450 reductase exists, but there are more than 40 different members of the human cytochrome P-450 superfamily and, collectively, they are probably the most significant enzymes for the metabolism of drugs, carcinogens, and corticosteroids.

Genes of the cytochrome P-450 superfamily encode a group of enzymes that share the following characteristics: they contain a noncovalently bound heme moiety; they are proteins bound to intracellular membranes, mainly the endoplasmic reticulum; and they use NADPH or occasionally nicotinamide adenine dinucleotide (NADH), and atmospheric oxygen (O_2) to oxygenate substrates. A second enzyme transfers the reducing equivalents from NADPH or NADH to cytochrome P-450. These physicochemical parameters suggest that the cytochrome P-450 genes share common structural features. The prosthetic group (a thiolate-bound heme) is identical in all, but the apoprotein structures differ, accounting for the different substrate specificities.

Nomenclature

Most nomenclature systems are based on global alignments of complete amino acid sequences. The cytochrome P-450 gene superfamily is subdivided into families, subfamilies, and individual genes. The italicized root symbol *CYP* (representing cytochrome P-450) is used for humans (*Cyp* is used for the mouse). Families are designated by Arabic numbers and share at least 40% amino acid sequence identity. Subfamilies are identified by capital letters and share more than 55% to 60% similarity. Individual forms of cytochrome P-450 within a subfamily are numbered sequentially. This system does not depend on cytochrome P-450 catalytic activities or function. Forms of cytochrome P-450 in separate subfamilies can have overlapping catalytic activities.

Evolution and Genetic Polymorphism

Various forms of cytochrome P-450 occur in prokaryotic and eukaryotic organisms. The evolution of cytochrome P-450 probably began 2 to 3 billion years ago, when only a few genes encoded forms of cytochrome P-450 that metabolized endogenous substrates such as corticosteroids, fatty acids, and eicosanoids. With evolutionary demand, cytochrome P-450 gene duplications and conversions increased, producing genes coding new forms of cytochrome P-450, which metabolized xenobiotics or endogenous substrates. One consequence of human cytochrome P-450 gene evolution is the polymorphism of drug metabolism, leading to marked differences in individual responses to the toxic and carcinogenic effects of drugs and other environmental chemicals. The differences among individuals, races, and ethnic groups are manifested in the varying levels of expression of forms of cytochrome P-450, as evidenced by differences in the metabolism of certain drugs. One well-known example of genetic polymorphism is *CYP2D6*, the activity of which is absent in 7% of whites, owing to numerous mutations. Perhexiline, a substrate of *CYP2D6*, causes peripheral neuropathy and cirrhosis only in persons deficient in *CYP2D6*. These genetic polymorphisms demonstrate typical mendelian inheritance.

Some forms of cytochrome P-450 show wide interindividual variability without genetic polymorphism. For example, a 20-fold interindividual variation in the activity of *CYP3A*, the main subfamily of cytochrome P-450 in man, accounts for almost 50% of human hepatic forms of cytochrome P-450. *CYP3A4* is the main isoenzyme metabolizing substrates, such as nifedipine, macrolide antibiotics, cimetidine, cyclosporine, FK506, and corticosteroids. Low levels of *CYP3A* in donor liver grafts increase cyclosporine and FK506 toxicity; conversely, high levels of *CYP3A* increase graft rejection, presumably because of an insufficient level of immunosuppressants. Knowledge of hepatic *CYP3A* activity before transplantation could guide immunosuppressive therapy.

Structure

Human forms of cytochrome P-450 are hydrophobic, intrinsic membrane proteins tightly associated with intracellular membranes. The cytochrome P-450 protein is a globular structure embedded into the membrane lipid bilayer by its amino-terminal peptide. The bulk of the enzyme is exposed to the cytoplasmic surface of the endoplasmic reticulum, and the heme iron is parallel with or at a slight angle to the membrane. This orientation is ideal for cytochrome P-450 interaction with hydrophobic and hydrophilic substrates and for cooperative association with NADPH-cytochrome P-450 reductase.

Reactions

The catalytic mechanisms of all forms of cytochrome P-450 appear to be similar. First, substrate binds to the oxidized cytochrome P-450, and the complex subsequently is reduced to the ferrous form in a reaction catalyzed by NADPH-cytochrome P-450 reductase in which one electron is transferred from NADPH to the hemoprotein. The reduced cytochrome P-450 substrate complex then binds oxygen, and the electron from the ferrous cytochrome P-450 is transferred to oxygen, forming a transient ferric-(O_2^-) substrate complex. A second electron then is transferred from the reductase (in some cases, the second electron is derived from NADH by cytochrome b_5), generating the ferric $(O_2^=)$ cytochrome P-450. The oxygen–oxygen bond is split, and one oxygen atom is released in water while the other remains bound to heme. This putative $(FeO)^{3+}$ species is a powerful oxidant responsible for the oxygenation of bound substrate. Oxygen transfer from the heme to the substrate involves initial abstraction of a hydrogen atom (or electron) from substrate, followed by oxygen "rebound" from the heme to the bound substrate radical. This produces the oxygenated product which then dissociates from the active site and completes the catalytic cycle. In addition to hydroxylation, other oxidative reactions, such as epoxidation, *N*-demethylation, *O*-dealkylation, and *N*-oxidation, are catalyzed similarly by forms of cytochrome P-450.

Sometimes, the products of cytochrome P-450–mediated reactions are more toxic than the parent compounds. These toxic products are electrophiles because they exhibit reactive centers that seek electrons. Therefore, covalent binding or alkylation of nucleophilic centers (electron-donating sites) on cellular constituents can ensue. Defense against electrophiles sometimes involves GSH conjugation. Phase 1 reactions may be "toxifying" and phase 2 reactions detoxifying.

For some reactions, many cytochrome P-450 enzymes overlap considerably in their catalytic efficiency; different forms of cytochrome P-450 catalyze the same reaction, although at different rates. However, in other cases, a single enzyme may be responsible for most of the activity, because of its much more rapid intrinsic rate or because other cytochrome P-450 enzymes are not plentiful. In vivo metabolism is a function of the efficiency of a cytochrome P-450 for a substrate and the abundance of that particular cytochrome P-450 relative to other forms of cytochrome P-450 in the cell.

Induction, Inhibition, and Drug–Drug Interactions

Multiple drugs induce different forms of cytochrome P-450. Sometimes exposure to specific substrates induces certain forms of cytochrome P-450, usually the forms that metabolize those substrates. Specific examples are phenobarbital (the *CYP2B* family), ethanol (*CYP2E1*), isoniazid (*CYP2E1*), clofibrate (*Cyp4* in rats), and corticosteroids (*Cyp3* in rats). In addition, smoking induces *CYP1A1* in human liver and extrahepatic tissues. Induction may be important in promoting hepatotoxicity if the form induced also activates a hepatotoxin, as in acetaminophen toxicity in chronic alcoholics. Chronic ethanol exposure induces *CYP2E1*, which oxidizes acetaminophen to an electrophilic toxic product. This is the predominant mechanism of enhanced susceptibility to acetaminophen hepatotoxicity in chronic alcoholics (see Acetaminophen-Induced Hepatotoxicity). Moreover, *CYP2E1* is preferentially expressed in the centrilobular zone, which may explain the histologic pattern of acetaminophen hepatotoxicity. Precise mechanisms of enzyme induction are poorly understood; increased transcription, messenger RNA or protein stabilization, or even selective translational enhancement may be involved.

Cytochrome P-450–associated activities in humans may vary on the basis of competitive or noncompetitive enzyme inhibition. Competitive inhibition occurs when two substrates compete, such as cimetidine and ketoconazole, or when one drug is a nonsubstrate inhibitor of a particular enzyme, such as quinidine and *CYP2D6*. Such interactions also may occur with food. An interesting example is grapefruit juice, which dramatically inhibits the oxidation of *CYP3A4* substrates such as nifedipine or cyclosporine. This may mandate dose reductions of these drugs or dietary counseling. A cytochrome P-450 also may oxidize a compound to a product, which then inhibits that enzyme. Certain antibiotics are nitrosylated and bind extremely tightly to the ferrous heme (e.g., troleandomycin). In other cases, the inhibition is truly mechanism-based, with a reactive intermediate covalently binding to the apoprotein or porphyrin. The effects of some of these inhibitors can be dramatic and produce clinical consequences.

Advanced liver disease suppresses some cytochrome P-450 apoproteins, leading to impaired drug elimination. The availability of the cosubstrates O_2 and NADPH also may be critical. Impaired hepatic perfusion, as in shock and congestive failure, may lead to decreased O_2 and interfere with drug elimination. Conversely, decreased O_2 may enhance the reductive metabolism of certain substrates, such as carbon tetrachloride and halothane. Sometimes the availability of the electron donor for cytochrome P-450, NADPH, is an important limiting factor. For example, ethanol metabolism in hepatocytes acutely interferes with mitochondrial NADPH production. Even minimal elevations in blood ethanol levels may inhibit cytochrome P-450 activities as a result of markedly decreased NADPH. High blood ethanol levels can lead to direct inhibition of forms of cytochrome P-450 by direct binding.

Drug–drug interactions often are associated with enzyme induction or inhibition by one of the drugs. Levels of *CYP3A4* are elevated by the administration of rifampin or barbiturates, resulting in more rapid elimination of 17α-ethinyl estradiol or cyclosporine and loss of contraceptive or immunosuppressive action, respectively. Oxidation of acetaminophen by cytochrome P-450 is inhibited by the coadministration of cimetidine.

Many of the cytochrome P-450 substrates are procarcinogens. Most of the activation of these chemicals in humans is attributable to only a few forms of cytochrome P-450: *CYP1A1* activates several polycyclic hydrocarbons; *CYP1A2* activates many arylamines; *CYP2E1* activates urethane, vinyl monomers, and small halogenated hydrocarbons; and *CYP3A4* activates aflatoxins, polycyclic hydrocarbon dihydrodiol, and some arylamines. Increased levels of these enzymes are associated with a higher incidence of cancer.

URIDINE DIPHOSPHATE-GLUCURONOSYLTRANSFERASE

Uridine diphosphate-glucuronosyltransferase (UGT) is a family of enzymes located in hepatic endoplasmic reticulum and various extrahepatic tissues, such as kidney, intestine, and olfactory epithelium. The UGT isoenzymes convert hydrophobic endobiotic and xenobiotic substances, such as bilirubin, steroid and thyroid hormones, and many drugs, into water-soluble glucuronides. In general, glucuronides are less toxic and active than their parent compounds and are excreted more readily in the bile. However, exceptions are discussed later, and the role of glucuronides in toxification has received increasing attention. As with other biotransformation processes, a family of enzymes with overlapping substrate specificities ensures the ability of the liver to eliminate many xenobiotics.

Nomenclature

Molecular biologic techniques are instrumental in the understanding of UGTs because conventional purification techniques failed as a result of the instability of these isoenzymes. Cloning of complementary DNAs and the expression of various isoenzymes has enabled classification of the UGT isoenzymes according to their genetic origin in a fashion analogous to the classification of forms of cytochrome P-450. More than 25 UGT complementary DNAs have been cloned. An international workshop in the Netherlands proposed a UGT classification scheme in which the root symbol UGT represents uridine diphosphate-glucuronosyltransferase in humans, an Arabic numeral denotes the family, a letter designates the subfamily, and a number represents the individual gene. Families share less than 50% amino acid sequence identity, whereas subfamilies share more than 60%.

Molecular Forms, Induction, and Deficiency

Human UGTs can be subdivided into two families. UGT family 1 consists of at least four members that catalyze the glucuronidation of phenols and bilirubin. These four isoenzymes are encoded on a single UGT gene on chromosome 2 and represent alternative splicing products of a common primary transcript. Although they are derived from the same primary transcript, they can be induced differentially and their perinatal development differs considerably. Clofibrate and phenobarbital induce bilirubin glucuronidation, whereas 3-methylcholanthrene induces planar phenol glucuronidation. Bilirubin UGTs are expressed after birth, whereas phenol UGTs are expressed before birth.

At least three UGT family 2 genes are on chromosome 4. Induction of this family has not been described.

Few "inborn errors" of glucuronidation have been discovered. Only deficiencies in bilirubin glucuronidation have been described in humans (the Crigler–Najjar syndrome and Gilbert's disease, which are discussed in Chapter 103).

Topology and Reactions

The UGTs are deeply embedded within membranes, particularly smooth endoplasmic reticulum, and are anchored by only one peptide fragment. Most of the enzyme is on the luminal side of the endoplasmic reticulum; only a small fragment of the protein is on the cytosolic side. The cosubstrate, UDPGlucA, interacts in the lumen of the endoplasmic reticulum. UDPGlucA is synthesized from UDP-glucose by the cytosolic enzyme UDP-glucose dehydrogenase. To gain access to UGT, therefore, UDP-GlucA is transported from the cytoplasmic to the luminal side of the endoplasmic reticulum.

Glucuronidation transfers the glucuronic acid group from UDPGlucA to a substrate acceptor group, forming ether, ester, thiol, N, and C glucuronides, and greatly enhancing water solubility. This is an S_N2 reaction in which a nucleophilic acceptor group on the substrate attacks the electrophilic C-1 atom of the glucuronic acid group. A high conjugation rate requires appreciable lipid solubility, possibly because the substrate-binding site is hydrophobic.

Many drugs are direct substrates of the various UGTs, including acetaminophen, morphine, oxazepam, and zidovudine. Most have a phenolic acceptor group, so sulfation is a competing reaction. Carboxylic acids such as ibuprofen, probenecid, and endogenous bilirubin are eliminated almost exclusively by glucuronidation. In addition, most other drugs can be metabolized by phase 1 reactions to generate acceptor groups for glucuronic acid. As a result, many drugs are excreted at least partially as glucuronides.

Determinants of Rate of Glucuronidation

A high rate of glucuronidation requires a sufficient supply of UDPGlucA, which fasting depletes. UDPGlucA is synthesized from UDP-glucose by a nicotinamide-adenine dinucleotide (NAD^+) –dependent dehydrogenase in the cytosol. Therefore, the availability of UDPGlucA is determined by the level of UDP-glucose, which depends on adenosine triphosphate (ATP) levels and glycogen stores. Severe liver disease impairs glucuronidation efficiency, although UGT activity in liver samples of such patients is hardly affected. An extrahepatic contribution to conjugation may ensure residual capacity if liver function is lost.

Role of Glucuronidation in Regulation of Biologic Activity of Drugs and in Toxification

Although glucuronidation is mainly a detoxifying and inactivating reaction, for several xenobiotics, the glucuronide is more toxic than the parent compound. In addition, glucuronide conjugates may mediate important pharmacologic activities. For instance, the glucuronide conjugate formed at the 6 position of morphine is a much more potent agonist than is morphine, whereas the glucuronide formed at the 3 position is an extremely potent antagonist. Glucuronidation at the 17β position leads to cholestatic conjugates of endogenous estradiol and the oral contraceptive ethinyl estradiol. The toxicity of drugs containing carboxylic groups may result from the formation of acyl glucuronides at those groups. These conjugates are reactive because of acyl bond instability, releasing electrophilic intermediates that may bind covalently to plasma proteins and present as haptens to the immune system. This happens with zomepirac, a muscle relaxant, and led to its withdrawal from clinical use.

SULFOTRANSFERASES

The human liver contains at least three well-characterized classes of sulfotransferase enzymes, dehydroepiandrosterone sulfotran-

sferase and two phenol sulfotransferases. At least 13 eukaryotic complementary DNAs of sulfotransferase enzymes and two human liver complementary DNAs of dehydroepiandrosterone sulfotransferase have been cloned. Dehydroepiandrosterone sulfotransferase catalyzes the sulfation of 3-hydroxysteroids, such as dehydroepiandrosterone, corticosteroid hormones such as estrone, bile acids such as lithocholic acid, the cardiac glycoside digitoxin, and even cholesterol. One of the two phenol sulfotransferases is thermostable, preferentially catalyzes the sulfation of "simple" planar phenols, and is inhibited by 2,6-dichloro-4-nitrophenol. The other phenol sulfotransferase is thermolabile, preferentially uses phenolic or catechol monoamines as substrates, and is resistant to 2,6-dichloro-4-nitrophenol inhibition. Levels of activity for dehydroepiandrosterone sulfotransferase and the two forms of phenol sulfotransferases vary widely among individuals, suggesting genetic polymorphism.

Reactions

The enzymes use 3'-phosphoadenosine-5'-phosphosulfate as a sulfate donor. 3'-Phosphoadenosine-5'-phosphosulfate is synthesized from two molecules of ATP and one sulfate that comes from dietary sources or hepatic cysteine degradation. The enzymes transfer sulfate mainly to hydroxyl groups, including simple alcohols, bile acids, and phenolic compounds such as thyroxine, isoproterenol, methyldopa, and acetaminophen.

Inhibition

Clinically significant inhibition is caused by limited 3'-phosphoadenosine-5'-phosphosulfate availability. 3'-Phosphoadenosine-5'-phosphosulfate production capacity is extremely limited. Many drugs or their cytochrome P-450 metabolites contain hydroxyl groups that can be sulfated or glucuronidated. In general, glucuronidation is a low-affinity and high-capacity reaction, whereas sulfation is a high-affinity and low-capacity reaction. At higher doses, glucuronidation predominates largely because of limited 3'-phosphoadenosine-5'-phosphosulfate availability. Conversely, at low drug levels, sulfation predominates because of higher sulfotransferase affinities. If both enzymes can catalyze a substrate, the substrate concentration will determine which pathway predominates.

Role of Sulfation in Toxification

Although sulfation usually results in inactive or less active compounds that are more water-soluble, the sulfate ester sometimes is more toxic than the parent molecule. For example, certain N-hydroxy sulfates of polycyclic hydrocarbons are more reactive than the parent N-hydroxy compounds.

GLUTATHIONE S-TRANSFERASES

Glutathione S-transferases play a selective but important role in hepatic biotransformation. The central molecule is GSH, which is involved in all reactions catalyzed by GSH S-transferases. In conjugation reactions, GSH reacts with any sufficiently electrophilic centers, which are potentially toxic. Although the liver conjugates with GSH far less frequently than it glucuronidates or sulfates to prepare substances for excretion, GSH conjugation is critical in detoxification.

Glutathione Metabolism

Glutathione is a tripeptide (γ-glutamylcysteinyl glycine) found in all mammalian tissues, with especially high hepatic concentrations that are essential for the survival of aerobic cells. GSH exists in thiol-reduced (GSH) and disulfide-oxidized (GSSG) forms, but the former predominates, existing in millimolar concentrations in most cells (about 5 mmol per liter in hepatocytes). The GSSG content is less than 1% that of GSH. Ninety percent of cellular GSH is cytosolic. The peptide bond linking the glutamate and cysteine of GSH is through the γ-carboxyl group of glutamate rather than the conventional α-carboxyl group. This unusual arrangement is hydrolyzed by only one known enzyme, γ-glutamyl transpeptidase, which occurs only on the external surfaces of certain cell types. Consequently, GSH resists intracellular degradation and is metabolized only outside the cell by organs with γ-glutamyl transpeptidase.

GSH serves several vital functions, one of the most important being detoxification of electrophiles. The liver has a large reserve of GSH for detoxification and maintains interorgan homeostasis of GSH by exporting nearly all the GSH it synthesizes into plasma and bile through carrier-mediated transport systems. In rats, plasma GSH comes almost entirely from sinusoidal efflux of hepatic GSH. The released GSH then is broken down by the ectoenzyme γ-glutamyl transpeptidase to amino acids such as cysteine, which can be taken up and reincorporated into GSH.

The synthesis of GSH from its constituent amino acids, L-glutamate, L-cysteine, and glycine, involves two sequential enzymatic steps requiring ATP. The first step of GSH biosynthesis, catalyzed by γ-glutamylcysteine synthetase, is rate-limiting and is regulated by feedback competitive inhibition by GSH. GSH synthesis is influenced significantly by the availability of intracellular cysteine. This is especially important when GSH is severely depleted (e.g., after massive acetaminophen overdose), because the synthesis rate will increase from loss of feedback inhibition. Cysteine normally is derived from diet, from protein breakdown, and, in the liver, from methionine through transsulfuration. Providing cysteine promotes GSH synthesis when GSH utilization is markedly increased. The most well-known example is the use of N-acetylcysteine to treat acetaminophen overdose (see Acetaminophen-Induced Hepatotoxicity).

Maintenance of normal hepatic γ-glutamylcysteine synthetase activity requires insulin and glucocorticoids. Hepatic γ-glutamylcysteine synthetase activity and GSH levels decrease 25% to 40% in insulin-deficient diabetic rats and in adrenalectomized rats, but remain normal with hormonal replacement. This small decrease in the hepatic GSH level is unlikely to affect GSH-dependent detoxification, but may predispose to toxicity after hepatotoxin overdose.

Another aspect of GSH metabolism is its redox cycle. GSH is a substrate for selenium-dependent GSH peroxidase, an important enzyme in the detoxification of hydrogen peroxide. Aerobic cells produce a small amount of hydrogen peroxide, and generate larger amounts under oxidant stress. GSH peroxidase reduces H_2O_2 to water while oxidizing GSH to GSSG, which is efficiently reduced back to GSH by NADPH-dependent GSSG reductase. GSSG also is transported into bile in direct proportion to its steady-state concentration. This reduction of H_2O_2 and the accompanying GSH redox cycle constitute the most important GSH function in the absence of xenobiotics and are especially critical in mitochondria.

Isozymes and Genetics

The GSH S-transferases are cytoplasmic enzymes made up of two subunits. As is common among biotransforming enzymes, the subunits of these enzymes represent multiple distinct gene products with broad, overlapping substrate specificity and constitute a superfamily. Three major families have been described: α, μ, and π. In humans, α is represented by at least three genes on chromosome 6; two are expressed in liver and one in skin. The α class enzymes exhibit GSH peroxidase activity and high-affinity organic anion binding. The major human a gene is on chromosome 1, whereas two related μ genes for muscle and brain enzymes are on chromosome 3. Expression of the μ enzyme is genetically polymorphic. About 50% of all whites and Asians do not express the hepatic and leukocyte μ enzyme. Preliminary evidence suggests that smokers lacking the μ enzyme have a higher risk for lung cancer. The human π class gene is on chromosome 11. The product encoded by this gene is expressed in placenta, intestine, and bile ducts but not in hepatocytes and its expression is increased in several human cancers. Accordingly, the π gene product may serve as a tumor marker and may contribute to resistance to chemotherapy.

A distinct microsomal form occurs in rodents and humans, which is structurally unrelated to the cytosolic enzyme. The importance of the microsomal form in detoxification is suggested by its activation by thiol alkylating agents, oxidized GSH, and superoxide anion.

Reactions

The GSH S-transferases all noncovalently bind GSH to an active site. The thiol of GSH can ionize; the pH of the thiol drops from pH 9.3 when GSH is free to 7.4 when it is bound. In addition, an adjacent site binds a wide variety of lipophilic xenobiotics. The enhanced affinity of GSH for nuclei and its proximity to bound electrophiles favor catalysis.

Three types of reactions occur: substitution, addition, and reduction. Substitution reactions involve GSH replacing a leaving group, such as bromide displaced from sulfobromophthalein. The product is a GSH conjugate. Additional reactions involve direct GSH conjugate formation with an electrophilic site, such as conjugation of leukotriene A_4 with GSH to form leukotriene C_4. These enzymes have few known endogenous substrates. GSH S-transferases also reduce organic peroxides, but not hydrogen peroxide. This peroxidase activity produces GSSG. Its importance in decreasing lipid peroxidation compared with selenium-dependent GSH peroxidase is uncertain.

The importance of GSH conjugation catalyzed by GSH S-transferases is illustrated by acetaminophen. Cytochrome P-450 converts the drug to an electrophile that readily reacts with thiols of proteins and GSH. However, despite this chemical nonselectivity, biologic preference for GSH is exhibited. This is the GSH threshold. Covalent binding to protein thiols occurs only after GSH levels fall near zero. The high preference for GSH is explained by GSH S-transferases catalyzing detoxification.

Role of Glutathione S-Transferases as Ligandins

The GSH S-transferases exhibit high binding affinity for certain endogenous substances that are not substrates, namely, bilirubin, heme, and bile acids. Certain forms of the enzymes from rats have separate binding sites for these ligands. In contrast, human transferases bind only heme with high affinity. Binding of lipophilic nonsubstrate ligands may facilitate the dissociation of these ligands from the plasma membrane or prevent their reflux by retaining these substances in the cell. Furthermore, the transferases may transfer heme from mitochondria to other cellular sites.

■ DRUG-INDUCED HEPATIC INJURY

GENERAL PRINCIPLES AND MOLECULAR MECHANISMS

Drug-induced hepatic injury can be predictable (usually dose-related) or unpredictable (usually unrelated to dose). In the former, typical injury usually can be produced in experimental animals and, if associated with liver cell necrosis, characteristically affects a particular region of the hepatic lobule (e.g., acetaminophen causes zone III necrosis). These hepatotoxins are "direct hepatotoxins" because of their predictability and dose-response relations. In contrast, most of the unpredictable or idiosyncratic forms of hepatic injury rarely can be produced in experimental animals. Their histologic patterns tend to be diffuse, usually with significant inflammation. Sometimes serum autoantibodies occur. Therefore, idiosyncratic hepatic injury may represent a drug allergy in which the immune response attacks the liver cell.

This classification undoubtedly is oversimplified. Many predictable hepatotoxins do not injure the liver directly, but only after biotransformation to toxic intermediates, which then interact with cell components. Although autoantibodies occur in many idiosyncratic reactions, the link to hypersensitivity is stronger in some (see Halothane-Induced Hepatotoxicity) than others. It appears in some cases that idiosyncrasy represents genetically determined differences in the relative rates of biotransformation by alternate pathways generating products of differing hepatotoxic potentials, or in the efficiencies of subsequent detoxification reactions.

The molecules responsible for drug-induced hepatotoxicity usually are electrophiles or free radicals. Although some drugs generate oxygen free radicals, the cytochrome P-450 system often generates reactive drug metabolites responsible for toxicity. In addition, redox cycling compounds generate oxygen free radicals. Electrophiles are substances (positive-charge-density nucleophiles) that seek electrons and form electron-sharing covalent bonds with substances that donate electrons (negative-

charge-density nucleophiles). They vary greatly in their inherent reactivity so that some preferentially attack thiol or amino groups on proteins and alter protein function. These metabolites are analogous to alkylating agents. A free radical is a chemical that has an unpaired electron and will remove an electron from other substances, leading to new free radicals. Drug free radicals preferentially attack unsaturated fatty acids in membrane phospholipids, causing lipid peroxidation. A chain reaction of free radical exchange ensues, ultimately breaking down the fatty acids. In addition, drug free radicals bind covalently, especially to unsaturated fatty acids. Oxygen free radicals also can cause lipid peroxidation, oxidize protein thiols, or attack other cellular constituents.

A series of cellular defense mechanisms counteracts these reactive drug metabolites. GSH detoxifies most electrophilic metabolites spontaneously or through a GSH S-transferase–catalyzed reaction. Scavengers defend against free radicals by interrupting the free radical chain reaction of lipid peroxidation. Endogenous scavengers include uric acid, bilirubin, ascorbic acid, vitamin A, and, perhaps most important, vitamin E (tocopherol), which is present in membranes.

Although the biochemical consequences of reactive metabolites, namely, covalent binding, lipid peroxidation, and protein–thiol oxidation, are important in mediating toxicity, the precise mechanism and the critical targets are undefined. Furthermore, the final common pathway leading to cell death is unclear. Disruption of cellular calcium homeostasis leading to a sustained rise in cytosolic calcium is one proposed final common pathway. A sustained rise in cytosolic calcium activates numerous degradative enzymes, such as proteases, phospholipases, and endonucleases and impairs mitochondrial function. However, some agents kill cells under calcium-free conditions by injuring the mitochondria directly. Conversely, the rise in cytosolic calcium may be a nonspecific terminal event in dying cells.

Two major modes of cell death occur: apoptosis and lytic necrosis. *Apoptosis,* also known as programmed cell death, turns certain genes on or off before cell death. Cells undergoing apoptosis have shriveled nuclei with characteristic chromatin condensation and eosinophilic condensation of the whole cell (Councilman's bodies). Molecular regulation of this active process requires messenger RNA and protein synthesis. In lytic necrosis, the toxic insult kills cells by disrupting mitochondrial integrity and inducing cytoskeletal changes leading to cell swelling and cell membrane lysis. Lytic necrosis usually causes secondary inflammation, whereas apoptosis does not. Toxic insults causing lytic necrosis tend to involve higher doses of toxins or anoxia, whereas lower doses of toxins or hypoxia probably kill by apoptosis.

Many drugs affect specific cellular functions and processes (e.g., rifampin interferes with organic anion uptake and estrogens alter the physical properties of membranes). Although the effects of many drugs are known, precise mechanisms are not. Table 122.2 summarizes postulated mechanisms of drug-induced hepatic injury.

HISTOLOGIC PATTERNS

Drug-induced hepatic injury encompasses many histologic changes. Because many drugs are associated with characteristic

TABLE 122.2. POSTULATED MECHANISMS OF DRUG-INDUCED HEPATIC INJURY

Mechanism	Drug Examples
Alteration of the physical properties of membranes	Estrogens
Inhibition of membrane enzymes (e.g., Na, K-ATPase)	Chlorpromazine metabolites
Interference with hepatic uptake	Rifampin
Interference with mitochondrial fatty acid oxidation	Valproate, fialuridine
Impairment of cytoskeletal function	Chlorpromazine metabolites
Formation of insoluble complexes in bile	Chlorpromazine
Toxicity mediated by toxic intermediates	
Electrophiles leading to covalent binding of proteins	Acetaminophen
Free radicals causing lipid peroxidation	Carbon tetrachloride
Redox cycling generating oxygen free radicals and protein thiol oxidation	Nitrofurantoin, menadione

ATPase, adenosine triphosphatase.
Adapted from Bass, NM, Ockner RK. Drug-induced liver disease, In: Zakim D, Boyer TD, eds. *Hepatology: a textbook of liver disease.* Philadelphia: WB Saunders, 1996:962.

histologic lesions, a classification scheme based on histologic patterns is conceptually and diagnostically useful (Table 122.3). However, although some drugs cause stereotypical reactions, many others cause a broad range of histologic responses. For example, oral contraceptives have been associated with bland cholestasis and various liver tumors. Similarly, isoniazid and methyldopa have been associated with acute and chronic hepatitis. The histologic features of drug-induced hepatic injury, although often relatively characteristic for a particular agent, rarely are specific. In addition, virtually all forms of drug-induced hepatic injury closely resemble other forms of liver disease.

Zonal Necrosis

Zonal necrosis usually is caused by predictable hepatotoxins. Agents that cause centrilobular necrosis include acetaminophen and carbon tetrachloride, whereas yellow phosphorus causes middle-zone necrosis, and allyl alcohol causes periportal necrosis. Usually, little or no inflammation results, and damaged cells may accumulate triglycerides. Clinically, patients may be asymptomatic or suffer fulminant liver failure. Biochemically, signs of liver cell dysfunction and necrosis, such as elevated serum transaminase levels and, in severe cases, elevated bilirubin levels and prolonged prothrombin times, occur. In most instances of acute injury of this type, the process resolves completely or terminates fatally without progression to chronicity.

The molecular basis for zonal selectivity for these agents is unclear, but probably reflects zonal differences in the determinants of injury. For example, zonal distribution of the different enzymes of biotransformation, defense mechanisms (e.g, GSH

levels), bioavailability of drugs, and even differences in oxygen tension probably play significant roles in determining these patterns.

Hepatitis

Nonspecific Hepatitis

In nonspecific hepatitis, an inflammatory response is the essential histologic feature. Typically, a few scattered foci of hepatocellular necrosis, usually associated with a mononuclear cell infiltrate, and variable portal inflammation are seen. The characteristic features of viral hepatitis, such as bile stasis, lobular disarray, and acidophil bodies, are missing. Nonspecific hepatitis occurs with a wide variety of drugs, virtually never produces serious or progressive hepatic injury, and reverses fully on discontinuation of the responsible agent.

Lesions Resembling Acute Viral Hepatitis

Many drugs can cause histologic lesions that are indistinguishable from viral hepatitis. Examples include isoniazid, methyldopa, and halothane. This form of injury often challenges clinicians. In some cases (e.g., phenytoin-induced hepatitis), prominent peripheral or tissue eosinophilia suggests a nonviral cause, but more often these features are absent. Note that drug-induced acute hepatitis carries a higher case fatality rate than does acute viral hepatitis; drug-induced acute hepatitis associated with overt jaundice carries a mortality rate of more than 10% compared with less than 1% in viral hepatitis. Possible reasons for the higher mortality rate include older patient age, more rapid disease progression, and often continuation of the unrecognized offending agent. As is true of most cases of acute drug-induced hepatic injury, recovery is the rule on discontinuation of the responsible agent. However, chronic hepatitis (see later in text) can develop with continued or repeated exposure.

Granulomatous Hepatitis

Drug-induced granulomatous hepatitis is characterized by noncaseating granulomas accompanied by variable numbers and types of inflammatory cells. The granulomas may contain abundant eosinophils, suggesting hypersensitivity-based injury. Typical offending agents are quinidine, allopurinol, phenylbutazone, sulfonamides, and sulfonylurea derivatives. Up to one-third of granulomatous hepatitis cases result from drugs.

Chronic Hepatitis

Drug-induced chronic hepatitis is a heterogeneous group of disorders differing in pathogenesis and histologic features. Chronic active hepatitis is associated with isoniazid and methyldopa, whereas focal nonspecific hepatic necrosis is associated with long-term aspirin use. In general, these hepatic injuries result from continued exposure rather than from a self-perpetuating process started by an acute insult. Often, the agent is taken in doses regarded as therapeutic rather than toxic. Careful inquiry

TABLE 122.3.	HISTOLOGIC CLASSIFICATION OF DRUG-INDUCED LIVER DISEASE
Histologic Finding	**Drug Examples**
Zonal necrosis	
Centrilobular (zone III)	Acetaminophen, halothane, carbon tetrachloride
Midzonal (zone II)	Yellow phosphorus
Periportal (zone I)	Allyl alcohol
Hepatitis	
Nonspecific hepatitis	Aspirin, oxacillin
Acute viral hepatitis-like	Isoniazid, α-methyldopa, phenytoin, halothane, diclofenac
Granulomatous hepatitis	Quinidine, allopurinol, phenylbutazone, sulfonylureas, procainamide
Chronic hepatitis	Isoniazid, α-methyldopa, nitrofurantoin, oxyphenisatin, sulfonamides, aspirin, propythiouracil, perhexilene maleate, amiodarone, dantrolene, ethanol, diclofenac, trazodone, fenfibrate, acetaminophen (rare)
Fatty liver	
Macrovesicular	Ethanol, corticosteroids, amiodarone, perhexilene maleate, 4,4′-diethylaminoethoxyhexrestrol
Microvesicular	Tetracycline, valproic acid, dideoxyinosine, tolmetin, piroxicam, pirprofen, salicylate, fialuridine
Alcoholic-like liver disease	
Hepatitis with fibrosis or cirrhosis	Amiodarone, perhexilene maleate, 4,4′-diethylaminoethoxyhexrestrol
Quiescent fibrosis or cirrhosis	Methotrexate, vitamin A, arsenicals, vinyl chloride
Cholestasis	
Inflammatory	Chlorpromazine, erythromycin estolate, captopril, methimazole, chlorpropamide, sulindac
Bland	Estrogens, anabolic steroids (C-17 alkyl steroids)
Vascular lesions	
Hepatic vein thrombosis	Estrogens
Veno-occlusive disease	6-Thioguanine, mitomycin C, doxorubicin (Adriamycin), dacarbazine, azathioprine, pyrrolizidine alkaloids, busulfan
Noncirrhotic portal hypertension	Vinyl chloride
Peliosis hepatis	Anabolic steroids, hydroxyurea, azathioprine
Hepatic tumors	
Adenoma	Estrogens, androgens
Focal nodular hyperplasia	Estrogens
Hepatocellular carcinoma	Androgens, estrogens
Angiosarcoma	Vinyl chloride, anabolic steroids

into the use of prescription and nonprescription drugs is essential in evaluating all patients with chronic liver disease.

Fatty Liver

The lipid that accumulates in the liver in almost all forms of hepatotoxicity is predominantly triglyceride. Two histologic patterns of fatty liver occur, macrovesicular and microvesicular steatosis. In macrovesicular fatty liver, the more common form, triglyceride deposits in relatively large globules, effectively filling the hepatocyte and displacing the nucleus and other intracellular constituents peripherally, making it appear adipocyte-like. This pattern is associated with ethanol abuse and various nutritional disorders such as obesity, malnutrition, diabetes mellitus, and jejunoileal bypass surgery. It also is associated with drugs such as amiodarone (see following section), methotrexate, and corticosteroids. Liver function is relatively well preserved unless other processes such as hepatitis are associated.

The other histologic form of fatty liver has small droplets of fat dispersed throughout the cytoplasm so that the nucleus remains central and the cell remains recognizable as a hepatocyte. This pattern is seen in a few unusual disorders, such as Reye's syndrome, fatty liver of pregnancy, Jamaican vomiting sickness, and certain rare inborn errors of metabolism in the urea cycle. Drugs associated with this hepatic injury include high doses of

intravenous tetracycline, valproic acid, and fialuridine (FIAU). Mitochondrial β-oxidation of fatty acid is impaired, leading to depletion of the ATP pool and disruption of cellular metabolism. This type of injury causes much more severe liver dysfunction and necrosis, with marked increases in serum transaminase and bilirubin levels, prolonged prothrombin times, and significant mortality rates.

Alcoholic-Like Liver Disease

Hepatitis with Fibrosis or Cirrhosis

Some of the drugs that can cause a histologic picture identical with alcoholic hepatitis are amiodarone (an antiarrhythmic agent), perhexiline maleate (an antianginal agent), and 4,4′-diethylaminoethoxyhexestrol (a coronary artery vasodilator). These drugs are structurally unrelated, but all are amphiphilic weak bases. This similarity may determine their hepatotoxicity.

Amiodarone, an iodine-containing benzofuran derivative, produces multisystem toxicity, including thyroid dysfunction, pulmonary fibrosis, and liver disease. Mild transaminase elevation occurs in 20% to 40% of patients receiving the drug. The histologic features on light microscopy are identical with alcoholic hepatitis, namely, Mallory bodies in hepatocytes, mixed inflammatory infiltration around proliferating bile ducts, macrovesicular fat, granular cytoplasm with foamy changes, and fibrosis with cirrhosis. On electron microscopy, prominent concentric lysosomal inclusions resembling those found with primary phospholipidoses, such as Fabry's, Niemann–Pick, or Tay–Sachs disease, are seen. The mechanism involves trapping amiodarone (a weak base) in its ionized form in acidic lysosomes, leading to inhibition of phospholipid breakdown because amiodarone is a potent competitive inhibitor of lysosomal phospholipase A1. How lysosomal phospholipidosis injures the liver is unclear.

Perhexiline maleate also is associated with lysosomal phospholipidosis and can produce the same histologic picture as amiodarone hepatotoxicity. Genetic polymorphism plays a significant role in determining susceptibility to perhexiline maleate hepatotoxicity (see Evolution and Genetic Polymorphism). Seven percent of caucasians lack *CYP2D6*, the isoform responsible for hydroxylating perhexiline maleate during its drug excretion. This phenotypic expression can be measured by the rate of hydroxylation of the test compound, debrisoquine, because perhexiline maleate hepatotoxicity occurs only in persons who hydroxylate debrisoquine poorly. The accumulation of unmetabolized perhexiline maleate in acidic lysosomes promotes secondary phospholipidosis.

Quiescent Fibrosis or Cirrhosis

Numerous drugs and chemicals can cause alcoholic-like quiescent fibrosis or cirrhosis. Classic examples are methotrexate, vitamin A, arsenicals, and vinyl chloride. Because the process can be indolent, without any significant inflammatory component, serum transaminase levels poorly reflect hepatic fibrosis. Liver histology reveals steatosis, hepatocyte ballooning with minimal necrosis, and perisinusoidal fibrosis leading to cirrhosis. Methotrexate hepatic fibrosis is related directly to the duration and mode of therapy. Small daily doses of methotrexate and alcoholism are associated with a significantly increased risk of hepatic fibrosis. The risk is minimal in nonalcoholics receiving weekly low-dose therapy. Although opinions vary, most hepatologists do not advocate pretreatment liver biopsy unless the patient has abnormal liver tests, is alcoholic, or has chronic hepatitis B or C infection. Some recommend liver biopsy after a cumulative dose of 3 to 4 g; others favor performing liver biopsy only if liver tests (transaminase and/or albumin levels) remain persistently abnormal.

Cholestasis

Drugs cause cholestasis by interfering with bile formation. Two histologic patterns occur. In one pattern, cholestasis accompanies variable hepatocellular necrosis, with inflammation occurring predominantly in the portal triads and, to a lesser extent, in the lobule. The inflammatory infiltrate is mostly mononuclear but may contain polymorphonuclear neutrophils or eosinophils. Typically, systemic manifestations such as fever, rash, and arthralgia occur. The prototypical drug is chlorpromazine, which inhibits membrane enzymes such as Na^+,K^+-ATPase, impairs cytoskeletal function, and forms insoluble complexes in bile. Chlorpromazine causes cholestatic jaundice in 1% of patients; 90% of these cases occur in the first 5 weeks of therapy. It usually resolves without sequelae 2 to 8 weeks after cessation of the drug. Rarely, jaundice persists despite discontinuation, and chlorpromazine-induced vanishing bile duct syndrome leads to biliary cirrhosis. Pregnancy apparently increases chlorpromazine toxicity.

A second type of cholestatic drug reaction is associated with the bland accumulation of bile in cells and canaliculi, principally in the centrilobular zone. This lesion can be caused by natural and synthetic estrogens and by all 17α-substituted anabolic and androgenic steroids. In contrast to the inflammatory type of cholestatic reaction, the bland type is accompanied by few systemic symptoms such as pruritus. Recovery is expected after drug cessation.

Vascular Lesions

Disorders Associated with Portal Hypertension

Four drug- or toxin-associated disorders cause portal hypertension independent of primary liver disease: hepatic vein thrombosis, associated with oral contraceptives; noncirrhotic portal hypertension after long-term exposure to vinyl chloride monomer; nodular regenerative hyperplasia, seen predominantly in patients treated with antimetabolite or antineoplastic drugs; and veno-occlusive disease, in which the major site of injury is the subendothelium of the small hepatic venules with necrosis around the terminal hepatic venule and secondary hepatic venular occlusion. Pyrrolidizine alkaloids from plants of the genera *Senecio* and *Crotalaria* ("bush tea poisoning") and numerous antineoplastic agents, such as 6-thioguanine, mitomycin C, doxorubicin (Adriamycin), dacarbazine, and azathioprine, cause veno-occlusive disease.

Peliosis Hepatis

Peliosis hepatis is characterized by blood-filled cavities, lined or unlined by sinusoidal cells, resulting from red blood cells leaking through the endothelial barrier, followed by perisinusoidal fibrosis. This lesion is associated with the long-term administration of androgenic and anabolic steroids, as well as with a variety of chronic wasting neoplastic and infectious diseases. Hydroxyurea and azathioprine also have been implicated. Portal hypertension in peliosis hepatis is rare because the condition usually is asymptomatic, although death occasionally results from a ruptured cyst and hemorrhage.

Hepatic Tumors

Benign (adenomas) and malignant (hepatocellular carcinomas) tumors have been described with estrogen and androgen use. Adenomas usually resolve with discontinuation of the agent, although large tumors may require resection. Hepatocellular carcinomas associated with estrogen use are rare and mostly occur after more than 5 years of treatment. They are found in noncirrhotic livers and are associated with other vascular lesions, such as peliosis hepatis. Focal nodular hyperplasia has been associated only with oral contraceptive use. Angiosarcoma has been linked to anabolic steroids, long-term exposure to vinyl chloride monomer, Thorotrast (a contrast dye), and inorganic arsenic.

TABLE 122.4.	ANALGESICS AND ANTI-INFLAMMATORY AGENTS	
Drug	**Histologic Pattern**	**Comment**
Acetaminophen	Centrilobular necrosis	Predictable toxin; chronic alcoholics more susceptible
Aspirin	Nonspecific hepatitis	Dose-dependent with substantial individual variabilty; groups at risk: JRA, SLE, RA
	Microvesicular steatohepatitis	Reye's syndrome
Phenylbutazone	Acute viral hepatitis-like most common	Overt hepatic injury seen in 0.25%
	Cholestasis	50% have fever, rash or arthralgia
	Noncaseating granuloma	
Allopurinol	Acute viral hepatitis-like with prominent eosinophils	Allergic features common; diuretic use and renal impairment predisposing factors
	50% have granulomas, similar to those seen in Q fever	
Gold	Cholestasis, noninflammatory	Onset usually within a few weeks of starting therapy
Dantrolene	Acute and chronic hepatitis	Predisposing factors: age >30, high dose (>30 mg/d), prolonged use (>2 months)
Nonsteroidal anti-inflammatory agents (NSAIDs):	Varied	Rarely associated with hepatotoxicity
		Risk factor: previous history of NSAIDs-induced hepatotoxicity resulting from cross-sensitivity
		Most are dose-independent
Examples of NSAIDs:		
Sulindac	Cholestatic hepatitis	Most common NSAID associated with liver injury
Diclofenac	Acute hepatitis	
	Chronic active hepatitis resembling autoimmune type	Some positive ANA, anti-Sm Ab; cross-sensitivity to ibuprofen; some responded to corticosteroid therapy

ANA, antinuclear antibody; *anti-Sm Ab,* anti–smooth muscle antibody; *JRA,* juvenile rheumatoid arthritis; *NSAIDs,* nonsteroidal anti-inflammatory drugs; *RA,* rheumatoid arthritis; *SLE,* systemic lupus erythematosus.

EXAMPLES OF DRUG-INDUCED HEPATIC INJURY

More than 800 drugs have been implicated in drug-induced hepatic injury, and a complete discussion of the topic is beyond the scope of this chapter. Instead, two classic examples, acetaminophen and halothane, are provided to highlight the principles of drug-induced hepatotoxicity. Tables 122.4 through 122.10 summarize several important classes of drugs and typical patterns of injury associated with them. Various herbal medicines also are associated with hepatotoxicity.

ACETAMINOPHEN-INDUCED HEPATOTOXICITY

Clinically, acetaminophen is perhaps the most important hepatotoxic drug. It also is one of the best-known predictable hepato-toxins; that is, it produces liver injury in all patients who ingest sufficient amounts. Most cases of acetaminophen hepatotoxicity result from large single overdoses as part of suicide attempts. Accidental overdoses and toxicity from therapeutic doses, especially in chronic alcoholics, have attracted more recent attention.

Mechanism of Injury

Eighty percent to 90% of therapeutic doses of acetaminophen normally are converted to nontoxic metabolites by glucuronidation or sulfation; only small amounts are metabolized by cytochrome P-450 to a toxic metabolite, *N*-acetyl-*p*-benzoquinone imine (NAPQI; Fig. 122.2). After massive ingestion (more than 15 g), glucuronidation and sulfation become saturated, and the absolute and relative production rates of NAPQI increase. NAPQI is an inherently reactive electrophile that binds covalently and highly selectively to nucleophilic cysteinyl thiol groups

TABLE 122.5.	ANTICONVULSANTS	
Drug	**Histologic Pattern**	**Comment**
Phenytoin	Acute viral hepatitis-like with prominent eosinophils	Serum sickness–like and pseudolymphoma-like features
Valproic acid	Microvesicular fatty liver, zone III necrosis, cholestasis	Dose-dependent increase in transaminases in 11–12% of patients after 10–12 wk of therapy
		Impairs mitochondrial oxidation of long-chain fatty acids
Carbamazepine	Granuloma, cholangitis, occasionally necrosis	
Phenobarbital	Hepatitis	May exhibit cross-sensitivity with phenytoin and carbamazepine

TABLE 122.6. ANTIMICROBIALS

Drug	Histologic Pattern	Comment
Oxacillin	Nonspecific hepatitis	Associated with large intravenous doses, onset usually after 1 wk of use; HIV-infected patients predisposed
Carbenicillin	Nonspecific hepatitis	
Cloxacillin	Cholestasis	Rare
Amoxicillin/clavulanic acid (Augmentin)	Cholestasis	Symptoms can develop up to 6 weeks after discontinuation; responsible moiety probably clavulanic acid; elderly males more susceptible
Erythromycin	Inflammatory cholestasis	Most common with estolate, but also reported with ethylsuccinate and lactobionate
Tetracyclines	Microvesicular fatty liver	Rare, usually with large intravenous doses in patients with impaired renal function
		Pregnant women at risk
Sulfonamides	Acute and chronic hepatitis	Allergic features common
		Slow acetylators of sulfonamide may be at risk
	Granuloma	
Nitrofurantoins	Cholestasis	Allergic features common
	Chronic active hepatitis with lupoid features	Patients with chronic active hepatitis often have positive serologies (ANA, anti-Sm Ab)
	Granuloma	
Clindamycin	Nonspecific hepatitis	20–50% incidence of increased transaminases with use
Ketoconazole	Nonspecific hepatitis	Estimated incidence 1:15,000
Isoniazid	Nonspecific hepatitis	10% of all recipients, regardless of age, develop mild increase in transaminases within first few months of therapy, which usually subsides despite continued use
	Acute and chronic hepatitis	1% develop severe overt hepatitis—age >50 and alcohol use are risk factors
		Higher incidence in patients also receiving rifampin
Rifampin	Acute hepatitis	Dose dependently impairs hepatic uptake of organic anions
P-aminosalicylic acid	Acute hepatitis	Serum sickness–like picture
	Cholestasis	Acute hepatitis 10% fatality rate
Dideoxyinosine (DDI)	Nonspecific hepatitis	Elevated transaminases reported in 17–35%
	Microvesicular fatty liver	
2′,3′-Didehydro-3′-deoxythymidine	Nonspecific hepatitis	Elevated transaminases reported in up to 10%
Pentamidine isethionate	Nonspecific hepatitis	Frequent mild increase in transaminases
Zidovudine (AZT)	Nonspecific hepatitis	Rare
	Macrovesicular steatosis	Associated with severe lactic acidosis and hepatic failure

ANA, antinuclear antibody; anti-Sm Ab, anti–smooth muscle antibody.

TABLE 122.7. ANTINEOPLASTIC AGENTS

Drug	Histologic Pattern	Comment
Methotrexate	Quiescent fibrosis, cirrhosis	Risk associated with cumulative dose (>1.5 g), liver biopsy before starting treatment recommended in high-risk patients
6-Mercaptopurine/azathioprine	Cholestasis, necrosis, veno-occlusive disease	Dose-dependent toxicity
6-Thioguanine	Veno-occlusive disease	
5-Fluorouracil	Sclerosing cholangitis, particularly at the common hepatic bifurcation	Only when given via constant infusion pump into hepatic artery, mechanism may be related to ischemia
L-Asparaginase	Macrovesicular fatty liver	50% incidence of hepatotoxicity
Mithramycin	Zone III necrosis	Dose-dependent toxicity
Doxorubicin (Adriamycin)	Veno-occlusive disease	
Cyclosporin	Cholestasis	Up to one-third of patients on high dose
Cyclophosphamide	Necrosis, veno-occlusive disease	Veno-occlusive disease usually when used in conjunction with radiation
Dacarbazine	Veno-occlusive disease	Usually follows the second cycle of treatment, often associated with eosinophilia, suggesting hypersensitivity reaction
Dactinomycin	Veno-occlusive disease, peliosis hepatis	

TABLE 122.8. CARDIOVASCULAR AGENTS

Drug	Histologic Pattern	Comment
α-Methyldopa	Acute or chronic hepatitis	Features of drug hypersensitivity common but eosinophilia rare
Hydralazine	Granulomatous hepatitis	Associated with systemic lupus erythematosus–like hydralazine disease
Captopril	Cholestatic hepatitis	Fever and eosinophilia common
Enalapril	Cholestatic hepatitis	Fever and eosinophilia common
Quinidine	Granulomatous hepatitis	
Amiodarone	Alcoholic hepatitis with fibrosis or cirrhosis	Lysosomal phospholipidosis
Perhexiline maleate	Alcoholic hepatitis with fibrosis or cirrhosis	Lysosomal phospholipidosis; patients with P4502D6 deficiency predisposed
Procainamide	Granulomatous hepatitis, cholestasis	
Aprinidine	Nonspecific hepatitis Cholestasis Granuloma	Dose-independent, idiosyncratic
Labetalol	Acute hepatitis	Female predonderance; up to 8% have elevated aminotransferases that resolve on continued treatment

TABLE 122.9. PSYCHOACTIVE DRUGS

Drug	Histologic Pattern	Comment
Chlorpromazine	Inflammatory cholestasis	Incidence estimated at 0.5–1% Most of the 0.5–1% of patients have eosinophilia, usually within 3–5 wk of starting therapy
Antidepressants		
Monoamine oxidase inhibitors		
Iproniazid	Acute hepatitis	
Tricyclic antidepressants		
Imipramine	Varies, both hepatitis and cholestasis reported	Possible cross-sensitization
Desipramine		
Amitriptylene		
Benzodiazepines		
Chlordiazepoxide	Cholestasis	Very low hepatotoxic potential
Diazepam		
Flurazepam		
Haloperidol	Cholestasis	Low incidence (<1%)

TABLE 122.10. HORMONES AND VITAMINS

Drug	Histologic Pattern	Comment
Hormones		
Estrogenic steroids	Bland cholestasis, hepatic tumors, hepatic vein thrombosis	Alters physical properties of membranes Estrogen-associated tumors highly vascular; occurs mostly in patients after treatment >5 yr
Androgens and anabolic steroids	Bland cholestasis, hepatic tumors, peliosis hepatitis	
Vitamins		
Vitamin A	Fibrosis, cirrhosis	Disease progress despite cessation of therapy
Synthetic analogues of vitamin A, etretinate and acitretin	Hepatitis	Allergic features common with etretinate Analogues not stored in liver so do not produce fibrosis

on proteins and GSH. The hepatocyte normally protects itself by conjugating NAPQI with GSH, and the GSH conjugate ultimately is excreted as mercapturic acid and cysteine derivatives in urine (Fig. 122.2). In addition, NAPQI is reduced back to acetaminophen by protein-SH (thiol) and GSH, forming disulfide, indicating that NAPQI is an oxidant and an electrophile. Hepatocyte injury occurs when hepatic GSH is depleted.

At least three isoenzymes of cytochrome P-450 oxidize acetaminophen: *CYP2E1*, *CYP1A2*, and *CYP3A4*. The K_m of *CYP3A4* for acetaminophen is low (0.25 mmol per liter, which corresponds to hepatic concentrations of the drug after therapeutic doses), whereas that of *CYP1A2* is high. One study using a bank of human liver microsomal fractions showed that *CYP3A4* contributed between 1% and 20% to total NAPQI formation; *CYP2E1* catalyzed the rest. This explains why long-term ingestion of alcohol (which induces *CYP2E1* and possibly *CYP3A4*) and use of anticonvulsants such as phenobarbital, phenytoin, and carbamazepine (which induce *CYP3A4*) increase susceptibility to acetaminophen hepatotoxicity, but cigarette smoking (which induces *CYP1A2*) does not. The histologic pattern of injury (zone III necrosis) corresponds to the distribution of *CYP2E1*.

There is considerable debate as to how acetaminophen causes cell death. Both covalent binding of NAPQI to critical protein-SH groups and oxidative stress secondary to the electrophilic properties of NAPQI and GSH depletion have been proposed. Covalent binding of NAPQI to critical mitochondrial targets may be responsible for cell death. However, this simply may reflect profound mitochondrial GSH depletion. Mitochondrial GSH is a critical requirement for the detoxification of normally produced oxygen free radicals; therefore, profound mitochondrial GSH depletion predisposes to cell death through oxidative stress. Oxidative stress causes many changes in the cell, but notably causes the oxidation of cysteine residues of many proteins, presumably resulting in their altered function, although the critical protein targets of oxidative attack are largely unknown. Finally, a provocative pathogenetic role for Kupffer cells has been proposed because inhibition of these cells attenuated acetaminophen-induced hepatotoxicity by a mechanism independent of NAPQI production.

Factors Influencing Acetaminophen-Induced Toxicity

Because the oxidation of acetaminophen is a cytochrome P-450–mediated reaction, inducers (e.g., ethanol, isoniazid or phenobarbital) and inhibitors (e.g., cimetidine) of cytochrome P-450 isoenzymes increase or decrease the risk of toxicity, respectively. Conditions decreasing the rate of glucuronidation or sulfation also increase the likelihood of toxicity (e.g., fasting may decrease both). Because hepatic GSH is critical in detoxifying NAPQI, conditions that lower GSH levels (e.g., starvation or chronic alcoholism) predispose to acetaminophen toxicity.

Therapeutic doses of acetaminophen can cause hepatotoxicity in chronic alcoholics. Their increased susceptibility is related to the induction of *CYP2E1* and, possibly, to decreased cytosolic and mitochondrial GSH levels. Even though chronic alcoholics are more susceptible to acetaminophen-induced injury, acute

alcohol administration in laboratory animals protects against acetaminophen hepatotoxicity because cytochrome P-450 may metabolize ethanol preferentially over acetaminophen, resulting in the production of less toxic metabolites. In addition, acute ethanol administration may decrease cytochrome P-450 activity by reducing the cellular concentration of NADPH, a required cofactor.

Clinical Presentation

The clinical course of acetaminophen toxicity is fairly predictable, occurring in four phases. In phase 1, acute gastrointestinal tract symptoms begin within a few hours of ingestion. The patient typically has nausea and occasional vomiting and may become moderately obtunded, particularly if sedatives were ingested with the acetaminophen. Phase 2, which lasts about 2 days, begins within 24 hours of ingestion when the nausea and vomiting abate and the patient feels relatively well. During this abatement of symptoms, biochemical evidence of hepatic injury appears; the patient also may experience pain and tenderness in the right upper quadrant and oliguria may develop. During phase 3, 3 to 5 days after ingestion, overt hepatic damage becomes clinically evident. Phase 4, or recovery, occurs in most patients 1 week after ingestion.

Biochemically, acetaminophen hepatotoxicity resembles other forms of acute liver necrosis. Within 24 to 48 hours after acetaminophen overdose, transaminase levels increase up to 10,000 IU per liter, and serum alkaline phosphatase and bilirubin levels rise to a lesser degree. Severe coagulation disturbances occur early in most severe cases. Leukocytosis, hypoglycemia, and metabolic acidosis also may occur. Serum bilirubin levels and prothrombin times are prognostic indicators.

The most important prognostic factor of acetaminophen toxicity is the plasma acetaminophen level, which correlates well with the severity of liver damage. A nomogram of the plasma level of acetaminophen measured 4 to 12 hours after ingestion predicts liver injury. Patients with drug levels above 300 μg per milliliter at 4 hours usually develop overt hepatic damage; those with values below 150 μg per milliliter usually do not. However, this nomogram applies only to single acetaminophen overdoses in nonalcoholics and requires knowledge of the time of ingestion. If the time is unknown, the toxic potential can be estimated by measuring levels 4 hours apart. An acetaminophen level that falls by at least half suggests normal metabolism; slower declines suggest toxic metabolite formation. However, levels may not peak until 4 hours after ingestion. In alcoholic patients with acute liver decompensation, acetaminophen toxicity must be considered in the differential diagnosis, regardless of the acetaminophen level.

Treatment

Treatment begins with gastric lavage in any patient suspected of overdose because gastric atony is common and acetaminophen can be recovered from the stomach even 48 hours after ingestion. This is followed by specific antidote therapy by the oral or intravenous route. *N*-acetylcysteine (Mucomyst) protects against acetaminophen hepatotoxicity by increasing GSH biosynthesis.

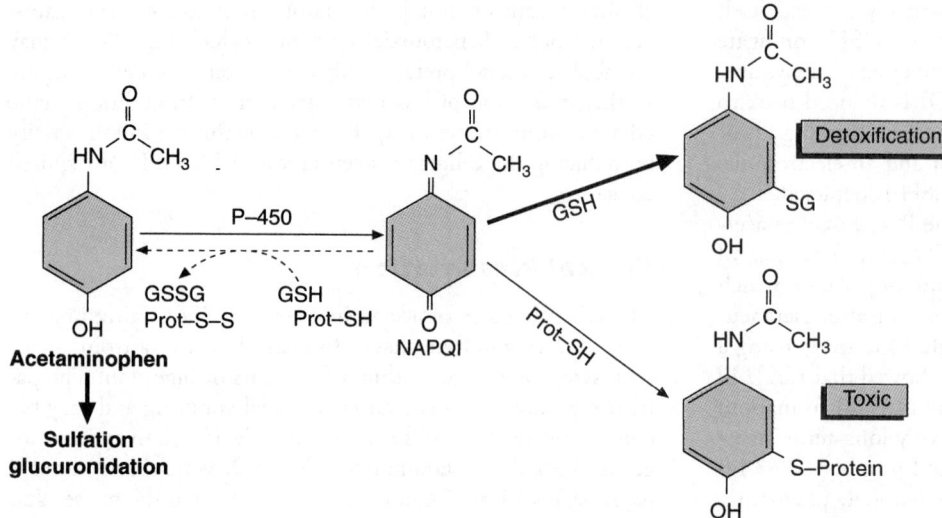

FIGURE 122.2. Hepatic acetaminophen metabolism. (From Kaplowitz N. Drug metabolism and hepatotoxicity. In: Kaplowitz N, ed. *Liver and biliary diseases.* Baltimore: Williams & Wilkins, 1992:673, with permission.)

When patients are treated within 16 hours, mortality is virtually abolished. Although the effectiveness of N-acetylcysteine therapy gradually is lost the longer therapy is withheld, benefit may occur even by the fourth day after overdose. This agent should be given to any patient strongly suspected of acetaminophen overdose, regardless of the time of ingestion, to try to abort liver failure.

Of patients who develop acute liver failure, the clinician must identify those likely to die; early referral for emergency hepatic transplantation may be life-saving. Several objective severity scores (e.g. King's or APACHE II) can help identify these patients. Early experience with bioartificial liver devices also suggests that transient support with these devices may allow patients to recover without hepatic transplantation.

HALOTHANE-INDUCED HEPATOTOXICITY

The overall incidence of halothane-induced hepatotoxicity is 1 in 10,000 recipients. However, the risk increases markedly with repeated exposure (1 in 3,000) and is especially high in obese women, perhaps because of the larger doses of halothane that are administered, with accumulation of the anesthetic in adipose tissue. Alternatively, obesity is associated with increased expression of *CYP2E1*, which mediates the oxidation of halothane and the generation of hepatotoxicity.

Mechanism of Injury

Halothane is metabolized by two different cytochrome P-450–mediated reactions (Fig. 122.3). With high O_2, halothane is oxidized to a trifluoroacetylhalide that can acetylate protein amino groups and induce an immune response. With low O_2, halothane undergoes reductive metabolism, generating a free radical that can cause lipid peroxidation. Toxicity appears to be immune-mediated. Fever, eosinophilia, and accelerated response after repeated exposure suggest a hypersensitivity reaction. Furthermore, circulating antibodies in patients recovering from halothane hepatotoxicity recognize trifluoroacetylated proteins (products of oxidative metabolism) and some nontrifluoroacetylated native proteins on the cell surface and in the microsomal fraction of hepatocytes. Antibody-dependent cell-mediated cytotoxicity has been demonstrated in vitro. Trifluoroacetylated microsomal proteins occur in all recipients of halothane, but overt liver disease is rare. Which of these proteins are antigenic and what determines autoimmunity are unknown.

Clinical Presentation

Fever, an early sign of halothane hepatotoxicity, almost always precedes jaundice. Symptoms usually appear within 7 to 14 days after initial exposure, but within 12 to 24 hours after subsequent

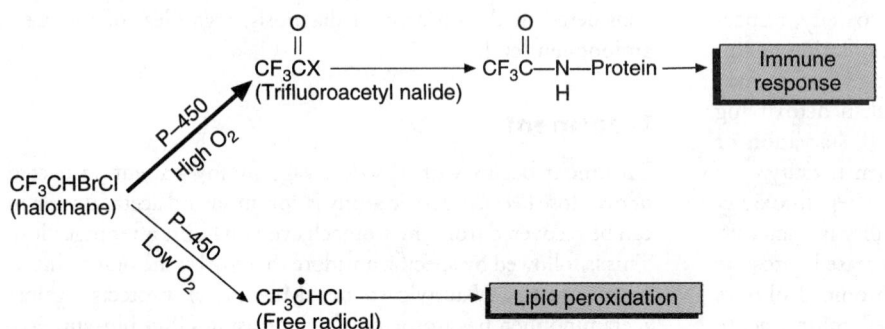

FIGURE 122.3. Oxidative and reductive halothane metabolism. (From Kaplowitz N. Drug metabolism and hepatotoxicity. In: Kaplowitz N, ed. *Liver and biliary diseases,* Baltimore: Williams & Wilkins, 1992:673, with permission.)

exposures. Jaundice appears within 10 to 14 days. A diffuse rash erupts in 10% of patients, and about 30% have myalgia. Rapid progression to fulminant liver failure occurs in some patients, requiring liver transplantation. No specific treatment is available other than general supportive care and, in fulminant cases, liver transplantation.

DIAGNOSIS AND TREATMENT OF DRUG-INDUCED HEPATIC INJURY

Drug-induced hepatic injury must be considered in any patient with acute or chronic hepatobiliary disease. A complete drug history, including prescription and nonprescription drugs (including vitamins and herbs), is essential. A history of any anesthetic exposure and the patient's reaction should be obtained. Signs of hypersensitivity such as fever, rash, and eosinophilia are particularly helpful. The development of symptoms within days or weeks of starting therapy with a new medication may suggest an acute drug reaction, especially when a rapid fall of more than 50% in transaminase levels follows its discontinuation. However, although some drugs induce hepatotoxicity soon after initiation (within 1 month with phenytoin and allopurinol), others have a long latency period (isoniazid and methotrexate). In addition, some drugs have delayed toxicity, developing after discontinuation. Liver histology usually is not diagnostic but may provide useful prognostic information in fulminant hepatitis.

In most cases, the only required therapy is withdrawal of the offending agent (except in acetaminophen hepatotoxicity, which has a specific antidote). Patients with fulminant liver failure may require liver transplantation. The efficacy of corticosteroids in patients with hypersensitivity has not been demonstrated, although they may suppress the marked features of systemic hypersensitivity associated with idiosyncratic reactions due to drugs such as allopurinol, diclofenac, and azulfidine.

Rechallenge with the offending agent would provide the most conclusive proof of drug toxicity, but should be avoided because it could be dangerous in patients with hypersensitivity-mediated injury. Often, patients are rechallenged inadvertently, so a careful review of the medical history may be valuable. Nevertheless, on occasion, the risk of rechallenge must be weighed against the potential therapeutic benefits of the drug. If rechallenge is considered, patients should be tested with a small initial dose and watched closely for the development of any sign of hepatic injury. Alternatively, studies of the effect of the drug on the in vitro integrity of lymphocytes from patients thought to have hypersensitivity drug reactions may prove promising. With improved understanding of the mechanisms of toxicity, the genetic polymorphism of key enzymes involved in biotransformation, and determinants of individual variability, methods soon may be developed to identify individuals who are susceptible to drug toxicity.

Although monitoring serum biochemical markers for liver injury would increase the detection of drug-induced hepatic injury, cost-benefit analysis does not justify its use in otherwise healthy persons. However, it may be reasonable to monitor groups of patients at special risk, such as those with alcoholic liver disease who are taking potentially hepatotoxic drugs (e.g., isoniazid, amiodarone, valproic acid, or methotrexate). The best way to prevent drug-induced hepatotoxicity is to teach clinicians to weigh the risks before prescribing drugs and to search for drug hepatotoxicity in any patient in whom liver disease develops.

BIBLIOGRAPHY

Ahern MJ, Smith MD, Roberts-Thomson PJ. Methotrexate hepatotoxicity: what is the evidence? *Inflamm Res* 1998;47:148–151.

Bass NM, Ockner RK. Drug-induced liver disease. In: Zakim D, Boyer TD, eds. *Hepatology: a textbook of liver disease.* Philadelphia: WB Saunders, 1996:962–1017.

Burchell B, Coughtrie MWH, Jansen PLM. Function and regulation of UDP-glucuronosyltransferase genes in health and liver disease: report of the seventh international workshop on glucuronidation, September 1993, Pitlochry, Scotland. *Hepatology* 1994;20:1622–1630.

Fernandez-Checa J, Lu SC, Ookhtens M, et al. The regulation of hepatic glutathione. In: Tavoloni N, Berk PD, eds. *Hepatic anion transport and bile secretion: physiology and pathophysiology.* New York: Raven Press, 1993:363–395.

Guengerich FP. Human cytochrome P-450 enzymes. *Life Sci* 1992;50:1471–1478.

Kaplowitz N. Drug metabolism and hepatotoxicity. In: Kaplowitz N, ed. *Liver and biliary diseases,* second edition. Baltimore: Williams & Wilkins, 1996:103–120.

Lewis D, Watson E, Lake BG. Evolution of the cytochrome P450 superfamily: sequence alignments and pharmacogenetics. *Mutation Res* 1998;410:245–270.

Makin, AJ, Williams R. Acetaminophen-induced hepatotoxicity: predisposing factors and treatments. *Adv Intern Med* 1997;42:453–483.

Mulder GJ. Glucuronidation and its role in regulation of biological activity of drugs. *Annu Rev Pharmacol Toxicol* 1992;32:25–49.

Otterness DM, Weinshilboum R. Human dehydroepiandrosterone sulfotransferase: molecular cloning of cDNA and genomic DNA. *Chem Biol Interact* 1994;92:145–159.

Kelley's Textbook of Internal Medicine, fourth edition. Edited by H. David Humes.
Lippincott Williams & Wilkins, Philadelphia © 2000.

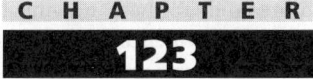

CHAPTER
123

METABOLIC, GRANULOMATOUS, AND INFILTRATIVE DISORDERS OF THE LIVER

BRUCE R. BACON

There are several metabolic diseases of the liver that should be understood by all physicians. In addition, granulomatous and infiltrative disorders of the liver must be well characterized because there may be specific treatments available. This chapter provides clarification of these disorders and recommendations for definitive diagnosis and management. Table 123.1 summarizes the features of these disorders.

TABLE 123.1.		EVALUATION FOR METABOLIC OR INFILTRATIVE LIVER DISEASE		
Disease	**Prevalence**	**Laboratory Tests**	**Liver Biopsy**	**Treatment**
Hereditary hemochromatosis	1 in 300	Transferrin saturation, ferritin, HFE mutation analysis	↑ Iron, often necessary	Therapeutic phlebotomy
Wilson's disease	1 in 30,000	Ceruloplasmin, 24-hour urine copper	↑ Copper, usually necessary	Copper chelation
Alpha₁-antitrypsin deficiency	1 in 1,700 (PiZZ)	A1AT level, Pi typing	A1AT globules, usually necessary	Transplantation
Porphyria cutanea tarda	Uncommon	Urine porphyrins, HFE, anti-HCV	May be helpful	Phlebotomy, avoidance of EtOH, estrogens
Nonalcoholic steatohepatitis	Common	↑ ALT > AST	Necessary	Weight loss, control of diabetes
Granulomatous hepatitis	Rare	Variable	Necessary	Occasionally prednisone
Hepatic amyloidosis	Rare	Variable	Necessary	None
Storage disease	Rare	Variable	May be necessary	Enzyme replacement

A1AT, α₁-antitrypsin; Pi, protease inhibitor; HCV, hepatitis C virus; ALT, alanine aminotransferase; AST, aspartate aminotransferase; EtOH, ethanol.

HEREDITARY HEMOCHROMATOSIS

Hereditary hemochromatosis (HH) is a common disorder of iron metabolism affecting approximately 1 in 200 to 400 individuals of northern European descent. HH results in increased absorption of iron from the proximal intestine, with deposition of iron in the liver, heart, pancreas, joints, skin, and endocrine organs. Complications of chronic liver disease, including hepatocellular cancer, can lead to premature death.

Methods are now available to detect HH in asymptomatic probands and in presymptomatic relatives of patients with the disease; therefore, the diagnosis can be applied legitimately to individuals who have not yet experienced any of the toxic consequences of iron overload in tissues. Accordingly, the diagnosis should not be confined only to those individuals who are symptomatic or who manifest evidence of organ damage, such as cirrhosis, diabetes, heart failure, arthritis, or skin pigmentation. Instead, all individuals who have inherited both alleles of the mutant hemochromatosis gene (*HFE*) and who have direct or indirect markers of iron overload should be regarded as homozygous for HH.

In 1996, the gene for hemochromatosis was identified and ultimately called *HFE*. *HFE* encodes for a major histocompatibility complex class I–like molecule that requires interaction with β₂-microglobulin for normal presentation to the surface of cells and binds with transferrin receptor. Two missense mutations have been identified in *HFE*. One results in a change of cysteine to tyrosine at amino acid position 282 (C282Y); the second results in a change of histidine to aspartate at amino acid position 63 (H63D). Approximately 85% to 90% of typical hemochromatosis patients are homozygous for C282Y. Compound heterozygotes are those patients who have one allele with the C282Y mutation and one allele with the H63D mutation. Approximately 3% to 5% of typical hemochromatosis patients are compound heterozygotes, but not all compound heterozy-

gotes experience significant degrees of iron loading. About 10% of patients who have a clinical syndrome that is phenotypically identical to HH do not have the C282Y mutation. These patients may have another condition causing iron overload, or they may have inherited another genetic abnormality.

HH is underdiagnosed, largely because physicians often think that it is a rare disorder manifested only by the classic triad of clinical findings consisting of increased skin pigmentation, diabetes, and cirrhosis (so-called bronze diabetes). In the 1990s, HH increasingly was identified by the evaluation of patients with abnormal iron results on routine serum chemistry panels or on screening iron studies for patients with a family history of HH. When patients are identified in this way, approximately 75% of them are without symptoms and do not exhibit any of the end-stage manifestations of hemochromatosis. Very few of these individuals have diabetes, cirrhosis, skin pigmentation, or arthropathy. About 25% of them have fatigue that improves with treatment. Because HH is a common disorder, it is important for clinicians to realize that any patient with an elevated transferrin saturation and/or an elevated ferritin level (see later discussion) might have HH.

When patients experience symptoms of fatigue, right-upper-quadrant abdominal pain, arthralgias, impotence, decreased libido, heart failure, or diabetes, the clinician should consider the possibility of HH. Similarly, findings of hepatomegaly, cirrhosis, extrahepatic manifestations of chronic liver disease, testicular atrophy, congestive heart failure, skin pigmentation, and arthritis should raise the suspicion of HH. Obviously, many of these symptoms and signs are indicative of a variety of medical illnesses, but HH should be part of the differential diagnosis.

Once the diagnosis of HH is considered—by evaluation of abnormal screening iron studies, in the context of family studies, in a patient with abnormal results on genetic testing, or in the evaluation of a patient with any of the cited symptoms or clinical findings—definitive diagnosis is relatively straightforward. To diagnose HH, fasting transferrin saturation (TS, serum iron ÷ by total iron binding capacity or transferrin × 100%) and ferritin levels should be obtained; both will be elevated in a symptomatic patient. TS should be measured in a fasting state, since serum iron levels have a diurnal variation and can be higher after a meal. Unfortunately, the diagnostic sensitivity and specificity of the TS and ferritin levels can be questionable when young individuals are being evaluated or when patients have abnormal results of iron studies in the context of other diseases. The advent of genetic testing (mutation analysis for C282Y and H63D in *HFE*) has helped clarify this situation. Thus, if TS and/or ferritin levels are elevated, then *HFE* mutation analysis should be carried out. If the patient is less than 40 years old, with normal liver enzyme levels but abnormal iron study results, and is homozygous for C282Y or compound heterozygous, then he or she should be considered to have HH and treated accordingly (Fig. 123.1). If the patient is older than 40 years or has abnormal liver test results, regardless of *HFE* test results, he or she should

undergo percutaneous liver biopsy for histologic interpretation and quantitative iron studies. Once the diagnosis of HH is confirmed either by genetic studies or by liver biopsy [more than 3+ iron stores, increased hepatic iron concentration, and/or hepatic iron index (measured as micromoles of iron per gram dry weight of liver divided by the patient's age)], treatment for HH should be commenced.

Treatment is weekly (or occasionally biweekly) therapeutic phlebotomy of 500 mL of whole blood. This is equivalent to approximately 200 to 250 mg of iron, depending on the hemoglobin concentration of the blood removed. Therapeutic phlebotomy is typically continued until the transferrin saturation is less than 50% and/or serum ferritin levels are less than 50 ng/mL. Most patients tolerate therapeutic phlebotomy quite well and have a sense of improved well-being after the initial phlebotomies have been completed. Once excess iron stores are depleted, therapeutic phlebotomy is replaced by maintenance phlebotomy of 1 u of blood, removed every 2 to 3 months for the patient's

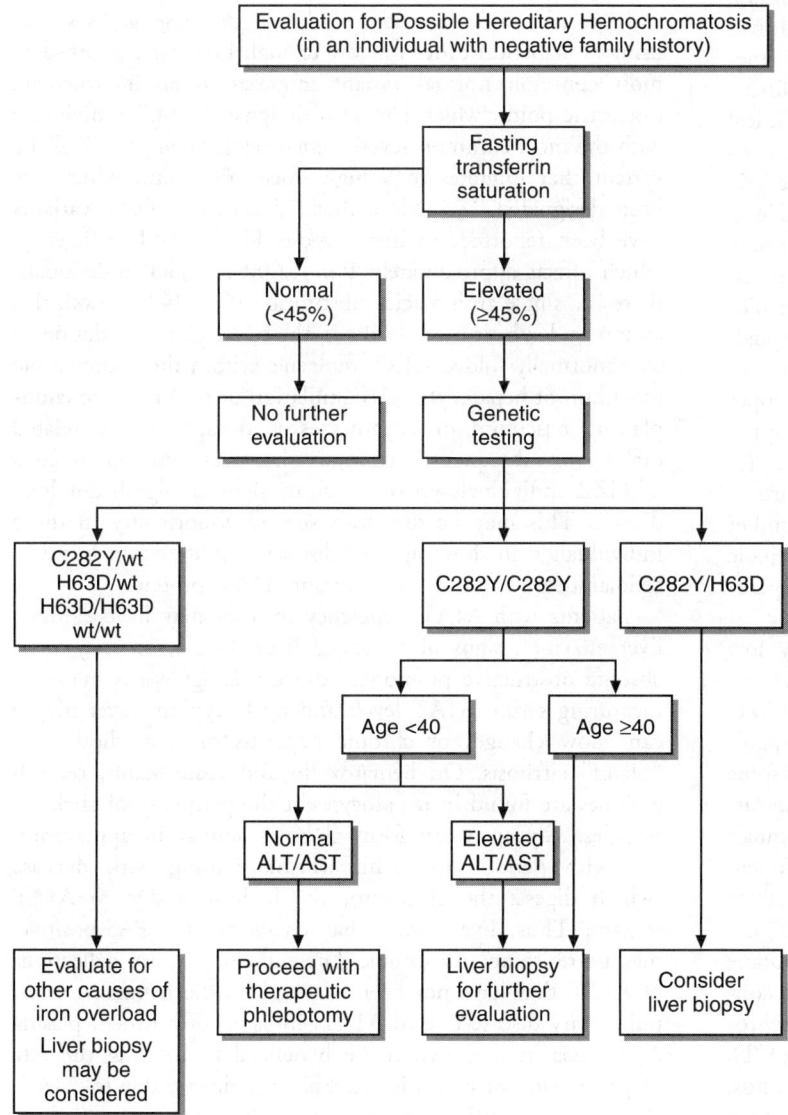

FIGURE 123.1. Proposed algorithm for evaluation for hereditary hemochromatosis.

lifetime. If treatment is initiated before complications of liver disease ensue, the prognosis is excellent and equal to an age- and sex-matched population. Family screening of all first-degree relatives should be done once a proband is identified. *HLA* typing is no longer used for family screening; instead, mutation analysis for C282Y and H63D in *HFE* is recommended.

WILSON'S DISEASE

Wilson's disease (WD) is a rare inherited disorder that occurs in 1 in 30,000 individuals. In WD, copper accumulates in the liver and brain in excess of normal metabolic needs. The defect in copper homeostasis in WD that leads to copper accumulation is a reduction in the biliary excretion of copper. Unrecognized and untreated, this disorder is progressive and fatal, with death due to neurologic deterioration and complications of end-stage liver disease. Patients can show signs of disease in childhood, adolescence, or young adulthood, among them, abnormal liver enzymes, complications of chronic liver disease, hemolytic anemia, or a variety of neurologic and neuropsychiatric disturbances. The diagnosis is established by a combination of clinical and biochemical findings. Copper deposition in Descemet's membrane in the periphery of the cornea shows characteristic Kayser-Fleischer rings. Laboratory studies show a decreased level of ceruloplasmin in approximately 85% of patients, and urinary copper excretion is elevated. Liver enzymes (alanine aminotransferase, aspartate aminotransferase) are typically high, and biochemical and hematologic signs of chronic liver disease (hypoalbuminemia, thrombocytopenia, elevated prothrombin time) can be present. Liver biopsy can show a rise in the level of copper using a variety of special stains; this increase in hepatic copper level (determined biochemically) is necessary for diagnosis. Hepatic steatosis is seen in early-stage disease; changes of chronic hepatitis occur later, and then cirrhosis develops. A small number of patients with WD have initial signs of fulminant hepatic failure, which is uniformly fatal unless emergency liver transplantation is successful.

Once the diagnosis is established (characteristic history, low ceruloplasmin level, increased urinary copper excretion, liver biopsy findings, elevated hepatic copper level), treatment of WD usually is initiated with copper chelation therapy using D-penicillamine. Side effects from D-penicillamine can occur, and some patients are better treated with trientine, another copper-chelating drug. The use of dietary zinc supplementation can impair the absorption of copper and also can induce metallothionein synthesis, which binds copper in the gut, decreasing the amount of copper that is absorbed. The gene for WD (called *ATP7B*) has been identified and codes for a P-type ATPase transmembrane protein that is involved in membrane copper transport. In contrast to the use of genetic markers for the diagnosis of hemochromatosis, the same opportunity does not exist for diagnosing WD, since there are more than 60 mutations in the WD gene. Thus, mutation analysis has not been considered practical. If WD is diagnosed before hepatic and neurologic complications ensue

and lifelong copper chelation therapy is instituted, the prognosis is excellent. Family screening of all first-degree relatives should be undertaken when a proband is identified. In this situation, genetic testing with mutation analysis may be helpful; serum ceruloplasmin levels and urinary copper excretion should be evaluated.

ALPHA₁-ANTITRYPSIN DEFICIENCY

Alpha₁-antitrypsin (A1AT) deficiency is a relatively uncommon autosomal disease predominantly seen in Whites, which can cause pulmonary disease or hepatic disease. A1AT is a normally occurring inhibitor of proteases and elastases that is synthesized predominantly by the liver. Structural variance of A1AT is classified according to the protease inhibitor (Pi) phenotype system, as defined either by agarose electrophoresis or isoelectrofocusing. The Pi classification system assigns a letter to each position of migration of A1AT in these gel systems, using alphabetical order for low to high isoelectric point. The most common normal variant migrates to an intermediate isoelectric point, which has been designated "M." Individuals with the most common severe deficiency have an A1AT allelic variant that migrates to a high isoelectric point, which has been designated "Z." More than 75 different allelic variants have been reported. In homozygous PiZZ A1AT deficiency, which affects approximately 1 in 1,600 to 1,800 individuals, there is a single amino acid substitution (Glu 342 → Lys); this amino acid substitution results in the selective accumulation of an abnormally folded A1AT molecule within the endoplasmic reticulum of hepatocytes. Accumulation of A1AT in the endoplasmic reticulum of hepatocytes is thought to be related directly to subsequent liver injury; however, only about 20% of PiZZ individuals go on to show signs of significant liver disease. This may be due to a second abnormality in those individuals who show signs of disease—an alteration in intracellular degradation of the mutant A1AT protein.

Patients with A1AT deficiency initially may have elevated liver enzymes, signs of advanced liver disease, or early-onset chronic obstructive pulmonary disease. Diagnosis is made by measuring serum A1AT levels and by Pi typing. Liver biopsy can show changes of chronic hepatitis or may show only "bland" cirrhosis. On hematoxylin and eosin stains, reddish globules are found in hepatocytes at the periphery of cirrhotic nodules. Glycogen can form globules similar in appearance, but with period acid–Schiff (PAS) staining with diastase (which digests the glycogen), the inclusions due to A1AT remain. Thus, liver biopsy has characteristic "PAS-positive, diastase-resistant" inclusions. These inclusions are collections of A1AT that have not been excreted by the hepatocyte. For pulmonary disease due to A1AT, infusion of purified, plasma A1AT has been shown to be beneficial in limiting the rate of progression of lung disease. For liver disease due to A1AT, there is no specific therapy short of liver transplantation. If liver transplantation is carried out, the recipient assumes the

A1AT phenotype of the donor. Once a proband with A1AT is identified, family screening should be undertaken. This is largely done to educate patients, because specific therapy is not available. In light of the fact that only about 20% of PiZZ individuals go on to experience liver disease due to A1AT, it is not clear how to evaluate siblings or children of individuals with A1AT what the nature of their risk of disease might be. While there are no clear-cut guidelines, simple screening with A1AT levels and Pi phenotype seems reasonable.

NONALCOHOLIC STEATOHEPATITIS

One of the most common causes of liver test abnormalities is the condition known as nonalcoholic steatohepatitis (NASH). The diagnosis of NASH is based on liver biopsy findings, which are similar to those seen in alcoholic hepatitis, and include steatosis, mixed inflammatory cell infiltration of the hepatic lobule, Mallory's hyalin, and perisinusoidal fibrosis that can progress to cirrhosis. The recognition of NASH as a diagnostic entity has evolved over the past 20 years as our understanding of liver disease in general has advanced. The pathogenetic basis of NASH is not known, but the disorder frequently is seen in obese, diabetic women, and the possibility of insulin resistance in a large proportion of patients has been considered. The diagnosis of NASH can be established only in the context of a carefully conducted clinical history, the most important feature of which is the exclusion of significant alcohol consumption. Thus, if patients consume more than 20 g of ethanol daily, it is inappropriate to consider a diagnosis of NASH; in this context, a diagnosis of alcoholic steatohepatitis is reasonable. In any patient with biochemical evidence of chronic liver injury, it is important to pursue the dietary history, the use of various medications, possible occupational exposure to toxins or solvents, and a family history of liver disease.

Liver biopsy is essential for the diagnosis of NASH and should be conducted for patients with unexplained elevations of liver enzymes unless there is reason to believe that a medication or an environmental factor is responsible, in which case, a diagnostic trial of avoidance is reasonable. The steatosis of NASH is typically macrovesicular. To actually visualize the fat, a frozen section must be stained with a fat-specific stain, such as oil red O. Involvement of hepatic lobules can be diffuse or localized to the centrilobular region. Inflammation is considered a necessary component of the biopsy findings in NASH. It is typically low grade and consists of a mixed neutrophilic and mononuclear cell infiltrate throughout the lobule. Glycogen nuclei are seen frequently, and Mallory's hyalin, which is usually less impressive than that seen in alcoholic liver disease, is present. Fibrosis typically occurs in the pericentral regions and is perisinusoidal; in more advanced cases, it can lead to the development of fully established cirrhosis.

Many patients who have NASH are asymptomatic and are identified in the process of an evaluation of abnormal liver enzymes. When patients are symptomatic, fatigue and vague right-upper-quadrant pain are most common. Similarly, physical examination findings frequently can be normal or show a slight increase in liver size and right-upper-quadrant tenderness with palpation. Changes of chronic liver disease (cutaneous manifestations) with portal hypertension are evident in advanced cases. Laboratory studies confirm elevated liver enzymes, typically with the alanine aminotransferase (ALT) being higher than the aspartate aminotransferase (AST) level. This is a useful feature distinguishing NASH from alcoholic liver disease—where the AST is typically higher than the ALT level. In the absence of advanced liver disease, serum albumin levels and bilirubin levels are normal. Gamma-glutamyltranspeptidase (GGT) levels are often elevated in patients with NASH. As mentioned previously, liver biopsy is necessary to establish a diagnosis in a suspect individual. Ultrasonography and abdominal computed tomography scanning can show images suggestive of fatty infiltration of the liver, but an assessment of fibrosis and/or severity is not possible.

The natural history of NASH is poorly understood, but generally it is thought that NASH can be a progressive disease leading to cirrhosis and liver failure in about 15% of cases. Because of this concern for disease progression, there has been growing interest in treatment over the past several years. Certainly, weight loss and control of serum glucose are recommended in the case of individuals who are overweight and/or diabetic. Patients with hyperlipidemia are urged to limit cholesterol and triglycerides with diet and/or lipid-lowering agents. Since the pathogenesis of NASH is so poorly understood, more specific therapy does not exist. Some investigators have tried vitamin E or ursodeoxycholic acid, with inconclusive results.

HEPATIC PORPHYRIAS

There are several types of porphyria that are broadly classified as *hepatic* or *erythropoietic*, based on the organ in which the major overproduction of heme precursors takes place. Alterations in various steps in the heme biosynthetic pathway can occur, causing each of the various types of porphyria. The most common hepatic porphyria is porphyria cutanea tarda (PCT); three subtypes have been identified. Of these subtypes, the most common, which makes up about 75% of cases, is provoked by an acquired or sporadic, and reversible, form of deficiency of hepatic uroporphyrinogen decarboxylase activity. Clinical findings of PCT include photosensitivity, usually on the sun-exposed areas of the hands and face, marked by blistering and ulcerating lesions. These lesions often are found in association with increased alcohol ingestion, mild to moderate iron overload, or, in women, exogenous estrogen use. Diagnosis is made by recognition of the characteristic skin lesions and by detection of increased amounts of uroporphyrins excreted in the urine.

Approximately 50% of PCT patients in North America have hepatitis C, and about 30% to 50% of PCT patients have one or both of the mutations found in the hemochromatosis gene, *HFE*. Thus, when a patient with PCT is identified, testing for anti–hepatitis C virus and mutation analysis for *HFE* should be carried out in addition to evaluating liver function. Liver biopsy usually is undertaken in patients with PCT, and characteristic abnormalities have been defined. Treatment consists of abstinence from alcohol, discontinuation of estrogens or other medications that have been shown to exacerbate porphyria, and therapeutic phlebotomy to lessen hepatic iron stores. Skin lesions usually respond to these measures, and if liver enzymes are elevated, improvement usually ensues. If hepatitis C is present, consideration should be given to antiviral treatment.

GRANULOMATOUS HEPATITIS

There are a number of sources of granulomatous reaction in the liver, the most important of which are the hepatic manifestations of sarcoidosis, certain drug reactions (e.g., allopurinol), and infections either with tuberculosis or with various fungi. Some patients with sarcoidosis can experience systemic symptoms of fever, weight loss, malaise, and fatigue, and liver tests show cholestatic enzyme abnormalities with a predominant increase in alkaline phosphatase and GGT activity. Liver biopsy shows noncaseating granulomata that have features characteristic of sarcoidosis. Occasionally, fibrosis is progressive, and cirrhosis with liver failure develops, though this is uncommon. Indication for treatment of granulomatous hepatitis with glucocorticoids depends on the presence of progressive fibrosis. It is critical that infectious causes of granulomatous infiltration be ruled out by tissue culture, by special stains for acid-fast bacilli (AFB) and for fungi, and by appropriate clinical evaluation.

HEPATIC AMYLOIDOSIS

Infiltration of the liver with amyloid is a complication of systemic amyloidosis and can be an end-stage manifestation of the disease. Symptoms of weakness, increased fatigue, weight loss, and joint pain are present. Liver test parameters (ALT, AST) may be slightly high or normal. The liver typically is enlarged, often massively, and signs of portal hypertension may be evident. In the past, liver biopsy was considered quite risky because of the concern of increased bleeding due to "hepatic fracture," but this complication has become less of a concern. Liver biopsy shows an amorphous infiltration of the protein in the perisinusoidal space of Disse, and special stains (Congo red) confirm the presence of amyloid. There is no specific treatment for hepatic amyloidosis, and the prognosis is very poor.

STORAGE DISORDERS

There are more than 40 distinct genetic diseases that can produce lysosomal storage disorders. Most are inherited in an autosomal recessive manner and are rare. Specific genetic deficiencies of particular lysosomal proteins have been identified for each disorder. Different phenotypic expression is related to various mutations in specific genes. The lysosomal storage diseases as a whole are found in approximately 1 per 8,000 births. Gaucher's disease is the most common, with a prevalence of approximately 1 per 60,000 births. In the Ashkenazi Jewish population, however, the prevalence of Gaucher's disease may be as high as 1 in 900. The typical clinical manifestations of Gaucher's disease are massive hepatomegaly with complications of portal hypertension. Onset is usually in childhood or early adulthood, and disease severity can vary considerably. In Gaucher's disease, there is a defect in β-glucocerebrosidase, which is required to catalyze the cleavage of glucocerebroside to glucoceramide. Deficiency results in the accumulation of glucocerebroside in tissue macrophages, which are known as Gaucher cells, with subsequent toxicity to these tissues. Affected macrophages are present in the liver in Kupffer cells, in the bone in osteoclasts, and in the spleen and lung. Complications of chronic liver disease can develop and cause premature death. Diagnosis is by clinical history, family history, and typical glucocerebroside-packed Gaucher macrophages seen either in the bone marrow or on liver biopsy. Treatment is largely symptomatic, but enzyme replacement therapy has been used and provides some benefit. This treatment is extremely expensive—a year of therapy costs more than $200,000. Advances in molecular genetics will help diagnosis this disorder early, and treatment may become less expensive.

BIBLIOGRAPHY

Bacon BR, Olynyk JK, Brunt EM, et al. *HFE* genotype in patients with hemochromatosis and other liver diseases. *Ann Intern Med* 1999;130: 953–962.

Bacon BR, Powell LW, Adams PC, et al. Molecular medicine and hemochromatosis: at the crossroads. *Gastroenterology* 1999;16:193–207.

Bacon BR, Schilsky M. New knowledge of the genetic pathogenesis of hemochromatosis and Wilson disease. *Adv Intern Med* 1999;44:91–116.

Bonkovsky HL, Poh-Fitzpatrick M, Pimstone N, et al. Porphyria cutanea tarda, hepatitis C, and *HFE* gene mutations in North America. *Hepatology* 1998;27:1661–1669.

Feder JN, Gnirke A, Thomas W, et al. A novel MHC class I–like gene is mutated in patients with hereditary haemochromatosis. *Nat Genet* 1996; 13:399–408.

Maier-Dobersberger T, Ferenci P, Polli C, et al. Detection of the His 1069Gln mutation in Wilson disease by rapid polymerase chain reaction. *Ann Intern Med* 1997;127:21–26.

Meikle PJ, Hopwood JJ, Clague AE, et al. Prevalence of lysosomal storage disorders. *JAMA* 1999;281:249–254.

Neushwander-Tetri BA, Bacon BR. Nonalcoholic steatohepatitis. *Med Clin North Am* 1996;80:1147–1166.

Wu Y, Whitman I, Molmenti E, et al. A lag in intracellular degradation of mutant alpha-1-antitrypsin correlates with liver disease phenotype in homozygous PIZZ alpha-1-antitrypsin deficiency. *Proc Natl Acad Sci USA* 1994;91:9014–9018.

Younossi ZM, Gramlich T, Liu YC, et al. Nonalcoholic fatty liver disease: assessment of variability in pathologic interpretations. *Mod Pathol* 1998; 11:560–565.

Kelley's Textbook of Internal Medicine, fourth edition. Edited by H. David Humes. Lippincott Williams & Wilkins, Philadelphia © 2000.

CHAPTER
124

GALLSTONES AND CHOLECYSTITIS

JOHN H. SEKIJIMA
SUM P. LEE

TABLE 124.1.	CONDITIONS PREDISPOSING TO GALLSTONE FORMATION
Cholesterol Gallstones	**Pigment Gallstones**
Obesity	Black
Ileal resection or disease	Chronic hemolysis
Pregnancy	Cirrhosis
Rapid weight loss	Total parenteral nutrition
Female gender	Advancing age
Spinal cord injury	
Drugs: estrogens, clofibrates	Brown
Advancing age	Chronic biliary infection
Cystic fibrosis	Biliary strictures and stasis

INCIDENCE AND EPIDEMIOLOGY

Cholelithiasis is a very common disorder in the United States, and it is estimated that more than 20 million Americans are afflicted with gallstones. Moreover, by age 75 approximately 35% of women and 20% of men have or have had gallstones. Although the majority of these individuals are asymptomatic, nearly 750,000 cholecystectomies are carried out each year, and there are 5,000 to 6,000 deaths annually as a direct result of gallstone-related disease.

Around the world, the prevalence rates for cholelithiasis vary widely depending on the specific geographic location and ethnic factors under consideration. Much of the data has been derived from either autopsy studies or screening ultrasonography surveys. Native Americans, in general, and the Pimas of southwestern North America, in particular, have extraordinarily high rates of gallstone formation, such that by age 30 approximately 70% of the women have had stones. Impressive prevalence rates are also seen in Chile, the United States (among whites), and northern Europe. Much lower rates are reported from Asia and Africa.

ETIOLOGY

In the United States, as in other Western countries, cholesterol stones comprise at least 75% to 80% of all gallstones, while the remainder are classified as pigment stones. Most cholesterol stones contain between 50% and 90% cholesterol in total weight. Some analyzed stones, however, are strikingly pure in cholesterol (more than 95%). Calcium salts of bilirubin pigment, carbonate, and various proteins account for the bulk of the remaining content. Risk factors for cholesterol lithogenesis include obesity, rapid weight loss, spinal cord injury, female gender (male to female ratio, 2:1), and, to a lesser extent, parity and estrogen use (Table 124.1). Pigment stones are categorized as either black or brown, depending on their chemical composition and gross appearance. These stones also differ with respect to their pathogenesis and associated clinical manifestations. Table 124.1 lists the conditions believed to be risk factors for pigment lithogenesis.

PATHOGENESIS OF CHOLESTEROL STONES

Cholesterol Solubilization

Cholesterol-enriched bile may be produced by absolute cholesterol hypersecretion or a diminished bile acid pool resulting from primary bile acid hyposecretion or intestinal losses. Previously, it was thought that biliary cholesterol was packaged and solubilized by bile salts and phospholipid cholesterol exclusively in the form of mixed micelles, and much attention was focused on the rigorous physicochemical characterization of these micellar structures. It has become clear that biliary lipid vesicles also play an important role in the solubilization of cholesterol. Collectively, these unilamellar vesicles, which range in size from 40 to 100 nm, are believed to represent the primary mode of cholesterol secretion into bile. Evidence suggests that biliary vesicles initially are constructed within the hepatocyte and consist of phospholipid and cholesterol. Once the vesicles are secreted into the canaliculi, bile salts adsorb onto them and remove or strip away phospholipid and cholesterol to form mixed micelles. Two distinct cholesterol transport systems (vesicular and micellar) apparently coexist in bile in a state of dynamic equilibrium. This lipid interchange is thought to take place throughout the biliary apparatus. When the bile salt concentration is dilute (hepatic bile), relatively more cholesterol is carried in the vesicular phase. Conversely, when the bile salt concentration is at its peak (gallbladder bile), a micellar shift is favored.

Nucleation of Cholesterol Crystals

The critical emergence and precipitation of solid cholesterol crystals from supersaturated bile is termed *nucleation*. This fascinating process appears to begin with the aggregation and fusion of unilamellar biliary vesicles into multilamellar liposomes. These multilamellar structures are birefringent and compressible under polarizing light microscopy and are referred to as *liquid crystals*. Under video-enhanced microscopy, solid cholesterol crystals appear to originate directly from aggregated or fused vesicles.

Not all vesicle populations have an equal propensity to participate in nucleation, however. Vesicles in gallbladder bile are observed to nucleate more readily than vesicles in dilute hepatic bile, which seem to be stable and fairly resistant to nucleation. This phenomenon can be explained in part by the differences in their respective cholesterol/phospholipid contents. In the concentrated environment of the gallbladder, bile salts remove preferentially greater amounts of vesicular phospholipid than cholesterol during the shift to the micellar phase. This results in a residual vesicle fraction that is relatively cholesterol enriched compared with phospholipid and therefore more likely to aggregate, fuse, and nucleate.

The importance of cholesterol supersaturation in bile to the process of nucleation cannot be overstated. It has long been recognized, however, that many individuals secrete cholesterol-saturated bile but never show signs of gallstones. Gallbladder bile harvested from patients with cholesterol stones was shown to nucleate crystals more rapidly than equally saturated bile taken from control subjects. These observations led investigators to search for factors in bile that can affect nucleation. Mucin and α_1-acid glycoprotein exhibit pronucleating properties, while immunoglobulin A, and apolipoproteins A1 and A11 are putative inhibitors. Efforts to purify other agents and to characterize their mechanisms of action are ongoing.

The striking variation in gallstone prevalence rates around the world and the identification of lithogenic genes in an inbred mouse model highlight the importance of genetic risk factors. Moreover, the apolipoprotein E-4 genotype in humans is associated with biliary cholesterol hypersecretion, rapid nucleation, and stone formation. Additional factors, such as infection, also may be important, since bacterial DNA now has been identified within cholesterol stones through molecular analyses. The precise role of bacterial infection in cholesterol lithogenesis remains unknown.

Biliary Sludge

No discussion on the pathogenesis of gallstone formation would be complete without addressing the relevance of biliary sludge. Such descriptive labels as microlithiasis, microcrystalline disease, and biliary gravel or sand have been attached to this entity. Biliary sludge is detected most often by ultrasonography. It may layer dependently within the gallbladder but, by definition, does not produce the postacoustic shadows that are pathognomonic of typical stones (Fig. 124.1). The chemical composition de-

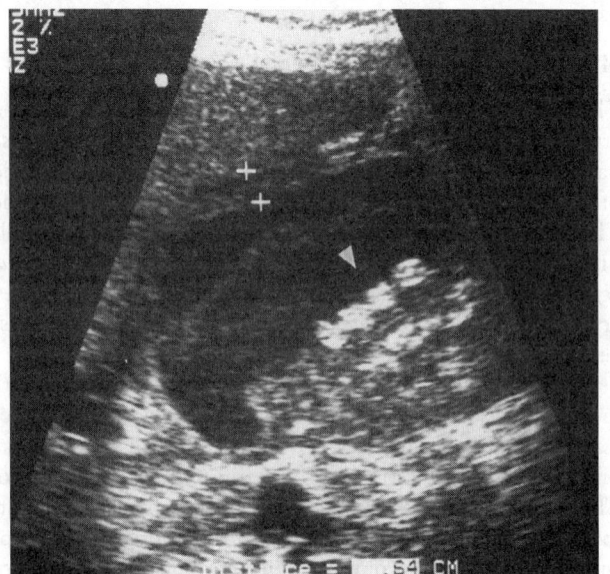

FIGURE 124.1. Ultrasonographic study showing tumefactive sludge within the gallbladder. Note the ball-like concretions of sludge that do not produce postacoustic shadows.

pends on the underlying clinical condition, but it typically consists of a conglomeration of calcium bilirubinate granules, cholesterol monohydrate crystals, and matrices of mucous gel in varying proportions. Sludge is believed to be a precursor of lithogenesis and is associated with many of the same risk factors as gallstones (Table 124.1). Other predisposing factors include bone marrow or solid organ transplantation as well as prolonged courses of ceftriaxzone or octreotide medications.

On prospective ultrasonography, gallbladder sludge can be documented to resolve spontaneously, to come and go over time, or to result in macroscopic stone formation. Although most patients remain clinically well, some unpredictably have signs and symptoms of disease. Sludge has been implicated convincingly as a cause of classic biliary pain, acute cholecystitis, and acute pancreatitis. Moreover, a normal result on gallbladder ultrasound does not exclude sludge as a cause of pancreaticobiliary disease. Bile microscopy is crucial in this context. Intravenous cholecystokinin (0.05 to 0.1 mg per kilogram) is given, and 5 to 15 mL of dark green gallbladder bile is aspirated from the duodenum at endoscopy or via a nasoduodenal tube. The sample is centrifuged at $3,000g$ for 15 minutes, and the sediment is suspended in 1 mL of distilled water and examined under a polarizing microscope. The findings of birefringent rhomboid plates typical of cholesterol crystals or reddish brown clumps of calcium/bilirubinate precipitates confirm the diagnosis of microscopic sludge. In these situations, biliary sludge can be treated as a gallstone equivalent, and, if there are no contraindications, cholecystectomy should be recommended.

Stone Formation

The spontaneous formation of biliary sludge or cholesterol gallstones is a multistep process in which several conditions and events are operative. At some point, the cholesterol concentration in bile must exceed the capacity of bile salts and phospholipid to hold it in solution. This results in the storage of gallbladder bile that is rich and supersaturated with cholesterol. As the bile is progressively concentrated, biliary vesicles aggregate and fuse into larger multilamellar vesicles. Crystals then begin to emerge when the balance of nucleator and antinucleator activity favors solid crystal formation (Fig. 124.2). The cholesterol crystals, along with precipitates of calcium bilirubinate pigment and viscoelastic gels of mucus, must be kept sequestered within the gallbladder. Gallbladder stasis is probably critical at this stage, and over time the retained sludge contents may evolve to form a solid concretion or stone.

PATHOGENESIS OF PIGMENT STONES

The pathogenesis of pigment stones remains incompletely understood, but some degree of elevation in the level of biliary unconjugated bilirubin appears to be important. Like cholesterol, bilirubin is essentially insoluble in water and must be glucuronidated to be secreted in bile. Disease states or disorders that lead to the handling of increased total bilirubin loads or to enzymatic hydrolysis of conjugated bilirubin to insoluble pigment raises the risk of pigment lithogenesis.

Black stones are formed within the gallbladder and often are

SOLUBLE FORMS	TRANSITIONAL FORMS	CRYSTALLINE FORMS

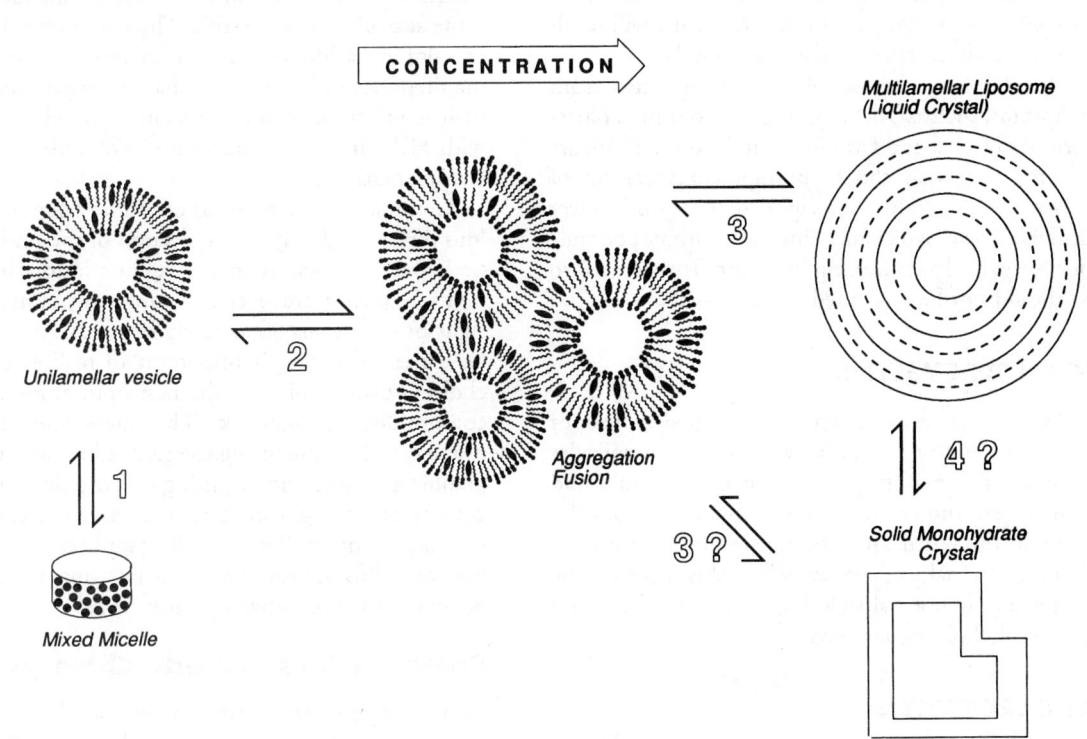

FIGURE 124.2. Schematic representation of cholesterol nucleation, as previously used.

associated with chronic hemolytic disorders. They are encountered more commonly in Western countries and are reported with increased frequency in patients with cirrhosis and those receiving long-term total parenteral nutrition. On gross inspection, black stones tend to be somewhat amorphous and easy to crush or fragment. From a biochemical perspective, they are believed to be composed primarily of bilirubin polymers, mucin glycoprotein, and calcium salts of phosphate and carbonate.

Brown stones consist of concentric layers of calcium bilirubinate alternating with complexes of calcium and fatty acids, such as palmitate. The pathogenesis likely involves some degree of biliary stasis and infection. Chronic bacterial infection is believed to be responsible for elevated activity levels of β-glucuronidases in bile. These enzymes may predispose to stone formation by cleaving glucuronic acid moieties from conjugated bilirubin. This results in a greater accumulation of unconjugated bilirubin, which may precipitate in bile as a calcium salt.

Brown stones rarely are found in the gallbladder, and in Western countries they are thought to form de novo in the common bile duct after cholecystectomy. In Asia, where they are encountered more often, they are found primarily within the intrahepatic ducts. Associated bile duct strictures and focal areas of marked dilatation and stasis often are described. Moreover, bouts of cholangitis have led to the use of such descriptive terms as *recurrent pyogenic cholangitis* or *oriental cholangiohepatitis*. Biliary cirrhosis and end-stage liver disease also may evolve as the result of the chronic and, at times, relentless nature of the disease.

CLINICAL FINDINGS

ASYMPTOMATIC STONES

The majority of gallstones remain clinically silent. In a long-term follow-up of asymptomatic gallstone patients, the cumulative risk that symptoms will develop over time was 10% at 5 years, 15% at 10 years, and 18% at 15 years. Put another way, the rates of biliary pain are approximately 1% to 2% per year soon after the diagnosis of cholelithiasis, and they appear to decline over time. Moreover, the appearance of a benign warning pain precedes the occurrence of serious complications in more than 90% of cases.

BILIARY COLIC

Classic biliary colic represents a discrete episode of steady, severe pain, typically located in the epigastrium or right-upper quadrant. It may radiate into the back or right shoulder region but usually does not fluctuate, as implied by the term *colic*. In general, the pain comes on rapidly, lasts from 30 minutes to 3 hours, and gradually subsides. Benign biliary colic is not associated with fever, leukocytosis, or acute peritoneal signs. The presence of these symptoms or biliary pain lasting longer than 4 to 6 hours should raise the suspicion of acute cholecystitis. On occasion, it may be difficult to differentiate biliary colic from cardiac chest pain or other intra-abdominal processes. Taking a careful history is absolutely critical, since an accurate description of the quality and character of the pain often is the only criterion on which to base the decision to operate. Moreover, an ill-advised cholecystectomy for atypical or vague symptoms frequently will result in the postoperative appearance of identical complaints.

True attacks of biliary pain should be distinguished from dyspeptic symptoms, such as belching, epigastric burning, bloating, heartburn, flatulence, and fatty food intolerance. These are nonspecific complaints that should prompt consideration of other diagnoses, such as gastroesophageal reflux, peptic ulcer disease, or irritable bowel syndrome. Similarly, chronic abdominal discomfort or pain that is fleeting in nature (less than 10 to 15 minutes) should not be attributed to gallstones.

CHRONIC CHOLECYSTITIS

Chronic cholecystitis arises as a result of repeated attacks of discrete biliary pain and/or acute cholecystitis. These episodes induce a chronic inflammatory process that may be mild and patchy or quite severe and extensive. Over time the gallbladder wall may become thickened and fibrotic, resulting in a contracted and nonfunctional gallbladder. When this happens, the gallbladder generally is not palpable on examination and will not opacify on oral cholecystography.

ACUTE CHOLECYSTITIS

Acute obstruction of the cystic duct by a stone leads to gallbladder distention and a host of potential injury-inducing mechanisms. Hydrolysis of lecithin to form lysolecithin can lead to epithelial toxicity; bile salts as well as inflammatory mediators, such as prostaglandins, are actively involved in the process. Histologic findings range from edema, erythema, and mild mucosal inflammation to gross infiltration of the wall with polymorphonuclear neutrophils and evidence of frank necrosis and perforation. Bacterial infection is not thought to be a primary or initiating step in the pathogenesis of acute cholecystitis. As a secondary event, however, superimposed bacterial infection seems to be critical in the development of such complications as empyema, emphysematous cholecystitis, or perforation.

At initial clinical examination, patients with acute cholecystitis often complain of continuous upper abdominal pain and a history of similar, but self-limited attacks. They may be nauseated but usually do not obtain relief by vomiting or changing positions. These patients typically run a fever in the range of 99°F to 101°F and exhibit right-sided subcostal tenderness and localized parietal pain because of progressive gallbladder inflammation. A classic Murphy's sign may be elicited when the patient's inspiration is halted abruptly as the result of painful palpation of the right-upper quadrant or gallbladder. Generalized rebound tenderness and an acute abdomen should raise the suspicion of a perforation.

Acute acalculous cholecystitis (cholecystitis in the absence of stone obstruction) accounts for approximately 5% to 10% of all cases of acute cholecystitis. This entity is associated most often with critical illness, major surgery, extensive trauma, or burn-related injuries. Elderly men with peripheral vascular disease or patients on prolonged total parenteral nutritional support also appear to be at greater risk. The pathophysiologic picture involves a combination of gallbladder stasis, inflammation, and ischemia. Primary infections of the gallbladder also can cause acute acalculous cholecystitis. These infections include rare cases of salmonella-induced disease in immunocompetent hosts or manifestations of cryptosporidia, microsporidia, and cytomegalovirus infection in immunocompromised patients (i.e., those with HIV disease or those who have undergone bone marrow transplantation).

Complications tend to be encountered more often in acalculous disease and may be a reflection of the underlying pathogenetic process, such as small-vessel occlusion and ischemia. Patients frequently are severely ill and may not manifest the typical signs or symptoms of acute cholecystitis. Although surgery can be contemplated, it is important to realize that percutaneous cholecystostomy often is the best option, given the significant comorbidity and high risks. This interventional radiologic technique calls for puncturing the gallbladder wall under ultrasonographic guidance and acquiring secure guide wire access. A percutaneous drainage catheter is then passed over the wire and put in place to drain. The overall complication rate is acceptably low with this approach and, in fact, may be lifesaving in the patient with prohibitive operative risks.

Complications of Acute Cholecystitis

Complications develop when severe gallbladder inflammation is allowed to progress to gangrene and necrosis. Perforation occurs in approximately 10% of cases and can result in diffuse peritonitis, localized abscess formation, or a cholecystenteric fistula. Free perforation is uncommon, but when it happens, it leads to generalized peritonitis and mortality rates approaching 30%. Fortunately, the inflamed gallbladder typically is effectively sealed off by omentum and adherent viscera. Organ rupture in this scenario results in a contained abscess or walled-off perforation.

The gallbladder also can erode and decompress its contents into a loop of bowel to form a cholecystenteric fistula. The duodenum is the most likely site, but in rare cases the colon, stomach, and jejunum also may be involved. When a particularly large gallstone passes through a fistula tract into the small bowel, it can become lodged (most typically in the distal ileum), which causes abdominal distention and vomiting. This is termed *gallstone ileus*, but it does not truly represent an ileus but rather a bonafide mechanical obstruction. Surgical retrieval of the offending stone is required. Depending on the overall stability of the patient, cholecystectomy and fistula repair may be attempted at the same operation.

Emphysematous cholecystitis results from secondary infection with gas-producing bacteria, such as clostridial organisms, *Escherichia coli*, or anaerobic streptococci. The diagnosis is suspected when gas is seen in the gallbladder wall or lumen on ultrasonography or computed tomography. Many cases are acalculous, and thus some element of underlying ischemia may be present. Diabetes is present 20% to 30% of the time.

CHOLEDOCHOLITHIASIS

Choledocholithiasis (formation of stones in the common bile duct) is found in approximately 10% to 15% of patients with

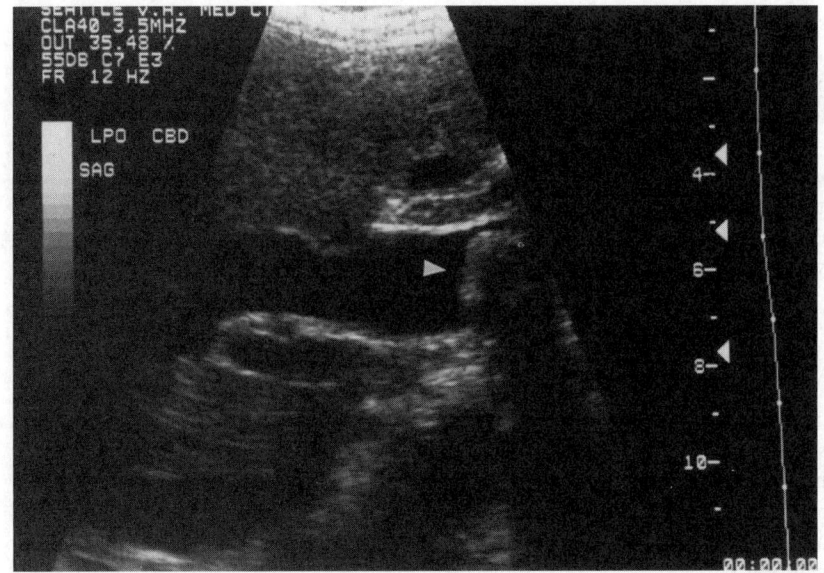

FIGURE 124.3. Ultrasonographic study showing a markedly dilated common bile duct with a distally obstructing stone (*arrowheads*).

symptomatic gallstones. Most of these stones originate in the gallbladder and pass through the cystic duct into the common bile duct. Although some stones pass uneventfully into the duodenum or reside in the duct without provoking apparent symptoms, the natural history of common duct stones is much less benign than that for incidental stones found in the gallbladder. Obstruction of stones in the distal duct or ampulla may give rise to serious complications of jaundice, cholangitis, or gallstone pancreatitis (Fig. 124.3).

The term *cholangitis* refers to the presence of bacterial infection behind an obstructed bile duct. Patients with cholangitis may have initial symptoms of biliary pain, fever with chills, and jaundice (Charcot's triad). Findings on examination often are less dramatic than the parietal pain and local tenderness associated with acute cholecystitis. The results of blood cultures usually are positive, and the organisms found include *E. coli*, *Klebsiella*, *Pseudomonas*, enterococci, and gut anaerobe species (15%). Some patients respond to aggressive broad-spectrum antibiotic treatment and intravenous fluids. True cholangitis should be viewed as a medical emergency, and hypotension, mental status changes, or severe sepsis should prompt immediate drainage of the biliary system by endoscopic sphincterotomy, percutaneous transhepatic drainage, or surgery.

LABORATORY FINDINGS

The laboratory evaluation of patients experiencing an attack of routine, uncomplicated biliary colic generally is unremarkable. In contrast, acute cholecystitis often is associated with leukocytosis in the range of 10,000 to 15,000. Mild jaundice is present in approximately 15% of patients, as a consequence of edema and compression of the common duct at the level of an inflamed and obstructed cystic duct. Bilirubin values of 2 to 10 mg per deciliter in a patient with upper abdominal pain are strongly suggestive of obstructive choledocholithiasis. Moreover, acute obstruction of the common duct occasionally gives rise to a high

transaminase level that peaks and then rapidly returns to baseline after directed treatment and drainage. The picture of abnormal serum liver test results and elevated amylase or lipase values is consistent with gallstone-induced pancreatitis. In jaundice due to choledocholithiasis, bilirubin levels rarely exceed 10 mg per deciliter. Substantially higher values should raise the suspicion of an underlying obstructive malignancy.

DIAGNOSTIC IMAGING STUDIES

Ultrasonography is the preferred imaging test in the evaluation of acute or recurrent biliary pain. It is performed easily, is readily available, and can detect the presence or absence of gallstones with a high degree of sensitivity and specificity (Fig. 124.4). Findings of gallbladder wall thickening (greater than 3 mm), pericholecystic fluid, and gallbladder tenderness elicited with a transducer (sonographic Murphy's sign) suggest the diagnosis of

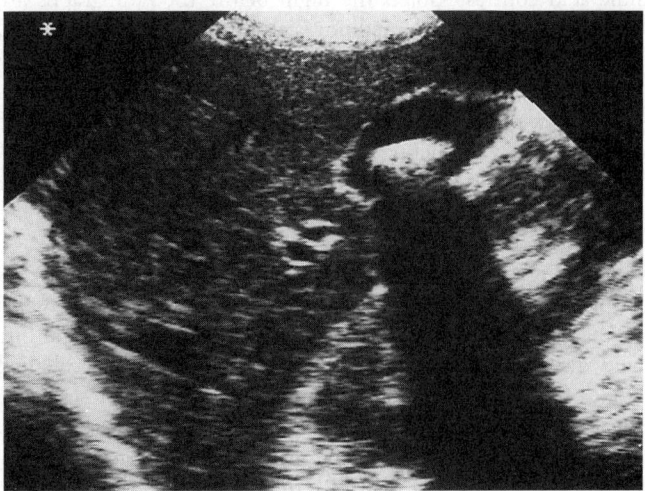

FIGURE 124.4. Ultrasonographic image of a gallbladder containing a single large stone. Note the classic postacoustic shadowing.

acute cholecystitis. Such complications as a gangrenous gallbladder may show irregular wall thickening and disruption, whereas findings of a dilated common bile indicate biliary obstruction and choledocholithiasis (Fig. 124.3). Ultrasonography also is quite useful in the simultaneous evaluation of other potential causes of acute abdominal pain. Although ultrasonography is superior to computed tomography in the primary detection of cholelithiasis and sludge, neither method is efficient in the diagnosis of common bile stones. Sensitivities in most cases are reported to be no better than 50%.

HEPATOBILIARY SCINTIGRAPHY

Radionuclide scanning of the biliary system is helpful in selected patients with symptoms and signs of acute cholecystitis and normal or inconclusive ultrasonography results. The patient is given an intravenous injection of a technetium Tc 99m–labeled iminodiacetic acid agent and undergoes scanning at regular intervals. Normally the gallbladder, common duct, and small bowel appear by 30 to 45 minutes. Failure to detect the gallbladder by 90 minutes, when the common duct and small bowel are visible, strongly points to acute obstruction of the cystic duct (Fig. 124.5). False-positive results can be caused by extremes of nonfasting or prolonged fasting states, chronic alcoholism, and chronic cholecystitis. Delayed images at 4 hours have been obtained routinely in an effort to decrease the incidence of false-positive results. The administration of intravenous morphine sulfate at 60 minutes has eliminated the need to acquire delayed images. Morphine increases the sphincter of Oddi pressure and acts to enhance isotope filling of the gallbladder through a patent cystic duct. After the morphine injection, the patient usually undergoes scanning for an additional 30 minutes, and then the films are interpreted. With very rare exceptions, a completely normal study virtually rules out the diagnosis of acute calculous cholecystitis.

ORAL CHOLECYSTOGRAPHY

Oral cholecystography involves the oral administration of iopanoic acid contrast tablets the night before the radiographs are obtained. The contrast medium is absorbed in the small bowel, conjugated in the liver, excreted into bile, and concentrated by the gallbladder. The day of the examination, multiple spot films of the right-upper quadrant are taken to assess the visibility of the gallbladder (cystic duct patency) as well as the size and number of stones. A double dose of contrast often is favored because the gallbladder cannot be seen in 15% to 50% of patients who are given a single dose.

Although it rarely is used in the routine evaluation of patients suspected of having gallstones, oral cholecystography is useful in the assessment of a few patients in anticipation of oral bile acid dissolution treatment. The finding of small noncalcified stones floating within a functioning gallbladder represents the ideal situation for this type of therapy (see later discussion). Direct cholangiography with either endoscopic retrograde cholangiopancreatography (ERCP) or percutaneous transhepatic cholangiography is used when additional delineation of the biliary tree is required or when such therapy as common duct stone

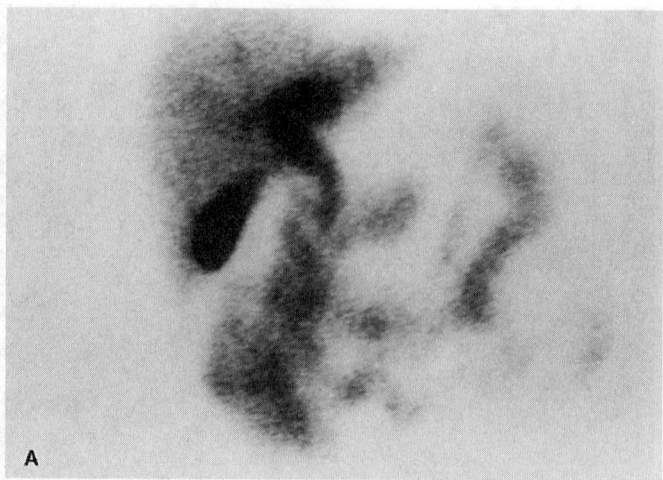

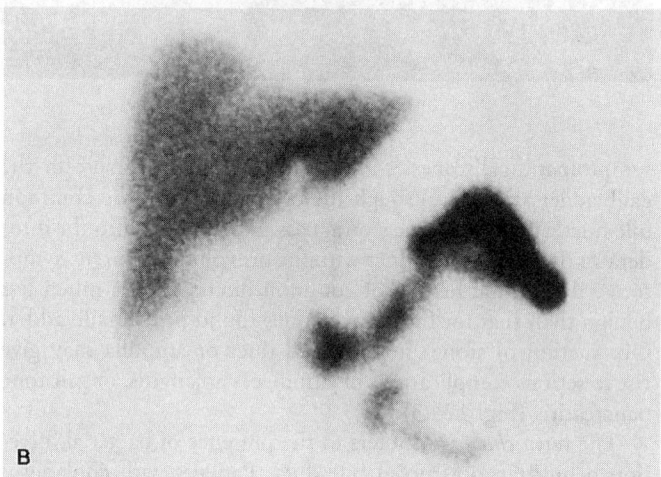

FIGURE 124.5. Hepatobiliary scintigraphy. **A:** Normal study at 60 minutes, showing the gallbladder, common bile duct, and small bowel. **B:** Abnormal study with no sign of the gallbladder. No effect was seen with morphine augmentation at 60 minutes in a patient with acute cholecystitis.

extraction or biliary stent placement is contemplated (Fig. 124.6).

■ TREATMENT OPTIONS

NONOPERATIVE TREATMENT

In the 1980s, considerable interest was generated in the evaluation of nonsurgical treatment strategies for gallstone disease. These efforts primarily consisted of attempts to dissolve the stones or to blast them into smaller fragments. The major drawback to these approaches was that they did not address or correct the underlying pathogenesis permanently. Hence, by leaving the original metabolic defects and gallbladder intact, nonoperative treatment methods were associated with high rates of long-term recurrence. These observations, in conjunction with the increasing popularity of laparoscopic cholecystectomy, eventually led to a decline in the demand and enthusiasm for nonsurgical alternatives. Nonoperative therapy now is limited to a highly select group of patients.

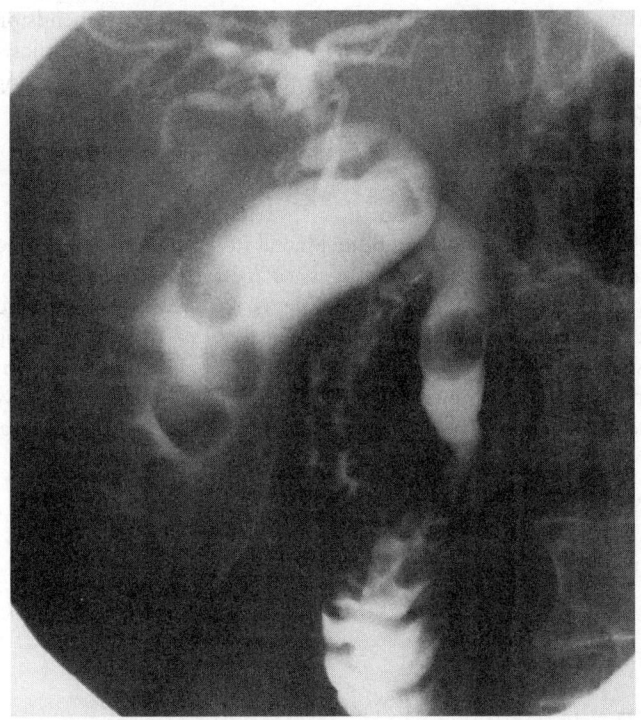

FIGURE 124.6. Endoscopic retrograde cholangiopancreatography examination showing both cholelithiasis and choledocholithiasis.

ORAL BILE ACID DISSOLUTION

Chenodeoxycholic acid, the first oral bile acid agent to be introduced for the dissolution of cholesterol gallstones, later was replaced by ursodiol (ursodeoxycholic acid) because of fewer side effects and greater efficacy. At a dosage of 8 to 10 mg per kilogram per day, ursodiol is thought to act by limiting the secretion of cholesterol in bile and by depleting or extracting cholesterol from nucleation-prone vesicles, multilamellar liposomes, and mature stones. Only 15% of patients with symptomatic, uncomplicated stone disease are potential candidates for this type of therapy. Prospective patients first undergo oral cholecystography to confirm cystic duct patency, adequate gallbladder function, and the size and number of stones. Ideally, the stones should be seen floating within the gallbladder and should measure less than 1 cm. Pigment stones or calcified stones are not amenable to this type of therapy.

The overall treatment efficacy varies greatly, but when appropriate selection criteria are adhered to strictly, dissolution rates range from 60% to 90%. Unfortunately, these successful results do not appear to hold up over time; nearly half the patients have stone recurrences within 5 years of therapy. Moreover, bile acid treatment is costly and lengthy, often requiring at least 6 to 12 months to complete.

CONTACT SOLVENTS

The instillation of contact solvents directly into the gallbladder has produced promising results in limited investigations. This technique uses a percutaneous transhepatic catheter or an endoscopically placed nasobiliary tube. The agent ethyl tert-butyl ether has received the most attention. It can be infused repeatedly and withdrawn through a catheter delivery system over several hours. This technique can be used to dissolve cholesterol stones in one or more sessions. Care must be taken to prevent the ether from leaking into the duodenum, where it can induce mucosal injury and can be absorbed into the systemic circulation. Nausea, vomiting, hemolysis, and renal injury have been reported with this form of therapy. Automated systems that rely on pressure sensors to prevent overdistention and spillover and other solvent candidates, such as ethylproprionate, also have been promoted for contact therapy. Direct dissolution therapy is still regarded as experimental.

EXTRACORPOREAL SHOCK WAVE LITHOTRIPSY

After the successes achieved in clearing renal calculi, shock wave lithotripsy was applied to the treatment of cholelithiasis. This approach uses high-energy shock waves to fracture stones into smaller bits and fragments. Shock wave pulses are generated and then targeted directly to a particular gallstone by a guiding ultrasonographic system. A functional gallbladder is mandatory, and ideally the stones should be few and small. Ursodiol is administered concomitantly to enhance the clearance rate of residual stone fragments. This technology is not approved by the Food and Drug Administration for the treatment of cholelithiasis. In the context of renal stone disease, shock wave lithotripsy can be used in selected patients to blast large common bile duct or pancreatic stones into fragments suitable for standard endoscopic removal.

LAPAROSCOPIC CHOLECYSTECTOMY

In a remarkably short time laparoscopic cholecystectomy has virtually replaced the traditional open approach to gallbladder resection. The potential advantages have been obvious, given the marked reduction in postoperative pain, shorter hospital stays, and more rapid return to usual activities and work. In fact, cholecystectomy rates were shown to rise from approximately 500,000 operations in 1987 to more than 700,000 in 1996. It has become clear that there is a substantial learning curve associated with laparoscopic surgery. The less experience and training a particular surgeon has, the higher the complication rate. In the context of laparoscopic cholecystectomy, cystic duct leaks and injuries to the common duct manifested by frank bile leakage or biliary obstruction have been seen with increasing frequency, at a rate of 0.95% versus 0.6% in open cholecystectomy. These observations have underscored the importance of establishing proper guidelines for training and granting credentials in the expanding field of laparoscopic surgery.

Conversion from a routine laparoscopic cholecystectomy to an open procedure is necessary in roughly 5% of cases, primarily when the anatomy is obscured, when the surgeon cannot retract the gallbladder or dissect it away because of inflammation or adhesions, or when there is excessive bleeding. Converting to an open approach under these circumstances reflects sound judgment and may serve to prevent a major bile duct injury or other complication. Patients who are not candidates for laparoscopic cholecystectomy include those who are in the last trimester of pregnancy and those who exhibit signs and symptoms of perforation, such as abscess, peritonitis, or fistula formation. End-stage liver disease with portal hypertension, severe coagulopathy, and suspected gallbladder malignancy are other contraindications.

OPTIMAL MANAGEMENT

Cholelithiasis is diagnosed in a variety of clinical circumstances. A patient may be asymptomatic, have a history of one or more uncomplicated biliary pain episodes, or have complications of acute cholecystitis, gangrene, jaundice, or even gallbladder cancer. Today, physicians and patients have myriad treatment op-

tions from which to choose. The optimal approach depends on the specific background and clinical circumstances. The following discussion highlights some of the salient features of treating patients with gallstone disease.

ASYMPTOMATIC STONES

Adult patients with silent or incidental stones should be observed and treated expectantly regardless of age or gender. The natural history of gallstones in these patients is generally benign, and the risk of a major complication is low. Moreover, warning symptoms of biliary pain usually manifest before a serious complication occurs, and there is no evidence to suggest that prophylactic cholecystectomy prolongs life expectancy. The potential

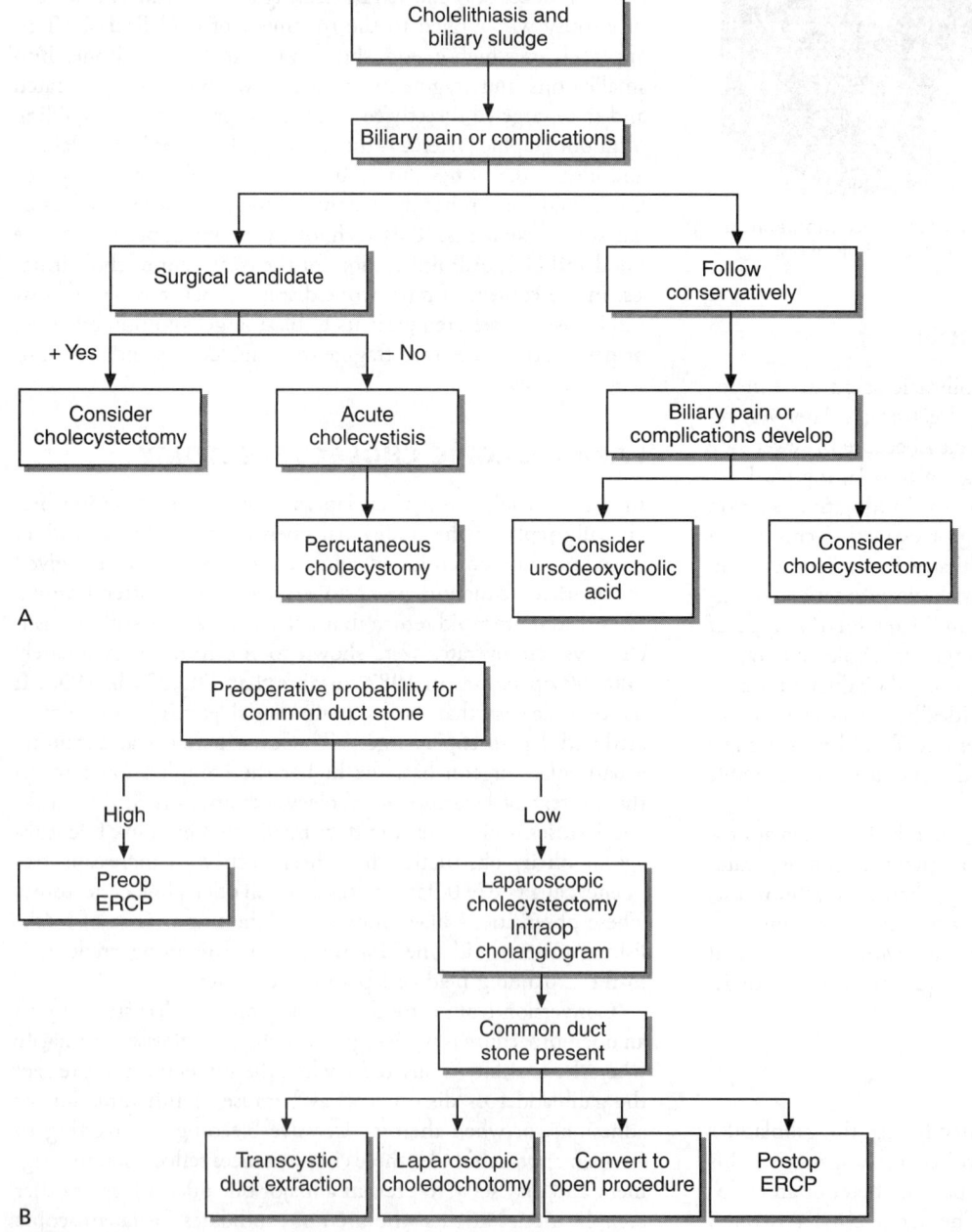

FIGURE 124.7. Management options for suspected choledocholithiasis. **A:** Cholelithiasis and biliary sludge. **B:** Preoperative probability of common duct stone.

exceptions to this recommendation relate to specific groups thought to be at higher risk of gallbladder carcinoma. These groups include individuals with calcified gallbladders (porcelain gallbladder), certain Native Americans, and perhaps patients with gallstones larger than 3 cm in size.

SYMPTOMATIC STONES

A patient with an episode of uncomplicated biliary pain has about a 30% to 50% chance of having a second attack within 1 to 2 years and approximately a 3% per year risk of complications. After the initial episode, however, as many as 30% of patients who are followed for the next 10 years will not experience further attacks. Therefore, the decision to proceed with laparoscopic cholecystectomy depends on the personal desires, attitudes, and surgical candidacy of each patient. For patients who do not want to risk the possibility of future attacks, laparoscopic cholecystectomy is recommended.

Nonoperative intervention, such as bile acid therapy, plays a limited role and is associated with a 50% recurrence rate. Moreover, it requires an initial oral cholecystogram to document adequate gallbladder function and subsequent follow-up ultrasonography studies. This costly and time-consuming form of therapy is best reserved for the symptomatic patient who declines surgery or is at high operative risk.

ACUTE CHOLECYSTITIS

Most physicians now agree that early laparoscopic cholecystectomy is indicated once the diagnosis of acute cholecystitis is secure and the patient's condition has been optimized. Selected patients are admitted, started on intravenous fluids and antibiotics, and then taken to laparoscopic surgery within 24 to 48 hours. Probably no more than one-third of the cases managed in this fashion have to be converted to an open procedure for technical reasons. Waiting longer than 72 hours increases the conversion rate to open cholecystectomy and the complication rate. For patients who have a major complication, such as a perforation, an urgent open laparotomy should be carried out. In addition, percutaneous cholecystostomy should be considered for patients with acute cholecystitis who are deemed to be at excessive risk for surgery (Fig. 124.7).

COMMON DUCT STONES

When a patient with known gallbladder stones has signs and symptoms of concomitant choledocholithiasis, the treating physician must select from among a variety of treatment options. The presence of obstructive jaundice, with or without fever and abdominal pain, generally leads to a preoperative ERCP examination with sphincterotomy and stone extraction, as indicated. Success rates for the endoscopic removal of common duct stones approach 90% to 95% in the hands of an expert surgeon; this procedure can be followed directly by routine laparoscopic cholecystectomy. A growing number of patients with a high probability of experiencing preoperative choledocholithiasis go directly to laparoscopic surgery. An experienced surgeon

cannulates the cystic duct to obtain a cholangiogram. If a common duct stone is present, it can be removed through the cystic duct with the use of choledochoscopes, balloon catheters, basket retrieval devices, or irrigation techniques. Success rates in most series range from 60% to 90%. If there is difficult biliary anatomy or the stone is too large, the common duct can be opened via a laparoscopic choledochotomy and then closed over a t-tube. Alternatively, the surgeon may elect to convert to an open common duct exploration or arrange for a postoperative ERCP (Fig. 124.7).

Whichever treatment option is ultimately pursued, it is important to stress that the chances for a successful clinical outcome are greatly enhanced by multidisciplinary participation and input. Any recommendations regarding the management of either suspected or confirmed choledocholithiasis depend largely on the local medical environment and the availability of appropriate radiologic, surgical, and endoscopic expertise.

BIBLIOGRAPHY

Hendry A, O'Leary JP. The history of cholelithiasis. *Am Surg* 1998;64: 801–802.
Howard DE, Fromm H. Nonsurgical management of gallstone disease. *Gastroenterol Clin North Am* 1999;28:133–144.
Hyser MJ, Chaudhry V, Byrne MP. Laparoscopic transcystic management of choledocholithiasis. *Am Surg* 1999;65:606–610.
Ko CW, Sekijima JH, Lee SP. Biliary sludge. *Ann Intern Med* 1999;130: 301–311.
Lanyi F. Percutaneous cholecystostomy: a valuable technique in high risk patients with presumed acute cholecystitis. *Br J Surg* 1996;83:428.
MacFadyen BV Jr, Passi RB. The Role of Endoscopic Retrograde Cholangiopancreatography in the Era of Laparoscopic Cholecystectomy. *Semin Laparosc Surg* 1997;4:18–22.
Ransohoff DF, Gracie WA. Treatment of gallstones. *Ann Intern Med* 1993; 119:606–619.
Rattner DW, Ferguson C, Warshaw AL. Factors associated with successful laparoscopic cholecystectomy for acute cholecystitis. *Ann Surg* 1993; 217:233–236.
Targarona EM, Marco C, Balague C, et al. How, when, and why bile duct injury occurs: a comparison between open and laparoscopic cholecystectomy. *Surg Endosc* 1998;12:322–326.
Tint GS, Dyrszka H, Sanghevi B, et al. Lithotripsy plus ursodiol is superior to ursodiol alone for cholesterol gallstones. *Gastroenterology* 1992;102: 2042–2049.

Kelley's Textbook of Internal Medicine, fourth edition. Edited by H. David Humes.
Lippincott Williams & Wilkins, Philadelphia © 2000.

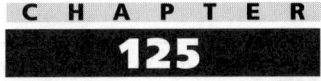

BILIARY TRACT DISEASE

JENNY HEATHCOTE

PRESENTATION

Biliary tract disease is often only intermittently symptomatic. In an asymptomatic patient, the clinician may have only abnormal results on liver biochemical tests (noted at the time of a routine checkup) to suggest that biliary tract disease is present (Chapter 104).

SYMPTOMS SUGGESTIVE OF BILIARY TRACT DISEASE

The three symptoms of right-sided upper quadrant pain, fever, and jaundice (Charcot's triad) suggest bacterial infection of the biliary tree, but symptoms of biliary tract disease are frequently intermittent and quickly forgotten (Table 125.1). Fever associated with rigors and chills may be transient and is often minimal, particularly in the elderly. Tachycardia and/or a high white blood cell count with neutrophilia may be all that indicates underlying infection. A history of biliary tract surgery in any patient with abdominal complaints should always prompt further investigation of the liver and biliary tract.

Dark urine and pale stools may be noted by patients just before the onset and during the course of jaundice. In the anicteric patient these symptoms are unreliable, since concentrated urine may appear dark and certain elements of dietary intake (e.g., lack of red meat) can produce stools that are paler than usual. Chalky white stools are seen only in the context of complete biliary obstruction, in which case obvious jaundice and symptoms of steatorrhea also will be present. Generalized pruritus, which is often most troublesome at night, may not be mentioned as a symptom by patients. There is no associated skin rash, and skin emollients or antihistamines bring only partial relief. Persistent severe pruritus causes secondary neurodermatitis. Sleep disturbance and severe emotional distress can be provoked by severe, prolonged pruritus.

Patients with biliary tract disease may have initial symptoms stemming from associated disorders, such as inflammatory bowel disease (IBD) and/or osteoporotic bone fractures in subjects with primary sclerosing cholangitis (PSC). Nephrolithiasis is associated with some congenital biliary disorders (Caroli's disease), and the appearance of kidney stones may precede that of the biliary disorder. Current excessive alcohol intake or a history of alcoholism can cause a silent form of chronic pancreatitis; abnormal results suggestive of biliary tract disease on biochemical testing may be the only indication of a biliary stricture resulting from chronic pancreatitis. A history of biliary tract surgery

TABLE 125.1.	BILIARY TRACT DISEASE
Symptoms	
Abdominal Pain	
Fever, chills, rigors	
Pruritus	
Jaundice	
Signs	
Fever	
Jaundice	
Weight loss	
Abdominal scars	

in a patient with blood tests indicating cholestasis suggests the possibility of strictures and/or recurrent stones.

EXAMINATION

PHYSICAL SIGNS OF BILIARY TRACT DISEASE

Not infrequently, biliary tract disease may be clinically silent for many years, and only laboratory tests indicate the presence of disease. In these cases, physical examination may yield normal findings. It is essential to examine closely any patient with a history suggestive of biliary tract disease, looking for signs of bacterial infection, including fever, tachycardia, and hypotension. Scleral icterus may not be obvious unless the patient is examined in natural light. Intermittent jaundice is not unusual in patients with incomplete biliary strictures or common bile duct stones and, occasionally, in patients who have lesions involving the ampulla of Vater. Overt jaundice stemming from biliary tract disease almost always is associated with weight loss. Hence, muscle wasting and loss of subcutaneous fat in the jaundiced patient does not necessarily indicate the presence of malignant disease, because profound malabsorption and/or maldigestion accompanying "benign" disease may do the same. Overwhelming intestinal parasitic infection causing weight loss and biliary obstruction is more commonly seen in the Far East than in North America. Abdominal scars from cholecystectomy may be quite small if surgery was performed laparoscopically. It is important to ascertain whether the patient with suspected biliary tract disease has undergone any previous gastric surgery, particularly since the presence of certain anastamoses may preclude endoscopic routes of investigation of the biliary tree.

Primary tumors of the hepatobiliary system usually are confined to the right-upper quadrant of the abdomen, but metastatic disease also can lead to biliary tract obstruction, particularly lymphoma and Kaposi's sarcoma. For this reason, lymphadenopathy should be sought, and the skin should be examined for lesions. It is unusual for systemic diseases to affect the biliary tract. In rare cases, symptoms mimicking sclerosing cholangitis can develop in patients with cystic fibrosis, paroxysmal hemoglobinuria, systemic mastocytosis, or retroperitoneal fibrosis. Acute cholecystitis has been described in patients with systemic vasculitis.

DIAGNOSTIC INVESTIGATIONS

Investigation of suspected biliary tract disease should begin with a complete blood count and serum alkaline phosphatase, γ-glutamyl transpeptidase, and total bilirubin levels (Fig. 125.1). It is wise to include testing for serum aminotransferase values (Chapter 104). It is essential to assess coagulation status, particularly when more invasive tests are planned; it may be profoundly, but reversibly affected by vitamin K deficiency stemming from obstructive jaundice.

It is rare for there to be clinically significant biliary tract disease when the liver biochemical test results are entirely normal, except in the case of a choledochal cyst. Even in patients with asymptomatic PSC and normal serum alkaline phosphatase

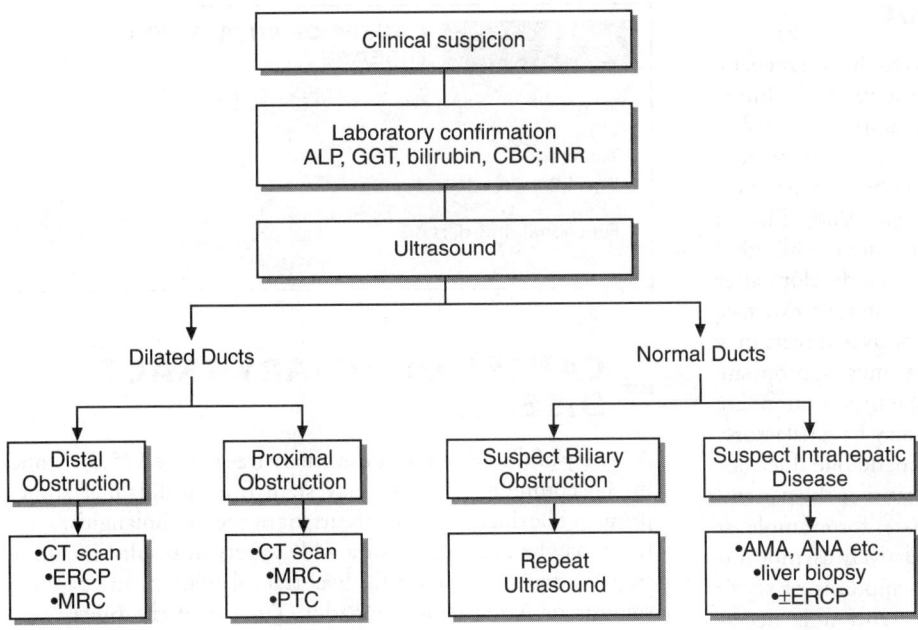

FIGURE 125.1. Investigative approach to biliary tract disease.

levels, it is usual for the γ-glutamyl transpeptidase level to be elevated. If the degree of hyperbilirubinemia does not correlate with the clinical picture, it may be worthwhile to fractionate the bilirubin, to assess whether the elevation is due in part to unconjugated bilirubin, which would cause more than the expected level of jaundice (Chapter 103).

Ultrasonography is the best noninvasive approach to examining the biliary tree. Overlying gas can impair interpretation, and the test may need to be repeated. If the clinical history is suggestive of extrahepatic biliary obstruction but ultrasonography does not show a dilated extrahepatic biliary system, it is necessary to conduct a second examination a week or so later. There are a number of conditions that cause biliary obstruction where dilatation of the ducts is either delayed or diminished (Table 125.2). The further investigation of patients suspected of having biliary tract disease very much depends on the results of ultrasonography, taken in concert with the clinical findings.

■ CARE OF THE PATIENT

DILATED COMMON BILE DUCT

In the icteric patient, a dilated common bile duct evident on ultrasonography most often implies biliary obstruction stemming from a stone, tumor, or stricture. Marked dilatation of the biliary tree in the absence of jaundice can be due to the same conditions, but the differential diagnosis would include choledochal cyst. The "post-cholecystectomy syndrome" and functional dysmotility of the biliary tree may be associated intermittently with mild common bile duct dilatation.

The finding of a dilated common bile duct on ultrasonography rarely provides a conclusive diagnosis, and further investigation is necessary in most but not all circumstances. For instance, the picture of a choledochal cyst on ultrasonography may be so typical that no further investigation before surgery is needed. In most instances, however, further analysis via magnetic resonance imaging (MRI) is advisable. If a pancreatic tumor is suspected, a computed tomographic (CT) scan would be the next appropriate investigation for staging. Should surgical intervention be contemplated, it is important to assess the patency of the portal vein (via ultrasonography) and nonocclusive venous involvement with a spiral CT scan.

In a patient with a history of cholecystectomy who subsequently is found to have common bile duct dilatation, MR cholangiography (MRC) is the next step; results of this test will decide if therapeutic endoscopy or surgery is required. Common bile duct stones are seen on ultrasonography only 50% of the time. Endoscopic retrograde cholangiopancreatography (ERCP) should be carried out only by a person trained to perform therapeutic procedures. If stones are present, papillotomy and stone removal will be necessary, and if a stricture is present, papillotomy followed by stent placement may be required. If the patient has stones in the gallbladder and common bile duct obstruction, immediate surgery may be appropriate, with examination of the common duct at the time of surgery. Most surgeons would recommend ERCP, papillotomy, and stone removal first—especially in the elderly. In young patients, subsequent laparoscopic cholecystectomy is required, whereas in the elderly or otherwise sick patient the option is to leave the gallstones alone and watch the patient.

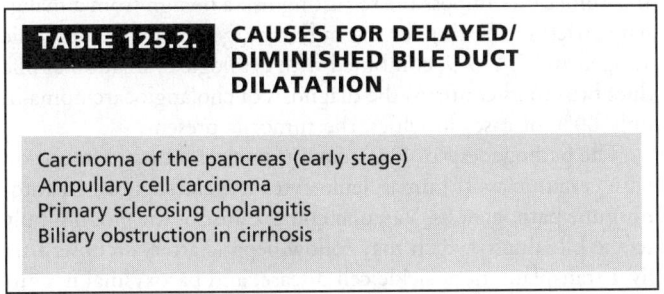

TABLE 125.2.	**CAUSES FOR DELAYED/ DIMINISHED BILE DUCT DILATATION**

Carcinoma of the pancreas (early stage)
Ampullary cell carcinoma
Primary sclerosing cholangitis
Biliary obstruction in cirrhosis

DILATED INTRAHEPATIC BILE DUCTS

When dilatation of the biliary tree is confined to the intrahepatic bile ducts, it generally indicates a tumor or stricture at the bifurcation of the common hepatic duct, for example, a Klatskin tumor if the patient is jaundiced. In rare cases, a gallbladder stone may erode through the cystic duct and obstruct the common hepatic duct high up (Mirizzi's syndrome). When dilation of the intrahepatic biliary tree is confined to one or the other side of the liver, intrahepatic stones, stricture that develops after cholecystectomy or, less often, a Klatskin tumor or extrinsic compression from hepatocellular carcinoma or liver abscess may be the cause. MRI plus MRC are probably the most appropriate investigations to define the specific diagnosis; if these options are not available, ultrasonography and CT scan may be satisfactory.

The best therapeutic approach to intrahepatic bile duct obstruction depends on the diagnosis and the status of the patient. On occasion, invasive therapy is inappropriate, for example, if the patient has an inoperable tumor but is relatively asymptomatic apart from jaundice. When there are symptoms of sepsis and/or pruritus, however, therapeutic intervention is necessary—even though surgery may be only palliative. Palliative procedures to the intrahepatic biliary tree can rarely be approached via ERCP; the percutaneous transhepatic approach is necessary unless surgical bypass or stenting is considered optimal. Curative procedures also can be conducted percutaneously—for example, removal of intrahepatic stones and stenting of benign biliary strictures—but surgical resection plus stone removal (when appropriate) may be the best choice, depending on the individual circumstances. It is therefore essential that there be adequate consultation between the surgical team and the interventional radiologists.

NORMAL BILE DUCTS

It can be very reassuring to find bile ducts that are of normal size on ultrasonography, but if this evidence does not fit the clinical picture, it is best to proceed further. A second ultrasonographic examination conducted after 2 weeks is generally sufficient to find conditions that may have delayed changes to bile duct size (Table 125.2). If any clinical suspicion remains, further delineation of the biliary tree via ERCP or MRC may be appropriate. There are, however, a number of conditions of intrahepatic cholestasis that may lead to initial symptoms suggestive of extrahepatic biliary obstructions—drug-induced jaundice being the most common. It may be difficult to be confident of the diagnosis in the case of patients who also are found to have gallstones on ultrasonography. Sepsis outside the biliary tree may cause persistent intrahepatic cholestasis with jaundice lasting several months (particularly in a patient with cirrhosis). MRC is the least invasive test to confirm a normal biliary tree, but it is not universally available. ERCP may be necessary in ambiguous cases. Liver biopsy may be helpful, but the pathologic characteristics are not always specific, for example, in the case of sepsis or drug-induced jaundice. In patients with anicteric cholestasis, it is useful to test for the autoantibodies [for example, antinuclear antibody, smooth muscle antibody (SMA) and antimitochondrial antibody (AMA)] before a liver biopsy.

TABLE 125.3.	CAUSES OF BILIARY TRACT DISEASE

Stones
Strictures
Tumors
Infections
Cysts
Functional disorders

CAUSES OF BILIARY TRACT DISEASE

A variety of disorders affect the biliary tree (Table 125.3). Stones in the common bile duct may stem from gallbladder stones, primary bile duct stones, or recurrent pyogenic cholangitis. Strictures may be due to PSC or a wide variety of insults, including surgery, trauma, pancreatitis, liver transplantation, and papillary stenosis or AIDS cholangiopathy. Tumors of the biliary tract include ampullary, pancreatic, and duodenal tumors; lymphoma; Kaposi's sarcoma; metastases; cholangiocarcinoma; and hepatocellular carcinoma (see Chapter 129). Among the infections that lead to biliary tract disease are bacterial cholangitis, parasitic invasion of the biliary tree, and liver abscess. Cysts (congenital choledochal cyst, Caroli's disease) also can lead to problems, as can such miscellaneous conditions as the so-called post-cholecystectomy syndrome, biliary dyskinesia, and hemobilia.

PRIMARY SCLEROSING CHOLANGITIS

PSC is likely an autoimmune disease that causes many strictures of the extra- and/or intrahepatic bile ducts. It is more common in males than females and can affect all ages from early childhood onwards. Because the disease is often asymptomatic and there are no specific serum markers, its true prevalence remains unknown. Between 50% and 70% of patients with PSC also have IBD, predominantly ulcerative colitis. The prevalence of PSC in patients with colitis is likely 5% to 10%, depending on the method of diagnosis. The main pathologic characteristic of this disease is progressive, irreversible fibrosis of the bile ducts, so that eventually the small intrahepatic ducts become obliterated and the larger ducts strictured and narrowed. There is an approximately 10% lifetime risk of cholangiocarcinoma in patients with PSC. It is sometimes impossible to distinguish a benign from a malignant stricture. Testing for the tumor antigens carcinoembryonic antigen and CA19-9, combined with cytologic evaluation of bile duct brushings confirms the diagnosis of cholangiocarcinoma in only 60% of cases in which the tumor is present.

The pathogenesis of PSC remains unclear, but an association with certain class II human leukocyte antigens suggests an autoimmune pathogenesis. Vascular compromise of the blood supply to the bile ducts, which may follow hepatic artery stenosis after liver transplantation, sickle cell disease, and paroxysmal nocturnal hemoglobinuria, can produce a strictured biliary tree almost indistinguishable from PSC. There is no evidence, however, that vasculitis is present in patients with PSC.

There is likely a long asymptomatic phase of PSC, and progression of the disease is slow. In one study, there was an 85% survival rate at 10 years for patients with asymptomatic PSC, whereas the 10-year survival rate in patients with symptomatic PSC was only 65%. In patients with associated IBD, there is a higher prevalence of colonic malignancy—greater than that seen in IBD not complicated by PSC. The diagnosis of PSC may precede that of IBD by many years. Alternatively, PSC may be noted only long after the initial diagnosis of IBD, even after total colectomy.

Symptoms include fatigue, right-upper-quadrant pain, and pruritus. Episodes of fever and chills suggest complicating bacterial cholangitis. Osteoporosis is frequently present, even in men. Occasionally, the pancreatic duct also is strictured, causing episodes of pancreatitis. The clinical course of PSC tends to be either recurrent episodes of cholangitis or slow, silent progression of cholestasis and liver fibrosis with eventual cirrhosis and liver failure. Portal hypertension develops early in the course of disease and may be present before the onset of cirrhosis as damage to the intrahepatic portal venous system in the portal triads takes place.

A complete blood count may show leukocytosis in those patients with an infected biliary system, and thrombocytopenia may complicate portal hypertension. The liver biochemical tests generally reflect cholestasis (see Chapter 104). The clinical, biochemical, and serologic pattern may be more in keeping with autoimmune hepatitis, particularly in children (elevation in serum aminotransferase levels, positive antinuclear antibody, and hypergammaglobulinemia). There are no biochemical or serologic tests specific to PSC. Rarely, thickened bile ducts are noted on ultrasonography, as is dilatation of the intrahepatic ducts. Until recently the diagnostic test of choice for this disease was ERCP (Fig. 125.2), but improvements in MRI technology indicate that MRC is equally reliable with high-quality machines (see Chapter 13). Liver biopsy is not a helpful diagnostic tool, but it is used to determine whether cirrhosis is present. Biopsies

from both lobes may be necessary, since the intrahepatic ducts can be affected unequally.

The management of PSC should include preventative, symptomatic, and therapeutic maneuvres. Preventive measures include checking for the presence of esophageal varices and using pharmacologic prophylaxis to lessen the chance of variceal hemorrhage. Bone mineral density should be checked regularly, and appropriate supplementation with calcium and vitamin D_3 (ergocalciferol) should be provided, as well as specific therapy for osteoporosis if necessary. There is no effective therapy for the fatigue associated with this disease. Pruritus usually can be controlled with the anion exchange resin cholestyramine. Patients who suffer recurrent bouts of bacterial cholangitis always should have a prescription for oral antibiotics on hand and carry the drug when traveling, since death from septicemia can occur within a few hours. No specific therapy has been shown to be helpful in the treatment of PSC. Dominant common duct strictures may benefit from balloon dilatation and stenting, but prolonged stent placement is not advised because any foreign body is a source of sepsis. Progressive hyperbilirubinemia in the absence of sepsis suggests the presence of complicating cholangiocarcinoma or simply progressive disease—the two may be very difficult to distinguish.

Randomized, controlled trials of the hydrophilic, dihydroxy bile acid ursodeoxycholic acid have shown that treatment improves serum biochemical test parameters without improving survival rates. Because the nature of this disease is fibrous stricturing of all the bile ducts, it is likely that medical therapy will be ineffective unless it is instituted very early in the course of the disease, before biliary stricturing and symptoms develop. Repeated therapeutic dilatation of strictures of the extrahepatic biliary tree are thought by some investigators to improve the course of this disease. There is, however, a significant risk of introducing infection into the biliary system with each invasive procedure. Since the only cure for this disease at present is liver transplantation and septicemia would preclude transplantation, septicemia is to be avoided at all costs. The post-transplant mortality rate for PSC patients is greatest in the first 3 months after surgery; death is mainly due to sepsis.

Survival rates for PSC patients after liver transplantation are higher than for patients with any other chronic liver disease. Recurrence of PSC in the transplanted liver is seen, but not to a degree that precludes consideration of liver transplantation. If a patient with PSC is found to have complicating cholangiocarcinoma at the time of transplantation, the procedure must be abandoned—the postoperative prognosis is very poor in this situation. Hence, there is a great need to develop more accurate tests to diagnose cholangiocarcinoma before liver transplantation. Colonoscopic surveillance for colorectal carcinoma in patients with associated colitis must continue after transplantation.

■ SECONDARY BILIARY STRICTURES

POSTOPERATIVE AND TRAUMATIC STRICTURE

Postoperative biliary strictures occur most frequently after cholecystectomy. If these strictures are recognized immediately after

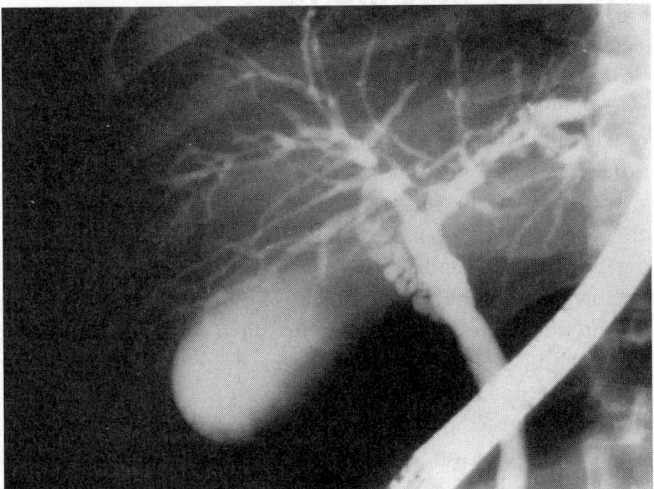

FIGURE 125.2. Endoscopic retrograde cholangiopancreatography (ERCP) in a patient with primary sclerosing cholangitis (PSC).

surgery and are incomplete, ERCP and temporary stent placement may be all that is necessary. Surgical repair is essential if complete ligation or transection of the bile duct is present and may be necessary with incomplete occlusion if enough time has elapsed that significant fibrous stricturing not amenable to balloon dilatation has taken place. The same approach applies to traumatic strictures.

STRICTURES RESULTING FROM PANCREATITIS

Narrowing of the biliary tree early in the course of acute pancreatitis is not unusual and generally improves spontaneously as the edema and inflammation of the pancreas resolve. Much more subtle is biliary stricture that complicates chronic alcohol-induced pancreatitis (see Chapter 123). The strictures are generally long and not amenable to therapeutic endoscopic manipulations, and corrective surgery may be necessary.

HEPATIC ARTERY THROMBOSIS AFTER LIVER TRANSPLANTATION

When the diagnosis of hepatic artery thrombosis is made within 1 week of placement of the allograft, re-transplantation is generally in order because of graft failure. Many strictures of the biliary tree result from the ischemic injury. Occasionally, they can be managed by bile duct reconstruction, but more often patients require retransplantation.

AIDS CHOLANGIOPATHY

Liver test abnormalities are found frequently in individuals infected with HIV. Biochemical alterations suggestive of icteric cholestasis most often are due to papillary stenosis with or without associated cholangiopathy, though they may be due to infiltration of the liver with tumor or opportunistic infections. AIDS cholangiopathy is seen only in patients with a very low CD4 count and takes the form of jaundice, often associated with pruritus. Leukopenia is the rule, particularly in patients whose cholangiopathy is due to cytomegalovirus infection. Ultrasonographic examination of the liver shows thickened and mildly dilated extra- and sometimes intrahepatic bile ducts (the pattern is very different from that seen with PSC). Symptomatic treatment for pruritus may be helpful. Papillotomy has been advocated when papillary stenosis is present.

◼ TUMORS AFFECTING THE BILIARY TREE

Malignant tumors external to the biliary tree may cause narrowing of the tree by invasion (metastases, lymphoma, Kaposi's sarcoma), by intermittent obstruction (ampullary cell carcinoma), or by circumferential compression (carcinoma of the pancreas or the duodenum). The clinical pictures are similar regardless of the source of the malignancy, including progressive jaundice,

pruritus, and weight loss. Involvement of the duodenum may cause upper small-bowel obstruction. It is most unusual for a malignant biliary stricture to be accompanied by cholangitis unless an invasive procedure, such as ERCP or PTC, is carried out. Pain may not always be present. After cholestatic signs have been identified on biochemical tests, the clue to diagnosis is a dilated bile duct system evident on ultrasonography. Abdominal nodes or a mass also may be seen. If a malignant tumor is suspected, it is best to stage the tumor with noninvasive imaging (for example, by CT scan with or without MRI) before undertaking any invasive procedure. Tissue diagnosis via so-called skinny needle aspiration is generally not appropriate because of the risk of pancreatitis or tumor seeding. It may be useful to plan alternative therapy, however, in the patient with an obviously incurable carcinoma of the pancreas. Direct visualization via upper panendoscopy is the appropriate diagnostic test if an ampullary or duodenal tumor is suspected from the history (intermittent biliary obstruction in the case of ampullary tumors or symptoms of upper small-bowel obstruction in the case of duodenal tumors).

Gastrointestinal Kaposi's lesions may be found at endoscopy in the patient at risk. Ampullary carcinoma may be diagnosed when it is still very small, causing only an intermittent biliary obstruction; unfortunately, however, this tumor more often is diagnosed late in its course. The early-stage lesion may not be seen on noninvasive radiologic imaging, and only very careful ERCP with good drainage pictures taken after the endoscope has been removed will confirm the diagnosis. Primary lymphoma within the pancreas is rare. Lymphomatous nodes in the portal tract in a patient with previously diagnosed lymphoma are more typically the cause of biliary obstruction. In young patients with night sweats, weight loss, and a small tumor mass seen on ultrasonographic or CT scan, a pancreatic mass might be a lymphoma and not the more common adenocarcinoma.

◼ INFECTIONS OF THE BILIARY TREE

BACTERIAL CHOLANGITIS

Bacterial cholangitis occurs only when there is impaired bile flow in the large bile ducts. Bacteria are found frequently in normal bile, and thus bacterial cholangitis may develop very rapidly after the onset of biliary obstruction. The patient may experience only short-lived symptoms before going into septic shock and may be unable to give a history on arrival in the emergency room. In a septic patient, laboratory findings suggesting obstructive jaundice and evidence of an abnormal biliary tree on ultrasonography (often with intrahepatic dilatation with or without stones) are enough to initiate urgent therapeutic ERCP and/or PTC. At the other end of the spectrum, it is not unusual for patients (generally the elderly) to have very nonspecific symptoms, though the blood glucose in diabetic patients will be out of control. In this situation abnormal liver biochemistry values with cholestatic features should prompt immediate investigation. If the biliary obstruction is confined to either the right or the left duct system, jaundice will be absent; cholangitis commonly is missed under these circumstances.

PARASITIC INVOLVEMENT OF THE BILIARY TRACT

Ascariasis, liver flukes, and ecchinococcus may all involve the biliary tree. Ascariasis is most common in areas of the world where hygienic conditions are substandard. Overwhelming gastrointestinal infection often is present when the biliary tract is affected. For this reason, symptoms of vomiting, abdominal cramps, and obstructive jaundice generally predominate. If endoscopic diagnosis cannot be made, a barium study will easily identify the worms, whose gastrointestinal tracts also take up barium. Therapy is with mebendazole or pyrantel pamoate.

In the Far East liver flukes are due to infection with *Clonorchis sinensis* and in the West to *Fasciola hepaticum*. Both are acquired from eating raw fish or fresh water. Patients experience right-upper-quadrant pain, fever, and possibly jaundice. The initial symptoms often are missed. In the case of *Clonorchis* infection, the diagnosis generally is made only when the parasites have induced chronic biliary tract inflammation and stricturing, which then causes bacterial cholangitis and/or intrahepatic stone disease. The primary infection responds well to common antiparasitic agents, for example, praziquantel.

It is unusual but not unknown for hydatid cysts to invade the biliary tree and provoke symptoms of biliary obstruction. Hydatid cyst disease within the liver always will be evident; depending on the age of the cysts, calcification may or may not be present. Hydatid disease is seen only in persons from rural areas where hygiene is poor and where animal (sheep, goat, moose) offal is fed to dogs and contamination of human food with dog feces has taken place. Ultrasonography is most helpful in identifying hydatid cysts. If these cysts are present in the biliary tree, surgery will be necessary once active infection has been eradicated. Percutaneous aspiration with a scolicidal agent (e.g., 95% alcohol) is being used with increasing frequency. Antiparasitic agents (e.g., abendazole) is only 40% effective.

LIVER ABSCESS

A liver abscess may be bacterial, amoebic, or fungal. The patient may have acute symptoms of severe right-upper-quadrant pain, fever, and mild jaundice or chronic symptoms of anorexia, weight loss, and mild fever and fatigue. Liver abscess due to bacterial infection spreads from the biliary tree, a colonic diverticulum, or an appendiceal abscess in two of three cases. In one-third of cases, no primary source is found. Unless the patient is immunocompromised, marked leukocytosis is present, and derangement of liver biochemistry values may be mild. In chronic cases it is usual for normocytic normochromic anemia and hypoalbuminemia to be present. Ultrasonography is the diagnostic test of choice. There may be a single or several abscesses. If there is a single abscess larger than 2 cm, aspiration and culture of the material should be undertaken and intravenous antibiotics given. When the abscesses are small and there are several, appropriate broad-spectrum intravenous antibiotics may be the only possible treatment, and the treatment may be prolonged. The prognosis of this once commonly fatal infection is now much improved, owing to excellent tissue penetration of the new antibacterial agents. Liver abscess may stem from intrahepatic stones or hepatic artery thrombosis after transplantation (Chapter 132).

Amoebic liver abscess is prevalent in parts of the world where amoebic dysentery is common. Right-upper-quadrant pain may be acute and severe enough to cause "splinting" of the diaphragm. The initial dysenteric infection itself may have gone unnoticed or been forgotten. "Punch" tenderness of the lower ribs is often detectable on the right side of the body. Confirmation with ultrasonography and immediate aspiration under ultrasonographic guidance are appropriate. The fluid obtained is said to look like anchovy sauce, since it is not pus but liquefied liver. Aspiration of all the contents is necessary, and it is the last aspiration that needs to be examined immediately under the microscope, because the amoeba hide in the wall of the abscess. Bacterial superinfection is typical, so culture of the aspirated material is necessary. Treatment with oral metronidazole (very well absorbed from the upper gastrointestinal tract) is sufficient for the abscess, but the bowel also must be treated with a 20-day course of Iodoquinol to completely eradicate the amoeba. Resolution of disease is generally rapid.

CYSTIC LIVER DISEASE OF THE BILIARY TREE

CONGENITAL CHOLEDOCHAL CYSTS

Congenital choledochal cysts most often develop in childhood and symptoms are likely prompted by proteinacious plugs; they are evidenced by abdominal pain, with or without fever and jaundice. These cysts also may be entirely asymptomatic and may be found at the time of abdominal ultrasonography conducted for an unrelated condition. Any part of the biliary tree may be involved. Surgical removal is mandatory, because malignancy complicates at least 10% of cases.

CAROLI'S DISEASE

Caroli's disease is a rare disorder of the biliary system, causing congenital cystic dilatation of the extrahepatic biliary tree. It is likely part of a spectrum of bile duct plate abnormalities that are responsible for polycystic liver disease and congenital hepatic fibrosis. It is common to find abnormalities of the kidneys as well—most often medullary sponge kidneys with or without nephrocalcinosis. Impairment of renal function may be present before any hepatobiliary abnormalities are recognized. Recurrent cholangitis complicates this disease. Liver fibrosis and hepatic decompensation may necessitate liver transplantation.

MISCELLANEOUS

Recurrent right-upper-quadrant pain after cholecystectomy suggests (a) that the original disorder for which the gallbladder was removed was not due to the patient's gallstones (e.g., irritable bowel syndrome/hepatic flexure syndrome) or (b) that there is recurrent biliary tract disease. Abnormal serum aminotransferase and/or alkaline phosphatase values suggest the latter possibility, in which case it is mandatory to examine the biliary tree. The post-cholecystectomy syndrome is considered only when common duct stones and biliary stricture have been ruled out. High intraluminal pressures are often recorded within the bile duct and are thought to be due to sphincter of Oddi dysfunction. Relief of symptoms may follow sphincterotomy. Such biliary dyskinesia may develop without previous cholecystectomy and is considered a functional motility problem of the biliary tree.

HEMOBILIA

Rarely, liver biopsy or trauma to the liver results in bleeding into the biliary tree, which causes severe right-upper-quadrant pain, anemia, and the passage of "silver" stools. If the bleeding does not stop spontaneously, surgical intervention and/or arterial embolization may be required. Extraction of the clot via endoscopy and a papillotomy are usually sufficient.

BIBLIOGRAPHY

Beuers U, Spengler U, Sackmann M, et al. Deterioration of cholestasis after endoscopic retrograde cholangiography in advanced primary sclerosing cholangitis. *J Hepatol* 1992;15:140–143.

Broome U, Olsson R, Loof L, et al. Natural history and prognostic factors in 305 Swedish patients with primary sclerosing cholangitis. *Gut* 1996; 38:610–615.

Broome U, Lofberg R, Veress B, et al. Primary sclerosing cholangitis and ulcerative colitis: evidence for increased neoplastic potential. *Hepatololgy* 1995;22:1404–1408.

Cello JP. The acquired immunodeficiency syndrome cholangiopathy: spectrum of disease. *Am J Med* 1989;86:539–546.

Davidson BR. Progress in determining the nature of bile duct strictures. *Gut* 1993;34:725–726.

Geenen JE, Hogan WJ, Dodds WJ, et al. The efficacy of endoscopic sphincterectomy after cholecystectomy in patients with sphincter of Oddi dysfunction. *N Engl J Med* 1989;320:82–87.

Kaneko K, Ardo H, Ho T, et al. Protein plugs cause symptoms in patients with choledochal cysts. *Am J Gastroenterol* 1997;92:1018–1021.

Lindor KD for the Mayo Primary Sclerosing Cholangitis–Ursodeoxycholic Acid Study Group. Ursodial for primary sclerosing cholangitis. *N Engl J Med* 1997;336:691–695.

Nashan B, Schlitt HJ, Tusch G, et al. Biliary malignancies in primary sclerosing cholangitis: timing for liver transplantation. *Hepatology* 1996; 23:1105–1111.

Rotstein LE, Makowka L, Harvey JC, et al. Caroli's disease: case report and management recommendation. *Can Med Assoc J* 1981;25:268, 273–274.

Sela-Herman S, Scharschmidt BF. Choledochal cyst: a disease for all ages. *Lancet* 1996;347:779.

Stiehl A, Rudolph G, Sauer P, et al. Efficacy of ursodeoxycholic acid treatment and endoscopic dilation of major duct stenoses in primary sclerosing cholangitis: an 8-year prospective study. *J Hepatol* 1997;26: 560–566.

Wiesner RH, Grambsch PM, Dickson ER, et al. Primary sclerosing cholangitis: natural history, prognostic factors and survival analysis. *Hepatology* 1989;10:430–436.

Kelley's Textbook of Internal Medicine, fourth edition. Edited by H. David Humes. Lippincott Williams & Wilkins, Philadelphia © 2000.

HEPATOBILIARY NEOPLASMS

ANDREW STOLZ

PRIMARY MALIGNANT HEPATIC NEOPLASMS

DEFINITION

Primary hepatocellular carcinoma (HCC), a malignant transformation of hepatocytes, is a well-recognized complication of longstanding liver disease of numerous causes, including alcohol abuse, chronic viral infection, toxin exposure, and inherited metabolic disorders. The diagnosis usually is made by percutaneous liver biopsy and histologic evaluation. Because HCC occurs in the context of chronic liver injury, small tumors can be difficult to differentiate from regenerating nodules and hepatic fibrosis associated with cirrhosis. Besides liver histologic examination, hepatic imaging by radiographic and ultrasonographic techniques and serum markers associated with HCC aid in identifying potential tumors.

INCIDENCE AND EPIDEMIOLOGY

Worldwide the incidence of HCC is correlated directly with the prevalence of chronic hepatitis B virus (HBV) infection. Vertical transmission at birth is the major factor contributing to the high incidence of chronic HBV infection, which is found in the distinct geographic locations of Southeast Asia, Japan, Korea, sub-Saharan Africa, and Alaska (among Native North Americans). With recognition of this mode of transmission and the availability of hyperimmune serum and effective vaccines against HBV, the incidence of HBV-associated HCC is predicted to decline significantly within the next one to two generations. In the United States and Europe, long-term alcohol abuse, alone or in combination with hepatitis C virus (HCV) co-infection, is associated with necro-inflammatory liver injury and recognized as a risk factor for HCC. Metabolic disorders, such as hemochromatosis, excess iron storage, tyrosinemia, α_1-antitrypsin deficiency disease, Wilson's disease, and type Ia glycogen storage disease, are other important risk factors for HCC. For unknown reasons, men are at increased risk for HCC stemming from all conditions in which cirrhosis develops, including chronic HBV infection. Exposure to the mycotoxin aflatoxin B1, a by-product of *Aspergillus flavus* and *Aspergillus parasiticus*, which infect grains, rice, and peanuts; C-17-alkylated androgenic steroids; estrogen; Thorotrast (a radiographic contrast agent used from the 1920s to the early 1950s); or vinyl chloride is also recognized as carrying the risk of HCC (Table 126.1).

TABLE 126.1. CONDITIONS PREDISPOSING TO THE DEVELOPMENT OF HEPATOCELLULAR CARCINOMA

Infections
   Chronic HBV infection
   Chronic HCV infection
Hereditary diseases
   Hemochromatosis
   α_1-Antitrypsin deficiency
   Hereditary tyrosinemia
   Glycogen storage disease (type I)
   Wilson's disease
Environmental hazards
Drugs
   Aflatoxin
   Chronic ethanol abuse
   Thorotrast
   ?Estrogens

HBV, hepatitis B virus; HCV, hepatitis C virus.
(From Schirmacher P, Rogler CE, Dienes HP. Current pathogenetic and molecular concepts in viral liver carcinogenesis. *Virchows Arch B Cell Pathol* 1994;63:71, with permission.)

PATHOGENESIS

Although the precise pathogenetic mechanisms involved in the development of HCC are not fully understood, advances in molecular biology and toxicology are helping identify critical steps required for HCC formation. Chronic inflammation of any cause exposes the liver to genotoxic free radicals, which presumably leads to a series of mutations culminating in HCC formation. In HBV infection, random integration throughout the host genome produces genetic instability, increasing the chance for a mutational event. Epidemiologic studies have shown that coinfection with HCV significantly contributes to the development of HCC in the context of chronic alcoholic liver injury. Hemochromatosis and other excess iron storage diseases, such as sporadic porphyria cutanea tarda, also are associated with a high risk of HCC, presumably because of increased free radical formation caused by excess iron. Metabolic disorders, such as Wilson's disease, type Ia glycogen storage disease, and tyrosinemia, are other examples of HCC-associated disease postulated to be mediated by free radical formation.

CLINICAL FEATURES

The clinical characteristics of HCC depend in part on the presence of an associated chronic liver disease. Patients may have nonspecific symptoms related to chronic liver disease, such as fatigue, jaundice, and weight loss, or they may complain of right-upper-quadrant pain. Occasionally, a liver mass is detected by self-palpation. On physical examination, there may be clinical evidence of chronic liver disease, such as ascites, peripheral edema, muscle wasting, and jaundice. Hepatomegaly caused by a mass or a firm, cirrhotic liver with discrete nodules may be found. A right-upper-quadrant vascular bruit can be heard, and dilated abdominal veins indicating portal hypertension may be found. Occasionally, HCC takes the form of a Budd-Chiari-like

syndrome—acute onset of progressive ascites without peripheral edema. HCC should be sought in patients with chronic liver disease who have hepatic decompensation with no identifiable precipitating factor.

On histologic examination, HCC looks like a liver cell cord-like structure (trabecular pattern) composed of hepatocytes of varying dedifferentiation and cytologic features. HCC is an aggressive tumor, with a median survival time of 7.1 months in one study. Fibrolamellar HCC (FL-HCC) is a distinct clinicopathologic variant of HCC with a less aggressive clinical course. On histologic evaluation, FL-HCC is composed of lamellar strands of fibrosis (typically absent in HCC) surrounding pseudoglands and cords of malignant cells. FL-HCC accounts for only 1% to 2% of all cases of HCC but up to half the cases diagnosed in patients younger than 40 years of age. FL-HCC usually is not accompanied by cirrhosis, has no male predominance, and is associated with a 50% 5-year survival rate. These tumors fail to secrete the tumor marker α-fetoprotein (AFP), which is associated with HCC, and can be treated by surgical resection or liver transplantation. The absence of cirrhosis and lack of association with chronic inflammatory liver diseases suggest a different pathophysiologic course for FL-HCC.

LABORATORY FINDINGS

Routine laboratory tests for liver injury and function; serum markers for specific diseases, such as hepatitis B and C, Wilson's disease (ceruloplasmin), and hemochromatosis (iron/total iron-binding capacity, ferritin); and α_1-antitrypsin are used in the evaluation of HCC. Serum HCC tumor markers, most notably AFP, also can be measured. Routine serum tests of liver injury assess levels of aspartate aminotransferase and alanine aminotransferase, which are markers for hepatocellular injury; alkaline phosphatase, which is elevated in infiltrative liver diseases or cholestatic injuries caused by obstruction of the biliary tree and is associated with elevation in γ-glutamyl transpeptidase, 5'-nucleotidase, or leucine aminopeptidase; bilirubin, which reflects the excretory capacity of the liver and the patency of major bile ducts; and albumin and clotting factors, which reflect the synthetic capacity of the liver. Polycythemia, hypercalcemia, and hypoglycemia also have been reported in the context of HCC stemming from the release of tumor-generated hormones. The development of a normal hematocrit in a previously anemic patient with cirrhosis may be the initial sign of HCC.

Serum Markers of Hepatocellular Carcinoma

Besides routine serum tests for liver disease, secreted HCC tumor markers can be used to detect disease and assess response to treatment. AFP, a glycosylated serum protein, usually is expressed exclusively during fetal development and declines gradually in the first year of life. Normally, less than 10 ng per milliliter is present in the serum. Other liver diseases, such as active viral hepatitis and cirrhosis, also may be associated with elevated AFP levels (10 to 100 ng per milliliter). In addition, higher serum levels have been reported during the course of aggressive viral hepatitis. Germline cell tumors, seminomas, ovarian and testicular teratomas, and, rarely, gastric and gallbladder carcinomas also secrete AFP.

AFP levels are elevated in 60% to 70% of all patients with HCC, and values above 400 ng per milliliter are uniquely associated with HCC. The percentage of HCC tumors that secrete AFP rises with tumor size, limiting the usefulness of this test in identifying tumors less than 2 cm in diameter, which have the best prognosis. AFP levels can be monitored after resection or other treatment of HCC to assess recurrence. In contrast to HCC, FL-HCC is not associated with increased serum AFP levels but with enhanced unsaturated B_{12} binding capacity. The use of AFP as a screening test for HCC should be reserved for patients with documented risk factors. Other serum tumor markers, such as carcinoembryonic antigen and C-19-9, also may be elevated in HCC, but they are nonspecific and also are found in patients with pancreatic, colonic, and biliary tumors.

Radiographic Evaluation

Radiographic evaluation is used to identify and characterize the features of a liver tumor, to direct percutaneous biopsy, and to assess the extent of disease. In a patient with proven HCC, radiographic imaging pinpoints the number of lesions and the

extent of liver resection necessary to effect a cure. The strategy for tumor evaluation depends on many factors, including cost and the availability of sophisticated radiographic equipment and experienced radiologists (Fig. 126.1). For the initial evaluation, ultrasonography (US) is widely available and can distinguish discrete nodules as small as 1 cm, especially those surrounded by a capsule. US can be used to locate intrahepatic metastasis and to guide percutaneous needle biopsy if hemangioma has been excluded. Alternatively, routine abdominal computed tomography (CT) can be carried out to evaluate the liver and the remainder of the abdominal cavity and to direct biopsy of suspicious lesions.

If an HCC nodule is found and resection is considered, or if there is a clinical suspicion of HCC but US or routine CT fails to confirm a tumor, rapid dynamic CT scanning coupled with intravenous infusion of contrast agents, known as helical CT (HCT), can facilitate the detection of small nodules in the liver. Besides increasing the sensitivity of detection of small tumors, HCT can image the portal and hepatic venous drainage systems, which often are the sites of intrahepatic metastasis. The addition of dynamic scanning to CT improved the sensitivity of detection of HCC from 35% to 81% in one study. Magnetic resonance imaging also can be used to complement HCT and

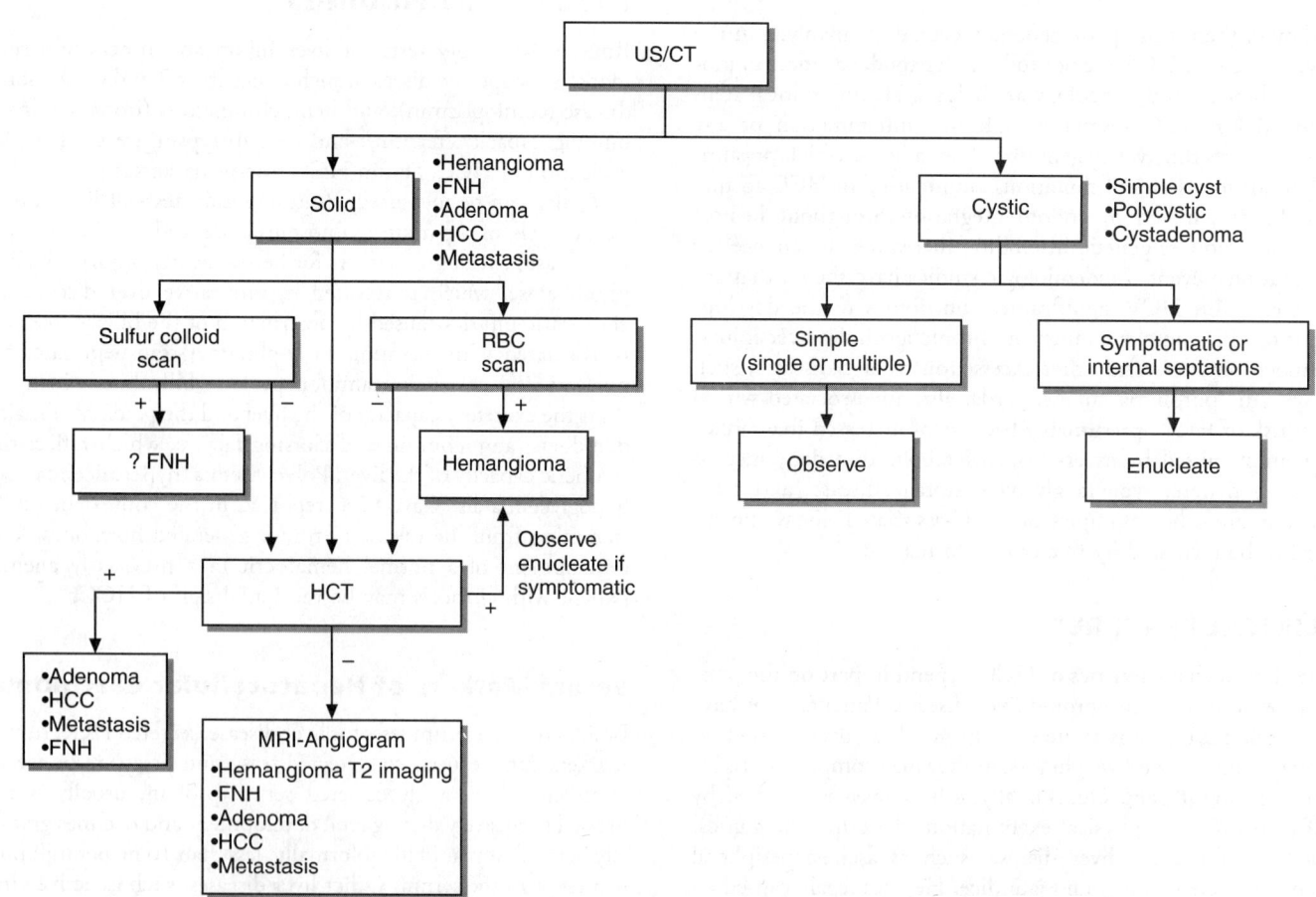

FIGURE 126.1. Evaluation and management of a liver mass. CT, computed tomography; HCT, helical computed tomography; FNH, focal nodular hyperplasia; HCC, hepatocellular carcinoma; MRI, magnetic resonance imaging; RBC, red blood cell; US, ultrasound. (From Jenkins RL, Johnson LB, Lewis WD. Surgical approach to benign liver tumors. *Semin Liver Dis* 1994;14:178–189, with permission.)

is especially useful for the detection of hemangiomas and fatty liver infiltrates and for patients with documented iodine allergy or renal insufficiency. When carried out by an experienced radiologist, this technique may be as sensitive as HCT for the detection of small hepatic nodules. Angiography is used only when other imaging methods have failed to pinpoint a lesion or to assess the vascular anatomy before resection. Intraoperative US remains the most sensitive technique for the detection of nodules smaller than 2 cm in diameter. It is recommended that imaging studies be repeated in 3 to 6 months for patients suspected of having HCC but in whom a tumor cannot be found.

OPTIMAL MANAGEMENT

Early detection and resection offer the best chance for cure, because incidental HCC found in resected liver after liver transplantation has the most favorable prognosis. Early detection of HCC nodules smaller than 2 cm followed by surgical resection for those patients with adequate hepatic reserve is the optimal approach for definitive cure, with a 5-year survival rate of 85% reported in one study. Five-year survival rates varying from 30% to 50% have been documented in other studies, depending on the size of the resected liver and the presence of underlying liver disease. US screening every 6 months in patients with longstanding cirrhosis (or every 3 months for patients with elevated AFP levels) is essential for early detection of disease. Because HCC develops in the context of chronic liver disease and metastasizes early in its course, careful preoperative evaluation is essential, to ensure that the patient can tolerate resection without experiencing liver failure or death from unsuspected extrahepatic or metastatic foci within the remaining liver. Occasionally, the extent of disease can be determined only at surgery; intraoperative US is the best technique for identifying small HCC nodules. For clinical situations in which resection is not feasible because of widespread disease, poor hepatic reserve, or evidence of metastatic foci, other noncurative therapeutic options are available, including intra-arterial chemo-embolization, percutaneous alcohol injection of the tumor, and cryosurgical ablation. In several case reports, these procedures significantly reduced tumor size and increased life expectancy.

With improvements in surgical technique and the development of effective therapy for organ rejection, orthotopic liver transplantation has been used successfully to treat HCC. The prognosis is best for patients who have incidental tumors and worst for those who have documented HCC before resection. Patients with cirrhosis who have nodules less than 2 cm in diameter have the best outcomes, but such cases are rare. Only certain patients with small HCC nodules who have no evidence of vascular invasion are candidates for transplantation. Orthotopic liver transplantation has been used in the context of unresectable FL-HCC because these slow-growing tumors appear in noncirrhotic livers, do not metastasize as early as HCC, and affect a younger population of patients. Recurrent disease after transplantation has been found in patients with FL-HCC, but survival is prolonged because of the slow progression of the disease. Adjuvant chemotherapy at the time of orthotopic liver transplantation may limit the development of metastatic disease. In patients with inherited metabolic disorders of childhood, such as

tyrosinemia or type Ia glycogen storage disease, transplantation before the development of liver failure and HCC also may be indicated.

BENIGN HEPATIC TUMORS

DEFINITION

There are several benign hepatic tumors composed of hepatocytes, cholangiocytes, or endothelial cells that can be confused with HCC (Table 126.2). In contrast to HCC, for which men are at greater risk, women are at increased risk of the two predominant benign hepatic tumors, hepatic adenoma (HA) and focal nodular hyperplasia (FNH). Although these tumors are not malignant, they can cause significant morbidity and mortality and must be differentiated from HCC.

INCIDENCE AND EPIDEMIOLOGY

The true incidence of benign hepatic tumors is unknown. As mentioned, women are at higher risk of HA, especially during the reproductive years and with the use of oral contraceptives. Patients with HA are divided into three groups: those taking oral contraceptives; those with associated diabetes mellitus or glycogen storage disease or those who are pregnant; and those with adenomatosis. Adenomatosis is a rare hepatic syndrome in

TABLE 126.2.	GENERAL CLASSIFICATION OF BENIGN LIVER TUMORS

Epithelial tumors
  Hepatocellular
    Nodular transformation
    Focal nodular hyperplasia
    Hepatocellular adenoma
  Cholangiocellular
    Bile duct adenoma
    Bile duct cystadenoma
  Nodular regenerative hyperplasia
Mesenchymal tumors
  Tumors of adipose tissue
    Lipoma
    Myelolipoma
    Angiomyelolipoma
  Tumor of muscle tissue
    Leiomyoma
  Tumor of blood vessels
    Infantile hemangioendothelioma
    Cavernous hemangioma
Mixed epithelial and mesenchymal tumors
  Mesenchymal hamartoma
  Benign teratoma
Miscellaneous tumors
  Adrenal nest tumors
  Pancreatic nests
  Inflammatory pseudotumors

(From Jenkins RL, Johnson LB, Lewis WD. Surgical approach to benign liver tumors. *Semin Liver Dis* 1994;14:178–189, with permission.)

which patients have 10 or more adenomas. This condition affects men and women equally and is not associated with estrogen use. These patients are at greater risk for malignant transformation of adenomas, which can be detected by increasing AFP levels. HA was a rare clinical entity until the introduction of oral contraceptives. The use of these agents is associated with a time-dependent increased risk of HA (up to a 25-fold increase in patients with more than 9 years of exposure) and a higher risk of intratumor bleeding or rupture. The relationship of these tumors to malignant transformation is unknown, though incidents of HCC transformation within HA have been reported. Epidemiologic studies in young women with HCC show that oral contraceptive use is an independent risk factor for HCC.

PATHOGENESIS

Significant differences exist in the pathologic appearance of HA and FNH. On gross examination, HA appears as a tan mass varying in size from 1 to 30 cm. It has a pseudocapsule and is located preferentially in the right hepatic lobe. On histologic evaluation, HA is made up of normal-appearing hepatocytes lining trabecular sinusoidal spaces in bland cords without portal triad elements and with microscopic and macroscopic evidence of hemolysis and necrosis. FNH is made up of all cell populations normally present in the liver and classically appears as a central vascular scar with fibrous septa radiating from it. This scar may be calcified on imaging tests, which is diagnostic of FNH. Twenty-five percent of patients with FNH have several lesions.

CLINICAL FEATURES

FNA and HA have two distinct clinical pictures. Patients with HA are of childbearing age and have histories of oral contraceptive use, whereas those with FNH are in their fifth to sixth decades and lack such histories. Eighty percent of patients with HA have symptoms, of which half are related to abdominal mass or pain and the rest to hemorrhage or rupture. Right-upper-quadrant abdominal pain may result from large tumor size, compression of the Glisson capsule, or displacement or compression of intra-abdominal organs. Patients without symptoms are identified by the presence of an asymptomatic mass noticed by the patient or palpated by the physician during routine physical examination. FNH often is discovered in asymptomatic patients during radiographic evaluation of the liver or as an incidental finding at laparotomy, with only 10% being accompanied by pain or appearing as an asymptomatic hepatic mass.

LABORATORY FINDINGS

Distinguishing benign hepatic tumors from HCC is a major diagnostic challenge (Table 126.3). Evidence of chronic liver disease should be sought through routine serum liver tests. Serologic markers for HBV and HCV should be measured if elevated transaminase levels or evidence of chronic liver disease is found. AFP levels are not elevated in patients with benign tumors and can be used to differentiate benign from malignant disease.

Hepatic imaging and biopsy are the primary tools used to discriminate benign from malignant disease. In HA, radio-

---

| TABLE 126.3. | COMPARISON OF COMMON HEPATIC MASS LESIONS |

Features	Hepatocellular Adenoma	Focal Nodular Hyperplasia	Hepatocellular Carcinoma	Metastatic Carcinoma	Cavernous Hemangioma
Incidence (per 100,000)[a]	3–4	3–4	1–4,800[b]	8–20	400–7,500
Solitary (%)	90	90	20–40	5–10	90
Characteristic gross appearance	Hemorrhage, necrosis	Central scar	Hemorrhage, necrosis, vascular invasion/ obstruction	Hemorrhage, necrosis, umbilicated	Blood-filled cyst
Characteristic microscopic features	"Neohepatocytes," normal cord structure, no portal structures	"Focal cirrhosis" with pseudoductules	"Thick" (>3–4 cells) trabeculae	Replacement of hepatocytes by malignant cells	Blood-filled spaces lined by single layer of flat endothelium
Previous liver disease	None	None	Hepatitis, cirrhosis, metabolic disorders	Usually not cirrhotic	None
Cause	Estrogens, anabolic steroids	None	HBV, HCV, aflatoxin, alcohol, cirrhosis	Extrahepatic cancer, primary	Varied

HBV, hepatitis B virus; HCV, hepatitis C virus.
[a] Based on autopsy studies.
[b] Dependent on geographic origin of patient.
(From LaBreque DR. Neoplasia of the liver. In: Kaplowitz N, ed. *Liver and biliary diseases*. Baltimore: Williams Wilkins, 1992:347, with permission.)

graphic evaluation should be undertaken first, because biopsy carries a significant risk of bleeding. Biopsy is safe in FNH. The presence of a stellate scar that may be calcified is diagnostic of FNH, but it is found in only 60% to 80% of cases. Scintigraphic studies also can help differentiate mass lesions that are not defined adequately by CT. Technetium sulfur colloid scanning also can distinguish FNH from HCC or HA; the absence of reticuloendothelial cells may appear as a photopenic area in HCC and HA, whereas these cells may accumulate radioactivity in FNH. False-positive and false-negative results have been reported with sulfur colloid scanning in HA and HCC, however, thus limiting the usefulness of this technique.

OPTIMAL MANAGEMENT

When a woman is found to have a hepatic mass, discontinuation of estrogen use is the first priority. Occasionally, large HAs shrink or resolve in the absence of hormone. Serum tests are used to identify chronic liver disease or other disorders associated with an increased risk of HCC. Radiographic imaging then is used to define the size, location, and characteristics of the lesion in preparation for potential surgical resection. Percutaneous biopsy carries a risk of significant bleeding with HA, and suspicious lesions should not be subjected to biopsy. Ultimately, exploratory laparotomy and resection may be needed to differentiate HA from other tumors. If HA is suspected, surgical resection is the preferred treatment because of the risk of rupture or hemorrhage and the documented potential for malignant transformation. If a benign tumor is not resected, its size must be monitored, because expansion of the tumor eventually may compromise normal tissue or signal malignant transformation. For FNH, no risk of bleeding or malignant transformation exists, and tumors can be removed by enucleation or wedge resection to release compression of normal liver or provide pain relief.

VASCULAR DISEASES OF THE LIVER

Vascular diseases of the liver are important entities that may appear on imaging studies as hepatic tumors. Hepatic hemangiomas, especially those larger than 3 cm (cavernous hemangiomas), may look like space-occupying lesions on hepatic imaging and now and then can be palpated. Biopsy is contraindicated because of a significant risk of bleeding. Benign hemangiomas are the most common liver tumors after metastatic disease and are estimated to be present in 0.7% to 7% of the population.

CLINICAL AND PATHOLOGIC FEATURES

On histologic examination, hemangiomas are characterized by dilated venous spaces lined by endothelial cells. Small hemangiomas appear with equal frequency in men and women, whereas large, symptomatic lesions are found more often in women taking oral contraceptives. Patients with benign hemangiomas rarely have symptoms, except in the case of cavernous hemangiomas, which can take the form of palpable, space-occupying lesions. Hemangiomas are detected most often as incidental findings during diagnostic hepatic imaging. Lesions smaller than 1.5 cm appear as echogenic masses on US, distinguishing them from primary or metastatic lesions. Larger lesions cannot be differentiated by US. Technetium-labeled blood pool scanning may identify hemangiomas larger than 3 cm if they are located in the periphery of the liver. On T2-weighted magnetic resonance imaging, hemangiomas routinely appear as lucent lesions with low attenuation, whereas on HCT, hemangiomas have a distinctive pattern of contrast filling from the periphery to the center. Ultimately, angiography may be necessary to confirm the diagnosis. Hemangiomas have a low probability of rupture (less than 5%) and are resected only when large lesions compromise normal tissue. Women with incidental hemangiomas should refrain from using oral contraceptives.

OTHER BENIGN HEPATIC NEOPLASMS

Focal fatty infiltrates or localized absences of fatty infiltrate in fatty liver may appear on imaging tests as focal tumors. Other mesenchymal elements may be present in these lesions, and rare malignant transformations have been reported. Other benign liver tumors include teratomas, hamartomas, adrenal rest tumors, and inflammatory pseudotumors.

BENIGN AND MALIGNANT DISEASES OF THE BILIARY TRACT

Benign and malignant transformations of the bile duct epithelium are rare clinical entities. Unlike HCC, there is no association between cirrhosis and cholangiocarcinoma.

DEFINITION

Cholangiocarcinoma is a malignant transformation of cholangiocytes lining the intrahepatic and common hepatic bile ducts. The location and caliber of bile duct involvement by cholangiocarcinoma influence its clinical picture. Cholangiocarcinoma can be divided into four subtypes, depending on the location and histologic features; the cholangiocarcinomas are different from the cystadenocarcinomas that arise from premalignant biliary cystadenomas.

INCIDENCE AND EPIDEMIOLOGY

The incidence of cholangiocarcinoma is 2% to 20% higher than that of HCC. This lesion affects older patients (fifth to sixth decades) and is strongly associated with chronic inflammatory disease of the bile ducts caused by primary sclerosing cholangitis, with or without associated inflammatory bowel disease (ulcerative colitis or Crohn's disease); lithostasis; parasitic infection of the biliary tract (eg., *Clonorchis sinensis*); congenital cystic diseases of the biliary tree; Caroli's disease; choledochocyst; and congenital hepatic fibrosis. Exposure to vinyl chloride and

Thorotrast are other recognized risk factors for cholangiocarcinoma.

ETIOLOGY AND PATHOGENESIS

Cholangiocarcinoma often develops at the site of chronic inflammatory disease and may appear as a stricture. Malignant transformation within these inflammatory lesions makes it difficult to differentiate tumor from fibrotic stricture. An increased incidence of cholangiocarcinoma also has been reported in patients with primary biliary cirrhosis. Little is known about the mechanism of malignant transformation of cholangiocytes other than its association with chronic inflammation of bile ducts.

CLINICAL FEATURES

The site and caliber of bile duct involvement play an important role in the clinical manifestations of cholangiocarcinoma. Small-duct disease may manifest as a hepatic mass with nonspecific right-upper-quadrant pain. Large-duct obstruction, especially from tumors at the bifurcation of the right and left hepatic ducts (so-called Klatskin tumors), often leads to jaundice and pruritus. Because of their strategic location, these tumors usually appear earlier than peripheral tumors.

LABORATORY FINDINGS

The location of the tumor and the size of the obstructed bile ducts influence the abnormalities in serum liver test results. Small-duct disease may show only elevated alkaline phosphatase levels and normal bilirubin levels, because most of the bile ducts are patent. Large-duct obstruction often is evidenced by elevated serum bilirubin (predominantly direct) and alkaline phosphatase levels. Minimal increases in transaminase levels are present without chronic liver disease.

OPTIMAL MANAGEMENT

Treatment of these patients requires localization of the disease and biopsy sampling or cytologic evaluation of the mass. US can identify potential mass lesions and effectively detect dilated intrahepatic ducts. Large-duct obstruction manifests as dilated intrahepatic ducts (depending on the position of the tumor) and normal extrahepatic ducts, whereas peripheral tumors often appear as mass lesions. CT also can identify the location of hepatic masses and detect dilated bile ducts, but this technique is unable to distinguish cholangiocarcinoma from HCC.

Contrast studies are used to define the anatomy of the biliary tree. With endoscopic retrograde cholangiopancreatography, the ampulla of Vater can be assessed visually and the pancreatic ducts and biliary tree examined by the retrograde injection of contrast media. Brushings of strictures, lesions, or biliary fluid also can be obtained for cytologic examination. Alternatively, percutaneous transhepatic cholangiography can be carried out in patients with normal coagulation and no ascites, if the intrahepatic ducts are dilated. Irregularity of the bile duct mucosa, stricture, or the appearance of a shelf on biliary contrast studies

suggest tumor, but histologic evaluation is required to distinguish cholangiocarcinoma from benign stricture. Biopsy of the mass ultimately may be required to confirm the diagnosis.

Unlike HCC, cholangiocarcinoma tends to be a slow-growing tumor that metastasizes at a later stage. Curative surgical resection is the primary treatment method. Preoperative radiation therapy to the region can minimize the metastatic potential. Cumulative 1-, 3-, and 5-year survival rates of 61.8%, 23.6%, and 23.6%, respectively, were reported in one study, and patients with hilar disease survived more than 2 years. For cholangiocarcinoma that is unresectable because of its location or size, adequate drainage of the biliary tree by dilatation or stent placement lowers the incidence of bacterial cholangitis and prevents the formation of secondary biliary cirrhosis. Cystadenocarcinomas are rare tumors arising from benign biliary cyst adenomas. Irregularities within the cyst wall or the presence of septa are radiographic findings of malignant transformation and indicate the need for surgical resection. These tumors are less aggressive than HCC or cholangiocarcinoma and have a better prognosis.

▎ BENIGN AND MALIGNANT DISEASES OF THE GALLBLADDER

BENIGN GALLBLADDER DISEASE

Benign gallbladder diseases that have aggressive clinical courses need to be discriminated from malignant diseases. Patients may have symptoms indistinguishable from cholecystitis, such as right-upper-quadrant pain, nausea, and vomiting. Adenomyosis is a form of benign hyperplasia of the gallbladder wall that involves the entire gallbladder or a single segment, usually the fundus. On US, this lesion appears as a focal area of thickening or a bandlike stricture. The appearance of a smooth wall differentiates this lesion from adenocarcinoma. The other major benign entity is cholesterolosis, which results from the accumulation of cholesterol within the connective tissue of the gallbladder wall and is not related to hypercholesterolemia or the presence of gallstones.

GALLBLADDER ADENOCARCINOMA

Gallbladder adenocarcinoma is an aggressive tumor found in about 1% of all patients with long-standing cholecystitis and gallstones. This lesion develops in the sixth to seventh decades of life and has a 4:1 female-to-male predominance. Chronic gallbladder inflammation caused by gallstones is the major risk factor for malignant transformation. A calcified gallbladder, so-called porcelain gallbladder, has an increased risk of harboring adenocarcinoma. Adenocarcinoma typically is an incidental finding in a gallbladder resected for chronic cholelithiasis.

Gallbladder adenocarcinoma spreads locally to the liver and metastasizes to local lymph nodes. On US, a thickened and irregular gallbladder wall, a complex mass in the gallbladder bed, and a polypoid lesion in the gallbladder (which must be distinguished from a benign polypoid lesion) are its distinguishing radiographic features. Adenopathy in the porta hepatis and para-aortic nodes is additional evidence of gallbladder carcinoma. The only treatment is surgical resection; most patients have metastatic disease, however, with a median survival time of only 6 months.

METASTATIC DISEASE OF THE LIVER

DEFINITION

Besides liver-specific benign and malignant tumors, tumor metastases from other sites favor the liver because of its portal system drainage and the unique vascular structure of the sinusoidal endothelial surface. Clinical studies show that resection of colorectal tumors that metastasize to the liver can improve mortality rates significantly in certain situations and warrants further evaluation.

INCIDENCE AND EPIDEMIOLOGY

The liver is a common site for the metastasis of pancreas, gallbladder, colon, and breast cancers; malignant melanomas; and neuroendocrine tumors, which have the best prognosis.

CLINICAL FEATURES

About 50% of patients with metastatic disease have hepatomegaly, and 15% have jaundice. Ascites is found in 50% of patients with metastatic gastric, ovarian, or gallbladder carcinomas. Patients with hepatic metastasis from primary tumors in the pancreas, stomach, or lung often have no symptoms. Patients with metastatic disease in the liver may have nonspecific symptoms of weight loss, anorexia, right-upper-quadrant pain, or cholestasis if there is obstruction of major bile ducts. On physical examination, firm, distinct nodules may be felt.

LABORATORY FINDINGS

In cases of metastatic disease of the liver, elevated alkaline phosphatase levels are common, and increased serum bilirubin levels may be a sign of large-duct obstruction. Serum markers for HCC, such as AFP, are not elevated in metastatic disease and are helpful in differentiating the two conditions.

OPTIMAL MANAGEMENT

As with benign and malignant hepatic tumors, anatomic localization with percutaneous biopsy to confirm the diagnosis is the first priority. CT can define the location and number of metastatic lesions and identify a primary, extrahepatic tumor within the abdomen. Resection of metastatic disease in the case of noncolorectal tumors has a dismal prognosis. In selected patients with colorectal carcinoma, resection of metastatic lesions has a better prognosis. Factors associated with a better prognosis (a 5-year survival rate greater than 30%) are the presence of three or fewer lesions, an interval of more than 1 year between bowel and liver resection, and a greater margin of normal resected liver around the tumor. Many metastatic colorectal tumors are slow growing; in considering surgery, the risk of death during surgery must be weighed against the potential for prolonged survival.

BIBLIOGRAPHY

Farmer DG, Rosove MH, Shaked A, et al. Current treatment modalities for hepatocellular carcinoma. *Ann Surg* 1994;219:236–247.

Ferrucci JT. Liver tumor imaging. Current concepts. *Radiol Clin North Am* 1994;32:39–54.

Gores GJ. Liver transplantation for malignant disease. *Gastroenterol Clin North Am* 1993;22:285–299.

Jenkins RL, Johnson LB, Lewis WD. Surgical approach to benign liver tumors. *Semin Liver Dis* 1994;14:178–189.

Karani J, Williams R. The staging of hepatocellular carcinoma. *Clin Radiol* 1993;47:297–301.

Lisker-Melman M, Martin P, Hoofnagle JH. Conditions associated with hepatocellular carcinoma. *Med Clin North Am* 1989;73:999–1009.

Robinson WS. Molecular events in the pathogenesis of hepadnavirus-associated hepatocellular carcinoma. *Annu Rev Med* 1994;45:297–323.

Roslyn JJ. Cancer of the gallbladder and bile ducts. In: Kaplowitz N, ed. *Liver and biliary diseases.* Baltimore: Williams & Wilkins, 1992:658.

Taketa K. Alpha-fetoprotein: reevaluation in hepatology. *Hepatology* 1990;12:1420–1432.

Vecchio FM. Fibrolamellar carcinoma of the liver: a distinct entity within the hepatocellular tumors. A review. *Appl Pathol* 1988;6:139–148.

Kelley's Textbook of Internal Medicine, fourth edition. Edited by H. David Humes. Lippincott Williams & Wilkins, Philadelphia © 2000.

DIAGNOSTIC AND THERAPEUTIC MODALITIES IN DIGESTIVE AND HEPATOBILIARY DISORDERS

ENDOSCOPIC DIAGNOSIS AND THERAPY

GREGORY G. GINSBERG

Clinicians are afforded an array of techniques for diagnosis and management of diseases of the digestive tract. These include esophagogastroduodenoscopy, small-bowel enteroscopy, colonoscopy, flexible sigmoidoscopy, endoscopic retrograde cholangiopancreatography (ERCP), and endoscopic ultrasonography (EUS). Flexible endoscopy allows direct imaging of the upper and lower digestive tracts. It is more sensitive and specific for most conditions than are indirect imaging techniques such as contrast radiography and allows directed tissue sampling for histologic assessment. It also allows direct curative and palliative measures.

EQUIPMENT

Gastrointestinal (GI) endoscopes are long, slim instruments capable of light and image transmission. Lengths and diameters vary according to purpose. Flexible endoscopes initially relied on fiber optic bundles to transmit light and images. Videoendoscopic images now are generated electronically by means of a charge coupled device (CCD chip) located at the tip of the endoscope. Digital photographs can be printed, and images can be stored and recalled from magnetic optical discs.

Endoscopes are equipped with an air-water channel to allow insufflation of the lumen and washing of the lenses. An accessory channel allows suctioning of air and fluid from the digestive tract and facilitates passage of instruments for tissue sampling and therapeutic applications. Bidirectional controls in the handpiece allow tip deflection for steering. An array of tissue sampling and therapeutic interventions can be performed (Tables 127.1,

127.2). Occupational Safety and Health Organization guidelines are followed to protect patients and medical staff from infectious hazards during endoscopic procedures. Endoscopes are cleaned manually and subjected to a high-level disinfection process to prevent patient to patient transmission of infectious disease through instrumentation.

PREPARATION, SEDATION, AND MONITORING

Most endoscopic examinations are performed as elective, outpatient procedures. Patients fast for 4 to 6 hours before the procedure. Patients undergoing colonoscopy also need a bowel purge to cleanse the colon of its contents. Screening flexible sigmoidoscopy requires administration of one or more enemas to cleanse the distal colon.

Other than screening flexible sigmoidoscopy, most endoscopic examination in the United States are performed with conscious sedation. Intravenously administered medications, typically a narcotic and a short-acting benzodiazepine, are used to induce relaxation, anxiolysis, and amnesia. Although not universally needed, sedation for diagnostic endoscopy allows toler-

TABLE 127.1.	TISSUE SAMPLING AND ENHANCED DIAGNOSTIC TECHNIQUES AVAILABLE THROUGH ROUTINE ENDOSCOPIC PROCEDURES

Forceps biopsy (directed or surveillance)
Excisional biopsy
Polypectomy
Brush cytology
Fine-needle aspiration
Campylobacter-like organism (CLO) test
pH Assessment
Biliary crystal analysis
Sphincter of Oddi manometry

TABLE 127.2. INTERVENTIONS COMMONLY PERFORMED DURING THERAPEUTIC ENDOSCOPIC PROCEDURES

Polypectomy (sessile and pedunculated polyps)
Hemostasis (nonvariceal, e.g., injection, electrocautery, laser coagulation; acute variceal bleeding and subsequent obliteration of varices, e.g., sclerotherapy, rubber band ligation)
Dilation (benign and malignant strictures
Management of achalasia (dilation, botulinum toxin injection)
Foreign body extraction
Bile duct stone extraction
Tumor ablation (electrothermal, laser photoablation, cytotoxic)
Insertion of endoprostheses (stents)
Biliary and pancreatic sphincterotomy
Placement of enteral feeding tube

TABLE 127.3. INDICATIONS FOR GASTROINTESTINAL ENDOSCOPIC PROCEDURES

Esophagogastroduodenoscopy
Abdominal distress
Dysphasia, odynophagia
Symptoms of gastroesophageal reflux
Surveillance of Barrett's esophagus
Suspected ulcer disease
Nausea, vomiting
Gastrointestinal bleeding
Iron deficiency anemia
Unexplained weight loss
Suspected neoplasm
Suspicion of esophagogastric varices
Evaluation of abnormalities seen on radiographic studies
Familial adenomatous polyposis
Assess extent of injury after ingestion of caustic substance

Colonoscopy
Colorectal cancer surveillance
  Positive result of fecal-occult blood test
  Finding of adenomatous polyps at flexible sigmoidoscopy
  Family history of colorectal cancer or adenomatous polyps
  Personal history of colorectal cancer or adenomatous polyps
Colorectal cancer screening (average risk)
Suspicion of polyps at radiologic examination
Iron deficiency anemia
Hematochezia
Diarrhea
Constipation
Change in bowel pattern
Abdominal pain
Inflammatory bowel disease

Flexible sigmoidoscopy
Screening of patients at average risk of colorectal cancer
Rectal bleeding
Rectal pain
Inflammatory bowel disease
Post treatment surveillance for rectal cancer

Endoscopic Retrograde Cholangiopancreatography
Biliary obstruction
Choledocolithiasis
Cholangitis
Abnormal liver tests
Postop bile duct complications
Postcholecystectomy pain
Severe acute biliary pancreatitis
Acute recurrent pancreatitis
Chronic pancreatitis
Pancreatic pseudocyst
Abnormal results at radiologic examination

Endoscopic Ultrasonography
Esophageal, gastric, and rectal tumors
Pancreatic, ampullary, and bile duct tumors
Submucosal lesions
Mediastinal, peritoneal and retroperitoneal lesions
Abnormal gastric folds

---

ance of otherwise unpleasant or uncomfortable procedures and makes most therapeutic procedures feasible.

GI endoscopy is generally safe and well tolerated. Major complications, such as bleeding or perforation, occur among less than 0.1% of patients. Complications are more apt to occur when therapeutic intervention is performed. Cardiorespiratory compromise associated with the use of intravenous sedation is the most common complication. For this reason, clinical and electronic monitoring is performed routinely by nurses. Heart rate, respiratory rate, blood pressure, continuous oxygen saturation, and electrocardiographic tracings commonly are monitored. The use of supplemental oxygen has become routine.

INDICATIONS FOR GASTROINTESTINAL ENDOSCOPY

GI endoscopy is indicated (a) when a change in management is apt to be based on results of endoscopy; (b) after empiric therapy for a suspected benign disorder of the digestive tract has been unsuccessful; (c) for further evaluation of abnormalities seen on radiographic images; and (d) when a primary therapeutic procedure is being considered (Table 127.3). GI endoscopy is generally not indicated when the results are not apt to contribute to management or for periodic follow-up evaluation of benign disease unless surveillance of a potentially malignant condition is warranted. GI endoscopy is contraindicated when comorbid disease causes the risks to outweigh the benefits; when perforation of a viscus is suspected; and when patient consent or cooperation cannot be obtained for elective procedures.

GASTROINTESTINAL ENDOSCOPIC PROCEDURES

ESOPHAGOGASTRODUODENOSCOPY

Esophagogastroduodenoscopy, or upper endoscopy, with a 1 m endoscope allows inspection of the upper digestive tract—the laryngopharynx to the descending duodenum. During this procedure the examiner can see the luminal esophagus, stomach, and proximal duodenum; upper and lower esophageal sphincters; esophagogastric junction; and pylorus.

FLEXIBLE SIGMOIDOSCOPY

Flexible sigmoidoscopy with a 60 cm endoscope is used to evaluate suspected anorectal disorders and distal colonic disease and in screening for colorectal neoplasia. The patient is not sedated for these procedures. Flexible sigmoidoscopes have largely replaced rigid sigmoidoscopes. Enema preparation is used to cleanse the rectum.

COLONOSCOPY

Colonoscopy allows direct inspection of the entire colon, anal canal, and terminal ileum. Total colonoscopy requires a bowel purge and is typically performed with sedation. The colonoscope is manually advanced under direct vision and steered by means of tip deflection. Careful inspection is performed during advancement and withdrawal. Colonoscopy is more sensitive and more specific than barium enema radiographic examination. Lesions identified at barium enema examination typically necessitate total colonoscopy for confirmation and management.

SMALL-BOWEL ENTEROSCOPY

For evaluation of the proximal small intestine beyond the descending duodenum, push enteroscopy with an extended-length instrument allows directed imaging and tissue sampling. It also allows a variety of therapeutic maneuvers in the horizontal duodenum and proximal to middle jejunum. Push enteroscopy is used in the evaluation of chronic GI bleeding when upper endoscopy and colonoscopy had failed to identify a source. Arteriovenous malformations in the small intestine are the most commonly identified causes of bleeding. When arteriovenous malformations in the small intestine are identified and managed with injection or electrocautery therapy, approximately 50% of patients have a marked reduction in bleeding and transfusion requirement. Other indications for push enteroscopy include small-bowel biopsy in the evaluation of celiac sprue and evaluation of abnormalities seen on contrast radiographic images.

For evaluation of the terminal ileum, colonoscopic intubation of the ileocecal valve can be achieved in 80% to 90% of attempts. Colonoscopic inspection of the terminal ileum is an effective means of assessing involvement of this segment of intestine by Crohn's disease, lymphoma, and other diseases of the ileum. Standard tissue sampling techniques can be performed.

Sonde enteroscopy allows visualization of the entire small bowel. The long, slim instrument is passed through the nose and advanced beyond the ligament of Treitz with endoscopic or fluoroscopic assistance. A water-filled balloon affixed to the tip allows the scope to be propelled by peristalsis. Unfortunately, depth of insertion is variable and there is no capability for tip control, tissue sampling, or application of therapy. Sonde enteroscopy is used to evaluate the presence and extent of arteriovenous malformations of the small intestine and to identify tumors beyond the reach of a push enteroscope or not seen on radiographic images.

Intraoperative enteroscopy is the ultimate means of examining the entire small bowel. After laparotomy, a push enteroscope or pediatric colonoscope is advanced through the mouth. The endoscopist and GI surgeon work together to manually advance the endoscope through the entire length of small bowel. Endoscopic and operative techniques can be used to identify mucosal and vascular lesions.

ENDOSCOPIC RETROGRADE CHOLANGIOPANCREATOGRAPHY

ERCP combines endoscopic and radiologic techniques to facilitate diagnosis and management of disorders of the biliary system and pancreas. A specialized side-viewing duodenoscope is negotiated into the second portion of the duodenum for *en face* viewing of the ampulla of Vater. Plastic catheters are passed through the accessory channel of the endoscope and directed selectively into the pancreatic duct or bile duct. Radiographic contrast medium is injected into the duct to produce opacification of the biliary or pancreatic ductal systems. Endoscopic retrograde pancreatography is the standard for biliary and pancreatic ductal imaging. Although magnetic resonance cholangiopancreatography is approaching parity for diagnostic accuracy, ERCP allows an array of therapeutic interventions. While it is generally safe and well tolerated, in addition to the standard risks associated with other endoscopic procedures, ERCP exposes patients to a 2% to 5% risk of pancreatitis.

ENDOSCOPIC ULTRASONOGRAPHY

EUS combines the technologies of endoscopy and ultrasonography. A fiber optic endoscope is modified with a microscopic ultrasound transducer affixed to the distal tip. The endoscopist advances the echoendoscope into the desired luminal location under endoscopic guidance. Bringing the ultrasound transducer close to the tissue or organ of interest circumvents the impediments of intervening bone, fat, and air and allows the use of high-frequency ultrasound waves that achieve high resolution. EUS is gaining broad acceptance. It is used for diagnosis and staging of abnormalities of the luminal GI wall and of periluminal organs, including the pancreas, biliary tree, and mediastinal, perigastric, and perirectal structures. Pulse Doppler ultrasound to assess vascular flow and real-time fine-needle aspiration of luminal and extraluminal lesions aligned with the endosonographic image can be performed.

EUS is used in the evaluation of focal intramural and extramural mass lesions identified at endoscopy or other imaging studies. It is used in the evaluation of biliary obstruction, pancreatic lesions, and neuroendocrine tumors when other imaging studies fail to yield a diagnosis. Its other principle role is as a staging tool. Compared with other imaging studies, EUS has been demonstrated superior for both tumor and node staging for esophageal, gastric, ampullary, biliary, and rectal carcinomas and gastric lymphoma (Fig 127.1). Once diagnosis and staging

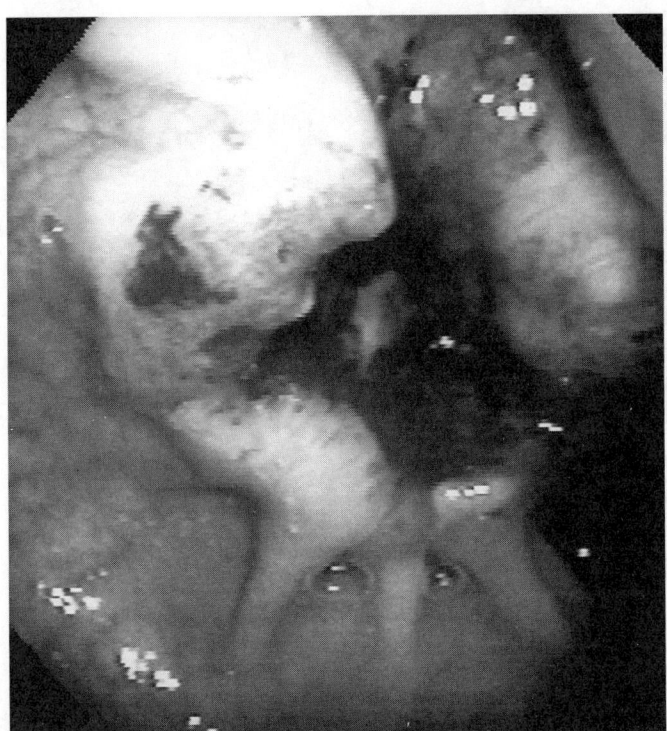

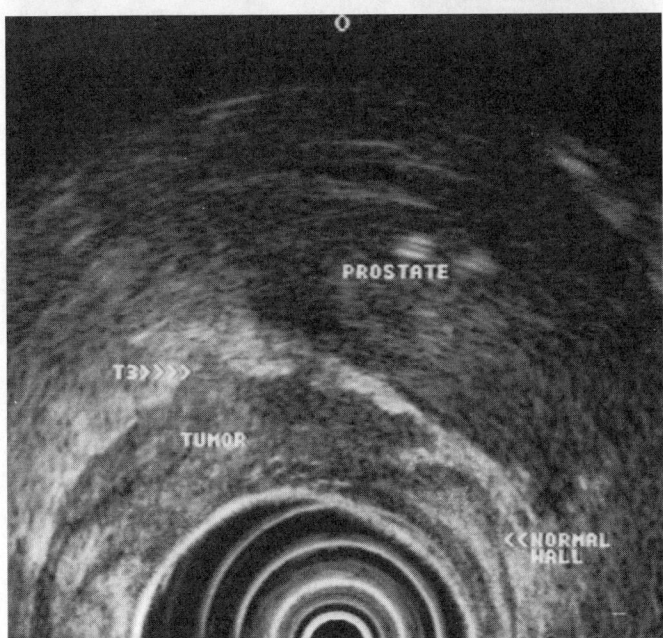

FIGURE 127.1. A: Colonoscopic view of ulcerated rectal carcinoma. **B:** Endoscopic ultrasound image shows the lesion as a hypoechoic mass disrupting the normal wall layer pattern with invasion into the perirectal fat and encroaching on but not directly invading the prostate gland. The multiple concentric circles are the echoscope in the lumen of the rectum.

have been achieved, EUS-guided fine-needle aspiration biopsy allows tissue diagnosis in as many as 95% of attempts, a yield superior to that of other tissue sampling techniques. EUS-guided fine-needle aspiration also is effective for biopsy of celiac and mediastinal lymph nodes (Fig 127.2).

ENDOSCOPIC APPROACH TO ESOPHAGEAL DISORDERS

DISORDERS

Gastroesophageal Reflux

Gastroesophageal reflux disease is the most common malady of the upper digestive tract (see Chapter 106). Episodic reflux of gastric acid into the esophageal lumen is normal. Excessive exposure of the esophagus to gastric acid causes symptomatic esophagitis. Esophageal ulceration, bleeding, and peptic stricture formation may complicate severe esophagitis. Most patients with symptoms of gastroesophageal reflux respond to empiric pharmacotherapy. Endoscopy is recommended for patients who do not respond to empiric therapy or have recurrence of symptoms when therapy is reduced or eliminated and those who need tissue sampling to clarify the diagnosis. Follow-up endoscopy for uncomplicated esophagitis usually is unnecessary. Endoscopy also is indicated when symptoms are accompanied by dysphagia, odynophagia, abnormalities on radiographs, GI blood loss, and compromised immune function.

Barrett Esophagus

Barrett esophagus is the replacement of normal squamous esophageal mucosa with specialized intestinal metaplasia in response to chronic acid reflux injury (see Chapters 106 and 115). Barrett mucosa is recognized at endoscopy as pink mucosa that can be differentiated from surrounding pale-white normal squamous epithelium. Forceps tissue biopsy allows histologic confirmation. Barrett mucosa is present among 5% to 15% of patients with frequent reflux symptoms. Identification of Barrett esophagus is important because this condition is associated with as much as 40-fold increased risk of esophageal adenocarcinoma. Adenocarcinoma arising from Barrett esophagus appears to emerge through grades of dysplasia that can be discriminated histologically. Patients with Barrett esophagus are advised to undergo periodic endoscopic examinations to detect dysplasia or early carcinoma. Because the prognosis for advanced carcinoma is so poor, the detection of precancerous lesions or early cancer is apt to have life-saving benefit. Endoscopic techniques for eradication of Barrett epithelium and superficial cancers by means of thermal, resection, and photochemical techniques are emerging.

Dysphagia and Odynophagia

Dysphagia, difficulty swallowing, and odynophagia, painful swallowing, are symptoms that require endoscopic investigation (see Chapter 94). Difficulty with swallowing can be caused by functional or mechanical disorders. An imaging study is needed to rule out structural lesions. Contrast radiography may be valuable in some instances to localize or characterize pathologic changes. Endoscopy is preferred, however, because it allows direct visualization, tissue sampling, and dilation therapy for mechanical processes.

Benign mechanical causes of dysphagia include peptic stricture, Schatzki's ring, congenital esophageal mucosal webs and rings, and strictures caused by radiation therapy, caustic ingestion, and surgical anastomoses. All respond to dilation therapy.

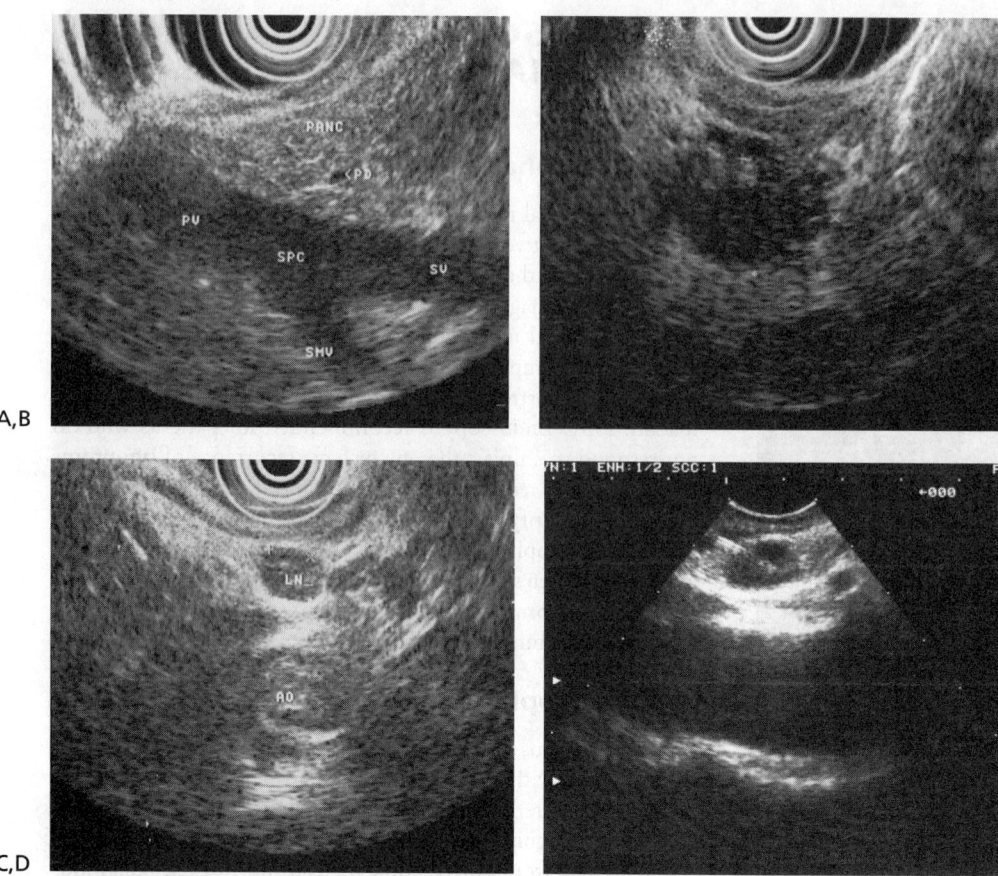

A,B

C,D

FIGURE 127.2. Endoscopic ultrasound (EUS) images of a pancreatic lesion. **A:** Normal endosonographic appearance of the pancreatic head (*panc*), pancreatic duct (*PD*), splenoportal confluence (*SPC*), portal vein (*PV*), splenic vein (*SV*), and superior mesenteric vein (*SMV*). **B:** A 1.8 cm hypoechoic mass in the genu (*between the markers*) has evidence of malignant growth. **C:** A 1 cm suspicious lymph node (*LN*) in the celiac region. **D:** Results of EUS-guided fine-needle aspiration biopsy confirmed metastatic pancreatic adenocarcinoma. Linear echoes represent the needle in the lymph node.

Dysphagia is the most common symptom of esophageal cancer. Achalasia is an acquired neuromuscular abnormality in which the esophagus loses normal peristaltic function and the lower esophageal sphincter is hypertensive and does not relax (see Chapter 108). These features can be demonstrated at esophageal manometry. Endoscopy is necessary to exclude a pseudoachalasia due to carcinoma at the esophagogastric junction.

Odynophagia occurs when injury to the esophageal mucosa causes ulceration. Because it may be a symptom of a serious pathologic condition, odynophagia should be investigated with endoscopy. Odynophagia may be caused by acid peptic ulceration, chemical injury, infection, or neoplasia. Among immunocompromised patients *Candida,* herpes, or cytomegalovirus infection can cause infectious esophagitis. In addition to these, idiopathic AIDS ulceration may occur among patients with HIV infection.

Esophageal Cancer

Esophageal cancer is highly lethal because most patients have advanced disease at diagnosis (see Chapter 115). The absence of a serosa surrounding the esophageal wall allows esophageal tumors to expand and spread hematogenously before symptoms of luminal compromise occur. Patients with suspected esophageal cancer should undergo endoscopy, including EUS, for confirmation and to assess appropriateness of treatment options.

Patients with advanced disease may benefit from endoscopic palliative therapy for dysphagia.

ENDOSCOPIC THERAPIES FOR ESOPHAGEAL DISEASE

Esophageal dilation is performed in the management of symptomatic benign and malignant esophageal strictures. Empiric dilation also may benefit patients who have dysphagia when eating solid foods and who have normal endoscopic findings. Esophageal dilation is performed most commonly with fixed-size, tapered, wire-guided, polyvinyl bougies (Savary dilators) or pneumatic balloon dilators. Savary dilators are passed over a guide wire that has been placed under endoscopic or fluoroscopic guidance. Pneumatic dilators are passed through the scope and inflated within the stricture. Published data suggest equal efficacy of dilation methods.

Dilation improves or resolves dysphagia for most patients with benign strictures (85% to 90%). Rings and webs are managed by means of disruption through passage of one large-caliber dilator. Adequate results usually are achieved in a single session. Malignant strictures respond to dilation, but relief of dysphagia is transient, and the degree and duration of relief typically diminish with progression of disease. Esophageal dilation for achalasia is unique in that it involves forceful disruption of the lower esophageal sphincter muscle. Lower esophageal sphincter dilation to 30 to 40 mm is performed with pneumatic dilators. Endoscopic injection of botulinum toxin into the lower esophageal sphincter area has been demonstrated to achieve short-term improvement.

Endoscopic Therapy for Esophageal Cancer

Endoscopic therapy for esophageal cancer is based on the individual tumor and patient characteristics. Simple endoscopic dilation achieves rapid but short-lived symptomatic improvement. Laser therapy, delivered through flexible fibers that can be passed through the accessory channel of the endoscope, destroys tumors by means of coagulative necrosis and vaporization. It is effective in reconstituting the lumens of patients with obstructing esophageal cancer 85% of the time and in achieving marked improvement in symptomatic dysphagia 75% of the time. Endoscopic laser therapy for esophageal cancer usually is safe and well tolerated, but perforation, bleeding, pain, and fever are possible complications. Multiple sessions may be needed to achieve satisfactory initial palliation. Repeated sessions are needed in response to regrowth of the tumor.

Esophageal stent placement achieves rapid and long-lasting palliation of dysphagia associated with esophageal cancer (Fig 127.3). Expandable, coated metal, mesh stents can be placed atraumatically under endoscopic and fluoroscopic guidance. When deployed, the stents expand to reconstitute the esophageal lumen. Synthetic membrane coating prevents tumor ingrowth and effectively seals esophagorespiratory fistulas.

An emerging technique for endoscopic management of esophageal cancer is photodynamic therapy. This technique entails systemic administration of a photosensitive chemical agent that is selectively retained by tumor tissue. The impregnated tumor tissue is exposed to laser light of a specific wavelength delivered through the endoscope to the involved area. Light energy absorbed into the tissue causes a cytotoxic photochemical reaction. Tumor tissue is selectively destroyed with limited injury to surrounding normal tissue. Photodynamic therapy is currently approved for palliation of advanced esophageal carcinoma. The more compelling application however, may be the use of photodynamic therapy as an alternative to surgical resection for cure of patients with superficial carcinoma and patients with Barrett and high-grade dysplasia.

ENDOSCOPIC APPROACH TO ABDOMINAL DISORDERS

DISORDERS

Dyspepsia

Abdominal discomfort has many and varied causes. The patient history and the findings at physical examination dictate the diagnostic approach. When dyspeptic symptoms predominate, endoscopy should be considered. Dyspepsia is pain or discomfort centered in the upper abdomen. Peptic ulcer disease (15% to 25% of instances) or reflux esophagitis (5% to 15%) may produce dyspeptic symptoms. Most patients have functional symptoms and normal endoscopic findings. Endoscopy also allows assessment for evidence of gastritis suggested by erythema or erosions in the gastric mucosa and the presence of *Helicobacter pylori* infection. Less common findings, such as atrophic gastritis, intestinal metaplasia, and gastric cancer, may be uncovered. If the decision is made to examine a patient with dyspepsia, endoscopy rather than upper GI contrast radiography should be performed. When dyspepsia is accompanied by so-called trigger symptoms (weight loss, early satiety, and evidence of GI bleeding), there is universal agreement on the need for endoscopy. Early endoscopy also may contribute to patient satisfaction, offering reassurance about the absence of more sinister disease and allowing directed therapy based on endoscopic and histologic diagnosis.

Upper Gastrointestinal Bleeding

For a patient with acute upper GI bleeding, the first priorities are stabilization and resuscitation (see Chapter 102). Once these efforts have been instituted, endoscopic inspection should be performed to localize and identify the bleeding source, assess the

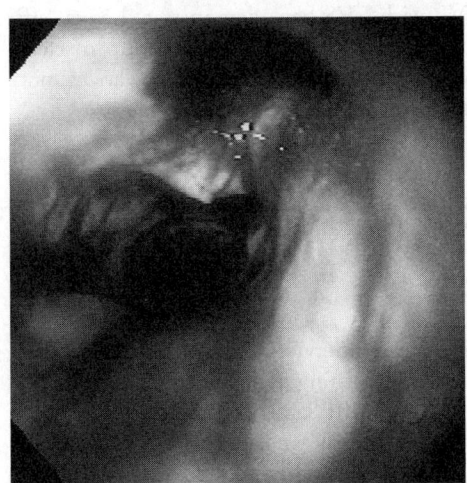
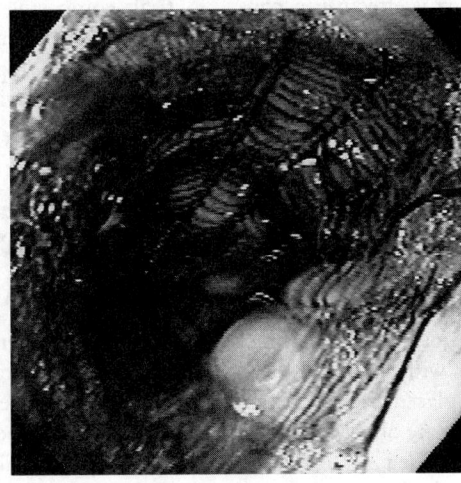

A,B

FIGURE 127.3. Endoscopic images demonstrate esophageal stricture due to carcinoma and esophagotracheal fistula before **(A)** and after **(B)** esophageal stent placement.

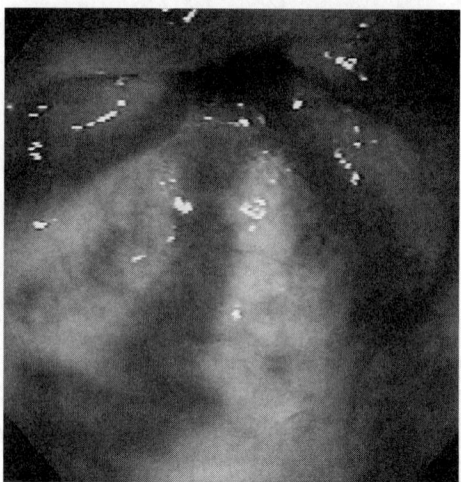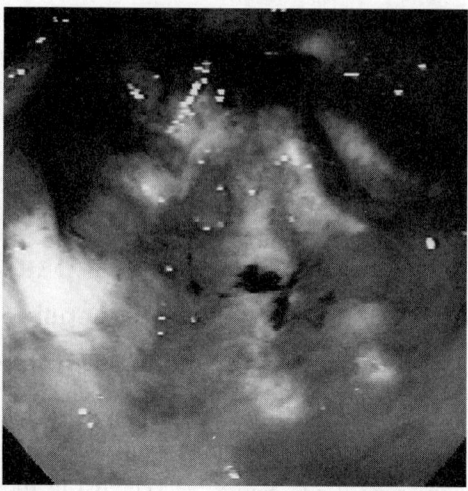

A,B

FIGURE 127.4. Endoscopic evaluation of iron deficiency anemia. **A:** Gastric antral vascular ectasia syndrome. The presence of multiple friable superficial vessels arrayed in a spoke-like pattern and emanating from the pylorus causes chronic gastrointestinal bleeding. **B:** The lesions are successfully managed with endoscopic laser photocoagulation.

persistence and rate of bleeding, and to determine the need for and administer endoscopic therapy. Esophagogastroduodenoscopy is highly accurate (95%) in identifying the source of acute upper GI bleeding. Accuracy decreases as the duration from presentation to endoscopy increases. Common causes of acute nonvariceal upper GI bleeding are gastroduodenal ulcer, erosive gastritis, and Mallory–Weiss tear. Endoscopy with hemostatic therapy has been demonstrated to stop active bleeding and to reduce the incidence of rebleeding, need for surgery, blood transfusion requirement, hospital mortality, and length of stay.

Chronic upper GI bleeding may be caused by an arteriovenous malformation, gastric antral vascular ectasia syndrome, portal gastropathy, erosive esophagitis, drug-induced or mechanical gastritis, or carcinoma. Endoscopy is indicated for diagnosis, and therapy is disease specific (Fig 127.4).

Although variceal hemorrhage accounts for only 15% of instances of acute upper GI bleeding, it accounts for 30% of major instances of upper GI bleeding and is associated with 50% mortality. Endoscopy is needed to confirm the source of bleeding because as many as 50% of patients with portal hypertension and acute upper GI bleeding may have bleeding from a source other than esophagogastric varices. The other sources include portal hypertensive gastropathy, Mallory–Weiss tear, and gastroduodenal ulcer disease. Endoscopic therapy is effective in controlling acute bleeding in as many as 80% of patients. Efforts to achieve hemodynamic resuscitation and stabilization are crucial. They include attempts to correct coagulopathy among patients with advanced liver disease. Once initial bleeding is controlled, follow-up endoscopic therapy to achieve obliteration of esophageal varices reduces the risk of rebleeding.

ENDOSCOPIC HEMOSTATIC THERAPY

Endoscopic therapies for acute nonvariceal bleeding include injection with epinephrine solution or a sclerosing agent, contact probe electrocautery, noncontact cautery with laser, and mechanical hemostasis with endoscopically placed metallic clips. When active bleeding or signs of rebleeding are observed, endoscopic therapy is effective in achieving sustained hemostasis in more than 90% of cases. Among patients who have evidence of

rebleeding after initial hemostasis, follow-up endoscopic therapy is favored over urgent surgery because the efficacy is similar and the morbidity and mortality are lower.

Endoscopic therapies for bleeding esophageal varices include sclerotherapy (EVS) and band ligation (EVL) (see Chapters 102 and 105). EVS is performed with a hollow-bore needle-tip catheter that is advanced through the accessory channel of the endoscope and inserted directly into or adjacent to the esophageal variceal column. A sclerosing agent is injected to produce thrombosis of the vessel, to stop active hemorrhage, and to reduce risk of rebleeding. Controlled trials of EVS for the primary prevention of initial esophageal variceal bleeding have not demonstrated benefit. Local and systemic complications may occur among as many as 30% of patients undergoing EVS. The complications include chest pain, ulceration, esophageal stricture, pleural effusion, and acute respiratory distress syndrome.

EVL has fewer complications than EVS and is supplanting it as the preferred initial endoscopic hemostatic therapy. EVL is performed by means of aspirating the variceal column into a vacuum chamber affixed to the tip of the endoscope and releasing a rubber band that effectively strangulates and thromboses the vessel. Use of a multiband delivery system improves the ease and speed of deployment. Numerous randomized prospective trials comparing EVL with EVS have demonstrated equal efficacy for cessation of active bleeding. EVL is superior to sclerotherapy with respect to complications, eradicating varices more rapidly, and having a lower rate of rebleeding.

ENDOSCOPIC APPROACH TO COLONIC DISORDERS

COLORECTAL CANCER AND POLYPS

The U.S. Preventive Health Services Task Force has recommended colorectal cancer screening or surveillance based on individual risk (see Chapter 116). Screening and surveillance are recommended because colorectal cancer arises from precancerous polyps, which are readily recognizable against the background of normal mucosa (Fig 127.5). The presence of adeno-

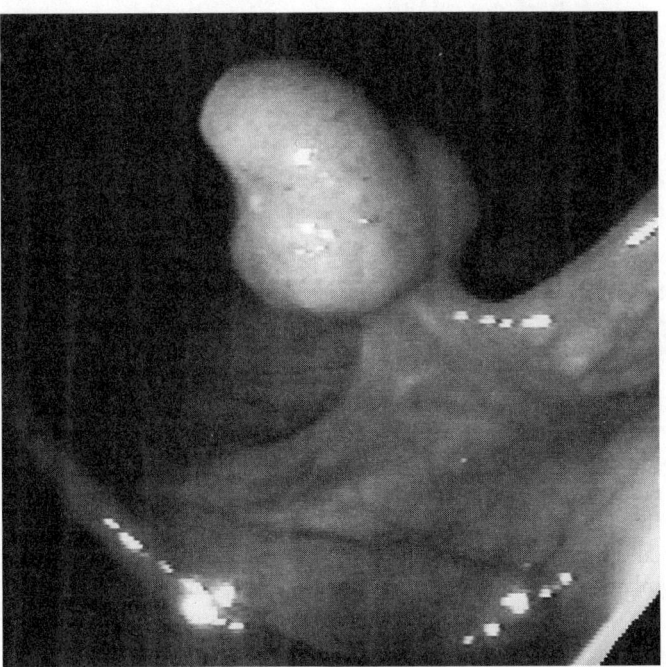

FIGURE 127.5. Adenomatous pedunculated colonic polyp found during surveillance colonoscopy for colorectal cancer. Curative resection is performed with colonoscopic electrocautery snare polypectomy.

matous colorectal polyps is associated with increased likelihood of the presence of or future development of colorectal cancer. Removal of adenomatous polyps by means of colonoscopic snare polypectomy followed by periodic surveillance colonoscopy prevents death due to colorectal cancer. Early cancer contained within polypoid lesions can be cured with simple endoscopic resection.

Most polyps seen during colonoscopy can be completely removed by means of electrocautery snare resection. Colonic polypectomy has been demonstrated to be safe and effective. Electrocautery snare polypectomy is performed with a wire loop passed through the working channel of the colonoscope. Monopolar current passed through the snare wire allows concomitant cutting and coagulation through the polyp base. The resected specimen can be retrieved and submitted to the pathology laboratory for histologic interpretation. In addition to patients with a known history of colorectal polyps, colonoscopy is recommended for patients with abnormalities seen on barium enema radiographs, patients with a family history of colorectal cancer or polyps, and patients with a history of gynecologic cancer, long-standing chronic ulcerative colitis, familial adenomatous polyposis, or nonhereditary colorectal cancer syndromes.

LOWER GASTROINTESTINAL BLEEDING

Most minor rectal bleeding (see Chapter 102) is caused by benign anorectal disease, such as internal hemorrhoids, anal fissures or anal tears. The patient's age and clinical history dictate management. In nearly all cases, flexible sigmoidoscopy or anoscopy should be performed at the minimum. A determination to evaluate the more proximal colon has to be individualized. Barium enema radiographic examination or total colonoscopy are effec-

tive options. Recurrent bleeding from internal hemorrhoids may be treated with injection sclerotherapy or rubber band ligation. Bleeding from unresectable colorectal cancers or radiation proctitis may be palliated with laser photocoagulation.

The most common causes of hemodynamically significant acute lower GI bleeding are diverticulosis, arteriovenous malformations, and, less commonly, acute colitis, ischemia, and carcinoma. Because rapid upper GI bleeding can manifest as hematochezia, upper gastrointestinal endoscopy should be considered irrespective of results of nasogastric tube aspiration biopsy. These results may be negative in as many as 15% of instances of upper GI bleeding due to duodenal ulcer disease. Because most lower GI bleeding is intermittent or self-limited, colonoscopic inspection with or without preparation of the colon can be performed once the patient's condition is stabilized. Colonoscopy is effective in identifying a source of bleeding in 70% to 80% of cases of acute lower GI bleeding. Furthermore, colonoscopy is likely to have a therapeutic application that is not obtained with other diagnostic studies such as radionuclide scanning and visceral angiography.

DIARRHEA

Most instances of diarrhea are self-limited. Chronic diarrhea, defined as that lasting more than 2 weeks, requires endoscopic evaluation (see Chapter 99). When initial history and stool studies do not help identify the likely source, flexible sigmoidoscopy should be performed to rule out proctosigmoiditis. When the diagnosis remains obscure, total colonoscopy with intubation of the terminal ileal should be performed, and multiple biopsy

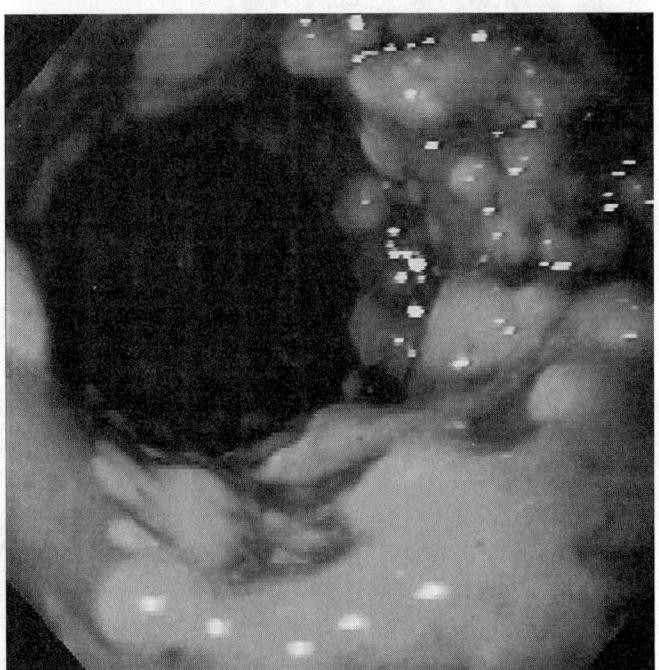

FIGURE 127.6. Images from flexible sigmoidoscopic examination of a patient with a 2-week history of diarrhea show pseudomembranous colitis associated with *Clostridium difficile* infection. The patient had been treated with antibiotics 1 month earlier for a pulmonary infection.

specimens should be collected throughout normal and abnormal mucosa. The colonoscopic findings confirm the diagnosis of Crohn's disease, ulcerative colitis, microscopic colitis, including lymphocytic and collagenous colitis, ischemia, colorectal cancer, and infectious colitis (Fig 127.6). Upper gastrointestinal endoscopy should be performed with small-bowel biopsy when sprue is considered. Duodenal aspiration should be performed when bacterial overgrowth is considered.

INFLAMMATORY BOWEL DISEASE

Colonoscopy is an important aid in the diagnosis and management of ulcerative colitis and Crohn's disease (see Chapter 111). Although many patients with inflammatory bowel disease do not need colonoscopic examination for initial diagnosis, colonoscopy frequently is necessary to differentiate ulcerative colitis and Crohn's disease. Colonoscopy is more sensitive than a barium enema in determining the anatomic extent of the inflammatory process. Colonoscopy with multiple biopsies or polypectomy frequently is necessary in the evaluation of polypoid lesions found at barium enema examination because the differential diagnosis includes inflammatory pseudopolyps, true polyps, and carcinoma. Colonoscopy is needed to determine the cause of strictures in discriminating inflammatory from neoplastic processes. Patients with pancolitis of more than 7 to 10 years' duration and patients with left-sided ulcerative colitis of more than

15 years' duration are are increased risk of carcinoma of the colon. These patients are advised to undergo surveillance colonoscopy with multiple biopsies to assess the presence of early carcinoma or dysplasia.

ENDOSCOPIC APPROACH TO PANCREATICOBILIARY DISORDERS

ERCP is indicated for the evaluation and management of suspected biliary disorders, including jaundice, cholestasis, postcholecystectomy pain, complications of biliary surgery, acute cholangitis, acute biliary pancreatitis, and confirmation of lesions demonstrated with other imaging techniques (see Chapters 103, 117, and 125). Suspected pancreatic disorders warranting ERCP include obstructive jaundice with pancreatic mass, chronic upper abdominal pain, increased serum amylase or lipase level, unexplained weight loss, malabsorption, unexplained gastric varices, recurrent pancreatitis, chronic pancreatitis of uncertain causation, and lesions found with other imaging techniques.

Findings at cholangiography include choledocholithiasis, benign and malignant stricture, ampullary tumor, primary sclerosing cholangitis, congenital abnormality of the biliary system, infestation with parasites, sphincter of Oddi dysfunction, bile duct leak, and hemobilia (Fig 127.7). Pancreatographic findings

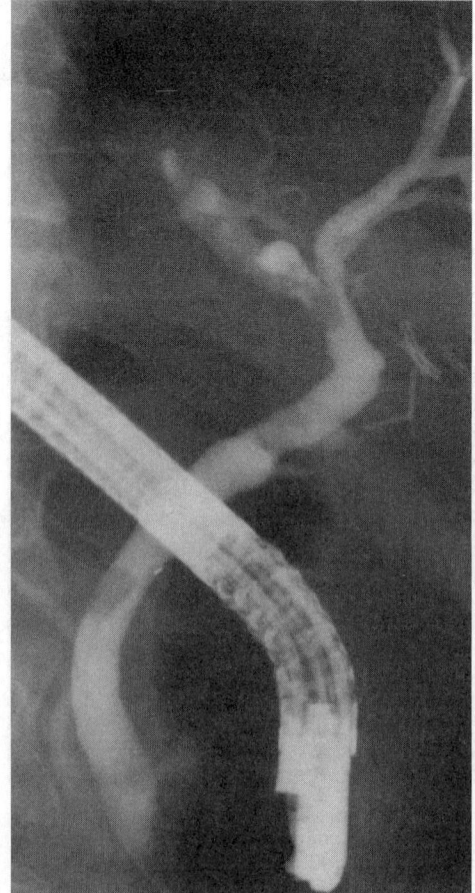
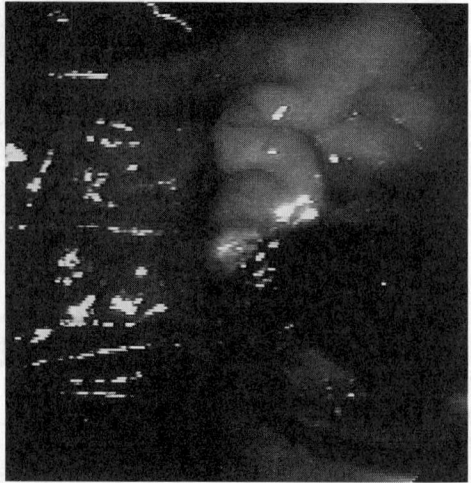

A,B

FIGURE 127.7. Endoscopic retrograde cholangiopancreatography. **A:** Retained common bile duct stone (relative lucency in duct) in a patient who had recently undergone cholecystectomy for chronic cholecystitis. **B:** After endoscopic biliary sphincterotomy, the stone is removed with a retrieval basket.

may include features of pancreatic carcinoma, chronic pancreatitis, pancreatic pseudocyst, nonmalignant pancreatic neoplasia, pancreas divisum, pancreatic duct disruptions, and pancreatic duct stones. Therapeutic maneuvers include biliary and pancreatic duct sphincterotomy, stone extraction including mechanical lithotripsy, tissue sampling techniques, dilation of malignant and benign strictures, drainage of obstructed biliary systems and pancreatic pseudocysts, and stenting with polyethylene and expandable metallic endoprostheses.

ENDOSCOPIC APPROACH TO ENTERAL FEEDING ACCESS

Enteral access can be a means of providing nutritional support to patients who are unable to maintain oral intake (see Chapter 130). Percutaneous endoscopic gastrostomy has become a commonly performed procedure in the care of patients who are unable to maintain oral intake because of compromise of mental status, swallowing dysfunction, or severe dysphasia. The endoscope is advanced into the stomach, and the light of the endoscope transilluminates the abdominal wall. A trocar is advanced through the abdominal wall into the inflated stomach under visualization through the endoscope. The newly established track allows insertion of a synthetic feeding tube. Internal and external bumpers prevent migration. In patients at risk of gastrorespiratory reflux, jejunal feeding tubes can be placed with endoscopic assistance beyond the ligament of Treitz, and enterorespiratory reflux is avoided.

ENDOSCOPIC APPROACH TO INGESTION OF FOREIGN BODIES

Ingestion of foreign objects, purposeful or accidental, is common among small children and among patients with mental status compromise due to psychiatric disease, mental retardation, or inebriation. Most foreign objects that reach the stomach pass through the digestive tract uneventfully. However, long objects, sharp objects, and objects lodged in the esophagus necessitate urgent removal. Flexible endoscopy has become the procedure of choice for diagnosis and for removal of foreign objects. A variety of devices can be used to remove all kinds of objects safely and effectively avoid laparotomy or thoracotomy.

THE FUTURE OF GASTROINTESTINAL ENDOSCOPY

The increasing miniaturization of technologic devices allows expansion of the diagnostic and therapeutic capabilities of endoscopy. Computer image analysis of cellular spectrofluorescence may enable discrimination of neoplastic potential. Early cancer detection and advancing endoscopic techniques will enable endoscopic therapies to replace many surgical procedures.

BIBLIOGRAPHY

Botet JF, Lightdale CJ. Endoscopic ultrasonography of the gastrointestinal tract. *Gastroenterol Clin North Am* 1995;24:385–412.

Consensus Conference: Therapeutic endoscopy and bleeding ulcers. *JAMA* 1989;262:1369–1372.

Faigel DO, Ginsberg GG, Bentz JS, et al. Endoscopic ultrasound-guided real-time fine-needle aspiration biopsy of the pancreas in cancer patients with pancreatic lesions. *J Clin Oncol* 1997;15:1439–1443.

Folsch UR, Nitsche R, Ludtke R, et al. Early ERCP and papillotomy compared with conservative treatment for acute biliary pancreatitis. *N Engl J Med* 1997;336:237–242.

Laine L, El-Newihi HM, Migikovsky B, et al. Endoscopic ligation compared with sclerotherapy for the treatment of bleeding esophageal varices. *Ann Intern Med* 1993;119:1–7.

Provenzale D, Kemp JA, Arora S, et al. A guide for surveillance of patients with Barrett's esophagus. *Am J Gastroenterol* 1994;89:670–680.

Scotiniotis I, Rubesin SE, Ginsberg GG. Imaging modalities in inflammatory bowel disease. *Gastroenterol Clin North Am* 1999;28:391–421.

Smith AC, Dowsett JF, Russell RCG, et al. Randomized trial of endoscopic stenting versus surgical bypass in malignant low bile duct obstruction. *Lancet* 1994;344:1655–1660.

Winawer SJ, Zauber AG, Ho MN, et al. Prevention of colorectal cancer by colonoscopic polypectomy. The National Polyp Study Workgroup. *N Engl J Med* 1993;329:1977–1981.

Zuccaro G Jr. management of the adult patient with acute lower gastrointestinal bleeding. Am J Gastroenterol 1998;93:1202–1208.

Kelley's Textbook of Internal Medicine, fourth edition. Edited by H. David Humes. Lippincott Williams & Wilkins, Philadelphia © 2000.

CHAPTER
128

ABDOMINAL AND ALIMENTARY TRACT IMAGING AND INTERVENTIONAL RADIOLOGY

STEPHEN TRENKNER

There are numerous imaging techniques for evaluating gastrointestinal disease. These vary from conventional radiographic techniques that have been used for decades to the latest applications of magnetic resonance (MR) imaging. The best yield from imaging studies is obtained when the radiologist is provided accurate clinical information. Knowledge of the clinical situation helps determine the best imaging modality and how it will be performed.

UPPER GASTROINTESTINAL TRACT

The widespread availability of endoscopy and the development of new drugs for the treatment of patients with peptic ulcer disease have resulted in a marked reduction in the number of barium radiographic studies of the upper gastrointestinal tract. Modified barium swallow and esophagram, however, maintain an important role in the evaluation of dysphagia (see Chapter 94). The purpose of a modified barium swallow examination is to identify a structural or functional abnormality of swallowing and to evaluate treatment options. The study often is performed jointly by a speech pathologist and a radiologist. Various consistencies of liquids and solids in various quantities are administered orally, and the study is recorded on videotape. Abnormalities such as aspiration or a prominent cricopharyngeous muscle are readily detected. The speech pathologist can vary the diet in conjunction with various swallowing maneuvers to help the patient eat safely.

If the cause of dysphagia is not identified with the swallowing study, the radiologist should obtain a complete barium esophagram. The point at which a patient perceives food sticking does not correlate well with the actual site of obstruction. Obstruction at the gastroesophageal junction is often felt in the neck. During esophagram the radiologist can evaluate the anatomic features of the esophagus, identify a hiatal hernia, observe esophageal peristalsis, and check for gastroesophageal reflux. With a modified barium swallow examination and esophagram the cause of

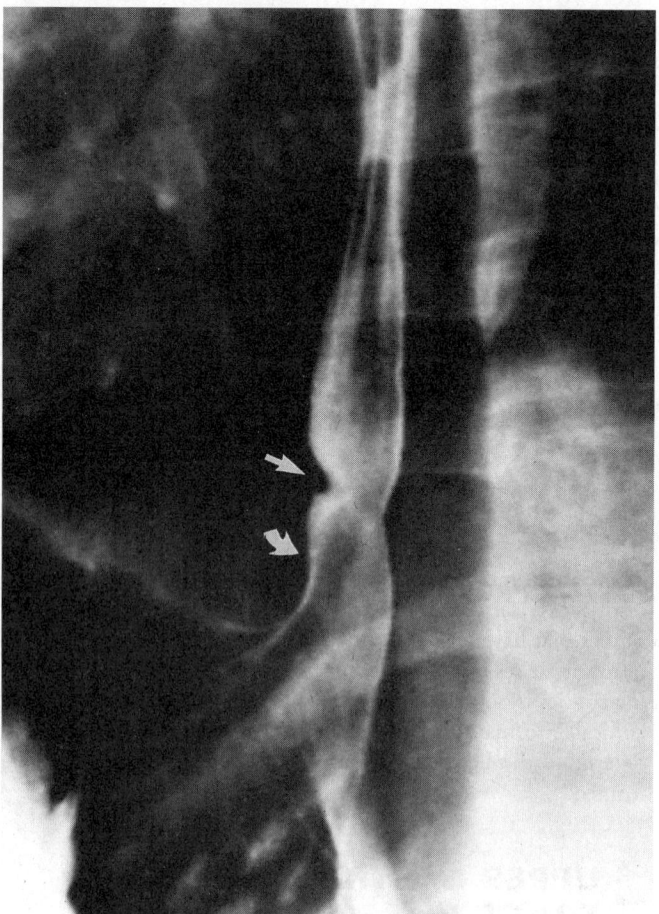

FIGURE 128.1. Prone esophagram performed after findings of modified barium swallow radiographic examination were normal. Dysphagia is caused by hiatal hernia (*curved arrow*), short stricture (*straight arrow*), and gastroesophageal reflux.

dysphagia frequently can be identified and the patient referred to the appropriate specialist (Fig 128.1)

SMALL BOWEL

Imaging plays a key role in the evaluation of small-bowel abnormalities. Although plain radiography and barium studies continue to be the major modalities, computed tomography (CT) is gaining in prominence.

There are a number of techniques for evaluating the small bowel with barium, including conventional small-bowel follow-through (SBFT) study, peroral pneumocolon, and enteroclysis. The preference of the radiologist often dictates the type of study performed. A conventional SBFT study with the addition of a peroral pneumocolon is especially helpful in examinations of patients with Crohn's disease. When orally administered barium reaches the cecum, a small catheter is passed into the rectum, and air is insufflated. The air distends the terminal ileum and gives a double contrast effect. In patients with Crohn's disease, narrowing of the ileum frequently is caused in part by spasm. Administration of air allows more accurate assessment of true luminal diameter. The double contrast effect also improves visualization of subtle abnormalities such as aphthous ulcers.

Enteroclysis allows the most detailed evaluation of the small bowel and may provide enough information for a diagnosis when findings of an SBFT study are normal. A catheter is passed through the nose or mouth and advanced to the duodenojejunal junction. Barium is administered through the tube and followed by methylcellulose. This study allows reliable distention of the small bowel and excellent depiction of the mucosal fold pattern (Fig 128.2). Indications for enteroclysis include gastrointestinal bleeding after endoscopy has failed to demonstrate an upper GI or colonic source, symptoms of intermittent or partial small-bowel obstruction, and strong suspicion of small-bowel disease.

As CT continues to improve, important small-bowel applications have become evident. CT has been especially helpful for evaluating small-bowel obstruction and ischemia. CT has a sensitivity of 94% in the diagnosis of small-bowel obstruction, allows correct prediction of the cause of obstruction in 73%, and is currently the best modality for detecting strangulation associated with closed-loop obstruction. The diagnosis of obstruction is based on demonstrating a transition point between dilated and decompressed bowel. When a transition point is found but there is no identifiable cause of obstruction, such as a tumor or abscess, an adhesion is suspected. Adhesions cannot be imaged directly with CT.

If a patient is believed to have acute mesenteric ischemia, angiography is the imaging study of choice. Vascular occlusion and vasoconstriction can be identified, and pharmacologic therapy can be provided through the catheter. The signs and symptoms frequently are nonspecific, however, and there is reluctance to perform an invasive procedure. Contrast-enhanced CT is an excellent tool for rapid evaluation of the entire abdomen. The sensitivity is 64% in the detection of acute mesenteric ischemia. Findings with a specificity of greater than 95% include arterial or venous thrombosis, pneumatosis intestinalis, portal venous

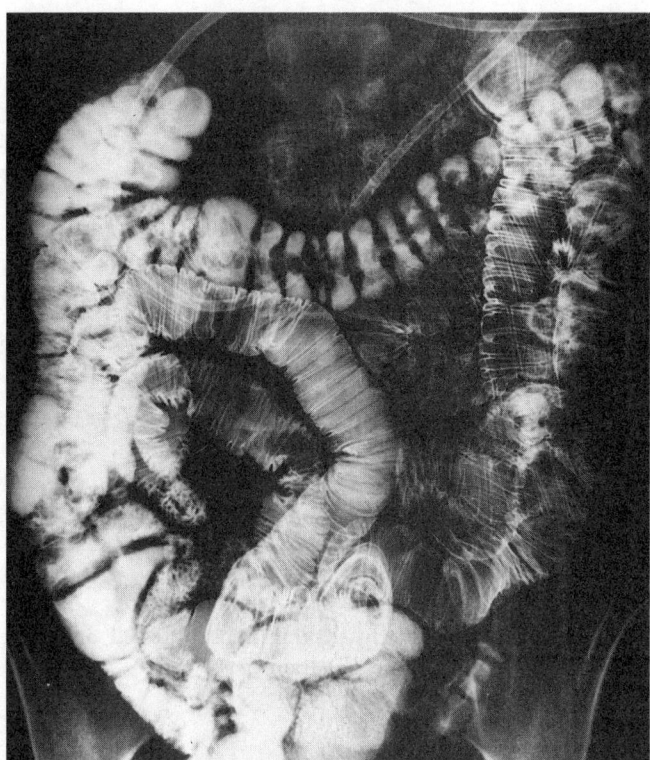

FIGURE 128.2. Normal enteroclysis. Normal fold pattern is well depicted.

gas, focal absence of bowel wall enhancement, and infarcts in other abdominal organs (Figure 128.3).

Chronic mesenteric ischemia is suspected when a patient has postprandial abdominal pain, weight loss, and an abdominal bruit (see Chapter 112). Most patients have thrombus at the origins of at least two of the three major visceral arteries (celiac axis, superior and inferior mesenteric arteries). Duplex sonography is a valuable tool for selecting patients who need angiography as the definitive test for this condition.

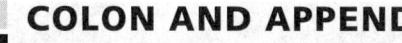

COLON AND APPENDIX

The widespread availability of colonoscopy and the development of cross-sectional imaging modalities have caused a reduction in the use of barium enema radiography. Contrast enema examination remains a valuable test with numerous important applications, including screening for polyps and colorectal cancer, evaluating obstruction, detecting fistulas, and evaluating the colon after a surgical procedure.

CT is an excellent modality in the diagnosis of diverticulitis or appendicitis. Many other colonic conditions also can be identified with CT that are not suspected clinically. It is not uncommon to find pseudomembranous colitis or ischemic colitis in a patient undergoing CT to evaluate a fever source or nonspecific abdominal pain.

DIVERTICULITIS

In direct comparison with barium enema radiography, CT is the best study for the diagnosis of diverticulitis. Diverticulitis is identified by the findings of stranding of the pericolic fat, thickening of the colonic wall, and abscess formation adjacent to the colon. CT can be used to guide percutaneous drainage of an abscess if clinically necessary. CT also may help identify an alternative diagnosis if diverticulitis is not present. Contrast enema examination still plays a role in the care of patients with diverticulitis when the CT findings are equivocal. The degree of obstruction and exact site and size of a fistula also are best demonstrated with a contrast enema examination.

The CT findings in pseudomembranous colitis (see Chapter 113) vary from normal in mild cases to marked, nodular colonic wall thickening in severe cases. Orally administered contrast material trapped between the thickened folds looks like an accordion. This sign is fairly specific for pseudomembranous colitis (Fig 128.4).

APPENDICITIS

Appendicitis is diagnosed clinically in most instances, but 20% of patients have atypical initial findings. This group of patients

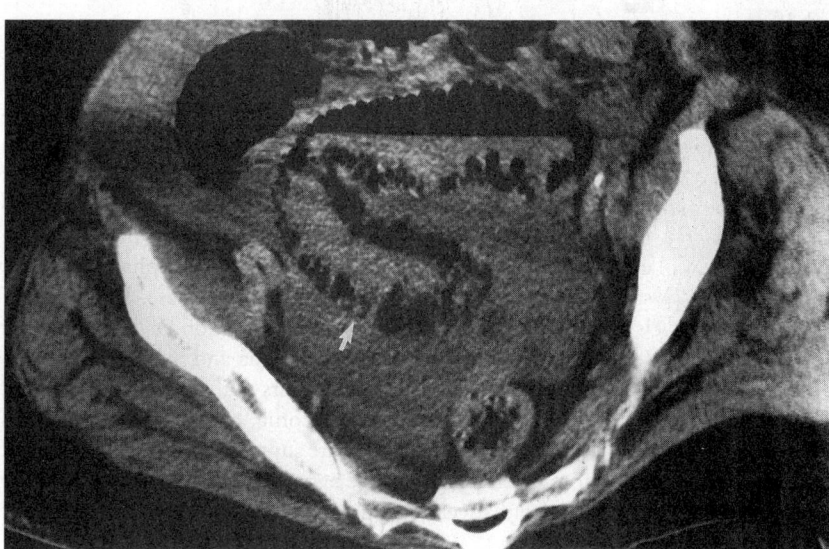

FIGURE 128.3. Extensive pneumatosis intestinalis (*arrow*) in a patient with acute mesenteric ischemia.

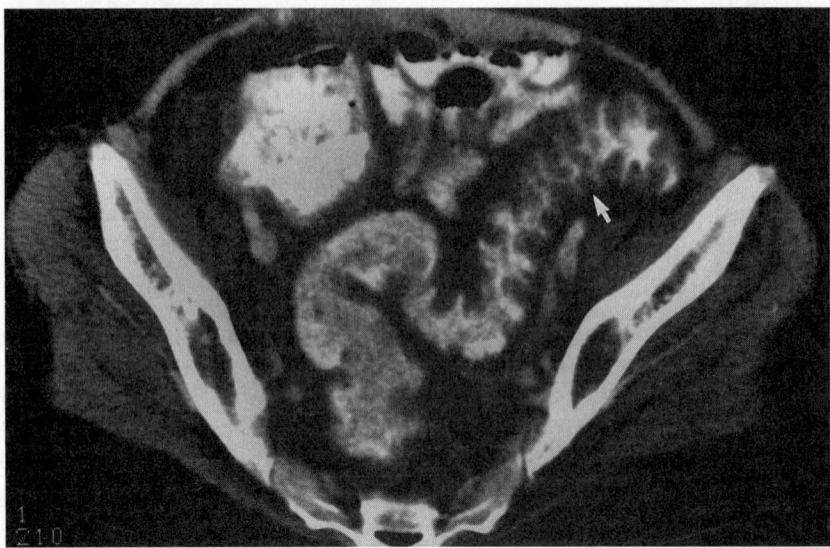

FIGURE 128.4. Pseudomembranous colitis with accordion sign in the sigmoid colon (*arrow*).

benefits most from imaging. Plain radiographs and a barium enema examination are of limited value. The most specific plain radiographic finding is an appendicolith, but one is seen in only 10% of cases. The diagnosis of appendicitis is made at barium enema radiography when there is incomplete filling of the appendix and a mass effect on the cecum. The appendix may not fill with barium in patients without appendicitis.

Ultrasound scanning and CT have become the two main imaging modalities for the evaluation of appendicitis. The ultrasound diagnosis is based on identifying a noncompressible appendix greater than 6 mm in diameter. If an appendicolith is seen at ultrasound examination, the result is considered positive even if the diameter is less than 6 mm. According to these criteria, appendicitis may be diagnosed with a sensitivity of 89.9% and a specificity of 96.2%. Ultrasonography is operator dependent and is difficult when the patient is obese and when the appendix is retrocecal. A normal appendix is infrequently seen with ultrasonography. The absence of appendicitis therefore is inferred when an appendix is not seen.

Appendicitis is diagnosed with CT when the appendix has a thickened wall, there are inflammatory changes in the fat surrounding the appendix, or an appendicolith is identified. If intravenous contrast medium is given, the wall of an abnormal appendix commonly becomes enhanced. CT also is excellent for detecting an appendiceal abscess. Sensitivities as high as 98% to 100% have been reported for the detection of appendicitis with CT. Among patients without appendicitis, CT allows an alternative diagnosis in as many as 62% of cases. In one series, CT scans were obtained of 100 patients consecutively hospitalized with the clinical diagnosis of appendicitis. CT findings led to changes in the treatment plan for 59 patients, prevented 13 unnecessary appendectomies, and showed a savings of $447 per patient.

Ultrasound and CT are both excellent tests for appendicitis. The expertise and experience of the radiologist should be taken into account when these studies are ordered. A reasonable approach is to perform ultrasound examinations of children and women of childbearing age. CT has advantages in examinations

of obese patients, the elderly, the immunosuppressed, and those with a palpable right lower quadrant mass.

COLORECTAL CANCER

The diagnosis of colorectal cancer typically is made by means of colonoscopy or barium enema radiography. Once the diagnosis is established, preoperative staging requires the evaluation of depth of tumor penetration, lymph node involvement, and presence of distant metastases, especially to the liver.

CT is superior to MR imaging in predicting tumor penetration beyond the muscularis propria but has a sensitivity of only 72%. Detecting a tumor in local lymph nodes is difficult with either CT or MR (sensitivity 49% and 23%, respectively). CT and MR depict liver metastases with a sensitivity of 62% and 70%, respectively. The ability to detect microscopic disease in lymph nodes and the liver with CT and MR imaging is limited.

■ LIVER AND BILIARY TRACT

CT is the dominant cross-sectional imaging modality for the liver and abdomen. With spiral or helical CT, the entire liver can be scanned during a single breath hold, eliminating misregistration due to breathing. The rapidity with which the scan can be performed allows imaging during different phases of contrast enhancement. The liver can be imaged twice during the intravenous administration of a single bolus of contrast material. The early scans depict the liver in the hepatic arterial phase, and later scans depict the liver in the portal venous phase. Biphasic CT is of particular importance in the evaluation of hypervascular tumors such as hepatocellular carcinoma and hypervascular metastases from renal cell tumors, tumors of the breast and thyroid, melanoma, carcinoid tumors, sarcoma, and pancreatic islet cell tumors. Hypervascular tumors are supplied by the hepatic artery. Therefore when imaged in the hepatic arterial phase, they appear as areas of enhancement against a relatively unenhanced liver

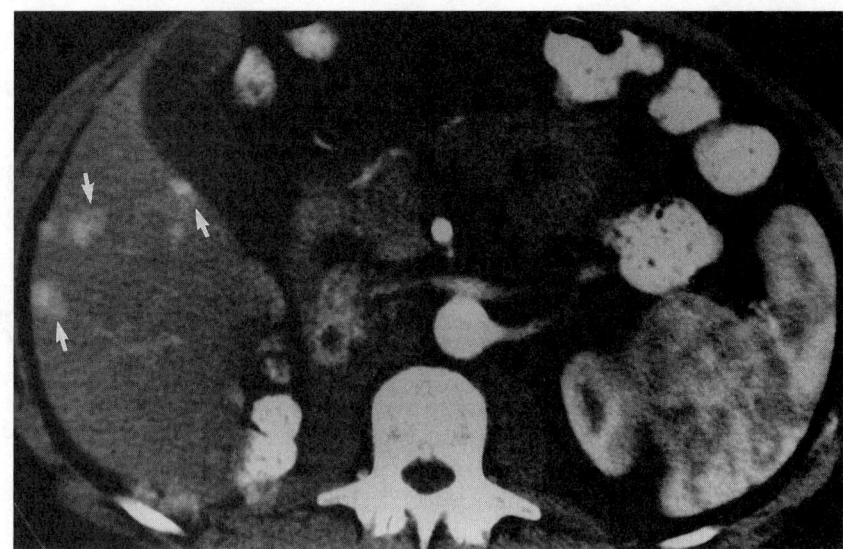

FIGURE 128.5. Metastatic renal cell carcinoma (*arrows*) imaged during the hepatic arterial phase.

(Fig 128.5). When imaged in the portal venous phase, hypervascular tumors may become the same density or less dense than normal liver. Hypovascular tumors such as metastases from the colon, lung, and pancreas are best imaged during the portal venous phase.

MR imaging is an excellent modality for hepatic imaging and often is used to characterize lesions that are equivocal at CT. MR imaging also provides an alternative to CT in examinations of patients for whom use of iodinated contrast material is contraindicated because of allergy or renal insufficiency (Fig 128.6). A new application of MR imaging is MR cholangiopancreatography (MRCP). This technique allows images acquired with MR to be projected in a manner similar to that of endoscopic retrograde cholangiopancreatography (ERCP). The spatial resolution of MRCP is inferior to that of ERCP, but many conditions such as choledocholithiasis and biliary strictures can be diagnosed reliably. MRCP provides a means for studying the bile ducts

and pancreatic duct of patients who have had unsuccessful ERCP or who have postoperative gastric anatomy that does not allow performance of ERCP. As MRCP continues to improve, it may replace diagnostic ERCP in many applications. ERCP will continue to have a strong role in therapeutic intervention.

Ultrasonography is the primary imaging modality for evaluating the gallbladder and for detecting biliary dilatation. Intraoperative ultrasonography also outperforms both CT and MR imaging in the detection of hepatic metastases and should be performed during partial hepatectomy.

The evaluation of transjugular intrahepatic portosystemic shunts (TIPS) is a recent application of ultrasonography. TIPS has become a valuable option in the management of complications of portal hypertension. Ultrasonography is helpful before and after TIPS placement. The preprocedure study consists of evaluation of the liver parenchyma and assessment of spleen size and the amount of ascites. A complete upper abdominal vascular

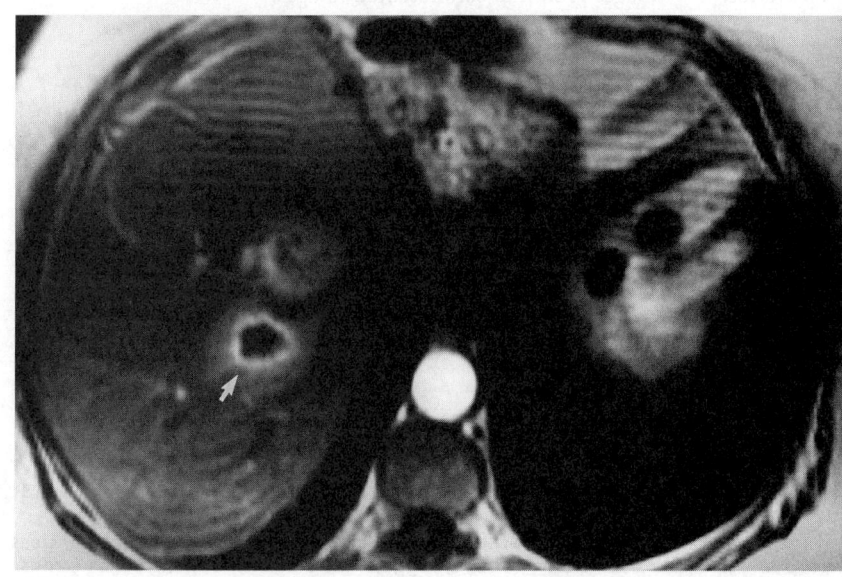

FIGURE 128.6. Gadolinium-enhanced magnetic resonance image shows liver metastases (*arrow*) from renal cell carcinoma in a patient allergic to iodinated contrast medium.

examination is performed to assure patency of the hepatic veins and to define portal venous anatomy and direction of blood flow. TIPS procedures are performed by an interventional radiologist. Vascular access is obtained through the internal jugular vein. A shunt is developed between a hepatic vein and the portal vein, which is kept open with a metallic stent. Postprocedure ultrasonography is used to assess shunt patency. The velocity of flow within the shunt is determined by means of evaluation of the Doppler signal. Stenosis of the shunt is usually caused by pseudointimal hyperplasia and is identified with either an increase or a decrease in shunt velocity compared with a baseline value.

Scintigraphy is important in hepatobiliary imaging. While conventional liver–spleen scanning rarely is used today, other techniques have taken its place. Technetium 99m HIDA scans are used to study the bile ducts and the gallbladder. When obstruction of the cystic duct is demonstrated, this study is more than 90% sensitive for the diagnosis of acute cholecystitis. Technetium 99m HIDA scans also can be used to detect bile leaks and biliary obstruction, especially in patients with postoperative anatomic features that preclude performance of ERCP.

Technetium 99m labeled red blood cell scintigraphy is an excellent study for confirming the diagnosis of hepatic cavernous hemangioma. Cavernous hemangiomas is the most common benign liver tumor and is a frequent incidental finding at ultrasound studies. When confirmation is needed, a ^{99m}Tc-labeled red cell study is an alternative to CT or MR imaging.

New imaging agents are being developed for specific indications. Indium 111 octreotide is a somatostatin analog that can be used to image neuroendocrine tumors, especially gastrinoma. Fluorodeoxy glucose (F-18FDG) has an affinity for colorectal neoplasms, and imaging with this agent may have a role in the evaluation of colorectal cancer when a patient has an elevated carcinoembryonic antigen level.

PANCREAS

CT is currently the best initial imaging study for evaluation of the pancreas. Two common indications for CT of the pancreas are pancreatic carcinoma and pancreatitis. The ability to obtain rapid contrast-enhanced images by means of spiral CT has improved the imaging of pancreatic carcinoma. Just as hepatic scanning has been improved by imaging during the arterial phase and the portal venous phase of contrast enhancement, pancreatic imaging has been improved by scanning during the pancreatic phase. The pancreatic phase falls between the arterial phase and the portal venous phase. At this time the difference in attenuation between hypovascular pancreatic cancer and contrast-enhanced normal pancreas is the greatest. Enhancement of surrounding vascular structures also is optimal during the pancreatic phase. For full staging of pancreatic carcinoma, the primary tumor must be imaged and assessed for local or distant spread. This is best done with imaging of the pancreas in the pancreatic phase and the liver in the portal venous phase.

Contrast-enhanced CT is the imaging study of choice for patients with pancreatitis. Lack of enhancement of portions of the pancreas indicates pancreatic necrosis, the presence of which is predictive of substantial morbidity and mortality (Fig 128.7). CT is useful for diagnosis of other complications of pancreatitis such as pseudocyst, abscess, hemorrhage, and pseudoaneurysm. CT also can be used to guide drainage of pseudocysts and abscesses.

THE FUTURE

The near future for abdominal radiology involves increasing applications for the noninvasive imaging of luminal structures. MRCP will continue to improve as an alternative to diagnostic ERCP. MR angiography is replacing conventional angiography. CT colography (virtual colonoscopy) may become the screening study of choice for the detection of polyps and colorectal cancer. This procedure is performed by means of imaging the colon with spiral CT. The data are reformatted into two- and three-dimensional images of the entire colon. The three-dimensional images look like colonoscopic images.

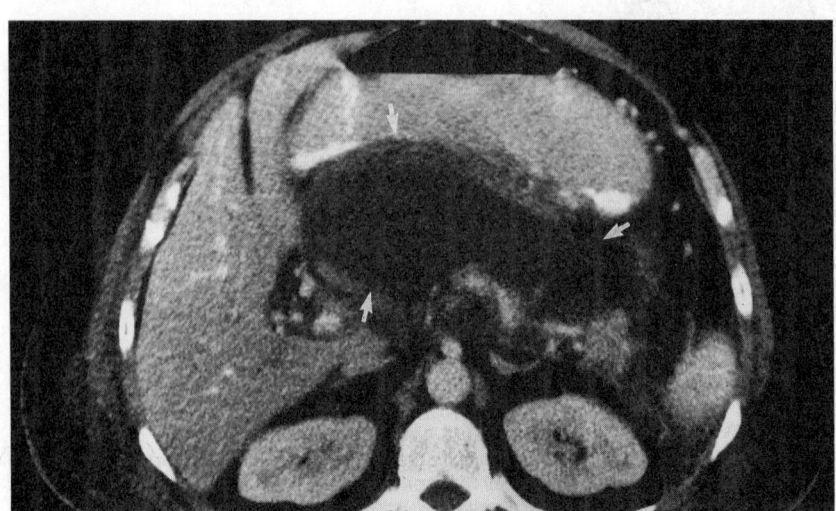

FIGURE 128.7. Lack of enhancement of the pancreas (*arrows*) suggests the diagnosis of pancreatic necrosis.

BIBLIOGRAPHY

Abbitt PL. Ultrasonography update on liver technique. *Radiol Clin North Am* 1998;36:299–307.

Balthazar EJ, Birnbaum BA, Yee J, et al. Acute appendicitis: CT and US correlation in 100 patients. *Radiology* 1994;190:31–35.

Boland GW, O'Malley ME, Saez M, et al. Pancreatic-phase versus portal vein–phase helical CT of the pancreas: optimal temporal window for evaluation of pancreatic adenocarcinoma. *AJR* 1999;172:605–608.

Cho KC, Morehouse HT, Alterman DD, et al. Sigmoid diverticulitis: diagnostic role of CT—comparison with barium enema studies. *Radiology* 1990;176:111–115.

Drane WE. Scintigraphic techniques for hepatic imaging: update for 2000. *Radiol Clin North Am* 1998;36:309–318.

Hara AK, Johnson CD, Reed JE, et al. Detection of colorectal polyps with CT colography: initial assessment of sensitivity and specificity. *Radiology* 1997;205:59–65.

Kemmerer SR, Mortele KJ, Ros PR. CT scan of the liver. *Radiol Clin North Am* 1998;36:247–260.

Logeman JA. *Evaluation and treatment of swallowing disorders,* 2 ed. Austin, TX: PRO-ED, 1998:168–189.

Paulson EK, Vitellas KM, Keogan MT, et al. Acute pancreatitis complicated by gland necrosis: spectrum of findings on contrast-enhanced CT. *AJR* 1999;172:609–613.

Rao PM, Rhea JT, Novelline RA, et al. Effect of computed tomography of the appendix on treatment of patients and use of hospital resources. *N Engl J Med* 1998;338:141–146.

Ros PR, Buetow PC, Pantograg-Brown L, et al. Pseudomembranous colitis. *Radiology* 1996;198:1–9.

Taourel PG, Deneuville M, Pradel JA, et al. Acute mesenteric ischemia: diagnosis with contrast-enhanced CT. *Radiology* 1996;199:632–636.

Trenkner SW, Hommeyer S. Practical imaging of the small bowel. *Radiologist* 1995;2:127–137.

Zerhouni EA, Rutter C, Hamilton SR, et al. CT and MR imaging in the staging of colorectal carcinoma: report of the radiology diagnostic oncology group II. *Radiology* 1996;200:443–451.

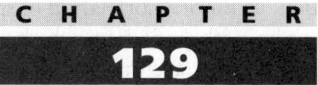

CHAPTER 129

DIAGNOSTIC TESTS IN GASTROINTESTINAL MOTILITY AND PHYSIOLOGY

WILLIAM L. HASLER

For many organic diseases of the gastrointestinal tract, structural evaluation with endoscopic or radiographic studies is needed for diagnosis. However, certain disorders of the gastrointestinal tract exhibit no visible abnormalities. To detect these conditions, a broad range of physiologic tests of visceral motor and secretory function can be performed.

GASTROINTESTINAL MOTILITY TESTING

Disorders of gastrointestinal motility may produce a variety of symptoms depending on the anatomic region involved and the severity of dysfunction (see Chapter 108). For each luminal segment, tests of motor function provide diagnostic information that can be used to direct treatment.

ASSESSMENT OF ESOPHAGEAL MOTOR FUNCTION

Common symptoms related to dysfunctional esophageal motor activity include dysphagia (see Chapter 94), noncardiac chest pain (see Chapter 95), and gastroesophageal reflux (see Chapter 106). Less common signs and symptoms of esophageal dysmotility include a globus sensation of fullness in the throat, pharyngeal irritation, and pulmonary complications such as asthma, recurrent bronchitis, and aspiration pneumonia.

Esophageal Manometry

Indications

Esophageal manometry is used most commonly to evaluate patients with unexplained dysphagia who have no evidence of esophageal obstruction. It is used specifically in the diagnosis of achalasia and other esophageal motor disorders. The test also is used to detect esophageal dysmotility among patients with chest pain after cardiac disease has been excluded. Esophageal manometry is performed on selected patients with gastroesophageal reflux, especially those being considered for surgical therapy.

Methods

After induction of topical anesthesia of the nasal cavity and throat with viscous lidocaine, a water-perfused or solid-state manometric catheter is passed so that all recording sites are initially in the stomach. The examiner slowly withdraws the catheter while looking for a positive deflection representative of lower esophageal sphincter (LES) pressure. After establishment of LES pressure, the catheter is left in place so that a distal recording site continuously measures LES pressure and three or more proximal sites record esophageal body pressure. The response to swallowing is assessed and should include generation of an aborally propagative peristaltic contraction and >90% reduction in LES pressure. Tone and relaxation of the upper esophageal sphincter (UES) and a crude assessment of pharyngeal peristalsis also can be measured for patients with cervical dysphagia; however, manometric evaluation of this region may be limited by patient tolerance and other technical factors.

Provocative testing can be performed during esophageal manometry for selected indications. Intravenous administration of edrophonium may increase esophageal contractions and reproduce symptoms in as many as 40% of patients with unexplained chest pain. Ergonovine and bethanechol also may reproduce chest pain; however, side effects are common with these agents.

An acid reflux test can be performed to assist in the diagnosis of gastroesophageal reflux. This provocation involves measuring esophageal pH 5 cm above the LES before and after maneuvers that increase intraabdominal pressure. The Bernstein test is performed by means of alternate infusion of hydrochloric acid and saline solution in the esophagus with the patient blinded. This test can be used to determine whether unexplained chest pain or heartburn is caused by acidification of the esophagus.

Clinical Findings

Lack of esophageal body peristalsis is a requirement for the diagnosis of achalasia, although low-amplitude simultaneous contractions often are present (Fig 129.1). Vigorous achalasia is a variant with high-amplitude (>80 mm Hg) nonperistaltic contractions. Incomplete LES relaxation is usually (>80% of cases) but not always present in achalasia; some early presentations have complete relaxations of very short duration. Some patients with achalasia may have elevated LES or intraesophageal pressure. The presence of simultaneous esophageal body contractions at more than two recording sites more than 10% of the time with normal LES relaxation is found with diffuse esophageal spasm. Nutcracker esophagus is characterized by high-amplitude (>180 mm Hg) peristaltic body contractions of long duration (>6 seconds). These conditions cause chest pain more often than they do dysphagia. Hypertensive LES is defined by an LES pressure >45 mm Hg. Low LES pressures are common among patients with scleroderma.

Impaired UES relaxation occurs with primary UES disorders such as cricopharyngeal achalasia and diffuse neuromuscular diseases such as central nervous system lymphoma, oculopharyngeal muscular dystrophy, and familial dysautonomia. UES hypertension may occur with gastroesophageal reflux. Low UES pressures occur with amyotrophic lateral sclerosis, myotonic dystrophy, and myasthenia gravis. Among patients with gastroesophageal

reflux, a low LES pressure is associated with a high rate of failure of medication therapy. Thus manometry may be useful in determining which patients might benefit from antireflux surgery. Preoperatively manometric assessment of esophageal body peristalsis also is important, because the presence of uncoordinated peristalsis can influence the type of surgical procedure chosen.

Twenty-four-hour pH Monitoring

Indications

Twenty-four-hour ambulatory esophageal pH monitoring is most commonly indicated to determine whether gastroesophageal reflux of acid is responsible for atypical symptoms, such as chest pain, cervical dysphagia, cough, pharyngitis, or pulmonary disorders such as asthma or bronchitis. The procedure also is performed to confirm that acid is the source of esophageal symptoms among patients being considered for antireflux surgery. Monitoring of pH may be performed during therapy with acid-suppressing medications to determine the adequacy of antireflux treatment among patients with persistent or atypical symptoms.

Methods

After topical anesthesia of the nasal cavity and throat, the catheter is passed through the nose until the pH electrode is determined to be 5 cm above the LES. Intraesophageal pH is recorded continuously with an electronic device worn on the belt or over the shoulder while the patient performs normal daily activities, including ingestion of meals, exertion, and sleep. An event recorder is included to correlate episodes of chest pain, heartburn, cough, or dysphagia with periods of gastroesophageal reflux of acid.

Clinical Findings

The maximal sensitivity and specificity of 24-hour pH monitoring are obtained by means of quantifying the percentage of time pH is greater than 4 and the number of episodes longer than 5 minutes in duration. Temporal correlation of specific symptoms on the event recorder with periods in which esophageal pH is greater than 4 enhances the accuracy of the test.

Cineradiography

Indications

Cineradiographic assessment of swallowing is indicated to determine whether impaired pharyngoesophageal coordination is the cause of cervical dysphagia, meal-related coughing, or pulmonary aspiration.

Methods

Cineradiography is performed to record the motor events in the mouth, pharynx, and upper esophagus that are associated with swallowing. Dynamic recordings are obtained in the lateral and posteroanterior projections after ingestion of thin and thick liquid barium and barium cookies.

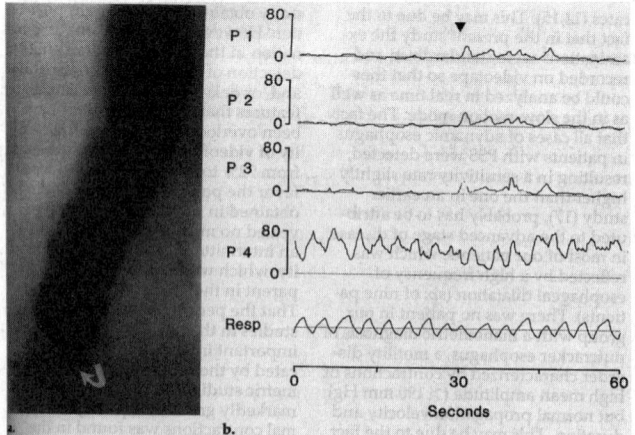

FIGURE 129.1. Videofluoroscopic and manometric findings for a patient with achalasia. **A:** Radiographic image shows a typical bird's beak appearance. **B:** Manometric tracing of the esophageal body (*P1-3*) shows a lack of peristalsis with swallowing water (*arrow*). There also is incomplete relaxation of the LES (*P4*). (From Schima W, Stacher G, Pokieser P, et al. Esophageal motor disorders: videofluoroscopic and manometric evaluation--prospective study in 88 symptomatic patients. *Radiology* 1992;185:487–491.)

Clinical Findings

Dysphagia among patients with neuromuscular disease may be caused by delayed initiation of bolus transfer or prolonged retention of the swallowed bolus in a pharyngeal recess. Delayed UES relaxation, as occurs with familial dysautonomia, also may produce dysphagia. Cricopharyngeal bars may be caused by muscular hypertrophy of the UES. Misdirected swallows with laryngeal or nasal penetration or tracheal aspiration are important abnormalities that may mandate initiation of enteral tube feedings for patients with symptoms of pulmonary aspiration.

ASSESSMENT OF GASTRODUODENAL MOTOR FUNCTION

Gastric motor dysfunction most commonly produces nausea, vomiting, early satiety, bloating, fullness, and abdominal discomfort. Gastric motor dysfunction also may be a predisposing factor for development of gastroesophageal reflux of acid. Symptomatic manifestations of small-intestinal dysmotility may be similar. When severe, small-intestinal motor dysfunction also may be a predisposing factor for the development of small-intestinal bacterial overgrowth, which can cause diarrhea, malabsorption of vitamins and nutrients, electrolyte disturbances, and weight loss.

Measurement of Gastric Emptying

Indications

Quantification of the rate of gastric emptying is most commonly indicated for the diagnosis of gastroparesis among patients with unexplained nausea and vomiting. Gastric emptying testing also is performed on patients with dysmotility-like functional dyspepsia, diabetes, and poor glycemic control. These disorders may be caused by gastroparesis, postgastrectomy syndrome, medically refractory gastroesophageal reflux, and chronic intestinal pseudoobstruction.

Methods

Scintigraphic assessment of gastric emptying of a solid meal is the most widely accepted test for the diagnosis of gastroparesis. Solid-phase scintigraphy is performed with a technetium Tc 99m sulfur colloid label mixed with a solid meal such as scrambled eggs, oatmeal, or chicken liver. Solid emptying shows a biphasic curve with an initial lag phase during which food is mixed in the stomach but not emptied. The lag phase is followed by a linear emptying phase that persists until the stomach is emptied. In general, 40% to 80% of a solid meal is emptied within 2 hours of ingestion. Liquid-phase gastric scintigraphy also may be performed after ingestion of water with an aqueous phase isotope such as indium In 111 diethylenetriamine pentaacetic acid (DTPA). Liquid emptying is rapid; the half-time is 8 to 28 minutes.

Other methods of quantification of gastric emptying are gaining favor. Breath tests after ingestion of octanoate or acetate preparations have been developed to assess emptying of both solids and liquids. The results correlate well with scintigraphic findings. With such tests, the nonradioactive isotope carbon C 13 is incorporated to provide the capability to study emptying among patients in whose care a radioactive tracer would be contraindicated, such as pregnant women. As the carbon C 13–labeled meal is delivered to the duodenum, the ligand is digested and liberates carbon dioxide C 13, which is absorbed into the bloodstream and exhaled in the breath. Ultrasonography and magnetic resonance imaging have been used to measure gastric emptying of liquids, but these techniques are poorly standardized. Ultrasonography depends heavily on the skill of the operator. Thus these modalities have not achieved widespread acceptance.

Clinical Findings

Gastroparesis is diagnosed when the time for emptying of either solids or liquids exceeds the maximal normal value (Fig 129.2). In general, solid-phase tests are more sensitive for the diagnosis of gastroparesis than are liquid-phase tests. However, liquid-phase emptying may be selectively accelerated among patients with postvagotomy dumping syndrome. The utility of gastric emptying testing in clinical decision making is unproved. Gastric symptoms often correlate poorly with delays in gastric emptying. Symptoms also may show drastic improvement during therapy with prokinetic drugs without acceleration of emptying. In the only study to date of the utility of gastric scintigraphy, emptying results did not influence clinical management.

Gastroduodenal Manometry

Indications

Gastroduodenal manometry is performed to detect gastric or small-intestinal dysmotility among patients with unexplained nausea, vomiting, or abdominal discomfort. Patients usually

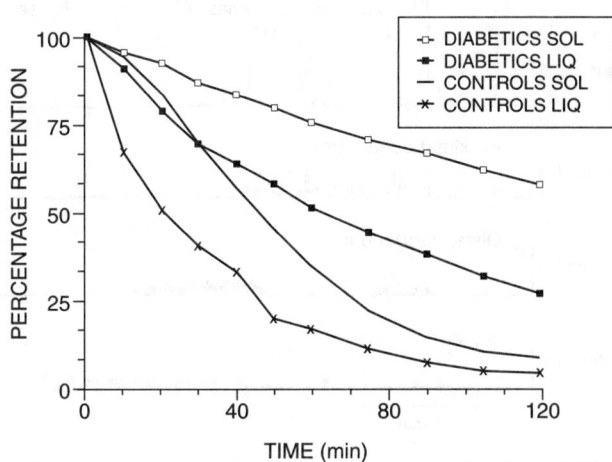

FIGURE 129.2. Gastric emptying profiles of solids and liquids measured by means of scintigraphy. Emptying is slower among patients with diabetes and gastroparesis than it is among healthy volunteers. (From Urbain JL, Vantrappen G, Janssens J, et al. Intravenous erythromycin dramatically accelerates gastric emptying in gastroparesis diabeticorum and normals and abolishes the emptying discrimination between solids and liquids. *J Nucl Med* 1990;31:1490–1493.)

have normal gastric emptying results or delayed emptying but do not respond to prokinetic agents. Manometry also may reveal specific motor patterns that can be used to differentiate myopathic and neuropathic intestinal pseudoobstruction and to detect a generalized dysmotility syndrome among patients with localized symptoms such as severe constipation. Intestinal manometry can be used to predict ability to tolerate enteral feeding.

Methods

Gastroduodenal manometry involves fluoroscopic placement of a water-perfused or solid-state catheter so that pressure ports span the antrum and duodenum (and in specialized cases, the pylorus, jejunum, and ileum). In the initial 4 to 6 hours fasting motility is recorded. During this time one or more cycles of the migrating motor complex (MMC) usually are observed. The MMC consists of three phases that cycle every 90 to 120 minutes, beginning in the stomach and propagating into the small intestine (Fig 129.3). Afterward the first phase, motor activity is measured for 2 hours after a solid meal, which should induce a fed pattern. Calculation of an antral motility index from the summed fed contractions has been shown to correlate with scintigraphic measurements of gastric emptying. Manometry affords the option of testing the effects of prokinetic drugs during recording. Advances in miniaturization have made it possible to record 24 hours of motor activity while the patient undertakes normal activity.

Clinical Findings

Absence of the MMC or a reduction in fed contractions in the antrum indicates gastroparesis. Some patients with gastroparesis have prolonged periods of increased tonic and phasic motor

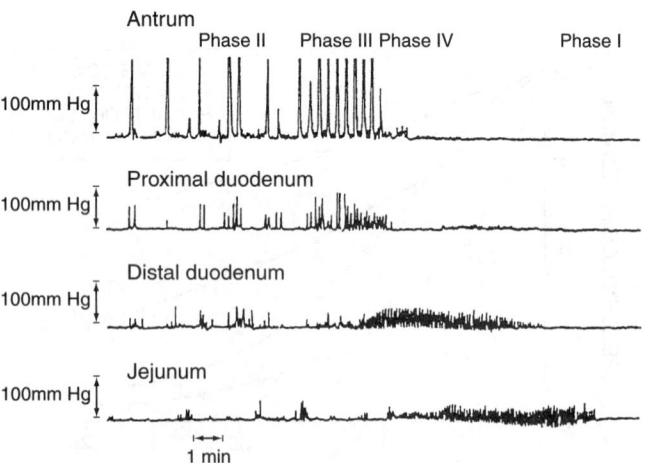

FIGURE 129.3. The migrating motor complex of a healthy person consistently shows three phases. Phase I is a period of motor quiescence. Phase II is a period of irregular contractions. Phase III is a brief complex of intense contractions that propagates from the stomach through the small intestine. Some studies show a transitional period, phase IV. (From Rees WDW, Malagelada JR, Miller LJ, et al. Human interdigestive and postprandial gastrointestinal motor and gastrointestinal hormone patterns. *Dig Dis* Sci 1982;27:321–329.)

activity in the pylorus, known as *pylorospasm.* Decreases in gastroduodenal contractile amplitude occur with myopathic disorders such as scleroderma, amyloidosis, and familial visceral myopathy. In contrast, intense uncoordinated intestinal bursts suggest familial visceral neuropathy, neuropathic forms of scleroderma or amyloidosis, or paraneoplastic intestinal pseudoobstruction. The minute rhythm, a regular pattern of intestinal bursts occurring every 1 to 3 minutes, occurs with mechanical obstruction, visceral neuropathy, and some cases of irritable bowel syndrome. In a study of the clinical utility of gastroduodenal manometry, management decisions were influenced by test results in 19% of cases, most commonly directing the choice of prokinetic drugs and feeding options.

Electrogastrography

Indications

The most common indication for electrogastrography is unexplained nausea and vomiting. Most patients have normal gastric emptying or delayed gastric emptying that has not responded to prokinetic medication. Electrogastrography has been proposed as a noninvasive test to predict gastroparesis among patients such as pregnant women in whose care use of a radioactive tracer would be contraindicated. Electrogastrography can be used to detect evidence of functional gastric impairment among patients with localized dysmotility syndromes such as severe gastroesophageal reflux or constipation.

Methods

Electrogastrography is used to measure gastric slow-wave activity acquired from cutaneous electrodes placed over the stomach for 15 to 60 minutes before and 60 to 120 minutes after a meal. The signal is carefully filtered to exclude cardiac (60 to 100 cycles per minute [cpm]), respiratory (10 to 25 cpm), and intestinal (10 to 12 cpm) electrical activity. The raw signal is analyzed with a computer program to produce a frequency spectrum of the dominant frequencies as a function of time (Fig 129.4). A normal gastric slow wave cycles at 2 to 4 cpm. Meal ingestion produces a physiologic increase in signal amplitude.

Clinical Findings

Tachygastria is diagnosed when a substantial fraction of the recording has a dominant frequency of >4 cpm. Bradygastria is diagnosed when the signal is <2 cpm. Such dysrhythmias are prevalent among patients with gastroparesis, dyspepsia, motion sickness, and the nausea of pregnancy. Some patients have no change or have a decrease in electrogastrographic amplitude after eating. This finding correlates with delays in gastric emptying.

ASSESSMENT OF COLORECTAL AND ANAL MOTOR FUNCTION

Impairment of colonic motility can cause inertia, a condition in which transit of feces is markedly delayed. The result is severe constipation. Contractile abnormalities of the rectum, anus, and

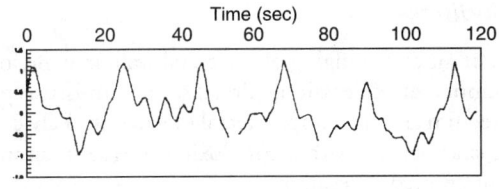

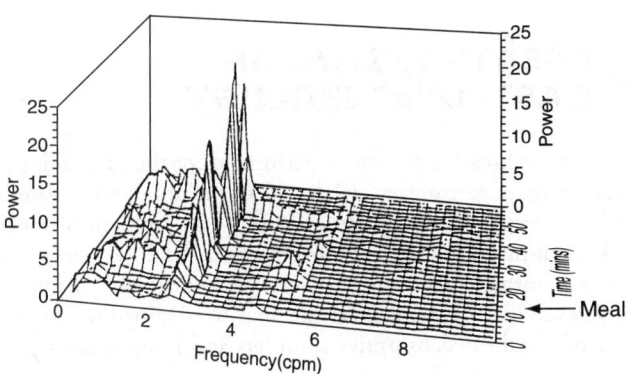

FIGURE 129.4. Electrogastrographic results of a healthy volunteer. *Top,* Raw slow wave signal exhibits rhythmic oscillation that cycles every 20 seconds. *Bottom,* Frequency spectral analysis of the slow wave. Throughout the recording, the dominant frequency is 3 cycles per minute. There is a physiologic increase in signal amplitude after eating. (From Kohagen KR, Kim MS, McDonnell WM, et al. Nicotine effects on prostaglandin-dependent gastric slow wave rhythmicity and antral motility in nonsmokers and smokers. *Gastroenterology* 1996;110:3–11.)

pelvic floor also may produce constipation. Other dysfunctional motor patterns in this region may promote development of fecal incontinence.

Colonic Transit Testing

Indications

Colonic transit testing is performed on patients with severe constipation to quantify the degree of colonic inertia. The most common indication is to determine whether inertia is so severe as to necessitate subtotal colectomy.

Methods

The most common method for assessing colonic transit is to obtain serial abdominal radiographs after ingestion of radiopaque markers. Calculation of markers remaining on each radiograph can generate a total colonic transit time (normal <68 hours). The radiopaque marker technique also can be used to estimate regional transit in the right, left, and rectosigmoid portions of the colon with use of bony landmarks on the radiographs. More detailed analysis of colonic transit can be performed with colonic scintigraphy. With this technique, a radioisotope is given orally or through an intestinal perfusion tube. The geometric center of the radioactive bolus is assessed as a function of time to calculate regional and total colonic transit times.

Clinical Findings

Some patients with severe colonic inertia respond poorly to laxative therapy. Demonstration of marked prolongation of colonic transit is predictive of a good response to subtotal colectomy. In selected instances, lesser resection can be performed for regional delays in colonic transit. Some patients who report severe constipation have normal colonic transit. Many of these patients have abnormal psychometric profiles and should not be considered for surgical treatment.

Anorectal Manometry

Indications

Anorectal manometry is indicated to exclude neuromuscular dysfunction of the defecation process among patients with fecal incontinence or with constipation caused by Hirschsprung's disease, reduced rectal sensitivity, or anismus (also known as *pelvic floor dyssynergia*) (see Chapter 100). Results of anorectal manometry also can be used to direct biofeedback therapy for defecation disorders.

Methods

A manometric catheter with a balloon on the tip and with anal-pressure recording sites is passed into the rectum. The catheter is slowly withdrawn to assess resting anal tone, a function of the internal anal sphincter. The patient is asked to squeeze maximally against the catheter to provide a measure of external anal sphincter pressure. The rectoanal inhibitory reflex is assessed by means of measuring relaxation of the internal anal sphincter during inflation of the rectal balloon (Fig 129.5). The rectal

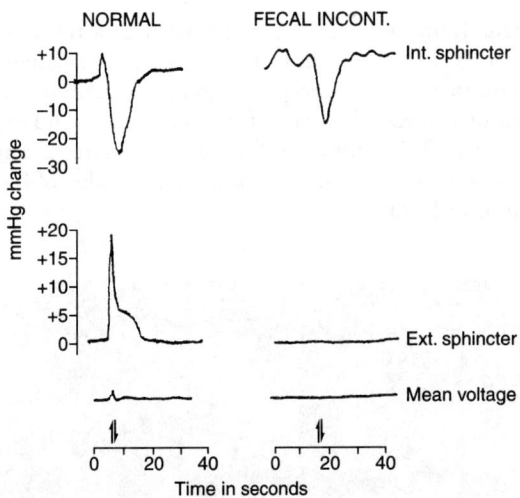

FIGURE 129.5. The rectoanal inhibitory reflex in response to rectal balloon inflation is demonstrated for a healthy volunteer (*left*) and a patient with fecal incontinence. For the healthy volunteer, rectal distention evokes relaxation of the internal anal sphincter with a compensatory increase in external pressure. In the patient with fecal incontinence, the rectoanal inhibitory reflex is preserved but the compensatory increase in external sphincter pressure does not occur. *Bottom,* Electromyographic recordings from the external sphincter that correlate with the contractile responses. (From Alva J, Mendeloff AI, Schuster MM. Reflex and electromyographic abnormalities associated with fecal incontinence. *Gastroenterology* 1967;53:101–106.)

balloon is gradually inflated with concurrent recording of rectal pressure to quantify rectal perception and compliance. With the balloon partly inflated, the patient may be asked to attempt to defecate the balloon.

Clinical Findings

Anorectal manometry can assist in the diagnosis of Hirschsprung's disease, a rare cause of constipation among adults, with the demonstration of a loss of the rectoanal inhibitory reflex. For confirmation of this disorder, however, a deep rectal biopsy specimen with a lack of ganglion cells is required. Patients with anismus may have a failure of relaxation of the external sphincter during attempts at defecation with an inability to expel the inflated balloon. Megarectum and megacolon may be characterized by impaired perception of rectal distention. Patients with fecal incontinence may have low resting anal tone or a failure of external sphincter pressure to increase with inflation of a rectal balloon (Fig 129.5). Patients with anismus can use biofeedback to retrain the external anal sphincter to relax during defecation. In biofeedback training for fecal incontinence, the patient is instructed learn to contract the external sphincter when a rectal stimulus is present.

Defecography

Indications

Defecography is a dynamic radiographic technique performed on patients with constipation to exclude structural abnormalities such as rectocele or rectal prolapse or functional disturbances such as anismus (pelvic floor dyssynergia) (see Chapter 100).

Methods

A paste made from 200 mL barium mixed with a thickening agent is inserted into the rectum with a syringe. The patient is asked to sit on an evacuation receptacle, and the resting anorectal angle is measured at rest. The patient is asked to strain and expel the barium paste. With normal defecation, the anorectal angle should show an increase from the normal resting value of 84 to 110 degrees (Fig 129.6).

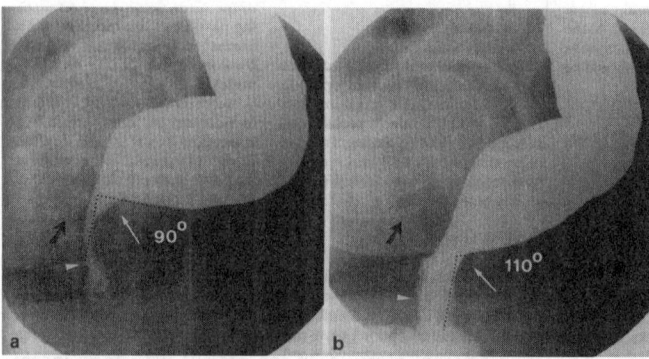

FIGURE 129.6. Normal results of defecography are shown at rest **(A)** and with defecation **(B)**. At rest, the anorectal angle is 90 degrees. With defecation, there is an increase in the anorectal angle to 110 degrees, which facilitates evacuation of the barium paste. (From Goei R. Defecography: principles of technique and interpretation. *Radiologe* 1993; 33:356–360.)

Clinical Findings

A rectocele, or anterior bulging of the rectal wall, may be found during attempts at defecation. Prolapse or intussusception within the rectum also may impair rectal evacuation. Pelvic floor dyssynergia is associated with a paradoxic decrease in anorectal angle with attempted defecation.

▮ BREATH TESTING IN GASTROENTEROLOGY

A variety of breath tests can be performed for the diagnosis of a broad range of gastrointestinal disorders, including gastroparesis, *Helicobacter pylori* infection (see Chapter 108), milk intolerance, and small-intestinal bacterial overgrowth. Each of these tests requires normal small-intestinal mucosal integrity and pulmonary gas transfer. Unreliable results may be obtained in the presence of certain malabsorptive disorders and lung diseases.

DIAGNOSIS OF LACTASE DEFICIENCY
Indications

Hydrogen breath testing for lactase deficiency is performed on patients with unexplained gas, bloating, abdominal discomfort, or diarrhea believed to caused by intolerance of dairy products.

Methods

After overnight fasting, the patient ingests 25 g lactose in water. Serial breath samples are obtained over 2 hours and analyzed for production of hydrogen. Patients should not smoke before testing. Mouthwash is given before lactose ingestion to prevent false-positive results caused by the presence of bacteria in the oral cavity.

Clinical Findings

Lactase deficiency is diagnosed when the breath hydrogen level rises to >20 ppm. The magnitude of the increase in hydrogen correlates semiquantitatively with the degree of malabsorption. False-positive test results occur with bacterial overgrowth. False-negative results may occur when a patient has colonic bacteria that do not produce hydrogen.

DIAGNOSIS OF SMALL-INTESTINAL BACTERIAL OVERGROWTH
Indications

Breath testing is performed to exclude small-intestinal bacterial overgrowth among patients with unexplained gas, bloating, discomfort, diarrhea, or malabsorption. Evaluation usually is considered for persons at risk for the condition, including those with intestinal dysmotility, hypochlorhydria, and small-intestinal diverticula, fistulas, or narrowing.

Methods

After overnight fasting, the patient ingests a carbohydrate solution in water. For ingested substrates such as lactulose or glucose, exhaled breath obtained serially over 2 hours is analyzed for hydrogen production. In some centers, carbon C 14 D-xylose is used as a substrate because of its minimal metabolism by the host. For this test, carbon dioxide C 14 is quantified in the exhaled breath. Radiolabeled bile acid breath tests are no longer used because of poor sensitivity and specificity.

Clinical Findings

Increases in breath hydrogen level after glucose or lactulose ingestion provide 62% to 68% sensitivity and 44% to 83% specificity for the diagnosis of bacterial overgrowth, whereas the carbon C 14 D-xylose test has 30% to 100% sensitivity and 89% to 100% specificity compared with quantitative intestinal fluid culture. Elevations in fasting breath hydrogen level occur among some patients with bacterial overgrowth. False-negative results occur among patients who have colonic flora that do not produce hydrogen. The most common reason for a false-positive test result is rapid small-intestinal transit, which delivers the ingested carbohydrate substrate to the colon before intestinal absorption.

■ SECRETORY TESTING IN GASTROENTEROLOGY

In some instances, assessment of secretory function can complement the findings of structural testing. Quantification of gastric acid production may be needed for the diagnosis of hypersecretory conditions and to ascertain vagal integrity among patients with unexplained ulcer disease. Determination of pancreatic output of bicarbonate or enzymes may be used in the diagnosis or direct management of chronic pancreatic insufficiency.

GASTRIC ACID ANALYSIS

Indications

Gastric acid analysis may be performed in the diagnosis of Zollinger–Ellison syndrome (ZES) to monitor the effectiveness of medication therapy for some patients with ZES that cannot be corrected with surgical resection, to provide important diagnostic information about unexplained hypergastrinemia, and to test for completeness of vagotomy among patients with recurrent ulceration who have undergone surgery for peptic ulcer disease (see Chapter 107).

Methods

After overnight fasting, a double-lumen perfusion catheter is passed into the stomach. Four 15-minute fasting gastric samples are withdrawn with perfusion of a nonabsorbable marker to ensure adequate recovery. Basal acid output (BAO) is determined by means of measuring the titratable acidity. Pentagastrin is administered intravenously, and four or more 15-minute acid sam-

ples are obtained and titrated to determine maximal acid output (MAO). To test for vagal integrity, acid output is measured after sham feeding, during which the patient chews and spits a meat meal without swallowing.

Clinical Findings

A BAO greater than 15 mEq per hour is found among more than 90% of patients with ZES, but 12% of duodenal ulcer patients also have this finding. A BAO/MAO ratio greater than 0.6 is highly specific for ZES, but many patients with ZES have lower ratios. Reduction in BAO to less than 10 mEq per hour with medical therapy for ZES confirms the adequacy of acid suppression. The presence of normal acid production in a patient with hypergastrinemia excludes pernicious anemia and atrophic gastritis. If a patient has undergone previous surgery for peptic ulcer disease, a BAO greater than 5 mEq per hour or a marked increase in acid output with sham feeding suggests that the vagotomy was incomplete.

TESTING OF PANCREATIC FUNCTION

Indications

Quantification of exocrine pancreatic secretion is indicated to document pancreatic insufficiency when structural evaluation with computed tomography, endoscopic retrograde pancreatography, and endoscopic ultrasound does not provide enough information for diagnosis. Assessment of exocrine function also is useful in the search for a pancreatic source of unexplained malabsorption or diarrhea. Pancreatic function testing also has been used to direct medication therapy for chronic pancreatic insufficiency.

Methods

After overnight fasting, a double-lumen perfusion tube is placed fluoroscopically in the descending duodenum. A gastric aspiration tube is placed to continuously aspirate gastric acid, which can stimulate duodenal secretion of bicarbonate and inactivate pancreatic enzymes. Pancreatic juice is aspirated from the duodenal tube during perfusion of a nonabsorbable marker to ensure adequate recovery. Duodenal fluid is collected for assay. Exocrine function is commonly measured in response to either secretin or cholecystokinin. With secretin stimulation, fasting and stimulated outputs of bicarbonate are measured. With cholecystokinin stimulation, fasting and stimulated outputs of trypsin and lipase are quantified.

Clinical Findings

Pancreatic function testing is 90% sensitive and 90% specific for the diagnosis of pancreatic insufficiency. It cannot, however, be used to determine the cause of impaired exocrine output. Quantification of exocrine output has been used to predict responses to medication therapy for pancreatic insufficiency. Patients with chronic pancreatitis with mild to moderate impairment of function have greater reductions in pain with administration of exogenous pancreatic enzyme supplements than do those with severe insufficiency.

BIBLIOGRAPHY

Baron JH. When should a clinician perform gastric analysis? *J Clin Gastroenterol* 1981;3:87–89.

Camilleri M, Hasler WL, Parkman HP, et al. Measurement of gastrointestinal motility in the GI laboratory. *Gastroenterology* 1998;115:747–762.

DiMarino AJ, Allen ML, Lynn RB, et al. Clinical value of esophageal motility testing. *Dig Dis* 1998;16:198–204.

Ekberg O, Wahlgren L. Dysfunction of pharyngeal swallowing. A cineradiographic study in 854 dysphagial patients. *Acta Radiol Diagn* 1985;26:389–395.

Goldberg DM, Durie PR. Biochemical tests in the diagnosis of chronic pancreatitis and in the evaluation of pancreatic insufficiency. *Clin Biochem* 1993;26:253–275.

King CE, Toskes PP. The use of breath tests in the study of malabsorption. *Clin Gastroenterol* 1983;12:591–610.

Logan RP. Urea breath tests in the management of *Helicobacter pylori* infection. *Gut* 1998;43[Suppl 1]:S47–S50.

Metcalf AM, Phillips SF, Zinsmeister AR, et al. Simplified assessment of segmental colonic transit. *Gastroenterology* 1987;92:40–47.

Meunier PD, Gallavardin D. Anorectal manometry: the state of the art. *Dig Dis* 1993;11:252–264.

Richter JE. Ambulatory esophageal pH monitoring. *Am J Med* 1997;103:130S–134S.

Yang XM, Partanen K, Farin P, et al. Defecography. *Acta Radiol* 1995;36:460–468.

Kelley's Textbook of Internal Medicine, fourth edition. Edited by H. David Humes. Lippincott Williams & Wilkins, Philadelphia © 2000.

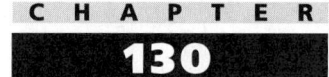

CHAPTER 130

PARENTERAL AND ENTERAL NUTRITION

WILLIAM F. STENSON
PATTI EISENBERG

■ NUTRITIONAL SUPPORT

WHO NEEDS NUTRITIONAL SUPPORT?

Protein calorie malnutrition impairs wound healing, is a predisposing factor for infection, and diminishes the functional capacity of every organ system. Patients who are not meeting their protein and calorie requirements through oral intake need nutritional support. Previously well-nourished patients who are at risk of protein-calorie malnutrition because of acute medical problems such as severe trauma or major surgery also need nutritional support. Nutrients can be provided through the veins (parenteral nutrition) or through the gastrointestinal tract (enteral nutrition). Nutrition provided through the gastrointestinal

tract can be administered by means of oral supplementation or feeding tubes (forced enteral nutrition).

The need for nutritional support is determined by means of comparing nutritional intake and protein and calorie requirements. If protein and calorie requirements exceed intake, nutritional needs are not being met. Intake can be estimated from a calorie count. As part of the determination of nutritional intake, remediable causes of diminished intake are assessed. Many patients have diminished nutritional intake as a result of oral and upper gastrointestinal problems such as poorly fitting dentures, esophagitis, and peptic ulcer disease. Medications can diminish nutritional intake by suppressing appetite or inducing nausea and dyspepsia. Depression is another common and remediable cause of diminished nutritional intake. Protein requirements for a healthy adult are 0.8 g per kilogram per day (56 g for a 70-kg person). Minimal energy requirements for a healthy adult are 25 kcal per kilogram per day (1750 kcal for a 70-kg person). Increased activity raises the calorie requirement; metabolic stress such as trauma or severe infection increases protein and calorie requirements (see Chapter 8).

If protein and calorie requirements exceed nutrient intake for a long time, protein and fat are depleted. The greater the degree of protein and fat depletion, the greater is the need for intensive nutritional support. A thorough patient history, including changes in weight, nutritional intake, functional capacity, and the presence and activity of disease, provides useful information regarding nutritional status. Loss of more than 15% of total weight suggests severe malnutrition. Interpretation of weight changes can be impeded by the development of edema. The physical examination also is useful for assessing malnutrition. Signs of muscle wasting, such as temporal wasting, and edema are especially important in evaluating nutritional status. Laboratory tests have a role in assessing nutritional status. Low levels of albumin, prealbumin, or transferrin raise the possibility of malnutrition. However, these test results also are affected by other factors, such as liver disease, the presence of infection, and urinary protein losses.

If protein calorie malnutrition already is established, the patient needs nutritional support. If the patient is well nourished but is about to enter a period of decreased nutrient intake or increased protein and calorie requirements, the need for nutritional support is determined by the expected duration of decreased intake or increased requirements. The longer the expected duration of decreased intake or increased requirements, the more pressing is the need to initiate nutritional support. Surgical procedures of moderate scope, such as appendectomy, cholecystectomy, or hysterectomy, are associated with predictable but relatively short periods of negative protein and calorie balance. An otherwise healthy person with normal protein and fat stores should not need intensive nutritional support when undergoing these procedures. However, the same person would be considered for intensive nutritional support if he or she had a condition that would cause negative protein and calorie balance. A patient with extensive burns or severe trauma needs to be considered for nutritional support event if baseline nutritional status is normal.

The last question to be addressed is whether nutritional support will markedly affect the patient's outcome. Some patients qualify for nutritional support on the basis of protein and calorie status, but intensive nutritional support would have no effect on clinical outcome. A patient in the last stages of AIDS or cancer may be in this group. The morbidity and expense of total parenteral nutrition (TPN) cannot be justified if the therapy will have no appreciable effect on longevity or clinical outcome.

DECIDING BETWEEN ENTERAL AND PARENTERAL NUTRITION

Most patients whose nutritional needs can be met orally should receive enteral nutrition rather than parenteral nutrition. Parenteral nutrition is much more expensive and is associated with a high incidence of major complications, including pneumothorax at central catheter insertion and line sepsis. Enteral nutrition provides nutrients directly to the epithelium of the gastrointestinal tract to support epithelial health and maintain barrier function. Glutamine, short-chain fatty acids, and nucleotides provided through the intestinal lumen support epithelial integrity. Enteral nutrition and parenteral nutrition are not mutually exclusive. Many patients can meet only some of their nutritional needs with enteral feeding. To help preserve the integrity of the gastrointestinal epithelium, those patients should receive a mixture of enteral and parenteral nutrition, rather than parenteral nutrition alone.

Some gastrointestinal disorders, such as ileus or obstructing small-bowel lesions, make any form of enteral nutrition impossible. Other disorders, such as impaired swallowing, make oral feeding impossible but have no effect on the feasibility of tube feeding. Other conditions, such as multiple small-intestinal strictures from radiation enteritis, make enteral administration of a regular diet impossible but allow the use of oral liquid supplements. The availability or lack of availability of the gastrointestinal tract usually is obvious, but in some cases, a trial of enteral feeding is necessary to determine whether this is a practical approach to nutritional support of a particular patient.

■ PARENTERAL NUTRITION

Parenteral nutrition is the process by which nutrients are administered to a patient through an intravenous catheter. By means of parenteral nutrition, it is possible to deliver part of a patient's macronutrient and micronutrient requirements (partial parenteral nutrition) or all of them (TPN). Nutrients can be delivered through a catheter into a peripheral vein (peripheral parenteral nutrition) or into a central vein, typically the superior vena cava (central parenteral nutrition). Most patients who receive TPN have protein calorie malnutrition, and their nutritional needs cannot be met with enteral nutrition. A few patients receive TPN as primary therapy for gastrointestinal disease. In these cases, TPN is given to provide nutrients and to rest the gastrointestinal tract.

PARENTERAL NUTRITION AS PRIMARY THERAPY

In a few clinical conditions, prolonged complete bowel rest is considered therapeutic. In these conditions, TPN is used to pro-

vide nutrients while the bowel is at rest. The two diseases in which complete bowel rest is used most commonly as a component of therapy are Crohn's disease and pancreatitis.

In Crohn's disease (see Chapter 111), the use of complete bowel rest is based on the theory that reducing the antigen load in the intestinal lumen reduces the level of immune activation in the affected bowel. Complete bowel rest eliminates introduction of dietary antigens into the intestine. Moreover, complete bowel rest reduces the amount of nutrients available for bacteria, decreasing the number of colonic bacteria and the load of bacterial antigens. TPN is more successful in inducing remission in small-bowel Crohn's disease than in colonic disease. Remission can be achieved in most patients with small-bowel Crohn's disease by treating them in the hospital with complete bowel rest and TPN. However, this approach does not appear to affect long-term remission rates. TPN also has proved useful in treating patients with fistulas from Crohn's disease. The reported success rate is 30% to 60%. Growth retardation, an important complication of Crohn's disease among children, can be reversed with TPN. Forced enteral nutrition often is successful and with far less cost and morbidity than TPN. Besides allowing complete bowel rest, TPN can reverse the nutritional deficiencies common with Crohn's disease. Enteral nutrition with an elemental diet has been used in the management of Crohn's disease for the same indications as has TPN.

In pancreatitis (see Chapter 117), complete bowel rest is used to prevent stimulation of pancreatic secretion by the presence of nutrients in the intestinal lumen. A regimen of complete bowel rest and TPN can reduce the duration and severity of pain and speed normalization of the serum amylase levels of persons with pancreatitis. This approach is most useful in the management of pancreatitis among patients with abscesses, fistulas, and other complications. When hypertriglyceridemia is part of the clinical presentation of pancreatitis, lipids should not be included in the TPN formula.

CENTRAL PARENTERAL NUTRITION AND PERIPHERAL PARENTERAL NUTRITION

Parenteral nutrition can be given centrally into the superior vena cava or peripherally into an arm vein. The amount of glucose and amino acids required to meet individual needs constitutes a massive osmotic load. To deliver this load in a reasonable volume, the formula must be hypertonic. Central administration of a hypertonic solution is possible because the solution is diluted rapidly in the high blood flow of the superior vena cava. However, in peripheral veins, which have low blood flow, hypertonic solutions cannot be diluted easily.

The limiting factor for peripheral parenteral nutrition is phlebitis induced by hypertonic solutions. Successful use of peripheral parenteral nutrition requires that osmolarity be kept at less than 800 to 900 mOsm per liter and glucose at less than 10%. Lipid emulsions, which have a high caloric density without a large osmotic load, allow delivery of a large number of calories through a peripheral vein without induction of phlebitis. However, an attempt to deliver all required nutrients through a peripheral vein would necessitate that about 70% of nonprotein calories be delivered in the form of lipids. Parenteral formulas with high lipid content have immunosuppressive effects and are associated with development of hyperlipidemia. For these reasons, the only practical route of delivery of parenteral nutrition among patients who must take all their nutrients parenterally is through a centrally placed catheter. Peripheral parenteral nutrition is useful, however, when only a fraction of a patient's total nutritional needs must be given parenterally. When applicable, peripheral parenteral nutrition has considerable advantages over central parenteral nutrition. Chief among them is reduced exposure to the risks of pneumothorax and other complications associated with placement of a central catheter.

NUTRIENT REQUIREMENTS AND SOURCES IN TOTAL PARENTERAL NUTRITION

CALORIES

A reasonable estimate of the minimal calorie needs for a healthy adult is 25 kcal per kilogram per day. With the stress of disease or surgery, the calorie requirement increases to 30 to 40 kcal per kilogram per day. Administration of the formula in Table 130.1 to a 50-kg person would yield 40 kcal per kilogram per day. The main calorie sources in TPN solutions are carbohydrate in the form of glucose and lipid in the form of soybean and safflower oils emulsified with egg phospholipids. Glucose monohydrate has 3.4 kcal per gram, 10% lipid emulsion has 1.1 kcal per milliliter, and 20% lipid emulsion has 2 kcal per milliliter. Glucose can be the sole calorie source, but the large load required can cause hyperglycemia, fatty liver, and fluid overload. The use of glucose as the only source of calories also leads to essential fatty acid deficiency. This condition can be prevented by means of providing 2% to 4% of nonprotein calories as linoleic acid. The triglycerides from soybean oil and safflower oil in TPN lipid emulsions are rich in linoleic acid. Almost all patients given TPN receive both glucose and lipid emulsion as calorie sources. In most TPN formulas, 25% to 50% of nonprotein calories are from lipids and the rest are from glucose. Lipids contribute 28% to 30% of nonprotein calories in standard formulas. Almost all patients can be treated with the standard distribution of lipids and carbohydrates. The metabolism of carbohydrates yields more carbon dioxide than does the metabolism of a calorically equivalent amount of lipids. For this reason, it has been suggested that patients with respiratory failure be given a high-lipid, low-carbohydrate formula. However, the total calorie load is more important than the lipid–carbohydrate distribution as a determinant of carbon dioxide production, so the first therapeutic approach to carbon dioxide retention among patients receiving TPN is to decrease the caloric load.

Risks are associated with administration of large amounts of carbohydrates or lipids. The more glucose administered in a given period, the more probable it is that hyperglycemia will develop, necessitating use of insulin. Fatty liver also develops when glucose is given in excessive amounts. The amount of glucose given per unit of time is enhanced by means of increasing the total caloric load, increasing the proportion of calories from carbohydrates, or using cycling to compress the time of adminis-

tration. A reasonable guideline for glucose administration is to limit the infusion to 7 mg per kilogram per minute or less. If a 50-kg patient receiving the formula in Table 130.1 (350 g glucose) were given cycled TPN, he or she would have to receive TPN at least 16 hours each day to stay within the recommended guidelines.

Risks of administration of excessive amounts of lipid include impairment of neutrophil function and increased risk of infection. Limiting the rate of lipid infusion to no more than 0.03 to 0.05 g per kilogram per hour has been recommended. Administration of the formula described in Table 130.1 (in which lipids provide 24% of total calories and 28% of nonprotein calories) to a 50-kg patient over 24 hours would necessitate a rate of lipid administration of 0.04 g per kilogram per hour.

PROTEIN

For nonstressed patients, the recommended dietary protein allowance is 0.8 g per kilogram per day. The recommendation increases to 1.5 g per kilogram per day for catabolic patients, such as those with burns or severe trauma or recovering from major surgery. Protein requirements also are increased among patients who lose protein, such as those with large open wounds or protein-losing intestinal diseases such as inflammatory bowel disease. Many standard TPN formulas deliver more protein than recommended. For example, administration of the standard formula in Table 130.1 to a 50-kg person would deliver protein at a rate of 1.6 g per kilogram per day.

The protein source in all TPN solutions is free amino acids. The standard amino acid mixture is formulated to achieve the same proportions of the various amino acids as are found in serum. The amino acids in TPN solutions have two metabolic fates. They can be incorporated into protein, or they can be converted to glucose and used for energy. How much of the administered amino acid load causes protein synthesis or is used for energy is determined by the patient's needs and the number of nonprotein calories administered. Positive caloric balance is necessary to establish positive nitrogen balance. For administered amino acids to be incorporated into new protein rather than undergo catabolism, the ratio of nonprotein calories to grams of nitrogen should approach 150:1. This ratio is based on the fact that 10% to 15% or more of caloric need during catabolism is derived from protein breakdown. One gram of nitrogen is the equivalent of 6.25 g of amino acids. Positive nitrogen balance can be established when the ratio of calories to nitrogen is less than 150:1; however, best use of the delivered amino acids occurs with the higher ratios of nonprotein calories to nitrogen. Almost all patients catabolize at least some of the administered amino acids, and many patients catabolize most of them. However, the exact amount catabolized is difficult to predict, so the contribution of amino acids to calorie expenditure also is difficult to predict.

Special amino acid formulas are available for patients with renal and hepatic diseases. The renal disease formulas contain high levels of essential amino acids and little or no nonessential amino acids. Use of these formulas allows patients to receive adequate amounts of essential amino acids without a large nitrogen load. These formulas are useful only to patients who have

| TABLE 130.1. | STANDARD 24-HOUR TOTAL PARENTERAL NUTRITION FORMULA |

Volume: 2594 mL
Total calories: 2000
Total nitrogen: 12.8 g
Nonprotein calories: nitrogen = 131:1

Macronutrients	Protein (Amino Acids)	Carbohydrates (Glucose)	Fats (20% Lipid Emulsion)
Percentage of total calories	16%	60%	24%
Total amount	80 g	350 g	240 mL

Electrolytes	Suggested Dose/24 h
Sodium	120 mEq
Potassium	80 mEq
Chloride	140 mEq
Acetate	20 mEq
Phosphorus	30 mmol
Calcium gluconate	9.2 mEq (2 g)
Magnesium sulfate	16.8 mEq (2 g)

Trace Elements	Daily Dose
Zinc	5 mg
Copper	1 mg
Chromium	10 μg
Manganese	0.5 μg
Selenium	60 μg

Vitamins	Daily Dose
A	3300 IU
D	200 IU
E	10 IU
B_1 (thiamine)	3 mg
B_2 (riboflavin)	3.6 mg
B_3 (niacin)	15 mg
B_5 (pantothenic acid)	40 mg
B_6 (pyridoxine)	4 mg
B_7 (biotin)	60 μg
B_9 (folacin)	400 μg
B_{12} (cobalamin)	5 μg
C (ascorbic acid)	100 mg
K	(5 mg/wk)

severe renal failure but are not yet undergoing dialysis. The amino acid formulas for patients with hepatic disease are high in branched-chain amino acids (leucine, isoleucine, valine). Branched-chain amino acids are oxidized outside the liver and serve as a fuel source for muscle. They also block protein breakdown in liver and muscle. These special hepatic amino acid formulas are most useful to patients who have encephalopathy when given conventional TPN formulas. The renal and hepatic amino acid formulas are expensive and should be reserved for those who clearly need them.

VITAMINS AND MINERALS

Vitamin requirements for most patients are met by adding a multivitamin preparation to the TPN formula (Table 130.1).

Vitamin K is not included in standard commercial multivitamin preparations because of the individual needs of patients receiving warfarin and must be ordered separately. Some trace minerals (zinc, copper, chromium, manganese, and selenium) are given every day. Iodine is of concern only for patients receiving long-term TPN. Iron is not given routinely and is not compatible with the lipids in three-in-one formulas. Iron–dextran solution can be given intramuscularly or intravenously at a dosage of 50 to 100 mg iron once a month. More iron should be given if there is a deficiency or excess loss.

FLUIDS AND ELECTROLYTES

Water requirements vary depending on the capability of the patient to excrete an osmotic load. The usual requirement is 30 to 35 mL per kilogram for a healthy adult, or about 1 mL per kilocalorie delivered. Additional water and electrolytes must be given to patients with increased losses, such as those with diarrhea, vomiting, or nasogastric suction. An additional 360 mL per day is recommended for each degree centigrade of temperature elevation. In addition, 300 to 400 mL of water per day may be necessary for new intracellular fluid if anabolism is being induced. Restriction of water is necessary during volume overload and in the presence of hyponatremia. Patients who become hyperosmotic may need additional free water every day. Regular laboratory monitoring and daily weight measurement help to detect abnormalities in water balance.

Electrolyte requirements are highly variable and are affected greatly by renal losses and losses from diarrhea, vomiting, and nasogastric suction. Potassium and phosphate requirements may be large when TPN is initiated because these electrolytes are driven into cells by infusion of glucose and reversal of the catabolic state. Electrolyte requirements also are affected by the underlying disease. For example, sodium may have to be restricted for patients with congestive heart failure, renal disease, or portal hypertension with ascites. For patients with renal disease, the potassium, phosphate, and magnesium content of the formula should be reduced.

The two major anions in TPN solutions are chloride and bicarbonate. The relative amounts of these two anions can be adjusted to accommodate the patient's acid–base balance. Acetate can be metabolized to bicarbonate; therefore, the acetate content of the TPN formula should be increased for patients with metabolic acidosis and reduced for patients with metabolic alkalosis.

MECHANICS OF TOTAL PARENTERAL NUTRITION

FORMULAS

In many institutions, TPN formulas are given with all the components in one bag. This form of administration is termed a *total nutrient admixture* or *three-in-one formula*, named for the three macronutrients (carbohydrates, protein, and lipids). The relative simplicity of administering a total nutrient admixture makes it a practical system for use in the hospital and at home. However, preparation of total nutrient admixture solutions requires expensive equipment, and this system is economically feasible only for institutions with many patients receiving TPN. Total nutrient admixtures are relatively unstable because the lipid droplets tend to coalesce into large particles, especially in the presence of vitamins and trace minerals. These formulas should be used within 24 hours of preparation. These admixtures are stable for longer periods if vitamins and minerals are withheld.

The alternative to use of a total nutrient admixture is a system in which the lipid emulsion is in one bag and all the other components are in a second bag. The two bags are connected with Y tubing, and the contents are combined just before they enter the patient. This system is easier for the pharmacy to prepare than are the three-in-one formulas, but administration requires more nursing time, more bags, and more tubing. These more stable formulas can be stored for up to 4 weeks before use.

CHOOSING A DELIVERY SYSTEM

TPN should be administered through a catheter placed directly into the central venous circulation because the formulas are hypertonic and would be damaging if administered through a small vessel. The type of central catheter selected depends on the expected duration of TPN. Catheters used to administer TPN for 6 to 8 weeks are relatively inexpensive and can be inserted percutaneously directly into the vein. When TPN is to be administered for more than 6 to 8 weeks, the catheter should be placed surgically and tunneled subcutaneously between the site of entrance through the skin and the site of entrance into the vein. Many of these catheters have a cuff at the point at which the catheter exits the vessel to promote stability. Subcutaneously placed catheters are less likely to be pulled out accidentally and allow the patient or caregiver to assume more responsibility and independence in daily care of the catheter. The subcutaneous tracking of these catheters serves as a barrier to the passage of skin bacteria, and the incidence of sepsis is reduced.

Another type of catheter is an implantable intravascular access device. The infusion site is implanted subcutaneously and accessed with a percutaneously inserted needle. This catheter allows even greater freedom of activity, because the patient has no tubing to manage when TPN is not being given. However, many patients object to the repeated needle sticks.

CATHETER CARE

The catheter should be flushed with heparin or normal saline solution on a routine schedule based on the recommendations of the manufacturer. The volume of the flush ranges from 0.5 to 5 mL and depends on the internal diameter of the catheter. Positive pressure is obtained by means of exerting pressure on the plunger in the syringe while closing the clamp on the lumen. This method is used to prevent reflux of blood into the tip of the catheter. The catheter insertion site should be inspected daily for early signs of catheter-related infection, such as erythema or drainage. The occlusive sterile dressing and catheter caps should be changed according to strict protocol to prevent or reduce catheter-related infections. With multilumen catheters, selection of the lumen to be used for TPN may be based on the policy of the institution or the recommendations of the manufacturer. The lumen through which TPN is administered should not be used for administration of drugs or blood products or for sampling of blood.

INITIATION, CYCLING, AND DISCONTINUATION

The first bag of TPN formula should be infused at an hourly rate determined by means of dividing the volume by 24 hours. The infusion rate is recalculated each day because the total volume of the formula varies with the volume of added electrolytes, medications, vitamins, and minerals. The formula can be administered at a slower rate and advanced to the calculated hourly infusion rate to allow adaptation to higher blood glucose levels. Gradual adjustment in the rate of administration is especially appropriate in the care of patients in unstable hemodynamic condition and those with type I diabetes.

Administration of a full day's TPN in less than 24 hours is called *cycling*, a practice that allows the patient freedom of movement for a portion of each day. Persons receiving TPN at home often are treated with shorter infusion schedules to allow greater independence. The shorter infusion schedule should be initiated before discharge from the hospital to determine whether blood glucose levels are controlled adequately during the accelerated infusion. The duration of infusion is limited by the amount of carbohydrates the liver can metabolize.

When TPN is interrupted unexpectedly, blood glucose level should be measured to determine whether hypoglycemia has developed as a result of continued secretion of insulin despite cessation of the glucose infusion. If the serum glucose level is 60 mg per deciliter or less, infusion with 5% or 10% glucose should be initiated. Hypoglycemia after abrupt discontinuation of TPN is especially likely to occur in a patient in unstable hemodynamic condition or with type I diabetes.

TPN can be discontinued when the patient's caloric needs can be met with oral or enteral feedings. TPN solutions, especially the lipid component, suppress appetite and promote a feeling of fullness. Reducing or withholding the lipid component for 1 to 2 days before discontinuing TPN often increases appetite and oral intake among patients who experience early satiety. Hypoglycemia should not occur with abrupt discontinuation of TPN after the initiation of oral or enteral intake because serum glucose level is maintained. Adequate intake of calories should be assessed with a calorie count. Identification of food preferences and use of oral supplements or enteral nutrition may be necessary to maintain caloric intake once TPN is stopped.

ADDING MEDICATION TO TOTAL PARENTERAL NUTRITION

Medication can be added to a TPN formula, but it is essential that the stability and activity of the medication in the formula be determined from the time of mixing to the completion of the infusion. Most of the data on drug stability are limited to two-in-one formulas (protein and carbohydrates) rather than three-in-one formulas (protein, carbohydrates, and lipids). Histamine 2 receptor antagonists, regular insulin, and heparin are stable in three-in-one TPN formulas. Iron–dextran can be added to two-in-one formulas but not to three-in-one formulas.

MONITORING TOTAL PARENTERAL NUTRITION

Administration of TPN initially induces shifts in electrolytes, especially potassium and phosphate, from the extracellular to the intracellular compartments. The magnitude of these shifts depends on the degree of starvation before the initiation of TPN. Frequent monitoring of electrolytes is recommended during the first few days of TPN until these shifts stabilize. The frequency of monitoring can be reduced as the body adapts to TPN (Table 130.2). Bedside blood glucose monitoring should be conducted every 4 to 6 hours until the glucose level is consistently less than 200 g per deciliter. Even after stable levels are achieved, daily glucose monitoring should be continued because an increase in glucose level may be the first indication of infection. Vital signs, including temperature, pulse, respiration, and blood pressure, should be assessed every 4 hours when TPN is initiated. The frequency can be reduced as the body adapts to TPN.

COMPLICATIONS OF TOTAL PARENTERAL NUTRITION

METABOLIC COMPLICATIONS

Metabolic complications associated with TPN are common and can occur immediately or after prolonged use (Table 130.3). Administration of glucose, especially at high rates of infusion, can produce hyperglycemia, which should be controlled promptly to prevent osmotic diuresis and dehydration. For patients with hyperglycemia, blood glucose level should be assessed every 4 hours with a bedside monitor until the level returns to

---

TABLE 130.2. MONITORING DURING TOTAL PARENTERAL NUTRITION

Before Initiation	Daily for 1–2 Days	Weekly for 2–3 Wk	Short-Term (up to 6 mo); Every 1–2 wk	Long-Term (>6 mo); Every 3–6 mo
Electrolytes (sodium, potassium, chloride, bicarbonate, phosphorus, calcium, magnesium)	Electrolytes	Electrolytes	Electrolytes	Electrolytes
	Bedside glucose	Liver enzymes and function	Liver enzymes and function	Liver enzymes and function
	Weight	Renal function	Renal function	Renal function
Bedside glucose	Intake and output	Weight	Weight	Weight
Liver enzymes and function (lactate dehydrogenase, aspartate aminotransferase, alanine aminotransferase, alkaline phosphatase, total bilirubin, albumin)		Intake and output		Triglycerides if previously elevated
		Triglycerides if previously elevated		
Triglycerides				
Renal function (urea nitrogen, creatinine)				
Weight				

TABLE 130.3.	METABOLIC COMPLICATIONS ASSOCIATED WITH TOTAL PARENTERAL NUTRITION

Early

Electrolyte abnormalities
  Sodium
  Potassium
  Calcium
  Magnesium
  Phosphate
Refeeding syndrome
Hyperglycemia
Hypoglycemia
Elevation of urea nitrogen
Adverse reactions to lipid emulsions
  Hyperlipidemia
  Poor lipid clearance
  Thrombocytopenia
Hypercapnia
Hyperammonemia
Fluid overload
Hyperosmolar nonketotic hyperglycemic coma
Acidosis
Alkalosis

Delayed

Lipid overload syndrome
Essential fatty acid deficiency
Metabolic bone disease
Liver dysfunction
Gallbladder disease
Mineral deficiency or excess
  Zinc
  Copper
  Chromium
  Selenium
  Molybdenum
  Iron
  Manganese

pulmonary dysfunction, neurologic symptoms, or death. When a patient is believed to have severe malnutrition, electrolyte monitoring should be performed every 4 to 6 hours for the first 24 to 48 hours of TPN. Aggressive intravenous replacement of electrolytes should be initiated for deficits when they are present.

Patients with impaired myocardial or renal function can have fluid overload during TPN. The volume administered can be minimized through use of TPN formulas with concentrated nutrients. Most TPN formulas can be mixed in 1.5 to 2 L, depending on the concentrations of the nutrients used. Restriction of fluids obtained from other sources, such as intravenous medications or oral and enteral intake, may reduce the incidence of cardiopulmonary complications, including congestive heart failure. Electrolyte levels, body weight, and total intake and output should be monitored to prevent these complications.

The calcium loss from bone that occurs with severe malnutrition causes metabolic bone disease. TPN also produces a negative calcium balance caused by hypercalciuria. Rapid weight gain associated with nutritional replacement in a patient with metabolic bone disease may cause vertebral compression or stress fractures of weight-bearing long bones.

NONMETABOLIC COMPLICATIONS

Nonmetabolic complications are related primarily to catheter placement or catheter-related infection (Table 130.4). The most common serious complication of insertion of a central venous catheter is pneumothorax. Other complications are caused by incorrect positioning of the catheter. The catheter can be displaced into the jugular vein or positioned outside the intravascular space. For these reasons, catheter position must be confirmed with radiography before TPN is initiated. Catheter thrombosis is a common complication, especially if blood is withdrawn through the catheter. Venous thrombosis at the site of catheter

normal. Insulin can be administered according to a sliding scale to control glucose level, and the daily insulin needs of individual patients can be determined by means of calculating the cumulative dose over 24 hours. When insulin is administered subcutaneously to patients with low oncotic pressures as a result of a decrease in albumin, absorption may be erratic. Therefore, blood glucose level is best controlled by means of intravenous administration of insulin as an infusion or a bolus. The use of intravenous insulin may necessitate more frequent bedside glucose monitoring (every 1 to 2 hours). Hypoglycemia can be caused by administration of too much insulin or by abrupt discontinuation of a TPN infusion in the care of a patient receiving insulin. Hypoglycemia also can occur with certain bacterial infections or severe hepatic disease.

Refeeding syndrome occurs among severely malnourished persons when protein, carbohydrates, fats, electrolytes, vitamins, and minerals are reintroduced. When patients chronically adapted to starvation are challenged with carbohydrate feedings, there are rapid shifts of electrolytes, especially phosphorus, magnesium, potassium, and calcium, from the extracellular to the intracellular compartment. This can induce arrhythmia, cardio-

TABLE 130.4.	NONMETABOLIC COMPLICATIONS ASSOCIATED WITH TOTAL PARENTERAL NUTRITION

Complications Related to Central Catheter Placement	Other Complications
Pneumothorax	Catheter thrombosis
Hematoma	Venous thrombosis
Undesirable catheter direction	Catheter-related infection
Arterial puncture	(common organisms)
Thoracic duct puncture	*Staphylococcus aureus*
Subcutaneous emphysema	*Candida* species
Air embolus	*Klebsiella pneumoniae*
Pulmonary embolus	*Pseudomonas aeruginosa*
Hydrothorax	*Staphylococcus albus*
Hydromediastinum	*Enterobacter* species
Hemothorax	
Brachial plexus injury	
Chylothorax	
Catheter fragment embolus	

entrance is a serious complication that can be associated with infection.

The incidence of catheter-related infection should not exceed 5% of the total number of catheters used annually for TPN. The organisms most commonly associated with catheter-related infection are listed in Table 130.4. The signs and symptoms of a catheter-related infection include fever, chills, increased blood glucose level, leukocytosis with a shift to the left, and the growth of organisms in blood cultures aspirated through the catheter, particularly if culture results from other sites, such as sputum, urine, and other drain sites, are negative. Catheter-related infection can be caused by infection at the insertion site or by translocation of organisms to the catheter from other sites in the body, such as infected surgical wounds or infected urine. Contamination of the central catheter dressing with pulmonary secretions can cause local catheter site infection, which can progress to bacteremia. When bacteremia develops among patients with central catheters, potential secondary sources of infection always must be considered. Specimens for blood cultures should be obtained from the lumen of the central venous catheter and from a peripheral site. Cultures of the TPN solution and of other intravenous solutions can be obtained to rule out bacterial contamination. When other sources of infection are not present, removal of the catheter may be necessary. The skin wound should be cleaned thoroughly with bactericidal cleansers, and the tip of the catheter should be sent for culture. Catheters used for long-term TPN should be evaluated carefully before removal because of the limited venous access of these patients.

ENTERAL NUTRITION

DELIVERING ENTERAL NUTRITION

Oral Supplementation

Oral supplementation can be implemented by means of increasing portion sizes, adding high-calorie foods to the diet, or giving commercial nutritional supplements. If the patient can eat and has an adequate appetite, oral supplementation can be an effective approach. Instituting multiple small meals, adding snacks, spreading nutrient intake throughout the day, and paying attention to taste and patient preference can help make this approach successful. Milk-based supplements such as Carnation Instant Breakfast are useful in the care of lactose-tolerant patients. Lactose-free supplements such as Ensure are available in a variety of flavors. Careful monitoring of calorie intake and periodic weight checks are needed to make sure that the food offered actually is consumed.

Forced Enteral Nutrition

If the gastrointestinal tract is available and functioning, and if the patient is not achieving adequate caloric intake even with oral supplementation, forced enteral nutrition is indicated. The choice of method of delivery of forced enteral nutrition is determined by the expected duration of nutritional support, the pa-

tient's clinical condition, and the availability of nursing support and equipment (Table 130.5).

For short-term nutritional support (less than 6 weeks), a nasogastric or nasointestinal tube commonly is used. Nasogastric tubes have large diameters that allow feeding without a pump and with an intermittent schedule. Although clogging is less of a problem than with smaller-diameter tubes, nasogastric tubes need to be irrigated regularly. The most common serious problem with nasogastric feeding is aspiration. The risk of aspiration can be reduced by means of elevating the patient's head during and after feeding and by monitoring residual volumes carefully before each feeding. Nasointestinal tubes are narrower than nasogastric tubes and require a pump with continuous infusion of formula. They clog easily, and replacement is more difficult than that of nasogastric tubes. Aspiration is less common with nasointestinal tubes but only if the tube is positioned properly. If a nasointestinal tube is displaced into the stomach, as commonly happens, the risk of aspiration is as high as with a nasogastric tube. Nasogastric and nasointestinal tubes are removed easily by uncooperative patients.

If nutritional support is needed for more than 6 weeks, a gastrostomy tube or, less commonly, a jejunostomy tube is the feeding method of choice. Gastrostomy tubes can be placed by a surgeon, endoscopist, or radiologist. Gastrostomy tubes allow intermittent feeding without a pump. Aspiration is a common problem with gastrostomy tubes. The patient's head should be elevated during and after feedings, and residual volumes should be monitored. The complication rate with placement of gastrostomy tubes is high because of the advanced age and debility of most patients who need them. Oversedation during the placement procedure and wound infections are common problems. Jejunostomy tubes are used when gastrostomy tubes are not practical, as in the care of patients undergoing gastric surgery or with duodenal obstruction, or when aspiration is a major problem. Jejunostomy tube feedings require continuous infusion with a pump. These tubes clog easily because of their small diameter, and they can be displaced into the peritoneal cavity.

Choosing an Enteral Formula

There are many commercial enteral formulas, and new formulas are introduced often. The rapid turnover of commercial formulas soon will make the list of products in Table 130.6 out of date. The most suitable formula for any patient is the one that provides the desired allowances of macronutrients and micronutrients and has appropriate restrictions for the patient's medical disorders. All the products listed in Table 130.6 can be used for tube feeding, although some are not suitable for small-diameter tubes. Many of the formulas also can be used as oral supplements. Products that are marketed as oral supplements are flavored, and many come in a variety of flavors. All the formulas in Table 130.6 include protein, carbohydrates, and lipids. In most of these products, the protein source is intact protein, often casein. The carbohydrate source can be a complex carbohydrate or an oligosaccharide. The fat source typically is vegetable oil. Almost all these formulas also contain electrolytes, trace metals, and vitamins. Many commercial formulas have similar features with minor variations. Table 130.6 groups commercial formulas

TABLE 130.5.   APPROACHES TO FORCED ENTERAL NUTRITION

Location and Indications	Procedure and Tube Selection	Special Considerations	Potential Complications
Nasogastric			
Used in patients with normal gastric and duodenal emptying for assessing tolerance of GI feeding before permanent tube; inability to maintain adequate nutritional status through oral route because of underlying illnesses. Short term (less than 3–6 wk).	Placement at bedside; length ranges 22–36 inches; size ranges 8–18F; composition may be silicone, polyurethane, or PVC. Obtain radiograph to confirm placement before using.	Elevate head of bed 30 degrees during feeding and 1 h after; check residuals before each feeding and hold if >50% of previous feeding; schedule irrigation every 4–8 h; intermittent feeding schedule; crush medications finely.	Aspiration; esophageal or gastric perforation; otitis media; sinusitis; sore throat; esophageal reflux; PVC tube stiffening with time; hemorrhage; strictures.
Nasointestinal			
Used in patients at risk of gastric aspiration; delayed gastric emptying; pancreatitis; gastroparesis; dysphagia; severe head injury; burns; sepsis	Placement at bedside, endoscopic or radiographic; tube is 43 inches long; size is 12F or smaller; composition may be silicone or polyurethane, weight is made of molded plastic or tungsten; may use stylet for stiffening of tube. Obtain radiograph to confirm placement before using.	Use elixirs to administer medication; use formula with viscosity designed for tube diameter; enteral pump with continuous infusion of formula; review compatibility, absorption, and action of medications given through tube.	Spontaneous displacement into stomach; diarrhea; laceration of pylorus or GE junction if tube pulled out too rapidly; clogging.
Gastrostomy			
Used in patients with functional GI tracts; neuromuscular impairment; facial or oral trauma; need for long-term enteral feedings (usually >6 wk); esophageal obstruction.	Placement is surgical, endoscopic, radiographic, or laparoscopic; may be done as an outpatient; length is 9–12 inches; size is 12–24F; anchor with balloon, mushroom, or disc; composition is latex, silicone, polyurethane, or rubber; balloon capacity is 5–30 mL; may convert to skin-level device for improved cosmetic image in the alert and active outpatient. Complications may be reduced with single dose of cephalosporin.	May use 24 h after placement; minimal tension on tube; keep head of bed elevated 30 degrees; if external bumper used, do not readjust, lift or occlude with a dressing; clean skin daily; observe site for bleeding, drainage, redness, and forward migration of tube into tract; contrast study to check placement if tube replaced in first 2 weeks; skin-level device contains an antireflux valve.	Gastric outlet obstruction from forward migration of tube; aspiration; wound infection; displacement of tube into the peritoneal cavity; closure of tract within 4–12 h if tube falls out; abscess; peritonitis; necrotizing fasciitis; gastrocolic fistula; may be contraindicated or extremely difficult in patients with ascites or previous surgery.
Jejunostomy			
Used in patients who cannot use upper GI tract; risk of chronic aspiration; total gastrectomy; obstruction of duodenum, esophagus, or gastric outlet; gastric surgery; abdominal trauma.	Placement is surgical or laparoscopic; size 5–28F; anchor with suture, slide ring, T fasteners, disc, or mushroom; composition is latex, silicone, polyethylene, polyurethane, or rubber. If patient's condition permits, may begin feedings 24–48 h after surgery; flush catheter every 4–6 h.	Continuous infusion of formula with an enteral pump, low-viscosity formula for smaller tube diameters; contrast study to verify placement if tube replaced or malposition suspected; do not administer medications in 5F tube.	Wound infection; clogging of tube; tube displacement into the peritoneal cavity; jejunal erosion; diarrhea; bowel obstruction if balloon overinflated.
Gastrojejunostomy			
Used in patients who need decompression of stomach and distal feeding; gastric atony; partial gastric obstruction; aspiration; GE reflux.	Placement is conversion of gastrostomy tube; size of G tube 18F with J tube 9–12F; composition is silicone or polyurethane.	Administer feeding through the J tube and medications in the G tube; irrigate regularly; if GJ adapter and tube become dislodged from the G tube, do not attempt to reinsert; continuous infusion of enteral formula.	Tube displacement from jejunum into duodenum or stomach; clogging of J-tube portion.

GI, gastrointestinal; PVC, polyvinyl chloride; GE, gastroesophageal.

| TABLE 130.6 | CLASSIFICATION OF COMMERCIALLY AVAILABLE ENTERAL NUTRITION PRODUCTS |

Intact Protein						
Standard (20–40 g/Kcal)	High Protein (41–59 g/Kcal)	Very High Protein (≥60 g/ Kcal)	Disease Specific	With Fiber	Milk Based	Elemental or Chemically Defined
Isocal	TraumaCal	NuBasics	Diabetes	Sustacal w/	Carnation	Criticare HN
Sustacal Basic	Isocal HN	VHP	Choice DM	fiber	Instant	Alitraq
Comply	Protain XL	Peptamen	Glucerna w/fiber	Ultracal	Carnation	Opimental
Deliver 2.0	IsoSource	VHP	Ensure Glucerna OS	Protain XL	Instant	Vital HN
Lacta/Care	1.5	PRO-	Nutra/Shake Free	Ensure Fiber	No Sugar	Peptamen
Sustacal Plus	ProBalance	Peptide	Glytrol	w/	Added	Crucial
IsoSource	Ensure Plus	VHN	Glutasorb	Nutraflora	Compleat	SandoSource
ReSource	HN	Sustacal	DiabetiSource	FOS	Regular	Peptide
Resource Plus	Impact	Replete HP	ReSource Diabetic	NuBasics w/	Ensure	Vivonex Plus
Compleat	Impact 1.5	Promote	Renal	fiber	Balanced	Vivonex TEN
Mod	Perative	Meritene	Nepro	Glucerna w/	Breakfast	Peptamen
Enlive	Osmolite HN	IsoSource	Suplena	fiber		VHP
Ensure	Osmolite HN	VHN	Re/Neph Free	FiberSource		Reabilan
Ensure Light	Plus		Re/Neph HP/HC	FiberSource		Reabilan HN
Ensure Plus	Ensure High		Magnacal Renal	HN		L-Emental
Introlite	Pro		Renalcal Diet	Impact w/fiber		PRO-Peptide
Pro/vide	Protain XL		Liver	Jevity		PRO-Peptide
Osmolite	TwoCal HN		Re/Heph LP/HC	Jevity Plus		VHN
Tolerex	Val/Shake		Hepatic-Aid II	Promote w/		
Nutra/Shake	Replete		NutriHep	fiber		
NuBasics Plus			L-Emental Hepatic	Juice Plus		
NuBasics			AIDS	Fiber		
NuBasics 2.0			Advera	Nutra/Shake		
Nutren 1.0			Pulmonary	w/fiber		
Nutren 1.5			Respalor	Nutren 1.0 w/		
Nutren 2.0			Oxepa	fiber		
Nutra/Shake			Pulmocare	Replete w/		
Citrus			NutriVent	fiber		
			Osteoporsis			
			Ensure High Calcium			

into classes based on the main features. The following is a series of descriptions of these classes of enteral products.

Standard formulas, which are the products of choice for most patients receiving forced enteral nutrition, have caloric densities of 1.2 kcal per milliliter or less and a protein content of 20 to 40 g per kilocalorie. *High-protein* formulas are designed for patients with high requirements for protein synthesis, such as those with severe trauma or healing wounds. These formulas have a protein content of 41 to 59 g per kilocalorie. *Very-high-protein* formulas are similar to high-protein formulas but have an even higher protein content of more than 60 g per kilocalorie.

Disease-specific formulas are promoted to meet the needs of patients with specific diseases, usually renal, hepatic, or pulmonary dysfunction. The renal formulas (Amin-Aid, Nepro, Suplena, and Travasorb Renal) are low in protein, high in essential amino acids, and low in electrolytes. These formulas are designed for patients with chronic renal failure who are not undergoing dialysis. Patients who are undergoing dialysis do not need special renal formulas and can be treated with standard enteral preparations. The hepatic formulas (Hepatic-Aid II and Travasorb Hepatic) are low in sodium, low in aromatic amino

acids, and high in branched-chain amino acids. These special hepatic formulas are justified in the care of patients who experience encephalopathy with standard formulas. Products for patients with pulmonary failure (Pulmocare and Nutrivent) are high in fat and low in carbohydrates because the metabolism of carbohydrates generates more carbon dioxide than does the metabolism of fat. However, the difference is small, and there are few patients with pulmonary disease for whom it would be clinically significant. All the disease-specific products are expensive, and use of these products is justified in the care of only a few patients.

Most commercial enteral products do not contain fiber. Several manufacturers, however, produce nonstandard formulas to which fiber has been added. The fiber source usually is soy–polysaccharide fiber, which is largely insoluble and increases stool bulk. Fiber-containing formulas may be useful to patients undergoing long-term tube feeding who have problems with constipation or diarrhea.

Commercial enteral formulas usually do not contain lactose because lactose causes diarrhea in many persons. Several milk-based dietary supplements are available, however. These products are used primarily as oral supplements rather than as tube feedings. As a group, they are better tasting and less expensive than any of the other enteral products. One of these products may be an excellent choice for patients who tolerate lactose.

In most commercial enteral formulas, the amino acid source is intact proteins. In elemental formulas, the amino acid source is free amino acids, and in chemically defined diets, the amino acid source is partially hydrolyzed proteins. In both elemental and chemically defined diets, the carbohydrate source is oligosaccharides. Elemental and chemically defined diets are promoted for patients with diminished ability to digest and absorb nutrients. Because of the large functional reserve of the pancreas and intestine, few patients are incapable of digesting and absorbing standard enteral formulas. The disagreeable taste of most elemental and chemically defined diets makes them unusable as oral supplements and confines their use to tube feeding. Moreover, elemental and chemically defined diets may be hyperosmolar and can cause gastric retention and diarrhea. These formulas also are considerably more expensive than standard formulas.

Enteral formulas are designed to meet nutritional needs. They may not, however, meet total water and electrolyte requirements, especially if vomiting, diarrhea, excessive urinary loss, or other factors increase fluid and electrolyte requirements. Different enteral formulas have different electrolyte contents. The choice of a formula with high levels of the appropriate electrolytes may compensate for urinary or fecal losses. Basal water requirements are 30 to 35 mL per kilogram per day. These requirements can increase greatly among patients with diarrhea or other sources of fluid loss. Enteral administration of water to supplement the enteral formula may be necessary.

COMPLICATIONS OF ENTERAL TUBES AND FEEDINGS

Metabolic Complications

Monitoring of patients receiving forced enteral nutrition is outlined in Table 130.7. The metabolic complications of enteral nutrition are similar to those of parenteral nutrition but typically are less common and less severe. Fluctuations in blood glucose level and serum electrolyte concentration are less common when nutrients are given enterally rather than intravenously. The electrolyte content is fixed in commercial enteral formulas. Patients may need additional supplementation, for example, of potassium, calcium, magnesium, or phosphorus. Monitoring of electrolytes during the initiation of enteral nutrition and periodically until the patient's condition is stable should help identify any abnormalities. The metabolic complications of enteral nutrition can be reduced with careful consideration of the enteral formula used and the rate of administration. Some formulas have lower sodium content than others and may be tolerated better by patients with sodium excess related to cardiac, renal, or hepatic disease. Refeeding syndrome (see earlier) also occurs among pa-

TABLE 130.7.	MONITORING DURING FORCED ENTERAL NUTRITION		
	Initially	**Week 1–2**	**After Week 3**
Nursing			
Gastric residuals	Every 4 h	Daily	Weekly and as needed
Elevation of head of bed	With each feeding	With each feeding	With each feeding
Intake and output	Daily	Daily	Daily if medically indicated
Weight	Daily	1 time/wk	Monthly
Vital signs	Every 4 h	Daily	Daily if medically indicated
Inspection of tube insertion site	Every 4 h	Daily	Daily
Laboratory			
Electrolytes Sodium Potassium Chloride Bicarbonate	Baseline	1 time/wk	Monthly or as medically indicated
Renal function Blood urea nitrogen Creatinine	Baseline	1 time/wk	Monthly or as medically indicated
Minerals Calcium Phosphorus Magnesium	Baseline	1 time/wk	Monthly or as medically indicated
Albumin	Baseline	1 time/wk	Monthly
Glucose			
Nondiabetic	Daily	3 times/wk	Weekly
Diabetic	Every 4–6 h until blood glucose is stable	As medically indicated	
Triglycerides	As indicated		
Cholesterol	As indicated		

tients receiving enteral nutrition. Care is the same as that of patients receiving parenteral nutrition.

Most commercially prepared formulas are fortified with trace minerals. Among the trace minerals, deficiencies in zinc and selenium are the most common and are caused by losses in stool and fistulas. Observation for these deficiencies should be part of the routine assessment of patients receiving long-term, defined enteral diets. Trace mineral supplements can be added to enteral formulas.

Nonmetabolic Complications

Diarrhea

The incidence of diarrhea among patients receiving enteral nutrition depends on how one defines diarrhea. One definition is an increase from one to more than four stools per day with a change in consistency from formed to loose or liquid. The common causes of diarrhea among patients receiving enteral nutrition include the following:

Medications such as antibiotics, elixirs containing sorbitol, laxatives, antacids, and electrolyte replacements

Infection of the gastrointestinal tract, such as pseudomembranous colitis

The presence of lactose in the formula (most commercially prepared formulas are lactose-free, but many homemade feedings contain lactose)

Infusion of the formula at too rapid a rate

Use of hypertonic formulas, which can cause an increase in stool output (switching to an isotonic formula may decrease the amount of diarrhea)

Ingestion of high-fat formulas by patients with pancreatic insufficiency, bile salt deficiency, or ileal resection

Bacterial contamination of the enteral formula or bag

The presence of hypoalbuminemia, which is associated with a higher incidence of diarrhea

Intermittent feedings into the small intestine (patients are more likely to tolerate the osmotic load of tube feedings introduced directly into the intestine if the feedings are spread throughout the day in a continuous infusion)

Underlying disease such as Crohn's disease or ulcerative colitis

Treatment of patients with diarrhea should begin with a review of all medications, formulas, infusion methods, infusion rates, handling techniques, and the potential for causing diarrhea. Stool cultures and tests for *Clostridium difficile* toxin should be obtained when indicated. Switching to a formula containing fiber or administering bulk-forming medications may reduce stool frequency but also may clog the tube.

Tracheobronchial Aspiration

Aspiration can occur when regurgitated stomach contents or food or secretions from the oropharynx enter the trachea. A decreased gag reflex, a swallowing disorder, or an altered level of consciousness increases the risk of aspiration. The presence of a nasogastric tube can increase the incidence of reflux and aspiration by interfering with the competence of the upper and lower esophageal sphincters. Although less common, aspiration also occurs when tubes are placed in the jejunum. The presence of a cuff on an endotracheal or tracheostomy tube does not necessarily protect a patient breathing with a ventilator from aspiration into the lungs, especially during tracheal suctioning. If aspiration is suspected or the patient is at high risk, testing of the sputum for glucose is indicated. The sputum also should be tested for blood, because the presence of blood in the sputum produces a positive test result for glucose.

Measures to reduce the incidence of aspiration include the following:

Verification of tube location in the stomach or small intestine

Elevation of the head of the bed to 30 degrees during feeding and for 2 hours after completion of feeding

In nasogastric tube feeding, monitoring the residual volume before each intermittent feeding (tube feeding should be withheld if the volume exceeds 50% of the previous feeding)

Assessment for delayed gastric emptying (this complication should be managed with erythromycin, metoclopramide, or cisapride)

Assessment for the presence of fever, tachycardia, tachypnea, or respiratory distress

Conversion of a temporary nasogastric tube to a gastrostomy to increase the competence of the upper and lower esophageal sphincters

Clogging of the Tube

Clogging of the tube is caused most often by administration of medications or the lack of routine flushing. Medications are more likely to cause clogging if they are poorly crushed or if they interact chemically with the formula residuals on the inner surface of the tube. Examples of medications that can react with formulas are calcium and magnesium supplements. The tube should be flushed every 4 to 6 hours with 20 to 30 mL water or sugar-free carbonated dark soda for both intermittent and continuous feedings. The tube also should be flushed before and after administration of each medication. Another cause of clogging is administration of a viscous formula through a small-bore tube.

BIBLIOGRAPHY

Alpers DH, Stenson WF, Bier D. *Manual of nutritional therapeutics,* 3d ed. Boston: Little, Brown, 1995.

ASPEN Board of Directors. Guidelines for the use of parenteral and enteral nutrition in adult and pediatric patients. *JPEN J Parenter Enteral Nutr* 1993;17:1SA–52SA.

Berger R, Adams L. Nutritional support in the critical care setting. *Chest* 1989;96:139–150, 372–380.

Fischer JE. *Total parenteral nutrition,* 2d ed. Boston: Little, Brown, 1991.

Klein S, Kinney J, Jeejeebhoy K, et al. Nutritional support in clinical practice: review of published data and recommendations for future research directions. *JPEN J Parenter Enteral Nutr* 1997;21:133–156.

Rombeau JL, Caldwell MD. *Clinical nutrition: parenteral nutrition,* 2d ed. Philadelphia: WB Saunders, 1993.

C H A P T E R
131

LAPAROSCOPIC SURGERY FOR GASTROINTESTINAL DISORDERS

C. DANIEL SMITH
TIMOTHY M. FARRELL

Laparoscopic surgery is the performance of abdominal operations through small incisions with the aid of rod-lens telescopes and fiberoptic light sources to project a view from within the abdomen to a video monitor. With this view the operating surgeon can manipulate intra-abdominal organs and viscera through additional small incisions. Sometimes called *minimal access surgery,* this operative technique has been embraced by the medical community and by the general public. In fact, the public sector often has been the primary influence driving the rapid development of laparoscopic surgery. Laparoscopy has revolutionized surgery of the gastrointestinal tract. In many ways, the development of laparoscopy is to gastrointestinal surgeons what the introduction and development of fiberoptic endoscopy has been to gastroenterologists. In both cases a technique-based specialty is aimed at minimizing the suffering of patients being treated for common gastroenterologic conditions.

Laparoscopic surgery is a technique-based concept and not a new therapy. Laparoscopic operations are not new procedures but are different techniques for realizing the same result. Performed by means of laparoscopy or laparotomy, cholecystectomy is completed with the same steps and degree invasiveness within the abdominal cavity. Laparoscopic surgery is changing not the nature of the procedure but the route of access to the abdominal cavity. The indications and considerations for operative intervention are the same for open and laparoscopic operations.

PHYSIOLOGIC ASPECTS OF LAPAROSCOPIC SURGERY

The laparoscopic approach introduces distinct and new physiologic concerns. Visualization of the abdominal viscera requires that the abdominal wall be lifted away from the abdominal organs. To accomplish this, gas is blown into the abdominal cavity to a pressure of 15 mm Hg to produce a space in which to operate. Carbon dioxide, the gas most commonly used for positive-pressure pneumoperitoneum, evokes physiologic derangements. Rapid absorption of carbon dioxide across the peritoneum causes respiratory acidosis. Although mild acidosis is not serious, severe acidosis may cause cardiac arrhythmia, tachycardia, or increased systemic vascular resistance with increased myocardial oxygen demand.

Among patients with underlying cardiopulmonary problems, even minor physiologic changes can be clinically significant. In most cases, these derangements can be avoided by means of intraoperative adjustments in respiratory minute ventilation. Increased intra-abdominal pressure, the use of dependent patient positioning, and the loss of lower extremity muscle tone may impede venous return and further affect cardiac function. To avoid this, sequential compression stockings are used routinely. Intraoperative oliguria is another complication. It does not typically indicate volume depletion but is an expected result of increased intra-abdominal pressure on the kidney and renal vein, and a transient increase in plasma renin and antidiuretic hormone levels.

Despite the potential disadvantages of laparoscopic surgery, the benefits to the patient—less postprocedural pain, earlier return of gastrointestinal function, a more rapid return to usual physical activity and work, and a better (external) cosmetic result—form the basis for its unequivocal success. This chapter reviews the indications for and outcome of common laparoscopic procedures performed on the gastrointestinal tract by means of laparoscopy.

ESOPHAGUS

Coincident with the growth of laparoscopic surgery, there has been a dramatic increase in the number of patients with diseases of the esophagus treated surgically (Table 131.1). A laparoscopic approach to the esophagus avoids the morbidity of an upper abdominal incision. In addition, the successful control of gastroesophageal reflux disease (GERD) with proton pump inhibitors has raised the awareness of patients and physicians of the effect GERD has on quality of life, and made effective long-term management of GERD very desirable.

GASTROESOPHAGEAL REFLUX DISEASE

GERD involves failure of the antireflux barrier (see Chapter 106). Operative management involves reconstructing the antireflux barrier by means of reinforcement of the lower esophageal sphincter (LES). The Nissen fundoplication (360-degree gastric wrap) is the most popular and successful operative technique. After a 1-day hospital stay, patients are able to return to their usual activities, including work, within 7 to 14 days of the laparoscopic procedure. The only postoperative restriction is maintenance of a soft diet for 3 weeks after surgery while operative edema at the fundoplication resolves. Complications common to open fundoplication, such as splenic injury and pneumonia, are almost completely eliminated with the laparoscopic approach. In centers with expertise in the techniques, 95% of patients have complete resolution of the reflux symptoms and are able to discontinue use of antisecretory medication and the lifestyle modifications necessary to control reflux. Patient satisfaction with this procedure is very high. Laparoscopic management of GERD results in marked improvement in quality of life among persons with GERD. Laparoscopic fundoplication has become the standard of care for operative management of GERD unless patients have contraindications to laparoscopy (previous upper abdominal operation or earlier failed open antireflux procedure).

TABLE 131.1.	**LAPAROSCOPIC SURGERY OF THE ESOPHAGUS**	
Indication	**Accepted Procedure**	**Procedure in Development**[a]
Gastroesophageal reflux disease	Antireflux procedures	
Normal esophageal body function	Nissen (360 degrees) fundoplication	
Impaired esophageal body function	Toupet (270 degrees) fundoplication	
Shortened esophagus		Esophageal lengthening (Collis gastroplasty)
Paraesophageal hiatal hernia	Repair, gastropexy, or fundoplication	
Primary motor disorders		
Achalasia	Operative myotomy (Heller)	
Spastic disorders		Long myotomy (esophagomyotomy)
Diffuse esophageal spasm		
Nutcracker esophagus		
Hypertensive lower esophageal sphincter		
Nonspecific motility disorder		
Esophageal diverticula		
Pharyngoesophageal (Zenker's)	Transoral endoscopic diverticulostomy	Diverticulectomy, myotomy
Midesophageal	Diverticulectomy (thoracoscopic)	
Epiphrenic	Diverticulectomy, myotomy	
Malignant tumor of esophagus		Esophagectomy, reconstruction

[a] Performed at selected centers with special interests or expertise; not widely available.

Success with laparoscopic surgery is changing the indications for operative management of GERD. Rather than controlling symptoms, the aim of modern management of GERD is permanent elimination of symptoms. Medical management remains the first-line therapy. However, the expense and psychological burden of a lifetime of medication dependence, undesirable changes in lifestyle, uncertainty about the long-term effects of newer medications, and the potential for persistent mucosal changes (Barrett changes and oncogenic potential) despite symptom control have prompted many patients to seek an alternative. Even third-party payers are recognizing the potential cost savings of a one-time intervention that could eliminate the lifetime expense of medication. Centers that would typically see only a few patients who would eventually undergo open antireflux procedures are now performing hundreds of laparoscopic operations each year. The success of both medical and surgical management of GERD is uncovering previously unrecognized indications for treatment. Increasing numbers of patients with atypical symptoms of GERD (asthma, laryngitis or hoarseness, chest pain) are found to have GERD and are responding well to antireflux procedures.

PARAESOPHAGEAL HERNIA

Through the use of laparoscopic approaches to GERD, surgeons have become more comfortable using laparoscopy to manage other esophageal conditions. Because of the risk of incarceration, bleeding, and respiratory compromise of some paraesophageal hernias, a laparoscopic approach is a natural extension of laparoscopic antireflux surgery. Laparoscopic paraesophageal herniorrhaphy has become the preferred approach to all but the largest of these hernias. Some physicians argue that the unmasking of GERD among patients with these hernias warrants a fundoplication in all cases.

MOTILITY DISORDERS

Primary motor disorders of the esophagus are being diagnosed with increasing frequency (see Chapter 108). Management of achalasia centers on ablation of the LES. The ineffectiveness and associated side effects of pharmacotherapy leaves only primarily mechanical means of disruption of the LES. Although pneumatic balloon dilation is effective, high rates of perforation have left many clinicians afraid to use this therapy. The newer approach of injection of botulinum toxin into the LES, while effective, does not often provide long-lasting relief of dysphagia. Operative myotomy is the standard of care. Laparoscopic esophagomyotomy has matured and is now routinely performed for the management of achalasia. Increasing numbers of patients are being referred for laparoscopic treatment soon after diagnosis. As many as 90% of patients have complete resolution of dysphagia and 98% have dramatic improvement in swallowing after laparoscopic esophagomyotomy. Postoperative recovery involves a 1 to 2 day hospital stay, rapid return to usual activity, and immediate improvement in quality of life.

Who should undergo operative myotomy? Long-term relief of symptoms by means of pneumatic dilation is clearly less effective in the treatment of younger patients, and the effect of injection of botulinum toxin is of short duration. These approaches therefore are less desirable in the care of young patients. After failing, pneumatic dilation or injection of botulinum toxin can be repeated with an increase in response with successive treatments. It seems reasonable, however, to offer laparoscopic myotomy to patients who have had two unsuccessful trials of either nonoperative therapy.

Previous nonoperative therapy complicates myotomy because of scarring of the tissue planes; thus some surgeons recommend myotomy as initial therapy if the patient is a good candidate for surgical treatment. Patients at excessive risk of esophageal perforation during pneumatic dilation, including those with a tortuous esophagus, esophageal diverticula, or previous operation on the gastroesophageal junction, may be best treated by means of laparoscopic myotomy. An increasing number of patients want to avoid multiple interventions and seek out minimally invasive therapies that have a low complication rate, fast recovery, and lasting results.

Motor disorders of the esophagus such as diffuse esophageal spasm and nutcracker esophagus can be managed with laparoscopic myotomy or an antireflux procedure. However, the rarity of the conditions and controversy surrounding the best treatment limit the use of laparoscopic techniques to centers with medical and surgical expertise in this area.

ESOPHAGEAL DIVERTICULA

Laparoscopic approaches to esophageal diverticula are limited to centers with programs in the management of esophageal diseases and minimally invasive surgery. Technical issues are related to the immaturity of instruments for these procedures, limitations in videoimaging (two-dimensional visual field), and concerns regarding the physiologic effect of laparoscopy on the mediastinum.

ESOPHAGEAL TUMORS

Laparoscopic techniques are not yet routine for curative resection of malignant tumors of the esophagus. However, the 10% of esophageal neoplasms that are benign, such as leiomyoma, may be amenable to laparoscopic resection. An endoscope often is needed for intraoperative location of the lesion. Most leiomyomas enucleate after longitudinal myotomy. If recent biopsy has induced inflammation, resection and closure may be necessary.

■ STOMACH AND DUODENUM

Laparoscopic procedures rarely are used to manage gastroduodenal disorders, mainly because most surgical disorders of the stomach necessitate some form of excision and reconstruction (Table 131.2). Management of peptic ulcer disease once was the most common indication for operations on the stomach and duodenum. The identification of *Helicobacter pylori* as the etiologic agent in peptic ulcer disease and the success of medical eradication of *H. pylori* have changed the spectrum of operations performed on the stomach and duodenum (see Chapter 107).

PEPTIC ULCER DISEASE

Although optimal management of peptic ulcer disease involves antisecretory therapy and antibacterial control of *H. pylori* infection, some patients do not respond to medical therapy or have complications of the disease, such as perforation, bleeding, gastric outlet obstruction, or recurrence. In these situations, an attractive concept is laparoscopic management of gastroduodenal ulcer disease. Early enthusiasm was devoted to laparoscopic vagotomy for intractable ulcer diathesis by means of parietal cell vagotomy (highly selective vagotomy) or thoracoscopic transthoracic vagotomy for recurrent ulcers after incomplete previous surgical vagotomy. However, surgical vagotomy rarely is indicated in this era of medical management of *H. pylori* infection.

More relevant to surgical management of peptic ulcer disease are the complications of perforation and pyloric obstruction. Perforated duodenal ulcers are almost always on the anterior surface of the postpyloric duodenum or within the pyloric channel and are thus readily accessible by a laparoscopic approach. Classic teaching in the management of perforated peptic ulcer disease dictated closure of the perforation and performance of a definitive antisecretory procedure (vagotomy). In the era of eradication of *H. pylori* and management of ulcers induced by nonsteroidal anti-inflammatory drugs, laparoscopic therapy to manage the acute complication (close the perforation) and deal later with the cause of the ulcer is appealing. The site of perforation can either be patched by means of sewing a piece of vascularized omentum over the hole or be closed by means of suture approximation and buttressing the closure with an omental patch. The extravasated duodenal secretions can be aspirated or irrigated from the peritoneal cavity laparoscopically. Patients with large, complex perforations typically are not good candidates for laparoscopic treatment. Perforated gastric ulcers, when easily accessible, may be amenable to a laparoscopic approach if gastric cancer can be excluded.

Bleeding gastric or duodenal lesions are difficult to approach

TABLE 131.2.   LAPAROSCOPIC SURGERY OF THE STOMACH

Indication	Accepted Procedure	Procedure in Development[a]
Leiomyoma	Wedge-type resection	—
Intractable duodenal ulcer disease	Parietal cell vagotomy	—
Complicated duodenal or gastric ulcer with perforation	Closure of perforation	Gastrectomy (partial)
Pyloric obstruction	Gastrojejunostomy bypass	—
Gastric cancer	—	Gastrectomy (partial, total)
Morbid obesity	Laparoscopic gastric banding	Roux-en-Y gastric bypass or vertical banded gastroplasty

[a] Performed at selected centers with special interest or expertise; not widely available.

laparoscopically. Laparoscopic endoluminal techniques (placement of trocars in the lumen of the stomach for direct visualization and oversewing of the bleeding site) have been used successfully but rarely. Endoscopically guided laparoscopic wedge resection of a bleeding area in the stomach may be successful. Laparoscopic duodenotomy and oversewing of a bleeding vessel in a duodenal ulcer can be performed by a surgeon expert in laparoscopic technique, but the advantages of such an approach are unproved.

Gastric outlet obstruction due to antropyloric ulcer disease is amenable to a laparoscopic approach. Considerations include classic pyloroplasty, although this requires extensive experience with laparoscopic suturing, or constructing a gastrojejunostomy accompanied by a truncal or highly selective vagotomy should a protecting vagotomy be deemed necessary to minimize the chance of a stomal ulcer.

GASTRIC TUMORS

Probably the most common gastric disorder managed laparoscopically is gastric stromal tumor (leiomyoma). Because they usually require only limited resection or when small and benign can be managed by means of simple enucleation, these neoplasms lend themselves to a laparoscopic approach. Large neoplasms (2 to 5 cm in greatest dimension) along the greater curvature or in the corpus or proximal antrum often can be wedged out with a laparoscopic stapling device without functional narrowing of the gastric lumen. Leiomyoma at the ends of the stomach (cardia or distal antrum) are best managed by means of enucleation with suture closure of the defect. When the stromal tumor exceeds 5 cm, the risk of sarcoma increases markedly, making a laparoscopic procedure less attractive, especially if more complex resection is needed.

Laparoscopic gastrectomy for gastric cancer or for gastric or duodenal ulcer disease (antrectomy with gastroduodenostomy [Billroth I] or gastrojejunostomy [Billroth II]) is in development. Although performed at some centers of expertise, this approach is certainly not generally available, experience is limited, and the use of this type of approach for gastric adenocarcinoma can be seriously questioned. Gastrectomy thus awaits further development.

MORBID OBESITY

Laparoscopic technique is under active development in the field of bariatric surgery—operations for clinically severe obesity. Severe obesity, defined as a body mass index (weight in kilograms divided by the square of height in meters) greater than 40 affects more than four million persons in the United States. Patients who do not respond to medical and behavioral weight control programs and have comorbid conditions such as hypertension, diabetes, atherosclerotic cardiovascular disease, pulmonary insufficiency, and osteoarthritis are candidates for bariatric operations. These procedures performed as open operations carry increased risk of incisional hernia (approximately 15%), wound infection (5% to 7%), and respiratory complications. A minimally invasive approach helps avoid these problems. One might find it difficult to believe that any major upper gastrointestinal

procedure can be performed laparoscopically on patients weighing more than 250 to 300 pounds (114 to 136 kg), but it is possible.

There are two NIH-sanctioned bariatric procedures—vertical banded gastroplasty and Roux-en-Y gastric bypass. In the former a gastrointestinal stapler is used to perform a gastroplasty to separate the stomach into a small upper compartment, which communicates with the rest of the stomach through a narrow channel, without any formal anastomosis. Technical developments in design and use of internal laparoscopic stapling devices make this procedure feasible with laparoscopy. A modification of the concept of gastroplasty has been introduced: an adjustable silicone gastric band is placed around the cardia for external induction of a form of gastroplasty similar to vertical banded gastroplasty. This technique is ideally suited to a laparoscopic approach because no anatomic rearrangement or anastomosis is necessary. This minimally invasive procedure has been used extensively in Europe with encouraging short-term results.

A minimally invasive approach to Roux-en-Y gastric bypass has been developed. This operation entails transection of the proximal stomach with construction of a gastrojejunostomy to the cardia of the stomach and a jejunojejunostomy to the Roux limb. Although preliminary experience is encouraging, whether this procedure will become widely performed remains to be seen.

■ SMALL BOWEL AND APPENDIX

APPENDICITIS

Laparoscopic approaches to diseases of the small (and large) intestine started with laparoscopic appendectomy (Table 131.3). The concept of laparoscopic appendectomy is attractive for the following reasons: (a) the procedure is technically easy, (b) it avoids the morbidity of a 4 to 10 cm right lower quadrant incision, (c) the incidence of wound infection should be low, (d) the pelvic adnexa of women of childbearing age can be examined should the appendix not prove to be inflamed, (e) the procedure and visualization are facilitated in operations on obese patients, and (f) disorders masquerading as appendicitis, such as Meckel's diverticulitis or ovarian cyst, can be found and managed laparoscopically, or formal celiotomy can be avoided if the disorder is a nonsurgical inflammatory condition such as simple acute

TABLE 131.3.	LAPAROSCOPIC SURGERY OF THE SMALL BOWEL AND APPENDIX
Indication	**Accepted Procedure**
Appendicitis	Appendectomy
Meckel's diverticulum	Diverticulectomy
Small-bowel obstruction	Adhesiolysis
Colonic diversion	Diverting loop ileostomy
Crohn's disease	Small-bowel resection with or without colectomy, stricturoplasty
Neoplasm	Resection

diverticulitis, regional enteritis (Crohn's disease), or mesenteric adenitis.

Despite these theoretical advantages, numerous feasibility studies followed by prospective, randomized studies have shown remarkably few clinically important objective benefits of laparoscopic appendectomy. The technique appears most beneficial when the diagnosis of acute appendicitis remains obscure, especially if the patient is a young woman with right lower quadrant or pelvic pain. Less clear benefit may be realized by patients sensitive to the presence of a right lower quadrant scar or by athletes who play rough sports and want an early return to full physical activity.

The indications for laparoscopic appendectomy depend on the surgeon's confidence in the diagnosis and the stage of appendicitis. If uncomplicated appendicitis is found, laparoscopic appendectomy is straightforward. If a normal appendix and no other pathologic condition are detected, or if the pathologic condition detected is likely to cause recurrent pain, such as terminal ileitis, the appendix is easily removed. Appendectomy is not performed if another surgical problem, such as acute cholecystitis, is apparent. If unsuspected advanced inflammatory conditions of the appendix (gangrene, phlegmon, and abscess) are found, conversion to laparotomy or antibiotic therapy and interval appendectomy is indicated. Perforation of the appendix can be managed laparoscopically if the inflammatory reaction is minimal and the base of the appendix is normal.

BOWEL OBSTRUCTION

The full length of the small bowel is available to laparoscopic assessment. Adhesive small-bowel obstruction sometimes can be managed by means of laparoscopic lysis of adhesions. If the patient has undergone a previous abdominal operation, achieving pneumoperitoneum and placing ports is challenging. If multiple dilated loops of bowel are present, as in distal obstruction, visualization may be impaired. Results with a laparoscopic adhesiolysis are better in operations on patients with early acute small-bowel obstruction (before marked abdominal distention occurs), nonacute, partial obstruction, or recurrent, intermittent obstruction. The offending adhesive band often represents a single, easily lysed adhesion readily accessible and visualized at laparoscopy. Complex adhesions fixing one segment of the small bowel to the abdominal wall, pelvis, or retroperitoneum, the presence of an internal hernia, or even an unrecognized abdominal wall hernia such as a femoral hernia also can be repaired. In general, success rates with a laparoscopic approach are better for intermittent partial obstruction, nonresolving partial obstruction, or chronic obstruction (60% to 80%) than they are for acute complete obstruction (approximately 50%).

SMALL-BOWEL TUMORS

Whether a primary neoplasm of the small intestine is amenable to a laparoscopic approach depends on the extent of mesenteric resection or lymphadenectomy needed. Stromal tumors, early adenocarcinoma, and primary small-bowel lymphoma seem to be amenable. Carcinoid tumors with known or highly suspected nodal metastases probably are best approached by means of open exploration because of a propensity for nodal metastases and mesenteric sclerosis or fibrosis. Small-bowel metastases to the intestine from extraintestinal neoplasms (carcinoma of the breast, lung, or kidney and melanoma) are ideal lesions for a laparoscopic approach. The lesion may be brought through a trocar site, the incision for which is enlarged to allow evisceration of the lesion. This allows resection of the lesion and extracorporeal anastomosis.

CROHN'S DISEASE

Many patients with small-bowel Crohn's disease are candidates for laparoscopic surgery. The involved segment often is quite mobile, even after previous resection, and lends itself well to directed exteriorization and resection or stricturoplasty. Ileocolonic Crohn's disease also allows relatively easy mobilization of the cecum and proximal ascending colon.

MISCELLANEOUS CONDITIONS OF THE SMALL BOWEL

Although rarely indicated, laparoscopic transmural biopsy of the small bowel is easy. A segment of jejunum or ileum can be exteriorized through one of the ports, the biopsy specimen obtained, the enterotomy closed by means of external hand suturing, and the segment placed back into the abdomen. When colonic or rectal diversion is necessary, as for distal colonic fistula or colonic dysmotility, loop ileostomy is easily performed with basic laparoscopic techniques. Less common situations in which laparoscopy might be performed include management of radiation enteropathy, inability to differentiate a primary small-bowel motility disorder from mechanical obstruction, or treatment of a patient younger than 40 years with chronic occult gastrointestinal bleeding when it is likely the cause can be found at exploration, for example, Meckel's diverticulum, leiomyoma, or a small carcinoid.

■ COLON AND RECTUM

Introduction of laparoscopic techniques to colorectal surgery has met with unique challenges that distinguish these procedures from other laparoscopic applications (Table 131.4). Use of laparoscopic colonic procedures has lagged behind other specialties for the following reasons: (a) resection of the colon requires advanced laparoscopic experience, (b) maintenance of oncologic principles may be difficult during resection of colorectal cancer, and (c) evidence of objective benefits of the approach are not obvious.

DIVERTICULITIS

Diverticulitis is a common benign indication for colectomy. The chief difficulty of laparoscopic resection is residual inflammation or scarring, which obliterates normal tissue planes, impedes iden-

TABLE 131.4.	LAPAROSCOPIC SURGERY OF THE LARGE INTESTINE	
Indication	**Accepted Procedure**	**Procedure in Development**[a]
Diverticulitis	Colectomy (segmental)	—
Large sessile polyp or mass	Transcolonic polypectomy or colectomy (segmental)	—
Colonic carcinoma (especially right-sided, left-sided, high rectum)	Colectomy (oncologic resection)	Colectomy (oncologic resection)
Colostomy	Laparoscopic colonic diversion or takedown of previous stoma	—
Inflammatory bowel disease (chronic ulcerative colitis, Crohn's disease)		Colectomy (partial, total abdominal)
Rectal prolapse	Colectomy, rectopexy	—
Hirschsprung's disease	Colectomy, anastomosis	—

[a] Performed at selected centers with special interest or expertise; not widely available.

tification of the left ureter, and often produces a bulky specimen that is difficult to manipulate. Laparoscopic techniques are most successful when used to treat patients with resolving or mild inflammation or contained perforation (abscess) without extensive surrounding inflammation. The degree of inflammation is difficult to predict preoperatively and explains the often higher rate of conversion to open laparotomy for diverticulitis. However, because patient-related benefits have been demonstrated in terms of shorter ileus and reduced analgesic requirements and lengths of stay, a laparoscopic approach should be considered in nearly all cases.

COLON CANCER

Because colorectal cancer is the most common intra-abdominal malignant tumor and the most common indication for colectomy, it is not surprising that colorectal cancer is one of the few malignant tumors resected with laparoscopic techniques. Issues surrounding the oncologic adequacy of a laparoscopic procedure have prompted caution in its use and led to performance of well-designed, randomized, prospective trials on a scale rare for evaluation of surgical procedures.

The primary issue in management of colorectal cancer is whether survival after treatment with a laparoscopic approach is equivalent to that after treatment with an open approach. Although the length of margins, number of lymph nodes removed, and ability to perform proximal ligation of the vascular pedicle are the same for the two approaches, the true oncologic end point is survival. Concerns have been raised through anecdotal reports of unexpected tumor recurrence in both the incision made to extract the specimen and in laparoscopic trocar sites. Results for large series of patients suggest that the rate of tumor recurrence is about 1%, which compares favorably with that for open colectomy. Current recommendations are that laparoscopic resection for cancer be performed in a clinical trial or with an equivalent form of follow-up study.

When colon or rectal polyps cannot be removed endoscopically, surgical resection is indicated. The procedure is performed most commonly on the right colon, where the thinner bowel wall precludes aggressive attempts at polypectomy. The extent of resection must not be compromised by the approach; the very indication for operation (size of the polyp) is also a risk factor for malignant growth within the polyp.

MISCELLANEOUS DISORDERS OF THE COLON AND RECTUM

Laparoscopy has been used for construction and reversal of stomas. Often only two trocar sites are needed, one becoming the stoma site. Such a minor procedure causes little interruption of bowel function. Colostomy closure can be performed laparoscopically. Success depends on the preceding operation and extent of adhesions. Laparoscopic management of ulcerative colitis requires proctocolectomy and either Brooke ileostomy or ileal pouch–anal anastomosis. These procedures require advanced laparoscopic skill. Anterior resection and rectopexy for rectal prolapse have been shown to be feasible laparoscopic procedures. Difficulties of the procedures lie in the complete rectal dissection necessary for full reduction of the prolapse. Current instrumentation does not fully address the challenges of working within the confines of the bony pelvis.

■ BILIARY TREE

Although gynecologic surgeons had been using laparoscopic techniques for years, an explosion in minimally invasive techniques in gastrointestinal circles occurred when the first laparoscopic cholecystectomy was reported (Table 131.5). Laparoscopic approaches to the biliary tree continue to be the most commonly performed laparoscopic operations.

CHOLELITHIASIS

The standard of care for elective cholecystectomy is a laparoscopic approach. Indeed, it is against the law not to mention a

TABLE 131.5.	LAPAROSCOPIC SURGERY OF THE HEPATOBILIARY–PANCREATIC AXIS	

Indication	Accepted Procedure	Procedure in Development[a]
Biliary tree		
Cholelithiasis	Cholecystectomy	—
Acute cholecystitis	Cholecystectomy	—
Choledocholithiasis	Common duct explorations	—
Liver		
Directed or high-risk liver biopsy	Liver biopsy	—
Peripheral mass	Limited wedge excision	—
Simple hepatic cyst	Partial cystectomy or fenestration	—
Hepatic neoplasm	—	Hepatectomy
Pancreas		
Palliation of pancreatic cancer	Cholecystojejunostomy with or without gastrojejunostomy	—
Distal gland disease	—	Distal pancreatectomy
Insulinoma	—	Enucleation
Pancreatic pseudocyst	—	Cystoenteric drainage[b]
Localized, organized pancreatic necrosis	—	Necrosectomy, drainage
Chronic pancreatitis	Thoracoscopic splanchnicectomy	—

[a] Performed at selected centers with special interest or expertise; not widely available.
[b] Combined endoluminal laparo-endoscopic approach

laparoscopic approach to a patient as an option. Hospitalization is minimized, usually less than 36 hours, and at some centers these operations are outpatient procedures. Pain is decreased, return to work is expedited, and overall cost, including convalescence and return to work, is decreased.

The laparoscopic approach initially was limited to elective surgery for biliary colic, unless the patient had acute cholecystitis. Now even acute cholecystitis is managed laparoscopically approximately 75% of the time. It would be difficult to argue a case for approaching cholecystectomy with a primary open incision without first performing a laparoscopic examination to assess the feasibility of a minimal access approach.

More than 95% of patients undergoing elective cholecystectomy should be able to undergo a successful laparoscopic procedure. Exceptions include rare patients with serious biliary anomalies not evident or clearly definable intraoperatively or patients with a stone impacted in the distal cystic duct with surrounding inflammation deemed too dangerous or too scarred to dissect. Early in the history (1990–1994) of laparoscopic cholecystectomy, serious biliary injuries were all too common whether the operation was performed by an experienced or an inexperienced surgeon. Some of the injuries were extremely serious and caused a plethora of problems that necessitated reconstruction of the biliary tree. This led to exponential growth in the number of lawsuits, many settled for large sums. These situations stimulated numerous teaching seminars and courses with hands-on laboratories designed to re-educate older surgeons in laparoscopic techniques of cholecystectomy. Since then, all general surgical residency programs have incorporated laparoscopy into the curriculum, and today open cholecystectomy is a rare operation.

With increasing experience and an intense nationwide educational program to highlight situations that predispose a patient to serious biliary complications, most tertiary referral centers are seeing fewer serious biliary injuries caused by laparoscopic cholecystectomy than in the first 5 years of the 1990s. Today patients should expect a success rate of laparoscopic cholecystectomy under elective conditions of approximately 95% with a risk of serious bile duct injury of 0.5% or less. However, the risk of bile duct injury is not zero, and preoperative discussion with the patient should emphasize the importance and possibility of conversion to an open procedure if the surgeon is unsure of the anatomic features. Such conversion should not be considered a failure by the patient or by the surgeon and should be acknowledged as such preoperatively. Conversion to open cholecystectomy or development of a complication, however serious, should be discussed immediately with the patient and family to minimize the chances of medicolegal confrontation.

A pregnant woman with cholecystitis presents a not uncommon problem. Pregnancy once was considered a contraindication to laparoscopic cholecystectomy because of unknown consequences of pneumoperitoneum for the woman and the fetus. Most surgeons now believe that an attempt at laparoscopic cholecystectomy may be warranted in the third trimester if necessary. Every reasonable attempt should be made to delay the procedure to the postpartum period.

CHOLEDOCHOLITHIASIS

Stones in the biliary tree (common bile duct, common hepatic duct, or intrahepatic ducts) have come under the technical realm of the laparoscopic surgeon. Common bile duct stones once were removed by an interventional endoscopist either before surgical exploration if the presence of the stones was known or suspected, or after exploration if the stones were found during intraoperative cholangiography. The technical development of a laparoscopic choledochoscope allows visualization of common bile duct stones and facilitates capture of stones with baskets introduced into the duct through the choledochoscope. Laparoscopic exploration of the common duct can be performed through the cystic duct if the ductal diameter is large enough after intraoperative dilation or even by means of direct choledochotomy and laparoscopic suture closure of the choledochotomy. If the laparoscopic procedure is technically unsuccessful, most patients can be treated with an endoscopic procedure the following day, avoiding open celiotomy and a long convalescence. Although the technical ability to perform laparoscopic common bile duct exploration is not yet widespread, many gastrointestinal surgeons are gaining the necessary experience and interest. Most laparoscopic surgeons soon should be able to perform common bile duct exploration.

■ LIVER AND PANCREAS

The bulkiness of the liver and pancreas, the rich and varied blood supply, the retroperitoneal and dorsal location in the abdomen, and the preponderance of malignant disease of these organs make laparoscopic approaches to the liver and pancreas limited at best (Table 131.5). Laparoscopic instruments and equipment are largely inadequate for laparoscopic management of diseases of these organs.

STAGING MALIGNANT TUMORS

With many forms of malignant gastrointestinal tumors, the surgeon operates with the intent to perform a curative procedure only to find small metastatic lesions in the peritoneum or liver or direct local extension of the tumor to another structure that either precludes curability or necessitates a much different approach. Laparoscopy and new evaluative procedures such as laparoscopic ultrasonography have fostered a more aggressive concept of staging of some malignant gastrointestinal tumors.

Preoperative staging laparoscopic examination of the intraperitoneal cavity has been suggested for adenocarcinoma of the esophagus, stomach, pancreas, liver, and biliary tree. In certain situations, the laparoscopic procedure should be performed as a separate, staged procedure one or more days before the proposed resection. In other instances, laparoscopy immediately precedes the proposed resection. The former approach may be used if the laparoscopist is not the surgeon performing the resection.

Performance of staging laparoscopy implies that treatment will be changed on the basis of the laparoscopic findings. Optimal use of this procedure would be in the care of a patient with what appears to be resectable pancreatic or liver cancer. The patient undergoes staging laparoscopy, which reveals unappreciated hepatic or peritoneal metastases, and cannot undergo resection for cure. The patient is spared the discomfort and requisite convalescence of a celiotomy to reveal such incurability. This approach allows the patient to proceed with palliative therapy if indicated and limit the time spent in the hospital.

LIVER TUMORS AND CYSTS

Resection of hepatic of tumors is in the developmental stage. Although they have been performed in highly specialized centers, more development of technique, hemostasis, and exposure is needed. Peripherally based, small lesions amenable to classic wedge hepatic resection are readily removed, but centrally situated masses within the hepatic parenchyma should be managed with open resection. One exception may be a neoplasm in the left lateral segment (Couinard segments 2 and 3), for which laparoscopic excision may be attempted by a highly experienced laparoscopic surgeon. Anatomic or nonanatomic segmental resection is fraught with the risk of hemorrhage and bile leak.

Symptomatic benign hepatic cyst is a hepatic disorder readily amenable to a laparoscopic approach. Most simple cysts that cause symptoms are quite large (more than 10 cm) and are not likely to be controlled with percutaneous sclerosis. Because they are so large, these cysts are present at the liver periphery and thus are easily accessible to a laparoscope. If these cysts meet the criteria for being a simple cyst (round, smooth internal wall, no associated eccentric mass component, lack of internal septa, and nonbilious content) and thus are differentiated from neoplastic or infectious cystic lesions, laparoscopic excision of the external wall is fairly easy and effective. The excised cyst wall should always be subjected to histologic review to exclude the rare unilocular cystic neoplasm of the liver (cystadenoma). Symptomatic polycystic liver disease can be managed with laparoscopy. All accessible cysts are unroofed and drained.

PANCREAS

Aside from staging of pancreatic cancer before open exploration, almost all laparoscopic operations directed at the pancreas itself, aside from simple biopsy, are in the developmental stage or are performed only at highly specialized centers.

Tumors

Although formal pancreatic resection for tumors has been accomplished successfully, such procedures remain in the developmental stage even at highly proficient laparoscopic centers. Of the resective techniques performed, distal pancreatectomy is the most realistic for a laparoscopic approach because no formal reconstruction (anastomosis) is needed, and closure of the proximal pancreatic stump and ligation of the splenic artery and vein can be accomplished with laparoscopic stapling devices. However, there are few indications for distal pancreatectomy, and few centers have sufficient experience in performing this procedure.

Another suggested pancreas-directed laparoscopic procedure is enucleation of insulinoma or other selected small, benign islet cell tumors. When the lesion is readily identifiable and accessible, a minimally invasive approach is reasonable if the lesion is not near the main pancreatic duct, which warrants formal pancreatectomy. In contrast, inability to palpate the pancreas of a patient without an obvious tumor or a patient with multiple endocrine neoplasia syndrome (risk of multiple tumors) is a limitation of the laparoscopic approach and may be a relative contraindication. Use of laparoscopic ultrasonography may play an important role in this situation.

Chronic Pancreatitis

Inflammatory disorders of the pancreas have been targeted with laparoscopic techniques. Laparoscopic internal drainage of pancreatic pseudocysts includes endoscopic cystogastrostomy and cystojejunostomy. In rare instances, when access to the gastric or duodenal region necessary for internal drainage is impossible with oral endoscopy, a combined laparoendoscopic approach may be possible. This technique allows laparoscopically directed insertion of trocars into the gastric and duodenal lumens to allow the laparoendoscopic procedure to be accomplished. This approach has been used for endoscopic excisions of polyps.

The visceral pain of chronic pancreatitis is amenable to a promising procedure that is yet to be established as a durable procedure—thoracoscopic splanchnicectomy. This minimal access thoracoscopic approach is designed to transect the greater splanchnic nerves believed to transmit visceral pain fibers from the pancreas to the central nervous system. Surgical history does not recall neurolytic procedures for chronic pancreatitis kindly, but this procedure has its advocates, especially when patients are selected with an epidural technique designed to differentiate visceral from nonvisceral pain. Whether a simultaneous bilateral procedure or unilateral left splanchnicectomy followed by staged right splanchnicectomy is optimal remains to be determined, as do the true success rate and duration of benefit.

BIBLIOGRAPHY

Bannon MP, Zietlow SP, Harmsen WS, et al. A prospective randomized comparison of laparoscopic appendectomy with open appendectomy. *Gastroenterology* 1997;112(4):A1429.

Conlon KC, Dougherty E, Klimstra DS, et al. The value of minimal access surgery in the staging of patients with potentially resectable peripancreatic malignancy. *Ann Surg* 1996;223:134–140.

Drucart ML, VanHee R, Etienne J, et al. Laparoscopic repair of perforated duodenal ulcer: a prospective, multicenter clinical trial. *Surg Endosc* 1997;11:1017–1020.

Fleshman JW, Nelson H, Peters WR, et al. for the Clinical Outcomes of Surgical Therapy (COST) Study Group. Early results of laparoscopic surgery for colorectal cancer: retrospective analysis of 372 patients treated by Clinical Outcomes of Surgical Therapy (COST) study group. *Dis Colon Rectum* 1996;39:S53–S58.

Katkhouda N, Hurwitz M, Gugenheim J, et al. Laparoscopic management of benign solid and cystic lesions of the liver. *Ann Surg* 1999;229: 460–466.

Park A, Schwartz R, Tandan V, et al. Laparoscopic pancreatic surgery. *Am J Surg* 1999;177:158–163.

Society of American Gastrointestinal Endoscopic Surgeons (SAGES). Guidelines for surgical treatment of gastroesophageal reflux disease (GERD). *Surg Endosc* 1998;12:186–188.

Spivak H, Smith CD, Phichith A, et al. Asthma and gastroesophageal reflux: fundoplication decreases need for systemic corticosteroids. *J Gastrointest Surg* 199;3:477–482.

Waters GS, Crist DW, Davoudi M, et al. Management of choledocholithiasis encountered during laparoscopic cholecystectomy. *Am Surg* 1996; 62:256–258.

Wittgrove AC, Clark GW. Laparoscopic gastric bypass, Roux-en-Y experience of 27 cases, with 3-18 months follow-up. *Obes Surg* 1996;6:54–57.

Kelley's Textbook of Internal Medicine, fourth edition. Edited by H. David Humes. Lippincott Williams & Wilkins, Philadelphia © 2000.

C H A P T E R
132

LIVER TRANSPLANTATION

CHRISTOPHER F. SCHULTZ
MICHAEL R. LUCEY

◼ HISTORICAL PERSPECTIVE

Surgical removal of a diseased liver and replacement with a donor organ in the same anatomic location is called *orthotopic liver transplantation* (OLT). The formidable complexities of the surgical technique, poor allograft quality, frequent rejection of transplanted organs, and a 1-year survival rate of only 30% produced a sense of skepticism about liver transplantation in the 1970s. Acceptance of the concept of brain-stem death in the 1970s and 1980s led to retrieval of organs from heart-beating donors, improving the viability of cadaveric livers offered for transplantation. The introduction of cyclosporin A in the early 1980s revolutionized immunosuppressant therapy of transplant recipients, which resulted in greater safety and efficacy in the prevention of rejection. In 1983, the National Institutes of Health Consensus Development Conference on Liver Transplantation declared that liver transplantation was a therapy that deserved broader application rather than experimental use. The introduction of the University of Wisconsin (UW) preservation solution in 1986 allowed longer cold ischemia time for donor allografts and resulted in improved outcomes.

◼ LIVER TRANSPLANTATION: AN OVERVIEW

Liver transplantation has become the preferred therapeutic approach to irreversible acute or chronic liver failure. More than 4,000 liver transplants are performed annually in the United States. Fifteen percent of recipients are younger than 18 years. The overall survival rate after liver transplantation currently approaches 80% to 90% at 1 year and 65% to 70% at 5 years.

Liver transplantation should be considered in the treatment of all patients (children and adults) with advanced acute or chronic hepatic failure or severe liver disease for which there are no satisfactory medical or surgical therapeutic options. Although many of the indications for liver transplantation for acute and chronic end-stage liver disease (ESLD) are now well established

TABLE 132.1. INDICATIONS FOR LIVER TRANSPLANTATION

Adults	Children
Chronic Liver Disease	
Primary parenchymal disease	
Postnecrotic cirrhosis	Congenital hepatic fibrosis
Chronic viral hepatitis	
Drug-induced cirrhosis	
Alcohol cirrhosis	
Hemochromatosis	
Autoimmune liver disease	
Steatohepatitis	
Cryptogenic cirrhosis	
Cystic fibrosis	
Cholestatic disease	
Primary biliary cirrhosis	Biliary atresia
Secondary biliary cirrhosis	Alagille syndrome
Primary sclerosing cholangitis	Byler disease
Caroli's disease	Neonatal hepatitis
Vascular disorders	
Hepatic venous thrombosis	
Veno-occlusive disease	
Acute Liver Failure	
A. Viral hepatitis (A, B, C, and D)	
B. Drug-induced and toxin-induced	
C. Metabolic disorder	
Wilson's disease	
Reye's syndrome	
D. Massive hepatic trauma	
Primary Hepatic Tumors	
Hepatocellular carcinoma	
Other primary hepatic malignant tumors	
	Hepatoblastoma
	Sarcoma
	Hemangioendothelioma
Hepatic adenoma	
Inborn Errors of Metabolism	
	Glycogen storage disease
	Tyrosinemia
	Lysosomal storage disease
	Crigler–Najjar syndrome type1
	Wilson's disease
	α_1-antitrypsin deficiency
	Protoporphyria
	Familial hypercholesterolemia
	Hereditary oxalosis
	Hemophilia
	Urea cycle deficiency

eric donors and suitable recipients has led to innovative approaches to expand the supply of donor organs, including dividing a cadaveric donor liver between two recipients and the use of partial grafts from living donors. Reduction in the size of donor allografts, use of living-related donor allografts, and split-liver transplantation have dramatically reduced waiting list mortality and improved overall survival among pediatric patients.

DONOR AND RECIPIENT FACTORS AFFECTING OUTCOME OF LIVER TRANSPLANTATION

Donor factors that reduce graft survival include donor age, transplantation of a liver allograft from a female donor into a male recipient, and total ischemia time. Steatosis of the donor liver influences early graft function, perhaps by facilitating the generation of reactive oxidative species.

Several recipient factors have been identified as independent predictors of outcome. The cause the underlying liver disease affects graft survival after OLT. Survival rates after OLT are best for chronic cholestatic liver diseases and slightly better than those for chronic hepatocellular disorders that cause cirrhosis. The outcome is somewhat worse among patients who undergo transplantation because of fulminant hepatic failure and markedly worse among patients with cancer. Retransplantation is less successful than primary grafting, especially among patients undergoing second OLT soon after the initial graft attempt. The outcome of liver transplantation is influenced by the severity of illness of the recipient before surgery. Patient and graft survival rates are markedly reduced among recipients cared for in intensive care units, those undergoing mechanical ventilation, and those with multisystem organ failure before transplantation.

TIMING OF LIVER TRANSPLANTATION

The minimal criterion for being placed on a waiting list is a predicted 1-year likelihood of survival without transplantation of less than 90%, that is, the 1-year survival rate with OLT is better than without OLT. The prognosis among patients with cirrhosis is assessed with the Child–Pugh classification (see Chapter 105). This empiric scoring scheme is a compilation of five features of chronic liver failure (ascites, encephalopathy, prothrombin time, serum bilirubin level, and serum albumin level). Likelihood of survival among patients with cirrhosis declines with worsening Child class. The Child–Pugh classification system is useful in the setting of evaluation for liver transplantation because a patient in Child–Pugh class B has crossed the threshold of probability of 1-year survival less than 90%.

A complementary approach is to consider end-stage liver disease as either compensated (stable) or decompensated cirrhosis. Stable cirrhosis is defined as cirrhosis without variceal hemorrhage, ascites, jaundice, or encephalopathy. Cirrhosis with at least one of these clinical phenomena is decompensated disease. The onset of decompensation in a patient with previously stable

(Table 132.1), the list continues to expand and generate controversy. More than 12,000 patients are awaiting liver transplantation in the United States alone, fueling debate over how best to allocate the limited number of suitable cadaveric livers available each year. The growing imbalance between the number of cadav-

TABLE 132.2.	**SPECIFIC CLINICAL INDICATIONS FOR CONSIDERATION OF LIVER TRANSPLANTATION IN PATIENTS WITH CHRONIC LIVER DISEASE**

Recurrent gastroesophageal variceal hemorrhage
Refractory ascites
Spontaneous bacterial peritonitis
Severe hepatic encephalopathy
Hepatorenal syndrome
Profound pruritis of cholestatic liver disease
Severe hepatic osteopathy
Progressive rise in serum α-fetoprotein without mass
Refractory bacterial cholangitis
Intractable coagulopathy
Severe fatigue and weakness
Severe malnutrition

cirrhosis is associated with a significantly reduced likelihood of survival and indicates the need for evaluation for OLT. Other life-threatening complications of end-stage liver disease, such as hepatorenal syndrome and spontaneous bacterial peritonitis, or an unacceptable quality of life because of hepatic disease, also warrant consideration of OLT (Table 132.2).

SPECIFIC INDICATIONS FOR LIVER TRANSPLANTATION

Cirrhosis due to viral hepatitis or alcohol-induced liver injury, is the leading indication for OLT among adults. Chronic hepatitis B virus infection historically was viewed as a relative contraindication to hepatic transplantation because of the reduced overall survival rate, particularly due to the development of a rapidly progressive form of recurrent hepatitis B virus infection known as fibrosing cholestatic hepatitis. In recent years, long-term administration of hepatitis B immune globulin has been shown to be effective in controlling recurrence of hepatitis B after liver transplantation, and outcomes are excellent. Lamivudine and famciclovir, antiviral agents with activity against hepatitis B, further expand the potential for control of post-transplantation hepatitis B infection and are undergoing clinical trials.

Chronic hepatitis C virus infection has become the most common underlying diagnosis among persons undergoing liver transplantation in the United States. The effect of chronic hepatitis C on the allograft is discussed later.

In North America and Europe, approximately 20% of all hepatic transplantation procedures are performed on patients with alcoholic liver disease. In addition to meeting minimal listing criteria, alcoholic patients being evaluated for liver transplantation should undergo formal psychosocial assessment and when feasible participate in alcoholism rehabilitation and counseling. Many transplantation programs and third-party payers demand abstinence for a specified time (6 months at most centers) before approving transplantation for candidates with alcoholism. Interesting is that the primary benefit of a mandated period of abstinence before transplantation is that it allows recovery from acute alcoholic hepatitis, which may obviate hepatic replacement. Al-

coholic patients need careful assessment of other sites of alcoholic end-organ damage. Among selected alcoholic patients, rates of graft and patient survival after liver transplantation are similar to those for other causes of end-stage liver disease.

Large hepatocellular carcinomas almost invariably recur after transplantation. Patients with this disease cannot be placed on the transplantation list, except within defined study protocols. Resection remains the treatment of choice among patients with small tumors without evidence of spread beyond the liver and with well-preserved hepatic synthetic function. Small hepatocellular carcinomas confined to the liver are amenable to transplantation, and the patients have excellent outcomes.

Primary biliary cirrhosis (PBC) and primary sclerosing cholangitis (PSC) are good indications for OLT. Together they account for approximately 20% of all liver transplantation procedures in the United States and Europe. Prognostic models of the natural history of PBC and PSC are a guide for the timing of transplantation. The Mayo mathematical model of PBC identified five independent variables from which a prognostic equation is derived (total bilirubin level, albumin level, age, prothrombin time, and amount of edema). The Mayo model is not time dependent and has not been validated for serial measurements. In contrast to models of PBC, prognostic models of PSC among patients with advanced disease are probably no better than Child–Pugh scores. Cholangiocarcinoma occurs among approximately 5% to 15% of patients with preexisting PSC. The prognosis among patients in whom cholangiocarcinoma develops is poor even with transplantation. The presence of cholangiocarcinoma usually is considered a contraindication to OLT. Patients with either PBC or PSC should be referred for formal evaluation for OLT when they meet minimal listing criteria for cholestatic liver disease (Child–Pugh score greater than 6), have life-threatening complications of cirrhosis, or have quality-of-life indications such as severe pruritus, severe hepatic osteopathy, profound fatigue, and recurrent cholangitis.

Fulminant hepatic failure, a term traditionally used to describe the condition of patients with hepatic encephalopathy that develops within 8 weeks of acute liver failure, and its clinical variant, submassive hepatic necrosis, are characterized by massive hepatocyte necrosis often resulting in dysfunction of multiple organ systems. The outcome with medical management is determined by the course of encephalopathy. Acute hepatic encephalopathy can progress rapidly. Table 132.3 lists the prognostic criteria developed at King's College Hospital, London, England, to assist in determining the necessity for liver transplantation for fulminant hepatic failure. The decision to place a patient with fulminant hepatic failure on the transplantation list is confounded by the difficulty of procuring a suitable donor organ quickly. Even when listed at the highest emergency status, it is not unusual for a patient in North America to wait 72 hours or longer. During this time further deterioration, especially worsening cerebral edema, may make transplantation impossible. The outcome of liver transplantation for fulminant hepatic failure is somewhat worse than that of liver transplantation for other causes. One-year survival rates of 50% to 60% are common.

Biliary atresia is the most common indication for OLT among children. It represents more than 50% of cases in most series. Metabolic liver disease is the second most common indica-

Cause of Liver Failure	Criteria

TABLE 132.3. CRITERIA FOR PREDICTING DEATH AND THE NEED FOR LIVER TRANSPLANTATION, KING'S COLLEGE HOSPITAL, LONDON[a]

Cause of Liver Failure	Criteria
Acetaminophen poisoning	pH <7.3 irrespective of grade of hepatic encephalopathy *or* International Normalized Ratio (INR) >6.5 and serum creatinine >3.4 mg/dl (300 μmol/L) in patients with grade 3 or 4 hepatic encephalopathy
All other causes	INR >6.5 irrespective of grade of hepatic encephalopathy *or* Any three of the following variables irrespective of grade of hepatic encephalopathy: Age <10 y or >40 y; Fulminant hepatic failure caused by non-A, non-B hepatitis, halothane-induced hepatitis, or idiosyncratic drug reactions; Duration of jaundice before onset of encephalopathy >7 days; INR >3.5; Bilirubin >17.5 mg/dL (300, μmol/L)

[a] Transplantation was considered if the likelihood of survival without it was less than 20%. Adapted from O'Grady JG, Alexander JG, Hayllar KM, et al. Early indicators of prognosis in fulminant hepatic failure. *Gastroenterology* 1989;97:439–445, with permission.

TABLE 132.4. CONTRAINDICATIONS TO LIVER TRANSPLANTATION

Absolute contraindications
Severe, uncontrolled infection outside the hepatobiliary system
Metastatic cancer
Extrahepatic cancer other than local skin cancer
Advanced cardiopulmonary disease
AIDS
Severe pulmonary hypertension
Relative contraindications
Active drug or alcohol abuse
Age older than 70 y
HIV infection
Inability to comply with immunosuppression protocol or participate in routine posttransplant medical follow-up care
Advanced chronic renal disease
Moderate pulmonary hypertension

tion for pediatric OLT, accounting for 21% of all hepatic transplantation procedures among children.

CONTRAINDICATIONS

The absolute and relative contraindications to OLT are listed in Table 132.4. Advanced age (greater than 65 years) is no longer considered to be a relative contraindication to OLT at many centers, but it necessitates more extensive preoperative cardiac evaluation.

COMPONENTS OF THE EVALUATION FOR LIVER TRANSPLANTATION

CARDIOPULMONARY EVALUATION

Prevention of life-threatening cardiac events in the perioperative period is one of the main objectives of the pre-OLT cardiac evaluation. All patients must undergo a complete history interview with special attention to risk factors for coronary artery disease, a thorough physical examination, baseline electrocar-

diography, and chest radiography. A history of systemic hypertension, angina pectoris, or myocardial infarction or age greater than 45 years necessitates a formal investigation of cardiac functional status that includes stress cardiography, echocardiography, and in selected cases coronary angiography. Perfusion imaging with pharmacologic stress testing is a reasonable alternative to exercise stress testing for debilitated patients.

Cardiac tolerance of hemodynamic stress, irrespective of the presence or absence of coronary artery atherosclerosis, is important in the evaluation and treatment of candidates for OLT. Patients with known valvular, hypertensive, or myopathic heart disease, as in alcoholic cardiomyopathy, must undergo estimation of left ventricular function. These data may be difficult to interpret because of reduced peripheral resistance and hyperdynamic circulation, which occur with advanced chronic liver disease.

Pulmonary hypertension, otherwise known as portopulmonary hypertension, occurs among 2% to 4% of patients with end-stage liver disease. Patients with symptoms of marked dyspnea, vascular abnormalities on chest radiographs, or electrocardiographic evidence of right ventricular strain or hypertrophy should undergo echocardiography. A possible diagnosis of pulmonary hypertension necessitates right heart catheterization for pressure measurements and assessment of reversibility. Patients with markedly elevated systolic pulmonary arterial pressure or irreversible portopulmonary hypertension have a high perioperative mortality and should not undergo hepatic transplantation.

The triad of liver disease, increased alveolar-arterial gradient on room air, and intrapulmonary shunting defines the hepatopulmonary syndrome. Although mild hypoxemia affects nearly one-third of patients with cirrhosis, severe hypoxemia in the absence of parenchymal lung disease is uncommon and suggests hepatopulmonary syndrome. The hepatopulmonary syndrome occurs among approximately 5% of patients with cirrhosis. Pulmonary symptoms should be evaluated with arterial blood gas measurements and either contrast-enhanced echocardiography or perfusion lung scanning. This syndrome is reversible in some patients after liver transplantation, but the process is often quite slow.

ASSESSMENT FOR MALIGNANT GROWTH

All candidates for OLT should undergo a careful evaluation for hepatocellular carcinoma that includes measurement of serum α-fetoprotein level and imaging of the hepatic parenchyma. Biopsy confirmation of a small tumor rarely is necessary, especially because there is a risk of spreading the tumor along the biopsy track. Patients with cholangiocarcinoma identified at evaluation before OLT are at high risk of recurrent disease after the operation. Malignant disease metastatic to the liver is considered an absolute contraindication to OLT with the possible exception of slowly growing neuroendocrine tumors.

A history of extrahepatic malignant disease is a difficult challenge for the OLT evaluation team. In general, patients with known recurrent disease are not candidates for OLT. Patients who have completed a curative treatment protocol should be considered on a case by case basis.

All patients older than 40 years should be screened for occult colorectal cancer by means of stool Hemoccult testing. Colonoscopy should be performed if the screening test result is positive. Digital rectal examination and testing for prostate-specific antigen should be included in the assessment of all men older than 45 years. All women need a gynecologic evaluation, including a Papanicolaou cervical cytologic smear. Women older than 40 years should undergo mammography.

ASSESSMENT FOR INFECTION

A standard screening protocol includes a chest radiograph and placement of purified protein derivative (PPD). Candidates who have a positive PPD result but have no evidence of active disease may be treated with antituberculosis monotherapy (isoniazid for 6 months) before transplantation, or treatment can be postponed until after OLT. Antibodies to cytomegalovirus (CMV), Epstein–Barr virus (EBV), and herpes simplex virus are routinely measured in baseline studies. In the case of CMV, the viral status of the donor and the recipient predicts the risk of CMV disease after transplantation. Candidates without circulating antibodies to hepatitis A or hepatitis B virus should receive appropriate vaccination. All patients should be screened for antibodies to HIV. HIV infection without AIDS is a relative contraindication to OLT; a diagnosis of AIDS is an absolute contraindication.

NUTRITIONAL ASSESSMENT

Many patients evaluated for liver transplantation are malnourished. The causes of poor nutritional status among patients with end-stage liver disease include reduced intake, metabolic alterations, malabsorption or maldigestion, effects of medications, and iatrogenic protein losses due to large-volume paracentesis. Severe malnutrition complicates OLT and results in higher perioperative morbidity and mortality. An aggressive approach to nutritional repletion is appropriate to improve metabolic reserves, potentially stabilize hepatic function, and improve outcome after OLT. Most patients with cirrhosis, even those with intermittent hepatic encephalopathy, can tolerate 80 g of protein daily.

SURGICAL ASSESSMENT

The presence of a surgical portacaval shunt, transjugular intrahepatic portosystemic shunt (TIPS), or previous surgical procedure on the right upper quadrant increase the surgical complexity of OLT but do not preclude liver transplantation. Extensive thrombosis of the portal venous system involving the confluence of the superior mesenteric vein and splenic vein and previous complex upper abdominal surgery may make transplantation technically impossible.

PSYCHIATRIC EVALUATION

Psychiatric symptoms are common among patients with advanced liver disease and must be sought in the pretransplantation evaluation. When informed that a liver transplant will be necessary, patients often have feelings of anger, grief, anxiety, and depression. Adjustment disorders occur among 20% to 25% of patients. Management of these symptoms should be initiated in the preoperative period. The preoperative evaluation also helps identify patients with psychiatric risk factors such as psychotic disorders and severe personality disorders, which may be predictive of postoperative difficulty with compliance or impulse control. The psychiatric evaluation is perhaps most important to patients with a history of illicit drug use or alcoholism. Assessing the prognosis for long-term abstinence from addictive substances both before and after transplantation is paramount. This assessment evaluates the patient's acceptance of the diagnosis of addiction, availability of social support to assist in maintaining abstinence, and use of behavior-modifying alcoholism treatment programs.

ASSESSING THE WISHES OF THE CANDIDATE

Prospective recipients and their families should be informed of the risks and benefits of liver transplantation. This includes providing the patient with the opportunity to withdraw from transplantation assessment. Patients considered unsuitable candidates should be given access to a second opinion regarding suitability for liver transplantation.

THE TRANSPLANTATION OPERATION

Donor and recipient are matched for ABO blood group compatibility and liver volume. The surgical approach to OLT consists of three steps: first, removal of the allograft from the heart-beating, brain-dead donor; second, perfusion and storage of the liver in cold UW preservation solution (cold ischemia) for transport to the transplantation center; and third, the recipient operation. The donor liver is inspected at the time of procurement. Cold ischemia times less than 12 hours are ideal. After 12 hours the risk of primary graft nonfunction and biliary complications increases. Younger allografts typically tolerate long cold ischemia times better than do older livers.

The recipient operation can be divided into three separate phases: recipient hepatectomy, the anhepatic phase, and reperfusion. Recipient hepatectomy is the most technically challenging part of the operation. The use of venovenous bypass allows decompression of the venous system below the diaphragm and less splanchnic congestion. The next phase is the anhepatic phase, during which the new graft is sewn into the recipient. Five anastomoses are needed: the suprahepatic inferior vena cava, the infrahepatic inferior vena cava, the portal vein, the hepatic artery, and the biliary anastomosis, most commonly a choledochocholedochostomy. In many centers, a percutaneous biliary drainage tube (T tube) is placed across the biliary anastomosis. This technique reduces bile leakage from the anastomosis, may reduce anastomotic stricturing, and allows monitoring of bile production in the immediately postoperative period. A choledochojejunostomy incorporating a Roux-en-Y loop is used to treat patients with an abnormal native common bile duct (as in PSC or biliary atresia) or patients with very small donor ducts. The third phase of the transplantation operation begins after the portal venous anastomosis. Hepatic reperfusion is a critical phase of the procedure and demands careful circulatory monitoring. Because of a sudden release of cold, hyperkalemic fluid, reperfusion syndrome may occur. This syndrome consists of hypotension, bradycardia, arrhythmias, and rarely, cardiac arrest.

POSTOPERATIVE CARE

NO COMPLICATIONS

The typical recipient of an orthotopic liver transplant remains in the intensive care unit for 24 to 48 hours. If the patient's hemodynamic condition is stable, the endotracheal tube can be removed within the first 24 hours. Doppler ultrasonography often is performed on the first postoperative day to confirm patency of vascular anastomoses. Early signs of satisfactory allograft function include correction of acidosis, improving urine output, normoglycemia without intravenous dextrose solutions, stable hemodynamic values, correction of coagulopathy without additional blood products, quality bile output if a T tube is present, and improving mental status. Daily liver enzyme studies are performed to assist in the monitoring of hepatic function. Serum transaminase levels peak 24 to 48 hours after transplantation and then decline as the ischemia and reperfusion injury resolves. No pattern of liver function abnormalities indicates a specific cause of allograft injury. Reperfusion injury, acute cellular rejection, and recurrent viral hepatitis produce overlapping biochemical profiles.

Recipients typically stay in the hospital for 10 to 14 days. Frequent office visits and serial measurements of liver enzymes and drug levels are needed. All patients receive immunosuppressive medications, initially in high doses and in gradually decreasing doses thereafter. Either cyclosporine or tacrolimus is the mainstay calcineurin inhibitor. The drug is used in combination with glucocorticoids and other immunosuppressive agents. There is no consensus on the best immunosuppressant regimen. Glucocorticoids typically are reduced to 5 mg per day or withdrawn within the first 6 months. All patients receive trimethoprim-sulfamethoxazole prophylaxis against *Pneumocystis carinii* pneumonia. Selected patients receive prophylaxis against CMV infection.

IMMEDIATE AND EARLY POSTOPERATIVE COMPLICATIONS

Unexplained failure of the allograft to function in the first 24 to 72 hours is called primary nonfunction. It is related to preexisting donor organ characteristics such as high fat content, poor graft preservation or prolonged cold ischemia time, or reperfusion injury. Primary nonfunction occurs among 5% to 10% of OLT operations on adults. The condition may mimic acute liver failure and is characterized by renal insufficiency, encephalopathy, coagulopathy, and jaundice. It is important to exclude technical problems such as intraperitoneal hemorrhage, vascular occlusion, or biliary anastomotic leak. Patients should be returned to the list for OLT when a diagnosis of primary nonfunction is made. A lesser degree of preservation injury is common after OLT and may cause a marked increase in transaminase levels and a delay in improvement. Intrahepatic cholestasis develops later and can be diagnosed by liver biopsy. Hepatic arterial thrombosis can cause a similar clinical and histologic appearance and must be excluded with Doppler ultrasonography.

After OLT, early infections are most commonly bacterial and often represent residual infection from the pretransplantation period or complications of mechanical ventilation. Biliary infections are common but must be differentiated from simple colonization of the biliary tract. The seronegative recipient of an allograft from a CMV-positive donor is at greatest risk of posttransplantation CMV infection. Prophylaxis with ganciclovir reduces both the frequency and the severity of CMV among liver allograft recipients. Invasive fungal infection is a serious development in the post-transplantation recovery period and frequently portends death.

Biliary problems are common after transplant, complicating 10% to 25% of cases. Anastomotic leakage usually occurs early in the postoperative course. The diagnosis is suggested by right upper quadrant abdominal pain, fever, and a biloma found at ultrasonography or computed tomography. Anastomotic stenosis and nonanastomotic strictures manifest as cholestasis and occasionally cholangitis. Biliary leaks or strictures may be caused by occlusion of the hepatic artery. Effective therapy for biliary leaks or strictures is dilation, stent placement, or surgical revision. The formation of biliary casts is a rare but devastating problem. Hepatic arterial thrombosis also may lead to the development of sterile hepatic abscesses. Hepatic arterial thrombosis usually necessitates retransplantation.

Failure of restoration of normal neurologic function in the first 24 to 48 hours is a particularly ominous development. The differential diagnosis includes primary nonfunction, cerebral injury due to intracranial hemorrhage in a patient with coagulopathy, or the consequences of cerebral edema in a patient with fulminant hepatic failure. Seizure activity in the first 7 to 14 days after transplantation may be caused by electrolyte disturbances, typically of calcium or magnesium, toxicity from cyclosporine or tacrolimus, or fungal infection of the central nervous system.

Central pontine myelinolysis due to a rapid change in serum sodium concentration is recognized as a later event after OLT.

Some patients have congestive heart failure in the early postoperative period. This is probably caused by occult cardiomyopathy previously masked by the hyperdynamic circulation and reduced systemic vascular resistance of end-stage liver disease.

ACUTE AND CHRONIC REJECTION

Despite immunosuppression, 50% of recipients of orthotopic liver transplants have at least one episode of acute cellular rejection that necessitates adjustment of immunosuppressive medications. Eighty percent of episodes of acute cellular rejection of liver allografts occur in the first 10 postoperative weeks. Curious is that an episode of acute cellular rejection that responds to adjustment in immunosuppression does not increase the risk of graft loss and may even protect the graft. In contrast, severe acute cellular rejection that does not respond to increased immunosuppression or recurs once immunosuppression is tapered may cause chronic ductopenic rejection and graft loss.

Acute cellular rejection is manifested by a disturbance in liver enzyme levels that sometimes is accompanied by a systemic illness with fever and malaise. It can be difficult to differentiate from other disorders, such as graft ischemia or viral hepatitis, such as hepatitis C or CMV infection. The diagnosis should be confirmed with a liver biopsy that demonstrates a mixed, predominately lymphocytic portal infiltrate, lymphocytic cholangitis (ductitis), and lymphocytic injury to the vascular endothelium (endotheliitis). The infiltrate often contains eosinophils. Standard therapy for acute cellular rejection is a short course of high-dose glucocorticoids, although patients with mild cases may not be treated. Clinical resolution of the elevated transaminase levels in response to increased corticosteroids supports the diagnosis. Failure of liver enzymes to respond to corticosteroids is called *steroid-resistant rejection*. Steroid-resistant rejection may be managed with conversion from cyclosporine to tacrolimus and the use of anti-CD3 monoclonal antibodies or agents such as mycophenolate mofetil.

Chronic ductopenic rejection (also known as chronic rejection or vanishing bile duct syndrome) is a serious sequela of acute cellular rejection. It consists of arteriopathy and bile duct loss. A liver biopsy shows loss of bile ducts. The clinical syndrome is cholestatic, consisting of elevated bilirubin and alkaline phosphatase levels, jaundice, and pruritus. It rarely responds to incremental immunosuppression and necessitates retransplantation. Fortunately, the incidence of chronic ductopenic rejection appears to be declining.

▌ LONG-TERM MANAGEMENT

RESTORATION OF LIFESTYLE

Recipients of a transplants should plan a return to work, school, and leisure activities as their condition allows. There should no restrictions on sexual activity. Patients should be encouraged to eat a well-balanced diet. Moderate use of alcohol is permitted except for patients with a history of alcoholism. Annual health

evaluations for adult recipients include cervical smears for all women, mammography for women 40 years or older, and measurement of prostate-specific antigen for all male recipients older than 45 years. All patients older than 45 years should perform annual screening for colorectal cancer using Hemoccult cards. Patients with a history of PSC or chronic ulcerative colitis (with the colon in situ) should undergo annual colonoscopy. Evidence of mucosal dysplasia is an indication for colectomy.

Most premenopausal female patients, even those who had prolonged amenorrhea before transplantation, menstruate within 3 months of successful OLT. Pregnancy should be avoided for at least 1 year after transplantation. Pharmacologic contraceptives and barrier contraceptives may be used. Use of intrauterine contraceptive devices, however, carries an unacceptable risk of infection. Successful pregnancy is possible after liver transplantation but should be considered a high-risk pregnancy and managed accordingly.

Live or attenuated vaccines such as bacille Calmette-Guérin, measles, mumps, rubella (MMR), varicella-zoster, yellow fever, oral typhoid, and oral polio vaccine (OPV) are not safe after transplantation and should be avoided. MMR is safe to administer to siblings or other household contacts of recipients, but OPV is not, and household contacts should receive inactivated polio vaccine (IPV) if immunization is necessary. Inactivated vaccines, capsular antigens, and toxoids are safe. These include immunization against hepatitis A, hepatitis B, *Haemophilus influenzae*, pneumococcus, and influenza. All older recipients should receive annual influenza vaccinations.

MEDICAL COMPLICATIONS OF IMMUNOSUPPRESSIVE THERAPY

Post-transplantation lymphoproliferative disorder (PTLD) is proliferation of lymphoid cells among patients taking high doses of immunosuppressants. The affected lymphocytes are infected with Epstein–Barr virus. PTLD manifests as a spectrum of features from a lymphocytic infiltrate that which resolves when immunosuppression is reduced to aggressive monoclonal non-Hodgkin's lymphoma. PTLD may manifest as a mass in the liver or an extrahepatic mass in the brain, intestine, or other solid organ. PTLD may occur soon after transplantation or be delayed for months or years of apparently successful graft survival. PTLD is more common among children than adults and among patients who have received high doses of immunosuppressive agents, especially anti-CD3 monoclonal antibody than patients who have not. These patients at high risk should undergo routine screening with an Epstein–Barr virus polymerase chain reaction. PTLD is managed by means of reducing immunosuppressant medications. When the disorder resembles lymphoma, PTLD is managed by means of chemotherapy. The outlook depends on the aggression of the tumor and the degree of improvement when immunosuppression is reduced or withdrawn.

Headache is the most common neurologic toxicity of immunosuppressive therapy and is most severe among patients with a history of migraine. It is equally common with cyclosporine- and tacrolimus-based treatment protocols. Tremor occurs with both cyclosporine and tacrolimus therapy and usually is a clinical manifestation of drug levels above the therapeutic range.

Many patients, especially those with a pretransplantation history of hypertension experience hypertension that necessitates medication. Cyclosporine, tacrolimus, and glucocorticoids are the main causes of hypertension. Post-transplantation hypertension should be controlled pharmacologically whenever immunosuppressants have been judiciously reduced. The calcineurin inhibitors (cyclosporine, tacrolimus) are the main causes of renal failure, which often accompanies hypertension and is in part dose dependent.

Insulin-dependent diabetes mellitus is related to use of glucocorticoids. There is a suggestion, that tacrolimus is more diabetogenic than cyclosporine. Weight gain is one of the most troubling metabolic complications of immunosuppression. Gout is another metabolic complication of immunosuppressants. Cyclosporine may cause hirsutism, gingival hyperplasia, and changes in facies. These phenomena may be sufficiently disabling to warrant conversion to tacrolimus-based immunosuppression. Hyperlipidemia complicates the use of cyclosporine and corticosteroids. Hypercholesterolemia may necessitate use of 3-hydroxy-3-methylglutaryl coenzyme A (HMG-CoA) reductase inhibitors.

Many patients, especially women, are osteopenic before transplantation. Bone loss is exacerbated by glucocorticoids in the first 6 to 12 months after transplantation. Thereafter bone density increases in concert with good allograft function. The desire to protect already thin bones is an indication to withdraw or reduce corticosteroids after transplantation. Calcium supplements, vitamin D repletion, hormone replacement therapy, and bisphosphonates all have a role in treating selected patients with osteopenia.

RECURRENCE OF THE UNDERLYING DISEASE

All patients with hepatitis B virus infection should undergo long-term administration of hepatitis B immune globulin after liver transplantation. With this regimen, fibrosing cholestatic hepatitis is very infrequent. Lamivudine or famciclovir or both may be used as additional agents.

Hepatitis C virus infection of the allograft is almost universal when patients with hepatitis C undergo liver transplantation. After transplantation hepatitis C is associated with a marked rise in circulating viral copy number. The clinical course of liver transplant recipients with hepatitis C is quite variable. Some data suggest that the circulating viral load before transplantation predicts the risk of post-transplantation graft injury. Aggressive hepatitis C, which rapidly leads to death or retransplantation, occurs among approximately 10% of patients. Perhaps another 50% of patients have moderately active chronic hepatitis with a natural history that is truncated compared with that of hepatitis C in the native liver. The remaining 40% of patients appear to have mild disease. Interferon alfa alone is ineffective. Combination therapy with interferon alfa and ribavirin is under study. It is probable that hepatitis C infection causes markedly higher rates of allograft loss, mortality, and retransplantation.

The grafted liver is the most common site of recurrence of hepatocellular carcinoma. No antitumor regimen, including systemic chemotherapy, chemoembolization, direct injection of alcohol, external beam radiation, or a combination of these treatments has been shown to control recurrent tumor after liver transplantation. Recurrence of alcoholism after liver transplantation occurs among 5% to 10% of transplant recipients who have alcoholism. Another 30% admit to "slips" defined as occasional drinking episodes. Alcoholic liver injury is rare in the first 5 years after transplantation. Recurrence of autoimmune liver disease, including PBC, PSC, and autoimmune hepatitis sometimes occurs after transplantation but is rarely clinically significant.

BIBLIOGRAPHY

Beresford T. Psychiatric assessment of alcoholic candidates for liver transplantation. In: Lucey MR, Merion RM, Beresford TP, eds. *Liver transplantation and the alcoholic patient.* Cambridge, UK: Cambridge University Press, 1994:24–49.

Gane EJ, Portmann BC, Naoumov N, et al. Long-term outcome of hepatitis C infection after liver transplantation. *N Engl J Med* 1996;334: 815–820.

Henley KS, Lucey MR, Appelman HD, et al. Biochemical and histopathological correlation in liver transplant: the first 180 days. *Hepatology* 1992; 16:688–693.

Lee WM. Acute liver failure. *N Engl J Med* 1993;329:1862–1872.

Lucey MR, Brown KA, Everson GT, et al. Minimal criteria for placement of adults on the liver transplant waiting list: a report of a national conference organized by the American Society of Transplant Physicians and the American Association for the Study of Liver Diseases. *Liver Transpl Surg* 1997;3:628–637.

Lucey MR, Carr K, Beresford TP, et al. Alcohol use after liver transplantation in alcoholics: a clinical cohort study. *Hepatology* 1997;25: 1223–1227.

Mazzaferro V, Regalia E, Doci R, et al. Liver transplantation for the treatment of small hepatocellular carcinomas in patients with cirrhosis. *N Engl J Med* 1996;334:693–692.

Samuel D, Muller R, Alexander G, et al. Liver transplantation in European patients with hepatitis B surface antigen. *N Engl J Med* 1993;329: 1842–1844.

Kelley's Textbook of Internal Medicine, fourth edition. Edited by H. David Humes. Lippincott Williams & Wilkins, Philadelphia © 2000.

4

NEPHROLOGY

H. David Humes, Editor

APPROACH TO THE PATIENT WITH RENAL AND ELECTROLYTE DISORDERS

CHAPTER

133

APPROACH TO THE PATIENT WITH RENAL DISEASE

H. DAVID HUMES

A patient with renal disease may have various initial signs and symptoms: symptoms directly referable to the kidneys, such as flank pain or gross hematuria; extrarenal signs and symptoms not directly related to the kidneys, such as hypertension or generalized edema; or no symptoms at all, but abnormal results on urinalysis or an elevated serum creatinine value discovered during a routine medical evaluation or in the diagnostic workup of another disorder.

Once renal disease is documented, the approach to the patient is twofold—to assess the severity of the renal process and to establish the correct diagnosis. The history and physical examination are useful, but the clinical evaluation of renal function primarily depends on laboratory data, especially the estimation of the glomerular filtration rate (GFR), the quantitation of urinary protein excretion, a careful urinalysis, and the assessment of urine electrolyte concentrations and osmolality. Radiologic studies and a renal biopsy may also aid in the diagnostic evaluation. These diagnostic tools are discussed in Chapters 163 and 164.

■ DIAGNOSTIC APPROACH TO RENAL DISEASE

Renal disease is often detected by abnormal urinalysis findings or an elevated plasma creatinine concentration (P_{cr}). Renal disease is always suggested if hematuria or abnormal amounts of protein are present on urinalysis. The diagnostic approach and pathophysiologic mechanisms responsible for hematuria and proteinuria differ substantially and are discussed in Chapters

134 and 135. The finding of an elevated P_{cr} should be confirmed by repeating the laboratory measurement. If it is verified and the history or physical examination suggests the presence of kidney disease, the laboratory evaluation should begin with an estimation of the GFR through a 24-hour urine collection for creatinine as a reasonable index of functioning renal tissue and of disease severity.

The first important assessment of structural renal disease is the determination of the duration of disease. This assessment is easiest to make if serial P_{cr} measurements rise during observation in the hospital, thus suggesting that the renal disorder is most likely acute. If previous data are unavailable, several clues can be helpful in determining the duration of disease. The presence of oliguria with a urine output less than 500 mL per day suggests an acute process, because prolonged oliguria rapidly results in renal failure and symptoms of uremia. Anemia is more common in advanced chronic renal disease than it is in acute disease of similar magnitude. The anemia of renal failure is due to diminished renal production of erythropoietin, which stimulates the production of red blood cells (RBCs) by the bone marrow. Because less than 1% of circulating RBCs turn over each day, in the absence of bleeding, hemolysis, or hemodilution stemming from fluid retention, the hematocrit in a patient with acute renal failure is usually normal or nearly normal because there has not been enough time for anemia to develop.

The second important assessment in the diagnosis of renal disease is the determination of whether the decline in GFR is due to prerenal, postrenal, or intrarenal disease (Table 133.1). The clinical and laboratory evaluations to diagnose the presence of prerenal functional or postrenal obstructive processes as the cause of a rise in blood urea nitrogen and P_{cr} are discussed in Chapters 138 and 140. If prerenal disease due to a decline in renal blood flow, with a concomitant reduction in GFR and urinary tract obstruction, has been excluded, some form of intrarenal structural disease must be present. Intrinsic renal disease is then best approached by categorizing the primary pathologic process into glomerular or nonglomerular disorders. The urinalysis is especially helpful in distinguishing between these two categories (Table 133.2).

Careful examination of the urine is the most important noninvasive diagnostic aid in the evaluation of renal disease. Mea-

TABLE 133.1.	MOST COMMON CAUSES OF RENAL DISEASE

Prerenal causes
    Absolute volume depletion
    Heart failure
    Hepatic cirrhosis with hepatorenal syndrome
    Nonsteroidal anti-inflammatory drugs
    Bilateral renal artery stenosis (particularly after use of an angiotensin-converting enzyme inhibitor)
Postrenal causes (obstructive uropathy)
    Prostatic disease
    Pelvic or retroperitoneal malignancy
    Calculi
    Congenital abnormalities
Intrarenal causes
    Glomerular disease
        Glomerulonephritis
        Nephrotic syndrome
    Vascular disease
        Acute
            Vasculitis
            Malignant hypertension
            Scleroderma
            Thromboembolic disease
        Chronic
            Nephrosclerosis
    Tubular disease
        Acute
            Acute tubular necrosis
            Multiple myeloma
            Hypercalcemia
            Acute uric acid nephropathy
        Chronic
            Polycystic kidney disease
            Medullary sponge kidney
            Medullary cystic kidney disease
    Interstitial disease
        Acute
            Interstitial nephritis (usually drug-induced)
            Pyelonephritis
        Chronic
            Pyelonephritis (due primarily to vesicoureteral reflux)
            Analgesic abuse

surements of electrolyte concentration, pH, and osmolality of the urine are common tests to assess renal tubular function and to evaluate fluid and electrolyte disorders; they are discussed in Chapter 163. Less quantitative analysis of the urine can be performed easily in the clinical setting, along with the urinalysis, and can provide substantial information as to the presence and type of renal disease.

GLOMERULAR DISEASE

Glomerular disease can appear as three distinctly different, but not mutually exclusive, clinical syndromes: the acute nephritic syndrome, the nephrotic syndrome, or chronic glomerulonephritis. The full diagnostic approach to glomerular disease is discussed in Chapters 150 and 164.

ACUTE NEPHRITIC SYNDROME

The acute nephritic syndrome complex reflects an acute inflammatory response within the kidney and is characterized by hematuria and RBC casts in the urine sediment along with other signs of acute inflammatory renal injury, including proteinuria, peripheral edema, hypertension, or renal insufficiency with or without oliguria. Hematuria alone is not sufficient to define this syndrome. Urinary bleeding may arise from various extrarenal and intrarenal disorders distinct from acute inflammatory processes. The finding of RBC casts in the urinary sediment clearly suggests a nephronal origin of bleeding and is thus of great importance. Because glomerular bleeding can originate from chronic as well as acute processes, it is important to look for other signs of acute inflammatory renal injury before diagnosing the syndrome of acute nephritis.

The hallmark of the acute nephritic syndrome is the finding of RBCs and RBC (as well as other) casts in the urine sediment. The finding of RBC casts in a patient with hematuria virtually ensures that the patient has a glomerular pathologic process. The urinary findings in acute glomerular disease vary, ranging from normal (usually seen in subclinical disease) to signs of proteinuria, hematuria, pyuria, lipiduria, and RBC and other casts. The severity of these abnormalities also varies, since hematuria can be either microscopic or grossly visible. The degree of proteinuria can range from just above the upper limit of normal to the nephrotic range.

The manner in which RBCs pass into the urine in glomerular disease has not been definitively clarified, but transit is probably due to focal disruptions in the glomerular capillary wall produced by the underlying inflammatory process. These focal disruptions along the glomerular capillary wall may contribute to proteinuria and may allow plasma proteins larger than albumin to escape into the urine.

Renal sodium and water retention resulting in generalized edema is common in the acute nephritic syndrome and develops because of poor renal perfusion stemming from a decline in renal blood flow and proteinuria, with resulting hypoalbuminemia and a decline in intravascular volume. Elevated blood pressure is an additional common clinical component of the acute nephritic syndrome. Both volume overload from inappropriate renal fluid retention and enhanced renin secretion from renal injury and resulting vasoconstrictor tone play important roles in this process.

The GFR is often reduced in the acute nephritic syndrome, resulting in a rise in blood urea nitrogen and P_{cr}. This reduction is a result of declines in glomerular blood flow, glomerular transcapillary hydraulic pressure gradients, and the glomerular permeability coefficient, which is a function of both porosity and surface area available for filtration of the glomerular capillary.

Often in this syndrome, renal insufficiency is transient, but it also can be progressive, leading to chronic glomerulonephritis and renal failure. Most patients with acute nephritis have a form of proliferative glomerulonephritis and, occasionally, acute tubulointerstitial nephritis; for this reason, renal biopsy is generally performed to determine the final diagnosis.

NEPHROTIC SYNDROME

Proteinuria above 3.5 g per day is usually classified as being in the nephrotic range, but the nephrotic syndrome complex usu-

TABLE 133.2.	URINARY FINDINGS AND CAUSES OF RENAL DISEASE

Urinary Findings	Etiology
Hematuria with red blood cell casts Heavy proteinuria (>3.5 g/d or >50 mg/kg/d)	Any of these findings, singly or in combination, is virtually diagnostic of glomerular disease or vasculitis. The absence of these changes, however, does not exclude these diagnoses.
Renal tubular epithelial cells with granular and epithelial cell casts	In acute renal failure, strongly suggests acute tubular necrosis, although marked hyperbilirubinemia alone can produce similar findings
Pyuria with white blood cell, granular, or waxy casts and no or mild proteinuria	Suggestive of tubular or interstitial disease or obstruction
Hematuria and pyuria with no or variable casts (excluding red blood cell casts)	May be seen in glomerular disease, vasculitis, obstruction, renal infarction, acute interstitial nephritis, or infection
Hematuria alone	Suggestive of vasculitis or obstruction in acute renal failure; may also be found with mild glomerular disease, polycystic kidney disease, or extrarenal problems, such as prostatic disease, calculi, or tumor
Normal or near normal (few cells with few or no casts or proteinuria; hyaline casts are not an abnormal finding)	Acute: May be found in prerenal disease, obstruction, hypercalcemia, myeloma, some cases of acute tubular necrosis, or vascular diseases with glomerular ischemia but not infarction (scleroderma, atheroemboli) Chronic: May be seen in prerenal disease, obstruction, tubular or interstitial disorders, and nephrosclerosis
Pyuria alone	Usually indicative of urinary tract infection (including tuberculosis); may occur with tubulointerstitial diseases

ally refers to the clinical triad of massive proteinuria, hypoalbuminemia, and edema. Hyperlipidemia and hypercoagulability may also be present. The nephrotic syndrome occurs in association with various primary renal diseases and systemic diseases, as discussed in Chapter 135.

Proteinuria in the nephrotic syndrome is due to an increase in glomerular permeability of serum albumin and arises in response to alterations in both the size and charge barriers of the glomerular filtration apparatus. As a consequence of proteinuria, the serum albumin concentration and therefore the plasma oncotic pressure fall. The generalized edematous state common to the nephrotic syndrome is largely caused by this drop in plasma oncotic pressure and the movement of fluid from the vascular to the interstitial fluid compartment, producing a decline in plasma volume that signals the kidney to retain sodium and water. Other sensing mechanisms may play a role in renal sodium retention, because many patients with this disorder have been reported to have normal rather than diminished plasma volumes.

Hyperlipidemia stemming from increased hepatic synthesis, along with lipiduria, also frequently occurs in this disorder. Two-thirds of patients have type IIa or IIb hyperlipoproteinemia; most others have type V. The nephrotic syndrome may accompany such systemic diseases as diabetes or amyloidosis or idiopathic processes. If no systemic disease is present and the P_{cr} value is not dramatically elevated, renal biopsy is often necessary to reach a final diagnosis.

CHRONIC GLOMERULONEPHRITIS

Many forms of glomerular disease can progress to chronic renal failure. On morphologic examination, this progression is charac-

terized by scarring of most of the glomeruli. Consequently, the urinalysis results are more benign, with less proteinuria and hematuria and with broad, waxy casts in the urine sediment. Occasionally, the urine may have characteristics of nephritic, nephrotic, and chronic patterns. This urinary finding has been called a "telescoped" sediment and is usually seen in severe glomerulonephritis or vasculitis.

NONGLOMERULAR DISEASES

When intrarenal disease processes are present and the laboratory evaluation does not suggest a glomerular disorder, nonglomerular disease processes should be considered in the differential diagnosis. Tubulointerstitial disease, the foremost cause of nonglomerular disease, is discussed in Chapter 151. Acute pyelonephritis, papillary necrosis, and hypersensitivity interstitial nephritis are the major causes of acute tubulointerstitial disease. The causes of chronic tubulointerstitial disease are numerous. It may be associated with essentially normal urinalysis results, although mild degrees of pyuria and proteinuria (less than 2 g per day) may be present. Vascular diseases are other major sources of nonglomerular disorders. Acute vascular intrarenal processes include vasculitis, scleroderma, coagulopathies, and renal infarction; chronic vascular processes include nephrosclerosis and renal artery stenosis. These disorders are discussed in Chapter 152.

BIBLIOGRAPHY

Fairley KF, Birch DF. Hematuria: a simple method for identifying glomerular bleeding. *Kidney Int* 1982;21:105.

Pankewyez OG, Sturgill BC, Bolton WK. Proliferative glomerulonephritis. In: Tisher CC, Brenner BM, eds. *Renal pathology with clinical and functional correlations.* Philadelphia: JB Lippincott, 1994:222.

Rodriguez-Iturbe B. Acute post-streptococcal glomerulonephritis. In: Schrier RW, Gottschalk CW, eds. *Diseases of the kidney,* fourth ed. Boston: Little, Brown, 1988:1929.

Rose BD. *Pathophysiology of renal disease,* second ed. New York: McGraw-Hill, 1987.

Kelley's Textbook of Internal Medicine, fourth edition. Edited by H. David Humes. Lippincott Williams & Wilkins, Philadelphia © 2000.

CHAPTER

134

APPROACH TO THE PATIENT WITH HEMATURIA

JOHN H. GALLA

Hematuria, the presence of an excessive number of red blood cells (RBCs) in the urine, may manifest dramatically as painful, gross hematuria or occultly as asymptomatic microscopic hematuria. Whatever the initial signs and symptoms, it can signal a process as ominous as an advanced malignancy or as innocuous as vigorous exercise. Because of its potentially grave implications, hematuria must always be thoroughly evaluated.

First, the presence of hematuria should be confirmed. Proper microscopic examination of the urine requires a freshly voided midstream specimen, preferably collected in the early morning. Contamination of the urine specimen with vaginal blood should be carefully avoided. Ten milliliters of urine is centrifuged at 2,000 rpm for 5 minutes in a conical centrifuge tube, about 9.5 ml of supernatant is decanted, and the infranatant is resuspended in the remaining 0.5 ml. A drop of this concentrated urine is placed on a clean glass slide and examined under a coverslip with a $\times 40$ objective. More than two to four RBCs per high-power field (hpf) is considered abnormal and corresponds to about 5,000 RBCs per milliliter of urine or between 500,000 and 600,000 RBC per 12 hours.

Gross hematuria can be confused with pigmenturia of hues from brown to red (Table 134.1). Except for the heme proteins, all of these pigments can be excluded by testing the urine with orthotolidine and peroxidase-impregnated paper strips, which have a high level of sensitivity (91% to 100%) and specificity (65% to 95%) and result in a positive test for blood for as few as three RBCs per hpf. A positive test in the absence of increased numbers of RBCs per hpf should prompt an investigation for intravascular hemolysis (hemoglobinuria) and rhabdomyolysis (myoglobinuria) (see Chapter 140). After confirming the presence of either gross or microscopic hematuria, clinical and laboratory evaluations should be carried out.

TABLE 134.1.	PIGMENTURIA AND OTHER SUBSTANCES THAT MAY CONFUSE THE DIAGNOSIS OF HEMATURIA

Drugs: Rifampin, sulfamethoxazole, phenazopyridine, ibuprofen, phenytoin, levodopa, nitrofurantoin, quinine
Foods: Beets, various food dyes
Bile pigments
Porphyrins
Hemoglobin or myoglobin
Ascorbic acid in high urinary concentration (heme false-negative result on dipstick)
Bacteriuria (heme false-positive result on dipstick)

DIFFERENTIAL DIAGNOSIS

The etiologic considerations for hematuria are myriad and most easily considered in an anatomical construct. This listing of the possibilities in differential diagnosis is not intended to be exhaustive; rather, broad categories provide a framework and then a focus for subsequent evaluation (Table 134.2). A specific etiologic diagnosis will frequently require tissue confirmation. Estimated rates of frequency of causes vary considerably, depending on age and whether the survey separates gross from microscopic hematuria or hematuria from concurrent proteinuria (Table 134.3). In adults between the ages of 20 and 40 years, the rates lie between these patterns. Urothelial tumors are rare before the age of 40 years.

EVALUATION

HISTORY AND PHYSICAL EXAMINATION

Important clues to a likely diagnosis will often be obtained from a thorough history and a physical examination and may direct subsequent testing. A number of elements in the history merit particular attention. The duration, timing, associations, and nature of hematuria should be established. Hematuria coincident with menses suggests endometriosis. Clots are more often seen with nonglomerular lesions. The presence of frequency, urgency, dysuria, or uretheral discharge suggests bladder or urethral involvement. Rectal or perineal pain or discomfort may occur in the context of prostatitis. Flank pain or colic may be seen with stones, acute obstruction, infarction, or polycystic kidneys; even if it is unilateral, severe and persistent flank pain may also be associated with intrinsic renal diseases, such as IgA nephropathy or sickle cell nephropathy. Weight loss may signal a malignancy.

Upper-respiratory-tract infections or gastroenteritis may trigger an exacerbation of IgA or mesangiocapillary glomerulopathy, in particular. Hemoptysis may indicate the presence of antiglomerular basement membrane or lupus glomerulonephritis. Environmental toxins or infectious exposures may be associated with glomerulonephritides and interstitial nephritides. Systemic symptoms, such as fever, arthralgias, easy bruising, and a host of indications of other organ system involvement, suggest lupus

TABLE 134.2.	CAUSES OF HEMATURIA

Systemic (not necessarily related to a specific renal lesion)
  Fever
  Anticoagulant therapy
  Hemoglobin S–related diseases
  Strenuous exercise
  Coagulopathies
  Toxins (cantharidin, djenkol bean)
Kidney
  Glomerulopathies (particularly IgA, proliferative and mesangi-
    ocapillary, C1q, thin-basement-membrane nephropathies)
  Interstitial nephritides (acute or chronic)
  Infarct
  Venous thrombosis (children)
  Tuberculosis
  Cystic diseases
  Papillary necrosis
  Neoplasms
  "Nutcracker" phenomenon
  Embolism
  Pyelonephritis
  Calculus (hypercalciuria hyperuricosuria)
  Trauma
  Cortical necrosis
  Vascular malformations
Urinary collecting system (renal pelvis, ureter, bladder, urethra,
  prostate, epididymis, and seminal vesicle)
  Calculus
  Foreign bodies
  Neoplasms
  Endometriosis
  Interstitial cystitis
  Congenital malformations
  Trauma
  Infections
  Vascular malformations
Other
  Essential benign or familial
  Loin pain–hematuria syndrome
  Factitious

TABLE 134.3.	ESTIMATED FREQUENCY RATES OF SOME CAUSES OF HEMATURIA[a]

Cause	Adults	Children Microscopic	Children Gross
Infection	30%		26%
Calculi/hypercalciuria	20%	26%	2%
Prostatic hypertrophy/ obstruction	10%		1%
Cancer	15%		<1%
Glomerulonephritis		13%	4%
Idiopathic		46%	14%
Perineal/penile irritation			18%
Trauma			7%
Coagulopathy			3%

[a] Categories do not sum to 100%.

erythematosus, Henoch–Schönlein purpura, or vasculitis. All medications should be noted; the loin pain–hematuria syndrome has been associated with oral contraceptives, and cystitis and bladder cancer have been noted with cyclophosphamide. Family history should focus on hematuria, such traits as deafness or ocular defects (Alport syndrome), urinary tract diseases, and bleeding disorders. Travel or residence in countries where such parasitic infections as malaria and schistosomiasis may be encountered is pertinent.

In view of the myriad possible causes, a complete, not a limited, physical examination should be performed, even though the urogenital tract is the major focus. Elevated blood pressure and peripheral edema may indicate a renal lesion. Fever, rash (lupus erythematosus), mucosal lesions, purpura (Henoch-Schönlein purpura, vasculitis), petechiae, cardiac murmur or rub (endocarditis, uremia), lymphadenopathy, or hepatosplenomegaly may direct the evaluation along a particular avenue toward the diagnosis of a systemic illness with or without a specific renal lesion. The kidneys and bladder should be carefully palpated for size and tenderness; the prostate examined for size, consistency, tenderness, and masses; and the external genitalia inspected and palpated for discharge, bleeding, or masses.

LABORATORY STUDIES

A complete urinalysis, the initial laboratory test, includes other important elements. RBC casts and heavy proteinuria point to a glomerular lesion; pyuria and bacteria or fungi indicate infection. Any significant proteinuria suggests other intrinsic renal diseases.

Additional maneuvers can enhance the diagnostic power of the urinalysis. In the "three-glass" test, the initial and final 15 ml of urine are examined separately from the midstream sample. Blood in the initial urine sample suggests bleeding in the urethra or male genital system; terminal hematuria is associated with bladder lesions. Second, examination of the urine by phase-contrast microscopy permits the determination of the proportion of dysmorphic RBCs, which, in contrast to the uniform size and shape of normal RBCs, show irregular outlines, blebs, and granular cytoplasm. When more than 75% of RBCs (at least 100 should be counted) are dysmorphic, renal (not solely glomerular) lesions are a possibility.

Initial blood studies should include a complete blood count (hemoglobin and white blood cell and platelet counts), prothrombin time, partial thromboplastin time, serum creatinine concentration, and hemoglobin electrophoresis or sickle cell screening in appropriate patients. Urinary calcium and uric acid excretion should be determined, particularly in children.

DIAGNOSTIC APPROACH

When the initial evaluation suggests a probable cause, that cause should be pursued until the diagnosis is either confirmed or excluded. Several approaches have been proposed to distinguish the etiologic possibilities in various subsets of patients or associated problems. The following approach for the adult seeks to balance the likely probabilities against the risks and costs of the evaluation (Fig. 134.1). This approach assumes a single cause, although hematuria may be multifactorial. If benign prostatic

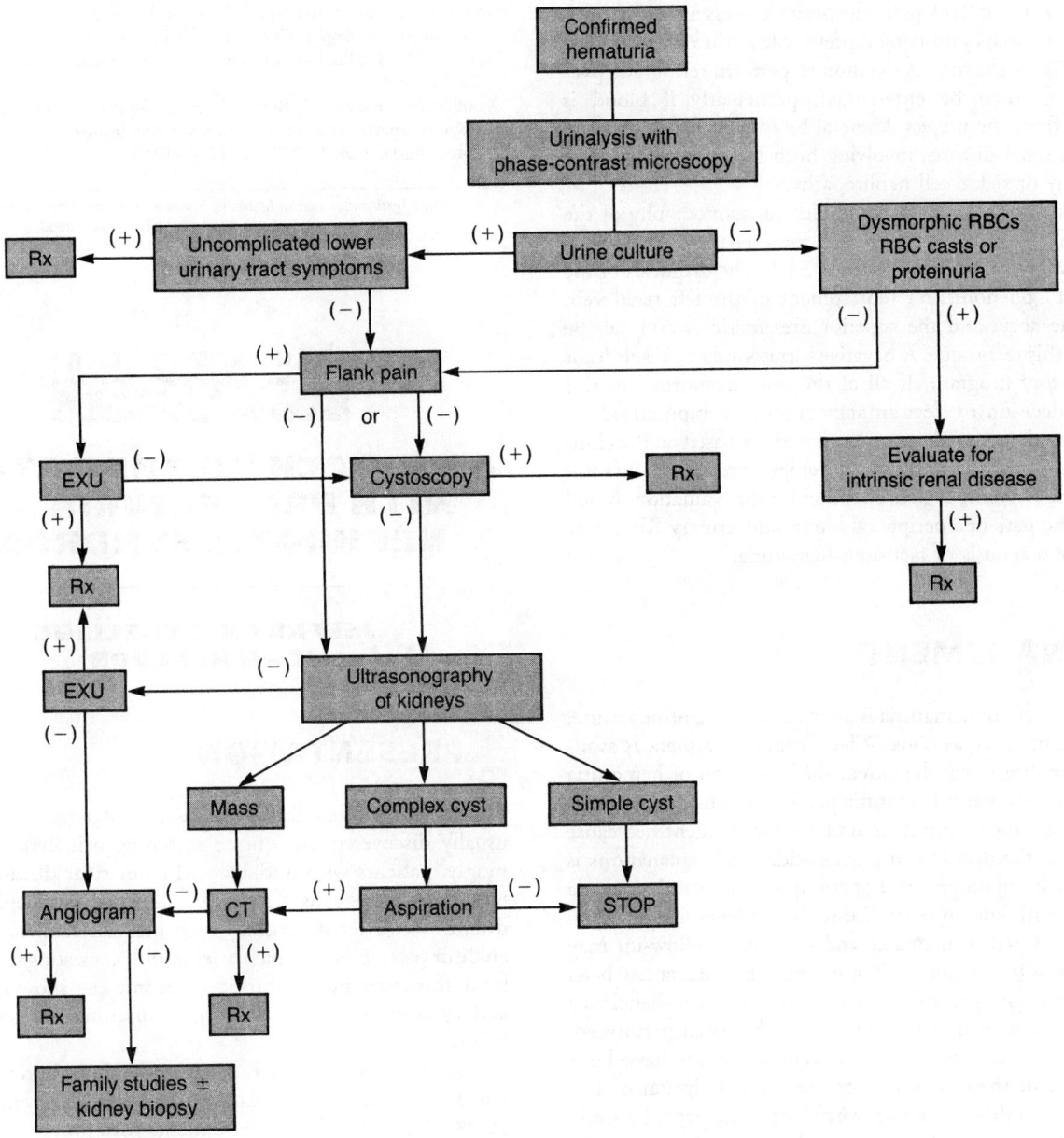

FIGURE 134.1. Approach to the evaluation of hematuria in the adult. Rx indicates the points at which appropriate therapy should be initiated, as discussed elsewhere. Cystoscopy can be deferred in children and young adults. EXU, excretory urogram; CT, computerized tomography; RBC, red blood cell.

hypertrophy or a coagulopathy is identified, further evaluation is mandatory to exclude alternative urinary tract lesions. Certain diseases may be associated with more than one cause, for example, analgesic nephropathy is associated with both papillary necrosis and urothelial tumors.

For a female patient with an uncomplicated urinary tract infection (a woman of childbearing age with her first episode of lower-urinary-tract symptoms and a urine culture positive for bacteria), specific treatment is initiated; all other urinary tract infections should be considered complicated and evaluated further. If the routine urine culture shows negative results in the context of lower-tract symptoms, special cultures (e.g., tuberculosis, chlamydia) should be obtained, as appropriate, and a tuber-

culin skin test performed. If lower-urinary-tract symptoms are absent and flank pain is present, an excretory urogram should be performed.

When the urinalysis or initial clinical and laboratory examination suggests intrinsic renal disease, the appropriate diagnostic evaluation, as outlined in Fig. 134.1, should be initiated; this evaluation may include some of the tests outlined. It is anticipated that an abundance of dysmorphic RBCs will be seen with IgA nephropathy and other mesangiopathic glomerular lesions in which asymptomatic or occasionally symptomatic gross hematuria occurs without significant proteinuria or an abnormal serum creatinine concentration. The decision to proceed to kidney biopsy is discussed in Chapter 164.

In the absence of flank pain, the problem is essentially asymptomatic hematuria; cystoscopy is preferable to the excretory urogram as a diagnostic tool. A decision to perform retrograde pyelography can then be entertained, particularly if blood is emanating from the ureters. Ureteral bleeding can be unilateral in intrinsic renal diseases involving both kidneys, such as IgA nephropathy or sickle cell nephropathy.

If cystoscopy shows negative results, ultrasonography of the kidney and its vessels begins a search for a renal mass, which, if found, is evaluated as shown in Fig. 134.1. The diagnosis of the "nutcracker" phenomenon (entrapment of the left renal vein between the aorta and the superior mesenteric artery) can be made with this technique. A negative ultrasound test result leads to an excretory urogram. If all of the tests are normal to this point, the decision to elect an angiogram or computerized tomography study with radiocontrast material is based on the clinical symptoms. In the young patient, benign or recurrent or familial hematuria is a more logical direction for the evaluation. Blood typing of the patient's peripheral blood and urinary RBC may assist in the diagnosis of factitious hematuria.

MANAGEMENT

The management of hematuria is directed at the identified cause, as indicated in other sections. When specific treatment is available and the disease can be cured, the resolution of hematuria should be confirmed; if hematuria persists, reconsider the diagnosis. If no specific treatment is available for the identified cause of hematuria, the decision to pursue additional explanations is a matter of clinical judgment. For example, new gross hematuria in a patient with known renal disease should be evaluated. If no cause is uncovered, reassurance and continued follow-up may be sufficient. On occasion, when essential hematuria has been recurrent, profuse, painful, or associated with iron-deficiency anemia, partial or complete nephrectomy has been performed, and small hemangiomas or patent venous sinuses have been found. Most of these reports antedate the description of IgA nephropathy. In these instances, when hematuria per se becomes the focus of treatment, thorough histologic examination of the kidney is mandatory before considering nephrectomy. Renal autotransplantation has been successfully employed for the loin pain–hematuria syndrome, but bilateral nephrectomy for this syndrome is to be decried.

BIBLIOGRAPHY

Bloom KJ. An algorithm for hematuria. *Clin Lab Med* 1988;8:577–584.
Copley JB. Isolated asymptomatic hematuria in the adult. *Am J Med Sci* 1986;291:101–111.
Corwin HL, Silverstein MD. Microscopic hematuria. *Clin Lab Med* 1988; 8:601–610.
Okada M, Tsuzuki K, Ito S. Diagnosis of the nutcracker phenomenon using two-dimensional ultrasonography. *Clin Nephrol* 1998;49:35–40.
Pollock C, Pei-Ling L, Gyory AZ, et al. Dysmorphism of urinary red blood cells: value in diagnosis. *Kidney Int* 1989;36:1045–1049.
Sheil AG, Chui AK, Verran DJ, et al. Evaluation of the loin pain/hematuria syndrome treated by renal autotransplantation or radical renal neurectomy. *Am J Kidney Dis* 1998;32:215–220.
Stapleton FB, Roy S III, Noe HN, et al. Hypercalciuria in children with hematuria. *N Engl J Med* 1984;310:1345–1348.
Sutton JM. Evaluation of hematuria in adults. *JAMA* 1990;263: 2475–2480.
Woolhandler S, Pels RJ, Bor DH, et al. Dipstick urinalysis screening of asymptomatic patients for urinary tract disorders. I. Hematuria and proteinuria. *JAMA* 1989;262:1214–1219.

Kelley's Textbook of Internal Medicine, fourth edition. Edited by H. David Humes. Lippincott Williams & Wilkins, Philadelphia © 2000.

C H A P T E R

135

APPROACH TO THE PATIENT WITH PROTEINURIA AND NEPHROTIC SYNDROME

JEFFREY R. SCHELLING
JOHN R. SEDOR

PRESENTATION

Proteinuria is often the first evidence of renal disease and is usually discovered on routine screening urinalysis. Less commonly, patients with undiagnosed glomerular disease and proteinuria that has caused hypoalbuminemia (i.e., nephrotic syndrome—see later discussion) seek medical care for new-onset ankle or periorbital edema. Patients with coexisting left ventricular dysfunction and nephrotic syndrome can show initial signs and symptoms of new-onset or worsening congestive heart failure.

The incidence of proteinuria identified on routine urinalysis screening varies in population-based studies from 0.6% to 10.7%. Careful evaluation of patients with proteinuria is necessary, since the underlying renal disease may be amenable to therapy. The quantity of urinary protein has both diagnostic and prognostic significance. Nephrotic proteinuria, defined as urinary protein excretion greater than 3.5 g per 24 hours, usually results from glomerular disease. If it is persistent and severe, nephrotic proteinuria is an independent risk factor for progression of the underlying renal disease. However, most proteinuric patients will have non-nephrotic proteinuria (less than 3.5 g per 24 hours), which is more typically associated with tubulointerstitial or glomerular diseases that do not progress, remit, or have an indolent clinical course. Proteinuria that is below the detection limits of standard reagent strips used for screening urinalysis, but which represents abnormally increased albumin excretion, is defined as microalbuminuria.

Both immunoassays and special reagent strips are available for detection of microalbuminuria. The prevalence of microalbuminuria varies in the population, ranging from 4% in healthy individuals to as high as 20% to 30% in diabetic and hypertensive patients. Microalbuminuria appears to be a marker of patients at risk of cardiovascular disease. Screening for microalbuminuria in the clinic is used most commonly in patients with diabetes mellitus, in whom this test has been validated to identify individuals at risk of nephropathy.

PATHOPHYSIOLOGY OF PROTEINURIA

Glomerular cells, matrix, and basement membrane are assembled to generate a highly selective filter that permits passage of water, electrolytes, and solutes with molecular weights of 10 kd or less but prevents movement of larger molecules into the urinary space. This property of the glomerular capillary wall, termed *glomerular permselectivity*, restricts solute filtration on the basis of both molecular size and ionic charge. Glomerular ultrafiltrate must pass through (a) negatively charged, fenestrated endothelial cells; (b) the glomerular basement membrane, which is composed primarily of anionic extracellular matrix components; and (c) slit diaphragms, which bridge negatively charged glomerular epithelial cell foot processes. Under normal circumstances, the net anionic charge of these three layers of the glomerular capillary membrane creates a barrier to passage of anionic proteins, such as albumin. The restrained filtration of larger molecules is also prevented by size constraints of the pores in the filtration barrier.

The molecular basis of glomerular permselectivity is beginning to be understood. Several glomerular epithelial cell proteins (podocalyxin, GLEPP1, and nephrin) have been cloned and appear to regulate glomerular permselectivity by as yet unknown mechanisms. Despite efficient restriction of protein from Bowman's space, small quantities of protein are filtered by the glomerulus in healthy individuals, but almost all of the filtered proteins are reabsorbed and catabolized by proximal tubule cells, so that the amount of protein measured in the urine is only a very small fraction of the amount filtered (less than 150 mg per day).

Increased proteinuria occurs in both glomerular and tubulointerstitial disease. Glomerular damage from disease eliminates both the charge and size barriers and results in loss of glomerular permselectivity. The ensuing leakage of plasma proteins into the glomerular ultrafiltrate in large amounts overwhelms tubular capacity for reabsorption and produces glomerular proteinuria. Interestingly, kidney biopsy samples from patients with many types of glomerular disease often also indicate significant tubulointerstitial disease. Several studies demonstrate that proteinuria can cause tubular epithelial cell injury by several mechanisms of action, which contributes to renal disease progression.

The composition of proteins lost in the urine reflects the extent of damage to the filtration barrier. Loss of glomerular basement membrane charge selectivity typically results in albuminuria, with little loss of larger proteins, such as globulins. This type of selective proteinuria occurs usually, but not exclusively, in patients with minimal-change nephropathy. Other glomerular diseases are characterized by more profound structural damage that destroys both size and charge barriers. Proteinuria in patients with these diseases tends to be nonselective (excretion of both albumin and larger-molecular-weight proteins). A subset

of multiple myeloma patients have glomerular proteinuria composed of immunoglobulin light chains. Because of their relatively small size (less than 25 kd) and neutral or cationic charge, these light chains, termed Bence Jones proteins, are freely filtered across the glomerular capillary wall with normal permselectivity. The quantity of filtered Bence Jones proteins frequently exceeds maximal tubular resorptive capacity. Unless glomeruli or tubules have undergone light chain–induced injury, albuminuria is absent, and screening with the urinary dipstick therefore will not identify these patients (see later discussion, Measurement of Urinary Protein Excretion and Urinalysis).

Primary or secondary tubular disorders, in the absence of glomerular disease, may cause tubular proteinuria by reducing the tubular capacity to reabsorb filtered proteins. Tubular proteinuria may result in urinary losses of albumin, low-molecular-weight globulins, and enzymes. Proteinuria in the context of inflammatory tubulointerstitial diseases may be due to decreased protein resorption, as well as secretion of IgA and uroepithelial mucoproteins. Tubular proteinuria rarely exceeds 2 g per 24 hours and usually is less than 1 g per 24 hours.

Mechanisms of microalbuminuria are less well understood and have been primarily explored in patients with diabetes. Careful morphologic analysis shows a diminished number of podocytes and increased glomerular volumes in diabetic Native Americans of the Pima tribe who have microalbuminuria. Since podocytes do not replicate, the remaining podocytes, though normal on ultrastructural examination, appear inadequate to maintain a normal filtration barrier. Microalbuminuria may also result from endothelial cell dysfunction, with leakage of protein across diseased glomerular capillary basement membranes.

HISTORY AND PHYSICAL EXAMINATION

After proteinuria is discovered, the patient should be carefully questioned for history or symptoms characteristic of systemic diseases that cause proteinuria (Table 135.1). Diabetes is the most common cause of proteinuria, and proteinuria rarely is the first indication of this disease in a patient with type II diabetes. While they are nonspecific symptoms, malaise, anorexia, and weight loss point to systemic illness or uremia. The patient's use of both prescribed and over-the-counter medications and street drugs should also be determined. Blood pressure levels may suggest the underlying disease source. For example, patients with minimal-change disease or membranous nephropathy less commonly are hypertensive. In contrast, hypertension is often associated with focal segmental glomerulosclerosis and proliferative glomerulonephritides. Orthostatic changes in blood pressure and other signs of extracellular fluid volume status should be assessed, because some patients with nephrotic syndrome exhibit intravascular volume depletion despite marked peripheral edema, findings that can alter subsequent management. Dependent or periorbital edema indicates the possibility of hypoalbuminemia from nephrotic syndrome. Lower-extremity skin rashes are characteristic of certain vasculitides, and a malar rash suggests systemic lupus erythematosus.

TABLE 135.1.   SOME SYSTEMIC DISORDERS ASSOCIATED WITH THE NEPHROTIC SYNDROME

Multisystem diseases
  Diabetes mellitus
  Collagen vascular disorders (systemic lupus erythematosus, systemic vasculitis)
  Amyloidosis
  Cryoglobulinemia
  Sarcoidosis
Neoplasms
  Solid tumors
  Lymphoma and leukemia
  Multiple myeloma
Infections
  Bacterial (poststreptococcal nephritis, endocarditis, shunt nephritis, syphilis)
  Viral (hepatitis B and C, human immunodeficiency virus)
  Protozoan (malaria, toxoplasmosis)
  Helminthic (schistosomiasis, trypanosomiasis)
Drugs and toxins
  Street heroin
  Heavy metals (gold, mercury)
  Nonsteroidal anti-inflammatory agents
  Penicillamine
  Captopril
Renal vascular conditions
  Unilateral renal artery stenosis
  Malignant hypertension
Hereditary disorders
  Alport's syndrome
  Sickle cell disease
  Nail–patella syndrome
  Congenital nephrotic syndrome
Miscellaneous conditions
  Preeclampsia
  Renal transplant rejection
  Vesicoureteral reflux with renal failure
  Analgesic abuse with renal failure

LABORATORY STUDIES AND DIAGNOSTIC TESTS

Initial laboratory studies and diagnostic tests for the proteinuric patient generally are limited to dipstick and microscopic urinalysis, quantification of urinary protein excretion, and measurement of serum creatinine and urea nitrogen to estimate renal function. A fasting blood sugar level and/or antinuclear antibody titer may be obtained to screen for undiagnosed diabetes or systemic lupus erythematosus. After this initial evaluation, as discussed later (see Differential Diagnosis), other laboratory and diagnostic tests may be ordered to determine the root cause of proteinuria and the presence of complications. For example, in patients with nephrotic-range proteinuria, serum total protein, albumin, triglycerides, cholesterol, calcium, and phosphate can be measured to assess for the presence of associated metabolic abnormalities.

MEASUREMENT OF URINARY PROTEIN EXCRETION AND URINALYSIS

Proteinuria often is detected initially by a dipstick examination of the urine. The dipstick does not detect albuminuria of less than 10 mg per deciliter and most reliably identifies patients with albuminuria that exceeds 20 to 30 mg per deciliter. Urinary dipsticks are quite insensitive in terms of detection of globulins, mucoproteins, and Bence Jones proteins. The presence of these proteins in the urine can be ascertained by semiquantitative techniques that depend on protein precipitation. Since urinary dipsticks measure protein concentrations, dipstick estimates of urinary protein quantity must be interpreted in the context of urine specific gravity. For example, in concentrated urine, protein determined by dipstick may be falsely elevated.

If a second urine dipstick evaluation yields results positive for protein, urinary protein should be quantified to distinguish between nephrotic and non-nephrotic proteinuria by either of two methods. First, the total urinary protein and creatinine excretion can be quantified by a 24-hour urine collection. Normal urinary protein excretion is less than 150 mg per 24 hours. Total urinary creatinine excretion also is used to assess the adequacy of the urine collection. Healthy men should excrete 20 to 25 mg creatinine per kilogram per 24 hours, and healthy women should excrete 15 to 20 mg creatinine per kilogram per 24 hours. Lower-than-predicted urine creatinine excretion may indicate inadequate urine collection that will falsely lower 24-hour urine protein measurements. Urinary creatinine excretion reflects muscle mass, however, and an adequate urine collection in an elderly or debilitated patient may contain significantly less creatinine than predicted. In these patients, replicate and consistent collections validate the accuracy of the protein measurements.

A second method to estimate total urinary protein excretion determines a urine protein (milligrams per deciliter)/urine creatinine (milligrams per deciliter) ratio from a single early-morning voided specimen. This ratio approximates the daily protein excretion rate (grams per 24 hours). This technique is ideal for use in the outpatient setting, and several studies suggest that this is the more accurate and preferred method of protein quantification, since patients are not required to collect urine over 24 hours. Repeated quantification of urinary protein excretion and serum albumin can be used to follow disease activity and to assess the efficacy of therapy. Although reductions in proteinuria usually indicate improvement in the underlying glomerulopathy, reduced protein excretion also can result from a diminished filtered load of protein due to a worsening glomerular filtration rate (GFR) or decreasing serum protein concentration. Changes in proteinuria on subsequent determinations must therefore be interpreted in association with other clinical and laboratory parameters.

Microscopic examination of the urine sediment from a centrifuged specimen can help in determining causes of proteinuria. For example, red blood cell casts almost always indicate underlying glomerulonephritis. Oval fat bodies (lipid-containing renal epithelial cells) and fatty casts often accompany nephrotic glomerular proteinuria. The absence of hematuria or fatty components and the presence of urinary leukocytes in conjunction with mild proteinuria are characteristic of tubulointerstitial disease. Proteinuric patients with azotemia and active urine sediment or with isolated, nephrotic-range proteinuria should be referred to a nephrologist for further evaluation. Those individuals with proteinuria less than 2 g per 24 hours and otherwise normal results on urinalysis and normal renal function can be carefully observed. Patients in the latter group with proteinuria greater than 2 g per 24 hours may benefit from consultation with a nephrologist.

ROLE OF BIOPSY

Although technologic advances in imaging techniques have reduced the morbidity and mortality of kidney biopsy, complications, usually significant bleeding, still develop in 1% to 5% of patients. Biopsy-related deaths occur in approximately 1 in 8,000 to 10,000 procedures. When biopsy is being considered, patients should be referred to a nephrologist for careful assessment of the information to be gained from this procedure.

Establishing a diagnosis in the patient with proteinuria eliminates both unnecessary diagnostic testing and potentially morbid empirical therapy. The indications for biopsy often depend on the quantity of proteinuria. We believe a biopsy should be strongly considered for a patient with non-nephrotic proteinuria who has azotemia, whose urine sediment contains red blood cells or red blood cell casts, or who has a systemic disease that has eluded diagnosis by clinical and noninvasive laboratory assessment. In addition, biopsy may be advised in this group of patients if urinary sediment is benign but proteinuria is persistent and increasing.

Routine renal biopsy is less controversial in adult patients with unexplained nephrotic syndrome or with an atypical presentation of a known condition resulting in nephrotic syndrome. For example, a diabetic patient with nephrotic syndrome would undergo renal biopsy only if proteinuria occurred soon after diagnosis or if there was evidence of co-existing disease. In the past, some investigators have advocated the empirical administration of glucocorticoids for treatment of adult idiopathic nephrotic syndrome before biopsy. More recent data suggest, however, that many adults with the most common condition associated with idiopathic nephrotic syndrome, membranous nephropathy, experience spontaneous remission and therefore would be needlessly exposed to steroid toxicities. In addition, for the substantial minority of patients with a progressive form of disease, a number of well-designed trials strongly suggest that therapy with cytotoxic agents should be used in addition to corticosteroids.

Biopsy should be considered early in the course of disease for a proteinuric patient with worsening renal function, since therapy, if indicated, needs to be initiated before widespread scar formation. A biopsy also can determine whether renal scarring has progressed to a degree that would make initiation or continuation of therapy futile, since serum creatinine poorly reflects underlying renal injury. Finally, unexplained acute renal failure remains an indication for biopsy in all patients. Biopsy results reported in two series of acute renal failure cases, which could not be attributed to volume depletion, obstruction, or acute tubular necrosis by clinical assessment, verified occult glomerulonephritis in approximately one-third of patients and tubulointerstitial diseases and unsuspected acute tubular necrosis in the remainder. Renal biopsy as a research tool remains critical to advancing our understanding of glomerular disease and, in certain instances, to evaluating the response to experimental therapies for proteinuric renal disease.

DIFFERENTIAL DIAGNOSIS

The amount of proteinuria stratifies patients for further laboratory assessment and suggests overlapping, but distinct differential diagnoses that often require more detailed history, physical examination, and laboratory analyses, as described in Fig. 135.1.

NON-NEPHROTIC PROTEINURIA

Non-nephrotic proteinuria is diagnosed in patients who excrete 150 mg to 3.5 g urinary protein per 24 hours, although non-nephrotic urine protein excretion characteristically is less than 1 g per 24 hours. In contrast to nephrotic proteinuria, a patient with non-nephrotic proteinuria is more likely to have a normal GFR, a normal urinalysis result, and absence of an associated systemic disease. Non-nephrotic proteinuria can reflect serious systemic disease, however, such as vasculitis or incipient diabetic nephropathy. Patients with non-nephrotic proteinuria, especially of more than 1 g per 24 hours, should be carefully screened for both glomerular and tubular diseases with detailed history, physical exam, and appropriate laboratory studies. In patients without serious systemic disease, non-nephrotic proteinuria can be classified as either benign (transient or orthostatic) or persistent (glomerular or tubular).

Benign Proteinuria

Transient proteinuria is defined as proteinuria that ultimately resolves with no identifiable harmful effects. Functional transient proteinuria is associated with fever, strenuous exercise, emotional stress, congestive heart failure, or other acute medical illnesses, whereas idiopathic transient proteinuria is proteinuria present in an otherwise healthy person. Orthostatic proteinuria occurs only when the patient is in the upright position and is diagnosed by quantitating proteinuria in daytime and nighttime urine collections. Approximately 90% of young men with proteinuria will have orthostatic proteinuria, which is usually associated with urinary protein excretion of less than 2 g per 24 hours. Orthostatic proteinuria spontaneously resolves in over 80% of cases.

Persistent Proteinuria

Persistent non-nephrotic proteinuria occurs in patients with either glomerular or tubulointerstitial disease. Glomerular diseases that cause non-nephrotic proteinuria can spontaneously remit, remain indolent, or rapidly progress from associated inflammation (see Chapter 150). Patients in the latter group usually have signs and symptoms of significant illness, and urinalysis generally shows hematuria and, occasionally, red blood cell casts. Patients with persistent proteinuria, but otherwise normal urinalysis results may eventually experience progressive renal failure and hypertension, although many patients' disease follows an indolent course. For this reason, follow-up investigation for renal disease may be warranted for at least some patients with persistent proteinuria. Many patients with persistent proteinuria without evidence of glomerular disease have tubulointerstitial disease

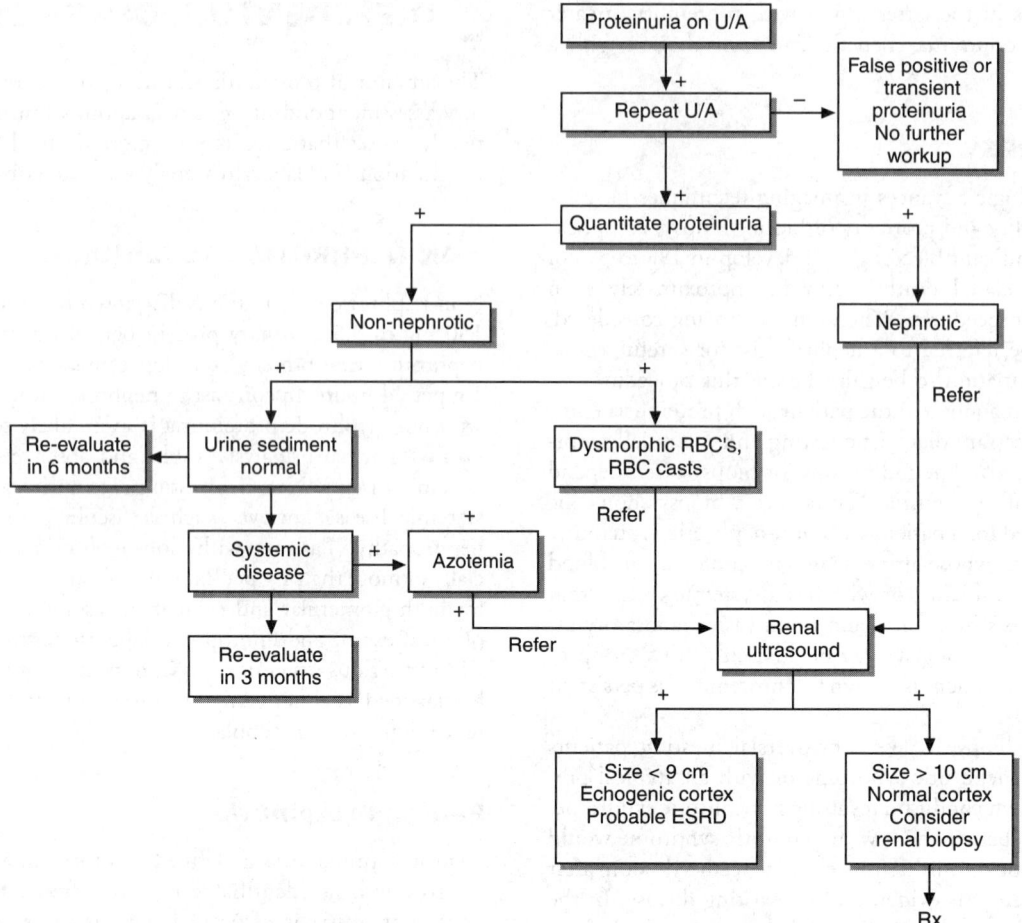

FIGURE 135.1. Approach to the evaluation of proteinuria in the adult. Urinalysis (U/A), Refer indicates where referral to a nephrologist is appropriate. Rx indicates points at which therapy can be initiated, as indicated in the text.

EVIDENCE LEVEL: B. Reference: Giatras I, Lau J, Levey AS. Effect of angiotensin-converting-enzyme inhibitors on the progression of nondiabetic renal disease: a meta-analysis of randomized trials. Angiotensin-Converting-Enzyme Inhibitor and Progressive Renal Disease Study Group. *Ann Int Med* **1997;127:337–345.**

as a primary disorder or as a result of a systemic illness (see Chapter 151).

NEPHROTIC SYNDROME

The nephrotic syndrome is a constellation of clinical and laboratory abnormalities common to a variety of primary and secondary kidney diseases, each characterized by increased permeability of the glomerular capillary wall to circulating plasma proteins. The defining clinical manifestation of filtration barrier dysfunction caused by these disorders is heavy proteinuria (more than 3.5 g per 24 hours) that leads to hypoalbuminemia. Secondary manifestations, such as edema, hyperlipidemia, and lipiduria, are common.

Proteinuria and Hypoalbuminemia

In the nephrotic syndrome, proteinuria results from a combination of defects in the size-selective and charge-selective sieving properties of the glomerular capillary membrane. Albumin is the predominant protein that is excreted, since it is the most abundant protein in plasma, but there may also be increased urinary loss of other proteins. Proteinuria and hypoalbuminemia are not necessarily directly related, since the serum albumin concentration reflects the composite effects of urinary protein loss, dietary protein intake, hepatic protein synthesis, protein catabolism, and the distribution of albumin between vascular and extravascular compartments. In the nephrotic syndrome, some or all of these regulatory factors may be altered. In the absence of coexisting liver disease or a systemic illness or malnutrition, hepatic synthesis of albumin is either normal or moderately high in nephrotic patients. The predominant cause of hypoalbuminemia appears to be a failure to enhance hepatic synthesis sufficiently to compensate for increased urinary losses and renal catabolism of albumin.

Edema

The mechanisms of edema formation in the nephrotic syndrome can vary and depend on the underlying glomerular abnormality. The classic view of edema formation is that hypoalbuminemia reduces plasma oncotic pressure, thereby promoting fluid transudation from the intravascular to the interstitial space. This theory may apply to some patients with minimal-change disease who exhibit signs of intravascular volume depletion. However, the observation that blood volume is increased in many other patients with nephrotic syndrome suggests that elevated hydrostatic pressure due to sodium and water retention mediated by intrarenal mechanisms (e.g., decreased GFR or enhanced tubular sodium reabsorption) may be a primary mechanism of edema formation. Patients with the nephrotic syndrome typically show signs of "pitting" edema in dependent areas where the imbalance of Starling forces is greatest, such as the lower extremities and periorbital and scrotal tissues. Transudative pleural effusions and ascites also may be present, but pulmonary edema is unusual in the absence of concomitant heart or renal failure.

Hyperlipidemia and Lipiduria

An increase in the serum concentrations of cholesterol and phospholipids is often a striking finding associated with nephrotic proteinuria. Reduction in plasma albumin concentration leads to enhanced hepatic synthesis of the cholesterol-transporting protein and apolipoprotein B, resulting in a higher serum concentration of very-low-density lipoproteins (VLDLs). The exact way in which apolipoprotein B synthesis is linked to hypoalbuminemia is unknown. Increasing oncotic pressure by infusion of albumin or dextran, however, causes a decrease in plasma lipid levels, suggesting that the reduction of serum oncotic pressure from hypoalbuminemia may be the primary signal for hyperlipidemia in a nephrotic patient. Increases in VLDLs are also caused by decreased VLDL clearance in the nephrotic syndrome.

In general, plasma concentrations of lipids are related inversely to the serum albumin concentration, but the specific plasma lipoprotein fractions that are elevated tend to vary with the severity of hypoalbuminemia. Early in the course of nephrotic syndrome, triglycerides of VLDL are hydrolyzed rapidly by lipoprotein lipase, causing low-density lipoproteins (LDLs) to form in excess without a rise in VLDL concentration. Thus, an increase in plasma LDL cholesterol levels is the first lipid abnormality to appear in nephrotic patients. Total serum high-density lipoprotein (HDL) levels vary, but the cardioprotective HDL_2 subfraction tends to be decreased. As the nephrotic syndrome progresses in severity, lipoprotein lipase activity diminishes in some patients, and hypertriglyceridemia results from overproduction of VLDL and defective lipolysis of triglyceride-rich lipoproteins. Lipiduria is common in the nephrotic syndrome and results from increased glomerular permeability to low-molecular-weight proteins, thus correlating better with the degree of proteinuria than with the degree of hyperlipidemia.

Other Metabolic Derangements

Patients with the nephrotic syndrome tend to experience arterial and venous thrombosis, especially renal vein thrombosis. Several mechanisms of action have been proposed for this hypercoagulable state. Minor elevations of the platelet count and plasma concentrations of fibrinogen and factors V, VII, VIII, and X have been reported. Urinary loss of antithrombin III, a potent anticoagulant protein with a molecular weight similar to that of albumin, may play a role in the thrombotic tendency of some patients. Decreased activity of protein S, a plasma protein that

serves as a cofactor for the anticoagulant effects of activated protein C, also has been described in patients with nephrotic syndrome. Nephrotic patients exhibit platelet hyperaggregability that is related inversely to the serum albumin concentration and reverses with infusion of albumin. Albumin binds arachidonic acid and limits its conversion to thromboxane, a potent stimulator of platelet aggregation. In addition, enhanced production of thromboxane in nephrotic patients with hypoalbuminemia may contribute to increased platelet aggregation.

In nephrotic patients with nonselective proteinuria, the serum concentrations of proteins other than albumin may be reduced through urinary losses. Loss of vitamin D–binding globulin may result in vitamin D deficiency, leading to hypocalcemia, osteomalacia, and secondary hyperparathyroidism. Loss of immunoglobulins may contribute to the increased rate of infections observed in nephrotic patients. Depletion of transferrin may lead to iron-deficiency anemia. Loss of thyroxine-binding globulin may affect certain thyroid function tests, but free thyroxine, triiodothyroxine, and thyroid-stimulating hormone levels are normal.

Etiology

The nephrotic syndrome either results from a primary glomerulopathy or is a manifestation of a systemic disorder. A partial list of such disorders is shown in Table 135.1, and they are discussed in Chapter 150. Most (50% to 70%) adult patients who show signs of the nephrotic syndrome have a related systemic illness. The most common multisystem diseases found in conjunction with this syndrome are diabetes mellitus, systemic lupus erythematosus and other collagen vascular diseases, and primary or secondary amyloidosis. Bacterial, viral, protozoan, and helminthic infections have been found to be related to the nephrotic syndrome, most often resulting in proliferative or membranous glomerulopathy. Chronic hepatitis C infection has been associated with cryoglobulinemia and proliferative glomerulonephritis and may be the most common infectious cause of nephrotic syndrome. Immunologic and virologic studies suggest that renal disease results from intraglomerular deposition of immune complexes containing hepatitis C. Infection with human immunodeficiency virus can cause a glomerular lesion that resembles focal segmental glomerulosclerosis, which usually leads to nephrotic syndrome and can cause rapidly progressive renal failure.

Neoplasms also are associated with the nephrotic syndrome. In the case of carcinomas, the histologic features are typical of membranous glomerulopathy, implicating an immune response to tumor antigens in the pathogenesis of this disease. Lymphomas and leukemias more often are associated with minimal-change disease. A variety of medications, particularly penicillamine and gold, have been linked to membranous glomerulopathy. Nonsteroidal anti-inflammatory drugs cause a syndrome of nephrotic proteinuria and acute renal failure. Pathologic examination in these cases usually reveals acute interstitial nephritis with minimal glomerular changes other than glomerular epithelial cell foot process fusion. Focal segmental glomerulosclerosis is a common lesion in nephrotic syndrome as a complication of intravenous heroin use. Subcutaneous drug abuse ("skin popping") more often is associated with amyloidosis.

Between 30% and 50% of adult patients with nephrotic syndrome do not show evidence of a systemic disorder and are identified as having idiopathic nephrotic syndrome. Histopathologic examination of biopsy material usually shows one of four pathologic entities: membranous glomerulopathy (30% to 40% of cases), focal segmental glomerulosclerosis (20% to 30%), minimal-change disease (10% to 20%), or membranoproliferative glomerulonephritis (10% to 20%). Focal segmental glomerulosclerosis is the most common lesion identified in biopsy specimens obtained from African Americans with nephrotic syndrome, and studies suggest that it is increasingly common in the general population. In contrast to the findings among adult patients, minimal-change disease accounts for more than 80% of all cases of nephrotic syndrome in children (less than 10 years of age).

STRATEGIES FOR OPTIMAL CARE

Specific management approaches to both glomerular and tubulointerstitial conditions related to proteinuria are discussed in Chapters 151 and 164. Supportive treatment of the patient with proteinuria is discussed here. Blood pressure should be optimally controlled in all patients, in an effort to slow progression of the underlying renal disease. A randomized, multicenter trial has shown that reduction of mean arterial blood pressure (MAP) to less than 92 mm Hg in patients with proteinuria and azotemia lowers the rate of decline in GFR compared with a control group of patients whose hypertension was treated to standard levels (MAP of 107 mm Hg). The benefit of blood pressure reduction is greatest in nephrotic patients and moderate in patients with protein excretions of 1 to 3 g per day.

Several classes of antihypertensives have been termed "renal protective" and may have beneficial effects on the rate of renal disease progression that are independent of blood pressure lowering. The renal-protective effects of angiotensin-converting enzyme (ACE) inhibitors are the best studied and most compelling, and a limited number of human studies have suggested that non-dihydropyridine calcium channel blockers (e.g., diltiazem and verapamil) and β-blockers may also belong in this category. Several multicenter trials, in diabetics and nondiabetics, have shown that treatment of both hypertensive and normotensive proteinuric patients with ACE inhibitors results in slower deterioration in renal function compared with control groups with equivalent blood pressure using a regimen that did not contain an ACE inhibitor. The greatest benefit has been confirmed in patients with nephrotic proteinuria, but use of these drugs in patients with lesser levels of proteinuria also appears to be warranted. Smaller trials similarly have suggested beneficial effects of angiotensin II receptor blockers on the rate of progression of renal disease and the level of proteinuria.

The renal protective effect of ACE inhibitors and other antihypertensive drugs seems to result from their "antiproteinuric" effects, which is in agreement with observations that proteinuria confers an independent risk of progressive kidney disease. ACE inhibitors are the most efficacious agents available to reduce proteinuria and are increasingly used in normotensive, nondiabetic nephrotic patients to prevent progression of the underlying nephropathy. Nonsteroidal anti-inflammatory drugs also have been administered in conjunction with sodium restriction (50 mEq per day) to limit protein excretion in patients with intractable hypoalbuminemia and edema, although the benefit on progression of renal disease has not been studied. The hemodynamic changes, which are induced by nonsteroidal anti-inflammatory agents and which contribute to the diminution of proteinuria, usually cause a stable but reversible decrease in GFR but also can precipitate ischemic acute renal failure in some nephrotic patients. Renal function and serum electrolytes of patients must therefore be carefully monitored if treatment with nonsteroidal anti-inflammatory agents or ACE inhibitors is initiated, particularly if the clinical status of the patient changes.

Management of diabetic proteinuria, the most common cause of the nephrotic syndrome, merits special comment. In addition to obtaining adequate blood pressure control, studies have demonstrated that aggressive blood glucose control delays progression of proteinuria in nonazotemic patients with type 1 diabetes and microalbuminuria. In one study, intensified insulin treatment regimens also prevented development of proteinuria in patients who entered the study with normal daily protein excretion rates. Studies to evaluate the advantage of tight glycemic control for end-organ complications in the context of type 2 diabetes are ongoing; most investigators believe that achieving normal serum glucose levels also should be a goal in this group of patients.

Nutritional therapy for all patients with chronic renal disease, including patients with the nephrotic syndrome, has generated great interest in the nephrology community for two reasons. First, adequate nutrition reduces morbidity and mortality in patients on dialysis. Patients with the nephrotic syndrome are at risk of malnutrition, particularly if urinary protein losses are persistent and appetite becomes suppressed owing to uremia. Adequate protein and calorie intake should be maintained to avoid malnutrition, and dietary management may require consultation with a dietician. Second, dietary protein restriction has been shown to delay the progression of renal disease in animal models. However, the applicability of these data to management of human disease remains controversial. In the multicenter Management of Diet in Renal Disease study, dietary protein restriction had no conclusive benefit on the decline in GFR, although progression in some subsets of patients may have minimally slowed. Protein restriction to slow progression in all patients with renal disease should be attempted only with adequate support from a dietician.

Other supportive therapies are directed primarily at alleviating edema. Dietary sodium restriction should be the initial maneuver to reduce edema. Usually, limiting a patient's sodium intake to 2 to 3 g per day is sufficient to lessen fluid retention, although patients with severe hypoalbuminemia may require further restriction of sodium intake. Diuretics can be added later, but they must be used judiciously to limit extracellular fluid volume while preserving intravascular volume. Although nephrotic patients usually have expanded extracellular fluid volumes, intravascular volume depletion also can be present in some patients if oncotic pressure becomes sufficiently low. Aggressive diuresis in these patients may precipitate acute renal failure as the result of further intravascular volume depletion. Bed rest alone or, more commonly, hospital admission for administration of intravenous albumin followed by a loop diuretic usually elicits diuresis in these patients. Low doses of dopamine (1 to 6 μg per kilogram per minute) increase renal blood flow and may be a useful adjunct to diuretics in the therapy of severe edema in the hospitalized patient. Finally, hemofiltration or continuous loop diuretic infusion can be employed to reduce extracellular fluid volume in the rare patient who is refractory to other therapies. In all cases, patients undergoing diuresis must be closely monitored for evidence of volume depletion.

Safe and effective modes of therapy are now available to lower serum lipid levels in nephrotic patients, but the association between hyperlipidemia, which often accompanies the nephrotic syndrome, and accelerated atherosclerosis has not been proved conclusively. Given the pro-atherogenic lipid profiles of most nephrotic patients, most nephrologists initiate appropriate lipid-lowering therapy in patients with persistent nephrotic proteinuria or other vascular risk factors. If lipid-lowering treatment is initiated, drug therapy will be required, because dietary modification is ineffective owing to the severity of hyperlipidemia in the nephrotic syndrome. Inhibitors of the rate-limiting enzyme in cholesterol synthesis (3-hydroxy-3-methylglutaryl coenzyme A reductase) are the most effective therapy for hypercholesterolemia. Fibric acids (e.g., clofibrate) lower triglyceride but not cholesterol levels in nephrotic patients. Combinations of lipid-lowering drugs from different categories also can be used if additive toxicities are avoided. Experimental evidence from animal studies has suggested that hyperlipidemia may hasten the progression of all types of renal disease, including those associated with the nephrotic syndrome, but further confirmation in human trials is warranted.

As described previously, the nephrotic syndrome is a hypercoagulable state, although estimates of the evidence of thromboembolic phenomena (most commonly renal vein thrombosis) vary widely. Anticoagulant therapy should be initiated if a thromboembolic complication is documented, but patients with the nephrotic syndrome may be relatively resistant to the effects of heparin as the result of losses of antithrombin III (the heparin substrate) in the urine. The duration of anticoagulation that is required after a thromboembolic event is unclear. In theory, anticoagulant therapy may need to be continued as long as nephrotic-range proteinuria persists, although the risk/benefit ratio of long-term anticoagulation in the nephrotic syndrome has not been established. Finally, doses of all drugs tightly bound to albumin may need to be reduced to avoid toxicities, because diminished albumin concentrations in nephrotic patients can lead to accumulation of the unbound fraction.

Indications for HOSPITALIZATION

Hospitalization is rarely necessary for evaluation of the patient with proteinuria. Renal biopsy can be performed in the outpatient setting if the patient can be monitored for at least 8 to 12 hours after the procedure. Several studies that analyzed biopsy complications suggest that major bleeding generally

occurs within that time period. Diuresis of the nephrotic patient with edema can generally be done in the clinic if the patient's weight is monitored daily. To prevent skin breakdown or anasarca, some patients with refractory edema will require hospitalization for intravenous diuretic therapy with or without intravenous albumin or low doses of dopamine. Finally, patients who require cytotoxic therapy may need hospitalization.

BIBLIOGRAPHY

Attman PO, Samuelsson O, Alaupovic P. Progression of renal failure: role of apolipoprotein-containing lipoprotein. *Kidney Int* 1997;52:S98–S101.
Diabetes Control and Complications Trial Research Group. The effect of intensive treatment on the development and progression of long-term complications in insulin-dependent diabetes mellitus. *N Engl J Med* 1993;329:977–986.
Giatras I, Lau J, Levey AS. Effect of angiotensin-converting enzyme inhibitors on the progression of nondiabetic renal disease: a meta-analysis of randomized trials. *Ann Intern Med* 1997;127(5):337–345.
Hricik DE, Chung-Park M, Sedor JR. Glomerulonephritis. *N Engl J Med* 1998;339(13):888–899.
Kloke HJ, Branten AJ, Huysmans FT, et al. Antihypertensive treatment of patients with proteinuric renal diseases: risks or benefits of calcium channel blockers? *Kidney Int* 1998;53(6):1559–1573.
Madaio MP. Renal biopsy. *Kidney Int* 1990;38:529–543.
Peterson JC, Adler S, Burkart JM, et al. Blood pressure control, proteinuria, and the progression of renal disease: the modification of diet in renal disease study. *Ann Intern Med* 1995;123:754–762.
Ponticelli C, Passerini P. Treatment of the nephrotic syndrome associated with primary glomerulonephritis. *Kidney Int* 1994;46:595–604.
Ruggenenti P, Gaspari F, Perna A, et al. Cross sectional longitudinal study of spot morning urine protein: creatinine ratio, 24 hour urine protein excretion rate, glomerular filtration rate, and end stage renal failure in chronic renal disease in patients without diabetes. *Br Med J* 1998;316(7130):504–509.
Ruggenenti P, Perna A, Gherardi G, et al. Renal function and requirement for dialysis in chronic nephropathy patients on long-term ramipril: REIN follow-up trial. *Lancet* 1998;352(9136):1252–1256.
Schieppati A, Mosconi L, Perna A, et al. Prognosis of untreated patients with idiopathic membranous nephropathy. *N Engl J Med* 1993;329:85–89.

Kelley's Textbook of Internal Medicine, fourth edition. Edited by H. David Humes. Lippincott Williams & Wilkins, Philadelphia © 2000.

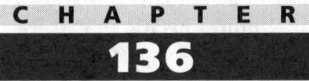

CHAPTER 136

APPROACH TO THE PATIENT WITH DYSURIA AND PYURIA

ERIC W. YOUNG

PRESENTATION

Dysuria and pyuria are common clinical problems and cardinal manifestations of diseases of the genitourinary tract. *Dysuria* refers to pain, burning, or other discomfort associated with urination and is often accompanied by urinary frequency, urgency, and suprapubic discomfort. *Pyuria* is the presence of abnormal numbers of white blood cells in the urine. Patients often present with both dysuria and pyuria. Infection is the most common cause of dysuria and pyuria, but other etiologies may need to be considered.

PATHOPHYSIOLOGY

In general, dysuria and pyuria indicate inflammation or irritation within the urinary bladder, urethra, or surrounding tissues. The specific cause of the inflammation depends on the cause, as detailed in the section Differential Diagnosis.

HISTORY AND PHYSICAL EXAMINATION

A patient with dysuria or pyuria should be asked about urinary frequency, urgency, cloudy or malodorous urine, urethral discharge, fever, and flank pain. Women should be asked about vaginal discharge or itching. It may be appropriate to inquire about recent sexual activity in the context of possible cystitis or a sexually transmitted disease. Pertinent aspects of the physical examination include the presence or absence of fever, suprapubic tenderness, and flank tenderness. If indicated by the clinical history, men should be examined for a urethral discharge and women should undergo a pelvic examination to detect vaginal discharge and inflammation.

LABORATORY STUDIES AND DIAGNOSTIC TESTS

A urinalysis should be done on patients with dysuria or other symptoms of lower-urinary-tract irritation. Quantitative measurements have established that pyuria is characterized by a leukocyte excretion rate of more than 200,000 cells per hour. For practical clinical purposes, however, pyuria is defined by the presence of at least five leukocytes per high-power field on the microscopic portion of a standard urinalysis. The leukocyte esterase dipstick test is quite specific (95%) for detecting pyuria, although its sensitivity is only fair (false-negative rate as high as 26%). The nitrite dipstick test detects the presence of bacteria, which reduce urinary nitrates to nitrites. Infection is unlikely if the leukocyte esterase and nitrite dipstick test results are both negative.

One reasonable cost-saving strategy is to screen urine with a dipstick and perform a microscopic examination only if the test for leukocyte esterase, nitrite, hemoglobin, or protein yields positive results. However, urine microscopy should be done for symptomatic patients regardless of the screening dipstick results. Finding bacteriuria on a urinalysis further supports a diagnosis of infection, whereas proteinuria or casts indicate renal disease. If acute renal interstitial nephritis is suspected, a Wright or Hansel stain of the urine should be done to detect eosinophils.

TABLE 136.1.	CAUSES OF DYSURIA
Acute cystitis	
Acute urethral syndrome	
Acute cystitis with pyelonephritis	
Acute vulvovaginitis with or without urethritis	
Idiopathic interstitial cystitis	
Genitourinary trauma	
Urethral irritants	
Allergic reaction	
Autoimmune diseases	

A urine culture may be ordered to establish or confirm a diagnosis of infection. Culture is mandatory for complicated, recurrent, or unclear cases, but it may be optional or even unnecessary for straightforward cases of cystitis. Vaginal or urethral cultures or smears should be done for suspected vaginitis or urethritis, as detailed later. Specific situations may call for more specialized tests, such as cystoscopy or kidney biopsy.

DIFFERENTIAL DIAGNOSIS

The major causes of dysuria (often accompanied by pyuria) are listed in Table 136.1 and the causes of pyuria in Table 136.2.

DYSURIA

Acute cystitis is the most common cause of dysuria in clinical practice. Women are particularly prone to cystitis, apparently owing to the ease with which the urethra can become contaminated with perineal flora. The risk of cystitis seems to be amplified with delayed bladder emptying following intercourse. Dysuria due to cystitis may also be seen in immunocompromised hosts. Cystitis in children or men might indicate an underlying structural urologic problem, particularly if infections are recurrent.

Coliform bacteria are the most common cause of infectious cystitis. *Escherichia coli* is the causative organism in approximately 85% of community-acquired infections; the rest are accounted for by *Proteus* and *Klebsiella* species and *Staphylococcus saprophyticus*. A much broader spectrum of resistant and unusual organisms are encountered in hospitalized patients and those with other complications.

A diagnosis of bacterial cystitis should be made in a patient

TABLE 136.2.	CAUSES OF PYURIA
Infection of the urinary tract	
Acute interstitial nephritis	
Chronic interstitial nephritis	
Acute glomerulonephritis or vasculitis	

with dysuria if pyuria is found on urinalysis. Other rapid laboratory indicators of cystitis include bacteriuria, the presence of bacteria on a Gram stain of the urine, and a positive dipstick reaction for leukocyte esterase or nitrite. The urine culture is usually considered positive with a bacterial density of more than 100,000 colony-forming units (CFU) per milliliter. Lower levels of growth, however, can occasionally indicate infection. A clean-catch urine culture specimen can be considered positive with as few as 100 CFU per milliliter in symptomatic women and 1,000 CFU per milliliter in symptomatic men.

Acute urethral syndrome refers to dysuria and frequency in the absence of significant bacteriuria. Many patients with this clinical picture have true bacterial cystitis with low bacterial counts on culture. Other patients have infections with chlamydia, *Ureaplasma*, or other fastidious organisms. Rarely, patients have no defined cause of dysuria.

Occasionally, a patient with subclinical pyelonephritis and cystitis may have isolated dysuria in the absence of fever and flank pain, which usually signals upper-urinary-tract infection. Various infectious sources are possible, as for cystitis. Silent pyelonephritis may be a reason for failure of short-term or oral antibiotic therapy directed at cystitis.

Vulvovaginitis is an important cause of dysuria in women. Dysuria may stem from accompanying urethritis or may be due to the contact of urine with inflamed external tissues. Burning toward the end of urination indicates the latter. If queried, patients with vaginitis usually complain of vaginal itching and discharge that may smell foul. On physical examination, there is inflammation and tenderness of the external genitalia and discharge. Urinalysis may show pyuria if there is coexistent urethral inflammation. The most common causes of vaginitis are *Candida albicans* and *Trichomonas vaginalis*. Candida vaginitis produces a thick white discharge. Candida infection may occur in any woman, but patients with diabetes or those who have recently undergone antibiotic treatment are particularly vulnerable. The diagnosis is made by finding fungal elements on a potassium hydroxide stain of vaginal secretions. Trichomonas vaginitis is characterized by a thin, watery discharge. Diagnosis is made by seeing trichomonads on a wet mount of vaginal fluid.

Urethritis may cause dysuria in women and men. Important causes of urethritis include *Neisseria gonorrhoeae*, *Chlamydia trachomatis*, and herpes simplex virus. In addition, *C. albicans* and *T. vaginalis* sometimes cause urethritis in women in the absence of symptoms of vaginitis. Urinalysis often shows pyuria without bacteriuria. Specific cultures must be obtained if these entities are suspected on clinical grounds.

Idiopathic interstitial cystitis appears to be a noninfectious cause of lower-urinary-tract symptoms, including dysuria, frequency, urgency, and nocturia. The origin of this condition is not well understood. Urinalysis often reveals pyuria without bacteriuria. The urine cultures are sterile. Cystoscopic examination classically documents very small petechial hemorrhages of the bladder wall. Dysuria may also arise from trauma, chemical or mechanical irritants, and autoimmune diseases.

PYURIA

Pyuria is most often caused by infection within the urinary tract, as detailed previously. Urine sediment showing white cells and white cell casts strongly suggests pyelonephritis. Pyuria usually resolves with successful treatment of urinary tract infections. Infectious agents that may require special efforts to culture and identify include chlamydia and *Mycobacterium tuberculosis*. The presence of "sterile pyuria" (as determined by standard culture techniques) should prompt the clinician to request multiple urine culture specimens for acid-fast bacilli. Sterile pyuria or isolated pyuria may also indicate renal parenchymal disease, particularly in patients with proteinuria or an elevated serum creatinine concentration.

Acute interstitial nephritis is a well-recognized cause of acute renal failure. The inflammatory response can be induced by drugs, autoimmune diseases, or infection (see Chapter 151). Drug-induced interstitial nephritis is characterized by eosinophilic pyuria in approximately 80% of cases. Other features can include hematuria, eosinophilia, fever, and rash. Many drugs have been reported to provoke acute interstitial nephritis, but the most common include penicillin and sulfa antibiotics, rifampin, allopurinol, loop diuretics, and cimetidine. The diagnosis is usually based on clinical findings and the presence of eosinophils in the blood or urine. A kidney biopsy may be needed to establish the diagnosis.

Chronic interstitial nephritis connotes chronic irreversible scarring of the renal interstitial space. Pyuria may be present, as well as increased serum creatinine concentration, renal tubular defects (diminished concentrating ability, renal tubular acidosis), hypertension, and papillary necrosis with sloughing of tissue into the urine. Prolonged exposure to analgesic agents has been implicated in this disease.

Pyuria may be seen in patients with acute glomerulonephritis or vasculitis, reflecting inflammation within the kidney. Usually, pyuria is eclipsed by other manifestations of renal disease, such as hematuria, red cell casts, proteinuria, azotemia, and hypertension. However, it is not uncommon for patients who are evaluated in the early stages of glomerulonephritis (e.g., Wegener's granulomatosis, Goodpasture's syndrome) to be mistakenly diagnosed as having urinary tract infection on the basis of pyuria and hematuria on urinalysis.

■ STRATEGIES FOR OPTIMAL CARE

Specific aspects of treatment are described in the chapters on specific entities. Usually, a patient with dysuria and pyuria should be started on antibiotics. A urine culture is unnecessary for uncomplicated cystitis, and treatment should not be delayed while awaiting the results of a urine culture. Uncomplicated infections are defined as those in adult, nonpregnant women without an accompanying condition that increases the risk or persistence of infection (e.g., diabetes, immunosuppression, and abnormalities of the urinary tract). Urinary infections in men, children, pregnant women, and hospitalized patients should be considered complicated. Short-course therapy (i.e., 1 or 3 days, as opposed to the traditional 7-day regimens) may be appropriate for uncomplicated cases. Appropriate antibiotic regimens include amoxicillin, trimethaprim-sulfamethoxazole, and quinolones (e.g., ciprofloxacin or norfloxacin). Specific antimicrobial therapy should be administered to patients with vulvovaginitis or urethritis, as guided by the diagnostic evaluation. Drug-induced interstitial nephritis is treated by withdrawing the putative agent. A short course of steroids is sometimes administered to dampen the inflammatory response.

BIBLIOGRAPHY

Barnett BJ, Stephens DS. Urinary tract infection: an overview. *Am J Med Sci* 1997;314:245–249.

Komaroff AL. Urinalysis and urine culture in women with dysuria. *Ann Intern Med* 1986;104:212–218.

Lipsky BA. Urinary tract infections in men: epidemiology, pathophysiology, diagnosis, and treatment. *Ann Intern Med* 1989;110:138–150.

Stamm WE, Hooten TM. Management of urinary tract infection in adults. *N Engl J Med* 1993;329:1328–1334.

C H A P T E R

137

APPROACH TO THE PATIENT WITH POLYURIA OR NOCTURIA

ROBERT M. A. RICHARDSON
SHELDON TOBE

■ POLYURIA

PRESENTATION

Polyuria is defined as the excretion of more than 2.5 to 3 L of urine per day. This definition is arbitrary and is based on the likelihood of a patient's being inconvenienced by the need to void frequently. It should be noted that much lower urine flow rates may be inappropriately high for a given clinical context but may not qualify as polyuria. Polyuria as a primary disorder stimulates thirst, leading to polydipsia. Because some patients have a primary increase in thirst or water intake, it may be difficult to determine whether polyuria is the cause or the effect of polydipsia.

PATHOPHYSIOLOGY

Polyuria may be caused by either water or solute diuresis. *Water diuresis* refers to the excretion of a large volume of dilute urine, with normal solute excretion. This may stem from a lack of antidiuretic hormone (ADH, vasopressin) or to failure of the kidney to respond to ADH. *Solute diuresis* is caused either by an excess of filtered solute, such as glucose, which disrupts the

concentrating mechanism, or by impaired tubular function, resulting in the excretion of large amounts of electrolytes, such as sodium chloride.

WATER DIURESIS

Water diuresis has three sources: failure of the posterior pituitary to secrete ADH (central or neurogenic diabetes insipidus), failure of the kidney to concentrate the urine despite the presence of adequate levels of ADH (nephrogenic diabetes insipidus), and excessive fluid intake, which includes psychogenic polydipsia and administration of fluids by physicians. When the lesions of nephrogenic diabetes insipidus (NDI) and central diabetes insipidus (CDI) are complete (total absence of ADH secretion or effect), they are easily recognizable in a patient with copious dilute urine. They may be incomplete, however, and have a more subtle clinical expression, making diagnosis much more difficult.

Central Diabetes Insipidus

CDI is caused by inadequate release of ADH from the posterior pituitary, resulting in the excretion of excessive urine volume (see Chapter 404). This loss of water leads to an increase in serum osmolality, triggering thirst and increased water intake to defend the normal limits of serum osmolality (285 to 295 mOsm per kilogram). A complete absence of ADH may lead to the daily excretion of 20 L or more of urine having an osmolality as low as 50 mOsm per kilogram. Incomplete CDI is a milder form of the condition; ADH secretion is present but still inappropriately low, causing less severe polyuria and a urine osmolality higher than minimum.

The causes of CDI are listed in Table 137.1. Congenital CDI is autosomal dominant, but rare. Acquired CDI most commonly arises from idiopathic causes, pituitary surgery, and hypothalamic-pituitary damage from neoplasia or infection. Pregnancy-induced CDI provoked by a vasopressinase responds to synthetic desmopressin (DDAVP).

ADH acts on V_1 and V_2 receptors present in different tissues. V_2 receptors mediate water resorption in the kidney and are present on the antiluminal surface (blood side) of cells lining the collecting ducts. ADH binding to V_2 receptors leads to activation of adenylate cyclase and production of cyclic AMP, which ultimately brings about an increase in permeability of the luminal membrane of the collecting duct to water by insertion of water channels into that membrane. The ADH-sensitive water channel in the collecting duct is called aquaporin 2; it is stored in the cytoplasm just beneath the luminal membrane in vesicles that merge with the luminal membrane on exposure of the cell to ADH. ADH receptors on endothelial cells mediate release of von Willebrand complexes, and infusion of the ADH analogue DDAVP can improve the defect in bleeding time found in patients with chronic renal failure.

Nephrogenic Diabetes Insipidus

NDI can be caused by resistance to ADH at the level of the collecting duct cell or by loss of ability to concentrate the renal

TABLE 137.1.   CAUSES OF POLYURIA

Water diuresis
  Central diabetes insipidus
    Idiopathic
    Traumatic
    Iatrogenic
      Surgery (i.e., hypophysectomy, radiation)
    Neoplasia-related
      Metastatic tumors (especially carcinoma of the breast),
        lymphoma, craniopharyngioma
    Vascular
      Stroke, aneurysm, Sheehan's syndrome
    Infection-related
      Encephalitis, meningitis
    Granulomatous
      Tuberculosis, sarcoidosis, histiocytosis
    Congenital (autosomal dominant)
    Pregnancy-related (from increased serum vasopressinase)
  Nephrogenic diabetes insipidus
    Drug-related
      Lithium-demeclocycline, amphotericin, aminoglycosides
    Metabolic
      Hypercalcemia, hypokalemia
    Tubulointerstitial disease–related (often solute diuresis as
      well)
    Congenital
      X-linked—abnormal V_2 receptor
      Autosomal recessive—abnormal aquaporin 2
  Excessive water intake
    Psychogenic polydipsia
    Iatrogenic
Solute diuresis
  Osmotic
    Glucose, mannitol, radiocontrast dye, urea
  Electrolyte
    Saline, diuretics
    Tubulointerstitial disease (obstructive uropathy, nonoliguric
      acute tubular necrosis, polyuric phase of acute tubular ne-
      crosis)

interstitium due to tubulointerstitial disease. The most common cause of resistance to the renal tubular effect of ADH is therapy of bipolar affective disorders with lithium, which causes polyuria in 20% to 30% of patients who take this drug. Lithium enters collecting duct cells from the lumen through amiloride-sensitive sodium channels and interferes with cyclic AMP formation. Hypercalcemia can induce NDI by blocking cyclic AMP production as well as through interstitial damage caused by chronic nephrocalcinosis.

Tubulointerstitial diseases lead to a loss of concentrating ability through the loss of the countercurrent mechanism responsible for producing a hypertonic renal interstitium. Most of these disorders are characterized by only modest degrees of polyuria (usually less than 4 L per day) and by urine that is roughly isotonic to plasma.

NDI is usually acquired, but there are congenital hereditary forms. The most common exhibits X-linked transmission with full penetrance in males and partial penetrance in females. The gene coding for the V_2 receptor has been localized to the X chromosome and has been shown to be defective in families with this rare congenital form of NDI. A less common form of hereditary NDI is an autosomal recessive disorder due to defects in the gene coding for aquaporin 2, causing failure of insertion of functional water channels into the lumen of the collecting duct cells. In both types of hereditary NDI, polyuria is present from birth.

Excessive Fluid Intake

Primary polydipsia results from the intake of large volumes of fluid. The most common form is psychogenic polydipsia, seen in many patients with chronic schizophrenia. The reason for the increased drinking behavior is unknown. Some of these patients experience recurrent episodes of severe hyponatremia that can result in serious acute and chronic neurologic dysfunction. Although it is not usually a diagnostic problem, inadvertent or unrecognized excess fluid therapy in a hospitalized patient can result in polyuria that is entirely physiologic. These patients have normal or expanded intravascular volume, low or low-normal serum osmolality, and resolution of polyuria when fluid administration is discontinued.

SOLUTE DIURESIS

Filtration of excessive amounts of osmotically active nonelectrolyte solutes, such as glucose, mannitol, or urea, overcomes the tubular resorptive capacity, resulting in excretion of an increased volume of water accompanying the solute. Osmotic diuresis is usually associated with a loss of sodium and chloride that is inappropriate to the (usually) reduced intravascular volume. The most common cause of osmotic diuresis is diabetes mellitus, with glucose acting as the solute. Mannitol administration, the use of contrast media, and urea-induced osmotic diuresis due to the administration of high-protein enteral diets are less common causes.

Electrolyte solute diuresis may be due to the use of diuretic drugs, the administration of large amounts of intravenous saline, and a wide variety of tubulointerstitial diseases, including relief of urinary tract obstruction (postobstructive diuresis) and the diuretic phase of acute tubular necrosis. The latter two may be associated with particularly large losses of water and electrolytes (i.e., more than 10 L per day of essentially isotonic saline).

HISTORY AND PHYSICAL EXAMINATION

The context in which polyuria occurs is important. Patients from the community are more likely to have diabetes mellitus; use drugs, such as diuretics or lithium; or have abnormal drinking habits. Polydipsia is suggested by episodic polyuria, absence of nocturia, and a plasma osmolality below 285. A history of head trauma, neoplasia, the sudden onset of unrelenting polyuria, a preference for ice water, and nocturnal polyuria suggest CDI. Hospitalized patients more often have solute diuresis. The main clinical contexts in which solute diuresis occurs are during the administration of large amounts of electrolyte solutions, relief of urinary tract obstruction, and the diuretic phase of acute tubular necrosis. The physical exam should focus on an evaluation of the intravascular volume to determine if it is diminished (i.e., low jugular venous pressure, postural hypotension, and tachycardia), since this will help determine if solute diuresis is appropriate.

LABORATORY STUDIES AND DIAGNOSTIC TESTS

A tiered approach to the workup of polyuria is found in Fig. 137.1. The presence of polyuria should be established with a 24-hour urine collection. Measurement of the urine osmolality separates patients with polyuria into two main categories. Those with hypotonic urine (less than 250 mOsm per kilogram) usually have water diuresis; a concentrated urine (more than 350 mOsm per kilogram) indicates solute diuresis. Patients with urine osmolality between 250 and 350 mOsm per kilogram may be more difficult to classify, but calculating the total daily solute excretion by multiplying urine volume in liters per day by the average urine osmolality is helpful. Patients who excrete normal amounts of solute (less than 1,000 mOsm per day, depending on diet) are likely to have water diuresis; patients with clearly high solute excretion (more than 1,200 mOsm per day) have solute diuresis.

If solute diuresis is diagnosed, the next step in determining the cause is to measure the urine electrolytes and compare their osmotic contribution to the total osmolality. If two times the sodium plus potassium (to represent the accompanying anions) is significantly less than the urine osmolality, then there is another solute in the urine. This solute is usually glucose, which is easy to measure. If there is no glucose, consider administering mannitol or radiocontrast dye or measure the urine urea. If the urine electrolytes are close to the urine osmolality, electrolyte diuresis is present. An alkaline pH indicates bicarbonaturia; a pH less than 7 indicates saline diuresis, as seen in intravenous saline loading, potent diuretics, and tubulointerstitial diseases, such as obstructive uropathy or the recovery phase of acute tubular necrosis.

Water diuresis of unclear cause should be investigated in the hospital. The first step is to measure the serum sodium concentration (Fig. 137.1). Patients who are hypernatremic usually have a coexisting disorder of thirst, because patients with even massive polyuria can usually maintain a normal serum osmolality by drinking fluid if their thirst center is intact and they have access to fluid. Hypernatremia is a medical emergency: these patients need to be watched very carefully, and referral to a specialist in fluid/electrolyte disorders is appropriate. Patients who are already hyperosmolar should not undergo a water-deprivation test but can immediately be given ADH or the synthetic analogue,

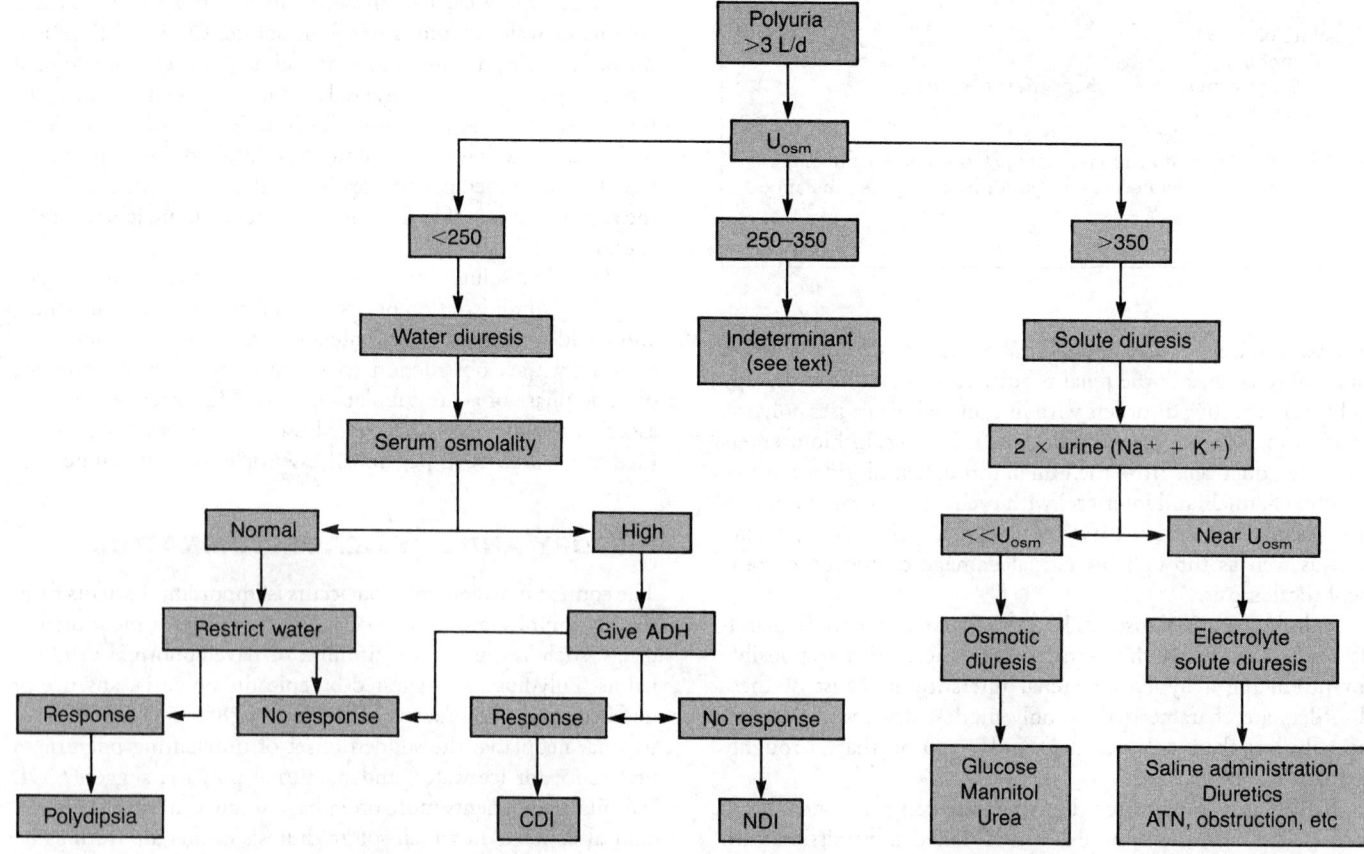

FIGURE 137.1. Approach to the diagnosis of polyuria. U_{osm}, urine osmolality; ADH, antidiuretic hormone; ATN, acute tubular necrosis; CDI, central diabetes insipidus; NDI, nephrogenic diabetes insipidus.
EVIDENCE LEVEL: C. Expert Opinion.

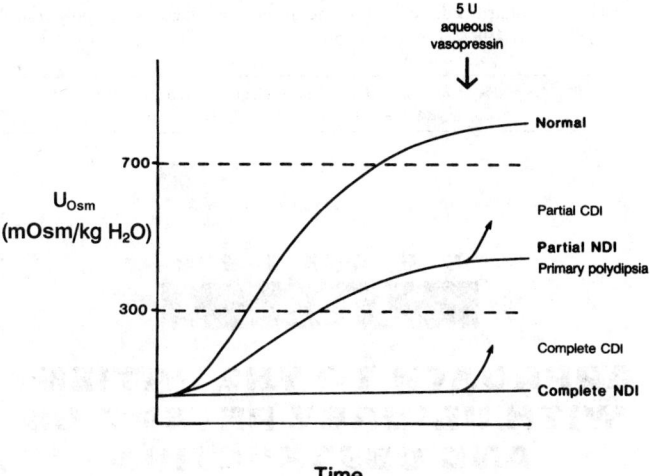

FIGURE 137.2. Idealized patterns of response of urine osmolality (U_{osm}) in the standard dehydration test. During dehydration, plasma osmolality and vasopressin levels rise, leading to a progressive increase in U_{osm} to more than 700 mOsm per kilogram in normal subjects. Patients with complete forms of diabetes insipidus have little or no increase in U_{osm} (U_{osm} less than plasma osmolality [P_{osm}]); patients with partial diabetes insipidus or primary polydipsia have intermediate rises in U_{osm} (maximal U_{osm} less than 700 mOsm per kilogram but more than P_{osm}). After the administration of 5 units of aqueous vasopressin, patients with partial or complete central diabetes insipidus (CDI) have large increases in U_{osm}, whereas normal subjects and patients with primary polydipsia have no increase in U_{osm}. Although shown as not responding to exogenous vasopressin, some patients with nephrogenic diabetes insipidus (NDI) experience an increase in U_{osm} in response to the pharmacologic plasma levels achieved.

DDAVP. If there is a response—that is, if the urine volume decreases and the urine osmolality increases (Fig. 137.2)—then the patient has CDI, and investigations should be directed toward establishing the cause. Computed tomography or magnetic resonance imaging of the hypothalamic area is indicated if the cause is not already known. If there is no response to ADH or DDAVP, then NDI is present, and appropriate investigations include assessment of renal function, urinalysis, and imaging of the urinary tract.

Dehydration Test

Patients who have water diuresis but are not hyperosmolar need to undergo a dehydration test to differentiate primary polydipsia from CDI or NDI. The idea behind a dehydration test is to restrict the water intake of the polyuric patient until the serum sodium has risen sufficiently to cause endogenous release of ADH; if the urine osmolality increases to a normal high value, the cause of polyuria is polydipsia. If there is no response, the possibilities are either CDI or NDI, which can be differentiated by the administration of ADH or DDAVP. Patients with CDI who have inadequate ADH secretion respond to ADH with an increase in urine osmolality, whereas patients with NDI, who already have endogenous release of ADH, do not.

Two important principles must guide the administration and interpretation of a dehydration test. The first is that patients with polyuria can become severely dehydrated if water deprivation is

carried out for too long, particularly if they do not respond with a reduction in urine volume. The second is that anyone with polyuria will have washed out the renal interstitial osmotic gradient, which may take days to regenerate.

With these principles in mind, the dehydration test is performed as follows. The duration of water deprivation before measurement of urine osmolality must be tailored to the patient and may range from only 4 to 6 hours in a patient with severe polyuria to the more usual 12 to 18 hours. Serum sodium, osmolality, and body weight should be measured frequently to assess the degree of water depletion, and no more than 3% of body weight should be lost. After the initial period of water deprivation, urine osmolality should be measured hourly; when the urine osmolality is no longer increasing by more than 30 mOsm per kilogram per hour, ADH (5 units of aqueous vasopressin subcutaneously) is given. Urine osmolality is again measured at 1 and 2 hours.

Characteristic responses to the dehydration test are shown in Fig. 137.2. A large increase in urine osmolality suggests CDI, whereas patients with either NDI or polydipsia have little increase. The urine osmolality does not rise to values seen in normal persons after water deprivation (more than 800 mOsm per kilogram) because of the time required to regenerate the interstitial osmotic gradient. This test clearly determines the diagnosis in most patients, but some are misdiagnosed; in ambiguous cases, measurement of plasma ADH levels may be required.

TREATMENT OF POLYURIA

Treatment of polyuria begins with diagnosing the underlying disorder and instituting both supportive and specific treatment. DDAVP is a V_2 receptor agonist that eliminates polyuria and polydipsia in CDI with few adverse effects. The dose required must be titrated to the individual but is given two or three times daily. The usual dose is 1 to 5 μg (0.03 to 0.15 μg per kilogram) intramuscularly or intravenously, 5 to 25 μg (0.15 to 0.75 μg per kilogram) intranasally, or 100 to 500 μg (3 to 15 μg per kilogram) orally. The main complication of DDAVP is water intoxication, manifesting as hyponatremia. If this occurs, DDAVP can be used at night to prevent nocturia and to allow polyuria and appropriate drinking during the daytime. Patients who are maintained on ADH therapy and who are admitted to the hospital should be continued on the same dose; their fluid intake needs to be adjusted to prevent erratic oscillations in urine output and plasma sodium concentration.

Partial CDI may be treated with DDAVP or chlorpropamide, which augments ADH release and its action on the collecting duct. The dose of chlorpropamide is 250 to 500 mg per day. The limiting side effect is hypoglycemia, and use of chlorpropamide should be avoided in patients with renal failure.

NDI is usually more difficult to treat but is often relatively mild and transient. Lithium-induced polyuria has been successfully treated with amiloride, which blocks lithium entry into collecting duct cells, and with indomethacin, which reduces prostaglandin inhibition of ADH action. Thiazide diuretics paradoxically improve many types of NDI, probably by lessening extracellular fluid volume and thereby limiting distal delivery of fluid by lowering the glomerular filtration rate and stimulating

TABLE 137.2.	CAUSES OF NOCTURIA

Nephrologic disorders
  Polyuria
  Nocturnal polyuria
  Chronic renal insufficiency
  Edematous state
    Congestive heart failure, cirrhosis, nephrotic syndrome
Urologic disorders
  Bladder outlet obstruction
    Urethral stricture, bladder or prostate carcinoma, benign
      prostatic hypertrophy
  Urinary tract infection
  Bladder calculi
  Bladder tumors

increased proximal resorption of salt and water. The treatment of polyuria in the recovery from acute renal failure or obstructive uropathy is to provide enough water and electrolyte solution until tubular function recovers.

NOCTURIA

Nocturia may be defined as urination at night with interruption of sleep. While it may occur at any age due to a variety of medical or surgical conditions affecting the kidney or lower urinary tract (Table 137.2), it is particularly common in the elderly. The prevalence may be as high as 80% by age 80. Nocturia in the elderly may be associated with impaired sleep quality, incontinence, and an increased risk of falls.

In normal adults, nocturia is avoided by an increase in ADH secretion at night, resulting in a lower urine flow rate. Nocturia arises as a result of either an increase in flow rate at night or reduced bladder capacity. Up to one-half of elderly patients with nocturia have an increase in nocturnal urine flow (without an increase in 24-hour urine flow), which has been attributed to loss of the normal circadian rhythm of ADH secretion and low ADH concentrations at night. In these patients, administration of DDAVP before bedtime may be successful in reducing nocturnal urine flow rates and alleviating nocturia.

BIBLIOGRAPHY

Asplund R, Sundberg B, Bengtsson P. Desmopressin for the treatment of nocturnal polyuria in the elderly: a dose titration study. *Br J Urol* 1998; 82:642–646.
Bichet DG. Nephrogenic diabetes insipidus. *Am J Med* 1998;105:431.
Donahue JL, Lowenthal DT. Nocturnal polyuria in the elderly person. *Am J Med Sci* 1997;314:232–238.
Oster JR, Singer I, Thatte L, et al. The polyuria of solute diuresis. *Arch Intern Med* 1997;157:721–729.
Richardson RMA. Water metabolism. *Curr Nephrol* 1994;17:81–120.
Robertson GL. Diabetes insipidus. *Endocrinol Metab Clin North Am* 1995; 24:549–572.
Zerbe RL, Robinson GL. A comparison of plasma vasopressin measurement

with a standard indirect test in the differential diagnosis of polyuria. *N Engl J Med* 1981;305:1539–1546.

Kelley's Textbook of Internal Medicine, fourth edition. Edited by H. David Humes. Lippincott Williams & Wilkins, Philadelphia © 2000.

C H A P T E R
138

APPROACH TO THE PATIENT WITH URINARY RETENTION AND OBSTRUCTION

NELSON LEUNG
AMIT K. GHOSH
KARL A. NATH

The presence of urinary tract obstruction, as for any disease process, is intimated by symptoms elicited from the medical history, signs detected during the physical examination, clues offered by laboratory and radiologic tests, and the appearance of syndromes of which urinary tract obstruction may be a contributing cause. Table 138.1 summarizes such varied signs and symptoms of urinary tract obstruction. These findings should lead the clinician to suspect the presence of underlying obstruction. By expeditiously securing the diagnosis, the condition can be effectively treated, thereby avoiding potentially irreversible renal failure and other complications. Chapter 158 provides further details regarding obstructive nephropathy.

DIFFERENTIAL DIAGNOSIS

Obstructive uropathy is caused by lesions that impede the flow of urine at any site along the tract, beginning at the renal calyxes and ending at the external urethral meatus. Congenital or developmental lesions account for the overwhelming majority of cases in children; however, a small percentage of such lesions escape detection in early life and may appear in the form of chronic renal insufficiency in adolescents or adults. Obstructive uropathy in adults, on the other hand, arises mainly from acquired lesions.

Obstruction of the upper tract can stem from lesions that are intrinsic or extrinsic to the urinary tract. Intrinsic lesions are further divided into intraluminal or intramural types (see Table 158.2). Intraluminal lesions may be located at either intrarenal or extrarenal sites. Causes of intraluminal obstruction include deposition of crystalline materials and proteinaceous casts. Medications can lead to obstruction either by intratubular precipitation (e.g., sulfonamide, acyclovir, indinavir, methotrexate) or by promotion of nephrolithiasis (e.g., acetazolamide, allopurinol, triamterene). Metabolic end products, such as uric acid, generated in excess, can provoke intraluminal obstruction, as occurs

TABLE 138.1.	PRESENTING FEATURES AND SYNDROMES OF URINARY TRACT OBSTRUCTION

Presenting Features and Syndromes	Possible Pathophysiological Implications
Symptoms	
Pain	
Ureteric colic	Acute obstruction usually due to calculus
Acute abdomen	Related to abdominal or pelvic diseases causing obstruction or to urinary calculi
Intermittent or low-grade pain	Chronic obstruction
Specific pain syndromes	Ureteropelvic junction obstruction or vesicoureteral reflux
Asymptomatic	Chronic obstruction
Urinary	
Hematuria	Stone, malignancy, mass, infection, papillary necrosis
Frequency, hesitancy, dribbling, incontinence, retention	Lower urinary tract obstruction
Alteration in urine output	
Oliguria/anuria	Acute renal failure, complete obstruction
Polyuria/nocturia	Partial obstruction
Oliguria alternating with polyuria	Intermittent obstruction
Systemic	
Fevers and chills	Urosepsis, papillary necrosis, extrarenal inflammatory conditions contributing to urinary tract obstruction
Uremic symptoms	Chronic obstruction causing renal failure
Signs	
Developmental/congenital lesions	Developmental lesions associated with obstruction
Abdominal/pelvic/rectal	
Abdominal/flank mass	Hydronephrotic kidney
Suprapubic mass	Palpable bladder
Abdominal or pelvic mass	Lesions causing obstruction
Enlarged prostate	Benign or malignant prostatic disease causing obstruction
Uremia-associated	
Fetor, asterixis, pigmentation, edema	Complete obstruction and renal failure
Malignancy-associated	
Cachexia, ascites, adenopathy, organomegaly	Pelvic mass or tumors
Neurologic deficit	Neurogenic bladder
Systemic hypertension	Volume overload or renin dependent
Systemic hypotension	Sepsis and associated urine tract obstruction, volume contraction from postobstructive diuresis
Laboratory findings	
Electrolyte abnormalities	
Hyperkalemic, hyperchloremic (type IV RTA) acidosis	Impaired acidification and tubular potassium secretion due to hypoaldosteronism or tubular resistance to aldosterone
Hyperchloremic acidosis without hyperkalemia	Acidification defect
Hyponatremia	Excessive free water intake in the context of renal insufficiency or salt-wasting nephritis
Hypernatremia	Postobstructive diuresis
Abnormal urinalysis	
Leukocyturia	Infection
Crystalluria	Stone, medications
Proteinuria	Vesicoureteral reflux
Other	
Polycythemia	Increased erythropoietin
Specific syndromes	
Acute or chronic renal failure	Bilateral obstruction or obstruction in solitary kidney
Acute or chronic renal failure	Bilateral obstruction or obstruction in solitary kidney diseased from other causes
UTI in males or recurrent UTIs in females	Chronic obstruction
Infection with unusual or urea-splitting organisms	Staghorn calculi and obstruction

UTI, urinary tract infection; RTA, renal tubular acidosis.

in acute uric acid nephropathy. Intraluminal renal obstruction may also be produced by casts due to paraproteins from plasma cell dyscrasias and casts formed from heme proteins and tubular epithelial cellular debris, as is seen in rhabdomyolysis.

Intraluminal causes in the upper tract include urinary calculi, blood clots, sloughed renal papillae, and fungus balls. Urinary calculi of a wide variety, including struvite, calcium oxalate, calcium phosphate, and cystine, can bring about urinary obstruction. Blood clots can arise from bleeding caused by trauma, calculi, tumors, or cysts or may develop as a complication of kidney biopsy. Sloughing of the renal papilla is a complication of analgesic abuse, diabetes mellitus, sickle cell disease, amyloid disease, tuberculosis, and acute pyelonephritis.

Intramural lesions may be functional, as in motility disorders affecting the ureteropelvic or the ureterovesical junctions, or structural, anchored within the walls (e.g., valves or strictures). Ureteropelvic junction obstruction originates from abnormalities in the architecture of the smooth muscle in the upper ureter and is a common cause of bilateral hydronephrosis in infants; this condition is usually unilateral when detected beyond the first year of life. This disorder should be considered in adults with obstruction, because many cases escape detection in childhood. Uncommon causes of obstructive uropathy in children are ureteral valves and strictures, conditions that usually affect the proximal and middle ureter, and ureteroceles that cause obstruction in the distal ureter. Ureteral strictures in adults are uncommon; they arise as a complication of radiation therapy, previous instrumentation, or surgery.

The ureterovesical junction is susceptible to a functional defect that causes obstructive uropathy infrequently in children. More common is vesicoureteral reflux, which may arise as either a primary or a secondary abnormality. In this disorder, there is reflux of urine from the bladder into the ureter during micturition. Such reflux does not normally occur, because of the oblique orientation of the ureter through the detrusor muscle and the arrangement of the muscle fibers of the ureterotrigonal unit. The primary disorder is congenital, and many cases resolve with age. Patients with vesicoureteral reflux are predisposed to recurrent infections; repeated episodes of infections involving the kidney in this context can lead to renal scarring. For unclear reasons, however, vesicoureteral reflux may also be associated with glomerulosclerosis and progressive renal insufficiency, despite treatment of infection and surgical correction of reflux.

Extrinsic lesions obstructing the upper tract can occur through five major mechanisms. *Vascular system* lesions include aberrant blood vessels at the ureteropelvic junction, perianeurysmal scarring from an abdominal aortic aneurysm, assorted vasculitides, and congenital "retrocaval" ureter obstructed by the vena cava. Lesions arising in the *female reproductive system* as a group are the most common causes of ureteric obstruction. By the end of the second trimester of pregnancy, most pregnant women show signs of dilatation of the collecting system. It usually involves the right ureter, generally does not perturb renal function, and abates in the postpartum period. Renal insufficiency due to urinary tract obstruction during pregnancy occurs very infrequently as a complication of such conditions as twin pregnancies and polyhydramnios. Cervical cancer is the most common malignant cause for obstructive uropathy in women; other uterine lesions that can obstruct the ureter include benign fibroids, malignancies, and uterine prolapse. Ureteral obstruction may also arise from ovarian tumors, ovarian abscesses, and endometriosis.

Lesions and pathologic conditions in the *gastrointestinal tract*, such as inflammatory bowel disease, diverticular disease, and malignancies, can also compress the ureters. Inflammatory bowel disease may predispose to obstruction because of associated nephrolithiasis. Crohn's disease and appendicular abscess may provoke right-sided hydronephrosis, whereas diverticular disease can obstruct the left ureter. Obstruction to the ureter also can originate in the *retroperitoneum*, as exemplified by idiopathic retroperitoneal fibrosis and assorted retroperitoneal tumors that develop de novo or as a consequence of metastatic disease. Retroperitoneal fibrosis can arise as a complication of radiation, malignancy, infection, perianeurysmal scarring, or scarring triggered by inflammatory processes in the intestinal tract. It also can come about as an adverse effect of medications such as methysergide, methyldopa, sotalol, and other β-adrenergic antagonist agents. Extrinsic compression of the ureters can develop as a result of inadvertent ligatures and other complications of *surgery*.

Obstruction of the lower tract can arise from such bladder lesions as blood clots, stones, tumors, foreign bodies, or infections or from neurogenic bladder. In males, lesions affecting this site include strictures, valves, stones, meatal stenosis, and phimosis. The bladder neck and urethra are constricted in older men by prostatic hypertrophy or carcinoma. Benign prostatic hyperplasia is a common and significant disorder because it provokes bladder outlet obstruction in more than 75% of men older than 50 years, necessitating surgery in 10% of these symptomatic patients. Prostate cancer can cause obstructive uropathy by occluding such sites as the bladder neck or the ureters as they enter the bladder.

A wide variety of neurogenic bladders can predispose to urinary tract obstruction. Reflex neurogenic bladder is found in patients with spinal cord injury or multiple sclerosis and is attended by high intravesical pressure, vesicoureteral reflux, and obstructive nephropathy. Patients with diabetes are often devoid of bladder sensation; this, in turn, leads to large bladder volumes before the micturition reflex is triggered and predisposes these patients to vesicoureteral reflux. Infrasacral neurogenic bladder arises from motor and sensory neural deficits and is seen as a complication of pelvic surgery.

Obstruction to the urethra occurs virtually exclusively in males and stems from posterior urethral valves or strictures as a result of complication from trauma, gonorrhea, or previous instrumentation. Bladder dysfunction can be an adverse effect of a number of medications, including anticholinergics, antihistamines, narcotic analgesics, and α-adrenergic agonists. In the transplanted kidney, urinary tract obstruction in the early postoperative period reflects blood clots, mechanical problems (e.g., twisting of the ureter), ischemia of the ureter, and extrinsic compression by a lymphocele. Later, obstruction may be due to ureteric fibrosis from ischemia or rejection.

■ HISTORY AND PHYSICAL EXAMINATION

The first step in evaluation is a detailed history and physical examination. A common initial complaint is pain. Acute obstruction arising from calculi and blood clots is often associated with severe flank and abdominal pain radiating into the groin. During these episodes, the patient is never pain-free and experiences intense paroxysms superimposed on a background of unremitting pain. Acute flank pain, low-grade fever, hematuria, and the passage of tissue in the urine are features of papillary necrosis. In contrast, chronic hydronephrosis may be associated with a dull ache or may be asymptomatic. Flank pain during micturition is characteristic of vesicoureteral reflux. Flank pain exacerbated by a large oral fluid intake or diuretics suggests ureteropelvic obstruction. Abnormalities in the urine, such as unusual discoloration or the presence of blood, stones, or tissue, should raise the suspicion of urinary tract obstruction.

Altered urine output may also be an initial feature. Complete obstruction leads to anuria, whereas partial obstruction can impose polyuria and nocturia; intermittent obstruction may appear as fluctuating urinary output. A single episode of urinary tract infection in males or recurrent urinary tract infections in females can also be a manifestation of underlying urinary tract obstruction. Patients should be asked about symptoms pointing to abnormalities of the lower urinary tract, including urgency, frequency, hesitancy, a poor urinary stream, terminal dribbling, dysuria, strangury, and nocturia.

Particular attention should be given to a personal or family history of kidney stones and cystic or other kidney diseases. Medications relevant to obstructive uropathy should also be carefully reviewed, including those that cause crystal formation in the urine, those that impair bladder function, and analgesics. Diseases that can predispose to obstructive uropathy, such as diabetes mellitus, multiple sclerosis, inflammatory bowel disease, and sickle cell disease, should be noted or specific inquires made as to their presence. A history of recurrent urinary tract infections, sexually transmitted infections, AIDS, and tuberculosis may also be relevant, since urinary tract obstruction can develop as complications of these disorders or their treatment.

A careful physical examination should be performed to ascertain the presence, cause, and complications of obstruction to the urinary tract. A general examination may uncover such features of the uremic syndrome as fetor, uremic pigmentation, and pallor of the mucous membranes or cachexia arising from an underlying malignancy. Systemic hypertension and signs of volume overload may reflect underlying high-grade obstructions, whereas signs of dehydration and orthostatic hypotension may develop in patients with postobstructive diuresis. Fever and rigors suggest a superimposed infection. Obstructive uropathy may be a complication of previous surgical procedures, and, for this reason, abdominal incisions should be noted.

The abdomen should be palpated for tenderness, guarding, bladder distention, enlargement and tenderness of the kidney, organomegaly, masses, and ascites. Abdominal aortic pulsations or abdominal bruits suggest an aortic aneurysm. Bowel sounds should be carefully auscultated, because several causes of obstructive uropathy can predispose to ileus. Rectal and pelvic examinations are essential components of the physical examination, since they can uncover pathologic conditions that lead to obstructive uropathy. The rectal examination may find an enlarged prostate, nodularity of the prostate, and rectal masses. During the pelvic examination, attention should be paid to any vaginal, pelvic, or

rectal mass or prolapse. Examination of the penis can disclose evidence of meatal stenosis or phimosis. Lymphadenopathy in the inguinal or other areas or tenderness over the bony skeleton raises the possibility of an underlying malignancy. A careful neurologic examination is also indicated, since neurogenic bladder can cause obstructive uropathy. Special attention should be paid to possible signs of diabetic neuropathy, spinal cord injuries, or multiple sclerosis, because these diseases can contribute to the development of neurogenic bladder.

■ LABORATORY STUDIES

Measurements of serum electrolytes and renal function must be obtained. Blood urea nitrogen (BUN) and serum creatinine levels may be elevated if there is bilateral obstruction, obstruction in a solitary kidney, or obstruction in one kidney with intrinsic disease in the other or both kidneys. In the absence of volume contraction or other conditions that disproportionately elevate the BUN, the ratio of BUN to serum creatinine is approximately $10:1$. Serum electrolyte measurements can show evidence of hyperchloremic metabolic acidosis accompanied by hyperkalemia, which usually bespeaks type IV renal tubular acidosis. Less commonly, hyperchloremic metabolic acidosis arises from a type I acidification defect in which the serum potassium level is normal or low.

Hyponatremia may be present and may reflect excess free water intake in the context of renal insufficiency; rarely, it may be due to renal salt wasting. Alternatively, hypernatremia may be present as the result of polyuria and excess free water loss. Acute obstruction may lead the fractional excretion of sodium to be less than 1 and cause urine osmolality to be more than 400 mOsm per kilogram of water, spuriously suggesting prerenal causes of renal failure. With chronic obstruction, the loss of concentrating ability leads to reduced specific gravity and osmolality of urine.

The urinary sediment is usually nondescript, showing trace to 1 + proteinuria and hyaline casts. Proteinuria of greater severity may accompany chronic renal insufficiency due to obstruction, and nephrotic-range proteinuria may occur in the context of vesicoureteral reflux and accompanying glomerulosclerosis. The presence of leukocytes and bacteria points to urinary tract infection. Red cells suggest bleeding, stones, malignancy, or papillary necrosis. Urinary crystals may indicate the presence and type of urinary calculi.

■ DIAGNOSTIC TESTS

Figure 138.1 shows an approach that can be used to evaluate patients in whom obstructive uropathy is suspected. The presence of symptoms and signs pointing to obstruction of the lower tract should lead to the assessment of the postvoid residual. A postvoid residual urine volume should be determined by catheterization of the urinary bladder; a volume above 100 ml suggests lower-tract obstruction. If insertion of a Foley catheter into the urinary bladder proves difficult or obstruction is encountered,

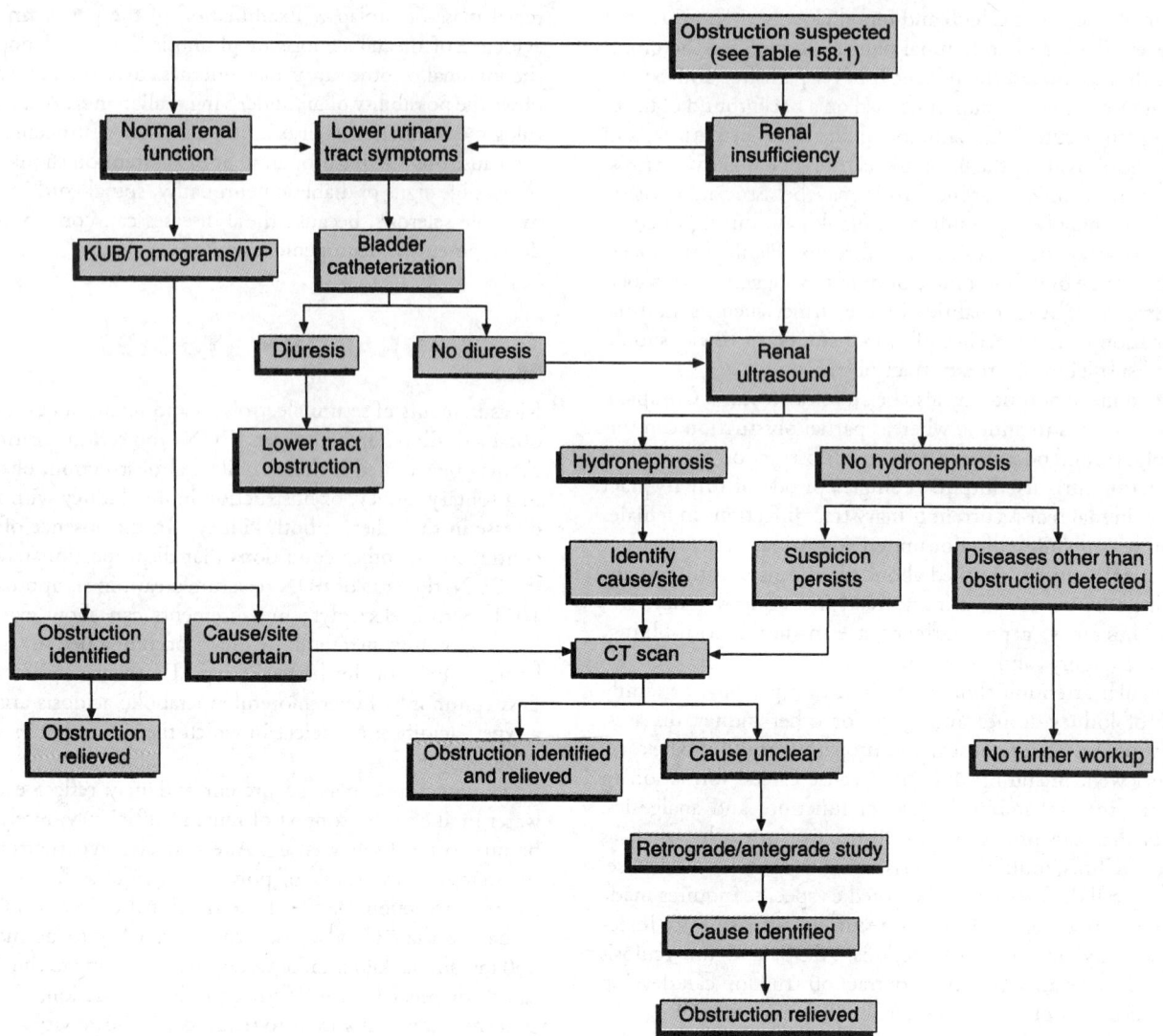

FIGURE 138.1. Approach to the patient with suspected urinary obstruction.
EVIDENCE LEVEL: C. Expert Opinion.

repeated attempts may traumatize the urethra or bladder. The expertise of urologists should be sought in such cases to catheterize the bladder or establish drainage of the urinary tract by a suprapubic catheter. If a large residual of urine is encountered, the bladder can be freely decompressed, because rapid decompression of the bladder does not predispose to hypotension or bladder hemorrhage.

Several visualization procedures are available. Each has its advantages and drawbacks. A plain film of the abdomen is usually obtained, because it can detect calculi (in approximately 80% to 90% of cases) and may provide information as to the size and shape of the kidneys and the presence of soft-tissue masses or bony metastatic disease. While it is inexpensive, a plain abdominal film is limited by its low sensitivity and specificity.

Ultrasonography is the recommended screening test for urinary tract obstruction. It relies on detecting dilatation of the urinary tract. It is noninvasive and does not require the use of intravenous contrast, making it particularly useful for patients with acute and chronic renal failure. The absence of radiation

makes ultrasonography safe for pregnant patients. This method has 90% sensitivity and 80% specificity in the diagnosis of obstructive uropathy. Nonobstructive dilatation of the upper tract can occur in several conditions, however; conversely, obstruction is not always detected by ultrasonography (Table 158.1 in Chapter 158).

An intravenous pyelogram (IVP) makes visible the kidney, calyxes, pelvis, and ureter and may localize the level of obstruction. It is the initial test of choice in examining the pyelocalyceal system and ureter in patients with normal renal function. The findings of an IVP depend on the degree and the duration of obstruction. In acute cases, the nephrogram is delayed but eventually attains a higher density than the normal kidney; the kidney is enlarged, and the collecting system is dilated above the obstruction. With chronic obstruction, the cortex is thin, the calyxes are dilated, the papilla is flattened and may be frankly concave, and the calyxes may have a clubbed appearance. In bladder outlet obstruction, both ureters are usually dilated, and bladder trabeculation or diverticula may also be present. An IVP may also suggest the presence of retroperitoneal fibrosis if there is medial deviation of the ureters. The adverse effects of IVP include allergic reactions to contrast dye and the nephrotoxicity of these agents. The latter is more likely to occur in patients with renal insufficiency, multiple myeloma, and diabetic nephropathy.

While intravenous pyelography and ultrasonography are typically employed as initial radiologic tests for urinary tract obstruction, computed tomography (CT) is increasingly utilized in this context. Improved anatomic imaging and lack of intravenous contrast are appealing features of CT scans, especially in patients with contrast dye allergy or poor renal function. Noncontrast CT scans can uncover calculi, dilatation of the collecting system, atrophy, and other changes of the renal parenchyma, and delayed excretion of contrast can be detected with contrast enhancement. CT scans can detect other abnormalities that impose urinary tract obstruction, including malignancies, abdominal lymphadenopathy, retroperitoneal fibrosis, hematomas, and calculi. Magnetic resonance imaging provides remarkable anatomic detail and renal functional measurements and does not require the use of contrast agents. Its expense and its inability to detect stones and parenchymal changes limit its uses, however. This imaging technique is not currently part of the routine evaluation of patients with suspected urinary tract obstruction.

Although diuretic scintigraphy is inferior to IVP in terms of anatomic detail, it is helpful in differentiating a dilated nonobstructed collecting system from true obstruction. In this test, renal scintigraphy is performed before and after the administration of a loop diuretic, such as furosemide. Diuresis facilitates washout of the isotope that accumulates in the dilated, nonobstructed renal pelvis but not in the pelvis with true anatomic obstruction.

Retrograde and antegrade pyelography calls for direct injection of contrast dye into the collecting system and may be indicated for patients suspected of having obstructive uropathy. It is particularly useful for patients with contrast dye allergy or those with renal insufficiency, in whom the administration of contrast dye can exacerbate renal dysfunction. These procedures usually allow identification of the site of obstruction and the presence of intraluminal and intramural lesions. Retrograde pyelography necessitates catheterization of the ureter after cystoscopy and may require general anesthesia. Antegrade pyelography allows entry into the renal pelvis via a percutaneous route under ultrasonographic guidance and local anesthesia. These tests also have therapeutic value, since they allow the placement of stents during a retrograde study or a percutaneous nephrostomy tube during an antegrade study.

The Whitaker test may be used to diagnose obstruction of the upper urinary tract when its presence is deemed uncertain using other diagnostic maneuvers. In this test, hydrostatic pressure differences between the renal pelvis and bladder are determined at ambient urinary flow and after the infusion of fluid into the renal pelvis at a defined rate. With significant ureteral obstruction, a pressure differential of more than 20 cm water usually indicates ureteral obstruction.

Lower-tract obstruction can be evaluated by cystoscopy and radiologic and urodynamic tests. Cystoscopy makes visible the entire urethra and bladder. The anterior urethra is assessed by retrograde urethrography. The posterior urethra can be seen by excretory or antegrade cystography. A voiding cystourethrogram is used to detect the presence of vesicoureteral reflux, the function of the bladder, and the presence of bladder neck and urethral abnormalities. Urodynamic evaluation is used in the diagnosis of neurogenic bladder dysfunction; this evaluation includes cystometrography, electromyography, a urethral pressure profile, and urine flowmetry.

■ MANAGEMENT

The aims of treatment of patients with obstructive uropathy include the relief of symptoms, the correction of fluid and electrolyte abnormalities, the restoration and preservation of renal function, and the prevention or effective treatment of complications, such as infection or stone formation. The therapeutic approach varies with the clinical circumstance: it may be conservative or may include the use of instrumentation, endourologic techniques, or surgical procedures. High-grade or total obstruction affecting both kidneys or high-grade obstruction in a solitary kidney must be relieved as soon as possible. Relief of obstruction of any severity should be promptly undertaken if there is concomitant urosepsis. In patients with renal failure as a complication of bilateral obstruction, dialysis may be indicated for fluid and electrolyte abnormalities. Severe volume overload, hyperkalemia, and acidosis mandate acute dialysis before relief of the obstruction. Surgical intervention for chronic partial low-grade obstruction can be delayed for several weeks, but such an obstruction should be expeditiously decompressed if there are repeated episodes of urinary tract infection, urinary retention, significant flank pain, and progressive renal insufficiency.

Decompression may be effected by percutaneous nephrostomy tubes or retrograde ureteral catheters. For lower-tract obstruction, relief is afforded by bladder catheterization or, rarely, suprapubic cystostomy. Complications of nephrostomy tubes include perirenal hematomas, acute obstruction due to blood clots, infection, and dislodgment of the tube. Indwelling stents may ensure patency of the collecting system for months, but their use can be complicated by blockage, migration into the bladder, urinary reflux, pain, hematuria, and infection. Indwelling ureteral stents minimize uremic symptoms and may be used instead of an ileal conduit in such poor-risk patients as those with advanced or incurable malignancy.

The prognosis after the relief of obstruction to the urinary tract depends on its underlying cause, severity, and duration and the development of complications during the obstructive and postobstructive phases. A remarkable recovery of the glomerular filtration rate, often to normal values, may take place in kidneys subjected to obstruction lasting several days. The longer the period of obstruction, the more attenuated is the regaining of renal function after decompression. As demonstrated by studies of experimental obstructive uropathy, however, obstruction of only 24 hours' duration in the rat leads to irreversible loss of a fraction of nephrons; thus, functional recovery does not reflect the irreversible damage inflicted on the kidney even with relatively short periods of obstruction. Defects in the concentrating ability and acidification mechanisms may persist for protracted periods after relief of obstruction.

The relief of bilateral obstruction or obstruction of a solitary kidney gives rise to a postobstructive diuresis characterized by polyuria and natriuresis and the loss of solutes, including potassium, magnesium, phosphate, and calcium. Natriuresis and diuresis may lead to marked contraction of the extracellular fluid and, depending on the relative losses, hyponatremia or hypernatremia; hypokalemia, hypomagnesemia, and hypophosphatemia may be present. This syndrome does not develop after the relief of unilateral obstruction. Postobstructive diuresis is multifactorial in origin and reflects the excretion of salt and water retained during the phase of obstruction, the renal effects of natriuretic factors, osmotic diuresis from retained urea, renal resistance to vasopressin, and defective tubular sodium absorption. If patients are euvolemic, half-normal saline should be infused at 50 to 75 ml per hour, with careful assessment of orthostatic changes in blood pressure and pulse, plasma electrolytes, and renal function. This regimen allows the excretion of salt and water retained during the obstructive phase and avoids excessive fluid administration that may sustain continued diuresis and natriuresis. If extracellular fluid volume contraction develops on this regimen such that orthostatic changes occur, additional amounts of fluid should be provided to repair the loss. Excessive administration of salt and water should also be avoided, however, since this will perpetuate diuresis. Serum potassium, calcium, magnesium, and phosphate levels should be carefully monitored, because replacement of these solutes may be required.

LOWER-TRACT OBSTRUCTION

Lower-tract obstruction should be relieved if it is complicated by urinary retention, recurrent episodes of urinary tract infection, hematuria, vesicoureteral reflux, or renal parenchymal damage. If such symptoms or complications arise from benign prostatic hyperplasia, transurethral resection of the prostate is the preferred procedure. This procedure has a mortality rate of less than 0.5%. Before prostatectomy, patients with urinary retention or compromised renal function should be treated with clean intermittent catheterization, which reduces the risks of perioperative urinary tract infections. Open prostatectomy may be required in patients with marked enlargement of the prostate.

Medical management of prostatic hyperplasia now includes such classes of drugs as 5α-reductase inhibitors (e.g., finasteride) and α-1-adrenergic receptor blockers (e.g., terazosin, doxazosin, and tamsulosin). The 5α-reductase inhibitors block the conversion of testosterone to dihydrotestosterone and thereby attenuate the humoral stimulus for prostatic hyperplasia; prostatic volume is thus reduced. The α-1-adrenergic receptor blockers decrease the tone of the internal urethral sphincter. Both classes of drugs relieve urinary tract obstruction and attendant symptoms. Cessation of either class of drug may lead to recrudescence of symptoms of lower-tract obstruction. Pharmacologic approaches should not be used in patients with urinary tract dilatation or renal insufficiency. In compromised or debilitated patients or patients with advanced malignancy, long-term indwelling catheters or prostatic stents may be considered. Lower-tract obstruc-

tion arising from strictures in males can be treated by urethral dilatation, endoscopic urethrotomy, or an open procedure.

Treatment of patients with neurogenic bladder depends, to some extent, on the cause. Clean intermittent catheterization is the basis of therapy for most forms of neurogenic bladder dysfunction. Reflex neurogenic bladder dysfunction, which occurs in patients with spinal cord injury and multiple sclerosis, is characterized by the release of the sacral reflex arc from inhibitory input, increased detrusor tone, and failure of the internal urethral sphincter to relax. This condition may be treated by clean intermittent catheterization in conjunction with anticholinergic agents. Attempting to decrease the tone of the internal urethral sphincter by using α-adrenergic blockers or skeletal muscle relaxants is another therapeutic approach. Patients with sensory neurogenic bladders experience an increase in bladder volume before contraction occurs; these patients are treated initially by voiding at regular intervals and subsequently by clean intermittent catheterization when they are unable to void. The use of cholinergic agents in these patients is the subject of debate. Clean intermittent catheterization is also used for patients with autonomous neurogenic bladder, a lesion characterized by motor and sensory deficits. Long-term indwelling catheters should be eschewed in patients with neurogenic bladder because of the risks of infection, stone formation, and carcinoma of the bladder. In patients with neurogenic bladder and other forms of lower-tract obstruction, surgical diversion using an ileal conduit may be required if there is progressive loss of renal function, refractory incontinence, or multiple bladder fistulas.

UPPER-TRACT OBSTRUCTION

Acute, high-grade, bilateral obstruction should be promptly decompressed, since delay increases the risk of irreversible loss of function. Acute partial obstruction is commonly caused by calculi in the renal pelvis or ureter. Patients with these stones can be treated as outpatients if they can tolerate large amounts of oral liquids, which are required to facilitate spontaneous passage of the stone. Relief of pain in acute renal colic usually requires intramuscular injection of narcotic analgesics. Stones smaller than 5 mm invariably pass spontaneously; ureteral stones 5 to 7 mm in size may require weeks to do so. Urine should be strained so that any calculi passed can be submitted for analysis. Stones larger than 7 mm usually necessitate intervention.

Extracorporeal shock-wave lithotripsy (ESWL) can be used for most types of kidney stones (except cystine stones) in the renal pelvis, upper ureter, and middle ureter. In this procedure, stones are pulverized by shock waves created by electrohydraulic, electro-acoustic, or ultrasonic means. Patients require anesthesia or sedation. Over subsequent weeks, the remains of the calculi are passed. Calculi distal to the pelvic brim are usually treated by ureteroscopy combined with stone extraction for smaller calculi or stone fragmentation for larger calculi. To secure the patency of the urinary tract and to ensure passage of the stone fragments, ureteral stents are often used in conjunction with ESWL. More details of renal stone disease are found in Chapters 139 and 159.

A surgical approach is used for several lesions. For example, intramural lesions, such as ureteropelvic junction obstruction, ureteral valves, or ureterovesical junction obstruction, can be surgically repaired; mass lesions of the renal pelvis or ureter are often amenable to resection. Surgical procedures, including ureterolysis, are also required to relieve obstruction caused by idiopathic retroperitoneal fibrosis or fibrosis stemming from such conditions as abdominal aneurysm. Sometimes repair is impossible, and urinary diversion may be necessary.

BIBLIOGRAPHY

Klahr S. Urinary tract obstruction. In: Schrier RW, Gottschalk CW, eds. *Diseases of the kidney.* Boston: Little, Brown, 1997:709–738.

Koch MO. Disorders of micturition. In: Jacobson HR, Striker GE, Klahr S, eds. *The principles and practice of nephrology.* St. Louis: Mosby, 1995: 315–321.

Lepor H, Williford WO, Barry MJ, et al. The efficacy of terazosin, finasteride, or both in benign prostatic hyperplasia. *N Engl J Med* 1996;335: 533–539.

McConnell JD, Bruskewitz R, Walsh P, et al. The effect of finasteride on the risk of acute urinary retention and the need for surgical treatment among men with benign prostatic hyperplasia. *N Engl J Med* 1998;338: 557–563.

Milam DF. Causes of upper urinary tract obstruction. In: Jacobson HR, Striker GE, Klahr S, eds. *The principles and practice of nephrology.* St. Louis: Mosby, 1995:298–306.

Walsh PC. Treatment of benign prostatic hyperplasia [Editorial]. *N Engl J Med* 1996;335:586–587.

Kelley's Textbook of Internal Medicine, fourth edition. Edited by H. David Humes. Lippincott Williams & Wilkins, Philadelphia © 2000.

CHAPTER
139

APPROACH TO THE PATIENT WITH NEPHROLITHIASIS

REBECA D. MONK
DAVID A. BUSHINSKY

PRESENTATION

The typical patient with an acute episode of renal colic is not difficult to identify. The discomfort is severe, described by many women as similar to that associated with childbirth. The pain often originates in the flank, radiating anteriorly toward the groin as the stone moves along the ureter toward the bladder. The patient also may experience dysuria, gross hematuria, urgency, and frequency. Stone passage confers almost instant relief of the pain. Associated urinary tract infection or obstruction contributes significantly to morbidity, but death related to nephrolithiasis is rare.

The lifetime risk of stone disease in industrialized nations approaches 20% in men, a rate three to five times greater than in women. The peak age of onset is in the twenties for both sexes. Professionals, despite better working conditions, are af-

fected more often than manual laborers and whites more often than Asian Americans or African Americans.

PATHOPHYSIOLOGY

Stone formation occurs only in the context of urine that is overly saturated with respect to the ionic components of the stone. When this oversaturation, which depends on chemical free-ion activity, reaches the so-called formation product, the relevant ions form clusters or small nuclei by a process termed *homogeneous nucleation.* More often, crystals form around different particles, such as sloughed epithelial cells, casts, or other types of crystals, by *heterogeneous nucleation.* For example, calcium oxalate crystals commonly nucleate around existing uric acid crystals, producing stones composed of both calcium oxalate and uric acid. Thus, when searching for the cause of stones, the urine must be carefully evaluated for concentrations of all relevant constituents, because several different ions may contribute to stone development.

Once nuclei are formed, they rapidly cluster together through a process termed *aggregation.* To prevent the nuclei from washing away in the urine flow before a sizable stone can be produced, the nuclei must anchor to the urothelial surface in a manner that is incompletely understood. Various proteins produced by the kidney (e.g., uropontin, nephrocalcin, Tamm-Horsfall mucoprotein) can inhibit distinct phases of stone formation. Deficiencies in any of these urinary inhibitors can potentiate nephrolithiasis.

Decreasing urinary oversaturation, which is possible through medical management, can prevent stone formation. To lessen the oversaturation of calcium oxalate crystals, for example, the solution volume in which the calcium and oxalate are suspended can be increased by drinking more fluids to expand urine volume or decreased by the concentrations of calcium and oxalate in the urine through dietary modifications or medications. The solubility of calcium also can be augmented by increasing the amount of citrate excreted with it. Manipulation of the urine pH also can affect ionic solubility, especially with respect to uric acid.

HISTORY AND PHYSICAL EXAMINATION

The approach to patients with a single episode of nephrolithiasis is outlined in Table 139.1. Additional studies for children and for patients with a second stone or multiple stones or with calculi that are increasing in size are outlined in Table 139.2. All patients with nephrolithiasis, even first-time stone-formers, should have a thorough history and physical examination to determine the cause of their stone disease and to formulate a management plan. Demographic data, such as age, sex, and race, are useful in determining whether a basic or a more complete evaluation is required. A patient in whom stone disease is unexpected (e.g., a child or an African American) must undergo a complete evaluation to exclude a significant underlying pathologic condition.

A stone history also provides essential data. The age at first

TABLE 139.1.   APPROACH TO PATIENTS WITH A SINGLE STONE

Collect and analyze all stones
History
  Medical risk factors
    Family history
    Malignant neoplasm
    Skeletal disease
    Inflammatory bowel disease
    Intestinal bypass
    Urinary tract infection
  Environmental risk factors
    Fluid restriction
    Urine volume
    Climate
    Occupation
    Immobilization
    Diet
    Medications
Physical examination
Laboratory
  Urinalysis ± culture
  Urine for cystine
  Blood
    Calcium ± parathyroid hormone
    Phosphorus
    Uric acid
    Electrolytes
    Creatinine
Radiologic
  Kidney, ureters, bladder
  Intravenous urography ± tomograms

stone formation, the number of stones present or passed, the size of calculi, and whether lithotripsy or surgery was required can help determine the severity and sometimes the source of nephrolithiasis. Calcium oxalate stones, for example, tend to grow no larger than 2 cm, whereas struvite and cystine stones can grow very large, forming staghorn calculi. The latter also

TABLE 139.2.   APPROACH TO PATIENTS WITH A SECOND OR MULTIPLE STONES OR GROWING STONES AND FOR ALL CHILDREN

As for single stone, plus
  24-h urine
    Volume
    pH
    Calcium
    Phosphate
    Sodium
    Uric acid
    Oxalate
    Citrate
    Creatinine
Repeat 24-h urine to monitor compliance and effectiveness of treatment.
Specialized testing is not recommended for most patients.

are distinctive in that they are refractory to fragmentation with extracorporeal shock-wave lithotripsy (ESWL) and often must be removed by percutaneous nephrolithotomy. Symptoms of hematuria and flank pain indicate active stone disease.

Exact chromosomal loci have not yet been discovered, but certain stone disorders exhibit clear hereditary patterns; thus, obtaining a family history is important. Idiopathic hypercalciuria is inherited, though the mechanism of inheritance is unclear. Cystinuria follows an autosomal recessive pattern. Uric acid lithiasis also may be associated with various genetic enzyme defects.

A complete medical history is crucial not only to diagnosing a particular stone type but also to elucidating important secondary causes of nephrolithiasis. In patients in whom hypercalcemia is a potential cause of hypercalciuria, evidence should be sought for systemic disorders that may lead to an elevated serum calcium concentration, such as malignancy, hyperparathyroidism, thyrotoxicosis, granulomatous disease, and immobilization. Uric acid stones may be associated with gout, inflammatory bowel disease, and various inborn errors of metabolism. A history of recurring urinary tract infections should alert one to the possibility of struvite stones. Nephrocalcinosis—the generation of numerous small calcifications within the kidney—often results from calcium phosphate precipitation in the high urinary pH associated with distal renal tubular acidosis.

A complete list of medications, both prescribed and over-the-counter drugs, must be obtained. Antacids and carbonic anhydrase inhibitors, such as acetazolamide, can raise the urinary pH, providing an optimal environment for calcium phosphate stone precipitation. Calcium-containing antacids can worsen stone generation by increasing the amount of calcium ingested and subsequently filtered by the kidneys. Loop diuretics (e.g., furosemide, bumetanide, torsemide) can diminish renal calcium reabsorption, thereby increasing urinary calcium concentration and producing oversaturation. Thiazide diuretics are often used to treat hypercalciuria because they lessen renal calcium excretion. They tend to diminish uric acid excretion, however, which may be detrimental to patients with complications of hyperuricemia. Certain medications can precipitate into crystals or stones. These include triamterene, a potassium-sparing diuretic; acyclovir, when rapidly administered intravenously; and indinavir, an antiretroviral medication used to treat HIV. Large doses of vitamin C (ascorbic acid) can potentially result in hyperoxaluria in some patients, as ascorbic acid is oxidized to oxalate. Excessive vitamin D ingestion can generate hypercalciuria by augmenting both intestinal calcium absorption and bone resorption.

Information on the patient's habits and occupation can provide important clues. For example, people with jobs that require commutes by car or who engage in intensive activity that allows little time for bathroom breaks, such as cardiothoracic surgeons, may limit their fluid intake to avoid having to urinate, resulting in very concentrated urine and marked oversaturation. Patients who exercise or work outdoors may have increased insensible losses that also result in more concentrated urine. Severely disabled, bedridden patients may become hypercalcemic and hypercalciuric as a result of immobilization-induced bone resorption.

Dietary factors have a significant effect on stone formation. Metabolism of animal protein induces mild metabolic acidosis that stimulates bone resorption, leading to an increased filtered load of calcium and a decline in tubular calcium reabsorption and hypercalciuria. Calcium solubility is further reduced by hypocitraturia, which may result from metabolic acidosis. Meats and other purine-containing foods also augment uric acid excretion, increasing the potential for both calcium-based and uric acid stones. A markedly excessive intake of oxalate-containing foods also can contribute to calcium oxalate nephrolithiasis. Foods rich in oxalate include certain leafy green vegetables, such as Swiss chard, kale, spinach, and mustard greens, as well as tea, chocolate, nuts, and rhubarb.

Calcium consumption should be assessed in hypercalciuric patients but should not be restricted unless intake is exorbitant. Diminished calcium intake in hypercalciuric patients can result in a net negative calcium balance, with ensuing bone resorption. A recent study also suggests that the rate of stone formation may be higher in patients with lower calcium intakes, possibly owing to enhanced oxalate absorption. Sodium intake and excretion directly correlate with calcium excretion.

To obtain accurate dietary information, it is useful to ask patients details about the contents of each meal, snacks, how many glasses of fluid they drink, consumption of fast foods or canned foods (both high in sodium), and rare food fetishes. The physical examination in patients with stone disease who are not experiencing renal colic is usually normal. Tophi, abdominal scars, and ileostomies or lymphadenopathy or other evidence of malignancy suggest metabolic abnormalities that can lead to stone formation.

LABORATORY STUDIES AND DIAGNOSTIC TESTS

The most common methods for analyzing stone composition are x-ray crystallography and infrared spectroscopy. Information on the constituents of the stone exterior and the core can be obtained, focusing therapy on measures that can lower the levels of those substances in the urine. Urinalysis is simple and inexpensive but often provides critical insights into the mechanisms of stone formation in a particular patient. An elevated urinary pH (more than 7) is associated with the formation of struvite and calcium phosphate stones; uric acid stones tend to form in more acid urine (pH less than 6). On microscopic examination, characteristic crystals may be noted. Bacteria and white blood cells, if present, may indicate the presence of infection stones, and hematuria suggests active stone disease. If pyuria is detected, a urine culture should be obtained, not only for proper antibiotic selection but also to determine whether urease-producing bacteria are responsible for both the calculi and the infection. Fewer than 100,000 colonies of urease-producing bacteria can still be responsible for producing infection stones. If struvite stones are suspected, the microbiology laboratory should be instructed to identify all organisms, regardless of colony count.

In all patients, even those with a single stone, the laboratory evaluation in Table 139.1 is warranted; the blood chemistry profile should include electrolytes, creatinine, calcium, phosphorus, and uric acid levels and, if the serum calcium is high, the parathyroid hormone level. Qualitative cystine screening of the urine should be performed on all patients.

Radiologic evaluation is an important step in determining the location and presence of stones. The size, location, number, and radiopacity of the calculi may be ascertained with a radiograph of the kidney, ureter, and bladder. Intravenous urography can provide additional information, such as the presence of anatomic abnormalities of the urinary tract, medullary sponge kidney, and obstruction. If roentgenographic examination is contraindicated, as in pregnancy, ultrasonography can be used. Although ultrasonography is safe for all patients, it can miss ureteral calculi and cannot distinguish between stones that are radiopaque (e.g., those containing calcium and cystine) and those that are radiolucent (e.g., those containing uric acid).

DIFFERENTIAL DIAGNOSIS

Acute renal colic must be distinguished from other conditions that result in severe pain in either the costovertebral angle (CVA) or the upper or lower quadrants of the abdomen. Pain due to appendicitis often occurs in the right-lower quadrant, but it usually originates in the periumbilical area rather than the CVA. Musculoskeletal pain or pain due to disk disease generally is not as severe as pain due to renal colic and is not associated with dysuria or urinary urgency. The presence of hematuria, crystalluria, or radiologic evidence of a calculus or urinary obstruction can further assist in making the correct diagnosis. Patients with stone disease who do not have severe pain or are not having active renal colic may have hematuria. If no urinary crystals are present, it is important to examine other causes of painless hematuria, such as malignancy, infection, or glomerulonephritis.

STRATEGIES FOR OPTIMAL CARE

Medical management is used to prevent further stone occurrence or growth in patients with nephrolithiasis. Treatment of stones that do not pass spontaneously and require surgical intervention is reviewed later in the chapter. All patients, regardless of stone number or type, can benefit from nonspecific therapy: increasing fluid intake to more than 2 L per day to lower or prevent oversaturation and decreasing dietary sodium and protein intake. Reducing sodium intake lessens sodium and thus calcium excretion. Decreasing protein intake lessens endogenous acid production and calcium excretion and increases citrate excretion. Citrate not only binds calcium, lowering its concentration, but also appears to inhibit crystallization. Calcium intake should not be restricted to less than approximately 1 g per day, to prevent bone demineralization. Specific therapy depends on the variety of stone passed or on the suspected origin of stones, based on the 24-hour urine collection. Computer programs that calculate saturation from measured concentrations can be used to determine the risk of stone formation.

CALCIUM STONES

If calcium stone formation stems from a systemic disorder resulting in oversaturation with respect to calcium salts, treatment of the underlying disease should abolish stone formation. For example, in a patient with primary hyperparathyroidism, parathyroidectomy should prevent further hypercalciuria. Calcium-containing stones can result from several metabolic abnormalities that can be detected by 24-hour urine collection. Therapy is directed by the findings of 24-hour urine collection, in conjunction with the results of stone analysis.

Hypercalciuria

Hypercalciuria is defined as urine calcium excretion greater than 300 mg in men and 250 mg in women (or 4 mg per kilogram per 24 hours in either sex). Several mechanisms of action have been proposed to explain the excessive calcium excretion in so-called idiopathic hypercalciuria. If a precise mechanism could be defined, optimal therapy could be specifically directed. For example, if hypercalciuria is secondary to increased intestinal calcium absorption, a low-calcium diet would be helpful, in theory; if there is a defect in renal calcium reabsorption, a thiazide diuretic should be effective. However, prescribing a low-calcium diet to a patient with a defect in renal calcium reabsorption would lead to a negative calcium balance and bone demineralization. Attempting to determine the source of hypercalciuria in individual patients has not proved helpful in directing treatment and is not recommended except in unusual circumstances.

After instituting nonspecific therapy, such as increasing fluid intake and reducing protein and sodium intake, we prescribe a long-acting thiazide diuretic, such as chlorthalidone, which can be taken once a day, starting at 25 to 50 mg. Indapamide (1.25 to 5.0 mg per day) is a preferable thiazide in patients at risk of coronary artery disease, because it does not tend to increase serum lipids. Since hypokalemia is often severe with long-acting thiazides and can lower the urinary citrate concentration, patients on thiazides should be monitored for hypokalemia and given potassium supplements; alternatively, a potassium-sparing diuretic, such as amiloride, can be added to the regimen. Triamterene should be avoided, because it can precipitate into stones.

Hypocitraturia

Acidosis leads to an increase in proximal renal tubular citrate reabsorption. Metabolic acidosis, often due to renal tubular acidosis or diarrhea, hypokalemia, androgens, strenuous exercise, and animal protein ingestion are common causes of diminished urinary citrate levels. Bacteria responsible for urinary tract infections also may utilize citrate and lower levels in the urine. Treatment with citrate, preferably as the potassium salt, is effective, but the liquid preparations are often not palatable. Patients often prefer tablets (e.g., Urocit-K, a wax matrix preparation, given 10 to 20 mEq two or three times a day). Potassium bicarbonate also is effective in reducing metabolic acidosis and increasing citrate excretion.

Hyperoxaluria

Excessive urinary oxalate excretion (more than 40 mg per day) can result from either increased endogenous production of oxalate or augmented intestinal absorption. The latter, often referred to as enteric oxaluria, can result from such conditions as inflammatory bowel disease, sprue, jejunoileal bypass, ileal resection, and other syndromes that can lead to malabsorption. Intestinal calcium normally combines with oxalate to form an insoluble, nonabsorbable complex that is excreted with the feces. In the context of malabsorption, excess fatty acids bind calcium and create a more permeable colonic membrane for absorption of the available free oxalate. This can result in urinary oxalate levels above 100 mg per day. A low calcium intake combined with excessive dietary oxalate can similarly result in enhanced intestinal oxalate absorption with mildly elevated urinary oxalate levels.

If a malabsorption syndrome is thought to be the cause of hyperoxaluria, a low-fat diet, calcium supplementation with meals to bind oxalate, and dietary oxalate restriction provide the core therapy. Both calcium carbonate (1 to 4 g three times a day in adults) and calcium citrate not only bind oxalate but also provide alkali. The resultant increase in urinary citrate excretion enhances calcium solubility and prevents calcium oxalate precipitation. Cholestyramine chelates bile salts, fatty acids, and oxalate and may further decrease urinary excretion of oxalate. Patients with malabsorptive syndromes typically have chronic diarrhea with pronounced losses of fluids, bicarbonate, potassium, and magnesium. Accordingly, the acidic, concentrated urine may result in other stone types, such as uric acid, and calcium stones may develop from insufficient excretion of inhibitors, such as citrate and magnesium, rather than from hyperoxaluria alone. Therefore, patients must ingest large quantities of fluid and replace losses of alkali, potassium, and magnesium (magnesium gluconate, 500 to 1,000 mg three times a day) as needed.

Primary hyperoxaluria, due to hereditary inborn errors of metabolism, can result in very high urinary oxalate levels in children and young adults. Some forms respond to vitamin B_6 supplementation, since pyridoxine is an important cofactor in the metabolic pathway that causes glyoxylate to form glycine, rather than oxalate. Orthophosphate also may be used to bind dietary oxalate in these patients with severe hyperoxaluria.

Hyperuricosuria

Excess urinary urate can provide nuclei for calcium oxalate aggregation. Urinary uric acid levels above 800 mg per day in men and 750 mg per day in women, urine pH above 5.5, normal serum calcium levels, and normal urinary calcium and oxalate levels are features associated with hyperuricosuric calcium nephrolithiasis. Nonspecific therapy, along with dietary purine restriction, can prevent further stone formation, but some patients require allopurinol (100 to 300 mg per day) to decrease the urinary excretion of uric acid adequately.

URIC ACID STONES

The three cardinal features of pure uric acid nephrolithiasis are low urine volumes, low urinary pH, and elevated urinary uric acid levels. By prescribing oral hydration to increase urine volumes to more than 3 L per day and alkalinizing the urine to pH 6.5 (a higher pH can result in calcium phosphate precipitation and should be avoided), existing uric acid stones may be dissolved and the formation of new ones prevented. In a urine pH of 6.5, even uric acid levels up to 1,000 mg per liter may be soluble. Higher levels of excretion, especially in conjunction with elevated serum levels, require the measures aimed at limiting uric acid formation. Dietary purine and protein restriction are valuable in preventing the production of uric acid and an acidic urine, respectively. Allopurinol effectively reduces the rate of uric acid excretion, but owing to side effects it should be used only if other measures fail. A dose of 100 mg should be used initially, increasing slowly to 300 mg as needed. If high doses of potassium citrate or other sources of alkali are insufficient to raise the urine pH, acetazolamide may be used, especially overnight.

STRUVITE STONES

Struvite stones also are called infection stones or stone cancer. The latter term refers to the high morbidity rate associated with these stones due to their rapid growth, difficult eradication, and large size and the potential need for nephrectomy. They are composed of three cations—magnesium, ammonium, and calcium (the latter as apatite)—complexed to phosphate; thus, they also are referred to as triple phosphate stones. The ammonium ions, trivalent phosphate, and high urine pH required for stone formation can exist simultaneously only in the presence of urease-producing bacteria. *Proteus* is the most common urease-producing bacterium associated with struvite stones, although *Pseudomonas, Providencia, Klebsiella, Serratia*, and *Enterobacter* also have been noted. Although *Escherichia coli* is common in urinary tract infections, it is not a urease producer and is never implicated in struvite stone formation. The presence of urease-producing bacteria, a urine pH above 7, and large stones is virtually pathognomonic.

After appropriate antibiotic therapy is instituted, ESWL or percutaneous nephrolithotomy is usually required, because the stones are large and frequently form staghorns. Chronic suppressive antibiotics are required to prevent stone recurrence because any infected stone particles remaining make eradication of the bacteria difficult. Urease inhibitors, such as acetohydroxamic acid, are theoretically efficacious, but their use is fraught with side effects.

CYSTINE

Cystinuria results from an autosomal recessive defect in proximal tubular reabsorption of certain dibasic amino acids. Because the solubility of cystine is low (300 mg per liter at a neutral pH) and most homozygous patients excrete more than 800 mg cystine per day, large volumes of fluid intake (close to 4 L per day) are required to prevent cystine precipitation. Therapy consists of water intake to match cystine excretion and increasing the solubility of cystine by raising the urinary pH above 7.5, as long as hypercalciuria is not present. If cystine excretion is so great that the required water intake is unmanageable, medications that

form soluble complexes with cysteine and decrease the production and excretion of cystine may be required. The most common agents used, D-penicillamine and tiopronin, are associated with numerous side effects. Cystine stones do not crush well with lithotripsy and require percutaneous nephrolithotomy for removal when they are large.

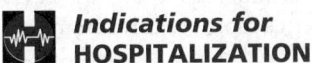

Indications for HOSPITALIZATION

Most stones less than 0.5 cm pass spontaneously. Larger stones, however, rarely advance through the narrow ureters without urologic intervention (Table 139.3). Although ESWL is associated with lower morbidity rates than percutaneous or open surgical nephrolithotomy, it is a relatively new technique, and the long-term side effects are not yet known. It is usually performed on an inpatient basis, since patients require anesthesia (local or general), intravenous hydration, and pain management for passage of the pulverized stone fragments.

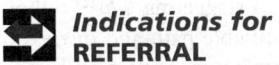

Indications for REFERRAL

Because the rate of stone recurrence in first-time stone-formers varies, the extent of the initial evaluation is the subject of controversy. Do patients with a first episode of nephrolithiasis merit the same workup as those with multiple stones? In 1988, a Consensus Conference on the Prevention and Treatment of Kidney Stones was convened by the National Institutes of Health (NIH) to explore such issues and to determine the direction of future research. The team resolved that

TABLE 139.3.	GUIDELINES FOR SURGICAL REMOVAL OF KIDNEY STONES

Proximal ureter (upper two-thirds): endoscopic placement of the stone into the renal pelvis, followed by ESWL

Distal ureter (lower third): endoscopic removal of the stone or in situ ESWL

Renal stones >0.5 cm, <2 cm: ESWL very effective; not as successful in lower-pole stones >1 cm or multiple stones

Renal stones >2 cm or lower-pole stones >1 cm: combination of ESWL and percutaneous nephrolithotomy

Cystine stones: percutaneous nephrolithotomy (poorly responsive to ESWL)

Large, infected stones: ESWL or nephrolithotomy; all stone fragments completely removed to prevent stone recurrence

Large stones that are not removed or do not pass with ESWL or percutaneous techniques may require open surgical removal.

Complex, large stones are best treated in hospitals with adequate facilities for ESWL, cystoscopy, and open surgery.

ESWL, extracorporeal shock-wave lithotripsy.

all patients, including first-time stone-formers, should undergo the basic evaluation outlined earlier. The combination of this evaluation and the institution of nonspecific therapy, also as outlined previously, can often prevent further stone formation. Patients who form additional stones or whose stones grow and all children require the more extensive, complete evaluation, including 24-hour urine collection. Patients with stones other than calcium oxalate may also have metabolic abnormalities that merit a more extensive examination. Referral to a nephrologist specializing in nephrolithiasis depends on the individual physician's proficiency in treating these patients and the complexity of each case. Surgical referral is warranted in patients who cannot pass stones, either spontaneously or with intravenous hydration.

COST-EFFECTIVENESS

With the advent of less invasive techniques for removal of renal calculi, such as percutaneous nephrolithotomy and ESWL, there is much reflection on the value of medical management. Is a complete metabolic evaluation cost effective? The yearly cost of stone disease in the United States is a staggering $2.39 billion, which does not include the unquantifiable pain and distress of renal colic. Medical evaluation and treatment, aimed at the prevention of stone recurrence, has been shown to decrease the direct cost of caring for these patients. With proper medical management, there is a $3,226 per year reduction in procedural costs, which far outweighs the estimated $1,068 yearly cost of complete medical treatment, resulting in a net saving of $2,158 per patient per year. Just as the medical evaluation cannot remove obstructing stones, surgical maneuvers cannot prevent further stone formation nor treat the underlying disorder. It is now generally accepted, and asserted by the NIH consensus conference, that medical and surgical interventions are not conflicting treatment strategies but rather valuable complementary approaches that are both required for comprehensive care of the stone-forming patient.

BIBLIOGRAPHY

Bushinsky DA, Monk RD. Calcium. *Lancet* 1998;352:306–311.

Coe FL, Parks JH, Asplin JR. The pathogenesis and treatment of kidney stones. *N Engl J Med* 1992;327:1141–1152.

Consensus Conference. Prevention and treatment of kidney stones. *JAMA* 1988;260:977–981.

Curhan GC, Willett WC, Rimm EB, et al. A prospective study of dietary calcium and other nutrients and the risk of symptomatic kidney stones. *N Engl J Med* 1993;328:833–838.

Monk RD. Clinical approach to adults. *Semin Nephrol* 1996;16:375–388.

Monk RD, Bushinsky DA. Pathogenesis of idiopathic hypercalciuria. In: Coe F, Favus M, Pak C, et al., eds. *Kidney stones: medical and surgical management.* New York: Lippincott–Raven Press, 1996:759–772.

Pak CYC. Pathophysiology of calcium nephrolithiasis. In: Seldin DW, Giebisch G, eds. *The kidney: physiology and pathophysiology.* New York: Raven Press, 1992:2461–2480.

Parks JH, Coe FL. The financial effects of kidney stone prevention. *Kidney Int* 1996;50:1706–1712.

Resnick MI, Persky L. Summary of the National Institutes of Arthritis, Diabetes, Digestive and Kidney Diseases conference on urolithiasis: state of the art and future research needs. *J Urol* 1995;153:4–9.

CHAPTER

140

APPROACH TO THE PATIENT WITH OLIGURIA AND ACUTE RENAL FAILURE

H. DAVID HUMES

PRESENTATION

Acute renal failure (ARF), a common clinical syndrome, is defined as an abrupt decline in renal function. Most nephrologists accept the definition of ARF as a rise in the serum creatinine concentration of 0.5 mg per deciliter per day and a rise in the blood urea nitrogen (BUN) level of 10 mg per deciliter per day over several days. The clinical manifestations of this disorder arise from the decline in glomerular filtration rate (GFR) and the inability of the kidney to excrete the toxic metabolic wastes produced by the body. It is recognized clinically by rising levels of BUN and serum creatinine concentration and may develop dramatically, with a patient progressing from normal renal function to uremia within a week. Most forms of ARF are reversible; correct diagnosis and management are necessary so that renal function can improve with minimal risk to the patient.

ARF is best understood when it is categorized according to the sequential process of urine formation and excretion. ARF may evolve from diminished renal blood flow (RBF), termed *prerenal functional ARF*; from a sudden, severe renal parenchymal insult, termed *intrarenal structural ARF*; or from obstruction to urine flow, termed *postrenal obstructive ARF*. The initial approach to treatment, therefore, is to localize the site of dysfunction (prerenal, intrarenal, or postrenal). If the process is restricted to prerenal or postrenal sites, the specific diagnosis and treatment are readily apparent, even though many diseases can alter renal perfusion or urine flow. If the process is confined to an intrarenal site, it is useful to categorize the pathogenetic process further into vascular, glomerular, interstitial, or tubular disease.

ETIOLOGY AND PATHOPHYSIOLOGY

PRERENAL FUNCTIONAL ACUTE RENAL FAILURE

Prerenal functional ARF, or prerenal azotemia, results from a persistent, significant decline in RBF. Because the GFR is highly

TABLE 140.1.	CAUSES OF PRERENAL FUNCTIONAL ACUTE RENAL FAILURE

Hypotension
Extrarenal sodium loss
   Gastrointestinal loss (vomiting, diarrhea, nasogastric suction, intestinal fistula, acute bleeding)
   Skin loss (heat exposure, burns, inflammatory diseases)
Renal sodium loss
   Extrinsic (osmotic diuresis, diuretic administration, mineralocorticoid deficiency)
   Intrinsic (salt-wasting nephropathy)
Third-space fluid accumulation
   Generalized edematous disorders (congestive heart failure, cirrhosis, nephrotic syndrome)
   Gastrointestinal (pancreatitis, peritonitis)
   Miscellaneous (crush injury, skeletal fracture)
Hepatorenal syndrome
Drug-induced
   Nonsteroidal anti-inflammatory drugs or aspirin
   Angiotensin-converting enzyme inhibitor
   Amphotericin B

dependent on RBF, a decline in RBF results in a decrease in GFR and rising levels of BUN and serum creatinine. It is labeled *functional* because the decline in GFR and renal excretory ability can be reversed rapidly if RBF is improved. A decline in renal perfusion is usually a component of a generalized condition involving poor tissue perfusion, such as myocardial failure, hypotension, and extracellular volume depletion (Table 140.1). This decline can evolve from true intravascular volume depletion, as in hemorrhage, diarrhea, or overdiuresis, or from redistribution of intravascular volume to a third space, as in the generalized edematous disorders, in which effective arterial volume is reduced because of fluid accumulation in ascites or peripheral edema. A decline in absolute or relative effective arterial blood volume leads to a decline in perfusion of vital tissues. In response to this decline, various vasoactive substances are released locally and systemically to promote arteriolar constriction, primarily in the renal, splanchnic, and musculocutaneous circulatory beds. At the renal level, sympathetic amines and angiotensin II are important hormones released locally for this response, resulting in substantial declines in RBF and thus in GFR.

Renal hypoperfusion also may stem from selective processes in which declines in RBF develop out of proportion to changes in blood flow to other tissues, as in the hepatorenal syndrome and drug-induced prostaglandin inhibition. The pathogenesis of the hepatorenal syndrome appears to be due to a functional decline in RBF. The hepatorenal syndrome is a form of ARF that occurs in hepatobiliary disease, in which no clinical, laboratory, or anatomic evidence of any recognized primary cause of renal failure is present. This syndrome most often is the result of alcohol-induced hepatic cirrhosis, but occasionally it complicates the course of fulminant acute viral hepatitis, biliary tract obstruction or surgery, hepatic malignancies, and partial hepatic resection. The basis of this functional secondary decline in renal function is increased renal vascular resistance and reductions in RBF. This severe renal vasoconstrictive response may well be

the result of many abnormalities, including hypoalbuminemia, peripheral vasodilatation, arteriovenous shunting, and sequestration of extracellular volume in the peritoneal cavity. All these processes manifest in hepatic cirrhosis and diminish the effective circulating plasma volume, resulting in lowered renal perfusion.

Prostaglandin inhibition by aspirin and nonsteroidal anti-inflammatory drugs (NSAIDs) is most likely to produce prerenal ARF in clinical disorders associated with declines in intravascular volume, as in dehydration and the generalized edematous disorders, including congestive heart failure, cirrhosis, and the nephrotic syndrome. In these disorders, the increased effects of vasoconstrictor hormones, including intrarenal angiotensin II, are counterbalanced by the enhanced production of vasodilatory compounds in the kidney, primarily prostaglandin E_2. Intrarenal prostaglandins help maintain GFR despite systemic vasoconstriction and hypoperfusion. Because of the important role renal vasodilatory prostaglandins play in maintaining RBF, and thus GFR, in these states of diminished effective arterial blood volume, prostaglandin inhibitors can significantly lower RBF and GFR and may produce functional ARF on a prerenal basis. Patients with underlying renal disease, such as lupus nephritis and chronic renal insufficiency, are also at higher risk of ARF with prostaglandin inhibitors.

The acute declines in renal excretory function associated with the use of the new immunosuppressant cyclosporine also are related to cyclosporine-induced declines in RBF. Long-term use of cyclosporine is reportedly associated with chronic tubulointerstitial nephritis. The use of angiotensin-converting enzyme inhibitors reportedly produces ARF in patients with bilateral renal artery stenosis, a condition in which intrarenal angiotensin II is required to maintain adequate glomerular capillary hydraulic pressure to drive the glomerular filtration process. Finally, amphotericin B increases renal vascular resistance acutely and results in prerenal azotemia; lowering the dosage ameliorates this effect.

INTRARENAL STRUCTURAL ACUTE RENAL FAILURE

Most cases of hospital-acquired intrarenal ARF result from ischemic or nephrotoxic processes. In many clinical settings, a combination of these two processes may be operating simultaneously to produce ARF. An ischemic insult often potentiates renal damage produced by nephrotoxins. Systemic vasculitis, atheroembolic disease, renal artery occlusion, rapidly progressive glomerulonephritis (RPGN), and acute hypersensitivity interstitial nephritis also can have initial symptoms of intrarenal structural ARF and must be considered in the differential diagnosis (Table 140.2). The clinicopathologic aspects and approach to diagnosis and treatment of these entities are detailed in Chapters 151, 152, and 164.

Acute tubular necrosis (ATN) is the most common name given to ARF stemming from either ischemic or toxic processes. Renal failure develops from tubular cell injury that produces necrosis limited to certain nephron segments within the kidney, so that only a patchy distribution of necrotic lesions is observed. Although tubule cell injury is limited to certain nephron segments, substantial renal excretory failure may still develop, since nephrons function as segmental units in series. Truly widespread

TABLE 140.2.	**CAUSES OF INTRARENAL STRUCTURAL ACUTE RENAL FAILURE**

Ischemic acute tubular necrosis
Nephrotoxic acute tubular necrosis
  Antibiotics (aminoglycosides, amphotericin B)
  Heavy metals (cisplatin)
  Radiocontrast agents
  Endogenous toxins (myoglobin, hemoglobin, myeloma light chains)
Vascular processes
  Atheroembolic disease
  Renal artery occlusion
  Vasculitis
Acute glomerulonephritis
Acute tubulointerstitial nephritis

tubular necrosis is associated with the entirely different entity of renal cortical necrosis, with causes and pathophysiologic signs quite different from those of nephrotoxic or ischemic ARF.

Progressive renal tubular cell injury initiates alterations at the nephron level that ultimately result in renal excretory failure. These alterations include intratubular obstruction, back-leakage of glomerular filtrate through damaged tubular epithelium, and primary reductions in the glomerular filtration of solutes and water. Of these factors, intratubular obstruction and back-leakage of filtrate appear to be major nephron mechanisms of GFR decline in ATN. The intratubular obstruction arises from casts composed of cellular debris from injured or necrotic renal tubular cells; these impede the flow of urine. The necrotic cells that are shed into the tubular lumen reduce renal excretory function by obstructing urine flow and by leaving gaps along the tubular epithelia through which glomerular filtrate can reenter the circulation.

Renal ischemia is a common cause of ATN. The length and severity of ischemic insults that produce ischemic ARF vary widely in clinical settings. In some patients, a period of a few minutes of ischemia leads to ATN; in others, prolonged renal ischemia generates only transient renal dysfunction. Any prerenal cause of renal excretory dysfunction, if prolonged and severe enough, can provoke progression to structural renal damage. Most cases of ischemic ARF, however, are associated with a period of frank hypotension. Postischemic ARF is more common in patients with sepsis or patients undergoing major surgery.

Nearly half of the clinical cases of ischemic ARF arise after surgery. Various processes, including preoperative and intraoperative fluid losses and anesthesia, result in intravascular volume depletion, with subsequent declines in RBF and GFR. If there is an additional hypotensive or hemolytic insult, susceptible patients may experience ATN. Abdominal aortic aneurysmal repair, open-heart surgery, and biliary tract surgery have the highest incidence of ischemic ARF. Each of these procedures is associated with a substantially greater decline in RBF than are other surgical procedures. The higher incidence of ATN in the septic patient may be related to the major hemodynamic effects

of endotoxins, which can produce systemic hypotension and secondary renal vasoconstriction.

Because the kidney is a major excretory organ for therapeutic agents, the list of drugs known to induce ARF is long, and as new agents are developed, the list will surely grow. For now, as detailed in Table 140.2, the causes of nephrotoxic ARF can be categorized into four major groups: antibiotics, heavy metals, radiocontrast agents, and endogenous toxins.

Aminoglycoside antibiotics are a mainstay of therapy in the clinical treatment of gram-negative infections. Approximately 10% of patients receiving parenteral therapy with aminoglycosides have significant declines in GFR. The kidney is the principal excretory route for the elimination of the aminoglycoside antibiotics, resulting in the accumulation of these antibiotics in the renal cortex. Aminoglycosides produce tubular cell necrosis, which is confined exclusively to the proximal tubule. Declines in effective GFR and elevations in serum creatinine usually are not seen clinically before 5 to 7 days of aminoglycoside treatment.

Various risk factors predispose to aminoglycoside nephrotoxicity, including the dose, duration, and dosage regimen; recent aminoglycoside therapy; elderly age; preexisting renal insufficiency; concomitant nephrotoxin administration; volume depletion; cirrhosis; potassium and magnesium depletion; and metabolic acidosis. The dose and duration of drug administration are probably the two most important factors in determining clinical nephrotoxicity. It has been suggested that there is a relationship of serum levels, renal parenchymal concentration, and nephrotoxicity for any given aminoglycoside.

Renal toxicity is a major side effect of amphotericin B, an antibiotic used to treat fungal infections. The cardinal features of renal toxicity due to amphotericin B are reduced GFR, distal renal tubular acidosis, renal potassium wasting, and antidiuretic hormone-resistant nephrogenic diabetes insipidus. Rapid declines in GFR are related to its renal vasoconstrictive effect and prerenal azotemia. Long-term declines in GFR with amphotericin B are due to tubulointerstitial injury.

Various heavy metals produce ARF with proximal tubule cell necrosis. Salts of mercury, platinum, arsenic, bismuth, silver, chromium, and uranium are potent nephrotoxins. ATN stemming from these agents is almost completely confined to occupational exposure or ingestion, either accidental or purposeful. Cisplatin, an inorganic antineoplastic compound containing platinum, is the most common heavy-metal agent of nephrotoxicity in the clinical setting. Several risk factors, including the total dose and duration of treatment, simultaneous administration of other nephrotoxic agents, and preexisting renal disease, increase the incidence of nephrotoxicity.

Radiocontrast-induced ARF appears to develop from the combined effects of radiocontrast-induced renal vasoconstriction with resulting ischemia, direct tubular cell toxicity, and intratubular precipitation of the contrast agent with proteins and membrane fragments, resulting in intratubular obstruction. Tubule toxicity of these agents in animal models is potentiated by a modest hypoxic insult. Preexisting renal impairment and long-standing insulin-dependent diabetes mellitus are the most important predisposing factors for radiocontrast-related ARF in humans. Renal insufficiency results in a higher plasma level and a longer plasma half-life of the contrast agent, with a greater exposure time to renal epithelial cells. Diabetes mellitus is a risk factor for this disorder because the common macrovascular and microvascular complications associated with this disease result in more prolonged renal ischemia after contrast administration, adding to the toxic potential of the contrast agent. Dehydration and multiple myeloma are additional important risk factors.

Several endogenous proteins have been associated with the development of ARF, including myoglobin, hemoglobin, and myeloma light chains. Myoglobinuric ARF can develop in the context of traumatic and nontraumatic muscle injury. Traumatic muscle injury occurs from crush syndromes and from postexertional, ischemic, and postseizure events. Nontraumatic rhabdomyolytic ATN has been associated with severe (especially alcohol-related) myopathies, drug overdose with pressure-induced myonecrosis, heat stroke, viral infections, potassium depletion, and phosphate depletion.

Hemolysis and release of free hemoglobin into the circulation appear to result in ATN only when they are associated with other systemic abnormalities, especially dehydration, shock, and acidosis. It is clearly established that hemoglobin-induced ATN is related to hemolysis resulting from exposure to various chemical compounds, snake and spider venoms, malarial infection, and transfusion reactions. Myeloma light chain–associated ARF is detailed in Chapter 154.

The pathophysiologic consequences of myoglobin- and hemoglobin-induced ARF relate both to the potential nephrotoxic effects of these heme pigments and to intratubular obstruction. Both myoglobin and hemoglobin can be filtered and reabsorbed by the proximal tubule epithelia, where toxic effects may manifest. The degree of reabsorption can be enhanced in volume depletion and poor renal perfusion states, so that these conditions can increase the risk of toxic renal cell injury and ATN. Because of its smaller molecular size, myoglobin is more readily filtered at the glomerulus than is hemoglobin. Consequently, in the clinical picture of pigment protein–induced ATN, the urine, but not the plasma, is pigmented during myoglobinuric states; both the urine and plasma are pigmented in hemoglobinuric events. Besides the direct nephrotoxic potential, these heme pigments may produce intratubular obstruction by local precipitation. This process can be promoted by acid urine in the distal segments of the nephron.

POSTRENAL OBSTRUCTIVE ACUTE RENAL FAILURE

ARF from obstructive disease can be the result of intrarenal and extrarenal processes (Table 140.3). Extrarenal processes leading to urinary tract obstruction are detailed in Chapters 138 and 158. ARF also may arise in the context of intrarenal obstruction from crystal formation and precipitation occurring diffusely within tubular lumina throughout the kidney, as seen in acute uric acid nephropathy and methotrexate-induced ARF. Acute uric acid nephropathy is most common during cytolytic therapy of diffuse lymphoma and acute leukemia. Renal failure is mainly due to tubule obstruction by uric acid crystals in the collecting ducts, especially in the context of low urine pH. Nephrotoxicity of the folate antagonist methotrexate (MTX) has become a sig-

TABLE 140.3.	CAUSES OF POSTRENAL OBSTRUCTIVE ACUTE RENAL FAILURE

Intrarenal
    Acute uric acid nephropathy
    Drugs (methotrexate)
Extrarenal
    Ureteral obstruction
    Bladder neck obstruction

nificant clinical problem with the institution of high-dose MTX (more than 50 mg per kilogram) treatment protocols that require citrovorum factor rescue. MTX or a metabolite precipitates in the renal tubules, causing intrarenal obstructive nephropathy. Direct tubule cell injury also may contribute to the complication.

CLINICAL FEATURES AND DIFFERENTIAL DIAGNOSIS

Correct identification of the source of ARF depends on the physician's ability to recognize key elements of data acquired by a careful history and physical examination (Table 140.4) and by diligent evaluation of appropriate laboratory tests, especially urinalysis results (Fig. 140.1). Using various diagnostic techniques, physicians in most cases can logically, rapidly, and accurately identify the event precipitating even the most complex forms of ARF.

PRERENAL ACUTE RENAL FAILURE

The predominant causes of prerenal ARF are myocardial failure and intravascular volume depletion. The signs and symptoms of heart failure are detailed in Chapter 66. In patients with absolute volume depletion, there may be a history of vomiting, diarrhea, or diuretic use. Physical examination may disclose poor skin turgor, orthostatic hypotension, and tachycardia. Postural tachycardia and hypotension usually become clinically apparent after loss of more than 5% of the extracellular fluid volume. Minor declines in cardiac function or mild decreases in intravascular volume can promote major declines in renal excretory function in patients with preexisting intrinsic renal disease. It is important to rule out these superimposed conditions in any patient with underlying renal disease, because it is critical to distinguish between a reversible prerenal cause of renal dysfunction and progression of the intrinsic renal disease.

Prerenal azotemia also may develop as the result of sequestration of extracellular volume into third spaces, with a consequent decline in effective arterial blood volume. This process is seen most often in the generalized edematous disorders of congestive heart failure, cirrhosis, and the nephrotic syndrome. These conditions are readily apparent on physical examination—peripheral edema or ascites is often present.

The diagnosis of hepatorenal syndrome should be considered

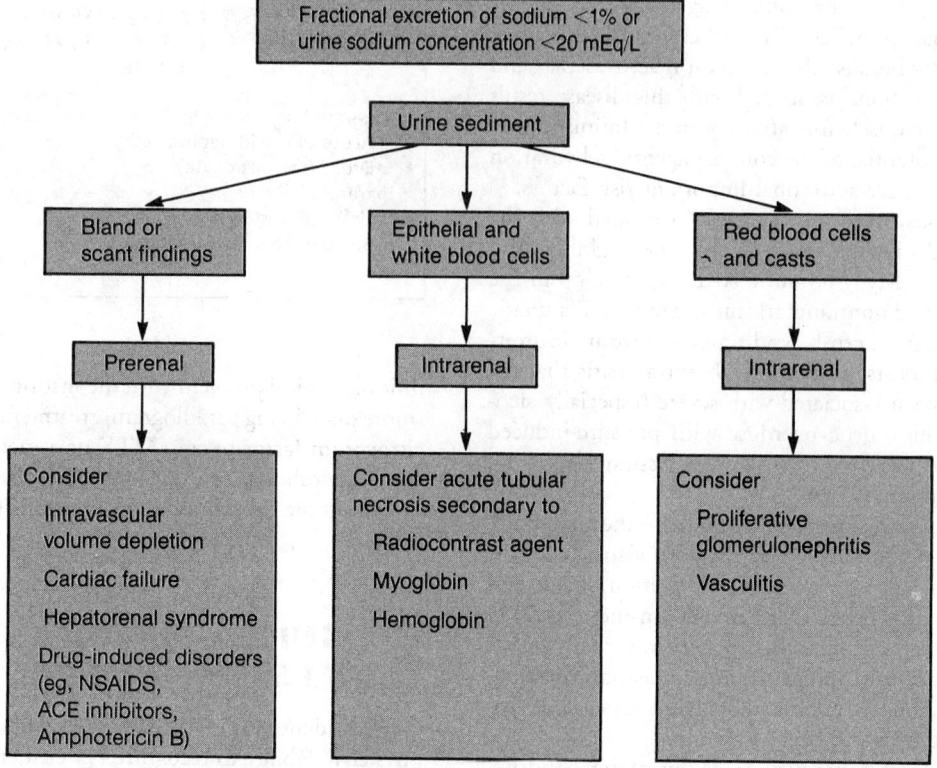

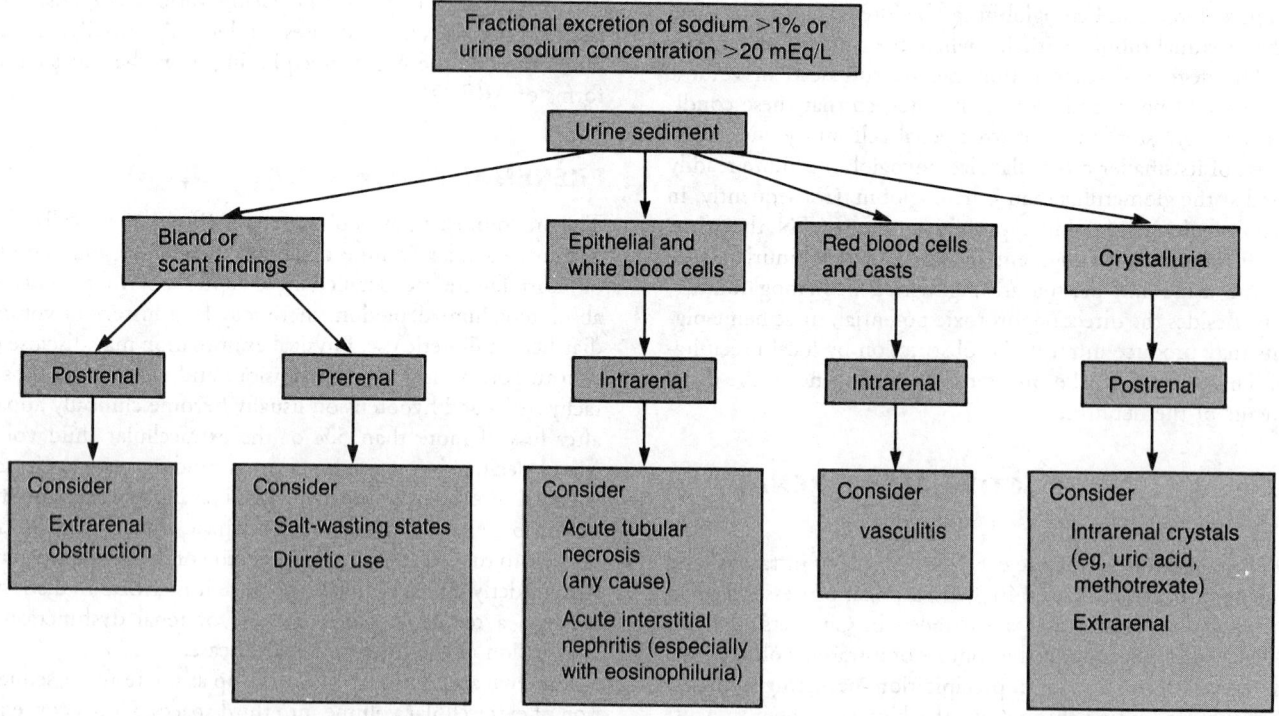

FIGURE 140.1. Use of urinary indexes and findings in the approach to the diagnosis of acute renal failure. NSAIDs, nonsteroidal anti-inflammatory drugs; ACE, angiotensin-converting enzyme.
EVIDENCE LEVEL: C. Expert Opinion.

TABLE 140.4.	THE DIAGNOSIS OF ACUTE RENAL FAILURE

Helpful facts in patient's history
  Intravascular volume depletion: recent weight loss, vomiting, diarrhea, hematemesis, melena, orthostatic dizziness, use of diuretics
  Cardiac failure: recent weight gain, edema, dyspnea or exertion, orthopnea
  Radiocontrast agent induction: recent radiocontrast exposure
  Pigment injury: excessive exercise, prolonged immobility, loss of consciousness, skeletal muscle trauma, seizure, excessive ethanol intake
  Vasculitis/proliferative glomerulonephritis: recent streptococcal infection, fevers or chills, skin rash, arthralgias, history of intravenous drug use
  Acute tubular necrosis: history of hypotension or shock, exposure to nephrotoxin
  Miscellaneous: change or addition of medications, methotrexate administration
Important physical examination findings
  Intravascular volume depletion: orthostatic hypotension, decreased skin turgor, dry mucous membranes, cool extremities
  Cardiac failure: jugular venous distention, rales, audible third heart sound, peripheral edema, hepatojugular reflux
  Hepatorenal findings: hepatomegaly, jaundice, spider telangiectasis, gynecomastia, ascites, caput medusae
  Obstruction: enlarged prostate, distended bladder by percussion
  Atheroembolism: distal extremity emboli, livedo reticularis, fever
  Rhabdomyolysis: muscle tenderness
  Interstitial nephritis: macular or maculopapular rash
  Vasculitis: skin rash, palpable purpura, arthritis
  Proliferative glomerulonephritis: nail splinter hemorrhage, new cardiac murmur, fever or chills, Osler's nodes, Janeway lesions, Roth's spots, impetigo

these underlying predisposing conditions and the continuing administration of these drugs.

Functional prerenal disease arises in a kidney that is not intrinsically diseased; for this reason, urinalysis results are usually unremarkable, except for the relatively nonspecific appearance of an increased number of hyaline and granular casts (Fig. 140.1). Chemical determinants of the urine, however, are extremely useful. The renal response to diminished perfusion is avid sodium and water reabsorption to protect the circulating blood volume. Accordingly, the urine in prerenal disease is relatively free of sodium and water, the urine sodium concentration is less than 10 mEq per liter, the FE_{Na} is less than 1%, and the urine osmolality is more than 450 mOsm per kilogram of water (Fig. 140.2).

In addition, the ratio of BUN to serum creatinine typically exceeds 20:1. This ratio normally is 10:1 to 15:1, but because urea reabsorption is coupled passively to sodium reabsorption in the kidney, the increase in renal sodium reabsorption in prerenal states is accompanied by an increase in urea reabsorption, a decline in urea clearance disproportionate to GFR alterations, and therefore a rise in BUN. Because creatinine reabsorption is independent of sodium reabsorption, the serum creatinine does not rise by an amount out of proportion to the decline in GFR. These processes lead to an increase in the ratio of BUN to serum creatinine, which often exceeds 20:1. This selective increase in

Diagnostic indices in acute renal failure

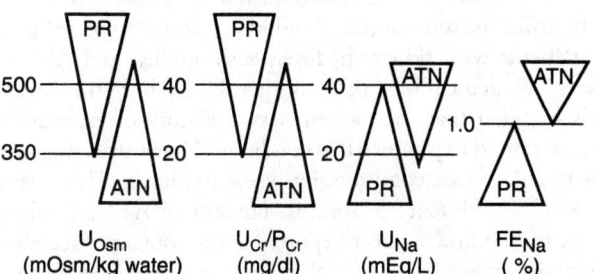

U_{Osm} (mOsm/kg water)	U_{Cr}/P_{Cr} (mg/dl)	U_{Na} (mEq/L)	FE_{Na} (%)

FIGURE 140.2. Common urinary indexes in acute renal failure. The horizontal axis displays four laboratory tests and the units used to differentiate functional prerenal (PR) azotemia from acute tubular necrosis (ATN). The vertical axis depicts values that define the nondiagnostic zones of overlap between the designated values and diagnostic areas of nonoverlap above and below the designated values. The derived urinary index, the fractional excretion of sodium (FE_{Na}), has essentially no nondiagnostic overlap zone. The fraction of the filtered sodium FE_{Na} can be calculated from a urine specimen:

FE_{Na} (%)

= (quantity of sodium excreted/quantity of sodium filtered) × 100

Because the quantity of sodium excreted is equal to the product of the urine sodium concentration (U_{Na}) and the urine volume (V), the quantity of sodium filtered is equal to the product of the plasma sodium concentration (P_{Na}) and the GFR (or creatinine clearance, $C_{Cr} = U_{Cr} \times V/P_{Cr}$):

$$FE_{Na} = \frac{U_{Na} \times V}{P_{Na} \times (U_{Cr}V/P_{Cr})} \times 100 = \frac{U_{Na} \times P_{Cr}}{P_{Na} \times U_{Cr}} \times 100$$

$$= \left(\frac{U}{P}\right)_{Na} \times \left(\frac{P}{U}\right)_{Cr} \times 100$$

(From Shayman JA, ed. *Renal pathophysiology.* Philadelphia: JB Lippincott, 1995:141, with permission.)

in a patient with hepatic failure. Typically, jaundice, ascites, and hepatic encephalopathy accompany this process. Because this syndrome is defined as renal failure resulting from secondary to primary hepatic disease, however, various processes that produce simultaneous primary hepatic and primary renal disease (see Chapter 105) must be excluded. Often the hepatorenal syndrome arises after decreases in extracellular volume due to gastrointestinal hemorrhage, aggressive diuresis, large-volume paracentesis, or diarrhea. Oliguria is usually evident, and early in the course of the syndrome, the fractional urinary excretion of sodium (FE_{Na}) is less than 1%. These values can rise with time and may reflect an element of structural renal damage produced by the persistent reduction in RBF that initially characterizes this disorder. Progressive renal insufficiency frequently ensues, though a few patients spontaneously recover, especially if liver function improves. Once renal failure develops, however, encephalopathy, gastrointestinal hemorrhage, or sepsis usually results, and the mortality rate is high. Because prostaglandin inhibitor–related prerenal azotemia occurs only in the context of diminished renal perfusion stemming from either absolute or relative declines in effective arterial blood volume or intrinsic renal disease, the diagnosis is made based on the presence of

BUN in these functional prerenal disease states is referred to as *prerenal azotemia.*

In several clinical situations, however, these diagnostic laboratory indexes can be misleading. Patients with preexisting renal disease lose the ability to conserve sodium below 10 mEq per liter and to concentrate the urine to levels above 400 mOsm per kilogram of water. Furthermore, if volume depletion is the result of renal salt wasting, the urine sodium concentration may be high. Finally, even in the context of prerenal disorders, the ratio of BUN to creatinine may be normal if urea production is reduced because of low protein intake or severe liver disease. On the other hand, the ratio may exceed 20:1 in obstructive renal disease because of the enhanced urea reabsorption arising from low rates of urine flow.

INTRARENAL ACUTE RENAL FAILURE

Certain acute, severe parenchymal insults can rapidly diminish renal excretory function. These processes include vascular, glomerular, interstitial, and tubular processes. Atheroembolic disorders, vasculitis, RPGN, and acute hypersensitivity interstitial nephritis are specific disorders that often produce ARF. These disorders are detailed in Chapters 151, 152, and 164. The combination of hypertension, proteinuria, and hematuria is most suggestive of acute glomerulonephritis, from either idiopathic processes or vasculitis. The absence of significant proteinuria, hematuria, and red blood cell casts virtually excludes this diagnosis. Patients with acute glomerulonephritis usually produce urine with low urine sodium (U_{Na}) and FE_{Na}, similar to prerenal ARF.

Patients with skin rash, fever, eosinophilia, and ARF most likely have acute interstitial nephritis. To establish the diagnosis, it is essential that the patient have a history of exposure to a drug reported to produce this condition. Hematuria, pyuria, and eosinophiluria are common. Urine eosinophiluria also are noted in RPGN and acute prostatitis, but not in ATN. Nephrotic-range proteinuria has been reported in the context of acute interstitial nephritis associated with the use of several NSAIDs. Renal biopsy is the only definitive way to diagnose this condition.

Once other acute parenchymal lesions have been excluded, a detailed investigation for causes of ischemic and nephrotoxic ATN can be made. A careful review of the clinical course before the development of ARF is necessary. Special attention should be paid to the temporal relations of fluid and electrolyte abnormalities, volume status, blood pressure, medication administration, surgical procedures, potential nephrotoxin exposure, and renal function parameters just before the development of ATN. This is particularly true for aminoglycoside, amphotericin B, cisplatin, and radiocontrast nephrotoxicity.

Various urinary findings can help the physician reach the correct diagnosis (Fig. 140.1). Measurement of the daily urine volume excreted from a patient with ARF can be useful. Anuria is the most severe reduction in urine volume (less than 100 mL per 24 hours) and may be the result of reversible urinary tract obstruction or the more ominous consequence of bilateral renal cortical necrosis, bilateral renal arterial or venous occlusion, or overwhelming acute glomerulonephritis. Prolonged anuria is rarely seen in simple, uncomplicated forms of prerenal ARF or

ATN. Oliguria, a reduced urine volume of 100 to 400 mL per 24 hours, may be the physiologic response to volume depletion or the pathophysiologic consequence of urinary tract obstruction or ATN. Nonoliguria is a urine volume exceeding 400 mL per 24 hours in the context of ARF. Most forms of ARF can be associated with nonoliguria. Anuria alternating with polyuria is an uncommon but classic occurrence in urinary tract obstruction.

The urine sediment in the early phase of ATN usually contains renal tubular epithelial cells and granular and epithelial cell casts. Because tubular function is impaired, the kidney's ability to conserve sodium and maximally concentrate the urine is diminished. These abnormalities can be of diagnostic value in patients with azotemia in differentiating between prerenal azotemia and ATN (Fig. 140.2). In patients with azotemia due to prerenal causes, the urinary indexes usually show a urinary osmolality greater than 500 mOsm per kilogram of water, a urine sodium concentration less than 20 mEq per liter, and a urine/plasma creatinine ratio above 40. In contrast, patients with ATN usually have urine osmolality less than 350 mOsm per kilogram of water, urinary sodium concentration greater than 40 mEq per liter, and a urine/plasma creatinine ratio less than 20:1. Although these ranges in urinary indexes are discriminating in about 80% of patients, about 20% have indexes in an intermediate, nondiagnostic zone. These two causes of azotemia can be distinguished further by the derived FE_{Na} parameter, which exceeds 1% in patients with ATN but is less than 1% in patients with prerenal ARF. Patients with radiocontrast-induced ARF often have FE_{Na} values less than 1%, even though ATN is present.

Consider the diagnosis of myoglobinuric rhabdomyolytic ARF if the patient has several laboratory findings unique to this disorder. This condition is commonly associated with pigmented granular casts (the pigmentation arises from the presence of myoglobin); a positive orthotolidine (Hematest) reaction in the urine supernatant or positive dipstick for heme in the absence of red blood cells in the spun urinary sediment, indicating the presence of myoglobin; and a marked elevation in the plasma level of creatine phosphokinase due to the release of this enzyme from damaged muscle cells. A definitive diagnosis can be made if there is evidence of myoglobin in the urine using counterimmunoelectrophoresis.

Because skeletal muscle is rich in creatinine and uric acid precursors, potassium, and phosphate, rhabdomyolysis releases large amounts of these compounds. Consequently, myoglobinuric rhabdomyolysis can result in a rate of rise of the serum creatinine level exceeding 2 mg per deciliter per day. The BUN/serum creatinine ratio is consequently lower than 10. Rhabdomyolytic ARF typically is associated with a serum uric acid concentration above 16 mg per deciliter. This finding should be differentiated from acute uric acid nephropathy. Hyperkalemia is often severe in this disorder; uncontrollable hyperkalemia is a common indication for dialysis. Hyperphosphatemia also results from the release of phosphate from necrotic muscle, and values exceeding 8 mg per deciliter are often seen. Resulting hypocalcemia, due in part to calcium deposition in damaged muscle, may accompany this abnormality. Although hypocalcemia may be present in the oliguric phase of myoglobinuric ARF, hypercalcemia can develop during the diuretic phase of this disorder.

The clinical diagnosis of hemoglobinuric ATN should be considered when a known hemolytic event is followed within minutes to hours by dark urine and a decline in urine output or renal excretory function. Chills and hypotension are common. Radiologic studies, including intravenous pyelography, ultrasonography, and retrograde and antegrade pyelography, are most useful in ruling out postrenal obstructive ARF. These procedures are rarely useful to diagnose intrarenal structural ARF except by exclusion. Similarly, radionuclide scans are infrequently helpful in the diagnosis of parenchymal ARF, but they can assess the possibility of complete renal artery occlusion as a cause of ARF. Renal biopsy is useful only when it is highly likely that patients have acute glomerulonephritis, vasculitis, or acute interstitial nephritis, as discussed in Chapter 164.

ARF is an uncommon but serious complication of pregnancy (see Chapter 162). Sources include severe preeclampsia, placental hemorrhage, septic abortion, and postpartum hemolytic-uremic syndrome. The HELLP syndrome (hemolysis, elevated liver enzymes, and low platelet count) is a severe complication of preeclampsia and has elements similar to the hemolytic-uremic syndrome. ARF also occurs frequently in patients who undergo bone marrow transplantation. Early ARF, within 5 days of transplantation, is due to a tumor lysislike syndrome. A hepatorenal-like ARF presentation stemming from hepatic veno-occlusive disease can develop up to a month after bone marrow transplantation.

POSTRENAL ACUTE RENAL FAILURE

Urine flow may be obstructed at any site along the urinary tract. ARF from obstructive disease can result from both intrarenal and extrarenal processes (see Chapters 138 and 158). In general, because extrarenal urinary tract obstruction is a reversible cause of renal failure, it always should be considered as part of the initial differential diagnosis in every patient who shows signs of renal insufficiency.

ARF may arise in the context of intrarenal obstruction from diffuse crystal formation and precipitation occurring within tubular lumina throughout the kidney (Table 140.1). Because most cases of intrarenal obstructive ARF have initial symptoms similar to those due to other causes of ATN and result from intrarenal rather than extrarenal obstruction, the diagnosis is not made with the commonly used urologic procedures of cystoscopy or retrograde pyelography. Usually the diagnosis is made because of an awareness of the contexts in which intrarenal crystal formation and precipitation can develop.

Acute uric acid nephropathy is characterized by the acute onset of oliguria, often leading to anuria with rapidly rising levels of BUN and creatinine. The level of serum uric acid usually exceeds 20 mg per deciliter. In the early phase, uric acid crystals and hematuria are often found on urinalysis. A uric acid/creatinine concentration ratio greater than 1 on a random urine sample may aid in the diagnosis. Recent exposure to high-dose MTX also must be excluded when intratubular precipitation of crystalline material is implicated as the cause of ARF.

STRATEGIES FOR OPTIMAL CARE

PRERENAL ACUTE RENAL FAILURE

Treatment of prerenal ARF depends on the underlying disorder. When volume depletion is the cause of prerenal azotemia, infusion of saline and plasma volume expanders, preferably albumin-containing solutions, is indicated. In the edematous disorders, prerenal azotemia usually results from excessive diuresis and diminished intravascular volume, even though peripheral edema and elevated total body sodium content persist. In these circumstances, gentle volume repletion improves renal function. In a critically ill patient with hemodynamic instability, more precise estimation of effective intravascular volume is indicated with the measurement of the pulmonary capillary wedge pressure by a Swan-Ganz catheter.

Therapeutic approaches to the hepatorenal syndrome have been relatively discouraging. The prognosis is extremely poor: once this process develops, renal function improves only if hepatic function improves, either spontaneously or after liver transplantation. Treatment therefore is directed toward improvement of liver function. Prevention or amelioration of the various forms of drug-induced prerenal functional ARF involves improvement in renal perfusion by withdrawal of the agent and treatment of the underlying disease. NSAIDs also can produce ARF resulting from acute hypersensitivity interstitial nephritis, with or without accompanying nephrotic-range proteinuria.

INTRARENAL ACUTE RENAL FAILURE

The approaches to management of ARF arising from vascular, glomerular, and interstitial processes are detailed in Chapters 151, 152, and 164. The therapy of ATN is to prevent or ameliorate renal injury during the developing phase of ARF and to treat established disease during the maintenance and recovery phases. Once ischemic or nephrotoxic ATN occurs, its treatment is similar to that of ARF that stems from other processes. The basic goals are to maintain fluid and electrolyte balance, to provide adequate nutrition, and to treat any infection and uremia. The use of mannitol or furosemide has been the subject of controversy. There is no good evidence that these diuretics can reverse ATN once it has developed, but it is reasonable to attempt a trial of furosemide (80 to 400 mg) or mannitol (12.5 to 25 g) by intravenous infusion in the early phase of oliguric ARF in the hope of inducing diuresis. This enhanced urine flow may lessen the need for dialysis by limiting hypervolemic and hyperkalemic complications, although that maneuver does not appear to improve renal function or mortality or to speed recovery from ATN. If there is no improvement in urine flow, the use of diuretics and mannitol should be discontinued, because the retention of mannitol in the extracellular space can lead to hyperosmolality, hyponatremia, and extracellular fluid overload; deafness, which can be irreversible, may follow the use of large doses of furosemide or, more often, ethacrynic acid.

Any condition associated with a decline in renal perfusion and functional prerenal azotemia, if prolonged and severe enough, can progress to structural ischemic renal damage. At this stage, return of RBF by hydration and reversal of underlying disease will fail to improve renal function. Mannitol and furosemide improve renal function in ischemic ARF if given before the injurious agent, but these maneuvers are usually no more beneficial than simple volume repletion. Clinical prevention of ischemic ARF is difficult with these interventions, since prophylactic therapy often is impossible.

Low-dose dopamine frequently has been employed to enhance renal perfusion to improve renal function and urine flow in ARF. At present there are no clinical data supporting its efficacy in terms of survival of patients and in obviating the need for dialysis in patients with ARF. Dopamine administration continues to be a valuable agent to support cardiovascular performance in critically ill patients, but its use solely to treat intrarenal ARF is not endorsed by current clinical evidence.

Prevention of nephrotoxic ARF requires a knowledge of the drugs with nephrotoxic side effects and their correct dosage, the careful selection of nephrotoxic agents only for clearly defined clinical indications, and the identification and modulation of the factors that increase the risk of nephrotoxic complications. Specific risk factors that contribute to the development of renal complications from drugs with nephrotoxic potential include preexisting renal disease, volume depletion, advanced age, and concomitant nephrotoxic drug administration. Even with the careful use of nephrotoxic agents, renal toxicity still occurs occasionally. When there is objective evidence of a decline in GFR along with a rising level of serum creatinine and BUN, the drug or drugs that may be responsible for nephrotoxicity should be discontinued if possible. Even after the drug responsible for renal damage is withdrawn, renal dysfunction may progress for several days as the toxic injury continues from the persistence of the toxin within the renal parenchyma. Careful monitoring of renal function is therefore necessary even after recognition of the insult.

The best approach to treatment of aminoglycoside nephrotoxicity is prevention. Because the aminoglycosides have a relatively low toxic therapeutic index, effective therapeutic doses for antibacterial activity are very near potentially toxic doses. Therefore, maintenance of serum antibiotic levels below toxic levels is the most important factor in reducing the clinical risk of nephrotoxicity (see Chapter 167). The patient receiving an aminoglycoside also should be well hydrated. Electrolyte and acid-base disturbances, such as potassium or magnesium depletion and metabolic acidosis, should be corrected. Finally, if therapy was begun empirically, culture results should be checked as quickly as possible to determine whether aminoglycoside therapy should be continued.

The renal side effects of amphotericin B have important clinical implications, since the degree of azotemia rather than the therapeutic response dictates the daily dosage and the duration of therapy. During therapy, serum electrolyte, BUN, and serum creatinine levels should be followed closely. If hypokalemia and acidosis develop, potassium and bicarbonate repletion is indicated. Most therapeutic regimens advise either discontinuance or alternate-day therapy when BUN exceeds 50 mg per deciliter. Once the BUN and, with it, the GFR improve, reinstitution of larger doses can be attempted.

There are several therapeutic maneuvers that minimize the nephrotoxic effects of cisplatin. Continuous infusion of cisplatin has resulted in much less renal toxicity than similar doses given as a daily intravenous bolus. Hydration with furosemide or mannitol (or both) before and during cisplatin administration has also been successful. Cisplatin should be avoided during treatment with other nephrotoxic agents, such as the aminoglycosides, and if the creatinine clearance rate is below 50 to 60 mL per minute.

Prevention of radiocontrast-induced ARF depends on identification of patients at high risk. Consideration must be given to alternative noninvasive diagnostic studies, including ultrasonography, isotopic scans, retrograde pyelography, and unenhanced computed tomography. If a contrast study cannot be avoided, volume repletion should be undertaken in patients with a serum creatinine level above 1.8 mg per deciliter before the contrast load. The development of new nonionic radiocontrast agents may lessen the incidence of contrast-induced nephrotoxicity and may be particularly useful in patients at high risk, if clinical studies confirm their lower nephrotoxicity.

The most important measure in treating rhabdomyolysis is early, aggressive replacement of the intravascular fluid lost into necrotic muscle. Administration of 4 to 12 L of normal saline solution intravenously in the first 24 hours may be necessary to maintain a high urine output. Administration of a single dose of mannitol (25 g) intravenously early in the course of volume replacement is also recommended. Early clinical trials using atrial natriuretic peptide or growth factors in established ATN have not supported the efficacy of these agents to improve the outcomes of patients with ARF despite evidence in experimental animal models.

POSTRENAL ACUTE RENAL FAILURE

Treatment of acute uric acid nephropathy is directed toward minimizing uric acid crystal formation within the collecting ducts. Raising urine pH by infusion of sodium bicarbonate and concomitant administration of the carbonic anhydrase inhibitor acetazolamide favors solubilization of uric acid. In patients with acute leukemia for whom combination chemotherapy is planned, pretreatment with allopurinol for at least 24 hours, and preferably for 3 days, diminishes the hyperuricemic response and the risk of this disorder. In patients with established renal failure or serum uric acid levels exceeding 25 mg per deciliter, hemodialysis is indicated to lower serum uric acid levels and to reverse ARF.

A similar approach to MTX-induced ARF has been established. Intratubular obstruction and ARF can be avoided by establishing and maintaining alkaline diuresis during and after MTX administration, increasing crystal solubility and thereby lessening the risk of crystal formation and deposition along the terminal segments of the kidney. Therapy of extrarenal obstructive postrenal ARF is detailed in Chapter 138.

CLINICAL COURSE AND OUTCOME

The decline in renal function observed in ATN may begin abruptly after an ischemic event or develop insidiously from nephrotoxic injury. Possible clinical problems during the developing phase of renal failure include volume overload, electrolyte disorders (such as hyponatremia, hyperkalemia, hyperphosphatemia, hypocalcemia, and acidemia), and the signs and symptoms of uremia (including pericarditis, lethargy, vomiting, and infection). Uremic symptoms, volume overload, intractable acidosis, and severe hyperkalemia are typical indications of the need for dialysis therapy in ATN (see Chapter 165). Peritoneal dialysis, hemodialysis, or continuous hemofiltration can be used. If the patient has oliguria and steadily rising levels of serum creatinine, dialysis or hemofiltration usually is initiated when the serum creatinine level reaches 8 to 10 mg per deciliter, to avoid major uremic problems, which would be immediately life-threatening.

During this maintenance phase of ATN, the patient usually experiences oliguria, but urine output above 500 mL per day or nonoliguria develops in 30% to 40% of patients with ATN. The urine output, therefore, cannot be used as an accurate reflection of GFR in developing ATN. Nonoliguric ATN has a better prognosis than oliguric ATN, perhaps because nonoliguric renal failure reflects lesser degrees of renal damage, with less frequent progression to symptomatic renal failure requiring dialysis.

Renal excretory failure usually persists for an average of 7 to 21 days, but cases lasting several months have been reported. ATN may result in irreversible renal failure, particularly in the clinical setting, where it has arisen from several causes in the critically ill patient. The potential reversibility is the result of the regenerative ability of surviving renal epithelial cells to repopulate the nephron. Renal function, therefore, may return completely, or nearly completely, to baseline levels. As renal function improves, urine output increases, and the serum creatinine level declines.

The prognosis of patients with ATN depends on the causative process. ATN after surgery or trauma has an overall mortality rate of 40% to 75%. The survival rate is much better among patients who do not experience other medical complications, such as infection, bleeding, or respiratory failure. Patients with nephrotoxic ATN have an average mortality rate under 10%. Because dialysis can correct most abnormalities associated with renal excretory failure, the fact that patients' survival depends on extrarenal disturbances is not surprising.

Indications for REFERRAL

Once ARF is diagnosed, an immediate and careful evaluation to rule out prerenal and postrenal causes is necessary. The possibility of a postrenal, obstructive source requires a urologic evaluation. If it appears likely that the culprit is an intrarenal structural process, the patient should be immediately referred to a nephrologist for an evaluation for glomerulonephritis, interstitial disease, renovascular events, and ATN, to clarify appropriate diagnostic and therapeutic approaches.

BIBLIOGRAPHY

Abassi ZA, Hoffman A, Better OS. Acute renal failure complicating muscle crush injury. *Semin Nephrol* 1998;18:558–565.

Chertow GM, Sayegh MH, Allgren RL, et al. Is the administration of dopamine associated with adverse or favorable outcomes in acute renal failure? *Am J Med* 1996;101:49–53.

Epstein M. Hepatorenal syndrome: emerging concepts. *Semin Nephrol* 1997;17:563–575.

Humes HD. Aminoglycoside nephrotoxicity. *Kidney Int* 1988;33:900–911.

Humes HD. Acute renal failure: prevailing challenges and prospects for the future. *Kidney Int Suppl* 1995;50:S26–S32.

Humes HD, MacKay SM, Funke AJ, et al. Acute renal failure: growth factors, cell therapy, and gene therapy. *Proc Assoc Am Physicians* 1997;109:547–557.

Humes HD, Paganini EP. Nephrology and the medical intensive care unit. *Semin Nephrol* 1994;14:1.

Paller MS. Acute renal failure: controversies, clinical trials, and future directions. *Semin Nephrol* 1998;18:482–489.

Palmer BF, Henrich WL. Clinical acute renal failure with nonsteroidal anti-inflammatory drugs. *Semin Nephrol* 1995;15:214–227.

Thadhani R, Pascual M, Bonventre JV. Acute renal failure. *N Engl J Med* 1996;334:1448–1460.

Kelley's Textbook of Internal Medicine, fourth edition. Edited by H. David Humes. Lippincott Williams & Wilkins, Philadelphia © 2000.

CHAPTER 141

APPROACH TO THE PATIENT WITH CHRONIC RENAL FAILURE

FUAD N. ZIYADEH

Chronic renal failure (CRF) is a slowly progressive and irreversible reduction in glomerular filtration rate (GFR). Chronicity implies that the disease process has been ongoing for a period of months to years. *Chronic renal insufficiency* is a term used to describe a mild to moderate reduction in GFR (usually not below 25 to 30 mL per minute) that has not reached the point at which uremic symptoms appear. The hallmark of uremia is evidence of widespread organ dysfunction, because loss of kidney function impairs metabolism and cell function as a result of abnormal regulation of body fluids, ions, and several hormones. Permanent nephron loss occurs as a consequence of irreversible scarring by any of a number of mechanisms of action and causes (Table 141.1). In general, whole-kidney GFR may be reduced through a decrease in the number of functioning nephrons, a marked decline in single-nephron GFR, or both.

The usual course of chronic renal insufficiency is inexorable progression to end-stage renal disease (ESRD). Sometimes, however, there is an element of reversibility, for one of two reasons. First, there may be ongoing activity of the process responsible for the loss of renal function, which can be treated or suppressed. Second, extrarenal reversible factors, such as hypovolemia, may be superimposed on the chronic process.

TABLE 141.1. CAUSES OF CHRONIC RENAL FAILURE

Glomerulopathies
  Primary glomerular diseases
    Focal and segmental glomerulosclerosis
    Membranous nephropathy
    Membranoproliferative glomerulonephritis
    IgA nephropathy
    Idiopathic crescentic glomerulonephritis
    Other
  Secondary glomerular diseases
    Diabetes mellitus
    Amyloidosis
    Postinfectious glomerulonephritis
    Heroin-abuse nephropathy
    Collagen vascular diseases (systemic lupus erythematosus, systemic sclerosis, polyarteritis nodosa, Wegener's granulomatosis)
    Sickle cell glomerulopathy
    HIV-related nephropathy
Tubulointerstitial renal diseases
  Nephrotoxic (antibiotics, nonsteroidal anti-inflammatory agents, heavy metals, diuretics)
  Analgesic nephropathy
  Reflux/chronic pyelonephritis
  Hypercalcemic nephropathy/nephrocalcinosis
  Renal tuberculosis
  Myeloma kidney
  Lymphoma/leukemia (with infiltration)
  Multisystem disorder (sarcoidosis, Sjögren's syndrome)
Hereditary diseases
  Polycystic kidney diseases
  Alport's syndrome
  Medullary cystic disease
  Fabry's disease
Vascular diseases
  Renal artery stenosis/obstruction
  Hypertensive nephrosclerosis
  Cholesterol embolization
  Chronic radiation nephritis
Obstructive nephropathy
  Prostatic disease
  Nephrolithiasis
  Retroperitoneal fibrosis/tumor
  Congenital
  Other

This chapter discusses current thoughts concerning the pathogenesis of the uremic syndrome and the causes of progression of renal insufficiency, reviews the clinical signs and symptoms, and describes an approach to the patient. The approach includes consideration of reversible factors or processes, establishment of a diagnosis, and institution of conservative management. Ultimately, a treatment plan requires consideration of the various therapeutic methods available for the long-term management of ESRD.

PROGRESSIVE NATURE OF CHRONIC RENAL FAILURE

A characteristic of most forms of CRF is the inexorable progressive deterioration of kidney function long after the initial insult is no longer present. The rate of loss of GFR is highly variable and depends on the patient, the type of renal lesion, the presence and severity of systemic hypertension, dietary factors, and concomitant complicating illnesses. For example, diabetic nephropathy tends to progress more rapidly and polycystic kidney disease more slowly than the glomerulonephritides or tubulointerstitial diseases. For any individual patient, however, the rate of decline in GFR is constant and can be predicted, in the absence of therapeutic interventions or complicating factors. The reciprocal of the serum creatinine concentration ($1/S_{Cr}$) declines in a linear fashion over a period of observation of months or years, at a rate characteristic of the individual patient.

The pathogenesis of the progressive nature of CRF remains puzzling, but several factors have been suggested. There may be persistent activity of the initiating insult (e.g., glomerulonephritis with ongoing glomerular injury) in some patients, but this does not explain the progression in most patients. Renal parenchymal calcifications (presumably caused by secondary hyperparathyroidism and a high calcium/phosphate product in plasma) may be detected in several forms of advanced renal failure and are thought to contribute to the progression of renal damage. Animal experiments and some human clinical studies have documented that dietary phosphate restriction halts the progression of renal failure and minimizes the severity of nephrocalcinosis. It has also been argued, however, that nephrocalcinosis may be a consequence, not a cause, of renal damage.

In many patients, long-standing, severe, and uncontrolled hypertension is generally believed to contribute significantly to the progression of renal failure. Another potentially important mechanism of action that could explain the inevitable progression of CRF relates to the development of glomerular hypertrophy, intraglomerular hypertension, and hyperfiltration. This last factor has been the subject of considerable investigation. In experimental animal studies, examination of remnant kidneys after subtotal nephrectomy shows compensatory intraglomerular hypertension, hyperperfusion, and hyperfiltration in surviving nephrons. This compensatory process is maladaptive, because it induces glomerulosclerosis and destruction of the surviving nephrons.

Experimental studies have shown that increased strain on the mesangial cells can stimulate them to produce cytokines, such as transforming growth factor-β, which can promote the synthesis and accumulation of extracellular matrix molecules. Mesangial matrix expansion can encroach on the capillary surface area and reduce the single-nephron GFR in surviving nephrons. Intraglomerular hypertension and the associated structural changes, such as glomerulosclerosis and tubulointerstitial fibrosis, can be prevented by feeding a low-protein diet or by administering angiotensin-converting enzyme inhibitors. Through unknown hemodynamic mechanisms of action, a low-protein diet increases afferent arteriolar tone, which leads to decrements in renal blood flow and intraglomerular hydrostatic pressure; this lowers the GFR in the surviving nephrons. Converting enzyme inhibitors diminish the circulating and intrarenal levels of angiotensin II, resulting in dilatation of the efferent arteriole and consequent reduction in glomerular filtration pressure. Both a low-protein diet and converting enzyme inhibitors also lessen the production and prosclerotic activity of transforming growth factor-β.

Both experimental and clinical studies have emphasized that the development of heavy proteinuria is an important risk factor for progression of CRF. Hemodynamic stress in the glomerulus can promote the development of proteinuria. Glomerular hypertension enlarges the radius of the pores of the glomerular membrane by a mechanism that is mediated at least in part by angiotensin II. In glomerular diseases, the excess filtration of proteins into the proximal tubule and their subsequent endocytosis may represent an important pathologic mechanism underlying renal scarring. Lysosomal degradation of proteins by epithelial cells incites a host of reactions, including the release of local vasoactive hormones and inflammatory cytokines, complement activation, and mononuclear cell infiltration. The resulting tubulointerstitial fibrosis and its severity correlate highly with the decline in GFR. A vicious cycle develops in which loss of nephrons leads to further hemodynamic stress in the glomeruli of surviving nephrons, increased proteinuria, and accelerated tubulointerstitial damage. In this view, heavy proteinuria provides a link between glomerulosclerosis and the development of tubulointerstitial fibrosis, and a decrease in proteinuria effected by angiotensin-converting enzyme inhibitors leads to an arrest of both glomerulosclerosis and tubulointerstitial fibrosis.

Whether progression of CRF in humans is also mediated by alterations in glomerular hemodynamics cannot be established with certainty. Nevertheless, in several long-term clinical trials, drug intervention to control systemic and intraglomerular hypertension, especially with converting enzyme inhibitors, has been shown to be effective in slowing the progression of most forms of CRF. Angiotensin-converting enzyme inhibitors are effective antiproteinuric agents, and this property can further protect from progressive renal damage in glomerular diseases characterized by nephrotic-range proteinuria. Also, large prospective clinical trials have confirmed that moderate dietary protein restriction (0.6 g per kilogram of body weight per day) delays the onset of the uremic syndrome and tends to reduce the rate of loss of renal function, at least in some patients.

■ PATHOPHYSIOLOGY OF THE UREMIC STATE

There are two categories of mechanisms that account for the uremic syndrome: those that have systemic or generalized effects due to accumulation of ill-defined uremic toxins normally eliminated by the kidney and those that stem from defects in a specific organ system.

UREMIC TOXINS

Many nitrogen-containing products of protein and amino acid metabolism accumulate in body fluids and tissues as putative uremic toxins. Although prolonged elevation of the blood urea nitrogen (BUN) concentration is associated with aggravation of the symptoms of uremia, no mechanism of action for this effect has been identified. Urea may be a minor toxin that contributes to some uremic symptoms, such as nausea and vomiting. Nevertheless, BUN can be taken as a surrogate for the true toxins, because urea production is closely related to catabolism of protein (both endogenous and dietary) in normal subjects and uremic patients, and the accumulation of urea reflects the accumulation of all products derived from the catabolism of protein and amino acids, including potential uremic toxins.

Nitrogen-containing uremic toxins include guanidines, polyamines, aliphatic or aromatic amines, some phenols, methylamines, and "middle molecules." Guanidines have been related to defective platelet function and the bleeding tendency of uremic patients. Spermine, a polyamine, has been shown to inhibit erythropoiesis, and its levels correlate inversely with the hematocrit levels of patients on hemodialysis therapy. The middle-molecule hypothesis states that uremic toxicity is caused by peptides and other nitrogen-containing compounds with molecular weights between 500 and 3,000 daltons. Because protein is the principal source of middle molecules, their concentrations can be reduced by restricting dietary protein or by various dialysis strategies. Most nitrogen-containing compounds are poorly characterized, however, and there is little proof that any particular agent exerts a specific toxicity. Moreover, because virtually none of the putative uremic toxins is measured in clinical laboratories, most physicians rely on the BUN concentration to estimate when uremia will become disabling. In general, a BUN concentration consistently above 100 mg per deciliter is a forerunner of uremic symptoms; however, it is not uncommon to encounter malnourished patients who have a lower BUN but also exhibit overt symptoms of uremia. One example of uremic toxicity due to a middle molecule in patients on long-term dialysis is the development of destructive spondyloarthropathy with β$_2$-microglobulin amyloid deposits.

TRADE-OFF HYPOTHESIS

A postulated systemic mechanism of development of many uremic symptoms is the trade-off hypothesis, which proposes that homeostatic factors activated in patients with renal failure permit a balance between intake and excretion, but the same homeostatic factors cause or exacerbate the uremic syndrome. This hypothesis is best illustrated by considering the dynamic effects of progressive renal failure on divalent ion metabolism and the development of secondary hyperparathyroidism (see Chapter 412). Stated simply, the release of parathyroid hormone is stimulated in an effort to normalize serum phosphate and calcium ion concentrations, but the persistent hyperparathyroid state promotes bone damage (Fig. 141.1). The details incorporated into this hypothesis have been greatly refined over the past two decades. As GFR decreases, renal excretion of phosphate is impaired.

Besides limiting phosphate excretion, kidney damage also reduces production of the most active form of vitamin D, calcitriol. Hyperphosphatemia directly inhibits the 1α-hydroxylation of calcifediol, further reducing calcitriol levels. Reduced production of calcitriol by the kidney limits intestinal calcium absorption, so that a higher level of parathyroid hormone is required to achieve a normal ionized calcium level. The mechanism of hyperphosphatemia-induced hypocalcemia involves the intermedi-

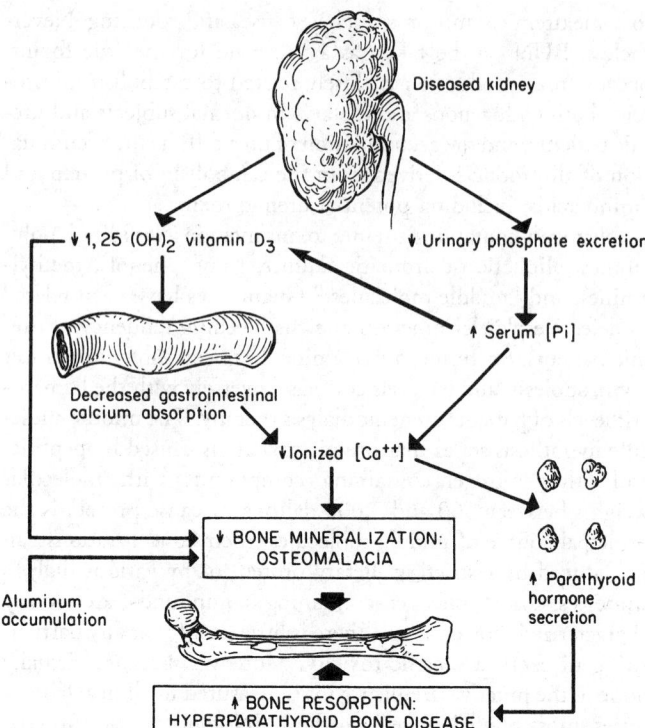

Diseased kidney

↓1, 25 (OH)₂ vitamin D₃   ↓ Urinary phosphate excretion

↑ Serum [Pi]

Decreased gastrointestinal
calcium absorption

↓Ionized [Ca⁺⁺]

Aluminum
accumulation

↓ BONE MINERALIZATION:
OSTEOMALACIA

↑ Parathyroid
hormone
secretion

↑ BONE RESORPTION:
HYPERPARATHYROID BONE DISEASE

FIGURE 141.1. Evolution of uremic osteodystrophy, showing the roles of calcitriol, parathyroid hormone, and aluminum accumulation.

ary development of calcitriol deficiency. More severe hyperphosphatemia can also lower the serum calcium concentration directly. Experimental evidence indicates that both calcitriol deficiency and hyperphosphatemia can stimulate parathyroid hormone secretion directly, further aggravating hypocalcemia-induced hyperparathyroidism.

Fortunately, parathyroid hormone increases renal phosphate excretion by inhibiting tubular reabsorption of phosphate and also increases the ionized calcium level by promoting bone resorption. Although serum phosphate and calcium concentrations are normalized, a high parathyroid hormone level is maladaptive; it promotes bone damage and renal osteodystrophy. Moreover, a low level of calcitriol leads to osteomalacia (a component of renal osteodystrophy) and also causes resistance of the skeleton to the action of parathyroid hormone, requiring progressively higher levels of the hormone to maintain a normal ionized calcium level. With further reductions in GFR, renal excretion of phosphate may not be augmented further. Thus, further loss of kidney function leads to repetition of the cycle of positive phosphate balance, deficiency of calcitriol, hypocalcemia, and stimulation of parathyroid hormone release that leads to progressively severe osteitis fibrosis cystica. Experimental studies suggest that parathyroid hormone can impair metabolism in many organs, possibly by changing intracellular calcium and cellular signaling pathways. Dysfunction of the skin, skeletal muscle, peripheral nerves, blood vessels, heart, and brain have been linked to secondary hyperparathyroidism.

ALTERATIONS IN FLUIDS AND ELECTROLYTES

SODIUM

The ability to balance sodium excretion with intake is usually maintained even when more than 90% of renal function is lost. This progressive adaptation of the failing kidney is usually attributed to increased function of individual surviving nephrons. Each glomerulus and its tubule are considered a unit (the intact nephron hypothesis), and each nephron increases sodium excretion sharply, either because of a circulating natriuretic hormone or "third factor" (e.g., putative inhibitors of Na, + K + -ATPase or atrial natriuretic peptide) or because glomerular filtration in each surviving nephron rises sharply with a corresponding adjustment in tubular reabsorption. Typically, patients with CRF maintain sodium balance even when sodium intake is relatively normal (i.e., 2 to 4 g per day or 86 to 172 mEq per day). What they cannot do is to respond rapidly to changes in dietary sodium. Sudden increases in dietary salt cause hypertension and edema (and, when severe, pulmonary edema). On the other hand, when dietary sodium is sharply restricted, sodium excretion continues, causing loss of extracellular volume and, often, loss of renal function.

WATER

The amount of water eliminated by the kidney becomes a greater proportion of the water filtered as the GFR declines. Consequently, the osmolality of the urine becomes relatively fixed at the same osmolality as serum (300 mOsm per liter), that is, the patient has isosthenuria. The limited ability to concentrate urine causes nocturia. Moreover, a limited capacity to excrete water may lead to hyponatremia and water intoxication if patients are given excessive hypotonic fluids or 5% dextrose in water intravenously.

POTASSIUM

In CRF, the amount of potassium secreted by each nephron is increased, in part through the action of aldosterone as well as an increase in urine flow in each nephron. The adaptation is remarkably efficient, and hyperkalemia is unusual until renal failure is advanced and urine volume falls below about 500 mL per day. This is a serious consequence of renal failure because hyperkalemia impairs cardiac conduction. Some patients may also have hyperkalemia when the serum creatinine concentration is relatively low (3 to 5 mg per deciliter) because of impaired secretion or the action of aldosterone on the collecting duct. Such patients are said to have hyporeninemic hypoaldosteronism or type IV renal tubular acidosis. In patients with advanced renal failure, including patients on dialysis, the capacity of the colon to secrete potassium rises sharply, so that as much as 25% to 40% of the potassium ingested each day is excreted in feces. In such patients, hyperkalemia can occur with constipation.

ACIDOSIS

Acidosis develops in uremic patients because of their inability to excrete the amount of acid generated each day with a normal diet (about 1 mEq hydrogen ion is generated per kilogram of body weight each day). A prominent factor that leads to this dysfunction in renal failure is the production of inadequate amounts of ammonia. Hyperchloremic metabolic acidosis evolves when the GFR is 30 to 60 mL per minute. High anion gap acidosis arises when the GFR falls below about 20 mL per minute, owing to the accumulation of nonvolatile acids generated during metabolism. The unexcreted acid is buffered principally by bone, leading to demineralization, which is characteristic of uremic osteodystrophy. Chronic metabolic acidosis also causes excessive catabolism of protein and amino acids, leading to protein wasting and negative nitrogen balance.

METABOLIC AND ENDOCRINE MANIFESTATIONS OF UREMIA

GLUCOSE AND INSULIN

Uremia is typically associated with impaired glucose metabolism. The sensitivity of muscle to the hypoglycemic action of insulin is reduced in uremic patients. Tissue sensitivity to insulin can be substantially improved by dialysis, which suggests the role of uremic toxins. Hepatic glucose production and uptake are normal in uremia. Other actions of insulin, such as promoting potassium uptake by cells and inhibiting proteolysis, are maintained in uremia. Some patients manifest mild hyperglycemia in response to glucose loading as a result of insulin resistance in skeletal muscle, while others are able to maintain normoglycemia by raising plasma insulin levels. Very rarely, spontaneous hypoglycemia can develop in severely malnourished or alcoholic patients who may also suffer from autonomic neuropathy and impaired release of counterregulatory hormones, such as catecholamines.

The kidney plays a central role in the metabolism of insulin in normal subjects. About 25% of the daily production of insulin by the pancreas is degraded in the kidney; it is also removed by muscle and liver. When the GFR declines to about 40 mL per minute, the half-life of insulin rises, but any benefit of a longer half-life is overcome by insulin resistance. Because the half-life is prolonged, administration of insulin without dose readjustment in diabetic patients with progressive renal insufficiency can lead to dangerous hypoglycemia.

LIPID METABOLISM

The incidence of atherosclerosis is higher in patients with CRF, and this condition is aggravated by hypertension. High-density lipoprotein cholesterol levels are usually reduced, but the levels of very low density and low-density cholesterol are higher in uremic patients.

THYROID METABOLISM

Patients with CRF often have low serum thyroxine levels because of decreased binding to thyroid-binding globulin due to the retention of binding inhibitors. Free thyroxine serum levels (measured by equilibrium dialysis) are usually normal, whereas total and free triiodothyronine serum levels are typically low. These low levels are the result of impaired conversion of thyroxine to triiodothyronine in peripheral tissues. In contrast to other causes of the euthyroid sick syndrome, the serum level of reverse triiodothyronine is normal rather than high. There is a higher incidence of goiter in patients with CRF, possibly owing to accumulation of an unidentified goitrogen. It may be difficult to separate the clinical symptoms of uremia from those of hypothyroidism. Both conditions may be characterized by cold intolerance, a puffy appearance, dry skin, lethargy, constipation, and a higher incidence of goiter. However, the serum concentration of thyroid-stimulating hormone is normal in the majority of patients with CRF. Treatment for hypothyroidism is necessary only for patients with distinct elevations in thyroid-stimulating hormone concentrations (above 10 mU per liter).

SEXUAL DYSFUNCTION

The incidence of impotence in patients with CRF is much greater than expected, compared with other chronic illnesses or states of depression, perhaps because of hormonal derangements and other factors, such as zinc deficiency. Testosterone levels are low because of decreased production; serum levels of dihydrotestosterone are also reduced. Follicle-stimulating hormone levels are usually normal, but this is an inappropriate response when there is a low circulating testosterone level. Luteinizing hormone levels are appropriately elevated; prolactin levels are usually abnormally high.

HEMATOLOGIC MANIFESTATIONS

The anemia of CRF is normochromic and normocytic and is caused principally by suppressed erythropoiesis, although shortened red cell survival may also play a minor role. Erythropoietin deficiency due to renal parenchymal damage is the predominant cause of suppressed erythropoiesis; inhibitors of erythropoiesis have also been implicated as contributory factors. The red cell survival is shortened by 25% to 30% as the result of extracellular factors: red blood cells from uremic patients have a normal life span when transfused into normal persons, but normal red blood cells have a shortened survival time when exposed to uremic serum.

The pathophysiologic cause of the increased tendency to bleeding is related to abnormal platelet function and impaired platelet/vessel wall interactions. There is often prolongation of the bleeding time, and this can be exaggerated by the severity of the anemia. The platelet count is usually normal or slightly low, and there is no prolongation of the prothrombin or partial thromboplastin time. The impairment in platelet adhesiveness may be due to an intrinsic dysfunction of GPIIb-IIIa, a platelet membrane glycoprotein complex that normally plays a role in platelet aggregation and adhesion by binding to von Willebrand's factor. Studies in uremic patients have shown that platelet nitric oxide synthesis is increased and that uremic plasma stimulates nitric oxide production by cultured endothelial cells. Nitric oxide is an inhibitor of platelet aggregation.

Altered membrane arachidonic acid metabolism may also contribute to platelet dysfunction in uremia; there is ineffective synthesis of thromboxane by platelets and excess prostacyclin production by blood vessels. Thromboxane is a potent vasoconstrictor and activator, whereas prostacyclin is a potent vasodilator and antagonist of platelet aggregation. Dialysis can correct the increased tendency to bleeding in part, implying that circulating uremic toxins are a major cause of platelet dysfunction. Desmopressin (DDAVP) has some therapeutic utility in most patients with uremic bleeding and appears to act by increasing the release of factor VIII:von Willebrand's factor multimers from endothelial storage sites. Conjugated estrogens are also of therapeutic benefit because they can increase platelet reactivity, possibly by limiting nitric oxide production. The neurologic, cardiovascular, and musculoskeletal manifestations of uremia are presented in Table 141.2 and are discussed in the subsequent sections.

◼ CLINICAL FEATURES

The symptoms of CRF depend on its severity, or the degree of reduction in GFR, and on the rapidity with which the reduction in GFR develops. In slowly progressive states, most patients remain virtually asymptomatic until far-advanced renal failure ensues (the acute discovery of chronic disease). The constellation of uremic symptoms that eventually develop is protean, reflecting malfunction of several organ systems, most notably the neuromuscular, cardiovascular, and gastrointestinal systems (Table 141.2). The initial symptoms may be so insidious that the patient is aware of them only in retrospect, after effective management has been instituted. In general, when uremic symptoms are present, the physician may conclude that the renal failure is advanced (GFR less than 10 to 15 mL per minute). Absence of symptoms, however, still may be associated with equally severe renal failure and may be life-threatening. One must then rely on physical signs and the laboratory evaluation to assess the severity of kidney damage.

HISTORY

In evaluating the chronicity of renal failure, the clinical history should document previous elevations in blood pressure, proteinuria, or hematuria. This information is usually available from school, life insurance, military service, or clinical records. Generalized manifestations of CRF include fatigue, malaise, and lassitude. Gastrointestinal symptoms, such as anorexia, nausea, vomiting, a metallic taste in the mouth, and hiccups, are common. Cardiovascular manifestations are sometimes prominent and consist of dyspnea, orthopnea, edema, and pericardial chest pain. Neuromuscular manifestations are typical and vary in severity; they include impaired mentation, diminished ability to concentrate, insomnia, irritability, headache, muscle cramps, and twitching. Severe encephalopathy can develop and progress to confusion, stupor, seizures, and coma. Peripheral neuropathy may manifest initially as paresthesias, with subsequent disturbances of motor function, including muscle weakness and atrophy. The restless leg syndrome refers to a persistent and ex-

TABLE 141.2.	MANIFESTATIONS OF THE UREMIC SYNDROME

Neurologic
  Central
    Daytime drowsiness
    Decreased attentiveness and cognitive function
    Imprecise memory
    Slurred speech
    Disorientation and confusion
    Asterixis and myoclonus
    Seizures
    Coma
  Peripheral
    Sensorimotor peripheral neuropathy
    Restless leg syndrome
    Increased muscle fatigability and muscle cramps
Cardiovascular
  Accelerated atherosclerosis
  Cardiomyopathy
  Pericarditis
Gastrointestinal
  Anorexia progressing to nausea and vomiting
  Stomatitis and gingivitis
  Parotitis
  Peptic ulcer diathesis
  Gastritis and duodenitis
  Enterocolitis
  Pancreatitis
  Arteriovenous malformations with bleeding
  Ascites
Musculoskeletal
  Renal osteodystrophy (osteitis fibrosa cystica, osteomalacia)
  Osteopenia and osteoporosis
  Extraskeletal calcifications
  Destructive spondyloarthropathy
  Carpal tunnel syndrome
Hematologic
  Anemia
  Altered neutrophilic chemotaxis
  Depressed lymphocyte function
  Bleeding diathesis with platelet dysfunction
Endocrinologic
  Secondary hyperparathyroidism
  Carbohydrate intolerance due to insulin resistance
  Hyperlipidemia
  Altered peripheral thyroxine metabolism
  Testicular atrophy
  Ovarian dysfunction (amenorrhea, dysfunctional uterine bleeding)
Pulmonary
  Atypical pulmonary edema
  Pneumonitis
  Fibrinous pleuritis
Dermatologic
  Pruritus
  Dystrophic calcification
  Changes in skin pigmentation
Ophthalmic
  Conjunctival or corneal calcifications

(From May RC, Kelly RA, Mitch WE. Pathophysiology of uremia. In: Brenner BM, Rector FC Jr, eds. *The kidney,* 4th ed. Philadelphia: WB Saunders, 1991, with permission.)

tremely uncomfortable sensation in the lower extremities that can be relieved by movements of the legs. Autonomic neuropathy, especially in the diabetic patient, can also develop and result in impaired bladder and bowel function. Skin manifestations include itching and bruising. Genitourinary complaints, such as nocturia, amenorrhea, and erectile dysfunction, also may be present.

PHYSICAL EXAMINATION

The signs of CRF are often multiple and nonspecific, and they usually do not appear until late in the course of the disease. The patient may appear chronically ill, with weight loss and muscle wasting. Dermal manifestations include pallor, yellow-brown discoloration, hyperpigmentation, ecchymosis, and petechiae. Inspection of the head may detect conjunctival or corneal calcifications, retinopathy characteristic of hypertension, and epistaxis. Cardiovascular findings include hypertension, cardiomegaly, edema, and, in the preterminal stages of renal failure, a pericardial friction rub. If they are present, Kussmaul's respirations reflect the severity of an underlying state of metabolic acidosis. Severe renal osteodystrophy can give rise to bone tenderness, fractures, and proximal muscle weakness.

Neuromuscular signs vary in intensity and severity during the course of the disease. Mental status findings include confusion, drowsiness, stupor, or coma. Myoclonic twitches and asterixis (uremic flap) are typical of advanced uremia. Uremic peripheral neuropathy is a distal, symmetric, mixed type of sensorimotor neuropathy. As in other neuropathies, injury is directly related to axon length; longer axons are affected first, resulting in symptoms that are more prominent in the lower extremities. Sensory abnormalities precede motor signs and may include loss of vibratory and position sense. If motor neuropathy develops, deep tendon reflex loss and footdrop may be evident. Mononeuropathies, such as carpal tunnel syndrome or peroneal palsy, will develop occasionally. Autonomic neuropathy can be detected by impaired cardiovascular reflexes, such as the Valsalva maneuver.

LABORATORY DATA

The diagnosis of renal failure is established by documenting an elevation in BUN and serum creatinine concentrations. With stable CRF, the BUN and serum creatinine rise proportionately, and a ratio of BUN to creatinine of 10:1 to 15:1 is typical. The BUN is disproportionately elevated to the creatinine with urinary obstruction, cardiac decompensation, high protein intake, catabolism associated with trauma, sepsis, corticosteroid therapy, or gastrointestinal bleeding. The creatinine is disproportionately elevated with malnutrition, liver disease, or rhabdomyolysis. When the GFR falls below 25 to 30 mL per minute, other laboratory abnormalities may be seen, including anemia (characteristically normochromic normocytic), metabolic acidosis, hyperphosphatemia, hypocalcemia, and hyperuricemia. Hyperkalemia, a late manifestation of CRF, typically occurs when the GFR falls below 10 to 15 mL per minute.

▎ PATIENT EVALUATION

A primary question in the evaluation of the patient with renal failure is whether the failure is chronic or acute. Chronicity

TABLE 141.3.	**POTENTIALLY REVERSIBLE FACTORS PRODUCING ACUTE DECOMPENSATION OF CHRONIC RENAL FAILURE**

Hypovolemia/hypotension
Hypertension
Reflux nephropathy
Congestive heart failure
Nephrotoxins
Pericarditis/tamponade
Hypercalcemia
Sepsis
Atheroembolic diseases

implies stability and thus presents less of an immediate threat to the patient than does acute renal failure. Acute renal failure implies reversibility; CRF is typically irreversible, although some specific forms of CRF are remediable or preventable. The approach to acute renal failure takes into account different considerations and is discussed in Chapter 140. A second question is whether there are recognizable factors that contribute to or aggravate renal failure (Table 141.3). Recognition and treatment of these complicating factors often proves valuable in halting the progression of kidney damage and may even result in improvement in renal excretory function.

A definite diagnosis should then be attempted, specifically considering disease processes that could be alleviated (Table 141.4). When the patient with advanced renal failure is first seen, it may be difficult or impossible to identify with certainty, even by histologic examination, the disease process responsible for initiating the damage. Nevertheless, some signs of the primary disease may persist and could be helpful in determining the cause of CRF. When remediable disorders or complicating conditions cannot be found, the physician must decide on a plan of maintenance therapy. Conservative management can be instituted for months or years and includes measures to slow the progression of CRF, prevention of complications, and therapy to avert or relieve the symptoms of uremia. Eventually, when ESRD ensues, conservative management may not suffice, and the next

TABLE 141.4.	**POTENTIALLY REMEDIABLE CAUSES OF CHRONIC RENAL FAILURE**

Malignant hypertensive nephrosclerosis
Renal artery stenosis
Wegener's granulomatosis
Systemic lupus erythematosus
Multiple myeloma
Obstruction
Reflux
Hypercalcemic nephropathy
Interstitial nephritis
Cholesterol embolization
Lead nephropathy

move is to refer the patient to a consulting nephrologist to institute replacement therapy by long-term dialysis (see Chapter 165) or renal transplantation (see Chapter 166).

DOCUMENTATION OF CHRONICITY

The best evidence that renal failure is chronic is documentation of a previous sustained reduction in GFR. This information is best obtained from records indicating elevations in BUN, serum creatinine, or both. Equally valuable are ancillary findings that reflect long-standing renal failure, such as small kidneys or renal osteodystrophy. Although radiographic or sonographic determination of shrunken kidneys is almost always associated with chronic rather than acute renal failure, normal-sized or even large kidneys can be associated with CRF caused by adult polycystic kidney disease, diabetic nephropathy, HIV nephropathy, malignant hypertensive nephrosclerosis, multiple myeloma, amyloidosis, and, occasionally, obstructive uropathy or glomerulonephritis. For patients who have normal-sized kidneys, a renal biopsy may be required to clarify the nature of the disease and to determine its chronicity.

Radiographic evidence of renal osteodystrophy, particularly osteitis fibrosa, is a reliable indication of long-standing renal failure, because significant hyperparathyroidism must be present for at least 1 year for diagnostic changes to appear on radiographic film. A long-standing history of nocturia or pruritus also may suggest chronicity. A family history of hereditary renal disease, such as polycystic kidney disease or Alport's syndrome, can be helpful in some patients. Anemia, hyperphosphatemia, hypocalcemia, and acidosis are relatively poor indicators of chronicity and often correlate better with the severity of renal failure; these manifestations frequently develop over a period of 10 days to 2 weeks in most cases of severe acute renal failure.

REVERSIBLE FACTORS COMPLICATING CRF

Recognizing and treating potentially reversible factors that can exacerbate renal failure (Table 141.3) are important steps in the attempt to delay the development of ESRD. If the information is available, it is useful to plot the relationship between $1/S_{Cr}$ and time. A steep deviation in the slope of the line at the time of initial evaluation of the patient may indicate the presence of reversible factors that are superimposed on the natural progression of the disease.

Hypovolemia

The inability to conserve sodium adequately when sodium intake is decreased and the impairment in maximal urine concentration may lead to excessive urinary losses of salt and water. The ensuing hypovolemia reduces renal perfusion, further worsening renal failure. This may be the most common exacerbating event in the course of CRF. Hypovolemia often develops because of poor salt intake related to uremic symptoms (anorexia and nausea), extrarenal salt losses (diarrhea, laxative intake, gastrointestinal hemorrhage, or vomiting), and renal electrolyte losses (excessive diuretic therapy or osmotic diuresis). Assessment of the

patient's hemodynamic status and institution of salt and water replacement are important steps to improving renal function.

Hypertension

Accelerated or malignant hypertension of any origin can impair renal function acutely but often reversibly. Hypertension may be a consequence of renal parenchymal diseases or renovascular disorders, or it may develop from nonrenal causes. The major factor that leads to hypertension in patients with renal disease, who were previously normotensive, is sodium retention. Increased peripheral resistance is another factor that contributes to hypertension, and this may be due to inappropriately high renin and angiotensin II production or activation of the sympathetic nervous system. Plasma levels of catecholamines are elevated primarily as the result of decreased renal clearance and reduced neuronal uptake and degradation. In general, severe hypertension that is poorly controlled can induce arteriolar nephrosclerosis and accelerate the progression of renal failure. Proper control of hypertension has been shown to slow the progression of renal damage and at times can lead to measurable improvement in renal function. Conversely, overzealous lowering of blood pressure using diuretics or vasodilators can compromise renal perfusion and further exacerbate renal failure.

The use of angiotensin-converting enzyme inhibitors or angiotensin II type 1 receptor antagonists to treat hypertension caused by bilateral renal artery stenosis or unilateral renal artery stenosis of a solitary functioning kidney is a well-recognized factor predisposing to the development of reversible acute renal failure. In the context of diminished renal blood flow due to arterial disease, the reduced GFR is maintained by the effect of angiotensin II on constricting the efferent arteriole. When production of angiotensin II is inhibited, efferent arteriolar dilatation results, which reduces glomerular hydraulic pressure and, in turn, glomerular filtration.

Congestive Heart Failure

Because sodium retention is common, congestive heart failure occurs frequently in patients with CRF. In addition to fluid overload, uremic patients can suffer from myocardial dysfunction because of concentric left ventricular hypertrophy from hypertension, an increased incidence of coronary artery disease, or ischemic cardiomyopathy. Finally, myocardial dysfunction can develop in diseases causing renal failure, such as diabetes, hypertension, atherosclerosis, or amyloidosis. Impaired cardiac function can lead to a precipitous decrease in GFR, which can be restored to its initial value if appropriate therapy of cardiac failure is instituted.

Pericarditis

Inflammation of the visceral and parietal pericardium often manifests in patients with slowly progressive severe uremia and may develop into hemorrhagic serositis. Pericarditis can be complicated by cardiac tamponade. This complication further impairs renal perfusion and function and often precipitates uremic symptoms. Pericardiocentesis can be lifesaving, and it improves cardiac output and renal function.

Infections and Catabolism

In the absence of associated obstruction, renal parenchymal infection rarely causes renal failure, except when the infection is fulminant or is complicated by multiple renal abscesses or papillary necrosis, particularly in the diabetic patient. Tuberculosis of the kidney is a well-known cause of renal failure, especially when ureteral constriction ensues. Extrarenal infections with septicemia, especially when they are associated with hypotension, can augment renal vascular resistance and impair renal blood flow, resulting in acute renal failure. Catabolic stresses of infection and surgery, gastrointestinal bleeding, or therapy with corticosteroids or tetracycline can result in marked azotemia and can be associated with the early development of uremic symptoms.

Obstruction

Obstruction of urine flow can contribute to impairment of renal function, particularly if it is associated with infection. The causes, diagnostic approach, and management of obstructive uropathy are outlined in Chapters 138 and 158. Relief of obstruction and treatment of any coexisting infection can be rewarding, because variable degrees of renal functional improvement can be achieved.

Reflux

Urine reflux, with or without urinary tract infection, can result in chronic pyelonephritis; it is the most common cause of CRF in children and adolescents. The prognosis is largely determined by the extent of kidney scarring at the time of evaluation. Surgical correction of reflux, especially if it is performed at an early age, can stabilize GFR and delay the development of ESRD.

Nephrotoxins

Various nephrotoxic agents are responsible for exacerbating renal failure in many patients with established chronic renal insufficiency. These agents include drugs (e.g., antibiotics, analgesics, nonsteroidal anti-inflammatory agents, diuretics), heavy metals (e.g., lead and cadmium), and radiographic contrast material. These agents produce renal injury through various mechanisms of action, such as acute interstitial nephritis (see Chapter 151), renal prostaglandin inhibition, diuretic-induced salt depletion, renal ischemia, or direct tubular injury. Usually, identification of the suspected agent and its early withdrawal can lead to stabilization or significant improvement in renal function.

Hypercalcemia

Sustained or severe hypercalcemia of any origin can result in impaired renal function through any of several mechanisms of action, including acute and reversible renal vasoconstriction leading to decreased GFR, hypovolemia from salt depletion (stemming from anorexia, nausea, vomiting, or diuretic therapy), water depletion (because of impaired concentration), chronic and irreversible renal parenchymal damage from nephrocalcinosis, and urinary obstruction from nephrolithiasis. Prompt reduction of an elevated serum calcium level, therefore, can improve renal hemodynamics, increase GFR, and halt the progression of renal parenchymal damage.

REMEDIABLE CAUSES OF CHRONIC RENAL FAILURE

When no potentially reversible complication can be identified as a contributor to acute decompensation in renal function, it generally is assumed that the GFR at the time of diagnosis of CRF is permanently and irreversibly depressed. There are a few specific causes of remediable CRF, however. With appropriate intervention in these situations, the GFR can be stabilized for months or years, modifying the need for long-term dialysis. These situations (Table 141.4) include malignant hypertensive nephrosclerosis (after prolonged, successful control of blood pressure and management of coexisting cardiac failure), bilateral renal artery stenosis (after successful angioplasty or corrective surgery), active Wegener's granulomatosis or lupus nephritis (with proper management using corticosteroids and cytotoxic drugs), multiple myeloma (after control of hypercalcemia and hyperuricemia and institution of effective chemotherapy), analgesic-abuse nephropathy (after withdrawal of analgesics), hypercalcemic nephropathy (with control of the elevated serum calcium level, such as that after parathyroidectomy), obstructive renal disease and reflux nephropathy (after relief of obstruction or antireflux surgery), and some cases of interstitial nephropathy (when drugs or toxins are removed).

In most cases, the diagnosis is made by the history and physical examination and standard diagnostic studies. Because the remediable causes are so important, it is useful to separate this list and to ensure that these diagnoses have been considered. Confirmation of the suspected diagnosis may require interventional studies. Renal biopsy is often of limited value in advanced renal disease, because end-stage histologic findings are relatively nonspecific. Nevertheless, if there is reason to suspect one of the vasculitides and if the kidney size is relatively normal, biopsy is indicated to guide therapy. Kidney biopsy may also provide useful prognostic information. For instance, the presence of severe tubulointerstitial fibrosis, independent of the primary etiologic lesion, implies irreversibility and a tendency toward progression of renal failure.

Renal artery stenosis may require interventional studies for diagnosis and management. This diagnosis can be pursued in a patient with renal insufficiency and in the absence of other definable causes, especially if there is accelerated or difficult-to-control hypertension, abdominal bruits, evidence of significant vascular disease elsewhere, and episodes of sudden-onset or "flash" pulmonary edema. The diagnosis can be established by digital subtraction angiography or magnetic resonance angiography. There are several published series of patients with renovascular disease with initial symptoms of moderate to advanced renal insufficiency in whom balloon angioplasty (often with stenting) or surgical reconstruction produced marked improvement in renal function and blood pressure control.

Another syndrome, lead nephropathy, has been reported to be both common and potentially reversible in patients without other obvious conditions that produce renal insufficiency. The diagnosis is suggested by the coexistence of renal insufficiency, arthritis resulting from gout, and a history of lead exposure and is confirmed by measurement of urinary lead excretion after administration of calcium ethylenediaminetetraacetic acid (EDTA). Treatment involves cessation of lead exposure and a course of EDTA chelation. Anecdotal reports have verified that chelation therapy can halt or partially reverse the course of chronic renal insufficiency. Studies to date are insufficient to warrant the diagnostic use of calcium EDTA infusions in the absence of the described disease characteristics.

■ DIFFERENTIAL DIAGNOSIS

CRF is the end result of damage to kidneys arising from a multiplicity of causes (Table 141.1). The initial factors leading to kidney failure are numerous and include immunologic insults, obstruction to urine flow, metabolic disturbances, infections, vascular disorders, hereditary diseases, neoplasia, trauma, and radiation. It is often useful to categorize the renal insult according to anatomic involvement that is predominantly glomerular, tubulointerstitial, obstructive, or vascular. Renal involvement also can be divided into either primary renal diseases (usually glomerular), in which the kidney is the sole afflicted organ, or renal disorders that accompany or complicate systemic illnesses.

The incidence of CRF in the community and the relative distribution of each of its causes remain difficult to establish. Data are available on the comparative importance of the various sources of renal failure in the population of adults with ESRD at the onset of maintenance dialysis. The glomerulopathies are the most important causes; they account for 30% of all cases. Diabetic glomerulosclerosis is the most common cause of renal failure among the systemic disorders and affects an increasing fraction (up to one-third) of the patients currently treated for ESRD. Interstitial renal disease and polycystic kidney disease account for about 20% and 10%, respectively, of cases of CRF among patients with ESRD. The relative contribution of hypertensive arteriolar nephrosclerosis varies with race. In blacks, it may affect a third of all ESRD patients, but it accounts for less than 10% of cases among the white population.

The exact cause of CRF is never established in many patients. This is usually the case even if histologic studies are available, because they may not be diagnostic in the context of far-advanced renal failure with bilaterally shrunken and scarred kidneys (see Chapter 164). Sometimes clues to the cause can be obtained from the history, physical examination, or specific laboratory studies.

HISTORY

A long-standing history of hypertension may suggest the diagnosis of arteriolar nephrosclerosis. Previous complaints of prostatism, stone passage, or bladder dysfunction may indicate obstructive uropathy. Recurrent urinary tract infection or analgesic abuse may reflect interstitial nephritis. A positive family history is often present in patients with polycystic kidney disease. Symptoms of long-standing diabetes mellitus often accompany the development of diabetic nephropathy. Symptoms of systemic lupus erythematosus or other vasculitides are also indicative in some patients with otherwise unexplained renal failure. HIV-associated nephropathy is typically present in patients with risk factors or symptoms of the infection. Chronic extrarenal infections or inflammation may indicate the presence of amyloidosis. A history of illicit alcohol abuse ("moonshine"), gout, and hypertension may suggest the diagnosis of lead nephropathy.

PHYSICAL EXAMINATION

Funduscopic findings of microaneurysms, exudates, and neovascularization strongly suggest the association of diabetic glomerulosclerosis. Palpable, irregularly enlarged kidneys are indicative of polycystic kidney disease. A large prostate or enlarged urinary bladder may be a sign of bladder outlet obstruction. A facial rash and arthritis can reflect lupus nephritis. Hearing loss and lenticular distortion often indicate the presence of hereditary nephritis (Alport's syndrome). The finding of angiokeratomas strongly supports the diagnosis of Fabry's disease. Dermal manifestations of scleroderma may point to the presence of kidney disease associated with progressive systemic sclerosis.

LABORATORY STUDIES

The urinalysis results are typically abnormal in most stages of renal failure and may show varying degrees of proteinuria, hematuria, pyuria, and casts. Heavy proteinuria and red blood cell casts are helpful in pinpointing glomerulonephritis. Broad and waxy casts are seen in CRF of almost any origin and reflect nonspecific dilatation of the renal tubules. In many forms of CRF (e.g., hypertensive nephrosclerosis, obstructive uropathy, polycystic kidney disease, hypercalcemic nephropathy), the urinalysis results can show minimal abnormalities and thus may be misleading. Other laboratory abnormalities may be more specific, because they can indicate the cause of CRF. Abnormal serum and urine electrophoresis results may suggest multiple myeloma. Urine immunoelectrophoresis is a very sensitive diagnostic test. A positive sickle cell test indicates sickle cell nephropathy, which is confirmed by performing hemoglobin electrophoresis. Renal disease stemming from infective endocarditis requires documentation by positive blood cultures. Positive urine cultures for mycobacteria point to renal tuberculosis. Depressed serum complement levels and positive tests for antinuclear and anti-DNA antibodies are important clues in diagnosing lupus nephritis. Antibodies for glomerular basement membrane are present in Goodpasture's syndrome and antiglomerular basement membrane nephritis; positive antineutrophil cytoplasmic antibodies are helpful in the diagnosis of Wegener's granulomatosis or other systemic vasculitides.

Radiographic studies often help establish the cause of renal failure. Renal ultrasonography, the primary approach for almost all patients, is a noninvasive, cost-effective procedure that provides valuable data, such as the presence of a solitary kidney, small kidneys with cortical atrophy, a dilated pelvicalyceal system, cystic diseases, and renal calculi. It is occasionally useful to include an ultrasonographic examination of the urinary bladder to detect outlet obstruction or other abnormalities. A plain abdominal radiographic film of good quality also may provide helpful clues on renal size and contour and show whether radiopaque calculi and nephrocalcinosis are present. The use of urography to evaluate advanced renal failure has been limited in recent years, partly because of the fear of precipitating contrast-induced acute renal failure in susceptible patients and partly because of the wide use of ultrasonography. It may still be indicated in some situations, however (e.g., establishing evidence of papillary necrosis in analgesic nephropathy). In reflux nephropathy, a voiding cystourethrogram can confirm the diagnosis and avoid intravenous administration of contrast medium. Unfortunately, renal biopsy is of limited value in determining the cause of renal failure, because the histologic findings may be too nonspecific to detect the initial insult. Nevertheless, in some forms of unexplained renal failure associated with normal-sized kidneys, renal histologic studies may be helpful, as discussed earlier.

■ CONSERVATIVE MANAGEMENT

After ruling out potentially treatable causes of renal failure and after looking for the reversible factors that can produce deterioration of renal function regardless of the underlying cause, it is appropriate to consider prophylactic and therapeutic methods that can improve the patient's quality of life, minimize symptoms, and prevent long-term complications. The following factors should be evaluated to generate a prescription tailored to each patient's needs.

CONTROL OF BLOOD PRESSURE

As renal failure progresses, hypertension, most often due to salt and water accumulation, inexorably develops. Hypertension can accelerate the progression of renal failure and can contribute to atherosclerotic cardiovascular disease. Meticulous blood pressure control, therefore, is an important goal of therapy. In part, this can be accomplished with regulation of sodium balance, as discussed later herein, but it often requires the addition of one or more antihypertensive agents to maintain the blood pressure in the normal range (see Chapter 30). Care should be taken not to lower the blood pressure too much, which may impair perfusion to vital organs, including the kidneys.

Treatment of hypertension is indicated at any stage of CRF. The superiority of angiotensin-converting enzyme inhibitors in slowing the progression of CRF has been documented in many large-scale studies both in diabetic and nondiabetic patients. The optimal level of blood pressure control is uncertain, but the results of long-term studies have indicated that systolic blood pressures of 125 to 130 mm Hg and diastolic pressures of 80 mm Hg or lower are desirable, particularly in patients excreting more than 2 to 3 g of urinary protein per day. Concurrent diuretic therapy will often be necessary, since fluid overload is present in most patients with CRF. Angiotensin II type 1 receptor antagonists are effective antihypertensive and antiproteinuric

agents, but it is still not known whether these agents can slow the progression of CRF. If specific side effects from angiotensin-converting enzyme inhibitors develop, such as cough, a receptor antagonist may be substituted.

PROTEINURIA

Heavy proteinuria can contribute to renal disease progression. For this reason, one aim of therapy is to diminish protein excretion by at least 50%, which may reflect reduced intraglomerular pressure and improved glomerular permselectivity. Even normotensive patients should be treated with antihypertensive agents if they have heavy proteinuria, preferably by angiotensin-converting enzyme inhibitors. Some clinical trials in patients with CRF and heavy proteinuria have established that verapamil, diltiazem, and angiotensin II type 1 receptor antagonists effectively diminish the amount of urinary protein excretion.

MINERAL METABOLISM

Owing to a combination of hyperphosphatemia and decreased production of calcitriol, hypocalcemia and secondary hyperparathyroidism always complicate renal insufficiency. Crippling bone disease in patients with ESRD can be prevented by prophylactic attention at earlier stages of the disease. The therapeutic goal is to maintain near-normal values for serum calcium, phosphate, and parathyroid hormone. This is accomplished in a series of steps. First, phosphate intake must not be excessive (less than 0.8 g per day). Protein restriction, which may be instituted for other reasons, as discussed later, reduces phosphate intake.

Second, when serum phosphate exceeds 5 to 5.5 mg per deciliter, it is appropriate to prescribe phosphate-binding agents with meals, preferably calcium carbonate or calcium acetate. Such therapy can also help maintain a normal level of serum calcium. Magnesium-containing antacids should be avoided by patients with impaired renal function, because of the risk of hypermagnesemia. Aluminum hydroxide is a potent phosphate-binding agent, but its use should be limited to a few days when severe hyperphosphatemia develops, in order to avoid aluminum toxicity. Sevelamer (Renagel®) hydrochloride is a novel non-aluminum- and non-calcium-containing phosphate binder that can be used if a patient shows signs of hypercalcemia (usually because of excess calcium supplements and vitamin D therapy) or if the calcium $\times$ phosphate product in the serum is above 75. Aluminum is absorbed from the gastrointestinal tract; thus, if urinary aluminum excretion is impaired, aluminum accumulates in the bone, brain, and other tissues. The most common toxic effect of aluminum is a type of adynamic osteomalacia that is resistant to treatment with calcitriol. The mechanism of action appears to be accumulation of aluminum in mineralizing bone, causing impaired calcification. Another syndrome linked to aluminum toxicity is dialysis dementia, characterized by seizures, aphasia, facial grimacing, paralysis, and, ultimately, coma. High aluminum levels have been associated with microcytic anemia.

Third, if the serum calcium level falls below 8.5 mg per deciliter despite well-controlled serum phosphate levels, it is reasonable to add calcitriol (0.25 to 1 μg per day) in conjunction with calcium supplements (more than 1 g per day of elemental calcium), which can be given between meals to optimize gastrointestinal calcium absorption.

SODIUM AND WATER INTAKE

With progression of renal disease, the kidney's capacity to adjust to marked variations in sodium and water intake becomes limited. The patient is at risk of sodium retention with high levels of intake (resulting in edema, congestive heart failure, and increased blood pressure) and is equally at risk of hypovolemia at low levels of intake (leading to hypotension and accelerated renal insufficiency). In general, the asymptomatic patient should be instructed to follow a diet that contains 4 to 6 g of sodium; this amount should be reduced to 2 to 4 g in the context of edema or significant hypertension and should be raised if hypotension, excessive renal or extrarenal salt wasting, or a sudden decline in GFR ensues. A few patients with interstitial nephritides, obstructive uropathy, or medullary cystic disease may excrete large amounts of salt and water. In these cases, dietary salt restriction leads to markedly negative sodium balance and loss of renal function.

The simplest method of avoiding these problems is to monitor body weight daily and to adjust dietary salt to maintain a constant weight. In patients with advanced renal insufficiency, water balance is generally governed by sodium balance, and patients who maintain a normal serum osmolality or sodium concentration can be left to their own instincts regarding water intake. They should be instructed, however, about the loss of adaptability with renal insufficiency and should avoid either severe water restriction or excess intake that is not stimulated by thirst.

POTASSIUM INTAKE

Despite significant loss of function, the kidney retains a remarkable capacity to excrete potassium until the GFR drops below 10 mL per minute. In the absence of iatrogenic manipulation, hyperkalemia is usually not seen before the development of ESRD. Hypokalemia is rare, except in situations of excess potassium losses (diuretics, diarrhea). Many superimposed factors can exacerbate problems with potassium balance, however. The patient may be placed on a low-salt diet with salt substitutes (which contain potassium chloride) or may develop intercurrent illnesses that increase potassium intake (gastrointestinal bleeding). Cellular potassium uptake may be impaired (hyperglycemia with insulin deficiency, β-blockers). Renal potassium excretion may also be limited (volume contraction, triamterene, amiloride, spironolactone, angiotensin-converting enzyme inhibitors, nonsteroidal anti-inflammatory agents). In addition, some renal diseases (diabetes, obstruction, interstitial nephritis) are complicated by hypoaldosteronism (with or without hyporeninism) or an impaired renal response to aldosterone, which can interfere with potassium secretion in the collecting duct. In these instances, avoidance of potassium-rich foods and potassium-sparing diuretics usually suffice; if not, addition of the ion-exchange resin sodium polystyrene sulfonate (Kayexalate) is helpful. As discussed later, the inability to control hyperkalemia in end-stage patients is an indication for dialysis.

ACID–BASE BALANCE

As the GFR falls below 15 to 20 mL per minute, the ability to excrete hydrogen ions becomes significantly limited, owing to the decreasing renal mass and consequent insufficient total renal ammonia production and excretion. At this point, significant metabolic acidosis may ensue. Many authors recommend therapy when the serum bicarbonate level falls below 20 mEq per liter. To the extent that chronic metabolic acidosis with a serum pH of less than 7.3 reduces bone density, increases respiratory work, impairs cardiovascular catecholamine responsiveness, and aggravates muscle protein catabolism, it is reasonable to begin alkali therapy at a bicarbonate level of 18 to 20 mEq per liter, rather than depending on respiratory compensation. Long-term alkali therapy to maintain a near-normal serum bicarbonate concentration may prevent bone resorption and muscle catabolism in patients with CRF. In the absence of edema or significant hypertension, sodium bicarbonate or citrate can be used.

Additionally, calcium carbonate or calcium acetate can be prescribed as adjunct alkali replacement, particularly in patients with a tendency toward hypocalcemia. Sodium citrate should be avoided when a patient is placed on aluminum-containing phosphate binders, because of the enhanced gastrointestinal absorption of aluminum and the increased risk of aluminum toxicity. Patients with advanced renal failure are susceptible to rapid worsening of acidosis when the demand for acid excretion is increased, as in the context of diarrhea. In these situations, larger amounts of alkali may be required to maintain near-normal serum bicarbonate levels.

DRUG DOSAGE

Many drugs depend on renal excretion, and the prescription of usual dosages may result in excessive serum levels and subsequent toxicity. Medications that may require dosage alteration include digoxin, many antibiotics, long-acting barbiturates, and insulin. A detailed listing of the necessary modifications is provided in Chapter 167, and tables published elsewhere should be consulted when reviewing the patient's medication list. Some drugs should be avoided because they are particularly dangerous to the patient with renal insufficiency. These include any magnesium-containing compounds, nonsteroidal anti-inflammatory drugs, potassium-sparing diuretics, and radiographic contrast materials.

PROTEIN INTAKE

Three issues merit consideration in designing the appropriate dietary program for a patient with CRF. The most obvious is the patient's complaint of common symptoms of uremia, which usually develop as the BUN exceeds 90 mg per deciliter. Reducing dietary protein intake improves anorexia, nausea, vomiting, worsening metabolic acidosis, and hyperkalemia. Simple limitation of protein intake, however, is insufficient. The second issue that must be considered is the adequacy of caloric intake and essential amino acids, which can be achieved by providing biologically useful protein mixtures. These issues have led to the development of reasonably palatable diets that provide symptomatic improvement without evidence of malnutrition. The usual protein-restricted diet supplies an intake of 0.6 g per kilogram of body weight of a mixed protein diet.

The third issue that has received considerable attention is the use of a low-protein diet early in the course of renal insufficiency, not to ameliorate uremic symptoms but to retard the progression of renal disease. This approach is based on the hyperfiltration hypothesis discussed earlier. There are scattered reports that dietary manipulation can slow the progression of CRF, including diabetic nephropathy. The results of the Modification of Diet in Renal Disease Study, a recently completed large-scale, randomized trial in nondiabetic patients, suggests that long-term adherence to the low-protein diet is well tolerated and tends to slow the progression of renal failure, although this effect is relatively small, requires at least 2 to 3 years of follow-up to become apparent, and has less of an impact on deterioration of GFR than does tight control of elevated blood pressure with antihypertensive agents that include converting enzyme inhibitors.

Thus, if attention is paid to compliance, palatability, and adequate intake of calories, essential amino acids, and vitamins, the prescription of a low-protein diet early in the course of renal insufficiency, in conjunction with strict control of hypertension, is a relatively safe and beneficial approach to reducing the rate of decline in GFR.

ANEMIA

The introduction of recombinant erythropoietin therapy has dramatically changed our approach to the management of anemia of CRF. This therapy is effective in correcting anemia in virtually all patients, even though red cell survival is shortened. Hormone replacement therapy imparts freedom from the complications of repeated blood transfusions, abatement of symptoms of anemia, and overall improvement in quality-of-life parameters, such as brain and cognitive function, sexual potency, and exercise tolerance. Patients should be screened for other causes of anemia, such as iron deficiency, blood loss, multiple myeloma, and vitamin deficiency. Because iron use is markedly augmented during therapy with erythropoietin, large amounts of iron supplements should also be administered.

◼ FOLLOW-UP AND REASSESSMENT

Because chronic renal insufficiency is almost invariably progressive, it is important to reassess the management program periodically to prevent and detect complications and to plan for eventual replacement therapy. The history and physical examination can provide evidence of uremia, sodium retention, or hypovolemia and the adequacy of blood pressure control. Electrolytes, calcium and phosphate, BUN, and creatinine levels should be assessed at 4- to 6-month intervals to determine when to alter dietary therapy or to add or subtract drugs. Bone roentgenograms and bone biopsy samples may furnish useful information regarding progressive osteodystrophy. A neurologic examination, supplemented by nerve conduction velocity studies, may be required to assess the progression of existing peripheral neuropathy.

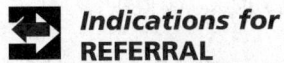

Indications for REFERRAL

With progression of renal insufficiency to end stage, conservative management becomes inadequate for the prevention of symptoms and the control of blood pressure. At this point, an end-stage renal program must be designed. Such symptoms as nausea, vomiting, anorexia, or weight loss may herald the need to initiate dialysis replacement therapy. Objective findings that indicate the need for dialysis include progressive peripheral neuropathy, pericarditis, inadequate nutrition, impaired cognitive function, general malaise and weakness that interfere with the ability to work, congestive heart failure, severe hypertension, significant hyperkalemia, and metabolic acidosis. Ideally, maintenance dialysis should be started when there is significant expectation that without dialysis, uremic symptoms would develop in a short time. Long-term dialysis is usually initiated when the creatinine clearance rate falls below 10 mL per minute. It therefore is prudent to begin planning at an earlier time, even in the absence of symptoms. Referral to a nephrologist is indicated to discuss the relative merits and advisability of various dialysis options or renal transplantation and to decide when to establish access to the circulation. Early referral is useful to prevent the development of severe uremic symptoms, to allow time for maturation of an arteriovenous fistula, to prepare the patient for kidney transplantation, and to allow preparation and evaluation of potential kidney donors.

BIBLIOGRAPHY

Eberst ME, Berkowitz LR. Hemostasis in renal disease: pathophysiology and management. *Am J Med* 1994;96:168–179.

Fraser CL, Arieff AI. Nervous system complications in uremia. *Ann Intern Med* 1988;109:143–153.

Gansevoort RT, Sluiter WJ, Hemmelder MH, et al. Antiproteinuric effect of blood-pressure-lowering agents: a meta-analysis of comparative trials. *Nephrol Dial Transplant* 1995;10:1963–1974.

Hruska KA, Teitelbaum SL. Mechanisms of disease: renal osteodystrophy. *N Engl J Med* 1995;333:166–174.

Ismail N, Becker BN. An opportunity to intervene: erythropoetin for the treatment of anaemia in pre-dialysis patients. *Nephrol Dial Transplant* 1998;13:14–17.

Klahr S, Levey AS, Beck GJ, et al. The effects of dietary protein restriction and blood-pressure control on the progression of chronic renal disease: Modification of Diet in Renal Disease Study Group. *N Engl J Med* 1994;330:877–884.

Llach F. Secondary hyperparathyroidism in renal failure: the trade-off hypothesis revisited. *Am J Kidney Dis* 1995;25:663–679.

Maschio G, Marcantoni C. Angiotensin converting enzyme inhibitors in nondiabetic renal disease. *Curr Opin Nephrol Hypertens* 1998;7:253–257.

Remuzzi G, Bertani T. Mechanism of disease: pathophysiology of progressive nephropathies. *N Engl J Med* 1998;339:1448–1456.

Rimmer JM, Gennari FJ. Atherosclerotic renovascular disease and progressive renal failure. *Ann Intern Med* 1993;118:712–719.

Vanholder R, De Smet R, Hsu C, et al. Uremic toxicity: the middle molecule hypothesis revisited. *Semin Nephrol* 1994;14:205–218.

Walser M. Progression of chronic renal failure in man. *Kidney Int* 1990; 37:1195–1210.

Ziyadeh FN. Evidence for the involvement of transforming growth factor-beta in the pathogenesis of diabetic kidney disease: Are Koch's postulates fulfilled? *Curr Pract Med* 1998;1:87–89.

Kelley's Textbook of Internal Medicine, fourth edition. Edited by H. David Humes.
Lippincott Williams & Wilkins, Philadelphia © 2000.

CHAPTER
142

APPROACH TO THE PATIENT WITH VOLUME DEPLETION AND DEHYDRATION

JAMES A. SHAYMAN

PATHOPHYSIOLOGY

Total body water comprises 50% to 70% of the total body weight. Fluid within the body distributes into three major compartments: intracellular, extracellular, and transcellular. The intracellular fluid compartment is the largest, accounting for approximately two-thirds of total body water. The extracellular fluid compartment consists of interstitial and intravascular compartments; approximately 75% of extracellular fluid is interstitial, and the rest is intravascular. Transcellular fluid includes cerebrospinal, intraocular, pleural, peritoneal, and synovial fluids. These fluid compartments are separated from the plasma fluid by a capillary endothelium and a specialized layer of epithelial cells.

The regulation of the size and composition of the body's fluid compartments is a primary requirement for survival. Water balance is a critical factor in determining the composition of the fluid compartment. Alterations in water balance manifest as changes in plasma osmolality and are detected as changes in plasma sodium concentration (see Chapters 144 and 145). In contrast, sodium balance is the critical factor in determining the size of the fluid compartment. Alterations in sodium balance are detected as changes in extracellular volume.

The regulation of sodium balance is a consequence of physical factors affecting fluid movement across cell membranes, of the renal handling of sodium, and of a complex affector and effector hormonal and neural network that maintains the volume in each fluid compartment (see Chapter 9). Physical factors that govern the distribution of fluid between the vascular and interstitial compartments can be understood on the basis of the hydrostatic and colloid osmotic pressures in the capillaries (Starling forces). The hydrostatic pressure of blood entering the capillary promotes the movement of fluid across the capillary endothelium into the interstitial space. This fluid movement is opposed by the plasma oncotic pressure and the hydrostatic pressure of the interstitial compartment. Changes in capillary hydrostatic, interstitial hydrostatic, or plasma oncotic pressure can contribute to a clinically significant redistribution of fluid between the interstitial and plasma compartments.

HISTORY AND PHYSICAL EXAMINATION

The intravascular, interstitial, and transcellular fluid compartments may each be evaluated for signs and symptoms of sodium depletion. The presence of signs and symptoms of sodium depletion depends on both the degree of depletion and on the rapidity of its development (Table 142.1). Acute decreases of less than 5% of the extracellular fluid volume produce minimal signs and symptoms. Losses of up to 10% of extracellular volume manifest as orthostatic changes in pulse and blood pressure. Fluid losses of 20% or more exceed the capacities of an individual's normal homeostatic defense mechanisms and are associated with shock.

The physical examination plays an important role in the assessment of volume depletion. However, a physical examination provides only a rough estimate of the extracellular volume status and may be difficult to interpret. Orthostatic changes in pulse and blood pressure may be absent in the presence of such sympatholytic agents as β-adrenergic receptor blockers or in patients with autonomic insufficiency, as is common in patients with long-standing diabetes mellitus. Skin turgor may be an unreliable sign in the elderly patient who has diminished skin elasticity. The oral mucosa may be dry in patients who respire through their mouths, independent of their volume status.

DIFFERENTIAL DIAGNOSIS

Volume depletion occurs when sodium losses exceed sodium gains. Because the kidneys are very efficient in their ability to conserve sodium, restriction of sodium intake alone is insufficient to produce sodium deficiency in healthy persons. Negative

TABLE 142.1.	PHYSICAL FINDINGS WITH EXTRACELLULAR VOLUME DEPLETION
Fluid Compartment	**Physical Findings**
Intravascular	Orthostatic fall in systolic blood pressure of >15 mm Hg
	Orthostatic rise in pulse rate >15 beats/min
	Hypotension while recumbent
Interstitial	Decreased skin turgor
Transcellular	Dry mouth, mucous membranes; decreased intraocular pressure

TABLE 142.2.	CAUSES OF SODIUM DEPLETION

Extrarenal sodium losses
  Gastrointestinal
    With metabolic alkalosis (vomiting, nasogastric suctioning)
    With metabolic acidosis (diarrhea, intestinal fistulas)
  Cutaneous
    Burns
    Inflammatory disease of the skin
    Excessive sweating
  Third-space sequestration
    Small-bowel obstruction
    Pancreatitis
    Peritonitis
Renal sodium losses
  With normal renal function
    Diuretics
    Hypoaldosteronism
  With renal impairment
    Salt-wasting nephropathy (medullary cystic disease, nephrocalcinosis, interstitial nephritis)
    Diuretic phase of acute tubular necrosis
    Chronic renal failure

sodium balance develops with excessive extrarenal or renal sodium losses (Table 142.2).

EXTRARENAL LOSSES

Gastrointestinal losses are a major cause of volume depletion due to extrarenal sodium loss. The composition of the fluid secretion varies along the gastrointestinal tract. Gastric secretions have a high hydrogen ion concentration; therefore, excessive sodium loss from vomiting or nasogastric suction tends to be associated with metabolic alkalosis. Biliary, intestinal, and pancreatic secretions have bicarbonate concentrations in excess of those found in plasma. Excessive fluid loss from these sources results in the net loss of bicarbonate and in metabolic acidosis. Gastrointestinal secretions at all levels are iso-osmotic relative to plasma, so hypo-osmolality (i.e., hyponatremia) does not develop unless hypotonic fluids (e.g., 0.45% sodium chloride) or isotonic glucose are replaced. Gastrointestinal secretions also have higher potassium concentrations than are found in plasma. Hypokalemia is a common feature of excess gastrointestinal fluid loss (see Chapter 146).

Clinically significant cutaneous sodium loss may accompany diaphoresis and burns. Because sweat is hypotonic, water loss from the skin is proportionately greater than sodium loss. For this reason, excess cutaneous sodium loss from perspiration (as with strenuous exercise) may result in hypernatremia in addition to significant hypovolemia. Burns and other inflammatory disorders of the skin are often associated with an increase in capillary permeability, resulting in the loss of plasma proteins in addition to sodium and water. The decline in plasma oncotic pressure results in contraction of the intravascular compartment in excess of that seen with an equivalent degree of sodium loss alone.

A significant volume of fluid can be sequestered within the body in a compartment where it cannot be exchanged readily with intravascular or interstitial fluid. Such accumulations can occur in the context of bowel obstruction (with fluid in the bowel lumen or wall), peritonitis (with fluid in the peritoneal cavity), or infection or hemorrhage (with fluid in such areas as the retroperitoneum or limbs).

RENAL LOSSES

Sodium depletion from renal losses can occur with a normally functioning kidney or in renal disease. Such diuretics as loop diuretics (furosemide) and thiazides act on the thick ascending limb of Henle's loop or distal tubule, respectively, to decrease sodium reabsorption. When sodium intake is less than sodium excretion, negative sodium balance results. Negative sodium balance is the desired therapeutic effect for hypervolemic patients, such as those with congestive heart failure. When diuretics are abused, are given at doses in excess of therapeutic requirements, or are active when another cause of volume depletion is present (e.g., vomiting or diarrhea), significant sodium depletion may result.

Osmotic diuretics also may produce sodium depletion. These diuretics may represent exogenously administered compounds (e.g., mannitol) or compounds endogenously present (e.g., glucose). In the latter case, a patient with poorly controlled diabetes may filter glucose in excess of his or her tubular capacity for tubular reabsorption. With both exogenously administered and endogenously produced osmotic diuretics, solutes that are not reabsorbed reduce water reabsorption and lower the luminal salt concentration in the tubule, limiting the concentration gradient for salt reabsorption.

Hypoaldosteronism is another cause of sodium depletion in the context of normal renal function. The modest increase in urinary salt excretion observed with hypoaldosteronism is usually compensated by moderate increases in dietary sodium chloride intake. Patients with hypoaldosteronism are susceptible to significant sodium depletion with extrarenal sodium losses, however, owing to lack of adequate renal compensation.

Renal losses of sodium occur in the context of several renal diseases (Table 142.2). Common to all these conditions is the inability of the renal tubules to reabsorb sodium at a normal level, even when maximally stimulated. In nonoliguric renal failure or during the diuretic phase of recovery from acute tubular necrosis, this inability is due to intrinsic defects in sodium transport. In chronic renal failure, the surviving nephrons may transport sodium efficiently but lack the collective capacity to handle the increased filtered load of sodium. Salt wasting is a feature of several types of renal disease, including medullary cystic disease, nephrocalcinosis, interstitial nephritis, and Bartter's syndrome.

◼ LABORATORY STUDIES

The serum sodium concentration may be normal, low, or high, depending on the concurrent state of water balance; for this reason, it is not a helpful parameter. The blood urea nitrogen (BUN) concentration is usually elevated disproportionately to the serum creatinine concentration. A ratio of BUN to creatinine of more than 20:1 is indicative of prerenal azotemia. In extrarenal sodium losses, the urinary sodium concentration is typically less than 10 mEq per liter. Urinary sodium concentrations are usually higher than 20 mEq per liter in conditions of volume depletion attributable to diuretics, hypoaldosteronism, or intrinsic renal disease with salt wasting.

STRATEGIES FOR OPTIMAL CARE

Regardless of the origin, volume depletion initially should be treated by restoring the vascular volume. Isotonic saline is typically infused so long as any evidence of hemodynamic compromise persists. Coexisting electrolyte abnormalities, such as metabolic acidosis or alkalosis, should be treated to correct the underlying acid–base disorder. When hemorrhage is the basis of the volume depletion, packed red blood cells should be transfused. After the circulatory hemodynamics are stabilized, the basis for the volume depletion must be established and treatment initiated. When the volume depletion is drug-induced (e.g., by diuretics), the offending agent is withheld. If the patient is deficient in aldosterone, mineralocorticoid therapy may be indicated. If volume depletion stems from salt-wasting nephropathy, increased dietary sodium chloride may be initiated.

BIBLIOGRAPHY

Aukland K. Is extracellular fluid volume regulated? *Acta Physiol Scand* 1989; 136(suppl 583):59–67.
Guyton AC. *Textbook of medical physiology*, eighth ed. Philadelphia: WB Saunders, 1991.
Shayman JA. Sodium. In Shayman JA, ed. *Renal pathophysiology*. Philadelphia: JB Lippincott, 1995:27–51.
Simpson FO. Sodium intake, body sodium, and sodium excretion. *Lancet* 1988;2:25–29.

C H A P T E R
143

APPROACH TO THE PATIENT WITH EDEMA

JAMES A. SHAYMAN

PATHOPHYSIOLOGY

Edema is the excessive accumulation of fluid within interstitial spaces. Interstitial fluid accumulation is largely determined by the distribution of fluid between intravascular and interstitial compartments or Starling forces. The distribution of fluid between the intracellular and extracellular compartments is determined by the osmotic forces operating across cell membranes, but the distribution of fluid between the intravascular and interstitial compartments is independent of fluid osmolality. This is because crystalloid solutes penetrate the capillary wall completely. In contrast, colloid solutes, such as plasma proteins, are almost completely confined to the vascular space and contribute an oncotic pressure that exerts a net force across the capillary wall. The colloid osmotic pressure (or oncotic pressure) favoring the movement of fluid into the vascular space is 25 to 30 mm Hg.

The distribution of fluid between the intravascular and interstitial compartments is also determined by hydrostatic forces. Blood entering the capillaries has a mean hydrostatic pressure of 40 to 45 mm Hg. At the arteriolar end of the capillaries, there is a net force of approximately 5 mm Hg, favoring movement of fluid into the interstitial space. The dissipation of pressure and the rise in capillary oncotic pressure by the end of the capillary favors the movement of fluid back into the capillary. The amount of intravascular fluid entering the venules from the capillaries is slightly less than that entering the capillary. This excess fluid is returned to the vascular space through the lymphatic circulation.

Based on the factors regulating the distribution of fluid between the intravascular and interstitial spaces, edema may develop as the result of four primary abnormalities: increased mean capillary hydrostatic pressure, decreased capillary oncotic pressure, increased capillary permeability to protein, or obstruction of lymphatic flow. Most disorders associated with edema are initiated by an alteration in the Starling forces and are perpetuated as a result of the retention of sodium by the kidney.

Normally, expansion of the extracellular fluid compartment results in natriuresis. In generalized edematous states, however, there is a stimulus for the retention of sodium by the kidney. This stimulus is a decline in the effective circulating arterial blood volume perfusing the kidney and other tissues. The decrease in effective tissue perfusion leads to increased release of renin, formation of aldosterone, and higher levels of antidiuretic hormone. The result is an increase in sodium and water retention. Three disorders are associated with generalized edema and renal sodium retention: congestive heart failure, the nephrotic syndrome, and cirrhosis. The decline in effective arterial blood volume in congestive heart failure stems from amplified hydrostatic pressure on the venous side and impaired cardiac output. Liver disease and the nephrotic syndrome cause a decrease in effective arterial volume due to a lowering of plasma oncotic pressure and a redistribution of plasma volume from the vascular to the interstitial space.

HISTORY AND PHYSICAL EXAMINATION

Sodium retention resulting in a generalized edematous state may be associated with pulmonary edema, peripheral edema, or ascites. Patients with pulmonary edema often complain of shortness of breath, dyspnea on exertion, or orthopnea. On physical examination, the patient may show signs of tachypnea and rales. A chest radiograph shows changes suggestive of interstitial edema or alveolar fluid accumulation (see Chapter 386). Peripheral edema is associated with swollen legs or the presacral accumulation of fluid in the patient at bed rest. Pitting edema is the persistence of a depression in the skin after 10 seconds of pressure applied with the fingers and is usually seen when at least 10 pounds of fluid has accumulated. Patients with ascites complain of increasing abdominal girth. The finding of shifting dullness or a fluid wave on physical examination is indicative of ascites. Ascites can be confirmed by abdominal ultrasonography.

DIFFERENTIAL DIAGNOSIS

Common disorders associated with generalized or localized edema can be categorized based on the primary factor affecting the distribution of fluid between the vascular and interstitial compartments (Table 143.1). Some disorders appear to produce edema as the result of the inappropriate retention of sodium by the kidney, independent of a primary alteration in Starling forces. These include primary aldosteronism, acute glomerulonephritis, and estrogen administration.

Generalized edematous states can be associated with pulmonary edema, ascites, or peripheral edema. Ascites and peripheral edema are common with right-sided ventricular heart failure. Right-sided atrial pressure is elevated; it is detected by distention of the jugular veins and can be confirmed by monitoring central venous pressure. Cirrhosis and the nephrotic syndrome are usually associated with normal or low central venous pressure. Patients with the nephrotic syndrome may have periorbital and peripheral edema; pulmonary edema is absent. These patients have proteinuria, with a 24-hour excretion of more than 3.5 g, and hypercholesterolemia. Diagnostic clues useful in distinguishing between generalized edematous disorders are summarized in Table 143.2.

STRATEGIES FOR OPTIMAL CARE

DIURETICS

Diuretics are a potent and useful alternative for the treatment of edema. Several classes of diuretics are available; the choice of

TABLE 143.1. PATHOPHYSIOLOGIC BASIS OF EDEMA

Increased hydrostatic pressure
   Generalized: congestive heart failure
   Localized: venous thrombosis
Decreased plasma oncotic pressure
   Nephrotic syndrome
   Cirrhosis
   Malnutrition
Increased vascular permeability
   Generalized: angioneurotic edema
   Localized: burns, histamine, pulmonary toxins, respiratory distress syndrome
Obstructed lymphatic flow
   Tissue irradiation, surgery, lymphatic spread of cancer

TABLE 143.2. DIAGNOSTIC CLUES IN EDEMATOUS DISORDERS

Disease	Source	Diagnostic Laboratory Values
Pulmonary edema	Left ventricular failure	Elevated pulmonary capillary wedge
	Increased pulmonary capillary permeability	Normal pulmonary capillary wedge pressure
Ascites	Right ventricular failure	Elevated central venous pressure
	Hepatic cirrhosis	Normal central venous pressure
Peripheral edema	Right ventricular failure	Elevated central venous pressure
	Hepatic cirrhosis	Normal central venous pressure
	Nephrotic syndrome	3.5 g proteinuria

agent is based on the degree of diuresis desired and the potential of any particular agent to induce untoward effects. Sulfonamide diuretics consist of two groups, the thiazides, including hydrochlorothiazide, and the nonthiazides, including chlorthalidone and metolazone. These agents act primarily at the distal tubule to inhibit the transport of sodium and chloride. Loop diuretics, including furosemide, bumetanide, and ethacrynic acid, act at the thick ascending limb of the loop of Henle to inhibit the Na-K-2Cl cotransporter. These potent agents may increase the urinary sodium excretion to more than 20% of the filtered sodium load. Potassium-sparing diuretics, including spironolactone, triamterene, and amiloride, act in the distal tubule to induce natriuresis and inhibit potassium excretion. Acetazolamide inhibits carbonic anhydrase in the proximal tubule, reducing bicarbonate reabsorption, and secondarily inhibits the reabsorption of sodium and water. In the absence of other diuretics, the sodium and water unabsorbed in the proximal tubule are reabsorbed more distally. Thus, acetazolamide is not a potent diuretic.

If mild diuresis is required, sulfonamide diuretics are often the agent of choice. These agents have poor efficacy in the context of renal insufficiency with glomerular filtration rates below 50 mL per minute. If more potent diuresis is required, a loop diuretic is chosen. Loop diuretics bind to plasma proteins, and their effectiveness depends on the plasma concentration of the unbound drug. Therefore, a single dose is more likely to be effective than a divided dose of the same total amount of diuretic. Diuretics acting in the proximal tubule are not typically used because of their poor natriuretic effects. Secondary hyperaldosteronism is common in cirrhosis. The diuretic of choice is therefore spironolactone, a competitive antagonist of aldosterone.

Diuretics alone often cannot eliminate generalized edema, owing to the secondary physiologic changes that accompany diuretic-induced diuresis. These changes include a decline in renal perfusion with a reduction in glomerular filtration rate, a stimulation of antidiuretic hormone and renin release and aldosterone production, and an increase in plasma protein concentration and peritubular oncotic pressure. These alterations result in the more avid reabsorption of sodium and water by the kidney. Because diuretics lead to the loss of salt and water from the vascular space, aggressive diuresis can bring about intravascular volume contraction and cardiovascular compromise. Finally, diuretics can produce untoward effects, such as hypokalemia, hyponatremia, and hyperglycemia.

DIETARY SODIUM AND WATER RESTRICTION

Restriction of dietary sodium and water intake is an important component in the treatment of generalized edema. In general, sodium and water restriction limits the further development of edema but has little effect on the resolution of edema. This is because the typical edema-forming patient excretes urine containing less than 10 mEq per liter of sodium, with a daily sodium excretion of less than 20 mEq. Because the most severe sodium-restricted diet may consist of 0.5 g (22 mEq) of sodium, it would take several days to lose even 1 L of excess fluid. Therefore, sodium restriction alone is unlikely to result in the resolution of edema and must be coupled with the use of diuretics or adjunctive therapy.

ADJUNCTIVE THERAPY

Elevation of the lower extremities or bed rest often improves the response to diuretics by increasing blood return to the heart and renal perfusion. The use of elastic stockings or bandages over edematous areas helps mobilize interstitial fluid and often promotes natriuresis and diuresis. Occasionally, patients with refractory edema require dialysis with ultrafiltration.

DISEASE-SPECIFIC TREATMENTS

The use of high-volume paracentesis for the treatment of ascites has become popular for patients with cirrhosis. This procedure can bring about a marked reduction in effective arterial blood volume, so patients should always undergo colloid expansion (usually with albumin) at the time of paracentesis. Patients with preexisting renal impairment may experience acute renal failure after high-volume paracentesis. This procedure should therefore be chosen carefully for patients with elevated creatinine levels.

The goal of diuretic therapy of patients with congestive heart failure is to lower the intravascular volume to the lowest level compatible with optimal cardiac output. This is best accomplished by monitoring cardiac filling pressures in the intensive care unit. In the outpatient setting, the physician must rely on measurements of central venous pressure, as assessed by jugular venous distention or hepatojugular reflux. In the patient on an optimal drug regimen, daily weight measurement is perhaps the best measure of volume status. In the compliant patient, a sliding regimen of loop diuretics can be instituted to maintain the weight within a desired range. Increasing cardiac output with the use of inotropic agents or vasodilators is an important factor in achieving the desired natriuresis and diuresis. Diuretics should be used cautiously in patients with the nephrotic syndrome, to avoid acute renal failure due to intravascular volume depletion. The use of salt-poor albumin in combination with a loop diuretic may initiate diuresis. Low-dose dopamine (1 to 2 μg per kilogram per minute) may also cause a diuretic response by promoting an increase in renal blood flow.

BIBLIOGRAPHY

Dzau VJ. Renal and circulatory mechanisms in congestive heart failure. *Kidney Int* 1987;31:1402–1415.
Kubo SH. Neurohormonal activity in congestive heart failure. *Crit Care Med* 1990;18:S39–S44.
Rocco VK, Ware AJ. Cirrhotic ascites: pathophysiology, diagnosis and management. *Ann Intern Med* 1986;105:573–585.
Schrier RW. Pathogenesis of sodium and water retention in high-output and low-output cardiac failure, nephrotic syndrome, cirrhosis and pregnancy. *N Engl J Med* 1988;319:1065–1134.
Schrier RW, Arroyo V, Bernardi M, et al. Peripheral arterial vasodilation hypothesis: a proposal for the initiation of renal sodium and water retention in cirrhosis. *Hepatology* 1988;8:1151–1157.
Shayman JA. Sodium. In: Shayman JA, ed. *Renal pathophysiology*. Philadelphia: JB Lippincott, 1995:27–51.

Kelley's Textbook of Internal Medicine, fourth edition. Edited by H. David Humes. Lippincott Williams & Wilkins, Philadelphia © 2000.

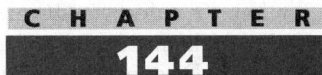

CHAPTER 144

APPROACH TO THE PATIENT WITH HYPONATREMIA

LAWRENCE S. WEISBERG
MALCOLM COX

 PRESENTATION

Hyponatremia (serum sodium concentration less than 135 mEq per liter) is one of the most common electrolyte disorders—it is found in approximately 3% of hospitalized patients and as many as 30% of patients in intensive care units. Although the exact prevalence is unknown, hyponatremia is also seen often in outpatient practice, especially among patients with underlying disorders of extracellular volume homeostasis. The clinical manifestations of hyponatremia can be attributed largely to intracellular volume expansion (cellular edema). Cellular edema occurs only when hyponatremia is associated with hypotonicity. Intracellular volume expansion is of greatest consequence in the brain, where it is translated into increased intracranial pressure because of the rigid calvarium.

Most cells—especially brain cells—have adaptive mechanisms for mitigating tonicity-related volume changes. Cell volume peaks 1 to 2 hours after the onset of acute hypotonicity. Thereafter, solute and water are lost from cells, and cell volume returns toward normal. Solute loss is initially rapid and consists mainly of electrolytes during the first 6 to 12 hours of adaptation. Over the next 24 to 72 hours, organic solutes (largely amino acids) are more slowly lost. After several days of sustained hypotonicity, cell volume is restored nearly to normal.

The morbidity and mortality associated with hypotonic hyponatremia are influenced by several factors, including the magnitude and rate of development of hypotonicity, the patient's age and gender, and the nature and severity of any underlying diseases. The very young and very old, women, and alcoholics appear to be at particular risk. Volume adaptation to hypotonicity may be deficient in premenopausal women, who suffer more frequent and more severe neurologic consequences than men with equivalent degrees of hypotonicity.

Neurologic symptoms usually do not develop until the serum sodium concentration falls below 125 mEq per liter, at which time the patient may complain of anorexia, nausea, and malaise. At a level between 120 and 110 mEq per liter, the patient experiences headache, lethargy, confusion, agitation, and obtundation. More severe symptoms (seizures, coma) may occur with levels below 110 mEq per liter. Focal neurologic findings are unusual, but they do occur, and transtentorial cerebral herniation has been described in severe cases, especially in young women.

Although symptoms generally resolve with correction of hypotonicity, there may be permanent neurologic deficits, particularly in cases of severe (serum sodium concentration less than 120 mEq per liter), acute hypotonicity, when the brain's volume-regulatory defenses can be overwhelmed. Hypotonicity of this magnitude that develops in less than 24 hours may be associated with residual neurologic deficits and has a 50% mortality rate. In contrast, when hypotonicity evolves more gradually, symptoms are both less common and less severe. Indeed, patients with chronic hyponatremia, even in the range of 115 to 120 mEq per liter, may be completely asymptomatic.

■ PATHOPHYSIOLOGY AND DIFFERENTIAL DIAGNOSIS

Sodium is the major cation in extracellular fluid and, along with its associated anions, accounts for almost all the osmolality of this body fluid compartment. Consequently, hypotonicity (low effective body fluid osmolality) always implies hyponatremia. In contrast, hyponatremia can coexist with normal (isotonic hyponatremia) or elevated (hypertonic hyponatremia) body fluid tonicity as well as with hypotonicity (hypotonic hyponatremia; Fig. 144.1).

Isotonic hyponatremia (also known as factitious or pseudohyponatremia) is a laboratory artifact seen with analytic techniques that measure the amount of sodium per unit volume of serum sampled. Normally, water constitutes approximately 93% of serum volume; the remaining 7% consists of solids, mostly lipids and proteins. In the presence of marked hypertriglyceridemia or paraproteinemia, when an increased volume of the serum is nonaqueous, the amount of sodium in the sample volume is reduced. This is reflected as a low serum sodium concentration, even though the concentration of sodium in serum water (and therefore plasma osmolality) is normal. Direct potentiometry (which uses an ion-selective electrode in undiluted serum) avoids this problem and has become the most common method for measuring the serum sodium concentration.

Hypertonic hyponatremia results from the presence in extracellular fluid of abnormal amounts of osmotically effective solutes other than sodium (glucose, mannitol). The osmotic pressure exerted by the nonsodium solute leads to redistribution of water from the intracellular to the extracellular fluid compartment and thereby to cellular dehydration and hyponatremia.

Hypotonic hyponatremia can arise from an isolated increase in total body water; deficits in both total body solute and water, with the water deficit being of lesser magnitude; or increases in both total body solute and water, with the water excess being of greater magnitude. Because water moves freely across cell membranes, hypotonic hyponatremia is always associated with cellular edema.

HYPOTONIC HYPONATREMIA

Hypotonic hyponatremia always reflects an inability of the kidney to excrete sufficient electrolyte-free water to match water intake (Table 144.1). The normal response to water ingestion (of sufficient magnitude to produce even slight hypotonicity) is the excretion of maximally dilute urine (urine osmolality less than 100 mOsm per kilogram). Hence, a urine osmolality less than 100 mOsm per kilogram in a patient with hypotonic hyponatremia points to excessive water intake as the cause (Fig. 144.1). In contrast, a urine osmolality above 100 mOsm per kilogram in the face of hypotonic hyponatremia signifies impaired renal electrolyte-free water excretion. In constructing a differential diagnosis, it is helpful to relate the causes of hypotonic hyponatremia to the patient's extracellular fluid volume status, which may be readily assessed at the bedside. Hypotonic hyponatremia may be associated with normal, decreased, or increased extracellular volume (Fig. 144.1).

EUVOLEMIC HYPONATREMIA

Because only one-third of total body water is extracellular in location (and only one-twelfth is intravascular), patients with pure water excess appear euvolemic; the only evidence of the increased total body water is low blood urea nitrogen and serum uric acid concentrations.

Patients with primary polydipsia usually have psychiatric disorders (hence, the use of such terms as psychogenic polydipsia and compulsive water drinking) and occasionally drink such large quantities of water that the kidney's ability to excrete electrolyte-free water is exceeded. The maximal rate of electrolyte-free water generation by the normal kidney is approximately 15 L per day, so that patients with primary polydipsia (and normal renal function) generally must ingest more than 15 L of water daily on an ongoing basis before hyponatremia develops. Because it is difficult to sustain such prodigious consumption for long periods, primary polydipsia is a distinctly unusual cause of hyponatremia in the context of normal renal diluting ability. Most

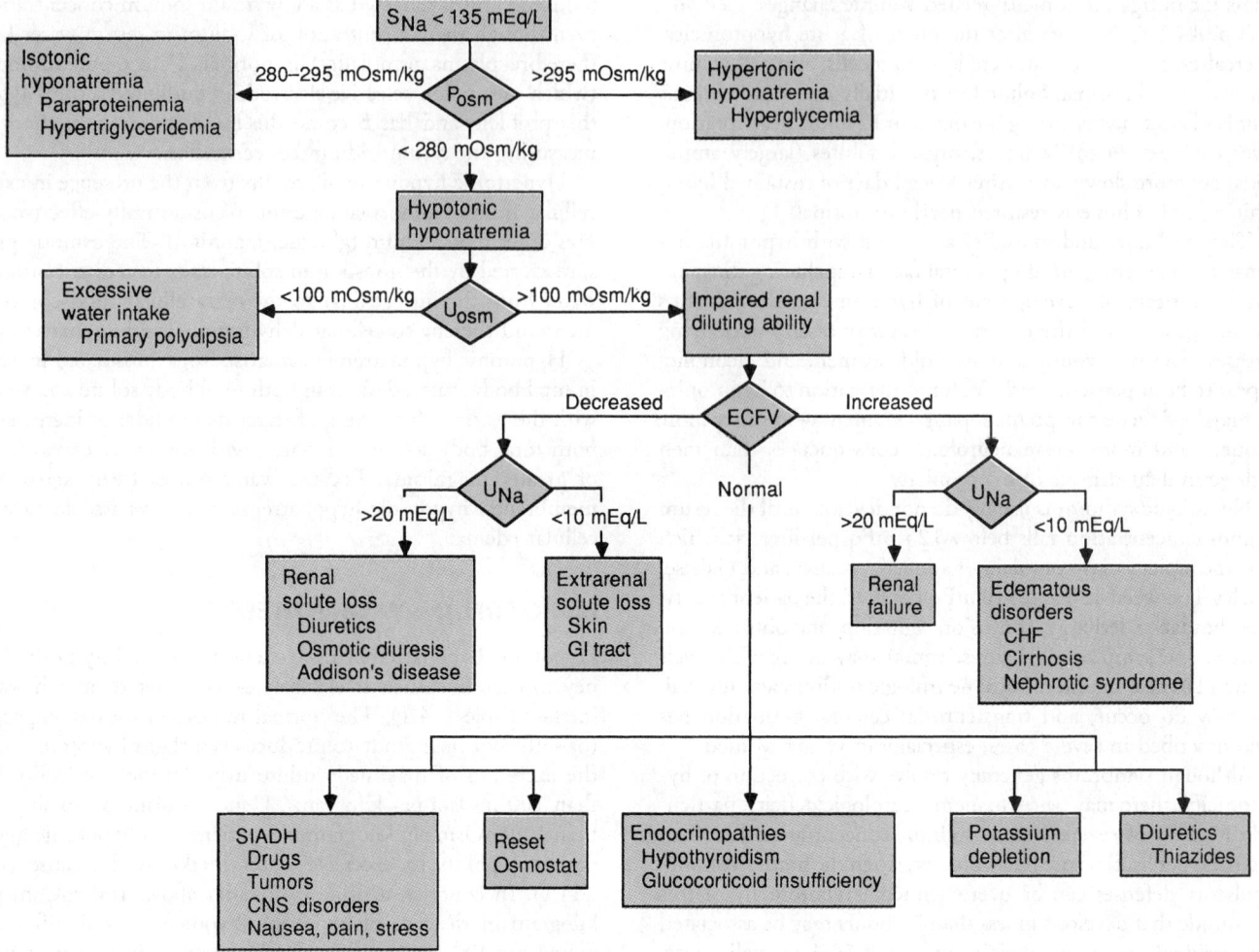

FIGURE 144.1. Approach to the patient with hyponatremia. S_{Na}, serum sodium concentration; U_{Na}, urine sodium concentration; P_{osm}, plasma osmolality; U_{osm}, urine osmolality; ECFV, extracellular fluid volume; GI, gastrointestinal; CHF, congestive heart failure; SIADH, syndrome of inappropriate antidiuretic hormone; CNS, central nervous system.

EVIDENCE LEVEL: C. Expert Opinion.

patients with psychogenic polydipsia who experience hyponatremia have concurrent diluting defects, either in association with the underlying mental illness (usually schizophrenia) or perhaps as a side effect of psychotropic or anticonvulsant medications.

The syndrome of inappropriate antidiuretic hormone (SIADH) is characterized by persistently elevated circulating vasopressin levels in the absence of physiologically appropriate (osmotic or hemodynamic) stimuli to vasopressin release (Fig. 144.2). The development of hypotonic hyponatremia in patients with SIADH depends on water ingestion in excess of that eliminated by insensible, gastrointestinal, and renal routes. Because the normal response to hypotonicity is the elaboration of maximally dilute urine (urine osmolality less than 100 mOsm per kilogram), the urine need only be inappropriately concentrated (i.e., more than 100 mOsm per kilogram in a hypotonic patient) to be compatible with a diagnosis of SIADH.

Although the diagnosis of SIADH is often entertained in any patient with hypotonic hyponatremia and an inappropriately concentrated urine, certain additional criteria must be met before the diagnosis is confirmed. Most important, the presence of a hemodynamic stimulus to vasopressin secretion must be rigorously excluded. Thus, clinical signs of extracellular volume depletion (tachycardia, hypotension) must be absent. In addition, because the pathologic edema-forming states (congestive heart failure, hepatic cirrhosis, the nephrotic syndrome) are all typically associated with effective arterial hypovolemia, cardiac and hepatic function must be normal, and proteinuria must be excluded. In more subtle cases, effective arterial blood volume is best assessed by measuring the urine sodium concentration. On a liberal sodium intake (more than 2 g per day) and in the absence of diuretic therapy or renal disease, a urine sodium concentration greater than 20 mEq per liter provides good evidence of a normal effective arterial blood volume.

Because hypothyroidism and glucocorticoid insufficiency may impair urinary dilution, patients in whom a diagnosis of SIADH is entertained should also undergo appropriate tests of thyroid and adrenocortical function. SIADH is discussed in

TABLE 144.1.	CONCEPT OF ELECTROLYTE-FREE WATER

The gain or loss of fluid with an electrolyte concentration equal to that of body fluids (isotonic) cannot change body fluid tonicity. To determine the magnitude of changes in body fluid tonicity caused by the gain or loss of a given fluid, it is helpful to divide that fluid conceptually into two parts: an isotonic component and an electrolyte-free water component. The perturbation in body fluid tonicity then can be calculated easily based solely on the contribution of the electrolyte-free water component.

Consider, for example, solution A, with a volume (V_A) of 2 L and an electrolyte concentration calculated as twice the sum of the sodium and potassium concentrations) (A_{elec}) of 70 mEq/L. Under most circumstances, body fluid tonicity can be estimated as twice the serum sodium concentration (S_{Na}). Thus, the isotonic component of solution A is:

$$A_{elec}/2 \times S_{Na} \times V_A = 70/2 \times 140 \times 2 = 0.5\ L$$

Solution A can therefore be considered to consist of 0.5 L of isotonic fluid and 2 − 0.5 L, or 1.5 L, of electrolyte-free water. The addition of the isotonic component (0.5 L) would not affect body fluid tonicity. In contrast, the addition of the electrolyte-free water component (1.5 L) would increase total body water (in a 70-kg man with a total body water of 42 L) from 42 to 43.5 L and reduce body fluid tonicity (at steady state) to 280 × 42/43.5, or 270 mOsm/kg. Since S_{Na} can be estimated as half body fluid tonicity, S_{Na} would decline to 135 mEq/L.

The urine volume also can be conceptually divided into two parts. Consider, for example, an individual with a daily urine volume (V_u) of 3 L with an electrolyte concentration (calculated as twice the sum of the urine sodium and potassium concentration, U_{elec}) of 35 mEq/L. The isotonic component of the urine is calculated as follows:

$$U_{elec}/2 \times S_{Na} \times V_u = 35/2 \times 140 \times 3 = 0.375\ L$$

The urine can therefore be considered to consist of 0.375 L of isotonic fluid and 3 − 0.375, or 2.625 L, of electrolyte-free water. The excretion of the isotonic component (0.375 L) would not affect body fluid tonicity. In contrast, the excretion of the electrolyte-free water component (2.625 L) would decrease total body water from 42 to 39.375 L and increase body fluid tonicity (at steady state) to 280 × 42/39.375, or 299 mOsm/kg.

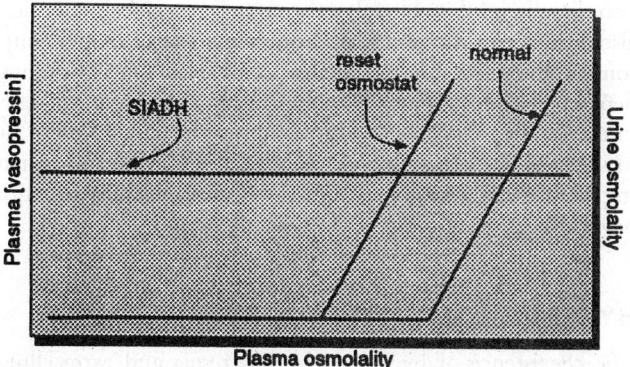

FIGURE 144.2. Relationships of plasma osmolality, plasma vasopressin concentration (plasma [vasopressin]), and urine osmolality in normal subjects, in patients with the reset osmostat variant of the syndrome of inappropriate antidiuretic hormone (SIADH), and in patients with classic SIADH. Patients with a reset osmostat can suppress vasopressin release and excrete dilute urine but only at a lower plasma osmolality than normal. Patients with classic SIADH have persistently elevated, although sometimes variable, vasopressin levels.

Hypovolemic hyponatremia generally arises when renal or extrarenal solute and water losses are replaced with electrolyte-free water. Because sodium deficits are always associated with intravascular volume contraction, tachycardia, hypotension, decreased central venous pressure, oliguria, and prerenal azotemia frequently accompany hypovolemic hyponatremia. The urinary diluting defect in this situation is mediated both by decreased delivery of fluid to the diluting segments of the nephron and by hemodynamically stimulated vasopressin release. Thus, the patient with volume contraction cannot excrete electrolyte-free water normally and readily becomes hyponatremic even in the face of modest water ingestion.

The cause of volume contraction is usually obvious (vomiting, diarrhea, diuretics). When it is not, the urine sodium concentration can be helpful in distinguishing between renal and extrarenal solute losses. Renal losses are usually reflected by sodium wasting, and extrarenal losses are typically accompanied by sodium conservation (Fig. 144.1). Exceptions occur in the recovery phase after diuretic therapy (in which solute losses are renal in origin, but the urine sodium concentration is appropriately low once the diuretic is discontinued) and in metabolic alkalosis due to vomiting (in which bicarbonaturia obligates urinary sodium loss). In the latter case, the urine chloride concentration, which is very low, is the best indicator of extracellular volume depletion.

DIURETIC-INDUCED HYPONATREMIA

The hyponatremia associated with diuretic treatment deserves special mention because it is the most common hypotonic state seen in outpatients. Its pathogenesis is multifactorial. Insofar as diuretics produce overt volume depletion, they can cause hyponatremia by the mechanisms of action discussed earlier. In addition, by blocking sodium reabsorption in the renal diluting segments, thiazide diuretics and loop diuretics, such as furosemide,

more detail in Chapter 404. An important variant of SIADH is the reset osmostat syndrome, in which vasopressin levels are suppressed by hypotonicity but at a lower plasma osmolality than normal (Fig. 144.2). This syndrome is seen most often in patients who are severely debilitated (e.g., those with malnutrition, metastatic cancer, advanced tuberculosis) and may account for up to one-third of cases of SIADH. The diagnosis of reset osmostat syndrome has important therapeutic implications, as will be discussed later.

HYPOVOLEMIC HYPONATREMIA

The coexistence of hypotonic hyponatremia and extracellular volume (salt) depletion implies the presence of both solute and water deficits, with the water deficit being of lesser magnitude.

also directly inhibit electrolyte-free water generation. Thiazides also have been associated with the development of severe, symptomatic hyponatremia in the absence of overt signs of volume depletion. The cause of this often alarming syndrome remains uncertain, but subclinical volume contraction, inhibition of diluting segment function, primary polydipsia in the context of impaired renal diluting ability, SIADH, and potassium depletion have all been implicated.

HYPERVOLEMIC HYPONATREMIA

The coexistence of hypotonic hyponatremia and extracellular volume expansion implies an excess of both salt and water, with the water surfeit being of greater magnitude. Consequently, hypervolemic hyponatremia is generally seen in patients who cannot excrete sodium normally because they have renal insufficiency or one of the pathologic edema-forming states (congestive heart failure, hepatic cirrhosis, the nephrotic syndrome; Fig. 144.1). These patients are characterized by extracellular volume expansion and impaired renal diluting ability. The effective arterial blood volume and absolute intravascular volume are normal or high in hyponatremic patients with renal insufficiency, whereas the hallmark of the pathologic edematous disorders is effective arterial hypovolemia.

Renal insufficiency, whether acute or chronic, can lead to hyponatremia for two reasons: the decreased glomerular filtration rate may prevent the excretion of sufficient water to match even a modest daily water intake, and the renal disease may directly limit electrolyte-free water generation. Because intrinsic diluting ability is normal in most patients with chronic renal failure, hyponatremia in this case is primarily due to the reduction in glomerular filtration rate. Treatment should be directed at restricting fluid intake to match ongoing losses.

Hyponatremia is common in the pathologic edema-forming states. Although extracellular and interstitial fluid volumes are higher by definition in these disorders, the effective arterial hypovolemia causes intense renal sodium retention. Such patients behave as if their intravascular volumes were low, even though the absolute intravascular volume may be normal or high. Because of the perceived intravascular volume depletion, renal diluting ability is compromised for reasons similar to those in hypovolemic hyponatremia, and hypotonicity may ensue with even modest levels of water ingestion.

Transurethral prostatic resection and hysteroscopic uterine ablation are performed using large volumes of nonelectrolyte (glycine, mannitol, or sorbitol) irrigating solutions. Hydrostatic pressure may force large amounts of these solutions through the surgical field into the systemic circulation during the operation, resulting in rapid intravascular volume expansion accompanied by profound hyponatremia.

■ HISTORY AND PHYSICAL EXAMINATION

Disorders of water homeostasis produce no specific clinical symptoms or signs and usually become evident only through screening laboratory examinations that find abnormalities in the serum sodium concentration. Otherwise unexplained neurologic abnormalities or a history or clinical findings of disorders commonly associated with hyponatremia, however, will often alert the experienced clinician to check the serum sodium concentration or plasma osmolality.

Given a diagnosis of hyponatremia, the history and physical examination should be guided by the associated alteration in body fluid tonicity. For the patient with isotonic hyponatremia, the history and physical examination generally reveal the telltale signs of severe hyperlipidemia or paraproteinemia, the presence of which then determines the path of further evaluation. The medication history may confirm iatrogenic paraproteinemia from the intravenous administration of immunoglobulin.

For the patient with hypertonic hyponatremia, the history should be directed at discovering the circumstances surrounding the development of the hypertonic state. Patients with hypertonic hyponatremia generally have a history or symptoms of diabetes mellitus, accounting for the hyperglycemia that is by far the most common cause of this disorder. If the patient is not hyperglycemic, documentation should be sought for the administration of an exogenous osmotic agent, usually mannitol.

In the case of hypotonic hyponatremia, the history and physical examination should first be directed at eliciting any neurologic symptoms or signs, the severity and duration of which are paramount in determining the aggressiveness of therapy (see later discussion). Thereafter, the history should be closely scrutinized for symptoms of hypovolemia or volume overload, for disorders of volume (sodium) homeostasis, and for the use of diuretics, the most common iatrogenic cause of salt depletion. Likewise, the physical examination should be directed at establishing the patient's volume status.

Further questioning of the patient with hypotonic hyponatremia is guided by subsequent laboratory results. For the patient with dilute urine, an attempt should be made to discover remediable causes of increased thirst, such as drugs that cause a dry mouth. For the patient with concentrated urine, the history follows directly from the differential diagnosis (Fig. 144.1). Patients in whom SIADH is suspected should be questioned about the diseases and conditions associated with that syndrome, with particular attention paid to intrathoracic and intracranial processes and to covert adrenal insufficiency and hypothyroidism. A thorough drug history must always be taken because of the many drugs that can cause SIADH (see Chapter 404).

■ LABORATORY STUDIES AND DIAGNOSTIC TESTS

The laboratory evaluation of hyponatremia is detailed in Fig. 144.1. Although the measurement of plasma osmolality readily segregates hyponatremia by body fluid tonicity, other laboratory tests often provide significant clues as well. For example, paraproteinemia of sufficient magnitude to produce pseudohyponatremia generally causes such significant hyperviscosity that it makes blood collection by standard venipuncture methods difficult. Hyperlipidemia is often suspected because of creamy or opalescent serum. A normal or only mildly elevated blood glucose concentration effectively excludes hypertonic hyponatremia.

Together with the history and physical examination, simple urinary indexes (urine osmolality and sodium concentration) can be used to divide hypotonic hyponatremia into hypovolemic, hypervolemic, and euvolemic categories (Fig. 144.1). The blood urea nitrogen, serum creatinine, and uric acid concentrations also can be useful in making this distinction. Prerenal azotemia and hyperuricemia often are present in patients with hypovolemic or hypervolemic hyponatremia, and hypouricemia is common in primary polydipsia and SIADH.

Before a diagnosis of SIADH can be made, adrenal insufficiency and hypothyroidism must be excluded (see Chapters 406 and 407). Once the diagnosis of SIADH is established, it is important to determine whether the patient has the reset osmostat variant. This diagnosis is often obvious because of the relative stability of the serum sodium concentration (usually 125 to 135 mEq per liter) despite unrestricted water ingestion. If the diagnosis is not apparent, it can be made by stressing the osmoregulatory system with a water load.

The standard oral water loading test is performed as follows. After several days on a liberal salt diet, the patient is instructed to drink tap water (20 mL per kilogram body weight over 15 to 30 minutes). For the next 5 hours, the urine is collected hourly, and its volume and osmolality are measured. Normally, during the peak of water diuresis, the urine osmolality is minimal (less than 100 mOsm per kilogram); in addition, over the 5 hours of the test, a normal subject excretes more than 80% of the administered water. Patients with a reset osmostat eliminate the water load normally once the plasma osmolality drops below their reset threshold for vasopressin release. In contrast, patients with classic SIADH cannot excrete the water load normally: minimal urine osmolality is not achieved, and less than 80% of the water is excreted over the 5 hours. The standard oral water load is designed to decrease the serum sodium concentration by no more than 3%, even if all the water is retained. Nonetheless, patients with severe hyponatremia (less than 120 mEq per liter) should not be water-loaded because of the risk of precipitating neurologic symptoms.

STRATEGIES FOR OPTIMAL CARE

MANAGEMENT AND COMPLICATIONS

Because the most important manifestations of disordered osmoregulation relate to alterations in body fluid tonicity rather than to the associated changes in serum sodium concentration, an assessment of plasma osmolality should accompany any diagnosis of clinically significant hyponatremia. Therapy can then be guided by this information. Thus, the treatment of isotonic hyponatremia should be directed at the underlying hyperlipidemia or paraproteinemia. Similarly, in patients with hypertonic hyponatremia, hypertonicity, not hyponatremia, must be addressed. Only when it is associated with hypotonicity, and therefore with cerebral edema, should hyponatremia receive specific attention.

Mild to moderate hypotonic hyponatremia is very common, especially in hospitalized patients. The vast majority of these persons are asymptomatic and should be treated conservatively. Severe hypotonicity (serum sodium concentration less than 120 mEq per liter), although much less common, can be life-threatening, and immediate therapy may be required.

The therapy of symptomatic hypotonicity, irrespective of cause, is directed at raising extracellular fluid tonicity to shift water out of the intracellular space, thereby ameliorating cerebral edema. The rate of correction, however, must be carefully regulated. Overly rapid correction, particularly in patients with chronic hyponatremia, in whom cell volume adaptations may be complete, can produce central pontine myelinolysis. This so-called osmotic demyelination syndrome is associated with a variety of irreversible neurologic deficits (dysarthria, dysphagia, incoordination, quadriplegia, coma), which typically develop 2 to 6 days after treatment.

Although the exact rate of correction remains the subject of controversy, in most circumstances the serum sodium concentration should be raised by no more than 10 mEq per liter in the first 24 hours and by no more than 20 mEq per liter in the first 48 hours. In grave situations (serum sodium concentration less than 105 mEq per liter), initial therapy can be more aggressive (targeting a change in the serum sodium concentration of 1 to 2 mEq per liter per hour for the first few hours), but the recommended daily target should not be exceeded.

Correction of severe symptomatic hypotonicity, regardless of cause, should be accomplished with hypertonic (3%) saline. The amount of solute required can be estimated as follows. First, calculate the amount of sodium to be administered by multiplying the target change in serum sodium concentration by the patient's total body water. Then calculate the volume of 3% saline that will supply that amount of sodium. For example, in a 70-kg man with a serum sodium concentration of 105 mEq per liter and a total body water of 42 L (60% of body weight), the amount of sodium needed to raise the serum sodium concentration by 10 mEq per liter is 10 $\times$ 42, or 420 mEq. Three percent saline has a sodium concentration of 513 mEq per liter; therefore, 420/513, or approximately 820 mL, would be required in the first 24 hours.

This calculation provides only a rough guideline, since it takes no account of ongoing solute and water losses, and the serum sodium concentration must be monitored frequently during treatment to adjust the rate of correction. Rapid extracellular volume expansion with hypertonic saline can precipitate pulmonary edema, particularly in patients with underlying heart disease. Thus, patients receiving 3% saline also should be assessed frequently for evidence of volume overload. A loop diuretic may be administered if necessary, recognizing that this will enhance electrolyte-free water clearance and accelerate the correction.

The treatment of chronic asymptomatic hypotonicity should be directed at correcting the pathophysiologic factors involved in generating the hypotonic state. Because euvolemic hyponatremia represents pure water excess, treatment depends on restricting water intake to less than daily water output. Patients with SIADH excrete little or no electrolyte-free water in the urine. Therefore, if water intake is limited to less than the amount of insensible water losses (approximately 10 mL per kilogram body weight per day), the serum sodium concentration will slowly rise. Progressive hypotonicity does not develop in patients with the reset osmostat variant of SIADH, and such patients rarely require therapy.

If the cause of SIADH cannot be corrected and if water restriction is poorly tolerated or ineffective, demeclocycline (a tetracycline antibiotic that increases electrolyte-free water excretion by inhibiting vasopressin-mediated water reabsorption in the collecting duct) can be used. Demeclocycline is contraindicated for patients with renal disease, hepatic cirrhosis, or congestive heart failure because drug-related renal insufficiency has been described in these situations. Urea (30 to 60 g per day, administered orally) has been used to increase electrolyte-free water clearance, but it is unpalatable, and gastrointestinal side effects limit its usefulness. Specific vasopressin (V_2) receptor antagonists, so-called aquaretic agents, are nearing approval for clinical use and are likely to change the treatment of patients with SIADH in the future.

Therapy of hypovolemic hyponatremia should be directed at restoring intravascular volume with intravenous saline and identifying and correcting the cause of the excessive solute loss. Volume repletion readily elicits water diuresis by increasing the delivery of fluid to the renal diluting segments and suppressing vasopressin release. As with all categories of hypotonic hyponatremia, the rate of correction must be carefully controlled. The treatment of diuretic-induced hyponatremia is straightforward: withdrawing the offending drug, liberalizing salt intake, and replenishing body potassium stores usually correct the disorder.

The treatment of hypervolemic hyponatremia is difficult and frustrating. Resolution of hyponatremia associated with any of the pathologic edematous disorders ultimately depends on effective treatment of the underlying disease. Regardless of the specific therapy of the underlying disorder, the mainstay of therapy for the hyponatremic edematous patient remains salt and water restriction. Diuretics are often a double-edged sword in a patient with hyponatremia and edema. They may be needed to treat pulmonary vascular congestion, peripheral edema, and ascites, but if they are used to excess, they can produce further decrements in effective arterial blood volume and exacerbate water retention. Strategies directed at increasing effective arterial blood volume (e.g., afterload reduction with angiotensin-converting enzyme inhibitors) have had some success in increasing electrolyte-free water excretion and ameliorating hyponatremia in patients with congestive heart failure.

The use of isotonic or hypertonic saline to treat hypotonicity in edematous patients provides at best only a transient increase in effective arterial blood volume. The sodium-containing fluid rapidly equilibrates throughout the extracellular fluid space, and the edema worsens. In addition, pulmonary edema is a serious threat when these solutions are administered to patients with underlying heart disease. Consequently, if hypertonic saline must be used in the emergency therapy of symptomatic hypotonicity in the edematous patient, potent diuretics should be administered simultaneously.

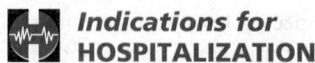

Indications for HOSPITALIZATION

Because neurologic deterioration is unpredictable and can proceed rapidly in patients with hypotonicity, the presence of any neurologic abnormality, irrespective of the degree of hyponatremia, is an absolute indication for immediate hospitalization. For the same reasons, hospitalization is also usually indicated if the serum sodium concentration is below 125 mEq per liter, regardless of signs or symptoms. If hyponatremia is known to be chronic and relatively stable, patients with more moderate, asymptomatic hyponatremia (serum sodium concentration 125 to 135 mEq per liter) can usually be treated as outpatients, but they may require admission for treatment of the underlying disorder.

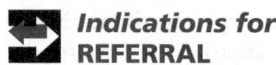

Indications for REFERRAL

Consultation, usually with a nephrologist or intensivist, is indicated for patients with severe hypotonicity, especially when aggressive therapy with hypertonic saline is contemplated. Consultation with a nephrologist can also be helpful when one is faced with establishing the diagnosis of SIADH or making the distinction between reset osmostat and classic SIADH. Psychiatric consultation may be required for the treatment of patients with primary polydipsia.

COST-EFFECTIVENESS

The evaluation of hyponatremia, for the most part, entails only a thorough history and physical examination and simple and inexpensive laboratory tests. Furthermore, the catastrophic consequences of severe hypotonicity can be prevented in most circumstances by simple prophylactic management (water restriction) or lessened by the judicious use of inexpensive crystalloid solutions in more critical situations. Although no formal cost/benefit analysis is available, common sense dictates the careful assessment and treatment of patients with severe hyponatremia (a serum sodium concentration less than 120 mEq per liter). Cost/benefit considerations would also be expected to favor the evaluation of patients with new-onset (or newly discovered) hyponatremia of any more than trivial magnitude.

BIBLIOGRAPHY

Illowsky BP, Kirch DG. Polydipsia and hyponatremia in psychiatric patients. *Am J Psychiatry* 1988;145:675–683.

Karp BI, Laureno R. Pontine and extrapontine myelinolysis: a neurologic disorder following rapid correction of hyponatremia. *Medicine* 1993; 72:359–373.

Kleeman CR. Metabolic coma. *Kidney Int* 1989;36:1142–1158.

Lauriat SM, Berl T. The hyponatremic patient: practical focus on therapy. *J Am Soc Nephrol* 1997;8:1599–1607.

Rose BD. New approach to disturbances in the plasma sodium concentration. *Am J Med* 1986;81:1033–1040.

Sterns RH, Capuccio JD, Silver SM, et al. Neurologic sequelae after treatment of severe hyponatremia: a multicenter perspective. *J Am Soc Nephrol* 1994;4:1522–1530.

Strange K. Regulation of solute and water balance and cell volume in the central nervous system. *J Am Soc Nephrol* 1992;3:12–27.

Szerlip H, Palevsky P, Cox M. Sodium and water. In: Rock RC, Noe DA, eds. *Laboratory medicine: the selection and interpretation of clinical laboratory studies.* Baltimore: Williams & Wilkins, 1994:692–731.

Weisberg LS. Pseudohyponatremia: a reappraisal. *Am J Med* 1989;86:315–318.

Kelley's Textbook of Internal Medicine, fourth edition. Edited by H. David Humes. Lippincott Williams & Wilkins, Philadelphia © 2000.

CHAPTER 145

APPROACH TO THE PATIENT WITH HYPERNATREMIA

HAROLD M. SZERLIP
MALCOLM COX

PRESENTATION

Hypernatremia (serum sodium concentration greater than 145 mEq per L) is found in about 1% of hospitalized patients. Because body fluid tonicity is tightly regulated in healthy persons, hypernatremia is generally a disorder of the very young, the very old, or the very ill, occurring most commonly in infants, debilitated elderly patients in chronic care facilities, and patients of all ages hospitalized with serious illnesses.

Irrespective of cause, hypernatremia always implies coexistent hypertonicity. Because almost all cell membranes are freely permeable to water, hypertonicity is associated with movement of water from the intracellular to the extracellular fluid compartment and intracellular volume contraction (cell shrinkage). Many of the symptoms of hypernatremia are the result of this change in cell volume. Of most significance are the neurologic manifestations associated with shrinkage of the brain.

The presenting symptoms and signs of hypernatremia typically are related to changes in the sensorium. In general, the higher the serum sodium concentration, the greater the depression of the sensorium, although there is considerable variation among individuals. Symptoms can range from agitation, restlessness, confusion, and lethargy to seizures, stupor, and coma. Brain pathology includes intracerebral, subarachnoid, and subdural hemorrhages.

Central pontine myelinolysis, a condition more commonly associated with rapid correction of hyponatremia, has also been reported in patients with hypernatremia. Other presentations of hypernatremia include muscle weakness, nausea, and vomiting.

The brain has well-developed regulatory mechanisms that mitigate tonicity-related changes in cell volume. Brain cells begin to adapt to hypertonicity by promptly increasing intracellular solute shortly after the onset of the disturbance. Extracellular sodium chloride provides some of this new solute, at least acutely. Over time, however, the brain adapts to hypertonic stress by generating organic osmolytes such as glutamine, glutamate, taurine, and myoinositol. Thus, brain cells do not act as true osmometers, as their shrinkage is less than that predicted by the degree of hypertonicity.

Because of this adaptive response, the manifestations of hypernatremia depend on the rapidity of the rise in the serum sodium concentration as well as the magnitude of the hypernatremia. Gradual development of hypertonicity provides time for the adaptive increase in brain solute, and cell shrinkage is less severe. In contrast, the rapid development of hypertonicity does not allow sufficient time for adaptation, and cerebral dehydration is unimpeded. Thus, acute changes in the serum sodium concentration are generally less well tolerated than more chronic changes.

Changes in extracellular fluid volume and the presence of comorbid conditions commonly modify the presentation of patients with hypernatremia and may dominate the clinical picture. For example, hypernatremia secondary to excess salt is often associated with symptoms of volume overload, whereas hypernatremia that results from the loss of hypotonic fluids is associated with signs of volume depletion. These changes in extracellular fluid volume may be of such import that their treatment might have to take priority over that of the hypernatremia.

PATHOPHYSIOLOGY AND DIFFERENTIAL DIAGNOSIS

Hypernatremia can arise from the gain of solute (sodium salts) in excess of water or the loss of water in excess of solute (pure water loss or hypotonic fluid loss). Pure water losses are associated with an isolated decrease in total body water. In contrast, hypotonic fluid losses produce both water and solute deficits, with the water deficit being of greater magnitude. Because hypernatremia is a potent stimulus to thirst, sustained hypernatremia always implies inadequate water intake. This may be due to impaired thirst (hypodipsia) or an inability to obtain adequate amounts of water (e.g., infants or bedridden adults).

HYPODIPSIA

In patients with free access to water, sustained hypernatremia is always associated with impaired thirst. Thirst is first stimulated at a plasma osmolality of approximately 295 mOsm per kg, a level at which urinary concentration has already been maximally stimulated by arginine vasopressin (antidiuretic hormone). Thus, whereas renal water conservation serves as the initial defense against hypernatremia, water intake provides the ultimate guarantee against death from progressive hypertonic dehydration.

Pure hypodipsia (i.e., a defect in thirst sensation in the absence of abnormalities in vasopressin secretion) is uncommon.

Although the hypothalamic center responsible for the regulation of thirst appears to be different from that regulating vasopressin release, defects in thirst most often coexist with disturbances in vasopressin secretion. For example, hypodipsia has been described in combination with partial hypothalamic diabetes insipidus; the osmotic thresholds for thirst and vasopressin release in these patients are normal, but the sensitivities of the two systems are depressed. Because of the concomitant defects in thirst and renal water conservation, hypernatremia can be particularly severe in such persons.

Other patients with hypodipsia are characterized by chronic, nonprogressive hypernatremia, euvolemia, and normal renal concentrating ability (for age). Those patients with so-called essential hypernatremia defend body fluid tonicity around a higher than usual osmolality (upward resetting of the osmolal set point) and have elevated thresholds for both thirst and vasopressin release. Upward resetting of the osmostat may also explain the mild hypernatremia seen in primary hyperaldosteronism.

Many elderly persons have impaired thirst. When dehydrated, even otherwise healthy elderly persons sense less thirst and drink less than younger subjects, putting them at increased risk for hypernatremia should intercurrent illness stress the osmoregulatory system. The cause of so-called geriatric hypodipsia has not been elucidated.

SOLUTE GAIN

The gain of solute in excess of water is a relatively uncommon cause of hypernatremia. However, two situations are typical: the accidental or purposeful ingestion of table salt, and the intravenous administration of hypertonic sodium-containing solutions.

A tablespoon of salt contains approximately 350 mEq of sodium chloride, and the ingestion of as little as one tablespoon can raise the serum sodium concentration by as much as 8 mEq per L in a 70-kg adult. Because of a lower body water content, elderly persons manifest similar increases in the serum sodium concentration with proportionately lesser amounts of salt. Fatal cases of hypernatremia resulting from the intentional ingestion of salt, the use of salt as an emetic, and the inadvertent administration of salt-containing (rather than sugar-containing) infant formula have been documented.

Hypernatremia due to the excessive administration of hypertonic salt solutions is restricted to hospitalized patients, where it usually presents as an iatrogenic complication of the treatment of hyponatremia or metabolic acidosis. The 3% saline solution commonly used in the treatment of severe hyponatremia contains 513 mEq sodium per liter. Even more hypertonic is the 7.5% sodium bicarbonate solution (890 mEq per L) routinely used during cardiopulmonary resuscitation: each 50-mL ampule contains 44.5 mEq sodium.

This type of hypernatremia is associated with expansion of the extracellular space. The magnitude of the increase in extracellular fluid volume depends on the size of the sodium load and the extent of the associated diuresis. With adequate renal function and in the absence of a stimulus for renal sodium retention, extracellular (and intravascular) fluid volume expansion is mitigated by a brisk diuresis. Edema and ascites may not be evident, but increased central venous pressure is almost invariable. If renal sodium excretion is limited, frank pulmonary edema may be present.

PURE WATER LOSS

Pure water deficits arise from inadequate water intake in the face of ongoing electrolyte-free water losses from skin, respiratory tract, or kidney. Isolated decreases in total body water, unless of very large magnitude, are not associated with significant extracellular (or intravascular) volume depletion. This is because only one third of a pure water deficit is derived from the extracellular fluid and only one twelfth from the intravascular compartment. Thus, patients with pure water deficits generally appear clinically euvolemic.

Cutaneous insensible losses are increased by fever or when the ambient temperature is high. Pulmonary insensible losses are increased in hot, dry environments and by hyperventilation. Excessive renal electrolyte-free water losses are the *sine qua non* of diabetes insipidus; this syndrome is characterized by impaired renal concentrating ability and results from either vasopressin deficiency (hypothalamic diabetes insipidus) or renal unresponsiveness to vasopressin (nephrogenic diabetes insipidus) (see Chapters 137 and 404).

HYPOTONIC FLUID LOSS

The most common cause of hypernatremia is the loss of hypotonic body fluids, which may occur through the kidney, gastrointestinal tract, or skin (Table 145.1). Because of the associated sodium loss, hypotonic fluid deficits lead to greater degrees of extracellular and intravascular volume depletion than do pure water deficits. Thus, patients with hypotonic fluid deficits usually manifest clinical symptoms and signs of intravascular volume depletion.

The chronic administration of potent diuretics (such as thiazides, metolazone, or furosemide), and especially combinations of such diuretics, is a notorious cause of excessive renal hypotonic fluid losses. So, too, is the prolonged polyuria that typically accompanies chronic hyperglycemia in patients with poorly controlled diabetes mellitus. In both situations, urinary water losses invariably exceed solute losses, and unless these water losses are

TABLE 145.1.	CAUSES OF HYPOTONIC FLUID LOSSES

Renal
  Diuretics
  Osmotic diuresis
    Hyperglycemia
Gastrointestinal
  Diarrhea
  Vomiting
  Nasogastric suction
Skin
  Sensible perspiration
  Burns

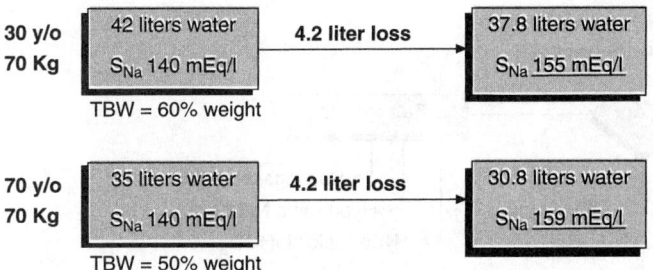

FIGURE 145.1. Differential effect of the same amount of water loss on S_{Na} in a young adult and an elderly subject. Because muscle mass decreases with age, total body water declines. Therefore, for any given water loss, the increase in S_{Na} is greater in the older than in the younger subject.

counterbalanced by increased water intake, hypernatremia is a predictable consequence.

Gastrointestinal fluid losses are also a common cause of hypernatremia. Except for biliary and pancreatic secretions, most gastrointestinal fluids are hypotonic in composition. Chronic watery diarrhea, extensive vomiting, and prolonged nasogastric suction account for the majority of these cases.

The skin may be a significant site of hypotonic fluid loss. Although only water is lost during insensible perspiration, sensible perspiration contains significant amounts of solute as well. In hot, humid environments, and especially when strenuous exercise produces profuse sweating, hypotonic fluid intake must be sufficient to counteract increased cutaneous water and solute losses. Extensive burns can also be associated with significant hypotonic fluid losses.

HYPERNATREMIA IN THE ELDERLY

Elderly persons are at special risk for developing hypernatremia. Because they have less muscle, total body water as a percentage of body weight is lower. Consequently, for any given degree of solute gain or water loss, hypernatremia is more severe than in young adults (Fig. 145.1). Furthermore, maximal urinary concentrating ability is lower in the elderly, so that their ability to conserve water is less than that of healthy young adults. In addition, because hypodipsia is relatively common in the elderly, they are less able to defend body fluid tonicity against progressive hypertonic dehydration. Likewise, chronically debilitated adults, especially the institutionalized elderly, depend on others for access to water. All of these factors combine to increase the incidence of hypernatremia in the elderly.

HISTORY AND PHYSICAL EXAMINATION

Hypernatremia produces no specific clinical symptoms or signs and usually becomes evident only through a screening laboratory examination. However, otherwise unexplained neurologic abnormalities or a history or clinical findings of diseases or disorders commonly associated with hypernatremia often alert the experienced clinician to check the serum sodium concentration.

Once a diagnosis of hypernatremia is established, the history and physical examination assume considerable importance in planning further evaluation and guiding therapy. The initial evaluation should include interviewing the patient (and any caregivers) and reviewing the medical records. Specific information regarding thirst, access to water, water intake, salt intake, urine volume, and medications (especially diuretics) should be sought, as should evidence of neurologic alterations, which are sometimes subtle. A history of fever, vomiting, diarrhea, or polyuria (or, more specifically, diabetes mellitus or diabetes insipidus) is also pertinent.

Extracellular volume status is helpful in segregating hypernatremia into its three main categories (Fig. 145.2). Moreover, the associated changes in extracellular fluid volume, rather than the hypernatremia itself, often dictate therapy as well, especially initial therapy. Consequently, the history should always be closely scrutinized for symptoms of hypovolemia or volume overload, especially intravascular volume overload. The physical examination should be used to establish volume status. Volume depletion generally indicates hypotonic fluid losses. In contrast, evidence of intravascular volume expansion is consistent with hypernatremia caused by solute gain.

◼ LABORATORY STUDIES AND DIAGNOSTIC TESTS

Laboratory studies are helpful in confirming extracellular volume status and in pinpointing the specific cause of hypernatremia. Prerenal azotemia and hyperuricemia generally imply extracellular volume depletion and therefore suggest hypotonic fluid losses. In contrast, the blood urea nitrogen and serum uric acid concentrations are typically normal or only trivially elevated in patients with pure water deficits.

The laboratory evaluation of hypernatremia is detailed in Figure 145.2. For the most part, simple urinary indexes (urine osmolality and sodium concentration) are used to distinguish between hypotonic and pure water deficits and between renal and extrarenal hypotonic fluid losses. In the absence of a stimulus to renal sodium retention, hypernatremia secondary to salt overload induces a rapid and marked natriuresis, resulting in very high urinary sodium concentrations (often greater than 100 mEq per L).

More specialized testing depends on the particular situation. Tests that evaluate the integrity of the vasopressin–renal axis (used to establish the diagnosis of diabetes insipidus) are discussed in Chapter 404. Although visual analog scales to quantify thirst are available, they are rarely used; clinicians generally rely on more subjective indexes of thirst.

◼ STRATEGIES FOR OPTIMAL CARE

MANAGEMENT AND COMPLICATIONS

The effective management of hypernatremia requires accurate knowledge of extracellular volume status and an appreciation of

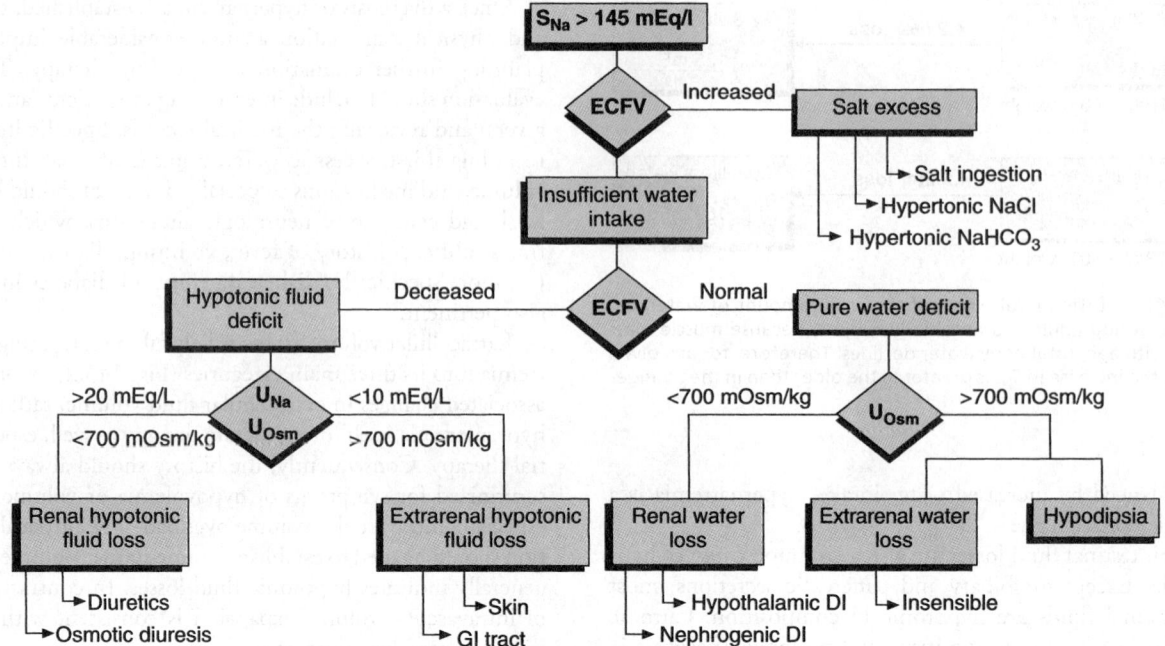

FIGURE 145.2. Approach to the patient with hypernatremia. S_{Na} and U_{Na}, serum and urine sodium concentrations, respectively; U_{Osm}, urine osmolality; ECFV, extracellular fluid volume; GI, gastrointestinal; DI, diabetes insipidus.

EVIDENCE LEVEL: C. Expert Opinion.

the cerebral adaptation to hypertonicity. Initial therapy should be directed at normalizing intravascular volume; thereafter, attention can be turned to correcting the hypernatremia itself.

When signs and symptoms of volume depletion are present, the restoration of adequate tissue perfusion is of paramount importance. Isotonic (0.9%) sodium chloride solutions generally provide the best means to this end and should be given intravenously at a rate sufficient to stabilize the blood pressure. Once blood pressure has been stabilized, the water deficit can be addressed.

Incipient or frank pulmonary edema is common in patients with hypernatremia caused by excess salt and may greatly complicate therapy. The rapid administration of large volumes of water to treat the hypernatremia will further expand extracellular volume, worsening pulmonary gas exchange. In this situation, therefore, initial therapy must include removal of the excess sodium as well as water administration. Potent diuretics (such as furosemide) are often effective in patients with intact renal function; otherwise, extracorporeal techniques (such as hemodialysis or hemofiltration) may be required to reduce extracellular volume rapidly.

Once the intravascular volume status has been addressed, attention can be turned to the treatment of the hypernatremia itself. Here consideration of the cerebral adaptation to hypertonicity assumes particular importance. Although the rate of new intracellular solute generation has not been precisely defined—and may vary considerably among persons and in different clinical situations—full adaptation can take several days. Consequently, acute hypertonicity is generally less well tolerated than hypertonicity that develops gradually, and it should be treated more aggressively.

Before a rapid correction regimen is begun, however, the hypertonicity must be determined to be acute in origin. This is usually straightforward in patients with hypernatremia secondary to solute gain (salt poisoning or iatrogenic hypertonic fluid administration) but may be more difficult in other situations. Because of the dangers that accompany the rapid correction of chronic hypertonicity (see below), aggressive therapy should never be used when the duration of the hypernatremia cannot be established with reasonable certainty.

The rate at which new brain solute is removed (or inactivated) during therapy is even less well understood than its rate of generation. In animal models, however, solute dissipation takes more than 24 hours. Because brain cells maintain their volume by an adaptive increase in solute, returning tonicity rapidly to normal may produce cerebral edema and may precipitate seizures, coma, permanent neurologic sequelae, or death. Consequently, the correction of chronic hypernatremia (or hypernatremia of unknown duration) should always proceed over a period of several days.

The treatment of hypernatremia should be directed at repleting total body water, matching ongoing losses with increased water intake, and eliminating any excessive insensible, gastrointestinal, or renal water losses. Calculation of the magnitude of an isolated water deficit is based on the fact that total body solute (or, more conveniently, total body sodium) remains constant, so that the resulting hypernatremia is directly proportional to the deficit in total body water (TBW). Thus:

$$\text{Current TBW} \times S_{Na} = \text{normal TBW} \times \text{normal } S_{Na}$$

In a 60-kg patient with S_{Na} 160 mEq per L:

$$\text{Current TBW} = (0.6 \times 60) \times 140/160 = 31.5 \text{ L}$$

The water deficit is therefore 36 − 31.5, or 4.5 L. Despite inherent inaccuracies in estimating normal total body water (current weight is used because the pre-dehydration or normal weight is rarely known, and it is assumed that total body water is 60% of body weight), this calculation provides an approximate value that can be used in planning therapy.

The same calculation is often used to estimate the water deficit in hypernatremic patients with hypotonic fluid losses, but because of the associated solute losses it may underestimate the true water deficit. However, an accurate reflection of the residual water deficit can be obtained once sodium (and any potassium) deficits have been corrected.

Because the rapid replacement of large water deficits in patients with chronic hypernatremia carries the risk of acute cerebral edema, no more than half of the estimated deficit should be replaced during the first 24 hours, with careful monitoring of the neurologic status and the serum sodium concentration. The rest of the deficit can then be replaced over the ensuing 24 to 48 hours. The oral route is always preferable, provided the patient is alert and there is no risk of pulmonary aspiration. In other cases, 5% dextrose in water should be administered intravenously.

Once water repletion is under way, consideration should be given to estimating and replacing ongoing water losses. Both insensible (cutaneous and pulmonary) and renal water losses must be considered. In addition, therapy for hypodipsia (prescription of an adequate water intake) and specific therapy for hyperthermia, hyperventilation, and diabetes insipidus (see Chapter 404) should be initiated.

In patients whose hypernatremia is caused by excess salt, the amount of water needed to correct the hypernatremia can be estimated in an analogous fashion. Of course, in this situation, there is no water deficit, and the water administered to correct body fluid tonicity increases total body water above normal. If the hypernatremia is clearly acute (less than 12 hours in duration), correction can be rapid; otherwise, the more conservative recommendations provided for the treatment of chronic hypertonicity should be followed. The rapid administration of electrolyte-free water should continue only until neurologic symptoms improve. Because many of these patients are also receiving potent diuretics, hemodialysis, or hemofiltration (treatment modalities that have their own unique effects on solute and water balance), close monitoring of neurologic status and the serum sodium concentration is mandatory, and frequent adjustments in the rate of water administration might be needed.

Indications for HOSPITALIZATION

Because neurologic deterioration is unpredictable in patients with hypernatremia, the presence of any neurologic abnormality, irrespective of the degree of hypertonicity, is an absolute indication for immediate hospitalization. Likewise, hospitalization for further evaluation is also usually indicated if the serum sodium concentration exceeds 155 mEq per L, regardless of signs or symptoms. If the hypernatremia is

known to be chronic and relatively stable (and extracellular fluid volume is neither compromised nor threatened), patients with more moderate, asymptomatic hypernatremia (serum sodium concentration 145 to 155 mEq per L) usually can be handled as outpatients. However, they may require admission for treatment of the underlying disorder.

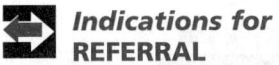

Indications for REFERRAL

Consultation, most often with a nephrologist or intensivist, is indicated in patients with severe hypernatremia, especially when aggressive therapy is contemplated. Consultation (with a nephrologist, endocrinologist, or neurologist) can also be helpful when one is faced with making the diagnosis of diabetes insipidus—and during the initial treatment of this disorder—or when confronted with otherwise unexplained hypodipsia.

COST EFFECTIVENESS

The evaluation of hypernatremia entails, for the most part, a thorough history and physical examination, as well as simple and inexpensive laboratory tests. Furthermore, in many situations the catastrophic consequences of severe hypernatremia can be prevented by simple and relatively inexpensive means (e.g., prescription of an adequate water intake, adequate enteral or intravenous electrolyte-free water administration in persons who cannot drink, hormone replacement therapy for hypothalamic diabetes insipidus). Thus, although no formal cost/benefit analysis is available, common sense dictates the careful assessment and treatment of patients with severe hypernatremia (serum sodium concentration greater than 155 mEq/L). Cost/benefit considerations would also be expected to favor the evaluation of patients with new onset (or newly discovered) hypernatremia of anything more than trivial magnitude.

BIBLIOGRAPHY

Baylis PH, Thompson CJ. Osmoregulation of vasopressin secretion and thirst in health and disease. *Clin Endocrinol* 1988;29:549–576.

Feig PU, McCurdy DK. The hypertonic state. *N Engl J Med* 1977;297:1444–1454.

Gullans SR, Verbalis JG. Control of brain volume during hyperosmolar and hypoosmolar conditions. *Annu Rev Med* 1993;44:289–301.

Miller PD, Krebs RA, Neal BJ, et al. Hypodipsia in geriatric patients. *Am J Med* 1982;73:354–356.

Palevsky PM, Bhagrath R, Greenberg A. Hypernatremia in hospitalized patients. *Ann Intern Med* 1996;124:197–203.

Palevsky PM. Hypernatremia. *Semin Nephrol* 1998;18:20–30.

Phillips PA, Rolls BJ, Ledingham JGG, et al. Reduced thirst after water deprivation in healthy elderly men. *N Engl J Med* 1984;311:753–759.

Snyder NA, Feigal DW, Arieff AI. Hypernatremia in elderly patients: a heterogeneous, morbid, and iatrogenic entity. *Ann Intern Med* 1987;107:309–319.

Szerlip H, Palevsky P, Cox M. Sodium and water. In: Rock RC, Noe

DA, eds. *Laboratory medicine: the selection and interpretation of clinical laboratory studies.* Baltimore: Williams & Wilkins, 1994:692–731.

Kelley's Textbook of Internal Medicine, fourth edition. Edited by H. David Humes.
Lippincott Williams & Wilkins, Philadelphia © 2000.

CHAPTER 146

APPROACH TO THE PATIENT WITH HYPOKALEMIA

MANUEL MARTINEZ-MALDONADO

The concentration of serum potassium is 3.5 to 5 mEq per L and total body potassium is about 50 mEq per kg, or about 3500 mEq for a 70-kg man. The relative distribution of potassium among various organs and extracellular fluid (ECF) is shown in Figure 146.1. The kidneys are responsible for the excretion of close to 95% of dietary potassium, but in the presence of diarrhea or impairment of renal function the gut may be a primary route of potassium excretion.

Several facts about potassium are important in understanding conditions in which serum K^+ is altered (Table 146.1). The abundance of intracellular K^+ (30 times higher than ECF K^+) should be a tip-off to the possible role of shifts of potassium as a cause of alterations in serum K^+. This is particularly the case in hyperkalemia (serum K^+ greater than 5 mEq per L); the fact that cells are a vast deposit for potassium can also lead to the development of hypokalemia.

Hypokalemia is defined as a value of serum K^+ lower than 3.5 mEq per L. Hypokalemia almost always results from abnormal losses of potassium or, rarely, from potassium shift into cells. Drugs are the most common cause of hypokalemia; therefore, review of the patient's drug record is essential.

POTASSIUM REDISTRIBUTION

Movement of potassium into cells, leading to hypokalemia, can be induced by various factors. Metabolic alkalosis decreases plasma K^+ by 0.3 mEq per L for each 0.1-unit increase in pH and can lead to a severe degree of hypokalemia. Respiratory alkalosis must be extremely severe (exaggerated and inappropriate mechanical ventilation) to cause substantial degrees of hypokalemia. Bicarbonate administration has only a slight effect on transcellular K^+ distribution in end-stage renal disease patients.

Exogenously administered insulin or that endogenously released in response to hyperglycemia stimulates K^+ uptake by muscle and liver cells. Hypokalemia inhibits whereas hyperkalemia stimulates insulin secretion. Drugs such as epinephrine and selective β_2-agonists (terbutaline, albuterol, salbutamol, ephedrine, and other bronchodilators) and tocolytic agents (ritodrine, nylidrin), can induce marked, if transient, hypokalemia. Endogenous release of catecholamines as a result of myocardial infarction, head injury, cardiac surgery, delirium tremens, and other stress-generating illnesses can lead to transient hypokalemia. Intoxication with several agents such as verapamil, chloroquine, theophylline, barium, and possibly toluene also shifts K^+ into cells.

A rare hereditary disorder, hypokalemic periodic paralysis, is the result of intracellular shifts of potassium, which may be spontaneous or induced by carbohydrate-rich diets or excessive acute intake of sugars. Most cases are familial, but sporadic cases occur as a complication of thyrotoxicosis, particularly in Asians. Thyroid hormone stimulates cellular uptake of K^+.

Hypothermia may lower plasma K^+ to below 3.0 mEq per L by inducing intracellular K^+ shifts. Potassium administration and rewarming may be associated with overshoot hyperkalemia.

Vitamin B_{12} therapy of megaloblastic anemia rapidly induces production of new blood cells that avidly extract potassium from the extracellular fluid; severe or lethal hypokalemia may ensue. Administration of washed frozen erythrocytes results in hypokalemia because the rewarmed low K^+ cells activate their Na^+,K^+-ATPase and feast on extracellular potassium. Reduction in plasma K^+ of as much as 1 mEq per L can be seen in delirium tremens, a phenomenon associated with the level of plasma epinephrine and, presumably, its β_2-agonist effects.

In circumstances in which cells proliferate and grow rapidly (e.g., acute leukemias, Burkitt's lymphoma), extracellular K^+ may also be sequestered, and hypokalemia may ensue. In vitro sequestration of potassium may occur in leukocytes rich blood

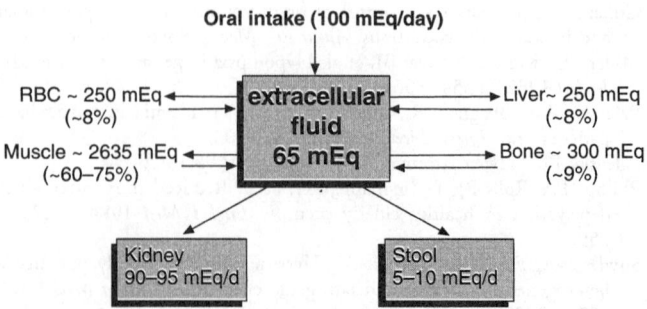

FIGURE 146.1. Internal and external potassium balance in humans.

(acute myelogenous leukemia) if sufficient time elapses before analysis. This leads to spurious reductions in K^+ that obviously need not be replaced.

POTASSIUM DEPLETION

DIETARY CAUSES

Reduced potassium intake (e.g., in the elderly person on a "tea-and-toast" diet and in sufferers of anorexia nervosa or bulimia) and states of protein/calorie malnutrition are associated with significant K^+ losses (3 mEq per gram of nitrogen loss in the latter). Induced vomiting and diuretic or laxative use often compounds the problem. Intravenous feedings of glucose solutions or the use of parenteral nutrition without appropriate potassium supplementation may result in hypokalemia. Geophagia (clay or dirt ingestion) results in hypokalemia if the clay is white (which binds intestinal K^+), but might lead to hyperkalemia, particularly in patients with renal insufficiency, if the clay is red (high K^+ content).

Uncomplicated body K^+ depletion lowers both intra- and extracellular K^+ concentration so that plasma K^+ decreases by 1 mEq for each 300-mEq deficit, up to a depletion of about 700 mEq. If losses exceed 1,000 mEq, plasma K^+ is usually less than 2 mEq/L. This relation between plasma K^+ and K^+ depletion may be altered if the factors determining transcellular distribution are offset simultaneously. For example, patients with diabetic ketoacidosis may have relatively normal K^+ levels as a result of lack of insulin, acidosis, and hyperosmolality (all of which promote extracellular shifts) yet may have marked K^+ depletion.

EXTRARENAL CAUSES

Diarrhea is a common cause of K^+ loss usually associated with metabolic acidosis (normal anion gap), which provides a clue to the underlying problem. Laxative abuse (usually surreptitious) can be uncovered by screening the stool and urine for phenolphthalein-containing compounds, which exhibit a reddish purple color on alkalinization. The discovery of melanosis coli on a proctoscopic examination can confirm this diagnosis. For unknown reasons, laxative abusers may present with metabolic alkalosis instead of metabolic acidosis. Two rare conditions, villous adenoma of the rectum and non-β-cell pancreatic islet tumors, lead to watery diarrhea of high K^+ content, hypokalemia, as well as metabolic acidosis.

Loss of gastric fluid from vomiting or drainage (K^+ 10 to 15 mEq/L) associated with renal potassium losses also leads to K^+ deficiency. Sweat losses from vigorous training in hot climates can deplete body stores, but for unknown reasons the kidney does not conserve potassium appropriately despite severe cellular depletion.

RENAL CAUSES

Urine potassium concentration above 20 mEq in the presence of hypokalemia is considered inappropriate. Almost invariably, hypokalemia of nonrenal origin is accompanied by reductions in potassium excretion below 20 mEq per day. Renal potassium wasting is principally found in states of high mineralocorticoid secretion or administration. For diagnostic purposes, the presence or absence of hypertension and the associated acid–base status can be used to classify hypokalemia.

METABOLIC ACIDOSIS

Because hypokalemia is usually associated with metabolic alkalosis or normal acid–base status, the presence of metabolic acidosis is an important diagnostic clue. Metabolic acidosis, renal potassium wastage, and hypokalemia—which may induce severe paralysis—are common in both distal (type I) and proximal (type II) renal tubular acidosis. In the latter, hypokalemia is particularly prominent during therapy with high doses of bicarbonate; in the former, alkali therapy curtails potassium loss. Acetazolamide (Diamox) and other carbonic anhydrase inhibitors can produce a combination of proximal and distal renal tubular acidosis and can lead to K^+ depletion. Metabolic acidosis and potassium deficiency is also found in diabetic ketoacidosis, in which, as already pointed out, the plasma K^+ level may be normal.

NORMOTENSIVE DISORDERS

Hypertension itself has little bearing on the development of alkalosis or hypokalemia, but its presence or absence is extremely helpful in establishing a cause for the disturbance. Chloride depletion is the most common cause of hypokalemic metabolic alkalosis and usually results from gastrointestinal fluid losses caused by vomiting, gastric drainage, or chloride-depleting diarrhea or from renal losses secondary to diuretic therapy.

Chloride depletion leads to contraction of the extracellular fluid and avid chloride retention by the kidney. As a consequence, urine concentration of chloride falls, but that of sodium, potassium, and bicarbonate may increase. The hypochloriduria (Cl^- less than 10 mEq per L) in a persistently alkalotic patient almost always indicates gastric fluid losses because the ion is clearly not wasted in the urine. Persistence of an inappropriate kaliuresis, in which increased aldosterone secretion plays a minor role, is partly responsible for the hypokalemia. Low chloride and high bicarbonate in the distal nephron directly stimulate K^+ secretion, with the former mechanism possibly playing the major role. Hypokalemia inhibits and alkalosis stimulates distal potassium secretion; if the latter predominates, it can perpetuate the kaliuresis.

The use of thiazides and loop diuretics is the most common cause of K^+ depletion and metabolic alkalosis. The increase in urine flow and distal sodium delivery in the presence of volume depletion and excess aldosterone secretion leads to marked kaliuresis. In patients taking prescribed diuretics, it may be easy to identify the cause of the hypokalemic (plasma K^+ rarely less than 3 mEq per L) alkalosis. Surreptitious diuretic use (e.g., weight loss schemes) must be suspected and excluded in normotensive patients in whom hypokalemic alkalosis or renal potassium wasting does not have a clear cause. The concomitant finding of high urine chloride is also suspicious, and proof can come from demonstrating the presence of diuretics by chromatographic analysis of the urine.

Bartter's syndrome is a rare disease characterized by hyperreninemia, hyperaldosteronism, hyperplasia of the juxtaglomerular apparatus, increased prostaglandin secretion, insensitivity to the pressor effect of angiotensin II, and normal blood pressure. The syndrome results from a defect of the loop of Henle's two chloride, sodium-potassium cotransporter, and is attended by hypokalemic alkalosis (see Chapter 149). Gitelman's syndrome is caused by a defect in the early distal tubule sodium chloride transporter and is characterized by a tendency to hypotension, metabolic alkalosis, hypomagnesemia, and hypokalemia.

Acute myelomonoblastic leukemias may present with renal potassium wastage (25% of cases), often associated with increased urine lysozyme excretion. Magnesium depletion may be accompanied by hypokalemia that is resistant to potassium replacement until the Mg^{2+} deficit is corrected. Drugs such as cisplatin, gentamicin, and levodopa can lead to potassium wasting.

HYPERTENSIVE DISORDERS

Hypertensive conditions usually result from excess mineralocorticoids or, less frequently, glucocorticoids. Extracellular fluid expansion is present so that the urine chloride level exceeds 10 mEq per L. Plasma renin assay can further help to classify these disorders.

Primary hyperaldosteronism (low renin, hypertension) can result from a solitary adenoma (65% of cases), bilateral adrenal hyperplasia, or carcinoma. Increased sodium delivery to the distal tubule in the presence of high aldosterone secretion leads to renal K^+ losses. A high salt intake, by increasing distal sodium for potassium exchange, worsens the kaliuresis. Moreover, salt loading (oral and intravenous) does not suppress aldosterone secretion, which in the presence of a low plasma renin level helps establish the diagnosis and distinguishes it from secondary hyperaldosteronism (edematous states such as heart failure and liver cirrhosis). Secondary hyperaldosteronism states (high renin, normotensive) often result in K^+ depletion, as when edematous patients are treated with diuretics, but in conditions such as renal artery stenosis, malignant hypertension, or rare renin-producing tumors (high renin, hypertensive), hypokalemia may be spontaneous.

Other mineralocorticoid excess conditions presenting with low renin hypertension and hypokalemic alkalosis include ingestion of compounds such as glycyrrhizic acid (present in licorice and some chewing tobacco) and carbenoxalone. Both of these inhibit 11β-hydroxysteroid dehydrogenase, an enzyme that converts cortisol to cortisone in mineralocorticoid-responsive cells (e.g., renal tubule). Cortisol, but not cortisone, interacts with the mineralocorticoid (aldosterone) receptor. Because cortisol in normal plasma is 100-fold greater than aldosterone, failure of conversion to cortisone permits it to occupy the mineralocorticoid receptor, resulting in salt retention, kaliuresis, and hypokalemia. Hypertension and hypokalemia characterizes a rare genetic abnormality that leads to 11β-hydroxysteroid dehydrogenase deficiency, also known as apparent mineralocorticoid excess, since plasma aldosterone is low or normal. The

use of fludrocortisone acetate (Florinef), intranasal corticosteroid with mineralocorticoid properties, or excessive deoxycorticosterone production as in adrenogenital syndromes (17α-hydroxylase or 11β-hydroxylase deficiencies) also are examples of low renin hypertension. In all of the nonaldosterone mineralocorticoid excess conditions, aldosterone secretion is suppressed.

Cushing's syndrome (excess endogenous production or exogenous administration of glucocorticoid) can lead to hypokalemia. Hypokalemia is more common when the syndrome is due to ectopic adrenocorticotropic hormone secretion by a tumor (small cell carcinoma of the lung). Plasma renin activity is usually normal, as is aldosterone, indicating that the most likely explanation for the development of K^+ depletion is increased fluid delivery to the distal nephron.

■ CONSEQUENCES OF K^+ DEPLETION

Potassium depletion reduces the extracellular K^+ concentration, and the ratio of intracellular to extracellular K^+ concentration increases. Cell membranes become hyperpolarized, reducing membrane excitability. Intracellular shifts of potassium (as in familial periodic paralysis) and other acute changes in extracellular K^+ affect the membrane potential more than do chronic changes, as the transmembrane potassium gradient is very steep.

The most important effects of hypokalemia (usually at values less than 3 mEq per L) are on the myocardium. Typical electrocardiographic changes result, including ST-segment depression, decreased amplitude or inversion of the T wave, and increased height of the U wave (more than 1 mm). With increases in severity, hypokalemia may lead to increased P-wave amplitude, prolongation of the PR interval, and widening of the QRS complex. Atrioventricular block and supraventricular and ventricular tachycardia, including ventricular fibrillation, can also occur, particularly in the setting of acute myocardial infarction. Hypokalemia also increases the incidence of digitalis toxicity.

Hypokalemia may lead to vague malaise, muscular weakness (usually proximal and in the lower extremities), and muscle cramps. Constipation and even intestinal ileus may occur from impaired smooth muscle function. Severe hypokalemia (less than 2 mEq per L) can cause marked weakness and life-threatening paralysis (respiratory arrest). Rhabdomyolysis may result from diminished exercise-induced vasodilatation in the presence of diminished muscle energy stores as a result of altered glycogen metabolism.

Endocrine complications of K^+ depletion include glucose intolerance secondary to defective pancreatic insulin secretion. Secretion of aldosterone, and possibly catecholamines, is also decreased, but these manifestations have no particular clinical significance. Prostaglandin and renin production is also increased by K^+ depletion.

Renal dysfunction in hypokalemia is characterized by impaired concentrating ability in combination with primary polydipsia and polyuria. Renal vasoconstriction reduces renal blood flow and the glomerular filtration rate, contributing further to the concentrating defect. These functional abnormalities are reversible on correction of the K^+ depletion. Nevertheless, prolonged severe K$^+$ depletion can lead to interstitial nephritis and to the development of chronic renal failure, can induce the development of renal cysts, can lead to vacuolar lesions in proximal and distal tubule cells, and can increase the sensitivity to nephrotoxic antibiotics (acute tubular necrosis). Metabolic alkalosis (increased bicarbonate reabsorption and increased acid excretion), abnormal sodium retention, and renal chloride wasting can develop because of low K$^+$ levels. Hyponatremia can occur from intracellular shifts of sodium to replace lost K$^+$. Defective tubular chloride handling in patients with severe K$^+$ depletion of any cause increases chloride concentration in the urine; it also results in increased renal ammonia production, which can induce encephalopathy in patients with hepatic disease.

◼ DIAGNOSTIC APPROACH

The cause of hypokalemia is usually apparent from the history and the clinical setting. The history should focus on medications; diet; the presence of vomiting, diarrhea, or other losses of body fluids; and a family history of hypokalemia. The physical examination may point to a condition that can account for the development of hypokalemia; however, with the exception of blood pressure, it is not particularly useful to help categorize hypokalemic disorders into diagnostic subsets. Blood acid–base parameters, urine potassium and chloride values, and, under certain conditions, measurements of renin and aldosterone levels are the most useful for diagnosis.

Figures 146.2 and 146.3 offer guidelines to the differential diagnosis of hypokalemic disorders. The first decision is whether the hypokalemia is a laboratory artifact, the result of redistribution, or a manifestation of actual K$^+$ depletion. Spurious hypokalemia can occur when a blood specimen with a very high white cell count (greater than 200,000 cells per L) stands at room temperature. Measurement of blood pH and an assessment of the clinical setting can usually determine whether redistribution is possible. Sometimes redistribution and K$^+$ depletion coexist, leading to a more complicated diagnostic problem.

In the presence of K$^+$ depletion, appropriate renal K$^+$ conservation points to an extrarenal source of the K$^+$ depletion. Systemic acid–base status may be helpful in this setting because the presence of metabolic acidosis would suggest diarrhea as the underlying cause.

Renal K$^+$ losses, in association with hypertension and altered acid–base status, provide useful clues. Metabolic acidosis accompanied by renal K$^+$ wasting narrows the diagnostic possibilities. When frank metabolic alkalosis is found, the determination of urine chloride excretion is valuable. High blood pressure, in combination with chloride excretion in excess of 10 mEq per day, suggests that hypokalemia results from an excess of either mineralocorticoid or glucocorticoid production. Measurements of plasma aldosterone, plasma renin, and possibly plasma cortisol levels can sort out the diagnostic possibilities as discussed earlier in this chapter and in the endocrine section of this text.

Normal blood pressure and high urine chloride excretion restrict the diagnostic possibilities to Bartter's syndrome and

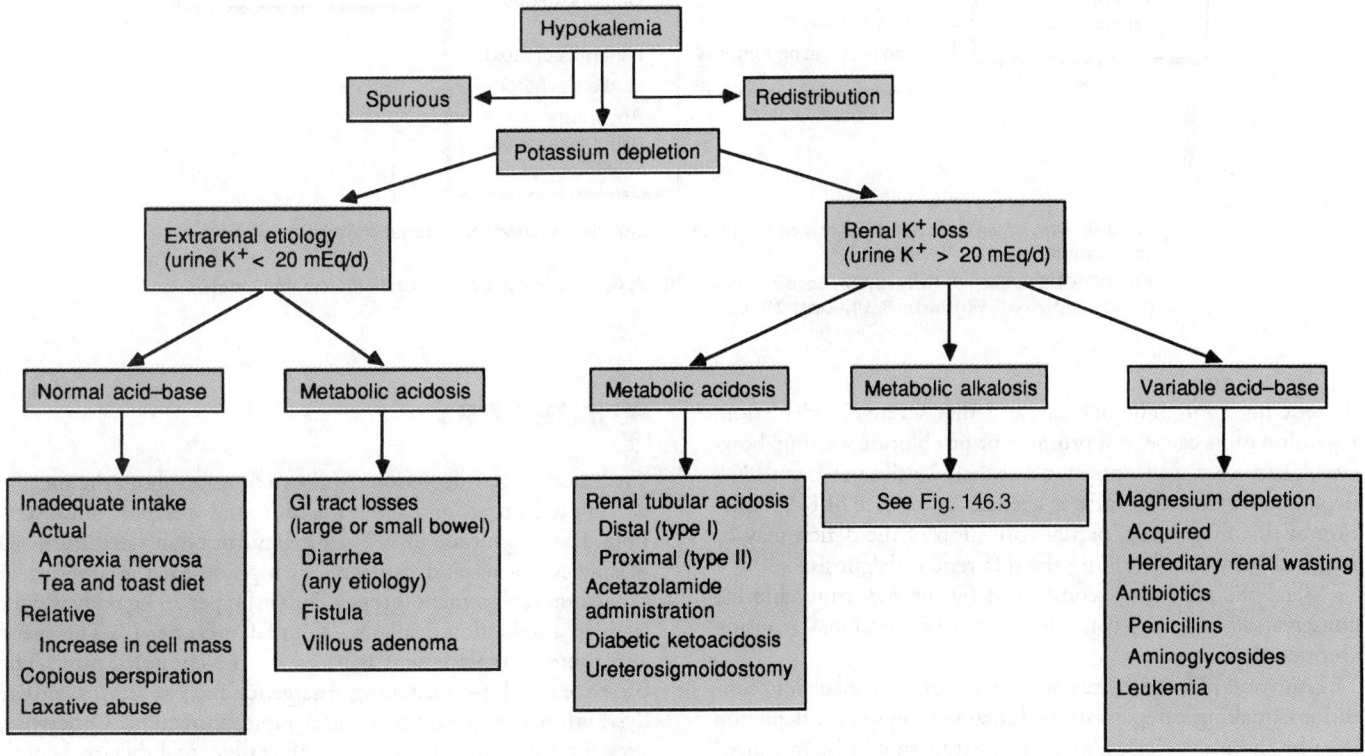

FIGURE 146.2. Diagnostic approach to hypokalemia.
EVIDENCE LEVEL: B. Reference: Seldin DW, Giebisch G, eds. *The Kidney, third edition*. Philadelphia: Lippincott Williams & Wilkins, 2000.

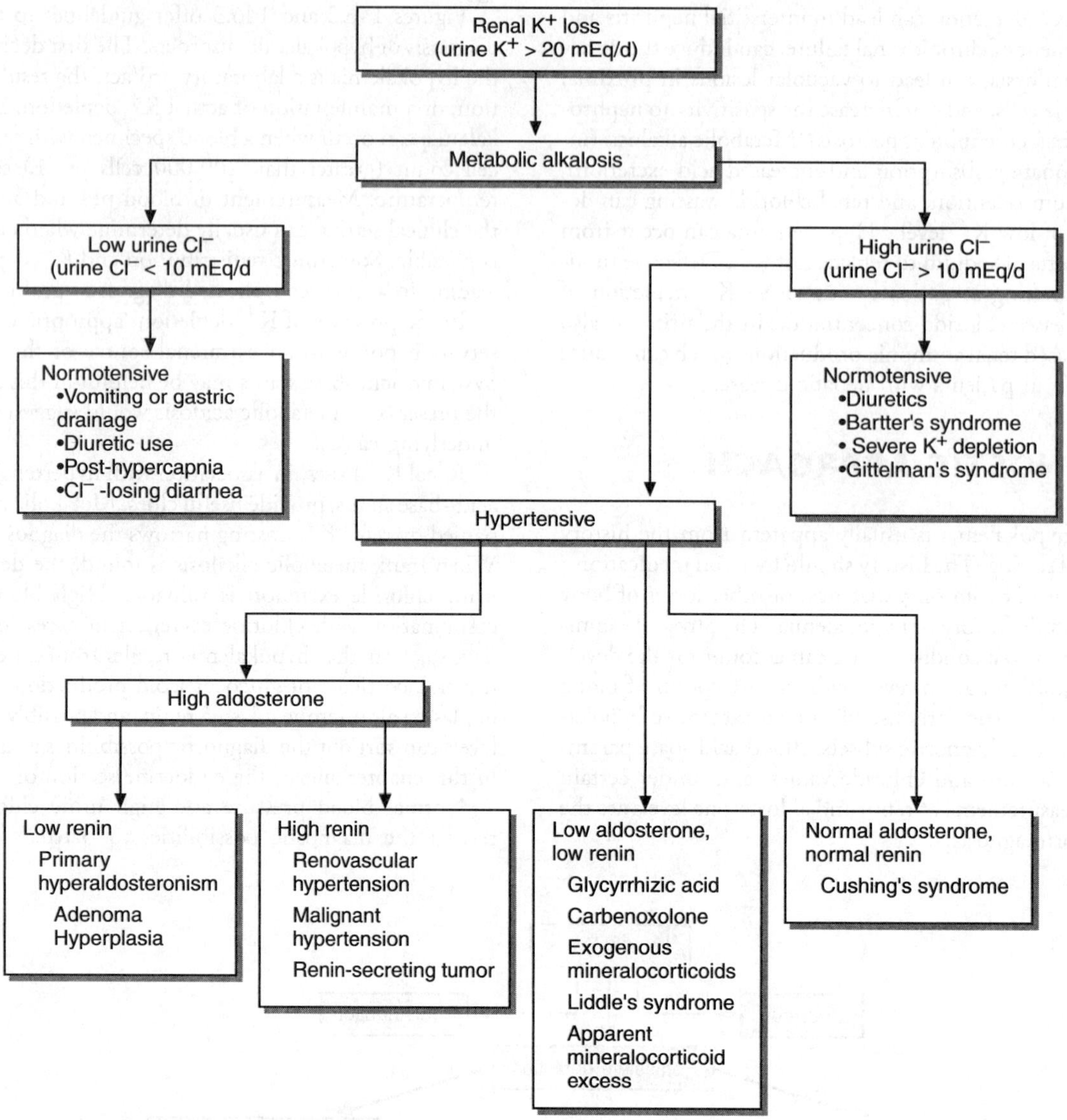

```
                        ┌─────────────────────────┐
                        │      Renal K⁺ loss       │
                        │ (urine K⁺ > 20 mEq/d)    │
                        └─────────────────────────┘
                                   │
                                   ▼
                        ┌─────────────────────────┐
                        │   Metabolic alkalosis    │
                        └─────────────────────────┘
```

Renal K⁺ loss (urine K⁺ > 20 mEq/d)

Metabolic alkalosis

Low urine Cl⁻ (urine Cl⁻ < 10 mEq/d)

High urine Cl⁻ (urine Cl⁻ > 10 mEq/d)

Normotensive
- Vomiting or gastric drainage
- Diuretic use
- Post-hypercapnia
- Cl⁻-losing diarrhea

Normotensive
- Diuretics
- Bartter's syndrome
- Severe K⁺ depletion
- Gittelman's syndrome

Hypertensive

High aldosterone

Low renin

Primary hyperaldosteronism

Adenoma Hyperplasia

High renin

Renovascular hypertension

Malignant hypertension

Renin-secreting tumor

Low aldosterone, low renin

Glycyrrhizic acid

Carbenoxolone

Exogenous mineralocorticoids

Liddle's syndrome

Apparent mineralocorticoid excess

Normal aldosterone, normal renin

Cushing's syndrome

FIGURE 146.3. Differential diagnosis of hypokalemic disorders secondary to renal potassium wasting that manifest metabolic alkalosis.

EVIDENCE LEVEL: B. Reference: Seldin DW, Giebisch G, eds. *The Kidney, third edition.* Philadelphia: Lippincott Williams & Wilkins, 2000.

diuretic ingestion. The one caveat is that severe K⁺ depletion, regardless of its cause, can promote urine chloride wasting; however, plasma K⁺ concentration less than 2 mEq per L with K⁺ depletion above 1,000 mEq is needed. In the face of K⁺ depletion of this magnitude, partial correction of the deficit may be required before undertaking the differential diagnosis.

Metabolic alkalosis accompanied by intense urine chloride conservation suggests conditions (mostly extrarenal) causing chloride depletion.

Equivocal pH values are common in some hypokalemic conditions, making categorization difficult. Magnesium depletion may be the most elusive, and magnesium should be measured in any patient with K⁺ depletion of unclear origin. Other conditions, such as drug-induced K⁺ depletion or leukemia, are usually readily apparent.

▌THERAPY

Treatment of K⁺ depletion requires a decision about the specific K⁺ salt to be used, and about the route and speed of administration. The magnitude of K⁺ depletion can be inferred from the plasma K⁺ level and can serve as a guide for the amount of potassium replacement (grossly, 300 mEq per 70 kg body weight leads to a reduction in plasma K⁺ of 1 mEq per L). The speed and route of replacement is based on the clinical setting. The presence of a life-threatening emergency such as serious cardiac dysrhythmia or paralysis requires rapid correction. Otherwise, slow intravenous replacement or, if feasible, oral therapy is preferable to avoid induction of hyperkalemia. Because estimates of potassium deficits are inexact, repeat measurements during treatment are wise if not mandatory. As normokalemia is approached, treatment, particularly intravenous, should be cut back.

The cause of K^+ depletion influences the choice of potassium salt. Potassium chloride replacement is effective in all circumstances and is required when chloride depletion accounts for the K^+ depletion. When the depletion is associated with acidosis, treatment with $KHCO_3$ or the potassium salt of a bicarbonate precursor such as citrate, acetate, or gluconate is a rational choice. Coexistence of K^+ and phosphate deficits, as in alcoholics and patients with diabetic ketoacidosis, can be treated with potassium phosphate.

Potassium chloride can be given orally as a liquid or as one of several slow-release tablets. Most patients because of the unpleasant taste of liquid KCl prefer tablets; however, the risk of enteric ulceration, although small, may be greater with slow-release preparations. To maintain a normal serum K^+ concentration, as in patients receiving diuretic therapy, an alternative to K^+ replacement is the use of the K^+-sparing diuretics such as spironolactone, triamterene, or amiloride. In general, the last two drugs are preferable because spironolactone inhibits only aldosterone-mediated K^+ secretion and, in addition, may induce gynecomastia.

There is considerable debate concerning the appropriate management of diuretic-induced hypokalemia. Many view the degree of depletion as typically mild and asymptomatic, making routine K^+ therapy inappropriate. Others believe that the risk of cardiac abnormalities is sufficient to warrant a more aggressive approach. A reasonable compromise is to recommend K^+ maintenance therapy (i.e., the maintenance of a normal serum K^+ level with either K^+-sparing diuretics or potassium chloride supplements) in patients treated with cardiac glycosides, those prone to hepatic coma, those whose serum K^+ levels decrease to less than 3 mEq per L, and those with underlying myocardial disease, diuretic-induced glucose intolerance, or symptoms attributable to hypokalemia. It must be understood that the safest way to minimize hypokalemia is to ensure adequate intake of dietary potassium. High potassium content is present in dry figs and molasses. Other K^+-rich foods include dried fruits, nuts, lima beans, tomatoes, carrots, potatoes, bananas, oranges, ground beef, veal, and lamb, to name some.

The major risk of the treatment of hypokalemia is overzealous therapy, with the development of life-threatening hyperkalemia. Conditions that predispose to this complication are detailed in Chapter 147.

BIBLIOGRAPHY

DeFronzo FA, Thier SO. Fluid and electrolyte disturbances in hypo- and hyperkalemia. In: Martinez-Maldonado M, ed. *Handbook of renal therapeutics.* New York: Plenum Publishing, 1983:25–55.

Gennari FJ. Hypokalemia. *N Engl J Med* 1998;339:451–458.

Schnaper HW, Freis ED, Fridman RG, et al. Potassium restoration in hypertensive patients made hypokalemic by hydrochlorothiazide. *Arch Intern Med* 1989;12:2677–2681.

Kelley's Textbook of Internal Medicine, fourth edition. Edited by H. David Humes.
Lippincott Williams & Wilkins, Philadelphia © 2000.

CHAPTER
147

APPROACH TO THE PATIENT WITH HYPERKALEMIA

MANUEL MARTINEZ-MALDONADO

Hyperkalemia, which refers to an elevated serum K^+ concentration, can result from a spurious laboratory value, redistribution from the intracellular to the extracellular compartment, or K^+ retention (a surfeit). Chronic hyperkalemia is invariably the result of a defect in renal potassium excretion.

SPURIOUS HYPERKALEMIA

Factitious elevation of serum K^+ can result from various factors (Fig. 147.1). Hemolysis of the specimen—rarely from an acquired or hereditary defect in the K^+ permeability of the erythrocyte membrane—can elevate K^+ concentration. Leukocytosis (white cell count >70,000/cm3) causes spurious hyperkalemia due to K^+ leakage from the cells when the specimen is allowed to clot, particularly if preserved in the cold. At room temperature, cellular K^+ uptake can cause artifactual hypokalemia. Therefore, leukemic blood specimens require rapid separation of cells from plasma or serum to avoid spurious K^+ determinations. Thrombocytosis (platelet counts >1,000,000/ cm3) can elevate serum K^+ levels as a result of K^+ release from the platelets during clotting. Obtaining a heparinized specimen can circumvent this. Excessively tight and prolonged tourniquet application, together with clenching of the fist, can also elevate the K^+ concentration by 2 mEq/L or more, by release from ischemic exercising muscle.

When spurious hyperkalemia is suspected, a repeat measurement is useful, applying the appropriate precautions. The clinical insignificance of factitious hyperkalemia is rapidly confirmed by normal electrocardiogram (ECG) results; unnecessary treatment should be avoided.

HYPERKALEMIA SECONDARY TO REDISTRIBUTION

Blocking K shifts into cells can result in hyperkalemia. Acidosis, insulin deficiency, and (β_2-blocking agents predispose to hyperkalemia secondary to cellular redistribution. The mechanism of acidosis-induced shifts is complex, as it appears that only mineral acid or hyperchloremic forms of acidosis result in K^+ shifts; organic forms of acidosis, such as lactic acidosis, do not. Organic acids are incompletely dissociated in solution and as such enter cells where they breakup into protons and the weak bases, thus the membrane potential is mostly unaffected which prevents

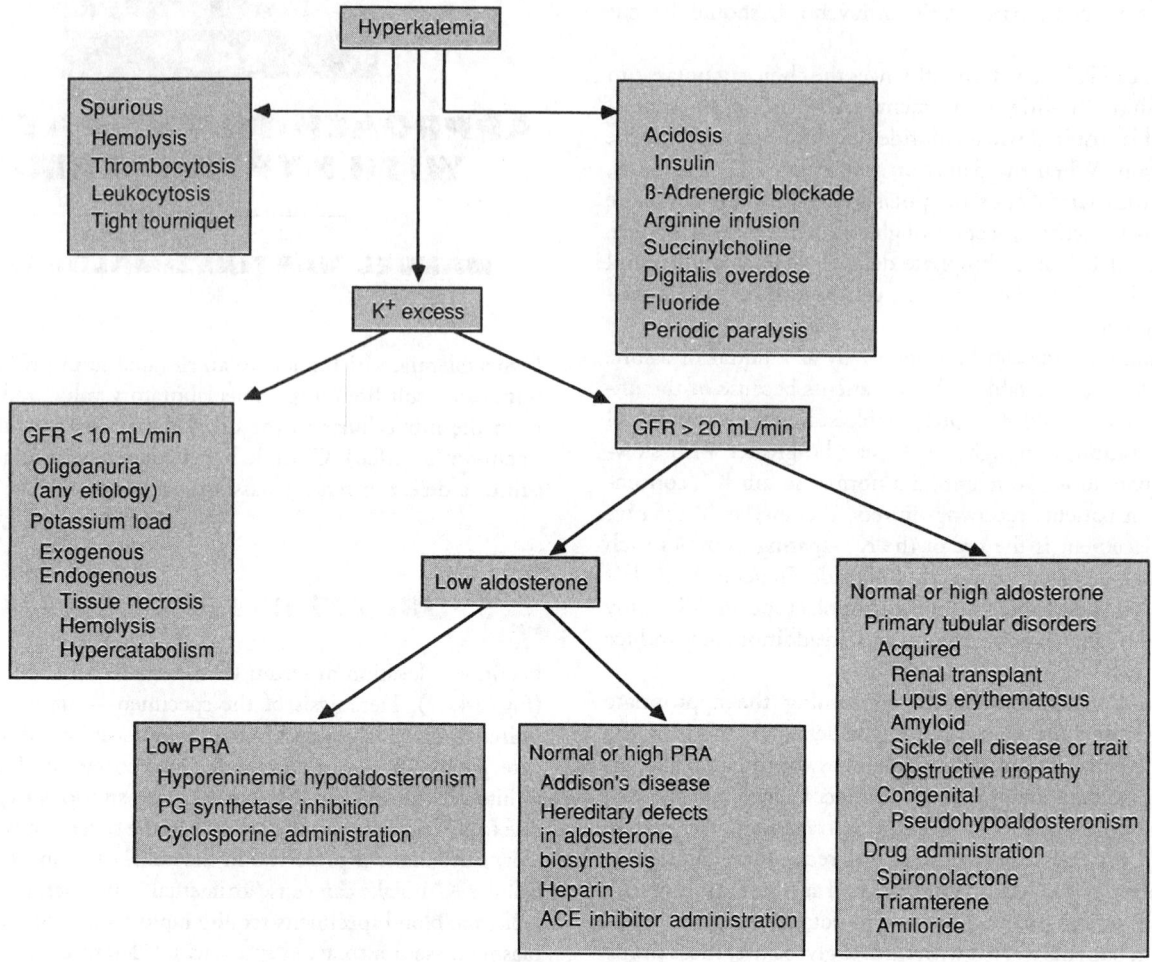

FIGURE 147.1. Diagnostic approach to hyperkalemia. GFR, glomerular filtration rate; PRA, plasma renin activity; PG, prostaglandin; ACE, angiotensin-converting enzyme.
EVIDENCE LEVEL: B. Reference: Weiner ID, Wingo CS. Hyperkalemia: a potential silent killer.
***J Am Soc Nephrol* 1998;9:1535–1543.**

conductive cellular postassium exit. Organic acidosis also stimulates insulin release, which by shifting K into cells may contribute to the absence of hyperkalemia. Thus, hyperkalemia may be seen in diabetic ketoacidosis as a consequence of insulin deficiency and hypertonicity from hyperglycemia, as high extracellular fluid (ECF) osmolality pulls both water and K+ from the intracellular space. The degree of K+ alteration is greater with metabolic than with respiratory acidosis, averaging 0.7 mEq/0.1 pH unit with metabolic and 0.1 mEq/0.1 pH unit with respiratory acidosis. Cell shifts are more likely to contribute to hyperkalemia than to hypokalemia, because cellular uptake is easier than cellular release of potassium.

Use of β-blockers predisposes toward hyperkalemia. If other K+ regulatory mechanisms are intact, only minimal increases in the serum K+ concentration occur; however, serious hyperkalemia can be provoked in patients otherwise prone to K+ abnormalities, such as those on chronic hemodialysis.

Redistribution hyperkalemia may be induced by the use of or intoxication with several drugs that can alter K+ distribution across cellular membranes, including cardiac glycosides, succinylcholine and other depolarizing muscle relaxants, arginine

HCl, and fluoride. K+ egress from contracting muscle can produce substantial hyperkalemia with acute, maximal, or very prolonged exercise, such as participation in marathons. Hyperkalemic periodic paralysis is an autosomal dominant hereditary disorder featuring episodic paralytic attacks accompanied by shifts of K from the cellular compartment. The attacks are precipitated by ingestion of small amounts of potassium or other unrelated stimuli (eg, excitement, cold, fasting, stress, infection, and general anesthesia). The attacks may be averted by eating sugar, to cause insulin release, or by using inhalers containing β2-adrenergic agonists.

■ HYPERKALEMIA SECONDARY TO K+ RETENTION

K+ excretion requires a normal number of functioning nephron units, adequate delivery of sodium and fluid to the distal nephron, an intact aldosterone system, and a distal tubular epithelium with an intact K+ secretory mechanism. Abnormalities in any of these parameters can lead to hyperkalemia secondary to K$^+$ retention.

ABNORMAL GLOMERULAR FILTRATION RATE

Decreases in the number of functioning nephron units curtails the kidney's capacity to excrete K$^+$. So long as K$^+$ intake is normal, however, a glomerular filtration rate (GFR) above 5 mL/min can usually sustain normokalemia. Preservation of K$^+$ balance occurs because the remaining nephrons adapt their K$^+$ secretory capacity, similar to the way normal kidneys do when confronted with an increase in dietary K$^+$. On the other hand, dependence on the kidney's adaptive capacity to sustain K$^+$ balance with a normal intake limits its ability to handle an increased K$^+$ load. Thus, when GFR is decreased significantly (ie, <20 mL/min), patients are at risk of hyperkalemia in response to an increased K$^+$ load. This can result from exogenous sources such as foods high in K$^+$, K$^+$ replacement therapy, or the use of salt substitutes (which contain K$^+$), or it may result from endogenous generation of a K$^+$ load. Release of K$^+$ from tissue breakdown, as in rhabdomyolysis and tissue trauma, red blood cell degradation in hematomas, or bleeding into the gastrointestinal tract, can produce life-threatening hyperkalemia in patients with a compromised GFR.

Hyperkalemia is a major potential complication of acute renal failure, whether oliguric or nonoliguric. Therefore, all patients with this diagnosis should have an ECG performed as early as feasible to rule out life-threatening hyperkalemia.

When the number of functioning nephron units is sufficient to sustain K$^+$ homeostasis (>20 mL/min), renal hyperkalemia results either from aldosterone deficiency or from a primary defect in K$^+$ secretion by the distal tubular epithelium.

HYPOALDOSTERONISM

Aldosterone deficiency, regardless of the underlying cause, predisposes to the development of hyperkalemia. Patients with low aldosterone levels are not always hyperkalemic if their renal function is normal; however, a decrease in distal salt and water delivery in these persons may induce overt hyperkalemia.

Combined aldosterone (mineralocorticoid) and glucocorticoid deficiencies result in the classical features of Addison's disease. The aldosterone deficiency leads to renal sodium wasting and potassium retention, and the glucocorticoid deficiency results in water retention and many of the constitutional symptoms. The defects lead to hypotension, hyponatremia, and hyperkalemia. Plasma renin levels are high, but plasma cortisol levels are low and unresponsive to adrenocorticotropic hormone (ACTH) stimulation. Addison's disease results from adrenal destruction (autoimmune disease, infection, or hemorrhage) or from bilateral adrenalectomy. Hereditary enzymatic defects in aldosterone biosynthesis, including the syndrome of congenital adrenal hyperplasia (C21 hydroxylase deficiency), or isolated abnormalities in aldosterone production secondary to a deficiency

in corticosterone methyloxidase I or II are less common causes of adrenal hormonal insufficiency. When a low aldosterone level results from a primary defect in adrenal steroid production, plasma renin levels are elevated.

Aldosterone deficiency in association with chronic renal disease has been recognized with increased frequency. These patients generally have tubulointerstitial forms of renal disease and often diabetes mellitus. A few appear to have an isolated defect in adrenal aldosterone production. Most, however, exhibit combined low renin and aldosterone levels, a syndrome referred to as hyporeninemic hypoaldosteronism. A defect in renin secretion seems to be responsible for the low aldosterone levels, although the precise pathophysiology of disordered renin metabolism is unresolved. Many of these patients also exhibit abnormal aldosterone release in response to potassium (usually a potent stimulus for aldosterone release), angiotensin II, or exogenous ACTH, suggesting that a primary defect in adrenal aldosterone production might coexist with the renal defect that causes low renin secretion. In addition to hyperkalemia, about half of these patients exhibit hyperchloremic metabolic acidosis, which appears to be secondary to hyperkalemia-induced suppression of renal ammonia production and perhaps also abnormal H$^+$ secretion as a result of low aldosterone levels (so-called type IV renal tubular acidosis). In contrast to patients with Addison's disease, persons with hyporeninemic hypoaldosteronism are fluid overloaded; hyponatremia is unusual because cortisol levels are normal.

Several medications can cause aldosterone deficiency that leads to hyperkalemia. Heparin directly impairs adrenal aldosterone biosynthesis. Prostaglandin synthetase inhibitors, such as indomethacin, reduce renin release and produce reversible hyporeninemic hypoaldosteronism, particularly in patients with chronic renal insufficiency. Angiotensin-converting enzyme inhibitors produce hypoaldosteronism by lowering angiotensin II levels, while angiotensin II receptor antagonists can do so through diminished aldosterone secretion. Cyclosporine produces hyperkalemia by suppressing renin levels, but it may also impair aldosterone secretion and directly interfere with tubular K$^+$ secretion.

In addition to the development of hyporeninemic hypoaldosteronism and acquired immune deficiency syndrome (AIDS)-related adrenal insufficiency, renal potassium excretion is impaired as a result of therapy with pentamidine or trimethoprim, both of which block the principal cell apical sodium channel, and thus potassium excretion, similar to amiloride. Pentamidine-induced hyperkalemia has been almost always observed in the setting of acute renal failure.

NORMAL ADRENAL FUNCTION

Several diseases, all of which can cause hyporeninemic hypoaldosteronism, can also produce hyperkalemia without a concurrent decrease in aldosterone levels. These conditions, which presumably interfere in some direct fashion with K$^+$ secretion by the distal nephron, include lupus erythematosus, amyloidosis, obstructive uropathy, sickle-cell disease, and postrenal transplantation. Patients with chronic renal failure may have increased levels of plasma aldosterone, suggesting some degree of resistance to mineralocorticoids.

Tubular hyperkalemia occurs in two hereditary conditions. Pseudohypoaldosteronism type I affects infants and presents with salt wasting and hyperkalemia suggestive of aldosterone deficiency. Aldosterone levels are normal or high, however, and a defect in the aldosterone receptor has been found in several aldosterone-responsive tissues. Pseudohypoaldosteronism type II presents in late childhood or in adults, with hypertension rather than salt wasting. Abnormally avid chloride reabsorption by the distal nephron may account for volume expansion, hypertension, and a defect in K^+ secretion.

The K^+-sparing diuretics all cause hyperkalemia through their effect on the renal tubule. Spironolactone interferes with the action of aldosterone; amiloride and triamterene inhibit K^+ secretion by an aldosterone-independent mechanism.

CONSEQUENCES OF HYPERKALEMIA

Hyperkalemia alters the function of excitable tissues by decreasing the K^+i/K^+e ratio. Because the intracellular K rises minimally or actually falls in hyperkalemia, the intracellular-to-extracellular ratio decreases, causing depolarization of the cell membrane and leading to clinically significant dysfunction of cardiac and skeletal muscle.

Severe hyperkalemia can produce cardiac arrest. The ECG manifestations of hyperkalemia parallel to some extent the severity of the rise in the K^+ level. An early manifestation is peaking or tenting of the T waves, which becomes most prominent with K levels of 6 mEq/L or more. More severe hyperkalemia flattens the P wave, prolongs the PR interval, and widens the QRS complex, with deepening of the S wave. The final event is a sine wave pattern (merging of the widening QRS complex with the T wave), followed by ventricular flutter, fibrillation, and cardiac arrest.

Hyperkalemia produces tingling, paresthesias, weakness, and even flaccid paralysis, particularly of the lower extremities but sparing the respiratory muscles. In most cases, this occurs when the plasma K level exceeds 8 mEq/L; thus, cardiac toxicity usually precedes these neurologic manifestations. Some of these symptoms (eg, weakness, tingling) may mimic hysteria and hyperventilation, which may transiently cloud the possibility of life-threatening hyperkalemia.

Hyperkalemia elevates plasma aldosterone levels by directly stimulating adrenal aldosterone release. A high K^+ level tends to suppress renin levels, but because a high K^+ intake is natriuretic, the volume contraction sometimes overrides the direct K^+ suppressive effects, elevating renin levels. Normal anion gap metabolic acidosis is commonly associated with hyperkalemia. This may be the result of a combination of hydrogen ion displacement from cells and the inhibitory effect of hyperkalemia on renal ammonia production. When aldosterone secretion is reduced, it contributes to the acidosis because renal hydrogen secretion is impaired.

DIAGNOSTIC APPROACH

SPURIOUS AND REDISTRIBUTION HYPERKALEMIA

The first step in the assessment of a hyperkalemic patient is to rule out a spurious laboratory value (see Fig. 147-1). If the K^+ level is severely elevated, an ECG should be performed promptly: it is helpful diagnostically and also indicates the need for rapid institution of therapy. Next, the possibility of hyperkalemia secondary to redistribution should be considered by reviewing the clinical situation, determining the acid-base status, and considering potential drug-induced conditions.

RENAL DYSFUNCTION

In the presence of oliguria or acute renal failure, the cause of hyperkalemia is usually apparent. On the other hand, in the presence of other renal diseases, it is essential to measure some index of renal function (plasma creatinine, blood urea nitrogen, or creatinine clearance). If the GFR exceeds 5 mL/min, the possibilities of excess K^+ intake and of a defect in tubule K^+ secretion must be considered. A practical approach is to obtain a 24-hour urine collection for K^+ and creatinine and to measure plasma K^+ and creatinine levels simultaneously. The total amount of K^+ in the urine indicates whether a hidden source of K^+ intake not detected in the history explains the hyperkalemia. The calculated fractional excretion of K^+ (FEK^+) in relation to the GFR indicates whether a defect in K^+ secretion accounts for the hyperkalemia. If the FEK^+ is low in relation to GFR, it is useful to measure plasma renin and aldosterone levels.

HORMONAL DEFICIENCIES

Low aldosterone levels and high renin levels suggest adrenal insufficiency, which can be confirmed by measuring plasma cortisol. If both aldosterone and renin are suppressed, the diagnosis of hyporeninemic hypoaldosteronism can be made; if the values are normal, the patient has a primary tubular defect. These two diagnostic possibilities can be confirmed by assessing the plasma K^+ response to mineralocorticoid replacement (fludrocortisone acetate [Florinef], 0.1 mg/d for 2 wk). This is usually unnecessary and should be carried out with caution, because salt retention with volume overload and hypertension are potential risks in patients with abnormal renal function.

THERAPY

Acute hyperkalemia is a life-threatening abnormality. The higher the plasma K^+ level and the more severe the ECG alterations and the clinical setting, the more urgent the need for treatment. When the correlation between potassium levels and clinical findings is uncertain, it is preferable to err on the side of overtreatment (Table 147.1). Calcium antagonizes the effects of hyperka-

TABLE 147.1. ACUTE THERAPY OF HYPERKALEMIA

	Mechanism	Dose	Onset	Duration of Hypokalemic Effect
Calcium gluconate (10%)	Membrane antagonism	10–12 mL IV	1–3 min	30–60 min
Albuterol (nebulized)	Redistribution	20 mg in 4 mL/saline inhaled over 10 min	15–30 min	1 h
Insulin plus glucose	Redistribution	20 units of regular insulin with 50 g glucose IV over 1 h	30 min	4–6 h
Cation exchange resin (Kayexalate)	Excretion	2–50 g PO or per rectum with sorbitol	1–2 h	4–6 h
Peritoneal or hemodialysis	Excretion	—	Within minutes after starting	Until dialysis is completed
Diuretics	Excretion		Within minutes of diuresis	Until diuresis ends
Furosemide		40 mg IV		
Ethacrynic acid		50 mg IV		

Modified from Martinez-Maldonado, ed. *Handbook of renal therapeutics*. New York: Plenum Publishing, 1983;39, with permission.

lemia on the heart by stabilizing the myocardium. The effects of hyperkalemia are reversed within seconds and ventricular fibrillation and arrest are averted. Calcium raises the threshold potential, reestablishes the difference between resting and threshold potentials and restores cell excitability, which is dramatically reduced by hyperkalemia.

Bicarbonate and insulin both drive K[+] into the intracellular compartment. Hyperkalemia is usually associated with a decrease in plasma bicarbonate concentration. Bicarbonate administration is effective in driving potassium into cells but the changes are small and unpredictable. The hypokalemic effects of insulin are dose-related; thus, an intravenous bolus should be given to achieve high plasma levels. Hypoglycemia should be prevented by infusing 50 g glucose per hour to accompany the repeated injections (every 15 min) of 5 units of insulin.

β$_2$-Adrenergic agonists, given intravenously or by inhalation (nebulized albuterol is particularly effective), also can rapidly induce cellular K[+] uptake, but they are not uniformly effective in patients with renal failure.

Diltiazem has been shown to reduce the rate of increase in plasma potassium in anuric patients with end-stage renal disease. The effect is independent of plasma aldosterone, cortisol, glucose, or magnesium. Diltiazem and other calcium channel blockers may enhance the cellular uptake of potassium secondary to inhibition of calcium-activated potassium channels in the cell membrane that normally permit diffusion of potassium out of cells.

In general, these maneuvers act rapidly and provide time to eliminate the excess K[+] burden from the body. The dose of albuterol used is usually too low to effect changes rapidly enough to be a first-line treatment in acute hyperkalemia. More delayed but effective action can be obtained from the cation exchange resin sodium polystyrene sulfonate (Kayexalate). It removes K[+] from the body most rapidly when given as a retention enema,

but is also effective orally in conjunction with a laxative (usually sorbitol). Colonic necrosis has been reported in postoperative patients treated with Kayexalate and sorbitol enemas, and animal studies suggest that sorbitol may be the offending agent.

Sometimes dialysis is necessary for K[+] removal. Hemodialysis is more efficient than peritoneal dialysis for this purpose.

Patients with hyporeninemic hypoaldosteronism exhibit chronic hyperkalemia. If the K[+] level is sustained below 5.8 mEq/L, no therapy other than counseling about high-K[+] foods and the avoidance of medications that can interfere with K[+] metabolism is required. Specific treatment options to increase K[+] excretion include the use of exogenous mineralocorticoid replacement, bicarbonate to correct metabolic acidosis, and thiazide or loop diuretics. The risks of mineralocorticoid replacement leading to volume depletion in patients with compromised renal function should be considered. If necessary, Kayexalate can be given on a chronic basis with a mild laxative, but most patients find this medication unpleasant for chronic use.

BIBLIOGRAPHY

Allon M. Treatment and prevention of hyperkalemia in end-stage renal disease. *Kidney Int* 1993;43:1197–1209.

Higham PD, Adams PC, Murray A, et al. Plasma potassium, serum magnesium and ventricular fibrillation: a prospective study. *Q J Med* 1993;9:609–617.

Solomon R, Dubey A. Diltiazem enhances potassium disposal in subjects with end-stage renal disease. *Am J Kidney Dis* 1992;5:420–426.

Tannen RL. Hypokalemia and hyperkalemia. In: Massry SG, Glassock RJ, eds. *Textbook of nephrology*, 3rd ed. Baltimore: Williams & Wilkins, 1994:313–326.

Weiner ID, Wingo CS. Hyperkalemia: a potential silent killer. *J Am Soc Nephrol* 1998;9:1535–1543.

Kelley's Textbook of Internal Medicine, fourth edition. Edited by H. David Humes. Lippincott Williams & Wilkins, Philadelphia © 2000.

APPROACH TO THE PATIENT WITH ALTERED MAGNESIUM CONCENTRATION

ANTON C. SCHOOLWERTH
GEORGE M. FELDMAN
R. MICHAEL CULPEPPER

Magnesium's vital intracellular functions are expressed through the formation of organometallic chelates involved in the function of approximately 300 cellular enzymes. Mg^{2+}-ATP (adenosine triphosphate) complex is essential for all phosphorylation reactions of ATP. Extracellular magnesium modulates contraction in smooth muscle and membrane potentials in excitable tissues through regulation of cellular or membrane calcium availability.

An interstitial pool and a small fraction of bone magnesium buffer changes in the serum magnesium concentration. Only a small fraction of the total intracellular magnesium (4.5 to 6 mEq per L) exists as free ion, which is maintained at a concentration below that of serum. The cellular magnesium content changes in relation to both cellular protein and potassium, rather than being freely exchangeable with extracellular magnesium. Recent evidence indicates that cell magnesium is regulated by intracellular organelles and is under hormonal control.

Gastrointestinal absorption of magnesium averages 30% to 40% of the dietary load and varies inversely with intake. The obligatory loss of magnesium in gastrointestinal secretions is usually trivial but may assume importance with excessive gastrointestinal fluid losses. Because body conservation of magnesium is imperfect, net gastrointestinal uptake of magnesium is necessary for maintaining body stores.

The serum magnesium concentration depends on renal handling and is determined by tubular absorption until the glomerular filtration rate (GFR) falls below 15 to 20 mL per minute, at which time filtration becomes the limiting determinant. Serum magnesium levels above the normal 1.4 to 2 mEq per L inhibit absorption in the thick ascending limb, leading to magnesuria. Though no single hormone controls renal magnesium balance, many hormones, such as parathyroid hormone, calcitonin, vasopressin, insulin, glucagon, prostaglandin E_2, and steroid hormones, plus metabolic alkalosis, have been shown to increase renal magnesium absorption and alter urinary magnesium excretion.

■ HYPOMAGNESEMIA

Extracellular fluid magnesium equilibrates differently with the magnesium content of bone and muscle (the major body depots). Hypomagnesemia, a fall in the serum magnesium concentration to less than 1.4 mEq per L (1.7 mg per dL or 0.7 mmol per L), may not be accompanied by a similar reduction in cellular magnesium content. Conversely, the large magnesium store of bone may prevent drastic falls in serum levels despite net losses of body magnesium. Overall, reduced levels of serum magnesium correlate best with bone content of the cation. Hypomagnesemia is common, especially in patients admitted to intensive care units. Recent studies have shown an association between hypomagnesemia and mortality in acutely ill medical patients, including patients with myocardial infarction.

ETIOLOGY

Virtually all cases of magnesium depletion stem from deficient gastrointestinal absorption or excessive renal loss. Acute cellular uptake of magnesium causes significant hypomagnesemia only in the setting of coexisting body magnesium deficits. Figure 148.1 provides a framework for sorting these disorders.

Gastrointestinal intake of magnesium is often marginal for optimal daily requirements. A higher intake is necessary during growth, pregnancy, and lactation. Although renal magnesium excretion can fall rapidly to below 1 mEq per day during reduced dietary intake, hypomagnesemia develops within days from the obligatory body losses. Absorption of the dietary load may increase to 75% to 80% with a low magnesium intake. Meat, whole grains, green vegetables, and seafood have relatively high magnesium contents, and water with a low mineral content (soft water) may contribute to low dietary intake. Patients on parenteral alimentation become hypomagnesemic without magnesium in the parenteral fluids.

Because most magnesium absorption occurs in the terminal small bowel, intestinal malabsorptive syndromes, jejunoileal bypass, or resection of a large portion of the small bowel lead to decreased uptake. In steatorrhea and acute pancreatitis, insoluble, nonabsorbable magnesium–fatty acid complexes (soaps) form and may lead to hypomagnesemia.

Intestinal secretions and large-bowel fluid generally have a low but fixed magnesium content. The continued loss of large volumes of such fluids through suction, fistulous drainage, or watery diarrhea eventually leads to a large net loss of body magnesium.

Renal loss of magnesium may be due to alterations in the physiologic factors that govern normal renal magnesium handling or may result from drug influences on the renal tubule. The tendency of magnesium reabsorption to parallel that of sodium, albeit at different rates, is key to a number of the causes of excess renal magnesium excretion.

Expansion of the extracellular fluid volume, either from parenteral fluids or from primary hyperaldosteronism, leads to decreased magnesium absorption in both the proximal tubule and the thick ascending limb. In both segments the reduction in magnesium absorption follows the reduction of sodium absorption. Osmotic diuretics reduce both sodium and magnesium absorption in those nephron segments, accounting for magnesuria in diabetics with glycosuria and in catabolic patients undergoing urea osmotic diuresis.

Although parathyroid hormone may have a slight direct effect to increase renal magnesium absorption, the hypercalcemia of

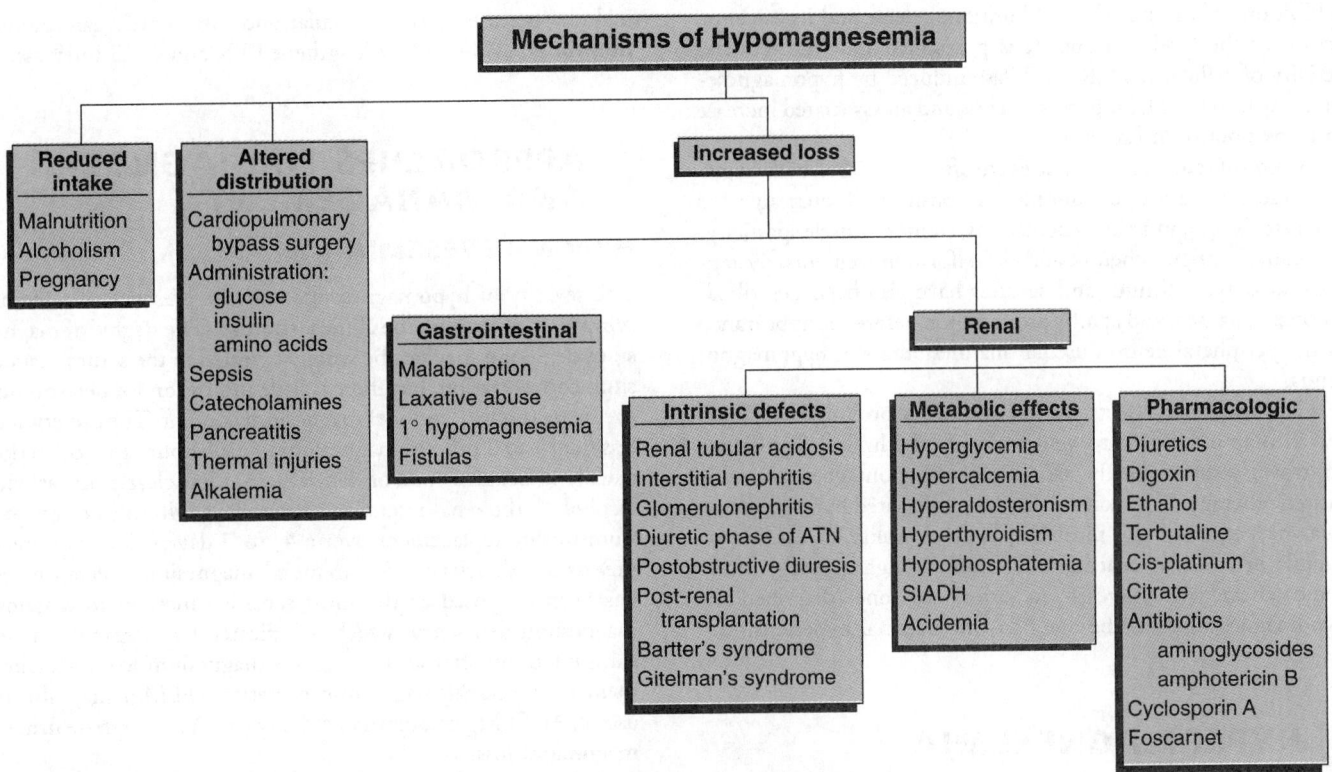

FIGURE 148.1. Mechanisms of hypomagnesemia.
EVIDENCE LEVEL:　C. Expert Opinion.

hyperparathyroidism strongly inhibits tubular reabsorption of magnesium, leading to excessive renal excretion.

Only free, ionized magnesium appears available for renal reabsorption, so magnesium complexed to absorbed organic anions is lost in the urine. Acute or chronic metabolic acidosis is associated with renal magnesium wasting. Such losses occur in diabetic ketoacidosis and in the lactic acidosis of alcoholism and starvation.

Figure 148.1 lists the mechanisms of hypomagnesemia. One of the most common causes is diuretic use. Loop diuretics such as furosemide and bumetanide inhibit both sodium and magnesium absorption in the thick ascending limb. Curiously, the thiazide diuretics, which act at a site of minimal magnesium reabsorption, are often associated with hypomagnesemia. Thiazide-induced hyperaldosteronism, hypokalemia, and hypercalcemia might converge to cause renal magnesium wasting. Similarly, Gitelman's syndrome, a familial disease due to mutations in the thiazide-sensitive cotransporter in the distal tubule, leads to hypokalemic alkalosis with hypocalciuria and hypomagnesemia. Drugs toxic to renal tubules, such as aminoglycoside antibiotics and the chemotherapeutic agent cisplatin, commonly lead to excess renal magnesium losses. The effect of cisplatin may persist for months. Pentamidine and foscarnet may also cause magnesium wasting.

Combined causes of hypomagnesemia are common in alcoholism and diabetes. In alcoholics, intake is often impaired by a magnesium-deficient diet, coupled with decreased uptake due to intestinal malabsorption. Cellular magnesium, potassium, and phosphorus are common losses in persons with alcoholics. Fi-

nally, renal conservation is compromised by increased urinary lactate excretion. Acute, but not chronic, alcohol ingestion directly increases urinary magnesium losses. Diabetics, especially those in poor metabolic control, tend to have a lower serum magnesium concentration. Both glycosuria and excretion of ketoacids enhance renal magnesium losses. Although uncommon, hypomagnesemia resulting from an acute intracellular shift may be seen after refeeding in the alcoholic or after insulin treatment of the diabetic with ketoacidosis.

PATHOGENESIS

The clinical syndromes seen with magnesium depletion must be differentiated with respect to the pool of magnesium most affected by the loss. For instance, a simple dietary deficiency of magnesium leads quickly to hypomagnesemia and, eventually, to reduced bone content of the cation, but uncommonly to muscle magnesium depletion. Conversely, diseases that lead to cellular wasting of protein, potassium, and phosphorus produce a decreased muscle magnesium content, but the patient may not exhibit hypomagnesemia.

CLINICAL FEATURES

The clinical effects of hypomagnesemia are strongly influenced by the frequent association with hypocalcemia or hypokalemia. Many of the signs and symptoms of hypomagnesemia are thought to be related to those associated electrolyte disturbances. Severe hypomagnesemia itself results in hypocalcemia due to an inhibition of both parathyroid hormone release and its calcemic action at the level of bone. It is postulated that the reduced activity of cellular Na^+,K^+-ATPase induced by hypomagnesemia may lead to cellular potassium loss and an associated increase in urine potassium excretion.

Neuromuscular abnormalities are often associated with hypomagnesemia—most commonly, a positive Trousseau's or Chvostek's sign, muscle fasciculations, tremor, muscle spasticity, or tetany. Vertigo, athetoid and choreiform movements, nystagmus, anxiety, delirium, and seizures have also been described. Anorexia, nausea, and apathy are common before the appearance of the peripheral neuromuscular manifestations of hypomagnesemia.

Cardiovascular effects, which include a prolonged QT interval, may predispose to ventricular dysrhythmias. Significant controversy surrounds the association of hypomagnesemia with diuretic therapy. Hypokalemia and the associated hypomagnesemia may enhance the morbidity and mortality of cardiac ischemia or acute myocardial infarction through a dysrhythmogenic effect. An increase in arteriolar tone described in hypomagnesemia may be one basis for essential hypertension.

HYPERMAGNESEMIA

With normal renal function, magnesium excretion can rise by more than fivefold to accommodate increased magnesium intake without changes in its serum concentration. In chronic renal insufficiency, reduced tubular absorption of magnesium maintains normomagnesemia until magnesium delivery becomes limited by the GFR (less than 15 mL per minute). Most cases of hypermagnesemia are seen in the setting of acute or chronic renal insufficiency with severe reductions in GFR. However, hypermagnesemia may occur without severe renal insufficiency in association with bowel disease, especially in elderly patients.

Clinically significant hypermagnesemia in these patients usually occurs as a consequence of ingestion of magnesium-containing antacids (which contain 7 to 14 mEq Mg^{2+} per 5 mL) or magnesium-based cathartics. Bone, but not cellular, magnesium is usually increased in chronic renal insufficiency. Acute hypermagnesemia may follow parenteral magnesium sulfate administration in obstetrics or after excess ingestion of magnesium sulfate (Epsom salt).

Clinical effects of hypermagnesemia are unusual until the serum magnesium exceeds 4 mEq per L. Pharmacologic doses of magnesium have a curare-like effect, increasing the stimulus threshold in nerve fibers and blocking synaptic transmission. Thus, hypermagnesemia may cause initial weakness that can progress to complete paralysis. Earlier, less specific findings include nausea, vomiting, cutaneous flushing, and diminished or absent deep tendon reflexes. Progressive elevations in the serum magnesium level may lead to respiratory muscle paralysis, requiring intubation. Intracardiac conduction abnormalities and hypotension may supervene. At a serum magnesium level above 8 to 10 mEq per L, flaccid quadriplegia, difficulties in talking or swallowing, and respiratory paralysis, coupled with hypotension and dysrhythmias, are imminent hazards. The ECG findings include increased atrioventricular and intraventricular conduction times, evidenced by lengthened PR and QRS intervals.

■ APPROACHES TO DIAGNOSIS AND MANAGEMENT

HYPOMAGNESEMIA

The severity of hypomagnesemia and the presence of referable symptoms determine the clinical strategy. The degree of magnesium depletion may not be wholly revealed in the serum magnesium concentration, but there is little indication for determining the tissue (bone or muscle) magnesium content. The excretion of less than 1 to 2 mEq of magnesium in a 24-hour urine collection usually indicates a state of deficiency. In less clear cases, as with alcoholics, the renal retention of more than 40 mEq of magnesium during replacement over a 4- to 5-day period indicates a preexisting deficiency. A parenteral magnesium tolerance test has been proposed as the most sensitive method to diagnose magnesium deficiency, which is indicated by increased magnesium retention after an intravenous magnesium load. Measurement of fractional magnesium excretion (FEMg) may also be useful. An FEMg greater than 4% suggests inappropriate urinary magnesium loss.

Generally, oral magnesium administration is safer and, thus, may be preferable in asymptomatic patients. Gastrointestinal absorption of an oral magnesium dose may be erratic, however, and magnesium salts are cathartic. For these reasons, particularly with significant hypomagnesemia, intravenous or intramuscular magnesium administration might be required. In persons with normal renal function, excess magnesium is promptly excreted into the urine. In the face of renal insufficiency, however, great care must be taken and a lower dose of magnesium used. Patients with advanced renal failure should receive magnesium infusions for urgent indications only. Monitoring of deep tendon reflexes (lost at a serum magnesium level greater than 5 mEq per L), the PR interval (prolonged at a serum magnesium level greater than 6 to 7 mEq per L), and blood pressure is critical to prevent serious complications. Simultaneous administration of potassium, phosphorus, and calcium may be needed to accompany magnesium repletion in recovery from diabetic ketoacidosis, in alcoholism, and during parenteral alimentation.

Figure 148.2 outlines an approach to magnesium repletion based on the mechanism of depletion and the magnitude of the existing or expected deficiency. Patients with chronic malabsorption and those on parenteral alimentation should be given magnesium prophylactically to avoid hypomagnesemia and hypocalcemia. In the early hospital stay for both diabetic ketoacidosis and alcoholism, daily requirements of magnesium may reach 30 to 50 mEq, with ongoing urinary losses with organic acids.

Magnesium supplementation may be warranted for patients receiving chronic diuretic therapy, particularly for patients given digitalis preparations. The goal is to prevent or reduce the incidence of significant ventricular dysrhythmias due to hypomagnesemia and hypokalemia. Such patients may be refractory to potassium repletion in the face of significant magnesium depletion. Oral magnesium plus potassium supplementation may suffice,

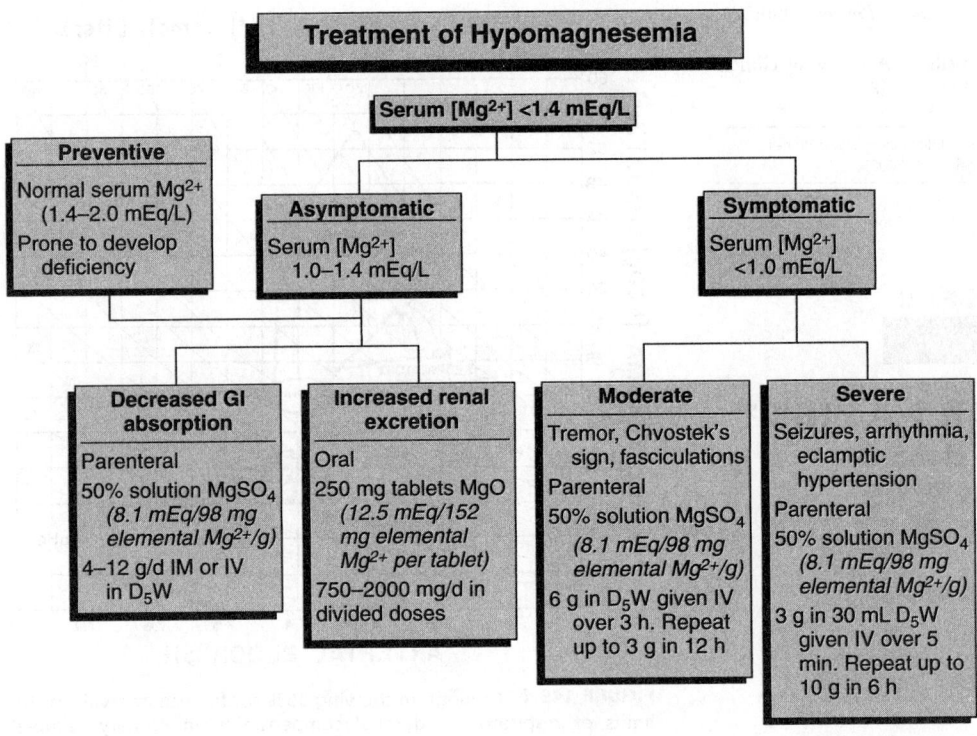

FIGURE 148.2. Treatment of hypomagnesemia.
EVIDENCE LEVEL: C. Expert Opinion.

but coadministration of potassium-sparing diuretics such as spironolactone or amiloride, which reduce urinary magnesium losses, is equally useful.

In asymptomatic mild hypomagnesemia (1.1 to 1.4 mEq per L), consumption of a normal diet containing adequate magnesium is often sufficient. This can be supplemented by oral magnesium, most effectively given as magnesium oxide, 250 to 500 mg, 3 or 4 times daily. Patients with more severe hypomagnesemia, particularly if symptomatic, should receive 3 g $MgSO_4·7H_2O$ in 5% dextrose in water given as an intravenous push over 5 minutes. This can be repeated up to a total dose of 10 g in 6 hours, but should be done with close ECG and blood pressure monitoring. In less severe situations, 6 g can be given over 3 hours, followed by another 6 g every 12 hours for 3 to 5 days until the magnesium deficiency is corrected. In general, dosages below 100 mEq per day are tolerated safely in the presence of normal renal function; rarely are more excessive dosages required.

HYPERMAGNESEMIA

Hypermagnesemia requires immediate assessment of neuromuscular and cardiac function, including bedside evaluation of motor and deep tendon reflex functions and performance of an ECG. Because cardiac arrest correlates poorly with blood levels, any serum magnesium level above 6 mEq per L should receive urgent attention.

Cessation of inadvertent magnesium administration is often sufficient in mild (less than 4 mEq per L) and asymptomatic hypermagnesemia. In patients with adequate renal function, the use of intravenous furosemide plus parenteral 0.45% saline replacement of urinary losses can augment magnesium excretion.

In the presence of life-threatening signs, usually at serum levels above 7 to 10 mEq per L, the acute administration of as little as 5 to 10 mEq of calcium can rapidly reverse a potentially lethal depression in respiration or cardiac dysrhythmias. A mild elevation of serum calcium after calcium administration might also enhance urinary magnesium excretion. In the presence of significant renal failure, dialysis using a magnesium-free dialysate is indicated. Hemodialysis is more efficient and is preferred in life-threatening conditions. If respiration is depressed, artificial ventilation may be necessary while the patient is undergoing dialysis for removal of magnesium.

BIBLIOGRAPHY

Al-Ghamdi SMG, Cameron EC, Sutton RAL. Magnesium deficiency: pathophysiologic and clinical overview. *Am J Kidney Dis* 1994;24: 737–752.

Colussi G, Rombola G, DeFerrari ME, et al. Correction of hypokalemia with antialdosterone therapy in Gitelman's syndrome. *Am J Nephrol* 1994;14:127–135.

de Rouffignac C, Quamme G. Renal magnesium handling and its hormonal control. *Physiol Rev* 1994;74:305–322.

Elisaf M, Panteli K, Theodorou J, et al. Fractional excretion of magnesium in normal subjects and in patients with hypomagnesemia. *Magnes Res* 1997;10:315–320.

Quamme GA. Renal magnesium handling: new insights in understanding old problems. *Kidney Int* 1997;52:1180–1195.

Rubeiz GJ, Thill-Baharozian M, Hardie D, et al. Association of hypomagnesemia and mortality in acutely ill medical patients. *Crit Care Med* 1993; 21:203–209.

Simon DB, Lifton RP. The molecular basis of inherited hypokalemic alkalo-

sis: Bartter's and Gitelman's syndromes. *Am J Physiol* 1996;271: F961–F966.
Tosiello L. Hypomagnesemia and diabetes mellitus. A review of clinical implications. *Arch Intern Med* 1996;156:1143–1148.

Kelley's Textbook of Internal Medicine, fourth edition. Edited by H. David Humes. Lippincott Williams & Wilkins, Philadelphia © 2000.

C H A P T E R
149

APPROACH TO THE PATIENT WITH ACID–BASE ABNORMALITIES

THOMAS D. DUBOSE, JR.

DIAGNOSIS OF ACID–BASE DISORDERS

Acid–base homeostasis is exemplified by the maintainence of systemic arterial pH between 7.35 and 7.45 pH units. This feat is accomplished by extracellular and intracellular chemical buffering in conjunction with regulatory responses by the respiratory and renal systems in concert. The initial defense of systemic pH is achieved by both extracellular and tissue buffers that serve to blunt changes in pH that would occur as a result of retention of acids or bases. Chemical buffers, in combination with respiration, and renal processes dispose of the physiologic daily load of carbonic acid (as volatile CO_2) and nonvolatile acids. The control of partial arterial CO_2 pressure ($PaCO_2$) by the central nervous and respiratory systems, as well as control of the plasma bicarbonate by the kidneys, constitutes the regulatory processes that act to stabilize the arterial pH by excretion or retention of acid or alkali.

Metabolic acidosis and alkalosis are disorders characterized by primary disturbances in the concentration of bicarbonate in plasma, whereas respiratory disorders primarily alter $PaCO_2$. Suspicion that an acid–base disorder exists is usually based on the finding of an abnormal blood pH, $PaCO_2$, or bicarbonate concentration. Arterial blood gases should be determined simultaneously with plasma electrolytes in all patients with acid–base disturbances. This is necessary since changes in plasma bicarbonate, potassium, and chloride do not allow precise diagnosis of specific acid–base disturbances. Care should be taken when measuring blood gases to obtain the arterial blood sample without using excessive heparin. A careful analysis of the blood gas indexes (pH, $PaCO_2$) should begin with a check to determine if the concomitantly measured plasma bicarbonates are all consistent. In the determination of arterial blood gases by the clinical laboratory, both pH and $PaCO_2$ are measured, whereas the reported bicarbonate concentration is calculated from the Henderson–Hasselbach equation:

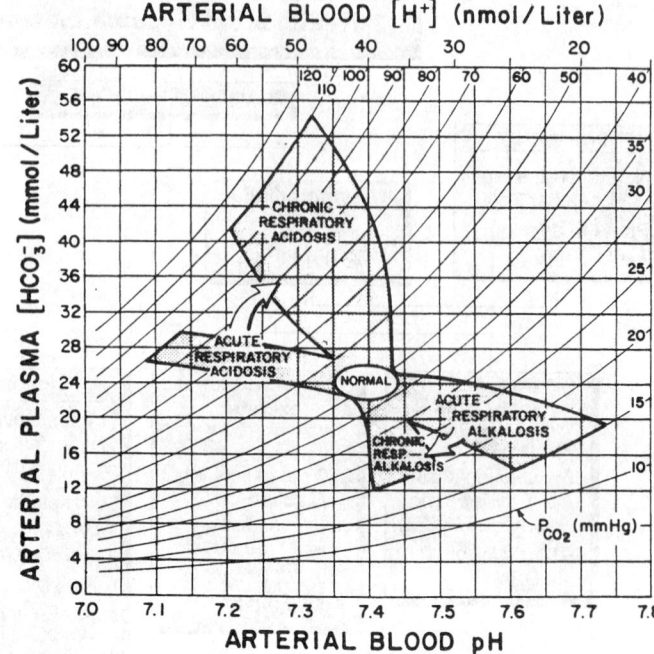

FIGURE 149.1. Nomogram showing 95% confidence intervals for the limits of respiratory and renal compensation in primary "simple" acid–base disturbances. Any two of three values for the pH, PCO_2, or $HCO_3{}^-$ should predict the third value. Failure of all three values to intersect means that either the patient's buffer systems are not at equilibrium or there is a laboratory error. If a given set of laboratory values falls within a stippled area, it is likely that the type of simple acid–base disturbance as designated in the figure exists. However, mixed acid–base disorders can also fall into these stippled areas, and care must be taken to distinguish a mixed from a simple acid–base disorder as discussed in the text. (From DuBose TD Jr. In: Brenner BM, Rector FC Jr, eds. *The kidney,* Vol. 1, 6th ed. Philadelphia: WB Saunders, 1999.)

$$pH = 6.1 + \log HCO_3{}^- / PaCO_2 \times 0.03$$

This calculated value reported with the blood gases with measured bicarbonate concentration within ±2 mEq per L should agree. After verifying the accuracy of the acid–base values in this manner, one can begin to define the precise acid–base disorder. Diagnosis may be aided by referral to an acid–base map or nomogram (Fig. 149.1); however, mixed disturbances, which are more common in critically ill patients, may not be diagnosed accurately using this nomogram. Therefore, additional steps to diagnose the acid–base disorder are necessary.

SIMPLE VERSUS MIXED ACID–BASE DISORDERS

The most commonly encountered clinical disturbances are *simple* acid–base disorders, that is, one of the four cardinal acid–base disturbances in a pure or simple form: *metabolic acidosis, metabolic alkalosis, respiratory acidosis,* and *respiratory alkalosis.* More complicated clinical situations, especially in severely ill patients, may give rise to *mixed* acid–base disturbances. The possible combinations of mixed acid–base disturbances are outlined in Table 149.1. In order to appreciate and recognize a mixed acid–base disturbance, it is important to understand the

TABLE 149.1.	CATEGORIES OF CLINICAL ACID–BASE DISTURBANCES

Simple Acid–Base Disorders
  Respiratory
    Acidosis (acute or chronic)
    Alkalosis (acute or chronic)
  Metabolic
    Acidosis
    Alkalosis
Mixed Acid–Base Disorders
  Mixed respiratory-metabolic disorders
    Respiratory acidosis + metabolic acidosis
    Respiratory acidosis + metabolic alkalosis
    Respiratory alkalosis + metabolic acidosis
    Respiratory alkalosis + metabolic alkalosis
  Mixed metabolic disorders
    Metabolic acidosis + metabolic alkalosis
    Anion gap acidosis + hyperchloremic acidosis
    Mixed anion gap acidosis
    Mixed hyperchloremic acidosis
  "Triple" disorders
    Metabolic acidosis + metabolic alkalosis + respiratory acidosis
    Metabolic acidosis + metabolic alkalosis + respiratory alkalosis

TABLE 149.2.	PREDICTION OF COMPENSATORY RESPONSES IN SIMPLE ACID–BASE DISTURBANCES

Disorder	Prediction of Compensation
Metabolic acidosis	$P_aCO_2 = (1.5 \times [HCO_3^-]) + 8$
	or
	P_aCO_2 will $\downarrow$ 1.25 mm Hg per mmol/L $\downarrow$ in $[HCO_3^-]$
	or
	$P_aCO_2 = [HCO_3^-] + 15$
Metabolic alkalosis	P_aCO_2 will $\uparrow$ 0.75 mm Hg per mmol/L $\uparrow$ in $[HCO_3^-]$
	or
	$P_aCO_2 [HCO_3^-] + 15$
Respiratory alkalosis	
Acute	$[HCO_3^-]$ will $\downarrow$ 2 mmol/L per 10 mm Hg $\downarrow$ in P_aCO_2
Chronic	$[HCO_3^-]$ will $\downarrow$ 4 mmol/L per 10 mm Hg $\downarrow$ in P_aCO_2
Respiratory acidosis	
Acute	$[HCO_3^-]$ will $\uparrow$ 1 mmol/L per 10 mm Hg $\uparrow$ in P_aCO_2
Chronic	$[HCO_3^-]$ will $\uparrow$ 4 mmol/L per 10 mm Hg $\uparrow$ in P_aCO_2

physiologic compensatory responses that occur in the simple acid–base disorders. The limits of the compensatory response to simple acid–base disorders are outlined in Table 149.2. To illustrate, metabolic acidosis, such as may occur from a gain of endogenous acids, will lower the concentration of bicarbonate in extracellular fluid and thus extracellular pH. As a result of the acidemia, medullary chemoreceptors will be stimulated and will invoke an increase in ventilation. In response to the hypocapnic response, the ratio of HCO_3^- to $PaCO_2$ and the subsequent pH will be returned toward, but not completely to, normal. The degree of compensation expected in simple metabolic acidosis can be predicted from the following relationship: $PaCO_2 = 1.5 \times HCO_3^- + 8 \pm 2$ mm Hg (Table 149.2). Alternately, in the range of pH from 7.2 to 7.55, the $PaCO_2$ can be predicted by adding 15 to the patient's bicarbonate (Table 149.2). Thus, a patient with metabolic acidosis and a plasma bicarbonate concentration of 12 mEq per L would be *expected* to have a $PaCO_2$ between 24 and 28 mm Hg. Values of $PaCO_2$ below 24 or greater than 28 mm Hg define a mixed disturbance (metabolic acidosis and respiratory alkalosis, or metabolic acidosis and respiratory acidosis, respectively). Therefore, by definition, mixed acid–base disturbances exceed the physiologic limits of compensation as predicted by the equations displayed in Table 149.2.

THE ANION GAP

All evaluations of acid–base disorders should include a simple calculation of the anion gap. The anion gap is defined as $Na^+ - (Cl^- + HCO_3^-)$. The anion gap represents those unmeasured anions normally present in plasma and is equal to 10 to 12 mEq per L. The anions normally present include anionic proteins (principally albumin), phosphate, sulfate, and organic anions. When acid anions, such as acetoacetate or lactate, are produced in excess endogenously, the anion gap increases above the normal value. Assuming that the serum albumin is within the normal range, for each milliequivalent per liter increase in the anion gap there should be an equal decrease in the plasma bicarbonate concentration. An *increase* in the anion gap may occur by a decrease in unmeasured cations or an increase in unmeasured anions. In addition, the anion gap may increase secondary to an increase in anionic albumin as a consequence of either an increased albumin concentration or alkalemia. The increased anion gap in alkalosis can be partially explained by the effect on albumin charge. A *decrease* in the anion gap can be generated by an increase in unmeasured cations or a decrease in the unmeasured anions (Table 149.3). A decrease in the anion gap can result from an increase in unmeasured cations (calcium, magnesium, potassium) or the addition to the blood of abnormal cations, such as lithium (lithium intoxication) or cationic immunoglobulins (IgG) as in plasma cell dyscrasias. The anion gap will also decrease if the quantity of the major plasma anionic substituent, albumin, is low, as in nephrotic syndrome, or if the effective anionic charge on the albumin is decreased by acidosis. Finally, laboratory errors can create a falsely low anion gap. Hyperviscosity and hyperlipidemia lead to an underestimation of the true sodium concentration, and bromide intoxication causes an overestimation of the true chloride concentration.

In the face of a normal serum albumin, elevation of the anion gap is usually due to addition to the blood of non-chloride-

TABLE 149.3. CLINICAL APPLICATIONS OF THE ANION GAP

$$\text{Anion gap} = Na^+ - (Cl^- + HCO_3^-) = 10 \text{ mEq/L}$$

Decreased Anion Gap
  Increased cations (not Na^+)
    ↑ Ca^{2+}, Mg^{2+}
    ↑ Li^+
    ↑ IgG
  Decreased anions (not Cl^- or HCO_3^-)
    ↓ Albumin concentration
    Acidosis
  Laboratory error
    Hyperviscosity
    Bromism

Increased Anion Gap
  Increased anions (not Cl^- or HCO_3^-)
    ↑ Albumin concentration
    Alkalosis
    ↑ Inorganic anions
    Phosphate
    Sulfate
    ↑ Organic anions
    Lactate
    Ketones
    Uremic
    ↑ Exogenously supplied anions
    Toxins: Salicylate
            Paraldehyde
            Ethylene glycol
            Methanol
    ↑ Unidentified anions
    Toxins
    Uremic
    Hyperosmolar, nonketotic states
    Myoglobinuric acute renal failure
  Decreased cations (not Na^+)
    ↓ Ca^{2+}, Mg^{2+}

Adapted from Emmett M, Narins RG. Clinical use of the anion gap. *Medicine* 1977;56(1):38–54, and from information appearing in Oh MS, Carroll HI. The anion gap. *N Engl J Med* 1977;297:814–817, with permission.

containing acids. The anions accompanying such acids include inorganic (phosphate, sulfate), organic (ketoacids, lactate, uremic organic anions), exogenous (salicylate or ingested toxins with organic acid production), or unidentified anions. The chloride concentration is not altered when the new acid anion is added to the blood; thus the "gap" increases. If the anion is not excreted by the kidney, the magnitude of the decrement in bicarbonate concentration will equal the increase in the unmeasured anion concentration and the anion gap. If the retained anion can be metabolized back to bicarbonate (e.g., ketones or lactate, after successful treatment), normal acid–base balance will be restored as the anion gap returns toward the normal value of 12 mEq per L.

METABOLIC ACIDOSIS

Metabolic acidosis occurs as a result of a marked increase in endogenous production of acid (such as lactic and ketoacids), loss of bicarbonate stores (diarrhea or renal tubular acidosis), or progressive accumulation of endogenous acids, the excretion of which is impaired because of renal insufficiency. The anion gap serves a useful role in the initial differentiation of metabolic acidoses. A metabolic acidosis with a *normal anion gap* (hyperchloremic) suggests that bicarbonate has been effectively replaced by chloride. This occurs when bicarbonate is lost from body fluids through gastrointestinal or renal mechanisms, or when

defective renal acidification results or renal failure impairs the excretion of metabolically produced acid. In contrast, metabolic acidosis with a *high anion gap* indicates addition of an acid other than hydrochloric acid or its equivalent to the extracellular fluid. If the attendant nonchloride acid anion cannot be excreted in relation to the rate of production, and is retained following bicarbonate titration, the anion replaces titrated bicarbonate without disturbing the chloride concentration. Hence, the acidosis is normochloremic and the anion gap increases.

HYPERCHLOREMIC METABOLIC ACIDOSIS

The diverse clinical disorders which may result in a hyperchloremic metabolic acidosis are outlined in Table 149.4. Hyperchloremic metabolic acidosis occurs most often as a result of loss of HCO_3^- from the gastrointestinal tract or as a result of a renal acidification defect. *Diarrhea* causes a loss of large quantities of HCO_3^- and HCO_3^- decomposed by reaction with organic acids. Since diarrheal stools contain a higher concentration of HCO_3^- and decomposed HCO_3^- than plasma, volume depletion and metabolic acidosis will develop. Hypokalemia exists because large quantities of K^+ are lost from stool and because volume depletion causes elaboration of renin and aldosterone, enhancing renal potassium excretion. Instead of an acid urine pH as anticipated with diarrhea, a pH of 6.0 or more may be found. This occurs because metabolic acidosis and hypokalemia increase renal ammonium synthesis and excretion, thus pro-

TABLE 149.4.	CAUSES OF HYPERCHLOREMIC METABOLIC ACIDOSIS

Gastrointestinal bicarbonate loss
  Diarrhea
  External pancreatic or small bowel drainage
  Uterosigmoidostomy, jejunal loop
  Drugs
    Calcium chloride (acidifying agent)
    Magnesium sulfate (diarrhea)
    Cholestyramine (bile acid diarrhea)
Renal acidosis
  Hypokalemia
    Proximal RTA (type II)
    Distal (classical) RTA (type I)
  Hyperkalemia
    Generalized distal nephron dysfunction (type IV)
      Mineralocorticoid deficiency
      Mineralocorticoid resistance
      ↓ Na^+ delivery to distal nephron
      Tubulointerstitial disease
      Ammonium excretion defect
    Drug-induced hyperkalemia
      Potassium-sparing diuretics (amiloride, triamterene, spironolactone)
      Trimethoprim
      Pentamidine
      ACE inhibitors and angiotensin II receptor blockers
      NSAIDs
      Cyclosporin A
  Normokalemia
    Early renal insufficiency
Other
  Acid loads (ammonium chloride, hyperalimentation)
  Loss of potential bicarbonate: ketosis with ketone excretion
  Expansion acidosis (rapid saline administration)
  Hippurate
  Cation exchange resins

RTA, renal tubular acidosis; ACE, angiotensin-converting enzyme; NSAIDs, nonsteroidal anti-inflammatory drugs.

viding more urinary buffer, which allows urine pH to increase above 6.0.

Thus, metabolic acidosis due to gastrointestinal losses with a high urine pH must be differentiated from *renal tubular acidosis (RTA)*. Urinary NH_4^+ excretion is typically low in RTA, whereas NH_4^+ excretion is high in patients with diarrhea. The adequacy of urinary ammonium excretion in metabolic acidosis can be assessed by calculating the urine anion gap (UAG): UAG $= (Na^+ + K^+)_u - Cl_u^-$. Since NH_4^+ can be assumed to be present if the sum of the major cations ($Na^+ + K^+$) is less than the sum of major anions in urine, a negative urine net charge is taken as evidence for ammonium in the urine. Urine containing little or no NH_4^+ will have more $Na^+ + K^+$ than Cl^- (urine net charge will be positive). This finding suggests a renal mechanism for the hyperchloremic acidosis, such as RTA. Conversely, if the urine $[Cl^-]$ exceeds the sum of $[Na^+ + K^+]$ in the urine, an extrarenal cause of the hyperchloremic acidosis should be considered. This test is only useful in the differential diagnosis of a hyperchloremic metabolic acidosis. If the patient

has ketonuria, or drug excreted as anions in large quantity (penicillins or aspirin), the test will not be reliable. Thus, the UAG or net charge allows the estimation of urine $[NH_4]$ on a spot urine and aids in distinguishing extrarenal from renal causes of hyperchloremic acidoses.

Dilutional acidosis (acidosis due to exogenous acid loads and the posthypocapnic state) can usually be excluded by history. When isotonic saline is infused rapidly, particularly in patients with temporary or permanent renal functional impairment, the plasma bicarbonate will decline reciprocally in relation to chloride. Addition of acid or acid equivalents to blood results in metabolic acidosis. Examples include infusion of arginine or lysine HCl during *parenteral hyperalimentation* or ingestion of NH_4Cl.

Loss of functioning renal parenchyma by *progressive renal disease* is known to be associated with metabolic acidosis. Typically, the acidosis is hyperchloremic when the glomerular filtration rate (GFR) is between 20 to 50 mL per minute but may convert to the typical high anion gap acidosis of uremia with more advanced renal failure (i.e., when the GFR is less than 20 to 50 mL per minute.

The majority of cases of *proximal RTA* occur in association with generalized proximal tubular dysfunction manifested by glycosuria, generalized aminoaciduria, hypercitraturia, and phosphaturia and referred to collectively as the Fanconi syndrome. The clinical disorders associated with proximal RTA are outlined in Table 149.5. Patients with proximal RTA generally present in the steady state with a chronic hyperchloremic metabolic acidosis, an acid urine pH, and a small amount of bicarbonate excretion. Upon infusion of $NaHCO_3$, and when the plasma HCO_3^- rises above the threshold, bicarbonaturia ensues and the urine becomes alkaline in patients with proximal RTA. The magnitude of the bicarbonaturia (more than 10% of the filtered load) requires that large amounts of bicarbonate be administered to correct the bicarbonate concentration. For example, 10 to 30 mEq per kg per day of bicarbonate or its metabolic equivalent (citrate) may be required to maintain the plasma bicarbonate concentration at normal levels. Supplementation with potassium is also often necessary because of the kaliuresis induced by high distal bicarbonate delivery when the plasma bicarbonate concentration is normalized. Thiazides may be useful in diminishing therapeutic requirements for bicarbonate supplementation by causing extracellular volume (ECV) contraction. Vitamin D and phosphate may be supplemented, and in some patients this might even improve the acidification defect. Fructose should be restricted in patients with fructose intolerance.

In contrast to proximal RTA, the hallmark finding in *classical hypokalemic distal RTA* is an inability to acidify the urine appropriately during spontaneous or chemically induced metabolic acidosis. The defect in acidification by the collecting duct impairs ammonium and titratable acid excretion, and can be detected easily since the UAG is usually positive (see above). The defect results in positive acid balance, hyperchloremic metabolic acidosis, and volume depletion. Moreover, medullary interstitial disease, which commonly occurs in conjunction with distal RTA, may impair ammonium excretion by interrupting the medullary countercurrent system for ammonium. Hypokalemia and hypercalciuria often accompany this disorder, but proximal

TABLE 149.5.	DISORDERS ASSOCIATED WITH PROXIMAL RTA

Selective (unassociated with Fanconi's syndrome)
  Primary
  Carbonic anhydrase deficiency, inhibition, or alteration
    Drugs
      Acetazolamide
      Sulfanilamide
      Mafenide acetate
  Carbonic anhydrase II deficiency with osteopetrosis (Sly's syndrome)
Generalized (associated with Fanconi's syndrome)
  Primary (without associated systemic disease)
    Genetic or sporadic
  Genetically transmitted systemic diseases
    Cystinosis
    Lowe's syndrome
    Wilson's syndrome
    Tyrosinemia
    Galactosemia
    Hereditary fructose intolerance (during fructose ingestion)
    Metachromatic leukodystrophy
    Pyruvate carboxylase deficiency
    Methylmalonic acidemia
  Dysproteinemic states
    Multiple myeloma
    Monoclonal gammopathy
Vitamin D deficiency or resistance
Drugs or toxins
  Ifosfamide
  Outdated tetracycline
  Streptozotocin
  Lead
  Mercury
Tubulointerstitial diseases
  Sjögren's syndrome
  Medullary cystic disease
  Renal transplantation
Other renal and miscellaneous diseases
  Nephrotic syndrome
  Amyloidosis
  Paroxysmal nocturnal hemoglobinuria

tubule reabsorptive function is preserved. The dissolution of bone is the result of chronic positive acid balance, which causes calcium, magnesium, and phosphate wasting. Since chronic metabolic acidosis also decreases renal production of citrate, the resulting hypocitraturia in combination with hypercalciuria creates an environment that is favorable for urinary stone formation and nephrocalcinosis. Nephrocalcinosis is a reliable marker of classical distal RTA since this disorder does not occur in proximal RTA or the generalized dysfunction of the nephron associated with hyperkalemia.

The disorders associated with classical distal RTA are displayed in Table 149.6. The vast majority of patients with distal RTA have distal RTA in association with a systemic illness. Conversely, distal RTA may occur as a part of an inherited defect in which there is no association with systemic disease. This autosomal dominant disorder has been demonstrated recently to be associated with a missense mutation of the *AE-1* gene, which encodes an abnormal HCO_3^-/Cl^- exchanger in the collecting duct.

In either inherited or acquired forms of distal RTA, the correction of chronic metabolic acidosis can usually be achieved in patients with classical distal RTA by administration of alkali in an amount sufficient to neutralize the production of metabolic acids derived from the diet. In adult patients with distal RTA, this is usually equal to no more than 13 mEq per kg per day.

TABLE 149.6.	DISORDERS ASSOCIATED WITH CLASSICAL HYPOKALEMIC DISTAL RTA

Primary (without associated systemic disease)
  Genetic
  Idiopathic
  Endemic (northeastern Thailand)
Secondary (with associated systemic disease)
  Genetically transmitted disease
    Ehlers–Danlos syndrome
    Hematologic disorders
      Hereditary elliptocytosis
      Sickle cell anemia
      Carbonic anhydrase I deficiency or alteration
    Medullary cystic disease
    Congenital nerve deafness
    Glycogenosis type III
  Autoimmune diseases
    Hypergammaglobulinemia
      Hyperglobulinemic purpura
      Cryoglobulinemia
    Sjögren's syndrome
    Thyroiditis
    Pulmonary fibrosis
    Chronic active hepatitis
    Primary biliary cirrhosis
    Systemic lupus erythematosus
    Vasculitis
  Diseases associated with nephrocalcinosis
    Primary hyperparathyroidism
    Vitamin D intoxication
    Hyperthyroidism
    Idiopathic hypercalciuria
      Hereditary
      Idiopathic
    Hyperoxaluria
    Hereditary fructose intolerance (after chronic fructose ingestion)
    Medullary sponge kidney
    Fabry's disease
    Wilson's disease
  Drug or toxic nephropathies
    Amphotericin B
    Toluene
    Glue
    Ifosfamide
    Analgesics
    Cyclamate
    Balkan nephropathy
  Tubulointerstitial diseases
    Chronic pyelonephritis
    Obstructive uropathy
    Renal transplant rejection
    Leprosy
  Miscellaneous
    Hepatic cirrhosis
    Empty sella syndrome

Larger amounts of bicarbonate must be administered to correct the acidosis and maintain normal growth in children. In patients with distal RTA, correction of acidosis with alkali therapy reduces urinary potassium excretion, and hypokalemia and sodium depletion may resolve with sustained correction of metabolic acidosis.

Generalized distal nephron dysfunction (or *type IV RTA*) is manifest as a hyperchloremic, hyperkalemic metabolic acidosis in which urinary ammonium excretion is invariably depressed and renal function is usually compromised. The UAG is always positive (see above). The transtubular potassium gradient $(TTKG) = K^+_u/K^+_p \div U/P_{osm}$, where "u" is the potassium concentration in the urine and "p" in plasma, and "osm" is the osmolality, is usually low in patients with this disorder, indicating that the collecting tubule is not responding appropriately to the prevailing hyperkalemia. Therefore, in such patients, a unique dysfunction of potassium and acid secretion by the collecting tubule coexists. This dysfunction can be attributed in many cases to hypoaldosteronism and in other cases to a decrease in the effectiveness of aldosterone (aldosterone resistance). A classification of the underlying disorders resulting in a generalized distal tubule dysfunction are outlined in Table 149.7. Hyperchloremic metabolic acidosis occurs in approximately 50% of patients with hyporeninemic hypoaldosteronism. This disorder is a common cause of hyperkalemic hyperchloremic metabolic acidosis and is most typically seen in older adults with diabetes mellitus or tubulointerstitial disease and renal insufficiency. Patients will usually have mild to moderate renal insufficiency and acidosis with modest elevation in plasma potassium (5.5 to 6.0 mEq per L), with concurrent hypertension and congestive heart failure. Drugs are important and common causes of hyperkalemia (Table 149.8). Although these agents do not cause hyperchloremic metabolic acidosis directly, they are frequently associated with this acid–base disorder in patients with moderate to severe renal insufficiency. The metabolic acidosis is the result of the suppression by hyperkalemia of renal ammonium production and thus a decrease in net acid excretion. The autosomal recessive form of pseudohypoaldosteronism type I (PHAI) occurs because of an inherited loss of function mutation in the gene that encodes the epithelial sodium channel protein (ENaC) of the cortical collecting duct principal cell. This defect impairs sodium absorption and potassium secretion; it also causes salt wasting, hyperkalemia, and acidosis, which are resistant to correction by aldosterone. Rather, these children respond to generous administration of NaCl supplements. This defect is more severe and persists throughout life, whereas, in contrast, the autosomal dominant form of PHAI is less severe and often resolves by puberty. Recent studies have revealed that autosomal dominant PHAI is due to a mutation of mineralocorticoid receptor gene (MLR) (Table 149.7).

Non-PHAI forms of type IV RTA are much more common. These patients respond to a cation exchange resin (sodium polystyrene sulfonate) and alkali therapy. Treatment with a loop diuretic (to induce renal potassium and salt excretion) and dietary potassium restriction are also helpful. The correction of the hyperkalemia is often associated with restoration of renal ammonium excretion and, thus, correction of the acidosis. Volume depletion should be avoided unless the patient is volume-

TABLE 149.7.	**DISORDERS ASSOCIATED WITH GENERALIZED ABNORMALITY OF DISTAL NEPHRON WITH HYPERKALEMIA**

Mineralocorticoid deficiency
Primary mineralocorticoid deficiency
  Combined deficiency of mineralocorticoids and glucocorticoids
    Addison's disease
    Bilateral adrenalectomy
    Bilateral adrenal destruction
      Hemorrhage or carcinoma
  Congenital enzymatic defects
    21-Hydroxylase deficiency
    3β-Hydroxydehydrogenase deficiency
    Desmolase deficiency
  Isolated (selective) aldosterone deficiency
    Chronic idiopathic hypoaldosteronism
    Heparin and/or hypoxemia in critically ill patient
    Familial hypoaldosteronism
      Corticosterone methyloxidase deficiency, types 1 and 2
  Angiotensin II–converting enzyme inhibitors and angiotensin II receptor antagonists
Secondary mineralocorticoid deficiency
  Hyporeninemic hypoaldosteronism
    Diabetic nephropathy
      Tubulointerstitial nephropathies
      Nephrosclerosis
      Nonsteroidal anti-inflammatory agents
      Acquired immunodeficiency syndrome
      IgM monoclonal gammopathy
Resistance to mineralocorticoid
  Pseudohypoaldosteronism type I—autosomal dominant form
Renal Tubular Dysfunction
  Loss of function mutation of Na⁺ channel in CCT
    Pseudohypoaldosteronism type I—autosomal recessive form
  Short circuit defects of CCT
    Pseudohypoaldosteronism type II
    Hyperkalemic distal RTA
  Drugs which interfere with Na⁺ channel function in CCT
    Amiloride
    Triamterene
    Trimethoprim
    Pentamidine
  Drugs that interfere with Na⁺, K⁺-ATPase in CCT
    Cyclosporin A
  Drugs that inhibit aldosterone effect on CCT
    Spironolactone
  Disorders associated with tubulointerstitial nephritis and renal insufficiency
    Methicillin nephrotoxicity
    Obstructive nephropathy
    Kidney transplant rejection
    Sickle cell disease
    Lupus nephritis

CCT, cortical collecting tubule.

TABLE 149.8.   CAUSES OF HIGH ANION GAP ACIDOSIS

I. L-Lactic acidosis
   Type A
      Poor tissue perfusion
      Shock
         Cardiogenic
         Hemorrhagic
         Septic
      Acute hypoxemia
      Carbon monoxide poisoning
   Type B
      Various common disorders
         Diabetes mellitus
         Renal failure
         Liver disease
         Infection (including HIV)
         Leukemia
         Anemia, pancreatitis
         Ingestion or administration of drugs or other toxic
         substances:

Metformin	Streptozotocin
Phenformin	Isoniazid
Ethanol	Cyanide
Salicylates	Nitroprusside
Sorbitol	Antiviral drugs (AZT and anlogues)

      Hereditary forms
         Glucose 6-phosphate deficiency (type I glycogenosis)
         Fructose 1,6-diphosphatase deficiency
         Pyruvate carboxylase deficiency
         Pyruvate dehydrogenase deficiency
         Oxidative phosphorylation deficiencies
         Methylmalonic aciduria
II. D-Lactic acidosis
   Short bowel syndrome
   Ischemic bowel
   Small bowel obstruction
III. Ketoacidosis
   Diabetic
   Alcoholic
   Starvation
IV. Intoxication
   Salicylates
   Ethylene glycol
   Methanol
V. Uremia (late renal failure)

HIV, human immunodeficiency virus; AZT, azidothymidine.
Adapted in part from Cohen RD, Woods HF. *Clinical biochemical aspects of lactic acidosis.* Oxford: Blackwell Scientific Publications, 1976; and Relman AS. Lactic acidosis. In: Brenner BM, Stein JH, eds *Contemporary issues in Nephrology. Acid–Base and Potassium Homeostasis,* Vol. 2. New York: Churchill Livingstone, 1978:65, with permission.

overexpanded or hypertensive. Supraphysiologic doses of mineralocorticoids may be necessary but should be administered cautiously, and only in combination with a loop diuretic to avoid volume overexpansion or aggravation of hypertension, and to increase potassium excretion.

HIGH ANION GAP ACIDOSES

Identification of the underlying cause of a high anion gap acidosis is facilitated by consideration of the clinical setting and associ-

ated laboratory values. The four most common categories of disorders that cause a high anion gap acidosis are outlined in Table 149.8 and include lactic acidosis, ketoacidosis, the toxin-induced acidoses, and uremic acidosis. Initial screening to differentiate the high anion gap acidoses should include (1) a history or other evidence for drug and toxin ingestion, (2) historical evidence of diabetes (diabetic ketoacidosis); (3) evidence of alcoholism or increased levels of β-hydroxybutyrate (alcoholic ketoacidosis); (4) observation for clinical signs of uremia and determination of the blood urea nitrogen (BUN) and creatinine (uremic acidosis); (5) inspection of the urine for oxalate crystals (ethylene glycol); and finally, (6) the recognition of the numerous settings in which lactate levels may be increased (hypotension, cardiac failure, leukemia, drugs, and cancer).

LACTIC ACIDOSIS

While lactate metabolism bears a close relationship to that of pyruvate, lactate is a metabolic dead-end pathway with pyruvate as its only outlet. The production of lactic acid can be increased with ischemia, during seizures, exercise, in some leukemic conditions, and in alkalosis. This increase in production occurs principally through enhanced phosphofructokinase activity. Decreased lactate consumption also leads to lactic acidosis. The principal organs for lactate removal are the liver, kidneys, and muscle. Hepatic utilization of lactate can be impeded by several factors: poor blood flow to the liver; defective active transport of lactate into cells; or inadequate metabolic conversion of lactate into pyruvate. Examples of impaired hepatic lactate removal include primary diseases of the liver, enzymatic defects, tissue anoxia or ischemia, severe acidosis, toxic levels of alcohol, fructose, phenformin, or nucleoside analog therapy for human immunodeficiency virus infection. Underutilization of lactate appears to be a more common cause of clinical lactate acidosis than lactate overproduction. *Type A lactic acidosis* is the result of tissue hypoperfusion or acute hypoxia, whereas *type B lactic acidosis* is associated with common diseases, drugs and toxins, and hereditary and miscellaneous disorders (Table 149.8). A lactate concentration of greater than 4 mEq per L (normal 1 mEq per L) is generally accepted as evidence that the metabolic acidosis is ascribable to net lactic acid accumulation.

d-Lactic acidosis has been described in patients with small bowel obstruction or hypomotility associated with overgrowth of abnormal gut flora. Treatment with a low-carbohydrate diet and oral antibiotics is often effective.

The basic principle of therapy for L-lactic acidosis is that the underlying condition initiating the disruption in normal lactate metabolism must first be corrected. Every attempt should be made to restore tissue perfusion when it is inadequate. Vasoconstricting agents are ill advised because they will potentiate the hypoperfused state. Alkali therapy should be provided as either intravenous sodium bicarbonate or Carbicarb (an equimolar solution of sodium bicarbonate and sodium carbonate) for acute, severe acidemia (pH less than 7.1). Use of agents such as tris(hydroxymethyl)-aminomethane (tromethamine; THAM), Tris buffer, or plasma expanders is not recommended. The use of alkali in states of moderate lactic acidemia is controversial, but it is generally agreed that attempts to normalize the pH or bicarbonate concentration by exogenous bicarbonate therapy is deleterious. Fluid overload occurs with bicarbonate therapy because the amount required is often massive when accumulation of lactic acid is relentless, necessitating diuretics, ultrafiltration, or dialysis against a bicarbonate dialysate. Volume administration is poorly tolerated because of central venoconstriction and decreased cardiac output. Carbicarb may offer potential advantages to sodium bicarbonate alone, since the $PaCO_2$ may not increase as much. If the underlying cause of the lactic acidosis can be remedied, blood lactate will be reconverted to bicarbonate. Bicarbonate derived from lactate conversion in addition to any new bicarbonate generated by renal mechanisms during acidosis and from exogenous alkali therapy are additive and might result in an overshoot alkalosis. When large doses of bicarbonate are administered, the goal should be to raise the pH to approximately 7.2 to 7.25, not higher. Recent reports suggest that continuous venovenous hemodialysis offers advantages in some patients although lactate-containing dialysate can increase blood lactate levels and remove bicarbonate.

KETOACIDOSIS

Diabetic Ketoacidosis

The pathophysiology of diabetic ketoacidosis is discussed in detail elsewhere in this text. Most, if not all, patients with diabetic ketoacidosis require correction of the volume depletion that almost invariably accompanies the osmotic diuresis and ketoacidosis. Initiate therapy with isotonic saline at a rate of 1,000 mL IV per hour. When the pulse and blood pressure have stabilized and the corrected serum sodium concentration is in the range of 130 to 135 mEq per L, switch to 0.45% NaCl. Ringer's lactate should be avoided. If the blood sugar declines below 300 mg per dL, 0.45% NaCl with 5% dextrose should be administered. Low-dose IV insulin therapy (0.1 unit per kg per hour) smoothly corrects the biochemical abnormalities and minimizes hypoglycemia and hypokalemia. Although regular insulin may also be administered intramuscularly (0.2 mg per kg initially, then 6 units every hour), it should be noted that IM insulin may not be effective in volume-depleted patients, as is often the case in ketoacidosis.

Total body potassium depletion is usually present, although the potassium level on admission may be elevated or normal. Since the plasma potassium concentration should increase by 0.6 mEq per L for each 0.1-unit decline in arterial blood pH, a normal or reduced $[K^+]$ on admission indicates severe potassium depletion. Administration of fluid, insulin, and alkali might cause the potassium level to decline further. When the urine output has been established, 20 mEq KCl should be administered in each liter of fluid as long as the $[K^+]$ is less than 4.0 mEq per L. Equal caution should be exercised in the presence of hyperkalemia, especially if the patient has renal insufficiency, since the usual therapy will not always correct hyperkalemia.

The routine administration of phosphate (usually as potassium phosphate) is not advised because of the potential for hyperphosphatemia and hypocalcemia. A significant number of patients with diabetic ketoacidosis will have significant hyperphosphatemia before initiation of therapy. However, in the volume-depleted, malnourished patient, a normal or elevated phosphate concentration on admission may be followed by a rapid fall in plasma phosphate levels within 2 to 6 hours of initiation of therapy.

Alcoholic Ketoacidosis

Chronic alcoholics may develop ketoacidosis when alcohol consumption is abruptly curtailed, usually as a result of vomiting, abdominal pain, starvation, and volume depletion. This disorder, which is more common in women who are binge drinkers, is frequently underdiagnosed and should be suspected in alcoholics presenting with an anion gap acidosis. Often the glucose concentration is low or normal, and the acidosis can be severe. The anion gap is expanded because of elevated ketones, which are predominantly β-hydroxybutyrate. The nitroprusside reaction (Acetest) detects acetoacetic acid preferential to β-hydroxybutyrate. Treatment consists of intravenous volume repletion and glucose administration (5% dextrose in 0.9% NaCl, not saline alone). Hypophosphatemia, hypokalemia, and hypomagnesemia often occur. Hypophosphatemia usually emerges 12 to 24 hours after admission, so that the need for therapy can be overlooked, especially if the serum phosphorus concentration on admission is normal.

RENAL FAILURE

Advanced renal failure (GFR below 15 mL per minute) will eventually convert the hyperchloremic acidosis of progressive chronic renal insufficiency to a high anion gap acidosis. The elevated anion gap is the result of retention of acid anions (e.g., phosphates and sulfates). Classical uremic acidosis is characterized by a reduced rate of ammonium production, primarily due to decreased renal mass. The bicarbonate concentration rarely falls below 15 mEq per L, and the anion gap rarely exceeds 20 mEq per L. Uremic acidosis requires oral alkali therapy to maintain the bicarbonate concentration above 20 mEq per L. This can be accomplished with relatively modest amounts of alkali (1.0 to 1.5 mEq per kg per day). Shohl's solution (sodium citrate) or sodium bicarbonate tablets are equally effective, but Shohl's solution may be better tolerated. Shohl's solution should never be administered to patients receiving aluminum-containing antacids because of the risk of aluminum intoxication.

TOXINS

Under most physiologic conditions, sodium, urea, and glucose together generate the osmotic pressure of plasma. Plasma osmolality (milliosmoles per kilogram) is calculated according to the following expression: $P_{osm} = 2Na^+ + Glu/18 + BUN/2.8$. The calculated and determined osmolality should agree within 10 to 15 mOsm per kg. When the measured osmolality exceeds the calculated osmolality by more than 15 to 20 mOsm per kg, one of two circumstances prevails. First, the serum sodium may be spuriously low, as occurs with hyperlipidemia or hyperproteinemia (pseudohyponatremia). Second, osmolytes other than sodium salts, glucose, or urea have accumulated in plasma. Examples include mannitol infusion, radiocontrast media, or the accumulation of other solutes including the alcohols, ethylene glycol, or acetone. In these examples, the difference between the osmolality as calculated above 40, and the measured osmolality is proportional to the concentration of unmeasured solutes. Such differences in these clinical circumstances have been referred to as the *osmolar gap*. With an appropriate clinical history and index of suspicion, the osmolar gap becomes a reasonable and helpful screening tool in poison-associated anion gap acidosis.

Ingestion of *ethylene glycol* leads to a metabolic acidosis in addition to severe central nervous system, cardiopulmonary, and renal damage. The increased anion and osmolar gaps can be attributed to ethylene glycol metabolites, especially oxalic acid, glycolic acid, and other incompletely identified organic acids. Lactic acid production also increases as a consequence of a toxic depression in the reaction rates of the citric acid cycle and altered intracellular redox state. Diagnosis is facilitated by recognizing oxalate crystals in the urine. Treatment includes prompt institution of osmotic diuresis, thiamine and pyridoxine supplements, ethanol administration, and dialysis. Ethanol serves to lessen toxicity because it competes (through alcohol dehydrogenase) with metabolic conversion with ethylene glycol and alters the cellular redox state.

Methanol ingestion causes metabolic acidosis in addition to severe optic nerve and central nervous system manifestations due to its metabolism to formic acid from formaldehyde. Lactic acids and ketoacids, as well as other unidentified organic acids, may contribute to the acidosis. Due to its low molecular weight, an osmolar gap is usually present. Therapy is generally similar to that for ethylene glycol intoxication, including general supportive measures, ethanol administration, and hemodialysis, as indicated.

The initial step in therapy of *salicylate intoxication* should include vigorous gastric lavage or induced vomiting followed by activated charcoal administration. Salicylate intoxication can result in several acid–base abnormalites: respiratory alkalosis, metabolic acidosis, or mixed metabolic acidosis–respiratory alkalosis. To facilitate removal of salicylate, intravenous sodium bicarbonate administration in amounts adequate to alkalinize the urine and to maintain urine output may be required (urine pH greater than 7.5). While this form of therapy is straightforward in acidotic patients, alkalemia from a respiratory alkalosis may make this approach hazardous. Hypokalemia may occur as a result of an alkaline diuresis from sodium bicarbonate or acetazolamide, and should be treated promptly. Glucose-containing fluids should be administered because of the danger of hypoglycemia. If renal failure prevents rapid clearance of salicylate, hemodialysis may be required against a bicarbonate dialysate.

The treatment of metabolic acidosis is summarized in Table 149.9.

METABOLIC ALKALOSIS

Metabolic alkalosis is a common primary acid–base disturbance that is manifest in a pure or "simple" form as alkalemia (elevated arterial pH), and an increase in $PaCO_2$ as a result of compensatory alveolar hypoventilation. It is often, but not always, accompanied by hypochloremia and hypokalemia. The patient with a high bicarbonate concentration and a low chloride concentration has either metabolic alkalosis or chronic respiratory acidosis. The arterial pH will establish the diagnosis, since the pH will be increased in metabolic alkalosis and decreased or normal in respiratory acidosis. Modest increases in the $PaCO_2$ are expected in

TABLE 149.9.	**TREATMENT OF METABOLIC ACIDOSIS**	
	Treatment	
Type of Acidosis	**Specific**	**Ancillary**
Anion gap acidosis		
Diabetic ketoacidosis	Volume replacement, insulin	K^+, $NaHCO_3$
Alcoholic ketoacidosis	Volume replacement, glucose	PO_4^{3-}
Lactic acidosis	Treat underlying disease, $NaHCO_3$	Hemodialysis, CRRT
Methanol	Ethanol, $NaHCO_3$, dialysis	$NaHCO_3$
Ethylene glycol	Ethanol, $NaHCO_3$, dialysis	$NaHCO_3$, thiamine
Salicylate intoxication	Diuresis, $NaHCO_3$, charcoal	Acetazolamide
Chronic renal failure	$NaHCO_3$ or Shohl's solution	Dialysis
Hyperchloremic acidosis		
Hypokalemia		
GI loss of bicarbonate	Volume, $NaHCO_3$, K^+	
Proximal RTA (III)	$NaHCO_3$, volume, K^+	Thiazide diuretic, vitamin D, PO_4
Distal RTA (III)	Shohl's solution or $NaHCO_3$	± K^+
Hyperkalemia		
Type IV RTA	± Fludrocortisone, furosemide	$NaHCO_3$, exchange resins

CRRT, chronic renal replacement therapy; GI, gastrointestinal; RTA, renal tubular acidosis.

metabolic alkalosis, and the expected increase in $PaCO_2$ can be approximated by simply adding 15 to the patient's bicarbonate concentration (Table 149.2). Metabolic alkalosis is also frequently observed, not as a pure or simple acid–base disturbance but in association with other disorders such as respiratory acidosis or alkalosis and even metabolic acidosis.

Under normal circumstances, the kidneys display an impressive capacity to excrete bicarbonate. The development of metabolic alkalosis represents a failure of the kidneys to eliminate bicarbonate in the usual manner. For bicarbonate to be added to the extracellular fluid, bicarbonate must be administered exogenously or gained through endogenously mediated events. The kidneys may be partially or entirely responsible for the generation of new bicarbonate, or the generation may be extrarenal.

The various causes of metabolic alkalosis are listed in Table 149.10. In attempting to establish the cause of metabolic alkalosis, it is necessary to assess the status of the ECV, blood pressure, serum potassium, and renin–aldosterone system. Determination

---

TABLE 149.10. CAUSES OF METABOLIC ALKALOSIS

Exogenous HCO_3^- loads
  Acute alkali administration
  Milk-alkali syndrome
Effective ECV contraction, normal blood pressure, K^+ deficiency, and secondary hyperreninemic hyperaldosteronism
  Gastrointestinal origin
    Vomiting
    Gastric aspiration
    Congenital chloridorrhea
    Villous adenoma
  Renal origin
    Diuretics (especially thiazides and loop diuretics)
    Edematous states
    Posthypercapnic state
    Hypercalcemia-hypoparathyroidism
    Recovery from lactic acidosis or ketoacidosis
    Nonreabsorbable anion
    Mg^{2+} deficiency
    K^+ depletion
    Bartter's syndrome
    Gitelman's syndrome
  Carbohydrate refeeding after starvation
ECV expansion, hypertension, K^+ deficiency, and hypermineralocorticoidism
  Associated with high renin
    Renal artery stenosis
    Accelerated hypertension
    Renin-secreting tumor
    Estrogen therapy
  Associated with low renin
    Primary aldosteronism
    Adrenal enzymatic defects
      11β-Hydroxylase deficiency
      17α-Hydroxylase deficiency
    Cushing's syndrome or disease
  Other
    Licorice
    Carbenoxolone
    Chewer's tobacco
    Lydia Pincham tablets

---

of urine electrolytes (especially the urine Cl^- concentration), and screening of the urine for diuretics might be helpful. If the urine is alkaline, with high values for sodium and potassium concentration but low values for the chloride concentration, the diagnosis is usually either active (continual) vomiting (overt or surreptitious), or alkali ingestion. If the urine is relatively acidic, with low concentrations of sodium, potassium, and chloride, the most likely possibilities are prior (discontinual) vomiting, the posthypercapnic state, or prior diuretic ingestion. If, on the other hand, neither the urine sodium, potassium, nor chloride concentration is depressed, one must consider magnesium deficiency, Bartter's syndrome, Gitelman's syndrome, or current diuretic ingestion.

Chronic administration of alkali to individuals with normal renal function results in minimal, if any, alkalosis. In patients with chronic renal insufficiency, overt alkalosis can develop following alkali administration, presumably because the capacity to excrete bicarbonate is exceeded, or because coexistent hemodynamic disturbances have caused enhanced fractional bicarbonate reabsorption. Alkali loads sufficient to develop alkalosis may be derived from oral or intravenous bicarbonate, acetate loads in parenteral hyperalimentation solutions, citrate loads (transfusions or infant formula), or antacids plus cation exchange resins. Another (but unusual) cause is a longstanding history of excessive ingestion of milk and antacids. Both hypercalcemia and vitamin D excess increase renal bicarbonate reabsorption. Patients with the "milk–alkali" syndrome are prone to develop nephrocalcinosis, renal insufficiency, and metabolic alkalosis. Discontinuation of alkali ingestion or administration is usually sufficient to repair the alkalosis.

Gastrointestinal loss of hydrogen ion results in retention of bicarbonate in the body fluids. The fluid and NaCl lost in vomitus or in nasogastric suction results in ECV contraction with an increase in plasma renin activity and aldosterone. These factors decrease GFR and enhance the capacity of the renal tubule to reabsorb bicarbonate. Upon cessation of vomiting, the plasma bicarbonate concentration falls to the bicarbonate threshold, which is markedly elevated by the continued effects of ECV contraction, hypokalemia, and hyperaldosteronism. The alkalosis will be maintained at a slightly lower level than during the phase of active vomiting, and the urine will be relatively acidic with low concentrations of sodium, bicarbonate, and chloride. Correction of the ECV contraction with sodium chloride and repair of the potassium deficit with potassium chloride corrects the acid–base disorder.

RENAL CAUSES OF METABOLIC ALKALOSIS

Drugs that induce chloriuresis without bicarbonaturia, such as thiazides and loop *diuretics* (furosemide, bumetanide, torsemide, and ethacrynic acid), diminish the ECV space without altering the total body bicarbonate content. The bicarbonate concentration in the blood and ECV will increase. Diuretics, by blocking chloride absorption in the distal tubule or by increasing proton pump activity, may also stimulate distal H^+ secretion. Maintenance of alkalosis can be ensured by the persistence of ECV contraction, secondary hyperaldosteronism, potassium deficiency, and the direct effect of the diuretic, provided diuretic administration continues. Repair of the alkalosis is achieved by cessation of the diuretic and by providing chloride (isotonic saline) to normalize the ECV deficit.

Prolonged *CO₂ retention* with chronic respiratory acidosis enhances renal bicarbonate absorption and the generation of new bicarbonate (increased net acid excretion). If the $PaCO_2$ is returned to the normal range, a metabolic alkalosis, due to the persistently elevated bicarbonate concentration, will emerge. Alkalosis develops immediately if the elevated $PaCO_2$ is abruptly returned toward normal by a change in mechanically controlled ventilation. Associated ECV contraction does not allow complete repair of the alkalosis by normalization of the $PaCO_2$ alone. Alkalosis will persist until chloride supplementation is provided.

When an underlying stimulus for the generation of lactic or ketoacidosis is removed, as occurs with repair of circulatory insufficiency or by insulin, the lactate or ketones can be metabolized to yield an equivalent amount of bicarbonate. Other sources of new bicarbonate are additive to the original amount of bicarbonate regenerated by organic anion metabolism to create a surfeit of bicarbonate. Such sources include (1) new bicarbonate added to the blood by the kidneys as a result of enhanced net acid excretion during the preexisting acidotic period and (2) alkali therapy during the treatment phase of the acidosis. The coexistence of acidosis-induced ECV contraction and potassium deficiency acts to sustain the alkalosis.

Administration of large amounts of *non-reabsorbable anions,* such as penicillin or carbenicillin, enhances distal acidification and potassium excretion. *Magnesium deficiency* also results in hypokalemic alkalosis by enhancing distal acidification through stimulation of renin and aldosterone secretion.

Bartter's syndrome is an uncommon cause of metabolic alkalosis associated with hypokalemia, juxtaglomerular apparatus hyperplasia, and hyperreninemic hyperaldosteronism. Young persons are most commonly affected, although the appearance of this syndrome in adults has been reported. Symptoms of the disorder are characteristically those of hypokalemia, including vascular hyporesponsiveness to pressors; a vasopressin-resistant inability to achieve maximal concentration of the urine; increased prostaglandin E_2 excretion; and, in some patients, hypercalciuria and hypomagnesemia. Recently, the defect in Bartter's syndrome has been localized to the thick ascending limb of Henle's loop. Loss of function mutations of both the Na^+-$2Cl^-$-K^+ cotransporter and the affiliated apical K^+ channel have been documented. Distinction from surreptitious vomiting, diuretic administration, and laxative abuse is necessary to make the diagnosis of Bartter's syndrome. The urine chloride concentration is elevated in Bartter's syndrome and depressed with vomiting. Treatment is generally focused on the repair of hypokalemia by inhibition of the renin–angiotensin–aldosterone or the prostaglandin–kinin systems. Potassium supplementation, magnesium repletion, propranolol, spironolactone, prostaglandin inhibitors, and angiotensin-converting enzyme inhibitors have all been advocated, but each has met with limited success.

While Bartter's syndrome is usually seen in children, similar findings are present in older children and adults with Gitelman's syndrome. This form of hypokalemic-hypochloremic metabolic alkalosis can be distinguished from Bartter's syndrome by the presence of both hypomagnesemia and hypocalciuria. These latter findings have led to the recent discovery that Gitelman's syndrome is the result of a loss-of-function mutation in the neutral Na^+-Cl^- cotransporter on the apical membrane of the distal tubule.

METABOLIC ALKALOSIS ASSOCIATED WITH HYPERTENSION AND MINERALOCORTICOID EXCESS

High Renin

Aldosterone elaboration by the adrenal gland occurs in response to angiotensin II, which is generated by renin release. States associated with inappropriately high renin levels may be associated with hyperaldosteronism and alkalosis. Renin levels are elevated, since a diminished effective circulating blood volume due to vascular disease is sensed by the kidney. Total ECV may not be diminished. Examples include *renovascular, accelerated,* or *malignant hypertension. Estrogens* increase renin substrate and, hence, angiotensin II formation. Primary *tumor* overproduction of renin is another rare cause of hyperreninemic hyperaldosteronemia-induced metabolic alkalosis.

Low Renin

In these disorders, primary adrenal overproduction of mineralocorticoid suppresses renin elaboration. Hypertension occurs as the result of mineralocorticoid excess with volume overexpansion.

Primary Aldosteronism

Tumor involvement (adenoma or, rarely, carcinoma) or hyperplasia of the adrenal gland is associated with aldosterone overproduction. The circadian pattern of aldosterone elaboration and response to posture is altered (morning aldosterone increases in hyperplasia and falls in adenoma). The diagnosis is made by evaluation of the plasma aldosterone/renin ratio, the clinical and biochemical response to administration of captopril or saline adrenal venography, [131]I-19-iodocholesterol scanning, and computed tomography. The treatment of primary aldosteronism is adrenalectomy or, if adrenalectomy is not indicated, spironolactone.

DIAGNOSIS OF METABOLIC ALKALOSIS

The diagnosis of metabolic alkalosis is summarized in Table 149.11. The diagnostic approach to metabolic alkalosis based on urine Cl^- concentration is outlined in Figure 149.2.

TREATMENT OF METABOLIC ALKALOSIS

Treatment is directed at removing the underlying stimulus for bicarbonate generation. If primary hypermineralocorticoidism is present, correction of the underlying cause will reverse the alkalosis. Stimuli that increase hydrogen ion loss by the stomach or kidneys can be improved by the use of an $H2^-$-receptor

TABLE 149.11.	DIAGNOSIS OF METABOLIC ALKALOSIS	

Saline-Responsive Alkalosis (Low Urinary [Cl⁻])	Saline-Unresponsive Alkalosis (High or Normal Urinary [Cl⁻])

Vomiting, nasogastric aspiration
Diuretics
Posthypercapnia
Bicarbonate therapy of organic acidosis
K⁺ deficiency
	Hypertensive
	  Primary aldosteronism
	  Cushing's syndrome
	  Renal artery stenosis
	  Renal failure plus alkali therapy
	Normotensive
	  Mg^{2+} deficiency
	  Severe K⁺ deficiency
	  Bartter's syndrome
	  Gitelman's syndrome
	  Diuretics

antagonist or discontinuation of diuretics. The second aspect of treatment is to eliminate factors that sustain bicarbonate reabsorption, such as ECV contraction or potassium deficiency (Fig. 149.2). Unusual cases, termed "saline-resistant," are associated with marked potassium deficits, magnesium deficiency, Bartter's

syndrome, Gitelman's syndrome, or primary autonomous hypermineralocorticoid states. Therapy in these cases must be directed toward the underlying pathophysiologic problem.

If warranted by associated conditions that preclude infusion of saline, accelerated renal bicarbonate loss can be achieved by

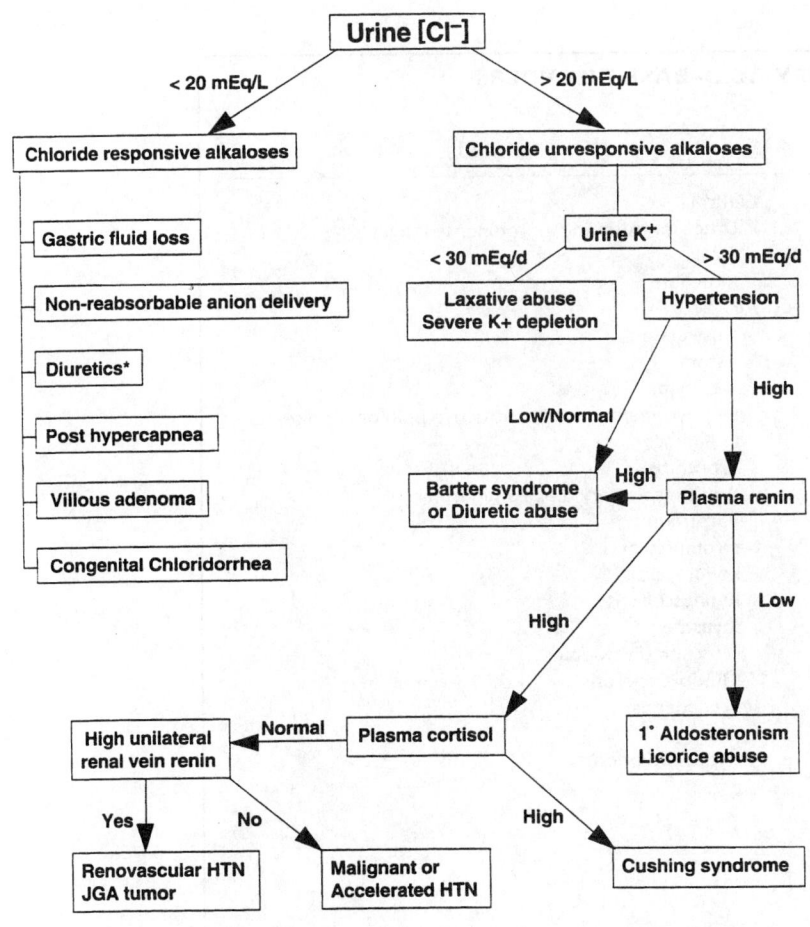

FIGURE 149.2. Diagnostic approach to metabolic alkalosis based on urine chloride and potassium concentrations.

EVIDENCE LEVEL: C. Expert Opinion.

* Post-diuretic therapy

administration of acetazolamide, a carbonic anhydrase inhibitor that is usually very effective in patients with adequate renal function. Dilute hydrochloric acid, while effective, can be dangerous and result in brisk hemolysis. Infusion of acidic amino acids, such as arginine hydrochloride, is safer and as effective. Acidification can also be achieved with oral ammonium chloride, which should be avoided in the presence of liver disease. Finally, hemodialysis against a dialysate that is low in bicarbonate and high in chloride can be effective when renal function is impaired .

RESPIRATORY ACIDOSIS

Respiratory acidosis occurs as the result of severe pulmonary disease, respiratory muscle fatigue, or depression in ventilatory control. The increase in $PaCO_2$ due to reduced alveolar ventilation is the primary abnormality leading to acidemia. In acute respiratory acidosis, there is an immediate compensatory elevation (due to cellular buffering mechanisms) in HCO_3^- that increases by 1 mEq per L for every 10 mm Hg increase in $PaCO_2$. In chronic respiratory acidosis (duration of more than 24 hours), renal adaption occurs and the HCO_3^- increases by 4 mEq per L for every 10 mm Hg increase in $PaCO_2$. The serum bicarbonate will usually not increase above 38 mEq per L. Renal compensation (increased reabsorption of HCO_3^-) requires 12 to 24 hours to take effect and is not fully completed until about 5 days.

The clinical features of respiratory acidosis vary according to severity, duration, the underlying disease, and whether there is accompanying hypoxemia. A rapid increase in $PaCO_2$ may result in anxiety, dyspnea, confusion, psychosis, hallucinations, and can progress to coma. Lesser degrees of dysfunction in chronic hypercapnia include sleep disturbances, loss of memory, daytime somnolence, and personality changes. Coordination may be impaired, and motor disturbances such as tremor, myoclonic jerks, and asterixis may develop. The sensitivity of the cerebrovasculature to the vasodilating effects of CO_2 helps to explain headaches and other signs that mimic raised intracranial pressure, such as papilledema, abnormal reflexes, and focal muscle weakness.

The causes of respiratory acidosis are displayed in Table 149.12. Reduction in ventilatory drive from depression of the respiratory center by a variety of drugs, injury, or disease can produce respiratory acidosis. Acutely, this may occur with general anesthetics, sedatives, β-adrenergic blockers, or head trauma. Chronic causes of respiratory center depression include the presence of sedatives, alcohol, intracranial tumors, and the syndromes of sleep-disordered breathing, including the primary alveolar and obesity–hypoventilation syndromes. Neuromuscular

TABLE 149.12.	**RESPIRATORY ACID–BASE DISORDERS**

Alkalosis	Acidosis
Central nervous system stimulation	Central
Pain	Drugs (anesthetics, morphine, sedatives)
Anxiety, psychosis	Stroke
Fever	Infection
Cerebrovascular accident	Airway
Meningitis, encephalitis	Obstruction
Tumor	Asthma
Trauma	Parenchyma
Hypoxemia or tissue hypoxia	Emphysema/coronary obstructive pulmonary disease
High altitude, ↓ P_aCO_2	Pneumoconiosis
Pneumonia, pulmonary edema	Bronchitis
Aspiration	Adult respiratory distress syndrome
Severe anemia	Barotrauma
Drugs or hormones	Neuromuscular
Pregnancy, progesterone	Poliomyelitis
Salicylates	Kyphoscoliosis
Nikethamide	Myasthenia
Stimulation of chest receptors	Muscular dystrophies
Hemothorax	Multiple sclerosis
Flail chest	Miscellaneous
Cardiac failure	Obesity
Pulmonary embolism	Hypoventilation
Miscellaneous	
Septicemia	
Hepatic failure	
Mechanical hyperventilation	
Heat exposure	
Recovery from metabolic acidosis	

disorders involving abnormalities or disease in the motor neurons, neuromuscular junction, and skeletal muscle can cause hypoventilation. Although a number of diseases should be considered in the differential diagnosis, drugs and electrolyte disorders should always be ruled out. Mechanical ventilation, when not properly adjusted and supervised, can result in respiratory acidosis. This occurs if carbon dioxide production suddenly rises (because of fever, agitation, sepsis, or overfeeding) or if alveolar ventilation falls because of worsening pulmonary function. High levels of positive end-expiratory pressure in the presence of reduced cardiac output may cause hypercapnia as a result of large increases in alveolar dead space.

Disease and obstruction of the airways when severe or long-standing cause respiratory acidosis. Acute hypercapnia follows sudden occlusion of the upper airway or the more generalized bronchospasm that occurs with severe asthma, anaphylaxis, and inhalational burn, or toxin injury. Chronic hypercapnia and respiratory acidosis occur in end-stage obstructive lung disease.

Restrictive disorders involving both the chest wall and the lungs can cause acute and chronic hypercapnia. Rapidly progressing restrictive processes in the lung can lead to respiratory acidosis because the high cost of breathing causes ventilatory muscle fatigue. Intrapulmonary and extrapulmonary restrictive defects present as chronic respiratory acidosis in their most advanced stages.

The diagnosis of respiratory acidosis requires, by definition, the measurement of arterial $PaCO_2$ and pH. Detailed history and physical examination often provide important diagnostic clues to the nature and duration of the acidosis. When a diagnosis of respiratory acidosis is made, its cause should be investigated. Pulmonary function studies, including spirometry, diffusing capacity for carbon monoxide, lung volumes, and arterial $PaCO_2$, and saturation usually provide adequate assessment of whether respiratory acidosis is secondary to lung disease. Workup for nonpulmonary causes should include a detailed drug history, measurement of hematocrit, and assessment of upper airway, chest wall, pleura, and neuromuscular function.

The treatment of respiratory acidosis depends on its severity and rate of onset. Acute respiratory acidosis can be life threatening, and measures to reverse the underlying cause should be simultaneous with restoration of adequate alveolar ventilation to relieve severe hypoxemia and acidemia. Temporarily this may necessitate tracheal intubation and assisted mechanical ventilation. Oxygen should be carefully titrated in patients with severe coronary obstructive pulmonary disease and chronic CO_2 retention who are breathing spontaneously. When oxygen is used injudiciously, these patients may experience progression of the respiratory acidosis. Aggressive and rapid correction of hypercapnia should be avoided because the falling $PaCO_2$ may provoke the same complications noted with acute respiratory alkalosis (i.e., cardiac dysrhythmias, reduced cerebral perfusion, and seizures). It is advisable to lower the $PaCO_2$ gradually in chronic respiratory acidosis, with the aim of restoring the $PaCO_2$ to baseline levels while at the same time providing sufficient chloride and potassium to enhance the renal excretion of bicarbonate.

Chronic respiratory acidosis often is difficult to correct, but general measures aimed at maximizing lung function with cessation of smoking, use of oxygen, bronchodilators, corticosteroids, diuretics, and physiotherapy can help some patients and can forestall further deterioration in most. The use of respiratory stimulants may prove useful in selected cases, particularly if the patient appears to have hypercapnia out of proportion to his or her level of lung function.

RESPIRATORY ALKALOSIS

Alveolar hyperventilation decreases $PaCO_2$ and increases the $HCO_3^-/PaCO_2$ ratio, thus increasing pH (alkalemia). Nonbicarbonate cellular buffers respond by consuming HCO_3^-. Hypocapnia develops whenever a sufficiently strong ventilatory stimulus causes $PaCO_2$ output in the lungs to exceed its metabolic production by tissues. Plasma pH and HCO_3^- concentration appear to vary proportionately with $PaCO_2$ over a range from 40 to 15 mm Hg. The relationship between arterial hydrogen ion concentration and $PaCO_2$ is about 0.7 nEq per L per mm Hg (or 0.01 pH unit per mm Hg), and that for plasma $[HCO_3^-]$ is 0.2 mEq per L per mm Hg.

Beyond 2 to 6 hours, sustained hypocapnia is further compensated by a decrease in renal ammonium and titratable acid excretion and a reduction in filtered HCO_3^- reabsorption. The full expression of renal adaptation may take several days and depends on a normal volume status and renal function. The kidneys appear to respond directly to the lowered $PaCO_2$ rather than the alkalemia per se. A 1 mm Hg fall in $PaCO_2$ causes a 0.4 to 0.5 mEq per L drop in HCO_3^- and a 0.3 nEq per L fall (or an 0.003-unit rise in pH) in hydrogen ion concentration.

The effects of respiratory alkalosis vary according to its duration and severity, but in general they are primarily those of the underlying disease. A rapid decline in $PaCO_2$ may cause dizziness, mental confusion, and seizures, even in the absence of hypoxemia, as a consequence of reduced cerebral blood flow. The cardiovascular effects of acute hypocapnia in the awake human are generally minimal; however, in the anesthetized or mechanically ventilated patient, the cardiac output and blood pressure may fall because of the depressant effects of anesthesia and positive-pressure ventilation on heart rate, systemic resistance, and venous return. Cardiac rhythm disturbances may occur in patients with coronary artery disease as a result of changes in oxygen unloading by blood from a left shift in the hemoglobin–oxygen dissociation curve (Bohr effect). Acute respiratory alkalosis causes minor intracellular shifts of sodium, potassium, and phosphate and reduces serum-free calcium by increasing the protein-bound fraction. Hypocapnia-induced hypokalemia is usually minor.

Respiratory alkalosis is the most common acid–base disturbance encountered in critically ill patients. When severe, it portends a poor prognosis. Many cardiopulmonary disorders manifest respiratory alkalosis in their early to intermediate stages. Hyperventilation usually results in hypocapnia. The finding of normocapnia and hypoxemia may herald the onset of rapid respiratory failure and should prompt an assessment to determine if the patient is becoming fatigued. Respiratory alkalosis is a common occurrence during mechanical ventilation.

The causes of respiratory alkalosis are summarized in Table 149.12. The hyperventilation syndrome may mimic a number of serious conditions and be disabling. Paresthesias, circumoral numbness, chest wall tightness or pain, dizziness, inability to take an adequate breath, and, rarely, tetany may themselves be sufficiently stressful to perpetuate a vicious cycle. Arterial blood gas analysis demonstrates an acute or chronic respiratory alkalosis, often with hypocapnia in the range of 15 to 30 mm Hg and no hypoxemia. Central nervous system diseases or injury can produce several patterns of hyperventilation with sustained arterial $PaCO_2$ levels of 20 to 30 mm Hg. Conditions such as hyperthyroidism, high caloric loads, and exercise raise the basal metabolic rate, but usually ventilation rises in proportion so that arterial blood gases are unchanged and respiratory alkalosis does not develop. Salicylates, the most common cause of drug-induced respiratory alkalosis, exert their effect by direct stimulation of the medullary chemoreceptor. The methylxanthine drugs, theophylline and aminophylline, stimulate ventilation and increase the ventilatory response to carbon dioxide. Progesterone increases ventilation and lowers arterial $PaCO_2$ by as much as 5 to 10 mm Hg. As a result of increased progesterone, chronic respiratory alkalosis is an expected feature of pregnancy. Respiratory alkalosis is a prominent feature in liver failure, and its severity correlates well with the degree of hepatic insufficiency and mortality. Respiratory alkalosis is common in patients with gram-negative septicemia, and it is often an early finding, prior to the development of fever, hypoxemia, and hypotension. It is presumed that some bacterial product or toxin acts as a stimulant, but the mechanism remains unknown.

The diagnosis of respiratory alkalosis relies on measurement of arterial pH and $PaCO_2$. The plasma potassium concentration is often reduced and the serum chloride concentration increased. In the acute phase, respiratory alkalosis is not associated with increased renal bicarbonate excretion, but within hours net acid excretion is reduced. In general, the bicarbonate concentration falls by 2.0 mEq per L for each 10 mm Hg decrease in $PaCO_2$. Chronic hypocapnia reduces the serum bicarbonate concentration by 5.0 mEq per L for each 10 mm Hg decrease in $PaCO_2$. It is unusual to observe a plasma bicarbonate concentration below 12 mEq per L as a result of a pure respiratory alkalosis. A detailed history and careful physical examination provide important clues to the nature and duration of any acid–base derangement.

When a diagnosis of hyperventilation or respiratory alkalosis is made, its cause should be investigated. The diagnosis of hyperventilation syndrome is made by exclusion. In difficult cases, it may be important to rule out other conditions such as pulmonary embolism, coronary artery disease, and hyperthyroidism.

The treatment of respiratory alkalosis is primarily directed toward alleviation of the underlying disorder. Since respiratory alkalosis is rarely life threatening, direct measures to correct it will be unsuccessful if the stimulus remains unchecked. If respiratory alkalosis complicates ventilator management, changes in dead space, tidal volume, and frequency can minimize the hypocapnia. Patients with the hyperventilation syndrome may benefit from reassurance, rebreathing from a paper bag during symptomatic attacks, and attention to underlying psychological stress. Antidepressants and sedatives are not recommended, although in a few patients β-adrenergic blockers may help to ameliorate distressing peripheral manifestations of the hyperadrenergic state.

BIBLIOGRAPHY

Bidani A, DuBose TD Jr. Cellular and whole-body acid–base regulation. In: Arieff AI, DeFronzo RA, eds. *Fluid, electrolyte, and acid–base disorders.* New York: Churchill Livingstone, 1995.

Cogan MG. *Fluid and electrolytes.* Norwalk, CT: Appleton & Lange, 1991.

DuBose TD Jr. Acid–base disorders. In: Brenner BM, ed. *The Kidney,* 6th ed. Philadelphia: WB Saunders, 1999:925–997.

DuBose TD Jr, Alpern RJ. Renal tubular acidosis. In: Scriver CR, Beaudet AL, Sly WS, Valle D, eds. *The metabolic bases of inherited diseases,* 8th ed. New York: McGraw-Hill *(in press).*

Emmett M, Alpern RF, Seldin DW. Metabolic alkalosis and metabolic acidosis. In: Seldin DW, Giebisch G, eds. *The kidney: physiology and pathophysiology,* 2nd ed. New York: Raven Press, 1992:2733–2836.

Halperin ML. *The acid truth and basic facts—with a sweet touch, an enlytenment.* Montreal: LetroMac, 1991.

Halperin ML, Goldstein MB. *Fluid, electrolyte and acid–base physiology.* Philadelphia: WB Saunders, 1994.

Madias NE, Cohen JJ. Respiratory alkalosis and acidosis. In: Seldin DW, Giebisch G, eds. *The kidney: physiology and pathophysiology,* 2nd ed. New York: Raven Press, 1992:2837–2872.

Narins RG, Kupin W, Faber MD, et al. Pathophysiology, classification and therapy of acid–base disturbances. In: Arieff AI, DeFronzo RA, eds. *Fluid, electrolyte, and acid–base disorders.* New York: Churchill Livingstone, 1995.

Rose BD. *Clinical physiology of acid–base and electrolyte disorders,* 4th ed. New York: McGraw-Hill, 1994.

Kelley's Textbook of Internal Medicine, fourth edition. Edited by H. David Humes. Lippincott Williams & Wilkins, Philadelphia © 2000.

DISORDERS OF THE KIDNEY

IMMUNE-MEDIATED GLOMERULOPATHIES

IAN R. RIFKIN
DAVID J. SALANT

Glomeruli are specialized capillary tufts that produce up to 180 L per day of cell- and protein-free plasma ultrafiltrate. These properties are attributable to the porous glomerular capillary wall composed of fenestrated endothelial cells, the underlying glomerular basement membrane (GBM), and the filtration slits between adjacent visceral epithelial cell foot processes, which allows the bulk flow of water and solutes while preventing the passage of cells and macromolecules based on their size and charge. In addition, the mesangial cells, which occupy the axial region between glomerular capillary loops, synthesize mesangial matrix and regulate the surface area available for glomerular filtration (see Chapter 164).

The clinical presentation of glomerular diseases in general, and immune-mediated glomerular diseases in particular, is a direct consequence of damage to one or more components of the filtration unit. This can impair glomerular filtration and/or alter permeability to cells or macromolecules. The decreased glomerular filtration rate (GFR) may lead to renal failure with accumulation of metabolic waste products (azotemia) and derangement in fluid and electrolyte balance (see Chapters 140 and 141). The alterations in permeability lead to the egress of cells and/or protein into the tubular lumen and then into the urine.

It is implicit in the above that glomerular damage can elicit only a limited number of functional outcomes. Therefore, the clinical presentation in terms of the urine sediment, proteinuria, or renal function is rarely specific for an individual disease. Nevertheless, although there are exceptions, the individual diseases present in a consistent manner, and two broad categories of clinical presentation are recognized: the *acute nephritic syndrome* and the *nephrotic syndrome* (Table 150.1). From a clinical standpoint, classification of patients into one of these two groups has proven extremely useful as a first step toward identifying the individual underlying disease. However, certain diseases present with features of both the acute nephritic syndrome and the nephrotic syndrome, and some produce only asymptomatic proteinuria and/or hematuria of varying degrees.

The *acute nephritic syndrome* is defined clinically and includes some or all of the following: hematuria with red blood cell casts, oliguria, azotemia, hypertension, mild to moderate proteinuria (1 to 3 g per day) and moderate edema. Of these, hematuria with red blood cell casts is diagnostically the most important. The underlying glomerular disease is inflammatory in nature and damages the glomerular capillaries allowing the passage of cells into the urinary space. The inflammation is generally accompanied by proliferation of resident cells and infiltration of leukocytes, thus making proliferative glomerulonephritis the histologic counterpart of the acute nephritic syndrome. The rapidity and intensity of the inflammatory response further subdivides the acute nephritic syndrome into clinically useful categories. Acute glomerulonephritis presenting with acute nephritic syndrome may be reversible, either spontaneously or with treatment. A subgroup of patients with rapidly progressive glomerulonephritis (RPGN) have a course that leads to end-stage renal disease in weeks to months unless it is halted with treatment. Others have only microscopic hematuria, sometimes punctuated by episodes of gross hematuria and accompanied by urinary red blood cell casts.

The *nephrotic syndrome* is defined by heavy proteinuria (more than 3 g per day), severe edema, and hypoalbuminemia, often accompanied by hyperlipidemia and hypercoagulability. Many patients have so-called "subnephrotic" proteinuria or heavy proteinuria without other features of the nephrotic syndrome. Hematuria may be present but is not a major feature, and there is frequently only minimal impairment of the GFR at initial presentation. The underlying glomerular pathologic process is generally noninflammatory but the nephrotic syndrome may accompany various inflammatory glomerular diseases (e.g., class IV lupus nephritis; see below). The major abnormality is seen in the visceral epithelial cells and subepithelial aspect of the GBM.

The immune-mediated glomerulopathies are a disparate group of diseases in which glomerular injury is thought to be caused directly by immunologic mechanisms. Glomerular diseases occurring in the context of an immune-mediated disease but where the glomerular disease itself is not due primarily to immunological mechanisms (e.g., diabetic nephropathy in type I diabetes mellitus), are not usually classified as immune-mediated glomerulopathies. The immunologic basis of many glomerular diseases was established by the advent of immunofluorescence microscopy, which documented the presence of immunoglobulins and complement components in the glomeruli of renal biopsy specimens. The pattern of immunofluorescence tends to define the underlying immunopathogenesis, with linear staining of the

TABLE 150.1.	CLINICAL SYNDROMES AND HISTOLOGIC LESIONS CAUSED BY IMMUNOLOGIC GLOMERULAR DISEASES	

Clinical Syndromes and Histology of Primary Glomerulopathy	Examples of Secondary Causes and Associations
Isolated proteinuria or nephrotic syndrome	
MCD	Hodgkin's lymphoma, NSAIDs
FSGS	Nephron loss, HIVAN
MN	SLE, HepB, cancer, various drugs
Isolated hematuria or acute nephritic syndrome	
Diffuse PGN	Poststreptococcal GN, SLE
Focal or mesangial PGN	IgAN/HSP, SLE, SBE
Crescentic GN (RPGN)	See Fig. 150.3
Mixed nephritic-nephrotic syndrome	
MPGN type I	HepC, cryo, SLE, lymphoma, infection
MPGN type II	C3NEF-partial lipodystrophy

Note that this table does not include nonimmunologic causes of proteinuric (e.g., diabetic and amyloid nephropathies) or hematuric (e.g., hereditary nephritis) syndromes.
MN, membranous nephropathy; FSGS, focal segmental glomerulosclerosis; MCD, minimal change disease; MPGN, membranoproliferative glomerulonephritis; PGN, proliferative GN; SLE, systemic lupus erythematosus; HepB, hepatitis B; HIVAN, HIV-associated nephropathy; HepC, hepatitis C; cryo, mixed cryoglobulinemia; IgAN/HSP, IgA nephropathy/Henoch-Schönlein purpura; SBE, infective endocarditis; C3NEF, C3 nephritic factor; NSAIDs, nonsteroidal anti-inflammatory drugs; RPGN, rapidly progressive glomerulonephritis.

GBM being characteristic of anti-GBM antibody disease, and granular deposits in the peripheral capillaries or mesangium representing immune complexes. However, not all glomerular diseases with an apparent immune basis are accompanied by glomerular immune deposits. Most notable examples are minimal change disease, the major cause of childhood nephrotic syndrome, and pauci-immune crescentic glomerulonephritis, an important cause of rapidly progressive glomerulonephritis. In addition, some diseases are included among the immune-mediated glomerulopathies by association because of similar clinical and/or pathologic features rather than by direct evidence of an immune basis. Indeed, the only glomerular disease in which the target antigen has been identified with certainty is anti-GBM disease/Goodpasture's syndrome. It is also noteworthy that certain nonimmune glomerulopathies may present with clinical syndromes that are indistinguishable from immune-mediated glomerular diseases. These are discussed elsewhere and include diabetic nephropathy (Chapter 153), hemolytic-uremic syndrome/thrombotic thrombocytopenic purpura (Chapter 152), amyloidosis (Chapter 154), the paraproteinemias (Chapter 154), human immunodeficiency virus (HIV)–associated nephropathy (Chapter 164), and hereditary nephritis (Chapter 157).

TERMINOLOGY

The following is a brief glossary of descriptions used in glomerular pathology. The term *diffuse* implies that all (or most) glomeruli are affected more or less uniformly, whereas *focal* and *segmental* means that some are partly abnormal. A *proliferative* lesion refers to a hypercellular inflammatory process involving infiltrating leukocytes and proliferation of intrinsic glomerular cells. *Sclerosis* describes a degenerative process in which there is an

increase in extracellular matrix accompanying the loss of glomerular cells and collapse of capillary loops. Thus, one may see a focal and segmental proliferative lesion give rise to a nephritic clinical presentation or find focal and segmental sclerosis underlying the nephrotic syndrome.

GLOMERULOPATHIES PRESENTING WITH ACUTE NEPHRITIC SYNDROME OR ISOLATED HEMATURIA

POSTSTREPTOCOCCAL GLOMERULONEPHRITIS

Definition

Poststreptococcal glomerulonephritis (PSGN) follows infection of the skin or pharynx with nephritogenic strains of Lancefield group A β-hemolytic streptococci. It is the classical example of an acute postinfectious glomerulonephritis.

Incidence and Epidemiology

Poststreptococcal glomerulonephritis remains endemic among children over the age of 2 years in certain developing countries where streptococcal pharyngitis and skin infection are common. Although it is now uncommon in developed countries, sporadic cases are still seen among children and younger adults, and occasional epidemics are reported, especially in groups housed in close quarters. Sporadic and epidemic PSGN may follow either streptococcal skin disease or pharyngitis.

Etiologic Factors

Only certain strains of streptococci are nephritogenic (such as M-protein type 12, associated with pharyngitis, and type 49, associated with impetigo). The reasons for this strain specificity have not been elucidated but the M-protein itself is probably not the pathogenic entity. Several other streptococcal antigens are being investigated as potential nephritogenic agents.

Pathogenesis

Poststreptococcal glomerulonephritis is thought to be an immune complex–mediated disease on the basis of the finding of glomerular capillary deposits of IgG and C3 on immunofluorescence. It is likely that early formation of subendothelial and mesangial immune complexes is responsible for the acute inflammatory component of the disease as manifest by proliferation and leukocyte recruitment. Although large hump-like subepithelial deposits on electron microscopy are characteristic of PSGN, they are probably not the cause of the inflammation but may contribute to proteinuria. It is also noteworthy that the alternate pathway of complement is activated to a greater extent than the classical pathway, which suggests that streptococcal cell wall components may have a direct role.

Clinical Findings

There is a latent period of about 10 days following streptococcal pharyngitis and 21 days following skin infection before the onset of glomerulonephritis. The classical clinical presentation is the sudden onset of the acute nephritic syndrome with oliguria, gross hematuria (appearing as smoky or dark urine), facial edema, hypertension, and azotemia. Flank or abdominal pain may be present. Pulmonary edema may occur, and some patients may have malignant hypertension accompanied by headache, nausea and vomiting, confusion, and seizures. It is important to note, however, that milder and even subclinical disease is common. The urine sediment reflects the nephritic process, with dysmorphic red blood cells and red blood cell casts. Proteinuria is usually in the subnephrotic range although a small minority of patients develop nephrotic range proteinuria, usually in the recovery phase as the GFR normalizes. Acute renal failure occurs in 1% to 2% of patients and may require temporary dialysis.

Laboratory Findings

Serum creatinine may rise rapidly but usually does not exceed 2 to 3 mg per dL before recovery begins. The diagnosis of PSGN is usually made on the basis of the clinical presentation in conjunction with antistreptococcal antibodies and low C3 with normal C4. Renal biopsy is reserved for cases with an atypical presentation or disease course. Bacteriologic culture is frequently negative at the onset of PSGN, especially in patients already receiving antibiotic therapy. Antibody levels start to rise after about 7 to 10 days and persist for several months. A rise in antistreptolysin O titer (ASO) is helpful in cases following pharyngeal infection, but titers fail to rise in as many as half of individuals with skin infections. Rising titers of antihyaluronidase (AHase), and antideoxyribonuclease B (ADNase B) are a good indicator of both pharyngeal and skin infection. Complement levels suggest preferential activation of the alternate complement pathway with low C3 and normal C1q, C2, and C4 and are helpful in supporting the diagnosis, as the only other glomerular disease commonly associated with this pattern of complement activation is type II membranoproliferative glomerulonephritis (Table 150.2). The C3 levels and total serum hemo-

TABLE 150.2.	SERUM COMPLEMENT PROFILE AND SEROLOGY IN GLOMERULAR DISEASES	
Disease	**Complement Profile**[a]	**Serology**
Poststreptococcal GN	Low (alternate)	Antistreptococcal antibodies
Other postinfectious[b]	Low (classical)	Blood or other cultures
SLE	Low (classical)	ANA, anti-dsDNA, anti-Sm
MPGN: Type I	Low (classical)	Idiopathic-none; secondary-anti-Hepatitis C
Type II	Low (alternate)	C3 nephritic factor
Mixed cryoglobulinemia	Low (classical)	IgG-IgM cryoglobulins, RF, anti-Hepatitis C
Anti-GBM nephritis	Normal	Anti-GBM antibodies
Wegener's granulomatosis	Normal	Antineutrophil cytoplasmic antibodies
Microscopic polyangiitis	Normal	Antineutrophil cytoplasmic antibodies
IgAN/HSP	Normal	None
MCD	Normal	None
FSGS	Normal	Idiopathic—none; secondary—HIV
MN	Normal	Idiopathic—none; secondary—ANA, HepB

[a] Pathway of complement activation: classical—low C2, C4, and C3; alternate—low C3, normal C2 and C4.
[b] Especially chronic bacteremia, e.g., infective endocarditis.
GN, glomerulonephritis; SLE, systemic lupus erythematosus; MPGN, membranoproliferative glomerulonephritis; IgAN/HSP, IgA nephropathy/Henoch–Schönlein purpura; MCD, minimal change disease; FSGS, focal segmental glomerulosclerosis; MN, membranous nephropathy; ANA, antinuclear antibodies; RF, rheumatoid factor; GBM, glomerular basement membrane; HIV, human immunodeficiency virus.

lytic complement (CH_{50}) levels are low in more than 90% of individuals by the second week of the disease, with normal levels being reestablished by about 8 weeks.

The histologic feature of PSGN by light microscopy is a diffuse proliferative glomerulonephritis with marked glomerular hypercellularity and a prominent infiltrate of leukocytes (Fig. 150.1A). Extensive crescent formation is rare and is generally limited to those cases that present with acute renal failure. Granular deposits of IgG and C3 are seen on the glomerular capillary walls on immunofluorescence microscopy with variable mesangial deposition (Fig. 150.1B). Different staining patterns may correlate with different patterns of clinical disease. C4 and C1q are absent. On electron microscopy large electron-dense subepithelial "humps" are most characteristic of PSGN (Fig. 150.1C), but subendothelial and mesangial deposits may be seen in early biopsies.

Optimal Management

Therapy for PSGN is predominantly supportive awaiting spontaneous resolution. Penicillin is usually given to prevent the spread of streptococcal infection to contacts and possibly to limit the severity of PSGN. Treatment is directed at the control of blood pressure and volume overload with diuretics, fluid and sodium restriction, and antihypertensive agents. The overall prognosis is excellent, with most patients recovering completely. A small subset of patients, particularly adults with sporadic disease, may be left with residual proteinuria, hypertension, or mild renal insufficiency, but progression to end-stage renal failure is very rare. In the 1% to 2% of patients who develop severe crescentic glomerulonephritis with acute renal failure, consideration should be given to a course of pulse corticosteroids, although there is no good evidence that this alters the natural history and spontaneous recovery is quite common.

OTHER POSTINFECTIOUS GLOMERULONEPHRITIDES

The acute nephritic syndrome and diffuse or focal proliferative glomerulonephritis can also be seen in association with many other bacterial, viral, fungal, or parasitic infections of which a few deserve emphasis.

Infective endocarditis, both acute and chronic, can present with a focal or diffuse proliferative glomerulonephritis (Table 150.1). The severity varies from microscopic hematuria to acute renal failure. Nephrotic syndrome is present in 25% of patients. Complement levels are usually low but, in contrast to PSGN, classical complement pathway activation is seen with low C4 as well as low C3 (Table 150.2). Circulating cryoglobulins and rheumatoid factor are often present, and glomerular deposits of IgG and C3 are found on immunofluorescence. The renal disease generally resolves with treatment of the endocarditis. A similar clinical presentation is seen in "shunt nephritis," a disease that may be seen in children with infection of ventriculoatrial shunts inserted for the treatment of hydrocephalus. Treatment involves appropriate antibiotics and frequently requires removal of the shunt. Recovery of renal function may be slow. Other deep-seated infections, including pulmonary, hepatic, and retroperitoneal abscesses, may be associated with acute proliferative glomerulonephritis. Renal dysfunction may be severe. In contrast to other postinfectious glomerulonephritides, complement levels are often normal and rheumatoid factor is negative although cryoglobulins are often present. Glomerular immune complex deposits may be scanty or absent. The pathogenesis of this disease is not well defined, but treatment involves eradication of the infection.

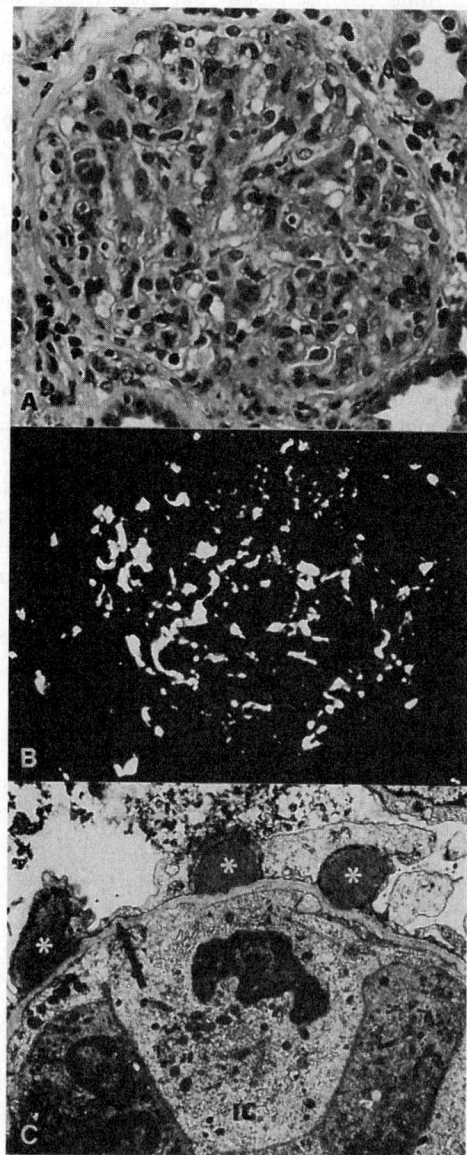

FIGURE 150.1. Acute poststreptococcal glomerulonephritis. **A:** The swollen glomerular tuft shows a prominent polymorphonuclear leukocytic infiltrate (hematoxylin-eosin, ×400). **B:** Granular immunofluorescent deposits of IgG are seen along the glomerular basement membrane and in the mesangial region (antihuman IgG, ×400). **C:** The electron micrograph shows a segment of basement membrane (*arrow*) with subepithelial "humps" (*asterisks*). Intracapillary inflammatory cells (IC) fill the capillary lumen (×5,400).

RAPIDLY PROGRESSIVE GLOMERULONEPHRITIS

Definition

Rapidly progressive glomerulonephritis is a syndrome of rapidly declining renal function accompanied by hematuria and red blood cell casts in the urine, and variable degrees of proteinuria and oliguria, with crescentic glomerulonephritis being the predominant pathologic lesion. In the absence of prompt and effective treatment, the disease frequently terminates in end-stage renal failure.

Incidence

Approximately 10% to 15% of patients with acute glomerulonephritis have a rapidly progressive course.

Etiologic Factors and Classification

The causes of crescentic glomerulonephritis can be conveniently classified according to the immunofluorescent staining pattern on renal biopsy and associated serologic findings (Figs. 150.2A–C and 150.3). There are three main categories. In anti-GBM nephritis, deposits of IgG decorate the GBM in a linear pattern. About 50% of patients with anti-GBM disease also have pulmonary hemorrhage (so-called Goodpasture's syndrome). Pauci-immune nephritis is characterized by few or no glomerular immune deposits and the presence of circulating antineutrophil cytoplasm antibodies (ANCA). The disease may be limited to the kidneys or associated with small-vessel vasculitis involving other organs (systemic vasculitis). The third group includes various renal limited and systemic diseases with abundant granular immune complex deposits on glomerular capillaries or in the mesangium.

Clinical Findings

Rapidly progressive glomerulonephritis generally presents with some or all of the typical features of the nephritic syndrome, including hematuria with red blood cell casts, oliguria, subnephrotic proteinuria, peripheral edema, mild hypertension, and renal impairment, which may progress to end-stage renal failure within weeks. Severe hypertension and nephrotic syndrome are unusual at initial presentation in anti-GBM and pauci-immune nephritis but may be present in the immune complex diseases causing RPGN. In addition to the renal manifestations, several causes of RPGN are associated with systemic symptoms and signs, including pulmonary hemorrhage (Table 150.3), cutaneous vasculitis (Table 150.3), and various rheumatologic manifestations as in systemic lupus erythematosus (SLE). These are discussed in more detail below (see also Chapters 178 and 181). Thus, a careful history and physical examination often provides clues to the diagnosis of the cause of RPGN and helps avoid extensive special investigation.

Histopathology

Glomerular crescents are the pathological hallmark of the various diseases that present with RPGN (Fig. 150.2D). The glomerular tuft itself may be the site of a diffuse or focal proliferative and necrotizing glomerulonephritis. Initially, the crescents are composed of macrophages and proliferating glomerular epithelial cells surrounded by a matrix of fibrinogen, fibronectin, and other plasma-derived proteins. Later, there is infiltration of fibroblasts and the crescents become fibrotic. With the formation of large, circumferential crescents in a high proportion of glomeruli, the glomerular tufts are compressed and GFR is impaired. There is frequently an associated periglomerular and interstitial inflammatory infiltrate, which gives rise to interstitial fibrosis and tubular atrophy, the harbingers of chronic renal failure. Immunofluo-

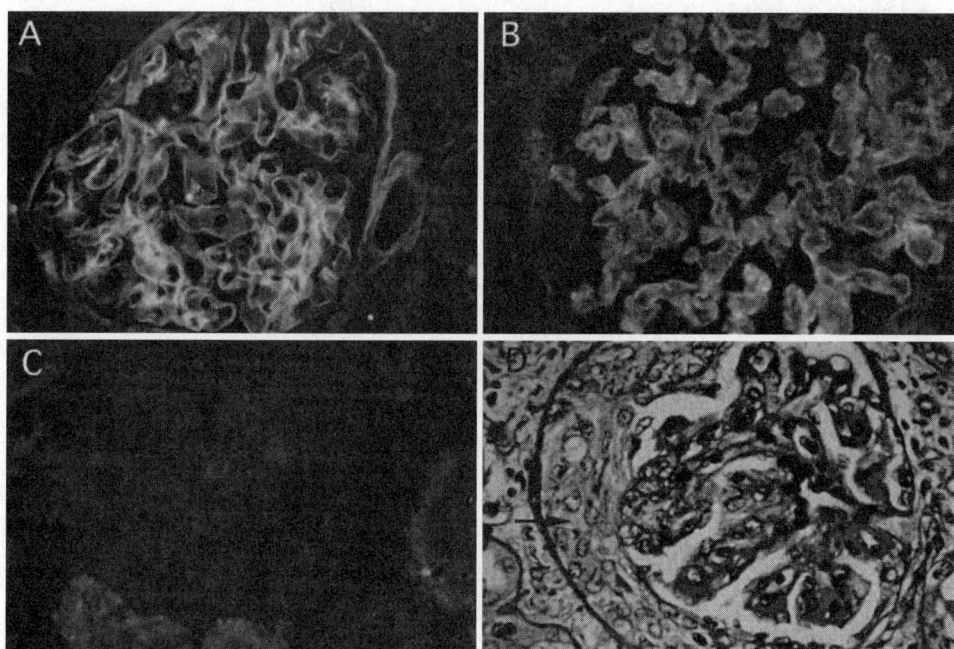

FIGURE 150.2. Rapidly progressive glomerulonephritis. **A:** A continuous (linear) pattern of immunofluorescence staining for IgG is seen along glomerular capillary basement membranes and in Bowman's capsule in a patient with Goodpasture's syndrome (antihuman IgG, ×400). **B:** Granular deposits are seen in the capillary walls in a patient with SLE (antihuman IgG, ×400). **C:** An absence of immunofluorescence staining indicating an absence of immune deposits is seen in the glomerulus of a patient with microscopic polyangiitis (antihuman IgG, ×400). **D:** A cellular crescent *(arrow)* compresses the adjacent glomerular capillary tuft in a patient with Wegener's granulomatosis (periodic acid–Schiff, ×400).

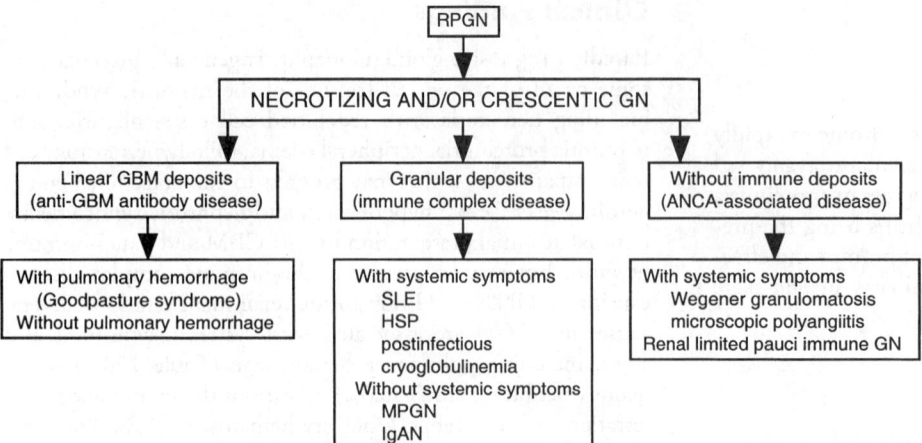

FIGURE 150.3. Immunopathologic classification of necrotizing and crescentic glomerulonephritis. The upper box indicates the typical histologic lesion in rapidly progressive glomerulonephritis; the next level represents the immunohistologic and serologic findings; the lowest level lists the etiologies of each. GBM, glomerular basement membrane; SLE, systemic lupus erythematosus; HSP, Henoch-Schönlein purpura; MPGN, membranoproliferative GN; IgAN, IgA nephropathy; ANCA, antineutrophil cytoplasmic antibody.

rescence reveals linear staining of the GBM, pauci-immune, or granular deposits. The granular deposits in the immune complex group are characteristic of the specific disease responsible; for example, mesangial IgA in IgA nephropathy and Henoch-Schönlein purpura (HSP), and diffuse IgG and C3 in lupus nephritis (see below). Electron microscopy discloses no immune deposits in anti-GBM and pauci immune nephritis, whereas immune deposits are seen in the locations characteristic of the various immune complex diseases. GBM disruption may be seen in all groups.

ANTI–GLOMERULAR BASEMENT MEMBRANE ANTIBODY DISEASE

Anti-GBM disease is caused by autoantibodies that recognize and bind to their target antigen in the noncollagenous 1 (NC1) domain of the α3 chain of type IV collagen, a major component of the GBM and alveolar basement membrane. As in other autoimmune diseases, the precise etiologic factors of the immune dysregulation is unknown, but glomerular and alveolar damage is due to the inflammatory response initiated by the binding of

anti-GBM autoantibodies to these basement membranes. Anti-GBM disease is uncommon, accounting for approximately 1% to 2% of cases of glomerulonephritis and about 10% to 15% of cases of RPGN. There appears to be a genetic susceptibility to disease, with individuals inheriting the gene for the major histocompatibility complex (MHC) class II molecule HLA-DRw15 being at increased risk. Goodpasture's syndrome tends to be more common in male patients under 40 years of age who may have a history of cigarette smoking, hydrocarbon exposure, or recent respiratory tract infection. Patients with renal-limited anti-GBM nephritis tend to be older and of either sex. Pulmonary involvement may precede nephritis by months or even years in Goodpasture's syndrome and is often accompanied by iron deficiency anemia due to subclinical intra-alveolar hemorrhage. Overt pulmonary hemorrhage ranges from mild to life threatening and is often accompanied by dyspnea, hemoptysis, and cough. Chest x-ray shows diffuse alveolar infiltrates in a "butterfly" pattern.

Diagnosis

The diagnosis is made by finding crescentic glomerulonephritis (Fig. 150.2D) with linear deposits of IgG on renal biopsy (Fig. 150.2A), and by detection of circulating anti-GBM antibodies (Table 150.2). Enzyme-linked immunosorbent assays that utilize a purified source of antigen for the detection of serum autoantibodies to the NC1 domain of type IV collagen α3 chain have a sensitivity and specificity in excess of 90%. Caution should be exercised to ensure that samples are sent to a laboratory that uses these assays and has a rapid turnaround time. Severe iron deficiency anemia is commonly present in patients with Goodpasture's syndrome. Between 10% and 30% of anti-GBM-positive patients are also positive for ANCA. It is not known at present whether these individuals have a different prognosis from those anti-GBM-positive individuals who are ANCA-negative. Complement levels are normal.

Differential Diagnosis

Pulmonary hemorrhage and glomerulonephritis with renal failure (pulmonary-renal syndrome) may also be seen in ANCA-

	TABLE 150.3.	DIFFERENTIAL DIAGNOSIS OF SYSTEMIC DISEASES ASSOCIATED WITH ACUTE GLOMERULONEPHRITIS, PULMONARY DISEASE, AND/OR CUTANEOUS VASCULITIS

Disease	Pulmonary Disease	Cutaneous Vasculitis
Goodpasture's syndrome	Present	Absent
Wegener's granulomatosis	Present	Present
Microscopic polyangiitis	Present	Present
Churg–Strauss allergic granulomatosis	Present	Present
Mixed cryoglobulinemia	Rare	Present
Henoch–Schönlein purpura	Rare	Present
Systemic lupus erythematosus	Rare	Unusual

positive pauci-immune vasculitides and less commonly in other systemic autoimmune diseases (including SLE, HSP, and cryoglobulinemia) (Table 150.3). In addition, acute renal failure from any cause may be complicated by superimposed pulmonary edema, infection, or embolism, which may be difficult to distinguish clinically from immune-mediated pulmonary hemorrhage. Serologic tests, if available rapidly, sometimes help with the diagnosis, but measurement of pulmonary capillary wedge pressure, pulmonary carbon monoxide transfer, and lung biopsy are sometimes required to make the distinction.

Optimal Management

Without treatment nearly all patients with anti-GBM disease either develop end-stage renal failure or die from pulmonary hemorrhage. The early initiation of treatment with plasmapheresis and immunosuppressive drugs is critical if long-term renal function is to be preserved. Progression to end-stage renal failure can usually be prevented if treatment is begun when the plasma creatinine concentration is less than 5 mg per dL and when the patient is not oliguric. On the other hand, if treatment is started when the plasma creatinine concentration is above 5 to 7 mg per dL or the patient is oliguric, progression to end-stage renal failure is almost inevitable. In this situation the risks of aggressive therapy are not warranted for the renal disease. However, if there is pulmonary involvement, treatment should be initiated irrespective of the level of plasma creatinine in order to prevent fatal pulmonary hemorrhage. The treatment of anti-GBM disease involves the removal of circulating anti-GBM autoantibodies with daily plasma exchange until circulating anti-GBM antibodies are no longer detectable, and concomitant immunosuppressive therapy. A typical immunosuppressive regimen includes corticosteroids (three daily doses of intravenous methylprednisolone 15 mg per kg per day followed by oral prednisone 1 mg per kg per day with gradual taper) and oral cyclophosphamide (2 to 3 mg per kg per day) with close monitoring to maintain the leukocyte count above 3,500/mm^3. Azathioprine (1 to 2 mg per kg per day) may be used instead if cyclophosphamide is contraindicated or in mild disease. Immunosuppressive therapy is continued for approximately a year. Relapses may occur and careful follow-up is necessary. Renal transplantation is a good therapeutic option for patients who develop end-stage renal failure provided the disease is in remission and circulating autoantibodies have been undetectable for 6 months or more using a reliable assay.

PAUCI-IMMUNE CRESCENTIC GLOMERULONEPHRITIS

Pauci-immune crescentic glomerulonephritis may occur in a renal-limited form or as part of a systemic vasculitis involving small vessels (see also Chapter 181). The clinical manifestations of the individual diseases within the group are determined by the size and location of the affected vessels. Within this subgroup of RPGN there are two diseases in which renal involvement is common and often severe. These are Wegener's granulomatosis and microscopic polyangiitis (including both a systemic and a renal-limited form). In the related Churg–Strauss syndrome,

renal involvement is less common and usually mild. The mean age of onset is approximately 50 years of age, with whites being affected sevenfold more commonly than blacks. Disease onset is more common in winter and early spring, and is preceded by a flu-like illness. Constitutional symptoms such as fever, anorexia, malaise, and weight loss frequently accompany the disease. The etiologic factors are unknown. Clinical renal involvement usually manifests as RPGN, but early cases may be detected with hematuria and red blood cell casts. Lower and/or upper airway involvement is almost always present in classical Wegener's granulomatosis, but the respiratory system may also be affected in microscopic polyangiitis. Pulmonary involvement spans the range from trivial infiltrates to life-threatening hemorrhage, and to more chronic conditions such as chronic interstitial pulmonary fibrosis and bronchiolitis obliterans. Upper respiratory tract involvement includes sinusitis, necrotizing lesions of the nose, eustachian tube blockage, and tracheal stenosis. Involvement of other organs is not unusual and includes the gastrointestinal tract (gastric ulceration, pancreatitis, gastrointestinal bleeding, bowel perforation), nervous system (most commonly mononeuritis multiplex), and eye (iritis, uveitis, sclerokeratitis).

Diagnosis

The diagnosis is made by finding crescentic glomerulonephritis (Fig. 150.2D) with scant or no immune deposits on renal biopsy (Fig. 150.2C), and by detection of circulating ANCA (Table 150.2). Antineutrophil cytoplasm antibodies are positive in about 90% of cases of active pauci-immune crescentic glomerulonephritis. However, ANCA are also found in certain nonvasculitic conditions; therefore, as with any laboratory test, a positive ANCA should be used in conjunction with clinical and pathologic data in making a diagnosis. It is not yet known whether ANCA are involved in disease pathogenesis. In Wegener's granulomatosis the ANCA target antigen is most often proteinase 3, which gives a diffuse cytoplasmic staining reaction on immunofluorescence (cANCA). In microscopic polyangiitis the ANCA antigen is most often myeloperoxidase and gives a perinuclear staining pattern (pANCA), but there is considerable overlap between groups. Serum complement levels are normal. Leukocytosis, thrombocytosis, and a normochromic, normocytic anemia are frequently seen. The erythrocyte sedimentation rate and serum C-reactive protein levels are typically elevated and may serve as imprecise markers of disease activity if ANCA assays are not available. In Wegener's granulomatosis, granulomatous inflammation is present in the upper and lower airways, with or without an accompanying necrotizing vasculitis. It is sometimes necessary to perform a lung biopsy to distinguish between Wegener's granulomatosis and infective causes of granulomas and vasculitis. This granulomatous inflammation is not a feature of microscopic polyangiitis. However, outside of the airways, the necrotizing vasculitis of Wegener's granulomatosis is identical to that of microscopic polyangiitis. Churg–Strauss syndrome is characterized by granulomatous vasculitis rich in eosinophils, peripheral blood eosinophilia, and a history of asthma.

Optimal Management

Corticosteroids combined with cyclophosphamide are the major form of therapy for the ANCA-associated small vessel vasculitides and pauci-immune crescentic glomerulonephritis. Initial immunosuppressive therapy is the same as in anti-GBM nephritis, but cyclophosphamide is continued for 12 to 18 months after clinical remission. Plasma exchange is not used routinely but may be considered in patients who are initially dialysis-dependent, have significant pulmonary hemorrhage, or have concurrent anti-GBM antibody disease. The relapse rate following discontinuation of immunosuppressive therapy is between 20% and 46%. Trimethoprim-sulfamethoxazole may be of use in preventing disease relapse in the upper airway or as sole therapy for mild upper airway disease. Although disease has been reported to recur following renal transplantation, this remains a good therapeutic option for patients who progress to end-stage renal failure.

CLASSIC POLYARTERITIS NODOSA

Polyarteritis nodosa is a necrotizing inflammation of medium-sized or small arteries. Typically, there is no glomerulonephritis or vasculitis of arterioles, capillaries, or venules; however, there may be overlap with microscopic polyangiitis. The renal injury is ischemic (as opposed to inflammatory) and arises as a consequence of necrotizing inflammation of renal arteries. The urine sediment is therefore often relatively normal and proteinuria, if present, is only modest. Renal failure is slowly progressive. Severe hypertension is common and is primarily mediated by ischemia-induced activation of the renin–angiotensin system. Multiorgan involvement, including the liver, gastrointestinal tract, heart, peripheral nerves, and skeletal muscle, is common. Evidence of hepatitis B virus infection may be found, but a causal link is not established. Antineutrophil cytoplasm antibodies are not detected and complement levels are normal. The finding of aneurysms of medium-sized arteries on angiography supports the diagnosis. Blood pressure control, corticosteroids, and cyclophosphamide are the mainstays of treatment. Antiviral therapy and intravenous immunoglobulin are indicated in selected cases.

IMMUNE COMPLEX–MEDIATED CRESCENTIC GLOMERULONEPHRITIS

Rapidly progressive glomerulonephritis due to crescentic glomerulonephritis is seen in a fraction of patients with one of the many renal-limited or systemic immune complex diseases shown in Figure 150.3. These are discussed in detail elsewhere in this chapter under the specific diseases. Associated nephrotic syndrome and hypertension are more common on initial presentation in this subgroup. Other clues to the diagnosis are the presence of granular immune deposits on immunofluorescence (Fig. 150.2B) and characteristic serologic abnormalities (Table 150.2).

IGA NEPHROPATHY AND HENOCH-SCHÖNLEIN PURPURA NEPHRITIS

Definition and Incidence

Immunoglobulin A nephropathy (IgAN) is a chronic glomerular disease with variable clinical presentation and characterized by mesangial deposits of IgA. It is the commonest form of primary glomerulonephritis, accounting for 8% to 50% of all cases with considerable geographic variability in incidence and severity. There are also ethnic differences, with blacks being relatively rarely affected in comparison to whites and Asians. All age groups may be affected, but it is particularly common in children and young adults. There is a male-to-female predominance of more than 2:1. It is usually a sporadic disease but familial cases have been reported. Certain polymorphisms of the angiotensinogen and angiotensin-converting enzyme (ACE) genes may influence the risk of progression and responsiveness to treatment in white patients with IgAN.

Clinical Findings

The most common clinical presentation is with asymptomatic microscopic hematuria (see Chapter 134), often found on routine physical examination. Proteinuria in these individuals is usually less than 1 g per day. Alternatively, and characteristically, IgAN can present with recurrent episodes of macroscopic hematuria, often coincident with an upper respiratory tract infection and commonly associated with flank pain. Proteinuria is often modest (1 to 3 g per day) and subsides after the acute episode passes. Nephrotic range proteinuria is not as common and signifies a less favorable prognosis. Red blood cell casts are often seen in the urine sediment but the full nephritic syndrome with hypertension, edema, and renal failure is rare. A third mode of presentation is as part of Henoch-Schönlein purpura (HSP) (see Chapters 164 and 181), which is a form of systemic vasculitis more common in children than in adults. The renal involvement in HSP is very similar to that seen in IgAN, and it is likely that they are part of the same disease spectrum. Systemic features of HSP are probably mediated by an IgA immune complex vasculitis and include the following: purpuric skin lesions usually on the extensor surfaces of the legs and forearms and buttocks but sparing the trunk; transient arthralgias of the large joints; and abdominal pain, ileus with vomiting, and bloody diarrhea. An unusual presentation of steroid-responsive nephrotic syndrome, with renal biopsy showing features of both IgAN and minimal change disease, has also been reported.

Differential Diagnosis

Other diseases that present with asymptomatic hematuria in young patients include thin basement membrane disease, Alport's hereditary nephritis (including female carriers), and hypercalciuria and hyperuricosuria (see Chapter 134). Immunoglobulin A nephropathy should also be distinguished from mesangial (class II) and focal and segmental lupus nephritis (class III), in which prominent IgA deposits may also be seen. In addition, there are several diseases in which mesangial IgA deposits are found in the absence of the typical clinical features of IgAN. They include chronic liver disease, gluten enteropathy, dermatitis herpetiformis, inflammatory bowel disease, cutaneous T-cell lymphomas, bronchial and laryngeal carcinoma, and spondyloarthropathies (including Reiter's syndrome and ankylosing spondylitis). It may not be coincidental that many of these are disorders of immune regulation with a prominent mucosal or skin component.

Diagnosis

Immunoglobulin A nephropathy is diagnosed by finding mesangial or focal proliferative glomerulonephritis with prominent mesangial IgA deposits in a patient with a compatible clinical presentation. Henoch-Schönlein purpura is distinguished from IgAN by its typical extrarenal symptoms. There are no diagnostic serologic markers in either disease (Table 150.2).

Histopathology

Light microscopy in IgAN and HSP demonstrates mesangial enlargement due to increased mesangial matrix and cellular proliferation (Fig. 150.4A). In more severe cases presenting with heavy proteinuria or RPGN there may be focal and segmental

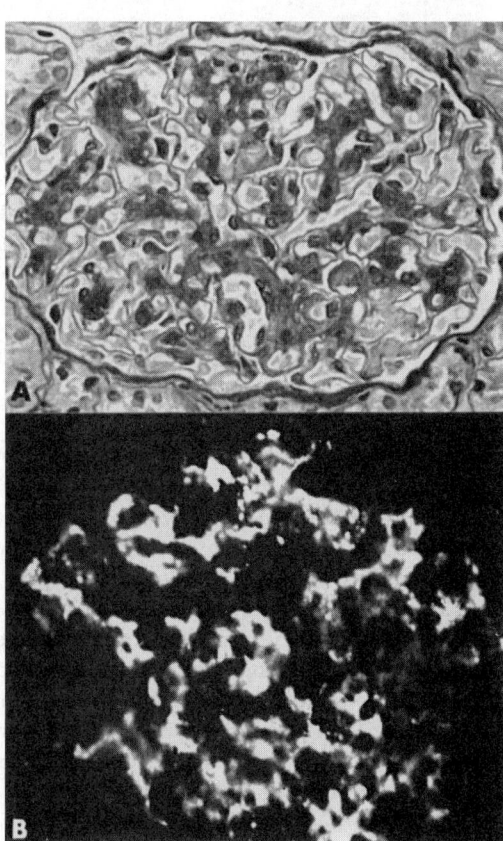

FIGURE 150.4. IgA nephropathy. **A:** Mesangial proliferation associated with normal peripheral capillary basement membranes (periodic acid–Schiff, ×400). **B:** Strong mesangial staining for IgA is present (×400).

proliferation and necrosis with crescents. Immunoglobulin A deposits, predominantly of the IgA1 subclass, are seen in the mesangium of all glomeruli on immunofluorescence (Fig. 150.4B). In addition, IgG or IgM may be seen. C3 is usually present with components of the alternate, but not the classical, complement pathway. Electron microscopy shows mesangial electron-dense deposits, sometimes extending into a subendothelial location in more severe cases.

Course and Prognosis

Despite its original designation as "benign recurrent hematuria," IgAN follows a chronic but not always benign course in the large majority of individuals. Ten-year renal survival ranges from 67% to 94%. About one third of patients follow a benign course with persistent microscopic and episodes of macroscopic hematuria. Renal function remains normal, and proteinuria is generally less than 1 g per day. Spontaneous clinical remission may occur in a small number of patients. About 10% have nephrotic syndrome, and a small number develop RPGN due to crescentic glomerulonephritis. Up to 40% of patients have a progressive course and develop end-stage renal failure within 20 years of presentation. Poor prognostic indicators include hypertension, heavy proteinuria, and reduced GFR at presentation; glomerular sclerosis, crescent formation, interstitial fibrosis, and vascular sclerosis on renal biopsy. The course in HSP nephritis is similar except that recurrent macroscopic hematuria is less common.

Optimal Management

Patients who present with the classical features of IgAN merit close follow-up but require no treatment if they have normal renal function and no hypertension or proteinuria. Pulse steroids, immunosuppressive therapy, and plasmapheresis are used in patients with RPGN due to crescentic glomerulonephritis, but the response is highly variable from patient to patient. In patients with heavy proteinuria, hypertension, and progressive renal insufficiency, blood pressure should be lowered well into the normal range with ACE inhibitors and other antihypertensive agents if necessary in an effort to decrease proteinuria and delay the progression toward end-stage renal failure. Individuals who are homozygous for the D allele of ACE may derive particular benefit. The ACE inhibitors may be of value even in normotensive patients with heavy proteinuria. Two out of four controlled studies showed that some patients with progressive IgAN have stabilization of renal function when treated with fish oils containing a high concentration of omega-3 fatty acids [eicosapentaenoic acid (EPA) 1.8 g per day and docosahexaenoic acid (DHA) 1.2 g per day]. Extended courses of alternate-day prednisone have also been found to stabilize renal function and modestly reduce proteinuria in some patients with progressive IgAN. Transplantation is a good therapeutic option for patients with end-stage IgAN; however, recurrence occurs in about one third of cases, with equal frequency in cadaveric and living related transplants. Such cases follow a slowly progressive course of allograft dysfunction, similar to that of the primary disease.

GLOMERULOPATHIES PRESENTING WITH THE NEPHROTIC SYNDROME OR ISOLATED PROTEINURIA

An approach to the patient with nephrotic syndrome, including differential diagnosis, metabolic complications, indications for renal biopsy, and general management, is given in Chapter 135. The following is a discussion of the specific immune-mediated diseases that cause nephrotic syndrome and isolated proteinuria (Table 150.1).

MINIMAL CHANGE DISEASE

Definition and Incidence

Minimal change disease causes severe nephrotic syndrome with essentially normal glomeruli on light and immunofluorescence microscopy (Fig. 150.5A). It accounts for about 90% of cases of nephrotic syndrome in children less than 10 years of age and for approximately 50% of cases in older children. In adults, about 20% of cases of nephrotic syndrome are due to minimal change disease. Boys are affected twice as frequently as girls, but the sex ratio is equal in adults.

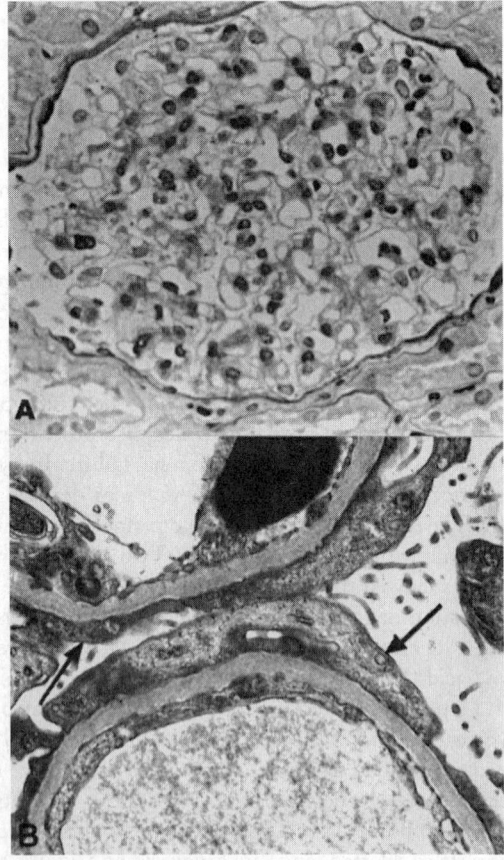

FIGURE 150.5. Minimal change disease. **A:** The glomerular capillary loops demonstrate no appreciable abnormalities (periodic acid–Schiff, ×400). **B:** The electron micrograph shows effacement of the visceral epithelial cell foot processes (*arrows;* ×11,000).

Etiologic Factors and Pathogenesis

Minimal change disease is nearly always idiopathic (primary), especially in children. An identical glomerular lesion with nephrotic syndrome may be seen rarely in association with Hodgkin's lymphoma and allergic reactions, especially to drugs. When caused by an idiosyncratic reaction to nonsteroidal anti-inflammatory drugs, minimal change nephrotic syndrome is accompanied by interstitial nephritis and acute renal failure. Association with T-cell lymphoma and responsiveness to steroids and immunosuppressive agents that interfere with T-lymphocyte function provide indirect evidence that immune-mediated mechanisms might be involved in the pathogenesis of idiopathic minimal change disease. Whatever the initiating pathogenic factors may be, the end result is damage to the visceral epithelial cells with consequent proteinuria.

Clinical Findings

The clinical presentation is dominated by the rapid onset of severe nephrotic syndrome with anasarca and associated hyperlipidemia. Severe hypertension and renal insufficiency are unusual, although creatinine clearance is mildly reduced. Urinalysis reveals lipiduria. Microscopic hematuria may be present in 20% of patients, but red blood cell casts are absent. Acute renal failure occurs occasionally, especially in adults after treatment with diuretics.

Histopathology

Glomerular morphology is normal on light microscopy (Fig. 150.5A) except for mild mesangial expansion in some cases. Immune deposits are absent on immunofluorescence microscopy. The characteristic and consistent feature on electron microscopy is diffuse effacement of the foot processes of visceral epithelial cells (Fig. 150.5B).

Diagnosis

There are no diagnostic laboratory tests (Table 150.2), and a definitive diagnosis can be made only on renal biopsy. However, because most children with nephrotic syndrome have minimal change disease, renal biopsy is reserved for those with an unusual clinical presentation or an inadequate response to treatment. In adults, the diagnosis is usually made on renal biopsy. When interpreting the finding of normal glomeruli on light microscopy in a patient with nephrotic syndrome, it is important to remember that early lesions of focal and segmental glomerulosclerosis may be missed due to sampling error in the biopsy. Similarly, early membranous nephropathy may appear normal on light microscopy, but the diagnosis is evident from the presence of granular glomerular deposits of IgG on immunofluorescence.

Optimal Management

In addition to general measures to control edema with diuretics and reduce proteinuria with ACE inhibitors, corticosteroids are particularly effective in the management of minimal change disease. They produce complete remission in about 90% of children within 8 weeks of starting treatment. Adults may take longer to remit. A typical dosing regimen in adults is to give prednisone at 1 mg per kg as a single daily dose for up to 12 weeks. A progressive shift to alternate day dosing, beginning at 1 mg per kg, is started 1 week after proteinuria remits and then tapered off over 2 to 3 months. If remission of proteinuria has not been achieved by 12 weeks, the disease is considered steroid-resistant. About 50% of adults relapse at least once after steroid therapy is discontinued, which requires retreatment with prednisone followed by a slower taper. Patients who relapse during steroid taper or shortly thereafter are said to be steroid-dependent. Those who relapse more than three times a year are termed frequent relapsers. Cytotoxic therapy with either cyclophosphamide (2 mg per kg per day for 8 to 12 weeks with a total cumulative dose of less than 200 mg per kg) or chlorambucil (0.1 to 0.2 mg per kg per day with a total cumulative dose of less than 10 mg per kg) is useful in the treatment of steroid-dependent, frequently relapsing, and some steroid-resistant individuals, and often induces long-lasting remissions. Cytotoxic therapy is usually started just after completing a course of steroids. Risk–benefit considerations are important in deciding whether to initiate cytotoxic therapy in an individual patient. Cyclosporin A (4 to 5 mg per kg per day for a year) is also effective in treating individuals who do not achieve lasting remission with steroids alone; however, relapse is common after cyclosporin A is discontinued and nephrotoxicity is a potential concern.

Course and Prognosis

Despite its relapsing course, the overall prognosis in minimal change disease is excellent. Complications are related to the nephrotic syndrome (see Chapter 135) in treatment-resistant individuals and to side effects of the medications.

FOCAL AND SEGMENTAL GLOMERULOSCLEROSIS
Definition

Focal and segmental glomerular sclerosis (FSGS) is a clinical-pathologic syndrome dominated by proteinuria, a high incidence of progressive renal failure, and focal and segmental sclerotic glomerular lesions.

Incidence, Etiologic Factors, and Pathogenesis

Focal and segmental glomerulosclerosis may be primary (idiopathic) or secondary to various causes. Primary FSGS is responsible for about 10% to 15% of cases of nephrotic syndrome in children and as many as 35% of cases in adults. It is the predominant cause of idiopathic nephrotic syndrome in African-Americans. The etiologic factors contributing to primary FSGS are unknown, although they appear to involve widespread injury to all visceral epithelial cells. It is speculated that clinical and histologic similarities between FSGS and minimal change nephropathy point to a common cause and pathogenesis, with FSGS

representing the more severe side of the disease spectrum. As in minimal change nephropathy, responsiveness of FSGS to immunosuppressive therapy, including cyclosporin A, suggests that immune mechanisms might be involved in the pathogenesis.

Secondary FSGS differs from primary FSGS in that visceral epithelial cell injury is limited to the sclerotic areas. Several factors are likely responsible for this, but glomerular hypertension plays an important role in many of the recognized causes. These include diseases causing substantial, longstanding nephron loss, such as unilateral renal agenesis and nephrectomy in childhood, and chronic renal diseases associated with areas of interstitial scarring and tubular atrophy. Examples of the latter include reflux nephropathy, analgesic nephropathy, chronic lithium toxicity, heroin abuse, and sickle cell disease. Glomerular hypertension may be directly responsible for FSGS associated with morbid obesity and sleep apnea. A severe variant of FSGS, termed collapsing glomerulopathy, is seen most commonly in HIV-associated nephropathy but may also occur in the absence of HIV infection. It is characterized clinically by massive proteinuria and a rapid decline in renal function, and histologically by segmental collapse and sclerosis of the glomeruli. Focal and segmental glomerular sclerosis can also be a relatively nonspecific consequence of previous focal and segmental proliferative glomerulonephritis.

Clinical and Laboratory Features

It is important to differentiate primary FSGS from secondary FSGS because the treatments differ. Primary FSGS usually presents with the acute onset of nephrotic syndrome, often accompanied by hypertension and microscopic hematuria. Reduced GFR is not unusual on presentation. A minority of patients are detected because of asymptomatic proteinuria. There is no history of antecedent renal, urologic, or other medical disorders, and serologic tests are normal (Table 150.2). Renal ultrasound shows symmetric, hyperechoic kidneys of normal or slightly reduced size. In secondary FSGS proteinuria is often in the subnephrotic range, and even when it is in the nephrotic range hypoalbuminemia and edema are not common. Symptoms and signs of one of the underlying causes can often be elicited, and renal imaging studies may show evidence of renal scarring, caliectasis, papillary necrosis, unilateral agenesis, or other clues to a previous urinary tract abnormality.

Histopathology

The diagnosis of FSGS is made on renal biopsy. Light microscopy reveals segmental sclerosis of a variable number of glomeruli with interstitial fibrosis and tubular atrophy in neighboring areas (Fig. 150.6). Acellular hyaline subendothelial deposits and adhesions to Bowman's capsule are common, and there may be associated capillary collapse. Deep cortical glomeruli are affected first, with subsequent progression to the outer cortex. Immunofluorescence microscopy shows focal deposits of IgM and C3 in sclerotic areas, which probably represent nonspecific entrapment. In primary FSGS, electron microscopy reveals diffuse effacement of visceral epithelial cell foot processes, whereas foot process effacement is limited mainly to the sclerotic areas in secondary FSGS. Collapsing glomerulopathy is characterized by

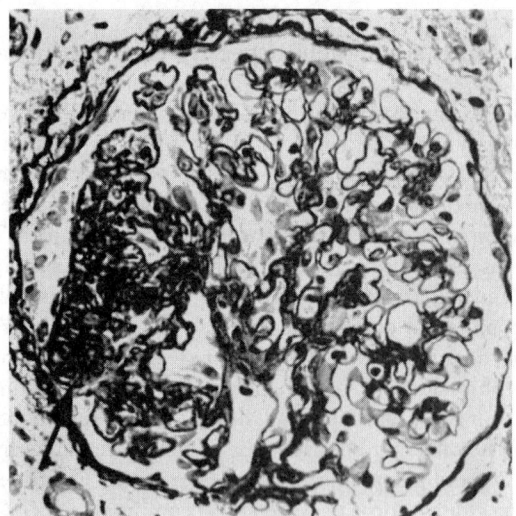

FIGURE 150.6. Focal segmental glomerulosclerosis. A segmental area of sclerosis *(arrow)* adheres to Bowman's capsule (periodic acid–Schiff, ×400).

visceral epithelial hyperplasia, marked capillary collapse, and, in HIV nephropathy, tubuloreticular structures in the endothelial cells.

Course, Prognosis, and Treatment

Most patients with untreated primary FSGS and nephrotic syndrome eventually progress to end-stage renal failure. The prognosis is worst in individuals with renal dysfunction at baseline or persistent heavy proteinuria, whereas the course is generally favorable in those with subnephrotic proteinuria and those who have partial or complete remission on treatment. Substantially longer courses of treatment with prednisone are required to induce remission in primary FSGS than in minimal change disease; even then, only about 40% of patients respond. Cytotoxic agents may be successful in steroid-resistant cases. Cyclosporin A effectively reduces proteinuria in primary FSGS, but relapse generally occurs when the drug is discontinued. Moreover, the incidence and severity of cyclosporin A nephrotoxicity is greater than in minimal change disease and is related to the extent of sclerosis and interstitial fibrosis. Primary FSGS may recur after renal transplantation. This occurs most often in children with severe and rapidly progressive FSGS and appears to be due to a circulating factor that can be removed by plasmapheresis.

Secondary FSGS is best treated by removing the cause, if possible, and by lowering intraglomerular pressure with ACE inhibitors. The addition of a low dose of diuretic appears to have a synergistic effect in reducing proteinuria, even in the absence of edema. Because of the protracted course in both forms of FSGS, general measures to limit the complications of nephrotic syndrome, control hypertension well into the normal range, and reduce proteinuria should be instituted early and pursued aggressively (see Chapter 135).

MEMBRANOUS NEPHROPATHY

Definition

Membranous nephropathy is a proteinuric disease characterized by subepithelial immune deposits and expansion of the GBM.

Incidence, Etiologic Factors, and Pathogenesis

Membranous nephropathy is responsible for approximately 25% to 35% of cases of idiopathic nephrotic syndrome in adults but less than 5% in children. Most cases occur between the ages of 30 and 60 years with a male-to-female predominance of 2:1. It is usually idiopathic (primary), but a secondary cause may be identified in up to 30% of cases. Notable secondary causes include membranous lupus nephritis, antirheumatic drugs (gold, penicillamine, nonsteroidal anti-inflammatory agents), and solid tumors of breast, colon, and other organs. It might also be associated with infections (hepatitis B, hepatitis C, schistosomiasis, congenital and secondary syphilis, leprosy, malaria, hydatid disease, filariasis), thyroiditis and other autoimmune diseases, sarcoidosis, and other miscellaneous disorders. Idiopathic membranous nephropathy itself is thought to be an autoimmune disease, probably caused by antibodies to antigenic determinants on the glomerular visceral epithelial cell with subsequent formation of the C5b-9 membrane attack complex of complement being responsible for cell damage.

Clinical Findings

Eighty percent of patients with idiopathic membranous nephropathy present with nephrotic syndrome. The remainder come to medical attention because of proteinuria. Microscopic hematuria is seen in up to 50% of adults and most children, but macroscopic hematuria and red blood cell casts are rare. Hypertension and impaired renal function are uncommon at initial presentation but become more common with disease progression. Complications of the nephrotic syndrome such as anasarca, hyperlipidemia, and growth retardation in children are common and might be severe. Hypercoagulability leading to deep vein and renal vein thrombosis and pulmonary embolism is a potential life-threatening complication. Rarely, anti-GBM-mediated RPGN may supervene.

Diagnosis

Membranous nephropathy is diagnosed by renal biopsy, as there are no clinical or laboratory features that distinguish it from other causes of the nephrotic syndrome. Serologic studies, including complement levels, are normal in idiopathic membranous nephropathy (Table 150.2). Once membranous nephropathy is diagnosed, secondary causes should be excluded where possible by careful history and selected laboratory tests, including antinuclear antibodies and screening for hepatitis B and C. Limited screening for occult malignancy with physical examination, chest X-ray, mammography, and stool tests for occult blood is warranted, particularly in patients over the age of 60 years, for whom the prevalence of malignancy in membranous nephropathy may be as high as 20%.

Histopathology

The histology of membranous nephropathy reflects the response of the glomerular basement membrane and visceral epithelial cell to the subepithelial immune complexes. Typically, light microscopy reveals diffuse thickening of the GBM with normal glomerular cellularity and absence of inflammation (Fig. 150.7A). Silver staining demonstrates characteristic spikes of newly synthesized basement membrane projecting between the subepithelial immune deposits (Fig. 150.7B). In early cases, the glomeruli may appear normal on light microscopy, but membranous nephropathy can be distinguished from minimal change disease by immunofluorescence, which reveals bright granular deposits of IgG and C3 along the capillary walls (Fig. 150.7C). As the disease progresses, the immune complexes may become totally enclosed by the newly synthesized basement membrane producing the typically expanded GBM. Electron microscopy reveals electron-dense immune deposits on the subepithelial surface of the GBM and effacement of adjacent visceral epithelial cell foot processes (Fig. 150.7D). Newly synthesized GBM is seen to extend between and around the deposits.

Course and Prognosis

The natural history of untreated idiopathic membranous nephropathy is uncertain in individual cases, and this complicates decisions about therapy. More than 50% of children and about 25% of adults will have a spontaneous complete remission within 5 years. An additional 25% of adults will have sponta-

neous partial remission with continuing subnephrotic proteinuria and stable renal function. The remaining 50% will have persistent nephrotic syndrome, and of these about 25% to 40% will develop end-stage renal failure or die within 5 years. Factors at presentation that are associated with a high risk for disease progression include male sex, older age, hypertension, impaired renal function, and nephrotic range proteinuria (particularly if greater than 10 g per day).

Optimal Management

An important part of treatment is general medical management to decrease complications of the nephrotic syndrome together with nonspecific measures to decrease the degree of proteinuria (see Chapter 135). These include the use of ACE inhibitors, control of hyperlipidemia with lipid-lowering agents, and control of edema with sodium restriction and diuretics. The treatment of idiopathic membranous nephropathy with immunosuppressive medication is controversial. Corticosteroid monotherapy has not been convincingly demonstrated to decrease proteinuria or to improve the long-term renal outcome. Addition of cyclophosphamide or chlorambucil appears to retard progression and diminish proteinuria in some patients. Cyclosporin A induces partial or complete remission of proteinuria in about 40% of patients, who then relapse when it is stopped. Given the uncertain natural history and the risks of long-term cytotoxic agents, a reasonable approach at this time is to reserve them, in combination with corticosteroids, for patients in a high-risk category with progressive renal dysfunction or severely debilitating nephrotic syndrome not responsive to conservative therapies. The cornerstone of treatment of secondary membranous nephropathy is treatment of the associated disease where possible or discontinuation of the offending drug. This usually, but not

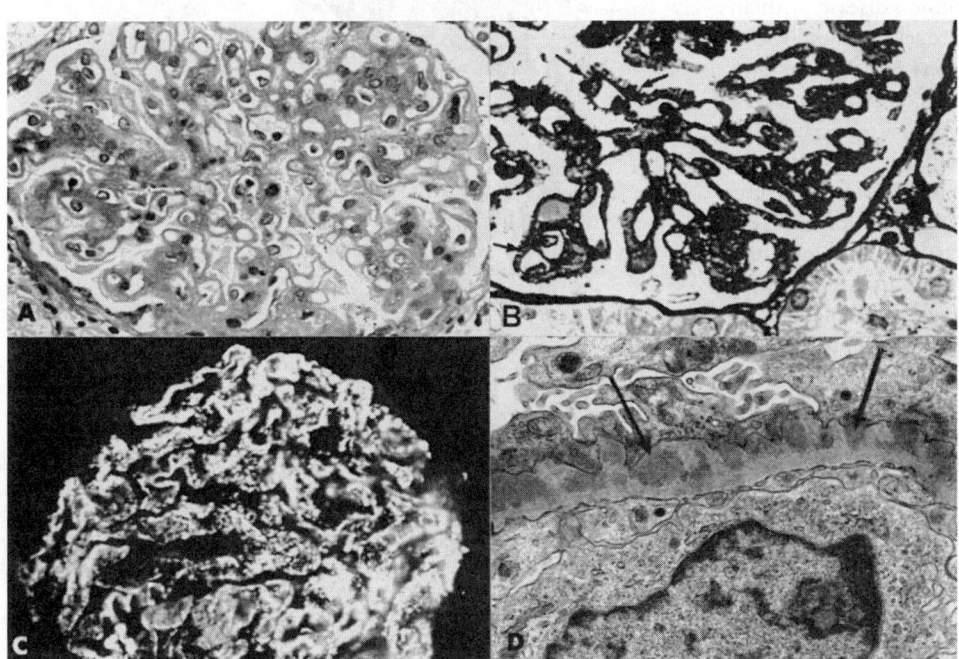

FIGURE 150.7. Membranous nephropathy. **A:** Thickened capillary basement membranes are seen throughout the glomerular tuft (periodic acid–Schiff, ×400). **B:** A silver methenamine stain shows prominent subepithelial spikes (*arrows*, ×625). **C:** Granular deposits of IgG are present along the glomerular capillary loops (antihuman IgG, ×400). **D:** The electron micrograph shows subepithelial deposits (*arrows*) between projections of glomerular basement membrane material (×12,000).

always, leads to resolution of the nephrotic syndrome over time. Membranous nephropathy may recur after renal transplantation, and it is a common cause of de novo nephrotic syndrome in kidneys transplanted into patients with renal failure from other diseases

GLOMERULOPATHIES PRESENTING WITH BOTH NEPHRITIC AND NEPHROTIC FEATURES

MEMBRANOPROLIFERATIVE GLOMERULONEPHRITIS

The membranoproliferative glomerulonephritides (MPGNs) are a heterogeneous group of glomerular diseases that present with nephritic and nephrotic features and have a similar histopathologic appearance at the light microscopic level. There are two main types of MPGN (I and II). Type I is further divided into idiopathic (primary) and secondary forms, the latter being far more common. In addition, some authorities recognize idiopathic MPGN type III as an overlap group having features of MPGN type I and membranous nephropathy. As with other types of glomerular diseases, it is essential to carefully exclude secondary causes using all available clinical, laboratory, and histopathologic data before making a diagnosis of idiopathic MPGN. Secondary causes of MPGN type I include chronic hepatitis C virus infection (discussed in greater detail below), other chronic infections (hepatitis B, HIV, infective endocarditis), systemic autoimmune diseases (SLE, Sjögren's syndrome), malignancy (chronic lymphocytic leukemia, non-Hodgkin's lymphoma), chronic liver disease, and hereditary deficiencies of complement (C1q, C2, C4, C3).

Idiopathic MPGN is a relatively uncommon disease, with an overall incidence of roughly 1% to 2% of renal biopsies. It usually occurs in children and young adults between the ages of 6 and 30 years. It is observed more frequently in whites than in other racial groups, but males and females are affected equally. MPGN type I most often presents with nephrotic range proteinuria or the nephrotic syndrome, accompanied by microscopic hematuria and red blood cell casts, and hypertension. The GFR is normal or only slightly decreased at first, and full-blown nephritic syndrome is unusual. C3 serum levels are low in up to two thirds of individuals together with low C4 (Table 150.2), which indicates classical pathway activation. MPGN type II can also present with nephrotic syndrome but, in addition, the acute nephritic syndrome and oliguric acute renal failure are quite common. The C3 serum levels are nearly always low and remain so for the duration of the illness, whereas classical pathway components (C4 and C2) are normal. This is due to a circulating IgG autoantibody called C3 nephritic factor (C3NeF) that binds to the alternative pathway C3 convertase, protecting it from inactivation by factor H and thereby causing continuous breakdown of C3. Partial lipodystrophy, the loss of fat in the upper half of the body including the face, is frequently present in patients with MPGN type II.

Histopathology

There are a number of characteristic features of MPGN on light microscopy. There is mesangial expansion due to an increase in both mesangial matrix and mesangial cellularity, which may cause a lobulated appearance of the glomerular tuft (Fig. 150.8A). The glomerular capillary wall appears thickened, and

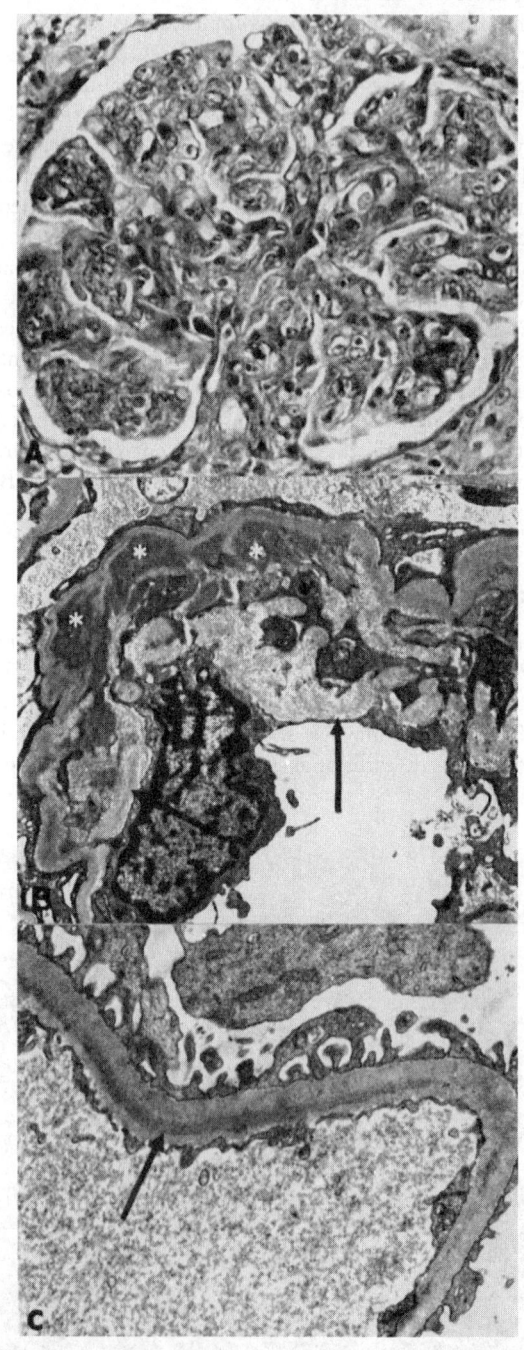

FIGURE 150.8. Membranoproliferative glomerulonephritis. **A:** Mesangial proliferation and basement membrane abnormalities result in an accentuated lobular architecture (periodic acid–Schiff, ×400). **B:** Subendothelial deposits (asterisks) and mesangial interposition (arrows) are seen in an electron micrograph of type I disease (×7,000). **C:** Electron micrograph of an intramembranous dense deposit (arrow) is diagnostic of type II disease (×9,800).

there may be reduplication of the GBM giving rise to the classical "double- contour" or "tram-track" appearance. In idiopathic MPGN type I, subendothelial and mesangial deposits are seen on electron microscopy (Fig. 150.8B). These can be shown by immunofluorescence microscopy to be immune complexes containing IgG and C3, sometimes accompanied by IgM and IgA. In MPGN type II (also known as "dense deposit disease") electron microscopy reveals distinctive ribbon-like, strongly electron-dense deposits in the GBM (Fig. 150.8C). These dense deposits stain for C3 at their margins, but immunoglobulins are absent and there is no evidence that the deposits are immune complexes.

Both the idiopathic and many secondary forms of MPGN type I have many features of immune complex–mediated diseases, including hypocomplementemia, circulating autoantibodies, and cryoglobulinemia. However, a similar morphology is seen in other diseases, such as chronic thrombotic microangiopathy, antiphospholipid antibody syndrome, and light chain deposition disease, in which endothelial injury or deposition of abnormal immunoglobulins is an etiologic factor rather than immune complex formation.

Optimal Management

Secondary causes of MPGN type I should be diligently sought and treated if possible. Idiopathic MPGN type I and MPGN type II in children and young adults is treated with a prolonged course of alternate-day prednisone if there is nephrotic syndrome or renal insufficiency. This sometimes causes severe hypertension, which should be treated to normalize the blood pressure. There is less information on the efficacy of such treatment of MPGN in adults. Diuretics are often required for control of edema, and an ACE inhibitor may help to diminish proteinuria. Initial promise with dipyridamole was not borne out in follow-up studies, and the role of newer platelet inhibitors, immunosuppressive agents, or anticoagulants in the treatment of MPGN is unclear. The MPGN types I and II frequently recur in renal allografts and may lead to graft failure.

HEPATITIS C-ASSOCIATED MPGN AND MIXED CRYOGLOBULINEMIA

Hepatitis C virus (HCV) infection has emerged as a common cause of adult MPGN type I and may be associated with mixed cryoglobulinemia. In the absence of cryoglobulinemia, HCV-associated MPGN presents as a renal-limited disease. Those with mixed cryoglobulinemia have a syndrome that includes weakness, cutaneous vasculitis causing purpura and leg ulcers, large joint arthralgias, and neuropathy. However, not all patients with HCV-related cryoglobulinemia actually develop renal disease. The clinical and laboratory features of MPGN secondary to HCV infection are very similar to those of idiopathic MPGN type I (see above), with the important additional findings of rheumatoid factor and/or mixed cryoglobulins (usually monoclonal IgMκ anti-IgG and polyclonal IgG). Clinical evidence of liver disease may or may not be present. Renal pathology is likewise very similar except that in cryoglobulinemic MPGN electron microscopy may reveal fibrillary "thumb-print" structures indicative of cryoglobulin deposition. The diagnosis of HCV infection is established by the finding of anti-HCV IgG

or HCV RNA in the serum or cryoprecipitates. If the renal failure is rapidly progressive or if the extrarenal disease is severe treatment with corticosteroids, cyclophosphamide and interferon-α is generally employed. In milder and more chronic disease, monotherapy with interferon-α is usually used. Adjunctive therapy with ribavirin is under investigation. Less commonly, cryoglobulinemic MPGN may be associated with lymphoma, myeloma, infective endocarditis, systemic autoimmune diseases, or hepatitis B infection.

SYSTEMIC LUPUS ERYTHEMATOSUS NEPHRITIS

Glomerulonephritis is one of the two most serious complications of SLE, the other being cerebritis (see Chapter 178). Approximately 40% to 80% of unselected patients with SLE have renal involvement as assessed by urinalysis or impairment of renal function, but often the disease is mild. Clinical assessment likely underestimates the actual frequency as histologic evidence of renal disease may be present even when urinalysis is essentially normal. The spectrum of lupus nephritis is wide, encompassing the acute nephritic syndrome, nephrotic syndrome, acute or chronic renal failure, and isolated abnormalities of the urinary sediment. However, proteinuria is the most constant feature, being present in almost every patient with clinical lupus nephritis. Although microscopic hematuria is common, it rarely occurs in isolation. The type of renal involvement may vary over time in an individual patient.

Histopathology and Clinical–Pathologic Correlation

Renal biopsy is an important component of the renal assessment of patients with SLE and is indicated in all cases involving abnormalities of the urine sediment or impaired renal function. There are two main reasons for this. First, it is not possible in an individual patient to predict the renal histology with any accuracy from the clinical presentation, although, in general, more severe histology tends to correlate with more severe clinical disease. Second, in untreated patients the renal histology, as classified by the World Health Organization (WHO), is a powerful predictor of eventual outcome.

Immune complexes are nearly always seen in diseased glomeruli. Although the basis for loss of self-tolerance and the precise composition and mechanism of glomerular immune deposit formation are still under intense investigation, it is likely that these complexes initiate the inflammatory pathways that lead to glomerular injury. It is important to emphasize that tubulointerstitial nephritis and involvement of the intrarenal vasculature (by immune complex deposition, vasculitis, or arteriolar thrombi) may coexist with the glomerular lesions and may be important contributors to renal failure.

The WHO classification recognizes six histologic classes. Although rarely performed, a class I biopsy is normal by light microscopy, sometimes associated with minimal mesangial deposits on immunofluorescence microscopy. Renal function and urinalysis are normal except for mild proteinuria in some cases. Class II (10% to 20% of cases) describes mesangial lupus nephritis in which immune complexes containing IgG, IgM, and C3 are seen only in the mesangium on immunofluorescence and electron microscopy. In Class IIA light microscopy is normal whereas in class IIB mesangial proliferation is seen. Moderate proteinuria is present with or without hematuria. Renal function is usually normal and the long-term prognosis is excellent unless there is transformation to a higher WHO class. Class III (30% to 40% of cases) describes a focal and segmental proliferative lesion on light microscopy, often with areas of necrosis (Fig. 150.9A). On immunofluorescence and electron microscopy there are diffuse mesangial and focal subendothelial immune deposits (Fig. 150.9B). IgG is usually predominant, but IgA and IgM can also be seen and C3, C4, and C1q are usually present. Focal tubulointerstitial nephritis may be present. Proteinuria is common and nephrotic syndrome occurs in about 30% of patients. Class IV (40% to 60% of cases) is diffuse proliferative lupus nephritis, the most aggressive lupus renal lesion. The nephrotic syndrome and impaired renal function are common. The histologic findings are similar to those of class III, except that nearly all of the glomeruli are involved and the lesions

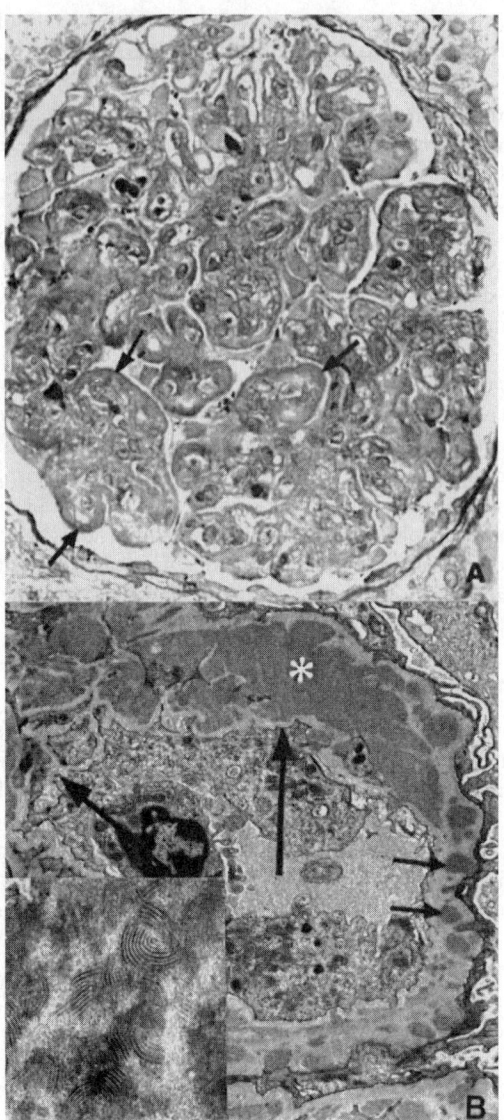

FIGURE 150.10. Diffuse proliferative glomerulonephritis in systemic lupus erythematosus. **A:** Extensive cellular proliferation and thickened glomerular basement membranes are present *(arrows)* giving a "wire loop" appearance (periodic acid–Schiff, ×400). **B:** The electron micrograph reveals large subendothelial *(asterisk)* and intramembranous *(short arrows)* deposits with mesangial interposition *(long arrow, ×5,200)*. A fingerprint pattern within the deposits *(inset)* is seen in some patients with lupus glomerulonephritis (×32,500).

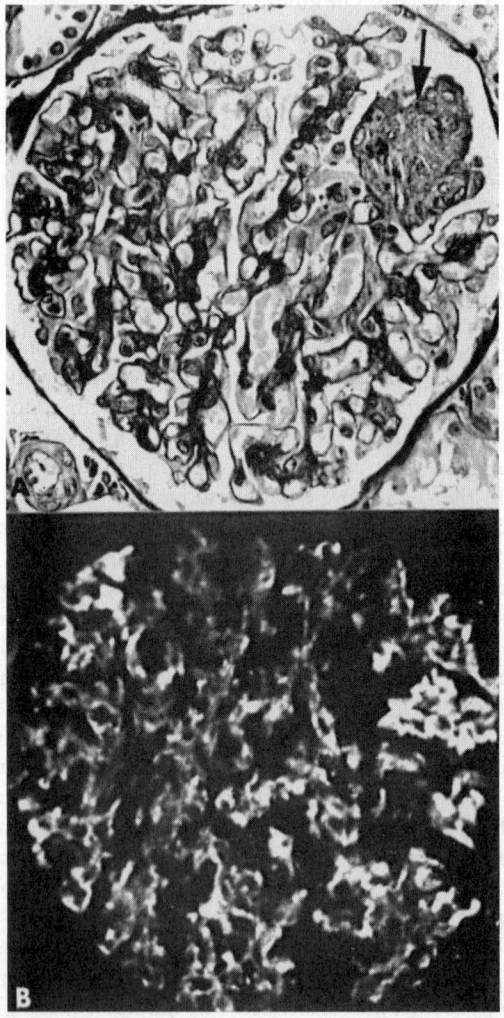

FIGURE 150.9. Focal proliferative glomerulonephritis in systemic lupus erythematosus. **A:** Segmental proliferation *(arrow)* is associated with mild mesangial expansion in a patient with class III glomerulonephritis (periodic acid–Schiff, ×400). **B:** Staining with antihuman IgG shows mesangial and peripheral capillary basement membrane deposits (×400).

themselves are more severe (Fig. 150.10A, B). Crescents may also be present, but inflammation and necrosis of the glomerular tuft is predominant. Tubulointerstitial nephritis is present in up to 75% of cases. Class V represents membranous lupus nephropathy (10% to 15% of cases), so named because of its close similarity both clinically and histologically to idiopathic membranous nephropathy. Glomerular pathology is identical to idiopathic membranous nephropathy, except that the presence of abundant mesangial immune deposits and multiple immunoglobulin isotypes (IgG, IgA, and IgM) on immunohistology favors a diagnosis of lupus nephritis. Tubuloreticular structures in the glomerular endothelial cells may be seen in all classes of lupus nephritis and, if present, strongly suggest the diagnosis of lupus nephritis. The other disease in which such structures are frequently seen is HIV-associated nephropathy. The usual presentation and course of lupus membranous nephropathy is similar to idiopathic membranous nephropathy (see above). Class VI describes a biopsy with diffuse glomerulosclerosis and tubulointerstitial disease. In addition to the above classification, each biopsy is usually assigned a semiquantitative score of activity and chronicity (scarring) based on certain defined histologic criteria. Some studies, but not all, have shown that these scores have predictive value in terms of renal outcome. It is not unusual for transformation to occur over time from one class to another either spontaneously or following treatment. Thus, a renal biopsy performed during an initial evaluation might not reflect the actual histologic lesion at a later time, and repeat biopsies may be required to guide therapy if the clinical presentation changes.

Diagnosis

The diagnosis of SLE as defined by criteria of the American Rheumatism Association is discussed in detail in Chapter 178. The large majority of patients with renal lupus will have SLE by these criteria at the time of diagnosis. An exception to this is membranous lupus nephropathy, which may predate by months the development of extrarenal and serologic features of lupus. Thus, one should exercise a high index of suspicion that a young woman with nephrotic syndrome and apparently idiopathic membranous nephropathy might have lupus nephritis. Separate and apart from the actual diagnosis of SLE is the question of whether there are laboratory tests (other than renal biopsy) that are helpful in determining renal lupus disease activity and predicting renal flares. Although no test is completely sensitive or specific in this regard, high titers of antibodies against double-stranded DNA appear to correlate best with active lupus nephritis. The development of hypocomplementemia with low levels of C3 and C4 might also indicate activity, but some patients have intermittently or chronically low levels without overt clinical activity.

Optimal Management

The optimal treatment of lupus nephritis remains controversial, in large part because controlled clinical trials have not been done comparing many of the treatment options. It is useful to consider treatment in two phases: acute and chronic. In the acute phase, the emphasis is on rapid reduction of disease activity. In the chronic phase, the emphasis is on maintaining suppression of low-grade disease activity and avoiding disease relapses while minimizing the potentially serious side effects associated with the long-term use of different immunosuppressive medications. Because the renal histology is the most powerful predictor of eventual outcome, treatment decisions are based largely on the renal biopsy result. Class II (mesangial) lupus nephritis is often treated with a course of corticosteroid monotherapy in the belief that prognosis might be improved, although no trial has been done to directly compare corticosteroid treatment with no treatment in this group. The optimal treatment of membranous lupus nephritis (class V) is not well defined in large part because of the unpredictable natural history of the disease. Nevertheless, oral corticosteroid therapy, often together with an ACE inhibitor, is frequently used both for symptomatic control of the nephrotic syndrome and for a potential but unproved benefit in delaying the progression of some patients to end-stage renal failure. Cyclophosphamide and cyclosporin A may also be of use in certain individuals. Untreated class III and IV lupus nephritis progress commonly to end-stage renal failure, and it is in these groups that immunosuppressive treatment is clearly indicated. The acute phase is initially treated with high-dose prednisone, sometimes administered intravenously as "pulse" methylprednisolone. This is then tapered to the lowest possible dose consistent with control of renal and systemic disease activity. Most patients with class III or IV lupus nephritis also receive cytotoxic therapy, generally given as monthly doses of intravenous cyclophosphamide for 6 months and then one dose every 3 months for 12 to 18 months. The purpose is to prevent lupus flares and preserve renal function in the long term. Such therapy requires intensive monitoring of the leukocyte count and dose adjustment to avoid excessive leukopenia. Azathioprine is sometimes substituted for cyclophosphamide if the latter is contraindicated or if the patient is unwilling to accept the risks associated with cyclophosphamide therapy, the most important of which are infertility, hemorrhagic cystitis, late neoplasia, and infection. There is no good evidence to support the use of other immunosuppressive agents or plasma exchange in class III and IV lupus nephritis. An important point to keep in mind is that the long-term survival of patients who develop end-stage renal failure secondary to lupus and who are treated with dialysis or transplantation is quite good and does not differ from the long-term survival of patients with lupus nephritis who do not develop end-stage lupus nephritis. Therefore, continued intensification of immunosuppression to improve renal function is not acceptable if it is accompanied by serious actual or potential treatment related side effects, or if there is evidence of advanced chronic renal disease. There is no single test to assess response to therapy; however, anti-double-stranded DNA levels, complement levels, urine sediment, proteinuria, and creatinine clearance are all of use. Despite optimal current therapy, approximately 10% to 20% of patients with proliferative lupus nephritis (class III or IV) will progress to end-stage renal failure. For reasons that are not clear the systemic activity of SLE decreases as patients develop end-stage renal failure, and both the systemic features of SLE and lupus nephritis are uncommon in patients after renal transplantation. Some patients with SLE have circulating antiphospholipid antibodies that can cause thrombotic microangiopathy and can further aggravate lupus nephritis or cause renal damage independently. This condition does not respond to immunosuppression and is best treated by long-term anticoagulation.

ACKNOWLEDGMENT

This work was supported by research grants DK 30932 (D. J. Salant) and DK 02597 (I. R. Rifkin)

BIBLIOGRAPHY

Brady HR, Wilcox CS, eds. *Therapy in nephrology and hypertension: a companion to Brenner and Rector's The Kidney*, 1st ed. Philadelphia: WB Saunders, 1999.

Cameron JS. Lupus nephritis. *J Am Soc Nephrol* 1999;10:413–424.

Cattran DC, ed. Evidence-based recommendations for the management of glomerulonephritis. *Kidney Int* 1999;70:S1–S2.

D'Amico G. Renal involvement in hepatitis C infection: cryoglobulinemic glomerulonephritis. *Kidney Int* 1998;54:650–671.

Donadio JV Jr, Grande JP. Immunoglobulin A nephropathy: a clinical perspective. *J Am Soc Nephrol* 1997;8:1324–1332.

Neilson EG, Couser WG, eds. *Immunologic renal disease*, 1st ed. Philadelphia: Lippincott-Raven Publishers, 1997.

Kelley's Textbook of Internal Medicine, fourth edition. Edited by H. David Humes.
Lippincott Williams & Wilkins, Philadelphia © 2000.

CHAPTER 151

TUBULOINTERSTITIAL DISEASES

CAROLYN J. KELLY
ERIC G. NEILSON

Tubulointerstitial disease has been described as a distinct pathologic entity for over 100 years. During that time, it has been called productive nephritis, granulating nephritis, pyelonephritis, and lymphomatous nephritis. However, none of these labels adequately describes the process or the lesion itself, and today it is commonly called interstitial nephritis. Primary forms of interstitial nephritis are those without identifiable glomerular disease, or lesions in which the interstitial pathology is far more significant than that in the glomerular compartment. Primary interstitial nephritis can be acute or chronic. Acute and chronic interstitial nephritis are typically associated with distinct etiologic factors and will be discussed separately in this chapter. Both acute and chronic forms of interstitial nephritis impair renal function. They can be distinguished on renal biopsy. The acute and chronic forms of interstitial nephritis may be points on a continuum in which an initial inflammatory, cell-mediated response is replaced by progressive fibrosis. In addition to primary forms of interstitial nephritis, most forms of glomerular injury associated with progressive decrements in glomerular filtration rate (GFR) also display significant interstitial pathology. These pathologic changes in the interstitium correlate more closely with the fall in GFR than do the glomerular abnormalities. Thus, interstitial nephritis, in addition to its role as a primary renal lesion, is a final common pathway of all forms of chronic renal failure. This chapter outlines the renal diseases that present as primary interstitial nephritis without significant concomitant glomerular injury.

ACUTE INTERSTITIAL NEPHRITIS

DEFINITION

Acute interstitial nephritis (AIN) is an inflammatory process involving the interstitial compartment of the kidney. This patho-logic abnormality is typically discovered because of the associated clinical findings of acute renal insufficiency.

INCIDENCE AND EPIDEMIOLOGY

Acute interstitial nephritis accounts for about 10% to 15% of cases of acute renal failure. This figure is based on a combination of presumptive and biopsy-proven diagnoses.

ETIOLOGY

The major etiologic categories of AIN are listed in Table 151.1. These include the interstitial nephritis associated with systemic infections or drug reactions, and the truly idiopathic cell-mediated interstitial lesion. Commonly used drugs such as the penicillin family, sulfonamides, some diuretics, cyclosporin A, allopurinol, cimetidine, and nonsteroidal anti-inflammatory drugs (NSAIDs) have all been associated with the development of AIN. Some of these interstitial reactions have been associated with the production of anti–tubular basement membrane (TBM) antibodies, although this is relatively uncommon. These drugs produce classic hypersensitivity reactions, and in many cases these adverse reactions can recur with related pharmacologic derivatives.

Although acute pyelonephritis is frequently associated with

TABLE 151.1.	CAUSES OF ACUTE INTERSTITIAL NEPHRITIS
Drugs	**Infection**
Anti-infectives	Bacteria
Penicillins	*Legionella*
Rifampin	*Streptococcus*
Sulfa derivatives	*Staphylococcus*
Vancomycin	*Brucella*
Ciprofloxacin	*Diphtheria*
Cephalosporins	*Yersinia*
Acyclovir	*Salmonella*
Ethambutol	*Escherichia coli*
Minocycline	*Campylobacter*
Indinavir	Viruses
Nonsteroidal anti-inflammatory drugs	Epstein-Barr
Diuretics	Cytomegalovirus
Thiazides	Hantaan virus
Furosemide	HIV
Triamterene	Herpes simplex
Other	Polyomavirus
Captopril	Hepatitis B
Cimetidine	Other
Ranitidine	*Mycoplasma*
Phenobarbital	*Rickettsia*
Phenindione	*Leptospira*
Phenytoin	Tuberculosis
Allopurinol	Idiopathic
Interleukin-2	Anti-TBM disease
	TINU syndrome

TBM, tubular basement membrane; TINU, tubulointerstitial nephritis with uveitis.

transient interstitial infiltrates containing neutrophils, uncomplicated pyelonephritis is rarely associated with acute renal failure or classic interstitial nephritis. When renal insufficiency develops in the setting of acute pyelonephritis, consideration should be given to the presence of urinary tract obstruction, papillary necrosis, volume depletion, or urosepsis with acute tubular necrosis as the explanation for diminished glomerular filtration. However, AIN can be seen in the setting of systemic infection.

Whereas drugs are clearly the most common etiologic agent for AIN in adults, infections are most important in children. Infections from streptococci and diphtheria are most provocative. Isolated lesions have also been seen with leptospirosis, leprosy, syphilis, toxoplasmosis, measles, infectious mononucleosis, brucellosis, *Mycoplasma* pneumonia, and Rocky Mountain spotted fever, and occasionally as a complication of Legionnaire's disease.

Although acute idiopathic interstitial nephritis is said to be an uncommon lesion, in as many as 30% of patients with AIN no etiologic factor can be identified. Such cases are typically discovered following a renal biopsy for an unexplained decrement in GFR. These patients are often asymptomatic. The interstitial nephritis is presumably autoimmune in etiology. One such group of patients, for example, consists of those with AIN and associated uveitis (TINU syndrome).

PATHOGENESIS

The nephritogenic immune response producing AIN can be arbitrarily divided into three domains. The first, the afferent or antigen-processing phase, begins with the introduction of recognizable antigen and the genetically determined ability to respond to that antigen. The second, the immunoregulatory phase, includes parameters that influence the amplitude and qualitative nature of that immune response. The third and final phase, the efferent or effector phase, includes the mechanisms directly responsible for producing tubulointerstitial damage by antigen-specific T cells, immune complexes, or tissue-specific antibodies.

Several possible immunogenic pathways can produce antigen recognition and immune activation. Several families of endogenous tubulointerstitial antigens can serve as target antigens in interstitial nephritis. Drugs such as penicillin, which bind tubulointerstitial structures, may render them immunogenic. Other drugs, such as sulfamethoxazole, may be able to bind directly to major histocompatibility complex–peptide complexes and thus activate helper T cells. Bacteria from urinary tract infections, which share cross-reactive determinants with renal structures, may direct an immune response to the kidney. Analgesics and heavy metals may initially damage interstitial structures through a toxic mechanism, inducing or exposing nephritogenic neoantigens with secondary immune-mediated damage. Interstitial disease associated with mechanical obstruction may alter structural determinants in the tubulointerstitium and force some of these moieties into renal lymphatics for processing by immunocompetent cells in regional lymph nodes.

Once the immune system is activated by recognition of a nephritogenic antigen, it comes under the control of regulatory processes that modulate the qualitative and quantitative nature of the immune response. The two major regulatory components

of the nephritogenic immune response are anti-idiotypic immunity and T-cell-mediated suppression or induced unresponsiveness. These regulatory processes typically downregulate antibody and cell-mediated responses to nephritogenic antigens and provide a basis for understanding their typically self-limiting nature. The failure to downregulate underlies many forms of experimental interstitial nephritis, which are progressive instead of self-limited. This failure of immune regulation in some instances also determines susceptibility to tubulointerstitial disease.

The effector phase, the final portion of the nephritogenic immune response, encompasses the processes that lead directly to renal injury. These processes are mediated by antibody, immune deposits, complement, and various cell-mediated subpopulations. The presence of a cellular infiltrate is required in the pathologic definition of interstitial nephritis, and mononuclear cells, particularly T lymphocytes, are thought to play a preeminent role in the immunopathogenesis of interstitial damage. The particular combination of cytokines and cytotoxic mediator proteins expressed by infiltrating T cells is important in determining the severity and phenotypic pattern of the resultant interstitial injury.

Although immune deposit–mediated interstitial nephritis was historically thought to be an important feature of parenchymal renal injury, it has been difficult to document this claim consistently by immunofluorescent analysis. Primary interstitial nephritis following the formation of tubulointerstitial immune deposits is unusual. Circulating immune complexes probably do not precipitate to cause immune deposit disease in primary interstitial nephritis because they would probably have precipitated first in glomeruli. Interstitial immune deposits are most consistently seen in "spillover" reactions stemming from immune deposit–mediated glomerulonephritis associated with progressive interstitial injury. Anti-TBM disease producing antibodies and cell-mediated infiltrates is one example of antibody- and cell-mediated processes that are codominantly expressed to produce injury. Complement components have been routinely observed along the TBM in anti-TBM disease. Anti-TBM antibodies can also act as an informational bridge between antigen and the cellular immune response through antibody-dependent, cell-mediated cytotoxicity reactions. Macrophage chemotactic factors are released by the deposition of anti-TBM antibodies. T cells and macrophages are subsequently found in these interstitial lesions. These cells probably damage tubular architecture via degradation of the basement membrane matrix by proteolysis or oxygen radical formation. Cytokines from tubular antigen-reactive T cells can also stimulate fibroblast proliferation and collagen synthesis. Therefore, progressive fibrogenesis may be directly linked to cell-mediated immunity in the overall pathogenesis of interstitial disease.

Most forms of interstitial nephritis, however, involve only the cell-mediated immune response, and T cells in particular probably play a major role. These T cells may alter the tubulointerstitial architecture by release of cytokines or through direct cytotoxic mechanisms of injury. In certain allergic drug reactions, eosinophils may predominate. Eosinophils can be chemotactically attracted to the kidney by T-cell cytokines or by soluble mediators released by mast cells.

CLINICAL FINDINGS

The presentation of AIN is typically that of a sudden decrease in renal function in an otherwise asymptomatic patient who has experienced an intervening illness or has been taking a new medication. Acute interstitial nephritis secondary to medications can occur in patients who have previously tolerated those medications. The clinical distinction among acute tubular necrosis, subtle glomerulonephritis, or AIN may be impossible without a renal biopsy. Several clinical features may help distinguish AIN from these other diagnoses. Factors in the patient's history, such as systemic infection or drug reaction, might suggest interstitial nephritis. The patient with drug-induced AIN commonly has systemic manifestations of an allergic process, including a maculopapular skin rash, fever, or eosinophilia. A prior allergic history is rarely obtained. Skin rash is present in less than 50% of patients, fever occurs in about 75%, and eosinophilia is found in 50% to 75%. The entire triad is present in less than 33% of drug-induced cases, and is distinctly uncommon in patients with AIN secondary to NSAID use. The onset of disease ranges from days (antibiotics) to months (NSAIDs) after initiation of therapy, and in most cases it appears to parallel the kinetics of a primary immune response. In patients previously sensitized to the offending drug, an anamnestic response may occur within several days. The reactivity usually peaks at about 2 weeks. Renal failure generally evolves over several days to several weeks. Bilateral or occasionally unilateral lumbar pain can occur and is probably due to distention of the renal capsule from swelling of the kidney.

LABORATORY FINDINGS

Urinalysis reveals nonnephrotic-range proteinuria, commonly with microscopic hematuria. Gross hematuria has been reported, although the sediment in about 75% of patients shows only moderate amounts of red and white blood cells. White cell casts can be observed (in the absence of infection), but red cell casts are so uncommon that their presence should suggest an alternative diagnosis of glomerulonephritis. The finding of eosinophils in the urine supports the diagnosis of allergic interstitial nephritis but is neither sensitive nor specific for this diagnosis. The absence of eosinophiluria should never preclude the diagnosis of AIN. The magnitude of proteinuria in AIN varies. Nephrotic-range proteinuria occasionally is seen when interstitial lesions are associated with minimal change lesions in the setting of NSAID use. Patients with AIN may be oliguric or nonoliguric and typically have a fractional excretion of sodium greater than 1%.

Although various specific renal tubular disorders, electrolyte abnormalities, and acid–base disturbances tend to occur in chronic interstitial nephritis, the metabolic complications of AIN are, in essence, the general complications associated with acute renal failure. Radiographic imaging procedures such as ultrasound can be performed if clinically indicated to rule out other causes of acute renal failure. There are no noninvasive imaging procedures that strongly indicate the presence of AIN. Gallium scanning, for example, has very limited predictive value.

Because many features of the history, presentation, urinalysis, and laboratory evaluation may lead to indefinite conclusions, a renal biopsy may be indicated in patients with acute renal failure presenting with signs or symptoms suggestive of an interstitial process, or in patients who lack a typical clinical picture for acute tubular necrosis and in whom obstructive nephropathy and prerenal azotemia have been ruled out. The decision to perform a renal biopsy must take into account whether the biopsy interpretation will influence clinical management (see below). Renal biopsy by experienced operators is generally safe, can provide valuable prognostic information, and can serve as a guide to therapy in defined clinical settings.

The most obvious histologic feature of AIN is the absence of glomerular injury and the presence of inflammatory cells in the cortical interstitium. These inflammatory cells are usually a mixture of T lymphocytes, macrophages, and an occasional plasma cell. Eosinophils, neutrophils, basophils, and natural killer cells may be present, and rarely eosinophils predominate. When infection is responsible for AIN, neutrophils are typically present in large numbers. Cellular infiltrates in AIN are profuse throughout the cortical interstitium in association with interstitial edema, disruption of the TBMs, and, in severe cases, the dissolution of normal interstitial architecture. Immune deposits in the interstitium are unusual in primary interstitial nephritis, although some forms of drug-associated AIN are associated with deposition of antibodies to the TBM. Immunofluorescent analysis is not used in the classification of interstitial disease as it is with forms of glomerulonephritis, as the presence of these reactants is uncommon and their pattern of deposition, when present, is not informative with regard to cause, clinical course, or therapy. Pathologic evaluation of the interstitium may reveal an active interstitial nephritis superimposed on preexisting renal injury. In such instances, it can be difficult to determine which is the primary process.

OPTIMAL MANAGEMENT

Most cases of AIN due to drugs or infection resolve after prompt discontinuation of the offending agent or treatment of the infection. The likelihood of full functional recovery, however, depends on the duration of renal failure. Serum creatinine levels at resolution average about 1.0 mg per dL in patients with acute renal failure of less than 2 weeks duration and 3.0 mg per dL in those diagnosed and treated after 3 weeks of acute renal failure. Prolonged, unrecognized interstitial injury usually leads to irreversible chronic interstitial fibrosis. The presence of scattered, patchy infiltrates in AIN is associated with a return of normal renal function, whereas diffuse involvement portends persistent functional impairment. Unless the offending agent can be identified and removed, progression to end-stage disease is likely.

The primary therapeutic principle in the treatment of AIN is to remove or treat any inciting factor. A limited course of high-dose prednisone is generally prudent for biopsy-proven AIN in which renal failure has persisted for more than a week after removal of any inciting factors. A general time frame exists for the use of steroids in AIN, usually after 1 week of rising serum creatinine levels but before several weeks of persistent renal failure. Steroids should be discontinued if no meaningful response is achieved after 3 to 4 weeks of therapy. Cytotoxic drugs may have a role in some treatment regimens, such as in patients with progressive renal failure who are not responding to corticosteroids. Plasmapheresis may be an effective adjuvant therapy in patients with anti-TBM antibodies. There is no reported clinical experience with drug desensitization regimens.

CHRONIC INTERSTITIAL NEPHRITIS

DEFINITION

Chronic interstitial nephritis (CIN) is pathologically defined as an abnormal process involving the interstitial compartment of the kidney characterized by increased interstitial fibrosis, abnormal tubulointerstitial architecture, and, at times, an infiltrate of chronic inflammatory cells. The glomeruli can additionally become sclerotic with advancing renal failure. The clinical characteristics are described below.

INCIDENCE AND EPIDEMIOLOGY

Primary CIN may account for as many as 10% to 20% of patients progressing to end-stage renal disease. In defined geographic areas, this figure may be significantly higher. Examples of geographic variation include the formerly higher incidence of analgesic nephropathy in Australia and some European countries, and the endemic interstitial nephropathy in the Balkans.

ETIOLOGY

Chronic interstitial nephritis is present in all forms of end-stage kidney disease producing interstitial fibrosis with diffuse glomerulosclerosis. The list of etiologies for primary CIN is lengthy (Table 151.2), so only the common causes are discussed below.

PATHOGENESIS

The pathogenesis of chronic interstitial nephritis is not well understood. The pathogenic mechanisms for different forms of chronic interstitial nephritis may not be the same. There is some experimental evidence that interstitial nephritis secondary to heavy metals may involve abnormal immune responses to induced heat-shock proteins.

CLINICAL FINDINGS

Physical impedance of urine flow by prolonged obstruction of the urinary tract can produce progressive interstitial injury and probably is the most common cause of primary CIN. Relief of this obstruction within several weeks of onset typically results

TABLE 151.2.	CAUSES OF CHRONIC INTERSTITIAL NEPHRITIS
Drugs and Toxins	
Analgesics	Lithium
Cadmium	Cyclosporine
Lead	Cisplatin
Nitrosoureas	Chinese "slimming" herbs
Germanium lactate citrate	
Obstructive and Mechanical Disorders	
Tumors	Vesicoureteral reflux
Stones	Outlet obstruction
Metabolic Disturbances	
Hypercalcemia/nephrocalcinosis	Hyperoxaluria
Hypokalemia	Hyperuricemia
Cystinosis	Methylmalonic acidemia
Immune-Mediated	
Renal allograft rejection	Systemic lupus erythematosus
Wegener's granulomatosis	Sjögren's syndrome
Sarcoidosis	Vasculitis
Hematologic Disturbances	
Multiple myeloma	Light-chain deposition disease
Sickle cell disease	Lymphoma
Infection	
HIV	Xanthogranulomatous pyelonephritis
Malacoplakia	Direct infection
Miscellaneous	
Endemic (Balkan) nephropathy	Aging
Radiation nephritis	Hypertension
Progressive glomerular disease	Ischemia
Extracorporeal shock wave lithotripsy	

HIV, human immunodeficiency virus.

in complete recovery of renal function without significant pathologic consequences. Obstructive nephropathy is discussed in more detail in Chapters 138 and 158.

Reflux nephropathy is the second most common anatomic abnormality associated with CIN (see Chapter 161). Although urinary tract infection or acute pyelonephritis alone is not considered a cause of interstitial nephritis, patients with reflux and recurrent urinary tract infection may develop chronic interstitial lesions. For their condition, the term *chronic pyelonephritis with cortical scarring* is most applicable. Reflux without concomitant urinary tract infection has not been shown to cause pyelonephritis in humans. Most persons with this form of CIN are young children. They often have hypertension, and, unless the injury is arrested early, progressive deterioration in renal function is the rule. Significant proteinuria is often present, usually associated with the histologic lesion of focal glomerulosclerosis. Prolonged antibiotic therapy with sterilization of the urinary tract is associated with the arrest of the pathologic process; surgical correction of reflux has an unclear effect on the progression of renal injury. Total unilateral nephrectomy is required only rarely.

Heavy analgesic use can be associated with renal failure and CIN. How commonly it occurs is controversial and may depend on the region or country of residence. To meet the criteria for this diagnosis, patients must have taken phenacetin, acetaminophen, or aspirin-containing compounds for at least several years, in total cumulative quantities of more than 1 kg and often more than 3 kg. Very often patients have ingested mixtures of these compounds, but because there are no pathognomonic clinical or laboratory findings, the diagnosis rests on a suggestive history and repeated questioning of the patient and family members. Many patients with analgesic nephropathy are women with chronic headaches. Many are anemic and have hypertension. Most patients have chronic persistent pyuria and a defect in urine concentrating ability. The most common radiographic findings are nonspecific (such as cortical scarring or shrunken kidneys), but the documentation of papillary necrosis with a relevant history can strongly suggest this diagnosis. Because abnormal serum creatinine levels associated with advanced renal failure are seen in fewer than 15% of patients followed for more than 10 years, the treatment of analgesic nephropathy requires only the withdrawal of the offending agents. Although this can be difficult to accomplish, it offers the best hope for stabilizing or improving renal function.

Environmental exposure to heavy metals is an important cause of CIN. Lead and cadmium are heavy-metal nephrotoxins that can damage proximal tubular cells and impair oxidative and phosphorylative functions. Many patients with heavy-metal poisoning develop a Fanconi-like syndrome with aminoaciduria, phosphaturia, and renal glycosuria. Prolonged moderate exposure seems to be a critical feature predisposing to renal damage. Lead nephropathy has been observed after exposure to lead-based paints or after ingestion of lead-containing "moonshine" whiskey. Cadmium nephropathy has been observed in battery production workers and those involved in zinc refining, plastics, pigment or alloy production, and steel-plating processes. Exposure to lead can be detected by measuring urinary lead excretion after ethylenediaminetetraacetic acid chelation or by monitoring

urinary porphyrins that may indicate altered globin metabolism. Cadmium may be monitored in the serum and urine and in hair samples. Determining the heavy-metal body burden using serum and urine tests is imprecise, however, and documentation of substantial exposure can be a diagnostic challenge in persons without an obvious exposure history. Therapy involves removal from the toxic source and, in selected patients, chelation therapy.

Arteriolar nephrosclerosis producing interstitial nephritis is associated with sustained, significant hypertension. Such hypertension can be benign or malignant, and some of the earliest and most pronounced lesions occur in the renal blood vessels. Malignant hypertension results in a subacute necrotizing arteriolar lesion, whereas the changes associated with benign nephrosclerosis include reduplication of the internal elastic lamina of the interlobular arteries, prominent afferent arteriolar wall thickening, and diffuse tubulointerstitial damage. The interstitial changes associated with these vascular lesions are thought to be secondary to ischemia. Ischemic sclerosis of glomeruli also occurs with advanced disease. Because the tubulointerstitium is more sensitive to diminished blood flow, changes there precede glomerular senescence. The treatment of this problem centers on blood pressure control.

LABORATORY FINDINGS

Because the process of CIN is subacute and indolent, there is time to observe specific abnormalities in tubular function that are not clinically obvious during the abbreviated course of acute interstitial injury. Patients with CIN are also more likely to develop clinical complications from one or more of these abnormalities in tubular function than are patients with the less chronic forms of renal failure.

The ability to concentrate the urine and thus conserve free water is universally impaired in patients with chronic interstitial disease, so that polyuria and nocturia are common clinical complaints. Hypernatremia does not usually develop because thirst mechanisms are intact. The ability to decrease urinary sodium excretion in response to a decrease in dietary sodium intake or volume depletion is often impaired in chronic interstitial disease. The most dramatic examples of this defect are the rare cases of salt-wasting nephropathy. The typical patient with chronic interstitial renal disease has a less severe disturbance in renal sodium conservation, but in some circumstances, clinically significant volume depletion can develop after vomiting, diarrhea, overzealous sodium restriction, or use of diuretics. When volume depletion occurs, a further decrease in renal function ensues.

Proximal tubular dysfunction producing a Fanconi syndrome with bicarbonate wasting, proximal renal tubular acidosis, glycosuria, phosphaturia, and aminoaciduria is most often associated with renal involvement caused by multiple myeloma and light-chain nephropathy. Other, less common etiologic factors include anti-TBM disease, heavy-metal nephropathy, paroxysmal nocturnal hemoglobinuria, and immune complex glomerulonephritis.

The distal tubule is responsible for urinary acidification, aldosterone responsiveness, and fine homeostatic adjustments in sodium and potassium balance. When dysfunction occurs at this level of the nephron, various clinical problems can appear. These include distal renal tubular acidosis, an aldosterone-resistant state with hyperkalemia and hyperchloremic metabolic acidosis, and apparent salt wasting. Any of these can be seen in obstructive nephropathy, either during or after relief of obstruction. Aldosterone resistance has also been reported in amyloidosis and sickle cell disease. Relative salt wasting is typically seen during postobstructive diuresis and medullary cystic disease. Isolated defects in concentrating ability, indicating disruption of the medullary gradient or dysfunction of the collecting tubule, have also been associated with certain tubulointerstitial nephropathies. These include analgesic abuse, sickle-cell disease, and cystic disease of the kidney.

The hyperchloremic metabolic acidosis associated with CIN is probably related to the progressive loss of interstitial mass and the associated impairment of renal ammonia production. If the GFR is not too low, the first morning urine in patients with a defect in ammonia production has a pH level below 6.0. Although there is poor ammonium excretion with a 24-hour acid load, these patients have normal fractional excretion of bicarbonate, excluding a proximal tubular defect. Eventually, progressive nephron loss results in an anion gap acidosis, and the hyperchloremia disappears. Hyperkalemia is typically present in these patients as well. The hyperkalemia is often out of proportion to the degree of renal failure and is probably related to a generalized impairment of distal tubular function.

In addition to regulating the transport properties of the renal tubules, the interstitium also plays a role in hormone metabolism. With progressive interstitial fibrosis, erythropoietin and renin secretion, as well as 1-hydroxylation of 25-hydroxyvitamin D, are impaired. There is a general impression that the anemia associated with CIN is more marked than that seen with primary progressive glomerular disease. Osteodystrophy may also be more severe in patients with chronic interstitial nephropathy.

OPTIMAL MANAGEMENT

By definition, CIN is an indolent, very slowly progressing form of interstitial nephritis that can evolve to end-stage renal disease after many years of follow-up. The treatment of the underlying disease or the elimination of inciting factors can contribute to the attenuation of progressive disease. Generally, there are no anti-inflammatory drugs or immunosuppressive agents that are appropriate to administer in this setting. Chronic fibrogenesis is probably irreversible, and the risk/benefit ratio of aggressive chemotherapy does not warrant its use. Good control of blood pressure may alter the rate of progression in hypertensive patients with CIN.

BIBLIOGRAPHY

Jones CL, Eddy AA. Tubulointerstitial nephritis. *Pediatr Nephrol* 1992;6: 572–586.
Kelly CJ, Tomaszewski J, Neilson EG. Immunopathogenic mechanisms of tubulointerstitial injury. In: Tisher CC, Brenner BM, eds. *Renal pathology*. Philadelphia: JB Lippincott, 1994:699–722.
Kleinknecht D. Interstitial nephritis, the nephrotic syndrome, and chronic renal failure secondary to nonsteroidal anti-inflammatory drugs. *Semin Nephrol* 1995;15:228–235.
Laberke H-G, Bohle A. Acute interstitial nephritis: correlations between clinical and morphological findings. *Clin Nephrol* 1980;14:263–273.
Michel DM, Kelly CJ. Acute interstitial nephritis. *J Am Soc Nephrol* 1998; 9:506–515.
Murray MD, Brater DC. Renal toxicity of the nonsteroidal antiinflammatory drugs. *Annu Rev Pharmacol Toxicol* 1993;33:435–465.
Neilson EG. Pathogenesis and therapy of interstitial nephritis. *Kidney Int* 1989;35:1257–1270.
Perneger TV, Whelton PK, Klag MJ. Risk of kidney failure associated with the use of acetaminophen, aspirin, and nonsteroidal antiinflammatory drugs. *N Engl J Med* 1994;331:1675–1679.
Sandler DP, Smith JC, Weinberg CR, et al. Analgesic use and chronic renal disease. *N Engl J Med* 1989;320:1238–1243.
Wedeen RP, Batuman V. Tubulointerstitial nephritis induced by heavy metals and metabolic disturbances. *Contemp Issues Nephrol* 1983;10: 211–228.

Kelley's Textbook of Internal Medicine, fourth edition. Edited by H. David Humes. Lippincott Williams & Wilkins, Philadelphia © 2000.

CHAPTER 152

VASCULAR DISEASES OF THE KIDNEY

WILLIAM L. HENRICH

EMBOLIZATION OF THE RENAL ARTERIES

The term *renal artery obstruction* refers to a heterogeneous group of diseases that cause obstruction to the main renal artery or its branches by embolic or atherothrombotic phenomena. Embolic diseases of the renal artery can cause silent and insidious loss of renal function or fulminant acute renal failure with oligoanuria, fever, flank pain, and hematuria.

ETIOLOGY, PATHOGENESIS, AND CLINICAL FEATURES

Emboli to the main renal artery or its branches most often occur in the setting of cardiac disease (myocardial infarction, valvular heart disease, or atrial fibrillation). The presence of a dilated left ventricle or a left ventricular aneurysm predisposes the patient to the formation of a mural thrombus, which may embolize. Rheumatic valvular disease also is associated with peripheral embolization, as is atrial fibrillation. Septic embolization from bacterial endocarditis used to be the most common cause of renal artery embolism. Chest, abdominal, flank, and back pain are present in most patients with emboli of cardiac origin, and nausea, vomiting, and fever occur in half the patients. Laboratory abnormalities may include leukocytosis, hematuria, proteinuria, azotemia, and increased levels of lactic acid dehydrogenase, serum glutamic oxaloacetic transaminase, serum glutamic pyruvic transaminase, and alkaline phosphatase.

Atheroembolism of the kidneys involves the embolization of small cholesterol crystals or microemboli from the surface of existing ulcerated plaques, or the detachment of atheromatous plaques from the intimal surface of the aorta. These emboli travel peripherally and cause occlusion of the microcirculation; the arcuate, interlobular, and terminal renal arteries, and even the glomeruli, may be affected. These cholesterol atheroemboli are seen in patients with extensive aortic atherosclerosis and may occur spontaneously or, more commonly, after aortic, carotid, or coronary angiography, especially if the femoral route for arterial puncture has been used. This disease also may be seen after aortic reconstructive surgery. The antemortem diagnosis is difficult to make, and autopsy studies suggest that the disease is more common than previously thought. Recent studies have suggested that some patients with extensive aortic and renal atherosclerosis have small showers of atheroemboli intermittently. This may contribute to a gradual loss of renal function in such patients.

The disease may present as an acute or catastrophic form with abdominal and back pain, acute hypertension, agitation, diarrhea (often bloody), foot and leg pain, extremity numbness or paralysis, skin discoloration (livedo reticularis, or "purple toes"), acute renal failure, and even hypotension and death. The chronic or noncatastrophic form also is called the *multiple cholesterol emboli syndrome* (MCES). This syndrome occurs most commonly after aortic surgery and is marked by slowly progressive renal failure. There may be episodic or malignant hypertension, acute pancreatitis, myopathy, peritonitis and ischemic colitis, livedo reticularis, and gangrene of the toes and feet (in as many as 30% of patients). Laboratory abnormalities may include leukocytosis, particularly eosinophilia (reported in as many as 70% of patients), an elevated erythrocyte sedimentation rate, decreased platelets (disseminated intravascular coagulation may be seen), and azotemia.

Multiple cholesterol emboli syndrome may be confused with polyarteritis nodosa, allergic vasculitis, subacute bacterial endocarditis, and left atrial myxoma. The cause of the eosinophilic response to MCES is not fully understood, but may be analogous to a foreign bodylike reaction in tissue. Atheroembolic disease should be suspected when the typical findings are seen after aortic surgery or angiography, especially if the patient has known atherosclerotic disease or widespread arterial bruits. Tissue demonstration of cholesterol crystals confirms the diagnosis, but these cannot always be obtained. The diagnosis may be suggested strongly by the finding of cholesterol crystals in the retinal arteries (Hollenhorst plaques).

Definitive diagnosis of renal embolic disease is made by renal angiography, but the less invasive dynamic ^{99m}Tc pertechnetate renal flow scan occasionally may prove diagnostic by demonstrating decreased flow to all or part of the kidney. Computed tomography of the kidneys with contrast medium enhancement may show focal or generalized decreased attenuation of the renal tomogram, or even a rim of cortical enhancement around the area of embolization. Magnetic resonance imaging with the use of paramagnetic contrast agents may be useful in defining the extent of tissue ischemia and disruption of blood flow. The degree of renal damage depends on the size of the embolus, the presence of collateral circulation, and the interval between diagnosis and therapy.

TREATMENT AND COURSE

The most efficacious treatment of embolization of the large renal arteries has not been established. No clear difference exists between medical therapy with anticoagulants and surgical embolectomy, with the exception that surgical mortality rates range from 11% to 25%. Fibrinolytic agents have been used successfully, as has percutaneous transluminal angioplasty in a few cases. Although the algorithm requires confirmation, one group has suggested that unilateral embolization with a functioning contralateral kidney is approached best by fibrinolytic therapy and the use of transluminal angioplasty, followed by anticoagulation. For patients with embolization to a single functioning kidney or those with bilateral embolization, initial therapy with fibrinolytic therapy and transluminal angioplasty is recommended; if there is no response, surgical embolectomy should be considered. Further study of this approach is needed.

■ RENAL VEIN THROMBOSIS

Renal vein thrombosis (RVT) is defined as thrombosis of the main renal vein or one of its tributaries.

ETIOLOGY, PATHOGENESIS, AND FREQUENCY

Renal vein thrombosis occurs most commonly as a complication of the nephrotic syndrome and usually is associated with membranous nephropathy, although it also may be seen with membranoproliferative glomerulonephritis, amyloidosis, renal allograft rejection, and minimal change disease. Cases also have been reported from the surgical literature in patients with no evidence of renal disease. The syndrome may be present as an acute or chronic problem; the chronic presentation predominates. The exact incidence cannot be established with certainty and ranges from 2% to 33% of cases of nephrotic syndrome. The duration of the nephrotic syndrome, amount of albuminuria, use of corticosteroid and diuretic therapy, and type of venography used to diagnose RVT all contribute to this wide range in incidence.

CLINICAL FEATURES

The nephrotic syndrome is associated with alterations in the coagulation system. These alterations lead to an increased incidence of thromboembolism, ranging from RVT to pulmonary thrombosis, deep venous thrombosis of the lower extremity, peripheral thrombophlebitis, and arterial occlusion. Elevated levels of factors V, VII, VIII, IX, and X and of fibrinogen may contribute to the hypercoagulable state seen in the nephrotic syndrome. In addition, thrombocytosis and enhanced platelet aggregation may be seen. Thromboplastin levels may be increased and antithrombin III levels may be low in some patients. Volume depletion caused by diuretics and an increase in the hypercoagulable state caused by corticosteroid therapy also may predispose to the development of RVT. In addition, RVT may occur after blunt abdominal trauma, dehydration in infants, and the use of oral contraceptive agents.

Renal vein thrombosis is most often a silent syndrome. Chronic RVT usually is not associated with loss of renal function and in the absence of pulmonary involvement gives little clue to its presence. Preservation of renal function depends on the degree of collateral blood flow to the kidney and the amount of recanalization of the renal vein. The presence of RVT should be suspected when pulmonary embolism, unexplained loss of renal function, or a large increase in proteinuria occurs.

DIAGNOSIS

Renal venography should be performed when there is a strong clinical suspicion of the diagnosis based on the foregoing findings. Renal venography remains the best test available to make the diagnosis. It is difficult to interpret, however, because of the large volume of blood that perfuses the kidney, making adequate renal vein contrast imaging difficult. Renal ultrasonic scanning and Doppler ultrasonography may prove to be useful and reliable diagnostic tests but require further study. Computed tomography with contrast media also is a promising diagnostic tool, but prospective studies are needed to evaluate its sensitivity and specificity.

TREATMENT AND COURSE

Anticoagulant therapy with heparin for 5 to 7 days followed by therapy with sodium warfarin is indicated in patients with RVT, particularly if pulmonary embolism has occurred. Long-term therapy is advocated by many for as long as the nephrotic syndrome is present because recurrent RVT and pulmonary emboli are seen shortly after discontinuation of anticoagulant therapy. Renal function in the setting of acute RVT typically improves with treatment, although this may require 6 months. There is no indication for surgical thrombectomy. The role of fibrinolytic therapy is intriguing but relatively unstudied. Similarly, the use of antiplatelet therapy in nephrotic patients with RVT probably is safe but its efficacy has not been tested rigorously.

■ HEMOLYTIC-UREMIC SYNDROME

Hemolytic-uremic syndrome (HUS) is a disease that is closely related to thrombotic thrombocytopenic purpura. It is characterized by renal failure, thrombocytopenia, and a microangiopathic hemolytic anemia. The kidney is the target organ of vascular endothelial damage in HUS; in thrombotic thrombocytopenic purpura, however, there is widespread vascular endothelial damage with extensive brain involvement. Hemolytic-uremic syndrome was first described in children but it also occurs in adults. The overall prognosis of HUS is better in children than in adults, and is better than that of thrombotic thrombocytopenic purpura.

ETIOLOGY, PATHOGENESIS, AND CLINICAL FEATURES

Childhood Hemolytic-Uremic Syndrome

The usual presentation of HUS in childhood typically follows an episode of acute nonfebrile gastroenteritis. Clinically, the dis-order presents abruptly with bleeding (melena, hematemesis, or hematuria) and oliguria, with anuria seen in 30% of patients. This is the most common cause of acute renal failure in children, and is more common in whites than blacks. Petechiae, scleral icterus, hyperbilirubinemia, hepatosplenomegaly, congestive heart failure, and hypertension also are common. The peripheral blood smear shows evidence of a microangiopathic hemolytic anemia. Hemolytic-uremic syndrome usually occurs in summer and fall, and may occur as single cases or as small clusters of cases. Although the exact pathogenesis of HUS is unknown, it is strongly believed that vascular endothelial cell damage is the primary pathologic event. However, thrombocytopenia, enhanced platelet aggregation, and the presence of an abnormal factor VIII level also contribute. A strong association has been established between HUS and veracytotoxin-producing *Escherichia coli* (VTEC). Veracytotoxins are potent protein exotoxins that can produce an irreversible cytopathic effect in certain cells, particularly endothelial cells. Hemolytic-uremic syndrome developed in 7% of a pediatric population with VTEC infection and in 24% of an elderly nursing home population with VTEC infection, most of whom died. The reservoir for VTEC is primarily animal intestinal tracts, and foods of animal origin probably are responsible for human infection. The toxin appears to bind to specific glycoprotein receptors on renovascular endothelial cells and then inactivates ribosomes, killing them.

Adult Hemolytic-Uremic Syndrome

Adult HUS has a more varied presentation and the diagnosis may not be obvious initially. The renal function may decline subacutely, there may be minimal evidence of hemolysis, and thrombocytopenia may be minimal. There also may be an acute presentation with a severe hemolytic anemia, profound thrombocytopenia, and rapid loss of renal function. Hemolytic-uremic syndrome may be seen after infection with VTEC or other bacterial agents, such as *Shigella, Salmonella typhi, Campylobacter, Yersinia, Streptococcus pneumoniae,* or *Legionella,* and after rickettsial, viral, or fungal infection. A strong association exists between HUS and the use of mitomycin C as anticancer therapy. Thirty-five percent of patients with HUS occurring after the use of mitomycin C are cancer-free at the time of diagnosis, and the development of HUS often coincides closely with the transfusion of blood products. Noncardiogenic pulmonary edema occurs in 65% of these patients. Hemolytic-uremic syndrome also is seen in patients using oral contraceptives and in women in the postpartum period. The presentation usually is acute, and the patient's condition deteriorates rapidly. Hemolytic-uremic syndrome has also followed cisplatin therapy and the disorder is recognized to occur during therapy with cyclosporin as an antirejection medicine. In this regard, recent reports point out that HUS has developed following liver, kidney, and heart transplantation. A hereditary form of HUS may appear in children and adults, occasionally causing recurrent episodes of disease in children, and typically follows an autosomal recessive inheritance pattern. An immunologic form of HUS also occurs that is associated with a low C3 complement concentration. Finally, HUS also has been seen in patients with scleroderma, systemic lupus erythematosus, and malignant hypertension, and in those who have received renal irradiation or immunosuppressive therapy with cyclosporin A.

LABORATORY AND PATHOLOGIC FINDINGS

Azotemia is present and the microangiopathic anemia usually is severe. There are obvious signs of hemolysis with anemia, fragmented helmet and burr cells, reticulocytosis, elevated lactic acid dehydrogenase and bilirubin levels, and a low haptoglobin value. Renal damage always is present and acute renal failure occurs in more than 90% of patients. Thrombocytopenia is a constant finding. The term *thrombotic microangiopathy* is used to describe the renal pathologic process, especially in children. There is widespread renal capillary wall thickening and capillary thrombi. In adults and older children, arteriolar necrosis and interlobular arterial thrombosis are seen. Pure glomerular disease, arterial disease, or a combination of the two may be seen.

TREATMENT AND COURSE

The most important part of the therapy for HUS is supportive, with vigorous control of blood pressure, fluid and electrolytes, hemorrhage, and azotemia, using dialysis as needed. There are no large prospective trials of therapy for HUS. Exchange transfusion, plasmapheresis, and corticosteroids have been associated with remission of the disease, with normalization of the hematologic abnormalities often occurring. Vitamin E therapy has been successful in children. The use of anticoagulant therapy with heparin has been proposed for the postpartum form of HUS but may worsen the hemorrhagic complications of the disease. Aggressive therapy with heparin, antiplatelet drugs, converting enzyme inhibitors, and plasmapheresis seems most justified in postpartum renal failure and HUS occurring after the use of oral contraceptives.

■ SCLERODERMA

Scleroderma is a collagen vascular disease in which the predominant pathologic event is progressive sclerosis of connective tissue and the vascular system (see Chapter 179). Patients with renal scleroderma usually have either an insidious or a rapidly progressive course. The insidious course is characterized by mild azotemia, hypertension, or nonnephrotic-range proteinuria. The rapidly progressive course is marked by severe hypertension and steady renal deterioration over weeks to months, finally progressing to end-stage renal disease. The hypertension may be accompanied by retinopathy, neurologic abnormalities (e.g., seizures, coma), or heart failure. These patients probably represent less than 10% of all patients with scleroderma. Rare reports have surfaced of a rapid decline in renal function without an elevation of blood pressure. In addition, a recent study has pointed out that black women appear more vulnerable to developing systemic complications than white women. The less severe or progressive form of renal involvement is seen in 15% to 37% of patients. The renin–angiotensin system appears to play a key role in the pathogenesis of renal failure and hypertension in renal

scleroderma. The kidney seems particularly vulnerable to the vasoconstrictive effects of angiotensin, which the vascular lesion is likely to stimulate. Once this cycle of angiotensin stimulation begins, more renal ischemia (and a decline in renal function) and more hypertension are likely to ensue.

In view of the accelerated decline in renal function produced by the renin–angiotensin system, it is not surprising that successful treatment of sclerodermatous renal crisis has involved angiotensin-converting enzyme inhibition (see Chapter 179). Blood pressure control constitutes the primary therapy in this disorder. Corticosteroid therapy has not proven helpful. Dialysis is useful in prolonging survival in those who progress to chronic renal failure. These patients have major difficulties with vascular access and continued severe hypertension. Bilateral nephrectomy has been used to control poorly responsive hypertension. Patients may undergo successful renal transplantation, but hypertension may be difficult to control. Recurrence of the disease in the allograft has been reported, but this is not a contraindication to transplantation.

■ ARTERIAL NEPHROSCLEROSIS

The term *arterial nephrosclerosis* refers to the progressive obliteration of the renovascular bed that occurs in systemic hypertension. As a cause of end-stage renal disease, hypertension and nephrosclerosis account for between 15% and 30% of new patients entering dialysis units. Hypertension accelerates the cessation of renal function in all primary renal diseases; hence, hypertension worsens the prognosis in primary and secondary nephropathies and in interstitial renal diseases. Hypertension occurs in up to 80% of patients with chronic renal insufficiency and may hasten the progression of renal disease in these patients. Nephrosclerosis is important both as a primary disease and as a disease that complicates other primary illnesses. Hypertension undoubtedly is the most important and treatable cause of renal insufficiency.

PATHOGENESIS

The kidneys of hypertensive patients usually are reduced in size and may weigh as little as 120 g. The cortex is thin and scars often are visible over the renal surface. Involved glomeruli may be completely hyalinized or wrinkled and shrunken in appearance. Larger blood vessels show fibroelastic thickening of the internal elastic lamina. A hyalinized thickening of the entire wall may occur in patches along the vessel. All this is accompanied by a fine fibrosis with or without chronic inflammatory cells. In malignant hypertension, the glomeruli show fibrinoid necrosis in the capillary tuft in continuity with a necrotic afferent arteriole. Epithelial crescents also may be present, depending on the duration of the disease. Fibrinoid necrosis of arterioles is the hallmark of malignant hypertension. In interlobular arteries, concentric thickening is seen. Recent studies suggest that hyalinization of renal arterioles may be a marker for development of atherosclerosis in other locations, particularly the coronary arteries.

TREATMENT AND COURSE

Antihypertensive therapy is beneficial in decreasing hypertension-related morbidity and mortality in patients with already existing end-organ damage or risk factors (black race, diabetes mellitus, hyperlipoproteinemia, cigarette smoking) and in patients with moderate to severe hypertension. The benefits of therapy in patients with mild hypertension and no risk factors are less clear. Although many physicians still use the stepped-care approach to therapy for hypertension, there is increasing emphasis on using drugs that have a favorable side effect profile (no alteration in lipid status, improvement in left ventricular compliance) and especially in monotherapy with calcium channel blockers, vasodilators, and angiotensin-converting enzyme inhibitors.

▊ SICKLE CELL NEPHROPATHY

ETIOLOGY AND INCIDENCE

The term *sickle cell nephropathy* refers to changes in the kidneys of patients who are heterozygous or homozygous for the hemoglobin S gene. These changes may cause acute or chronic symptoms and signs. About 8% of African-Americans are heterozygotes and 0.2% are homozygotes. American whites and persons of Italian, Greek, or Middle Eastern descent may carry the hemoglobin S gene.

PATHOGENESIS AND CLINICAL FEATURES

Hemoglobin S polymerizes during deoxygenation, internal red blood cell viscosity increases, and an irregular sickle-shaped red blood cell shape occurs. Hypertonicity accentuates this process. These conditions of deoxygenation and hypertonicity exist in the renal medulla; hence, sickling of red blood cells is prominent in this location. Renal function related to an intact medulla, such as renal concentration and acidification, is impaired in this disorder. Even worse, scarring may result from ischemia to the region; therefore, interstitial fibrosis and papillary necrosis are features of the disease. Medullary changes also include local edema, tubular atrophy, and round cell infiltrates. Several clinical consequences of sickle cell disease are listed in Table 152.1.

One interesting feature of the pathology of sickle cell nephropathy is the association of the disease with glomerular lesions. Proteinuria (including the nephrotic syndrome), hypertension, and hematuria are present in many patients, particularly children. One study observed that about 25% of patients with sickle cell disease have proteinuria. Glomerular enlargement and perihilar focal sclerosis were common lesions. Membranoproliferative glomerulonephritis with granular capillary deposits has been reported. Cryoprecipitable deposits of renal tubular epithelial antigen–antibody complexes have been detected in the circulation of some patients. An immune complex, normocomplementemic glomerulonephritis, may occur that is related to the deposition of renal tubular antigen–antibody complexes. The hypothesis that initial damage to the tubular structures of the medulla incites this reaction has been entertained. Other typical lesions described in patients with sickle cell nephropathy who

TABLE 152.1.	RENAL INVOLVEMENT IN SICKLE CELL DISEASE

Medullar and Tubular Disorders

Polyuria: Decreased maximum urinary concentration ability. Renal tubular acidosis type IV, incomplete; type IV and type I also described

Papillary necrosis: May be exacerbated by use of nonsteroidal anti-inflammatory drugs

Hematuria

Small infarcts

Cortical and Glomerular Disorders

Nephrotic syndrome: Due to glomerular sclerosis (? from hyperfiltration); membranous, membranoproliferative, and nil lesions also described (immune complex lesions)

Chronic renal failure: Unusual, progressive sclerosis

Acute renal failure: Clinical course similar to that of rhabdomyolysis; nonsteroidal anti-inflammatory drugs may provoke this

Hematuria: Possibly due to hyperfiltration

have proteinuria or the nephrotic syndrome are focal sclerosis and mesangial proliferation.

Glomerular filtration and renal blood flow in patients with sickle cell nephropathy are highly dependent on the presence of vasodilator prostaglandins. As a result, these patients may be vulnerable to the effects of nonsteroidal anti-inflammatory agents, even when renal function is normal. Type I, type IV, and incomplete type IV renal tubular acidosis also have been described. Continued intramedullary sickling eventually leads to a loss of concentrating ability. This complication may be seen in school-aged children but is more prominent in older persons. As long as the glomerular filtration rate is preserved, renal sodium wasting is rare and free water clearance remains normal. The loss in concentrating ability is believed to be related to the washout of medullary solute secondary to damage of the vasa recta, decreased water permeability in the distal tubule, or both. Exogenous vasopressin administration has no effect on improving the concentrating ability.

Other clinical features of sickle cell nephropathy include hematuria in homozygotes (11%), in heterozygotes (62%), and in patients with hemoglobin SC disease (27%). Hematuria most commonly occurs from the left kidney and is not necessarily bilateral. The presence of asymptomatic bacteriuria is increased in pregnant women with sickle cell disease, but the incidence of pyelonephritis is not increased. Oligoanuric acute renal failure may occur during the course of a crisis; this may be secondary to pigment damage. Complete renal artery occlusion during a sickle cell crisis also has been reported. Asymptomatic papillary necrosis may occur in as many as 40% of patients with SS disease. Only 30% of patients with SS disease have a normal excretory urogram. Deterioration of renal function leading to dialysis does occur, and its incidence probably is underestimated. Finally, an association has been made between sickle cell trait and renal medullary carcinoma. The origin of this tumor is believed to be calyceal epithelium; the lesion is highly malignant and the prognosis is poor.

TREATMENT AND COURSE

Hematuria has been managed most effectively by ε-aminocaproic acid. The nephrotic syndrome is unresponsive to corticosteroids and immunosuppressive agents, although corticosteroids may be useful if a biopsy lesion of minimal change disease is found. The use of angiotensin-converting enzyme inhibitors has been tested in patients with mild to moderate proteinuria. In these studies, a 57% decrease in protein excretion was observed after treatment with an angiotensin-converting enzyme inhibitor. Nonsteroidal anti-inflammatory agents should be avoided. Bicarbonate therapy occasionally may be required for the treatment of a renal tubular acidosis. Dialysis can be performed safely in these patients, and extracorporeal hemodialysis and peritoneal dialysis with hypertonic dextrose solutions do not lead to increased sickle cell crises. Renal transplantation is successful in these patients, although the experience is limited.

BIBLIOGRAPHY

Berns JS, Kaplan BS, Machow RC, et al. Inherited hemolytic uremic syndrome. *Am J Kidney Dis* 1992;19:331–334.

Falk RJ, Scheinman J, Phillips G, et al. Prevalence and pathologic features of sickle cell nephropathy and response to inhibition of angiotensin-converting enzyme. *N Engl J Med* 1992; 326:910–915.

Harrington JT, Kassirer JP. Renal vein thrombosis. *Annu Rev Med* 1982; 33:255–262.

Haviv YS, Safadi R. Normotensive scleroderma renal crisis: case report and review of the literature. *Ren Fail* 1998; 20(5):733–736.

Henrich WL. Medical considerations in the evaluation of the obstructed renal artery. *Am J Med Sci* 1990;300:53–58.

Krieg T, Meurer M. Systemic sclerosis: clinical and pathophysiologic aspects. *J Am Acad Dermatol* 1988;18:457–481.

Ponticelli C, Rivolta E, Imbasciati E, et al. Hemolytic uremic syndrome in adults. *Arch Intern Med* 1980;140:353–357.

Singh N, Gayowski T, Marino IR. Hemolytic uremic syndrome in solid-organ transplant recipients. *Transpl Int* 1996;9(1):68–75.

Tracy RE, Strong JP, Newman WP III, et al. Renovasculopathies of nephrosclerosis in relation to atherosclerosis at ages 25 to 54 years. *Kidney Int* 1996;49(2):564–570.

Kelley's Textbook of Internal Medicine, fourth edition. Edited by H. David Humes.
Lippincott Williams & Wilkins, Philadelphia © 2000.

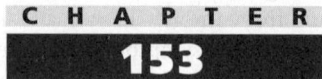

CHAPTER 153

DIABETES AND THE KIDNEY

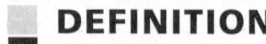
FRANK C. BROSIUS III
CHARLES W. HEILIG

DEFINITION

Diabetic nephropathy is characterized by the development of proteinuria followed by a progressive decline in renal function in patients with either type 1 or type 2 diabetes, who usually have some degree of diabetic retinopathy. Although the natural history of diabetic nephropathy is that of an inexorable reduction in renal function until end-stage renal disease (ESRD) is reached, there is increasing evidence that such progression can be indefinitely forestalled in many patients by aggressive medical intervention.

INCIDENCE AND EPIDEMIOLOGY

Diabetic nephropathy occurs in only a minority of both type 1 and type 2 diabetic patients. Approximately 30% of patients with type 1 diabetes ultimately develop nephropathy. Although it was originally felt that nephropathy was less common in type 2 patients, more recent data suggest that the prevalence in type 2 patients is similar to that of type 1 patients. However, there is heterogeneity among type 2 patients with some ethnic groups being at much higher risk of developing nephropathy (see below). Diabetic kidney disease is by far the most common cause of ESRD in the United States, accounting for over 39% of all patients reaching ESRD in the 1990s. Of these, approximately two thirds have type 2 diabetes, given the higher prevalence of type 2 disease. Unfortunately, the prognosis for diabetic patients with end-stage renal disease on dialysis is significantly worse than for other ESRD patients.

ETIOLOGY AND PATHOGENESIS

The specific cause or causes of diabetic nephropathy remain unidentified. However, a number of factors are clearly important for the development of diabetic nephropathy. Many of these factors can be best understood in the context of the pathologic features of the disease. Early pathologic features that are predictive of progressive diabetic nephropathy can occur within the first few years of diabetes, well before there is any clinical manifestation of the process. A prominent finding early during the course of either type 1 or type 2 diabetes is enhanced renal growth. The glomeruli and other structures increase in size, and total renal size (often gauged by the longitudinal diameter) is frequently significantly greater than normal. The increase in renal size occurs in most patients with diabetes, whether or not they ultimately develop nephropathy.

Within 5 years after onset of diabetes, pathologic changes can be found that do correlate with progressive diabetic kidney disease. These changes are mostly, though not exclusively, confined to the glomerulus. The initial pathologic changes that best correlate with progressive disease are widening of the glomerular basement membrane and expansion of the extracellular portion of the mesangial space by extracellular matrix proteins. Gradually, over years, these lesions evolve into those of advanced diabetic nephropathy: nodular glomerulosclerosis (the Kimmelstiel–Wilson lesion), diffuse intercapillary glomerulosclerosis, and arteriolar hyalinization. It appears that accumulation of extracellular matrix in the mesangium best predicts development of clinical nephropathy. Thus, many of the studies on the patho-

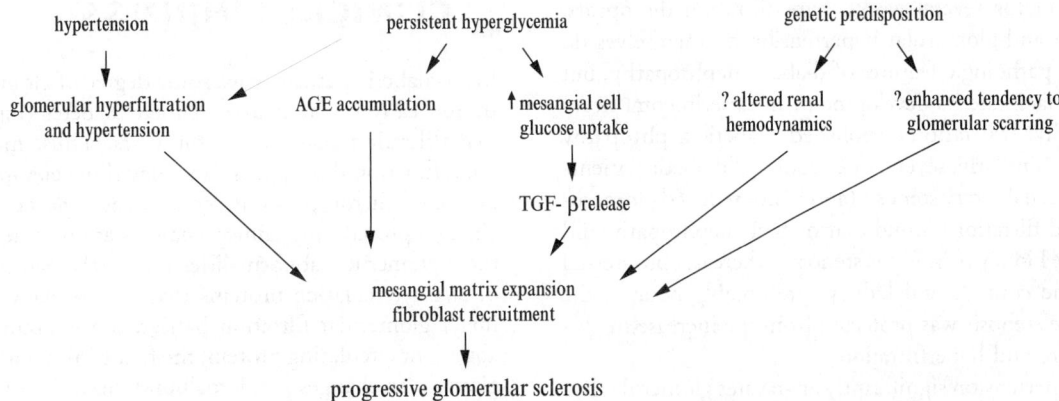

FIGURE 153.1. Proposed scheme for the pathogenesis of diabetic nephropathy. Present therapies are aimed at interruption of hemodynamic *(left)* and metabolic *(middle)* factors. The genetic factors *(right)* that predispose to nephropathy have yet to be defined precisely, but they appear to play a significant role in determining outcomes.

genesis of diabetic nephropathy have concentrated on abnormalities that can promote such accumulation.

Although the causes of the glomerular changes are still a matter of intense investigation, recent basic and clinical research findings have identified, at least in broad strokes, many of the factors that are important in the pathogenesis of the disease. Figure 153.1 shows a pathway of progression of diabetic nephropathy that outlines, albeit simplistically, those factors that appear to ultimately result in the pathological lesions of diabetic nephropathy. This formulation implies that interruption of any of the abnormalities in the pathway could retard or potentially prevent progression of diabetic kidney disease.

Clinical studies and recent genetic analyses have strongly suggested that there is a genetic predisposition to nephropathy among certain type 1 and type 2 patients. There are significant familial-associated risks of developing nephropathy in type 1 patients and similar genetic influences exist in the type 2 population, as the risk of developing nephropathy is several fold greater in African-American, American Indian, and Hispanic patients with type 2 diabetes than it is in other type 2 populations. Many recent studies have examined potential candidate genes to determine whether differences in these genes could predispose diabetic patients to develop nephropathy. One area of focus has been on genes that encode components of the renin–angiotensin–aldosterone system. At this point, none of the genes in this system, or any other genes, have been unequivocally linked to development of nephropathy in patients with diabetes. Although there are no genetic alterations that have been unequivocally shown to lead to an increased risk of developing diabetic nephropathy, various genetic loci have been identified that may contain such genes. It seems likely that specific genes that increase (or decrease) the risk of developing nephropathy will be identified in the near future for at least some populations with diabetes. It has been suggested that these genetic alterations are likely to alter renal hemodynamics in a way that potentiates the abnormalities found in most diabetic patients (see below), or may predispose to enhanced scarring responses to glomerular

injury by increasing extracellular matrix protein deposition and enhancing recruitment of fibroblasts into the glomerulus.

Another factor that appears to be a critical component of the pathogenetic progression to diabetic glomerulosclerosis is glomerular hyperfiltration. During the first few years of diabetes, the glomerular filtration rate is usually increased above normal in both type 1 and type 2 diabetic patients (Fig. 153.2). This hyperfiltration is most pronounced in the postprandial period but can persist for hours after eating. In animal models, this hyperfiltration is due to enhanced glomerular pressure resulting from abnormal vasodilatation of the glomerular afferent arteriole. Although the specific causes of these abnormalities have not been clearly identified, it is certain that poor glycemic control predisposes to this phenomenon. In patients who have good

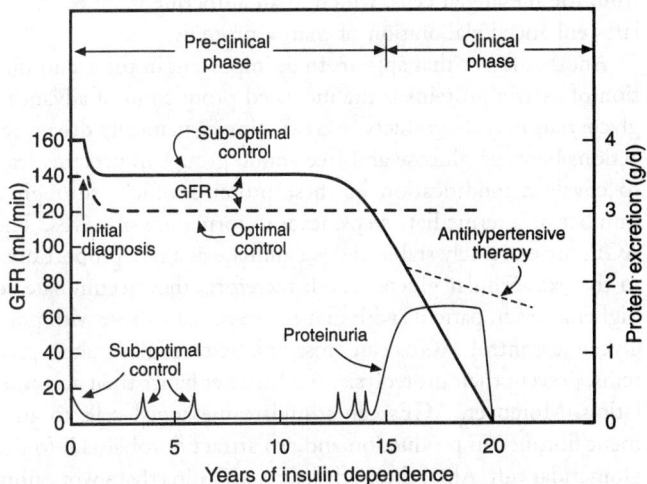

FIGURE 153.2. The natural history of diabetic nephropathy in type 1 patients. Type 2 patients appear to follow a similar course, although the time scale may be somewhat more compressed in type 2 patients with nephropathy. (From Hostetter TH. Diabetic nephropathy. In: Brenner BM, Rector F, eds. *The kidney,* third edition. Philadelphia: WB Saunders, 1986, with permission.)

glycemic control for several weeks, hyperfiltration disappears. Hyperfiltration and glomerular hypertension by themselves do not lead to the pathologic features of diabetic nephropathy, but they appear to facilitate its development. In experimental situations in which hyperfiltration is abolished, diabetic nephropathy does not occur. Similarly, several case reports of diabetic patients with unilateral renal artery stenosis (and hence reduced glomerular pressure and filtration) found that diabetic nephropathy did not occur in the kidney behind the stenosis, whereas it progressed unabated in the contralateral kidney, presumably because the kidney with the stenosis was protected from the increase in glomerular pressure and hyperfiltration.

Systemic hypertension significantly aggravates glomerular hypertension. Normal kidneys respond to elevated systemic blood pressure by vasoconstriction of the renal afferent arterioles thereby preventing transmission of elevated blood pressure to the glomerulus. However, in diabetes, the renal afferent arteriole is abnormally dilated (in animals and presumably in humans) and does not constrict in response to an increase in systemic blood pressure. Therefore, glomerular pressures increase substantially in the presence of systemic hypertension. This phenomenon may partly explain why systemic hypertension is such an important risk factor for progression of diabetic nephropathy.

A final set of factors that are critical for the evolution of diabetic nephropathy are responsible for enhanced accumulation of extracellular matrix proteins in the glomerular tuft. Experimental studies have suggested that the enhanced matrix expansion is due to both increased secretion of extracellular matrix proteins (such as fibronectin and collagen IV) by glomerular mesangial cells as well as reduced degradation of secreted extracellular matrix proteins. It appears that mesangial cells exposed to abnormally high glucose levels take up more glucose, perhaps due to an increase in the number of glucose transport proteins on the cell surface. This in turn leads to a number of abnormalities including enhanced transforming growth factor–β secretion from the mesangial cells, which in an autocrine manner stimulates enhanced elaboration of matrix proteins.

Another factor that appears to be important in the accumulation of matrix proteins is the increased production of advanced glycosylation end-products (AGEs). Nonezymatically driven reactions between glucose and free amino groups in proteins lead to covalent modification of these proteins which, through a number of intermediate steps, leads to formation of AGEs. The AGEs are extremely stable and accumulate at a rate proportional to the extracellular glucose level; therefore, they accumulate to higher levels in patients with diabetes, especially those with poor glycemic control. AGEs can cross-link extracellular matrix proteins, prevent their proteolysis, and hence enhance their accumulation. Moreover, AGEs can stimulate mesangial cells to augment fibronectin production and can attract fibroblasts into the glomerular tuft. All of these effects can lead directly to worsening of typical diabetic glomerular pathology. Both AGE levels and glucose effects on mesangial cells are enhanced by hyperglycemia and are reduced by normalization of blood sugar, again implicating glycemic control as a critical determinant of the development of diabetic nephropathy.

CLINICAL FINDINGS

Most diabetic patients have some degree of glomerular hyperfiltration early in the course of their diabetes (Fig. 153.2). This hyperfiltration may persist for years. Thus, measurements of renal function during this time may show elevated function. As described in the previous section, early glomerular pathologic changes precede any clinical manifestation of nephropathy, but these glomerular abnormalities ultimately lead to increased loss of larger circulating proteins that are normally retained by an intact glomerular filtration barrier. Since albumin is the most abundant circulating protein, the first clinical indication of these glomerular changes is microalbuminuria, the presence of small but abnormal amounts of albumin in the urine (discussed more fully under "Laboratory Findings," below). This abnormality is usually not detectable in type 1 patients until 5 or more years after the onset of diabetes. In type 2 patients, microalbuminuria can occur sooner after diagnosis because the onset of diabetes may go undetected for some time and because the progression of disease may be faster in type 2 than in type 1 patients. It has been clearly demonstrated that the great majority of type 1 diabetic patients who develop microalbuminuria, and therefore have so-called incipient nephropathy, will progress to overt diabetic nephropathy (Fig. 153.2). For type 2 patients, the situation is more complex because older patients can develop microalbuminuria independently of diabetes. However, the finding of microalbuminuria in a patient with type 2 disease is associated with a significantly increased likelihood of developing overt nephropathy, and most experts suggest that screening and intervention should be tailored similarly in both type 1 and type 2 patients. Approximately 90% of type 1 patients have some degree of diabetic retinopathy by the time they develop nephropathy. Although the prevalence of retinopathy is lower in type 2 patients with nephropathy, most type 2 patients will have evidence of retinopathy at the time of diagnosis of nephropathy. Therefore, the presence of clinically detectable renal disease in the absence of retinal abnormalities (especially in type 1 patients) raises the possibility that the kidney disease is due to some cause other than diabetes.

After onset of microalbuminuria, most patients will have a 5- to 10-year period of relative stability with few other clinical manifestations of nephropathy (Fig. 153.2). This period can be extended in many patients, perhaps indefinitely, if they receive aggressive intervention at this point. However, in the absence of aggressive treatment and in some patients who are aggressively managed, the degree of albuminuria tends to gradually increase until it is detectable on routine urinary dipstick evaluation. At this point, overt diabetic nephropathy is present. Peripheral edema is likely to occur and may be the first symptom of nephropathy noted by many patients. Moreover, by this stage, hypertension is likely to be present in both type 1 and type 2 patients. Hypertension is almost universal in type 2 patients with overt nephropathy. Thereafter, the glomerular filtration rate, previously elevated above normal, begins to fall. Uncontrolled hypertension accelerates the deterioration of renal function in patients with overt nephropathy. With the onset of overt nephropathy, patients who do not receive aggressive treatment will progress inexorably to ESRD over a 5- to 15-year period.

The presence of overt nephropathy also correlates with a much higher risk of cardiovascular disease. The relative morbidity and mortality in diabetic patients with overt nephropathy are increased many fold when compared to age-matched diabetic patients without albuminuria. This finding is true for both type 1 and type 2 patients, but the relative increase in mortality conferred by nephropathy may be up to 40-fold in type 1 patients, whereas it is less than 10-fold in type 2 patients. Most of this increase in mortality is attributable to accelerated cardiovascular disease. Because other risk factors for cardiovascular disease, such as hypertension and hyperlipidemia, are prevalent among these groups, aggressive management of all risk factors is required to ameliorate the profound increase in cardiovascular risk. It is noteworthy that microalbuminuria itself, even in the absence of diabetes, is associated with an increased risk of progressive vascular disease. Thus, any patient with microalbuminuria, with or without diabetes, should be managed aggressively.

LABORATORY FINDINGS

As noted above, the first laboratory indication of diabetic kidney involvement is microalbuminuria. The diagnostic algorithm for the approach to screening for microalbuminuria is shown in Figure 153.3. Microalbuminuria is defined as the urinary excretion of more than 30 mg, but less than 300 mg, of albumin in a 24-hour period (more than 300 mg per day is detectable by conventional dipsticks and is defined as overt nephropathy). Over the past decade, a number of sensitive assays for urinary albumin have been developed and have been validated as good screening tests. Microalbuminuria can be most easily tested on spot urine samples by determining the albumin-to-creatinine ratio. This is usually expressed as a ratio of milligrams of albumin to grams of creatinine. A ratio of between 30 and 300 usually signifies microalbuminuria for most laboratories (since approximately 1 g—or 1,000 mg—of creatinine is excreted daily, a ratio of 30 would correspond to a daily excretion of 30 mg of albumin). In order to make the diagnosis of persistent microalbuminuria and hence of incipient diabetic nephropathy, other causes of a transient increase in urinary albumin excretion, such as severe hyperglycemia, severe hypertension, urinary tract infection, fever, recent exercise, and congestive heart failure, should be excluded. The test should be performed at least three times over a 3- to 6-month period and must be abnormal on at least two of those occasions to indicate persistent microalbuminuria. Otherwise, screening should continue yearly (Fig. 153.3). Once the diagnosis is made, it might be helpful to continue monitoring the albumin-to-creatinine ratio to help determine responses to treatment (see below). Screening for microalbuminuria should begin 5 years after onset of diabetes in type 1 patients and at the time of diagnosis for type 2 patients.

Because diabetes is associated with renal growth, especially during the first several years of diabetes, radiographic studies will often show enlarged kidneys. The presence of bilateral small

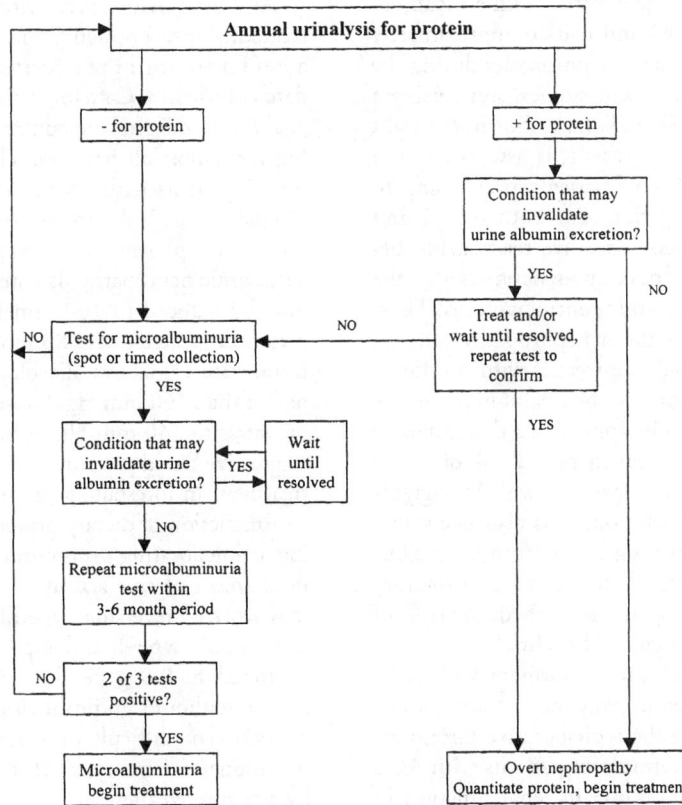

FIGURE 153.3. Algorithm for screening for microalbuminuria in both type 1 and type 2 patients. (From American Diabetes Association. Diabetic nephropathy. *Diabetes Care* 1999;22[Suppl 1];S66, with permission.)

kidneys in a type 2 patient might suggest the presence of significant renovascular disease associated with so-called ischemic nephropathy. The presence of one small kidney and one normal-sized or enlarged kidney in a type 2 patient with severe hypertension could suggest unilateral renal artery stenosis.

There are usually no other significant laboratory abnormalities directly related to diabetic nephropathy until overt nephropathy occurs. Patients will then tend to have a gradual decline in renal function, detectable by decreased creatinine clearances or increases in serum creatinine. Hypercholesterolemia may become manifest if not previously present, and hypoalbuminemia can develop as proteinuria worsens. As renal function worsens, patients with diabetic nephropathy will experience the plethora of metabolic and laboratory abnormalities that occur with progressive chronic renal insufficiency of any cause. Hyperkalemia tends to occur earlier, however, in diabetic patients due to hyporeninemic hypoaldosteronism (type IV renal tubular acidosis), insulin resistance, hypoinsulinemia, and/or hyperglycemia. This may limit intervention with angiotensin-converting enzyme (ACE) inhibitors (see below).

OPTIMAL MANAGEMENT

The Diabetes Complication and Control Trial (DCCT), published in 1993, demonstrated unequivocally that glycemic control was critical for preventing diabetic complications, including nephropathy. In that study, patients who received intensive insulin treatment achieved tight glycemic control (with a mean hemoglobin$_{A1C}$ of approximately 7%) and had an approximately 50% decrease in the risk of developing nephropathy during the 9-year study period. A number of recent studies, some using a design very similar to that of the DCCT, have shown that tight glycemic control in type 2 diabetic patients is associated with a similar reduction in the number of patients progressing to nephropathy over a several year period. For both type 1 and type 2 patients, there is a continuous positive relationship between glucose levels and the risk of developing nephropathy; the risk of nephropathy increases as glycemic control worsens. Thus, both type 1 and type 2 patients without nephropathy (i.e., no abnormal microalbuminuria) should be treated with insulin or other hypoglycemic agents to achieve a hemoglobin$_{A1c}$ of 7% or lower whenever possible. It must be appreciated that intensive insulin treatment is associated with an increased risk of severe hypoglycemic episodes, and its use in patients with hypoglycemia unawareness requires special caution. It is also likely that tight control helps prevent or delay progression from microalbuminuria to overt nephropathy, but there are no confirmatory data at present. Once overt nephropathy is reached, the risks of tight glycemic control may outweigh the benefits.

After microalbuminuria is confirmed, treatment with ACE inhibitors should be initiated, even in patients who are normotensive. Several studies, including the Collaborative Group report in 1993, have shown that treatment of patients with ACE inhibitors can reduce progressive decline in renal function in patients with diabetic nephropathy, independent of the level of blood pressure control. These agents reduce hyperfiltration and glomerular hypertension by (relatively) selectively dilating the efferent arteriole. They may also have a salutary effect on renal cell growth by inhibiting the intrarenal renin–angiotensin system and may reduce matrix protein accumulation by blocking angiotensin II effects on mesangial cells. In normotensive patients, treatment should begin at the lowest dose and then gradually be increased to levels that approximate those of the various published studies (e.g., enalapril or lisinopril of 20 mg per day). Major side effects include cough, orthostatic hypotension, angioedema, and hyperkalemia. Acute renal failure can occur in patients with bilateral renal artery stenosis who begin ACE inhibitor treatment, since these patients are dependent on efferent arteriolar constriction to achieve an intraglomerular pressure compatible with filtration. Therefore, all patients should have serum potassium and creatinine checked within the first few days of initiating therapy. A relatively small percentage rise (less than 40%) in serum creatinine does not signify bilateral renal artery stenosis and should not prevent continuation of therapy. Many patients develop a dry cough due to accumulation of bradykinin (which is metabolized by ACE). The cough is not dangerous, but can be irritating and prevent continuous therapy. In those patients, it is recommended that angiotensin II receptor blockers be utilized, though there are no clinical data available to demonstrate renal protection similar to that achieved with ACE inhibitors. Finally, it is imperative that ACE inhibitors not be used during pregnancy due to severe toxic effects on the fetus. These effects are manifested in the second and third trimesters. Therefore, ACE inhibitors should be used cautiously in women of child-bearing age.

Any time that hypertension occurs it should be aggressively treated. The recommendations of the American Diabetes Association for treatment of hypertension are contained in the "Standards of Medical Care for Patients with Diabetes Mellitus." The goal for blood pressure control should be less than 130/85 mm Hg for almost all patients. The only exceptions should be for type 2 patients with severe vascular disease in whom perfusion of vital organs is dependent on a higher blood pressure, and in type 1 or 2 patients with severe orthostatic hypotension due to autonomic neuropathy. Isolated systolic hypertension should be initially reduced to 160 mm Hg for those with systolic blood pressures greater than 180 mm Hg, reduced by 20 mm Hg for those with initial systolic blood pressures lower than 180 but higher than 160 mm Hg. Subsequent reduction of systolic blood pressures to 140 mm Hg or lower can be achieved as tolerated. Aggressive blood pressure control may be the single most critical treatment in forestalling progressive diabetic nephropathy.

Restriction of dietary protein may also be helpful in preventing or ameliorating the progression of diabetic nephropathy. The mechanism of this action is uncertain, but protein restriction may work by reversing hyperfiltration and glomerular hypertension. Adult type 1 and type 2 patients can usually be safely restricted to 0.8 g per kg per day (plus any urinary protein losses), without significant risk of protein malnutrition. Further restriction is difficult to achieve and may be accompanied by nutritional deficiency. Such restricted diets require monitoring by a registered dietitian.

Other treatment modalities to retard progression of nephropathy are less well defined, but there are increasing data which suggest that hyperlipidemia promotes progression whereas reduction of low-density lipoprotein cholesterol with the use of β-hydroxy-β-methylglutaryl coenzyme A reductase inhibitors can delay or prevent progression of nephropathy. Other suggested treatments include use of spironolactone to block the effects of aldosterone and cessation of smoking, which has a salutary effect on all microvascular disease.

Patients with diabetic nephropathy with elevated creatinines are at especially high risk of developing acute renal failure when exposed to radiocontrast media. If radiologic evaluation with radiocontrast materials is necessary, one should consider use of nonionic contrast agents in this group.

Finally, in patients who progress toward end-stage renal disease, despite all efforts, early transplant evaluation is indicated. For diabetic patients who are acceptable candidates for transplant, this is clearly the preferred modality of renal replacement therapy. Patient survival, at least over the first several years, for diabetic patients receiving either cadaveric or living donor transplants is now virtually identical to that of nondiabetic patients. The U.S. Renal Data System has reported that 1-year survival for diabetic patients receiving cadaveric allografts was 91.3% in 1995, compared with 92.6% for the nondiabetic population. Survival is even better for recipients of living donor allografts (95.4% for diabetic patients and 96.3% for nondiabetic patients). Renal allograft survival has also improved for diabetic patients and is now identical to that of the nondiabetic population. Excellent glycemic control, the use of ACE inhibitors, and aggressive blood pressure management all help to prevent recurrence of diabetic kidney disease in the transplanted kidney. Over the past few years, the use of combined kidney–pancreas transplants has increased. This procedure, when successful, has cured a growing number of type 1 patients. Short-term morbidity and mortality is greater for kidney–pancreas recipients than for type 1 diabetic patients receiving kidney allografts alone. However, it appears that long-term patient and kidney allograft survival is comparable to those type 1 patients receiving kidneys alone. Better long-term evaluation of combined kidney–pancreas will be forthcoming in the next several years.

BIBLIOGRAPHY

American Diabetes Association. Diabetic nephropathy. Clinical practice recommendations. *Diabetes Care* 1999;22(Suppl 1);S66–S69.

Diabetes Control and Complications Trial Research Group. The effect of intensive treatment of diabetes on the development and progression of long-term complications in insulin-dependent diabetes mellitus. *N Engl J Med* 1993;329:977–986.

Ellis D, Lloyd C, Becker DJ, et al. The changing course of diabetic nephropathy: low density lipoprotein cholesterol and blood pressure correlate with regression of proteinuria. *Am J Kidney Dis* 1996;27:809–818.

Lewis EJ, Hunsicker LG, Bain RP, et al. The effect of angiotensin-converting enzyme inhibition on diabetic nephropathy. *N Engl J Med* 1993; 329:1456–1462.

Pedrini MT, Levey AS, Lau J, et al. The effect of dietary protein restriction on the progression of diabetic and nondiabetic renal diseases: a meta-analysis. *Ann Intern Med* 1996; 124:627–632.

U.S. Renal Data System. USRDS 1998 annual report. National Institutes of Health, National Institute of Diabetes, Digestive and Kidney Diseases, Bethesda, MD, 1998.

Kelley's Textbook of Internal Medicine, fourth edition. Edited by H. David Humes. Lippincott Williams & Wilkins, Philadelphia © 2000.

CHAPTER 154

DYSPROTEINEMIAS AND THE KIDNEY

PAUL W. SANDERS

▬ RENAL LESIONS ASSOCIATED WITH MONOCLONAL IMMUNOGLOBULIN LIGHT-CHAIN DEPOSITION

Renal lesions related to deposition of monoclonal immunoglobulin or fragments of immunoglobulin represent about 2.7% of all morphologic abnormalities identified by kidney biopsy. They have in common abnormal accumulation in the kidney of monoclonal immunoglobulin fragments: light chains alone or, more rarely, a combination of light and heavy chains or heavy chains alone. Deposition of light chains in the various compartments of the kidney produces several clinicopathologic syndromes (Table 154.1). The presence of monoclonal light chains in the kidney confirms a plasma cell dyscrasia. The most common underlying diseases are multiple myeloma and primary amyloidosis (Table 154.2).

PATHOGENESIS

Light chains of immunoglobulins are 22-kD proteins that have two independent globular domains derived from a multigene family. The constant region is a homogeneous 105- to 107-polypeptide chain that is the product of genes located on chromosome 2 for the kappa light chain and on chromosome 22 for the lambda light chain. The variable region makes up the remaining 110 to 120 amino acids of the light chain and forms part of the antigen binding site. Multiple gene segments are

TABLE 154.1.	RENAL LESIONS RELATED TO MONOCLONAL LIGHT-CHAIN DEPOSITION

Glomerulopathies
  Amyloidosis, type AL
  Light-chain—related glomerulopathy of systemic light-chain deposition disease
Tubulointerstitial lesions
  Fanconi's syndrome
  Isolated hyperphosphaturia
  Proximal tubule necrosis (acute tubular necrosis, or "tubulopathy")
  Cast nephropathy ("myeloma kidney")
  Tubulointerstitial nephritis
Vascular lesions
Asymptomatic (Bence Jones proteinuria)

TABLE 154.2.	CAUSES OF MONOCLONAL LIGHT-CHAIN PROTEINURIA AND ASSOCIATED RENAL MORPHOLOGIC LESIONS			
		Type of Renal Involvement		
Disease	**Neoplastic Infiltration**	**Glomerular**	**Tubulointerstitial**	**Vascular**
Multiple myeloma	Rare	Light-chain—related glomerulopathy; AL-type amyloid	Cast nephropathy Acute tubulopathy interstitial nephritis	Infiltration of arterioles/arteries
Primary amyloidosis	No	AL-type amyloid	Acute tubulopathy	Infiltration of arterioles/arteries
Systemic light-chain deposition disease	No	Light-chain—related glomerulopathy	Acute tubulopathy	Infiltration of arterioles/arteries
Waldenström's macroglobulinemia	Common	IgM-associated glomerulopathy	Cast nephropathy (rare)	No
Heavy-chain disease	Uncommon	AL-type amyloid (μ-chain disease only); AH-type[a] amyloid	No	No
Chronic lymphoproliferative disease	Uncommon	AL-type amyloid	Cast nephropathy (rare)	No
Rifampin therapy	No	No	Cast nephropathy (rare)	No

[a] Rarely, heavy chains polymerize to form amyloid.
AL, amyloid, light-chain; AH, amyloid, heavy-chain.

rearranged to produce the variable polypeptide region. Thus, despite similar chemical properties, no two light chains are identical. Once synthesized and released into the plasma, light chains are cleared from the circulation by glomerular filtration. The glomerular filter serves as a minimal restrictive barrier for these low molecular weight proteins. After appearance in the tubule fluid, light chains are reabsorbed by the proximal tubule. When this process is saturated, light chains appear in distal tubule fluid and urine as Bence Jones proteins. Bence Jones protein is the original term for monoclonal light chain in the urine in amounts sufficient to demonstrate the unique thermal solubility properties of light chains (precipitation on heating to 45°C to 60°C, followed by solubilization after continued heating to 100°C). Thus, during transit through the kidney, light chains may interact with the glomeruli, proximal tubules, and distal nephron. In doing so, different renal lesions may develop, depending on the intrinsic physicochemical properties of the light chain.

In the glomerulus, some light chains bind to mesangial cells and stimulate these cells to produce transforming growth factor-β, a fibrogenic growth factor that in turn stimulates matrix production by these resident glomerular cells. The result is light-chain-induced glomerulosclerosis (light-chain-related glomerulopathy of systemic light-chain deposition disease). Other light chains can deposit in glomeruli and under proper environmental conditions can polymerize to form AL-amyloid (A for amyloid, L for light chains), in contrast to AA-amyloid, named after amyloid A protein, which occurs secondary to an underlying inflammatory or chronic infectious process. The amyloid replaces the normal architecture of the glomeruli and results in glomerular damage. After filtration through the glomerulus and subsequent

reabsorption into the proximal tubule epithelium, light chains ordinarily are hydrolyzed and the amino acid components are returned to the circulation by the basolateral circulation. However, some light chains appear to be poorly hydrolyzed. They congest and disrupt the endolysosomal system of these cells, producing proximal tubule cell toxicity. Other light chains escape absorption into the proximal tubule and appear in the lumen of the distal nephron where they bind to a specific site on Tamm–Horsfall glycoprotein, which is synthesized by the thick ascending limb of the loop of Henle. With binding, these proteins aggregate to form dense casts in the distal nephron. A subsequent inflammatory response with giant cell formation around the cast is typical. Cast nephropathy or "myeloma kidney" appears to be the direct result of the interaction between these proteins.

Finally, some of these proteins transit the kidney without consequences and produce no evident clinical manifestations. The physicochemical properties of the light chain that confer toxicity remain poorly defined, but changes as subtle as alteration of one amino acid can cause toxicity.

CLINICAL FINDINGS

The diagnosis of renal disease related to deposition of monoclonal light chain has traditionally been confirmed by the setting in which it developed. For example, over half of patients who present with clinical features of multiple myeloma have concomitant renal failure related to light-chain overproduction. However, renal failure can be the presenting feature of a plasma cell dyscrasia. Demonstration of monoclonal light-chain deposition in the kidney can thus uncover a hematologic disorder. The clinical manifestations of these renal lesions vary, depending on which compartment of the kidney is involved. Usually a progressive chronic loss of renal function is observed, but acute renal failure might be seen. A clinical syndrome reminiscent of rapidly progressive glomerulonephritis might also occur, particularly in the glomerulopathy associated with systemic light-chain deposition disease. Clinical findings of a glomerular lesion include hematuria with or without red blood cell casts, nephrotic syndrome, and nephrotic-range proteinuria. In the absence of an overt nephrotic syndrome, it is important to quantify the albumin component of proteinuria. Ordinarily, heavy proteinuria suggests a glomerular lesion, but because filtration of light chains is not restricted significantly by the normal glomerulus, large amounts of protein may be present in the urine of these patients, and yet no glomerular pathology is present. Associated albuminuria suggests AL-type amyloidosis or light-chain-related glomerulopathy of systemic light-chain deposition disease. The AL type of amyloidosis develops in about 10% of patients with multiple myeloma, less frequently with Waldenström's macroglobulinemia. The clinical presentation and type and degree of organ infiltration are similar between primary and myeloma-associated amyloidosis.

LABORATORY FINDINGS

Several electrolyte abnormalities may result from the presence of abnormal γ-globulins in serum. By displacing water in the volume of serum used to quantify sodium by flame photometry, large quantities of circulating protein produce pseudohyponatremia, a laboratory phenomenon. Correction for the portion of serum displaced by protein usually reveals that the serum sodium concentration is not altered. Plasma osmolality and serum sodium measured by ion-selective electrodes are normal in these circumstances. Hypercalcemia is the most common electrolyte disturbance in myeloma. Myeloma proteins may bind phosphate and produce spurious hyperphosphatemia. Rarely, abnormal protein binding of copper causes hypercupremia and Kayser–Fleischer–like rings. Multiple myeloma may be associated with a low anion gap because the immunoglobulin, particularly IgG, may have a net positive electrostatic charge, thereby reducing the normal anion gap by increasing the amount of counterbalancing anions in the serum. The result may be an anion gap of less than 5 mEq per L (normal, 12 mEq per L). Isolated damage to the proximal tubule can produce renal tubular acidosis, along with derangement of other sodium-coupled transport processes. The result is Fanconi's syndrome, which is characterized by hyperchloremic metabolic acidosis, glycosuria, and aminoaciduria. Fanconi's syndrome may be the presenting manifestation of multiple myeloma. Isolated hyperphosphaturia with attendant hypophosphatemia can occur in myeloma and can improve with successful treatment.

Diagnosis and classification of a plasma cell dyscrasia generally depend on the identification and quantification of the abnormal immunoglobulin molecule. Often, this is accomplished by electrophoretic analysis of proteins in the serum and urine. In over two thirds of patients, a monoclonal gammopathy is detected in the serum. Quantitative assay of the abnormal immu-

noglobulin ("M" component) is one of the best indexes used to follow the progression of the disease and the response to treatment. Examination of the urine further supports the diagnosis. Polyclonal light chains may appear normally in the urine, but in very small amounts (less than 2.5 μg per mL). The urinary light-chain concentration generally ranges from 0.02 to 0.5 mg per mL in patients with monoclonal gammopathies of undetermined significance, but the concentration is usually much higher (0.02 to 11.8 mg per mL) in patients with multiple myeloma or Waldenström's macroglobulinemia. Routine protein electrophoresis is too insensitive as a screening test and has been replaced by antibody detection assays, which confirm the presence and monoclonal nature of the immunoglobulin and light chain. Immunofixation electrophoresis, which is very sensitive, detects monoclonal light chains even in very low concentrations. However, occasionally the amount of monoclonal light chain is very small and can be masked by coexistent tubulointerstitial disease, which produces significant proximal tubule damage and therefore results in increased excretion of low molecular weight proteins, including polyclonal light chains.

Despite problems with detection, a diagnostic hallmark of plasma cell dyscrasias has been Bence Jones proteinuria. The causes of monoclonal light-chain proteinuria are listed in Table 154.2. Rifampin can rarely induce Bence Jones proteinuria and renal failure from cast nephropathy. Light-chain overproduction resolves by stopping this antibiotic. Because of difficulties with currently available detection techniques, renal monoclonal light-chain deposition may be diagnosed by kidney biopsy despite the absence of detectable paraprotein in serum or urine. Thirty to fifty percent of patients with documented systemic light-chain deposition disease have normal serum and urine immunoelectrophoretic profiles.

Bone marrow biopsy may reveal that plasma cells make up more than 20% of the total nonerythroid cells. When these cells appear vacuolated, bizarre, and multinucleated, a diagnosis of multiple myeloma is strongly supported. Immunophenotyping to document a monoclonal population of plasma cells may be useful when other findings are ambiguous. Nevertheless, a "negative" bone marrow biopsy does not exclude the existence of abnormal light-chain-producing plasma cells as a cause of renal failure. Patients with renal failure from documented systemic light-chain deposition disease but without diagnostic criteria for myeloma may develop overt multiple myeloma over time. Patients with monoclonal gammopathy of undetermined significance and normal renal function on presentation should also be closely followed because as many as one fourth will develop overt myeloma, amyloidosis, macroglobulinemia, or malignant lymphoproliferative disorder.

OPTIMAL MANAGEMENT

The mainstay of therapy is to abolish production of immunoglobulin light chains, the pathogenic feature of all of these renal lesions. As a group, these lesions belong to an unusual class of potentially reversible renal failure. The standard chemotherapeutic regimen, including melphalan and prednisone, ameliorates renal failure in over half of patients presenting with renal failure and multiple myeloma.

TREATMENT OF GLOMERULAR DISEASES

Although successful chemotherapy decreases the bone marrow biosynthesis of abnormal monoclonal light chains in systemic light-chain deposition disease, light-chain-related glomerulopathies are particularly resistant to chemotherapy. Uncontrolled trials of chemotherapy in systemic light-chain deposition disease have suggested benefit in some patients by preventing progression and occasionally improving renal function. Although most studies examining the role of chemotherapy in the management of glomerular lesions of systemic light-chain deposition disease are uncontrolled, given the inexorable progression of these glomerular lesions when untreated and the proven pathogenic role of monoclonal light chains in these glomerulopathies, a trial of chemotherapy should be considered, especially if the serum creatinine concentration at the time of diagnosis is less than 2 mg per dL. To identify these early lesions, however, a careful and comprehensive evaluation must be performed early in the course of the disease. The cumulative dose of melphalan and clinical response should be monitored during treatment.

Alkylating agents and prednisone decrease proteinuria, ameliorate nephrotic syndrome, and improve renal dysfunction in some patients with AL-type amyloidosis. Chemotherapy appears to prolong survival, although the overall response rate to chemotherapy approaches only 20% in amyloidosis. Generally, however, progressive systemic amyloid deposition continues, and deterioration of renal function is the rule. Unlike amyloidosis in familial Mediterranean fever, treatment of AL-type amyloidosis with colchicine alone has been disappointing.

TREATMENT OF CAST NEPHROPATHY ("MYELOMA KIDNEY")

Reducing the plasma concentration of monoclonal light chain generally improves renal function in cast nephropathy. Plasmapheresis to clear circulating light chains rapidly may be used initially in acute renal failure. However, despite chemotherapy, progressive loss of renal function subsequently occurs in many patients with cast nephropathy. Thus, other potential treatments designed to disrupt coprecipitation of Tamm–Horsfall glycoprotein with cast-forming light chains should be implemented. Factors known to aggravate nephrotoxicity of light chains by facilitating coprecipitation with Tamm–Horsfall glycoprotein in the distal nephron include hypercalcemia, an acidic urine, furosemide, radiocontrast material, low tubule fluid flow rates, and a high sodium chloride concentration in tubule fluid. Correction of hypercalcemia usually improves renal function. Alkalinization of the urine prevents renal failure from Bence Jones proteins in rats. In one inadequately controlled trial in humans, however, alkalinization of the urine by itself was not readily beneficial. Thus, alkalinization should be used only in conjunction with other measures, especially those aimed at enhancing hydration and keeping the urine flow rate high and the sodium chloride concentration in the distal nephron low. It is prudent to recommend a daily intake of 2 to 3 L of dilute fluids, as long as no significant defect in plasma osmoregulation coexists with renal failure. The detrimental effect of radiocontrast agents on

renal function has been shown in several studies, so that radiocontrast agents should be avoided in patients with multiple myeloma. Nonsteroidal anti-inflammatory agents produce a significant incidence of renal failure in myeloma and should be avoided. Because furosemide aggravated cast formation in an experimental animal model and facilitates coprecipitation of Tamm–Horsfall glycoprotein and light chains in vitro, this loop diuretic should be used with caution, particularly when extracellular fluid depletion is present.

CLINICAL COURSE

The clinical course of patients who have a monoclonal light-chain-related renal disease varies depending on the type of renal lesion. If untreated, however, virtually all of the renal lesions cause progressive loss of renal function and contribute to mortality because renal insufficiency predisposes to infection, the major cause of death in myeloma. For all patients with myeloma, median survival approaches 25 months. When significant renal failure coexists (creatinine concentration at least 180 μmol per L, or 2 mg per dL), median survival decreases to 4.3 months. In general, systemic light-chain deposition disease that shows a nodular glomerulopathic morphologic pattern has a poor renal prognosis, with most patients progressing rapidly to end-stage renal failure. Along with the glomerulopathy, proximal tubule injury (acute tubulopathy) contributes to progressive loss of renal function in systemic light-chain deposition disease. Adequate control of light-chain proteinuria promotes resolution of the proximal tubule injury. Overall, patients with myeloma and amyloidosis also have a poor prognosis, with median survival of less than 12 months. However, in patients with remissions induced by chemotherapy, survival can be prolonged and amyloid deposits might regress.

Renal replacement therapy in the form of hemodialysis or peritoneal dialysis is generally recommended in patients with renal failure from monoclonal light-chain-related renal diseases, especially if the renal failure is of recent onset. Recovery of renal function sufficient to survive without dialysis occurs in as many as 5% of patients with multiple myeloma but requires months in some patients. In addition, although multisystem involvement and advanced age at the time of diagnosis of myeloma shorten the life span (death often occurs early in the course of treatment), some patients, particularly those with disease limited mostly to the kidney, achieve functional rehabilitation and survive for more than 2 years.

Renal transplantation may also be considered for patients with myeloma, AL-type amyloidosis, or systemic light-chain deposition disease after the extrarenal manifestations of the disease have been absent for more than a year. Renal transplantation in these patients may be particularly beneficial if the disease has remained limited to the kidney. Transplant experience is limited, but glomerular light-chain deposition may also recur in the allograft and cause renal failure. Despite careful screening, myeloma may also recur after transplantation.

WALDENSTRÖM'S MACROGLOBULINEMIA

About 12% of patients with monoclonal gammopathy have Waldenström's macroglobulinemia, a B-cell line neoplastic transformation distinct from multiple myeloma. This condition behaves more like a lymphoma, and clinical manifestations are related primarily to organ infiltration, anemia, and hyperviscosity of blood. Osteolytic lesions are typically absent. The neoplastic cell, a large plasmacytoid lymphocyte, secretes monoclonal IgM (macroglobulin). Some of these immunoglobulins can bind autologous IgG (rheumatoid factor) and behave as cryoglobulins, producing cryopathic signs and symptoms. Direct neoplastic infiltration of the kidneys is more common in macroglobulinemia than in multiple myeloma. Plasmacytoid cells have been recovered from the urine sediment in patients with massive renal infiltration, and IgM in the urine supports the diagnosis of renal involvement. A peculiar glomerular lesion that is relatively common in macroglobulinemia is associated with massive subendothelial deposits of IgM. The glomerular capillary loops occasionally are filled with occlusive thrombi that contain IgM. These deposits must be differentiated from amyloid by Congo red staining and immunofluorescence and electron microscopy. Other immunoglobulins and complement are usually absent. The AL type of amyloid deposition occurs in about 5% of these patients. Although Bence Jones proteinuria is often detected, cast formation and "myeloma kidney" are rare.

The most dramatic, and usually initial, manifestation of macroglobulinemia is hyperviscosity syndrome related to the presence of large amounts of the abnormal macroglobulin in the circulation. Symptoms and signs attributable to hyperviscosity and hypervolemia are present in most patients with macroglobulinemia at some time during the illness. Characteristics of hyperviscosity syndrome include fatigue, weakness, bleeding diathesis, confusion, headache, visual disturbances, and circulatory congestion. In addition, renal dysfunction is usually present and manifested by impaired urine concentration, azotemia, and, occasionally, hematuria. The acute renal failure that may occur is typically reversible with treatment. The diagnosis of hyperviscosity syndrome rests on demonstration of the typical "M" spike in the serum, venous congestion (best observed by marked dilatation of retinal veins), and an elevated "relative" serum viscosity, although this latter parameter does not correlate linearly with the serum concentration of abnormal immunoglobulins. A relative serum viscosity of more than 4 and a serum concentration of abnormal immunoglobulin of more than 5 g per dL are usually encountered when symptoms of hyperviscosity are present. In contrast to macroglobulinemia, less than 5% of patients with IgG- and light-chain-secreting multiple myeloma show symptoms attributable to increased serum viscosity. This difference is probably related to the high molecular weight and structure of multimeric IgM, which permits slow removal from the circulation and accumulation in the intravascular compartment.

In patients with macroglobulinemia and hyperviscosity, emergent plasmapheresis is the treatment of choice, and it should be continued until symptoms have resolved. Chemotherapy in the form of alkylating agents and prednisone helps to maintain a stable serum viscosity. Many patients with macroglobulinemia have an indolent course; the overall median survival (5 years) is much higher than in multiple myeloma.

CRYOGLOBULINEMIA

Cryoglobulins are circulating proteins that precipitate on cooling. They are usually immunoglobulins or their fragments (light chains) but also may contain other components, including complement (C1q, C3, C4), fibronectin (cold-insoluble globulin), and endogenous (DNA) or exogenous (hepatitis B virus, hepatitis C virus, bacteria, or fungi) antigens. Cryoglobulinemic states are traditionally divided into three types. In type I cryoglobulinemia, the cryoprotein is a monoclonal immunoglobulin or light chain. Such patients typically have an associated plasma cell or lymphocytoid neoplasia, such as multiple myeloma or Waldenström's macroglobulinemia. Renal disease may result from precipitation of the cryoprotein in the glomerular capillaries. The cryoprotein in type II (mixed IgM and IgG) cryoglobulinemia consists of two or more distinct immunoglobulin classes, one of which is a monoclonal paraprotein, usually IgM. The IgM component has rheumatoid factor activity and binds to the Fc portion of polyclonal IgG. This type is associated with a plasma cell or lymphocytoid neoplasia, certain infections (especially hepatitis B and C), or autoimmune disease, or occurs as a primary (essential) disorder. The incidence of essential mixed cryoglobulinemia declined when hepatitis C infection was shown to account for the cryoglobulinemia in many of these patients. Presenting features can include purpura, fever, arthralgias, splenomegaly, and liver disease. Serum C4 levels are often decreased more than C3 levels. Renal disease may be severe and progressive, and is usually due to glomerulonephritis in which glomerular capillary deposits of the cryoprotein and complement components are accompanied by an intense monocytic infiltrate. Vasculitis and crescents may also occur. Renal failure and nephrotic syndrome are common. In type III cryoglobulinemia, the cryoprotein consists of two or more immunoglobulin classes, both polyclonal. The cryoglobulins are believed to be immune complexes that are insoluble at low temperatures. Type III cryoglobulinemia occurs in autoimmune and inflammatory disorders, including poststreptococcal glomerulonephritis, systemic lupus erythematosus, chronic infections, and neoplasias. An unidentifiable (essential) etiology is found in about 40% of patients with type III cryoglobulinemia.

Treatment of cryoglobulinemia depends on the underlying etiology. General measures should include avoidance of exposure to cold temperatures, particularly when peripheral necrotizing and purpuric skin lesions are present. In essential cryoglobulinemia, intensive plasma exchange or cryopheresis, glucocorticoids, and cytotoxic agents may be beneficial, especially when the plasma level of cryoglobulins is very high. Recent evidence suggests that interferon-α therapy can improve hepatitis C–induced cryoglobulinemia and associated renal injury and hypertension in some patients.

BIBLIOGRAPHY

Buxbaum JN, Chuba JV, Hellman GC, et al. Monoclonal immunoglobulin deposition disease: light chain and light and heavy chain deposition diseases and their relation to light chain amyloidosis. *Ann Intern Med* 1990;112:455–464.

Ganeval D, Noel LH, Preud'Homme JL, et al. Light-chain deposition disease: its relation with AL-type amyloidosis. *Kidney Int* 1984; 26:1–9.

Ganeval D, Rabian C, Guérin V, et al. Treatment of multiple myeloma with renal involvement. *Adv Nephrol* 1992;21:347–370.

Heilman RL, Velosa JA, Holley KE, et al. Long-term follow-up and response to chemotherapy in patients with light-chain deposition disease. *Am J Kidney Dis* 1992;20:34–41.

Huang ZQ, Sanders PW. Localization of a single binding site for immunoglobulin light chains on human Tamm-Horsfall glycoprotein. *J Clin Invest* 1997;99:732–736.

Misiani R, Bellavita P, Fenili D, et al. Interferon alfa-2a therapy in cryoglobulinemia associated with hepatitis C virus. *N Engl J Med* 1994;330: 751–756.

Sanders PW, Herrera GA. Monoclonal immunoglobulin light chain–related renal diseases. *Semin Nephrol* 1993;13:324–341.

Sanders PW, Herrera GA, Kirk KA, et al. Spectrum of glomerular and tubulointerstitial renal lesions associated with monotypical immunoglobulin light chain deposition. *Lab Invest* 1991;64:527–537.

Kelley's Textbook of Internal Medicine, fourth edition. Edited by H. David Humes. Lippincott Williams & Wilkins, Philadelphia © 2000.

CHAPTER 155

RENAL TUBULAR ACIDOSIS AND FANCONI SYNDROME

PETER C. BRAZY

DISTAL RENAL TUBULAR ACIDOSIS

Distal renal tubular acidosis (RTA) is characterized by hyperchloremic (normal anion gap) metabolic acidosis in association with a urine that is less than maximally acidic (Table 155.1). Acid is produced in the body (at a rate of 1.0 to 1.5 mEq/kg body wt/day) by acids in the diet, cellular metabolism and alkali losses in the stool. In steady state conditions, H^+ excretion by the kidney as free ions and buffered acid (with ammonia and anions such as phosphate) equals H^+ production from the processes mentioned above. Normal distal tubules can generate a H^+ concentration gradient (>100:1) between urine and blood, and the urine pH will fall to less than 5.4 during the excretion of an acid load. This lower pH increases the amount of H^+ excreted as free ions and as buffered acid. In distal RTA, the H^+ gradient is not achieved because of an impairment of the H^+ secretory mechanism or an increased back-diffusion of H^+ from urine to blood. This distal tubular defect reduces the absolute rate of acid excretion (both free and buffered H^+). The kidney fails to replace completely the bicarbonate that has neutralized ingested acid, and the serum bicarbonate level falls. In some cases, associated defects in distal tubule function may increase potassium excretion, leading to hypokalemia. Proximal tubules respond to distal RTA with increased reabsorption of sodium chloride producing hyperchloremia. Chronic metabolic acidosis stimulates skeletal buffering mechanisms and increases calcium mobilization from bone. Patients develop hypercalciuria, nephrocalcinosis and bone disease.

Distal RTA is rare. In children it may occur as a familial trait with several modes of inheritance. In some families, idiopathic hypercalciuria appears to be the inherited trait and the distal RTA develops later. In adults, distal RTA usually occurs as a secondary event in association with autoimmune disorders (systemic lupus erythematosus, Sjogren's syndrome), hypercalciuria (hypervitaminosis D, hyperparathyroidism), drugs (amphotericin B, ifosfamide) and tubulo-interstitial disease (pyleonephritis, obstructive uropathy). In these cases it goes away with resolution of the primary disorder. Children with distal RTA present with failure to thrive and grow; adults present with symptoms of nephrocalcinosis, nephrolithiasis, or hypokalemia. Hypokalemic symptoms include muscle weakness, cardiac arrhythmias, and inability to form a concentrated urine. Laboratory values include a urine pH of greater than 5.4 when the patient is acidemic. Serum bicarbonate is reduced (may be less than 10 mg/dl), the serum chloride level is increased, and often there is hypokalemia. Patients with chronic distal RTA have hypercalciuria with nephrocalcinosis or nephrolithiasis at some point in the disease. Bone pain and pathological fractures may occur. This disorder is characterized by slowly progressive renal insufficiency. Effective treatment includes neutralizing the daily acid load with oral preparations of sodium bicarbonate or sodium citrate (1 to 2 mEq/kg/d). Potassium citrate may be used if hypokalemia is present.

PROXIMAL RENAL TUBULAR ACIDOSIS

Proximal RTA is caused by a decrease in the maximum capacity (Tm) of the proximal tubule to reabsorb bicarbonate; it presents as a hyperchloremic, hypokalemic metabolic acidosis. The urine pH may be less than 5.4. The serum bicarbonate level is usually between 12 and 20 mEq/L. The proximal tubule reclaims about 85 to 90% of filtered bicarbonate by a process that involves the exchange of cellular H^+ for urine sodium, the activity of the enzyme carbonic anhydrase in the brush border and the cell, and the activity of the sodium, potassium ATPase in the basolateral membrane of the tubular cell. The defect in proximal RTA is unknown, but may be related to an abnormality in one of the above parameters. With this defect, bicarbonate is lost into the urine (reduced Tm) until the filtered load of bicarbonate (serum concentration times filtration rate) is less than the reabsorptive capacities of proximal and distal tubules. Because distal acidification is normal, the urine pH may be appropriately low (less than 5.4) when all the bicarbonate has been reabsorbed. Reduced reabsorption of sodium bicarbonate by proximal tubules results in volume contraction, increased activity of the renin-angioten-

TABLE 155.1.   **FEATURES OF RENAL TUBULAR ACIDOSIS**

	Distal	Proximal	Type IV
Basic defect	No H+ gradient in distal tubule	Reduced bicarbonate reabsorption	Decreased K secretion by distal tubule
Urine pH after acid load	>5.4	<5.4	Usually <5.4
Diagnostic test	NH$_4$Cl load	Maximum capacity for HCO$_3$	Urinary K excretion, renin, aldosterone
Serum K before treatment	Low	Low	High
Serum K after bicarbonate	Normal	Lower	Toward normal
Long-term complications	Renal stones, renal insufficiency	Osteomalacia, growth retardation	None
Associated diseases	Autoimmune	Fanconi syndrome	Diabetes mellitus, interstitial nephritis

sin-aldosterone system, increased reabsorption of sodium chloride (hyperchloremia) and increased secretion of potassium by distal tubules (hypokalemia).

Proximal RTA is rare. It may be an inherited disorder, either as an isolated defect or as a part of a more generalized defect in proximal tubular function (i.e. a Fanconi syndrome). Acquired forms of proximal RTA are associated with the Fanconi syndrome and the conditions listed under that heading. Familial cases present with growth retardation. Patients may have symptoms of hypokalemia and reduced extracellular fluid (ECF) volume. They do not have problems with nephrolithiasis or bone disease (unless the disorder is part of a Fanconi syndrome). Urine pH may be maximally acid when plasma levels of bicarbonate are significantly reduced. Hypokalemia is usually present and worsens with sodium bicarbonate therapy. In some inherited forms, the child outgrows the disorder.

In secondary proximal RTA, treatment of the primary disorder may improve proximal tubular function; otherwise, the disorder is difficult to treat. Huge doses of sodium bicarbonate result in large urinary losses of bicarbonate and increased urinary losses of potassium. Replacement therapy should include a mixture of sodium and potassium salts (bicarbonate or citrate) at about 1 to 2 mEq/kg/day. Modest volume depletion enhances proximal reabsorption, minimizes potassium losses from distal tubule and may reduce symptoms.

TYPE IV RENAL TUBULAR ACIDOSIS

Type IV RTA is characterized by hyperkalemia and a hyperchloremic metabolic acidosis. It results from an aldosterone deficiency or an unresponsiveness of the renal tubule to aldosterone. Aldosterone stimulates the reabsorption of sodium and the secretion of potassium and H+ by the distal nephron. Patients with type IV RTA have either a defect in renin and aldosterone release or an alteration in the structure or function of distal tubules rendering them unresponsive to normal levels of aldosterone. A functional decrease in aldosterone activity reduces distal tubular reabsorption of sodium and reduces secretion of potassium and

H+. Acidosis occurs because hyperkalemia inhibits ammonium production by the renal tubules and thereby reduces the buffer capacity for H+ in the urine.

Type IV RTA, the most common type of RTA, is often seen in patients with diabetes mellitus and mild to moderate renal insufficiency; in some patients taking nonsteroidal antiinflammatory drugs, angiotensin-converting enzyme inhibitors, cyclosporine, or potassium-sparing diuretics; and in some patients with interstitial renal diseases such as systemic lupus erythematosus, obstructive uropathy, and sickle cell disease or HIV nephropathy. Patients are usually asymptomatic and the abnormality is discovered during routine laboratory studies. Laboratory findings include mild renal insufficiency and hyperkalemia. Hyperchloremic acidosis occurs in about half of the patients. The urine pH is usually normal.

Type IV RTA usually requires no therapy if contraction of ECF volume is avoided. Volume contraction with reduced delivery of sodium and fluid to the distal tubule reduces the renal excretion of potassium and exacerbates the hyperkalemia. Some patients require discontinuation of the offending drug or addition of a potassium-wasting diuretic, such as furosemide. A few patients need mineralocorticoid replacement therapy to correct the hyperkalemia and often require supraphysiologic doses.

FANCONI SYNDROME

The Fanconi syndrome results from a generalized defect in proximal tubular function that may reduce transport rates for glucose, phosphate, amino acids, bicarbonate, uric acid and sodium. The transport of glucose, phosphate, amino acids and urate across brush-border membranes of proximal tubules is coupled to sodium transport. The Fanconi syndrome can be produced by factors which reduce the favorable sodium gradient, such as a reduction in the availability of ATP, inhibition of Na+, K+-ATPase activity, or an alteration in membrane permeability. Decreased proximal tubular reabsorption of filtered solute usually results in low serum levels and high urinary excretion rates. The magnitude of the defect varies because transport mechanisms may be incompletely inhibited, more than one transport mecha-

TABLE 155.2.	Inherited Defects in Tubular Transport		
	Tubule Site	**Involved Solute**	**Clinical Expression**
Fanconi syndrome	Proximal	Phosphate glucose amino acids, bicarbonate	Hypophosphatemia, metabolic acidosis, bone disease
Nephrogenic diabetes insipidus	Distal	Water	Polyuria, hypernatremia
Vitamin D–resistant rickets	Proximal	Phosphate	Poor growth, bone disease
Hartnup disease	Proximal	Tryptophan histidine	Rash, mental retardation
Bartter's syndrome	Loop of Henle	Sodium chloride	Metabolic alkalosis, hyperaldosteronism
Renal glycosuria	Proximal	Glucose	Glycosuria without hyperglycemia

nism may exist for a solute, and increased rate of distal tubular reabsorption may reduce the impact of a proximal transport defect.

Fanconi syndrome rarely occurs as a primary disorder (Table 155.2); more often it is associated with other disorders of renal tubule structure and metabolism. These include genetic diseases (cystinosis, galactosemia, fructose intolerance and some glycogen storage diseases), dysproteinemic states (multiple myeloma, amyloidosis), drugs and toxins (heavy metals, outdated tetracycline) and tubulo-interstitial diseases (Sjogren's syndrome, medullary cystic disease, Balkan nephropathy). Children with Fanconi syndrome present with growth failure, osteomalacia or rickets, and symptoms related to hypokalemia. Adults present with abnormal laboratory values. Serum levels of potassium, bicarbonate, phosphorus and uric acid are reduced and urinary excretion rates of these same solutes are increased. Bones may show evidence of osteomalacia. Plasma creatinine levels are elevated, usually as a result of renal damage from the underlying disease.

Chronic hypophosphatemia causes growth retardation and progressive bone disease, osteomalacia and pathological fractures. The associated diseases may cause tubular necrosis, interstitial inflammation and scaring, and progressive decline in all renal functions. Therapy is directed toward the underlying disease and includes providing supplements of phosphate, bicarbonate, and potassium to replace excess urinary losses. Vitamin D therapy with calcitriol may be needed to treat osteomalacia.

NEPHROGENIC DIABETES INSIPIDUS

Nephrogenic diabetes insipidus is characterized by an unresponsiveness of renal tubules to antidiuretic hormone (ADH). The action of ADH on the collecting ducts of the kidney involves binding to specific V2 receptors on the basolateral membrane, activation of adenylate cyclase and generation of intracellular cAMP, cAMP-dependent phosphorylation of membrane proteins in the cell and the insertion of the aquaporin-2 water channel into the urinary membrane. These events increase the membrane permeability to water, sodium and urea and are modified by calcium and prostaglandin E2. In the presence of ADH and an osmotic gradient, water and solutes are reabsorbed and the urine becomes more concentrated. In the absence of an ADH

response, the urine leaves the kidney as dilute as it was when it entered the collecting tubule. Nephrogenic diabetes insipidus is associated with defects in the V2 receptor or with the insertion of aquaporin-2 into the membrane. Thus, patients with nephrogenic diabetes insipidus have increased volumes of urine and increased losses of water and sodium. Water losses are proportionally greater than sodium losses (as compared to plasma).

Nephrogenic diabetes insipidus has familial and acquired forms. The familial form is rare. One type of defect in the V2 receptor is carried on the X chromosome and this inherited trait is X-linked recessive. Affected males present in infancy, and incomplete forms of the disease occur in female carriers of the gene. An autosomal recessive form of nephrogenic diabetes insipidus occurs when there is a defect in the function of the aquaporin-2 water channel. Acquired forms of the disorder occur in adults or children and are most commonly associated with the therapeutic use of lithium (for manic-depressive diseases) or with hypercalcemia or hypokalemia. The acquired forms are more prevalent, but often have an incomplete expression of the defect; they are recognized only during episodes of water deprivation. The presenting symptoms are polydipsia, polyuria, and a marked impairment in the ability to form a concentrated urine. In the familial form, affected males present shortly after birth with polyuria, dehydration if fluids are withheld, unexplained fever, failure to gain weight and constipation. In the females of affected families, the disorder has a variable expression and the polydipsia and polyuria may not be sufficient to bring them to medical attention. People with acquired forms of this disorder are usually asymptomatic. The disorder presents clinically when they are stressed with a solute diuresis or can not regulate their water intake.

Laboratory findings are hypernatremia, hypertonicity and normal or elevated values of serum ADH. Glomerular filtration rates may be reduced with dehydration, but all laboratory abnormalities should return to normal with administration of adequate fluid. The X-ray examination in severely affected patients may show dilated ureters and bladder, presumably from chronic polyuria. Nephrogenic diabetes insipidus is distinguished from central diabetes insipidus and primary polydipsia with a water deprivation test. This test measures the response of the kidney (in urine osmolality) to an increase in serum osmolality and to an injection of exogenous ADH after the urine osmolality has reached a plateau. In nephrogenic diabetes insipidus, the maximum urine osmolality is reduced (<800 mOsm/kg) and the response to ADH is blunted (an increase of <50 mOsm/kg).

Therapy should be aimed at correcting any underlying disorder such as dehydration, lithium use, or an electrolyte disorder. A second approach for patients with chronic dysfunction is to induce a mild degree of volume depletion with amiloride and a thiazide diuretic. This maneuver limits the water delivery to the ADH-sensitive segments of the nephron and minimizes potassium losses. A low sodium diet may also reduce the daily urine excretion. In patients with recurring episodes of severe dehydration, renal injury and reductions in glomerular filtration rate occur over time.

HYPOPHOSPHATEMIC VITAMIN D–RESISTANT RICKETS

Hypophosphatemic vitamin D-resistant rickets results from a defect in renal phosphate transport and is characterized by hypophosphatemia and osteomalacia that are unresponsive to standard doses of vitamin D. In this disorder the maximum rate of phosphate transport by the renal proximal tubules is decreased, phosphate is lost into the urine and hypophosphatemia develops. Additionally, there is a defect in vitamin D metabolism by these same proximal tubules. Serum levels and production rates of 1,25-dihydroxy-vitamin D3 by the renal tubules are abnormally low for the degree of hypophosphatemia. The genetic basis of this abnormality is being characterized. The gastrointestinal tract has reduced rates of calcium and phosphorus absorption, but these defects respond to vitamin D treatment. The bone disease (rickets or osteomalacia) occurs because of chronic hypophosphatemia and a blunted response to metabolites of vitamin D. Parathyroid hormone excess appears to enhance the clinical manifestations of the disorder (the phosphaturia) but does not have a primary role in the pathogenesis of the disease.

Several subtypes exist. The most common type is familial, with an X-linked dominant pattern of inheritance and a frequency of about 1 in 25,000 live births. Another type, which is not familial, is associated with the presence of specific tumors, such as giant cell tumors of bone, sarcomas, hemangiomas, breast carcinoma and prostate carcinoma. Children present with rickets and short stature in the first year of life. Later skeletal changes include lateral curvature of femora and tibia. There is no muscle weakness, tetany or convulsions which accompany vitamin D-responsive rickets. Adults have inactive rachitic deformities such as bowed legs or short stature. A few have active osteomalacia with pseudofractures, coarsened trabeculation and rarified areas of bone. Affected females have a lower incidence of bone disease than males. Hypophosphatemia is the biochemical marker of this disease. Affected individuals have increased urinary phosphate excretion. The serum calcium level is normal, but urinary calcium level is low due to poor intestinal absorption. Serum alkaline phosphatase activity is elevated and correlates roughly with the activity of bone disease. Serum levels of 1,25-dihydroxy-vitamin D3 are in the normal range, but should be higher in the presence of hypophosphatemia. Serum parathyroid hormone levels are normal or slightly elevated.

In patients with hypophosphatemia, bone disease is present

in 95% of affected males and 53% of affected females. Bone disease and growth retardation are the major concerns of patients and their families. Treatment with pharmacologic doses of vitamin D fails to correct the disease process and may produce vitamin D intoxication. Better results have been achieved with a combination of oral phosphate (1-4 g/d in divided doses) and 1,25-dihydroxy-vitamin D3 (0.5 to 2.0 μg/d). This treatment improves hypophosphatemia, bone histomorphology and growth. This therapy may be associated with hypercalciuria, hypercalcemia and reduced renal function, so patients should be followed closely for these complications.

SELECTIVE DISORDERS OF AMINO ACID TRANSPORT

Disorders involving defects in the renal transport mechanisms for specific amino acids or groups of amino acids are inherited, usually as autosomal recessive traits. Plasma levels of the affected amino acids may be low as a consequence of decreased absorption from the intestinal tract and increased losses into the urine. Usually an adequate diet can maintain plasma levels of these amino acids near normal despite the specific transport defects, because amino acids can be absorbed by the intestine by other transport mechanisms. These disorders are rare and often have no specific clinical features. Symptoms may occur if the diet is poor or deficient in the critical amino acids. Examples of these inherited defects in amino acid transport are Hartnup disease (neutral amino acids, such as tryptophan, histidine, and methionine), iminoglycinuria (proline, hydroxyproline, and glycine), dicarboxylic amino-aciduria (aspartic and glutamic acids), and cystinuria (see Chap. 414).

BARTTER'S SYNDROME

Bartter's syndrome is a rare disorder characterized by hypokalemia, metabolic alkalosis, and hyperplasia of the juxtaglomerular apparatus (the source of renin) with hyperaldosteronism. The genetic defects appear to involve the sodium, potassium, chloride transporter in the tubules of the thick ascending limb of the loop of Henle. Hypokalemia and metabolic alkalosis are explained by increased urinary sodium losses leading to mild volume depletion, increased renin-angiotensin-aldosterone system activity, increased secretion of potassium and hydrogen ions by the distal nephron and increased reabsorption of sodium bicarbonate by the proximal nephron. Hypertension is not present. Increased release of prostaglandins (PGE2 and prostacyclin) may oppose the hypertensive action of other hormones. Patients usually have an impaired ability to dilute urine, consistent with a defect in the thick ascending limb of the loop of Henle. There appears to be several genetic variants of Bartter's syndrome. One of these variants is now called Gitelman's syndrome. The genetic defect in Gitelman's syndrome is in the sodium chloride transporter in the distal nephron (the site of action of thiazide diuretics). This syndrome differs from the classic Bartter's syndrome in that magnesium wasting in the urine and hypomagnesemia are present, and the concentrating ability of the kidney is maintained (normal loop of Henle function).

Most cases are sporadic, but the syndromes can have a familial pattern which is transmitted usually as an autosomal recessive trait. Patients usually present in childhood with symptoms of hypokalemia such as muscle cramps, weakness, ileus, nocturia and polyuria. There is no hypertension or edema. They often have delayed growth and may have mental retardation. Presentation of the syndrome in adults is less common and may be mimicked by diuretic abuse or surreptitious vomiting. The prominent biochemical findings are described above. Additional biochemical abnormalities may include hypomagnesemia (Gitelman's syndrome), hyperuricemia and increased urinary excretion of PGE2 (Bartter's syndrome). Renal biopsy reveals hyperplasia of the juxtaglomerular apparatus.

This syndrome must be distinguished from surreptitious vomiting or unreported diuretic abuse. The urine chloride is low (<20 mEq/L) with vomiting. Diuretic use may be detected by assays for the drug in urine. Therapy is aimed at minimizing the effects increased prostaglandin and aldosterone production. The combination of a nonsteroidal antiinflammatory drug and a potassium-sparing diuretic (e.g., spironolactone or amiloride) can raise serum potassium levels and reverse the metabolic alkalosis. The use of angiotensin-converting enzyme inhibitors can also improve the electrolyte abnormalities but produces a lower blood pressure. Most patients require oral potassium and magnesium supplements in addition to drug therapy.

RENAL GLYCOSURIA

Renal glycosuria is an isolated abnormality of glucose transport by renal tubules, in which glucose appears in the urine when plasma concentrations are normal. The clinical expression and pattern of inheritance of renal glycosuria are variable; thus, the syndrome may result from more than one defect in renal glucose transport. The disorder is asymptomatic and is detected on a routine urinalysis. The Joslin Clinic found only 94 cases of renal glycosuria in 50,000 cases evaluated for diabetes mellitus. Patients have a negative evaluation for diabetes mellitus, (i.e. normal storage and use of glucose), excrete 800 mg to several grams of glucose a day (normal people excrete <300 mg/d) in their urine, and have no other abnormality in renal function. Intestinal transport of glucose is usually normal. These patients have the disorder for many years without developing other signs of renal or metabolic disease.

BIBLIOGRAPHY

Bichet DG, Oksche A, Rosenthal W. Congenital nephrogenic diabetes insipidus. *J Am Soc Nephrol* 1997;8:1951–1958.
Caruana RJ, Buckalew VM Jr. The syndrome of distal (type 1) renal tubular acidosis. Clinical and laboratory findings in 58 cases. *Medicine* 1988;67:84–99.
DeFronzo RA. Hyperkalemia and hyporeninemic hypoaldosteronism. *Kidney Int* 1980;17:118–134.
Drezner MK. Clinical disorders of phosphate homeostasis. In: Feldman D, Glorieux FH, Pike JW, eds. *Vitamin D.* San Diego: Academic Press, 1997:733–754.
Rose BD. Metabolic acidosis. In: Rose BD, ed. *Clinical physiology of acid–base and electrolyte disorders,* 4th ed. New York, McGraw-Hill, 1994:540–603.
Simon DB, Karet FE, Hamdan JM, et al. Bartter's syndrome, hypokalemic alkalosis with hypercalcuria, is caused by mutations in the Na-K-2CL cotransporter NKCC2. *Nature Genet* 1996;13:183–188.
Simon DB, Nelson-Williams C, Bia MJ, et al. Gitelman's variant of Bartter's syndrome, inherited hypokalemic alkalosis, is caused by mutations in the thiazide-sensitive sodium-chloride cotransporter. *Nature Genet* 1996;12:24–30.
Verge CF, Lam A, Simpson JM, et al. Effects of therapy in X-linked hypophosphatemic rickets. *N Engl J Med* 1991;325:1843–1848.

Kelley's Textbook of Internal Medicine, fourth edition. Edited by H. David Humes. Lippincott Williams & Wilkins, Philadelphia © 2000.

C H A P T E R

156

RENAL CYSTS AND CYSTIC DISEASES

WILLIAM D. KAEHNY

The advent of sensitive and minimally invasive imaging techniques presented clinicians with the problem of managing largely asymptomatic renal cysts. More recently, molecular biology has provided the potential for presymptomatic diagnosis of autosomal dominant polycystic kidney disease (ADPKD), the most common inherited disease in the United States. Thus, the well-prepared internist will be familiar with the more common causes and effects of these fluid-filled sacs lined by epithelium and located within renal parenchyma. All cysts probably arise as dilatations or diverticuli of renal tubules. Some are connected, such as early (small) cysts in ADPKD and the ectatic tubular cysts of medullary sponge kidneys. Most become disconnected as they enlarge, as do simple cysts and larger ADPKD cysts.

SIMPLE RENAL CYSTS

Simple renal cysts develop with aging and can be detected in one-third of persons aged 60 years and older. The incidence is low in persons younger than 40 years of age, although simple cysts do occur rarely in infants and children. Simple cysts may be single or multiple, and enlarge with time. Most simple cysts are asymptomatic and are detected fortuitously. Occasionally, the cysts may cause abdominal masses, abdominal or back pain from bleeding, sepsis from infection (uncommon), and (even more uncommonly) erythrocytosis or hypertension (case reports).

More commonly, the clinician must decide whether single

or multiple cysts are simple or are due to renal cell carcinoma, ADPKD, or other disorders. This problem is statistically small but highly important for the individual patient. Single cysts with smooth walls by ultrasonography require no further evaluation. Simple cysts are present in up to 3% of kidneys containing renal cell carcinoma, but renal cell carcinoma occurs rarely (less than 0.1%) in the walls of simple cysts. Perhaps 15% of renal cell carcinomas are cystic. Thick and irregular cyst walls and cyst fluid abnormalities allow diagnosis in almost all instances. Multiple simple cysts cannot be distinguished from the cysts of ADPKD by appearance and location. The presence of multiple but not many (about five) cysts in a 70-year-old asymptomatic patient with a family history of ADPKD is not likely to be ADPKD, whereas this presentation is highly likely to be ADPKD in a 20-year-old. Time is the best diagnostic tool in most cases.

Treatment is rarely needed. Infection of a cyst, pain, or hypertension may be alleviated by cyst puncture, drainage, and instillation of antibiotics or sclerosing agents. If the unlikely prospect of renal cell carcinoma is suspected, surgical exploration is required.

AUTOSOMAL DOMINANT POLYCYSTIC KIDNEY DISEASE

Autosomal dominant polycystic kidney disease is a hereditary disease that occurs in 1 in 200 to 1,000 of the world's population. The more common type (ADPKD1) appears to be caused by an abnormal gene on the short arm of chromosome 16. A second type (ADPKD2; 10%) is related to a gene on the long arm of chromosome 4. A third genotype is proposed. ADPKD may be found in fetuses, infants, children, and adults. ADPKD causes advanced renal failure in about 50% of affected persons, thus accounting for about 10% of cases of end-stage renal failure.

A cause for excitement is the potential for linking the genetic, molecular, cellular, anatomical, and physiologic defects in this disease. The products of PKD1 and PKD2 genes are the large integral membrane proteins polycystin 1 and 2, respectively. These two proteins interact in normal epithelial growth and proliferation programs. All cells contain the mutated gene in ADPKD, but the expression of disease in tissue may require a second mutation or injury. The renal cysts develop anywhere along the tubule, and the epithelium may retain the functional properties of its origin. Perhaps only 2% of nephrons develop cysts that appear to disconnect from the parent tubules as their size increases with time. Cysts may grow to diameters larger than 10 cm, but most measure 2 to 5 cm. The kidneys enlarge such that they are palpable in about half of patients. Progressive renal failure is not due to the cysts, which are markers of the disease. Rather, enlargement of the interstitium with matrix deposition and cellular infiltrates seems to lead to loss of normal noncystic parenchyma.

Back or flank pain (60%) and gross hematuria (30%) are the major causes of distress. Renal stones (20%), cyst infections, and retroperitoneal hemorrhage also occur. Extrarenal manifestations are diverse and often important. Hypertension develops in 60% of patients before the onset of measurable renal failure. The

mechanism probably includes a role for the renin–angiotensin system induced by vascular compression. Liver cysts begin to appear in 30-year-old patients and increase in size and number in parallel with renal cyst progression, reaching an overall peak prevalence of about 60%. Sex hormones may account for more liver involvement in women. Liver function is well preserved, and complications are unusual. Mitral valve prolapse occurs in about 25% of patients with ADPKD, with significant regurgitation in about one third of these. Intracranial aneurysms occur in about 10% of patients, with an uncertain but important frequency of rupture. Colonic diverticulosis, ovarian cysts, and inguinal hernias appear to develop with increased frequency.

The diagnosis is usually readily established by renal ultrasonography; computed tomography is more sensitive but also more costly. In the absence of the typical image of many cysts in both kidneys, the presence of any renal cysts in persons younger than 40 years with a family history of ADPKD or liver cysts should be considered to indicate ADPKD. If clinically desirable, gene linkage analysis of multiple family members may provide a high level of inferential likelihood of the presence or absence of the gene in problematic cases, but this test is not recommended for screening or random testing. Screening of all patients with ADPKD for intracranial aneurysms is excessive, but magnetic resonance imaging angiography of the brain is reasonable if the patient has a family history of ruptured intracranial aneurysm. The timing and need for repetition are uncertain.

Treatment starts with genetic counseling to reduce the incidence of the disease. Blood pressure control with angiotensin-converting enzyme inhibitors and eradication of cyst infections are directed at preserving renal function. Infected cysts require the use of antibiotics that penetrate into cyst fluid, such as ciprofloxacin and trimethoprim-sulfamethoxazole. Severe pain or massive renal enlargement that compromises physical functioning may be treated by surgical cyst unroofing or percutaneous cyst drainage and ethanol sclerosis without apparent compromise, but also without improvement, of renal function. Patients with large kidneys should avoid potentially traumatic situations. Gross hematuria abates with rest; hydration and pain control are comfort measures. Once the diagnosis of ADPKD is established, imaging studies of the kidneys need not be performed routinely unless new symptoms require evaluation.

The prognosis is variable and difficult to predict. Renal function usually remains normal until after age 30 years. In about 90% of patients, some degree of renal failure develops, progressing to end-stage disease by age 70 in 50%. Factors associated with a worse prognosis include later age at diagnosis, male gender, hypertension, increased left ventricular mass, and larger renal volumes. ADPKD diagnosed before the age of 1 year may progress to renal failure during childhood, whereas ADPKD detected during childhood seems to follow a clinical course identical to that of patients diagnosed as adults.

MEDULLARY SPONGE KIDNEY

The intriguing disorder of medullary sponge kidney was so named because of a controversial gross resemblance to the sea sponge. Medullary sponge kidney has a strong association with calcium nephrolithiasis and medullary nephrocalcinosis, does not cause renal failure, and is distinctly different from renal medullary cystic disease, a variant of the nephrophthisis–cystic renal medulla complex.

This disorder is found in 1 in 100 to 200 persons who undergo routine excretory urography; the true prevalence is unknown. Medullary sponge kidney affects only the renal medulla, with development of ectasia of the papillary and medullary collecting ducts and formation of many tiny cysts (under 7.5 mm in diameter). The pathogenesis is unknown because of the lack of formal tissue studies and because of the difficulty in making the diagnosis. Provocative reports support the hypothesis that medullary sponge kidney is an autosomal dominant genetic disorder.

Many persons with medullary sponge kidney have no symptoms. The most common symptoms are renal or ureteral colic, gross hematuria, and dysuria. Calcium stones occur in perhaps half of patients. Twenty percent of idiopathic calcium stone formers have medullary sponge kidney, with probably a higher frequency in women. The stones are composed of calcium oxalate or a calcium oxalate/phosphate mixture. The most likely cause appears to be hypercalciuria, which is found in 45% of men and 26% of women with medullary sponge kidney. The mechanism of hypercalciuria is unclear, but evidence exists supporting intestinal hyperabsorption and renal leak in different persons. Gross hematuria occurs in a few patients, with or without stones. Infection is common in women with medullary sponge kidney but uncommon in men. Several unusual or rare disorders accompany medullary sponge kidney, but congenital hemihypertrophy appears to have a nonrandom association. In the absence of secondary problems such as obstruction and pyelonephritis, the glomerular filtration rate remains normal. Incomplete distal renal tubular acidosis occurs in 40% of patients, and renal concentrating defect occurs in almost all patients.

Diagnosis depends exclusively on the characteristic appearance demonstrated by excretory urography. The opacification of the ectatic collecting ducts makes them look like a brush, and the cysts resemble grapelike clusters. If at least three papillae are affected, medullary sponge kidney is present. The interpretation of localized findings and papillary blush appearance is problematic.

Treatment is simple and usually highly successful. Thiazide diuretics effectively prevent stone formation. Vigorous treatment of infection is essential. The prognosis for patient and renal survival should approach that of unaffected persons.

MEDULLARY CYSTIC DISEASE

Medullary cystic disease is a rare disease that is one variety of an entity renamed the nephronophthisis–cystic renal medulla complex. The three major variants of this complex are juvenile nephronophthisis (50%), renal-retinal dysplasia (17%), and medullary cystic disease of adult onset (18%). Medullary cystic disease is characterized by progressive renal insufficiency terminating in renal failure in about 4 years. An early urine concentrat-

ing defect appears to be invariable; renal salt wasting with volume depletion occurs much less often. It is an autosomal dominant genetic disorder of uncertain pathogenesis. Small cysts are present in the medulla and corticomedullary areas of the shrunken, fibrotic kidneys. Diagnosis is based on family history and demonstration of corticomedullary or medullary cysts in small kidneys by imaging, biopsy, or nephrectomy analysis. The role of the cysts in the renal failure and their necessity for diagnosis are uncertain. Treatment is supportive.

ACQUIRED RENAL CYSTIC DISEASE

Many patients on chronic hemodialysis (40% to 90%) have multiple bilateral renal cortical and medullary cysts. Such cysts are much less common in chronic peritoneal dialysis patients (5%) and undialyzed patients with chronic renal failure. These acquired cysts are much more common in men than in women.

The clinical importance of these cysts is based on two features: the potential for renal cell carcinoma to develop in the cysts and the potential for serious hemorrhage from the cysts. As many as 7% of patients with acquired cysts develop renal cell carcinoma, although several large imaging studies have failed to find tumors in any patient. Part of the difficulty is distinguishing between renal adenomas and carcinomas in the absence of metastases. Masses with diameters exceeding 3 cm are considered malignant and should be removed. Another difficulty is the lack of firm guidelines to determine surveillance programs. Regular computer tomographic scanning, the preferable study, appears excessive. The clinician should use the symptoms to instigate investigation. Hemorrhage into a cyst or from cyst rupture can cause severe pain, gross hematuria, blood loss anemia, and even shock. Usually conservative observation, volume maintenance, and analgesia suffice, but occasionally nephrectomy or arterial embolization is necessary. The pathogenesis is unknown, but the resemblance of the renal cysts to ADPKD is intriguing.

OTHER RENAL CYSTIC DISEASES

Chronic hypokalemia causes tubular hyperplasia, hypertrophy, and dilatation. In one study, 44% of patients with primary hyperaldosteronism and hypokalemia were found to have renal cysts; about half of patients had more than two. Cysts appear common in other chronic hypokalemic states. Correction of the hypokalemia appears to cause cyst regression. This exciting observation demonstrates a humoral influence on renal cystogenesis.

Autosomal recessive polycystic kidney disease is a rare disorder affecting 1 in 14,000 newborns. Four varieties occur, dominated by the manifestations of either progressive renal failure or liver failure due to fibrosis. End-stage renal failure appears inevitable, although it may be delayed until early childhood. Glomerular cystic disease bears clinical resemblance to this disorder, but it spares the liver and might have variable forms of heredity.

| TABLE 156.1. | FEATURES OF MAJOR RENAL CYSTIC DISORDERS |

Disorder	Simple Cysts	Autosomal Dominant Polycystic Disease	Medullary Sponge Kidney	Medullary Cystic Disease	Acquired Renal Cystic Disease
Frequency	33% over 60 y	1:200–1000	20% of stone formers	Rare	50% in hemodialysis
Pathogenesis	Uncertain	Inherited autosomal dominant	Inherited autosomal dominant probable	Inherited: autosomal dominant, autosomal recessive	Unknown
Symptoms	Usually none	Hypertension, pain	Hematuria	Variable	Pain, mass
Complications	Rare	Liver cysts, aneurysms mitral valve prolapse	Stones, nephrocalcinosis	Salt wasting	Hemorrhage, tumor
Diagnosis	Ultrasound	Ultrasound, gene linkage	Excretory urography	Clinical course	Computed tomography
Prognosis	Excellent	End-stage renal failure in 50% at 60 y	Excellent	End-stage renal failure in 4 y	0–7% cancer

Congenital multicystic kidney is the most common cause of abdominal mass in the newborn (1 in 2,000 hospitalized infants). It is more often unilateral. It is not functional and is often removed surgically. This disorder is one of the causes of unilateral functioning kidney in adults (1 in 1,000). It and related dysplastic disorders are associated with many other developmental abnormalities and rare syndromes.

Tuberous sclerosis and von Hippel–Lindau disease are inherited systemic disorders that involve the kidneys, occasionally with cysts.

The important features of the more important cystic disorders are listed in Table 156.1.

BIBLIOGRAPHY

Avasthi PS, Erickson DG, Gardner KD. Hereditary neural-retinal dysplasia–nephronophthisis complex. *Ann Intern Med* 1976;84:157–161.

Fick GM, Gabow PA. Natural history of autosomal dominant polycystic kidney disease. *Annu Rev Med* 1994;45:23–29.

Fick GM, Gabow PA. Hereditary and acquired cystic disease of the kidney. *Kidney Int* 1994;46:951–964.

Ginalski JM, Portmann L, Jaeger PH. Does medullary sponge kidney cause nephrolithiasis? *AJR* 1990;155:299–302.

Grantham JJ. Mechanisms of progression in autosomal dominant polycystic kidney disease. *Kidney Int* 1997;52(Suppl 63):S93–S97.

Johnson AM, Gabow PA. Identification of patients with autosomal dominant polycystic kidney disease at highest risk for end-stage renal disease. *J Am Soc Nephrol* 1997;8:1560–1567.

Marple JT, MacDougall M, Chonko AM. Renal cancer complicating acquired cystic kidney disease. *J Am Soc Nephrol* 1994;4:1951–1956.

Murcia NS, Sweeney WE Jr, Avner ED. New insights into the molecular pathophysiology of polycystic kidney disease. *Kidney Int* 1999;55:1187–1197.

Ravine D, Gibson RN, Doulan J, et al. An ultrasound renal cyst prevalence survey: specialty data for inherited renal cystic diseases. *Am J Kidney Dis* 1993;22:803–807.

Torres VE, Young WF Jr, Offord KP, et al. Association of hypokalemia, aldosteronism, and renal cysts. *N Engl J Med* 1990;322:345–351.

Watson ML. Complications of polycystic kidney disease. *Kidney Int* 1997;51:353–365.

Kelley's Textbook of Internal Medicine, fourth edition. Edited by H. David Humes.
Lippincott Williams & Wilkins, Philadelphia © 2000.

CHAPTER 157

HEREDITARY NEPHROPATHIES

MARTIN C. GREGORY

Hereditary renal disease is more common than is generally realized. Underdiagnosis results in part from subtleties of inheritance. Whereas the familial pattern is readily apparent in autosomal dominant conditions such as adult polycystic disease, recessive or X-linked conditions can be much harder to spot. A classic example is Alport's syndrome (hereditary nephritis). Although best defined by hematuria as an X-linked dominant trait, the penetrance and severity of the condition are both usually greater in males. This means that if renal failure is used to define affectedness, Alport's syndrome appears to behave as an X-linked recessive. An affected man is likely to have a family history of renal failure only in his mother's male relatives—further afield than the family history may be known.

Many renal diseases not generally considered hereditary disorders occasionally run in families. This is particularly noteworthy in the case of vesicoureteral reflux, which can show autosomal dominant transmission with variable penetrance. The significance of this familial clustering is that the children of a parent with familial reflux are at risk for urinary tract malformations and should be screened by radionuclide cystography, or at least watched closely for urinary infections.

ALPORT'S SYNDROME

Alport's syndrome is progressive hereditary hematuric glomerulonephritis that generally affects male individuals much more severely than female individuals. There is a juvenile form of the disease in which boys develop renal failure at a mean age of 18 years, and an adult type in which renal failure occurs in men around the age of 35. Alport's syndrome is often associated with progressive hearing loss and, occasionally, with other nonrenal defects.

GENETICS

Inheritance is X-linked dominant in 85% of families. Over 300 different mutations of the COL4A5 gene, which codes for the α_5 chain of type IV collagen, have been described. COL4A5 is located on the X chromosome at Xq22. In 15% of families, typically those with early development of renal failure in both genders, autosomal recessive Alport's syndrome results from mutations of COL4A3 or COL4A4, both on chromosome 2 at 2q36. About 1% of patients, particularly those with associated hematologic abnormalities, display autosomal dominant inheritance, with as yet obscure mutations.

PATHOGENESIS

The fundamental lesion in most variants of Alport's syndrome is a defect in one of the genes coding for the α_3, α_4, or α_5 chains of type IV collagen in the glomerular basement membrane (GBM). Fetal GBM is composed of collagen α_1 and α_2 chains. Around birth, a developmental switch to collagen composed of α_3, α_4, and α_5 heterotrimers occurs. If one of these α chains is defective, normal assembly of a α-chain heterotrimers cannot occur. This is believed to lead to formation of imperfect collagen. The defect of basement membrane collagen may be more susceptible to proteolysis or less capable of orderly repair. The glomerular basement membrane becomes irregularly thickened and splits into multiple lamellae.

INCIDENCE AND EPIDEMIOLOGY

Alport's syndrome occurs worldwide. The incidence is probably 1 in 5,000 but many cases go unrecognized.

CLINICAL FEATURES

With X-linked disease, all hemizygous males have uninterrupted microscopic hematuria from birth, as do affected males and females with autosomal disease. In contrast, most heterozygous females with an X-linked gene show early but milder signs, and a few are clinically normal.

In childhood, hematuria may be episodically macroscopic, often after minor infections, and this may cause confusion with post-infectious and other forms of glomerulonephritis. Microscopy of the urine sediment shows dysmorphic erythrocytes with occasional tubular cells and erythrocytic, blood, and granular casts. Proteinuria is variable.

Some families with Alport's syndrome have associated abnormalities; the most common is high-frequency sensorineural hearing loss. This was true of Alport's original kindred, but overt hearing loss is not found in all families. When present, premature hearing loss in many family members is a valuable clue to the

diagnosis, but requiring it as a condition for diagnosing Alport's syndrome results in many cases being overlooked. Hearing impairment worsens roughly in step with increasing renal dysfunction and becomes profound in severe cases. Tinnitus troubles some patients.

Less common than hearing loss but nearly pathognomonic of Alport's syndrome is anterior lenticonus. It occurs in families with juvenile type Alport's syndrome and is readily apparent if the examiner uses a series of strong convex lenses in the ophthalmoscope to examine the anterior structures in the eye through a dilated pupil. The "oil drop" seen on the anterior surface of the lens explains the severe refractive error that impairs vision and prevents a clear view of the fundus. In many families, white or yellowish retinal flecks are seen, particularly near the macula.

LABORATORY FINDINGS

Renal biopsy shows a mixture of glomerular and tubular lesions with progressive scarring as the disease advances. Foam cells may be prominent but are not diagnostic, and glomerular crescents can occur in juvenile type nephritis. Routine immunofluorescence is negative, but examination of the biopsy with fluoresceinated anti-GBM sera or with monoclonal antibodies to the α_3 chain of type IV collagen reveals striking findings. The normal distinct linear staining of the GBM is usually absent in males who are hemizygous for an X-linked gene and often shows interrupted staining in heterozygous females. Electron microscopy of early cases may show thinning of the GBM. More advanced cases show a characteristic thickening of the GBM, which is frayed into several lamellae, often separated by small electron-dense granules. Basement membrane splitting is not pathognomonic of Alport's syndrome because similar appearances can occur in many glomerular diseases; however, only in Alport's syndrome is the splitting prominent and widespread at a time when there are few other changes in the kidney. A renal biopsy is unnecessary for diagnosis in a patient with hematuria if he or she has an extensive family history of hematuria and of renal failure in male relatives.

The blood in advanced cases shows the findings expected with renal insufficiency. Rare families have thrombocytopenia with giant platelets or pale blue, peripheral, cytoplasmic Fechtner inclusions in granulocytes.

Specific genetic tests are available for identifying the more than 300 known mutations of COL4A5. At present, these are of value to perhaps 50% of known families with Alport's syndrome. It is likely that the number of identified mutations will increase and that genetic screening and diagnosis will become increasingly practicable. Some adult type families, both with and without overt hearing loss, contain many hundreds of known gene carriers and there are likely many more undiscovered. Tests for the more common mutations may be appropriate in adults with familial or unexplained glomerulonephritis.

COURSE AND PROGNOSIS

All affected males eventually develop renal failure, at varying ages in different kindreds. The few women with X-linked disease who develop renal failure are mostly elderly. Boys and girls with homozygous autosomal recessive disease commonly develop renal failure in childhood or early adult life.

TREATMENT

There is no specific treatment. Control of hypertension is important, and modest protein restriction could be advised when renal function begins to deteriorate. Surprisingly, preliminary trials have not shown benefit from angiotensin-converting enzyme inhibitors, but in one small uncontrolled study, cyclosporin appeared to retard deterioration.

Appropriate plans should be made for dialysis or transplantation. Rarely, anti-GBM nephritis may develop in the renal allograft of a patient with Alport's syndrome, but this is not a bar to transplantation unless other members of the same family have lost grafts to anti-GBM nephritis. As in any familial nephropathy, great care should be taken in the selection of living donors.

Hearing aids help the hearing loss to some degree. If vision becomes severely impaired by lenticonus, intraocular lens implantation is feasible. Genetic counseling is vital but is complicated by the genetic heterogeneity of Alport's syndrome. For this reason, it is desirable to assemble as complete a pedigree as possible and perhaps to attempt molecular diagnosis before counseling the patient.

THIN BASEMENT MEMBRANE DISEASE

Thin basement membrane disease differs from Alport's syndrome in that hearing loss and renal failure rarely occur, even at advanced ages. Inheritance is autosomal dominant in most families, although many sporadic cases occur. Some studies have indicated that up to 3% of the population might have thin GBMs. The term *benign familial hematuria* is sometimes used to encompass both these patients and those who have unexplained glomerular hematuria with GBMs of normal thickness. Thin basement membrane disease is important to recognize so that unnecessary alarm, cystoscopies, and usurious insurance premiums can be avoided.

Many families with thin GBM disease have mutations in COL4A3 or COL4A4. Cases have been described in which homozygotes or mixed heterozygotes in these families have all the manifestations of Alport's syndrome.

Electron microscopy of a renal biopsy shows uniform thinning of the GBM to about half its normal thickness. Although this finding is highly characteristic, similar appearances occur in early cases of Alport's syndrome, so that a careful family history for longevity of affected males is at least as important as the biopsy in reaching a precise diagnosis of familial thin basement membrane disease.

NAIL PATELLA SYNDROME

Nail patella syndrome is an uncommon but striking autosomal dominant condition marked by abnormalities of bones, joints,

nails, and sometimes the kidney. Partial dysplasia of the nails, most marked in the thumb and index finger, and absence or hypoplasia of the patella with a tendency to genu valgum and recurrent subluxation are the most obvious features. On radiographs bilateral posterior iliac horns are visible; these can be palpated in thin subjects. About 30% of gene-carrying persons have proteinuria and some become uremic.

Nail patella syndrome arises from dominant mutations (haploinsufficiency) of the LIM homeodomain gene LMX-1B at 9q34. There is a very characteristic ultrastructural lesion of the GBM, which is thickened and irregularly fenestrated or "moth-eaten." High-resolution pictures of these lucent areas and of the subendothelial space show fibers of collagen with regular 64-nm periodicity. There is no specific treatment, but dialysis and transplantation are appropriate.

FABRY'S DISEASE

Fabry's disease is an X-linked disorder of sphingolipid metabolism that affects about one in 40,000; manifestations are much more common and severe in males. The disease arises from mutations of the α-galactosidase A gene at Xq21. Deficiency of α-galactosidase A permits accumulation of ceramide trihexoside in many tissues. Characteristic dark red macules and papules (angiokeratomata) may be found on the abdomen and scrotum, and subtle whorled corneal opacities occur in most patients. Glycolipid-laden macrophages are shed in the urine and are easily recognized by their "Maltese cross" appearance under crossed polarization. Electron microscopy shows remarkable lamellated "zebra bodies" in the cytoplasm of glomerular epithelial cells. Renal impairment begins in early adulthood in affected males and progresses to renal failure. Dialysis controls uremia but may not relieve the limb pains that torment many patients. Successful renal transplantation replaces the missing enzyme and might bring about regression of nonrenal manifestations.

OTHER CONDITIONS

CYSTINOSIS

Homozygous or mixed heterozygous mutations in the CTNS gene on chromosome 17 that codes for cystinosin, the putative cystine transporter, impair cystine transport out of liposomes. This allows cystine to accumulate in many tissues, including renal tubules, interstitium, and glomerular epithelial cells. Fanconi's syndrome develops in infancy or childhood; uremia soon follows. In adult forms of cystinosis, glomerular lesions may be severe and tubular damage mild. Deposits of cystine in the superficial layers of the cornea and conjunctiva can be seen on slit-lamp examination or by careful direct ophthalmoscopy. Renal rickets is a deforming consequence of acidosis, hypophosphatemia, and renal failure. Excessive intracellular cystine stores can be depleted to a degree by therapy with reducing reagents such as ascorbic acid, cysteamine, or dithiothreitol, but it is too early to judge the long-term benefits of these treatments. Rickets should be treated with alkali, calcium, and vitamin D analogs, and uremia with transplantation.

PRIMARY HYPEROXALURIA

Rare recessively inherited deficiency of either of two enzymes, alanine-glyoxalate aminotransferase or D-glyceric dehydrogenase, results in overproduction, generalized deposition, and overexcretion of oxalate. Urolithiasis and renal failure are the important sequelae. About one third of all patients respond to large doses of pyridoxine. Results of dialysis are poor as have been those of renal transplantation, although greater success may be obtained with vigorous peritransplantation dialysis and treatment with pyridoxine, orthophosphate, and magnesium starting immediately after transplantation. Hepatorenal transplantation is effective, but hepatic transplantation before widespread oxalate deposition occurs may be the best option.

BIBLIOGRAPHY

Barker DF, Hostikka SL, Zhou J, et al. Identification of mutations on the COL4A5 collagen gene in Alport's syndrome. *Science* 1990;248: 1224–1227.

Desnick RJ, Astrin KH, Bishop DF. Fabry disease: molecular genetics of the inherited nephropathy. *Adv Nephrol* 1989;18:113–127.

Govan JAA. Ocular manifestations of Alport's syndrome: a hereditary disorder of basement membranes? *Br J Ophthalmol* 1983;67:493–503.

Gregory MC, Atkin CL. Alport's syndrome. In: Schrier RW, Gottschalk CW, eds. *Diseases of the kidney,* 6th ed. Boston: Little Brown & Co, 1997:561–590.

Kelley's Textbook of Internal Medicine, fourth edition. Edited by H. David Humes. Lippincott Williams & Wilkins, Philadelphia © 2000.

C H A P T E R

158

OBSTRUCTIVE NEPHROPATHY

NELSON LEUNG
AMIT K. GHOSH
KARL A. NATH

In its role of defending the constancy of the internal milieu, the kidney elaborates urine of appropriate chemical composition and volume. The egress of urine from the kidney, its unimpeded flow through the urinary tract, and its excretion are the subsequent and essential steps critical to processes in the kidney that maintain homeostasis. Excretion of urine requires a patent urinary tract, effective ureteral peristalsis, a hydrostatic pressure gradient in the urinary tract, and normal micturition. Impairment in any of these requirements by lesions at any site from the renal calyx to the external urethral meatus—conditions des-

TABLE 158.1.	CLINICAL CIRCUMSTANCES IN WHICH DILATATION AND URINARY TRACT OBSTRUCTION MAY NOT COEXIST
Dilatation without Obstruction	**Obstruction without Dilatation**
Pregnancy	Low-grade obstruction
Any state of high urinary output	Intermittent obstruction
Vesicoureteral reflux	Early obstruction
Congenital megaureters	Anuric renal failure
After relief of obstruction	Severe volume contraction
Acute pyelonephritis	Restrictive processes such as retroperitoneal fibrosis
Bladder distention	Masking of dilatation on ultrasound because of acoustic shadowing from staghorn calculi

ignated as obstructive uropathies—can exert damaging effects locally within the urinary tract and also systemically, by virtue of impairment of renal function.

Obstructive nephropathy is defined as the functional and structural changes in the kidney sustained by obstructive uropathy. Obstruction is thus an important and potentially reversible cause for renal insufficiency. Delay in considering or securing this diagnosis incurs the risk of irreversible loss of renal function and enhances the susceptibility to such complications as infection and stone formation. Upper tract obstruction refers to lesions proximal to the bladder; obstruction at the level of the bladder and urethra is referred to as lower tract obstruction. Obstruction may be acute or chronic, intermittent or sustained, complete (or high-grade) or incomplete (low-grade). Renal failure arises if high-grade obstruction involves both kidneys or a solitary kidney, or if one kidney is obstructed and there is intrinsic disease in one or both kidneys.

Dilatation is designated by the prefix *hydro,* so hydroureter refers to dilatation of the ureter and hydronephrosis refers to dilatation of the renal pelvis and calyces. Dilatation of the urinary tract usually indicates underlying obstructive uropathy because the caliber of the urinary tract increases when obstructed. However, dilatation may exist without true obstruction to the urinary tract and, conversely, obstructive uropathy may be present with little or no dilatation (Table 158.1).

▓ INCIDENCE AND ETIOLOGY

Urinary tract obstruction in children is overwhelmingly due to congenital or developmental lesions, but in adults the causes are acquired and depend on the patient's age and sex. In persons ages 20 to 60 years, obstructive uropathy is more likely to afflict women than men, largely as a consequence of pregnancy and pelvic malignancies. Malignant obstruction in women is most commonly caused by carcinoma of the cervix; less common malignant causes are endometrial and ovarian carcinoma. In young to middle-aged adults, especially men, renal and urinary calculi are relatively common causes of obstructive uropathy, and these calculi usually consist of calcium oxalate; patients with recurrent infections may progress to struvite stones, which are prone to form staghorn calculi and cause obstruction. In patients older than 60, obstructive uropathy predominates in men because of the mounting incidence of benign prostatic hypertrophy and prostatic carcinoma. Indeed, transurethral resection of the prostate is the most common operation performed in men. Prostatic carcinoma is the most commonly diagnosed non–skin cancer in males, with approximately 200,000 new cases diagnosed in 1998.

Obstructive nephropathy contributed 5,358 cases of end-stage renal disease in the United States from 1993 to 1997. This number represents 2% of the total patients with end-stage disease. Of these, a little more than 75% were men. Similarly, in European studies, about 4% of patients with end-stage renal disease exhibited obstructive nephropathy, largely as a consequence of prostatic disease. In autopsy studies, the incidence of urinary tract obstruction is about 4%; many such lesions may remain undetected in older, relatively asymptomatic patients.

The causes of obstructive uropathy are summarized in Table 158.2. Lesions may be intrinsic or extrinsic to the urinary tract, and intrinsic lesions are subdivided into intraluminal and intramural causes. Intraluminal lesions, in turn, may either be intrarenal or extrarenal. Intrarenal intraluminal obstruction may arise from the deposition of crystalline material such as uric acid in uric acid nephropathy or medications such as acyclovir; intraluminal obstruction may also occur from casts due to paraproteins from plasma cell dyscrasias. Intraluminal causes in the upper tract include urinary calculi, blood clots, sloughed renal papillae, and fungus balls. Intramural lesions may be functional, as in motility disorders affecting the ureteropelvic or the ureterovesical junctions, or structural lesions anchored within the walls of the ureter. Extrinsic lesions obstructing the upper tract may originate in several major sites, including vascular lesions, diseases involving the female reproductive system, disorders of the gastrointestinal tract, and retroperitoneal processes. Obstruction to the lower tract in older patients may arise from mass lesions in the bladder, prostatic hypertrophy, or carcinoma. In younger men, lower tract obstruction may be due to strictures, valves, stones, meatal stenosis, or phimosis.

TABLE 158.2.	DIFFERENTIAL DIAGNOSIS OF OBSTRUCTION TO THE URINARY TRACT

Upper Tract Obstruction

Intrinsic

Intraluminal
 Tubules: urate, paraproteins, sulfonamide, triamterene, methotrexate, acyclovir, indinavir,
 Pelvis/ureter: stones, blood clots, papilla, fungus ball

Intramural
 Ureteropelvic junction obstruction, vesicoureteric reflux, ureteral stricture or valve, ureterocele, tumors involving the urinary tract

Extrinsic

Female reproductive system
 Pregnancy, uterine enlargement from tumors or fibroids, uterine prolapse, endometriosis, carcinoma cervix, ovarian tumors, tubo-ovarian abscesses

Gastrointestinal tract
 Crohn's disease, malignancy, abscesses, diverticular disease, appendiceal masses, pancreatic disease

Vascular disease
 Aortic aneurysms, aberrant blood vessels, retrocaval ureter, assorted vasculitides

Retroperitoneal disease processes
 Idiopathic or radiation-induced fibrosis, drug-induced fibrosis (e.g., methysergide, sotalol, methyldopa) retroperitoneal malignancy, hematomas, lipomatosis, retroperitoneal inflammation (e.g., granulomatous inflammation from tuberculosis, sarcoid), urinoma

Postsurgical
 Inflammatory scarring after surgery, inadvertent ligature, lymphocele

Lower Tract Obstruction

Bladder
 Blood clots, stone, tumor, foreign body, drug-induced neurogenic bladder (e.g., tricyclic antidepressants, anticholinergic agents, narcotic analgesics, α adrenergic agents), disease-associated neurogenic bladder (e.g., diabetes mellitus, spinal cord injury, demyelinating conditions, cerebrovascular disease)

Bladder neck and urethra
 Prostatic hypertrophy, prostatic carcinoma, stricture, valves, meatal stenosis, phimosis

---

FUNCTIONAL CHANGES IN OBSTRUCTIVE NEPHROPATHY

ALTERATIONS IN RENAL HEMODYNAMICS

Acute total unilateral ureteral obstruction elevates renal pelvic and intratubular pressures. Renal blood flow is initially increased owing to dilatation of the afferent arteriole, a process that probably reflects increased production of vasodilatory prostaglandins. During the first few hours after the onset of obstruction, the tendency for increased intratubular pressures to decrease the glomerular filtration rate (GFR) is counteracted by increased glomerular capillary pressure and glomerular plasma flow rates, so GFR is not appreciably decreased. As obstruction persists, vasoconstrictive autacoids (thromboxanes and angiotensin II) are in-creasingly produced by the kidney, leading to the normalization and then the reduction in renal blood flow rates; GFR is now severely compromised as vasoconstriction is maintained. By 24 hours, sustained reductions in renal blood flow and GFR occur, although tubular pressures are relatively normal.

Acute bilateral complete obstruction is characterized by changes in GFR and renal blood flow directionally similar to those occurring in unilateral obstruction and more marked elevations in tubular hydrostatic pressures. When vasoconstriction supervenes in bilateral obstruction, the postglomerular vasculature is preferentially affected. In chronic partial obstruction, the degree to which GFR is diminished is determined by the severity of obstruction and any deficits in extracellular fluid volume. With adequate extracellular fluid volume, GFR is preserved by elevations in the glomerular capillary pressure, which is achieved by preferential efferent arteriolar constriction.

When bilateral ureteral obstruction is relieved, there is pronounced postobstructive diuresis and natriuresis and a slow recovery of GFR. The duration of obstruction determines the extent of recovery of renal function. A remarkable recovery of GFR, often to normal values, may occur in kidneys subjected to obstruction lasting several days. The longer the period of obstruction, the more attenuated is the regain of renal function after decompression. However, as demonstrated by studies of experimental obstructive uropathy, obstruction for as little as 24 hours incurs a loss of up to 15% of nephrons. The recovery of function that occurs, as assessed by GFR or serum creatinine, is partly due to hyperfunction in functioning remnant nephrons and does not truly reflect the irreversible scarring imposed by even relatively short periods of obstruction.

Vesicoureteral reflux provides a functional form of obstructive uropathy and nephropathy in which alterations in glomerular hemodynamics may contribute to the progressive glomerulosclerosis and renal insufficiency seen in some of these patients. In this disorder, there is reflux of urine from the bladder into the ureter during micturition. Such reflux does not normally occur because of the oblique course of the ureter through the detrusor muscle and the arrangement of the muscle fibers of the ureterotrigonal unit. Vesicoureteral reflux predisposes to recurrent infections, and infected urine refluxing into the kidney is the chief determinant of scar formation. Reflux also induces obstruction, albeit temporarily and intermittently; as described previously, obstruction is associated with renal hyperemia followed by vasoconstriction. Such repetitive cycles of glomerular hyperemia and vasoconstriction during vesicoureteral reflux may predispose to glomerulosclerosis.

ALTERATIONS IN TUBULAR FUNCTIONS

Alterations in tubular function are also determined by the chronicity of obstruction of the urinary tract. During acute partial obstruction, the fractional excretion of sodium may decrease. With chronic obstruction, however, sodium reabsorption by the kidney is reduced, as is the concentrating ability of the nephron. Reduction in concentrating ability reflects diminished responsiveness of the collecting duct to antidiuretic hormone, in conjunction with decreased interstitial medullary tonicity. The causes of decreased interstitial medullary tonicity include the washout of solute owing to persisting medullary blood flow in the face of diminished delivery of solute to the thick ascending limb of Henle. Additional mechanisms arise from the impaired reabsorption of solute by the thick ascending limb of Henle. High concentrations of solutes in the medullary interstitium are maintained by continued reabsorption of sodium chloride by the thick ascending limb of Henle, a reabsorptive process that is inhibited by prostaglandins and requires intact Na-K-ATPase activity. In the obstructed kidney, Na-K-ATPase activity is diminished but prostaglandin production is increased: these two biochemical alterations may impair the reabsorption of solute by the thick ascending limb, and in turn the maintenance of high concentrations of solute in the medullary interstitium. Prostaglandins also render the collecting ducts resistant to antidi-

uretic hormone, and such effects may provide an additional mechanism by which enhanced production of prostaglandins impairs concentrating ability.

Obstruction impairs urinary acidification. This may take the form of a type IV renal tubular acidosis (RTA) that results from resistance to the effects of aldosterone or from hyporeninemic hypoaldosteronism. In type IV RTA, hyperkalemia is a characteristic feature and arises because of the deficiency of aldosterone or the refractoriness of the potassium-secreting sites in the distal nephron to aldosterone. The inability of the chronically obstructed kidney, in some instances, to produce renin and to respond to aldosterone may represent the injurious effects of sustained obstruction or the effects of the interstitial infiltrate in the obstructed kidney. Obstruction may also impose a type I or classic distal RTA in which the distal nephron cannot initiate or maintain a maximal pH gradient. Studies in experimental models of obstructive nephropathy have uncovered defects in the proton ATPase, an enzyme critical in urinary acidification. With type I RTA, there is a tendency to urinary potassium wasting; the serum potassium level is normal or low. Tubular defects may persist for several months after the release from an obstructing lesion.

The relief of bilateral obstruction of a solitary kidney usually gives rise to postobstructive diuresis, but this does not occur after the relief of unilateral obstruction. Postobstructive diuresis can result in striking urinary output and natriuresis. Several mechanisms contribute to postobstructive diuresis, including the appropriate natriuresis for salt and water retained during the phase of compromised renal function and in excess of that required for adequate expansion of the extracellular fluid, the effects of a natriuretic factor accumulated during the anuric/oliguric phase, osmotic diuresis due to increased luminal concentrations of urea, resistance of the collecting duct to antidiuretic hormone, and impaired tubular reabsorption of sodium in the thick ascending limb of Henle and the medullary collecting ducts.

PATHOLOGIC CHANGES IN OBSTRUCTIVE NEPHROPATHY

Complete occlusion to the ureter dilates the pelvis and flattens the papillae. Increased water content in the acutely obstructed kidney accounts for increased kidney weight. Calyces dilate at the expense of the progressively thinning cortex, and it is such pelvicalyceal dilatation that enlarges the chronically obstructed kidney. On histologic examination, the medullary tubules are dilated and the epithelia of the distal nephron are flattened and simplified. An interstitial leukocytic infiltrate appears soon after the onset of obstruction. Proximal tubules exhibit dilatation and atrophy; the latter accounts for cortical thinning. The end-stage chronically obstructed kidney may be grossly cystic.

Such changes reflect the combined effects of ischemia due to sustained renal vasoconstriction, disuse atrophy, and the interstitial cellular infiltrate. Disuse atrophy is thought to occur in renal tubular epithelia that are reabsorbing less solute and water—and are thus metabolically less active—because of decreased GFR. The overriding importance of the interstitial infiltrate as a determinant of renal functional and structural impairment is supported by considerable recent evidence. Obstruction provokes the synthesis and release of chemotactic substances from the renal tubular epithelium that recruit the interstitial cellular infiltration engendered by urinary tract obstruction. The interstitial infiltrate produces various autacoids (e.g., prostanoids), cytokines, degradative enzymes, and reactive oxygen species that exert vascular effects, effects on tubular transport, and effects that are ultimately damaging to the kidney. This infiltrate may produce such fibrogenic cytokines as TGF-β1, which could contribute to scarring of the kidney. Upregulation of the renin angiotensin system within the acutely obstructed kidney, and, in turn, activation of the transcription factor NFκB by angiotensin II, are assigned critical roles in the initiation of the inflammatory events after obstruction to the urinary tract. Another mechanism by which injury arises may involve Tamm-Horsfall protein, a large-molecular-weight protein produced by the distal nephron and a major constituent of urinary casts. Tamm-Horsfall protein is detected in the interstitium in urinary tract obstruction, and the inspissation of protein in the interstitium may incite an inflammatory response.

CLINICAL FEATURES

The presenting features of obstructive uropathy depend on the cause of the obstruction, location, severity, and duration. Acute obstruction arising from calculi and blood clots is often associated with severe abdominal pain radiating into the groin. During these episodes, the patient experiences intense paroxysms superimposed on a background of unremitting pain. Such pain arises from acute distention of the renal capsule. Chronic hydronephrosis may be asymptomatic or may cause low-grade discomfort. With chronic obstructive conditions, the circumstances that surround the exacerbation of pain may suggest the underlying condition. For example, flank pain occurring after a large intake of fluid or diuretics intimates the presence of obstruction at the ureteropelvic junction, but pain in this area during micturition points to vesicoureteral reflux.

Alterations in urine output may also be a presenting feature. Complete bilateral obstruction may impose anuria, partial obstruction may underlie polyuria and nocturia, and intermittent obstruction may lead to oliguria alternating with polyuria. Bladder neck obstruction may present with a palpable bladder, suprapubic pain, frequency, urgency, hesitancy, and a weak urinary stream with terminal dribbling. Symptoms of dysuria, urgency, and discolored or cloudy urine may indicate underlying urinary tract infection.

Other clinical findings suggestive of obstructive uropathy are abdominal fullness or an abdominal mass, gross hematuria, or the presence of tissue or gravel in the urine. Patients may also present with hypertension that is dependent in part on impaired sodium excretion or activation of the renin–angiotensin system. Uremic symptoms may be the presenting feature in patients with advanced renal insufficiency due to obstructive uropathy.

In addition to these presenting features that directly result from the complications of obstructive uropathy, patients may display local or systemic manifestations of the disease or condition provoking obstruction to the urinary tract.

A careful physical examination should be performed, in particular attempting to ascertain the presence, cause, and complications of obstruction to the urinary tract. General examination may reveal such features of the uremic syndrome as fetor, pigmentation and pallor of the mucous membranes, or cachexia arising from an underlying malignancy. Hypertension and signs of volume overload may be present. Superimposed infection may be suggested by fever. Abdominal, rectal, and pelvic examinations should be done with special care. Obstructive uropathy may complicate prior surgical procedures, so abdominal incisions should be noted. The abdomen should be palpated for the presence of tenderness, enlargement of the bladder, organomegaly, masses, and ascites. The abdomen should be auscultated, as obstructive uropathy may present as an ileus. Rectal and pelvic examinations are essential components of the physical examination in patients suspected of having underlying obstructive uropathy. The rectal examination may reveal an enlarged prostate, nodularity of the prostate, or rectal or pelvic masses. The pelvic examination may reveal a vaginal, pelvic, or rectal mass.

LABORATORY FEATURES

Patients with obstructive nephropathy may present with hyperkalemia and hyperchloremic normal anion metabolic acidosis due to type IV RTA. Plasma bicarbonate concentrations may also be decreased because of type I RTA. Hyponatremia may arise from excess free-water intake in the setting of renal insufficiency or renal salt wasting. Alternatively, hypernatremia results from polyuria and excess free-water loss. Compromised GFR elevates blood urea nitrogen and serum creatinine levels. The serum calcium concentration may be decreased along with an elevation in the serum phosphate level. With progressive renal disease, normochromic, normocytic anemia is observed, but rarely polycythemia may be a complication of hydronephrosis.

Urinalysis may reveal hyaline and granular casts. Proteinuria is absent or present in trace to 1+ amounts. The presence of leukocytes and bacteria points to an underlying infection. Hematuria suggests calculi, blood clot, tumors, or a sloughed papilla. In patients with calculi, crystals of calcium oxalate, calcium phosphate, or cystine can be detected on urinalysis.

Acute urinary tract obstruction may decrease the fractional excretion of sodium and increase urine osmolality, thereby mimicking prerenal causes of renal insufficiency. However, in chronic obstructive nephropathy, sodium reabsorption is reduced, as is the kidney's concentrating ability.

RADIOGRAPHIC TECHNIQUES

These clinical and laboratory findings raise the suspicion of urinary tract obstruction, but establishing the diagnosis invariably requires procedures that visualize the kidneys and urinary tract.

PLAIN ABDOMINAL FILM

A kidney-ureter-bladder (KUB) film detects calculi along the course of the ureter in 80% to 90% of cases. A KUB may provide information on the size and shape of the kidneys and any differences in kidney size. Tomograms may provide better visualization of the renal size and shape and small areas of calcification. Other germane findings—such as the presence of bladder enlargement, abdominal or pelvic masses, or bony metastatic disease—may be revealed on a KUB.

ULTRASONOGRAPHY

Ultrasound is the screening procedure of choice in assessing the presence of obstructive uropathy. It is noninvasive and especially suitable for demonstrating obstruction in the setting of renal insufficiency because it does not depend on renal function. In the normal kidney, the relatively hypoechoic parenchyma surrounds a hyperechoic central complex comprising peripelvic fat, blood vessels, and the renal pelvis. Hydronephrosis is diagnosed on ultrasound by a dilated intrarenal central collecting system containing anechoic fluid. Cortical thinning, which may arise in chronic obstructive nephropathy, is also readily detected. Ultrasound examination has 90% sensitivity and 80% specificity in the diagnosis of obstructive uropathy. A false-positive diagnosis of urinary obstruction may occur in nonobstructive dilatation of the upper tract; on the other hand, obstruction may be present without ultrasound-detectable dilatation. Calculi can also be detected by ultrasound.

Although useful as a screening procedure, ultrasound examination is limited by its inability to define the site and cause of obstruction. Obtaining such information often requires other procedures.

INTRAVENOUS PYELOGRAPHY

Intravenous pyelography (IVP) visualizes the kidney, calyces, pelvis, and ureter and may detect the site of obstruction. It should be used in the initial assessment of patients suspected of having obstructive uropathy and in whom renal function is normal. The chronicity and severity of obstruction determine the findings on IVP. In acute cases, the nephrogram is delayed but is of higher density, because contrast medium is concentrated to a greater extent. The calyces, renal pelvis, and ureter are dilated above the obstruction, and the renal contour may be increased in size. The calyceal fornices promptly dilate after obstruction. With the persistence of urinary tract obstruction, the papillae are blunted and become frankly concave, the calyces assume a clubbed contour, and the overlying cortex progressively thins. Such structural derangement is accompanied by functional impairment leading to a faint nephrogram. In some cases, the kidney subjected to sustained obstruction is contracted and reduced in size. Whatever the size of the chronically obstructed kidney, the contralateral, uninvolved kidney undergoes hypertrophy. Retroperitoneal fibrosis causes a characteristic medial deviation of the ureters on IVP. Bladder neck obstruction causes dilatation of the bladder and ureters, bladder trabeculation, and sometimes the formation of bladder diverticula and tortuosity of both ureters.

The adverse effects of IVP include allergy to contrast dye and the nephrotoxicity of these agents. The latter is more likely to occur in patients with renal insufficiency, multiple myeloma, or diabetes mellitus, or in older patients.

RETROGRADE AND ANTEGRADE PYELOGRAPHY

Retrograde and antegrade pyelography involves direct injection of contrast dye into the collecting system. It may be indicated in patients suspected of having obstructive uropathy in whom the diagnosis is not secured by other means, or in patients in whom IVP is contraindicated because of dye allergy or renal insufficiency. These procedures can localize the level of obstruction, determine whether obstruction is intraluminal or intramural, and decompress the urinary tract.

Retrograde pyelography involves catheterization of the ureter after cystoscopy and may require general anesthesia. The absence of contrast 10 minutes after retrograde injection argues against the presence of underlying obstruction. Antegrade pyelography involves entry into the collecting system by a percutaneous route under local anesthesia. This procedure also allows immediate relief of unilateral obstruction, urodynamic studies, and sampling of urine and tissue. The risks include bleeding, infection, and extravasation of urine.

RADIONUCLIDE IMAGING

Although it lacks the anatomical clarity of IVP, renal scintigraphy allows assessment of renal function, especially the relative function of the two kidneys, and allows monitoring of the recovery of renal function in a previously obstructed kidney. Diuretic renography is helpful in differentiating a dilated nonobstructed collecting system from true obstruction. In this test, renal scintigraphy is performed, a loop diuretic such as furosemide is administered, and additional scans are obtained. Diuresis facilitates washout of the isotope that accumulates in the dilated nonobstructed renal pelvis but not in a renal pelvis with true anatomical obstruction.

ABDOMINAL COMPUTED TOMOGRAPHY

Although not usually used in the initial evaluation of the patient suspected of having obstruction, computed tomography (CT) is particularly useful in determining the cause of obstruction because of the remarkable anatomical visualization it provides. In addition, CT is especially useful in evaluating patients in whom IVP is contraindicated because of dye allergy or renal insufficiency. Features that may be present on CT scans are dilatation of the collecting system, delayed excretion of dye in studies using contrast, and atrophy of the renal parenchyma. CT scanning of the abdomen is particularly useful in determining such causes of obstruction as retroperitoneal fibrosis and malignancies, abdominal lymphadenopathy, abdominal and pelvic masses, hematomas, and calculi.

MAGNETIC RESONANCE IMAGING

The exact role magnetic resonance imaging (MRI) will play in diagnostic evaluation is currently being defined. MRI provides enhanced soft-tissue contrast resolution, freedom from adverse effects of contrast material, and, in combination with gadolinium compounds, determination of GFR. It may thus assess obstruction structurally and functionally. MRI allows visualization of the kidney, even without any function, and dilatation of the urinary tract, the site of obstruction, and the presence of urinary tract infection. Lesions such as malignancies, enlarged lymph nodes, other mass lesions, and processes in the retroperitoneum (e.g., fibrosis, masses) may also be detected by MRI.

OTHER DIAGNOSTIC PROCEDURES

The Whitaker test may be used to diagnose obstruction of the upper urinary tract if other diagnostic tests are unclear. In this test, the hydrostatic pressure difference between the renal pelvis and bladder is determined at ambient urinary flow rates and again after fluid is infused into the renal pelvis at a specific rate. A pressure differential greater than 20 cm H_2O usually indicates ureteral obstruction. A voiding cystourethrogram is used to investigate the presence of vesicoureteral reflux and the function of the bladder. Obstruction to the lower urinary tract may be evaluated by cystoscopy, contrast studies, and urodynamic tests. Cystoscopy inspects the urethra and bladder. The anterior and posterior urethra can be assessed by contrast studies. Urodynamic evaluation is used in the diagnosis of neurogenic bladder dysfunction and includes cystometrography, electromyography, a urethral pressure profile, and urine flowmetry.

◼ OPTIMAL MANAGEMENT

The goals of management are the relief of symptoms, the correction of fluid and electrolyte abnormalities, the restoration and preservation of renal function, and the prevention or effective treatment of complications such as infection or stone formation. The clinical circumstances determine management, so the therapeutic approach may be conservative or may require instrumentation, endourologic techniques, or surgical procedures. High-grade obstruction involving both kidneys or high-grade obstruction in a solitary kidney should be relieved as soon as possible, using retrograde ureteral catheters or percutaneous nephrostomy tubes. Obstruction of any severity should be promptly relieved if there is concomitant urosepsis. In some patients with renal failure as a complication of bilateral obstruction, the severity of volume overload, hyperkalemia, or acidosis may mandate acute dialysis before the relief of obstruction.

Acute obstruction to the upper tract is commonly caused by calculi. Stones less than 7 mm usually pass spontaneously, and patients can be managed on an outpatient basis if they can tolerate large amounts of oral liquids. Larger stones usually necessitate intervention. Extracorporeal shock-wave lithotripsy can be used for most types of kidney stones lying in the pelvis and the upper and mid-ureter. Calculi distal to the pelvic brim are usually treated by ureteroscopy combined with stone extraction or stone fragmentation. A surgical approach is used for some lesions that cause upper tract obstruction, including intramural lesions, ureteropelvic junction obstruction, mass lesions of the renal pelvis or ureter, retroperitoneal fibrosis, or fibrosis secondary to such

conditions as an abdominal aneurysm. Sometimes repair is impossible, and urinary diversion may be necessary.

Lower tract obstruction may require prostatectomy, urethral dilatation, endoscopic urethrotomy, or an open procedure, depending on the underlying cause. Occasionally, suprapubic cystostomy is required before definitive correction. Clean intermittent catheterization is indicated for most forms of neurogenic bladder; for certain types of dysfunction, pharmacologic therapy may be beneficial. Chronic indwelling catheters should not be used in patients with neurogenic bladder because of the risks of infection, stone formation, and bladder carcinoma. In patients with neurogenic bladder and other forms of lower tract obstruction, surgical diversion using an ileal conduit may be required.

Postobstructive diuresis may lead to marked contraction of the extracellular fluid and, depending on the relative losses, hyponatremia or hypernatremia; hypokalemia, hypomagnesemia, and hypophosphatemia may also occur. If patients are euvolemic, half-normal saline should be infused at 50 to 75 mL per hour, with careful assessment of orthostatic changes in blood pressure, pulse, plasma electrolytes, and renal function. This regimen usually allows the excretion of salt and water retained during the obstructive phase and avoids excessive fluid administration, which may sustain continued diuresis and natriuresis. If extracellular fluid volume contraction develops on this regimen, then additional amounts of fluid, and solutes where appropriate, should be provided to repair the loss.

BIBLIOGRAPHY

Bander SJ, Buerkert JE, Martin D, Klahr S. Long-term effects of 24-hour unilateral ureteral obstruction on renal function in the rat. *Kidney Int* 1985;28:614–620.

Batlle DC, Arruda JAL, Kurtzman NA. Hyperkalemic distal renal tubular acidosis associated with obstructive uropathy. *N Engl J Med* 1981;304: 373–380.

Klahr S. Urinary tract obstruction. In: Schrier RW, Gottschalk CW, eds. *Diseases of the kidney*. Boston: Little, Brown, 1997:709–738.

Klahr S, Morrissey JJ. The role of growth factors, cytokines, and vasoactive compounds in obstructive nephropathy. *Semin Nephrol* 1998;18: 622–632.

Kelley's Textbook of Internal Medicine, fourth edition. Edited by H. David Humes.
Lippincott Williams & Wilkins, Philadelphia © 2000.

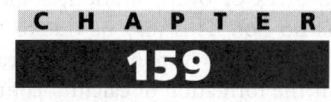

CHAPTER
159

RENAL LITHIASIS

DAVID A. BUSHINSKY

The incidence of renal lithiasis (kidney stones), although difficult to determine precisely, appears to be slightly over 1 case per 1,000 hospitalized patients per year and has been slowly increasing in recent decades. Stones lead to considerable morbidity, often requiring hospitalization, shock-wave lithotripsy, or surgery. Understanding the mechanisms of stone formation leads to rational treatment and a decreased incidence of stone disease and its associated morbidity.

Kidney stones are generally composed of calcium salts, uric acid, magnesium ammonium phosphate (struvite), or cystine. They develop from urine that is oversaturated with the components of the stone. Saturation depends on chemical free-ion activity. The chemical free-ion activity of the components of a stone, in a solution in which the stone will neither grow nor dissolve, is said to be at the equilibrium solubility product. If the free-ion activity decreases, the urine becomes undersaturated and the stone does not grow and may even dissolve. If the free-ion activity increases, the solution becomes oversaturated, and the stone may grow.

The chemical free-ion activity is influenced by many factors, including the concentration of the relevant ions, the urine pH, and complexation with substances in the urine. The chemical free-ion activity is directly related to the ion concentration, a function of how much of the particular ion is excreted in a specific volume of urine. Increased ion excretion and decreased urine volume increase free-ion activity. Urine pH is particularly important with respect to uric acid oversaturation. Citrate forms soluble complexes with calcium and thus reduces its free-ion activity.

Kidney stones can form and grow through homogeneous or heterogeneous nucleation. With homogeneous nucleation, increasing chemical free-ion activity leads to oversaturation with respect to a solid phase. Once this oversaturation reaches the formation product, the relevant ions form small clusters, which can grow to form a permanent solid phase. With heterogeneous nucleation, crystals grow on the surface of a dissimilar but complementary crystal or on another, often foreign, substance. *In vivo*, heterogeneous nucleation predominates over homogeneous nucleation, as the presence of a solid phase allows for crystal growth at a lower level of oversaturation (a so-called metastable solution) than if no solid phase is present. Microscopic crystals take longer to grow into clinically significant stones than the passage time for fluid through the renal tubule. It is thought that crystals must adhere to tubular cells, allowing time for further growth.

Urine from stone-formers is generally more oversaturated than urine from persons who do not form stones. However, despite similar degrees of oversaturation, some persons form stones but others do not. This may be due to the presence of inhibitors of crystallization. Uropontin, nephrocalcin, and pyrophosphate inhibit the formation of calcium-containing crystals. Some studies have shown a decrease in inhibitor activity when the urine of stone-formers is compared with that of controls, but the influence of abnormalities in the composition or quantity of inhibitors on the occurrence or frequency of stone formation is unclear.

Clinicians generally determine the lithogenic potential of urine by measuring the rates of solute excretion, in mass per unit time, of the principal components of stones, but the critical determinant of crystallization is oversaturation. Computer programs that calculate saturation from measured ion concentra-

tions are available and will increasingly be used for more accurate determination of the lithiasis risk. Even with sophisticated calculations of saturation, because of variations in hourly urine output of both water and solute, any mean collection underestimates the maximum oversaturation.

CALCIUM STONES

About 70% of all kidney stones contain calcium and are composed of calcium oxalate or calcium phosphate or a combination (Table 159.1). Pure calcium oxalate stones are more common than pure calcium phosphate stones. In general, once a patient forms a calcium-containing stone, he or she will form another in less than 7 years, with a decreasing time interval to subsequent stone events. Although pregnancy causes an increase in urine calcium excretion, it does not accelerate stone formation. Calcium stones may form secondary to excess calcium, oxalate, or uric acid excretion, or they may be idiopathic.

EXCESS CALCIUM EXCRETION
Idiopathic Hypercalciuria

Patients with idiopathic hypercalciuria have a normal serum calcium concentration, but their urine calcium excretion rate exceeds 300 mg per 24 hours (men) or 250 mg per 24 hours (women), or 4 mg per kilogram in either sex. These patients lack an apparent disorder that would elevate urine calcium excretion. Idiopathic hypercalciuria tends to be familial and is more prevalent in men, and initial stone formation often occurs in the third decade of life. The cause of idiopathic hypercalciuria is not known, but it may result from disordered regulation of calcium handling at sites where large fluxes of calcium must be tightly regulated. This disordered regulation may occur in the intestine, the kidney, or the bone, resulting in an increase in urine calcium excretion (Table 159.2). Increased intestinal calcium absorption may occur either by a direct mechanism or through excess calcium absorption mediated by 1,25-dihydroxyvitamin D_3.

The increase in intestinal calcium absorption results in a slight increase in the serum calcium level, a fall in the parathyroid hormone (PTH) level, and an increase in the amount of calcium filtered by the glomerulus and entering the renal tubule. Because PTH increases renal tubule calcium reabsorption, a fall in PTH, combined with an increase in the filtered load of calcium, results

TABLE 159.1.	TYPE AND PERCENTAGE OF RENAL STONES
Type	**%**
Calcium oxalate and calcium phosphate	37
Calcium oxalate	26
Calcium phosphate	7
Uric acid	5
Struvite	22
Cystine	2

TABLE 159.2. EXPECTED SERUM AND URINE VALUES IN ALTERNATIVE MECHANISMS OF IDIOPATHIC HYPERCALCIURIA

Parameter	Increased Intestinal Ca Absorption		Decreased Renal Reabsorption		Enhanced Bone Demineralization
	Direct	Excess 1,25(OH)$_2$D$_3$	Calcium	Phosphorus	
Ca absorption	Primary ↑	↑	↑	↑	↓
Serum 1,25(OH)$_2$D$_3$	↓	Primary ↑	↑	↑	↓
Serum PTH	↓	↓	↑	↓	↓
Bone Ca	nl	nl to ↓	nl to ↓	nl to ↓	Primary ↓
Fasting serum Ca	nl to ↑	nl to ↑	↓	nl to ↑	nl to ↑
Fasting serum P	nl	nl to ↑	nl to ↑	↓	nl to ↑
Fasting urine Ca	nl	↑	Primary ↑	↑	↑
Urine Ca after low Ca diet	nl	nl to ↑	↑	nl to ↑	↑

Ca, calcium; 1,25(OH)$_2$D$_3$, 1,25 dihydroxyvitamin D$_3$; PTH, parathyroid hormone; P, phosphorus; nl, normal.

in hypercalciuria. Decreased renal reabsorption of either calcium or phosphorus (the latter through a hypophosphatemia-induced increase in 1,25-dihydroxyvitamin D$_3$) results in hypercalciuria. A primary increase in bone mineral resorption increases the serum calcium level, suppresses PTH, and results in hypercalciuria.

Patients with idiopathic hypercalciuria have eluded efforts to be characterized into any of these specific diagnostic groups. Although there are expected serum and urine values for the alternative mechanisms of hypercalciuria, in formal metabolic studies there has been enough day-to-day variation among individual patients to preclude specific categorization. Among large numbers of patients, there appear to be smooth transitions in these metabolic parameters between patients, again precluding meaningful grouping. However, several general concepts have emerged from studies of patients with idiopathic hypercalciuria. Most investigators agree that patients have an increase in net intestinal calcium absorption, have increased 1,25-dihydroxyvitamin D$_3$ levels, have increased intestinal calcium absorption relative to the 1,25-dihydroxyvitamin D$_3$ levels, and have mild decreases in bone mineral density. These abnormalities appear to point to a systemic dysregulation of the effect of 1,25-dihydroxyvitamin D$_3$ acting on the intestine, bone, and possibly kidney. Studies in a genetic hypercalciuric rat model support this concept.

Reducing urine calcium excretion, especially with long-acting thiazide diuretics, and increasing fluid intake are the cornerstones of treatment. Limiting sodium and protein intake are advantageous in decreasing urine calcium excretion and stone formation.

Hyperparathyroidism

Patients with hyperparathyroidism have an elevated serum calcium concentration, elevated urine calcium excretion, and decreased serum phosphorus concentration, all associated with an increase in the serum level of PTH. The elevation in serum calcium can be very mild, and measurement of ionized calcium

may be helpful for diagnosis. The disorder is more common in elderly females, and generally a single parathyroid adenoma is found at surgery. Patients generally form hydroxyapatite or calcium oxalate stones.

PTH increases renal tubule calcium reabsorption, increases net bone resorption, and increases the synthesis of 1,25-dihydroxyvitamin D$_3$. Thus, excess, unregulated secretion of PTH results in hypercalcemia, which increases the renal filtered load of calcium. When this increased filtered load exceeds tubule calcium reabsorption, which is increased by PTH, hypercalciuria ensues. PTH also decreases renal tubule phosphate reabsorption, resulting in hypophosphatemia despite the increased phosphate absorption mediated by increased 1,25-dihydroxyvitamin D$_3$. A reduction in serum phosphate results in further elevations of 1,25-dihydroxyvitamin D$_3$, and thus calcium absorption, worsening the hypercalcemia and hypercalciuria.

Other hypercalcemic disorders occasionally lead to stone formation. The granulomatous tissue found in sarcoidosis and tuberculosis may convert 25-hydroxyvitamin D$_3$ to 1,25-dihydroxyvitamin D$_3$, resulting in hypercalcemia and hypercalciuria; however, PTH levels are depressed. Excess vitamin D supplementation, especially with ample calcium intake, results in hypercalciuria, and PTH levels again are depressed. Lithium therapy may directly increase the PTH level and result in hypercalcemia and hypercalciuria. Malignant cells can secrete PTH-related peptide, which acts in a manner similar to PTH but is not detected on standard PTH assays. Specific assays for PTH-related peptide are available.

Renal Tubular Acidosis

Two thirds of patients with classic distal renal tubular acidosis (type I RTA), either of the spontaneous or inherited variety, have nephrocalcinosis or nephrolithiasis; the stones are generally composed of calcium phosphate. Patients with proximal RTA (type II) generally do not have nephrocalcinosis or stones.

The mechanism of stone formation in patients with distal RTA is multifactorial. These patients have increased urinary excretion of calcium and phosphate, a high urinary pH, and decreased excretion of citrate. Increased urinary calcium excretion is due to a direct effect of acidosis, which reduces renal tubule calcium reabsorption. There is no concomitant increase in intestinal calcium absorption, so the increased urinary calcium must be derived from bone stores. The increased urinary pH decreases the solubility of calcium phosphate complexes, resulting in greater urinary oversaturation at any urinary calcium and phosphorus concentration. Citrate, the most prevalent organic anion in the urine, is freely filtered by the glomerulus and reabsorbed in the proximal tubule. Acidosis increases proximal tubule citrate reabsorption and decreases its excretion. Citrate binds calcium, lowering its concentration, and appears to inhibit crystallization. Thus, an acidosis-induced reduction in urinary citrate excretion increases the available calcium, raising oversaturation with respect to calcium phosphate complexation, and decreases an important crystallization inhibitor. Alkali administration, best given as the potassium salt, is thought to reduce nephrocalcinosis and nephrolithiasis, despite maintenance of an elevated urinary pH.

DECREASED CITRATE EXCRETION

Urinary citrate is decreased in many patients who form calcium stones. The decreased citrate excretion may be secondary to excessive protein intake, which leads to increased production of endogenous acid and increased net acid excretion. Decreasing dietary acid intake or ingesting potassium bicarbonate or potassium citrate increases citrate excretion and may help prevent stone formation.

EXCESS OXALATE EXCRETION

Most patients who form calcium oxalate stones excrete amounts of urinary oxalate (less than 40 mg per day) similar to those who do not. However, some excrete excessive oxalate, leading to calcium oxalate oversaturation and stone formation.

Oxalate is an end product of metabolism. Excessive urinary oxalate comes either from enhanced intestinal absorption or production. Normal humans absorb less than 5% of dietary oxalate. However, foods rich in oxalate, such as spinach and rhubarb, chocolate, peanuts, and cocoa, can increase urinary oxalate by 25% to 50%. Intestinal oxalate absorption, mainly in the colon, is increased by a reduction of dietary calcium, as oxalate forms insoluble and unabsorbable salts with calcium. Conversely, absorption is decreased by the use of oral calcium carbonate. Gastrointestinal disorders such as Crohn's disease, celiac sprue, and intestinal bypass surgery, which result in dietary fat malabsorption, lead to enhanced oxalate absorption, because the long-chain fatty acids and bile increase colonic permeability to oxalate. Binding the fatty and bile acids with cholestyramine decreases oxalate absorption.

Glycolate oxidation produces the bulk of urinary oxalate. There are two types of hereditary hyperoxaluria; in both cases, oxalate production is increased. The more common type, type I, is an autosomal recessive disease in which the excretion of glyoxylate, glycolate, and oxalate is increased. In type II, excretion of L-glyceric acid and oxalate is increased. Pyridoxine administration decreases oxalate excretion in some patients with type I.

A not uncommon cause of acute calcium oxalate crystal deposition, in the form of nephrolithiasis or nephrocalcinosis, is the accidental or intentional ingestion of ethylene glycol, used as an antifreeze, which is metabolized to oxalate.

EXCESS URIC ACID EXCRETION

Calcium stone-formers have an increased frequency of hyperuricosuria (more than 800 mg per day in men, more than 750 mg per day in women) than do persons who do not form stones. In general, excess uric acid excretion is a consequence of increased dietary purine intake derived from meat, poultry, and fish. Reducing uric acid excretion with allopurinol decreases the formation of calcium oxalate stones.

The mechanism by which hyperuricosuria promotes calcium oxalate stones is uncertain. The dimensions of uric acid crystals closely match those of calcium oxalate, and uric acid crystals appear to promote heterogeneous nucleation of calcium oxalate from a metastable urine. Alternatively, the excess uric acid may adsorb inhibitors of calcium oxalate crystallization, allowing stone formation to occur at modest degrees of oversaturation.

IDIOPATHIC

Even after extensive evaluation, in some patients a clear cause of stone formation cannot be found. Excretion of calcium, oxalate, and uric acid is normal, and the urine is not oversaturated with respect to solid phases of calcium oxalate or calcium phosphate. It is impossible to determine a mechanism for stone formation, so decisions regarding treatment to prevent another stone are speculative. The results of stone analysis, if available, can guide treatment.

URIC ACID STONES

Urine pH is a major determinant of uric acid oversaturation and subsequent stone formation. Uric acid is a weak acid in which two H^+ may, in theory, be dissociated. However, as the pK of the first H^+ dissociation is 5.4 and of the second is 10.0, only the first can be dissociated at an attainable urine pH. Uric acid (with two H^+) is far less soluble than urate (with one H^+), indicating that solubility increases with increasing urine pH. At an acid urine pH of 5, even the normal uric acid excretion of less than 800 mg per 24 hours (in men) in 1 L of urine may result in oversaturation and potential stone formation. Urine pH is determined by endogenous acid production and the proportion of net acid excreted as NH_4^+ compared with that excreted as titratable acidity. The more net acid that can be excreted as the base NH_4^+, the higher the urine pH. Several studies indicate that uric acid stone-formers excrete less net acid as NH_4^+ and more as titratable acidity, lowering the urine pH.

Other than urine pH, the main determinants of urinary saturation with respect to uric acid are uric acid production and excretion and urinary volume. In normal persons, uric acid production is a direct function of dietary purine intake from meat, poultry, and fish. Increasing purine intake (especially more than 4 mg per kilogram per day) increases uric acid excretion. Some patients with gout have mild overproduction of uric acid; others with genetic defects of purine reuse, such as the Lesch–Nyhan syndrome, have massive overproduction of uric acid. Patients with myeloproliferative disorders often overproduce uric acid and during treatment may have massive release of preformed uric acid.

The kidneys are responsible for over 50% of daily uric acid excretion, with the rest degraded in the intestine. Some patients have a relative decrease in renal tubule uric acid reabsorption, resulting in increased uric acid excretion and decreased intestinal degradation. Up to 25% of patients with clinical gout have uric acid nephrolithiasis. These patients tend to have excess uric acid excretion, even when they consume a low-purine diet and have a very acidic urine pH. Patients with chronic diarrhea are particularly at risk for uric acid stones, because they tend to be dehydrated and the alkaline diarrheal fluid causes metabolic acidosis and an acidic urine. Probenecid and large doses of salicylates promote uric acid excretion and predispose to stone formation.

The main tenets of treatment are hydration, dietary purine moderation, urinary alkalization, and, if necessary allopurinol. Increasing fluid intake and decreasing the amount of dietary purine decrease urinary oversaturation. Alkalinization with bicarbonate or a bicarbonate precursor such as citrate should be aimed at maintaining a urine pH over 6.0 throughout the day and night. During the day, multiple doses of bicarbonate—to match the endogenous acid production of about 1 mEq kilogram per 24 hours—can be used. If the nocturnal urine pH falls, acetazolamide can be used. If these measures are unsuccessful, allopurinol can be instituted.

MAGNESIUM AMMONIUM PHOSPHATE (STRUVITE) STONES

Magnesium ammonium phosphate stones form only when the urinary tract is infected with urea-splitting bacteria. Most *Proteus* and *Providencia* species have urease that splits urea, as do some species of *Klebsiella pneumoniae* and *Serratia marcescens*. Bacterial urease hydrolyzes urea to form NH_3, CO_2, and H_2O, consuming H^+ during the hydrolysis; the urine pH rises. NH_3 spontaneously hydrolyzes to form NH_4OH, and the CO_2 is hydrated to form HCO_3^-, which becomes $CO_3^=$ in the alkaline urine. Concentrations of NH_4OH and $CO_3^=$ are elevated, and any phosphate present is deprotonated (PO_4^{3-}). The struvite ($MgNH_4PO_4 \cdot H_2O$) stones are readily formed on the PO_4^{3-} backbone, as are carbonate apatite [$Ca_{10}(PO_4)_6 \cdot CO_3$] stones due to the presence of $CO_3^=$. The carbonate apatite is usually present within the struvite and can even be the predominant species.

Without bacterial urease, this cascade of events cannot occur. Infection often occurs in the presence of structural abnormalities, either congenital or acquired. Struvite stones may form secondary to another stone that causes infection and obstruction.

In the presence of bacteria, local oversaturation occurs and crystals form around the bacteria. The infection is difficult to control because normal urine flow, which can wash away bacteria, is disrupted. The stones rapidly grow and can fill the renal collecting system, resulting in staghorn calculi. Hematuria is common, and renal failure can result from obstruction and infection. Surgical stone removal is difficult, because any retained stone fragment often contains bacteria and can be the nidus for new calculi formation.

CYSTINURIA

Cystinuria is a rare hereditary disorder in which a tubular defect in dibasic amino acid transport results in increased cystine, ornithine, lysine, and arginine (COLA) excretion. The stone disease often presents by the fourth decade. Owing to the sulfur content of the cystine molecule, the stones are apparent on plain radiographs and often present as staghorn calculi or multiple bilateral stones. Cystinuria, in which cystine accumulates only in the lumen of the renal tubules, is distinct from cystinosis, in which there is widespread intracellular cystine deposition.

Cystine is poorly soluble, at about 300 mg per liter at neutral pH. Thus, the normal cystine excretion of about 30 to 50 mg per day is readily soluble in the daily urine output. However, homozygote cystinurics generally excrete 250 to 1,000 mg of cystine per day, with heterozygotes excreting an intermediate amount. There are at least three distinct types of cystinuria, which can be classified by intestinal transport studies.

Treatment must be directed at decreasing the urinary cystine concentration below the limits of solubility. The dietary precursor of cystine, methionine, is an essential amino acid, and it is impractical to reduce intake and thus excretion. Increasing urinary volume so that cystine remains below the limits of solubility is often practical, but sometimes 4 L of urine is necessary. Increasing urine pH above 7.5 increases the solubility of cystine, but this is often difficult on a chronic basis. D-penicillamine or tiopronin bind cystine and reduce urinary oversaturation, but side effects limit their use.

BIBLIOGRAPHY

Asplin JR, Favus MJ, Coe FL. Nephrolithiasis. In: Brenner BM, ed. *The kidney.* Philadelphia: WB Saunders, 1996:1893–1935.

Bushinsky DA, Krieger NS. Integration of calcium metabolism in the adult. In: Coe FL, Favus MJ, eds. *Disorders of bone and mineral metabolism.* New York: Raven Press, 1992:417–432.

Bushinsky DA, Monk RD. Calcium. *The Lancet* 1998;352:306–311.

Coe FL, Parks JH. New insights into the pathophysiology and treatment of nephrolithiasis: new research venues. *J Bone Miner Res* 1997;12:522–533.

Coe FL, Bushinsky DA. The pathophysiology of hypercalciuria. *Am J Physiol* 1984;247:F1–F13.

Consensus Conference. Prevention and treatment of kidney stones. *JAMA* 1988;260:977–981.

Curhan GC, Willett WC, Rimm EB, et al. A prospective study of dietary calcium and other nutrients and the risk of symptomatic kidney stones. *N Engl J Med* 1993;328:833–838.

Monk RD, Bushinsky DA. Pathogenesis of idiopathic hypercalciuria. In: Coe F, Favus M, Pak C, et al, eds. *Kidney stones: medical and surgical management.* New York: Raven Press, 1996:759–772.

Pak CYC. Pathophysiology of calcium nephrolithiasis. In: Seldin DW, Giebisch G, eds. *The kidney: physiology and pathophysiology.* New York: Raven Press, 1992:2461–2480.

Parks JH, Coe FL. Pathogenesis and treatment of calcium stones. *Semin Nephrol* 1996;16:398–411.

Kelley's Textbook of Internal Medicine, fourth edition. Edited by H. David Humes.
Lippincott Williams & Wilkins, Philadelphia © 2000.

C H A P T E R

160

TUMORS OF THE KIDNEY, URETER, AND BLADDER

JIA BI
DEREK RAGHAVAN

■ CANCER OF THE KIDNEY

DEFINITION

Renal neoplasms are uncommon, accounting for 3% of all adult malignancies in Western society. Most of these cancers are renal cell carcinomas, although other rare tumors of the kidney have been described, including transitional cell carcinoma, sarcoma, adult Wilms' tumor, and germ cell tumor (teratoma).

INCIDENCE AND EPIDEMIOLOGY

Renal cell carcinoma (RCC) affects 30,600 people in the United States annually, and the incidence is steadily rising. More than 10,000 deaths occur each year. Patients with this cancer usually present during the fifth to seventh decades of life; the median age at diagnosis is 60. Men are affected twice as frequently as women. RCCs are found in all ethnic groups with no racial predilection. Most RCCs occur sporadically; however, about 4% of cases are an inherited pattern. Such familial renal cancers include von Hippel–Lindau disease (VHL) and familial papillary renal cell cancers. Approximately 1.6% of RCCs are part of the autosomal dominant VHL disease, characterized by retinal and central nervous system hemangioblastoma, pheochromocytoma, pancreatic cyst, and RCC. Compared with sporadic cases, RCCs in the von Hippel–Lindau syndrome tend to be multifocal and bilateral and appear at a younger age in life. RCC and malignant angiomyolipoma are also associated with tuberous sclerosis complex, an autosomal dominant disorder of unknown cause characterized by seizures, mental retardation, and hamartomas.

ETIOLOGY

The cause of RCC remains largely undefined. Smoking is linked to an increased risk of renal cell carcinoma in men, but the association is somewhat weaker in women. Obesity and hypertension are two other independent risk factors. The relation between RCC and the use of antihypertensive agents such as calcium channel blockers and diuretics remains unclear. Patients with autosomal dominant or recessive polycystic kidney disease do not have an increased risk for RCC compared with the general population. However, a 3- to 6-fold higher incidence of RCC has been found in the chronic dialysis population as well as in renal transplant recipients, presumably owing to the development of acquired cystic kidney disease. Occupational exposure to chemicals appears to have little consistent significance, although a range of different occupations has been implicated in isolated case-control studies. Data are inconsistent on the role of diet in the development of RCC.

The isolation of the VHL gene in 1993 on chromosome 3p25 came as a breakthrough in the area of molecular genetics of RCC. Subsequently, the gene was found to encode for a tumor suppressor protein. This protein competes with elongin A in binding with elongin B and C, thus preventing the formation of a transcriptional elongation complex and thereby inhibiting the transcription of certain target genes in cell proliferation. At the molecular level, both copies of the VHL gene must be inactivated for tumors to develop; therefore, the first mutation in the VHL gene is inherited in the germline, and inactivation of the remaining wild-type allele occurs as a somatic event. Inactivation of the VHL gene could also be responsible for the nonhereditary forms of RCC, since somatic mutation of the VHL gene has been found in 75% to 80% of sporadic RCC cases. To date, the VHL gene does not appear to be involved in the development of papillary renal carcinomas.

PATHOGENESIS

Recent immunohistochemical studies suggest that RCCs arise from the proximal convoluted tubular cells. Therefore, "hypernephroma" is a misnomer because Grawitz, who introduced the term to describe the clear cell variant of RCC, thought the tumor originated from heterotopic adrenal (hypernephroid) rests in the kidney.

Most RCCs are solitary lesions affecting either kidney with equal frequency. However, the tumors can be multicentric in the same kidney (4%) or bilateral (3%). Grossly, the tumors are often well-demarcated round masses protruding from the cortex. The clear cell tumors are usually yellow owing to high lipid content. On cross section, areas of necrosis, cystic degeneration, hemorrhage, and calcification are commonly present. Histologically, RCCs are classified into clear cell type (75% to 85%), chromophilic type (12% to 14%), chromophobic type (5%), oncocytic type (2% to 4%), and collecting duct type (1%).

CLINICAL FINDINGS

With the increasing application of ultrasonography and computed tomography (CT) scans for the diagnosis of nonspecific abdominal symptoms and other conditions, 20% to 30% of cases are discovered incidentally as small tumors in a clinically asymptomatic stage. The classic triad of hematuria, flank pain, and a palpable mass is seen only in less than 10% of patients with

RCC and usually portends an unfavorable outcome. However, presentation with one or two of these three symptoms is common, since about 70% of patients with RCC have gross or microscopic hematuria, 50% have abdominal or flank pain, and 40% have a palpable mass. An approach to the investigation of hematuria is summarized in Figure 160.1. When the tumor grows, it may extend into and invade surrounding structures, such as the perinephric fat, posterior abdominal wall, inferior vena cava, ureter, adrenal gland, spleen, liver, and pancreas. Patients with left-sided RCC can present with acute left varicocele from obstruction of the spermatic vein. Hypertension may occur if the tumor compresses the parenchymal vasculature, causing increased renin production. Renal failure may result from tumor replacing the normal kidney tissue or from secondary amyloidosis. Constitutional symptoms, such as fever, night sweats, anorexia, and weight loss are common.

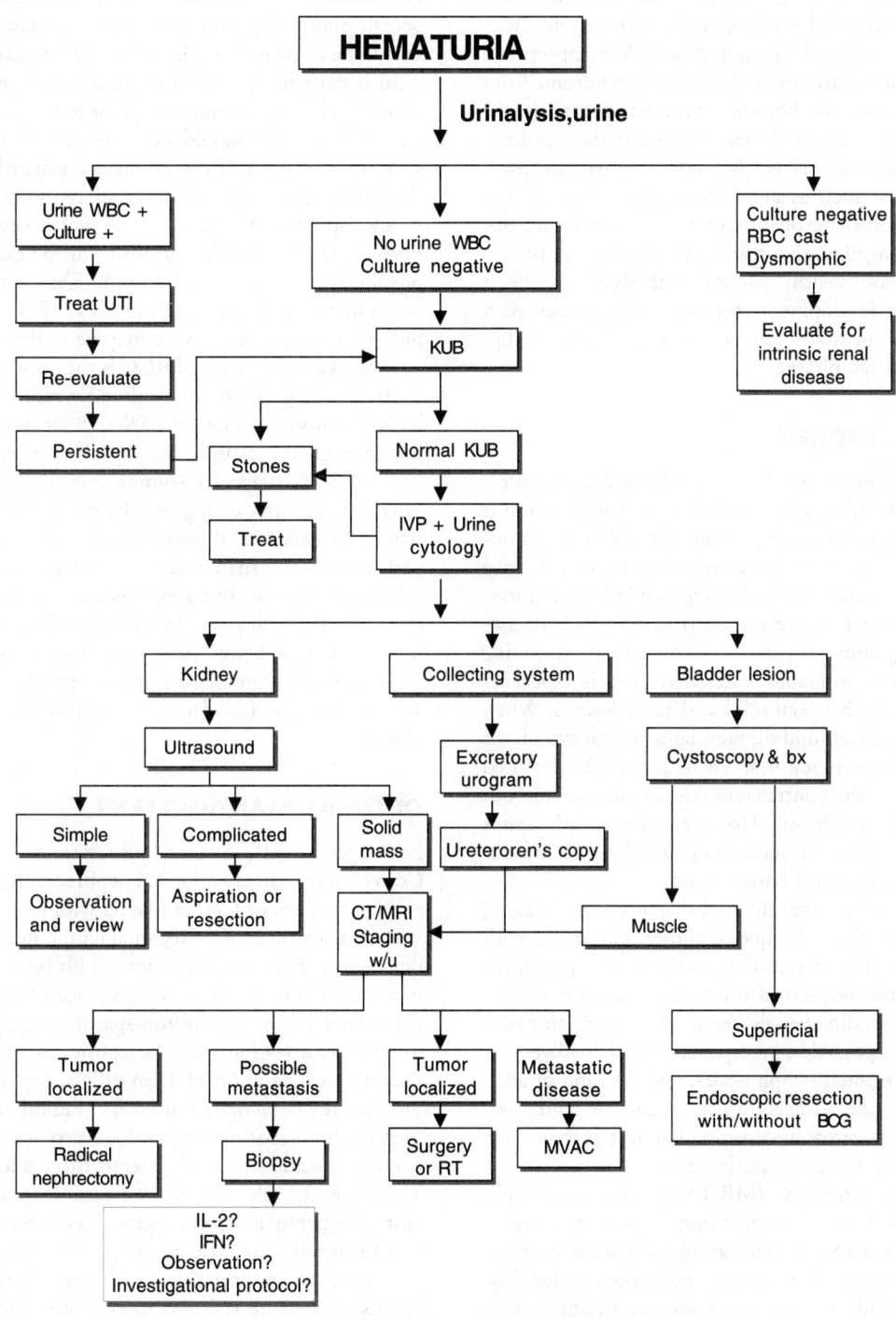

FIGURE 160.1. Approach to the investigation of hematuria.
EVIDENCE LEVEL: C. Expert Opinion.

Because the renal bed is a clinically silent area, only 40% of patients have disease confined to the kidney at diagnosis, and over 20% of patients present with symptoms of metastatic lesions. Tumor spreads by either hematogenous or lymphatic routes. The common sites of distant metastasis are the lungs, lymph nodes, liver, bone, and brain, although metastatic lesions have been described in virtually every organ of the body.

Paraneoplastic syndromes are relatively common features in RCC, the most notable ones being hypercalcemia and erythrocytosis, from the tumor secretion of parathyroid hormone-like immunoreactive protein and erythropoietin, respectively. Anemia may often be present. Hyponatremia with inappropriate secretion of antidiuretic hormone and Cushing's syndrome from ectopic adrenocorticotrophic hormone production can also be seen. Hypercoagulable states with venous thrombosis or pulmonary emboli have been described. Moreover, other rare paraneoplastic syndromes, such as amyloidosis, nonmetastatic hepatic dysfunction, limbic encephalitis, erythema gyratum repens, myopathy, and polymyalgia rheumatica, have been reported.

For reasons that are unclear, patients with RCC may be at increased risk for the development of second malignancies, such as those of the breast, prostate, colorectum, and bladder, malignant melanoma, and lymphoma.

LABORATORY FINDINGS

In a patient with a history or physical findings that suggest a renal malignancy, the initial characterization of a mass lesion is usually achieved with intravenous pyelography (IVP) or ultrasonography. IVP is a simple, noninvasive screening test. It may differentiate between renal cysts and malignant lesions and may reveal complications such as ureteral obstruction and hydronephrosis. Ultrasonography is another convenient screening method to evaluate a suspicious renal mass and is especially useful in differentiating between solid and cystic lesions. When combined with IVP, ultrasound differentiates benign cysts from solid masses with an accuracy near 98%. It can also be used to evaluate the size of the contralateral kidney and to rule out obstruction and hydronephrosis. However, ultrasound cannot be reliably used to assess the renal vein, intrahepatic inferior vena cava, and retroperitoneal lymph nodes.

CT scan is the most commonly used diagnostic and staging modality and remains the technique of choice. Performed with intravenous contrast, it accurately defines the renal topographic anatomy, the size and location of the tumor, and the relation of tumor to the surrounding vessels (renal vein and inferior vena cava). It also evaluates possible extracapsular spread, involvement of blood vessels or regional lymph nodes, and invasion of adjacent organs, such as the adrenals, spleen, pancreas, and liver. However, CT is less sensitive in detecting lesions less than 2 cm or tumor extension to the perinephric fat.

Magnetic resonance imaging (MRI) may have some additional benefit over CT in detecting tumors less than 2 cm or extracapsular extension and in delineating local anatomy more clearly. However, because of its expense and limited availability, MRI is often reserved for patients with known contraindications to iodine contrast or for patients whose CT results are equivocal. The role of positron-emission tomography (PET) has not been

defined in the context of renal tumors. Because 80% of RCCs are hypervascular, angiography is sometimes used to depict the lesion and provide a vascular map for the surgeon. Angiography is expensive and invasive and should therefore be used only for tumors in a solitary kidney, for vascular mapping before surgery, or for tumors in which angioinfarction is planned.

The staging process of RCC should include a detailed history and physical examination, basic hematologic parameters, liver and kidney functions, serum electrolytes, and a chest radiograph. CT scanning of the chest is sometimes necessary to rule out occult pulmonary and mediastinal metastasis. A bone scan should be obtained to rule out skeletal metastasis, although the yield is particularly low in asymptomatic patients with normal blood levels of serum alkaline phosphatase. Imaging of the brain with CT or MRI should be done in patients with neurologic symptoms or signs. If the tumor is apparently localized only to the kidney, the patient should undergo surgical resection. Fine-needle aspiration (FNA) is usually not necessary, because if the FNA is negative the lesion must still be excised owing to the possibility of a false-negative result. On the other hand, if there is extrarenal involvement of tumor, a CT- or ultrasound-guided biopsy of the primary lesion may be indicated.

The pathologic stage of RCC is the most important prognostic factor. Stage I (tumor confined within the kidney capsule) has a 5-year survival rate of 65% to 85%, stage II (tumor invading through the capsule but confined within Gerota's fascia) 45% to 80%, stage III (tumor invading into the renal vein, inferior vena cava, or regional lymph node) 15% to 35%, and stage IV (metastatic disease) 0% to 10%. In the past, patients with tumors less than 3 cm in diameter were thought to have a better prognosis, but some recent studies have contradicted this view. It is still generally held that those with asymptomatic tumors have a better prognosis than those with significant tumor-related symptoms. Other important prognostic factors are microscopic vascular invasion, nuclear grade, and DNA ploidy.

OPTIMAL MANAGEMENT

For stages I to III, the standard treatment is surgical resection. Conventional surgery is radical nephrectomy, which involves the en bloc removal of Gerota's fascia with its contents and usually ipsilateral adrenectomy. Regional lymph nodes are resected during surgery. However, in patients with bilateral tumors, tumors in a solitary kidney or in the presence of a poorly functioning contralateral kidney, nephron-sparing surgery (partial nephrectomy or enucleation) may be considered. Recent studies have shown that for tumors of 4 cm or less, nephron-sparing surgery provides the same rate of survival as radical nephrectomy. However, nephron-sparing surgery does carry some risk of postoperative complications, namely, hemorrhage and fistula formation. Therefore, the selection of candidates for this surgery is important. Preoperative or postoperative radiation does not add any benefit in reducing local recurrence or improving survival.

The outcome for patients with stage IV disease is very poor, because RCCs are resistant to chemotherapy in general. Most clinical studies in the past have shown response rates of less than 6%. Continuous infusion of floxuridine has reportedly produced response rates between 14% and 27%, although the responses are usually partial and short lived. Surgical intervention is recommended in patients with solitary metastatic lesions that are resectable. Radiation can be used to palliate symptoms from metastases to the bone or brain and to reduce spinal cord compression.

Spontaneous regression of metastatic RCC lesions has been reported in the literature, with an incidence of 0.8% to 3%. This has been reported for metastatic sites, including the brain, bone, regional and distant lymph nodes, liver, and most commonly the lungs. Complete and durable disappearance of tumors has been documented. The mechanism for this phenomenon is unknown, although immunologic factors have been postulated. Many of the spontaneous regressions were associated with surgical removal of the primary tumor, but nephrectomy does not appear to be the crucial event, because regression has been observed without primary tumor manipulation. Therefore, for patients with stage IV RCC, nephrectomy should not be recommended for the sole purpose of achieving spontaneous regression. It should be considered only when palliation of local symptoms such as pain and hematuria is required.

During the last decade, extensive research has been conducted to evaluate the role of immunomodulators in the treatment of metastatic RCCa. Interleukin-2 (IL-2) works through the activation of cytotoxic T-cell subgroups and stimulation of cytokine release. In a multicenter trial, IL-2 demonstrated 4% complete response rate and 8% partial response rate, with median duration of response of 23 months. However, the toxicities of high-dose intravenous IL-2 is substantial, mainly from a capillary leak syndrome, which can cause cardiovascular ischemia, renal failure, and shock. Supportive measures such as vasopressors and intensive care unit monitoring are often needed. Interferon-α is found to have an overall response rate of 12%, but with less common complete responses. A recent randomized study comparing IL-2, interferon-α, and both found a significantly higher response rate in the combination group (18.6% compared with 6.5% and 7.5%). Event-free survival at 1 year was also higher in the combination group, although there was no difference in overall survival. However, other studies using similar combinations have failed to show any benefit over IL-2 used alone.

▪ CANCER OF THE BLADDER

DEFINITION

Bladder cancer is the sixth most common cancer in the United States, causing over 10,000 deaths each year. It accounts for more than 90% of urinary tract malignancies. Management of this disease—which exhibits stem cell function, is associated with expression of several common oncogenes, and is responsive to surgical intervention, radiation, and chemotherapy—has become one of the recent paradigms of our approach to solid tumor malignancy.

INCIDENCE AND EPIDEMIOLOGY

Cancer of the bladder affects 50,000 people annually in the United States. Its incidence rises with age and peaks during the seventh decade of life. The male:female ratio is about 4:1. It is seen more often in the white than in the black population. The incidence of bladder cancer is higher in urban areas, suggesting a possible role of environmental factors in carcinogenesis. Cigarette smoking is by far the leading risk factor, with a confirmed dose- and time-response relation for both sexes. Occupational exposure to carcinogenic compounds found in dye, rubber, paint, plastics, metal, and motor vehicle exhaust significantly raises the risk of bladder cancer. Other established risk factors are chronic infection of the lower urinary tract, history of external-beam radiation to the pelvis, chronic indwelling urinary catheter, the use of cyclophosphamide, and high-fat diet. In the Mediterranean basin, schistosomiasis is still the main causative agent of bladder cancer and is classically associated with squamous cell carcinoma.

PATHOGENESIS

Most bladder cancers are transitional cell carcinomas (90%). The less common cell types are squamous cell carcinoma (7%), adenocarcinoma (1% to 2%), and small cell carcinoma; rare histologic types such as sarcoma, lymphoma, and melanoma comprise less than 1% of cases. Although the histogenesis is not fully understood, it is clear that there is a stem cell tumor of origin, and dominant transitional cell carcinoma may coexist with squamous and glandular differentiation. Bladder cancer is often associated with a field defect of the urinary mucosa, with the result that the entire lining of the urinary tract may be at risk for malignancy. Transitional cell carcinoma may be classified into two prognostic groups. Superficial tumors are those that occur at the level of the bladder mucosa, including carcinoma in situ (Tis), papillary lesions (Ta), and those that invade into (but not through) the lamina propria (T1). These superficial tumors constitute 80% of incident bladder cancers. They can be solitary but are often multifocal with a strong tendency to recur.

Recurrence can occur at the same site or any other site along the urothelial tract. Invasive tumors penetrate into (T2) and beyond (T3, T4) the muscularis propria. They are aggressive and tend to metastasize early. About 20% of patients have invasive cancer at presentation. The most important prognostic factor is the depth of tumor invasion (stage). Tumor grade is also an important factor. Low-grade (I) tumors rarely progress, whereas most high-grade (III) tumors progress and are associated with a rate of poor survival. Vascular or lymphatic invasion predicts an increased risk of invasion and metastasis. The presence of a Tis tumor significantly increases the risk of invasion when identified in association with other foci of superficial disease. Other prognostic factors are the absence of expression of blood group antigens on the tumor cell surface, DNA ploidy, expression of epidermal growth factor receptor, and p53 mutations.

CLINICAL FINDINGS

Most patients with bladder cancers present with painless, gross or microscopic hematuria, which can occur suddenly and intermittently. Symptoms of urinary frequency and urgency can be the result of bladder wall irritation or volume loss due to space-occupying lesions and is often misdiagnosed as "chronic interstitial cystitis." Abdominal discomfort, flank pain, or a palpable mass can occasionally be the first clinical evidence of invasive bladder cancer. Obstruction of the ureteral orifice with subsequent hydronephrosis and renal insufficiency is possible from an invasive tumor, although it can remain clinically silent until locally advanced. Invasive bladder cancer may extend locally into the prostate, seminal vesicles, rectum, uterus or vagina, sacral vertebra, and the retroperitoneal soft tissue. It spreads through the lymphatics and blood vessels to distant lymph nodes, the lungs, the liver, and the bones and may even cause brain metastases or carcinomatous meningitis. Five to 20% of patients present with symptoms from metastatic lesions. Constitutional symptoms may occur with disseminated disease, but paraneoplastic syndromes are rare in transitional cell cancers.

LABORATORY FINDINGS

Routine urinalysis almost invariably shows hematuria, the degree of which does not correlate with the extent of the lesion or lesions. Intravenous urography reveals an intravesical filling defect in 60% of cases. It also provides anatomical information about the urinary tract, such as hydronephrosis or hydroureter. Ultrasound is sometimes used to assess the bladder wall and to evaluate the kidneys and ureters. Urine cytology is a convenient and inexpensive method of obtaining a tissue diagnosis and provides a specificity and sensitivity of 80% in grade III tumors but relatively low sensitivity for grade I and II tumors (10% and 50%, respectively). Direct visualization and biopsy of the tumor are usually achieved by cystoscopy, which has been facilitated in recent years by the introduction of flexible instrumentation.

The staging process for bladder cancer should include a thorough history and physical examination, laboratory studies with complete blood cell count and hepatic and renal functions. Chest radiograph should be obtained in all patients. CT scan of the abdomen and pelvis is the standard noninvasive diagnostic modality to evaluate lymphadenopathy and other organ involvement.

OPTIMAL MANAGEMENT

For superficial papillary bladder cancer, the initial treatment is endoscopic resection of the tumor or tumors. For patients at high risk for recurrence, bacille Calmette-Guérin (BCG) may be administered into the bladder through a catheter as an adjuvant to transurethral resection. A common schedule is weekly administration of BCG for 6 weeks, followed by monthly doses for 6 to 12 months. The mechanism of action is incompletely understood, but there is evidence that the attachment of the bacillus to bladder cells elicits an immune response, which eradicates the malignant cells; or, the effect may simply be due to nonspecific immune stimulation with alteration of local suppressor:helper T-cell ratios. The adjuvant treatment has been proved to reduce the rate of recurrence and prolong disease-free time but may not affect the ultimate frequency of disease progression to invasive stage. During BCG treatment, the patient may experience dysuria, frequency, hematuria, or a general flulike syndrome. Because BCG is a living organism, it can produce local, regional, and systemic infections. Granulomatous infections can occur at extravesical sites, including the prostate, epididymis,

testes, kidney, liver, and lungs. BCG sepsis is the most serious complication and can be life threatening. When the diagnosis of extravesical involvement is made, combination antituberculous antibiotic therapy should be given for 6 months.

For patients with organ-confined invasive bladder cancer, cystectomy is viewed as the standard treatment in North America and Europe. Radical cystectomy involves the en bloc removal of the anterior pelvic organs, which includes the bladder, prostate, and seminal vesicles in men and the bladder, urethra, uterus, ovaries, and vaginal cuff in women. Bilateral pelvic lymph node dissection is often performed. The ureters are reconnected to an intestinal conduit as a urinary diversion. Traditionally, the conduit drains into an external collecting bag attached to the abdominal wall. Recently, continent reservoirs such as Koch's pouch (using the ileum) and Indiana pouch (using ileocecal segment) have become popular. The procedures involve the creation of an internal conduit with an antireflux mechanism that is either brought to the abdominal wall or sutured to the urethra, thus allowing patients to self-catheterize or void in the normal position, which greatly improves their self-image and increases acceptance rates. Also, the technology for creating orthotopic (artificial) bladders has improved. Radical cystectomy results in a 60% to 75% 5-year survival rate with T2 disease and 20% to 40% with T3 or T4 disease.

For patients with localized invasive disease, who are not surgical candidates, radiation is the alternative definitive therapy in North America, although radical radiation therapy is used as definitive treatment in some British and European centers. To date, there have not been any well-designed, randomized studies comparing radiation with surgery among patients with similar characteristics. Toxicities of radiation are dermatitis, proctitis that is occasionally complicated by bleeding and obstruction, cystitis or bladder fibrosis, impotence, incontinence, and development of secondary malignancies in the radiation field.

Combined-modality approaches, incorporating systemic chemotherapy with definitive local modalities, have been studied extensively in the past few years in the hope of sparing the bladder or improving overall survival. This has been predicated on the concept that systemic chemotherapy may reduce the extent of local tumor while controlling occult metastases. In a randomized, prospective trial assessing the benefit of concurrent chemoradiation, a protocol of single-agent cisplatin administered during the period of radiation therapy resulted in a 67% rate of sustained pelvic tumor control compared with 45% from radiation alone; however, overall survival was not significantly different. The role of neoadjuvant (first-line) systemic chemotherapy, followed by definitive radiation therapy or cystectomy, is still being investigated. Although earlier studies with the combination of cisplatin, methotrexate, and vinblastine (with or without adriamycin) demonstrated higher local tumor response, recent randomized trials have failed to show any survival benefit from the combination approach, although one major North American trial has not yet been analyzed.

Adjuvant (postoperative) chemotherapy has shown some promise in improving the outcome of definitive treatment. Randomized trials assessing the usefulness of combination regimens (e.g., the combination of methotrexate, vinblastine, adriamycin, and cisplatin, or MVAC), administered after radical cystectomy for patients with involved lymph nodes, have suggested that improved disease-free survival may be achieved. However, in the extant trials, which have been flawed by poor design and inadequate sample size, overall improvement in rate of survival has not been demonstrated.

For patients with metastatic bladder cancer, chemotherapy is the treatment of choice. A landmark study, conducted by an international consortium, compared the MVAC regimen with single-agent cisplatin. The MVAC regimen produced a response rate of 39% with a median survival of 12.5 months, which was statistically superior to the response rate of 12% and an overall survival of 8.2 months in the group that received cisplatin alone. The survival benefit persisted after a minimum follow-up of 6 years. Newer agents are being actively studied; in recent years, paclitaxel, gemcitabine, docetaxel, and ifosfamide have been shown to produce response rates of 20% to 40% as single agents. Combination of these agents has resulted in response rates of 50% to 80%, with apparently less toxicity than the conventional combination MVAC regimen. A phase III trial comparing gemcitabine and cisplatin with the standard MVAC regimen has been completed and awaits analysis.

CANCER OF THE RENAL COLLECTING SYSTEM

DEFINITION

The renal pelvis and the ureters form the upper collecting system. Histologically, they share the same transitional cell epithelium as that of the bladder. Therefore, neoplasms arising in these structures differ very little from their bladder counterparts, with the exception that the upper tracts do not have the investing tissues, such as fat and muscle, characteristic of the bladder.

INCIDENCE AND EPIDEMIOLOGY

Cancers of the renal pelvis and ureters are uncommon, constituting about 5% of all urinary system neoplasms. Men are affected more than women (4:1), and median age of onset is 65 years (range 32 to 88).

Cigarette smoking is the primary risk factor for the development of cancers of the renal collecting system, with a clear dose-response relationship. Occupational exposure to carcinogenic chemicals, such as those found in petroleum, plastics, coal, asphalt, and tar products, is another well-documented risk factor. Heavy use of analgesics, especially phenacetin, can cause analgesic nephropathy with papillary necrosis, which leads to a 2- to 6-fold higher risk of urothelial malignancy. Ten to 50% of patients with bladder cancer can have synchronous or metachronous cancers of the upper collecting system, due to field defect or to intraluminal seeding or both. Other reported risk factors are a history of external-beam radiation, prior use of cyclophosphamide, chronic urinary calculi, and chronic interstitial nephritis from urinary stasis. A particularly high incidence of urothelial cancers is found in populations at risk for the Balkan endemic nephropathy—a unique familial kidney disease of unknown cause that appears in restricted rural areas of the Balkans.

PATHOGENESIS

Neoplasms of the ureter and renal pelvis can appear at any part of the upper collecting system, but the distal third of the ureter and the extrarenal portion of the pelvis are affected more often. Tumors are usually solitary, although multiple lesions are not rare. Pathologically, these epithelial malignancies do not differ from those of the bladder. Most are transitional cell carcinomas. Other histologic types, including squamous cell carcinoma, adenocarcinoma, and soft-tissue sarcoma, have also been reported.

CLINICAL FINDINGS

Painless hematuria, macroscopic or microscopic, is the most common presenting symptom (over 75%). Flank pain or palpable mass occurs less frequently. About 15% of patients present with symptomatic urinary tract infection. Ureteral obstruction or hydronephrosis often remains clinically silent until late-stage disease. Hypertension results from vascular compression leading to increased renin secretion. Local invasion causing ureterocolic fistula, thrombosis of the inferior vena cava, and unilateral lower extremity edema due to lymphatic obstruction are other less common presentations. Paraneoplastic syndromes such as hypercalcemia and amyloidosis have been reported, although this may reflect misreporting of RCCs. Common sites of metastasis are regional lymph nodes, lungs, liver, lumbar vertebrae, and peritoneal cavity.

LABORATORY FINDINGS

The common initial screening test for cancer of the renal collecting system is intravenous urography, which may reveal a filling defect, calyceal obliteration, hydronephrosis, or hydroureter. Retrograde pyelography may define more clearly the morphologic features of tumors visualized on IVP, may identify a tumor missed on IVP, and may help to evaluate a nonfunctioning kidney. Ultrasonography is useful to differentiate tumors from non-opaque calculi. CT scanning may confirm the presence of a tumor and may provide staging information. MRI is useful in its ability to detect vascular invasion and in defining local anatomy more clearly. For tissue diagnosis, urine cytology has a sensitivity of 50%. Fluoroscopic guided brush cytology has a sensitivity and specificity of approximately 90%. With the introduction of ureterorenoscopy, direct visualization of the tumor as well as endoscopic biopsy is now possible.

OPTIMAL MANAGEMENT

Tumors arising from the renal pelvis and calyces are treated with nephroureterectomy, including excision of a cuff of the bladder. For patients with solitary kidney, multifocal lesions, or poor function of the contralateral kidney, renal-sparing surgery may be indicated. Recent studies have focused on endoscopic ablation of low-grade tumors, with adjuvant topical instillation of agents such as BCG or mitomycin C, a cytotoxic agent. For locally extensive or metastatic disease, combination chemotherapy with MVAC or equivalent regimens has a response rate of 40% to 50%, with a median survival of 12.5 months, an outcome not different from that achieved for transitional cell carcinoma of the bladder. As yet, the role of adjuvant chemotherapy has not been determined.

BENIGN AND MISCELLANEOUS TUMORS

Papillary renal adenomas are the most common benign neoplasms arising from the renal tubular epithelium, occurring in up to 40% of adults. Metanephric adenoma and metanephric adenofibroma are closely related benign tumors, affecting all age groups and with a slight female predominance, and are often accompanied by polycythemia. Tuberous sclerosis is known to associate with hamartoma and angiomyolipoma. The latter often grows rapidly in pregnancy and can be complicated by hemorrhage. Other rare benign tumors are hemangioma, lipoma, leiomyoma, myxoma, and neurofibroma. These tumors are usually diagnosed incidentally and require intervention only when they become clinically symptomatic.

As mentioned earlier in this section, rare malignancies of the urinary tract include sarcoma, melanoma, and teratoma. They should be managed in the same fashion as their counterparts from other primary sites and have been reviewed in detail elsewhere. Metastatic cancers to the kidney are usually derived from primary cancers of the breast, lung, pancreas, liver, or gastrointestinal tract or may be due to malignant lymphoma or leukemia. These are frequently asymptomatic, especially in the context of metastatic solid tumors, and are mostly found during autopsies.

BIBLIOGRAPHY

Boccardo F, Rubagotti A, et al. Interleukin-2, interferon-alpha and interleukin-2 plus interferon-alpha in renal cell carcinoma. A randomized phase II trial. *Tumori* 1998;84(5):534–598.

Brooks JD, Marshall FF. Transitional cell carcinoma of the upper urinary tract. In: Raghavan D, Scher HI, Leibel SA, et al., eds. *Principles and practice of genitourinary oncology.* Philadelphia: Lippincott-Raven, 1997: 337–346.

Eschwege P, Saussine C, Steichen G, et al. Radical nephrectomy for renal cell carcinoma 30 mm or less: long term follow-up results. *J Urol* 1966; 155:1196–1199.

Fyfe G, Fisher RI, Rosenberg SA, et al. Results of treatment of 255 patients with metastatic renal cell carcinoma who received high-dose recombinant interleukin-2 therapy. *J Clin Oncol* 1995;15:688–696.

Linehan WM, Lerman MI, Zbar B. Identification of the von Hippel-Lindau (VHL) gene: its role in renal cancer. *JAMA* 1995;273:564–570.

Loehrer PJ, Einhorn LH, Elson PJ, et al. A randomized comparison of cisplatin alone or in combination with methotrexate, vinblastine, and doxorubicin in patients with metastatic urothelial carcinoma: a cooperative group study. *J Clin Oncol* 1992;10;1066–1073.

Negrier S, Escudier B, Lasset C, et al. Recombinant human interleukin-2, recombinant human interferon alfa-2a, or both in metastatic renal cell carcinoma. *N Engl J Med* 1998;338:1272–1278.

Raghavan D, Shipley WU, Garnick MB et al. Biology and management of bladder cancer. *N Engl J Med* 1992;322:1129–1133.

Sternberg CN, Swanson DA: Non-transitional cell bladder cancer. In: Raghavan D, Scher HI, Leibel SA, et al., eds. *Principles and practice*

of genitourinary oncology. Philadelphia: Lippincott-Raven, 1997:315–330.

Kelley's Textbook of Internal Medicine, fourth edition. Edited by H. David Humes. Lippincott Williams & Wilkins, Philadelphia © 2000.

C H A P T E R
161

CONGENITAL ANOMALIES OF THE KIDNEY, URETER, AND BLADDER

PATRICK BROPHY
JEAN E. ROBILLARD

Congenital abnormalities of the kidneys, urinary collecting system, and bladder are seen first and primarily in children. The widespread application of prenatal ultrasonography has led to the in utero detection of genitourinary (GU) abnormalities, especially after 28 weeks of gestation, at an incidence of roughly 1% of total births. With such early identification, prenatal diagnosis of urinary tract anomalies will probably continue to decrease the number of uncorrected anomalies discovered de novo in older children and in adults. However, because some apparent abnormalities appear to be developmental without clinical importance after birth, multidisciplinary consultation is wise before any intervention.

EMBRYOLOGY OF THE KIDNEY

The development of the kidney in mammals proceeds in three stages with three sets of kidneys developing successively: the pronephros, the mesonephros, and the metanephros. The first stage (pronephros) is characterized by the emergence of paired tubules that arise from the cephalic end of the nephrotomes to form the pronephros, a rudimentary organ that appears at about the third week of gestation and undergoes complete involution within 2 weeks. The mesonephros develops more caudally on about day 24 of gestation in humans. The mesonephros is induced by the pronephric duct and consists of approximately 20 pairs of glomeruli and thick-walled tubules. By the fifth week of gestation, the mesonephric kidneys are able to form urine, which drains into the mesonephric duct and in turn opens into the cloaca. The mesonephros, the permanent kidney in amphibians, degenerates by the eleventh to twelfth week of gestation in humans. The most important role of the mesonephros is to induce the formation of the ureteric bud, which is required for the formation of the metanephros. Failure of mesonephric differentiation often leads to renal agenesis and renal hypoplasia, as well as to anomalous development of the gonads and adrenal glands. The metanephros begins to develop around the seventh week of gestation and is the result of reciprocal inductive interactions between the metanephric blastema and the ureteric bud. Renal tubular function begins in the human metanephric kidney by the ninth week of gestation. By the fourteenth week, the loop of Henle is functional and tubular reabsorption occurs. Nephron formation ceases by the thirty-sixth week of gestation in humans.

Several genes have now been implicated in the development of the kidney. One of the earliest genes responsible for lateral mesoderm differentiation and mesonephric development is the homeobox gene *Lim1.* Homozygous *Lim1* mutant newborn mice completely lack kidney and gonads. Other genes such as *Pax2* and *WT1* have been identified as essential for development of the metanephric mesenchyme and differentiation of the renal epithelium. *Pax2,* a transcription factor of the paired box family, is normally expressed in the mesonephric duct, the ureteral bud, and metanephric mesenchyme. Heterozygous *Pax2* mutant newborn mice often present with hypoplastic kidney with reduced calyces and upper parts of the ureters, suggesting defects in branching of the ureteric bud and in epithelial transformation of metanephric mesenchyme. Heterozygous *Pax2* mutation in humans is associated with optic colobomas and vesicoureteral reflux. Homozygous *Pax2* mutant mice present with complete lack of kidneys, ureters, and genital buds.

The Wilms' tumor suppressor gene, *WT1,* a transcription factor with zinc finger binding domains, is expressed in mesonephric tubules and in derivatives of the metanephric mesenchyme. Mutations in the tumor suppressor function of the *WT1* gene are found in 10% to 20% of patients with Wilms' tumor and are associated with the Denys–Drash syndrome, a triad of pseudohermaphroditism, nephropathy, and Wilms' tumor. Heterozygous for null mutations of the *WT1* gene in humans may also present with the WAGR syndrome (Wilms' tumor, aniridia, GU malformation, and mental retardation).

C-ret, a gene encoding a tyrosine urinase receptor, is expressed at the tip of the ureteric bud and is required for ureter bud growth. Homozygous c-*ret* mutant exhibits a high degree of renal agenesis and often a complete absence of ureters. In addition to c-ret, the development and growth of the ureteric bud is also dependent on GDNF (glial cell line–derived neurotrophic factor), a member of the transforming growth factor-β (TGF-β) super family. GDNF, which is expressed in the metanephric mesenchyme, has been identified as the ligand for the c-*ret* receptor and is essential for the development and branching of the ureteric bud. Another gene, the *ld* (limb deformity) gene, also plays an important role in ureteric bud and metanephric development. Absence of *ld* expression is associated with renal agenesis secondary to a failure of the ureteric bud to induce the metanephric mesenchyme.

Wnt4, a member of the Wnt family of secreted glycoproteins, plays an important role in condensing metanephric mesenchyme cells and in transforming these cellular aggregates into epithelial vesicles. Mutant mice lacking Wnt4 fail to form peritubular cell aggregates, although other aspects of mesenchymal and ureteric development are preserved.

In addition to these important genes, many other genes are involved in kidney development. Among these, insulin-like growth factors (IGF-I, IGF-II), transforming growth factor-β, and fibroblast growth factors have been shown to be involved in renal epithelium differentiation and renal growth and maturation.

SYNDROMES INVOLVING CONGENITAL ANOMALIES OF THE KIDNEY, URETER, AND BLADDER

Abnormalities of the urinary tract are noted in approximately 1 in 500 routine obstetric sonographic studies. There are now well over 100 syndromes involving some abnormality of the GU system. Table 161.1 provides a summary of our current understanding of the genetic underpinnings responsible for some of the phenotypic presentations of GU abnormalities. Discussion of these is beyond the scope of this chapter. Readers are referred to the review by Woolf (1998). Many of these syndromes are evident in the neonatal period and require full investigation (Table 161.2). Renal function and urinary abnormalities, electrolyte disturbances, growth and development issues, and coexisting deformities (i.e., ear/umbilical) should alert the clinician to the potential underlying pathologic condition.

RENAL ABNORMALITIES

Renal abnormalities or renal malformations encompass a large group of anatomical defects of the kidney. These abnormalities include aplasia or anatomical absence of kidneys, hypoplasia resulting from a reduction in the number of nephrons and leads to small kidneys, and dysplasia resulting from abnormal differentiation of the metanephros.

Bilateral renal agenesis (Potter's syndrome) is rare and is incompatible with survival. However, unilateral renal agenesis often is not even diagnosed unless there are other symptoms in early life or unless a renal ultrasound is done. The incidence of unilateral renal agenesis is about 1 in every 500 to 1,000 births. Nonurologic abnormalities, however, are often associated with unilateral renal abnormalities.

Multicystic dysplastic kidney is usually unilateral and consists of multiple cysts of varying sizes without normal structure to the kidney. Glomeruli, if present, are primitive, and there is usually an atretic ureter. Whether this anomaly is due to maldevelopment of both the ureteric bud and renal blastema is unclear. The condition often presents with a unilateral flank mass observed in the fetus or newborn. Abnormalities are seen frequently in the contralateral kidneys. Most multicystic dysplastic kidneys involute; surgical removal is performed only if there are complications such as hypertension, vomiting with failure to thrive, or chronic infection. Malignant transformation had been thought to be a risk, but this possibility now seems remote.

In general, most renal malformations observed during the newborn period are sporadic. However, a small number of renal malformations appear to be familial or occur as part of a syndromic presentation. Specific genetic mutations that play a functional role in nephrogenesis have been linked to different kidney malformations (Table 161.1).

TABLE 161.1. **SOME GENETIC MUTATIONS ASSOCIATED WITH RENAL MALFORMATIONS**

Disease Entity	Mode of Inheritance	Mutations or Genetic Locus
VUR and optic nerve coloboma	Autosomal dominant	*PAX2* mutation
Apert syndrome	Autosomal dominant	*FGF 2* receptor mutation
Hydronephrosis, digital and cranial malformations		
Kallman's syndrome	X-linked recessive	KAL mutation
Renal agenesis, olfactory bulb, and hypothalamic defects		
Zellweger syndrome	Autosomal recessive	Peroxisome factor-1 mutation
Renal cysts and dysplasia with neurologic and hepatic defects		
Bardet–Biedle syndrome	Autosomal recessive	Locus on 11q13
Renal dysplasia with obesity hypogonadism, and polydactily		
Brachio-otorenal syndrome	Autosomal dominant	Locus on 8q
Di George syndrome		Locus on 221
Meckel syndrome	Autosomal recessive	Locus on 17q21–24
Multicystic dysplastic kidney with neural tube defect		
Isolated renal dysplasia	Autosomal dominant	Unknown
Isolated vesicoureteral reflux	Autosomal dominant	Unknown

(From Woolf AS. Molecular control of nephrogenesis and the pathogenesis of kidney malformations. *Br J Urol* 1998;81:1–7.)

COLLECTING SYSTEM ABNORMALITIES

Structural ureteral malformations that occur during fetal development can manifest as single defects (i.e., vesicoureteral reflux [VUR], ureteropelvic/ureterovesicular junction obstruction, duplicated ureters [DU] or bifid pelvis) or as a combination of several abnormalities.

Ureteral duplication is one of the more common abnormalities of the GU system with an incidence of 1 in 125 patients based on nonselected autopsy series. Clinical incidence suggests a 2:1 female predominance. Duplication is generally unilateral and has a genetic predisposition of approximately 10% in parents or siblings of an affected individual. Complete duplication can occur if two separate buds arise from the mesonephric duct, with the more cephalad-placed bud tending to drain the upper pole of the kidney and the more caudally placed draining the lower pole. Based on migration and fetal rearrangement, the ureteric segment draining the upper renal pole ultimately drains into the bladder more caudally than the segment draining the lower pole. A variety of associated anomalies may coexist with complete duplication and affect one or both ureteral orifices. VUR, ureteral ectopy, and ureteroceles all may associate with a duplicated system.

VUR, when associated with ureteral duplication, is classically seen in the lower pole system. This occurs because of the lateral positioning of the lower pole orifice in the bladder. Once diagnosed (usually in conjunction with a urinary tract infection), management includes prophylactic antibiotics and thorough sonographic, radiologic, and nuclear medicine studies to accurately characterize the lesion.

Ureteral ectopy occurs when the ureteral bud originates at a position more craniad than normal. It follows the course of the mesonephric duct for a longer period of time and fails to separate from the duct, thereby terminating in a structure derived from the duct.

Ectopic ureters may insert into the trigone, bladder neck, or urethra of either sex at its lower end and be surrounded by dysplastic tissue at its upper end. Men can also have the ectopic ureter end in the vas deferens, ejaculatory ducts, or seminal vesicles, whereas in women ectopic ureters may open in the lateral vaginal wall and be associated with continuous incontinence. A thorough radiologic, sonographic, and nuclear imaging workup is required, along with renal function assessment. Surgical intervention is predicated based on the extent of associated clinical symptoms, anatomical abnormalities, and degree of VUR.

Ureteroceles occur as a cystic dilatation of the intravesical or submucosal ureter. Although more common on the left, ureteroceles are observed bilaterally 10% of the time. There is a 4:1 female predominance, with an overall incidence of 1 in 500 to 1 in 4,000. The embryology of ureteroceles is incompletely understood. Current theories suggest that there is a delayed union between the developing ureter and the urogenital sinus. Ureteroceles can be associated with ectopic ureters and thereby potentially present as a bladder outlet obstruction. The primary presentation is with a urinary tract infection, although some have abdominal masses and others are diagnosed on prenatal ultrasonography.

URETEROPELVIC JUNCTION OBSTRUCTION

Ureteropelvic junction obstruction (UPJO) contributes to the array of GU abnormalities collectively known as the obstructive uropathies. UPJO posterior urethral valves, cloacal anomalies, urethral atresia, and cystic renal disease represent the most commonly detected GU obstructing lesions. These lesions may be unilateral or bilateral. Obstructive uropathy is frequently found on prenatal ultrasound, with an estimated incidence of 1 in 500 fetuses imaged.

UPJO accounts for 80% of cases of congenital hydronephrosis and is a common cause of urinary tract obstruction in neonates (Fig. 161.1). It is more common in male infants, with a

TABLE 161.2.	Syndromes with Renal Structural Components Identifiable in the Neonatal Period	
Syndrome	**General Features**	**Renal Abnormalities**
Skeletal Malformations		
Spina bifida	Meningomyelocele	Double ureter, horseshoe kidney, hydronephrosis
Hemihypertrophy	Hemihypertrophy	Wilms' tumor, hypospadias
Potter's syndrome	Abnormal facies; lung, cardiac, and skeletal anomalies	Renal agenesis
Meckel's syndrome	Encephalocele, polydactyly	Polycystic kidneys
Cerebrohepatorenal syndrome (Zellweger syndrome)	Hepatomegaly, glaucoma, brain anomalies, chondrodystrophy	Polycystic kidneys
Jeune's syndrome	Thoracic asphyxiating dystrophy	Medullary necrosis, proteinuria, hydronephrosis, horseshoe kidneys
VATER syndrome	Vertebral abnormalities, anal atresia, tracheoesophageal fistula, radial dysplasia	Renal dysplasia
VACTERL syndrome	Same as VATER, plus additional cardiac and limb abnormalities	Renal dysplasia
MURC5 syndrome	Mullerian duct aplasia, cervicothoracic somite dysplasia	Renal aplasia
Visceral Abnormalities		
Prune-belly syndrome	Hypoplasia of abdominal muscles, cryptorchidism	Urinary tract dysplasia
Tuberous sclerosis	Tuberous sclerosis, adenoma sebaceum	Cystic kidneys, kidney tumors
Beckwith–Wiedemann syndrome	Macroglossia, hypoglycemia	Renal dysplasia, nephroblastoma
Williams syndrome	Peripheral pulmonic stenosis, coarctation of the aorta, vascular stenoses, eye abnormalities, hypercalcemia	Horseshoe kidney, single-kidney renovascular disease, genitourinary reflux
Laurence–Moon–Biedl syndrome	Obesity, polydactyly, retinal anomalies	Fetal lobulations of kidneys, renal failure
Facial or Eye Abnormalities		
Aniridia–Wilms syndrome	Aniridia, cryptorchidism	Wilms' tumor
Johanson–Blizzard syndrome	Hypoplastic alae nasi, hypothyroidism, deafness	Hydronephrosis, caliectasis
Meckel–Gruber syndrome (dysencephalia splanchnocystica)	Encephalocele, polydactyly, cryptorchidism, cardiac anomalies, liver disease	Polycystic kidneys
Melnick–Fraser syndrome (branchio-otorenal syndrome)	Preauricular pits, brachial clefts, deafness	Renal dysplasia
Oral–facial–digital (OFD) syndrome, type I	Oral frenula and clefts, hypoplastic alae nasi, digital asymmetry (cross-linked, lethal in male)	Renal microcysts
Chromosomal Abnormalities		
Down syndrome (trisomy 21)	Abnormal facies, brachycephaly, congenital heart disease	Cystic kidney and other renal abnormalities in 7%
Turner's syndrome	Small stature, congenital heart disease, amenorrhea, XO sex chromosomes	Horseshoe kidney; duplications and malrotations of the urinary collecting system occur in 60%
Trisomy 13 (Patau's syndrome)	Abnormal facies, cleft lip and palate, congenital heart disease	Cystic kidneys and other renal anomalies in 60%
Trisomy 18 (Edwards syndrome)	Abnormal facies, abnormal ears, overlapping digits, congenital heart disease	Cystic kidneys, horseshoe kidney, or duplication occurs in 70%
Partial trisomy 10q	Abnormal facies, limb and cardiac abnormalities	Renal anomalies
Triploidy syndrome	Abnormal facies, cardiac defects, hypospadias and cryptochidism in male, brain anomalies	Renal anomalies
Congenital Infection		
Congenital rubella	Cataracts, cardiac anomalies, deafness, microcephaly	Various renal anomalies, renal artery stenosis with late hypertension
Miscellaneous Syndromes		
Rokitansky sequence	Failure of paramesonephric ducts, vaginal atresia, absent or hypoplastic uterus	Renal hypoplasia, agenesis, or double ureters
Rubinstein–Tayhi syndrome	Broad thumbs and toes, slanted palpebral fissures, hypoplastic maxilla	Renal anomalies

(From Woolf AS. Molecular control of nephrogenesis and the pathogenesis of kidney malformations. *Br J Urol* 1998;81:1–7.)

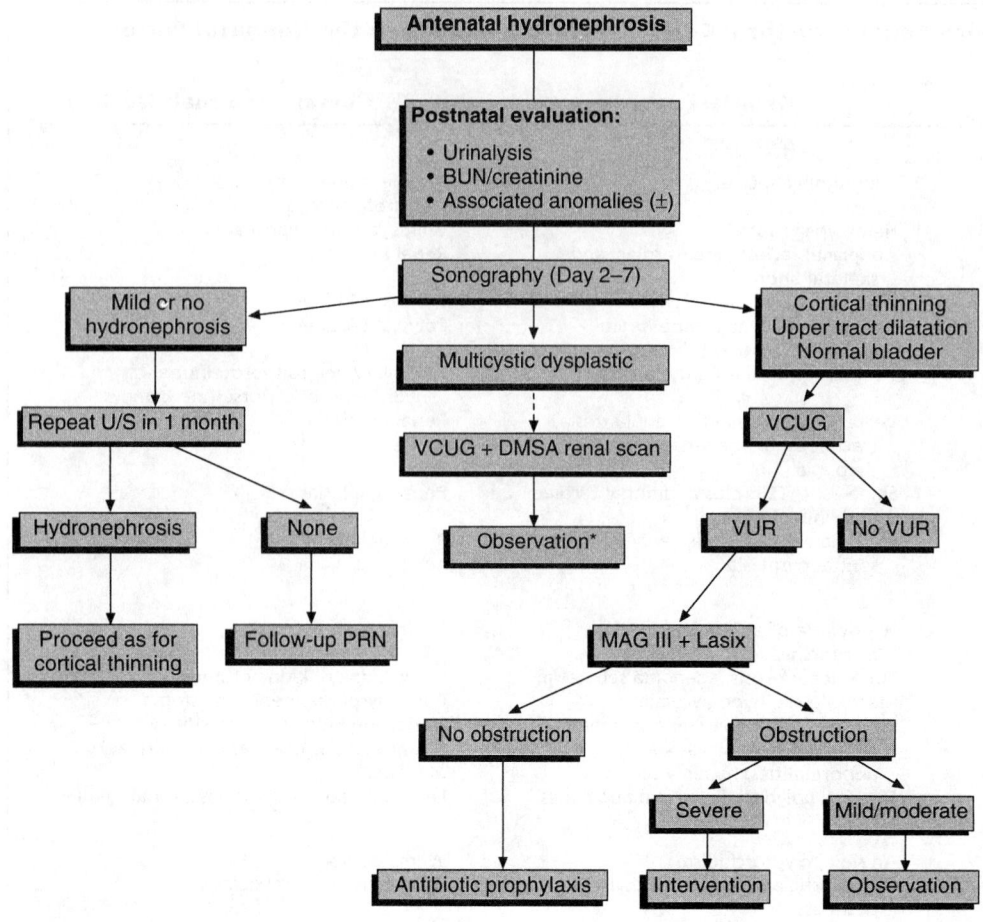

FIGURE 161.1. Flow diagram for postnatal monitoring of fetal hydronephrosis. VUR, vesicoureteral reflux; VCUG, voiding cystourethrogram; U/S, ultrasound; MAGIII, Tc-99m Mertiatide, a radiopharmaceutical product used in renal imaging. Surgery has been advocated in the past for therapy of unilateral multicystic kidney disease, but this is not current general practice. (Adapted from Cedron M, D'Alton ME, Crombleholme TM. Prenatal diagnosis and management of the fetus with hydronephrosis. *Semin Perinatol* 1994;18:163–181.)

2:1 predominance. Although approximately 60% of cases involve the left side only, 10% to 40% are bilateral. Familial presentation of UPJO has also been reported and is often associated with other anomalies, including Hirschsprung's disease and imperforate anus.

Current classification of UPJO is based on the following anatomical criteria:

- Intrinsic stenosis/valves—this results in functional absence of peristalsis and inadequate luminal distention
- Insertional anomalies—the ureter inserts abnormally high, and often obliquely, into a dilated renal pelvis
- Fibrous bands/adhesions—dense periureteral fibrosis likely secondary to inflammatory processes
- Crossing vessels—blood vessels that erroneously cross at the UPJ level resulting in obstruction

The initial diagnosis and treatment of UPJO can be difficult. The functional obstructions can be particularly hard to define and may be volume dependent. Most cases of UPJO are found in childhood, with an abdominal mass being the most common clinical presentation. Other presentations are abdominal pain secondary to hydronephrosis, hematuria, and increased renal susceptibility to minor trauma. Assessment of renal function, electrolytes, urinary concentrating ability and imaging are very important in the initial workup. Nuclear renal scanning with

diuretic is also a particularly valuable tool in assessment of UPJO.

Early neonatal intervention by experienced pediatric nephrologists and urologists may help to maintain or restore renal function in a GU system that would otherwise be destined to become nonfunctional. This is especially true in patients with confirmed bilateral involvement.

OTHER TYPES OF URETERAL OBSTRUCTION

Ureteric vesical junction obstruction (UVJO) with megaureter is less common than UPJO. This malformation appears to be sporadic, with a male predisposition. UVJO also has been associated with other anomalies, including duplicated renal collecting system, ectopic ureterocele, VUR, contralateral renal agenesis, multicystic kidney disease, and Hirschsprung's disease. Megaureter usually occurs secondarily to UVJO and in the absence of a dilated bladder. Diagnosis is often made by ultrasound in the prenatal period. There may or may not be associated pelvic dilation, depending on the severity and duration of the UVJO and megaureter.

Vesicoureteral Reflux

VUR can be defined as regurgitation of urine from the bladder into the ureters and in some cases the kidneys themselves. This

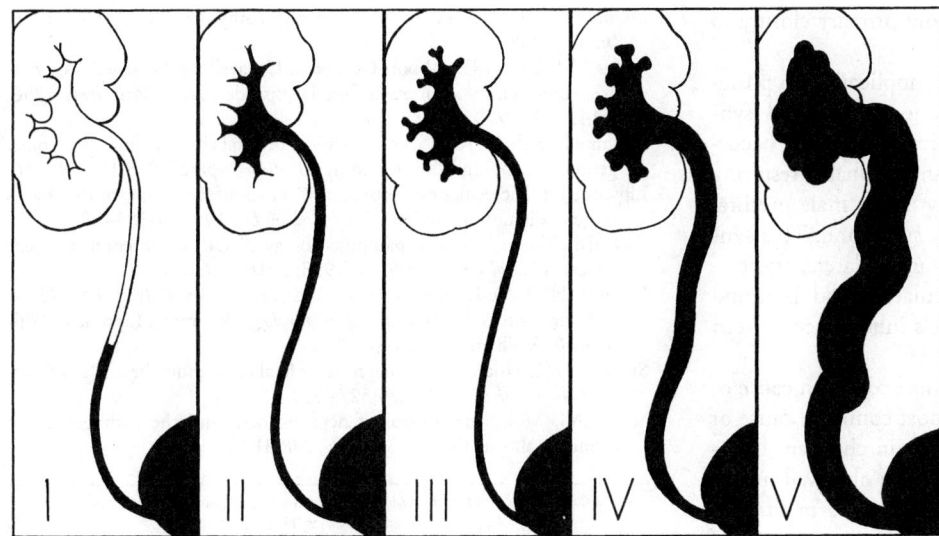

FIGURE 161.2. Classification of vesicoureteral reflux by the international grading system. I, lower ureteral filling only; II, ureteral and pelvicalyceal filling without dilatation; III, ureteral and pelvicalyceal filling with mild dilatation of renal pelvis and mild blunting; IV, moderate dilatation and/or tortuosity of ureter, dilated renal pelvis, and blunted calyces; V, gross dilatation of ureter, renal pelvis, calyces, with intrarenal reflux.

occurs through the vesicoureteral junction, which is either aberrantly placed, lax, or immature. The defect is essentially an insufficient valve mechanism, owing to an abnormality in the diameter, length, innervation, or musculature of the submucosal intravesicular ureter. The specific cause of the abnormality is likely related to an abnormal morphogenesis of the ureteric bud, resulting in a congenital lateral ectopia of the ureteric orifice.

VUR can be divided into primary and secondary groups. Primary VUR is not associated with any underlying obstructive or nervous system/muscular abnormality or with pathologic bladder dynamics, whereas secondary VUR is associated with those factors. The degree of VUR is graded I through V, with grade V reflux being the most severe (Fig. 161.2). Patients may remain clinically quiescent, with VUR resolving on its own or proceeding to end-stage renal disease with scar formation.

Most persons with VUR are asymptomatic, making it difficult to determine the exact incidence. General estimates place the incidence to be 1 in 100 to 1 in 1,000. Epidemiologic data available for VUR are equally unclear. The prevalence in healthy persons is unknown, because most primary cases of VUR have been demonstrated in patients being evaluated for urinary tract infections. Certainly, the most important and controversial fact is that VUR is an inherited trait. It is consistently demonstrated in approximately 30% of siblings of patients with VUR and appears to be present in an even higher percentage in offspring of those with known VUR. The type of inheritance is unclear but has been demonstrated in most kindreds to follow an autosomal dominant pattern with variable expression and reduced penetrance. Some have suggested sex-linked transmission, but the evidence for this is less clear. The specific genetic aberrations causing isolated VUR remain to be defined, although the incidence of the gene has been estimated at 1 in 600, which would make it the most common dominantly inherited condition in mankind. VUR associated with other disease entities (coloboma-ureteral-renal syndrome, prune-belly syndrome, Apert's disease, chromosome 8 and 10 short arm abnormalities, among many) has been attributed to developmental pathway gene mutations, more specifically, a *Pax2* gene mutation. Mutations in other

genes required for nephrogenesis, such as FGF receptor (FGFR2) and the GDNF receptor (RET), known to be expressed in the developing ureter, have been excluded as the cause of primary VUR. Although it appears that primary VUR has genetic heterogeneity, severity of scar formation and subsequent end-stage renal disease/reflux nephropathy appear to be related to angiotensin-converting enzyme gene polymorphism, with homozygosity conferring the greatest risk of scarring on its carriers.

Diagnosis and management of VUR are becoming more homogeneous. Most persons presenting with a urinary tract infection in early childhood have a renal sonogram performed, with a subsequent voiding cystourethrogram in conjunction with renal function blood work. Nuclear renal scan is also performed to evaluate the kidneys for scarring after the infection is cleared. Depending on the severity of the VUR, clinicians have a variety of options available for further patient management. These include prophylactic antibiotics with regularly scheduled follow-up imaging studies, and close observation by or referral to a urologist for potential surgical intervention. The usefulness of screening in siblings or offspring of affected persons is still debated.

ANOMALIES OF THE BLADDER AND URETHRA

The urinary bladder arises from the primitive urogenital sinus, and bladder anomalies are relatively rare. Structural abnormalities range from agenesis to megacystasis secondary to distal obstruction. These conditions are primarily associated with other GU anomalies or severe developmental abnormalities. Bladder extrophy is one of the more notable anomalies of this structure. It has a male predominance and refers to an anteriorly open bladder from a lack of abdominal wall closure. This anomaly may result from interference with inferolateral abdominal mesenchymal closure by an overdeveloped cloacal membrane. Thus, upon rupture of the cloacal membrane, the bladder cavity is exposed because the inferior abdominal wall has not completely closed. Surgical intervention in the neonatal period is the treatment of choice. Surgical options range from primary closure to full bladder reconstruction.

Urethral defects range from agenesis to duplication to posterior urethral valves. Each defect has various associated syndromes. Both urethral agenesis and duplication are rare occurrences and tend to have a male predominance probably resulting from the increased embryonic complexity of the male urethra. Both can be demonstrated in prune-belly syndrome. This syndrome involves a triad of dilated urinary tracts, bilateral cryptorchidism, and deficient abdominal musculature and is found mainly in males. However, the syndrome's inheritance pattern is uncertain.

Posterior urethral valve (PUV) is the most common cause of distal urinary tract obstruction and the most common cause of obstructive uropathy leading to renal failure in children. It appears to arise sporadically, although it has been observed in siblings and twins. PUV is thought to arise from abnormalities of two normal folds in the posterior urethra that are remnants of the mesonephric ducts. However, the specific pathologic lesion is not clear. PUV can often be found by routine prenatal ultrasound in the form of proximal urethral dilation with a thick-walled bladder. Potential outcome and intervention depends on prenatal age, renal function, and the presence or absence of other GU abnormalities or syndromes (i.e., prune-belly syndrome), which are observed in 25% of patients with PUV. Patients that survive the prenatal period (primarily those diagnosed postnatally or after 24 weeks of gestation) have 5% mortality, and approximately 25% progress to chronic renal failure. Urinary tract decompression is the initial treatment choice, followed by endoscopic fulguration of the PUV.

HYPOSPADIAS AND EPISPADIAS

Hypospadias, or failure of the penile meatus to develop ventrally, is common, with an incidence of about 8 in 1,000 male births. Most cases are mild (87%), with glandular or coronal abnormalities. Only 3% of hypospadias is the severe penoscrotal type. In hypospadias, the prepuce is abnormally formed on its ventral surface, so the phallus itself often has a ventral curvature called a *chordee*. Ventral foreskin development is usually deficient, and circumcision should be avoided so that the foreskin may be used in repair. Renal anomalies are not more common in those with hypospadias. If cryptorchidism is associated with hypospadias, the possibility of an intersex problem should be considered. Parental counseling or corrective surgery of the hypospadias is required.

Epispadias, or failure of the dorsal surface of the penile urethra to form normally, is rare, occurring in 1 of every 140,000 live births. This anomaly may be associated with dorsal penile curvature caused by penile deformity and separation of the pubis. Evaluation of the upper and lower GU tract is essential; ureteral reflux and incontinence are possible associated problems. Staged surgical procedures may be necessary. Complications are similar to those seen in hypospadias.

BIBLIOGRAPHY

Decter RM. Renal duplication and fusion anomalies. *Pediatr Clin North Am* 1997;44:1323–1341.

Dillon MJ, Goonasekera CD. Reflux nephropathy. *J Am Soc Nephrol* 1998; 9:2377–2383.

Eccles MR, Bailey RR, Abbott GD, et al. Unravelling the genetics of vesicoureteric reflux: a common familial disorder. *Hum Mol Genet* 1996; 5:1425–1429.

Klemme L, Fish AJ, Rich S, et al. Familial ureteral abnormalities syndrome: genomic mapping, clinical findings. *Pediatr Nephrol* 1998;12:349–356.

Lipschut JH. Molecular development of the kidney: a review of the results of gene disruption studies. *Am J Kidney Dis* 1998;31:383–397.

Park JM, Bloom DA. The pathophysiology of UPJ obstruction. Current concepts. *Urol Clin North Am* 1998;25:161–169.

Rushton HGJ. Vesicoureteral reflux and scarring. In: Barratt TM, Avner ED, Harmon WE, eds. *Pediatric nephrology*. Baltimore: Lippincott Williams & Williams, 1999:851–871.

Stamilio DM, Morgan MA. Diagnosis of fetal renal anomalies. *Obstet Gynecol Clin North Am* 1998;25:527–552.

Woolf AS. Molecular control of nephrogenesis and the pathogenesis of kidney malformations. *Br J Urol* 1998;81:1–7.

Kelley's Textbook of Internal Medicine, fourth edition. Edited by H. David Humes. Lippincott Williams & Wilkins, Philadelphia © 2000.

C H A P T E R

162

PREGNANCY, THE KIDNEY, AND HYPERTENSION

MARSHALL D. LINDHEIMER
ADRIAN I. KATZ

The renal system has a distinctive place in the history of obstetric care. Long before recognition of the marked anatomical and functional changes in the urinary tract characteristic of gestation, physicians diagnosed pregnancy by the sweet taste of the urine (due to increased filtration and excretion of glucose), and demonstration of proteinuria was among the first signs identified in the diagnosis of preeclampsia, at first believed to be a form of Bright's disease. This chapter reviews the striking changes in the renal system and the control of blood pressure in pregnancy, stressing their relevance to the diagnosis and management of pregnant women with kidney disorders or with hypertension complicating pregnancy.

Both kidney volume and length increase—the latter by ~1 cm—and there is substantial dilation of the calyces, pelves, and ureters, most prominently on the right. These changes, which have been ascribed to both hormonal factors and mechanical obstruction, begin in early pregnancy. They are most pronounced in the last trimester and may persist through the third postpartum month. The clinical relevance of these changes includes the difficulty in obtaining timed urine collections from pregnant women, a rare "overdistention" syndrome, characterized by abdominal pain, hydronephrosis (more marked than the usual degree of physiologic dilation), and hypertension, which may require the placement of ureteral stents. Elective assessment of the urinary tract should be deferred until ≥12 weeks postpartum. These changes may also complicate management of pregnant women with underlying reflux nephropathy or chronic pyelonephritis of infectious origin.

Functional changes during pregnancy are even more striking. Glomerular filtration rate (GFR) and renal plasma flow (RPF) rise ~50%, ascribed mainly to humoral changes (e.g., increased circulating relaxin levels). These changes begin during the luteal phase of the last menstrual cycle and progress rapidly thereafter, reaching maximum values by mid-trimester. The relevance of the hormonal changes is that values considered normal in nonpregnant women may be ambiguous in pregnancy; for example, a $P_{creatinine}$ and $P_{urea\ N'}$ exceeding 0.8 mg per deciliter (70 μmol per liter) and 13 mg per deciliter (5 mmol per liter), respectively, are associated with abnormal renal function in a pregnant woman. Furthermore, increased filtered loads of many solutes (e.g., glucose and amino acids) as well as proteins results in increments in their urinary excretion (e.g., the excretion of up to 300 mg per day of protein is considered normal).

There are also changes in tubular function, the most clinically relevant relating to urate and acid–base metabolism. Both the absolute and fractional clearance of urate rise and plasma levels exceeding only 5 mg per deciliter (298 μmol per liter) are abnormal. Blood pH, which is ~7.40 in the nonpregnant state, averages 7.44 in pregnancy, the mild alkalemia being attributed to the effect of progesterone on respiration that results in a decrement in P_{CO_2} to ~30 mm Hg, as well as alterations of renal proton handling, so that plasma HCO_3 falls to about 20 mEq per liter. Thus, a pregnant woman with a blood pH of ~7.38 is already acidemic, whereas a P_{CO_2} of 40 mm Hg signals substantial carbon dioxide retention.

Pregnancy affects volume regulation and the control of body tonicity. Pregnant women gain an average of 12.5 kg, and total body water increases 6 to 9 L. Four to seven of these liters are in the plasma (~1.2 L) and interstitial spaces, so that edema, observed in over 50% of normotensive pregnancies, is *a normal occurrence of gestation*. The osmotic thresholds for both thirst and vasopressin (AVP) release decrease by ~10 mOsm per liter. These changes are maximal between the eighth and tenth gestational week and are accompanied by a decrement in P_{Na} of 5 mEq per deciliter. Thus, if P_{Na} exceeds 140 mEq per liter, a search for causes of hypernatremia is warranted. Pregnant women experience a fourfold increase is the metabolic clearance of AVP, ascribed to the placental production of vasopressinase, yet they concentrate their urine normally. There is, however, a rare syndrome of transient diabetes insipidus of pregnancy that includes women with subclinical partial central diabetes insipidus whose disease is unmasked by the increments in AVP disposal during pregnancy and other women whose placentae produce excessive amounts of vasopressinase or who experience reductions in hepatic inactivation of the enzyme (as occurs in some women with preeclampsia). These patients can be treated with DDAVP (desmopressin acetate), an analogue resistant to inactivation by vasopressinase.

Finally, profound cardiovascular changes occur during pregnancy. Mean blood pressure decreases soon after conception, with diastolic levels falling by ~10 mm Hg to a nadir by midgestation. Pressures then rise slowly approaching nongravid levels near term and may transiently rise above preconception values in the puerperium. Simultaneously, cardiac output rises 30% to 50%. Given the magnitude of this increment, the simultaneous decline in pressure must be due to a striking decrease in peripheral vascular resistance, making gestation *a markedly vasodilated state*. The causes of these changes are incompletely understood, but are believed to relate to alterations in the production of vasodilatory prostanoids, as well as to enhancement of the activity of endothelium-derived relaxing factors (both nitric oxide-dependent and oxide-independent in origin).

■ APPROACH TO THE PREGNANT PATIENT WITH RENAL DISEASE

ASSESSMENT OF RENAL FUNCTION

Pregnancy may be the first time a woman's urine is monitored and abnormalities uncovered, another cogent reason for practitioners to be familiar with the normal changes of gestation. Urinary excretion of red blood cells rises so that a urinalysis demonstrating two to three red blood cells per high-power field can still be regarded as normal. Whether leukocyturia also increases normally is unclear. Proteinuria up to 300 mg per day is still considered normal, and in the absence of timed collections protein:creatinine ratios performed on spot urine samples are acceptable. Urine concentration and dilution are similar in nongravid and gravid populations, but one should be aware that an upright or supine position interferes with the ability of pregnant women to produce a maximally dilute urine, whereas lateral recumbency interferes with optimal concentration. In addition, the lower limit of normal for endogenous creatinine clearance in nongravid populations should be increased by 30% to 110 to 120 mL per minute. Finally, although renal biopsy for most indications may be deferred until after delivery, the procedure can be performed on pregnant women and should be considered in the following situations: sudden deterioration of function without apparent cause; the appearance of symptomatic nephrotic syndrome (or when its biochemical abnormalities are marked); and, rarely, when there is need to differentiate an acute glomerular disorder (e.g., lupus nephritis) from preeclampsia. The procedure is not indicated after gestational week 31 because its risk:benefit ratio increases markedly at this time.

URINARY TRACT INFECTION

This topic is discussed in detail in Chapter 271, but the following caveats are pertinent to pregnancy. Pregnant women should be screened for covert bacteriuria, and if present it should be treated, because there is a greater propensity for asymptomatic urinary tract infections to progress to symptomatic upper and lower tract infections in gestation. Pyelonephritis tends to be more virulent in gestation and more apt to be associated with sepsis, including acute respiratory distress syndrome, renal failure, and intravascular coagulation, as well as fetal loss. Thus, many practitioners treat covert bacteriuria for 10 to 14 days, and symptomatic infections for 3 weeks, although recent studies suggest that shorter periods of treatment may suffice.

ACUTE RENAL FAILURE

Acute renal failure (ARF) is an extremely rare complication in pregnancy, acute tubular necrosis severe enough to require dialysis having an incidence of 1 in 10,000 to 20,000, and cortical necrosis 1 in 70,000. Maternal mortality, once considerable in pregnant women with ARF, is practically nonexistent in the industrial world, primarily because women seeking abortion early in pregnancy now have easy access to sterile terminations.

The cause of ARF in pregnant women is often similar to that in nonpregnant populations (see Chapter 140), but there are also several pregnancy-specific causes. As noted, septic abortions (illegal; nonsterile) were once a major cause of ARF and were associated with high lethality, especially when due to *Clostridia* sepsis (see Chapter 290). In late gestation, acute fatty liver and a variant of preeclampsia known as the HELLP syndrome (see Preeclampsia-Eclampsia) are associated with ARF. Although very rare, cortical necrosis occurs more readily in pregnancy, and it is often linked to placental abruption, especially in the presence of a concealed hemorrhage. Another rare complication unique to the gravid state is labeled idiopathic postpartum renal failure, which may be manifest 24 hours to several weeks after delivery. It is irreversible and is associated with a surprisingly high incidence of maternal morbidity and death. The renal pathologic character of the lesion has been described as being similar to the adult hemolytic-uremic syndrome when biopsies are performed early in the course of the disease and to scleroderma kidney when tissue is obtained at a later period. Its cause remains unknown and has been linked to mechanisms similar to those postulated for the thrombotic microangiopathies, that is, dysfunction of the vascular endothelium with a deficiency in endothelium-derived relaxing factor or the prostanoid system. Idiopathic postpartum renal failure is the cause of ARF related to pregnancy most often resulting in end-stage renal disease.

CHRONIC RENAL DISEASE

Table 162.1 summarizes the relation of pregnancy to several specific renal diseases. The following are general guidelines for the management of pregnant women with preexisting renal disease (Table 162.2): (a) Women who before conception have only mildly decreased and stable kidney function (creatinine ≤1.4 mg per deciliter; 125 μmol per liter), do well in pregnancy—live births exceeding 95%. Exacerbation of the underlying kidney disorder is unusual, and the pregnancy does not influence adversely its long-term prognosis. Fetal growth is adequate in more than 75%, but these women have an increased incidence of superimposed preeclampsia. (b) Women whose renal dysfunction is moderate ($P_{creatinine}$ between 1.5 and 3 mg per deciliter; 133 to 275 μmol per liter) or worse have a more guarded prognosis, with one third or more experiencing renal functional deterioration or the appearance of hectic hypertension after mid-pregnancy (often superimposed preeclampsia), or both. Prognosis is better for the pregnancy, of which ~90% succeed, but growth restriction and preterm deliveries occur in more than 50%. (c) Women with advanced or end-stage renal disease (especially those requiring renal replacement therapy), although relatively infertile, do occasionally conceive and therefore require contraceptive counseling. Only about 50% of these pregnancies succeed and are accompanied by considerable maternal risk, including cardiac failure, severe hypertension with cerebrovascular accidents, and maternal death.

The above précis of pregnancy in women with preexisting renal disease requires the following qualifications: (a) These guidelines are based on retrospective data, and more definitive strategies require prospective studies. (b) Prognosis at all stages of renal dysfunction is more guarded when pregnant women have poorly controlled hypertension. (c) Certain specific entities appear to be adversely affected by gestation. These are renal

---

TABLE 162.1.	**PREGNANCY IN WOMEN WITH RENAL DISORDERS**

Renal Disease	**Effects**
Diabetic nephropathy	Gestation does not appear to accelerate functional loss; more covert bacteriuria and increased incidence of nephrotic-range proteinuria and hypertension after mid-gestation
Chronic glomerulonephritis (GN) and focal glomerulosclerosis (FGS)	Increased incidence of hypertension in late pregnancy, but no apparent adverse effects if function preserved and hypertension absent before conception
Systemic lupus erythematosus	More problems than in most glomerular disorders, but prognosis favorable if disease is in remission ≥6 months before conception; maternal and fetal outcomes poorer when antiphospholipid antibodies or lupus anticoagulant present
Scleroderma and periarteritis nodosa	Many reports of accelerated hypertension, maternal deaths, and poor fetal prognosis; thus therapeutic abortion should be considered in both conditions
Reflux nephropathy and chronic (infectious) interstitial nephritis	Prognosis favorable when function is preserved, but patients require frequent urine cultures and may need chronic suppressive antibiotic therapy
Polycystic kidney disease	Pregnancy tolerated well when function is preserved; liver cysts may enlarge; more gestational hypertension and/or preeclampsia
Urolithiasis	Prognosis good except for a greater risk of urinary tract infections; patients with calcium oxalate stones do best; those with struvite stones more problematic; stents placed successfully in gravidas

TABLE 162.2.	**GUIDELINES FOR MANAGING RENAL DISEASE AND HYPERTENSION IN PREGNANCY**

1. Determine renal function in all patients with known disorders and in women demonstrating abnormal proteinuria in early gestation. Counsel patients regarding prognosis (see text).
2. Examine patients at biweekly intervals (and weekly after gestational week 32). Routine antenatal observations and tests should be supplemented by (a) assessing creatinine clearances (or at least P$_{creatinine}$) and proteinuria at 4- to 6-week intervals and ruling out bacteriuria once during each trimester, (b) careful monitoring of blood pressure for early detection and treatment of hypertension.
3. Establish a database early in pregnancy for all women with renal disease or chronic hypertension to aid in the differential diagnosis of superimposed preeclampsia. Suggested tests: quantitative proteinuria, platelet count, serum creatinine, uric acid, albumin, lactic acid dehydrogenase, and aspartate (or alanine) aminotransferase levels.
4. Presence of moderate or severe hypertension resistant to treatment before or during gestation is indication for screening for renal artery stenosis and pheochromocytoma (and other causes of secondary hypertension as dictated by index of suspicion).
5. Antihypertensive drug treatment should be instituted when diastolic levels are chronically ≥100 mm Hg or pressure rises rapidly to ≥105 mm Hg. Some initiate therapy when levels are ≥95 mm Hg before mid-gestation (see text for drugs of choice and *Physicians Desk Reference* for pregnancy safety classification).
6. Pregnant women with end-stage renal disease or acute renal failure requiring renal replacement therapy can be managed with *either* peritoneal or hemodialysis. The dialysis prescription should be intensified, sometimes to daily or 5× weekly treatments, and erythropoietin requirements rise substantially.

scleroderma and periarteritis (in which most practitioners proscribe or interrupt pregnancy), some instances of severe lupus nephritis, and perhaps instances of membranoproliferative glomerulonephritis. Some investigators also believe that gestation exacerbates IgA nephropathy, focal glomerulosclerosis, and reflux nephropathy, even when function is preserved. However, careful review of the literature regarding these entities supports a favorable prognosis conforming to the general guidelines previously described.

RENAL TRANSPLANTATION

The maternal and fetal prognosis in women with renal transplants is similar to those in women with disease in their native kidneys. Allograft recipients with preserved function do well, but the prognosis for graft and pregnancy is more guarded when hypertension is present and the functional loss is greater. Recipients are counseled to wait 2 years after transplantation before attempting conception to ensure kidney function stability. Concerning immunosuppression, abundant retrospective data suggest that corticosteroids and azathioprine at dose schedules used in transplant patients do not appear to have serious fetal effects.

Cyclosporin A is associated with more hypertension and possibly a greater degree of fetal growth restriction. There are insufficient data to rate the newer agents. Finally, although the issue is still disputed, most investigators failed to find an adverse effect of gestation on long-term allograft survival.

APPROACH TO THE PREGNANT PATIENT WITH HYPERTENSION

Hypertension complicates 5% to 10% of all pregnancies and is a major cause of morbidity and death for both mother and unborn child, especially in underdeveloped parts of the world. Most of these adverse outcomes are due to preeclampsia, either pure or superimposed on another form of hypertension or on renal disease. This is because preeclampsia is more than hypertension. It is a multisystem disease, with complications in various organs often being the cause of the morbidity rather than the high blood pressure per se. There is considerable confusion in the literature concerning detection, classification, and management of the hypertensive disorders of gestation. Much of the text that follows is in accordance with the views and recommendations of the 1999 Working Group Report on High Blood Pressure in Pregnancy issued by the National High Blood Pressure Education Program (NHBPEP).

DETECTION AND CLASSIFICATION

Hypertension is defined as a systolic and diastolic pressure of ≥140 and ≥90 mm Hg, respectively, using the fifth Korotkoff sound (disappearance) to determine the diastolic level. Nevertheless, considering the physiologic decrease in blood pressure that occurs early in pregnancy, women with levels of 75 mm Hg before mid-gestation or 85 mm Hg at any time in pregnancy require close scrutiny, because a number of epidemiologic studies demonstrate that patients with such findings are at risk. Similarly, pregnant women manifesting increments of 15 and 30 mm Hg in diastolic and systolic pressures, respectively, should be closely observed even when their levels remain below 140/90 mm Hg.

There are many classification schemes, a major source of confusion in the literature. We believe that terms such as toxemia, pregnancy-induced or pregnancy-associated hypertension, and gestosis, often misunderstood or misinterpreted by the reader should be discouraged, and we endorse the most recent Working Group definition. The definition is concise, separates accurately the more benign from the serious disorders, and uses only four categories: chronic hypertension (of whatever cause), preeclampsia-eclampsia, preeclampsia superimposed on chronic hypertension, and gestational hypertension.

Chronic Hypertension

Most pregnant women with chronic hypertension (defined as high blood pressure before gestational week 20 or persisting after the puerperium) have the essential variety (accounting for 50% of all high blood pressure in pregnancy). In most pregnant women and especially in younger patients (under 35 years), blood pressure elevations are mild, there is little evidence of end-organ damage, and pregnancies are uneventful. However, 25% of these women develop superimposed preeclampsia with more guarded outcomes (see next section, Preeclampsia-Eclampsia). Secondary hypertension in pregnancy is extremely rare, but must be considered in pregnant women with moderately severe hypertension resistant to therapy. Such women should be screened for underlying kidney disease, renal artery stenosis, pheochromocytoma, and other disorders, as directed by the degree of suspicion. Pheochromocytoma may be particularly lethal in pregnancy, but risks decline dramatically when it is detected and the patient is managed appropriately.

Preeclampsia-Eclampsia

As noted, the pregnancy-specific disorder of preeclampsia-eclampsia is the complication with manifestations most likely to imperil mother and fetus, especially when superimposed on renal disease or chronic hypertension (category 3). It occurs mainly in nulliparas (7% to 10%), most often after mid-trimester and mainly near term. Its cardinal features are hypertension and proteinuria, and the more severe forms are associated with disordered coagulation (primarily thrombocytopenia) and liver function abnormalities. Preeclampsia may rapidly progress to a convulsive phase (eclampsia), whose premonitory signs and symptoms include hemoconcentration, severe headaches, visual disturbances, hyperreflexia, and epigastric and right upper quadrant pain. Eclampsia is particularly ominous and life-threatening (often because of concomitant cerebral bleeds) as is another variant of the disorder, termed the HELLP syndrome (Hemolysis, usually with schistocytes on the peripheral smear, Elevated Liver enzymes, Low Platelet counts). Both entities should be treated by rapid termination of the pregnancy.

Gestational Hypertension

Women with gestational hypertension have mild, or rarely moderate, nonproteinuric hypertension late in gestation or in the immediate puerperium. Blood pressure normalizes rapidly postpartum, when the diagnosis is changed to transient hypertension of pregnancy. The gestations are usually uneventful, the difficulty being in differentiating this entity from early manifestations of the more ominous preeclampsia. Women in this category are most apt to have essential hypertension later in life, for which pregnancy acts as a predictor.

PATHOGENESIS, PREDICTION, DIFFERENTIAL DIAGNOSIS, AND PREVENTION

Preeclampsia is the most common complication with potentially ominous additional complications in pregnancy. Knowing its cause, the pathogenesis of its manifestations and how to anticipate it should lead to better strategies that include prediction, prevention, and ideal management. Unfortunately, these goals have not yet been achieved. One major hypothesis attributes a key role in pathogenesis to placental ischemia, which results in the excessive production of cytokines deleterious to the endothelium. Other investigators consider preeclampsia a heterogeneous disorder, implicating genetic traits in susceptible populations. These include those with aberrations of the angiotensin gene, those with genes responsible for a variety of thrombophilic disorders, and those said to have a genetic disposition toward lipid and carbohydrate abnormalities, as well as early atherosclerosis (syndrome X).

Searches for tests to predict imminent preeclampsia or to distinguish the disease from other hypertensive disorders of pregnancy have included measurements of a variety of circulating hormones, autacoids, serum lipids, and oxidant and antioxidant activity; markers of endothelial dysfunction; evidence of neutrophil activation, adhesion molecules, a host of circulating cytokines; and measurement of urinary excretion of kallikrein, calcium, and albumin. All are based on plausible hypotheses as well as known pathophysiologic aspects of preeclampsia. However, to date the sensitivity of all these approaches is too weak to recommend them for clinical practice. Similarly, several large randomized, placebo-controlled and blinded multicenter studies regarding the ability of low-dose aspirin or calcium supplementation to prevent preeclampsia (in either low- or high-risk populations) have produced only marginal or negative results. Therefore, such strategies cannot be recommended.

MANAGEMENT

Suspicion of preeclampsia is grounds for hospitalization, given the unpredictably explosive nature of this disorder. Near term, induction of labor is the treatment of choice, but earlier in pregnancy ($\leq$34 gestational weeks) temporization may be attempted. Delivery, regardless of gestational age, is indicated when hypertension is severe and cannot be controlled within the first 24 to 48 hours or if ominous signs are present that include evidence of cerebral irritability, progressing liver and coagulation abnormalities (especially signs and symptoms of the HELLP syndrome), and fetal jeopardy. Parenteral magnesium should be used to prevent or treat eclampsia, an approach once disputed but now supported by the results of randomized clinical trials.

Antihypertensive Therapy

Few, if any, studies are available that demonstrate the complete fetal safety of any antihypertensive drug prescribed to pregnant women. Methyldopa remains the agent with the longest post-market history of safety, and results of a randomized study with a 7.5-year follow-up of the neonates are the reasons why the Working Group considers it the drug of choice for hypertension during pregnancy. Because of remaining uncertainties regarding drug safety, women whose hypertension is mild (diastolic levels between 90 and 100 mm Hg for most and up to 110 mm Hg for some) are not treated if they are asymptomatic and have no evidence of end-organ damage.

When methyldopa is unsuccessful, oral hydralazine can be used as a second drug, and labetalol (a combined α- and β-receptor antagonist) also has a relatively good safety record. β-blocking drugs may be associated with fetal growth restriction.

Although the use of calcium channel blocking agents looks promising, the synergism of these agents used with $MgSO_4$ may lead to precipitous decreases in pressure and even respiratory arrest. Most other drugs have insufficient pregnancy data to discuss, with two exceptions. Diuretics, when prescribed before pregnancy in patients with chronic hypertension may be continued during gestation, especially in patients with volume-sensitive hypertension. However, such drugs should not be used in those with preeclampsia in whom intravascular volume and placental perfusion are already compromised. Angiotensin-converting enzyme inhibitors are associated with neonatal renal failure, which is at times irreversible, and are therefore contraindicated in pregnancy. On theoretical grounds, a similar contraindication has been assigned to angiotensin receptor-blocking agents.

Parenteral hydralazine is the drug of choice for treating acute hypertension, especially at term or during delivery. This drug is prescribed when pressures rise to ≥ 105 mm Hg, with a goal of maintaining pressures below these levels, but preferably above 90 mm Hg to avoid fetal distress. Experience is growing with parenteral labetalol, used in the rare instance in which blood pressure control cannot be achieved with hydralazine.

BIBLIOGRAPHY

Hou S, ed. Pregnancy in end-stage renal disease. *Adv Ren Replace Ther* 1998;5:1–63.

Jungers P, Chauveau D. Pregnancy in renal disease. *Kidney Int* 1997;52: 871–885.

Lindheimer MD, Katz AI: Renal physiology and disease in pregnancy. In: Seldin DW, Giebisch G, eds. *The kidney: physiology and pathophysiology,* third ed. Philadelphia: Lippincott Williams & Wilkens (in press).

Lindheimer MD, Roberts JM, Cunningham FCG, eds. *Chesley's hypertensive disorders of pregnancy,* second ed. Stamford, CT: Appleton & Lange, 1999.

National High Blood Pressure Education Working Group: consensus report on high blood pressure in pregnancy. *Am J Obstet Gynecol* 1990;163: 1689. 1999 update NIH document (in press).

Pertuiset N, Grüunfeld J-P. Acute renal failure in pregnancy. *Clin Obstet Gynaecol* (Baillières) 1994;8:333–351.

Poppas A, Shroff SG, Korcaz CE, et al. Serial assessment of the cardiovascular system in normal pregnancy: role of arterial compliance and pulsatile arterial load. *Circulation* 1997;95:2407–2415.

Sibai BM. Treatment of hypertension in pregnant women. *N Engl J Med* 1996;335:257–265.

Sturgiss SN, Davison JM. Effect of pregnancy on long-term function of renal allografts. An update. *Am J Kidney Dis* 1995;26:54–56.

Kelley's Textbook of Internal Medicine, fourth edition. Edited by H. David Humes. Lippincott Williams & Wilkins, Philadelphia © 2000.

DIAGNOSTIC AND THERAPEUTIC MODALITIES IN RENAL AND ELECTROLYTE DISEASES

LABORATORY EVALUATION OF RENAL DISORDERS

MAJD I. JARADAT
BRUCE A. MOLITORIS

Clinical laboratory and radiologic tests are of paramount importance in the diagnosis and management of patients with renal disorders. This chapter reviews tests that are useful to the internist for evaluating renal function and disease processes.

■ URINALYSIS

Since the earliest microscopic observation of urine in the early 1600s, urinalysis has evolved immensely and remains an extremely important diagnostic tool. Nevertheless, it is underutilized in clinical practice, although it can reflect and provide important clues to the presence of specific diseases. A complete urinalysis consists in visual inspection of the urine (Table 163.1), dipstick examination, and then microscopic examination of the urinary sediment.

URINE PH

The dipstick is a practical tool for determination of urine pH and is accurate to ± 0.5 pH units. pH is determined by two classic indicators: methyl red and bromothymol blue. The most accurate measurement of urinary pH requires a metered determination on urine collected under oil to protect loss of HCO_3 via CO_2. The normal value for urine pH is 4.5 to 6.5. A high value almost always reflects bicarbonaturia (with the exception of the presence of urease-releasing organism in the urine, e.g., *Proteus* and *Klebsiella*). For example, an alkaline urine in the presence of metabolic acidosis may be seen when hydrogen ion secretion

by the kidney is impaired, indicating renal tubule acidification problems.

URINE SPECIFIC GRAVITY

The specific gravity of urine is the mass of 1 mL of urine compared with 1 mL of distilled water; a specific gravity near 1.010 indicates isosthenuria, with a urine osmolality matching plasma. Urine specific gravity is used to determine whether the urine is or can be concentrated. It is elevated when urine is concentrated or when dense solutes such as protein, glucose, or radiographic contrast are present.

GLYCOSURIA

Dipstick glucose testing is both specific (95%) and sensitive (90%) to the concentration of approximately 50 mg per deciliter. Glycosuria occurs in the setting of excessive filtered load of glucose that exceeds the capacity for tubular reabsorption (diabetes mellitus). Blood glucose spills into urine variably, depending on individual renal thresholds. Hence, urine glucose concentration correlates poorly with serum levels. Glycosuria can also occur with a normal filtered load of glucose when there is a proximal

TABLE 163.1.	URINE COLORS AND THEIR CAUSES
Color	**Common Cause(s)**
Yellow	Normal
Red	Hemoglobinuria, myoglobinuria, hematuria, beets, rifampin, levodopa, methyldopa, phenolphthalein, deferoxamine
Orange	Bilirubin, Pyridium (phenazopyridine)
Brown	Bilirubin, methemoglobin (Hb in acid urine), levodopa, methyldopa
Black	Melanin, hemoglobinuria, homogentisic acid (alkaptonuria)
Blue, blue-green, green	Amitriptyline, methylene blue, vitamin B complex, triamterene
White	Chyluria, pus

tubule defect in glucose reabsorption (isolated glycosuria of Fanconi's syndrome). Any time that the patient is spilling glucose in the urine and yet has normal serum glucose, chronic tubulointerstitial disease should be considered.

PROTEINURIA

Detection of proteinuria is an important part in the evaluation of every patient with a renal disorder. For example, the detection of microalbuminuria is a useful predictor of subsequent nephropathy in diabetic patients. Microalbuminuria and albuminuria have been shown to be associated with increased cardiovascular disease risk in patients both with and without diabetes mellitus. The most widely used screening test for proteinuria is the dipstick, which detects primarily albumin and is 95% sensitive to the 30 mg per deciliter upper limit of normal albumin excretion. The protein reaction may be scored from trace to 4+; the equivalence is as follows: trace, 5 to 20 mg per deciliter; 1+, 30 mg deciliter; 2+, 100 mg per deciliter; 3+, 300 mg per deciliter; 4+, greater than 2,000 mg per deciliter. The disadvantages of the dipstick test are that it misses proteinuria when excretion is less than 300 to 500 mg per day. Therefore, it cannot distinguish between physiologic and low-grade pathologic protein excretion (microalbuminuria). In addition, dilute samples may be falsely negative, whereas false-positives occur in very alkaline, concentrated, or bloody specimens.

The dipstick results must be confirmed with a 24-hour urine collection for quantification of proteinuria. The normal value is less than 150 mg per day, and patients excreting more than 3 g per day are considered to have nephrotic-range proteinuria. Collections obtained over a shorter period of time (8 to 12 hours) are subject to alterations in protein excretion induced by postural changes and other fluctuations in daily protein excretion. The adequacy of urine collection should be examined by measuring the urinary creatinine excretion in the same collection, because urinary creatinine excretion is relatively constant (20 to 25 mg per kilogram per day for men, 15 to 20 mg for women). The disadvantages of this test are inconvenience and the difficulty of accurately collect a complete 24-hour specimen. One can eliminate these two disadvantages by calculating the protein: creatinine ratio milligram per milligram in a random (preferably upright) untimed urine specimen. A value greater than 0.02, for example, suggests a protein excretion of greater than 20 mg per day. This method provides a convenient, reliable, and inexpensive method for monitoring proteinuric patients. Finally, urine negative by dipstick but positive with use of sulfosalicylic acid is likely to have proteins other than albumin (i.e., multiple myeloma proteins).

HEMATURIA

Testing for hematuria by dipstick is based on the pseudoperoxidase activity of hemoglobin. Red blood cells (RBCs) are lysed on the test pad resulting in a colorful dot, whereas free pigment distributes color evenly. The sensitivity is 78% to 99%. However, this test is not specific and also detects myoglobin, which has intrinsic peroxidase activity. A urine that is positive for heme pigments by dipstick, but shows no RBCs on microscopic examination, is suspect for myoglobinuria or hemoglobinuria resulting from RBC rupture. False-negatives occur with acidic, highly concentrated, or protein-rich samples and with improper storage (air exposure of strips).

Hematuria should be confirmed by microscopic examination. The presence of more than two to three erythrocytes per high-power field usually indicates a pathologic condition. In glomerular disease, erythrocytes are dysmorphic, with spicules, blebs, submembrane cytoplasmic precipitations, membrane folding, and vesicles. These dysmorphic RBCs are reportedly easier to distinguish using phase-contrast microscopy. Note, however, that osmolality and pH significantly influence RBC morphology; a change toward eumorphism and lysis of erythrocytes in the urine occurs at less than 700 mOsm per kilogram and at a pH of 7 or higher. A three-tube urine collection test is used to locate the source of bleeding within the urinary tract. The first few milliliters of urine, a midstream sample, and the last few milliliters are collected. A urethral lesion is most likely if the hematuria occurs primarily in the first sample, and a lesion near the trigone is likely with terminal hematuria. Intrinsic renal, ureteric, and diffuse bladder lesions result in equivalent degrees of hematuria in all three specimens. The presence of casts and significant proteinuria in a patient with hematuria indicates a nephritic picture and glomerular disease.

LIPIDURIA

In the nephrotic syndrome, tubular cells reabsorb filtered lipids composed of cholesterol esters to form oval fat bodies in sloughed tubular cells in the urine. Fatty casts contain lipid-laden tubular cells or free lipid droplets. By light microscopy, lipid droplets appear round and clear with a green tinge. Cholesterol esters are anisotropic; cholesterol-containing droplets rotate polarized light, producing a Maltese-cross appearance. Lipiduria requires increased glomerular permeability and indicates glomerular disease. However, in polycystic kidney disease, lipid droplets may be seen both in the urine and in cyst fluid samples.

EOSINOPHILURIA

The presence of eosinophils requires clinical investigation. Wright's stain is the most commonly used stain for detection, but it is not a sensitive method. Hensel's stain greatly improves identification of eosinophils by their brilliant red to pink granules. Urine specimens should be fresh, because leukocytes lyse with aging of the urine. Eosinophiluria is seen in patients with acute interstitial nephritis, rapidly progressive glomerulonephritis, atheroembolic disease, and prostatitis (in some cases).

WHITE BLOOD CELLS

Granulocyte esterase can cleave pyrrole amino acid esters producing free pyrrole that reacts with a dipstick chromagen. The dipstick threshold is 5 to 15 white blood cells (WBCs) per high-power field. False-negatives occur with glycosuria and high specific gravity. The polymorphonuclear neutrophils in urine signify inflammation in the kidney or urinary tract. The actual number correlates poorly with the degree of inflammation. Pyuria often indicates urinary tract infection, especially when associated with bacteriuria, and urine culture should be obtained. Sterile pyuria might be seen in partially treated infection, urinary tract tuberculosis, tubulointerstitial disease, and glomerular diseases.

LEUKOCYTE ESTERASE AND NITRITE

Unique to granulocytes are esterases that can hydrolyze an intermediary, which then couples to a diazo compound causing a characteristic color change. This reaction can be inhibited by high concentrations of glucose, albumin, and some antibiotics such as cephalosporins, but bacteria and blood do not interfere. Sensitivity for urinary tract infection of the leukocyte esterase (LE) test is 76% to 96%, and specificity is 79% to 98%. Urine tests positive for LE when granulocytes are present, regardless of their source. Nitrite is more specific than LE but a far less sensitive dipstick test for urinary infection. Gram-negative bacteria convert excreted dietary nitrates to nitrites, which react with aromatic amines and diazo indicators in a color reaction similar to that seen with LE. Sensitivity ranges from 25% to as high as 70% for first morning-voided samples. Specificity for gram-negative organism is superb (92% to 98%). False-negative results can occur with decreased dietary nitrates or recent-onset infections. False-positives occur with improper storage (air exposure) of the strips.

CASTS

Tamm–Horsfall protein is a mucoprotein with unclear function, which is secreted by the thick ascending limb of Henle. It represents the matrix of all urinary casts. The casts may contain only the matrix (hyaline casts). These casts are nonspecific and occur in normal concentrated urine as well as numerous pathologic conditions. When casts include degenerated cells or filtered proteins, they are called *granular casts,* which can have fine granules (derived from altered serum proteins) or coarse granules (resulting from degeneration of embedded cells). Granular casts are nonspecific and may be seen after exercise or with simple volume depletion, glomerulonephritis, and tubulointerstitial disease. Large muddy-looking granular casts are found in acute tubular necrosis. Waxy casts are made of hyaline material with a much greater refractive index than hyaline casts; hence, their waxy appearance. These casts usually form in tubules that are atrophic owing to chronic parenchymal disease. Cellular casts contain intact cells. RBC casts are the hallmark of glomerulonephritis. They may exhibit intact erythrocytes or may be composed of erythrocytes in various stages of degeneration. They also have been described along with hematuria in healthy persons after exercise.

Phase-contrast microscopy is helpful in distinguishing erythrocyte membranes within the casts. WBC casts consist of white cells in a protein matrix. They are characteristic of those with pyelonephritis and are useful in distinguishing it from lower tract infection. WBC casts may also be seen with interstitial nephritis, other tubulointerstitial disorders, and glomerular diseases.

Tubular cell casts consist of sloughed epithelial cells in a hyaline matrix. They occur in concentrated urine, but are more frequently seen with sloughing tubular cells in patients with acute tubular necrosis, pyelonephritis, renal transplant rejection, and interstitial nephritis.

CRYSTALS

Urinary crystals do not always indicate pathologic condition; they may be present spontaneously or may precipitate with refrigeration of the specimen. The most distinctive crystal forms are calcium oxalate (often described as envelope-shaped), uric acid (diamond-shaped) triple phosphate (coffin lid–shaped), and cystine crystals (hexagonal plates). Urinary pH is a useful clue; the only stones made more likely by alkaline urine are apatite (calcium phosphate) and struvite (magnesium ammonium phosphate). They occur with infection by urease-producing organisms. Massive oxalate crystalluria is seen with ethylene glycol (antifreeze) poisoning.

■ MEASUREMENT OF RENAL FUNCTION

GLOMERULAR FILTRATION RATE

Glomerular filtration rate (GFR) is the rate at which an ultrafiltrate of plasma is produced per unit of time (milliliter per minute). It is dependent on the permeability of the glomerular membrane barrier and the difference between the hydraulic and oncotic pressures (Starling forces). In healthy persons, GFR is approximately 125 mL per minute per 1.73 m^2 or 180 L per day per 1.73 m^2. It averages 8% lower in women than in men. The level of GFR is the sum of the filtration rates of all the nephrons:

$$GFR = n \cdot sglGFR$$

where n is the number of nephrons and sglGFR is single-nephron GFR.

When renal mass is lost during disease processes, remaining nephrons hyperfiltrate to maintain adequate GFR and renal function. If a substance is freely filtered across the glomerular capillary wall and excreted only by glomerular filtration, its rate of filtration is equal to its rate of urinary excretion. Therefore, the ideal substance to measure GFR accurately would be a substance freely filtered but not secreted, reabsorbed, or metabolized, meaning that GFR would equal the urinary clearance of the marker after its intravenous infusion. Inulin and ^{131}I (iodine)-iothalamate are such substances. However, they require constant intravenous infusion, which is time-consuming and expensive.

Nuclear medicine techniques are also available to measure GFR; ^{99m}technetium (Tc)-diethylene triaminopentaacetic acid (DTPA) is excreted by glomerular filtration, and GFR can be estimated after a single injection of the radioisotope by determining the amount in plasma samples obtained 60 and 180 minutes after injection. Imaging clearances are obtained by measuring the increase in counts over the kidney for 3 to 6 minutes.

SERUM CREATININE

Creatinine is an end product of muscle metabolism and is excreted solely by the kidneys. The production rate is relatively stable over time for an individual because it is proportional to muscle mass. The normal range for plasma creatinine is 0.8 to 1.3 mg per deciliter (70 to 114 μmoles per liter) in men and 0.6 to 1.0 mg per deciliter in women. Serum creatinine is used as an endogenous marker of GFR because it is freely filtered across glomeruli—not metabolized or reabsorbed—and it has constant generation. However, it is secreted by proximal tubular cells. In healthy persons, creatinine secretion accounts for 5% to 10% of urinary creatinine; hence, creatinine clearance exceeds GFR by approximately 10 mL per minute per 1.73 m^2. This is important for evaluating patients with reduced GFR, because enhanced secretion of creatinine in these patients leads to a greater disparity between creatinine clearance and GFR. Therefore, with reduced GFR, the value for creatinine clearance can markedly overestimate the GFR. In addition, significant renal function is lost before the plasma creatinine rises, and, with early renal dysfunction, relatively small changes in P_{Cr} reflect large decrease of GFR (Fig. 163.1).

Many substances can affect P_{Cr}. It can rise acutely without a change in GFR because of decreased creatinine secretion or interference with the plasma assay. Creatinine is secreted by the organic cation pump in the proximal tubule. Trimethoprim and the H_2-blocker cimetidine can inhibit this pump causing a rise in serum creatinine by as much as 0.4 to 0.5 mg, but the effect is reversible with discontinuation of the drug.

Because of differences among individuals in creatinine generation and excretion, creatinine clearance provides a more accurate estimate of GFR than does serum creatinine. Creatinine clearance is defined as the volume of plasma that is cleared of creatinine by the kidney per unit time and is calculated from a 24-hour urine collection for creatinine:

$$GFR = Cr\ clearance = (U_{Cr} \cdot V) / P_{Cr}\ [mL/min]$$

This method of estimating GFR from creatinine clearance does not require a steady state, in contrast to measuring GFR from serum creatinine which is only valid in a steady state:

$$GFR = ([140 - age] \cdot weight) / (P_{Cr} \cdot 72) (\cdot\ 0.85\ for\ women)$$

In patients with moderate to severe renal dysfunction, an alternative method for estimation of GFR is to take the average of the creatinine and urea clearances. Urea clearance underestimates GFR, because about 40% to 50% of the filtered urea is reabsorbed. Because the magnitude of the two errors tends to be similar but in opposite directions, the average is more accurate.

BLOOD UREA NITROGEN

Urea is synthesized primarily by the liver and is the end product of protein catabolism. One third of synthesized urea is metabolized in the intestine to carbon dioxide and ammonia. The generated ammonia returns to the liver, where it is converted to urea. Urea is also excreted principally by glomerular filtration. In a steady state, urea level varies inversely with GFR. However, it is not a useful marker of changes in the GFR owing to the renal reabsorption and the various factors affecting the serum level (Table 163.2). The normal serum value is 8 to 12 mg deciliter; therefore, the normal ratio of blood urea nitrogen (BUN) to creatinine is approximately 10:1. This ratio is useful to indicate alterations in urea reabsorption or generation, because a reduction in GFR would lead to a rise in BUN but would not alter the BUN:creatinine ratio. Urea reabsorption occurs in proximal and distal nephrons and is influenced by the patient's volume status in the medullary collecting duct, which is relatively impermeable to urea in the absence of antidiuretic hormone

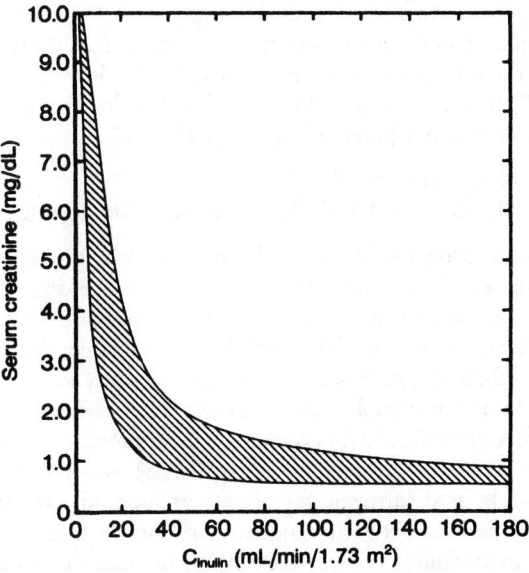

FIGURE 163.1. The shaded area represents the variation in GFR, measured by inulin clearance, which corresponds to a given level of serum creatinine. A serum creatinine of 2 mg/dL may reflect a GFR from 18 to 45 mL/min. At lower levels of serum creatinine concentration, this variability increases. (Adapted from Shemesh O, Golbetz H, Kriss JP, et al. Limitations of creatinine as a filtration marker in glomerulopathic patients. *Kidney Int* 1985;28:830–838.)

TABLE 163.2.	CAUSES OF CHANGES IN BLOOD UREA NITROGEN (BUN) INDEPENDENT OF RENAL FUNCTION
Increased BUN	**Decreased BUN**
Increased catabolic rate	Decreased catabolic
Trauma	rate
Fever	Liver disease
Cell lysis	Decreased protein
Infection	intake
Hyperthermia	
Therapy with tetracycline or corticosteroids	
Increased protein intake	
Gastrointestinal bleeding (with volume depletion)	
Reduced renal perfusion (volume depletion, congestive heart failure)	

(ADH). In volume depletion, ADH stimulation raises the duct's permeability to urea. Subsequently, BUN is reabsorbed and serum BUN rises out of proportion to the decline in GFR.

EVALUATION OF TUBULAR FUNCTION

Tests of tubular function reflect the ability of the kidney to maintain homeostasis.

URINARY SODIUM AND FRACTIONAL EXCRETION OF SODIUM

Normally, the 24-hour urine sodium excretion equals 24-hour sodium intake minus small losses in stool and sweat. Urinary Na^+ concentration reflects both Na^+ and H_2O intake. In volume-depleted states, the kidney conserves sodium; hence, the U_{Na} level is useful in assessing volume status. A low urine sodium concentration (less than 20 mEq per liter) suggests the diagnosis of volume depletion, whereas a high value points toward Na^+ wasting, which can be appropriate or inappropriate. Variations in the rate of water reabsorption can result in a U_{Na} between 20 and 40 mEq per liter, even in volume-depleted patients. Therefore, a more dependable index is the fractional excretion of sodium FE_{Na} defined as the fraction of filtered sodium that is excreted in the urine.

$$Na\ absorption = filtered\ Na - urinary\ Na\ excretion$$
or,
$$Na\ absorption = (GFR \cdot P_{Na}) - (V \cdot U_{Na})$$

where U_{Na} is the urinary sodium concentration, P_{Na} is the plasma sodium concentration. FE_{Na} is equal to $(U_{Na}/P_{Na}) / (U_{Cr}/P_{Cr})$.

Sodium reabsorption is appropriately enhanced in hypovolemic states, and the FE_{Na} is usually less than 1% (i.e., more than 99% of the filtered Na has been reabsorbed). In contrast, tubular damage leads to a FE_{Na} of more than 2% in most cases of acute tubular necrosis.

Several conditions other than hypovolemia (prerenal azotemia) present with an elevated serum creatinine and a low FE_{Na}. Moreover, several factors can interfere with sodium conservation and may result in a high FE_{Na} in the setting of prerenal azotemia (Table 163.3).

The FE_{Na} is most useful in oliguric states after ruling out obstruction. It should be noted that a high FE_{Na} cannot be interpreted in patients who received diuretics, but a low value can be. Chloride is another urinary electrolyte that is very useful in determining volume status in patients with metabolic alkalosis. A value less than 15 mEq per liter implies decreased effective or absolute arterial blood volume or very low salt intake. It differentiates chloride-responsive metabolic alkalosis (contraction alkalosis) from other causes (e.g., hyperaldosteronism, severe hypokalemia, alkali loading) in which the urine chloride is usually higher than 20 mEq per liter, provided that the patient is not receiving diuretics.

TABLE 163.3.	**CAUSES OF HIGH OR LOW FE_{Na} AND U_{Na} IN PATIENTS WITH ACUTE RENAL FAILURE**
$FE_{Na} < 1\%$, $U_{Na} < 20$ mEq/L	$FE_{Na} > 1\%$, $U_{Na} > 40$ mEq/L
Prerenal azotemia	ATN (90%)
Acute urinary tract obstruction (few hours)	Chronic urinary tract obstruction (days to months)
Acute glomerulonephritis	Poorly reabsorbable solute (glycosuria, bicarbonaturia, mannitol diuresis)
Contrast-induced acute tubular necrosis (ATN) (early)	Preexisting chronic renal failure
Rhabdomyolysis with myoglubinuria-induced ATN (sometimes)	Diuretic administration
Early sepsis	
Nonoliguric ATN (10%)	

URINARY ACIDIFICATION

The typical Western diet yields a net of close to 1 mmol of H^+ per kilogram of body weight per day. These H^+ ions are removed for the most part by combining with bicarbonate ions (HCO_3^-) forming H_2O and CO_2 (which is exhaled). As a result, the body is left with an overall deficit of HCO_3^-. To maintain acid–base balance, the kidney must not only reclaim all filtered HCO_3^-, but also generate new bicarbonate. This latter task is achieved by excreting $H_2PO_4^-$ and NH_4^+. The rate of excretion of $H_2PO_4^-$ and NH_4^+ must exceed that of HCO_3^- to have a positive renal balance of HCO_3^-; hence, the principle of net acid excretion. Renal tubular acidosis occurs when there is excessive excretion of HCO_3^-, low excretion of NH_4^+, or excessive excretion of metabolizable organic anions, which represent a potential source of HCO_3^-.

$$Net\ acid\ excretion = NH_4^+ + H_2PO_4^- - HCO_3^- - metabolizable\ organic\ anions.$$

The fractional excretion of bicarbonate can provide useful information. In general, a high FE_{HCO3} could be due to either a very large defect in H^+ secretion in the proximal tubule, or a smaller defect in proximal tubule H^+ secretion combined with a reduced distal capacity for H^+ secretion or lastly, normal proximal but a near complete defect in distal H^+ secretion.

The kidney's ability to excrete H^+ as ammonium is the basis for the concept of urinary anion gap (UAG), which is the most commonly used surrogate for urinary ammonium excretion. It is the difference between major urinary cations ($Na^+ + K^+$) and urinary anions ($Cl^- + HCO_3^-$). Because the amount of bicarbonate is very small in acid urine (pH < 6.5), the difference between urinary ($Na^+ + K^+$) and Cl^- reflects the ammonium, and the UAG would equal: $[Na^+ + K^+]_u - [Cl^-]_u$. In an extrarenal cause of acidosis (e.g., gastrointestinal bicarbonate wasting), the excretion of NH_4^+ (and of Cl^- to maintain electroneutrality) increases several-fold (intact renal acidification), resulting in a negative UAG (urinary $Na^+ + K^+$ is less than Cl^-). In contrast, NH_4^+ excretion remains low in renal tubular acidosis, resulting in a positive UAG. Urine pH in patients with RTA is useful when such patients are found to have a low rate of excretion of NH_4^+. A low urine pH in this setting suggests a decreased NH_3 availability in the renal medullary interstitium to match the increased H^+ secretion by the distal nephron, whereas a high value suggests a defect in distal or proximal H^+ secretion ($H^+ + NH_3 \leftrightarrow NH_4^+$).

WATER BALANCE

Under ADH control from the posterior pituitary, the kidney can achieve a wide range of osmolality (50 to 1,200 mOsm per kilogram), resulting in water excretion (diuresis) or conservation, with a target serum osmolality of 280 to 290 mOsm per kilogram. A urine of 300 mOsm per kilogram osmolality is called *isosmotic*. Hypotonic urine would then represent a urine that has all the solute excreted with free water added that would make the urine dilute; hence, the concept of free-water clearance (C_{H2O}), which is the difference between the amount of water excreted and the amount of water needed to excrete the urinary solute load in isotonic urine.

$$V = C_{osm} + C_{H2O},$$

where C_{osm} is the osmolal clearance ($[U_{osm} \cdot V]/P_{osm}$).

$$C_{H2O} = V \cdot (1 - [U_{osm}/P_{osm}]),$$

where P_{osm} is the plasma osmolality and V is urine vol (liters per day).

C_{H2O} is inappropriately increased in patients with diabetes insipidus, causing a dilute urine and hypernatremia, and is appropriately increased after a water load. Conversely, hypertonic urine would represent a urine containing all the urinary solute in an isotonic solution with free water removed from this urine by tubular reabsorption, resulting in a hyperosmotic value; hence, the concept of free-water reabsorption (T^C_{H2O}):

$$V = C_{osm} - T^C_{H2O} \Rightarrow T^C_{H2O} = C_{osm} - V$$
$$= V \cdot ([U_{osm}/P_{osm}] - 1)$$

T^C_{H2O} is appropriately increased in volume depletion and is inappropriately increased in the syndrome of inappropriate ADH secretion, resulting in hyponatremia.

Water handling by the kidney may be evaluated by the water deprivation test, which involves following the changes in plasma and urine osmolality for 12 to 24 hours. At plasma osmolality of 295 to 300 mOsm per kilogram (osmolality at which stimulation of ADH is maximum), 5 units of aqueous vasopressin is given subcutaneously and urine osmolality is measured. Patients with central diabetes insipidus have a concentrated urine, whereas patients with nephrogenic diabetes insipidus maintain a dilute urine. Patients with primary polydipsia have a maximally concentrated urine at the end of water deprivation and do not need to receive ADH.

RENAL BLOOD FLOW

An estimation of renal blood flow (RBF) can be derived from the renal clearance of any compound that is totally cleared (ex-

creted) by a single pass through the kidney and completely eliminated into the urine. Para-aminohippurate (PAH) is an organic acid that is both filtered at the glomerulus and extensively secreted by the proximal tubule, with a first-pass clearance approaching 100%. PAH is experimentally used to calculate RBF by measuring its clearance in a fashion similar to creatinine or inulin clearance: infusing PAH to achieve a steady-state plasma level and carefully collecting timed urine samples:

$$RBF = (U_{PAH} \cdot V)/P_{PAH}$$

RADIOLOGIC EVALUATION OF THE RENAL SYSTEM

Radiologic tests evaluate renal morphology and function (Table 163.4).

SONOGRAPHY

On plain abdominal x-ray, a normal kidney is the height of 3.5 vertebrae. However, this overestimates the kidney length by 10% to 15%, and the renal outline is sometimes difficult to discern. Ultrasound is a good test for evaluating renal size and ruling out obstruction. It provides precise measurement of the length and volume and can differentiate cortex from medulla. It can also identify cortical thinning and increased echogenicity, which indicate chronic renal disease. In general, an ultrasound is also the first investigation performed to evaluate renal cysts and masses. It can detect cysts as small as 1 to 1.5 cm in diameter and can differentiate a simple cyst from a carcinoma or abscess in most cases. Simple cysts are sharply demarcated, with smooth walls and a strong posterior wall echo due to strong transmission through the cyst.

Duplex Doppler ultrasonography in experienced hands is valuable in detecting renal hypoperfusion. It has also proved to be valuable in assessment of patients with acute renal failure, most of whom show elevated renal resistive index. Patients with acute tubular necrosis have markedly abnormal Doppler flow profiles, with increased pulsatility and loss of diastolic flow. A renal resistive index (RI) value of 0.75 has been reported as optimal in attempting differential diagnosis between renal and prerenal acute renal failure. In addition, in kidneys with a dilated collecting system, a RI value of 0.70 or more is suggestive for obstruction, whereas lower values are suggestive of nonobstructive dilation. Duplex Doppler ultrasonography can also have some predictive value for subsequent development of kidney dysfunction and hepatorenal syndrome in patients with liver disease when the RI value is elevated.

COMPUTED TOMOGRAPHY

Computed tomography (CT) scan is a useful test to evaluate renal masses and cysts. It can detect simple cysts as small as 0.5 cm. Cysts are characterized by smooth, thin walls and cystic fluid with a consistency similar to that of water. Simple cysts do not enhance after radiocontrast. Enhancement implies vascularity and strongly suggests a tumor. Unenhanced CT adds clini-

TABLE 163.4.	TESTS FOR EVALUATION OF RENAL SYSTEM AND THEIR USES

Test	Primary Uses
Ultrasonography	Kidney size, renal cysts and masses, hydronephrosis, chronic cortical disease, calculi
Abdominal flatplate	Kidney size
Excretory urogram	Scan of entire renal and excretory system; evaluating hematuria, screen for stones and renal masses, medullary sponge kidney
Antegrade pyelogram	View upper tract in cases of obstruction
Retrograde pyelogram	Evaluate obstruction; obtain image of ureters
CT	Evaluate renal masses, cysts and renal morphology, renal vein thrombosis, examine retroperitoneum
Spiral CT	Ureteral calculi, obstruction, morphology and masses, mild hydronephrosis and kidney volume (unenhanced), pyelonephritis (enhanced)
MRI and MRA	RVT, renal masses, RAS, corticomedullary differentiation in obstruction
Magnetic resonance renography	Renal excretory function
Arteriogram	RAS, RVT, evaluation of renal masses
Venogram	RVT
Scintigraphy (usefulness depending on agent used)	GFR, perfusion (RBF), split renal function, obstruction, morphology, pyelonephritis
ACE inhibitor scintigraphy	Functionally significant RAS
^{67}Ga (gallium) citrate scintigraphy	Infection, interstitial nephritis, renal abscess
Voiding cystourethrogram	Gold standard for vesicoureteral reflux

CT, computed tomography; MRA, magnetic resonance angiography; MRI, magnetic resonance imaging; RVT, renal vein thrombosis; RAS, renal artery stenosis; RBF, renal blood flow; GFR, glomerular filtration rate

cally important information when sonograms are indeterminate. CT is as sensitive as ultrasonography in detecting hydronephrosis and is much more sensitive in detecting ureteral calculi. Dilated ureters can be traced to the point of obstruction. ARF induced by iodinated contrast media accounts for about 10% of all hospital cases of renal failure, especially in azotemic patients. Nonionic, low-osmolarity media should be used in high-risk patients because these media have been shown to be significantly less nephrotoxic than ionic contrast media—in patients with and without renal insufficiency. Spiral CT scan is superior to conventional CT. It minimizes artifacts and reduces the amount of contrast needed. Non–contrast spiral CT is 97% accurate in detecting ureteral calculi and obstruction and is even more sensitive than intravenous pyelograms. It is superior for precise evaluation of renal volume and detection of mild hydronephrosis. Contrast-enhanced spiral CT has become the major initial study in acute pyelonephritis in addition to detecting structural abnormalities.

MAGNETIC RESONANCE IMAGING

The images produced by magnetic resonance imaging (MRI) are higher in contrast resolution than those from a CT scan. Unlike CT, multiplanar imaging is possible, and although contrast medium is used, no significant nephrotoxicity was reported for paramagnetic contrast agents, either ionic or nonionic, with the concentrations used in common clinical practice. Sensitivity reactions have been extraordinarily rare. Corticomedullary differentiation is shown best with this modality. Magnetic resonance is exquisitely sensitive to blood flow and produces superb depiction of the larger renal vessels. Therefore, magnetic resonance angiography has been an important modality in the evaluation of renal artery and vein obstructions from any cause.

Indications for renal MRI are evaluation and characterization of renal masses and fluid collections, accurate staging of renal cancer, semiquantitative evaluation of renal function using contrast-enhanced dynamic studies (magnetic resonance renography), and evaluation of renal vessels using magnetic resonance angiography (MRA). It can also be used as an alternative imaging modality to CT for patients allergic to iodine or patients with an inconclusive CT study, in addition to patients at high risk for contrast nephrotoxicity. MRA is rapidly becoming the most useful screening test for significant renal artery stenosis, with a sensitivity of 87% and a specificity of 97%, which compare favorably with those of conventional angiography. However, it cannot detect distal or intrarenal stenoses, and is therefore not recommended when fibrodysplastic stenosis is suspected.

MRI is the method of choice for the diagnosis of renal vein thrombosis in patients with impaired renal function. Dynamic functional MRI allows the evaluation of renal excretory function, even in patients with diffuse functional impairment. Dynamic examinations can be quantitatively evaluated by plotting the signal intensity values in the renal cortex and medulla as a function of time. MRI can also differentiate between acute and chronic obstruction and hydronephrosis. In acute obstruction, the corticomedullary demarcation is preserved, and the renal cortex shows enhancement similar to that of a normal kidney after injection with gadolinium-DTPA (diethylenetriamine pentaacetic acid), but medullary enhancement is greater and sustained. In chronic obstruction, the demarcation is often absent, and cortical enhancement is lower than in the normal kidney, with a prolonged tubular phase.

SCINTIGRAPHY (RADIONUCLIDE IMAGING)

The flow of radioisotopes through the kidney may be monitored, resulting in imaging of vascular perfusion, parenchymal integrity and outflow tract anatomy. Radiopharmaceuticals available for assessing renal function and anatomy are grouped into three categories: those excreted by glomerular filtration (^{99m}Tc-DTPA), those excreted by tubular secretion (iodine orthoiodo-hippurate [^{131}I-OIH] and ^{99m}Tc-mercaptoacetyltriglycine [MAG$_3$]), and those retained in the renal tubules for long periods of time (^{99m}Tc-dimercaptosuccinic acid [DMSA]). DTPA is used to measure GFR. It has a low extraction fraction, which limits its use in patients with renal impairment. Extraction of ^{99m}Tc-MAG$_3$ requires delivery of the compound to the kidney (renal plasma flow) and extraction from the plasma (proximal tubules) and has a higher extraction fraction, which provides better images than ^{99m}Tc-DTPA, particularly in patients with impaired renal function. DMSA is an excellent cortical imaging agent and is used when high-resolution anatomical images are required, as in detecting pyelonephritis. Scintigraphy, then, is useful in measuring renal function (GFR) and renal plasma flow in addition to the measurement of each kidney's contribution to the total renal plasma flow and total GFR (split renal function).

Captopril-scintigraphy is useful in diagnosing functionally significant renal artery stenosis. This is done by obtaining a baseline scan, followed by a scan after its administration. The angiotensin-converting enzyme (ACE) inhibitor, by causing efferent arteriole vasodilation, induces a decline in the GFR in the kidney on the side of the stenosis, thus enhancing the difference in the function of the two kidneys. An ACE inhibitor renogram is considered positive if there is decreased uptake of the radioisotope by one kidney such that the GFR of that kidney accounts for less than 40% of the total GFR. Another criterion is delayed peak of uptake of isotope by the kidney. However, the test has a sensitivity of only 70%, which can be higher in high-risk patients, but is 90% specific for high-grade stenotic lesions. Scintigraphy is useful in providing valuable functional information about the significance of obstruction in obstructive nephropathy (diuresis renography). This is important in the differentiation of hydronephrosis (dilated, obstructed tract) from hydroureteronephrosis (dilated, nonobstructed tract). In this test, a diuretic during dynamic scintigraphy can induce a rapid washout of the tracer from a dilated, nonobstructed, renal pelvis, but not from an obstructed one.

ANGIOGRAPHY

Renal angiography can be diagnostic in patients with suspected renal artery stenosis or occlusion, most of whom are hypertensive or thought to be at high risk for renal artery occlusive disease. It is also diagnostic in suspected arteritis, renal vein thrombosis, and persistent unexplained hematuria. This test has therapeutic applications in angioplasty, angio-occlusion, and thrombolysis. Complications of angiography include thrombosis, aneurysm, and bleeding and are rare in experienced hands. However, the major concern is deterioration of renal function in patients with renal insufficiency. This can be minimized by using the minimal amount of low-ionic-strength contrast media and proper hydration before the test.

PYELOGRAPHY

Intravenous pyelography (IVP) is commonly requested when an obstructive calculus or lesion is suspected. It is also the study of

choice in medullary sponge kidney disease. Contrast stasis and delayed excretion of contrast material into collecting system after IV injection are indicative of obstruction. A standing column of contrast within the ureter and dilatation of the collecting system are signs of ureteral obstruction. Direct retrograde and antegrade injection of contrast into the renal collecting system or ureter is considered when precise anatomical information is required, which is particularly valuable when the IVP is suboptimal owing to poor renal function and inadequate contrast excretion. Retrograde and antegrade pyelography are also used for defining level and degree of obstruction and whether or not the obstruction is intraluminal or not. They are particularly useful in planning interventions such as stenting and percutaneous nephrostomy.

BIBLIOGRAPHY

Davison AJ, Hartman DS, Choyke PL, et al. Radiologic assessment of renal masses. *Radiology* 1997;202(2):297–305.

Hierholzer K, Hierholzer J. Renal imaging techniques. *Am J Nephrol* 1997; 17(3-4):369–381.

Jou WW, Powers RD. Utility of dipstick urinalysis as a guide to management of adults with suspected infection or hematuria. *South Med J* 1998; 91(3):266–269.

Gonin J, Molitoris BA. Laboratory evaluation of renal disorders. In: *Kelley's textbook of internal medicine*, third edition. Philadelphia: Lippincott-Raven, 1997:1042–1048.

Kamel KS, Briceno LF, Sanchez MI, Brenes L. A new classification of renal defects in net acid excretion. *Am J Kid Dis* 1997;29(1):136–146.

Mucelli RP, Bertolotto M. Imaging techniques in acute renal failure. *Kidney Int* 1998;66:S102–S105.

Peredy TR, Powers RD. Bedside diagnostic testing of body fluids. *Am J Emerg Med* 1997;15(4):400–407.

Platt JF. Urinary obstruction. *Radiol Clin North Am* 1996;34(6): 1113–1129.

Pugia MJ, Lott JA, Clark LW. Comparison of urine dipsticks with quantitative methods for microalbuminuria. *Eur J Clin Chem Clin Biochem* 1997; 35(9):693–700.

Taylor A Jr, Nally JV. Clinical applications of renal scintigraphy. *Am J Roentgenol* 1995;164(1):31–41.

Kelley's Textbook of Internal Medicine, fourth edition. Edited by H. David Humes. Lippincott Williams & Wilkins, Philadelphia © 2000.

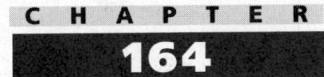

C H A P T E R

164

RENAL BIOPSY AND TREATMENT OF GLOMERULAR DISEASE

RONALD J. FALK

RENAL BIOPSY

INDICATIONS

Many indications exist for renal biopsy in a patient with glomerular disease. The most common of these is to establish the diagnosis for a renal-limited process or a systemic disease that has renal involvement (e.g., systemic vasculitis). A renal biopsy diagnosis provides insight into the natural history of the disease and guides the initiation of choice of therapy. Renal biopsy results provide an estimation of prognosis based on the type of disease identified and the pathologic aggressiveness and chronicity of the renal injury. A biopsy frequently relieves uncertainty in the patient and the physician regarding the nature of the patient's illness. A specific pathologic diagnosis also obviates further investigations that would be necessary in the absence of a conclusive diagnosis. For example, in patients with persistent hematuria of uncertain cause, a renal biopsy diagnosis of IgA nephropathy or thin basement membrane nephropathy renders unnecessary repetitive urologic evaluations such as cystoscopy and intravenous pyelography.

Table 164.1 lists the major clinical manifestations of glomerular diseases that prompt renal biopsy. The many glomerular diseases in Table 164.1 have differing natural histories, and affected patients have different responses to therapy. Most therapies for active, progressive forms of glomerulonephritis require anti-inflammatory or immunosuppressive agents, or both. Because these agents have significant side effects, some of which are life-threatening, their use is justified only if the risk:benefit ratio is favorable. This chapter focuses on the use of renal biopsy in specific clinical syndromes that suggest underlying glomerular disease, the possible diagnosis in each of these syndromes, and therapeutic options that are indicated by the renal biopsy findings. Renal biopsies also are useful in the management of some forms of tubulointerstitial and vascular disease, but these are considered in Chapters 151 and 152.

METHOD

Percutaneous needle biopsies of the kidney usually are performed using real-time ultrasonography guidance to localize the lower pole of the kidney. When the biopsy needle is close to the renal capsule, the patient is asked to hold his or her breath, and the biopsy is performed. A variety of biopsy needles were used in the past, but new spring-loaded devices, or "biopsy guns," have improved the yield of renal tissue, especially when 15-gauge needles are used. These devices may improve patient safety because no more than three attempts are usually necessary to obtain a sufficient tissue sample.

The major complications of renal biopsy are bleeding and

TABLE 164.1. CLINICAL MANIFESTATIONS OF GLOMERULAR DISEASES AND REPRESENTATIVE DISEASES THAT PRESENT WITH THESE MANIFESTATIONS

Asymptomatic microscopic hematuria
  Thin basement membrane nephropathy
  IgA nephropathy
  Mesangioproliferative glomerulopathy
  Alport's syndrome
Recurrent gross hematuria
  Thin basement membrane nephropathy
  IgA nephropathy
  Alport's syndrome
Acute nephritis
  Acute diffuse proliferative GN
    Poststreptococcal GN
  Focal or diffuse proliferative GN
    IgA nephropathy
    Lupus nephritis
Asymptomatic proteinuria
  Focal segmental glomerulosclerosis
  Mesangioproliferative glomerulopathy
Nephrotic syndrome
  Minimal-change glomerulopathy
  Membranous glomerulopathy
    Idiopathic
    Secondary
  Focal segmental glomerulosclerosis
  Mesangioproliferative glomerulopathy
  Type I membranoproliferative GN
  Type II membranoproliferative GN
  Diabetic glomerulosclerosis
  Amyloidosis

Acute renal failure
  Acute diffuse proliferative GN
    Poststreptococcal GN
  Crescentic GN
    Anti-GBM GN
    Immune complex GN
    ANCA-associated GN
Rapidly progressive renal failure
  Crescentic GN
    Anti-GBM GN
    Immune complex GN
    ANCA-associated GN
Pulmonary-renal vasculitic syndrome
  Anti-GBM GN (Goodpasture's syndrome)
  Immune complex GN
    Lupus
    Henoch–Schönlein purpura
  ANCA-associated GN
    Microscopic polyangiitis
    Wegener's granulomatosis
    Churg–Strauss syndrome
Chronic renal failure
End-stage renal disease

ANCA, antineutrophil cytoplasmic autoantibody; GBM, glomerular basement membrane; GN, glomerulonephritis.
(Adapted from Jennette JC, Falk RJ. Glomerular clinicopathologic syndromes. In: Greenberg A, ed. *Primer of kidney diseases*, second ed. San Diego, CA: Academic Press, 1998:127.)

infection. A sterile technique must be used to prevent infectious complications. The kidney is a vital organ that filters about 180 L of plasma per day. Some bleeding into the surrounding tissue is unavoidable; however, clinically significant retroperitoneal bleeding, or bleeding into the urinary tract, occurs in only 1% to 2% of patients. Careful measurement of coagulation and bleeding parameters typically is performed before biopsy. An abnormality in any of these parameters is a contraindication to renal biopsy. Anatomical abnormalities can present potential problems, especially if the kidney is congenitally abnormal (horseshoe kidney) or the patient has only one kidney. Operator experience and patient compliance are major factors associated with a safe biopsy.

CLINICAL PATTERNS OF GLOMERULAR DISEASE

Although there are many causes of glomerular injury, demographic characteristics such as age, gender, and race provide clues to its underlying nature. For example, in patients with nephrotic-range proteinuria, certain diseases are more common among young people and others occur more often in the elderly (Fig. 164.1). Most glomerular diseases affect males and females equally, but some diseases are more common in women than

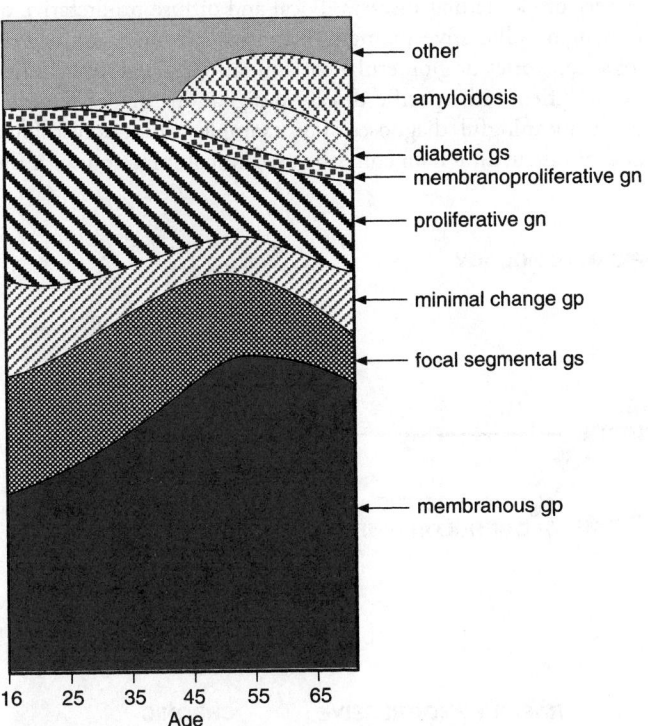

other
amyloidosis
diabetic gs
membranoproliferative gn
proliferative gn
minimal change gp
focal segmental gs
membranous gp

16   25   35   45   55   65
Age

FIGURE 164.1. Diagram demonstrating the approximate frequency of different renal diseases in patients with nephrotic-range proteinuria whose renal biopsy samples were evaluated in the University of North Carolina Nephropathology Laboratory. Note the variation in frequency with age. *Gn*, glomerulonephritis; *gp*, glomerulopathy; *gs*, glomerulosclerosis. (Jennette JC, Mandal AK. The nephrotic syndrome. In: Mandal AK, Jennette JC, eds. *Diagnosis and management of renal disease and hypertension.* Durham, NC: Carolina Academic Press, 1994:243.)

in men (e.g., lupus erythematosus). Some glomerular diseases have clear racial predilections. However, these data indicate only which disease is most probable statistically. Renal biopsy is necessary to obtain a definitive diagnosis.

Clinical patterns also suggest which glomerular disease is the most probable cause of renal dysfunction (Fig. 164.2). Clinicopathologic syndromes include asymptomatic microscopic hematuria with or without recurrent gross hematuria, asymptomatic proteinuria, nephrotic syndrome, acute nephritis, rapidly progressive glomerulonephritis with or without systemic illness, pulmonary–renal vasculitic syndrome, and chronic nephritis.

The clinical course of a glomerular disease can be acute and self-limited (e.g., acute poststreptococcal glomerulonephritis), persistent and indolent (e.g., focal segmental glomerulosclerosis [FSGS]), or fulminant (e.g., rapidly progressive glomerulonephritis, pulmonary–renal vasculitic syndrome). The clinical manifestations of a glomerular disease can change over time. For example, any form of proliferative glomerulonephritis can present with asymptomatic hematuria and proteinuria. Later, a more acute or even rapidly progressive nephritic picture may emerge (Fig. 164.3). Certain glomerular diseases, such as anti–glomerular basement membrane (GBM) crescentic glomerulonephritis, usually progress to severe failure within weeks to months. Others, such as lupus nephritis, tend to cause focal or diffuse proliferative glomerulonephritis, which may progress to end-stage disease over several years. Diseases such as IgA nephropathy tend to begin as mild mesangioproliferative lesions and progress into more severe lesions over several decades, whereas diseases such as poststreptococcal glomerulonephritis initially cause an active proliferative glomerulonephritis and then resolve through a mesangioproliferative phase to normal. Because the treatment of most of these diseases involves immunosuppressive agents or other expensive and inherently dangerous modalities (i.e., plasma exchange), a precise renal biopsy diagnosis is imperative.

RENAL BIOPSY EVALUATION

For optimum clinical value, a renal biopsy specimen should be evaluated by a pathologist with extensive experience in renal pathology. Renal biopsy specimens should be examined by light, immunofluorescence, and electron microscopy when a glomerular disease is suspected. These three modalities are always complementary or confirmatory, and, in particular diseases, each is essential for making a diagnosis. For example, IgA nephropathy cannot be diagnosed without immunohistology, and thin basement membrane nephropathy cannot be diagnosed without electron microscopy. A detailed discussion of the histologic patterns of various forms of glomerulonephritis is presented in Chapter 150.

Light microscopic evaluation of glomerular diseases begins with the identification of structural changes in glomeruli, which then must be characterized with respect to type and distribution. Glomerular lesions are considered focal if 50% or fewer glomeruli are involved and considered diffuse if more than 50% of glomeruli are involved. A segmental lesion affects only a portion

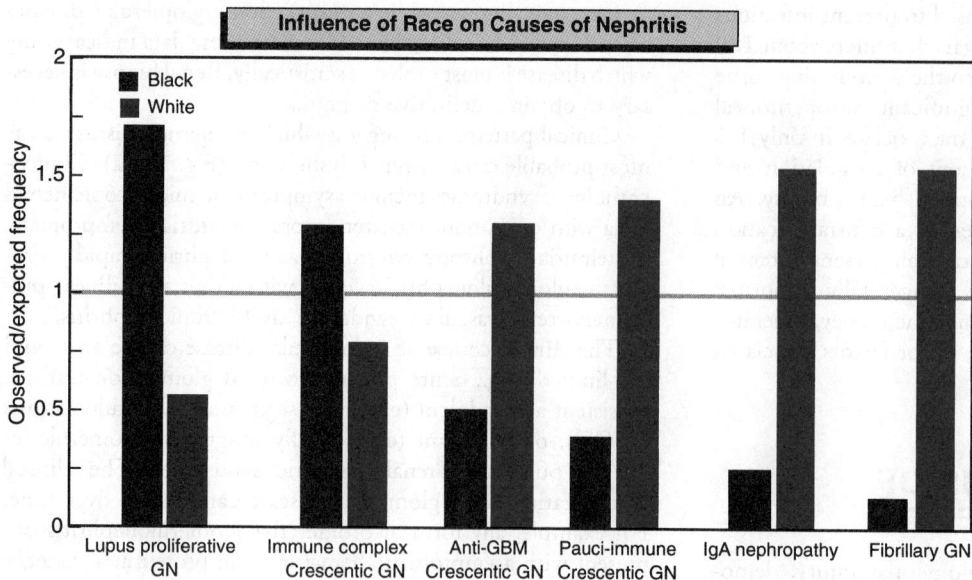

FIGURE 164.2. An estimation of the frequency of glomerular lesions by race. A value of "1" indicates the expectation that the white:black ratio will be equivalent. *GBM*, glomerular basement membrane; *GN*, glomerulonephritis.

of a glomerular tuft, whereas a global lesion affects the entire tuft.

Glomerular changes that can be identified by light microscopy include glomerular hypercellularity, capillary wall thickening, sclerosis, and necrosis. For example, normal glomeruli by light microscopy are consistent with minimal change glomerulopathy, early membranous glomerulopathy, or thin basement membrane nephropathy. Thick capillary walls without hypercellularity suggest membranous glomerulopathy, whereas thick walls with hypercellularity suggest some form of membranoproliferative glomerulonephritis or, possibly, diffuse proliferative

lupus glomerulonephritis. Diffuse global hypercellularity with conspicuous neutrophils strongly suggests acute postinfectious (especially poststreptococcal) glomerulonephritis. Focal or diffuse hypercellularity indicative of a focal or diffuse proliferative or mesangioproliferative glomerulonephritis can be caused by a variety of glomerular diseases. Focal and diffuse proliferative or mesangioproliferative glomerulonephritis are merely morphologic categories of glomerular inflammation. These terms must be modified with specific disease designations before they become meaningful diagnoses. For example, immunohistologic and ultrastructural data could be used in combination with the

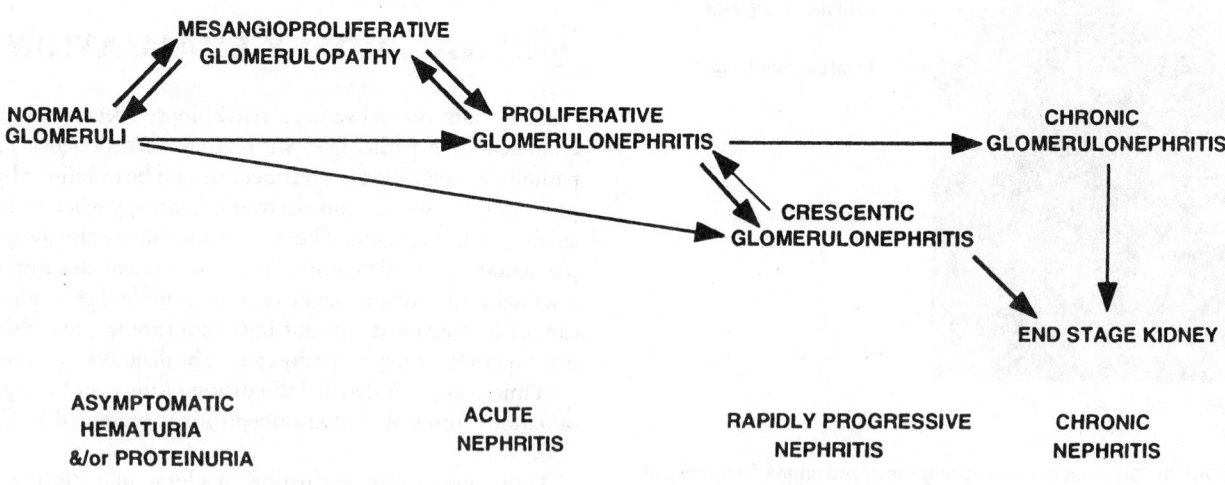

FIGURE 164.3. Morphologic stages of proliferative glomerulonephritis **(top)** aligned with the usual clinical manifestations **(bottom)**. (Jennette JC, Mandal AK. Syndrome of glomerulonephritis. In: Mandal AK, Jennette JC, eds. *Diagnosis and management of renal disease and hypertension,* second ed. Durham, NC: Carolina Academic Press, 1994:207.)

light microscopic pattern of glomerular hypercellularity to reach a diagnosis, such as focal proliferative IgA nephropathy or diffuse proliferative lupus glomerulonephritis.

Focal segmental glomerular scarring raises the possibility of FSGS, but other causes, such as the sclerotic phase of a focal proliferative glomerulonephritis or hereditary nephritis, must be ruled out by immunohistology and electron microscopy before this diagnosis can be made.

Light microscopic evaluation of glomerular diseases should include an evaluation of histologic features that indicate the activity and chronicity of the disease. For example, glomerular necrosis and crescents are indicators of active aggressive inflammatory disease, whereas glomerular sclerosis, interstitial fibrosis, and tubular atrophy are indicators of chronic injury.

Crescents result from the rupture of glomerular capillaries with the release of proinflammatory plasma constituents into Bowman's capsule. This causes the accumulation of macrophages and the proliferation of epithelial cells, that is, crescent formation. Therefore, crescent formation is an indicator of severe capillary injury; however, crescent formation can be caused by many different types of glomerular disease and is etiologically nonspecific. The term *crescentic glomerulonephritis* is not a specific diagnosis until it is modified by additional information derived from other pathologic, serologic, or clinical data (i.e., anti-GBM, antibody-mediated crescentic glomerulonephritis, antineutrophil cytoplasmic autoantibodies [ANCA]-associated crescentic glomerulonephritis, or crescentic type I membranoproliferative glomerulonephritis associated with cryoglobulins). The pathologic term crescentic glomerulonephritis usually is reserved for specimens with crescents in more than 50% of glomeruli. When fewer crescents are present, this is indicated in the diagnosis as a percentage, such as focal proliferative IgA nephropathy with 25% crescents.

Immunofluorescence or immunoenzyme microscopy is essential for optimum examination of renal biopsy specimens. The presence or absence of staining for various immunoglobulins and complement components is important for differentiating among most of the diseases in Table 164.1. The pattern (e.g., granular, linear, band-like), distribution (e.g., mesangial, capillary wall, both), and composition (e.g., IgA-dominant, C3-dominant) of glomerular immune deposits is characteristic, if not diagnostic, for many antibody-mediated glomerulonephritides. The absence of immunohistologic evidence for immune deposits can be as useful as positive staining in pointing to the appropriate diagnosis. For example, no granular or linear glomerular immunoglobulin staining in a specimen with crescentic glomerulonephritis is about 90% predictive of ANCA-associated crescentic glomerulonephritis.

Examination of renal biopsy specimens by electron microscopy may be required for diagnosis or may add complementary data to a diagnosis made by light and immunofluorescence microscopy. For example, electron microscopy is required for making a pathologic diagnosis of fibrillary glomerulonephritis, immunotactoid glomerulopathy, collagenofibrotic glomerulopathy, or thin basement membrane nephropathy. Occasionally, the electron microscopic observations constitute the feature in a biopsy specimen that guides the pathologist to a diagnosis that otherwise might have been overlooked, such as

hereditary nephritis, type II membranoproliferative glomerulonephritis, and Fabry's disease. Sometimes, the electron microscopic findings do not alter the basic diagnosis but provide additional refinement or insight into the patient's disease. For example, the finding of mesangial immune deposits in a patient with membranous glomerulopathy increases the likelihood of secondary membranous glomerulopathy, such as hepatitis B–induced membranous glomerulopathy. The finding of microtubular configurations in a specimen with type I membranoproliferative glomerulonephritis increases the likelihood of hepatitis C–induced cryoglobulinemic glomerulonephritis.

The light, immunofluorescence, and electron microscopy data from a renal biopsy specimen should be correlated and integrated with clinical data to yield a final pathologic diagnosis. Individual uncorrelated reports of each microscopic procedure should be avoided. Any time that the pathologist feels that the report might be confusing to the clinician or the clinician is not absolutely certain about the reported pathologic diagnosis, it is important for the pathologist and clinician to discuss the findings personally.

RENAL BIOPSY AND THE TREATMENT OF PATIENTS WITH ISOLATED HEMATURIA

Asymptomatic hematuria is caused most often by a urologic disease, such as urinary tract infection, urolithiasis, or a tumor of the urinary epithelium or renal parenchyma. Occasionally, however, asymptomatic microscopic hematuria is the harbinger of glomerular injury. The morphology of the red blood cells in the urine is useful for differentiating between bleeding derived from the glomerulus and that derived from the urinary tract. Glomerular hematuria typically is dysmorphic. For example, the red blood cells in the urine include many acanthocytes and other misshapen cells rather than biconcave discs. This is one of the most specific manifestations of glomerular injury. The association of asymptomatic hematuria with proteinuria or formed elements such as casts (especially red blood cell casts) provides supportive evidence for glomerular injury. In the absence of these findings, patients with asymptomatic hematuria without urinary tract infection usually undergo excretory urograms and cystoscopy in search of a cause for the hematuria (Chapter 134). If no cause is found, a renal biopsy may be performed. Of patients with hematuria, a serum creatinine level of less than 1.5 mg per deciliter, and proteinuria of less than 1 g per day who undergo renal biopsy, about 85% are relatively evenly divided among patients with IgA nephropathy, thin basement membrane disease, and normal glomeruli. The other 15% have miscellaneous other glomerular lesions (Table 164.1).

Thin basement membrane nephropathy is a group of conditions in which there is thinning of the GBM. The clinical course typically is benign, manifested by occasional bouts of macroscopic hematuria with viral infections. Commonly, first-degree relatives also have microscopic hematuria. There is no known therapy for this condition, and renal failure is uncommon. A more severe variant of hereditary basement membrane nephropathy that is associated with hearing loss is known as Alport's syndrome. At the time of diagnosis, this disease usually manifests with proteinuria and renal insufficiency along with hematuria. These patients progress to end-stage renal disease and there is no known treatment.

IGA NEPHROPATHY

IgA nephropathy is the most common form of glomerulopathy in the world. The renal biopsy findings in IgA nephropathy include conspicuous glomerular IgA-dominant or IgA-codominant mesangial immunostaining. Electron microscopy reveals electron-dense deposits corresponding to the immune deposits seen by immunohistology. Light microscopic lesions range from mild mesangial hypercellularity to diffuse inflammation with necrosis and crescent formation (Fig. 164.3). Consistent with the relapsing nature of this disease, renal biopsy specimens often have areas of glomerular and tubulointerstitial scarring, suggesting prior acute inflammation adjoining regions of active ongoing inflammation. Once mistakenly considered a uniformly benign disease, IgA nephropathy has many different clinical expressions, including mild asymptomatic hematuria, acute nephritis, rapidly progressive glomerulonephritis, chronic nephritis, and even the nephrotic syndrome. In most patients, the disease process follows a course of exacerbation and remission.

End-stage renal disease develops in 15% to 20% of patients after 10 years and in 20% to 40% of patients after 20 years. Should all patients with IgA nephropathy receive treatment? In this disease that waxes and wanes, should therapy be aimed at aggressive episodes of disease? Should patients who have mild disease be treated in the same way as those who have aggressive IgA nephropathy with crescent formation? Patients who have substantial proteinuria and an elevated creatinine level are more likely to undergo renal biopsy. These patients probably have more severe structural changes than patients who do not undergo biopsy and tend to have a worse long-term prognosis. Should these patients be selected for special study? Unfortunately, there are few answers for these questions.

Several treatment protocols have been suggested for IgA nephropathy, usually for patients with proteinuria or renal insufficiency. There are few data that support the use of daily corticosteroid therapy. Anecdotal data in children suggest that alternate-day therapy for 1.5 to 3 years is associated with less proteinuria and, perhaps, preservation of renal function. In the absence of firm positive data, no compelling reason supports this therapy in light of the potential adverse consequences of long-term prednisone treatment. However, prednisone treatment is effective in IgA nephropathy coexisting with minimal change glomerulopathy. In this condition, the renal biopsy shows typical immunohistologic features of IgA nephropathy, no or mild glomerular changes by light microscopy, and diffuse foot process fusion of glomerular epithelial cells by electron microscopy. Proteinuria is diminished rapidly by prednisone therapy in a manner consistent with its response in minimal change disease. A renal biopsy is crucial to identify this combined process.

More aggressive treatment of IgA nephropathy has been tried, including concurrent therapy with cyclophosphamide, warfarin, and dipyridamole. Although this approach is associated with a reduction in proteinuria, no significant preservation of renal function has been observed.

Treatment with omega-3 fatty acid products is gaining favor. A controlled trial has been performed comparing fish oil with placebo. In this study of patients with at least 1 g of proteinuria, 55 patients received omega-3 fatty acid and 51 received placebo. Treatment consisted of about 1.6 g of eicosapentaenoic acid per day. Hypertension was controlled in both groups. Decline in renal function was significantly more rapid in the placebo group than in the fish oil group. Forty percent of the placebo group reached end-stage disease after 4 years, compared with only 10% of the fish oil group. IgA nephropathy may be ameliorated by this simple, relatively nontoxic therapy. However, two smaller studies using omega-3 fatty acids in similar patients did not find preservation of renal function. The nature of the discrepancy in these studies is not clear, but may relate to the complete lack of uniformity of this form of treatment. Omega-3 fatty acid preparations are not controlled by the Food and Drug Administration. These preparations contain varying amounts of eicosapentaenoic acid, and many are laden with vitamins E, A, and D. Whether this treatment stabilizes renal function in all patients with IgA nephropathy or just those with proteinuria and progressive renal insufficiency is not known. Lifelong therapy with even this benign agent is cumbersome and marked by gastrointestinal complaints. Patients should know that their hematuria and proteinuria is a consequence of biopsy-proven IgA nephropathy before embarking on such a program.

Because anti-inflammatory agents have shown few beneficial effects, other potentially less toxic regimens have been considered. These include angiotensin-converting enzyme (ACE) inhibitors, which have a salutary effect, at least to diminish proteinuria and perhaps to sustain renal function.

RENAL BIOPSY AND THERAPY IN THE NEPHROTIC SYNDROME

MEMBRANOUS GLOMERULOPATHY

Membranous glomerulopathy is the most common cause of nephrotic syndrome in persons older than 30 years of age. Membranous glomerulopathy can be an idiopathic disease (no specific cause), or it can result from infections, toxins, drugs, autoimmune diseases, neoplastic diseases, renal transplantation, or many other conditions (Table 164.2). The issue of malignant tumors associated with membranous glomerulopathy is especially pertinent for patients older than 55 years. In these patients, the tumors may precede the membranous glomerulopathy by 18 to 24 months. In some cases, simultaneous detection of tumors and renal disease occurs, whereas in others, tumors develop only 18 to 24 months after the membranous glomerulopathy is first detected. Therefore, in elderly patients with the nephrotic syndrome, a renal biopsy diagnosis of membranous glomerulopathy mandates vigilant screening for cancer with tests, such as chest radiography, mammography, pelvic examination, and colonic evaluation.

Idiopathic membranous glomerulopathy has a variable clinical course. The prognosis of patients with this disease depends

TABLE 164.2.   SECONDARY CAUSES OF MEMBRANOUS NEPHROPATHY

Drugs and Toxins
Nonsteroidal anti-inflammatory drugs
Captopril
Gold
Penicillamine
Probenecid
Hydrocarbons

Autoimmune Disease
Systemic lupus erythematosus
Rheumatoid arthritis
Primary biliary cirrhosis
Thyroiditis

Infectious Disease
Syphilis
Malaria
Quartan malaria
Filariasis

Neoplastic Disease
Solid carcinomas
  Lung
  Breast
  Gastrointestinal (especially colon)
  Melanoma
Lymphoproliferative disease
  Chronic lymphocytic leukemia
  Non-Hodgkin's lymphoma

Post-transplantation Glomerulopathy

on their geographic location in the world. Ten-year renal survival rates vary from as low as 50% to as high as 90%. Data at 20 years reflect the continued loss of renal function in this chronic disease. Many patients who progress to end-stage renal disease do so within the first 3 years after diagnosis. Fortunately, 20% to 35% of patients have a spontaneous remission within 1 to 4 years after diagnosis.

Several factors that portend a worse prognosis are hypertension, renal insufficiency, male gender, older age, and persistent proteinuria for more than 8 months. Massive proteinuria is an additional independent risk factor. Some genetic phenotypes, such as DRW 3, are associated with a rapid downhill course. Young women with membranous glomerulopathy who do not have nephrotic-range proteinuria have a better prognosis.

A variable clinical course complicates the evaluation of treatment regimens. In many patients, the disease is relatively benign, whereas in others, end-stage renal disease rapidly ensues. For more than a decade, the standard therapy for membranous glomerulopathy was based on an American collaborative placebo-controlled study suggesting that high-dose, alternate-day, oral corticosteroids decreased the number of patients in whom renal failure developed. Although the amount of proteinuria improved transiently in the prednisone-treated group, the long-term effects on proteinuria were the same regardless of whether patients received corticosteroids.

This trial has been subject to much criticism. The serum creatinine level doubled in more than 40% of the control pa-

tients during 2 years of follow-up—a more rapid decline in renal function than is typical of patients with membranous glomerulopathy. Because of this criticism, two other long-term prospective trials have evaluated the use of corticosteroid therapy in patients with membranous glomerulopathy. The Toronto collaborative group tested corticosteroid therapy for 6 months. In this study, both the control group and the corticosteroid group fared well, with no differences in renal dysfunction. In a study performed in the United Kingdom, patients were treated with corticosteroids or placebo; progressive renal insufficiency developed in both groups of patients and corticosteroids did not have a beneficial effect. A meta-analysis and pooled analysis confirms these findings and suggests that prednisone therapy does not alter renal survival and has only a minimal effect on the nephrotic syndrome.

More aggressive therapies for membranous glomerulopathy have been proposed. One protocol for patients with new-onset membranous glomerulopathy involves a combination of pulse methylprednisolone (Medrol) and oral prednisone for 1 month, followed by oral chlorambucil for another month. This 2-month cycle is repeated for three cycles (a total of 6 months). In a controlled prospective trial with 5 years of follow-up, treated patients had a substantial stabilization in renal function when compared with control patients, and complete remission of the nephrotic syndrome was observed in 57% of treated patients but only 23% of control patients. Whether this effect is a consequence of the pulse methylprednisolone or the chlorambucil by itself has been examined. In a separate study, treatment with methylprednisolone and chlorambucil led to an improvement in the number of patients who had remission of membranous glomerulopathy for at least 3 years. By 4 years, however, the effect of the alkylating therapy over that of methylprednisolone alone dissipated. Methylprednisolone alone resulted in the same degree of preservation of renal function as did methylprednisolone and chlorambucil together.

The controversy remains. Corticosteroids by themselves do not appear to be efficacious, whereas alkylating therapy may improve the chances of remission of nephrosis. These drugs are associated with significant side effects, including life-threatening infections and the development of malignant tumors (Table 164.3).

The current focus of treatment is aimed at detecting patients with poor prognostic signs at the outset of disease who are destined to have renal failure. Several trials have examined the effect of alkylating therapy and corticosteroids in patients with renal insufficiency. Data suggest that patients with renal insufficiency who are given intravenous cyclophosphamide and corticosteroids for 6 months do not experience any additional benefit over those who receive corticosteroids alone. Whether other protocols for salvage therapy, such as a year of oral cyclophosphamide or chlorambucil, produce improved results is still under study.

Alkylating therapy and corticosteroid treatment should be reserved for patients who have a poor overall prognosis. In young women who have membranous glomerulopathy and a minimal amount of proteinuria, general supportive care may be the best approach.

Supportive care is essential in the treatment of all patients with glomerular disease, including membranous glomerulopa-

TABLE 164.3.	COMPLICATIONS OF IMMUNOSUPPRESSIVE THERAPY		
Corticosteroids	**Cyclophosphamide**	**Plasmapheresis**	
Infections	Infections	**Immediate**	
Fluid and electrolyte disturbances	Hemorrhagic cystitis	Hypotension	
Sodium retention	Mutagenesis	Hypocalcemia	
Fluid retention	Impairment of fertility	Disequilibrium syndrome (hypotension,	
Potassium loss	Nausea and vomiting	sweating, pallor, nausea-vasovagal	
Hypertension	Leukopenia	reaction)	
Musculoskeletal	Interstitial pulmonary fibrosis	Vascular access problems	
Steroid myopathy	Alopecia	Hypothermia	
Osteoporosis		Allergic reactions to soluble proteins	
Aseptic necrosis of femoral and humeral heads		and fresh frozen plasma	
Gastrointestinal		Prolonged clotting times	
Peptic ulcer		Thrombocytopenia	
Pancreatitis		Cardiac arrhythmia	
Dermatologic		Dyspnea	
Impaired wound healing		Convulsions	
Petechiae and ecchymoses		**Long-term**	
Endocrine		Infections	
Development of cushingoid state		Vascular thrombosis and sclerosis	
Adrenocortical and pituitary unresponsiveness			
Diabetes mellitus			
Ophthalmic			
Posterior subscapular cataracts			
Glaucoma			

thy. Hypertension must be controlled, hyperlipidemia treated, and volume removed as needed. Substantial support has been garnered for the use of ACE inhibitors in patients with proteinuria with or without mild to moderate renal insufficiency. These agents decrease the amount of proteinuria and retard the progression of renal insufficiency. Whether the angiotensin II receptor antagonists have a similar salutary role is not certain.

MINIMAL CHANGE DISEASE

Minimal change glomerulopathy is characterized by the lack of alterations in glomerular architecture seen on light microscopy. Immunofluorescence microscopy shows an absence of immunoglobulin and complement deposition or only mild mesangial IgM or C3. On electron microscopy, characteristic fusion of epithelial foot processes is observed without immune complex–type electron-dense deposits. In most cases, children are treated with a course of corticosteroids before renal biopsy. Renal biopsy is reserved for children who prove to be corticosteroid-resistant or those in whom a complicated clinical presentation or course of disease requires histopathologic identification. A renal biopsy is performed in the initial management of minimal change glomerulopathy in adults with the nephrotic syndrome.

Corticosteroids are the mainstay of therapy for minimal change disease. No other cause of the nephrotic syndrome is as sensitive to treatment with prednisone. Disappearance of proteinuria is rapid, especially in children, who usually respond within 4 to 6 weeks. Adults with minimal change disease usually are sensitive to prednisone therapy, but may require up to 16 weeks of daily corticosteroids to induce remission. The response

to treatment is heralded by diuresis and decrement in proteinuria. The usual starting dosage of prednisone is 2 mg per kilogram body weight per day not to exceed 60 mg per day. A response rate of 80% to 90% has been documented in both children and adults.

One of the most useful ways of monitoring patients is to teach them to perform dipstick analysis of their own urine. Daily dipstick analysis allows precise documentation of the onset of protein-free urine—at which point prednisone therapy should be tapered, usually over the course of 3 to 4 weeks.

Several patterns of response to corticosteroid therapy have been observed (Table 164.4). Patients with frequently relapsing or corticosteroid-dependent minimal change disease pose some of the most difficult treatment dilemmas. Sudden massive nephrosis results in morbid complications and requires urgent attention. Bursts of high-dose corticosteroid therapy, even of relatively short duration, result in large cumulative doses in patients who relapse more than four times per year. In these persons, remission may be maintained on long-term, low-dose corticosteroid therapy. In others, cyclophosphamide has proved effective. Prednisone is used to induce remission, then cyclophosphamide is added (2 mg per kilogram per day) for 8 to 12 weeks. Long-term remission has been reported in 40% to 50% of patients. Cyclophosphamide often is useful in patients who are corticosteroid-dependent and occasionally in patients who are resistant to corticosteroid therapy.

In some patients who are corticosteroid-resistant, a second renal biopsy must be considered. In these, a diagnosis of FSGS may have been missed in the original biopsy. FSGS is a focal lesion. It involves only a few glomeruli at the outset of the dis-

TABLE 164.4.	PATTERNS OF STEROID RESPONSE IN MINIMAL CHANGE DISEASE

Steroid-Responsive

Complete remission of proteinuria with infrequent relapses

Frequently Relapsing

Relapses more than 4 times per 12 months

Steroid-Dependent

Relapses during the taper of steroids
Relapses within 2 weeks of cessation of therapy

Steroid-Resistant

Failure to obtain complete remission within 12 to 16 weeks

(Adapted from Siegel NJ. Minimal change nephropathy. In: Greenberg A, ed. *Primer of kidney diseases.* San Diego: Academic Press, 1994:69.)

TABLE 164.5.	CAUSES OF FOCAL SEGMENTAL GLOMERULOSCLEROSIS

Focal Segmental Glomerulosclerosis (The Clinicopathologic Syndrome)

Primary (idiopathic)
  With glomerulopathy
  Without glomerulopathy
Secondary
  With glomerulopathy
    Morbid obesity
    Sickle cell disease
    Cyanotic congenital heart disease
    Reduced renal functional mass
      Unilateral renal agenesis
      Oligomeganephronia
      Reflux/interstitial nephropathy
      Focal cortical necrosis
      Nephrectomy

Glomerular Tip Lesion

With foot process effacement only
With other glomerulopathy (e.g., FSGS, membranous)

Focal Glomerulosclerosis with Epithelial Changes

HIV-associated nephropathy
IV drug abuse nephropathy
Collapsing glomerulopathy

FSGS, focal segmental glomerulosclerosis; HIV, human immunodeficiency virus; IV, intravenous.

ease. The biopsy sample may miss one of the involved glomeruli, and a diagnosis of minimal change disease may be rendered. Because patients with FSGS do not usually respond to corticosteroid therapy, the clinician may wonder whether the patient has corticosteroid-resistant minimal change disease. A second renal biopsy will change the therapeutic strategy.

FOCAL SEGMENTAL GLOMERULOSCLEROSIS

FSGS is a glomerular lesion that can be idiopathic or result from many recognized causes (Table 164.5). The disease is more common in African Americans than in whites. The pathologic diagnosis depends on the identification in some glomeruli (focal) of areas of glomerular sclerosis in only parts of the glomerular tuft (segmental). The remainder of the glomerulus is not affected, although some degree of foot process effacement usually is observed on electron microscopy.

Several patterns of idiopathic FSGS have been described, but there is controversy over whether they represent significantly different diseases or simply different morphologic variants of little clinical significance. One of these idiopathic conditions, called the *collapsing variant of FSGS,* is more common in African Americans and results in a much more rapid decline in renal function than do other forms of FSGS. Collapsing FSGS is associated with a substantial increase in the amount of protein excretion. Another variant, called the *glomerular tip lesion variant of FSGS,* is characterized by cytoplasmic vacuolation, sclerosis, and hyalinosis in the portion of the glomerulus that is opposite the hilus and adjacent to the origin of the proximal tubule. This lesion is more common in older whites and may be more responsive to corticosteroid therapy. These patterns of FSGS with differing natural histories can be discovered only by renal biopsy.

A biopsy also may provide clues to secondary forms of FSGS. For example, in human immunodeficiency virus (HIV) nephropathy, a collapsing form of FSGS is found by light microscopy that differs from idiopathic collapsing glomerulopathy because of the presence in HIV-affected patients of numerous tubuloreticular inclusions in endothelial cells that can be identified by electron microscopy. Enlarged glomeruli associated with FSGS may suggest morbid obesity or a condition in which there is decreased oxygenation (sickle cell anemia or congenital cyanotic heart disease) or reduced functional renal mass (unilateral renal agenesis or aplasia).

Therapy for FSGS is controversial. Only one controlled trial has been performed, and it indicated the ineffectiveness of immunosuppressive therapy in children. Unfortunately, only a few patients experience spontaneous remission. In general, patients with FSGS and the nephrotic syndrome progress to end-stage renal disease. Patients with spontaneous remission of nephrosis, those with less than 3 g of proteinuria, and those who experience remission with therapy tend to have a better course. Only 10% to 30% of patients respond to corticosteroids with complete remission of proteinuria. The relapse rate after treatment is high. Reports suggest that up to 50% of patients respond to long courses of oral corticosteroids (i.e., between 4 and 5 months of daily therapy). In view of the common occurrence of corticosteroid resistance in patients with FSGS, several trials have evaluated therapy with low-dose cyclosporin A (4 to 6 mg per kilogram per day) for 2 to 6 months. Although patients do respond to this treatment, most experience a relapse when therapy is stopped. The hazard of interstitial fibrosis associated with long-term cyclosporin A therapy decreases the usefulness of this approach.

Except for administering ACE inhibitors, most clinicians do

not treat patients with FSGS who have less than nephrotic-range proteinuria. In patients with substantial nephrotic syndrome, a trial of corticosteroid therapy may be considered. If remission is not induced after 4 to 5 months, this form of therapy should be discontinued.

The collapsing variant of FSGS and the glomerular tip lesion variant of FSGS may require different forms of therapy. Collapsing FSGS without evidence of HIV disease has a strong predilection for African Americans and is associated with massive proteinuria and rapid progression to renal insufficiency. Many of these patients have extrarenal signs of a systemic illness that appears viral in nature. Anecdotal experience with corticosteroids in this population indicates that they are ineffective and may be contraindicated. In contrast, older whites with glomerular tip lesions discovered on renal biopsy may respond to corticosteroid therapy. Patients with FSGS secondary to a process such as sickle cell disease or obesity typically have less proteinuria (less than 3 g per day). In this population, therapy with ACE inhibitors may reduce proteinuria substantially. Whether it will result in long-term preservation of renal function is a matter of ongoing investigation.

RENAL DISEASE AND DYSPROTEINEMIA

Dysproteinemia, or paraproteinemia, encompasses a group of disorders characterized by the overproduction of immunoglobulin proteins or their components, which result in tissue damage (Chapter 154). The most common renal manifestation of glomerular involvement by dysproteinemia is proteinuria, often in the nephrotic range. Some patients with glomerular injury caused by immunoglobulin paraproteins have overt multiple myeloma, whereas others have dysproteinemia without other evidence of myeloma. Still others have no evidence of a paraprotein dyscrasia except for the abnormal glomerular deposits.

Sometimes, dipstick methods detect little proteinuria, whereas 24-hour urine collection indicates substantial proteinuria. Dipsticks are designed to detect anionic proteins such as albumin. Immunoglobulin light chains are commonly cationic and therefore are not detectable on dipsticks. In patients older than 60 years with renal insufficiency and mild proteinuria by dipstick analysis but with substantial proteinuria by sulfosalicylic acid analysis, renal biopsy is warranted. In such patients, immunoglobulin deposition diseases are found. These diseases include light-chain deposition disease, heavy-chain deposition disease, AL amyloidosis, and immunotactoid glomerulopathy. The renal biopsy is critical in determining the nature of the renal disease that is caused by immunoglobulin dysproteinemia. For example, amyloidosis is characterized by the deposition of fibrillar proteins and characteristic β-pleated sheet configurations. AL amyloidosis (primary) is caused by a plasma cell dyscrasia, whereas AA amyloidosis (secondary) is associated with high levels of nonimmunoglobulin serum amyloid protein (SAA).

Multiple myeloma often causes the overproduction of immunoglobulins or immunoglobulin fragments. Many lesions can be found on renal biopsy specimens from patients with multiple myeloma. Cast nephropathy is characterized by numerous para-

protein-containing casts in tubular lumina and usually manifests as acute renal failure. Light-chain deposition disease is the result of overproduction of a monoclonal immunoglobulin light chain. On deposition, these proteins do not form β-pleated sheets and do not stain with Congo red. Whereas AL amyloidosis usually is caused by lambda light chains, light chain deposition disease usually is caused by kappa light chains.

The treatment of paraproteinemia varies according to the biopsy findings. There is no specific therapy for AL amyloidosis. Chemotherapy and colchicine have been tried with varying degrees of success. The usefulness of ablative chemotherapy with stem cell transplantation is under investigation. In contrast, therapy for multiple myeloma and light-chain deposition disease initially is aimed at improving urine flow and decreasing the production of immunoglobulins with corticosteroids and chemotherapy. Plasma exchange, when added to chemotherapy, lowers myeloma protein levels more rapidly and may improve renal function. Patient survival has been better with plasmapheresis. Treatment with chemotherapy for light-chain deposition disease is similar to that for myeloma; however, long-term survival is poor.

TREATMENT OF NEPHRITIS

Glomerular inflammation (glomerulonephritis) often manifests clinically as acute, rapidly progressive, or chronic nephritis. In general, the aggressiveness of treatment is tailored to the aggressiveness of the glomerulonephritis. Renal biopsy evaluation is important for identifying the type of lesion that is causing the nephritis and for determining the activity and chronicity of the process, which influence the prognosis and treatment.

The treatment of glomerulonephritis usually involves the use of anti-inflammatory drugs such as corticosteroids, and alkylating agents such as cyclophosphamide, chlorambucil, or azathioprine. In patients who have pulmonary hemorrhage with the pulmonary renal vasculitic syndrome, plasma exchange is useful. In the following sections, we review each of these forms of treatment.

PREDNISONE

Therapy with prednisone remains as much an art as a science in that there is no appropriate means of assessing the pharmacokinetics of this drug. First, the dosage must be tailored to the individual patient, based on body weight or surface area and response to therapy. Second, the amount of corticosteroid used depends on the disease being treated. For example, the treatment of minimal change disease may require considerably less total prednisone than the treatment of lupus nephritis or systemic vasculitis. In rapidly progressive glomerulonephritis, much higher dosages of corticosteroids usually are required for longer periods. Patients are treated with 1 mg per kilogram of prednisone for 1 to 2 months; then the dosage is tapered during months 2, 3, and 4. Tapering schedules usually involve changing to alternate-day therapy, so that a patient receiving 60 mg of prednisone every day starts taking 60 mg on 1 day and 50 mg the next day. Each week, the alternate-day prednisone is reduced by

10 mg, so that within 4 to 6 weeks, the patient is not taking any prednisone on alternate days. The dosage then can be tapered by 10 mg per day for the next 6 weeks. If this protocol is followed, the patient is no longer receiving prednisone therapy by the end of the fourth month. Switching to alternate-day prednisone therapy at the beginning of the second month of treatment takes advantage of the reduced side effects associated with this approach.

For most glomerular diseases, prednisone tapering continues until the drug is discontinued altogether. There are exceptions to this approach. For example, in patients with lupus nephritis, the prednisone should not be discontinued altogether. Most patients with lupus nephritis require a dosage between 10 and 15 mg per day with slow tapering to prevent extrarenal lupus flares.

Intravenous methylprednisolone is warranted in at least two circumstances. First, oral corticosteroids are not effectively absorbed by the edematous bowel wall in patients with massive nephrosis, and intravenous methylprednisolone should be considered at a dosage equivalent to that of oral prednisone. Second, intravenous methylprednisolone should be used in patients who have rapidly progressive glomerulonephritis with crescentic disease. Pulse methylprednisolone is administered at a dose of 7 mg per kilogram, with a maximum dose of 1 g per day over 3 days or, alternatively, every other day for 6 days. The rationale for using pulse methylprednisolone stems from its rapid obliteration of inflammation and edema in areas of reduced blood flow. This form of therapy has never been subject to a large-scale trial. Pulse methylprednisolone has been used in diseases other than crescentic glomerulonephritis. For example, in the regimen for membranous nephritis, pulse methylprednisolone is given on alternate months, cycling with chlorambucil (see Membranous Glomerulopathy).

Complications of corticosteroid therapy are numerous (Table 164.3) and include life-threatening infections with bacteria, viruses, and unusual, opportunistic agents such as mycobacteria, *Pneumocystis carinii,* and fungi. The likelihood of infection increases with the duration of treatment. Patients following protocols using an alternate-day schedule have fewer associated side effects than those using daily high-dose (1 mg per kilogram) treatment. Divided daily doses of prednisone (e.g., two or three times a day) have the strongest anti-inflammatory action, but also the most side effects. The musculoskeletal complications of corticosteroid therapy are significant. Osteoporosis is accelerated, which commonly results in vertebral collapse. The most dreaded complication of long-term corticosteroid therapy, however, is aseptic necrosis of the femoral head. This crippling process requires joint replacement. Other complications of corticosteroid therapy include the development of diabetes mellitus, posterior subcapsular cataracts, glaucoma, gastritis, and pancreatitis.

CYCLOPHOSPHAMIDE AND CHLORAMBUCIL

Cyclophosphamide and chlorambucil are alkylating agents. Cyclophosphamide is converted in the liver to an active metabolite. Both drugs cross-link the nucleic acid that interferes with cell division and transcription. The usual oral dosage used for the treatment of glomerular disease reduces the leukocyte count to

about 3,000 cells per microliter. At this dosage, the immune response to newly presented antigens is suppressed, although the cutaneous inflammatory response is unchanged.

Cyclophosphamide is administered orally or intravenously. Oral cyclophosphamide typically is given at a dosage of 2 mg per kilogram per day. Although the starting dosage may be prescribed, the maintenance dosage must be adjusted constantly based on the total leukocyte count. Cyclophosphamide therapy is targeted to lower the leukocyte count to between 3,000 and 5,000 cells per microliter. The dosage must be decreased continually to prevent leukopenia and, especially, neutropenia. The efficacy of cyclophosphamide may be limited by its toxicity.

Monthly intravenous administration of cyclophosphamide at a starting dosage of 0.5 g per square meter of body surface has been popularized for the treatment of lupus nephritis. This therapy has been used in other diseases, especially systemic ANCA vasculitis. The prescription is altered on the basis of the 2-week leukocyte nadir. During the second month of therapy, the dosage is increased to 0.75 g per square meter, and if the 2-week leukocyte nadir is greater than 5,000 cells per microliter, a final dosage of 1 g per square meter is used in subsequent months. Therapy is typically discontinued after 6 months. The advantages of intravenous cyclophosphamide include the certainty of drug administration, smaller total drug dose (about one third to one half the equivalent monthly dose of oral cyclophosphamide), and reduced incidence of infection and hemorrhagic cystitis.

The dreaded complications of cyclophosphamide therapy are life-threatening infections and hemorrhagic cystitis (Table 164.3). Hemorrhagic cystitis is observed primarily with oral cyclophosphamide. Adequate hydration and the use of intravenous cyclophosphamide have decreased its incidence substantially. The risk of ovarian and testicular failure is associated with the use of any alkylating drug. Because the incidence of ovarian failure increases with age, perimenopausal women or those older than 35 years are most likely to be affected. The potential for decreasing the rate of ovarian and testicular failure with agents such as leuprolide acetate is under investigation. Mutagenesis is one of the most serious complications of cyclophosphamide therapy. Long-term treatment of Wegener's granulomatosis with oral cyclophosphamide is associated with a nearly 15% incidence of transitional cell carcinoma of the bladder. Whether this will occur with intravenous cyclophosphamide is not clear. Lymphoproliferative diseases occur at a rate at least 2.4 times above normal in patients taking cyclophosphamide. These long-term risks must be considered when therapy is initiated. A renal biopsy that identifies a lesion responsive to alkylating therapy provides the rationale for the use of this drug.

Chlorambucil usually is given at a dosage of 0.1 to 0.2 mg per kilogram per day. It is slower acting than cyclophosphamide and takes longer to produce myelosuppression. Like cyclophosphamide, chlorambucil induces life-threatening infections and malignant tumors. The unusual side effects of chlorambucil are pulmonary fibrosis, hepatic toxicity, and seizures.

AZATHIOPRINE

Azathioprine has been used to treat renal allografts for decades. It is an analogue of the purine-based hypoxanthine. Metabolites of azathioprine inhibit enzymes required for DNA synthesis. Azathioprine typically is used to treat aggressive glomerular diseases (lupus nephritis) or relapsing systemic vasculitis at a starting dosage of 1 to 3 mg per kilogram. Careful attention must be paid to leukopenia, especially in the setting of renal insufficiency. The leukocyte count should remain above 5,000 cells per microliter. Pancreatitis is an uncommon but concerning complication of therapy. Abdominal discomfort must be evaluated with serum amylase and lipase tests and careful history and physical examination. In the setting of allopurinol therapy or renal insufficiency that reduces clearance of the active drug, the major side effect is bone marrow suppression. Because this suppression primarily takes the form of neutropenia, infection is a major side effect. Azathioprine also carries a mutagenic potential, with some form of tumor (primarily dermal carcinomas) developing in up to 5% of transplant recipients.

CYCLOSPORIN A

The use of cyclosporin A in glomerular disease is an experimental therapy. Cyclosporin A is reserved for conditions in which other forms of anti-inflammatory or immunosuppressive therapy have failed. It is useful in patients with corticosteroid-resistant minimal change disease and massive nephrosis, in some patients with nephrosis and FSGS or membranous nephropathy who have not responded to other forms of therapy. The starting dosage is 5 mg per kilogram per day. Cyclosporin A levels must be measured regularly and the dosage titrated based on the serum creatinine level. Like other immunosuppressive drugs, cyclosporin A is associated with life-threatening infections. The major long-term complication of cyclosporin A therapy for glomerular disease is interstitial fibrosis resulting from chronic cyclosporin A toxicity. Cyclosporin A causes chronic, irreversible renal dysfunction and should be used for no more than a year.

PLASMAPHERESIS

Plasmapheresis is used in the treatment of pulmonary hemorrhage with anti-GBM disease, pulmonary hemorrhage with ANCA-associated systemic vasculitis, and thrombotic thrombocytopenic purpura. It usually is prescribed as one or two volume exchanges given daily for the first 5 days, then on alternate days for a total of 14 days. The efficacy of plasma exchange can be documented by the decrease in anti-GBM or ANCA titers during the course of therapy. The primary complications of plasma exchange occur immediately and are associated with hypocalcemia and allergic reactions. Albumin replacement is useful in the setting of anti-GBM disease. For the treatment of thrombotic microangiopathy, fresh frozen plasma or cryoprecipitate has been suggested. Allergic reactions to these proteins are more common. Long-term complications usually are associated with vascular thrombosis and sclerosis as a consequence of venous access.

■ RENAL BIOPSY AND THE TREATMENT OF SPECIFIC FORMS OF NEPHRITIS

POSTINFECTIOUS GLOMERULONEPHRITIS

Postinfectious glomerulonephritis is an episodic form of glomerulonephritis, especially poststreptococcal glomerulonephritis.

TABLE 164.6.	**CAUSES OF POSTINFECTIOUS GLOMERULONEPHRITIS**

Bacterial

β-hemolytic streptococci
Diplococcus pneumoniae
Staphylococcus aureus
Staphylococcus epidermidis
Leptospirosis

Viral

Hepatitis B
Hepatitis C
Cytomegalovirus
Varicella
Enteroviral infection

Parasites

Malaria
Toxoplasmosis
Schistosomiasis
Treponemiasis
Filariasis

Many infectious agents are associated with acute immune complex glomerulonephritis (Table 164.6).

The common clinical manifestations of acute poststreptococcal glomerulonephritis are hematuria, edema, hypertension, oliguria, and pulmonary congestion manifested by dyspnea and cough. Other systemic features are fever, nausea, and abdominal pain, with occasional central nervous system confusion, headache, somnolence, and, rarely, convulsions. A renal biopsy usually is not performed in patients with typical poststreptococcal glomerulonephritis because the diagnosis is apparent from clinical and laboratory data. Most renal biopsies that demonstrate postinfectious glomerulonephritis are performed in the setting of acute renal failure of uncertain cause that has not recovered in more than 3 to 4 weeks. In this setting, the diagnosis usually comes as a surprise.

In acute poststreptococcal glomerulonephritis, diffuse proliferation of endothelial and mesangial cells is found in association with infiltrates of leukocytes, especially numerous neutrophils. Rarely, there is crescent formation. The finding of more than 30% crescents by light microscopy portends a poor long-term prognosis. During the acute phase, immunohistology usually demonstrates coarsely granular capillary wall and mesangial staining for complement, with or without IgG. The finding of humplike subepithelial electron-dense deposits by electron microscopy is characteristic of this disease, although mesangial and small subendothelial deposits also are present and may be more important in the cause of glomerular inflammation.

The course of poststreptococcal glomerulonephritis usually is self-limited, and hematuria disappears within 6 months in most patients. Proteinuria resolves in one third of patients by 1 year and in two thirds by 2 years. The prognosis is less favorable in adults than in children. The development of crescentic glomerulonephritis appears to be more common in adults and may portend progression to end-stage renal disease. Nonetheless, long-term follow-up of adult patients for as long as 20 years indicates that recovery usually is complete. Therapy for poststreptococcal glomerulonephritis is largely symptomatic, aimed at treating hypertension and fluid overload with diuretics and dialysis as needed. Antibiotic therapy has no influence on the course of the disease.

In contrast to the treatment of postinfectious glomerulonephritis, antibiotics are the mainstay of therapy for subacute subendocardial bacterial endocarditis with associated glomerulonephritis. Endocarditis-induced glomerulonephritis has a variable pathologic and clinical expression. The course of the glomerulonephritis parallels that of the infective endocarditis. Active acute endocarditis usually causes an acute diffuse proliferative glomerulonephritis with numerous neutrophils that can be pathologically identical with the acute poststreptococcal glomerulonephritis caused by pharyngitis. More indolent (subacute) endocarditis usually causes a membranoproliferative (type I) or proliferative glomerulonephritis.

Therapy must be directed at eradication of the infection with bactericidal antibiotics. In patients with only mild to moderate renal insufficiency (a serum creatinine less than 3 mg per deciliter), antibiotic therapy usually results in the recovery of renal function and amelioration of glomerular inflammation. In patients with substantial renal failure associated with endocarditis, several forms of therapy have been suggested, including pulse methylprednisolone, plasma exchange, and even the use of immunosuppressive agents such as cyclophosphamide. These reports are only anecdotal. Because there may be a considerable delay from the initiation of antibiotic therapy and the recovery of renal function, it appears counterintuitive to use immunosuppressive therapy in the setting of severe endocarditis.

MEMBRANOPROLIFERATIVE GLOMERULONEPHRITIS AND CRYOGLOBULINEMIA

Membranoproliferative glomerulonephritis is a relatively uncommon form of glomerular injury. There are three types of membranoproliferative glomerulonephritis. Type I is the most common and has been associated with mixed essential cryoglobulinemia with hepatitis C virus infection. This association may have important therapeutic implications. An increasing number of reports suggest that long-term antiviral therapy with interferon-α and other agents have a beneficial effect in patients with membranoproliferative glomerulonephritis type I and mixed cryoglobulinemia. In a large prospective trial of 53 patients with serologic evidence for hepatitis C and cryoglobulinemia who were randomly assigned to interferon-α or conventional therapy, 60% of patients treated with antiviral therapy demonstrated improvement in cryoglobulin titers, plasma creatinine concentrations, and even cutaneous vasculitis. With cessation of therapy, a relapse in cryoglobulinemia was evident. Many patients with membranoproliferative glomerulonephritis do not have cryoglobulinemia or hepatitis C. Some of these patients have lymphoproliferative disease, but most appear to have an idiopathic condition. In general, one third of these patients has a spontaneous remission, one third has an indolent course, and one third will develop end-stage renal disease. As of yet, there is no useful treatment option.

HENOCH–SCHÖNLEIN PURPURA

Henoch–Schönlein purpura is a systemic disease, usually of children and adolescents, characterized by glomerulonephritis, a purpuric rash, arthritis, and gastrointestinal bleeding. Transient episodes of asymptomatic hematuria and proteinuria accompany self-limited cases of Henoch–Schönlein purpura. The pattern of this renal–dermal syndrome mimics that of systemic vasculitides, including microscopic polyangiitis (see ANCA-Associated Glomerulonephritis and Systemic Vasculitis). A renal biopsy is useful to determine whether the disease process is Henoch–Schönlein purpura characterized by IgA deposition in the kidney. Henoch–Schönlein purpura typically is associated with a focal or diffuse proliferative glomerulonephritis, although a crescentic form of glomerulonephritis can occur and usually portends an unfavorable prognosis. Anti-inflammatory and immunosuppressive therapy usually is not warranted in Henoch–Schönlein nephritis unless there is severe proliferative disease and crescents. In such cases, therapy with pulse methylprednisolone, prednisone, and cytotoxic drugs may prove useful.

▪ RENAL BIOPSY AND THE TREATMENT OF LUPUS NEPHRITIS

Renal biopsy rarely is necessary for the diagnosis of lupus nephritis, particularly in patients with long-standing extrarenal systemic lupus erythematosus. It may be useful in patients with new onset of systemic inflammatory diseases who have positive antinuclear antibodies but no other manifestations of systemic lupus erythematosus. In this setting, a renal biopsy may provide a diagnosis of lupus nephritis or indicate a completely different diagnosis. Another benefit of a renal biopsy in lupus is the information a biopsy specimen provides regarding the form of lupus nephritis and its level of activity. The World Health Organization has categorized lupus nephritis into five general subsets: class I with no abnormalities; class II with mild mesangial proliferation or mesangial immune deposits; class III with focal and segmental proliferative glomerular injury; class IV with diffuse proliferative glomerulonephritis; and class V with membranous glomerulonephritis. Patients with class I and II lesions have a better prognosis than do patients with class III and IV lesions. Patients with membranous lupus (class V) without proliferative changes have excellent long-term renal survival. Renal biopsy also is used by some pathologists to calculate a disease activity and chronicity score. The usefulness of these scores is controversial. The chronicity score has proved to be more useful than the activity score in assessing long-term renal prognosis (Table 164.7).

The clinical manifestations of lupus nephritis are variable and include mild asymptomatic hematuria, acute nephritis, rapidly progressive nephritis, and chronic nephritis leading to end-stage renal disease (see Chapter 178). These patterns of injury are typical of any process in which there is a proliferative glomerulonephritis (Fig. 164.4). The heterogeneity of the clinical and pathologic course in this condition makes therapy more difficult and has caused significant controversy.

What are the indications for therapy? Patients who have acute nephritis or rapidly progressive glomerulonephritis and who have a diffuse proliferative glomerulonephritis with or without

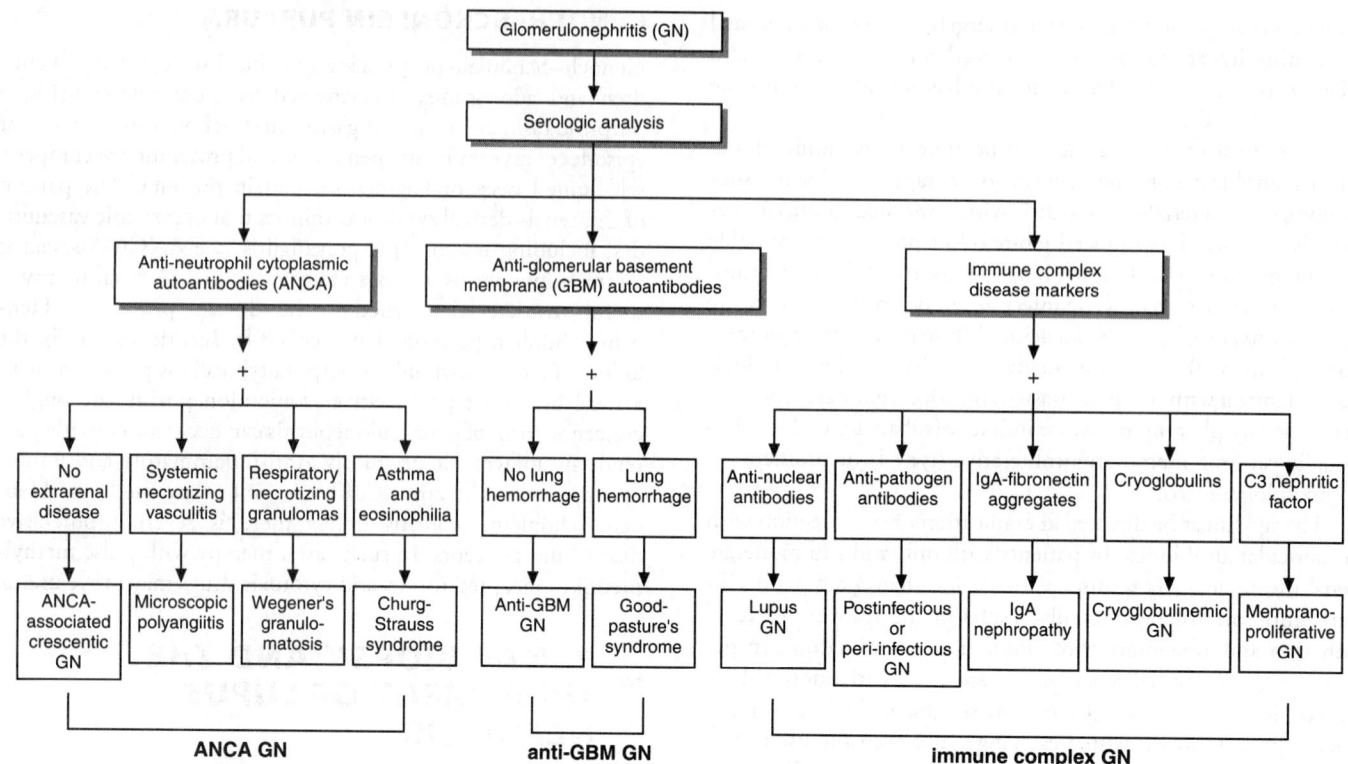

FIGURE 164.4. Diagram depicting the serologic analysis of patients with glomerulonephritis. *ANCA*, anti-neutrophil cytoplasmic antibodies; *GN*, glomerulonephritis; *GBM*, glomerular basement membrane. (Modified from Jennette JC, Falk RJ. Diagnosis and management of glomerulonephritis and vasculitis presenting as acute renal failure. *Med Clin North Am* 1990:893.)

EVIDENCE LEVEL: C. Expert Opinion.

necrosis and crescent formation on biopsy should be treated. In general, treatment is initiated with intravenous methylprednisolone (7 to 15 mg per kilogram per day). A reasonable approach to combined cytotoxic and corticosteroid therapy in acute disease is outlined in Table 164.8. Nearly all such patients receive cytotoxic drugs in combination with oral corticosteroids. In patients

with severe lupus nephritis, the 5-year renal survival rate is 70% to 80% for those with glucocorticoid treatment alone compared with 30% for those without therapy. This improved survival is attributable to many factors, including earlier diagnosis based on serologic findings, more careful and rational use of glucocorticoid therapy, substitution of antimalarial drugs, and aggressive control of hypertension. The additive effects of cyclophosphamide or cyclophosphamide plus azathioprine have improved appreciably the long-term survival of patients with aggressive lupus nephritis. These agents have significant side effects, however, including life-threatening infection, neoplasia (especially transitional cell carcinoma of the bladder and lymphoproliferative disorders), gonadal failure, and hemorrhagic cystitis (Table 164.4).

Transformation from one morphologic class of lupus nephritis to another (i.e., from milder focal proliferative glomerular disease [class III] to more aggressive diffuse proliferative glomerulonephritis [class IV]) is a well-established phenomenon. Glucocorticoid therapy may transform an aggressive proliferative glomerulonephritis into a pattern of membranous nephropathy. Transformation from one histologic class to another occurs in up to 30% of cases.

Systemic lupus erythematosus is subject to frequent relapses that are extrarenal in manifestation and recurrence of glomerular inflammation. Unless the urinary sediment is typical of a proliferative process, serum complement studies such as the C3 and CH50 decline, and double-stranded DNA titers rebound, a renal

TABLE 164.7.	LUPUS NEPHRITIS INDICES OF ACTIVITY AND CHRONICITY
Activity[a]	**Chronicity**[a]
Glomeruli	Glomerulosclerosis
Hypercellularity	Fibrous crescents
Fibrinoid necrosis/karyorrhexis[b]	Interstitial fibrosis
Cellular crescents[b]	Tubular atrophy
Hyaline thrombi	
Leukocyte infiltration	
Tubule/interstitium	
Mononuclear cell	
Infiltration	

[a] Score 0 to 3 for each item.
[b] Multiply score by 2.
(Modified from Austin HA, Muenz LR, Joyce KM, et al. Prognostic factors in lupus nephritis: contribution of renal histological data. *Am J Med* 1982;75:382.)

TABLE 164.8. COMBINED PREDNISONE AND INTRAVENOUS CYCLOPHOSPHAMIDE TREATMENT PROTOCOL

1. Administer pulse methylprednisolone 7 mg/kg (to a maximum single dose of 1 g) IV over 20 minutes for 3 consecutive days.
2. Within 48 hours after initiation of final dose of pulse therapy, begin oral prednisone, 1 mg/kg/d (not to exceed 80 mg per single dose) for 4 weeks.
3. Within 1 week after start of pulse methylprednisolone therapy, begin giving monthly IV cyclophosphamide (Cytoxan) for 6 total monthly doses as follows:
   a. IV Cytoxan is given at an initial dosage of 0.5 g/m² (range 0.5–1.0 g/m²) to induce a leukocyte nadir no lower than 3,000 cells/mm³.
   b. Each infusion is administered over a period of 1 hour and preceded and accompanied by frequent voiding of dilute urine for 24 hours after drug administration.
   c. After 4 to 6 weeks, the dosage of oral prednisone should be decreased to 0.5 mg/kg/d for 1 month, then tapered over the next 4 to 6 weeks.

(Adapted from Falk RJ, Jennette JC. Systemic vasculitis. In: Glassock RJ, ed. *Current therapy in nephrology and hypertension*, third ed. St. Louis: Mosby-Year Book, 1992:171.)

biopsy may be considered to restage the lesion and determine whether a relapse of proliferative glomerulonephritis has occurred. From a clinical perspective, it is not always clear whether the transformation and subsequent rise in creatinine level are consequences of relapsing active disease or progressive scarring. Enthusiasm for treating a patient a second time may be tempered by a biopsy specimen that shows globally sclerotic glomeruli with little potential for preserving renal function.

Patients with advanced renal failure and severe chronic changes in lupus nephritis should not be treated further. These patients must be prepared for dialysis or transplantation because continued aggressive immunosuppressive therapy will result in life-threatening complications.

Patients who have membranous lupus nephritis with little proliferative change or chronicity have an excellent long-term prognosis and should be treated conservatively. Although some of these patients respond to corticosteroid therapy with a decrement in proteinuria, most do not. Antimalarial drugs such as hydroxychloroquine (Plaquenil) may be effective in controlling extrarenal manifestations of the disease in patients who have mild symptoms. In such patients, cyclophosphamide is considered primarily for extrarenal manifestations of the disease.

RENAL BIOPSY AND THERAPY IN RAPIDLY PROGRESSIVE GLOMERULONEPHRITIS

USEFULNESS OF SEROLOGIC TESTING IN RAPIDLY PROGRESSIVE GLOMERULONEPHRITIS

Three major types of crescentic glomerulonephritis cause the clinical syndrome of rapidly progressive glomerulonephritis.

These can be divided on the basis of renal biopsy findings into immune complex–mediated glomerulonephritis (e.g., lupus nephritis); anti-GBM–mediated glomerulonephritis, including Goodpasture's syndrome; and pauci-immune glomerulonephritis, which usually is associated with ANCA and frequently is a component of a systemic small vessel vasculitis. Serologic studies are useful in differentiating these diseases (Fig. 164.4). In patients with immune complex glomerulonephritis, there may be evidence of antinuclear antibodies, anti–double-stranded DNA antibodies suggestive of lupus nephritis, or cryoglobulins indicative of cryoglobulinemia or antistreptococcal antibodies such as anti-streptolysin O (ASO) or anti-DNase antibodies. The presence in renal biopsy specimens of linear staining for IgG along GBM is strong evidence for anti-GBM glomerulonephritis, but serologic demonstration of anti-GBM antibodies is useful to confirm this diagnosis.

A close association exists between ANCA and pauci-immune necrotizing glomerulonephritis. This form of glomerulonephritis may occur as a process limited to the kidney or as part of a systemic small vessel vasculitis, such as Wegener's granulomatosis, microscopic polyangiitis, or Churg–Strauss syndrome. ANCA are found in 90% of patients with pauci-immune systemic necrotizing vasculitis. They are detected in serum by indirect immunofluorescence microscopy using alcohol-fixed normal human neutrophils as a substrate. Two patterns of neutrophil staining—perinuclear (P-ANCA) and cytoplasmic (C-ANCA)—discriminate between the two major subtypes of ANCA. The major antigen for P-ANCA is myeloperoxidase, which is located within the primary granule of normal human neutrophils and monocytes. Most C-ANCA are specific for a neutrophil and monocyte proteinase called proteinase 3.

ANTI–GLOMERULAR BASEMENT MEMBRANE DISEASE

Anti-GBM antibodies are found in patients with Goodpasture's syndrome and with anti-GBM antibody–mediated glomerulonephritis. Goodpasture's syndrome initially was defined as the coexistence of pulmonary hemorrhage and glomerulonephritis. This term now is reserved for the coexistence of pulmonary hemorrhage and glomerulonephritis mediated by anti-GBM antibodies. Renal biopsy reveals characteristic linear immunostaining of the GBM with anti-GBM antibodies associated with a necrotizing and crescentic glomerulonephritis. Many rapid immunoassays have been developed for the detection of anti-GBM antibodies because the major antigen, the noncollagenous NCI domain of type IV collagen, appears to be the major reactive moiety of anti-GBM autoantibodies.

Goodpasture's syndrome requires immediate and aggressive therapy. Patients with severe pulmonary hemorrhage need intensive care unit support. Initial therapy is with pulse methylprednisolone (7 to 15 mg per kilogram per day) for 3 days. Corticosteroid treatment is continued using prednisone (1 mg per kilogram of body weight). Plasma exchange is especially beneficial in patients with pulmonary hemorrhage. Total body plasma exchange should be performed daily for 5 days, then on alternate days for 2 weeks. The usual replacement fluid is 5% albumin or normal plasma. To prevent the rebound of autoantibodies after induction therapy is complete, immunosuppressive therapy with cyclophosphamide (2 mg per kilogram) is instituted. The starting dosage is adjusted according to the leukocyte nadir, and the response to therapy is monitored by measurement of anti-GBM titers. Patients with serum creatinine levels of less than 7 mg per deciliter or with fewer than 30% to 50% crescents are more likely to respond to this regimen than are patients with higher creatinine levels or widespread crescentic disease. The latter patients usually progress quickly to end-stage renal disease. Because of the need for rapid therapy, renal biopsy must be performed promptly. Induction therapy with Medrol and plasma exchange need to be instituted even before the biopsy data are available if the patient follows a typical course of rapidly progressive renal failure with pulmonary hemorrhage.

ANCA-ASSOCIATED GLOMERULONEPHRITIS AND SYSTEMIC VASCULITIS

The most common form of aggressive glomerulonephritis is pauci-immune necrotizing glomerulonephritis, which is associated with circulating ANCA in about 90% of patients. By immunohistologic techniques, there is no evidence for immune complex localization or direct antibody binding in the glomerulus. This lesion is associated with systemic vasculitides such as microscopic polyangiitis, Wegener's granulomatosis, and Churg–Strauss syndrome. Pauci-immune necrotizing glomerulonephritis also occurs as a renal-limited process.

Typically, patients with pauci-immune glomerulonephritis have rapidly progressive disease. However, some patients have milder disease with asymptomatic hematuria, and others have acute nephritis. Renal biopsy is essential for the diagnosis of these conditions. Focal necrotizing lesions may be present in few sampled glomeruli, or widespread crescentic disease may be found.

Many extrarenal manifestations of systemic vasculitis are apparent. Most patients have a flulike syndrome heralded by arthralgia and myalgia. The arthralgia typically is migratory, moving from joint to joint. More than 50% of these patients have a pulmonary–renal vasculitic syndrome characterized by pulmonary infiltrates or nodules and cavities. These patients usually have granulomatous inflammation indicative of Wegener's granulomatosis. One third of patients with microscopic polyangiitis or Wegener's granulomatosis have upper respiratory tract symptoms, including otitis media, necrotizing sinusitis, and nasal ulcerations. Gastrointestinal disease is manifest by nonhealing gastric ulcers and the catastrophic development of perforated abdominal viscus. Pancreatitis also may develop. It can be difficult to determine whether the pancreatitis is the consequence of vasculitis or corticosteroid/immunosuppressive therapy. Other extrarenal manifestations of vasculitis are iritis and uveitis and the neurologic deficit of mononeuritis multiplex.

These systemic vasculitides cause a renal–dermal syndrome. Palpable purpura, necrotizing ulcerative lesions, and even allergic reactions are observed in patients with ANCA-associated systemic vasculitis. The renal–dermal syndrome also is found in patients with cryoglobulinemia, Henoch–Schönlein purpura, and systemic lupus erythematosus. A renal biopsy is most useful in determining which of these conditions is present. For example, a biopsy is necessary to determine whether a patient with palpable purpura and hematuria has Henoch–Schönlein purpura or an ANCA-associated vasculitis and necrotizing glomerulonephritis. Patients with Henoch-Schönlein purpura usually are managed conservatively, whereas those with the renal–dermal vasculitic syndromes associated with lupus or ANCA must be managed with aggressive anti-inflammatory and immunosuppressive therapy.

Pulmonary–renal vasculitic syndromes are caused by ANCA-associated vascular inflammation, anti-GBM disease, and systemic lupus erythematosus. A renal biopsy must be performed in these conditions to prescribe appropriate therapy. These conditions require corticosteroid treatment and, if there is pulmonary hemorrhage, necessitates plasmapheresis in anti-GBM disease and ANCA-associated small vessel vasculitis.

Renal biopsy is useful in evaluating the long-term prognosis of patients with anti-GBM disease and ANCA-associated glomerulonephritis. In patients with Goodpasture's syndrome, a serum creatinine level higher than 7 mg per deciliter and widespread crescents on renal biopsy is associated with almost universal progression to end-stage renal disease and long-term dialysis. In contrast, ANCA-associated necrotizing glomerulonephritis and a creatinine level of 7 mg per deciliter may be associated with recovery of renal function and a prolonged dialysis-free interval. Given equally high initial serum creatinine levels, patients with ANCA-associated crescentic glomerulonephritis have a better prognosis than do those with anti-GBM disease.

High-dose corticosteroids (pulse methylprednisolone) and cytotoxic agents such as cyclophosphamide are used to control the major end-organ damage caused by systemic vasculitis and renal-limited pauci-immune necrotizing and crescentic glomerulonephritis (Table 164.8). Patients usually are treated with tapering dosages of corticosteroids over 3 months and with oral or intravenous cyclophosphamide. Substantial controversy has surrounded the optimal route of cyclophosphamide administration. Typically, patients with Wegener's granulomatosis have been treated with oral cyclophosphamide for 1 to 2 years. However, intravenous cyclophosphamide appears to be equally efficacious. In inducing a remission, oral cyclophosphamide may be a better modality to decrease the relapse rate. Oral cyclophosphamide is associated with a substantially higher rate of infection and other complications. Its use must be tempered by the consideration of the patient's risks and benefits. The optimal duration of therapy also is controversial. Patients with microscopic polyangiitis may require as little as 6 months of treatment, because 75% never have a relapse. Patients with Wegener's granulomatosis have been treated with intravenous cyclophosphamide with similar results. Because transitional cell carcinoma of the bladder develops in up to 15% of patients who undergo long-term treatment of Wegener's granulomatosis with oral cyclophosphamide, research is underway to determine the shortest effective duration of therapy in patients with systemic vasculitis. Plasmapheresis may be useful in the treatment of massive pulmonary hemorrhage associated with systemic vasculitis, but it has no other indications in this condition.

Up to 25% of patients with these systemic vasculitides have a relapse after the initial therapy is completed. Defining a relapse can be difficult. For example, a patient with a rise in creatinine

TABLE 164.9.	THROMBOTIC MICROANGIOPATHY

Hemolytic-uremic syndrome
Thrombotic thrombocytopenic purpura
Systemic sclerosis
Malignant hypertension
Eclampsia
Toxic drugs
Anticardiolipin antibodies
   Cyclosporin A
   Mitomycin
   Cisplatin

level of 2 mg per deciliter or more may have relapsing necrotizing glomerulonephritis or progressive glomerulosclerosis. A renal biopsy is essential in this circumstance to document the presence of an active necrotizing glomerulonephritis before anti-inflammatory and immunosuppressive therapy is reinstituted.

RENAL BIOPSY AND THE TREATMENT OF THROMBOTIC MICROANGIOPATHY

The renal lesions of thrombotic microangiopathy are glomerular consolidation with expansion of the subendothelial zone, arteriolar fibrinoid necrosis, and edematous intimal expansion in small arteries. These angiopathic lesions also can have superimposed thrombi. The pathologic changes in the kidney are similar in all types of thrombotic microangiopathy (Table 164.9). The clinical features of these diseases often resemble those of glomerulonephritis and include proteinuria, hematuria, hypertension, and renal insufficiency. Thrombocytopenia and microangiopathic hemolytic anemia distinguish thrombotic microangiopathy from glomerulonephritis, but are not always present. Thrombotic microangiopathy manifests as a variety of clinical syndromes, including childhood and adult hemolytic–uremic syndrome, acute postpartum renal failure, malignant hypertension, thrombotic thrombocytopenic purpura, and systemic sclerosis renal crisis. Childhood hemolytic–uremic syndrome typically presents as acute renal failure, often after a diarrheal enteritis caused by virotoxin-producing *Escherichia coli*. The renal crises of progressive systemic sclerosis should be suspected when there are serologic and clinical manifestations of systemic sclerosis. However, the diagnosis may be detected only on renal biopsy if the patient does not have conspicuous skin changes. Most recently, antibodies to von Willebrand's factor–cleaving protease have been found in patients with thrombotic thrombocytopenic purpura. These antibodies may directly participate in causing the disease and should be removed by plasmapheresis.

The initial treatment of thrombotic microangiopathy is directed at the control of hypertension. This is especially true for systemic sclerosis, in which ACE inhibitors play a prominent role. In postdiarrheal childhood hemolytic–uremic syndrome, the disease process usually abates spontaneously and supportive care is in order. In contrast, plasma exchange with fresh frozen plasma or cryoprecipitate is the appropriate treatment in thrombotic thrombocytopenic purpura. The survival rate is greater than 90% when plasma exchange is used in conjunction with corticosteroid therapy.

RENAL BIOPSY IN ACUTE RENAL FAILURE

Renal biopsy is useful in a patient with acute renal failure when the cause cannot be determined by a careful history, physical examination, and laboratory evaluation. It is particularly helpful when acute renal failure is associated with nephrosis or nephritis, or when it does not resolve after 3 to 4 weeks. In this circumstance, renal biopsy can be used to look for aggressive glomerulonephritis, systemic vasculitis, thrombotic microangiopathy, minimal change disease with acute renal failure, tubulointerstitial nephritis, or acute tubular necrosis. The treatment of acute renal failure is different in the setting of acute tubular necrosis compared with glomerulonephritis or thrombotic microangiopathy.

A small subset of adult patients with minimal change disease have acute renal failure. These patients typically are older and have evidence of systolic hypertension and atherosclerosis. The cause of the acute tubular dysfunction is uncertain, but the condition improves with corticosteroid therapy or diuresis. Affected patients can be identified by their massive proteinuria. Anecdotal data suggest that other forms of nephrotic syndrome in older patients are accompanied by renal insufficiency that resolves with corticosteroid therapy.

CONCLUSION

Renal biopsy is indicated in the diagnosis and management of most forms of glomerular injury. Numerous glomerular diseases produce similar clinicopathologic syndromes but require different types of treatment. The cause and pathogenesis of many forms of glomerular disease are not clearly understood. Until the specific causes of glomerular injury are determined, therapeutic options are limited and often involve anti-inflammatory and immunosuppressive drugs. Because most of these agents carry substantial morbid and even mortal complications, they should be used only after careful consideration of the risks and benefits to the patient. Renal biopsy is an essential tool in this process because it enables a more definitive diagnosis, helps elucidate the natural history of the disease, and reveals the response to treatment.

BIBLIOGRAPHY

D'Amico G. Influence of clinical and histological features of actuarial renal survival in patients with idiopathic IgA nephropathy, membranous nephropathy, and membranoproliferative glomerulonephritis: survey of recent literature. *Am J Kidney Dis* 1992;20:315–323.

Donadio JV Jr, Bergstralh EJ, Offord KP, et al. A controlled trial of fish oil in IgA nephropathy. *N Engl J Med* 1994;331:1194–1199.

Furlan M, Robles R, Galbusera M, et al. von Willebrand factor-cleaving protease in thrombocytopenic purpura and the hemolytic-uremic syndrome. *N Engl J Med* 1998;339:1578–1584.

Hogan SL, Muller KE, Jennette JC, et al. A review of therapeutic studies of idiopathic membranous glomerulopathy. *Am J Kidney Dis* 1995;25: 862–875.

Iskandar SS, Falk RJ, Jennette JC. Clinical and pathological features of fibrillary glomerulonephritis. *Kidney Int* 1992;42:1401–1407.

Jennette JC, Falk RJ. Small vessel vasculitis. *N Engl J Med* 1997;337: 1512–1523.

Korbet SM, Schwartz MM, Lewis EJ. Primary focal segmental glomerulosclerosis: clinical course and response to therapy. *Am J Kidney Dis* 1994; 23:773–783.

Madaio MP. Renal biopsy. *Kidney Int* 1990;38:529–543.

Ponticelli C, Altieri P, Scolari F, et al. A randomized study comparing methylprednisolone plus chlorambucil versus methylprednisolone plus cyclophosphamide in idiopathic membranous nephropathy. *J Am Soc Nephrol* 1998;9:444–450.

Kelley's Textbook of Internal Medicine, fourth edition. Edited by H. David Humes. Lippincott Williams & Wilkins, Philadelphia © 2000.

C H A P T E R

165

RENAL SUBSTITUTION TREATMENT IN ACUTE AND CHRONIC RENAL FAILURE

PAUL SAKIEWICZ
EMIL PAGANINI

Renal dysfunction has been shown to enhance morbidity and mortality at all levels of patient care. Total renal failure—acute or chronic—is an absolute life-threatening situation, which fortunately can be attenuated somewhat by means of renal substitution treatment, also called renal replacement therapy. Unlike other organ failures, which require transplantation for successful support, the kidneys can also be substituted by artificial mechanical measures that have stood the test of time in both the acute and chronic failure arena.

The functions of the normal kidney are multiple, involving both the well-known aspects of solute and water excretion and balance, participation in acid–base regulation, erythrocyte production through bone marrow erythropoietin stimulation, and the lesser known aspects of hormone and cytokine regulation and bone metabolism. Current methods to "replace" renal function in acute or chronic renal failure aim at achieving fluid and solute balance and azotemic control but do little to replace the more sophisticated renal participation in metabolic balance. Experimental renal substitution treatments are presently being developed, which may address these shortcomings of current dialytic support. Clearly, those techniques that are capable of replacing some of the renal physiologic functions have several limitations and cannot achieve the efficiency of normal renal function. Occasionally, extracorporeal "renal replacement" therapies are used in the treatment of life-threatening intoxications and are frequently undertaken even in the absence of renal dysfunction.

RENAL SUBSTITUTION TREATMENT

The preservation of any residual renal function should be the goal of all renal therapy. Thus, the use of supportive measures for renal replacement should be considered an adjunct to whatever residual function that exists. This concept is of utmost importance because an aggressive therapy outline may compromise residual renal activity. There are indeed indications for aggressive support, especially in the acute renal failure population, but the overall premise to preserve underlying renal function while adding solute and fluid control with dialysis should be standard practice. Thus, a dose-delivery concept of dialysis has become popular in the description and ordering of therapy. This dose considers not only the patient variables such as size, volume, or state of catabolism and diet, but also the renal reserve present and the effect of dialytic management upon its preservation.

In the normal kidney, solute and water clearance occurs by first producing a large volume of plasma ultrafiltrate (approximately 170 to 180 L per day) through application of arteriolar hydrostatic pressure across the glomerular membrane. This primary ultrafiltrate is then altered along its path through the renal tubuli such that ideal water and solute homeostasis in the whole organism results. Glomerular filtration is thus a convective process forcing fluid into Bowman's space. This fluid has the constituents of what was presented to the basement membrane up to the size that is allowed to pass through that membrane.

In standard dialytic treatment, however, solute and water are balanced across a semipermeable membrane with a dialysate solution. The dialysate content can be altered to achieve differing balance characteristics and end points. This process is predominantly a diffusive method. During extracorporeal therapy, the semipermeable membrane is a manufactured substance, such as cellulose acetate or polysulfone. On the other hand, peritoneal dialysis uses the peritoneal membrane as the barrier between blood and dialysate fluid. In a broad sense, the term "dialysis" can be described as a process in which a solute composition of one fluid compartment is changed by exposing it to a second solution in another fluid compartment. Transfer of solutes and water takes place by different physiologic principles: passive diffusion of molecules (diffusive transport) and ultrafiltration through the semipermeable membrane (convective transport). A third process of solute movement can be attributed to adsorption. Although this third process may be minimal in certain diffusive modalities, membrane composition and pressure differentials also play a role in adsorptive properties. Adsorption is also the primary method of solute clearance when applied with resin or activated charcoal during hemoperfusion.

Dialysis efficiency has been centered on the effective removal of small substances such as urea, which are thought to be surrogate indicators for the state of "uremia." As discussed later in this chapter, dialysis doses have been based on the removal rates of blood urea nitrogen (BUN) or serum creatinine. Although there is ample clinical evidence that this approach is both practical and effective, one must not lose sight of other potential "toxins" that may be important. For example, other "small" molecular substances, such as guanidine and phenolic compounds, aliphatic amines, or ammonia, as well as higher-molecular-weight (1300 to 10,000 daltons) toxins known as "middle molecules," such as β_2-microglobulin, have been shown to have potential pathologic effects.

DIFFUSIVE TRANSPORT

Defined as the passive transfer of solutes through a membrane in the absence of net solvent transfer, diffusion remains the basis for the most efficient form of dialytic intervention when addressing small molecular substances. The amount of solute crossing a membrane by diffusion depends on (a) the mean concentration gradient of the substance, (b) the effective dialysis surface area (A) exposed to the differing fluids, and (c) the resistance of solute movement through the various layers established by the blood, membrane, and dialysate solution, known as the *dialyzer permeability coefficient* (Ko).

A concentration gradient between compartments is necessary for passage of a given solute from one compartment to the other. Molecular size, protein binding, molecular charge, and membrane pore size and material affect transfer of solutes as well. Small molecules with a molecular weight of less than 200 daltons have a higher transport rate through the membrane than molecules with a molecular size of more than 1,000 daltons. Highly negatively charged molecules such as inorganic phosphate ($PO_4^=$) may have more difficulty in moving through a membrane than molecular size might predict. Other influences such as fluid temperature, blood and dialysate flow rates, and artificial kidney design also influence diffusive characteristics.

CONVECTIVE TRANSPORT

Ultrafiltration is the movement of water and permeable solutes through a semipermeable membrane. This process occurs either through the application of hydrostatic pressure (positive or negative respectively) to the blood or dialysate side of the semipermeable membrane (hemodialysis), or through plasma water transfer from one compartment to the other after a high osmotic gradient (peritoneal dialysis). Solvent drag caused by frictional forces between water and solutes leads to convective transfer of small and mid-size molecular substances in the same direction. In hemodialysis, the hydrostatic pressure gradient between the blood and dialysate compartment of the artificial dialyzer causes the plasma water movement from blood to dialysate. The rate of convective movement depends on: (a) the solvent filtration rate that is created by the pressure difference between compartments, (b) the sieving coefficient of the substance directly related to the permeability (porosity) and the surface area of the dialyzer, and (c) the blood concentration of the substance. In peritoneal dialysis, ultrafiltration occurs because of osmotic intraperitoneal pressure.

Solute removal can be achieved through diffusion and/or convection (ultrafiltration), and water removal can be achieved through ultrafiltration. The importance of convection and diffusion varies considerably, depending on the molecular weight of solutes. Diffusive transfer predominates convective transport for small molecules, whereas higher-molecular-weight substances move through the membrane principally by convection. Naturally, in renal replacement therapy both physiologic principles are active in solute balance. Diffusive transport is the primary means of metabolic waste removal in both hemodialysis and peritoneal dialysis. The technique of hemofiltration, defined as a plasma water exchange, relates to the use of high ultrafiltration rates as a means of removing larger-sized solutes, whereas hemodiafiltration is a combination of both aggressive diffusive and high-rate convective treatment, creating the most effective method of large and small solute balance. It is, however, limited by cost and technical challenge.

ADSORPTIVE MECHANISM

An alternative way to remove solutes from the bloodstream is through hemoperfusion, where anticoagulated blood is brought into close contact with an adsorptive substance like activated charcoal or resins. Hemoperfusion relies on the physical process of solute adsorption for its efficiency, and in many instances drug removal in terms of clearance is far better than what could be done with hemodialysis, peritoneal dialysis, or forced diuresis. Activation of carbon is the formation, induced by chemical or physical processes, of pores within the carbon structure. Hemoperfusion is used mainly in the acute treatment of drug poisoning but has been used in such areas as iron and aluminum intoxication. Some attempts at utilizing the adsorptive properties of some dialysis membrane types for cytokine removal have also found their way into the treatment of the septic patient with acute renal failure, but the data are preliminary.

▌ HEMODIALYSIS

HEMODIALYSIS APPARATUS AND CIRCUIT

Dialysis technology has made great strides not only in the use of equipment and techniques but also in the understanding of the various conditions and issues that are both created and resolved by the dialytic process itself. Dialysis times have varied from a long (8-hour) process in the early years to the short dialysis times (2.5 hours) of the valiant experiments of the late 1980s and the more standard time/clearance ratio of modern prescription dialysis therapy. Although technology has made the process easier to perform, it still consists of a basic dialytic circuit, and principles remain the same.

During hemodialysis, blood is pumped at a fairly high flow rate (300 to 400 mL per minute) from the patient through the dialysis apparatus and then returned to the patient. Basic technical components of hemodialysis include the hemodialysis machine, which consists of pump systems for both blood and dialysate fluid paths and pressure-monitoring devices within those circuits. The artificial kidney is added to the middle of both flow circuits, thus creating an "arterial" or "to" line and a "venous" or "from" line. It is within these lines that the measurements of pressure and the adjustment of anticoagulation occur. Heparin, if used, is usually added to the arterial line, prior to the kidney to ensure that the blood entering the dialyzer does not clot, thus avoiding a lower efficiency of the therapy and reducing the obligatory blood loss of the dialysis session. Nonheparin techniques also are available for use in patients who either cannot tolerate heparin or in whom anticoagulation would be contraindicated.

The dialysate fluid is prepared through a series of proportioning mechanisms, combining dialysate concentrate with a steady supply of purified (treated) water. This highly purified water is then combined with the dialysate concentrate, which contains the solutes required for a balanced dialysis session. It is in this proportioning that the various solute concentrations (sodium, potassium, calcium, bicarbonate) can be altered as dictated by patient need and physician desire. Altering the pressure differences across the semipermeable membrane of the dialyzer will alter the amount of fluid lost (ultrafiltrated) during the session. This difference is set by the machine operator, and volume loss is precisely controlled over time.

The dialyzer is the part of the dialysis circuit in which solute and water transfer actually occur. It consists of a shell containing the semipermeable membrane that separates blood from dialysate fluid. The membrane can consist of a variety of plastic materials (polysulfone, cellulose acetate, poliamide, and others) that have been manufactured to yield a certain fluid porosity and diffusive characteristic. Membrane types differ in several characteristics, such as surface area, porosity, biocompatibility, and charge. The rate of whole blood pumped through the dialyzer is usually between 250 to 500 mL per minute. Dialysate fluid flows at a rate of 500 to 800 mL per minute.

Another prerequisite for hemodialysis is a functioning vascular access that allows for sufficient blood flow. Blood access types may be percutaneous double-lumen venous catheters (mostly tunneled), natural arteriovenous fistulas, or arteriovenous bypass grafts. Percutaneous double-lumen catheters are usually placed in a major vein (internal jugular, femoral vein), because these vessels already support high blood flows. The subclavian vessels were used at one time as a primary site of entry, but recent data showing a strong correlation between subclavian access and subsequent venous stenosis have drastically changed practice. Fistulas and grafts are surgically created arteriovenous malformations that connect an artery and a vein. They increase both venous blood flow and pressure substantially, thereby thickening (arterializing) the venous wall and allowing for a more consistent, stable, and repetitive venous needle entry, while also ensuring an adequate blood flow for dialysis. Most commonly, the radiocephalic natural fistula of the nondominant arm is attempted, followed by the brachiocephalic bypass anastomosis approach. A fistula can take several weeks to months to "mature" from placement to a point at which it can be used for dialysis. Grafts can be used earlier, are usually placed either in the forearm or upper arm, and can have either a straight or loop configuration. For practical purposes, the arteriovenous fistula is the preferred hemodialysis access for chronic hemodialysis because it has a lower complication rate and the longest survival after successful maturation. Grafts are technically easier to place; however, their long-term complications, including stenosis and thrombosis, cause higher morbidity and cost. Potential complications of arteriovenous fistulas or grafts are limb ischemia through a "steal syndrome" that shunts blood away from the limb, venous stenosis and thrombosis, aneurysm formation, and infection. Thrombosis of the hemodialysis access renders it unusable for dialysis and thus should be considered an urgent situation requiring relatively rapid correction. Angioplasty and thrombolysis can be used to attempt recanalization and continued use of the access. Percutaneous double-lumen catheters are the least preferred chronic dialysis access choice, because of lower blood flows and a higher rate of complications caused by catheter-related infections and malfunction. They can be either tunneled or nontunneled and are used mainly in the acute setting. For chronic dialysis, central catheters may be used transiently while awaiting maturation of a fistula or graft. Chronic use of catheters, however, is sometimes seen in dialysis patients only if all other available access sites have been exhausted.

FORMS OF HEMODIALYSIS

Current dialysis techniques are intermittent and continuous hemodialysis. Table 165.1 reflects the current definitions, primary method, and abbreviations commonly used. Intermittent hemodialysis became widely available in 1972 for support of the otherwise fatal condition of end-stage renal disease (ESRD). The usual frequency of intermittent hemodialysis in ESRD is three times weekly, with an average duration of 3 to 5 hours each session. Alternative forms are home hemodialysis, in which the patient dialyzes at home, usually with the help of a relative, and nocturnal hemodialysis, in which longer hemodialysis sessions at slower blood and dialysate flows are used.

Continuous hemodialysis is a form of renal replacement therapy that is used mainly for acute renal failure support. It applies the principles of hemodialysis in a slow and continuous manner, ideally providing solute and fluid removal 24 hours per day. The gradual solute and fluid removal is thought to be especially beneficial for hemodynamically unstable patients in whom conventional hemodialysis may exacerbate hypotension. The nomenclature and abbreviations applied to continuous dialysis techniques are complex (Table 165.2). Just as in conventional hemodialysis, vascular access is necessary to provide blood flow in the continuous hemodialysis circuit. Vascular access can be either venovenous (when a double-lumen venous catheter is used, meaning that blood is being drawn from one lumen of the catheter by means of a blood pump and returned through the other lumen of the catheter) or arteriovenous (when one single-lumen catheter is inserted into each femoral artery and femoral vein).

In the arteriovenous form of continuous dialysis, the arterial pump provides blood flow through the dialyzer. The dialytic techniques applied continuously through the mentioned accesses can be either diffusional or convectional in nature, or consist of a combination of both. For example, CVVHD means that the renal replacement is continuous, access is venovenous, and solute clearance is achieved with hemodialysis. CAVHF means that the technique is continuous, arteriovenous access is used, and solute clearance is achieved through purely convective solute transport. Another frequently used term is SCUF, which refers to slow and continuous ultrafiltration (usually 100 to 200 mL per hour); the access can be either venovenous or arteriovenous. No dialysate or replacement fluid is present, and the sole purpose of SCUF is fluid removal without significant solute removal.

TABLE 165.1.	DEFINITIONS AND PHYSIOLOGY BEHIND VARIOUS EXTRACORPOREAL THERAPY INTERVENTIONS	
Procedure	**Definition**	**Underlying Physical Principle of Operation**
Ultrafiltration	Removal of plasma water	*Hydrostatic pressure* Isolated ultrafiltration During hemodialysis During hemofiltration *Osmotic pressure* During peritoneal dialysis using glucose as the determinant osmotic variant
Dialysis	Movement of solute across a semipermeable dialysis membrane from blood to dialysate or vice versa following gradients. Countercurrent blood flow and dialysate flow rates determine therapy dosage	*Solute diffusion* across a membrane. Controlled by temperature, charge, molecular size, and flow characteristics. Membrane is either a plastic variant (hemo-) or natural (peritoneal); best "small" molecule solute movement
Hemofiltration	Movement of solute across a semipermeable dialysis membrane following the flow of fluid during a plasma water exchange. Exchange rates determine therapy dosage	*Solute convection* following the rapid flow of fluid across a membrane; size, charge, temperature have less influence up to membrane pore size; best "middle" molecule solute movement
Hemodiafiltration	Combination of dialysis and hemofiltration aspects in a single therapy session	*Convection and diffusion* flows. Most efficient form of extracorporeal dialytic support; maximum small and middle molecular solute movement
Hemoperfusion	Flow of whole blood or plasma over substances such as charcoal or resin with specific desired surface characteristics	*Adsorption* from perfusate on to surface structures of material contained in the cartridge; system material saturation limits therapy

GOALS AND MONITORING OF THERAPY

Perhaps one of the most significant advances in the delivery of dialysis therapy to ESRD patients has been the establishment of a dialysis dose. On the basis of both a prospective national cooperative dialysis trial and later on the United States Renal Data System (USRDS) results, there seems to be a close association with patient outcome and amount of dialysis delivered. The surrogate marker used for dosing the session is the control of BUN. This control can be expressed either as a clearance of the therapy delivered using terms that relate to both the patient and the therapy session or as a total amount of marker removed as determined by measurement of a percent change from pre- and postdialysis blood levels of BUN.

The clearance method uses the dialyzer clearance (K) during a dialysis session, the actual length of the session in minutes (t), and the volume of urea present in the body determined from the patient's total fluid content (V). The ratio established (Kt/V) should express a ratio of 1.2 to 1.4. Dialysis ratios of less than 1.2 are associated with a higher mortality. The usual ESRD patient requires three times weekly hemodialysis with a duration of 3 to 5 hours per session to achieve this urea reduction requirement. Wide variations in time on dialysis are due to differing patient size, dietary intake, comorbidities, and access type. Furthermore, the clinician also evaluates nutritional status, calcium and phosphorus balance, weight gains between dialysis sessions, choice of anticoagulation dose on dialysis, hypertension control and medication schedule, and anemia management, including iron and erythropoietin therapy, to arrive at the optimal dialysis dose for each patient.

In acute renal failure support, an optimum dialysis dose has not been established. These patients are varied and present with a myriad of problems that may have much more influence on mortality than does an individually delivered dialysis dose. Both intermittent and continuous hemodialysis techniques are used for support, with the more hemodynamically unstable patient generally being treated with continuous techniques. Controversy exists with respect to the dose of dialysis, such that it is not clear whether adequacy parameters from chronic renal failure support can be extrapolated to acute renal failure support, and to the survival benefit of either intermittent or continuous hemodialysis. It is, however, customary to target a urea reduction of 65% per intermittent dialysis session and to achieve a steady urea concentration of less than 60 mg per deciliter when using continuous hemodialysis. Overall, it appears that daily intermit-

TABLE 165.2.	FORMS OF CONTINUOUS RENAL REPLACEMENT THERAPY	
Time Frame	**Access Type**	**Renal Replacement Form**
Continuous (C)	Venovenous (VV)	Hemodialysis (HD)
	Arteriovenous (AV)	Hemofiltration (HF) Hemodiafiltration (HDF)

Possible Forms–CVVHD, CAVHD, CVVHF, CAVHF, CVVHDF, CAVHDF
SCUF, Slow continuous ultrafiltration (can be VV- or AV-SCUF)

tent hemodialysis may be the optimal technique for most acute renal failure patients, who can hemodynamically tolerate it. Prospective studies to evaluate outcome, modality choice, and dialysis dose in acute renal failure are currently underway.

COMPLICATIONS

The most common hemodialysis complication is hypotension, followed by cramps, nausea and vomiting, headache, chest and back pain, itching, fever, and chills (Table 165.3). These complications can be multifactorial, but in general they relate to the many physiologic and unphysiologic factors that the patient is exposed to during rapid fluid and solute removal. The contact of blood with synthetic material can elicit an inflammatory response, which can be somewhat modulated by choosing so-called biocompatible membranes. Those biocompatible membranes usually elicit the least amount of inflammatory response, and their influence on morbidity and mortality seems positive, although not conclusively proved. Hematologic abnormalities during hemodialysis are transient initial leukopenia, enhanced extracorporeal platelet aggregation, and hemolysis.

Frequent long- or short-term access-related complications include infection, thrombosis, limb ischemia through steal syndrome, and malfunction. Chronic complications and associated conditions in chronic renal failure are abnormal lipid profile, anemia, iron loss, β_2-microglobulin amyloidosis with carpal tunnel syndrome, elevations of homocysteine levels, depression, sexual dysfunction, and a general preponderance for morbidity and mortality from cardiovascular disease. These complications are probably inherent in the pathologic state of renal failure rather than to the dialysis modality alone. Aluminum accumulation in ESRD patients can cause aluminum bone disease and dementia. The source of aluminum can be either the dialysate water supply or the use of aluminum-based phosphate binders, a practice now largely abandoned. Upon initiation of hemodialysis, a dramatic symptom constellation can occasionally be observed, called *dialysis dysequilibrium syndrome*. Central nervous system solute and water shifts causing cerebral edema are responsible for this rarely observed syndrome, and prevention of rapid solute and fluid shifts are the mainstay of therapy. Patients can exhibit headache, cramps, nausea, vomiting, mental status changes, seizures, and, in extreme cases, death. Patients who are new to dialysis are particularly at risk, and gradual, slow removal of solutes and fluid should therefore be attempted initially. Anticoagulation is required for efficient dialysis to prevent clotting of the extracorporeal circuit, and patients are obviously exposed to all its inherent risks, like bleeding and anemia. Recombinant erythropoietin therapy has greatly facilitated anemia management in ESRD patients, and the previously observed iron overload from long-term transfusions is now rather rare. Indeed, the opposite effect, iron deficiency, is prevalent among hemodialysis patients and is probably related to the blood loss experienced during the dialysis sessions.

Other inherent risks associated with hemodialysis are exposure to infectious viral hepatitis, and the potential for exposure to dialysate water contaminants such as bacterial pyrogens, chlorines, chloramines, aluminum, and fluorides. The practice of reusing dialyzers can occasionally cause severe reactions like hemodynamic collapse and death when dialyzer rinsing is incomplete and sterilant is flushed into the patient. Diligent attention to dialysate water preparation and reuse practices is of utmost importance, and those complications have fortunately become rare.

PERITONEAL DIALYSIS

In the adult population, peritoneal dialysis is mostly used as a means to replace renal function in chronic renal failure. It can, however, be used as an alternative to hemodialysis in acute renal failure. Peritoneal dialysis uses the peritoneal membrane as barrier and exchange medium between blood and dialysate fluid. Usually 1 to 3 L of a dialysis solution containing dextrose and solutes in a physiologic concentration are instilled into the peritoneal cavity. The principles of diffusion and convection achieve equilibration between dialysate fluid and blood in mesenteric capillaries and therefore solute and water removal. Fluid removal is achieved osmotically through a high osmotic gradient in the dialysate fluid. After dwelling for a certain period of time (widely different, but usually 4 to 6 hours in continuous ambulatory peritoneal dialysis), the dialysate fluid is then drained and a new cycle is started. Peritoneal dialysis can be performed either continuously, in which dialysate solution is constantly present in the peritoneal cavity, or cycler-assisted, in which usually nocturnal cycles are being performed automatically with a programmable machine.

APPARATUS FOR PERITONEAL DIALYSIS

A peritoneal dialysis catheter must be placed percutaneously through either a midline or, preferably, a lateral abdominal entry

TABLE 165.3.	POTENTIAL COMPLICATIONS OF HEMODIALYSIS
Probable Cause	**Symptoms**
Solute and fluid removal	Hypotension, cramps, nausea, vomiting, headache, chest pain, back pain, dialysis dysequilibrium syndrome
Contact of synthetic materials and dialysate fluid with blood	Fever, chills, itching, transient leukopenia, anemia, thrombocyte aggregation, pyrogen reactions, aluminum deposition
Vascular access-related	Infection, thrombosis, stenosis, aneurysm formation, limb ischemia and steal syndrome, high cardiac output heart failure
Dialyzer sterilant use—inadequate rinsing	Formaldehyde/ethyleneoxide: hemodynamic collapse, chest pain, burning sensation
Anticoagulation	Bleeding
Miscellaneous conditions associated with chronic renal failure	Carpal tunnel syndrome, dyslipidemia, hyperhomocysteinemia, anemia, depression, sexual dysfunction, dementia, risk for viral hepatitis infection

site. The ideal internal location is between the anterior abdominal wall and the omentum and bowel loops. The catheter is usually a silicone or polyurethane cuffed catheter, which has to allow for adequate dialysate fluid inflow and outflow. The dialysate fluid is usually a lactate-based dialysate solution with differing solute dextrose levels. Available dextrose concentrations are 1.5%, 2.5%, and 4.25%, which allow for targeted ultrafiltration and solute removal (4.25% providing the highest rate of fluid removal).

Dialysate filling and draining are achieved by using exchange tubing, which is connected to the patient's catheter. Utmost diligence is required when handling the connections because of a high infection risk otherwise. Exchanges of dialysate fluid can be achieved manually or cycler assisted. When performing cycler-assisted peritoneal dialysis, the tubing is attached to a programmable cycler apparatus, which performs instillation, dwell and drain functions, and ultrafiltration measurements automatically.

GOALS AND MONITORING OF THERAPY

The usual peritoneal dialysis prescription (continuous ambulatory peritoneal dialysis) involves exchanging between 1 and 3 L up to four to six times daily. Physiologic differences in peritoneal membrane characteristics of individual patients influence the rate of solute and fluid removal. Occasionally, these individual differences require a change from peritoneal to hemodialysis based on inadequacy of solute or fluid removed. Adequacy of peritoneal dialysis is mostly measured by determining the amount of urea removal and the creatinine clearance provided with dialysis. The ideal dose of peritoneal dialysis is unknown; however, certain adequacy parameters can serve as guides to achieve adequate fluid and uremia control. Peritoneal dialysis can certainly achieve results similar to those of hemodialysis with respect to patient morbidity, mortality, and solute and fluid control. The overall cost on average is significantly less for peritoneal dialysis, and comparative studies with hemodialysis have been controversial but have proved peritoneal dialysis to be comparable to hemodialysis and a viable option as renal replacement therapy for chronic renal failure.

COMPLICATIONS

Infection of the peritoneal dialysis catheter with peritonitis remains the most significant complication of peritoneal dialysis and is frequently the limiting factor in its application. The incidence of catheter-related peritonitis is approximately 1 episode every 18 to 24 months, and the most common causative organisms are *Staphylococcus epidermidis* and *S. aureus.* Depending on the severity of the infection, either intravenous or intraperitoneal antibiotics can be used; occasionally, the catheter must be removed and the patient changed to hemodialysis. Several interventions have been attempted in counteracting catheter infections, and the combination of diligent attention to the catheter exit site and exchange techniques and preventive local antibiotic treatment has decreased the incidence of catheter-related peritonitis.

Catheter malfunction can occur either through fibrinous deposits around the catheter or through obstruction of the catheter holes. Metabolic complications such as hyperglycemia with increased insulin requirements and abdominal wall hernias and pleural leak can occur. Abdominal distention can impair pulmonary function, and gastrointestinal reflux disease can be exacerbated. Loss of protein in the dialysate fluid can be substantial (10 to 15 g per day), requiring adequate oral supplementation. As with all ESRD patients, comprehensive management of lipid and volume status, anemia and hypertension, calcium and phosphorus metabolism, nutrition, and psychological well-being need to be ascertained when managing peritoneal dialysis patients.

GUIDELINES FOR INITIATION OF RENAL SUBSTITUTION THERAPY

Although anyone can start dialysis support, it is much more difficult to know when not to start. There are only vague and general rules on the initiation of dialytic support in the chronic renal failure population, and those rules are even further blurred in patients with acute renal failure.

Absolute indications for initiating renal replacement therapy are the clear presence of signs or symptoms of the uremic syndrome, severe and refractory hyperkalemia, severe acidosis, fluid overload, and severe life-threatening substance intoxications. Another way to remember these is to use the mnemonic AEIOU, standing for **a**cidosis, **e**lectrolyte abnormalities, **i**ntoxications, **o**verload, and **u**remia. An absolute level of BUN or serum creatinine alone is rarely an indication for dialysis in the patient with either acute or chronic renal failure, because symptoms vary from patient to patient. High levels of BUN can be used as a factor in the decision to initiate therapy but should not be used as the only indication for dialysis. Also, small patients with poor nutritional status or small muscle mass may not generate serum creatinine to a level indicative of their degree of renal dysfunction. Indeed, it is not unusual to see serum creatinine levels of 1.5 to 2.0 mg per deciliter in patients with a glomerular filtration rate of less than 10 mL per minute. Thus, the laboratory findings are to be used as aids in the search for an appropriate starting time for dialysis, but must be taken in the context of the whole constellation of signs and symptoms.

The initiation of chronic renal replacement therapy is somewhat controversial but replacement should be started when the patient's glomerular filtration rate drops to less than 10 mL per minute per square meter or, in diabetics, to less than 15 mL per min^2. This rate should be used as the threshold to avoid major uremic and other complications and to ensure an uncomplicated transition into life with renal replacement therapy. In addition, significant medical and psychological care, most effectively achieved through a multidisciplinary approach involving patient and family, primary and renal physicians, dialysis nurse, social worker, and dietitian, needs to be ascertained. The adequate frequency, duration, and dose of renal replacement therapy is still a matter of intense debate. The usual frequency of maintenance hemodialysis is three times weekly for 3 to 5 hours depending on patient variability, and the frequency and mode of peritoneal dialysis is highly variable but averages about six times per week either as daytime or night-time peritoneal dialysis or a combination of both.

ACUTE RENAL FAILURE

Acute renal failure is still a life-threatening disease with high mortality (on average 50%) despite significant technical advances in the field of renal replacement therapy, including the development of continuous forms of dialysis. Acute renal failure is heterogeneous in nature and invariably complicates patient management by increasing the risk for sepsis, bleeding, mental status changes, and respiratory and cardiac failure. Theoretically, renal replacement therapy should facilitate management of these conditions through solute and fluid control. Renal replacement therapy in acute renal failure can be achieved with either intermittent or continuous forms of hemodialysis. Peritoneal dialysis is used mainly in the pediatric population, but in the adult patient it has the disadvantage of insufficient removal of solutes and volume. Factors and considerations in the choice and frequency of modality are comorbidities and hemodynamic stability. Uncertain factors in the renal replacement treatment of acute renal failure are the time of initiation and the frequency and the dose of dialysis. The mode of hemodialysis is also a matter of debate with respect to patient outcome.

A theoretical advantage of continuous renal replacement therapy is the gradual rate of solute and fluid removal, which minimizes hypotension. Solute and fluid removal is usually greater than in intermittent hemodialysis, and intuitively continuous dialysis is preferred for patients with a greater risk for hemodynamic instability. A specific form of continuous renal replacement therapy, *continuous hemofiltration* (using solely convective solute removal), has been invoked in being able to remove adverse inflammatory cytokines. Because of this theoretical advantage, continuous forms of dialysis intuitively should lead to improved patient outcome. This theoretical advantage, however, has not been corroborated in clinical trials, and currently intermittent and continuous forms of dialysis are equivalent methods for acute renal failure treatment. The approach to renal replacement therapy in acute renal failure should therefore include a proactive approach toward renal replacement therapy, meaning earlier initiation, more frequent (possibly daily) dialysis, usage of biocompatible dialysis membranes and an overall increase in dialysis dose.

A common error in management of acute renal failure is to underestimate its extent by considering the level of BUN or creatinine, as well as by ignoring the fact that a "normal" urine output of 2 to 3 L per day can be easily achieved with a glomerular filtration rate well below 10 mL per minute per square meter. A prolonged delay in renal replacement therapy in this situation can have devastating consequences by allowing the effects of uremia to continue unabated. At the same time, one must consider that renal replacement therapy can cause hypotension, exacerbate renal damage, and slow renal recovery. Other potential side effects are the risk of bleeding with the use of anticoagulants and infections caused by the placement of temporary dialysis access.

Management of the patient with acute renal failure should involve early nephrologic subspecialty consultation, because the above-mentioned approach is best achieved with the thoughtful judgment of the renal consultant with respect to the application of medical and interventional means that are most likely to benefit the patient.

CHRONIC RENAL FAILURE

Medical care for the chronic renal failure patient on renal replacement therapy (called ESRD by the Health Care Financing Administration) involves several factors: providing sufficient dialysis, special attention to ensuring adequate nutrition, maintaining a healthy dialysis access, correcting hormone deficiencies, treating comorbidities, and practicing an overall excellent general practice of medicine. This approach results in prolonged patient survival, decreased hospitalization, and enhanced patient well-being. In ESRD, there are three choices for chronic renal substitution treatment: standard intermittent hemodialysis, peritoneal dialysis, and renal transplantation. Although peritoneal dialysis is primarily a home dialysis technique, intermittent hemodialysis can be "in-center" (carried on in a dialysis facility), hospital-based (dialysis in the hospital as an outpatient), or home-based method of delivery. Further, home hemodialysis can be performed either nightly or daily or can follow the more traditional thrice-weekly treatment schedule.

The overall life expectancy of patients with ESRD has improved over the last several years, but it is still well below that of the general population. According to the 1999 United States Renal Data System Annual Report, "The expected lifetimes of the ESRD population are between 16 and 38 percent of an age-race-sex matched U.S. population, while lifetimes of all ESRD patients are reported to be 19 to 47% the corresponding US population." Although it is possible for individuals to live with dialytic renal replacement therapy for over 20 years, the average annual mortality rate for all dialysis patients was 23.3% in 1997 (Health Care Financing Administration Annual Facility Survey, 1998).

Survival is best with living-related renal transplantation, whereas overall among dialysis patients mortality increases with age, diagnosis of diabetes, and the addition of other comorbid entities. The main cause of death in dialysis patients is cardiovascular complications. There seems to be no overall survival benefit for either hemo- or peritoneal dialysis, even though in general a larger amount of solute clearance can be achieved with hemodialysis. Several current studies have examined patient outcome with respect to dialysis modality and are controversial, but suggest a slight advantage for continuous ambulatory peritoneal dialysis (CAPD) in young nondiabetic patients. With respect to the selection of modality of renal replacement therapy, several patient- and modality-specific variables must be considered. A patient's home situation, preference, practical availability, and convenience are important factors. Considerations in the decision-making process are also large patient size, prior intra-abdominal operations, and presence of intra abdominal infections, which directs therapy away from CAPD.

Once a patient initiates dialytic renal replacement one must ensure further quality medical management, but in addition one must direct attention to healthy maintenance of vascular access (the lifeline of hemodialysis), aggressive treatment of hypertension and anemia (with erythropoietin and iron substitution), and achieving sufficient dialysis.

Dialysis dose is specifically measured by observing the influence of dialysis on blood urea levels (Kt/V_{UREA}, URR_{UREA}), which are used as surrogate markers for the solute control achieved with renal replacement. There are certain minimum treatment goals that the nephrologist attempts to achieve during dialysis therapy, and usually a minimum URR of 68% or a Kt/V of 1.2 is attempted with dialysis. One must be clearly aware of the limitations associated with such practice, knowing that the blood urea level can vary greatly based on nutritional protein intake and other factors. For example, a relatively high blood urea level (60 to 80 mg per deciliter) does not necessarily imply poor patient health or poor dialysis delivery; occasionally, a very low urea and creatinine level can indicate severe malnutrition and underdialysis. Additional clinical signs of dialysis adequacy are calcium and phosphorus metabolism, hypertension control, anemia control, interdialytic weight gain, control of metabolic acidosis, control of hyperkalemia, nutritional status as measured with albumen, transferrin, prealbumin levels, increase in non-water weight, and subjective patient well-being. Hemodialysis factors that may play a role in patient outcome include dialyzer membrane type, the practice of dialyzer reuse, and the so-called high-flux dialysis. It is abundantly clear that inadequate dialysis, late referral to the nephrologist, and the presence of malnutrition at initiation of dialysis lead to poorer survival independent of the modality of renal replacement therapy. Currently it is recommended to refer patients for renal consultation when the serum creatinine level reaches 2 mg/dl for men and 1.5 mg/dl for women recognizing that serum creatinine is a relatively inaccurate indicator of glomerular filtration rate. These thresholds however are attempting to recognize significant renal failure in otherwise asymptomatic patients, in order to assure proper preparation for the possibility of renal replacement therapy and also optimized chronic renal failure management. The recent improvement in patient survival in the United States is encouraging and it suggests that improved dialysis is being delivered and that several of the important management factors mentioned above are being adequately applied.

ROLE OF RENAL SUBSTITUTION TREATMENT IN INTOXICATION

Renal replacement therapy in the form of hemodialysis or hemoperfusion can be used as adjunctive treatment to enhance poison elimination even in the absence of renal failure. Hemoperfusion is an extracorporeal technique by which toxins are adsorbed to either a charcoal or resin hemofilter in a circuit setup similar to hemodialysis. Toxin properties affecting dialytic clearance are molecular weight, protein binding, volume of distribution, lipid solubility, membrane binding and charge. Extracorporeal removal of toxins is necessary when conservative poisoning management cannot adequately assure the patient's well-being. Significant benefit from renal replacement therapy is most frequently achieved in overdoses of lithium, ethylene glycol, methanol, salicylates, and theophylline.

BIBLIOGRAPHY

CANUSA Peritoneal Dialysis Study Group. Adequacy of dialysis and nutrition in continuous peritoneal dialysis: association with clinical outcomes. *J Am Soc Nephrol* 1996;7:198–207.
Forni LG, Hilton PJ. Continuous hemofiltration in the treatment of acute renal failure. *N Engl J Med* 1997;336:1303–1309.
Hakim R. Assessing the adequacy of dialysis. *Kidney Int* 1990;37:822–832.
Ifudu O. Care of patients undergoing hemodialysis. *N Engl J Med* 1998;339:1054–1062.
Kierdorf HP, Sieberth HG. Continuous renal replacement therapies versus intermittent hemodialysis in acute renal failure: what do we know? *Am J Kidney Dis* 1996;28:S90–S96.
Leblanc M, Tapolyai M, Paganini EP. What dialysis dose should be provided in acute renal failure? A review. *Adv Ren Replace Ther* 1995;2:255–264.
Paganini EP, Tapolyai M, Goormastic M, et al. Establishing a dialysis therapy/patient outcome link in intensive care unit acute dialysis for patients with acute renal failure. *Am J Kidney Dis* 1996;28:S81–S89.
Ronco C, Bellomo R. Complications with continuous renal replacement therapy. *Am J Kidney Dis* 1996;28:S100–S104.
Star RA. Treatment of acute renal failure. *Kidney Int* 1998;54:1817–1831.
United States Renal Data System 1999 Annual Data Report. Treatment modalities for ESRD patients, Chapter 3:39–56; Patient mortality and survival, Chapter 5:73–88.

Kelley's Textbook of Internal Medicine, fourth edition. Edited by H. David Humes. Lippincott Williams & Wilkins, Philadelphia © 2000.

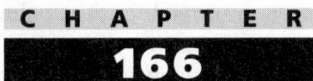

CHAPTER 166

RENAL TRANSPLANTATION

CHRISTOPHER Y. LU
MIGUEL A. VAZQUEZ
MARIUSZ KIELAR
D. ROHAN JEYARAJAH
XIN J. ZHOU

A successful kidney transplantation may completely reverse the uremic state in a patient with end-stage renal disease (ESRD). Advances in basic and clinical research have progressively improved the results. One-year renal allograft survival rates are 84% for first cadaveric renal transplants and 96% for two-haplotype-identical transplants from a sibling. The corresponding 1-year patient survival rates are 94.6% and 98%. This chapter takes the perspective of a general practitioner caring for a transplant recipient in concert with a transplant center.

The care of a patient undergoing renal transplantation may be divided into phases: evaluation of the potential transplant recipient, the immunologic evaluation of the patient and potential donor, management of the early post-transplantation course, and management and prevention of late complications. Although the problems of one phase can overlap those of another, we discuss each phase separately and then address related topics: the interpretation of the allograft biopsy, the immunosuppressive agents used to treat and prevent rejection, and the donor (living *versus* cadaveric) of the renal allograft.

EVALUATION OF THE POTENTIAL TRANSPLANT RECIPIENT

The major objectives of the evaluation phase are to determine whether the risk of complications from transplantation surgery and immunosuppression is acceptable; to identify and, if possible, correct any underlying diseases; and to educate the patient about transplantation.

The physician and patient must determine whether transplantation or dialysis is the best treatment for ESRD for that individual patient. For some patients, coexisting illnesses, such as cardiovascular disease, cause an excessive risk of morbidity or mortality from the transplantation surgery or the immunosuppressive regimen. Transplantation is a treatment but not a cure for ESRD; a few patients will not accept the risks of the transplantation surgery and the complications of the immunosuppressive medications that must be taken for the life of the transplant. However, for many patients, transplantation is the optimal treatment for ESRD and markedly improves their quality of life.

Many centers exclude patients with recent or disseminated cancer or with severe, untreatable cardiac, pulmonary, or vascular disease. However, patients with diabetes mellitus or inactive systemic lupus erythematosus may receive a transplant if they are in good general physical condition. Infections, peptic ulcers, and active gallbladder and diverticular disease should be identified and treated before transplantation. Patients with symptomatic heart disease, older patients, those with diabetes mellitus, and others with significant risk factors for atherosclerosis require a cardiac evaluation. The specific tests vary among transplant centers. The possible adverse effects of long-term immunosuppression on chronic viral hepatitis remain unsettled. Many centers perform a liver biopsy and discourage transplantation if severe chronic active hepatitis is found. Some patients may benefit from treatment with interferon before transplantation. Such treatment after transplantation may precipitate rejection. Functional integrity of the urinary tract may need to be confirmed, particularly in patients with histories of recurrent urinary tract infection, reflux, or kidney stones. Patients should be intellectually and emotionally capable of managing the stresses that accompany many of the post-transplantation complications and should be willing to comply with the medical regimen.

Many types of primary glomerulopathy and secondary renal disease recur in the allograft. However, rejection remains the major cause of allograft loss. Recurrent disease rarely results in allograft failure. An exception is focal segmental glomerulosclerosis, which has a high rate of recurrence in the allograft and can lead to transplant failure. Diabetic nephropathy, type II membranoproliferative glomerulonephritis, IgA nephropathy, and Henoch–Schönlein purpura recur frequently in the allograft, but the long-term prognosis for allograft function remains good. Some centers perform simultaneous kidney and pancreas transplantations to ameliorate the complications of type I diabetes mellitus.

In choosing between dialysis and transplantation, patients and their physicians must understand the risks associated with the surgery and the long-term immunosuppression. Despite the progress made in this field, many problems remain unsolved. Although the 1-year survival of transplanted organs is excellent, only 50% of all first-time recipients of a kidney from a cadaver donor have a functioning transplant after 9 years. There are many late complications (discussed under Management of Late Post-Transplantation Complications). Compared with patients receiving dialysis, transplant recipients have a higher risk of mortality and morbidity during the first months after transplantation. Only after 3 years is the cost-effectiveness of transplantation over dialysis demonstrable.

IMMUNOLOGIC EVALUATION OF THE PATIENT AND POTENTIAL RECIPIENT

About 75% of transplant recipients in the United States obtain their kidneys from cadavers. The donors are brain dead from trauma or acute illness but have functioning kidneys. The legal criteria for brain death are rigorous and indicate irreversible absence of brain function. Prospective studies, before the era of cadaveric transplantation and in countries where there is no legal definition of brain death, indicate that people who satisfied these criteria also inevitably suffered a cardiovascular death as well, despite continued aggressive intensive care. Although the number of patients waiting for transplant has tripled from 1985 to 1995, the number of transplantations performed annually has remained constant and is severely limited by the shortage of cadaver organs. Misconceptions about brain death prevent many families from allowing recovery of kidneys from the brain dead. Because of the shortage of cadaver organs, it is not uncommon for a patient to wait years for a transplant. Therefore, patients should be encouraged to explore the possibility of receiving a kidney from a living donor—a blood relative or a spouse—as discussed at the end of this chapter.

When their pretransplantation evaluations are complete, all patients awaiting cadaver kidneys are placed on a national waiting list maintained by the United Network for Organ Sharing (UNOS). UNOS is authorized by the federal government to distribute all cadaveric organs in the United States according to a computerized algorithm. This algorithm allows transplantations only between donors and recipients with compatible blood groups. It attempts to maximize the match between the human leukocyte antigen (HLA) genotype of the donor and recipient. However, these gene loci are extremely polymorphic, and the average match between donor and recipient in the United States is only two out of a possible six HLA antigens. A kidney with no HLA mismatches with a recipient will be shipped anywhere in the United States to that recipient; kidneys with lesser mismatches are used locally because the damage suffered by the kidney during the "cold ischemia" time required for the long-distance shipment outweighs the benefits of better HLA matching.

Approximately 10% to 20% of patients waiting for transplant have antibodies against 80% or more of a panel of all possible HLA genotypes. These patients have a "high panel reactivity" or PRA. These antibodies arise in patients who have previously rejected kidney transplants within 1 year of transplantation, received numerous blood transfusions, or borne several children. If a patient has antibodies against the HLA antigens of the donor kidney, the transplant will be destroyed shortly after transplantation. Thus, patients with a high PRA cannot receive transplants from 80% of the population and often wait many years longer than the average patient before obtaining a transplant. The UNOS algorithm gives these patients an advantage when an appropriate cadaver kidney does become available. Even when laboratory testing indicates that patients with a high PRA do not have antibodies against a cadaver kidney (negative cross-match), there is still an increased likelihood of rejection. Many transplant centers prefer a better HLA match and perform special cross-match tests (such as flow cytometry or B-cell cross-matches) for these high-risk patients to improve outcomes.

The UNOS algorithm also takes other factors into account. For example, patients with uncommon HLA genotypes would be disadvantaged by an algorithm that placed too great an emphasis on matching HLA genotypes of the donor and recipient. Therefore, the algorithm gives some consideration to patients solely based on the time they have waited for a transplant.

Although patients are waiting for their cadaver transplant, they may develop new, active medical problems, such as severe infection, myocardial disease, or gastrointestinal bleeding. There is no evidence that earlier transplantation prevents these complications. The primary physician should keep the transplant center informed about any new medical problems and resolve any treatable illnesses so that the patient is ready for transplantation when the organ finally becomes available.

MANAGEMENT EARLY AFTER TRANSPLANTATION

During the first 2 months after transplantation, the most common complications center around dysfunction of the renal allograft, the recent surgery, and medications. Most infections involve conventional pathogens at this phase after transplantation.

Several electrolyte abnormalities are common early after transplantation. Hyperkalemia is associated with cyclosporin A or tacrolimus and can occur in patients with excellent serum creatinine and therapeutic serum levels of drug. Dangerous hyperkalemia can occur with dietary indiscretion and the use of nonsteroidal anti-inflammatory agents, β-blockers, and angiotensin-converting enzyme (ACE) inhibitors. Hypophosphatemia may require treatment with phosphate supplements. Hypercalcemia can result from hyperparathyroidism associated with the uremic state before transplantation; it is usually mild and remits spontaneously. Some patients with type I diabetes mellitus receive combined kidney–pancreas transplants. If the exocrine pancreas is drained into the bladder, these patients may develop profound hypovolemia and acidosis owing to the losses of bicarbonate and sodium in the exocrine pancreatic secretions into

the bladder. These losses should be prevented by ingestion of sodium and bicarbonate.

Although immunosuppressive protocols vary among transplant centers, most patients receive a regimen of prednisone, cyclosporin A, and mycophenolate mofetil. To reduce the adverse effects of these agents, their dosages are tapered gradually, which may allow the development of acute rejection. Rejection occurs in about 20% to 30% of transplant recipients, and the highest incidence is during the first several weeks after transplantation. Successful treatment depends on expeditious diagnosis, often by renal biopsy. This invasive diagnostic procedure should be performed only after the diagnoses in Table 166.1 have been excluded by following the approach shown in Figure 166.1.

Inadequate salt and fluid intake is a common cause of allograft dysfunction because transplant recipients are trained to limit their salt and fluid intake during dialysis. In addition, after the ischemic insult of transplantation, the kidney is unable to conserve salt and water optimally. After diarrhea, vomiting, or sweating, hypovolemia may occur. The serum creatinine level improves quickly after salt and water are replenished by the oral or intravenous route.

Anatomical problems can be detected by ultrasonography or renal flow scans of the allograft. Lymphoceles may occur because the lymphatic system is disrupted during the transplantation surgery. A diagnostic tap may be necessary to exclude the more uncommon diagnoses of urinoma (the creatinine level of the fluid should be high), hemorrhage, or abscess. In addition to routine bacteriologic cultures, the specimen should be cultured for fungi, *Mycobacterium tuberculosis,* and atypical mycobacteria. Lymphoceles frequently reaccumulate after a diagnostic tap. If

TABLE 166.1.	COMMON CAUSES OF EARLY TRANSPLANT DYSFUNCTION

Decreased effective arterial blood volume
    Inadequate volume replacement
    Congestive heart failure
    Myocardial ischemia
    Excessive antihypertensive medications
    Postoperative hemorrhage
Anatomical problems
    Bladder dysfunction, particularly in diabetics
    Obstructive lymphocele or hematoma
    Ureteral obstruction
    Urine leak
    Vascular embolism/thrombosis
Drug nephrotoxicity
    Cyclosporin A
    Antibiotics
    Nonsteroidal anti-inflammatory drugs
    Angiotensin-converting enzyme inhibitors
    Other
Infection
    Urinary tract infection
    Sepsis
    Cytomegalovirus
Acute tubular necrosis
Acute rejection
Recurrent or de novo renal disease

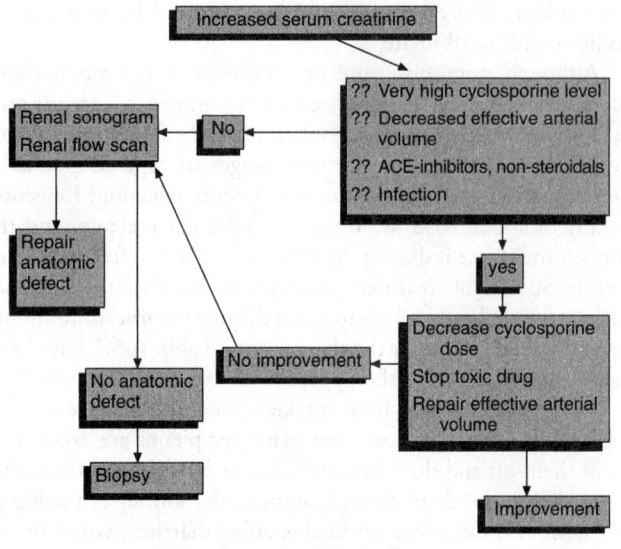

Complete algorithm rapidly

FIGURE 166.1. A simplified approach for renal allograft dysfunction during the early phase after transplantation. *ACE,* angiotensin-converting enzyme.

the lymphocele does not compromise allograft function by obstructing the ureter or blood vessels, it usually resolves spontaneously over months without treatment. If the lymphocele does obstruct the allograft ureter or blood vessels, chronic catheter drainage or surgical drainage into the peritoneal cavity may be necessary. These invasive procedures may be performed best at the transplant center by experienced surgeons and radiologists. Bladder dysfunction is another common cause of allograft dysfunction, particularly in patients with diabetes, who may develop neurogenic distention of the bladder. Other, less common, anatomical problems are listed in Table 166.1.

The renal allograft often is sensitive to nonsteroidal antiinflammatory agents and ACE inhibitors during the first weeks after transplantation. The serum creatinine level should return to baseline rapidly after these agents are withdrawn. The use of a combination of trimethoprim and sulfamethoxazole (Bactrim) is recommended by many transplant centers to prevent *Pneumocystis* and urinary tract infections. These agents may cause a rise in creatinine but not in blood urea nitrogen.

After these conditions have been excluded, three other complications must be considered: acute tubular necrosis in the allograft, nephrotoxicity due to either cyclosporin A or tacrolimus, and acute rejection. A biopsy may be necessary to differentiate these conditions. The allograft may fail to achieve a normal serum creatinine level because of acute tubular necrosis. This injury results from ischemia occurring in the donor kidney during organ procurement and storage and during the surgery.

Cyclosporin A is the mainstay of most immunosuppressive regimens. However, cyclosporin A itself causes renal dysfunction. It can be difficult to distinguish allograft dysfunction caused by cyclosporin A nephrotoxicity from that caused by rejection. Although high blood or serum levels of cyclosporin A often are associated with nephrotoxicity, rejection occasionally occurs in patients with high levels, and toxicity sometimes occurs

in patients with low levels. Oliguria, fever, graft tenderness, or more than 50% elevation of the serum creatinine level suggest rejection. If the cyclosporin A level is markedly elevated and none of these findings is present, it may be appropriate to decrease the cyclosporin A dosage and observe the patient for 24 to 48 hours. If a favorable response does not occur, biopsy may be necessary. Rarely, cyclosporin A and tacrolimus are associated with a hemolytic uremic syndrome that may respond to decreasing or discontinuing these agents.

Several points deserve emphasis. Successful treatment of acute rejection requires early diagnosis. The diagnostic and therapeutic maneuvers outlined herein are usually completed within 24 to 48 hours. In patients receiving cyclosporin A, rejection generally occurs without fever and allograft tenderness. Most often, the only finding is an elevated serum creatinine level detected during a routine clinic visit. The presence of fever may indicate infection or rejection, particularly if localized findings of pneumonia, urinary tract infection, or sore throat are absent. Finally, reducing the cyclosporin A or tacrolimus dosage to treat nephrotoxicity may result in drug levels that are too low to prevent rejection. Careful follow-up is necessary whenever the immunosuppressive regimen is changed.

The diagnosis of acute rejection is made by allograft biopsy in the setting of deteriorating allograft function. The biopsy, treatment, and prognosis of the different types of acute rejection are discussed in the section on the allograft biopsy.

■ MANAGEMENT OF LATE POST-TRANSPLANTATION COMPLICATIONS

RENAL ALLOGRAFT FUNCTION

Late deterioration in renal function may result from factors unique to transplantation or from diseases common to all kidneys. Acute transplant rejection is rare in the late post-transplantation period unless the immunosuppressive regimen has been recently tapered to reduce side effects or the patient has been noncompliant. The most common cause of late allograft loss is chronic allograft nephropathy. This manifests as a slow, progressive rise in the serum creatinine. The precise mechanisms responsible for chronic allograft nephropathy are unknown. Many authors divide its causes into alloantigen-dependent and alloantigen-independent causes. Alloantigen-dependent causes include chronic rejection; however, chronic rejection is not known to respond to currently available immunosuppressive agents. Previous episodes of acute rejection increase the risk for subsequent chronic rejection. Alloantigen-independent causes include chronic cyclosporin A toxicity, the maladaptive response to nephrons lost during the transplantation procedure or previous rejections, insufficient nephron mass due to transplanting small or aged kidneys into large recipients, hypertension, and hyperlipidemia. Anatomical problems such as renal artery stenosis or obstruction also can appear long after transplantation.

Treatment of chronic allograft nephropathy is problematic because its cause is not understood. However, the patient and allograft may benefit from aggressive treatment of hyperlipidemia and blood pressure, as discussed in the text that follows, and from optimal doses of cyclosporin A or tacrolimus.

CARDIOVASCULAR DISEASE

Cardiovascular disease is the leading cause of death among renal transplant recipients. Risk factors are pretransplantation ischemic heart disease, diabetes, male gender, hypertension, smoking, hypercholesterolemia, older age, and high cumulative doses of corticosteroids. Disease of the native kidneys, suboptimal allograft function, preexisting hypertension, cyclosporin A, and corticosteroids all can contribute to hypertension. Allograft artery stenosis is rare given the use of modern surgical techniques. Calcium channel blockers may offer some protection against cyclosporin A–induced afferent arteriolar vasoconstriction. Diuretics are effective, but volume contraction should be avoided. ACE inhibitors may be effective but may cause an acute deterioration of the glomerular filtration rate, particularly if renal allograft artery stenosis is present. These agents also are associated with hyperkalemia and are avoided early after transplantation in some centers. Impaired renal function, the nephrotic syndrome, diabetes, obesity, and both cyclosporin A and corticosteroids increase the risk for hyperlipidemia. Treatment of hypercholesterolemia may require HMG-CoA reductase inhibitors (statin drugs). Patients should be observed closely after the initiation of HMG-CoA reductase inhibitors because rhabdomyolysis can occur when they are given in combination with cyclosporin A. Resin binders such as cholestyramine may prevent the absorption of cyclosporin A and should be given more than 2 hours after the cyclosporin A dose, if at all.

INFECTION

Recipients of renal transplants are susceptible to more infections than affect the general population. Furthermore, they differ from other persons in their increased susceptibility to opportunistic infections and in the greater severity and more subtle physical findings of their illnesses. During the early post-transplantation period, conventional pathogens cause pneumonia, urinary tract infections, and catheter and wound infections. Most opportunistic infections occur following the first month after transplantation. Pathogens include herpesviruses, *Candida* and other fungi, *M. tuberculosis,* atypical mycobacteria, and parasites. Dysphagia can indicate a fungal or viral esophagitis, and endoscopy may be indicated.

Candida growth limited to the oral pharynx is common and responds to oral nystatin. Persistent diarrhea should prompt an investigation for parasites or invasive cytomegalovirus (CMV) colitis. Headache may indicate the presence of *Listeria,* cryptococcal meningitis, or lymphoma. "Cold" swelling of the joints or skin should prompt a consideration of fungal or atypical mycobacterial infection. Immunosuppression plus preexisting peripheral vascular disease and neuropathy predispose patients with diabetes to osteomyelitis and amputation of their extremities. These patients must be instructed carefully in the proper care of their feet and hands to prevent this complication.

CMV infection is common, and many transplant recipients who are not ill shed virus into their urine and other secretions.

Occasionally, CMV causes disease. Patients with CMV infection may present with a mild illness with fever, leukopenia, thrombocytopenia, and small elevations in liver function test results, or they may have a severe disease with pneumonitis, gastrointestinal ulcerations, and a high mortality rate. Rapid diagnosis involves the use of polymerase chain reaction or monoclonal antibodies against viral proteins expressed on the surfaces of infected cells. CMV disease predisposes to superinfection with other pathogens and has been associated with graft dysfunction and, possibly, rejection. Transmission of CMV by the donor kidney into a recipient not previously immunized against CMV may predispose the recipient to severe disease. Patients receiving antilymphocyte antibodies to treat rejection also are at high risk. Some studies indicate that severe CMV disease can be prevented in high-risk patients by high-dose acyclovir, ganciclovir, or CMV hyperimmune immunoglobulin. Established CMV disease is treated with ganciclovir or foscarnet.

Pneumonia is the leading cause of death secondary to infection in transplant recipients. In addition to conventional pathogens, organisms such as *Pneumocystis carinii, Nocardia,* and *M. tuberculosis* must be considered. An aggressive diagnostic approach is necessary to guide therapy effectively. Many transplant centers recommend prophylactic therapy with a combination of trimethoprim and sulfamethoxazole to prevent *P. carinii* pneumonia.

MALIGNANCY

Renal transplant recipients are at higher risk than the general population for some malignancies. The most common are skin cancers; these are common in white patients with significant sun exposure. Squamous cell carcinomas are more common than basal cell carcinomas and may be aggressive and metastasize earlier than in immunocompetent persons. Post-transplantation lymphoproliferative disease can occur after intensive immunosuppressive therapy. It usually involves B lymphocytes and is extranodal. The most common locations are the central nervous system, the renal allograft, and the gastrointestinal tract. Epstein–Barr virus often is found in the abnormal B lymphocytes. Kaposi's sarcoma is more common in transplant recipients, can manifest as mucocutaneous lesions, and may progress to visceral involvement. Hepatobiliary tumors and anogenital cancers also are more common.

LIVER DISEASE

Chronic infections with hepatitis B or C virus are a leading cause of long-term morbidity and mortality in the transplant population. Transplant recipients who have evidence of active hepatitis B viral replication at the time of transplantation are at high risk for cirrhosis and ESRD. Patients with chronic hepatitis may have mild elevations in their transaminase levels and progress silently to cirrhosis. Reduction of immunosuppressive therapy and administration of interferon-α have been used to treat chronic hepatitis, with variable results.

BONE DISEASE

Patients with ESRD have renal osteodystrophy and osteomalacia. Patients with successful renal transplants also experience significant morbidity secondary to bone disease. Progressive osteopenia is a common problem in many renal transplant recipients who are taking corticosteroids. Osteonecrosis usually affects the femoral head in adults and can lead to significant pain and impaired mobility. Magnetic resonance imaging aids in the early diagnosis of hip osteonecrosis. Total hip arthroplasty is occasionally required. Hypercalcemia due to hyperparathyroidism may complicate administration of calcium and vitamin D supplements. Some patients may benefit from oral bicarbonate to treat any metabolic acidosis caused by cyclosporin A or tacrolimus or by any renal insufficiency.

POST-TRANSPLANTATION ERYTHROCYTOSIS

Post-transplantation erythrocytosis is self-limited, occasionally requires phlebotomy, and generally responds to the inclusion of ACE inhibitors in the hypotensive regimen. Affected patients should be screened for other causes of erythrocytosis, such as pulmonary disease and polycythemia vera. In addition, the native kidneys should be imaged. Patients with ESRD develop acquired cystic disease of the kidneys, which may undergo malignant transformation to renal cell carcinoma.

■ INTERPRETATION OF THE TRANSPLANT BIOPSY

The interpretation of the renal allograft biopsy has been standardized by the Banff 97 working classification. This classification results from a multicenter collaborative effort and multiple revisions since 1991. Parts of this classification are summarized in Table 166.2.

Two types of acute allograft rejection are mediated predominantly by antibodies. Immediate or hyperacute rejection occurs shortly after the blood supply to the allograft is established. The kidney becomes dusky and cyanotic immediately, and there is no urine output. By light microscopy, neutrophils and platelets are found in the glomeruli, arterioles, small arteries, and peritubular capillaries. These lesions often result in cortical necrosis.

TABLE 166.2.	COMMON BIOPSY FINDINGS IN PATIENTS WITH RENAL ALLOGRAFT DYSFUNCTION

Banff 97 Classification	Prognosis After Treatment
Antibody-mediated rejection	
Immediate (hyperacute)	Very poor
Delayed (accelerated acute)	
Acute rejection	
Type I: interstitial inflammation, tubulitis, no arteritis	Good
Type II: intimal arteritis	Fair
Type III: transmural arteritis	Poor
Chronic/sclerosing allograft nephropathy	Long-term, poor

Preformed antibodies in the recipient against the donor HLA molecules are responsible for this form of rejection. Hyperacute rejection is rare because modern cross-match techniques usually detect these antibodies in the recipient before transplantation, and the kidney is not allocated to that patient. Immediate nephrectomy is necessary when this form of rejection occurs. Delayed antibody-mediated (or accelerated acute) rejections occur in the first weeks after transplantation. Often, the patient had a high PRA before transplantation. Rejection mediated predominantly by antibodies has a very poor prognosis. By light microscopy, antibody-mediated rejection is differentiated from acute rejection by the type of inflammatory cells (neutrophils and platelets *versus* mononuclear cells).

Acute rejection is divided by Banff 97 into three major types. In type I, there is a mononuclear inflammation of the interstitium and tubules. The prognosis after therapy with high-dose corticosteroids is good. In type II acute rejection, there is also mononuclear inflammation involving the arterial intima. The prognosis after therapy with high-dose corticosteroids or polyclonal or monoclonal anti–T-cell antibodies is fair. (Agents used to treat rejection are discussed in the following text). In type III rejection, the endarteritis of mononuclear cells is more severe and involves not only the intima but the entire arterial wall, which may be necrotic. The prognosis of this lesion is poor.

CYCLOSPORIN A NEPHROTOXICITY

Acute cyclosporin A or tacrolimus nephrotoxicity usually has no definitive pathologic findings and is associated with an improvement in allograft function after the doses of these drugs are decreased. Previous reports indicate that isometric tubular vacuoles occurred with much higher doses of cyclosporin A than are commonly used today. Rarely, there may be glomerular thrombi, which are associated with a hemolytic uremic syndrome. Chronic cyclosporin A toxicity is associated with characteristic apoptosis of the medial smooth muscle cells of arterioles and small arteries; these cells are replaced by nodular protein deposits. In addition, there may be interstitial fibrosis, glomerular sclerosis, and tubular atrophy common to chronic allograft nephropathy.

■ IMMUNOSUPPRESSIVE AGENTS

Different immunosuppressive agents, detailed below, are used at different times after transplantation:

■ To prevent rejection, many protocols use low-dose corticosteroids and either cyclosporin A or tacrolimus. In addition, these protocols may include either azathioprine or mycophenolate mofetil.
■ To treat rejection, high-dose corticosteroids, polyclonal anti-lymphocyte antibodies, or monoclonal antibodies to the CD3 ε molecule on T cells are used.
■ In addition, during the days immediately after transplantation, some centers use agents that are otherwise used to treat rejections, or monoclonal antibodies against the interleukin-2 receptor α chain.

Several immunosuppressive regimens are available. In general, the primary physician should follow the transplant center's protocol and consult the center if adjustments are necessary.

CYCLOSPORIN A AND TACROLIMUS

Cyclosporin A and tacrolimus (FK506) are generally used to prevent rejection. They have many similarities in their actions and side effects. The active intracellular forms are the drug bound to intracellular proteins called *immunophilins*. The drug–immunophilin complex prevents the dephosphorylation of the nuclear factor of activated T cells and its translocation into the nucleus, where it would activate lymphokine gene transcription. Many drugs affect the pharmacokinetics of cyclosporin A. For example, the antifungal agents, fluconazole and ketoconazole, can increase cyclosporin A levels sufficiently to cause acute renal failure if appropriate dosage adjustments are not made. Rifampin, dilantin, and phenobarbital dramatically decrease cyclosporin A levels such that rejection can occur unless the cyclosporin A dosage is adjusted appropriately. Common side effects of cyclosporin A and tacrolimus are hepatotoxicity, neurotoxicity, hyperlipidemia, hirsutism, and gingival hyperplasia. Tacrolimus and cyclosporin A have similar nephrotoxicity. Tacrolimus causes more hyperglycemia and neurotoxicity, but less hirsutism, gingival hyperplasia, and hyperlipidemia. The different preparations of cyclosporin A have different pharmacokinetics, and patients must be observed carefully for rejection and toxicity if they are switched from one preparation to another.

CORTICOSTEROIDS

Corticosteroids continue to play an important role in many immunosuppressive regimens. They are used in combination with cyclosporin A or azathioprine to prevent allograft rejection. High doses of corticosteroids may reverse acute rejection and are also used immediately after transplantation. Corticosteroids inhibit inflammation by inhibiting the production of tumor necrosis factor-α, interleukin-1, eicosanoids, and adhesion molecules. Finally, some data suggest a role for corticosteroids in preventing transcription of interleukin-2.

Corticosteroids have many side effects, including infections, hypertension, glucose intolerance, obesity, cosmetic changes, bone loss, growth retardation in children, cataracts, gastrointestinal disturbances (pancreatitis, ulcers), and psychiatric disturbances. Dosages should be minimized.

AZATHIOPRINE

Azathioprine is used to prevent rejection. It is converted in red blood cells to 6-mercaptopurine, which is metabolized into thioinosinic acid. This molecule interferes with the synthesis of purines, especially adenosine nucleotides. The side effects of azathioprine are bone marrow suppression, infection, malignancy, and hepatotoxicity. Although gout is common in transplant recipients, allopurinol should not be used in patients receiving azathioprine. Allopurinol interferes with the metabolism of azathioprine, and severe leukopenia may result.

MYCOPHENOLATE MOFETIL

Mycophenolate mofetil is metabolized to mycophenolic acid. Like azathioprine, mycophenolate mofetil inhibits purine synthesis. However, it inhibits the enzyme inosine monophosphate dehydrogenase. This enzyme is required for the de novo synthesis of guanosine nucleotides, which are important for the proliferation of lymphocytes and the production of adhesion molecules. The main side effects of this agent are nausea, vomiting, diarrhea, and bone marrow suppression.

POLYCLONAL ANTIBODIES

Polyclonal antilymphocyte antibodies are an effective treatment for acute rejection and are also used by some transplant centers immediately after transplantation surgery, particularly when there is post-transplant acute tubular necrosis and the allograft is susceptible to cyclosporin A nephrotoxicity. There are major differences in the recommended doses of the various approved preparations. Common side effects are fever, leukopenia, and thrombocytopenia. Serum sickness and anaphylaxis can occur. An increased incidence of infection and lymphoma has been observed in some patients.

MUROMONOAB-CD3 (OKT3)

Muromonoab-CD3 (OKT3) is a mouse monoclonal antibody against the ϵ chain of the CD3 complex of the T-cell receptor. It is more effective than corticosteroids in the treatment of first rejection episodes and is also effective in cases of corticosteroid-resistant rejection. In addition, muromonoab-CD3 can be used immediately after transplantation as induction therapy to delay the introduction of cyclosporin A and avoid an additional nephrotoxic insult in the early post-transplantation period. The administration of muromonoab-CD3 may precipitate a first-dose reaction. This ranges from fever, headache, and diarrhea to life-threatening pulmonary edema secondary to increased capillary permeability. To ameliorate the latter, patients should be at their "dry weight" before administering the first dose. Aseptic meningitis can occur early in the course. An increased risk of infection and lymphoma has been observed in some patients after therapy with muromonoab-CD3. Because it is a murine product, some patients form antimouse antibodies, which may interfere with the action of the drug.

BASILIXIMAB AND DACLIZUMAB

Basiliximab and daclizumab (anti–interleukin-2 receptor) are monoclonal antibodies that are genetically engineered to contain the antigen-binding sites of murine antibodies placed into the framework of human immunoglobulin. Thus, the first-dose response seen with muromonoab-CD3 is ameliorated, and the patient does not make antibodies against these agents. Basiliximab and daclizumab both bind to the α chain of the interleukin-2 receptor. The α chain is found only on activated T cells. Blocking this receptor decreases further activation of these cells and thus decreases the likelihood of rejection. These antibodies should be started before the transplantation surgery. At this time, they are not used for treatment of rejection.

KIDNEY TRANSPLANT DONORS

In the United States, about one fourth of all kidney transplantations involve living donors, both blood relatives and spouses. The main benefit of living related donor kidney transplantation is better short- and long-term allograft survival. Donors should have two normal kidneys as confirmed by anatomical and functional studies. They should be free of any medical problems and emotionally and intellectually able to understand the preoperative evaluation and kidney donation process. The perioperative mortality risk to the carefully selected donor is extremely low (0.03% to 0.6%), and significant perioperative morbidity is seen in less than 2% of cases. Long-term follow-up of kidney donors has revealed no evidence of progressive loss of renal function when compared with control patients. Hypertension also is no more common than in control patients. A higher incidence of proteinuria has been reported in some series. Life expectancy is not affected by kidney donation.

Cadaveric renal transplantation is the only option available for most transplant candidates with ESRD. Cadaver donors used in transplantation have suffered brain death most frequently secondary to head injuries, central nervous system vascular events, localized brain tumors, or severe cerebral anoxia. As the number of patients awaiting renal transplantation continues to increase (more than 40,000), the criteria for donor acceptability have been revised. Nevertheless, certain conditions, such as extremes of age, most infections and malignancies, underlying advanced medical illnesses, and renal diseases or dysfunction, preclude the use of cadavers as donors. A history of behavior in the donor that may result in a high risk for AIDS or hepatitis and technical or logistical aspects that result in prolonged ischemia time for the kidney also are considered relative contraindications.

BIBLIOGRAPHY

Colvin RB. Renal transplant pathology. In: Jennette JC, Olson JL, Schwartz MM, et al, eds. *Heptinstall's pathology of the kidney*, fifth ed. Philadelphia: Lippincott-Raven, 1998:1409–1540.

Danovitch GM. *Handbook of kidney transplantation*. Boston: Little, Brown, 1996.

Fishman JA, Rubin RH. Infection in organ-transplant recipients. *N Engl J Med* 1998;338:1741–1751.

Held PJ, Kahan BD, Hunsicker LG, et al. The impact of HLA mismatches on the survival of first cadaveric kidney transplants. *N Engl J Med* 1994; 331:765–770.

Kasiske BL and the Patient Care & Education Committee of the American Society of Transplant Physicians. The evaluation of renal transplant candidates: clinical practice guidelines. *J Am Soc Nephrol* 1995;6:1–34.

Kasiske BL and the Ad Hoc Clinical Practice Guidelines Subcommittee of the Patient Care and Education Committee of the American Society of Transplant Physicians. *J Am Soc Nephrol* 1996;7:2288–2313.

Kasiske BL and the Patient Care & Education Committee of the American Society of Transplant Physicians. Recommendations for the outpatient surveillance of renal transplant recipients (in press).

Norman DJ, Suki WN. *Primer on transplantation*. Thorofare, NJ: American Society of Transplant Physicians, 1998.

Racusen LC, Solez K, Colvin RB, et al. The Banff 97 working classification of renal allograft pathology. *Kidney Int* 1999;55:713–723.

Terasaki PI, Cecka JM, Gjertson DW, Takemoto S. High survival rates of kidney transplants from spousal and living unrelated donors. *N Engl J Med* 1995;333:333–336.

Kelley's Textbook of Internal Medicine, fourth edition. Edited by H. David Humes. Lippincott Williams & Wilkins, Philadelphia © 2000.

CHAPTER

167

ADJUSTMENT OF DRUG DOSAGE IN PATIENTS WITH RENAL INSUFFICIENCY

SUZANNE K. SWAN

Normal renal function is required for the metabolism and elimination of many pharmacologic agents from the body. Likewise, pharmacologically active metabolites of many drugs depend on the kidney for removal from the body. Many compounds, whether excreted by renal or nonrenal means, exert toxic effects in the setting of reduced renal function. Renal function often declines with advanced age, and the increase in adverse drug reactions in geriatric populations is attributable, in part, to drug accumulation by the kidney. In this chapter, basic pharmacologic principles are reviewed and applied to the clinical setting of renal insufficiency. Guidelines for dosage adjustments appear in tabular form. However, clinicians should not rely heavily on dosing tables or nomograms when treating patients with impaired renal function. Rather, they should maintain a heightened awareness of the pharmacologic alterations that occur in this setting while closely monitoring their patients' clinical courses to help guide dosimetry.

PHARMACOKINETICS

Pharmacokinetic factors can be altered by renal insufficiency (Table 167.1). Drug absorption can be affected by gastrointestinal dysfunction and the concurrent medications often used in the setting of renal failure. For example, uremia-induced vomiting,

TABLE 167.1.	PHARMACOKINETIC FACTORS AFFECTED BY RENAL INSUFFICIENCY
Absorption	
Volume of distribution	
Protein binding	
Biotransformation (metabolism)	

delayed gastric emptying, and decreased intestinal motility may contribute to decreased drug absorption. In addition, the concurrent ingestion of phosphate binders, both aluminum- and calcium-containing, can lead to the formation of insoluble compounds with drugs such as ferrous sulfate or tetracycline, blocking absorption. Bowel wall edema, often encountered in congestive heart failure and hypoalbuminemic states such as nephrosis or cirrhosis, also can slow drug absorption.

The volume of distribution can be altered in the setting of renal failure, but not in a predictable manner. The volume of distribution for a specific drug is derived by dividing the total amount of drug in the body by its plasma concentration. It does not refer to a specific anatomical compartment; instead, it is used mathematically to determine the dose of a drug necessary to achieve a desired concentration. Volume contraction tends to decrease and ascites and edematous states tend to increase the volume of distribution for hydrophilic compounds such as aminoglycosides. As a general rule, serum or plasma concentrations of a drug correlate inversely with its volume of distribution.

Changes in the protein binding of various pharmacologic agents can be expected with significant renal impairment. The organic acids and bases that accumulate in azotemic patients can displace acidic and basic drugs, respectively, from their binding proteins. This, in turn, results in a greater proportion of unbound or "active" drug being available at tissue sites.

Finally, the biotransformation or metabolism of pharmacologic agents can be altered in patients with renal insufficiency. Although renal impairment usually has little effect on drug metabolism by hepatic mechanisms, exceptions do exist. For example, more rapid oxidation of phenytoin, digitoxin, and propranolol has been reported. This may be attributable to the observation that a larger proportion of a given compound can exist in its unbound or free form in uremic serum. Conversely, quinidine is oxidized more slowly in patients with renal insufficiency. Acetylation, hydrolysis, and reduction also may be impaired in such patients. In addition, agents with active metabolites that are dependent on renal excretion may require dosage adjustment even when parent compound pharmacokinetics are unaffected by the presence of renal impairment.

◼ DOSING REGIMENS

When the glomerular filtration rate (GFR) is reduced, the elimination of many compounds and pharmacologically active metabolites falls proportionately. In other words, the prolongation of a drug's elimination half-life (the time required for the plasma drug concentration to be reduced by half) is proportional to the reduction in the GFR. Although drug accumulation can occur at any level of renal insufficiency, such adverse events are relatively uncommon when the GFR remains greater than 40 to 50 mL per minute. If dosage restrictions are excessive because of fears of toxicity, inadequate therapy may result. This is particularly important when prescribing anticonvulsants, antiarrhythmics, and antibiotics. Patients with impaired renal function must be maintained within a narrow therapeutic window, avoiding drug accumulation and toxicity on one hand and subtherapeutic dosing on the other. A stepwise process can aid clinicians in estab-

TABLE 167.2.	APPROACH TO DOSING REGIMENS IN RENAL INSUFFICIENCY

1. Perform initial assessment
2. Calculate creatinine clearance
3. Choose a loading dose
4. Choose a maintenance dose
5. Monitor therapy

lishing drug dosage regimens for patients with renal insufficiency (Table 167.2).

INITIAL ASSESSMENT

A history and physical examination constitute the first step in assessing dosimetry in a patient with renal impairment. Previous drug toxicity or intolerance should be ascertained if possible. The patient's current medication list (both prescription and non-prescription formulations) must be reviewed to identify potential drug interactions and nephrotoxins. Physical findings indicate the patient's volume status, provide the height and weight data used in calculating ideal body mass, and reveal whether extrarenal disease states such as hepatic dysfunction exist, which require additional dosage adjustment.

CALCULATING CREATININE CLEARANCE

An estimate of renal function is necessary because the elimination rate of most drugs is related to the GFR. Because blood urea nitrogen and serum creatinine (SCr) values themselves are insensitive measures of renal function, creatinine clearance (C_{cr}) conventionally is used to estimate the GFR. The Cockcroft-Gault formula for calculating Ccr is convenient and appropriate for clinical use because age and lean body mass correlate with C_{cr}:

$$C_{cr} = \frac{[140 - \text{age}] \, [\text{lean body weight in kg}]}{[72] \, [\text{SCr in mg/dL}]}$$

In women, 85% of this calculated value should be used. The lean body weight in men is about 50 kg plus 2.3 kg per inch of height over 5 feet, whereas in women it is 45.5 kg plus the same height adjustment factor. These calculations assume that renal function is stable. In the setting of oliguric acute renal failure, SCr values should be ignored and a C_{cr} of less than 10 mL per minute used for drug dosing adjustment. Likewise, an SCr value that falls within the "normal" range cannot be presumed to reflect normal renal function. Particularly in elderly or debilitated patients with reduced muscle mass, this erroneous assumption frequently results in overdose and adverse drug reactions.

CHOOSING A LOADING DOSE

In general, rapid achievement of therapeutic, steady-state drug concentrations is sought. A standard loading dose should be administered to patients with renal insufficiency to achieve therapeutic drug levels rapidly. The loading dose can be calculated by the following formula:

$$\text{Loading dose} = \text{Vd} \times \text{IBW} \times \text{Cp}$$

where Vd is the volume of distribution (in liters per kilogram), IBW is the ideal body weight (in kilograms), and Cp is the desired plasma concentration (in milligrams per liter).

If a drug with a particularly narrow therapeutic window is being used, such as digoxin or an aminoglycoside, and its volume of distribution is predictably low in uremic or volume-contracted patients, reducing the loading dose by 25% to 30% may be prudent.

CHOOSING A MAINTENANCE DOSE

After a loading dose has been administered, a maintenance regimen in patients with renal insufficiency can be determined by one of two methods. One approach involves lengthening the dosing interval as follows:

$$\text{Dosing interval} = \frac{\text{normal } C_{cr}}{\text{patient's } C_{cr}} \times \text{normal interval}$$

Alternatively, the dose can be reduced but administered at the standard interval:

$$\text{Dose} = \frac{\text{patient's } C_{cr}}{\text{normal } C_{cr}} \times \text{normal dose}$$

The varying interval method can lead to periods of inadequate drug concentrations, whereas the varying dose method allows for more constant drug levels but risks toxicity resulting from higher trough levels. The interval method is preferred for aminoglycosides, which demonstrate concentration-dependent bactericidal properties, whereas the dosage method is more appropriate for anticonvulsant or antiarrhythmic agents. A combination of these methods also can be used to individualize pharmacotherapy.

MONITORING DRUG LEVELS

Measurement of plasma drug concentrations is helpful in assessing the success of a dosing regimen, especially in patients with multiple problems. It is imperative that the relations among the measured level, efficacy, and toxicity of the drug are known and that attention is paid to the details of sample collections. For example, an aminoglycoside drug level within the therapeutic range would indicate major drug accumulation and toxicity if the sample were obtained 48 hours after the last dose. In general, blood levels should be determined after three or four doses to ensure steady-state conditions. For some drugs, maximum and minimum concentrations are useful. Peak levels obtained after the rapid distribution phase are helpful in ensuring that an adequate concentration to provide efficacy has been reached. The trough concentration measured before the next dose is an index of drug elimination during the dosing interval; it measures drug accumulation in the setting of renal failure. Because therapeutic drug monitoring is expensive, it should be limited to pharmaco-

logic agents with narrow therapeutic windows and those with pharmacologic actions that are difficult to assess clinically.

For patients receiving hemodialysis, peritoneal dialysis, or continuous renal replacement therapy, attention must be paid to dose scheduling and the need for supplemental doses to replace lost body stores. Dialysis clearance of a drug depends primarily on its molecular weight, degree of protein binding, and water solubility. As protein binding increases, dialysis clearance decreases. The smaller and more hydrophilic the compound, the more drug is removed during a dialysis treatment. In general, scheduled doses should be given after dialysis if possible. In addition, if a drug undergoes significant dialyzer clearance, supplemental doses should be given after each dialysis treatment or, in the case of continuous therapy, dosage reductions may need to be limited given the continuous clearance provided.

■ NARCOTIC PAIN MANAGEMENT

The number of options are limited for narcotic pain management in patients with renal impairment because of an increase in adverse reactions to this class of compounds as well as excessive sedation and respiratory depression. This is due in part to active metabolites of the parent compound as well as to prolonged elimination half-lives of both parent drug and metabolite. In addition, many narcotic agents are not readily removed from the body by dialysis, thus compounding the problem of prolonged or increased sedation. Unfortunately, little data regarding the use of narcotics in patients with reduced renal function exist in the literature.

One approach is to categorize narcotic use in renal failure on the basis of relative safety recommendations (Fig. 167.1). For example, meperidine is a narcotic that should be avoided in patients with renal failure. Meperidine is metabolized to normeperidine, which has little analgesic effect but has an excitatory effect on the central nervous system. Normeperidine is also eliminated from the body by the kidneys. Thus, in patients with renal

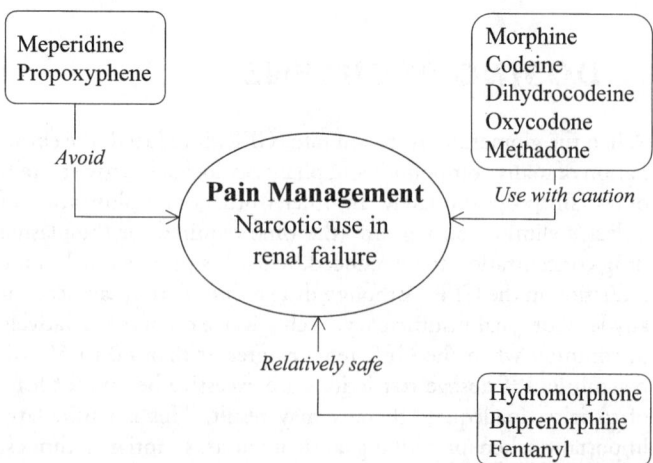

FIGURE 167.1. Flow chart showing the relative safety of narcotic therapy for pain management in patients with end-stage renal disease. (Adapted from Lewis MJ, Swan SK. A potpourri of drug idiosyncrasies in ESRD. *Semin Dial* 1997;10:278–281.)

TABLE 167.3. DOSAGE ADJUSTMENTS FOR PATIENTS WITH RENAL FAILURE

Drug	Elimination & Metabolism	Method	Adjustment for Renal Failure GFR (mL/min)		Supplement for Dialysis	Toxicity Notes
			10–50	<10		
Antimicrobial Agents						
AMINOGLYCOSIDE ANTIBIOTICS						
Ototoxic, nephrotoxic; rare respiratory paralysis; serum levels to ensure efficacy. Posthemodialysis dose is 2/3 of normal maintenance dose or 1/2 of loading dose. 50% to 90% absorbed from peritoneum. Volume of distribution larger with obesity, edema, or ascites.						
Gentamicin	Renal	D, I or 100% q24–48h	30–70 q12h or 100% q48–72h	20–30 q24–48h	Yes (He, P)	Concurrent penicillins may result in subtherapeutic blood levels
Netilmicin	Renal	D, I or 100% q24–48h	20–60 q12h or 100% q48–72h	10–20 q24–48h	Yes (He, P)	May be less ototoxic than other members of this class
Tobramycin	Renal	D, I or 100% q24–48h	30–70 q12h or 100% q48–72h	20–30 q24–48h	Yes (He, P)	Concurrent penicillins may result in subtherapeutic blood levels
CEPHALOSPORIN ANTIBIOTICS						
Rare allergic interstitial nephritis; absorbed well when administered intraperitoneally; may cause bleeding in patients with renal failure from impaired prothrombin biosynthesis						
Cefamandole	Renal	I	6–8	12	Yes (He, P)	
Cefazolin	Renal	I	12	24–48	Yes (He, P)	
Cefoxitin	Renal	I	8–12	24–48	Yes (He, P)	May raise creatinine by interference with assay
Ceftazidime	Renal	I	24–48	48	Yes (He, P)	
Ceftriaxone	Renal (hepatic)	I	Unchanged	12–24	Yes (He, P)	Monitor levels in dialysis patients
Cefuroxime	Renal	I	8–12	24	Yes (He) No (P)	
Cephalothin	Renal	I	6–8	12	Yes (He) No (P)	
MISCELLANEOUS ANTIBACTERIAL ANTIBIOTICS						
Aztreonam	Renal	D	50–75	25	Yes (He) No (P)	
Chloramphenicol	Hepatic	D	Unchanged	Unchanged	No (He, P)	Half-life markedly prolonged with combined liver and kidney dysfunction
Ciprofloxacin	Renal (hepatic)	D	50–75	50%	Yes (He, P)	Poorly absorbed with antacids or phosphate binders; IV dose 1/3 of oral dose
Clindamycin	Hepatic		Unchanged	Unchanged	No (He, P)	
Erythromycin	Hepatic		Unchanged	50–75	No (He, P)	
Imipenem	Renal	D	50	25	Yes (He)	Ototoxic in high doses in ESRD
Fleroxacin	Renal (hepatic)	D	50–75	50	Yes (He, P)	Seizures in ESRD
Lomefloxacin	Renal	D	50–75	50	No (He, P)	

TABLE 167.3. *Continued*

Drug	Elimination & Metabolism	Method	Adjustment for Renal Failure GFR (mL/min)		Supplement for Dialysis	Toxicity Notes
			10–50	<10		
Metronidazole	Hepatic	D	Unchanged	50	Yes (He)	Rare drug-induced lupus
Norfloxacin	Hepatic	I	12–24	Avoid	No (He)	
Spectinomycin	Renal	I	Unchanged	Unchanged	No (He, P)	
Sulfamethoxazole	Renal	I	18	24	Yes (He)	Antifolate activity; can cause hyperkalemia
Trimethoprim	Renal	I	18	24	Yes (He)	
Vancomycin	Renal	I or D, I	1g q24–96	1g q4–7 d	No (He, P)	Ototoxic at serum level >50 mg/mL, 40% to 70% absorbed from peritoneum; monitor levels.
PENICILLINS						
Agents in this group cause allergic interstitial nephritis; seizures and coagulopathy at high blood levels.						
Amoxicillin	Renal	I	8–12	12–24	Yes (He, P)	
Ampicillin	Renal	I	6–12	12–24	Yes (He, P)	
Dicloxacillin	Renal		Unchanged	Unchanged	No (He, P)	
Mezlocillin	Renal		6–8	8	No (He, P)	3 mEq Na⁺/g
Nafcillin	Hepatic (renal)		Unchanged	Unchanged	No (He, P)	1.9 mEq Na⁺/g; Coagulopathy
Penicillin G	Renal	D	75	25–50	Yes (He)	Potassium salt has 1.7 mEq/million units; convulsions, false-positive urine protein reactions; 6 million units/d upper limit dose in ESRD
Piperacillin	Renal	I	6–8	8	Yes (He)	1.9 mEq Na⁺/g
Ticarcillin	Renal	D, I	1–2 g q8h	1–2 g q12h	Yes (He), No (P)	5.2 mEq Na⁺/g
TETRACYCLINE ANTIBIOTICS						
Agents in this group potentiate acidosis, raise blood urea nitrogen and phosphorus, and increase catabolism. Use of tetracycline should be avoided in renal failure.						
Doxycycline	Hepatic		Unchanged	Unchanged	No (He, P)	Group drug of choice for decreased renal function, not antianabolic
ANTIFUNGAL ANTIBIOTICS						
Amphotericin	Nonrenal		24	24–36	No (He, P)	Nephrotoxic, renal tubular acidosis, hypokalemia, nephrogenic diabetes insipidus; toxicity lessened by saline loading; colloidal dispersion form less nephrotoxic
Fluconazole	Renal	D	Unchanged	50–100	Yes (He)	May increase blood cyclosporine levels
Flucytosine	Renal	I	12–24	24	Yes (He, P)	Hepatic dysfunction, marrow suppression more common in azotemic patients
Ketoconazole	Hepatic		Unchanged	Unchanged	No (He, P)	
ANTIMYCOBACTERIAL ANTIBIOTICS						
Ethambutol	Renal	I	24–36	48	Yes (He)	Decreased visual acuity, peripheral neuritis
Isoniazid	Hepatic	D	Unchanged	Unchanged	Yes (He)	Supplement with 50–100 mg pyridoxine qd to prevent neurotoxicity
Pyrazinamide	Hepatic	D	100%	50–100%	Dose 24° prior to HD	Can precipitate gout
Rifampin	Hepatic	D	50–100	50	No (He)	May cause acute interstitial nephritis, potassium wasting, and renal tubular defects; biologically active metabolite, desacetyl-rifampicin
ANTIVIRAL ANTIBIOTICS						
Acyclovir	Renal	D, I	5 mg/kg q12–24h	2.5 mg/kg q24h	Yes (He)	Neurotoxic in patients with renal failure; may cause acute renal failure if injected rapidly, intravenously
Amantadine	Renal	I	48–72	168 (7 days)	No (He, P)	
Didanosine	Hepatic (renal)	D, I	24	50% q24h	Yes (He), No (P)	
Foscarnet	Renal	D	15 mg/kg q8h	6 mg/kg q8h	Yes (He), No (P)	Nephrotoxic; seizures, hypokalemia, hypocalcemia, hypomagnesemia
Ganciclovir	Renal	I	24–48	48–96	Yes (He), No (P)	Marrow toxicity

Antihypertensive Agents (In This Group, Blood Pressure Is the Best Guide to Dose and Interval)

ADRENERGIC AND CARDIOVASCULAR MODULATORS

Drug	Route (Hepatic/Renal)	Method			Dialysis	Toxicity / Comments
Clonidine	Hepatic (renal)		Unchanged	Unchanged	No (He, P)	Rebound hypertension if drug is abruptly withdrawn; tricyclic antidepressants decrease efficacy; potentiates central nervous system depressant effects of alcohol, sedatives
Methyldopa	Hepatic (renal)	I	8–12	12–24	Yes (He)	Orthostatic hypotension; retroperitoneal fibrosis; prolonged hypotension caused by retained active metabolites; interference with serum creatinine measurement
Prazosin	Hepatic		Unchanged	Unchanged	No (He, P)	May produce profound hypotension with first dose
Terazosin	Hepatic		Unchanged	Unchanged	?	

ANGIOTENSIN-CONVERTING ENZYME INHIBITORS

Hypotensive effect magnified by natriuretic agents or sodium depletion; hyperkalemia; acute renal dysfunction with bilateral or transplant renal artery stenosis. Dry cough 5% to 10%.

Drug	Route	Method			Dialysis	Toxicity / Comments
Benazepril	Hepatic (renal)	D	75–100	25–50	Yes (He), No (P)	
Captopril	Renal (hepatic)	D, I	75 q12–18h	50 q24h	Yes (He), No (P)	Rare proteinuria, nephrotic syndrome, dysgeusia, granulocytopenia; can increase serum digoxin levels
Cilazapril	Renal (hepatic)	D	50	25–50	Yes (He)	
Enalapril	Renal (hepatic)	D	75–100	50	Yes (He), No (P)	Enalaprilat, the active moiety formed in liver
Lisinopril	Renal	D	50–75	25–50	Yes (He), No (P)	

AII RECEPTOR ANTAGONISTS

Losartan	Hepatic		Unchanged	Unchanged	?	Similar precautions as ACEI class

β-BLOCKERS

Drug	Route	Method			Dialysis	Toxicity / Comments
Atenolol	Renal	D, I	50 q48h	50 q96h	Yes (He), No (P)	Significant accumulation in ESRD
Labetalol	Hepatic		Unchanged	Unchanged	No (He, P)	
Metoprolol	Hepatic		Unchanged	Unchanged	Yes (He), No (P)	
Propranolol	Hepatic		Unchanged	Unchanged	No (He, P)	Metabolites may accumulate; increases bilirubin by assay interference; less frequent doses in some patients with ESRD; hypoglycemia reported in ESRD

CALCIUM BLOCKING AGENTS

Headache, flushing, and dizziness in patients with renal disease; may increase serum digoxin and cyclosporine levels.

Drug	Route	Method			Dialysis	Toxicity / Comments
Amlodipine	Hepatic		Unchanged	Unchanged	No (He, P)	
Diltiazem	Hepatic		Unchanged	Unchanged	No (He, P)	
Isradipine	Hepatic		Unchanged	Unchanged	No (He, P)	
Nifedipine	Hepatic		Unchanged	Unchanged	No (He, P)	Active metabolites; acute renal dysfunction reported
Nisoldipine	Hepatic		Unchanged	Unchanged	No (He, P)	Active metabolites; edema; acute renal dysfunction reported
Verapamil	Hepatic		Unchanged	Unchanged	No (He, P)	Active metabolites; acute renal dysfunction reported

CARDIAC GLYCOSIDES

Add to uremic gastrointestinal symptoms; serum levels guide to therapy; toxicity enhanced by dialysis potassium and magnesium removal.

Drug	Route	Method			Dialysis	Toxicity / Comments
Digitoxin	Hepatic (renal)	D	Unchanged	50–75	No (He, P)	Protein binding decreased by dialysis; volume of distribution reduced by uremia
Digoxin	Renal	D, I	25–75 q36h	10–25 q48h	No (He, P)	Radioimmunoassay may overestimate serum levels in uremia; clearance reduced by spironolactone, quinidine, verapamil; hypokalemia, hypomagnesemia enhance toxicity. Volume of distribution decreased in ESRD. Serum level 12 hours after first dose is best guide in ESRD.

TABLE 167.3. *Continued*

Drug	Elimination & Metabolism	Method	Adjustment for Renal Failure GFR (mL/min)		Supplement for Dialysis	Toxicity Notes
			10–50	<10		
ANTIARRHYTHMIC AGENTS						
Blood levels most often the best guide to therapy. Half-life may be prolonged in heart failure or with reduced hepatic blood flow.						
Adenosine	Hepatic		Unchanged	Unchanged	No (He, P)	
Amiodarone	Hepatic		100%	100%	No (He, P)	Hepatotoxicity. Thyroid dysfunction. Peripheral neuropathy. Pulmonary fibrosis. Active metabolite. Increased plasma digoxin. Increases cyclosporine levels
Bretylium	Renal	D	25%–50%	25%	No (He, P)	Hypotension. Active metabolites
Cibenzoline	Renal	D, I	100% q24h	66% q24h	No (He, P)	Urinary retention. Protein binding concentration dependent
Disopyramide	Renal	I	q12–24h	q24–40h	No (He, P)	Volume of distribution decreased in ESRD
Flecainide	Hepatic	D	100%	50%–75%	No (He, P)	Excretion enhanced in acid urine
Lidocaine	Hepatic	D	100%	100%	No (He, P)	
Mexiletine	Hepatic (renal)	D	100%	50%–75%	No (He, P)	Increased renal excretion in acid urine
Moricizine	Hepatic		100%	100%	No (He, P)	
N-acetyl-procainamide	Renal	D, I	50% q8–12h	25% q12–18h	Yes (He), No (P)	Hemofiltration useful in poisoning
Procainamide	Renal	I	50% q6–12h	q8–24h	No (He, P)	Half-life acetylator phenotype dependent. Active metabolite is N-acetyl-procainamide. Lupus-like syndrome. Hemofiltration useful in poisoning
Propafenone	Hepatic		100%	100%	No (He, P)	Half-life acetylator phenotype dependent
Quinidine	Hepatic (renal)	D	100%	75%	Yes (He), No (P)	Increased plasma levels of digoxin and digitoxin. Excretion enhanced in acid urine. Hemodialysis useful in poisoning
Tocainide	Hepatic (renal)	D	100%	50%	Yes (He), No (P)	Excretion decreased in alkaline urine

Analgesics

Drug	Elimination & Metabolism	Method	Adjustment for Renal Failure GFR (mL/min)		Supplement for Dialysis	Toxicity Notes
			10–50	<10		
NARCOTICS AND NARCOTIC ANTAGONISTS						
Alfentanil	Hepatic		100%	100%	NA	
Butorphanol	Hepatic	D	75%	50%	?	
Codeine	Hepatic	D	75%	50%	?	
Fentanyl	Hepatic	D	75%	50%	NA	
Meperidine (Demerol)	Hepatic	D	75%	50%	No (He, P)	Normeperidine, an active metabolite, accumulates in ESRD and may cause seizures; protein binding reduced in ESRD; 20% to 25% excreted unchanged in acidic urine
Methadone	Hepatic	D	100%	50%–75%	No (He, P)	Fecal elimination increased in ESRD
Morphine	Hepatic	D	75%	50%	No (He)	Increased sensitivity to drug effect in ESRD
Naloxone	Hepatic		100%	100%	NA	
Pentazocine (Talwin)	Hepatic	D	75%	50%	No (He)	
Propoxyphene (Darvon)	Hepatic	D	100%	Avoid	No (He, P)	Active metabolite norpropoxyphene accumulates in ESRD
Sufentanil	Hepatic		100%	100%	NA	
NONNARCOTIC DRUGS						
Acetaminophen	Hepatic	I	q6h	q8h	No (He, P)	Nephrotoxic in overdoses because of a reactive alkylating metabolite. Metabolites may accumulate in ESRD; drug is major metabolite of phenacetin
Acetylsalicylic acid (aspirin)	Hepatic (renal)	I	q4–6h	Avoid	Yes (He), No (P)	Nephrotoxic in high doses; may decrease GFR when renal blood flow is prostaglandin dependent; excretion enhanced in alkaline urine; may add to uremic gastrointestinal and hematologic symptoms; protein binding reduced in ESRD; 5% excreted unchanged in acidic urine, 85% in alkaline urine

Sedatives, Hypnotics, Drugs Used in Psychiatry

Drug	Route	Method			Dialysis	Comments
ANTIDEPRESSANTS						
Amoxapine (Asendin)	Hepatic		100%	100%	?	Half-life of active metabolite is 30 hours
Bupropion	Hepatic		100%	100%	?	Half-life of active metabolite is 21 hours
Fluoxetine	Hepatic		100%	100%	?	Half-life of active metabolite is 7–9 days
Maprotiline	Hepatic		100%	100%	?	
Sertraline	Hepatic	D	Unknown	Unknown	?	Active metabolite
Trazodone	Renal	D	Unknown	Unknown	?	
BARBITURATES — May cause excessive sedation, increase osteomalacia in ESRD. Charcoal hemoperfusion and hemodialysis more effective than peritoneal dialysis for overdose.						
Hexobarbital	Hepatic		100%	100%	No (He)	
Pentobarbital	Hepatic		100%	100%	No (He)	Protein binding decreased in ESRD
Phenobarbital	Hepatic (renal)	I	q8-12h	q12-16h	Yes (He, P)	Up to 50% unchanged drug excreted in urine with alkaline diuresis
Secobarbital	Hepatic		100%	100%	No (He, P)	
Thiopental	Hepatic	D	100%	75%	NA	
BENZODIAZEPINES — May cause excessive sedation and encephalopathy in ESRD						
Alprazolam	Hepatic		100%	100%	No (He)	Active metabolite
Chlorazepate (Tranxene)	Hepatic (renal)		100%	100%	?	Active metabolite
Chlordiazepoxide (Librium)	Hepatic	D	100%	50%	No (He)	
Clonazepam (Klonopin)	Hepatic		100%	100%	No (He)	
Diazepam (Valium)	Hepatic		100%	100%	No (He)	Active metabolite; protein binding decreased in ESRD; volume of distribution increased in ESRD
Estazolam	Hepatic		100%	100%	?	
Flurazepam (Dalmane)	Hepatic		100%	100%	No (He)	Active metabolite
Lorazepam (Ativan)	Hepatic		100%	100%	No (He)	
Midazolam	Hepatic	D	100%	50%	NA	Protein binding decreased in ESRD
Oxazepam (Serax)	Hepatic		100%	100%	No (He)	Glucuronide metabolite increased in ESRD; protein binding decreased and volume of distribution increased in ESRD
Temazepam (Restoril)	Hepatic		100%	100%	No (He)	Protein binding decreased in renal disease
Triazolam (Halcion)	Hepatic		100%	100%	No (He, P)	Protein binding correlates with α_a-acid glycoprotein concentration
BENZODIAZEPINE ANTAGONIST						
Flumazenil	Hepatic		100%	100%	No (He)	
PHENOTHIAZINES — Anticholinergic. Urinary retention. Orthostatic hypotension. Confusion. Extrapyramidal symptoms.						
Chlorpromazine	Hepatic		100%	100%	No (He, P)	Plasma levels rebound after oral dose
Promethazine	Hepatic		100%	100%	?	Excessive sedation
SELECTIVE SEROTONIN REUPTAKE INHIBITORS (SSRIs)						
Fluoxetine	Hepatic		Unchanged	Unchanged	?	
Paroxetine	Hepatic		50–75%	50%	?	
Sertraline	Hepatic		Unchanged	Unchanged	?	
TRICYCLIC ANTIDEPRESSANTS — Anticholinergic. Urinary retention. Orthostatic hypotension. Confusion. Excessive sedation.						
Amitriptyline	Hepatic		100%	100%	No (He, P)	Reduce dose in elderly
Desipramine	Hepatic		100%	100%	No (He, P)	Active metabolites
Doxepin	Hepatic		100%	100%	No (He, P)	Protein binding decreased in ESRD
Imipramine	Hepatic		100%	100%	No (He, P)	Active metabolites
Nortriptyline	Hepatic		100%	100%	No (He, P)	
Protriptyline	Hepatic		100%	100%	No (He, P)	

TABLE 167.3. Continued

Drug	Elimination & Metabolism	Method	Adjustment for Renal Failure GFR (mL/min) 10–50	<10	Supplement for Dialysis	Toxicity Notes
Miscellaneous Agents						
ANTICOAGULANTS						
Alteplase	Unknown		100%	100%	?	(Tissue-type plasminogen activator [tPa])
Anistreplase	Unknown		100%	100%	?	
Dipyridamole	Unknown		100%	100%	?	
Heparin	Nonrenal Nonhepatic		100%	100%	No (He, P)	Half-life increases with dose
Low–molecular-weight heparin	Unknown	D	100%	50%	?	
Iloprost	Unknown	D	100%	50%	?	
Indobufen	Unknown	D	50%	25%	?	
Streptokinase	Nonrenal Nonhepatic		100%	100%	NA	
Sulfinpyrazone	Renal	D	100%	Avoid	No (He, P)	Occasional acute renal failure; uricosuric effect at low GFR
Solutroban	Renal	D	30%	10%	?	
Ticlopidine	Hepatic		100%	100%	?	
Tranexamic acid	Renal	D	25%	10%	?	
Urokinase	Unknown Nonrenal	D	Unknown	Unknown	?	
Warfarin	Nonhepatic		100%	100%	No (He, P)	Monitor prothrombin time; decreased protein binding in uremia
ANTICONVULSANTS Monitor serum levels						
Carbamazepine	Hepatic		100%	100%	No (He, P)	May cause inappropriate antidiuretic hormone secretion
Ethosuximide	Hepatic		100%	100%	No (He)	
Gabapentin	Renal	D, I	300 mg q12–24h	300 mg QOD	Yes (He), No (P)	
Lamotrigine	Hepatic		100%	100%	?	
Oxcarbazepine	Hepatic		100%	100%	?	
Phenytoin	Hepatic		100%	100%	No (He, P)	Measure free levels; protein binding decreased and distribution volume increased in renal failure; may cause folate deficiency; interstitial nephritis; saturable metabolism
Primidone	Renal	I	q8–12h	q12–24h	Yes (He)	Partially converted to phenobarbital and other metabolites with long half-life; excessive sedation; nystagmus, folate deficiency
Sodium valproate	Hepatic		100%	100%	No (He, P)	Decreased protein binding in uremia; concurrent phenytoin, phenobarbital, and primidone shorten half-life
Trimethadione	Hepatic	I	q8–12h	q12–24h	?	Active metabolites with long half-life; nephrotic syndrome
H₂ ANTAGONISTS						
Cimetidine	Renal	D	50%	25%	No (He, P)	Increases serum creatinine and decreases creatinine clearance by inhibition of tubular creatinine secretion; mental confusion in patients with renal or hepatic disease; acute renal failure reported (applies to cimetidine only)
Famotidine	Renal	D	25%	10%	No (He, P)	
Nizatidine	Renal	D	50%	25%	?	
Ranitidine	Renal	D	50%	25%	Yes (He), No (P)	

ESRD, end-stage renal disease; GFR, glomerular filtration rate; He, hemodialysis; P, peritoneal dialysis; D, dosage reduction method wherein the percentage of the standard dose to be given at the usual interval is listed; I, interval extension method wherein the number of hours between the standard dose is listed.

failure, seizure activity may result because of the accumulation of normeperidine. Despite the relative safety categorizations of different compounds in Figure 167.1, *no narcotic agent is truly considered safe in the presence of renal failure.* Thus, close monitoring of this patient population during narcotic analgesic therapy to detect the earliest sign of drug accumulation in addition to minimizing drug exposure to this class of compounds is imperative.

GUIDELINES FOR DRUG DOSAGE IN RENAL FAILURE

The preceding text has presented the theoretical aspects of dosimetry adjustments that may be required in the presence of renal insufficiency. Table 167.3 provides rough guidelines and recommendations on which to base therapy for drugs commonly used in clinical practice. The prescribing physician is responsible for assessing individual patient factors; the data presented are simply starting points. Individualization of therapy is mandatory, and adjustments in these guidelines should be made as frequently as clinically necessary. More complete compilations are available but are beyond the scope of this book (see Bibliography).

BIBLIOGRAPHY

Aronoff GA, Berns JS, Brier ME, et al. *Drug prescribing in renal failure: dosing guidelines for adults,* fourth ed. Philadelphia: American College of Physicians-American Society of Internal Medicine, 1999.

Bennett WM, Aronoff GA, Golper TA, et al. *Drug prescribing in renal failure: dosing guidelines for adults.* Philadelphia: American College of Physicians, 1994.

Cockcroft DW, Gault MH. Prediction of creatinine clearance from serum creatinine. *Nephron* 1976;16:31–41.

Lewis MJ, Swan SK. A potpourri of drug idiosyncrasies in ESRD. *Semin Dial* 1997;10:278–281.

Swan SK. Diuretic strategies in patients with renal failure. *Drugs* 1994;48: 380–385.

Swan SK, Bennett WM. The use of cardiovascular drugs in chronic renal failure. In: Parfrey PS, Harnett JD, eds. *Cardiac dysfunction in chronic uremia.* Boston: Kluwer Academic Publishers, 1992:267–282.

Turnheim K. Pitfalls of pharmacokinetic dosage guidelines in renal insufficiency. *Eur J Clin Pharmacol* 1991;40:87–93.

Kelley's Textbook of Internal Medicine, fourth edition. Edited by H. David Humes.
Lippincott Williams & Wilkins, Philadelphia © 2000.

5

RHEUMATOLOGIC, ALLERGIC, AND DERMATOLOGIC DISEASES

Edward D. Harris, Jr., Editor

APPROACH TO THE PATIENT WITH RHEUMATOLOGIC AND ALLERGIC DISORDERS

APPROACH TO THE PATIENT WITH MUSCULOSKELETAL COMPLAINTS

ERIC L. RADIN

Musculoskeletal complaints constitute the second most common problem seen in a general medical practice, just after respiratory problems. This chapter presents an overall approach to these patients; the presentation and treatment of specific clinical entities are discussed in subsequent chapters.

GUIDELINES FOR THE GENERAL EVALUATION OF PATIENTS WITH MUSCULOSKELETAL COMPLAINTS

APPRECIATION OF THE MUSCULOSKELETAL SYSTEM AS AN INTERACTIVE ORGAN COMPLEX

The musculoskeletal system is composed of several interrelated organs: bones, joints, muscles, and a complex neuromuscular control system. As in all organ systems, aberrations of one organ sequentially affect the other organs. For example, the clinical presentation of muscle weakness about the shoulder may arise from a pathologic condition within the muscles themselves, the shoulder joint, the proximal humerus, the upper scapula, the distal clavicle, or nerves, plexus, cervical roots, or central nervous system. Problems in one muscle affect nearby organs. As an example, hip abductor weakness affects the hip joint, the proximal femur, and the gait. Atrophy from disuse of the muscles of

a limb causes osteopenia (loss of mineral) in trabecular bone in that limb and eventually leads to cortical bone depletion. A displaced fracture of a bone causes painful muscle spasms in the muscles spanning the fracture. The point is that to make the correct diagnosis, the physician cannot focus only on the first sign of a clinical abnormality, but must perform a complete organ system evaluation.

DIFFERENTIATION OF THE MECHANICAL, METABOLIC, AND INFLAMMATORY CAUSES OF MUSCULOSKELETAL PAIN

The initial underlying cause of most musculoskeletal problems is metabolic, inflammatory, or mechanical in nature. The biologic processes within cells of the musculoskeletal organs can be controlled by feedback mechanisms from their matrix, acting through the cells, and by deformation or damage of the cells themselves. A primary mechanical abnormality can be expected to create secondary metabolic and inflammatory changes. The reverse is true as well. Metabolic and inflammatory changes in a musculoskeletal tissue, because they alter the material properties of that tissue, have secondary mechanical effects. For example, a patient may have an inflammatory joint effusion, but the underlying cause may be mechanical. A mechanical abnormality of a joint (e.g., loss of part of its articular load-bearing surface) creates secondary local inflammatory and metabolic reactions in the joint. These secondary symptoms may be the patient's chief complaint. On the other hand, a patient may have inflammation of a muscle tendon sheath, eventually leading to rupture of the tendon and resulting in loss of joint motion, but the underlying cause is inflammatory.

Mechanical aberrations in musculoskeletal tissues can be the result of congenital, developmental, traumatic, inflammatory, or metabolic circumstances (Table 168.1). Although mechanical problems often involve trauma, the initiating injury need not be a memorable incident. It can be the end product of small, repetitive, unrecognized incidents that accumulate over years. The cumulative damage to connective tissue eventually overwhelms the body's capacity to heal. Hitting a tree while skiing and breaking a leg would be a memorable incident. Attrition

TABLE 168.1.	GENERAL TYPES OF MUSCULOSKELETAL CONDITIONS	
Mechanical	**Inflammatory**	**Metabolic**
Osteoarthrosis (C/DH)	Rheumatoid arthritis (I)	Gout (H/D)
Congenital dysplasia of the hip (C)	Systemic disseminated lupus erythematosus (I)	Ochronosis (H/D)
Slipped capital femoral epiphysis (D/T)	Dermatomyositis (I)	Gaucher's disease (H/D)
After staphylococcal pyarthrosis (INF)	Polyarteritis nodosa (I)	Paget's disease (H/D)
Stress fracture (T)	Scleroderma (I)	Type II collagen defect and
Evident fracture of bone (T)	Infectious arthritis (Inf)	osteogenesis imperfecta (H)
Epiphyseal dysplasia (H)	Ankylosing spondylitis (H/I)	Osteoporosis (H/D)
	Muscular dystrophies (H/C/I)	Osteomalacia (D)
		Drug-induced: myopathies, bone diseases (D)

C, congenital; D, development; H, hereditary; I, immunologic and inflammatory; INF, infectious; T, traumatic. These distinctions may not be absolute.

and eventual tearing of the rotator cuff conjoin tendon of the shoulder in late middle age is an example of small, unrecognized cumulative trauma. Small repetitive trauma, accumulating over years, can cause bursitis, tendinitis, tendon rupture, osteoarthrosis, stress fracture, and other "overuse" syndromes.

EFFECTS OF CUMULATIVE INJURY

Cumulative microdamage has become accepted only recently as a cause of significant musculoskeletal problems. As the use of computers in the workplace has grown, employees who work at keyboards all day have complained of chronic wrist pain. In most of these cases, there are no objective findings. Similar keyboards, used by typists for years, generated few complaints.

Nevertheless, cumulative microdamage can occur and has been implicated in the cause of idiopathic osteoarthrosis. Data indicate that microfractures of the subchondral calcified bed are increased significantly in osteoarthrosis. The healing of these microfractures leads to remodeling and thickening of the calcified bed at the expense of its overlying articular cartilage. The process of healing this damage thickens the subchondral plate at the expense of the articular cartilage. It thins. This leads to progressive deterioration of the cartilaginous weight-bearing surface. Osteoarthrosis is not related to hard work; the condition affects many sedentary persons. Laboratory tests have revealed that impulsive loads of short duration are most deleterious to connective tissue matrix. The mystery of how this damage could occur in normal joints was solved when it was shown that about one-third of the population lacks the appropriate natural neuromuscular mechanisms that prevent repetitive peak loads from being applied to joints in the course of normal activities. These sharp, transient forces occur in just a few thousandths of a second, much too quickly to be seen by the naked eye or by conventional motion analysis techniques. For this reason, patients so affected are referred to as "microklutzes." They have a minor

aberration of neuromuscular control that cannot be observed by the human eye; such an aberration allows the heel to strike the ground during gait in less than .05 second, compared with a usually much longer time. The creation of microdamage is related less to the amount of the load and more to the speed and impact with which the load is applied. These findings have led to an entirely new way of thinking about this common and debilitating musculoskeletal problem that is responsible for most of the musculoskeletal disability in the industrialized world.

Metabolic conditions that affect the musculoskeletal system include Paget's disease, gout, postmenopausal status, osteoporosis, rickets, Gaucher's disease, dwarfism, gigantism, and hyperparathyroidism. Congenital, developmental, infectious, traumatic, and tumorous conditions can initiate secondary mechanical or inflammatory reactive processes. Inflammation can result from an uncontrollable and persistent immunologic response (e.g., rheumatoid arthritis), from articular cartilage breakdown in a joint (e.g., osteoarthrosis), or from an acute (e.g., pyarthrosis from staphylococcal septicemia) or chronic (e.g., low-grade joint prosthesis infection) infectious process (Table 168.1).

To cure any pathology, treatment of the primary cause and not just the secondary reactive processes is a more reliable approach. This is referred to as *causative therapy*. Treatment that is not directed at the initial cause of a condition addresses only its symptoms. The clinical problem is likely to persist or recur. For example, treating a primary mechanical joint problem such as osteoarthrosis with nonsteroidal anti-inflammatory drugs may provide symptomatic relief but will not positively affect the progression of the condition. Treating gout with nonsteroidal anti-inflammatory drugs will not change the persistent abnormality in uric acid metabolism, which will continue to cause the problem. Treating a knee joint that is deformed from rheumatoid involvement with realignment by osteotomy has no good rationale, because the underlying problem is inflammatory and will erode the surgical result.

Before causative therapy can be prescribed, it must be determined whether the cause of the patient's complaints is primarily mechanical, metabolic, or inflammatory. This can usually be accomplished mainly by obtaining and analyzing the history of the problem. By way of illustration of this, metabolic processes usually involve the whole body and are symmetric, chronic, and long-standing. Metabolic conditions commonly are hereditary, and a family history may be significant. The symptom constellation itself may be diagnosable. For example, Paget's disease of bone should be suspected from a history of localized, unremitting pain with slow progression, unrelated to position or activity.

To distinguish between inflammatory and mechanical pain, it is important to discover what aggravates the pain and what relieves it. Pain from both inflammatory and mechanical aberrations worsens with use. Mechanically generated pain improves at rest, whereas pain from inflammation tends to persist. The physician should inquire whether certain positions, movements, or activities reliably alleviate or aggravate the symptoms. Severe, chronic immunologic and inflammatory responses, such as rheumatoid arthritis, are global enough that a patient's activities may have little effect on the symptoms. Such joints are usually most comfortable when held in a position that maximizes the volume of the joint, reducing the tension in the joint's capsule and synovial membrane.

Pains from inflammatory conditions persist at rest and frequently are associated with joint stiffness after immobilization as a result of the associated edema that collects around the joint during rest. In contrast, pain from mechanically caused problems usually is relieved by rest, is better in bed, and often is least noticeable first thing in the morning. On physical examination, inflamed joints are swollen and diffusely tender. Mechanically damaged tissues usually are focally tender and not very warm.

Chronic inflammatory musculoskeletal problems that are not obviously infectious or metabolic usually involve immunopathologic pathways. Chronic inflammation can follow an injury that is slow to heal. Persistent inflammation of soft tissues that are in constant use, such as tendons and bursae, eventually can cause self-sustaining chronic inflammation and a proliferation of fibroblasts and macrophages that can lead to secondary mechanical problems, such as rupture of a tendon or a calcific deposit in a bursa.

The ability to move an injured part of the body after significant trauma does not exclude the possibility of fracture. Pain may not increase on use with an undisplaced impacted fracture. Radiographs are required to make this diagnosis, which should be suspected from the nature of the force involved and localized tenderness. Tendinitis and bursitis resulting from accumulated microtrauma are usually limited to a single structure.

The possibility of neoplasm must be included in the differential diagnosis, particularly when the patient's symptoms are localized and the physical signs do not fit the usual pattern for a musculoskeletal abnormality of mechanical or inflammatory origin. A history of symptom onset in association with trivial trauma is common in nontraumatic conditions. About 30% of patients with osteogenic sarcoma, a rapidly growing malignant bone tumor, report the onset of symptoms after trivial trauma. Fractures can result from trivial trauma to pathologically weakened bone; from infectious, congenital, or metabolic problems; or from metastatic cancer. If the trauma is inconsistent with the symptoms, the examiner must be suspicious of pathologically

involved structural tissues and cognizant that infection mimics tumorous or metabolic involvement of bone. Infection of bones and joints does not require a break in the skin.

■ LOCALIZATION OF THE PROBLEM TO A PARTICULAR ORGAN

Next, the physician must identify the structure (organ) involved. Locating the source of the problem is critical to the use of causative therapy. Pain of musculoskeletal origin actually may be generated in organs distal to the pathology. Pain can be referred to more distant regions because of the sensory distribution of the nerves that innervate the pathologically involved part. Failure to recognize referred pain is a major cause of misdiagnosis.

The physician should be able to isolate the structures involved through physical examination of the musculoskeletal system. A knowledge of surface anatomy is crucial, and an anatomy text is a useful adjunct in the examining room. For example, direct tenderness over the lateral malleolus of the ankle suggests a fracture, whereas tenderness just distal, anterior, or posterior to the lateral malleolus suggests a ligamentous sprain. Combined palpation and range-of-motion testing often are useful to differentiate tendon and ligamentous injuries. Pathologic condition of the hip with referred pain to the knee can be identified by putting the hip and knee, separately, through a full range of motion to determine which joint motion provokes the symptoms. Osteomyelitis of bone near a joint can be differentiated from pyarthrosis (infection in a joint) by precisely locating the tenderness and determining whether gentle motion of the joint aggravates the pain.

With an appropriate physical examination, differentiation of the pain's origin—from joints, bones, or soft tissues and muscles—should be possible. Imaging studies are helpful to confirm the diagnostic conclusions of the history and physical examination but should not be used as the primary means of diagnosis.

■ ORIGINS OF MUSCULOSKELETAL PAIN

Physicians often are inclined to use radiographs, computed tomography, magnetic resonance imaging, bone scanning, and other imaging procedures to screen patients with musculoskeletal complaints. They assume that the diagnosis can be made on the basis of these studies. Individual structures show up well. Harried practitioners often believe that such technology is a superb substitute for the history and physical examination. This philosophy has led to many therapeutic disasters.

Artifacts of normal aging are common and are difficult or impossible to visually differentiate from pathologic conditions. The pathophysiology of most musculoskeletal pain cannot be demonstrated by imaging. Musculoskeletal pain is caused by inflammation or swelling of periarticular soft tissues, by muscle spasm, or by increased interosseous venous pressure. None of this is visible on imaging studies. It takes 10 to 14 days for bone infection to become visible on radiographs. Joints with arthritis or arthrosis can appear normal on radiographs for years. Increased fluid in the joint (effusion) from synovitis can be seen on radiographs, but it is identified better in most joints by a careful physical examination. The correlation between musculoskeletal pain and radiographic images is poor.

Natural tissue remodeling occurs with aging. Some manifestations are bulging, thinning, and rupture of intervertebral disks; softening and fibrillation of articular cartilage; attrition of knee meniscal cartilages, soft tissue, and fat; and osteopenia and bony remodeling. These processes affect everyone and usually do not cause symptoms. Other changes seen on imaging may have caused symptoms at one time but are no longer painful; a previous pathologic condition leaves anatomical artifacts that are not associated with the patient's present symptoms. A diagnosis based solely on imaging studies can lead to misdirected therapy.

Similar difficulties are common when joint arthroscopy, particularly of the knee, is performed in the absence of an adequate history and physical examination, routine radiographs, and laboratory studies. Considerable arthroscopic surgery of the knee may be inappropriate, focusing on artifactual and age-related changes of articular cartilage and menisci that never have been or no longer are symptomatic. In some cases, arthroscopic surgical procedures work to the detriment of the patient, accelerating osteoarthrotic change.

To avoid diagnostic and therapeutic pitfalls, the findings from radiographic imaging and interventional procedures must be interpreted in context with the patient's complaints and physical examination. Before therapeutic intervention is attempted, all the data must be collected and must fit together pathophysiologically.

ARTHRITIS VERSUS ARTHROSIS

In evaluating joint complaints, arthritis and arthrosis must be differentiated if causative therapy is to be recommended. Arthritis is caused by inflammation of the synovium, the lining of the joint cavity. A general list of such problems appears in Table 168.1 and includes conditions resulting from infections, chronic immunologic responses, and metabolic abnormalities causing chemical irritations. Arthrosis is created by a mechanical problem of the joint, such as traumatic injury or cumulative microdamage. Inflammation of the synovium in arthrosis always results from intra-articular sulfated proteoglycan and articular cartilage and bony debris.

In early arthritis and arthrosis, no radiographic changes can be seen, and "baseline" radiography probably is of little benefit. Later in the inflammatory or degenerative process, radiography is associated with loss of cartilage space (joint-space narrowing) as the articular cartilage disappears. In arthritis, the bone surrounding a joint is osteopenic, and bony erosions associated with synovial inflammation are common. In arthrosis, the bones tend to be normal or more dense than normal. Subchondral bony sclerosis is evident, and osteophytes almost always are present.

In recommending causative therapy, arthrosis must not be

thought of as a primarily inflammatory condition, even though its symptoms (pain and joint stiffness) frequently result from the secondary synovial inflammation. The unfortunate term for this condition, *osteoarthritis,* suggests an inflammatory cause. For the purposes of causative therapy, it is best to think of the condition as *osteoarthrosis.*

A SYSTEMATIC APPROACH TO LOW BACK PAIN

The treatment of low back pain is a persistent problem in medical practice and is discussed in detail in Chapter 171. Low back pain can be acute and self-limiting or chronic and refractory. Causative therapy is difficult to apply because the diagnosis is so challenging. Psychogenic overlay is common, and entire professional groups have been organized to treat the symptoms without addressing the underlying cause. The results of the physical examination in such patients can be nonspecific and can change from day to day.

Healers of low back pain by manipulation usually can relieve the patient's symptoms temporarily. Spinal manipulation interrupts paraspinal muscle spasm, a common reason for pain. No data suggest that spinal manipulation "rearranges" any tissue. Spinal manipulation can effect a cure only when the problem is strictly muscle spasm. If there is a persistent underlying pathologic condition, such as spondylosis, osteoarthrosis, spinal instability, disk herniation, or neurapraxia, symptoms usually recur. Occasionally, spinal manipulation aggravates symptoms.

In evaluating patients with low back pain, two important determinations should be made. The first is whether the pain is primarily muscular in origin. Muscular pain results from muscle spasm and can be caused by a partially torn muscle, bone or joint pathologic lesion, or neurapraxia of the spinal roots. Ninety-five percent of all cases of acute low back pain are the result of pulled muscles. The muscles of the back are torn when they are contracted and the patient moves suddenly, stretching them. The symptoms of a spinal muscle tear can be acute and incapacitating. It is useful to think of the condition as a "charley horse" of the paraspinal muscles. It doesn't last more than a few days.

The diagnosis of a torn paraspinal muscle or muscles is made by a history and physical examination. Lifting of a heavy object usually is not the inciting factor. Rather, the most common onset is from reaching or bending to pick up a smaller object or a sudden motion in another direction, as when trying to keep a carried object from falling. The entire back goes into spasm. There is no localizing tenderness; the whole back is tender and the pain is incapacitating. These muscle tears are self-limited and improve within 1 or 2 weeks. Rest is not mandatory for healing.

After the possibility of a torn paraspinal muscle (i.e., acute low back strain) is ruled out, the physician must determine whether the back pain is mechanical or neurogenic in origin. Mechanical problems such as vertebral fracture can occur, particularly in postmenopausal women. The pain associated with this is acute, well localized, and associated with characteristic radiographic findings. In the case of a pathologic fracture (e.g., a vertebral body fracture with a metastasis from a lung tumor or a fracture in a thin malnourished woman with a long-standing malabsorption syndrome), the trauma may have been as mild as putting on underwear. In contrast, damage to intervertebral ligaments or dislocation of the spine requires high-velocity trauma, such as being thrown out of a car or off a horse.

Mechanically caused low back pain, from spondylosis or arthrosis of the intervertebral facet joints, is common in middle-aged and older persons. It is the most common cause of chronic low back pain with radiation to the lower extremities in males in these age groups. Sometimes there is no low back component to the pain. Spinal instability can result from congenital and developmental problems. Symptoms of claudication (pain and cramping in the buttocks or below that occurs during walking and is relieved by rest) imply stenosis of the spinal canal and frequently are arthrotic in cause. In such cases, arterial claudication of the lower extremities must be ruled out.

Neurogenic pain is associated with the clinical signs of neurapraxia: motor weakness, sensory loss, and reflex diminution. It is not appropriate to make a diagnosis of neurogenic pain on the basis of pain alone without these physical findings. Neither the nature of the pain (e.g., sharp, dull) nor its pattern of radiation differentiates reliably between mechanical and neurogenic causes. Acute ruptured disks are rare, but chronic ruptured disks are common and frequently asymptomatic. Bulging intervertebral disks are normal with aging. Magnetic resonance imaging evidence of an old ruptured disk in a patient with low back pain radiating to the lower extremities may be a false-positive finding. Treatment of persistent low back pain with surgical excision of previously ruptured disks in the absence of objective signs of neurapraxia usually is ineffective.

The cause of low back pain remains an enigma because the spine is buried within muscle, making it impossible to palpate each spinal component individually. It is difficult to determine which structure of the spinal complex is involved through physical examination. All that can be done is to isolate the spinal segment that is the source of the symptoms by localized tenderness. The history and physical examination should indicate whether the pain is mechanical or neurogenic in origin. Magnetic resonance imaging and computed tomography are capable of demonstrating the entire spinal and neurologic anatomy, but these findings must be consistent with the history and physical examination before a causative diagnosis can be made. Advanced imaging studies should be performed only after a presumptive diagnosis has been made, based on the history, physical examination, and x-rays.

Psychogenic overlay may potentiate musculoskeletal symptoms, especially because physical disability has become a socially acceptable way to hide from harsh reality. In the case of psychogenic musculoskeletal problems, complaints are vague and generalized, are unrelated to activity or time of day, and wax and wane unpredictably. The diagnosis is made by history in the absence of objective physical signs. It is unfortunate that costly advanced imaging techniques frequently are used to ensure that nothing has been overlooked. Instead, careful social histories should be obtained to elicit those factors in patients' lives that can precipitate such pain, often without their awareness. Primary care physicians see many such patients. The diagnosis should not be one of exclusion, but should be made on the basis of a consistent history and physical examination.

BIBLIOGRAPHY

Blaha JD, Radin EL. Arthritis and arthrosis. In: Radin EL, ed. *Orthopaedics for the medical student.* Philadelphia: JB Lippincott, 1987:93–112.

Eyring EJ, Murray WR. The effect of joint position on the pressure of intra-articular effusion. *J Bone Joint Surg* 1964;46A(6):1235–1241.

Frymoyer JW, Gordon SL, eds. *New perspectives on low back pain.* Park Ridge, IL: American Academy of Orthopaedic Surgeons, 1989.

Handler NM, Bunn MD, eds. *Occupational problems in medical practice.* New York: Lawrence Dellacorte, 1990.

Pauwels F. *Biomechanics of the normal and diseased hip: theoretical foundation, technique and results of treatment. An atlas.* (translated by Furlong RJ, Maquet P). New York: Springer-Verlag, 1976.

Radin EL, Burr DB, Fyhrie, et al. Characteristics of joint loading as it applies to osteoarthrosis. In: Mow VC, Ratcliffe A, Woo SY, eds. *Biomechanics of diarthrodial joints.* New York: Springer-Verlag, 1990:437.

Radin EL, Rose RM, Blaha JD, et al. *Practical biomechanics for the orthopaedic surgeon,* second ed. New York: Churchill Livingstone, 1992.

Sokoloff L. *The biology of degenerative joint disease.* Chicago: University of Chicago Press, 1969.

Wright V, Radin EL, eds. *Mechanics of human joints: physiology, pathophysiology and treatment.* New York: Marcel Dekker, 1993.

Kelley's Textbook of Internal Medicine, fourth edition. Edited by H. David Humes. Lippincott Williams & Wilkins, Philadelphia © 2000.

C H A P T E R

169

APPROACH TO THE PATIENT WITH PAIN IN ONE OR A FEW JOINTS

ALISA E. KOCH

APPROACH TO THE PATIENT AND PRESENTATION

Most patients with joint disorders present with symptoms of monarticular arthritis (pain and swelling of a single joint), which creates a diagnostic challenge for clinicians. Some of these disorders, such as septic arthritis, require immediate attention and possible hospitalization. The clinician is initially faced with the problem of localizing the pain to the joint itself or surrounding structures.

In contrast to what happens with arthritis in which pain can be elicited on active motion of the joint, patients with tendinitis or bursitis often present with local tenderness with active motion on one side of the joint. Pain of the biceps tendon, for instance, can be elicited by direct palpation of the tendon itself. Identification of a septic bursitis is particularly important, because it is critical not to introduce microorganisms into the joint by performing an arthrocentesis through the infected area.

Soft tissue infections can masquerade as arthritis. For instance, perirectal abscesses may be referred to the sacroiliac joint. Psoas abscesses may manifest as hip pain. Fever and the acute onset of symptoms with normal synovial fluid findings suggest nonarthritic processes. Computed tomography or magnetic resonance imaging may be helpful in diagnosing these conditions.

Bone pain results from involvement of the periosteum or marrow, which contains sensory nerves. Bone pain may result from fractures, malignancy, infiltrative processes, or new bone formation. Typically, bone pain is elicited by tenderness to palpation of the involved periosteum or pain on weight-bearing. Often, minimal pain is elicited while performing active range-of-motion exercises of a nearby joint. Radiographs of the involved areas may be helpful if the process is long-standing.

Neuropathic pain is due to irritation of a peripheral nerve and may radiate to a joint. Carpal tunnel syndrome, or compression of the median nerve, may radiate to the wrist or even to the elbow. Neuropathic pain often occurs at night and follows the distribution of the involved nerve. Percussion over the median nerve at the wrist may result in tingling in the nerve distribution (first four digits) in patients with carpal tunnel syndrome (Tinnel's sign). Generally, the distribution of the pain is not localized to the nearby joint. Nerve conduction velocities may be useful in distinguishing this type of pain.

Compartment syndromes can occur when locally increased pressure occurs in a closed muscle compartment and compromises vascular and neuromuscular function. These syndromes may arise with limb trauma, ischemia, and physical exertion. Typically, patients with compartment syndrome present with severe pain (particularly on stretch of the muscles in the compartment), muscle weakness, and altered sensation in the distribution of the nerves coursing through the compartment. These syndromes can occur in the thigh, buttocks, hand, forearm, and arm. Treatment is aimed at minimizing neurologic deficits and often involves surgical intervention.

LABORATORY STUDIES AND DIAGNOSTIC TESTS

After a thorough history and physical examination to determine the presence of monarticular arthritis, initial laboratory evaluation should include a complete blood with differential count, urinalysis, hepatic and renal function tests, and serum uric acid. If infection is likely and the patient is febrile, blood cultures should be obtained. The white count is often elevated, and a left shift is seen in the differential count in cases of septic arthritis. If the clinician suspects gonococcal arthritis, then genital, oral, anal, and blood cultures should be obtained because synovial fluid cultures for *Neisseria gonorrhoeae* are positive in less than 25% of cases. Hyperuricemia is suggestive of gout, but does not establish it. Similarly, normouricemia does not rule out gout. It is important for the patient to have normal or near-normal renal function if a nonsteroidal anti-inflammatory medication is prescribed, as in the case of pseudogout.

Perhaps the most useful test for a patient with joint pain is *synovial fluid aspiration,* with culture and crystal analysis. In nongonococcal bacterial arthritis, the synovial fluid cultures are positive in 95% of cases. These tests can generally be performed using a few drops of synovial fluid. If enough fluid is available, a white cell count should be obtained. Synovial fluid findings in some common causes of monarticular arthritis are found in Table 169.1. In addition to the white cell count, the percentage of neutrophils is high in those with acute inflammatory and septic forms of arthritis, but low in those with noninflammatory forms of arthritis. Synovial fluid glucose values are low in patients with inflammatory and septic forms of arthritis, but not in those with noninflammatory forms of arthritis. The more the sample resembles pus, the greater the urgency to determine whether infectious or crystalline disease is the cause of the effusion.

Radiographs are useful in helping establish the diagnosis of the cause of joint pain. Even if the radiographs are normal, the initial studies serve as a baseline for future examinations. Linear cartilage calcification can be seen in chondrocalcinosis, suggesting that pseudogout may be the diagnosis. Medial joint space narrowing of the knee is often seen in patients with osteoarthritis. Patients with osteochondritis dissecans may present with sclerotic lesions separated from the surrounding bone by a radiolucent line. Periarticular osteopenia, joint space narrowing, and marginal bony erosions may suggest an inflammatory process such as rheumatoid arthritis. Destructive bony changes may indicate a chronic infectious arthritis such as that seen with tuberculosis or fungal disease. Alternatively, tumors may result in bony destruction.

Radionuclide scans may be used to search for a hidden site of infection. In some instances, computed tomography or magnetic resonance imaging may be useful. In compartment syndromes, these tests may help establish the diagnosis. In mechanical injury, such as a meniscal tear of the knee, the latter examinations can indicate the site of damage, thus helping make the diagnosis.

If chronic destructive changes are present on x-ray or if the patient continues to have a recurrent hemarthrosis or undiagnosed condition, a synovial biopsy may be indicated. This biopsy may be performed blind, during an open surgical procedure, or through an arthroscope. Recently, office-based arthroscopy often replaces the need for an open surgical procedure. The synovial sample should be examined for routine histology and also sent for culture. A biopsy is often useful in diagnosing tumors as well as chronic fungal or tuberculous arthritis.

DIFFERENTIAL DIAGNOSIS

After the clinician has determined that the patient does not have a nonarticular process, he or she should ask several key questions.

Is the arthritis chronic or acute? Pain that occurs over minutes suggests an internal derangement, trauma, or fracture. *Is the arthritis truly monarticular?* It is important to rule out additional joint involvement, such as may occur in migratory polyarthralgias, since this may signal a noninfectious cause such as rheumatoid arthritis.

| TABLE 169.1. | SYNOVIAL FLUID FINDINGS IN SOME COMMON CAUSES OF MONOARTICULAR ARTHRITIS |

Condition	Gross Characteristics	Viscosity	WBC/mm	PMNs (%)	Glucose Concentration	Crystals
Noninflammatory arthritis						
Trauma	Clear to turbid, straw to red	High	<2000, many RBCs	<25	Normal	Negative
Osteoarthritis	Clear yellow	High	0–2000	<25	Normal	Negative
Inflammatory arthritis						
Pseudogout	Cloudy, yellow	Low	10,000–150,000	<50	Low	Positively birefringent crystals
Gout	Cloudy, yellow to milky white	Low	10,000–150,000	60–70	Low	Negatively birefringent crystals
Rheumatoid arthritis	Cloudy, yellow	Low	5,000–50,000	60–70	Low	Negative
Reiter's syndrome	Cloudy; yellow	Low	5,000–50,000	60	Low	Negative
Septic arthritis						
Tuberculosis arthritis	Turbid, purulent	Low	50,000–50,000	50–60	Very low	Negative
Bacterial arthritis[a]	Turbid, purulent	Low	10,000–150,000 (usually > 100,000)	75	Very low	Negative

[a] Synovial fluid cultures are positive; in gonococcal arthritis, 20% to 25% of the cultures are positive. *PMNs,* polymorphonuclear leukocytes (neutrophils); *RBC,* red blood cells; *WBC,* white blood cells.

Once the clinician has determined that the condition is indeed a monarticular arthritis, it is important to determine whether the arthritis is inflammatory or noninflammatory (Fig. 169.1). The American College of Rheumatology has recently proposed guidelines for the workup and therapy of monarticular arthritis. Often, the best way to determine this is to perform an arthrocentesis and synovial fluid analysis.

If the synovial white blood cell count is over 5,000 cells per cubic millimeter, one should suspect an inflammatory arthritis. Synovial fluid Gram stain and culture should be performed to rule out infection. Joint sepsis can lead to rapid destruction of cartilage and bone and can be the harbinger of a severe systemic infection. An infected joint is often red, swollen, and extremely tender upon active motion. Large joints, particularly the knees, are more likely to be infected than are small joints. Often, the patient experiences fever, rigors, and leukocytosis. Patients at risk for joint sepsis include those on systemic immunosuppressive agents, such as glucocorticoids. Also at risk are patients with immunodeficiency syndromes and those who are drug abusers. Inflammatory arthritis, such as rheumatoid arthritis, particularly in sites of joint prostheses, can predispose patients to septic arthritis. Patients with penetrating joint trauma also may develop joint infections. Staphylococcal and streptococcal infections are among the most common causes of bacterial monarticular joint infections in otherwise healthy adults. Synovial fluid Gram stains are positive in approximately 50% to 75% of cases of nongonococcal arthritis. Gram-negative microorganisms, such as *Escherichia coli,* are found in patients with underlying medical conditions such as sickle cell anemia, drug abuse, or immunosuppressed states.

The most common infectious arthritis of sexually active adults is due to *N. gonorrhoeae,* which produces septic arthritis

of the small joints of the hands, wrists, elbows, knees and ankles, and rarely the axial skeletal joints. This form of arthritis is often accompanied by a rash, tenosynovitis, and sterile synovial fluid cultures. Tuberculous and fungal arthritis often present with a more indolent course.

If the patient gives a history of recurrent, self-limited attacks in the same joint, a crystal-induced arthritis is likely. Monosodium urate crystals are found in those with acute gout. These intracellular, needle-shaped, negatively birefringent crystals can be visualized by polarized microscopy in 95% of gouty joint effusions and even in some asymptomatic joints by polarized microscopy. Patients with acute gout generally present with pain so severe that "even the bed sheets hurt my joints." Approximately 75% of patients with acute gout have inflammation of the great toe, *podagra,* during the course of their disease. Often, the joints of the lower extremities are involved. Typically, patients are middle-aged and may have recent predisposing factors such as alcohol intake, diuretic use, vigorous exercise, or recent surgery.

Calcium pyrophosphate dihydrate deposition disease may manifest as acute monarticular arthritis (*pseudogout*). This form of crystalline arthritis often is associated with osteoarthritis. The knee joint is the most commonly affected joint. Attacks, although self-limited, tend to last longer than gout attacks, often resolving within 1 week after initial symptoms. The diagnosis is made by visualizing positively birefringent, rhomboid-shaped crystals within white blood cells under polarizing microscopy.

Hydroxyapatite deposition disease, due to the deposition of basic calcium phosphate crystals, presents a particular diagnostic problem. Affected patients often are on dialysis and present with shoulder pain and immobility, called the *Milwaukee shoulder.* These calcium phosphate crystals cannot be seen by polarized

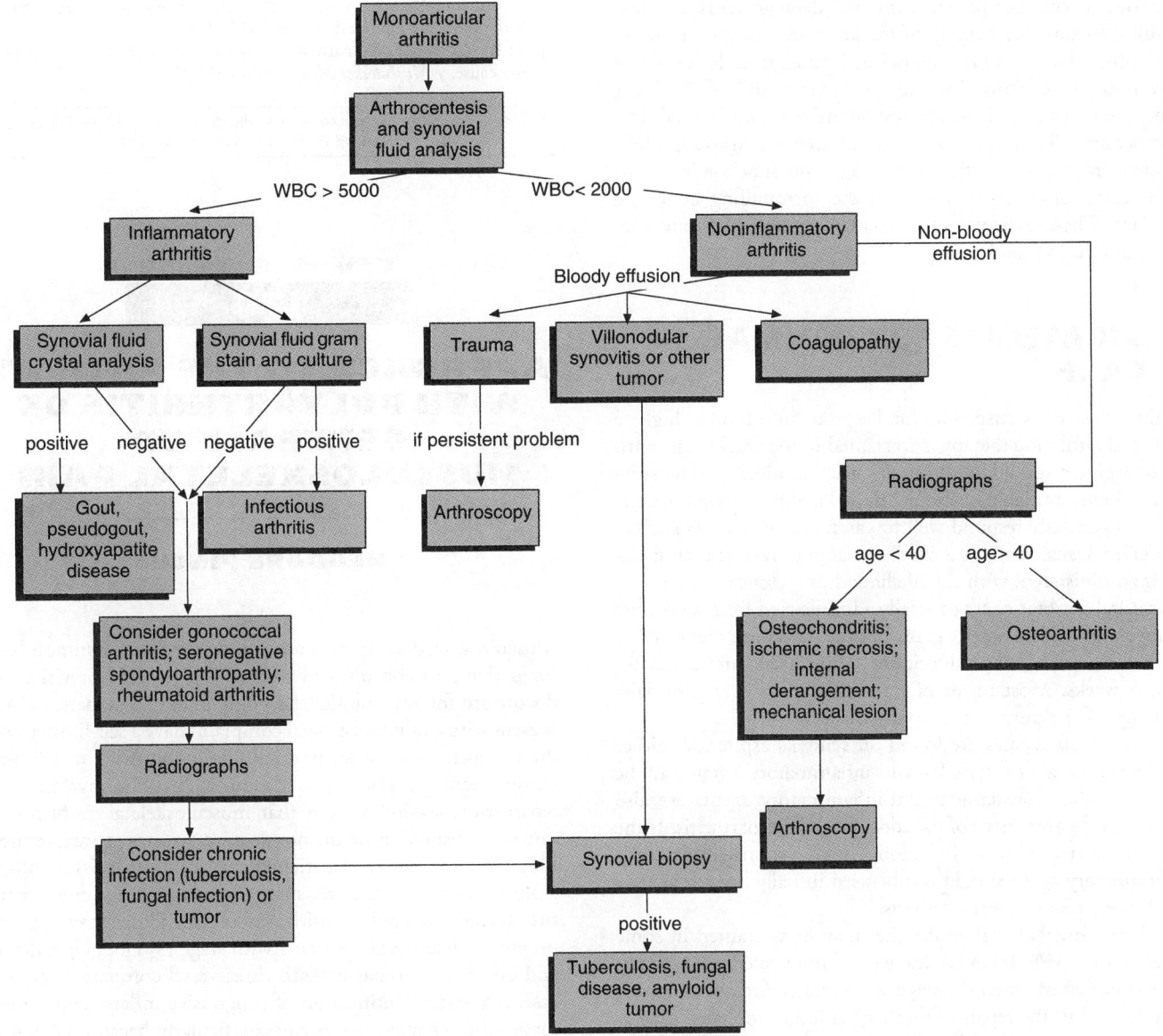

FIGURE 169.1. The flowchart shows the steps in determining whether monarticular arthritis is inflammatory or noninflammatory.
EVIDENCE LEVEL: A. Reference: Guidelines for the initial evaluation of the adult patient with acute musculoskeletal symptoms. American College of Rheumatology Ad Hoc Committee on Clinical Guidelines. *Arthritis Rheum* 1996;39:1–8.

microscopy, but must be visualized with an electron microscope or under light microscopy using Alizarin red stain.

If the synovial fluid culture and crystal examination are both negative, a physician should consider other disorders. Patients with rheumatoid arthritis present with an acute monarticular arthritis in approximately 20% of patients. This disease generally becomes polyarticular with time. Seronegative spondyloarthropathies, which include ankylosing spondylitis, psoriatic arthritis, enteric-associated arthritis, and Reiter's disease can manifest as monarticular arthritis. Patients with rheumatoid arthritis as well as those with seronegative spondyloarthritis complain of morning joint stiffness.

If the synovial fluid white blood cell count is under 2,000 cells per cubic millimeter, the patient probably has a noninflam-

matory monarthritis. If the synovial effusion is bloody, the physician should consider joint trauma, villonodular synovitis or other tumors, and coagulopathies.

Joint trauma is a major cause of acute joint pain and swelling. The synovial effusion can be bloody. The physician must be certain to rule out fracture. If a patient presents with hemarthrosis, the clinician should consider tumors, particularly pigmented villonodular synovitis. Patients with coagulopathies, such as hemophilia and von Willebrand's disease, also present with hemarthroses.

If the synovial effusion is nonbloody with a white blood cell count under 2,000 cells per cubic millimeter, osteoarthritis should be considered in patients over 40 years of age. These patients may also present with monarticular pain without joint effusion. In younger patients, internal derangements and mechanical lesions, particularly of the knee, may occur and result in a joint effusion. Torn menisci or ligaments or loose bodies may result in clicking, locking, or "giving out" of the knee. Symptoms are often elicited by testing the knee joint for stability. Osteochondritis dissecans occurs in children and in young adults when a fragment of articular cartilage and subchondral bone demarcates, often separating from the surrounding bone and cartilage. These patients may present with decreased joint motion, an effusion, and a limp.

STRATEGIES FOR OPTIMAL CARE

If the physician's suspicion for bacterial infection is high, a course of antibiotic therapy is warranted immediately. The antibiotic regimen should be adjusted, since the culture and sensitivity results are available in about 2 days. Patients with gonococcal arthritis generally respond well to parenteral antibiotics such as penicillin. Usually, a 1- to 2-week course of intravenous antibiotics is administered, with the likelihood of a clinical response in days. Oral antibiotics are generally administered for a week after intravenous antibiotics. If gram-positive cocci are identified, a penicillinase-resistant antibiotic should be given parenterally for 2 to 4 weeks. Most forms of infectious arthritis require daily drainage of the purulent synovial effusions.

If uric acid crystals are found on synovial aspiration, either colchicine or a nonsteroidal anti-inflammatory agent can be given acutely. Nonsteroidal anti-inflammatory agents are also helpful in the treatment of pseudogout and osteoarthritis. If the physician's suspicion for infection is high, a nonsteroidal anti-inflammatory agent should not be used initially because it may mask the patient's febrile response.

Therapeutic surgical approaches may be warranted in some cases of joint pain. If closed drainage of an infected joint cannot be accomplished, open drainage is necessary. Arthroscopic surgery can aid in the repair of mechanical joint problems, such as knee meniscal tears and ligamentous injuries.

BIBLIOGRAPHY

American College of Rheumatology Ad Hoc Committee on Clinical Guidelines. Guidelines for the initial evaluation of the adult patient with acute musculoskeletal symptoms. *Arthritis Rheum* 1996;39:1–8.
Baker DG, Schumacher HR Jr. Acute monoarthritis. *N Engl J Med* 1993; 329:1013–1020.
Bomalaski JS, Lluberas G, Schumacher HR Jr. Monosodium urate crystals in the knee joints of patients with asymptomatic nontophaceous gout. *Arthritis Rheum* 1986;29:1480–1484.
Goldenberg DL. Bacterial arthritis. *Curr Opin Rheumatol* 1995;7:310–314.
Goldenberg DL, Reed JI. Bacterial arthritis. *N Engl J Med* 1985;312: 764–771.
McCune WJ, Golbus J. Monarticular arthritis. In: Kelley WN, Harris EDJ, Ruddy S, Sledge CB, eds. *Textbook of rheumatology,* fifth ed. Philadelphia: WB Saunders, 1997;371–380.
Pioro MH, Mandell BF. Septic arthritis. *Rheum Dis Clin North Am* 1997; 23:239–258.
Rose CD, Eppes SC. Infection-related arthritis. *Rheum Dis Clin North Am* 1997;23:677–695.
Schumacher HR. Monarticular joint disease. In: Klippel JH, Weyand CM,
Wortmann RL, eds. *Primer on the rheumatic diseases,* eleventh ed. Atlanta: Arthritis Foundation, 1997;116–118.
Spiera RF, Crow MK. Monarticular pain and inflammation: tracking down the cause. *J Musculoskel Med* 1997;14:10–22.

Kelley's Textbook of Internal Medicine, fourth edition. Edited by H. David Humes. Lippincott Williams & Wilkins, Philadelphia © 2000.

C H A P T E R
170

APPROACH TO THE PATIENT WITH POLYARTHRITIS OR GENERALIZED MUSCULOSKELETAL PAIN

THEODORE PINCUS

Musculoskeletal symptoms are among the most common bases for patients to consult a physician. Up to 20% of visits to a doctor are for musculoskeletal complaints. Most patients who present with a musculoskeletal complaint have a self-limited condition, such as a transient tendinitis or bursitis, or a limited chronic noninflammatory condition, such as fibromyalgia or osteoarthritis, leaving a sense that musculoskeletal problems are not life-threatening or do not require an urgent intervention. However, a minority of patients have connective tissue inflammatory rheumatic diseases, such as systemic lupus erythematosus, scleroderma, polymyositis, vasculitis, and may have a poorer prognosis than that of patients with stage IV Hodgkin's disease and other lymphomas or with three-vessel coronary artery disease. Accurate identification of progressive inflammatory rheumatic diseases may be difficult, particularly because laboratory tests and imaging procedures often are not definitive. Therefore, the approach to a patient with generalized musculoskeletal pain is governed by the following principles:

1. The definitive diagnosis in most patients generally emerges primarily from the history and physical examination. Laboratory tests, radiographs, and other imaging procedures are generally used to confirm the diagnosis, and only a limited number are needed.
2. The most common cause of generalized musculoskeletal pain is fibromyalgia, found in 5% of women over the age of 50. Patients with fibromyalgia are often easily recognized, and elaborate evaluations to rule out specific diseases are generally unproductive and are often harmful to a patient's reassurance that there is no life-threatening disease.
3. At least 50% of patients who present with an inflammatory arthritis, even those who meet criteria for rheumatoid arthritis, have a self-limited process rather than a progressive disease. The distinction between self-limited or progressive generally is accomplished primarily by observation of the

patient's clinical course rather than by extensive laboratory or other tests.

4. Blood tests in patients with rheumatic diseases are often not precise guides to a diagnosis, unlike those tests for many diseases, such as a blood glucose in diabetes or a serum creatinine in renal failure. Blood tests identify higher probabilities of certain diagnoses, such as rheumatoid arthritis or systemic lupus erythematosus, but usually are not definitive. For an individual patient, probabilities are often only marginally useful, because of a high rate of false-positive and false-negative results.

5. False-positive results, in which blood tests are abnormal in people who do not have a disease, are common in tests for rheumatic diseases. For example, more than 5% of people in the population have a positive antinuclear antibody (ANA) test, elevated uric acid level, or *Borrelia burgdorferi* antibodies found in Lyme disease, and most who have a positive test do not have systemic lupus erythematosus, gout, or Lyme disease, respectively. This phenomenon would not be a clinical problem if blood tests were performed only in patients who had clinical evidence of these diseases. However, because musculoskeletal symptoms are so common and evoke considerable uncertainty in many physicians, blood tests are performed on a large number of persons whose clinical picture is uncertain, but does not suggest a specific rheumatic disease. Many, if not most, people who are given labels of systemic lupus erythematosus, gout, or Lyme disease do not have these diseases, but merely a positive laboratory test.

6. The problem of false-negative laboratory test results, in which patients have a certain disease but a normal laboratory test, is less common, but nonetheless leads to important errors in diagnosis. For example, 20% of patients with rheumatoid arthritis do not ever have rheumatoid factor in their serum, and 50% of patients whose sera eventually become positive for rheumatoid factor have negative results during the first 6 months of disease. Therefore, a test for rheumatoid factor is least useful when it is clinically needed most—in early disease—when the patient may have either a self-limited inflammatory polyarthritis or progressive rheumatoid arthritis. Most positive rheumatoid factor tests are performed in patients known to have rheumatoid arthritis, resulting in an unnecessary or inappropriate medical expense.

7. Abnormal findings on radiographs, bone scans, or magnetic imaging resonance scans are common, particularly in most people over age 40. However, these findings often do not explain the patient's musculoskeletal symptoms. Symptoms of fibromyalgia, soft tissue rheumatism, back pain, and other conditions are frequently incorrectly attributed to osteoarthritis, often on the basis of common radiographic abnormalities. By contrast, radiographs may be minimally abnormal in early rheumatoid arthritis at a time when aggressive intervention might provide optimal therapeutic benefit.

8. The importance of establishing a precise diagnosis to direct treatment usually is not as urgent for patients with subacute and chronic musculoskeletal pain as for those with acute diseases. In patients with generalized musculoskeletal pain, it is usually possible to easily recognize fibromyalgia, soft tissue rheumatism, osteoarthritis, or other noninflammatory condi-

tions and thereby be reasonably certain that a patient does not have progressive inflammatory connective tissue disease, such as rheumatoid arthritis, systemic lupus erythematosus, vasculitis, subacute bacterial endocarditis, or polymyositis, which are seen in a very small minority of patients with generalized musculoskeletal pain.

9. A rheumatology consultation is often the most cost-effective test for diagnosis of a person with musculoskeletal pain, provided that it does not include irrelevant extensive laboratory and imaging data.

▌ HISTORY AND PHYSICAL EXAMINATION

A systematic, careful history and physical examination can effectively be used to determine whether patients have a noninflammatory condition such as soft tissue rheumatism, osteoarthritis, or fibromyalgia, or an inflammatory condition such as a self-limited inflammatory polyarthritis, progressive inflammatory articular or nonarticular condition, or connective tissue disease (Table 170.1). Diffuse connective tissue diseases, such as systemic lupus erythematosus, scleroderma, polymyositis, and vasculitis, are rare, defined as occurring in fewer than 1 in 2,000 persons. A physician in general practice may expect to see only two or three cases of some of these diseases during a 40-year career. Affected patients should generate an appropriate sense of urgency, but an expert rheumatologist is often more helpful than extensive testing.

▌ LABORATORY STUDIES AND DIAGNOSTIC TESTS

A diagnosis at the first visit may be difficult in some patients, even for the experienced rheumatologist, and it may be reasonable to observe a patient over two or more visits to establish a diagnosis. Laboratory tests should be used sparingly. A screening complete blood count and erythrocyte sedimentation rate may provide clues to the presence of inflammatory diseases, although all tests may be normal in the presence of inflammatory disease, as discussed in the text that follows.

▌ DIFFERENTIAL DIAGNOSIS

NONINFLAMMATORY CAUSES OF GENERALIZED MUSCULOSKELETAL PAIN

A classification of patients with musculoskeletal symptoms (Table 170.1) is based primarily on information elicited from the history and physical examination.

Localized Musculoskeletal Soft Tissue Conditions

The most common cause of acute musculoskeletal symptoms is soft tissue rheumatism, including tendinitis, bursitis, and back

TABLE 170.1.	CLASSIFICATION OF RHEUMATIC DISEASES BASED ON THE LIKELIHOOD OF BEING SEEN IN A GENERAL PRACTICE SITUATION

Noninflammatory Conditions

1. Soft tissue rheumatism (tendonitis, bursitis, back pain)
   Pain limited to one joint or a few joint areas
   Generally associated with discomfort in only certain planes of joint movement, rather than all planes seen in patients with arthritis
2. Osteoarthritis
   Pain generally localized to one or a few joints with limited motion and/or with discomfort in all planes of joint movement (osteoarthritis tends to be polyarticular but pauciarticular)
   Accompanied by evidence of structural damage such as joint space narrowing or bone cysts
3. Fibromyalgia (myofascial pain)
   Diffuse, noninflammatory musculoskeletal pain
   Not characterized by any abnormalities of laboratory tests, radiographs, or other imaging studies. However, may be seen in the presence of any other rheumatic conditions and is frequently seen in patients with osteoarthritis, rheumatoid arthritis, and other conditions.
4. Other noninflammatory articular conditions
   Myofascial syndromes, reflex sympathetic dystrophy, amyloidosis, hypertrophic pulmonary osteoarthropathy, sickle cell crisis

Inflammatory Conditions

5. Self-limited inflammatory arthritis
   Requires supportive care only; most commonly occurs after viral infection
   Many persons experience joint swelling that is not progressive and generally resolves within 4–8 weeks
6. Chronic and progressive interventions
   Requires aggressive interventions
   Rheumatoid arthritis, gout, ankylosing spondylitis, gout, psoriatic arthritis. Reiter's syndrome
7. Nonarticular inflammatory conditions
   Polymyalgia rheumatic, giant cell arteritis, diffuse fasciitis with eosinophilia, eosinophilia-myalgia syndrome
8. Connective tissue diseases
   Systemic lupus erythematosus, vasculitis, polymyositis, dermatomyositis, scleroderma

by most textbooks, if the physician has solid reasons for making the diagnosis (Table 170.2), it is not necessary nor desirable to perform exhaustive laboratory tests to rule out possible diagnoses with a lower probability of being the problem.

Two important problems are associated with the "rule-out" approach. First, common abnormalities such as radiographic osteoarthritis of the cervical spine, found in most people between the ages of 30 and 60 years, or a positive ANA or Lyme disease test (i.e., antibodies to *B. burgdorferi*), found in 5% of the population, may lead to an erroneous diagnosis. Second, the process of extensive testing often renders it difficult to reassure a patient that there is no progressive or life-threatening disease.

The differential diagnosis of fibromyalgia may be difficult, in part because this condition may mimic early rheumatoid arthritis. The absence of specific signs of rheumatoid arthritis can be used to exclude this diagnosis, although for some patients, it is unclear whether the primary problem is early rheumatoid arthritis or fibromyalgia, in which case an "n of 1" clinical trial of treatment for one disease sequentially with the second is sometimes helpful in establishing a diagnosis and helping the patient.

Other Noninflammatory Articular Conditions

Localized myofascial syndromes are similar to fibromyalgia but may be seen in specific joint areas, such as the shoulder, knee, and hip. These conditions are manifested by pain without a recognized structural source of the pain.

Reflex sympathetic dystrophy syndrome manifests as diffuse and burning pain involving a single extremity, although this

TABLE 170.2.	Diagnosis and Treatment of Fibromyalgia

History

Widespread pain not limited to joints; may be "all over"
Frequent report of other somatization problems such as headaches, gastrointestinal distress, chest pain, dyspnea
Dysfunctional sleep

Physical Examination

Muscle spasm
Tender points
No joint swelling or limited motion

Radiographs

Osteoarthritis seen, but nonexplanatory, especially for the cervical spine

Laboratory Tests

Generally normal, but 5% may have positive results for antinuclear antibiotic and elevated uric acid levels

Treatment

Frank discussion
Pain is real
Exercise program
Better sleep
Drugs: tricyclic antidepressants, nonsteroidal antiinflammatory drugs: avoid narcotics

pain, which tends to be localized. In some patients, soft tissue rheumatism may progress to a chronic, significant, but localized, long-term problem.

Osteoarthritis

Osteoarthritis is probably the most common form of structural damage manifested as arthritis. Osteoarthritis is usually localized to one or a few joints, but it may be generalized. A diagnosis of osteoarthritis should include radiographic evidence of joint space narrowing and joint destruction.

Fibromyalgia

Fibromyalgia is the most common basis for generalized musculoskeletal pain. Although referred to as a diagnosis of exclusion

condition may be bilateral. Patients generally have a history of trauma preceding development of this syndrome.

Amyloidosis is a relatively unusual infiltrative rheumatic disease in which infiltration involving the hands, wrists, elbows, and shoulders may mimic the swelling of synovitis.

Hypertrophic pulmonary osteoarthropathy presents with diffuse musculoskeletal pain in persons with pulmonary neoplastic or infectious disease. The pain is generally pronounced in the distal bones of the limbs near the wrists and ankles. The digits may or may not be clubbed. Radiographs reveal periosteal separation. A search for pulmonary disease is indicated in patients with this clinical or radiographic finding.

Sickle cell crises may lead to joint effusions, most commonly involving the knees and elbows with a noninflammatory synovial fluid.

INFLAMMATORY MUSCULOSKELETAL CONDITIONS

The term "inflammatory" refers to conditions characterized by a host response that involves release of cytokine mediators from polymorphonuclear leukocytes. The presence of an inflammatory condition is established by clinical evidence of a systemic disease, including the presence of widespread symmetric polyarthritis and morning stiffness, often accompanied by constitutional symptoms of fatigue and malaise. The physical examination indicates joint tenderness, swelling, or other signs of inflammation.

Self-Limited Inflammatory Arthritis

Classification criteria established by the American College of Rheumatology for rheumatoid arthritis are useful to identify relatively homogeneous patients for research studies. However, many persons who manifest an inflammatory arthritis and meet these criteria do not have a progressive disease. In population surveys, only about 25% of persons who meet criteria for rheumatoid arthritis have evidence of disease 3 to 5 years later. Most self-limited inflammatory polyarthritis is resolved within 6 months of onset.

Acute-phase reactants such as the erythrocyte sedimentation rate (ESR) or C-reactive protein (CRP) determinations may be elevated in both self-limited and early progressive inflammatory arthritis. The presence of rheumatoid factor suggests a higher likelihood of a progressive disease, but the absence of rheumatoid factor does not exclude rheumatoid arthritis, because rheumatoid factor is not found in more than 50% of persons with rheumatoid arthritis during the first 6 months of their disease. Radiographs are usually normal or show minimal soft tissue swelling and osteopenia for patients with both self-limited or progressive inflammatory arthritis.

Patients with self-limited inflammatory arthritis may have a variety of diagnoses, such as postinfectious arthritis, reactive arthritis, inflammatory polyarthritis, or benign polyarthritis of the elderly. Note that patients who meet criteria for rheumatoid arthritis may have a self-limited process rather than a progressive disease. Often, the exact cause remains unknown. One of the primary reasons to establish a viral cause is to assess the strong probability of a self-limited course. Patients who are improving significantly when first seen are likely to have a self-limited form of inflammatory arthritis.

If a polyarticular arthritis persists longer than 30 or 60 days, it is likely that some form of progressive arthritis such as rheumatoid arthritis is present, rather than a reactive or postinfectious inflammatory polyarthropathy. Observation over 30 to 90 days is usually the most effective and most cost-effective approach to differentiate self-limited from progressive inflammatory arthritis.

Progressive Inflammatory Arthritis

Rheumatoid Arthritis

The prototypical form of inflammatory arthritis is rheumatoid arthritis, characterized by symmetric polyarthritis, morning stiffness, and systemic symptoms of fatigue, malaise, and weight loss. The physical examination in early-stage disease indicates tenderness, swelling, and limited motion of joints, most commonly the metacarpophalangeal and proximal interphalangeal joints of the hand, wrists, and feet. Other signs of inflammation such as erythema and warmth are uncommon.

Early rheumatoid arthritis is characterized by disease activity, seen as tenderness and swelling, which leads to long-term tissue damage, seen as joint deformity and radiographic malalignment, and poor long-term outcomes, such as work disability and premature death. Inflammatory activity is reversible and amenable to drug therapies, whereas long-term damage is generally irreversible and not affected by drug therapy. Unfortunately, inflammation may persist indefinitely, and therefore treatment to reduce inflammation is needed even after damage is present.

Crystal-induced arthritis such as gout is described as the great masquerader because it can mimic any rheumatic disease, including rheumatoid arthritis. The classic podagra of acute gout affects the great toe, although gout may affect the ankle or any joint. A search for tophi in the ear and urate nodules, which may mimic rheumatoid nodules, is valuable. The definitive test for the diagnosis of gout is identification of negatively birefringent uric acid crystals in the synovial fluid, but this test often is not done or is done poorly. Gout tends to be overdiagnosed in persons with elevated uric acid levels and musculoskeletal symptoms on the basis of other rheumatic conditions. The diagnosis of gout also is missed in some persons who have normal uric acid levels.

Calcium pyrophosphate deposition disease, also called *pseudogout,* is often seen in the knee or ankle, commonly in a hospitalized patient with recent surgery for an acute illness. This disease is also diagnosed definitively on the basis of positively birefringent crystals in synovial fluid.

Seronegative Spondyloarthropathies

Seronegative spondyloarthropathies include ankylosing spondylitis, Reiter's syndrome, the arthritis of inflammatory bowel disease, and some forms of psoriatic arthritis. These conditions are characterized by inflammation involving the enthesis (i.e., structure that connects a tendon to bone), in contrast to the synovitis seen in rheumatoid arthritis, which involves a generalized synovial inflammation. This distinction is important in at least two respects. First, patients with enthesitis generally do not experience constitutional symptoms at a level as high as patients with synovitis, as seen in rheumatoid arthritis. Second, patients with enthesitis are more likely to respond to indomethacin than to other nonsteroidal anti-inflammatory drugs (NSAIDs), but patients with synovitis are more likely to respond to salicylates than to other NSAIDs.

Patients with seronegative spondyloarthropathies are likely to have the HLA-B27 antigen on the surface of their lymphocytes. Although this phenomenon is considerably helpful in understanding pathophysiology, it is of little clinical usefulness because 6% of normal persons are HLA-B27–positive. In fact, only one of three persons who have back pain and are HLA-B27–positive have ankylosing spondylitis.

Ankylosing spondylitis is manifested primarily by involvement of the spine, with limited motion detected on physical examination. The radiograph may indicate syndesmophytes of the spine, culminating in the appearance of a "bamboo spine." In more severe cases of ankylosing spondylitis, hip, knee, shoulder, and other large joints may become involved, often before a person reaches the age of 20 years.

Reiter's syndrome classically includes the triad of arthritis, urethritis, and conjunctivitis. Various manifestations of "incomplete" Reiter's syndrome have been described, including an oligoarthritis involving several large joints, such as one or both ankles, wrists, or knees. Reactive arthritis has been associated with several enteric bacterial entities, including *Yersinia, Helicobacter, Shigella,* and *Salmonella.* Reiter's syndrome and reactive arthritis may occur as a single episode, as infrequently recurring episodes, or as a chronic arthritis.

Psoriatic arthritis is probably second to rheumatoid arthritis in prevalence among the progressive inflammatory rheumatic diseases. It may be seen in several forms, including a symmetric polyarthritis, which appears almost identical with rheumatoid arthritis; an asymmetric oligoarthritis, which appears similar to Reiter's syndrome; and a severe deforming type called *arthritis mutilans.*

The *arthritis associated with inflammatory bowel disease* tends to be nondestructive, involving large joints of the knees and ankles.

Rheumatic fever is a relatively unusual condition that was thought to be disappearing, but it has reappeared in some small epidemics.

Lyme disease is an important new rheumatic disease described over the last two decades. It begins with a rash known as *erythema chronicum migrans,* and the disease may progress to produce arthritis, carditis, and neurologic inflammation. The diagnostic test involves identification of antibodies to *B. burgdorferi* in the serum. As is the case in most rheumatic diseases, this diagnostic test is overused, if not abused. Fewer than 1 of 100 individuals with a positive Lyme antibody titer actually have evidence of Lyme disease.

The *arthritis of sarcoidosis* often produces a characteristic picture of swelling in the ankles. In classic cases, erythema nodosum, hilar adenopathy, and fever may be manifestations of sarcoidosis, but arthritis may occasionally be the primary manifestation of sarcoid. Although sarcoid arthritis usually is self-limited, in some cases, it may be relapsing and may lead to cystic destructive lesions of bone.

Polyarthritis and Fever

Theoretically, all forms of inflammatory arthritis may include fever. However, fever is unusual in rheumatoid arthritis and most forms of polyarthritis and raises a concern about infection. Fever is seen in several forms of arthritides: juvenile rheumatoid arthritis (Still's disease), subacute bacterial endocarditis, septic arthritis involving a bacterial, mycobacterial, or fungal cause. Fever may accompany a postinfectious or reactive arthritis, vasculitis, systemic lupus erythematosus, and several unusual diseases, including familial Mediterranean fever, Behçet's disease, Kawasaki's disease, and pyoderma gangrenosum. Familial Mediterranean fever generally appears in childhood with brief episodes of fever, arthritis, and abdominal and pleuritic pain.

Vasculitis may present as a polyarticular arthritis that appears similar to rheumatoid arthritis. Other manifestations of vasculitis are generally seen, including palpable purpura, postprandial abdominal pain, and mononeuritis multiplex.

Diffuse Connective Tissue Diseases

Diffuse connective tissue diseases are rare diseases seen in fewer than 1 in 2,000 patients. They can life threatening and are associated with as high a 5-year mortality rate as in many types of cardiovascular or neoplastic diseases.

Systemic lupus erythematosus is a multisystem disease, which may include a rash, serositis, Raynaud's phenomenon, oral ulcers, pleuritis, pericarditis, anemia, leukopenia, thrombocytopenia, and possible evidence of pulmonary, cardiac, gastrointestinal, renal, or central nervous system involvement. More than 90% of these patients have arthritis. The arthritis tends to mimic that of rheumatoid arthritis but is not as destructive. The natural history of systemic lupus erythematosus with renal, cardiac, or central nervous system involvement includes mortality rates of 50% over 5 years. Considerable evidence suggests preservation of renal function and longer survival with use of cytotoxic therapy, rendering a sense of urgency in making a correct diagnosis.

The diagnosis is established through a positive ANA test, but, as previously noted, many persons have positive high-titer ANA tests and no evidence of a multisystem disease. A positive ANA test result may be considered analogous to an enlarged lymph node. In most persons, this finding is not of any pathologic significance (e.g., benign hyperplasia), although it may indicate a relatively urgent problem (e.g., lymphoma) in a few. A biopsy is required to establish the pathologic significance of an enlarged lymph node. By contrast, the pathologic significance of a positive ANA test result is established by a careful history and physical examination.

In most cases, a physical examination generally reveals evidence of multisystem disease. Antineutrophil cytoplasmic antibodies (ANCA) may be detected in patients with Wegener's granulomatosis and other forms of vasculitis, but clinical evidence from the history and physical examination remains the primary guide to diagnosis and therapy.

Polymyositis and dermatomyositis are diseases that present

with muscle weakness. A useful finding is evidence that a patient cannot arise from a chair without help, which indicates a problem affecting joints, muscles, or nerve structures. The diagnosis can be made on the basis of a triad of elevated muscle enzymes (creatine phosphokinase and aldolase), a muscle biopsy, and electromyographic results. Polyarthritis is unusual but may be a component of the initial presentation, although muscle weakness emerges as the primary symptom.

Scleroderma may manifest as generalized musculoskeletal pain. Patients occasionally have diffusely puffy hands, but may have pain associated with skin thickening and contractures. Scleroderma is diagnosed on the basis of a physical examination by an experienced physician. A skin biopsy is rarely needed to the make the diagnosis.

Generalized Inflammatory Musculoskeletal Syndromes Without Arthritis

Polymyalgia rheumatica is seen almost exclusively in persons older than 50 years of age who have discomfort of the hip and shoulder girdles. Constitutional symptoms of malaise, fatigue, and weight loss are often seen, similar to findings in patients with early rheumatoid arthritis. The diagnosis is established by the finding of a substantially elevated ESR, usually at least 50 mm per minute.

■ DIAGNOSIS OF INFLAMMATORY RHEUMATIC DISEASES

Figure 170.1 summarizes information used to establish a diagnosis for a patient with musculoskeletal pain. It outlines the four major sources of data, including the history and physical examination, laboratory tests, radiographs and imaging procedures, and synovial fluid analysis. A box surrounds the most important information required to establish a diagnosis.

The top half of Figure 170.1 includes the four most prominent inflammatory rheumatic diseases—rheumatoid arthritis, systemic lupus erythematosus, gout, and ankylosing spondylitis. Critical data for a diagnosis of rheumatoid arthritis is derived from the history and physical examination; for systemic lupus erythematosus, from a laboratory test, the ANA, although with a requirement for multisystem disease; for gout, from a synovial fluid examination; and for ankylosing spondylitis, from a radiograph. Figure 170.1 may clarify why the practice of ordering a battery of blood tests and radiographs is rarely definitive in establishing a diagnosis of an inflammatory rheumatic disease or other inflammatory condition.

The bottom half of Figure 170.1 includes two other common conditions seen in usual practice, osteoarthritis and fibromyalgia, and two unusual diseases, scleroderma and polymyositis. As noted previously, a diagnosis of osteoarthritis should require a radiograph to document joint space narrowing and other changes. Fibromyalgia is seen in about 3% of the population. In certain cases, even experienced rheumatologists have difficulty differentiating fibromyalgia from inflammatory musculoskeletal disease, but distinguishing these problems is generally not resolved through laboratory tests. Patients with fibromyalgia often

have more extensive testing than patients with rheumatoid arthritis, systemic lupus erythematosus, or other potentially life-threatening rheumatic diseases.

The diagnosis of scleroderma can generally be established from a physical examination. Similarly, polymyositis includes a test of creatine phosphokinase and muscle biopsy, but, again, patients in whom this diagnosis is considered should be seen by a rheumatologist. The clinician might consider an early referral to a specialist in patients in whom a problem appears complex. The author suggests that the primary basis for referral to a rheumatologist should involve symptoms that remain unexplained or with poor response to therapy, rather than laboratory tests or radiographs.

A COST-EFFECTIVE APPROACH TO DIAGNOSIS

The clinician seeing a patient with musculoskeletal symptoms seeks to identify an accurate diagnosis. In view of the likelihood that laboratory and radiographic data will not be helpful in many, if not most cases, a cost-effective approach is outlined here.

The history provides most of the important information. A thorough review is not possible, and a simple set of questions generally suffices:

1. Is there pain, stiffness, swelling, limited motion, or weakness in any joint, bone, muscle, or supporting structure, or unusual fatigue? (If the answer is "no," no further musculoskeletal history is needed.)
2. Where is the pain (localized or widespread)?
3. How severe is the pain, stiffness, or swelling?
4. When is the discomfort most difficult (early morning, after activities, late in the day)?
5. How did the pain, stiffness, or swelling begin (acute or chronic)?

Widespread pain and report of morning stiffness suggest fibromyalgia or an inflammatory disease. Inflammatory arthritis is suggested by polyarthritis, pain localized to joints, and the absence of diffuse symptoms. Fibromyalgia is suggested by poor sleep, generalized pain with absence of localization to joints, and a history of somatization in other organ systems, such as irritable bowel syndrome, headaches, and floppy mitral valve.

A brief physical examination can identify most problems of the musculoskeletal system. Examination of affected areas should involve palpation for tenderness and swelling and a check of range of motion; generally, the examiner can serve as a "control." Arthritis is suggested by pain in all motions of a joint. Tendinitis or bursitis is suggested by point tenderness and pain in only one plane of motion. Fibromyalgia is suggested by diffuse muscle spasm and tender points. A brief, gentle "squeeze" of each proximal interphalangeal (PIP) and metacarpophalangeal (MCP) joint requires no more than 30 seconds and can detect subtle inflammation, as seen in early rheumatoid arthritis.

The patient can be asked to squeeze the finger of the examiner to assess hand strength and then move his or her arms above the head, behind the back, and in a wing-span position to test for shoulder flexion, abduction, and internal and external rota-

Source of data	Rheumatoid arthritis	Systemic lupus erythematosus	Ankylosing spondylitis	Gout
History and physical exam	Symmetrical polyarthritis Morning stiffness	Multisystem disease	Back pain Axial involvement	Recurrent attacks
Blood tests	Latex test + in approx. 80% Elevated ESR in 50 – 60%	ANA-screening + in >99% DNA antibodies + in 60 – 75%	Approx. 90% of patients are HLA-B27	Uric acid elevated in 75 – 90%
Radiographs	Demineralization Erosions Joint space narrowing	Generally non-destructive	Sacroiliitis Vertebral squaring	Erosions Cysts
Synovial fluid	Inflammation, WBC > 10,000	Mild inflammation	Inflammation WBC 5 – 20,000	Negatively birefringent crystals

Source of data	Osteoarthritis	Fibromyalgia	Scleroderma	Polymyositis
History and physical exam	Pain ± swelling ± limited motion	Chronic pain "all over" No swollen joints Muscle spasm	Skin tightness dorsum of hand Facial skin tightening	Muscle weakness ± pain
Blood tests	Nonspecific abnormalities	No abnormalities may have +ANA (2-5%); uric acid >8.0(2-5%)	+ANA, up to 90% with Hep-2 cells	CPK elevated in 80% +ANA in 33%
Radiographs	Joint space narrowing Osteophytes	No severe abnormalities (may have cervical osteoarthritis)	± Pulomary fibrosis ± Esophageal dysmotility ± Calcinosis	Not helpful
Synovial fluid	Non-inflammatory WBC < 10,000	None	Not specific	Not specific

FIGURE 170.1. Diagnosis of rheumatic diseases. Clinical data from different sources, with the source of the most valuable data boxed. *ANA*, antinuclear antibodies; *WBC*, white blood cell count.
EVIDENCE LEVEL: C. Expert Opinion.

tion. The trapezius muscle should be palpated for spasm and tender points characteristic of fibromyalgia. Clinicians may not recognize that a patient cannot walk when the patient is evaluated only on an examining table or a bed; therefore, it is worthwhile to include asking the patient to arise from a chair without holding on to anything and walk to a wall. A patient who cannot arise from a chair without holding on to a support has an abnormality, which may exist in the joints, muscles, or nerves. It is more important to recognize an abnormality than to characterize it precisely.

Laboratory tests should be ordered sparingly. A complete blood count is often as helpful as any specific "rheumatology" test. If evidence points to rheumatoid arthritis, a test for an acute-phase protein, such as an ESR or a C-reactive protein, and a test for rheumatoid factor may be ordered. If systemic lupus erythematosus is suggested on the basis of multisystem disease, an ANA should be ordered; an ANA with no multisystem disease will yield 5% or more false-positive results. If the patient is

acutely ill, a urinalysis, chemistry profile, anti-DNA test, and a test for complement, C3 and C4, or CH50 (but only one of the three) should be ordered.

If the patient is weak and might have polymyositis, testing of creatine phosphokinase and aldolase is indicated. In cases of suspected vasculitis, an ANCA may be ordered, although diagnosis and treatment are determined by clinical criteria. In case of recurrent miscarriages or clotting tendencies, an anticardiolipin antibody is appropriate. Ordering additional subsets of ANAs or rheumatology screens is discouraged.

In general, the radiographic investigation of most patients with arthritis requires only an anteroposterior view of joints. The lateral and oblique views are included routinely in radiologic evaluation and are appropriate for possible fractures, but are rarely useful in screening joints for arthritis other than the knee. Radiographs should be limited to affected areas, although an elderly patient with hip or knee pain should have two radiographs, an anteroposterior view of the pelvis and an anteroposterior view of both knees standing, to screen for severe osteoarthritis, which may be more effectively treated by means of total joint replacement surgery than with any medication.

If a radiographic explanation for widespread musculoskeletal pain is sought, a set of four radiographs may include (a) an anteroposterior view of the hands and wrists, (b) an anteroposterior view of the pelvis, (c) an anteroposterior view of both knees standing, and (d) an anteroposterior view of both feet. If these radiographs do not point to a specific diagnosis, such as rheumatoid arthritis or gout, it is most unlikely that extensive imaging procedures will prove helpful. In most situations, even this radiographic evaluation is beyond what is needed; this is especially true in the diagnosis of back pain.

BIBLIOGRAPHY

Callahan LF, Pincus T. Mortality in the rheumatic diseases. *Arthritis Care Res* 1995;8:229–241.

Kovarsky J. Serologic testing in SLE. *J Musculoskel Med* 1986;3:55.

Lichtenstein MJ, Pincus T. How useful are combinations of blood tests in "rheumatic panels" in diagnosis of rheumatic diseases? *J Gen Intern Med* 1988;3:435–442.

Pincus T. A pragmatic approach to cost-effective use of laboratory tests and imaging procedures in patients with musculoskeletal symptoms. *Prim Care Clin North Am* 1993;20:795–814.

Shmerling RH, Delbanco TL. How useful is the rheumatoid factor? An analysis of sensitivity, specificity and predictive value. *Arch Intern Med* 1992;152:2417–2420.

Kelley's Textbook of Internal Medicine, fourth edition. Edited by H. David Humes. Lippincott Williams & Wilkins, Philadelphia © 2000.

CHAPTER

171

APPROACH TO THE PATIENT WITH BACK PAIN

GLEN S. O'SULLIVAN

Lower back pain is one of the most common reasons for medical visits. Two of every three people have suffered from lower back pain at some time in their lives; the annual incidence is 2% to 5%. Lower back pain is becoming a growing problem in industrialized countries, accounting for up to $50 billion spent per year in the United States alone. Ninety percent of that budget is spent on 10% of those patients, who have persistent chronic pain lasting longer than 3 months. In 85% of cases, an underlying cause for lower back pain is not established.

A detailed history and examination will help determine the presence or threat of neurologic compromise. The clinical conditions of herniated disc with sciatica and spinal stenosis have a clearly different set of initial signs and symptoms, natural history, and treatment course compared with backache alone. Infections,

tumors, or fractures must be ruled out before settling on a diagnosis related to aging or degenerative processes. As physicians, we must diagnose and treat our patients with lower back pain in a cost-effective manner without adding to morbidity. This chapter focuses on the key elements of the history and physical examination, when and what type of imaging studies are appropriate, and specific common clinical conditions, such as backache (sprain/strain), herniated discs, cauda equina syndrome, spinal stenosis, and spondylolisthesis.

HISTORY

The initial encounter with a patient with lower back problems may be the most important factor affecting his or her outcome. The patient should be observed for any nonorganic signs suggestive of psychological problems or underlying psychosocial disorders. Care must be taken to prevent the patient from falling into the sick role or becoming dependent on the medical system for medications, excessive tests, permission not to perform work, and continual therapy. It is important to instill confidence and foster attitudes of independence from the outset. The cause for lower back pain is rarely known; a precise symptom-related diagnosis might be made only 10% to 15% of the time. The patient may become confused by conflicting diagnoses and different terms used by various caregivers, including chiropractors, osteopaths, medical doctors, and physiotherapists.

AGE

The age of the patient at the onset of lower back symptoms is critical. When adults complain of back pain, the diagnosis and management may be difficult and frustrating because of subjective complaints, the coexistence of degenerative diseases, and the frequent involvement of psychological, medical, and legal compensation issues. In contrast, children and adolescents complain of back pain infrequently. When they do complain, the history and clinical examination usually show objective findings, a differential diagnosis becomes clear, and therapeutic interventions are often effective. The diagnosis and treatment of back pain in young patients is generally a much more rewarding experience for the physician. Typically, one-third of children with back pain have spondylolysis or spondylolisthesis, one-third have Scheuermann's disease, and about 20% of patients have either tumors or spinal infections. Older patients are more likely to have underlying neuropathy, degenerative disease, metabolic disorders, or malignancy. Adolescents with back pain frequently fall midway between adults and children, reflecting socioeconomic and cultural factors.

MEDICAL REVIEW

A thorough general medical review is particularly important in older patients. Metabolic and systemic conditions that might play a role include infection, tumors, diabetes mellitus, osteoporosis, pancreatitis, and hyperthyroidism. It is imperative to rule out any neurologic deficit, particularly changes in bowel or bladder habits, such as urinary retention with overflow incontinence. Perianal paresthesia or pain is a clue to the symptoms of possible cauda equina syndrome. A history of trauma or transient paresis is important, particularly in elderly patients with underlying osteoporosis.

PAIN

The onset, duration, quality, severity, and location of the pain are all important in a detailed history. One should distinguish between the ubiquitous human experience of acute lower back pain lasting up to 6 weeks, from which 80% of patients usually recover, and chronic pain, which persists beyond 3 months and evades specific diagnosis in most cases. It is essential to differentiate mechanical lower back pain from nonmechanical pain that is present at rest. The red flags that may indicate a serious problem warranting a more thorough diagnostic evaluation include pain at rest, no positional relief, night pain, fever, weight loss, history of malignancy, and morning stiffness lasting more than 30 minutes. The nonmechanical serious causes of lower back pain are very rare, accounting for only 1% of cases; they comprise infection, tumors, and fractures. When they are suspected, a comprehensive workup is necessary, including erythrocyte sedimentation rate, serum protein electrophoresis, radiographs, bone scan, and, possibly, further imaging with magnetic resonance imaging (MRI) or computed tomography (CT).

Chronic pain lasting longer than 3 months should alert the treating physician to reconsider the initial diagnosis. Workers' compensation, job dissatisfaction, previous lower back disorders, and personal problems, including psychosocial issues and narcotic addiction, all contribute to the disability of lower back pain. Other causes for mechanical back pain include degenerative disc disease with a collapsing spine, resulting in an instability pattern, such as scoliosis or spondylolisthesis. Systemic causes include seronegative spondyloarthropathy, metabolic bone disease, osteoporosis, osteomalacia, fibromyalgia, and polymyalgia rheumatica.

Besides quantifying the intensity of the pain and the accompanying degree of disability, it is important to determine the location and the relative ratio of back pain to leg pain. A pain diagram and visual analog scale can be helpful. Patients often describe a dull, deep pain radiating into the posterior buttock and thigh. This is typically referred pain and occurs in structures with the same mesodermal origin. Neurocompressive pain can be felt as sharp, lancinating pain radiating below the knee into the foot. This radicular pain can be associated with radiculopathy, weakness, and reflex changes in the distribution of a specific nerve root due to mechanical compression or inflammation of the nerve root itself. True sciatica or radicular pain develops in a small percentage (~1%) of patients with lower back pain. Extraspinal nerve compression stemming from intrapelvic tumor or aneurysms, trochanteric bursitis, pathologic conditions of the hip, neuralgia paresthesia, diabetes, and piriformis syndrome, in addition to disc herniation, should all be considered in the differential diagnosis of sciatica. Claudication pain can take the

TABLE 171.1.	LOWER BACK PAIN: SYMPTOMS AND CAUSES
Symptom	**Possible Cause**
Sharp, narrow band of pain radiating below the knee	Herniated disc
"Stocking-glove" numbness	Referred pain, nonorganic pain
Night pain unrelieved by positional change	Tumor
Fever, chills, sweats	Infection
Long-standing back pain aggravated by activity	Deconditioning
Pain increased by sitting	Discogenic disease
Leg pain worsened by walking, unaffected by standing, but relieved by sitting	Neurologic claudication
Chronic spinal pain in patient with unsatisfying job or home life	Stress
Global pain	Nonorganic pain
Morning stiffness that improves as day goes on	Inflammatory arthritis
Unremitting, throbbing lumbar pain	Aortic aneurysm
Abdominal pain radiating to midback	Pancreatitis, gastrointestinal reflux disease, peptic ulcer disease
Back pain in athletic teenager	Epiphysitis, juvenile discogenic disease, spondylolysis, or spondylolisthesis
Back pain dating to a specific injury	Strain or sprain

form of diffuse fatigue or heaviness in the legs developing in the context of ambulation, relieved by rest, and accompanied by a forward flexed stooped change in position of the lumbar spine (see Table 171.1).

Efforts should be made to distinguish between vascular and neurogenic provocation and to assess the possibility of peripheral neuropathy due to other disease processes (Tables 171.1 and 171.2). Typically, the difference between neurogenic claudication symptoms and vascular claudication symptoms is that neurogenic pain is severe in the leg after walking a short distance. The patient is forced to stop and bend forward or sit. Pain due to vascular compromise, on the other hand, may occur at rest or in the standing position; this pain usually dissipates quickly. A noninvasive vascular workup may be necessary.

OCCUPATIONAL AND SOCIAL FACTORS

It is important to establish whether the patient was injured on the job. A detailed account should be made of the tasks performed and the mode of injury. The patient may be unhappy with the work environment. The accident process may provide a solution, especially when injury compensation can provide income. These patients may have a poor prognosis for recovery.

TABLE 171.2.	SPECIFIC DIAGNOSES ASSOCIATED WITH BACK PAIN	
Diagnosis	**Symptoms**	**Signs**
Degenerative spinal stenosis	Diffuse leg(s) pain aggravated by standing and walking downhill	Limited lumbar range of motion, weakness only after excercise
Hip disease (degenerative)	Groin and/or anterior thigh pain	Limited hip rotation range, especially loss of internal rotation
Peripheral vascular disease	Distal leg pain relieved by standing	Check for bruits and diminished pulses
Diabetic neuropathy	Glove and stocking diffuse distal bilateral burning pain	Reflexes diminished or absent
Tumor or infection	Constant pain at rest, location of pain varying	Weight loss, increased ESR, positive bone scan

(From Mooney, LM. Lumbosacral spine. In: *Southwestern Orthopaedic Review Course.* 1989:152, with permission.)

Social factors that should be taken into consideration include excessive alcohol intake, use of drugs, and cigarette smoking, which can all adversely affect the prognosis.

PHYSICAL EXAMINATION

GENERAL EXAMINATION

The patient's vital signs should be assessed, to rule out fever indicating infection. Skin involvement may suggest an underlying systemic illness, such as psoriasis, inflammatory bowel disease, or sarcoidosis. Pathologic lesions of the eye include conjunctivitis (Reiter's syndrome) or iriditis (ankylosing spondylitis). Lymphadenopathy or thyroid dysfunction may be evident from the neck examination. Costovertebral inflammation or cardiac disease can induce back pain. Limitation of chest expansion to less than 2 inches in women and 3 inches in men suggests ankylosing spondylitis. A detailed abdominal examination is important, to rule out visceral causes for back pain, including gallbladder disease, abdominal masses, and the presence of aneurysms. A rectal exam and a fecal Hemoccult test should be performed on all men over the age of 50, to rule out prostatic and bowel disease. A detailed neurologic assessment for perianal function, including rectal tone, also must be made.

EXAMINATION OF THE SPINE

One should examine the patient from a distance to see how easily the patient moves and whether he or she requires assistive devices, such as walking canes, lumbosacral orthoses, or corsets. Patients should be examined standing, kneeling, and sitting as well as bending forward. With the patient standing, abnormalities in posture should be noted, including the presence of scoliosis and asymmetry in the shoulder and pelvic height as well as spinal range of motion. The spinous processes, sacroiliac joints, and paraspinous musculature should be palpated to look for signs of muscle spasm or atrophy. The patient should be examined walking on toes, walking on heels, and tandem walking (sequential heel to toe walking as by a tightrope walker). To test for sacroiliac joint movement, place one thumb on the posterior superior iliac spine and the other on the sacrum, and ask the patient to flex the ipsilateral hip. If the iliac spine moves up, the sacroiliac joint is fixed.

The character of motion is as important as the range of motion of the lumbosacral spine. An increase in pain while bending to the ipsilateral side (lateral flexion) suggests facet articular disease or a herniated disc lateral to the nerve root. The same symptoms on the contralateral side suggest a herniated disc medial to the nerve root. The tender points of fibromyalgia should be assessed quickly. The amount of pressure applied is the amount that begins to induce a pain sensation on one's own ulnar styloid process, usually about 4 kg (10 lb of force). One should look for control points (the lateral forehead and dorsal surface of the lower midforearm). If the patient overreacts to these control points, one should suspect psychogenic pain. If these control points are not painful, proceed to palpate the fibromyalgia tender points. Coccyodynia frequently can arise in association with lower back pain felt to be due to pain in a sacral coccygeal joint.

POSITIONAL EXAMINATIONS

Kneeling

Ask the patient to kneel on a chair facing the backrest, to test for the S1 ankle (Achilles tendon) reflex. An absent ankle reflex is not necessarily a pathologic sign; it must be compared with the contralateral limb. To test for malingering, have the patient kneel on a chair, grasp the chair back with one hand, and reach forward and down to the floor with the outside hand. Acute flexion of the knee and hip does not aggravate spinal disease. If the pain is exacerbated, malingering might be considered. Other findings related to nonorganic causes for lower back pain include increased lower back pain with light pressure on the vertex of the skull, exacerbated lower back pain with motion of the lumbosacral spine and pelvis in unison (holding the patient's torso and pelvis and rotating both together), and diffuse nondermatomal global glove and stocking pain or numbness involving one or more extremities.

Sitting

Have the patient sit on a chair with feet on the floor and apply steady downward pressure on the dorsum of the foot. Genuine weakness of the muscles supplied by the L5 nerve root is felt as uniform resistance to pressure that is gradually and smoothly overcome. The patient who feigns weakness will often resist the pressure briefly and then suddenly let go. This is described as *collapsing strength.* With the patient seated, begin manual muscle testing for motor strength and control, first of the upper extremities and then of the lower extremities, including hip flexion, extension, abduction and adduction; knee flexion and extension; and ankle dorsiflexion, plantar flexion, inversion, and eversion. Examine radicular and cortical dermatomal function and responses and deep tendon reflexes.

Bending Forward

With the patient flexed at the waist over the examination table, one should inspect the spine for asymmetry and palpate the sacroiliac joint, ischiatic tuberosities, and sciatic notch. Look for tenderness, masses, and defects. When patients with radiculopathy lie supine, certain maneuvers tighten the sciatic nerve and further compress an inflamed lumbar root against a herniated disc or bony spur. These maneuvers are generally termed "tension signs" or a straight-leg-raising test. The examiner slowly elevates the supine patient's leg by the heel with the knee straight. The test result is considered positive if leg pain occurs below the knee, not just in the back and buttocks. The pain is aggravated by dorsiflexion of the foot. The reliability of this test may be age dependent. With the patient in a supine position, test hip range of motion—the straight-leg-raise test. Look for hamstring tightness by measuring the popliteal angle with the leg elevated and palpate the pelvis. Hip abduction and extension and the femoral nerve stretch test (L3 and L4 nerve root irritation) are best done with the patient in a lateral position.

DIAGNOSTIC STUDIES

A challenge to the physician in the assessment of lower back pain is to select tests that can lead to the correct diagnosis at the lowest cost and morbidity. Because of the high potential for false-positive results, these tests are not performed for screening purposes and should not be used in an isolated context for making management decisions, particularly surgery. Treatment options must be based on a careful assessment of the history and clinical findings and interpretation of imaging studies.

ROENTGENOGRAPHY

Plain x-ray films are useful for surveying the bony structures of the spine, particularly such instability patterns as spondylolisthesis, scoliosis, fractures, tumors, and infections. They do not display the soft tissues, including the neuroelements and discs. The presence of degenerative changes, such as disc space narrowing with vacuum phenomenon, traction osteophytes, and endplate sclerosis, though common, do not correlate well with clinical symptoms. Radiographs should be performed early in patients younger than 20 or older than 50 who are experiencing pain. When spondylolysis is suspected, oblique views are helpful. To follow the progression of spondylolisthesis, a spot lateral view of the area in question, usually the L5-S1 segment, may be better than lateral views of the entire lumbar sacral spine. An anteroposterior view of the pelvis should incorporate both hips, to rule out pathologic hip conditions.

COMPUTED TOMOGRAPHY AND MYELOGRAPHY

CT scans provide the greatest information about osseous lesions and less specific information about periosseous soft-tissue swelling. They can be particularly helpful in evaluating spondylolysis, infection, or tumor associated with bony destruction. Using myelography in conjunction with CT allows for more precise viewing of pathologic anatomy and enhances diagnostic accuracy.

MAGNETIC RESONANCE IMAGING

MRI is an excellent noninvasive imaging method for the lumbar spine. MRI best evaluates soft tissue, such as the disc, nerve roots, thecal sac, and paraspinous soft tissues. It is especially helpful when spine infection or soft-tissue tumors are suspected. Gadolinium contrast enhancement helps distinguish recurrent disc herniations from scar tissue.

NUCLEAR MEDICINE STUDIES

The technetium Tc 99m bone scan can be very helpful in elucidating any underlying sinister cause for back pain, including occult spondylolysis, primary and metastatic tumors, discitis, and vertebral osteomyelitis as well as some visceral causes for back pain. The single-photon-emission CT scan has been particularly helpful in detecting occult spondylolysis.

ELECTRODIAGNOSTIC TESTING

Electromyelography is performed by placing needles into muscles to determine the integrity of the nerve supply. Results can establish impaired nerve transmission to a specific muscle and can isolate the involved nerve root. Fibrillation potentials confirm the presence of denervation. This study can help distinguish radiculopathy from other neuropathic conditions that cause leg pain, such as diabetes. Both electromyelography and nerve conduction studies are helpful when the correlation between clinical signs and imaging is equivocal.

CLINICAL CONDITIONS

Several conditions can show initial symptoms of lower back pain. The following are the most common and important conditions that are seen in primary practice settings.

BACK SPRAIN/STRAIN

The vast majority of people with lower back pain without radiation into the lower extremities have what is described as a back strain, or lumbago. Following an acute back injury, 70% of patients are significantly improved after 2 weeks, and 90% recover within 2 to 3 months. Typically, the patient has no findings of nerve root compression (sciatica). Physical examination may pinpoint both lumbar tenderness and muscle spasms, with restricted range of motion of the lumbosacral spine. These attacks can vary in intensity. Radiographic findings are usually normal; these tests should be obtained only if the patient does not improve over a course of 2 to 3 months or if the patient is younger than 20 or older than 50 and has history or physical examination findings that suggest a nonmechanical, serious cause for lower back pain.

The Agency for Health Care Quality and Research convened a 23-member multidisciplinary panel to establish basic guidelines for treatment of acute back pain in adults. They defined an acute lower back problem as limitation of activity stemming from symptoms in the lower back and/or back-related leg symptoms of less than 3 months' duration. The guideline provided numerous conclusions about the safety and efficacy of current options for treating acute lower back pain in adults (Table 171.3).

A comprehensive treatment plan is important for these patients, not just in terms of addressing the acute situation but also for incorporating preventive measures. Initial treatment includes supportive measures to control pain, with the goal of early return to maximum function. The patient should not stay at bed rest for longer than 3 days, to avoid deconditioning. Medication used to treat lower back pain includes analgesics, anti-inflammatory drugs (occasionally for chronic pain), and such mood-altering medications as antidepressants. Short-term use of opiates is appropriate and is unlikely to lead to habituation or abuse. It is important to involve the patient in as active a program as possible in the early phases of management. The patient should start in a physical therapy program and be instructed in posture techniques (Table 171.4). In the early phases of acute pain, such passive treatments as heat, ultrasonography, manual manipulation, and mobilization techniques may be helpful, but ultimately the patient should be instructed in a stretching and conditioning program that can be performed at home as well as with the

therapist (Table 171.5). The most common techniques are dynamic stabilization and the use of muscle-strengthening exercise equipment. All require instruction by trained therapists for maximal benefit. Each has a specific rationale, and a combination of these techniques may be beneficial (Table 171.6).

If the symptoms do not resolve over a 12-week period, the treating physician should reconsider the diagnosis. Psychosocial issues, including narcotic addiction and workers' compensation, should be considered as possible causes of persistent back pain. After other causes of mechanical pain have been eliminated, such as degenerative disc disease, scoliosis, and spondylolisthesis, one must consider systemic causes in the differential diagnosis, such

---

TABLE 171.4.   POSTURE TECHNIQUES THAT HELP AVOID LOWER BACK PAIN[a]

Standing
   Maintain good abdominal tone; keep abdomen flattened while standing.
   When prolonged standing is necessary, place one foot on a step for a few minutes.
   Wear cushion-soled shoes for prolonged standing.
Bending, lifting, carrying
   Bend at the knees not at the waist.
   Lift with the thighs (keep heavy objects centered close to abdomen).
   Flex knees while bending.
   When carrying heavy objects, turn with the feet, not by twisting the trunk.
Sitting and lying
   Sit on straight-backed, firm, supportive chair.
   Sit only for short periods.
   Sleep on back, with knees bent, or on side on a firm mattress.

---

[a] Avoid prolonged standing, prolonged sitting, and improper lifting.

TABLE 171.3.   GUIDELINES OF THE AGENCY FOR HEALTH CARE QUALITY AND RESEARCH

Bed rest for more than 4 days may lead to debilitation and is not recommended.
Low-stress aerobic exercise can prevent debilitation due to inactivity during the first month of symptoms. Thereafter it may help return patients to the highest level of functioning.
Acetaminophen, NSAIDs, muscle relaxants, and opioid analgesics are all options.
Lumbar corsets and belts beneficial only when used prophylactically.
Manipulation can be helpful in patients without radiculopathy, but only within the first month of symptoms.
Epidural injections are an option only for short-term relief of radicular pain after conservative therapy.
Back schools in the workplace that offer worksite-specific education may be effective adjuncts.
Oral steroids and antidepressants are not recommended.
Transcutaneous electrical nerve stimulation is not recommended.
Spinal traction is not recommended.
Trigger point and facet joint injections are not recommended.

NSAIDs, nonsteroidal anti-inflammatory drugs.

TABLE 171.5.   GUIDELINES FOR TREATMENT OF A PATIENT WITH LUMBAR SPINE COMPLAINTS

Most patients with back pain improve. If a back problem cannot be cured, function should at least be optimized.
Imaging abnormalities are common in persons with and without back problems.
Explain to the patient that "hurt" does not equal "harm." Back pain is common and does not necessarily signify a permanently impaired life.
The key decision point in treatment is 6 weeks after injury. Back pain should spontaneously improve in this time. If improvement has not occurred, reassess the patient and refer him or her to an active physical therapy program, emphasizing functional restoration rather than pain relief.
Reserve expensive imaging studies for those patients not responding to an active rehabilitation program or at risk of progressive neurologic compromise.
Surgery is a last resort for most patients, considered only for one who has failed a good, active, functional restoration program or shows signs of progressive neurologic injury.

TABLE 171.6.	STRATEGIES TO IMPROVE BACK PAIN		
	Definition	**Technique**	**Outcome**
McKenzie program	With symptom-specific treatment, the patient responds favorably to mechanical forces applied to the spine	Careful analysis of the patient's movements characterize directional preference. In the *centralization* phenomenon, pain moves toward the center of the spine or is abolished with repeated end-range spinal movements. Centralization is a predictor of successful outcomes with mechanical therapy and reliably determines the appropriate direction of the treatment.	Patient self-treatment program avoids dependency on passive interventions and may prevent recurrent episodes of back pain.
Dynamic stabilization	Develops adequate musculoligamentus control of the lumbar spine to limit repetitive microtrauma by promoting muscular coordination, endurance, and aerobic fitness.	Gym-based and functional training instruction in symmetric strength, flexibility, balance, proprioception, and trunk control	Learned techniques become automatic and ingrained, leading to independence of the patient
Guided exercises with equipment	Strength training improves neuromuscular control. Specialized exercise equipment isolates and evaluates certain target weak-link muscle groups (lumbar extensors)	With the patient in a sitting position use of specialized equipment prevents pelvic motion and gives consistent standardized exercises that isolate the lumbar extensors.	Treatment is complete when isometric strength testing confirms muscular function and strength has returned to normal or has reached a plateau.

as seronegative spondylarthropathy, metabolic bone disease (osteoporosis, osteomalacia), fibromyalgia, and polymyalgia rheumatica. If the workup at this point generates negative results, it is important to keep in mind that a specific anatomic source is clearly identifiable in only 10% to 20% of patients with chronic lower back pain. The advice of a spine specialist should be sought if the patient suffers chronic lower back pain (Fig. 171.1).

HERNIATED DISC

True sciatica or radicular pain related to nerve root compression occurs in a small percentage of patients with lower back pain, roughly 1%. A herniated disc is defined as a herniation of the nucleus pulposus through the torn fibers of the annulus fibrosis. This takes place most often in the third and fourth decades of life. Eighty percent of cases arise at the L4-5 and L5-S1 levels, compressing the fifth lumbar and first sacral nerve roots, respectively. Typically, the patient has localized pain radiating down the leg in the distribution of the affected nerve root. The symptoms may be severe enough to prevent the patient from standing and walking and may be associated with loss of range of motion of the spine. A dynamic list away from the affected side is noticeable as the patient bends forward. The patient may avoid bearing weight on the extremity in an attempt to avoid stretching the sciatic nerve. A neurologic examination may detect findings of nerve root compression, including sensory, motor, and reflex changes (Table 171.7). The straight-leg-raise test is very important in eliciting nerve root irritation.

MRI is the study of choice to determine the extent of disc herniation and the level affected. CT can be used alone or with myelography. The herniation may be either contained or extruded, with nuclear pulposus contents passing beyond the posterior longitudinal ligament or even sequestered completely free in the spinal canal. Ninety percent of patients respond to conservative efforts, usually an exercise program. Occasionally, a spinal epidural injection or selective nerve root block can help diminish the pain and allow further exercises to be performed. If radiculopathy persists, as occurs in 10% to 25% of cases, or if there is progressive neurologic compromise with increasing weakness, the patient may become a candidate for a surgical decompressive procedure. The surgical treatment of choice is microdiscectomy, involving a minimal incision and the use of a microscope to enhance visibility of the neurological tissues. The surgical success rate with this procedure is about 92%. There is a 10% incidence of recurrent herniation and a 10% to 15% incidence of ongoing disabling back pain.

CAUDA EQUINA SYNDROME

Only a small percentage of patients with lower back pain have cauda equina syndrome; the incidence is one in 10,000. One should inquire about changes in bowel or bladder habits. A large midline disc herniation may compress several roots of the cauda equina, resulting in lower back pain, bilateral motor weakness of the lower extremities, bilateral sciatica, saddle anesthesia, and even frank paraplegia with bowel and bladder incontinence. Patients with suspected cauda equina syndrome require immediate imaging, such as MRI or myelography. A missed diagnosis can

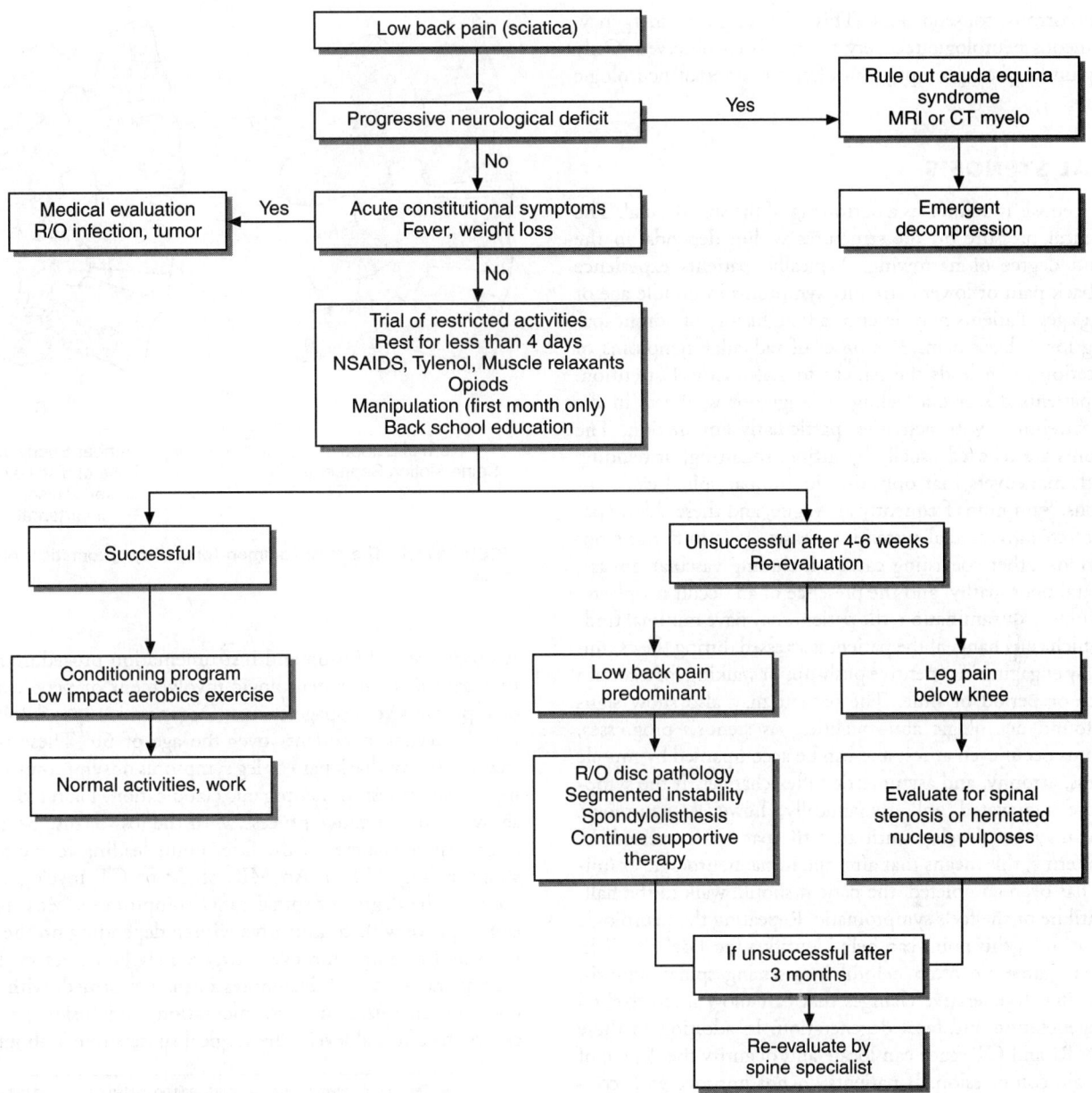

FIGURE 171.1. Algorithm for assessment of low back pain.
EVIDENCE LEVEL: B. Reference: Mooney V. Treating low back pain with exercise. *J Musculo-skeletal Med* 1995;12:24–36.

TABLE 171.7.	RADICULAR SYMPTOMS AND SIGNS		
Disc space	**L3-4**	**L4-5**	**L5-S1**
Root compressed	L4	L5	S1
Reflex diminished	Knee jerk	No reflex	Ankle jerk
Motor weakness	Knee extension	Great toe dorsiflexion	Ankle plantiflexion
Sensory deficit	Medial ankle and foot	Dorsal foot at the first web space	Lateral foot
Pain	Anterior thigh	Posterior leg	Posterior leg

have disastrous consequences. This is a surgical emergency. Spontaneous neurologic recovery has not been observed. Only surgery undertaken promptly can offer any hope of neurologic recovery.

SPINAL STENOSIS

Spinal stenosis is defined as a narrowing of the spinal canal. The mechanical pressure on the structures within depends on the rate and degree of narrowing. Typically, patients experience lower back pain or lower extremity symptoms in middle age or at older ages. Patients may describe a long history of nonincapacitating lower back pain. The onset of radicular symptoms or claudication often leads the patient to seek medical attention. Some patients describe a feeling of fatigue or weakness in the lower extremities with activities, particularly ambulation. The symptoms are relieved usually by sitting, squatting, or bending forward, maneuvers that optimize the lumbar spinal canal dimensions. Symptoms frequently are vague, and these elderly patients often have several systemic diseases. It is important not to overlook other coexisting causes, including vascular disease, peripheral neuropathy, and the presence of an occult neoplasm.

On physical examination, the patient may have minimal findings, which can change if the patient is stressed during the examination by engaging in repetitive push-ups or walking for a certain distance or period of time. The patient may also show signs of profound neurologic abnormalities. As stenosis progresses, symptoms occur even at rest and can be accompanied by muscle weakness, atrophy, and asymmetric reflex changes. If the symptoms are aggravated only dynamically, however, neurologic changes may not develop until after the patient is stressed. In clinical terms, this means that after the initial neurologic examination has been completed, the patient should walk in the hallway until he or she feels symptomatic. Repeating the neurologic examination at this point can help identify a focal deficit. Plain roentgenograms are often helpful in assessing spinal stenosis, pinpointing degenerative changes that can show intervertebral disc degeneration and facet degeneration. In addition to these films, MRI and CT scans can locate and quantify the degree of neurologic compression. If patients do not improve with conservative efforts, a surgical decompressive procedure might be considered. Usually the success rate is approximately 70%.

SPONDYLOLISTHESIS

Spondylolisthesis is defined as slippage forward of one vertebral body onto another (Fig. 171.2). The amount of displacement varies and has been graded from 1 (minimal) to 5 (severe). There are five types of spondylolisthesis, which can be differentiated with proper imaging techniques. A lateral radiograph of the lumbar spine can show the degree of forward displacement (percentage of slip) and the angular relationships between the lower lumbar vertebrae and the sacral vertebrae (angle of slip). The oblique views disclose the actual pars defect.

A child typically has symptoms of lower back pain, tight hamstrings, and exaggeration of lumbar lordosis, with a palpable step-off at the level of the slippage. A growing child may be at risk of progressive slippage and should be carefully monitored.

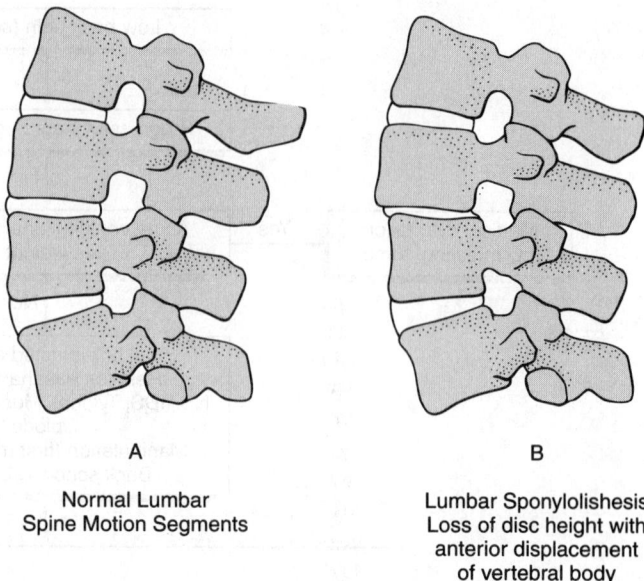

A
Normal Lumbar
Spine Motion Segments

B
Lumbar Sponylolishesis
Loss of disc height with
anterior displacement
of vertebral body

FIGURE 171.2. The most common form of symptomatic spondylolisthesis.

A surgical spinal fusion and instrumentation procedure may be necessary if there is neurologic involvement or persistent pain or if progressive slippage occurs. Degenerative spondylolisthesis usually occurs in patients over the age of 60. These patients frequently have back pain or leg symptoms or symptoms suggesting spinal stenosis or neurogenic claudication. Plain radiographs show the degenerative process, with the loss of disc height and degenerative changes in the facet joints leading to the forward slippage (Fig. 171.2). An MRI study or CT myelogram will confirm the degree of spinal canal compromise. Most patients can improve with conservative efforts; depending on the symptoms and findings, however, surgery may be necessary. In that case, posterior spinal decompression is performed, with a concomitant stabilization, instrumentation, and fusion procedure across the affected level. The surgical success rate is about 70%.

Kelley's Textbook of Internal Medicine, fourth edition. Edited by H. David Humes. Lippincott Williams & Wilkins, Philadelphia © 2000.

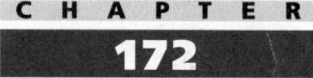

CHAPTER
172

APPROACH TO THE PATIENT WITH ANERGY

ABBA I. TERR

Anergy is the inability of the T or B lymphocyte to respond immunologically to an antigen or a bacterial superantigen, such as *Streptococcus pyogenes* erythrogenic toxin A or *Staphylococcus aureus* enterotoxins. In the normal immune response, the antigen is phagocytized and processed by the monocyte/macrophage, known as the antigen-presenting cell (APC). Antigen processing generates peptide fragments that are presented to the CD4$^+$ T-cell receptor (TCR) in association with products of the major histocompatibility complex expressed on the APC surface. T-cell activation and clonal expansion also requires co-stimulating signals from the APC to the CD4$^+$ T cell. The activated T cell then synthesizes and releases cytokines and expresses interleukin-2 receptors. The profile of the released cytokines determines the nature of the immune response. For example, a predominant interleukin-4 response that characterizes the helper T-cell subtype 2 cytokine profile favors IgE antibody production by B cells, which, in turn, leads to an allergic response to the antigen.

T-CELL ANERGY

T lymphocytes are rendered anergic in vivo by exposure of an antigen or an antigenic peptide fragment to the TCR without the co-stimulatory signals from the APC necessary for activation of the T cell. The resulting T-cell anergy is both peptide specific and major histocompatibility complex restricted. The anergic T cell, however, retains the ability to respond to mitogen and to interleukin-2. CD4$^+$ and CD8$^+$ T cells made specifically anergic to an antigenic peptide or to a bacterial superantigen fail to proliferate when stimulated with antigen or bacterial superantigen, do not produce interleukin-2 or interferon-α, and do not express interleukin-2 receptors.

B-CELL ANERGY

When occupied by an antigenic molecule, the B-cell receptor for antigen, like the TCR, activates the cell to cause differentiation and proliferation with ultimate production and secretion of specific antibody by the plasma cell, or it induces a state of specific tolerance to the antigen. The former scenario is the probable outcome for foreign antigens, and the latter is the preferred pathway for self-antigens. T cell–B cell interactions and the secreted cytokine profile of the activated T cell are important determinants of B-cell immunity versus anergy. Antigen-specific B-cell anergy is an important feature of theories that explain the normal tolerance to self-antigens. In vitro experiments show that immature cells in the B-lymphocyte lineage are the most susceptible to this phenomenon, and susceptibility is related to the preferential use of particular V$_\beta$ gene families.

TESTING METHODS

Skin testing for the absence of delayed hypersensitivity to a standard panel of recall antigens is the procedure for detecting a state of global T-cell anergy (lack of T-cell immunity). The test antigens are selected on the basis of an expected high prevalence delayed skin hypersensitivity because of frequent natural expo-sure in the general healthy population. These usually include streptococcal, fungal, tuberculous, and vaccine antigens. The absence of delayed hypersensitivity in an adult to all antigens in such a panel would be presumptive evidence of T-cell immunosuppression.

The skin tests are applied to the volar surface of the forearm and read in 48 hours. There are two accepted procedures for performing these tests. The standard one is the intradermal injection of 0.1 mL of each antigen at separate skin sites at least 3 cm apart. This is the procedure known as the Mantoux test for tuberculosis. For large-scale epidemiologic studies, a prick test method often is used. In this case, a plastic device delivers eight superficial skin pricks for individual antigens simultaneously, according to a preset pattern.

CAUSES OF GLOBAL T-CELL ANERGY

CONGENITAL CELLULAR IMMUNODEFICIENCIES

There are three categories of congenital immunodeficiencies: B-cell (antibody) deficiencies, T-cell (cellular) deficiencies, and combined immunodeficiencies. Representative examples are shown in Table 172.1.

INFECTIONS

The anergy that occurs in patients infected with the human immunodeficiency virus is the best-known example of acquired arrest of immune system function caused by a viral infection. Skin testing with the panel of recall antigens described earlier in this chapter correlates inversely with the clinical status of the disease but even more closely with the peripheral blood CD4 cell count. Transient T-cell anergy may develop during the course of

TABLE 172.1.	SELECTED CONGENITAL IMMUNODEFICIENCY DISORDERS

B-cell immunodeficiency
  Common variable immunodeficiency
  Selective IgA deficiency
  Selective IgG subclass deficiencies
  X-linked hypogammaglobulinemia
  Immunodeficiency with hyper-IgM
T-cell immunodeficiency
  DiGeorge syndrome (congenital thymic aplasia)
  T-cell deficiency with purine nucleoside phosphorylase deficiency
  Chronic mucocutaneous candidiasis
Combined T-cell and B-cell immunodeficiency
  Severe combined immunodeficiency disease
  Wiskott–Aldrich syndrome (T-cell deficiency, eczema, and thrombocytopenia)
  Nezelof syndrome (T-cell deficiency with abnormal immunoglobulin synthesis)
  Immunodeficiency with ataxia–telangiectasia
  Immunodeficiency with thymoma
  Immunodeficiency with adenosine deaminase deficiency

acute infectious mononucleosis. Cellular immunity is depressed significantly, but transiently, during acute measles infection. Both skin test reactivity and in vitro lymphocyte activation by antigens and mitogens reflect this state and should suggest the possibility of reactivation of dormant tuberculosis or other infections.

MALNUTRITION

Protein-calorie malnutrition of dietary origin or from chronic debilitating disease reduces the number of CD4 cells and the activity of CD8 cells. Patients with this form of malnutrition are functionally anergic with respect to their cell-mediated immunity.

TRAUMA

Severe physical trauma causes transient suppression of delayed skin tests for cell-mediated immunity. In children there also is a temporary depletion of circulating B cells.

OTHERS

Jaundice from liver disease is associated with anergy, regardless of whether the underlying pathologic condition is benign or malignant. Advanced age itself does not cause anergy, though the intensity of the skin test reaction is lessened, suggesting waning of the inflammatory phase of immunity. Splenectomy attenuates the IgM antibody response, and patients who have had their spleens removed are especially susceptible to pneumococcal infections. Acquired immunodeficiency also has been associated with cancer, chronic infection, chronic renal disease with azotemia, primary biliary cirrhosis, drug abuse, and many transfusions.

Sarcoidosis is a disease with active local immune responsiveness at sites of disease activity, hypergammaglobulinemia, and tissue granulomas but paradoxically diminished cellular responses in vitro to antigens and mitogens, peripheral blood lymphopenia, and delayed skin test anergy. The cause of this disease remains unknown. In terms of immunologic features, it bears some resemblance to asbestosis, a noninfectious disease of known origin that also exhibits skin anergy, lymphopenia, and evidence of diminished lymphocyte activity measured in vitro.

CAUSES OF ANTIGEN-SPECIFIC ANERGY

About 10% of patients with pulmonary tuberculosis have anergy, as shown by the absence of delayed skin test reactivity to tuberculin. Compared with infected patients who have positive skin test results, they tend to be older and to have more extensive pulmonary disease, especially miliary tuberculosis, but they do not necessarily have a higher prevalence of extrapulmonary disease. Furthermore, they tend to be less symptomatic, which probably reflects lessening of inflammation in the anergic state. The skin test result may revert to positive with effective antituberculosis therapy. A similar state of antigen-specific T-cell unre-

sponsiveness occurs in certain clinical manifestations of parasitic diseases, such as filariasis and leishmaniasis.

THERAPEUTIC INDUCTION OF ANERGY

Immunosuppressant regimens to prevent transplant rejection and to treat certain connective tissue or autoimmune disorders are nonspecific and, therefore, subject the patient to opportunistic infections. A potential new approach to immunotherapy for autoimmune or allergic diseases, involving an attempt to induce antigen-specific anergy, is being pursued actively in several diseases. The challenge to the use of this method in autoimmune disease is the identification of the pathogenetic autoantigen. Patients with multiple sclerosis have autoantibodies to myelin basic protein, and oral administration of this antigen has been used in therapeutic trials.

BIBLIOGRAPHY

Belfer MH, Stevens RW. Sarcoidosis: a primary care review. *Am Fam Physician* 1998:58:2041–2055.
Bianco NE. The immunopathology of systemic anergy in infectious diseases: a reappraisal and new perspectives. *Clin Immunol Immunopathol* 1992; 62:253–257.
Fletcher JP, Little LM, Walker PJ. Anergy and the severely ill surgical patient. *Aust N Z J Surg* 1986;56:117–120.
Jenkins MK, Miller RA. Memory and anergy: challenges to traditional models of T lymphocyte differentiation. *FASEB J* 1992;6:2428–2433.
Markowitz N, Hansen NI, Wilcosky TC, et al. Tuberculin and anergy testing in HIV-seropositive and HIV-seronegative persons. *Ann Intern Med* 1993;119:185–193.
Wilson NW, Gooding A, Peterson B, et al. Anergy in pediatric head trauma patients. *Am J Dis Child* 1991;145:326–329.

Kelley's Textbook of Internal Medicine, fourth edition. Edited by H. David Humes.
Lippincott Williams & Wilkins, Philadelphia © 2000.

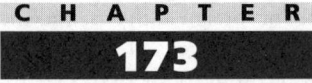

CHAPTER 173

APPROACH TO THE PATIENT WITH ALLERGY

ABBA I. TERR

Allergy refers to both a pathogenetic mechanism and the resulting diseases. In these diseases, immunologically induced inflammation is triggered by environmental antigens, referred to as *allergens*. In most cases, the allergens themselves are innocuous. Allergy is common and can be local or systemic, depending, in part, on the mode of exposure to the allergen. Allergic rhinitis, asthma, and allergic contact dermatitis are the most prevalent

TABLE 173.1.	GELL AND COOMBS CLASSIFICATION OF ALLERGIC DISEASES	
Type	Immunologic Mechanism of Action	Representative Diseases
I	IgE antibody–mast cell mediator release	Atopy (allergic rhinitis, asthma, atopic dermatitis) Anaphylaxis
II	IgG antibody-complement activation-cytolysis	Drug-caused immune-mediated hemolytic anemia, neutropenia, thrombocytopenia
III	Immune complex–mediated, complement-dependent inflammation	Serum sickness
IV	T cell-mediated inflammation	Allergic contact dermatitis

manifestations and are responsible for significant morbidity. Accurate diagnosis and appropriate treatment can significantly curtail the pathologic manifestations and disability of the disease. Because of the variety of pathways by which the immune response can generate inflammation, allergic diseases are classified by their underlying immunologic pathogenesis. A commonly used scheme is the Gell and Coombs classification shown in Table 173.1.

PRINCIPLES OF ALLERGY DIAGNOSIS

The diagnosis of any allergic disease is dependent on an accurate and thorough history and physical examination. Laboratory tests and specific allergy testing should be selective and based on the clinical history. The important elements in the history are a detailed description of the patient's symptoms and the time and place of their occurrence, to establish the relationship between symptoms and specific environmental exposures. Respiratory symptoms suggest the role of airborne allergens, such as pollens, dusts, fungi, animal dander, and materials and substances found in the workplace. Allergic contact dermatitis often is caused by plants, perfumes, cosmetics, clothing, topical medications, and substances encountered on the job and in association with hobbies. Other cutaneous reactions may implicate ingested allergens in foods or drugs. Finally, a complete medical history is necessary to rule out nonallergic diseases in the differential diagnosis.

Physical signs of active tissue inflammation, such as rhinitis, asthma, or dermatitis, will be detected if the patient is examined during a period of disease activity. These signs may be absent between active episodes, so a normal physical examination does not preclude a diagnosis of allergy. Depending on the results of the history and physical examination, tests for target organ dysfunction, such as pulmonary function testing, imaging of the paranasal sinuses, and stool examination for eosinophils, may be indicated.

LABORATORY TESTS FOR ALLERGY (TABLE 173.2)

SKIN TESTS FOR IGE ALLERGY

Atopy, anaphylaxis, and urticaria are mediated by IgE antibodies, which respond to the allergen by prompt local release of vasoactive and inflammatory mediators. Challenge of the skin vasculature to the allergen results in an immediate wheal-and-flare reaction, which has been well validated as an accurate test for diagnosis. The epicutaneous test involves pricking the skin with a needle through a drop of aqueous allergen extract applied to the skin site. In a patient with IgE antibodies to the test allergen, a cutaneous wheal-and-flare reaction appears in 15 to 20 minutes and is pruritic. Intracutaneous testing gives the same response to the injection of 0.005 to 0.020 mL of a properly diluted sterilized allergen extract. It is used selectively to supplement prick testing for atopy.

IN VITRO TESTS FOR IGE ALLERGY

The detection of circulating IgE antibodies uses such techniques as the radioallergosorbent test or the enzyme-linked immunosorbent assay, which are sensitive enough to detect and measure allergen-specific antibody levels in picograms per milliliter. Nevertheless, their diagnostic sensitivity is lower than that of skin testing. Measurement of total serum IgE concentration does not determine allergen specificity and has only limited value for diagnosis. Compared with nonallergic controls, levels are higher, on average, in patients with atopy, especially those with atopic dermatitis and asthma, but many patients have normal levels. Total serum IgE is markedly elevated in allergic bronchopulmonary aspergillosis, especially during exacerbations.

TABLE 173.2.	PRINCIPLES OF ALLERGY TESTING

Allergy tests detect the presence of a response through a particular immune pathway to a specific allergen.

The type of test must be selected to be consistent with the patient's disease.

The allergens selected for testing must be consistent with those to which the patient might have been exposed at the appropriate time interval in relation to symptoms.

The existence of a specific immune response, as detected by a positive allergy test result, is not in initself sufficient to cause an allergic reaction on exposure to that allergen.

A positive allergy test result may indicate past, present, or future disease.

There are varying degrees of diagnostic sensitivity and specificity.

Allergy test results are diagnostically useful only in relation to the clinical examination.

SKIN PATCH TEST

In testing for allergic contact dermatitis, a predetermined concentration of allergen is taped on a patch of skin for 48 hours. A positive test result consists of localized erythema, papules, and vesicles, which usually are present at the skin test site when the patch is removed; in some cases, the result may not be seen for up to 96 hours.

■ PRINCIPLES OF ALLERGY TREATMENT

The three cardinal principles of allergy treatment are avoidance of the allergen, medications to control symptoms, and immunotherapy with specific allergens. Although it may not be necessary to implement all three treatments in every case, effective therapy requires accurate diagnosis and follow-up monitoring of the recommended regimen.

AVOIDANCE

Avoiding inhaled aeroallergens requires various environmental control maneuvers. Exposure to outdoor pollens and fungal spores usually can be minimized by staying indoors but at the sacrifice of a lifestyle change that may be undesirable. Indoor mold exposure can be partly abated through cleaning and dehumidification. Animal dander from household pets can be avoided only by removing the animals from the house. Treatment of the animals, such as frequent washing, is of unproven benefit. House dust control is directed toward elimination of the dust mite from its principal habitat: mattresses, pillows, and bedroom carpets. Food and drug allergens must be avoided.

MEDICATIONS

Drug therapy for allergic diseases is aimed at reversing or preventing target organ inflammation and its effects on organ function. These drugs do not alter allergic sensitivity itself. Glucocorticoids are especially powerful in suppressing every known form of allergic inflammation. Their usefulness is limited by side effects and long-term toxicity, but these effects can be significantly lessened by using one or more of the many topical forms available for skin, nasal, and bronchial application.

The H_1 histamine receptor-blocking drugs (antihistamines) often are effective in minimizing or eliminating the symptoms of allergic rhinitis and may relieve the pruritus of atopic dermatitis and urticaria. They are not helpful for asthma, but they are not contraindicated if needed for other purposes. Nonsedating H_1 histamine receptor antagonists lack the major adverse effect of older antihistamines. Nevertheless, they retain the undesirable drying effect on mucous membranes, and patients must be cautioned against overdose because of reports of cardiac arrhythmias associated with some of these agents.

Drugs that modify the inflammatory effect of leukotrienes are effective for asthma, but to date they have not been shown to be useful for other allergic diseases. Both 5-lipoxygenase inhibitors and leukotriene receptor antagonists are available. Other drugs with proven efficacy include inhaled or systemic β_2-adrenergic agonists and anticholinergic drugs, α-adrenergic agonists, theophylline (because of its bronchodilator action), and cromolyn and nedocromil, which have a poorly defined mast cell–stabilizing property.

ALLERGY IMMUNOTHERAPY

Immunization to induce clinical tolerance to the effects of environmental allergens is accomplished by repeated subcutaneous injections of the allergen at frequent intervals in increasing dosage. The treatment is tailored to each patient, to ensure that the amount of allergen administered each time is small enough to avoid initiating an allergic reaction but sufficient to stimulate ongoing protective immunity. Patients with multiple atopic allergies can be treated with a mixture of all relevant allergens simultaneously. Numerous controlled clinical trials over the past 30 years prove that this form of therapy is effective, without long-term toxicity in most patients with allergic rhinitis to the major inhaled allergens. Effectiveness of immunotherapy for allergic asthma is less well established. There is no documented role for this form of treatment in improving atopic dermatitis.

Immunization of patients with *Hymenoptera* venom anaphylaxis is highly successful. Short-term desensitization of penicillin allergy has been established, but the effect may be transient and therefore unreliable for a future course of the drug. Oral desensitization for cutaneous reactions to other drugs, especially sulfonamides, is frequently efficacious, but it should not be attempted in patients with an exfoliative reaction to the drug. There is no role for its use in the context of food allergy.

■ ALLERGIC DISEASES

ALLERGIC RHINITIS

Atopy is the term used to denote an inherited tendency toward the development of IgE antibodies to a variety of inhaled and ingested organic substances commonly encountered in everyday life. Allergic rhinitis is the most common manifestation of atopy (see Chapter 366). The other atopic diseases are allergic asthma and atopic dermatitis. Overall, 10% to 20% of the US population is affected. The onset of symptomatic disease can occur at any age, but most cases begin in childhood. The illness persists for many years, though it may remit spontaneously. Both sexes are affected equally.

A typical attack of allergic rhinitis consists of paroxysmal sneezing; clear, watery rhinorrhea; nasal congestion; red, watery eyes; itching of the eyes, nose, and palate; and postnasal drainage. Malaise is common when symptoms are severe. Headache accompanies sinus congestion, and pain in the neck may ensue from sneezing spasms. Symptoms are triggered on exposure to allergen, so the illness follows a seasonal pattern in patients with pollen allergy. Allergy to indoor dust mites, dander, and fungi can cause year-round symptoms. Although the problem is not life-threatening, morbidity and disability can be significant. Complications are otitis media, especially in children, and sinusitis at any age.

Physical findings during symptomatic periods are red, swollen conjunctivae; pale blue, swollen nasal mucosa with excessive clear secretions; and edema of the mucosa of the soft palate and posterior oral pharynx. The diagnosis is made by history, physical examination, and specific allergy skin testing. The differential diagnosis includes infectious rhinitis (usually viral), chronic nonallergic (vasomotor) rhinitis, rhinitis medicamentosa, sinusitis, and, rarely, a cerebrospinal fluid leak from fracture of the cribriform plate. Routine laboratory studies are not necessary in uncomplicated cases, but the presence of eosinophilia in blood and nasal secretions is helpful in differentiating this disease from nonallergic forms of rhinitis.

Every effort should be made to avoid those allergens that are avoidable, especially indoor allergens. Antihistamines long have been helpful in minimizing or alleviating symptoms, and the development of nonsedating antihistamines (fexofenadine, astemizole, loratadine, cetirizine) makes this therapeutic option more attractive than previously. The addition of oral sympathomimetic decongestants occasionally is warranted, but topical nasal decongestants should not be used. Topical nasal corticosteroids are beneficial and safe. Cromolyn sodium by nasal spray is an effective prophylactic medication for some patients, and it has the advantage of producing no side effects or long-term toxicity.

Allergic conjunctivitis almost always accompanies allergic rhinitis, and the same allergens are responsible for both conditions. In addition to avoidance of allergens, treatment consists of oral antihistamines, conjunctival antihistamines or cromolyn, and immunotherapy. Glucocorticoid eyedrops may provide temporary relief, but the potential for glaucoma, corneal ulcers, or other complications must be monitored.

ASTHMA

The pathophysiologic characteristics and treatment of asthma are discussed in detail in Chapter 363. Some patients with asthma have atopy, and their attacks can be triggered by environmental allergens. The immunologic mechanism of action is the same as that described for allergic rhinitis. Allergic asthma can accompany allergic rhinitis, especially in patients with symptomatic pollen allergy. Certain allergens, such as the house dust mite, airborne fungi, and animal dander, can cause asthma preferentially, without significant nasal symptoms. Childhood asthma may remit during adolescence and then recur later in life. A search for the presence of immune responses to specific inhaled allergens, preferably by prick or intradermal skin testing, is important when the history points to an allergic component of asthma. Seasonal or diurnal variations in disease activity, worsening in certain physical locations, and the presence of pets in the home are examples of factors that warrant an allergy evaluation.

The treatment of asthma requires special attention to the elimination of environmental allergens because of the considerable morbidity associated with respiratory obstruction and the potential for a fatal outcome in a severe asthma attack. Environmental avoidance measures also must include protection against nonallergic respiratory irritants, including a variety of dusts, fumes, and vapors to which all patients with asthma are susceptible because of the nonspecific bronchial hyperirritability that

characterizes the disease. Immunotherapy is indicated for patients who experience significant exacerbation of the disease by airborne allergens that cannot be avoided effectively.

ATOPIC DERMATITIS

Atopic dermatitis is a chronic skin disease with the primary features of pruritus and an eczematous eruption that occurs on scratching of the skin (see Chapter 196). The term *eczema* refers to any inflammatory skin disease, including atopic dermatitis, that is characterized by erythema, papules, and scaling. Because of repeated scratching, the lesions undergo lichenification, and scarring results. As signified by its name, atopic dermatitis is the cutaneous manifestation of atopy. It affects less than 1% of the population and can coexist with allergic rhinitis and asthma in the same patient or in other family members.

ANAPHYLAXIS

Anaphylaxis is a systemic allergic reaction that begins rapidly on exposure to an allergen and can be fatal because of irreversible shock, bronchospasm, and laryngeal angioedema. The interaction of allergen and IgE antibody triggers mediator release, which affects several target organs almost simultaneously. Anaphylactic shock is caused by vasodilatation and vascular leakage, resulting from enhanced permeability of the postcapillary venules in the vascular beds of visceral organs, skin, and mucous membranes. Bronchial and gastrointestinal muscle spasms produce acute airway obstruction and colicky abdominal pain. Increased vascular permeability in the skin results in pruritus, urticaria, and angioedema. Uterine muscle contractions and various effects on the intrinsic coagulation pathway are less common manifestations.

Anaphylaxis is not common, but prevalence and incidence figures are unavailable because it is not a reportable disease. The diagnosis must be made on the basis of clinical findings and treatment initiated with the greatest urgency, because the mortality rate approaches 10% in patients with anaphylactic shock. The first sign or symptom typically occurs within a few minutes to an hour of contact with the allergen. A latent period of more than 2 hours is unusual. The list of reported allergens causing anaphylaxis is extensive, but the most common ones are foods, drugs, and *Hymenoptera* insect venom. The most frequently encountered food triggers are seafoods, nuts, legumes (especially peanuts), berries, buckwheat, and seeds. Penicillin, other β-lactam antibiotics, and injected protein drugs, such as antisera, enzymes, and vaccines, lead the list of medication triggers. Among health care workers, exposure to latex in gloves and other medical devices is becoming a growing cause of anaphylaxis and a range of other allergic diseases.

The term *anaphylactoid* is used to designate reactions that are indistinguishable from anaphylaxis but lack a demonstrable IgE allergic element. Some anaphylactoid reactions are triggered by an identifiable agent, such as a drug that possesses the pharmacologic property of causing nonimmunologic release of mast cell mediators. Aspirin and nonsteroidal anti-inflammatory drugs, opiates, and iodinated contrast media used in radiography are the most common agents with this property. In other cases, the reaction is triggered by a physical activity, such as exercise, and a few patients have recurrent idiopathic "anaphylaxis." Details concerning the treatment of acute attacks can be found in Chapter 60.

Permanent desensitization can be achieved in virtually all cases of *Hymenoptera* venom anaphylaxis through the subcutaneous injection of 100 mg of venom at monthly intervals, after a build-up period of increasing amounts starting at a dose lower than that capable of causing a local or systemic allergic response. After 5 years of such treatment, most patients are permanently protected from future reactions to natural stings, whereas the untreated disease carries a 50% risk of systemic reaction to subsequent stings. A temporary state of tolerance to penicillin can be achieved in some patients with anaphylaxis to the drug by "rush" desensitization, permitting therapeutic use of the drug. In this case, the allergic sensitivity returns at the termination of treatment.

URTICARIA AND ANGIOEDEMA

Urticaria is a common disease that occurs most often as a single episode recognized easily as an allergic reaction. The disease is provoked by the same types of allergens that are responsible for systemic anaphylaxis (drugs, foods, and insect stings). As in the case of anaphylaxis, some drugs, such as aspirin and the nonsteroidal anti-inflammatory agents, and some foods, most notably mollusks, crustaceans, and berries, contain certain chemicals that trigger nonimmunologic mast cell mediator release. In some individuals urticaria also can result from physical triggers, such as exercise, cold, heat, or local skin pressure. In addition, emotional stress is a fairly common initiator. Angioedema is a variant of urticaria in which the target blood vessels that undergo enhanced permeability are located subcutaneously.

The typical lesions of urticaria are intensely pruritic and evanescent. The individual lesions clear completely within hours without side effects, though recurrences can be frequent or even continuous. The chronic form of urticaria (continuously recurring lesions over many weeks or months) is a nonallergic, idiopathic disease in most cases. Angioedema consists of localized, nondependent, and usually nonpruritic, areas of edema with a particular predilection for the eyelids, lips, and buccal mucosa, but they may appear anywhere. Urticaria-like lesions that persist for days and are characterized by skin discoloration, purpura, or tenderness are likely to be caused by cutaneous vasculitis. This may be a manifestation of a systemic disorder, such as infection (especially hepatitis B) or autoimmune disease.

SERUM SICKNESS

Serum sickness is a systemic immune complex–mediated allergic disease. High-dose administration of a potent allergen, such as foreign serum, elicits a brisk IgM and IgG antibody response, resulting in the formation of circulating antigen–antibody complexes that deposit in various target organs. The immune complexes induce local and systemic inflammation through the action of various complement-derived proinflammatory mediators. Although it was a much more common disease in the past, serum sickness is now encountered rarely, because the therapeutic use of foreign serum protein is limited to antilym-

phocyte or antithymocyte globulin and a few antivenins. The exceptions to this rule are some of the recombinant products (anti-tumor necrosis factor α). A mild form of serum sickness occurs occasionally with injected nonprotein drugs, especially penicillin. There is a latent period of several days to weeks after drug administration because of the time required for specific antibody production and immune complex formation. Dermatitis, fever, lymphadenopathy, and arthritis are the cardinal manifestations. The rash can be erythematous, morbilliform, or urticarial. Peripheral neuritis and central nervous system involvement are rare. The disease remits spontaneously and usually without permanent tissue damage. Treatment can be directed toward alleviation of symptoms. The diagnosis is made on the basis of clinical findings, because there are no pathognomonic laboratory tests and because evidence of circulating immune complexes and complement consumption may come and go before symptoms and signs appear.

ALLERGIC BRONCHOPULMONARY ASPERGILLOSIS

Allergic bronchopulmonary aspergillosis is a unique allergic disease caused by *Aspergillus fumigatus* (see Chapter 369). It develops in patients who produce IgE antibodies to an allergen from the spore and IgG antibodies to a different allergen of the organism's mycelial phase. Patients typically are young adults with atopic allergy or children with cystic fibrosis. The IgE antibody causes asthma, which usually is chronic, because airborne allergens from *Aspergillus* spores are ubiquitous in the environment. Organisms persisting in the mucus of proximal airways stimulate the production of IgG antibodies, which then form localized immune complexes that activate complement and induce focal immune-mediated inflammation. This accounts for the acute episodes interspersed in ongoing chronic asthma. Repeated bouts lead to bronchiectasis and pulmonary fibrosis.

Allergic bronchopulmonary aspergillosis should be suspected in a patient with asthma who has repeated episodes of fever, productive sputum, and pulmonary infiltrates on chest radiography. The diagnosis requires appropriate laboratory confirmation. The result of an immediate wheal or erythema skin prick test to *A. fumigatus* almost always is positive. IgG antibodies often can be detected by the precipitin test. Total serum IgE levels typically are elevated during acute episodes and fall after the attack subsides. Blood eosinophilia is present, as it is in any case of symptomatic asthma.

HYPERSENSITIVITY PNEUMONITIS

An uncommon form of allergic pulmonary disease in which acute high-dose inhalation of an airborne allergen produces a specific immune inflammatory response in the lung parenchyma is known as hypersensitivity pneumonitis. Numerous allergens and their environmental sources have been identified, though many have been discovered as single cases or in only a few patients. Some of the more common causes are listed in Table

TABLE 173.3.	ALLERGENS THAT CAUSE HYPERSENSITIVITY PNEUMONITIS

Bacteria
   Thermophilic actinomycetes
   Bacillus subtilis
   Streptomyces albus
Fungi
   Aspergillus species
   Aureobasidium species
   Graphium species
   Cryptostroma corticale
   Penicillium species
   Alternaria species
Insects
   Sitophilus granarius
Miscellaneous
   Animal fur proteins
   Rat urine proteins
   Pituitary snuff
   Coffee bean protein

173.3. In most cases, the allergen is a protein, inhaled in the form of fumes, vapors, dusts, or intact microorganisms.

The immunopathogenesis of hypersensitivity pneumonitis, as confirmed by extensive clinicopathologic studies and experimental disease models in animals, is complex, but the disease principally is a T cell–mediated response to the allergen causing localized alveolar inflammation on contact with the inhaled allergen. Repeated acute or long-term exposure leads to chronic granulomatous inflammation and fibrosis. Reaction of allergen with precipitating antibody is involved in the acute form of the disease, analogous to the Arthus reaction. Genetic predisposition and immunoregulatory effects of the allergens themselves are additional factors in pathogenesis.

The diagnosis is made on the basis of clinical findings and evidence of host immune response to the suspected allergen. This requires that the clinician be acutely aware and vigilant and that a searching environmental history be taken, with particular emphasis on occupational exposures. Although specific serum precipitins correlate with exposure to the organic allergens causing hypersensitivity pneumonitis, the test lacks disease-related specificity. Therefore, a positive test result cannot diagnose the disease without clinical confirmation. The differential diagnosis and treatment of acute hypersensitivity pneumonitis are discussed in Chapter 372.

ALLERGIC CONTACT DERMATITIS

Allergic contact dermatitis is a T cell–mediated allergic disease expressed on the skin at the area of contact with the allergen. It is a common form of allergy and is reviewed in Chapter 196. Both sensitization and elicitation of the reaction result from skin contact. Once sensitized, later contact with the allergen anywhere on the skin surface will produce the eruption, which consists of erythema, swelling, papules, and vesicles at the site of exposure. Because this is a nonantibody cellular immune inflammatory reaction, there is a delay of 24 to 48 hours or even longer for mild reactions before the lesions are apparent. Sensitivity usually is permanent.

DRUG ALLERGY

Allergy is one of several adverse drug effects (Table 173.4). The clinical manifestations of drug allergy reflect the inflammation induced by the patient's immune response to an antigenic determinant from the drug. The determinant can be the drug itself, a drug metabolite, a product of a drug (or one of its metabolites) conjugated with a host protein, or an autoantigen elicited by the drug. The immune response can be mediated through the IgE–mast cell route, the IgG complement–immune complex pathway, or the T cells. Cytotoxic reactions from complement activation by IgG or IgM antibodies to drugs also can be considered a form of drug allergy. Cutaneous drug reactions are discussed in detail in Chapter 199.

Because almost all therapeutic agents are "foreign" to the body, an immune response after exposure to any drug is an expected event and usually has no clinical consequence. Allergy to a drug requires additional factors, such as dose, route of administration, genetic predisposition, nature of the underlying disease, and probably others. The manifestations of drug allergy are consistent with the immune pathway involved. IgE responses and T cell–mediated allergic contact dermatitis are the most common. IgE responses usually take the form of anaphylaxis, urticaria, or angioedema. Asthma and rhinitis are rare and restricted to protein drugs given by inhalation or nasal insufflation.

An erythematous or maculopapular rash from a drug, usually an antibiotic, is a particularly common problem, which is encountered by most physicians. This condition presumably is an allergic one when the intensity of the skin eruption is greater and the latency period shorter with each succeeding course of the drug. In most such cases, there is no validated skin or in vitro test to identify the relevant immune response. In some cases, an empiric course of "desensitization" has permitted the patient to tolerate therapeutic doses of the drug, at least transiently, further supporting an allergic cause.

The basic immunologic concepts of allergen determinant specificity and cross-reactivity are clinically relevant in drug allergy. For example, the immunologic specificity in penicillin allergy usually is to the β-lactam heterocyclic ring structure and not to its side chain. An individual with allergy to penicillin G usually reacts similarly to all β-lactam penicillin derivatives and occasionally to a cephalosporin, but not to a monolactam, such as aztreonam.

The diagnosis of drug allergy requires a history to explore the symptoms, timing, previous experience with the drug and

TABLE 173.4.	ADVERSE DRUG REACTIONS

Allergy
Side effects
Toxicity
Idiosyncracy

potentially cross-reacting drugs, other drug use, other allergies, and the nature of the patient's disease. In spite of continuing research efforts to devise specific diagnostic tests for any drug and for each type of allergic reaction, reliable tests are few. Immediate wheal-and-flare skin testing with protein drugs usually is diagnostic for cases of suspected IgE reactions. The patch test is appropriate for drug-caused allergic contact dermatitis. Because most drugs used today in clinical practice are low-molecular-weight organic molecules, the drug or one of its metabolites functions as a hapten in drug allergy. In the case of penicillin, penicilloic acid is the major determinant of most nonanaphylactic IgE reactions. Penicilloyl-polylysine is a polyvalent skin test reagent that predicts future IgE-mediated penicillin reactions with a high degree of sensitivity and specificity, except for systemic anaphylaxis. Skin testing with a mixture of penicillin, penicilloic acid, and penicillamine, the so-called minor determinant mixture, is predictive of penicillin anaphylaxis, though this product is not marketed for general clinical use. Similar testing reagents for allergy to other drugs are not available.

The treatment of drug allergy is avoidance of the drug and all cross-reacting compounds. When there is no alternative therapy, desensitization can be attempted. This is performed by administering increasing doses of the drug at about 30-minute intervals, beginning with an appropriately low initial dose. Desensitization has been used successfully in many cases of penicillin allergy. It lowers the level of circulating IgE and increases the level of IgG antibodies to the drug, but these changes and clinical tolerance to the drug eventually disappear, and the procedure may have to be repeated for a later course of the drug.

BIBLIOGRAPHY

Adams RM. *Occupational skin disease*. Philadelphia: WB Saunders, 1999.

Fink JN, Zacharisen MC. Hypersensitivity pneumonitis. In: Middleton E Jr, Reed CE, Ellis EF, et al., eds. *Allergy: principles and practice*. St. Louis: Mosby, 1998.

Janssens MM-L, Howarth PH. The antihistamines of the nineties. *Clin Rev Allergy* 1993;11:111–153.

Kurup VP, Apter AJ. Allergic bronchopulmonary aspergillosis. *Immunol Allergy Clin North Am* 1998;18:471–715.

Lenfant C, Sheffer AL. Guidelines for the diagnosis and management of asthma. *J Allergy Clin Immunol* 1991;88(suppl):425–534.

Nicklas RA, Bernstein IL, Li JT, et al. The diagnosis and management of anaphylaxis. *J Allergy Clin Immunol* 1998;101:S465–S528.

Pope AM, Patterson R, Burge H, eds. *Indoor allergens: assessing and controlling adverse health effects*. Washington, D.C.: National Academy Press, 1993.

Szefler SJ: Leukotriene modifiers: What is their position in asthma therapy [Editorial]? *J Allergy Clin Immunol* 1998;102:170–172.

Skoner DP, Doyle WJ, Fireman P, et al. Nasal physiology and inflammatory mediators during natural pollen exposure. *Ann Allergy* 1990;65:206–210.

Tilles SA, ed. Drug hypersensitivity. *Immunol Allergy Clin North Am* 1998;18:717–934.

Kelley's Textbook of Internal Medicine, fourth edition. Edited by H. David Humes. Lippincott Williams & Wilkins, Philadelphia © 2000.

DISORDERS OF THE RHEUMATOLOGIC AND ALLERGIC SYSTEMS

RHEUMATOID ARTHRITIS

GARY S. FIRESTEIN

Rheumatoid arthritis (RA) is a chronic symmetrical polyarthritis of the small joints of the hands and feet as well as the larger appendicular joints. In addition to articular manifestations, patients with RA can suffer from a variety of extra-articular complications, such as nodule formation and vasculitis.

INCIDENCE AND EPIDEMIOLOGY

RA is the most common form of inflammatory arthritis, affecting about 1% of people worldwide. This incidence is surprisingly constant regardless of ethnic or racial origin, with a few notable exceptions. For example, RA develops in 3% to 6% of the Yakima Indians. Females are affected two to three times more often than males. The disease can begin at any age, but the peak onset is in the fifth decade of life. Susceptibility to RA has a genetic component, and the risk is approximately doubled (2% to 4%) if an individual has a first-degree relative with the disease, including a fraternal twin. The rate of concordance for monozygotic twins is considerably higher, approaching 30% to 50%. The fact that the concordance is not 100% implicates as yet undefined environmental factors.

Of the several genes that likely contribute to RA susceptibility (probably six or more), the class II major histocompatibility complex (MHC) plays a particularly prominent role. These cell-surface molecules bind to antigenic peptides and present the antigens to $CD4^+$ helper T cells. Early studies confirmed a higher prevalence of HLA-DR4 in patients with RA compared with controls. After a variety of DR4 subtypes were identified, however, it became clear that only selected ones were associated with RA. Furthermore, in some ethnic and racial populations

there were different associations. The discrepancies were resolved in part using molecular biology techniques to sequence the respective HLA-DR genes. These studies showed that susceptibility to RA is associated with a specific sequence of amino acids (amino acids 70-74: Glu-Lys-Arg-Ala-Ala, sometimes called QKRAA) in the third hypervariable region of the β chain of HLA-DR. However, it is important to appreciate that the association is still weak or nonexistent in many ethnic and racial groups, even when this sequence is considered. In addition, some data suggest that the DR associations define the severity of RA rather than susceptibility to disease.

QKRAA is strategically located near the antigen-binding site in HLA-DR that is responsible for initiating immune responses by T cells, suggesting that the association between RA and HLA-DR is somehow related to the ability of a putative "rheumatoid antigen" to bind specific MHC proteins. This could result in an immune response by the appropriate antigen-specific T cells. There are also several alternative explanations for the HLA-DR associations. For instance, it is possible that this specific sequence results in a "hole" in the immune response that permits an arthrotrophic pathogen to proliferate and cause arthritis in the absence of an appropriate T-cell response. Also, the effect on T cells could be due to the fact that class II MHC genes help shape the repertoire of T-cell receptors in the thymus, thereby indirectly altering T-cell responses. Finally, the sequence of MHC genes can alter trafficking of DR proteins in the cell cytoplasm and alter antigen presentation.

ETIOLOGY

Despite an intensive search for transmissible agents that might cause RA, an infectious source has yet to be proved. Occasional associations with nonbacterial pathogens, such as chlamydia or mycoplasma, are intriguing but far from conclusive. Sensitive reverse transcriptase–polymerase chain reaction studies of synovial tissue have detected bacterial DNA in RA as well as other inflammatory types of arthritis. The types of bacteria identified are nonspecific and could merely reflect the phagocytic capacity of synovial macrophages as they clear live or dead organisms from the blood. It is also possible that nonbiodegradable bacterial cell walls play a key role in the disease. This is amply illustrated in a model of inflammatory arthritis in which purified streptococcal cell walls induce an RA-like disease in rats; similar antigens have not been detected in human articular samples. Inflammatory arthritis in animals also can be caused by live microorganisms. For instance, in caprine arthritis/encephalitis disease, a lentivirus infects macrophage precursors in the bone marrow that subsequently migrate to the joint and cause synovitis. Mycoplasma can produce arthritis in a variety of species.

In humans, various viruses are known to cause arthritis. Rubella virus can lead to a rheumatoid-like syndrome after either wild-type rubella infection or vaccination with attenuated virus. In some cases, the virus can be cultured from synovial tissue or synovial fluid. However, rubella arthritis is generally self-limited, and viral cultures in RA are usually negative. Parvovirus B19 has also been associated with inflammatory arthritis; B19 proteins and infective virus have been reported in RA synovial tissue. Serologic studies in RA suggest that some individuals with new-onset RA have experienced recent B19 infection, but this represents a small fraction of patients.

Epstein–Barr virus (EBV) has also been implicated in RA. Patients with RA have higher serum antibody titers for EBV proteins, and rheumatoid peripheral blood lymphocytes have a specific defect in the immune response to EBV. Moreover, one of the EBV coat proteins contains the QKRAA sequence that is found in HLA-DR4, suggesting that molecular mimicry might link EBV and RA (see later discussion). There is also a suspicion that patients with RA have increased EBV shedding in their saliva. Despite these tantalizing data, there is no compelling evidence that EBV can initiate RA, and its role in chronic disease is uncertain at best.

An immune response against autoantigens is another mechanism for initiating arthritis. Several self-antigens can potentially serve as autoimmune targets. Type II collagen (which is a major component of hyaline cartilage), heat-shock proteins, the cartilage protein gp39, cartilage link protein, proteoglycans, or even class II MHC proteins could serve as autoantigens. Several of these autoantigens, such as gp39 and type II collagen, can induce inflammatory arthritis when particular strains of mice are immunized with them. The basis for the claims regarding the etiologic role of such antigens in RA is serologic (anti–type II collagen or anti-proteoglycan antibodies in the serum of some RA patients) or related to cell-mediated responses (increased proliferative responses of synovial fluid T cells to heat-shock proteins). Evidence of the direct role of these antigens as initiators of RA is circumstantial, however, and the immune responses could be epiphenomena related only to the destruction of articular tissue with the release of neo-antigens.

While it is not known exactly how one initiates immunity to these articular antigens, one possibility is molecular mimicry. In this paradigm, an immune response can be mounted against an exogenous antigen bearing structural homology to a normal human antigen. The normal tissue, though it is an innocent bystander, could ultimately be the target of an immune attack and be damaged. Adjuvant arthritis in the rat is one example of molecular mimicry in an animal model of inflammatory arthritis. In this model, animals are immunized against nonviable mycobacteria and mount a brisk immune response directed against mycobacterial proteins (especially heat-shock proteins). Never-

theless, some T cells that respond to mycobacteria also recognize an epitope on proteoglycans and might serve as a link between the robust response to mycobacteria and destruction of cartilage in this model.

PATHOGENESIS

The synovium serves two major functions in the joint: to provide oxygen and nutrients to cartilage, which lacks its own blood supply; and to produce lubricants that permit the articular surfaces to glide smoothly across one another. The normal synovium in diarthrodial joints is a delicate tissue made up of a synovial intimal lining and a sublining region supported by an underlying fibrous capsule. The intimal lining, which is in direct contact with synovial fluid, is typically a discontinuous structure one to two cell layers deep containing macrophage-like and fibroblast-like cells (referred to as type A and type B synoviocytes, respectively). The sublining contains bland fibrous tissue with scattered mononuclear cells or fibroblasts, a few blood vessels, and fat cells.

In RA the synovium is a transformed into a hyperplastic, chronically inflamed tissue. The intimal lining dramatically increases in size and is sometimes more than a dozen cell layers deep. This change is due to local proliferation of fibroblast-like cells and an even greater increase in the number of macrophage-like synoviocytes. Macrophage-like cell accumulation is mainly due to migration of new cells from the bone marrow via the bloodstream. The sublining is marked by a prominent mononuclear cell infiltrate that is composed mainly of T cells, B cells, and macrophages. The T cells, which are primarily CD4$^+$ helper cells, can accumulate diffusely through the synovium or collect into lymphoid aggregates. These aggregates are occasionally so prominent that the synovium looks like a lymph node. Local proliferation appears to account for only a very small fraction of T-cell accumulation; most T cells migrate into the joint under the nonspecific stimulus of local adhesion molecule and cytokines. Macrophages, B cells, and plasma cells are scattered throughout the sublining.

The degree of mononuclear cell infiltration varies considerably between patients and even between different regions of the same joint. Some biopsy specimens have only a minor inflammatory infiltrate despite significant symptoms, and even asymptomatic joints in patients can have synovial-lining hyperplasia and characteristic infiltration with lymphocytes. While neutrophils are abundant in synovial fluid, they are conspicuously absent in synovium in the context of RA. Angiogenesis is prominent in RA, because the number of blood vessels is greater than normal; careful capillary morphometry suggests, however, that the increase in the number of blood vessels is not commensurate with the increase in tissue mass, resulting in local ischemia. Surprisingly, the histopathologic characteristics of the synovium in early RA (within a few weeks after symptoms begin) can be very similar to chronic disease, including abundant cytokines and metalloproteinase expression.

Various aspects of humoral immunity dominated early paradigms of RA, beginning in the 1940s with the initial descriptions of rheumatoid factor in the serum of patients with RA. Rheumatoid factors are antibodies that bind to the $C_\gamma 2$ and $C_\gamma 3$ regions of the Fc portion of IgG and can lead to the formation of immune complexes in the joint or in the blood. Standard clinical tests for rheumatoid factors mainly detect IgM antibodies, though other types (especially IgG) are also produced and can be more phlogistic. Rheumatoid factors found in patients with RA are distinct from those detected in other diseases, such as cryoglobulinemia and Waldenstrom's macroglobulinemia. For instance, distinct germ line genes are used in constructing the RA rheumatoid factors. In addition, the autoantibodies have higher affinity for IgG in RA and have distinct mutations in the hypervariable regions, suggesting that their production is driven by a specific antigen(s).

In addition to being present in blood, rheumatoid factors are synthesized in the synovium and can be detected in synovial fluid. Rheumatoid factor–containing immune complexes are found in synovial fluid as well as in synovial tissue and cartilage. These complexes activate complement with the subsequent generation of a variety of chemotactic factors, including C5a, that serve to recruit additional inflammatory cells to the joint. Neutrophils, in particular, are summoned by this mechanism and, upon arrival in the joint, they can ingest the immune complexes and disgorge their full panoply of degradative enzymes to act upon the cartilage and extracellular matrix. Other chemotactic mediators in synovial fluid, like interleukin-8 (IL-8), also draw inflammatory cells into the articular cavity.

The types of T cells in synovial fluid differ from those of synovial tissue: there is a greater number of $CD8^+$ lymphocytes in synovial fluid. In light of the preponderance of neutrophils and the differences in T-cell subsets in synovial fluid, it is clear that effusions do not simply mirror the synovium but are, in fact, a distinct compartment. Synovial fluid also contains many cytokines, small molecule mediators of inflammation (prostaglandins and leukotrienes), and proteolytic enzymes. The synovium itself appears to be the source of many of these factors in synovial effusions. In contrast to the synovium (see later discussion), the cytokine milieu of synovial fluid seems to favor cytokine antagonists, with very substantial concentrations of IL-1Ra, soluble tumor necrosis factor (TNF) receptors (which can bind and neutralize synovial fluid TNF-α), and suppressive cytokines like IL-10 and transforming growth factor β.

While synovial fluid was the focus of early studies, the synovium itself, with its own distinct mechanisms of inflammation, has garnered increasing scrutiny in recent years. Many studies strongly implicate cell-mediated immune responses in rheumatoid synovium rather than the acute inflammatory processes that predominate in the intra-articular cavity. The prominent helper T-cell synovial infiltrate and class II MHC associations in RA have suggested to many that RA is an antigen-specific T cell–mediated response in the joint. In this model, an arthrotrophic agent in the joint activates local T cells, causing in situ proliferation and release of soluble mediators known as cytokines that subsequently induce adhesion molecules and activate other cell types in the vicinity. Some studies examining T-cell receptor gene rearrangement in rheumatoid joints support this hypothesis owing to the suggestion of T-cell oligoclonal expansion. Other studies, however, have not confirmed a T-cell receptor bias, so this is by no means established. In fact, depending on the technique used and the population of patients studied, highly conflicting results have been reported.

How, then, does one account for the accumulation of T cells within the synovium? As was mentioned earlier, local proliferation does not seem to be the answer. Instead, the local cytokine milieu induces adhesion molecules on synovial endothelium. Molecules like ICAM (intercellular adhesion molecule) and VCAM-1 (vascular cell adhesion molecule) are overexpressed on endothelial cells in the RA joint. These bind to counterreceptors known as integrins on circulating leukocytes, especially the $\beta 2$ and $\alpha 4$ integrin families (e.g., VLA-4). The combination of increased adhesion molecule expression in the joint and local chemokine production serves as a siren song to summon cells into the synovium, where they can take up residence. Hence, the populations of T cells that accumulate in the joint are probably determined by antigen-independent forces.

While the abundance of T cells in the joint is striking, a variety of antigen-independent forms of arthritis evidence a similar histologic picture, and T cells accumulate at sites of chronic inflammation regardless of the cause. Another perplexing aspect is the relative lack of cytokines typically associated with T-cell activation in the joint. In normal immune responses, T cell–derived factors like IL-2, IL-3, IL-4, TNF-β, or immune interferon (IFN-γ) orchestrate the inflammatory response. These cytokines are readily detected at the site of disease in T cell–mediated diseases like tuberculous pleuritis or asthma. The levels of T-cell cytokines are conspicuously low in the rheumatoid joint, however.

Helper T cells have been divided into specific subsets based on their cytokine profile; $T_h 1$ cells produce IFN-γ and IL-2 but not IL-4, IL-5, or IL-10, whereas $T_h 2$ cells express the opposite profile. While levels of most T-cell cytokines are rather low in the joint, the profile of those that have been detected using very sensitive techniques suggest a $T_h 1$ bias in the synovium. This is similar to the situation in animal models of autoimmunity, where $T_h 1$ cells are responsible for disease initiation, whereas $T_h 2$-cell activation correlates with disease regression.

In contrast to T-cell cytokines, macrophage and fibroblast cytokines are abundant. These include cytokines IL-1, IL-6, TNF-α, granulocyte–macrophage colony stimulating factor, macrophage colony stimulating factor, and a family of chemoattractants known as chemokines as well as prostaglandins, complement proteins, and proteolytic enzymes. The plethora of macrophage/fibroblast products in the rheumatoid joint suggests that they might play a key role in disease perpetuation. Moreover, a complex network of factors that stimulates macrophages and fibroblasts in an autocrine or paracrine fashion could contribute to the pathogenesis of RA. It is not certain how the cytokine cascade is initiated, nor is it clear whether it requires intermittent stimulation from an outside source, such as infectious agents, or low levels of T-cell activation. Current models of RA suggest that the initiation phase of the disease might result from an antigen-specific T-cell response, but the late chronic phase is quite complex and might involve T cell–independent processes in addition to T-cell responses.

In the synovium, degradative enzymes are mainly produced by intimal lining fibroblasts and are responsible for much of the tissue destruction associated with long-standing RA. In situ hybridization studies of RA synovial tissue show massive amounts of messenger RNA (mRNA) for such metalloproteinases as collagenase and stromelysin in the intimal lining, along with smaller amounts of the natural inhibitors of metalloproteinases known as TIMPs (tissue inhibitors of metalloproteinases). Protease gene induction takes place very early in the disease, with significant mRNA detected in synovial biopsy specimens obtained a few weeks to months after onset. The production of metalloproteinases is regulated by the cytokine network, with macrophage-derived factors like IL-1 and TNF-α acting as the major inducers. One major determinant of net extracellular matrix destruction is related to the ratio of natural inhibitors like TIMP to the active enzymes. Studies of synovial gene expression indicate that relatively subtle imbalances between these inhibitors can lead to net tissue damage over long periods of time. In addition, cysteine proteases called cathepsins are also expressed in RA synovium. Cathepsin K, in particular, has been associated with bone resorption and is produced by synovial cells near sites of bone destruction.

New evidence suggests that chronic erosive RA might be perpetuated by partial transformation of synoviocytes in the joint. The proliferative tissue in the synovial intimal lining contains pleomorphic mesenchymal cells that express genes typically associated with transformation, such as the oncogenes c-*jun* and c-*fos*. Furthermore, cultured synovial tissue fibroblasts, under some circumstances, can proliferate under anchorage-independent conditions, a phenotype that is characteristic of transformed cells. Finally, somatic mutations in key regulatory genes, like H-*ras* and the p53 tumor suppressor gene, can occur in RA synovium and synoviocytes. The mutations do not cause arthritis but might be the result of long-standing exposure to genotoxic oxygen and nitrogen radicals in the inflamed joint. The altered cells can then behave more aggressively by proliferating and invading cartilage.

CLINICAL FINDINGS

The American College of Rheumatology revised 1987 criteria are shown in Table 174.1. These guidelines can be useful in

TABLE 174.1.	1987 AMERICAN COLLEGE OF RHEUMATOLOGY REVISED CRITERIA FOR RHEUMATOID ARTHRITIS[a]

Morning stiffness (>1 hr before maximal improvement)
Arthritis of three or more joint areas (e.g., MCPs, wrists, knees)[b]
Arthritis of the hands
Symmetrical arthritis
Rheumatoid nodules
Serum rheumatoid factor
Radiographic changes typical of RA (e.g., marginal erosions, periarticular osteopenia)

MCP, metacarpal phalangeal joints.
[a] Four or more criteria must be satisfied for at least 6 weeks to diagnose RA.
[b] Must be observed by a physician.

TABLE 174.2.	CLASSIFICATION OF DISEASE SEVERITY IN RHEUMATOID ARTHRITIS

Class I: No restriction of ability to perform normal activities
Class II: Moderate restriction, but adequate for normal activities
Class III: Marked restriction, inability to perform most duties related to occupation or self-care
Class IV: Incapacitation or confinement to wheelchair or bed

some situations, though patients with the classic symptoms are usually not difficult to distinguish from those with other forms of arthritis. A scale to grade the clinical severity of RA also has been established to guide clinical evaluation, determine prognosis, and provide guidelines for quantifying treatment responses (Table 174.2).

MODE OF ONSET AND GENERAL FINDINGS

The onset of RA varies greatly. Typically, it begins insidiously, in the form of symmetric polyarticular arthritis involving the small joints of the hands and feet. This picture is by no means universal, and patients can show initial signs of monoarthritis or oligoarthritis that persists for weeks or months before disseminating to a more characteristic pattern. Signs and symptoms may wax and wane during the early stages of the disease, making the diagnosis difficult to establish owing to a paucity of physical findings. The average time from the onset of symptoms to diagnosis is about 6 months to 1 year. In some cases, the onset can be explosive, with an abrupt onset of polyarthritis associated with constitutional signs such as fever and weight loss. In addition to joint pain, patients with RA experience generalized fatigue and often require naps in the afternoon. Morning stiffness lasting longer than 30 minutes is particularly prominent and can persist for several hours or even all day during disease exacerbations. A similar "gelling" phenomenon occurs when patients remain in a single position for a prolonged period of time, such as on an airplane or simply sitting in a chair to read a book. Once established, the course of RA varies considerably. About 70% of patients have a chronic remitting course, while 10% to 20% express a very aggressive and destructive form of disease with few clinical remissions. The remaining patients have spontaneous, long-lasting remissions after the initial diagnosis; patients experiencing an abrupt onset of symptoms might be more likely to fall into this group.

ARTICULAR MANIFESTATIONS

The distribution of arthritis in RA is usually symmetrical and diffuse. The small diarthrodial joints of the hands are classically involved early in the course. The proximal interphalangeal joints (PIPs) and metacarpal phalangeal joints (MCPs) are usually tender and swollen. Physical examination shows loss of the usual contours across the MCPs, with palpable synovium between and over the bony prominences. Distal interphalangeal joint (DIP) disease can arise, but it is usually very mild. If it is prominent, alternative diagnoses should be considered, especially psoriatic

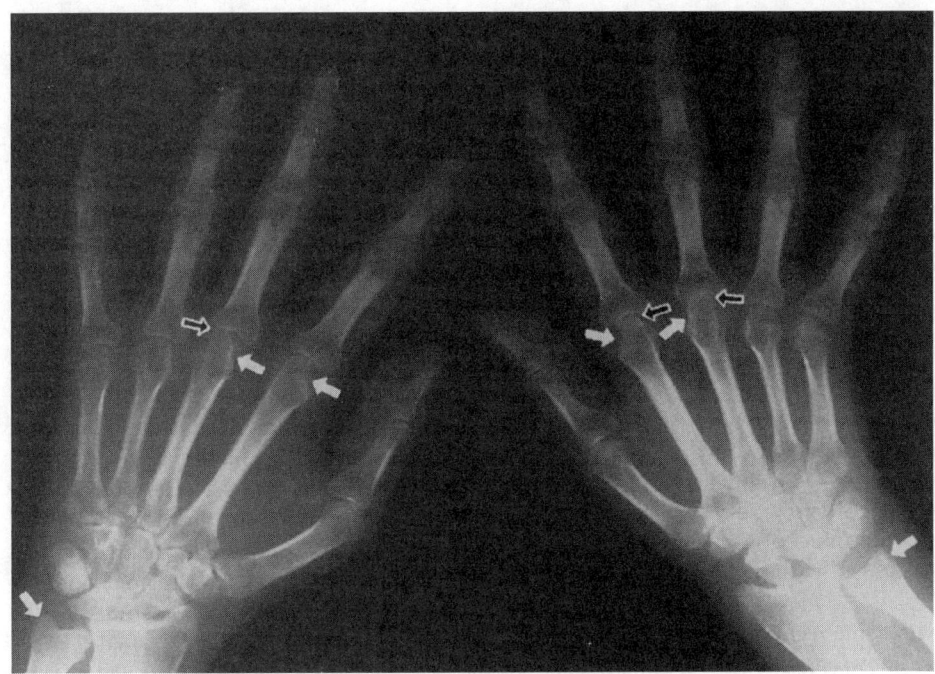

FIGURE 174.1. Typical hand radiographic findings in RA. This 34-year-old female patient had had RA for 2 years and was being treated only with NSAIDs. In addition to soft-tissue swelling and periarticular osteopenia, there is also evidence of cartilage damage with joint space narrowing (◊) and destruction of bone with marginal erosions (◆). Note the bilateral destruction of the ulnar styloid, which is a common location for early erosive disease.

arthritis or osteoarthritis. Wrist disease is quite common in RA, with resultant pain, tenderness, and decreased range of motion. Deformities of the hands and wrists are prevalent and can develop relatively early in the disease. One of the earliest deformities is radial deviation at the wrist, where the normal obtuse angle formed by the fifth metacarpal bone and the ulna increases to 180°. This deformity causes torque across the MCPs and contributes to the ulnar deviation at the MCPs, which is the most characteristic and obvious deformity of RA (Fig. 174.1). Swan neck deformities (hyperextension of the PIP and flexion of the DIP) and boutonniere deformities (flexion of the PIP and hyperextension of the DIP) are also very common after years of unabated synovitis. Similar pathologic manifestations can develop in the small joints of the feet, with synovitis of the metatarsal phalangeal joints as well as the PIPs of the toes. Common deformities of the feet include cock-up toes, loss of arches due to chronic midfoot disease, and hallux valgus.

The larger proximal joints are also affected in RA. Chronic elbow synovitis frequently leads to mild flexion contractures. Arthritis in the shoulder joint can cause pain, decreased range of motion, and chronic rotator cuff tears. Abduction is especially restricted in long-standing RA, and marked atrophy of the shoulder girdle muscles is a frequent accompaniment. Difficulty in sleeping due to pain is a very common complaint in patients with significant shoulder arthritis. In the lower extremities, disease of the knees and hips can be quite debilitating. Because of the weight-bearing responsibilities of the cartilage and ligaments, progressive cartilage destruction and ligamentous laxity can lead to difficulty in walking, pain, and, ultimately, joint replacement surgery. In the most severe cases, the femoral head migrates medially and superiorly and, with tissue remodeling, can protrude through the acetabulum into the pelvis ("petrusio acetabulum").

Cervical spine disease, with neck pain and decreased range of motion due to synovitis of the facet joints, is a prevalent complication of RA. One insidious and dangerous complication is myelopathy due to subluxation of the atlantoaxial joint. Atlantoaxial disease is especially important to note in patients undergoing surgical procedures, since forced flexion during intubation can be complicated by a neurologic catastrophe if the anesthesiologist is not appropriately forewarned. The presence of myelopathy due to cervical spine disease is a clear indication for surgical intervention and stabilization. In long-standing disease, the odontoid process can be eroded so severely that it is reduced to a mere spicule of bone, thereby increasing the risk of subluxation. The thoracic and lumbar spine is relatively spared in RA, although back pain from vertebral compression fractures can occur after years of inactivity and chronic glucocorticoid use in postmenopausal women. Other joints can be affected in RA and present special problems, including the temporomandibular joint and the cricoarytenoid joint. With RA of the temporomandibular joint, chewing food can be painful and lead to weight loss from malnutrition, while RA of the cricoarytenoid joint can cause throat pain or hoarseness.

EXTRA-ARTICULAR MANIFESTATIONS

Articular symptoms are the primary clinical manifestations of RA in the majority of patients. Extra-articular complications also occur with some regularity. Rheumatoid nodules are especially common and are caused by the formation of extra-articular granulation tissue. They are found in about 20% of patients, almost all of whom are seropositive for rheumatoid factor and have erosive disease. Nodules can appear anywhere, but they are most prevalent on bony prominences, pressure points, and tendon sheaths. They are rubbery or granular in texture and can be indistinguishable from gouty tophi. In some cases, such as in the olecranon bursa, rheumatoid nodules can be large and highly mobile; they also can be fixed to the surface of the bone (such as the ulna) or to tendons. On histologic examination, nodules have a central area of fibrinoid necrosis, a middle zone of palisading histiocytes, and an outer layer of dense fibrous tissue with a mononuclear cell infiltrate. While they are usually of only cosmetic significance, rheumatoid nodules can sometimes arise in the vocal cords, nervous system, lungs, or heart (particularly the conduction system). Nodules tend to wax and wane over time, with new nodule formation sometimes paralleling exacerbations of disease. Treatment is usually conservative, since surgical removal can be followed promptly by formation of new nodules in the same location.

Compression neuropathy is also a typical extra-articular manifestation of RA. Carpal tunnel syndrome is the most common, with proliferative synovitis compressing the median nerve as it passes through the wrist. Numbness or paresthesias of the thumb, index, and middle finger are suggestive symptoms; weakness and muscular atrophy occur late. The tarsal tunnel of the ankle also can be affected by compression neuropathy, though this is less common.

Synovial cysts or herniation also form with some regularity. Particularly troublesome are popliteal cysts, known as Baker's cysts. They can sometimes rupture and lead to extravasation of synovial fluid into the calf, causing signs and symptoms resembling deep venous thrombosis. Cysts also can appear as periarticular masses in the elbow (particularly in the forearm), shoulder, or the small joints of the hand.

Pleuropulmonary disease is a relatively typical accompaniment of RA. Asymptomatic effusions are frequently noted on routine chest roentgenograms and can vary in size from a minor radiographic curiosity to a massive effusion. On occasion, effusions can cause shortness of breath or pleuritic chest pain. Aspiration of the pleural space yields exudative fluid, typically with a mildly elevated leukocyte count (less than 5,000 cells per cubic millimeter), low glucose level, and low complement levels. Pleural biopsies can show nonspecific chronic inflammation or rheumatoid nodules. Pulmonary parenchymal disease in RA ranges from mild fibrosis to progressive interstitial lung disease that is indistinguishable from idiopathic pulmonary fibrosis. Rheumatoid nodules also can form in lung parenchyma. They are usually of little functional significance, but because of their resemblance to solitary metastases, they present a diagnostic dilemma.

Other major organ systems also can be involved in RA. For instance, symptomatic cardiac disease is uncommon, though pericardial thickening has been found in 40% of patients at autopsy. Asymptomatic pericardial effusions occur with even greater frequency. In rare cases, pericardial effusions can be quite large and result in pericardial tamponade. Conduction system abnormalities from rheumatoid nodules in or about the atrioventricular node can cause heart block with syncope. Rarely, dilatation of the aortic root due to local inflammation or nodule formation can lead to aortic regurgitation. Ocular disease has also been noted in RA. Episcleritis is a common inflammatory eye condition in RA that causes mild discomfort and can be treated conservatively. Scleritis, however, is more serious and can be accompanied by severe eye pain; if left untreated, it can cause scleral perforation. The sicca syndrome (dry eyes and dry mouth) can result from lymphocytic infiltration into lacrimal and salivary glands (as in primary Sjögren's syndrome). Severe cases can lead to corneal erosion or ulceration in the eye, dental carries, and oral thrush.

Among the most feared complications of RA is systemic rheumatoid vasculitis. This syndrome is very similar to idiopathic polyarteritis nodosa and appears to result from immune complex–mediated inflammation in small and medium-size arteries. As with polyarteritis, the signs and symptoms depend on the location and caliber of the involved vessels. Mononeuritis multiplex with prominent motor dysfunction (such as wrist- or foot-drop) as well as sensory deficits are present, as is evidence of cutaneous vasculitis with palpable purpura. Systemic rheumatoid vasculitis is a life-threatening disease that is associated with elevated circulating immune complexes in the blood and hypocomplementemia. Its presence does not correlate with activity of RA, since it is characteristically found in older men with relatively inactive arthritis. Patients are almost invariably seropositive for rheumatoid factor and have rheumatoid nodules. Small nail-fold infarcts are also evident and sometimes can be a harbinger of impending systemic vasculitis. Nail-fold infarcts, due to small vessel vasculitis, can also be found in the absence of systemic rheumatoid vasculitis. Treatment of fulminant vasculitis typically consists of high-dose glucocorticoids with or without such cytotoxic drugs as cyclophosphamide.

A variety of other diseases are associated with RA. For instance, the incidence of bacterial infections in rheumatoid joints is higher than normal. Establishing the diagnosis can sometimes be difficult if patients have very active disease or several septic joints. Diagnostic clues favoring infection include a relatively abrupt onset (though it can be insidious in patients taking immunosuppressive drugs or corticosteroids) and a synovial fluid analysis with a positive gram stain result and a low level of synovial fluid glucose. Nevertheless, the gram stain often gives negative results in septic arthritis. Other complications of RA or its treatment (particularly corticosteroids) include osteoporosis, vertebral compression fractures, and avascular necrosis, primarily in the femoral head. Tendon rupture, especially of the extensor tendons of the wrist and finger, can also occur as the result of overgrowth of synovium and might be forestalled by wrist synovectomy.

The overall mortality rate of patients with RA is modestly higher than that of the normal population. For the most part, people with RA die of the same causes as the general public, albeit earlier. In severely disabled patients with stage IV disease, however, mortality is equivalent to stage IV Hodgkin's disease. Such statistics dispel the myth that advanced RA is a benign disease and leads one to the conclusion that aggressive management is warranted. When RA patients are taken as a group, cardiovascular diseases are responsible for about 40% to 45% of deaths, followed by cancer (about 15%) and infection (about 10%). Lymphoproliferative diseases are somewhat more prevalent in the context of RA; non-Hodgkin's lymphoma, leukemia, multiple myeloma, and Hodgkin's disease account for most excess malignancies. A slight increase in renal deaths is caused by amyloidosis, which is an uncommon side effect of long-standing RA. It is often difficult to single out RA itself as the cause of death, rather than to assign the blame to complications of treatment.

LABORATORY FINDINGS

There are no specific tests to confirm the diagnosis of RA (Table 174.3). Hematologic parameters are usually notable for mild normochromic, normocytic anemia and an elevated platelet count. In fact, the degree of thrombocytosis is useful as a clinical manifestation and is often an indicator of disease activity. The leukocyte count is generally normal, though neutropenia occurs in association with splenomegaly in Felty's syndrome. Neutropenia may stem from a number of factors and appears to be related to antineutrophil antibodies, splenic sequestration, and/or cell-mediated damage to bone marrow precursors. Some cases of Felty's syndrome are associated with oligoclonal or monoclonal expansion of large granular lymphocytes in the blood and represent a form of chronic leukemia. The erythrocyte sedimentation rate and C-reactive protein level are usually elevated in active RA and can be used to monitor disease activity and response to disease-modifying drugs. Results of serum chemistry studies are normal, though liver enzymes can be elevated either by nonsteroidal anti-inflammatory drugs (NSAIDs) or, more commonly, by methotrexate or leflunomide.

While there is no specific diagnostic test, a variety of serologic tests have some usefulness in RA. By far the most useful is the rheumatoid factor test. As noted, rheumatoid factors are antibodies that bind to the Fc portion of immunoglobulins. This propensity for aggregation is used to perform the latex or sheep red blood cell agglutination test. Latex particle or red cells coated with IgG are incubated with various dilutions of patient's serum, and the degree of agglutination is assessed. The results are most often reported as the greatest dilution of serum that still causes agglutination. About 85% of patients with RA are "seropositive" for rheumatoid factor, usually at a dilution of $\geq 1:80$. New quantitative assays are also available, though determination of seropositivity depends on the standards established by an individual clinical laboratory. The presence of rheumatoid factor in the blood portends more aggressive disease, and its absence might identify a subset of patients with milder disease or with a syndrome similar to polymyalgia rheumatica. The test result can be positive for many years before arthritis develops, but only a relatively small percentage of individuals with a positive rheumatoid factor test result ultimately develop RA. Seropositivity, if it is going to develop in a patient with RA, usually does so before the end of the first year of disease.

In spite of its name ("rheumatoid" factor), this test is relatively nonspecific. In fact, 1% to 5% of normal individuals show positive latex agglutination test results, the higher percentage found in the elderly. Many other chronic inflammatory conditions are also associated with a positive result on a rheumatoid factor test, though the titers are usually somewhat lower than those observed in seropositive nodular RA. Patients with subacute bacterial endocarditis, tuberculosis, other connective tissue diseases (such as systemic lupus erythematosus), and noninflammatory diseases (like cirrhosis of the liver and sarcoidosis) can have positive test outcomes.

Other serologic tests that are used often to diagnose various connective tissue diseases are of limited value in RA. Tests for antinuclear antibodies usually show negative results, or else antibodies are present at low titers (though some patients have high

---

TABLE 174.3.   LABORATORY TESTS IN ACTIVE RA

Test	Typical Finding
Complete blood count	Normochromic, normocytic anemia
Platelet count	Elevated (usually 350,000–500,000 platelets/mm³)
Erythrocyte sedimentation rate	Elevated (usually 30–60 mm/hr)
C-reactive protein	Elevated
Chemistry panel	Normal
Urinalysis	Normal
Synovial fluid	2,000–20,000 leukocytes/mm³, predominantly polymorphonuclear leukocytes
	Normal glucose
	No crystals
	Low complement
Rheumatoid factor	Positive
Antinuclear antibody	Variable
Anti–double-stranded DNA antibody	Negative
Serum complement	Normal
Hand and feet radiographs	Soft-tissue swelling
	Periarticular osteopenia
	Marginal erosions
	Joint space narrowing
Synovial tissue biopsy	Synovial lining hyperplasia
	Mononuclear cell infiltration
	Lymphoid aggregates
	Negative cultures

titers of antinuclear antibodies). If anti-DNA antibodies are detected, they are almost always directed against single-stranded DNA rather than native double-stranded DNA. Other specialized serology tests, such as those for anti-Sm and anti-RNP antibodies, typically generate negative results. SSA and SSB antibodies are variably positive, and serum complement levels are normal in uncomplicated RA. Serologic tests for other viruses can be helpful in the differential diagnosis and can aid in distinguishing post-rubella arthritis or parvovirus B19 from RA. Hepatitis B and C serology tests can also furnish useful information, since these infections can cause a self-limited symmetrical polyarthritis. The usefulness of EBV serology is limited.

Analysis of synovial fluid can provide supportive data but is rarely, if ever, diagnostic. Synovial fluid is most frequently aspirated from the knee, though virtually any diarthrodial joint can contain an increased volume of fluid in RA. On gross examination, synovial fluid in RA is generally straw-colored and mildly turbid. If a wide-bore needle is used to aspirate fluid, gelatinous particles called "rice bodies" can also be withdrawn. These particles are composed of fibrin, collagen, and, occasionally, small fronds of synovium. White counts in synovial fluid are moderately elevated (between 2,000 and 20,000 cells per cubic millimeter), with varying differential counts. Usually, 50% to 75% of cells are neutrophils. The balance of cells are lymphocytes (mainly T cells) and monocytes.

In some cases, synovial fluid leukocyte counts exceed 100,000 cells per cubic millimeter with more than 90% neutrophils, which causes difficulty in ruling out pyogenic infection or crystal-induced arthropathy. A normal synovial fluid glucose level helps distinguish RA from acute infections. Complement levels are usually low in inflamed rheumatoid joints despite abundant production of complement proteins by synovium. A variety of other studies are frequently ordered on synovial fluid, but they are rarely useful. Rheumatoid factors are often present in RA synovial fluid, but they might not be detected by standard assays because they can be of the IgG isotype. Rheumatoid factor tests on synovial fluid are rarely indicated. Other traditional studies, such as the mucin clot test, do not provide significant additional clinical information.

Despite the well-documented MHC associations in RA and other forms of inflammatory arthritis, tests to determine the HLA phenotype of patients are not indicated, owing in part to the high prevalence of HLA-DR4 and other susceptibility markers in the normal population. Rarely, tests to determine the presence of HLA-B27 might be useful, if there is concern that polyarticular seronegative arthritis could be a form of seronegative spondyloarthropathy, such as psoriatic arthritis or Reiter's syndrome, rather than RA.

There is considerable overlap in the synovial histologic features of various forms of inflammatory arthritis. Hence, synovial biopsies provide little useful information. They occasionally can be used to rule out mycobacterial or fungal infections. Surrogate markers for disease activity or for prognosis, in general, have been disappointing. The degree of macrophage infiltration in early arthritis might be a predictor of radiographic progression.

Bone radiographs in RA can help with diagnosis and can be used to follow the progression of erosions and the response to therapy. Hand and wrist radiographs (as well as radiographs of other areas disproportionately affected) should be obtained early in the course of disease as a baseline determination. The presence of erosions at this time would be a clear indication to advance therapy rapidly to a second-line agent. Typically, the first changes in the hand are periarticular osteopenia and soft-tissue swelling, especially of the PIPs and MCPs. The source of osteopenia is not certain; it could be due to immobilization or disuse. Alternatively, the local cytokine milieu might favor increased osteoclast activity. Synovial effusions sometimes can be detected in joint radiographs, owing to subtle changes in fat pads. As RA progresses, cartilage loss causes joint space narrowing, particularly at the second and third MCPs, the PIPs, and between the carpal bones in the wrist. Bone erosions often first appear at the "bare areas" located in the recesses of joints, where bone is not protected by cartilage and is in direct contact with synovium or synovial fluid (Fig. 174.1). It is here that pannus forms and begins to erode into the extracellular matrix. Pannus, which is unique to RA, is the aggressive leading edge of synovium and is composed of pleomorphic mesenchymal cells that express oncogenes and proteases. In the later stages of disease, the erosions and joint space narrowing become more prominent, and a variety of nonreducible deformities can be seen on radiographs, such as ulnar deviation of the fingers. Intra-osseous cysts can also develop, especially in the wrist. Ultimately, the carpal bones can fuse, causing ankylosis.

Radiographs of the lower extremities show a similar progression from osteoporosis to erosions/joint space narrowing to deformity. In the knees, tricompartmental narrowing and cartilage loss are evident. This picture differs from that of osteoarthritis, where medial joint space narrowing is the most prominent. The hip also shows symmetric joint space narrowing in RA, with medial and superior migration of the femoral head, whereas superior joint space narrowing predominates in osteoarthritis. Radiographs of the cervical spine can be used to identify and quantify atlantoaxial subluxation, erosions of the odontoid process, and erosive disease of the facet joints.

There are no established criteria for determining the frequency of radiography in RA. Most of the erosions occur during the first 5 years of disease, but it is unusual to see significant progression at intervals of less than 6 months. If the radiographs will help guide therapy, it is reasonable, at least during the earliest phases of RA, to obtain films of significantly affected joints or of the hands every 1 to 2 years, to assess progression.

THERAPY

NONSTEROIDAL ANTI-INFLAMMATORY DRUGS

The treatment of RA in large part addresses the symptoms; few drugs alter the natural history of the disease. For decades the mainstays of therapy have been NSAIDs, including aspirin and newer selective and nonselective cyclo-oxygenase inhibitors. Sufficient aspirin must be given in order to achieve anti-inflammatory blood levels (10 to 20 mg per deciliter). At lower concentrations, patients can experience analgesia, albeit without significant anti-inflammatory effects. The typical daily dose of aspirin in patients with RA ranges from 2 to 6 g of aspirin in divided doses. At the higher doses, clearance mechanisms can be saturated, and a relatively small increase in dose can be accompanied by a marked increase in blood levels. Because of gastrointestinal toxicity (including dyspepsia, erosive gastritis, and peptic ulcer disease), the large number of pills required, and skillful marketing, aspirin use has declined in recent years in favor of newer NSAIDs. Nonselective NSAIDs like ibuprofen or indomethacin provide little additional benefit besides improved pharmacokinetics, however, and exhibit a similar toxicity profile. Because aspirin inhibits platelet function and prolongs bleeding time, some physicians prescribe nonacetylated salicylates or salicylsalicylate instead. These are generally tolerated better than aspirin.

Production of prostaglandins in the rheumatoid synovium is dependent on two distinct cyclooxygenase enzymes, known as COX-1 and COX-2. The former is constitutively expressed and is responsible for normal endogenous production of prostaglandins in many tissues, including cytoprotective prostaglandins in the stomach. COX-2, on the other hand, is induced by such inflammatory cytokines as IL-1 and TNF-α and regulates increased prostaglandin synthesis in RA synovium. Most NSAIDs, including indomethacin, naproxen, and ibuprofen, inhibit both COX-1 and COX-2. It appears that most of the anti-inflammatory activity and analgesia result from inhibition of the latter. Selective COX-2 inhibitors, such as celecoxib and rofecoxib, are as effective as the nonselective inhibitors in RA, suggesting that COX-1 inhibition does not add appreciably to the therapeutic benefit.

A vast array of newer NSAIDs are now available, some of which can be purchased without prescription in the United States (ibuprofen and naproxen). No single drug can be recommended as clearly superior, and patients frequently try a number of agents to determine the most effective. For unclear reasons, some patients seem to respond better to one NSAID compared with the others. To avoid an unending cycle of NSAID experimentation, a physician should become familiar with a limited number of these agents and individualize therapy. The role of the selective COX-2 inhibitors in the treatment of RA is still evolving. In general, they probably should be used by patients with contraindications to standard NSAIDs, including bleeding diatheses, a history of peptic ulcer disease, or gastrointestinal intolerance. Because COX-2 is not expressed in platelets, the selective COX-2 inhibitors potentially can be used in patients with platelet dysfunction. If patients respond well to generic NSAIDs, however, and do not experience adverse effects, there is no specific indication for switching to the more expensive agents. It is hoped that pharmaco-economic studies evaluating the relative costs of nonselective NSAID toxicity and selective COX-2 inhibitors will provide additional guidance.

There are few reasons to favor one drug over another. Because of the long half-life of piroxicam, it should be used with care in the elderly, in whom clearance might be diminished. Sulindac is said to have less kidney toxicity in patients with mild renal insufficiency, though the clinical relevance of this observation remains unclear. None of the nonselective NSAIDs have a clearcut benefit over others with regard to gastrointestinal toxicity. Some gastrointestinal side effects can be minimized if pills are taken with food. Antacids, sucralfate, H_2 blockers, or proton pump inhibitors can also be symptomatically helpful, though they may not protect against drug-induced gastric erosions or ulcers. Prostaglandin analogues (e.g., misoprostol) appear to limit mucosal damage, but they need to be taken three to four times a day and can cause diarrhea. The selective COX-2 agents may have a lower incidence of asymptomatic gastric erosions and ulcers associated with their use.

Doses of NSAIDs in RA can be advanced quickly to the maximum recommended dose (500 mg naproxen taken orally twice a day or 600 to 800 mg ibuprofen taken orally four times a day), which frequently exceeds analgesic doses or doses used in osteoarthritis. Celecoxib, a selective COX-2 inhibitor, is given at 100 to 200 mg in oral doses twice a day and rofecoxib is administered at doses of 12.5 to 25 mg once a day. While some improvement might be noted within days after starting a new drug, a fair therapeutic trial should be 2 to 4 weeks before switching to another compound. If pain relief is not achieved with NSAIDs, judicious use of narcotics, such as codeine, can be appropriate on occasion, but they should be used with caution, owing to the obvious problems of tolerance and addiction that can arise in patients with chronic pain.

SECOND-LINE AGENTS

In traditional paradigms of RA treatment, advancement from NSAIDs to second-line agents is recommended if a patient does not have sufficient symptomatic improvement after an adequate therapeutic trial of NSAIDs; if a patient has aggressive seropositive disease, especially with rheumatoid nodules; or if there is radiographic evidence of erosions or joint destruction. The second-line agents are sometimes called DMARDs, or disease-modifying antirheumatic drugs, though their ability to slow progression of RA is not fully established. An alternative name for this class of drugs is SAARDs, or slow-acting antirheumatic drugs. There are many available SAARDs, and each has advantages and disadvantages. As a group, they tend to have relatively low response rates (usually about 30%), comparatively high toxicity levels, and a significant delay before onset of action (3 to 6 months). Some of the newer agents have more favorable profiles. A typical paradigm for treating patients whose pain is not adequately controlled by NSAIDs is shown in Fig. 174.2.

The most commonly used second-line drug is the folic acid antagonist methotrexate. Originally designed to inhibit dihydrofolate reductase, low-dose weekly methotrexate has unique efficacy in RA. Unlike the results with other second-line drugs, the majority of patients benefit, with a response rate of 70% to 80%. Moreover, the benefit occurs relatively rapidly compared with the other drugs, and improvement is sometimes observed after only 4 to 8 weeks of therapy. Treatment is usually initiated at 7.5 mg taken orally as a single dose 1 day a week. The dose is usually advanced (increasing by 2.5 to 5 mg per week each month) to 15 mg per week or until clinical benefit is achieved. Occasionally, higher doses (20 to 25 mg per week) or parenteral therapy (intramuscular or intravenous injections) are required for clinical improvement. When a sufficient clinical response is achieved, the dose sometimes can be modestly diminished without loss of benefit. The majority of patients have less morning stiffness, fewer signs of synovitis (swelling, warmth, erythema),

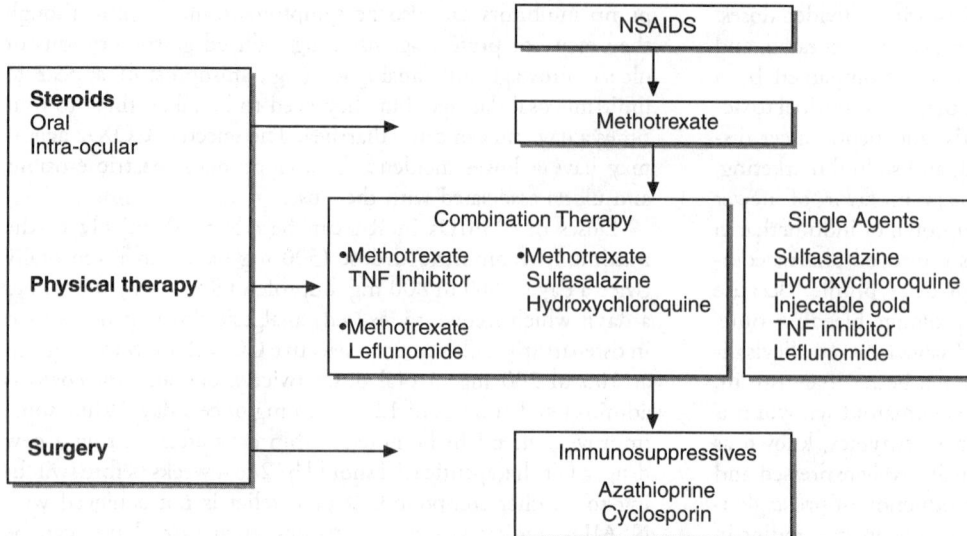

FIGURE 174.2. Suggested schema for RA treatment. In the past, patients whose disease was not adequately controlled by NSAIDs were treated with SAARDs (slow-acting antirheumatic drugs), such as gold. Many rheumatologists today bypass these drugs in favor of methotrexate as the initial second-line treatment. Superimposed on this paradigm is the judicious use of various glucocorticoid preparations, physical therapy, and surgery.

less pain, and improved energy levels while taking methotrexate. Complete remissions are uncommon, and discontinuation of the drug usually leads to a flare-up within a few weeks. Methotrexate is very well tolerated, and about 50% of patients continue to take the medicine for at least 5 years. It is difficult to be certain whether methotrexate has true disease-modifying action or simply improves symptoms and quality of life. Radiographic studies suggest that erosions heal in a subset of patients, perhaps owing to a selective decrease in synovial collagenase gene expression.

The mechanism of action of methotrexate is still a matter of conjecture. At the doses used in RA, there are at most only very modest immunosuppressive effects. In adjuvant arthritis in the rat, methotrexate inhibits IL-1 production by macrophages. In addition, some acute anti-inflammatory activities appear to be mediated by increasing endogenous adenosine production. It is not clear whether the anti-inflammatory activities are in any way related to inhibition of dihydrofolate reductase, since coadministration of methotrexate with folic acid or folinic acid decreases gastrointestinal toxicity (especially oral ulcers) without affecting efficacy.

The primary safety concern with methotrexate is hepatotoxicity. Prolonged use of methotrexate can cause hepatic fibrosis and, rarely, cirrhosis with portal hypertension. This problem was particularly prominent in the 1950s and 1960s, when methotrexate was administered daily to treat patients with psoriasis. The advent of pulse methotrexate therapy (once a week) appears to have alleviated many of these problems. Several studies of liver biopsies from RA patients taking weekly methotrexate suggest that significant hepatic fibrosis is very uncommon. For this reason, it is no longer standard practice to perform serial liver biopsies (formerly recommended after every 1 to 2 g of total dose) unless specific risk factors dictate, such as preexisting liver disease or a history of excessive alcohol intake.

A complete blood count and liver enzyme profile should be obtained before initiating therapy and every 4 to 6 weeks thereafter to monitor toxicity. Renal insufficiency is a relative contraindication, since it can delay excretion and exacerbate the poten-

tial for bone marrow toxicity, leading to leukopenia or thrombocytopenia. Concomitant use of other folic acid antagonists, such as trimethoprim or trimethoprim-sulfamethoxazol is contraindicated, owing to possible synergistic marrow and mucosal toxicity. A mild increase in liver enzymes (usually the transaminases) in patients taking methotrexate is often rapidly reversed by temporarily discontinuing the drug and restarting it at a lower dose after the blood test results normalize. The relationship between serum transaminase elevation and hepatic fibrosis is tenuous at best. Nevertheless, it seems prudent to maintain liver enzymes within the normal range. The best-known risk factor for liver toxicity is the use of alcohol; it should be avoided. Methotrexate can also cause allergic pneumonitis marked by dyspnea and a eosinophilic infiltrate. In addition, it is a potent teratogen and abortifacient. Women of childbearing years must be advised of the reproductive consequences and should take appropriate precautions to avoid becoming pregnant. In men, methotrexate can cause mild azospermia.

If patients fail to have an adequate response to methotrexate, one can either add therapeutic agents (combination therapy) or switch to another single agent. Injectable gold, sulfasalazine, or antimalarial agents have been widely used individually as SAARDs. For many years, injectable gold was the first line of therapy after the failure of NSAIDs. Its effectiveness was established in prospective double-blind studies, and it is one of the few drugs with documented disease-modifying properties (albeit mild). Gold is available in two forms, an aqueous formulation (gold sodium thiomalate) and an oil-based preparation (aurothioglucose). The aqueous form is used preferentially, and the oil-based form is given to patients who experience "nitritoid" reactions with gold sodium thiomalate (episodes of flushing, diaphoresis, and hypotension shortly after injection).

To initiate gold therapy, a test dose of 10 mg gold sodium thiomalate is usually given intramuscularly, followed 1 week later by 25 mg. If it is well tolerated, the intramuscular dose is increased to 50 mg per week until a total dose of 1 g is reached. Before each dose, a urinalysis should be performed and a complete blood count taken (including a platelet count). Patients should be questioned about side effects, particularly oral ulcers and skin rash, which can occur in up to 30% of patients. The skin rash of injectable gold is usually intensely pruritic and can develop virtually anywhere on the body. If the rash resolves quickly upon cessation of therapy, injectable gold can sometimes be restarted at a lower dose and gradually increased without recurrence. Other adverse effects, such as thrombocytopenia, leukopenia, or proteinuria from membranous glomerulonephritis, are indications to discontinue gold permanently. Severe glomerulonephritis or thrombocytopenia might respond to high-dose corticosteroids.

Antimalarial drugs are second-line agents that, like gold, require 3 to 6 months of continuous therapy to determine efficacy. As with many other slow-acting drugs, any clinical response observed before about 1 to 2 months of therapy must be considered coincidental rather than evidence of response. The most commonly used antimalarial agent in RA is hydroxychloroquine (200 mg administered orally twice a day). The response rate is similar to that observed with injectable gold; its primary advantage over gold is relative safety and ease of administration. The general tendency has been to administer injectable gold to patients with more aggressive disease and to use hydroxychloroquine in patients with milder RA. The major toxicity of antimalarial agents is ocular; retinal deposits develop after administration of high doses for years. Visual problems that can ultimately lead to blindness, such as loss of fine color distinction, can be monitored easily at home by patients, and periodic funduscopic examination can be used to confirm the lack of toxicity. Retinal disease due to the interaction of the drug with melanin in the pigmented epithelial layer and damage to the rods and cones should be distinguished from benign corneal deposits that can produce a halo effect around bright lights; the latter condition is not an indication to discontinue the drug. At the therapeutic doses used today, hydroxychloroquine is very safe, and discontinuation for retinal toxicity is rare. Other potential side effects include dyspepsia, increased skin pigmentation, and myopathy.

Sulfasalazine is used by many physicians to treat RA, especially in Great Britain; it is probably as effective as antimalarial drugs. Sulfasalazine is usually started at low doses (500 mg orally twice a day), and the dose is increased over several weeks to a maximum of 3 g per day, taken in divided doses. Gastrointestinal intolerance and lack of efficacy are the major reasons for discontinuing therapy. The active moiety in arthritis appears to be the sulfapyridine portion of the molecule. The mechanism of action is not known, but it might be inhibition of leukotriene B4 production by neutrophils, scavenging of reactive oxygen species, blocking activation of the transcription factor NF-κB, or increasing production of the anti-inflammatory autocoid adenosine.

Instead of using a series of individual agents to treat refractory RA, some clinicians use combination therapy. One possible approach is to add sulfasalazine and hydroxychloroquine to methotrexate (triple therapy), and there are data that suggest that this treatment is more effective than any of these agents used alone.

Specific anticytokine approaches have been successfully tested in RA. TNF inhibitors, in particular, have shown striking efficacy. Both an anti-TNF-α antibody (infliximab) and a soluble TNF receptor/Fc fusion protein (etanercept) have been con-

firmed to be effective in clinical studies and both are approved for use in the United States. Although both can be used as single agents, considerable success has also been achieved in combining them with methotrexate. Etanercept has been approved for use in RA as a subcutaneous injection twice a week (25 mg per dose). The response rate is 50% to 70%, and clinical improvement can occur within weeks of initiating therapy. Toxicity seems limited to local irritation at injection sites. In addition, acute phase reactants, such as the erythrocyte sedimentation rate and C-reactive protein, also decrease rapidly. Infliximab is administered intravenously at a dose of 3 mg/kg every 8 weeks. It is generally used in combination with oral methotrexate since this appears to diminish production of human antimouse antibodies. TNF-α inhibition does not cure RA; symptoms quickly return if the inhibitors are discontinued. It appears that they delay progression of RA, as evidenced on radiography, perhaps through the capacity of TNF-α to induce metalloproteinase production. Long-term safety of TNF inhibition remains uncertain, especially with regard to infections, and there is concern about antibody development to components of the compounds, particularly IgG, and tumor immunology. Studies with etanercept suggest safety comparable to methotrexate after at least 3 years of continuous treatment. Nevertheless, this therapy represents a truly effective alternative to the SAARDs.

IMMUNOSUPPRESSIVE AGENTS

Patients that fail treatment with standard second-line agents can advance to immunosuppressive drugs. Some are approved for use in RA in the United States, though they are used somewhat sparingly. Azathioprine, which is metabolized to the active metabolite 6-mercaptopurine, is modestly effective at doses from 1 to 2 mg per kilogram per day. Alkylating agents (such as chlorambucil and cyclophosphamide) are efficacious, but they are rarely used because of the potential for toxicity (especially the increased risk of malignancy). Cyclosporin (2.5 to 5 mg per kilogram per day) appears to provide modest benefit for a subset of patients, often at the expense of renal toxicity. Combinations of antimetabolites, like azathioprine and methotrexate, seem to have marginal additional benefit and a higher risk of side effects. Leflunomide is an inhibitor of *de novo* pyrimidine synthesis recently approved for use in RA. Because of its long half-life, a loading dose usually is required (100 mg/dx5), followed by 20 mg/d. Leflunomide also appears to block radiographic progression. Its major target for toxicity is the liver, although preliminary studies suggest that it can be given safely with methotrexate.

GLUCOCORTICOIDS

Superimposed on this strategy for treating RA are a variety of other treatment methods. The most prominent is the judicious use of oral prednisone. In general, the dose should not exceed 10 mg per day. Alternate-day treatment, with a view to limiting side effects, is generally not successful, owing to worsening of symptoms during the "off" day. Steroid therapy should be started with some trepidation, because it can be difficult to wean patients once it has been initiated. Glucocorticoids are indicated for patients who are unable (or unwilling) to wait for the benefit of a second-line drug or whose disease is so severe that it jeopardizes their livelihood or their ability to care for themselves or others (especially their children). The clinical response is usually gratifyingly rapid (within a few days). Once the decision has been made to begin tapering prednisone, patience is a key virtue. One should be satisfied with very small decreases in the dose at intervals of 2 to 4 weeks, particularly when the dose is less than 5 mg per day.

Corticosteroids should be used with particular care in postmenopausal women because of the increased risk of osteoporosis. It is often advisable to initiate preventive therapy for osteoporosis, such as estrogen replacement or bisphosphonates. In men, low-dose steroids can be used with somewhat greater assurance, though care should still be taken to monitor patients periodically for evidence of declining bone density, such as vertebral compression fractures. In particular, bone densitometry should be performed on postmenopausal women to determine whether they are candidates for hormone replacement therapy or bisphosphonates. At the doses used in RA, diabetes, mood changes, sleep disturbances and other serious side effects are not common. Cataracts and skin atrophy, with easy bruising, do occur with some frequency.

Intra-articular steroids represent an effective alternative in treating RA of the individual joints that flares up out of proportion to the rest of the disease. Care must be taken, of course, to rule out an infectious source for a monarticular flare-up. The amount of corticosteroid injected depends on the size of the joint. A useful guideline is 40 mg or the equivalent of an insoluble salt of triamcinolone (triamcinolone hexacetonide) in large joints (hips, shoulders, knees), 20 mg in medium-size joints (elbows and ankles), 10 mg in small joints (wrists), and 5 mg in the joints of the fingers and toes. If a soluble steroid preparation is injected instead of an insoluble form, the response is generally more limited and transient. Many physicians recommend immobilizing the injected joint for 1 to 2 days to enhance and prolong the response. Improvement after injection is usually relatively rapid, with a significant response in less than a week (usually after a day or two).

Occasionally, short-term flare-ups develop within a few hours after injection, perhaps because of the phlogistic properties of the steroid crystals themselves. The duration of the response varies, but it averages about 6 months. Sometimes joints remain quiescent for well over a year. Improvement occasionally can be observed in other joints, possibly due to small amounts of the active compound leaking into the circulation or activated immune cells trafficking through the injected joint and being suppressed by the local glucocorticoid effect before recirculating to other active joints. Repeated injections into the same joint have few demonstrable adverse effects, though it is probably inadvisable to inject an individual joint more than two or three times in a year.

PHYSICAL THERAPY AND SURGERY

Physical therapy and other nonpharmacologic treatments are often prescribed but rarely are shown to be effective in well-controlled studies. Most physical measures, like whirlpool baths,

heated wax treatments, ultrasonography, and diathermy, certainly make patients feel better during the procedure and perhaps for a short time afterward. This, in and of itself, is a worthy outcome. Nevertheless, such methods have not been shown to provide significant long-term functional, anti-inflammatory, or disease-modifying benefit. Many patients become disillusioned with these treatments after varying degrees of experimentation. It is important for patients to maintain an active life, and guidance from physical therapists with range-of-motion exercises and aerobic training is probably beneficial. Swimming or other water exercises are especially valuable for patients with significant pain in weight-bearing joints. Exercise programs might help delay or prevent joint contractures and muscular atrophy. Too much activity can exacerbate arthritis; a good balance must be struck. Temporary immobilization of some joints by splinting can provide significant relief in these cases. In fact, in years past, bed rest was an effective anti-inflammatory regimen for generalized RA flare-ups. Splinting might also lessen the progression of nonreducible deformities, especially in the hands and wrists.

Surgical treatment has become an important therapeutic option. Improvement in surgical techniques, antibiotic prophylaxis, and the development of new polymers have revolutionized the care of surgical patients, particularly those with total knee and total hip replacements. These procedures can transform a patient from wheelchair bound to ambulatory. With increased activity after surgery, new problems can arise, and previously unrecognized foot disease or other problems can suddenly become limiting. Long-term complications include loosening of the prostheses and bacterial infection. Despite such problems, joint replacement surgery has had a major impact on the quality of life for RA patients.

The indications for surgical interventions vary from patient to patient. A primary reason is amelioration of intractable pain, especially for joint replacement surgery. The relief achieved by total joint replacement or even less radical approaches is nothing short of remarkable. A second indication for surgery is severely impaired function. Completely eroded cartilage (resulting in bone-on-bone articulation), ruptured ligaments, and progressive destruction of bone matrix can lead to severe functional derangement that is amenable only to surgical correction. In addition to weight-bearing joints, impairment due to severe deformities in the hands also can be helped by surgery. For instance, dislocation and subluxation of the MCPs can render the hands useless, while implantation of artificial joints or merely arthrodesis (joint fusion) can improve grip and lead to dramatic functional improvement. Synovectomy in aggressive wrist disease may delay rupture of the extensor tendons of the hand. Arthroscopic synovectomy is also useful if symptoms in one joint, especially the knee, are particularly disabling in the absence of structural abnormality. This is a temporizing procedure, however, since the synovium can grow back over a period of a few years. Occasionally, surgery is indicated for cosmetic reasons, either to correct a deformity or to remove strategically located rheumatoid nodules.

Conclusion

Future therapeutic interventions in RA are being guided by increased understanding of the mechanisms of disease. In addition to the TNF inhibitors, IL-1 inhibitors are also being developed. For instance, IL-1Ra, which is a naturally occurring antagonist of IL-1, has been evaluated as a therapeutic agent. Preliminary data suggest that modest anti-inflammatory activity is accompanied by decreased bone destruction. Small-molecule inhibitors of signal transduction pathways involved in cytokine gene expression, such as the mitogen-activated protein (MAP) kinases, could lead to novel oral agents to block cytokine production. Treatment with immunosuppressive T_h2 cytokines, such as IL-10 and IL-4, might have usefulness in RA. Attempts to inhibit cellular trafficking through the synovium by interfering with adhesion molecule function are also under investigation, including specific inhibitors and integrins. While antibodies directed at specific T-cell subsets (including anti-CD4 and anti-CD5) have generally been a disappointment in clinical trials, newer, more specific reagents designed to remove cells expressing specific combinations of α and β T-cell receptor genes might have greater success. Moreover, it is hoped that such rationally designed agents will be able to achieve something that empirical treatment has not: arresting the progression of RA as well as providing symptomatic relief.

BIBLIOGRAPHY

Albani S, Carson DA, Roudier J. Genetic and environmental factors in the immune pathogenesis of rheumatoid arthritis. *Rheum Dis Clin North Am* 1992,18:729–740.

Brennan FM, Maini RN, Feldmann M. Role of pro-inflammatory cytokines in rheumatoid arthritis. *Springer Semin Immunopathol* 1998;20:133–147.

Firestein GS, Zvaifler NJ. How important are T cells in chronic rheumatoid synovitis? *Arthritis Rheum* 1990;33:768–773.

Firestein GS, AM Manning. Signal transduction and transcription factors in rheumatic diseases. *Arthritis Rheum* (in press).

Fox DA. The role of T cells in the immunopathogenesis of rheumatoid arthritis: new perspectives. *Arthritis Rheum* 1997;40:598–609.

Koopman WJ: Moreland LW. Rheumatoid arthritis: anticytokine therapies on the horizon. *Ann Intern Med* 1998,128:231–233.

Weinblatt ME. Efficacy of methotrexate in rheumatoid arthritis. *Br J Rheumatol* 1995;34(suppl 2):43–48.

Weyand CM, Goronzy JJ. HLA-DRB1 alleles as severity markers in RA. *Bull Rheum Dis* 1994;43:5–8.

Kelley's Textbook of Internal Medicine, fourth edition. Edited by H. David Humes. Lippincott Williams & Wilkins, Philadelphia © 2000.

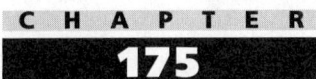

175

OSTEOARTHRITIS AND POLYCHONDRITIS

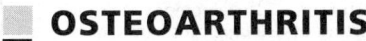

MARC C. HOCHBERG

OSTEOARTHRITIS

Osteoarthritis, formerly referred to as degenerative joint disease, is the most common form of arthritis. In 1986, a comprehensive definition of osteoarthritis was published in the proceedings of a conference on the etiopathogenesis of osteoarthritis, sponsored by the National Institutes of Health; this definition summarized the clinical, pathophysiologic, biochemical, and biomechanical changes that characterize osteoarthritis:

> Clinically, the disease is characterized by joint pain, tenderness, limitation of movement, crepitus, occasional effusion, and variable degrees of local inflammation, but without systemic effects. Pathologically, the disease is characterized by irregularly distributed loss of cartilage more frequently in areas of increased load, sclerosis of subchondral bone, subchondral cysts, marginal osteophytes, increased metaphyseal blood flow, and variable synovial inflammation. Histologically, the disease is characterized early by fragmentation of the cartilage surface, cloning of chondrocytes, vertical clefts in the cartilage, variable crystal deposition, remodeling, and eventual violation of the tidemark by blood vessels. It is also characterized by evidence of repair, particularly in osteophytes, and later by total loss of cartilage, sclerosis, and focal osteonecrosis of the subchondral bone. Biomechanically, the disease is characterized by alteration of the tensile, compressive, and shear properties and hydraulic permeability of the cartilage, increased water, and excessive swelling. These cartilage changes are accompanied by increased stiffness of the subchondral bone. Biochemically, the disease is characterized by reduction in the proteoglycan concentration, possible alterations in the size and aggregation of proteoglycans, alteration in collagen fibril size and weave, and increased synthesis and degradation of matrix macromolecules.

In 1994, a revised definition of osteoarthritis was proposed at a conference sponsored by the American Academy of Orthopaedic Surgeons and National Institutes of Health:

> Osteoarthritis (OA) is the result of both mechanical and biologic events that destabilize the normal coupling of degradation and synthesis of articular cartilage and subchondral bone. Although it may be initiated by multiple factors including genetic, developmental, metabolic and traumatic; OA involves all of the tissues of the diarthrodial joint. Ultimately, OA is manifested by morphologic, biochemical, molecular and biomechanical changes of both cells and matrix which lead to a softening, fibrillation, ulceration and loss of articular cartilage, sclerosis and eburnation of subchondral bone, osteophytes and subchondral cysts. When clinically evident, OA is characterized by joint pain, tenderness, limitation of movement, crepitus, occasional effusion, and variable degrees of local inflammation.

EPIDEMIOLOGY

Osteoarthritis is the most common form of arthritis, with a worldwide distribution; indeed, age-specific prevalence rates of osteoarthritis by groups of joints are strikingly similar in all populations studied. Most epidemiologic studies of osteoarthritis have used the presence of radiographic changes as illustrated in the *Atlas of Standard Radiographs* for the purpose of case definition. Population-based studies in the United States, reviewed by the National Arthritis Data Workgroup in 1998, show that approximately one-third of US adults aged 25 to 74 had radiographic evidence of osteoarthritis involving at least one joint group; the prevalence was greatest in the hands and then the feet, knees, and hips in declining order of frequency. The prevalence rises with increasing age in all joint groups and is generally

TABLE 175.1.	RISK FACTORS FOR OSTEOARTHRITIS

Increasing age
Female sex
Genetic predisposition
Overweight[a]
Trauma (joint injury)[a]
Occupations (farmers, weavers, dockworkers, elite athletes)[a]
Congenital and developmental bone and joint disorders[a]
Abnormal joint biomechanics (joint malalignment)[a]
Previous inflammatory joint disease[a]
Metabolic disorders (hemochromatosis, ochronosis, acromegaly, calcium pyrophosphate deposition disease)[a]

[a] Potentially modifiable or treatable.
(From Hochberg MC. Epidemiology of osteoarthritis: current concepts and new insights. *J Rheumatol* 1991;18(suppl 27):4–6, modified and reproduced with permission.

higher in women than men. Gender-specific rates vary by age and site, especially at the knee and hip.

Factors associated with the development of osteoarthritis are listed in Table 175.1. Age is the strongest determinant of osteoarthritis; indeed, radiographic changes of osteoarthritis are almost universal in at least one joint group in persons older than 75. Gender is also associated with variations in the rate of development of osteoarthritis; the disorder is more common in men younger than 45 and in women older than 55. Furthermore, the clinical subset of nodal generalized osteoarthritis (see "Classification" below) is seen almost exclusively in middle-aged and elderly women. In the United States, osteoarthritis of the knee is both more common and more severe in African-American women than in white women, even after adjustment for other known risk factors.

Heredity

Hereditary factors have been recognized as important in the development of Heberden's nodes for more than 40 years. New studies have presented significant evidence of familial aggregation of polyarticular osteoarthritis, and twin studies have established significant heritability for the radiographic features of osteoarthritis, including osteophytes and joint space narrowing. In several families, a single base mutation at position 419 in the *COL2A1* gene, resulting in a single amino acid change from cysteine to arginine, has been found to be linked to a syndrome of mild chondrodysplasia with polyarticular osteoarthritis. Other mutations in the *COL2A1* gene as well as in genes for type IX and XI collagen and the aggrecan protein also have been associated with osteoarthritis.

Obesity

Data from prospective epidemiologic studies show a causal association between obesity and the development of osteoarthritis of the knees. This association is most likely explained on a biomechanical basis, though the role of an underlying metabolic

disturbance cannot be completely excluded. The association of obesity with knee osteoarthritis is stronger than that with osteoarthritis of the hip; furthermore, obesity is more strongly associated with bilateral than unilateral disease at both the hip and knee.

Mechanical Stress

Biomechanical stresses, as reflected by repetitive occupational joint use or a history of significant joint trauma, are also associated with the development of osteoarthritis. Persons with jobs that require frequent knee bending and greater strength demands are at higher risk of knee osteoarthritis, while those with jobs that require heavy bending and lifting are at increased risk of hip osteoarthritis. Persons with a history of unilateral knee or hip trauma are at increased risk of ipsilateral but not contralateral knee or hip osteoarthritis, respectively. The role of avocational exercise, including running, as a risk factor for osteoarthritis, in the absence of injury, remains the subject of controversy.

Other Factors

Other risk factors for osteoarthritis include congenital and developmental disease of bones and cartilage (congenital hip subluxation, slipped capital femoral epiphysis), previous inflammatory joint disease (rheumatoid arthritis), selected metabolic and endocrine disorders (ochronosis, hemochromatosis, acromegaly), and calcium pyrophosphate deposition disease.

CLASSIFICATION

Based on the occurrence of osteoarthritis in various populations and the risk factors that have been identified from epidemiologic studies, several classification schema have been developed. One such schema, modified from the one proposed by the American College of Rheumatology, is shown in Table 175.2. Idiopathic

TABLE 175.2.	CLASSIFICATION OF OSTEOARTHRITIS

Idiopathic
    Localized (hands, feet, knee, hip, spine, and other single sites)
    Generalized (includes three or more areas listed above)
Secondary
    Posttraumatic
    Congenital or developmental diseases
        Localized (hip disease)
        Generalized (bone dysplasias and metabolic diseases, such as ochronosis, hemochromatosis)
    Calcium deposition disease
    Other bone and joint disorders (avascular necrosis, rheumatoid arthritis, Paget's disease)
    Other diseases
        Endocrine diseases (acromegaly, hyperparathyroidism)
        Neuropathic arthropathy
        Miscellaneous

(From Altman RD, Asch E, Bloch D, et al. Development of criteria for the classification and reporting of osteoarthritis. *Arthritis Rheum* 1986;29:1038–1049, modified and reproduced with permission.)

osteoarthritis manifests either in a localized form, affecting one or two joint groups (usually the distal interphalangeal, proximal interphalangeal, and first carpometacarpal joints of the hands; the cervical or lumbar spine, or the first metatarsophalangeal joints of the feet, knees, and hips), or in a generalized form, involving three or more joint groups. This generalized form is frequently associated with Heberden's nodes; in this instance, it most often affects middle-aged or elderly women and is inherited in an autosomal dominant fashion. In patients with osteoarthritis of atypical joints (metacarpophalangeal joints of the hands, wrists, elbows, shoulders, and ankles), the physician should search for an underlying disorder (e.g., hemochromatosis) as a cause of secondary osteoarthritis.

ETIOLOGY AND PATHOGENESIS

Osteoarthritis is thought to be primarily a disease of the articular cartilage and subchondral bone, with mild secondary inflammation of the synovial membrane. In idiopathic osteoarthritis, it is not known whether the primary abnormality occurs in the articular cartilage or the subchondral bone; in most cases of secondary osteoarthritis, however, it appears that the primary defect is in the articular cartilage.

The articular cartilage has two major functions in health: minimizing contact stress by deforming under conditions of mechanical load and providing a smooth load-bearing surface to permit motion of the joint with minimal friction and wear. Articular cartilage is composed of chondrocytes imbedded in an extracellular matrix of collagen and proteoglycans. The major structural protein in articular cartilage is type II collagen, other minor collagens include types IX and XI. It is believed that these minor collagens are involved in cross-linking of adjacent bundles of type II collagen and interactions between proteoglycan molecules and type II collagen. Proteoglycan molecules are composed of hyaluronic acid and an aggrecan molecule attached by link protein; the aggrecan molecule is composed of a core protein to which are attached glycosaminoglycans, including keratin sulfate, chondroitin-4-sulfate, and chondroitin-6-sulfate.

The earliest biochemical changes in articular cartilage are an increase in water content, presumably due to weakening of the type II collagen network, and accompanying decreases in proteoglycan concentration, aggregation, and size. These changes result in other changes in the biomechanical properties of the cartilage, with increased hydraulic permeability and decreased ability to bear load. Remodeling of the subchondral bone leads to advancement of the tidemark region of calcified cartilage and a decline in the volume of articular cartilage. Proliferation of cartilage at the margins of the joint, followed by endochondral ossification, leads to the formation of the osteophyte, the radiologic hallmark of osteoarthritis.

As noted earlier, osteoarthritis reflects a disturbance in the homeostasis of synthesis and degradation of articular cartilage. The chondrocyte, under stimulation by interleukin-1 and other cytokines as well as by mechanical deformation, increases synthesis of degradative enzymes, including matrix metalloproteases (collagenase, gelatinase, stromelysin) and aggrecanase; these enzymes degrade the structural components of articular cartilage, hastening its biomechanical failure. Although synthesis of normal cartilage extracellular components remains intact and is even increased early in the course of disease, in later stages synthesis declines, and the cartilage cannot be repaired. Data from numerous laboratories suggest that inhibitors of interleukin-1 and inhibitors of the synthesis of matrix metalloproteases may alter the development and progression of osteoarthritis in animal models of this disease. Trials of these agents in humans are in progress.

CLINICAL FINDINGS

Typically, the patient with osteoarthritis is middle-aged or elderly and experiences gradual onset of pain and stiffness accompanied by loss of function. This gradual or insidious pain is usually moderate in intensity, worsened by use of the involved joints, and improved or relieved with rest. While pain at rest or nocturnal pain are felt to be features of severe disease, they also may be markers of local inflammation. The onset of pain in patients with osteoarthritis stems from several possible factors; pain may result from periostitis at sites of bony remodeling, subchondral microfractures, capsular irritation from osteophytes, periarticular muscle spasm, bone angina due to decreased blood flow and elevated intraosseus pressure, and synovial inflammation accompanied by the release of prostaglandins, leukotrienes, and various cytokines, including interleukin-1. Articular cartilage itself has no nerves.

Morning stiffness is common in patients with osteoarthritis. The duration of morning stiffness, however, is significantly shorter (often less than 30 minutes) than in patients with active rheumatoid arthritis. A gelling phenomenon, or stiffness after periods of inactivity, is also common and resolves within several minutes. Both pain and stiffness are modified by weather changes in the majority of patients; symptoms worsen in damp, cool, and rainy weather and improve when the weather improves. Patients with osteoarthritis of the knees also may complain of a sense of instability or buckling, especially when descending stairs or curbs.

On physical examination, evidence of disease usually is found to be localized to symptomatic joints. Bony enlargement is common, with tenderness at the joint margins and attachments of the joint capsule and periarticular tendons. Limitation of motion of the affected joint frequently is related to osteophyte formation and/or severe cartilage loss. Signs of local inflammation may be present, including warmth and soft-tissue swelling due to joint effusion. The presence of a hot, erythematous, markedly swollen joint should suggest either a superimposed microcrystalline process, such as gout or pseudogout, or septic arthritis. Instability can be detected by excess joint motion; locking of a joint during range-of-motion testing is likely due to loose bodies. Crepitus, which can be felt on passive range of joint motion and is due to irregularity of the opposing cartilage surfaces, is present in more than 90% of patients with osteoarthritis of the knee. Malalignment is evident in almost 50% of patients with osteoarthritis of the knee; a varus deformity (e.g., bowlegs) due to loss of articular cartilage in the medial compartment is more common than a valgus deformity.

LABORATORY FINDINGS

The clinical diagnosis of osteoarthritis is usually confirmed with radiographs. The radiographic features of osteoarthritis are illus-

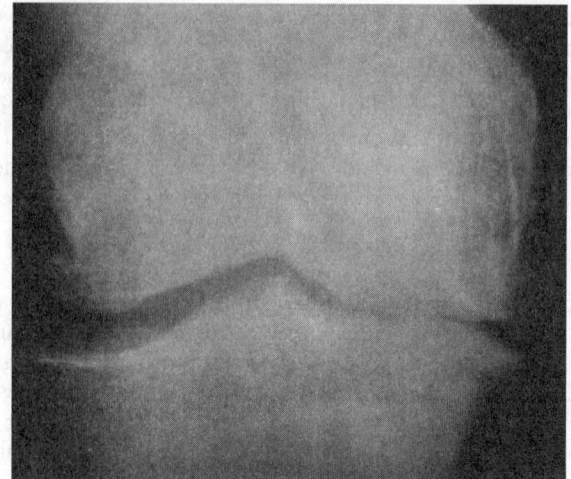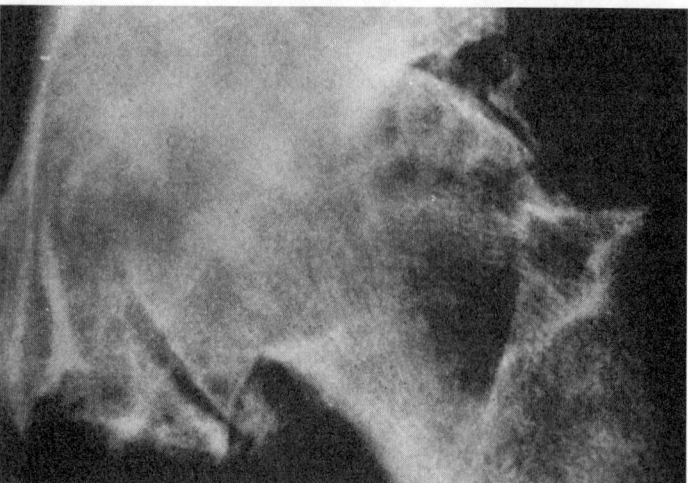

A

B

FIGURE 175.1. A: Radiograph of the knee showing osteoarthritis. Note the marked narrowing of the joint space in the medial compartment, osteophyte formation, sclerosis of subchondral bone, and attrition of bone in the medial tibial plateau. **B:** Radiograph of the hip showing osteoarthritis. Note the marked loss of joint space, osteophyte formation, subchondral sclerosis, subchondral cyst formation, and deformity of the femoral head.

trated in Fig. 175.1. The classic radiographic finding is marginal osteophyte formation. Subchondral bone sclerosis and asymmetric joint space narrowing due to loss of articular cartilage develop with progression of disease. Joint space narrowing may be due to actual degradation of articular cartilage and/or progression of the tidemark region of calcified cartilage toward the surface during bone remodeling. Later changes include the formation of subchondral cysts with sclerotic walls and bone remodeling with alteration in the shape of the bone ends. Bone demineralization (periarticular osteoporosis) and marginal erosions are not a radiographic feature of osteoarthritis; their presence should strongly suggest the diagnosis of a form of inflammatory arthritis, such as rheumatoid arthritis.

Routine laboratory tests, including complete blood count, erythrocyte sedimentation rate, chemistry panels, and urinalysis, generally show normal results in patients with osteoarthritis. These studies, especially the complete blood count and chemistry panel, should be obtained at the time of baseline evaluation of patients with osteoarthritis—before instituting therapy with nonsteroidal anti-inflammatory drugs (NSAIDs)—and at 3- to 6-month intervals during therapy. Tests for rheumatoid factor, commonly performed in the evaluation of patients with arthritis, may show positive results in low titer in up to 20% of elderly individuals; therefore, the presence of rheumatoid factor does not exclude a diagnosis of osteoarthritis if the clinical picture and radiographic changes are most suggestive of this disorder. Synovial fluid analysis usually reveals type I, noninflammatory fluid. The finding of inflammatory fluid with an elevated white cell count suggests either a superimposed microcrystalline process (gout, pseudogout, or basic calcium apatite crystals) or septic arthritis.

Optimal Management

The principles of the treatment of patients with osteoarthritis are listed in Table 175.3. Treatment should be individualized

based on the distribution and severity of joint involvement as well as the presence of comorbid conditions. Educational materials, including pamphlets published by the Arthritis Foundation, provide basic information that allows the patient to understand and cope with his or her disease. Patients should be encouraged to participate in the Arthritis Self-Help Course, administered by local chapters of the Arthritis Foundation; this course includes educational sessions supervised by a lay coordinator with professional speakers.

Patients with osteoarthritis are likely to suffer from physical disability characterized by difficulty in performing activities of

TABLE 175.3.	APPROACH TO THE TREATMENT OF PATIENTS WITH OSTEOARTHRITIS

Nonpharmacologic therapy
  Education of the patient
  Self-management programs
  Social support
  Physical and occupational therapy
  Range-of-motion and muscle-strengthening exercises
  Aerobic conditioning
  Weight loss
Pharmacologic therapy
  Simple analgesics (acetaminophen)
  Topical analgesics (capsaicin cream)
  Nonsteroidal anti-inflammatory drugs
  COX-2-specific inhibitors
  Intra-articular corticosteroid injections
  Intra-articular hyaluronate injections
  Closed tidal joint irrigation
  Narcotic analgesics
Surgical therapy
  Arthroscopic debridement and joint irrigation
  Osteotomy
  Total joint arthroplasty

daily living, including bathing, dressing, eating, grooming, and toileting, and limitation in mobility. The occupational therapist will evaluate the patient's ability to perform activities of daily living, provide assistive devices as needed, and teach joint protection techniques and energy conservation skills. In addition, splints can be designed either to stabilize or to reduce inflammation in finger joints, especially the thumb base. The physical therapist also will teach the patient the therapeutic use of heat and massage and devise an individualized exercise program. This exercise program will stress muscle strengthening to provide stability to weight-bearing joints. In addition, braces, canes, and other ambulation aids and devices can be furnished, if needed. Physical therapy also plays a key role in the pre- and postoperative care of patients who undergo reconstructive orthopaedic surgery, including total joint arthroplasty.

Overweight patients should be encouraged to lose weight; referral for dietary instruction and enrollment in an aerobic exercise program, either supervised fitness walking or aquatic swimming, may be helpful. Studies have verified that weight loss is associated with improvement in both pain and disability. The main indication for drug therapy in patients with osteoarthritis is pain relief. Simple analgesics, such as acetaminophen, are the drug of choice for initial therapy in patients with mild to moderate pain. Patients who fail to achieve adequate pain relief with acetaminophen should be treated with an NSAID; these drugs are approximately equally effective, and the choice of a specific NSAID is largely influenced by differences in toxicity profiles and costs. It is preferable for patients who are at high risk of adverse upper-gastrointestinal-tract effects to receive a COX-2-specific inhibitor, such as celecoxib or rofecoxib, rather than an NSAID that inhibits both isoforms of the cyclooxygenase enzyme. COX-2-specific inhibitors have an incidence of adverse upper-gastrointestinal-tract effects similar to that of placebo and significantly less than that of nonselective NSAIDs.

Intra-articular corticosteroid injections have a role in the treatment of patients whose symptoms are limited to one or a few joints that have effusions and signs of local inflammation. Local injections are beneficial as an adjunct to NSAID therapy or for the patient who is unable either to take or to tolerate NSAIDs. Care should be taken to use aseptic technique when injecting joints; in addition, fluid aspirated at the time of injection always should be sent for appropriate bacteriologic culture. Other medical treatments include topical analgesic creams (capsaicin) and intra-articular preparations of hyaluronic acid in patients with osteoarthritis of the knee who have failed to respond to or who are intolerant of other therapies, .

Patients whose symptoms are not adequately controlled with medical therapy and who have severe pain and functional impairment are candidates for reconstructive joint surgery. Total joint arthroplasty has markedly altered the quality of life of patients with osteoarthritis of the knees and hips and is thought to be the major advance in the treatment of patients with osteoarthritis over the past 30 years. Short-term outcomes include moderate to marked pain relief; in the long-term, the majority of patients experience significant improvement in function. The perioperative mortality rate is generally below 1%, and short-term complications, including thromboembolic disease and infection, occur in less than 5% of patients. A major concern is the long-term

development of loosening due to deterioration of the bone–cement interface; the development of porous coated prostheses, which allow fixation by bone ingrowth, and newer techniques for cementing of noncoated prostheses may lead to a reduction in the rate of revision surgery due to loosening.

RELAPSING POLYCHONDRITIS

Relapsing polychondritis is a rare multisystem disease characterized by episodic inflammation of cartilaginous structures, resulting in tissue destruction. Little is known of the epidemiology of relapsing polychondritis; no reliable data are available on incidence and prevalence. Proposed diagnostic criteria for relapsing polychondritis are based on the clinical manifestations (see Clinical Findings).

ETIOLOGY AND PATHOGENESIS

The cause of relapsing polychondritis remains unknown. Tissue destruction results from release of degradative enzymes, including matrix metalloproteases, from chondrocytes and other cells. The release of these enzymes likely stems from immune-mediated activation of the chondrocytes and inflammatory cells; data supporting the role of the immune system include the association of relapsing polychondritis with autoimmune diseases—among them, rheumatoid arthritis, systemic lupus erythematosus, and systemic vasculitis—the presence of antibodies to type II collagen in the serum samples of patients with relapsing polychondritis, and the finding of immunoglobulins suggestive of immune complexes in tissue lesions from patients with relapsing polychondritis.

CLINICAL FINDINGS

Relapsing polychondritis can develop at any age, though the majority of cases are diagnosed in patients between ages 40 and 59. The sex distribution is equal; the disorder, however, has been reported mainly among whites. Clinical features are listed in Table 175.4. The most common feature of this disease is bilateral auricular chondritis, with redness, swelling, and tenderness in the acute phase and development of so-called cauliflower ears in the later phase. Hearing impairment, due to closure of the external auditory meatus, serous otitis media, eustachian tube obstruction, inflammation of the middle ear and a neurosensory hearing loss, and vestibular dysfunction, may accompany the ear symptoms. Involvement of the nasal cartilage is typical, with redness, swelling, and tenderness in the early phase and a "saddle nose" deformity in the later phase. Ocular inflammation manifests as episcleritis, scleritis, iritis, and keratitis in the majority of patients. Joint symptoms include peripheral inflammatory, nonerosive, and nondeforming polyarthritis and costochondritis. Involvement of the larynx and tracheobronchial tree is accompanied by complaints of hoarseness, dyspnea, wheezing, and stridor. Airway collapse is a major cause of death in these patients. Cardiovascular symptoms include aortic insufficiency, usually due to aortitis with dilatation of the aortic ring rather

TABLE 175.4.	CLINICAL MANIFESTATIONS OF RELAPSING POLYCHONDRITIS

Ears
  Bilateral auricular chondritis
  Auditory and/or vestibular dysfunction
Nose
  Nasal chondritis
Eyes
  Episcleritis, scleritis
  Nongranulomatous uveitis
  Keratitis with corneal perforation
Joints
  Parasternal arthropathy
  Peripheral nondeforming, nonerosive polyarthritis
Respiratory tract
  Laryngeal chondritis
  Tracheobronchial chondritis
  Airway collapse
Cardiovascular
  Aortic insufficiency
  Aortic aneurysms
  Small-, medium-, and large-vessel vasculitis
  Arterial and venous thrombosis
Kidney
  Crescentic glomerulonephritis
Skin
  Cutaneous vasculitis

than valvular changes; aneurysms of the ascending and descending aorta have also been described. Renal symptoms are rare. Small-vessel vasculitis may produce palpable purpura.

LABORATORY FINDINGS

Results of laboratory tests generally show nonspecific changes suggestive of chronic inflammation, including elevation of the erythrocyte sedimentation rate, mild normochromic/normocytic anemia, leukocytosis, thrombocytosis, and polyclonal hyperglobulinemia. Tests for antinuclear antibodies and rheumatoid factor usually generate positive results in patients with coexistent connective tissue diseases. Positive test results for antinuclear cytoplasmic antibodies and antiphospholipid antibodies have been reported in a minority of patients. Antibodies to both native and denatured type II collagen and a cell-mediated immune response to type II collagen and cartilage proteoglycans have been found in some patients. On biopsy of tissue lesions, the cartilage shows loss of basophilic staining of matrix, suggesting proteoglycan depletion, focal or diffuse infiltration by mononuclear inflammatory cells (predominantly CD4$^+$ lymphocytes), and replacement of normal cartilage structure by fibrous granulation tissue. Focal calcification may be present.

OPTIMAL MANAGEMENT

There is no standard therapy for relapsing polychondritis. Generally, patients with signs of acute inflammation are treated with prednisone, in doses equivalent to 0.75 to 1 mg per kilogram per day. When the acute inflammation subsides, doses are tapered to a maintenance level, as tolerated; alternate-day therapy is not recommended. Diaminodiphenyl sulfone (Dapsone), in doses of 50 to 200 mg per day, has also been used for patients without respiratory or cardiovascular involvement. In patients who are unresponsive to or intolerant of corticosteroids or who require higher than acceptable maintenance doses of corticosteroids, such immunosuppressive agents as azathioprine, cyclophosphamide, cyclosporine, and methotrexate may be useful. Patients with upper-airway involvement may require tracheostomy for relief of symptoms of airway collapse; those with laryngeal symptoms may need endotracheal intubation or surgical stabilization of the trachea. Patients with aortic insufficiency should be considered for valve replacement in conjunction with replacement of the aortic root.

BIBLIOGRAPHY

Bellamy N. Osteoarthritis. *Baillieres Clin Rheumatol* 1997;11(4):657–840.
Brandt KD. Osteoarthritis. *Rheum Dis Clin North Am* 1999;25(2): 257–488.
Creamer P, Flores R, Hochberg MC. Management of osteoarthritis in older adults. *Clin Geriatr Med* 1998;14(3):435–454.
Creamer P, Hochberg MC. Osteoarthritis. *Lancet* 1997;350:503–508.
Eccles M, Freemantle N, Mason J, for the North of England Non-Steroidal Anti-Inflammatory Drug Guideline Development Group. North of England evidence-based guideline development project: summary guideline for non-steroidal anti-inflammatory drugs versus basic analgesia in treating the pain of degenerative arthritis. *Br Med J* 1998;317: 526–530.
Hochberg MC, Altman RD, Brandt KD, et al. Guidelines for the medical management of osteoarthritis. I. Osteoarthritis of the hip. *Arthritis Rheum* 1995;38:1535–1540.
Hochberg MC, Altman RD, Brandt KD, et al. Guidelines for the medical management of osteoarthritis. II. Osteoarthritis of the knee. *Arthritis Rheum* 1995;38:1541–1546.
Keuttner KE, Goldberg V, eds. *Osteoarthritic disorders.* Rosemont, Ill.: American Academy of Orthopaedic Surgeons, 1995.
McAdam LP, O'Hanlan MA, Bluestone R, et al: Relapsing polychondritis: prospective study of 23 patients and a review of the literature. *Medicine* 1976;55:193–216.
Michet CJ, McKenna CH, Luthra HS, et al. Relapsing polychondritis: survival and predictive role of early disease manifestations. *Ann Intern Med* 1986;104:74–78.
Trentham DE, Le CH. Relapsing polychondritis. *Ann Intern Med* 1998; 129:114–122.

Kelley's Textbook of Internal Medicine, fourth edition. Edited by H. David Humes. Lippincott Williams & Wilkins, Philadelphia © 2000.

C H A P T E R
176

SPONDYLOARTHROPATHIES

FRANK C. ARNETT

The spondyloarthropathies encompass a family of chronic inflammatory disorders primarily affecting peripheral and axial joints. Although they have been considered variants of rheumatoid arthritis, these diseases now are classified as distinct entities based on clinical, epidemiologic, and immunogenetic differences. Unifying features include the following:

- A tendency for the disease to affect sacroiliac and other spinal joints (sacroiliitis and spondylitis)
- Peripheral arthritis, typically asymmetrical and oligoarticular
- Inflammatory lesions of tendon and fascial insertions (enthesopathy) at peripheral and axial sites
- Extra-articular complications affecting the eye (anterior uveitis) or heart (aortitis and conduction disturbance)
- Disease onset in young adults, especially men
- Absence of rheumatoid factor and other autoantibodies
- Strong associations with the class I histocompatibility antigen HLA-B27

Despite these common characteristics, each spondyloarthropathy manifests unique clinical and immunogenetic features, suggesting etiologic diversity. In clinical features, these differences usually permit precise diagnosis, which is important for management and prognosis. At times, overlapping clinical manifestations or incomplete expression make diagnosis difficult. Members of the spondyloarthropathy family include the following:

- Ankylosing spondylitis, a predominantly axial form of arthritis that usually begins in the sacroiliac joints and slowly progresses to spinal fusion
- Reiter's syndrome, or reactive arthritis, an acute peripheral type of arthritis associated with nongonococcal urethritis, conjunctivitis, or other mucocutaneous features, which typically occurs after enteric or genitourinary infections
- Psoriatic arthritis, a slowly progressive peripheral variety of arthritis, with or without axial disease, that occurs in the context of cutaneous psoriasis
- Enteropathic arthritis, a type of peripheral or axial arthropathy accompanying the idiopathic inflammatory bowel diseases, ulcerative colitis, and Crohn's disease

ETIOLOGY AND PATHOGENESIS

An atypical immune response to certain specific bacteria, mediated by HLA-B27, other major histocompatibility complex genes (HLA-B60, -DR1, and -DR8 and tumor necrosis factor α), and additional unidentified genetic loci, is believed to underlie the pathogenesis of most of the spondyloarthropathies (Table 176.1). The strongest evidence for this model is provided by Reiter's syndrome, or reactive arthritis, in which genitourinary infections caused by *Chlamydia trachomatis* and, possibly, *Ureaplasma urealyticum* and gastroenteritis caused by *Shigella flexneri*, many *Salmonella* species, *Yersinia enterocolitica* and *Yersinia pseudotuberculosis*, and *Campylobacter jejuni* have been shown in epidemiologic studies to incite the disease, primarily in individuals with HLA-B27. Accumulating data suggest that there is bacterial persistence at the primary sites of infection and dissemination of living microbes or their products to the joints and other extra-articular structures.

TABLE 176.1.	**ETIOLOGIC AND PATHOGENETIC FACTORS IN REACTIVE ARTHRITIS AND POSSIBLY OTHER SPONDYLOARTHROPATHIES**

Infections
  Enteric pathogens
    Shigella flexnari
    Salmonella species
    Yersinia species
    Campylobacter jejuni
  Venereal pathogens
    Chlamydia trachomatis
    ? *Ureaplasma urealyticum*
  Other pathogens
    ? *Chlamydia pneumoniae*
  Evidence for bacterial persistence
    Bacterial antigens (? living organisms) in synovial fluid/tissue
    Specific proliferative response of synovial fluid T cells against causative bacteria
    Serum IgA antibodies to causative bacteria
    Asymptomatic bowel inflammation (? site of bacteria)
    Clinical response to specific antibiotic treatment
    Animal model of spondyloarthropathy (B27 transgenic rat) does not develop disease in germ-free environment.
Genetic
  Strong association of diseases across ethnic lines with class I HLA-B27
  Transgenic rats with human HLA-B27 spontaneously develop manifest spondyloarthropathy.
  High concordance rate of ankylosing spondylitis in monozygotic versus dizygotic twins
  Genetic modeling in families shows ankylosing spondylitis to be predominantly genetic in origin
  Genetic mapping in families shows linkage to HLA-B27 as well as several other chromosomal regions

Bacterial antigens, especially lipopolysaccharides, from most of these intracellular pathogens have been found in synovial fluid phagocytes or synovial cells from patients with reactive arthritis using electron microscopy or fluorescent monoclonal antibodies. Although attempts to culture living bacteria from the joints have been unsuccessful, studies using the polymerase chain reaction have detected chlamydial RNA or DNA in synovial tissue, suggesting the presence of viable microorganisms. In addition, synovial fluid T lymphocytes from patients with reactive arthritis proliferate specifically when challenged with bacterial antigens from the causative agent, whereas peripheral blood mononuclear cells show this response less often. Moreover, serum IgA antibodies to the triggering microbe often are found for many months or even years in patients with reactive arthritis, suggesting ongoing mucosal immunity to a chronic infection. Asymptomatic bowel inflammation has been verified by ileocolonoscopy in most patients with postenteric reactive arthritis and ankylosing spondylitis, but it is not known whether these bowel lesions represent sites of persisting bacterial infection. Finally, several controlled clinical trials suggest that reactive arthritis and other spondyloarthropathies are responsive to certain antibiotics, especially tetracycline or sulfasalazine.

The exact role of HLA-B27 in the pathogenesis of the spondyloarthropathies is not known (Table 176.1). A direct effect of the HLA-B27 molecule seems certain, because diarrhea with inflammatory bowel lesions, peripheral and axial arthritis, and psoriasiform skin and nail lesions resembling human disease develop spontaneously in transgenic rats that express high copy numbers of the human B27 and β_2-microglobulin genes. Underscoring the requirement for bacteria, the bowel and joint lesions do not develop when these animals are reared in a germ-free environment. Additional studies in HLA-B27 transgenic animals have shown that T lymphocytes are required for spondyloarthropathy, that the disease can be transferred to nontransgenic animals by bone marrow–derived cells from affected transgenes, and that experimental *Yersinia* infection is more severe and persistent in these HLA-B27–positive animals.

Three major hypotheses concerning the possible role of HLA-B27 in human spondyloarthropathies are being explored. The first is that the HLA-B27 class I molecule fails to mount an effective immune response, presumably cytotoxic T cells, to certain bacteria, permitting microbial persistence and dissemination. The second hypothesis states that HLA-B27 presents an arthritigenic bacterial or self-peptide (presumably cross-reactive) to cytotoxic T cells that then incites an autoimmune response in the joints and other tissues. In each of these models, the normal function of HLA-B27 (peptide presentation) might or might not have a role. Molecular mimicry between HLA-B27 and bacteria, in theory, could result in either possibility, and HLA-B27 has been shown to share sequence homology with *Klebsiella pneumoniae*, an *S. flexneri* plasmid, and other enteric bacteria. The third hypothesis, which is supported by experimental evidence, is that the HLA-B27 molecule might promote bacterial invasiveness and/or persistence in cells.

Studies of the immunology of synovial fluid in reactive arthritis show predominantly helper T cells, especially those with the T_h2 cytokine profile, reacting to bacterial products and restricted by HLA class II molecules. HLA-B27 (class I)–restricted, cytotoxic T-cell responses to triggering bacteria also have been found, but it is unclear whether they are relevant to the underlying cause of the disease. A causative agent for ankylosing spondylitis has not been identified, though *K. pneumoniae* has been proposed as a possibility. Some cases definitely evolve from reactive arthritis. Whether bacterial antigens or viable organisms are present in sacroiliac and other spinal joints is unknown; this question awaits further study. Similarly, modern bacteriologic investigations of psoriasis and enteropathic arthritis have not been reported. New genomic mapping studies of twins and multiplex families with ankylosing spondylitis have established a strong polygenic mode of inheritance, and several non-HLA regions that may correspond to those regions linked to inflammatory bowel disease and psoriasis have been linked tentatively to the disease.

The inflammatory lesions of joints and entheses in the spondyloarthropathies are made up primarily of mononuclear cells, including T cells and macrophages, and cytokines, including tumor necrosis factor α and transforming growth factor β, which invade the synovium, cartilage, subchondral bone, joint capsule, or bony periosteum. There is a striking tendency for fibrosis and ossification leading to bony and periarticular fusion around peripheral and axial joint structures, resulting in the characteristic roentgenographic findings.

PREVALENCE AND EPIDEMIOLOGY

The prevalence of spondyloarthropathies, especially ankylosing spondylitis and reactive arthritis, generally parallels the prevalence of HLA-B27 in different populations. Ankylosing spondylitis affects about 0.1% to 0.2% of American and European whites, or about 2% of such HLA-B27–positive individuals. HLA-B27 occurs in about 6% to 14% of whites, depending on the ethnic background. American blacks have an HLA-B27 prevalence of only 2% to 3% and are affected less often by the disease. Ankylosing spondylitis and HLA-B27 are rare in African blacks and Japanese but common among certain Native American tribes. Men appear to be affected more often than women (3:1), and the disease usually begins in young adulthood.

Family studies indicate that about 15% of patients with ankylosing spondylitis will have at least one affected relative with both the disease and HLA-B27. It appears that HLA-B27–negative relatives are at no risk of this disease. However, HLA-B27–positive relatives of a patient with ankylosing spondylitis have a 25% to 45% risk of disease development, in contrast to the only 2% risk of HLA-B27–positive individuals with a negative family history. Concordance rates for ankylosing spondylitis are 63% in monozygotic twins and 13% in dizygotic twins.

The prevalence of Reiter's syndrome in most populations is unknown, primarily because of its sporadic occurrence and usually self-limited course. A high prevalence has been reported in Navajo Native Americans and both Alaskan and Greenland Inuits, who have high prevalence rates of HLA-B27 and who reside in areas endemic for shigellosis or venereal infections. Reiter's syndrome appears to be the most common cause of inflammatory peripheral arthritis in young adult men in the military; however, its frequency has fallen significantly since the introduction of safer sexual practices dictated by the AIDS epidemic. Women acquire the disease less frequently than men, usually after an enteric infection. The risk that reactive arthritis will develop after exposure to each of the causative bacterial infections has been estimated at 1% to 2% overall for whites and 20% for HLA-B27–positive individuals. Reiter's syndrome has been reported often in men infected with the human immunodeficiency virus, especially those with AIDS, in whom it appears to pursue a more severe course.

Cutaneous psoriasis affects nearly 2% of whites, but psoriatic arthritis develops in only 5% to 7% of patients with psoriasis. Men and women, usually young adults, are affected equally. Streptococcal infections, trauma, and stress have been implicated as triggers for psoriasis. Several HLA class I antigens are associated with susceptibility to psoriasis but the strongest is HLA-Cw6, which also shows genetic linkage in families. Other non-HLA genes also appear to be necessary. Peripheral arthritis occurs in 20% and spondylitis in 10% of patients with ulcerative colitis or Crohn's disease. Men and women are affected equally.

CLINICAL FEATURES

The clinical features of the spondyloarthropathies are summarized in Table 176.2.

TABLE 176.2.	CONTRASTING CLINICAL AND IMMUNOGENETIC FEATURES AMONG THE SPONDYLOARTHROPATHIES			
Feature	**Ankylosing Spondylitis**	**Reiter's Syndrome (Reactive Arthritis)**	**Psoriatic Arthritis**	**Enteropathic Arthritis**
Male-to-female ratio	3:1	9:1	1:1	1:1
Mode of onset	Insidious, usually lower back pain	Acute urethritis, conjunctivitis, and peripheral arthritis	Insidious, usually peripheral arthritis	Acute peripheral arthritis and bowel symptoms or insidious lower back pain
Patterns of peripheral arthritis	Infrequent, except hips and shoulders	100%, asymmetrical, oligoarticular, lower extremities, "sausage" digits, heel pain	95%; asymmetrical or symmetrical; oligoarticular or polyarticular; upper and lower extremities, especially distal interphalangeal joints; "sausage" digits	20%; migratory, asymmetric; knees, ankles, wrists
Spinal involvement	100%	20%	20%	10%
Sacroiliitis	Bilateral	Unilateral or bilateral	Unilateral or bilateral	Bilateral
Syndesmophytes	Symmetrical	Asymmetrical	Asymmetrical	Symmetrical
Extra-articular features				
Fever	Rare	Frequent	Rare	Frequent
Uveitis	25%	20%	Rare	Occasional
Carditis	5%	5%	Rare	Rare
Mucocutaneous	Rare	Keratoderma, balanitis, painless oral ulcers	Psoriasis Nail pitting and dystrophy	Erythema nodosum, pyoderma, painful oral ulcers
Amyloid	4%	Rare	Rare	Rare
Prevalence of HLA-B27[a]	90%	75%	Not increased in peripheral arthritis 50% with spondylitis	Not increased in peripheral arthritis; 50% with spondylitis
Other HLA associations	B60, DR1, DR8	None definite	Cw6, B38, B39	None

[a] Based on white population prevalence rates of 6%–14%.

ANKYLOSING SPONDYLITIS

Ankylosing spondylitis typically shows initial features of chronic lower back pain or stiffness in an adolescent or young adult. The discomfort usually localizes to the sacroiliac regions of the buttocks; however, a more generalized lumbar or thoracic stiffness may dominate. Typically, symptoms are worse during periods of rest and improve with increasing physical activity. Sciatica-like pains may occur but are not associated with neurologic deficits. As the disease progresses, normal lumbar lordosis is lost, and spinal mobility in all planes is restricted. The thoracic spine may assume an accentuated kyphosis, and fusion of costovertebral joints results in diminished chest expansion. Cervical motion may become severely restricted, with eventual head fixation in a flexed position. Although the disease usually progresses slowly over many years, spinal deformity, at times of a grotesque degree, occasionally develops rapidly. Peripheral joints are involved infrequently, except for the shoulders or hips.

Atypical forms of the disease, with peripheral arthritis, occur commonly in children, usually boys who have oligoarthritis of the lower-extremity joints and enthesopathy. Later, spinal symptoms emerge and pursue the usual course. Similarly, women often have a predominantly peripheral or cervical pattern of involvement, with few or no lower spinal symptoms. Extra-articular complications include episodes of acute anterior uveitis in 25% of patients, which occur independently of arthritis activity. Aortic regurgitation or varying degrees of atrioventricular conduction disturbance eventually develop in 5% of patients from inflammatory involvement of aortic valve cusps, proximal aortic root, and adjacent atrioventricular nodal tissue. Apical pulmonary fibrosis, often mimicking tuberculosis, is rare, as are amyloidosis and cauda equina syndrome. IgA nephropathy may develop.

The diagnosis is based on clinical features, supporting physical findings, and, most specifically, pelvic radiographs showing sclerosis, erosions, or fusion of sacroiliac joints (sacroiliitis) (Fig. 176.1). Computed tomography and magnetic resonance imaging of sacroiliac joints are more sensitive than conventional radiographs in the early stages of disease, but rarely are they necessary. In advanced cases, spinal radiographs show inflammatory erosions of vertebrae, resulting in a squared appearance; ossified ligamentous structures originating at vertebra; and bridging intervertebral discs (syndesmophytes), bony fusion of apophyseal joints, and spinal osteopenia (Fig. 176.1). Distinguishing ankylosing spondylitis from diffuse idiopathic skeletal hyperostosis

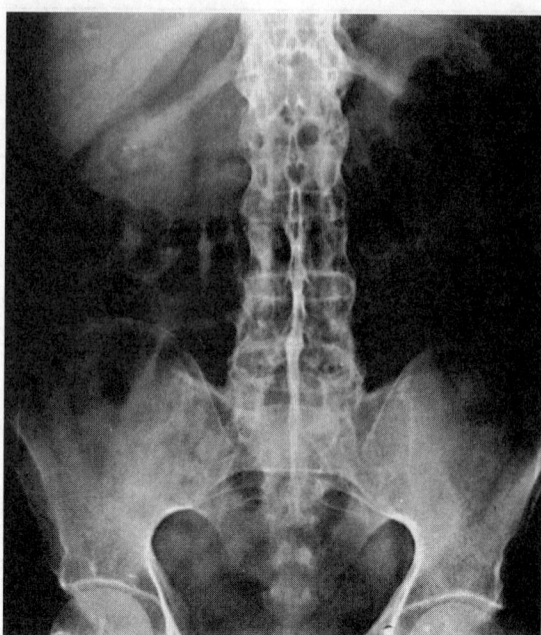

FIGURE 176.1. Roentgenogram of the pelvis in advanced ankylosing spondylitis. Both sacroiliac joints have undergone bony fusion, and previous sacroiliac sclerosis and erosions are now gone. Bilateral syndesmophytes bridge intervertebral disks at multiple lumbar levels, and there is marked osteopenia.

can be difficult, though sacroiliitis is not present in the latter condition. Determination of HLA-B27 sometimes is diagnostically useful in disease that is not evident on radiography and in the atypical forms commonly seen in children and women.

REITER'S SYNDROME (REACTIVE ARTHRITIS)

Reiter's syndrome typically begins 2 to 4 weeks after a diarrheal illness or venereal exposure. Mild dysuria and a mucopurulent urethral discharge, along with conjunctivitis, usually herald by several days the development of acute arthritis, enthesitis, fever, and other mucocutaneous features. The knees, ankles, and small joints of the feet are affected most often in an asymmetrical and oligoarticular pattern. Diffuse swelling of the digits, especially the toes, results in a "sausage" appearance. Enthesopathy produces pain over nonarticular bony areas; heel pain (Achilles or plantar tendonitis) is a common and disabling symptom. Back pain is common, but sacroiliitis eventually develops in only 20% of patients. In addition, more than half of all patients have one or more mucocutaneous lesions, such as keratoderma blennorrhagicum, a papulosquamous eruption indistinguishable from pustular psoriasis usually over the soles or palms; painless oral ulcers on the tongue or palate; circinate balanitis on the penile glans or shaft; or dystrophic nails.

Incomplete forms of Reiter's syndrome are common—urethritis and conjunctivitis often are absent. Nevertheless, the distinctive pattern of arthritis, enthesopathy, and mucocutaneous involvement should strongly suggest the diagnosis. Exclusion of septic arthritis is mandatory, and typing for HLA-B27 may prove useful. Even more limited clinical syndromes of HLA-B27 diathesis have been reported, including uveitis, pustular psoriasis

(keratoderma), circinate balanitis, "sausage" digits, chronic heel pain, monoarthritis, and heart block, all of which have been associated with HLA-B27. Reiter's syndrome, or reactive arthritis, is a self-limited disease that lasts 3 to 12 months in most patients. Relapses occur in up to one-third of patients. Persistent and progressive joint or skin disease ensues in about 15% to 20% of patients. Distinctive radiographic features are found most often in the latter group of patients, including joint destruction, bony fusion across joints, and periosteal reactions at sites of enthesopathy, especially the calcaneus.

PSORIATIC ARTHRITIS

Psoriatic arthritis typically emerges long after or concurrently with cutaneous psoriasis, though arthritis may appear first, especially in children. Several forms have been described, including a type with distal interphalangeal involvement; arthritis with an asymmetrical, oligoarticular pattern; symmetrical polyarthritis; arthritis mutilans (similar to serious cases of rheumatoid arthritis); and sacroiliitis and spondylitis. Overlap among these patterns is the norm, and "sausaging" of digits and pitting of nails occur frequently. The disease usually is indolent and progresses slowly. Radiographic changes include "pencil-in-cup" deformities and bony fusion similar to that of chronic Reiter's syndrome.

Acne arthritis, or the SAPHO syndrome (synovitis, acne, pustulosis, hyperostosis, osteitis), is a rare disorder with features of reactive and psoriatic arthritis. It typically takes the form of oligoarthritis with or without bony lesions or palmoplantar pustulosis (resembling psoriasis) in patients with severe types of acne (acne fulminans, acne conglobata, hidradenitis suppurativa, and dissecting cellulitis of the scalp). Sacroiliitis and syndesmophytes have been described, but there appears to be no association with HLA-B27. Microbiologic studies have failed to identify a causative bacterium, and antibiotic therapy usually is ineffective. Low-dose corticosteroids, along with vigorous local treatment of the acne, are the best approach in most cases.

ENTEROPATHIC ARTHRITIS

Peripheral arthritis and the extra-articular features (Table 176.1) of inflammatory bowel disease reflect active gut involvement. Asymmetric arthritis of the knees, ankles, feet, and wrists is the typical pattern and results in no radiographic changes or permanent deformities. Sacroiliitis and spondylitis occur independently of active bowel inflammation. Although it resolves peripheral arthritis, colectomy for ulcerative colitis does not alter the progression of axial disease. The radiographic changes in this type of spondylitis are indistinguishable from those of idiopathic ankylosing spondylitis, in contradistinction to Reiter's syndrome and psoriatic arthritis, in which sacroiliitis and syndesmophytes are more asymmetrical.

Whipple's disease is a rare systemic condition that most often affects middle-aged white men and is characterized by diarrhea with malabsorption, weight loss, fever, lymphadenopathy (especially mesenteric), skin hyperpigmentation, and, occasionally, cardiac or nervous system involvement. Peripheral arthritis, usually symmetrically affecting the knees, ankles, or wrists, occurs in about 60% of cases and may precede the other symptoms by many years. Sacroiliitis and spondylitis have been documented, and about one-third of patients have been reported to possess HLA-B27 regardless of spinal involvement. The disease appears to be caused by widespread dissemination of a bacillus that is positive on periodic acid–Schiff staining and is found in biopsy samples of most affected tissues, including synovium but especially the small bowel. The bacterium has not been cultured, but it has been identified in tissue samples and peripheral blood by polymerase chain reaction as a gram-positive actinomycete and has been named *Tropheryma whippelii*. Long-term treatment with tetracycline or sulfonamide antibiotics seems to be curative.

LABORATORY FINDINGS

Laboratory abnormalities are few in the spondyloarthropathies. Mild normocytic, normochromic anemia and elevation of the erythrocyte sedimentation rate and total serum IgA level are common. Modest leukocytosis and thrombocytosis are seen most often in acute Reiter's syndrome and enteropathic arthritis. Tests for serum rheumatoid factors and antinuclear antibodies render uniformly negative results. The incidence rates of class I HLA are shown in Table 176.2; HLA-B27 may serve as a useful test in early-stage or atypical ankylosing spondylitis or Reiter's syndrome, but not when there is either a high or very low probability that one of these conditions is present. Synovial fluid findings include leukocyte counts ranging from 5,000 to 50,000 per microliter, with the highest counts found in Reiter's syndrome; elevated protein levels; normal glucose levels; and an absence of organisms on Gram stain and culture.

OPTIMAL MANAGEMENT

Therapy for the spondyloarthropathies involves pharmacologic suppression of joint inflammation in conjunction with physical therapy to preserve axial and peripheral joint function and prevent deformity. Unlike rheumatoid arthritis, these arthritides usually do not respond to salicylates, proprionic acids, corticosteroids, or long-acting drugs, such as gold salts, D-penicillamine, or hydroxychloroquine. Instead, the nonsteroidal anti-inflammatory agents indomethacin, tolmetin, piroxicam, and others are more effective in suppressing symptoms of pain and stiffness, and signs of inflammation. A rational basis for the concomitant use of certain antibiotics has been established (see Etiology and Pathogenesis). Sulfasalazine (2 to 3 g per day) has been shown to be effective in relieving joint symptoms and signs and improving acute phase reactants in all the spondyloarthropathies. Tetracycline therapy may shorten the duration of *Chlamydia*-induced reactive arthritis and may prevent recurrences when used early to treat venereal infections. In all patients with reactive arthritis, an attempt should be made to identify the causative microorganism so that the most appropriate antibiotic trial can be initiated (Fig. 176.2). Quinolone antibiotics do not appear to be effective in acute or chronic reactive arthritis caused by enteric pathogens.

Immunosuppressants, such as methotrexate or azathioprine, are needed occasionally, but they should be used sparingly in patients with reactive arthritis in view of the possibility of promoting further bacterial persistence, and they should not be used at all in those with human immunodeficiency virus infection. Methotrexate is a more useful agent for psoriatic arthritis. The presence of peripheral arthritis in inflammatory bowel disease indicates active bowel inflammation, and treatment of the bowel with corticosteroids or other drugs (or colectomy in the case of ulcerative colitis) usually results in resolution of the peripheral, but not axial, joint disease. Physical therapy exercises to preserve range of motion in affected spinal and peripheral joints and habits that promote good posture are important in preventing contractures and spinal deformities. Swimming is an excellent recreational exercise. With these measures, less than 20% of patients have permanent disability. Death occurs in less than 5% of patients and results primarily from spinal (especially cervical) fractures, cardiac complications, and amyloidosis.

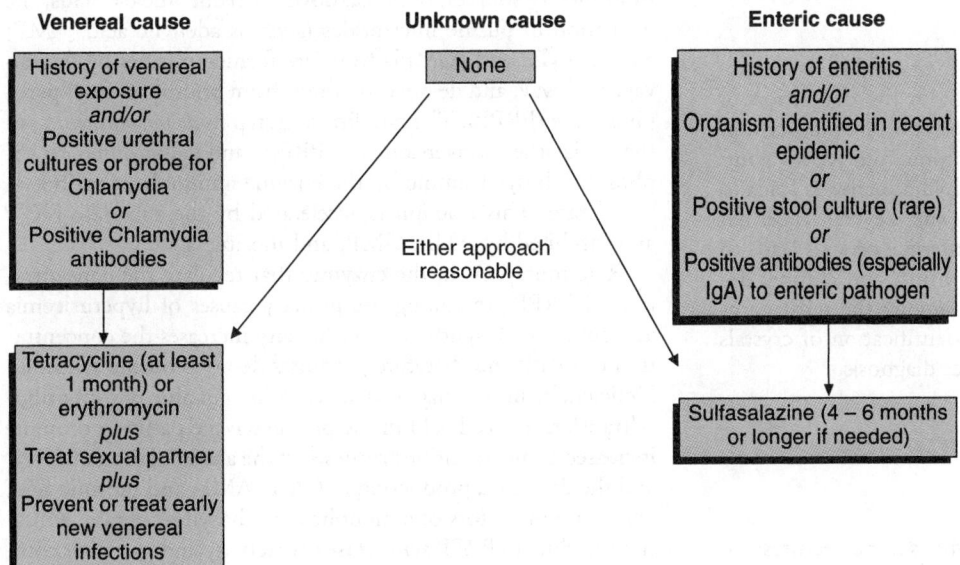

FIGURE 176.2. Rational approach to antibiotic treatment of reactive arthritis.

BIBLIOGRAPHY

Arnett FC. Seronegative spondyloarthropathies. *Bull Rheum Dis* 1987;37: 1–12.

Brown MA, Kennedy LG, MacGregor AJ, et al. Susceptibility to ankylosing spondylitis in twins: the role of genes, HLA, and the environment. *Arthritis Rheum* 1997;40:1823–1828.

Carette S, Graham D, Little H, et al. The natural disease course of ankylosing spondylitis. *Arthritis Rheum* 1983;26:186–190.

Dougados M, van der Linden S, Leirisalo-Repo M, et al. Sulfasalazine in the treatment of spondyloarthropathy: a randomized, multicenter, double-blind, placebo-controlled study. *Arthritis Rheum* 1995;38:618–627.

Granfors K, Jalkanen S, von Essen R, et al. *Yersinia* antigens in synovial-fluid cells from patients with reactive arthritis. *N Engl J Med* 1989;320: 216–221.

Hammer RE, Maika SD, Richardson JA, et al. Spontaneous inflammatory disease in transgenic rats expressing HLA-B27 and human β2m: an animal model of HLA-B27–associated human disorders. *Cell* 1990;63: 1099–1112.

Hermann E. T cells in reactive arthritis. *APMIS* 1993;101:177–186.

Khan MA. Spondyloarthropathies. *Rheum Dis Clin North Am* 1992;18: 1–14.

Lauhio A, Leirisalo-Repo M, Lähdevirta J, et al. Double-blind, placebo-controlled study of three-month treatment with lymecycline in reactive arthritis, with special reference to *Chlamydia* arthritis. *Arthritis Rheum* 1991;34:6–14.

Nanagara R, Beutler FLA, Hudson A, et al. Alteration of *Chlamydia trachomatis* biologic behavior in synovial membranes: suppression of surface antigen production in reactive arthritis and Reiter's syndrome. *Arthritis Rheum* 1995;38:1410–1417.

Kelley's Textbook of Internal Medicine, fourth edition. Edited by H. David Humes. Lippincott Williams & Wilkins, Philadelphia © 2000.

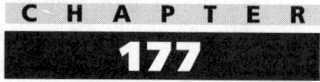

CHAPTER 177

CRYSTAL-INDUCED SYNOVITIS

MICHAEL M. WARD

Crystal-induced synovitis refers to a group of conditions characterized by acute or chronic arthritis due to the deposition of crystals in and around joints. The deposition of monosodium urate crystals leads to acute gout and chronic tophaceous gout; deposition of calcium pyrophosphate dihydrate crystals leads to chondrocalcinosis, acute pseudogout, and several types of chronic arthritis; and deposition of apatite-like crystals leads to calcific tendinitis, periarthritis, acute arthritis, and chronic destructive arthritis. These conditions are among the most common causes of inflammatory arthritis. Identification of crystals in synovial fluid is the key to the correct diagnosis.

◼ GOUT

DEFINITION

Gout is a chronic metabolic disease with several features: an elevated serum urate concentration (hyperuricemia), intermit-tent episodes of acute arthritis induced by monosodium urate monohydrate crystals, extracellular deposition of masses of urate crystals in and around joints or in soft tissues (tophi), uric acid nephrolithiasis, and renal disease due to the deposition of urate or uric acid crystals in the renal interstitium, tubules, or collecting system. Hyperuricemia is a necessary precursor of each of the clinical features. Individual patients may experience one or more of the clinical features.

INCIDENCE AND EPIDEMIOLOGY

Hyperuricemia, defined as a serum urate concentration of more than 7 mg per deciliter in men and more than 6 mg per deciliter in women, is found in 2% to 10% of adults. Serum urate concentrations increase with age, body size, blood pressure, decreased renal function, and alcohol intake and are higher in men and in persons of Pacific Islander ethnicity. Fewer than 20% of all persons with hyperuricemia experience clinical consequences.

Acute gouty arthritis primarily affects middle-aged and elderly men and, less often, elderly women. The incidence of acute gouty arthritis in the general population ranges from 0.20 to 0.35 per 1,000 person-years. Among adult men, the incidence is about 10 times higher (two to three per 1,000 person-years). The incidence of gouty arthritis rises with age and with serum urate concentration, from one per 1,000 person-years at serum urate concentrations of less than 7 mg per deciliter to 49 per 1,000 person-years at serum urate concentrations of 9 mg per deciliter or more. It is the most common type of inflammatory arthritis in adult men, with a prevalence of 1.4% to 5%. Tophaceous gout develops in up to 25% of patients with recurrent attacks of acute gouty arthritis who are not treated with hypouricemic medications.

ETIOLOGY

Hyperuricemia can result from either overproduction or underexcretion of uric acid (Table 177.1). Uric acid is the end product of purine metabolism (Fig. 177.1). The purine pool is derived from dietary sources, the breakdown of tissue nucleic acids, the formation of purine nucleotides (such as adenylic acid [AMP] and guanylic acid [GMP]) from pre-formed purines by the salvage pathway, and de novo synthesis from phosphoribosyl pyrophosphate (PRPP). The rate-limiting step in *de novo* purine synthesis is the conversion of PRPP and glutamine to 5-phosphoribosyl-1-amine by the enzyme amidophosphoribosyltransferase. This reaction is accelerated by the substrate PRPP and inhibited by AMP, GMP, and inosinic acid.

Rare mutations in the enzymes that regulate the concentration of PRPP are among the primary causes of hyperuricemia and gout. PRPP synthetase overactivity increases the concentration of PRPP and therefore promotes de novo purine synthesis. Deficiencies in the enzyme hypoxanthine-guanine phosphoribosyltransferase (HGPRT) in the purine salvage pathway promote increased de novo purine synthesis by the accumulation of PRPP and the decreased production of GMP, AMP, and inosinic acid, which are inhibitors of amidophosphoribosyltransferase. Mutations leading to PRPP synthetase overactivity and partial or complete HGPRT deficiency are X linked, and patients with these

TABLE 177.1. CAUSES OF HYPERURICEMIA

Increased urate production
  Primary
    Idiopathic
    Complete hypoxanthine-guanine phosphoribosyltransferase deficiency (Lesch–Nyhan syndrome)
    Partial hypoxanthine-guanine phosphoribosyltransferase deficiency (Kelley–Seegmiller syndrome)
    Phosphoribosylpyrophosphate synthetase overactivity
  Secondary
    Increased catabolism of ATP
      Glycogen storage disease (types I, III, IV, and VII)
      Tissue hypoxia
      Ethanol intake
      Exercise and metabolic myopathy
    Increased turnover of nucleic acid
      Myeloproliferative and lymphoproliferative diseases
      Intravascular hemolysis
      Psoriasis
      Paget's disease
    Excessive dietary purine intake
Decreased urate excretion
  Primary
    Idiopathic decrease in tubular secretion
  Secondary
    Renal insufficiency
    Increased tubular reabsorption
      Dehydration
      Diabetes insipidus
      Diuretic use
    Decreased tubular secretion
      Increased levels of β-hydroxybutyrate and acetoacetate (starvation, diabetic ketoacidosis)
      Lactic acidosis (alcohol intake, toxemia of pregnancy)
    Mechanisms incompletely understood
      Lead nephropathy
      Hypertension
      Polycystic kidney disease
      Hyperparathyroidism
      Medications (diuretics, low-dose salicylates, cyclosporine, ethambutol, pyrazinamide, nicotinic acid)

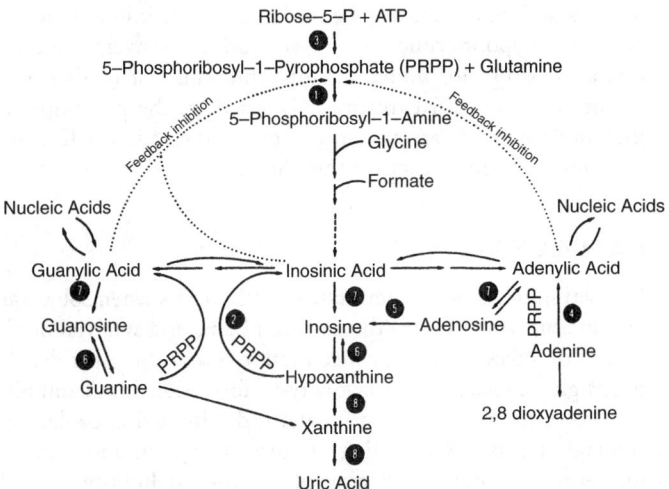

FIGURE 177.1. Human purine metabolism. Inosinic acid is synthesized by the pathway of purine biosynthesis de novo. This purine nucleotide can be converted to adenylic acid or guanylic acid. Purine nucleotides may be degraded to uric acid following initial dephosphorylation to adenosine, inosine, or guanosine. Inosine or guanosine is then converted to hypoxanthine or guanine, respectively. These compounds are further degraded to xanthine and uric acid. Purine bases may be salvaged to purine nucleotides by the reutilization pathways. Hypoxanthine and guanine are converted to inosinic acid and guanylic acid, respectively, while adenine can be converted to adenylic acid. Reaction 1, amidophosphoribosyltransferase; reaction 2, hypoxanthine-guanine phosphoribosyltransfere; reaction 3, phosphoribosylprophosphate synthetase; reaction 4, adenine phosphoribosyltransferase; reaction 5, adenosine deaminase; reaction 6, purine nucleoside phosphorylase; reaction 7, 5'-nucleotidase; reaction 8, xanthine oxidase. PRPP, phosphoribosylpyrophosphate; ATP, adenosine triphosphate. (From Palella TD, Kelley WN. Purine and deoxypurine metabolism. In: Kelley WN, Harris ED Jr, Ruddy S, et al., eds. *Textbook of Rheumatology.* Philadelphia: WB Saunders, 1985:337, with permission.)

mutations have severe and premature gout. Patients with complete HGPRT deficiency (Lesch–Nyhan syndrome) also have neurologic signs of growth and mental retardation, spasticity, choreoathetosis, and self-mutilation. Among the secondary causes of increased urate production are conditions that increase the catabolism of ATP or cell turnover and high dietary purine intake (Table 177.1).

Urate excretion occurs mainly via the kidney (up to 75%); the remainder is excreted in the intestines and metabolized by gut bacteria. In the kidney, urate undergoes glomerular filtration (100%), proximal tubular reabsorption (98%), tubular secretion (50%), and postsecretory tubular reabsorption (40%), so that about 10% of filtered urate is excreted in the urine. Conditions that affect any of these processes can lead to hyperuricemia (Table 177.1). For example, renal insufficiency may diminish urate filtration, dehydration increases proximal tubular reabsorption of urate (and may decrease glomerular filtration), and elevated levels of organic acids compete with urate for tubular secretion. In the vast majority of patients, however, diminished urate

excretion results from primary undefined defects in tubular secretion. In these patients, urate excretion is 40% lower than that of normal individuals at any given plasma urate concentration.

Alcohol may cause hyperuricemia by both increased urate production through accelerated catabolism of ATP in the liver and decreased urate excretion by competition from lactate. Beer is also rich in purines. Diuretics raise serum urate concentrations by increasing its proximal tubular reabsorption and possibly by lessening glomerular filtration. Up to 80% of transplant patients treated with cyclosporine have hyperuricemia, owing in part to impaired fractional urate clearance and irreversible tubular damage; coexisting renal insufficiency and hypertension may also be contributory.

In 90% of patients, hyperuricemia is due to diminished urate excretion, and in 10% it is due to urate overproduction. Those patients with hyperuricemia due to urate overproduction can be identified by quantitation of the urinary excretion of uric acid. Excretion of more than 600 mg of uric acid per 24 hours while consuming a purine-free diet or excretion of more than 800 to 1,000 mg per 24 hours on an unrestricted diet is an indication of urate overproduction. Collections should not be obtained during acute attacks. The sensitivity of this test is lower in the context of renal insufficiency or incomplete collections, and its specificity is lessened by the use of medications that increase urate excretion. Results may be used to guide the initial choice of long-term hypouricemic therapy (allopurinol for overproducers; uricosuric drugs for underexcretors), but this test is often not performed, and initial treatment is based on the presumption that most patients are underexcretors. Other clinical features may also have an impact on this choice.

PATHOGENESIS

Formation of monosodium urate crystals occurs when solutions become supersaturated with urate. In plasma and synovial fluid, saturation takes place at a concentration near 7.0 mg per deciliter. Higher concentrations favor crystal formation. Urate solubility also varies with temperature and is diminished at cooler peripheral joints. Solubilizing factors likely inhibit crystal formation in plasma and may play a role in limiting crystal formation in supersaturated synovial fluids. In most cases, 20 to 30 years of sustained hyperuricemia is required before sufficient urate becomes deposited in joint tissues, leading to acute gout.

Acute gouty arthritis develops when monosodium urate monohydrate crystals are shed from the synovium or cartilage into the joint space, where they produce local inflammation, or when crystals form in supersaturated synovial fluid. Shedding may be promoted by local trauma or abrupt declines in serum urate levels. Crystal precipitation may occur with abrupt increases in urate levels (either systemically or within joints as a result of preferential resorption of free water) or with changes in temperature, pH, or the concentration of local inhibitory factors.

The inflammatory response to crystals depends on their size and surface character, including the types of proteins bound to them. Urate crystals have a strong affinity for immunoglobulin. Immunoglobulin-coated crystals are highly phlogistic. They attract and activate neutrophils, which perpetuate inflammation by activating the complement, kinin, prostaglandin, and leukotriene pathways and generating reactive oxygen species. Phagocytosis of crystals by neutrophils can cause rupture of these cells and their lysosomes, releasing intracellular enzymes. Urate crystals also stimulate synovial lining cells to produce interleukin-1, interleukin-6, interleukin-8, tumor necrosis factor α, prostaglandin E_2, leukotriene B_4, and reactive oxygen species, further increasing local inflammation. The natural processes that terminate acute attacks or prevent inflammation on occasions when urate crystals are shed into joints are not well understood.

Tophi are compact extracellular collections of monosodium urate crystals surrounded by a chronic inflammatory cell infiltrate and foreign-body granuloma. They incite a low-grade local inflammatory reaction mediated by interleukins, tumor necrosis factor α, and prostaglandins derived from macrophages or adjacent synovial fibroblasts, which causes bone and cartilage damage.

CLINICAL FINDINGS
Acute Gout

Acute gouty arthritis typically affects one joint, though 10% of attacks may be polyarticular. Podagra, or inflammation at the first metatarsophalangeal joint, is the initial sign of gout in 50% of patients and occurs at some time in 90% of patients. Other commonly affected joints are the midfoot, ankle, knee, wrist, finger joints, and elbow. Olecranon or prepatellar bursitis may also occur. The affected joint is intensely painful, swollen, erythematous, and warm. Fever and chills may ensue, raising concern about the possibility of septic arthritis. Attacks often happen at night. Patients may report that the weight of the bedsheet causes severe pain, or they may become aware of symptoms only on rising from bed in the morning. Attacks can be precipitated by local trauma, dehydration, surgery, severe illness, alcohol intake, dietary indiscretion, or certain medications (most often diuretics). Symptoms usually peak within 24 hours. With treatment, attacks can last 2 to 7 days, but untreated attacks may last several weeks.

Intercritical Gout

Patients are asymptomatic, and joints appear normal between attacks. This period is called interval, or intercritical, gout. Recurrence of acute gouty arthritis is common: two-thirds of patients experience a second attack within 1 year, 75% within 2 years, and 90% within 5 years. A second attack usually marks someone as being at risk of frequent recurrences, which may be reduced or eliminated with hypouricemic treatment. Without treatment, the interval between attacks often declines over time.

Tophaceous Gout

Tophaceous gout develops more often in persons with persistent severe hyperuricemia. Tophaceous gout can affect either joints or primarily soft tissues (Fig. 177.2). Chronic gouty arthritis develops in patients with tophaceous deposits of urate in synovium, cartilage, and bone. These deposits cause low-grade inflammatory synovitis in many joints, often in the hands and feet, that is slowly progressive and leads to severe deformity and disability. Rarely, patients have chronic gouty arthritis in the absence of a recalled history of acute attacks. Tophi in soft tissue and skin typically develop over the first metatarsophalangeal joint, the ulnar forearm, olecranon, finger pads, or external ear. Tophi

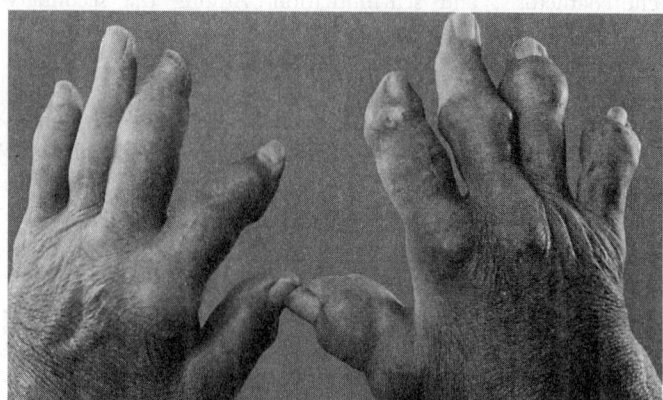

FIGURE 177.2. Chronic tophaceous gout. Deformities of the hands are related to tophaceous deposits.

over finger joints are common in elderly women treated with diuretics. Tophi are painless firm masses that distend the skin and show mottled hypopigmentation. Overlying skin may occasionally ulcerate and drain urate chalk. Tophi may resorb with treatment, but residual joint damage is not repaired.

Nephrolithiasis

Uric acid nephrolithiasis develops in 10% to 25% of patients with gout. The annual incidence is 0.27% in those with asymptomatic hyperuricemia and 1.0% in those with a history of acute gouty arthritis. The risk increases with the level of hyperuricemia and urinary uric acid excretion. Acute uric acid nephropathy is acute renal failure due to the precipitation of uric acid crystals in the distal tubules and collecting system. It occurs most commonly in patients with very high serum urate levels, those with leukemia or lymphoma with high cell turnover, after chemotherapy (acute tumor lysis syndrome), and with the initiation of uricosuric medications. Urate nephropathy, the deposition of urate crystals in the kidney interstitium, is rarely thought to cause clinically significant renal disease.

LABORATORY FINDINGS

The diagnosis of acute gouty arthritis depends on the identification of monosodium urate monohydrate crystals in leukocytes in synovial fluid from an inflamed joint. Urate crystals are needle-shaped. Under polarizing microscopy, they are highly birefringent (bright) and evidence negative elongation (they appear yellow when aligned parallel to the orientation of the red compensator). Crystals are most numerous early in an attack. Extracellular crystals can be seen in synovial fluid obtained during intercritical periods. Sheets of urate crystals also may be seen on aspirates of tophi.

Synovial fluid leukocyte counts during episodes of acute gouty arthritis range from 5,000 to 100,000 per cubic millimeter; these cells are mostly neutrophils. Peripheral leukocytosis and elevation of acute phase reactants are common, making the distinction from septic arthritis more difficult. Septic arthritis and acute gout can coexist. During episodes of acute gouty arthritis, serum urate levels can be spuriously normal or low and are unreliable for diagnosis. Mildly inflammatory synovial fluid may be present in patients with chronic gouty arthritis, but evidence of systemic inflammation is absent. Radiographs in acute gouty arthritis usually show only soft-tissue swelling or joint effusions. Radiographs in tophaceous gout often show large cystic erosions of bone near affected joints, with sclerotic margins and overhanging edges.

OPTIMAL MANAGEMENT

Hyperuricemia without associated clinical features of gouty arthritis or uric acid nephrolithiasis does not require treatment. Prophylaxis with allopurinol is indicated before chemotherapy for patients at risk of acute uric acid nephropathy due to tumor lysis syndrome. Acute gouty arthritis is treated by resting the affected joint (using splints or crutches) and taking anti-inflam-

matory medications, including nonsteroidal anti-inflammatory drugs (NSAIDs), glucocorticoids, *or* colchicine. NSAIDs are the optimal choice for most patients. Although indomethacin is often used, any NSAID at a sufficiently high dose will likely be effective. Salicylates should be avoided because they decrease urate excretion. Treatment should be stopped when the acute episode resolves. Glucocorticoids (GCs) may be used when NSAIDs are contraindicated. Intra-articular injections of GCs are preferred when one or two joints are affected. Parenteral GCs may be used for severe polyarticular attacks. Oral colchicine can be given hourly until symptoms abate, side effects occur, or a maximum of 6 mg is consumed. Because this treatment often causes diarrhea, abdominal pain, and vomiting, NSAIDs are preferred. Intravenous colchicine is not recommended, owing to the risk of serious morbidity and mortality. It should be noted that a clinical response to colchicine is not specific to acute gouty arthritis.

Long-term treatment to lower serum urate concentrations is indicated for patients who have had two or more attacks of acute gouty arthritis, both to lessen the frequency of recurrences and to prevent chronic tophaceous gout. Uricosuric medications, such as probenecid or sulfinpyrazone, which lower serum urate levels by blocking renal tubular reabsorption and therefore increasing excretion, should be used in patients when hyperuricemia is known or suspected to be due to defects in renal urate excretion. This group includes 90% of patients with idiopathic hyperuricemia.

Allopurinol is a competitive inhibitor of xanthine oxidase, the enzyme that catalyzes the two terminal steps in uric acid production (Fig. 177.1). Inhibition of this enzyme by allopurinol and its metabolite oxypurinol decreases the conversion of hypoxanthine to xanthine and of xanthine to uric acid. Hypoxanthine and xanthine are excreted readily in the urine, and uric acid production is diminished. Treatment with allopurinol is indicated for patients who are known overproducers of urate, for those who fail treatment with uricosurics, for those with renal insufficiency (creatinine clearance of less than 60 ml per minute), and for those with uric acid nephrolithiasis. Initiation of treatment with either uricosurics or allopurinol may precipitate acute gouty arthritis, the risk of which may be lessened by delaying the start of treatment 4 to 6 weeks after an attack and by using NSAIDs or daily oral colchicine concomitantly. The goal of treatment is to maintain serum urate concentrations at less than 6.8 mg per deciliter. Lifelong treatment is usually necessary. Symptoms of chronic gouty arthritis can be treated with analgesics or NSAIDs. Tophi often resolve faster with the use of allopurinol than with uricosurics and when serum urate concentrations are less than 5 mg per deciliter.

■ CALCIUM PYROPHOSPHATE DIHYDRATE DEPOSITION DISEASE

DEFINITION

Calcium pyrophosphate dihydrate (CPPD) deposition disease is a chronic metabolic disease that results from the local overproduction of pyrophosphate (PP_i) in cartilage, which causes the deposition of crystals of CPPD ($Ca_2P_2O_7 \cdot 2H_2O$) and a group of associated joint conditions. CPPD deposition disease has several manifestations, including asymptomatic chondrocalcinosis, episodes of acute arthritis (pseudogout), and chronic arthritis.

INCIDENCE AND EPIDEMIOLOGY

CPPD deposition disease is a disease of aging. The prevalence of chondrocalcinosis in radiographic surveys of the general population is less than 1%, but the rate increases to 10% in those aged 60 to 75 and to 30% or more in those age 80 or older. Premature disease may develop in rare familial forms. Men and women are equally affected. Symptomatic acute or chronic arthritis develops in more than 75% of cases. In the general population, acute pseudogout has a prevalence of 0.1%.

The prevalence of CPPD deposition disease is higher in patients with hyperparathyroidism (20% to 30%), hemochromatosis (20% to 50%), hypophosphatasia, hypomagnesemia, and several other conditions (Table 177.2). Screening for these conditions is indicated when CPPD deposition disease occurs before age 60. Severe myxedema also may be associated with CPPD deposition disease, but mild hypothyroidism is not. Chondrocalcinosis is associated with osteoarthritis, but its presence does not predict the later development of osteoarthritis, suggesting that chondrocalcinosis may be a consequence of osteoarthritic changes in cartilage.

ETIOLOGY

CPPD crystals form in cartilage as a result of excess production by chondrocytes of PP_i. PP_i is produced in the metabolism of most major macromolecules; nucleoside triphosphates are the major source. Nucleoside triphosphates (such as ATP) are metabolized to nucleoside monophosphates (such as AMP) and PP_i. In chondrocytes, this reversible reaction is catalyzed by a group of enzymes, the nucleoside triphosphate pyrophosphohydrolases (NTPPPHase), present on the external surface of the cell membrane. The activity of these enzymes, which is enhanced by trans-

forming growth factor β and inhibited by interleukin-1, results in the extracellular accumulation of PP_i. Calcium salts of PP_i develop in areas of focal high concentrations. Systemic levels of PP_i are normal in patients with CPPD crystal deposition disease.

Formation of CPPD crystals is favored by conditions that increase the extracellular concentration of PP_i, including high concentrations or overactivity of NTPPPHases, high local concentrations of ATP (the enzyme substrate) or transforming growth factor β, or decreased activity of enzymes that metabolize PP_i, such as inorganic pyrophosphatases and alkaline phosphatases. The activity of NTPPPHases is high in cartilage affected by CPPD crystal deposition disease. Elevated levels of calcium and iron and low levels of magnesium inhibit inorganic pyrophosphatases and may account for the accumulation of PP_i and the development of CPPD crystal deposition disease in patients with hyperparathyroidism, hemochromatosis, and hypomagnesemia. In hypophosphatasia, deficiency of alkaline phosphatase may also lead to the accumulation of PP_i.

PATHOGENESIS

Episodes of acute pseudogout occur when CPPD crystals are shed from the articular cartilage, a process that can stem from a decrease in the concentration of either calcium or phosphate in synovial fluid (as after surgery), from direct trauma to the joint, or from joint inflammation. The inflammatory response to crystal shedding is similar to that which occurs in acute gout. CPPD crystals also stimulate synovial cells to produce and release metalloproteinases, including collagenase, stromelysin, and gelatinase, which degrade cartilage and periarticular tissues. Ongoing exposure to these degradative enzymes may contribute to the chronic form of arthritis associated with CPPD crystal deposition disease.

CLINICAL FINDINGS

Chondrocalcinosis is evident on radiographs as fine, stippled calcifications in fibrocartilage (knee menisci, triangular cartilage of the wrist, symphysis pubis, glenoid and acetabular labra) and, less often, in hyaline cartilage of joints. Acute pseudogout develops in 25% of patients with CPPD deposition disease and may be present in joints without radiographic evidence of chondrocalcinosis. Acute pseudogout usually appears as the sudden onset of swelling, warmth, and pain in one joint, typically the knee (in 50% of attacks), wrist, or ankle. The degree of joint inflammation may be less than that seen in gout. Polyarticular attacks may occur. This condition may be accompanied by fever, particularly in the elderly. Episodes can be precipitated by trauma, surgery, or severe illness. Joint inflammation peaks on day 2 or 3 and can last from 7 to 14 days, with subsequent complete resolution. Recurrent attacks are more common in patients with more extensive chondrocalcinosis.

A chronic form of arthritis that mimics osteoarthritis, with pain and deformity, develops in 50% of patients with CPPD deposition disease. The knees are affected most often, but joints that are not usually affected by idiopathic osteoarthritis, such as the wrists, elbows, shoulders, ankles, and metacarpophalangeal joints, may also be involved. Chronic arthritis may develop in patients who have not experienced previous episodes of acute

TABLE 177.2.	**CONDITIONS ASSOCIATED WITH CALCIUM PYROPHOSPHATE DIHYDRATE DEPOSITION DISEASE**

Hyperparathyroidism
Familial hypocalciuric hypercalcemia
Hemochromatosis
Hemosiderosis
Hypomagnesemia
Hypophosphatasia
Osteoarthritis
Gout
Amyloidosis
Bartter's syndrome
Neuropathic joints
Osteochondrodysplasias

pseudogout. A chronic type of symmetrical inflammatory polyarthritis that mimics rheumatoid arthritis develops in 5% of patients.

LABORATORY FINDINGS

Synovial fluid in acute pseudogout can evince intracellular and extracellular CPPD crystals, which are rod-shaped or rhomboid crystals. Under polarizing microscopy, the crystals are weakly birefringent (dull), show positive elongation (they appear blue when aligned parallel to the orientation of the red compensator), and may be sparse and difficult to locate. Synovial fluid leukocyte counts are elevated, but they are usually less than 50,000 per cubic millimeter; these cells are mainly neutrophils. Peripheral leukocytosis and elevation of acute phase reactants may be seen. CPPD crystals also may be found in synovial fluids of joints affected by chronic CPPD-associated arthritis. Serum chemistry tests give normal results in patients with idiopathic CPPD deposition disease.

OPTIMAL MANAGEMENT

Chondrocalcinosis requires no treatment. Episodes of acute pseudogout are treated in the same manner as episodes of acute gout. If episodes are frequent, daily oral colchicine may help limit their number. Aspiration of the affected joint often provides relief, even without additional therapy. Chronic arthritis is treated symptomatically with analgesics, NSAIDs, and colchicine and is generally slowly progressive.

BASIC CALCIUM PHOSPHATE CRYSTAL DEPOSITION DISEASES

Basic calcium phosphate (BCP) crystals include crystals of carbonate-substituted apatite, octacalcium phosphate, tricalcium phosphate, and other rare types. Shedding of crystals from deposits in cartilage, tendons, bursae, and soft tissues surrounding joints leads to acute inflammation. Clumps of apatite crystals, the most common crystal of this group, appear on microscopic examination of synovial fluids as shiny but non-birefringent globules that stain with alizarin red S stain. Individual apatite crystals are too small to be distinguished by light microscopy, and specific identification requires electron microscopy or x-ray diffraction. Because of the difficulty of precise identification of these crystals, the diagnosis of BCP crystal deposition diseases often rests on the recognition of typical clinical and radiographic features.

BCP crystal deposition diseases include calcific tendinitis and bursitis, acute arthritis, and a type of chronic destructive noninflammatory arthritis. Calcific tendinitis is an acute, painful tendinitis, most often of the rotator cuff tendons, associated with periarticular calcifications on radiographs. It occurs most often in young adults and in diabetics. Calcific bursitis or periarthritis is an acute inflammatory reaction in a bursa or near a joint, associated with local calcific deposits on radiographs. Typical

sites include the areas around the first toe, shoulder, greater trochanter, elbow, wrist, and knee. Affected areas are painful, swollen, and erythematous, mimicking acute gout or cellulitis. Acute inflammatory arthritis due to BCP crystals may develop in joints affected by osteoarthritis or in patients with chronic renal failure. The treatment for each of these conditions includes NSAIDs, local glucocorticoid injection, and colchicine.

Rarely, destructive arthritis associated with apatite crystals develops in the shoulder (Milwaukee shoulder) or knee. Elderly women are affected most often. Large, cool effusions with abundant apatite crystals and leukocyte counts less than 500 per cubic millimeter are common, as is disruption of the rotator cuff, subluxation of the humerus, and destruction of cartilage and bone. Joint damage may progress rapidly. Pain may be present only with use of the joint. Treatment includes rest, administration of analgesics or NSAIDs, and joint replacement.

BIBLIOGRAPHY

Emmerson BT. The management of gout. *N Engl J Med* 1996;334: 445–451.

Kelley WN, Wortmann RL. Gout and hyperuricemia. In: Kelley WN, Harris ED, Ruddy S, et al., eds. *Textbook of rheumatology*, fifth ed. Philadelphia: WB Saunders, 1997:1313–1351.

Ryan LM, McCarty DJ. Calcium pyrophosphate crystal deposition disease, pseudogout, and articular chondrocalcinosis. In: Koopman WJ, ed. *Arthritis and allied conditions*, thirteenth ed. Baltimore: Williams and Wilkins, 1996:2103–2125.

Kelley's Textbook of Internal Medicine, fourth edition. Edited by H. David Humes. Lippincott Williams & Wilkins, Philadelphia © 2000.

CHAPTER

178

SYSTEMIC LUPUS ERYTHEMATOSUS AND OVERLAP SYNDROMES

RONALD F. VAN VOLLENHOVEN

DEFINITION

Systemic lupus erythematosus (SLE) is a chronic, multisystem disease of unknown origin that exhibits wide variations in its clinical expression and disease course. A cardinal feature of the disease is laboratory-based evidence for autoimmunity, as reflected by the positive fluorescent antinuclear antibody (FANA) test result found in virtually all patients and a range of other autoantibodies that are present in varying percentages of patients. The clinical picture of SLE can change over time, in terms of both disease activity and organ involvement. The immunopathogenesis of SLE is complex and parallels the wide variation in

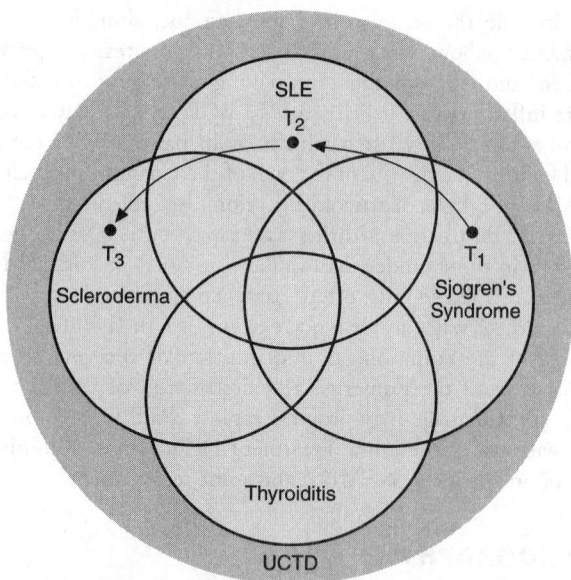

FIGURE 178.1. SLE and overlap syndromes. Patients may have simultaneous symptoms and signs of more than one autoimmune disease, that is, an overlap syndrome. Another possibility is that the patient's clinical course over time reflects a change from one disease to another. For example, the patient plotted here had characteristic keratoconjunctivitis sicca, xerostomia, SSA and SSB antibodies, and a positive lip biopsy result at time point T1, with a diagnosis of Sjögren's syndrome. Several years later, at time point T2, she showed signs of arthritis and nephritis, with anti-DNA antibodies and low complement levels, giving a diagnosis of SLE. Many years later, at time point T3, she experienced a characteristic tightening of the skin, severe Raynaud's phenomenon, esophageal dysmotility, and lung fibrosis; a skin biopsy confirmed the diagnosis of scleroderma. SLE, systemic lupus erythematosus; UCTD, undifferentiated connective tissue disease.

clinical symptoms. No single mechanism of action applies to all cases, and the initial triggering events remain largely unknown.

The finding of the lupus erythematosus (LE) cell in the 1940s and of FANA and anti-DNA antibodies in the 1950s and 1960s enhanced clinicians' ability to properly diagnose and classify patients with SLE and several related immunologic multisystem disorders. Several syndromes akin to SLE but with distinct clinical and immunologic features have also been identified, including subacute cutaneous LE (SCLE), mixed connective tissue disease (MCTD), and the antiphospholipid antibody syndrome. Patients exhibiting features of both SLE and one or more other autoimmune disorders are often classified as having "overlap syndromes" (Fig. 178.1). The development of diagnostic criteria for SLE in 1971 (revised in 1982 and again in 1997) has permitted the classification of patients for purposes of research, epidemiology, and clinical trials (Table 178.1). Although the American College of Rheumatology (ACR) criteria provide a useful reference frame, the diagnosis in an individual patient does not strictly depend on meeting these criteria but rather on a consistent diagnostic impression by a qualified clinician.

INCIDENCE AND EPIDEMIOLOGY

The prevalence rate of SLE in the United States remains unclear, in part owing to difficulties in ascertaining diagnoses made in

varying clinical settings; the most reliable estimates are 0.05% to 0.1% of the population. SLE occurs infrequently among prepubertal children but frequently has its onset during the second and third decades of life; some studies suggest a second peak of new (incident) cases around the age of 50. The sex distribution of SLE is distinctly biased; SLE develops in women of childbearing age approximately 10 times more often than in men of a similar age. At lower and higher ages, women are affected 3 to 4 times more frequently than men. In the United States, blacks and other minorities appear to be at higher risk of SLE and may have more severe disease as well, which can be explained in part by socioeconomic factors. While SLE is reported worldwide, it is significantly less prevalent in developing countries.

ETIOLOGY

The cause of SLE is unknown. Three distinct areas contribute to the development of lupus: genetic, environmental, and hormonal. In each patient, the relative contributions of the three factors may differ. Thus, some patients may have a largely genetically determined disease that reaches clinical expression irrespective of other factors. Other genetically susceptible individuals may require just one additional trigger to acquire full-blown SLE, and still others who are less genetically susceptible may contract the disease only with the interaction of several factors.

GENETIC FACTORS

Family studies suggest that the likelihood of acquiring SLE can be explained to a significant extent by heredity. Genetic studies have identified several genetic markers, and intense research is under way to identify what are probably at least a half dozen genes conferring increased risk of SLE. The best-described genetic factors are deficiencies in complement factors. Deficiencies of all complement components have been linked to SLE, but most of them are very rare (see Chapter 187). Complete (homozygous) deficiency of C2 or C4, while it is uncommon, is encountered in clinical practice and confers a high risk of SLE. Incomplete (heterozygous) deficiencies of C2 and C4, which are quite prevalent in the US population, also increase the risk of SLE. Among whites, the human leukocyte antigen (HLA) DR2 as well as the shared haplotype that includes HLA-B8 and HLA-DR3 also impart increased risk of SLE (as well as various other autoimmune diseases).

Determinants of risk for SLE have been localized to a segment of chromosome 1 that includes many genes of importance to the immune system, including genes encoding various cytokines and growth factors. Among them, the gene encoding interleukin (IL)-10 and the *bcl-2* gene may be of particular importance, and it has been suggested that an individual possessing the high-risk form of both genes is at particularly high risk of acquiring SLE. Family studies have confirmed that genetically encoded strong expression of IL-10 is a powerful risk factor for SLE. Inasmuch as SLE develops in a subset of patients during the first two decades of life, these individuals may have a largely genetically determined disease, the expression of which occurs after maturation of the immune system or in response to endo-

TABLE 178.1.	**THE AMERICAN COLLEGE OF RHEUMATOLOGY CLASSIFICATION CRITERIA FOR SLE, UPDATED IN 1997**[a]
Item	**Description**
Malar rash	Fixed erythema, flat or raised, over the malar eminences, sparing the nasolabial folds
Discoid rash	Erythematous raised patches with adherent keratotic scaling and follicular plugging; possible atrophic scarring in older lesions
Photosensitivity	Skin rash as a result of unusual reaction to sunlight, by patient's history or physician observation
Oral ulcers	Oral or nasopharyngeal ulceration, usually painless, observed by a physician
Nonerosive arthritis	Involving two or more peripheral joints, characterized by tenderness, swelling, or effusion
Pleuritis or pericarditis	Pleuritis—convincing history of pleuritic pain or rub heard by a physician or evidence of pleural effusion, OR
	Pericarditis—documented by electrocardiography or rub or evidence of pericardial effusion
Renal disorder	Persistent proteinuria of >0.5 g/d or $>3+$ if quantitative analysis of proteinuria is not performed, OR
	Cellular casts—red cell, hemoglobin, granular, tubular, or mixed
Seizures or psychosis	Seizures—in the absence of offending drugs or known metabolic derangement, e.g., uremia, ketoacidosis, or electrolyte imbalance, OR
	Psychosis—in the absence of offending drugs or known metabolic derangement, e.g., uremia, ketoacidosis, or electrolyte imbalance
Hematologic disorder	Hemolytic anemia with reticulocytosis OR
	Leukopenia—$<4,000/mm^3$ on two occasions OR
	Lymphopenia—$<1,500/mm^3$ on two occasions OR
	Thrombocytopenia—$<100,000/mm^3$ in the absence of offending drugs
Immunologic disorder	Anti-DNA—antibody to native DNA in abnormal titer OR
	Anti-Sm—presence of antibody to Sm nuclear antigen OR
	Positive finding of antiphospholipid antibodies based on an abnormal serum level of IgG or IgM anticardiolipin antibodies, a positive test for lupus anticoagulant using a standard method, or a false-positive test for ≥ 6 months and confirmed by *Treponema pallidum* immobilization or fluorescent treponemal antibody absorption test
Positive antinuclear antibody	An abnormal titer of antinuclear antibody by immunofluorescence or an equivalent assay at any point in time in the absence of drug

[a] For classification purposes, the diagnosis of SLE is said to be present if at least four of the listed 11 findings are present. Note that the purpose of these criteria is primarily as an instrument for epidemiologic and other clinical investigations, not as a diagnostic tool in clinical practice.
Sm, Smith antigen.

crine changes. From a practical point of view, the occurrence of overt SLE among relatives of patients is seen infrequently, and the role of triggering factors and other environmental influences that may be responsible for disease initiation and/or perpetuation must therefore be considered.

ENVIRONMENTAL FACTORS

Among triggers for lupus disease activity, ultraviolet light stands out as the most undisputed and widely recognized. Many patients with SLE experience photosensitive rashes, frequently accompanied by general malaise, fever, and other signs of systemic inflammation. The mechanism of disease activation by ultraviolet light may include induction of antigenic epitopes in the dermis or epidermis, the release of nuclear material by light-damaged skin cells, or dysregulation of immune cells in the skin. Clinical observations suggest that in some patients ultraviolet light exposure plays a role in first acquiring SLE as well.

Various other environmental factors also have been implicated in lupus. Such medications as procainamide and hydralazine—and, rarely, minocycline (used in patients with rheumatoid arthritis)—can cause drug-induced LE (DILE), a disease with similarities to but also notable differences from SLE (see "Drug-Induced Lupus Erythematosus"). Perhaps more interest-

ing is the observation that some antirheumatic drugs, such as sulfasalazine, can induce an illness that is akin to SLE in clinical and serologic features. Whether a new class of antirheumatic agents that antagonize tumor necrosis factor (TNF) also belong to this group is not yet clear.

Diverse chemicals, particularly aromatic amines, have been implicated as the cause of lupus-like syndromes. These syndromes are usually more similar to drug-induced than to systemic lupus and resolve after the exposure ends. Hair care products, such as hair dyes, and silicone breast implants have been largely cleared from suspicion of causing SLE after extensive epidemiologic research. A few reports regarding geographic clusters of lupus, suggesting an environmental factor, have not been confirmed.

The nonessential amino acid L-canavanine has come under suspicion, owing to the development of a lupus-like disease in monkeys after ingestion of large quantities of alfalfa sprouts, which contain L-canavanine. Exposure to this amino acid has been implicated in a few instances of transient autoimmune manifestations in humans as well. The presence in the environment of increasing quantities of plant-derived estrogens (phytoestrogens) has been proposed as an explanation for the apparent increase in the incidence of SLE over the past 30 years.

Infectious agents may play a role in disease activation. Once a patient has SLE, common infections of the respiratory or urinary tract are frequently followed by flare-ups of disease activity. Animal studies suggest that retroviruses may induce autoimmune phenomena akin to SLE. A recent study in children with SLE suggests that infection with the Epstein–Barr virus is a necessary prerequisite, but certainly not a sufficient cause, for SLE. Cases of SLE arising in the wake of physical or chemical exposures, accidents, or physical and psychological trauma are encountered fairly often in clinical practice. No distinct pattern has emerged, and the causality of these associations remains speculative.

HORMONAL INFLUENCES

Clinical observations suggest the role of sex steroids as a source of SLE. These observations include the higher incidence of SLE in women of childbearing age, increased SLE disease activity during pregnancy, and a slightly higher risk of acquiring SLE among postmenopausal women who take estrogen supplements. Moreover, subtle hormonal abnormalities have been found in patients with SLE, including preferential hydroxylation of estrone at the 16α position, resulting in more immunologically active metabolites; accelerated oxidation (inactivation) of testosterone in female patients; and generally lower serum levels of androgens, including the adrenal androgen dehydroepiandrosterone (DHEA). The net result of these findings implicates a relative excess of estrogens and deficiency of androgens in the pathogenesis of SLE.

Sex steroids have immunoregulatory properties that may put some of these observations into context. Estrogen has several immunomodulating effects, including a general immunostimulating effect on antibody formation and more ambivalent effects with respect to cellular immunity. Prolactin has powerful immunostimulating properties, while progesterone tends to be more immunosuppressive. Androgens may have mild immunosuppressive properties, antagonizing some of estrogen's up-regulatory effects with respect to humoral immunity. In animal models, DHEA has been implicated in a change in the phenotype of T cells away from the T_h2 phenotype characterized by the production of IL-4, IL-5 and IL-10; this T-cell phenotype would result in an environment more likely to produce pathogenetic autoantibodies than the T_h1 phenotype characterized by production of IL-2 and interferon-γ. In summary, many clinical as well as experimental observations suggest that a high-estrogen, low-androgen state may be conducive to SLE in predisposed individuals and that hormone levels can influence disease activity and expression in the patient via their immunomodulatory effects.

▬ PATHOGENESIS

The pathologic characteristics of SLE are those of an inflammatory disorder with evidence of self-reactivity (autoimmunity). The most important immunologic abnormalities seen in SLE reflect the presence of antibodies that target self-antigens. Virtually all patients have antinuclear antibodies (ANAs), which is really a large family of antibodies that target nuclear antigens.

While ANAs are helpful in clinical terms, only some of them are believed to be important from a pathophysiologic perspective. About half of all patients have anti-DNA antibodies, which are very specific and may be pathogenetic (see "Laboratory Findings"). Many other autoantibodies are seen in SLE, including anti-Smith (anti-Sm), anti-Ro, anti-La, anti-ribonucleoprotein (anti-RNP) and anti–proliferating cell nuclear antigen antibodies as well as autoantibodies more typically associated with other diseases, such as rheumatoid factor. Whether the formation of these autoantibodies reflects an abnormality of the target autoantigen, a primary defect in B cells, or a defect in regulatory T cells remains the subject of debate. Autoantibodies may lead to disease manifestations through at least three pathophysiologic mechanisms of action: the formation of immune complexes, the direct effects of pathogenetic autoantibodies on their targets, and antibody-mediated thromboembolic phenomena.

IMMUNE COMPLEXES

Many SLE manifestations are reflected at the histopathologic level by immune complex deposition, subsequent complement activation, and chronic lymphocytic inflammation. Thus, the skin lesions in SLE frequently contain immune complexes at the dermal–epidermal junction, and the glomerular lesion of lupus nephritis is defined to a great extent by the granular deposits that contain immunoglobulins and complement factors. The origins of these immune complexes are uncertain. Even in the best-studied situation, namely, the immune complexes containing anti-DNA antibodies in lupus nephritis, considerable uncertainty persists as to whether the antibodies bind antigen (DNA) in the circulation or within the target tissue and even as to whether they bind DNA or a cross-reacting antigen. It is also not clear whether the primary defect is the excessive formation of immune complexes or the ineffective clearance of such complexes. Evidence for the latter theory includes the association of SLE with complement deficiencies and the relatively low expression of complement receptor CR1 in patients with SLE.

AUTOANTIBODIES

Some SLE disease manifestations are the result of pathogenetic autoantibodies acting directly on their targets. They include autoimmune thrombocytopenia, hemolytic anemia, leukopenia, and possibly even some of the neurologic manifestations of lupus. Cell-specific autoantibodies can cause complement-mediated cytolysis or, through opsonization, can induce phagocytosis of the cell in the reticuloendothelial system. Whether antibody-mediated cellular cytotoxicity, antibody-induced apoptosis, or other mechanisms also play a role is unclear. Neonatal lupus, a disease provoked by maternal anti-Ro (SSA) antibodies reaching the infant's circulation through the placenta, is a remarkable "experiment of nature" that proves that this antibody can be the direct cause of various lupus manifestations, including skin lesions, pleuropericarditis, arthritis, alopecia, and heart block.

THROMBOEMBOLIC PHENOMENA

Several of the classic characteristics of lupus, such as Libman–Sacks endocarditis, are now known to be primarily thrombotic manifestations of the hypercoagulability seen in the anti-phospholipid antibody syndrome. This syndrome is encountered as a concomitant condition in a sizable subset of patients with SLE as well as in a primary form (without SLE). Hypercoagulability is believed to be the result of antibodies binding to coagulation factors or cofactors, platelets, or endothelium.

Several manifestations of SLE appear to be independent of the presence of immune complexes and cannot be attributed to specific autoantibodies or thromboembolism. The pathologic substrate for such diverse disease manifestations as pulmonary alveolar hemorrhage, organic brain syndrome, or myalgias cannot be identified in many instances. Vasculopathy induced by cytokines (Shwartzman phenomenon) is one of the proposed mechanisms of development.

Finally, the cytokine tumor necrosis factor α (TNF-α) has come under scrutiny as a therapeutic target in a variety of autoimmune diseases, including rheumatoid arthritis and Crohn's disease. It is therefore of importance to recognize the ambiguous findings regarding TNF-α in SLE. Although TNF-α is broadly proinflammatory, it is beneficial in the NZB/NZW animal model of SLE. IL-10 is known to down-regulate TNF-α, yet high levels of IL-10 appear to be a risk factor for SLE. Moreover, patients treated with TNF-α antagonists sometimes form autoantibodies reminiscent of SLE, and at least one patient developed transient SLE-like symptoms following such treatment.

CLINICAL FINDINGS

The clinical picture of SLE is extremely variable, both in terms of actual organ involvement in the disease at any particular point in time and the severity of disease manifestations in that organ. In addition, the chronological course of the disease varies considerably from patient to patient. Thus, lupus can be visualized as myriad possibilities along the dimensions of organicity and severity, evolving along the dimension of time. The severity can range from mild or moderate to severe or even life-threatening. Because of the multisystem diversity of its clinical manifestations, lupus has replaced syphilis as the "great imitator." A selection of SLE manifestations is given in Table 178.2.

Most patients with SLE have mild to moderate disease with chronic smoldering symptoms, punctuated by gradual or sudden increases in disease activity (flare-ups). The disease course in a smaller percentage of patients is characterized by alternating flare-ups and complete clinical remissions. Rarely, a patient has a single episode of active SLE followed by a sustained remission. The clinical description of SLE is complicated further by two issues. First, while SLE can cause many symptoms and signs, not all symptoms and signs in a patient with SLE are the result of the disease. Many intercurrent illnesses, particularly viral infections, can mimic SLE. Second, side effects of medication, particularly those of long-term glucocorticoid use, must be distinguished from the symptoms and signs of SLE.

CONSTITUTIONAL MANIFESTATIONS

Fever is present in most patients with active SLE, but infectious causes always must be considered as well, particularly in patients under immunosuppressive therapy. Weight loss may occur early in the course of disease, whereas weight gain, especially in glucocorticoid-treated patients, may be more typical later. Fatigue and general malaise are among the most common and often most debilitating symptoms of the disease. The exact origin of these symptoms is often uncertain—disease activity itself, medication side effects, subtle neuroendocrinologic disturbances, and psychogenic factors all play a role.

MUCOCUTANEOUS MANIFESTATIONS

The classic butterfly rash, an erythematous rash over the malar area of the cheeks and the bridge of the nose that spares the nasolabial folds, is seen in about half of all patients. It may be raised and very inflammatory, persisting for weeks or months. It resolves without scarring. In contrast, the lesion of discoid lupus can result in disfiguring scars. It is found in 20% to 25% of patients with SLE but is usually seen without any other lupus manifestations. These erythematous plaques with adherent scale and telangiectases develop mostly on the face, neck, and scalp. Acute cutaneous lupus in the form of intense inflammatory erythema can be triggered by exposure to ultraviolet light. Subacute and chronic lupus lesions are frequently found on the areas of the skin that have long been exposed to the sun (forearms, V-region around the neck), but without immediately preceding sun exposure. Many other skin lesions are encountered from time to time in SLE, including livedo reticularis, periungual erythema, palmar erythema, palmar nodules, vesicular or even bullous lesions, acute or chronic urticaria, panniculitis, vasculitic purpura, and non-healing vasculitic ulcers.

Alopecia may develop as the result of typical lupus lesions on the scalp, but it is much more common as a nonspecific feature of a lupus flare-up, often following a period of intense disease activity. Alopecia tends to be reversible, except when there are discoid lesions on the scalp. Its specificity for SLE is higher when it appears in patches rather than as diffuse loss. Oral and nasal ulcers are fairly common and may be either painless or painful; the latter ulcers must be distinguished from fungal and viral lesions. Dry eyes and dry mouth (sicca syndrome) can result from autoimmune lacrimal and salivary gland inflammation, which can be considered an overlap with Sjögren's syndrome. More frequently, dry eyes and dry mouth are the result of medication side effects.

MUSCULOSKELETAL MANIFESTATIONS

The arthritis of SLE is typically inflammatory and accompanied by synovitis and pain, but it is nonerosive and nondeforming. Rarely, patients have Jaccoud's deformities, which resemble rheumatoid arthritis but are reducible and not associated with radiographic evidence of cartilage or bone destruction. Whereas muscle weakness is often seen in SLE as the result of glucocorticoid or antimalarial therapy, true myositis with elevated muscle enzyme levels is rare and suggests an overlap syndrome. Tenosynovitis and bursitis are seen frequently. Tendon rupture may be a complication of long-term glucocorticoid treatment. Osteonecrosis (avascular necrosis) is a major concern in patients with SLE, since both the disease itself and treatment with gluco-

TABLE 178.2.   SELECTED MANIFESTATIONS OF SLE AND TREATMENT RECOMMENDATIONS

Manifestation	General Therapy	Specific Therapy	Experimental Therapy
Mild			
Constitutional (fever, fatigue, weight loss)	Topical corticosteroids for rash and mucous lesions	Calcium channel blockers for Raynaud's phenomenon	Dehydroepiandrosterone (DHEA)
Mucositis	Antimalarial agents	Tricyclic antidepressants and exercise for myalgias	
Mild cutaneous disease	NSAIDs	for myalgias	
Arthralgia, arthritis, myalgia	Low-dose corticosteroids (5–10 mg/day) if other therapy ineffective	Dapsone or thalidomide for refractory skin lesions	
Mild serositis		Antimigraine therapy if migraines predominate	
Lymphadenopathy, splenomegaly			
Minor cytopenias			
Moderate			
Refractory cutaneous disease	Moderate-dose corticosteroids (15–40 mg/d)	Anticonvulsants for seizures	DHEA
High fever		Antipsychotics for psychosis	Cyclosporin A
Hemolytic anemia (hematocrit <30)	Azathioprine	Methotrexate for arthritis, serositis	
Thrombocytopenia (platelets <50,000)		Anticoagulation for thrombosis	
Myositis		Intravenous immunoglobulin, danazol, or splenectomy for unresponsive thrombocytopenia	
Membranous nephritis			
Pleuropericarditis			
Polyarthritis			
Neurologic disease			
Thrombosis			
Severe			
Pneumonitis	High-dose corticosteroids (1–2 mg/kg/d)	Angiotensin-converting enzyme inhibitor or cyclosporin A for nephrotic syndrome	IVIG
Vasculitis			Plasmapheresis
Diffuse proliferative glomerulonephritis	Pulse corticosteroids (1,000 mg i.v./d × 3 days)		Total lymphoid irradiation
Membranous nephritis with nephrotic syndrome	Cyclophosphamide i.v.		High-intensity chemotherapy
Severe neurologic disease			Autologous stem-cell transplant
Recalcitrant multiorgan disease			
Diffuse pulmonary hemorrhage			
Myocarditis			

NSAIDs, nonsteroidal anti-inflammatory drugs; DHEA, dehydroepiandrosterone; IVIG, intravenous immunoglobulin.

corticoid contribute to the risk. The femoral head, humoral head, tibial plateau, and talus are the sites most often affected. Joint pain without objective evidence of inflammation (arthralgia) and myalgia are among the most common symptoms of SLE. They may be related to the disease itself, medication side effects, the "glucocorticoid withdrawal syndrome," endocrinopathies, or psychogenic factors. The diagnosis of fibromyalgia is best reserved for patients in whom all these causes have been ruled out.

CARDIOVASCULAR MANIFESTATIONS

Pericarditis is a typical symptom, with positional substernal chest pain and sometimes a rub. Echocardiography may show an effusion or, in chronic cases, a thickened, fibrotic pericardium. Tamponade or constrictive hemodynamics are rare. Myocarditis is unusual, but it must be suspected in any patient with active SLE and atypical chest symptoms, minimal electrocardiographic changes, arrhythmias, or hemodynamic changes. Myocarditis can lead to dilated cardiomyopathy, with signs of left ventricular failure. Echocardiography or thallium perfusion scintigraphy are useful diagnostic tests to rule out subclinical lupus myocarditis.

Noninfectious thrombotic endocarditis (Libman–Sacks) is uncommon and often asymptomatic, but in rare cases it can cause valvular dysfunction of the mitral or aortic valve or embolization. Premature arteriosclerosis with angina pectoris and myocardial infarction has emerged as one of the most serious long-term sources of morbidity and mortality in patients with SLE. The disease itself, hypercoagulability, chronic glucocorticoid therapy, premature menopause, and dietary and lifestyle factors may all contribute to arteriosclerosis. Raynaud's phenomenon, that is, cold-induced reversible vasospasm of the fingers and toes, is common in SLE and is rare in rheumatoid arthritis. Irreversible arterial narrowing in the hands and feet is sometimes seen in overlap syndromes with features of scleroderma. A similar pathologic picture in the pulmonary circulation may give rise to pulmonary hypertension, an unusual but frequently fatal complication of SLE.

PULMONARY MANIFESTATIONS

Pleurisy is very prevalent in SLE. Pleuritic chest pain, a rub, and effusions are evident on radiography in some patients, while others may have convincing symptoms without objective findings. Inflammation in the lung parenchyma, referred to as pneumonitis or alveolitis and evidenced by cough, hemoptysis, and pulmonary infiltrates, is uncommon but possibly life-threatening. It requires an aggressive and expeditious workup to rule out infectious causes and institution of glucocorticoid and immunosuppressive therapy. Diffuse alveolar hemorrhage may be present with or without acute pneumonitis and carries a very high mortality rate. Chronic lupus pneumonitis with mostly fibrotic lung changes behaves similarly to idiopathic pulmonary fibrosis, with a slowly progressive course and, ultimately, a poor prognosis. Restrictive lung disease also may be caused by long-standing pleuritic changes, myopathy, or fibrosis of the respiratory muscles, including the diaphragm, and even neuropathy of the phrenic nerve. Recurrent pulmonary emboli resulting from antiphospholipid antibodies must be ruled out in all patients with unexplained pulmonary symptoms.

RENAL MANIFESTATIONS

Lupus nephritis is present in about half of all patients with SLE. The spectrum of pathologic involvement can vary from almost completely asymptomatic mesangial proliferation to aggressive, diffuse membranoproliferative glomerulonephritis that progresses to renal failure. The World Health Organization (WHO) classification scheme for lupus nephritis (Table 178.3) has been very useful in categorizing the histopathologic features. The clinical picture of lupus nephritis can be characterized by minimal findings, including mild proteinuria and microscopic hematuria; the nephrotic syndrome, with high-level proteinuria, hypoalbuminemia, peripheral edema, hypertriglyceridemia, and hypercoagulability; or the nephritic syndrome, with hypertension, erythrocytes and erythrocyte casts in the urine sediment, and a progressively declining glomerular filtration rate with rising serum creatinine and uremia. The nephrotic syndrome is often seen with membranous nephritis (WHO class V), and the nephritic syndrome usually accompanies membranoproliferative disease (WHO class IV); the latter condition is often associated with high-titer anti-DNA antibody and low complement levels. The most important point is that the renal histopathologic characteristics *cannot* be predicted accurately by the clinical manifestations alone. Transition from one form of glomerulonephritis to another in the course of SLE is not uncommon.

NEUROLOGIC AND PSYCHIATRIC MANIFESTATIONS

Central nervous system (CNS) involvement occurs in 5% to 15% of patients with lupus and is sometimes referred to as neuropsychiatric SLE or lupus cerebritis. It can have such objective manifestations as aseptic meningitis or meningoencephalitis, seizures, chorea, ataxia, stroke, and transverse myelitis. In such patients, the diagnosis can be supported by abnormal findings on cerebrospinal fluid (CSF) analysis, such as elevated protein levels, pleiocytosis, and/or characteristic autoantibodies; on computerized tomography scanning or magnetic resonance imaging, such as inflammatory white and gray matter lesions; or even on leptomeningeal biopsy, with evidence of inflammation (usually indicated only if an alternative diagnosis is also suspected). Infectious

---

TABLE 178.3. **THE WORLD HEALTH ORGANIZATION (WHO) CLASSIFICATION OF LUPUS NEPHRITIS**[a]

Class	Description	Clinical Findings	Prognosis	Treatment
I	Minimal change	None	Excellent	None
II	Mesangial glomerulonephritis	Few erythrocytes Mild proteinuria	Good	None
III	Focal proliferative glomerulonephritis	Microscopic hematuria and mild to moderate proteinuria	Variable	Low to moderate doses of corticosteroids ?Azathioprine
IV	Diffuse membranoproliferative glomerulonephritis	Nephritic syndrome: hypertension, hematuria with erythrocyte casts, progressive uremia	Poor (without therapy)	High-dose corticosteroids plus cyclophosphamide (or azathioprine)
V	Membranous glomerulonephritis	Nephrotic syndrome: high-level proteinuria, peripheral edema, hypertriglyceridemia, hypercoagulability	Fair to poor	(Corticosteroids?) (Azathioprine?) Angiotensin-converting enzyme inhibitors Cyclosporin A
VI	End Stage	Progressive renal failure	Poor	Prepare for dialysis/ transplantation

[a] The classification is represented in simplified form. Therapeutic decisions need be directed by complete histopathologic and clinical evaluation.

causes must always be ruled out, as must drug-induced disease, for example, aseptic meningitis induced by ibuprofen.

An alternative picture of CNS lupus is a major psychiatric disorder, that is, psychosis. In this case, CSF and imaging studies may show normal results, and the differential diagnosis from primary psychogenic disease and/or drug reactions can be very difficult to determine. Compounding the problem is the relatively large group of patients with milder cognitive and personality disturbances. Some studies of neuropsychologic functioning indicate that more than half of all patients with SLE have impaired memory, attention, concentration, reasoning, executive skills, and so on. These symptoms occur largely in the absence of any demonstrable abnormalities on CSF analysis or conventional imaging, but they can be verified by neuropsychologic testing. Whether they represent subtle organic manifestations of the disease in the form of CNS inflammation below the threshold of detection, CNS changes in response to chronic stress, long-term treatment effects, or psychological adjustments to chronic disease remains unclear; a combination of all of these factors seems most likely.

Headaches are common in patients with SLE and can be as easy or as difficult to manage as they are in the general population. The particularly severe, often migraine-like "lupus headache" that responds only to glucocorticoids is unusual, and most headaches in patients with SLE should be addressed as they would be in other individuals. Cranial and peripheral neuropathies are encountered now and then in patients with SLE; they may represent small-vessel vasculitis or infarction.

GASTROINTESTINAL MANIFESTATIONS

Nonspecific gastrointestinal symptoms, including diffuse abdominal pain and nausea, are typical in patients with SLE. Sterile peritonitis with ascites is an uncommon but serious abdominal complication. Many upper-gastrointestinal symptoms are related to therapy, in the form of nonsteroidal anti-inflammatory drug (NSAID) and/or glucocorticoid-related gastropathy. Duodenitis can become symptomatic. In rare cases, vasculitis of the bowel in SLE can provoke an acute surgical emergency. On occasion, pancreatitis can be a manifestation of lupus itself, but it results more frequently from the use of glucocorticoids or azathioprine. Liver enzyme elevations are sometimes associated with SLE in the form of noninfectious hepatitis, which is indistinguishable in histologic features from chronic autoimmune hepatitis. To confuse the issue further, the latter disease is sometimes called "lupoid hepatitis." Liver enzyme elevations can also occur with the use of NSAIDs, azathioprine, or methotrexate, and long-term glucocorticoid use can result in "fatty liver" changes with mildly elevated transaminases.

HEMATOLOGIC MANIFESTATIONS

Splenomegaly and diffuse lymphadenopathy are common, nonspecific findings in active SLE. Anemia is a typical feature of SLE, often stemming from several sources. Lupus may cause anemia through hemolysis, with a positive Coombs test result, low haptoglobin levels, and high lactate dehydrogenase levels, or through autoimmune myelosuppression. Indirect mecha-

nisms of action include decreased erythropoietin synthesis and uremic myelosuppression in patients with lupus nephritis. The picture may be complicated further by occult blood loss and dietary insufficiency. Leukopenia and lymphopenia are very common in lupus but rarely reach levels of clinical concern. Leukocytosis can be caused by glucocorticoids, but this symptom should raise concerns about infections. Mild thrombocytopenia (platelet count 100,000 to 150,000/μL) is seen frequently, particularly in patients with antiphospholipid antibodies. Severe autoimmune thrombocytopenia (platelet count less than 50,000/μL), caused by antiplatelet antibodies, may predate the diagnosis of SLE and may be diagnosed initially as idiopathic thrombocytopenic purpura.

OPHTHALMOLOGIC MANIFESTATIONS

Cotton-wool exudates and retinal infarcts ("cytoid bodies") are relatively uncommon and nonspecific findings. Conjunctivitis and episcleritis are sometimes seen in active disease. Dry eyes may represent an overlap with Sjögren's syndrome. Transient or permanent blindness can be the result of optic neuritis or occlusion of the retinal arteries or veins.

◼ LATE LUPUS SYNDROME

Patients with SLE who have had the disease for decades frequently suffer a set of symptoms that are partly the result of end-organ damage caused by SLE and partly due to medication side effects, particularly from chronic glucocorticoid use. This "late lupus syndrome" is characterized by widespread arteriosclerotic disease, skin atrophy, osteoporosis, osteonecrosis, diabetes mellitus, chronic renal failure, adrenal insufficiency, cognitive impairment, depression, and deconditioning. It is likely that the long-term survival and the quality of life of patients with lupus are limited to a great extent by this constellation of symptoms.

◼ SPECIAL PRESENTATIONS OF SYSTEMIC LUPUS ERYTHEMATOSUS

Several clinical syndromes within the spectrum of SLE have been defined more clearly as information regarding specific autoantibody involvement, course, and outcome has evolved (Table 178.4). Other patients manifest symptoms, signs, and laboratory test abnormalities that are suggestive of SLE as well as another autoimmune disease: such patients can properly be considered to have an overlap syndrome. Finally, some patients have incontrovertible evidence of autoimmune disease, but their conditions defy all attempts at classification; they can be identified as having "undifferentiated connective tissue disease."

SUBACUTE CUTANEOUS LUPUS ERYTHEMATOSUS

SCLE represents a subset of patients with primarily cutaneous disease in the form of a papulosquamous, psoriasiform, or annu-

TABLE 178.4. **CLINICAL SUBSETS OF SYSTEMIC LUPUS ERYTHEMATOSUS**

Discoid lupus	Inflammatory skin lesion resulting in atrophic scar	ANA may be positive but other lab results negative
Subacute cutaneous lupus erythematosus	Characteristic rash, mild systemic disease	Anti-Ro (SSA), anti-La (SSB)
Mixed connective tissue disease	Overlap features of SLE, polymyositis and scleroderma, nephritis/CNS disease uncommon	High-titer anti-RNP
Drug-induced lupus erythematosus	Pleuropericarditis, arthritis, no nephritis or anti-DNA	Antihistone antibodies
Neonatal lupus	Rash, serositis, cytopenias, conduction disorder (rare)	Anti-Ro (SSA) acquired passively from the maternal circulation
Antiphospholipid antibody syndrome	Arterial and/or venous thrombosis, obstetrical complications, thrombocytopenia	May occur with or without SLE, anticardiolipin antibodies, lupus "anticoagulant," false-positive VDRL

SLE, systemic lupus erythematosus; CNS, central nervous system; ANA, antinuclear antibody; RNP, ribonucleoprotein.

lar rash, mostly on the routinely sun-exposed areas of the body (face, neck, V-region, lower arms). Bouts of arthritis and serositis may occur episodically. Anti-Ro (SSA) and anti-La (SSB) antibodies are very common in this group of patients, and they have a favorable prognosis.

NEONATAL LUPUS

Soon after birth, the baby born to a mother with anti-Ro (SSA) antibodies (whether in the context of SLE, Sjögren's syndrome, or another rheumatic disorder) may experience a syndrome of arthritis, photosensitive skin eruption, alopecia, serositis, cytopenias, and, rarely, cardiac conduction disorders, including heart block. This disease, termed neonatal lupus, is almost certainly the result of the maternal autoantibodies that have passed across the placenta and exert their effects in the neonate. Over time, as the antibodies are cleared and replaced by the neonate's own, the disease subsides; however, the conduction disorder may be permanent. Whether anti-La (SSB) or other antibodies can cause the same syndrome is unclear.

DRUG-INDUCED LUPUS ERYTHEMATOSUS

Several medications have been implicated as the cause of DILE, a clinical and immunologic syndrome similar to SLE (Table 178.5). The data are strongest for hydralazine and procainamide, which have been the subject of large prospective studies. These agents do not appear to cause disease flare-ups when taken by patients with SLE. There are several important differences between DILE and SLE:

- The sex ratio for DILE is equal, whereas SLE is found predominantly in women.
- The symptoms of DILE tend to be milder and primarily involve the skin, joints, and serous membrane.
- DILE is reversible after discontinuation of the drug.
- Renal and CNS disease is rare in DILE.
- Anti-DNA and low complement are uncommon in DILE, though DILE induced by sulfasalazine is an exception to this rule.

- DILE is almost invariably associated with antihistone antibodies.

ANTIPHOSPHOLIPID ANTIBODY SYNDROME

A subset of patients with SLE, as well as otherwise healthy individuals, may have a history of recurrent venous and/or arterial thromboembolism and obstetrical complications, particularly intrauterine growth retardation and fetal demise. Such patients may also have moderate thrombocytopenia, livedo reticularis, migraine headaches, and Libman–Sacks endocarditis. The presence of antiphospholipid antibodies can be established by enzyme-linked immunosorbent assay for anticardiolipin (ACL) an-

TABLE 178.5. **SELECTED MEDICATIONS ASSOCIATED WITH DRUG-INDUCED LUPUS ERYTHEMATOSUS[a]**

Definite Association	Possible Association
Procainamide	Quinidine
Hydralazine	Propylthiouracil
Isoniazid	Sulfonamides
Minocycline	β-blockers
Chlorpromazine	Phenytoin
Methyldopa	Carbamazepine
Sulfasalazine[b]	Other anticonvulsants
D-penicillamine	L-dopa
	Lithium
	Tetracyclines
	Thiazide diuretics
	Affliximab[b]
	Etanercept[b]

[a] More than 100 medications or even categories of drugs have been implicated in drug-induced lupus; most of these associations are very rare.
[b] Can cause anti-DNA positivity in patients with rheumatoid arthritis.

tibodies (which is a special class of antiphospholipid antibodies), a false-positive test result for syphilis, or evidence of the "lupus anticoagulant" (which is a misnomer—see "Laboratory Findings"). These patients are in a hypercoagulable state and should be treated accordingly. Frequently, the treatment of the two conditions—SLE and the antiphospholipid antibody syndrome—must be pursued completely separately in the same patient.

OVERLAP SYNDROMES

Patients with SLE may have features suggestive of other rheumatic diseases as well (Fig. 178.1). Patients who clearly exhibit features of more than one disease can be said to have an overlap syndrome. It is important to emphasize to the patient that this is hardly likely to represent a chance occurrence of two disorders simultaneously! Instead, it illustrates the failure of our somewhat arbitrary categories to fit each patient's unique disease characteristics. Equally important is the recognition that patients may not remain in one particular diagnostic category; some patients may have classic symptoms of more than one autoimmune disease at different points in time (Fig. 178.1). The most common overlap syndromes are MCTD, SLE combined with Sjögren's syndrome, SLE with scleroderma, SLE with thyroiditis, and SLE with microangiopathic hemolytic anemia.

Mixed Connective Tissue Disease

MCTD is the most well-defined overlap syndrome, a clinical entity with features of SLE, scleroderma, and myositis. Typical manifestations include Raynaud's phenomenon, sclerodactyly, chronic dermatitis of sun-exposed skin, arthritis, serositis, esophageal dysmotility, and myositis. The finding of high-titer anti-RNP (1:100,000 or more) antibodies identifies this subset of patients. CNS and renal involvement is uncommon. These patients generally do well, but lung fibrosis and/or pulmonary hypertension mark a poorer prognosis.

Systemic Lupus Erythematosus and Sjögren's Syndrome Overlap

Sjögren's syndrome is autoimmune inflammation of the lacrimal and salivary glands, which may be associated with systemic features. The characteristic symptoms and signs are recurrent keratoconjunctivitis of the eyes, recurrent problems with dental and periodontal disease, and difficulty in swallowing; symptoms of dry eyes and dry mouth are by far too nonspecific to permit diagnosis. Anti-Ro (SSA) and anti-La (SSB) antibodies are common in patients with Sjögren's syndrome, as is rheumatoid factor. A minor salivary gland biopsy (lip biopsy) can help establish the diagnosis. Patients with Sjögren's syndrome may be at higher risk of interstitial lung disease and peripheral neuropathies.

Systemic Lupus Erythematosus and Scleroderma

The combination of SLE and scleroderma is suggested by a characteristic hardening of the skin, severe Raynaud's phenomenon,

and esophageal dysmotility. Inasmuch as the pathologic lesion of scleroderma is a merging of fibrosis and arterial hyperplasia, neither of which is likely to respond to glucocorticoid therapy, the distinction is important to make from a clinical point of view. For example, both SLE and scleroderma can cause severe renal disease, but the treatments are very different. Frequently, renal biopsy is needed to make the distinction.

Systemic Lupus Erythematosus with Autoimmune Thyroiditis

Autoimmune thyroiditis occurs often in the course of SLE; the condition may be hypothyroid, euthyroid, or hyperthyroid. As a general rule, the workup of any new set of symptoms in a patient with SLE should include thyroid function tests. Antithyroglobulin and antimicrosomal antibodies may support the diagnosis of autoimmune thyroiditis.

Systemic Lupus Erythematosus with Microangiopathic Hemolytic Anemia

SLE with microangiopathic hemolytic anemia is present when a patient with severe, active SLE and kidney, CNS, and hematologic symptoms also manifests evidence of significant microangiopathy, such as can be found on peripheral blood smear or by histopathologic examination. The clinical syndrome thus resembles thrombotic thrombocytopenic purpura or hemolytic-uremic syndrome. Evidence suggests that this overlap may be caused by antibodies directed against von Willebrand's factor–cleaving serum protease. Treatment for such patients should include plasma exchange.

Undifferentiated Connective Tissue Disease

Patients who do not fit into any of the disease categories discussed, but who nevertheless have clear evidence of a systemic autoimmune disorder, can be said to have undifferentiated connective tissue disease (Fig. 178.1). If the symptoms have been present for a relatively short period of time (less than 1 year), the disease may eventually declare itself. On the other hand, a number of patients will continue to exhibit the same set of limited symptoms for many years and never progress to a more well-defined rheumatic illness.

■ LABORATORY FINDINGS

A routine complete blood cell count often shows evidence of systemic inflammation, such as normocytic, normochromic anemia (anemia of chronic disease) and thrombocytosis. Modest leukocytosis is a general feature of most inflammatory diseases, but patients with SLE more often exhibit leukopenia and lymphopenia; the former tends to be obscured once glucocorticoid therapy is begun. Renal function is usually preserved in early-stage disease, even if active nephritis is present, but urinalysis may show evidence of proteinuria and microscopic hematuria. Erythrocyte casts are a sign of severe glomerulonephritis. Liver function test results are usually normal; a small subset of patients may have autoimmune liver inflammation with elevated transaminase levels. Widely used markers for inflammation include the erythrocyte sedimentation rate and C-reactive protein. The erythrocyte sedimentation rate can be markedly elevated in patients with severe disease, but on occasion it may be within the normal range despite convincingly active SLE. C-reactive protein levels are usually elevated more modestly in SLE and more significantly in the case of acute infections, helping to differentiate the two.

Immunologic studies are of cardinal importance in the correct diagnosis of SLE and other related disorders. The ANA test result is virtually always positive in patients who have SLE. The converse is not true: many individuals with a positive ANA test result do not have SLE! The titer of positivity (the highest dilution of serum at which the immunofluorescent stain is seen) does not by itself say much about the diagnosis. It should be borne in mind, however, that a low-positive titer can well be false-positive (by definition, at least 2.5% of the population ought to fall outside the "normal" range). On the other hand, a high-positive titer probably has an explanation, though the explanation does not have to be SLE. The pattern of staining on occasion can provide a diagnostic clue: for example, a nucleolar pattern points to a diagnosis of scleroderma. Most ANAs, however, give a diffuse (homogeneous) or speckled (heterogeneous) staining pattern, and these patterns do not provide further helpful information. A possible way of evaluating a positive ANA result is given in Fig. 178.2.

The presence of antibodies against double-stranded (native) DNA is the most helpful confirmatory test for SLE. In a reasonable clinical context, a positive result all but proves the diagnosis. This is particularly true if an immunofluorescent method (Crithidia test) is used. Tests for anti–single-stranded or denatured DNA are not very helpful from a clinical perspective. A positive anti–double-stranded DNA antibody test also increases the likelihood that the patient has or will have lupus nephritis. These antibodies, in fact, may have pathogenetic significance. In some patients, anti-DNA titers may reflect disease activity accurately, and a sudden increase in titer may even predict impending flare-ups. Anti-Sm and anti–proliferating cell nuclear antigen antibodies are also very specific for SLE, but are found infrequently. Antiribosomal P antibodies and antineuronal antibodies support a diagnosis of CNS lupus. Antihistone antibodies are seen in virtually all cases of DILE.

Anti-Ro (SSA) and anti-La (SSB) are two autoantibodies originally described in patients with Sjögren's syndrome. They are found in up to half of all patients with lupus and indicate a higher likelihood of cutaneous manifestations, photosensitivity, and neonatal lupus in the offspring of women of childbearing age. Anti-RNP at a low titer is a nonspecific finding in SLE, while anti-RNP at extremely high titers (1 : 1,000,000) suggests the diagnosis of MCTD. Many other autoantibodies can be found in patients with SLE, but they are more typically associated with other diseases, including rheumatoid factors and antithyroid antibodies. An overview of autoantibodies found in SLE is given in Table 178.6.

Low complement levels, particularly C3, C4, and CH50 (total hemolytic complement), are important both in the diagno-

TABLE 178.6.	AUTOANTIBODIES FOUND IN SYSTEMIC LUPUS ERYTHEMATOSUS
Antibody Specificity	**Disease Association**
Native (ds) DNA	SLE, nephritis
Denatured (ss) DNA	Nonspecific; various autoimmune diseases, including SLE
Sm antigen	SLE
Ribonucleoprotein	MCTD (very high titer), SLE (low to moderate titer)
Ro (SSA)	Sjögren's syndrome, SLE, SCLE, neonatal lupus
La (SSB)	Sjögren's syndrome, SLE, SCLE
Histone	Drug-induced lupus erythematosus
Proliferating cell nuclear antigen	SLE
Ribosomal P antigen	CNS lupus with psychosis
Neuronal	CNS lupus
Thyroglobulin	Autoimmune thyroiditis
Rheumatoid factor	Rheumatoid arthritis, SLE (low titer)
Cardiolipin	Antiphospholipid antibody syndrome
Centromere	CREST syndrome

Sm, Smith; SLE, systemic lupus erythematosus; MCTD, mixed connective tissue disease; SCLE, subacute cutaneous lupus erythematosus; CNS, central nervous system; CREST, calcinosis, Raynaud's, esophageal dysmotility, sclerodactyly, teleangiectasias; ds, double-stranded; ss, single-stranded.

sis of lupus and in monitoring disease activity. Low C4 levels may reflect disease activity but also can be the result of a (partial) deficiency of this complement product, whereas low C3 nearly always implies activation of complement. It has been suggested that measuring complement split products (e.g. C3d) is even more helpful in monitoring SLE—higher levels imply complement activation as a result of the disease process.

Various tests can indicate a thromboembolic tendency, including those for ACL antibodies and the so-called lupus anticoagulant; while these features can be found in otherwise healthy individuals, they are distinctly more common in patients with SLE. The term *lupus anticoagulant* is a misnomer: patients with this abnormality are at risk of venous and arterial embolism. The reason for the misnomer is that the activated partial thromboplastin time in these patients is prolonged. The lupus anticoagulant is therefore an anticoagulant in vitro but a procoagulant in vivo. This abnormality can be confirmed by mixing and platelet absorption studies. ACL antibodies also imply increased risk of thromboembolic events, particularly if they are of the IgG isotype. The risk correlates with the titer of the antibody. ACL antibodies are a special example of the larger group of antiphospholipid antibodies; laboratories can screen for a whole range of antiphospholipid antibodies, but their clinical significance is not always clear. ACL antibodies will result in a false-positive VDRL or rapid plasma reagin test for syphilis; a negative fluorescent treponemal antibody absorption test helps rule out true syphilis.

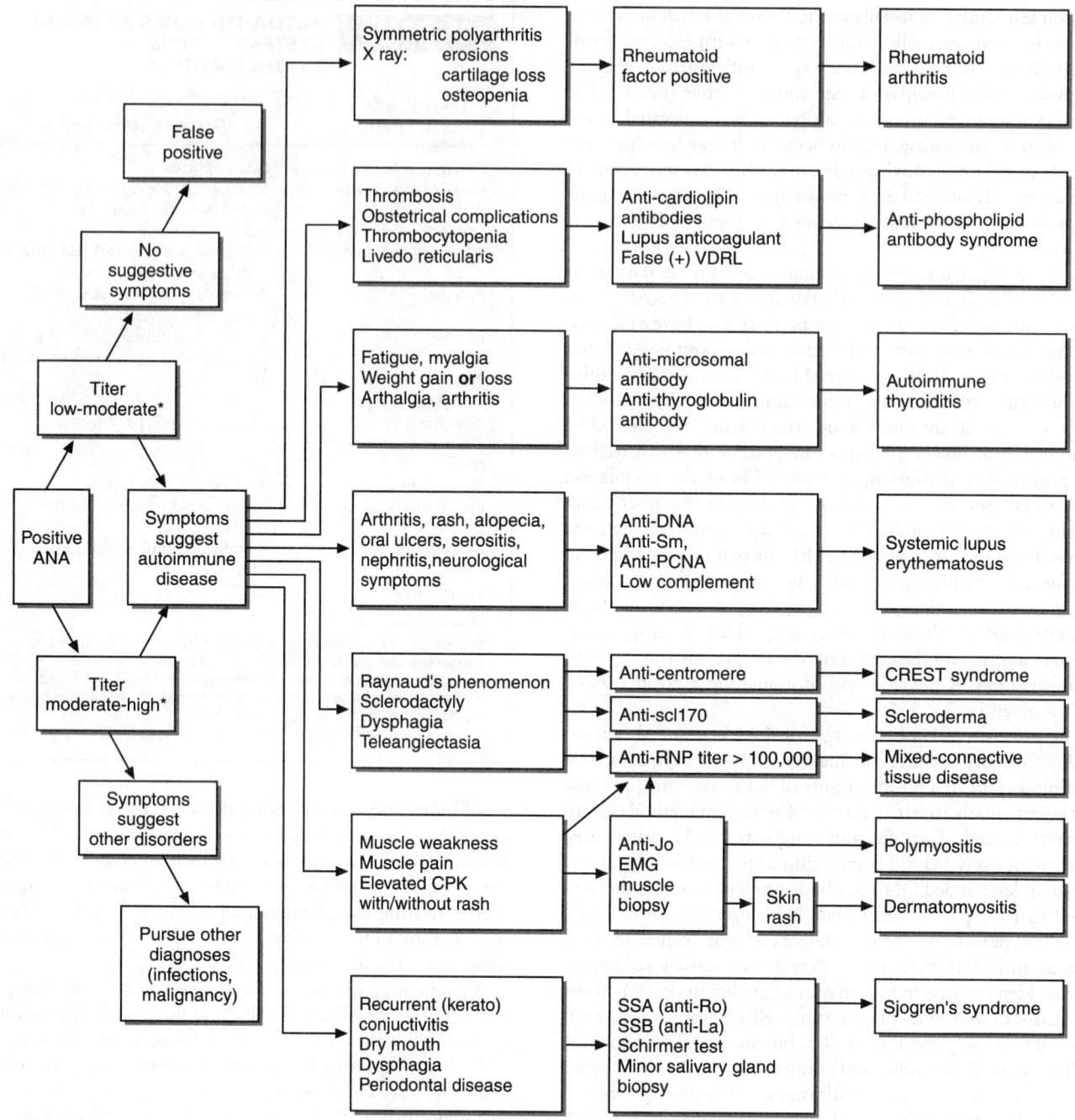

*low-moderate-high titer depends on the specific laboratory used; an example would be: low = 1: 80, moderate = 1: 160-320, high = 1: 640 or greater

FIGURE 178.2. Evaluating a positive antinuclear antibody (ANA) result.
EVIDENCE LEVEL: C. Expert Opinion.

Cerebrospinal fluid in patients with overt CNS lupus can show pleiocytosis and elevated protein levels, and antiribosomal P and antineuronal antibodies can be found in some patients' CSF even when results are negative in serum. Ancillary diagnostic studies are of great importance in the evaluation of patients with suspected or confirmed SLE. These tests generally can be guided by the symptoms, signs, and findings on laboratory studies. They include radiographs of heart, lungs and affected joints; echocardiography for the evaluation of peri-, myo-, and endocar-

dial involvement; high-resolution computed tomography of the lungs to define parenchymal lung disease; and magnetic resonance imaging of the CNS to evaluate patients with CNS lupus. Specialized diagnostic studies of the CNS are under investigation because of the difficulties in correlating CNS symptoms with objective findings in some patients, but positron emission tomography, single-positron emission computerized tomography, magnetic resonance spectroscopy, and others are still largely experimental.

Biopsies are invaluable in the evaluation of skin and kidney disease. The skin biopsy result of patients with SLE shows the "lupus band test," deposition of immune complexes and complement products in a granular pattern at the dermal–epidermal junction. This pattern can be seen even in clinically unaffected skin. The kidney biopsy in SLE may evince any of a number of histopathologic changes; they have been distinguished as WHO classes I to VI, the higher classes reflecting more serious disease (Table 178.3). Both immunofluorescence and electron microscopy are necessary for correct interpretation of the renal histopathologic features of SLE.

OPTIMAL MANAGEMENT

DIAGNOSIS

The time when a patient is first diagnosed with SLE marks a watershed in the individual's life and should be treated with due respect. The failure to diagnose SLE when it is present is usually of less dramatic consequence than the mistake of diagnosing SLE incorrectly. A false diagnosis of SLE results in great distress for the patient, and a common practical problem is that it is very difficult to reverse this incorrect diagnosis, particularly in those individuals who experience symptoms for which no other explanation has been found.

Figure 178.3 indicates a suggested path to follow when considering the diagnosis of SLE. The diagnosis of SLE should be considered only when suspicion is aroused by an appropriate set of symptoms. In such individuals, a positive ANA test result can strengthen the suspicion, whereas a negative test result should direct the evaluation toward other, more likely diagnoses. A positive ANA result also opens up the possibility of finding more disease-specific autoantibodies, such as anti-DNA. After completion of this evaluation, one can take stock of the net result in terms of positive and negative findings. The ACR criteria can serve as a useful reference frame, but many other symptoms

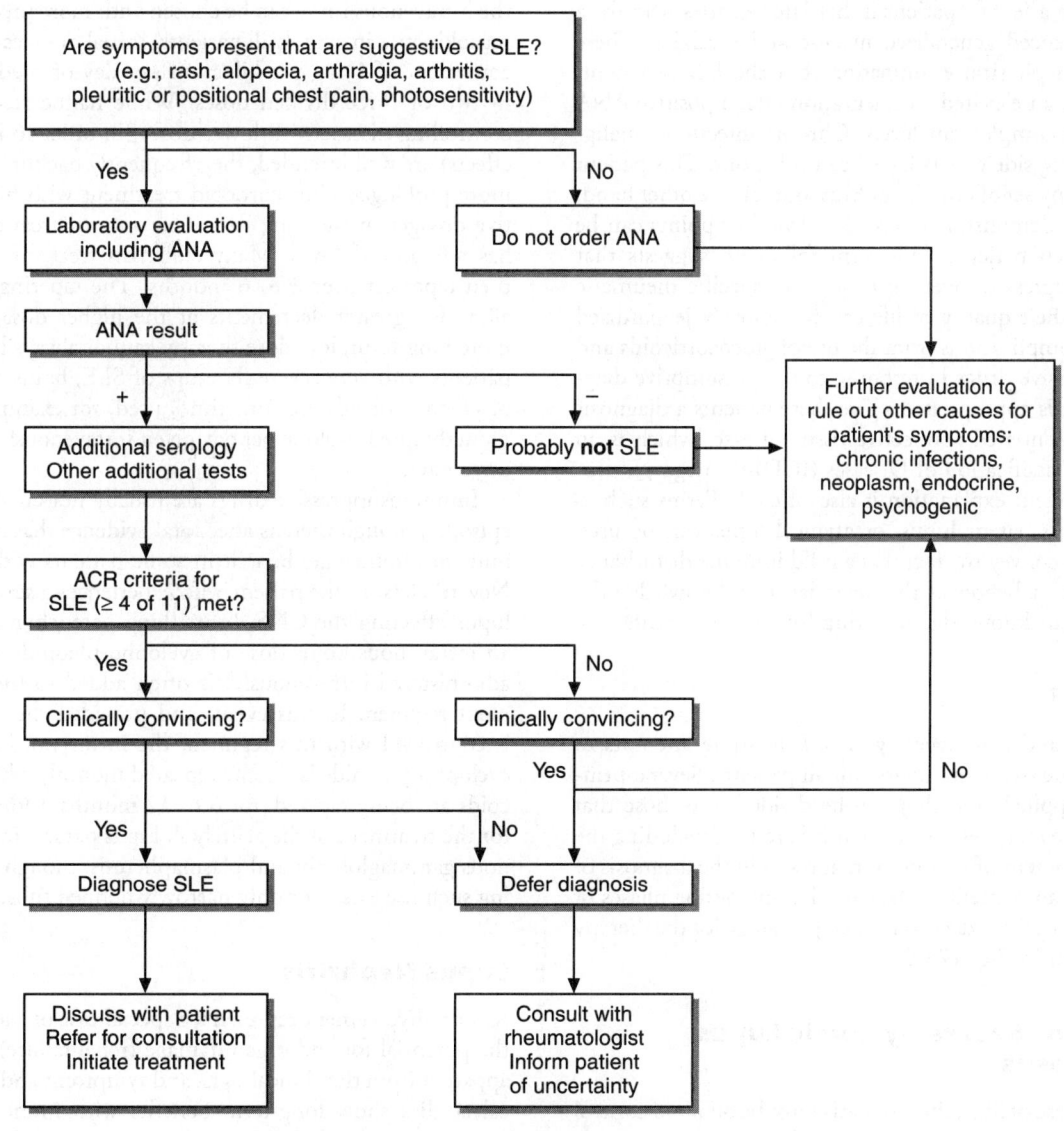

FIGURE 178.3. Diagnosis of sytemic lupus erythematosus (SLE).
EVIDENCE LEVEL: C. Expert Opinion.

and signs can be present or absent in patients under evaluation. Important clues that SLE is the correct diagnosis include previous episodes in the patient's history of unexplained inflammatory disease (arthritis, pleurisy, pericarditis, aseptic meningitis) or obstetrical complications, persistent subtle markers of systemic inflammation (non–iron deficiency anemia, elevated erythrocyte sedimentation rate), unexplained leukopenia, photosensitivity, hair loss, nonspecific rashes, lymphadenopathy, and temperature elevations. Conversely, the absence of all these symptoms should prompt due hesitation about the diagnosis.

If such a rigorous workup uncovers four or more ACR criteria plus a host of other consistent findings, the diagnosis should be made and discussed with the patient. More frequently, uncertainty will persist even when the diagnosis is likely correct. In either instance, confirmatory consultation with a rheumatologist (second opinion) is appropriate. Unless there is abundant evidence to suggest SLE, the diagnosis probably should be deferred. A relatively common situation arises when patients have objective evidence of chronic mild systemic inflammation and some evidence of autoimmunity, without other explanation. One example would be a female patient in her late twenties who for a year has experienced generalized malaise and myalgias. There are no signs on physical examination, but she has persistent, modest anemia; an elevated sedimentation rate; a positive ANA result, and low complement levels. Chronic infections, malignancies, and drug side effects have been ruled out. This patient does not meet any set of criteria for SLE, but, on the other hand, she does have a demonstrable disorder. Two key points can be made about such patients: long-term follow-up suggests that they do not progress to overt SLE or other specific rheumatic disorders, and their quality of life can be seriously jeopardized by iatrogenic complications from the use of glucocorticoids and immunosuppressive drugs in response to the presumptive diagnosis of SLE. It is appropriate to give these patients a diagnosis such as undifferentiated connective tissue disease [which is an International Classification of Diseases (ICD)-9 category], provided that sufficient explanation is also offered. Terms such as incomplete lupus, latent lupus, or atypical lupus can be used with caution to convey the fact that a mild immune disturbance may be present. It behooves the physician to acknowledge the limitations of our knowledge in caring for such a patient.

TREATMENT

The variability and heterogeneity of SLE frustrate attempts to prescribe any one treatment course for all patients. Several principles can be applied, and they can be divided into those that should guide the treatment of acute SLE flare-ups, including the de novo development of symptoms that result in the diagnosis of SLE, and the management of the chronic, smoldering phases of the disease. A simplified decision-making strategy for the therapy of lupus is given in Fig. 178.4.

Acute and/or Severe Systemic Lupus Erythematosus

In the active phase of SLE, the emphasis must be on rapid control of disease symptoms tailored to the individual patient. The medications chosen to accomplish this goal must be adapted to the organs involved and the activity of the disease in those organs (Table 178.2), taking into account the potential for end-organ damage. For example, the patient with an acute flare-up of arthritis, pleurisy, or pericarditis can sometimes be treated with NSAIDs. This class of agents is not easy to use in lupus patients, because several toxicities can interact unfavorably with lupus manifestations per se. For example, the nephritis and hypertension common to SLE can be aggravated by NSAIDs, and some NSAIDs, including ibuprofen, can cause aseptic meningitis, particularly in patients with SLE. There are no rules that predict which NSAID would be of most benefit for which patient. The development of new COX-2-selective NSAIDs may limit toxicity, but data as to efficacy in patients with SLE are lacking.

The mainstay of therapy in active SLE is glucocorticoids. The efficacy of glucocorticoids and their rapid onset of action make them particularly suitable for treatment of newly developed severe lupus manifestations, whether at the first presentation of the illness or as a flare-up punctuating a more chronic course. Glucocorticoids are usually effective when taken orally, though the intravenous route can be chosen with more predictable pharmacokinetics in acutely ill patients. Initial dosages should be the equivalent of 1 mg per kilogram per day of prednisone, given in two or three divided doses. While halfhearted attempts at controlling disease with lower doses (in order to minimize side effects) are well intended, they frequently backfire by leading to more prolonged glucocorticoid treatment with higher cumulative dosages in the long run. The optimal treatment duration has not been defined. Many clinicians treat for 1 month and then taper off over 2 to 6 months. The tapering regimen can allow for greater decrements at the higher dosage levels, but more long-term, low-dose therapy cannot always be avoided. In patients with very severe flare-ups of SLE, bolus or pulse doses of glucocorticoids are sometimes used, for example, 1,000 mg of methylprednisolone per day given intravenously for 3 consecutive days.

Immunosuppressive drugs are usually not effective for acute episodes, though there is anecdotal evidence that cyclophosphamide has immediate benefit in some patients with CNS lupus. Nevertheless, in the patient who experiences a severe flare-up of lupus affecting the CNS, heart, lung parenchyma, or kidneys, an intravenous bolus dose of cyclophosphamide (0.5 to 1.0 g, administered intravenously) is often added to the initial treatment regimen. In this event, and provided the lupus flare-up is controlled with this regimen, the intravenous bolus dose of cyclophosphamide is usually repeated monthly while glucocorticoids are being tapered, for 6 to 12 months. Other agents used for the treatment of the acutely ill lupus patient include intravenous gammaglobulin and plasmapheresis, though data supporting such use exists for only narrowly defined subsets of patients.

Lupus Nephritis

Kidney involvement represents a special case of therapy, because the potential for end-organ damage (renal failure) is not always apparent from the clinical signs and symptoms and because clinical studies show long-term benefits with immunosuppressive treatment, particularly with cyclophosphamide. Management of

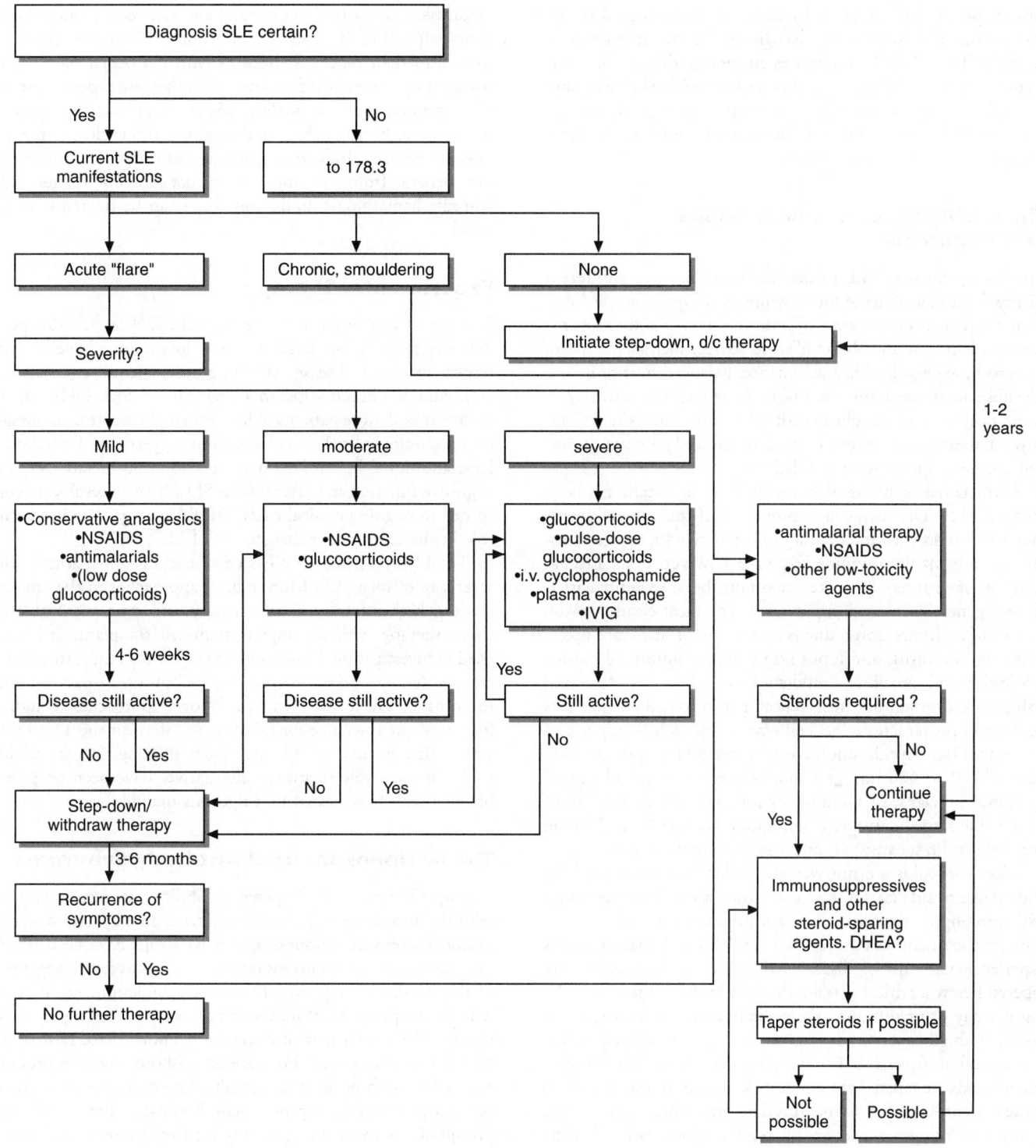

FIGURE 178.4. Treatment of systemic lupus erythematosus (SLE).
EVIDENCE LEVEL: C. Expert Opinion.

lupus nephritis depends critically on the renal histologic features, and consultation with a nephrologist and a rheumatologist is essential. Table 178.3 summarizes current guidelines for treatment of lupus nephritis. Note that patients with SLE who have reached end-stage renal disease and are undergoing dialysis often have very little active SLE and can be good candidates for renal transplant if a donor is available.

Chronic Phase of Systemic Lupus Erythematosus

The management of SLE in the chronic phase is of a different nature from that of acute lupus symptoms. Prevention of long-term consequences, in terms of both the disease and iatrogenic damage, is paramount. Basic lifestyle advice, such as the use of sunscreen, general health maintenance, balanced nutrition, and psychosocial support, must not be neglected. Conservative treatment options include glucocorticoid creams for skin lesions, physical therapy and splints for mild muscle and joint symptoms, and analgesic agents when needed.

Antimalarial agents are very useful in the long-term management of SLE. The therapeutic properties of this class of agents may have to do with their ability to interfere with antigen-processing steps in the immune response; however, other mechanisms of action may be more important, because antimalarials are not generally immunosuppressive. The most clearly proven benefit of hydroxychloroquine is prevention of SLE flare-ups; a lessening of arthritis and lupus skin lesions, diminished photosensitivity, and, possibly, a mild cholesterol-lowering effect and a slight antithrombotic effect may all play a role. Some patients perceive improvements in general symptoms, such as fatigue and lassitude. Hydroxychloroquine is administered as a single daily dose of 200 to 400 mg, and routine eye exams are advocated by some clinicians, to monitor for the very rare eventuality of irreversible retinal damage. Chloroquine given at 60 to 250 mg per day can be substituted, but it may be more retinotoxic.

Glucocorticoids are not well suited for long-term use. The wide range of side effects, many of which are a virtual certainty with prolonged treatment, makes it imperative to try to minimize glucocorticoid exposure. On the other hand, many patients experience flare-ups of disease activity when these agents are tapered below a critical threshold, often in the range of 5 to 15 mg per day of prednisone. To facilitate tapering, alternate-day dosing with glucocorticoids is advocated by some clinicians, but it is not often successful. The symptoms encountered when glucocorticoids are tapered are sometimes difficult to classify: while some patients experience true SLE flare-ups, others have diffuse, nonspecific symptoms that are the result of glucocorticoid-withdrawal syndrome or even adrenal insufficiency.

Joint and muscle pain without objective inflammation, that is, arthralgias and myalgias, should be treated as conservatively as possible. The patient's expectations may need to be addressed, since some degree of joint or muscle discomfort may be impossible to avoid. Nonpharmacologic interventions, including physical therapy, are preferable. Some patients respond well to mild analgesics or low doses of antidepressants. Vigilance is needed to rule out other causes of noninflammatory pain, especially since thyroid abnormalities and psychogenic causes of pain (depression, somatization disorder) are relatively common in patients with SLE. If patients consistently fail to gain sufficient control of their disease symptoms with glucocorticoids and/or consistently experience flare-ups when they are tapered, the use of immunosuppressive medications as steroid-sparing agents is appropriate. Azathioprine, methotrexate, and cyclosporin A are possible choices. Individual patients with chronic skin lesions can benefit from treatment with dapsone or thalidomide. Chronic hematologic lupus sometimes can be treated with danazol.

Experimental Therapy

In patients with mild to moderate SLE, DHEA at a dosage of 200 mg per day has been reported to produce benefits with respect to overall disease activity, glucocorticoid requirements, and reduction in flare-ups. In a large clinical trial, DHEA treatment allowed more patients to lower their glucocorticoid dosages to a physiologic level. Smaller studies suggest that DHEA may have additional benefits with respect to bone metabolism and cognitive function in patients with SLE. If these results are confirmed in ongoing clinical trials, DHEA may gain an important role in the long-term management of SLE.

Total lymph irradiation has been used in some patients with severe, refractory SLE. More radical approaches to therapy, including high-intensity chemotherapy and even myeloablative chemotherapy with autologous stem-cell transplant, are being tried in investigational studies in several centers; these treatments are clearly appropriate for only a small group of patients with the most severe forms of disease. Novel approaches to induce immunologic tolerance for DNA or to interrupt the T-cell activation that occurs in SLE are under investigation in clinical trials. Innumerable treatment alternatives have been proposed, but few have been tested in a rigorous manner.

The Antiphospholipid Antibody Syndrome

Attempts to control the hypercoagulability state seen in patients with the antiphospholipid antibody syndrome by administering glucocorticoids or immunosuppressive drugs have been largely unsuccessful, and the current recommendations for management of this syndrome rely entirely on anticoagulation. For patients who have experienced thromboembolic events, lifelong anticoagulation with warfarin at an international normalized ratio of 3.0 to 4.0 is recommended. For patients without any such previous events but with positive test results, low-dose aspirin seems to be a reasonable form of prophylaxis. Pregnant women with antiphospholipid antibodies generally require treatment with heparin, low-molecular-weight heparin, and/or aspirin; they should be treated by an obstetrician who is experienced in high-risk pregnancies.

Preventive Therapy

Patients with SLE will want to know how to prevent lupus flare-ups. Although there are no proven ways of doing so, the following list gives common-sense recommendations that are valid for most patients:

- Avoid ultraviolet light exposure not only through the use of sunscreens but by staying out of the sunlight or wearing protective clothing.
- Avoid exercising to exhaustion. Whereas a solid cardiovascular workout is very beneficial, the effects of extreme physical efforts are likely to trigger increased lupus activity, possibly through the release of nuclear material from damaged cells into the circulation or through the release of cytokines.
- Avoid infections. Many common respiratory infections can be prevented by frequent washing of the hands and other simple hygiene measures.
- Pregnancy may entail a slightly increased risk of a lupus flare-up, and the patient facing the highly personal decision of becoming pregnant is entitled to know this. She also should be informed that breast-feeding may increase the risk of a postpartum flare-up (through the proinflammatory effects of prolactin).

Prevention of disease-related as well as treatment-related long-term consequences of SLE is very important. Risk factors for arteriosclerotic disease should be identified and treated aggressively. Most patients on prolonged treatment with glucocorticoids have some degree of dyslipidemia, hypercholesterolemia, or hypertriglyceridemia. Appropriate dietary advice and, if necessary, lipid-lowering therapy should be provided. An elevated serum homocysteine level is an independent risk factor for arteriosclerosis and may be present to an even higher degree in patients with SLE. Diagnosis of this condition and treatment with vitamins B_6 and B_{12} and folic acid is likely to minimize morbidity and mortality.

Patients on moderate- to high-dose glucocorticoids and immunosuppressive agents, such as cyclophosphamide, have a higher risk of infection. Common-sense avoidance of potential sources of infection (hand washing, use of disinfectants) can be discussed with each patient. Prophylaxis against *Pneumocystis carinii* pneumonia can be considered. Immunizations have been scrutinized with regard to the potential of inducing SLE flare-ups; on balance, vaccines against influenza and pneumococcus are appropriate for patients with lupus, whereas live/attenuated vaccines should be avoided in a person with immunosuppression.

Prevention of osteoporosis should begin before bone is lost, that is, at the inception of glucocorticoid therapy. Calcium (1,000 to 1,500 mg per day) and vitamin D supplementation should be prescribed to all patients, and the benefits of weight-bearing activities must be explained. Patients at higher risk of osteoporosis may be candidates for antiresorptive medications (bisphosphonates, calcitonin). Whether postmenopausal women with SLE should receive hormone replacement therapy is the subject of controversy; it seems that the slight risk of enhanced SLE activity could be outweighed readily by advantages with respect to arteriosclerotic disease and bone metabolism. The adrenal androgen DHEA, which is under investigation for the treatment of SLE, may have benefits for bone metabolism as well.

Treatment of Overlap Syndromes

The treatment of patients with overlap syndromes as well as those with undifferentiated connective tissue disease is targeted to the specific organ systems involved. For example, the manifestations of Sjögren's syndrome seen in the context of SLE can be treated as they would in the primary disease: artificial tears for the eyes, pilocarpine or saliva substitutes (which are less successful than was hoped), and increased dental care. Sclerodermatous features often respond poorly to immunosuppressive therapies and may require more conservative measures. On the other hand, scleroderma renal disease responds well to angiotensin-converting enzyme inhibitors, and, in the case of gastrointestinal scleroderma, the use of pro-motility agents can improve quality of life.

COURSE AND PROGNOSIS

The 5- and 10-year survival rates of SLE have improved considerably over the past several decades. Renal disease can be treated more effectively, but SLE affecting the CNS, lungs, heart, and gastrointestinal tract can still be frustrating at times. The prognosis for the individual patient depends on many factors, including the clinical symptoms, affected organ systems, and comorbid conditions. The long-term consequences of SLE, including the late lupus syndrome, are of concern. Nevertheless, the closing years of the twentieth century have seen an unprecedented increase in our knowledge and understanding of SLE as well as the introduction of large-scale clinical trials of several new therapeutic agents with new and, in some instances, unique modes of action that, if successful, will herald a new era in the treatment of SLE.

BIBLIOGRAPHY

Canadian Hydroxychloroquine Study Group. A randomized study of the effect of withdrawing hydroxychloroquine sulfate in systemic lupus erythematosus. *N Engl J Med* 1991;324:150–154.

Carbotte RM, Denburg SD, Denburg JA. Prevalence of cognitive impairment in systemic lupus erythematosus. *J Nerv Ment Dis* 1986;174: 357–364.

Hochberg MC. Updating the American College of Rheumatology revised criteria for the classification of systemic lupus erythematosus. *Arthritis Rheum* 1997;40:1725.

James JA, Kaufman KM, Farris AD, et al. An increased prevalence of Epstein–Barr virus infection in young patients suggests a possible etiology for systemic lupus erythematosus. *J Clin Invest* 1997;100:3019–3026.

Mehrian R, Quismorio FP, Strassmann G, et al. Synergistic effect between IL-10 and *bcl-2* genotypes in determining susceptibility to systemic lupus erythematosus. *Arthritis Rheum* 1998;41:596–602.

Nesher G, Hanna VE, Moore TL, et al. Thrombotic microangiographic hemolytic anemia in systemic lupus erythematosus. *Semin Arthritis Rheum* 1994;24:165–172.

Sharp GC, Irvin WS, Tan EM, et al. Mixed connective tissue disease—an apparently distinct rheumatic disease syndrome associated with a specific antibody to an extractable nuclear antigen (ENA). *Am J Med* 1972;52: 148–159.

Steinberg AD, Gourley M. Cyclophosphamide in lupus nephritis. *J Rheumatol* 1995;22:1812–1815.

Tsao BP, Cantor RM, Kalunian KC, et al. Evidence for linkage of a candidate chromosome 1 region to human systemic lupus erythematosus. *J Clin Invest* 1997;99:725–731.

Van Vollenhoven RF, Engleman EG, McGuire JL. Dehydroepiandrosterone (DHEA) in systemic lupus erythematosus: results of a double-blinded, placebo-controlled, randomized clinical trial. *Arthritis Rheum* 1995;38:1826–1831.

Kelley's Textbook of Internal Medicine, fourth edition. Edited by H. David Humes. Lippincott Williams & Wilkins, Philadelphia © 2000.

179

SCLERODERMA AND RAYNAUD'S SYNDROME

JAMES R. SEIBOLD

Systemic sclerosis (scleroderma) is characterized by thickening and fibrosis of the skin (scleroderma) and by distinctive forms of internal organ involvement. The cause and pathogenesis are unknown, and effective disease-modifying treatment is lacking. Morbidity and mortality are related directly to the extent and severity of visceral involvement, which in turn are related closely to the pace of disease progression and the extent of skin involvement. The recognition of well-defined subgroups within the diagnosis of scleroderma is important in determining prognosis and planning therapy.

INCIDENCE AND EPIDEMIOLOGY

Modern studies have suggested an annual incidence of scleroderma of 1 to 2 per 100,000 population. The onset of scleroderma is highest in the fourth and fifth decades of life, and the disease is four times more common in women. It is likely that many cases of scleroderma are misdiagnosed as isolated Raynaud's phenomenon (RP), primary pulmonary hypertension, or primary biliary cirrhosis, particularly in individuals with limited and subtle skin changes. The development of scleroderma is not linked to race or geography in any consistent fashion, and familial occurrence is uncommon. Genetic contribution is suspected from studies of a case cluster in Choctaw Indians of Oklahoma. Case reports and series linking silicone gel breast implants and occupational exposures to organic solvents have not been supported by epidemiologic surveys.

ETIOLOGY AND PATHOGENESIS

Any hypothesis concerning the pathogenesis of scleroderma must account for the heterogeneity of patterns of disease progression and extent, the common and somewhat characteristic immunologic abnormalities, the accelerated rate of accumulation of collagen and other extracellular matrix components, and the prominent and characteristic abnormalities of vascular structure and function. The sporadic occurrence of scleroderma and the absence of strong genetic or environmental causative factors have prevented recognition of a "prescleroderma" state. Therefore, reasonable information on early pathogenesis is lacking.

Raynaud's phenomenon is the initial complaint in about 70% of patients and results largely from narrowing of digital arterial

lumina secondary to intimal accumulation of ground substance and collagen. Similar fibrotic and arteriosclerotic changes occur in the vasculature of the heart, lungs, kidneys, and gastrointestinal tract and contribute to the dysfunction of these organs. Swelling and disruption of the endothelium of the arteriolar and capillary beds occur at the earliest recognizable stages of disease. Examination of the nail fold tissues by in vivo wide-field microscopy reveals enlargement and tortuosity of capillary loops interspersed with areas of capillary obliteration. Similar changes occur in the microvasculature of the internal organs. The factors responsible for this vascular injury are unknown. Chronic, ongoing endothelial injury and repair is suggested by the finding of increased levels of factor VIII/von Willebrand's factor and adhesion molecules as well as by measures of *in vivo* platelet activation. Vascular inflammation is uncommon.

The biology of established disease has been more amenable to study. Early tissue lesions feature the ingress of immigrant inflammatory cell populations, including helper–inducer T lymphocytes, monocytes, and mast cells. These cells in turn release proinflammatory and profibrotic growth factors/cytokines locally. Autocrine effects of growth factors such as transforming growth factor β from nonlesional cell populations such as circulating platelets also are implicated. The net effect of this complex array of cells and signals is the accumulation of extracellular matrix, predominantly collagen but also glycosaminoglycan, fibronectin, adherence molecules, and tissue water (edema). Cytokine-driven selection of hypersecretory and hyperproliferative dermal fibroblast subpopulations in involved skin of patients with scleroderma results in excessive accumulation of the principal skin collagens, types I and III. The collagen is biochemically normal, and the proportion of type I to type III collagen is that of normal skin. Studies with clonal DNAs have demonstrated increased transcription of messenger RNA for types I and III collagen and no evidence of a disease-associated genomic polymorphism for collagen. Dermal collagenase activity appears to be unaffected.

Elevated levels of serum interleukin-2, interleukin-6, and soluble interleukin-2 receptors are present in scleroderma and are linked to the clinical progression of disease. This evidence of T-cell activation suggests a role for lymphokines that stimulate collagen production or that stimulate other cells, such as monocytes or mast cells. Human chronic graft-versus-host disease is associated with similar dermal fibrotic changes. There is evidence of fetal microchimerism both in peripheral blood and involved skin of patients with scleroderma lending credence to the hypothesis that scleroderma may be partially graft-vs.-host in mechanism. Mast cell infiltrates and evidence of local mast cell degranulation are present in skin and internal organs. Marked and persistent reduction of collagen accumulation by scleroderma dermal fibroblasts in response to interferon-γ has focused attention on the potential role of the monocyte. Transforming growth factor β and other platelet-derived growth factors are released during platelet activation and may mediate fibroblast proliferation and further endothelial injury in scleroderma.

Tissue injury in internal organs is centered around the small arteriole and, as in the skin, features varying contributions of fibrosis, inflammation, and obliterative vascular change.

Serum antinuclear antibodies are present in 90% of patients with scleroderma and disease-specific serologic abnormalities have been defined. About 60% to 70% of patients with limited scleroderma have serum antibodies to centromeric and kinetochore proteins. About 30% to 40% of patients with diffuse or generalized disease have serum antibodies to DNA topoisomerase I (previously known as Scl-70). The antigenicity of DNA topoisomerase I resides in an 11-amino-acid sequence closely homologous to that of a group-specific antigen of some mammalian retroviruses. An additional 30% to 40% of patients with diffuse scleroderma have antibodies to RNA polymerases I and III. Cell injury in conditions of hypoxemia/reperfusion leads to selective release of scleroderma-specific antigens.

CLINICAL FINDINGS

EARLY DIAGNOSIS

Scleroderma is variable in extent and progression but can be grouped into two principal syndromes of prognostic and therapeutic importance. Patients with diffuse or generalized scleroderma are at risk for rapidly progressive and widespread skin involvement and the early development of the full complement of internal organ abnormalities. A nearly equal number of patients have slowly progressive skin changes that usually are restricted to the fingers, hands, and face, and may have an extended course of illness before the development of visceral abnormalities. Historically termed the CREST syndrome variant of scleroderma (subcutaneous calcinosis, Raynaud's phenomenon, esophageal dysmotility, sclerodactyly, telangiectasia), these patients have limited scleroderma.

RAYNAUD'S PHENOMENON

Raynaud's phenomenon is the clinical syndrome of episodic color changes of the digits in response to cold and, in some patients, emotional stress. Although not all patients have the complete syndrome, the typical sequence is pallor (arterial constriction), followed by cyanosis (venospasm and desaturation of hemoglobin), followed by reactive hyperemia.

The exact incidence of RP is not known but may be as high as 10% in selected populations, such as premenopausal women. Most patients with RP have structurally normal blood vessels and no evidence of an underlying disease process (primary RP). Within this larger group are individuals whose presentation is indicative of structural vascular disease and hemorheologic abnormalities (secondary RP). Blood flow to the skin is 10 to 20 times that required for oxygenation and nutrition; alterations of perfusion to the skin are a principal homeostatic mechanism of thermoregulation. Irrespective of cause, patients with RP have undue intolerance to environmental cold. No single pathophysiologic mechanism explains cold-induced vasospasm in all forms of the syndrome, and there is no single form of RP in which the cause is completely understood. Table 179.1 classifies the diverse clinical syndromes associated with RP according to the

TABLE 179.1.	A MECHANISTIC CLASSIFICATION OF RAYNAUD'S PHENOMENON

Vasospastic

Primary (idiopathic) Raynaud's phenomenon
Drug-induced
β-Adrenergic blockers
Ergot
Methysergide
Pheochromocytoma
Variant angina
Migraine

Structural

Vibration syndrome
Arteriosclerosis
Thromboangiitis obliterans
Cold injury (frostbite, pernio, immersion foot)
Neurovascular compression (thoracic outlet syndrome, carpal tunnel syndrome, crutch pressure)
Chemotherapy (bleomycin, vinblastine)
Polyvinyl chloride disease
Connective tissue disease
   Systemic sclerosis
   Systemic lupus erythematosus
   Overlap syndrome
   Polymyositis/dermatomyositis
   Rheumatoid arthritis

Hemorrheologic

Cryoglobulinemia
Cryofibrinogenemia
Cold agglutinin disease
Paraproteinemia (plasma cell dyscrasia)
Polycythemia (essential thrombocythemia polycythemia vera)

assumed principal mechanism: vasospastic, structural, or hemorrheologic.

RAYNAUD'S PHENOMENON AND SCLERODERMA

The typical sequence of clinical events in all forms of scleroderma is RP, followed by finger and hand edema, followed by tightening and thickening of the skin. The order of events and their temporal association are important clues to clinical classification. In diffuse scleroderma, RP may be concomitant in onset or may be preceded by finger edema, skin thickening, polyarthralgia, or signs of specific internal organ involvement. In limited scleroderma, patients may have RP alone for years, even decades, before more specific manifestations of scleroderma develop.

The assessment of RP as an isolated clinical complaint forces the consideration of a wide range of seemingly unrelated conditions (Table 179.1). Much information can be obtained from a directed history and physical examination. The criteria for primary RP include the presence of at least two of the three characteristic color changes in response to cold, bilateral involvement, normal radial artery pulsations, absence of digital ischemic injury, and absence of clinical evidence of an underlying causal disease.

TABLE 179.2.	CLINICAL FEATURES HELPFUL IN DISTINGUISHING PRIMARY RAYNAUD'S PHENOMENON FROM RAYNAUD'S PHENOMENON OF EARLY CONNECTIVE TISSUE DISEASE	

Clinical Feature	Primary Raynaud's Phenomenon	Raynaud's Phenomenon Secondary to Connective Tissue Disease
Sex	Overwhelmingly female	Male and female
Age of onset	Menarche	Mid-20s and later
Extent	Usually all digits	Often begins in a single digit
Symptoms	Mild to moderate	Moderate to severe
Attacks with emotional stress	Yes	Unusual
Ischemic injury	No	Yes
Finger edema	Rare	Common
Periungual erythema	Rare	Common
Evidence of other vasomotor syndromes (e.g., migraine)	Yes	No

A special area of concern is the recognition of early connective tissue disease, particularly in patients suspected of having early limited scleroderma. The age of onset is an important clue because primary RP typically begins in the teens to early 20s, whereas secondary forms of RP begin later in life. Raynaud's phenomenon in men usually is a secondary form of the syndrome (Table 179.2).

SKIN INVOLVEMENT

The initial skin edema of the fingers and other sites typically is painless but may be accompanied by symptoms of morning stiffness, arthralgia, and carpal tunnel syndrome, suggesting the diagnosis of early rheumatoid arthritis or systemic lupus erythematosus. As the edema lessens, tightening and thickness of the skin develops, usually beginning on the fingers. In diffuse scleroderma, this transformation usually ensues within weeks to a few months, whereas in limited scleroderma, the edematous phase may persist for years before actual skin thickening occurs. Rare patients have *systemic sclerosis sine scleroderma,* in which typical vascular and internal organ features of scleroderma are seen but skin changes never develop.

MUSCULOSKELETAL FEATURES

As skin thickening worsens, the underlying joints become tethered and restricted in motion. Patients with diffuse disease may have painful involvement of tendon sheaths, which can mimic inflammatory arthritis. Leathery friction rubs may be palpated during active or passive motion of involved areas. Arthritic complaints are common and erosive arthropathy occasionally occurs. Restricted motion leads to disuse atrophy of the muscles, and weakness may be worsened by accompanying skeletal muscle inflammation. Ischemic ulcerations of the fingertips occur in 10% to 20% of patients per year and the fingers themselves may shorten and atrophy from disuse and ischemic resorption of the

phalanges. Skin tightening on the face may restrict the ability to open the mouth and impair adequate dental hygiene.

GASTROINTESTINAL INVOLVEMENT

The gastrointestinal tract is involved in all forms of scleroderma. Atrophy of the muscularis is followed by submucosal fibrosis. Weakness of the lower esophageal sphincter is associated with chronic reflux esophagitis. Hypomotility of the lower esophagus causes symptoms of dysphagia for solid foods, which may be worsened significantly by lower esophageal stricture secondary to chronic reflux. Ease of satiety and dyspepsia may occur as a result of impaired motility of the stomach. Small bowel involvement presents as intermittent abdominal cramping and diarrhea. Malabsorption can occur and weight loss is seen in virtually all patients. Bacterial overgrowth in areas of intraluminal stagnation is an important cause of diarrhea and cramping in some patients. Colon involvement is typified by complaints of constipation. Wide-mouthed diverticula may occur but seldom are a source of bleeding. Pseudo-obstruction is common, although hypomotile areas of large and small bowel also can lead to intussusception and volvulus. Gastrointestinal bleeding most commonly results from erosive esophagitis, but "watermelon stomach" also must be considered. Although hepatic involvement is uncommon, patients with limited scleroderma may have primary biliary cirrhosis.

CARDIAC INVOLVEMENT

Patchy fibrosis of the myocardium occurs in as many as 80% of patients with scleroderma. Contraction band necrosis has been reported, suggesting intermittent myocardial ischemia. A Raynaud's-like reactivity of the coronary microvasculature is suspected from studies demonstrating thallium perfusion abnormalities in most patients. Exertional dyspnea and palpitations are common, whereas chest pain and clinical congestive heart failure are not. Although pericardial fluid is demonstrable by echocardiography in 30% to 40% of patients, pericardial rubs and clinical presentations of pericarditis and tamponade are uncommon. Supraventricular and ventricular arrhythmias are seen in 60% to 70% of patients, and the latter are strongly associated with mortality, including sudden death. Involvement of the conduction system and bradyarrhythmias are encountered less commonly.

PULMONARY INVOLVEMENT

Pulmonary involvement is a major cause of morbidity and mortality in scleroderma. No organ illustrates the diversity of pathologic processes operative in scleroderma as well as the lung, in which any combination of interstitial inflammation, fibrosis, and pulmonary vascular injury may be present. Patients with diffuse scleroderma are more likely to have interstitial lung disease typified by basilar rales, abnormal chest radiographs, and loss of lung volume on pulmonary function testing. Patients with limited scleroderma are at risk for progressive pulmonary hypertension in the absence of interstitial lung disease and are more likely to demonstrate a disproportionate loss of pulmonary diffusing capacity. Gallium scanning is relatively insensitive in recognizing pulmonary inflammation. Nonetheless, bronchoalveolar lavage reveals increased numbers of neutrophils, lymphocytes, and, occasionally, eosinophils in 40% to 60% of patients, suggesting that inflammatory alveolitis precedes the interstitial fibrotic change.

RENAL INVOLVEMENT

The sudden onset of accelerated to malignant hypertension and progressive renal insufficiency, usually accompanied by microangiopathic hemolytic anemia, constitutes the syndrome of scleroderma renal crisis. Patients with diffuse scleroderma are at highest risk for this complication, which most often occurs in the first 2 to 3 years of illness, while skin involvement is the most progressive. Obliterative vasculopathy with cortical infarction is present and marked hyperreninemia is the principal mechanism of hypertension. The onset peaks during the cold-weather months. A Raynaud's-like mechanism overlying renal intimal fibrotic arteriosclerosis is supported by the demonstration of transient renal cortical perfusion abnormalities and increases in plasma renin activity during cold pressor tests. If scleroderma renal crisis is not recognized early, progression to irreversible renal failure and death is the rule.

ENDOCRINE AND EXOCRINE FEATURES

Hypothyroidism occurs in up to 50% of patients with scleroderma and often is occult. Although many patients have antithyroid antibodies, lymphocytic infiltration of the thyroid is uncommon and fibrotic replacement is typical. Dryness of the eyes and mouth is common and attributable to fibrosis of the lacrimal and salivary glands. Vaginal dryness and dyspareunia are common. Impotence is recognized as a presenting feature in men and is believed to be vascular in cause. Fertility is decreased in women, probably because of the severity of the illness. Increased fetal wastage and low birth weights are reported, but there is no specific evidence that pregnancy affects the mother's scleroderma.

LABORATORY FINDINGS

Specific laboratory tests that are useful in the assessment of internal organ involvement are discussed later. Nonspecific serologic abnormalities are common in scleroderma, including antinuclear antibodies in around 90% of patients (usually nucleolar in pattern), rheumatoid factor in 30%, and polyclonal hypergammaglobulinemia in 20% to 40%. Many patients have moderate elevations of the erythrocyte sedimentation rate and anemia of chronic disease, although neither abnormality has proven useful in monitoring disease activity. Anticentromere antibody is found in 50% to 60% of patients with limited scleroderma but rarely in those with diffuse disease. Its presence is useful in the classification of scleroderma and in the differential diagnosis of RP. Antibodies to DNA topoisomerase I and RNA polymerases I and III are of low sensitivity, being present as mutually exclusive findings in 20% to 40% of patients with diffuse scleroderma but are highly specific for this diagnosis.

COURSE AND PROGNOSIS

The natural history of systemic sclerosis has not been described adequately. Most of the clinical information has been derived from point prevalence surveys of specific features of the illness. Retrospective studies have suggested that patients with diffuse scleroderma typically have inexorable progression in the extent and severity of skin involvement during the first 2 to 3 years. The risk of new internal organ involvement is highest during this period. The disease then seems to plateau in many patients and skin involvement lessens slowly in later stages of the disease. The risk of new visceral involvement also is reduced, although spontaneous improvement of previously involved organs is unusual. Patients with limited scleroderma progress continually in skin disease and accrual of visceral involvement. Clinical change sometimes is so slow as to be unrecognizable from year to year. At late stages (more than 10 years), improving diffuse scleroderma and worsening limited scleroderma are nearly indistinguishable. Morbidity and mortality are related to visceral involvement. The early accrual of visceral involvement in diffuse scleroderma is responsible for a 5-year survival rate of 60%.

APPROACH TO ASSESSMENT

Once the diagnosis of scleroderma has been established, the clinician faces two principal issues. The first is classification of the disease as diffuse or limited, and the second is assessment of the presence, extent, and type of visceral involvement. Table 179.3

TABLE 179.3.	CLASSIFICATION AND ASSESSMENT OF SYSTEMIC SCLEROSIS	
	Diffuse Scleroderma	**Limited Scleroderma**
Onset of Raynaud's phenomenon	<2 y	>2 y
Initial symptoms	Finger edema	Raynaud's phenomenon
	Arthralgia	(>90%)
	Raynaud's phenomenon	
	Visceral complaint	
Tendon friction rubs	60%	<1%
Extent of skin involvement	Extremities and trunk	Extremities only
Pace of skin involvement	Rapid in first 2 y	Minimal
Visceral involvement[a]		
Gastrointestinal	90% early	70% early
Lung	70% early	60% late
Heart	50% early	50% late
Kidney	25% early	Rare
Anticentromere antibody	<5%	60–70%
Anti–topoisomerase I antibody	30–40%	<5%
Anti–RNA polymerase antibodies	20–30%	<5%

[a] Type of visceral involvement, total percentage risk, peak incidence of onset (early = first 3 years; late = after 3 years).

outlines the clinical and laboratory features that should be considered in the classification. Clinical assessment of the extent of skin involvement in scleroderma is the key determinant. The presence of skin thickening proximal to the elbows or knees, or on the chest or abdomen, indicates diffuse scleroderma. Restriction of skin changes to sites distal to the elbows, knees, and clavicles suggests limited disease. Because skin changes always begin on the extremities, a patient with early diffuse disease may have somewhat limited skin changes at the first assessment. Repeated, closely spaced clinical evaluations are necessary at this early, unclassifiable stage of disease.

Baseline determinations of internal organ involvement are important to follow-up care and recognition of changing status. Esophageal function can be assessed by a thin barium recumbent cinesophagraphy, manometry, or radionuclide esophagraphy. Small bowel involvement is studied best by D-xylose absorption. Barium enemas usually have no clinical value in scleroderma. Pulmonary function studies, including measures of diffusing capacity, and chest radiography are essential. The presence of alveolitis is determined by bronchoalveolar lavage or high-resolution computerized tomography. Ambulatory electrocardiography is believed to be the most sensitive and clinically valuable test of cardiac involvement. Urinalyses and measures of creatinine clearance should be performed. No reliable laboratory tools for the assessment of scleroderma activity are available. Serum-soluble interleukin-2 receptor levels are useful in predicting disease progression and mortality.

OTHER CLINICAL SYNDROMES

Scleroderma means "hard skin," and several clinical disorders are included in this differential diagnosis (Table 179.4). All of these disorders should be suspected in patients who do not have RP and in whom the skin changes begin at locations proximal to the digits. Eosinophilia–myalgia syndrome linked to contaminated L-tryptophan supplements and the closely related eosinophilic fasciitis syndrome are characterized by rapidly developing inflammation and induration of the arms, legs, and trunk. The

TABLE 179.4.	DIFFERENTIAL DIAGNOSIS OF SYSTEMIC SCLEROSIS (SCLERODERMA)

Disorders Characterized by Scleroderma

Eosinophilic fasciitis
Eosinophilia—myalgia syndrome
Scleredema adultorum
Scleromyxedema (papular mucinosis)
Bleomycin therapy
Chronic reflex sympathetic dystrophy
Chronic graft-versus-host disease
Subcutaneous morphea
Localized scleroderma
Carcinoid skin change
Overlap syndromes
Chronic diabetes mellitus

Disorders Characterized by Similar Internal Organ Involvement

Primary pulmonary hypertension
Primary biliary cirrhosis
Intestinal pseudo-obstruction
Collagenous colitis
Infiltrative cardiomyopathies
Idiopathic pulmonary fibrosis

Disorders Characterized by Raynaud's Phenomenon (see Table 179.1)

involved skin typically has an "orange-peel" appearance, and warmth and erythema are common. Joint contractures, neuromyopathy, and interstitial lung disease develop early. The diagnosis is established by full-thickness biopsy (skin to skeletal muscle) demonstrating inflammation and fibrosis centered in the deep fascia. Peripheral eosinophilia and an elevated erythrocyte sedimentation rate are present at early stages. Corticosteroid therapy is palliative and improvement to clinical resolution may occur in 2 to 5 years. Scleredema and scleromyxedema present as nonpitting edema and brawny induration of the face, upper back, chest, and shoulder girdles. Both conditions have been linked to underlying plasma cell dyscrasias, and about half of all adults with scleredema have associated diabetes mellitus. Scleroderma localized to the skin as linear scleroderma in children or as morphea in adults and children is not associated with visceral involvement. The subtle clinical features of limited scleroderma may be overlooked in patients believed to have "primary" biliary cirrhosis and pulmonary hypertension.

■ OPTIMAL MANAGEMENT

RAYNAUD'S PHENOMENON

All patients with RP, irrespective of cause, benefit from simple behavioral changes. Cessation of cigarette smoking is an absolute necessity. Careful planning of cold-weather activities can obviate the need for drug therapy. Dress can be important. In addition to warm mittens and footwear, hats and layered clothing on the trunk can minimize reflex responses to central body cold stimuli.

The choice of drug therapy is complicated by the wide range of available agents and the diverse mechanisms of RP. Many reported clinical trials lack careful definitions of the cause of RP or do not stratify by cause in their data analyses. Measures of therapeutic outcome are without standardization and include subjective parameters such as patient diaries, visual analogue ratings of the severity of RP episodes, and intermittent interviews focused on patient ratings of frequency, severity, and precipitating circumstances of attacks. Response rates to placebo typically are 30% to 40%. Physiologic measures of drug effect include tests of digital perfusion during cold challenge and indirect measures such as time of digital temperature recovery, the latter in effect monitoring only the phase of reactive hyperemia. It is common to encounter favorable subjective response in the absence of physiologic improvement.

Calcium channel blockers cause vascular smooth muscle relaxation by interfering with the transmembrane influx of calcium through membrane channels termed *slow channels*. Their antivasoconstrictive actions are well suited to intermittent vasospastic disorders such as RP, and agents active at receptor-operated calcium influx channels, including nifedipine, isradipine, and amlodipine, seem to be the most effective. Adverse effects include headache, dyspepsia, and fluid retention, but these can be minimized by the use of newly available time-release preparations of these agents. Inhibition of smooth muscle contractility may worsen intestinal dysmotility in patients with scleroderma.

Sympatholytic agents include reserpine, guanethidine, and prazosin. The peripheral vasodilative effects of prazosin, an orally active selective antagonist of α_1-adrenoceptors, are accompanied by little reflex tachycardia or increases in plasma renin and norepinephrine levels. Controlled studies suggest excellent responses in primary RP and in RP secondary to lupus; this agent is less effective in RP secondary to severe structural changes such as scleroderma. Nitroglycerin preparations are of little use, particularly in disorders typified by endothelial injury or by the concomitant use of cyclooxygenase inhibitors.

Antiplatelet agents, including low-dose aspirin and dipyridamole, often are used in scleroderma and other forms of RP resulting from intimal hyperplasia with endothelial injury and platelet activation. Although they are ineffective for RP itself, their use is associated with a reduction in digital ulceration. Similar effects are reported with pentoxifylline, an aminophylline derivative that enhances red blood cell flexibility and microvascular perfusion. Intravenous prostaglandin E_1 and carbaprostacyclin (Iloprost) are useful in the treatment of digital ulcerations complicating scleroderma but are unavailable in the United States.

Compromised ischemic digits require prompt diagnosis and aggressive treatment. Angiographic studies are useful for localizing sites of vascular occlusion and recognizing arterial emboli. The use of intra-arterial tolazoline in the assessment of reversible vasoconstriction guides subsequent therapeutic choices. Patients who are likely to benefit from sympathectomy can be chosen on the basis of their short-term responses to sympathetic ganglion instillation of bupivacaine.

Precision in clinical diagnosis leads to reasoned selection of therapy. Patients with functional vasospasm in the absence of structural narrowing of their digital arteries (primary RP) are at low risk for ischemic injury and typically have insufficiently severe subjective complaints to warrant therapy with vasoactive agents. Such patients often claim that emotional stress provokes attacks, and physiologic studies support the importance of peripheral adrenergic tone in these cases. Biofeedback and relaxation techniques are therapeutic options for these patients. Patients with secondary RP, including those with scleroderma or arteriosclerosis, commonly have functional evidence of diminished peripheral sympathetic tone. These patients are at high risk for digital ischemic injury.

SCLERODERMA

A successful disease-modifying therapy for scleroderma would enhance survival and reduce disability and comorbidity from the disease. These effects are equated with the behavior of internal organ involvement. An effective therapy for lung involvement would improve survival whereas an effect on skin involvement would likely enhance quality of life and function.

AN APPROACH TO THERAPY

The goals of therapy in scleroderma include prevention of disease worsening and/or reversal of accomplished tissue injury. At present, no therapies have emerged that influence the vascular component of disease although prostacyclin preparations are under study for scleroderma pulmonary hypertension. Modern prevention approaches utilize immunosuppressants with the theoretic goal of slowing development of fibrotic tissue injury. Well-controlled trials of methotrexate, chlorambucil, 5-fluorouracil, interferon-alpha and extracorporeal photoactivated methoxypsoralen have proven their lack of benefit. Uncontrolled studies of cyclophosphamide hint at efficacy for alveolitis and slower loss of forced vital capacity. Immunoablation with stem cell transplantation, thalidomide, and oral toleralization to Type I collagen are the subjects of ongoing trials.

Reversal of fibrosis would be expected to benefit patients with scleroderma. D-penicillamine has been used for its known effects in inhibiting intermolecular and intramolecular cross-linking of collagen. However, a multicenter comparison of 1,000 mg per day versus 125 mg every other day failed to demonstrate effect on survival, skin thickening, or internal organ status. Recombinant human relaxin, a pregnancy-related hormone with antifibrotic effects, is the subject of ongoing trials.

There are currently no therapies proven effective for the basic fibrotic features of scleroderma and none that could be described as disease-modifying.

Supportive Therapy

The range of potential clinical problems facing patients with scleroderma is broad and requires attentive and individualized monitoring.

Musculoskeletal Features

Impaired hand function is seen in all patients with scleroderma. Skin thickening and tendon involvement restrict the ability to extend the fingers and to close the fist. Raynaud's phenomenon combined with ischemic injury to the digital pulp results in impaired tactile sensibility. Arthralgia and arthritis can be present, as can median nerve compression. In addition to ischemia of the digital tip, traumatic ulcerations are common over flexion-contracted interphalangeal joints and in areas of spontaneously extruding subcutaneous calcinosis. Vigorous, long-term occupational and vocational therapy are important in maintaining hand function. Nonsteroidal anti-inflammatory drugs are useful in relieving pain. Ulcerations of all types should be treated promptly with wound care and topical or systemic antibiotics. Physical therapy for proximal joint contractures and gentle aerobic conditioning programs should be considered. Skeletal muscle inflammation often responds to corticosteroid therapy.

Gastrointestinal Involvement

Reflux esophagitis is common in scleroderma and often responds to simple measures such as elevating the head of the bed and avoiding postprandial recumbency, large meals, and clothing that is tight around the waist. Postprandial antacids and cimetidine, ranitidine, famotidine, or nizatidine are useful in reducing symptoms and may help to delay or prevent secondary lower esophageal stricture. Omeprazole is dramatically effective for symptoms of pyrosis. Agents to enhance lower esophageal

sphincter tone or to improve lower esophageal motility, such as cisapride, urecholine, and metoclopramide, are effective mainly in the early stages of the disease before esophageal smooth muscle is lost. There is a clear correlation between the degree of lower esophageal dysmotility and the prevalence and severity of erosive esophagitis. Stricture can be managed with periodic dilatation. The small bowel symptoms of diarrhea and cramping sometimes respond to broad-spectrum antibiotics for presumed bacterial overgrowth but otherwise are not amenable to therapy.

Cardiac and Pulmonary Involvement

Although heart and lung involvement are independently important causes of mortality in scleroderma, little is known about effective treatment. Ventricular arrhythmias are associated with sudden death and overall mortality, but no studies are available regarding the usefulness of antiarrhythmic therapy. Hypoxemia, if present, should be corrected with nocturnal or continuous ambulatory supplemental oxygen. Pulmonary hypertension has been recognized increasingly in late limited scleroderma and may be responsive to prostacyclin preparations.

Renal Involvement

The availability of angiotensin-converting enzyme inhibitors for controlling the accelerated hypertension of scleroderma renal crisis has revolutionized the management of this complication. Before the development of these agents, rapidly progressive renal insufficiency and early death were the expected outcome. If treatment is begun at an early stage, arrest of renal insufficiency and occasional improvement in renal function results. In those patients with more advanced renal insufficiency, dialysis may be required and eventual renal transplantation considered.

BIBLIOGRAPHY

Arnett FC, Howard RF, Tan F, et al. Increased prevalence of systemic sclerosis in a Native American tribe in Oklahoma. Association with an Amerindian HLA haplotype. *Arthritis Rheum* 1996;39:1362–1370.

Artlett CM, Smith JB, Jimenez SA. Identification of fetal DNA and cells from skin lesions from women with systemic sclerosis. *N Engl J Med* 1998;338:1186–1191.

Casciola-Rosen L, Wigley F, Rosen A. Scleroderma autoantigens are uniquely fragmented by metal-catalyzed oxidation reactions: implications for pathogenesis. *J Exp Med* 1997;185:71–79.

Clements PJ, Furst DE, Wong W-K, et al. High-dose versus low-dose D-penicillamine in early diffuse systemic sclerosis: analysis of a two-year, double-blind, randomized, controlled clinical trial. *Arthritis Rheum* 1999;42:1194–1203.

Lacey JV, Garabrant DH, Laing T, et al. Petroleum distillate solvents as risk factors for undifferentiated connective tissue disease (UCTD). *Am J Epidemiol* 1999;149:761–770.

Sjogren RW. Gastrointestinal motility disorders in scleroderma. *Arthritis Rheum* 1994;37:1265–1282.

Strehlow D, Korn JH. Biology of the scleroderma fibroblast. *Curr Opin Rheumatol* 1998;10:572–578.

Wells AU, Hansell DM, Rubens MB, et al. Fibrosing alveolitis in systemic sclerosis: indices of lung function in relation to extent of disease on computed tomography. *Arthritis Rheum* 1997;40:1229–1236.

IDIOPATHIC INFLAMMATORY MYOPATHIES

ROBERT L. WORTMANN

The idiopathic inflammatory myopathies are a heterogeneous group of conditions characterized by symmetrical proximal muscle weakness, elevated serum levels of enzymes derived from skeletal muscle, electrophysiologic changes consistent with myopathy, and evidence of nonsuppurative inflammation in skeletal muscle tissue. Traditionally, the term *polymyositis* has been used to represent all of the noninfectious inflammatory myopathies, including adult and childhood forms of polymyositis and dermatomyositis, myositis associated with other defined connective tissue diseases, myositis associated with malignancies, inclusion body myositis, and other rare conditions. Today it is more appropriate to use the term *idiopathic inflammatory myopathy* to represent the entire group and to reserve the term *polymyositis* to represent a specific subset of patients (Table 180.1).

INCIDENCE AND EPIDEMIOLOGY

Inflammatory myopathies are rare diseases, with estimates of incidence ranging between 0.5 and 10 cases per million population. The age of onset for the group as a whole has a bimodal distribution, with a peak at 10 to 15 years of age and another at about 50 years of age. The onset of myositis associated with other connective tissue diseases is similar to that of the associated disorders. Myositis associated with malignancy and inclusion body myositis are more common after 50 years of age. Both childhood and adult forms of these diseases tend to affect blacks more than whites. Overall, women are affected twice as frequently as men, with the exception of inclusion body myositis, in which the ratio is reversed. Female predominance is greatest between 15 and 44 years of age.

ETIOLOGY AND PATHOGENESIS

IMMUNOGENETICS AND CAUSATION

Although the cause of the idiopathic inflammatory myopathies is unknown, they are believed to develop in genetically susceptible individuals as a result of immune-mediated processes that may be triggered by environmental factors. The immunologic basis for these diseases is evidenced by the mononuclear leukocyte infiltration present in skeletal muscle. In polymyositis and inclusion body myositis, lymphocytes are seen surrounding and invading non-necrotic muscle fibers. They are mostly CD89[+], major histocompatibility complex (MHC) class I–restricted T

lymphocytes, indicating that T-cell-mediated cytotoxicity plays a pathogenic role. The invading T cells are activated (HLA-DR[+]), antigen-primed memory (CD45 Ro[+]) cells. Measures of cytokines reveal high levels of interleukin-4 (IL-4) and low levels of transforming growth factor β1 (TGF-β1). Intercellular adhesion molecule 1 (ICAM-1) adhesion molecules have been induced on the surface of non-necrotic muscle fibers. In polymyositis, the T-cell receptor repertoire expressed is oligoclonal in the Vβ region with restriction in CDR3 usage. This suggests a conventional antigen as the target of the immune response. Findings are similar in inclusion body myositis, except there is heterogeneity in the CDR3 domain, indicating that a superantigen may be involved in the process. Histologically, muscle from patients with inclusion body myositis is further characterized by occasional angulated fibers and by the presence of lined vacuoles. These vacuoles contain abnormally accumulated β-amyloid and ubiquitin. It is not clear as to whether these deposits are primary to the disease, secondary to the inflammatory response, or related to a superantigen-mediated process. Election microscopy reveals intracytoplasmic or intranuclear filamentous or tubular inclusions and mitochondrial abnormalities.

In dermatomyositis, humoral immune mechanisms appear to play a prominent role. The cellular infiltrate includes macrophages, T cells, and B cells and is localized to perivascular areas. B cells outnumber T cells, and the T cells are primarily CD4[+] helper lymphocytes. Vasculopathy is a prominent feature in dermatomyositis, especially in the childhood variety. Early in the process, microangiopathy causes a net reduction of capillaries per muscle fiber. This is associated with the deposition of immunoglobulins and complement components, including the C5b, 6, 7, 8, and 9 membrane attack complex, in capillaries. High levels of TGF-β1 are present, but little IL-4 is found in the tissue and ICAM-1 adhesion molecules are expressed on endothelial cells of perimysial arterioles and venules and perifascicular capillaries. Later in the course of the disease, ischemic involvement of larger intramuscular blood vessels develops, resulting in perifascicular atrophy.

MUSCLE METABOLISM

Studies using magnetic resonance spectroscopy have shown that patients with polymyositis, dermatomyositis, and inclusion body myositis have altered skeletal muscle energy metabolism. This noninvasive technique, which can measure levels of high-energy phosphate compounds, shows that adenosine triphosphate levels are lower, become depleted more rapidly with exercise, and take longer to return to baseline in patients with myositis than in control subjects. Therefore, it is likely that altered energy metabolism disturbs the mechanisms of muscle contraction and contributes to the weakness.

VIRAL INFECTIONS

It is attractive to consider viral infections as possible causes of inflammatory myopathies. Some viruses, such as coxsackievirus A9, adenovirus 21, and influenza viruses A and B, can cause myositis in humans. Enteroviral genomes have been identified in muscle from some patients with polymyositis and dermato-

TABLE 180.1. AUTOANTIBODIES IN INFLAMMATORY MYOPATHIES		
Name	**Antigen**	**Clinical Features**
Myositis-Specific Autoantibodies		
Antisynthetase antibodies		
Jo-1	Histidyl-tRNA synthetase	Polymyositis, dermatomyositis, interstitial lung
PL-7	Threonyl-tRNA synthetase	disease, Raynaud's phenomenon, mechanic's hands
EJ	Glycyl-tRNA synthetase	
OJ	Isoleucyl-tRNA synthetase	
PL-12	Alanyl-tRNA synthetase and tRNA^{a1a}	
KS	Asparaginyl-tRNA synthetase	
Nonsynthetase anticytoplasmic antibodies		
SRP	Signal recognition particle	Treatment-resistant polymyositis of rapid-onset cardiac involvement
Nonsynthetase antinuclear antibody		
Mi-2	CHD3 and CHD4 helicase components of histone deacetylase complexes	Dermatomyositis
Associated Myositis Antibodies		
RNP (ribonucleoprotein)	U1 small nuclear RNA protein	Mixed connective tissue disease, systemic lupus erythematosus, scleroderma, myositis
Sm	(Smith antigen)	Systemic lupus erythematosus, myositis
Ro (SSA)	RNA-protein	Sjögren's syndrome, myositis
PM-Scl	Unidentified	Scleroderma, myositis
Ku	DNA-binding proteins	Scleroderma, systemic lupus erythematosus, myositis
KJ	Unidentified translocation factor	Polymyositis, interstitial lung disease, Raynaud's phenomenon

myositis, and some patients with myositis have elevated antibody titers to viruses. In addition, two animal models support the hypothesis that viral infections are causative. A chronic myositis with changes characteristic of juvenile dermatomyositis develops in neonatal Swiss mice injected with coxsackievirus B1, and a polymyositis-like disease develops in adult BALB/c mice injected with encephalomyocarditis virus 221A. In each case, the muscle inflammation persists after virus can be cultured or demonstrated to be present by in situ techniques.

AUTOANTIBODIES

The autoimmune nature of these diseases is supported by the finding of myositis-specific autoantibodies in many patients. These autoantibodies are heterogeneous and do not cross-react with one another. The myositis-specific autoantibodies tend to identify groups of patients that have common clinical and genetic features (Table 180.2). The most commonly recognized myositis-specific autoantibodies are directed at aminoacyl-tRNA synthetases, which are cytoplasmic enzymes that catalyze the binding of an amino acid with its specific tRNA. The most common of these is anti-Jo-1, an autoantibody directed against histidyl-tRNA synthetase. Because these autoantibodies are found only in patients with inflammatory myopathies and identify clinically distinct subsets of patients, it is possible that they play a pathogenic role.

The association of different class II immunohistocompatibility antigens with different disease subsets indicates a role for genetic factors. Individuals with HLA-DR3 are at increased risk for the development of polymyositis and dermatomyositis. All patients with anti-Jo-1 antibodies have HLA-DR52, and whites with anti-Jo-1 also have a higher prevalence of HLA-DR3 and DR6. HLA-DR5 is associated with anti–signal recognition particle (SRP) antibodies and DR7 plus DRw53 with anti-Mi2. In inclusion body myositis, the prevalence of HLA-DR1 is significantly increased.

CLINICAL FINDINGS

Symmetrical proximal muscle weakness is the dominant feature of all idiopathic inflammatory myopathies. Although strength can be essentially normal at the time of presentation, with rare exception, significant weakness develops during the course of the disease. The weakness can be accompanied by myalgia and tenderness. Atrophy can develop over time. The inflammatory myopathies are systemic diseases, and patients may complain of malaise, fatigue, morning stiffness, arthralgia, and anorexia. These symptoms may be accompanied by weight loss and low-grade fever.

POLYMYOSITIS IN THE ADULT

Adult-onset polymyositis begins insidiously with no identifying precipitating event. An abrupt onset associated with clinically

TABLE 180.2.	CONDITIONS THAT CAN MIMIC IDIOPATHIC INFLAMMATORY MYOPATHIES

Neurologic Disorders

Muscular dystrophies
  Limb-girdle
  Becker's dystrophy
Myasthenia gravis
Amyotrophic lateral sclerosis
Eaton–Lambert syndrome

Infectious Diseases

Toxoplasmosis
Viral infections
  Influenza A and B
  Coxsackieviruses A9, B2, B3, B5
  Adenoviruses 2, 21
  Epstein–Barr virus
  Human immunodeficiency virus
Trichinosis

Electrolyte Disorders

Hyponatremia
Hypokalemia
Hypercalcemia
Hypophosphatemia
Hypomagnesemia

Toxic or Drug-Related Conditions

Alcohol
Choroquine and hydroxychloroquine
Clofibrate
Cocaine
Colchicine
Corticosteroids
Cyclosporine
D-Penicillamine
Gemfibrozil
Gold salts
Heroin
L-Tryptophan
Lovastatin, dravastatin, and simvastatin
Zidovudine (AZT)

Inborn Errors of Metabolism

Glycogen storage diseases
  Myophosphorylase deficiency
  Phosphofructokinase deficiency
Carnitine deficiency
Mitochondrial myopathies

Miscellaneous

Sarcoidosis
Myopathy with eosinophilia
Chronic fatigue syndrome

Additional systems become involved in some patients. Periorbital edema may occur. Pulmonary manifestations may include interstitial fibrosis with fine, dry rales heard on chest auscultation, or interstitial pneumonitis with dyspnea, a nonproductive cough, and hypoxia. Cardiac involvement is uncommon and usually restricted to clinically insignificant changes identified only on the electrocardiogram. However, heart block, supraventricular arrhythmia, or cardiomyopathy may develop, causing palpitations, syncope, or congestive heart failure. Esophageal dysmotility may be associated with epigastric pain or swallowing difficulties. This problem and pharyngeal muscle weakness may lead to aspiration pneumonia. Arthralgia is common, but frank synovitis is rare. Raynaud's phenomenon is reported as an early finding. The neurologic portion of the physical examination is normal except for motor function, although deep-tendon reflexes may appear diminished because of severe muscle weakness.

These manifestations can develop at any time during the course of the illness and can occur in any combination. The presence of a circulating myositis-specific autoantibody tends to identify patterns of involvement (Table 180.2). For example, compared with patients who have no autoantibody, those with antisynthetase antibodies have a significantly higher prevalence of interstitial lung disease, arthritis, Raynaud's phenomenon, and fever.

DERMATOMYOSITIS IN THE ADULT

The clinical picture of dermatomyositis includes all of the manifestations described for polymyositis plus cutaneous features. At times, rash is the presenting complaint and may predate the onset of weakness by as much as 4 years. Rarely, the cutaneous manifestations of dermatomyositis occur without evidence of muscle involvement. The terms *dermatomyositis sine myositis* and *amyopathic dermatomyositis* are applied to this condition.

Skin involvement varies widely from patient to patient. Some patients have a variety of cutaneous manifestations. Some have only one type. In others, the rash can change from one variety to another during the course of the illness. In some, the rash and muscle weakness tend to flare and remit together. In others, the activities of the two processes have no apparent connection.

The classic skin changes of dermatomyositis are Gottron's papules. These are pink to violaceous scaly areas usually seen over the knuckles, elbows, and knees. Other characteristic changes include heliotrope (red–lilac) discoloration of the eyelids or periorbital regions; macular violaceous erythema covering the dorsal aspects of the hand, extensor aspects of the forearms, posterior shoulders, and neck (shawl sign), a "V" area of the anterior chest and neck, or face; and capillary nail fold changes with periungual telangiectasia and dystrophic cuticles. Linear erythematous discoloration may develop around nail beds. Over time, the cutaneous lesions can develop scaling, become hypopigmented or hyperpigmented, or turn brawny and indurated. Darkened or dirty-appearing horizontal lines can be seen across the lateral and palmar aspects of the hands. These changes are termed *mechanic's hands* because they are similar to changes seen in the hands of individuals who perform heavy, manual labor.

evident rhabdomyolysis is unusual. Initially, weakness occurs in the shoulder and pelvic girdles, with the latter slightly more involved. Distal weakness is seen only late in the course of severely afflicted patients. The neck flexors become involved in about half of all cases. Pharyngeal muscle weakness may cause dysphonia, hoarseness, and difficulty swallowing, each a poor prognostic sign. Facial and bulbar muscle weakness are rare and ocular muscle involvement does not occur.

JUVENILE (CHILDHOOD) DERMATOMYOSITIS

Although children may have myositis with clinical pictures similar to those seen in adults, more often the usual inflammatory myopathic process has a highly characteristic pattern. As in adults, the general features of juvenile dermatomyositis are rash and weakness. However, the process differs from that of the adult form because of the coexistence of vasculitis, ectopic calcification, flexion contractures, and lipodystrophy.

MYOSITIS WITH OTHER CONNECTIVE TISSUE DISEASES

Muscle weakness is found in many patients with connective tissue diseases, including systemic lupus erythematosus, scleroderma, mixed connective tissue disease, Wegener's granulomatosis, polyarteritis nodosa, giant cell arteritis, hypersensitivity vasculitis, and Sjögren's syndrome. In some cases, the myopathic features, which may be indistinguishable from those of polymyositis, dominate the clinical picture. More commonly, however, the signs and symptoms of the other condition predominate.

MYOSITIS AND MALIGNANCY

Malignancy and inflammatory myopathy can occur together, but the relationship between the two is unclear. If there is a connection, the greater association probably is with dermatomyositis. The two conditions often develop within a year of each other. The clinical features of the myositis in patients with malignancy are not unique and the activities of the myositis and the malignancy usually do not coincide. The incidence of malignancy in patients with myositis increases with age. With the exceptions of ovarian cancer in women with dermatomyositis, and nasopharyngeal cancer in parts of the world where it is prevalent, the sites and types of tumors are the same as those found in other patients of the same age and gender.

INCLUSION BODY MYOSITIS

Inclusion body myositis is similar to polymyositis in many ways but different in others. Inclusion body myositis usually begins more insidiously, often progressing slowly for 2 to 6 years before being diagnosed. Proximal muscles are involved in a symmetrical fashion, but lower extremity weakness tends to predominate, especially early in the course. The most distinctive clinical feature is the involvement of distal muscles. Distal muscle weakness is present in about 50% of patients at the time of diagnosis and develops in a higher percentage over time. Dysphagia is a prominent feature in about one-third of patients and is attributed to weakness of the cricopharyngeus muscle. Myalgia is uncommon and muscle tenderness is rare. Diagnosis can be made on histologic and electron microscopic sections.

FOCAL OR LOCALIZED MYOSITIS

Occasionally, weakness or myalgia is present in only one limb or in a focal nodular area. In some cases, the findings remain localized for several years. In others, this is an atypical presenta-

TABLE 180.3.	IDIOPATHIC INFLAMMATORY MYOPATHIES

Polymyositis
Dermatomyositis
Myositis with an associated connective tissue disease
Myositis with an associated malignancy
Inclusion body myositis
Localized or focal myositis

tion of polymyositis and progresses to a more typical distribution after a few days to weeks. These lesions must be differentiated from a skeletal muscle tumor or myositis ossificans.

DIFFERENTIAL DIAGNOSIS

If the response to glucocorticoid therapy is poor, and especially if there is no response at all, the accuracy of the diagnosis should be questioned. The criteria for idiopathic inflammatory myopathy are nonspecific and the diagnosis always should be made by excluding other potential causes. A wide variety of conditions that may not respond to glucocorticoids can satisfy some or all of the criteria for an inflammatory myopathy (Table 180.3).

LABORATORY FINDINGS

Proximal muscle weakness in patients with idiopathic inflammatory myopathy is associated with elevated serum levels of enzymes derived from skeletal muscle and evidence of inflammation by electromyographic and muscle tissue examinations. Changes in these parameters can occur in a variety of patterns or combinations with no single finding being specific or diagnostic. Consequently, the diagnosis of an inflammatory myopathy is made by recognizing characteristic combinations of findings and excluding other causes for the abnormalities (Table 180.3).

SERUM TESTS

Serum levels of enzymes released as a result of muscle cell damage are elevated in all types of inflammatory myopathy. These enzymes include creatine phosphokinase, aldolase, glutamine-oxaloacetic transaminase, glutamic-pyruvic transaminase, and lactate dehydrogenase. However, high levels of these enzymes are not specific for inflammatory myopathy. The creatine phosphokinase level is the most sensitive and is elevated in almost every patient with an inflammatory myopathy at some time during the course of the illness. In most patients the creatine phosphokinase level is a helpful indicator of the severity of muscle damage and can be used to gauge disease activity and response to therapy. Normal creatine phosphokinase levels are encountered in patients who are seen early in the disease course, in patients with severe disease late in the course after significant atrophy and fibrosis have developed, in patients with active disease who have a circulating inhibitor of creatine phosphokinase activity, and in some patients with myositis and malignancy. However, elevated creatine phosphokinase levels are not specific for inflammatory muscle diseases. They can be encountered as a result of a variety of disorders.

HEMATOLOGIC STUDIES

The erythrocyte sedimentation rate is abnormal in 50% of patients with inflammatory myopathy and exceeds 50 mm per hour in less than 20%. The sedimentation rate usually does not correlate well with disease activity. Anemia is not a common finding in polymyositis, and leukocytosis occurs in about 15% of patients.

IMMUNOLOGIC STUDIES

Most patients with idiopathic inflammatory myopathy have circulating autoantibodies. Antinuclear antibody testing is positive at low titers in a few patients with polymyositis, about 60% of patients with juvenile dermatomyositis, and almost all patients with an associated connective tissue disease. The last of these patients also may have the antibodies indicative of the associated disease. Myositis-specific autoantibodies have been reported in approximately 40% of patients with inflammatory myopathies in research studies (Table 180.2).

ELECTROMYOGRAPHY

No electromyographic changes are diagnostic of an inflammatory myopathy. However, some are suggestive. Classic findings include the triad of increased insertional activity, fibrillations, and sharp positive waves; spontaneous, bizarre, high-frequency discharges; and polyphasic motor unit potentials of low amplitude and short duration. There is significant variability because the complete triad is found in only about 40% of patients; 10% of patients have normal examinations. In some patients, changes are localized (limited to the paraspinal muscles) despite widespread weakness. Typically, the only electromyographic changes are those consistent with a myopathic process. The exception occurs in patients with inclusion body myositis, one-third of whom also have neuropathic features.

MAGNETIC RESONANCE IMAGING

Magnetic resonance imaging is a noninvasive method of identifying abnormal muscle. Regions of high signal intensity indicative of inflammation can be observed using a standard T2-weighted or fat-suppressive technique. Magnetic resonance imaging can be used to establish the extent of the disease process and to localize sites for biopsy. It also can be valuable in selected cases for evaluating the response to therapy, particularly in dermatomyositis.

MUSCLE HISTOLOGIC STUDIES

Muscle histologic studies are extremely helpful in the evaluation of patients with inflammatory myopathy. However, no change

is truly pathognomonic and wide variations can be seen both in the tissue of an individual patient and between different patients.

The characteristic histologic changes of polymyositis include an endomysial inflammatory infiltrate with lymphocytes surrounding and invading non-necrotic fibers, degenerating and regenerating fibers, areas of fibers necrosis, and fibrosis. In some cases, changes are minimal and type II fiber atrophy is the only identifiable abnormality. In dermatomyositis, the infiltrate includes lymphocytes, plasma cells, and macrophages localized to perivascular areas. Fiber necrosis may be minimal, but perifascicular atrophy may be prominent. The diagnosis of inclusion body myositis is defined by histologic changes similar to those seen in polymyositis (with angulated fibers in patients with a neuropathic component), by the characteristic changes of lined vacuoles on histology, and by tubular or filamentous inclusions on electron microscopy.

■ OPTIMAL MANAGEMENT

The management of an inflammatory myopathy begins with an objective assessment of the patient's clinical status. Pretreatment testing of muscle strength can be performed by manually grading the strength of various muscle groups. A timed-stands test (measuring the amount of time it takes a patient to rise 10 times from a chair without using his or her arms) can be used to assess lower extremity strength. Without an accurate baseline assessment, it may be difficult to differentiate between the subjective and objective effects of therapy or to detect small changes in strength. Blood pressure measurement, chest examination, chest radiography, and pulmonary function studies should be performed. Fluoroscopic studies with contrast material may be important if the patient has swallowing problems or dysphonia. Serum levels of muscle enzymes and laboratory tests that might be affected by the medications used should be measured.

PHYSICAL THERAPY

Physical therapy can play an important role in the treatment of inflammatory myopathy. When the disease activity is severe, bed rest is used and passive range-of-motion exercises are performed to prevent joint contractures and overuse of regenerating muscle bundles. A soft cervical collar may be helpful for patients with significant neck involvement. Active exercises can be prescribed as improvement is observed, even in the presence of elevated creatine phosphokinase levels.

GLUCOCORTICOIDS

Glucocorticoids are the first drugs used in patients with any type of idiopathic inflammatory myopathy. Initially, prednisone is prescribed in a single oral morning dose of about 1 mg per kg. In severe cases, the daily dose can be divided and up to 2 mg per kg can be given. Once instituted, high-dose daily prednisone therapy is continued until muscle strength improves. Improvement may occur in the first weeks or gradually over 3 to 6 months. The variability in improvement is related to the timing of treatment and the specific inflammatory process. In general, the earlier in the course medication is given, the more satisfying is the result. Inclusion body myositis is more refractory to therapy than other forms of idiopathic inflammatory myositis.

Patients should be followed up with regular objective evaluations of muscle strength and measurements of serum enzyme levels. The prednisone dosage is maintained at high levels for 6 weeks as improvement occurs, then gradual tapering is performed over many months on an individualized basis.

Glucocorticoids have a beneficial effect in 90% of patients and produce complete remission in 50% to 75%. If remission is not evident after 6 to 12 weeks of high-dose prednisone therapy, a second agent should be added. Both azathioprine and methotrexate have been used successfully in this situation. In adults, azathioprine usually is prescribed to be taken by mouth at dosages up to 3 mg per kg per day. Methotrexate is taken on a weekly basis, with dosages ranging between 7.5 mg by mouth and 50 mg by intravenous or intramuscular routes.

With therapy, some patients who have experienced varying degrees of improvement actually lose strength. This is usually a flare-up of the basic disease or the development of steroid myopathy. Laboratory tests, electromyography, and muscle biopsy are not helpful in differentiating the cause. The situation can be resolved only by giving a provocative challenge with higher dose glucocorticoids or tapering the dosage rapidly and assessing the clinical response.

In refractory cases, the combination of prednisone, azathioprine, and methotrexate has proven beneficial in some patients. Cyclophosphamide, cyclosporine, chlorambucil, and tracolimus have been variably beneficial. Although intravenous immune globulin has been used early in treatment, it is perhaps best employed as a "bridging therapy" when initiating one of these agents in refractory cases.

Special consideration should be given to patients within certain groups. The cutaneous manifestations of dermatomyositis (but not the myositis) may respond to hydroxychloroquine. The myositis in patients with associated connective tissue diseases may respond dramatically to glucocorticoid therapy, even at lower dosages. Emphasis should be placed on treating the neoplasms in patients with associated malignancies. Removal, debulking, or cure of the cancer may be accompanied by remission of the myositis. Inclusion body myositis may be refractory to therapy; in many patients, strength declines progressively despite therapy. Patients with interstitial lung disease and myositis also tend to have a poor prognosis. The presence of densities on chest radiography consistent with aspiration pneumonia in these patients portends an unfavorable outcome.

BIBLIOGRAPHY

Bohan A, Peter JB, Bowman RL, et al. A computer-assisted analysis of 153 patients with polymyositis and dermatomyositis. *Medicine (Baltimore)* 1977;56:255–286.
Calabrese LH, Chou SM. Inclusion body myositis. *Rheum Dis Clin North Am* 1994;20:955–972.
Callen JP. Relationship of cancer to inflammatory muscle diseases: dermatomyositis, polymyositis, and inclusion body myositis. *Rheum Dis Clin North Am* 1994;20:943–953.
Hicks JE. Role of rehabilitation in the management of myopathies. *Curr Opin Rheumatol* 1998;10:548–555.
Euwer RL, Sontheimer RD. Dermatologic aspects of myositis. *Curr Opin Rheumatol* 1994;6:583–589.
Hohlfeld R, Engel AG. Cellular immune mechanisms in inflammatory myopathies. *Curr Opin Rheumatol* 1997;9:520–526.
Kagen LJ. Polymyositis/dermatomyositis. In: McCarty DJ, Koopman WJ, eds. *Arthritis and allied conditions*, twelfth ed. Philadelphia: Lea & Febiger, 1993:1225.
Love LA, Leff RA, Fraser DD, et al. A new approach to the classification of idiopathic inflammatory myopathy: myositis-specific autoantibodies define useful homogeneous patient groups. *Medicine (Baltimore)* 1991; 70:360–374.
Lundberg IE, Nyberg P. New developments in the role of cytokines in inflammatory myopathies. *Curr Opin Rheumatol* 1998;10:521–529.
Oddis C. Idiopathic inflammatory myopathy. In: Wortmann RL, ed. *Clinical disorders of skeletal muscle*. Philadelphia: Lippincott Williams & Wilkins *(in press)*.
Targoff IN, Autoantibodies. In: Wortmann RL, ed. *Clinical disorders of skeletal muscle*. Philadelphia: Lippincott Williams & Wilkins *(in press)*.
Wortmann RL. Inflammatory muscle disease. In: Kelley WN, Harris ED Jr, Ruddy S, et al, eds. *Textbook of rheumatology*, fifth ed. Philadelphia: WB Saunders *(in press)*.
Wortmann RL. Idiopathic inflammatory diseases of muscle. In: Weisman MH, Weinblatt ME, eds. *Treatment of the rheumatic diseases*, second ed. Philadelphia: WB Saunders *(in press)*.

Kelley's Textbook of Internal Medicine, fourth edition. Edited by H. David Humes.
Lippincott Williams & Wilkins, Philadelphia © 2000.

C H A P T E R

181

VASCULITIS: ITS MANY FORMS

GARY S. HOFFMAN
BRIAN F. MANDELL

■ DEFINITION AND CLASSIFICATION

Classification of the vasculitides remains a work in progress. Despite the publication of diagnostic guidelines and proceedings of consensus conferences, areas of controversy remain. The benefits of an accurate classification scheme for the vasculitides include (a) facilitation of communication about disorders that share certain traits or etiologies; (b) recognition that certain systemic vasculitides have distinct prognoses and may respond to particular therapies; (c) assurance that patients enrolled in clinical studies have the same disease; and (d) generation of diagnostic guidelines that aid clinicians in the recognition of patients with alternative illnesses that may mimic specific vasculitides. A definitive classification scheme should be based on an understanding of the pathogenesis of the diseases under study and the presence of pathognomonic clinical, laboratory, imaging, or histopathologic features that make distinctions between categories unambiguous. Because these conditions are uncommonly met in vasculitis, classification systems have utilized various combinations of these features.

When applying pathology criteria to an individual patient, the physician must recognize that biopsy-derived data are subject to sampling error and site selection bias, and that a biopsy represents a picture of an evolving disease process at only a single point in time. Because vasculitic lesions often occur in a seemingly random pattern of "skip lesions" within a particular vessel or organ, false-negative biopsy results may occur. Vasculitis may be present, but the histology of the tissue sample being evaluated may reveal only nonspecific inflammation or ischemic changes, whereas more characteristic features (e.g., granulomata, arteritis) may be present in a contiguous area. In addition, if a biopsy is obtained in an area in which the predominant vessel size is arterioles, capillaries, and venules (e.g., skin, nasal, or enteric mucosa), one may make the diagnosis of a small-vessel vasculitis or ischemic necrosis and not recognize additional involvement of larger vessels because they have not been evaluated. Similar concerns apply to arteriography, which has adequate resolution to evaluate large and medium-size vessels, but not microscopic vessels.

Classification guidelines derived from patient data have generally included patients who have established, well-differentiated vasculitis. Patients with diseases that are in an early stage of evolution or have ambiguous features are often excluded from these analyses, although such presentations may not be uncommon in a clinical practice. Thus, published criteria may achieve the desired goal of having high degrees of specificity but have limited sensitivity in identifying the entire spectrum of disease. Early in the disease course, patients may not express sufficient characteristic features of a vasculitic disorder to warrant a specific diagnostic label.

Published criteria for classification of the vasculitides have not been thoroughly evaluated for their ability to distinguish vasculitis mimics from primary systemic vasculitis, and the diagnosis must always be made with the proviso that multisystem disorders, including infections, coagulopathies, drug reactions, and malignancy, are excluded. The American College of Rheumatology (ACR) 1990 Criteria for Classification of Vasculitis provided the cautionary note that classification systems cannot include the full spectrum of disease features and are therefore not appropriate for diagnosis of individual patients. A more recent effort to refine nomenclature (Table 181.1) was initiated at the Chapel Hill Consensus Conference (CHCC). Emphasis was placed on the clinical pattern of disease and the presence or absence of demonstrable tissue immune complexes, and associations with antineutrophil cytoplasmic autoantibodies (ANCAs). Specific recognition of microscopic polyangiitis (MPA), distinct from classical polyarteritis (PAN), was emphasized. An increasing number of studies have demonstrated the important association between certain viral infections and specific vasculitic syndromes, especially disease phenotypes that mimic MPA and PAN.

CLINICAL FINDINGS

For most physicians, recognition and treatment of the systemic vasculitides is difficult. There are multiple distinct forms of primary systemic vasculitis. Each is uncommon and likely to be confused with other systemic illnesses. Processes that may be confused with a primary vasculitis include sepsis (particularly bacterial endocarditis), drug toxicities and poisonings (especially with agents that are likely to produce vasospasm), coagulopathies, malignancies, cardiac myxomas, generalized atherosclerosis, and multifocal emboli from large-vessel aneurysms.

The pattern and degree of critical organ involvement and the rate of disease progression determines the intensity and pace of the diagnostic evaluation, the ultimate diagnosis, and treatment decisions. The physician may be confronted by a patient with rapidly deteriorating clinical condition in whom suggestive features of systemic vasculitis cannot be distinguished from occult infection or malignancy. Under such circumstances, one may be forced to treat multiple possible diagnoses prior to achieving a final diagnosis. To minimize the risk implied with such an approach, the evaluation should be insightful and aggressive.

The diagnostic process is best facilitated by recognizing clinical patterns of competing diagnoses, rather than by depending on nonspecific serologic and immunologic studies. The greatest certainty in the diagnosis of a specific vasculitic disorder results from combining compatible clinical features with pathologic proof of vasculitis. Certain types of systemic vasculitis may present with a characteristic clinical phenotype. For example, the presence of upper and lower airway inflammation, inflammatory eye disease, and red blood cell casts in the urine sediment, suggests Wegener's granulomatosis (WG). Hypertension, constitutional features, subclavian bruits, and extremity claudication in a girl or young woman should suggest Takayasu's arteritis. Unfortunately, many patients with vasculitis do not present with such characteristic features. Instead, one often has to depend on combinations of less specific clues. A patient with fever, an active urine sediment, and peripheral neuropathy is likely to have vasculitis, especially if competing diagnoses (Table 181.2) have been excluded; however, the specific type of vasculitis may not be immediately evident. Such features occurring in the setting of an established autoimmune disease, such as rheumatoid arthritis, systemic lupus erythematosus (SLE), Sjögren's syndrome, or relapsing polychondritis, further enhance the likelihood of vasculitis being present, although in this setting the vasculitis is likely related to the underlying systemic autoimmune disorder and not to a primary vasculitic syndrome. A patient with active hepatitis B or C infection and a similar clinical syndrome very likely has vasculitis, with or without cryoglobulinemia.

Concern for the presence of a systemic vasculitic disorder should be increased in a patient with multisystem symptoms or findings, constitutional features, or otherwise unexplained tissue ischemia or infarction. The presence of purpura is extremely suggestive of cutaneous vasculitis. However, there is a broad

TABLE 181.1. **NOMENCLATURE OF THE VASCULITIDES ADAPTED FROM THE CHAPEL HILL CONSENSUS CONFERENCE**[a]

Large-vessel vasculitis[b]	
Giant cell (temporal) arteritis	Granulomatous arteritis of the aorta and its major branches, with a predilection for the extracranial branches of the carotid artery. *Often involves the temporal artery. Usually occurs in patients older than 50 and often is associated with polymyalgia rheumatica.*
Takayasu's arteritis	Granulomatous inflammation of the aorta and its major branches. *Usually occurs in patients younger than 50.*
Medium-size vessel vasculitis	
Polyarteritis nodosa	Necrotizing inflammation of medium-size or small arteries without glomerulonephritis or vasculitis in arterioles, capillaries, or venules.
Kawasaki's disease	Arteritis involving large, medium-size, and small arteries, and associated with mucocutaneous lymph node syndrome. *Coronary arteries are often involved. Aorta and veins may be involved. Usually occurs in children.*
Small-vessel vasculitis	
Wegener's granulomatosis	Granulomatous inflammation involving the respiratory tract, and necrotizing vasculitis affecting small to medium-size vessels (e.g., capillaries, venules, arterioles, and arteries). *Necrotizing glomerulonephritis is common.*
Churg–Strauss syndrome	Eosinophil-rich and granulomatous inflammation involving the respiratory tract, and necrotizing vasculitis affecting small to medium-size vessels, and associated with asthma and eosinophilia.
Microscopic polyangiitis[c] (microscopic polyarteritis)	Necrotizing vasculitis, with few or no immune deposits, affecting small vessels (i.e., capillaries, venules, or arterioles). *Necrotizing arteritis involving small and medium-size arteries may be present. Necrotizing glomerulnephritis is very common. Pulmonary capillaritis often occurs.*
Henoch–Schönlein purpura	Vasculitis, with IgA-dominant immune deposits, affecting small vessels (i.e., capillaries, venules, or arterioles). *Typically involves skin, gut, and glomeruli, and is associated with arthralgias or arthritis.*
Essential cryoglobulinemia vasculitis	Vasculitis, with cryoglobulins and immune deposits, affecting small vessels (i.e., capillaries, venules, or arterioles), and associated with cryoglobulins in serum. *Skin and glomeruli are often involved.*
Cutaneous leukocytoclastic angiitis	Isolated cutaneous leukocytoclastic angiitis without systemic vasculitis or glomerulonephritis.

[a] Jennette JC, et al. *Arthritis Rheum* 1994;37:187–192.
[b] *Large vessel* refers to the aorta and the largest branches directed toward major body regions (e.g., to the extremities and the head and neck); *medium-size vessel* refers to the main visceral arteries (e.g., renal, hepatic, coronary, and mesenteric arteries); *small vessel* refers to venules, capillaries, arterioles, and the intraparenchymal distal arterial radicals that connect with arterioles. Some small- and large-vessel vasculitides may involve medium-size arteries, but large- and medium-size vessel vasculitides do not involve vessels smaller than arteries. Essential components are represented by normal type; italicized type represents usual.
[c] Preferred term.

TABLE 181.2. **MIMICS OF PRIMARY SYSTEMIC VASCULITIS**

Infection[a]
  Endocarditis, *Neisseria*
  Mycotic aneurysms, histoplasmosis, syphilis
Drug toxicity/poisoning[a]
  Cocaine, sympathomimetics, allopurinol, diphenylhydantoin, arsenic
Coagulopathy
Malignancy[a]
Cardiac myxoma[a]
Generalized atherosclerosis[a]
Cholesterol embolization syndrome[a]
Calciphylaxis/end-stage renal disease[a]

[a] Vasculitis may or may not occur as a secondary event.

differential diagnosis for purpura (Table 181.3), and even when leukocytoclastic angiitis is documented by histopathology, the complete diagnosis may not yet be identified. Documenting the presence of cutaneous vasculitis is not equivalent to diagnosing a systemic vasculitis, and its presence does not mandate immediate systemic immunosuppressive therapy. As in all patients with possible multisystem disease, a very detailed history and physical examination must be obtained. Particular attention should be paid to the ocular, upper respiratory tract, neurologic, vascular, and lymph node examinations. We view the examination of a fresh sample of urine sediment by the physician as an *absolutely necessary* component of the evaluation. Glomerulonephritis is generally asymptomatic until the onset of uremia; early diagnosis will only be made by a carefully performed urinalysis. The history and physical examination may strengthen or weaken the clinician's suspicion of a specific primary vasculitis and thus direct the appropriate laboratory testing to support the most reasonable diagnoses. Laboratory tests alone should not generate initial suspicion of systemic vasculitis. Elevated acute phase reactants, elevated rheumatoid factor levels, or hypocomplementemia do not necessarily indicate the presence of a primary vascu-

TABLE 181.3.	PURPURIC SKIN LESIONS

Leukocytoclastic angiitis, infection-associated
Kaposi's sarcoma
Bacterial emboli
Fungal emboli
Steroid therapy (steroid purpura)
Amyloidosis
Senile purpura
Coumadin necrosis
Calciphylaxis
Trauma (e.g., following vigorous needle-prick sensory examination)

litis. Anemia, leukocytosis, and thrombocytosis are commonly present in patients with systemic vasculitis but are not specific findings. Eosinophilia may occur in Churg–Strauss syndrome (CSS) or WG, but it may also be found in patients with atherosclerotic embolization and some malignancies. Leukopenia and thrombocytopenia are not characteristic of any of the primary vasculitic syndromes, although they may occur in patients with polyarteritis associated with hairy cell leukemia, sarcoidosis, SLE, Felty's syndrome, and in the setting of hypersplenism associated with chronic hepatitis.

PROVING THE DIAGNOSIS

Definitive diagnosis requires the visualization of vasculitic lesions in affected tissue. In patients with proven vasculitis, the yield from biopsies of clinically normal sites is considerably less than 20%. Therefore, a biopsy of apparently normal tissue is not recommended. Biopsies of abnormal organs provide diagnostically useful information in over 65% of cases. Biopsy results must be coupled with the clinical pattern of disease to define the disorder. A 100% yield is not observed because involvement of vessels in systemic vasculitis is not uniform. Heterogeneity of pathology occurs within vessels as well as throughout solid organs. This has been convincingly demonstrated in the serial sectioning of temporal arteries in patients with giant cell arteritis, in angiographic imaging of large vessels in Takayasu's arteritis, and in chest radiographs of patients with WG. These observations are compatible with the clinical experience that larger excisional biopsies of abnormal tissue provide a greater yield than needle biopsies.

A biopsy may not be practical in certain circumstances. Consider the patient with symptoms of visceral ischemia, carotidynia, and findings of unequal extremity blood pressures. Biopsy of large vessels or diagnostic laparotomy in the absence of an acute abdomen is impractical. In this setting, angiography may be helpful. Evidence of vascular injury may be apparent from areas of vascular stenosis and/or aneurysm formation, but these findings must be distinguished from atherosclerotic injury. Angiography is not generally adequate to detect vascular injury of the smaller arterioles, capillaries, and venules, as might occur in Henoch–Schönlein purpura.

Angiography is particularly useful for patients with diseases that involve large (Takayasu's arteritis, giant cell arteritis of the elderly) and medium-size vessels (e.g., polyarteritis nodosa). Angiographic abnormalities may not indicate *active* arteritis. Certain caveats need to be considered before one can assume that suspicious angiographic images are confirmatory of vasculitis or that a negative study indicates the absence of vasculitis:

- Angiographic changes are not as specific as histopathologic abnormalities.
- Inflammation of blood vessels may produce symptoms before observable changes occur in the vascular lumen.
- Angiographic lesions that may be confused with primary vasculitis have been described in patients who (a) have used drugs that produce vasospasm (e.g., cocaine, amphetamines), (b) have embolic injury from cardiac myxomas, (c) have been afflicted with peritoneal carcinomatosis, (d) have fibromuscular dysplasia, and (e) have vascular infections. Infection due to slow-growing organisms (e.g., tuberculosis, syphilis, fungi) may not produce the usual systemic features that one might expect from acute bacterial infections.

Once the diagnosis of vasculitis is clearly established, based on the strongest of circumstantial evidence or biopsy documentation of vascular inflammatory injury, one must still determine whether the disorder is due to *secondary vasculitis* from bacterial, fungal, or viral infection (e.g., parvovirus, hepatitis B or C, HIV, or cytomegalovirus) or malignancies. Paraneoplastic vasculitis should be considered on the basis of a suspicious history; in the setting of significant adenopathy, leukopenia, or thrombocytopenia; and in patients who fail to respond to usually effective aggressive immunosuppressive therapy. Aggressive diagnostic efforts are warranted, since potentially life-threatening immunosuppressive therapy is frequently used in the treatment of the systemic vasculitides.

SPECIFIC FORMS OF VASCULITIS

TAKAYASU'S ARTERITIS

Takayasu's arteritis is a large-vessel vasculitis of unknown cause that involves the aorta and its major branches. It affects young women about ten times more often than men. Morbidity results from arterial stenosis and organ ischemia (extremity claudication, cerebral ischemia, renal artery hypertension, congestive heart failure, coronary syndromes, mesenteric vascular insufficiency). Stenotic lesions are characteristic, but aneurysms may also form, particularly in the aortic root, which may produce aortic regurgitation. Mortality is primarily due to hypertensive or primary cardiac, renal, and central nervous system (CNS) vascular disease. Estimates of mortality range from 3% at 8 years to 35% at 5 years after diagnosis. The presence of symptoms or findings of large-vessel obstruction or hypertension in young patients, necessitates careful examination of pulses and blood pressures in all four extremities, and a search for vascular bruits. Rarely will Takayasu's arteritis present as unexplained fever alone.

Symptoms of increasing extremity or visceral ischemia may indicate active disease. When these occur in the setting of an elevated erythrocyte sedimentation rate (ESR), along with malaise, myalgias, arthralgias, night sweats, and fever, active disease is likely and should be evaluated by angiography to establish the initial diagnosis and to provide a baseline vascular image. In known cases of Takayasu's arteritis, repeat angiography is useful to assess the degree of disease progression. A significant number of patients may have a normal ESR, not have constitutional or new vascular symptoms, and still experience progressive disease. Until we are better able to accurately judge the degree of disease activity in Takayasu's arteritis, outcomes will continue to be compromised. Studies are currently under way to evaluate refinements in ultrasound and magnetic resonance techniques that may enable the clinician to detect qualitative abnormalities in the vessel wall that imply inflammatory change. Active disease, as indicated by vascular pain (e.g., carotidynia), constitutional symptoms, fever, and high ESR, may also occur in the absence of angiographic progression. This would suggest that vascular inflammation may need to be present for an extended period to produce structural changes. Although rarely reported, skin lesions, pulmonary infiltrates, and glomerulonephritis are not characteristically present. There are no specific diagnostic serologic tests. Isolated involvement of the abdominal aorta and lower extremities is uncommon. Sarcoidosis with vasculitis and giant cell arteritis of the elderly may mimic Takayasu's arteritis.

Approximately 60% of patients with Takayasu's arteritis will achieve remission with glucocorticoid therapy (e.g., prednisone 1 mg per kilogram per day). However, tapering of glucocorticoid therapy has been associated with disease relapse in over 40% of patients. Glucocorticoid-resistant or relapsing patients may respond to the addition of daily therapy with low doses (approximately 2 mg per kilogram) of cyclophosphamide (CP) or weekly therapy with methotrexate (15 to 25 mg per week). About 40% of patients who are treated with a cytotoxic agent and glucocorticoids will achieve remission, but about half of these patients will also relapse, leading to the requirement for chronic immunosuppressive therapy in about one-fourth of all patients.

A discussion of only anti-inflammatory strategies ignores the significant hemodynamic effects of vascular lesions and other potentially useful interventions. Patients may suffer clinical deterioration due to fixed critical stenoses or aneurysms. This is most evident with regard to hypertension that may affect 21% to 90% of patients. In Asia and Mexico, Takayasu's disease is one of the more common causes of hypertension in the young adult population. Inadequately treated hypertension may lead to cerebral, cardiac, and renal injury. One of the most common errors in clinical management of Takayasu's arteritis relates to the physician not knowing which extremity is representative of aortic root pressure. Because over 90% of patients have stenotic lesions, and the most common site of stenosis is the subclavian artery(ies), blood pressure recordings in one or both arms may not reflect even critically elevated pressures in the aorta. If aortic root pressure is elevated, unrecognized, and untreated, the risk of hypertensive complications is enhanced. Thus, angiographic procedures must include intravascular pressure recordings (Fig.

181.1). In the setting of renal insufficiency, the potential of contrast agents to cause further renal impairment may limit exploring the extent of all possible vascular lesions. However, if contraindications are not present, patients with Takayasu's arteritis should have the entire aorta and its primary branches included in vascular imaging studies. Magnetic resonance angiography lacks the ability to measure intravascular pressures in patients with stenoses that may have created clinically significant pressure gradients. However, if the clinical examination does not suggest that extremity lesions are present and extremity pressures are equal, a magnetic resonance study may be sufficient for routine follow-up evaluations. Whenever feasible, anatomical correction of clinically significant lesions should be considered, especially in the setting of renal artery stenosis and hypertension. In about 20% of patients, aortic root involvement may lead to valvular insufficiency, angina, and congestive heart failure. Severe or progressive changes may require aortic surgery, with or without valve replacement. Since disease activity may be difficult to determine, all such surgeries should include sending vascular specimens for histopathologic evaluation. Occasionally, the diagnosis of Takayasu's arteritis is first made at time of aortic surgery. If arterial bypass procedures are planned, it is advisable to avoid placing grafts that originate from the subclavian or inominate arteries, which are at high risk of becoming stenosed in the future. The most suitable origin for carotid or subclavian bypass procedures is the aortic root.

GIANT CELL ARTERITIS OF THE ELDERLY

Giant cell arteritis (GCA) and Takayasu's arteritis are the principal diseases that are associated with sterile granulomatous inflammation of large and medium-size vessels. Whereas Takayasu's arteritis has a predilection for young women of childbearing age, GCA occurs in people older than 50 years. The mean age for patients in most series is 70 years. Women are affected more often than men, but the degree of female predominance (2–3:1) is not as striking as in Takayasu's arteritis. The demographic characteristics of patients with GCA is the same as for patients with polymyalgia rheumatica (PMR), and 30% to 50% of patients with GCA may concurrently have features of PMR. The most common characteristics of GCA are represented in Table 181.4. Some patients may exhibit only systemic features, but this is uncommon. Occasionally, patients have inflammatory arthritis of peripheral joints. The new onset of severe headaches, scalp or temporal artery tenderness, acute visual loss, and claudication of the muscles of mastication are among the most compelling features to suggest the diagnosis. When such abnormalities are present in conjunction with marked elevations in the ESR, a clinical diagnosis of GCA can be presumed and treatment initiated, even without the benefit of a temporal artery biopsy. However, because biopsy generally does not cause significant morbidity, it is often performed when clinical features are not entirely classical (Fig. 181.2). The yield of positive temporal artery biopsies in patients strongly suspected to have GCA has been estimated to be about 50% to 80%, depending on the size of the biopsy, the clinical features of the illness, and whether bilateral samples have been obtained. These data are obviously affected by whether the practice of the clinical investigator is to

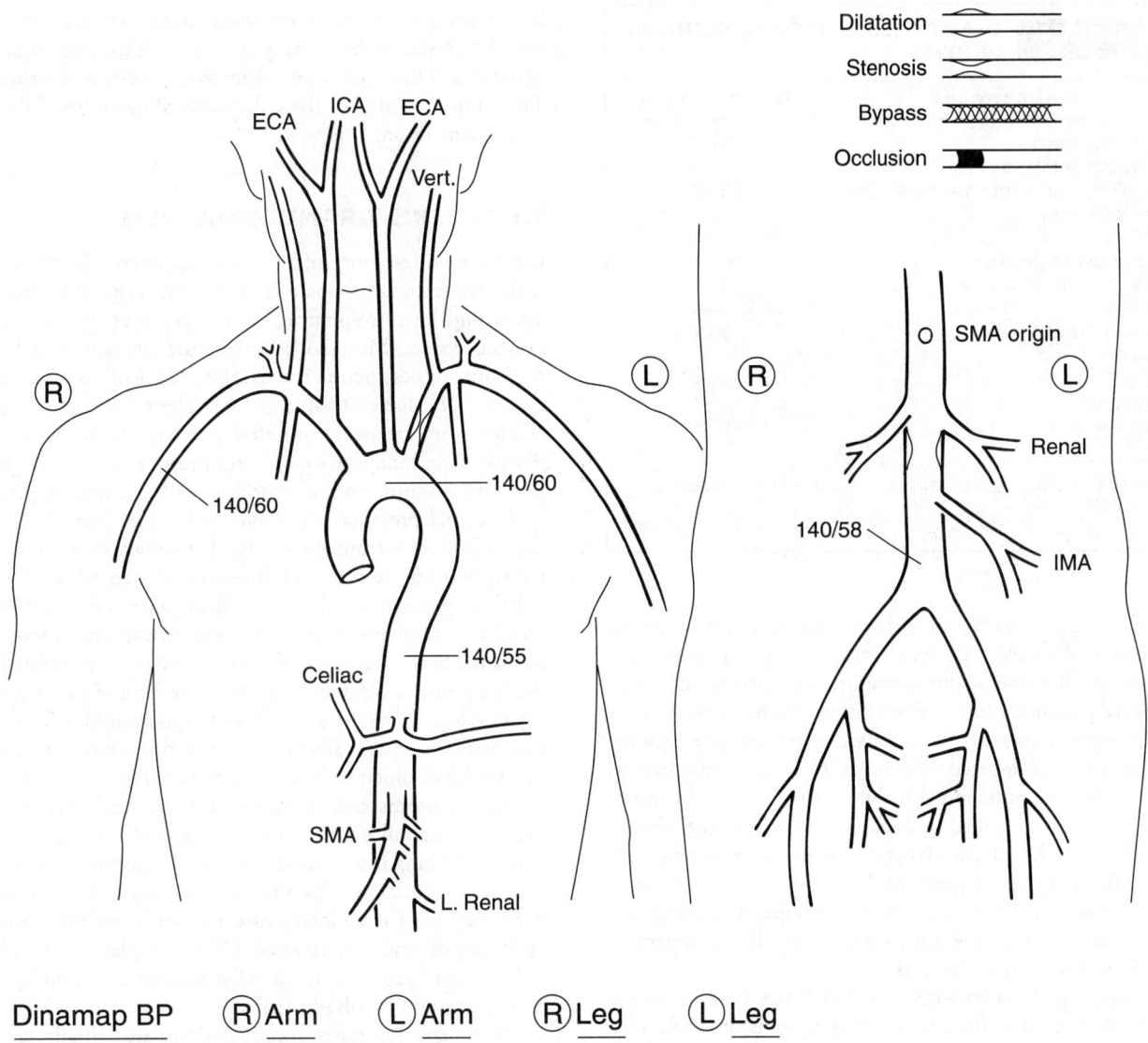

Dilatation

Stenosis

Bypass

Occlusion

ECA   ICA   ECA

Vert.

ⓇDinamap BP   ⓇArm   ⓁArm   ⓇLeg   ⓁLeg

FIGURE 181.1. Standard vascular diagram used by the authors to summarize angiographic and blood pressure data in patients with Takayasu's arteritis. An ascending thoracic aortic aneurysm is present in this 21-year-old woman. Blood pressure in the right arm is a reliable measure of aortic root pressure, but left arm blood pressure by either catheter or cuff recordings is not. Hemodynamically insignificant abdominal aortic stenosis is present. Right-arm blood pressure (BP), 135/60; left-arm BP, 80/−; right-leg BP, 145/65; left-leg BP, 145/65.

biopsy patients with classic features (as opposed to only individuals with vague or nonspecific systemic symptoms). A diagnostic biopsy may be obtained even after more than a week of glucocorticoid therapy. The clinical diagnosis should be questioned if dramatic improvement does not occur within 24 to 72 hours of initiating high-dose glucocorticoid therapy.

Aortitis may be part of GCA in at least 15% of cases. The primary branches of the aorta are affected in a similar number of individuals. Consequently, some patients present with features resembling those of Takayasu's disease. Among the elderly with large-vessel inflammatory disease, the same considerations and precautions must be applied in GCA as in Takayasu's arteritis. Recent studies have demonstrated that patients with GCA were more than 17 times more likely than age-matched controls to

have thoracic aortic aneurysms, and about 2.5 times more likely than aged matched controls to have abdominal aortic aneurysms. Because such aneurysms were found either in the course of routine care or at post mortem, these may be conservative estimates. The finding of large-vessel disease, including aortic aneurysms, in elderly persons with GCA should not be assumed to be secondary to atheromatous disease.

Glucocorticoids are the most effective therapy for GCA. Prednisone (0.7 to 1 mg per kilogram per day) will reduce symptoms within 1 to 2 days and often eliminate symptoms within a week. About a month after clinical and laboratory parameters, particularly tests (e.g., ESR or C-reactive protein) for acute phase reactants, have normalized, tapering of glucocorticoid therapy can begin. Unfortunately, the ESR does not always normalize

TABLE 181.4.	GIANT CELL ARTERITIS: CLINICAL PROFILE	
Abnormality		**Frequency (%)**
Atypical headache		60–90
Tender temporal artery		40–70
Systemic symptoms not attributable to other diseases		20–50
Fever		20–50
Polymyalgia rheumatica		30–50
Acute visual abnormalities		12–40
Blindness		5–17
Transient ischemic attack		5–10
Claudication		
"Jaw"		30–70
Extremities		5–15
Aortic aneuysm		15–20

Dramatic response to glucocorticoids ~ 100. Positive temporal artery biopsy ~ 50+.

even with disease control, so it should not be relied on as the only measure of disease activity. Steroids may also lower the ESR even if elevation is due to alternative etiologic factors (infection, monoclonal gammopathy). Patients either may not achieve complete remission or may experience a flare-up in their disease as the glucocorticoids are tapered. Cytotoxic or immunosuppressive agents are often recommended for such patients, but the utility of these agents in controlled trials has not been adequately investigated. Some authors have advocated initiation of therapy with less than 0.5 mg per kilogram of daily prednisone in patients without severe visual symptoms with the hope of limiting side effects of steroid therapy. Large, prospective, dose comparison studies have not been performed.

As many as 40% of patients with PMR may have histologic proof of GCA, even in the absence of symptoms of GCA. This has continued to fuel controversy about whether all patients with PMR should be initially treated with high doses of glucocorticoids. This issue is not likely to be resolved any time soon. The clinical overlap of these disorders obligates careful vascular evaluations of patients with PMR.

WEGENER'S GRANULOMATOSIS

Disease manifestations of WG result from aseptic inflammation with necrosis, granuloma formation, and vasculitis affecting the upper and lower respiratory tracts, ears, eyes, kidneys, skin, or nervous system. Musculoskeletal features are common, but joint deformity or destruction is rare. About 25% of cases have peripheral or CNS disease (Table 181.5). The most common sources of morbidity are related to airway, renal, auditory, and ocular disease. Combination immunosuppressive therapy is generally very effective but is often associated with serious complications.

At initial presentation, about 80% of patients do not have renal involvement and about 50% do not have overt lung disease. However, over the course of illness, more than 80% will develop pulmonary and/or renal disease. Most patients first seek medical care because of upper and/or lower airway symptoms. Nasal, sinus, tracheal, and/or ear abnormalities are responsible for initial symptoms in 73% of patients. Over 90% of patients eventually develop upper airway and/or ear abnormalities. These problems may be acute, subacute, or most often indolent, and may initially be assumed to be secondary to allergy or infection. Persistent symptoms and complications, especially recurrent epistaxis, mucosal ulcerations, nasal septal perforation, nasal deformity, or hearing loss, should lead to suspicion of WG and more extensive evaluation. The findings of asymptomatic hematuria (especially with red blood cell casts) on urinalysis, pulmonary infiltrates or nodules, elevated ESR, unexplained anemia, and ANCAs may prompt pursuit of definitive diagnosis by biopsy of one or more involved organs.

Pulmonary infiltrates and/or nodules are initially present in about 50% of patients (Fig. 181.3). Symptoms may include cough, dyspnea, hemoptysis, and/or pleuritis. Bronchospasm is not common. Wheezing and stridor should prompt evaluation

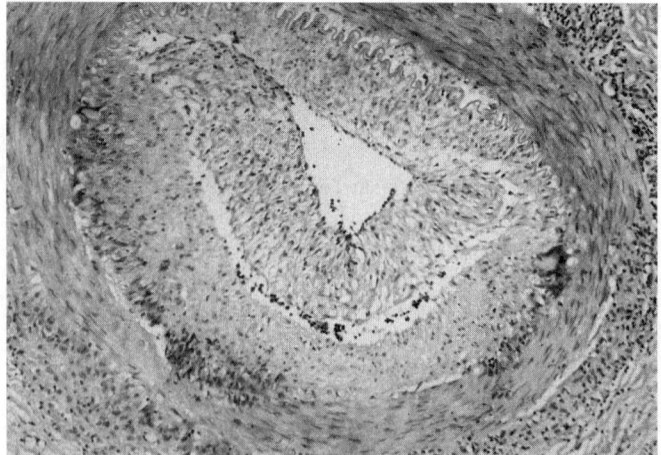

FIGURE 181.2. Temporal artery biopsy in a 64-year-old woman with new onset severe headaches, scalp tenderness, and polymyalgia rheumatica. Note the intense inflammatory changes in the adventitia and media, where giant cells are present. Intimal proliferation has caused luminal narrowing.

TABLE 181.5.	WEGENER'S GRANULOMATOSIS: CLINICAL PROFILE	
Abnormality	**Frequency at Presentation (%)**	**Frequency During Disease Course (%)**
Upper airways	73	92
Lower airways	48	85
Kidneys	18	75
Joint	32	67
Eye	15	52
Skin	13	46
Nerve	1	20

(Data from Hoffman GS, et al. *Ann Intern Med* 1992;116:488–498.)

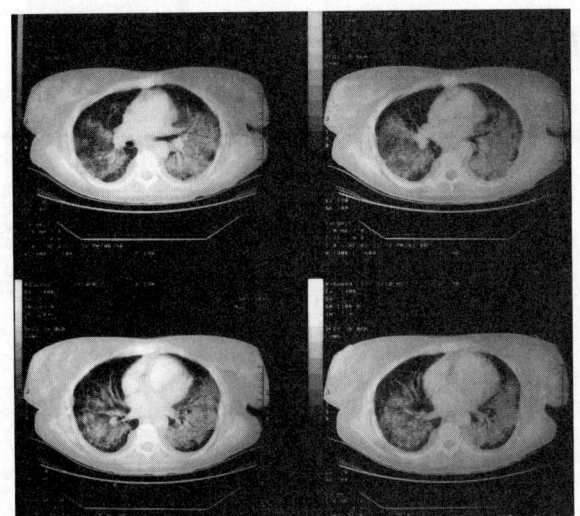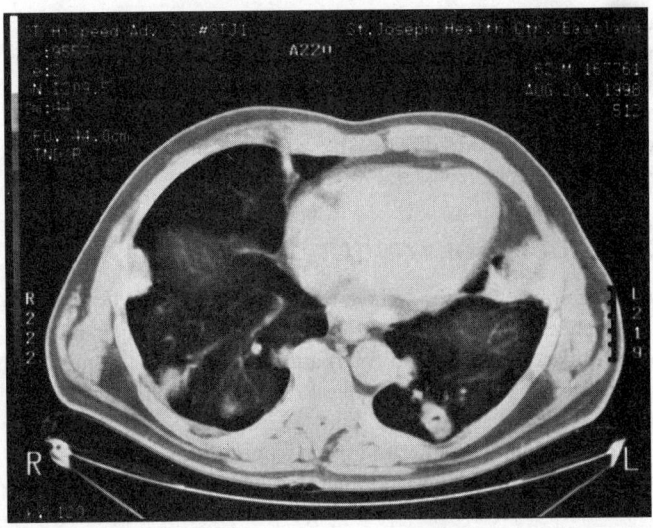

FIGURE 181.3. Wegener's granulomatosis pulmonary disease may present as diffuse pulmonary hemorrhage **(A)** or pulmonary nodules, which may cavitate **(B)**.

of subglottic stenosis or main stem bronchial stenoses. About 85% of patients will eventually develop lung disease. About 33% of patients may have asymptomatic pulmonary involvement. We periodically evaluate patients with chest computed tomography (CT) scans to aid in therapeutic decisions regarding the tapering of medication; CT scans are more sensitive than chest radiographs in demonstrating nodules and infiltrates. Auditory and ocular problems are common. The latter may include scleritis, tear duct obstruction, or orbital pseudotumor.

Less than 20% of patients have glomerulonephritis at presentation. Until the point of uremia, renal disease is generally asymptomatic. This is a critically important observation that necessitates frequent evaluation of the urine to detect glomerulonephritis as early as possible because such discovery warrants intensification of therapy. About 75% of WG patients eventually develop glomerulonephritis. Thus, the concept of "limited" WG (not involving the kidney) in a given patient must be recognized as a description of disease status at one point in time that carries no guarantees about organ involvement in the future.

Ideally, the diagnosis of WG should be suspected on clinical grounds and confirmed by histopathologic examination. Lung tissue is the most likely to yield an unequivocal diagnosis. Open-lung biopsy usually demonstrates areas of geographic necrosis with giant cells, vasculitis, and often some eosinophils. Transbronchial biopsy specimens are often inadequate to diagnose WG but are useful in excluding infection. Nasal biopsies may be "consistent with" the diagnosis in one-third of cases but may not have all classical features. Renal biopsy may provide evidence of glomerulonephritis, with little or no evidence of immune complex deposition.

A positive immunofluorescence test for ANCAs is present in approximately 90% of patients with active generalized disease. In patients with milder forms of WG, without renal involvement, positive tests may only occur in 50% to 70% of cases. In a majority of WG patients antibody specificity is to proteinase 3 (PR3), but in others the antibodies may be directed to myeloperoxidase (MPO). Anti-PR3 specificity usually produces a

cytoplasmic pattern (C-ANCAs) and MPO antibodies usually produce a perinuclear pattern (P-ANCAs), by indirect immunofluorescence techniques. Tissue diagnosis should be aggressively pursued if there are atypical clinical features, including a slow response to therapy, reasons to suspect possible malignancy or infection, or comorbid processes that may require alternative or additional therapy. ANCA titers should not be used as the only guide to adjusting therapy.

Prior to the 1970s, only 50% of patients with WG survived for 5 months from the time of diagnosis and 82% of patients died within a year. In 1973, Fauci and Wolff noted that 13 of 15 WG patients who were treated with glucocorticoids plus an adequate trial of daily low-dose cyclophosphamide (CP) (14 patients) or azathioprine (1 patient) experienced remissions. As of 1991, the National Institutes of Health (NIH) WG cohort included 158 patients followed for 6 months to 24 years (mean = 8 years). Among all patients treated with daily CP and glucocorticoids, 143 (91%) patients had marked improvement, and 118 patients (75%) achieved remission. Unfortunately, 50% of remissions were later associated with at least one relapse. Ninety-nine patients were followed for more than 5 years, of whom 44% had remissions of more than 5 years' duration. Over a mean follow-up period of 8 years, mortality from disease and/or treatment was 13%—a dramatic improvement over historical series in which 50% mortality occurred over 5 months. Initial treatment of severe generalized WG should include glucocorticoid therapy in conjunction with CP. After substantial improvement has occurred, usually within 1 month, high-dose glucocorticoids can be tapered over several months. Cytotoxic therapy should be continued for at least a year following the induction of remission. For patients who do not have severe, immediately life-threatening or critical organ-threatening disease, weekly methotrexate therapy has been successfully used in place of CP during the initial phase of treatment. Methotrexate has also been effectively utilized as maintenance therapy after induction of remission with CP. Daily treatment with trimethoprim–sulfamethoxazole has been shown to decrease the frequency of upper airway flare-ups in WG, without influencing the course of renal or pulmonary disease. The mechanism for this effect may relate to alteration of staphylococcal or other bacterial flora in the upper airway, and it may be a useful adjunct in patients with smoldering upper airway disease. It should not be relied on as a primary treatment for visceral WG.

MICROSCOPIC POLYANGIITIS

Microscopic polyangiitis, as defined by the Chapel Hill Consensus Conference, is a systemic necrotizing vasculitis, with sparse or no immune complex deposition. It affects small vessels (capillaries, venules, or arterioles) but, like PAN, can also affect medium-size arteries (Table 181.1). Like WG and CSS, MPA has a predilection to involve the lungs (e.g., pulmonary infiltrates and hemorrhage), the kidneys (glomerulonephritis), and the peripheral nervous system. The pathologic process of MPA does not include granulomas, which are more characteristic of WG and CSS. MPA may pose an immediate threat to life in the setting of pulmonary hemorrhage and rapidly progressive renal failure. Once diagnosed, MPA necessitates aggressive treatment.

Because MPA and PAN have only recently been differentiated from one another, there exists a sparse historical literature on the incidence of clinical characteristics of MPA beyond glomerulonephritis and pulmonary capillaritis. Most patients with MPA experience myalgias, arthralgias, or arthritis, and a significant minority may have purpuric skin lesions, symptoms of intestinal ischemia, and axonal peripheral neuropathy. Diffuse alveolar hemorrhage and rapidly progressive renal failure may be reversible with aggressive therapy but nevertheless are poor prognostic markers. It is critical to note that the clinical expression of idiopathic PAN, MPA, and cryoglobulinemic vasculitis can be the same as that seen with viral infections complicated by vasculitis (e.g., hepatitis B and C, or HIV). Proof of viral infection in these disease phenotypes would support the use of antiviral therapies, which may minimize immunosuppressive treatment and their inherent toxicities.

Diagnosis of MPA should be confirmed pathologically whenever possible. Transbronchial biopsy may not provide sufficient tissue to confirm the diagnosis, even in the setting of alveolar hemorrhage. Renal biopsy in the clinical setting of an active urine sediment may confirm suspicion of necrotizing crescentic glomerulonephritis. P-ANCA, usually specific for MPO in this setting, occurs in 40% to 80% of patients with MPA. The specificity of this test is *not* 100%. Cases of infection-related or drug-induced ANCAs have also been described.

Treatment is often similar to that described for WG. The usefulness of apheresis in the treatment of MPA has not been demonstrated convincingly. However, in the setting of acute, life-threatening alveolar hemorrhage, with or without renal failure, apheresis therapy should be considered especially if anti–basement membrane disease has not yet been excluded.

POLYARTERITIS NODOSA

Descriptions of PAN are quite variable because a consistent disease definition has not been utilized by all authors. What some authors have in the past called PAN, with pulmonary vasculitis

TABLE 181.6. POLYARTERITIS NODOSA: CLINICAL PROFILE[a]

Abnormality	Frequency (%)
Fever	36–76
Weight loss	30–71
Hypertension	25–70
Kidney	8–77
Gastrointestinal	14–78
Cardiac	10–56
Nervous system	
Peripheral	23–60
Central	3–41
Musculoskeletal	
Arthralgias/arthritis	33–58
Myalgia	8–77
Skin	28–65
Eye	1–47
Testicular pain	1–4

[a] Incidence represents a compilation of data from several series prior to recent acceptance of the concept of microscopic polyangiitis being distinct from polyarteritis nodosa.

or glomerulonephritis, would today be considered MPA. If one is guided by the CHCC nomenclature, PAN is a disease of medium-size or small arteries that can affect patients of any age. Glomerulonephritis and pulmonary capillaritis are not present based on this definition. Significant gender preferences are not appreciated. Affected patients may have fever, musculoskeletal symptoms, skin findings of livedo, nodules, ulcers or gangrene (but not palpable purpura), neurological abnormalities (peripheral more than central), cardiac disease and GI vasculitis (Table 181.6). Glomerulonephritis is not a feature of CHCC-defined PAN, but patients may experience renal failure or hypertension due to involvement of renal arteries. Peripheral neuropathy may have a pattern of mononeuritis multiplex or symmetrical polyneuropathy.

Diagnosis is ideally achieved by biopsy of symptomatic or abnormal structures. If this approach is impossible or unrewarding, and visceral or systemic symptoms are present, angiography should be considered. To maximize the diagnostic yield, a complete study should include the celiac artery and its principal branches, the superior and inferior mesenteric and renal arteries (Fig. 181.4). Angiographic abnormalities may be present even without apparent clinical compromise of the perfused organ. Symptomatic GI, cardiac or renal vasculitis with hypertension, are poor prognostic markers. ANCAs are generally absent in PAN.

Untreated PAN has a >85% mortality rate at 5-year-followup. Treatment with high-dose glucocorticoids may improve this figure to 48%, and the combination of glucocorticoids plus cytotoxic agents may lead to about 80% 5-year survival. Indications for the use of initial concurrent therapy with glucocorticoids and CP, as opposed to glucocorticoids alone have not been fully defined. However, most authorities agree that critical organ involvement should be treated with glucocorticoids plus a cytotoxic agent, usually CP during the initial phase of therapy. Any concerns regarding the effects of glucocorticoids on wound heal-

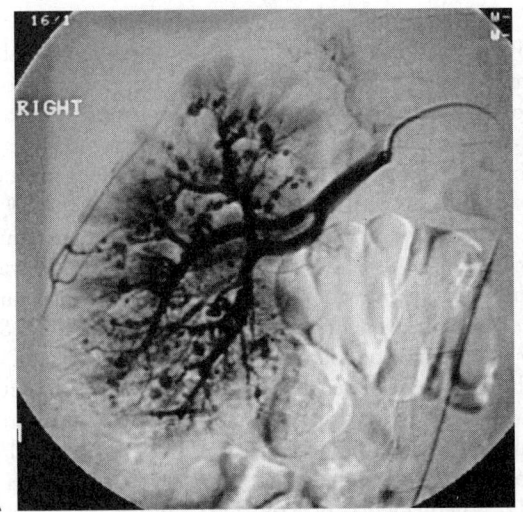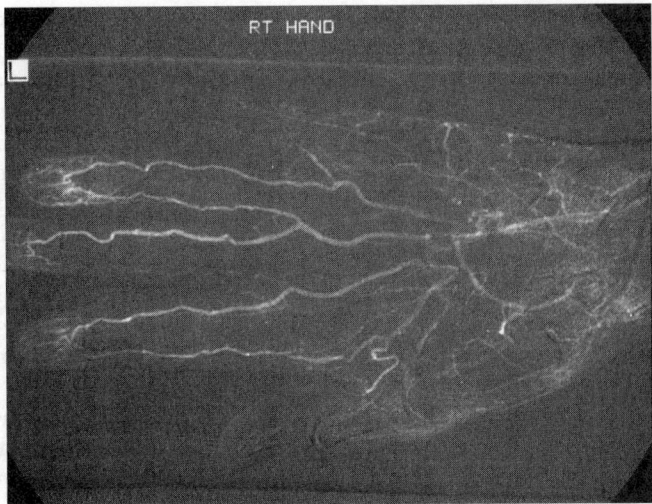

FIGURE 181.4. **A:** Polyarteritis nodosa. Renal angiogram. Multiple vascular stenoses and aneurysms are noted in this patient with new onset severe hypertension, abdominal pain and mononeuritis multiplex. **B:** Angiography reveals occlusion of multiple digital arteries that lead to gangrene of the distal thumb and fifth digit.

ing or risk of infection should be secondary to the need for suppression of the inflammatory process that is the cause of gut ischemia, ulceration, and/or hemorrhage. This concept would appear to be valid for ischemia due to any form of vasculitis involving critical organs.

CHURG–STRAUSS SYNDROME (ALLERGIC ANGIITIS AND GRANULOMATOSIS)

Churg–Strauss syndrome is a rare, hypereosinophilic, granulomatous disorder that affects small and medium-size vessels, with a predilection for smaller arteries, arterioles, capillaries, and venules. There is no clear sexual preference, and persons of any age may be affected. This syndrome differs clinically from PAN, MPA. and WG in that the systemic vasculitis occurs in the setting of asthma and/or allergic rhinitis. Apart from asthma and eosinophilia, it is similar to WG in that it can affect the upper and lower airways and kidneys. Pathologic studies reveal intra- and/or extravascular granulomas and inflammatory lesions rich in eosinophils. Asthma usually precedes the clinical features of vasculitis by months to many years; but in up to 20% of cases both processes begin simultaneously. Unlike WG, allergic nasal and sinus disease of CSS is generally not a destructive process, pulmonary nodules are less common than fleeting infiltrates, and nodules, when they do occur, usually do not cavitate, as often occurs in WG. The degree of blood and tissue eosinophilia in CSS is usually more marked than in WG and renal involvement is usually milder. Coronary arteritis, myocarditis, and gut involvement is more common in CSS.

Churg–Strauss syndrome is generally more responsive to glucocorticoid therapy alone than are MPA, PAN, or WG. Response to high doses of prednisone (1 mg per kilogram per day) is often prompt. Cytotoxic agents should be reserved for severe, progressive, or acute critical organ-threatening (e.g., CNS, heart, renal, gut) or life-threatening disease.

SMALL-VESSEL VASCULITIS

Vasculitis that exclusively involves arterioles and predominantly postcapillary venules can occur as a limited cutaneous disease or be part of a more severe systemic vasculitic process. Limited cutaneous vasculitis, often purpuric, has been termed "hypersensitivity vasculitis" even though a triggering antigen is not usually identifiable. Biopsy of the skin usually demonstrates leukocytoclastic angiitis, with or without immune complex deposition. The presence of cutaneous vasculitis does not necessarily imply a systemic, visceral vasculitic process, but warrants evaluation for visceral disease. Cutaneous vasculitis may also occur in association with infections (bacterial endocarditis, *Neisseria, Rickettsia,* hepatitis B and C, cytomegalovirus, HIV), malignancies (predominantly myeloproliferative and lymphoproliferative, but also "solid" tissue carcinomas), drug allergic reactions, cryoglobulinemia (which may be secondary to malignancy or infection, particularly hepatitis C) and other systemic autoimmune disorders such as rheumatoid arthritis, SLE, or Sjögren's syndrome. Rarely, small-vessel vasculitis may present as urticarial vasculitis. Nonvasculitic causes of purpura and chronic urticaria should be excluded (Table 181.3).

If cutaneous vasculitis is mild and of recent onset, skin integrity is not compromised, and careful evaluation does not reveal a precipitant (e.g., new drug, recent infection) that can be eliminated or treated, only cautious observation may be warranted. However, progression or visceral involvement would require treatment. Extremity edema associated with the skin lesions can be treated with the use of compressive stockings. Pharmacologic therapy with nonsteroidal anti-inflammatory drugs, colchicine, dapsone, or pentoxyfylline can be tried. Unfortunately, the benefits of such therapy are inconsistent at best. Glucocorticoids should be used sparingly and cytotoxic therapy generally avoided for isolated cutaneous disease. If extremely high levels of cryoglobulins are present, apheresis may be of benefit. Controlled studies of apheresis in this setting have not been performed.

HENOCH–SCHÖNLEIN PURPURA

Henoch–Schönlein purpura (HSP) is a systemic small-vessel vasculitis that predominantly affects postcapillary venules. Children of any age may be affected (peak age 4 to 6 years). Less often, adults may suffer from HSP as well. Neither sex is particularly favored. Non-thrombocytopenic palpable purpura is characteristic. Skin lesions may also be nonpurpuric. Mild glomerulonephritis, heme-positive stools (often with abdominal pain), and arthralgias are common components of the syndrome. In typical cases, the skin lesions all appear to be at the same stage of development, and they may recur in "crops" (Fig. 181.5). When measured early in the course of illness, circulating immune complexes can be found in serum and immunoglobulin and complement identified in vessel walls. Although IgA is the predominant immunoglobulin noted in circulating and tissue deposited immune complexes, IgG and IgM may be found as well.

In more than two-thirds of patients, an upper respiratory infection will have preceded HSP by 1 to 3 weeks. The syndrome is characterized by an urticarial or purpuric rash (100%) that is most striking in gravity-dependent areas, fever (75%), musculoskeletal symptoms (68%), GI pain and/or bleeding (70%), and glomerulonephritis (45%). Diagnosis is more difficult if rash is not an initial feature, which is the case in 10% to 30% of patients. Most children with HSP experience one episode of illness that usually lasts less than 4 weeks. However, up to 40% may

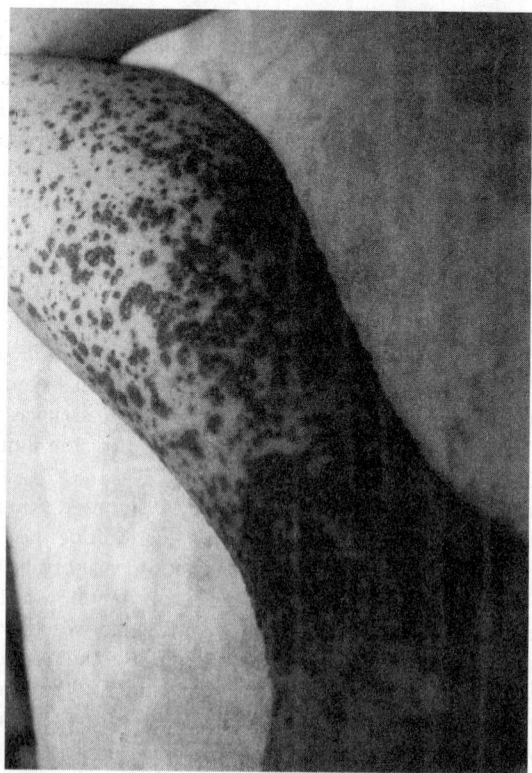

FIGURE 181.5. Henoch–Schönlein purpura. Skin lesions in this 14-year-old girl are particularly striking. Fever, polyarthralgias, and purpura cleared without glucocorticoid therapy. However, several recurrences followed a period of wellness.

have recurrences following a period of well-being. Recurrences usually occur during a 3-month period after the initial episode but may rarely persist for years. The majority of patients do well without glucocorticoids or other immunosuppressive treatment. A minority will have serious GI complications including massive hemorrhage, intussusception, infarction, perforation, or obstruction. Treatment with glucocorticoids usually achieves prompt relief of nonsurgical GI symptoms. At what point glucocorticoids should be used is a matter of judgment, but we usually institute such therapy for GI bleeding, peritoneal inflammation, severe abdominal or testicular pain, and renal failure. Such patients should also be followed closely by surgical staff.

About 40% of patients have mild renal involvement, half of whom will have elevations of blood urea nitrogen or creatinine. Renal biopsy is seldom necessary but if done will reveal IgA and complement deposition. Progressive renal failure occurs uncommonly. Whether glucocorticoid and cytotoxic therapy effectively alter the course of progressive renal disease is uncertain. Until definitive data are available, it would seem prudent to treat progressive glomerulonephritis with aggressive immunosuppressive therapy.

In adults, acute leukocytoclastic vasculitis resembling HSP of children can occur and may be associated with recent respiratory infection, medication hypersensitivity, or parasitic infection. However, in most cases no significant association is apparent. The GI manifestations are less common in adults, being noted in about 25% as compared with 66% of children. If a coincidental infectious process is present it should be treated, and if an exogenous antigen is suspected, such as a medication, it should be eliminated.

BEHÇET'S DISEASE

Behçet's disease (BD) can occur in people of any age, with the mean age being about 35 years. Sex ratios favor men (2:1) in Asia and eastern Mediterranean countries, where the disease is most prevalent, but a more even distribution between the sexes occurs in the United States. Behçet's disease is a very unusual vasculitic process; it affects vessels of all sizes, from capillaries and venules to the aorta and vena cava. It may resemble the small-vessel leukocytoclastic vasculitides, PAN, or Takayasu's arteritis. Diagnosis of BD is confounded by the observation that typical features of this illness may be separated from each other in time, over months to years. It is best recognized by a combination of features including recurrent aphthous stomatitis (without which the diagnosis cannot be made), genital aphthous ulcers, uveitis, cutaneous vasculitis, arthritis, GI disease, and meningoencephalitis. The pathergic response, an exaggerated local inflammatory reaction to trauma such as a needle stick, is perhaps more common in patients in the Middle and Far East than in North America (Table 181.7). Gastrointestinal Behçet's may affect any site in the GI tract, from the mouth to the anus. Distinction from Crohn's disease may at times be difficult. Mucosal ulcers are the most common finding. In most cases, ulcers are well marginated, like those in the mouth or on the genitalia, and intervening GI mucosa usually appears normal. Ulcer depth varies from superficial to complete penetration and perforation,

TABLE 181.7.	BEHÇET'S DISEASE: CLINICAL PROFILE

Abnormality	Frequency (%)
Aphthous oral ulcers	100
Aphthous genital ulcers	67–74
Uveitis	50–80
Cutaneous vasculitis	56–84
Arthritis	30–50
Meningoencephalitis	10–30
Gastrointestinal inflammation/ulcers	~50

(Data from Shimizu T, et al. Semin Arthritis Rheum 1979;8: 223–260; O'Duffy JD, Chapter 69, *Textbook of Rheumatology,* Third ed., 1989; Baba SM, et al., *Dis Colon Rectum* 1976;19: 428–440.

which may occur in up to half of patients with GI involvement, or 25% of all BD cases. Gastrointestinal ulcers are usually multiple and most often located in the ileocecal region and right colon. Multiple perforations and potential perforations and fistulas may be present, increasing the risk of recurrent acute abdominal events and reoperation. Surgery for "apparently" limited ileal, cecal, or right colonic ulceration should consider at least a 1-m resection from the terminal ileum to healthy mucosa, beyond visible ileocecal abnormalities. Transmural inflammation, including noncaseating granuloma, oral ulcers, ocular problems, arthritis, and skin lesions, are seen in both BD and Crohn's disease. The presence of genital ulcers and CNS abnormalities favors the diagnosis of BD.

The treatment of BD is far from satisfactory. Spontaneously relapsing and remitting features make evaluation and treatment complex and confusing. Controlled studies using colchicine have yielded conflicting results. Thalidomide may be effective in reducing oral and genital ulcers. Mucocutaneous lesions have been shown to respond to thalidomide, although relapses usually follow drug discontinuation. Thalidomide use is limited to men and women who do not have reproductive potential. Treatment may be complicated by sedation or neuropathy. Because of neurotoxicity and teratogenicity its use is restricted and consent forms are required. Pentoxifylline has been reported to be effective in the treatment of mucosal ulcers, as has therapy with interferon-alpha 3 to 7 times weekly. Glucocorticoids have provided dramatic improvement in some cases, but temporary or no improvement in others. Some of the best treatment studies have been conducted in ocular BD. Visual complications may affect up to 85% of patients and lead to blindness in 25%.

Controlled studies of azathioprine and cyclosporine have convincingly demonstrated that each of these agents provides palliation for ocular BD, beyond that achieved with only glucocorticoids or colchicine. Although not specifically analyzed, extraocular features of BD also improved in most patients. CP and weekly methotrexate have been less well studied in BD, but appear to be efficacious and may be considered for severe systemic disease. Death directly attributed to BD occurs in about 4% of cases. Major contributing causes include GI perforation, vascular rupture of aneurysms, and CNS disease.

COGAN'S SYNDROME

Cogan's syndrome is a rare disorder of young adults (peak ages 15 to 30 years). There is no sexual predilection. Characteristic features include acute episodic interstitial keratitis that may eventually impair vision in 25% of cases and vestibulo-auditory dysfunction that may cause permanent severe hearing loss in 60% of cases. Vestibulo-auditory dysfunction may be indistinguishable from that of Ménière's disease. Eye and ear disease may occur and recur independently of each other. The dominant ocular lesion in some cases may not be interstitial keratitis. Other ocular features include scleritis, episcleritis, retinal artery occlusion, chorioretinitis, and retinal hemorrhages. A small number of postmortem examinations have revealed vasculitis of small vessels of the optic and acoustic nerves, and of large vessels including the aorta and its branches. However, most specimens from sensory organs do not reveal features of vasculitis. Aortitis, which occurs in approximately 10% of cases, may mimic Takayasu's disease both angiographically and histologically. Aortitis, coronary arteritis, and myxomatous inflammatory changes of the aortic valve may lead to life-threatening events. About 33% of patients develop abdominal pain, some of whom have associated GI bleeding. Although such features have been demonstrated to be the result of vasculitis, limited histologic and angiographic data preclude making conclusions regarding the frequency with which GI bleeding is due to vasculitis as opposed to other forms of inflammatory injury.

Systemic glucocorticoid therapy is indicated for severe ocular disease, vestibulo-auditory dysfunction, and vasculitis. As would be expected for any inflammatory disorder, the sooner glucocorticoids are provided, the greater the likelihood of preserving function. Whether cytotoxic therapies have a role in glucocorticoid-resistant disease is uncertain, but we offer this therapy to patients with life- or organ-threatening glucocorticoid-resistant disease. Cochlear implants have restored hearing for patients who have had severe bilateral sensory neural deafness.

KAWASAKI'S DISEASE

Kawasaki's disease (KD) is an acute febrile illness that primarily affects children less than 4 years old. It is extremely rare in children older than 8 years (mean age in Japan is 12 months and in the United States 2.8 years). The most prominent features are included in the case definition guidelines of the U.S. Centers for Disease Control and are provided in Table 181.8. The illness is usually self-limiting within 4 to 8 weeks, and mortality is 2%. Deaths are usually due to acute thrombosis of coronary artery aneurysms, the result of prior vasculitis. Using noninvasive techniques, coronary artery aneurysms are noted in 20%, compared with 60% of cases studied by angiography. Data from postmortem studies have also demonstrated vasculitis of the aorta, celiac, carotid, subclavian, and pulmonary arteries. Rare case reports of gut vasculitis in KD exist; GI morbidity may result from small- rather than large-vessel disease. The conjunctivitis is nonpurulent. Adenopathy is most prominent in the cervical nodes. Oral mucous membrane changes should be sought on physical examination. Desquamation of hands or feet may begin several days into the illness or be delayed. This is not specific to Kawasaki's

TABLE 181.8.	CDC CASE DEFINITION OF KAWASAKI'S SYNDROME

Fever ≥5 days without other explanation, plus at least four of the following:
1. Bilateral conjunctival injection
2. Mucus membrane changes: injected or fissured lips; injected pharynx or "strawberry" tongue
3. Extremity abnormality: erythema of palms/soles, edema of hands/feet, or generalized or peripheral desquamation
4. Rash
5. Cervical lymphadenopathy

Note: 80% cases < 4 years old; rare > 8 years old.
CDC, U.S. Centers for Disease Control and Prevention.

disease and may follow staphylococcal or streptococcal infections with toxic shock syndrome.

Treatment with high doses of aspirin (30 mg per kilogram per day) or intravenous γ-globulin may prevent aneurysms or hasten their regression. Glucocorticoids have been felt to be of little value, perhaps even exacerbating the coronary artery disease. Nonetheless, in cases that do not respond rapidly to the initial therapy with intravenous γ-globulin and aspirin, glucocorticoids are often added and have appeared to be beneficial.

POLYANGIITIS OVERLAP SYNDROMES

The term polyangiitis overlap syndrome has been applied to patients who have had typical features of vasculitis common to more than one diagnostic entity. An example would be a patient with arteriographic features of PAN and biopsy or angiographic evidence of Takayasu's arteritis. Some patients who cannot be easily classified may be best served with the tentative diagnosis of undifferentiated systemic vasculitis. These individuals may evolve to have a more clearly defined syndrome. Assessment of disease severity, anatomical distribution of disease, rate of progression, and comorbid conditions should determine the aggressiveness of therapy.

ANTINEUTROPHIL CYTOPLASMIC AUTOANTIBODIES

Antineutrophil cytoplasmic autoantibodies have become a prominent part of the literature of vasculitic disease over the past 15 years and thus warrant specific discussion as to their utility and limitations. Certain types of ANCAs have been recognized to be useful adjuncts to clinical diagnosis. Currently, two types of assays are commonly used for the detection of ANCAs: the indirect immunofluorescence technique and antigen-specific enzyme-linked immunosorbent assay (ELISA).

C-ANCA and P-ANCA are patterns of immunofluorescence that result from antibodies binding to antigens that are widely distributed in the cytoplasm (C-ANCA) or antigens that have been artifactually displaced, by ethanol fixation, to the perinuclear region (P-ANCA). Fluorescence is produced by using an antihuman immunoglobulin with a fluorescein tag. The charac-

teristic C-ANCA pattern is usually caused by antibodies against PR3, a neutral serine protease present in the azurophil granules of neutrophils. Differentiating the characteristic centrally accentuated granular C-ANCA fluorescence from other diffuse types of cytoplasmic fluorescence may at times be difficult. In addition, autoantibodies against PMN cytoplasmic antigens other than PR3 can occasionally also cause cytoplasmic fluorescence. It is the anti-PR3/C-ANCA pattern that has the greatest specificity for patients with WG.

ELISA techniques have identified many antigens that are associated with autoantibodies causing P-ANCA fluorescence. MPO is the P-ANCA target antigen with the greatest clinical utility because of the frequent association of MPO–ANCA with MPA and necrotizing crescentic glomerulonephritis with few or no immune complexes. However, autoantibodies against elastase, cathepsin G, lactoferrin, lysozyme, and azurocidin have all been identified as causing the P-ANCA phenomenon. In a significant proportion of P-ANCA-positive sera the target antigens have not been characterized. The significance of finding P-ANCAs with specificities other than MPO is not defined.

The clinician should know how the laboratory determines ANCA or at least be able to contact someone in the laboratory who is knowledgeable about the limitations of the assays and can advise how to proceed in situations where the clinical findings are inconsistent with the reported ANCA test result. The indirect immunofluorescence technique results should be corroborated with antigen-specific testing for PR3 and MPO.

Since the first descriptions of ANCA, the number of diseases in which ANCA may occur has continued to increase. In addition to the systemic vasculitides, the list now includes rheumatic autoimmune diseases, inflammatory bowel disease (40% to 80% of ulcerative colitis patients), autoimmune liver diseases, infections, malignancies, myelodysplastic processes, and many others. Increasing numbers of case reports and small series have associated diseases and certain drug reactions with the presence of ANCAs. The following drugs have been linked to ANCA production and autoimmune syndromes, including vasculitis: allopurinol, hydralazine, propylthiouracil, and minocycline. Therefore, a positive ANCA test does *not* equate to a diagnosis of a primary vasculitis.

TREATMENT OF SYSTEMIC VASCULITIS

GENERAL COMMENTS

The NIH protocol for WG has become a standard treatment approach for other forms of vasculitis, such as PAN, when critical organ involvement is present. For this reason, the principles of this protocol will be reviewed in depth. Initial treatment consists of CP 2 mg per kilogram per day orally, simultaneously with prednisone (1 mg per kilogram per day orally). Daily prednisone is continued for approximately 4 weeks. If marked improvement has occurred, prednisone is gradually (over 3 months) converted to an alternate-day regimen (60 mg on alternate days). After conversion to an alternate-day regimen, the dose is gradually tapered for several months until the patient is no longer receiving prednisone and is maintained solely on CP. The CP is continued for at least a full year after the patient is in complete clinical remission. After this period, which varies among patients, a tapering schedule is begun in which the dose of CP is lowered by 25-mg decrements every 2 to 3 months. The drug is then either discontinued or a dosage is reached below which the patient may have a flare-up of disease activity. When patients are critically ill with presenting symptoms that include severe alveolar hemorrhage or rapidly progressing renal failure due to glomerulonephritis, "pulse" dosing of glucocorticoids (1 g daily of intravenous methylprednisolone for 3 days in single or divided doses) is frequently utilized. CP is concurrently provided in a dose of 3 to 5 mg per kilogram per day for 2 to 3 days and then reduced to 2 mg per kilogram per day. This latter practice has evolved through experience, without controlled trials. During periods of intense immunosuppression, antibiotic prophylaxis against *Pneumocystis carinii* should be provided.

The peripheral leukocyte count should be used as a guide in adjusting the CP dosage to avoid undue risks of toxicity. It is desirable to not allow the leukocyte count to drop below 3,000 to 3,500 per cubic millimeter or the neutrophil count to drop below 1,000 to 1,500 per cubic millimeter. Observation of the slope of decrease of the leukocyte count is essential to the proper adjustment of dosage. The effect of a given dose of CP on the leukocyte count is generally seen within 1 to 2 weeks after it is administered. If the leukocyte count approaches neutropenic levels, dose reductions should be made. In the early induction phase of therapy, it is advisable to follow the leukocyte count about every 2 to 3 days and, after the leukocyte count stabilizes, to follow the counts at intervals no greater than every week until a stable dose has been achieved. It cannot be over-emphasized that therapeutic benefits do not require leukopenia or neutropenia. Patients undergoing long-term CP therapy must be reminded to sustain excellent hydration to maintain dilute urine so that acrolein, the principal bladder-irritating metabolite of CP, will exert minimal toxicity. The appropriate degree of dose adjustment of CP in the setting of renal failure is unclear, but it seems prudent to decrease the dose when the glomerular filtration rate is decreased by 50% in all but the most life-threatening circumstances. Following the peripheral white blood cell count is crucial. Occasionally in the setting of profound leukopenia, neutrophil growth factors may be briefly required as supportive therapy.

Treatment Toxicity and Changing Strategies

In recent years, several prospective studies have evaluated the utility of alternative therapies to daily CP. These studies have included use of glucocorticoids plus intermittent high-dose intravenous ("pulse") CP, or weekly low-dose (15 to 25 mg) methotrexate (MTX) therapy. Preliminary results indicate that pulse CP and glucocorticoids may provide substantial initial improvement but are not as effective as daily low-dose CP therapy in maintaining improvement. There is also concern regarding the inflexibility of dose modification following the initial "pulse" in the severely ill patient; neutropenia may occur while the patient is still in an intensive care unit and at high risk for nosocomial infection. The role for pulse CP therapy remains a subject of controversy and continued study.

The use of MTX (with glucocorticoids) in systemic vasculitis has been under study at the NIH for over 10 years. One protocol enrolled 42 patients with WG without life-threatening pulmonary or rapidly progressive renal disease (or serum creatinine more than 2.5 mg per deciliter). Initiation of treatment was with 0.3 mg per kilogram once weekly, followed by a gradual increase in dose to the maximum tolerated, not to exceed 25 mg per week; folic acid supplementation was also prescribed. Seventy-one percent of these patients achieved remission within a mean period of 4.2 months. Thirty-six percent of patients subsequently relapsed over a mean period of 29 months and required retreatment. These results compare quite favorably to those with daily CP, but concurrent comparisons of these agents in comparable patients were not made. MTX and azathioprine have also been successfully employed as maintenance agents for patients in whom marked improvement or remission has been achieved with CP during the first 3 to 6 months of treatment. The hope in using MTX instead of CP is that there will be decreased late toxicity from the CP. MTX is cleared rapidly following each dose by the kidney, and administration of MTX to a patient with significant renal insufficiency (or on dialysis) may result in severe bone marrow suppression. MTX use is contraindicated in advanced renal failure.

Daily CP therapy produces transient hair loss in about 20% of patients. MTX-induced hair loss is much less common. Examples of persistent morbidity include CP cystitis (50%), bladder cancer (16% at 15-year follow-up), myelodysplasia (2%), and commonly recognized toxicities of glucocorticoids such as cataracts (21%), osteoporosis-related fractures (11%), and aseptic necrosis (3%). Less often, CP may cause thrombocytopenia, profound anemia, or prolonged leukopenia, even after the drug is discontinued. A marrow examination is appropriate in this setting. The malignancy rate in WG patients in the NIH cohort was compared to that in the National Cancer Institute Registry for adults in the general population. The results indicate a 2.4-fold overall increase in malignancies, a 33-fold increase in bladder cancer, and an 11-fold increase in lymphomas. The latency period from the start of CP therapy to detection of transitional cell carcinoma of the bladder varied from 7 months in one man who was receiving daily CP for active WG to 12 years in another who was in remission and had not received CP for 10 years. Almost all patients who had CP-associated bladder cancer were previously noted to have had either microscopic or gross hematuria. If hematuria is not due to glomerulonephritis, cystoscopy should be performed. Urine cytology is a relatively insensitive screening test in this setting. Once CP cystitis is demonstrated by the cystoscopic appearance of either mild to severe mucosal erythema, erosion(s), hemorrhage, pallor, and/or telangiectases, follow-up surveillance cystoscopy should be routinely instituted at intervals of about a year, depending on the degree of abnormality and the quality of subsequent urinalyses and cytologic evaluations. CP therapy should be avoided when CP cystitis has been recognized.

Infection remains a serious and common complication of intense immunosuppressive therapy. Of the patients with WG treated at the NIH, 50% developed serious infections. Eleven of 180 patients (6%) developed *Pneumocystis carinii* pneumonia. All of the *Pneumocystis*-infected patients had been receiving glucocorticoids plus a cytotoxic agent, were in the earliest phase of treatment for disease exacerbation, and were lymphopenic (mean lymphocyte count 303 per cubic millimeter). We and others now recommend chemoprophylaxis for *Pneumocystis* during periods of intense immunosuppressive therapy.

Although chronic therapy with CP has dramatically altered outcomes for many types of severe vasculitis, long-term toxic effects have lead to numerous ongoing studies of alternative protocols.

REFERENCES

Agnello V, Chung RT, Kaplan LM. A role for hepatitis C virus infection in type II cryoglobulinemia. *N Engl J Med* 1994;327:1490–1405.

Blanco R, Martinez-Taboada VM, Rodriguez-Valverde V, et al. Cutaneous vasculitis in children and adults. Associated diseases and etiologic factors in 303 patients. *Medicine* 1998;77:403–418.

Evans JM, O'Fallon WM, Hunder GG. Increased incidence of aortic aneurysm and dissection in giant cell (temporal) arteritis. *Ann Intern Med* 1995;122:502–507.

Guillevin L, Cohen P, Gayraud M, et al. Churg–Strauss syndrome. Clinical study and long-term follow-up of 96 patients. *Medicine* 1999;78:26–37.

Hoffman GS, Kerr GS, Leavitt RY, et al. Wegener's granulomatosis: an analysis of 158 patients. *Ann Intern Med* 1992;116:488–498.

Hoffman GS. Classification of the systemic vasculitides: antineutrophil cytoplasmic antibodies: consensus and controversy. *Clin Exp Rheumatol* 1998;16:111–115.

Hunder GG. Giant cell arteritis and polymyalgia rheumatica. *Med Clin North Am* 1997;81(1):195–219.

Kerr GS, Hallahan CW, Giordano J, et al. Takayasu's arteritis. *Ann Intern Med* 1994;120:919–929.

Lhote F, Guillevin L. Polyarteritis nodosa, microscopic polyangiitis and Churg–Strauss syndrome. Clinical aspects and treatment. *Rheum Dis Clin North Am* 1005;21:911–947.

Mandell BF, Hoffman GS. Differentiating the vasculitides. *Rheum Dis Clin North Am* 1884;20:409–442.

Sneller MC, Hoffman GS, Talar-Williams C, et al. An analysis of 42 Wegener's granulomatosis patients treated with methotrexate and prednisone. *Arthritis Rheum* 1995;38:608–613.

Kelley's Textbook of Internal Medicine, fourth edition. Edited by H. David Humes. Lippincott Williams & Wilkins, Philadelphia © 2000.

CHAPTER

182

INFECTIOUS ARTHRITIS

MARY M. STIMMLER

BACTERIAL ARTHRITIS

Infection of the joint with a bacterial organism is a medical emergency. Prompt diagnosis and initiation of treatment is necessary to avoid excessive morbidity and mortality.

TABLE 182.1.	RISK FACTORS FOR INFECTIOUS ARTHRITIS
Risk Factor	**Specific Disease**
Extremes of age	Infants, elderly
Joint injury or manipulation	Arthrocentesis, intra-articular injection
Chronic debilitating disease	Cirrhosis, alcoholism, diabetes, cancer, uremia
Altered joint integrity	Rheumatoid arthritis, osteoarthritis, hemophilia
Immunosuppression	Human immunodeficiency virus, hypogammaglobulinemia, systemic lupus erythematosus, systemic steroids, cytotoxics
Intravenous drug use	—
Prosthetic joint	—

NONGONOCOCCAL INFECTIONS

Incidence and Epidemiology

No decrease in the frequency of septic arthritis has been noted in spite of advances in antibiotic therapy and sophisticated methods of detecting infection. Most patients have one of the risk factors listed in Table 182.1.

Etiologic Factors

Most organisms reach the joint by the hematogenous route from transient bacteremia or prolonged sepsis. Direct inoculation occurs following trauma and arthrocentesis. Infection can extend from adjacent tissue such as bone, bursa, tenosynovium, or abscess. Cartilage is rapidly destroyed and joint integrity altered by direct effects of the bacteria, proteolytic effects of the polymorphonuclear leukocytes, an intrasynovial immune response, and cytokine release.

The age of the patient and presence of comorbid conditions aid in identifying the infecting organism. Most infections in neonates are caused by *Staphylococcus aureus* and gram-negative bacilli. *Haemophilus influenzae* infection is now almost nonexistent in children who have received *Haemophilus influenzae* type b vaccine. The organisms seen in children are *S. aureus* and *Streptococcus* species, and affect knees and hips. Gram-positive cocci predominate in healthy adults, the elderly, and the immunosuppressed.

Polyarticular infection is usually caused by *S. aureus* and occurs more often in rheumatoid arthritis, hemophilia, and immunocompromised states. *Staphylococcus aureus* is the most common infecting organism after joint aspiration and injection. Anaerobes may accompany *S. aureus* and other organisms in a traumatized joint. Gram-negative bacilli (*Pseudomonas* species) and *S. aureus* reflect the skin and oral flora of intravenous drug users who lick and share needles. *Staphylococcus epidermidis* is found in early postoperative prosthetic joint infection, and gram-positive cocci and anaerobes are found in late infections. *Salmonella* species are associated with sickle cell disease and systemic lupus erythematosus. Joint infection in hemophilia is becoming more common as patients self-inject coagulation factor. *Staphylococcus aureus* accounts for 50% of these cases, followed by streptococci and gram-negative bacilli. Ureaplasma urealyticum should be considered in hypogammaglobulinemia, and *Brucella* species are found in patients who drink unpasteurized milk.

Clinical Findings

Patients present acutely with decreased range of motion in a painful, warm, swollen joint. Signs of inflammation are often less impressive in patients with chronic disease. Most infections are monarticular and involve the knees (42%), hips (13%), ankles and shoulders (10% to 12%). Polyarticular disease in the immunocompromised host involves the knees, elbows, shoulders, and small joints more frequently than the hips. Fibrocartilaginous joints of the axial skeleton (sternoclavicular, sacroiliac, symphysis pubis, and intervertebral disc spaces) are involved in intravenous drug abusers. The patient keeps the infected joints immobilized in a flexed position to relieve elevated intra-articular pressure. Signs of systemic infection may be lacking in diabetics, the elderly, and patients taking immunosuppressive drugs. Fever may be high (more than 39°C), but 20% are afebrile and only 63% of rheumatoid patients with polyarticular infection have fever. Diagnosis of infection is frequently delayed in patients with rheumatoid arthritis when inflamed joints are mistaken for flaring joints with active disease and should be suspected when one or two joints are more inflamed than the remaining joints.

Laboratory Findings

Diagnostic evaluation includes a complete blood count, cultures of blood and other possible sites of infection, arthrocentesis, and baseline joint radiographs. The peripheral white blood cell (WBC) count is normal in as many as 40% to 50% of cases. The C-reactive protein (CRP) and erythrocyte sedimentation rate (ESR) are usually strikingly elevated. Blood cultures are obtained before antibiotics are started and often are the only means of identifying the offending organism. They are positive 30% to 50% of the time, and may be positive in as many as 75% of cases of polyarticular sepsis. When all possible sites of infection are cultured, the source is identified in up to two-thirds of cases.

The most valuable information comes from analysis of the synovial fluid, and all suspect joints should be aspirated before antibiotic therapy is begun. Typical findings are outlined in Table 182.2. A cell count higher than 50,000 WBC per cubic millimeter is usually indicative of infection, although lower cell counts are seen in 30% to 60% of cases. Glucose in septic joint fluids is moderately low. A positive (50%) Gram stain can be helpful in selecting antibiotics. Both aerobic and anaerobic cultures are requested, along with Thayer–Martin media if gonococcal infection is suspected. Use of blood culture bottles may increase the chance of identifying the infecting organism. Bacterial cultures are frequently positive (up to 95%) and should be requested on all joints aspirated. The polymerase chain reaction assay has been used on synovial fluid and tissue in selected cases to detect specific bacterial nucleic acid base sequences.

Radiographs of the involved joints may show only soft tissue swelling and effusion early in the disease but should be obtained to rule out an underlying osteomyelitis. Technetium and gallium bone scanning may be helpful in diagnosing osteomyelitis and evaluating structures that are difficult to visualize, such as the sacroiliac, sternoclavicular, and facet joints. Computed tomography is useful in delineating areas with bony overlap and to look for abscesses. Magnetic resonance imaging is the method of choice for evaluating the hip and can be used to look for soft tissue infection and to confirm the presence of osteomyelitis.

Optimal Management

Treatment consists of parenteral antibiotics and drainage of the affected joint. Initial antibiotic therapy is directed to the most likely organism given the clinical setting, age of the patient, underlying disease, and results of Gram stain and cultures. Therapy is modified when the organism is identified and antibiotic sensitivities are available. Specific recommendations are given in Table 182.3. Nonsteroidal anti-inflammatory drugs (NSAIDs) can confuse the picture and should not be used until response to antibiotics has been documented.

Drainage is accomplished by daily aspiration of the joint with a large-bore needle until the effusion is minimal and WBC counts are less than 50,000 per cubic millimeter. Reaccumulation of the effusion and failure to respond to therapy may be due to lack of sensitivity to the antibiotics, the presence of multiple organisms, or loculation of fluid. Treatment failure has occurred when blood or synovial fluid cultures remain positive after 72 hours or symptoms persist after 5 days of therapy.

Immediate surgical intervention is required for infections of the hip and shoulder, and for unresponsive organisms in a damaged joint. Arthroscopy with lavage of the joint and removal of bacterial and cellular debris can be used in easily accessible joints

TABLE 182.2.	SYNOVIAL FLUID CHARACTERISTICS IN INFECTIOUS ARTHRITIS				
Organism	Appearance	WBC/mm³	% PMN	% Positive Smear	% Positive Culture
Bacterial	Opaque/turbid	>50,000	>90	50	30–50
Gonococcal	Opaque/turbid	30,000–100,000	>80	<25	50
Tuberculous	Opaque	10,000–20,000	>50	20	80

WBC, white blood cell; PMN, polymorphonuclear neutrophil leukocyte.

TABLE 182.3.	ANTIBIOTIC THERAPY FOR NONGONOCOCCAL INFECTIOUS ARTHRITIS	
Bacteria	**Patient Characteristics**	**Antibiotics**
Staphylococcus aureus	Children, adults, polyarticular, rheumatoid arthritis, immunocompromised	Nafcillin 2 g q4h IV × 2–4 wk, *then* oral × 2 wk
Streptococcus pneumoniae Group A Non–group A (enterococcal)	Elderly, children, immunocompromised Prosthetic joints	Penicillin G 2 million U q4h IV Ampicillin 1–2 g q4h IV *plus* gentamicin 1 mg/kg q8h × 2–4 wk, *then* oral × 2 wk
Gram-negative bacilli *Escherichia coli, Pseudomonas* *Salmonella* *Haemophilus influenzae*	Neonates, elderly, intravenous drug abusers Sickle cell, systemic lupus erythematosus Nonimmunized children	Gentamicin 1 mg/kg q8h IV or third-generation cephalosporin *plus* nafcillin 2 g q4h IV (pending cultures) × 2–4 wk, *then* oral × 2 wk

IV, intravenous.

and in patients who are poor surgical candidates. Infection of a joint prosthesis requires removal of the prosthesis, extensive debridement, and prolonged antibiotic treatment. Timely initiation of physical therapy is important in maintaining range of motion.

Parenteral antibiotics are given for 2 to 4 weeks depending on the underlying disease and response to therapy, followed by oral antibiotics for an additional 2 to 4 weeks. Indolent organisms, polyarticular infection, and treatment of prosthetic joint infections may require a longer course of treatment.

Prognosis

Outcome is related to the time elapsed from onset to diagnosis, host defenses, virulence of the organism, and integrity of the joint. Complete function is recovered in 50% to 70% of cases. Poor outcome is associated with a delayed diagnosis in infants or the elderly, polyarticular infection, an unknown organism, and previously damaged joints. Mortality has changed little since the 1960s (5% to 10%) and is as high as 29% in polyarticular infection. In patients with rheumatoid arthritis, complete recovery occurs in only 35%, and the mortality is as high as 56% in those with polyarticular infection.

GONOCOCCAL ARTHRITIS

Incidence and Epidemiology

Neisseria gonorrhoeae is the most common organism causing bacterial arthritis, accounting for almost 75% of infections in healthy, sexually active young adults. Disseminated gonococcal infection (DGI) follows spread of infection from mucosal surfaces. Characteristics of the cell wall proteins and antigenic structure of the pili have been associated with virulence and dissemination. DGI is more common in women than men. Pregnant women, women in the immediate postpartum period, or those within 1 week of their menses are at increased risk for dissemination. Also at risk are those with complement component deficiencies, especially the terminal C5 to C8 components, owing

to their inability to form the membrane attack complex that is necessary for bacterial killing.

Etiologic Factors

Gonococcal bacteremia results in spread of the organism to the joint. Viable organisms have been cultured from the blood and synovial fluid. There is also evidence that arthritis may occur in the absence of viable organisms.

Clinical Findings

Two forms of DGI have been described that may represent either separate entities or two different ends of a spectrum. The *bacteremic form*, resembling serum sickness, occurs in about two-thirds of patients and consists of a triad of polyarthralgia, tenosynovitis, and dermatitis. It begins with migratory polyarthralgias, fevers, chills, and constitutional symptoms. A tendinitis or tenosynovitis may affect the wrists, fingers, ankles, or toes. Skin lesions are papular or pustular on an erythematous base (Fig. 182.1). They are usually found on the extremities and trunk and may continue to appear for up to 48 hours on antibiotics. Aspiration reveals sterile fluid.

The second form consists of a nonerosive, *suppurative arthritis* that is usually monarticular (75%) and affects the knees, feet, and ankles. The patient may be febrile, but rash and tenosynovitis are usually absent at this stage. Synovial fluid is inflammatory (Table 182.2).

Other features of DGI may include sore throat (gonococcal pharyngitis), urethral or vaginal discharge, dysuria, pericarditis, and hepatitis.

Laboratory Findings

A mild leukocytosis may be present, as well as a mild to moderate increase in the ESR. During the bacteremic phase there may be a transient elevation of the transaminases. Circulating immune complexes, if present, are found in the early bacteremic phase.

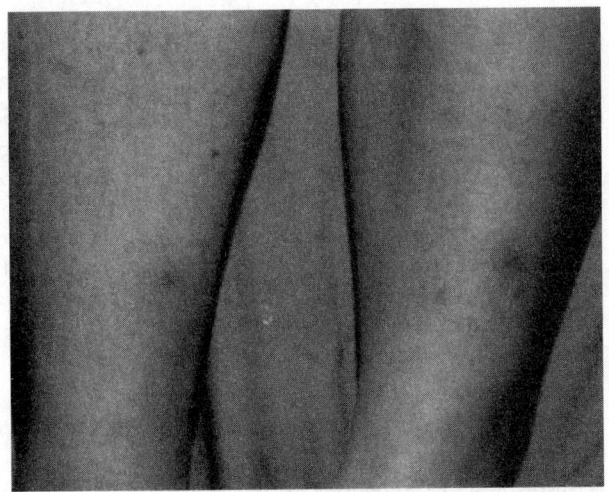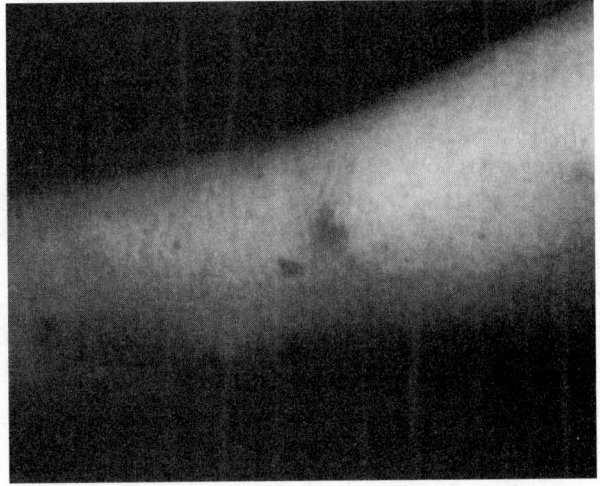

FIGURE 182.1. Disseminated gonococcal infection. **A:** Multiple skin lesions on lower extremities. **B:** Papule on hemorrhagic base. (Courtesy of Thomas H. Rae, MD.) See color figure 182.1.

There may be a small, bland joint effusion that becomes inflammatory once the arthritis is well established.

The diagnosis of gonococcal arthritis is made by demonstrating the organism on culture of body fluids. Handling of specimens is of utmost importance. Swabs for Gram stain and culture are obtained from all mucosal surfaces that could yield bacteria and immediately plated on antibiotic-impregnated culture medium that will inhibit the growth of the other organisms colonizing these areas. Thayer–Martin medium is used for swabs of the urethra, endocervix, rectum, and pharynx. Blood and synovial fluid are plated on chocolate agar. Plates should be kept for 7 days. Blood cultures are positive in up to 30% of cases in the bacteremic phase and are negative in the purulent phase localized in joints. Synovial fluid cultures are positive in about 50% of cases of purulent arthritis. The yield on urogenital cultures is much higher, with best results obtained on cervical culture (80% to 90%). DNA probes are sensitive and specific for bacterial rRNA but do not allow for testing of antibiotic sensitivity. Cultures are also sent for *Chlamydia trachomatis*, which is a coinfection in as many as 40% of cases of gonorrhea. A Venereal Disease Research Laboratory test is obtained and repeated in 6 weeks to rule out incubating syphilis.

Optimal Management

Patients improve dramatically within 48 hours of beginning treatment with appropriate antibiotics. Therapy is initiated in the hospital with intravenous antibiotics until the fever has resolved and symptoms are controlled, followed by a week of oral antibiotics. Typically, 3 to 4 days of intravenous therapy is adequate in the dermatitis–tenosynovitis form and 7 to 10 days in purulent arthritis. Although the arthritis usually is not destructive, daily aspirations may be required for the first few days to ensure adequate response to therapy. The hip also does well with closed-needle aspiration.

Therapy is initiated with a penicillinase-resistant cephalospo-

rin as outlined in Table 182.4. All patients, except pregnant women, should also receive 1 week of doxycycline 100 mg twice daily for *C. trachomatis* coinfection.

MYCOBACTERIAL INFECTIONS

Mycobacterium tuberculosis

Although the prevalence of tuberculosis in the United States and western Europe had been steadily decreasing since the 1960s, there has been a significant resurgence of tuberculosis since the mid-1980s, related to the worldwide epidemic of HIV infection. The prevalence of extrapulmonary tuberculosis (15%) remains the same, with bone and joint infections accounting for 15%

TABLE 182.4.	ANTIBIOTIC THERAPY IN GONOCOCCAL INFECTIOUS ARTHRITIS
Patient Characteristics	**Antibiotics**
Healthy, young, sexually active	Ceftriaxone 1 g IM/IV/d × 2–3 d, *then* cefuroxime or ciprofloxacin 500 mg po b.i.d. × 7 d *plus* doxycycline 100 mg b.i.d.
Penicillin-sensitive	Penicillin G 10 million units/d IV, *then* ampicillin 500 mg/clavulanic acid 125 mg po t.i.d. × 7 d *plus* doxycycline 100 mg b.i.d.
Penicillin-allergic	Spectinomycin 2 g IM q 12 h, *then* ciprofloxacin 500 mg po b.i.d. *plus* doxycycline 100 mg b.i.d.
Pregnancy[a]	Spectinomycin 2 g IM q 12 h, *then* erythromycin *base* 500 mg po q.i.d.

[a] Erythromycin stearate and ciprofloxacin are contraindicated in pregnancy.
IV, intravenous; IM, intramuscular.

to 20% of the extrapulmonary cases or about 1% to 3% of cases overall. Infection reaches the joint by either the hematogenous route or direct extension from adjacent osteomyelitis. Three forms of joint involvement are seen. Tuberculosis of the spine (Pott's disease), which formerly occurred commonly in children and young adults, is now seen most frequently in patients older than 40 years. Collapse of the anterior vertebral bodies gives the characteristic "gibbous deformity" on x-ray. Extension to the disc space and adjacent vertebral bodies occurs along the anterior longitudinal ligament. Paraspinous abscess formation is common (50% to 95%). Involvement of the sacroiliac joint is unusual. Diagnosis is made by identifying organisms obtained in biopsy of the involved bone.

Peripheral joint infection with tuberculosis is manifested by a chronic monarticular arthritis of a weight-bearing joint and usually is seen in males. The knee is most commonly involved. The infection is indolent and delay in diagnosis is common. Palpation of the joint reveals a doughy synovial thickening. The purified protein derivative test is usually positive, but pulmonary involvement is seen in only 50% of cases of tuberculous arthritis. Synovial fluid is mildly inflammatory (Table 182.2) and culture of synovial fluid is positive (80%). Radiographs may be normal or show bony involvement.

An unusual presentation is an acute, recurrent, sterile polyarthritis of hands, knees, and ankles associated with visceral tuberculosis (Poncet's disease).

Treatment of tuberculous arthritis begins with isoniazid, rifampin, and pyrazinamide. Ethambutol is added in areas of endemic drug resistance. Pyrazinamide can be stopped after 2 months and the other medications continued for 10 to 24 months, depending on the clinical response. Surgical debridement may aid in healing when extensive bony involvement is present.

Atypical Mycobacteria

Indolent and chronic infection with atypical mycobacteria occurs more frequently in patients who have had previous manipulation of a joint or who are immunocompromised (Table 182.1). Tenosynovitis, arthritis, and osteomyelitis are often accompanied by cutaneous lesions. The joints and tendon sheaths of the hand are frequently involved (50%), followed by the knee. *Mycobacterium marinum*, *M. kansasii*, and *M. avium* complex are the most common organisms in the HIV-negative host. *Mycobacterium marinum* is associated with aquatic hobbies and is frequently resistant to therapy; a five-drug regimen, including either azithromycin or clarithromycin, is usually required.

▆ VIRAL ARTHRITIS

RUBELLA

An acute, painful, symmetrical polyarthritis occurring during rubella infection affects 30% to 50% of women but is rare in men or children. The fingers, knees, and wrists are painful and stiff, without heat or swelling. The arthritis occurs within 5 to 6 days of the morbilliform rash and follows the usual prodrome of malaise, fever, coryza, and posterior cervical adenopathy. Joint effusions are small and synovial fluid is inflammatory (15,000 to 60,000 WBCs per hpf). It is self-limited and resolves within a month. The arthritis becomes chronic in 15% to 30% of women. Viral particles have been identified in the synovial fluid and in mononuclear cells of blood and synovial fluid, suggesting that the virus directly infects the synovial membrane. Aspirin and NSAIDs provide symptomatic relief.

A causal role of rubella vaccine in both acute and chronic polyarticular arthritis has been established in 5% to 10% in women receiving the RA 27/3 strain. Acute arthralgias and arthritis occur 1 to 6 weeks after vaccination with live attenuated virus.

HEPATITIS

One-third of patients with acute hepatitis B infection have arthritis, often accompanied by an urticarial rash. The arthritis is usually symmetrical and polyarticular. It affects the small joints of the hands, knees, shoulders, ankles, and elbows in the preicteric phase and resolves when jaundice becomes apparent. Demonstration of circulating immune complexes containing hepatitis B surface antigen, immunoglobulins, and complement components suggests that the rash and arthritis is an immune complex–mediated phenomenon. The synovial fluid is noninflammatory with lymphocytic predominance. The arthritis is self-limited and responds to NSAIDs. A reactive arthritis can follow hepatitis B vaccination and last for up to 6 months. Other rheumatologic conditions associated with hepatitis B infection include *polyarteritis nodosa* and *mixed cryoglobulinemia*.

Hepatitis C infection is associated with polyarthralgias and polyarthritis in both the acute and chronic stages and may be difficult to differentiate from rheumatoid arthritis. Autoimmune phenomena include the presence of autoantibodies [antinuclear antibodies (10% to 30%), anti–smooth muscle antibodies (60% to 70%) and rheumatoid factor (60% to 80%)], mixed cryoglobulinemia, glomerulonephritis, sialoadenitis, and induction of thyroid disease. Many of the autoimmune features respond to treatment with interferon-α, but relapse when treatment is stopped.

ARBOVIRUS

A number of arboviruses cause sporadic outbreaks of polyarthritis. Epidemics commonly follow heavy rainfall in endemic areas where mosquitoes multiply. They are characterized clinically by severe but self-limited polyarthralgias, rash, and varying degrees of fever and constitutional symptoms. Diagnosis is confirmed by seropositive tests. Treatment consists of aspirin and narcotic analgesics. Arthritis rarely lasts longer than 2 weeks.

Ross River virus affects adults and is endemic in Australia, Fiji, and other South Pacific islands.

Chikungunya virus is a cause of hemorrhagic fever and is endemic in Africa, Southeast Asia, and the Philippines.

O'nyong-nyong is endemic in Africa and affects older children and adults.

PARVOVIRUS (ERYTHEMA INFECTIOSUM)

An acute symmetrical polyarthritis resembling rheumatoid arthritis occurs in about 50% of adult women with parvovirus infection. The "slapped cheek" rash seen in children is often lacking. Arthritis begins after a flulike prodrome coincident with the antibody response, suggesting an immune-mediated mechanism. The serum B19-IgM response lasts for 1 to 3 months and is diagnostic of recent infection. Anti-IgG is found in 40% to 60% of adults. B19-DNA has been detected in serum, bone marrow, and synovial fluid using polymerase chain reaction but is not diagnostic of infection. The arthritis is nonerosive and usually is self-limited. A mild but definite exfoliation of skin on the hands is occasionally seen. Symptomatic treatment with NSAIDs is helpful. There is some evidence that B19 DNA can be found in synovium of patients with rheumatoid arthritis. A definite causal role of the virus has not been established.

Other viruses occasionally associated with arthritis include mumps, smallpox, adenovirus, and the herpesviruses (varicella-zoster, herpes simplex virus 1, Epstein–Barr, and cytomegalovirus).

HUMAN IMMUNODEFICIENCY VIRUS

Musculoskeletal manifestations are found in 5.5% to 72% of patients with HIV infection (Table 182.5).

Articular Syndromes

Arthralgias are seen in patients with acute HIV infection along with sore throat, fever, and malaise. Up to one-third of patients may have nonspecific generalized arthralgias of mild to moderate degree that recur intermittently and respond to NSAIDs.

A *painful articular syndrome* is characterized by severe, debilitating oligoarticular pain without synovitis. It occurs suddenly, is unresponsive to NSAIDs, and requires narcotic analgesics. The joint pain resolves within 48 hours without sequelae.

Reiter's syndrome is the most frequently observed inflammatory arthritis associated with HIV infection. It can precede the diagnosis of HIV. An incomplete form is seen more frequently than the classic triad. The arthritis is usually severe, persistent, and oligoarticular, involving primarily the large joints of the lower extremities. Extra-articular manifestations include urethritis, conjunctivitis, circinate balanitis, keratoderma blennorrhagicum, enthesopathies, and oral ulcers. Some cases appear reactive in nature, precipitated by culture-negative urethritis or diarrhea. Reiter's syndrome is frequently described in homosexuals, in whom the disease is usually human leukocyte antigen (HLA)–B27 related. It is not seen commonly in intravenous drug abusers, and it is not related to HLA-B27 in Africans who acquire HIV through heterosexual contact. The arthritis responds poorly to NSAIDs and variably to sulfasalazine.

Psoriasis was the first rheumatic syndrome described in HIV infection. The skin disease can be severe and arthritis seen in less than half of patients. The arthritis is asymmetrical, oligoarticular, and frequently accompanied by enthesopathy. It can be erosive, rapidly progressive, and refractory to treatment.

HIV-associated arthritis is a nonerosive, oligoarticular arthritis affecting knees and ankles. It is characterized by moderate to severe pain, mildly inflammatory synovial fluid, and a mild chronic synovitis. Some relief is seen with NSAIDs, and the arthritis resolves in 6 weeks to 6 months.

Septic arthritis in AIDS is uncommon. Involvement is usually monarticular with *S. aureus* or *Candida albicans*. Multiple joints may be involved with fungal or mycobacterial organisms later in the disease when CD4 counts are low. *Mycobacterium haemophilum, M. kansasii,* and *M. avium* complex are the most common organisms. Septic arthritis appears to be related to the intravenous drug abuse and its complications, just as Reiter's syndrome appears to be related to homosexual behavior. Hemophiliacs seem to be at particular risk for septic joints.

Myopathies

Myalgias can be generalized or confined to the thighs. They are a common finding, tend to recur, and respond well to analgesics. Inflammatory polymyositis is indistinguishable from idiopathic polymyositis and patients respond to treatment with systemic corticosteroids.

Zidovudine (azidothymidine, AZT) therapy has been associated with an inflammatory myositis with muscle tenderness, weakness, and elevated creatine phosphokinase. Some cases resolve when the AZT is stopped. *Staphylococcus aureus* is the organism most commonly identified in *pyomyositis*. Other myopathies reported are nemalin rod myopathy, myositis ossificans, and a necrotizing myositis.

Sjögren's Syndrome

A seronegative Sjögren's syndrome (keratoconjunctivitis sicca and xerostomia) described in AIDS tends to predominate in men and consists of significant parotid swelling and lymphadenopathy in the absence of arthritis.

Vasculitis

Several types of vasculitis can be seen in HIV disease, including a systemic necrotizing vasculitis of the polyarteritis nodosa type, peripheral neuropathy, mononeuritis multiplex, and hypersensitivity vasculitis.

TABLE 182.5.	**MUSCULOSKELETAL MANIFESTATIONS OF HIV INFECTION**

Articular syndromes
  Arthralgias
  Painful joint syndrome
  Reiter's syndrome
  Psoriatic arthritis
  HIV-associated arthritis
  Septic arthritis
Myopathies
  Polymyositis
  Zidovudine-associated myositis
  Pyomyositis
  Subclinical myopathy
  Myositis ossificans
Sjögren's syndrome
Vasculitis
Autoimmune manifestations

Autoimmune Manifestations

There is a striking similarity between HIV-related disease and many of the autoimmune diseases. Clinical findings are often identical and autoantibody production is common.

FUNGAL ARTHRITIS

Fungal arthritis is increasing in incidence and affects the compromised host. A self-limited hypersensitivity reaction with polyarthritis may accompany initial pulmonary infection (erythema nodosum in histoplasmosis, acute valley fever in coccidioidomycosis) or the fungus may directly infect the joint. Fungal infections typically present as a chronic monarticular arthritis, with an indolent course that results in a delay in diagnosis.

Coccidioides immitis is found in the soil of the desert areas of the southwestern United States, northern Mexico, and Central and South America. Fever is common and arthritis affects the weight-bearing joints, especially the knees. The organism can be seen in synovial fluid. Serologic testing of serum and synovial fluid by complement fixation may be helpful in establishing the diagnosis.

Blastomyces dermatitidis is endemic in the midwestern and southeastern United States and affects outdoor workers who have contact with the soil. It is one of the few fungal infections that presents with an acute monarthritis, affecting the knee, ankle, elbow, or wrist. Organisms are easily seen in joint fluid.

Arthritis is rare in *sporotrichosis,* occurring after cutaneous inoculation. It is an occupational disease seen in people working in agricultural jobs with exposure to soil or plants. Arthritis affects the knees, wrists, and hands and may mimic rheumatoid arthritis. Systemic symptoms are present in the polyarticular form but absent with monarthritis. Synovial fluid is inflammatory and cultures are frequently negative.

Monarticular arthritis occurs after introduction of atypical species of *Candida* (*C. parapsilosis, C. guilliermondi*) into the knee during aspiration and articular injection, or by contamination of the knee or hip at surgery with *C. albicans, C. tropicalis,* or *C. parapsilosis.* A monarticular or polyarticular arthritis results from hematogenous spread in immunocompromised patients. Intravenous drug abusers have involvement of the knee or fibrocartilaginous joints with *C. albicans.* Brown heroin use is associated with a triad of ocular and cutaneous lesions and arthritis of the costochondral joints.

OPTIMAL MANAGEMENT

Intravenous amphotericin B is the drug of choice in critically ill patients. Flucytosine is an useful adjunct in recalcitrant *Candida* and *Cryptococcus* infections. Fluconazole can be used as first-line therapy in *Candida* or *Cryptococcus* arthritis and itraconazole in *Blastomyces* and *Aspergillus* arthritis. Either drug can be used for maintenance therapy following amphotericin. Treatment should continue for at least 6 weeks, combined with surgical synovectomy and debridement.

BIBLIOGRAPHY

Balkhy HH, Sabella C, Goldfarb J. Parvovirus: a review. *Bull Rheum Dis* 1998;47:4–9.

Bisbe J, Miro JM, Latorre X, et al. Disseminated candidiasis in addicts who use brown heroin: report of 83 cases and review of the literature. *Clin Infect Dis* 1992;15:910–923.

Cucurull E, Espinoza LR. Gonococcal arthritis. *Rheum Dis Clin North Am* 1998;24:305–322.

Cuellar ML. HIV infection–associated inflammatory musculoskeletal disorders. *Rheum Dis Clin North Am* 1998;24:403–421.

Dubost JJ, Fis I, Denis P, et al. Polyarticular septic arthritis. *Medicine* 1993; 72:296–310.

Hirsch R, Miller SM, Kazi S, et al. Human immunodeficiency virus associated with atypical mycobacterial skin infections. *Semin Arthritis Rheum* 1996;25:347–356.

McMurray RW, Elbourne K. Hepatitis C virus infection and autoimmunity. *Semin Arthritis Rheum* 1997;26:689–701.

Munoz-Fernandez S, Cardenal A, Balsa A, et al. Rheumatic manifestations in 556 patients with human immunodeficiency virus infection. *Semin Arthritis Rheum* 1991;21:30–39.

Kelley's Textbook of Internal Medicine, fourth edition. Edited by H. David Humes. Lippincott Williams & Wilkins, Philadelphia © 2000.

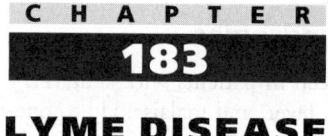

LYME DISEASE

LEONARD H. SIGAL

DEFINITION

Lyme disease (LD) is a multisystem inflammatory condition caused by spirochetes, known collectively as *Borrelia burgdorferi,* that are spread by *Ixodes* ticks. It was first described in studies of an outbreak of presumed juvenile rheumatoid arthritis in Connecticut, which led to the identification of Lyme arthritis. As nonarticular features were identified, the full spectrum of LD became clear.

Early localized LD occurs days to weeks after the tick bite and is characterized by a distinctive rash known as *erythema migrans* at the site of the bite and associated symptoms. Early disseminated LD develops within a similar period as a result of spirochetemia and can include multiple lesions of erythema migrans, cardiac disease, and neurologic problems. Late LD occurs weeks to months after infection and features the often insidious development of arthritis or neurologic problems. Patients do not always progress smoothly through each phase of LD. Some have erythema migrans and no further disease, whereas others never have the rash and the first manifestations of LD may be late features. In addition, rarely in the United States but more commonly in Europe, two other cutaneous features of LD are observed: *lymphadenosis benigna cutis (lymphocytoma)* in early disseminated LD and *acrodermatitis chronica atrophicans* in late LD.

TABLE 183.1.	CDC CRITERIA FOR LYME DISEASE

Presence of erythema migrans
OR
Cases with at least one late manifestation and laboratory confirmation of infection. The late manifestations include any of the following *when an alternate explanation is not found:*

1. *Musculoskeletal system:* Recurrent brief attacks of objective joint swelling in one or a few joints, *sometimes* followed by chronic arthritis in one or a few joints. Manifestations not considered to be criteria for diagnosis include chronic progressive arthritis not preceded by brief attacks and chronic symmetric polyarthritis. In addition, arthralgias, myalgias, or fibromyalgia syndromes alone are not accepted as criteria for musculoskeletal involvement.
2. *Nervous system:* Lymphocytic meningitis, cranial neuritis, particularly facial palsy (may be bilateral), radiculoneuropathy, or, rarely, encephalomyelitis alone or in combination. Encephalomyelitis must be confirmed by showing antibody production against *Borrelia burgdorferi* in the CSF, demonstrated by a higher titer of antibody in CSF or serum. Headache, fatigue, paresthesia, or mild stiff neck alone is not accepted as a criterion for neurologic involvement.
3. *Cardiovascular:* Acute-onset, high-grade (second- or third-degree) atrioventricular conduction defects that resolve in days to weeks and sometimes are associated with myocarditis. Palpitations, bradycardia, bundle-branch block, or myocarditis alone is not accepted as a criterion for cardiovascular involvement.

CDC, U.S. Centers for Disease Control and Prevention; CSF, cerobrospinal fluid.

The U.S. Centers for Disease Control and Prevention (CDC) has developed an epidemiologic definition of LD (Table 183.1). Because the definition is epidemiologic, it should not be used in clinical practice as a set of diagnostic criteria; however, it is useful insofar as LD must be reported to the CDC. Much has been made about how difficult it is to diagnose LD. However, a complete history and physical examination, proper use of testing, an unbiased synthesis of the information obtained, and familiarity with LD allow easy diagnosis and treatment.

INCIDENCE AND EPIDEMIOLOGY

Lyme disease is spread by the bite of infected *Ixodes* ticks (*I. scapularis* in the eastern and north central United States, *I. pacificus* in the western United States, *I. ricinus* in Europe, and *I. persulcatus* in Asia). The areas where LD is found are those where ixodid ticks abound. About 90% of U.S. cases occur in the following nine states: Massachusetts, Connecticut, Rhode Island, New York, New Jersey, Pennsylvania, Minnesota, Wisconsin, and California. Within each state, there are hot spots of disease (i.e., the incidence is not uniform across the state). In New Jersey in 1991, the incidence of LD in urban Hudson County was 0.36 per 100,000 population; in suburban/rural Ocean, Atlantic, Somerset, and Hunterdon counties, the incidence was 30 to 50 per 100,000. Obtaining a travel history from

the patient is crucial; even if a patient does not reside in an endemic area, he or she may have vacationed in one.

Ixodid tick larvae hatch from the egg mass in the summer and then search for a blood meal, usually from mice (or small mammals or birds). About 99% of ticks are born uninfected, even in hyperendemic areas; the ticks acquire the organisms during their first blood meal from spirochetemic (but healthy) mice. Having fed, the ticks molt and reemerge in the spring as nymphs, which then seek a blood meal, usually from the same type of host that fed the larvae. The vast majority of LD is spread by infected nymphs, which explains the seasonal variation in incidence: nymphs are looking for a blood meal in the late spring, summer, and early fall: "LD season." Once fed, the ticks drop off the hosts and molt to adults in the fall. Adults seek a blood meal in the late fall, winter, and even spring, and their preferred hosts are white-tailed deer, although other mammals are used. LD can be acquired from adult ticks, but they are more easily seen and felt, and more protective clothing is worn in the fall and winter than in the summer. Females lay their eggs in the leaf clutter on the forest floor and the 2-year life cycle repeats itself. Ticks seeking a meal reside on the undersides of low-lying shrubs or grass; ticks do not jump, hop, fly, or descend from trees. Ticks sense a warm body exhaling carbon dioxide and latch on if it brushes against them. Therefore, when walking along a deer path, the main area of risk is the foliage at the edges; an individual should walk in the center of the path.

In unfed ticks, *B. burgdorferi* resides on the midgut wall. Shortly after the blood meal, which occurs 24 hours or more after attachment, the organism multiplies and disseminates, eventually reaching the salivary glands. The tick excretes excess water from the blood meal back into the host throughout its meal, and this is how the organism invades the host. It takes 48 hours or more after tick attachment for *B. burgdorferi* to spread to the unwitting host of the tick. This helps explain why so few individuals contract LD after known tick bites. A study suggests that in an area where 40% of adult ixodid ticks carry *B. burgdorferi*, LD develops in only about 1% of individuals who were bitten.

Lyme disease may be obtained on vacation, on the job, or near home. Homes with properties sculpted from surrounding forest provide a perfect "eco-niche" of low-lying shrubs and grasses for white-footed field mice. Old stone fences can serve as "apartment complexes" for mice. Mice are often attracted to the seeds spilled from bird feeders kept near suburban homes. Deer wandering across the property also suggest an increased risk in that environment. Ticks do not survive on open lawns and fields for long because they desiccate rapidly; ticks prefer the higher humidity of the leaf clutter at the forest floor.

ETIOLOGY

Lyme disease is caused by three closely related genospecies, all of which are included in the term *B. burgdorferi sensu lato* ("in the general sense"). *Borrelia burgdorferi sensu stricto* ("in the strict sense") is the cause of LD in the United States and also is found in Europe and Asia. *Borrelia afzelii* and *B. garinii* cause LD in

Europe and Asia. Lyme disease is found across Europe and Asia, including Japan, Korea, and China. It has been suggested that the differences between European and American LD (a greater incidence of arthritis and multiple erythema migrans lesions and a lower incidence of neurologic disease in the United States) may be the result of differences in the organisms, as well as differences in the immunogenetics of the human victims.

Borrelia burgdorferi is a microaerophilic, fastidious organism that grows in Barbour–Stoener–Kelly medium. A paucity of organisms in tissue makes histologic or immunologic staining a low-yield diagnostic test. Likewise, low yields in culturing the organism make this a poor diagnostic tool.

PATHOGENESIS

The way in which *B. burgdorferi* causes LD and may cause disease of long duration is a matter of debate. The organism does not make exotoxins or directly cause local tissue damage. There is evidence to suggest that the organism can bind and activate the host's proteolytic enzymes, which may facilitate tissue invasion and dissemination. *Borrelia burgdorferi* has been identified in erythema migrans lesions, myocardium, spinal fluid, and synovial fluid by culture, polymerase chain reaction, and histologic examination. Local inflammation at these sites presumably results from the immune response to the organism. It is likely that persistence of dead or effete organisms can cause ongoing inflammation. A mechanism much like that seen in the antigen-induced model of rheumatoid arthritis may be at work. In this model, persistence and resistance to proteolytic degradation of an antigen causes the antigen to be a focus of inflammation; as long as the antigen persists, the inflammation persists, and every time there is a "boost" in the systemic immune response to that antigen, there is a flare-up of arthritis. Persistence of antigen also may result in ongoing production of cytokines, which may cause local and nonspecific systemic symptoms. Vasculitis has been implicated in some cases of peripheral neuropathy. Finally, there is in vitro evidence implicating molecular mimicry as a mechanism in neurologic and articular LD. The organism's flagellin contains an epitope that cross-reacts with a human axonal protein, and a monoclonal antibody to this epitope can modify neural cell tumor lines in vitro. Chronic, antibiotic-resistant arthritis is linked to the presence of HLA-DR-B*0401 and the emergence of measurable anti–outer surface protein A (OspA) antibody, which suggested that autoimmunity might play a role in the immunopathogenesis of Lyme arthritis. Recent studies have shown that an epitope in OspA of *B. burgdorferi* cross-reacts with one on human lymphocyte function–associated protein (LFA-1); how this cross-reactivity can be implicated in the pathogenesis of chronic arthritis is not yet clear.

CLINICAL FINDINGS

EARLY LOCALIZED DISEASE

Early localized disease includes erythema migrans and associated findings. Erythema migrans occurs in 50% to 90% of patients,

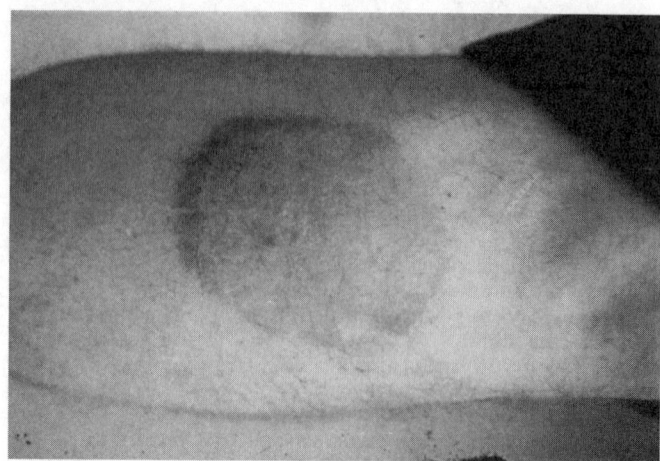

FIGURE 183.1. Lyme disease, erythema chronicum migrans. (Courtesy of Pfizer Central Research.) See color figure 183.2.

usually less than 1 month after the tick bite. About 30% of patients recall having been bitten by a tick. In adults erythema migrans is typically found in or near the axilla or inguina; in children, the neck and hairline are common sites of erythema migrans. The lesion is usually asymptomatic, but it may burn or itch.

Erythema migrans expands over the course of a few days, often with central clearing, although it can be uniformly red or have a more complex "bull's eye" appearance (Figure 183.1); the bull's-eye lesion is classic for LD but constitutes less than 30% of all erythema migrans lesions. About 10% of all patients with erythema migrans have multiple lesions, as a result of spirochetemia; satellite lesions are less likely to have central clearing. Early localized disease may be associated with nonspecific complaints resembling a viral syndrome. In the absence of erythema migrans, there is nothing about this syndrome that is diagnostic of LD. Further details of the syndrome are listed in Table 183.2.

EARLY DISSEMINATED DISEASE

Early disseminated disease (Table 183.2) develops days to months after the tick bite and can occur in the absence of any features of localized LD. Early disseminated LD can be the initial presentation of *B. burgdorferi* infection, with no antecedent erythema migrans or documented tick bite. Neurologic findings are seen in about 10% of untreated patients and include lymphocytic meningitis; cranial nerve palsy, especially of cranial nerve VII (which may be bilateral); and radiculoneuritis. The neurologic features of early disseminated LD usually resolve spontaneously, although there are rare cases of irreversible neurologic damage, e.g., persisting seventh nerve palsy, focal encephalopathy with seizure disorder, persisting weakness due to radiculoneuropathy. Therapy is directed at preventing progression to later features of LD or hastening their resolution. About 8% of patients with untreated LD (Table 183.2) have carditis that can include any degree (or combination of degrees) of heart block and mild myopericarditis (including subclinical congestive heart failure detected by reversible echocardiographic and/or radio-

TABLE 183.2.	CLINICAL MANIFESTATIONS OF LYME DISEASE

Early Localized Disease: Occurring a Few Days to a Month After the Tick Bite

Erythema migrans (in 50–70% of patients; multiple lesions in 10% of patients)[a]
Fatigue/malaise/lethargy
Headache
Myalgia/arthralgia
Regional/generalized lymphadenopathy

Early Disseminated Disease[b]: Occurring Days to 10 Months After the Tick Bite

Carditis
 About 8–10% of *untreated* patients
 Conduction defects[a]
 Mild cardiomyopathy/myopericarditis[a]
Neurologic disease
 About 10–12% of *untreated* patients
 Lymphocytic meningitis[a]
 Encephalitis
 Cranial neuropathy (most often facial, can be bilateral)[a]
 Peripheral neuropathy/radiculoneuropathy[a]
 Myelitis
Musculoskeletal
 About 50% of *untreated* patients
 Migratory polyarthritis and/or polyarthralgia[a]
 Fibromyalgia
Other
 Skin: lymphadenosis benigna cutis (lymphocytoma),[a] erythema nodosum
 Lymphadenopathy: regional and/or generalized
 Eye: conjunctivitis, iritis, choroiditis, vitritis, retinitis
 Liver: liver function test abnormalities, hepatitis
 Kidney: microhematuria, proteinuria

Late Chronic Disease[b]: Occurring Months to Years After the Tick Bite

Musculoskeletal
 About 50% of *untreated* patients have migratory polyarthritis
 About 10% of *untreated* patients have chronic monoarthritis, usually of the knee
 Fibromyalgia, often in adequately treated patients
Neurologic disease
 Chronic (often subtle) encephalopathy, encephalomyelitis, and/or peripheral neuropathy[a]
 Ataxia, dementia, sleep disorder
Cutaneous
 Acrodermatitis chronica atrophicans[a]
 ?Morphea/localized scleroderma–like lesions

[a] Features included as part of the defined clinical syndrome of Lyme disease referred to in Table 183.1.
[b] Can occur in the absence of any prior features of Lyme disease.
(From Sigal LH, Academy of Medicine of New Jersey Lyme Disease Task Force. *Lyme disease in New Jersey: a practical guide for New Jersey clinicians.* 1993, with permission.)

graphic changes). *Borrelia burgdorferi* has been implicated in chronic congestive cardiomyopathy in Europe, but this association has not been substantiated in the American experience. Cardiac features of LD usually begin to resolve during or even before the initiation of antibiotic therapy, although there have been a few cases of permanent heart block requiring insertion of a pacemaker.

LATE DISEASE

Late disease occurs months to years after the onset of infection and may not be preceded by other features of LD. About 80% of patients with untreated LD will develop musculoskeletal symptoms, including arthralgia (20%), intermittent episodes of arthritis (50%), and chronic monarthritis (10%), usually of the knee. Patients with chronic monarthritis usually complain more about knee stiffness than pain; they often develop very large effusions that reaccumulate quickly after aspiration. Many patients with arthritis had previous arthralgia. Oral antibiotic therapy is usually effective for the arthritis, with intravenous antibiotics reserved for refractory cases; synovectomy and disease-modifying treatment (e.g., hydroxychloroquine) occasionally are necessary. The other feature of late LD is tertiary neuroborreliosis, a term that refers to tertiary neurosyphilis, to which it bears some resemblance. Encephalopathy, neurocognitive dysfunction, and peripheral neuropathy are characteristic. The two neurologic stages of LD are compared in Table 183.3.

Other medical problems have been ascribed to LD, often on the basis of only a positive blood test result; such "proof" is not enough to ensure causality. Some less well established features of LD include ophthalmologic findings (inflammation of all eye structures has been described), liver dysfunction (mild hepatitis in early LD), splenitis, and myositis. Established cutaneous features of *B. burgdorferi* infection, more common in Europe than in the United States, are lymphocytoma and acrodermatitis chronica atrophicans.

Nonspecific complaints (e.g., headache, fatigue, arthralgia) may persist after the treatment of LD, often lingering for months with slow, spontaneous resolution. In the absence of objective evidence of LD, there is no justification for antibiotic therapy in such patients. Fibromyalgia syndrome is common after LD. The aches of fibromyalgia should not be mistaken for Lyme arthritis, and fatigue and forgetfulness should not be misdiagnosed as central nervous system LD. There is an ongoing controversy in regard to "chronic LD." Lack of response to therapy can occur, although there are no isolates of *B. burgdorferi* shown to be resistant to the standard antibiotics used for LD. Cases of refractory LD are uncommon and should prompt a search for objective evidence of inflammation and/or tissue dysfunction in order to document damage of true ongoing infection. The most common cause for lack of response to therapy is initial misdiagnosis, i.e., the patient never had LD in the first place! Competent clinicians should search assiduously for alternate explanations for such patients' complaints.

■ LABORATORY FINDINGS

The widely available immunologic tests used in LD are the enzyme-linked immunosorbent assay (ELISA) and the Western blot, but neither should be referred to as a Lyme disease test; they are actually measurements of anti–*B. burgdorferi* antibodies. The diagnosis of LD should be made on clinical grounds (objective signs of inflammation and/or tissue dysfunction), with testing used only for confirmation. Thus, they are more properly

TABLE 183.3. CONTRASTS BETWEEN EARLY DISSEMINATED AND TERTIARY NEUROBORRELIOSIS

	Early Disseminated Neuroborreliosis	Tertiary Neuroborreliosis
Time since EM manifestations	Weeks to months Facial palsy Peripheral nerve palsies Meningitis Meningoencephalitis	Months to years Encephalopathy Myelitis Peripheral neuropathy
Associated manifestations	EM Cardiac disease	Lyme arthritis
Cerebrospinal fluid	Lymphocytic pleocytosis Intrathecal antibody production	Intrathecal antibody production
Serologic testing	May be positive, occasionally IgM	Routinely seropositive

EM, erythema migrans.

used as seroconfirmatory tests rather than serodiagnostic tests. False-positive ELISA results can occur in other spirochetal diseases (e.g., syphilis, other borrelioses, gingivitis); in rheumatologic diseases (e.g., rheumatoid arthritis); and in other infections (e.g., endocarditis, Epstein–Barr virus). Specific antibodies made to other organisms (e.g., the flagellin of *Escherichia coli*) also may bind the *B. burgdorferi* flagellin, so that antibodies binding to *B. burgdorferi* in ELISA do not necessarily indicate prior infection. All positive and equivocal ELISA results must be corroborated by Western blot. ELISA results may not become positive for 6 to 8 weeks, although seroconversion may become apparent within 2 weeks; in general the more sensitive Western blot can detect seroconversion earlier than ELISA. ELISA and Western blot may never become positive if the patient receives antibiotic therapy early in the course of LD, even if the total dose received is inadequate to cure the infection. There is no role for follow-up testing of asymptomatic patients because antibody levels (even IgM) may stay elevated for years. There may be a transient rise in antibody levels following the treatment of early LD, pre-sumably representing the momentum of the immune response; with resolution of the infection the antibody levels will either fall or stabilize.

In patients with LD, a further rise in ELISA level or an increase in the number of bands in the Western blot test in the presence of lingering complaints may indicate persistent LD. The finding of higher antibody levels in inflammatory (e.g., spinal, synovial) fluids relative to serum is definitive evidence that the neurologic or joint disease is caused by *B. burgdorferi* (Fig. 183.2). Modifications of the criteria developed by Dressler and Steere for the interpretation of Western blot tests (Table 183.4) are now generally accepted. Studies suggest that the polymerase chain reaction, which identifies the nucleic acids of the organism, may be useful in the diagnosis of LD, but this has not been proven in clinical practice. There is no established role for measurement of borrelial antigens in the urine. Neuropsychological testing, electrophysiologic testing (cardiac and neurologic), brain magnetic resonance imaging, and single photon emission computed tomography (SPECT) can be helpful in

TABLE 183.4. CRITERIA FOR POSITIVE WESTERN BLOT (IMMUNOBLOT) ANALYSIS IN THE SEROLOGIC CONFIRMATION OF INFECTION WITH *BORRELIA BURGDORFERI* (LYME DISEASE)

Disease	Isotype Tested	Bands To Be Considered
First few weeks of infection	IgM	Two of the eight following: 18, 21, 28, 37, 41, 45, 58, 93 OR Two of the three following: ospC (23), 39, 41[a]
After first weeks of infection	IgG	Five of the ten following: 18, 21, 28, 30, 39, 41, 45, 58, 66, 93

Alternate criteria for IgM reactivity, proposed by a Centers for Disease Control and Prevention conference. Other points noted at that conference were the need for standardization of antigen preparation and techniques used.
Adapted from Dressler F, Whalen JA, Reinhardt BN, et al. Western blotting in the serodiagnosis of Lyme disease. *J Infect Dis* 1993;167:392.

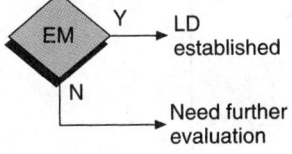

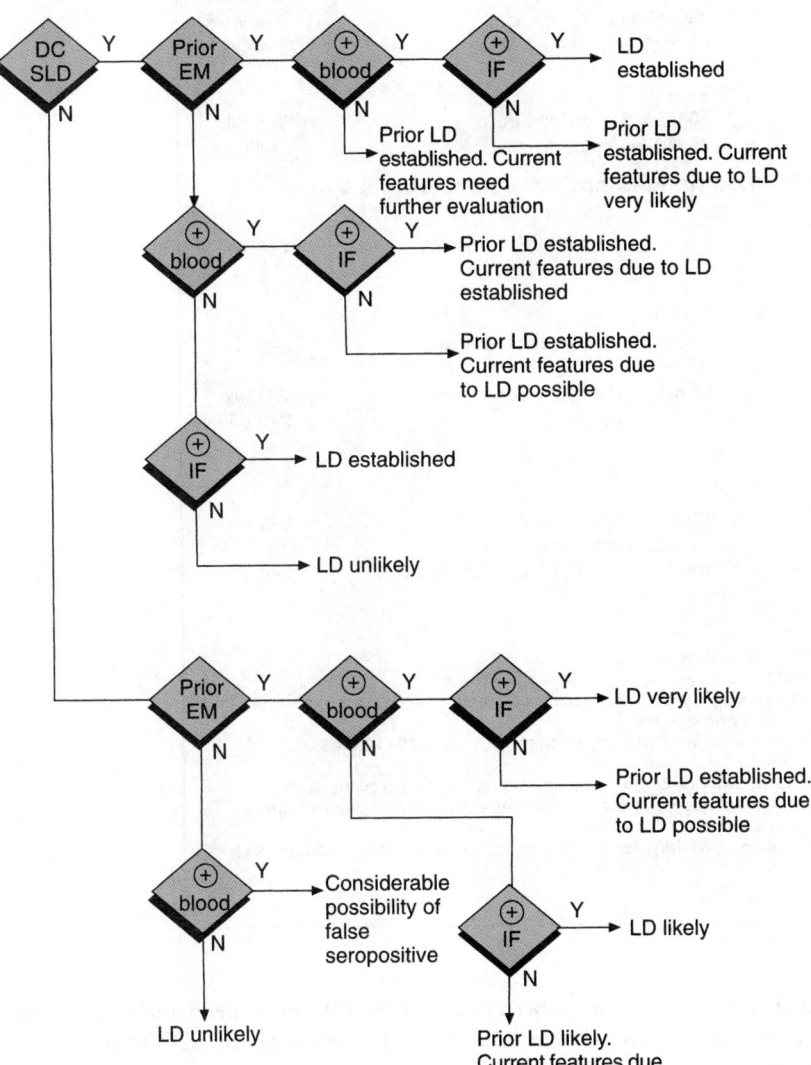

FIGURE 183.2. Algorithm for diagnosis of Lyme disease. +blood, blood test containing antibodies to *Borrelia burgdorferi;* DCSLD, defined clinical syndrome of Lyme disease (Table 183.2); EM, erythema migrans; +IF, inflammatory fluid (synovial or spinal fluid) containing antibodies to *Borrelia burgdorferi.*

EVIDENCE LEVEL: A. Reference: Nadelman RB, Wormser GP. Erythema migrans and early Lyme disease. *Am J Med* **1995;98:15S–24S.**

documenting objective abnormalities but are not specific markers of damage caused by *B. burgdorferi;* there is no pattern in any of these tests unique for or diagnostic of LD.

OPTIMAL MANAGEMENT: TREATMENT AND PREVENTION

Antibiotics are the appropriate therapy for LD. Timely treatment prevents progression to later disease stages, although it may not decrease the duration or severity of many of the symptoms of early LD. Suggested drug regimens for each feature of LD are given in Table 183.5. There is no evidence that oral therapy in follow-up of intravenous therapy, more prolonged or higher dose treatment, use of combinations of different antibiotics, or any other changes in these regimens are helpful. Five percent to 10% of patients with early LD have a Jarisch–Herxheimer reaction within the first days of therapy (a worsening of many of the signs and symptoms of LD). This usually lasts for less than a day and has never been reported as fatal in LD; there is no documentation of recurrent "Herxheimer-like reactions" and such reports must be investigated on a case-by-case basis. Pregnant patients with LD should be treated as appropriate for the features of the disease, although some clinicians recommend the

TABLE 183.5.   CURRENT RECOMMENDATIONS FOR THERAPY IN LYME DISEASE

Oral Therapy for Early Localized Lyme Disease

ADULTS

Doxycycline[a]		
100 mg PO b.i.d.	3–4 wk[d]	
Tetracycline[a,b]	250–500 mg PO q.i.d.	3–4 wk[d]
Amoxicillin[b,c]	250–500 mg PO q.i.d.	3–4 wk[d]
	40 mg/kg/d, divided dose	3–4 wk[d]

CHILDREN

Amoxicillin		
Erythromycin	30 mg/kg/d, divided dose	3–4 wk[d]
Penicillin G	25–50 mg/kg/d, divided dose	3–4 wk[d]

Intravenous Therapy for Early Disseminated and Late (or Chronic) Lyme Disease[e]

ADULTS

Third-generation cephalosporins:	2 g q.d. or 1 g b.i.d.	2–4 wk
Ceftriaxone		
Cefotaxime	3 g b.i.d.	2–4 wk
Penicillin	20 million U in 4 divided doses	2–4 wk
Penicillin G		
Chloramphenicol	50 mg/kg/d in 4 divided doses	2–4 wk
	75–100 mg/kg/d	2–4 wk

CHILDREN

Third-generation cephalosporins:		
Ceftriaxone		
Cefotaxime	90–180 mg/kg/d, in 2 or 3 divided doses	2–4 wk
Penicillin	300,000 U/kg/d in 6 divided doses	2–4 wk
Penicillin G		

[a] No studies comparing doxycycline with tetracycline have been done.
[b] Dosage determined by weight of patient.
[c] No studies comparing amoxicillin with amoxicillin plus probenecid have been done; cefuroxime-axetil and azithromycin also have been studied in Lyme disease.
[d] There is no proof that this is the optimal duration of therapy or that more than 10–14 days of treatment are necessary.
[e] There is no proof that isolated facial nerve palsy or carditis must be treated with intravenous therapy. Oral doxycycline for early Lyme neuroborreliosis has been shown to be effective in European studies. Especially in children, oral therapy for Lyme arthritis may suffice.
(From: Sigal LH. Current drug therapy recommendations for the treatment of Lyme disease. *Drugs* 1992; 43:683, with permission.)

use of parenteral therapy for all pregnant patients; there is no proof that this practice provides a better outcome for mother or fetus. There have been adverse outcomes reported in cases of pregnancy complicated by LD, but there is no firm proof that in utero infection with *B. burgdorferi* occurs or that it causes congenital anomalies or prematurity. Lack of response to antibiotic therapy should suggest the possibility that the current problems are not due to LD: either the initial diagnosis was in error or the LD has been successfully treated and the patient either has a "post-LD syndrome" (e.g., fibromyalgia) or another medical problem totally unrelated to *B. burgdorferi*. Because studies suggest that the risk of contracting LD from a known tick bite is small, prophylactic therapy is not recommended. A human outer surface A protein vaccine has been approved for use in adults. It may be a useful adjunct in the prevention of LD, but persons at risk for LD must take personal precautions (e.g., tick checks after time spent in an endemic area). In many LD-endemic areas, coinfection with *Babesia microti* or the human granulocytic *Ehr-lichia* has been documented. Of course, neither of these *I. scapularis*-borne infections is prevented by the LD vaccine.

BIBLIOGRAPHY

Lightfoot RW Jr, Luft BJ, Rahn DW, et al. Empiric parenteral antibiotic treatment of patients with fibromyalgia and fatigue add a positive serologic result for Lyme disease. A cost-effectiveness analysis. *Ann Intern Med* 1993;119:503–509.

Rahn DW, Malawista SE. Treatment of Lyme disease. In: Mandel GL, Bone RC, Cline MJ, et al, eds. *Year book of medicine, 1994.* St. Louis: Mosby–Year Book, 1994:xxi–xxxvi.

Sigal LH. Lyme disease: testing and treatment. Who should be tested and treated for Lyme disease and how? *Rheum Dis Clin North Am* 1993;19: 79–93.

Sigal LH. Persisting complaints attributed to Lyme disease: possible mechanisms and implications for management. *Am J Med* 1994;96:365–374.

Sigal LH. The Lyme disease controversy. Social and financial costs of misdiagnosis and mismanagement. *Arch Intern Med* 1996;156:1493–1500.

Sigal LH. Lyme disease: a review of aspects of its immunology and immunogenesis. *Annu Rev Immunol* 1997;15:63–92.

Sigal LH. Special article: Diagnostic and management pitfalls in Lyme disease. *Arthritis Rheum* 1998;41:195–204.

Sigal LH. Lyme arthritis. *Rheum Dis Clin North Am* 1998;24:323–351.

Sigal LH, Zahradnik JM, Lavin P, et al. A vaccine consisting of recombinant *Borrelia burgdorferi* outer surface protein A to prevent Lyme disease. Recombinant Outer-Surface Protein A Lyme Disease Vaccine Study Consortium. *N Engl J Med* 1998;339:216–222.

Steere AC. Lyme disease. *N Engl J Med* 1989;321:586–596.

Steere AC, Sikand VK, Meurice F, et al. Vaccination against Lyme disease with recombinant *Borrelia burgdorferi* outer-surface lipoprotein A with adjuvant. Lyme Disease Vacine Study Group. *N Engl J Med* 1998;339:209–215.

Kelley's Textbook of Internal Medicine, fourth edition. Edited by H. David Humes. Lippincott Williams & Wilkins, Philadelphia © 2000.

TABLE 184.1.	RHEUMATIC MANIFESTATIONS OF SARCOIDOSIS

Acute

Ankle arthritis and periarthritis

Erythema nodosum (bilateral hilar adenopathies on chest radiographs)

Chronic

Indolent arthritis and tenosynovitis

Skin lesions

Bone lesions

Myositis, focal subclinical or nodular (fibrosis and/or adenopathy on chest radiographs)

CHAPTER 184

INFILTRATIVE, NEOPLASTIC, AND ENDOCRINOLOGIC CAUSES OF MUSCULOSKELETAL COMPLAINTS

JUAN J. CANOSO

Many illnesses that originate in tissues outside the joint affect articular structures or simulate arthritis at some time in the course of the disease. Occasionally, these musculoskeletal manifestations provide the physician with diagnostic clues.

INFILTRATIVE CONDITIONS

SARCOIDOSIS

Rheumatic manifestations of sarcoidosis include arthropathy, myopathy, and bone lesions (Table 184.1). Sarcoid arthropathy can be acute or chronic. Acute cases, which are the most common, are characterized by abrupt, bilateral, inflammatory lower leg edema with painful limitation of ankle and subtalar motion. Often there is a periarthritis involving tissues around the joint without true synovial involvement. Erythema nodosum is common in these patients. Joint fluid analysis and synovial biopsy are nonspecific. Bilateral hilar adenopathy shown by chest radiography or, when this is negative, computed tomography (CT) confirms the diagnosis of sarcoidosis. When doubt exists, transbronchial, lymph node, or liver biopsy can be used to exclude other disease processes. (Systemic sarcoid is discussed in Chapter 373.) Nonsteroidal anti-inflammatory drugs usually are effective in treatment. Colchicine occasionally has nonspecific beneficial effects.

Episodic, or indolent, sarcoid arthritis is less common, occurring in patients with chronic pulmonary interstitial disease. It often is associated with skin and bone lesions, and assays of synovial biopsy specimens often are positive. Clinical sarcoid myopathy is rare in patients with chronic pulmonary interstitial disease. However, noncaseating granulomas are found on random muscle biopsy in more than half of these patients. Proximal muscle weakness resembling polymyositis and palpable intramuscular nodules with little change in strength are unusual manifestations of chronic sarcoidosis. In bone sarcoidosis, expansion of intraosseous granulomas leads to pain and fusiform enlargement of the digits. Typical radiographic findings consist of focal cystic rarefaction and coarse trabeculation in the bones of the hands. Other bones rarely are affected. The treatment of chronic sarcoidosis is described in Chapter 373.

CROHN'S DISEASE

Synovium, muscle, bone, and skin granulomas all can occur in patients with Crohn's disease. Pathologically, the lesions resemble sarcoidosis; extraintestinal granulomatous involvement is limited in Crohn's disease, however, and transmural bowel inflammation is not a feature of sarcoidosis.

HEMOCHROMATOSIS

An arthropathy that looks like rheumatoid arthritis but feels like osteoarthritis is seen in about half of all patients with hemochromatosis. Pain on motion is severe but morning stiffness is minimal. Synovial proliferation is missing, although knobby bone enlargement at joint margins can be palpated directly under the skin. Pathologic changes include massive hemosiderin deposits in the synovial lining, cartilage loss, and osteophytosis. Calcium pyrophosphate dihydrate (CPPD) and basic calcium phosphate crystals often are present in cartilage. Radiographic findings are consistent with a diagnosis of osteoarthritis; lesions at the metacarpophalangeal joint of the index and middle fingers, wrists, and knees are particularly prominent. Chondrocalcinosis is present in about 20% of patients. The arthropathy of hemochromatosis can occur with few other symptoms of the disease. Treatment of the excess iron stores has little effect on the arthropathy.

AMYLOIDOSIS

Amyloid arthropathy resulting from synovial and capsular deposits of light-chain amyloid is an uncommon complication of multiple myeloma and nonmyelomatous plasma cell dyscrasias (see Chapter 235). Amyloid arthropathy resembles rheumatoid arthritis, but the soft-tissue swellings observed are rubbery and more firm than is the rheumatoid synovium. Amyloidosis is suggested further by manifestations such as macroglossia, bilateral carpal tunnel syndrome, cardiomyopathy, prominence of the shoulders ("shoulder pads" sign), osteolytic masses (amyloidomas) at single or multiple bone sites, and a negative rheumatoid factor in serum. A monoclonal spike usually is present on serum or urine electrophoresis. The diagnosis is confirmed by the presence of amyloid in abdominal fat pad, rectal, synovial, or other tissue biopsy specimens.

In patients undergoing hemodialysis and peritoneal dialysis, synovial and bone amyloid deposits often lead to carpal tunnel syndrome, tenosynovitis, painful limitation of the shoulders, and bone cyst formation. The constituent of this amyloid (AH) is β_2-microglobulin, a serum protein that normally is excreted by the kidney. Because this protein is poorly filtered out by cellulosic membranes, high plasma levels occur in patients receiving hemodialysis. Visceral deposition in AH amyloidosis is minimal, and abdominal fat biopsies usually are negative.

NEOPLASTIC AND RELATED CONDITIONS

Musculoskeletal complaints are common in patients with malignancies. Although these complaints may result from tumor extension, metastasis, or nonmetastatic manifestations of malignant disease, other possible causes of arthritis are more probable and should not be overlooked.

The diagnosis of malignancy usually precedes rheumatic complaints, but musculoskeletal manifestations can appear first. For example, in one patient with recent-onset polyarthritis, digital clubbing prompted a chest radiograph that revealed lung cancer. The following atypical manifestations suggest the possibility of underlying malignant disease: excessive nonhemorrhagic anemia (hematocrit less than 20%) or thrombocytopenia in a patient with juvenile rheumatoid arthritis (acute leukemia); bone lysis in a patient with monarthritis (metastatic disease); a Baker's cyst that remains hard when the knee is flexed (sarcoma); tender bones in a patient with polymyalgia rheumatica (metastases, multiple myeloma); thrombocytosis in a patient with dermatomyositis (cancer); thrombocytosis in a patient with lupus (ovarian tumor); acute Dupuytren's contractures, hand swelling, and joint restrictions (ovarian, tubal, lung carcinoma); and digital vasculitis with gangrene in a patient without ergot ingestion, evidence of cryoglobulins, or connective tissue disease.

METASTATIC ARTHRITIS

Carcinomatous joint involvement is relatively rare, given the frequency of solid tumors in the general population. There is evidence that articular cartilage inhibits angiogenesis and interferes with the articular penetration of bone metastases. Metastatic arthritis usually is monarticular and subacute, and tends to involve the knee in patients with known malignant disease.

LYMPHOMA

Bone involvement in lymphoma can be primary (5% of all non-Hodgkin's lymphomas), or it can develop in the course of disseminated disease. In some patients, bone deposits lead to pain and nonspecific joint effusion. Lymphomatous infiltration of the synovium is rare.

LEUKEMIC SYNOVITIS

Leukemic synovitis occurs predominantly in acute myelogenous leukemia and in the blastemic phase of chronic myelogenous leukemia. Synovial involvement also has been reported in T-cell leukemia. Clinically, leukemic synovitis can be distal and symmetrical, or it can be asymmetrical, involving large joints. Bone tenderness often is present. In synovial fluid, in contrast to the peripheral blood, mature polymorphonuclear cells predominate. Leukemic cell infiltration is found inconsistently on synovial biopsy specimens. The process is rapidly reversible with successful chemotherapy.

MALIGNANT SPINAL DISEASE

Nocturnal predominance and spinal point tenderness characterize the back pain of metastatic disease, multiple myeloma, lymphoma, primary (benign and malignant) tumors of the spine, spinal osteomyelitis, and osteoporotic fractures. Clinical differentiation of these lesions can prove difficult. The erythrocyte sedimentation rate is high in patients with malignant lesions and osteomyelitis, and normal (barring associated diseases) in those with benign tumors and osteoporotic fractures. Seen on radiographs, areas of bone lysis (or sclerosis) indicate malignancy, whereas disc narrowing and end-plate erosions are features of spinal osteomyelitis. Unfortunately, all of these changes appear late. Bone scans are useful in the initial assessment, except in patients with multiple myeloma. Magnetic resonance imaging (MRI) detects early disease, and the findings usually are diagnostic. More important, because it provides direct evidence of peridural or intradural involvement, MRI has become essential in the evaluation of back pain in patients with cancer. Bone needle biopsy may be required for culture or to establish cell type in malignant lesions of unknown origin.

HYPERTROPHIC OSTEOARTHROPATHY

Hypertrophic osteoarthropathy is a poorly understood arthropathy that complicates lung cancer, pulmonary metastases, intrathoracic lymphomas, pleural tumors, and mediastinal malignancies. Nonmalignant causes of hypertrophic osteoarthropathy include pulmonary granulomas, chronic lung abscesses, congenital heart diseases with right-to-left shunts, and subacute bacterial endocarditis. Hypertrophic osteoarthropathy occasionally results from a miscellany of extrathoracic conditions, and there also is a hereditary familial form. Characteristic manifestations of hypertrophic osteoarthropathy include digital clubbing, long-bone tenderness (particularly near joints), and arthritis affecting predominantly the knees and ankles. Leg edema and finger and toe paresthesia also occur. Synovial fluid findings include high viscosity, low leukocyte count (less than 800 cells per liter), and predominance of mononuclear cells. Periosteal new bone formation, a salient feature of the disease, usually is seen on radiography. Earlier lesions can be detected by bone scintigraphy. Pain in hypertrophic osteoarthropathy is well controlled by indomethacin. Complete, predictable resolution follows resection of the intrathoracic mass if present, or even from a thoracotomy alone.

PRIMARY TUMORS IN JOINTS

Persistent monarticular swelling should suggest the possibility of a tumorous condition. The diagnostic challenge is to differentiate an articular swelling caused by synovial effusion or proliferation from an extra-articular mass that is cystic (bursa, ganglion, meniscal cyst), adipoid, vascular, or neoplastic. As an example, in the knee, joint effusions bulge medial, proximal, and lateral to the patella, and fluid can be freely displaced. In contrast, effusions in the prepatellar bursa occur superficial to the patella while the previously described areas remain flat. Localized swelling distal to the patella is investigated while the quadriceps is isometrically contracted; a tense patellar ligament allows the differentiation of subcutaneous bursitis from deep swelling caused by hypertrophy of the fat pad or deep infrapatellar bursitis. Swelling in the lateral aspect of the knee usually indicates a meniscal cyst; typically, the bulging is prominent when the joint is in partial flexion and decreases with further flexion or extension. Popliteal (Baker's) cysts occur in the medial third of the popliteal fossa in the cleft between the semimembranosus tendon and the medial head of the gastrocnemius.

Unlike other popliteal swellings, Baker's cysts soften with knee flexion (Foucher's sign). Masses that remain firm in flexion include sarcomas, ganglions, and popliteal artery lesions such as aneurysms and cystic degeneration of the vessel wall.

Relatively localized areas of thickening within a joint may represent pigmented villonodular synovitis (PVNS), synovial chondromatosis, or, less commonly, angiomas, lipomas, or fibromas; arthroscopy is the preferred method of diagnosis. Extra-articular masses can be evaluated by ultrasonography, CT, or MRI. Ultrasonography is confirmatory in Baker's cysts and assists in the diagnosis of popliteal artery lesions, in which flow can be detected by a Doppler effect. Solid masses are investigated best by MRI and, subsequently, biopsy.

PIGMENTED VILLONODULAR SYNOVITIS

Pigmented villonodular synovitis is a locally invasive process that can affect a joint, a deep bursa, or a tendon sheath. Polyarticular cases are rare and often associated with congenital malformations. The lesions can be nodular or diffuse; diffuse lesions have a tendency to invade bone. Histologically, both forms feature giant cells, macrophage aggregates, foam cells, and hemosiderin deposits.

Collagenase and stromelysin genes are expressed abundantly in lining cells and deep cellular infiltrates in diffuse PVNS. It is not known as to whether PVNS represents a benign neoplasm or a chronic infection. Clinically, nodular cases are characterized by intermittent joint swelling and locking, whereas diffuse cases behave as a chronic, often destructive monarthritis. The erythrocyte sedimentation rate is normal. Synovial fluid is hemorrhagic or chocolate-colored, with a variable leukocyte content. Although the diagnosis of PVNS has been facilitated by MRI, which shows thickened synovium with a peculiar intermediate signal, biopsy is required to rule out chronic infection. Treatment is by arthroscopic or open resection. Unfortunately, PVNS has a tendency to recur. Total joint arthroplasty is useful in recurrent disease and as a definitive form of treatment.

SYNOVIAL CHONDROMATOSIS

Multifocal, self-limited synovial cartilaginous metaplasia characterizes the monarticular condition known as synovial chondromatosis. In rare cases, the site of the lesion is a bursa or a tendon sheath. The cartilaginous nodules may remain in the synovium or be released into the joint cavity. Ossification is common. Clinically, synovial chondromatosis features intermittent joint locking and noninflammatory synovial effusions. Multiple intra-articular bodies with stippled calcification on radiography are pathognomonic of the condition. The differential diagnosis includes osteoarthritis and chondrocalcinosis, both of which can lead to secondary osteochondromas. Most cases must be treated by synovectomy.

SYNOVIAL SARCOMA

Synovial sarcoma is a highly malignant tumor that rarely originates in joints; most cases appear in the soft tissues of the limbs, sometimes in the proximity of a joint. The adjective *synovial* denotes histologic similarities with the inner lining of joints. However, certain electron microscopic, immunohistologic, and chromosomal findings in synovial sarcoma are not present in normal or diseased synovium. The synovial histogenesis of this tumor is uncertain.

ENDOCRINOLOGIC CAUSES OF MUSCULOSKELETAL COMPLAINTS

Endocrine diseases often have prominent rheumatic manifestations (Table 184.2). Although musculoskeletal findings usually occur in the context of florid disease, they are the presenting features in some patients. When faced with patients with peripheral arthritis, fibromyalgia, aseptic necrosis of bone, crystal synovitis, disseminated idiopathic skeletal hyperostosis, back symptoms, myopathy, carpal tunnel syndrome, frozen shoulder, certain fibrotic syndromes, and neuropathic arthropathy, the clinician should include endocrine disease in the differential diagnosis.

TABLE 184.2.	**RHEUMATIC FEATURES OF ENDOCRINE DISORDERS**

Acromegaly
  "Polyarthritis"
  Back pain (degenerative disease)
  Carpal tunnel syndrome
  Myopathy
Hyperthyroidism
  Fibromyalgic pain
  Back pain (osteopenia)
  Frozen shoulder
  Myopathy
  Sicca syndrome
  Periodic paralysis
  Myasthenia gravis
  Antithyroid (methimazole) arthritis
Hypothyroidism
  Fibromyalgic pain
  "Polyarthritis"
  Carpal tunnel syndrome
  Frozen shoulder
  Myopathy
  Sicca syndrome
  Myasthenia gravis
Hyperparathyroidism
  Pseudogout (calcium pyrophosphate dihydrate chondrocal-
    cinosis)
  Back pain (osteopenia)
  Brown tumors
Chronic adrenal insufficiency (also steroid reduction)
  Fibromyalgic pain
  Arthralgia
  Joint effusions
Cushing's syndrome (also exogenous glucocorticoid administra-
    tion)
  Back pain (osteopenia)
  Osteonecrosis
  Myopathy
  Joint effusions (massive doses)
Diabetes
  Cheirarthropathy
  Dupuytren's contracture
  Trigger finger
  Frozen shoulder
  Diffuse idiopathic skeletal hyperostosis
  Diabetic osteoarthropathy (Charcot joint, diabetic osteolysis)

SERONEGATIVE "POLYARTHRITIS"

Articular symptoms resembling those of rheumatoid arthritis can occur in hypothyroidism and acromegaly. Certain clinical characteristics should suggest the diagnosis of endocrine disease. Myxedematous arthropathy occurs in the context of weight gain, cylindrical leg edema, and profound carpal tunnel syndrome. There may be little morning stiffness, and the erythrocyte sedimentation rate is normal or minimally elevated. Joint effusions in myxedema are extremely viscous and noninflammatory. Resolution of symptoms with thyroid replacement is slow and often incomplete.

Acromegalic arthropathy is characterized by joint pain and stiffness in the shoulders, elbows, knees, and back. Unexpectedly severe degenerative changes are found on radiographs, particularly in the shoulders. The height of the intervertebral discs and the width of the joint spaces (hyaline cartilage) in the hand may be increased, leading to a larger glove size. These changes in association with bilateral carpal tunnel syndrome strongly indicate acromegaly.

FIBROMYALGIC PAIN

A diffuse myalgic syndrome resembling fibromyalgia can occur in patients with hypothyroidism, hyperthyroidism, or chronic adrenal insufficiency, and in those undergoing rapid reduction of long-term glucocorticoid therapy. Glucocorticoid reduction fibromyalgia can be confused with enteropathic arthritis in patients with inflammatory bowel disease and interpreted as polymyalgia rheumatica in patients with temporal arteritis. The diagnosis is based on the presence of multiple tender points on physical examination, a normal erythrocyte sedimentation rate, and resolution of symptoms with resumption of a higher glucocorticoid dosage. Slower dosage reduction often circumvents this problem.

OSTEONECROSIS

The protracted use of glucocorticoids often results in osteonecrosis, a condition that is comparatively uncommon in patients with endogenous Cushing's syndrome. Important pathogenic factors include expansion of intramedullary fat, leading to tissue hypertension with hypoperfusion and subsequent tissue death. Disease susceptibility varies among patients; in systemic lupus erythematosus risk factors for osteonecrosis include high steroid doses, Cushing's syndrome, the presence of IgG anticardiolipin antibodies, and findings of thrombophlebitis or vasculitis. In retrospective studies, most patients with osteonecrosis received high, protracted daily dosages of oral glucocorticoids. The first symptomatic joint usually is the hip, and osteonecrosis should be suspected immediately when patients receiving long-term glucocorticoid therapy complain of hip pain. A high index of suspicion is required when the underlying condition features synovitis; hip pain that develops while the remaining joints are stable, improving, or in remission should prompt investigation. In early cases, radiographs are normal; the classic radiographic findings of osteonecrosis appear late. Bone scintigrams initially show hypoperfusion followed by increased uptake around the wedge of dead bone. Magnetic resonance imaging is extremely useful in the detection of early lesions. There is controversy regarding the treatment of early cases with core decompression biopsy. This procedure consists of drilling a tunnel through the trochanter into the femoral head to relieve osseous hypertension and promote epiphyseal revascularization. In advanced cases, collapse of the necrotic portion of the femoral head leads to secondary osteoarthritis, and arthroplasty eventually is required in most patients. In contrast, osteonecrosis of the shoulder is well tolerated.

CRYSTAL ARTHRITIS

Occasionally, patients with CPPD deposition disease are found to have hyperparathyroidism. Removal of the parathyroid adenoma does not affect the chondrocalcinosis and may be followed transiently by an increased frequency of pseudogout. Colchicine prophylaxis should be used in this setting.

DIFFUSE IDIOPATHIC SKELETAL HYPEROSTOSIS

About half of all patients with diffuse idiopathic skeletal hyperostosis (DISH) have non–insulin-dependent diabetes mellitus. The basic pathologic finding is ossification of paraspinal ligaments and tendons at the attachment sites. Little is known about the pathogenesis of this disorder. There is an absence of inflammation. In diabetes, DISH tends to occur more frequently in patients with dyslipidemia and hyperuricemia. Vitamin D–resistant rickets, fluorosis, and prolonged retinoid therapy for severe acne are associated with tendon and ligament ossification resembling DISH.

The usual form of DISH, occurring in about 10% of the elderly, is manifested by subclinical ossification of the anterior longitudinal ligament in the thoracic spine. More extensive cases feature prominent neck and lower back pain, spinal rigidity, and decreased joint motion closely resembling the findings in younger men with ankylosing spondylitis. Anterior cervical osteophytes may cause dysphagia. Cord compression may result from involvement of the posterior longitudinal ligament or from nonunion of a traumatic fracture across an ankylosed segment of the spine. The treatment of DISH includes analgesics and physical therapy; neck lesions may require surgery.

BACK PAIN AND OSTEOPENIA

Back pain based on compression fractures with osteopenia on radiographs is a prominent manifestation of endogenous and exogenous Cushing's syndrome and some cases of hyperthyroidism, hyperparathyroidism, and hypogonadism. The importance of measures to prevent steroid-induced osteoporosis cannot be overemphasized.

MYOPATHY

Hyperthyroidism and hypothyroidism can be attended by myopathic (proximal) weakness. In patients with hypothyroidism, myopathic weakness, elevation of creatine kinase levels, carpal tunnel syndrome, and arthralgia may suggest the erroneous diagnosis of polymyositis. Myopathy, sometimes profound, complicates endogenous Cushing's syndrome and long-term glucocorticoid therapy. In this setting, iliopsoas muscle weakness precedes diffuse myopathic weakness, and serum creatine kinase levels are normal. Resistive exercises, begun early on, are believed to be important in the prevention of steroid-induced myopathy. Finally, proximal weakness is common in acromegaly. Diabetes mellitus may result in muscle infarction, which usually affects the thigh and is manifested by focal swelling and tenderness. Patients are afebrile and regression occurs in weeks.

CARPAL TUNNEL SYNDROME

Carpal tunnel syndrome sometimes complicates diabetes, is commonly associated with late pregnancy, and is a classic finding in myxedema and active acromegaly (see Chapter 185).

FROZEN SHOULDER

Frozen shoulder is seen in diabetes, hyperthyroidism, and hypothyroidism (see Chapter 185).

FIBROTIC SYNDROMES

Diabetes results in a variety of fibrotic syndromes that include Dupuytren's contracture (fibrosis involving the palmar fascia), so-called trigger finger (fibrosis at the proximal flexor tendon sheath), frozen shoulder (capsular fibrosis), and a unique syndrome known as *cheirarthropathy*. Diabetic cheirarthropathy (palmar and digital fibrosis) correlates with microangiopathy and is characterized clinically by thickened, waxy skin and incomplete contact of the palms in the praying position.

NEUROPATHIC ARTHROPATHY

Neuropathic arthropathy, also known as a Charcot joint, is the mechanical failure of a joint in a patient whose sensory input is impaired. Charcot's joints develop in patients with peripheral neuropathy, such as in diabetes, leprosy, amyloidosis, and chronic renal failure; syringomyelia; tabes dorsalis; and congenital indifference to pain. The process initially may be painful, but the degree of pain falls short of the degree of anatomical distortion, which can be extreme. Neuropathic arthropathy is characterized by a lack of involuntary fixation that is the rule in severely damaged joints, a range of motion that is normal or increased, coarse bone-on-bone crepitation, and joint swelling that represents synovial effusion at first, and synovial, cartilage, and bone overgrowth late in the disease. Synovial fluid usually is hemorrhagic and noninflammatory; CPPD crystals have been found in some joints. As in other peripheral neuropathies, Charcot joints in patients with diabetic neuropathy involve the midfoot or the forefoot. Occasional cases involve the knee or the spine. Diabetic osteolysis, an aseptic destructive lesion of metatarsal heads, is another complication of the diabetic denervated foot. In syringomyelia, neuropathic arthropathy classically occurs in the shoulder. In tabes dorsalis, the knee and the spine are more likely to be involved. Because the treatment of Charcot joints is unsatisfactory, emphasis should be placed on prevention. Full attention should be paid to seemingly minor injuries in a hypoesthetic limb. In the foot, the principles developed for the treatment of patients with leprosy are applied: aggressive treatment of early ulcers and shoes designed to spread the strain of weight bearing equally over the foot. Braces are useful in the neuropathic knee and spine. Total joint replacement, initially considered ineffective, has produced favorable results in neuropathic knees.

BIBLIOGRAPHY

Canoso JJ. Tumors of joints and related structures. In: Koopman WJ, ed. *Arthritis and allied conditions*, thirteenth ed. Philadelphia: Williams & Wilkins, 1997:1867–1886.

De Ruiter EA, Ronday HK, Markusse HM. Amyloidosis mimicking rheumatoid arthritis. *Clin Rheumatol* 1998;17:409–411.

Farrell J, Bastani B. Beta 2–microglobulin amyloidosis in chronic dialysis patients: a case report and review of the literature. *J Am Soc Nephrol* 1997;8:509–514.

Koo KH, Kim R, Ko GH, et al. Preventing collapse in early osteonecrosis of the femoral head. A randomised clinical trial of core decompression. *J Bone Joint Surg* 1996;78:870–874.

Martínez-Lavín M. Hypertrophic osteoarthropathy. In: Klippel JH, Dieppe PA, eds. *Rheumatology,* second ed. London: Mosby, 1998:8.46.1–4.

Pettersson T. Rheumatic features of sarcoidosis. *Curr Opin Rheumatol* 1998; 10:73–78.

Rosembloom AL, Silverstein JH. Connective tissue and joint disease in diabetes mellitus. *Endocrinol Metab Clin North Am* 1996;25:473–483.

Sinigaglia L, Fargion S, Fracanzani AL, et al. Bone and joint involvement in genetic hemochromatosis: role of cirrhosis and iron overload. *J Rheumatol* 1997;24:1809–1813.

Schumacher HR Jr. Arthropathy in hemochromatosis. *Hosp Pract (Off ed)* 1998;33:81–86, 89–90, 93–94.

Vezyroglou G, Mitropoulos A, Antoniadis C. A metabolic syndrome in diffuse idiopathic skeletal hyperostosis. A controlled study. *J Rheumatol* 1996;23:672–676.

Kelley's Textbook of Internal Medicine, fourth edition. Edited by H. David Humes. Lippincott Williams & Wilkins, Philadelphia © 2000.

C H A P T E R

185

FIBROMYALGIA (FIBROSITIS), CHRONIC FATIGUE SYNDROME, BURSITIS, AND OTHER NONARTICULAR RHEUMATIC COMPLAINTS

JUAN J. CANOSO

FIBROMYALGIA

A typical patient with fibromyalgia complains of chronic widespread pain, fatigue, and stiffness. She may have received diagnoses such as hypochondria, chronic fatigue syndrome, psychogenic rheumatism, or undetermined connective tissue disease. The condition may have been attributed to a local pain syndrome, such as Tietze's syndrome, costochondritis, tennis elbow, or trochanteric bursitis. Many surgical procedures may have been performed. The results of laboratory tests have been entirely normal. On direct questioning, she reports a sleep disturbance that involves repeated awakening and greater fatigue on rising in the morning than on retiring at night. She also may complain of depression, migraine, irritable bowel, temporomandibular joint pain, and orthostatic intolerance. The diagnosis of fibromyalgia is confirmed by a physical examination that reveals multiple symmetrical tender points (Table 185.1).

In contrast to normal tenderness, the tenderness of fibromyalgia is characterized by an exaggerated emotional response, withdrawal of the tender part, and worsening of pain after examination. Examination often reveals the presence of previously unknown tender areas. Fibromyalgia is believed to be a multifac-

TABLE 185.1.	**SITES OF TENDERNESS IN FIBROMYALGIA**[a]

Lateral epicondyle (R & L): The tennis elbow sites, actually 1–2 cm distal to the epicondyle

Trapezius (R & L): The midpoint of the upper trapezius in a somewhat firm portion of the muscle

Supraspinatus origin (R & L): Above the scapular line, near the medial border of the scapula

Occiput (R & L)

Low cervical (R & L): At the anterior aspect of the intertransverse ligaments C4–5 or C5–6

Second costochondral junction (R & L): Close to the origin of the pectoralis major

Buttock (R & L): In the midportion of the outer quadrant of the buttock, in the anterior portion of the gluteus medius

Greater trochanter (R & L)

Knee (R & L): In the fat pad medial to the knee

[a] Fibromyalgia criteria: widespread pain (axial plus upper and lower segment plus left- and right-sided pain) in combination with tenderness at 11 or more of the 18 specified sites yielded a sensitivity of 88.4% and a specificity of 81.1% in a study of 293 patients with fibromyalgia and 265 control subjects.
R, right; L, left.
(From Wolfe F, Smythe HA, Yunis MB, et al. The American College of Rheumatology 1990 criteria for the classification of fibromyalgia. *Arthritis Rheum* 1990;33:171, with permission.)

torial neurophysiologic disturbance in which environmental or endogenous stress deteriorates the non–rapid eye movement sleep. This disturbed sleep results in perceptual (mainly pain) amplification, depression, and fatigue. These, in turn, lead to additional stress plus physical and cardiovascular deconditioning. Fibromyalgia may present alone or in association with conditions such as systemic lupus erythematosus, rheumatoid arthritis, osteoarthritis, hypothyroidism, metastatic cancer, AIDS, and Lyme disease. In addition, a transient fibromyalgic state is not uncommon during acute viral and bacterial illnesses, corticosteroid withdrawal, or alcohol and narcotic withdrawal. Fibromyalgia should be distinguished from myofascial pain, a regional pain condition in which pressure to a trigger point causes the pain to radiate to the entire painful area.

The treatment of fibromyalgia includes tricyclic medications, an exercise program, and measures to reduce stress. Low doses of amitriptyline (25 mg at night) or cyclobenzaprine (20 to 30 mg per day) tend to improve the sleep pattern; patients wake up with less fatigue and less pain. Tramadol may be used as an interval or adjunct medication. To further decrease pain and restore endurance, a structured aerobic exercise program including stretching and flexibility exercises is recommended. Relaxation techniques such as yoga are a helpful adjunct to the overall treatment program. Patients must understand that fibromyalgia is not a crippling disease and should be encouraged to move away from beliefs and behaviors that may be perpetuating symptoms and disability.

CHRONIC FATIGUE SYNDROME

Chronic fatigue syndrome (CFS) affects predominantly young women. The onset is abrupt, often in the aftermath of a viral-

TABLE 185.2.	**CHRONIC FATIGUE SYNDROME: DIAGNOSTIC CRITERIA**

A. Clinically evaluated, unexplained, persisting, or relapsing fatigue that is of new or definite onset; is not the result of ongoing exertion; is not substantially alleviated by rest; and results in substantial reduction in previous levels of occupational, educational, social, or personal activities;

AND

B. Four or more of the following concurrent and persistent symptoms:

1. Impaired short-term memory or concentration
2. Sore throat
3. Tender cervical or axillary lymph nodes
4. Muscle pain
5. Multijoint pain without arthritis
6. Headaches of a new type, pattern, or severity
7. Unrefreshing sleep
8. Postexertional malaise lasting more than 24 h

Note: Chronic fatigue denotes self-reported, persistent, or relapsing fatigue lasting for 6 or more consecutive months; prolonged fatigue denotes self-reported persistent fatigue lasting for a month or longer.
(From Fukuda K, Straus SE, Hickie I, et al. Chronic fatigue syndrome: a comprehensive approach to its definition and study. *Ann Intern Med* 1994;121:953, with permission.)

like illness. Profound fatigue, sore throat, tender adenopathy (by history rather than documented on examination), headache, general achiness, and an array of neurologic complaints ranging from mild memory impairment to sensory disturbances characterize the condition. Unrefreshing sleep and depression often are present. The 1994 Consensus Criteria for the Diagnosis of CFS are shown in Table 185.2. The reported prevalence of chronic fatigue in the general population is 1% to 3%, whereas in general medical practices it may reach 10%. Medical conditions to be ruled out in patients complaining of chronic fatigue include anemia, chronic infection including HIV infection, liver disease, chronic adrenal insufficiency, hypothyroidism, and systemic lupus erythematosus. Physical examination often reveals fibromyalgic tenderness, which, if absent, may appear in subsequent visits at times of greater psychological distress. Laboratory investigation should include a complete blood count; an erythrocyte sedimentation rate; measurements of liver enzymes, thyroid-stimulating hormone, and antinuclear antibody; cortisol levels before and after adrenal stimulation in some cases; and, possibly, screening for HIV. A chest radiograph also should be obtained. In CFS, all test results should be normal. Chronic fatigue syndrome bears similarities to the neurasthenia of the nineteenth century, the obscure epidemic neuromyasthenia seen early this century, the postwar syndromes seen in Vietnam and Persian Gulf veterans, and today's fibromyalgia.

A critical review of published data would suggest that CFS and fibromyalgia basically describe the same entity: a cluster of fatigue, pain, depression, and dysautonomia that is probably caused by chronic stress and is clearly modulated by psychological distress. Internists, based on the analysis of patients who predominantly complain of fatigue, call it CFS. Rheumatologists, because they see patients who are in pain, call it fibromyalgia. Chronic fatigue syndrome and fibromyalgia are treated simi-

larly, the mainstays being reassurance, tricyclic antidepressants, physical exercise, and stress management. Cognitive behavior therapy has been used in CFS with variable success. Low-dose hydrocortisone has been somewhat effective in short-term controlled trials, but subsequent hypoadrenalism, plus unavoidable long-term side effects, outweigh any reported benefits of glucocorticoids in CFS. Acyclovir treatment has failed to improve patients' symptoms.

BURSITIS

Bursae are synovium-lined sacs located in the subcutaneous tissue (subcutaneous bursae) or between tendons, muscles, and bones (deep bursae) to promote tissue gliding.

SUBCUTANEOUS BURSITIS

The olecranon bursa and prepatellar bursa are the most common sites of bursitis in adults and children, respectively. Adventitious bursae, which are acquired sacs in areas of abnormal stress, such as prominent bunions or amputation stumps, also can be involved. Usual causes of subcutaneous bursitis include trauma, bacterial infection, gout, and rheumatoid arthritis. Most septic cases are caused by *Staphylococcus aureus* followed by *Streptococcus hemolyticus;* other agents, such as anaerobic bacteria, mycobacteria, fungi, and algae *(Prototheca),* rarely are involved. Most infections occur through the skin; hematogenous bursitis is rare. Bacteremia is uncommon, but toxic shock can occur.

Subcutaneous bursitis usually is manifested as a cystic lump. However, confusion arises when the inflammation is severe or bursal rupture occurs. Acute arthritis and bursitis can be differentiated on the basis of passive motion. In acute arthritis of the elbow or knee, the limb is held in partial flexion, and full passive extension or flexion is prevented by pain; in acute bursitis, however, passive extension is painless. Bursal rupture is characterized by massive forearm and hand edema, suggesting extensive cellulitis or axillary vein thrombosis. The correct diagnosis is indicated by fluctuation at the elbow tip and is confirmed by bursal aspiration.

The macroscopic appearance of bursal fluid can be deceiving; clear fluids with low leukocyte counts are common in septic bursitis and gout, and turbidity may result from cholesterol crystals. Routine analysis must include a cell count and differential, crystal search by polarizing microscopy, Gram stain, and cultures. Findings in the various types of bursitis are summarized in Table 185.3.

Most cases of traumatic bursitis resolve spontaneously within 3 months if repetitive trauma is avoided. Refractory cases can be treated by glucocorticoid injection. Septic bursitis is treated with repeated bursal aspirations and systemic antibiotics, which are administered orally in routine cases involving the olecranon bursa. Intravenous antibiotics are used in patients with prepatellar bursitis, in weakened hosts (diabetes, alcoholism, AIDS, immunosuppressant therapy), and in patients with suspected bacteremia. A 10-day course usually is sufficient.

TABLE 185.3.	BURSAL FLUID FINDINGS IN SUBCUTANEOUS BURSITIS			
	Leukocytes (per μL)	Polymorphonuclear Cells (%)	Crystals	Culture
Traumatic (n = 115)	350 (0–24,500)	5 (0–98)	None	Negative
Septic (n = 51)	13,500 (1,000–425,000)	94 (30–100)	None	Positive[a]
Gout (n = 25)	2,375 (650–12,000)	40 (2–98)	MSU in all	Negative
Rheumatoid arthritis (n = 13)	2,500 (200–25,200)	30 (2–86)	Cholesterol in 6	Negative

[a] *Staphylococcus aureus* = 45; *Staphylococcus epidermidis* = 1; hemolytic streptococci = 5.
n, number of observations; MSU, monosodium urate crystals.
(Modified from Canoso JJ. Bursal membrane and fluid. In Cohen AS, ed. *Laboratory diagnostic procedures in the rheumatic diseases,* third ed. Orlando: Grune & Stratton, 1985:55.)

DEEP BURSITIS

The only clinically significant bursae are the subacromial, trochanteric, anserine, gastrocnemius-semimembranosus, and retrocalcaneal bursae. Subacromial bursitis (a misnomer for rotator cuff tendinitis) is diagnosed in patients with acute lateral shoulder pain featuring pain on resisted motion and a relatively normal passive motion. The injection of glucocorticoids produces prompt relief of symptoms; these agents should be administered skillfully and never abused. Alternatively, high doses of a nonsteroidal anti-inflammatory drug can be used. Ancillary measures include the use of a sling for 24 hours, pendular exercises, and abduction and rotation exercises, which are initiated promptly once pain is brought under control.

Trochanteric and anserine bursitis often represent tendinous strain rather than bursal inflammation. Trochanteric bursitis is characterized by lateral hip pain and greater trochanter tenderness, and pain prevents the patient from lying in bed on the affected side. This syndrome results from abnormal stresses generated by hip or knee disease, leg-length discrepancy, and scoliosis, among other conditions. Anserine bursitis is characterized by medial knee pain on walking up or down stairs. There is tenderness in the medial upper tibia corresponding to the pes anserinus insertion. This syndrome commonly results from knee osteoarthritis. Both trochanteric and anserine bursitis respond well to glucocorticoid infiltration; an attempt should be made to correct the primary abnormality of gait.

Baker's cysts occur when excessive fluid formation in knee processes leads to the distention of communicating gastrocnemius-semimembranosus bursae. Baker's cysts may present clinically in several ways: local pain; compression of the popliteal artery, the deep veins, and or the tibial nerve or its branches; or acute inflammation in the calf (pseudothrombophlebitis) from rupture of the cyst. Pseudothrombophlebitis is suggested by the presence of knee effusion, a history of knee pathology, knee swelling or pain just preceding the calf symptoms, or point tenderness between the gastrocnemius and the semimembranosus. Unruptured Baker's cysts can be palpated and the diagnosis confirmed by echography if necessary. In patients with a tender, swollen calf echo imaging is extremely useful to distinguish a ruptured Baker's cyst from thrombophlebitis. In the occasional patient both conditions are present. Heparin treatment insti-tuted on the basis of an erroneous diagnosis of thrombophlebitis can result in massive calf hematoma in patients with ruptured Baker's cysts. Baker's cysts regress with the successful treatment of synovitis in the knee. Rupture of tense, tender cysts can be prevented with intra-articular glucocorticoids and splinting of the knee in partial flexion.

Retrocalcaneal bursitis, or inflammation of the bursa located between the calcaneus and the Achilles tendon, occurs commonly in the spondyloarthropathies, often in association with Achilles tendinitis and plantar fasciitis. The diagnosis can be made clinically on the basis of posterior heel pain plus medial and lateral swelling in the angle between the Achilles tendon and the calcaneus. Retrocalcaneal bursitis is treated with the general treatment of the underlying condition, a higher heel, and, in some cases, a walking cast.

OTHER NONARTICULAR RHEUMATIC COMPLAINTS

CARPAL TUNNEL SYNDROME

The tight boundaries of the carpal tunnel make the traversing median nerve vulnerable to compression. Compressive neuropathy of the median nerve at the carpal tunnel is characterized by nocturnal (then permanent) pain and paresthesia in the palmar aspect of the radial half of the hand. Shaking the hand relieves the symptoms and allows the patient to fall asleep again. Increased interstitial fluid explains the syndrome in pregnancy, myxedema, and vascular shunts, whereas tissue growth is the culprit in rheumatoid arthritis and other synovitides, repetitive trauma, amyloidosis, diabetes, acromegaly, leprosy, anomalous muscle, ganglions, and lipomas. Helpful in diagnosis are Tinel's sign (paresthesia produced or accentuated by light percussion of the median nerve at the wrist) and Phalen's sign (symptoms elicited or accentuated by maximal passive wrist flexion maintained for 1 minute). Electromyographic and nerve conduction studies are used in atypical cases and in the preoperative evaluation of patients with refractory disease.

The treatment of carpal tunnel syndrome consists of wrist splinting with additional measures that depend on the cause. Resting splints help because carpal tunnel pressures are lowest when the wrist is held in the neutral position. Glucocorticoid infiltration may be required. Resistant cases must be relieved by open or endoscopic surgery to prevent permanent nerve damage.

FROZEN SHOULDER

Frozen shoulder, also known as shoulder capsulitis or periarthritis, is characterized by deep pain in the lateral aspect of the upper arm, limitation of passive shoulder motion in all planes, absence of laboratory evidence of inflammation, and radiographic films showing normal findings or (late) osteopenia. Pathologically, there is capsular fibrosis and retraction; early cases may exhibit synovial inflammation. Frozen shoulder may be primary (idiopathic); may occur in the aftermath of stroke, myocardial infarction, or upper extremity cardiac catheterization; and may complicate diabetes and untreated thyroid disease. Primary cases, and those that follow stroke, myocardial infarction, and cardiac catheterization, usually are unilateral and have a regressive course.

Predominantly nocturnal pain and rapid loss of glenohumeral joint motion characterize the initial 4 to 8 weeks of disease. As nocturnal symptoms subside, pain on motion becomes the salient complaint; joint motion remains restricted, with painful end points. After several months, all pain ceases and motion improves gradually over 1 to 2 years. Frozen shoulder is treated with low-dose oral corticosteroids (e.g., prednisone, 10 mg per day) for 4 to 6 weeks or a single dose of intra-articular corticosteroids (e.g., triamcinolone hexacetonide, 40 mg) preferably administered under fluoroscopic control, and pendular exercises every 2 hours while awake until maximal improvement has been achieved. The diabetic frozen shoulder is less likely to undergo spontaneous resolution. Arthroscopic release surgery is usually effective in these and other unyielding cases.

STENOSING TENOSYNOVITIS

Stenosing tenosynovitis is a fibrotic constriction of the tendon sheath that interferes with the free gliding of the tendon within the sheath. In the digits, the lesion results in the familiar "trigger finger," which is characterized by snapping on finger action. When the abductor pollicis brevis sheath is involved in the lateral aspect of the wrist, the condition is known as de Quervain's syndrome. Overuse of the hand and diabetes mellitus are important risk factors in the development of stenosing tenosynovitis. Multicentric cases, which should be differentiated from rheumatoid tenosynovitis, may be primary or may complicate diabetes, acromegaly, ochronosis, and amyloidosis. Glucocorticoid infiltrations are highly effective in stenosing tenosynovitis.

DUPUYTREN'S CONTRACTURE

Dupuytren's contracture is characterized by fibrosis and retraction of the palmar fascia, leading in severe cases to finger contractures. Dupuytren's contracture is common among the elderly; the prevalence is close to 30% in individuals older than 65 years of age. There is a strong genetic influence. Risk factors include tobacco smoking, diabetes mellitus, alcoholism, and possibly microtrauma. Disabling Dupuytren's contracture can be treated surgically.

BIBLIOGRAPHY

Canoso JJ. Musculoskeletal conditions (regional rheumatic diseases). In: Canoso JJ, ed. *Rheumatology in primary care.* Philadelphia: WB Saunders, 1997:209–296.

Fukuda K, Straus SE, Hickie I, et al. Chronic fatigue syndrome: a comprehensive approach to its definition and study. *Ann Intern Med* 1994; 121:953–959.

Benson LS, Williams CS, Kahle M. Dupuytren's contracture. *J Am Acad Orthop Surg* 1998;6:24–35.

Levine PH, Guest Editor. Recent developments in chronic fatigue syndrome. *Am J Med* 1998;105(3A):1S–124S.

Ogilvie-Harris DJ, Myerthall S. The diabetic frozen shoulder: arthroscopic release. *Arthroscopy* 1997;13:1–8.

Macfarlane GJ, Morris S, Hunt IM, et al. Chronic widespread pain in the community: the influence of psychological symptoms and mental disorder on healthcare seeking behavior. *J Rheumatol* 1999;26:413–419.

McDermid AJ, Rollman GB, McCain GA. Generalized hypervigilance in fibromyalgia: evidence of perceptual amplification. *Pain* 1996;66: 133–144.

Sibbitt WL Jr, Eaton RP. Corticosteroid responsive tenosynovitis is a common pathway for limited joint mobility in the diabetic hand. *J Rheumatol* 1997;24:931–936.

Wigers SH, Stiles TC, Vogel PA. Effects of aerobic exercise versus stress management treatment in fibromyalgia. A 4.5 year prospective study. *Scand J Rheumatol* 1996;25:77–86.

Wolfe F, Smythe HA, Yunus MB, et al. The American College of Rheumatology 1990 criteria for the classification of fibromyalgia. Report of the Multicenter Criteria Committee. *Arthritis Rheum* 1990;33:160–172.

Kelley's Textbook of Internal Medicine, fourth edition. Edited by H. David Humes.
Lippincott Williams & Wilkins, Philadelphia © 2000.

CHAPTER
186

HERITABLE DISORDERS OF CONNECTIVE TISSUE

UTA FRANCKE

Connective tissue is present in all organ systems. Therefore, inherited disorders that affect its composition and stability are characterized by multisystem involvement. Depending on whether the molecular defect resides in a gene for collagen, fibrillin, elastin, or other matrix protein, the bones, ligaments, joints, blood vessels, eyes, or skin are affected to various degrees. This chapter focuses on the more common clinical entities that often are not diagnosed until adulthood.

Inheritance patterns usually are autosomal dominant, but there is considerable heterogeneity with respect to organ involvement and disease severity both between and within families. The family history may be negative because many cases occur as new mutations.

Autosomal recessive inheritance patterns usually are associated with defects in an enzyme, such as homocystinuria resulting from cystathionine β-synthase deficiency, the kyphoscoliosis type of Ehlers–Danlos syndrome resulting from lysyl hydroxylase deficiency, and the dermatosparaxis type of Ehlers–Danlos syndrome resulting from procollagen *N*-proteinase deficiency.

Although the literature contains reports of occasional autosomal recessive inheritance disorders that usually are autosomal dominant (e.g., osteogenesis imperfecta), disease recurrence in siblings born to unaffected parents frequently results from gonadal mosaicism in one parent. In such cases, the mutation occurred in an early embryonal or gonadal precursor cell and gave rise to a carrier individual who may display no or only minimal somatic features of the disorder but is identified as a mosaic by having more than one affected offspring.

Systemic connective tissue abnormalities also occur as secondary manifestations of primary defects in copper metabolism, as in X-linked cutis laxa, Menkes' syndrome, and occipital horn disease. Furthermore, systemic connective tissue disorders are not always genetic but can have an autoimmune basis.

Considerable phenotypic overlap exists between the nosologically defined disease entities (Table 186.1). For example, fragmented elastic fibers are the hallmark of the disorders in the cutis laxa group but also are seen in the aortas of patients with

---

TABLE 186.1. CHARACTERISTICS OF HERITABLE DISORDERS WITH PRIMARY DEFECTS IN CONNECTIVE TISSUE COMPONENTS

Syndrome	Inheritance and Incidence	Principal Clinical Features	Therapy	Molecular Pathology
Disorders of Fibrillin				
Marfan Syndrome	AD with high rate of new mutations 1/10,000	Tall stature; long, thin extremities; decreased subcutaneous fat; arm span >8 cm excess of height; upper to lower segment ratio ~0.85; arachnodactyly; long, narrow face; high-arched palate; dental crowding; scoliosis; pectus excavatum or carinatum; pes planus; protrusio acetabuli; joint laxity; striae distensae; contractures; dural ectasia; hernias	Corrective surgery for scoliosis; orthodontia	Mutations in gene for fibrillin-1 (*FBN1*) on chromosome 15q21.1 lead to abnormalities in microfibrillar assembly and stability; reduced microfibrils in elastic and nonelastic tissues
		Aneurysmal dilatation of ascending aorta; aortic regurgitation; aortic dissection; mitral valve prolapse	β-Adrenergic blockade Composite aortic graft	
		Ectopia lentis; myopia; flat cornea; retinal detachment	Corrective lenses	
Congenital contractural arachnodactyly (CCA or Beal syndrome)	AD (rare)	Tall stature; arachnodactyly; long, thin face; flexion contractures involving large and small joints; "crumpled ear deformity"; osteopenia; severe kyphoscoliosis Variable ocular lesions Mitral valve regurgitation	Corrective surgery for scoliosis	Family linkage studies have mapped *CCA* gene to 5q23–q31 near gene for fibrillin-2 (*FBN2*) Mutations in *FBN2* have been reported
Homocystinuria	AR 1/100,000	Long, slender extremities; light-colored hair; malar flush and thin skin; crowded teeth; high-arched palate; pectus carinatum or excavatum; kyphoscoliosis Ectopia lentis; myopia; glaucoma; spontaneous retinal detachment	Administration of oral pyridoxine in pyridoxine-responsive cases and/or low-methionine, cystine-supplemented diet	Deficiency of cystathionine β-synthetase (CBS) resulting from mutation in the gene (*CBS*) on 21q22.3, may contribute to endothelial cell damage, increased platelet adhesiveness, and smooth muscle cell growth, and inhibition of cross-linking of fibrillin
		Osteoporosis	Folate supplementation	The most common mutation in the *CBS* gene is Gly308Ser
		Myocardial infarction; major artery or vein thrombosis	Betaine in pyridoxine-unresponsive cases	
		Seizures; mental retardation (in two-thirds of patients)	Anticoagulation for occlusion	

TABLE 186.1. *Continued*

Syndrome	Inheritance and Incidence	Principal Clinical Features	Therapy	Molecular Pathology
Disorders of Collagen				
Ehlers–Danlos syndromes				
Type I (severe)	AD (common)	Hyperextensible joints leading to osteoarthritis; reversal of spinal curves	Supportive: to protect joints while building muscle mass	Unknown defects of collagen or other matrix proteins contribute to abnormal collagen fiber
		Hypotonic, floppy infants; born prematurely, often with hernias		Fragility of connective tissue
		Parrot-like facies; broad nasal root; epicanthal folds; floppy ears; hyperextensible skin with soft, velvety or doughy texture, dystrophic scarring after even minor trauma		
		Easy bruising; varicose veins		
		Pulmonary lesions; blebs, emphysema, pneumothorax		
		Mitral valve prolapse; bladder diverticulum		
Type II (mild)	AD (common)	Same manifestations as type I but fewer and less severe		
Type III (benign hypermobility syndrome)	AD (common)	Joint hypermobility, rarely dislocation of joints		Gly637Ser mutation in the type III collagen (*COL3AI*) gene in one family
		Moderate skin hyperextensibility		
		Minimal scarring		
Type IV (ecchymotic or arterial)	AD (apparently rare, but probably undiagnosed)	Acro-osteolysis	Early diagnosis and subsequent vigilance	Mutations in the *COL3A1* gene that result in the production of a defective molecule; the effects of the mutations are analogous to those in type I collagen genes that result in osteogenesis imperfecta
		Pinched nose, thin lips		
		Hypermobility of distal interphalangeal joints		
		Spontaneous arterial rupture leading to massive hematomas or sudden death		
		Thin, soft, transparent skin with prominent venous patterns; fragile skin, easy bruising		
		Rupture of viscera, including bowel, diverticula, and the gravid uterus		
		Spontaneous pneumothorax		
		Friable tissues in surgery		
		Mitral valve prolapse		
Type VI-A (ocular)	AR (rare)	Severe scoliosis; joint dislocations	High doses of ascorbic acid (to increase lysyl hydroxylase affinity for substrate)	Decreased hydroxylysine content in type I collagen of skin and bone (type II collagen is normal) resulting from defective lysyl hydroxylase activity; a consequence of low hydroxylysine level is altered cross-linkage of collagen
		Hyperextensible skin and joints; diminished muscle mass		
		Microcornea		
		Retinal detachment; glaucoma		
Type VI-B	AR	Corneal fragility; keratoglobus; blue sclerae		Ultrastructural changes: fiber-free spaces filled with amorphous material
		Joint hyperextensibility		Normal lysyl hydroxylase activity
		Other changes similar to type VI-A		

TABLE 186.1.	*Continued*			

Syndrome	Inheritance and Incidence	Principal Clinical Features	Therapy	Molecular Pathology
Type VII (arthrochalasis multiplex congenita)	AD	Pronounced joint hypermobility Moderate cutaneous elasticity Moderate bruising; round facies; short stature Multiple dislocations of large joints; friable tissues in surgery		Abnormal accumulation of procollagen I in tissue resulting from defective enzymatic cleavage of the precursor to mature form caused by mutations in *COL1A1* OR *COL1A2* involving the cleavage site or mutations elsewhere in the molecule that cause misalignment of the three chains at the cleavage site
	Subclassified into VII-A [α1(I)] and VII-B [α2(I)] depending on the collagen I chain involved			
Type VII-C	AR	Dermatosparaxis		Procollagen *N*-protease deficiency
Type VIII	AR (rare)	Severe resorption peridontitis with loss of teeth Moderate fragility of skin Mild to moderate dermal and joint hyperextensibility		Normal collagen studies
Osteogenesis imperfecta: Type I (mild)	AD 50% of cases	Scoliosis, biconcave vertebrae Blue sclerae Sensorineural or mixed hearing loss after age 20 y Usually no fracture at birth but 5–15 fractures before puberty, fewer in adulthood; fractures heal well Hyperextensible joints; joint dislocations	Rehabilitative therapy for muscle strength Careful surgery Estrogen for postmenopausal women	Null *COL1A1* allele, possibly caused by a defect in mRNA splicing, premature stop codon, or frameshift mutation; net effect is reduced collagen synthesis of the affected allele; the collagen that accumulates in tissues arises from the remaining normal allele; bone disease is mild because the collagen in the matrix is reduced in quantity but its structure is normal
Type II (lethal)	Most result from new dominant mutations (rarely recessive) 10% of all cases	Soft calvaria (wormian bones) Multiple intrauterine fractures Blue sclerae Death within 1 wk of birth, usually from diminished respiratory function		Deletions or substitutions in *COL1A1* or *COL1A2* chain genes leading to destabilization of collagen triple helix
Type III (severe deforming)	AD (rarely recessive) 20% of all cases	Severe limb deformity with marked kyphoscoliosis and stunted growth Frontal bosselation and occipital "overhang" Platybasia may cause brain damage (hydrocephalus, cranial nerve palsy) White sclerae in adults Hearing impairment (in 10%) 20 or more fractures in the first 3 y of life, but fewer after puberty Dentinogenesis imperfecta	Bracing for scoliosis Orthopedic surgery; spinal fusion	Deletions or substitutions in *COL1A1* or *COL1A2* collagen genes In recessively inherited forms, collagen type I genes have been excluded by linkage studies

TABLE 186.1. *Continued*

Syndrome	Inheritance and Incidence	Principal Clinical Features	Therapy	Molecular Pathology
Type IV (moderate deforming)	AD (may be variant of type I) 20% of all cases	Variable deformity of long bones and spine White sclerae Dentinogenesis imperfecta Progressive hearing loss, otosclerosis Hernias		Mutations in the type I collagen genes
Stickler syndrome	AD 1/10,000	Osteochondrodysplasia, cleft palate, micrognathia; prominent large joints; hyperextensibility changing to joint stiffness; early degenerative arthritis; midface hypoplasia Progressive sensorineural hearing loss Progressive myopia, occasional cataracts; vitreoretinal degeneration, retinal detachment Mitral valve prolapse		Premature termination mutations in the type II collagen gene (COL2A1) on 17q21 Heterogeneous, some families not linked to COL2A1
Kniest dysplasia	AD	More severe than Stickler syndrome Disproportionate dwarfism Limb deformities		Mutations in COL1A2

Disorders of Elastin

Syndrome	Inheritance and Incidence	Principal Clinical Features	Therapy	Molecular Pathology
Cutis laxa	AD	Lax, redundant, inelastic skin with loose folds No hyperextensible joints	Plastic surgery	Fragmented elastic fibrils Acquired form resulting from autoimmune mechanism
	AR type I	More severe skin manifestations Pulmonary emphysema; pneumothorax Hernias; gastrointestinal diverticula; tortuous arteries; arterial aneurysms and stenoses; early death from cardiopulmonary complications		Fragmented, reduced elastic fibers
	AR type II	Growth retardation; lax skin; joint hypermobility; hip dislocation Mental retardation		Heterogeneous
Pseudoxanthoma elasticum	AD (rare)	Thickened, yellowish, nodular, or reticular skin (like flat xanthomas) in flexural skin folds (e.g., neck, axilla)	Plastic surgery	Frayed, swollen, clumped, and calcified elastic fibers Linkage to the elastin gene on 7q11.23 has been excluded in one AD family
	AR (more common) 1/100,000	Angioid streaks in fundus oculi reflect breaks in Bruch's membrane; retinal hemorrhage; blindness Damaged elastic laminae and calcification of the media of many arteries leading to occlusion and rupture; coronary artery disease; restrictive cardiomyopathy		
Supravalvular aortic stenosis syndrome	AD	Arterial dysplasia involving aorta and pulmonary artery, but also peripheral pulmonary stenoses	Surgical correction	Total or partial deletion or disruption of elastin gene in 7q11.23 by translocation (deletion of elastin gene as part of Williams syndrome)

AD, autosomal dominant; AR, autosomal recessive.

Marfan-like disorders and those with dominant and recessive forms of pseudoxanthoma elasticum. Redundant and lax skin, as seen in cutis laxa, also is one of the distinctive features of severe Marfan syndrome of prenatal onset that leads to early infantile death. Whereas ascending aortic aneurysms typically are associated with Marfan syndrome, they may also be present in the vascular type of Ehlers–Danlos syndrome (formerly type IV) and forms of osteogenesis imperfecta.

The molecular pathology of disorders caused by mutations in structural molecules of the extracellular matrix, such as collagen or fibrillin, involves dominant-negative interference of the abnormal products of the mutant alleles in the formation of the matrix, despite the presence of a normal allele. Fundamental differences in the phenotypic consequences of different types of mutations have to be considered. For intracellular proteins, such as enzymes, a null mutation that does not generate a mutant product (because of gene deletion, disruption, promoter mutation, premature termination codon that leads to messenger RNA instability, or missense mutation that leads to instability of the mutant polypeptide), if present in the homozygous state, causes a more severe phenotype than does a point mutation that yields a partially functioning molecule. The opposite is true for connective tissue disorders that are dominantly inherited and in which the primary defect involves the gene for a structural protein. When the mutant product is synthesized in the cell, secreted, and incorporated into the extracellular matrix by interacting with other molecules (fibrillar collagens or fibrillin), the consequences of null mutations are less severe, whereas heterozygous expression of a structurally abnormal protein is more severe (dominant-negative or poison protein). Homozygosity (or compound heterozygosity) for missense mutations has the most severe clinical consequences.

This point is illustrated by the fact that in osteogenesis imperfecta and Marfan syndrome, a distinct correlation exists between mutations that cause absent or low levels of expression of the mutant allele and a mild phenotype. In contrast, certain point mutations that are associated with normal levels of expression of the mutant allele are correlated with severe neonatal lethal forms that result from new mutations.

The practical consequences of these considerations are manifold. One is the realization that identification of the gene in which the disease-causing mutation resides is not likely to provide a definitive clinical diagnosis. In the study of connective tissue disorders, more than in any other field, different disorders have been shown to arise from different types of mutations in the same gene. Molecular defects in specific extracellular matrix components may cause phenotypes that are clearly separated on nosologic grounds (e.g., COL1A1 and COL1A2 mutations lead to various types of osteogenesis imperfecta, Ehlers–Danlos syndrome, and osteoporosis). COL2A1 defects are responsible for numerous bone dysplasias with a wide range of clinical severity, including achondrogenesis type II, hypochondrogenesis, spondyloepiphysial dysplasia congenita, Kniest dysplasia, Stickler syndrome, and osteoarthritis with mild skeletal dysplasia. Fibrillin-1 mutations are common in Marfan syndrome but also have been identified in familial isolated aortic aneurysm and familial ectopia lentis. Heterozygous deletion or disruption of the gene for tropoelastin is responsible for autosomal dominant supraval-

var aortic stenosis, while frameshifts resulting in synthesis of a truncated tropoelastin molecule cause autosomal dominant cutis laxa. The elastin gene also is deleted in most patients with Williams–Beuren syndrome that includes supravalvar aortic stenosis and results from a 1.6 mega base pair deletion of chromosome band 7q11.23.

The presentation of disease nosology provided in Table 186.1 must be considered preliminary. The group of Ehlers–Danlos syndromes that are characterized by loose-jointedness, stretchable skin, and easy bruising has recently been reclassified. Molecular defects have been identified in both chains of collagen type V (COL5A1 and COL5A2) in the classic type of Ehlers–Danlos syndrome, in collagen type III (COL3A1) in the vascular type, and in genes encoding collagen-processing enzymes in the kyphoscoliosis, arthrochalasia, and dermatosparaxis types.

The clinical classification of osteogenesis imperfecta subtypes (the Sillence classification in Table 186.1) is not entirely satisfactory; considerable overlap exists, particularly in types I and IV. One-fourth to one-third of all patients cannot be classified into one of the subtypes listed, suggesting a phenotypic continuum. Because most osteogenesis imperfecta subtypes involve mutations in one of the two α chains of collagen type I (gene symbols COL1A1 and COL1A2), the type of molecular defect is likely to determine the phenotype associated with a particular mutation. The clinical findings range from minimal (e.g., benign joint hypermobility, occasional fractures) to significant (e.g., intrauterine fractures with neonatal lethal presentation, adult-onset forms with life-threatening consequences). Therefore, accurate clinical classification is important for counseling patients in regard to prognosis and for instituting prophylactic therapy.

Mutations in nonfibrillar collagen genes have been found in other disorders, such as collagen type VII mutations in dystrophic epidermolysis bullosa and involvement of genes for collagen types IV and V in Alport syndrome.

The clinical treatment of patients with heritable connective tissue disorders requires ongoing contributions from multiple specialists and is coordinated best through a multidisciplinary clinical center. The rapid progress being made in gene identification and mutational analysis may lead to major revisions in the classification of these disorders. However, the specific diagnoses will continue to be made in the clinic rather than the molecular genetics laboratory.

Therapy is directed at preventing complications through the use of protective orthopedic measures, β-adrenergic blockade for aortic disease, and cardiovascular, orthopedic, or plastic surgical procedures. If the connective tissue manifestations are caused by an inborn error of metabolism, such as in homocystinuria resulting from cystathionine synthetase deficiency, early diagnosis and systemic treatment can prevent some of the clinical complications. Treatment with intravenous bisphosphonates (such as pamidronate) appears to reduce the number of fractures in children with severe osteogenesis imperfecta type I.

BIBLIOGRAPHY

Beighton P, De Paepe A, Steinmann B, et al. Ehlers–Danlos syndromes: revised nosology, Villefranche, 1997. *Am J Med Genet* 1998;77:31–37.
Byers PH. Disorders of collagen biosynthesis and structure. In: Scriver CR,

Beaudet AL, Sly WS, et al, eds. *The metabolic and molecular bases of inherited disease*, vol 3, seventh ed. New York: McGraw-Hill, 1995: 4029–4077.

De Paepe A, Devereux RB, Dietz HC, et al. Revised diagnostic criteria for the Marfan syndrome. *Am J Med Genet* 1996;62:417–426.

Glorieux FH, Bishop NJ, Plotkin H, et al. Cyclic administration of pamidronate in children with severe osteogenesis imperfecta. *N Engl J Med* 1998;339:947–952.

Ramirez F, Godfrey M, Lee B, et al. Marfan syndrome and related disorders. In: Scriver CR, Beaudet AL, Sly WS, et al, eds. *The metabolic and molecular bases of inherited disease*, vol 13, seventh ed. New York: McGraw-Hill, 1995:4079–4094.

Royce PM, Steinmann B, eds. *Connective tissue and its heritable disorders: molecular, genetic, and medical aspects.* New York: Wiley-Liss, 1993.

Kelley's Textbook of Internal Medicine, fourth edition. Edited by H. David Humes. Lippincott Williams & Wilkins, Philadelphia © 2000.

CHAPTER 187

INHERITED DEFICIENCIES OF COMPLEMENT AND IMMUNOGLOBULINS

GEORGE F. MOXLEY

While younger normal children have episodic otitis, gastroenteritis, and upper respiratory infections, repeated serious bacterial infections are distinctively uncommon in older children and adults. Older children or young adults with repeated serious pyogenic infections (e.g., with *Staphylococcus aureus, Streptococcus pneumoniae, Escherichia coli, Neisseria gonorrhoeae,* or *N. meningitidis*) may have an underlying predisposition from an inherited complement or immunoglobulin deficiency. Except for selective IgA deficiency, all are rare.

■ INHERITED COMPLEMENT DEFICIENCIES

Complement deficiencies typically predispose to bacterial infections. An outline is presented in Table 187.1. The complement system aids host defense by linking immunoglobulin recognition of pathogens with specific protective effects. C3 cleavage fragments that are covalently bound to immune complexes prevent immune complex precipitation in tissues, dissolve precipitated complexes, and attach immune complexes to cell surface receptors, resulting in clearance of immune complexes and microbial invaders. Such immune adherence also helps to localize such complexes to immune cells such as follicular dendritic cells and B lymphocytes, with subsequent activation of T cells. Other consequences are vascular effects through release of anaphylatoxins, contraction of smooth muscle, and attraction of inflammatory cells through generation of chemotactic factors. Complement kills some pathogenic microorganisms, such as *Neisseria* species, by lytic mechanisms.

Except for properdin deficiency (X-linked recessive inheritance) and the control protein C1 inhibitor (C1-INH) (autosomal dominant), total complement protein deficiencies are inherited as autosomal recessives. The alleles are expressed codominantly, and carriers of null alleles typically have about half-normal levels. For complement deficiencies other than C1-INH, the spectrum of clinical manifestations includes recurrent serious bacterial infections and immune complex–mediated diseases (systemic lupus erythematosus, glomerulonephritis, and others). For deficiencies in complement proteins of the classic pathway (C1q, C1r, C1s, C4, and C2), inflammatory rheumatic and renal diseases predominate. With deficiencies of the alternative pathway (factor B, factor D, and properdin), infections with encapsulated organisms are most common. For C3 and its control proteins, factor H and factor I, deficiencies result in severe bacterial infections and nephritis. In a deficiency of the membrane attack complex (C5, C6, C7, C8, and, to some extent, C9), recurrent infections with *Neisseria* species (*N. gonorrhoeae* and *N. meningitidis*) are most prominent. In C1-INH deficiency, subcutaneous and mucosal edema is the major feature; C1-INH deficiency also has been associated with a higher than usual frequency of immune complex diseases.

Homozygous C2 deficiency is associated with recurrent pyogenic infections and systemic lupus erythematosus with prominent skin manifestations, including photosensitivity and a lower frequency of serious renal disease.

The most common homozygous complement deficiency in humans is C2 deficiency, which occurs in about 0.01% of all whites. The *C2* gene is between the HLA-B and HLA-D region genes of the human major histocompatibility complex. Defects in C2 deficiency include nonfunctional C2 genes and absent secretion of C2. About half of all C2-deficient individuals have no symptoms, but others have manifestations of inflammatory rheumatic and renal diseases. These include systemic lupus erythematosus, discoid lupus, juvenile rheumatoid arthritis, polymyositis, Henoch–Schönlein purpura, and vasculitis. The clinical picture of systemic lupus erythematosus associated with homozygous C2 deficiency differs from that of idiopathic systemic lupus erythematosus by milder renal disease, more skin manifestations, and lower titers of antinuclear antibody (ANA). The ANA specificities include anti–Sjögren syndrome A (SSA) (Ro) and anti-SS-B (La). Recurrent serious infections with pyogenic organisms also can occur.

C1-INH deficiency results in hereditary angioneurotic edema with episodic swelling of subcutaneous tissues, intestinal pain and obstruction from gut swelling, and sometimes respiratory obstruction from swelling of the upper respiratory tissues.

C1-INH is a serine protease inhibitor that controls not only the C1r and C1s proteases of the complement system but also kallikrein of the contact system and factors XIa, XIIa, and plasmin of the clotting system. Genetic C1-INH defects lead to the syndrome of angioneurotic edema. The illness is characterized by 2- to 3-day-long episodes of nonpitting subcutaneous edema (angioedema) and intestinal and respiratory obstruction caused by edematous mucosal tissue. Although most such indi-

TABLE 187.1.	INHERITED COMPLEMENT DEFICIENCIES		

Complement Deficiency	Mode of Inheritance, Chromosomal Location[b]	Consequence of Deficiency to Function	Major Clinical Features
C1q (>40 cases)[a]	Autosomal recessive, C1q A, B, and C chains 1p34.1–1p36.3	Inability to initiate classical pathway activation	Most have severe systemic lupus erythematosus, glomerulonephritis, infections
C1r, C1s (rare)	Autosomal recessive, 12p13	C1r and C1s deficiency always combined. Inability to form classical pathway C3 convertase	SLE > infections
C4A	Autosomal recessive, 6p21.3 in MHC region	C4A deficiency probably results in diminished ability to deposit cleaved C3b on immune complexes	Null alleles at C4A are frequent in most populations (up to 25%) and associated with SLE. Complete C4A deficiency (due to 2 null alleles) is associated with SLE, insulin-dependent diabetes mellitus, Henoch–Schönlein purpura, and autoimmune chronic active hepatitis
C4B	Autosomal recessive, 6p21.3 in MHC region	C4B mutation results in synthesis of C4B-like protein with diminished lytic function	C4B null alleles are also frequent (up to 20%, depending on the population) and associated with Felty's syndrome and IgA nephropathy
Combined C4A and C4B deficiency (17 cases)		Complete C4A and C4B deficiency results in inability to form classical pathway C3 convertase	Complete C4B deficiency is associated with SLE and bacterial meningitis. Complete C4 deficiency due to 4 null alleles at C4A and C4B loci is rare but associated with SLE often with anti-Ro autoantibodies, glomerulonephritis, and infections
C2 (>100 cases)	Autosomal recessive, 6p21.3 in MHC region often on A25 B18 DR2 haplotype	Inability to form classical pathway C3 convertase	Recurrent pyogenic infections, polymyositis, Henoch–Schönlein purpura, SLE often with anti-Ro autoantibodies
C1 esterase inhibitor	Autosomal dominant, 11q11–11q13.1	Deficient inhibition of C1r and C1s, contact system, and clotting system. Unbridled complement consumption. Low C4, normal C1 level. Edema possibly due to C2 kinin or bradykinin	Hereditary angioedema. Episodic nonpitting subcutaneous edema (angioedema), intestinal edema, laryngeal edema, SLE, glomerulonephritis
P (>50 cases)	X-linked, Xp11.4–11.23	Diminished stabilization of alternative pathway C3 convertase	Recurrent Neisseria and pyogenic infections > discoid lupus
D (1 case)	Autosomal dominant vs. X-linked	Diminished ability to form alternative pathway C3 convertase postulated	Recurrent Neisseria infections
C3 (16 cases)	Autosomal recessive, 19p13.2–19p13.3	Absence of anaphylatoxin effects, immune complex precipitation and diminished immune complex removal	Recurrent pyogenic infections, membranoproliferative glomerulonephritis, partial lipodystrophy. IgG anticomplement antibodies
I (15 cases)	Autosomal recessive, 4q25	Inability to limit turnover of C3 and consequent C3 depletion	Recurrent pyogenic infections, urticaria
H (12 cases)	Autosomal recessive, 1q32	Same consequence as factor I deficiency	Recurrent pyogenic infections, IgA nephropathy, hemolytic uremic syndrome, vasculitis
C5 (19 cases)	Autosomal dominant vs. recessive, 9q34.1	Absence of anaphylatoxin effects and bacterial lysis	Recurrent Neisseria infections, seborrheic dermatitis, wasting, SLE
C6 (>50 cases)	Autosomal recessive, 5p13	Diminished bacterial lysis by membrane attack complex	Sometimes healthy, or recurrent Neisseria infections
C7 (>25 cases)	Autosomal recessive, 5p13	Diminished bacterial lysis by membrane attack complex	Recurrent Neisseria infections
C8$\alpha\gamma$	Autosomal recessive, C8A at 1p32, γ on 9q	Diminished bacterial lysis by membrane attack complex	In blacks and Japanese. Recurrent Neisseria infections, SLE
C8β (>30 cases)	Autosomal recessive, C8B at 1p32	Diminished bacterial lysis by membrane attack complex	In whites. Recurrent Neisseria infections, SLE. Juvenile chronic arthritis

TABLE 187.1.	*Continued*			
Complement Deficiency	**Mode of Inheritance, Chromosomal Location**[b]	**Consequence of Deficiency to Function**	**Major Clinical Features**
C9 (5 white cases, many Japanese cases)	Autosomal recessive, 5p13	Diminished bacterial lysis by membrane attack complex	Usually asymptomatic, sometimes recurrent *Neisseria* infections
CR1 (C3b receptor, rare) CD35	Autosomal codominant, 1q32	Lower clearance of C3b-coated bacteria and immune complexes	Possible association of low numbers of CR1 with SLE, but low CR3 levels are likely a consequence of SLE
CR3 (rare)	Autosomal recessive, CR3a 16p, CR3b 21q22.3, β-2 integrin, ITGB2	Absence of β chain of LFA-1 p150,95 and CR3 causes abnormal adhesion-dependent activities of neutrophils, mononuclear cells, and lymphocytes	Leukocyte adhesion deficiency syndrome. Delayed umbilical cord separation, recurrent bacterial infections, impaired wound healing
Decay accelerating factor (rare) CD55	Autosomal recessive, 1q32	Less dissociation of C3 convertases	Episodic intravascular hemolysis (PNH)
CD59, protectin (rare)	Autosomal recessive, 11p13	PNH reflects defective glycolipid anchoring of several proteins in cell membrane because of absent phosphatidylinositol glycan. CD59 absence causes inability to limit complement damage to host erythrocytes	Episodic intravascular hemolysis (PNH)

[a] Case frequencies from Morgan BP, Walport MJ. Complement deficiency and disease. *Immunol Today* 1991;12:301–306.
[b] Chromosomal locations and individual allelic mutations may be found in Online Mendelian Inheritance in Man (OMIM). Center for Medical Genetics, Johns Hopkins University (Baltimore, MD) and National Center for Biotechnology Information, National Library of Medicine (Bethesda, MD), 1997. World Wide Web URL: http://www.ncbi.nlm.nih.gov/omim/.
>, more frequently than; MHC, major histocompatibility complex; SLE, systemic lupus erythematosus; PNH, paroxysmal nocturnal hemoglobinuria; LFA, leukocyte-function associated.

viduals with C1-INH have an affected relative, about 1 in 10 persons with C1-INH deficiency has an apparently new mutation. The more common pattern in C1-INH deficiency is relative inhibitor absence, but about 15% of cases result from mutations with normal levels of a dysfunctional C1-INH protein. Because of complement consumption from uncontrolled activation, C4 and C2 levels are low, even between episodes. Episodes of hereditary angioneurotic edema may occur spontaneously or after trauma. During an attack, C1-INH, C4, and C2 levels are depressed even more than between attacks.

One may suspect an inherited complement deficiency in the context of recurrent, serious bacterial infections with pyogenic bacteria or *Neisseria*. To screen for inherited complement deficiencies other than C1-INH deficiency, the total hemolytic complement (50%) should be measured on a specimen properly collected and stored at −70°C. For angioedema with respiratory or intestinal tract obstruction, the appropriate screening test for C1-INH deficiency is the C4 level antigen followed by a C1-INH test if the C4 level is low. For most complement deficiencies, no replacement is necessary. For hereditary angioedema, supportive care such as maintenance of a patent airway and fluid administration may be necessary until the episode subsides. C1-INH plasma concentrate (or if not available, fresh frozen plasma)

is available for serious acute attacks. Attenuated androgens increase levels of normal C1-INH and may lengthen the period between acute attacks. However, long-term use of these androgens can cause liver damage, masculinization, and diminished growth.

INHERITED IMMUNOGLOBULIN DEFICIENCIES

Immunoglobulin deficiency also predisposes to recurrent bacterial infections. Antibodies normally contribute to immunity by neutralizing bacteria, viruses, and toxins and serving as surface receptors for certain cells of the immune system.

The clinical spectrum of inherited immunoglobulin deficiencies ranges from incidental asymptomatic findings (such as some persons with selective IgA deficiency or certain IgG subclass deficiencies) to life-threatening infections. An outline is presented in Table 187.2. Some antibody deficiencies are accompanied by defects in cellular immunity. Many antibody deficiency syndromes are associated with autoimmune diseases (e.g., Bruton's agammaglobulinemia, Wiskott–Aldrich syndrome, selective IgA deficiency, common variable immunodeficiency), and

TABLE 187.2. INHERITED IMMUNOGLOBULIN DEFICIENCIES

Immunoglobulin Deficiency	Mode of Inheritance, Gene Defect, Chromosomal Location[a]	Immune Consequences	Major Clinical Features
Bruton's agammaglobulinemia	X-linked recessive, Bruton tyrosine kinase (Btk), Xq21.3–Xq22 Autosomal recessive form, unknown gene and location	Mutant Btk results in failure of B-cell development and of heavy-chain rearrangement. Absence of plasma cells and mature B cells. Normal T-cell-mediated immunity. IgG <200, IgA and IgM low.	Onset after age 6 mo. Severe bacterial infections, particularly respiratory, *Campylobacter,* and *Salmonella. Giardia* infections. Severe CNS viral infections. Lymphatic and colorectal malignancies. Often arthritis like rheumatoid.
Wiskott–Aldrich syndrome	X-linked recessive, Wiskott–Aldrich syndrome protein (Wasp) involved in tyrosine phosphorylation, Xp11.23–p11.22	Mutant Wasp leads to poor B-cell activation. Normal IgG, IgA, and IgM levels but impaired response to polysaccharides.	Thrombocytopenia, eczema, and bloody diarrhea. Lymphatic malignancies, autoimmune diseases. Recurrent infections.
Ataxia-telangiectasia	Autosomal recessive, unknown genes involving DNA repair or DNA processing enzymes, 11q22.3	Thymic hypoplasia. Typically selective IgA deficiency and IgG2 deficiency. Cutaneous anergy.	Cerebellar ataxia, conjunctival telangiectasias, chronic sinus and respiratory infections, high frequency of malignancies. Abnormal sensitivity to radiation.
X-linked lymphoproliferative syndrome (Duncan's disease)	X-linked recessive, SH2 domain protein 1A (SH2D1A), Xq25	Extreme sensitivity to EBV with uncontrolled polyclonal expansion of T and B cells. Low IgG, IgA, and IgM. Natural killer cell deficiency.	Severe infectious mononucleosis, then agammaglobulinemia, aplastic anemia, and lymphoma.
X-linked hyper IgM syndrome	X-linked recessive, gp39 or CD40, Xq26	Mutant CD40 ligand gp39 present on T-cell surface, or mutant receptor CD40 on B-cell surface, interferes with signaling during B-cell growth and differentiation. Impaired immunoglobulin heavy-chain switch. High IgM, low or absent IgG and IgA.	Onset <2 y, *Pneumocystis carinii* pneumonia, *Cryptosporidium* diarrhea; autoimmune neutropenia, hemolytic anemia, and thrombocytopenia; respiratory infections and lymphoid hyperplasia.
X-linked severe combined immunodeficiency	X-linked recessive, IL-2 receptor γ chain, Xq13	Mutant γ chain that is shared among lymphocyte receptors for IL-2, IL-4, IL-7, IL-9, and IL-15 depresses B- and T-cell immunity. Mutant Zap-70 protein leads to deficient T-cell activation. Deficient ADA leads to B- and T-cell dysfunction. Thymic hypoplasia, no T cells, normal or increased B cells. Low IgG, IgA, and IgM.	Onset <6 months of age. Bacterial, viral, and fungal infections.
Autosomal severe combined immunodeficiency (Swiss-type agammaglobulinemia)	Autosomal recessive, Zap-70 at 2q12, Janus kinase-3 at 5p13, DNA-dependent protein kinase at 8q11, IL-2 receptor at 5p13, and others, or ADA at 20q13.11		
Selective IgA deficiency (common, 1 in 800)	Genetically heterogeneous, possibly MHC region gene. Found in some individuals with deletion of one arm of human chromosome 18 and of 21. Associated with HLA A1 B8 DR3 haplotype bearing null allele for C4A.	Normal IgG and IgM, IgA <5 mg/dL. Absent neutralization of toxins, bacteria, and viruses. Often have anti-IgA antibodies of IgE class. Both serum and secretory IgA absent.	Some are asymptomatic. Others, particularly with accompanying IgG2 subclass deficiency, have recurrent sinus and pulmonary infections. Autoimmune diseases, atopy, malabsorption. Propensity to anaphylaxis upon exposure to blood products and most γ globulin preparations.

TABLE 187.2. *Continued*

Immunoglobulin Deficiency	Mode of Inheritance, Gene Defect, Chromosomal Location[a]	Immune Consequences	Major Clinical Features
IgG subclass deficiency	Autosomal recessive, sometimes due to gene deletions, 14q32.33	May result in diminished response to antigen.	Often with Wiskott–Aldrich syndrome, complement deficiency, or selective IgA deficiency. IgG1 deficiency results in infections like agammaglobulinemia, IgG2 with infections from encapsulated bacteria, IgG3 with recurrent sinus and lung infections.
IgM deficiency	X-linked recessive, unknown gene and location	IgM <10% of normal, normal IgG and IgA	Recurrent sinus and pulmonary infections, gram-negative septicemia, meningococcal meningitis.
κ light chain deficiency	Autosomal recessive, κ constant segment, 2p12	Only λ light chains in immunoglobulins	None
Common variable immunodeficiency	Genetically heterogeneous, some X-linked, gp39 at Xq26.3–Xq27.1. Associated with HLA A1 B8 DR3 haplotype bearing null allele for C4A.	Normal number of B cells, but failure of B-cell differentiation. 25% B-cell defect, 75% T-cell defect. IgG <250, IgA and IgM low. Blunting of antigen-specific antibody responses.	Onset after age 10 y, recurrent bacterial infections of respiratory and GI tracts, as well as viral, fungal, and parasitic infections, including *Pneumocystis carinii*. Autoimmune diseases, arthritis, pernicious anemia, hemolytic anemia, thrombocytopenia, neutropenia. Gastric carcinoma, lymphoma.
Transient agammaglobulinemia of infancy	Unknown	Low IgG, IgA, and IgM, but normal natural antibodies and response to immunization.	Resolution by age 1–2 y.
Hyper-IgE syndrome	Autosomal dominant, unknown gene and location	Markedly increased IgE, high IgD. Normal IgG, IgA, and IgM. Deficient specific immune response.	Recurrent staphylococcal abscesses, pruritic dermatitis, eosinophilia.
Hyper-IgE syndrome (Job)	Autosomal recessive, unknown gene and location		

[a] Chromosomal locations and individual allelic mutations may be found in Online Mendelian Inheritance in Man (OMIM). Center for Medical Genetics, Johns Hopkins University (Baltimore, MD) and National Center for Biotechnology Information, National Library of Medicine (Bethesda, MD), 1997. World Wide Web URL: http://www.ncbi.nlm.nih.gov/omim/.
MHC, major histocompatibility complex; HLA, human leukocyte antigen; IL, interleukin; ADA, adenosine deaminase; EBV, Epstein–Barr Virus.

some also are associated with malignancies (e.g., Bruton's agammaglobulinemia, Wiskott–Aldrich syndrome, ataxia-telangiectasia, Duncan's disease).

As a rule, persons with inherited immunoglobulin deficiencies tend to have recurrent infections with encapsulated bacteria. The exceptions are hyperimmunoglobulinemia M syndrome and common variable immunodeficiency, which may also have opportunistic infections associated with them. Most are inherited as autosomal recessives or X-linked recessives.

The most common inherited immunoglobulin deficiency is selective IgA deficiency. Persons with selective IgA deficiency tend to have recurrent episodes of sinus and lung infections as well as urinary tract and gastrointestinal infections.

IgA is the major immunoglobulin normally found in the secretions on mucosal surfaces, and it contributes to protection against external toxins and pathogens. Some individuals with selective IgA deficiency are entirely asymptomatic. Others, particularly those with accompanying IgG2 subclass deficiency, have recurrent infections of the paranasal sinuses and lungs. Gastrointestinal manifestations include giardiasis, idiopathic inflammatory bowel disease, and a sprue-like syndrome. Atopy and various organ-specific autoimmune diseases also can occur. Individuals with selective IgA deficiency typically have circulating and cell-bound anti-IgA antibodies that may predispose to anaphylaxis on exposure to whole blood or blood constituents contaminated with IgA. Because most preparations of immune serum globulin contain trace amounts of IgA and may cause anaphylaxis, and because immune serum globulin does not restore the deficient mucosal IgA, most authorities consider immune serum therapy to be unwarranted.

Screening tests for inherited immunoglobulin deficiencies may include blood counts and differential counts of leukocytes. Although IgG subclass determinations are usually not helpful, quantitation of IgG, IgA, and IgM may aid in diagnosis. One may also measure antibodies directed to defined antigens such as blood group antigens. One may also test for antibodies prior to and after immunization with specific immunogens such as diphtheria and tetanus toxoids and polysaccharide antigens from *Haemophilus influenzae* or *S. pneumoniae.*

Infections in inherited immunoglobulin deficiencies are treated with appropriate antimicrobial therapy. In addition, for persons lacking the ability to generate protective IgG antibody responses directed to organisms causing systemic infections, intravenous administration of γ-globulin may be indicated. Because globulin replacement therapy does not prevent serious respiratory infections, chronic antimicrobial therapy is typically required. The use of vaccines with live organisms (e.g., bacille Calmette–Guérin, attenuated polio) should be avoided in individuals with suspected antibody deficiency syndromes.

BIBLIOGRAPHY

Burrows PD, Cooper MD. IgA deficiency. *Adv Immunol* 1997;65:245–276.

Cicardi M, Bergamaschini L, Cugno M, et al. Pathogenetic and clinical aspects of C1 inhibitor deficiency. *Immunobiology* 1998;199:366–376.

Infante AJ, Kamani NR. The evaluation of suspected immune deficiency by the primary care physician. *Compr Ther* 1997;23:89–94.

Puck JM. Primary immunodeficiency diseases. *JAMA* 1997;278: 1835–1841.

Ratnoff WD. Inherited deficiencies of complement in rheumatic diseases. *Rheum Dis Clin North Am* 1996;22:75–94.

Sicherer SH, Winkelstein JA. Primary immunodeficiency diseases in adults [clinical conference]. *JAMA* 1998;279:58–61.

Kelley's Textbook of Internal Medicine, fourth edition. Edited by H. David Humes. Lippincott Williams & Wilkins, Philadelphia © 2000.

DIAGNOSTIC AND THERAPEUTIC MODALITIES IN RHEUMATOLOGIC AND ALLERGIC DISEASES

USE OF LABORATORY TESTS IN RHEUMATOLOGY AND CLINICAL IMMUNOLOGY

JOHN A. HARDIN

Numerous tests are relevant in the evaluation of connective tissue diseases. Some of them are helpful diagnostically, particularly when applied to a patient population enriched in the disease in question, and others are useful for estimating disease activity.

ERYTHROCYTE SEDIMENTATION RATE AND ACUTE PHASE PROTEINS

Many different processes, including surgical wounds, bacterial infection, necrosis of tumors, tissue ischemia, myocardial injury, and inflammation secondary to connective tissue diseases, are associated with characteristic alterations in the protein components of plasma. All of these conditions share features of tissue injury or inflammation. They lead to the generation of a variety of cytokines capable of altering the metabolic activity of hepatocytes. The result is that plasma proteins, such as C-reactive protein and serum amyloid A, increase 1,000-fold or more in a matter of a day, whereas others, such as fibrinogen, complement components, and haptoglobin, increase one- to fourfold over several days. In contrast, other proteins such as transferrin and, especially, albumin exhibit a decrease in the circulation because of a reduction in their synthesis by hepatocytes. These alterations are referred to as the *acute phase plasma protein response*.

The erythrocyte sedimentation rate (ESR) is a simple method for evaluating the extent of this response, and it is helpful to understand the responsible mechanisms. Red blood cells (RBCs) suspended in plasma normally repel each other because of their surrounding net negative charge. Large asymmetrical molecules in the supporting plasma act as dipoles and bridge charges between individual cells. Fibrinogen is especially effective in this regard. As the concentrations of such molecules increase, RBCs aggregate more readily to form rouleaux structures that fall through plasma at an accelerated rate.

Measurement of the ESR usually is carried out by the Westergren or Wintrobe method. Because the former is not affected by the packed volume of RBCs, it is considered superior. Normal ESRs usually range slightly higher in women than in men, and aging is associated with a moderate increase. Normal values at 50 years of age are considered to be 20 mm per hour for men and 30 mm per hour for women. Many individuals older than 70 years of age have ESRs in the range of 40 to 50 mm per hour without any apparent tissue injury or inflammation. This should be remembered when treating elderly patients with diseases such as temporal arteritis or polymyalgia rheumatica. In some cases, even with adequate therapy, ESRs do not fall below this range. Occasionally, an unusually low ESR (less than 1 mm per hour) is observed and may be associated with abnormal immunoglobulins that form cryogels. Chronic liver disease or other illnesses that can generate low serum albumin and a high globulin fraction produce high ESR measurements.

Measurement of the ESR is useful diagnostically and as a guide to treatment in selected clinical circumstances. The ESR can supplement clinical efforts to differentiate inflammatory from noninflammatory joint disease (e.g., rheumatoid arthritis from osteoarthritis). In addition, marked elevations in the ESR (greater than 100 mm per hour) are associated particularly with severe deep-tissue infections, systemic lupus erythematosus (SLE), polymyalgia rheumatica, giant cell arteritis, and malignancy. Most patients with polymyalgia rheumatica or giant cell arteritis have ESRs greater than 50 mm per hour. However, 8% to 20% of patients with either condition have been noted to have ESRs less than 30 to 40 mm per hour. In several rheumatic diseases, longitudinal ESRs reflect relative disease activity and may be helpful for adjusting therapy. Fibrinogen and many other acute phase proteins that contribute to the ESR have half-lives of 3 to 5 days, limiting the rate at which effective therapy can alter the ESR. In addition, patients with rheumatoid arthritis and SLE occasionally have obvious active disease but normal ESRs.

The ESR is not useful as a screening test for occult disease. It can be within normal limits even when a serious disease is obvious. Conversely, with the exception of transient elevations in otherwise normal individuals, a high ESR almost always is accompanied by a clinically apparent disorder.

Information about the acute phase response can be supplemented by measurement of the C-reactive protein level. Acute inflammation, such as intercurrent infection, causes the concentration of this protein in the circulation to increase rapidly. In contrast, chronic inflammation, such as that which accompanies rheumatoid arthritis or SLE, may be associated with lesser elevations in C-reactive protein. As a marker, the C-reactive protein level rises sooner after the onset of bacterial infection and declines more rapidly after successful therapy than does the ESR. Unlike the ESR, C-reactive protein is not influenced by circulating levels of albumin, immunoglobulins, or rheumatoid factor. For this reason, C-reactive protein may provide a more accurate assessment of inflammation per se in diseases such as rheumatoid arthritis.

■ SYNOVIAL FLUID EXAMINATION

The examination of synovial fluid often is the most informative part of the evaluation in patients with arthritis. The aim is to distinguish between inflammatory and noninflammatory joint diseases and to detect the presence of such causative agents as bacteria and crystals. The small joints of the hands and feet, the wrists, the elbows, the shoulders, the knees, and the sternomanubrial joints are readily accessible for aspiration in the physician's office. Usually, as much fluid as possible should be removed. Its color and viscosity should be observed, and separate samples should be reserved for a leukocyte count (citrate tube), a crystal examination (no anticoagulant), culture, and Gram stain. Sometimes only a few hundred microliters of fluid can be obtained from small joints. In such cases, it often is best to express a small amount onto a swab for culture and the remainder onto a glass slide, where it can be examined for crystals and used for Gram and Wright stains.

Normal synovial fluid is an ultrafiltrate of plasma to which synovial cells add elements, most notably hyaluronic acid (a macromolecule that accounts for the high viscosity of synovial fluid). Fibrinogen and other large molecules do not enter the joint space readily, and normal synovial fluid does not clot. With mild inflammation, however, some clot formation may be noted. With severe inflammation, proteolysis may degrade clotting factors, so that no clot forms.

In addition to a routine leukocyte count, culture, Gram stain, and crystal examination, several special analytic studies may be indicated. Synovial fluid glucose levels normally are slightly lower than those of peripheral blood, but in infectious arthritis and in rheumatoid arthritis, they may be less than half as high. For these measurements to be meaningful, the samples must be obtained after at least 6 hours of fasting. Occasionally, neoplastic processes involving joints can be diagnosed through cytologic examinations of synovial fluid. In most clinical settings, measurements of complement and other plasma proteins rarely provide much additional information. The mucin clot test is not a useful diagnostic test.

The diagnostic implications of various synovial fluid findings are presented in Fig. 188.1. One of the most important findings is whether the synovial fluid is inflammatory or noninflammatory. In most patients with osteoarthritis or traumatic joint disease, the total number of leukocytes is less than 2,000 cells per microliter. Occasionally, osteoarthritis accompanied by mild inflammation is associated with leukocyte counts as high as 5,000 cells per microliter. Systemic lupus erythematosus, scleroderma, and related overlap syndromes usually are associated with relatively non-inflammatory synovial fluids, even when joint inflammation is clinically striking. Synovial fluid leukocyte counts vary widely in rheumatoid arthritis, juvenile rheumatoid arthritis, psoriatic arthritis, Lyme disease, and Reiter's syndrome but typically are in the range of 20,000 to 40,000 cells per microliter. Sometimes, leukocyte counts in rheumatoid joint fluid are in excess of 100,000 cells per microliter. All of these disorders are associated with about 75% to 90% polymorphonuclear neutrophil leukocytes.

Leukocyte counts also vary widely in crystal-induced arthritis but average about 20,000 cells per microliter. Cell counts do not help distinguish between gout and pseudogout. The diagnosis of crystal-induced disease usually can be established with polarizing microscopy. Sodium urate crystals appear as relatively large, needle-shaped structures and are seen more readily than the smaller, more rhomboid-shaped crystals of calcium pyrophosphate. Hydroxyapatite and calcium phosphate crystals can be associated with synovitis, especially in patients with underlying osteoarthritis. These crystals are too amorphous to be visualized with light microscopy; special electron microscopy studies are needed for their demonstration. Occasionally, synovitis is associated with the presence of calcium oxalate or cholesterol crystals, or with crystalline forms of corticosteroids used for joint injections. Other debris in synovial fluid also may be helpful in making the diagnosis. Cartilage fragments suggest degenerative arthritis or chondromalacia. Free globules of fat in a hemorrhagic specimen can indicate fracture of the subchondral bone.

■ RHEUMATOID FACTORS

Rheumatoid factors are autoantibodies that are directed against epitopes on the Fc portion of other immunoglobulin molecules. They occur within the IgM, IgG, IgA, and IgE classes and usually bind their target epitopes with low affinity. In clinical settings the term rheumatoid factor generally refers to an IgM class autoantibody because most hospital-based assays selectively detect this type of rheumatoid factor. While a number of genetic and environmental mechanisms are involved in the generation of rheumatoid factors, a fundamental component is the chronic exposure of the immune system to circulating immune complexes. These complexes are selectively ingested and processed by B lymphocytes that are capable of secreting anti-Ig antibodies.

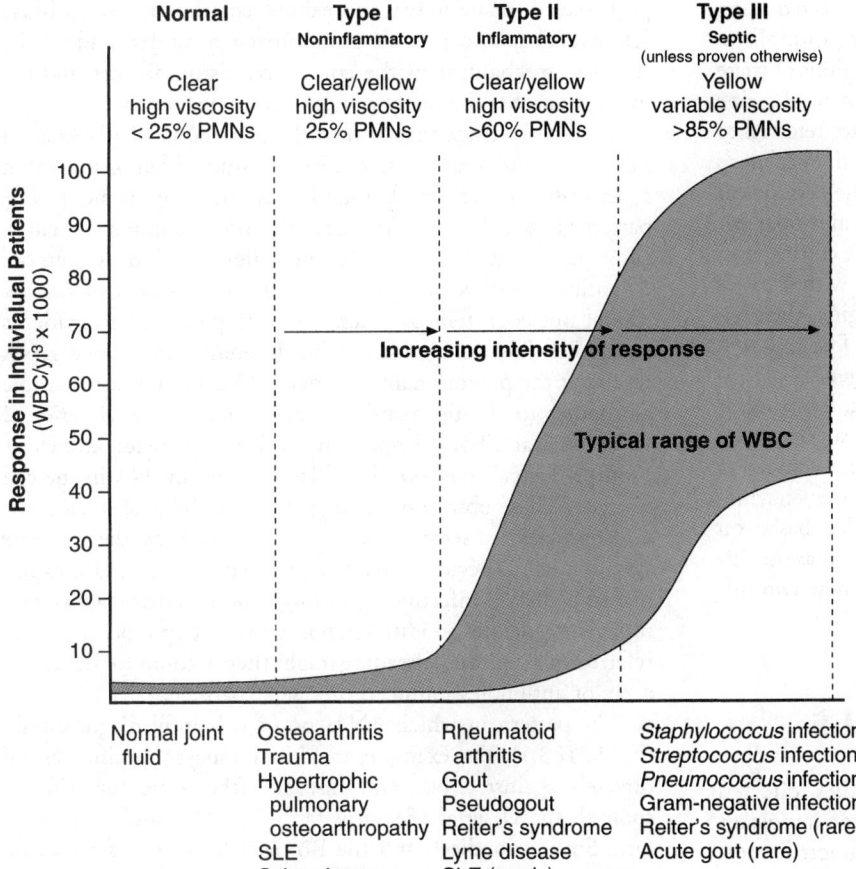

FIGURE 188.1. Characteristic changes in synovial fluid that accompany diseases of joints. Synovial fluid can be categorized as normal, type I, type II, or type III according to physical features and white blood cell (WBC) count. Specific diseases are associated with each category as shown. The shaded area indicates the typical range of WBC count in each type, with higher counts corresponding to increasing degrees of severity of each process. PMN, polymorphonuclear neutrophil leukocyte; SLE, systemic lupus erythematosus.

In selected patients, notably those with rheumatoid vasculitis, rheumatoid factor–Ig complexes reach high levels and mediate tissue injury, but more often it is not possible to identify specific pathogenetic roles for these autoantibodies.

In standard clinical assays, test sera are combined with RBCs or particles of latex or bentonite coated with rabbit or human IgG, and the degree of agglutination is observed. Because most rheumatoid factors from patients with rheumatoid arthritis bind epitopes shared by both types of IgG, either substrate is acceptable. These agglutination assays detect almost exclusively rheumatoid factors of the IgM class, which are about 1,000-fold more potent as agglutinators than are antibodies of the IgG class. More recently, ELISA methods for detecting rheumatoid factors have been developed. In these tests, the solid phase substrate consists of monomeric IgG to which test sera are exposed and bound antibody is detected with a labeled second antibody. These tests can be conducted at high dilutions of patient sera, thus minimizing interference from circulating immune complexes or the patient's own IgG, which can act as a competitor if present at high concentrations.

Rheumatoid factors occur in a broad range of diseases. For example, the results of latex agglutination tests are positive in about 13% of patients with active tuberculosis, 40% of patients with subacute bacterial endocarditis, 50% of patients with nodu-

lar pulmonary silicosis, 60% of patients with idiopathic pulmonary fibrosis, 80% of patients with rheumatoid arthritis, most patients with Sjögren's syndrome, and virtually all patients with essential mixed cryoglobulinemia. Rheumatoid factors also are observed transiently in patients with a variety of viral infections, including mononucleosis. Among normal blood donors, their prevalence increases with age and ranges from 1% to 4% among younger individuals to as high as 20% among individuals older than 5 years. When present in normal individuals, rheumatoid factors are usually found at lower levels. Their specificity for rheumatoid arthritis increases in conjunction with high titers, reactivity with both human and rabbit IgG, and distribution among the IgM, IgG, and IgA classes. Rheumatoid factors do not appear to occur with increased frequency among patients with juvenile rheumatoid arthritis, Lyme disease, or uncomplicated psoriatic arthritis.

ANTINEUTROPHIL CYTOPLASMIC AUTOANTIBODIES

Antineutrophil cytoplasmic autoantibodies (ANCAs) are autoantibodies directed against a number of different enzymes found in neutrophils. Historically, these antibodies were detected using indirect immunofluorescence with ethanol-fixed neutrophils as substrate. Sera that stain the central cytoplasmic regions of these cells usually contain antibodies to proteinase 3, a neutral serine protease in azurophil granules. These antibodies are referred to as C-ANCAs. They are most strongly associated with Wegener's granulomatosis. In contrast, antibodies that stain the perinuclear regions of ethanol-fixed cells contain antibodies to myeloperoxidase and sometimes other positively charged granule constituents of neutrophils. These antibodies are associated with various forms of vasculitis including microscopic polyangitis, rheumatoid arthritis, SLE, primary biliary sclerosis, etc. The reported sensitivity of C-ANCAs for detecting cases of Wegener's granulomatosis ranges from 28% to 92% in various studies, whereas the specificity is 80% or better. Some evidence suggests that C-ANCA titers may be useful in estimating disease activity in patients with Wegener's granulomatosus. The newer enzyme-linked immunosorbent assays (ELISAs) for ANCAs based on purified proteinase 3 (C-ANCA) and myeloperoxidase 3 (P-ANCAs) provide improved ability to distinguish these two different antibody classes.

ANTINUCLEAR ANTIBODIES

Antinuclear antibodies (ANAs) are autoantibodies directed against normal constituents of cell nuclei. They are an important feature of the connective tissue diseases and the common denominator that unites nearly all patients with SLE. They are also found to some extent in normal individuals where there is no association with an evident disease process. This group of autoantibodies is important for several reasons. Clinically, they are useful in diagnosis because of correlations with specific disease syndromes (Table 188.1). Some ANAs, particularly anti-DNA,

play roles in tissue injury and exhibit correlations with disease activity. They also provide an approach to understanding the etiologic mechanism in the connective tissue diseases and are useful as probes for many cellular components.

The mechanisms that lead to the generation of ANAs are a subject of considerable interest. Recent studies demonstrate that a permissive genetic background is an enabling element. The patterns in which the ANAs occur also provide important clues. Most patients with SLE exhibit high titers of a limited number of antibodies directed against various components of one or several nucleoprotein particles. For example, in many patients antibodies directed against the five different histones and DNA represent the predominant specificity. Others produce multiple antibodies to the polypeptide components of the U series of small nuclear ribonucleoprotein (snRNP) particles known as "snurps," which mediate the splicing of pre-mRNA in the cell nucleus. These observations suggest that individual nucleoprotein particles are selected as targets for attack by the immune system much as occurs with a foreign infecting agent. One explanation is that an infecting agent might bear a cross-reactive epitope that generates an initial response to a self-epitope. A process referred to as epitope spreading might then account for the entire array of antibodies found to the "self" particle.

The pattern in which ANAs occur is helpful diagnostically (Table 188.1). For example, in SLE the major specificities are directed against DNA and histones (the antichromatin response), the U series of snurps [anti–UI RNP and anti-Smith (anti-Sm) antibodies], and the Ro particle (which is a specific RNA-protein particle of unknown function). In scleroderma, the predominant targets are nucleolar components such as topoisomerase I (scl-70 antigen), the RNA polymerases (which synthesize pre–messenger and ribosomal RNAs and a variety of small RNAs), and the U3 ribonucleolar particle (which processes rRNA). Scleroderma contrasts with the CREST (calcinosis, Ray-

TABLE 188.1.		ANTINUCLEAR ANTIBODIES IN VARIOUS DISEASES									
Antibody	**Normal (%)**	**SLE (%)**	**DLE (%)**	**Drug LE (%)**	**MCTD (%)**	**Sjögren's (%)**	**SCL (%)**	**CREST (%)**	**DM/ PM (%)**	**RA (%)**	**Mono (%)**
FANA	1–10	95	95	100	95	70	80	80	80	50	15
Anti-nDNA[a]	—	60	—	—	—	30	—	—	—	—	—
Antihistones[b]	—	60	—	90	—	—	—	—	—	—	—
Anti–UI RNP[b]	—	40	—	—	90	—	15	10	15	—	—
Anti-Sm[b]	—	40	—	—	—	—	—	—	—	—	—
Anti-Ro[c]	—	40	—	—	—	50	—	—	—	5	—
Anti-La[b]	—	15	—	—	—	60	—	—	—	—	—
Anti-Scl-70[c]	—	—	—	—	—	—	20	10	—	—	—
Anti-Ku[b]	—	10	—	—	—	—	—	—	—	—	—
Anticentromere[d]	—	—	—	—	—	—	30	80	—	—	—

[a] Farr assay.
[b] Immunoblotting assay.
[c] Immunodiffusion.
[d] Immunofluorescence.
SLE, systemic lupus erythematosus; DLE, discoid lupus erythematosus; CREST, subcutaneous calcinosis, Raynaud's phenomenon, esophageal dysmotility, sclerodactyly, telangiectasia; drug LE, drug-induced lupus erythematosus; MCTD, mixed connective tissue disease; SCL, scleroderma; DM/PM, dermatomyositis/polymyositis; RA, rheumatoid arthritis; Mono, mononucleosis; FANA, fluorescent antinuclear antibody; nDNA, nuclear DNA; RNP, ribonucleoprotein; Sm, Smith antigen; —, no apparent increase over normal levels.

naud's phenomenon, esophageal motility disorder, sclerodactyly, and telangiectasia) variant because the latter is much more likely to be accompanied by antibodies that bind components of the chromosomal centromere. In polymyositis, the major antibodies are directed against tRNA synthetase complexes such as tRNA-histidyl synthetase (the Jo-1 antigen) and, less commonly, against the signal recognition particle (SRP) and the U2 RNP particle. Sjögren's syndrome is characterized by the presence of anti-La antibodies, which bind a protein associated with RNA polymerase III transcripts. These antibodies are usually accompanied by the anti-Ro specificity. High titers of ANAs that are restricted in specificity to polypeptide components of the U1 snRNP (particularly the 70-kd polypeptide) are typical of mixed connective tissue disease. An uncommon ANA known as anti-Ku is of special interest because its target, the Ku protein, has turned out to be the regulatory component of the nuclear enzyme known as DNA-dependent protein kinase. This enzyme plays a central role in double-stranded DNA break repair and in V(D)J recombination of immunoglobulin and T-cell receptor genes.

Initial screening for the presence of ANAs should be carried out with the fluorescent antinuclear antibody assay (FANA). Several considerations apply to interpretation of the FANA assay results. Determination of positive end-point titers is subjective and there is considerable test-to-test variability, particularly when individual sera are examined in different laboratories. A recent multilaboratory study demonstrates that nearly one-third of normal individuals have FANA titers of 1:40 but less than 5% have titers of 1:160 or greater. In SLE, scleroderma, and Sjögren's syndrome, FANA titers of 1:160 were found in 94.7%, 86.5%, and 73.7% of individuals, respectively. Other studies have noted that asymptomatic individuals with positive FANAs do not generally progress to overt connective tissue disease. In other words, a positive FANA in the absence of signs and symptoms of inflammation should not be regarded as evidence for a lurking connective tissue disease. A negative FANA argues strongly against the diagnosis of SLE. A notable exception occurs with sera that contain only antibodies to the Ro antigen, which can be difficult to detect because of its limited quantity in cells. Therefore, if the clinical situation suggests connective tissue disease but the FANA result is negative, antibodies directed at the Ro particle or cytoplasmic antigens such as ribosomes and Jo-1 should be sought by specialized assays such as those based on ELISA or immunoprecipitation.

When the FANA result is positive, the pattern of staining yields important information. *Homogeneous* staining is associated with antibodies to chromatin (histones and DNA) and occurs with sera from patients with SLE and many other diseases. This is the only pattern that is consistent with the diagnosis of drug-induced lupus because patients with this disorder usually produce antibodies to histones exclusively. The *rim* pattern, which is associated with antibodies directed at DNA, correlates most strongly with SLE. Although DNA is distributed throughout the nucleus, sera containing anti-DNA antibodies produce preferential staining at the nuclear margin because the chromatin is packaged more densely in this region, and because these sera tend to contain associated antibodies directed at components of the nuclear membrane and the nuclear lamin proteins that reside just underneath the nuclear membrane and to which the chromatin fibers are anchored. The *speckled* pattern results largely

from antibodies directed at RNPs, such as the U series of snRNP particles. This pattern is consistent with anti–U1 RNP antibodies that bind exclusively the U1 snRNP particles, and with anti-Sm (anti-Smith) antibodies, which bind the U1, U2, and U4–6 snRNP particles. Anti-Sm antibodies are found almost exclusively in patients with SLE, whereas anti–U1 RNP antibodies occur in both SLE and its variants, such as mixed connective tissue disease. The *nucleolar* pattern is associated with a variety of autoantibodies that bind components of nucleoli, including the Pm/Scl antigen (which is a complex of multiple proteins found in nucleoli) and other nucleolar components. This pattern is most common among patients with scleroderma. Individual sera often produce homogeneous or rim patterns at low dilutions and speckled or nucleolar patterns at high dilutions; such variable patterns reflect the presence of multiple ANA specificities.

ANTIBODIES TO CARDIOLIPIN

Antibodies to cardiolipin and other phospholipids are found in about 25% of patients with documented SLE and in certain patients characterized as having a *primary* antiphospholipid antibody syndrome, manifested by recurrent fetal loss and thrombosis of venous and arterial vessels in the absence of criteria for lupus. These antibodies also occur occasionally in a wide range of other diseases including rheumatoid arthritis, scleroderma, temporal arteritis, Sjögren's syndrome, Behçet's syndrome, various infections, and in association with drug therapy (especially phenothiazines, hydralazine, procainamide, and phenytoin).

Historically, antiphospholipid antibodies were detected as the lupus anticoagulant that produced a prolonged activated partial thromboplastin time that did not correct when test plasma was combined with normal plasma (so-called mixing study). Subsequently, this factor was shown to be an autoantibody to phospholipid (platelet factor III) that interfered with the generation of the prothrombin activator complex (comprising clotting factors III, V, X, and calcium). Typically, in an in vitro assay, this interference results in a relatively normal prothrombin time but a prolonged partial thromboplastin time. Most of the antibodies that give positive results in this test and some additional specificities can be readily detected in ELISAs using phospholipids (e.g., cardiolipin) as substrate. The addition of β_2-glycoprotein 1 enhances the binding of many sera in these assays. IgM class anticardiolipin antibodies are responsible for the biologically false-positive test result for syphilis (Venereal Disease Research Laboratory). Comprehensive testing for the lupus anticoagulant syndrome should be carried out with a functional clotting assay, such as the activated partial thromboplastin time, kaolin clotting time, or dilute Russell viper venom time, in combination with a specific antibody test, such as an ELISA based on cardiolipin and, possibly, additional negatively charged phospholipids.

It seems reasonable to test all patients who have had recurrent miscarriages or unexplained thrombotic events for antiphospholipid antibodies because positive individuals are candidates for therapeutic interventions. However, the isolated finding of anticardiolipin antibodies in asymptomatic individuals is not an indication of high risk for future thrombosis. In the cardiolipin ELISA, it may be worthwhile to determine whether the autoantibodies are of the IgM or IgG class because individuals with high

---

TABLE 188.2.	**LABORATORY TESTS IN RHEUMATOLOGY: SUMMARY OF KEY POINTS**

The ESR and Acute Phase Response

ESR is an indirect measure of the acute phase response.
ESR rises moderately with age.
ESR is not useful as a screening test for serious disease.
Elevated ESR values usually are limited to serious, clinically apparent diseases.
C-Reactive protein rises and falls more closely in concert with active inflammatory processes.

Synovial Fluid Examination

Key studies are the leukocytes, percentage of polymorphonuclear cells, glucose, crystal examination, and culture.

Rheumatoid Factors

Occur in many diseases, about 5% of normal population, and about 70% of patients with rheumatoid arthritis.
IgM, but not IgG or IgA, class rheumatoid factors are detected with agglutination assays.

Antinuclear Antibodies

FANA is the most useful screening test.
ANAs occur in virtually all patients with SLE and in most patients with scleroderma, Sjögren's syndrome, and polymyositis.
Anti–native DNA antibodies are strongly diagnostic for spontaneous SLE, represent a marker for patients at risk for renal disease, and typically fluctuate with disease activity.
Specific antibodies correlate with specific diseases and certain organ involvement, as described in the text.

Antibodies to Cardiolipin

The lupus anticoagulant is an antibody that binds phospholipid, inhibits formation of the clotting factor V–X complex, and prolongs clotting times in vitro.
Antibodies associated with the lupus anticoagulant syndrome can be detected in ELISA based on cardiolipin and other negatively charged phospholipids.
Diagnosis should combine clotting assays and ELISA because some patients are identified by only one of these assay systems.

Antineutrophil Cytoplasmic Autoantibodies

C-ANCA (anti–proteinase 3) correlates most strongly with Wegener's granulomatosis and may vary with disease activity
P-ANCA (antimyeloperoxidase) is associated with various forms of vasculitis, particularly microscopic polyarteritis

---

ANA, antinuclear antibody; ELISA, enzyme-linked immunosorbent assay; ESR, erythrocyte sedimentation rate; FANA, fluorescent antinuclear antibody; SLE, systemic lupus erythematosus.

---

titers of antibodies of the latter class are thought to be at the greatest risk for thrombotic complications (Table 188.2).

APPROACH TO THE EVALUATION OF PATIENTS WITH SPECIFIC RHEUMATIC SYNDROMES

For diagnostic purposes, it usually is most cost-effective to formulate an initial impression on the basis of the history and physical examination and to attempt to support that diagnostic hypothesis with a limited array of applicable laboratory tests. A *rheumatology screen* is not necessary, and often results in needless costs and reliance on imprecise assay methods.

MONARTHRITIS OR POLYARTHRITIS

As a first approximation, a patient with monarthritis may be considered to have infection, crystal-associated arthritis, or traumatic joint disease, whereas one with polyarthritis may be considered to have rheumatoid arthritis, osteoarthritis, some form of reactive arthritis, or a systemic connective tissue disease that is not fully expressed. In this setting, the ESR or C-reactive protein is useful as supplemental information about the presence of inflammation. Synovial fluid examination and culture are indicated to confirm or exclude from further consideration infection and crystal-associated arthritis, and as another means of identifying inflammatory joint disease. A test for rheumatoid factor helps to confirm a clinical impression of rheumatoid arthritis and yields information about the potential for this disease to cause tissue injury. If the patient has had a tick bite and lives in an endemic area, an assay for antibodies to *Borrelia burgdorferi,* the causative agent of Lyme disease, should be considered.

Radiologic studies usually are helpful for identifying the characteristic changes of osteoarthritis and chondrocalcinosis, for excluding fractures, and for determining whether the disease produces purely periarticular osteopenia and bone erosions (e.g., rheumatoid arthritis) or both erosive and proliferative changes of bone (e.g., Reiter's syndrome, inflammatory bowel disease, ankylosing spondylitis), usually without associated osteopenia. Changes in bone evolve slowly. The earliest sign in inflammatory synovitis often is periarticular osteopenia, which may appear within weeks after onset of disease. Bone erosions and proliferative changes usually are not seen until the disease process has been present for several months. Patients with erosive disease should be followed up with serial radiographs because progression of bone injury warrants more aggressive therapy. Technetium bone scans are useful for identifying metastatic disease, bone infections, and aseptic necrosis, and often yield clues to these diagnoses earlier than do conventional bone radiographs.

BACK PAIN

When a patient's main complaint is back pain, the first goal is to establish on clinical grounds the likelihood of a mechanical injury such as a herniated nucleus pulposus, an inflammatory spine disease such as ankylosing spondylitis, a neoplasm, or an infectious process. It is helpful to determine the mode of onset of the pain, whether there is a history of trauma or evidence of neurologic impingement, whether the pain is exacerbated by activity (suggesting a mechanical lesion) or by rest (suggesting inflammatory disease), and whether motion is limited in all planes (inflammatory) or predominantly in one plane (mechanical). After this initial assessment, laboratory studies should be used judiciously with the aim of confirming or denying the initial clinical hypothesis.

In most cases, the clinical evaluation suggests a mechanical or inflammatory disorder. In such cases, ESR can provide data that further distinguish these two categories. Human leukocyte antigen phenotyping provides an approach to identifying patients who fall into higher risk categories for the development of reactive arthritis. The HLA-B27 phenotype occurs in about 8% of healthy whites and is present in at least 90% of patients with ankylosing spondylitis, 80% of patients with reactive arthritis caused by *Yersinia*, *Shigella*, or *Salmonella* infections, 70% of patients with Reiter's syndrome, and 50% of patients with psoriatic spondylitis. This phenotype is not increased in patients with inflammatory bowel disease or psoriasis, and is increased only marginally in patients with peripheral arthritis uncomplicated by spondylitis.

Plain radiographs are of limited use for detecting intervertebral disc disease. Many patients exhibit disc space narrowing without having symptoms, and most surgically proven herniated discs are not associated with disc space narrowing. Similarly, hypertrophic changes such as osteophyte formation around the vertebral bodies do not correlate with pain. Degenerative changes of the apophyseal joints, however, do correlate with symptoms. Technetium Tc 99 diphosphonate bone scans can demonstrate early evidence for inflammatory spine disease and are helpful for excluding tumors and infection. These studies are limited by the fact that any process associated with bone proliferation, including hypertrophic osteoarthritis, produces increased uptake. After affected spinal levels have been identified, computed tomography and magnetic resonance imaging can provide highly accurate means of documenting a herniated nucleus pulposus and spinal stenosis.

DIFFUSE CONNECTIVE TISSUE DISEASE

Patients with connective tissue diseases (e.g., SLE, scleroderma, dermatomyositis, polymyositis, Sjögren's syndrome) often have evidence of multiple organ involvement. Signs and symptoms involving the skin and joints are particularly common. These diseases share certain important pathogenetic features, including prominent autoimmune responses to nucleoproteins. The analysis of ANAs often is an important step in their diagnosis (Table 188.1).

The FANA assay result is positive in about 95% of patients with SLE. When the result of this test is negative, it rarely is profitable to order specialized tests for individual nuclear autoantigens such as DNA. However, some patients mainly produce autoantibodies to cytoplasmic nucleoproteins. If a certain connective tissue disease is suggested strongly, it may be worthwhile to test specifically for individual ANA specificities.

Low levels of C3 and C4 can indicate active complement fixation at sites of immune complex deposition in SLE. A normal C3 but a low total hemolytic complement (CH_{50}) can indicate a deficiency of one or more other components of complement. C3 levels are usually normal in rheumatoid arthritis, scleroderma, and polymyositis.

In patients with suggested inflammatory muscle diseases or muscle weakness, it is important to determine whether serum levels of enzymes derived from muscle tissue are elevated. The serum creatine kinase level is elevated in about 90% of patients with polymyositis or dermatomyositis. This enzyme, a dimer made up of polypeptide subunits known as M and B, is found within brain and muscle tissue and exists in three isoenzymatic forms, referred to as MM (skeletal and cardiac muscle), MB (cardiac muscle), and BB (brain and smooth muscle). In cardiac muscle, the MB form constitutes 20% to 30% of the total amount of this enzyme. Although only a minute portion of the creatine kinase in normal skeletal muscle is of the MB form, regenerating skeletal muscle may contain considerable amounts of this isoenzyme fraction, and levels may reach 20% or more in some patients with inflammatory muscle diseases or muscular dystrophy. Moderate exercise in untrained individuals also can lead to elevated serum levels of creatine kinase. In addition, other enzymes, such as aldolase and lactate dehydrogenase, are released from muscle tissue, but these enzymes also are found in other tissues.

VASCULITIS

When vasculitis is suspected, measurements of the ESR or C-reactive protein and of complement components can provide information about the presence of humoral alterations. One straightforward method that is available to nearly all clinicians is examination of serum for cryoglobulins. Cryoglobulins form when serum is chilled. In practice, blood for cryoglobulin assays can be drawn at room temperature, but it should be clotted at 37°C to prevent cryoprecipitable proteins from becoming incorporated into the fibrin clot. After storage at 4°C for 48 hours, the serum should be observed for a precipitate. Tiny amounts of cryoprecipitable proteins are present even in normal serum but usually are barely visible; precipitate that is grossly visible can be measured. Large amounts of cryoglobulins accompanied by high titers of rheumatoid factor are present in virtually all patients with essential mixed cryoglobulinemia, a condition that often is accompanied by palpable purpura. Smaller amounts are found in patients with many other inflammatory conditions and are often associated with hepatitis C infections. The correlation of these cryoprecipitates with circulating immune complexes can be improved by demonstrating that they contain immunoglobulins.

Antibodies against leukocyte serine proteases or myeloperoxidase are measured as ANCAs and are useful in patients suspected of having Wegener's granulomatosis or other vasculitides. However, tissue biopsy often is essential for correct diagnosis of these conditions (see Chapter 181).

BIBLIOGRAPHY

Alper CA. Plasma protein measurements as a diagnostic aid. *N Engl J Med* 1974;291:287–290.

Carson DA. Rheumatoid factor. In: Kelley WN, Harris ED, Ruddy S, et al., eds. *Textbook of Rheumatology*, fourth edition. Philadelphia: WB Saunders, 1993:155–163.

Greaves M. Antiphospholipid antibodies and thrombosis. *Lancet* 1999;353:1348–1353.

Hardin JA. The lupus autoantigens and the pathogenesis of systemic lupus erythematosus. *Arthritis Rheum* 1986;29:457–460.

Hoffman GS, Specks U. Antineutrophil cytoplasmic antibodies. *Arthritis Rheum* 1998;41:1521–1537.

Sox HC Jr, Liang MH. The erythrocyte sedimentation rate: guidelines for rational use. *Ann Intern Med* 1986;104:515–523.

Tan EM. Antinuclear antibodies: diagnostic markers for autoimmune diseases and probes for cell biology. *Adv Immunol* 1989;44:93–151.

Tan EM, Feltkamp TE, Smolen JS, et al. Range of antinuclear antibodies in "healthy" individuals. *Arthritis Rheum* 1997;40:1601–1611.

Kelley's Textbook of Internal Medicine, fourth edition. Edited by H. David Humes. Lippincott Williams & Wilkins, Philadelphia © 2000.

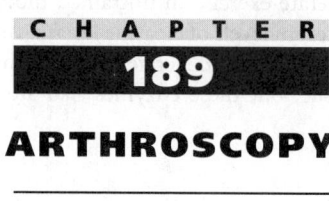

CHAPTER 189

ARTHROSCOPY

WILLIAM J. ARNOLD

In the last 20 years the widespread availability of arthroscopy has revolutionized the diagnosis and therapy of articular disorders. Sophisticated fiberoptic arthroscopes of various sizes and angulations allow for a thorough and precise inspection of all intra-articular structures. Minimally invasive arthroscopic inspection of the joint has provided direct evidence for the relation of symptoms and abnormal joint anatomy, particularly in the shoulder. Simultaneous videotaping of the procedure provides a permanent visual record for subsequent analysis and also for comparison at the time of a follow-up arthroscopy. In response to this remarkable ability to visualize intra-articular structures, a growing array of specifically designed motorized shavers, forceps, burs, staples, sutures, and other tools have been developed to permit a variety of therapeutic interventions to be performed. Precise removal of only the damaged (symptom-producing) portion of a structure (e.g., partial meniscectomy) with arthroscopic techniques preserves joint integrity. Reconstruction techniques for ligaments and menisci can preserve joint function, allow return to athletic activity, and potentially prevent the subsequent development of degenerative arthritis.

Although today the indications for arthroscopy can be divided into diagnostic and therapeutic categories, the future promises a role for arthroscopy in following new therapies directed at regrowth or preservation of articular cartilage, restoration of joint surfaces with flowable polymers cured in situ, and genetic or immunomodifying therapy of inflammatory arthritis.

DIAGNOSTIC ARTHROSCOPY

Specific indications for use of arthroscopy to diagnose articular disorders includes tuberculous or fungal monoarthritis, pigmented villonodular synovitis, and synovial chondromatosis. In patients with bacterial arthritis, arthroscopic debridement and lavage of the infected joint can assist in both the diagnosis and management. Also, chronic knee pain due to arthrofibrosis and adhesions after total knee replacement (TKR) is best evaluated and treated with arthroscopy.

Although it initially requires general anesthesia and an operating room, knee arthroscopy can often be performed under regional or local anesthesia in an ambulatory surgery center or in the physician's office. In the knee, local skin infiltration at portal sites and intra-articular anesthesia provides excellent patient comfort for routine diagnostic arthroscopy. Almost every joint in the body is amenable to arthroscopic inspection with the appropriate-size arthroscope. Even microarthroscopy of the metacarpophalangeal joint and the proximal interphalangeal joint is now possible. However, arthroscopy is most frequently performed for the knee and shoulder. This is both because the ease of access and frequency of involvement by either trauma or arthritis are greater for these two joints.

Standard 3- to 4-mm diameter, 30-degree fore-oblique, glass rod arthroscopes provide the best visualization in most circumstances, even in smaller joints such as the elbow and wrist. The lavage of 1 to 3 L of saline usually performed during diagnostic arthroscopy has been reported to improve symptoms in patients with osteoarthritis of the knee. Arthroscopy is not indicated for the diagnosis of inflammatory or degenerative arthritis. A thorough history and physical with appropriate laboratory studies and x-rays establish the diagnosis of arthritis in most of these patients.

Arthroscopy is extremely useful in the diagnosis of a joint that is painful after trauma. Arthroscopy permits direct visualization and probing of intra-articular structures while moving the joint. With the advent of magnetic resonance imaging (MRI), diagnostic arthroscopy can be more precisely directed to a possibly damaged structure or sometimes avoided altogether. Damage to the rotator cuff or glenoid labrium in the shoulder and the cruciate ligaments and menisci of the knee can be suspected clinically and usually confirmed by MRI. However, the presence and extent of damage to the articular cartilage, inflammation of the synovium and some meniscal tears in the knee can best be determined by direct arthroscopic inspection and probing.

THERAPEUTIC ARTHROSCOPY

With the excellent visualization provided by the arthroscope, therapeutic techniques have evolved to match the needs of the patients, the understanding of the relation among pain, joint anatomy, and function, the skill of the arthroscopist, and the available technology.

RECONSTRUCTIVE PROCEDURES

In patients with sports injuries, reconstructive procedures have preserved important articular structures and allowed return to full athletic function. Thus, although rupture of the anterior cruciate ligament (ACL) was previously a career-ending injury, modern ACL reconstructive techniques with a B-T-B (bone-tendon-bone) or gracilis/semitendinosis graft often can return a player to competition. Suturing of knee menisci torn during sporting activity can also return function and preserve a vital joint structure. Since degenerative arthritis occurs over time in patients with a torn ACL or surgically absent meniscus, these reconstructive procedures are likely to also prevent the subsequent development of osteoarthritis. In the shoulder, repair of tears of the glenoid labrum and rotator cuff due to trauma are possible.

In swimmers, recurrent dislocation of the shoulder due to capsular laxity can be disabling. Recent evidence suggests that the use of low levels of thermal energy to "shrink" the collagen in the articular capsule can tighten the capsule and decrease the tendency for recurrent dislocation.

For patients with arthritis, reconstructive techniques are not effective for damaged menisci or cruciate ligaments. However, reconstructive techniques for articular cartilage have been attempted in these patients. In patients with osteoarthritis of the knee, abrasion of the subchondral bone on the tibial plateau with a bur or microfracture with a specially designed awl has been attempted to stimulate the formation of articular cartilage from primordial (stem cells) bone marrow cells just under the bony surface. These techniques can be successful in relieving knee pain in some patients. However, the results are unpredictable, particularly in patients over age 60 years with large areas of bare bone and angular deformity of the knee. In addition, subsequent arthroscopic inspection reveals coverage of the tibial plateau by fibrocartilage characterized by the presence of type I collagen, not hyaline cartilage with type II collagen.

In younger patients (under age 30) with isolated chondral defects due to trauma in the medial femoral condyle, transplantation of cultured autologous chondrocytes under a periosteal covering of the defect has been reported to restore the surface of the articular cartilage and relieve symptoms for up to 5 years of follow-up. Another approach is to fill chondral defects with plugs of cartilage obtained from donor sites in the knee.

DEBRIDEMENT PROCEDURES

Debridement procedures are usually performed for patients with chronic pain or mechanical symptoms, such as locking or giving away owing to arthritis, or in patients over 40 years with traumatic injuries in whom reconstructive techniques are not considered appropriate. Local or regional pain in a specific joint due to osteoarthritis should first be managed with a comprehensive medical program consisting of a balance of rest and exercise with the use of thermal modalities, splints and assistive devices (e.g., a cane), analgesics and nonsteroidal anti-inflammatory drugs (NSAIDs), and judicious use of intra-articular glucocorticoid injections. A series of intra-articular injections of a hyaluronic acid preparation may also be useful in relieving pain due to osteoarthritis of the knee. If these measures fail, then arthroscopic debridement may be indicated. Use of motorized shavers and hand instruments, removal of damaged menisci and inflamed synovium, smoothing of articular cartilage flaps, and removal of loose bodies may produce prolonged therapeutic benefit while delaying or avoiding knee replacement surgery. In general, patients with minimal or moderate x-ray changes of osteoarthritis, meniscal tears, and preserved joint alignment experience the greatest benefit from arthroscopic debridement of the knee. In the shoulder, arthroscopic debridement with decompression by release of the coracoacromial ligament can often provide significant relief to elderly patients with osteoarthritis and elevation of the humeral head due to chronic rotator cuff tears. In addition, the saline lavage that accompanies these procedures also augments the pain relief.

Synovectomy

The role of arthroscopic synovectomy in the management of patients with inflammatory arthritis remains controversial. In such patients (e.g., those with rheumatoid or psoriatic arthritis), the medical management regimen plays a critical role in determining the success of the synovectomy, whether measured by pain relief, preservation of function, or halt in the progression of destructive disease. The optimum outcome of arthroscopic synovectomy is likely to occur in patients who are well controlled on a medical regimen (e.g., with NSAIDs or disease-modifying antirheumatic drugs [DMARDs]), have pain caused by inflammation in a single joint (usually the knee or shoulder) and have minimal evidence of joint destruction on radiograph. These patients should also have at least one joint aspiration and glucocorticoid injection before considering arthroscopic synovectomy.

■ THE FUTURE

Arthroscopy can provide a method for monitoring the efficacy of new therapies designed to prevent cartilage destruction and reduce synovial inflammation. Serial arthroscopic inspection and grading of articular cartilage damage under local anesthesia in patients with osteoarthritis of the knee (chondroscopy) have been proposed as the optimal method to gauge the efficacy of chondroprotective agents now under development. Quantitation of inflammation in arthroscopically directed synovial biopsies taken during immunomodulator or gene therapy will be useful in monitoring the synovium-specific effect of these interventions. In both of these situations, rheumatologists with appropriate education and skills may provide these procedures as part of a continuum of services to their patients with arthritis.

Driven by the economic impact of the growing number of patients with osteoarthritis and capitalizing on the minimally invasive and cost-effective nature of arthroscopic techniques, new technology to restore articular cartilage or its function will be developed. Restoration of the impact absorption and low coefficient of friction by flowable polymers that can be administered under arthroscopic guidance and cure in situ to form a new surface on denuded bone is now being studied.

Cartilage cell regrowth on joint surfaces from stem cell precursors in the presence of growth factors may provide another option. Since direct visualization and manipulation are always important in developing and evaluating new therapies, arthroscopy is likely to occupy a central and growing position in the management of articular disorders.

BIBLIOGRAPHY

Ayral X, Dougados M. Rheumatological arthroscopy or research arthroscopy? *Br J Rheumatol* 1998;37(10):1039–1041.

Ayral X, Guegen A, Ike RW, et al. Inter-observer reliability of the arthroscopic quantification of chondropathy of the knee. *Osteoarthritis Cartilage* 1998;6:160–166.

Bresnihan B, Cunnane G, Youssif P. Microscopic measurement of synovial membrane inflammation. *Br J Rheumatol* 1998;37(6):636–642.

Broy S, Schmid FR. A comparison of medical drainage (needle aspiration) and surgical drainage (arthrotomy or arthroscopy) in the initial treatment of infected joints. *Clin Rheum Dis* 1986;12(2):501–522.

Chang RW, Falconer J, Stulberg D, et al. A randomized, controlled trial of arthroscopic surgery versus closed-needle joint lavage for patients with osteoarthritis of the knee. *Arthritis Rheum* 1993;36(3):289–296.

Clancy WG Jr. Anatomic endoscopic ACL reconstruction with autogenous patellar tendon graft. *Orthopedics* 1997;20(5):397, 399–400.

Gilbert J. Current treatment options for the restoration of articular cartilage. *Am J Knee Surg* 1998;11(1):42–54.

Goldman RT, Scuderi GR, Kelly MA. Arthroscopic treatment of the degenerative knee in older athletes. *Clin Sports Med* 1997;16(1):51–68.

Ogilvie-Harris DJ, Weisleder L. Arthroscopic synovectomy of the knee: is it helpful? *Arthroscopy* 1995;11(1):91–95.

Szachnowski P, Wei N, Arnold W, Cohen L. Complications of office-based arthroscopy of the knee. *J Rheumatol* 1995;22(9):1722–1725.

Kelley's Textbook of Internal Medicine, fourth edition. Edited by H. David Humes. Lippincott Williams & Wilkins, Philadelphia © 2000.

C H A P T E R
190

IMAGING TECHNIQUES FOR RHEUMATOLOGIC DIAGNOSIS

CURTIS W. HAYES
AVINASH A. BALKISSOON

Radiologic imaging plays a pivotal role in the effective diagnosis and management of patients with suspected or known rheumatologic disease. The plain radiographic examination remains the primary imaging test under almost all circumstances. However, choices for secondary imaging studies have increased dramatically in the past several decades. Tomography, arthrography, and radionuclide imaging were previously used to supplement radiographs when necessary. Computed tomography (CT), ultrasonography, and especially magnetic resonance imaging (MRI) are increasingly used to achieve more sensitive and more specific diagnoses for many musculoskeletal disorders. To make the appropriate choice of techniques, the physician must understand the strengths and weaknesses of available imaging examinations, as well as the way in which test results may influence management.

■ IMAGING TECHNIQUES

Imaging tests may be classified as survey or specific studies. A survey study usually includes a large anatomical area and should be sensitive, although not necessarily specific. A specific study is usually tailored to the symptomatic area and ideally should be specific for diagnosis of a suspected disease.

RADIOGRAPHY

The radiographic examination should be the primary imaging study performed in almost all cases of known or suspected rheumatologic disease. Radiographs provide superb spatial resolution of bony structures and are particularly useful for assessing the hands and feet, erosions, periosteal changes, and soft-tissue calcifications (Fig. 190.1).

Standard radiographic views include anteroposterior (AP) and lateral projections. Specialized projections are added for some areas or when a particular pathologic process is suspected. For the lower extremities, weight-bearing views provide more accurate assessment of the joint space and alignment than non–weight-bearing views (Fig. 190.2). Radiographs performed with stress applied across the joint allow assessment of ligamentous stability, particularly for the wrist, thumb, and ankle.

Fluoroscopy of a joint allows the operator to assess joint motion dynamically. Subtle abnormalities not seen on static radiographs can sometimes be detected with this technique.

ARTHROGRAPHY

Arthrography is a radiographic technique for the evaluation of joints through the intra-articular injection of contrast agent. The

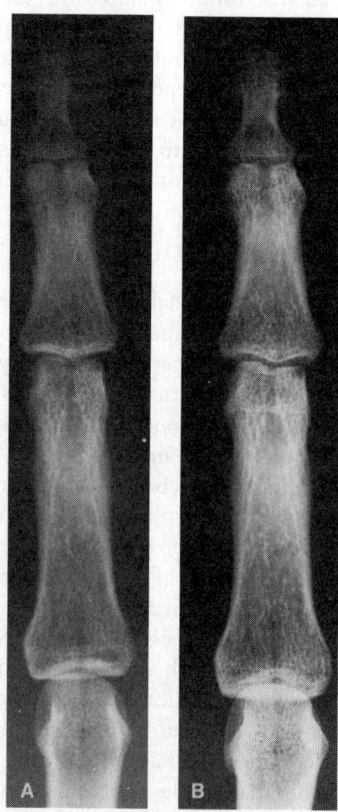

FIGURE 190.1. A: Conventional radiograph of the finger compared with **(B)** high-resolution radiograph. Magnification has been adjusted for comparison.

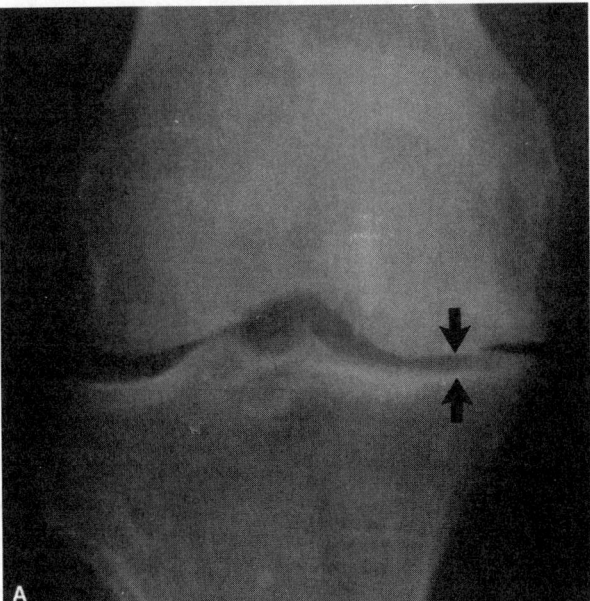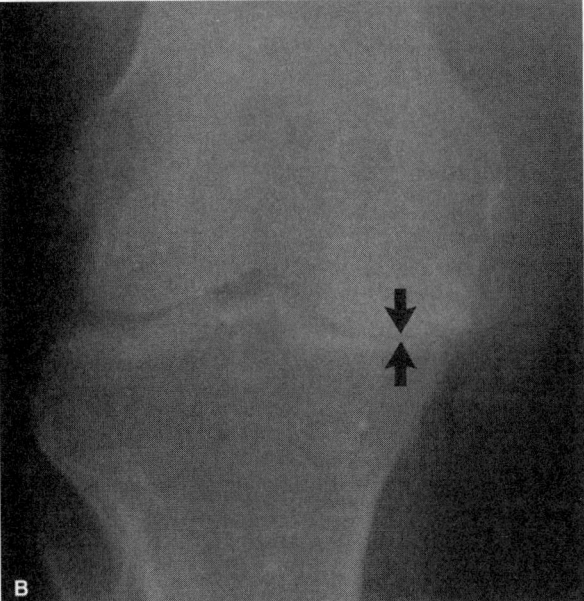

FIGURE 190.2. A: Non–weight-bearing anteroposterior radiographic projection of the knee fails to show the true severity of medial compartment narrowing of the knee (*arrows*) compared with (**B**) the weight-bearing view (*arrows*). (From Hayes CW, Conway WF. Evaluation of articular cartilage: radiographic and cross-sectional imaging techniques. *RadioGraphics* 1992;12:409, with permission.)

major strength of arthrography is that it outlines the synovial lining, articular cartilage, and other intra-articular structures. There is an opportunity to aspirate joint fluid and to inject intra-articular drugs under accurate fluoroscopic guidance. Studies have shown the safety of arthrography to be high, with serious contrast reactions or infection quite rare.

Arthrography continues to be valuable for assessment of some joints, remaining competitive with more sophisticated techniques such as MRI. Diagnostic arthrography is particularly useful for the shoulder, elbow, and wrist joints, and is an excellent method for evaluating joint prostheses (which cause serious artifacts with MRI). Arthrography is useful for evaluating abnormal communications to a joint, such as synovial cysts. Fluoroscopically guided injection of local anesthetic can provide useful information when one is attempting to localize the source of unexplained periarticular pain, particularly around the hip, ankle, and foot.

COMPUTED TOMOGRAPHY

The development of CT in the 1970s and its subsequent refinement have produced significant advances in all areas of radiology. Fundamentally, CT is based on the principle that the internal structure of a body part can be reconstructed from radiologic data acquired from multiple angles. An x-ray tube rotates in a circular fashion around a body part, as a highly collimated x-ray beam passes through the part from all directions. Image data are reconstructed into a cross-sectional image with greatly improved ability to discriminate between tissue densities. CT has gone through many technical refinements. Spiral CT now provides improved multiplanar images, with comparatively lower radiation dose.

In patients with rheumatologic disease, CT is useful for showing detailed anatomy of irregular or complex joints, such as the sacroiliac joint, subtalar joints, wrist, and spine. The combination of CT after arthrography (arthroCT) has proved useful in the assessment of several joints, including the shoulder and ankle.

ULTRASONOGRAPHY

Ultrasonography is a relatively inexpensive and noninvasive imaging technique. Significant operator experience is required to achieve technical proficiency. A joint may be examined during motion, which is particularly useful in the shoulder and foot.

Ultrasonography is highly sensitive for the detection of fluid in the soft tissues, including joints, bursae, and around tendons. Aspiration can be performed under ultrasound guidance. In large joints affected by an inflammatory arthritis, ultrasonography provides discrimination of effusion from adjacent proliferative synovium, similar to that of an expert physical examination. It may demonstrate complications of rheumatic disease such as tendinitis or tendon ruptures and can help evaluate periarticular soft-tissue masses by differentiating solid masses from cystic lesions.

Ultrasonography has been used effectively by some authors for the evaluation of rotator cuff and biceps tendon abnormalities in the shoulder. Reports also have demonstrated the usefulness of ultrasonography in the evaluation of carpal tunnel syndrome, pigmented villonodular synovitis, and synovial osteochondromatosis.

MAGNETIC RESONANCE IMAGING

MRI has evolved as an invaluable diagnostic tool in the assessment of musculoskeletal disease. The main advantage of MRI

TABLE 190.1.	MAGNETIC RESONANCE APPEARANCES OF SELECTED TISSUE		
Tissue Type		**T1-Weighted Image**	**T2-Weighted Image**
Cortical bone		VL	VL
Red (hematopoietic) marrow		I	I
Yellow (fatty) marrow		H	I
Fat		H	I
Muscle		I	I
Ligaments, tendons		L	L
Fluid		L	H

H, high signal white; I, intermediate signal, light gray; L, low signal, dark gray; VL, very low signal, black.

stems from its superb soft-tissue contrast discrimination and the ability to produce images in any plane. MRI is particularly useful in the evaluation of bone marrow, periarticular, and soft-tissue abnormalities (Table 190.1).

Disadvantages of MRI include low sensitivity in detecting small calcifications and relatively low spatial resolution for cortical bone. Because of the high magnetic field used with MRI, patients with cardiac pacemakers, cerebral aneurysm clips, and shrapnel near critical organs should not be imaged. Claustrophobic and obese patients are also problematic because of the small aperture of high-field strength in MRI units. Open configurations and low-field strength dedicated extremity units are an alternative for these patients, but image quality is inferior.

MRI has proved to be effective in evaluating many joints, including the knee, shoulder, and hips and is the preferred modality for assessing the spine. It is recommended for assessing possible osteonecrosis and other marrow or trabecular bone abnormalities. MRI is useful in the evaluation of osteochondral lesions and focal cartilage abnormalities. Contrast-enhanced

MRI can aid in the differentiation of hypertrophied synovium from an effusion and in the assessment of articular cartilage and joint disease (Fig. 190.3). Intra-articular MR contrast injection (MR arthrography) provides excellent contrast between the fluid and articular structures and has been shown to be valuable in the assessment of the shoulder and knee.

RADIONUCLIDE IMAGING

Standard bone scintigraphy uses a phosphate compound labeled with technetium Tc 99m, which, when injected intravenously, is bound to the crystal lattice of bone with distribution dependent on blood flow and osteoblastic activity. Images are routinely obtained approximately 4 hours after injection, but can be modified if information on the vascularity of a lesion is important.

Bone scintigraphy is a sensitive but nonspecific indicator of disease activity in joints and in the spine. It therefore can be used to assess the distribution of arthritis and identify joints that subsequently can be radiographed. Three-phase Tc 99m phosphate imaging alone or with gallium citrate Ga 67 or indium In 111-labeled leukocyte imaging are useful and sensitive techniques for the diagnosis of septic arthritis but are no substitute for examination and culture of synovial fluid. Studies have demonstrated mixed results in the use of bone scintigraphy for the differentiation of prosthetic joint loosening from infection.

IMAGING OF SPECIFIC ANATOMICAL SITES

HAND AND WRIST

Rheumatologic diseases that commonly affect the hand and wrist are osteoarthritis, rheumatoid arthritis, spondyloarthropathies, scleroderma, systemic lupus erythematosus, crystal deposition diseases, and infection. The radiographic examination should be the initial and often only examination performed. The routine

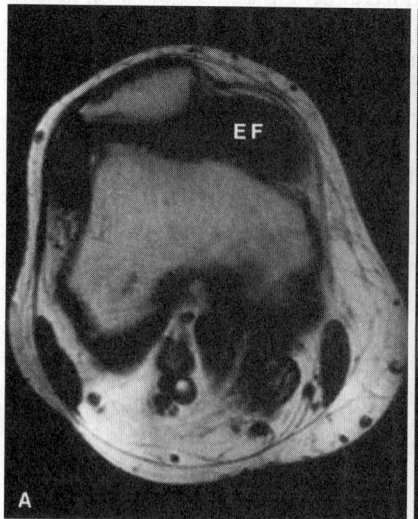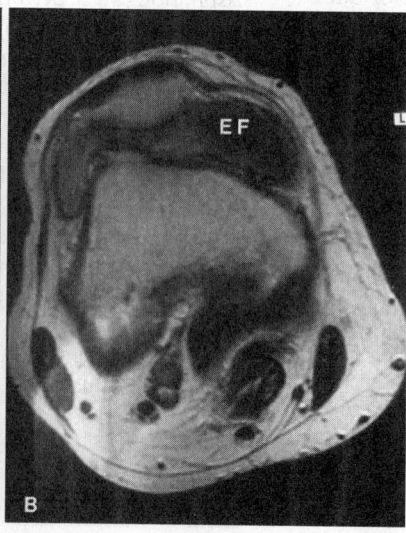

FIGURE 190.3. T1-weighted axial images of the knee (**A**) before and (**B**) 20 minutes after intravenous infection of gadopentetate dimeglumine show enhancement of the large joint effusion (*EF*) in a patient with rheumatoid arthritis.

TABLE 190.2.	CARDINAL RADIOGRAPHIC FEATURES OF RHEUMATOLOGIC DISEASE

Joint space narrowing
Bone erosions
Bone formation (sclerosis, osteophytosis, periostitis)
Bone mineralization
Alignment
Soft-tissue swelling
Soft-tissue calcifications
Distribution

study usually consists of two to four projections. Radiographs obtained during radial and ulnar deviation or with a clenched fist are useful in the evaluation of wrist instability. Specialized views are available for better demonstration of the first carpometacarpal joint and carpal tunnel.

Radiographs of any joint should be evaluated carefully for several cardinal radiographic features of arthritis: soft-tissue swelling, joint deformity, joint space narrowing, periarticular osteopenia, erosions, sclerosis, and new bone formation (periostitis, osteophytes; Table 190.2).

Based on the observation that different arthritides tend to involve predictably different joints, the "target approach" to radiographic interpretation is particularly useful in the hand and wrist (Fig. 190.4). Most often, osteoarthritis affects the distal interphalangeal joints, the proximal interphalangeal joints, the first carpometacarpal joint, and the radiocarpal joint. Characteristic sites of involvement of rheumatoid arthritis include symme-

tric involvement of the metacarpophalangeal joints, the proximal interphalangeal joints, the carpus, and the ulnar styloid. Psoriasis and Reiter's syndrome tend to have asymmetric distribution, classically involving the distal interphalangeal joints. With calcium pyrophosphate dihydrate deposition disease, the radiocarpal joint and second and third metacarpal joints are commonly affected.

Wrist arthrography is most frequently used for assessing the integrity of the intercarpal ligaments, but it may also be helpful for indicating the presence and extent of synovial inflammation. Ultrasonography can be used to evaluate carpal tunnel syndrome, ganglion cysts, and tenosynovitis. MRI is useful in the evaluation of patients with carpal tunnel syndrome, soft-tissue masses, and suspected avascular necrosis of the wrist.

ELBOW

Common rheumatologic diseases of the elbow include juvenile chronic arthritis, rheumatoid arthritis, secondary osteoarthritis, and gout.

The standard radiographic series consists of AP and lateral projections. The lateral radiograph allows identification of the important fat pads, which are useful indicators of elbow joint effusion. Additional radiographic projections are available to improve visualization of the radial head, capitellum, and coronoid and olecranon processes. CT is useful in the evaluation of complex fractures, bony erosions, and loose bodies.

Arthrography of the elbow is useful for detection of intraarticular loose bodies, assessment of articular cartilage surfaces, and evaluation of synovial abnormalities.

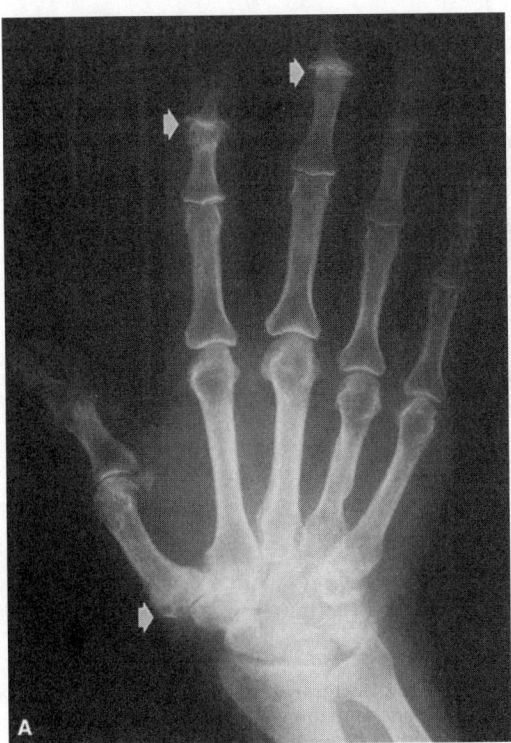 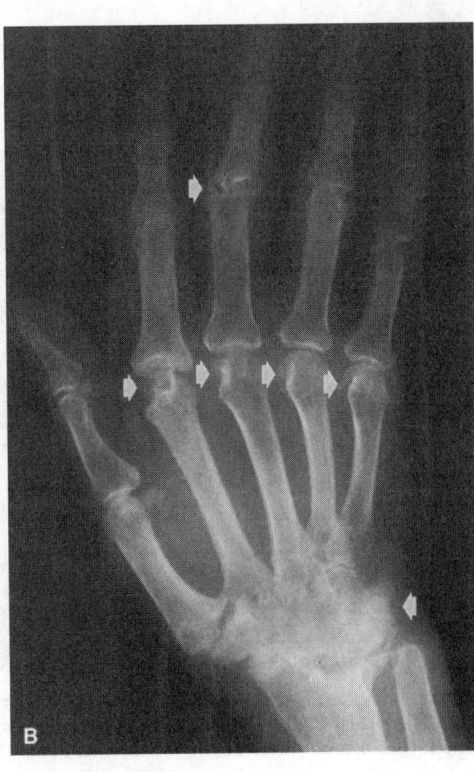

FIGURE 190.4. Posteroanterior radiographs of the hand and wrist showing typical pattern of involvement for (**A**) osteoarthritis (*arrows*) and (**B**) rheumatoid arthritis (*arrows*).

MRI can display tendon and ligament avulsions and strains, osteochondral lesions, and synovial lesions such as pannus, pigmented villonodular synovitis, or osteochondromatosis.

SHOULDER

Common rheumatologic diseases affecting the glenohumeral joint include rheumatoid arthritis, crystal-induced arthropathies, neuroarthropathy, and infection. Primary osteoarthritis of the shoulder is unusual but degenerative changes may be secondary to any of the arthritides or trauma. Osteonecrosis of the humeral head may mimic articular disease.

The radiographic shoulder series usually includes frontal views with the humerus in internal and external rotation and an axillary or lateral scapular view. Radiographs remain most valuable for showing bony erosions, degenerative change, and periarticular calcium deposition. Chronic, complete tears of the rotator cuff can be inferred by a narrow acromiohumeral distance and superior subluxation of the humeral head.

Shoulder arthrography is a safe procedure that can reliably reveal complete and deep surface partial tears of the rotator cuff. Other uses are the identification of loose intra-articular bodies and adhesive capsulitis.

With ultrasonography, experienced operators can reliably show full-thickness rotator cuff tears and biceps tendon abnormalities.

MRI is quickly becoming the technique of choice for the evaluation of the rotator cuff and for the demonstration of synovial disease around the shoulder. It provides information on the site and extent of a rotator cuff tear, although differentiating partial tears from tendinitis may be difficult. MRI can identify erosion of bone, loss of cartilage, synovitis, pigmented villonodular synovitis, synovial osteochondromatosis, amyloid deposition, and osteonecrosis. MR arthrography is accurate in the diagnosis of full and partial rotator cuff tears and in the evaluation of glenohumeral instability.

SPINE

Major rheumatologic diseases affecting the spine include degenerative disc disease, facet joint osteoarthritis, the spondyloarthropathies, infection, and rheumatoid arthritis.

Frontal and lateral radiographs, often supplemented by obliques, may be the only imaging required for the evaluation of rheumatologic disease. Careful assessment of the alignment, disc spaces, and facet joints frequently leads to a specific diagnosis. However, since radiographically visible osseous changes are relatively late sequelae of degenerative disc disease and discitis, sophisticated imaging is necessary when radiographs have negative findings but clinical suspicion is high.

Discography is a controversial technique of contrast injection directly into the nucleus pulposus of an intervertebral disc under fluoroscopic guidance. Discography remains popular among some advocates as an adjunct to newer imaging modalities for the evaluation of equivocal disc disease. The added diagnostic value of discography, based on the reproduction of pain on injection, remains a controversy and rarely is indicated.

Spinal facet joint injection is advocated by some authors as

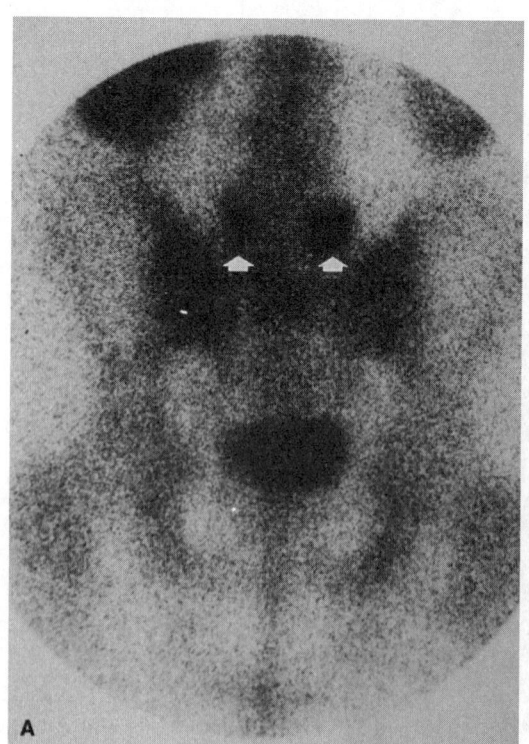
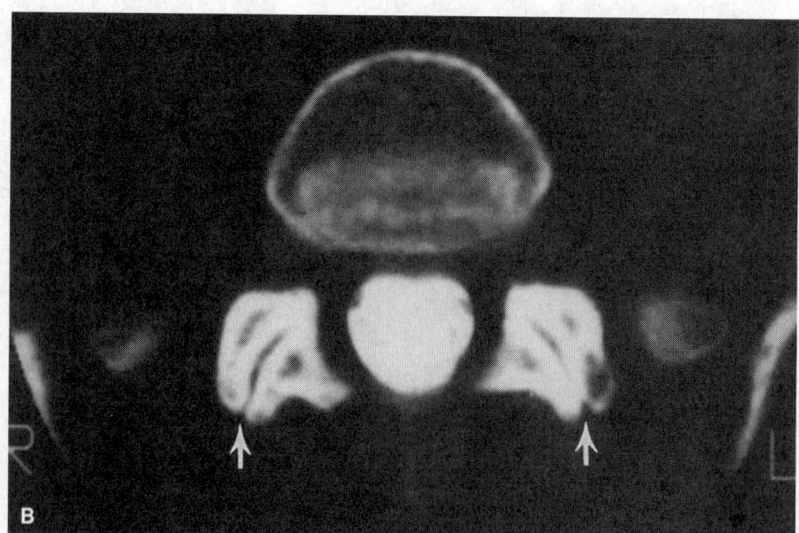

FIGURE 190.5. **A:** Pelvic image from a radionuclide bone scan shows two areas of focal increased uptake at approximately the L4–L5 level (*arrows*). This appearance is nonspecific. **B:** Axial computed tomography image clearly shows severe osteoarthritis of the facet joints at L4–L5 (*arrows*).

both a diagnostic and therapeutic study in the management of patients with suspected painful facet joint arthritis.

Increased uptake of radionuclide isotope in spinal articulations and at entheses are early observations in patients with active inflammatory arthritis. For the detection of vertebral infection, three-phase Tc 99m phosphate scans and Ga 67 citrate imaging approximate MRI in accuracy; however, MRI provides greater spatial resolution and is therefore the procedure of choice for suspected spinal infection.

Myelography, the previous standard for intradural and extradural spinal disease, has been largely replaced by MRI in many institutions.

CT is the imaging technique of choice for the assessment of spinal fractures and facet joint arthritis (Fig. 190.5)

MRI has become the preferred method for the evaluation of spinal cord, bone marrow, and intervertebral disc lesions (Fig. 190.6).

SACROILIAC JOINTS

Rheumatologic diseases commonly affecting the sacroiliac joints are the spondyloarthropathies, osteoarthritis, and infection.

The sacroiliac joints are obliquely oriented and slightly sigmoid shaped, making tangential visualization on the standard

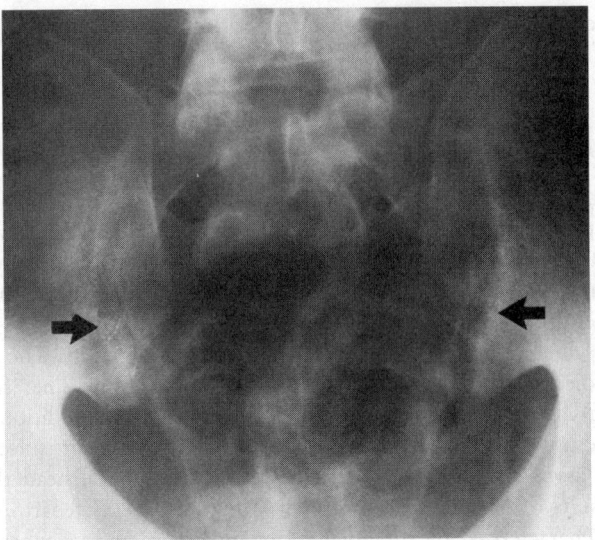

FIGURE 190.7. Ferguson view of the pelvis showing bilateral sacroiliitis (*arrows*).

AP projection impossible. Overlying stool and bowel gas further complicate the evaluation. Oblique projections or the Ferguson projection (AP with 30-degree cephalic angulation) are often necessary for effective delineation (Fig. 190.7). Cardinal features to assess include joint space width, erosions, sclerosis, and symmetry.

CT, MRI, and bone scintigraphy have been evaluated for usefulness in establishing a diagnosis of sacroiliitis when radiographs are equivocal. The cross-sectional display of CT is ideally suited for evaluating early bony changes (Fig. 190.8). Although MRI does not image cortical bone as effectively as CT, the superior soft-tissue and marrow contrast of MRI make it promising for sacroiliac joint evaluation. Conventional bone scintigraphic

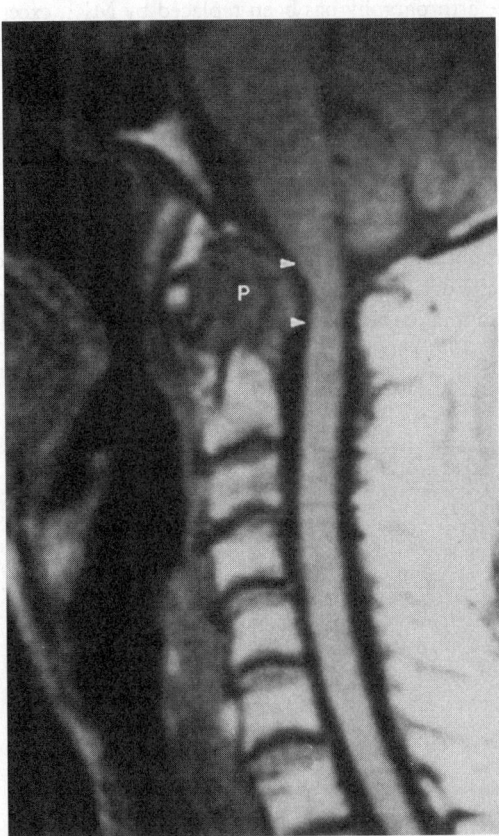

FIGURE 190.6. Midline sagittal T1-weighted magnetic resonance image of the cervical spine shows replacement of the odontoid process of C2 with pannus (*P*), producing deformity of the adjacent spinal cord (*arrowheads*). (From Hayes CW, Jensen ME, Conway WF. Non-neoplastic lesions of the vertebral bodies: findings in magnetic resonance imaging. *RadioGraphics* 1989;9:883, with permission.)

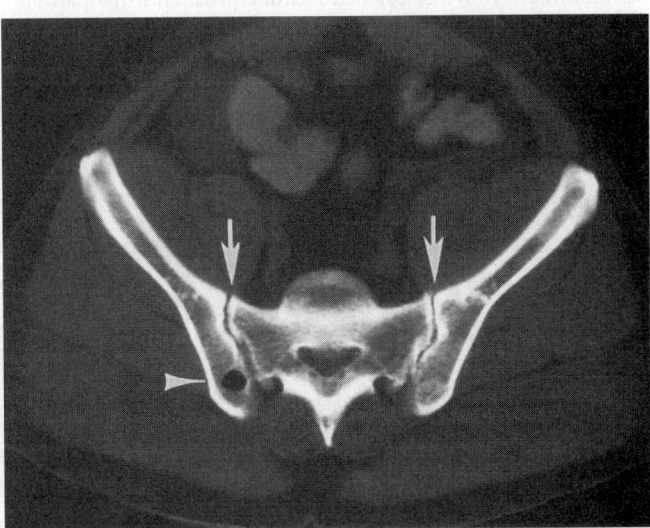

FIGURE 190.8. Axial computed tomography image through the sacroiliac joints provides optimal visualization of the joints (*arrows*). Note the pneumocyst in the right ilium (*arrowhead*), resulting from osteoarthritis.

techniques are sensitive but not specific for sacroiliitis because of a wide range of normal variability.

HIP

Rheumatologic diseases that commonly affect hip joints include osteoarthritis, rheumatoid arthritis, spondyloarthropathies, crystal arthropathies, and infection. Osteonecrosis, stress fractures, bursitis, tendinitis, and muscular injuries are also common at the hip.

The hip joints can be evaluated well by radiography. The AP projection should include both hips for comparison. The "frog leg" lateral projection should also be performed. In addition to the usual cardinal features of rheumatologic disease, it is useful to assess the direction of migration of the femoral head that results from joint space narrowing (Fig. 190.9). Osteoarthritis is characterized by superolateral or medial migration, whereas inflammatory arthritides produce uniform cartilage loss that results in axial movement of the femoral head.

Arthrography of the hip joint is valuable in the assessment of complications related to joint prostheses. Arthrography with fluoroscopically directed joint aspiration is the single most useful test to evaluate possible loosening or infection of a hip prosthesis. Bone scintigraphy is useful when one of the following conditions is suspected: osteonecrosis, occult fracture, or transient regional osteoporosis.

When radiographs are nondiagnostic, MRI is our preferred second-line imaging examination. MRI is arguably the most sensitive imaging modality for the detection of osteonecrosis. The volume of osteonecrotic bone in the femoral head can be estimated, which correlates well with the likelihood of subchondral collapse. MRI is a sensitive test for the detection of occult fractures, which can be clinically confused with true articular abnormalities. MRI can help to identify other processes around the hip such as effusions, synovitis, bursitis, tendinitis, pigmented villonodular synovitis, osteochondromatosis, and myopathy.

KNEE

The knee joint is commonly affected by osteoarthritis, rheumatoid arthritis, crystal deposition arthropathies, neuroarthropathy, and infection. Occult fractures, soft-tissue injury, and osteonecrosis may mimic articular disease.

Plain radiographs are frequently all that is necessary to evaluate the knee for rheumatologic disease. In addition to standard AP and lateral projections, a weight-bearing AP view is useful in assessing joint space narrowing and alignment. The tangential or "sunrise" view of the patella is used for assessing patellofemoral arthritis and alignment. The intercondylar posteroanterior (tunnel) view reveals the posterior aspect of the femorotibial joint, commonly the earliest area of localized cartilage loss in primary osteoarthritis of the knee.

In addition to the cardinal radiologic features of rheumatologic disease, it is useful to note the distribution of joint space narrowing in the knee. Osteoarthritis typically results in narrowing of one or two compartments (medial, lateral, or patellofemoral). Inflammatory arthritis affects the joint diffusely, eventually producing narrowing of all three compartments. Isolated patellofemoral involvement is typical of calcium pyrophosphate dihydrate deposition disease. The periarticular soft tissues should be assessed for chondrocalcinosis, loose bodies, and dystrophic calcifications.

Knee arthrography has been replaced by MRI, except in the following situations: contraindication to MRI, evaluation of knee joint prostheses, and evaluation of suspected dissecting Baker's cyst (Fig. 190.10). Ultrasonography is useful in detecting synovial cysts and other fluid collections around the knee.

MRI is the modality of choice for the evaluation of suspected internal derangements of the knee and has been shown to be accurate for the evaluation of menisci and ligaments, joint effusions, abnormalities of the periarticular soft tissues, and radiographically occult fractures. The value of MRI in the evaluation of nontraumatic rheumatologic disease has been studied less extensively (Fig. 190.11). Preliminary reports suggest that MRI is

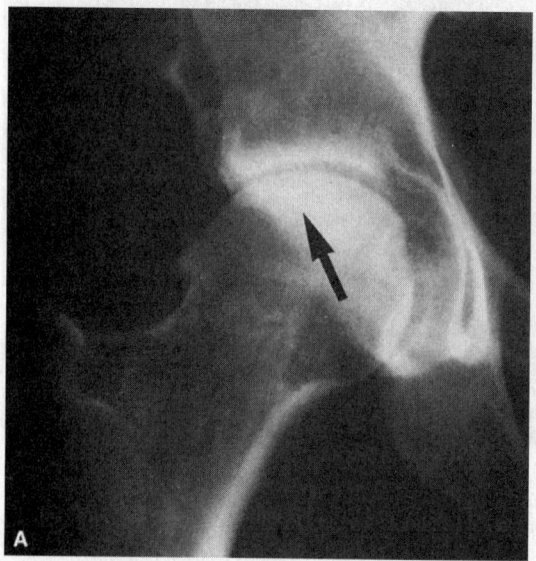
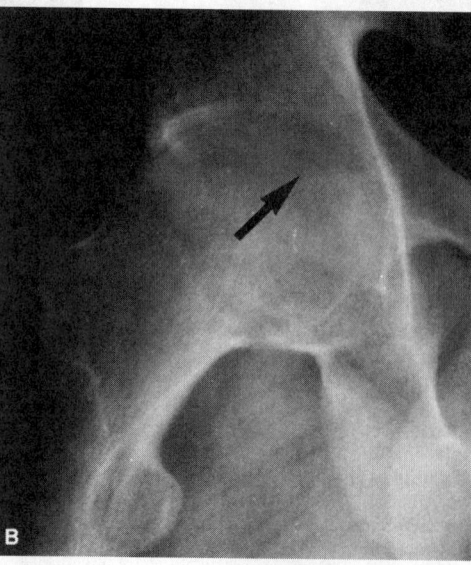

FIGURE 190.9. Anteroposterior radiographs of the hip in patients with (**A**) osteoarthritis and (**B**) rheumatoid arthritis showing typical superolateral (**A,** *arrow*) and axial (**B,** *arrow*) migration of the femoral heads.

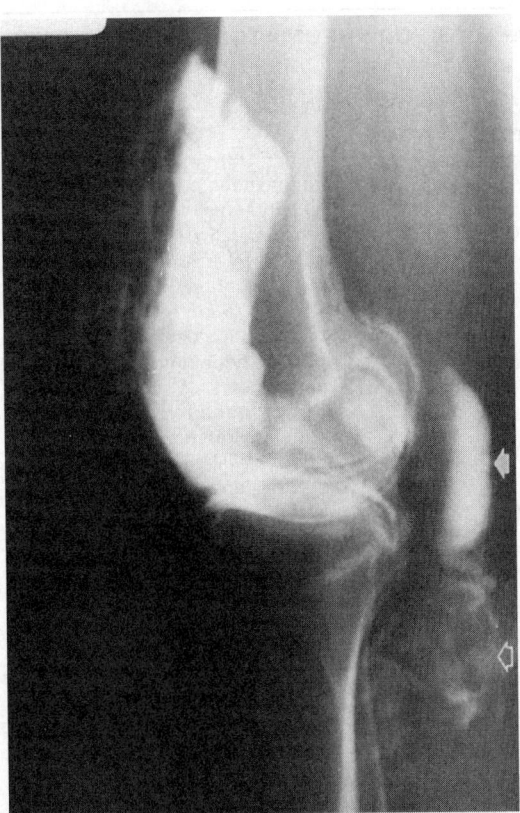

FIGURE 190.10. Lateral radiograph from a single-contrast knee arthrogram showing a ruptured popliteal cyst (*solid arrow*) with contrast dissecting distally into the gastrocnemius muscle (*open arrow*).

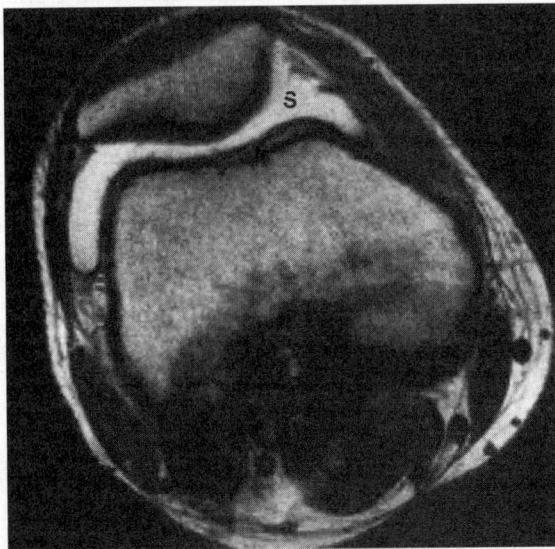

FIGURE 190.12. Axial T1-weighted magnetic resonance arthrogram image of the patellofemoral compartment of the knee shows the joint space (*S*) distended with high-signal contrast agent. This technique is useful for precise evaluation of the articular cartilage.

capable of showing small bone erosions with greater accuracy than radiographs. The signal intensity of synovial fluid is enhanced after intravenous injection of gadolinium.

Numerous studies have shown that MRI is accurate at showing moderate and advanced cartilage abnormalities such as chondromalacia or osteochondritis dissecans. MR arthrography is advocated by some as the most sensitive imaging examination to evaluate the thickness of articular cartilage (Fig. 190.12).

ANKLE AND FOOT

Rheumatologic diseases affecting the ankle and foot include osteoarthritis, rheumatoid arthritis, spondyloarthropathies, infection, and gout. Neuroarthropathy commonly involves the intertarsal and tarsometatarsal joints. Stress fractures involving the metatarsals and tarsals are also common.

As with the hand and wrist, high-quality radiographs are most valuable in assessing the ankle and foot. Weight-bearing views of the foot are useful in assessing alignment and for the evaluation of the arch of the foot. The target approach for arthritis, similar to that used for the hand and wrist, is useful for the foot. Osteoarthritis most commonly affects the first metatarsophalangeal joint, the tarsometatarsal joints, and the intertarsal joints. The most characteristic site of involvement for early rheumatoid arthritis is the fifth metatarsophalangeal joint. With gout, the first metatarsophalangeal joint is characteristically affected. Reiter's and psoriatic arthritis tend to involve the distal interphalangeal joints; Reiter's arthritis also commonly affects the posterior and plantar aspects of the calcaneus. Neuropathic joint disease affects the ankle and tarsometatarsal joints.

CT may be useful in showing tarsal coalitions or stress fractures in the feet. Ultrasonography can be used to evaluate the tendons and ligaments supporting the ankle and foot. MRI can be useful in the evaluation of tarsal tunnel syndrome, refractory

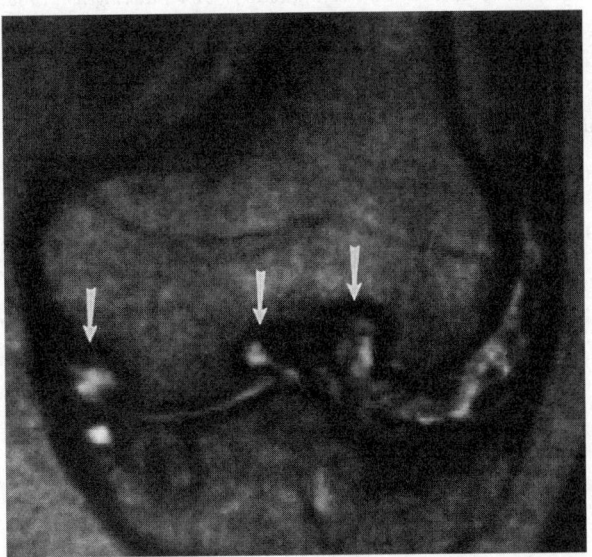

FIGURE 190.11. Coronal T2-weighted magnetic resonance image of the knee showing multiple erosions (*arrows*) in a patient with chronic juvenile arthritis.

TABLE 190.3.	SUMMARY COMPARISON OF IMAGING MODALITIES FOR RHEUMATOLOGIC EVALUATION					
Modality	**Cost**	**Invasiveness**	**Bone**	**Soft Tissue**	**Joint Space**	**Comments**
Radiography	+	0	+ +	+	+	Recommended primary examination for all joints
Tomography	+ +	0	+ + +	0	0	Limited usefulness for complex fractures, adjunct to arthrography
Anthrography	+ +	+	+ +	+	+ + +	Direct evaluation of joint space Allows aspiration for analysis, culture Useful for shoulder, wrist, prostheses
Computed tomography (CT)	+ + +	0	+ + + +	+ +	+	Useful for defining complex bones and joints ArthroCT useful for shoulder, elbow, and patellofemoral joint
Ultrasound	+ +	0	0	+	+	Useful for evaluating possible cysts Operator dependent for shoulder evaluation
Magnetic resonance imaging	+ + + +	0	+ +	+ + + +	+ + +	Most sensitive modality for bone marrow and soft tissues Fine resolution of cortical bone limited for small joints
Radionuclide imaging	+ + +	0	+	+	0	Sensitive but nonspecific overview Useful for infection, osteonecrosis

plantar fasciitis, occult fractures, and tendon abnormalities. MRI has been reported to be useful in the evaluation of infection, especially in the setting of the diabetic patient in whom the distinction between foot infection and neuroarthropathy may be difficult. Three-phase bone scintigraphy, Ga 67 imaging, and In 111-labeled leukocyte scans are also useful in this setting.

SUMMARY

Radiologic imaging can be indispensable in the identification and follow-up of patients with musculoskeletal manifestations of rheumatologic disease. The radiographic examination is the initial study of choice in all circumstances. Making the most effective choice for more sophisticated imaging is less straightforward and requires background knowledge of available modalities. Table 190.3 is a comparative summary of the strengths and weaknesses of commonly available imaging modalities.

BIBLIOGRAPHY

Brower AC, Kransdorf MJ. Imaging of hip disorders. *Radiol Clin North Am* 1990;28:955–974.

Chan WP, Lang P, Stevens MP, et al. Osteoarthritis of the knee: comparison of radiography, CT and MR imaging to assess extent and severity. *Am J Roentgenol* 1991;157:799–806.

Forrester DM, Brown JC. *The radiology of joint disease,* third ed. Philadelphia: WB Saunders, 1987.

Jacobson JA, van Holsbeeck. Musculoskeletal ultrasonography. *Orthop Clin North Am* 1998;29:135–167.

McCauley TR, Disler DG. MR imaging of articular cartilage. *Radiology* 1998;209:629–640.

Resnick D. Common disorders of synovium-lined joints: pathogenesis, imaging abnormalities, and complications. *Am J Roentgenol* 1988;151:1079–1093.

Resnick D. Target approach to articular diseases. In: Resnick D, ed. *Diagnosis of bone and joint disorders.* Philadelphia: WB Saunders, 1994:1755–1780.

Sauser DD, Thordarson SH, Fahr LM. Imaging of the elbow. *Radiol Clin North Am* 1990;28:923–940.

Stiles RG, Otte MT. Imaging of the shoulder. *Radiology* 1993;188:603–613.

Vande Streek PR, Carretta RF, Weiland F. Nuclear medicine approaches to musculoskeletal disease. *Radiol Clin North Am* 1994;32:227–253.

Kelley's Textbook of Internal Medicine, fourth edition. Edited by H. David Humes. Lippincott Williams & Wilkins, Philadelphia © 2000.

DERMATOLOGY

SECTION

I

APPROACH TO THE PATIENT WITH DERMATOLOGIC DISEASES

CHAPTER
191

APPROACH TO THE PATIENT WITH SKIN LESIONS

CHRISTOPHER M. BARNARD

This chapter is an overview of the essential elements an internist needs for the accurate diagnosis and treatment of the patient with skin lesions. Knowledge of the structure and function of normal skin is crucial to the understanding of cutaneous disease and is presented first in this chapter. To describe cutaneous findings accurately, the vocabulary and language of the dermatologist are also presented. The final section provides many useful therapeutic strategies in treating selected dermatologic diseases.

■ SKIN: CELLS, MATRIX, AND FUNCTION

The skin is the primary site of interface between the human organism and the environment. This fact dictates the need for enormous diversity and adaptability within the organ system. The barrier function of the skin alone serves a multiplicity of functions, including protection from physical injury, infectious organisms, and natural or man-made environmental pollutants. This same barrier function helps to ensure the integrity of the organism by its preservation of internal fluids, electrolytes, and proteins and by serving as the major thermoregulatory effector organ through sweating and vasoregulation. Although these functions have been known for decades, only recently have the profoundly important immunologic, endocrine, and paracrine functions of the skin been understood. The importance of each of the components of the skin is further emphasized by the fact that, after physical damage, the skin manifests its remarkable capacity for regeneration into a nearly perfect, anatomically and functionally diverse organ system.

STRUCTURE AND FUNCTION

The skin is composed of two major layers: the epidermis, of ectodermal origin, and the dermis, of mesodermal origin (Fig. 191.1). The subcutaneous layer beneath the dermis, although morphologically and functionally different, is of the same origin. The subcutaneous fat serves as a reservoir for fluid and energy and as a means of protecting underlying tissues.

Epidermis

The epidermis consists of a stratified keratinizing epithelium that makes an interface at mucous membrane junctions. Typically, the epidermis is divided into the basal cell layer, which is the germinative layer; the spinous layer, which comprises several layers of cells above the basal layer; and the granular layer, which is a layer of nucleated cells containing cytoplasmic inclusions called *keratohyalin granules*. This layer is important because it is the zone in which cells become devoid of nuclei. Cells become nonviable in the cornified layer (stratum corneum), which is of such importance in the barrier effect. The epidermal cells are attached to each other through desmosomes and to the dermis at least partly through hemidesmosomes. These two structures are important in some hereditary and autoimmune diseases of epidermal dyshesion.

Constant regeneration of the epidermis requires that the terminally differential keratinized outer cells be shed continuously. Although variable, transit times from the basal layer to the stratum corneum are 4 or 5 weeks, and about 2 more weeks are required for shedding the cornified cells. Each of these kinetic parameters can be disrupted in certain proliferative and keratinizing diseases of the skin, such as psoriasis and ichthyosis.

The keratins are the principal protein products of the epidermis. The expression of this family of fibrous proteins, ranging in size from 47 to 65 kd, differs in various cornified structures, such as the epidermis, hair, and nails. There are biochemical differences among the keratins of these structures. The differences are, like the kinetic variations, of importance in such diseases as psoriasis and the ichthyoses.

The keratins are organized into structures called *intermediate filaments* (formerly, tonofilaments) whose quantity increases as the cell moves outward. In the granular layer, the filaments associate with the keratolinin granules. These granules also contain

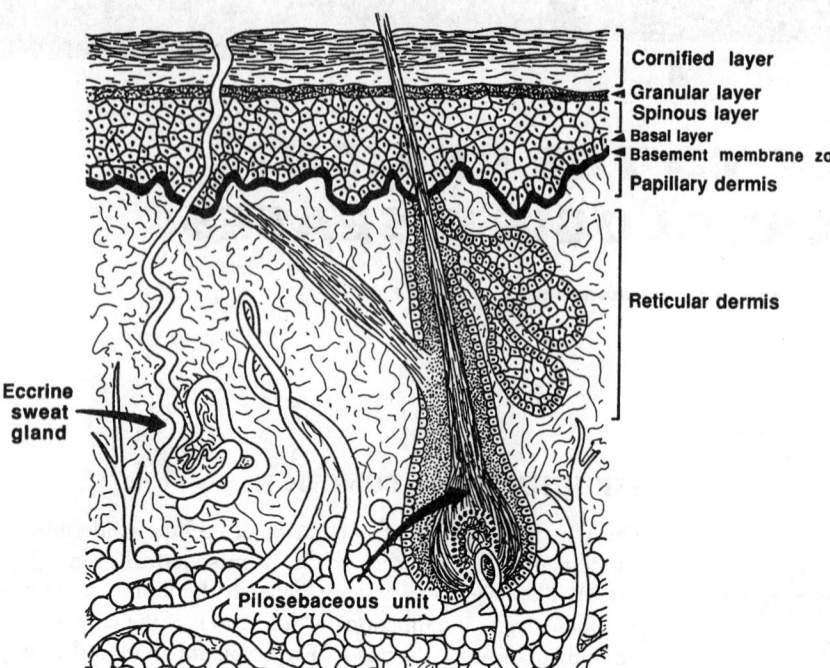

Cornified layer
Granular layer
Spinous layer
Basal layer
Basement membrane zone
Papillary dermis

Reticular dermis

Eccrine sweat gland

Pilosebaceous unit

FIGURE 191.1. Diagrammatic representation of the major structures of the skin.

the histidine-rich protein filaggrin. The keratins and filaggrin, together with the envelope proteins involucrin and keratolinin, are major cellular proteins in the epidermal barrier. In the stratum corneum, the intercellular space is filled with a variety of lipids. During the transition from the granular layer to the stratum corneum, cells discharge their lipids through lamellar bodies. Among the lipids are long-chain saturated fatty acids that subserve the barrier function. This barrier can be disrupted mechanically or in diseases of the epidermis. Lipophilic substances cross the stratum corneum more readily than water and ions. Indeed, topical application of various materials may exert effects on the entire body. For example, under certain circumstances, percutaneous absorption of glucocorticoids can have significant systemic effects, and certain cardiovascular drugs are now often delivered through the skin.

The epidermis is the major source of photoprotection. In addition to the stratum corneum itself, the melanin synthesized by the melanocyte population of the epidermis absorbs radiant energy and protects the skin from the harmful effects of ultraviolet light. All skin contains pigment-forming cells, regardless of the racial derivation of the individual. Melanocytes synthesize melanin and transfer it to regional keratinocytes through dendritic processes. The racial differences in pigmentation are caused by differences in the packaging of melanin by the melanocytes, rather than by differences in numbers of melanocytes. Decreased or absent pigmentation can be acquired (e.g., after chemical insult or other inflammatory process) or hereditary (e.g., albinism).

The epidermis also harbors important components of the immune system. Cells within the epidermis are important for antigen processing. The Langerhans' cells, once thought to be effete melanocytes, possess both crystalloid fraction and complement receptors and immune-associated surface antigens. These

cells operate in the afferent limb of the cutaneous immune system. In addition, epidermal keratinocytes synthesize certain cytokines, including interleukin-1, thus suggesting a role in cutaneous inflammation and repair. The dermis also contains dendritic cells and migrating populations of lymphocytes that participate in both afferent and efferent mechanisms.

Epidermal–Dermal Junction

The interface between the epidermis and the dermis, termed the *epidermal–dermal junction* or the *basement membrane zone,* is under normal conditions an undulating border. This zone, which consists of three morphologically easily identifiable zones—the plasma membrane of the basal cells on the outside, the lamina lucida in the middle, and the lamina densa on the dermal side—in fact comprises additional structures such as hemidesmosomes, anchoring filaments, and anchoring fibrils. Several proteins that anchor the epidermis to the dermis have been defined biochemically. Among these are laminin I, basement membrane proteoglycan, and type IV collagen. In addition, other proteins of importance in hereditary and autoimmune blistering diseases have been identified, including the 230- and 180-kd bullous pemphigoid antigens, laminin V, and type VII collagen. The anchoring fibril complex consists of type VII collagen, which forms loops into the papillary dermis and presumably can interact with other types of interstitial collagens and cells, possibly through domains of fibronectin.

Dermis

The dermis is divided into two major portions, the papillary and the reticular dermis. The biologic function of the dermis is to provide the major structural framework underlying the epidermis and supporting the cutaneous vascular network. The papillary dermis consists of rather fine collagen fibrils and is located outermost. It closely hugs the undulating epidermis and contains the small vasculature. The reticular dermis lies beneath the papillary dermis and makes up the bulk of the dermis with coarse bundles of collagen and elastin. These structures provide strong functional support and resilience to the skin.

Fibroblasts are the major cell type characteristic of the dermis. Interstitial collagen (types I and III) constitutes more than 70% of the dry weight of the skin. The requirement for tensile strength is served by collagen, whereas elasticity, resilience, and hydration are conferred in part by the other connective tissue components, elastin and the proteoglycans. The remaining collagenous components and basement membrane components are found in minor amounts.

The elastic elements of the dermis are made up of two components: *microfibrils,* which are tubular, and an amorphous component, called *elastin.* These, too, are synthesized by the dermal fibroblasts. If the integrity of dermal elastin is compromised, as in cutis laxa, the skin hangs loosely in folds. A much more common phenomenon is the wrinkling of the skin resulting from loss of elasticity due to actinic irradiation.

The dermal proteoglycans are synthesized also by the fibroblasts. Their functional importance is poorly defined, but probably involves water trapping within the skin. Their presence in the basement membrane zone further implies a role in the complex interactions of adhesive macromolecules.

Skin Appendages

The skin appendages are the pilosebaceous units and the sweat glands, both eccrine and apocrine. The pilosebaceous unit is the hair follicle with its associated sebaceous gland. These glands secrete complex oils that may function in addition to the lipids released by the keratinocytes in cutaneous lubrication and protection. The distribution of sebaceous glands varies significantly in density over the body. For example, the excessive oiliness of acne or rosacea is often concentrated in areas of the highest number of sebaceous glands.

Similarly, terminal hairs (those that are medullated) do not grow in equal density over the entire body. Indeed, hair growth itself is not continuous; instead, hair grows in cycles. The growth phase is termed *anagen;* the resting phase is *telogen.* At any given time, most of the scalp hair is in the anagen or growth phase. Profound illness, or changes in metabolic states (e.g., at the end of pregnancy) can alter the relative proportion of growing and resting hairs and lead to hair loss (effluvium).

Eccrine sweat glands are found over the entire body and function in thermoregulation. Indeed, their diminished numbers in hypohidrotic ectodermal dysplasia lead to failure of the evaporative cooling effect and to fevers from poor cutaneous heat exchange. In contrast, the apocrine glands are of more restricted distribution and are found principally in the axillae, the inguinal folds, and the breasts. Likewise, they are functionally more restricted, with intermittent rather than continuous secretion.

Aging Skin

Perhaps no situation so dramatically emphasizes the interactive nature of all the components of the skin as the aging process.

Although it may be impossible to separate effects of aging from effects of actinic damage, the end results appear in many cases to be similar; decreased keratinocyte proliferation and epidermal atrophy result from years of sun damage. With increasing age, there is an overall decrease in the number of melanocytes. Despite the frequent occurrence of somewhat increased pigmentation in chronically sun-exposed regions, which might be expected to exert a protective effect, there is typically also loss of dermal cellularity and elasticity. This in turn results in loss of vascular support and in large cutaneous ecchymoses.

Loss of hair occurs with aging, and other epidermal appendage structures become attenuated. Sebaceous glands may increase in size, but their secretion of oils decreases. The decreased epidermal proliferation may contribute to one of the most vexing problems of aging, *xerosis,* or dry skin. This problem affects most elderly people. The characteristic loss of skin turgor and resilience may lead to chronic pruritus, scratching, and self-induced skin damage, all of which further compromise the barrier function of the skin.

■ CUTANEOUS MANIFESTATIONS OF INTERNAL DISEASE

Many systemic diseases have cutaneous findings that may appear before, or concurrently with, the onset of the underlying disorder. These findings are particularly helpful in obtaining a diagnosis when the systemic manifestations of a disease may be difficult to elucidate. The following brief descriptions serve to provide a reference for identifying these cutaneous clues.

ENDOCRINE DISORDERS

Adrenal Disorders

Addison's Disease

Hyperpigmentation of the palmar creases and a generalized darkening of the skin and of the skin covering the joints may occur in persons with Addison's disease. Pigmented macules may develop on the tongue, gingiva, and oral mucous membranes. Longitudinal pigmented bands may be seen within the nails, and the hair may darken in color. Areas that are normally the darkest (areola, axilla, genitalia, perineum, and the skin folds) become even more hyperpigmented.

Cushing's Disease

Striae, atrophy, telangiectasia, purpura, petechia, ecchymoses, poor wound healing, and acne all may develop in persons with Cushing's disease. Subcutaneous body fat increases over the upper back and abdomen and decreases on the extremities in this disorder.

Diabetes

Many cutaneous changes have been associated with diabetes, some of which are seen with a number of other diseases as well. Diabetic dermopathy, a poorly understood phenomenon at best, typically appears as depressed, brown plaques or flat patches over the pretibial surfaces. In long-standing diabetes, bullae (bullous diabeticorum) may develop over the extremities and feet. Necrobiosis lipoidica diabeticorum, which consists of yellowish-brown, telangiectatic, waxy, scaly plaques on the pretibial surfaces, often begins as red papules or nodules and is seen in 0.3% of all diabetics. The face, trunk, and upper extremities may also be involved. Acanthosis nigricans, brown, velvety plaques located around the neck and within the axillary, inframammary, and inguinal folds, can be seen with endocrinopathies such as diabetes, obesity, or with an underlying malignancy. Increased cutaneous fungal infections, especially *Candida*, and bacterial infections may be seen with diabetes. Vitiligo also occurs more frequently in diabetics. Diabetic neuropathy can result in neuropathic ulcers in areas with decreased sensation.

Parathyroid Disease

Hyperparathyroidism is associated with pruritus. Hypoparathyroid disease is associated with xerosis, brittle nails, coarse hair, and chronic mucocutaneous candidiasis.

Pituitary Disease

Hyperpituitary disease may manifest as hyperhidrosis, increased skin folds on the face, thickening of the lips and eyelids, increased pore size, and generalized thickening of the skin. Hyperpigmentation, coarsening of the hair, and increased oiliness of the skin are also noted. Hypopituitary disease manifests as dryness and thinning of the skin, thinning and loss of hair, and pallor.

Thyroid Disease

Hyperthyroidism

Soft, warm, moist skin is typical in persons with hyperthyroidism, with easy flushing and erythema of the face and palms. Increased nail growth with an upward curvature may occur, a condition known as "Plummer's nails." Thinning of the hair is also seen. Pretibial myxedema can occur with Graves' disease. Both hyperpigmentation and hypopigmentation may occur, as well as vitiligo.

Hypothyroidism

Dry, cool, rough, pale skin that bruises easily, along with slowly growing, dry, brittle hair and nails, is seen in persons with hypothyroidism.

RHEUMATOLOGIC AND IMMUNOLOGICALLY MEDIATED DISORDERS

Behçet's Syndrome

Persons affected with Behçet's syndrome have oral aphthae, genital aphthae, and pustular vasculitis are the cutaneous findings in this disease.

CREST/Scleroderma

CREST syndrome includes cutaneous **c**alcinosis, **R**aynaud's phenomenon, **e**sophageal dysmotility, **s**clerodactyly, and numerous **t**elangiectasias. Systemic sclerosis shows the same changes as CREST syndrome, as well as a cutaneous fibrosis that may be localized or generalized in distribution. Ulcerations of the distal fingertips may result in "pitting scars." Breakdown or trauma to contractures or areas of calcinosis may also produce ulcers. Hyperpigmentation can be widespread or alternating with hypopigmented patches. The proximal nail folds reveal enlarged capillary loops, and telangiectatic mats are commonly seen on the hands.

Dermatomyositis

The most characteristic features are a heliotrope rash (periorbital violaceous rash), malar erythema, and Gottron's papules (e.g., violaceous papules located over the metacarpophalangeal and interphalangeal joints). Similar red to violaceous scaly plaques may be seen over the elbows and knees. The proximal nail folds may show telangiectasia and periungual erythema. Erythema may be widespread and appear with a blotchy pattern over the trunk and extremities. Atrophy, hypopigmentation, and ulcerations may appear at involved sites. Cutaneous calcinosis may be seen in adults but is more often a finding in children with dermatomyositis.

Graft-Versus-Host Disease

In acute graft-versus-host disease, pruritus, palmar erythema, and red macules or papules, which may become confluent and progress to an exfoliative erythroderma, are seen. Chronic graft-versus-host disease may begin with a lichen planus–like eruption of violaceous papules. Localized, and later generalized, sclerosis may develop over the trunk and extremities.

Lupus Erythematosus

The cutaneous lesions of lupus erythematosus may be divided into acute, subacute, and chronic forms. In acute lupus erythematosus, malar erythema and photosensitivity are commonly seen. Erythematous rashes are often maculopapular and pruritic and may involve any area of the body. Other findings may include vasculitis, oral ulcerations, periungual erythema, telangiectasia, and alopecia. With subacute cutaneous lupus, annular, erythematous, scaly patches or psoriasiform papules and plaques may be present. Photosensitivity is common. In chronic discoid lupus, atrophic scarring is usually present after the appearance of erythematous scaly plaques. The typical lesions are hypopigmented atrophic scars surrounded by hyperpigmentation.

Polyarteritis Nodosum

Cutaneous polyarteritis nodosum typically reveals tender nodules or a livedo (reticulated)-pattern vasculitis of the skin only. Systemic polyarteritis nodosum reveals tender nodules of the lower extremities, livedo reticularis, cutaneous ulcerations, urticaria, and digital infarcts.

Vasculitis

Patients with small-vessel vasculitis present with palpable purpura. Large-vessel vasculitis may appear as necrosis, ulcerations, purpura, cutaneous or nail-fold infarcts, subcutaneous nodules, and hemorrhagic bullae.

GASTROINTESTINAL DISORDERS

Biliary Obstruction

In biliary obstruction, cholestasis from all causes can result in significant pruritus, and jaundice may be seen with hyperbilirubinemia.

Celiac Sprue

Gluten-sensitive enteropathy and malabsorption can be seen in association with dermatitis herpetiformis, a vesicular eruption characterized by grouped vesicles located on extensor surfaces. Common locations are the elbows, forearms, shoulders, knees, and buttocks. Crusts and erosions are commonly seen after rupture of the vesicles. Symmetric distribution and pruritus are characteristic features.

Cirrhosis

Spider angiomas and telangiectasias frequently appear on the trunk and face in patients with cirrhosis. Distended abdominal vessels are visible in patients with portal hypertension. Palmar erythema is present in several chronic diseases and may be related to elevated estrogen levels. Dysfunctional synthesis of clotting factors results in purpura and ecchymoses. White nails, or Terry's nails, are typically bright white from the proximal nail fold forward and pink at the distal edge. Pruritus may be severe, particularly when caused by primary biliary cirrhosis. Thinning and loss of body hair are common.

Crohn's Disease

Perineal fissures and fistulas, cutaneous and oral granulomas, pyoderma gangrenosum, oral ulcerations, pustular vasculitis, and erythema nodosum all are seen with Crohn's disease, an inflammatory bowel disease.

Hemochromatosis

Hemochromatosis is associated with generalized brown or bronze hyperpigmentation with accentuation of the sun-exposed areas and genitalia.

Hereditary Hemorrhagic Telangiectasia

Telangiectatic mats can be found on the mucous membranes, particularly of the lips, tongue, and nose. Progression of the disease results in telangiectasias of the face, palm, and soles.

Hyperlipidemia

Xanthomas associated with hyperlipidemia may be classified into tuberous, tendinous, planar, and eruptive. Tuberous xanthomas appear as pink to yellow nodules over the elbows and knees. Tendinous xanthomas may be seen as skin-colored nodules along the extensor tendons of the elbows, hands, and knees, and the Achilles tendon. Planar xanthomas typically appear within the palmar creases as yellow patches. Eruptive xanthomas are usually yellow to red pruritic papules and may be distributed over any area of the body. Xanthelasma, a soft yellow plaque, may appear over the eyelids.

POLYPOSES

Cowden's Disease

Pseudofissures of the tongue (the so-called scrotal tongue), trichilemmomas (smooth, flesh-colored papules around the nose and face), keratotic papules on the face and hands, and a cobblestone grouping of papules on the oral mucosa are found in persons with Cowden's disease.

Gardner's Syndrome

Multiple epidermal cysts and subcutaneous fibromas in addition to desmoid tumors and osteomas are findings in those with Gardner's syndrome.

Peutz–Jeghers Syndrome

Hyperpigmented macules may appear on the lips, oral mucous membranes, and over the hands and feet of persons with Peutz–Jeghers syndrome.

Ulcerative Colitis

Oral ulcers, pustular vasculitis, pyoderma gangrenosum, and erythema nodosum are seen with ulcerative colitis, an inflammatory bowel disease.

ENDOCARDITIS, RENAL FAILURE, AND SARCOIDOSIS

In persons with *endocarditis,* splinter hemorrhages may appear in the nail plate; Osler's nodes are painful or tender red nodules, which may be present on the fingerpads or toepads; Janeway's lesions are painless red macules on the palms and soles; and petechiae, the most common finding, may be found anywhere on the skin or mucous membranes.

Pruritus, hyperpigmentation, pallor secondary to anemia, xerosis, and cutaneous calcification may be seen in those with *renal failure.* "Half-and-half" nails may be present and consist of a white proximal nail plate and a distal reddish-brown portion.

The cutaneous manifestations of *sarcoidosis* are divided into specific (containing granulomas) and nonspecific (lacking granulomas). Specific lesions include red, brown, or purple papules, plaques, and nodules. Infiltration of scars, ichthyosiform patches, hypopigmented areas, atrophy, and ulcerations are also types of specific lesions. Nonspecific lesions include erythema nodosum, erythema multiforme, pruritus, and erythroderma.

MANAGEMENT OF ACUTE AND CHRONIC DISEASES OF THE SKIN

The proper approach to therapy of skin disorders should be founded on a thorough understanding of the pathophysiology of skin disease and confidence in making one's diagnostic skills. The most common error made by nondermatologists is the choice of improper therapy based on an incorrect diagnosis. After the proper diagnosis is established, excellent references are available that can provide insight into proper therapy. The following section highlights the important aspects of dermatologic therapy and gives examples of the treatment of selected acute and chronic dermatoses.

TOPICAL THERAPY

Compresses and Soaks

Compresses are usually used to clean or debride a wound. They are also commonly used to dry acutely exudative dermatoses, such as those seen in acute contact dermatitis. Wet-to-dry dressings debride more thoroughly than wet dressings. Solutions for wet dressing are numerous; the most common are aluminum acetate (Burow's solution) diluted 1:10 to 1:40, normal saline, and 0.25% acetic acid. Care must be taken not to overuse the compresses, which can cause excessive drying.

Antipruritic Agents

Topical antipruritics are rarely useful enough to replace systemic agents in the treatment of pruritic dermatoses. When combined with emollients, however, they may have a role in the treatment of asteatotic eczema, the dry, erythematous, finely fissured skin that is sometimes seen in elderly patients. Care must be taken to avoid topical antihistamine agents that can sensitize the skin. Useful agents include doxepin cream, pramoxine lotion, and combinations of agents containing menthol, phenol, and camphor.

Antimicrobials

Topical antimicrobial drugs are useful in the prophylaxis and treatment of selected cutaneous bacterial and fungal infections. Numerous purely antibacterial and combination preparations are available. Neosporin contains polymyxin B sulfate, zinc bacitracin, and neomycin sulfate. The potential problem of neomycin sensitivity is avoided by the use of Polysporin, which contains only polymyxin B and bacitracin or mupirocin (Bactroban). The most common use of these agents is in prophylaxis against wound infections after cutaneous surgical procedures or around vascular access sites. They have little role in the treatment of

true cutaneous bacterial infections; systemic antibacterial agents are usually required in this setting.

Topical antifungal drugs are widely used for the treatment of cutaneous dermatophyte infections (nail infections respond poorly) and superficial candidiasis. The most effective topical antifungal agents are the synthetic imidazoles (12% miconazole nitrate, 1% clotrimazole, 1% econazole nitrate), all of which are effective against tinea versicolor, dermatophyte infections, and superficial candidiasis. Clotrimazole in troche form is effective for oral candidiasis. Nystatin, a polyene antimicrobial agent that is also effective against *Candida albicans,* can be used as an oral suspension for thrush or as a powder for the candidal infections that develop in bed-ridden patients in skin occluded by the bedsheets. The newer synthetic allylamines (1% naftifine and 1% terbinafine) are effective against most cutaneous dermatophyte infections as well as superficial candidiasis, but are not useful in the treatment of tinea versicolor.

Corticosteroids

Corticosteroids are potent antiproliferative and anti-inflammatory agents; their use has revolutionized dermatologic therapeutics. The dermatoses listed in Table 191.1 are those that are the most responsive to topical corticosteroid therapy.

The potencies of different topical corticosteroids vary widely, depending on the concentration of the active drug and on structural changes, including fluorination of certain key positions in the basic corticosteroid molecule (Table 191.2). In general, treatment should be started with low- to intermediate-potency drugs and progress to high-potency agents only if necessary. This is particularly true in infants or small children, in whom the potential for significant systemic absorption is greater. Furthermore, high-potency fluorinated topical corticosteroids should be used with extreme caution on the face, genitals, and intertriginous areas. In these locations, long-term use often results in adverse effects (e.g., corticosteroid acne and atrophy on the face and striae in intertriginous locations).

Corticosteroid potency is also influenced by the vehicle in which the drug is compounded or the manner in which it is applied. The use of occlusive wraps (e.g., plastic wraps, nylon sauna suits) or ointments, rather than less occlusive creams, gels, lotions, or sprays, results in increased warmth and humidity of the skin, with consequent increased penetration into the skin.

TABLE 191.1. DERMATOSES RELATIVELY RESPONSIVE TO TOPICAL CORTICOSTEROIDS

Eczematous dermatitis
  Allergic contact dermatitis
  Irritant contact dermatitis
  Dyshidrotic eczema
  Atopic dermatitis
  Stasis dermatitis
Psoriasis
Seborrheic dermatitis
Exfoliative erythroderma (secondary to psoriasis or other steroid-responsive disorders)

TABLE 191.2.	CLASSIFICATION OF SELECTED TOPICAL CORTICOSTEROIDS BY POTENCY

Highest Potency

Betamethasone-dipropionate (C, O), 0.05% (Diprolene)
Clobetasol propionate (C, O), 0.05% (Temovate)

High Potency

Amcinonide (C, O), 0.1% (Cyclocort)
Desoximetasone (C, O, G), 0.25% (Topicort)
Fluocinonide (C, O, G, L) 0.05% (Lidex)
Halcinonide (C, O, L) 0.1% (Halog)

Intermediate Potency

Betamethasone valerate (C, O, L), 0.1% (Valisone)
Flurandrenolide (C, O), 0.05% (Cordran)
Halcinonide (C), 0.05% (Halog)
Triamcinolone acetonide (C, O, L) 0.1% (Aristocort, Kenalog)

Low Potency

Desonide (C, O), 0.05% (Desowen, Tridesilon)
Hydrocortisone valerate (C, O), 0.2% (Westcort)
Triamcinolone hexacetonide (C, O, L), 0.025% (Aristocort, Kenalog)

Lowest Potency

Hydrocortisone (C, O, L), 1% (Cort-Dome, Hytone)
Hydrocortisone (C, O, L), 2.5% (Syancort, Hytone)

C, cream; O, ointment; G, gel; L, liquid solution.

TABLE 191.4.	ADVERSE REACTIONS TO TOPICAL CORTICOSTEROIDS

Systemic

Hypothalamic-pituitary-adrenal axis suppression
Iatrogenic Cushing's syndrome
Growth retardation
Avascular bone necrosis

Local

Cutaneous atrophy
Striae
Telangiectasia
Impaired wound healing
Steroid rosacea
Perioral dermatitis
Hypertrichosis
Hypopigmentation
Glaucoma
Cataracts
Aggravation of local bacterial or fungal infections
Exacerbation of psoriasis

Adverse reactions to topical corticosteroids are listed in Table 191.4. The more prolonged the course of treatment and the more potent the drug, the greater is the risk of these complications. Unfortunately, certain of these adverse effects (e.g., posterior subcapsular cataracts, striae) are sometimes irreversible even after discontinuation of the drug.

An additional problem is that of corticosteroid addiction, which is observed most commonly with the potent, fluorinated, topical corticosteroids. In this situation, the patient may initially experience improvement in the dermatosis, but then experience a rebound effect requiring the more frequent use of the corticosteroid for prolonged periods. Often a vicious cycle ensues, resulting in more profound side effects (e.g., atrophy, steroid rosacea, or striae).

SYSTEMIC THERAPY

The most common systemic agents used in the treatment of skin diseases are the antihistamines, the systemic glucocorticoids, certain antimetabolites, the synthetic retinoids, and selected systemic antibiotics.

Antihistamines

Antihistamines are widely used in dermatologic conditions for the control of pruritic dermatoses such as eczema or urticaria. These agents function as competitive antagonists of histamine tissue receptor sites and may be of the H_1 or H_2 type. The different types of antihistamines are listed in Table 191.5. If a patient fails to respond to one class or type, an agent from a different class should be selected. It is occasionally necessary to use H_1 and H_2 blockers simultaneously to obtain optimal clinical results. Tricyclic antidepressants, which also have antihistaminic activity, can be used instead of, or in addition to, the classic antihistamines.

Adverse effects of antihistamines include sedation and other

Care must be exercised when using long-term occlusion of potent topical corticosteroids, because this may lead to systemic absorption with consequent hypothalamic–pituitary–adrenal axis suppression. Solutions and gels are often best tolerated in hair-bearing areas, whereas creams and ointments are most commonly used in glabrous skin. Occlusive ointment-based drugs should be avoided in intertriginous areas.

Topical corticosteroids are usually applied two or more times daily. Given the risk of tachyphylaxis, however, less frequent use may be indicated. A common practical problem in the use of these drugs has been the underestimation by nondermatologists of the quantity of drug required to treat a particular dermatosis. Table 191.3 provides some realistic guidelines.

TABLE 191.3.	DISPENSING OF TOPICAL CORTICOSTEROIDS

Area to Be Treated	Each Application (g)	Weekly Dose With Two Daily Applications (g)
Hands, head, face, or anogenital area	2	28
One arm or anterior or posterior trunk	3	42
Entire body	30–60	420–840

TABLE 191.5.   **SUMMARY OF ANTIHISTAMINES**

Class	Examples	Oral Dosage	Comments
H$_1$ Antagonists			
Ethanolamine	Diphenhydramine (Benadryl)	25–50 mg q 4–6 hr	Marked sedation; significant anticholinergic activity
Ethylenediamine	Tripelennamine hydrochloride	50 mg q 4 hr	Avoid ethylenediamine-sensitive patients; moderate gastrointestinal irritant
Piperazine	Hydroxyzine hydrochloride (Pyribenzamine)	10–25 mg q 4–6 hr	Most effective drug in histamine-induced pruritus; cross-reacts with ethylenediamine, sedation
Alkylamine	Brompheniramine maleate (Dimetane)	4 mg q 4 hr	Lower incidence of sedation but higher incidence of stimulation than other H$_1$ antagonists
	Chlorpheniramine maleate (Chlor-Trimeton)	4–8 mg q 4 hr	
Phenothiazine	Promethazine hydrochloride	12.5 mg q 4–6 hr	Sedation; anticholinergic effects; may produce photosensitivity
Piperidine	Cyproheptadine hydrochloride (Periactin)	4 mg q 4 hr	Antiserotonin activity
	Terfenadine	60 mg q 12 hr	Nonsedating, torsades de pointes
Other	Astemizole (Hismanol)	10 mg q d	Coadministration of erythromycin, ketoconazole, and itraconazole is contraindicated
H$_2$ Antagonist			
Thioguanidine	Climetidine (Tagamet)	300 mg q 6 hr	Primarily useful in peptic ulcer disease

central nervous system manifestations, such as paradoxical hyperexcitability, gastrointestinal intolerance, dry mouth, urinary retention, diplopia, and other anticholinergic effects. Terfenadine, an H$_1$ antihistamine, is uniquely able to block peripheral H$_1$ receptors while sparing central ones. This drug may thus be better tolerated than many other H$_1$-blocking agents. Topical antihistamines should be avoided because of their potential for eliciting contact sensitization.

Corticosteroids

Systemic corticosteroids (usually prednisone) are frequently given orally in the management of acute inflammatory dermatoses, such as acute contact dermatitis. In this setting, prednisone is typically started at a dosage of 0.5 to 1.0 mg per kilogram per day, which is tapered over a 2-week period. Certain other dermatologic disorders may require the administration of varying doses of systemic corticosteroids. Table 191.6 lists selected skin disorders in which systemic corticosteroids are a major therapeutic option. Other disorders (e.g., urticaria, alopecia areata, psoriasis, atopic dermatitis) may respond temporarily to these drugs but are often significantly exacerbated by tapering or discontinuation of the corticosteroids. It is difficult to rationalize the long-term use of corticosteroids for these disorders.

Retinoids

The synthetic retinoids represent an option for selected cutaneous disorders. Isotretinoin is most frequently used for severe, recalcitrant cystic acne. Administration of this drug in a daily dose of 0.5 to 1 mg per kilogram per day for 4 months can produce dramatic long-term remission. Acitretin, the main metabolite of etretinate, has been approved for the management of

recalcitrant pustular or exfoliative psoriasis, but must be used with extreme caution because of its long half-life in vivo.

Adverse reactions to the retinoids are numerous and include dry skin and mucous membranes, hair loss, paronychia, exuberant granulation tissue, pseudotumor cerebri, teratogenesis, liver disorders, blood lipid abnormalities, and musculoskeletal abnormalities, including skeletal hyperostoses, premature epiphyseal closure, and extraspinal tendon and ligament calcification. The teratogenicity of these agents must be underscored; retinoids should not be given to women of childbearing age who are not practicing effective contraception.

TABLE 191.6.   **DERMATOLOGIC DISORDERS RESPONSIVE TO SYSTEMIC CORTICOSTEROIDS**

Disorders Requiring Short-Term Therapy Only[a]
Acute contact dermatitis (e.g., Rhus dermatitis)
Erythema multiforme
Toxic epidermal necrolysis
Drug eruption
Herpes zoster (prophylaxis of phostherpetic neuralgia)
Dyshidrotic eczema

Disorder Usually Requiring Long-Term Therapy
Lichen planus
Pemphigus vulgaris
Bullous pemphigoid
Systemic lupus erythematosus
Dermatomyositis
Widespread eczematous dermatitis
Pyoderma gangrenosum

---

[a] Therapy of less than 3 weeks' duration.

Cytotoxic and Immunosuppressive Agents

Methotrexate is the antimetabolite most widely used in dermatology for the treatment of severe psoriasis. The drug is usually administered orally or intramuscularly in small (15 to 25 mg) weekly doses. A liver biopsy may be indicated before treatment as well as periodically thereafter (every 1- to 2-g cumulative dose). The adverse effects of methotrexate include hepatic fibrosis, bone marrow suppression, teratogenesis, skin ulceration, mucositis, azotemia, and pulmonary disorders. Cyclosporin A and hydroxyurea have also been used in the management of psoriasis. Success is variable.

Antibiotics

Antibiotics such as tetracycline and erythromycin are often given on a long-term basis to patients with acne vulgaris or acne rosacea. Griseofulvin, ketoconazole, itraconazole, terbinafine, and fluconazole are the most frequently given systemic antifungal agents. Whereas griseofulvin is effective only against dermatophytes, ketoconazole and itraconazole are useful for dermatophyte, candidal, and selected deep fungal infections with cutaneous manifestations. Terbinafine is effective against cutaneous dermatophyte and candidal infections. Fluconazole is reserved for systemic and cutaneous candidiasis.

TREATMENT OF SELECTED ACUTE DERMATOSES

A selected number of dermatoses may present in a dramatic fashion and require expeditious initiation of therapy. Some of these disorders serve as examples of how the therapeutic principles outlined previously can be applied.

Acute contact dermatitis, such as that seen after poison ivy exposure, is manifested by vesicles and surrounding erythema and edema. For reactions limited to small areas of the body, treatment with an intermediate- or high-potency topical corticosteroid can be helpful. Systemic antihistamines (e.g., hydroxyzine, 10 to 25 mg every 4 to 6 hours) are often advisable, depending on the degree of pruritus. In widespread reactions, best results are obtained by the addition of systemic corticosteroids. The initial dosage of 0.5 to 1.0 mg per kilogram per day of prednisone can be tapered over a 2-week period. A rebound of clinical symptoms is often observed if corticosteroids are tapered too rapidly. For weeping lesions, compresses of Burow's solution or 0.25% acetic acid solution for 20 to 30 minutes three or four times a day are helpful.

Exfoliative erythroderma has a number of possible causes. Clinically, patients present with generalized erythema and exfoliation of the skin without frank denudation. Patients with exfoliative erythroderma often demonstrate systemic toxicity, including difficulties with temperature regulation, high-output cardiac failure, anemia, hypoalbuminemia, and fluid and electrolyte abnormalities.

Treatment of patients with exfoliative erythroderma is largely supportive, with efforts made to maintain temperature control and replace fluid and nutritional deficits. While efforts are underway to establish the cause, skin care can be initiated with intermediate-potency topical corticosteroids (e.g., triamcinolone, 0.1% cream or ointment) occluded with a nylon sauna suit. Systemic corticosteroids can be used in selected circumstances, depending on the presumed cause of the exfoliation (e.g., drug allergy, contact dermatitis). Every effort (e.g., skin biopsies, patch tests) should be made to establish a causal diagnosis and to direct care accordingly.

TREATMENT OF SELECTED CHRONIC DERMATOSES

Chronic *eczematous dermatitis,* which can be either widespread or localized, may be caused by a number of factors, including atopic eczema and chronic contact dermatitis. Although an effort should always be made to identify the cause, many cases of chronic eczema remain idiopathic. Effective control can often be achieved with topical corticosteroids, beginning with a non-occlusive intermediate-potency topical corticosteroid. Especially on the hands and feet, higher-potency topical corticosteroids (Table 191.2) with plastic glove or plastic wrap (e.g., Saran Wrap) occlusion may be needed. Systemic corticosteroids can be used for severe exacerbations, but chronic long-term use should be avoided. The management of chronic *psoriasis* can be specialized, and most patients with this disorder should be evaluated by a dermatologist. For chronic plaque-type psoriasis, the most efficacious therapy is ultraviolet light. Potent topical corticosteroids can be beneficial but occasionally lead to pustular flare-ups of the disease. In some locations (e.g., scalp and other hair-bearing areas), topical corticosteroids in a solution vehicle are helpful. Topical anthralin (Dritho-Creme) in various concentrations can be applied but can lead to skin irritation and reversible, purplish staining. Topical tar preparations can also be used (e.g., crude coal tar 0.5% to 3% [Estargel]).

BIBLIOGRAPHY

Arndt KA. *Manual of dermatologic therapeutics: with essentials of diagnosis,* fifth ed. Boston: Little, Brown, 1995.
Callen JP, Jorizzo JL, Greer KE, et al, eds. *Dermatological signs of internal disease,* second ed. Philadelphia: WB Saunders, 1995.
Clark RAF. Cutaneous tissue repair: basic biologic considerations. *J Am Acad Dermatol* 1985;13:701–725.
Clark RAF. Overview and general consideration of wound repair. In: Clark RAF, Henson PM, eds. *Molecular and cellular biology of wound repair.* New York: Plenum Press, 1988:3.
Eaglstein WH, ed. Wound healing. *Clin Dermatol* 1984;2:1.
Fenske NA, Lober CW. Structural and functional changes of normal aging skin. *J Am Acad Dermatol* 1986;15:571–585.
Fine RM. Systemic corticosteroids in dermatology. *Semin Dermatol* 1983; 2:250.
Freedberg IM, Eisen AZ, Wolff K, et al, eds. *Dermatology in general medicine,* fifth ed. New York: McGraw-Hill, 1999.
Goldsmith LA. *Physiology, biochemistry, and molecular biology of the skin.* New York: Oxford University Press, 1991.
Kastrup EK, Hebel SK, Rivard R, et al. *Drug facts and comparisons,* fifty-third ed. St Louis: Facts and Comparisons, 1999.
Lowe NJ. *Practical psoriasis therapy.* Chicago: Year Book Medical Publishers, 1986.
Rook AJ, Maibach HI. Dermatologic therapeutics. *Semin Dermatol* 1987; 6:1.
Shalita AR, Cunningham WJ, Leyden JJ, et al. Isotretinoin treatment of acne and related disorders: an update. *J Am Acad Dermatol* 1983;9: 629–638.

Shelley WB, Shelley ED. *Advanced dermatologic therapy.* Philadelphia: WB Saunders, 1987.

Kelley's Textbook of Internal Medicine, fourth edition. Edited by H. David Humes. Lippincott Williams & Wilkins, Philadelphia © 2000.

CHAPTER

192

APPROACH TO THE PATIENT WITH ALOPECIA OR BALDING

SUSAN M. SWETTER

Hair loss may be acquired or congenital, scarring or nonscarring, patchy or diffuse, temporary or permanent, and influenced by heredity, nutrition, illness, and aging. The two most common forms of alopecia are alopecia areata and androgenetic alopecia, the latter of which is commonly referred to as "male pattern" or "female pattern" baldness.

NORMAL HAIR CYCLE

The three phases of the normal hair cycle are anagen, catagen, and telogen. Approximately 90% of scalp hair is in a growing phase, termed *anagen.* This phase usually lasts between 2 and 6 years, with an average length of 1,000 days. Scalp hair normally grows at a rate of 0.35 mm per day, which slows with age. Less than 1% of hair is in the involuting stage, or *catagen,* at any time. The average length of this phase is 10 to 15 days. Ten percent of scalp hairs are in *telogen,* or resting phase, which lasts about 3 months (average, 100 days). Telogen hairs show a distinctive white bulb or "club" proximally. Forty to 100 telogen hairs are normally shed every day as growing hair involutes and rests over a period of several years. Hair washing results in the loss of 200 to 300 hairs in the normal range.

ANDROGENETIC ALOPECIA

Androgenetic alopecia occurs in both men and women. It is the most common type of nonscarring hair loss and typically affects the crown, or vertex, as well as the frontal scalp and bitemporal areas in men. The parietal and occipital portions of the scalp are often spared. Hair thinning occurs without symptoms, inflammation, or scaling of the scalp. It may begin at any time after puberty in men, and the incidence increases with age; that is, 25% of men 25 years of age show hair loss compared with 50% of men age 50 years. Hair loss may be gradual and continuous or episodic. The cause of androgenetic alopecia involves a shortening of the anagen phase of the hair cycle, which is the active growing phase, in response to androgen exposure and genetic factors.

The onset of androgenic alopecia in women is later, typically occurring between 25 and 35 years of age. Hair loss is usually less extensive than in men, with involvement usually limited to the frontal scalp and vertex. The frontal hairline is almost always preserved in women. Diffuse, central thinning may be subtle and preceded by a telogen effluvium in which increased numbers of hairs in the resting phase show synchronized shedding. Both male and female androgenetic alopecia result from a genetically determined end-organ sensitivity to androgens. Thus, family history of common baldness should be obtained in the patient presenting with either localized or diffuse hair loss.

OPTIMAL MANAGEMENT

The options for therapy for androgenetic alopecia have increased in recent years. Surgical scalp reduction may be performed after significant hair loss has occurred on the frontal scalp or vertex. Hair transplantation using grafts from the occiput results in long-term hair regrowth because transplanted hair plugs show site-specific androgen sensitivity from their location of origin; thus, occipital plugs do not develop vertex or frontal scalp androgen sensitivity. Improved techniques in hair grafting have resulted in increased cosmesis with a more natural-appearing hairline.

Only two medical treatments are approved for the treatment of androgenetic alopecia in the United States: the topical application of minoxidil (2% or 5%) or systemic treatment with finasteride 1 mg. Minoxidil (or, rather, its vasoactive metabolite, minoxidil sulfate) works by stimulating the hair follicle to remain in anagen phase for a longer period of time. It has no antiandrogen activity and is not absorbed in significant enough amounts to result in hypotension or other systemic side effects.

A 6-month trial of minoxidil on a twice-daily basis is required to assess response, which may present clinically as cessation of hair shedding or visible hair regrowth, usually of the vellus type. Approximately 30% of patients experience some hair regrowth, although up to 80% notice a reduction or complete cessation of hair loss. Topical minoxidil must be continued indefinitely to remain effective.

Finasteride is a 5-α-reductase type II inhibitor that causes reduction in the androgen, dihydrotestosterone, and has recently been approved as a 1-mg daily dose for men with androgenetic alopecia. It is contraindicated in pregnant women because it may cause feminization of a male fetus. Antiandrogen drugs such as spironolactone and flutamide have been tried for androgenetic alopecia in women, although they tend to be more useful in patients with underlying endocrine dysfunction. Finally, complete or partial hairpieces are available and may be custom-fitted and dyed to achieve a more natural appearance.

ALOPECIA AREATA

Alopecia areata is common, occurring in 1% of the population by 55 years of age. All ages are affected, although the incidence is increased in younger age groups. A family history of alopecia areata is present in more than 30% of patients with onset before age 30 years, compared with only 7% in patients with later onset. Clinical findings include well-demarcated patches devoid of hair and with visible follicles, indicative of a nonscarring process. Alopecia areata involving the entire scalp is termed *alopecia totalis,* whereas progression to involve the eyebrows, body, and pubic hair is called *alopecia universalis.* These two types are associated with a worse prognosis in terms of eventual hair regrowth.

Alopecia areata is believed to be an autoimmune disease and has been associated with other autoimmune diseases such as Hashimoto's thyroiditis, vitiligo, pernicious anemia, and early-onset diabetes mellitus. Abrupt onset of inflammation at the base of the hair follicle is believed to cause a dysfunction of the hair growth cycle with subsequent acute hair loss. Although this process is reversible (i.e., no scarring or loss of follicles occurs), hair regrowth does not always occur.

Most patients with new-onset alopecia areata are healthy. Routine laboratory testing usually is not useful unless there is a family history of thyroid disease. Thyroid function tests may also be helpful in the workup of young children presenting with alopecia areata. Recurrent episodes of alopecia areata are not uncommon and cannot be prevented by prior treatment.

OPTIMAL MANAGEMENT

Treatment options for alopecia areata include intralesional or systemic corticosteroids, production of allergic contact dermatitis with dinitrochlorobenzene, diphenlycyclopropenone, squaric acid dibutylester, or anthralin short-contact therapy, photochemotherapy with psoralin and ultraviolet A light (PUVA), and topical minoxidil. Appropriate treatment depends on the extent of disease, and alopecia may improve or worsen with or without therapy. There is no therapy proven efficacious for diffuse disease, and the likelihood of hair regrowth decreases with increased degree and duration of hair loss.

▎ TRACTION ALOPECIA

Traction alopecia may manifest similarly to alopecia areata with discrete areas of scalp hair loss. When associated with habitual hair pulling or psychological stress, traction alopecia is termed *trichotillomania* and often reverses when a person has psychological counseling. Traction alopecia may also be acquired in the setting of tight braids, hairclips, or ponytails worn for many years and is usually seen in young children or adult women. A chronic folliculitis along the temporal and frontal hairline may result in permanent scarring with loss of visible hair follicles. Reversible traction alopecia occurs if the problem is recognized and corrected early.

▎ TELOGEN EFFLUVIUM

Telogen effluvium is an important cause of hair loss in adults. It is caused by a disruption of the normal hair cycle that synchro-

nizes an increased number of hairs to enter the telogen phase. Those hairs are usually shed 2 to 3 months after the inciting event (the average length of the normal telogen phase) and are thus perceived as a period of increased hair loss. Marked hair shedding may occur with or without evidence of clinical hair thinning.

The most recognizable cause of telogen effluvium occurs in the postpartum period, typically 2 to 3 months after delivery. It is usually self-limited and resolves over 6 months, although normal hair growth equal to that before pregnancy does not always occur. Other causes of telogen effluvium include reduction in protein intake due to "crash dieting," hyperthyroidism or hypothyroidism, severe chronic illness, or drugs such as β-blockers, coumarin, sodium valproate, lithium carbonate, sulfasalazine, or oral contraceptives with increased progestational activity. It is important to obtain a medical history related to these possible causes for the 2 to 3 months preceding the onset of telogen effluvium. Correction of thyroid disease, increased protein intake, or discontinuation of the offending drug usually results in complete reversibility and cessation of increased hair shedding.

TABLE 192.1.	**APPROACH TO THE PATIENT PRESENTING WITH HAIR LOSS**

History

Onset and duration of hair loss
How much hair lost daily and when? (hair count may be necessary)
Does hair come out "by the roots" or is it breaking?
Family history of hair loss, baldness
Medical history—medications (oral contraceptives, β blockers, anticoagulants, cancer chemotherapeutic agents); history of thyroid disease, pregnancy, normal menses, menopause
Dietary changes, history of abrupt weight loss or "crash dieting"

Clinical Examination

Hair length and texture—damage from hair cosmetics?
Pattern and distribution of hair loss
Presence or absence of follicles within areas of hair loss
Other changes to suggest scarring process—scalp atrophy, pigmentary change
Hair "pull test"—more than six hairs with firm tugging denotes active hair loss
Hair mount to examine hair bulb and shaft, assess for telogen versus anagen hairs

Laboratory Tests

Scalp biopsy—helpful in diagnosis of most alopecias (scarring inflammation?)
VDRL in setting of "moth-eaten" alopecia seen with secondary syphilis
Complete blood count, thyroid function tests, serum iron—usually not useful in workup of alopecia areata, unless clinical signs of anemia or thyroid dysfunction are present
Androgen studies (serum testosterone and dihydroepiandrosterone levels)—particularly in women with scalp hair loss, hirsuitism or virilization, acne, and ovarian dysfunction

---

VDRL, test for syphilis.

TABLE 192.2.   **ALGORITHM FOR SCARRING AND NONSCARRING ALOPECIA**

Scarring			Nonscarring		
Inflammatory		**Noninflammatory**	**Inflammatory**		**Noninflammatory**
Patchy	*Diffuse*	*Patchy or Diffuse*	*Patchy*	*Diffuse*	*Patchy or Diffuse**
Lupus erythematosus	All patchy,	Trichotillomania/	Alopecia areata	Alopecia	Androgenetic
Folliculitis decalvans	inflammatory,	traction alopecia	Follicular mucinosis	areata	alopecia
Lichen planopilaris	scarring	(chronic process	Secondary syphilis		Telogen effluvium
Pseudopelade of	processes	may result in			Trichotillomania
Brocq	may also be	eventual scarring)			Traction alopecia
Tinea capitis with	diffuse	Morphea (chronic			Anagen arrest
kerion		process shows no			Trichodystrophies
Acne keloidalis		inflammation)			(Structural hair
Morphea (acute)					abnormalities)

* Often with specific pattern.

ANAGEN ARREST

Anagen arrest occurs in the setting of cancer chemotherapy because hair bulb cells show the greatest mitotic activity of any cells in the human body. Chemotherapeutic agents cause narrowing of the hair shaft and subsequent hair breakage within 1 to 3 weeks. The process is entirely reversible after cessation of chemotherapy. Patients should be warned about the expected time course and abrupt onset of alopecia, and cosmetic hairpieces may be advisable before the onset of hair loss.

LUPUS ERYTHEMATOSUS

The most important disease causing a scarring scalp alopecia is lupus erythematosus. Discoid lupus erythematosus manifests as erythematous, scaly telangiectatic plaques on the malar areas of the face, and up to 50% of patients have similar discoid lesions in the scalp. Pigmentary alteration, including hyperpigmentation and hypopigmentation, telangiectasia, and atrophy of the plaques, occurs with time. Potent topical corticosteroids, intralesional corticosteroids, or systemic immunosuppressive agents such as prednisone or hydroxychloroquine may be used for treatment. Approximately 15% of patients with systemic lupus erythematosus show classic discoid lesions and have possible scalp involvement over the course of their disease. Treatment is similarly directed to prevent permanent scarring and hair loss.

Tables 192.1 and 192.2 represent a specific approach to the workup and diagnosis of patients presenting with hair loss.

BIBLIOGRAPHY

Chen W, Zouboulis CC, Orfanos CE. The 5 alpha-reductase system and its inhibitors. Recent developments and its perspective in treatment androgen-dependent skin disorders. *Dermatology* 1996;193:177–184.

DeVillez RL, Jacobs JP, Szpunzar CA, Warner ML. Androgenetic alopecia in the female. Treatment with 2% topical minoxidil solution. *Arch Dermatol* 1994;130:303–307.

Fiedler VC. Alopecia areata: a review of therapy, efficacy, safety, and mechanism. *Arch Dermatol* 1992;128:1519–1529.

Headington JT. Telogen effluvium. *Arch Dermatol* 1993;129:356–363.

Kaufman KD, Olsen EA, Whiting D, et al. Finasteride in the treatment of men with androgenetic alopecia. Finasteride male pattern hair loss study group. *J Am Acad Dermatol* 1998;39:578–589.

Propecia and Rogaine Extra Strength for Alopecia. *Med Lett Drugs Ther* 1998;40:25–27.

Reitschel RL, Duncan SH. Safety and efficacy of topical minoxidil in the management of androgenetic alopecia. *J Am Acad Dermatol* 1987;16:677–685.

Sawaya ME. Clinical updates in hair. *Dermatol Clin* 1997;15:37–43.

Shapiro J, Price VH. Hair regrowth. Therapeutic agents. *Dermatol Clin* 1998;16:341–356.

Templeton SF, Solomon AR. Scarring alopecia: a classification based on microscopic criteria. *J Cutan Pathol* 1994;21:97–109.

Kelley's Textbook of Internal Medicine, fourth edition. Edited by H. David Humes.
Lippincott Williams & Wilkins, Philadelphia © 2000.

DISEASES OF THE DERMATOLOGIC SYSTEMS

PSORIASIS, LICHEN PLANUS, AND PITYRIASIS ROSEA

CHRISTOPHER M. BARNARD

PSORIASIS

Psoriasis is a primary disease of the skin characterized by well-demarcated inflammatory papules and plaques, which are typically covered by thickened, silvery scales.

ETIOLOGY

Psoriasis is a disease of increased proliferation of epidermal cells, the precise cause of which is unknown. Evidence that a genetic (familial) predisposition is a major factor in the clinical expression of psoriasis is supported by the greater than normal incidence in patients with psoriasis of certain human leukocyte antigen (HLA) markers, especially HLA-A1, B13, B17, Cw6, DRw6, and DR7. It has been further suggested that the presence of HLA-DR$^+$ keratinocytes in psoriatic plaques correlates with disease activity. Linkage to a gene for familial psoriasis susceptibility has recently been localized to the distal end of chromosome 17q in a study of several kindreds. An incomplete autosomal dominant pattern of inheritance seems most likely; however, a polygenic, multifactorial pattern is also possible.

PATHOGENESIS

Traditional investigations into the pathogenesis of psoriasis have focused on the increased proliferation and hyperplasia of the epidermis. In normal skin, the time for a cell to move from the basal layer through the granular layer is 4 to 5 weeks. In psoriatic lesions, the time is decreased seven to ten times because of a shortened cell cycle time, an increase in the absolute number of cells capable of proliferating, and the fact that, among those cells, an increased proportion of cells are actually dividing. The

hyperproliferative phenomenon is also expressed, although to a substantially smaller degree, in the clinically uninvolved skin of psoriatic patients.

Several biologic aberrations have been proposed to account for the enhanced proliferation of keratinocytes. T-cell–mediated immune responses appear to be responsible for the inflammation and hyperproliferation seen in psoriasis. Cytokine production elicited by the dermal immune reaction stimulates abnormal epidermal cell (keratinocyte) proliferation and differentiation. The possibility that a superantigen (e.g., microbial antigen) might activate cutaneous T cells has been studied but not conclusively shown to trigger psoriasis.

Psoriasis is an inflammatory disease in which neutrophils are found within psoriatic lesions. Arachidonic acid, the levels of which are much higher than normal in psoriatic plaques, and its metabolites are probably important in this aspect of the disease because they can act as vasodilators and chemoattractants for neutrophils. The cause, or possibly the effect, of this may be increased levels of plasminogen activator in psoriatic lesions. Enhanced plasminogen activator may lead to neutrophil accumulation through direct complement activation and to enhanced activation of proteases.

Normal skin contains capillary loops within the dermis, which have intact basement membranes. In contrast, psoriatic skin has multiple gaps in endothelial cells that appear to lead to increased vascular permeability. These gaps can be seen in both involved and uninvolved psoriatic skin. It is not clear how the gaps occur, but they may represent cellular injury from the inflammatory responses or abnormalities in other cells in the dermis.

Other cells of the psoriatic dermis also display abnormalities. Psoriatic fibroblasts have increased levels of enzymes involved in collagen synthesis. This phenomenon is probably secondary to expansion of the papillary dermis required to support the hyperproliferative epidermis, rather than a primary abnormality. When fibroblasts are cultured from the skin of unaffected people, 1,25-dihydroxyvitamin D$_3$ inhibits proliferation; in contrast, fibroblasts from either involved or uninvolved skin of psoriatic patients display a relative resistance to this effect. Vitamin D$_3$ analogues have been shown to successfully clear psoriatic plaques, although the exact mechanism of action is unknown. Furthermore, when psoriatic fibroblasts from either involved or uninvolved skin are incorporated in vitro into a collagen lattice that functions as a dermal equivalent, they induce hyperproliferation in normal keratinocytes.

Primary immunologic mechanisms have been implicated in initiating the proliferative process of psoriasis. HLA-DR$^+$ keratinocytes and Langerhans' cells and activated T lymphocytes with increased numbers of interleukin-2 receptors have been found in active psoriatic plaques. In addition to these laboratory observations, in several well-controlled clinical studies, dramatic clearing of recalcitrant, severe psoriasis has been achieved by using cyclosporin A. The major mechanism of action of cyclosporin A is to inhibit the release of lymphokines produced by activated T lymphocytes. Thus, a hypothesis is that the activated T cells, in response to autologous or exogenous antigens, may release factors that directly result in inflammation and epidermal proliferation or indirectly produce these effects by activating macrophages or keratinocytes, which then release cytokines, mediators of inflammation, or growth factors that can elicit the pathologic condition of psoriatic plaques.

INCIDENCE AND EPIDEMIOLOGY

The incidence of psoriasis in the United States is about 2% of the population. About 3% of whites and 1% of blacks are affected. Occurrence is extremely low in Native Americans. Psoriasis affects both sexes equally. It occurs in about 2.5% of HIV-infected patients and is severe in 25% to 30% of the HIV-infected population.

CLINICAL FEATURES

The typical lesion of psoriasis is a well-demarcated erythematous plaque covered by thick, silvery scales (Fig. 193.1). A characteristic finding is the isomorphic response (Koebner's phenomenon), in which new psoriatic lesions arise at sites of cutaneous trauma. Lesions are often localized to the extensor surfaces of the extremities, and the nails and scalp are also commonly involved. The entire body, including mucosal, genital, and perineal skin, can be involved. Nail involvement in psoriasis is usually manifested by pitting of the surface or by onycholysis (distal separation of the nail plate from the nail bed).

Psoriasis can become so extensive as to cause exfoliative eryth-

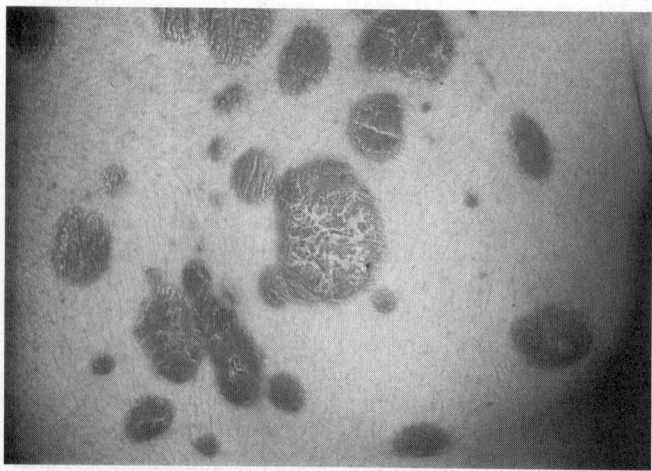

FIGURE 193.1. Chronic plaque-type psoriasis.

roderma, in which the entire epidermal surface is in a state of hyperproliferation. In this condition, many of the critical barrier functions of the skin are lost: The cutaneous microvasculature is dilated, leading to heat loss and hypoproteinemia; there is increased transepidermal water loss; and patients often experience profound chilling. Prolonged exfoliation can also lead to anemia, presumably due to iron and folate loss through the skin.

In *guttate psoriasis,* a form of the disease that often erupts after streptococcal pharyngitis, lesions are characteristically 1 to 3 cm in diameter and widely distributed over the body. The course is unpredictable; the disease may go into remission or be a prologue to a more chronic form of psoriasis.

A third form is *pustular psoriasis,* which is characterized by numerous sterile pustules, often 2 to 5 mm in diameter, on the palms and soles or distributed over the body. When they involve the palms and soles, the pustules are associated with hyperkeratosis. In other parts of the body, the pustules may form clusters on oval plaques with an erythematous inflammatory base, which can spread and leave a fine superficial scale. In pustular psoriasis, there may be acute, often explosive, life-threatening episodes in which the patient experiences fever, chills, leukocytosis, hypoalbuminemia, and hypocalcemia. Hypovolemia can also occur. This form of psoriasis demands immediate, vigorous therapy.

Acute exacerbations of previously stable, typical plaque-type psoriasis may occur in patients who acquire HIV infection. These exacerbations may become more refractory to conventional therapy. New-onset psoriasiform dermatitis may signal the possibility of underlying HIV infection. This form of psoriasis, which develops after the onset of HIV infection, tends to appear in association with palmoplantar psoriasis.

Psoriatic arthritis is divided into five types and is described in further detail with the seronegative spondyloarthropathies (Chapter 176).

LABORATORY FINDINGS

The major procedure required for the diagnosis of psoriasis is skin biopsy. The specimen reveals hyperkeratosis with parakeratosis, which indicates the retention of nuclear fragments, increased proliferation, and defective keratinization. Elongation of the rete ridges (acanthosis) and thinning of the epidermis above the dermal papillae are found. The dermal capillaries are often dilated, and there is a chronic inflammatory infiltrate. Frequently, neutrophils migrate into the stratum corneum to form microabscesses. In pustular psoriasis, the microabscesses are a predominant feature.

COURSE, THERAPY, AND PROGNOSIS

Untreated psoriasis typically follows a chronic course, with some fluctuation in severity. Patients frequently report improvement during the summer, probably from the beneficial effects of natural ultraviolet light. Conversely, exacerbation of psoriasis is common in the winter, possibly owing to low humidity and xerosis, leading to epidermal damage and an isomorphic response. Other modalities that traumatize the skin—abrasion, infection, and various types of dermatitis—also can worsen the disease. As

TABLE 193.1. DRUG-RELATED EXACERBATION OF PSORIASIS		
Drug	**Possible Mechanisms of Exacerbation**	**Types of Exacerbation**
Lithium	Inhibition of adenylate cyclase	Exacerbation of preexisting psoriasis
	Enhanced release of inflammatory mediators	New-onset psoriasis
	from neutrophils	Therapeutic resistance
β-Adrenergic blockers	Decreased β-adrenergic receptor activity with	New-onset psoriasis
Propranolol	decreased adenylate cyclase activity	
Oxyprenolol		Generalized pustular psoriasis
Pindolol		preexisting plaque psoriasis
Alprenolol		
Atenolol		
Metoprolol		
Antimalarials	Unknown	Exacerbation of preexisting psoriasis
Chloroquine		
Hydroxychloroquine		Exfoliative erythroderma
Quinacrine		Therapeutic resistance
Corticosteroids	Unknown	Therapeutic resistance
		Generalized pustular psoriasis in
		preexisting plaque psoriasis
Nonsteroidal anti-inflammatory agents	Inhibition of cyclooxygenase with arachidonic	Exacerbation of preexisting psoriasis
Indomethacin	acid accumulation, shunting metabolism to	Pustular psoriasis
Phenylbutazone	the lipoxygenase pathway, and increased	
Meclofenamate	leukotrienes (LTB_4)	

Modified from Abel EA, Dicicco LM, Orenberg EK, et al. Drugs in exacerbation of psoriasis. *J Am Acad Dermatol* 1986;15:1007.

noted, guttate psoriasis can be precipitated by streptococcal pharyngitis.

Several commonly used drugs exacerbate preexisting psoriasis by inducing new types of lesions in patients with psoriasis (e.g., pustular psoriasis in a patient with plaque-type disease), by eliciting new psoriasis in patients without a history of the disease, or by inducing treatment resistance (Table 193.1). With most of these drugs, the incidence of exacerbation appears to be low, but no prospective studies have been carried out. The most worrisome features of drug-related exacerbation of psoriasis are the unpredictability of its occurrence, the long latent periods (up to several months), and the possibility of severe manifestations, such as exfoliative erythroderma and acute pustular psoriasis.

Therapeutic efforts in psoriasis are aimed at decreasing the proliferative rate of the epidermis, either by direct action on cell division or through agents that reduce the inflammatory response or vascular permeability. For patients with localized, limited psoriasis, administration of topical corticosteroids is the most convenient outpatient therapy. Rapid improvement may be seen with this approach, but the beneficial short-term efficacy is limited and long-term topical corticosteroid treatment is not advisable. Side effects from long-term topical corticosteroid therapy can include atrophy of the skin, development of a tolerance to the agent used (tachyphylaxis), and serious exacerbation of the disease after discontinuation. Pituitary–adrenal suppression is a potential and serious complication of potent topical corticosteroid therapy, particularly when the agent covers a large portion of the body surface and is used under occlusive dressings. Despite these potential drawbacks, topical corticosteroid therapy, in combination with emollients or used alone, remains the most commonly prescribed treatment for psoriasis.

Calcipotriene 0.005% ointment is a vitamin D_3 derivative, which may be applied topically twice daily to improve plaque-type psoriasis. At recommended dosages, calcium metabolism appears to be minimally affected, although hypercalcemia has been seen in patients using excessive amounts of the topical ointment. The safety and efficacy of this treatment have been established for up to 52 weeks of therapy if dosages are maintained below 100 g per week.

Tazarotene gel (0.05% and 0.1%) is a topical retinoid recently introduced for once-a-day treatment of plaque-type psoriasis. Mild to moderate psoriasis can be controlled after 1 to 12 weeks of treatment, and improvement has been noted to remain for up to 12 weeks after discontinuation of therapy. Local skin irritation has been reported to occur with tazarotene therapy and can be minimized with concomitant topical corticosteroid therapy. As with all retinoids, tazarotene is contraindicated in women who are or who may become pregnant.

Topical coal tar preparations have been effective when used alone to clear psoriatic plaques; however, the unpleasant odor and propensity to stain fabrics reduce their acceptance by patients. Hospitalization may be required for patients with more extensive disease, who are treated with topical coal tar preparations followed by irradiation with B-spectrum ultraviolet light (290 to 320 nm). This regimen, known as *Goeckerman's regimen,* can be modified to include the use of topical corticosteroids.

For patients with extensive disease, systemic antimitotic agents such as methotrexate can be used. Methotrexate is usually administered on an intermittent basis and should not be given more frequently than once weekly. Patients receiving it should be monitored for hematologic and liver toxicity; because methotrexate-induced cirrhosis is a risk, especially after a cumulative dose of 1.5 g has been reached, liver biopsy may be indicated. Treatment with methotrexate in HIV-positive patients has been studied, although its safety has not been clearly established.

Extensive psoriasis can also be treated with photochemotherapy. In this regimen, oral 8-methoxypsoralen produces photosensitization, which is followed by exposure to ultraviolet A (psoralen ultraviolet light A [PUVA], 320 nm). Like Goeckerman's regimen, this therapy inhibits mitotic activity in the epidermis, and it produces remissions in up to 80% of patients with plaque-type psoriasis. It seems to be less useful in patients with pustular psoriasis. Major complications of PUVA therapy are acute sunburn and the risk of corneal damage. Eyes must be protected for up to 24 hours after ingestion of the psoralens. PUVA therapy may cause retinal damage in aphakic persons and is therefore contraindicated in these patients. Although skin cancer develops in 2% of patients on PUVA, it also occurs in patients on Goeckerman's regimen who have had intensive tar and ultraviolet B exposure. Fair-skinned people with long histories of exposure to ultraviolet irradiation are at highest risk.

The retinoids, particularly acitretin (the major metabolite of etretinate), either alone or in combination with PUVA, also constitute an effective treatment for psoriasis. Acitretin is especially useful in the exfoliative and pustular varieties. Several major potential complications must be monitored in patients placed on retinoids. As a class, the retinoids are potent teratogens and should not be given to women of childbearing age who are not using adequate contraception. Acitretin, like other retinoids, can produce elevations in cholesterol and triglyceride levels, so dietary regulation may be necessary. In addition, because acitretin can induce hepatotoxicity, liver function tests should be performed before and at regular intervals during use of the drug. The half-life of acitretin is about 49 hours, considerably shorter than its parent compound of etretinate with a half-life of about 6 months. For HIV-positive patients with severe psoriasis, acitretin may be the best therapeutic strategy.

During acute attacks of pustular psoriasis, systemic corticosteroids have been the therapy of choice. Acitretin can also produce rapid remission or can be used for maintenance therapy after initial control has been achieved with systemic corticosteroids. Except in life-threatening pustular psoriasis, systemic corticosteroids have no place in the therapy of psoriasis; indeed, acute severe flare-ups of psoriasis can result when systemic corticosteroids are withdrawn (Table 193.1).

In view of the postulated immunologic mechanisms in psoriasis, it is interesting that cyclosporin A has been shown to be an effective treatment. The results of the clinical trials using low-dose (3 to 7 mg per kilogram) cyclosporin A are impressive, because the time required to achieve complete remission ranges from 1 to 4 weeks. The major adverse effects of cyclosporin A with short-term, low-dose usage include potential renal dysfunction and hypertension. The renal toxicity is usually reversible at low doses on discontinuing therapy; however, irreversible damage may occur with a prolonged treatment course. Patients who have previously received extensive phototherapy, particularly PUVA, must be monitored for the development of invasive squamous cell carcinomas of the skin. The use of cyclosporin A should be reserved for patients with recalcitrant, debilitating

psoriasis when the benefits outweigh the potential risk of complications.

 LICHEN PLANUS

Lichen planus (LP) is a common inflammatory dermatosis characterized by pruritic, angular, purple papules on the skin and small, white papules forming netlike patterns on mucosal surfaces.

ETIOLOGY AND PATHOGENESIS

The cause of LP is unknown, but a cell-mediated immune response appears to play a major role in its pathogenesis. Early LP lesions reveal increased CD4$^+$ T cells in the dermal infiltrate; later lesions show CD8$^+$ T cells in the epidermis. This pattern suggests that antigen presentation to helper T cells activates a cytokine response to recruit cytotoxic T cells, which results in damage to the keratinocytes of the epidermis. More recently, infection with hepatitis C virus has been found in association with LP in some cases. However, a significant causal relation has not been definitively established.

INCIDENCE AND EPIDEMIOLOGY

The incidence of LP is reportedly 0.1% to 1.4% in dermatology clinics. Most patients are between ages 30 and 60, with both sexes affected equally.

CLINICAL FEATURES

LP is a pruritic inflammatory dermatosis that affects the skin and mucous membranes. The flat-topped, polygonal, purple, scaly papules characteristic of LP appear most commonly on the trunk and the flexor surfaces of the extremities. Very fine, white reticulate lines on the surface of the papules, known as *Wickham's striae*, are a helpful diagnostic feature. The dorsal hands, flexor surfaces of the forearms, wrists, and ankles are areas of predisposition. Oral lesions on the lips or buccal mucosa, consisting of fine, lacy, or netlike reticulate patterns of small white papules or plaques, are present in over 50% of patients with cutaneous LP and may be the only finding in up to 25% of patients. In addition, the genitalia, nails, and scalp may be affected with specific forms of the disease. There are many variations in the morphology of LP, including hypertrophic, bullous, erosive, and atrophic types.

The differential diagnosis includes LP-like eruptions secondary to medications such as antimalarial agents, captopril, gold, methyldopa, penicillamine, phenothiazines, propranolol, tetracyclines, and thiazides. Chemical exposure to para-phenylenediamine in color photographic film developer can result in an eruption similar to LP. In graft-versus-host disease, an LP-like eruption may develop and can be distinguished histologically on skin biopsy. The lichen planus–lupus erythematosus overlap syndrome exhibits features of both disorders and may simply represent the coexistence of these two diseases.

LABORATORY FINDINGS

Skin biopsy, the only valuable diagnostic laboratory test for LP, reveals a classic "sawtooth" pattern to the epidermis, with hypergranulosis and hyperkeratosis at the surface. Keratinocyte degeneration at the lower epidermis results in eosinophilic or colloid bodies (e.g., Civatte bodies), which are positive for IgM antibody on direct immunofluorescence. Basal cell layer degeneration results in separation, or clefting, between the dermis and epidermis. Below the dermal–epidermal junction, a lichenoid or band-like infiltrate of lymphocytes is present.

COURSE, THERAPY, AND PROGNOSIS

The onset of LP may be gradual or sudden. With acute, sudden eruptions, the course is usually shorter, and clearing may occur within several months. The papules in localized forms of LP usually resolve within 6 to 18 months, resulting in hyperpigmentation at the sites of involvement. In the more generalized forms, the eruption may persist for several years or longer. Involvement of the mucous membranes also prolongs the course.

Moderate to severe pruritus is reported by most patients. Koebner's phenomenon, similar to that seen with psoriasis, results in new papules of LP at sites of trauma to the skin.

Topical or intralesional corticosteroids are effective treatment for most cases of localized lesions of LP. Antihistamines are also beneficial in relieving pruritus. For patients with more widespread involvement, oral corticosteroids may be required to control severe pruritus and to slow or halt progression of the disease. Oral LP may be treated with topical corticosteroids in combination with an adhesive base such as Orabase for better adhesion to the mucous membranes. In particularly recalcitrant cases, retinoids, cyclosporin A, and photochemotherapy all have been used with varying success.

LP recurs in 10% to 20% of patients; recurrence is more common after generalized eruptions. The erosive and hypertrophic types are particularly difficult to treat and may also result in a protracted course or recurrence.

PITYRIASIS ROSEA

Pityriasis rosea (PR) is a common, acute, inflammatory skin eruption that manifests as oval, erythematous, scaly papules and plaques. It begins with a single red, scaly "herald patch" followed by a generalized eruption. The course of the disease is self-limited, and it is of unknown origin.

ETIOLOGY AND PATHOGENESIS

Many studies have attempted to identify an infectious agent responsible for the PR eruption, which has a similar onset, course, and resolution to a viral exanthem. However, no conclusive evidence for this mechanism has ever been obtained. A PR-like eruption has been reported to be caused by numerous drugs, particularly captopril and gold therapy. Barbiturates, metronidazole, isotretinoin, and several other medications all have been implicated as well. An immune mechanism has been postulated

in the pathogenesis of PR. HLA-DR$^+$ helper T lymphocytes and keratinocytes have been found in the cellular infiltrate of the inflammatory plaques, suggesting a cellular immune reaction.

CLINICAL FEATURES

The classic presentation of PR involves the onset of a single red, oval patch, commonly on the trunk and several centimeters in diameter. This initial lesion, the herald patch, precedes the generalized eruption by 1 to 2 weeks. The herald patch is usually scaly at the borders, with clearing toward the center of the lesion. The generalized eruption that follows is distributed over the trunk, abdomen, neck, and proximal extremities, with sparing of the palms and soles. Typical lesions are pink, oval, 1- to 2-cm thin plaques or patches with an inwardly pointed collarette of scale. Individual oval lesions may be oriented along their long axes in line with the skin tension lines of the trunk, creating a "Christmas tree" pattern characteristic of PR. The herald patch may resolve before the secondary generalized eruption, which generally subsides after 1 to 3 months without treatment. Mild to severe pruritus is noted in up to 75% of patients with PR. Resolution of the inflammatory patches may result in hypo- or hyperpigmentation.

The differential diagnosis of PR may include widespread superficial tinea infections, nummular eczema, drug eruptions, and, most important, secondary syphilis. Tinea can be excluded by mycology culture or potassium hydroxide examination for hyphae. Nummular eczema is much more persistent than PR and is characteristically annular with thicker, scaly plaques. Drug eruptions can be difficult to distinguish, particularly if they are related to the medications mentioned previously. Secondary syphilis can be differentiated by the presence of scaly, erythematous palmar and plantar papules, a history of a genital chancre, and a positive serologic test for syphilis.

LABORATORY FINDINGS

Biopsy of the characteristic oval patch reveals a spongiotic dermatitis with a lymphocytic infiltrate and patchy parakeratosis. Extravasated red blood cells into both the dermal papillae and epidermis may be seen. There are no helpful blood tests to identify this disorder, although elevated white blood cell counts have been reported.

MANAGEMENT

Because PR is generally self-limited within 6 to 8 weeks, symptomatic relief with topical midpotency corticosteroids and emollients may be beneficial. Ultraviolet B light therapy has been used with success but has also been reported to result in greater postinflammatory changes. Avoiding irritation of the lesions is helpful in preventing further pruritus. Recurrence occurs in less than 2% of patients.

BIBLIOGRAPHY

Anderson TF, Voorhees JJ. Psoriasis. In: Thiers BH, Dobson RL, eds. *Pathogenesis of skin disease.* New York: Churchill Livingstone, 1986:67.

Bjornberg A. Pityriasis rosea. In: Fitzpatrick TB, Eisen AZ, Wolff K, et al, eds. *Dermatology in general medicine,* fourth ed. New York: McGraw-Hill, 1995:1117.

Daoud MS, Pittelkow MR. Lichen Planus. In: Freedberg IM, Eisen AZ, Wolff K, et al, eds. *Dermatology in general medicine,* fifth ed. New York: McGraw-Hill, 1999.

Greaves MW, Weinstein GD. Treatment of psoriasis. *N Engl J Med* 1995; 332:581–588.

Madison KL. Lichen planus, pityriasis rosea, pityriasis rubra pilaris, and related conditions. In: Sams WM, Lynch PJ, eds. *Principles and practice of dermatology.* New York: Churchill Livingstone, 1990:325.

Ramsay CA. 1997. Management of psoriasis with calcipotriol used as monotherapy [Review]. *J Am Acad Dermatol* 1997;37(Pt 2):S53–S54.

Weinstein GD. Tazarotene gel: efficacy and safety in plaque psoriasis. *J Am Acad Dermatol* 1997;37:S33–S38.

Kelley's Textbook of Internal Medicine, fourth edition. Edited by H. David Humes. Lippincott Williams & Wilkins, Philadelphia © 2000.

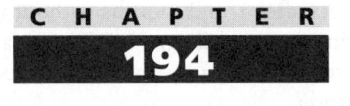

INFECTIONS OF SKIN

GARY L. DARMSTADT

■ BACTERIAL INFECTIONS

MECHANISM OF PYOGENIC BACTERIAL INFECTION

Skin microflora is composed primarily of resident bacteria that are attached to the skin and are present in relatively stable numbers and transient flora that attach and cause disease only when the integrity of the skin is disturbed. The most important of the transient bacteria are the group A β-hemolytic streptococci (*Streptococcus pyogenes;* GABHS) and *Staphylococcus aureus.*

IMPETIGO

Clinical Findings

Nonbullous impetigo accounts for more than 70% of cases of impetigo. Lesions of nonbullous impetigo usually begin on skin that has been traumatized. A vesicle or pustule forms initially and develops rapidly into a honey-colored, crusted plaque. Regional adenopathy is found in up to 90% of patients, and leukocytosis is present in approximately 50%. Without treatment, lesions generally resolve spontaneously without scarring within about 2 weeks.

Bullous impetigo manifests most commonly with flaccid, transparent bullae on the face, buttocks, trunk, perineum, and extremities. Rupture of bullae occurs easily, leaving a narrow rim of scale at the edge of a shallow, moist erosion. Surrounding erythema and regional adenopathy usually are absent.

Complications

Cellulitis has been reported in approximately 10% of patients with nonbullous impetigo but rarely follows the bullous form. Lymphangitis, suppurative lymphadenitis, guttate psoriasis, and scarlet fever may occasionally follow streptococcal disease. Infection with nephritogenic strains of GABHS may result in acute poststreptococcal glomerulonephritis. The most commonly affected age group is school-age children 3 to 7 years old. Impetigo-associated epidemics of poststreptococcal glomerulonephritis are caused by M groups 2, 49, 53, 55, 56, 57, and 60. Strains of GABHS associated with endemic impetigo in the United States have little or no nephritogenic potential. The clinical character of impetigo lesions does not differ between those that lead to poststreptococcal glomerulonephritis and those that do not. Acute rheumatic fever does not occur after impetigo.

Etiology

S. aureus is the predominant organism of nonbullous impetigo in the United States. Staphylococci usually spread from the nose to normal skin and then may colonize and possibly infect the skin. The staphylococcal types that cause nonbullous impetigo usually are not from phage group II, the group associated with scalded skin and toxic shock syndromes. GABHS are implicated in the development of some lesions of nonbullous impetigo. In contrast to what happens with *S. aureus* infection, the skin is colonized directly with GABHS an average of 10 days before impetigo develops. Several serotypes of GABHS, termed "impetigo strains," are found most frequently in lesions of nonbullous impetigo and are different from those that cause pharyngitis.

Bullous impetigo is always caused by coagulase-positive *S. aureus;* lesions of bullous impetigo are a manifestation of localized staphylococcal scalded skin syndrome and develop on grossly intact skin.

Diagnosis and Optimal Management

Diagnosis of impetigo is usually made on clinical grounds. Culture of fluid from an intact blister should yield the causative organism. When the patient appears ill, blood cultures should also be obtained.

Mupirocin applied three times daily for 7 to 10 days is equal to or greater in effectiveness and with fewer side effects than oral erythromycin ethylsuccinate for 7 to 10 days for treatment of localized, uncomplicated impetigo. Mupirocin may be preferable in areas with a high prevalence of erythromycin-resistant strains of *S. aureus.* In patients with widespread or deep involvement, including cellulitis, furunculosis, abscess formation, or suppurative lymphadenitis, systemic therapy with a β-lactamase–resistant oral antibiotic (e.g., cephalexin, dicloxacillin) should be prescribed. If a satisfactory clinical response is not achieved within 7 days, a culture should be taken by swabbing beneath the lifted edge of a crusted lesion. If a resistant organism is detected, an appropriate antibiotic should be given for an additional 7 days.

ECTHYMA

Clinical Findings

Ecthyma resembles nonbullous impetigo in onset and appearance but gradually develops into a deeper, more chronic infection. The initial lesion is a vesicle that erodes through the epidermis into the dermis to form a crusted ulcer. Lesions occur most commonly on the legs. Predisposing factors include pruritic lesions, such as insect bites, scabies, or pediculosis, which are subject to frequent scratching; poor hygiene; and malnutrition. Complications include lymphangitis, cellulitis, scar formation, and, rarely, poststreptococcal glomerulonephritis.

Etiology

The causative agent of ecthyma is usually GABHS. *S. aureus* is also cultured from most lesions but is probably a secondary pathogen.

Optimal Management

Crusts should be softened by warm compresses and removed. Systemic antibiotic therapy, as for impetigo, is indicated.

Ecthyma Gangrenosum

Ecthyma gangrenosum is a descriptive term for a necrotic ulcer covered with a gray-black eschar. Classically, it is a sign of *Pseudomonas aeruginosa* sepsis and usually occurs in immunosuppressed patients. The lesion begins as a red or purpuric macule that vesiculates and then ulcerates. There is a surrounding rim of pink to violaceous skin. The punched-out ulcer develops raised edges with a dense, black, depressed, crusted center. Clinically similar lesions may also develop as a result of infection with other bacilli, such as *Pseudomonas cepacia, Xanthomonas maltophila, Escherichia coli, Serratia marcescens,* and *Aeromonas hydrophila,* and with *Candida* species. Blood cultures and skin biopsy for culture should be obtained, and empirical intravenous broad-spectrum antibiotic therapy, including antipseudomonal agents, should be initiated as soon as possible.

STAPHYLOCOCCAL SCALDED SKIN SYNDROME

Clinical Findings

Staphylococcal scalded skin syndrome occurs predominantly in infants and children younger than 5 years. A wide range of presentations may occur, from localized bullous impetigo to generalized cutaneous involvement with systemic toxicity. Onset of the rash may be preceded by malaise, fever, and cutaneous tenderness. Scarlatiniform erythema develops diffusely and is accentuated in flexural and periorificial areas. The conjunctivae are inflamed and occasionally become purulent, but oral mucosal surfaces are spared. In severe cases, sterile, flaccid blisters and erosions develop diffusely. Circumoral erythema is prominent, as is radial crusting and fissuring around the eyes, mouth, and nose. At this stage, areas of epidermis may separate in response

to gentle shear force (Nikolsky's sign). Secondary problems of cutaneous superinfection and cellulitis, sepsis, fluid and electrolyte disturbances, and pneumonia may cause increased morbidity. Desquamation follows cutaneous erythema by a few days, and healing occurs without scarring within approximately 2 weeks.

Etiology

Staphylococcal scalded skin syndrome is caused predominantly by phage group II staphylococci, particularly strains 71 and 55, which are present at localized sites of infection such as the nasopharynx, skin, urinary tract, and conjunctivae. The clinical manifestations of staphylococcal scalded skin syndrome are mediated by hematogenous spread of staphylococcal epidermolytic or exfoliative toxins A or B.

Diagnosis and Optimal Management

Intact bullae are consistently sterile, unlike those of bullous impetigo, but cultures should be obtained from all suspected sites of localized infection and from the blood to identify the source for elaboration of the epidermolytic toxins. The subcorneal, granular layer split can be identified on skin biopsy or by examination of the exfoliated corneal layer on a frozen biopsy specimen.

Systemic therapy should be initiated with a β-lactamase–resistant antistaphylococcal antibiotic. The skin should be cleansed with Burow's or Dakin's solution, and an emollient should be applied during the resolution phase.

FOLLICULITIS

Clinical Findings

Folliculitis is a superficial infection of the hair follicle caused most often by *S. aureus*. The lesions are typically small, discrete, dome-shaped pustules with an erythematous base, located at the ostium of the pilosebaceous canals. Favored sites include the scalp, buttocks, and extremities. Poor hygiene, maceration, and drainage from wounds and abscesses are predisposing factors.

Etiology and Optimal Management

The causative organism of folliculitis can be identified by Gram's stain and culture of purulent material from the follicular orifice.

Treatment for folliculitis includes topical antibiotic cleansers such as chlorhexidine or hexachlorophene. In chronic recurrent folliculitis, daily topical application of a benzoyl peroxide lotion or gel may facilitate resolution. Topical therapy is usually all that is required for mild cases, but more severe cases may require β-lactamase–resistant systemic antibiotics such as dicloxacillin or cephalexin.

Gram-Negative Folliculitis

Folliculitis due to gram-negative organisms occurs primarily in patients with acne vulgaris who have been treated long-term with broad-spectrum systemic antibiotics. A superficial pustular form, caused by *Klebsiella* species, *Enterobacter* species, *E. coli*, or *P. aeruginosa*, occurs around the nose and spreads to the cheeks and chin. A deeper, nodular form of folliculitis on the face and trunk is caused by *Proteus* species. Culture of infected follicles is necessary to establish the diagnosis. Treatment consists of incision and drainage of the deeper, larger cysts; topical antibiotics; or selection of an oral antibiotic based on the sensitivity profile of the pathogenic organism. For severe, recalcitrant cases, 13-*cis*-retinoic acid 1 mg per kilogram per day has been helpful.

Sycosis Barbae

Sycosis barbae is a deeper, more severe, recurrent, inflammatory form of folliculitis due to *S. aureus* infection, which involves the entire depth of the follicle. Erythematous follicular papules and pustules develop on the chin, upper lip, and angle of the jaw, primarily in young black men. Papules may coalesce into plaques, and healing may occur with scarring. Those affected are frequently found to be *S. aureus* carriers. Treatment with warm saline compresses and topical antibiotics such as mupirocin usually clears the infection. More extensive, recalcitrant cases may require therapy with β-lactamase–resistant systemic antibiotics, as well as elimination of *S. aureus* from sites of carriage.

FUNGAL INFECTIONS

TINEA VERSICOLOR

Clinical Findings

Tinea versicolor often begins with perifollicular macules that enlarge to form confluent, scaling patches, most commonly on the neck, upper chest, back, and upper arms. The lesions are typically reddish-brown in whites; in blacks, they may be either hypopigmented or hyperpigmented. Pruritus is variable but usually minimal. Involved areas do not tan after sun exposure.

Etiology

Tinea versicolor is a chronic infection of the stratum corneum caused by the dimorphic yeast *Malassezia furfur*. Names used previously to identify the causal organism are *Pityrosporum ovale* and *Pityrosporum orbiculare*. *M. furfur* is part of the normal flora, predominantly in the yeast form and particularly in areas of skin that are rich in sebum production. Predisposing factors include a warm, humid environment; excessive sweating; occlusion; high plasma cortisol levels; immunosuppression; malnourishment; and genetically determined susceptibility. Tinea versicolor is most prevalent in adolescents and young adults.

Diagnosis and Optimal Management

A potassium hydroxide (KOH) preparation of scrapings is diagnostic of tinea versicolor, demonstrating groups of thick-walled spores and numerous short, thick, angular hyphae, resembling "spaghetti and meatballs."

Given that *M. furfur* is a normal human saprophyte, the organism is not eradicated from the skin after treatment. Consequently, the disorder tends to recur in predisposed persons. Appropriate topical therapy may include twice-daily application of one of the following for 2 to 4 weeks: selenium sulfide 2.5% lotion; 25% sodium hyposulfite or thiosulfate lotion; lotions, ointments, or creams containing 3% to 6% salicylic acid; or miconazole, clotrimazole, ketoconazole, or terbinafine cream. Recurrent episodes continue to respond promptly to these agents. Oral therapy may be more convenient and may be achieved successfully with ketoconazole or fluconazole 400 mg, repeated in 1 week, or itraconazole 200 mg per day for 5 to 7 days.

DERMATOPHYTE INFECTIONS

Dermatophyte infections of the stratum corneum, hair, or nails are caused primarily by *Trichophyton*, *Microsporum*, and *Epidermophyton* species. The severity of disease tends to be greater in persons with diabetes mellitus, lymphoid malignancies, immunosuppression, and states with high plasma cortisol levels such as Cushing's syndrome. Local factors that predispose to infection include trauma to the skin, hydration of the skin with maceration, occlusion, and elevated temperature. Some degree of immunity is acquired by most infected people and may be associated with a delayed hypersensitivity response.

Tinea Capitis

Tinea capitis is a dermatophyte infection of the scalp, most often seen in children and due to infection with *Trichophyton tonsurans* and *Microsporum canis*. In *M. canis* infections, the spores are distributed in a sheathlike fashion around the hair shaft (ectothrix infection), whereas *T. tonsurans* produces an infection within the hair shaft (endothrix). Endothrix infections such as those caused by *T. tonsurans* can create a pattern known as "black dot ringworm," characterized by multiple, small, circular patches of alopecia in which hairs are broken off close to the hair follicle. Another clinical variant presents with diffuse scaling and minimal hair loss secondary to traction. A severe inflammatory response produces elevated, boggy, granulomatous masses (kerions), which are often studded with sterile pustules. Permanent scarring and alopecia may result.

In *Microsporum*-infected lesions, a characteristic bright green fluorescence is seen at the base of each hair on examination with the Wood lamp, whereas lesions caused by *T. tonsurans* fail to fluoresce. Microscopic examination of a KOH preparation of infected hair from the active border of a lesion discloses tiny spores surrounding the hair shaft in *Microsporum* infections and chains of spores within the hair shaft in *T. tonsurans* infections. Fungal culture is the most reliable method for diagnosis of tinea capitis. A specific causal diagnosis of tinea capitis may be obtained by planting broken-off infected hairs on Sabouraud's dextrose agar; growth of the dermatophyte may take 2 weeks or more.

Oral administration of griseofulvin microcrystalline is recommended for all forms of tinea capitis. Treatment may be necessary for 8 to 12 weeks or more and should be terminated only after fungal culture shows negative results. Itraconazole or terbinafine are useful in instances of griseofulvin resistance, intolerance, or allergy. Adult household contacts of infected children may be asymptomatic carriers and should be treated with ketoconazole shampoo daily until the infected child is clear clinically.

Tinea Corporis

Dermatophyte infection of the glabrous skin, excluding the palms, soles, and groin, can be caused by most of the dermatophyte species, although *Trichophyton rubrum* and *Trichophyton mentagrophytes* are the most prevalent causal organisms.

The most typical clinical lesion begins as a dry, mildly erythematous, elevated, scaly papule or plaque. The lesion spreads centrifugally as it clears centrally to form the characteristic annular lesion recognized as "ringworm." Some lesions may contain grouped pustules. Most lesions clear spontaneously within several months, but some become chronic.

Microscopic examination of KOH wet mount preparations and cultures should always be obtained when fungal infection is considered.

Tinea corporis usually responds to treatment with a topical antifungal agent in the imidazole or allylamine families, or cyclopirox olamine twice daily for 2 to 4 weeks. Itraconazole or terbinafine have produced excellent results, in many cases with a relatively short 1- to 2-week course of therapy.

Tinea Cruris

Dermatophyte infection of the groin occurs most often in adolescent boys and men and is usually caused by infection with *Epidermophyton floccosum* or *T. rubrum*, but occasionally by *T. mentagrophytes*.

The initial lesion is a small, raised, scaly, erythematous patch on the inner aspect of the thigh, which spreads peripherally, often developing multiple tiny vesicles at the advancing margin. It eventually forms bilateral, irregular, sharply bordered patches with hyperpigmented, scaly centers. In some cases, the infection may spread beyond the crural region. The penis is usually not involved in the infection, which is an important sign differentiating it from *Candida* infection. Pruritus may be severe initially but abates as the inflammatory reaction subsides. Bacterial superinfection must be excluded when there is a severe inflammatory reaction. *Tinea cruris* is more prevalent in obese people and in those who perspire excessively and wear tight-fitting clothing.

The patient should be advised to wear loose cotton underwear. Topical therapy with an imidazole or allylamine antifungal agent is recommended for severe infection, especially because these agents are effective in mixed candidal–dermatophytic infections. Pure dermatophytic infection may also be treated with tolnaftate.

Tinea Pedis

Dermatophyte infection of the toe webs and soles of the feet is caused primarily by *T. rubrum, T. mentagrophytes,* and *E. floccosum*. Most commonly, the lateral toe webs (third/fourth and fourth/fifth interdigital spaces) and the subdigital crevice are fissured, and the surrounding skin is macerated. Severe tenderness, itching, and a persistent foul odor are characteristic. Chronic infection is multifactorial, and involves overgrowth of bacterial flora, including *Micrococcus sedantarius, Brevibacterium epidermidis,* and gram-negative organisms. Diffuse hyperkeratosis and mild erythema of the soles of both feet and the palm of one hand is more refractory to treatment and tends to recur. A number of factors, such as occlusive footwear and warm, humid weather, predispose to infection. Tinea pedis may be transmitted in shower facilities and swimming pool areas.

Occasionally, a secondary skin eruption, referred to as a *dermatophytid* or "id" reaction appears in sensitized people and has been attributed to circulating fungal antigens derived from the primary infection. The eruption occurs most frequently on the extremities, especially the lower legs, and is characterized by grouped papules and vesicles and occasionally by sterile pustules. Id reactions are most often associated with tinea pedis but also occur with tinea capitis.

Simple measures such as avoidance of occlusive footwear, careful drying between the toes after bathing, and the use of an absorbent antifungal powder may suffice for management of milder infections. Topical antifungal therapy is curative in most cases. Several weeks of therapy may be necessary; low-grade, chronic infections, particularly those caused by *T. rubrum*, may be refractory. In such patients, oral itraconazole or terbinafine therapy may effect a cure, but recurrences are common.

Tinea Unguium

Dermatophyte infection of the nail plate occurs most often in people with tinea pedis but may occur as a primary infection. It can be caused by a number of dermatophytes, of which *T. rubrum* and *T. mentagrophytes* are the most common. The most superficial form of tinea unguium (white superficial onychomycosis) is often caused by *T. mentagrophytes* infection; it is manifested by irregular, single or multiple white patches on the surface of the nail unassociated with paronychial inflammation or deep infection. More commonly, *T. rubrum* causes a more invasive, subungual infection (distal subungual onychomycosis) that is initiated at the lateral distal margins of the nail and often preceded by mild paronychia. The nail initially develops a yellowish discoloration and slowly becomes thickened, brittle, and loosened from the nail bed.

Subungual debris and thin shavings of the infected nail should be examined microscopically with KOH and cultured. Repeated attempts may be required to demonstrate the fungus.

The long half-life of itraconazole in the nail has led to promising trials of intermittent short courses of therapy such as 400 mg per day, 1 week per month for 2 to 4 months.

■ CANDIDAL INFECTIONS

Candida albicans is not a member of the normal skin flora, but may colonize the skin, as well as the alimentary tract and the vagina as a saprophytic organism. Certain environmental conditions, notably elevated temperature and humidity, are associated with an increased colonization of the skin. Many bacterial species inhibit the growth of *C. albicans,* and alteration of the normal flora by use of antibiotics may promote overgrowth of the yeast.

INTERTRIGINOUS CANDIDOSIS

Intertriginous candidosis occurs most often in the axillae and the groin, under the breasts, under pendulous abdominal fat folds, in the umbilicus, and in the gluteal cleft. Typical lesions are confluent, moist, denuded, erythematous plaques with an irregular, macerated border. Satellite lesions are characteristic and consist of small vesicles or pustules on an erythematous base. With time, intertriginous candidal lesions may become lichenified, dry, scaly plaques. The lesions develop on skin subjected to irritation and maceration. Candidal superinfection is more likely to occur under conditions that lead to excessive perspiration, especially in the obese and in those with underlying disorders such as diabetes mellitus.

Interdigital candidosis commonly presents with fissures between the fingers of people whose hands are constantly immersed in water. Similar lesions between the toes may be secondary to occlusive footgear.

PERIANAL CANDIDOSIS

Perianal dermatitis is caused by irritation of the skin from occlusion, constant moisture, and poor hygiene. Superinfection may occur with *C. albicans,* especially in those who are receiving oral antibiotic or corticosteroid medication. The involved skin becomes erythematous, macerated, and excoriated, as with candidal intertrigo. Application of a topical antifungal agent (e.g., imidazole, allylamine, cyclopirox olamine, polyene) in conjunction with improved hygiene is usually effective for treatment of intertriginous or perianal candidosis.

CANDIDAL PARONYCHIA

Candidal paronychia is characterized by tenderness, erythema, and edema at the posterior nail fold. Purulent material is discharged occasionally. If the lesion becomes chronic, the nail may be invaded secondarily and become brittle and thickened, initially in the proximal portion but subsequently over the entire nail plate. The nail may manifest a brownish discoloration and prominent transverse ridges or grooves, or it may be completely destroyed. Associated infection with *Pseudomonas* species imparts a green color to the nail plate.

C. albicans can usually be cultured from the posterior nail fold and can often be identified on a KOH preparation of nail scrapings. Effective management includes keeping the finger as dry as possible and applying a topical antifungal agent three times daily for weeks to months until the nail plate grows out normally.

BIBLIOGRAPHY

Darmstadt GL. Oral antibiotic therapy for uncomplicated bacterial skin infections in children. *Pediatr Infect Dis J* 1997;16:227–240.

Darmstadt GL, Lane AT. Impetigo: an overview. *Pediatr Dermatol* 1994; 11:293–303.

Degreef HJ, DeDoncker PRG. Current therapy of dermatophytosis. *J Am Acad Dermatol* 1994;31:S25–S30.

Faergemann J. Pityrosporum infections. *J Am Acad Dermatol* 1994;31: S18–S20.

Frieden IJ, Howard R. Tinea capitis: epidemiology, diagnosis, treatment, and control. *J Am Acad Dermatol* 1994;31:S42–S46.

Kaaman T, Torssander J. Dermatophytid: a misdiagnosed entity? *Acta Derm Venereol (Stockh)* 1983;63:404–408.

Odom R. Pathophysiology of dermatophyte infections. *J Am Acad Dermatol* 1993;5:S2–S7.

Rezabek GH, Friedman AD. Superficial fungal infections of the skin: diagnosis and current treatment recommendations. *Drugs* 1992;43: 674–682.

Roth RR, James WD. Microbiology of the skin: resident flora, ecology, infection. *J Am Acad Dermatol* 1989;20:367–390.

Kelley's Textbook of Internal Medicine, fourth edition. Edited by H. David Humes. Lippincott Williams & Wilkins, Philadelphia © 2000.

CHAPTER 195

BULLOUS DISEASES OF SKIN AND MUCOUS MEMBRANES

MARK C. UDEY

Bullous diseases of skin and mucous membranes, although uncommon, are particularly significant because patients with these disorders may experience considerable morbidity from the disease process itself or as a consequence of therapy. These conditions are characterized by clinically apparent vesicles, bullae (blisters), erosions, or crusts when lesions are present on skin, and erosions when lesions are present on mucous membranes. In considering bullous diseases, it is useful to differentiate between the rare, inherited, noninflammatory mechanobullous diseases that are seen at birth or early in life (termed *epidermolysis bullosa*) and the more common, acquired, immune-mediated blistering disorders that form the basis for the discussion in this chapter. Disorders typified by microscopic (often subclinical) intraepidermal vesicles are termed "eczema" (or dermatitis) and are considered in other chapters.

■ PEMPHIGUS

The term "pemphigus" refers to several disorders that result from decreased adhesion between keratinocytes. Lesions of pemphigus vulgaris result because suprabasal keratinocytes fail to adhere to basal cells (keratinocytes that are anchored to the epidermal basement membrane) and to each other. In contrast, pemphigus foliaceus is a manifestation of the failure of the most superficial keratinocytes (cells of the granular layer) to adhere to underlying suprabasal cells. Lesions of paraneoplastic pemphigus may reflect more complex adhesive defects. Pemphigus vulgaris is an unremitting disease characterized by erosive lesions of oral and other mucous membranes, and blisters and erosions on skin. Pemphigus foliaceus is characterized by crusted lesions and rarely involves mucous membranes. Paraneoplastic pemphigus is characterized by severe stomatitis, conjunctival erosions, and polymorphic skin lesions and occurs in patients with known (usually lymphoid) neoplasms. These disorders are important to recognize because they cause significant morbidity and mortality. Before the use of glucocorticoids, pemphigus vulgaris was frequently a fatal disease. Patients with paraneoplastic pemphigus rarely recover despite aggressive therapy.

ETIOLOGY AND PATHOGENESIS

The cause of pemphigus is unknown. In the case of pemphigus vulgaris, genetic predisposition may be an important causal factor. Pemphigus vulgaris (but not pemphigus foliaceus) is more common among people of Jewish or Mediterranean descent. Among patients with pemphigus vulgaris, the frequency of human leukocyte antigen (HLA)-DR4 and DRw6 haplotypes is markedly increased. Furthermore, essentially all patients with the DR4 haplotype share a rare allele (DRB1*0402) that encodes the β chain of one of the HLA-DR antigens. Similarly, patients with the DRw6 haplotype share an allele (DQB1*0503) that encodes a β chain of HLA-DQ antigens. Although genetic predisposition is not known to play a role in the pathogenesis of pemphigus foliaceus, one form (fogo selvagem or "wild fire") is endemic in inland river valleys of rural Brazil, where an arthropod has been implicated as a vector (an agent that predisposes to development of disease) in transmission of disease. Paraneoplastic pemphigus may develop as a consequence of cancer-associated immune dysregulation.

Lesions of pemphigus vulgaris, pemphigus foliaceus, and paraneoplastic pemphigus are caused by IgG antibodies that react with adhesion molecules called *desmogleins*. These cadherin-like transmembrane glycoproteins localize in desmosomes of stratified squamous epithelial cells, where they likely constitute an important adhesive mechanism. Antibody titers may correlate with disease activity in individual patients. Anti-desmoglein 1 antibodies in sera of patients with pemphigus foliaceus and anti-desmoglein 3 antibodies in patients with pemphigus vulgaris and paraneoplastic pemphigus cause blisters after adoptive transfer into newborn mice. Pemphigus vulgaris sera often also contain anti-desmoglein 1 antibodies, but these antibodies do not cause lesions in adoptive transfer studies. Pemphigus has also been described in neonatal children born to mothers with pemphigus as a result of passive transfer of pathogenic autoantibodies in utero. In this setting, the disease improves with disappearance of the maternally derived autoantibodies in the postnatal period. Some desmoglein 3–derived peptides that stimulate T-cell clones expanded from the peripheral blood of pemphigus vulgaris patients bind specifically to major histocompatibility complex (MHC) class II antigens encoded by the genes that appear to predispose to development of disease. Patients with paraneoplastic pemphigus have circulating antibodies that react with several members of the plakin family of desmosomal plaque proteins as well as desmoglein 3. The multiple reactivities present in the sera of these patients may contribute to the morphologic variation in paraneoplastic pemphigus lesions.

INCIDENCE AND EPIDEMIOLOGY

Sporadic pemphigus is an uncommon disease primarily of middle-aged and elderly people, although younger people can also be affected. Among Jews, pemphigus vulgaris is more common than pemphigus foliaceus. Pemphigus vulgaris and foliaceus are similarly infrequent in non-Jewish populations. In contrast to sporadic disease, endemic pemphigus foliaceus (fogo selvagem) frequently affects children and adolescents. Pemphigus foliaceus has been reported with increased frequency in patients treated with penicillamine, captopril, and structurally related drugs, and a number of patients with pemphigus foliaceus and thymic abnormalities (including thymoma) have been described. Paraneoplastic pemphigus is a rare disorder, which usually develops in association with lymphoid neoplasms.

CLINICAL FINDINGS

Generalized blisters and erosions are the clinical hallmarks of pemphigus. Considerable burning and pain may be present in lesional skin. Cutaneous pemphigus lesions may manifest as vesicles, blisters, erosions, or crusts. Patients with pemphigus vulgaris commonly present with oral erosions, and almost all patients have oral lesions at some time during the course of their disease. Conjunctivae, genital mucosae, and the esophagus may also be involved. In contrast, mucosal lesions are uncommon in pemphigus foliaceus. Cutaneous lesions of pemphigus vulgaris are typically erosive. When present, blisters do not have a prominent inflammatory component, may be flaccid, and are fragile. During periods of disease activity, blisters may be extended with gentle lateral traction (positive Nikolsky's sign). The scalp represents an area of common involvement in pemphigus vulgaris, but lesions are often present on the trunk and extremities. Scalp lesions and lesions in intertriginous areas may have a vegetative appearance. Mucosal predominant disease apparently occurs in patients with only anti-desmoglein 3 antibodies, whereas patients with mucosal and skin lesions produce antibodies reactive with desmoglein 1 and desmoglein 3. Cutaneous lesions of pemphigus foliaceus are more crusted than those of pemphigus vulgaris and intact blisters may be infrequent. Lesions of pemphigus foliaceus commonly are present in a seborrheic distribution (central chest, back, and face) and may remain localized for years. Mucosal lesions are rarely seen.

The differential diagnosis of pemphigus vulgaris includes other immune-mediated blistering diseases such as pemphigus foliaceus, bullous pemphigoid, erythema multiforme (Stevens–Johnson syndrome), drug eruptions, and other less common diseases. The differential diagnosis of pemphigus foliaceus includes pemphigus vulgaris, impetigo, and other bullous and pustular diseases. Patients with paraneoplastic pemphigus exhibit painful, recalcitrant erosions of oral and other mucous membranes and polymorphic cutaneous lesions. Cutaneous lesions of paraneoplastic pemphigus may resemble those of sporadic pemphigus, erythema multiforme, or even papulosquamous disorders.

LABORATORY FINDINGS

Laboratory features of pemphigus are distinctive. Routine histopathologic sections of biopsy specimens obtained from lesional skin reveal an intraepidermal separation immediately above the basal keratinocyte layer (suprabasal cleft formation) without evidence of abnormal keratinocyte differentiation in the case of pemphigus vulgaris, and a subcorneal cleft in the case of pemphigus foliaceus. Biopsies from patients with paraneoplastic pemphigus show intraepidermal separations and prominent, often lichenoid, inflammation in the dermis.

The histopathologic diagnosis of pemphigus should be confirmed by searching for immunoreactants in the skin and sera. Most patients have deposits of IgG on the surfaces of keratinocytes in perilesional as well as nonlesional skin. In addition, circulating autoantibodies can be detected and quantitated. Pemphigus vulgaris and pemphigus foliaceus autoantibodies cannot be differentiated with certainty by indirect immunofluorescence. Sera from patients with paraneoplastic pemphigus react with keratinocytes and also desmosomes in other tissues (such as rodent urinary bladder epithelia).

OPTIMAL MANAGEMENT

Without therapy, pemphigus vulgaris is a progressive, life-threatening disease. Extensive oral lesions may preclude adequate caloric intake, and widespread cutaneous lesions predispose to sepsis. The diagnosis of pemphigus foliaceus portends a somewhat better prognosis, although extensive untreated disease can also be fatal. Paraneoplastic pemphigus is resistant to therapy. Systemic glucocorticoid therapy is the mainstay of treatment for pemphigus. Prednisone (0.5 to 2 mg per kilogram per day) is used to achieve control, although higher doses may be required. The initial goal of therapy is to suppress the formation of new lesions. After control has been achieved, prednisone doses are decreased as the disease activity permits. Alternate-day dosing with prednisone is preferred if control can be maintained. Drugs such as azathioprine and cyclophosphamide are frequently used as steroid-sparing agents, especially in elderly patients with intercurrent medical problems. Mycophenolate mofetil has recently been reported to be efficacious, and other drugs such as gold salts and cyclosporine (and related agents) may also have a role. Plasmapheresis in conjunction with glucocorticoid and immunosuppressive therapy has been used in the treatment of patients with severe disease. Remissions can occur, but are not the rule. Topical or intralesional glucocorticoids may be of benefit in the treatment of pemphigus foliaceus if disease is localized.

■ BULLOUS PEMPHIGOID

Bullous pemphigoid is an uncommon disease of elderly people characterized by tense blisters and vesicles with a prominent inflammatory component. Pruritus is a common manifestation of active disease; mucous membrane involvement is not. Lesions result because basal keratinocytes fail to adhere to the epidermal basement membrane. In otherwise healthy patients, bullous pemphigoid is not a life-threatening disease.

ETIOLOGY AND PATHOGENESIS

The cause of bullous pemphigoid is unknown, but the pathogenesis of lesion development is relatively well understood. Sera from patients with bullous pemphigoid contain IgG autoantibodies that commonly react with a hemidesmosomal component (the 230-kd bullous pemphigoid antigen; BPAG1) that is homologous to desmoplakin, an intracellular component of desmosomes. Many sera also react with a transmembrane protein that has homology to collagen (the 180-kd bullous pemphigoid antigen; BPAG2; type XVII collagen). In neonatal mice, rabbit antimurine BPAG2 antibodies cause lesions similar to those that occur in patients with pemphigoid. The matrix metalloproteinase gelatinase B (MMP-9) also appears to play a role in lesion formation in this experimental model. Complement components are universally present in the perilesional skin of bullous pemphigoid patients, and complement-dependent recruitment of neutrophils into lesional skin is required for blister formation in the bullous pemphigoid mouse model.

CLINICAL FINDINGS

Characteristic lesions of bullous pemphigoid are tense blisters or vesicles with surrounding erythema. Early lesions may resemble urticaria; late lesions may manifest as erosions. Common sites of involvement include the trunk and flexor surfaces of extremities. Lesions are localized to the legs in some patients. A few patients have oral erosions at some time during the course of their disease. Pruritus is a common feature of bullous pemphigoid, and increased pruritus may herald an exacerbation. It is important to differentiate bullous pemphigoid from cicatricial pemphigoid. Although skin lesions may be indistinguishable, cicatricial pemphigoid is a mucosal-predominant disease characterized by desquamative gingivitis (marginal gingival erosions) and frequent conjunctival erosions that may result in scarring and blindness. Acquired epidermolysis bullosa can mimic bullous pemphigoid as well as cicatricial pemphigoid. Several common disorders that must be distinguished from bullous pemphigoid include erythema multiforme, drug eruptions, and acute contact dermatitis. Linear IgA bullous dermatosis is less common and can be distinguished from bullous pemphigoid on the basis of immunofluorescence studies. Herpes gestationis is a rare bullous disease of pregnant and postpartum women that is a variant of bullous pemphigoid.

LABORATORY FINDINGS

Biopsy of a newly formed vesicle or blister reveals a subepidermal separation with a prominent underlying polymorphous inflammatory infiltrate that is often eosinophil-rich. The blister fluid itself may also contain inflammatory cells (including eosinophils). Immunoreactants (including complement components and, in most cases, IgG) are present in a linear pattern along the basement membrane of perilesional skin, and most patients also have circulating autoantibodies. The sensitivity of indirect immunofluorescence testing can be increased if NaCl-split human skin, in which an epidermal–dermal separation is induced, is used as the substrate. Cicatricial pemphigoid, acquired epidermolysis bullosa, and linear IgA bullous dermatosis all can be differentiated from bullous pemphigoid using clinical criteria in conjunction with a combination of these techniques. Autoantibody titer does not correlate well with disease activity in patients with bullous pemphigoid.

OPTIMAL MANAGEMENT

Although bullous pemphigoid may remit, most patients are affected for several years or longer. Topical fluorinated glucocorticoids are not usually of benefit in the treatment of bullous pemphigoid unless disease is localized. Most patients respond well to prednisone, 0.5 to 1.5 mg per kilogram per day. However, because patients are often elderly and may have intercurrent medical illnesses, unwanted side effects of systemic corticosteroid therapy are a serious problem. Azathioprine and cyclophosphamide are commonly used as steroid-sparing agents. Dapsone may also be of benefit in some patients. Therapy with broad-spectrum antibiotics (including tetracycline and erythromycin) or niacinamide may be helpful. In most patients, bullous pemphigoid is not a life-threatening disease. Thus, it is important to minimize the side effects of systemic immunosuppressive therapy.

■ DERMATITIS HERPETIFORMIS

Dermatitis herpetiformis is an uncommon chronic disease typified by the appearance of intensely pruritic vesicles on extensor surfaces of the extremities, sacrum, buttocks, back, and neck. It affects men and women with equal frequency and is rare in blacks.

ETIOLOGY AND PATHOGENESIS

The cause of dermatitis herpetiformis is unknown, and the pathogenesis of lesion formation is not well understood. Focal collections of IgA and complement can almost always be demonstrated at the tips of dermal papillae in involved as well as uninvolved skin, but the role that these immunoreactants play in lesion development is unknown. Most patients with dermatitis herpetiformis have subclinical gluten-sensitive enteropathy that can be demonstrated by small-bowel biopsy. In addition, patients who can adhere to a strict gluten-free diet often experience amelioration of their cutaneous symptoms. HLA-B8, HLA-DR3, and HLA-DQw2 antigens are present in 80% to 90% of patients with dermatitis herpetiformis. Dermatitis herpetiformis may represent a cutaneous manifestation of an IgA-predominant immune response directed at antigens encountered in the gastrointestinal tract of genetically predisposed people.

CLINICAL FINDINGS

Dermatitis herpetiformis is a distinctive disorder characterized by frequently excoriated, intensely pruritic papules and vesicles on the elbows, knees, scalp, back, sacrum, and buttocks. Lesions may occur individually or in groups. It frequently presents in young and middle-aged adults, but children may also be affected. The differential diagnosis of dermatitis herpetiformis includes scabies, acute eczematous dermatitis, erythema multiforme, pemphigoid, and linear IgA bullous dermatosis. Although subclinical gluten-sensitive enteropathy is almost universally present, symptomatic gastrointestinal disease is uncommon.

LABORATORY FINDINGS

Biopsies of early lesions reveal collections of neutrophils in the tips of dermal papillae with subepidermal cleft formation, and perivascular lymphohistiocytic inflammation in the dermis. Late lesions reveal more extensive subepidermal separation and may be difficult to differentiate from linear IgA bullous dermatosis, bullous pemphigoid, and acquired epidermolysis bullosa. Direct immunofluorescence testing of perilesional or normal skin is diagnostic and shows deposition of IgA and complement components in a granular pattern in the tips of dermal papillae. Circulating immunoreactants are not routinely detected.

OPTIMAL MANAGEMENT

Although dermatitis herpetiformis is a chronic disease with a remitting and relapsing course, the prognosis is excellent. Therapy with dapsone and related drugs has a uniquely favorable effect on the disease course. Institution of dapsone (100 to 150 mg per day) often results in cessation of lesion formation and decreased pruritus in less than 24 hours. Patients who adhere to a strict gluten-free diet often require lower doses of medication or may not need drug therapy at all. Nonsteroidal anti-inflammatory drugs may exacerbate dermatitis herpetiformis.

BIBLIOGRAPHY

Anhalt GJ. Paraneoplastic pemphigus. *Adv Dermatol* 1997;12:77–97.
Lin MS, Mascaro JM, Liu Z, et al. The desmosome and hemidesmosome in cutaneous autoimmunity. *Clin Exp Immunol* 1997;107(Suppl 1): 9–15.
Katz SI. Dermatitis herpetiformis. In: Freedberg IM, Eisen AZ, Wolff K, et al, eds. *Dermatology in general medicine.* New York: McGraw-Hill, 1999:709–715.
Katz SI. Herpes gestationis (pemphigoid gestationis). In: Freedberg IM, Eisen AZ, Wolff K, et al, eds. *Dermatology in general medicine.* New York: McGraw-Hill, 1999:686–689.
Stanley JR. Bullous pemphigoid. In: Freedberg IM, Eisen AZ, Wolff K, et al, eds. *Dermatology in general medicine.* New York: McGraw-Hill, 1999: 666–673.
Stanley JR. Pemphigus. In: Freedberg IM, Eisen AZ, Wolff K, et al, eds. *Dermatology in general medicine.* New York: McGraw-Hill, 1999:654.
Udey MC, Stanley JR. Pemphigus: diseases of anti-desmosomal autoimmunity. *JAMA* 1999;282:572–576.
Yancey KB. Cicatricial pemphigoid. In: Freedberg IM, Eisen AZ, Wolff

K, Austen KF, Goldsmith LA, Katz SI, et al, eds. *Dermatology in general medicine.* New York: McGraw-Hill, 1999:674–679.

Kelley's Textbook of Internal Medicine, fourth edition. Edited by H. David Humes. Lippincott Williams & Wilkins, Philadelphia © 2000.

CHAPTER

196

ATOPIC AND CONTACT DERMATITIS

TERESA A. BORKOWSKI
MARK C. UDEY

ATOPIC DERMATITIS

Atopic dermatitis is a chronic, relapsing, inflammatory dermatosis with lesions characterized by pruritus, erythema, and lichenification. It occurs most frequently in patients with a personal or family history of allergic disease and comprises one leg of the atopic triad (asthma, allergic rhinoconjunctivitis, and atopic dermatitis).

INCIDENCE AND EPIDEMIOLOGY

Atopic dermatitis affects 5% to 10% of children and is slightly more prevalent in boys than girls (1.2:1). There is no racial predisposition to atopic dermatitis within a geographic area. Approximately 60% of patients experience onset of symptoms within the first year of life, and 85% have disease symptoms by 5 years of age. The onset of atopic dermatitis in late adulthood is unusual.

ETIOLOGY AND PATHOGENESIS

Atopic dermatitis is a familial and, most likely, polygenic disease. Although the cause is unknown, the frequent coincidence of atopic dermatitis and allergic rhinitis or asthma suggests that IgE-mediated hypersensitivity may be involved in disease pathogenesis. Approximately two-thirds of patients have a family or personal history of asthma or allergic rhinitis, and 80% have elevated levels of serum IgE that may correlate with disease activity. In some pediatric patients, food allergens reproducibly induce acute pruritus in lesional skin. Atopy has been linked to polymorphisms in genes encoding the high-affinity IgE and β_2-adrenergic receptors, as well as interleukin-4 (IL-4) gene regulatory regions.

Studies of immunologic abnormalities in atopic dermatitis may provide insight into disease pathogenesis. Cutaneous immune responses to environmental antigens are Th2 (IL-4–secreting T cell) predominant in atopic skin, and responses to infectious agents are blunted during periods of disease activity. Epicutaneous patch tests to allergens frequently show increased numbers of allergen-specific (Th2 cells) in atopic dermatitis patients. IL-4 enhances IgE production and suppresses production of the Th1 cytokine interferon (IFN)-γ. A relative deficiency in Th1 immunity may account for the attenuated delayed type hypersensitivity responses to contact and viral antigens that are characteristic of atopic dermatitis and may explain the increased susceptibility of patients to cutaneous viral infections such as herpes simplex and molluscum contagiosum.

Aberrant immune responses could reflect abnormalities in T cells or antigen-presenting cells. Atopic epidermal Langerhans' cells (members of the dendritic cell lineage) express high levels of the high-affinity IgE receptor and may play a role in the initiation (or perpetuation) of Th2-predominant responses to allergens. Excessive production of prostaglandin E_2 (PGE_2) by atopic monocytes may also foster Th2 responses by inhibiting IFN-γ production.

CLINICAL FINDINGS

The most consistent feature of atopic dermatitis is pruritus, often accompanied by generalized xerosis (dry skin). Acute skin lesions are erythematous patches and papules, often with excoriation, vesiculation, and crusting. With persistent scratching, acute lesions evolve into lichenified patches that are characteristic of chronic atopic dermatitis. Papulovesicular and lichenified lesions may be present in the same patient. Atopic dermatitis typically involves the flexural areas of the extremities and neck in older children and adults. Extensor surfaces of the extremities are more frequently involved in 2- to 10-year-old children, and infants often develop lesions on the cheeks, scalp, and buttocks. In severe cases, involvement may be generalized, resulting in exfoliative erythroderma. The clinical course is chronic with periodic exacerbations and remissions. Most patients experience a decrease in disease severity by adulthood.

Associated clinical features include Dennie–Morgan folds (transverse creases below the lower eyelids), hyperlinear palms, and keratosis pilaris (keratotic follicular papules on the extensor surfaces of arms and legs). Patients with severe atopic dermatitis may be at increased risk for cataracts.

Infection with *Staphylococcus* aureus is a common complication of atopic dermatitis, and disease exacerbation may result. Impetiginized lesions manifest as crusting and sometimes vesiculation. Crusting and vesiculation in a patient with atopic dermatitis may also result from herpes simplex infection. Patients with severe atopic dermatitis are predisposed to generalized herpes simplex (eczema herpeticum or Kaposi's varicelliform eruption). Patients may present with malaise, fever and lymphadenopathy, and disseminated papulovesicular (or papulopustular) lesions that may become hemorrhagic or evolve into painful punched-out erosions. Secondary bacterial infection is common. Eczema herpeticum is a potentially life-threatening complication of atopic dermatitis and warrants immediate treatment with antiviral and antibacterial agents. Concern regarding the possibility of ocular involvement should prompt immediate evaluation by an ophthalmologist.

LABORATORY FINDINGS

No serologic tests are diagnostic of atopic dermatitis. However, 80% of patients exhibit elevated levels of serum IgE. Skin and radioallergosorbent tests are often positive but may not correlate with clinical symptoms. Skin biopsies of acute lesions of atopic dermatitis display epidermal hyperplasia, microvesicles and intracellular edema, and a primarily dermal mononuclear cell infiltrate comprising lymphocytes, monocytes, and macrophages with occasional neutrophils or eosinophils. Chronic lesions show hyperkeratosis with variable intracellular edema and a mononuclear cell infiltrate. Chronic lesions may also contain increased numbers of mast cells.

OPTIMAL MANAGEMENT

Adequate skin hydration is an essential component of therapeutic regimens for atopic dermatitis, regardless of the severity of the disease. Frequent soaking baths followed by the immediate application of fragrance-free emollients are helpful in most cases. When pruritus is moderate to severe or interrupts sleep, oral antihistamines may be necessary. Topical corticosteroids are indicated when inflammation is present. In general, the least potent effective topical corticosteroid should be used, and potency or total dose should be tapered as soon as possible to prevent cutaneous thinning secondary to chronic use. Absorption may lead to systemic side effects in young children treated with potent topical corticosteroids and in older persons with extensive involvement. Application of potent topical corticosteroids to facial or periorbital skin may predispose to cataract formation. Flare-ups of atopic dermatitis are often associated with secondary *S. aureus* infections, and appropriate antibiotic therapy is usually efficacious.

During severe flare-ups of atopic dermatitis, oral corticosteroid therapy may be warranted. Systemic corticosteroids should be used judiciously, however, because prolonged remissions will not result and an alternative chronic therapy with its attendant side effects will be required. Ultraviolet light therapy, methotrexate, cyclosporine, and azathioprine may be useful for difficult-to-treat patients. Investigational drugs include IFN-γ and phosphodiesterase inhibitors. Children (not adults) may benefit from evaluation for food and inhalant allergies.

■ CONTACT DERMATITIS

Contact dermatitis is an eczematous dermatitis that develops as a consequence of exposure to an external and usually noninfectious agent. Two varieties of contact dermatitis exist: primary irritant dermatitis, which is not immunologically mediated and occurs in almost all who are exposed, and allergic contact dermatitis, which is antigen-specific and occurs only in those who have been previously sensitized.

ETIOLOGY AND PATHOGENESIS

Primary irritant dermatitis results when substances disrupt the barrier function of the stratum corneum and elicit cutaneous inflammatory responses by causing injury to underlying epidermal and perhaps dermal constituents. Irritant responses can be induced in most people, but the threshold for injury may vary considerably. Examples of common irritants include acids, alkalis, detergents, and organic solvents. In contrast, allergic contact dermatitis develops only in those who have been exposed and become sensitized to a particular agent, and then only after reexposure.

Allergic contact dermatitis is a clinically important example of a delayed-type hypersensitivity phenomenon. The events leading to development of allergic contact dermatitis can be divided into the sensitization and elicitation phases. The process begins when antigen penetrates the stratum corneum and encounters resident Langerhans' cells or similar dendritic cells in the dermis. After an incompletely understood activation process, these class II major histocompatibility complex antigen-bearing cells migrate to regional lymph nodes, where the initial presentation of antigen to T cells probably occurs. After clonal expansion and differentiation, some antigen-specific memory T cells circulate systemically. During subsequent exposure to antigen, antigen associated with epidermal cells (including Langerhans' cells and perhaps keratinocytes) is presented locally to sensitized T cells, evoking proinflammatory cytokine release and perhaps T-cell proliferation within the skin. Antigen-nonspecific elements (macrophages, other lymphocytes, and perhaps basophils, mast cells, and eosinophils) are also recruited to the involved area by cytokines and chemoattractants to participate in the inflammatory response.

Primary irritant dermatitis, which is extremely common, often results from the improper or excessive use of detergents or organic solvents. True allergic contact dermatitis, although seen less frequently, is also common. Frequent contact sensitizers include *Rhus* antigen (a pentadecylcatechol found in poison ivy, oak, and sumac), para-phenylenediamine, nickel, rubber compounds, ethylenediamine, certain local anesthetics (such as benzocaine), chromate, and neomycin.

CLINICAL FINDINGS

The typical primary lesions of acute allergic contact dermatitis are papulovesicles with surrounding erythema, often occurring in linear patterns as a result of direct exposure to antigen. Weeping and crusted lesions develop and may become secondarily infected. Lesions of chronic contact dermatitis exhibit prominent scaling and lichenification.

The most helpful features in determining the cause of contact dermatitis are patient history and physical examination. For example, nickel dermatitis is commonly seen in areas where metal and skin are apposed (e.g., in association with snaps, buckles, watchbands, and earrings). Beauticians with hand dermatitis may be sensitive to para-phenylenediamine in hair dyes. This chemical, which is also used in leather processing, photographic work, and rubber manufacture, cross-reacts with azo- and aniline dyes, printing inks, and several medications, including benzocaine, procaine, para-aminobenzoic acid, hydrochlorthiazide, and sulfonamides. An eczematous dermatitis involving exclusively the waistline or the dorsum of the feet suggests rubber sensitivity. Chromates used in cement may cause contact dermatitis of the dorsa of the hands in construction workers but spare the feet, particularly in workers who wear impermeable protective boots.

LABORATORY FINDINGS

The closed patch test is most commonly used to identify the allergen in allergic contact dermatitis. A nonirritating concentration of the compound is applied to the patient's skin in an area with no preexisting dermatitis. The test material is then covered by an occlusive dressing for 48 hours, after which the dressing and the compound are removed and the skin examined for redness, edema, and vesicles. In every case, the reaction caused by the test substance should be compared with that elicited by vehicle alone. Patch test results are most useful when they are obtained under standard conditions, replicated, and interpreted in a clinical context. The most common chemical allergens and the preferred testing concentrations can be found in Fisher's classic text (see Bibliography).

OPTIMAL MANAGEMENT

For localized contact dermatitis, moist compresses and simple drying antipruritic lotions (e.g., calamine lotion) applied several times daily suffice. Potent topical corticosteroids may also decrease pruritus and inflammation. Systemic antihistamines decrease pruritus and may provide symptomatic relief. Topical antihistamines and anesthetics should be avoided because of their sensitizing potential. For widespread contact dermatitis, a short course of systemic corticosteroids should be used. Relatively high doses of prednisone (0.75 to 1.5 mg per kilogram per day) are given initially and then tapered off over 14 days. Severe cases may require a more protracted course, but chronic systemic corticosteroid therapy is inappropriate.

If the substance causing contact dermatitis can be identified, avoidance is the simplest therapy. If the agent is an irritant, reexposure under modified conditions (shorter time, less frequent intervals, or lower concentrations) can sometimes be tolerated. True sensitization to a chemical, however, essentially precludes its use unless exposure areas can be shielded (e.g., with gloves). Barrier creams or ointments usually are not effective.

BIBLIOGRAPHY

Adams RM. Occupational skin disease. In: Freedberg IM, Eisen AZ, Wolff K, et al, eds. *Dermatology in general medicine.* New York: McGraw-Hill, 1999:1609–1632.

Belsito DV. Allergic contact dermatitis. In: Freedberg IM, Eisen AZ, Wolff K, et al, eds. *Dermatology in general medicine.* New York: McGraw-Hill, 1999:1447–1461.

Cooper KD. Atopic dermatitis: recent trends in pathogenesis and therapy. *J Invest Dermatol* 1994;102:128–137.

Fisher AA. *Contact dermatitis,* third ed. Philadelphia: Lea & Febiger, 1986.

Hanifin J, Chan SC. Diagnosis and treatment of atopic dermatitis. *Dermatologic Ther* 1996;1:9–18.

Hebert A, Mays S. Atopic dermatitis of infancy. *Dermatol Ther* 1996;1:61–74.

Leung DYM, Tharp M, Boguniewicz M. Atopic dermatitis (atopic eczema). In: Freedberg IM, Eisen AZ, Wolff K, et al, eds. *Dermatology in general medicine.* New York: McGraw-Hill, 1999:1464–1480.

Reinhold U, Pawelec G, Wehrmann W, et al. Cytokine release from cultured peripheral blood mononuclear cells of patients with severe atopic dermatitis. *Acta Derm Venereol* 1989;69:497–502.

Walley AJ, Cookson WO. Investigation of an interleukin-4 promoter polymorphism for associations with asthma and atopy. *J Med Genet* 1996; 33:689–692.

Kelley's Textbook of Internal Medicine, fourth edition. Edited by H. David Humes.
Lippincott Williams & Wilkins, Philadelphia © 2000.

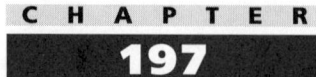

CHAPTER 197

URTICARIA AND ERYTHEMA MULTIFORME

CHRISTOPHER M. BARNARD

URTICARIA AND ANGIOEDEMA

Allergic urticaria and angioedema are manifestations of an immediate hypersensitivity reaction resulting from the antigen-driven release of vasoactive products from IgE-sensitized mast cells (and perhaps basophils). Complement-mediated urticaria, hereditary or acquired, may result from serum complement abnormalities. Identical reactions also can result from direct mast cell degranulation through nonimmunologic mechanisms.

ETIOLOGY AND PATHOGENESIS

A variety of triggering mechanisms can result in mast cell degranulation (Chapter 6). Among these are IgE-mediated immediate hypersensitivity reactions, complement-dependent immune complex–induced release of vasoactive mediators, and release resulting from modulation of arachidonic acid metabolism by certain drugs (aspirin or other nonsteroidal anti-inflammatory agents). Stimuli such as pressure, exercise, and cold also may provoke mast cell degranulation, but a discussion of the physical urticarias is beyond the scope of this chapter.

Allergic urticaria develops only in persons who previously have encountered and formed IgE (reaginic) antibodies directed against the offending antigen (e.g., drug, venom, food). Mast cells and basophils concentrate IgE on their cell surfaces through specific receptors that bind the Fc fragment of IgE with high affinity, becoming sensitized to antigen. When individual IgE molecules are cross-linked on the surface of mast cells by multivalent antigen, a multitude of biochemical events occurs that rapidly culminates in the release of preformed (e.g., histamine) and newly synthesized (e.g., leukotrienes) vasoactive mediators and chemoattractants. Urticarial skin lesions then result from local vasodilatation and extravascular fluid accumulation (edema) with minimal cellular infiltrate.

INCIDENCE AND EPIDEMIOLOGY

Urticaria and angioedema are among the most common skin disorders and occur with the highest incidence in young adults. Although 15% to 20% of the population may have urticaria during their lifetime, it is probable that only a small percentage of this group has true allergic urticaria. Nonimmunologic urticaria is perhaps more common. For example, among agents that directly cause degranulation of mast cells, radiologic contrast media produce urticaria in 5% to 8% of the population, and aspirin, nonsteroidal anti-inflammatory agents, and tartrazine may cause reactions in 1% to 2%.

CLINICAL FEATURES AND LABORATORY FINDINGS

The lesions of urticaria (hives) can be polymorphic. Faintly erythematous well-circumscribed edematous papules (wheals), annular lesions, and polycyclic lesions all are typical (Fig. 197.1). Often, an erythematous halo (flare) surrounds the raised portion of the lesions. Urticarial lesions usually are pruritic and transient, disappearing over a 12- to 24-hour period. Alternatively, an individual lesion may appear to migrate. Persistent urticarial lesions with purpura or residual hyperpigmentation should undergo biopsy to exclude urticarial vasculitis. Angioedema represents a deeper dermal or subcutaneous edematous reaction and may occur with or without urticaria. The face, tongue, and extremities are the most commonly involved areas with angioedema; however, laryngeal edema with respiratory symptoms may occur and require immediate intervention.

Skin biopsy reveals dermal edema and a variable perivascular infiltrate of mononuclear cells and eosinophils. Specific antigen IgE-mediated sensitivity may be revealed by scratch tests, intradermal skin testing, or radioallergosorbent tests (RAST). Patients with chronic urticaria (persisting for 2 to 6 months) should be evaluated not only for allergic problems, such as food, drug, pollen, and insect sting sensitivity, but also for other underlying causes. Some of the more common factors in the last category are occult infection (e.g., dental abscess, sinusitis, helminth infestation); physical urticaria (e.g., pressure, cold, light, cholinergic);

and collagen vascular diseases. The workup should be systematic and complete to avoid repeated partial evaluations.

COURSE, THERAPY, AND PROGNOSIS

Acute urticaria usually resolves in less than 6 weeks. Although identification and elimination of the specific causative agent are desirable, these are not always possible. In about 70% of patients with chronic urticaria, a specific cause cannot be elucidated, and avoidance or elimination of a specific agent is not possible. Antihistamines are useful in the treatment of urticaria, regardless of its duration or cause. Many H_1 antagonists are available, and individual patients may tolerate or respond to certain drugs better than to others. Nonsedating H_1 antagonists, such as cetirizine, loratadine, fexofenadine, or astemizole, may be especially useful as first-line therapy. Concomitant administration of astemizole with erythromycin, ketoconazole, or itraconazole poses a rare, but potential, risk of serious cardiovascular side effects. Cetirizine, a metabolite of hydroxyzine, is a potent, nonsedating, selective H_1 antagonist with a rapid onset of action and the unique ability to inhibit eosinophil chemotaxis. Cetirizine appears to be the most efficacious of the nonsedating histamine H_1 antagonists currently available. An H_1 antagonist in combination with an H_2 antagonist may be efficacious in cases in which the same H_1 antagonist alone has been ineffective. Doxepin, a highly potent H_1 and H_2 antagonist, is a tricyclic antidepressant that is effective in controlling chronic idiopathic urticaria complicated by agitated clinical depression at relatively low doses. The sedating H_1 antihistamines, hydroxyzine and diphenhydramine, are helpful in reducing restlessness and anxiety in addition to controlling urticaria and facilitating sleep at night. Ketotifen, a mast cell stabilizer and H_1 antagonist, is effective in refractory cases of cholinergic urticaria but still awaits approval for use in this country. It is best to continue an effective regimen for 1 or 2 weeks after control has been achieved before decreasing dosages or changing the frequency of administration. Short courses of systemic corticosteroids may be appropriate in severe cases, but the side effects of chronic corticosteroid therapy outweigh the benefits.

ERYTHEMA MULTIFORME: STEVENS–JOHNSON SYNDROME AND TOXIC EPIDERMAL NECROLYSIS

Erythema multiforme is a spectrum of acute, self-limited, cutaneous and mucosal inflammatory syndromes, the hallmark of which is a persistent erythematous, annular, target lesion.

ETIOLOGY AND PATHOGENESIS

A wide variety of agents have been implicated in the cause of erythema multiforme. The most common of these are infections and drugs. Drugs commonly associated with erythema multiforme major and minor include sulfonamides (and sulfonamide derivatives), phenylbutazone, phenytoin, and the penicillin de-

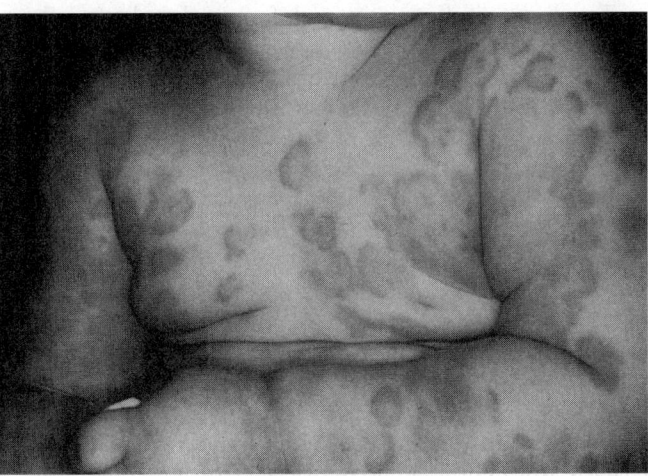

FIGURE 197.1. Urticaria.

rivatives. Two infectious agents, recurrent herpes simplex and *Mycoplasma,* cause most cases of infection-associated erythema multiforme. Physical agents (e.g., x-radiation), immunizations and hyposensitizations, malignancies (e.g., carcinoma, lymphoma), contact allergies (e.g., as part of a vigorous response to poison ivy or poison oak), and various autoimmune diseases also have been associated with erythema multiforme, but not as frequently. Although specific pathogenic mechanisms remain to be defined, erythema multiforme appears to be an immunologically mediated syndrome. For example, typical lesions of erythema multiforme have been induced with intradermal injections of formalin-killed herpes simplex virus. In addition, viral antigens have been demonstrated in circulating immune complexes and in perilesional deposits of immunoreactants in patients with herpes simplex virus–associated erythema multiforme.

INCIDENCE AND EPIDEMIOLOGY

Erythema multiforme occurs in about 0.2% of patients with dermatologic disorders and in 0.01% to 0.1% of hospital inpatients. Most patients are 20 to 40 years of age, but children and elderly also may be affected. Recurrent episodes of erythema multiforme are common and may be associated with episodes of recurrent herpes simplex virus.

CLINICAL FEATURES AND LABORATORY FINDINGS

Erythema multiforme has been divided into major (involving skin and mucous membranes, such as Stevens–Johnson syndrome and toxic epidermal necrolysis) and minor (involving only one surface) forms. In reality, a continuum of disease exists. Often, lesions become acute after a prodrome of fever, malaise, and sore throat. Diagnostic lesions are typical erythematous, annular, target lesions with concentric rings of color and a symmetric distribution (Fig. 197.2). Bullae often develop in the center of target lesions and evolve into erosions that eventually crust. Mucosal involvement, particularly of the mouth or con-

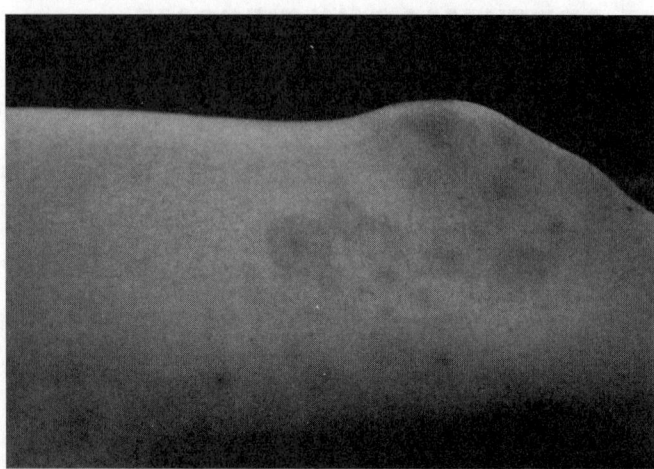

FIGURE 197.2. Erythema multiforme.

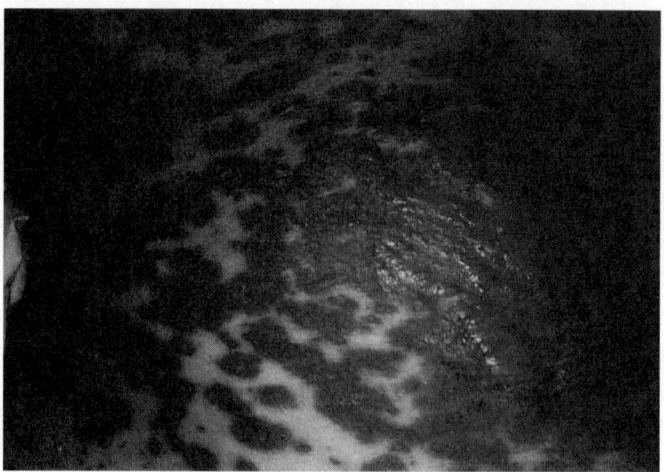

FIGURE 197.3. Toxic epidermal necrolysis.

junctiva, occurs in up to 50% of patients. Widespread bulla formation, often on a background of large erythematous plaques, can result in the loss of substantial amounts of the epidermis.

Stevens–Johnson syndrome, or erythema multiforme major, represents the intermediate form of the disease and is more likely to be triggered by drugs than by infectious agents. At least two mucosal surfaces (e.g., oral, labial, conjunctival, anogenital) must be involved in addition to the usual cutaneous findings of erythematous targetlike or bullous lesions to make the diagnosis of Stevens–Johnson syndrome. The mucosal lesions may precede the cutaneous erythema or bullae and can be painful in contrast to the skin lesions, which usually are nontender.

Toxic epidermal necrolysis probably is the most extreme form of erythema multiforme major (Fig. 197.3). This entity usually is caused by drugs and occurs in adults. It is characterized by the acute onset of generalized cutaneous inflammation with bulla formation that may involve most of the body surface. Oral and conjunctival involvement is common, and involvement of the respiratory tract, gastrointestinal tract, and vaginal mucosa is not unusual. Patients with toxic epidermal necrolysis often are febrile and toxic-appearing and complain of skin tenderness.

The diagnosis of erythema multiforme is based primarily on clinical findings. Skin biopsy shows a predominantly mononuclear cell infiltrate with a variable number of neutrophils and eosinophils around blood vessels and the dermal–epidermal junction, with vacuolization of the basal cell layer. Subepidermal edema is characteristic, and bulla formation may occur. Widespread full-thickness epidermal necrosis is characteristic of toxic epidermal necrolysis. Frozen-section examination of the sloughed skin, combined with cytologic examination (Tzanck preparation) of the denuded base or frozen-section examination of a punch biopsy specimen, may aid in the rapid diagnosis of this life-threatening disorder. Tissue sections in the staphylococcal scalded skin syndrome reveal intraepidermal separation beneath the granular layer, whereas full-thickness epidermal necrosis with separation at the dermal–epidermal junction is characteristic of drug-induced toxic epidermal necrolysis. In addition, cytologic examination of cells from the denuded surface shows keratinocytes in the case of staphylococcal scalded skin syndrome and inflammatory cells in drug-induced toxic epidermal necrolysis.

Depending on the symptoms and severity of the disease, other laboratory studies may be indicated. The leukocyte count may be elevated. Patients with respiratory symptoms should undergo a chest radiograph to search for *Mycoplasma pneumoniae*.

COURSE, THERAPY, AND PROGNOSIS

Both minor and major erythema multiforme are self-limited, the former resolving in 1 to 2 weeks and the latter in 3 to 6 weeks. If the oral involvement is severe, food and fluid intake may be compromised. Ophthalmologic (keratitis and perforation) and respiratory (obstruction or pneumonia) problems and progression to toxic epidermal necrolysis with associated fluid and protein loss, internal organ involvement, and predisposition to septicemia are major complications. Death may occur in up to 20% of patients with severe erythema multiforme major and in up to 50% of patients with toxic epidermal necrolysis.

The mainstay of therapy is nutritional and fluid support and local care (compresses or whirlpool baths) to provide gentle debridement and prevent infection. Erythema multiforme major with widespread bullae formation and toxic epidermal necrolysis probably can be treated most effectively in a burn unit, where requirements for aggressive fluid and nutritional support are recognized and local care is routine.

Systemic corticosteroid therapy for erythema multiforme is controversial. If prednisone is given early in the course of the illness, mortality may be diminished. The use of high doses of corticosteroids (e.g., prednisone, 1 to 2 mg per kilogram per day) in toxic epidermal necrolysis can decrease morbidity and may halt progression of cutaneous inflammation, but may not alter the high mortality rate seen in severely affected patients. For patients with recurrent erythema multiforme secondary to recurrent herpes simplex infection, chronic oral administration of acyclovir in suppressive doses has been helpful.

BIBLIOGRAPHY

Davidson AE, Miller SD, Settipane G, et al. Urticaria and angioedema. *Cleve Clin J Med* 1992;59:529–534.

Goldsmith P, Dowd PM. The new H_1 antihistamines. Treatment of urticaria and other clinical problems. *Dermatol Clin* 1993;11:87–95.

Millikan SB, Atkinson JP. Urticaria. In: Theirs BH, Dobson RL, eds. *Pathogenesis of skin disease.* New York: Churchill Livingstone, 1986.

Monroe EW. Nonsedating H_1 antihistamines in chronic urticaria. *Ann Allergy* 1993;71:585–591.

Ormerod AD. Urticaria: recognition, causes and treatment. *Drugs* 1994; 48:717–730.

Schafer T, Ring J. Epidemiology of urticaria. *Monogr Allergy* 1993;31: 49–60.

Soter NA. Treatment of urticaria and angioedema: low-sedating H_1-type antihistamines. *J Am Acad Dermatol* 1991;24:1084–1087.

Soter NA. Urticaria and angioedema. In: Fitzpatrick TB, Eisen AZ, Wolff K, et al, eds. *Update: dermatology in general medicine.* New York: McGraw-Hill, 1995.

Kelley's Textbook of Internal Medicine, fourth edition. Edited by H. David Humes.
Lippincott Williams & Wilkins, Philadelphia © 2000.

CHAPTER
198

APPROACH TO THE MANAGEMENT OF SKIN CANCER

SUSAN M. SWETTER

GENERAL INCIDENCE AND EPIDEMIOLOGY

Skin cancer is best divided into two groups: melanoma and nonmelanoma. Nonmelanoma skin cancer includes basal cell carcinoma (BCC) and squamous cell carcinoma (SCC), and it accounts for more than one-third of all cancers in the United States, with over 1 million cases detected annually. Melanoma, on the other hand, develops in over 44,000 Americans each year, and approximately 7,300 will die from metastatic disease.

BASAL CELL CARCINOMA

EPIDEMIOLOGY AND CLINICAL FINDINGS

Basal cell carcinoma arises from basal keratinocytes of the epidermis and adnexal structures. It is the most common skin cancer in humans and is primarily induced by ultraviolet B irradiation. Unlike SCC, BCC has no precursor lesion. It typically presents as a "pearly" or translucent, telangiectatic papule, although several distinct morphologic and histologic subtypes exist.

Superficial BCC is usually an erythematous, thin plaque on the trunk and extremities and may clinically resemble SCC in situ (Bowen's disease), psoriasis, or nummular eczema. Nodular BCC has the classic appearance of translucent, rolled borders and possible ulceration. Infiltrative BCC may appear as a depressed or ulcerated plaque and tends to behave more aggressively with a higher local recurrence rate if incompletely excised. Skin biopsy establishes the diagnosis and specific subtype of BCC.

OPTIMAL MANAGEMENT

Primary surgical excision is the mainstay of treatment for BCC. Surgical margins of 2 to 3 mm show cure rates over 95%. Larger clinical lesions, aggressive-growth subtypes, and lesions located in areas of higher local recurrence (nasolabial folds, preauricular and posterior auricular areas, and inner canthi) are excised with wider surgical margins (5 to 10 mm) or by means of Mohs' micrographic surgery.

Superficial BCC is confined to the epidermis and may be adequately treated with curettage and electrodesiccation, liquid nitrogen cryotherapy, or topical 5-fluorouracil, although recurrence rates are slightly higher compared with primary surgical excision. Most BCC is cured after surgery or destructive therapy. Recurrent tumors respond similarly to therapy, although cure rates tend to decrease with each unsuccessful procedure.

Mohs' micrographic surgery is indicated for recurrent tumors, large tumors (larger than 2.5 cm in diameter), tumors with poorly defined clinical margins, and those with aggressive histologic features, as just described. Mohs' micrographic surgery allows intraoperative assessment of tumor margins to ensure complete excision. In addition, it is a tissue-sparing technique that provides maximum tissue preservation in cosmetically sensitive areas such as the face.

Metastatic BCC is extremely rare, occurring in less than 1 per 4,000 cases (0.003% to 0.55% of all patients). Metastatic tumors occur most commonly on the scalp, head, and neck and are usually detected more than 10 years after treatment of the primary tumor. The most common site of metastasis is the regional lymph nodes, with lung, bone, and liver also possible. Metastatic BCC carries a poor prognosis, with average survival of 1.5 years after diagnosis and despite aggressive therapy.

SQUAMOUS CELL CARCINOMA

EPIDEMIOLOGY AND PRECURSOR LESIONS

Squamous cell carcinoma is the second most common form of skin cancer in whites, occurring in over 160,000 Americans each year. SCC arises from epidermal keratinocytes, as do its precursor lesions. Common precursor lesions for invasive nonmucosal SCC include actinic keratoses (AKs) and SCC in situ (Bowen's disease). AKs occur on sun-exposed sites as scaly or hyperkeratotic, erythematous papules. Although only a small percentage of AKs progress to invasive SCC (less than 0.2%), patients with numerous preexisting AKs are at significantly greater risk for development of SCC over a lifetime. Therefore, AKs are treated prophylactically with either liquid nitrogen cryotherapy or topical 5-fluorouracil. The regular use of sunscreen may also result in regression of AKs.

Bowen's disease typically presents as a well-demarcated, erythematous, thin plaque on sun-exposed sites of the body, although it may occur on nonexposed sites as well (e.g., on the glans penis as *erythroplasia of Queyrat*). An estimated 5% of untreated SCC in situ progresses to invasive SCC over many years, and thus treatment is similar to that for AKs. Therapeutic options include cryotherapy, topical 5-fluorouracil, curettage and electrodesiccation, or excision for recurrent lesions.

RISK FACTORS AND CLINICAL FINDINGS

Risk factors for SCC include fair complexion, increased ultraviolet B exposure, and decreased host immunity. Immunosuppressed organ transplantation patients have shown a significantly greater risk for development of cutaneous SCC with an increased likelihood for regional and distant metastasis. SCC typically presents as an erythematous, scaly papule, nodule, or plaque and may have central ulceration.

OPTIMAL MANAGEMENT

Treatment for invasive SCC is similar to that for BCC and includes excisional surgery, cryosurgery, topical chemotherapy, and radiation therapy. No uniform recommendation exists for surgical margins, although 3 to 5 mm is generally considered adequate for small, well-defined lesions. Wider margins may be necessary for large or histologically aggressive tumors, and Mohs' micrographic surgery is often performed in these cases.

Metastasis from cutaneous SCC occurs in 3% to 10% of cases, with increased incidence on mucosal surfaces and in immunosuppressed patients. Eighty-five percent of metastases from cutaneous SCC occur in the regional lymph nodes, with liver, lung, bone, and brain metastases also reported. Five-year survival rates remain low (14% to 39%).

Because approximately 50% of patients with nonmelanoma skin cancer have new primary lesions in the first 5 years after treatment, careful follow-up with regular skin examinations is recommended. In addition, sun protection and the use of sunscreens may help to prevent new precancerous and cancerous lesions.

PRIMARY CUTANEOUS MELANOMA

EPIDEMIOLOGY AND PRECURSOR LESIONS

By the year 2000, an estimated 1 in 75 Americans will develop melanoma over the course of a lifetime. Despite the increased incidence of melanoma, the case-based fatality rate has steadily fallen over the past 50 years, presumably because of earlier detection and treatment of thinner melanomas, which lack the potential to metastasize. Melanoma may arise de novo or from precursor melanocytic lesions, including congenital melanocytic nevi, common acquired melanocytic nevi, dysplastic nevi (also referred to as "atypical moles"), and melanoma in situ (lentigo maligna, superficial spreading melanoma in situ, and acral lentiginous melanoma in situ).

CONGENITAL MELANOCYTIC NEVI

Congenital melanocytic nevi are present at birth or within the first few months of life and are estimated to occur in 1% to 2% of newborns. Most nevi are small (less than 1.5 cm in diameter) and solitary. Giant congenital melanocytic nevi (larger than 20 cm in diameter) occur in approximately 1 in 20,000 newborns and show increased risk of developing into melanoma over a lifetime (5% to 15% lifetime risk). Because of the large size of these lesions, the presence of frequent "satellite" melanocytic nevi, and the fact that nevus cells may extend to the underlying muscle and fascia, complete surgical excision is difficult, if not impossible. In addition, an estimated 50% of melanomas in these patients develop in extracutaneous sites, so excision of pigmented skin alone may not affect melanoma risk, although it may have significant cosmetic and psychosocial benefits for the child.

The actual risk of malignant transformation in small (less than 1.5 cm) and intermediate-size (1.5 to 20 cm) congenital melanocytic nevi is not known, but appears to be no greater than the risk for common acquired nevi. In addition, progression to melanoma is extremely rare in the prepubertal period, unlike melanoma arising within giant congenital melanocytic nevi. Therefore, surgical excision of smaller congenital melanocytic nevi can be deferred until the second decade of life, or permanently, if the lesion is clinically stable or removal will result in cosmetic or functional impairment.

Acquired melanocytic nevi may develop from early childhood into the fourth decade. Increased numbers of common acquired nevi (more than 100) are a risk factor for the development of melanoma, and patients should be examined periodically as well as educated in the warning signs of malignant change (change in color, size, or diameter, or onset of itching or bleeding in preexisting moles).

Dysplastic Nevi/Atypical Moles

Dysplastic nevi were initially described in the late 1970s in families with large numbers of clinically atypical moles and an increased incidence of melanoma. They may develop throughout life, unlike common acquired nevi. Dysplastic nevi show larger size than normal melanocytic nevi (more than 6 mm in diameter), variegated pigmentation (tan, brown, pink), irregular borders, and topographic asymmetry (central raised portion). Although any or all of these clinical features suggest a dysplastic nevus, histologic examination is necessary for confirmation.

Patients with the rare *familial atypical mole/melanoma syndrome* have atypical moles and have two or more first-degree relatives with dysplastic nevi and a history of melanoma. The estimated lifetime risk in affected persons approaches 100% by the age of 70. However, dysplastic nevi also occur sporadically, in a nonfamilial form, in up to 10% of the general population, and the risk of malignant transformation in these persons is difficult to assess. Most congenital, common acquired, and clinically atypical moles do not progress to melanoma, and histologic studies have established that only 30% to 50% of cutaneous melanomas are associated with precursor nevi. Thus, atypical moles are best considered markers for increased melanoma risk, rather than precursor lesions that will progress to melanoma. For this reason, patients should be taught to examine their moles periodically and to seek medical attention for any suspicious changes in existing nevi.

Melanoma In Situ

Melanoma arises from melanin-producing cells of the basal layer of the epidermis. Superficial spreading melanoma, lentigo maligna melanoma, and acral lentiginous melanoma have an in situ phase of intraepithelial, radial growth that may last for months to years before progressing to more invasive, vertical growth within the dermis. Nodular melanoma, on the other hand, is characterized by lack of an in situ phase and is typically thicker at the time of diagnosis.

Clinical Findings

Superficial spreading melanoma is the most common subtype of melanoma, occurring in about 70% of cases. Superficial spreading melanoma presents most commonly on the trunk in men and women and on the legs in women as a flat or slightly elevated nevus, with variegated pigmentation or irregular borders. A history of recent change in the nevus (size, color, shape, or onset of bleeding or pruritus) is reported by 80% of melanoma patients at the time of diagnosis.

Nodular melanoma occurs in 15% to 20% of patients and also is most commonly seen on the legs and trunk. Rapid growth over weeks to months is characteristic. Nodular melanoma presents as a dark brown to black nodule, which may ulcerate and bleed with minor trauma.

Lentigo maligna melanoma makes up 4% to 15% of cutaneous melanoma. Like BCC and SCC, lentigo maligna melanoma is closely linked to cumulative sun exposure, and it is usually located on the head and neck of older people (mean age, 65 years). Lentigo maligna is the specific in situ precursor lesion, although only 5% to 8% are estimated to progress to invasive melanoma. In these cases, the precursor lesion is usually large (3 to 6 cm in diameter), present for at least 10 to 15 years, and shows areas of dark brown to black macular pigmentation or raised blue-black nodules.

Acral lentiginous melanoma is the least common subtype of melanoma, accounting for only 2% to 8% of melanoma in whites. However, it makes up a high percentage of melanoma in African Americans, Asians, and Hispanics (35% to 90%). It is typically located on the palms or soles or beneath the nail plate. Subungual melanoma manifests as diffuse nail discoloration or a longitudinal pigmented band within the nail plate and must be differentiated from a benign junctional melanocytic nevus of the nail bed, which may present similarly. Involvement of the proximal or lateral nail folds (Hutchinson's sign) is a hallmark of acral lentiginous melanoma.

If melanoma is suspected clinically, excisional biopsy with 2- to 5-mm margins should be performed to allow optimal histologic examination and estimation of prognostic features. The most important determinant of prognosis is tumor thickness (also known as Breslow depth). Increased tumor thickness confers a higher metastatic potential and thus a poorer prognosis (Table 198.1). Clark's levels measure tumor invasion anatomi-

TABLE 198.1.	CORRELATION OF TUMOR THICKNESS AND SURVIVAL RATE IN MALIGNANT MELANOMA (VERTICAL GROWTH PHASE)
Thickness of Tumor (mm)	**8-Year Survival (%)**
Melanoma in situ	100
<0.76 mm	93.2
0.76–1.69	85.6
1.70–3.60	59.8
>3.60	33.3

Radial growth phase tumors <1.0 mm in depth show 100% survival at 8 years.
Data from Clark WH Jr, Elder DE, Guerry DN, et al. Model predicting survival in Stage I melanoma based on tumor progression. *J Nat'l Center Inst* 1989;81:1893.

TABLE 198.2.	AMERICAN JOINT COMMITTEE ON CANCER/UNION INTERNATIONALE CONTRE LE CANCER pTNM STAGING SYSTEM FOR MALIGNANT MELANOMA (1988)

Stage	Criteria
0	Primary melanoma in situ (Clark level I)
Ia	Primary melanoma <0.75 mm thick and/or Clark level II (pT1, N0, M0)
Ib	Primary melanoma 0.76–1.5 mm thick and/or Clark level III (pT2, N0, M0)
IIa	Primary melanoma 1.51–4.0 mm thick and/or Clark level IV (pT3, N0, M0)
IIb	Primary melanoma >4.0 mm thick and/or Clark level V (pT4, N0, M0)
III	Regional lymph node and/or in-transit metastasis (any pT, N1 or N2, M0)
IV	Distant skin, nodal, or systemic metastasis (or any combination) (any pT, any N, M1)

Tumor thickness should take precedence over Clark level and be used for pT staging when differences arise, according to the American Joint Committee on Cancer Melanoma Committee. Data from American Joint Committee on Cancer. *Manual for staging of cancer.* 4th ed. Philadelphia. JB Lippincott, 1922:143.

cally and appears to affect prognosis only in thinner (less than 1 mm) melanomas. The melanoma staging system currently accepted by the American Joint Committee on Cancer (AJCC) incorporates tumor thickness and anatomical level of invasion, with the recommendation to follow Breslow depth over Clark's level when any discordance arises (Table 198.2). Revisions in the AJCC melanoma staging system to incorporate histologic ulceration and number of lymph nodes involved are currently underway.

OPTIMAL MANAGEMENT

Surgery is the primary mode of therapy for localized cutaneous melanoma. Recommendations for surgical margins have evolved dramatically over the past century with the realization that wider margins for deep tumors do not prevent metastatic disease. Although narrow surgical margins (less than 1.5 cm) may result in a higher local recurrence rate (or "persistent disease") for thicker melanomas, they do not affect metastatic potential or survival rate. Five-millimeter surgical margins are recommended for melanoma in situ and 1-cm margins for melanomas up to 1 mm in depth (low-risk primaries). Randomized, prospective studies suggest that 2-cm margins are appropriate for tumors in the intermediate-risk group (1 to 4 mm in Breslow depth), although 1-cm margins have been proposed for tumors 1 to 2 mm thickness. Margins of at least 2 cm are recommended for cutaneous melanomas greater than 4 mm in thickness (high-risk primaries) to prevent potential local recurrence on the skin.

Elective Lymph Node Dissection

Prophylactic lymph node dissection for primary cutaneous melanoma of intermediate thickness was initially believed to confer a survival advantage for patients with tumors 1 to 4 mm in depth. However, subsequent prospective, randomized clinical trials have shown no survival benefit for elective lymphadenectomy for melanomas of varying thicknesses on the extremities and have shown marginal to no benefit for nonextremity melanomas.

The use of lymphatic mapping and the "sentinel node" biopsy has effectively solved the dilemma of whether to perform regional node dissection in the absence of clinically palpable nodes in patients with thicker melanomas (more than 1 mm in depth). This procedure involves preoperative radiographic mapping (lymphoscintigraphy) and biopsy of the initial draining regional node to assess for the presence of micrometastasis, in which case a therapeutic lymph node dissection is performed.

Adjuvant Therapy

Numerous trials of adjuvant chemotherapy, nonspecific, passive immunotherapy, radiation therapy, and biologic therapy have been performed to assess survival benefit in patients with localized cutaneous disease. No increase in patient survival has yet been found with these adjunctive therapies. Adjuvant interferon alfa-2b and various experimental melanoma vaccines show promise in persons with high-risk primary cutaneous melanoma.

METASTATIC MELANOMA

Metastatic melanoma may occur locally, within or around the primary site, in regional lymph node basins, or distally, including remote skin, lymph node, visceral, skeletal, or central nervous system sites. Initial sites of disease relapse are most frequently seen in the skin, subcutaneous tissue, and lymph nodes. In these cases, surgical excision of isolated metastasis may result in long-term survival (up to 61% reported). Regional lymph node metastasis is associated with a 36% to 40% 5-year survival rate, although adjuvant interferon-α and melanoma cell vaccines show promise in prolonging survival.

The prognosis for persons with untreated distant metastatic disease is extremely poor, with a median survival of only 6 to 9 months and a 5-year survival rate between 5% and 7%. Systemic chemotherapy is the mainstay of treatment, despite low response rates (less than 20%). Use of modified concurrent biochemotherapy (with interleukin-2 and interferon) has shown increased response rates in some randomized trials and is being further investigated. In addition, specific active immunotherapy with experimental melanoma-derived, autologous, peptide, and dendritic cell vaccines has been shown to mediate tumor regression and is being intensively studied. Despite advances in the treatment of metastatic disease, however, detection and treatment of cutaneous melanoma in its thin, early phase remains the best chance for cure.

BIBLIOGRAPHY

American Cancer Society. *Cancer facts and figures–1999.* Atlanta: American Cancer Society, 1999.

Balch CM, Urist MM, Karakcusis CP, et al. Efficacy of 2 cm surgical margins for intermediate-thickness melanomas (1–4 mm): results of a multi-institutional randomized surgical trial. *Ann Surg* 1993;218: 262–269.

Kirkwood JM, Strawderman MH, Ernstoff MS, et al. Interferon alfa-2b adjuvant therapy of high-risk resected cutaneous melanoma: the eastern cooperative oncology group trial EST 1684. *J Clin Oncol* 1996;14:7–17.

Koh HK. Cutaneous melanoma. *N Engl J Med* 1991;325:171–182.

Morton DL, Wen DR, Cochran AJ. Management of early-stage melanoma by intraoperative lymphatic mapping and selective lymphadenectomy: an alternative to routine elective lymphadenectomy or "watch and wait." *Surg Oncol Clin North Am* 1992;1:247–259.

NIH Consensus Statement on the Diagnosis and Treatment of Early Melanoma. Bethesda: US Department of Health and Human Services, 1992.

Preston DS, Stern RS. Nonmelanoma cancers of the skin. *N Engl J Med* 1992;327:1649–1662.

Swetter SM. Malignant melanoma from the dermatologic perspective. *Surg Clin North Am* 1996;76:1287–1298.

Thompson SC, Jolley D, Marks R. Reduction of solar keratoses by regular sunscreen use. *N Engl J Med* 1993;329:1147–1151.

Williams ML, Sagebiel RW. Melanoma risk factors and atypical moles. *West J Med* 1994;160:343–350.

Kelley's Textbook of Internal Medicine, fourth edition. Edited by H. David Humes. Lippincott Williams & Wilkins, Philadelphia © 2000.

TABLE 199.1.	ALLERGIC SKIN REACTION RATES
Drug	**Reaction Rate**[a]
Amoxicillin	52
Trimethoprim-sulfamethoxazole	34
Ampicillin	33
Blood	22
Semisynthetic penicillin	21
Penicillin G	19
Cephalosporins	21
Erythromycin	20
Dihydralazine hydrochloride	19
Quinidine	13
Cimetidine	13

[a] Reaction rate per 1000 recipients.
(From Bigby M, Jick S, Jick H, et al. Drug induced cutaneous reactions: a report from the Boston Collaborative Drug Surveillance Program on 13,438 inpatients, 1975–1983. *JAMA* 1986; 256:3358, with permission.)

CHAPTER 199

CUTANEOUS REACTIONS TO DRUGS

MARTIN VAZQUEZ

Drug eruptions are a heterogeneous group of cutaneous reactions due to medications. Although difficult to determine, cutaneous drug reactions are reported to occur in 0.3% to 2.2% of hospitalized patients, with antibiotics accounting for at least 40% of reactions (Table 199.1). Morbilliform reactions and urticaria are the most common manifestations. Other reactions are angioedema, erythema multiforme, exfoliative dermatitis, photosensitivity, vasculitis, and erythema nodosum. Risk factors include increased number of medications and AIDS.

DIAGNOSIS

Mislabeling a dermatosis as a drug eruption may unnecessarily limit future use of specific medications. To help minimize this, the differential diagnosis should include dermatosis not associated with drug use, such as allergic contact dermatitis, viral exanthems, and atopic dermatitis.

Although no algorithm is universally practiced, the following approach is recommended:

1. Classify the morphology and pattern of the eruption (e.g., morbilliform, urticarial, palpable purpura), including associated symptoms. Features of cutaneous skin eruptions with potential morbidity include skin pain, necrosis, and blisters; confluent erythema; palpable purpura; mucosal involvement; angioedema; high fever and lymphadenopathy; and cardiopulmonary compromise.

2. Obtain a detailed history, including prescription and over-the-counter medications, eye drops, suppositories, topical medications, herbal treatments, and other remedies currently or recently taken.

3. List previous allergies to medications, because reexposure may have occurred.

4. Note the temporal relation between the onset of the eruption and the ingestion of the drug or drugs. Most cutaneous drug eruptions occur within 7 to 14 days after beginning a new medication.

5. Determine the probability that a suspected drug is causing a particular eruption based on reports (this may require reference to the medical literature).

6. The response to stopping medication (i.e., "dechallenge") needs to be followed. After discontinuation of the offending agent, resolution of the eruption may take as long as 4 to 6 weeks. In certain cases when the medication is strongly indicated for a given patient, rechallenge may be performed. This, however, is not usually recommended.

Table 199.2 outlines important primary drug-induced cutaneous eruptions with their key clinical features, differential diagnoses, implicated drugs, and management principles. Only the statistically most common causative drugs are listed. The list is otherwise extensive, and consulting the referenced text is advised.

In general, treating through a drug eruption (i.e., continuation of a possibly offending drug) is advised only for life-saving medications for which there are no substitutes. However, this is contraindicated when evolving erythema multiforme, toxic epidermal necrolysis, or exfoliative erythroderma is suspected.

TABLE 199.2. **PRIMARY CUTANEOUS DRUG ERUPTIONS**

Lesion	Clinical Features	Differential Diagnosis	Drugs Implicated	Management
Morbilliform reaction	Flat/papular Symmetrical Begins head and neck and goes down Time of onset: first 2 wk	Viral exanthem Cutaneous eruption of lymphocytic recovery Graft-versus-host disease Toxic shock syndrome	Ampicillin Penicillin Sulfonamides	Varies Dechallenge (ie, stop drug) depending on severity, need for medication, availability of substitutes Adjunctive 1. Topical steroids 2. Topical antipruritics 3. Antihistamines

Urticaria	Pruritic red wheals that last ≤24 hr
	Urticarial vasculitis that lasts >24 hr
	Time of onset: minutes to hours
		Other causes of urticaria:
		  Idiopathic
		  Foods
		  Physical contact
		  Cholinergic
			Antibiotics
			Aspirin
			Blood
			Captopril
			NSAIDs
			Activation: ethanol, aspirin, opiates, aminoglycosides
				1. Stop drug(s)
				2. Antihistamines
				No substitutes
				Rechallenge not recommended
				Medicalert

Fixed drug reaction	Dusky violaceous-brown plaque Appears same site w/each exposure Distribution: face, glans, limbs, hands, feet Time of onset: 30 min–8 hr	Erythema multiforme	Ampicillin Aspirin Barbiturates Metronidazole NSAIDs Birth control pills Phenolphthalein Sulfonamides Tetracycline	1. Stop medication 2. May rechallenge 3. Potent topical steroids

Angioedema	Urticaria or swelling of central part of face
	Respiratory distress
	Cardiovascular collapse
	Time of onset: varies
	  Minutes: penicillin
	  Days: NSAIDs
	  Weeks (<4): Angiotensin-converting enzyme inhibitors
		Insect stings
		Food
		Hereditary angioedema
			IgE-mediated
			  Penicillin
			  Anesthetics
			  Radiocontrast
			Non-IgE–mediated
			  Angiotensin-converting enzyme inhibitors
			  NSAIDs
			  Radiocontrast
			  Opiates
			  Curare
				1. Stop medication
				2. 0.1–1.0 mL of 1:1,000 epinephrine (0.01 mL/kg) subcutaneously
				3. Antihistamines

Exfoliative erythroderma	Starts with erythema and exudation on flexural skin and progresses to generalized erythema and scaling Spares palms/soles ++ Shivers/febrile Time of onset: several weeks	Psoriasis Atopic dermatitis Contact dermatitis Seborrheic dermatitis Cutaneous T-cell lymphoma	Barbiturates Captopril Carbamazepine Cimetidine Furosemide Gold Isoniazid Lithium NSAIDs Penicillamine Phenytoin Quinidine Sulfonamides Thiazide diuretics Allopurinol	1. Skin biopsy 2. Wet compresses 3. Topical steroids 4. Oral steroids if needed

| TABLE 199.2. | *Continued* | | | |

Lesion	Clinical Features	Differential Diagnosis	Drugs Implicated	Management
Vasculitis (small vessel)	Purpuric papules/ palpable purpura Distribution: Extremities (lower > upper) Time of onset: 1–3 wk May involve gastrointestinal kidney, nervous system, liver	Petechiae—not raised Pigmented purpuric eruption Schönlein-Henoch purpura Other causes Infection Cryoproteins Collagen vascular disease Malignancies	Allopurinol Animal antisera Antibiotics Furosemide Gold NSAIDs Phenytoin Thiazide diuretics Prophylthis uracil Radiographic contrast Sulfonamides	1. Skin biopsy 2. Cryoproteins 3. Immunofluorescent study of biopsy for IgA (Schönlein–Henoch purpura) 4. Stool guaiac and urinalysis 5. Complete blood count (infection) 6. Antinuclear antibody, rheumatoid factor 7. Stop medication if possible
Hypersensitivity syndrome	Widespread maculopapular eruption or exfoliative erythroderma Fever Hepatitis Eosinophilia Worsening renal function Arthralgias Lymphadenopathy Time of onset: 8 d–6 wk	Infectious illness Serum sickness	Antiepileptics Phenytoin Carbamazepine Phenobarbital Sulfonamides Allopurinol Gold Dapsone	1. Rule out infection 2. CBC, GSP, UA 3. Stop medication 4. Systemic corticosteroid (0.5 mg/kg)
Erythema multiforme/ Stevens–Johnson syndrome	Targetoid lesion 3 cm, round with 3 color zones Morphology may vary Distribution: distal extremities Dorsal hands and arms ± Palms/trunk, mucosa Time of onset: 1–3 wk Fever and respiratory tract lesions in 10–30%	Toxic epidermal necrolysis (see below) Erythema multiforme secondary to: Herpes simplex *Mycoplasma* pneumonia	Allopurinol Anticonvulsants Barbiturates Carbamazepine Estrogen Gold Sulfonamides NSAIDs Penicillamine Piroxicam	1. Corticosteroids— controversial—early with high dose and pulse 2. Supportive care 3. Ophthalmologic consult 4. Do not rechallenge 5. Rule out infection
Toxic epidermal necrolysis	Morbilliform eruption Rapid progression to confluent "burning" and painful erythema, blistering, and denudation Systemic symptoms: flu-like symptoms + Nikolsky's sign (pressure denudation) + Mucosa involvement Time of onset: 1–3 wk	Staphylococcal scalded skin syndrome (requires frozen section biopsy) Staphylococcal infection: subcorneal split Toxic epidermal necrolysis: subepidermal split	Allopurinol Sulfonamides Phenytoin Phenobarbital NSAIDs Ampicillin/amoxicillin Pentamidine	1. Stop medication 2. Metabolic/fluid May require burn unit Prevent skin infection Eye care

TABLE 199.2. *Continued*

Lesion	Clinical Features	Differential Diagnosis	Drugs Implicated	Management

Serum sickness	Urticaria
	Angioedema
	Systemic
	  Arthralgias
	    (hands/feet)
	  Lymphadenopathy
	  ± Nephritis,
	    endocarditis,
	    neuritis, fever,
	    eosinophilia
	Time of onset: 5 d–3 wk
		Urticaria and angiodema
		Serum sickness occurs much
		  later after drug ingestion
			Heterologous serum
			Aspirin
			Penicillin
			Streptomycin
			Thiouracils
			Globulin preparations
				1. Antihistamines
				2. Systemic corticosteroids
				3. Ephedrine (if indicated)

Coumarin necrosis (anticoagulant necrosis)	Tender ecchymoses
	  progressing to
	  hemorrhagic
	  blisters, necrosis,
	  and eschar
	  formation
	Distribution:
	  buttocks, breasts,
	  and thighs
	Time of onset:
	  warfarin: 3–5 d
	  heparin: 5–10 d
		Disseminated intravascular
		  coagulopathy
		Septicemia
			Coumarin
			Heparin
				Laboratory tests
				  1. Protein C deficiency
				  2. Platelet count
				Treatment
				  1. Surgical debridement
				  2. For warfarin (one
				    source)
				      Stop warfarin
				      Give vitamin K
				      Give heparin
				      Give protein C
				        concentrate

Photosensitivity	Varies: erythema,
	  edema, blisters,
	  weeping,
	  desquamation
	Distribution (key):
	  face, dorsa of
	  hands, anterior
	  neck, upper chest
	Spares: under chin
	  and nose, upper
	  eyelids
		Polymorphous light eruption
		Systemic lupus erythematosus
		Porphyria cutaneatarda
		Photoallergic contact
			Phototoxic
			  Tetracycline
			  Doxycyclin
			  Chlorpromazine
			  Sulfonamides
			  Furosemide
			  NSAIDs
			  Psoralens
			  Amiodarone
			Photoallergic
			  Phenothiazines
			  Sulfonamides
			  Thiazide diuretics
			  Oral hypoglycemics
			  Griseofulvin
			  Quinidine
				1. Stop medication
				  (dechallenge)
				  If no change, then:
				2. Biopsy, rule out other
				  disease
				3. Phototesting
				4. Serologic evaluation for
				  systemic lupus
				  erythematosus if
				  indicated
				5. Sunscreen
				Note: photosensitivity may
				last weeks to months after
				discontinuation of the
				offending medication

Lichenoid drug eruption	Multiple, violaceous,
	  polygonal,
	  discrete flat-
	  topped papules
	Distribution: light-
	  exposed areas,
	  oral
	Time of onset:
	  weeks, months to
	  years
		Lichen planus
		Chronic graft-versus-host
		  disease
			Gold
			Thiazide diuretics
			Quinidine
			Phenothiazines
			Methyldopa
			Furosemide
			Chlorpropamide
			Antimalarials
				1. Stop medication—may
				  take months to resolve
				2. Medium- to high-potency
				  topical steroids

Erythema nodosum	Tender, red
	  subcutaneous
	  nodules
	Distribution: shins,
	  thighs
		Panniculitis
		Fat necrosis
		Infection
		Systemic vasculitis
		Trauma
		Phlebitis
		Other causes
		  Infection
		  Sarcoidosis
		  Malignancies
		  Enteropathies
			Antibiotics
			Amiodarone
			Estrogen/progesterone
			Gold
			NSAIDs
			Opiates
			Sulfonamides
				1. Rule out infection
				2. Potassium iodide
				3. Bed rest
				4. Leg elevation
				5. NSAIDs
				6. Potassium iodide

TABLE 199.2. *Continued*

Lesion	Clinical Features	Differential Diagnosis	Drugs Implicated	Management
Pityriasis rosea	Multiple round-oval patches with collarette of scale, trunk > extremities	Secondary syphilis (check palms/soles/mucosa) Check serologies	Barbiturates Bismuth compounds Captopril Clonidine Gold Griseofulvin Isotretinoin Labetalol Metronidazole Penicillins	1. Rule out syphilis 2. Decrease or stop medication
Acneiform eruptions	Paupular and pustular acneiform lesions No comedones Distribution: head, neck, upper trunk, extremities Comedonal with chloracne	Acne vulgaris Folliculitis	Adrenocorticotropic hormone Androgens Bromides Corticosteroids Halothane Iodides Isoniazid Lithium Phenytoin Vitamins B_2, B, B_{12}	1. Stop medication 2. Antiacne medication

CBC, complete blood count; GSP, general survey panel; NSAIDs, nonsteroidal-anti-inflammatory drugs; UA, urinalysis.

BIBLIOGRAPHY

Bigby M, Jick S, Jick H, et al. Drug induced cutaneous reactions. A report from the Boston Collaborative Drug Surveillance Program on 15,438 inpatients, 1975–1982. *JAMA* 1986;256:3358–3363.

Goldstein S, Wintroub B. *A physician's guide: adverse cutaneous reactions to medication.* New York: CoMedica, 1994.

Goldstein S. Cutaneous drug reactions: a practical approach. *Resident Staff Phys* 1992;38(4):41–47.

Litt J, Pawlak W Jr. *Drug eruption reference manual 1997.* New York: Parthenon Publishing Group, 1997.

Roujeau J, Stern R. Severe adverse cutaneous reactions to drugs. *N Engl J Med* 1994;331:1272–1285.

Kelley's Textbook of Internal Medicine, fourth edition. Edited by H. David Humes. Lippincott Williams & Wilkins, Philadelphia © 2000.

DIAGNOSTIC AND THERAPEUTIC MODALITIES IN DERMATOLOGIC DISEASES

CHAPTER

200

DERMATOLOGIC DIAGNOSIS: FUNDAMENTALS FOR THE INTERNIST

JULIE ANNE WINFIELD

It is almost impossible to practice current internal medicine without some working knowledge of dermatology. These two specialties are very closely intertwined. Just as a dermatologist cannot fully treat a patient's cutaneous problem without a full understanding of the underlying disease process, neither can an internist ignore cutaneous findings as a clue to the patient's disease. The two specialties work hand in hand.

The first goal of this chapter on basic aspects of dermatologic diagnosis is to develop a common language of communication between the specialties of dermatology and internal medicine. Dermatology is a descriptive specialty and, by means of a common language to describe the entities found, provides internists with a valuable tool to aid in evaluation of their patients. This language also helps to "paint a picture," which will be very helpful in the communication between the two specialties. Keep in mind that a combined group of descriptors, along with a complete history, typically leads to a diagnosis or series of diagnostic possibilities.

Although dermatologists sometimes categorize lesions as primary (those that develop as part of the pathologic process, such as a vesicle of bullous pemphigoid) or secondary (those that derive or evolve from the primary lesions, such as a crusted excoriation resulting from scratching a vesicle), for the purpose of this chapter no such division will be made.

The goal here is to develop a small working common vocabulary that can be used in clinical circumstances ranging from bedside to long-range (even telemedicine) consultations to a problem-oriented algorithm.

Annular—occurring in a ring, such as in tinea corporis or a nodular annular lesion of sarcoidosis (Fig. 200.1)

Atrophy—loss of substance of the skin; in the epidermis (loss of skin markings) or in the dermis or subcutis, creating a hollowed-out appearance such as in lipoatrophy (Fig. 200.2, with blue-yellow discoloration and increase in visibility of vasculature, and necrobiosis lipoidica diabeticorum (Fig. 200.3)

Bulla—an elevated fluid-filled lesion larger than 0.5 cm, such as in bullous pemphigoid (Fig. 200.4)

Crust—a conglomeration of serum, blood, and inflammatory debris that develops after a spontaneous or induced break in the skin (scab), such as over an erosion or ulcer (Fig. 200.24) and in impetigo with characteristically "honey colored" crust

Cyst—an often well-circumscribed, compressible lesion filled with semisolid material; most likely an epidermal cyst if a central punctum or pore is visible

Erosion—a well-circumscribed, often oval, moist lesion that results from a superficial break within the skin, most commonly resulting from a vesicle or blister, such as porphyria cutanea tarda (Fig. 200.5)

Erythema—redness, as a primary event, as in nevus flammeus

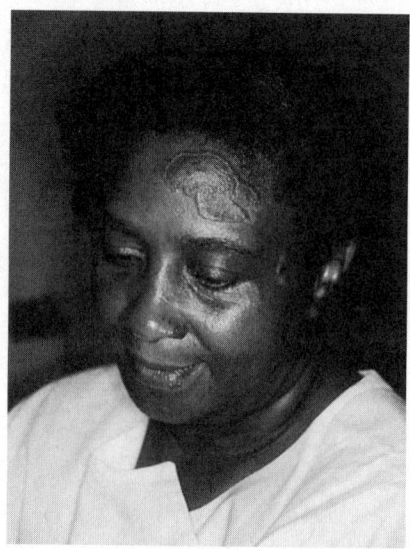

FIGURE 200.1. Annular: sarcoidosis. See color figure 200.1.

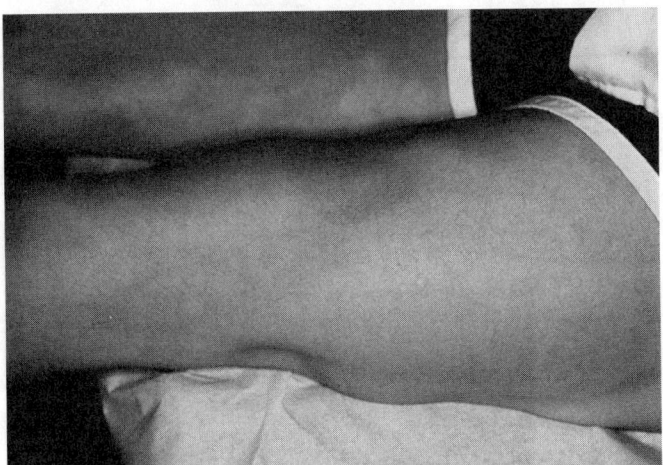

FIGURE 200.2. Atrophy: lipoatrophy. See color figure 200.2.

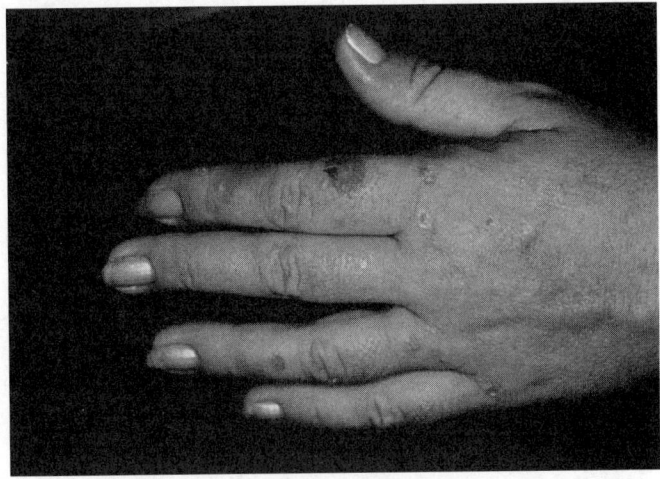

FIGURE 200.5. Erosion: porphyria cutanea tarda. See color figure 200.5.

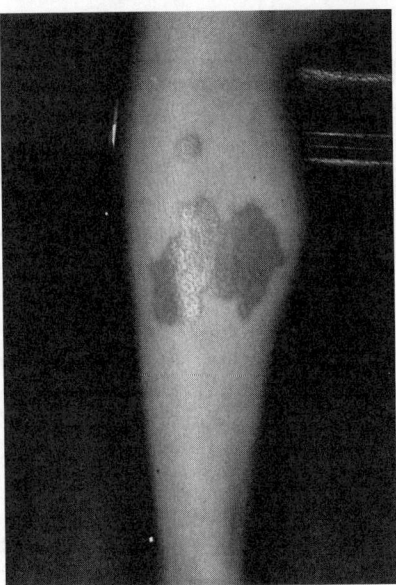

FIGURE 200.3. Atrophy: necrobiosis lipoidica diabeticorum. See color figure 200.3.

(stork bite) or as a secondary event, as in inflammation (Color Fig. 200.7)

Exfoliative—diffuse shedding of scales (essentially involving the entire epidermis as an exfoliative dermatitis in erythrodermic psoriasis (Fig. 200.6), pityriasis rubra pilaris, and ichthyosis

Fissure—a linear, moist lesion that results from a superficial spontaneous break in the skin, as may result from underlying edema and inflammation in eczematous dermatitis of the hand (Fig. 200.7)

Herpetiform—grouped or clustered lesions often on an erythematous base, as in herpes simplex (Fig. 200.8)

Hyperpigmentation—localized or generalized increase in pigmentation, as occurs in postinflammatory hyperpigmentation from an inflammatory process such as inflammatory acne lesion, eczema, and discoid lupus erythematosus (Fig. 200.9)

Hypopigmentation—a decrease in normal pigmentation, again usually as a result of a chronic inflammatory process, such as discoid lupus erythematosus, eczema, or psoriasis (Fig. 200.9)

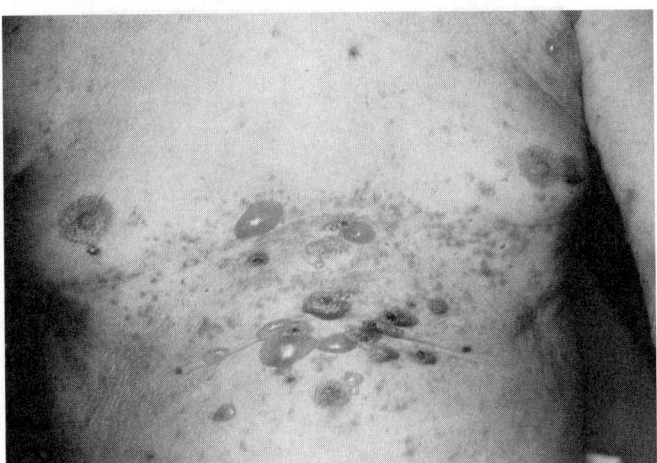

FIGURE 200.4. Vesicle and bulla: bullous pemphigoid. See color figure 200.4.

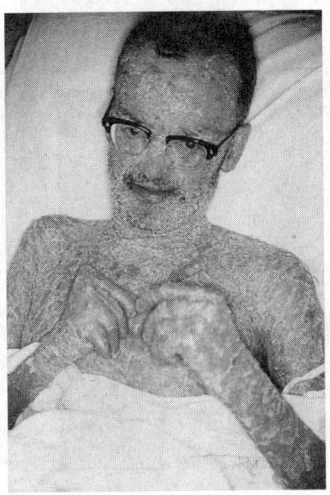

FIGURE 200.6. Exfoliation: psoriasis. See color figure 200.6.

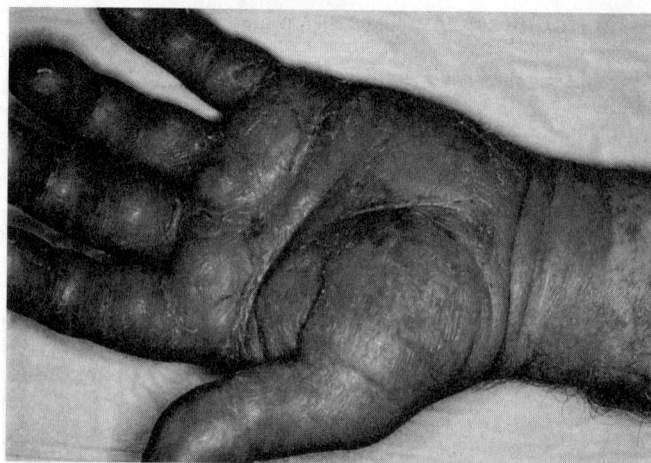

FIGURE 200.7. Fissure: hand eczema with erythema. See color figure 200.7.

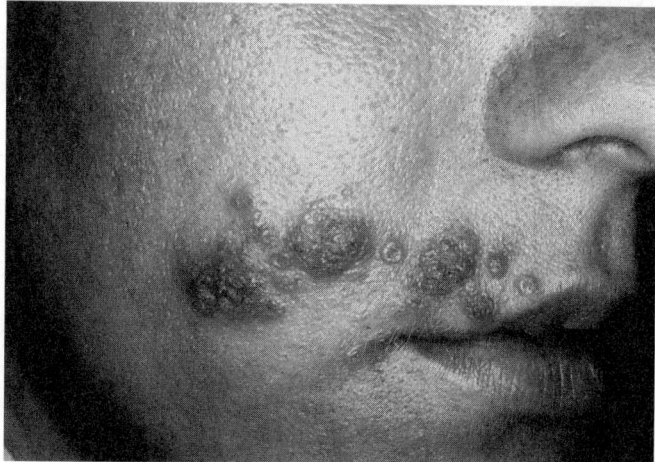

FIGURE 200.8. Herpetiform: herpes simplex with umbilicated vesicles. See figure 200.8.

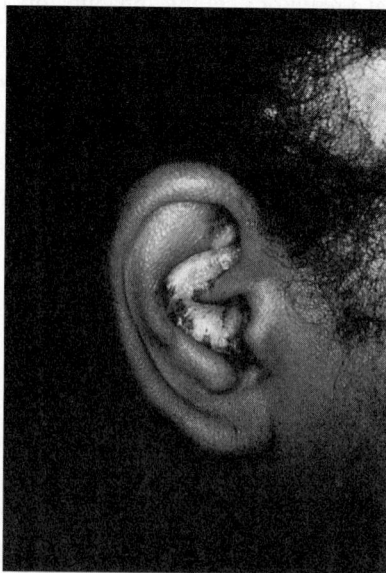

FIGURE 200.9. Hyperpigmentation/hypopigmentation: discoid lupus erythematosus with atrophic, hypopigmented center and hyperpigmented border. See color figure 200.9.

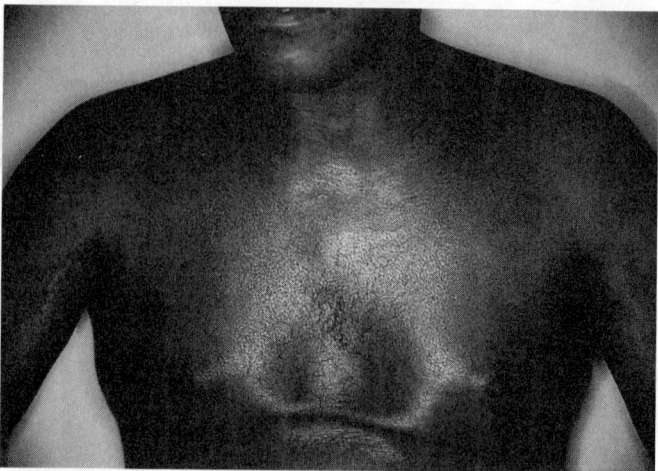

FIGURE 200.10. Indurated: scleroderma with diffusely shiny, taut skin. See color figure 200.10.

Indurated—thickened, often plaquelike area, as seen in mycosis fungoides (cutaneous T-cell lymphoma) and scleroderma (Fig. 200.10)

Lichenification/lichenoid—proliferation of the keratinocytes and stratum corneum forming a thickened plaquelike structure as a result of chronic rubbing of the skin and occurring typically in chronic eczematous dermatosis (Fig. 200.11), but also in psoriasis and other pruritic conditions, as in lichen planus with the white Wickham striae overlying (Fig. 200.15)

Linear—occurring in a line, as in contact dermatitis from poison ivy and in excoriation (Fig. 200.12)

Macule—a circumscribed area of color change in normal skin without elevation or depression, as in vitiligo (Fig. 200.13) or a port wine stain

Nodule—a palpable lesion deeper than a papule, often more than 2 cm in diameter, as in squamous cell carcinoma (Fig. 200.14) (Persistent nontender nodules are important signs of underlying systemic disease and should be considered for biopsy,

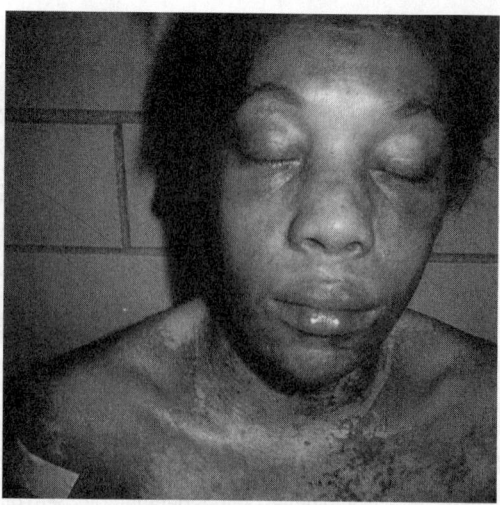

FIGURE 200.11. Lichenification: chronic eczematous dermatitis with hyperpigmentation. See color figure 200.11.

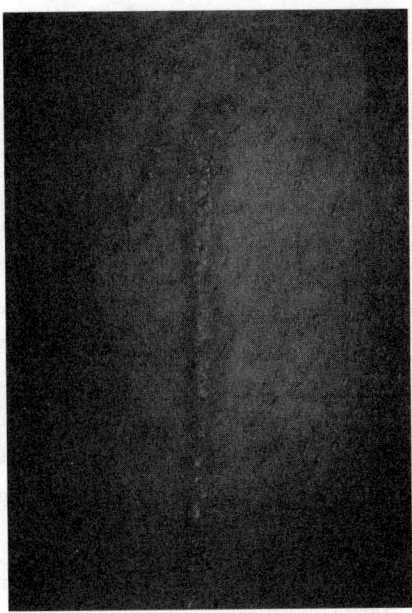

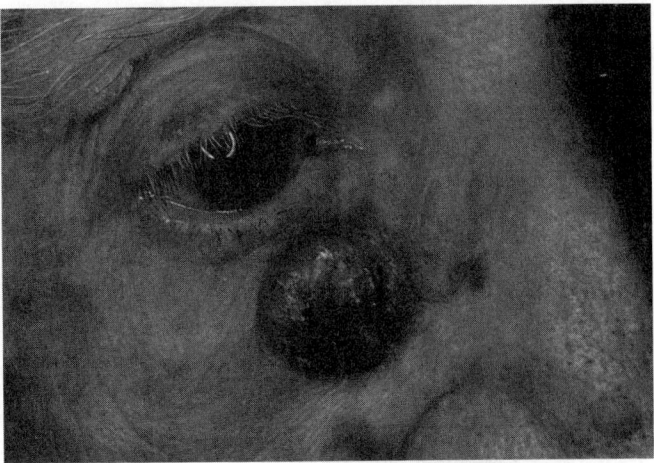

FIGURE 200.14. Nodule: squamous cell carcinoma. See color figure 200.14.

FIGURE 200.12. Linear: poison ivy contact dermatitis. See color figure 200.12.

also possibly sending half of a sterile biopsy specimen for culture if clinically indicated.)

Papule—a raised palpable, often well-circumscribed lesion less than 0.5 cm in diameter (usually arising from surrounding tissue, not from deep within the skin like a nodule), as in lichen planus (Fig. 200.15)

Plaque—a raised area larger than 0.5 cm, which may be the result of confluence of papules, as in plaque psoriasis or erythema nodosum (Fig. 200.16)

Polygonal—having discernible sides and angular corners, as in lichen planus (Fig. 200.15)

Purpura—red-violet discoloration resulting from cutaneous hemorrhage, as in ecchymosis in autoerythrocyte sensitization (Fig. 200.17) and in petechiae (palpable purpura) in leukocytoclastic vasculitis (Fig. 200.18)

Pustule—a fluid-filled lesion that contains purulent exudate

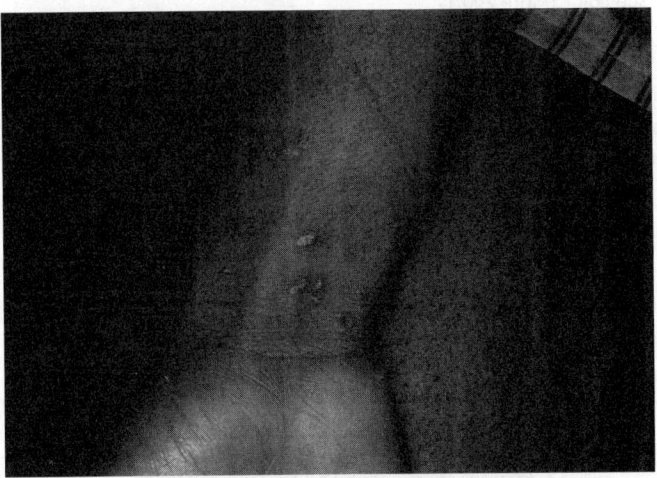

FIGURE 200.15. Papule: lichen planus. See color figure 200.15.

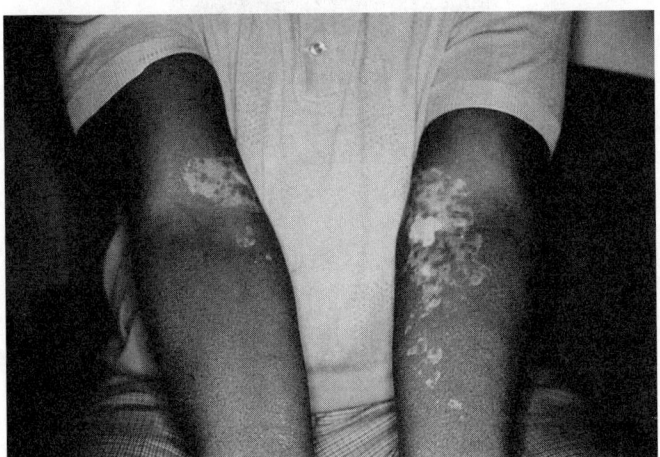

FIGURE 200.13. Macule: vitiligo. See color figure 200.13.

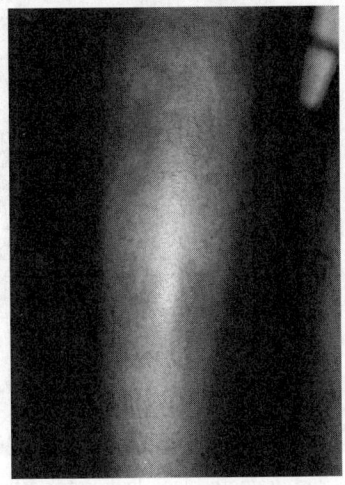

FIGURE 200.16. Plaque: erythema nodosum. See color figure 200.16.

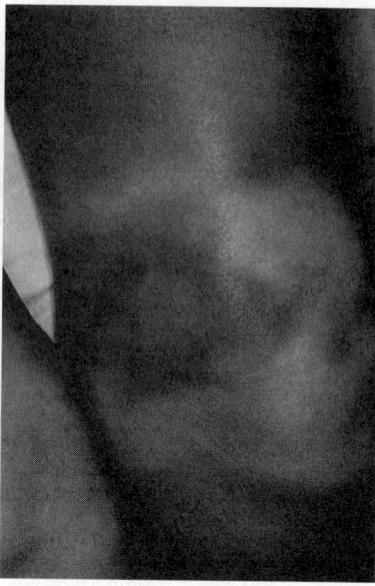

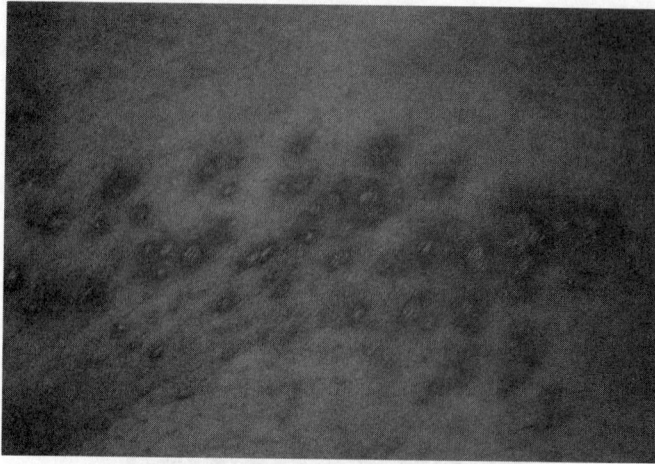

FIGURE 200.19. Pustule: pustular psoriasis. See color figure 200.19.

FIGURE 200.17. Purpura/ecchymosis: autoerythrocyte sensitization. See color figure 200.17.

that may be white, yellow, or green, as in pustular psoriasis (Fig. 200.19). (A pustule surrounding a hair follicle with a central hair is called *folliculitis.* Also, many of the vesicular lesions of some viral diseases can secondarily become pustules, as in herpes and varicella. If indicated clinically, a Gram's stain and culture should be done to identify an infectious agent.)

Reticulated—a lacelike or network pattern, as in prominent vascular pattern in cutis marmorata

Scaling/desquamation—flesh-colored flakes of skin that represent the outermost terminally differentiated epidermis and may be enhanced as a primary event, as in ichthyosis (Fig.

200.20), or as a secondary event, as in chronic eczematous dermatitis (Fig. 200.21); also *scaly.*

Serpiginous—moving in a curvilinear fashion, as in cutaneous larva migrans (Fig. 200.22)

Targetoid/iris—like a bullseye, a series of concentric rings, often with central clearing, as in erythema multiforme (Fig. 200.23)

Ulcer—a deep marginated lesion that results from destruction of the epidermis and dermis, such as stasis ulcer (Fig. 200.24)

Umbilicated—having a central dell or indentation suggesting a viral cause, as in molluscum contagiosum or herpes simplex (Fig. 200.8)

Verrucous—having an irregular, rough, warty surface, as in seborrheic keratosis (Fig. 200.25)

Vesicle—an elevated fluid-filled lesion less than 0.5 cm, as in bullous pemphigoid (Fig. 200.4)

Violaceous—dusky red-violet/purple discoloration characteristic in the heliotrope rash of dermatomyositis (Fig. 200.26)

Wheal—often pale red papule or plaque that usually feels indurated and is characteristically evanescent, changing in size,

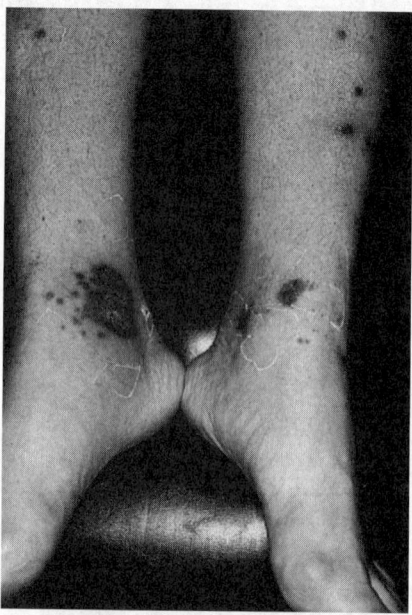

FIGURE 200.18. Purpura/petechiae: leukocytoclastic vasculitis. See color figure 200.18.

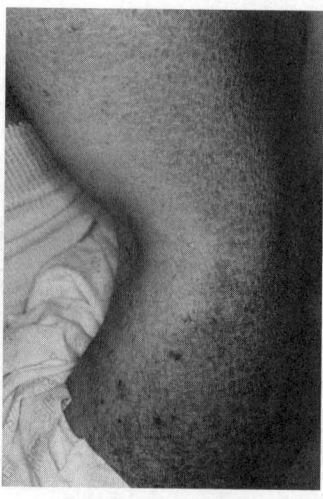

FIGURE 200.20. Scale: X-linked ichthyosis. See color figure 200.20.

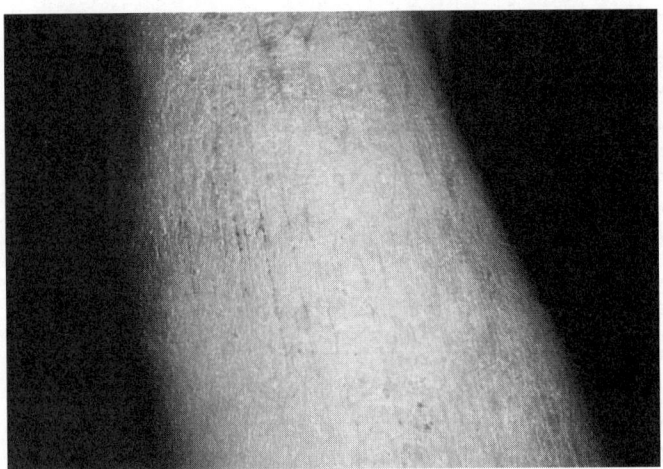

FIGURE 200.21. Excoriation: atopic dermatitis. See color figure 200.21.

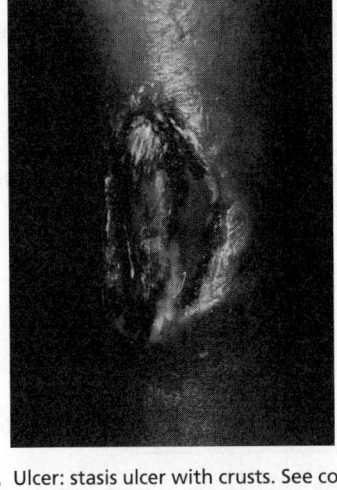

FIGURE 200.24. Ulcer: stasis ulcer with crusts. See color figure 200.24.

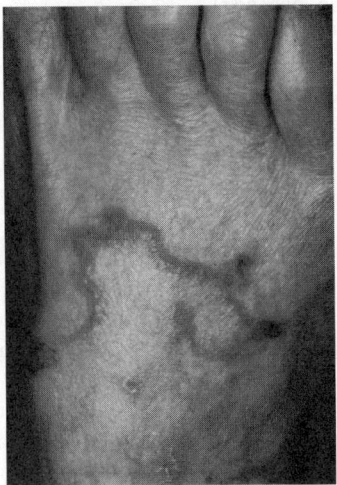

FIGURE 200.22. Serpiginous: cutaneous larva migrans. See color figure 200.22.

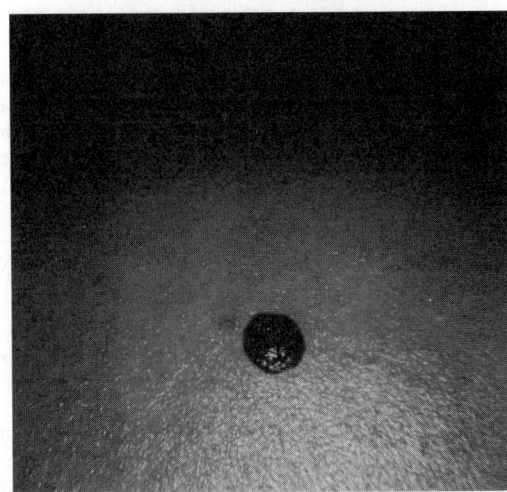

FIGURE 200.25. Verrucous: seborrheic keratosis. See color figure 200.25.

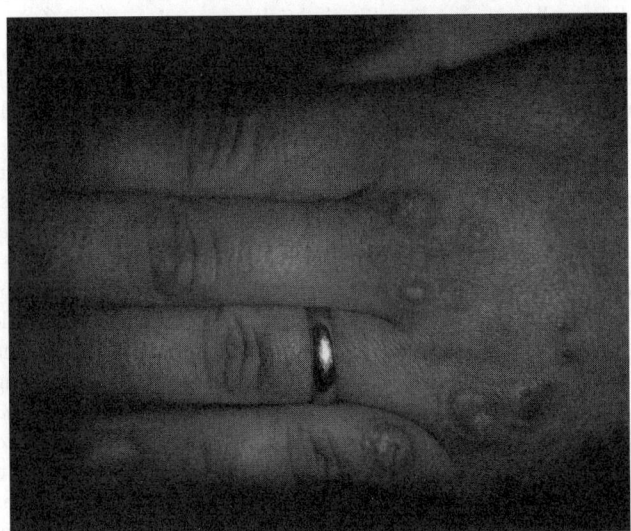

FIGURE 200.23. Target/iris: erythema multiforme. See color figure 200.23.

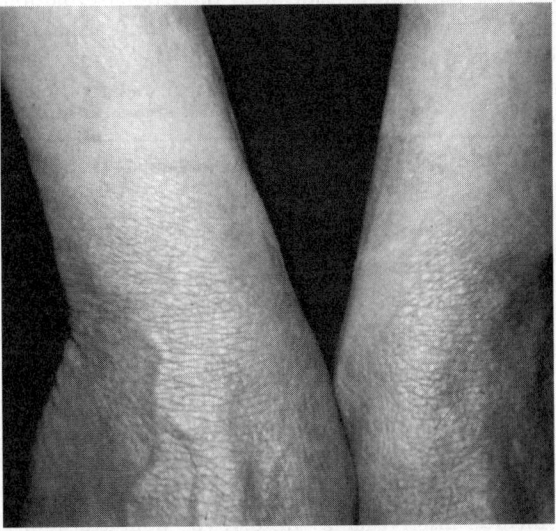

FIGURE 200.26. Violaceous: heliotrope discoloration of dermatomyositis. See color figure 200.26.

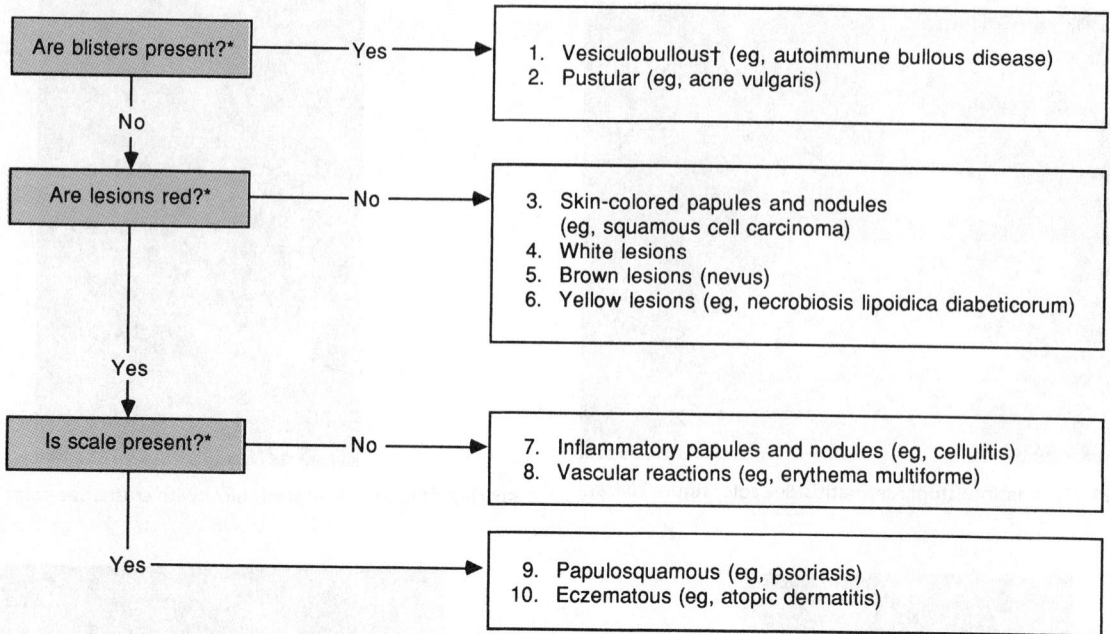

FIGURE 200.27. Problem-oriented dermatologic algorithm. Only one example is taken from each category. Please refer to the text for an expanded list of diagnoses. (Adapted from Lynch PJ. *Dermatology for the house officer.* Baltimore: Williams & Wilkins, 1982.)
EVIDENCE LEVEL: C. Expert Opinion.

shape, and location within hours; may be very pruritic. (Wheals fixed to a particular spot or that do not disappear within 72 hours may indicate urticarial vasculitis. If clinically appropriate, a biopsy with direct immunofluorescence fluoroscopy should be considered.)

The above-defined terms, as well as others, can be used for the basis of a diagnostic algorithm. An example of this is seen in Figure 200.27. Here, ten morphologic groups of dermatologic diseases are proposed based on a problem-oriented approach. This scheme has the advantage of giving an inexperienced observer a way of approaching an unknown dermatologic problem. It does not take into consideration the natural evolution of a problem nor any resultant changes in the cutaneous characteristics over this evolution. In addition, this scheme may be redundant, resulting in the placement of a particular problem into more than one category.

■ FOLLOWING THE DERMATOLOGIC CLUES

The process of evaluating the dermatologic aspects of a patient's disease is similar to that for other problems. The advantage with cutaneous signs is the visual correlation with the history, which helps to "paint a picture" of the underlying process. The complete dermatologic history is of paramount importance in elucidating the problem and should include the following: prodrome, onset, rapidity of progression, general symptoms, dermatologic symptoms, medication history including any known drug allergies, medical history, family history, vocation, avocations, and known exposures. With this information as well as the physical examination, the physician can then develop a list of differential

diagnoses. The morphologic characteristics of the lesions and their distribution are very important clues for the physician. Specific diagnostic techniques may also be added to the history and physical examination, which will aid in an accurate diagnosis.

Table 200.1 emphasizes several important techniques that can be used with ease. *Diascopy,* the application of pressure to a lesion with a magnifying lens or microscope slide, allows the differentiation of erythema, which blanches with pressure, from purpura, which persists. This simple physical diagnostic tool can allow the physician to distinguish relatively unimportant erythematous papular lesions from palpable purpura, which implies an allergic vasculitis. Similarly, diascopy allows the differentiation of solely epidermal processes (e.g., psoriasis) from those deeper lesions that involve the dermis (e.g., sarcoidosis, which occasionally has a psoriasis-like scale overlying the dermal nodules).

The skin-punch biopsy deserves particular emphasis. This technique, in which a core of tissue is removed under local anesthesia, can be accomplished at the bedside or in the office. Smaller biopsies (2 to 3 mm) do not require suturing for hemostasis and healing. However, for most punch biopsies of 4 mm and greater, simple interrupted suturing is recommended. Indications for use of a punch biopsy specimen are several: for routine histopathologic diagnosis, for direct immunofluorescence testing in the autoimmune bullous diseases or lupus erythematosus, and for obtaining an adequate amount of tissue to allow cultures to be done (e.g., in a case of ulcerative nodules on an extremity in which the identical clinical picture can be caused by sporotrichosis, nocardiosis, or an atypical *Mycobacterium*). The necessity of sterile technique and the choice of transport medium depend on the type of study to be performed.

TABLE 200.1.   TECHNIQUES IN DERMATOLOGIC DIAGNOSIS

Procedure	Indication	Interpretation
Diascopy—pressure on lesion through magnifying lens or microscopic slide	Differentiate inflammatory from hemorrhagic lesions (e.g., erythema from petechiae or purpura)	Pressure fails to blanch purpura or petechiae
	Differentiate epidermal from dermal nodules (e.g., tinea corporis from annular cutaneous sarcoid)	Epidermal papules disappear, but dermal nodules are enhanced; "Apple jelly" with diascopy
Wood's lamp—low-energy black light	Detect hypopigmentated macules of vitiligo or tuberous sclerosus	Lesions become more prominent under black light
	Detect tinea capitis (e.g., *Microsporum* species)	Infected areas show blue-green fluorescence
KOH preparation—microscopic examination of scales or hairs after solubilization with 20% KOH	Establish diagnosis of superficial fungal infection	Fungal and yeast elements are not dissolved by KOH; look for branching hyphae
Scabies preparation—microscopic examination of skin scrapings suspended under coverslip in mineral oil	Establish scabies mite infestation	Diagnosis is confirmed by mite, feces, or eggs
Tzanck preparation—microscopic examination of cells scraped from floor of vesicle or pustule after staining with Wright's or Giemsa stain	Differentiate viral from nonviral pustules (e.g., herpes simplex from folliculitis)	"Balloon" cells and multinucleate giant cells support viral cause
	Differentiate pemphigus from subepidermal bullous disease (e.g., pemphigus from pemphigoid)	Acantholytic epidermal cells are present in pemphigus, whereas inflammatory cells occur in other diseases
Fungal culture—culture of skin scrapings on Sabouraud's or Mycosel agar medium at room temperature for 2–4 wk	Establish fungal or yeast cause	Mycelial or yeast elements confirm diagnosis
Patch test—exposure of possible contact allergen (e.g., nickel) to skin under an occlusive dressing for 48 hr	Establish cause of contact dermatitis	Pruritic, erythematous papules or vesicles support an allergic contact origin
Skin-punch biopsy—surgical removal of a small (3–4 mm) core of tissue under local anesthesia	Establish histopathologic diagnosis	Pathologic confirmation of diagnosis often requires clinical correlation
	Tissue for direct immunofluorescence (e.g., in bullous pemphigoid or lupus erythematosus)	Immunofluorescence patterns may depend on site of biopsy
	Tissue for culture by sterile technique (e.g., in systemic fungal infections such as North American blastomycosis or sporotrichosis)	This technique is important but underused for obtaining a sufficient amount of material for many types of cultures (e.g., bacterial, microaerophilic, mycobacterial, fungal) from a single source

KOH, potassium hydroxide.

ILLUSTRATIVE CASES

The importance of the interplay of history, physical examination, and diagnostic techniques is illustrated best by several clinical cases studies. These case studies also show the way terms are used to make subtle distinctions between two problems of similar history or morphologic characteristics. The important points in the diagnostic process are described.

CASE STUDIES 1 AND 2

The history for Case 1 is helpful (Table 200.2; Fig. 200.28). A respiratory tract infection treated with ampicillin with an abrupt onset of a pruritic eruption, suggests a drug allergy. The physical

examination confirms a diffuse, maculopapular, erythematous (morbilliform) eruption. The blanching on diascopy suggests that there is no vasculitis. In contrast, for Case 2 (Fig. 200.29), despite the rapid onset, the history is relatively uninformative. Fatigue, excessive thirst, and frequent urination provide the only clues to the underlying problem. In this case, the physical examination is most important. It reveals red papules with yellow centers in rosettes that do not blanch on diascopy. These features are typical of eruptive xanthomas, a finding confirmed by biopsy. The final diagnosis was diabetes mellitus.

CASE STUDIES 3 AND 4

Cases 3 and 4 illustrate how subtle differences in distribution can lead to the proper diagnosis (Table 200.3; Figs. 200.30 and

TABLE 200.2.   CASES 1 AND 2: ERYTHEMATOUS ERUPTIONS OF THE TRUNK

	Case 1 (*Fig. 200.28*)	Case 2 (*Fig. 200.29*)
History		
Onset	Rapid onset of truncal eruption 24 hours earlier	Same
General symptoms	None	Fatigue
Cutaneous symptoms	Pruritus	None
Systems review	Respiratory tract infection 1 wk earlier	Excessive thirst, frequent urination
Medications	Ampicillin	None
Preliminary assessment	Drug allergy	Unknown
Examination		
General skin	Diffuse, erythematous papular and coalescent lesions on trunk	Diffuse, erythematous papular lesions on trunk; some have faintly yellow centers and coalesce into clusters or rosettes
Diascopy	Lesions blanch, leaving no erythema or dermal nodules	Lesions accentuated, revealing dermal nodules
Preliminary assessment	Drug allergy to ampicillin	Eruptive xanthomas secondary to diabetes mellitus
Special Techniques or Tests		
Fasting blood glucose	Not done	Significantly elevated
Triglycerides	Not done	Significantly elevated
Skin biopsy	Not done	Compatible with eruptive xanthoma
Final Assessment	Drug allergy to ampicillin	Eruptive xanthomas secondary to diabetes mellitus

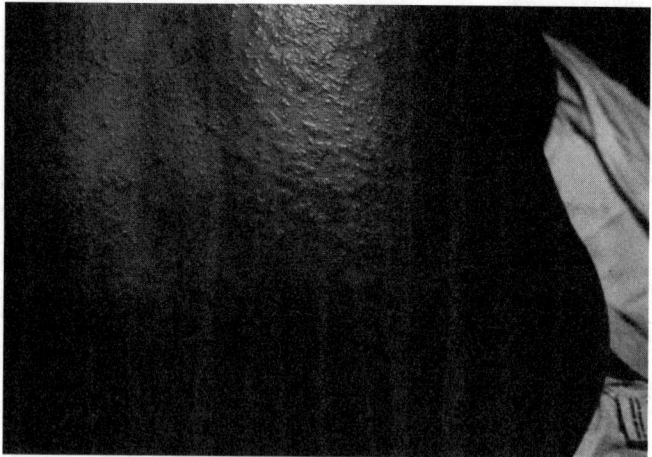

FIGURE 200.28. Case 1—Drug allergy secondary to ampicillin. See color figure 200.28.

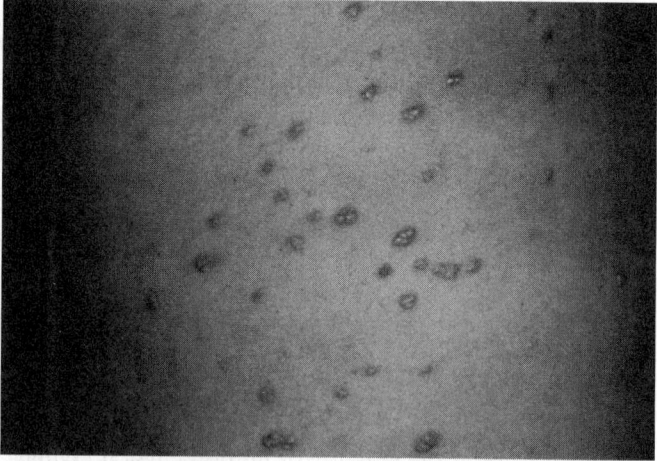

FIGURE 200.29. Case 2—Eruptive xanthomas secondary to diabetes mellitus. See color figure 200.29.

TABLE 200.3.	CASES 3 AND 4: ERYTHEMATOUS ERUPTIONS OF THE FACE	
	Case 3 (Fig. 200.30)	**Case 4 (Fig. 200.31)**
History		
Onset	Onset and slow progression of eruption of face during past month	Same
General symptoms	Fatigue, arthralgia	None
Cutaneous symptoms	Cosmetic only	Same
Medications	None	None
Family history	Not helpful	Not helpful
Preliminary assessment	Possible light-induced eruption	Same
Examination		
General skin	Sharply marginated, erythematous oval plaques with peripheral scales on face and upper trunk; spares submental region and nasolabial folds	Sharply marginated erythematous, oval plaques of forehead, eyebrows, glabella, and nasolabial folds
Diascopy	Erythema blanches	Same
Preliminary assessment	Lupus erythematosus or other light-related eruption	Seborrheic dermatitis, discoid lupus erythematosus, or tinea faciei
Special Techniques or Tests		
KOH preparation	No hyphal element	Same
ANA	Markedly positive	Nonreactive
Skin biopsy	Compatible with lupus erythematosus	Not done
Final Assessment	Lupus erythematosus	Seborrheic dermatitis

KOH, potassium hydroxide; ANA, antinuclear antibody.

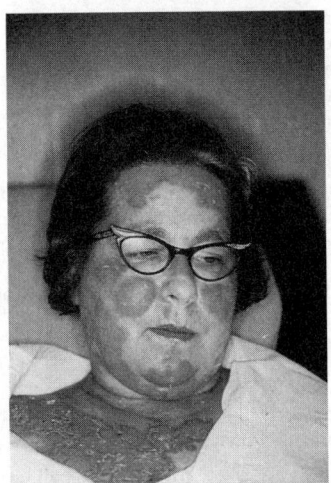

FIGURE 200.30. Case 3—Systemic lupus erythematosus. See color figure 200.30.

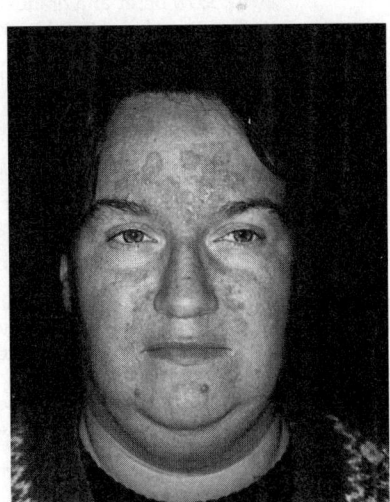

FIGURE 200.31. Case 4—Seborrheic dermatitis. See color figure 200.31.

200.31). Except for the fatigue and arthralgia, the history for Case 3 is relatively unrevealing. The morphologic characteristics and the distribution of the lesions (in light-exposed areas, sparing the submental region) suggest lupus erythematosus. In contrast, the distribution of the lesions in Case 4 is typical of seborrheic dermatitis, because it involves the eyebrows, glabella, and naso-labial folds, but spares other light-exposed regions. In both cases, the sharp, scaly borders require at least the consideration of a superficial fungal infection (excluded by the negative potassium hydrochloride preparations). A skin biopsy for hematoxylin-eosin (H&E) and direct immunofluorescence, along with hematologic studies in Case 3 will confirm the diagnosis of lupus erythematosus.

CASE STUDIES 5 AND 6

Cases 5 and 6 illustrate the problems of dealing with ulcerated nodules on extremities and elucidating whether there is an infectious basis (Table 200.4; Figs. 200.32 and 200.33). The history for Case 5 points to a joint problem of undetermined cause involving both hands, whereas the history of gardening and the ipsilateral spread of the lesions for Case 6 suggest an infectious basis. The physical findings provide strong evidence of this origin because sporotrichosis, nocardiosis, and atypical mycobacterial infections all can produce this picture. Typically, the potassium hydroxide preparation does not reveal the organism, but purulent drainage and tissue samples are adequate sources for culture. A biopsy for H&E can supply additional information for diagnosis. The key to Case 5 is the physical finding of tan and violaceous nodules overlying the metatarsophalangeal and proximal inter-

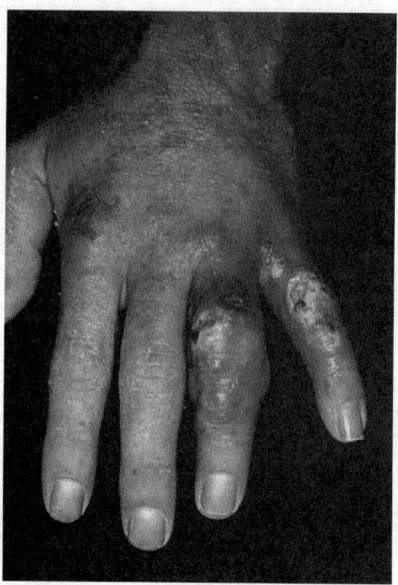

FIGURE 200.32. Case 5—Multicentric reticulohistiocytosis. See color figure 200.32.

TABLE 200.4.	**CASES 5 AND 6: ULCERATIVE NODULES OF THE UPPER EXTREMITIES**	

	Case 5 (*Fig. 200.32*)	Case 6 (*Fig. 200.33*)
History		
Onset	Slow onset and gradual progression to ulceration over knuckles of both hands	Onset of single boil on hand 6 wk earlier with progression to ulceration and proximal spread up the arm of additional ulcerative nodules
General symptoms	Painful joints of the hands	None
Cutaneous symptoms	Open, weeping blisters	Same
Medication	None	None
Family history	Not helpful	Not helpful
Occupation	Office work	Carpenter
Avocation	Sailing	Gardening
Preliminary assessment	Possible infection (e.g., sporotrichosis)	Same
Examination		
General skin	Multiple, poorly dermarcated erythematous and violaceous nodules over dorsum of both hands and fingers; some ulcerated; fusiform swelling of three digits of left hand	Multiple erythematous ulcerated nodules in linear array from dorsum of right hand to just proximal to right elbow; left arm spared
Preliminary assessment	Infection (e.g., sporotrichosis), destructive arthritis (e.g., multicentric reticulohistiocytosis)	Infection (e.g., sporotrichosis, atypical *Mycobacterium*, or *Nocardia*)
Special Techniques or Tests		
KOH preparation	No hyphae seen	Same
Radiograph	Destructive arthritis of hands	Not done
Wound culture	No growth of routine, acid-fast fungal, or microaerophilic organism	Sporotrichosis
Skin biopsy	Histology: multicentric reticulohistocytosis Culture: no growth	Histology: dense inflammation, no organisms Culture: sporotrichosis
Final Assessment	Multicentric reticulohistiocytosis	Sporotrichosis

KOH, potassium hydroxide.

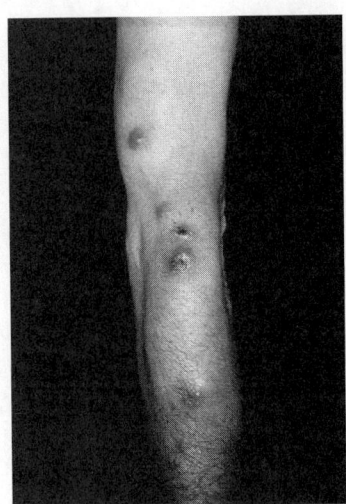

FIGURE 200.33. Case 6—Sporotrichosis. See color figure 200.33.

phalangeal joints and the swelling of the proximal interphalan-

geal joints. These lesions, combined with the destructive arthritis, suggest multicentric reticulohistiocytosis. A skin biopsy would help confirm the diagnosis.

ACKNOWLEDGMENT

I would like to thank and acknowledge Dr. Eugene Bauer for allowing me to use his examples and the text from his chapter in the third edition of *Kelley's Textbook of Internal Medicine* for use in this updated edition.

BIBLIOGRAPHY

Dobson RL, Abele DC. *The practice of dermatology.* Philadelphia: Harper & Row, 1985.

Epstein E. *Regional dermatology: a system of diagnosis.* Orlando: Grune & Stratton, 1984.

Freedberg IM, Fitzpatrick TB. *Fitzpatrick's dermatology in general medicine,* fifth ed. New York: McGraw-Hill, 1999.

Lazarus GS, Goldsmith LA. *Diagnosis of skin disease.* Philadelphia: FA Davis, 1980.

Lynch PJ. *Dermatology for the house officer.* Baltimore: Williams & Wilkins, 1994.

Kelley's Textbook of Internal Medicine, fourth edition. Edited by H. David Humes. Lippincott Williams & Wilkins, Philadelphia © 2000.

6

ONCOLOGY AND HEMATOLOGY

Robert F. Todd III, Editor

APPROACH TO THE PATIENT WITH ONCOLOGIC AND HEMATOLOGIC DISORDERS

APPROACH TO THE PATIENT WITH LYMPHADENOPATHY

DAVID J. VAUGHN

■ PRESENTATION

Evaluation of the patient with lymphadenopathy or lymph node enlargement is common in clinical practice. The enlarged lymph node may have been noticed by the patient or discovered on routine physical examination by the physician. Lymph node enlargement may be a result of significant disease such as infection or malignancy. A careful history and physical examination and an understanding of the pathophysiology and differential diagnosis of lymph node enlargement are crucial in the evaluation of such patients.

■ PATHOPHYSIOLOGY

Lymph nodes are discrete organs of the lymphatic system (Fig. 201.1). Afferent lymphatics passively carry lymph that contains lymphocytes, macrophages, and antigens and sometimes carries microorganisms to the node for processing, passing through the subcapsular sinus to enter the cortex.

The cortex consists of the primary and secondary lymphoid follicles. The primary follicles, which contain antibody-bearing B cells and T cells, give rise to secondary follicles after antigenic stimulation. Secondary follicles consist of an outer mantle zone of B cells and an inner germinal center, where macrophages, antigen-presenting dendritic reticulum cells, T cells, and B cells interact. This results in dramatic B-cell proliferation, differentiation, and antibody production.

The paracortex, found between the cortex and medulla, is the primary location for T cells in the node, with a predominance of the CD4 (helper or inducer T cell) phenotype. The paracortex also serves as the site where B cells, T cells, and macrophages, sometimes actively transporting antigens, reenter the node from the venous circulation through postcapillary venules.

The medulla, the innermost zone of the node, contains the medullary sinuses that converge on the hilum to form the efferent lymphatics. The lymph node architecture is well designed to facilitate its principal function: allowing the complex interaction of the cells of the immune system to process, respond to, and ultimately eliminate antigen. During the normal immune response, antigenic stimulation often results in lymphadenopathy from dramatic B-cell and T-cell proliferation and marked accumulation of lymphocytes and macrophages from increased blood flow to the node.

Lymphadenitis is the infiltration of inflammatory cells into the lymph node. Acute lymphadenitis results from direct microbiologic drainage; the nodes histologically demonstrate prominent germinal centers and neutrophilic infiltration, sometimes with abscess formation. Chronic lymphadenitis due to ongoing antigenic stimulation may manifest distinct histologic patterns. Follicular hyperplasia, resulting from various processes such as HIV infection or autoimmune disorders, manifests as marked enlargement and prominence of the germinal centers. In paracortical lymphoid hyperplasia such as that seen with some viral infections (e.g., Epstein–Barr virus) and in drug-induced reactions (e.g., from phenytoin), expansion of paracortical zones by means of immunoblastic proliferation results in a "pseudolymphomatous" pattern. Granulomatous lymphadenitis resulting from tuberculosis, sarcoidosis, and histoplasmosis typically results in lymphadenopathy.

Lymph node enlargement can result from the malignant transformation and proliferation of cells indigenous to the lymph node. Malignant lymphomas are neoplasms that arise from lymphocytes and their precursors. Lymphadenopathy can also result from infiltration of the node by leukemic cells. Many cancers of epithelial and sarcomatous origin metastasize to lymph nodes, where the milieu allows the neoplastic cells to thrive, resulting in nodal enlargement.

Lymph node enlargement may be caused by an accumulation of benign cells or substances in the node parenchyma. In some hereditary disorders such as lipid storage diseases, histiocytes laden with excess metabolites accumulate and result in nodal

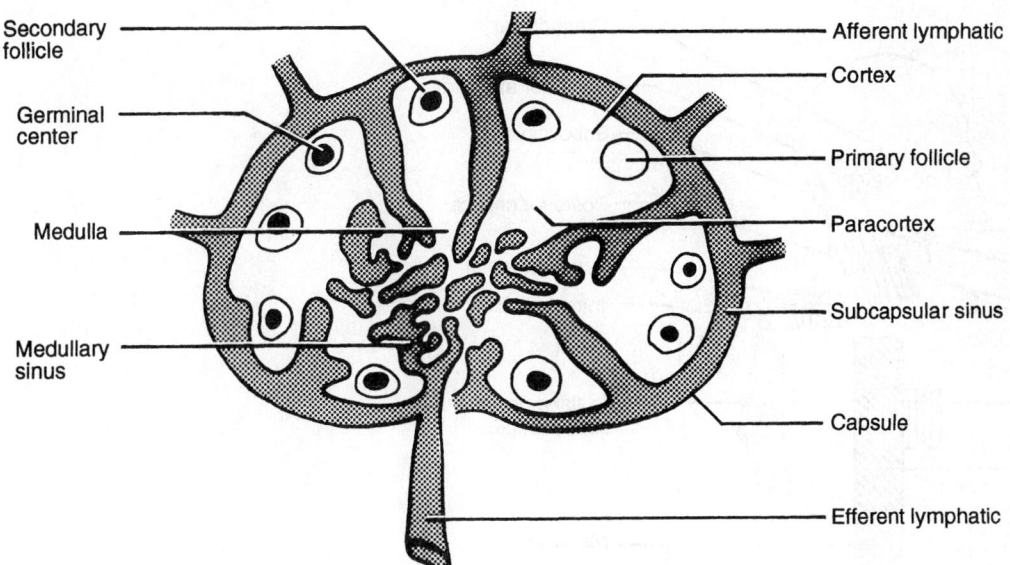

FIGURE 201.1. Structure of the lymph node.

enlargement. In amyloidosis, the excessive deposition of the fibrillar protein can cause enlargement of the lymph node.

HISTORY AND PHYSICAL EXAMINATION

The history of the patient presenting with lymphadenopathy may provide clues to the cause of the lymph node enlargement. The age of the patient is important. In patients younger than 30 years of age, most cases of lymphadenopathy are benign and frequently are caused by infection. A typical example is the college-age student presenting with tender cervical nodes and fever who may have a viral upper respiratory infection, bacterial pharyngitis, or infectious mononucleosis. However, in patients older than 50 years, lymphadenopathy results from benign conditions only 40% of the time, and malignancy must be aggressively excluded. A careful review of risk factors for HIV infection, such as high-risk sexual activity or intravenous drug use, is important for the patient presenting with generalized lymphadenopathy of more than 3 months' duration. Symptoms accompanying the lymphadenopathy may also help the clinician formulate a differential diagnosis. Fever may be a component of infectious and malignant causes of lymphadenopathy. Fever and lymphadenopathy may be accompanied by signs of a localized infection such as pharyngitis. However, when ongoing low-grade fevers are accompanied by night sweats or weight loss, these constitutional symptoms suggest lymphoma, HIV infection, or tuberculosis.

Lymph nodes are best examined by palpating with the fingertips in a circular motion to determine the physical characteristics of the node. These characteristics include size, mobility of the lymph node versus fixation to underlying tissue, tenderness, and consistency. In adults, the normal lymph node is usually soft and can vary in size from a few millimeters for most regions to 1 cm in diameter for inguinal nodes. In acute infections, nodes may be tender, localized, and matted. Chronic infections may result in less tender, more generalized nodes. Lymphoma nodes are often large, rubbery, and nontender. Metastatic carcinoma results in localized, hard, fixed nodes. Only with experience does the clinician develop the ability to differentiate normal from abnormally enlarged nodes.

A thorough knowledge of the anatomical regions and drainage patterns of normal nodal groups is important (Fig. 201.2) because the location of the abnormally enlarged nodes can help the clinician to determine the diagnosis (Table 201.1). The cervical lymph nodes drain the head and neck. To examine the cervical nodes, the clinician can stand behind or in front of the patient. The submental nodes are located under the chin; submandibular nodes are found under the angle of the jaw. These nodes drain the mouth and the associated salivary glands. The anterior cervical nodes lie anterior to the sternocleidomastoid, and the posterior cervical nodes are posterior. The suboccipital nodes are located in the apex of the posterior cervical triangle. The preauricular and posterior auricular nodes are in front of and behind the pinna of the ear, respectively.

In younger patients, cervical lymphadenopathy is common. Infectious mononucleosis frequently causes enlargement of posterior cervical nodes; bacterial or viral pharyngitis commonly results in enlargement of the anterior and posterior cervical nodes. Unilateral cervical node enlargement in an older patient, especially with a history of tobacco or alcohol abuse, may represent metastatic head and neck carcinoma.

In addition to draining head and neck structures, the supraclavicular nodes that lie posterior to the midclavicle drain the thorax and abdomen. Enlarged supraclavicular nodes may indicate a malignancy, such as lymphoma or metastatic cancer. *Virchow's node* refers to an enlarged left supraclavicular node as a result of metastatic gastrointestinal carcinoma.

Axillary lymph nodes are divided into central and lateral groups. The central axillary nodes are located near the middle of the axillary chest wall, with lateral groups along the upper humerus. These nodes are best examined by having the patient drop his or her arm in a relaxed position to the side of the body, allowing the examiner to more easily palpate the axilla by putting

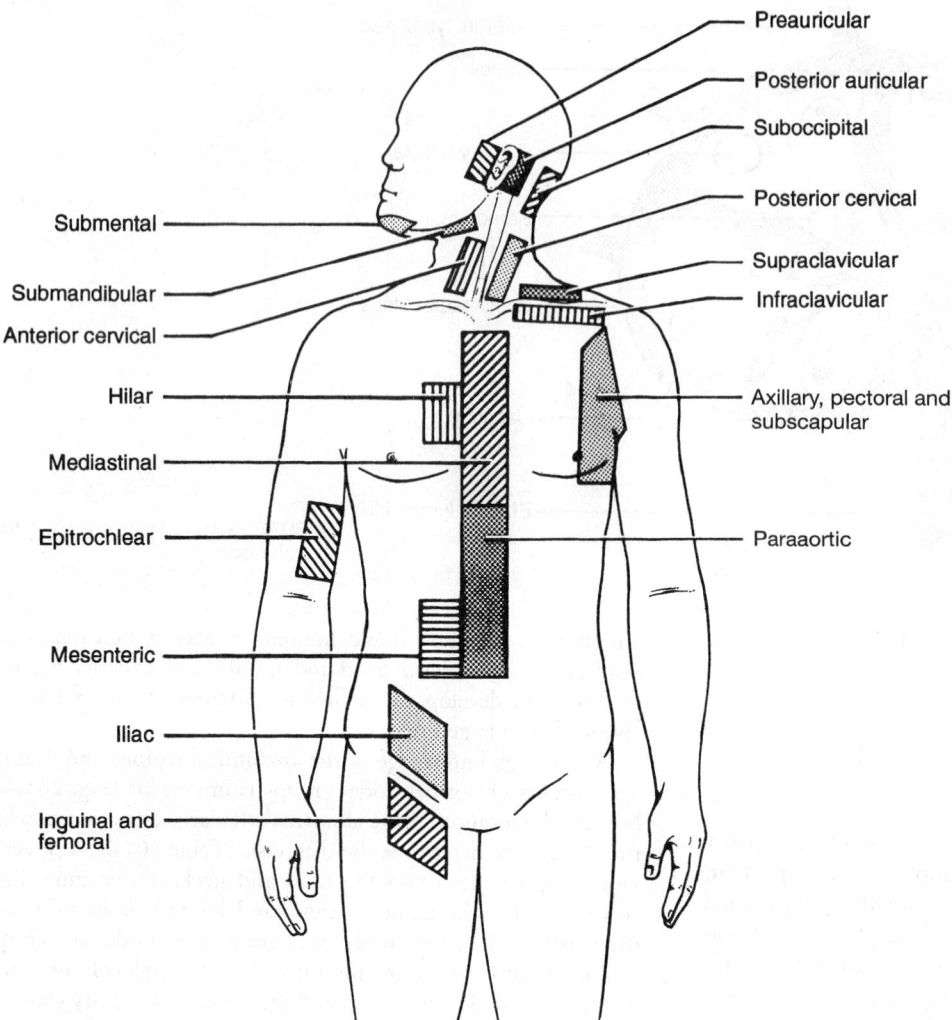

FIGURE 201.2. Anatomical lymph node regions.

pressure against the chest wall and moving the examining hand downward from the apex. Axillary lymph nodes drain the upper extremity, chest wall, breast, and intrathoracic organs. Bilateral small, soft axillary nodes may be benign; tender unilateral enlarged nodes in this site may be the result of cat-scratch disease or upper extremity infections. Rubbery or firm nodes in the axilla may indicate lymphoma or metastatic breast carcinoma.

The chest wall, breast, and intrathoracic structures are also drained by the subscapular nodes that lie anterior to the latissimus dorsi, the pectoral nodes found beneath the lateral edge of the pectoralis major, and the infraclavicular nodes located under the distal clavicle. Epitrochlear nodes lie just proximal to the medial epicondyle of the humerus. These nodes may be difficult to examine, and they are best approached by palpating across this region in a posterior direction.

The inguinal lymph nodes located along the inguinal ligament drain the lower extremity and the genitalia. The external iliac and femoral nodes located in the femoral triangle drain structures in the pelvis. Benign inguinal lymph node enlargement is common, and small palpable nodes less than 1 cm in diameter are found in many patients. Sexually transmitted diseases such as syphilis and lymphogranuloma venereum may cause unilateral inguinal node enlargement. Progressive enlargement of inguinal lymph nodes or association with femoral or iliac lymphadenopathy suggests malignancy, such as lymphoma or metastatic cervical or anal carcinoma.

In addition to the superficial lymph nodes that may be palpated by the examiner, the history and physical examination may yield clues concerning lymphadenopathy in the deeper regions of the chest, abdomen, and pelvis. Hilar or mediastinal lymph node enlargement due to malignancy or other causes may produce symptoms caused by compression of thoracic structures. These include cough, dyspnea, and wheezing due to tracheobronchial compression; dysphagia due to esophageal compression; swelling of the face, neck, and arms due to superior vena cava or subclavian vein compression; and hoarseness due to recurrent laryngeal nerve compression. Mediastinal and hilar lymphadenopathy may also be discovered as a result of radiographic investigation (e.g., computed tomography [CT] scanning) of clinically evident superficial lymphadenopathy.

The abdomen and pelvis may harbor deep lymphadenopathy, such as that caused by lymphoma. Because of the physical charac-

TABLE 201.1.	TYPICAL CAUSES OF LYMPHADENOPATHY ACCORDING TO THE ANATOMIC SITE OF ENLARGEMENT

Location of Lymphadenopathy	Common Causes
Suboccipital nodes	Infection of the scalp (bacterial)
	Systemic viral infection
Cervical nodes	Infections of the head and neck (including scalp, pharynx, eyes, ears)
	Infectious mononucleosis syndrome
	Tuberculosis
	Lymphoma
	Carcinoma of the head and neck
Supraclavicular nodes	Lung, gastrointestinal, or breast carcinoma
	Lymphoma
	Thoracic or retroperitoneal infection (bacterial, fungal)
Axillary nodes	Infection of the hand and arm (bacterial)
	Cat-scratch disease
	Tularemia
	Breast carcinoma
	Melanoma
	Lymphoma
Epitrochlear nodes	Infection of the hand and arm (bacterial)
	Lymphoma
	Sarcoidosis
Inguinal nodes	Infections of leg and foot (bacterial)
	Venereal disease (chancroid, herpes simplex, lymphogranuloma venereum, syphilis)
	Lymphoma
	Metastasis (anal and pelvic malignancy)
Hilar nodes	Sarcoidosis
	Tuberculosis
	Systemic fungal infections
	Lung carcinoma
	Lymphoma
Mediastinal nodes	Sarcoidosis
	Tuberculosis
	Systemic fungal infections
	Lung and breast carcinoma
	Lymphoma
	Germ cell tumor
Abdominopelvic nodes (includes retroperitoneum)	Tuberculosis
	Lymphoma
	Germ cell tumor
	Prostate carcinoma
	Pelvic malignancies
Generalized	Human immunodeficiency virus infection
	Infectious mononucleosis syndromes (Epstein–Barr, cytomegalovirus, toxoplasmosis)
	Miliary tuberculosis
	Disseminated fungal infections
	Drug reaction
	Sarcoidosis
	Immunologic disorders
	Leukemia and lymphoma

teristics of this cavity, large asymptomatic lymph node masses may arise in the retroperitoneum and pelvis. Occasionally, a large mesenteric or abdominopelvic lymph node mass may be palpable on physical examination. Clues to the presence of internal iliac or pelvic nodes include swelling of the lower extremities due to lymphatic or vascular compression by these nodes.

The spleen may be important in the evaluation of patients with lymphadenopathy. Splenomegaly that is tender may be seen in infectious mononucleosis syndromes. Patients with lymphoma and acute and chronic lymphocytic leukemia may manifest splenomegaly as well as lymphadenopathy. Infiltrative disease such as lipid storage diseases or amyloidosis may manifest with splenomegaly, as can autoimmune disease such as systemic lupus erythematosus.

LABORATORY STUDIES AND DIAGNOSTIC TESTS

The ancillary workup of the patient with lymphadenopathy is often directed by the clinical setting and the data obtained from performing a thorough history and physical examination. There is no prescribed battery of tests that all patients should undergo. The clinician should carefully select ancillary testing based on the differential diagnosis. A complete blood count may be helpful for patients suspected of having infection or malignancy. The blood smear may provide important clues to a hematologic malignancy such as chronic lymphocytic leukemia or acute leukemia. The young patient suspected of infectious mononucleosis may have circulating atypical lymphocytes on a blood smear. However, this patient should also undergo a confirmatory Monospot (heterophile antibody) test. If suspected of a bacterial pharyngitis, a simple throat culture can be diagnostic. A patient with known risk factors for HIV infection can have generalized lymphadenopathy explained by performing a diagnostic serologic test for HIV. Serologic titers for other infectious agents such as cytomegalovirus or toxoplasmosis may be helpful. An elevated erythrocyte sedimentation rate is nonspecific and usually does not further a differential diagnosis. Titers for antinuclear antibody or rheumatoid factor may be diagnostic for patients suspected of autoimmune illnesses.

Ancillary radiographic testing of the patient presenting with lymphadenopathy should be guided by the suspected diagnosis. A chest x-ray film and CT scans of the chest, abdomen, and pelvis may demonstrate lymphadenopathy in the deeper nodal groups and are especially useful for patients suspected of having lymphoma. However, many patients with superficial lymphadenopathy need no radiographic testing.

A lymph node biopsy is appropriate in several clinical situations. The patient with persistent, unexplained, localized, or generalized lymphadenopathy should undergo biopsy, especially if the node is firm, rubbery, or fixed. If lymphadenopathy is accompanied by fevers, night sweats, or weight loss and no source of infection is identified, a lymph node biopsy is indicated. Any patient suspected of having a malignant lymphoma should undergo immediate lymph node biopsy. In patients with a known malignancy, a lymph node biopsy may alter the therapeutic approach. For example, the patient with a gastric mass and a supraclavicular lymph node that is diagnostic of adenocarcinoma on biopsy might not need to undergo radical surgery. Lymph node biopsy can also be useful in the diagnosis of recurrent malignancy.

For patients with generalized lymphadenopathy, the largest node that is accessible should be biopsied to ensure that adequate tissue is available for pathologic diagnosis. Lymph nodes larger than 2 cm in diameter are preferred for biopsy. Abnormalities of inguinal lymph nodes are likely to represent reactive hyperplasia. Concern should be given to cosmetic issues; for example, the incisional scar from a resected axillary lymph node is less apparent than that from a node excised from the neck. Lymph node biopsy is diagnostic in about one half of the cases for which it is performed. Of the patients with a nondiagnostic biopsy, approximately 25% develop a disease, often a lymphoma, within 1 year. Patients with nondiagnostic biopsies need to be followed up closely and rebiopsy performed if nodes persist or worsen over time or if constitutional symptoms develop.

After the decision is made to perform a lymph node biopsy, the physician, surgeon, and pathologist need to communicate to be certain that the specimen is properly handled and appropriate testing performed (Table 201.2). An initial frozen section or "touch prep" histologic examination of the node may direct further studies. Patients who thought to have an infection such as tuberculosis should have the specimen properly cultured. The biopsied node should be delivered fresh to the pathology department, with instructions concerning the differential diagnosis of the suspected disorder.

If a lymphoma is suspected, the diagnostic workup includes standard formalin fixation with histologic examination of the node and immunophenotyping by flow cytometry or immunohistochemistry. Freezing part of the specimen for potential molecular diagnostic studies such as analysis of immunoglobulin or T-cell receptor gene rearrangement is prudent. Fresh tissue can be analyzed for cytogenetic abnormalities, such as the translocation of chromosomes 14 and 18 seen in follicular lymphomas. If breast cancer is suspected, the node can be analyzed for estrogen and progesterone hormone receptor expression. In cases of malignancy of undetermined site, the fixed node can be processed for immunohistochemical analysis to help determine the site of origin. For example, a supraclavicular node that is histologically malignant and demonstrates cytokeratin and mucicarmine positivity on immunohistochemical stains suggests an adenocarcinoma, raising the possibilities of carcinoma of the lung, breast, or gastrointestinal tract.

Lymph node aspiration may occasionally be performed in lieu of a biopsy. Fine-needle aspiration (FNA) is particularly useful in diagnosing metastatic carcinoma or infectious lymphadenitis. FNA may be useful in diagnosing lymphoma in patients without easily accessible lymphadenopathy and in those who cannot tolerate an open biopsy. The major drawback of aspiration is obvious: no tissue is obtained for histopathologic review, which is critical in the classification of the lymphomas. Inconclusive results from FNA frequently necessitate open biopsy.

◼ DIFFERENTIAL DIAGNOSIS

The differential diagnosis of lymphadenopathy is summarized in Table 201.3. The diseases responsible for the enlargement of lymph nodes can be classified as infection, malignancy, inflammation, nonmalignant infiltration, endocrine abnormalities, and miscellaneous disorders including the histiocytoses.

Infectious causes of lymphadenopathy are best approached by considering the types of infectious agents. Viral infections are important causes of lymphadenopathy. Epstein–Barr virus and cytomegalovirus can result in lymphadenopathy, as in the infectious mononucleosis syndromes (Chapters 313 and 314). HIV is an important cause of lymphadenopathy (Chapter 341). Persistent generalized lymphadenopathy is a clinicopathologic entity in which the HIV-infected patient develops generalized lymphadenopathy, especially in the cervical, axillary, occipital, and inguinal regions. The development of persistent generalized lymphadenopathy may be a harbinger to progression to AIDS. Patients with HIV infection also have a markedly increased risk of malignant lymphoma, usually a high-grade non-Hodgkin's type. Rapidly progressive lymphadenopathy in the HIV-infected patient should alert the physician to the diagnosis of malignancy.

Acute bacterial infections such as that caused by *Staphylococcus* species may cause a suppurative lymphadenitis. Chronic bacterial infections may also result in enlargement of lymph nodes. Cat-scratch disease is caused by infection with a very small gram-negative bacillus. This disease occurs most commonly in children and young adults and manifests as enlargement of the superficial nodes that drain the site of entry of the organism. Although the patient's history may or may not give a clue of a recent cat bite, most affected patients live in homes with cats.

Lymphogranuloma venereum, caused by a chlamydial organism, results in enlarged matted inguinal lymph nodes that may become fixed to the skin and form sinuses. Syphilis is the most important spirochetal infection that results in lymphadenopathy. It is seen principally in the primary and secondary stages, often in the inguinofemoral regions.

Mycobacterial infections such as tuberculosis can result in lymphadenopathy, especially in primary tuberculosis in which the nodes draining the portal of entry are enlarged. Endemic fungal infections may also result in lymphadenopathy. For example, histoplasmosis of the lung may be accompanied by hilar lymphadenopathy.

Parasitic infections may cause lymphadenopathy. *Toxoplas-*

TABLE 201.2.	DIAGNOSTIC EVALUATION OF THE BIOPSIED LYMPH NODES

1. Perform initial frozen section or touch prep histologic examination.
2. If infection is suspected, perform standard fixed histologic examination, as well as special stains and cultures for bacteria, fungus, or mycobacteria.
3. If malignancy is suspected, perform standard histologic examination, as well as immunohistochemical stains if needed.
4. If lymphoma is suspected, perform immunophenotyping (flow cytometry or immunohistochemistry) and, if needed to subclassify, cytogenetic analysis and immunoglobin and T-cell receptor gene rearrangement studies.

TABLE 201.3.	DIFFERENTIAL DIAGNOSIS OF LYMPHADENOPATHY
Cause	**Possible Diagnoses**
Infection	
Viral	Infectious mononucleosis (Epstein–Barr virus, cytomegalovirus), upper respiratory viruses (adenovirus, influenza), human immunodeficiency virus (HIV), rubella, herpes zoster (varicella), vaccinia, infectious hepatitis viruses
Bacterial	Streptococcus, Staphylococcus, Salmonella, Brucella, tularemia, Listeria monocytogenes, Pasteurella pestis, Haemophilus ducreyi, cat-scratch disease
Fungal	Histomosis, coccidiomycosis
Mycobacterial	Tuberculosis, leprosy
Chlamydial	Lymphogranuloma venereum, trachoma
Spirochetal	Syphilis, leptospirosis
Parasitic	Toxoplasmosis, trypanosomiasis, filariasis
Malignancy	
Hematologic	Hodgkin's and non-Hodgkin's lymphoma, acute lymphocytic and myelogenous leukemia, chronic lymphocytic and myelogenous leukemia, Waldenström's macroglobulinemia, malignant histiocytic disorders
Metastatic	Carcinomas of the breast, gastrointestinal tract, gynecologic tract, head and neck, kidney, lung, prostate, testis; germ cell neoplasms; melanoma; neuroblastoma; sarcoma
Inflammation	Rheumatoid arthritis, systemic lupus erythematosus, Sjögren's syndrome, dermatomyositis, serum sickness, angioimmunoblastic lymphadenopathy, drug reactions, posttransplant lymphoproliferative disorder
Infiltration	Amyloidosis, Gaucher's disease, Niemann–Pick disease
Endocrine	Hyperthyroidism
Miscellaneous	Sarcoidosis, dermatopathic lymphadenitis, Castleman's disease (giant follicular lymph node hyperplasia), Kawasaki's disease (mucocutaneous lymph node syndrome), lymphomatoid granulomatosis, benign histiocytic disorders, vascular transformation of the sinus, inflammatory pseudotumor of the node

mosis gondii infection, acquired by contamination with cat feces, may present with an enlarged node or group of nodes in the cervical, posterior auricular, suboccipital, or parotid regions that may persist for months. Biopsy demonstrates a distinctive histologic picture of follicular hyperplasia, clusters of epithelial histiocytes, and accumulation of monocytoid B cells in the nodal sinuses. Serologic confirmation should be obtained.

The malignant lymphomas comprise Hodgkin's disease and the non-Hodgkin's lymphomas (Chapters 232 and 233). Hodgkin's disease most commonly begins as a painless enlargement of superficial lymph nodes, most frequently the cervical and supraclavicular nodes. The patient may also have involved mediastinal and hilar nodes found on the chest x-ray film. The patient may have classic "B" symptoms such as fever, night sweats, or weight loss. Non-Hodgkin's lymphoma may also manifest as painless lymphadenopathy. The clinical presentation of patients with non-Hodgkin's lymphoma depends on the histologic subtype.

Primary malignancies of the bone marrow may manifest with lymphadenopathy. For example, patients with acute lymphocytic leukemia may have extensive generalized lymphadenopathy or a large mediastinal mass. Patients with chronic lymphocytic leukemia often have generalized lymphadenopathy and splenomegaly. Waldenström's macroglobulinemia is a disease of the older patient characterized by lymphadenopathy, splenomegaly, and a monoclonal IgM protein spike.

Abnormally enlarged lymph nodes may result from malignant infiltration by metastatic cancer. These nodes are usually hard and may be fixed. A variety of adult tumors can metastasize to superficial lymph nodes. Malignant melanoma and carcinomas of the breast, lung, and stomach are most likely to produce lymphadenopathy that is clinically evident. Occasionally, a lymph node biopsy demonstrates a poorly differentiated malignancy (Chapter 226). The clinician relies on the pathologist for performing immunohistochemical, flow cytometric, and molecular diagnostic studies to determine the diagnosis. It is crucial to differentiate lymphoma from metastatic carcinoma, because the prognosis and treatment are different.

Lymphoid hyperplasia may occur in a variety of inflammatory disorders. Autoimmune diseases such as systemic lupus erythematosus, rheumatoid arthritis, and Sjögren's syndrome may manifest with generalized lymphadenopathy. Angioimmunoblastic lymphadenopathy affects mainly elderly persons and is characterized by generalized lymphadenopathy often associated with fever, hepatosplenomegaly, Coombs'-positive hemolytic anemia, and polyclonal hypergammaglobulinemia. Some patients have a history of an autoimmune illness, but, in most, the disease arises de novo. This benign disease may transform into malignant lymphoma.

Patients with organ transplants maintained on immunosuppressant therapy may develop post-transplantation lymphoproliferative syndrome (Chapter 23). This disorder may present with generalized lymphadenopathy and constitutional symptoms. It is often caused by Epstein–Barr virus infection and can resolve with the discontinuation of immunosuppressants; however, some cases are rapidly progressive and may require chemotherapy.

Lymphoid hyperplasia and lymphadenopathy may be a result of drug reaction, such as to phenytoin, hydralazine, and allopurinol.

Nonmalignant infiltration of the lymph node may result in lymphadenopathy. Amyloidosis (Chapter 235) may have lymphadenopathy as a prominent symptom. The fibrillar protein material may be deposited in lymph nodes and other organs. This disorder may be associated with malignancy or inflammatory disorders or may be primary. Occasionally, enlarged nontender lymph nodes are the first manifestation of the disease. In lipid storage diseases such as Gaucher's and Niemann–Pick disease (Chapter 12), lipid-laden histiocytes accumulate in the lymph nodes, resulting in enlargement. This most commonly occurs in the abdomen, and patients may have associated involvement of the liver and spleen.

Nonmalignant thyroid disorders may involve lymphadenopathy. Patients with Graves' disease or Hashimoto's thyroiditis occasionally have associated lymphadenopathy. Pathologically, these nodes demonstrate reactive hyperplasia.

Although most patients who present with lymphadenopathy have an infectious, neoplastic, or inflammatory disorder, there are miscellaneous disorders of unclear cause that result in prominent lymphadenopathy. Patients with sarcoidosis (Chapter 373) may present with bilateral hilar lymphadenopathy; patients may also have generalized peripheral lymphadenopathy. Castleman's disease, or giant follicular lymph node hyperplasia, is an idiopathic disorder that may manifest as localized or generalized lymphadenopathy. Frequently, mediastinal or hilar nodes are involved. Patients with the multicentric subtype of the disease may present with a rapidly progressive course that may lead to death.

Kawasaki's disease, or mucocutaneous lymph node syndrome, is seen in children and young adults. This disease is characterized by fever, conjunctivitis, a desquamative truncal exanthem, and cervical lymphadenopathy. Patients may develop a fatal coronary arteritis.

Lymphomatoid granulomatosis (Chapter 374) is characterized by the infiltration of the vessels of various organs by atypical lymphocytes and macrophages. Lungs, skin, and the central nervous system are most frequently affected. Forty percent of cases have mediastinal lymphadenopathy, but only 10% of cases have peripheral node enlargement. A significant proportion of these patients develop a malignant lymphoma, often of the T-cell phenotype.

The histiocytic disorders include an interesting array of diseases that may present with prominent lymphadenopathy. These diseases include benign and malignant proliferation of the two main classes of histiocytes: antigen-presenting cells such as Langerhans' cells and antigen-processing histiocytic cells, including monocytes and macrophages. The Langerhans' cell histiocytoses (formerly known as histiocytosis X) includes three syndromes of reactive histiocytic proliferation: eosinophilic granuloma, a benign disease that may present in children or adults, often with only a localized bone lesion; multifocal eosinophilic granuloma including the Hand–Schüller–Christian disease, manifesting in young children with a triad of exophthalmus, diabetes insipidus, and lytic bone lesions; and disseminated Langerhans' cell histiocytosis or Letterer–Siwe disease, a disease of infants, with fever, lymphadenopathy, hepatosplenomegaly, rash, and cytopenias.

Dermatopathic lymphadenitis occurs in patients with chronic skin disorders such as exfoliative dermatitis. These patients develop enlargement of superficial lymph nodes that pathologically demonstrate paracortical expansion of the antigen-presenting interdigitating reticulum cells. The lymphadenopathy may regress with appropriate treatment of the skin condition. Dermatopathic lymphadenopathy may also be associated with mycosis fungoides and cutaneous T-cell lymphoma. Malignant transformation of lymph node reticulum cells may rarely occur. These uncommon malignancies usually manifest as localized lymphadenopathy and frequently recur after chemotherapy.

Persons with benign proliferative disorders of antigen-processing cells such as macrophages also present with lymphadenopathy. Sinus histiocytosis with massive lymphadenopathy or Rosai–Dorfman disease occurs predominantly in young adults, who present with fever, leukocytosis, and bulky matted lymphadenopathy, often in the cervical region. The reactive hemophagocytic syndromes occur in the setting of infectious and neoplastic conditions, and patients may present with enlargement of lymph nodes in addition to pancytopenia and hepatosplenomegaly. In familial erythrophagocytic lymphohistiocytosis, a rare autosomal recessive disorder, patients presenting with lymphadenopathy, hepatosplenomegaly, pancytopenia, and frequently with fatigue and fever demonstrate a unique pathologic finding: phagocytized red blood cells in the bone marrow or lymph nodes.

Histiocytic medullary reticulosis is characterized by lymphadenopathy, hepatosplenomegaly, and constitutional symptoms, and a biopsy demonstrates proliferation of histiocytes and immature monocytoid cells. Kikuchi's disease, or histiocytic necrotizing lymphadenitis, is a benign, self-limited disease that occurs throughout the world. This disorder usually affects those younger than 40 years of age, and patients present with fever and symptoms of a flulike illness. The lymphadenopathy of this disorder may be generalized or, more commonly, localized to the cervical region. Pathologically, proliferation of histiocytes and immunoblasts is demonstrated, with marked necrosis and karyorrheatic debris.

Malignant disorders of mononuclear phagocytes include acute monocytic leukemia and true histiocytic lymphoma. The latter is an uncommon subtype of non-Hodgkin's lymphoma, in which patients present with lymphadenopathy as well as bone, skin, and gastrointestinal tract involvement.

Vascular transformation of the sinuses (nodal angiomatosis or stasis lymphadenopathy) may occur in any age group and can manifest as localized or generalized lymphadenopathy, although usually this is an incidental finding in lymph nodes surgically obtained for other reasons. Pathologically, the lymph node sinuses demonstrate expansion and sclerosis with vascular proliferation.

Young adults with inflammatory pseudotumor of lymph nodes may present with constitutional symptoms and lymphadenopathy of the superficial and deep groups. Pathologically, the connective tissue elements of the node such as the hilum, trabeculae, and capsule demonstrate proliferation of spindled histiocytes and fibroblasts, as well as vascular proliferation. This disease demonstrates spontaneous remission in most cases.

■ STRATEGIES FOR OPTIMAL CARE

MANAGEMENT

The management of the patient with unexplained lymphadenopathy is based on an understanding of the pathophysiology of lymph node enlargement and clinical expertise in obtaining

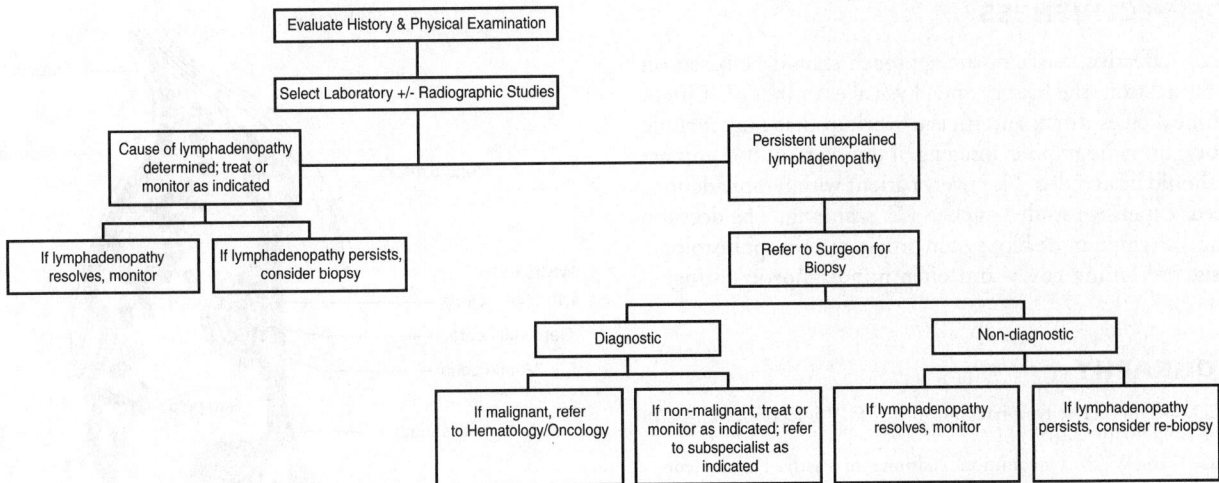

FIGURE 201.3. Algorithm for the evaluation of lymphadenopathy. Empiric antibiotics or corticosteroids should not be given. If biopsy performed, coordinate with the surgeon and pathologist to ensure proper processing of specimen.
EVIDENCE LEVEL: C. Expert Opinion.

a history, performing a physical examination, and obtaining a differential diagnosis–directed ancillary battery of tests. If an infectious cause is strongly suspected, a period of observation or a trial of antimicrobial therapy can be instituted. HIV testing should be considered for patients with persistent generalized lymphadenopathy. However, if the nodes manifest characteristics suggesting malignancy or if unexplained lymphadenopathy persists, patients should undergo biopsy (Fig. 201.3).

COMPLICATIONS AND PITFALLS

Several important errors may be made in evaluating a patient with lymphadenopathy. The unjustified use of antibiotics should be avoided. If the physician strongly suspects an infectious cause of the enlarged lymph nodes or if the diagnosis is established, prompt institution of specific antibiotics is indicated. However, the use of antibiotics in an attempt to treat unexplained lymphadenopathy delays diagnosis and is costly. It also places the patient at risk of having a drug reaction. Patients suspected of infectious mononucleosis should not be given antibiotics such as ampicillin because of a high incidence of rash, and lymph node biopsy should be avoided in these patients because the pathology of the lymph node may mimic that of malignant lymphoma.

The empiric use of corticosteroids should also be avoided. Unexplained lymphadenopathy demands an explanation, and empiric corticosteroid therapy can distort lymph node histopathology by its lympholytic effect. Corticosteroids can occasionally worsen infection.

The biopsy of a lymph node is important in the diagnosis of unexplained lymphadenopathy. However, lymph node biopsy may have potential problems that should be avoided. The physician, surgeon, and pathologist must communicate clearly concerning suspected causes of lymphadenopathy. Inappropriate handling of the specimen, such as submitting the entire node in fixative, which may preclude potentially important immuno-

phenotyping and molecular analysis, or forgetting to send the tissue for appropriate cultures may result in nondiagnostic biopsies.

If a "watch and wait" approach is indicated, patients should be monitored closely (e.g., every 2 to 4 weeks), because unexplained, persistent lymphadenopathy or increasing enlargement of nodes requires biopsy. Patients with nondiagnostic biopsies need careful observation, because some will develop clinically significant disease over time. HIV testing should be considered for patients with nondiagnostic biopsies that have persistent generalized lymphadenopathy.

Indications for HOSPITALIZATION

Most patients with lymphadenopathy undergo evaluation and treatment as outpatients. However, patients with rapidly enlarging lymphadenopathy accompanied by significant symptoms, such as bulky mediastinal adenopathy and shortness of breath, and patients with debilitating constitutional symptoms require hospital admission for close observation, support, and diagnostic evaluation. Occasionally, patients require admission for the diagnostic biopsy of enlarged deep nodes, such as those in the retroperitoneum or thorax.

Indications for REFERRAL

Most cases of lymphadenopathy are managed by the primary care physician. Referral to a general or plastic surgeon for lymph node biopsy is often made by the internist. Sometimes, referral to an oncologist or hematologist is indicated, especially if the diagnosis of malignancy is strongly suspected.

COST-EFFECTIVENESS

To be cost-effective, a diagnostic approach should be based on data obtained from the history and physical examination. Often, these clinical clues direct an efficient workup that may include laboratory or radiographic imaging. However, indiscriminate testing should be avoided. Not every patient with lymphadenopathy needs expensive studies such as CT scanning. The decision to perform a lymph node biopsy can provide a prompt histologic diagnosis, precluding costly and often nondiagnostic testing.

BIBLIOGRAPHY

Baroni CD, Uccini S. The lymphadenopathy of HIV infection. *Am J Clin Pathol* 1993;99:397–401.
Chan JKC, Tsang WYW. Uncommon syndromes of reactive lymphadenopathy. *Semin Oncol* 1993;20:648–657.
Gonzalez CL, Jaffe ES. The histiocytoses: clinical presentation and differential diagnosis. *Oncology* 1990;4:47–60.
Greenfield S, Jordon MC. The clinical investigation of lymphadenopathy in primary care practice. *JAMA* 1978;240:1388–1393.
Lee Y, Terry R, Lukes RJ. Lymph node biopsy for diagnosis: a statistical study. *J Surg Oncol* 1980;14:53–60.
Pangalis GA, Vassilakopoulos TP, Boussiotis VA, et al. Clinical approach to lymphadenopathy. *Semin Oncol* 1993;20:570–582.
Sinclair S, Beckman E, Ellman L. Biopsy of enlarged, superficial lymph nodes. *JAMA* 1974;228:602–603.
Stansfeld AG, d'Ardenne AJ. *Lymph node biopsy interpretation,* second ed. London: Churchill Livingstone, 1992.

Kelley's Textbook of Internal Medicine, fourth edition. Edited by H. David Humes.
Lippincott Williams & Wilkins, Philadelphia © 2000.

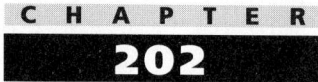

C H A P T E R

202

APPROACH TO THE PATIENT WITH SPLENOMEGALY

LYNN M. SCHUCHTER

ANATOMY AND FUNCTION

The spleen is the largest lymphoid organ in the body; in a healthy adult, it weighs between 75 and 100 g. The organ is located in the left upper quadrant, protected anteriorly, laterally, and posteriorly by the lower portion of the rib cage.

The spleen consists of a fibrous capsule and radiating fibrous trabeculae that enclose the white and red pulp (Fig. 202.1). The splenic vasculature and the intricate meshwork of splenic reticulum provide a unique environment for the primary function of the spleen—filtration—which results in removal of aging and defective erythrocytes, antigens, and microorganisms from

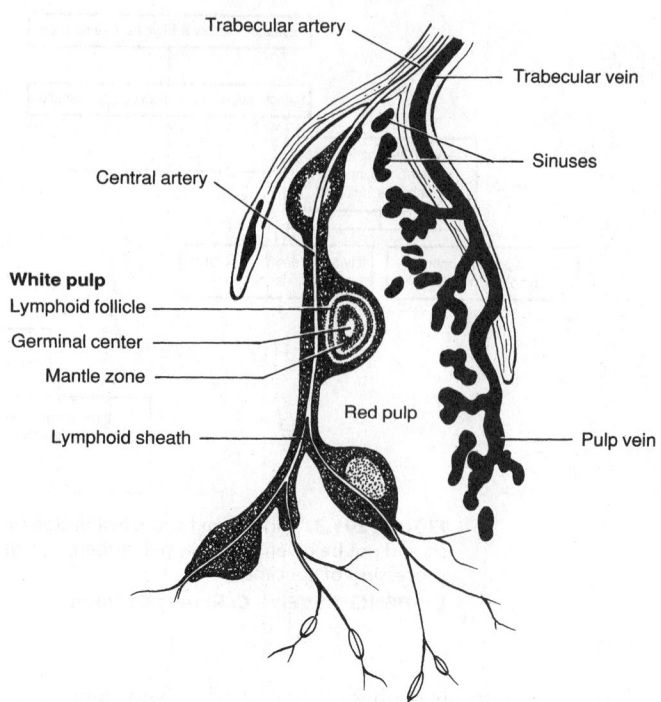

FIGURE 202.1. The structure of the spleen.

the blood. Accessory spleens, which result from the failure of the spleen to develop into a single tissue mass, have been reported in 14% to 30% of patients.

Arterial blood enters the spleen through the splenic artery, a branch of the celiac artery. Most blood from the splenic central and trabecular arterioles flows into the sinuses and cords, which are lined with macrophages. Blood from the red pulp sinuses and cords empties directly into the splenic venous system. The major venous drainage of the spleen is the splenic vein, which joins the superior mesenteric vein to form the portal vein.

The spleen is conventionally divided into three zones: the white pulp, the red pulp, and the marginal zone, which is located between the red and white pulp. The white pulp is further subdivided into a T-cell domain (predominantly CD4+ helper T lymphocytes), which surrounds the central arteriole and forms the periarteriolar lymphoid sheath, and a B-cell domain, which comprises the follicles and perifollicular mantle zone. Similar to the lymph node, the follicles are inactive or activated, the latter being associated with germinal center formation. The white pulp is responsible for the immunologic functions of the spleen. It contains a concentration of immunologically active cells, captures circulating antigens, provides an arena for their interaction, and is a major site for the production of opsonizing IgM antibody. The marginal zone, another predominantly B-cell layer in the periphery of the white pulp, contains the sinuses that filter material from the white pulp and blends into the red pulp area.

The red pulp occupies the largest portion of the spleen, and it is within the red pulp that the primary function of the spleen, filtration of defective or foreign cells, is carried out. The principal sites of red blood cell entrapment in the spleen are fenestrations in the wall of splenic sinuses, where blood from the splenic cords of the red pulp enters the venous circulation. Blood cells must squeeze through small slits in the cord lining before returning to the venules. Aging changes the biophysical properties of the red cell, making splenic entrapment of the red blood cells that have circulated for 105 to 120 days more likely. Damaged, defective, and aging erythrocytes are less deformable and are therefore retained in the cords, where they are phagocytized by splenic macrophages. During the course of a day, approximately 20 mL of aging red blood cells are removed.

Pitting, the ability of the spleen to remove particulate inclusions from red cells without destroying the cell itself, is also performed by these phagocytes. This pitting function removes Howell–Jolly bodies (nuclear remnants), Heinz bodies (denatured hemoglobin), and erythrocytic parasites such as *Plasmodium. Culling* refers to phagocytosis by splenic macrophages of abnormal whole red blood cells that have been damaged physically or immunologically.

The spleen also serves as a reservoir for platelets. One-third of the total platelet pool is normally sequestered in the spleen, but the role of the spleen in the final removal of normal platelets has not been precisely defined. Additional functions of the spleen include removal of bacteria from the circulation, especially pneumococci, and production of blood components if the bone marrow is unable to meet demands (i.e., extramedullary hematopoiesis). The spleen plays an important role in the generation of an immunologic response to certain pathogens.

PATHOPHYSIOLOGY

Although many conditions are associated with splenic enlargement or splenomegaly, limited types of pathologic mechanisms cause splenomegaly. Splenomegaly can result from infiltration of the spleen by reactive lymphoid cells or proliferating macrophages due to inflammation or infection or from infiltration by neoplastic cells in hematologic malignancies. Infiltration of the spleen with abnormal material, as in amyloidosis or Gaucher's disease, can produce splenomegaly. Hypertrophy or hyperplasia of the spleen usually is caused by reticuloendothelial hyperplasia resulting from underlying hematologic disorders such as hereditary spherocytosis and thalassemia or from extramedullary hematopoiesis in primary bone marrow disorders. Vascular congestion as a result of decreased venous drainage due to portal hypertension is associated with an increase in the size of the spleen and is called *congestive splenomegaly.* Splenomegaly can result from space-occupying lesions such as cysts, abscesses, or hemangiomas.

The pathologic action of the spleen—the reduction of circulating blood elements—has been attributed to three possible mechanisms: excessive splenic cellular elements (e.g., phagocytes), splenic production of an antibody that results in the destruction of hematopoietic cells, and overactivity of splenic function, leading to accelerated removal of any or all of the circulating blood elements. This action, referred to as *hypersplenism,* results

in anemia, leukopenia, or thrombocytopenia, alone or in combination. The cytopenias associated with hypersplenism are the result of splenic pooling in the enlarged spleen with resultant sequestration of platelets, red blood cells, and granulocytes.

HISTORY AND PHYSICAL EXAMINATION

Disorders of the spleen usually are part of a generalized pathologic disorder, and the initial presentation depends on the underlying disease. The most common symptom directly related to the spleen is pain in the left upper quadrant. Pain may result from stretching of the splenic capsule or from splenic infarction, which is most commonly seen in patients with sickle cell anemia. A persistent dull ache or fullness in the left upper quadrant is often reported by patients with a massively enlarged spleen. Patients with disorders of the spleen may also present with signs and symptoms of shock due to splenic rupture and resultant intraperitoneal bleeding. Rupture of the spleen is most frequently associated with penetrating trauma, nonpenetrating trauma, or operative trauma, and rupture occasionally complicates infectious diseases. Splenic rupture is rarely a spontaneous event.

The history of exposure to potential sources of infection and constitutional complaints such as fever, malaise, fatigue, and weight loss that accompany hematologic malignancies and systemic infections are important. The duration of symptoms and signs is suggestive: in patients with a prolonged history, splenomegaly is often associated with a neoplastic process, and in patients with infection or inflammatory conditions, the symptoms often develop over days. Because splenomegaly may result from portal hypertension caused by cirrhosis of the liver, a history of alcoholism or previous liver disease is relevant to the evaluation.

Physical examination of the spleen should include auscultation, percussion, and palpation. Under normal circumstances, the spleen is not palpable on abdominal examination, but the organ may be felt in about 2% of healthy adults. In one study, the spleen was palpable in only 3% of students entering an American college and was a persistent finding in only one-third. In healthy persons, no significant dullness is elicited by percussion over the spleen anteriorly or laterally. As the organ enlarges, dullness may be detected at the level of the ninth intercostal space in the left anterior axillary line. Palpation of the spleen is best identified during deep inspiration. A palpable spleen usually signifies an enlarged spleen. However, patients may have significant splenomegaly without a palpable spleen. The enlarged spleen is generally not tender except when the peritoneum is inflamed from infection or infarction. Auscultation over the spleen may reveal a friction rub or bruit, suggestive of splenic infarct or aneurysm, respectively. Because most conditions that cause splenomegaly may also cause lymphadenopathy, the physical examination should include careful examination for enlarged lymph nodes. Similarly, physical signs of liver dysfunction and portal hypertension should be included as part of the physical examination.

TABLE 202.1.	DISEASES ASSOCIATED WITH SPLENOMEGALY

Infectious Diseases

Infectious mononucleosis
Cytomegalovirus
Echinococcus
Human immunodeficiency virus infection
Toxoplasmosis
Viral hepatitis
Salmonellosis
Relapsing fever
Tularemia
Syphilis
Malaria
Subacute bacterial endocarditis
Tuberculosis
Schistosomiasis
Response to infection (viral, bacterial)
Bacterial septicemia
Splenic abscess
Histoplasmosis
Leishmaniasis
Trypanosomiasis

Inflammatory Disease

Felty's syndrome
Systemic lupus erythematosus
Rheumatic fever
Serum sickness
Sarcoid

Congestive Diseases

Intrahepetic
  Cirrhosis
  Venoocclusive disease
  Congenital hepatic fibrosis
Portal vein obstruction or hypertension
Splenic veinobstruction or splenic artery aneurysm
Hepatic vein occlusion (Budd–Chiari syndrome)
Congestive heart failure

Primary Hematologic Diseases

Spherocytosis
Early sickle cell anemia
Ovalocytosis
Thalassemia major
Hemoglobinopathies
Paroxysmal nocturnal hemoglobinuria
Nutritional anemias
Immunothrombocytopenia
Polycythemia vera
Myeloid metaplasia with
  myelofibrosis
Primary thrombocytosis
Chronic myelogenous leukemia

Infiltrative Disease

Leukemia
Lymphoma
Hodgkin's disease
Malignant histocytosis
Hairy cell leukemia
Metastatic cancer
Primary tumors: hemangioma,
  hamartoma fibroma
Angiosarcomas
Angioimmunoblastic
  lymphadenopathy
Eosinophilic granuloma

Storage Diseases

Gaucher's disease
Neimann–Pick disease
Amyloidasis Tangier disease
Hyperlipedemia
Hurler's syndromes
Other muco-polysracchariodoses

Miscellaneous Conditions

Tropical splenomegaly
Primary splenic hyperplasia
Drug reactions
Extramedullary hematopoiesis

DIFFERENTIAL DIAGNOSIS

Table 202.1 lists the principal conditions associated with splenomegaly. Any condition that causes generalized lymphadenopathy can cause splenomegaly, including chronic infections such as mononucleosis, inflammatory and immunologic diseases such as sarcoidosis and collagen vascular diseases, and hematologic malignancies such as lymphoma, chronic lymphocytic leukemia (CLL), and chronic myelogenous leukemia (CML).

The differential diagnosis of splenomegaly as a function of splenic size is summarized in Table 202.2. In general, the larger the spleen, the greater the likelihood that the pathogenesis is a serious medical problem. The causes of massive splenomegaly (greater than 3000 g) are somewhat limited, most commonly to myeloproliferative disorders and malignant lymphoma. The spleen is greatly enlarged in patients with CML and myelofibro-

sis. Malignant tumors such as Hodgkin's disease and non-Hodgkin's lymphoma are usually not primarily in the spleen but rather part of a generalized process. Splenomegaly due to metastatic cancers is usually observed late in the course of a widely metastatic tumor, most often associated with metastatic breast cancer, stomach cancer, and malignant melanoma. Splenomegaly may also be caused by nonmalignant hematologic disorders such as immune hemolytic anemias and conditions associated with abnormal erythrocytes as in hereditary spherocytosis and hemoglobinopathies (e.g., thalassemia, sickle cell anemia).

Systemic infections are the most common causes of moderate and transient splenomegaly. This condition is frequently seen in patients with mononucleosis due to Epstein–Barr viral infections, but it may also occur with other viral infections such as cytomegalovirus and adenovirus infection and in cases of acquired toxoplasmosis. Modest splenomegaly is seen in patients

TABLE 202.2.	DIFFERENTIAL DIAGNOSIS OF SPLENOMEGALY AS A FUNCTION OF SIZE		
Category	**Centimeters Below Left Coastal Margin**	**Spleen Weight (grams)**	**Diseases**
Not palpable	None	100–200	None
Minimal	Tip–4 cm	200–500	Acute splenitis
			Hypersensitivity reactions
			Lupus
			Bacterial endocarditis
Moderate	4–8 cm	500–1000	Cirrhosis and congestive diseases
			Acute leukemias
			Mononucleosis
			Hemolytic anemia
			Thalassemia
			Idiopathic thrombocytopenic purpura
			Spherocytosis
			Polycythemia vera
			Niemann–Pick disease
			Histiocytosis X
			Tuberculosis
			Sarcoidosis
			Metastatic tumors
Marked	>8 cm	>1000	Chronic myelogenous leukemia
			Chronic lymphocytic leukemia
			Lymphomas
			Hairy cell leukemia
			Myelofibrosis with myeloid metaplasia
			Malaria
			Gaucher's disease
			Primary tumors

with HIV infection but is more often related to hepatic or infectious complications of the disease. Bacterial infections associated with splenomegaly include secondary syphilis, acute bacterial endocarditis, and acute brucellosis. Malaria, schistosomiasis, and leishmaniasis result in splenomegaly and are common in tropical populations. Hematogenous spread of tuberculosis or histoplasmosis can involve the spleen as well. Rickettsial infection can cause splenic enlargement, with a palpable spleen found in 40% of patients who have Rocky Mountain spotted fever.

Chronic congestive splenomegaly due to portal hypertension is associated with gastrointestinal bleeding and pancytopenia. It is usually secondary to cirrhosis of the liver or, less commonly, to portal vein thrombosis. Splenomegaly due to cysts or primary tumors is uncommon. The most common primary benign tumors of the spleen are hemangiomas and lymphangiomas.

Acute splenic sequestration can complicate sickle cell anemia, most commonly in young children with hemoglobin SS disease and patients of all ages with hemoglobin SC and sickle cell disease or β-thalassemia. Acute splenic sequestration is characterized by acute worsening of anemia, by reticulocytosis, and by a tender, enlarging spleen; 15% of attacks are fatal. Because splenic sequestration recurs in 50% of cases, splenectomy is often recommended after resolution of the acute episode.

Miscellaneous conditions are also associated with splenomegaly. In patients with sarcoidosis, involvement of the liver and spleen may produce hepatomegaly and splenomegaly in about 25% of cases. Splenomegaly occurs in 10% to 20% of patients with systemic lupus erythrocytosis. In patients with rheumatoid arthritis, splenomegaly is associated with thrombocytopenia or, more often, leukopenia and is designated Felty's syndrome. The cytopenia often responds to splenectomy. Gaucher's disease is a familiar disorder characterized by abnormal storage or retention of glycolipid cerebrosides in reticuloendothelial cells. Proliferation and enlargement of these cells produce enlargement of spleen, liver, and lymph nodes. Modest splenomegaly is associated with deficiency diseases, such as megaloblastic anemias and, rarely, iron deficiency.

Splenomegaly is often accompanied by the syndrome of hypersplenism, consisting of a large spleen, anemia, leukopenia, or thrombocytopenia and hyperplastic bone marrow. About 20% of patients with splenomegaly develop manifestations of hypersplenism. In hypersplenism, the platelet count is usually 50 to 150×10^9 per liter, and only rarely are platelet counts below 20×10^9 per liter. Anemia and neutropenia associated with hypersplenism are usually moderate and asymptomatic. The severity of cytopenias does not correlate with the degree of splenic enlargement. Because the splenomegaly and hypersplenism are secondary pathologic processes, treatment usually is directed toward the underlying condition. However, splenectomy often corrects persistent and significant cytopenias.

Not all left upper quadrant masses are related to splenomegaly. Other causes of a left upper quadrant mass include gastric or colon tumors and pancreatic or renal cyst or tumors.

LABORATORY STUDIES AND DIAGNOSTIC TESTS

Splenomegaly is common, but a palpable spleen in an adult is almost always clinically significant and requires evaluation. In general, diagnostic tests to evaluate splenomegaly are not performed on the spleen itself; they are oriented toward diagnosis of disease states that result in splenomegaly. However, a determination of splenic size can begin with a plain abdominal radiograph that may demonstrate an enlarged splenic shadow. Computed tomography (CT), ultrasonography, and magnetic resonance imaging (MRI) of the left upper quadrant can depict the spleen, define abnormalities in size and shape, and delineate parenchymal pathology. Radioisotopic scanning with a technetium Tc 99m sulfur colloid scan is another technique, although less sensitive than CT or MRI, to determine the size and shape of the spleen and to look for defects suggesting tumors, cysts, or extrasplenic masses displacing the spleen. This test can also be used as an indicator of splenic function.

The major laboratory abnormalities associated with splenomegaly are determined by the underlying disease. The most valuable laboratory tests in the differential diagnosis of splenomegaly are the complete blood cell count and a differential count, examination of the peripheral blood smear, and liver function tests. Bone marrow aspiration and biopsy are often useful in the diagnosis of leukemia, lymphoma, lipid storage disorders, and disseminated fungal and mycobacteria infections. For patients presenting with anemia, Coombs' test and hemoglobin electrophoresis are sometimes useful. Hemolytic anemia is detectable by routine laboratory tests for anemia and for hemolysis, including a reticulocyte count and determinations of serum bilirubin and serum haptoglobin levels. Erythrocyte counts may be elevated in patients with polycythemia vera, but in most presentations, the erythrocyte count is normal or decreased. Leukocyte counts may be elevated (e.g., in chronic leukemias), normal, or decreased (e.g., in Felty's syndrome, hairy cell leukemia). Platelet counts also may vary; they are often increased in patients with polycythemia vera or normal or decreased in patients with idiopathic thrombocytopenic purpura (ITP). In cases of primary marrow failure, the spleen may be enlarged and undergo myeloid metaplasia in an effort to generate more cells to compensate for the abnormal marrow.

For patients with fever, blood and bone marrow cultures are valuable, as are the tests for viral disease with specific viral titers. Laboratory abnormalities consistent with liver dysfunction or radiologic evidence of esophageal varices suggest portal hypertension. Serologic tests for collagen vascular diseases may be useful. Because many conditions associated with splenomegaly also cause lymphadenopathy, biopsy of a palpable lymph node often discloses the cause of the splenomegaly. When systemic symptoms accompany splenomegaly, but no lymphadenopathy is found, a laparotomy with biopsies of the liver and lymph nodes is sometimes indicated, as is splenectomy itself.

STRATEGIES FOR OPTIMAL CARE

The most common emergency indication for splenectomy is traumatic or iatrogenic splenic rupture. The medical indications for splenectomy include two broad categories: diagnostic splenectomy and splenectomy to alleviate the consequences of splenomegaly, principally cytopenias. Splenectomy is a part of the staging laparotomy in patients with Hodgkin's disease; however, with improvements in radiologic imaging, this is no longer routinely performed. Occasionally, splenectomy is indicated to establish the diagnosis of isolated splenomegaly. More recently, laparoscopic splenectomies have been performed, which appear to have advantages over the open operation.

Splenectomy is useful for symptom control in patients with CML and hairy cell leukemia. Although the overall survival rates for patients with CML treated with splenectomy are not different from those treated without splenectomy, removal of the spleen usually makes patients more comfortable and makes management somewhat easier by reducing transfusion requirements. Splenectomy is an effective treatment for patients with CLL in selective clinical situations, including patients with extensive splenomegaly that is refractory to chemotherapy and patients with autoimmune cytopenias as a complication of CLL.

HIV infection is associated with thrombocytopenia that is similar to classic ITP. However, unlike results for patients with classic ITP, splenectomy has been highly effective in producing a sustained increase in platelet counts in approximately 90% of HIV-infected patients. Although the data are limited, most reported series show no significant increase in the incidence of infection after splenectomy in patients with AIDS nor acceleration in the clinical progression of AIDS.

Splenectomy is indicated for the management of autoimmune hemolytic anemia in patients who fail to respond to corticosteroids. Approximately 50% to 60% of patients with autoimmune hemolytic anemia have an excellent response to splenectomy. Cytopenias associated with hypersplenism are frequently corrected by splenectomy. Splenomegaly associated with increased destruction of red blood cells, as in hereditary spherocytosis, responds dramatically to splenectomy.

The main contraindication to splenectomy is marrow failure, because the enlarged spleen is the only source of hematopoietic cells for these patients. It is critically important in the setting of an enlarged spleen and cytopenias to differentiate extramedullary hematopoiesis from increased cell destruction. Hypersplenism is suggested by a cellular marrow and signs of increased peripheral destruction (e.g., reticulocytes, band forms, and large platelets). Extramedullary hematopoiesis is suggested by the presence of bizarre erythrocyte sizes and shapes.

The main complication associated with splenectomy is the risk of infection, particularly by encapsulated bacterial organisms. The precise reason for enhanced susceptibility to infection in asplenic patients or in patients with splenic dysfunction is not entirely clear, but a variety of immunologic defects have been reported. These include diminished responses to intravenous immunization with particular antigens; defects in the production of antibodies to T-cell–independent antigens, such as the polysaccharide components of the bacterial capsules; a deficiency in tuftsin, a phagocytosis-promoting peptide; decreased serum levels of IgG and IgM; and an inability to remove opsonized bacteria from the bloodstream. As a consequence, patients who have had splenectomy have an increased risk of septicemia with encapsulated bacteria, including *Streptococcus pneumoniae, Neisseria meningitidis,* and *Haemophilus influenzae.* Septicemia in these patients is characteristically fulminant.

The risk of serious infection depends somewhat on the cause of the abnormal splenic function, the age of the patient, and the presence of other immunologic abnormalities. Patients who have undergone splenectomy after trauma have a lower risk of infection. Because septicemia is more common in children and adolescents, it is reasonable to delay splenectomy for hematologic disorders in very young children. Infection occurs most frequently within the first 3 years after splenectomy. Patients with sickle cell anemia are functionally asplenic as a result of repeated infarctions and are particularly susceptible to *Salmonella* infections. Patients who have had splenectomy are also more susceptible to the parasitic disease, babesiosis, which is caused by *Babesia microti;* such patients should avoid areas where this parasite is endemic (e.g., Cape Cod, Massachusetts). Splenectomy does not appear to enhance the risk of nonbacterial infections.

All patients undergoing splenectomy should receive as prophylaxis a pneumococcus vaccine and a vaccine against *H. influenzae,* if available. Vaccination is best performed about 10 days before elective splenectomy and preoperatively in traumatized patients in whom splenectomy is anticipated.

After splenectomy, characteristic changes in blood composition occur. Howell–Jolly bodies are found in almost all patients, and siderocytes, nucleated red blood cells, and Heinz body inclusions are common as a result of the loss of the pitting and culling functions of the spleen. Splenectomy results in an increase in platelets, which sometimes reach levels greater than 1 million cells per cubic millimeter. Postsplenectomy thrombocytosis is often transient but may persist. In patients with marked thrombocytopenia before splenectomy, the platelet count often returns to normal within 2 days, but peak levels may not be reached for 2 weeks. The white blood cell count usually is elevated the first day and may remain persistently elevated for several months.

BIBLIOGRAPHY

Alonso M, Gossot D, Bourstyn E, et al. Splenectomy in human immunodeficiency virus-related thrombocytopenia. *Br J Surg* 1993;80:330–333.

Aquino VM, Norvell JM, Buchanan GR. Acute splenic complications in children with sickle cell-hemoglobin C disease. *J Pediatr* 1997;130(6): 961–965.

Eichner ER, Whitfield CL. Splenomegaly: an algorithmic approach to diagnosis. *JAMA* 1981;246:2858–2861.

Hambelton J. Hematologic complications of HIV infection [Review]. *Oncology* 1996;10(5):671–680.

McAneny D, LaMorte WW, Scott TE, et al. Is splenectomy more dangerous for massive spleens? *Am J Surg* 1998;175(2):102–107.

O'Reilly RA. Splenomegaly in 2,505 patients at a large university medical center from 1913 to 1995. *West J Med* 1998;169(2):88–97.

Rege RV, Merriam LT, Joehl RJ. Laparoscopic splenectomy [Review]. *Surg Clin North Am* 1996;76(3):459–468.

Sheth SG, Amarapurkar DN, Chopra KB, et al. Evaluation of splenomegaly in patients with hypertension. *J Clin Gastroenterol* 1996;22(1):28–30.

Tallman MS, Hakimian D, Peterson L. Massive splenomegaly in hairy cell leukemia. *J Clin Oncol* 1998;16(3):1232–1233.

Weiss L. Barrier cells in the spleen. *Immunol Today* 1991;12:24–29.

Kelley's Textbook of Internal Medicine, fourth edition. Edited by H. David Humes.
Lippincott Williams & Wilkins, Philadelphia © 2000.

CHAPTER
203

APPROACH TO THE PATIENT WITH A MEDIASTINAL MASS

KEVIN R. FOX

PRESENTATION

The mediastinum is the anatomic space that separates the left and right pleural sacs of the thorax. The development of a mediastinal mass may occur in any of the compartments of the mediastinum. The traditional anatomic compartmentalizations of the mediastinum are varied; the division of the mediastinum into three compartments—anterior, middle, and posterior—simplifies the diagnostic process for the internist or medical oncologist (Fig. 203.1).

The *anterior* mediastinum contains the thymus gland, fat, and lymph nodes. The *middle* mediastinum, which encompasses the superior mediastinum at the thoracic inlet, includes the trachea with its bifurcation, aortic arch and great vessels, subcarinal and paratracheal nodes, pericardium, heart, and upper esophagus. The *posterior* mediastinum includes most of the esophagus,

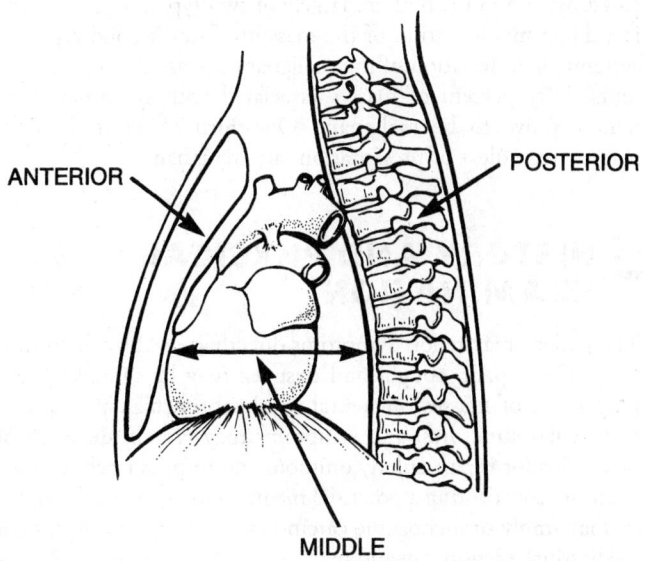

FIGURE 203.1. Anatomic subdivision of the mediastinum.

TABLE 203.1.	DIFFERENTIAL DIAGNOSIS OF MEDIASTINAL MASSES ACCORDING TO LOCATION	
Anterior Compartment	**Middle Compartment**	**Posterior Compartment**
Thymoma and benign thymic disorders	Germ cell tumors	Neurogenic tumors
Germ cell tumors	Teratoma	Lymphoma
Teratoma	Teratocarcinoma	Non-Hodgkin's lymphoma
Teratocarcinoma	Seminoma	Hiatal hernia
Seminoma	Lymphoma	Meningocele
Thyroid gland and thyroid tumors	Hodgkin's disease	Mediastinal cysts
Lymphoma	Non-Hodgkin's lymphoma	Bronchogenic
Hodgkin's disease	Mediastinal cysts	Enteric
Non-Hodgkin's lymphoma	Bronchogenic	Thoracic duct
Lipoma	Pericardial	Esophageal cancer and diverticula
Soft-tissue tumors	Enteric	Aortic aneurysms and vascular
Benign tumors	Hiatal hernia	malformations
Sarcomas	Granulomatous diseases	Soft tissue tumors
Pericardial cysts	Aneurysms and vascular malformations	Benign tumors
Lymph nodes enlarged by benign conditions	Lipoma	Sarcomas
Parathyroid tumors		

the descending aorta, the nerve chains of autonomic origin, and lymph nodes. The presentation of a mediastinal mass varies greatly from one patient to another, given the wide array of potentially affected structures and the wide variety of benign and malignant illnesses that may involve the mediastinum. Mediastinal masses usually are manifestations of diseases that have a predilection for one of the three mediastinal compartments and are thereby differentiated from diseases that involve two or more mediastinal compartments, such as acute and chronic mediastinitis, hemorrhage, or pneumomediastinum.

An understanding of the clinical presentation of mediastinal masses is best derived from a review of the broad differential diagnosis associated with these masses (Table 203.1). Approximately one-half of mediastinal masses are asymptomatic and are found incidentally at chest radiography performed for different reasons. Of the asymptomatic masses, approximately 10% prove to be malignant. The other 50% of mediastinal masses are heralded by symptoms that are largely of two types. The first type is a direct manifestation of the mass itself; the second type is a systemic manifestation of the malignant disease the mass represents. Fifty percent of masses associated with symptoms ultimately prove to be malignant. One-third of all mediastinal masses, regardless of presentation, are malignant.

HISTORY AND PHYSICAL EXAMINATION

The patient may report symptoms directly caused by the tumor mass. Chest pain, cough, and dyspnea may be caused by impingement of masses on neural, tracheobronchial, pericardial, or vascular structures, and symptoms may vary in duration of onset. Stridor is particularly ominous and implies tracheal compromise, constituting a potential medical emergency. Hemoptysis may imply bronchogenic carcinoma giving rise to malignant mediastinal adenopathy and may be an important clue in directing the diagnostic evaluation. Hoarseness implies paralysis of the recurrent laryngeal nerve in its course through the mediastinum, and dysphagia suggests intrinsic esophageal abnormality or extrinsic compression of the esophagus and directs attention to the posterior mediastinum. Dyspnea, cough, and head pain or fullness that occur while the person is supine may herald superior vena cava obstruction and imply a pathologic condition in the middle mediastinum.

Systemic symptoms of a malignant mediastinal tumor may predominate in the clinical presentation. Fever, weight loss, and night sweats are the classic B symptoms that may accompany Hodgkin's disease or non-Hodgkin's lymphoma, or they may rarely accompany other malignant lesions such as lung cancer or thymoma. Thyrotoxicosis, symptoms of weight loss, agitation, and irritability may be a manifestation of an enlarged, substernal thyroid gland. Because most malignant tumors of the posterior mediastinum are of neurogenic origin, a few patients have the hypertensive crises of pheochromocytoma or the episodic flushing and diarrhea of carcinoid-like tumors. Myasthenia gravis and its attendant symptoms of weakness, dyspnea, and double vision are present at diagnosis among a small percentage of patients with thymoma. A history of tobacco abuse and passive exposure to cigarette smoke always should be sought.

The physical examination is directed toward signs that may lend evidence to the diagnosis, make feasible diagnosis by relatively noninvasive means, or serve as harbingers of cardiopulmonary compromise that necessitates emergency hospitalization. Examination of the vital signs should seek unexplained tachycardia, pulsus alternans, or an increase in the pulsus paradoxus, all of which in addition to the mediastinal mass may suggest pericardial involvement. Careful examination of the neck may disclose auscultatory signs of stridor or tracheal deviation, which may constitute emergency airway obstruction. Marked enlargement of the thyroid may be the only physical finding that accompanies substernal thyroid that becomes apparent as a superoanterior mediastinal mass. The characteristic facial swelling and dilatation of the superficial veins of the neck, thorax, and scalp that are signs of the superior vena cava syndrome occur among patients with lung cancer or, less often, lymphoma.

Perhaps nowhere can the physical examination benefit the patient more than in establishing sites for diagnosis that do not require invasive thoracic procedures. A thorough lymph node examination of the neck, supraclavicular fossae, and axillae may disclose lymphadenopathy and a site for biopsy. This approach is particularly relevant for patients with Hodgkin's disease, because most patients with mediastinal disease also have cervical or supraclavicular lymphadenopathy. Careful examination of the testes of young men with anterior mediastinal masses may disclose a testicular mass associated with a germ cell tumor of the mediastinum. A thorough neurologic examination always should be performed; weakness and oculomotor dysfunction may suggest myasthenia gravis if the patient has thymoma and may increase the risk of invasive diagnostic surgical procedures.

LABORATORY STUDIES AND DIAGNOSTIC TESTS

ROUTINE EVALUATION

Routine laboratory studies and various tumor markers are not fail-safe substitutes in establishing the diagnosis of mediastinal masses. Because most patients with such masses ultimately undergo invasive diagnostic or therapeutic procedures, routine evaluation of serum electrolytes, a complete blood cell count, liver function tests including lactate dehydrogenase determination, and coagulation studies should be undertaken. Measurements of β-human chorionic gonadotropin (β-hCG) and α-fetoprotein (AFP) can be justified in the care of any patient younger than 40 years with an anterior mediastinal mass. Whether the elevation of one or both of these markers obviates tissue diagnosis is controversial. Because germ cell tumors represent a minority of mediastinal masses, it is usually prudent to proceed with the diagnostic evaluation rather than waiting for the results of these assays.

In rare instances laboratory evaluation circumvents invasive biopsy procedures. This occurs occasionally for patients with lymphoblastic lymphoma, a relatively uncommon high-grade lymphoma of the non-Hodgkin's type with a predilection for the mediastinum. This lymphoma sometimes manifests itself with circulating lymphoblasts detectable on a peripheral blood smear. For this reason, a young patient with a mass in the anterior mediastinum should undergo careful examination of the peripheral blood film by an experienced hematopathologist. If any suspicion of such malignant lymphocytosis is raised, oncologic consultation for bone marrow aspiration and biopsy should be obtained immediately.

Patients with malignant posterior mediastinal masses usually have tumors of neural origin, which may include pheochromocytoma or carcinoid-like tumors. Measurements of urinary catecholamines or 5-hydroxyindoleacetic acid are useful if either of these diagnoses is suspected on the basis of clinical presentation.

RADIOLOGIC EVALUATION

For almost every patient the mass of interest is first found on posteroanterior and lateral chest radiographs. However, the requisite diagnostic study for every patient with a mediastinal mass is contrast-enhanced computed tomographic (CT) scanning of the chest. This study should be performed with intravenous contrast and oral contrast media; oral contrast medium better delineates the esophagus. The CT scan should extend from the thoracic inlet to the most caudal extent of the posterior diaphragmatic recesses.

The value of thoracic CT scanning cannot be understated. The scan localizes the mediastinal mass and directs further diagnostic studies. It can help differentiate vascular abnormalities, benign collections of fat, cysts, and hiatal hernias, and it may allow the evaluation to cease if these anomalies necessitate no therapeutic intervention. The proximity of masses to critical vascular structures, large airways, and the pericardium is easy to evaluate.

Magnetic resonance imaging (MRI) should not be considered a substitute for CT scanning of the mediastinum. MRI is more expensive and more inconvenient for the patient than is CT scanning, and it provides the same information. MRI is justified when no form of iodine-containing contrast material can be safely administered to a patient in preparation for CT scanning. MRI of the thoracic spine should be considered if a patient with a posterior mediastinal mass has back pain in a radicular distribution or has CT evidence of foraminal invasion by the mass. These findings herald epidural space involvement by tumor and may alter surgical strategy. Other diagnostic studies rarely are indicated before the biopsy procedure. A barium swallow examination is indicated if the patient has dysphagia and the CT scan suggests an esophageal mass or malformation.

DIFFERENTIAL DIAGNOSIS

Table 203.1 provides a comprehensive list of diagnostic possibilities based on the anatomic location of the mass of interest. Some confusion in organizing such a list may occur with the inclusion of the "superior" mediastinum in the anterior or middle mediastinal compartments. Such rigid adherence to anatomic lines is relatively impractical, because many diseases occur in more than one of these arbitrarily designated compartments.

The relative frequency of primary mediastinal tumors can be derived from review of the records of large groups of patients and is shown in Table 203.2. At least one-half of mediastinal

TABLE 203.2.	RELATIVE FREQUENCY OF MEDIASTINAL TUMORS	
Tumor	Overall Frequency (%)	Anterior Compartment Frequency (%)
Thymoma and thymic lesions	19	47
Lymphoma	13	23
Germ cell tumors	11	15
Soft-tissue tumors	7	<10
Endocrine tumors and masses	6	16
Neurogenic tumors	21	<1

neoplasms among adults are thymoma, lymphoma, and germ cell tumors, which are likely to be situated in the anterior or middle mediastinum. When anterior mediastinal masses are considered separately, thymoma predominates, followed by lymphoma, germ cell tumors, and masses and tumors of thyroid and parathyroid origin (Table 203.2).

Hodgkin's disease is more likely to manifest itself with a mediastinal mass than is non-Hodgkin's lymphoma. Approximately 60% of patients with Hodgkin's disease have mediastinal masses as part of their clinical presentations; this is more than twice the frequency of patients with such masses caused by non-Hodgkin's lymphoma. Lymphoblastic lymphoma and diffuse large-cell lymphoma constitute most types of non-Hodgkin's lymphomas associated with such masses.

The neurogenic tumors that predominate in the posterior mediastinum compose a broad array of rare tumor types that may arise from nerve tissue or from the nerve sheath. Neurofibroma, neurilemoma, schwannoma, pheochromocytoma, and paraganglioma may be encountered in the posterior mediastinum. Many of these lesions are benign and nonfunctional, and they are easily managed by means of surgical extirpation.

STRATEGIES FOR OPTIMAL CARE

DIAGNOSTIC MANAGEMENT

The approach to a patient with a mediastinal mass culminates in the invasive procedure that carries the greatest likelihood of establishing the diagnosis with the least morbidity. The CT finding of fat, a benign-appearing cyst, or a vascular anomaly or aneurysm generally necessitates no further intervention, although referral to a cardiothoracic surgeon may be warranted for final diagnostic and therapeutic intervention.

All other lesions require a tissue diagnosis. The temptation to render a diagnosis by means of fine-needle aspiration biopsy under CT guidance is great because of the low morbidity of this procedure. In many circumstances, however, such a diagnostic step is inaccurate, inadequate, or unnecessary. Fine-needle aspiration biopsy often is inadequate for the diagnosis of Hodgkin's disease and non-Hodgkin's lymphoma, because it does not provide the architectural information necessary for precise subclassification of these disorders. It may be more reliable in the diagnosis of germ cell tumors and may be considered in the evaluation of a young man with a mediastinal mass and dramatically elevated (more than 500 units) AFP and β-hCG levels.

Bronchoscopy should be considered for any patient with disease in the middle mediastinum, especially in the paratracheal and subcarinal nodes, who is a smoker and is older than 40 years, particularly if there is a history of hemoptysis or radiographic evidence of lobar or segmental atelectasis. Transtracheal biopsy of the mediastinal nodes may provide an accurate diagnosis of lung carcinoma if no endobronchial lesion is located. Esophagoscopy is appropriate if the CT scan suggests posterior mediastinal or esophageal disease and if barium swallow results confirm the CT findings.

Most mediastinal masses ultimately require the diagnostic or therapeutic services of a thoracic surgeon. The internist should incorporate the thoracic surgeon in the diagnostic team at the earliest possible moment. The surgeon can use full thoracotomy, limited thoracotomy, mediastinoscopy, or video thoracoscopy with biopsy for diagnostic purposes. Mediastinoscopy, performed with general anesthesia, is performed through an incision in the suprasternal notch to evaluate tissues in the upper middle mediastinum along the course of the trachea to its bifurcation. It is probably not the optimal diagnostic procedure for truly anterior tumors, nor can it always be used to assess subcarinal or aortopulmonary window nodes. Thoracotomy through a standard thoracotomy or for anterior lesions through a limited incision in the left second or third interspace (Chamberlain procedure) allows direct inspection of mediastinal lymph nodes and allows removal of the largest quantities of tissue for pathologic review. Video thoracoscopy through a paramediastinal incision or lateral chest wall incision may be particularly useful for the diagnosis of posterior lesions and may occasionally be used for anterior mediastinal lesions that extend into the adjacent pulmonary parenchyma.

Figure 203.2 provides an algorithm for the evaluation of a mediastinal mass. This diagram begins with acquisition of a contrast-enhanced CT scan of the chest. It is assumed that a basic laboratory evaluation has been performed that includes serum markers for germ cell tumors and that a detailed physical examination has been performed. Any evidence of symptomatic large-airway compromise demands hospitalization and urgent surgical and oncologic consultation.

The CT scan may suggest a purely vascular, cystic, or fatty mass. The need for diagnostic or therapeutic surgical intervention depends on the nature and location of the anomaly and the related symptoms. All other masses should be directed toward the most reliable means of diagnosis. Biopsy should be performed on enlarged cervical nodes. Suspect circulating lymphocytes, such as lymphoblasts, should be characterized by means of bone marrow evaluation. Elevated serum AFP or β-hCG levels should prompt oncologic consultation and a careful testicular examination.

Most mediastinal masses seen in clinical practice do not lend themselves to easy diagnosis by noninvasive means. The final branches in Figure 203.2 outline the most reliable diagnostic maneuvers. CT-guided fine-needle aspiration biopsy should be considered if there is a high likelihood of bronchogenic carcinoma or malignant germ cell tumor but cannot obviate subsequent diagnostic or therapeutic thoracotomy or mediastinoscopy in most situations. The indications for esophagoscopy or bronchoscopy discussed previously have almost no application for patients with anterior lesions. Thoracotomy provides the most reliable means of diagnosis and allows simultaneous surgical resection of thymoma, benign teratoma, most neural tumors, and most endocrine tumors. Surgical resection of malignant germ cell tumors, Hodgkin's disease, and non-Hodgkin's lymphoma constitutes inappropriate management, because these diseases often are curable with chemotherapy, external beam irradiation, or both modalities.

COMPLICATIONS AND PITFALLS

The two greatest pitfalls in the evaluation of a mediastinal mass are failure to recognize the potentially life-threatening nature of

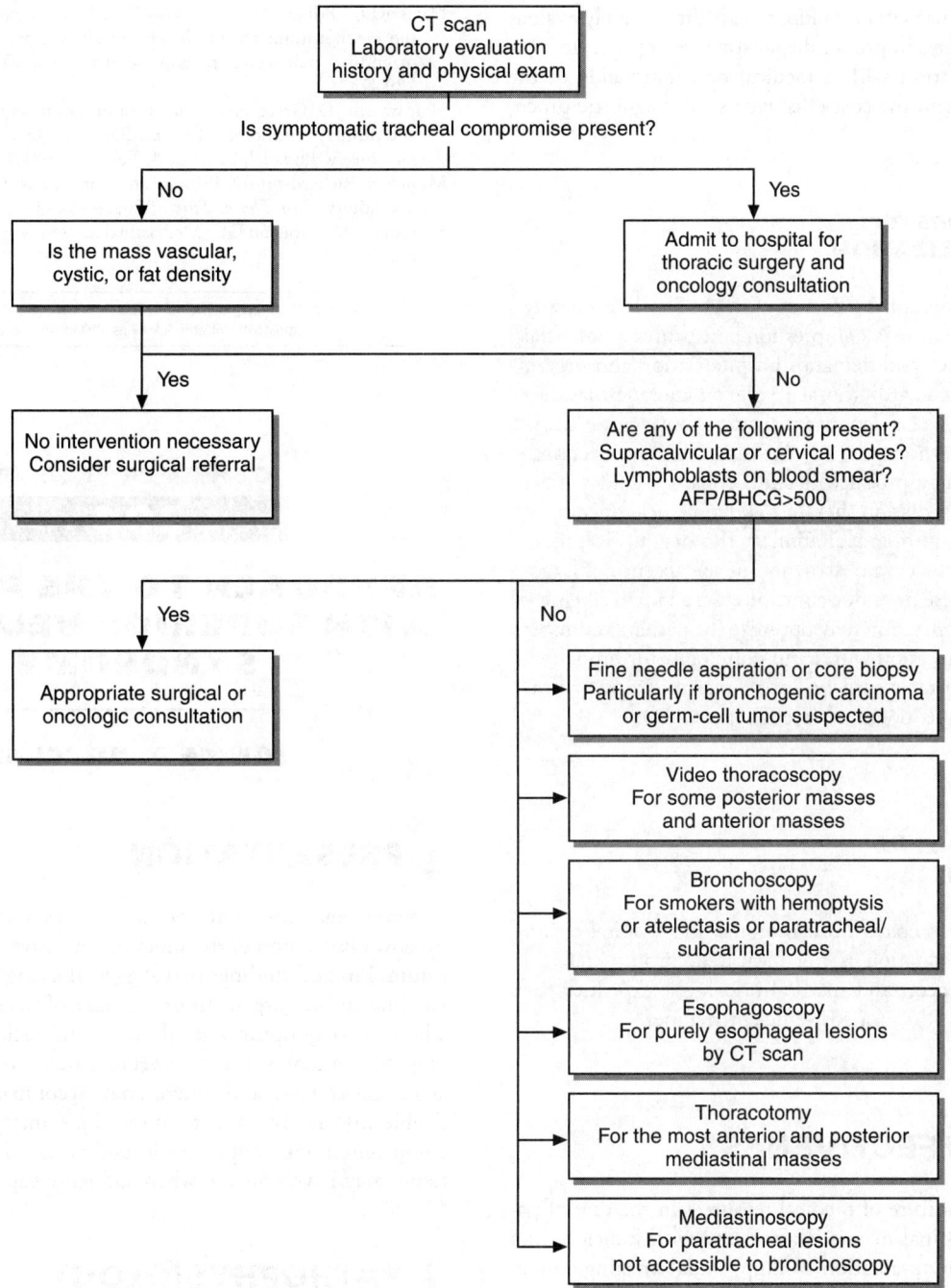

FIGURE 203.2. Algorithm for evaluation of mediastinal masses. *AFP*, α-fetoprotein; *BHCG*, β-human chorionic gonadotropin; *CT*, computed tomography.
EVIDENCE LEVEL: C. Expert Opinion.

some mediastinal masses and failure to expedite a timely evaluation because of delays in proper diagnostic intervention. In general, early consultation with a medical oncologist aids in the prompt diagnosis and the cost-effective use of diagnostic procedures.

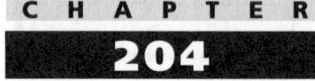 Indications for HOSPITALIZATION

Clinical and radiographic evidence of tracheal or large-airway compromise by extrinsic compression constitutes a potential medical emergency and demands hospitalization and urgent consultation with a cardiothoracic surgeon and anesthesiologist. If intubation is needed for ventilatory failure or for delivery of general anesthesia, the act of extubation may be hazardous, because it may produce tracheal collapse. Under these circumstances, a radiation therapist and a medical oncologist should be called into consultation at the diagnostic procedure. Superior vena cava obstruction in the absence of large-airway compromise does not constitute a true medical emergency, but hospitalization may optimize the patient's comfort while rapid consultation with a pulmonologist for bronchoscopy or cardiothoracic surgeon for mediastinoscopy or limited thoracotomy is obtained (see Chapter 204).

Indications for REFERRAL

Most patients do not have dire symptoms, and hospitalization for diagnostic evaluation is not indicated. Prompt referral to a thoracic surgeon and medical oncologist expedites the diagnostic evaluation in a cost-efficient manner.

COST-EFFECTIVENESS

Appropriate expenditure of medical resources in the care of patients with mediastinal masses is associated with judicious and truncated laboratory evaluation workup, initial imaging evaluation with a radiograph and CT scan of the chest, and avoidance of diagnostic procedures that carry a low likelihood of obviating more invasive but necessary interventions. The role of fine-needle aspiration of anterior and posterior masses should be carefully considered; this procedure frequently constitutes an unnecessary step if the patient ultimately needs a more detailed histologic diagnosis. Hospitalization should not be necessary for most patients with asymptomatic or minimally symptomatic masses before appropriate triage for the diagnostic procedure.

BIBLIOGRAPHY

Blossom GB, Steiger Z, Stephenson LW. Neoplasms of the mediastinum. In DeVita VT, Hellman S, Rosenberg SA, eds. *Cancer: principles and practice of oncology,* 5th ed. Philadelphia: JB Lippincott, 1997:951–969.

Davis RD, Oldham HN, Sabiston DC. Primary cysts and neoplasms of the mediastinum: recent changes in clinical presentation, methods of diagnosis, management, and results. *Ann Thorac Surg* 1987;44:229–237.

Hainsworth JD, Greco FA. General features of malignant germ cell tumors and primary seminomas of the mediastinum. In: Shields T, ed. *Mediastinal surgery.* Philadelphia: Lea & Febiger, 1991:211–218.

Mullen B, Richardson JD. Primary anterior mediastinal tumors in children and adults. *Ann Thorac Surg* 1986;42:338–345.

Silverman NA, Sabiston DC. Mediastinal masses. *Surg Clin North Am* 1980;60:757–777.

Kelley's Textbook of Internal Medicine, fourth edition. Edited by H. David Humes. Lippincott Williams & Wilkins, Philadelphia © 2000.

CHAPTER 204

APPROACH TO THE PATIENT WITH SUPERIOR VENA CAVA SYNDROME

JANICE P. DUTCHER

PRESENTATION

Superior vena cava syndrome usually is a subacute process caused by slow obstruction of the superior vena cava within the mediastinum. Physical findings that suggest the diagnosis include facial swelling and engorgement of the veins of the neck or chest wall. The earliest symptoms are dyspnea and tachypnea. There also may be hoarseness, tongue swelling, nasal congestion, or headache. Chest pain and cough may accompany this syndrome (Table 204.1). In rare instances there may be hemodynamic compromise with hypotension and severe dyspnea. These patients may have syncope when suddenly supine.

PATHOPHYSIOLOGY

The development of superior vena cava syndrome usually is insidious as obstruction progresses, leading to engorgement of veins that feed into the superior vena cava and decreasing venous return to the heart. Venous thrombus may develop progressively within the superior vena cava. The most common cause of this obstructive process is an intramediastinal malignant tumor that produces external compression with or without direct extension into the vena cava. Because superior vena cava syndrome may be the initial presentation of a previously undiagnosed malignant tumor, the management of symptoms and the diagnosis of underlying disease are important. Superior vena cava syndrome may be a manifestation of recurrent or metastatic tumor or occasionally indicate a nonmalignant process.

TABLE 204.1.	PHYSICAL FINDINGS AND SYMPTOMS OF SUPERIOR VENA CAVA SYNDROME

Sign or Symptom	Percentage of Patients Affected (n = 370)
Venous distention, neck	66
Dyspnea	63
Venous distention, chest	54
Facial swelling or edema	46–50
Cough	24
Cyanosis	20
Plethora of face	19
Arm swelling or edema	14–18
Chest pain	15
Dysphagia	9

Source: Data from Armstrong BA, Perez CA, Simpson JR, et al. Role of irradiation in the management of superior vena cava syndrome. *Int J Radiat Oncol Biol Phys* 1987;13:531–539; Bell DR, Woods RL, Levi JA. Superior vena cava syndrome. *Med J Aust* 1986;145: 566–568; Parish JM, Marschke RF, Dines DE, et al. Etiologic considerations in superior vena cava syndrome. *Mayo Clin Proc* 1981;56:407–413; and Yahalom J, ed. *Cancer: principles and practice of oncology*, 5th ed. Philadelphia: JB Lippincott, 1997: 2469–2476.

HISTORY AND PHYSICAL EXAMINATION

The patient frequently has no symptoms and first notices the engorged veins on the chest and neck or facial swelling. Some patients report increasing dyspnea and tachypnea or even chest pain (Table 204.1). Because the most common cause of the syndrome is a malignant tumor (in 78% to 86% of series), lung cancer being the most common cause (65% of cases in one series), a history of cigarette smoking often is obtained, as is a history of prior chronic pulmonary disease. Because recurrent metastatic cancer can cause superior vena cava syndrome, a history of prior malignant disease should be obtained.

Physical examination confirms venous engorgement of the superficial veins of the chest and neck and possibly edema of the face and arms. In severe cases, there may by cyanosis. Examination of the lungs may reveal the distant breath sounds of a patient with chronic obstructive pulmonary disease, the unilaterally absent breath sounds of a patient with a pleural effusion, or normal findings. The cardiac examination reveals normal heart sounds, but sinus arrhythmias are common among this patient population.

LABORATORY STUDIES AND DIAGNOSTIC TESTS

The most important diagnostic study is chest radiography, the result of which often suggest the cause of the problem, showing mediastinal widening or a hilar mass (80%) (Fig. 204.1). There may be a pleural effusion. The radiograph occasionally appears normal. Other laboratory tests that may be helpful include those for serum electrolytes, arterial blood gases, and serum lactate

dehydrogenase. A computed tomographic (CT) scan of the chest obtained with contrast is important in assessing the extent of the mass. The scan also may demonstrate the apparent absence of central blood vessels caused by obstruction. If the differential diagnosis of superior vena cava syndrome is uncertain, a venogram through the upper extremity can help confirm the diagnosis when the clinical findings are subtle.

DIFFERENTIAL DIAGNOSIS

Despite the potential clinical significance of the signs and symptoms, the diverse causes of superior vena cava syndrome make it imperative to obtain a precise pathologic diagnosis to direct disease-specific treatment. Rarely are the symptoms immediately life threatening. The three most common tumors that cause superior vena cava syndrome are small-cell cancer of the lung, non–small-cell cancer of the lung, and non-Hodgkin's lymphoma. Less commonly, mediastinal germ cell tumors, malignant thymoma, and Hodgkin's disease can produce superior vena cava syndrome, as can metastatic cancers such as breast cancer involving the mediastinal lymph nodes.

Most patients with superior vena cava syndrome have a readily apparent hilar or mediastinal tumor with superior mediastinal widening revealed on a chest radiograph. In the case of primary lung cancer, sputum cytologic analysis often is diagnostic and can help differentiate the histologic subtype, allowing caregivers to specify the treatment approach. For patients who also have a pleural effusion, such as those with lung cancer or lymphoma, thoracentesis with cytologic evaluation of the fluid may provide a histologic diagnosis. If results of neither of these modalities help confirm the diagnosis, bronchoscopy with biopsy or CT-guided fine-needle aspiration or core biopsy should yield a diagnosis in cases of lung cancer or germ cell cancer (Fig. 204.1). However, needle biopsy usually does not provide enough information for diagnosis of lymphoma and yields an inadequate pathologic specimen.

A surgical procedure may be necessary to obtain sufficient tissue for an accurate pathologic diagnosis of the type of tumor causing compression. Procedures that must be considered include mediastinoscopy and mediastinotomy (paramediastinal incision or Chamberlain procedure). The approach used is based on the level of concern about engorged mediastinal vessels. An indication of severity may be obtained from the CT scan. Open biopsy with direct visualization of the vessels often is safer than mediastinoscopy and may be the procedure of choice. Mediastinoscopy, however, can be safely performed in more subtle clinical situations.

In some cases, biopsy can be performed on other sites of disease to obtain a pathologic diagnosis. For example, in the case of small-cell carcinoma or lymphoma, bone marrow biopsy may demonstrate systemic involvement and provide a diagnosis. For patients with palpable supraclavicular lymph nodes, biopsy often yields a diagnosis.

The other cause of superior vena cava syndrome that can develop among patients with known malignant disease is venous thrombosis due to the presence of a central venous catheter, such as an access device. This can also be associated with cardiac

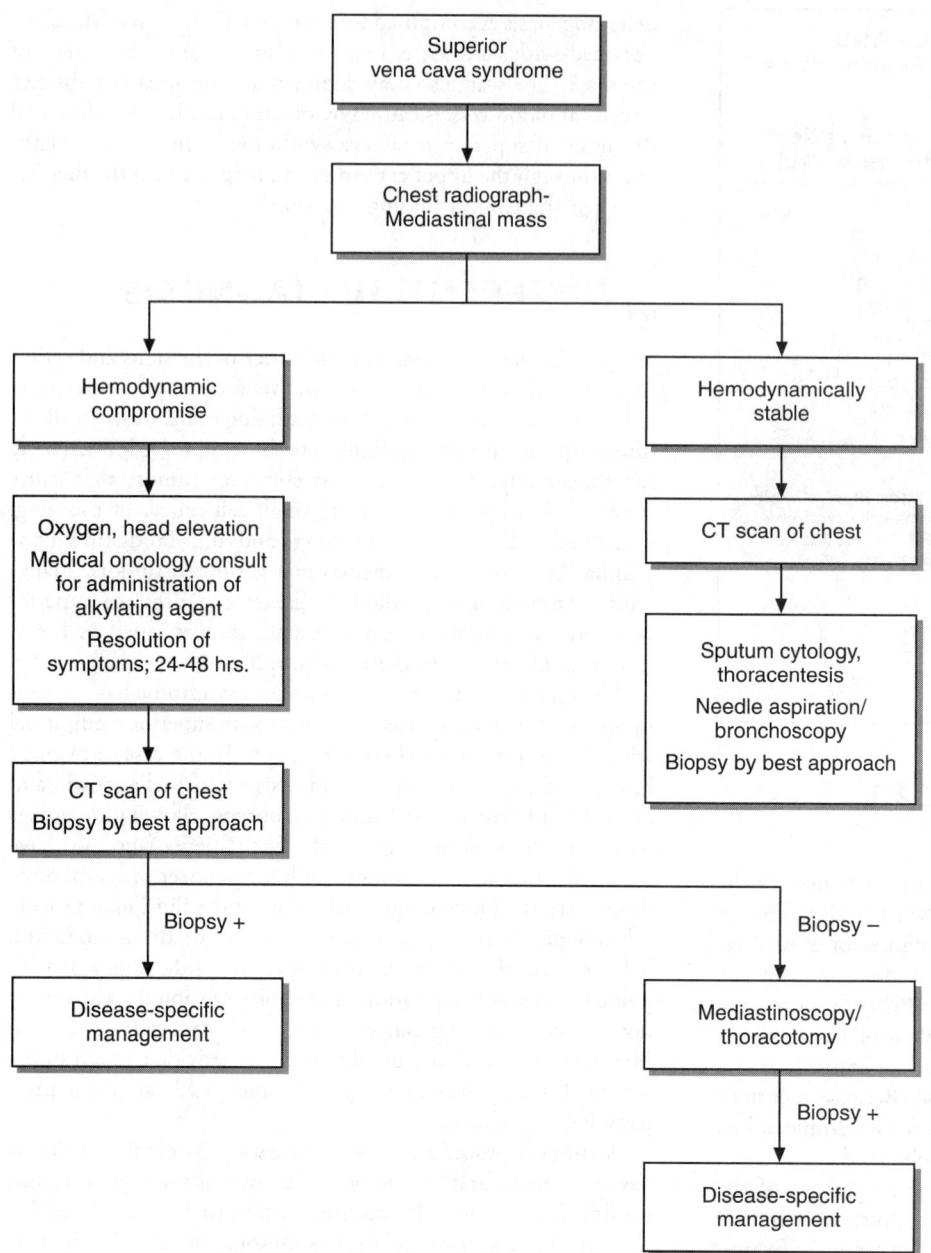

FIGURE 204.1. Algorithm for the evaluation of superior vena cava syndrome, utilizing chest radiography.

pacemakers. This cause should be considered in the evaluation of a patient with superior vena cava syndrome, an access device, and no apparent mediastinal tumor. Although thrombolytic agents may be helpful early in the thrombotic process, this complication usually necessitates removal of the catheter in conjunction with anticoagulation to prevent embolization. A nonmalignant and rare cause of superior vena cava compression to be considered in the differential diagnosis is idiopathic mediastinal fibrosis or histoplasmosis.

■ STRATEGIES FOR OPTIMAL CARE

MANAGEMENT

In the care of a patient with superior vena cava syndrome, the goals are to relieve symptoms and to obtain a histologic diagno-

sis. Initial symptomatic relief can be obtained with bed rest with head elevation and oxygen administration (Fig. 204.1). This reduces cardiac output and decreases venous pressure. The diagnostic evaluation previously described then proceeds as expeditiously as possible.

If the clinical situation is considered an emergency because of hemodynamic compromise, every attempt should be made to obtain a correct histologic diagnosis, and the most direct approach to obtaining tissue should be considered. If emergency treatment is deemed necessary before biopsy, irradiation should be avoided because it adversely affects the integrity of the tissue at subsequent biopsy. An alternative approach to induce rapid decompression of the vena cava that has a high likelihood of preservation of the histologic features of the tumor at biopsy is administration of a single, large dose of an alkylating agent. This approach should be used only to relieve life-threatening signs and symptoms and only under the guidance of a medical oncologist. It is exceedingly rare that such an emergency situation would arise.

After obtaining an accurate diagnosis of the cause of new-onset superior vena cava syndrome, which presumably is caused by a malignant tumor, management involves complete staging of the disease followed by disease-specific therapy. Non–small-cell lung cancer frequently is localized to the chest and mediastinum. However, small-cell cancer or lymphoma frequently is systemic and necessitates a comprehensive diagnostic evaluation followed by chemotherapy. Radiation therapy to the mediastinal tumor is to the management of most of these diseases. When superior vena cava syndrome is a manifestation of a known previously managed malignant tumor, irradiation usually is the therapy of choice. In the care of patients with recurrent obstruction after radiation, placement of an expandable wire stent or balloon angioplasty has been successful in maintaining patency.

COMPLICATIONS AND PITFALLS

The most common complication is inability to obtain a histologic diagnosis in the apparent urgency to manage superior vena cava syndrome. Careful assessment of hemodynamic status determines the rapidity with which the diagnostic evaluation must be concluded. A careful history interview and physical examination and rapid biopsy of lymph nodes, bone marrow, or mediastinal mass leads to rapid diagnosis and treatment. Complications of mediastinal biopsy have led to hesitancy in pursuing mediastinoscopy in the setting of dilated intrathoracic blood vessels. However, biopsy guided by CT scanning usually can be accomplished safely, as can an open biopsy. Concern about the safety of mediastinoscopy or the efficacy of needle biopsy for a given patient should prompt immediate consideration of open biopsy with direct visualization to enable acquisition of adequate tissue for diagnosis.

An additional potential complication of superior vena cava syndrome is tracheomalacia, which may develop from prolonged tracheal compression by the mediastinal mass. This may lead to complications such as trauma, edema, or rupture of the trachea during intubation for anesthesia. During extubation, there may be tracheal collapse with acute respiratory distress. These potential complications must be considered when patients are undergoing diagnostic surgical procedures.

In the care of patients for whom superior vena cava syndrome is a manifestation of a recurrent malignant tumor, the situation may be more ominous, because primary therapy already may have been exhausted. Such patients are at much greater risk for local complications from invasion of adjacent structures such as the trachea, esophagus, and pericardium. If not previously used, radiation therapy is the therapy of choice for such local complications.

Patients with superior vena cava syndrome usually need to be admitted to the hospital for assessment of hemodynamic status, diagnostic evaluation including biopsy, and initial treatment with radiation therapy or chemotherapy. After the acute problem resolves, completion of the diagnostic evaluation and therapy can be accomplished on an outpatient basis.

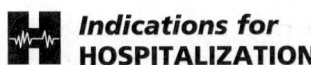

Indications for HOSPITALIZATION

Patients with malignant superior vena cava syndrome should be treated by experienced medical oncologists, who can direct the diagnostic evaluation and intervene with chemotherapy if necessary. Thoracic surgeons familiar with the anatomic features of engorged vessels and the physiologic mechanisms of this syndrome are consulted if biopsy of a supraclavicular node or the mediastinum is anticipated.

COST-EFFECTIVENESS

Despite the drama of the initial clinical presentation, newly diagnosed lymphoma, germ cell cancer, and in some cases, small-cell lung cancer are potentially curable, and the appropriate pathologic diagnosis and management can return otherwise healthy persons to their optimal level of activity.

BIBLIOGRAPHY

Chen JC, Bongard F, Klein SR. A contemporary perspective on superior vena cava syndrome. *Am J Surg* 1990;160:207–211.

Gray BH, Olin JW, Grador RA, et al. Safety and efficacy of thrombolytic therapy for superior vena cava syndrome. *Chest* 1991;99:54–59.

Hennequin LM, Fade O, Fays JG, et al. Superior vena cava stent placement: results with the Wallstent endoprosthesis. *Radiology* 1995;196: 353–361.

Urschel HC Jr, Razzuk MA, Netto GJ, et al. Sclerosing mediastinitis: improved management with histoplasmosis titre and ketoconazole. *Ann Thorac Surg* 1990;50:215–221.

Yedlicka JW, Schultz K, Moncada R, et al. CT findings in superior vena cava obstruction. *Semin Roentgenol* 1989;24:84–90.

Yahalom J. Superior vena cava syndrome. In: DeVita VT, Hellman, S, Rosenberg SA, eds. *Cancer: principles and practice of oncology*, 5th ed. Philadelphia: JB Lippincott, 1997:2469–2476.

Kelley's Textbook of Internal Medicine, fourth edition. Edited by H. David Humes. Lippincott Williams & Wilkins, Philadelphia © 2000.

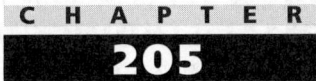

C H A P T E R
205

APPROACH TO THE PATIENT WITH A PALPABLE MASS AND/OR AN ABNORMAL MAMMOGRAM

HELEN PASS
MARK HELVIE
SOFIA D. MERAJVER

The advent of mammographic screening for early detection of breast cancer among women older than 40 years has been shown in randomized trials to decrease mortality from this disease 15% to 30%. As the number of women undergoing screening increases, larger numbers of clinically occult radiographic abnormalities of the breast are being evaluated. The increase in the practice of routine monthly breast self-examination and yearly clinical breast examination likewise leads to early detection of palpable abnormalities of the breast. The evaluation of an abnormal mammogram and a palpable mass is focused on establishing the distinction between breast cancer and a multitude of nonmalignant conditions. The evaluation centers on the triad of physical examination, radiologic evaluation, and tissue sampling. Because delays in diagnosis of breast cancer are likely to have an adverse effect on the quality and length of life of the patient, the algorithms described herein are specifically designed to execute an efficient and cost-effective evaluation in light of the untoward consequences of a missed cancer diagnosis.

PATHOPHYSIOLOGY

The normal breast tissue of an adult is highly heterogeneous to palpation and radiologic imaging throughout life. Among premenopausal women, changes in the hormonally responsive ducts and lobules during the menstrual cycle are reflected in cyclical differences in the findings at physical examination of the breasts. Individual differences in the proliferative capacity of the epithelial tissue of the breast and the abundance of fibrous connective tissue are reflected in density on mammograms and affect the sensitivity and specificity of this imaging modality. Use of exogenous estrogens (oral contraceptives, hormone replacement therapy, fertility treatments), lean body mass, diet, and heredity all are thought to contribute to the fibroglandular content of breast tissue and to mammographic density. Given the intrinsic heterogeneity of breast tissue appreciated during both physical and radiologic examinations, criteria have been developed to help clinicians discern malignant causes of masses and mammographic abnormalities.

APPROACH TO A PATIENT WITH ABNORMAL FINDINGS AT CLINICAL BREAST EXAMINATION

It is estimated that at some point in her life one of every two women will see a physician for a breast problem. Although breast cancer is the most common malignant tumor among U.S. women, 80% to 90% of clinical evaluations for breast disorders are for benign conditions. Thus the goal of the evaluation after abnormal findings have been obtained at clinical breast examination is to avoid missing the diagnosis of malignant disease while providing reassurance if the diagnosis is a benign condition.

HISTORY AND PHYSICAL EXAMINATION

Evaluation begins with a history interview and physical examination to identify the patient's area of concern (if the abnormality was discovered at self-examination) and to assess the clinician's degree of suspicion of malignancy. The initial impression whether the abnormality represents a vague area of thickening or nodularity as opposed to a true dominant mass should be recorded.

Salient points of history about the mass or abnormality are the timing of appearance with respect to the menstrual cycle, rate of change, associated signs such as redness, pruritus, or nipple discharge (which may no longer be present), history of trauma, and present hormone and other drug use. Family history, previous breast biopsy, reproductive history, and hormonal exposures help place the present mass or abnormality in the context of the patient's breast cancer risk profile.

Accurate interpretation of the findings at clinical breast examination can be challenging. In a study of concordance for the need for biopsy, diagnostic accuracy was 73% among four experienced surgeons in examinations of 15 patients with malignant lesions. Therefore, in the evaluation of a palpable breast mass, the diagnostic triad of physical examination, mammography, and fine-needle aspiration biopsy (FNA), known as the *triple test,* should be used. In Europe successful use of the triple test for many years has decreased the need for excisional biopsy. When results with all three diagnostic components are benign, the triple test has a greater than 99% positive predictive value for benign disease. Nevertheless, for many practitioners, the safest and most expeditious method of practice is excisional biopsy of any breast mass. The triple test is useful only for the evaluation of a dominant mass, because FNA is unreliable in the evaluation of thickening or nodularity.

ALGORITHM FOR THE EVALUATION OF BREAST THICKENING OR NODULARITY

The initial step in the evaluation of diffuse thickening or nodularity is to compare the affected site with the mirror image area of the opposite breast (Fig. 205.1). Symmetrical areas are seldom pathologic, and reassurance with follow-up clinical evaluation is appropriate. Postmenopausal women should undergo a follow-up examination in 6 weeks, and premenopausal women on day 5, 6, or 7 (follicular phase) of the menstrual cycle. If at reexamination, the area is clinically stable, the patient should undergo routine follow-up examinations according to her health maintenance schedule. If the area seems to progress in this period, further evaluation with mammography, ultrasonography of the breast, or both depending on the patient's age, and referral to a breast specialist should be obtained. A radiologic abnormality with only a vaguely palpable abnormality should be managed by means of image-guided biopsy (see later). A distinct, palpable abnormality (dominant palpable mass) should be evaluated further (see later).

Persistent asymmetric thickening or nodularity should be evaluated by means of breast imaging. If findings at radiologic assessment are normal and are concordant with the findings at physical examination, a 6-week clinical follow-up examination is indicated. Any patient with an abnormality that shows progression at the short-term follow-up examination should be referred for biopsy. Patients with stable areas may be treated conservatively with reinforcement of breast self-examination and

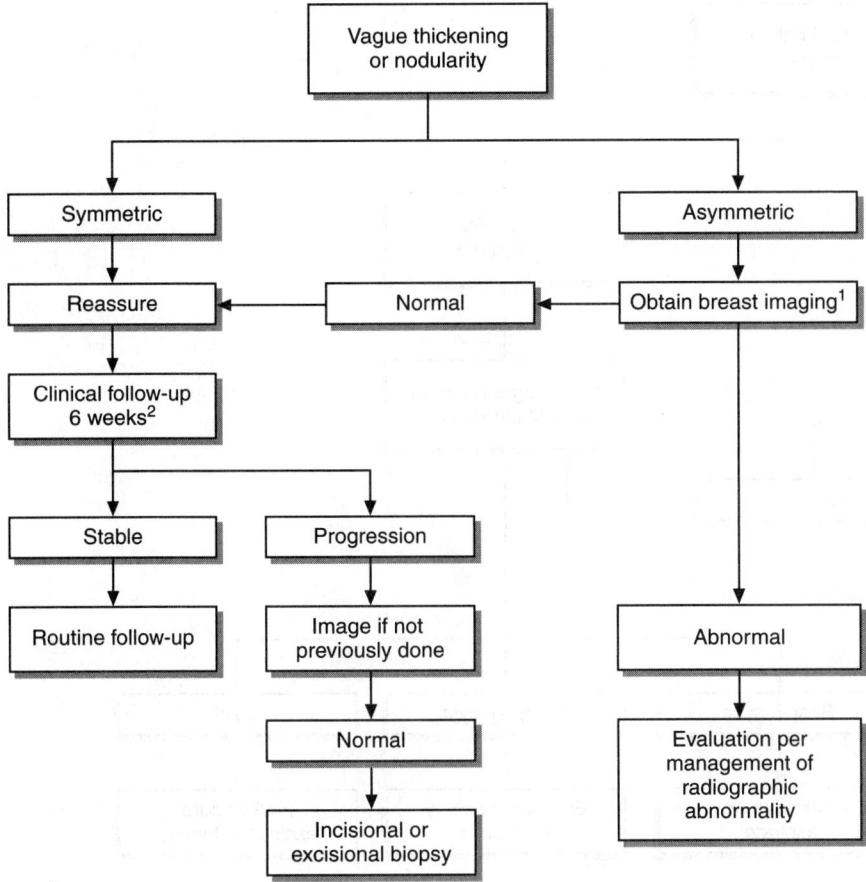

FIGURE 205.1. Algorithm for the assessment of thickening or nodularity of the breast. The objective is to focus the invasive diagnostic assessment on asymmetric findings and to provide adequate short-term follow-up care to ensure stability of symmetric findings.
EVIDENCE LEVEL: C. Expert Opinion.

1. Age < 30: Consider ultrasound
   Age ≥ 30: Obtain diagnostic mammogram ± ultrasound
2. Or one week post menses in premenopausal women

education about the need to return before the next scheduled health maintenance evaluation if the area changes.

The most common cause of nodularity, especially when the nodule is tender, is fibrocystic changes. Among younger women, the upper outer quadrants and axillary tail are common areas of these changes. Older women often have a bilateral thickened ridge along the inframammary folds. Symmetry and stability over time help avoid overaggressive evaluation of these frequent findings.

ALGORITHM FOR THE EVALUATION OF A DOMINANT PALPABLE BREAST MASS

The initial step in the evaluation of a dominant palpable mass is to determine degree of suspicion (Fig. 205.2). Breast cancer generally becomes apparent as a hard, nontender, irregular mass; it is impossible, however, to rule out cancer on the basis of clinical evaluation alone. A premenopausal patient may be observed if the clinician has low index of suspicion regarding malignancy of the lesion. The patient should be reexamined on day

5, 6, or 7 of her next menstrual cycle. A dominant mass that persists through one cycle requires further evaluation (see below).

For a dominant mass that persists through one menstrual cycle or a lesion that the primary care provider is concerned is not a simple cyst, additional evaluation and referral to a breast specialist are indicated. Urgent radiologic evaluation (within 1 week) followed by FNA is appropriate. There are advantages to performing imaging studies first. Even when performed by experienced physicians, FNA results in tissue disruption and hematoma formation that may interfere with mammography or ultrasonography. If a malignant lesion is diagnosed through FNA, mammography still is needed to evaluate the remainder of the breast parenchyma and the contralateral breast. Negative mammographic findings in the setting of a clinically dominant mass should not delay biopsy because 10% of breast cancers are mammographically occult. If, however, imaging is delayed one needs to consider proceeding with FNA in the interest of timely assessment.

A clinician's skill and experience with FNA should guide whether aspiration is performed in the primary care setting or

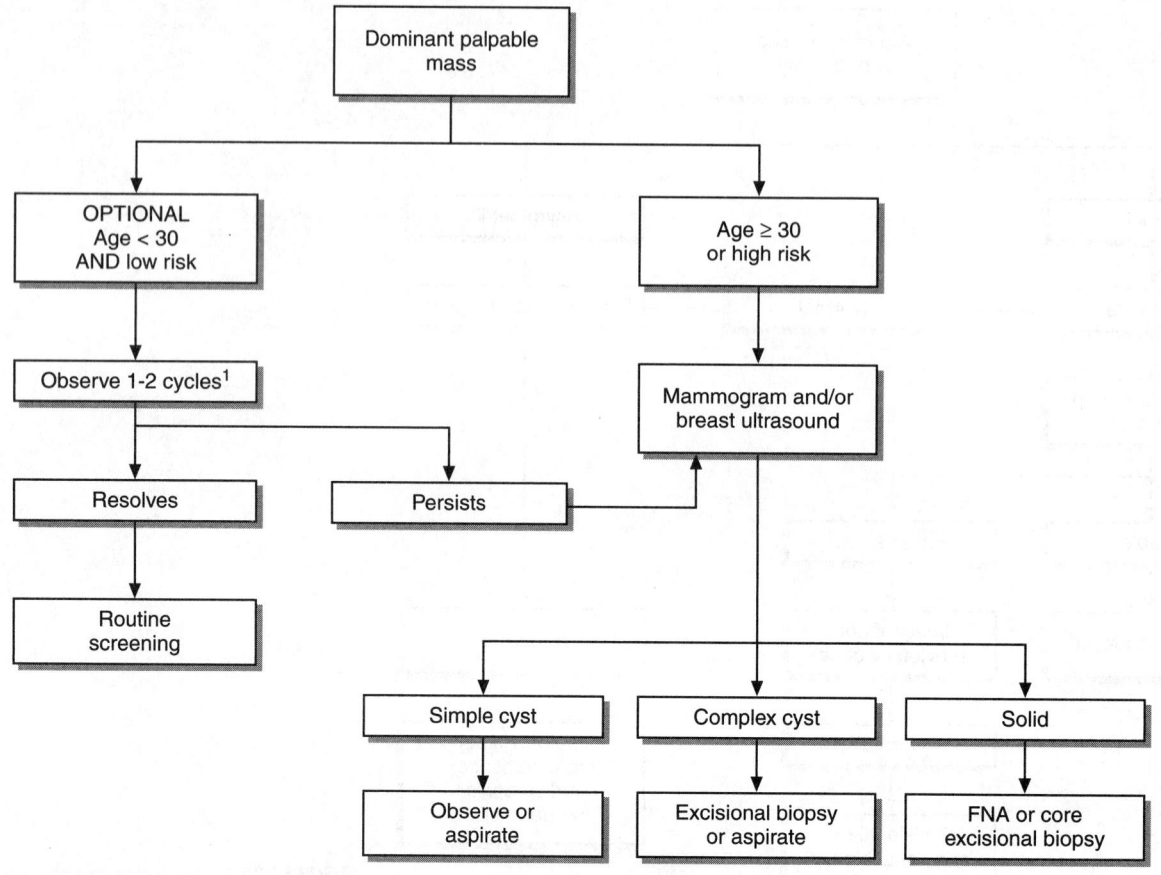

1. Re-examine day 5-7 of menstrual cycle

FIGURE 205.2. Algorithm for assessment of a palpable dominant breast mass. The objective of this evaluation is to differentiate benign and malignant causes with the triad of physical examination, imaging, and tissue sampling.
EVIDENCE LEVEL: C. Expert Opinion.

referral to a breast care specialist is obtained. FNA is a simple office procedure that requires readily available equipment (a 10 cc syringe, 22 gauge needle, and cytology solution). The most significant risk of FNA performed by an inexperienced practitioner is that the FNA may yield an inadequate sample, thereby delaying diagnosis. Repeat FNA, possibly under image guidance, or excisional biopsy should be obtained by a breast specialist after FNA does not provide enough information for diagnosis. Other potential side effects of FNA include hematoma and, rarely, pneumothorax. In general, unless the clinician is very experienced, it is recommended that FNA be performed by a breast care specialist.

If a cyst is suspected after clinical examination (smooth, mobile, possibly tender mass) or documented at ultrasonography, FNA can be both diagnostic and therapeutic. Observation alone may be chosen only if a lesion meets all of the sonographic criteria for a simple cyst. The lesion must be a round, well-circumscribed, smooth-walled structure that is anechoic (with-

out internal echoes) and is enhanced through transmission. If the lesion does not meet all of these criteria, is painful, or interferes with performance of an adequate examination, FNA should be performed. The abnormal area should be well localized in case excisional biopsy is necessary after cyst aspiration. Indications for excisional biopsy after cyst aspiration include the recovery of grossly bloody or turbid cyst fluid, the presence of residual mass after aspiration, or recurrence of a cyst in the same location two or three times after aspiration. A follow-up physical examination always should be performed 2 to 3 months after cyst aspiration. Cytologic analysis of clear, straw-colored fluid is neither necessary nor helpful. If, however, the character of the fluid is atypical, cytologic analysis must be performed.

DIAGNOSTIC PITFALLS

Unlike that of a cyst, FNA of a solid mass produces little or no fluid. Aspiration of a solid lesion requires more skill than simple cyst aspiration to obtain an accurate diagnosis. Nevertheless FNA of a solid mass is less invasive than excisional biopsy and allows rapid diagnosis. If malignant growth is diagnosed, treatment may be reduced to a one-step operative procedure with frozen-section confirmation. Any patient for whom an FNA reveals atypical or insufficient sampling should be referred for biopsy without delay. Concordance must be established among the physical examination, imaging, and FNA results because the false-negative rate of FNA has been reported to range between 0.4% and 35% with a much lower false-positive rate of 0.17%. False-negative FNA results are most often caused by inadequate tissue sampling, aspiration of a tumor less than 1 cm in diameter, or tumors with a large degree of fibrosis. A critical element of FNA that produces enough information to confirm a diagnosis is the availability of a skilled cytopathologist.

In summary, a palpable abnormality must be adequately explained through a multimodality approach. It is impossible to rule out cancer on clinical or radiologic grounds alone, and two-thirds of women with breast cancer have no identifiable risk factors. Therefore radiologic or pathologic assessment or both must be obtained for any dominant palpable abnormality. Even when performed correctly, the triple test is only 99% accurate; thus patients who are unwilling to accept a 1% false-negative rate should undergo open biopsy. Referral to a breast care specialist should be initiated when the diagnostic requirements exceed the skills or experience of the clinician.

APPROACH TO A PATIENT WITH AN ABNORMAL MAMMOGRAM

EVALUATION OF THE MAMMOGRAM

The primary purpose of mammography is detection of clinically occult breast cancer at an early stage. Mammographic evaluations frequently are categorized as *screening* or *diagnostic*. Screening mammography is performed on women who do not have symptoms and generally includes two views (crandiocaudal and mediolateral oblique) of each breast. The goal of screening mammography is detection, not characterization of an abnormality. Diagnostic mammography is performed on patients who have abnormal screening mammograms, palpable clinical findings, or complex surgical or medical histories. Diagnostic mammography often entails additional mammographic views and adjunctive modalities such as ultrasonography. Correlation with physical findings is essential. The goal of diagnostic mammography is to characterize a potential mammographic abnormality. After completion of diagnostic mammography for a patient who has no symptoms, a final assessment is rendered regarding the need for biopsy or follow-up mammography. Evaluation after abnormal mammographic results are obtained is summarized in Fig. 205.3.

Mammographic images are obtained by means of passing low-energy x-rays (25 to 28 kilovolts peak [kVp]) through a compressed breast onto an image receptor, typically film. The resolution of mammography is higher than that of almost all

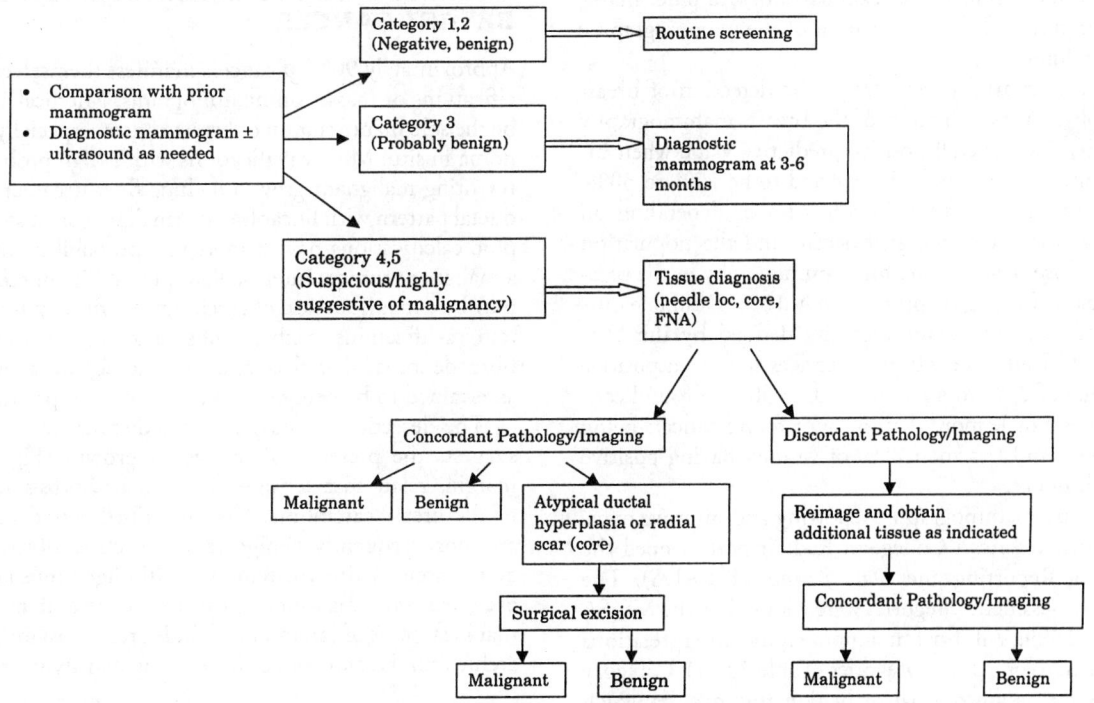

FIGURE 205.3. Algorithm for assessment after abnormal mammographic results are obtained. The objective of this evaluation is to help identify lesions that have moderate or high probability of being malignant and to assist in the procurement of accurate tissue diagnosis. (Adapted from *National Comprehensive Cancer Network breast cancer screening guidelines,* version 1. Rockledge, PA: National Comprehensive Cancer Network, 1999, with permission.)
EVIDENCE LEVEL: B. Adapted from the NCCN Breast Screening Guideline.

other medical imaging systems. Since the passage of the Mammography Quality Standards Act (MQSA) in 1992, all mammographic facilities and personnel have been federally regulated. The U.S. Food and Drug Administration provides yearly on-site inspection of mammographic equipment, quality processes, and personnel. Interpreting radiologists are required to provide documentation of continuing education, tracking of positive results, and demonstration of minimal yearly interpretative volume (480 studies). MQSA also regulates reporting of mammographic findings.

Interpretation of mammograms depends on perception or detection of an abnormal finding and characterization of an abnormality once detected. Mammographic analysis entails skillful, thorough evaluation of high-quality images by a trained and experienced radiologist. There is a high rate of interobserver variation. Double reading by two independent radiologists may improve sensitivity. Once an abnormality is detected with a screening study, additional diagnostic images usually are needed before final characterization. Five to ten percent of women who undergo screening need additional evaluation of potential abnormalities found at screening. Most women who need additional evaluation have normal results and can return to undergoing routine screening examinations without biopsy.

Magnification views with smaller focal spots define the number and morphologic features of microcalcification particles. *Spot compression views* and *angled views* are used to assess the margins of masses. *Incremental* mammographic views are used to determine whether a potential abnormality seen on only one view truly represents a three-dimensional mass or is merely a summation shadow found on one view. Comparison with older mammograms is important for interpretation of the mammographic stability of findings.

Although it is relatively sensitive in the detection of breast cancer, like physical examination of the breast, mammography lacks specificity. The overall positive predictive value when biopsy is recommended generally is reported to be 15% to 30%. There is considerable variation in this number depending on factors such as the interpreting physician and the population screened. The false-negative rate for mammography in the presence of a palpable finding is approximately 10%. Desirable outcome goals of screening mammography defined by the U.S. Department of Health and Human Services include a positive predictive value of 25% to 40%, more than 50% of found cancers being stage 0 or I, more than 30% of found cancers being minimal cancer, and less than 25% of women having positive axillary lymph nodes.

To standardize mammographic reporting and improve communication, the American College of Radiology developed the Breast Imaging Reporting and Data System (BIRADS). The BIRADS final assessment categories were adopted by the MQSA beginning in 1999. All final mammographic interpretations must be assigned to one of six categories (Table 205.1). Category 1 and 2 assessments are normal or benign findings for which routine care is recommended. Category 4 and 5 assessments indicate a probability of malignancy high enough that biopsy is warranted. Category 3 assessments ("probably benign") indicate findings that have a very low probability of malignancy. Experienced centers have reported the probability of malignancy of

TABLE 205.1.	FOOD AND DRUG ADMINISTRATION AND AMERICAN COLLEGE OF RADIOLOGY BIRADS FINAL ASSESSMENT OF MAMMOGRAPHIC FINDINGS

1. Negative
2. Benign
3. Probably benign
4. Suspicious
5. Highly suggestive of malignancy
0. Incomplete, need additional imaging evaluation

(Source: From American College of Radiology. *Breast Imaging Reporting and Data System*, 3rd ed. Reston, VA: American College of Radiology, 1998, with permission.)

category 3 lesions to be 1% to 2%. Women receiving category 3 mammographic assessment are counseled to undergo short-term follow-up mammography, usually in 3 to 6 months. It is assumed that a corresponding physical abnormality does not exist. Informed patients or their physicians unwilling to accept this very low risk for malignancy may be referred for surgical consultation. Category 0 is used only to describe abnormal screening mammograms awaiting further diagnostic investigation. The Food and Drug Administration requires that as of 1999 patients receive a written summary mammographic report directly from the radiologist.

MAMMOGRAPHIC CHARACTERISTICS OF BREAST CANCER

Approximately 90% of cancers manifest themselves as microcalcifications or masses on mammograms. Microcalcifications may be the sole manifestation of breast cancer, especially ductal carcinoma in situ. Microcalcifications with a high probability of representing malignant growth include fine, irregular particles in a ductal pattern with linear forms. Small foci of clustered pleomorphic calcifications have a moderate probability of representing a malignant tumor. Intermediate-probability microcalcifications may be a manifestation of carcinoma or fibrocystic change. Certain calcifications, such as those associated with degenerating fibroadenoma, ductal ectasia, or microcystic adenosis, can be ascertained to be benign on the basis of the specific appearance.

The detection of masses with indistinct or spicular margins suggests the presence of malignant growth (Fig. 205.4). The margins relate to extension of tumor or fibrosis at the margins of the breast carcinoma. Circumscribed round or oval masses are most frequently benign lesions such as fibroadenoma or a cyst. Circumscribed carcinoma, although unusual, cannot be excluded with mammography. Less common mammographic manifestations of carcinoma include areas of asymmetric density, architectural distortion, or developing density from year to year.

ULTRASONOGRAPHY AS AN ADJUNCT IN THE EVALUATION OF AN ABNORMAL MAMMOGRAM

Ultrasonography is used to further characterize a mammographic mass. The primary role of ultrasonography is to differentiate a

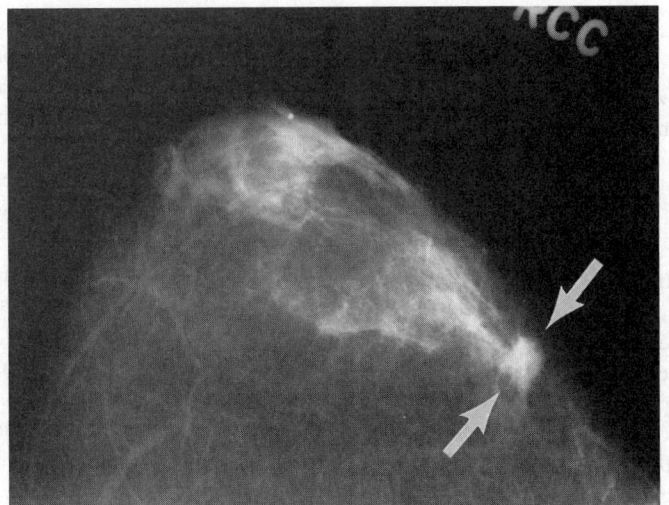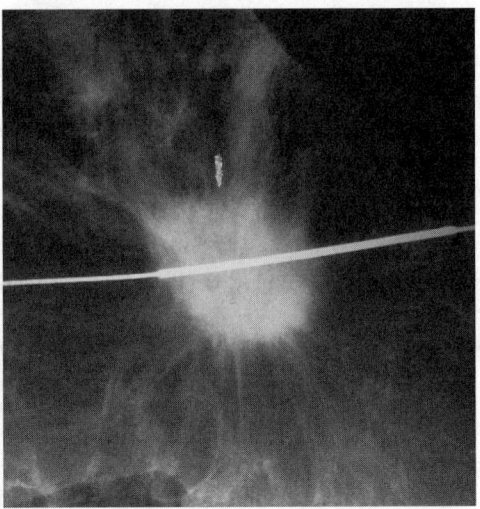

FIGURE 205.4. A: Craniocaudal mammogram shows a 1 cm spicular nonpalpable mass (*arrows*) in the lateral aspect of the breast. **B:** Specimen radiograph of excised tissue shows spicular margins to better advantage. Metallic hook wire (*white line*) had been placed to guide surgical excision. Invasive carcinoma was diagnosed by means of pathologic examination of this specimen.

fluid-filled cyst from a solid mass. Geographic correlation between the mammographic mass and ultrasound finding is essential. Masses fulfilling criteria for a simple cyst, such as smooth-walled, circumscribed, anechoic masses with increased through transmission, are classified as benign and necessitate no further management unless they are painful (Fig. 205.5). Solid masses usually require tissue biopsy because ultrasonography cannot conclusively differentiate benign from malignant solid masses. Ultrasonography also is used for imaging examinations of women with palpable findings even in the absence of mammographic abnormality to differentiate a solid from a cystic mass.

This is especially helpful to women with dense breasts. Normal findings of a sonographic evaluation in the presence of a palpable mass does not exclude carcinoma; clinical management is needed.

TISSUE DIAGNOSIS OF AN ABNORMAL MAMMOGRAPHIC LESION

Biopsy options for women with nonpalpable category 4 or 5 assessments include wire localization with open surgical biopsy, image-directed core-needle biopsy, and less commonly FNA with cytologic analysis. Needle localization procedures involve the placement of a localizing needle and a hook wire at the site of the mammographic abnormality. The procedure is performed with mammographic or sonographic guidance. Open surgical biopsy is performed by means of excision of tissue around the hook wire. A specimen radiograph of the excised tissue obtained with mammographic technique confirms successful removal before pathologic analysis (Fig. 205.4B). Core biopsy of nonpalpable lesions gained wide acceptance in the 1990s. This method involves placing a core breast biopsy needle (11 to 14 gauge) into a breast abnormality with the patient under local anesthesia and obtaining repeated samples. Image guidance may be accomplished with either stereotactic mammography or ultrasonography. The sensitivity and specificity of core-needle biopsy are reported to be higher than 95%. Because core biopsy is a sampling technique, lesions are not typically completely excised. Areas of atypical ductal hyperplasia or radial scarring should be surgically re-excised because some patients are found to have associated carcinoma. Core biopsy specimens showing ductal carcinoma in situ are, in a minority of cases, found to contain invasive carcinoma when more tissue is excised. The results of all biopsies must be correlated with the mammographic findings. Discordant results between mammographic and pathologic evaluations necessitate imaging in 4 to 6 weeks and possible re-excision.

FIGURE 205.5. Ultrasound image obtained to characterize a mass found on a mammogram. Image shows a simple cyst with smooth margins and anechoic (*black*) center with enhanced through transmission.

DIAGNOSTIC PITFALLS

Breast density or composition influences the sensitivity of mammography. A very dense mammographic pattern occurs when the breast composition is primarily fibroglandular and has minimal adipose tissue. In extremely dense breasts, carcinoma may be masked or camouflaged by the overlying dense tissue, which markedly limits mammographic sensitivity. A fat density pattern, however, allows higher sensitivity. Breast density varies from person to person and may be increased with hormone replacement therapy.

Mammography cannot be used to rule out breast cancer in a patient with a palpable finding. Because patients may derive false assurance from a normal mammographic report in the presence of a palpable finding, it is the clinician's responsibility to ensure that these patients have complete evaluation. After thorough diagnostic evaluation, sound clinical and surgical judgment is needed to integrate the palpable findings with the imaging results. Any patient with clinically suspect findings should be referred for surgical consultation regardless of the breast imaging results.

UNCOMMON PRESENTATIONS

The symptoms of approximately 3% to 5% of breast cancers are erythema, edema, and peau d'orange. After 1 week of unsuccessful antibiotic treatment, these patients should undergo immediate mammography and biopsy of either the affected skin or a mammographic abnormality if one is detected. These patients should be considered to have inflammatory breast cancer and urgently referred to the care of a surgical oncologist to expedite diagnosis and initiation of chemotherapy.

Nipple discharge is a relatively common presenting symptom of breast disease and is most often of nonneoplastic causation. The evaluation for nipple discharge centers on discerning whether benign or malignant neoplasia is the cause, because both are likely to necessitate surgical intervention to excise a neoplasm or to control the symptoms. Serous, serosanguineous, bloody, or watery discharge is evaluated with mammography to find an associated mass or calcification, which increases the likelihood of neoplasia as an etiologic factor. Unilateral and spontaneous discharge, confinement to one duct at expression of the breast, association with a mass, and male sex are characteristics used by the surgeon to decide on intervention. Bloody discharge is most often caused by intraductal papilloma. Persistent nipple discharges that exhibit any of the characteristics listed warrant referral to a breast specialist. Bilateral galactorrhea unexplained by lactation or pregnancy is assessed by means of prolactin level, visual field testing, and computed tomography or magnetic resonance imaging of the sella turcica region to ascertain the presence of a pituitary adenoma. Other causes of bilateral galactorrhea, such as hypothyroidism and syndromes associated with amenorrhea, generally are best evaluated by an endocrinologist.

An isolated enlarged axillary node should be considered for biopsy if the node is not easily movable, is larger than 2 cm in diameter, or appears other than benign on a mammogram in the absence of other mammographic abnormalities. If adenocarcinoma is diagnosed in an isolated lymph node, special stains

for estrogen and progesterone receptors and mucin should be performed on the biopsy specimen, and serum tumor markers (cancer antigens CA 27.29, CA 125, and CA 19–9 and carcinoembryonic antigen [CEA]) should be evaluated to help identify the organ of origin of the cancer.

Although risk for breast cancer increases with age, breast cancer does occur among the very young. A family history of breast or ovarian cancer or known *BRCA* mutation carrier status are major risk factors for early-onset breast cancer. Women with a family history of breast or ovarian cancer who have a palpable mass or abnormal mammogram should undergo aggressive diagnostic evaluation, regardless of age. Mammographic screening generally is begun when a woman is 5 years younger than the family member who had the earliest case of breast cancer. Women who have undergone radiation therapy to the chest for lymphoma or another condition before they are 20 years of age also are at high risk for bilateral breast cancer and need special consideration. These women should start mammographic screening by 25 years of age. Abnormalities found at physical examination or mammography should be thoroughly evaluated.

Breast cancer rarely develops in pregnant or lactating women. An asymmetric, enlarging mass should be evaluated, even in the absence of unusual risk factors, because breast cancers that arise under these conditions tend to grow rapidly and thus carry a poor prognosis. There is no known contraindication to mammographic evaluation or tissue sampling of a suspicious mass in a pregnant or lactating patient.

BIBLIOGRAPHY

American College of Radiology. *Breast Imaging Reporting and Data System (BIRADS),* 3rd ed. Reston, VA: American College of Radiology, 1998.

Bassett L, Winchester DP, Caplan RB, et al. Stereotactic core-needle biopsy of the breast: a report of the joint task force of the American College of Radiology, American College of Surgeons, and College of American Pathologists. *CA Cancer J Clin* 1997;47:171–190.

Boyd NF, Sutherland HJ, Fish EB, et al. Prospective evaluation of physical examination of the breast. *Am J Surg* 1981;142:331–334.

Elmore JG, Wells CK, Lee CH, et al. Variability in radiologists' interpretations of mammograms. *N Engl J Med* 1994;331:1493–1499.

Larsson LG, Andersson I, Bjurstam N, et al. Updated overview of the Swedish Randomized Trials on Breast Cancer Screening with Mammography: age group 40–49 at randomization. *J Natl Cancer Inst Monogr* 1997;22:57–61.

Layfield LJ, Glasgow BJ, Cramer H. Fine needle aspiration in the management of breast masses. *Pathol Annu* 1989;24:23–62.

National Comprehensive Cancer Network breast cancer screening guidelines, version 1. Rockledge, PA: National Comprehensive Cancer Network, 1999.

Sickles EA. Periodic mammographic follow-up of probably benign lesions: results in 3,184 consecutive cases. *Radiology* 1991;179:463–468.

US Congress. Quality mammography standards: final rule. *Federal Register* 1997 October 28:62:55852.

US Department of Health and Human Services. Quality determinants of mammography. In: *Clinical practice guideline,* no. 13. Rockville, MD: US Department of Health and Human Services; 1994; AHCPR 95-0632.

Kelley's Textbook of Internal Medicine, fourth edition. Edited by H. David Humes. Lippincott Williams & Wilkins, Philadelphia © 2000.

C H A P T E R

206

APPROACH TO THE PATIENT WITH A TESTICULAR MASS

STEPHEN D. WILLIAMS

■ PRESENTATION

The initial symptom of cancer of the testis typically is a scrotal mass. The mass may be tender or painless. Many patients first notice the mass after minor trauma, and the injury commonly is considered by the patient the cause of the mass. In reality, the injury draws attention to the mass, or the abnormal testis is more susceptible to trauma. In the past, some men were reluctant to seek medical attention when they noticed a scrotal mass. This delay still occurs, but it does seem that various public education efforts have been responsible for a heightened awareness of testicular cancer. Similar efforts have led to more awareness by primary physicians and earlier consideration of the presence of testicular neoplasia.

■ HISTORY AND PHYSICAL EXAMINATION

A logical approach to the initial evaluation of a scrotal mass is imperative. The patient should be questioned carefully about his symptoms, including duration, the presence of pain, fever, dysuria, urethral discharge, a history of trauma, and antecedent urologic conditions, particularly a history of an undescended testis or prior scrotal or inguinal operation. The age of the patient is important, because the likely diagnosis varies according to age. Other symptoms that should be sought include those specifically related to potential areas of metastatic spread of testicular cancer. These include back pain, which indicates retroperitoneal nodal involvement, dyspnea or cough, weight loss, or gynecomastia, which indicates tumor production of human chorionic gonadotropin (hCG).

Physical examination of the scrotum carefully delineates the size and character of the mass and its consistency. A normal testis is ovoid, smooth, tense, and sensitive to pressure. A normal epididymis is posterior to the testis and is separated from the testis by a thin groove. It is flaccid and slightly sensitive to palpation. The relation of the mass to the testis, epididymis, and spermatic cord is critical. A mass clearly separable from the testis suggests epididymitis, and a mass within the parenchyma of the testis suggests neoplasia.

Transillumination of the mass should be attempted. Masses that readily transilluminate are cystic and not likely to be malignant. Masses that do not transilluminate and are not clearly separable from the testis should be assumed to be neoplastic until proved otherwise. Other important aspects of the physical examination include palpation for an abdominal mass, organomegaly, and inguinal or supraclavicular lymphadenopathy.

■ LABORATORY STUDIES AND DIAGNOSTIC TESTS

The choice of laboratory and radiographic studies is dictated by the findings derived from the history and physical examination. If a neoplasm is suspected, testicular ultrasonography should be considered. Ultrasonography can better define the anatomic structures in the scrotum, show specifically whether the mass is cystic, and show whether the mass is of testicular or paratesticular origin. Figure 206.1 is a testicular ultrasound scan that shows a hypoechoic parenchymal testicular mass. This patient underwent radical inguinal orchiectomy; it was confirmed that the lesion was a malignant germ cell tumor of the testis.

Diagnostic studies should include determination of the tumor markers β-hCG and α-fetoprotein (AFP). These marker levels are useful only if elevated; an elevated β-HCG or AFP level in this clinical situation confirms the diagnosis of a neoplasm of testicular germ cell origin. However, normal marker levels in no way exclude malignancy. Patients with testicular seminoma usually have normal levels of markers, and many patients with germ cell tumors other than seminoma have normal marker levels, particularly if the tumor is localized to the testis. Neoplasms that rarely involve the testis or paratesticular structures, such as lymphoma, stromal tumors, or sarcoma, do not have elevated levels of germ cell tumor markers. Other diagnostic tests

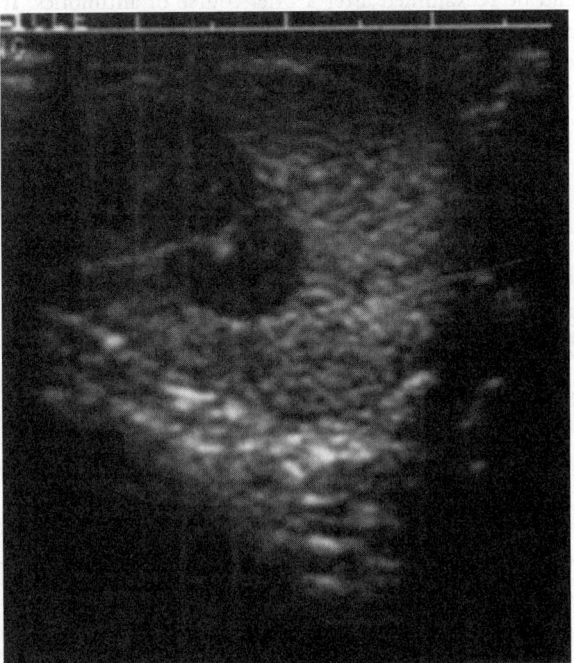

FIGURE 206.1. Ultrasound scan of the testis shows a well-defined, hypoechoic mass, proven at orchiectomy to be a nonseminomatous testicular tumor.
EVIDENCE LEVEL: C. Expert Opinion.

that may be appropriate include urinalysis and smear and culture of urethral discharge, if present.

DIFFERENTIAL DIAGNOSIS

The critical issues that define the differential diagnosis for a given patient are duration and severity of the symptoms, whether the scrotal mass is of testicular or paratesticular origin, and whether the mass is cystic or solid. Differential diagnostic considerations and a decision tree are shown in Fig. 206.2. Scrotal masses of acute onset and associated with severe symptoms usually are acute epididymitis or testicular torsion. Differentiating these two processes may be quite difficult for an acutely ill patient. Although malignant neoplasms of the testis may be thought by the patient to be of abrupt onset, the severity of the illness is not ordinarily that of these two conditions.

Cystic masses revealed with transillumination or ultrasonography usually are hydroceles. Hydroceles may surround the testis (except the posterior aspect) or may be localized to the spermatic cord. Some have a relatively acute onset. Some acute-onset hydroceles may be reactive in nature and may be associated with a testicular tumor. If this is the case, ultrasonography can help confirm the presence of a testicular mass.

The most common misdiagnosis of testis tumor is epididymitis. This differential diagnosis occasionally may be difficult. At examination, the epididymis is thick, tense, and tender. The groove between the testis and epididymis is obliterated, and the epididymis fits over the posterior aspect of the testis like a crescent. Unless a diagnosis of epididymitis is certain, the patient should be reexamined after a brief course of antibiotics. If the enlargement is not resolving, the diagnosis of epididymitis may be erroneous, and inguinal exploration should be considered.

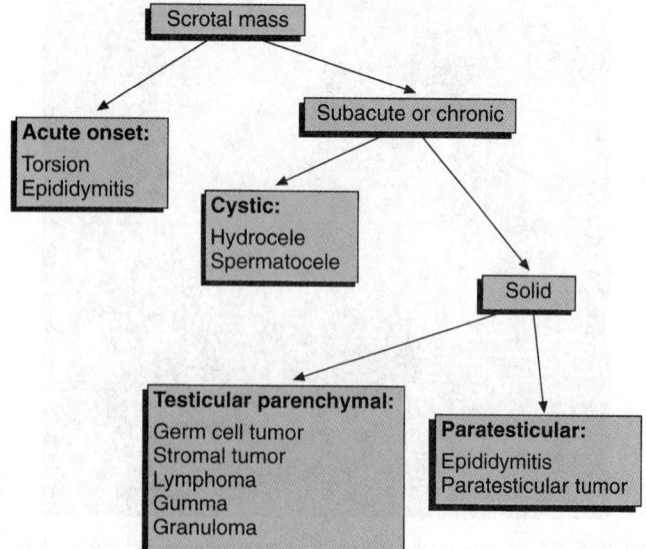

FIGURE 206.2. Differential diagnosis of a scrotal mass.
EVIDENCE LEVEL: C. Expert Opinion.

STRATEGIES FOR OPTIMAL CARE

MANAGEMENT

The choice of diagnostic studies is dictated by the clinical findings. The management of a testicular mass thought to be a neoplasm is outlined in Chapter 222. In brief, results of inguinal exploration and orchiectomy confirm the diagnosis and initiate therapy.

COMPLICATIONS AND PITFALLS

A testicular neoplasm must not be erroneously diagnosed as a benign condition. As discussed in Chapter 222, these tumors are sometimes rapidly progressive, and the likelihood of cure correlates strongly with tumor stage and volume at diagnosis.

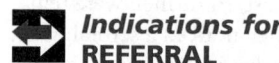 ***Indications for*** **REFERRAL**

Low-grade epididymitis ordinarily does not necessitate urologic consultation, and many causes of scrotal masses, such as hydrocele, spermatocele, and varicocele, usually necessitate no specific management. Testicular tumors do necessitate urologic consultation, and acute, severe epididymitis and testicular torsion are urologic emergencies.

COST-EFFECTIVENESS

The widespread availability of testicular ultrasonography has added to the cost of the evaluation of a scrotal mass. However, the information gained from such a procedure may have a substantial effect on the treatment of these patients, and the study frequently is justified in the diagnostic evaluation of many patients. The most costly aspect of the evaluation of these patients is erroneous diagnosis of a lesion that proves to be a testicular tumor. The resultant delay in diagnosis may mandate much more aggressive therapy and reduce the likelihood of cure.

BIBLIOGRAPHY

Bosl GJ, Bajorin DF, Sheinfeld J, et al. Cancer of the testis. In: DeVita VT, Hellman S, Rosenberg SA, eds. *Cancer: principles and practice of oncology.* Philadelphia: Lippincott-Raven; 1997:1397–1426.

Foster RS, Bihrle R, Donohue JP, et al. Testicular tumor. In: Stein BS, ed. *Clinical urologic practice.* New York: WW Norton, 1995:1027.

Kalota SMJ, Greene LF, Parsons CL. Evaluation of the urologic patient. In: Stein BS, ed. *Clinical urologic practice.* New York: WW Norton, 1995:257.

Kelley's Textbook of Internal Medicine, fourth edition. Edited by H. David Humes. Lippincott Williams & Wilkins, Philadelphia © 2000.

APPROACH TO THE PATIENT WITH A PROSTATE NODULE OR ELEVATED PROSTATE-SPECIFIC ANTIGEN LEVEL

DAVID C. SMITH
JAMES E. MONTIE

PRESENTATION

Because of the widespread ability to measure prostate-specific antigen (PSA), it is not uncommon for male patients to request assistance in the interpretation of a serum PSA level. Although many patients with prostate cancer have only an abnormal elevation in PSA level, an isolated elevation in PSA is not enough information to confirm a diagnosis of prostate cancer. A thorough understanding of the interpretation of this serum marker is needed to appropriately advise patients.

Patients also may have urinary symptoms, including frequency, urgency, decreased flow, nocturia, urinary tract infection, or signs of prostatic inflammation. These symptoms may be caused by both benign and malignant causes of prostatic enlargement that lead to obstruction of urinary flow. Measurement of PSA and digital rectal examination (DRE) are commonly used in the initial evaluation of these symptoms. DRE is mandatory for patients with urinary symptoms and should be a component of the routine physical examination of any male patient older than 40 years. Palpation of the entire prostate sometimes is difficult, but most men can be thoroughly examined by an experienced clinician. The presence of a prostate nodule or abnormally firm prostate gland mandates further evaluation.

PATHOPHYSIOLOGY

Prostate-specific antigen is a 34 kd glycoprotein with serine protease activity. Its main biologic role appears to be liquefaction of coagulated semen after ejaculation. PSA has also been shown to activate growth factors; the implication is that PSA has a regulatory role in epithelial growth in the prostate. PSA is produced almost exclusively by prostatic epithelial cells. In the setting of neoplasia or inflammation, breakdown of epithelial barriers causes release of PSA into the blood stream, where it is complexed to circulating proteins. Total PSA levels roughly correlate with prostate volume.

Prostate cancer is typically multifocal in distribution throughout the gland. Although an index lesion often is present, even these areas typically contain more than one histologic grade of tumor and often are mixtures of tumor with benign prostatic

hyperplasia (BPH). Most tumors arise in the peripheral zone of the gland, and a minority occur in the transitional and central zones. The peripheral zone is easily accessible because this is the portion of the gland typically palpated during DRE. Unfortunately, many tumors become clinically significant before a palpable nodule or area of induration develops.

HISTORY AND PHYSICAL EXAMINATION

The first element of the history and physical examination is a discussion of urinary symptoms. Voiding dysfunction such as decreased stream and nocturia suggest enlargement of the prostate gland. These findings may be associated with benign conditions, particularly in the absence of a palpable abnormality. Dysuria, hematuria, and hematospermia are relatively rare as initial signs of prostate cancer and should prompt a thorough evaluation of the urinary tract, including excretory urography and cystoscopy. Both prostatitis and benign enlargement of the gland may elevate serum PSA level.

Family history is an important historical element. Evidence suggests that only 9% of prostate cancers are caused by inherited factors. Men with first- and second-degree relatives with prostate cancer are at increased relative risk for prostate cancer, particularly if the relative was found to have prostate cancer at a young age. Race and ethnicity also appear to be important factors. African American men have a higher incidence and death rate of prostate cancer than do white men. Familial risk also appears to be more important among African American men. Race and ethnicity also play a role through environmental and dietary exposures. The clearest indication of this is increased risk for prostate cancer among Asian men immigrating to the United States. Asians typically have low levels of clinically significant prostate cancer; however, this rate increases in subsequent generations after immigration.

Documentation of current medications is a critical component of the history. The 5α-reductase inhibitor finasteride decreases serum PSA levels as much as 50%. Patients taking exogenous androgens to manage sexual dysfunction and symptoms associated with aging may have an elevated PSA level. Phytoestrogens are present in a number of commonly used nutritional supplements, including soy products and some herbal preparations. These may have the effect of lowering PSA levels.

Urologic instrumentation such as catheterization or cystoscopy may cause an elevated PSA. Prostate biopsy can markedly elevate serum PSA; a 4 to 6 week period is needed after biopsy before a baseline PSA level is determined. Ejaculation and strenuous exercise also have been reported to cause transient increases in serum PSA level.

Although patients presenting with metastatic disease are becoming rare with the advent of widespread PSA testing, a thorough review of systems and physical examination are necessary for patients with an elevated PSA level or a prostate nodule. All patients should undergo DRE. A normal prostate has two lobes, a median crease, and easily palpable lateral lobes. The seminal vesicles usually are not palpable. A normal prostate gland has a firm, rubbery consistency commonly likened to the thenar eminence of the palm. Areas of induration and nodules are hard. The presence of these features, obliteration of any of the normal landmarks, or any asymmetry is a sign of prostate carcinoma. It is important to record the location, character, size, and margins of any palpable abnormality and its relation to any of the normal landmarks. An enlarged gland with a normal consistency typically is associated with a benign condition such as BPH.

LABORATORY STUDIES AND DIAGNOSTIC TESTS

An abnormal finding at DRE is a clear indication for measuring PSA if this has not already been done. Although there are several assays for serum PSA, the most commonly used is the Tandem-R assay, which has a normal range of less than 0.2 to 3.9 ng per milliliter. Ultrasensitive PSA assays have been developed that allow detection of PSA levels as low as 0.01 ng per milliliter, but the usefulness of such information is not known. Assays also have been developed to differentiate free PSA from PSA bound to circulating serum proteins.

The definitive diagnostic procedure for patients in this setting is transrectal ultrasound (TRUS)–guided needle biopsy of the prostate gland. Performed by an experienced examiner and after appropriate preparation, this diagnostic study has minimal morbidity. When no palpable abnormality is found at DRE and no lesion is clearly seen on a TRUS scan, sextant biopsy in which all portions of the gland are sampled is also performed. When an abnormality can be palpated or seen on an imaging study, specific biopsy of the abnormal area is also performed. By itself TRUS biopsy is nonspecific as a screening modality, although it does allow estimation of prostate volume, which may be useful in estimating PSA density (see later).

TRUS biopsy is an outpatient procedure that is generally well tolerated. A Fleet enema and prophylactic oral antibiotics usually are given before the procedure. Patients with indications for full intravenous prophylactic antibiotic coverage, such as artificial heart valves or a prosthesis, or anticoagulation for cardiac conditions need more extensive intervention before TRUS biopsy. Complications of this procedure include a relatively low risk for urosepsis, a 1% to 2% risk for urinary retention caused by swelling, and possible hematuria and local discomfort. Bleeding typically is not a problem, although patients taking nonsteroidal anti-inflammatory agents should discontinue these 1 week before the biopsy is performed. Radionuclide bone scans and pelvic imaging such as computed tomography or magnetic resonance imaging are appropriate before pathologic diagnosis only when the PSA level is markedly elevated or abnormal findings at physical examination suggest dissemination of disease.

DIFFERENTIAL DIAGNOSIS

An elevation in serum PSA level is not enough information to confirm a diagnosis of prostate cancer. Men with BPH, prostatitis, prostatic infarction, or urologic manipulation and those who exercise strenuously can have an elevated PSA level. In rare in-

TABLE 207.1.	DIFFERENTIAL DIAGNOSIS
Elevated Prostate-Specific Antigen	**Prostate Nodule**
Prostate cancer	Prostate cancer
Benign prostatic hyperplasia	Benign prostatic hypertrophy (nodular)
Prostatis	
Prostatic infarction	Prostatitis (granulomatous)
	Prostatic infarction
Urologic manipulation	Previous biopsy
Exercise (minimal)	
Ejaculation (minimal)	
Other malignant lesion (rare)	

stances elevations in serum PSA level have been associated with undifferentiated cancers such as breast cancer.

A palpable nodule found at DRE may be caused by infarction or inflammation, nodular BPH, or an earlier biopsy. Tenderness at DRE suggests ongoing inflammation or infection. Induration, asymmetry of the gland, or obliteration of the typical landmarks is more often associated with the presence of a malignant tumor than with a benign condition. The differential diagnosis of conditions associated with an elevated PSA level or palpable abnormality at DRE is summarized in Table 207.1.

STRATEGIES FOR OPTIMAL CARE

The most important decision to be made concerns the timing of biopsy of the prostate. This decision must take into account the overall condition of the patient. Establishing a diagnosis of localized prostate cancer for a patient whose life span is limited because of comorbid conditions may be of minimal benefit. These factors ideally are considered before serum PSA is measured. Most patients and physicians, however, do not consider how the information will be used until after the value is obtained. Screening is controversial. Several groups, including the American Cancer Society and American Urologic Association, recommend screening for men older than 50 years (40 years for men with a family history of prostate cancer and for African Americans). The American College of Physicians and other groups do not recommend screening given the lack of evidence that screening influences mortality from prostate cancer. Despite these conflicting recommendations, many men have PSA levels measured, and a large percentage have elevations in these levels. Data from several clinical series indicate that as many as 20% of men who have PSA levels measured have elevated values and that as many as 25% of these men undergo further evaluation. Most of the cancers detected in this way are clinically significant. Even in the setting of a T1c lesion (TNM staging system; elevated PSA level, normal DRE findings), 85% to 95% of cases of cancer detected are of clinically significant volume. Studies suggest that most cancers detected through screening are potentially harmful, confined to the organ, and potentially curable.

An isolated elevated PSA level in a patient who has no symptoms is problematic. The criteria used to refer these men for biopsy is a major issue. PSA cutoff levels at 4 and 10 ng per milliliter provide the best levels of sensitivity and specificity. Patients with levels less than 4 ng per milliliter are at very low risk for prostate cancer, whereas those with levels greater than 10 ng per milliliter are at high enough risk to justify biopsy in most instances. Decisions for the patient with a PSA level between 4 and 10 ng per milliliter remain problematic. Several strategies have been developed to refine this approach.

AGE-SPECIFIC REFERENCE RANGES FOR SERUM LEVEL OF PROSTATE-SPECIFIC ANTIGEN

The prostate gland enlarges with age, and prostatic inflammation is most common among older men. Because of these factors more tissue is available to produce PSA, and there is more leakage of PSA into the circulation. Older men without prostate cancer therefore have higher PSA levels than do younger men. Several studies have examined age-specific PSA ranges. With lower ranges of PSA for men younger than 60 years, sensitivity for detection of prostate cancer increases. Analyses have suggested that the effect of using the lower range will be limited and that there will be only a 2% to 4% increase in the rate of detection of curable cancer. The number of additional younger men who would undergo biopsy was not predicted. In contrast, wider PSA reference ranges for older men increase the specificity for detecting prostate cancer. The increased specificity would cause a decrease in the number of these men referred for biopsy. Analysis of one large practice suggested that this broader range would cause a 6% decrease in biopsy rate. Less than 1% of men who actually had cancer would not have been referred for biopsy, and most of these had well-differentiated organ-confined cancers that posed little threat to their lives. Other analyses have suggested that as many as 10% of organ-confined cancers would not be detected with use of the age-specific rages for older men. Race also has been incorporated into this approach. Mean serum PSA concentrations are significantly higher among African American men in both populations with and populations without cancer, and these levels increase with age. The age-specific reference ranges for both whites and African Americans are shown in Table 207.2.

TABLE 207.2.	AGE-SPECIFIC REFERENCE RANGES FOR PROSTATE-SPECIFIC ANTIGEN (PSA)

| Age Range (yr) | Appropriate PSA Range (ng/mL) | |
	Whites	African Americans
40–50	0.0–2.5	0.0–2.0
51–60	0.0–3.5	0.0–4.0
61–70	0.0–5.5	0.0–4.5
>70	0.0–6.5	0.0–5.5

FREE AND PROTEIN-BOUND PROSTATE-SPECIFIC ANTIGEN

Prostate-specific antigen circulates in both free and protein-bound forms, with approximately 70% bound to serum proteins, primarily α1-antichymotrypsin. Patients with prostate cancer have a lower percentage of free PSA than do patients with BPH. Results of initial studies suggest that a free PSA percentage less than 18% suggests the presence of prostate cancer and may increase the specificity of PSA testing. The combination and potential interactions of free PSA percentage and the age-specific reference ranges have not been evaluated, although at least one study has shown that free PSA values are not age dependent.

PROSTATE-SPECIFIC ANTIGEN DENSITY AND VELOCITY

Prostate-specific antigen density is an attempt to differentiate BPH from prostate cancer by means of assessing PSA production per unit volume of the prostate gland. The ratio between serum PSA level and prostate volume as estimated with TRUS suggests that patients with a PSA density greater than 0.15 have a much greater rate of having detectable cancer. Prostate volume is difficult to determine in clinical practice, making this a less than useful measure.

PSA velocity relies on serial measurements of PSA to determine the rate of rise of PSA level over time. Data suggest that patients with organ-confined prostate cancer have a rise of approximately 0.5 ng per milliliter per year compared with 0.18 ng per milliliter per year among men with BPH. Unfortunately, the variability in the PSA assay itself often approaches the level of change associated with the presence of malignancy. This and variability among laboratories performing the assay make using the assay somewhat difficult.

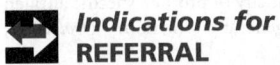

Indications for REFERRAL

The most important decision concerns referral of patients for biopsy. The decision to proceed with evaluation ideally is made before the PSA level is measured, because only patients who will benefit from the diagnosis of or current therapy for prostate cancer should undergo biopsy. Once PSA has been measured and shown to be elevated, it is unlikely that the evaluation will stop short of biopsy of the prostate gland. Patients with PSA values greater than the age-specific ranges might benefit from TRUS-guided biopsy whether or not an abnormality is found at DRE. Any patient in generally good medical condition who has a palpable nodule should be referred for biopsy. Patients with symptoms of urinary outflow obstruction and either a normal or elevated PSA level who can tolerate therapy should consult with a urologist. A strategy for the detection of early prostate cancer is outlined in Table 207.3.

TABLE 207.3.	DETECTION OF EARLY PROSTATE CANCER FOR APPROPRIATE PATIENTS	
Prostate-Specific Antigen	Digital Rectal Examination	Action
Normal age specific	Negative	Annual PSA and DRE
Elevated age specific	Negative	TRUS: biopsy-visualized lesions and sextant biopsy
Any	Positive	TRUS: biopsy-visualized and palpable lesions and sextant biopsy

PSA, prostate-specific antigen; DRE, digital rectal examination; TRUS, transrectal ultrasonography.

COST-EFFECTIVENESS

Economic grounds often have been used to criticize the use of measurement of PSA in prostate cancer screening. A comparison of the cost of PSA screening with that of mammographic screening for breast cancer shows that prostate cancer compares quite favorably. On average, the cost per case of prostate cancer detected is approximately $3,000 compared with $15,000 for each case of breast cancer detected. The main difference is that screening for breast cancer has been shown to reduce mortality, whereas no similar data exist for prostate cancer. Data addressing this question will be available at the completion of large, randomized screening trials within the next few years.

BIBLIOGRAPHY

Bangma CH, Rietbergen JB, Kranse R, et al. The free-to-total prostate specific antigen ratio improves the specificity of prostate specific antigen in screening for prostate cancer in the general population. *J Urol* 1997; 157:2191–2196.

Benoit RM, Naslund MJ. The economics of prostate cancer screening. *Oncology* 1997;11:1533–1548.

Carter HB, Epstein JI, Partin AW. Influence of age and prostate-specific antigen on the chance of curable prostate cancer among men with non-palpable disease. *Urology* 1999;53:126–130.

Catalona WJ, Smith DS, Ornstein DK. Prostate cancer detection in men with serum PSA concentrations of 2.6 to 4.0 ng per milliliter and benign prostate examination: enhancement of specificity with free PSA measurements. *JAMA* 1997;277:1452–1455.

Collins MM, Barry MJ. Controversies in prostate cancer screening. Analogies to the early lung cancer screening debate. *JAMA* 1996;276: 1976–1979.

Fowler FJ Jr, Bin L, Collins MM, et al. Prostate cancer screening and beliefs about treatment efficacy: a national survey of primary care physicians and urologists. *Am J Med* 1998;104:526–532.

Morgan TO, Jacobsen SJ, McCarthy WF, et al. Age-specific reference ranges for prostate-specific antigen in black men. *N Engl J Med* 1996;335: 304–310.

Oesterling JE, Jacobsen SJ, Chute CG, et al. Serum prostate-specific antigen in a community-based population of healthy men: establishment of age-specific reference ranges. *JAMA* 1993;270:860–864.

Smith JR, Freije D, Carpten JD, et al. Major susceptibility locus for prostate cancer on chromosome 1 suggested by a genome-wide search. *Science* 1996;274:1371–1374.

Thiel R, Pearson JD, Epstein JI, et al. Role of prostate-specific antigen velocity in prediction of final pathologic stage in men with localized prostate cancer. *Urology* 1997;49:716–720.

Kelley's Textbook of Internal Medicine, fourth edition. Edited by H. David Humes. Lippincott Williams & Wilkins, Philadelphia © 2000.

CHAPTER 208

APPROACH TO THE PATIENT WITH AN ADNEXAL MASS

IVOR BENJAMIN
STEPHEN C. RUBIN

PRESENTATION

The word *adnexa* is the plural of *adnexum,* which means "connected part" or "appendage." In gynecology, the term *adnexa* is used to include the ovaries, the fallopian tubes, the broad ligament, and the structures in it that are derived from embryonic remnants of the wolffian ducts or from peritoneal inclusions. Any one of these structures can be called an *adnexum,* but this term is seldom used.

The most common presentation of an adnexal mass is the incidental finding of a tumor adjacent to the uterus during a routine pelvic examination of a woman who has no symptoms. An adnexal mass also may become apparent with pelvic or abdominal pain. These may be caused by complications of the mass, such as torsion, infection, or hemorrhage, or symptoms due to pressure on adjacent organs. The symptoms may depend on the origin of the adnexal mass. Menstrual disorders such as menorrhagia or dysmenorrhea due to ovarian endometrioma or pelvic inflammatory disease (PID) may prompt the pelvic examination that elicits the mass. Bowel symptoms such as diarrhea, constipation, or the passage of mucus or blood may lead to the discovery of an adnexal mass due to diverticulitis or colon cancer. Urinary symptoms such as dysuria, hematuria, or incontinence may occur if the mass originates in the urinary tract.

PATHOPHYSIOLOGY

An adnexal mass may arise from the gynecologic organs themselves or be caused by disease in adjacent anatomic structures. Most adnexal masses are of gynecologic origin, arising from the ovary, fallopian tube, broad ligament, or uterus. The various gynecologic conditions that can account for the finding of an

TABLE 208.1.	GYNECOLOGIC ADNEXAL MASSES
Structure	**Mass**
Ovary	Functional cyst
	Follicle cyst
	Corpus luteum cyst
	Theca lutein cyst
	Neoplasm
	Benign
	Malignant
	Endometrioma
	Inflammatory disease
	Adhesive disease (subacute or chronic infection)
	Abscess (ovarian or tuboovarian)
Fallopian tube	Tuboovarian abscess
	Pyosalpinx
	Hydrosalpinx
	Ectopic pregnancy
	Neoplasm
	Carcinoma
	Sarcoma
	Choriocarcinoma
Broad ligament	Cyst from wolffian duct remnants
	Gartner duct cyst
	Peritoneal inclusion cyst
	Malignant tumor of the broad ligament
Uterus	Pedunculated or intraligamentous leiomyoma
	Pregnancy in horn of bicornuate uterus

adnexal mass are listed in Table 208.1. Adnexal masses also can originate in the intestine, urinary tract, abdominal wall, or retroperitoneum (Table 208.2.)

During the reproductive years, the most common adnexal enlargement found at pelvic examination is a functional cyst of the ovary. These non-neoplastic cysts form as a result of minor aberrations in the normal process of ovulation. If ovulation does not occur (anovulatory cycle), the follicle continues to enlarge and may reach a size of 10 cm or more in diameter, resulting

TABLE 208.2.	NONGYNECOLOGIC ADNEXAL MASSES
Structure	**Mass**
Intestine	Feces or gas
	Diverticulitis
	Enteritis
	Pelvic appendicitis
	Carcinoma of the colon
Urinary tract	Distended bladder
	Bladder neoplasm or calculus
	Pelvic kidney
Abdominal wall	Hematoma
	Abscess
	Desmoid tumor
Retroperitoneal cavity	Lymphoma
	Sarcoma
	Teratoma

in a follicular cyst. Less commonly, a functional cyst may arise from the corpus luteum. Formation of the corpus luteum is a normal postovulatory event. On occasion, however, the corpus luteum may become palpably enlarged because of hemorrhage, and a corpus luteum cyst forms. Because normal corpus lutea are cystic, the term *corpus luteum cyst* should be reserved for those larger than 3 cm in diameter. Functional ovarian cysts of either follicular or luteal origin usually regress spontaneously within one or two menstrual cycles.

If the ovarian follicle is overstimulated by excess luteinizing hormone, as occurs in Stein–Leventhal (polycystic ovary) syndrome, or by excess human chorionic gonadotropin (hCG), as occurs with hydatidiform mole, theca lutein cysts form. These cysts resolve spontaneously when the underlining pathophysiologic process has been corrected. While present, however, the cysts must be differentiated from primary adnexal neoplasms or other adnexal disorders.

The most important concern in finding an adnexal mass is that it might represent a malignant neoplasm. Most adnexal neoplasms are of ovarian origin. Neoplasms of the fallopian tube and parametrium are rare. Ovarian neoplasms can be cystic or solid. The most common benign cystic tumors are serous cystadenoma, mucinous cystadenoma, and cystic teratoma. Malignant epithelial tumors of the ovary usually are serous or mucinous cystadenocarcinoma. Less common histologic types are endometrioid, clear-cell, or mixed epithelial tumors. The common benign solid ovarian tumors are fibroma, adenofibroma, thecoma, and Brenner tumor. All usually are firm to palpation. Solid malignant ovarian neoplasms usually are primary adenocarcinoma of the ovary. Metastatic lesions to the ovary usually originate in the uterus, gastrointestinal tract, or breast.

Endometriosis is a frequently encountered gynecologic cause of an adnexal mass. The hallmark of this disease is ectopic endometrial tissue. Although endometriosis may be found in distant sites such as the pleura and gastrointestinal tract, it is most commonly found on peritoneal surfaces in the pelvis. Endometriotic implants on the ovarian surface may coalesce and form a hemorrhagic cyst known as *endometrioma*. These cysts have a complex, loculated appearance on ultrasound scans and therefore may mimic ovarian cancer.

PID commonly becomes apparent as a tender adnexal mass. This may be the result of a tuboovarian abscess, hydrosalpinx, or chronic adhesions and scarring from resolved PID. Uterine disease also can manifest itself as an adnexal mass—pedunculated, intraligamentous, or cervical leiomyoma. Ectopic pregnancy in a rudimentary or well-developed horn of a bicornuate uterus also can become apparent as a palpable adnexal mass.

Although most adnexal masses are of gynecologic origin, it is important for the clinician to be cognizant that masses in the region of the adnexa may originate in the intestine, urinary tract, abdominal wall, or retroperitoneal cavity. Feces or gas in the colon or a distended neurogenic bladder may mimic an adnexal mass of ovarian origin. It is prudent to ensure that the patient has evacuated her bowel and voided before a pelvic examination for a suspected adnexal tumor. Diverticulitis, appendicitis, inflammatory bowel disease, and tumors arising in the intestine are examples of gastrointestinal disorders that cause a mass in the region of the adnexa. Urinary tract disease, including bladder calculus and neoplasia of the kidney, ureter, bladder, or urethra, also may cause an apparent adnexal mass. A pelvic kidney from congenital malformation or transplantation may be palpable in the adnexal region. Abdominal wall masses (hematoma, abscess, hernia, or desmoid tumor) can develop caudad to the umbilicus and may be diagnosed as adnexal masses. The most common tumors of retroperitoneal origin that may cause adnexal masses are lymphoma, sarcoma, or teratoma.

HISTORY AND PHYSICAL EXAMINATION

Because of the wide array of gynecologic and nongynecologic diseases that can be responsible for the clinical finding of an adnexal mass, a comprehensive gynecologic and medical history is mandatory. Most ovarian neoplasms, unless advanced, are not associated with pain or menstrual disturbances. The association of pain with a mass in the region of the adnexa suggests torsion, infection, leiomyomatous degeneration, PID, or endometriosis. Rapidly growing germ cell tumors of the ovary can cause pain from stretching of the ovarian capsule. Menstrual disorders such as oligomenorrhea, dysmenorrhea, or menorrhagia also should alert the clinician to the possibility of the presence of a functional ovarian cyst, endometriosis, leiomyoma, granulosa cell tumor, or ectopic pregnancy. Because masses in the adnexal region may be caused by intestinal or urinary tract disease, the history interview must elicit any symptoms pertaining to these systems. A history of nausea, vomiting, anorexia, constipation, diarrhea, or the passage of blood through the rectum may be relevant. Disturbances in micturition may point to urinary tract disease. In rare instances hematuria or blood in the stool may be caused by endometriotic implants involving the wall of the bladder, colon, or rectum.

The physical examination should include general medical surveillance, a breast examination, examination for enlarged supraclavicular nodes, and abdominal examination for masses, ascites, or organomegaly. The initial identification of an adnexal mass usually is made by means of pelvic examination. During the pelvic examination, the location, consistency, size, laterality, and tenderness of the mass are assessed. These facts should be interpreted in the context of the age of the patient to formulate an appropriate differential diagnosis. The pelvic examination must include both vaginal and rectovaginal examinations. The latter affords the best assessment of the rectum, posterior pelvis, and parametrium. Stool on the glove should be examined for occult blood. Cross contamination from vaginal blood must be avoided. If tenderness or fever is present, cervical cultures for gonorrhea and chlamydia should be obtained.

LABORATORY STUDIES AND DIAGNOSTIC TESTS

A pregnancy test (urine or serum β-hCG) should be performed whenever there is a mass in the adnexal region of a woman of reproductive age. If β-hCG level is elevated, it must be assumed that the patient is pregnant. Patients with an adnexal mass in addition to an elevated β-hCG level should be immediately referred to an obstetrician–gynecologist for further treatment. Evaluation of these patients may lead to the diagnosis of ectopic pregnancy, theca lutein cyst associated with gestational trophoblastic disease, ovarian choriocarcinoma, embryonal carcinoma, or endodermal sinus tumor of the ovary. All these are life-threatening conditions without timely diagnosis and treatment. However, the most likely diagnosis is physiologic enlargement of the corpus luteum during the first trimester of a normal intrauterine pregnancy. Because many of these patients may have normal pregnancies, the use of diagnostic studies with ionizing radiation should be avoided.

Pelvic ultrasonography is a safe and useful diagnostic test. In most cases, it can be used to determine the position, size, and structure of an adnexal mass. Transvaginal ultrasonography provides enhanced resolution of the adnexa compared with transabdominal sonography. Therefore, use of the transvaginal probe has become a routine component of ultrasound examination of the pelvis. In addition to size and location, knowledge of the internal morphologic features of the mass are critical for diagnosis. Benign follicle cysts have distinct borders with little or no internal septation. Cysts with a complex internal architecture that might include septa, solid components, papillary formations, and vessels present a diagnostic challenge. Gas-fluid levels suggest tuboovarian abscess, pelvic abscess, or ruptured viscus. A pelvic hematoma in the vicinity of the adnexa is likely to have a more homogeneous appearance. Benign cystic teratoma (dermoid cysts) often exhibit a highly specific sonographic findings. Benign ovarian teratomas typically have both cystic and solid components. The former usually contains oily and sebaceous material, whereas the latter may include bone, teeth, and hair. Certain sonographic findings suggest ovarian cancer. These include a high proportion of solid areas, a complex internal structure with thick septa separating cystic loculations, papillary formations, and the presence of ascites. Color-flow Doppler analysis of the vessels within an adnexal mass can provide additional information regarding the likelihood of malignancy.

Computed tomography (CT) of the abdomen and pelvis can be helpful in confirming the presence of a pelvic mass and is useful for assessment of the retroperitoneal cavity. Magnetic resonance imaging (MRI) is expensive and rarely provides information beyond that obtained with CT. A simple radiographic examination of the abdomen and pelvis may be useful in detecting the teeth of a benign cystic teratoma or calcifications within a degenerating uterine leiomyoma. When gastrointestinal symptoms are elicited, sigmoidoscopy or contrast radiographic studies of the gastrointestinal tract are indicated. Urinary tract symptoms may warrant cystoscopy and intravenous pyelography.

Tumor markers may be used to aid in diagnosis. The level of cancer antigen CA 125 may be elevated in epithelial ovarian cancer. Germ cell tumors may be associated with elevations in serum β-hCG or α-fetoprotein level. Sex cord–stromal tumors of the ovary, granulosa cell tumor, and Sertoli–Leydig cell tumor may produce excess estrogens and androgens, respectively. Steroid cell tumors are exceedingly rare neoplasms that may produce androgens, estrogens, progestins, or corticosteroids. In rare instances patients with steroid cell tumors of the ovary have Cushing's syndrome.

Some physicians advocate serum CA 125 measurement as a screening test for ovarian cancer. However, CA 125 determination has an unacceptably low positive predictive value even when a reference value is selected to provide relatively low sensitivity. Therefore, serum CA 125 determination is not a valid screening test for ovarian cancer. It is, however, an appropriate component of the evaluation for an adnexal mass. Markedly elevated levels of serum CA 125 (more than 200) have a positive predictive value of more than 75% and therefore usually indicate the presence of epithelial ovarian cancer. However, moderately elevated levels (less than 200) are common in association with benign ovarian tumors, endometriosis, PID, and pregnancy. Level of CA 125 also may be elevated in association with pancreatitis, cirrhosis, peritonitis, peritoneal tuberculosis, or malignant disease of the pancreas, lung, breast, or colon. Conversely, some instances of ovarian cancer (as many as 25%) may not elevate serum CA 125 level. An elevated peripheral white blood cell count (WBC) and erythrocyte sedimentation rate may support the diagnosis of PID.

DIFFERENTIAL DIAGNOSIS

Arriving at a precise diagnosis is important because many adnexal masses may respond to nonsurgical management (e.g., functional ovarian cysts, tuboovarian abscess, or endometriosis), whereas others necessitate surgical removal (e.g., benign or malignant neoplasms or ectopic pregnancy). The differential diagnosis of an adnexal mass includes all the conditions listed in Tables 208.1 and 208.2. A careful and thorough history interview is necessary to support a differential diagnosis. An adequate history must include a menstrual history, bowel and bladder function, and any symptoms of direct or referred pain, abdominal bloating, nausea, vomiting, or diarrhea.

Physical examination aids in diagnosis when special attention is paid to the abdominal and pelvic findings. In most cases, laboratory studies and special diagnostic tests are needed, including a pregnancy test, complete blood cell count, pelvic ultrasonography, and possibly a CT of the abdomen and pelvis. If the history and physical findings point to a possible gastrointestinal or urinary tract origin of the mass, laboratory studies and diagnostic tests aimed at these areas are warranted. When the cause of an adnexal mass is unclear after the aforementioned evaluation, diagnostic laparoscopy may be helpful. For example, laparoscopy enables one to differentiate readily between uterine leiomyoma and an ovarian neoplasm.

STRATEGIES FOR OPTIMAL CARE

MANAGEMENT

An algorithm for care of a patient with an adnexal mass is outlined in Fig. 208.1. Before a pelvic examination, it is prudent to request that the patient void and evacuate. If a mass is felt and there is a possibility of retained feces, an enema may be necessary before a second examination. Adnexal masses that are not retained stool or urine necessitate further scrutiny. Postmenopausal or premenarchal women with a palpable adnexal mass have a reasonably high likelihood of having malignant pelvic disease and therefore should be referred to a gynecologic oncologist for additional evaluation. This evaluation would probably include pelvic ultrasonography and serum CA 125 measurement. For women of reproductive age urinary β-hCG should be measured. If the test result is positive, the patient is either pregnant (highly likely) or has a β-hCG–secreting neoplasm (rare) that is probably of gynecologic origin. The adnexal mass may represent normal corpus luteum, which often is palpable during the first trimester of a normal pregnancy or during ectopic pregnancy. If any of these diagnoses is likely, the patient should be referred to a gynecologist.

If the urine pregnancy test result is negative, transvaginal ultrasonography should be performed. If the adnexa appear normal, an evaluation workup for tumor of other pelvic structures should be undertaken. A simple ovarian cyst 5 cm or less in diameter in a nonpregnant woman of reproductive age probably is functional. These cysts are likely to resolve spontaneously. Repetition of the pelvic examination and ultrasonography in 6 weeks is reasonable. Ultrasonically simple cysts that persist for more than 10 to 12 weeks should be surgically removed to exclude malignant growth and prevent the development of adnexal torsion.

If the pelvic ultrasound scan depicts an adnexal mass with irregular borders or a complex internal architecture (septa, papillary formations, cystic and solid components), then medical or surgical intervention is likely to be needed. Often an experienced ultrasonographer is able to discriminate between infectious (tuboovarian abscess), benign (endometrioma, cystic teratoma), and malignant (ovarian carcinoma) conditions with fair accuracy. However, there is considerable overlap in the appearance of complex adnexal masses. Overall, approximately 70% of multilocular solid ovarian masses are malignant. The other 30% are likely caused by infection (tuboovarian abscess) or endometriosis (endometrioma). Both these nonmalignant diagnoses occur almost exclusively among women of reproductive age. Therefore, a complex adnexal mass in a premenarchal or postmenopausal woman is highly likely to be malignant. Malignant ovarian tumors should be managed by a gynecologic oncologist. Standard management of ovarian cancer involves surgical staging and cytoreduction. Preoperative evaluation usually includes complete blood cell count, serum chemical analysis, measurement of CA 125, barium enema radiography, and abdominal and pelvic CT with oral and intravenous contrast. The management of ovarian cancer is discussed in Chapter 221.

Complex adnexal masses in women of reproductive age that are associated with tenderness during pelvic examination or a fever likely represent a tuboovarian abscess. Blood, urine, and cervical cultures should be performed for gonorrhea and chlamydia. Serologic testing for syphilis and HIV infection also are are indicated. Antibiotic therapy in accordance with treatment guidelines of the Centers for Disease Control and Prevention should be initiated during the wait for culture results (Table 208.3). Persistent symptomatic tuboovarian abscess refractory to combination antibiotic therapy may necessitate surgical management. The operation usually includes exploratory laparot-

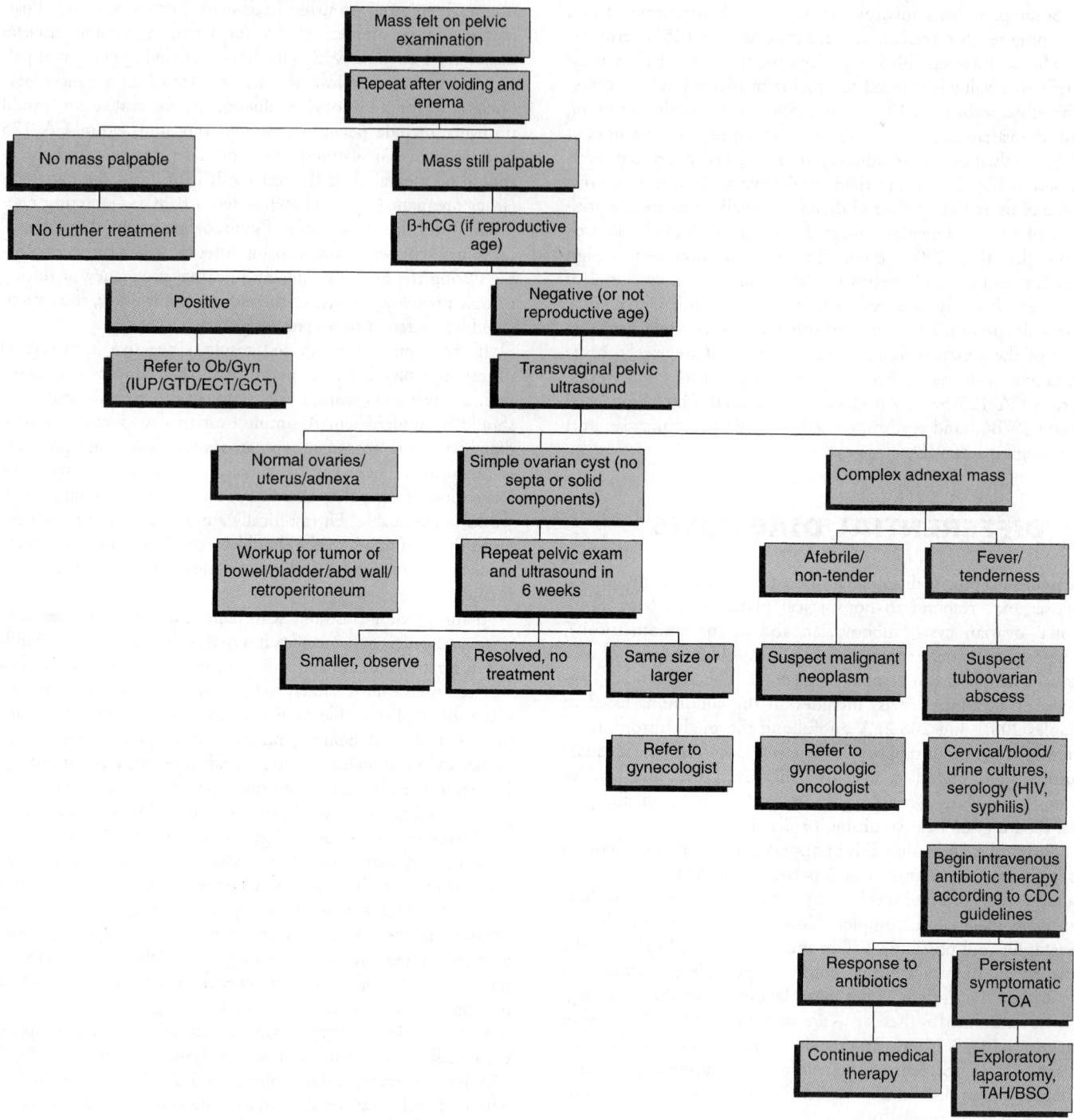

FIGURE 208.1. Algorithm for management of an adnexal mass. *β-hCG,* β-human chorionic gonadotropin; *BSO,* bilateral salpingo-oophorectomy; *CDC,* Centers for Disease Control and Prevention; *ECT,* ectopic pregnancy; *GCT,* germ cell tumor; *GTD,* gestational trophoblastic disease; *HIV,* human immunodeficiency virus; *IUP,* intrauterine pregnancy; *TAH,* total abdominal hysterectomy; *TOA,* tuboovarian abscess.
EVIDENCE LEVEL: C. Expert Opinion.

TABLE 208.3.	1989 CDC TREATMENT GUIDELINES FOR PELVIC INFLAMMATORY DISEASE

Inpatient Treatment

Regimen A
  Cefoxitin 2 g i.v. every 6 hr or cefotetan 2 g i.v. every 12 hr
  Doxycycline 100 mg i.v. or by mouth every 12 hr
Regimen B
  Clindamycin 900 mg i.v. every 8 hr
  Gentamicin loading dose (2 mg/kg) i.v. or i.m. followed by
    maintenance dose (1.5 mg/kg) every 8 hr
Either regimen should be given for at least 48 hr after clinical
  improvement.
Doxycycline (100 mg by mouth two times per day) or clindamycin
  (450 mg by mouth five times per day) should be continued for
  a total of 10 to 14 days.

Outpatient Treatment

Cefoxitin 2 g i.m., probenecid 1 g by mouth, or ceftriaxone 250
  mg i.m.
plus
Doxycycline 100 mg by mouth two times per day or tetracycline
  500 mg by mouth four times per day for 10 to 14 days

omy, total abdominal hysterectomy, and bilateral salpingo-oophorectomy.

Findings at pelvic ultrasonography may suggest that the adnexal mass is not of ovarian origin. Leiomyomas uteri (fibroid tumors) are a common finding in the region of the adnexa. These masses appear solid and usually do not require medical or surgical intervention even if quite large (5 cm in diameter or more). However, any adnexal mass, cystic or solid, in a premenarchal or postmenopausal woman mandates further investigation. Adnexal neoplasms are more commonly malignant among premenarchal patients. Management usually leads to surgical exploration for staging and cytoreduction by a gynecologic oncologist.

COMPLICATIONS AND PITFALLS

The important pitfalls in the care of patients with adnexal masses involve either being too aggressive, as in managing functional ovarian cysts surgically, or being too conservative and delaying surgical management of an adnexal mass that may be malignant. The key to avoiding such errors is thorough evaluation with early and accurate diagnosis. The likelihood that an adnexal mass is a malignant neoplasm is highly age dependent. In cases that elude diagnosis with noninvasive tests, diagnostic laparoscopy often is a reasonable approach. The patient must be adequately informed that the procedure may be converted to exploratory laparotomy depending on the intraoperative findings.

A woman of reproductive age with complex adnexal masses presumed to be tuboovarian abscesses may have ovarian cancer. Pain or fever may be associated with an ovarian cancer when tumor necrosis, ovarian torsion, chronic PID, or intestinal obstruction from carcinomatosis is present. These clinical scenarios may further blur the distinction between an underlying infectious and a malignant condition.

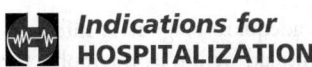

Indications for HOSPITALIZATION

Any patient with an adnexal mass that might be malignant should be hospitalized for exploratory laparotomy with possible surgical staging and cytoreduction. Women of reproductive age who have complex adnexal masses believed to be tuboovarian abscesses associated with pain or fever should be hospitalized for appropriate intravenous antibiotic therapy. Most adnexal masses resulting from other causes may be managed in an outpatient setting. Hospitalization might be needed only if surgical intervention is needed. However, in many of these cases, laparoscopic removal of small (likely benign) adnexal masses may be performed in a same-day surgery unit.

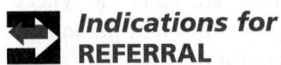

Indications for REFERRAL

The need for surgical intervention or obstetric care is a common indication for referral of a patient with an adnexal mass. Any woman of reproductive age who has a positive urine β-hCG test result and an adnexal mass should be referred to an obstetrician–gynecologist. A normal intrauterine pregnancy or diagnosis and management of ectopic pregnancy are likely outcomes. However, a premenarchal or postmenopausal woman with an elevated β-hCG level should be referred to a gynecologic oncologist for evaluation of a probable malignant tumor. A persistent simple adnexal cyst in a woman of reproductive age is an indication for referral to an obstetrician–gynecologist. Surgical removal by means of laparoscopy or laparotomy usually is appropriate. A postmenopausal or premenarchal woman with an adnexal mass should be referred to a gynecologic oncologist. Exploratory laparotomy for surgical staging and cytoreduction often is needed.

COST-EFFECTIVENESS

The evaluation and management of an adnexal mass may be cost-effective without diminution in the quality of patient care. Appropriate selection of patients with adnexal masses for outpatient medical and surgical management will result in substantial cost savings. Appropriate selection of diagnostic imaging studies for these patients also may further reduce costs.

We are in the midst of a technological explosion. With MRI, CT, and ultrasonography, noninvasive imaging of the deepest recesses of the body can be performed. Although these advanced, expensive imaging modalities often are invaluable for diagnosis and surveillance of an adnexal mass, they may greatly increase health care costs and afford little benefit over lower-cost alternatives. Inappropriate use may be caused by failure to select the least expensive test that provides adequate diagnostic information. For example, use of MRI instead of ultrasonography for surveillance of a simple ovarian cyst in a woman of reproductive age is inappropriate. Costs may be increased by frequent use of inappropriate imaging tests for documentation of a persistent adnexal cyst. Combination of expensive imaging modalities that provide overlapping diagnostic information (CT and MRI) often is inappropriate.

Too often a postmenopausal woman with a large pelvic mass and greatly elevated CA 125 level is referred to a gynecologic oncologist after normal results are obtained at pelvic ultrasonography, CT, and MRI. A strong argument can be made that the findings at pelvic examination alone mandate hospitalization and exploratory laparotomy. For this hypothetical patient, limiting the evaluation to CT of the abdomen and pelvis, barium enema radiography, mammography, and measurement of CA 125 and carcinoembryonic antigen (CEA) provides more useful diagnostic information. This battery of tests would discriminate with acceptable accuracy between tumors arising in the gynecologic organs, intestine, urinary tract, breast, or retroperitoneum at lower overall cost than would laparotomy.

Benign processes that become apparent as adnexal masses also may be diagnosed and managed in a cost-effective way. Tuboovarian abscess often is diagnosed with a combination of assessment of vital signs, pelvic examination, cervical culture, blood culture, and pelvic ultrasonography. CT, MRI, and nuclear isotope scans are expensive and usually are unnecessary. The appropriate selection of outpatient as opposed to inpatient surgical management of adnexal masses may greatly reduce costs. Women of reproductive age who have persistent simple ovarian cysts often are excellent candidates for laparoscopic surgery in a same-day surgical unit.

BIBLIOGRAPHY

Bailey CL, Land GL, DePriest PD, et al. The malignant potential of small cystic ovarian tumors in women over 50 years of age. *Gynecol Oncol* 1998;69:3–7.

Barnhart K, Mennuti MT, Benjamin I, et al. Prompt diagnosis of ectopic pregnancy in an emergency department setting. *Obstet Gynecol* 1994; 84:1010–1015.

Benjamin I, Rubin SC. Management of early-stage epithelial ovarian cancer. *Obstet Gynecol Clin North Am* 1994;21:107–119.

Centers for Disease Control. 1989 Sexually transmitted diseases: treatment guidelines. *MMWR Morb Mortal Wkly Rep* 1989;38:1–43.

Fleischer AC. Transabdominal and transvaginal sonography of ovarian masses. *Clin Obstet Gynecol* 1991;34:433–442.

Jacobs I, Bast RC. The CA 125 tumor associated antigen: a review of the literature. *Hum Reprod* 1989;4:1–12.

Maiman M, Seltzer V, Boyce J. Laparoscopic excision of ovarian neoplasms subsequently found to be malignant. *Obstet Gynecol* 1991;77:563–565.

Nezhat F, Nezhat C, Welander CE, et al. Four ovarian cancers diagnosed during laparoscopic management of 1011 women with adnexal masses. *Am J Obstet Gynecol* 1992;167:790–796.

Wilson JR. Ultrasonography in the diagnosis of gynecologic disorders. *Am J Obstet Gynecol* 1991;164:1064–1071.

Young RF, Scully RE. Sex cord-stromal and steroid-cell tumors. In: Rubin SC, Sutton GP, eds. *Ovarian cancer.* New York: McGraw-Hill, 1993: 153–172.

Kelley's Textbook of Internal Medicine, fourth edition. Edited by H. David Humes. Lippincott Williams & Wilkins, Philadelphia © 2000.

C H A P T E R

209

APPROACH TO THE PATIENT WITH AN ABNORMAL PAPANICOLAOU SMEAR

ANDREW W. MENZIN
STEPHEN C. RUBIN

In the 1940s, Dr. George Papanicolaou introduced techniques for interpreting cytologic specimens from the vagina and cervix to detect cervical cancer and its precursors. More than 50 years later the Papanicolaou (Pap) smear is the prime example of cancer prevention through community-based screening programs. Epidemiologic data from British Columbia reveal a threefold decrease in the incidence of cervical cancer during the three decades after institution of widespread use of Pap smears. In the United States, an 80% decrease in the incidence of cervical cancer and a fall in the death rate occurred during the same period. Although cervical cancer ranks as the second most common cancer among women worldwide, it is only seventh most common in countries with established screening programs. Almost 50 million Pap smears are performed each year in the United States. As a screening test, the Pap smear is performed on women who do not have symptoms. Through a joint effort of the American College of Obstetricians and Gynecologists (ACOG), the American Cancer Society, and several other organizations, recommendations have been outlined to guide primary care physicians in screening for cervical cancer (Table 209.1).

PATHOPHYSIOLOGY

The normal cervix is covered with nonkeratinized squamous epithelium. The cervical canal is lined with mucinous columnar cells. The transition between these epithelial types is the squamocolumnar junction. The region in which the columnar epithelium is gradually covered and replaced by squamous epithelium is called the *transformation zone*. Metaplastic change is a normal

TABLE 209.1.	GUIDELINES FOR CERVICAL CANCER SCREENING

Annual pelvic examination and Pap smear for
  All women who have been sexually active
  All women who have reached the age of 18 years
After three consecutive normal and satisfactory[a] Pap smears performed on a yearly basis, the interval between Pap smears may be extended (e.g., from 1 to 3 years) at the discretion of the physician and on the basis of the patient's risk factors.

[a] See Table 209.2.

finding in this area, but most cases of cervical neoplasia also are found in the transformation zone.

Intraepithelial neoplasia precedes cervical cancer. The mean age of a patient at diagnosis of cervical cancer is 54 years. Carcinoma in situ is generally detected in women in their early forties. Dysplastic lesions usually occur among women in their twenties and thirties. However, a consistent trend toward earlier development of preinvasive and invasive lesions has been observed.

Preinvasive and invasive forms of cervical neoplasia are associated with sexual contact. Women who abstain from intercourse are thought not to be at risk. Specific associations include young age at first intercourse, a large number of partners, and relations with partners who have been promiscuous. Changing sexual practices may be responsible in part for the increasing incidence of preinvasive cervical neoplasia.

Investigators are searching for a transmittable agent that is passed during intercourse. Most of the known sexually transmitted diseases have at one time been implicated, included gonorrhea, syphilis, chlamydia, and trichomonas vaginalis. Considerable work has targeted the role of herpes simplex virus 2 (HSV-2). Women with preinvasive and invasive disease are more likely to have HSV-2 serum antibody titers. Though HSV-2 DNA and antigens have been detected in cervical neoplastic specimens, the prevalence rates have been low. Doubt exists about the role of HSV-2 as the primary causative agent in cervical neoplasia.

More extensive and convincing information implicates the human papillomavirus (HPV), the most common sexually transmitted infection. HPV DNA can be demonstrated in more than 90% of intraepithelial and invasive lesions. Considerable molecular evidence is emerging to support the notion that HPV actively participates in the oncogenic cascade of cervical epithelium. Epidemiologic data also support this association.

Other factors may play a role. Immunosuppressed patients, such as those taking steroids or those with AIDS, are at increased risk for preinvasive and invasive cervical neoplasia. Cigarette smoking increases a woman's risk; nicotine metabolites have been detected in the cervical mucous. Use of oral contraceptive also may play a role, as may deficiencies in vitamins A and C.

HISTORY AND PHYSICAL EXAMINATION

The Pap smear is only one component of cancer screening and prevention. Before a cytologic sample is obtained, a detailed history should be obtained and a physical examination performed. During the pelvic examination, careful, systematic inspection and palpation with accurate documentation allow proper assessment and interpretation of subsequent tests, including cytologic sampling.

The reliability of any screening test is related to the ability to obtain proper samples for analysis. Much effort has been directed at development of the optimal technique to obtain a Pap smear. Samples should not be obtained during the menses. Specimens are obtained before a manual examination is performed. Using a wooden spatula and a moistened endocervical cotton swab or brush, the examiner samples the portio and canal of the cervix to include cells from the transformation zone. The

use of an endocervical brush has improved the sampling of endocervical cells, reducing the rate of unsatisfactory smears. The endocervical brush is safe for use during pregnancy.

Cytologic specimens must be transferred to a glass slide, and fixative is applied immediately to avoid air-drying artifacts, which can occur even in a matter of seconds. This effect of delayed fixation can severely limit accuracy and confound diagnosis. Endocervical and ectocervical sample material may be placed on a single slide without altering cytologic interpretation. Techniques with a liquid dispersion medium into which the cytologic sample is placed are becoming widely available. This process removes some of the background artifact before the final smear is produced. Although the background can obscure the underlying cytologic processes, it also can aid in interpretation of these processes. Though available, the technique has not been embraced by all cytopathologists or clinicians.

Despite an overall sensitivity of more than 90% with these sampling techniques, the false-negative rate remains in the range of 20%. In an effort to decrease false-negative rates, re-screening programs have gained acceptance. Whether performed manually or with computer assistance (Papnet), re-screening efforts supplement the quality-control criteria applied to Pap smear evaluation.

LABORATORY STUDIES AND DIAGNOSTIC TESTS

The criteria for describing cytologic findings have evolved considerably since Papanicolaou proposed a five-category system. However, a lack of reproducibility has hampered most classification schemes, and this ambiguity has led to inconsistent diagnoses and difficulty in management. In an effort to improve Pap smear reporting, the National Cancer Institute (NCI) sponsored a workshop to refine Pap smear classification into more consistent, reproducible guidelines, which became known as the Bethesda system. Changes included the use of diagnostic categories, descriptive diagnoses, and a statement regarding the adequacy of the sample (Table 209.2).

Diagnoses are divided into benign cellular changes and epithelial cell abnormalities. The former category includes cytologic evidence of infection, as with *Candida* organisms, herpesvirus, or *Trichomonas vaginalis*, or reactive change from atrophy, irradiation, or inflammation. The latter category includes squamous and glandular changes. They are characterized on the basis of nuclear hyperchromasia and enlargement. Perinuclear clearing and smudging of chromatin are typical of koilocytes, which are cells infected with HPV. Squamous abnormalities (Fig. 209.1) are further categorized as low grade, including HPV-associated lesions and mild dysplasia; high grade, which represents moderate and severe dysplasia; or carcinoma in situ. Glandular cell abnormalities may include endocervical, endometrial, or extrauterine lesions. The finding of benign or atypical endometrial cells on a Pap smear from a postmenopausal woman warrants further investigation. Squamous and glandular cell changes may include atypical cells of undetermined importance that are abnormal but do not provide enough information to confirm the diagnosis of dysplasia.

TABLE 209.2.	THE BETHESDA SYSTEM, REVISED 1991

Adequacy of Specimen

Satisfactory for evaluation
Satisfactory for evaluation but limited by [specify reason]
Unsatisfactory for evaluation [specify reason]

General Categorization (Optional)

Within normal limits
Benign cellular changes: See descriptive diagnoses
Epithelial cell abnormalities: See descriptive diagnoses

Descriptive Diagnoses

Benign cellular changes
  Infection
    Trichomonas vaginalis
    Fungal organisms morphologically consistent with Candida species
    Predominance of coccobacilli consistent with shift in vaginal flora
    Bacteria morphologically consistent with Actinomyces species
    Cellular changes associated with herpes simplex virus
    Other[a]
Reactive changes, cellular changes associated with
  Inflammation (includes typical repair)
  Atrophy with inflammation ("atrophic vaginitis")
  Radiation therapy
  Presence of intrauterine contraceptive device
  Other
Epithelial cell abnormalities
  Squamous cell
    Atypical squamous cells of undetermined significance: qualify[b]
    Low-grade squamous intraepithelial lesion (LG-SIL) encompassing HPV[b]; mild dysplasia/CIN 1
    High-grade squamous intraepithelial lesion (HG-SIL) encompassing moderate and severe dysplasia (CIN 2 and CIN 3/CIS)
    Squamous cell carcinoma
  Glandular cell
    Endometrial cells, cytologically benign, in a postmenopausal woman
    Atypical glandular cells of undetermined significance: qualify[b]
    Endocervical adenocarcinoma
    Endometrial adenocarcinoma
    Extrauterine adenocarcinoma
    Adenocarcinoma, NOS
  Other malignant neoplasms: specify
  Hormonal evaluation (applies to vaginal smears only)
    Hormonal pattern compatible with age and history
    Hormonal pattern incompatible with age and history: specify
    Hormonal evaluation not possible due to: specify

---

[a] Cellular changes of HPV previously termed koilocytosis, koilocytic atypia, or condylomatous atypia are included in this category of low-grade squamous intraepithelial lesion.
[b] Atypical squamous or glandular cell of undetermined significance should be further qualified, if possible, as to whether a reactive or a premalignant or malignant process is favored.
CIN, cervical intraepithelial neoplasia; CIS, carcinoma in situ; HPV, human papillomavirus; NOS, non–organ specific.

The Bethesda system is an attempt to better correlate cytologic and histologic findings. It provides a basis for more consistent management (Table 209.2). Not all clinicians, however, favor the Bethesda system, particularly because of the inclusion of HPV changes with mild intraepithelial neoplasia and inclusion of moderate dysplasia as high grade. Some cytopathologists have continued to use the three-part classification of mild, moderate, and severe dysplasia, which correlates with the frequently used terms, *cervical intraepithelial neoplasia (CIN) 1, 2,* and *3.* Anderson reviewed data from Canada that refute concerns about the reproducibility of this classification and its accuracy when it is used for large-scale screening.

STRATEGIES FOR OPTIMAL CARE

MANAGEMENT

When a normal Pap smear result is obtained, a woman should continue to follow the recommended schedule for preventive health care and cancer screening (Table 209.1). Cytologic abnormalities are managed according to the type of finding. Infections require appropriate therapy and follow-up care. Certain types of reactive changes may be managed expectantly, such as that following radiation therapy or use of an intrauterine device. Others, including atrophic changes associated with hormonal deficiency, may be reversed with appropriate intervention.

Because a Pap smear serves as a screening test, the management of epithelial cell abnormalities next focuses on diagnosis. ACOG recommendations for the evaluation of an abnormal Pap smear include inspection of the lower genital tract and colposcopy. In this technique, introduced in 1925, almost 20 years before the development of the Pap smear, a microscope is used to detect and sample lesions not readily visible without magnification. If a lesion is identified at gross inspection, biopsy should precede colposcopy.

After application of a dilute solution of acetic acid, a colposcope is used to examine the cervix. The squamocolumnar junction and transformation zone are identified. Attention is directed at abnormal areas, such as white epithelium (acetowhite) and vascular changes (punctation, mosaicism, abnormal vascular patterns). Biopsy with colposcopic guidance should be performed on these areas. Sampling usually includes endocervical curettage, particularly if a glandular cell abnormality is detected on the Pap smear. Although some physicians advocate biopsy of only the most severe abnormalities, liberal sampling is encouraged, especially for less experienced colposcopists.

Higgins et al. investigated the accuracy of different methods to evaluate abnormal Pap smears. They found that visual colposcopic impression was not a reliable determinant of histologic abnormality. However, colposcopically directed cervical biopsies have a reported accuracy of about 90%. The multimodality approach, incorporating information from cytologic and histologic sampling with an overall visual impression provides the most complete information for planning the appropriate care of these patients.

Evaluation of an abnormal Pap smear for a pregnant patient

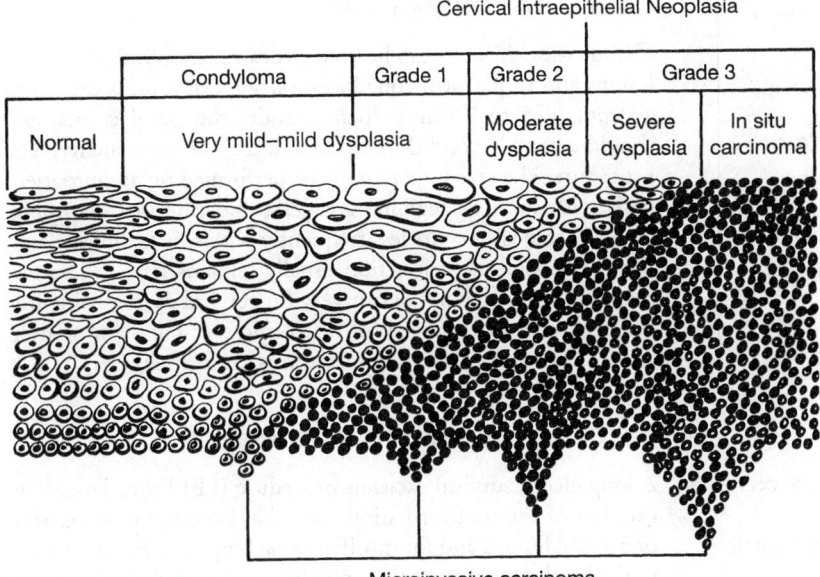

FIGURE 209.1. Schematic representation of cervical premalignant lesions shows the level of infiltration with dysplastic cells for each grade of dysplasia. The notion that microinvasive cancer may follow each grade of dysplasia also is depicted. (Adapted from Kurman RJ, ed. *Blaustein's pathology of the female genital tract,* 4th ed. New York: Springer-Verlag, 1994:229–277.)

deserves special consideration. Pregnancy may cause hyperplastic changes that may appear atypical. Biopsy and curettage usually are deferred unless the colposcopic impression raises concern for carcinoma, though such sampling may be performed safely during pregnancy. Less severe abnormalities may be closely observed during gestation and more complete histologic assessment conducted in the postpartum period. However, if the presence of an invasive lesion is suspected, appropriate sampling (including conization if needed) is mandatory to avoid hazardous delays in treatment.

Appropriate follow-up care of a patient whose Pap smear reveals atypical squamous cells of undetermined significance (ASCUS) is unclear. Several guidelines were suggested by Kurman et al. at the 1992 NCI workshop. If the cytopathologist favors a reactive or inflammatory process, a repeat smear in 4 to 6 months may be advised. If neoplasia is suspected, a management plan similar to that for a clearly defined epithelial cell abnormality is more appropriate. Some clinicians advocate HPV typing to identify the so-called high-risk types. The NCI is sponsoring a trial to examine the effectiveness of a triage system based on HPV typing among women with ASCUS and low-grade smears. An NCI-sponsored clinical trial also is underway to examine use of molecular markers to identify neoplastic lesions among women whose Pap smears contain atypical glandular cells of undetermined significance. The results of these studies may improve the cost-effectiveness of Pap smear evaluation algorithms.

Management after review of all diagnostic results is outlined in (Fig. 209.2). If findings at cytologic, colposcopic, and histologic assessment agree, a treatment plan is developed. If the diagnostic information is not in agreement, particularly if histologic confirmation of a high-grade abnormality is not obtained, further diagnostic evaluation with cervical cone biopsy is appropriate. Other indications for conization are given in Table 209.3. Usually performed in an outpatient surgical setting, conization may require regional or general anesthesia. Complications in-

clude bleeding (10% or less of patients), which may occur perioperatively or after 10 to 14 days, when the cervical eschar is shed; cervical stenosis, caused by scarring of the external cervical os; and subsequent pregnancy loss related to an incompetent cervix caused by excision of large volumes of tissue. Conization

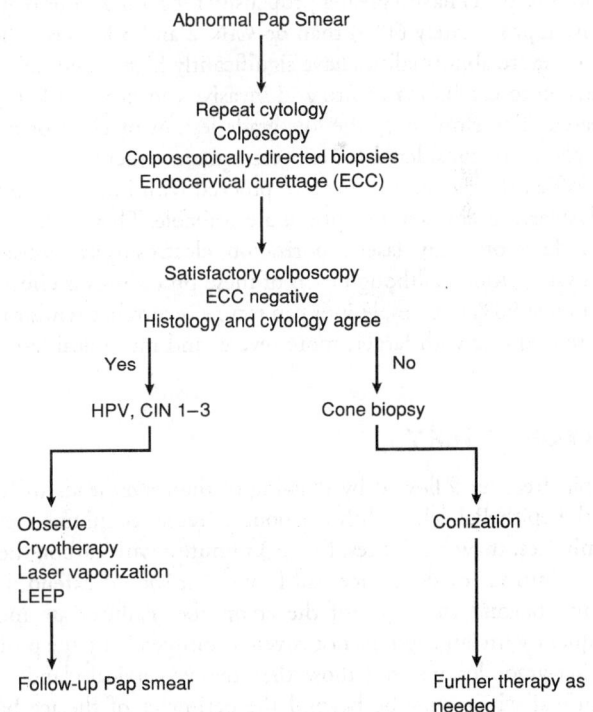

FIGURE 209.2. Algorithm for evaluation of an abnormal Pap smear. *LEEP,* Loop electrosurgical excision procedure. (Modified from Giuntoli RL, Atkinson BF, Ernst CS, et al. *Atkinson's correlative atlas of colposcopy, cytology, and histopathology.* Philadelphia: JB Lippincott, 1987:233.) **EVIDENCE LEVEL: B. Reference: Cervical cytology: evaluation and management of abnormalities.** *ACOG Technical Bulletin* **1993;183:1–8.**

TABLE 209.3.	INDICATIONS FOR CONE BIOPSY

Unsatisfactory colposcopy (failure to completely visualize the squamocolumnar junction or a cervical abnormality)
Identification and evaluation of early invasive carcinoma (micro-invasion)
Excision of a lesion that extends into the endocervical canal
Cellular abnormality found on specimen from endocervical curettage
Glandular neoplasia identified at cytologyic or histologic sampling
Disparity between cytologic, colposcopic, and histologic (biopsy) results

remains the standard of care for the histologic diagnosis of cervical neoplasia.

The management of subclinical HPV infection (abnormalities detected only at cytologic or histologic examination) emphasizes the reality that eradication of the virus is not possible. Ablative or excisional intervention is reserved for more severe abnormalities. The patient should be informed that the abnormality may persist or regress intermittently. Follow-up examinations at 6- to 12-month intervals are recommended because of the association between the presence of HPV and cervical neoplasia.

In longitudinal studies of the natural history of CIN, mild lesions (CIN 1) have a greater propensity for spontaneous regression (approximately 60%) than do CIN 2 and 3 lesions. These more severe abnormalities have significantly higher rates of progression to carcinoma in situ and invasive cancer when left untreated. Therefore, only the low-grade lesions of HPV or mild dysplasia are considered for expectant management.

When the decision is made to proceed with intervention for a dysplastic lesion, several options are available. These modalities include cryotherapy, laser vaporization, electrosurgical excision, or hysterectomy. Although each of these procedures is effective in almost 90% of cases, lesions can recur. Recurrence tends to be more frequent with larger, more severe, and multifocal lesions.

CRYOSURGERY

Rapid freezing followed by thawing of the cervix leads to lysis of the epithelial cells. With the double-freeze technique (freeze 3 minutes, thaw 5 minutes, freeze 3 minutes) with carbon dioxide or nitrous oxide, an ice ball forms that should extend 4 to 5 mm beyond the edges of the cryoprobe. Failures are more frequent with large lesions not covered completely by the probe, higher-grade lesions, and those that involve cervical glands the depth of which may be beyond the perimeter of the ice ball. This technique is not appropriate for lesions that extend into the endocervical canal. Cramping is common during the procedure. A watery discharge usually occurs for several weeks after therapy. Cervical stenosis may occur in as many as 5% of cases as the cervix heals, and the squamocolumnar junction frequently assumes an endocervical location.

LASER VAPORIZATION

Carbon dioxide lasers can be used to destroy dysplastic and HPV lesions and to perform cone biopsies. Vaporization is carried to a depth of 5 to 7 mm, which includes the gland crypts, and should extend beyond the colposcopic area of abnormality. The procedure, like cryosurgery, may be performed on an outpatient basis with local or regional analgesia and minimal cramping. Cervical stenosis occurs less frequently with this technique, and the squamocolumnar junction usually remains visible. The primary disadvantages of laser surgery for cervical dysplasia include the high cost and the lack of histologic specimens for analysis and confirmation (unless conization is performed).

ELECTROSURGICAL EXCISION

A loop electrosurgical excision procedure (LEEP), or large-loop excision of the transformation zone, has been used for excision of cervical lesions and for in-office cone biopsy. With the patient under local anesthesia, a thin wire loop connected to a generator is passed through cervical tissue to remove the entire transformation zone. A blend of cutting and coagulation current minimizes the bleeding complications, which occur in 1% to 2% of procedures. For additional hemostasis, the base of the site is cauterized. This procedure may destroy residual dysplastic cells that remain after excision and reduce recurrence. LEEP has become widely practiced. Because deeper endocervical tissue can be removed, this technique may replace operative conization in certain cases. The success of LEEP is directly related to the cost-effectiveness of the equipment compared with that of laser technology, to the availability of a histologic specimen produced with minimal cauterization artifact, and to ease of use and safety. Cervical stenosis is unusual (less than 1% of cases), and healing typically is associated with easy identification of the squamocolumnar junction.

HYSTERECTOMY

When childbearing has been completed, women with high-grade dysplasia may choose hysterectomy. The procedure also can be used to treat patients with recurrent disease or those with lesions not otherwise amenable to less invasive procedures. Even after "definitive" treatment with hysterectomy, surveillance for lower genital tract dysplasia is important because of the field effect of intraepithelial and invasive neoplasia.

COST-EFFECTIVENESS

Economic issues are increasingly affecting patterns of care. The guidelines for management after abnormal findings are obtained at cytologic examination of the cervix are no exception. The appropriate interval between Pap smears is at the forefront of this debate. Data from Europe suggest that although screening decreases the incidence of cervical cancer, the benefit improves little as the interval between smears is shortened from 3 years to 2 years to 1 year (90.8%, 92.5%, 93.5%, respectively). This information comes from a population whose demographics differ from those in the United States, and it is predicated on complete compliance throughout the study population. Current guidelines from the ACOG remain those in Table 209.1.

The algorithm in Fig. 209.2 is under review on economic grounds. In an effort to reduce the expenditure on colposcopy and cervical biopsies, consideration is being given to evaluation with repeat cytologic smears only for low-grade lesions. A study by Flannelly et al. cautioned against this plan. They reported a high prevalence of severe dysplasia among women whose initial Pap smear revealed only mild or moderate dysplasia.

"See and treat" is a proposed management plan for patients with an abnormal Pap smear. In one visit, colposcopy and LEEP are performed if dysplasia is confirmed by the colposcopic impression. The advantages of a reduced number of visits, fewer treatment failures due to lack of compliance, and elimination of the expense and delay from colposcopic biopsy are championed. Concerns about inappropriate use, excessive treatment of many women because of the stated inaccuracy of colposcopic impressions, and the potential long-term sequelae of more excisional procedures make this treatment option still investigational.

The cornerstone of optimal care with regard to cervical cancer screening is communication and education. Patients need to be informed about the indications for screening and subsequent treatment options. When abnormalities exist on a Pap smear, communication between the clinician and the cytopathologist may clarify ambiguities.

BIBLIOGRAPHY

American College of Obstetricians and Gynecologists. Cervical cytology: evaluation and management of abnormalities. Technical bulletin no. 183. Washington, D.C.: American College of Obstetricians and Gynecologists, 1993:1–10.

Anderson G. Bethesda system of reporting: a Canadian viewpoint. *Diagn Cytopathol* 1991;7:559–561.

Flannelly G, Anderson D, Kitchener HC, et al. Management of women with mild and moderate cervical dyskaryosis. *BMJ* 1994;308:1399–1403.

Giuntoli RL, Atkinson BF, Ernst CS, et al. *Atkinson's correlative atlas of colposcopy, cytology, and histopathology.* Philadelphia: JB Lippincott, 1987.

Herbst A. Intraepithelial neoplasia of the cervix. In: Herbst AL, Mishell DR Jr, Stenchever MA, et al., eds. *Comprehensive gynecology,* 2nd ed. St. Louis: Mosby, 1992:821–859.

Higgins RV, Hall JB, McGee JA, et al. Appraisal of the modalities used to evaluate an initial abnormal Papanicolaou smear. *Obstet Gynecol* 1994; 84:174–178.

International Agency for Research on Cancer, Working Group on Evaluation of Cervical Cancer Screening Programmes. Screening for squamous cervical cancer: duration of low risk after negative results of cervical cytology and its implication for screening policies. *Br Med J* 1986;293: 659–664.

Kurman RJ, Henson DE, Herbst AL, et al. 1992 National Cancer Institute workshop: interim guidelines for management of abnormal cervical cytology. *JAMA* 1994;271:1866–1869.

Melnikow J, Nuovo J, Willan, et al. Natural history of cervical squamous intraepithelial lesions: a meta-analysis. *Obstet Gynecol* 1998;92: 727–735.

Wright TC, Kurman RJ, Ferenczy A. Precancerous lesions of the cervix. In: Kurman RJ, ed. *Blaustein's pathology of the female genital tract,* 4th ed. New York: Springer-Verlag, 1994:229–277.

Kelley's Textbook of Internal Medicine, fourth edition. Edited by H. David Humes. Lippincott Williams & Wilkins, Philadelphia © 2000.

APPROACH TO THE PATIENT WITH A PATHOLOGIC FRACTURE

JANICE P. DUTCHER

PRESENTATION

Patients with cancer metastatic to bone may have disability from pain and loss of function caused by pathologic fractures or impending fractures through lytic lesions. The initial presentation usually is pain but may be the classic presentation of a fracture; the exact clinical manifestations depend on the site. Development of increasing bone pain in a patient with known cancer of a type that frequently produces lytic metastases in bone, such as breast cancer, renal cell cancer, lung cancer, or multiple myeloma, should suggest fracture. In contrast, although they have bone pain, patients with prostate cancer usually have blastic lesions in bone that are much less likely to fracture.

PATHOPHYSIOLOGY

Metastatic bone disease occurs most frequently in the axial skeleton and lower extremities, affects weight-bearing structures, and often limits activity. The bones most often affected by metastatic cancer include the vertebrae, pelvis, femur (especially the hip), and skull. The upper extremity is much less commonly involved (10% to 15% of cases). Despite the frequency of bony involvement by metastatic cancer, pathologic fractures requiring surgical intervention occur among only approximately 10% of patients with metastatic bone disease. However, such fractures are much more likely to occur in the weight-bearing bones.

The strength of a bone depends on the continuity of the cortex and on the underlying medullary structure. A lytic metastatic lesion of a long bone usually destroys the cortex and the underlying bone. Evaluations of the biomechanical strength of bone have shown that a defect the length of which is less than the diameter of the bone decreases strength 70%, but a defect larger than the diameter of the bone (most common) produces a 90% reduction in strength. Predictions of the types of lesions in long bones that will fracture are based on clinical factors such as anatomic site, pain pattern, type of lesion, and size of lesion (Table 210.1) and show an 81% risk for fracture in lesions larger than two-thirds of the diameter of the bone and greater risk in lower extremities than in upper extremities.

HISTORY AND PHYSICAL EXAMINATION

The initial history is that of the events surrounding the fracture. Often there is no trauma, but the stress of normal activity leads

TABLE 210.1.	SCORING SYSTEM FOR PATHOLOGIC FRACTURES		
	Score		
Variable	1	2	3
Site	Upper limb	Lower limb	Peritrochanter
Pain	Mild	Moderate	Functional
Lesion	Blastic	Mixed	Lytic
Size[a]	<⅓	⅓–⅔	>⅔

[a] In relation to the diameter of the bone.
Source: Mirels H. Metastatic disease in the long bones. A proposed scoring system. *Clin Orthop* 1989;249:256–264.

to fracture through the weakened bone. A history of known malignant disease in such a patient, particularly one of the four types previously listed, should prompt a potential diagnosis of fracture, not just pain from bony involvement by tumor. Physical examination may reveal the classic findings of a hip fracture, obvious dislocation of a shoulder, or minimal alteration in structure, as in a patient with collapse of the thoracic vertebrae.

LABORATORY STUDIES AND DIAGNOSTIC TESTS

Radiographs are the most useful studies for evaluating fractures. Computed tomography (CT) or magnetic resonance imaging (MR) sometimes help to differentiate progressive bone involvement from fracture. However, patients with a high likelihood of having cancer metastatic to bone should be examined periodically before symptoms occur to identify areas of involvement. These areas usually can be found with a bone scan followed by radiography of areas of increased isotope uptake. CT or MRI can be used to delineate the degree of bone destruction, particularly in the pelvis. In the case of myeloma, a bone survey is much more helpful than a bone scan, because the lack of osteoblastic reaction in this disease produces no areas of isotope uptake on a bone scan, but the usual lytic disease and osteoporosis are obvious on radiographs. Radiographs of patients with prostate cancer frequently demonstrate blastic rather than lytic lesions, and these are much less likely to cause fractures. Cancer antigen CA 27.29 is a tumor marker used in following metastatic bone disease from breast cancer; measurement of this marker can be useful in assessing response to therapy for bone disease.

DIFFERENTIAL DIAGNOSIS

If the chief symptom is sudden onset of bone pain with loss of function and clinical findings of fracture–dislocation, the diagnosis is based on examination and radiographic results. If the patient is known to have malignant disease, the fracture is almost certainly pathologic. If the patient has no known malignant disease, but the radiograph shows a lytic lesion and a fracture, biopsy or other evaluation is necessary to provide a tissue diagno-

sis. For a patient with less obvious physical findings but increasing bone pain, as in the back or pelvis, CT or MRI may be necessary to differentiate progressive bone disease or spinal cord compression from a fracture.

STRATEGIES FOR OPTIMAL CARE

MANAGEMENT

The role of surgical intervention in metastatic bone disease has increased because of improved orthopedic techniques and systemic treatment approaches to many of these tumors. Patients are living longer, and function must be maintained. The tumors that most commonly involve bone are also those that are most likely to heal after intervention with a combined-modality approach.

Newer materials such as polymethyl methacrylate (PMMA) function as bone cement and can be used to replace and stabilize large segments of abnormal bone. Because abnormal bone does not heal through a pathologic fracture, replacement with PMMA and external or internal fixation with metal hardware provides stabilization and time for healing. In many cases, irradiation may enhance bone healing in areas of normal bone surrounding the previous lesion. The technique curettage of tumor, defect filling with PMMA, and fixation is called *composite osteosynthesis,* and it is used to manage fractures of the long bones. The metal component is a bone plate placed parallel to the bone and attached to normal bone with screws or an intramedullary rod that provides fixation of the healing cavity. These procedures are most commonly used to repair damaged long bones (Fig. 210.1).

With newer techniques and materials, it is possible to replace extensive bone involved with metastatic disease in the hip area, including hemijoint replacement, and provide enough support to allow walking. Depending on the site of tumor in the trochanteric region, other prosthetic devices may be used with PMMA. Lesions in the pelvis are managed with local irradiation and sometimes with embolization without surgery. These types of restorative approaches are particularly important because they allow rapid return of function without the disability of prolonged bed rest.

Vertebrectomy through anterior or posterior approaches to manage metastatic cancer in isolated vertebrae is becoming common; PMMA is used for replacement and rods for stabilization. Careful preoperative assessment makes this operation an alternative method to preserve function. Embolization of vertebral tumors followed by radiation therapy or surgery also has been effective in the short term. All such interventions eventually depend on the effectiveness of systemic treatment.

In breast cancer, treatment with systemic therapy (hormones or chemotherapy) frequently is beneficial for generalized bone disease. Irradiation usually is effective in treating patients with localized, painful lesions. Surgical management is indicated for pending or actual fractures, particularly in weight-bearing bones. For patients with breast cancer with bone-only disease, aggressive management of skeletal metastases is indicated to maintain func-

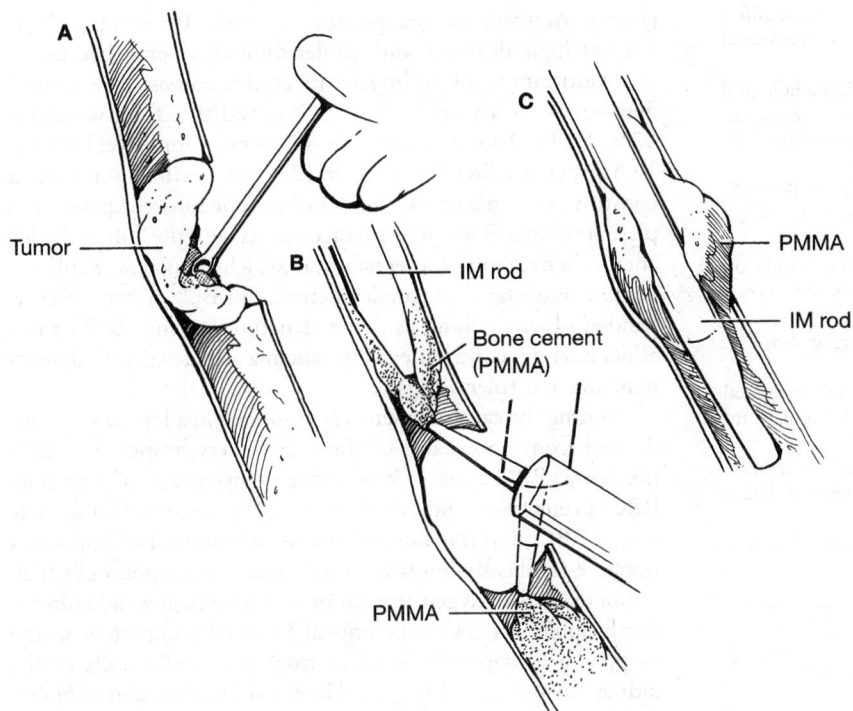

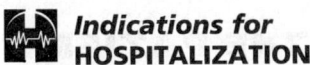

FIGURE 210.1. Diaphyseal reconstruction for metastatic cancer. Long bones (femur and humerus) with metastatic tumors of the shafts (diaphysis) are reconstructed by means of intramedullary (IM) rod fixation combined with application of polymethyl methacrylate (PMMA). **A:** Curettage of tumor. **B:** Placement of PMMA proximal and distal to the site of the tumor or fracture or both in addition to filling the tumor defect. **C:** Stable fixation depends on this combined fixation. Small diaphyseal tumors can be managed prophylactically with fluoroscopic control without opening of the fracture site.

tion to the greatest degree possible over the course of several years. Bisphosphonates have been found to be effective in preventing new bone problems and in reducing the development of new lesions. This has been shown in breast cancer and myeloma, both diseases with generalized bony involvement. Prolonged treatment is indicated. The results for other bone-tropic tumors are not known.

Patients with renal cell cancer also are likely to have bony metastases, particularly in the pelvis and vertebrae. Surgical intervention is somewhat more difficult because of the location and because of the vascular nature of the tumor. In large pelvic tumors, vascular embolization sometimes is indicated to reduce blood flow, shrink the tumor, and obtain pain relief. Irradiation of this tumor is effective in about 50% of cases, and effective treatment promotes bone healing. The goals of managing bone disease are to maintain function as long as possible and to reduce pain. Surgical stabilization of lesions in weight-bearing bones usually is indicated to allow walking.

In lung cancer, skeletal metastases rarely lead to pathologic fractures, in part because bone lesions are fewer and usually are managed successfully with radiation therapy. Because of the blastic nature of the bone metastases in prostate cancer, fractures also are rare.

COMPLICATIONS AND PITFALLS

The most important complication of pathologic fractures among patients with metastatic cancer is permanent loss of function. Fractures can lead to medical problems that progressively impair function and disable the patient. Attempts to improve function with surgical intervention are not always successful, but risks and benefits must be assessed on a case by case basis, determined

by each patient's clinical and functional status and the potential to relieve pain and suffering and maintain function.

Indications for HOSPITALIZATION

A patient with a new fracture of the lower extremity needs hospitalization to assess the extent of injury and to provide initial pain relief. If the decision is to pursue a surgical approach, an experienced orthopedic surgeon or neurosurgeon should be consulted.

COST-EFFECTIVENESS

As techniques improve and surgical morbidity lessens, the benefit of preventing and managing fractures among patients with otherwise good prognoses outweighs the risk of surgery. Aggressive assessment and maintenance of function become the goals in the management of bone metastases in keeping with the overall status of the patient's underlying disease. Even with limited intervention, there is opportunity to relieve pain and suffering. After appropriate intervention, patients with isolated fractures and an indolent course of disease may continue to function for years with abnormal bone lesions.

BIBLIOGRAPHY

Bauer HC, Wedin R. Survival after surgery for spinal and extremity metastases: prognostication in 241 patients. *Acta Orthop Scand* 1995;66: 143–146.

Borel Rinkes IH, Wiggers T, Bouma WH, et al. Treatment of manifest and impending pathological fractures of the femoral neck by cemented hemiarthroplasty. *Clin Orthop* 1990;260:220–223.

Dijstra S, Wiggers T, van Geel BN, et al. Impending and actual pathological fractures in patients with bone metastases of the long bones: a retrospective study of 233 surgically treated fractures. *Eur J Surg* 1994;160: 535–542.

Healey JH. Metastatic cancer to the bone. In: DeVita VT, Hellman S, Rosenberg SA, eds. *Cancer: principles and practice of oncology*, 5th ed. Philadelphia: JB Lippincott, 1997:2570–2586.

Martoni A, Guaraldi M, Camera P, et al. Controlled clinical study on the use of dichloromethylene diphosphonate in patients with breast carcinoma metastasizing to the skeleton. *Oncology* 1991;48:97–101.

Mirels H. Metastatic disease in long bones: a proposed scoring system. *Clin Orthop* 1989;249:256–264.

O'Reilly GV, Kleefield J, Klein LA, et al. Embolization of solitary spinal metastases from renal cell carcinoma: alternative therapy for spinal cord or nerve root compression. *Surg Neurol* 1989;31:268–271.

Orr FW, Kostenuik P, Sanchez-Sweatman OH, et al. Mechanisms involved in the metastasis of cancer to bone. *Breast Cancer Res Treat* 1993;25: 151–163.

Rock MG, Harrington KD. Pathologic fractures of the pelvis and acetabulum. *Orthopedics* 1992;15:569–576.

Kelley's Textbook of Internal Medicine, fourth edition. Edited by H. David Humes.
Lippincott Williams & Wilkins, Philadelphia © 2000.

C H A P T E R

211

APPROACH TO THE PATIENT WITH ANEMIA

THOMAS P. DUFFY

■ PRESENTATION AND PATHOPHYSIOLOGY

Anemia is a reduction in normal red blood cell (RBC) mass within the body. It is found with measurement of the hematocrit and hemoglobin content of peripheral blood samples. Hematocrit was originally determined by means of centrifugation of a sample of whole blood within a capillary tube; the hematocrit represented the ratio of packed RBC volume to plasma volume within the tube after centrifugation. Alterations in either component affected the ratio, plasma volume changes elevating or depressing a stable red cell volume. Hematocrit now is derived from the calculated product of electronically generated values for RBC number and the average size or mean corpuscular volume (MCV) of the RBCs; the hemoglobin content of the same sample is measured with a chromogenic assay performed with the electronic counter.

Normal values have been established for these hematologic measurements through the study of large populations of healthy controls. The values vary according to atmospheric pressure and gender. Ambient oxygen pressure accounts for elevated RBC mass at high altitudes, and gender differences exist because of the contribution of androgens to erythropoiesis. The normal hematocrit for a man is 47% ± 7%, and that for a woman is 42% ± 5%. A lower hematocrit or a hemoglobin level less than 13.5 g per deciliter for men or 12 g per deciliter for women constitutes anemia unless there is disproportionate expansion in plasma volume. This circumstance occurs with the "physiologic" anemia or hydremia of pregnancy, in which an increase in plasma volume outdistances a parallel increase in RBC volume. Overexpanded plasma volume is the explanation for anemia for some athletes, and it contributes to the anemia associated with dysproteinemia and splenomegaly.

Finding the cause of anemia is grounded in a logical sequence derived from knowledge of the cycle of erythropoiesis within the body. RBC mass is kept constant by means of matching RBC production with destruction of senescent RBCs. The body's RBC mass is maintained within circumscribed limits by a negative-feedback stimulatory mechanism the set point of which responds to the oxygen tension of blood perfusing the kidneys. Erythropoietin (EPO), the critical humoral component in the loop, is a glycoprotein released from peritubular cells of the kidneys in amounts determined by the oxygen tension of blood. A fall in this level, whether caused by hypoxemia or by anemia, results in increased secretion of EPO in an attempt to increase RBC production to compensate for the reduced availability of oxygen. EPO directly stimulates the proliferation and differentiation of erythroid precursors, leading to erythroid hyperplasia of the bone marrow. The presence of the hormone accelerates release of increased numbers of young RBCs, or reticulocytes, from the marrow. The normal cycle of erythropoiesis requires coordination of EPO stimulation with the necessary precursor cells and building blocks in a conducive microenvironment to maintain production. Normal RBC structure and function determine the life span of an RBC. Lesions in any component of this cycle may cause anemia of variable severity.

If shortened RBC survival causes anemia, as occurs with bleeding or hemolysis, an intact EPO feedback mechanism causes increased secretion of EPO. The EPO surge leads to erythroid hyperplasia, amplification of the marrow erythroid pool, and release of increased numbers of reticulocytes from the marrow. Measurement of an elevated reticulocyte count identifies an insult outside the marrow as the source of anemia (Table 211.1). This elevated reticulocyte count indicates that the marrow is attempting to respond to a peripheral lesion that has caused anemia. An inadequate reticulocyte count implicates an abnormality within the marrow or EPO deficiency as the cause of the anemia. Because reticulocyte count allows a division of anemic states into the two broad categories of medullary or extramedullary causes, counting reticulocytes is an essential initial step in the evaluation of any patient with anemia (Fig. 211.1).

For an anemic patient with an elevated reticulocyte count, pursuit of the cause of this hyperregenerative anemia entails an investigation for evidence of hemolysis or bleeding. Because the final common pathway in all types of hemolytic anemia involves alterations in RBC structure, examination of a peripheral blood smear for any morphologic abnormalities is the single most important task in the diagnosis of hyperregenerative anemia. The

TABLE 211.1.	HYPOREGENERATIVE AND HYPERREGENERATIVE ANEMIA	
Characteristics	Lesion in the Marrow	Lesion outside the Marrow
Site of lesion	Stem cell disorders (e.g., aplasia, leukemia, myelodysplastic syndrome); building block disorders (e.g., Fe, B_{12}, folate deficiencies); erythropoietin deficiency	Blood loss; hemolysis; hypersplenism
Reticulocytosis[a]	Absent	Present
Type of anemia[b]	Hyporegenerative	Hyperregenerative

[a] Absolute reticulocyte count is calculated as % reticulocytes $\times$ red blood cell count, given in millions of cells/mm^3. Reticulocytosis is defined as $>100,000$/mm^3.
[b] Anemia is defined as a hematocrit less than 40% for men and less than 37% for women.

focus in determining the cause of a reticulocytopenic or hyporegenerative anemia is the marrow, the presumed site of deficient production of RBCs. Bone marrow examination provides a window onto this aspect of erythropoiesis, although serum measurements of essential factors such as iron, folate, and vitamin B_{12} may provide enough information to prove the existence of the lesion without a painful bone marrow examination. Radioimmunoassay can be used to measure EPO levels to complete the information necessary to address the cause of hyporegenerative anemia. A low EPO level in the presence of anemia indicts this humoral deficiency as a cause of the anemia.

A second broad categorization of anemia is based on the size of RBCs. This value is generated with a Coulter electronic counter as part of the standard blood count. On the basis of RBC size, anemia can be classified as microcytic (MCV less than 80 fL), macrocytic (MCV greater than 95 fL), or normocytic (MCV of 80 to 95 fL) (Table 211.2). The microcytic types of anemia originate in iron or hemoglobin deficiencies; most macrocytic anemia is caused by folate and vitamin B_{12} deficiencies. The normocytic types of anemia have more heterogeneous origins; they include all types of hemolytic anemia and the EPO-deficient states. All types of anemia are initially normocytic, because

the original normocytic RBC population outnumbers the burgeoning abnormal cell population and is only slowly diluted by abnormal cells of a different size.

An additional measurement generated by the electronic counter is RBC distribution width (RDW), a visual display of the range of RBC sizes. This is an important determination for patients with more than one population of RBCs, a circumstance that occurs after transfusion and in mixed-deficiency types of anemia. A combination of folate and iron deficiencies is a not uncommon cause of anemia during pregnancy and in alcoholic states; this mixed deficiency may generate a normal MCV although microcytic and macrocytic RBCs are present. The RDW allows recognition of this dual population of RBCs and the contribution of a mixed lesion to a normocytic anemia.

The electronic counter also measures white blood cell (WBC) and platelet counts as part of a complete blood cell count. Reduction in all three cell lines constitutes the condition called *pancytopenia*. This entity is caused by a defect in a shared precursor cell, such as a deficiency of stem cells in aplastic anemia or a lesion in nucleic acid metabolism in megaloblastic processes. Pancytopenia also may be caused by hypersplenism, a state in which an enlarged spleen prematurely removes cells from the

TABLE 211.2.	CATEGORIZATION OF ANEMIA ACCORDING TO SIZE OF RED BLOOD CELLS	
Microcytic Anemia (MCV $<$ 80 fL)	Normocytic Anemia (MCV $=$ 80 to 95 fL)	Macrocytic Anemia (MCV $>$ 95 fL)
Iron deficiency	Initial stage of all types of anemia	Megaloblastic anemia
Anemia of chronic disease	Erythropoietin deficiency	Vitamin B_{12} or folate deficiency
Thalassemia	Anemia of chronic disease	Myelodysplasia
Sideroblastic anemias	Stem cell disorders	Purine or pyrimidine metabolism abnormalities
	Myelophthisic anemia	Nonmegaloblastic anemia
	Endocrine disorders	Liver disease
	Dysproteinemia	Hypothyroidism
		Reticulocytosis
		Red blood cell agglutinins

MCV, mean corpuscular volume of erythrocytes.

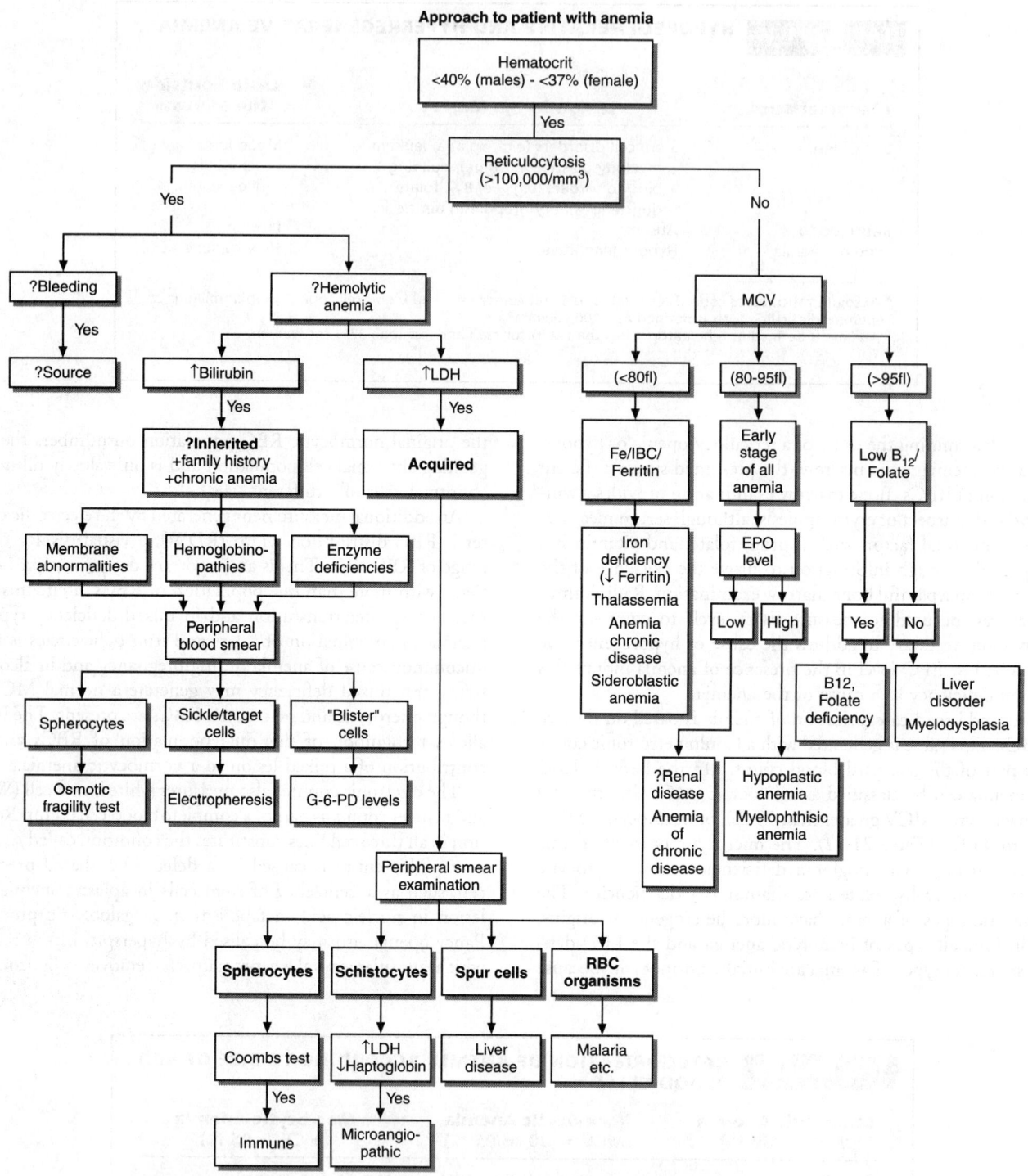

FIGURE 211.1. Algorithm for the approach to the care of a patient with anemia.
EVIDENCE LEVEL: C. Expert Opinion.

peripheral blood. Recognition of anemia as a component of a more generalized process of pancytopenia necessitates recasting of the differential diagnosis to explain the trilineage reduction; a lesion in the stem cell usually is found in this situation.

The initial approach to the problem of anemia requires information derived from the electronic counter–generated complete blood cell count (hematocrit, hemoglobin level, MCV, WBC count, platelet count, RDW), reticulocyte count, and examination of a peripheral blood smear (Fig. 211.1). The reticulocyte count allows assignment of the anemia to a hyporegenerative or hyperregenerative process, that is, whether the cause is within or outside the marrow. The MCV of the RBCs is a second determinant that allows characterization of the anemia as microcytic, macrocytic, or normocytic anemia on the basis of cell size. These measurements dictate the evaluation necessary to identify the specific cause of anemia.

DIFFERENTIAL DIAGNOSIS

MICROCYTIC ANEMIA

All microcytic types of anemia involve a deficiency in hemoglobin synthesis within the developing RBC. Because hemoglobin production requires coordinated synthesis of heme and globin, deficiencies in either of these two components of hemoglobin may produce microcytic RBCs. Absolute lack of iron is the leading cause of deficient hemoglobin synthesis, although abnormalities in iron transport (e.g., anemia of chronic disease) or heme synthesis (e.g., sideroblastic anemia) also may cause a reduction in RBC hemoglobin content and size.

Differentiation of the varied causes of microcytic anemia is possible by means of direct inspection of marrow iron stores or measurement of serum iron indices. Because iron deficiency anemia does not occur until mobilization of marrow iron stores is complete, the absence of iron in a bone marrow specimen is the absolute determinant of iron deficiency anemia. Marrow stores of iron are paralleled by serum levels of ferritin, a storage form of iron that circulates in small amounts in the peripheral blood. Radioimmunoassay can be used to measure ferritin levels, which can substitute for the marrow examination in uncomplicated instances of iron deficiency anemia. Serum levels of iron and its transport protein, transferrin, also mirror the availability of iron for hemoglobin synthesis; a decrease in serum iron level and elevation of transferrin level to that associated with transferrin saturation of less than 15% are evidence that a deficiency of iron is rate limiting for hemoglobin synthesis.

All other causes of microcytic anemia represent deficient hemoglobin synthesis (sideropenic anemia) in the face of adequate to increased amounts of iron stores. In the anemia of chronic disease, the vector of iron delivery is directed away from its specific target of the developing RBC, and iron becomes closeted within reticuloendothelial cells. This reorientation of iron transport is a reaction to the effect of cytokines released in response to the challenge of infection, inflammation, or malignancy within the body. Iron-deficient erythropoiesis in the anemia of chronic disease represents a form of nutritional immunity in which a small amount of hemoglobin synthesis is sacrificed while invading microorganisms and malignant cells are deprived of iron, an essential nutrient for all cellular growth and proliferation. Iron indices in the anemia of chronic disease reveal a low serum iron level and a low transferrin level. Transferrin saturation also may be reduced, although not usually to levels as low as those associated with iron deficiency anemia. Serum ferritin level, a mirror of iron stores, is increased in the anemia of chronic disease and differentiates this form of microcytic anemia from iron deficiency anemia.

Iron accumulation characterizes the sideroblastic types of anemia. Iron accumulates on and around the mitochondria of developing RBCs within the marrow. All sideroblastic types of anemia share this morphologic feature, which requires bone marrow examination for identification. Iron accumulates in this location because sideroblastic types of anemia represent a defect in protoporphyrin ring synthesis, a multistep process that occurs in the mitochondria surrounding the nucleus of the developing RBC; this feature determines the "ringed" designation of this type of anemia, because the mitochondria are distributed in necklace-like manner around the nuclei of the RBCs.

Near-total saturation of transferrin with an elevated serum iron level occurs in sideroblastic types of anemia; elevated ferritin levels are additional evidence of this iron-overload state. Iron stains of the marrow readily show the ringed distribution of iron or siderotic granules around the erythroblast nucleus. The causes of these types of anemia include inherited deficiencies of enzymes essential in protoporphyrin ring synthesis and lesions resulting from toxins, such as alcohol, and drugs, such as chloramphenicol and isoniazid. Sideroblastic anemia is a component of myelodysplastic syndromes, which may presage an ultimate transformation into leukemia.

Another major cause of microcytic anemia, thalassemia, is a more prominent consideration when microcytic anemia occurs among persons of Mediterranean ancestry. Defective globin chain synthesis of various degrees determines the severity of this inherited form of faulty hemoglobin synthesis. Hemoglobin electrophoresis, family documentation of similar anemia, and globin chain synthesis ratios can help ascertain whether a person has this form of microcytic anemia.

The cause of a hypochromic microcytic anemia may be identified with a trial of iron therapy. When modest microcytic or normocytic anemia is found, correction of the anemia after ferrous sulfate administration confirms the role of iron deficiency in producing the anemia. The response of an iron-deficient patient to iron therapy is manifested initially in reticulocytosis that occurs 5 to 7 days after initiation of therapy. Measurement of ferritin before iron therapy provides an essential baseline value for iron stores that can be used to gauge replenishment of these stores.

Identification of iron deficiency as the source of anemia is only the initial step in managing the problem. This type of anemia commonly is caused by a malignant tumor; anemia may be the initial sign that unmasks a lesion, often in the gastrointestinal tract, that is still localized and potentially curable. A physician who discovers iron deficiency incurs the responsibility to investigate and define the source of blood loss that has produced the iron deficiency.

MACROCYTIC ANEMIA

Macrocytic anemia can be categorized according to the presence or absence of megaloblastic hematopoiesis; the latter condition is a morphologic manifestation of nuclear–cytoplasmic asynchrony caused by a disorder in DNA synthesis in hematopoietic elements. Deficiencies in folate or vitamin B_{12} metabolism are the most frequent causes of a megaloblastic state. Measurement of serum vitamin B_{12} and RBC folate provides a means of documenting the contribution of these substances to macrocytic anemia (Fig. 211.1). Drugs such as zidovudine and methotrexate induce megaloblastic anemia by interfering with nucleic acid synthesis.

A megaloblastic lesion is not restricted to cells of the erythroid lineage alone, and involvement of all three cell lines within the marrow leads to varying degrees of pancytopenia in the peripheral blood. Disordered DNA synthesis causes markedly ineffective hematopoiesis; the involved cell lines self-destruct within the marrow. The marked elevation in serum lactate dehydrogenase levels that occurs in megaloblastic states is caused by this intramedullary death of hematopoietic precursor elements. Another characteristic of megaloblastic processes is an alteration in WBC structure. Hypersegmentation of polymorphonuclear cells is the earliest peripheral blood manifestation of a megaloblastic process. Examination of a peripheral blood smear for neutrophils containing more than five lobes is a critical component of the evaluation of macrocytic anemia.

Megaloblastic maturation is not restricted to vitamin deficiencies or to the effects of drugs. Inherited abnormalities in purine and pyrimidine metabolism also may compromise nucleic acid synthesis as a rare cause of megaloblastic anemia. Less pronounced megaloblastic transformation accompanies the myelodysplastic–myeloleukemic disorders in which alterations in nuclear function are attributable to acquired chromosomal or genetic abnormalities.

Megaloblastic types of anemia, especially those caused by folate or vitamin B_{12} deficiency, are associated with the most exaggerated macrocytosis. An MCV of more than 115 fL usually is the result of a vitamin deficiency rather than of myelodysplasia. If a megaloblastic process is believed to be the cause of anemia, therapy with both vitamins should be initiated after measurement of baseline serum vitamin B_{12} and RBC folate levels. Vitamin B_{12} and folate should be administered until the specific deficiency is identified, because the morphologic alterations in hematopoiesis with vitamin B_{12} and folate deficiency are indistinguishable from one another. Vitamin B_{12} deficiency also causes a neurologic disorder characterized by the loss of vibratory and position sensation in the lower extremities, and such neurologic findings help to support the diagnosis of vitamin B_{12} deficiency.

Nonmegaloblastic macrocytic types of anemia may have multiple causes. Liver disease, hypothyroidism, and alcoholism independent of any vitamin deficiency cause macrocytic anemia through poorly understood mechanisms that increase the RBC membrane surface. Because these macrocytic types of anemia do not involve the other hematopoietic elements, pancytopenia is not a feature, as it is in megaloblastic macrocytic states. Hypoplastic and aplastic types of anemia may produce a slight increase in MCV. Another cause of macrocytosis is the elevated reticulocyte count that accompanies hemolytic anemia. The elevation in MCV is explained by the increased size of the reticulocytes. Spurious macrocytosis often exists in the presence of cold agglutinins or cryoglobulins. These cold-reactive plasma proteins cause agglutination of RBCs in the electronic counter, producing a false reading of increased RBC size. Heating the blood sample helps unmask this contribution to macrocytosis.

NORMOCYTIC HYPOREGENERATIVE ANEMIA

Normocytic types of anemia with no compensatory reticulocytosis may be caused by a primary defect within the marrow or represent a secondary process from an absolute or functional deficiency of EPO. Renal disease is commonly complicated by anemia through the latter pathway, as is the anemia of chronic disease, which may be normocytic or microcytic, caused by cytokine-mediated suppression of the EPO pathway. Measurement of EPO may document the contribution of this deficiency to anemia, and a recombinant form of EPO is available to reverse the process.

Mature RBCs represent a final step in the differentiation that has its shared origin with WBCs and platelets in stem cells within the marrow. In aplastic and hypoplastic types of anemia, stem cell deficiencies give rise to a parallel reduction in peripheral counts. Selective elimination of erythroid precursors, as occurs with parvovirus infection of the marrow and immune disorders produces pure RBC aplasia. Infiltrative disorders of the marrow caused by tumor, infection, or fibrosis cause myelophthisic anemia, which has leukoerythroblastic blood features of teardrop-shaped RBCs and nucleated RBCs as well as some immature WBCs revealed on the peripheral blood smear. Malignant hematologic diseases also are complicated by normocytic anemia as the malignant process suppresses the production of normal marrow elements.

NORMOCYTIC HYPERREGENERATIVE ANEMIA

Hemolytic types of anemia are normocytic or slightly macrocytic if marked reticulocytosis is present. The two broad categories of hemolytic anemia are inherited and acquired (Table 211.3). An important clue to the presence of inherited hemolytic anemia is a family history of anemia or a history of chronic anemia. Lesions of the RBC membrane, abnormalities in the enzymatic pathways necessary for energy metabolism within the RBC, and defects in hemoglobin structure and function produce the inherited hemolytic types of anemia. The acquired forms are predominantly immune in origin, whereas RBC trauma is another mechanism of hemolysis (microangiopathic anemia). Infectious organisms may parasitize the RBC, as in malaria, or secrete substances that disrupt the RBC membrane, as in clostridial sepsis. Severe liver and kidney disease may be complicated by hemolytic anemia. Hypersplenism also leads to shortened RBC survival, often with leukopenia and thrombocytopenia.

The shortened RBC survival in hemolytic anemia can be quantified with chromium-labeling techniques that allow calculation of RBC half-life and document the role of the spleen in sequestering RBCs. More indirect evidence of hemolysis is the hyperbilirubinemia that often accompanies the excessive breakdown of RBCs by hemolysis. Hemolysis frequently is expressed in alterations of RBC structure. Examination of a peripheral blood smear still is the most important and productive pursuit in the evaluation of a patient with hemolytic anemia (Fig. 211.1).

Hyperregenerative anemia is not synonymous with hemolysis, because marrow that responds to bleeding or to administration of a missing nutrient displays reticulocytosis. Withdrawal of a toxin such as alcohol may be followed by reticulocytosis. The clinical setting in which reticulocytosis occurs strongly influences the importance of these contributions to anemia.

TABLE 211.3.	**TYPES AND CAUSES OF HEMOLYTIC ANEMIA**
Inherited Forms	**Acquired Forms**

Membrane abnormalities
  Spherocytosis
  Pyropoikilocytosis
  Stomatocytosis
  Elliptocytosis
Hemoglobinopathies
  Abnormal variants (e.g., hemoglobin S, C)
  Defective synthesis (e.g., thalassemia)
Unstable hemoglobins
Red blood cell enzyme deficiencies
  Glucose-6-phosphate dehydrogenase
  Pyruvate kinase
	Membrane abnormalities
	  Paroxysmal nocturnal hemoglobinuria
	  Spur cell anemia (e.g., liver disease)
	Immune hemolytic anemias
	  Autoimmune forms
	  Drug-induced forms
	  Isoimmune forms (transfusion reaction,
	    hemolytic disease of newborn)
	Traumatic (microangiopathic) hemolysis
	  Thrombotic thrombocytopenic purpura
	    syndrome
	  Eclampsia
	  Malignant hypertension
	  Scleroderma renal crisis
	  Mechanical prosthetic valves
	  Disseminated intravascular coagulation
	Infection
	  Malaria
	  Clostridia
	  Bartonellosis
	  Babesiosis
	Miscellaneous
	  Burns
	  Toxins
	  Drugs
	  Wilson's disease
	Hypersplenism

STRATEGIES FOR OPTIMAL CARE

Although laboratory findings define anemia, it is often only by integrating hematologic data with the clinical signs and symptoms and history that the correct diagnosis can be made. The family history, social and travel history, and history of occupational exposures may contain vital information and clues to the cause of anemia. Laboratory data from previous hospitalizations or examinations may help in placing a current episode of anemia into perspective. Anemia frequently is not the primary lesion but is a manifestation of an underlying disorder. Anemia often serves as a "sickness index" of the body that calls attention to the primary disorder and narrows the diagnostic possibilities on the basis of the type of anemia.

BIBLIOGRAPHY

Duffy TP. Hematologic aspects of systemic disease. In: Hardin R, Lux S, Stossel T, eds. *Blood: principles and practice of hematology*. Philadelphia: JB Lippincott, 1995:1925–1944.

Lux S. Introduction to anemia In: Hardin R, Lux S, Stossel T, eds. *Blood: principles and practice of hematology*. Philadelphia: JB Lippincott, 1995: 1383.

Williams W, Morris M, Nelson D. Examination of the blood. In: Beutler E, Lichtman M, Coller B, et al., eds. *Williams' hematology*. New York: McGraw-Hill, 1995:8.

Duffy T. Hematology. In: Braunwald E. *Atlas of internal medicine*. Philadelphia: Current Medicine,1998:10.2–10.16.

Toh BH, van Driel IR, Gleeson PA. Pernicious anemia. *N Engl J Med* 1997;337:1441–1448.

Kelley's Textbook of Internal Medicine, fourth edition. Edited by H. David Humes. Lippincott Williams & Wilkins, Philadelphia © 2000.

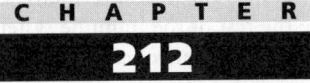

CHAPTER 212

APPROACH TO THE PATIENT WITH LEUKOPENIA

LAURENCE A. BOXER

Leukopenia is defined as a reduction in total white blood cell count to less than 4,000 cells per microliter. *Neutropenia* is an absolute blood neutrophil count (total leukocyte count per microliter multiplied by the percentage of neutrophils and bands) more than two standard deviations below the normal mean. Normal neutrophil levels should be stratified for age and race. For whites, the lower limit for normal neutrophil count is 1,500 cells per microliter, and it may reflect a reduction in neutrophils and lymphocytes. Blacks have somewhat lower neutrophil counts, and the lower limit of normal is approximately 1,200 cells per microliter. These relatively low counts among blacks probably reflect a relative decrease in neutrophils in the storage compartment of the bone marrow.

Individual patients may be characterized as having mild neutropenia with cell counts of 1,000 to 1,500 per microliter, moderate neutropenia with counts of 500 to 1,000 per microliter, or severe neutropenia with counts less than 500 per microliter. This stratification is useful in predicting the risk for infection, because only patients with severe neutropenia have increased susceptibility to life-threatening infections.

Normal lymphocyte count for adults is 1,000 to 4,900 cells per microliter. Approximately 80% of normal adult blood lymphocytes are CD3+ T lymphocytes, and almost two thirds of blood T lymphocytes are CD4+ (helper) T lymphocytes. Most patients with lymphocytopenia have reductions in the absolute number of T lymphocytes and reductions in numbers of CD4+ T lymphocytes in particular. The average absolute number of CD3+ T lymphocytes in normal adult blood is 1,800 per microliter, ranging from 1,000 to 2,300 per microliter. The average absolute number of CD4+CD3+ T lymphocytes is 1,100 per microliter, ranging from 300 to 1,300 per microliter. The average absolute number of cells of the other main T-cell subgroup, CD8+CD3+ T lymphocytes, is 600 per microliter, ranging from 100 to 900 per microliter. Lymphocytopenia is defined as a total lymphocyte count of less than 2,000 per microliter, but among children the lower limit of normal is less than 1,500 per microliter.

PRESENTATION

Persons with neutrophil counts lower than 500 per microliter are at substantially greater risk for infection, largely from their own endogenous flora, but colonization with various nosocomial organisms also occurs. Some patients with isolated chronic neutropenia with an absolute neutrophil count (ANC) of fewer than 200 cells per microliter do not have many serious infections, probably because the rest of the immune system remains intact. In contrast, patients with neutropenia caused by acquired disorders of production, such as patients receiving cytotoxic therapy, immunosuppressive drugs, or irradiation, particularly as management of malignant disease, are more likely to contract serious bacterial infections because the overall immune system is compromised.

Leukopenia associated with neutropenia and accompanied by monocytopenia and lymphocytopenia often is more serious than neutropenia alone. The integrity of the skin and mucous membranes, the vascular supply to tissue, and the nutritional status of the patient also influence risk for infection. The most frequently occurring types of pyogenic infections among patients with profound neutropenia cause a fever higher than 101°F, cutaneous cellulitis, abscesses (including liver), furunculosis, pneumonia, and septicemia. Stomatitis, gingivitis, perirectal inflammation, colitis, sinusitis, and otitis media also may occur.

Isolated neutropenia does not heighten a patient's susceptibility to parasitic, viral, or fungal infections or to bacterial meningitis. The most common pathogens isolated from patients with neutropenia are *Staphylococcus aureus* and gram-negative organisms. The usual signs and symptoms of local infection and inflammation, such as exudate, fluctuation, and regional lymphadenopathy, are generally less evident among patients with than among those without neutropenia because of the inability of a patient with neutropenia to form pus. However, the neutropenic patient can feel pain at a site of infection.

PATHOPHYSIOLOGY

Attempts have been made to classify neutropenia on a pathophysiologic basis, such as disorders of production, maturation, accelerated use, or a combination of these mechanisms. Unfortunately, kinetic methods of characterizing neutropenia are not sufficiently refined to allow unambiguous delineation. The neutropenic disorders are classified herein according to whether there appears to be an intrinsic defect in the myeloid progenitors or whether neutropenia is caused by factors extrinsic to marrow myeloid cells (Table 212.1).

Acute neutropenia often develops when there is rapid neutrophil use and impaired production. Cytotoxic drugs are particularly likely to induce neutropenia because of the high proliferative rate of neutrophil precursors and the rapid turnover of blood neutrophils. Chronic neutropenia usually arises from reduced production or excessive splenic sequestration of neutrophils.

TABLE 212.1.	**CLASSIFICATION OF NEUTROPENIA**

Secondary Neutropenia Caused by Factors Extrinsic to Bone Marrow Myeloid Cells (Common Disorders)

Bone marrow replacement by malignant tumor, fibrosis, granuloma, Gaucher's cells
Neutropenia following irradiation, cytotoxic chemotherapy, or immunosuppression
Neutropenia associated with folate or vitamin B$_{12}$ deficiency
Alcoholism
Infection
Autoimmune neutropenia
Tγ lymphoproliferative disease
Drug-induced neutropenia
Hypersplenism

Neutropenia Arising from Intrinsic Defects in Myeloid Cells or Their Precursors (Rare Disorders)

Cyclic neutropenia
Severe congenital neutropenia (Kostmann's syndrome)
Idiopathic neutropenia including benign neutropenia
Neutropenia associated with dysgammaglobulinemia
Syndrome-associated neutropenia (e.g., Shwachman–Diamond syndrome, cartilage-hair hypoplasia, Chédiak–Higashi syndrome, dyskeratosis congenita, glycogen storage disease type 1b)
Myelodysplasia
Paroxysmal nocturnal hemoglobinuria

HISTORY AND PHYSICAL EXAMINATION

Evaluation begins with a thorough clinical history to establish the onset of neutropenia; the type, frequency, and severity of infections; drug, animal, or toxic exposures; and family history of recurrent infection or unexplained infantile deaths. The examiner also assesses the locations of infections and complications of these infections, the means by which infections were documented, the presence or absence of a symptom-free interval, including febrile episodes, the microbiologic report on any isolates, and the response to antibiotic therapy.

The physical examination may provide clues to the basis of the underlying condition that predisposes the patient to recurrent infections. Height and weight measurements of children are essential to identify failure to thrive or recent weight loss. Other important physical findings include scarred tympanic membranes and postnasal drip or cervical adenopathy, which suggests chronic respiratory infection. Recurrent cough, wheezing, or chest deformity suggests pulmonary disease. Lymphadenopathy, hepatosplenomegaly, pallor, wasting, or recent weight loss suggest systemic disease. Gingivitis and oral ulcers often accompany chronic neutropenia. Documentation of fever is important, but taking the rectal temperature of a patient with neutropenia should be avoided to avoid injury to the rectal mucosa and spread of bacteria to the circulation.

LABORATORY STUDIES AND DIAGNOSTIC TESTS

In the appropriate setting, the diagnosis of neutropenia is not difficult. Isolated absolute neutropenia has a limited number of causes (Table 212.1). The duration and severity of neutropenia greatly influence the extent of laboratory evaluation. Patients with chronic neutropenia since infancy and a history of recurrent fever and chronic gingivitis should have white blood cell counts and differential counts obtained three times a week for 6 weeks to evaluate the periodicity that suggests cyclic neutropenia. Bone marrow aspiration and biopsy should be performed on selected patients to aid in diagnosis and to assess cellularity. Additional marrow studies, such as cytogenetic analysis and special stains for detecting leukemia and other malignant disorders, should be performed for patients who might have intrinsic defects in myeloid cells or their progenitors and for patients who might have malignant disease. Selection of additional laboratory tests is based on the duration and severity of neutropenia and the findings at physical examination (Fig. 212.1).

The presence of antineutrophil antibodies is associated with immune neutropenia. A variety of known neutrophil antibody assays have been used to evaluate suspected autoimmune neutropenia, but all assays directly measure antibody on the patient's own neutrophils or indirectly measure antibody in the patient's serum.

DIFFERENTIAL DIAGNOSIS

NEUTROPENIA CAUSED BY FACTORS EXTRINSIC TO MARROW MYELOID CELLS

Secondary neutropenia is caused by factors extrinsic to bone marrow myeloid cells.

BONE MARROW REPLACEMENT

Bone marrow replacement with leukemia, myeloma, lymphoma, or metastatic solid tumors (e.g., breast, prostate) that infiltrate the bone marrow may produce leukoerythroblastic peripheral blood smears. Tumor-induced myelofibrosis may further accentuate the neutropenia. Myelofibrosis also can be caused by granulomatous infection, Gaucher's disease, or radiation therapy.

NUTRITIONAL DEFICIENCIES

Neutropenia is an early and consistent feature of megaloblastic anemia caused by vitamin B_{12} or folate deficiency, although it is usually accompanied by macrocytic anemia and sometimes by mild thrombocytopenia. Alcohol may suppress the marrow and inhibit the response of the marrow to infection when patients have diseases such as pneumococcal pneumonia. Mild neutropenia can occur among patients with anorexia nervosa, but neutropenia is generally not a feature of kwashiorkor or starvation.

INFECTION

Transient neutropenia is commonly caused by viral infection (Table 212.2). Neutropenia associated with common childhood viral illnesses develops during the first 1 to 2 days of illness and may persist for 3 to 8 days. This usually corresponds to the period of acute viremia and may be related to virus-induced redistribution of neutrophils from the circulating to the marginating pool. Sequestration or increased neutrophil use after tissue damage by the viruses also may occur. Acute transient neutropenia often occurs during the early stages of infectious mononucleosis.

Chronic neutropenia often accompanies infection with HIV-1 associated with AIDS. Neutropenia associated with AIDS arises from a combination of impairment of neutrophil production and the accelerated destruction of neutrophils by antibodies. Neutropenia also may be associated with bacterial, protozoal, rickettsial, and severe fungal infections. Sepsis is a particularly serious cause of neutropenia.

DRUG EFFECTS

Drugs can induce severe neutropenia through immune, toxic, or hypersensitivity reactions (Table 212.3). Drug-induced neutropenia should be differentiated from that associated with viral infection and from the severe neutropenia that occurs after administration of large doses of cytotoxic drugs or after radiation therapy. Drug-induced neutropenia may be asymptomatic despite the presence of absolute neutropenia, especially among pa-

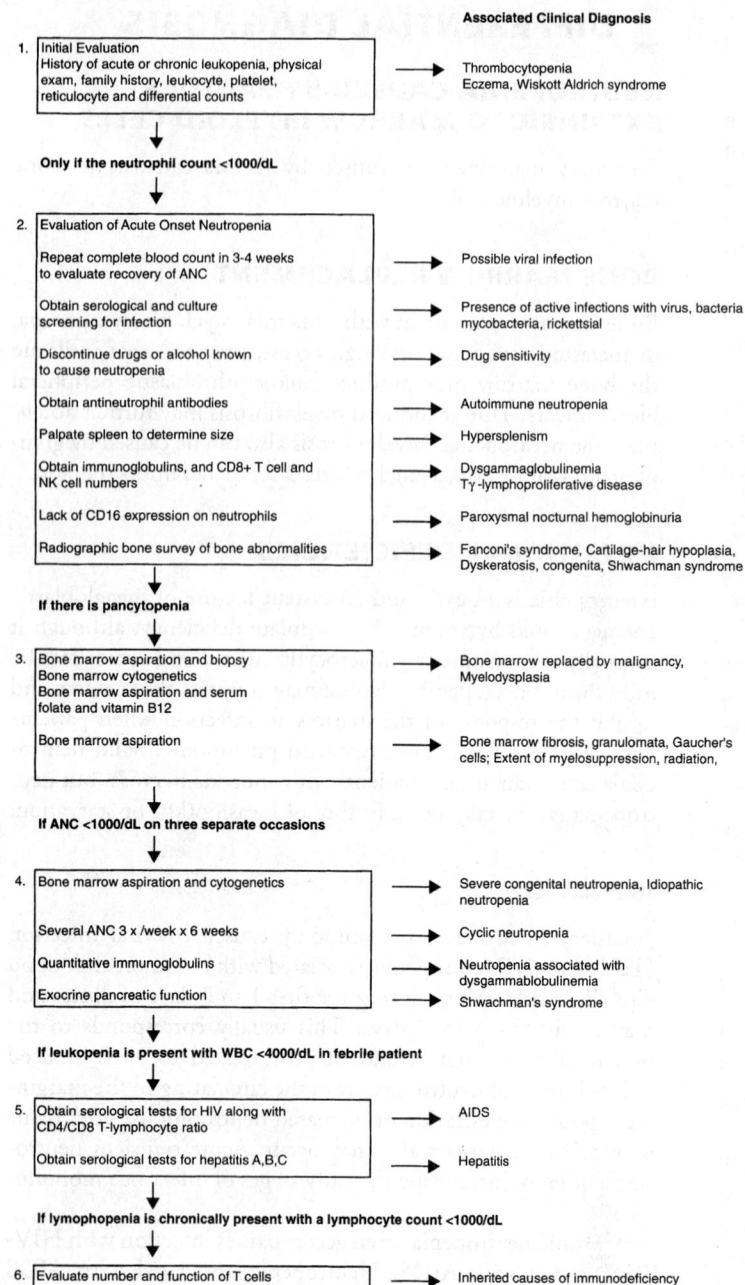

Associated Clinical Diagnosis

1. **Initial Evaluation**
History of acute or chronic leukopenia, physical exam, family history, leukocyte, platelet, reticulocyte and differential counts

→ Thrombocytopenia
Eczema, Wiskott Aldrich syndrome

Only if the neutrophil count <1000/dL

2. **Evaluation of Acute Onset Neutropenia**

Repeat complete blood count in 3-4 weeks to evaluate recovery of ANC → Possible viral infection

Obtain serological and culture screening for infection → Presence of active infections with virus, bacteria mycobacteria, rickettsial

Discontinue drugs or alcohol known to cause neutropenia → Drug sensitivity

Obtain antineutrophil antibodies → Autoimmune neutropenia

Palpate spleen to determine size → Hypersplenism

Obtain immunoglobulins, and CD8+ T cell and NK cell numbers → Dysgammaglobulinemia
Tγ-lymphoproliferative disease

Lack of CD16 expression on neutrophils → Paroxysmal nocturnal hemoglobinuria

Radiographic bone survey of bone abnormalities → Fanconi's syndrome, Cartilage-hair hypoplasia, Dyskeratosis, congenita, Shwachman syndrome

If there is pancytopenia

3. Bone marrow aspiration and biopsy
Bone marrow cytogenetics
Bone marrow aspiration and serum folate and vitamin B12 → Bone marrow replaced by malignancy, Myelodysplasia

Bone marrow aspiration → Bone marrow fibrosis, granulomata, Gaucher's cells; Extent of myelosuppression, radiation,

If ANC <1000/dL on three separate occasions

4. Bone marrow aspiration and cytogenetics → Severe congenital neutropenia, Idiopathic neutropenia

Several ANC 3 x /week x 6 weeks → Cyclic neutropenia

Quantitative immunoglobulins → Neutropenia associated with dysgammablobulinemia

Exocrine pancreatic function → Shwachman's syndrome

If leukopenia is present with WBC <4000/dL in febrile patient

5. Obtain serological tests for HIV along with CD4/CD8 T-lymphocyte ratio → AIDS

Obtain serological tests for hepatitis A,B,C → Hepatitis

If lymophopenia is chronically present with a lymphocyte count <1000/dL

6. Evaluate number and function of T cells → Inherited causes of immunodeficiency

FIGURE 212.1. Algorithm for the evaluation of a patient with leukopenia. *ANC,* absolute neutrophil count; *WBC,* white blood cell count.

EVIDENCE LEVEL: B. Reference: Dr. Laurence A. Boxer. Guidelines for evaluation for patients with neutropenia: Severe Chronic Neutropenia International Registry Guidelines.

tients whose blood cell counts are regularly monitored during drug therapy. The annual incidence of drug-induced neutropenia is 3.4 cases per 1 million persons. The incidence of drug-induced neutropenia rises precipitously with age; only 10% of cases occur among children and young adults, and more than 50% of cases develop among older persons. Idiosyncratic reactions are unpredictable and occur with administration of drugs such as chloramphenicol.

Clinical observation and laboratory studies have suggested that drug-induced neutropenia has as least three underlying mechanisms. Acute hypersensitivity drug reactions may last for only a few days, but chronic idiosyncratic reactions may last for months or years. Immune-mediated neutropenia usually lasts

for 1 week. After neutropenia occurs, the most important therapeutic measure is withdrawal of all drugs that are not essential, particularly drugs that might be myelotoxic.

Immune neutropenia is associated with the presence of circulating antineutrophil antibodies and may occur in isolation or with associated disease (Table 212.4). The antibodies may mediate neutrophil destruction by means of complement-mediated lysis or splenic phagocytosis of opsonized neutrophils. Antineutrophil antibodies cause transfusion reactions and may cause a variety of neutropenic disorders in later life. Lymphoproliferative neutropenia may be associated with the presence of circulating large granular lymphocytes (suppressor Tγ cells). Because reliable methods to measure neutrophil-specific antibodies or to as-

TABLE 212.2.	INFECTIONS ASSOCIATED WITH NEUTROPENIA

Bacterial

Typhoid fever
Paratyphoid fever
Tuberculosis (disseminated)
Brucellosis
Tularemia
Gram-negative sepsis

Viral

Infectious hepatitis
Infectious mononucleosis
Influenza
Measles
Rubella
Roseola
Varicella
Respiratory syncytial virus
Dengue fever
Colorado tick fever
Yellow fever
Sand-fly fever
Psittacosis
Mumps
Cytomegalovirus
Lymphocytic choriomeningitis
   virus
Human immunodeficiency
   virus type 1

Rickettsial

Rocky Mountain spotted fever
Typhus fever
Rickettsial pox

Fungal

Histoplasmosis (disseminated)

Protozoal

Malaria
Leishmaniasis (kala-azar)

TABLE 212.4.	AUTOIMMUNE NEUTROPENIA

Systemic lupus erythematosus
Seropositive rheumatoid arthritis
Felty's syndrome
Sjögren's syndrome
Immune thrombocytopenic purpura
Coombs'-positive autoimmune hemolytic anemia
Chronic active hepatitis
Hypogammaglobulinemia
Dysgammaglobulinemia (hyper IgM)
Lymphoproliferative disease
Graves' disease
Hashimoto's thyroiditis
Cyclical neutropenia and Tγ lymphocytosis
Infectious mononucleosis
Hodgkin's disease
Pure white cell aplasia

INTRINSIC DEFECTS IN MYELOID PROGENITORS

Neutropenia uncommonly is caused by intrinsic defects in myeloid cells or their progenitors.

CONGENITAL NEUTROPENIA

Cyclic neutropenia is a rare congenital granulopoietic disorder. It may be inherited in an autosomal dominant manner and is characterized by regular, periodic oscillations in the number of peripheral neutrophils from normal to neutropenic values. The mean oscillatory period is 21 ± 3 days. During the neutropenic phase, most patients have oral ulcers, stomatitis, or pharyngitis associated with lymph node enlargement. Serious infections occur occasionally and may lead to pneumonia, recurrent ulceration of the oral, vaginal, and rectal mucosa, and death. Pneumonia and chronic periodontitis often occur, and sepsis may arise from *Clostridium perfringens* infection. Cyclic neutropenia arises from a regulatory abnormality involving early hematopoietic precursor cells, but the exact nature of the defect remains unknown.

sess neutrophil survival in vivo have been difficult to develop, the pathophysiologic and clinical importance of these antibodies among patients who might have an immune disorder frequently remains unclear.

Splenic enlargement is associated with a variety of disorders (see Chapter 202). The neutropenia often is accompanied by moderate thrombocytopenia and anemia. In some cases, splenectomy may be necessary to restore neutrophil count to normal, but splenectomy predisposes the patient to infection by encapsulated organisms and should be used sparingly in treating neutropenic patients.

TABLE 212.3.	IMMUNE, TOXIC, AND HYPERSENSITIVITY-MEDIATED NEUTROPENIA

Characteristic	Immunologic Form	Toxic Form	Hypersensitivity Form
Paradigm drugs	Aminopyrine, propylthiouracil, penicillin	Phenothiazine	Phenytoin, phenobarbital
Time to onset	Days to weeks	Weeks to months	Weeks to months
Clinical appearance	Acute, often explosive symptoms	Often asymptomatic or insidious onset	May be associated with fever, rash, lymphadenopathy, hepatitis, nephritis, pneumonitis, or aplastic anemia
Rechallenge	Prompt recurrence with small test dose	Latent period; high doses required	Latent period; high doses required
Laboratory findings	Antibody test results positive	Evidence of direct toxicity to cells	Evidence of metabolite-mediated damage to cells

Severe congenital neutropenia, also called *Kostmann's syndrome,* is a rare disorder characterized by an arrest in myeloid maturation at the promyelocyte stage of the bone marrow, resulting in an ANC of less than 200 cells per microliter. In the United States, this disorder occurs sporadically. Patients typically have monocytosis and eosinophilia. Beginning in early infancy, they have recurrent, severe pyogenic infections, especially of the skin, mouth, and rectum. Platelet count is normal, and these patients typically have anemia associated with chronic inflammatory disease. With supportive therapy alone, only a few patients with severe congenital neutropenia have survived to adolescence. Sixteen percent of patients now treated with granulocyte colony-stimulating factor (G-CSF) have had acute myelogenous leukemia or myelodysplasia associated with monosomy 7 and revealed at cytogenetic analysis of the bone marrow.

CHRONIC IDIOPATHIC NEUTROPENIA

Chronic idiopathic neutropenia is a group of uncommon, poorly understood disorders involving committed stem cells of the myeloid series. Normal numbers of red cell and platelet precursors are present. The monocyte count often is moderately elevated. There is no splenomegaly. The degree of susceptibility to infection associated with chronic idiopathic neutropenia is roughly proportional to the blood neutrophil count, and patients with an ANC less than 500 cells per microliter are more susceptible to infection. Bone marrow examination shows a spectrum of abnormalities from normal cellularity to selective hypoplasia of the neutrophilic series. Neutropenia can be caused by bone marrow failure, as in rare syndrome-associated processes (Table 212.1). Neutropenia also is a prominent feature of myelodysplasia and is accompanied by megaloblastoid features in the bone marrow (see Chapter 230).

HEREDITARY AND ACQUIRED LYMPHOCYTOPENIA

Inherited causes of lymphocytopenia may be associated with inherited immunodeficiency diseases (Table 212.5). Inherited immunodeficiency disorders may be accompanied by a quantitative or qualitative stem cell abnormality that causes ineffective lymphocytopoiesis. Other conditions, such as Wiskott–Aldrich syndrome, may be accompanied by lymphocytopenia arising from accelerated destruction of T cells. A similar mechanism is present in patients with adenosine deaminase deficiency and purine nucleoside phosphorylase deficiency.

Acquired lymphocytopenia defines syndromes associated with depletion of blood lymphocytes that are not caused by inherited diseases. AIDS is the most common infectious disease associated with lymphocytopenia. The lymphocytopenia is caused by destruction of CD4 + T cells infected with HIV-1 or HIV-2. Lymphocytopenia also may reflect impaired lymphocyte production and proliferation caused by destruction of the normal thymic or lymphoid architecture. Patients with AIDS or inherited dysfunction of lymphocytes have recurrent infections. They often have unusual responses to usually benign infectious agents, or they have infections with unusual organisms. *Pneumocystis carinii* infection, cytomegalovirus infection, rubeola, and

TABLE 212.5.	CAUSES OF LYMPHOCYTOPENIA

Acquired Causes

Infectious diseases including AIDS, hepatitis, influenza, tuberculosis, typhoid fever, and sepsis

Iatrogenic conditions after administration of immunosuppressive therapy, glucocorticoids, high-dose PUVA therapy, cytotoxic chemotherapy, irradiation, and thoracic duct drainage

Systemic disease associated with autoimmune diseases, including systemic lupus erythematosus, myasthenia gravis, Hodgkin's disease, protein-losing enteropathy, renal failure, sarcoidosis, thermal injury, and aplastic anemia

Dietary deficiency associated with ethanol abuse and zinc deficiency

Inherited Causes

Aplasia of lymphopoietic stem cells

Severe combined immunodeficiency associated with defect in IL-2 receptor γ-chain, deficiency of ADA or PNP, or unknown

Ataxia telangiectasia

Wiskott–Aldrich syndrome

Immunodeficiency with thymoma

Cartilage-hair hypoplasia

Idiopathic CD4 + T lymphocytopenia

ADA, adenosine deaminase; PNP, purine nucleoside phosphorylase; IL-2, interleukin-2; PUVA, psoralen and ultraviolet A irradiation.

varicella often cause fatal pneumonia among these patients. Pneumonitis with any of these agents should suggest a potential immunodeficiency. These patients also have a higher incidence of malignant disease and autoimmune disorders. Other viral and bacterial diseases may be associated with lymphocytopenia (Table 212.5). In some instances of acute viremia, lymphocytes may undergo accelerated destruction from active infection with the virus, may be trapped in the spleen or nodes, or may migrate to the respiratory tract.

IATROGENIC AND AUTOIMMUNE LYMPHOPENIA

Iatrogenic lymphopenia is caused by cytotoxic chemotherapy, radiation therapy, and the administration of antilymphocyte globulin. During long-term treatment of patients with psoriasis with psoralen and ultraviolet irradiation, T lymphocytes may be destroyed. Glucocorticoids can cause lymphopenia through induced cell destruction. Systemic diseases associated with autoimmunity may lead to lymphocytopenia. These include systemic lupus erythematosus, rheumatoid arthritis, and myasthenia gravis. Conditions such as protein-losing enteropathy may be associated with lymphocyte depletion. An algorithm for the evaluation of a patient with leukopenia, neutropenia, or lymphopenia is presented in Fig. 212.1.

■ STRATEGIES FOR OPTIMAL CARE

MANAGEMENT

The management of acquired, transient neutropenia characteristically associated with malignant disease, myelosuppressive chemotherapy, or immunosuppressive therapy differs from that of congenital or chronic forms of neutropenia. Among patients with acquired neutropenia, infection sometimes heralded only by fever is a leading cause of death. The clinician therefore must have a high index of suspicion. Early recognition and management of infection may be lifesaving.

Therapy for chronic neutropenia is dictated by the patient's history. For patients with benign neutropenia, including those with neutropenia after an acute viral illness without evidence of repeated bacterial infection or chronic gingivitis, no specific therapy is needed. For patients with life-threatening infection, broad-spectrum intravenous antibiotics should be started promptly.

Recombinant technology has produced effective therapy for severe congenital neutropenia, chronic symptomatic idiopathic neutropenia, and cyclic neutropenia. A randomized, controlled trial involving patients with severe chronic neutropenia in which recombinant human G-CSF (rhG-CSF) was administered subcutaneously at dosages ranging from 3.4 to 11.50 µg per kilogram per day, dramatic increases in neutrophil counts occurred among patients with these disorders, resulting in marked attenuation of infection and inflammation. Recombinant human G-CSF also has been used successfully in the treatment of some patients with drug-induced neutropenia whose neutrophil count did not increase after cessation of the offending drug.

The management of chronic autoimmune neutropenia is dictated by the patient's medical history. Many patients with autoimmune neutropenia have associated diseases or have drug-associated antibodies. Among patients with more severe neutropenia (less than 500 cells per microliter), infection may become an increasing problem. They often respond to prednisone (60 to 100 mg per day). A modest increase in blood neutrophil count occurs within 1 to 2 weeks after the initiation of therapy. The prednisone should be administered daily, followed in 1 month by alternate-day steroid therapy at a reduced dose (e.g., 20 to 30 mg per day). For patients with autoimmune neutropenia who have not had success with glucocorticoid therapy, results of several uncontrolled studies have shown responses with cytotoxic drugs such as cyclophosphamide, azathioprine, or vincristine, intravenous γ-globulin therapy, and plasmapheresis. The approach to the treatment of patients with Felty's syndrome remains controversial. Splenectomy has been the mainstay of therapy, but the ANC commonly increases only temporarily. Fortunately, some patients with Felty's syndrome have responded to rhG-CSF.

COMPLICATIONS AND PITFALLS

All of the long-term effects of rhG-CSF therapy remain unknown, but they do include a propensity for development of moderate splenomegaly. Some patients who have preleukemia disorders, such as severe congenital neutropenia and Shwachman–Diamond syndrome, while receiving rhG-CSF have had myelodysplasia or acute myelogenous leukemia. Such patients should be monitored with frequent blood counts and annual bone marrow cytogenetic analyses. If patients with preleukemia disorder do eventually have myelodysplasia or acute myelogenous leukemia, bone marrow transplantation is the only effective

treatment. On a short-term basis, administration of rhG-CSF has been associated with elevation of serum lactate dehydrogenase, uric acid, and alkaline phosphatase levels. Some patients have had transient erythematous rashes, alopecia, thrombocytopenia, and vasculitis. These clinical complications resolved promptly after cessation of rhG-CSF therapy. Twenty percent of patients receiving rhG-CSF before the increase in the circulating neutrophil count have bone pain, which presumably reflects myeloid expansion. The pain is easily relieved with nonsteroidal anti-inflammatory drugs and usually lasts only 1 day.

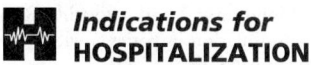

Indications for HOSPITALIZATION

Patients with acute neutropenia (less than 500 cells per microliter) who are immunosuppressed should be hospitalized at the onset of fever (temperature greater than 38.2°C) and treated with broad-spectrum antibiotics after the diagnostic evaluation for the source of the fever (see Chapter 267). Patients with chronic neutropenia who have life-threatening infections also should be hospitalized and treated with broad-spectrum antibiotics. A patient with chronic neutropenia with a superficial infection or low-grade fever can be treated with oral antibiotics outside the hospital.

Indications for REFERRAL

All patients with chronic neutropenia who might have an intrinsic disorder of the myeloid or precursor cells should undergo bone marrow and cytogenetic analyses by a hematologist. A patient with severe congenital neutropenia found to have myelodysplasia or a cytogenetic abnormality is best treated by a hematologist. Patients with autoimmune neutropenia who do not respond to glucocorticoids also are probably best treated by a hematologist.

COST-EFFECTIVENESS

Therapy with rhG-CSF has proved to be cost-effective in the treatment of patients with severe congenital neutropenia or cyclic neutropenia, because these patients have fewer hospitalizations and need reduced amounts of intravenous antibiotics. Therapy with rhG-CSF is not cost-effective for patients with idiopathic neutropenia if the primary benefit is to prevent recurrent mouth ulcers and gingivitis. For many patients with idiopathic neutropenia, rhG-CSF can be administered every other day. Therapy with rhG-CSF should be used primarily for patients with chronic neutropenia who have symptoms and have had recurrent infections.

BIBLIOGRAPHY

Boxer LA. Autoimmune leukopenia. In: Lichtenstein LM, Fauci AS, eds. *Current therapy in allergy, immunology and rheumatology,* 4th ed. Philadelphia: BC Decker, 1992:294–297.

Boxer LA, Todd RF III. Therapeutic modulation of neutrophil number and function. In: Wheeler JG, Abramson JS, eds. *The natural immune system: the neutrophil.* Oxford, England: Oxford University Press, 1991: 263–302.

Dale DC, Bonilla MA, Davis MW, et al. A randomized controlled phase III trial of recombinant human G-CSF for treatment of severe chronic neutropenia. *Blood* 1993;81:2496–2502.

Jones EA, Bolyard AA, Dale DC. Quality of life of patients with severe neutropenia receiving long-term treatment with granulocyte colony-stimulating factor. *JAMA* 1993;270:1132–1133.

Kalra R, Dale D, Freedman M, et al. Monosomy 7 and activating RAS mutations accompany malignant transformation in patients with congenital neutropenia. *Blood* 1995;86:4579–4586.

Laurence J. T-cell subsets in health, infectious disease, and idiopathic CD + T lymphocytopenia. *Ann Intern Med* 1993;119:55–62.

Moses A, Nelson J, Bagby GC Jr. The influence of human immunodeficiency virus-1 on hematopoiesis. *Blood* 1998;91:1479–1495.

Welte K, Boxer LA. Severe chronic neutropenia: pathophysiology and therapy. *Semin Hematol* 1997;34:267–278.

Kelley's Textbook of Internal Medicine, fourth edition. Edited by H. David Humes. Lippincott Williams & Wilkins, Philadelphia © 2000.

CHAPTER 213

APPROACH TO THE PATIENT WITH THROMBOCYTOPENIA

DOUGLAS B. CINES

Advances in medical technology over the past two decades have markedly increased the frequency with which thrombocytopenia is detected. This has meant changes in both the typical presentation and the relative prevalence of predisposing disorders. Twenty years ago, thrombocytopenia, often severe, was typically diagnosed when a patient had bleeding. Today, with platelets included in automated blood cell counting, it is far more common for mild to moderate thrombocytopenia to be detected as an incidental finding, especially among patients admitted to a hospital for other conditions. Thus thrombocytopenia often is a clue to an underlying medical disorder in addition to being a risk factor for bleeding.

When it does occur, bleeding due to thrombocytopenia usually begins in the skin or mucous membranes. Spontaneous bleeding is rare at platelet counts greater than 30,000 per microliter. Risk for bleeding increases as the platelet count falls below 20,000 per microliter, at which point patients may begin to bruise easily. Spontaneous bruising and petechiae, generally starting in dependent areas, gingival bleeding after brushing, menorrhagia, and epistaxis become progressively more common

if platelet count falls below 10,000 to 20,000 per microliter. At platelet counts less than 5,000 per microliter, persistent gastrointestinal bleeding may occur, and there is risk for spontaneous intracranial hemorrhage. Bleeding may occur at higher platelet counts when qualitative platelet defects, such as those caused by medications that impair platelet function, have been superimposed or when underlying anatomic defects that predispose to bleeding are present.

PATHOPHYSIOLOGY

Physiologic recruitment of platelets to sites of bleeding (see Chapter 218) does not by itself cause thrombocytopenia, because the bone marrow can increase platelet production about fivefold in otherwise healthy persons. Thrombocytopenia develops when there is a disequilibrium between platelet production, distribution, and destruction. This conceptual approach to understanding platelet function also provides a convenient means to categorize the disorders that cause thrombocytopenia.

IMPAIRED PLATELET PRODUCTION

Platelets are formed when the cytoplasm of mature megakaryocytes undergoes fragmentation. Megakaryocytes develop from pluripotent stem cells under the coordinate influence of several soluble peptides, including c-Mpl ligand (thrombopoietin) and interleukin-3, -6, -11, and possibly others (see Chapter 256). Conditions that cause physical or toxic injury to the megakaryocytes or their progenitors, that consume requisite growth factors, or that disrupt their interaction with the marrow stroma and vasculature may impair platelet production (Table 213.1). Examples include chemotherapy, ethanol ingestion, exposure to

TABLE 213.1.	THROMBOCYTOPENIA DUE TO DECREASED PLATELET PRODUCTION

Acquired

Marrow infiltration: metastatic cancer, hematologic malignant disease (e.g., leukemia, lymphoma, myeloma), myelofibrosis, Gaucher's disease, granulomatous processes, others

Aplastic anemia (idiopathic or immune), chemotherapy, radiation therapy

Amegakaryocytic thrombocytopenia (autoimmune; drug-induced, including chemotherapy, alcohol, thiazides; myelodysplasia; viral [e.g., congenital rubella, parvovirus infection, HIV infection])

Ineffective thrombopoiesis: folate and vitamin B_{12} deficiency; paroxysmal nocturnal hemoglobinuria; myelodysplasia and other clonal hematologic disorders; iron deficiency (rare)

Congenital

Normal-size platelets: thrombocytopenia with absent radius, Wiskott–Aldrich syndrome and variants, miscellaneous autosomal dominant and recessive syndromes

Giant platelets: Bernard Soulier syndrome, May–Hegglin anomaly, Alport's syndrome and variants, miscellaneous types of autosomal dominant macrothrombocytopenia

radiation, and viral infection (e.g., HIV, parvovirus) that can propagate within these cells. Platelet production is impaired in some patients with pernicious anemia or folate deficiency, in clonal disorders such as myelodysplasia and paroxysmal nocturnal hemoglobinuria, and in some congenital thrombocytopenic conditions, including those characterized by the production of abnormally large or small platelets.

INCREASED PLATELET POOLING

About one-third of platelets exist in the splenic circulation, from which they emerge without discernible impairment of function. The size of this pool is roughly proportional to that of the spleen itself. Any disorder that causes clinically detectable splenic enlargement may reduce the number of circulating platelets. However, the life span of these platelets is not necessarily lessened, and bleeding is uncommon. In contrast, platelet clearance within the spleen may be accelerated in some of these conditions as well, a situation known as *hypersplenism*. It remains unclear why platelets are prematurely removed in hypersplenic conditions or why erythrocytes and leukocytes often are spared. The causes of splenomegaly and hypersplenism are considered in Chapter 202.

INCREASED PLATELET DESTRUCTION

It is convenient to divide the causes of platelet destruction into immunologic and nonimmunologic disorders (Table 213.2).

TABLE 213.2.	THROMBOCYTOPENIA DUE TO INCREASED PLATELET DESTRUCTION

Immune Platelet Destruction

Autoimmune thrombocytopenia
  Idiopathic (occasionally accompanied by autoimmune hemolytic anemia)
  Secondary autoimmune thrombocytopenia (e.g., chronic lymphoblastic leukemia, systemic lupus erythematosus, thyroid dysfunction, hypogammaglobulinemia, antiphospholipid syndrome, bone marrow transplantation)
  HIV infection[a]
Drug-dependent immune thrombocytopenia
Posttransfusion purpura
Sepsis[a]
Neonatal alloimmune thrombocytopenia

Nonimmunologic Platelet Destruction

Disseminated intravascular coagulation
Cardiopulmonary bypass surgery
Sepsis[a]
Thrombotic thrombocytopenic purpura or hemolytic-uremic syndrome
Preeclampsia
Acute or hyperacute allograft rejection
Hemophagocytic syndrome[a] (postinfectious, neoplastic)
Hypersplenism

_____

[a] Multifactorial thrombocytopenia due to decreased production and increased destruction involving both immunologic and nonimmunologic factors.

Immunologic Factors

Platelets can become the target of autoantibodies, alloantibodies, or immune complexes. In idiopathic autoimmune thrombocytopenia (ITP), platelets are sensitized by autoantibodies directed to one or more cell-specific glycoprotein complexes, such as IIb/IIIa or Ib/IX/V. ITP is most common among children. Most patients are otherwise healthy, but ITP occurs with increased frequency among patients with systemic lupus erythematosus, primary antiphospholipid syndrome, chronic lymphocytic leukemia, hypogammaglobulinemia, and thyroid dysfunction, among others. Platelets coated with IgG antibodies are recognized by specific receptors expressed by tissue macrophages, leading to their internalization and destruction. Some antibodies also may bind to megakaryocytes, impeding a compensatory increase in platelet production. During pregnancy, IgG autoantibodies can cross the placenta and cause transient neonatal thrombocytopenia.

Posttransfusion purpura (PTP) is a rare disorder that affects primarily multiparous women or persons who have received previous transfusions. Affected persons have profound thrombocytopenia 1 to 2 weeks after exposure to a blood product containing platelet antigens that they lack, most commonly in the form of soluble antigens in the plasma that accompanies packed erythrocytes. PTP may be mediated by alloantibodies that destroy both the transfused platelets and, through undefined mechanisms, the host's platelets. Binding of immune complexes to platelets may accelerate platelet destruction in some patients with bacterial sepsis, during certain systemic viral infections, and after exposure to drugs such as heparin.

Nonimmunologic Factors

Platelets may be cleared more rapidly when they are activated or when macrophage function is stimulated. Such activation may initiate translocation of normally cryptic determinants (e.g., anionic phospholipids) to the cell surface, which can be recognized by macrophages. In disseminated intravascular coagulation (DIC), platelets are activated by thrombin and by traversing fibrin clots in the microcirculation. Platelets become activated at the interface between blood and artificial surfaces during cardiopulmonary bypass. In sepsis, activation may be caused by immune complexes or soluble microbial products. In thrombotic thrombocytopenic purpura (TTP), hemolytic-uremic syndrome (HUS), preeclampsia, and hyperacute allograft rejection, platelets may be activated as a result of endothelial cell injury. Seemingly normal platelets (as well as erythrocytes and granulocytes) may be subject to phagocytosis by splenic macrophages in hypersplenic conditions and in hemophagocytic syndrome, in which it is presumed that macrophages are "activated" by excessive production or an exuberant response to cytokines.

HISTORY AND PHYSICAL EXAMINATION

A directed history interview should establish the severity and duration of bleeding if present, identify anatomic lesions that may be predisposed to bleed, identify the presence of comorbid conditions known to cause thrombocytopenia, and include or exclude known causes of thrombocytopenia. Bleeding caused by thrombocytopenia ranges in onset, distribution, and severity from chronic, localized, and mild to acute, generalized, and profound. Bleeding may be superimposed on the clinical features of numerous other disorders (considered elsewhere).

Although most patients seek medical attention within days of the onset of bleeding, it is by no means uncommon for patients to have an exacerbation of intermittent or mild bleeding that had been present for several weeks, months, or even years. Some patients may recall an untoward frequency or severity of epistaxis in childhood. Others report severe menorrhagia or excessive bleeding after tooth extraction, giving birth, or other minor trauma or surgical procedures. Evidence of chronicity often is a valuable clue to the cause of thrombocytopenia. A diligent search must be conducted to find previous platelet counts or to identify events such as hospital admissions during which such a determination was likely to have been made. The patient should also be asked about family members who may have a history of excessive bleeding or bruising.

When bleeding is of recent onset, it is important to consider the possibility that thrombocytopenia is part of a multisystem disorder. Questions related to changes in the patient's general health, including fatigue, fever, and changes in weight, as well as a search for symptoms attributable to dysfunction of specific organs, may provide insight. A search should be conducted for specific factors known to cause thrombocytopenia, including prescribed and over-the-counter medications, especially those taken for the first time, resumed within the previous 3 weeks, or taken intermittently. Attention should be given to ingestion of alcohol, the use of illicit drugs, unusual dietary habits, or recent vaccinations or infections.

A separate category involves patients in whom thrombocytopenia is detected during the investigation of a thrombotic event. The specific disorders in which thrombosis and thrombocytopenia occur coincidentally are considered in detail below.

The physical examination is directed initially at assessment of the extent of bleeding and then at specific findings that favor or tend to exclude the more common causes of thrombocytopenia. The extent of cutaneous bleeding provides some guidance in gauging risk for internal bleeding. A thorough ophthalmologic examination is mandatory, as is examination of stool and urine for evidence of occult bleeding. Although no organ may be overlooked, because it may provide a clue to causation, special attention is paid to the liver, spleen, and lymphatic tissue.

▮ LABORATORY STUDIES AND DIAGNOSTIC TESTS

A complete blood cell count and analysis of the peripheral blood with a light microscope should be performed for every patient for several reasons. First, the presence of thrombocytopenia must be confirmed. Platelets from about 0.01% of all persons agglutinate in the presence of EDTA, the anticoagulant in which blood is collected routinely for automated blood counts. This phenomenon is caused by autoantibodies that bind to platelets only at

concentrations of ionized calcium less than those that occur in vivo. The clumped platelets are ignored by automated counters, and falsely low values are obtained. The disparity between the number of platelets evident on a blood smear and the recorded value is readily evident by visual examination, as is the presence of platelet clumps. The patient's actual platelet count can then be determined in other anticoagulants or whole-blood specimens.

Second, examination of a peripheral blood smear may reveal abnormalities in the erythrocytes or leukocytes that provide clues to the cause of thrombocytopenia and that may indicate other clinical features necessitating immediate treatment. For example, the presence of schistocytes and nucleated red blood cells provide a clue to the presence of TTP. Leukoerythroblastic findings (immature granulocytes and nucleated erythrocytes) may suggest infiltration of the bone marrow. The blood smear may reveal myeloblasts, lymphoblasts, circulating lymphoma cells, large granular lymphocytes, or dysplastic changes indicative of a myelodysplastic disorder or atypical lymphocytes, suggesting a systemic viral disorder. Deficiencies of folate or vitamin B_{12} produce characteristic changes in the erythroid and myeloid cells that occur early in the course of each disease.

Third, the size of the platelets may provide a clue to the cause of thrombocytopenia. Mean platelet volume increases more commonly in disorders that accelerate peripheral destruction, in those that infiltrate the bone marrow, and in myeloproliferative conditions such as essential thrombocythemia and agnogenic myelofibrosis or myeloid metaplasia. A predominance of giant platelets approaching or exceeding the size of erythrocytes may be a clue to hereditary thrombocytopenia.

Bone marrow aspiration and biopsy may be indicated when the cause of thrombocytopenia remains uncertain despite careful history taking, physical examination, and evaluation of the peripheral blood smear, especially when the thrombocytopenia is severe or progressive or when abnormalities in multiple cell lineages are present. The presence of a normal number, distribution, and appearance of megakaryocytes in the marrow suggests that platelet destruction or pooling or loss of platelets in the peripheral circulation is more likely, although these features do not exclude impaired production as a contributing feature. Examination of the bone marrow may reveal the extent of marrow cellularity and is therefore required to make the diagnosis of aplastic anemia or to identify the rare case of isolated amegakaryocytic aplasia. Examination of the bone marrow also is necessary when an infiltrative or dysplastic process is suspected. In dysplastic conditions, there may be subtle alterations in megakaryocyte structure, including the presence of micro- or hypolobulated megakaryocytes; in myeloproliferative disorders, the megakaryocytes may be found in clusters. In a few patients, chromosomal abnormalities or clonal genetic rearrangements may be identified that are of diagnostic or prognostic importance.

In many patients with thrombocytopenia, a bone marrow examination is performed reflexively, without careful consideration as to its utility or necessity. The probability that bone marrow examination will help in making a diagnosis varies widely, depending on the cause of thrombocytopenia. Therefore, the decision to perform a bone marrow examination should be based on the likelihood that the suspected cause is one in which diagnostic morphologic abnormalities are likely to be found.

Other tests that should be ordered as part of the initial evaluation depend on the clinical setting. For example, among patients with sepsis or cancer, it may be appropriate to consider a diagnosis of DIC and to measure fibrin split products. In others, it may be appropriate to perform a more detailed biochemical evaluation of liver function and spleen size. No single paradigm for subsequent testing is suitable for all clinical situations. Tests useful to make the diagnosis of specific disorders are as follows.

■ DIFFERENTIAL DIAGNOSIS

IMPAIRED PLATELET PRODUCTION

Impairment of platelet production usually is part of a multilineage process, and bone marrow examination usually is needed for definitive diagnosis. The most common causes are aplasia (drug induced, autoimmune, myelodysplasia, congenital, paroxysmal nocturnal hemoglobinuria); infiltration (neoplastic, granulomatous, infectious, fibrosis, necrosis); nutritional (folate or vitamin B_{12}) (see Chapter 243); and clonal disorders, such as myelodysplasia or hypoproliferative leukemia (see Chapters 229 and 231). Isolated amegakaryocytic thrombocytopenia is a rare condition caused by ethanol ingestion, antibody- or cell-mediated immune suppression, or myelodysplasia.

INCREASED SPLENIC SEQUESTRATION

Any disorder that enlarges the spleen increases the splenic pool of platelets and proportionately reduces the number of circulating platelets. Some disorders also accelerate platelet destruction within the spleen; the most prevalent example is portal hypertension due to cirrhosis. The specific disorders that cause splenomegaly and hypersplenism are discussed in Chapter 202.

INCREASED PLATELET DESTRUCTION

Immunologic Causes

Idiopathic Thrombocytopenic Purpura

Idiopathic thrombocytopenic purpura is a diagnosis of exclusion. The diagnosis requires the absence of other hematologic abnormalities unless readily explained, such as iron deficiency anemia, and failure to detect other potential causes, such as drugs known to cause thrombocytopenia. Patients are in their usual state of health with the exception of bleeding, and the physical examination should reveal only petechiae or ecchymoses. Bone marrow analysis, if performed, should have entirely normal findings or show increased numbers of megakaryocytes. Although antibodies to individual platelet glycoproteins often are found, the positive and negative predictive values of such tests in clinical practice remain to be established. One of the associated disorders listed in Table 213.2 may be present. HIV testing is indicated for patients at risk because the progress and approach to therapy differ among these patients and because of the social implications.

Drug-induced Thrombocytopenia

Prescribed, over-the-counter, and illicit drugs have become the most common causes of thrombocytopenia among patients who are not in hospitals or long-term care facilities. Although medications initiated within the 1 to 4 weeks before the patient seeks medical attention usually are responsible, all drugs should be suspected, especially when the medication is taken intermittently or was recently resumed. The list of medications implicated as causing thrombocytopenia is extensive. The utility of laboratory tests to include or exclude a diagnosis of drug-induced thrombocytopenia has been established only for heparin. Suspected medications should be discontinued or a chemically unrelated drug substituted whenever possible.

Posttransfusion Purpura

The diagnosis of PTP should be considered for any multiparous woman or any person who has undergone a transfusion who has severe thrombocytopenia 7 to 10 days after receiving a blood product containing platelet antigens. Most affected persons lack human platelet antigen HPA-1a, which is present on the platelets of 99% of the general population. A few cases have been attributed to other polymorphic antigens. The diagnosis should be suspected on clinical grounds but can be corroborated in many cases when the patient's serum lyses platelets from most donors. Antibody specificity can be established with a panel of platelets that lack individual alloantigens, and the genotype of the patient's platelets can be established on recovery with molecular biologic techniques.

Nonimmunologic Causes

Disseminated Intravascular Coagulation

Disseminated intravascular coagulation is a complex coagulation disorder in which platelets and clotting factors are activated by thrombin and are then consumed. Most patients with DIC are gravely ill and have a fulminant bleeding diathesis when they come to medical attention. The most common cause is sepsis, but acute DIC also can follow massive trauma, thermal injury or trauma to the brain, and various obstetric disorders, including placental abruption, retention of fetal parts, and eclampsia. Patients with acute DIC have thrombocytopenia, consumption of coagulation proteins leading to prolonged prothrombin and partial thromboplastin times, and evidence of secondary fibrinolysis that entails rapid lysis of thrombi within the microvasculature. Schistocytes caused by residual fibrin clots are found on peripheral blood smears in about 25% of cases, but overt hemolysis is rare.

The diagnosis of acute DIC usually is obvious on the basis of the clinical signs and symptoms, profound thrombocytopenia, and prolonged clotting times. The diagnosis is confirmed when D-dimers are found in the patient's plasma; these represent the effect of sequential cleavage of fibrinogen by thrombin and plasmin. About 5% of patients have a more indolent disorder characterized by recurrent arterial or venous thrombi, generally in the setting of malignant disease. Elevation of fibrinogen and fibrin degradation products or D-dimers may be the only clue to diagnosis in these cases.

Thrombotic Thrombocytopenic Purpura

Thrombotic thrombocytopenic purpura is an uncommon disorder; the incidence is about 1 case among 500,000 persons per year. It is characterized by an onset over several days to weeks when a previously healthy person has fluctuating neurologic signs, fever, weakness, anorexia, or other gastrointestinal problems. TTP also may occur during or immediately after pregnancy, after a systemic viral illness, among patients with HIV infection, and among persons with underlying vascular disorders such as systemic lupus erythematosus or progressive systemic sclerosis. The neurologic signs and symptoms, such as headache, visual disturbances, seizures, and stupor, may wax and wane initially, but eventually they predominate in most cases. Some patients have myocardial or mesenteric ischemia or respiratory distress syndrome. Almost every patient has thrombocytopenia, and more than 90% have evidence of microangiopathic hemolytic anemia when they seek medical attention. Nucleated red blood cells disproportionate to the number of reticulocytes usually are evident in the peripheral blood smear, serum lactate dehydrogenase level usually is markedly elevated, and about one-half of patients have evidence of mild renal insufficiency, although urinalysis may show only hematuria and proteinuria.

The signs and symptoms of TTP are caused by platelet thrombi that produce diffuse microvascular occlusion, a finding evident in histologic sections from affected organs. The disease may be caused by an autoantibody to an enzyme involved in the physiologic processing of ultralarge von Willebrand's factor multimers released from activated endothelium. Persistence of these ultralarge multimers may promote platelet agglutination. A deficiency of the processing enzyme may be present in some cases of familial or multiple relapsing disease. As yet, no laboratory test can be used to confirm or exclude a diagnosis of TTP. The diagnosis rests on the clinical and laboratory features. The diagnosis is progressively more difficult to confirm when fewer features are present, and a trial of therapy (see later) often is needed in atypical cases when the disorder is suspected.

Hemolytic-Uremic Syndrome

Patients with HUS have the signs and symptoms of renal failure. About 90% of cases occur among children after 6 months of age, typically several days to a week after a gastrointestinal disorder characterized by bloody diarrhea. The endemic form of the disease prevalent among children is generally caused by Shiga-like toxins (SLT) secreted by certain serotypes of *Escherichia coli* (0157:H7 accounts for half the cases in the United States) that damage glomerular endothelial cells and initiate platelet adhesion within the glomerular arterioles and capillaries. In the United States, HUS occurs episodically, especially among young children and persons living in nursing homes, through exposure to SLT-producing *E. coli* in food. HUS also occurs among some patients treated with mitomycin C, cyclosporine, quinine, or ticlopidine, after irradiation to the kidney, after pregnancy, and perhaps among women taking oral contraceptives. Autosomal dominant and recessive forms of the disease have been described that may be insidious in onset and refractory to treatment.

In endemic areas, the diagnosis of HUS is evident when a young child has renal insufficiency, thrombocytopenia (which may be mild or absent in one-third of cases), and microangiopathic hemolysis a week after a diarrheal illness. On occasion, however, extraglomerular manifestations predominate, including gastrointestinal pain or bleeding, respiratory distress, and neurologic symptoms, making the differentiation from TTP difficult, especially among adults in nonendemic areas. Detection of SLT-1 in the stool or antibodies to SLT-1, or isolation and speciation of *E. coli* may be helpful in such settings.

Hemophagocytic Syndrome

Hemophagocytic syndrome is a rare disorder characterized by pancytopenia caused by phagocytosis of hematologic cells by macrophages. The disorder may follow diverse microbial infections and occurs among children with a genetic inability to contain Epstein–Barr virus infection and occasionally among patients with T-cell lymphoma or histiocytic malignant disease. Patients are generally profoundly ill from the underlying systemic inflammatory disorder. The diagnosis is confirmed when bone marrow aspiration biopsy or tissue section shows erythrophagocytosis or macrophages containing nuclear debris.

THROMBOSIS AND THROMBOCYTOPENIA

The differential diagnosis for patients with thrombosis and thrombocytopenia (Table 213.3) differs from that for patients with bleeding. TTP, HUS, and DIC are considered earlier. Sufficient platelets may be consumed within acutely rejected renal allografts to cause thrombocytopenia. Thrombocytopenia usually is a late finding in preeclampsia and rarely necessitates specific therapy, but sometimes it can precede other manifestations of the disease. When thrombocytopenia is severe or progressive or persists longer than 3 to 5 days after delivery, additional diagnoses should be considered, including DIC, TTP, and HELLP syndrome (hemolysis, elevated liver function test results, and thrombocytopenia).

TABLE 213.3.	DISORDERS ASSOCIATED WITH SIMULTANEOUS ONSET OF THROMBOSIS AND THROMBOCYTOPENIA

Heparin-induced thrombosis or thrombocytopenia
Thrombotic thrombocytopenic purpura, hemolytic-uremic syndrome
Systemic lupus erythematosus
Primary antiphospholipid syndrome
Disseminated intravascular coagulation
Preeclampsia
Hyperacute renal allograft rejection
Paroxysmal nocturnal hemoglobinuria

Heparin-induced Thrombocytopenia and Thrombosis

About 1% of patients treated with heparin have thrombocytopenia, usually starting 5 to 7 days after therapy begins. Some of these patients have arterial or venous thrombosis, especially at sites of indwelling peripheral catheters. Patients also may have myocardial, cerebrovascular, or mesenteric infarction or pulmonary emboli. Heparin-induced thrombocytopenia and thrombosis (HIT) is more common among patients with cardiovascular disease, but it can occur in any setting. The diagnosis should be suspected when any patient receiving heparin (including subcutaneous heparin, infusion to maintain the patency of intravenous lines, and heparin-bonded central venous catheters) is found to have thrombocytopenia or a platelet count that decreases 40% to 50% without another explanation. Sera from most patients with HIT contain antibodies to complexes between heparin and platelet factor 4 that are presumed to cause platelet activation and possibly endothelial cell injury. Laboratory confirmation can be made in about 90% of cases either by means of measuring antibodies to heparin–platelet factor 4 complexes with enzyme-linked immunosorbent assay (ELISA) or by means of detecting heparin-dependent antiplatelet antibodies through the release of serotonin from normal platelets in the presence of the patient's plasma and heparin. The diagnosis is confirmed with a response to heparin withdrawal (see later).

Primary Antiphospholipid Syndrome

About 15% of patients with primary antiphospholipid syndrome have thrombocytopenia, which is generally mild and not associated with bleeding. Patients typically have arterial or venous thrombosis, which may be recurrent, in the absence of known risk factors. There may be a history of unexplained, recurrent spontaneous abortions, or the disorder may be found incidentally when the patient is found to have a prolonged partial thromboplastin time. Antiphospholipid (e.g., cardiolipin) antibodies may be found by ELISA or when they prolong phospholipid-dependent clotting (so-called lupus inhibitor or lupus anticoagulant). However, antiphospholipid antibodies also may be detected after various infections (e.g., HIV infection), after exposure to certain medications (e.g., phenothiazines), and in some persons who do not have symptoms. Antibodies to phospholipid-binding proteins such as β_2-glycoprotein I, annexin V, or prothrombin may be more specific and play a role in pathogenesis through activation of platelets or through vascular injury.

Paroxysmal Nocturnal Hemoglobinuria

Paroxysmal nocturnal hemoglobinuria is a rare disorder in which patients may have episodes of intravascular hemolysis and hemoglobinuria. Hemolysis is caused by enhanced sensitivity of the erythrocytes to the lytic actions of complement caused by a deficiency of the complement regulatory proteins CD55 (decay-accelerating factor) and CD59 (membrane inhibitor of reactive lysis). Hemolysis is part of a general defect in the expression of proteins linked to cell membranes by a glycosyl-phosphatidylinositol (GPI) anchor caused by a deficiency in hematopoietic cells of an enzyme, α-1,6-N-acetylglucosaminyl-transferase, required for anchor synthesis. Thrombocytopenia, which occurs among about one-third of the patients, is part of a general impairment in hematopoiesis rather than being caused by accelerated platelet destruction. It is unclear which GPI-linked protein is responsible for impaired platelet production or why these patients are susceptible to thrombosis.

The diagnosis paroxysmal nocturnal hemoglobinuria should be suspected when the classic features of periodic hemolysis and hemoglobinuria are present, but it also should be considered in patients with arterial thrombi or venous thrombi at atypical sites (e.g., mesenteric, hepatic, or superior sagittal veins) and for patients with a hypoplastic bone marrow. The diagnosis is confirmed when the erythrocytes have enhanced sensitivity to complement-mediated lysis initiated by low-ionic-strength or acidic media. The diagnosis is made with greater precision when flow cytometry shows the erythrocytes or leukocytes have reduced expression of GPI-linked proteins.

◾ STRATEGIES FOR OPTIMAL CARE

The first step in treating a patient with thrombocytopenia is to assess the magnitude and sites of bleeding or the risk for bleeding. Spontaneous bleeding is uncommon among otherwise healthy persons with platelet counts greater than 20,000 per microliter. The risk increases as the platelet count falls below this level. In general, hospitalization should be considered for patients with bleeding at sites other than the skin, patients with platelet counts less than 10,000 per microliter, and patients with platelet counts less than 20,000 per microliter who are perceived to be at increased risk for bleeding because of concomitant medical problems or social conditions (e.g., elderly patients living alone). Platelet counts of 50,000 to 100,000 per microliter generally are required for invasive and most surgical procedures (other than simple dental extractions), as are platelet counts in excess of 100,000 per microliter for patients undergoing cardiopulmonary bypass.

General measures that reduce the risk or severity of bleeding should not be overlooked. These include avoidance of trauma, including placement of central venous catheters, avoidance of medications that impair platelet function, control of hypertension, correction of medical problems that may predispose to bleeding (e.g., control of acid secretion for patients with a history of peptic ulcer disease), and red blood cell transfusions, which may improve platelet function. Administration of ϵ-aminocaproic acid, which inhibits fibrinolysis, may help reduce mucosal bleeding for patients with thrombocytopenia but should be avoided if there is evidence of DIC.

Platelet transfusions may be indicated to manage active bleeding outside the skin when the underlying cause of thrombocytopenia is not readily reversible. Transfusion also is indicated for prophylaxis in the care of patients at high risk of bleeding because of mucosal damage (e.g., patients with leukemia undergoing induction therapy) or those predisposed to bleed from identified structural lesions. Although platelet transfusion often is initiated when platelet counts fall below 20,000 per microliter, it appears safe to use a lower threshold (e.g., 10,000 per microliter) in the care of patients whose condition is clinically stable and afebrile. Transfusion of platelets confers a higher risk for allergic, pyogenic, and infectious complications and graft-versus-host disease among immunocompromised persons than does erythrocyte transfusion, because multiple donors often are needed and because cytokines accumulate in the accompanying plasma. Mechanical depletion or irradiation of leukocytes and shortened storage time may decrease the incidence of noninfectious complications, but about 40% of patients still will develop alloantibodies that ultimately make them resistant to platelet support, even when HLA-matched platelets are used. Moreover, platelet transfusions are contraindicated in the management of TTP and HIT in the absence of life-threatening hemorrhage, because they may exacerbate the thrombotic manifestations with disastrous consequences. Therefore platelet transfusions should be used judiciously in the care of all patients while attempts are made to correct the underlying disease.

MANAGEMENT OF IMMUNE THROMBOCYTOPENIA

Idiopathic Autoimmune Thrombocytopenia

Idiopathic autoimmune thrombocytopenia among children is distinct from the disease of the same name among adults. Children commonly have severe thrombocytopenia and an abrupt onset of petechiae or purpura. Despite the sometimes florid onset, the disorder generally is self-limited. Platelet counts generally exceed 30,000 to 50,000 per microliter within a week, even in the absence of treatment. Complete remission within 6 to 12 months is the rule for more than 80% of children. Spontaneous intracranial hemorrhage is the main fear, but this complication is too uncommon for an effect of therapy to be proven.

Treatment with glucocorticoids or intravenous immunoglobulin (IVIG) lessens the number of days the platelet count is less than 20,000 per microliter, but the medical importance of this outcome is controversial. Therapy is indicated in the care of severely thrombocytopenic children who have a chronic course, those with diffuse or internal bleeding, and perhaps older adolescents, among whom the clinical course is less predictable.

Unlike children, adults rarely have a spontaneous remission. Therefore adults with bleeding are treated with prednisone (1 mg per kilogram per day). Between 50% and 70% of patients will respond to this treatment within 3 weeks with a rise in the platelet count to greater than 50,000 per microliter. Bleeding may stop within days, even before a rise in platelet count is detected. Patients with profound thrombocytopenia and bleeding and those who do not respond to prednisone should be treated with IVIG (1 g per kilogram per day for 1 or 2 consecutive days), which has a success rate greater than 80%. Platelet transfusions may be surprisingly successful in emergencies. Adults with platelet counts greater than 30,000 to 40,000 per microliter rarely need immediate treatment in the absence of concomitant hemostatic problems, trauma, or surgery.

Despite the success of initial therapy, most adults relapse when corticosteroids are withdrawn and within 3 to 4 weeks of IVIG administration. Therefore, most adults with platelet counts persistently below 40,000 to 50,000 per microliter are candidates for splenectomy, which has an initial success rate of about 60% to 70%. Patients should receive Pneumovax vaccine and vaccinations against *H. influenza* and meningococcus before the procedure, but a lifelong risk for sepsis remains.

Numerous options exist for treatment of patients with severe thrombocytopenia refractory to splenectomy. These include a search for an accessory spleen, use of danazol, use of vinca alkaloids, immunosuppression with azathioprine or cyclophosphamide, use of high-dose dexamethasone, reinstitution of the initial therapy with corticosteroids and IVIG at lower doses, and a combination of these approaches, among others.

Pregnancy presents a special problem. There is a weak correlation between maternal and fetal platelet counts, and there has been no demonstration that a maternal response to any therapy lessens the risk for severe neonatal thrombocytopenia. Fetal platelet count can be obtained by means of percutaneous umbilical blood sampling near term, but the need for this measurement and the benefits of cesarean section when fetal thrombocytopenia is found are unproven. Most hematologists currently do not favor either intervention for most patients.

Posttransfusion Purpura

The course of PTP can be prolonged and severe in the absence of therapy. IVIG has replaced plasmapheresis as the treatment of choice with a success rate greater than 90%. Some patients need a second course of treatment. Limitation of subsequent transfusions to antigen-negative cells is logical but unproven.

Drug-induced Thrombocytopenia

Management of drug-induced thrombocytopenia is to discontinue all nonessential medications for at least 3 weeks and to substitute chemically distinct medications when necessary. Some patients need ancillary measures like those used to manage ITP or PTP when thrombocytopenia is unusually severe or bleeding occurs.

MANAGEMENT OF NONIMMUNE AND THROMBOTIC THROMBOCYTOPENIA

Acute DIC has a high mortality because the prognosis of the underlying disorders is generally poor. Mortality is generally unaffected by heparin despite improvement in coagulation measurements. Heparin nevertheless is indicated in the treatment of patients with thrombotic complications and may prolong the life span of transfused platelets and fresh frozen plasma in specific instances.

TTP is uniformly fatal without therapy, but the mortality rate has been lowered to about 20% with the advent of plasmapheresis. The value of adding prednisone is uncertain. Plasmapheresis should be performed daily until platelet count and the serum lactate dehydrogenase level have returned to normal. Plasmapheresis should not be discontinued because the patient's condition appears clinically improved unless the results of these two laboratory tests corroborate the impression. It may take as long as 3 weeks of daily plasmapheresis to see improvement.

About 15% of patients have a relapse within the first few weeks and another 15% sometime thereafter. Patients with relapses almost always respond to reinstitution of plasmapheresis, although a chronic relapsing course develops in a few. Failure to respond to plasmapheresis is ominous, but about 40% to 50% of such patients respond to splenectomy. Anecdotal responses have been reported with the use of cryosupernatant, vinca alkaloids, prednisone, antiplatelet drugs, staphylococcal protein A columns, IVIG, and immunosuppressive therapy.

There is no evidence that any intervention, including antibiotics, prevents the development of end-stage renal disease among children with postdiarrheal HUS. The evidence that plasmapheresis, or indeed any therapy, alters the course of atypical childhood or adult-onset HUS is far less convincing than it is for TTP.

IVIG has been proved to be of benefit in the care of some patients with hemophagocytic syndrome, which once was almost universally fatal. Anecdotal responses to cyclosporine have been reported.

The critical decisions in the management of HIT involve proper diagnosis and scrupulous avoidance of subsequent exposure to even small amounts of heparin. Risk for thrombosis decreases during the first 36 hours after heparin is discontinued, but it persists for several days among some patients. Improvement in platelet count generally takes 2 to 5 days. Management of preexisting or heparin-induced thrombi is a particular problem, because additional exposure to the drug exacerbates the thrombocytopenia and may precipitate new thrombotic events. Low-molecular-weight heparin should be avoided because most HIT antibodies are cross-reactive. The treatments of choice are the thrombin inhibitors lepirudin and danaparoid, a mucopolysaccharide complex with anti–factor Xa activity; approximately 7% of patients with HIT have antibodies that cross-react with danaparoid in vitro, but their clinical significance is uncertain. Ancrod, dextran, warfarin sodium, plasma exchange, antiplatelet agents, and iloprost (a prostacyclin analogue) have been used successfully in individual cases.

Therapy for primary antiphospholipid syndrome and thrombosis involves immediate and long-term anticoagulation. Immunosuppression may be added in refractory cases, and plasma exchange has been used in life-threatening circumstances. Heparin or antiplatelet drugs are used commonly to treat women with recurrent spontaneous abortion, although efficacy has yet to be proved through placebo-controlled trials.

Corticosteroids may ameliorate the rate of hemolysis for patients with paroxysmal nocturnal hemoglobinuria, but they have relatively little effect on platelet count among most patients. Danazol has been helpful in a few cases, but the mainstay of therapy is antithymocyte globulin and bone marrow transplantation.

BIBLIOGRAPHY

Berkman N, Michaeli Y, Or R, Eldor A. EDTA-dependent pseudothrombocytopenia: a clinical study of 18 patients and a review of the literature. *Am J Hematol* 1991;36:195–201.

Burstein SA. Thrombocytopenia due to decreased platelet production. In: Hoffman R, Benz EJ Jr, Shattil SJ, et al., eds. *Hematology: basic principles and practice*, 3rd ed. New York: Churchill Livingstone, 2000: 2115–2125.

Bussel J, Cines DB. Immune thrombocytopenic purpura, neonatal alloimmune thrombocytopenia and post-transfusion purpura. In: Hoffman R, Benz EJ Jr, Shattil SJ, et al., eds. *Hematology: basic principles and practice*, 3rd ed. New York: Churchill Livingstone, 2000:2096–2114.

Colman RW, Robboy SJ, Minna JD. Disseminated intravascular coagulation: a reappraisal. *Annu Rev Med* 1979;30:359–374.

George JN, El-Harake MA, Raskob GE. Chronic idiopathic thrombocytopenic purpura. *N Engl J Med* 1994;331:1207–1211.

Harker LA, Finch CA. Thrombokinetics in man. *J Clin Invest* 1969;48: 963–974.

Hillmen P. Natural history of paroxysmal nocturnal hemoglobinuria. *N Engl J Med* 1995;333:1253–1258.

McCrae KR, Cines DB. Drug-induced thrombocytopenias. In: Loscalzo J, Schaeffer AI, eds. *Thrombosis and hemorrhage*, 2nd ed. Baltimore: Williams & Wilkins, 1998:617–642.

McCrae KR, Cines DB. Thrombotic thrombocytopenic purpura and the hemolytic-uremic syndrome. In: Hoffman R, Benz EJ Jr, Shattil SJ, et al., eds. *Hematology: basic principles and practice*, 3rd ed. New York: Churchill Livingstone, 2000:2126–2137.

Warkentin TE, Kelton JG. Thrombocytopenia due to platelet destruction and hypersplenism. In: Hoffman R, Benz EJ Jr, Shattil SJ, et al., eds. *Hematology: basic principles and practice*, 3rd ed. New York: Churchill Livingstone, 2000:2138–2153.

Kelley's Textbook of Internal Medicine, fourth edition. Edited by H. David Humes. Lippincott Williams & Wilkins, Philadelphia © 2000.

CHAPTER 214

APPROACH TO THE PATIENT WITH PANCYTOPENIA

JOEL RAPPEPORT

Pancytopenia is defined as a decrease in all cellular elements of the circulating blood, including erythrocytes, leukocytes, and platelets. The degree of decrease in any one of these elements may vary at any time in the course of the illness. Some disorders that cause pancytopenia may initially come to attention as single-cell cytopenia. Anemia is a red blood cell (RBC) count two standard deviations below the age- and sex-appropriate RBC level. Thrombocytopenia is a platelet count less than 150,000 per microliter, and leukopenia is a white blood cell count less than 4,500 per microliter. Although leukopenia may be caused by lymphopenia or neutropenia, the most common finding is neutropenia with an absolute neutrophil count less than 1,500 per microliter.

■ PRESENTATION

Mild pancytopenia may be asymptomatic, the patient manifesting findings associated with the primary underlying disorder. Patients with severe pancytopenia come to medical attention with pancytopenia in an explosive, life-threatening clinical scenario. Patients with granulocyte counts less than 500 per microliter may have overwhelming sepsis. A patient with a platelet count less than 20,000 per microliter may have life-threatening, spontaneous hemorrhage. Acquired or congenital qualitative platelet dysfunction may cause increased hemorrhage. Patients may have simultaneous severe bleeding and infection. Symptoms associated with anemia often are more insidious because of the usual gradual onset of anemia. In addition to the findings of the underlying disease, findings at physical examination often are pallor, fever, necrotic abscess, and spontaneous petechiae and ecchymoses.

Severe pancytopenia is a medical emergency. Because this condition is life threatening, immediate supportive care, rapid diagnosis, and definitive and preventive treatment should be instituted. Pancytopenia is a symptom complex of an underlying disorder in which there is an absolute or relative decrease in effective hematopoietic production of peripheral blood cell elements.

PATHOPHYSIOLOGY

In general pancytopenia results from one of four pathophysiologic processes. Absence of hematopoietic progenitors that cause aplastic anemia is thought to be synonymous with pancytopenia. However, pancytopenia may be caused by other pathologic states. A decrease in normal hematopoiesis may be caused by replacement of the bone marrow cavity, the site of adult hematopoiesis, through a pathologic process that may be hematopoietic in origin or be caused by invasion by extrahematopoietic cells. Reactive myelofibrosis may be present. This process is called *myelophthisis*. Ineffective hematopoiesis results in progenitors that produce normal to increased numbers of cellular elements that are incapable of normal maturation and succumb to intramedullary destruction. This situation is manifested in severe folate or vitamin B_{12} deficiency or myelodysplasia. Pancytopenia may be caused by increased peripheral destruction of cellular elements with a hypercellular marrow incapable of adequate compensatory production. Some disorders, such as HIV infection, that cause pancytopenia may do so by more than one mechanism.

HISTORY AND PHYSICAL EXAMINATION

The history and physical examination often lead to the diagnosis of pancytopenia (Table 214.1). Because of the diversity of manifestations and causes of pancytopenia, an extensive and careful history and physical examination are required. Anemia may cause increasing fatigue and dyspnea on exertion, but because of the gradual onset of symptoms, it may be insidious. Among elderly patients, increasing signs and symptoms of congestive heart failure may be evident. Despite severe anemia, the blood volume may be increased. Leukopenia and neutropenia may cause unexplained high fevers, shaking chills, and repeated, persistent infections. Thrombocytopenia may come to attention as increasing ecchymoses and petechiae, particularly in the lower

TABLE 214.1.	**DIFFERENTIAL DIAGNOSIS OF PANCYTOPENIA**

Hypocellular bone marrow
  Aplastic anemia (acquired or congenital)
  Myelodysplastic syndrome (10–15%)
  Anorexia nervosa
Cellular bone marrow with ineffective hematopoiesis
  Megaloblastic anemias (vitamin B_{12}, folate deficiency)
  Myelodysplastic syndrome
Myelophthisic bone marrow
  Hematologic malignant disease
    Acute leukemia
    Hairy cell leukemia
    Multiple myeloma
    Lymphoma (Hodgkin's and non-Hodgkin's)
    Chronic lymphocytic leukemia
  Nonhematologic malignant disease
    Breast cancer
    Prostate cancer
    Stomach cancer
    Thyroid cancer
    Lung cancer
    Neuroblastoma
  Myelofibrosis
  Lipid storage disorders
  Osteopetrosis
  Granulomatous disorders
Normocellular or hypercellular bone marrow
  Acute leukemia
  Hypersplenism
  Immune pancytopenia
  Paroxysmal nocturnal hemoglobinuria
  AIDS
  Sepsis
  Reactive hemophagocytosis

extremities. Patients with severe thrombocytopenia may report bleeding from their gums or oral mucosa or visual changes caused by retinal hemorrhage. Patients may have the signs and symptoms of life-threatening intracranial hemorrhage. Women of childbearing age may have severe menorrhagia.

The history often determines the duration of pancytopenia. Some patients notice the gradual onset of increasingly severe symptoms, but for others, the onset is sudden and fulminant. Evaluation may include results of earlier laboratory tests. The history may show the cause of the pancytopenia. The history of illnesses, medications, and surgical procedures is important. That a patient has undergone gastrectomy or ileal resection suggests the possibility of vitamin B_{12} deficiency. A careful drug history, including the months before the onset of symptoms, is important in ascertaining whether the patient has drug-induced aplastic anemia. Administration of chemotherapy or high-dose radiation therapy to the bone marrow often causes expected pancytopenia of finite duration. A history of collagen vascular disease or rheumatoid arthritis suggests aplastic anemia or a lymphoproliferative disorder. The patient should be asked specifically about the presence of dark urine at the initial morning void, which suggests the presence of paroxysmal nocturnal hemoglobinuria.

A history of a malignant disease metastatic to bone marrow suggests the possibility of a myelophthisic process. The primary malignant tumor may be remote in time; recurrence comes to attention as bone marrow involvement or a more generalized process accompanied by constitutional symptoms such as weight loss and night sweats, although fever also may be symptomatic of infection due to neutropenia. Secondary hematopoietic malignant diseases or myelodysplastic syndromes may be caused by earlier chemoradiation therapy.

The history should include an adequate dietary evaluation that includes alcohol ingestion. The possibility of HIV infection should be entertained, and the history should include potential risk factors. To determine the possibility of a genetic disorder such as lipid storage disease or congenital aplastic anemia, a complete family history should be obtained. Although primarily diagnosed in childhood, these disorders may occur in young adulthood or later. A travel history should be established, because infectious diseases may cause pancytopenia.

The physical examination is important in determining the severity and consequences of pancytopenia and possibly in establishing the underlying diagnosis. In mild pancytopenia, only pallor may be observed. With serious thrombocytopenia, ecchymosis and petechiae may be noticed, particularly on the lower extremities and pressure points. In cases of severe thrombocytopenia, petechiae and bleeding also may be seen in the oral mucosa and retina. The latter findings indicate an emergency. High, spiking fevers may indicate the presence of potentially life-threatening infection. Careful examination for the source of the infection must be undertaken. In the absence of neutrophils, an infected site contains necrotic ulcers. Important cutaneous microemboli and rashes may be present. Sinuses should be percussed for tenderness. A careful, noninvasive examination of the perirectal area should be performed. In the absence of adequate neutrophils, the findings of pneumonia may be subtle.

The physical examination should be an attempt to determine the cause of the pancytopenia. In many disorders, there may be no further physical findings. However, splenomegaly may indicate that pancytopenia has been caused by hypersplenism or a myelophthisic state with extramedullary splenic hematopoiesis. With massive splenomegaly, the spleen extends into the lower abdomen, and the examination should begin in the lower abdomen and carefully proceed cephalad. Massive splenomegaly occurs in Gaucher's disease, myelofibrosis, hairy cell leukemia, and lymphoma. Splenomegaly usually does not occur with aplastic anemia, acute nonlymphocytic leukemia, ineffective hematopoiesis, and myelodysplastic syndromes.

Lymphadenopathy may indicate the presence of lymphoma, acute or chronic lymphocytic leukemia, or metastatic carcinoma. Examination of the breasts should be performed, because pancytopenia may accompany metastatic breast carcinoma. Skin and joint findings suggesting collagen vascular disease or arthritis may indicate the presence of immunologically mediated pancytopenia.

LABORATORY STUDIES AND DIAGNOSTIC TESTS

Laboratory studies are the most definitive aspect of the evaluation for pancytopenia (Fig. 214.1). An immediate and careful

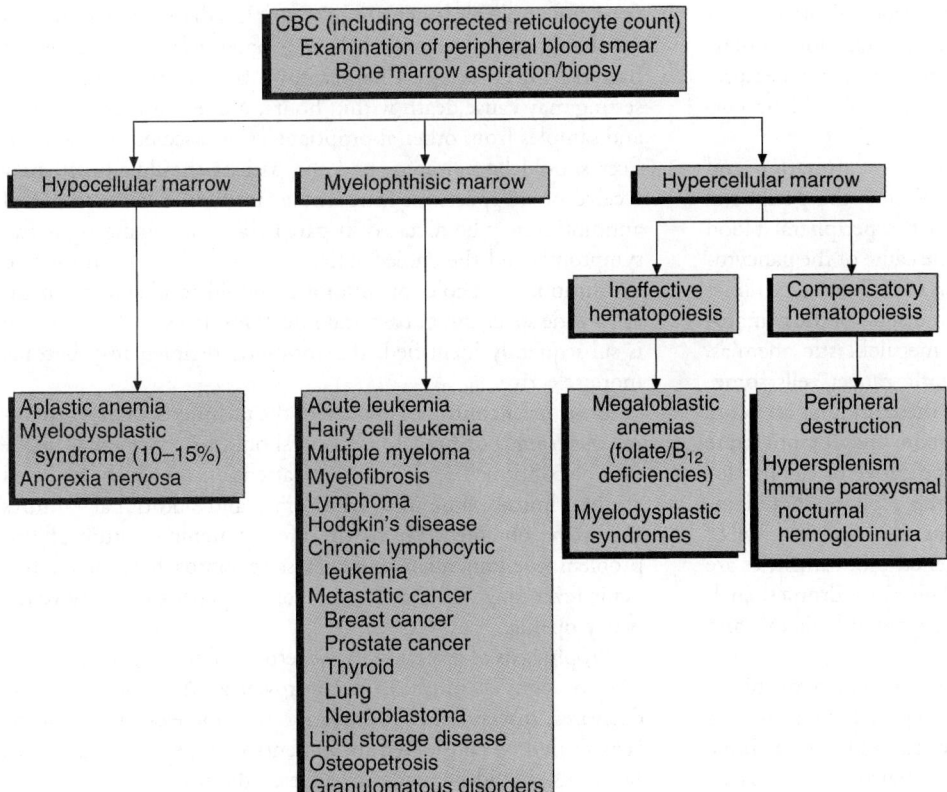

FIGURE 214.1. Algorithm for the evaluation of pancytopenia.

EVIDENCE LEVEL: C. Expert Opinion.

examination of a good-quality peripheral blood smear is mandatory. The complete blood cell count and differential count may indicate that some cell lines are more severely affected than others. Cell lines should be individually examined.

Erythroid macrocytosis may indicate ineffective hematopoiesis, as in vitamin B_{12} or folate deficiency, or the defect may occur as leukoerythroblastosis in myelophthisic disorders. The latter condition may be associated with poikilocytosis, nucleated RBCs, and teardrop-shaped cells. Nucleated RBCs are findings of stress erythropoiesis. Although aplastic anemia is classified as normochromic normocytic anemia, macrocytosis indicative of terminal stress erythropoiesis may be present. Polychromatophilia is indicative of erythroid production.

Rouleaux formation may indicate lymphoma or multiple myeloma. Blasts may indicate an underlying leukemia or myelodysplastic syndrome. Hairy cell leukemia, chronic lymphocytic leukemia, and non-Hodgkin's lymphoma may be associated with the finding of circulating cells the presence of which is enough information to confirm a diagnosis. In some bone marrow failure syndromes, such as aplastic anemia, an absence of myeloid cells causes relative lymphocytosis. A leukoerythroblastic smear has a few immature myeloid cells in addition to the RBC changes. Pelger–Huet anomaly and hypogranulation of the myeloid cells suggest an underlying myelodysplastic syndrome. Hypersegmentation of polymorphonuclear leukocytes is associated with megaloblastic anemia. An almost normal differential count and percentage of myeloid cells may indicate peripheral destruction caused by hypersplenism. Decreased numbers of small platelets indicate decreased platelet production, and the presence of giant platelets is associated with a myelophthisic process or compensatory thrombopoiesis.

Most important, examination of the peripheral blood must include a reticulocyte count with a supravital stain for numeric assessment of erythroid production. For more accurate measurement of erythropoiesis, the reticulocyte count should be corrected for an abnormal hemoglobin level.

In all cases of pancytopenia, bone marrow aspiration and biopsy should be performed immediately after the peripheral blood examination. In conjunction with the peripheral blood findings, these studies can help identify the cause of the pancytopenia in most cases. Aspirate examination of individual cell lines and cells allows the diagnosis of malignant disease of the hematopoietic system, lipid storage disorders, megaloblastic anemias, and myelodysplastic syndromes. Metastatic cancer cells sometimes are found in the aspirate, although these findings are more frequent in core biopsy. Prussian blue stains may demonstrate the presence of the ringed sideroblasts indicative of the myelodysplastic syndromes. Examination of the aspirate should include flow cytometry, which may aid in the identification of clonal abnormal cell populations. Cytogenetic abnormalities are found in the congenital bone marrow failure syndromes, such as Fanconi's aplastic anemia, and in some types of leukemia and myelodysplastic syndrome.

Extremely important in the evaluation of pancytopenia is core bone marrow biopsy, especially if a hypocellular aspirate is obtained. The biopsy provides the only true estimate of bone marrow cellularity. Although hypocellular marrow usually is associated with aplastic anemia, the possibility of a hypocellular myelodysplastic syndrome must be considered, and the core biopsy should be carefully correlated with the aspirate biopsy and cytogenetic studies. Bone marrow biopsy allows the diagnosis of myelofibrosis and increases the yield of diagnosis of metastatic carcinoma, mycobacterial infection, lymphoma, and hairy cell leukemia. No specific marrow findings are associated with HIV infection, although some of the secondary consequences such as granuloma or lymphoma may be demonstrated in the marrow. Bone marrow aspiration and biopsy often establish the diagnosis among patients with an enlarged spleen, particularly if the splenomegaly is caused by an infiltrative disorder or extramedullary hematopoiesis.

Careful evaluation of the peripheral blood and bone marrow often establish the cause of the pancytopenia. The need for further laboratory testing is dictated by the results of these examinations.

STRATEGIES FOR OPTIMAL CARE

MANAGEMENT OF PANCYTOPENIA

The care of a patient with pancytopenia involves four simultaneous issues. The first two are complete evaluation of the underlying disorder and institution of appropriate treatment (see elsewhere). The third issue involves management of complications, which may represent a medical emergency. The fourth aspect involves prophylaxis of future complications of pancytopenia.

Patients with mild to moderate pancytopenia may need no immediate care other than diagnostic evaluation. A patient with fever and an absolute neutrophil count less than 500 per microliter should be considered to have a potentially life-threatening bacterial infection (see Chapter 267). Because infection in this setting may cause death within hours, numerous blood samples and samples from other appropriate lesions, secretions, and orifices should be cultured, and the patient should immediately receive broad-spectrum intravenous antibiotics. The choice of antibiotics may be dictated in part by accompanying signs and symptoms, and the choice varies somewhat from institution to institution. The choice of antibiotics should be adequate to manage a wide spectrum of bacterial infections. If a specific organism is subsequently identified, the antibiotic regimen may become more selective.

If the fever continues unabated, the possibility of *Staphylococcus epidermidis* or fungal infection should be considered. In the case of continued fever, constant attention should be directed at the clinical signs and symptoms, and additional cultures should be obtained. Given the life-threatening nature of this problem, the immediate and aggressive approach to the neutropenic fever may well dictate whether the patient will survive the pancytopenia.

Prophylaxis of infection in the setting of neutropenia without fever or signs of infection is controversial. As neutrophil level decreases, susceptibility to infection may increase, and prophylaxis should be considered for patients with severe neutropenia. Attempts should be made to decrease the patient's exposure to potential sources of exogenous infection, including fresh fruit, vegetables, flowers, and plants, all of which may contain a heavy burden of soil organisms and fungal spores. Patients should be hospitalized in single rooms, and careful hand washing by hospital personnel may decrease acquisition of nosocomial infections. Patients with potential respiratory illnesses should avoid large crowds, and ill personnel should wear high-filtration masks.

The patient should be carefully examined for the presence of oral fungal infection and may be treated prophylactically with oral antifungal agents. Although some patients have been treated with prophylactic antibiotics, this must be undertaken with the knowledge that a selective infection, often with resistant organisms, may develop. Careful attention should be paid to personal hygiene that includes daily bathing with particular attention to intertriginous areas. Skin breaks should be avoided or promptly treated. A careful dental evaluation may be in order. In the setting of some causes of pancytopenia, the underlying disorder may cause an additional immunosuppressed state, leaving the patient susceptible to viral, fungal, and parasitic infections. Consideration should be given in these situations to *Pneumocystis carinii* prophylaxis.

Complete microbial isolation of the patient in a protective environment and decontamination of the gastrointestinal flora with nonabsorbable oral antibiotics are controversial. A patient with only mild to moderate neutropenia and immunosuppression does not need this type of treatment. Use of these limited facilities often is expensive, the procedure isolates the patient, and the oral antibiotics taste bad. Such facilities usually are limited to hematopoietic stem cell transplant recipients with prolonged severe neutropenia and immunosuppression.

MANAGEMENT OF HEMORRHAGE

Patients with pancytopenia most frequently have hemorrhage. A patient with hemorrhage and thrombocytopenia, especially with a platelet count less than 50,000 per microliter, should be treated with platelet transfusions (see Chapters 213 and 218). Each platelet unit ideally causes an increment of 10,000 platelets per microliter per square meter of body surface area. An aggressive approach should be taken to life-threatening hemorrhage, especially in the gastrointestinal tract, oral cavity, retina, or central nervous system. Increased increments are found among patients who have undergone splenectomy, and less than ideal responses occur among patients with splenomegaly. Patients with sepsis, disseminated intravascular coagulation, microangiopathic states, and active bleeding may have blunted responses. Patients alloimmunized to HLA antigens or platelet-specific antigens may have little or no response and may need transfusions with HLA-compatible platelets. Alloimmunization may be caused by prior transfusions and pregnancies. Medications that interfere with platelet function should not be used. Myelodysplastic syndromes or myeloproliferative disorders may cause qualitative platelet dysfunction and increased bleeding. Coincidental congenital platelet dysfunctional disorders may require a higher platelet count for active bleeding or as prophylaxis.

Prophylaxis of hemorrhage is a more controversial issue. Activities conducive to trauma should be avoided, and for women of childbearing potential, menses should be suppressed. In many centers, a platelet count of 20,000 per microliter mandates a platelet transfusion, even in the absence of active bleeding. However, decisions to transfuse platelets prophylactically should be made on the basis of laboratory data and clinical assessment. For patients with active production of platelets but increased consumption, little value is derived from platelet transfusions, even in severe thrombocytopenia, except in rare circumstances. Patients who have stable thrombocytopenia because of decreased production in the absence of active bleeding probably need transfusions at levels less than 5000 per microliter or as preparation for an invasive procedure.

Suboptimal posttransfusion increments necessitate additional evaluation. In the absence of nonimmune reasons for a poor response, patients should be evaluated for alloimmunization by means of HLA antibody testing. Certain causes of pancytopenia, such as aplastic anemia, more frequently cause such sensitization. HLA-compatible donors should be sought, and transfusion of single-donor platelets treated with pheresis should be attempted. When results are appropriate, attempts should be made to use the same donor repeatedly. In the absence of an identified donor, a cross-match test should be performed to identify potential donors. Avoidance of alloimmunization among patients who need long-term platelet support is attempted through the judicious use of blood products and the use of leukocyte-depleted products.

Erythrocyte transfusions should be given after consideration of the clinical situation and the laboratory results. Younger patients with anemia that developed over long periods tolerate lower hemoglobin levels than do older persons. RBC transfusions among older persons with pancytopenia from megaloblastic anemia should be administered cautiously, because the blood volume may be expanded, and transfusions may precipitate congestive heart failure. Long-term transfusion may cause transfusion hemosiderosis, and iron chelation may have to be considered.

In the setting of pancytopenia, any transfusion must be administered judiciously, especially until it is established whether the patient has aplastic anemia. Transfusions, particularly in cases of aplastic anemia, may cause sensitization to non-HLA minor histocompatibility antigens, resulting in nonengraftment of transplanted hematopoietic stem cells. Transfusions from family members should be avoided. Because many of the conditions that cause pancytopenia may lead to therapy with hematopoietic stem cell transplantation, immediate evaluation of the patient's cytomegalovirus (CMV) history should be undertaken with measurement of CMV antibody. Before these results are obtained, patients should receive CMV-negative blood products if possible. If the patient is CMV-naive, CMV-negative products should be used. For patients with immunosuppressed states resulting from the underlying disease or its therapy, blood products should be irradiated to prevent potentially fatal transfusion-associated graft-versus-host disease.

Few of the conditions previously described necessitate use of exogenous hematopoietic cytokines. Under most circumstances, measured levels are appropriately elevated. In some disorders, granulocyte colony-stimulating factor or granulocyte-macrophage colony-stimulating factor can be detrimental because they stimulate the underlying hematopoietic malignant lesion. However, these cytokines have aided therapy for neutropenic infections. Although these agents have not been demonstrated to cure aplastic anemia, the infection rate appears to be diminished among responders. A variety of agents and combinations of agents are under study (see Chapters 212 and 213).

BIBLIOGRAPHY

Aboulafia DM, Mitsuyasu RT. Hematologic abnormalities in AIDS. *Hematol Oncol Clin North Am* 1991;5:195–214.

Alter BP, Young NS. The bone marrow failure syndromes. In: Nathan DG, Oski FA, eds. *Hematology of infancy and childhood.* Philadelphia: WB Saunders, 1993:216–316.

Beutler E. Platelet transfusions: the 20,000/μL trigger. *Blood* 1993;81: 1411–1413.

Pizzo PA. Management of fever in patients with cancer and treatment-induced neutropenia. *N Engl J Med* 1993;328:1323–1332.

Robinson BE, Quesenberry PJ. Review: hematopoietic growth factors—overview and clinical applications. *Am J Med Sci* 1990;300: 163–321.

Rosse W. Evolution of clinical understanding: paroxysmal nocturnal hemoglobinuria as a paradigm. *Am J Hematol* 1993;42:122–126.

Kelley's Textbook of Internal Medicine, fourth edition. Edited by H. David Humes. Lippincott Williams & Wilkins, Philadelphia © 2000.

C H A P T E R
215

APPROACH TO THE PATIENT WITH AN ELEVATED HEMOGLOBIN LEVEL

EUGENE P. FRENKEL

■ PRESENTATION

An increase in hemoglobin concentration, hematocrit, or red blood cell (RBC) number may reflect a decrease in plasma volume or indicate an absolute increase in the number of RBCs. *Polycythemia* is the term used to designate an absolute increase in circulating RBC mass. Because a reduction in plasma volume with normal numbers of RBCs results in a relative increase in RBC mass, such clinical events have been called *relative polycythemia* or *spurious polycythemia.* The increased RBC mass can be primary (polycythemia vera), which defines an autonomous underlying mechanism, or secondary, indicating that the increase in RBCs is caused by an identifiable mechanism, tissue hypoxia, or increased production of erythropoietin (EPO).

■ PATHOPHYSIOLOGY

The forms of polycythemia (Table 215.1) have limited pathophysiologic mechanisms. In relative polycythemia, plasma vol-

ume is constricted, and RBC mass is normal or high normal. Although fluid loss is the acute cause, the pathogenesis of chronic relative polycythemia is unknown.

In the absolute or true types of polycythemia, different pathophysiologic mechanisms exist. In (primary) polycythemia vera an autonomous clonal expansion of EPO-independent hematopoietic stem cells occurs. The autonomy is consistent with the evidence that polycythemia vera is a neoplastic disease. The growth advantage of the neoplastic clone appears to relate to alterations in the bcl-2 oncogene family with deregulated and increased expression of bcl-X (an important inhibitor of apoptosis) in the EPO-independent clone. In the other forms of polycythemia, increased RBC production is caused by a physiologic increase in EPO secretion (e.g., high altitude, cardiopulmonary causes of hypoxia), a pathologic increase (e.g., aberrant sites of EPO production), or increased responsiveness of erythroid progenitor cells to physiologic amounts of EPO (e.g., familial, congenital lesions of the EPO receptor).

EPO is the normal regulator of RBC production, and cellular hypoxia is the primary stimulus to its production and release. EPO, the first identified cytokine, is an approximately 35-kd glycoprotein that is an obligatory growth factor for erythroid development. It is produced by interstitial cells of endothelial or fibroblast lineage, which are present primarily in the renal cortical peritubular site. Approximately 10% of EPO is extrarenal in origin, largely from the liver. Hypoxia stimulates prostaglandin release, which recruits new cells to produce EPO. The enhanced EPO production is caused by an increase in the number of these cells not from more EPO derived from extant cells.

The gene for human EPO is on chromosome 7. Renal interstitial cell hypoxia causes gene activation with increased transcription and messenger RNA (mRNA). A "hypoxic-responsive element" at the 3′ tail of the gene appears to serve as the activator of transcription, and mRNA synthesis increases. EPO does not induce the hematopoietic stem cell to its primary commitment to the erythroid compartment. The mechanism for the initial commitment to a given cell lineage (e.g., erythroid, myeloid, megakaryocytic) is unknown. However, EPO receptors (approximately 200 per cell) are present on the erythroid progenitor cells, and as a result, EPO serves as a lineage-specific cytokine to enhance growth, differentiation, and amplification of these cells into the erythroid cell pool. Truncated mutations of the EPO receptors (particularly at exon 8, which encodes the c-terminal region) have been associated with familial (congenital) polycythemia. Hyperresponsiveness of erythroid progenitor cells to EPO has been shown to be caused by these mutations, although the true mechanism in this form of polycythemia may be altered signal transduction of downstream elements, such as *JAK2* and *STATS.*

The physiologic half-life of EPO is not known, but studies with transgenic mice that express the human EPO gene have shown that even a slight increase in hormone secretion sustained over a long period produces polycythemia. A pulse of EPO transforms undifferentiated erythroid-committed precursors to proerythroblasts, accelerates the cells in the maturation sequence, and causes reticulocyte formation within 5 days.

Any alteration in ambient oxygen content (e.g., high altitude), disorders associated with decreased arterial oxygen tension

TABLE 215.1.	CAUSES OF POLYCYTHEMIA

Clinical Pathophysiologic Mechanisms	Salient Laboratory Features
Normal RBC mass (relative polycythemia)	Normal measured (^{51}Cr) RBC mass
Acute: hemoconcentration (e.g., dehydration)	Decreased plasma volume
Chronic: relative (spurious, stress, Gaisböck's syndrome)	
Increased RBC mass (absolute polycythemia)	
Neonatal: physiologic	Increased measured (^{51}Cr) RBC mass
Familial: altered hemoglobin structure or function altered (truncated) EPO receptor	Decreased P_{50} of whole blood
Decreased 2,3-DPG	Left shift in oxygen dissociation curve
DPG mutase deficiency	Decreased P_{50} of whole blood
Hereditary high adenosine triphosphate level	
Autonomous EPO production	
Acquired	
Primary: polycythemia vera	Increased EPO
	Splenomegaly
	Increased platelets and white blood cells
	Increased vitamin B_{12} and B_{12}-binding proteins
Secondary to decreased arterial oxygen	Arterial oxygen saturation tension less than 92%
High altitude	
Pulmonary diseases with hypoventilation	Pao_2 less than 65 mm Hg
Cardiovascular shunts	
Secondary to decreased oxygen-carrying capacity	Direct measurement
Elevated carboxyhemoglobin (e.g., smoker's polycythemia)	Carboxyhemoglobin
Methemoglobinemia	Methemoglobin
Secondary to decreased oxygen delivery	
Hemoglobin with altered structure of function: high oxygen affinity for hemoglobin	Decreased P_{50} of whole blood
Secondary to aberrant (inappropriate) EPO production	Increased EPO
Renal: renal artery stenosis, cystic disease, renal cell carcinoma, transplant rejection	
Liver: hepatoma	
Uterus: leiomyoma	
Adrenal: pheochromocytoma	
Secondary to blood transfusion (i.e., blood doping)	Hormone assays
Secondary to administration of EPO	
Secondary to other hormones	
Cushing's syndrome	
Androgens	

DPG, diphosphoglycerate; EPO, erythropoietin; RBC, red blood cell.

(e.g., cardiac or arteriovenous shunting), reduced oxygen-carrying capacity of the blood (e.g., elevated carboxyhemoglobin levels caused by smoking), or altered oxygen delivery to tissues (e.g., high-oxygen-affinity hemoglobin) increases EPO production and causes secondary polycythemia. In the absence of hypoxia, familial or acquired secondary polycythemia may be caused by aberrant or inappropriate EPO production (Table 215.1).

HISTORY AND PHYSICAL EXAMINATION

The clinical history can define some of the clinical states associated with elevated hemoglobin concentration. The familial forms of polycythemia (e.g., high-affinity hemoglobin, altered diphosphoglycerate) often are first recognized in adulthood

when family members become dedicated blood donors. A smoking history is important, because cessation is a prerequisite for the delineation of other possible mechanisms.

Patients with relative polycythemia have definable clinical features. They are usually middle-aged white men with moderate obesity, hypertension, and a history of smoking and alcohol use. The symptoms commonly include nervousness, headaches, and dizziness. These patients have a high prevalence of thromboembolic cardiac and cerebral vascular episodes and often a family history of cerebral and cardiovascular disease.

The symptoms and signs of true polycythemia, such as headaches, vertigo, visual disturbances, and mental confusion, are caused by the increase in RBC mass and the concomitant increase in blood viscosity and total blood volume. Studies of residents of high altitudes have shown adaptive tolerance; few symptoms are expressed despite hemoglobin concentrations as high as 25 g per deciliter. The acclimatization process is associated with a shift to the right of the oxygen dissociation curve, which enhances the unloading of oxygen to the tissue. Because a variety of events can cause tissue hypoxia, the clinical correlations with elevated hemoglobin levels can be broad (Table 215.1).

LABORATORY STUDIES AND DIAGNOSTIC TESTS

The initial diagnostic evaluation for a patient with an elevated hemoglobin concentration, hematocrit, or RBC count is measurement of RBC mass. This should be done, ideally in the nonsmoking state, for men with a stable hematocrit higher than 51% and for women with a hematocrit higher than 48%. Unless the body habitus is unusual, an RBC mass of 36 mL per kilogram or greater for a man and 32 mL per kilogram for a woman is enough information to confirm a diagnosis of polycythemia. A more accurate expression of normal involves surface area; this is particularly critical in the diagnostic evaluation for obese patients.

Arterial blood gases and carboxyhemoglobin should be measured; methemoglobin should be measured in cases of cyanosis. Hypoxia with resultant increased EPO production occurs at an arterial oxygen saturation of less than 92% and a PaO$_2$ of less than 65 mm Hg. Carboxyhemoglobin decreases oxygen-carrying capacity and must be directly measured; because this value increases during the course of smoke exposure, it is best obtained late in the day. A normal value for nonsmokers is $0.9 \pm 0.5\%$. Levels in moderate smokers are in the range of 3% to 5%. Among heavy smokers, concentrations are in the range of 5% to 7%. Methemoglobin need not be measured unless cyanosis is present; concentrations greater than 1.5 g per deciliter are associated with cyanosis.

If high-oxygen-affinity hemoglobin is suspected, the oxygen dissociation curve and P$_{50}$ are measured. The classic pattern is a hyperbolic curve shifted to the left. Because most hemoglobin variants have normal electrophoretic patterns, peptide mapping and amino acid analysis may be needed for final diagnosis.

An EPO assay can be used in the differential diagnosis of polycythemia. Because much overlap exists between clinical entities, the physician must be cautious in interpreting results obtained from any single sample. The range among healthy persons is 4 to 16 (immunoradiometric method). Among most untreated patients with polycythemia vera it is less than 4 mU per milliliter or in the lower range of normal. Most patients with secondary polycythemia have a level in the high normal range or above. In polycythemia vera the EPO level is not greatly influenced by phlebotomy therapy. The basis for the reduced levels in polycythemia vera is unknown, but the reductions may be caused by down-regulation of normal EPO secretion. Spontaneous EPO-independent in vitro endogenous erythroid colony growth characterizes the peripheral blood (sample) in polycythemia vera. In secondary polycythemia an absolute EPO requirement exists for growth. In many parts of the world, this differential feature is included in the diagnostic criteria for polycythemia; such assays are not readily available in the United States.

DIFFERENTIAL DIAGNOSIS

The primary mechanisms of elevated hemoglobin level and the focused diagnostic tests are outlined in Table 215.1. A sequential diagnostic approach is displayed in Fig. 215.1. Measurement of RBC mass separates relative from absolute polycythemia. When the hematocrit is significantly greater than 60%, RBC mass is almost always abnormal; the measurement can be bypassed in certain cases.

Because the most common cause of true polycythemia is decreased oxygen delivery, the next step in evaluation is measurement of arterial blood gases and carboxyhemoglobin. If the values are abnormal, the diagnosis is easily defined through evaluation of the causes of the low arterial oxygen tension or high carboxyhemoglobin or methemoglobin level.

If blood gases are normal, three diagnostic categories exist. The first is autonomous drive to hematopoiesis. Associated findings of splenomegaly and elevated platelet and white blood cell counts support this diagnosis. The second is defective oxygen delivery system to tissues (e.g., high-affinity hemoglobin, alteration in diphosphoglycerate binding). An oxygen dissociation curve and P$_{50}$ measurement are required for diagnosis of these lesions. Third, inappropriate secretion of EPO may cause polycythemia. A variety of organs have been implicated in cases of aberrant or inappropriate secretion of EPO, although most cases are caused by kidney or liver lesions. If no other specific symptoms or signs exist, it is wise to perform abdominal ultrasonography or computed tomography.

STRATEGIES FOR OPTIMAL CARE

MANAGEMENT

Relative Polycythemia

Although the RBC mass is not increased in relative polycythemia, risk for cardiac and cerebrovascular complications is increased. Because the pathophysiologic mechanisms are unknown, therapy is directed at weight reduction, cessation of alcohol use and smoking, control of hypertension, and an attempt at alteration of lifestyle. These supportive measures have produced an improved clinical outlook.

Secondary Polycythemia

Because secondary polycythemia is physiologic compensation, the proper clinical approach is to identify and manage the primary cause. This is particularly true for aberrant or inappropriate secretion of EPO, for which correction of the lesion often is curative. If repair of the primary lesion is impossible, the nature

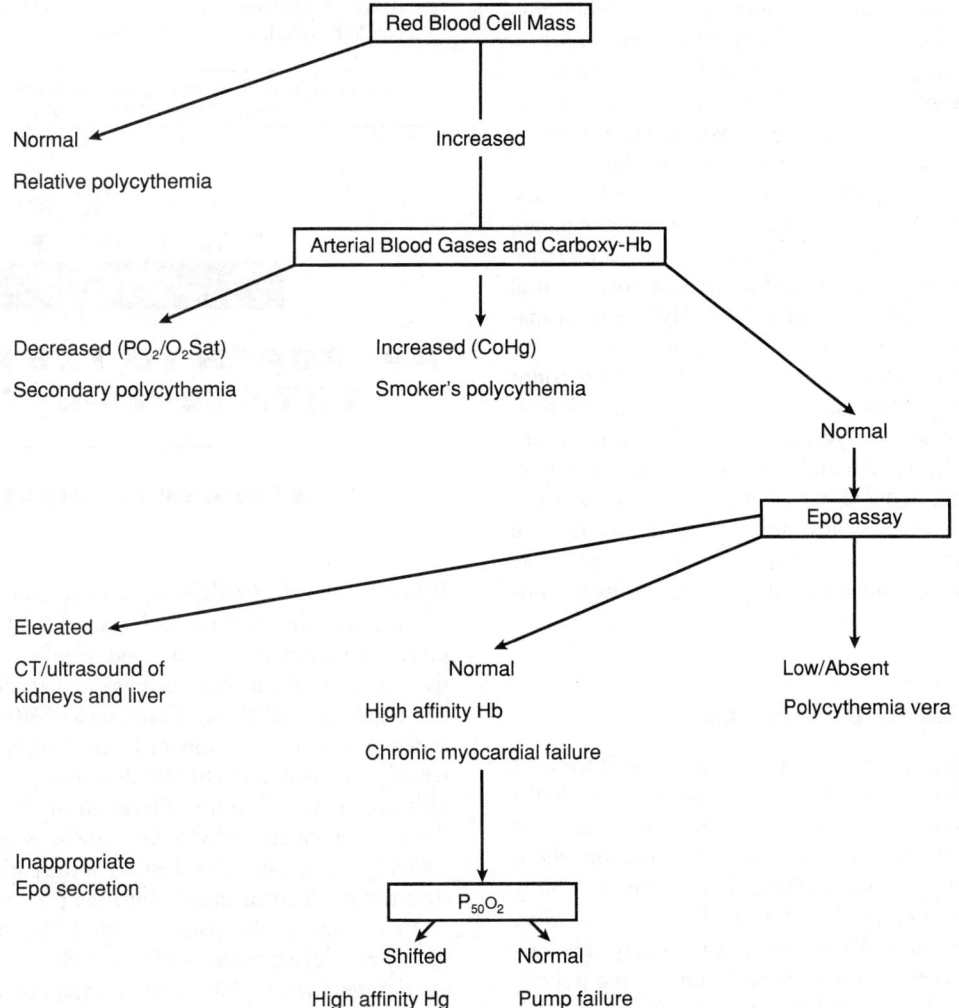

FIGURE 215.1. Algorithm for evaluation of patient with an elevated hemoglobin level. Carboxyhemoglobin is measured only for smokers or when there is potential industrial exposure. Bone marrow culture to separate normal EPO-dependent growth from EPO-independent growth in polycythemia vera is of value, but relatively unavailable. A patient with a normal EPO level and no other findings should be considered for $P_{50}O_2$ measurement to identify very rare high-affinity hemoglobin, more than 40 of which are recognized. Long-standing myocardial failure also can produce these findings.
EVIDENCE LEVEL: C. Expert Opinion.

of the physiologic burden of the increased RBC mass must be considered. Clinical wisdom is that the increase in RBCs provides needed compensation for the underlying hypoxia-related disease and that therapy should not perturb this compensatory status.

Because blood viscosity is directly related to RBC mass, concern has focused on the potential cardiovascular burden. Work capacity improves after phlebotomy reduction of hematocrit from 63% to 48% among patients with secondary polycythemia. Patients with obstructive lung disease whose hematocrit is reduced to normal have a decrease in pulmonary artery pressure, total pulmonary vascular resistance, and right ventricular work. This supports the view that RBC production frequently overcompensates for physiologic needs and that a phlebotomy program using the patient's symptoms as therapeutic criteria is appropriate. Most patients with secondary polycythemia have

maximum cardiopulmonary function with a hematocrit maintained in the range of 47% to 50%.

Polycythemia Vera

Because polycythemia vera evolves through several stages, therapy is focused on the critical clinical issues in the specific phase (see Chapter 231). In the pre-erythrocytic phase, histamine H_1- and H_2- blocking agents provide relief from the primary symptom of pruritus. Recombinant interferon-alfa also has been effective in controlling pruritus. Phlebotomy therapy has substantially prolonged median survival time, and it is the primary therapeutic modality used during the erythrocytic phase, when RBC mass and whole-blood viscosity are mainly responsible for the clinical findings. The therapeutic target is a hematocrit of 44% to 50%.

Hydroxyurea has been used to reduce risk for phlebotomy-related thrombotic events during the initial 2 to 3 years of therapy. This chemotherapeutic agent appears to have the least mutagenic and leukemogenic potential of the vast number of agents tried. Recombinant interferon-alfa has proved effective at reducing RBC values. Iron deficiency does supervene during serial phlebotomy, but iron replacement should be avoided, because high iron levels stimulate RBC production. Patients with a high phlebotomy requirement or those who enter the proliferative phase, in which the associated thrombocythemia poses clinical risk, should be treated with suppressive drugs. Hydroxyurea anagrelide and interferon are effective (see Chapter 231).

The primary aims of therapy are to maintain platelet count at less than 500,000 per microliter and hematocrit at less than 48%. Late in the course of polycythemia vera, the clinical problems are related to the anemia and progressive splenomegaly of the postpolycythemic myeloid metaplasia phase. Transfusions and, for those with relatively low serum EPO levels, the use of EPO are supportive measures. For patients with late-stage leukemic transformation, the therapy is that used for any secondary acute leukemia.

COMPLICATIONS AND PITFALLS

The primary complication in the care of a patient with elevated RBC values is risk for cerebral ischemia or the cardiac arrhythmias or ischemia associated with a phlebotomy program. This is particularly true of patients older than 60 years, for whom the volume shifts may produce dramatic changes. Small-volume (100 to 200 mL) phlebotomy should be used, particularly when treatment begins; volume replacement increases safety. The primary diagnostic pitfall is failure to identify underlying polycythemia in a patient who has had recent bleeding and who has normal or borderline RBC values and a decreased mean corpuscular volume that provides evidence of iron-deficient erythropoiesis with a drive to increased RBC production.

BIBLIOGRAPHY

de la Chapelle A, Traskelin AL, Juvonen E. Truncated erythropoietin receptor causes dominantly inherited benign human erythrocytosis. *Proc Natl Acad Sci USA* 1993;90:4495–4499.

Frenkel EP, McCall MS, Reisch JS, et al. An analysis of methods for the prediction of normal erythrocyte mass. *Am J Clin Pathol* 1972;58:260–271.

Hocking WG, Golde DW. Polycythemia: evaluation and management. *Blood Rev* 1989;3:59–65.

Hsia CCW. Respiratory function of hemoglobin. *N Engl J Med* 1998;338:239–247.

Kralovics R, Sokol L, Broxson Jr EH, et al. The erythropoietin receptor gene is not linked with the polycythemia phenotype in a family with autosomal dominant primary polycythemia. *Proc Assoc Am Physicians* 1997;6:580–585.

Michiels JJ. Diagnostic criteria of the myeloproliferative disorders (MPD): essential thrombocythemia, polycythemia vera and chronic megakaryocytic granulocytic metaplasia. *Neth J Med* 1997;51:57–64.

Silva M, Richard C, Benito A, et al. Expression of Bcl-X in erythroid precursors from patients with polycythemia vera. *N Engl J Med* 1998;338:564–571.

Weinreb NJ. Relative polycythemia. In: Wasserman LR, Berk PD, Berlin NI, eds. *Polycythemia vera and the myeloproliferative disorders.* Philadelphia: WB Saunders, 1995:226–258.

Kelley's Textbook of Internal Medicine, fourth edition. Edited by H. David Humes. Lippincott Williams & Wilkins, Philadelphia © 2000.

CHAPTER

216

APPROACH TO THE PATIENT WITH LEUKOCYTOSIS

STEPHEN G. EMERSON

White blood cells (WBCs) are mobile agents of infectious surveillance and tissue repair. Each class of WBC, including neutrophils, monocytes, eosinophils, and lymphocytes, makes a distinctive contribution to host defense and repair. The production and regulated trafficking of each class of WBC, whether orchestrated by the bone marrow or by the lymph nodes, is extremely sensitive to acute and chronic demands produced by infection, inflammation, and injury. Elevation in the WBC count above the normal range, called leukocytosis, is extremely common. Careful and thoughtful evaluation of the patient with leukocytosis can provide great insight into the patient's health.

In evaluating the patient with leukocytosis, the clinician should ask three questions. First, which class or classes of WBCs are elevated: neutrophils, lymphocytes, monocytes, eosinophils, basophils, or monocytes? The causes of leukocytosis are quite distinctive, depending on which class of white cells is elevated, and pinpointing which class of cells is too numerous is the critical first step. Second, how high is the elevation? All normal ranges are really the mean plus or minus two standard deviations of a large population sampling, and in the course of a medical practice, many normal individuals with "abnormally" elevated WBC counts will be encountered. Conversely, the higher the WBC count, the less likely it is that the elevation is a normal Gaussian variation. Third, for how long has the particular subset of WBCs been elevated? The differential diagnoses of acute elevations of each class of leukocytes are different from those of chronic elevations, and lifelong elevations are distinctive altogether.

Once the clinician has determined the specific cell type that is elevated, the degree of elevation, and the chronicity of the problem, a specific list of likely differential diagnoses should be generated. With this list in hand, the next step is to review or repeat the history and physical examination of the patient, focusing on those features that can differentiate the specific diagnoses under consideration. It is frequently important to repeat the initial interview and examination because the clinician may not ask the critical questions or may miss a subtle physical finding without the elevated WBC count in hand. After this process is completed, the clinician reevaluates the list of likely diagnoses, effectively reorganizing the list from most to least likely.

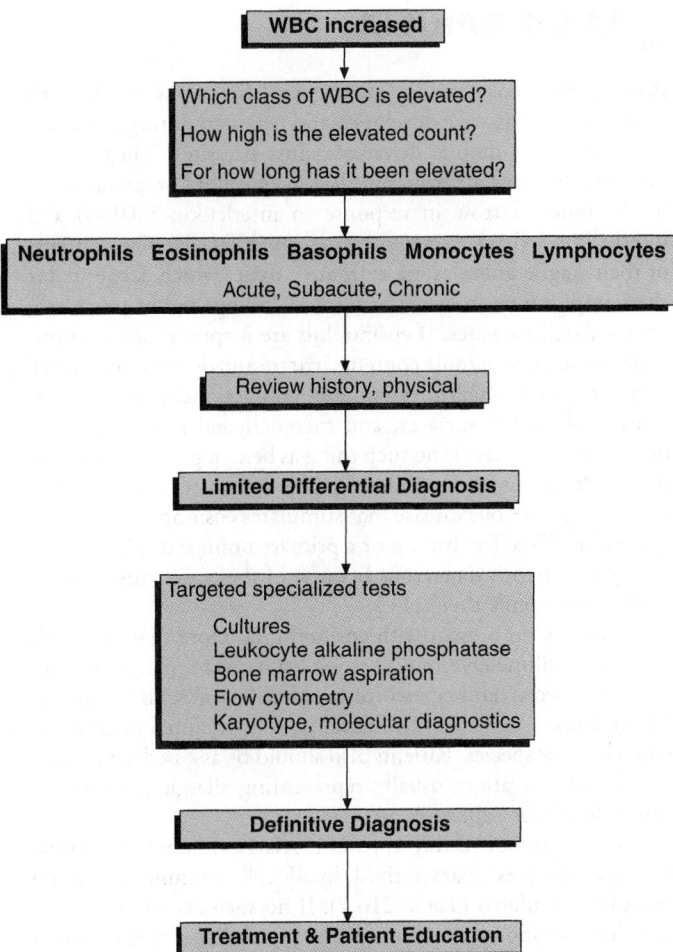

FIGURE 216.1. Algorithm for evaluation of the patient with leukocytosis.

With the newly organized list of differential diagnoses in hand, specialized tests can be ordered if necessary. These can include hematology cytochemical stains, such as leukocyte alkaline phosphatase; serologic tests for viral illnesses; flow cytometric analyses of circulating blood cells; and bone marrow aspiration. Results of the appropriate focused tests usually pinpoint the diagnosis. Following this evaluation algorithm leads directly and efficiently to accurate diagnoses (Fig. 216.1).

■ NEUROPHILIA

In the adult, the neutrophils usually constitute most of the circulating WBCs. What makes evaluation of neutrophilia interesting is that the neutrophils measured by phlebotomy are only 5% of the total body neutrophil pool at any one time, and they are being measured during only 2% to 3% of their lifetime, in rapid transit from the bone marrow to the tissues. Because the neutrophil count normally varies widely within a broad range, a single sampling can be confusing. A single circulating neutrophil count is a snapshot of one corner of a rapidly changing cellular population.

CONSTITUTIONAL NEUTROPHILIAS

Some individuals are totally normal but have neutrophil counts above the "normal range." Five percent of individuals tested have neutrophil counts above the mean plus two standard deviations (approximately 8,000 per cubic millimeter) in any laboratory. Although sometimes high neutrophil counts are found to be normal when repeated, in other individuals the neutrophil count is always high. Individuals have been followed for as long as two decades with elevated neutrophil counts, without known causes or consequences. Such *chronic idiopathic neutrophilia* can be an isolated occurrence in an individual or can rarely be hereditary. The only important caveat is that patients with otherwise obscure neutrophilia should have congenital asplenia excluded by ultrasonography.

Uncommon genetic disorders that are accompanied by neutrophilia include leukocyte adhesion deficiency, familial myeloproliferative disease, and Down's syndrome, but these are invariably diagnosed in childhood.

ACUTE ACQUIRED NEUTROPHILIA

Neutrophilia is an acquired disorder in most patients in whom it is detected. Because neutrophils are the infantry of the inflammatory and immune systems, frequently employed in any and all combat theaters, neutrophilia is a common finding with any infection, inflammation, injury, or stress. Acute or chronic bacterial infection, acute myocardial infarction (usually paralleling the rise and fall of aspartate aminotransaminase levels), pulmonary embolism, and trauma or surgery are probably the most common causes seen in clinical practice.

Although neutrophilia follows the stress of many surgical procedures temporarily, splenectomy can result in prolonged or even lifelong neutrophilia as high as 20,000 to 25,000 per cubic millimeter. Heat stroke, burns, hemolysis, diabetic ketoacidosis, acute thyrotoxicosis, and acute gout are additional stresses that often result in neutrophilia. A clinician discovering new-onset neutrophilia should carefully evaluate the patient for these common occurrences (Table 216.1).

Patients should be questioned about drug treatments that commonly cause neutrophilia, including epinephrine, corticosteroids, and lithium, as well as the recombinant pharmaceuticals granulocyte colony-stimulating factor (G-CSF) and granulocyte–macrophage colony-stimulating factor (GM-CSF). Epinephrine releases into the circulation a sequestered pool of mature neutrophils that normally adhere to the vascular endothelium. Patients receiving subcutaneous epinephrine for bronchospasm, for example, develop neutrophilias in the range of 10,000 to 20,000 per cubic millimeter. Corticosteroids accelerate the release of neutrophils and bands from a large storage pool within the bone marrow, resulting in neutrophilia often accompanied by an increase in band forms. Lithium, usually prescribed for bipolar affective disorders, also raises the neutrophil count by an unknown mechanism. G-CSF and GM-CSF are parenteral pharmaceuticals that are prescribed by hematologists and oncologists, and their use should be easily identified.

SUBACUTE AND CHRONIC NEUTROPHILIA

For patients in whom neutrophilia is acquired but has a longer history or does not disappear when potential common causes are

TABLE 216.1.	COMMON CAUSES OF NEUTROPHILIA

Acute neutrophilia
  Infection (esp. bacteria)
  Trauma
  Tissue infarction: pulmonary embolism, myocardial infarction, sickle cell crisis, burns
  Labor and delivery
  Hypoxia
  Drugs (esp. adrenergic agonists, corticosteroids, lithium, granulocyte–macrophage colony-stimulating factors)
  Diabetic ketoacidosis
  Acute gout
  Renal failure, hepatic coma
  Hemolytic anemia
  Hemorrhage
Chronic but acquired neutrophilia
  Infections (esp. osteomyelitis, sinusitis)
  Vasculitis (esp. polyarteritis nodosum)
  Chronic pulmonary emboli
  Pericarditis, pleuritis
  Carcinomas, malignant lymphomas, Hodgkin's disease
  Chronic myelogenous leukemia
  Polycythemia vera
  Myelofibrosis and myeloid metaplasia
  Splenectomy
Life-long neutrophilia
  Chronic idopathic neutrophilia
  Hereditary neutrophilia
  Asplenia

remedied, a more extensive and slightly different list of diagnoses needs to be considered. These include chronic infections, recurrent pulmonary emboli, vasculitis (especially polyarteritis nodosa), chronic pleuritis or pericarditis, Hodgkin's disease, and a variety of tumors, including carcinomas (especially bladder and pancreatic tumors) and lymphomas. Although acute myelogenous leukemia rarely presents with neutrophilia, circulating blasts with any mature neutrophil count necessitates bone marrow aspiration to rule out acute myelogenous leukemia. Persistently elevated neutrophil counts can be the presenting sign of chronic myelogenous leukemia or, if accompanied by elevations in platelet counts, eosinophils, basophils, or polycythemia vera.

In evaluating persistent neutrophilia, the clinician must review the patient's history, physical examination results, and laboratory studies for indexes of these infectious, inflammatory, and neoplastic conditions. In pursuing this differential diagnosis, the leukocyte alkaline phosphatase cytochemical stain of circulating WBCs is often most useful. The result is uniformly near zero in chronic myelogenous leukemia, and it is normal to elevated in reactive secondary neutrophilias and in polycythemia vera. If the result is low, bone marrow aspiration for karyotyping to detect t(9:22) or molecular diagnostic evaluation for the presence of abnormal P210 BCR/ABL mRNAs should be performed to confirm the diagnosis of chronic myelogenous leukemia. If the leukocyte alkaline phosphatase result is normal or elevated, specific measures to identify or rule out the causes of persistent reactive neutrophilia should be vigorously pursued because they are all serious.

EOSINOPHILIA

Rose-staining eosinophils (*eos* means "dawn," as in Homer's "rosy-fingered dawn") developed and persisted during evolution as a specialized mobile defense against parasites. They are induced to differentiate from multilineage myeloid progenitor cells in the bone marrow in response to interleukin-5 (IL-5) and interleukin-3 (IL-3) secreted by activated T cells. The contents of their fragile granules are extremely toxic, which accounts for their importance in penetrating and killing highly protected, encapsulated parasites. If eosinophils are inappropriately stimulated, these same granule contents irritate and deform the normal structures with which they come in contact, including vascular walls, endocardial surfaces, and mesenchymal tissues. Because of these effects, there is no such thing as benign persistent eosinophilia. Persistent eosinophilia signifies a serious parasitic infection or other serious disease that stimulates eosinophilia through generalized T-cell activation or a primary nonreactive hypereosinophilia, which is dangerous because of the toxic consequences of the eosinophils themselves.

Patients who present with eosinophilia (more than 450 cells per cubic millimeter) should first be evaluated for parasites, especially hookworm and tapeworm, and for *Ascaris*, schistosomiasis, *Strongyloides* (roundworm), filarial worms, trichinal infestation, and *Toxocara* species. Patients also should be assessed for overactive T-cell activation, usually representing allergic reactions to drugs, foods, or exposures.

If these are not readily apparent, a large number of unusual systemic diseases characterized by T-cell immune activation must be considered (Table 216.2). If no such causes are found, the clinician should evaluate for the possibility that the patient has a clonal T-cell lymphoproliferative disorder in which the abnormally expanded clone autonomously secretes IL-5 or

TABLE 216.2.	COMMON CAUSES OF EOSINOPHILIA

Acute eosinophilia
  Allergic reactions: drugs, food exposures
  Parasites
  Arthropod infestations (esp. scabies)
  Protozoan infections: *Pneumocystis, Plasmodium, Entamoeba histolytica, Toxoplasma*
Chronic eosinophilia
  Addison's disease
  Vasculitis: Wegener's granulomatosis, Churg–Strauss disease, Loffler's endocarditis, polyarteritis nodosum, Goodpasture's syndrome
  Sarcoidosis
  Postinfectious eosinophilia (esp. poststreptococcal infections)
  Eosinophilic gastroenteritis
  Inflammatory skin diseases: eczema, dermatitis herpetiformis, ichthyosis, pityriasis
  Chronic myelogenous leukemia
  Pernicious anemia
  Polycythemia vera
  Hodgkin's disease
  Carcinomas, lymphomas
  T-cell chronic lymphocytic leukemia
  Idiopathic hypereosinophilic syndrome

IL-3 and therefore should pursue T-cell gene rearrangement studies of peripheral blood mononuclear cells. Chronic myeloid leukemia should also be considered if neutrophilia is present as well.

If no specific diagnosis can be made to direct treatment, the patient is left with the diagnosis of idiopathic hypereosinophilic syndrome, at which point anti-eosinophilic treatment is initiated to prevent vasculitic and mesenchymal toxicities.

BASOPHILIA

Basophilia is rare and should prompt the clinician to consider many of the conditions that trigger eosinophilia. However, persistent basophilia (more than 100 cells per cubic millimeter) is a common sign of myeloproliferative diseases such as chronic myelogenous leukemia, or polycythemia vera and myelodysplasia (preleukemia). Patients with undiagnosed basophilia should undergo bone marrow aspiration for morphologic and karyotyping studies.

MONOCYTOSIS

Monocytes serve as the initiators of the immune response through antigen presentation, through secretion of activating cytokines such as IL-1α and tumor necrosis factor α, and as effectors of ingestion of invading organisms. Monocytosis (more than 1,000 cells per cubic millimeter) is most often the sign of an acute bacterial, viral, protozoal, or rickettsial infection. Monocytosis in the absence of significant neutrophilia occurs especially in cases of tuberculosis, syphilis, brucellosis, and typhoid fever, and these diagnoses should be considered and evaluated. Chronic inflammatory conditions can stimulate sustained monocytosis.

Unexplained persistent monocytosis should raise the suspicion of occult leukemia, especially acute monocytic leukemia, and should be evaluated by bone marrow aspiration.

LYMPHOCYTOSIS

Most circulating lymphocytes are T cells, and their numbers increase as the normal response to any viral infection. The most common cause of lymphocytosis is an acute viral illness. In many cases, the numerous lymphocytes appear large and vacuolated, a sign of their activation against viral antigens on infected target cells, such as the Epstein–Barr virus–infected B lymphocytes of infectious mononucleosis.

Persistent lymphocytosis is unusual as a sign of infectious disease. Much more commonly, lymphocytosis is a sign of a clonal lymphoproliferative disease. If persistent lymphocytosis (more than 6,000 cells per cubic millimeter) is detected, chronic lymphocytic leukemia should be considered first in the differential diagnosis. The clinician should reinterview the patient, with particular attention to eliciting complaints of fevers, weight loss, and night sweats, and reexamine the patient, concentrating on the lymph nodes, liver, and spleen. The peripheral blood smear

should be examined for the presence of many broken "smudge" cells, a sign of B-cell chronic lymphocytic leukemia, or large lymphocytes with fine granules, a sign of T-cell chronic lymphocytic leukemia. In cases of persistent, significant lymphocytosis, peripheral blood should be evaluated by flow cytometry for patterns of lymphocyte cell surface proteins diagnostic of T-cell or B-cell chronic lymphocytic leukemia.

BIBLIOGRAPHY

Hoffman R, Benz EJ, Shattil SJ, et al. *Hematology: basic principles and practice.* New York: Churchill Livingstone, 1994.
Israels MCG, Delamore IW. *Haematological aspects of system disease.* London: WB Saunders, 1976.

Kelley's Textbook of Internal Medicine, fourth edition. Edited by H. David Humes. Lippincott Williams & Wilkins, Philadelphia © 2000.

C H A P T E R
217

APPROACH TO THE PATIENT WITH THROMBOCYTOSIS

ALAN M. GEWIRTZ

PRESENTATION

Thrombocytosis is defined as a sustained elevation in platelet count. As will be discussed below, a variety of mechanisms may result in this condition, and presentation largely depends on the cause of the platelet count increase. In the vast majority of cases, thrombocytosis is asymptomatic and therefore comes to the attention of a physician only when a routine blood count reveals its presence. The likely reason for this will be discussed below. In those patients who do have symptoms directly referable to their elevated platelet count, the most common presenting complaints are related to occlusive phenomena of the microcirculation of the central nervous system and/or the peripheral vasculature. Headache, dizziness, or episodes consistent with transient ischemic attacks are common, as are paresthesias and acrocyanosis of the digits. A particularly dramatic presenting complaint is a syndrome known as erythromelalgia. It is characterized by erythema, burning, and intense pain of the fingers and toes, and it is often dramatically improved by a single dose of aspirin. Thrombosis of larger arteries or veins is less common but may be found in approximately 2% to 20% of patients at the time of diagnosis. Although it is not unusual for a patient to have thrombotic and bleeding complaints simultaneously, bleeding in the absence of thrombosis is several times less common. When an isolated hemorrhagic diathesis is present, it typically manifests itself in the form of epistaxis, hematuria, or gastrointestinal bleeding.

PATHOPHYSIOLOGIC FACTORS

Since platelets are derived from megakaryocytes it seems self-evident that a basic understanding of megakaryocyte developmental biology and thrombopoiesis would aid in the understanding of the pathogenesis of quantitative platelet production disorders. This subject is reviewed briefly below.

Megakaryocytes, like all hematopoietic cells, are ultimately derived from an undifferentiated pluripotent hematopoietic stem cell (Fig. 217.1). By mechanisms still unknown, a stem cell gives rise to a daughter cell that is committed to development within the megakaryocyte lineage. Subsequent development is characterized by progenitor cell proliferation, followed by terminal maturation of non-dividing cells. The proliferative step is necessary to produce the requisite numbers of megakaryocytes needed for daily platelet production. Terminal maturation is concerned with carrying out the steps needed for actual thrombopoiesis. These focus on cytoplasmic maturation, as well as on increasing cellular DNA content by a process known as endoreduplication in which multiple rounds of DNA synthesis occur in the absence of cell division. Endoreduplication is a development characteristic that is unique to megakaryocytes.

Thrombopoiesis is also poorly understood. Platelets are formed within the megakaryocyte cytoplasm and may then be shed by a variety of mechanisms. For example, they may be released like seeds from a pod into vascular sinuses in the bone marrow. Alternatively, megakaryocytes may extend long pseudopods into the vascular sinusoids and then fracture into platelets as a result of flow-induced shear stress. It has also been postulated that entire cells migrate into the vascular sinusoids where they then travel to the lung. Cell fracturing and platelet release take place as the cells traverse the pulmonary vasculature.

The gene that encodes the major protein regulator of megakaryocyte development, thrombopoietin *(TPO)*, has recently been cloned. It is perhaps not surprising that the human gene maps to the long arm of chromosome 3 (3q26–27) since inversions, insertions, and translocations involving the long arm of chromosome 3 have been associated with megakaryocyte hyperplasia and thrombocytosis. The *TPO* gene encodes a 322-amino-acid protein. The biological activity of the protein appears to reside in the amino terminus, which, interestingly, has significant homology to erythropoietin, the principal regulator of red cell production.

Although *TPO* appears to play a major role in regulating megakaryocyte and platelet production, other cytokines, including interleukins 3, 6, and 11, stem cell factor, and fetal liver kinase-2 (flk-2) ligand also influence this process.

HISTORY AND PHYSICAL EXAMINATION

Thrombocytosis may result from an intrinsic proliferative abnormality of megakaryocyte progenitor cells or an abnormal stimu-

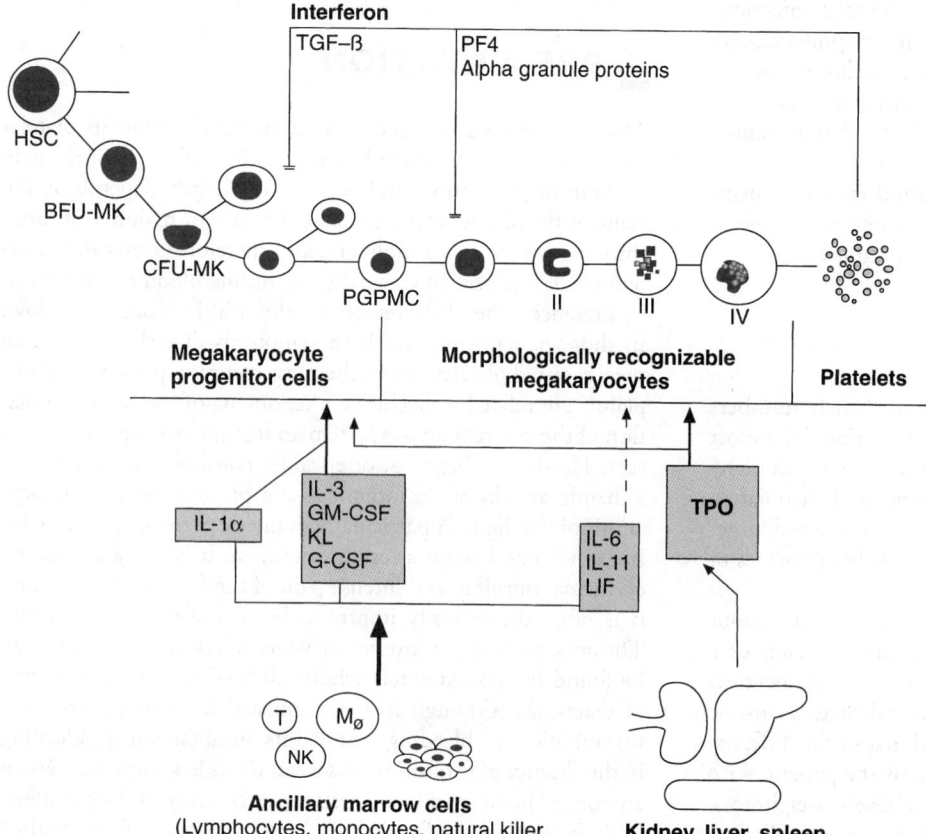

FIGURE 217.1. Human megakaryocytes are derived from a pluripotent hematopoietic stem cell. Human megakaryocyte progenitor cells, the burst-forming unit and colony-forming unit megakaryocyte, give rise to platelet glycoprotein–bearing mononuclear cells, which are the immediate progenitors of mature, platelet-producing megakaryocytes. Megakaryocytes evolve through four morphologically recognizable stages that are characterized on the basis of their nuclear morphology and nuclear/cytoplasmic ratio. When maturation is complete, the megakaryocytes give rise to platelets. Positive and negative regulators of this process are depicted in the figure.

TABLE 217.1. FEATURES HELPFUL IN DIFFERENTIATING ESSENTIAL FROM REACTIVE THROMBOCYTOSIS		
Diagnostic Features	Reactive Thrombocytosis	Essential Thrombocytosis
History		
Chronic inflammatory disorder or infection	+	−
Nonhematologic malignancy	+	−
Acute blood loss or trauma	+	−
Splenectomy	+	−
Easy bruising; abnormal bleeding	−	+
Thromboembolic phenomena	−	+
Physical Examination		
Petechiae, ecchymoses	−	+
Splenomegaly	+/−	+
Hepatomegaly	+/−	+
Laboratory Evaluation		
Platelet count >600,000/μL	+	+
Elevated ESR, C-reactive protein, fibrinogen, interleukin-6 level	+	−
Morphologic abnormalities on blood or bone marrow smear	−	+
Absent marrow irion, normal or elevated serum ferritin, MCV normal	+	−
Increased marrow reticulin or marrow fibrosis	−	+/−
Abnormal cytogenetics	−	+/−, bcr/abl (−)
Increased bleeding time	−	+
Diminished platelet aggregation in response to epinephrine	−	+
Spontaneous megakaryocyte or erythroid colony formation	−	+

+, consistent with; −, feature not observed; +/−, feature observed inconsistently or mildly; ESR, erythrocyte sedimentation rate; MCV, mean corpuscular volume.

lus that drives otherwise normal megakaryocyte progenitor cells to proliferate. The former mechanism leads to primary, or essential, thrombocytosis (ET), whereas the latter leads to a secondary, or reactive, thrombocytosis (RT). Either circumstance leads to an increase in megakaryocyte mass and a rise in platelet count. The primary task for the physician evaluating a patient with thrombocytosis is to determine which mechanism is operative because the course, prognosis, and treatment of each form varies considerably (Table 217.1).

A detailed history can be useful in attempting to differentiate ET from RT. RT is commonly observed in a diverse array of clinical conditions that have an accompanying inflammatory component. Acute and chronic tissue infections, rheumatoid arthritis, inflammatory bowel disease, malignancies, and injury or surgically related trauma may be accompanied by thrombocytosis. Recent splenectomy is particularly likely to produce thrombocytosis. The spleen serves as an important storage site for platelets, and counts are transiently elevated after the spleen is removed, although mild elevations can persist in about one third of these patients. Iron-deficiency anemia is commonly associated with RT and should be suspected in young female patients with a history of heavy menstrual bleeding. A history compatible with any of the above mentioned conditions should initially suggest a diagnosis of RT. Nevertheless, 20% to 30% of patients

with ET may also have constitutional symptoms, including fever, weight loss, and night sweats. As bleeding or thrombotic complications are exceptionally rare in patients with RT, any such history should immediately suggest that the elevated platelet count is caused by ET. The results of previous blood tests are helpful in documenting duration and trend of the thrombocytosis and should be sought.

Although the physical examination is rarely definitive, it may at times be helpful in determining the cause of thrombocytosis. Neurologic findings and erythromelalgia would certainly suggest a diagnosis of ET. On the other hand, pale skin and conjunctiva, suggestive of recent blood loss or anemia, would be consistent with RT. Enlarged lymph nodes, spleen, or mass lesions are suggestive of an underlying malignancy as the cause of the elevated platelet count, as are the joint deformities common to rheumatoid arthritis. Nevertheless, the liver and spleen are enlarged in about 20% to 40% of ET patients, respectively. Accordingly, the physical examination may be very ambiguous.

LABORATORY STUDIES AND DIAGNOSTIC TESTS

As neither the history nor the physical examination is conclusive, the diagnosis of ET or RT often depends on the results of laboratory testing. Since ET typically becomes a diagnosis of exclusion, the goal of testing is to exclude abnormalities known to be associated with RT, other myeloproliferative disorders associated with elevated platelet counts, in particular polycythemia vera and chronic myelogenous leukemia. From this perspective, evaluation of the peripheral blood smear and a bone marrow aspirate or biopsy can be helpful.

White blood cell counts may be elevated in both RT and ET and are not discriminatory unless morphologic abnormalities, such as immature or dysplastic myeloid precursors, are noted. The presence of such forms are suggestive of a myeloproliferative disorder or myelodysplastic syndrome. Anemia in the absence of other hematologic abnormalities suggests an RT. Platelet morphology is helpful only if megathrombocytes or large, bizarre-looking cells are present. Such abnormalities are associated with myeloproliferative disorder. Platelet counts per se are of little use in differentiating primary from reactive thrombocytosis. The pervasive notion that counts greater than $1,000 \times 10^9$ per liter signify the presence of ET is incorrect. Personal observation and published reports document that RT patients may have counts that exceed $2,000 \times 10^9$ per liter. Unfortunately, duration of platelet count elevation may not discriminate between RT and ET because many of the conditions associated with RT tend to be chronic.

In ET and RT patients, the bone marrow may be hypercellular, with an increase in the megakaryocyte-to-erythrocyte ratio. As was true in the peripheral blood, absence of morphologic abnormalities does not reliably discriminate between ET and RT. However, if such abnormalities are demonstrable, it becomes unlikely that the condition is reactive. Much attention is typically paid to cells of the megakaryocyte lineage. Hematopathologists look for dysplastic megakaryocytes, which are characterized by unusually large or small sizes and by abnormally lobulated nuclei. Small, hypolobulated megakaryocytes are thought to be typical of chronic myelogenous leukemia. Megakaryocyte clusters or aggregates are often associated with ET, but they are not specific because such formations may be found in as many as 25% of RT patients. Marrow reticulin is not increased in RT, and there is no fibrosis. In ET, marrow reticulin ranges from normal to slightly increased in essential thrombocytosis to grossly fibrotic in myelofibrosis with myeloid metaplasia.

It is difficult to diagnose ET in the absence of stainable marrow iron because polycythemia vera characteristically has absent marrow iron and RT is associated with iron deficiency. Nevertheless, absent marrow iron may result from artifact. Helpful clues to discern such artifact would be normal or increased serum ferritin and normal red blood cell mean corpuscular volume. In addition, recent studies suggest that a hematocrit greater than 60 is always due to polycythemia vera and never ET.

Marrow cytogenetics are not often diagnostic because they are normal in RT and in more than 95% of cases of ET. Despite this, cytogenetic testing may be worthwhile because it occasionally detects an abnormality consistent with a myelodysplastic syndrome (5q−) or the Philadelphia chromosome t(9:22) of chronic myelogenous leukemia.

Platelet function tests are commonly employed to differentiate ET from RT. Results of these tests, which typically include a bleeding time and aggregation in response to various agonists,

are normal in patients with RT. For ET patients, prolonged bleeding time, spontaneous aggregation, and impaired aggregation, especially in response to epinephrine, have been widely reported. Unfortunately, spontaneous aggregation is an unreliable test, and some otherwise normal patients (15%) have impaired aggregation in response to epinephrine or other aggregating agents, thereby lessening the test's discriminatory power. The common use of aspirin, nonsteroidal anti-inflammatory drugs, and other agents that impair platelet function is also problematic because they obviously render platelet function tests uninterpretable. The physician should be certain that the patient has not used these drugs or over-the-counter preparations containing these medications before carrying out platelet function studies.

Several cytokines may augment megakaryocytopoiesis and thrombopoiesis. Of these, IL-6 has been shown to be particularly active in vitro. This cytokine has several other activities, the most important of which may be its B-cell-stimulatory activity. Interleukin-6 production is augmented in acute inflammatory responses and in a variety of chronic inflammatory states. Plasma levels of IL-6 have been reported to be elevated in patients with RT but not in those with ET. The C-reactive protein levels parallel IL-6 levels and therefore give similar, but less expensive, information. Plasma fibrinogen levels in excess of 500 mg per deciliter have been reported to be sensitive and reasonably specific for RT. Least expensive of all these options, and one that probably yields qualitatively similar information, is the erythrocyte sedimentation rate. It is a sensitive, although nonspecific, test for inflammatory states.

With the recent cloning of the *TPO* gene and its receptor, c-*mpl*, it has been natural to explore the relationship between expression and/or mutation of these genes and the development of thrombocytosis. A number of publications suggest that *TPO* levels are elevated in ET but not in RT. One investigation of familial ET suggested that there were no mutations present in the c-*mpl* receptor. It is of interest, however, that a splice donor mutation in the *TPO* gene resulting in higher levels of *TPO* has been reported in a kindred with hereditary ET. The practicality and reliability of these assays remain to be determined.

In many cases, none of the standard tests can differentiate RT from ET, and it may be useful to contact a laboratory that is capable of cloning hematopoietic progenitor cells. My colleagues and I reported several years ago that patients with ET have dramatically increased numbers of assayable megakaryocyte colony-forming units (CFUs-MK) compared with normal controls or patients with RT. The CFUs-MK from ET patients had significantly increased proliferative capacity and the ability to form colonies without an exogenous source of growth factors. This observation has been confirmed by several groups and may therefore be of use in diagnosing particularly difficult cases. However, colony assays are not standardized, and long-term follow-up studies correlating colony-forming ability with disease status have not been reported. These factors, combined with the limited availability of such testing, suggest that CFU-MK assays should not be considered part of the routine workup of these patients.

DIFFERENTIAL DIAGNOSIS

The differential diagnosis of an elevated platelet count has been suggested by the discussion in the preceding paragraphs. The major decision is whether the condition is secondary or primary. As discussed in previous sections, there are multiple secondary causes of an elevated platelet count, and treatment of the underlying cause normalizes the platelet count in virtually all cases; this is a major differential point. As was mentioned above, several primary marrow disorders may manifest with a prominent thrombocytotic component. These conditions include myeloproliferative disorders, myelodysplastic syndrome associated with the 5q− syndrome, and even some acute leukemias. The latter are associated with inversion of chromosome 3.

Although it has been estimated that as many as one-third of cases of thrombocytosis will ultimately be found to have an underlying myeloproliferative disorder, more recent reports cast doubt on this figure. A recent study of 280 hospitalized patients found that even when the platelet count exceeded 1×10^9 per liter, approximately 80% had a nonhematologic condition as underlying cause of their elevated platelet count, and only 14% had a myeloproliferative disorder. Modern clonality studies using molecular analytical techniques suggest that this figure may be even lower.

STRATEGIES FOR OPTIMAL CARE

Management depends on whether the cause of the platelet count elevation is primary or secondary. Since bleeding or thrombotic complications directly attributable to the platelet count elevation are quite rare in patients with secondary thrombocytosis, intervention (other than identifying and treating the underlying cause, and advising patients who smoke to quit) is rarely indicated.

Patients with essential thrombocytosis have an excellent long-term prognosis. Although extended follow-up studies are few, the disease appears to be highly compatible with a normal life expectancy. ET rarely transforms into acute leukemia, and only about one-third of patients experience a major bleeding or thrombotic complication. Unfortunately, neither bleeding nor thrombosis can be predicted on the basis of platelet count elevation or platelet function abnormalities. Accordingly, it is not always clear as to who should be treated and when such treatment should be initiated. In a young, asymptomatic patient with no history of coronary or peripheral vascular disease, it is defensible to observe the patient only. In older individuals, in particular those with vascular disease, treatment is likely indicated. Recent studies suggest that thrombotic complications are uncommon in individuals with platelet counts below 600×10^9 per liter. Many hematologists therefore use this value as a goal when initiating treatment.

In the acute setting, such as significant bleeding or a major thrombotic event, platelet pheresis combined with myelosuppressive therapy, typically administration of hydroxyurea, rapidly lowers the platelet count. The usual dosage of hydroxyurea in this setting is 2 g per day or higher. The clinical goal again is to bring the platelet count below the level of 600×10^9 per liter.

For long-term control, hydroxyurea has been the drug of choice. Studies of a relatively large number of patients suggest that this drug may be particularly useful in patients who are at high risk of developing thrombotic complications. Hydroxyurea is inexpensive and generally well tolerated. When carefully monitored, its side effects usually are limited to gastrointestinal upset and dermatologic manifestations, especially hyperpigmentation. It is important to note, however, that this agent is not without risk. There are data to indicate that hydroxyurea is leukemogenic in myeloproliferative disorder patients. Having said this, however, the Polycythemia Vera Study Group's final report on ET indicates that leukemia only developed in patients who received hydroxyurea followed by another myelosuppressive agent, such as phosphorus 32, busulfan, or cyclophosphamide. In those treated with hydroxyurea only, there was no increased incidence of acute leukemia. Accordingly, the drug remains recommended. Usual doses are from 500 mg to 2 g per day, and the goal is to reduce the platelet count to less than 600×10^9 per liter without inducing leukopenia.

In addition to hydroxyurea, long-term control of platelet count can be maintained with anagrelide or interferon-α. Anagrelide, a quinazoline derivative, has been extremely effective in the management of thrombocytosis. The drug appears to affect thrombopoiesis at the level of the maturing megakaryocyte and to have no other significant effects on hematopoietic progenitor cells. When given in the usual doses of 1 to 4 mg per day, it is effective in more than 75% of patients. Its usual side effects include palpitations, headache, nausea, and fluid retention, which may be encountered in 20% to 30% of patients. This drug has recently received Food and Drug Administration approval, so that reports of its use in larger numbers of patients should become available before too long. Interferon-α is also effective. Typical doses are 3 to 5×10^6 units per day for 3 to 7 days a week. The drug is injected subcutaneously, which is problematic for some patients. In addition, it is expensive and is often poorly tolerated because of its side effects, which include fatigue, musculoskeletal pain, headache, and other flulike symptoms.

Symptoms due to erythromelalgia are easily managed with aspirin (300 to 500 mg per day) or nonsteroidal anti-inflammatory drugs. However, many authorities recommend that these agents be avoided, except for the indication previously discussed, because their use is associated with increased hemorrhagic complications.

As was noted above, the management of asymptomatic patients is somewhat controversial. Several studies of individuals younger than 40 years suggest that it is appropriate to manage such patients expectantly and to initiate treatment only when a patient develops vasomotor symptoms or a major bleeding or thrombotic episode. The long-term prognosis for these patients is excellent, and this must be balanced with the known and unknown risks of long-term administration of drugs such as hydroxyurea and anagrelide. In older patients, especially those with a history of thrombotic disease, it is probably wise to keep the platelet count below 600×10^9 per liter.

Pregnant patients are also problematic. The incidence of fetal wastage, probably caused by placental infarction, is not known with certainty; however, in one series the incidence was reported to be 45% of the 34 pregnancies observed in 18 patients. In this series, the outcome of the pregnancy could not be predicted from the height of the platelet count, the history of complications or lack thereof, or the treatment administered. Not giving any treatment appeared to be an acceptable alternative. Other series report that aspirin administration has been associated with successful pregnancies, although aspirin may increase the mother's risk of serious bleeding at the time of delivery.

Hydroxyurea and busulfan have been administered to a small number of patients during the first trimester without incident, but other physicians have reported an increase in fetal malformations. In patients who require chemotherapeutic agents for control of their platelet count, the most conservative course would be to advise against pregnancy. Attempts to control platelet counts with interferon may be an alternative strategy in this selected subset of patients. The teratogenic risk of interferon in human patients is unknown, but it has been administered to rhesus monkeys at 20 to 500 times the therapeutic dose without apparent teratogenic effect. However, in rhesus monkeys interferon had abortifacient activity.

The management of surgical patients can be complicated and should involve consultation with a hematologist–oncologist. In general, drugs that interfere with platelet function should be avoided because patients receiving agents such as aspirin are more likely to have bleeding complications. Suppressing the platelet count to less than 600×10^9 per liter is probably also indicated, especially for patients older than 60 years or those with previous thrombotic complications.

BIBLIOGRAPHY

Cortelazzo S, Finazzi G, Ruggeri M, et al. Hydroxyurea for patients with essential thrombocythemia and a high risk of thrombosis. *N Engl J Med* 1995;332:1132–1136.

Gewirtz, A. Megakaryocytopoiesis: the state of the art. *Thromb Haemost* 1995;74:204–209.

Gilbert HS. Long term treatment of myeloproliferative disease with interferon-alpha-2b: feasibility and efficacy. *Cancer* 1998;83:1205–1213.

Metcalf D. Thrombopoietin—at last. *Nature* 1994;369:519–520.

Murphy S, Peterson P, Illand H, et al. Experience of the Polycythemia Vera Study Group with essential thrombocythemia: final report on diagnostic criteria, survival, and leukemic transition by treatment. *Semin Hematol* 1997;34:29–39.

Neimer SD. Essential thrombocythemia: another "heterogeneous" disease better understood? *Blood* 1999;93:415.

Silverstein MN, Tefferi A. Treatment of essential thrombocythemia with anagrelide. *Semin Hematol* 1999; 36(1 Suppl 2):23–25.

Tefferi A, Hoagland HC. Issues in the diagnosis and management of essential thrombocythemia. *Mayo Clin Proc* 1994;69:651–655.

Wang JC, Chen C, Novetsky AD, et al. Blood thrombopoietin levels in clonal thrombocytosis and reactive thrombocytosis. *Am J Med* 1998; 104:451–455.

Wiestner A, Schlemper RJ, va der Maas AP, et al. An activating splice donor mutation in the thrombopoietin gene causes hereditary thrombocythemia. *Nature Genet* 1998;18:49–52.

Kelley's Textbook of Internal Medicine, fourth edition. Edited by H. David Humes. Lippincott Williams & Wilkins, Philadelphia © 2000.

APPROACH TO THE PATIENT WITH BLEEDING

KEITH R. McCRAE

PRESENTATION

Excessive bleeding complicates many medical and surgical illnesses. Patients requiring evaluation for a bleeding disorder usually present in a manner reflecting their underlying medical conditions, as well as the specific defect responsible for their hemorrhagic diathesis. For example, an apparently healthy woman with previously undiagnosed von Willebrand disease may present with a chief complaint of progressive fatigue, with hematologic evaluation revealing iron deficiency anemia. Further questioning may reveal a history of long-standing menorrhagia, with directed laboratory studies confirming the diagnosis of the coagulopathy. Such a presentation contrasts sharply with that of an elderly patient with no prior bleeding history who develops acute hemorrhage as a result of a vascular defect incurred during a surgical procedure.

Because of this wide array of clinical presentations, evaluation of the patient with excessive bleeding depends on a basic understanding of normal hemostatic mechanisms and the specific clinical symptoms resulting from their disruption. In this chapter, we review normal hemostatic pathways as well as the pathophysiology of some of the more common defects in this system that are associated with bleeding.

PATHOPHYSIOLOGIC FACTORS

Coagulation may be considered as two interdependent processes, referred to as primary and secondary hemostasis. Primary hemostasis is characterized by the formation of a platelet plug at the site of vascular trauma. This involves the adhesion of circulating platelets to subendothelial matrix components such as collagen, fibronectin, and von Willebrand factor, which are exposed after vessel damage. Platelet adhesion is mediated through specific cellular receptors such as the collagen receptor (platelet glycoprotein Ia/IIa) and the platelet glycoprotein Ib/IX/V complex, which binds von Willebrand factor incorporated into the subendothelial matrix. Adhesion to the damaged vessel wall induces platelet activation, a complex process that involves "outside-in" signaling responses transmitted by platelet integrin receptors. As a consequence, platelets undergo shape change, secrete the contents of their α and dense granules, and expose and activate fibrinogen receptors (platelet glycoprotein IIb/IIIa). Exposure of fibrinogen receptors facilitates the recruitment of additional platelets to the platelet plug by allowing the dimeric fibrinogen molecule to bridge receptors on adjacent platelets and induce platelet aggregation.

Platelet activation also results in rearrangement of membrane phospholipid, with increased expression of anionic phospholipid on the platelet surface and the release of anionic phospholipid–enriched platelet microparticles. Exposed anionic phospholipid provides a surface that supports the binding and activation of circulating coagulation factors, particularly those most important in the assembly of key coagulation complexes such as the "tenase" and prothrombinase complexes (see below). Thus, the surface of the activated platelet provides a fertile site for the generation of thrombin. In turn, thrombin promotes the direct activation of additional platelets through its binding and proteolytic activation of the platelet thrombin receptor.

Although primary hemostasis usually leads to the cessation of bleeding, the shear forces associated with flowing blood are sufficient to cause the eventual dissolution of the platelet plug. The role of secondary hemostasis, which involves the sequential activation of soluble coagulation factors, is to solidify the platelet plug through the formation of a stable, cross-linked fibrin clot. Secondary hemostasis has been conceptually subdivided into three major pathways: the intrinsic, extrinsic, and final common pathways (Fig. 218.1).

Although the physiologic activators of the intrinsic pathway remain controversial, factor XII (FXII) may be activated (FXIIa)

following contact with negatively charged substances (e.g., collagen) exposed as a result of vascular trauma. Activation of FXII to FXIIa leads to the activation of FXI (in a reaction catalyzed by high molecular weight kininogen) and prekallikrein (Fletcher factor). Newly activated FXI then activates FIX, and in the final reaction of the intrinsic pathway, FIXa activates FX through the formation of the tenase complex, which consists of FIXa, FX, calcium, phospholipid, and FVIII. This reaction constitutes a particularly important regulatory step in the coagulation cascade. However, the proximal steps in the intrinsic pathway are not essential for normal hemostasis, since individuals deficient in FXII, prekallikrein, or high molecular weight kininogen do not have a bleeding diathesis.

The extrinsic pathway is characterized by the direct activation of FX by a complex formed between FVIIa and tissue factor. This pathway is of central importance in initiation of the hemostatic response. Tissue factor, the only cell-associated, noncirculating coagulation factor, is produced by endothelial and other cells of the vascular wall. This factor is normally deposited in the subendothelial matrix but not expressed on the luminal aspect of the vessel wall under static conditions. After vessel damage, the exposure of tissue factor promotes the binding of FVIIa and the subsequent activation of FX. The activity of tissue factor is rapidly quenched through the action of a naturally occurring coagulation inhibitor, the tissue factor pathway inhibitor (TFPI). However, since the tissue factor/FVII complex also activates FIX, limited FXa generation may still occur through the assembly of the tenase complex.

The final common pathway represents convergence of the intrinsic and extrinsic pathways. In this pathway, FXa activates prothrombin to form thrombin, in a reaction involving the formation of the "prothrombinase" complex. This complex is analogous to the tenase complex, with FVa performing a catalytic role similar to that performed by FVIIIa in the latter. Newly generated thrombin cleaves fibrinogen to form fibrin monomers; these monomers self-associate to form mature fibrils, which are subsequently cross-linked by FXIIIa, leading to the formation of insoluble fibrin.

From the discussion above, it is evident that normal hemostasis involves numerous reactions, beginning with interactions of platelets with damaged vessel walls and proceeding through platelet activation and aggregation, the expression of platelet procoagulant activity, and the activation of soluble coagulation factors. Defects in any of these processes may lead to a bleeding diathesis.

Some of the more common congenital bleeding disorders are von Willebrand disease, hemophilia A, and hemophilia B. von Willebrand disease is inherited in an autosomal dominant manner, and results from either diminished production or the production of a functionally abnormal von Willebrand factor protein. Because von Willebrand factor plays a critical role in the adhesion of platelets to exposed subendothelium, particularly at sites of high-shear stress (such as the arterial circulation), its deficiency leads to impaired formation of the platelet plug and clinical manifestations similar to those caused by disorders of primary hemostasis. Conversely, impairment of the activity of the tenase complex in the hemophilias leads to defects of secondary hemostasis and clinical manifestations that are distinct from those attributable to platelet dysfunction (see below).

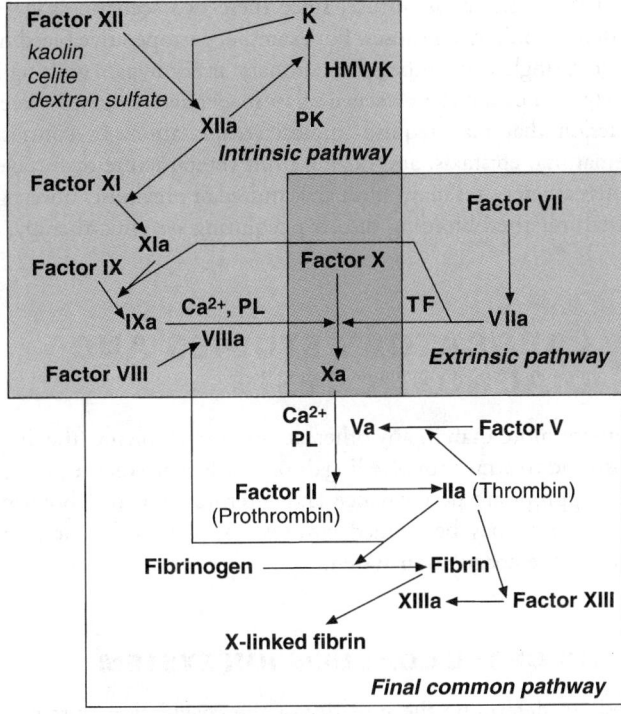

FIGURE 218.1. The coagulation cascade. The intrinsic *(lightly shaded)* and extrinsic *(more densely shaded)* pathways converge at the activation of factor X *(densely shaded)*. The reactions of the final common pathway are enclosed in the box without shading. HMWK, high molecular weight kininogen; K, kallikrein; PK, prekallikrein. (Reproduced from Feldman MD, McCrae KR. Applications of the clinical coagulation laboratory in the perioperative period. In: Lake CL, Moore RA, eds. *Blood: hemostasis, transfusion, and alternatives in the perioperative period.* New York: Raven Press, 1995:155, with permission.)

The majority of patients with bleeding do not have congenital or acquired coagulation defects. Bleeding in these individuals may result from a myriad of acquired conditions ranging from traumatic defects in the vascular wall, which may be of sufficient size that bleeding is not controlled by normal hemostatic mechanisms, to deficiencies in the levels of coagulation factors resulting from hepatic dysfunction.

HISTORY AND PHYSICAL EXAMINATION

BLEEDING HISTORY

The bleeding history must be carefully obtained, and the answers to only specific, directed questions designed to probe for truly abnormal bleeding events should be sought. Vague questions such as "Do you have heavy menstrual bleeding?" or "Do you bruise easily?" should be avoided since the responses to these queries are highly subjective. Similarly, the number of pads used in the course of a typical menstrual period may depend as much on the personal habits of the patient as on the amount of bleeding. Instead, questions such as "How many days do your menstrual periods last?" or "Do you frequently notice bruises larger than a quarter in areas where you do not remember receiving any trauma?" should be substituted.

The characteristics of bleeding in individual patients provide insight into the nature of the bleeding disorder. Defects in primary hemostasis are usually characterized by superficial bleeding involving the skin or mucous membranes, particularly those of the gastrointestinal or female genital tracts. Bleeding most often occurs immediately after trauma and usually does not recur after it is stopped. In contrast, bleeding that results from defects in secondary hemostasis, such as hemophilia, usually involves deeper tissues and may result in intramuscular hematomas, hemarthroses, or retroperitoneal hemorrhages. Bleeding events such as these may be delayed by a variable period after initial trauma, reflecting the inability of the platelet plug to be appropriately stabilized through activation of the coagulation cascade and the generation of cross-linked fibrin.

In all cases, it is essential to inquire about whether the patient has undergone previous surgical procedures (including dental extractions) and, if so, whether they were complicated by excessive hemorrhage. Subjective reports concerning a history of surgical bleeding may be misleading, and the physician should determine whether such episodes required a return to the operating room or blood transfusion through the direct review of the patient's records. Another critical aspect of the history is whether any immediate or first-degree family members have experienced excessive bleeding. In many cases, the patient's recollection of such events is vague, and in such circumstances direct questioning of the family member should be pursued. If a family history of bleeding exists, careful documentation may allow the pattern of inheritance to be established, providing information that will be useful in determining the nature of the bleeding disorder.

PHYSICAL EXAMINATION

A thorough physical examination is mandatory during the evaluation of a patient for a potential bleeding diathesis. Specific attention should be devoted to examination of the skin for petechiae (pinpoint hemorrhagic lesions occurring primarily in dependent areas, which are characteristic of quantitative or qualitative platelet dysfunction). Although nonpalpable purpura may also reflect quantitative or qualitative platelet abnormalities, other causes of such lesions, such as senile purpura, scurvy, corticosteroid excess, cholesterol or fat emboli, systemic infections, and dysproteinemias and defects in secondary hemostasis, should be considered. The finding of lax, velvety skin in a patient with a history of bleeding suggests Ehlers–Danlos syndrome, a disorder of collagen synthesis leading to weakened vessel walls. The mucous membranes, particularly the oropharynx, should also be closely inspected because this is another site where petechiae are frequently observed. Examination of these areas may also reveal lesions such as the arteriovenous malformations of Osler–Weber–Rendu disease (hereditary hemorrhagic telangiectasia), which occur throughout the gastrointestinal tract and may cause chronic gastrointestinal blood loss. The latter has recently been shown to result from mutations in the gene for endoglin, or *ALK1*.

The physical examination is of particular importance when evaluating the hospitalized patient with acute hemorrhage. In many cases, such patients are too ill to provide a reliable bleeding history, and the relevant history may not have been obtained at the time of admission. In this situation, the physical examination should focus on determining whether the bleeding is localized to a single site or is diffuse, since these two scenarios suggest different underlying causes. For example, postoperative bleeding from a single chest tube after coronary artery bypass grafting is likely to indicate the presence of an inadequately ligated vessel, a lesion that may require surgical reexploration. In contrast, hematuria, epistaxis, and oozing from venipuncture or intravenous catheter sites may reflect an acquired or previously unrecognized inherited bleeding disorder requiring systemic therapy.

LABORATORY STUDIES AND DIAGNOSTIC TESTS

Perhaps more than in any other situation in medicine, the diagnosis and treatment of bleeding disorders depends on the prompt and appropriate performance and interpretation of laboratory tests. These may be divided into tests of platelet function and tests of the coagulation system.

TESTS OF THE COAGULATION SYSTEM

Tests to determine the integrity of the coagulation system include, among others, the prothrombin time (PT), activated partial thromboplastin time (aPTT), thrombin time (TT), mixing studies (inhibitor screen), and specialized studies such as those used to evaluate the levels and function of specific coagulation factors. The two tests most commonly performed to evaluate the integrity of intrinsic and extrinsic coagulation pathways, respectively, are the aPTT and the PT. The techniques used to

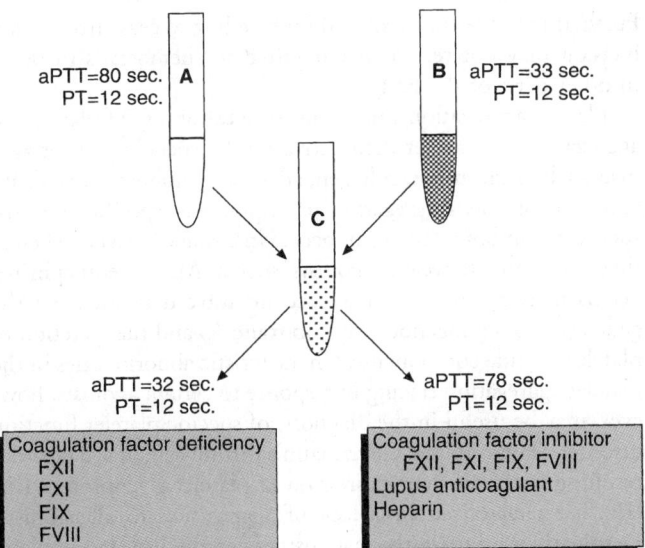

FIGURE 218.2. The inhibitor screen. In this example, the activated partial thromboplastin time (aPTT) of sample A is prolonged at 80 seconds (normal range, 30 to 36 seconds). Sample B represents normal plasma, and sample C represents a 1:1 mixture of A and B. A normal aPTT of sample C would demonstrate that the prolonged aPTT of sample resulted from a coagulation factor deficiency *(box on left)*. If the aPTT of sample C remained abnormal, it would be assumed that sample A contains a coagulation inhibitor *(box on right)*.

perform the PT and aPTT are outlined in Fig. 218.2. The PT measures the time required for plasma to clot after the addition of calcium and tissue thromboplastin. Tissue thromboplastin is an aqueous extract, generally prepared from rabbit brain, which is rich in anionic phospholipid and tissue factor. When added to plasma in the presence of calcium, thromboplastin preferentially supports the activation of coagulation through the reactions of the extrinsic pathway. For this reason, an isolated prolongation of the PT is most often caused by deficiencies of FVII. However, because this test is more sensitive than the aPTT to deficiencies of final common pathway factors, prolongation of the PT may also result from mild to moderate deficiencies of FX, prothrombin, or fibrinogen.

In the 1980s, it was realized that the use of different commercial thromboplastin preparations among clinical coagulation laboratories often led to discrepant PT values in individual patients tested at different locations. To address this problem, the World Health Organization developed a reference thromboplastin reagent, against which all manufacturers of such reagents were required to standardize their products. Hence, all commercial thromboplastins now are assigned a specific ISI (International Standardized Index) number. These values are used to translate a specific PT value to an INR (international normalized ratio), which is defined as:

$$INR = (patient\ PT/control\ PT)^{isi}$$

Common clinical settings associated with a prolonged PT (INR) include vitamin K deficiency, which causes functional deficiencies of the vitamin K–dependent coagulation factors (prothrombin, FVII, FIX, and FX), and disseminated intravascular coagulation, which leads to consumption of fibrinogen. In addition, the anticoagulant warfarin (Coumadin) induces functional vitamin K deficiency by preventing regeneration of oxidized vitamin K. Therapeutic INR values for patients on warfarin range from 2.0 to 4.0, depending on the indication for anticoagulation.

In contrast to the PT, the aPTT measures the time required for plasma to clot after the addition of calcium, phospholipid, and an FXII activator (kaolin), which induces coagulation through the intrinsic pathway. The aPTT is prolonged in situations characterized by deficiency of any of the proteins involved in this pathway (FXII, FXI, FIX, FVIII, prekallikrein, or high molecular weight kininogen). Hence, the aPTT is prolonged in hemophilia A and B. The aPTT may also be prolonged by deficiencies of final common pathway factors (although in this situation a prolonged PT would be expected as well) and by standard preparations of unfractionated heparin that stimulate the inhibitory activity of antithrombin III toward thrombin and other coagulation proteases. In contrast, low molecular weight heparin preparations have more potent inhibitory activity toward FXa and do not cause significant prolongation of the PTT. Hence, these agents must be monitored (if monitoring is deemed necessary), through measurement of plasma anti-FXa activity. Common causes of an abnormal PT and/or aPTT are listed in Table 218.1. The clinician should be aware, however, that the most common cause of a prolonged PTT is a lupus anticoagulant, which is paradoxically associated with an increased risk of thrombosis.

When a prolonged aPTT or PT is detected, the first test that should be performed to evaluate the abnormality is an inhibitor screen. This test is based on the principle that only 30% to 50% of the normal levels of any coagulation factor are required to yield a normal PT or aPTT, and is performed by repeating the abnormal test using a 1:1 mixture of patient and normal plasma (Fig. 218.2). Even if the patient's plasma is completely deficient in a specific factor, a 1:1 mixture of this and normal plasma should contain at least 50% of the normal amount of the deficient factor, a quantity sufficient to correct the clotting time. If the PT and/or PTT value of the mixture is normal (the inhibitor screen is negative), the cause of the initial prolongation is presumed secondary to a factor deficiency. However, if the patient's plasma contains a coagulation inhibitor (usually an antibody that neutralizes the activity of a specific coagulation factor), mixing of patient and normal plasma does not correct the clotting time because the inhibitor neutralizes the factor supplied by normal plasma. In this case, the inhibitor screen is said to be positive—a result with important therapeutic implications.

The TT measures the time required for plasma to clot after the addition of thrombin and reflects the levels of functional fibrinogen. The TT should be performed when a patient has concurrent prolongation of the PT and aPTT, a pattern that may result from deficiencies of fibrinogen, FX, FV, or prothrombin. Prolongation is consistent with a deficiency of fibrinogen, whereas a normal result suggests that deficiencies of other final common pathway factors may be present. The TT may also be prolonged by contamination of the plasma sample with heparin. This is a common problem when coagulation studies are drawn from indwelling catheters, a practice that should be avoided. To evaluate a sample for heparin contamination, plasma may be

TABLE 218.1.	COMMON CAUSES OF ELEVATED PROTHROMBIN AND PARTIAL THROMBOPLASTIN TIME		
Etiologic Factors		**PT**	**PTT**
Poor-quality sample[a]		↑>↓	↑>↓
Heparin[b]		–/↑	↑↑↑
Warfarin[b]		↑↑↑	–/↑
Liver disease or vitamin K deficiency[c]		↑↑↑	–/↑
von Willebrand disease[d]		–	–/↑
DIC[e]		↑↑	–/↑
Hemophilia A		–	↑↑↑
Hemophilia B		–	↑↑↑
Acquired inhibitors (most often factor VIII or IX)[f]		–	↑↑↑
Lupus anticoagulant		–/↑	↑

[a] Samples are considered inadequate if they are clotted or are contaminated by heparin. An inappropriate blood-to-anticoagulant ratio (normally 4.5:0.5 using 3.8% citrate) can falsely elevate the PT or PTT. A traumatic venipuncture can release thromboplastin and cause the generation of thrombin in the collection tube, falsely lowering the PT/PTT.
[b] The effect of heparin is most pronounced on the PTT, but large amounts may also interfere with the PT. Conversely, warfarin principally affects the PT but large amounts may also elevate the PTT.
[c] The prothrombin time is elevated first, followed by the PTT if the liver disease or vitamin K deficiency is severe.
[d] Depending on the type of von Willebrand disease, the PTT may be affected if the factor VIII levels are sufficiently decreased.
[e] The PT is a more sensitive marker for DIC than the PTT.
[f] Acquired inhibitors to factor VIII and IX (abnormal PTT) are more common than inhibitors to factors II, VII, and X (elevated PT).
(From Feldman MD, McCrae KR. Applications of the clinical coagulation laboratory in the perioperative period. In: Moore RA, Lake CL, eds. *Blood: hemostasis, transfusion, and alternatives in the perioperative period.* New York: Raven Press, 1995:153–178, with permission.)
PT, prothrombin time; PTT, partial thromboplastin time; DIC, disseminated intravascular coagulation.

adsorbed with a heparin-binding cationic resin and the clotting time repeated; alternatively, a reptilase time may be performed. Reptilase is a snake venom protease that directly converts fibrinogen to fibrin in a heparin-insensitive manner.

TESTS OF PLATELET FUNCTION

The two most common tests of platelet function are the bleeding time and platelet aggregation studies. The bleeding time, which ranges from 2 to 9 minutes in normal individuals, measures the time for bleeding to cease from a standardized skin wound and reflects the formation of the platelet plug at the site of vessel damage. This test was designed to assess the adequacy of primary hemostasis and in the appropriate setting may be useful. However, for several reasons, the predictive value of the bleeding time is poor, particularly in individuals with a low pretest probability of a congenital or acquired defect in primary hemostasis. The bleeding time is influenced by minor technical variations in its performance, such as the orientation of the forearm incision, and is prolonged for up to 7 days after ingestion of aspirin or aspirin-containing compounds, as well as other medications.

Furthermore, the time required for bleeding to cease from a skin incision may not reflect that required for hemostasis to occur in other parts of the body.

Platelet aggregation studies measure the ability of platelets to aggregate in vitro after their activation by specific platelet agonists such as thrombin, collagen, adenosine diphosphate (ADP), and epinephrine. Aggregation in response to specific agonists, such as thrombin or collagen, occurs in a single "wave," whereas that in response to weaker agonists, such as ADP or epinephrine, occurs in two waves, with the second wave dependent on the generation of endogenous thromboxane A_2 and the secretion of platelet granule components. Characteristic abnormalities in the platelet aggregation tracing in response to certain agonists, however, may be useful in the diagnosis of specific platelet function disorders. For example, Glanzmann's thrombasthenia, a disorder resulting from deficient expression of platelet glycoprotein IIb/IIIa, is characterized by a lack of aggregation to all agonists. Despite their utility in the diagnosis of certain disorders of platelet function, platelet aggregation results are usually normal in patients with prolonged bleeding times who have no bleeding history, again demonstrating the lack of specificity of a prolonged bleeding time in such circumstances. Because of their expense and the complexity of their interpretation, platelet aggregation studies should only be obtained on the recommendations of a consultant with expertise and experience in the evaluation of bleeding disorders.

Recently, an automated assay for analyzing platelet function in whole blood has become available through the use of the Platelet Function Analyzer (PFA-100) system. The PFA-100 measures the time required for blood to occlude an aperture (defined as the closure time, CT) in the membrane of a collagen/epinephrine (CEPI) or collagen/ADP-coated test cartridge (CADP). A potential advantage of the PFA-100 is its ability to detect aspirin-induced platelet dysfunction versus that due to congenital thrombocytopathies through differences in closure times of a given sample on CEPI or CAPD cartridges. Though the PFA-100 has not yet achieved widespread clinical use, recent studies suggest that its sensitivity and specificity for determination of aspirin-induced platelet function defects is similar to that of the bleeding time and that it may be superior to platelet aggregometry for detection of congenital thrombocytopathies such as von Willebrand disease.

DIFFERENTIAL DIAGNOSIS

The differential diagnosis of hemorrhage must be tailored to the individual case and is based on several factors, such as the site and intensity of bleeding, whether bleeding was spontaneous or occurred in response to trauma, and whether the affected individual has a history of prior hemorrhagic events. Although discussing all possible causes of hemorrhage is beyond the scope of this chapter, it is instructive to consider the differential diagnosis for a limited number of patients with common symptoms.

One example is a young woman with menorrhagia and a history of easy bruisability and epistaxis (Fig. 218.3). These symptoms are most consistent with a disorder of primary hemostasis, and several causes must be considered in attempting to

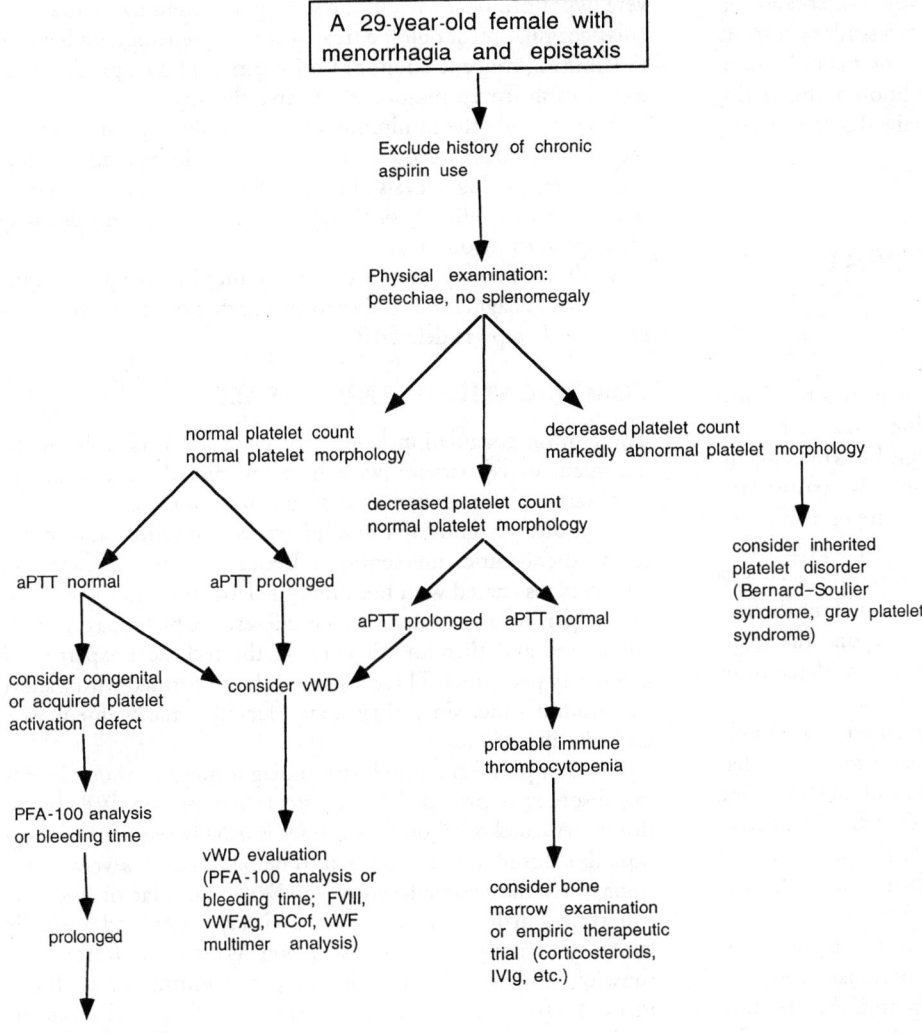

FIGURE 218.3. Hypothetical evaluation of a young woman with menorrhagia and epistaxis. aPTT, activated partial thromboplastin time; FVIII, factor VIII; vWD, von Willebrand disease.

explain the symptoms. First, the possibility of a thrombocytopenic disorder, most likely immune-mediated in this setting, should be evaluated by obtaining a platelet count and examining the peripheral blood film. Thrombocytopenia in the presence of reduced numbers of normal-appearing to slightly large platelets is most consistent with a diagnosis of immune thrombocytopenic purpura. However, because individuals with specific subtypes of von Willebrand disease may also be thrombocytopenic, an aPTT should also be assessed in this situation, with any observed prolongation pursued by a directed evaluation for von Willebrand disease. In contrast, if this individual was found to have reduced numbers of large, abnormal-appearing platelets, an inherited disorder of platelet function, such as the Bernard–Soulier syndrome or a platelet storage pool disease (see Chapter 239), must be considered.

If the initial evaluation of this individual revealed a normal platelet count with normal-appearing platelets, von Willebrand disease would be the most likely diagnosis. Such a patient should be fully evaluated for this disorder, regardless of the aPTT, by obtaining a bleeding time (or PFA-100 analysis), assays for FVIII

activity and antigen, von Willebrand factor antigen, and ristocetin cofactor activity. A platelet activation defect should also be considered in this setting, particularly if the aPTT is normal. Evaluation for such a disorder includes a bleeding time (or PFA-100 analysis) followed by specific platelet aggregation studies and/or measurement of platelet cyclic nucleotide content.

An entirely different differential diagnosis must be generated for the patient with excessive postoperative bleeding. The most common cause of postoperative bleeding is a vessel that was not adequately ligated during surgery. Bleeding of this nature is often localized and may present, for example, as hemorrhage from a single surgical drain. In contrast, postoperative bleeding from systemic causes, such as a dilutional coagulopathy (transfusion of multiple units of packed red blood cells without replacement of plasma and platelets) or unrecognized sepsis leading to disseminated intravascular coagulation, is usually associated with diffuse bleeding. A systemic cause of bleeding should thus be suspected in the presence of symptoms such as excessive oozing after venipuncture or around vascular access sites, mucous membrane or gastrointestinal bleeding, or hematuria.

An inherited bleeding disorder such as von Willebrand disease, mild hemophilia, or a platelet function disorder occasionally presents for the first time after surgery or major trauma. However, the initial discovery of such a condition in this setting is rare, particularly if a bleeding history is obtained before elective surgical procedures have been done.

STRATEGIES FOR OPTIMAL CARE

MANAGEMENT

Appropriate management of the bleeding patient requires identification and understanding of the underlying cause of hemorrhage. Comprehension of the pathophysiologic basis of congenital and acquired hemorrhagic syndromes is particularly important for employing the expanding repertoire of hemostatic agents in a cost-effective manner. Selection of appropriate therapy depends on the nature of the immediate bleeding event and the underlying bleeding diathesis. A full discussion of the therapy of inherited or acquired bleeding disorders is beyond the scope of this chapter, but several guidelines should be considered prior to initiating procoagulant therapy (Table 218.2).

First, the cause of the bleeding must be discerned as accurately as possible. The patient's history alone is rarely sufficiently reliable to allow for the design of a specific plan of therapy. The author has personally observed several instances when inaccurate information from either medical personnel or the patient led to that individual inappropriately receiving plasma-based therapy for a bleeding disorder that he or she did not have. A laboratory-documented diagnosis must be obtained prior to institution of coagulant therapy in all but the most urgent circumstances. Furthermore, the specific set of events that triggered the bleeding episode in question must be understood in the context of the patient's underlying diagnosis.

Second, the goals of therapy should be accurately defined. For example, infusion of plasma into a patient with advanced hepatic disease in order to transiently decrease the hemorrhagic risk of liver biopsy may be justified, although achieving a complete and sustained correction of the coagulopathy in such a patient would be unlikely.

Third, the product most appropriate for the optimal management of bleeding should always be employed. For example, se-vere hypofibrinogenemia in the setting of disseminated intravascular coagulation should be treated with cryoprecipitate because the limiting concentrations of fibrinogen in plasma preclude the use of fresh-frozen plasma as effective therapy.

Fourth, only the minimum amount of blood product that is required to induce adequate hemostasis should be used. Achieving supraphysiologic levels of coagulation factors in plasma does not increase the efficacy of therapy and in some conditions may predispose to thrombosis.

Fifth, all therapy should be closely monitored by appropriately timed coagulation studies to ensure that pertinent and cost-effective therapy is delivered.

COMPLICATIONS AND PITFALLS

The clinical coagulation laboratory plays a central role in the management of patients with bleeding disorders. The ability to obtain reliable coagulation studies promptly is essential in appropriately diagnosing causes of excessive bleeding and monitoring therapeutic interventions. Because of the vast array of disorders associated with bleeding, the laboratory must be capable of performing many specialized tests, which may not be automated and therefore depend on the technical expertise of laboratory personnel. These tests must be performed with a short turnaround time, since they may affect the management of a critically ill patient.

An example of the complexity of diagnosing a common bleeding disorder is provided by consideration of von Willebrand disease. A panel of laboratory studies is usually required to diagnose this disorder and may need to be repeated on several occasions, since the plasma levels of von Willebrand factor fluctuate over time. Furthermore, individuals with type O blood normally have significantly lower levels of von Willebrand factor than those of patients with other blood types, requiring the establishment of separate normal ranges. Hence, to offer a service capable of diagnosing von Willebrand disease accurately, a laboratory must be able to perform several sophisticated assays with a high degree of reproducibility. A competent clinical coagulation laboratory should also maintain an accurate and facile system for prompt retrieval of the results of prior coagulation studies.

In attempts to reduce health care costs, the staffs of many clinical laboratories have been reduced, and in some cases technicians have been asked to perform assays with which they have little training and experience. Although this may not be inappropriate for certain automated assays, technicians who perform specialized coagulation analyses must have a thorough understanding and extensive familiarity with the technical aspects of these studies. Thus, although common automated studies such as the aPTT and PT may be performed during non-peak hours in a consolidated general clinical or "stat" laboratory, complex and/or nonroutine coagulation studies should be performed only by highly trained and experienced personnel (who should be available to perform such studies as patient needs dictate).

Indications for HOSPITALIZATION

The mode of presentation of the patient with excessive bleeding is highly variable. The evaluation of patients who present

---

TABLE 218.2. GUIDELINES FOR USE OF PROCOAGULANT THERAPY IN THE BLEEDING PATIENT

1. Accurately discern the cause of bleeding using clinical and laboratory data.
2. Define the goals of therapy prior to its administration.
3. Employ the product that is optimal for treatment of the specific patient.
4. Use the minimum of product required to achieve adequate hemostasis.
5. Monitor the efficacy of therapy closely.

for investigation of a chronic bleeding diathesis can be performed in the outpatient setting. Similarly, patients with milder forms of von Willebrand disease or platelet function disorders who present with non–life-threatening bleeding events such as epistaxis usually can be managed without hospital admission. The use of agents such as intranasally administered arginine vasopressin [desmopressin acetate (DDAVP)], which has efficacy equal to that of intravenous DDAVP in the therapy of mild hemophilia and von Willebrand disease, has facilitated the outpatient management of such individuals.

Uncontrolled, spontaneous bleeding of any type is an absolute criterion for hospital admission and occurs most commonly in patients with known bleeding diatheses, such as hemophilia. Despite the efficacy of prophylactic home therapy in such individuals, therapy of active and significant bleeding in patients with hemophilia should be administered and monitored in the hospital, with the length of stay depending on the nature of the bleeding episode. Similar considerations must be applied to patients with bleeding diatheses who require minor surgical procedures, for which normal individuals are generally not hospitalized. In such cases, hospitalization ensures that hemostatic therapy is delivered on an appropriate schedule designed to minimize the risk of intraoperative and postoperative hemorrhage. However, most patients with mild or moderately severe bleeding disorders can usually undergo minor dental procedures in the outpatient setting, since bleeding related to such procedures can usually be well controlled by the direct application of highly effective local hemostatic agents to the bleeding site.

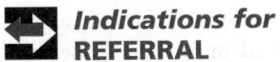

Indications for REFERRAL

The diagnosis and management of bleeding disorders is a complex issue that requires the expertise of appropriately trained physicians. Any patient suspected of having a congenital or acquired bleeding disorder should be evaluated by a hematologist prior to surgical intervention. Similarly, the management of patients with acute hemorrhage, including those with postoperative bleeding, warrants hematologic consultation. However, appropriate management of surgical patients, or patients with hemorrhage in specialized settings such as the puerperium, requires close collaboration between the hematologist and the appropriate specialist.

COST-EFFECTIVENESS

Significant changes in the practice of medicine have occurred in the United States in the past decade. These primarily reflect the financial stresses faced by hospitals and physicians in response to diminished reimbursement for inpatient and outpatient care. Since severe hemorrhage attributable to coagulopathy

is an uncommon event, there has been a tendency on the part of many hospitals to divert scarce resources to programs with a greater potential for revenue generation. Though this may be a fiscally sound approach, the quality of patient care will ultimately suffer in the absence of a carefully conceived institutional strategy to the management of patients with congenital and acquired coagulopathies.

Despite these concerns, a significant proportion of the studies performed in most clinical coagulation laboratories are indeed unnecessary, resulting in poor utilization of technician time and avoidable expenditures. One example of this practice is the continued utilization of the bleeding time, an extremely labor-intensive assay, in patients without a clear history of bleeding (and thus with a low pretest probability). A particular example of this practice is the routine measurement of preoperative bleeding times. The bleeding time has no predictive value in this setting; in fact, the predictive value of a carefully obtained bleeding history is superior not only to that of the bleeding time but also to that of routine coagulation assays. Detection of a clinically insignificant abnormality in a screening coagulation assay (particularly the bleeding time) in a patient without a bleeding diathesis forces the performance of additional and costly studies to exclude an underlying hemorrhagic disorder.

Education of physicians with regard to the ordering of screening coagulation assays does not seem to be an effective means of altering their test ordering behavior. Only through education coupled with restrictions on the ordering of specific assays can the volume of such studies be reduced. One approach to this dilemma may be the use of a questionnaire developed by physicians with expertise in coagulation, in collaboration with surgical staff, which would be completed by patients scheduled for elective surgical procedures at the time of preadmission testing. A predetermined threshold of positive responses would prompt further evaluation of selected patients by a hematologist, potentially leading to substantial savings.

BIBLIOGRAPHY

Bowie EJW, Owen CA Jr. Hemostatic failure in clinical medicine. *Semin Hematol* 1977;14:341–364.

De Caterina R, Lanza M, Manca G, et al. Bleeding time and bleeding: an analysis of the relationship of the bleeding time test with parameters of surgical bleeding. *Blood* 1994;84:3363–3370.

Feldman MD, McCrae KR. Applications of the clinical coagulation laboratory in the perioperative period. In: Lake CL, Moore RA, eds. *Blood: hemostasis, transfusion, and alternatives in the perioperative period.* New York: Raven Press, 1995:153–178.

Hirsh J. Oral anticoagulant drugs. *N Engl J Med* 1991;324:1865–1875.

Lind SE. The bleeding time does not predict surgical bleeding. *Blood* 1991; 77:2547–2552.

Mammen EF, Comp PC, Gosselin R, et al. PFA-100 system: a new method for assessment of platelet dysfunction. *Semin Thromb Hemost* 1998;24: 195–202.

Mannucci PM. Hemostatic drugs. *N Engl J Med* 1998;339:245–253.

March CM. Bleeding problems and treatment. *Clin Obstet Gynecol* 1998; 41:928–939.

Rodgers RPC, Levin J. A critical reappraisal of the bleeding time. *Semin Thromb Hemost* 1990;16:1–20.

Schafer AI. Approach to bleeding. In: Loscalzo J, Schafer AI, eds. *Thrombosis and hemorrhage.* Boston: Blackwell Scientific, 1998:459–475.

APPROACH TO THE PATIENT WITH THROMBOSIS

JOEL S. BENNETT

PRESENTATION

Thrombosis is among the most common problems encountered by physicians and is the leading cause of death in the United States. Thrombosis can be segregated into arterial and venous disease based on differences in clinical presentation and pathophysiology.

Arterial thrombosis is principally a manifestation of arteriosclerosis, and patients present with coronary ischemia and with cerebrovascular and peripheral vascular disease. The substrate for an arterial thrombosis is usually an arteriosclerotic lesion, and thrombosis may be the first indication of such a lesion.

Venous thrombosis occurs most often in the veins of the lower extremities, where it presents as thrombophlebitis, a syndrome of pain and swelling in the lower leg. A diagnosis of venous thrombosis in the lower extremities may be difficult to make on clinical grounds alone. As many as 70% of patients with pulmonary emboli have asymptomatic venous thrombi in their legs, and 50% of patients for whom the diagnosis of thrombophlebitis is considered are found to have an alternate diagnosis.

PATHOPHYSIOLOGIC FACTORS

Arterial thrombi are composed primarily of aggregated platelets (white thrombi) and form when the endothelial lining of an artery is breached, allowing platelets in the circulating blood to interact with subendothelial connective tissue. Thrombi form on the surfaces of arteriosclerotic plaques when their surfaces are denuded of endothelial cells or when a plaque is physically disrupted, exposing platelets to highly thrombogenic material in the plaque interior. A detailed description of the formation of platelet thrombi is presented in Chapter 240.

Venous thrombi are composed primarily of fibrin and trapped red cells (red thrombi). Fibrin is produced by a series of biochemical reactions that culminate in the activation of coagulation factor X, the cleavage of prothrombin by activated factor X (FXa) to liberate thrombin, and the cleavage of fibrinogen by thrombin to yield fibrin monomer. Sensitive assays have shown that small amounts of FXa and thrombin are continuously being generated in normal individuals but that the activity of these enzymes is sufficiently controlled by proteins such as antithrombin III and the complex of protein C with protein S to prevent the formation of thrombi. As discussed in Chapter 240, venous thrombi can form in regions of venous stasis when conditions such as immobilization, malignancy, pregnancy, oral contraceptive use, nephrotic syndrome, or the presence of anticardiolipin antibodies shift the coagulation–anticoagulation balance toward the generation of procoagulant coagulant activity. This shift is further enhanced when the control of FXa and thrombin activity is impaired by hereditary deficiencies of antithrombin III and proteins C and S or inherited resistance to the anticoagulant effect of protein C.

HISTORY AND PHYSICAL EXAMINATION

Because arterial thrombi obstruct the flow of oxygenated blood, they result in tissue ischemia and manifest most often as acute myocardial infarction and stroke. When arterial thrombosis complicates a myeloproliferative disorder such as polycythemia vera, essential thrombocythemia, or heparin-associated thrombocytopenia, it is likely to occur in arteries involved by arteriosclerosis. The hyaline thrombi characteristic of thrombotic thrombocytopenic purpura obstruct normal arterioles, producing waxing and waning symptoms of tissue ischemia that often involve the central nervous system.

Venous thrombosis occurs most often as thrombophlebitis in the lower extremities, as superficial thrombophlebitis usually involving varicosities, or as potentially more serious deep venous thrombosis. Deep venous thrombosis in the leg can be complicated by pulmonary embolism. Thrombi that result in clinically significant pulmonary embolism are almost invariably located in the proximal veins of the legs, but many begin as calf vein thrombi that extend into the proximal veins in the thigh.

The symptoms of venous thrombosis result from obstruction of venous outflow and from accompanying local inflammation. Classically, leg vein thrombosis presents as a triad of calf pain, edema, and pain on dorsiflexion of the foot (Homans's sign). However, this presentation is observed in less than one-third of patients, and more often, symptomatic leg vein thrombosis presents as calf discomfort or tenderness or as unexplained leg edema. Moreover, when leg vein thrombosis is considered on clinical grounds alone, it can be confirmed by objective testing in fewer than 50% of cases. Conditions confused with deep venous thrombosis in the legs include muscle strains and tears, swelling of a paralyzed leg, lymphatic obstruction, Baker's cyst, cellulitis, internal derangements of the knee, and the postphlebitic syndrome. Of particular concern, asymptomatic deep venous thrombosis has been found in 70% of patients with confirmed pulmonary embolism. Conversely, asymptomatic pulmonary embolism has been detected in 50% of patients with proximal deep venous thrombosis.

Venous thrombi usually arise in the large venous sinuses in the calf, in the pockets of valves in the deep veins in the calves, and at sites of vascular damage. Although small calf vein thrombi usually resolve completely, complete lysis of larger thrombi is uncommon. Instead, these thrombi may organize and recanalize. The resulting venous obstruction and venous valve destruction can result in a postphlebitic syndrome of chronic calf pain associated with brawny edema, hyperpigmentation, induration, and ulceration of the lower leg.

Clinically significant thrombosis can involve the axillary, mesenteric, hepatic, renal, and cerebral veins, but these forms of thrombosis are considerably less common than thrombi of the calf venous sinuses. Hepatic vein thrombosis (Budd–Chiari syndrome) is feature of the myeloproliferative disorders and paroxysmal nocturnal hemoglobinuria. Acute and chronic forms of renal vein thrombosis occur in the nephrotic syndrome, especially when the nephrotic syndrome is secondary to membranous glomerulonephritis. Mesenteric and cerebral venous thromboses have been reported in patients with the inherited causes of thrombosis discussed in Chapter 240, myeloproliferative disorders, paroxysmal nocturnal hemoglobinuria, or the antiphospholipid antibody syndrome, and after estrogen administration.

LABORATORY STUDIES AND DIAGNOSTIC TESTS

Evaluation of patients with thrombosis should be tailored to their clinical situations. Because most cases of arterial thrombosis result from arteriosclerosis and not from abnormalities of platelet function or blood coagulation, studies should focus on the extent of the arteriosclerosis and on factors that may contribute to its progression. However, when arterial thrombosis occurs in the absence of significant arteriosclerosis, the possibility of hemostatic abnormalities must be considered.

Venous thrombosis is a common occurrence, especially in immobilized medical and surgical patients. However, because tests to detect a specific cause of the thrombosis are expensive and unlikely to change the management of a patient after the first episode of thrombosis, such testing should be restricted to patients with recurrent thrombosis, unless the patient has a family history that strongly suggests a hereditary disorder. Moreover, measurement of the proteins associated with familial thrombosis (antithrombin III, protein C, and protein S) may not be reliable after an acute thrombotic episode. It is preferable to wait several weeks before obtaining these studies. Meaningful measurements of protein C and protein S, both of which are vitamin K–dependent proteins, cannot be performed when patients are receiving the oral anticoagulant warfarin. Consequently, measurement of the levels of these proteins should be delayed until warfarin has been discontinued for several weeks.

Venous thrombosis associated with malignancy occurs more frequently in patients with advanced disease. The biochemical basis for the procoagulant effect of tumors is not always apparent and may be different for different types of tumors. For example, some tumors express tissue factor, others produce activators of factor X, and still others produce fibrinolytic inhibitors. The continuous elaboration of procoagulant activity by tumors can produce chronic disseminated intravascular coagulation (DIC). Although acute DIC generally produces thrombocytopenia, prolongation of the prothrombin and partial thromboplastin times, depletion of fibrinogen, and increased concentrations of fibrin-split products, tumor-associated chronic DIC may manifest as only recurrent thromboembolism and persistent elevation of fibrin-split products.

Venous thrombosis can be a presenting symptom of malignancy, particularly when patients have mucin-producing carcinomas (Trousseau's syndrome). Venous thrombosis in an otherwise healthy patient raises concern about the possibility of an occult malignancy. When this issue was studied prospectively, malignancy was found in 3% to 10% of patients presenting with venous thrombosis and was discovered in 7% to 11% of patients in the ensuing 6 to 24 months. Malignancy was found most often in patients without an obvious cause for venous thrombosis, in patients with recurrent idiopathic thrombosis, and in patients older than 60 years. However, it was not apparent from these studies that an extensive workup to detect occult malignancy in these patients resulted in improved survival. A reasonable approach to the evaluation of patients with venous thrombosis and in whom malignancy is a possibility is to supplement routine studies with multiple fecal samples for occult blood loss, prostate-specific antigen measurements in men, and mammography in women.

A diagnosis of deep venous thrombosis in the lower extremities is difficult on clinical grounds alone and should be supplemented by objective tests. Objective testing to rule out the presence of thrombosis is cost-effective because the costs of hospitalization substantially exceed the costs of testing. The standard for venous thrombosis is *venography,* against which all other tests for the detection of venous thrombosis are compared. Venography detects thrombi in the deep veins of the calf and in the popliteal, femoral, and iliac veins. However, venography is an invasive study that is not suitable for serial studies. It is associated with a 2% to 3% incidence of chemical phlebitis.

Several noninvasive studies can detect venous thrombi with variable degrees of success. *Impedance plethysmography* (IPG) measures changes in electrical impedance in the calf after deflation of a pressure cuff around the thigh and detects impairment in venous outflow from the leg. IPG can detect venous thrombi in the thigh, but it is insensitive to isolated calf vein thrombi. Although initial reports indicated that IPG was highly sensitive and specific for proximal thrombi, later studies suggest that IPG is far less sensitive than previously thought and that it may fail to detect occlusive and nonocclusive proximal thrombi. Consequently, IPG cannot be recommended as a noninvasive test to rule out the presence of venous thrombi in symptomatic or asymptomatic patients.

Real-time B-mode ultrasonography uses very high frequency sound waves to produce two-dimensional images. It is purported to be 97% sensitive and 97% specific for detecting proximal deep venous thrombosis in symptomatic patients. The most sensitive finding is failure of a vein to collapse under gentle pressure (compression ultrasonography). B-mode ultrasonography can be supplemented by Doppler flow detection (duplex scanning), but the contribution of the latter to the diagnostic accuracy of the test is not clear. Like IPG, ultrasonography is not sensitive to calf vein thrombosis, and its sensitivity drops considerably in asymptomatic patients.

An increased concentration of the D-dimer fragment of fibrin in plasma has been used as an indication of the presence of venous thrombosis. A D-dimer results from the degradation of cross-linked fibrin by plasmin and serves as a marker for the activation of coagulation. Although an increased concentration of D-dimer in plasma correlates highly with venous thrombosis (sensitivity of 97%), its sensitivity is low (specificity of 35%).

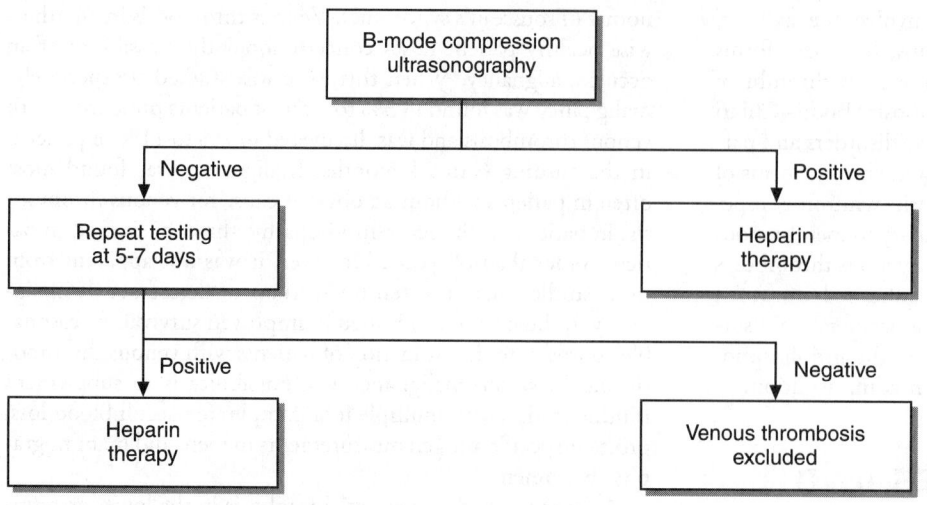

FIGURE 219.1. Algorithm for the diagnosis and treatment of suspected deep venous thrombosis of the lower extremity using B-mode compression ultrasonography. If this noninvasive test is unavailable, venography should be performed to rule out venous thrombosis. Venography should also be performed to resolve ambiguous studies.

Absence of an increased D-dimer concentration cannot rule out venous thrombosis.

Because of cost and availability, the roles of *computed tomography* and *magnetic resonance venography* in the routine management of venous thrombosis are likely to be limited.

For a patient with symptoms suggesting venous thrombosis, most recent studies suggest it is safe to withhold anticoagulant therapy in the face of normal serial real-time B-mode ultrasonographic examinations, and an abnormal test result is an indication for treatment (Fig. 219.1). There is no satisfactory objective test to screen asymptomatic patients for venous thrombosis.

STRATEGIES FOR OPTIMAL CARE

MANAGEMENT

The pharmacology of agents employed in the medical management of arterial and venous thrombosis is discussed in Chapter 240.

Except for specific circumstances, such as early acute myocardial infarction or selected cases of peripheral arterial thrombosis for which thrombolytic therapy is effective, the goal for the medical management of arterial thrombosis is prevention of recurrence. Drugs that inhibit platelet function such as aspirin and ticlopidine help to prevent thrombosis in patients with arteriosclerotic vascular disease. Aspirin, a drug that prevents platelet prostaglandin synthesis, decreases the risk of myocardial infarction and death in patients with unstable angina; reduces the risk of recurrent cardiovascular complications in patients with myocardial infarction, transient cerebral ischemia, and stroke; and decreases the risk of cardiovascular events in healthy patients or patients with chronic stable angina. Ticlopidine, an alternative to aspirin that primarily inhibits adenosine diphosphate–induced platelet aggregation, reduces the risk of nonfatal and fatal thrombotic strokes in patients with transient attacks of cerebral ischemia or completed thrombotic stroke, and is as effective as aspirin in preventing myocardial infarction in patients with

unstable angina or intermittent claudication in patients with peripheral vascular diseases.

Heparin, administered in small subcutaneous doses, is frequently used to prevent venous thrombosis in immobilized medical and surgical patients and in patients congenitally predisposed to thrombosis at times of increased risk. The basis for low-dose heparin therapy is the ability of the drug to inhibit excess FXa that could shift the normal hemostatic balance toward thrombosis. Prophylactic heparin is given at a dose of 5,000 units every 12 hours, and it usually has no effect on the activated partial thromboplastin time (aPTT). When given in this way to surgical patients, the incidence of venous thrombosis and fatal pulmonary emboli is decreased by 60% to 70%. However, low-dose heparin has been less effective as prophylaxis after orthopedic surgery or trauma in which the stimulus for thrombosis may be greater. In these patients, subcutaneous heparin adjusted to maintain a top normal aPTT, low molecular weight heparin, or moderate-dose warfarin therapy has been more efficacious therapy. Although a patient given low-dose heparin is free from the risk of serious bleeding, because of the potential for minor bleeding, it should not be used in patients undergoing cerebral, spinal, or ophthalmologic surgery. Despite the lower dosage, prophylactic heparin remains a cause of heparin-associated thrombocytopenia.

Heparin at a dose sufficient to prolong the aPTT to 1.5 to 2.5 times the mean of the control aPTT is the treatment of choice for active venous thrombosis. Achieving this dose within the first 24 hours of treatment minimizes treatment failure and recurrent thrombosis. There is essentially no difference in the efficacy and incidence of complications for heparin given by continuous intravenous infusion or by intermittent subcutaneous injection, although the latter requires a larger heparin dosage to reach the therapeutic range within 24 hours. Generally, an initial bolus of 5,000 units followed by more than 30,000 units within 24 hours is required to achieve and maintain the therapeutic range when heparin is given intravenously, and more than 33,000 units within 24 hours is required when it is given subcutaneously. Given in this way, the incidence of bleeding is 2% to 7%.

Low molecular weight heparin (see Chapter 240) preferentially catalyzes the inhibition of FXa over thrombin and has potential advantages of greater bioavailability at low dosage and longer duration of action than standard heparin. Given at a fixed dosage subcutaneously once or twice daily and without laboratory monitoring, low molecular weight heparin has been found to be at least as effective and safe as standard heparin in prophylaxis against thrombosis and in the treatment of thrombi. These results suggest that low molecular weight heparin may be useful for the outpatient management of venous thrombosis, bypassing the considerable costs of hospitalization. However, issues of efficacy, neutralization of low molecular weight heparin by protamine, safety in pregnancy, and incidence of osteoporosis and thrombocytopenia must be resolved.

Following initial treatment with heparin, patients are treated with oral anticoagulants (warfarin, see Chapter 240) to prevent the recurrence of thromboembolism. Current practice is to treat with heparin for at least 5 days, starting warfarin on day 1. Warfarin dosage is adjusted using the prothrombin time and the INR (International Normalized Ratio) calculated from it. An INR of 2.0 to 3.0 is recommended to prevent recurrent venous thrombosis. Treatment with warfarin is overlapped with heparin for at least 2 days to ensure that patients are adequately anticoagulated when the heparin is stopped and to prevent the rare occurrence of warfarin-induced skin necrosis. The duration of warfarin therapy depends on the inciting cause of the venous thrombosis. In patients with reversible risk factors for venous thrombosis such as recent surgery, 6 weeks of therapy may be sufficient. However, in patients with idiopathic thrombosis, the risk for recurrence may be as high as 18% at 2 years, 25% at 5 years, and 30% at 8 years. Accordingly, more prolonged treatment with warfarin is necessary. Although the optimal duration remains to be established, a trial of treatment for 3 months versus more prolonged treatment revealed a recurrence rate of 27.4% per patient year in the group treated for 3 months compared to 1.3% per patient year in patients treated for an average of 12 months, suggesting that treatment for 3 months is inadequate.

When there are contraindications to the use of anticoagulant drugs such as active bleeding or if thrombosis recurs despite adequate anticoagulation, interventions to prevent pulmonary embolization by interrupting the inferior vena cava should be considered. The most popular device is the Greenfield filter, which is associated with a caval patency rate of 95% and an overall incidence of recurrent pulmonary embolization of less than 5%. Migration of the filter and perforation of the caval wall have been rare occurrences. Other types of filters have been devised, but as yet there is no clinical evidence that they are superior to the Greenfield filter. Nevertheless, a long-term follow-up of high-risk patients with filters revealed that their initial benefit was counterbalanced by a significant increase in deep vein thrombosis and no change in mortality.

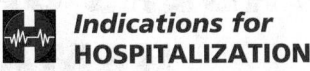

Indications for HOSPITALIZATION

Treatment of established thrombotic disease requires hospitalization for the administration of medication and monitoring of drug dosage. Patients with suspected deep venous thrombosis of the lower extremity can be safely followed as outpatients if serial B-mode ultrasonographic examinations remain negative. A caveat to this practice is that it was previously thought safe to follow outpatients with negative IPG studies, although we now know that this is not the case. Further clinical experience will determine if serial B-mode ultrasonographic examination is as specific and sensitive as currently thought. Whether replacement of standard heparin with low molecular weight preparations will permit outpatient treatment of established thrombosis is a question that cannot be answered until clinical trials have been carried out.

BIBLIOGRAPHY

Bounameaux H, de Moerloose P, Perrier A, et al. Plasma measurements of D-dimer as diagnostic aid in suspected venous thromboembolism: an overview. *Thromb Haemost* 1994;71:1–6.

Heijboer H, Büller HR, Lensing AWA, et al. A comparison of real-time compression ultrasonography with impedance plethysmography for the diagnosis of deep-vein thrombosis in symptomatic outpatients. *N Engl J Med* 1993;329:1365–1369.

Hirsh J, Levine MN. Low molecular weight heparin. *Blood* 1992;79:1–17.

Hull R, Hirsh J, Sackett DL, et al. Cost effectiveness of clinical diagnosis, venography, and noninvasive testing in patients with symptomatic deep-vein thrombosis. *N Engl J Med* 1981;304:1561–1567.

Hull RD, Raskob GE, Rosenbloom D, et al. Heparin for 5 days as compared with 10 days in the initial treatment of proximal venous thrombosis. *N Engl J Med* 1990;322:1260–1264.

Kearon C, Hirsh J. Factors influencing the reported sensitivity and specificity of impedance plethysmography for proximal deep vein thrombosis. *Thromb Haemost* 1994;72:652–658.

Litin SC, Gastineau DA. Current concepts in anticoagulant therapy. *Mayo Clin Proc* 1995;70:266–272.

Prandoni P, Lensing AWA, Büller HR, et al. Deep-vein thrombosis and the incidence of subsequent symptomatic cancer. *N Engl J Med* 1992; 327:1128–1133.

Stewart JH, Grubb M. Understanding vascular ultrasonography. *Mayo Clin Proc* 1992;67:1186–1196.

Weinmann EE, Salzman WE. Deep vein thrombosis. *N Engl J Med* 1994; 331:1630–1641.

Kelley's Textbook of Internal Medicine, fourth edition. Edited by H. David Humes.
Lippincott Williams & Wilkins, Philadelphia © 2000.

DISORDERS OF ONCOLOGY AND HEMATOLOGY

BREAST CANCER

TERESA GILEWSKI
LARRY NORTON

DEFINITIONS

Several different types of malignancies are found in the human breast, each defined by a specific histologic appearance. The term *breast cancer* usually refers to adenocarcinoma. This is the most common malignant neoplasm of mammary tissue and, with lung cancer, one of the two most common cancers of women in the developed world. The rare primary malignancies of the breast include cystosarcoma phyllodes, various sarcomas, and lymphomas. Cancers from other primary sites, such as the skin (i.e., melanoma), lung, ovary, cervix, prostate, and bladder, may sometimes metastasize to the breast, and metastases of breast cancer to the contralateral breast are not uncommon.

Breast cancer is occasionally diagnosed in men, at a rate that is approximately 1% of its incidence in women. Female breast cancer is one of the oldest diseases in the medical literature, having been described in ancient Egyptian texts. It has also been one of the most studied of human cancers and remains a major focus of much contemporary science. Although significant progress has been made in the understanding, diagnosis, and clinical management of breast cancer, universal cure has not yet been attained. Although most individuals diagnosed with breast cancer in high-incidence areas such as North America and Europe will now be cured, it is one of the most common causes of cancer fatality among women in these same areas.

Normal breast anatomy consists of specialized epithelial breast tissue, the outer layer of skin, subcutaneous adipose and connective tissues, nerves, blood and lymph vessels, and other supportive stroma. The specialized breast tissue itself largely consists of numerous ducts, arranged in intertwined treelike (fractal) structures rooted at the nipple and connecting terminally to secretory lobules. The nipple is surrounded by a cutaneous hyperpigmented areola. Because the development of breast tissue is influenced positively by female hormones, including progesterone as well as estrogen, the male breast is anatomically complete but grossly hypoplastic compared with that of postpubertal women.

Most breast adenocarcinomas are thought to arise from the ductal epithelial cells close to or at the juncture of a duct and a lobule. These cancers may be *in situ* or *infiltrating* (also called *invasive*). The in situ carcinomas are further classified as *lobular carcinoma in situ (LCIS)* or *ductal carcinoma in situ (DCIS)*. DCIS is also called *intraductal carcinoma*, a term often and erroneously confused with *infiltrating ductal carcinoma*. DCIS and LCIS do not invade the parenchyma or stroma of the breast and have a very low potential for generating metastases. Invasive breast adenocarcinomas, which do infiltrate into surrounding normal tissues, also fall into ductal and lobular types, with the ductal types predominating. About 15% of breast cancers have "special" histopathologic patterns, including mucinous, papillary, medullary, tubular, and adenoid cystic types.

The ability of cancer cells to grow into normal breast parenchyma and stroma is called *invasion*. This property is correlated with the ability of these cells to grow in sites other than the breast itself, including noncontiguous sites—a process called *metastasis*. Cancer cells gain access to foreign tissues through the flow of blood and lymph. The most common site of metastasis is the axillary lymph nodes. The number of lymph nodes containing breast cancer cells is a good indicator of that primary cancer's propensity for metastasizing to more distant anatomical sites such as bone, lung, liver, and brain.

Breast cancer is staged by assessing tumor (T) size, nodal (N) involvement, and presence or absence of distant metastasis (M). The TNM classification for breast cancer developed by the Union International Contra le Cancrum and the American Joint Committee on Cancer Staging (AJCC) is shown in Table 220.1. Proper staging is achieved by pathologic examination of the breast tissue and the axillary lymph nodes, physical examination, chest radiograph, and assay of serum markers such as liver transaminases and the various alkaline phosphatases. Physical examination is not a reliable way of assessing axillary nodal involvement because nodes can be involved without being palpable and not all palpable nodes are positive histologically for cancer. Recently, a technique for assessing axillary involvement called *sentinel lymph node mapping* has been developed and popularized. This technique was pioneered in the treatment of melanoma. It introduces a radioactive tracer or a dye or both into the breast

TABLE 220.1.	TNM CLASSIFICATION FOR BREAST CANCER

T Tumor Size

Tis	In situ
T1	≤2 cm
T2	>2–5 cm
T3	>5 cm
T4	Extension to chest wall or skin

N Nodal Involvement

N0	None
N1	Movable, ipsilateral axillary
N2	Fixed, ipsilateral axillary
N3	Internal mammary

M Metastases

M1	(includes supraclavicular nodes)

Stages

0	Tis
I	T1 N0
IIA	T1 N1
	T2 N0
IIB	T2 N1
	T3 N0
IIIA	T3 N1
	Any N2
IIIB	Any N3
	Any T4
IV	M1

at the time of tumor resection and dissects the one to several nodes that first take up the substance. If these sentinel nodes are free of cancer, the overwhelming likelihood is that the rest of the axilla will be free as well. This saves the patient unnecessary axillary surgery and allows the pathologist to concentrate (using immunohistochemistry and molecular techniques in addition to routine histology) on the few nodes removed.

Most patients in North America and Europe present with disease in stages I and II. Stage I cancers, small and without axillary lymph node involvement, have the best prognoses. A greater risk of eventual systemic recurrence is associated with stage II cancers. These can be of any size up to 5 cm in diameter with axillary lymph nodes that are movable but histologically positive. Stage II also includes cancers without axillary lymph node involvement if the tumors are larger than 2 cm in diameter. In practice, many clinicians classify breast cancers as "node-negative" or "node-positive," crossing TNM categories; a node-negative case could be in stage I, II, or even IIIA.

Nodal involvement is quantified by the number of involved nodes, with the denominator (total number of nodes examined) serving to indicate that an adequate dissection has been performed. Nodes are also described by their level; level I nodes are lateral to the pectoralis minor muscle, level III nodes are medial, and level II nodes are between levels I and III. The level of nodal involvement is important only because it correlates with the number of involved nodes. Skip metastases (e.g., level II being positive when level I is negative) do occur rarely and may indicate sampling error in the examination of the level I nodes.

Hence, the wider use of sentinel lymph node mapping may make these cases even more unusual.

Locally advanced breast cancers (mostly stage III) are either larger than 5 cm in diameter, invade into the skin or chest wall, or are associated with fixed, histologically positive axillary nodes. Their prognosis is worse than those in the earlier stages, but the outcome is still largely a function of the number of involved axillary lymph nodes. Stage III is a common presentation in economically underdeveloped parts of the world, largely because of the failure of early diagnosis rather than rapidly growing disease.

Stage IV tumors demonstrate evidence of metastatic spread to regions outside the breast and axilla, including, since reclassification in 1988, supraclavicular lymph nodes.

The TNM staging system evolved primarily to aid surgical decisions. This is because most stage I cancers, many stage II cancers, and some stage III cancers can be cured with local therapy alone. Patients with more advanced stage III cancers and with stage IV disease are not curable by surgery alone, although an operative procedure to achieve local control may be indicated. Medical oncologists use classic TNM staging but they also commonly categorize patients by the number of involved axillary lymph nodes. This has guided and continues to facilitate decisions regarding systemic adjuvant drug therapy, although modern chemotherapies are becoming effective enough that we may soon reach a point where all patients will receive the same treatment regardless of axillary status.

Toward the end of the nineteenth century, William Halsted promulgated the idea that breast cancer spreads in an orderly fashion from the breast to the axillary lymph nodes and then to distant sites if the cells are not arrested in the axillary "filter." This concept supported the use of aggressive local surgery to remove all of the cancerous cells before they could spread, as well as the evolution of more extensive operations, culminating in Jerome Urban's extended radical mastectomy, which resected parts of the chest wall. A more modern idea, associated with the work of Bernard Fisher and colleagues, is that cancer cells have anatomical access to the entire body even when the primary tumor is very small. These cancer cells may grow in sites other than the breast because of the fertility of these fields rather than mere mechanical access. Applying this concept, axillary nodal involvement is only a sign of the potential for systemic disease. An emerging composite hypothesis, associated with the writings of Samuel Hellman, is that both anatomical and biochemical factors are important. Axillary nodes are often involved because they are fertile fields biochemically and because they are accessible by virtue of the pattern of lymph flow. The fact that sentinel lymph node mapping works supports this latter view. By the composite hypothesis, local control is insufficient to ensure cure but is necessary for optimal management. Recent data showing that radiotherapy to the chest wall after complete mastectomy increases long-term cure rates are consistent with this idea.

INCIDENCE AND EPIDEMIOLOGIC FACTORS

Breast cancer and lung cancer are the most common malignancies in women in the economically developed world. In 2000, an estimated 182,800 women will be diagnosed with breast cancer in the United States, and 40,800 women will die of this disease. One of the strongest risk factors for the development of breast cancer in women is advancing age. Between 1994 and 1996, the probability of an American woman presenting with infiltrating breast cancer was 0.43% before the age of 40, 4.06% from 40 to 59 years of age, and 6.88% from 60 to 79 years, giving an overall risk of 12.56%. Women with a personal history of breast cancer develop contralateral disease at a rate of a little over 1% per year. This risk, however, is not equally spread among the members of this population; women with specific hereditary predispositions, or those who received prior radiation exposure (such as in treatment of Hodgkin's disease), clearly carry higher risks.

Breast cancer is becoming more common, although it remains unclear as to whether this is due to the increasing age of the population, the efficiency of mammographic diagnosis, or a true change in the character of the disease. Europe, Canada, the United States, Australia, and the developed parts of South America have higher rates than most Asian countries. Germ line differences in predisposition alone cannot account for these observations, and environmental and lifestyle factors—including diet—are under intense scrutiny. Although there is no convincing evidence that dietary fat (or total calories, which is inextricably linked to fat content) is etiologic within a country, societies composed of individuals who consume less fat, fewer calories, and more vegetables also have less breast cancer. Because the range of fat intake between countries in these studies is greater than that between subjects in the studies within one culture, the fat–breast cancer link has not yet been disproved. Daily alcohol consumption of one drink or more per day is associated with an increased risk of breast cancer, especially among younger women. The relationship is not linear, however, and rises more quickly with more alcohol consumed.

ETIOLOGIC FACTORS

The etiology of breast cancer is clearly multifactorial (Table 220.2). Family history is a major component of the overall risk profile. A woman's family history of breast cancer in a first-degree relative (mother or sister) increases her risk by up to threefold. This risk is highest in association with a family history of bilateral disease or of premenopausal cancer. Nevertheless, it is estimated that only 10% of breast cancers are related to a hereditary predisposition. Henry Lynch and others have long described a familial association between breast and ovarian cancers, and links with colon, salivary gland, skin (melanoma), and, especially, prostate cancers are also under study. Although some of these familial patterns may be associated with factors other than hereditary predisposition, genetic epidemiology is revolutionizing our view of the cause of breast cancer.

Germ line deleterious mutations of the gene *BRCA1*, identified on chromosome 17, and the gene *BRCA2*, mapped to chromosome 13, are associated with a higher risk of breast and ovarian cancer. Although these genes have characteristics similar to those of tumor suppressor genes, and their function is not completely clear, there is growing evidence that they may be involved

TABLE 220.2.	POTENTIAL ETIOLOGIC FACTORS FOR BREAST CANCER

Family history
  Germ line mutations
Hormonal exposure
  Age at menarche
  Age at menopause
  Age at first full-term pregnancy
  Exogenous estrogen
    Oral contraceptives
    Estrogen replacement
Radiation exposure
Hyperproliferative benign breast lesions
Prior breast cancer
Diet
Alcohol intake

in the cell's response to DNA damage. Following Knudson's multistep paradigm, inactivating germ line mutations coupled with the random loss of the other allele may be catastrophic to the individual. Mutations of these genes are more common in those with a family history of early-onset breast cancer and ovarian cancer. *BRCA1* and *BRCA2* mutations account for a significant proportion of hereditary breast cancers, perhaps as high as 90%, but there is evidence that other as yet unidentified genes also contribute to this syndrome. Rarer breast cancer–related familial syndromes, thought to be inherited in an autosomal dominant pattern, include Cowden's disease (multiple hamartomas), Muir's syndrome (skin and gastrointestinal tumors), and Li–Fraumeni or SBLA syndrome (soft tissue and bone sarcomas, brain tumors, leukemia, adrenocortical carcinoma, and others). Li–Fraumeni syndrome is associated in many cases with germ line *p53* mutations.

Men who are heterozygous in BRCA1 do not carry an increased risk of developing breast cancer. Men who are heterozygous in BRCA2 have a higher risk than normal men but a lower risk than women with these lesions. Hence, estrogen plays a role in the expression of familial breast cancer. Similarly, for sporadic cases, about 90% of the total cases, estrogen seems to be implicated in etiology. The disease is rare in women with congenital absence of ovarian function. Men who are homozygous normal in BRCA1 and BRCA2 seldom develop breast cancer unless they are hyperestrogenemic by virtue of Klinefelter's syndrome, liver disease, massive obesity, or exogenous hormone use. In women, the early onset of menarche (≤ 12 years) and a greater number of ovulatory cycles are associated with increased risk. Nulliparous women or those with their first pregnancy after age 35 have a higher incidence of breast cancer. An early full-term pregnancy may be partially protective. Intense physical activity on the positive side and malnutrition on the negative side can delay menarche or decrease the number of ovulatory cycles; both situations also diminish risk, as does natural menopause before age 45 or a bilateral oophorectomy before age 50. Moderate levels of physical activity, particularly in childhood, are also somewhat protective. There is some evidence that the beneficial effect may be mediated by factors other than the suppression of ovarian function.

All ductal hyperproliferations of breast tissue seem to increase the risk of carcinogenesis, although not all carry the same degree of negative impact. Atypical ductal hyperplasia, for example, is associated with increased subsequent risk, especially if coupled with a positive family history. Benign lesions not involving hyperproliferation, such as cysts, most fibroadenomas, or mastitis, are not predisposing. It is likely, therefore, that the hyperproliferative lesions carry some genetic changes that are necessary but not sufficient for full neoplastic transformation. Consistent with this view is the fact that exposure to ionizing radiation, by radiotherapy or secondary to radiation accidents, increases the risk of breast cancer, particularly if the event occurs before 20 years of age. Links to chemical exposure from pesticides or industrial contamination, some of which is known to be mutagenic, have been suggested by some studies, and more work is needed in this area.

Considering the importance of estrogen in breast cancer etiology, it would seem reasonable that exposure to exogenous estrogens in the form of birth control pills or postmenopausal replacement would be deleterious. Evidence is accumulating that both treatments are associated with slightly increased risk, especially after prolonged use, although it is possible that the breast cancers that arise secondary to estrogen use tend to be positive for estrogen receptors and may carry a better prognosis for this reason. Recommendations in regard to the use of exogenous estrogens are controversial largely because the beneficial effects of such treatment may outweigh the increased risk of breast cancer in certain individuals. At present, the physician and patient must weigh the risks and benefits carefully and make individual, independent decisions regarding use of these treatments. As newer estrogens (such as raloxifene for the prevention of osteoporosis) come into wider use, the controversies may diminish because these agents may actually reduce the risk of breast cancer. Currently, these topics are under intense scrutiny.

PATHOPHYSIOLOGIC FACTORS AND PATHOGENESIS

Ductal carcinoma in situ comprises a heterogeneous group of lesions that are usually regarded as a unilateral, very early, preinvasive form of true breast cancer. Future, further subclassifications of this entity will probably be based on molecular analysis. One type is characterized by comedo necrosis, high mitotic rate, and pleomorphic nuclei. This form of DCIS often overexpresses the ligandless receptor protein tyrosine kinase HER2 (also designated as *neu* and c-*erb*B2). It more commonly transforms or progresses into microinvasive or frank invasive cancer than the noncomedo types: solid, papillary, or cribriform types. DCIS is commonly multifocal or even diffuse throughout the breast, and it often appears as microcalcifications on mammograms.

Lobular carcinoma in situ is often thought of as a marker of carcinogenic potential rather than a true cancer. It is characterized by a proliferation of small, uniform cells and often is multifocal. A patient with a biopsy showing LCIS carries a risk of developing invasive cancers of ductal or lobular types of 1% to 2% per year. Both breasts are at equal risk. LCIS lesions rarely form microcalcifications and are usually invisible by mammography.

Among the invasive cancers the most common histologic type, accounting for approximately 75% of tumors, is infiltrating ductal carcinoma (not to be confused with intraductal carcinoma, which is DCIS). Infiltrating ductal cancers tend to grow as discrete masses, sometimes with microcalcifications, and more commonly as solitary rather than multiple lesions. Good nuclear grade (i.e., graded from 1 to 3, with grade 3 the least differentiated) is associated with a better prognosis. Histologic grading is inverse, with grade 1 indicative of a well-differentiated tumor with better prognosis. The absence of cancer cells in lymphatic channels or blood vessels is also relatively favorable.

Infiltrating lobular carcinoma constitutes approximately 10% of breast cancers. They usually grow as spreading sheets with indistinct edges. Because they tend not to calcify and not to form distinct masses, they are more difficult to diagnose by palpation or mammogram. Some reports associate lobular invasive cancer with bilaterality and multicentricity, but this observation is not universal. Infiltrating lobular carcinomas generally have the same prognosis as infiltrating ductal carcinomas of the same size and number of involved axillary lymph nodes. However, infiltrating lobular carcinomas have a greater tendency to metastasize to the meninges and serosal surfaces, such as the peritoneum.

The less common, special types of invasive breast cancer—mucinous (invasive colloid), papillary, medullary, tubular, and adenoid cystic—seem to have particularly good prognoses if they are small and do not involve the axillary lymph nodes. However, if they are large or node-positive, they may be very aggressive, especially if the medullary type.

Paget's disease of the nipple occurs in 1% to 2% of patients with breast cancer. The usual presentation is an eczematoid change of the nipple, such as scaling or a bloody discharge. This lesion is associated with a cancer involving the breast ductal parenchyma under the nipple. The prognosis for Paget's disease depends on its histologic type and other features of the underlying cancer. Intraductal Paget's disease is quite curable with complete excision, which usually means mastectomy.

Inflammatory breast cancer is an especially aggressive form of invasive disease, accounting for fewer than 5% of breast cancers in North America. It is seen more frequently in women in other parts of the world, especially in North Africa. Typical findings include diffuse swelling of the breast, erythema and warmth of the skin, breast pain, and peau d'orange type of edema of the skin. Because these changes bear a superficial resemblance to bacterial infection, it may be misdiagnosed as mastitis. The essential feature of this presentation, discoverable only on histopathologic examination, is dermal lymphatic invasion. However, the disease may be diagnosed on clinical grounds even if dermal lymphatic invasion is not found on biopsy as the result of a sampling error.

PROGNOSTIC FACTORS

The major factors reported to predict the prognosis of breast cancer are listed in Table 220.3. Of these, only a few are suffi-

TABLE 220.3.	FACTORS EVALUATED IN BREAST CANCER TO AID IN PROGNOSTICATION

Established

Number of positive axillary lymph nodes
Tumor size
Histologic tumor type
Histologic features, including grade
Estrogen and progesterone receptor status
Patient's age
S-phase fraction

Investigational

Ploidy
Proliferative indexes
   Thymidine labeling index
   Topoisomerase II
   Histones
   Ki-67
   Cyclins
Growth factors
   Transforming growth factors
   Epidermal growth factor receptor
   Insulin-like growth factors
Genes (e.g., *neu, ras, p53, myc, int2, brca1, brca2, nm23*)
Cathepsin D
Angiogenesis factors
Aromatase in tumor and stroma
Laminin receptor
Heat-shock proteins

ciently well characterized to be useful for clinical guidance. The number of positive axillary lymph nodes is the most reliable prognostic factor. Survival rates decrease, and relapse rates increase as the number of involved lymph nodes rises.

A less favorable outcome is usually associated with larger tumors, more poorly differentiated lesions, and absence of receptors for estrogen and progesterone in the cancer cells. The hormone receptor status can be determined by the older dextran-coated charcoal biochemical assay, which requires fresh-frozen and abundant tissue, or by the newer method of immunohistochemistry. This can be performed on lesions of any size or on archival (paraffin-embedded) specimens, and is subject to fewer false-negative results because of handling errors. The biochemical assay, however, provides a quantitative result, which has prognostic importance. Hence, there is value in both techniques.

Several studies indicate that development of breast cancer at a young age (less than 35 years) is associated with a higher risk of relapse, although this effect may not be independent of other prognostic factors such as tumor size, hormone receptor status, and nodal positivity. Many of the other prognostic factors, while profoundly interesting, remain experimental. Much of the data are preliminary, many of the assays are not standardized, some of the reports are contradictory, and reliable corroboration is often lacking. DNA ploidy measures the amount of DNA in cells, with diploidy being normal and aneuploidy abnormal. Aneuploidy, which usually means too much DNA per cell, tends to correlate with differentiation. The S-phase fraction, measured

by flow cytometry or by thymidine labeling index, estimates the percentage of cells preparing for mitosis. This also correlates positively with differentiation and with tumor size, and is felt by many investigators to be a reliable and independent prognostic factor. However, variations in the technical aspects of this assay can make comparisons between studies difficult.

There has recently been a surge of interest in growth factors and their receptors, such as the epidermal growth factor receptor (EGFR) and HER2, and in mitosis regulators such as p53, which may play an important role in carcinogenesis and in the clinical course of the disease. Tumors that overexpress HER2 and involve axillary lymph nodes tend to behave more aggressively, as do HER2-positive metastatic lesions. It remains controversial as to whether HER2 status is prognostic in node-negative disease. However, recent data indicate that tumors that overexpress HER2 may be more sensitive to doxorubicin-based chemotherapy regimens and perhaps paclitaxel as well. Therefore, some of the factors studied for their prognostic value may be as or more useful in terms of their ability to predict response to certain types of therapy. The classic example of this phenomenon is the estrogen receptor, which was developed to predict response to hormonal therapy but has some prognostic value as well.

CLINICAL FINDINGS

PREOPERATIVE EVALUATION

As in all fields of medicine, good practice demands a thorough history and physical examination. The history should ascertain potential risk factors as discussed previously and disclose symptoms associated with local or systemic disease. These include changes in the breast or axilla: erythema, edema, masses, dimpling of the skin, nipple discharge, or pain. A complete review of systems should focus on possible metastatic indicators such as bone pain or respiratory difficulties.

The physical examination should be complete while focusing on the breast, axilla, and supraclavicular areas. These sites are evaluated for the presence of erythema, edema, dimpling, masses, skin nodules, ulceration, and skin discoloration. Abnormalities in the breast are better described by using a clock distribution than by specifying the quadrant. Although clinical assessment of axillary node palpability is important, it is notoriously inaccurate regarding actual histologic involvement. The supraclavicular nodal examination is crucial because the presence of nodal involvement is an indication of metastatic disease, dramatically altering the patient's prognosis and treatment. Evaluation of this area may be facilitated by asking the patient to shrug her or his shoulders forward.

POSTOPERATIVE EVALUATION

Guidelines for the follow-up of patients after primary therapy remain somewhat controversial. The American Society of Clinical Oncology surveillance recommendations include a history and physical examination every 3 to 6 months for 3 years, then every 6 to 12 months for 2 years, and then annually. Symptomatic patients should undergo further evaluation promptly in all cases, and all abnormal laboratory findings, discussed subsequently, should be thoroughly investigated.

SCREENING

The only screening technique available is mammography. There is considerable controversy regarding the timing of this study. The American Cancer Society and most professional groups recommend that women 50 years of age and older undergo yearly mammograms, with mammograms every 1 to 2 years starting at age 40 for those younger than 50. The value of breast self-examination has been questioned, but it has no significant deleterious effects except possibly for causing increased patient anxiety, which should be correctable by patient education. Women should be encouraged to perform monthly self-examinations, and they should have an annual professional manual breast examination. These examinations should be in addition to routine screening for gynecologic and gastrointestinal tumors.

LABORATORY AND RADIOGRAPHIC FINDINGS

PREOPERATIVE EVALUATION

A mammogram is useful in evaluating the remainder of the abnormal breast and the contralateral breast for masses or calcifications before definitive surgery. A negative mammogram does not rule out malignancy. A persistent mass must be biopsied regardless of the mammogram findings.

Evaluation of a palpable breast mass and abnormal mammograms are further discussed in Chapter 205. Bone scans and liver scans are not routinely performed preoperatively in asymptomatic patients with normal laboratory values because the probability of detecting occult metastases in these women is less than 2%. Chest radiographs are obtained routinely, primarily because they are required for surgical anesthesia.

A complete blood count and chemistry profile are routinely obtained before surgery. Persistent elevation of bone or hepatic enzymes, specifically alkaline phosphatase or aspartate transaminase, warrant further evaluation with scans to rule out metastatic disease. However, these laboratory tests are nonspecific and frequently reflect a benign problem. There is no definite role for preoperative assessment of tumor-associated antigens such as carcinoembryonic antigen (CEA) or serum glycoprotein CA 15-3.

POSTOPERATIVE EVALUATION

A yearly mammogram is obligatory. Due to lack of evidence to suggest clinical benefit, the American Society of Clinical Oncology does not recommend routine bone scans, chest x-rays, or liver imaging. Many medical oncologists obtain complete blood counts, liver transaminase levels, and alkaline phosphatase levels on a routine basis, although available data do not support this practice. The value of other serum markers, such as CEA and CA 15-3, is also controversial. An isolated abnormal value is not necessarily an indication of recurrent disease, but a persistent or rising level is worrisome. The CEA level may be increased because of smoking or other benign or malignant disease of the liver, lung, gastrointestinal tract, ovary, or breast. Almost half of patients with documented metastatic breast cancer have increased CEA values, and the CA 15-3 level is elevated in as many as 80% of these patients. The CA 15-3 test is thought to have greater sensitivity than the CEA level, but an abnormal result may also be attributed to benign and malignant conditions similar to those associated with an elevated CEA level, except for smoking. There is, however, no doubt that assessment of the trend of CEA and CA 15-3 levels may be useful in following the clinical course of disease after metastases have been documented.

OPTIMAL MANAGEMENT

Because clinical breast cancer is conspicuously heterogeneous, the best guidelines are general, with excellent care often requiring marked variances from specified pathways. This is especially so because psychosocial factors often dominate the clinical setting in a disease as emotionally stressful as breast cancer. Nevertheless, certain principles have been established by clinical experience and by prospective, randomized clinical trials, and these form a basis for decision making and the evaluation of therapeutic practices.

The therapy of primary breast cancer is aimed at local control and the prevention of the appearance of systemic recurrence (metastatic spread). Local therapeutic modalities include surgery and radiation therapy. Established systemic therapies are chemotherapy and hormonal therapy. An immunotherapeutic approach is also emerging as a potentially effective treatment.

The first step in planning good treatment is to verify the histology of the tumor. In situ and infiltrating tumors are managed differently, and for both types of breast cancer, the histologic features may affect the prognosis and therapeutic decisions. For invasive lesions, knowledge of the status of receptors for estrogen (and progesterone, if available) is also key.

DUCTAL CARCINOMA IN SITU

Ductal carcinoma in situ can present as a mass, but it is more commonly found by biopsy of abnormal calcifications seen on a mammogram. The diagnosis of DCIS has increased during the past several decades, probably because of the increased use of mammographic screening. The optimal management of this condition is not yet established. In former years, the standard therapy was a mastectomy, which is so effective that there is a paucity of information on the natural history of this disease. Axillary dissection is usually not recommended for DCIS unless microinvasion is present. However, some surgeons are now offering sentinel lymph node mapping at the time of surgery for DCIS.

Local excision of a DCIS lesion leaves the rest of the breast at risk for recurrence. This risk is influenced by the extent of the DCIS (diameter of involved breast tissue), the presence of comedo necrosis, and the status of the margins of resection. Half of recurrences in the breast are infiltrating cancers, rather than DCIS. The National Surgical Adjuvant Breast and Bowel Project (NSABP) reported that radiation therapy to the remaining breast after local excision reduces the local recurrence rate by 50%, with more efficacy in preventing invasive recurrences than recurrent DCIS. Therefore, most patients receive radiation therapy after undergoing local excision. However, there may be some who do not require radiation therapy. The identification of patients at an extremely low risk of relapse remains an active area of research, with several ongoing trials.

Even with the best therapy for DCIS, recurrences do occur and postsurgical follow-up is necessary. In addition, very long-term research will be needed to determine if the local failure rate of breast-conserving surgery plus irradiation for DCIS is acceptable. The likelihood of systemic metastases occurring from true DCIS is extremely small, and there has been no clear role for systemic adjuvant drug therapy. However, recent preliminary results from the NSABP indicate that tamoxifen can decrease the risk of invasive breast cancer in patients treated with lumpectomy and radiation. Further follow-up is necessary to determine an effect on overall survival. Therefore, tamoxifen may be appropriate therapy in patients with DCIS and may be useful to decrease the incidence of contralateral intraductal and invasive disease, as discussed below.

LOBULAR CARCINOMA IN SITU

Because lobular carcinoma in situ is usually not palpable and is invisible by mammography, the diagnosis of LCIS is commonly incidental to a breast biopsy performed for another reason. Because LCIS is an indicator of a propensity for developing invasive cancers and because both breasts are at equal risk, treatment options include observation alone or bilateral simple prophylactic mastectomies. There is no role for radiation therapy. Ipsilateral mastectomy with a contralateral biopsy has been performed in the past, but it is not advised because a negative contralateral biopsy does not rule out the risk of subsequent cancer occurring in the contralateral breast. Prophylactic mastectomy surely decreases the risk of the patient later presenting with invasive cancer. However, the magnitude of benefit is not certain because no mastectomy is absolutely complete, and patients have had recurrences in residual breast tissue in the chest wall or axilla after this procedure. Hence, current standard practice includes careful observation, with a growing movement toward the use of chemoprevention. Until recently there was also no clear-cut role for systemic drug therapy in the treatment of LCIS. However, recent data from the NSABP Breast Cancer Prevention Trial P-1 demonstrate an approximately 50% reduction in the risk of infiltrating breast cancer in patients with a history of LCIS after the administration of tamoxifen.

INFILTRATING TUMORS

Local Therapy

Local treatment of breast cancer involves surgery and radiation therapy. In the late nineteenth century, Halsted popularized the radical mastectomy (RM). This operation resected the breast, all axillary lymph nodes, a significant amount of skin, and the pectoralis major and minor muscles. Motivated by the prevailing biologic hypotheses of his time, Urban's *extended radical mastec-*

tomy added dissection of the internal mammary lymph nodes to Halsted's operation.

Largely because of public demand, to circumvent the disfigurement caused by these operations, the modified radical mastectomy (MRM) was investigated, starting in the 1940s. This operation removes the breast tissue, overlying skin, and axillary lymph nodes without resection of the muscle of the chest wall. Randomized studies have demonstrated no significant difference in disease-free or overall survival after RM or MRM, thereby establishing the less mutilating procedure as the standard. These results raised questions about the validity of the biologic concepts that motivated the more extreme resection.

Based on some of the newer concepts mentioned above, and in response to patients' concerns, Bernard Fisher in the United States, Umberto Veronesi in Milan, and subsequently others led investigations of even less mutilating surgery. These studies have established that breast-conserving surgery (BCS)—quadrantectomy or lumpectomy—plus axillary dissection plus radiation therapy to the remaining breast was as curative as MRM. Axillary dissection, when performed, should include the lymph nodes lateral to and underneath the pectoralis minor muscle. Fisher's group, the NSABP, demonstrated that the risk of local relapse exceeds 40% without radiation therapy. With radiation and good surgery (margins free of cancer), the national average for local control is in excess of 90%. However, BCS is not appropriate for all patients. Potential contraindications include multicentric tumors, large cancer-to-breast ratio, history of previous irradiation of the breast (for breast cancer or for treatment of lymphoma or other cancers), scattered malignant calcifications throughout the breast, very young age, extensive DCIS involving the lumpectomy margins, or anatomical factors that may predispose to a poor cosmetic result. It has long been felt that a history of connective tissue disease would contraindicate breast irradiation, for fear of a poor cosmetic result, but recent experience has raised doubts about this point.

When mastectomy is indicated, some surgeons are now performing a procedure called skin-sparing mastectomy. This leaves much of the skin overlying the breast intact, which facilitates reconstruction using the patient's own tissues.

It is also notable that sentinel lymph node mapping is now standard in many hospitals, being used instead of routine axillary dissection, especially in conjunction with BCS. However, major questions regarding this procedure are still unanswered, prompting much ongoing research by the American College of Surgeons and other groups.

When systemic adjuvant chemotherapy is used, radiation therapy is usually administered after chemotherapy. While this is still a point of some controversy, most radiation is being delivered in this sequence. Radiation therapy to the chest wall may also be administered after MRM in patients with large tumors or in those with a large number of positive nodes. In these cases the risk of local recurrence is high. In addition, several recent studies have demonstrated decreased mortality in premenopausal patients treated with radiation therapy after MRM. These results have generated much discussion. In general, based on these data, radiation therapy should be considered following MRM for most patients with four or more positive axillary nodes. Some patients with fewer positive nodes may also be considered candidates, largely because of factors that increase the likelihood of local recurrence, although specific treatment guidelines are in evolution.

Toxic effects from surgery and radiation therapy include self-limited pain, rare and usually treatable infection, disfigurement, and lymphedema. The availability of breast reconstruction using tissue expanders and saline-filled implants or using myocutaneous flaps should be discussed with the patient before local therapy. Lymphedema is a persistent problem that afflicts about 10% of patients undergoing axillary dissection. One of the advantages of sentinel lymph node mapping is that it may decrease the risk of the development of this complication. If the sentinel node is positive, then a complete axillary dissection is performed. If the sentinel node is negative, further axillary surgery is not performed because there is a low chance of there being positive axillary lymph nodes. While this procedure is now widely used, it clearly requires considerable expertise to be successful, and its ultimate reliability is still being studied.

Systemic Therapy

The drug treatment of breast cancer involves the use of several different types of therapy. For many decades the mainstays of treatment were chemotherapy and hormonal therapy, but these were recently joined by antibody therapy following approval of the drug trastuzumab. Drugs are used in three settings. The first setting is as an adjunct to the local therapies described previously. The intention is to damage micrometastatic cells that are likely to be present but are not yet apparent on physical examination or by laboratory tests. The second setting is in the treatment of overt metastatic disease. A third setting is primary therapy for locally advanced breast cancer, used to render the local disease amenable to surgical and radiotherapeutic approaches. A variant on this third setting, which remains investigational, is to shrink resectable breast cancer to make BCS feasible in cases that otherwise would require mastectomy. For all of these uses, detailed knowledge of the drugs, their indications, toxicities, and interactions is essential (see Chapter 254). Chemotherapeutic drugs, designed to attack mitosis or biochemical precursors to mitosis, are notable for their toxicity as well as their efficacy. Many normal tissues—gastrointestinal mucosa, hematopoietic cells, hair follicles—do have high mitotic rates and are therefore susceptible to chemotherapeutic damage. Granulocytopenia used to be a common life-threatening emergency caused by the use of chemotherapy drugs, but it can now be ameliorated in most cases by the use of recombinant granulocyte colony-stimulating factor (G-CSF).

Hormonal therapies are rooted in the incidental observation made in the nineteenth century that oophorectomy was beneficial to women with metastatic breast cancer. This is based on the fact that many breast cancer cells need estrogen to grow and to remain viable. The biochemical correlate of this need is the presence of hormone receptors. Since progesterone receptor is induced by activated estrogen receptor, estrogen receptor negativity plus progesterone receptor positivity in the same tumor means that the estrogen receptor negativity must be a false result. Hormone therapies work by the disruption of growth factor loops mediated by estrogen. Because they are so targeted, they are generally associated with less acute toxicity than chemotherapy.

TABLE 220.4.	COMMONLY USED DRUGS IN THE TREATMENT OF BREAST CANCER

Hormonal Therapy
Tamoxifen
Anastrozole, letrozole
Megestrol acetate

Chemotherapy
Alkylating agents
  Cyclophosphamide (C)[a]
  Melphalan
  Thiotepa (T)
Antimetabolites
  Methotrexate (M)
  5-Fluorouracil (F, 5-FU)
  Capecitabine
Antitumor antibiotics
  Doxorubicin (A)
  Epirubicin
  Mitomycin C (Mito-C)
  Mitoxantrone
Vinka alkaloids
  Vinblastine
  Vincristine
  Vinorelbine
Taxanes
  Docetaxel
  Paclitaxel
Others
  Gemcitabine

[a] Commonly used abbreviations are given in parentheses.

Chemotherapy Agents

Most of the chemotherapy drugs used as postoperative adjuvant therapy were first employed in the treatment of metastatic disease. The most common chemotherapies used in breast cancer are listed in Table 220.4 according to their presumed primary mechanism of action. Almost all of these agents can be administered in an outpatient setting. Cyclophosphamide (C), methotrexate (M), 5-fluorouracil (F), doxorubicin [Adriamycin] (A), and the taxanes, paclitaxel and docetaxel, are the most commonly used drugs, often in various combinations (Table 220.5).

TABLE 220.5.	COMMONLY USED DRUG COMBINATIONS

CMF (cyclophosphamide, methotrexate, 5-fluorouracil)
CAF (cyclophosphamide, doxorubicin, 5-fluorouracil)
CMFVP (cyclophosphamide, methotrexate, 5-fluorouracil, vincristine, prednisone)
AC (doxorubicin, cyclophosphamide)
VAT (vinblastine, doxorubicin, thiotepa)
VATH (vinblastine, doxorubicin, thiotepa, halotestin)
Mitomycin C + vinblastine
Doxorubicin followed by CMF
AC followed by paclitaxel

One of the most frequently prescribed adjuvant regimens has been CMF (cyclophosphamide, methotrexate, 5-fluorouracil), which is usually administered for a total of 6 months. Doxorubicin is used alone or in combination with other drugs (e.g., AC, CAF). The adjuvant AC regimen is four cycles of intravenous drugs every 3 weeks and hence is of shorter duration than CMF. An overview analysis has suggested that doxorubicin (and similar drugs, called anthracyclines) in combination is slightly more active than CMF, but this benefit may be restricted to certain subsets of patients, a topic of intense current study.

A toxicity common to CMF, taxanes, and the doxorubicin-based regimens is myelosuppression (anemia, leukopenia, and thrombocytopenia). These hematologic values are transiently reduced, with their nadir occurring 1 to 2 weeks after the administration of chemotherapy. Platelet transfusions are rarely required, erythrocyte transfusions are somewhat more common, and antibiotics are only occasionally needed to treat neutropenic fevers. The use of G-CSF is mentioned above. Nausea and vomiting from CMF or the doxorubicin regimens are usually well controlled by the use of the antiemetics granisetron and ondansetron. Mucositis, diarrhea, and severe weight gain are unusual toxicities. The CMF and CAF regimens are associated with a slightly increased incidence of thromboembolic events, which are somewhat more likely when prednisone or tamoxifen is added. Alopecia requiring the wearing of a wig occurs in almost all patients treated with doxorubicin or a taxane, but CMF causes this in only a minority of patients.

Irreversible amenorrhea is induced by the drugs in approximately half of premenopausal patients. It is much more common in older premenopausal patients than in younger patients (up to their mid-thirties). Several studies have suggested that adjuvant AC causes less amenorrhea than CMF, but this lack of amenorrhea is not associated with an inferior response to therapy. The mortality rate from standard adjuvant chemotherapy in expert hands is much less than 1%. Life-threatening complications from chemotherapy are more common in the setting of metastatic disease, probably because of multiple organ impairment from the disease itself. Secondary leukemia is a theoretical concern with the use of adjuvant chemotherapy, but more than 20 years of experience with the CMF regimen has uncovered no higher rate than the expected background incidence. In contrast, the AC combination seems to be associated with a small but real incidence of drug-induced leukemia, and cytogenetic changes have been reported more commonly in patients who received very high doses of chemotherapy with autologous stem cell infusions as hematologic support. There is still no evidence that adjuvant chemotherapy increases the risk of any type of secondary cancer other than leukemia.

Hormonal Therapy

Among their many biologic effects, estrogens are known to stimulate production of growth factors such as transforming growth factor α, which can increase breast tumor proliferation in an autocrine (acting on the cell itself) and paracrine (acting on adjacent cells) manner. The hormonal manipulation of breast cancer involves the inhibition of estrogen's actions by lowering estrogen levels or interfering with the actions of estrogen on the cellular level.

Ovarian Ablation

The classic hormonal therapy for premenopausal breast cancer is ovarian ablation. This is achieved by surgical oophorectomy, by irradiation (which is slow and often incomplete), or by the administration of a gonadotropin-releasing hormone agonist. Adrenalectomy and hypophysectomy are rarely performed today because of their morbidity and their lack of therapeutic advantage over other hormonal therapies. The luteinizing hormone–releasing hormone analogues leuprolide or goserelin provide reversible medical castration by reducing the levels of follicle-stimulating hormone and luteinizing hormone. Ovarian ablation produces postmenopausal symptoms such as hot flashes, vaginitis, and sexual dysfunction.

Antiestrogens

The most commonly used drug for the hormonal therapy of breast cancer is tamoxifen, which is commonly classified as an *antiestrogen*, although this is an incomplete description of the drug's actions. The exact mechanisms by which tamoxifen exerts its antitumor effect remain unclear, but it is clearly not just by interference with estrogenic cell stimulation. In cultured cells, the binding of tamoxifen to estrogen receptors causes a cytostatic rather than a cytocidal effect, with cells piling up in the cell cycle phase (G1) just before DNA synthesis. Estrogen receptors are required for tamoxifen to work. Because cells that seem progesterone receptor–positive but estrogen receptor–negative are really falsely negative for the estrogen receptor, tamoxifen will usually work in these cases as well. Yet the clinical response rates are highest when the tumors express both estrogen and progesterone receptors. Tamoxifen is administered orally at a dose of 20 mg per day. Higher dose levels are not more effective but are more toxic. The most common toxicities are hot flashes, irregular menses, vaginal discharge, depressed mood, and, rarely, thromboembolic events. In general, however, the drug is extremely well tolerated.

Ocular changes and thrombocytopenia do occur but are uncommon. Postmenopausal patients who have received tamoxifen in the adjuvant setting have a slightly higher rate of presenting with uterine cancer, including rare excess fatalities. Screening methods including serial endometrial biopsies and pelvic ultrasound examinations for the early detection of uterine abnormalities in this setting are under investigation, but so far no screening program has proven useful. Meanwhile, women receiving tamoxifen should have a clinical pelvic examination at least yearly. In terms of ancillary positive benefits, tamoxifen's estrogenic effects produce a decrease in cholesterol levels and an improvement in bone mineral density.

Antiestrogens, such as tamoxifen, that have an estrogenic effect on some cells but an antiestrogenic effect on others are now commonly classified as selective estrogen receptor modulators (SERMs), a term first used to describe the antiosteoporosis drug raloxifene. Like tamoxifen, raloxifene seems to decrease the incidence of new breast cancers, at least in postmenopausal women being treated for osteopenia. Unlike tamoxifen, raloxifene does not seem to stimulate growth of the uterine lining. A prospective randomized comparison of tamoxifen and raloxifene as cancer prevention agents is currently under way. The search for better hormonal agents that have an antitumor effect on breast cancer cells and endometrial cells, an estrogenic effect on bone cells and serum lipids, and fewer toxicities is ongoing.

Progestational Agents

Medroxyprogesterone acetate and megestrol acetate are the most frequently used progestational agents in the treatment of advanced breast cancer. They are seldom used in the adjuvant setting. Possible mechanisms of action include a direct cytotoxic effect and indirect effects on the hormonal axis and on tumor growth factors. Megestrol acetate is usually preferred because of its lower rate of toxicity, but it does cause weight gain, fluid retention, and, sometimes, mild hyperglycemia. The standard dosage of megestrol acetate is 160 mg daily. Although higher dosages have been used to treat cachexia, they offer no additional anticancer benefit. Megestrol acetate in lower dosages (20 to 40 mg per day) is often used to treat hot flashes in postmenopausal women.

Aromatase Inhibitors

In postmenopausal women, aromatase in adipose and liver cells catalyzes the rate-limiting step by which adrenal androstenedione is converted to estrone, the major estrogen. Aminoglutethimide and related drugs inhibit this reaction, but they also impair adrenal biosynthesis. Several newer aromatase inhibitors, with proven superior activity/toxicity ratios, are now available, and others are in development. Examples are anastrozole and letrozole. These are usually used as second-line therapies for recurrent breast cancers that are no longer responsive to tamoxifen. A role in the adjuvant setting is under investigation.

Estrogens and Androgens

Pharmacologic doses of estrogens themselves can produce clinical responses in breast cancer, although the actual mechanism is uncertain. Diethylstilbestrol is the prototypic drug, but it is almost never now used because of a significant incidence of troubling toxicities such as nausea, vaginal bleeding, fluid retention, and thromboembolic events. Androgens such as fluoxymesterone have been used to treat breast cancer, although these drugs produce unpleasant virilization.

Adjuvant Therapies

The goal of adjuvant drug therapy is to prevent the growth of microscopic metastatic cells that may have disseminated from the primary tumor. Most patients with primary breast cancer have no clinical evidence of metastatic disease at the time of initial presentation. However, many patients eventually demonstrate metastatic disease. The probability of systemic recurrence varies largely as a function of tumor histopathology and the number of involved axillary lymph nodes. A patient with a small (less than 1 cm in diameter) infiltrating ductal or lobular carcinoma and no involvement of the axillary lymph nodes has an almost 90% chance of being recurrence-free at 20 years. In contrast, a patient with 10 or more involved axillary lymph nodes has less than a 15% chance of being disease-free at 10 years. Adjuvant drug therapy has been proven to improve these odds. It is of theoretical as well as practical interest to recognize that patients with the worst prognoses are the ones who benefit most from adjuvant drug therapy.

Most adjuvant drug therapy is initiated several weeks after the completion of primary breast surgery. A prospective randomized trial by the International Breast Cancer Study Group found that patients receiving at least 6 months of adjuvant chemotherapy fared equally well if they started the treatment immediately after surgery or about 5 weeks later. In the treatment of inoperable stage III disease, chemotherapy drugs are commonly applied before definitive local treatment, an approach termed *primary* or *neoadjuvant chemotherapy*. In the treatment of stage II and operable stage III disease this approach has proven capable of rendering large primaries suitable for BCS. A prospective randomized trial in this setting has been completed by the NSABP and has concluded that preoperative and postoperative AC produce equivalent benefits in such patients in terms of disease-free and overall survival. Long-term results in terms of local control rates are awaited.

Historically, adjuvant chemotherapy was first investigated in the late 1960s and early 1970s in patients with positive axillary lymph nodes. It was thought to be more ethically justifiable to apply potentially toxic treatments to patients with relatively poor prognoses. As the efficacy of adjuvant chemotherapy became clearer, patients without involved nodes were studied, confirming the positive impressions regarding benefits gained from the node-positive trials. Adjuvant hormonal therapy, largely with tamoxifen, has also been studied in node-negative and node-positive patients.

Adjuvant Chemotherapy

The impetus for the widespread study of adjuvant chemotherapy throughout the world were two classical controlled trials. One was the study of L-phenylalanine mustard by the NSABP and the other was the study of the CMF combination by the National Cancer Institute in Milan, led by Gianni Bonadonna and supported by the U.S. National Cancer Institute. Both trials, which treated node-positive patients only, demonstrated real clinical benefit and created a level of excitement that has been the motivation behind hundreds of trials to this day. Topics that have been studied over the years include various combinations of drugs, various dose levels and schedules, and various durations of treatment.

Until recently, 6 months of CMF was the most widely used regimen in general practice. Both the four-cycle AC combination and 6 months of CAF have also proven popular. However, doxorubicin is associated with a real but low incidence of cardiac damage and of drug-induced leukemia. These toxicities have not been seen with CMF. Until recently, there was a lack of data to support the superiority of a doxorubicin-based regimen over CMF for most patients. However, a recent overview (meta-analysis) of all randomized trials has identified a small additional benefit from anthracycline-containing combinations such as AC and CAF. A prospective randomized trial by the Cancer and Leukemia Group B (CALGB) has found that reductions in dose of doxorubicin below 40 mg per square meter are associated with worse outcome. The most dramatic beneficial effects of doxorubin were seen in patients whose tumors overexpressed HER2 and who received doxorubicin at 60 mg per square meter. Hence, reductions in doses of standard adjuvant chemotherapy regimens or significant delays in treatment courses are not justified by the available evidence.

The concept of *dose intensity,* which is the amount of drug administered per unit of time, was formulated by William Hryniuk and colleagues. Based on retrospective analyses, these researchers proposed that the more dose-intensive regimens would result in improved outcome. Dose intensity is properly subdivided into *dose escalation* (increasing the dose level) and *dose density* (decreasing the time between administrations). In this regard, the NCI–Milan group conducted a now classic study of patients with four or more involved lymph nodes. They found that a regimen of doxorubicin for four 3-week cycles followed by CMF for eight 3-week cycles provided significantly decreased relapse and death rates, in comparison with an equally well-tolerated regimen giving the same drugs in an alternating pattern. The doxorubicin followed by CMF is more dose-dense than CMF alternating with doxorubicin because in the superior regimen the same amount of doxorubicin is given over a much shorter interval. However, dose escalation above standard dose levels was not employed in this regimen. The question of whether escalation of dose levels over the standard levels is beneficial or not remains open. As an ultimate application of dose escalation, a short course of chemotherapy can be given at such a high dose level that the reinfusion of autologous hematopoietic stem cells and/or granulocyte colony-stimulating factor (G-CSF) is necessary to accomplish adequate hematopoietic recovery. Based on promising pilot studies, the concept that clinical results of treating high-risk primary breast cancer can be improved by giving such treatment is undergoing extensive evaluation in prospective randomized trials. Preliminary results in several studies in the United States and Europe have indicated no benefit of high-dose chemotherapy and stem cell support over conventional therapy. However, these studies have been either of insufficient size or too short follow-up duration, so that definitive conclusions await longer follow-up. One South African trial was positive and awaits confirmation. Pending the results of these trials, adjuvant high-dose chemotherapy, popularly called autologous bone marrow (or stem cell) transplantations, remains investigational.

A recent study by CALGB has demonstrated that AC followed by paclitaxel was more effective than AC alone in women with node-positive breast cancer. This trial was based on the same concept of sequential dose-dense therapy as the study of doxorubicin and CMF from Milan. Ongoing trials will determine the optimal sequencing, dose, and schedule of administration of these agents, whether docetaxel has any advantages over paclitaxel in this setting, and if trastuzumab (see below) can safely augment the activity of the taxane.

Adjuvant chemotherapy has found its place in the treatment of node-negative and node-positive disease. In 1990, more than three-fourths of all newly diagnosed breast cancers were in stage I or II. Almost two-thirds of these women had node-negative disease. About one-fourth of the patients with node-negative disease would eventually have recurrences in the form of systemic metastases within 10 years of diagnosis if they were treated with local therapy alone. By 1988, studies from several U.S. and European cooperative groups had demonstrated that recurrence rates could be decreased by adjuvant chemotherapy in these patients, as had been previously shown for those with node-positive disease. However, some of these patients are at a sufficiently low risk of developing recurrent disease that the advantages of adjuvant chemotherapy do not outweigh the disadvantages of acute toxicity. Hormonal therapy may also offer these patients significant benefit, as it may for those with node-positive disease. Guidelines for offering adjuvant drug therapy follow the discussion of adjuvant hormonal therapy.

Adjuvant Hormonal Therapy

The hormonal therapies in common use in the adjuvant setting are tamoxifen and ovarian ablation. Ovarian ablation, applicable only in premenopausal patients, is the oldest of adjuvant therapies. Indeed, a trial of this treatment was initiated in 1948 by the Christie Hospital in England. Tamoxifen, with its low toxicity rate and ease of administration, is the most studied drug, with trials beginning in the 1970s. Premenopausal and postmenopausal patients have participated in tamoxifen trials. Major benefits are associated with the use of 5 years of tamoxifen in premenopausal and postmenopausal patients with estrogen receptor–positive cancers. Its use in other patients has been a subject of several worldwide meta-analyses.

There had been concern about the possible deleterious effects of the hyperestrogenemia that can accompany the use of tamoxifen in young premenopausal patients. However, this has not been shown to have significant clinical impact. The optimal duration of adjuvant tamoxifen use has yet to be determined with certainty, although most oncologists prescribe 5 years of the drug based on data summarized below. Longer durations are under study. In cultured cells, tamoxifen, by causing a cell cycle arrest before DNA synthesis, interferes with the cytotoxicity of some chemotherapy drugs, but it synergizes with others. There is no clinical evidence of any adverse interaction of tamoxifen with chemotherapy, but the optimal timing of chemotherapy and hormone therapy remains a subject of ongoing clinical trials. Because chemotherapy and tamoxifen can increase the incidence of thrombotic complications, their sequential use (chemotherapy followed by 5 years of tamoxifen) is advised by many. There is also significant ongoing research regarding ovarian ablation in premenopausal patients, as either an alternative to chemotherapy or an adjunct to chemotherapy and/or tamoxifen.

■ WORLDWIDE TRIALS

A meta-analysis by the Early Breast Cancer Trialists' Collaborative Group, published in 1992, retrospectively analyzed data on 75,000 women who participated in randomized trials before 1985. This approach provides a means by which to use large numbers of patients to find benefits that may escape notice in smaller, individual clinical trials. A major innovation was that the benefit to patients was expressed as the percent reduction in the annual odds of recurrence or death. The results, modified by the further analyses of Gelber and colleagues, are summarized in Table 220.6. This analysis indicates that female patients of all ages benefit from tamoxifen and chemotherapy; however, the benefit of chemotherapy is greater in those who are less than 50 years old, whereas tamoxifen has a greater impact in those who are older than 50. Tamoxifen, as expected, is particularly active against cancers rich in estrogen receptors. Ovarian ablation in those younger than 50 years resulted in an approximately 25% reduction in the annual risk of relapse and death. Tamoxifen was also found to decrease the risk of contralateral breast cancer.

To use this overview to help make individual clinical decisions, the meaning of "percent reduction in the rates of recurrence or death" must be clarified. A patient at high risk of such events, such as a woman with numerous involved axillary lymph nodes, would benefit considerably from a therapy that gives even a moderate reduction in the rates. However, a patient at very low risk of recurrence and hence death, such as a woman with a cancer smaller than 1 cm in diameter and without axillary nodal involvement, might not benefit appreciably, even from a therapy with a relatively strong impact on these rates.

An update of the overview analysis in 1998 reevaluated the role of tamoxifen in early breast cancer. The use of tamoxifen (in estrogen receptor–positive or estrogen receptor–unknown tumors) for 5 years resulted in a greater effect on recurrence and mortality than its use for approximately 2 years. The impact on survival continued to increase for at least 10 years. The benefit in estrogen receptor–negative tumors was minimal. However, tamoxifen decreased the risk of contralateral breast cancer by nearly 50% after 5 years of use, regardless of the estrogen receptor status.

On the basis of data from large, prospective, randomized individual trials and the overview analysis, several sets of guidelines have emerged for the use of adjuvant drug therapy. One respected proposal, based on a consensus conference held in St. Gallen, Switzerland, in 1998, is paraphrased in Table 220.7. For node-positive disease, chemotherapy is clearly indicated for

TABLE 220.7.	TREATMENT OPTIONS FOR ADJUVANT THERAPY OF BREAST CANCER[a]

Axillary Node–Negative Disease
Premenopausal and postmenopausal women
  No therapy
  Chemotherapy (CMF, AC, AC followed by paclitaxel) ± tamoxifen
  Tamoxifen alone

Axillary Node–Positive Disease
Premenopausal women
  Chemotherapy (CMF, AC, AC followed by paclitaxel) ± tamoxifen
  Chemotherapy (CMF, AC, AC followed by paclitaxel) ± ovarian ablation
  Ovarian ablation ± tamoxifen
Postmenopausal women
  Chemotherapy (CMF, AC, AC followed by paclitaxel) ± tamoxifen
  Tamoxifen alone

---

[a] Treatment decisions are based on evaluation of prognostic factors, the patient's overall medical condition, and consideration of the potential risk and benefits. Patients should also be offered investigational protocols if available. Ovarian ablation remains investigational.
Note that the regimens in parentheses are in common use but are not completely inclusive.
CMF, cyclophosphamide, methotrexate, 5-fluorouracil; AC, doxorubicin, cyclophosphamide.
(Data from Goldhirsch A, Glick JH, Gelber RD, et al. Meeting highlights: international consensus panel on the treatment of primary breast cancer. *JNCI* 1998;90:1601–1608.)

premenopausal and most postmenopausal patients, whereas tamoxifen is indicated for all patients with estrogen or progesterone receptor–positive tumors. Most patients who are at high risk of recurrence will benefit from both types of therapy. For node-negative disease, the same guidelines generally apply. Some patients at very low risk would receive inconsequential benefit from adjuvant therapy in terms of prevention of recurrent disease, but these same patients might benefit considerably from adjuvant tamoxifen in terms of prevention of contralateral disease. This latter point is particularly relevant to patients with very tiny cancers and with special histologic subtypes, as discussed previously. One subtle point to be kept in mind, however, is that the Southwest Oncology Group has presented preliminary data suggesting that young patients with estrogen receptor–negative tumors are actually harmed, in terms of disease recurrence, by the use of tamoxifen. Hence, even chemopreventive use of tamoxifen may be inadvisable in this subgroup. Confirmatory analyses using other data sets are under way.

The major type of chemotherapy represented by the overview analysis and subsequent analyses is 6 months of CMF or an equally effective variant. However, some of the newer chemotherapy regimens, such as the doxorubicin- and taxane-based regimens, may offer more benefit, at least in patients at high risk of recurrence. Many ongoing trials are investigating innovative regimens that vary the dose or schedule, use combinations of chemotherapy and hormonal therapies (including ovarian ablation), and apply immunotherapeutic agents such as monoclonal

TABLE 220.6.	BENEFIT OF ADJUVANT THERAPY IN BREAST CANCER		
Age	**Type of Therapy**	**Recurrence**[a]	**Death**[a]
<50	TAM vs. no drug	27 ± 07	STS
	CMF vs. no drug	37 ± 05	27 ± 06
	CMF + TAM vs. CMF	NS	NS
	CMF + TAM vs. TAM	STS	STS
≥50	TAM vs. no drug	30 ± 2	19 ± 03
	CMF vs. no drug	22 ± 04	14 ± 05
	CMF + TAM vs. CMF	28 ± 03	20 ± 05
	CMF + TAM vs. TAM	26 ± 05	NS

---

[a] Percent reduction (+/− SD) in the annual odds.
STS, sample too small for firm conclusions; NS, not significant; TAM, tamoxifen; CMF, cyclophosphamide, methotrexate, 5-fluorouracil.
(Data from Early Breast Cancer Trialists' Collaborative Group. Systemic treatment of early breast cancer by hormonal, cytotoxic, or immune therapy. *Lancet* 1992;339:1; and Gelber RD, Goldhirsch A, Coates AS for the International Breast Cancer Study Group. Adjuvant therapy for breast cancer: understanding the overview. *J Clin Oncol* 1993;11:580–585.)

antibodies against HER2 and vaccines. This field is evolving rapidly and is already sufficiently complex that treatment decisions must be made by consultation with experienced specialists. As in all areas of internal medicine, patient-directed goals and lifestyle concerns are also essential in the decision making process. They are especially relevant when the benefits of relatively toxic treatments are slight.

LOCALLY ADVANCED DISEASE

In most parts of the world, locally advanced breast cancer is not an uncommon stage at presentation. However, in the United States and Europe, only 5% to 20% of patients present at this stage of disease. This range reflects socioeconomic and geographic differences. Before chemotherapy, decades of experience with aggressive surgery and high-dose radiation therapy alone were profoundly disappointing. Most patients are now treated with preoperative chemotherapy, followed by modified radical mastectomy, additional chemotherapy, and radiation therapy. Tamoxifen is also used thereafter when appropriate.

METASTATIC DISEASE

Because stage IV breast cancer is not curable with conventional therapy, the primary goal of treatment is palliation of symptoms. Prognosis varies widely. Patients with most of their disease in soft tissues fare better than those who have primarily bone involvement; those with visceral metastases fare worse; and those with brain metastases have the worst prognosis. Patients with a large number of sites involved do more poorly than those with one site, and estrogen receptor–positive cancers tend to have more indolent growth rates and respond much better to both hormonal therapy and chemotherapy. Involvement of certain sites may create complications that are best managed by surgery and, in particular, radiotherapy, in addition to systemic drug treatment.

■ SITES OF RECURRENT DISEASE

When breast cancer recurs in metastatic sites, it is inapparent by signs or symptoms in about one-half of cases. The most common sites of initial presentation of stage IV disease are the skin and soft tissues of the chest wall, axilla, or supraclavicular areas (regional recurrence) and bone. Osseous recurrences are usually painful and are frequently associated with elevated alkaline phosphatase levels. Less common locations for the first sites of metastatic disease are the lung, liver, and, most uncommonly, the central nervous system. Most patients with initial stage IV disease have one or at most two different organ systems involved. As the disease progresses, involvement of multiple sites usually becomes evident. At autopsy, metastatic cancer is usually more widespread than could be suspected from clinical examination. Metastases at autopsy have been found in nearly every organ of the body, including heart, kidneys, ovaries, thyroid gland, and gastrointestinal tract.

■ HORMONAL THERAPY FOR METASTATIC DISEASE

About one-third of unselected patients benefit from the initial administration of a wide spectrum of hormonal treatments, listed in Table 220.8. The median duration of response is 1 to 2 years. Patients whose tumors have strongly positive estrogen or progesterone receptors experience a higher response rate, and those with truly receptor-negative cancers rarely benefit. Ovarian ablation is only effective in premenopausal patients, and aromatase inhibition is only effective in those who do not have ovarian estrogen secretion. Otherwise, the choice of initial hormonal therapy is based primarily on considerations of feasibility and tolerance. Tamoxifen, one of the least toxic drugs, is commonly the first therapy offered to postmenopausal patients. It can also be effective in premenopausal patients but is more active in the absence of ovarian function. The response to tamoxifen in this group of patients predicts good response to subsequent ovarian ablation. The best candidates for hormonal therapy as the first treatment of metastatic disease are those with slow-growing cancers as manifest by a long interval between initial presentation in the breast and the first appearance of stage IV disease. Because falsely negative estrogen receptor determinations can occur, hormonal therapy may be attempted in patients with indolent tumors even if the biochemistry of the specimens would seem to predict a poor response rate. Because responses to hormonal therapy tend to be slow, an observation period of as long as 16 weeks may be necessary to see substantial tumor regression.

If a patient's tumor shrinks in response to hormonal therapy but later regrows, the cancer may respond again if a second hormonal therapy is tried. Third-line responses are also seen, but the odds of response decrease with each new episode, the durations of response become shorter, and eventually most breast cancers become refractory to hormonal manipulation. Some patients who demonstrate progression of the disease on tamoxifen may show tumor shrinkage after withdrawal of the drug for at least 6 weeks. Although best described for diethylstilbestrol (almost never used) and tamoxifen, all hormonal therapies may cause bone pain or the appearance of transiently rapid growth

TABLE 220.8.	HORMONAL THERAPY OPTIONS FOR METASTATIC BREAST CANCER

Premenopausal and postmenopausal women
  Tamoxifen
  Progestins
  Androgens
  Adrenalectomy
Premenopausal women
  Oophorectomy
  LHRH analogues
Postmenopausal women
  Aromatase inhibitors
  Estrogens

LHRH, luteinizing hormone–releasing hormone.

of soft tissue involvement within the first month of administration (a phenomenon called *flare*). This is a good prognostic sign because it often portends a good subsequent response. However, considerable skill must be exercised to differentiate flare from frank tumor progression.

CHEMOTHERAPY FOR METASTATIC DISEASE

For patients with hormone-refractory stage IV disease, de novo or after initial response, chemotherapy is the best option. It may also be used instead of hormonal therapy if the patient's degree of visceral involvement or the rapidity of tumor growth does not permit a sufficiently long observation time to monitor a hormonal treatment.

Chemotherapy is not curative at standard doses. The patient's quality of life is a very important consideration in the choice of regimen and time to initiate treatment. Doxorubicin, paclitaxel, and docetaxel are the most effective single agents for the treatment of metastatic disease. Doxorubicin combinations are more active than CMF, although at the price of greater toxicity. A standard taxane combination has not yet been established. Some studies indicate a higher than expected incidence of cardiac toxicity with the combination of paclitaxel and doxorubicin. In the past, combination chemotherapy produced longer durations of response than single agents; however, high response rates have been observed with the use of single-agent taxanes. Newer drugs with real activity in breast cancer have recently expanded the therapeutic options and are now often used after the failure of the primary drugs listed above. These newer drugs include capecitabine, vinorelbine, and gemcitabine.

The median duration of response and survival rates are given in Table 220.9. Chemotherapy is often useful in controlling the symptoms of cancer, but it may make an asymptomatic patient ill with toxic effects. The optimal duration of chemotherapy is unclear. There is little evidence to suggest that prolonged courses beyond the time needed to achieve stable tumor volume regression are beneficial. One plan that has been widely used is to treat the patient with a regimen to the point of maximal tumor response and then administer one additional cycle of chemotherapy, followed by observation. Chemotherapy should be reinstituted at the time of documentation of progressive disease. As with hormonal therapy, when chemotherapy fails, other regimens may be used to good effect, but the chance of response decreases with each episode.

The administration of high-dose chemotherapy with bone marrow or peripheral stem cell support plus G-CSF has been used widely in the United States in the treatment of metastatic breast cancer, usually in patients whose cancers are responding to conventionally dosed treatments. This usage was motivated by the results of uncontrolled, single-institution pilot studies, which have demonstrated that approximately 20% of patients remain free of disease for at least 5 years after such treatment. High-dose chemotherapy is toxic, both acutely and chronically, and is associated with a small but reproducible mortality rate. Some oncologists have claimed that the long-term disease-free percentages seen may be the consequence of the careful selection of patients for inclusion in these programs rather than the therapy itself. Others are convinced that these results indicate that such treatment is effective, if only for properly chosen patients. Such controversy can only be settled by prospective, randomized clinical trials, several of which are in progress.

IMMUNOTHERAPY FOR METASTATIC DISEASE

One of the most exciting developments in the past few years has been the discovery of the monoclonal antibody trastuzumab. This agent binds with the extracellular domain of the transmembrane glycoprotein HER2. Several trials have demonstrated modest clinical benefit when trastuzumab was used alone in patients with HER2-overexpressing disease who had ceased to benefit from chemotherapy. Of greater interest, a randomized trial found the drug to be most effective when used in conjunction with chemotherapy (AC or paclitaxel) in patients with HER2-overexpressing disease who had received no chemotherapy for metastatic disease. Significant cardiac toxicity has been observed with the combination of trastuzumab and doxorubicin. Hence, the combination of trastuzumab and paclitaxel has now become standard in the treatment of HER2-overexpressing metastatic breast cancer. Numerous trials are ongoing to evaluate the optimal use of this antibody with a variety of chemotherapeutic agents. In addition, the evaluation of other antibodies and vaccines remains a particularly active area of investigation. Several large national trials are testing the activity of trastuzumab plus paclitaxel in the adjuvant setting.

SPECIAL THERAPEUTIC SITUATIONS

MALE BREAST CANCER

Because of the small size of the normal male breast, physical examination should disclose primary tumors of relatively small size. Nevertheless, many male patients have presented with advanced local disease because of their lack of knowledge regarding the possibility of developing breast cancer. The prognosis for

TABLE 220.9.	CHEMOTHERAPY FOR METASTATIC BREAST CANCER

First-line regimens
  CMF
  CAF, AC, doxorubicin alone
  Paclitaxel, docetaxel
Response data after first-line regimens
  Time to first response (median): 4–8 wk
  Response duration (median): 5–13 mo
  Survival of responders (median): 15–33 mo

A, doxorubicin; C, cyclophosphamide; F, 5-fluorouracil; M, methotrexate.
(Response data from Harris, Morrow M, Bonadonna G. Cancer of the breast. In: DeVita VT Jr, Hellman S, Rosenberg SA, eds. *Cancer: principles and practice of oncology,* fourth ed. Philadelphia: JB Lippincott, 1993.)

a man with breast cancer seems to be equivalent to that of a postmenopausal woman with breast cancer of the same TNM stage. Modified radical mastectomy is the acceptable local treatment. The systemic therapy in the adjuvant setting or for stage IV disease should follow recommendations for postmenopausal female breast cancer.

PREGNANCY

Breast cancer is reported to complicate approximately 1 in 4,000 pregnancies. Although most patients present with a breast mass, delays in diagnosis are common because of the density of the breast in these patients. Although pregnant patients experience the same prognoses stage for stage as their nonpregnant counterparts, they tend to present at more advanced stages or, within the stage II category, with more involved axillary lymph nodes. This may be because of delay in diagnosis, but a growth-stimulatory role of the high levels of female hormones and growth factors associated with pregnancy cannot be excluded. Breast biopsies can be performed safely during pregnancy and should be followed, if a diagnosis of invasive malignancy is confirmed, by mastectomy in most cases. Breast conservation in the first two trimesters is ordinarily contraindicated because the obligatory breast radiation therapy is precluded by its potential for harming the fetus. BCS can be performed in the last trimester, with chemotherapy and especially radiation therapy delayed until delivery. If indicated, chemotherapy can be administered after the first trimester, but antimetabolites, being teratogenic, are best avoided. For this reason, many oncologists prescribe the combination of doxorubicin and cyclophosphamide as adjuvant chemotherapy. Tamoxifen should not be given during pregnancy.

Considerable controversy exists regarding the safety of a subsequent pregnancy in a woman with a personal history of breast cancer. There are no conclusive data to indicate that prognosis is worsened by this event, but some researchers advise caution because the available information is scanty. Following the model established for Hodgkin's disease, patients are often counseled to avoid pregnancy for at least 2 years after the therapy of primary breast cancer. This is to allow for the recovery of normal organs from the toxicity of drug therapy and to eliminate the possibility of rapid recurrence of aggressive disease. Metastatic spread in pregnant women tends to follow the same anatomical distribution as in other patients. Metastases to the placenta are rare, and fetal metastases have not been reported.

BONE METASTASES

Pain is commonly associated with osseous metastases, and pain relief is a good indication of the anticancer efficacy of drugs or irradiation. For impending or frank pathologic fractures, especially of the weight-bearing bones of the spine, pelvis, and lower extremities, surgical stabilization is often necessary (see Chapter 210). Vertebral fractures unresponsive to radiation therapy, especially when the integrity of the neural canal is threatened, may sometimes be amenable to surgical approaches even though this is technically challenging. A back brace and physical therapy can be useful. Bisphosphonates, in particular pamidronate, have

routinely been used for treatment of hypercalcemia. However, several studies have shown a decrease in bone pain and skeletal complications with monthly doses of pamidronate. The role of bisphosphonates in the adjuvant setting remains investigational.

LUNG METASTASES

Malignant pleural effusions, usually exudates, are often associated with dyspnea, pain, and cough. Thoracentesis may provide temporary relief of symptoms, but pleurodesis with a sclerosing agent (e.g., tetracycline, talc, bleomycin) is preferable for longer term control. Lymphangitic involvement of the lung commonly presents suddenly and, if unresponsive to systemic therapy, progresses rapidly. It is characterized by dyspnea and cough, appears as diffuse reticulonodular infiltrates on radiographs and especially on computed tomography (CT) scans, and often causes hypoxemia. Infectious and other nonmalignant causes must be ruled out. Biopsy by means of bronchoscopy or thoracoscopy is often helpful, but lymphangitic disease can be a diagnosis of exclusion. Chemotherapy rather than hormonal therapy is the treatment of choice. The use of corticosteroids and inhaled oxygen may temporarily decrease symptoms.

LIVER METASTASES

Liver metastases are primarily treated with systemic chemotherapy. There is usually no role for radiotherapy in this setting. Attempts at increasing response rates or reducing systemic toxicity by infusing chemotherapy directly into the hepatic circulation have so far been disappointing. Surgical resection of hepatic lesions after an initial chemotherapy response and in the absence of other sites of metastases has been used in special cases, but it is not recommended for routine management.

CENTRAL NERVOUS SYSTEM METASTASES

Epidural compression of the spinal cord or the cauda equina may result in permanent neurologic damage if these are not treated promptly. Pain is the most common presenting symptom, followed by sensory and motor deficits with loss of sphincter control. Lesions may be located by a thorough neurologic examination plus spinal imaging, particularly the use of magnetic resonance imaging (MRI). Treatment usually involves corticosteroids to decrease localized edema plus radiation therapy. Decompressive surgery is sometimes appropriate.

Brain metastases commonly manifest with headaches or neurologic symptoms. The diagnosis can be confirmed with CT or MRI. Corticosteroids are used to decrease edema, and anticonvulsants are prescribed to control seizure activity. Radiation therapy is recommended for the treatment of multiple metastases, but it is associated with considerable toxicity, including hair loss and loss of cognitive function. Surgery, alone or followed by radiation therapy, has been used for solitary lesions. There is increasing experience with the use of radiosurgery (i.e., the use of very carefully designed, highly specifically localized radiation fields) in the management of brain involvement with a few dominant masses. This can be used in conjunction with whole-brain radiotherapy.

Leptomeningeal involvement (carcinomatous meningitis) is best diagnosed by lumbar puncture, although radiographic imaging may also be helpful. Patients may present with a variety of symptoms, including headache, alteration of mental status, nausea, and neurologic deficits. Radiation therapy, corticosteroids, and chemotherapy by the intrathecal or intraventricular route provide the mainstays of therapy.

HYPERCALCEMIA

Hypercalcemia is a common complication of very advanced stage IV breast cancer, and it generally denotes bone involvement, which usually is already apparent. In the treatment of less advanced metastatic disease, the serum calcium level may rise acutely in response to hormonal therapy, especially associated with the flare reaction. In these cases, the hypercalcemia is transient, often preceding a good therapeutic response. Hypercalcemia causes mental status changes, nausea, vomiting, and constipation. Acute therapy consists of intravenous hydration and bisphosphonates (e.g., pamidronate). The longer term management of hypercalcemia depends on the control of the metastatic process with anticancer drugs.

LOCAL RECURRENCE

Patients who have disease recurring on the chest wall after mastectomy have a very high rate of systemic relapse. Treatment options in the absence of other sites of stage IV disease have included local resection and radiation therapy, which can be considered standard management. A variety of other treatments have been used—including standard-dose chemotherapy, high-dose chemotherapy, and hormonal therapy—but no clear advantages of such approaches are apparent. Patients who have recurrent disease in the breast after breast conservation are usually treated with mastectomy. The role of systemic therapy in this situation is not yet established, but adjuvant chemotherapy or hormone therapy is often applied. Patients with local recurrences are often ideal candidates for investigational therapies such as vaccines.

▪ PREVENTION

Interest in preventing breast cancer, a goal of obvious intrinsic merit, has been heightened by several observations hinting at potentially profitable lines of investigation. The association between breast cancer incidence and various states of altered estrogen levels has led to some trials seeking to simulate early pregnancy. Other trials seek to deny breast tissue estrogenic stimulation while maintaining beneficial estrogenic effects on end organs such as bone and blood vessels. The largest of these is the P-1 trial of the NSABP, discussed below. Other large, randomized, controlled trials of tamoxifen are under way in Europe. These trials were explicitly motivated by the observation of decreased contralateral primary disease in patients taking tamoxifen as adjuvant therapy.

Recent data from a randomized trial by the NSABP clearly demonstrate a 49% decrease in the risk of invasive breast cancer and a 50% reduction in the risk of noninvasive disease with tamoxifen versus placebo. The impact was exclusively on the appearance of estrogen receptor–positive cases, with no differences noted between tamoxifen and placebo in estrogen receptor–negative disease. Eligibility criteria included age 60 years or more, or age 35–59 years with a high risk of developing breast cancer based on a mathematical epidemiologic model or because of a personal history of LCIS. A small increased risk of early-stage endometrial cancer and thrombotic events was found in the patients receiving tamoxifen. This may not be a problem if only women at considerable risk of breast cancer take the drug, but it could be a problem if tamoxifen is prescribed for women at borderline or average risk. Two European trials were not able to confirm the results of the NSABP trial although these studies differed from the U.S. trial due to allowance of hormone replacement therapy, smaller numbers of patients, and patient noncompliance. Therefore, the findings of the large NSABP trial are important. They have led to the approval of tamoxifen by the U.S. Food and Drug Administration as a preventive agent for breast cancer in women who fit the above eligibility criteria. It is important to note that the potential benefits and toxicities for any given patient need to be evaluated on an individual basis.

As described above, in a large, prospective randomized trial with the primary end point of determining its effects on bone mineral density, the SERM raloxifene was shown to decrease breast cancer incidence in postmenopausal women with osteopenia by about 75%. This has led to the P-2 trial of the NSABP in which volunteer postmenopausal women with increased risk, or women aged 60 or greater, are randomly allocated to receive tamoxifen or raloxifene. Effects on the endometrium as well as the breast will be ascertained. Since many postmenopausal women with osteopenia and osteoporosis are now taking raloxifene, an incidental but considerable lowering of breast cancer incidence may be noted.

Attention is being paid to possible environmental causes of high breast cancer risk, in addition to the personal behaviors associated with diet, exercise, and childbearing. Except for unnecessary radiation exposure, which should clearly be avoided, these studies are too preliminary to lead to specific recommendations. Nevertheless, efforts to limit exposure to potentially carcinogenic chemicals such as pesticides and industrial pollutants are commendable on a variety of health grounds. Exercise and a healthy diet are standard medical prescriptions.

As genetic analysis of breast cancer susceptibility becomes part of our available options, many questions will be posed for the individual, for the implicated family, and for society as a whole. We do not know the roles of lifestyle changes, exogenous hormone ingestion, more intense surveillance, or prophylactic resection of the breasts or ovaries on cancer incidence and mortality in carriers of mutant *BRCA1* or other such altered genes. Allele-specific penetrance in terms of incidence and virulence is also unknown. The lack of a specific *BRCA1* or *BRCA2* mutation does not imply that there is no increased risk of cancer because other genes may be mutated. Nevertheless, many women want to know the best estimate of their risk, and formal genetic counseling must become a common part of standard oncologic practice. The availability of hereditary predisposition testing raises ethical and legal issues, including the so far theoretical potential for employment and insurance discrimination, that must be addressed. Despite these problems, a growing knowledge of the genetic basis for breast cancer, both hereditary and acquired, offers real hope for a fundamental improvement in our ability to control and even eradicate this common disease.

BIBLIOGRAPHY

American Society of Clinical Oncology. 1998 update of recommended breast cancer surveillance guidelines. *J Clin Oncol* 1999;17:1080–1082.

Carter CL, Allen C, Henson DE. Relation of tumor size, lymph node status, and survival in 24,740 breast cancer cases. *Cancer* 1989;63:181–187.

Early Breast Cancer Trialists' Collaborative Group. Systemic treatment of early breast cancer by hormonal, cytotoxic, or immune therapy. 133 radomised trials involving 31,000 recurrences and 24,000 deaths among 75,000 women. *Lancet* 1992;339:1–15, 71–85.

Early Breast Cancer Trialists' Collaborative Group. Tamoxifen for early breast cancer: an overview of the randomised trials. *Lancet* 1998;351: 1451–1467.

Fisher B, Costantino JP, Wickerham DL, and other National Surgical Adjuvant Breast and Bowel Project investigators. Tamoxifen for prevention of breast cancer: report of the National Surgical Adjuvant Breast and Bowel Project P-1 Study. *JNCI* 1998;90:1371–1388.

Fisher B, Dignam J, Wolmark N, et al. Lumpectomy and radiation therapy for the treatment of intraductal breast cancer: findings from National Surgical Adjuvant Breast and Bowel Project B-17. *J Clin Oncol* 1998; 16:441–452.

Goldhirsch A, Glick JH, Gelber RD, et al. Meeting highlights: international consensus panel on the treatment of primary breast cancer. *JNCI* 1998; 90:1601–1608.

Greenlee RT, Murray T, Bolden S, et al. Cancer statistics, 2000. *CA Cancer J Clin* 2000;50:7–33.

Krag D, Weaver D, Ashikaga T, et al. The sentinel node in breast cancer: a multicenter validation study. *N Engl J Med* 1998;339:941–946.

Overgaard M, Hansen PS, Overgaard J, et al. Postoperative radiotherapy in high-risk premenopausal women with breast cancer who receive adjuvant chemotherapy. *N Engl J Med* 1997;337:949–955.

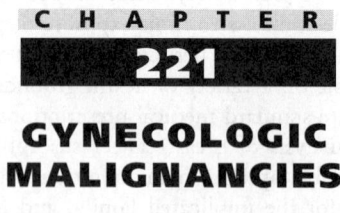

C H A P T E R

221

GYNECOLOGIC MALIGNANCIES

MARK A. MORGAN

■ CERVICAL CANCER

DEFINITION

Invasive squamous cell carcinoma is the most common malignancy of the uterine cervix. Histologic subtypes include both large cell keratinizing and nonkeratinizing cancer as well as poorly differentiated and small cell cancer with neuroendocrine features. The latter two have a worse prognosis. Adenocarcinoma accounts for 10% to 20% of invasive cervical cancers. The clear cell variant is associated with diethylstilbestrol exposure in utero but may occur in the absence of such exposure.

INCIDENCE AND EPIDEMIOLOGIC FACTORS

The incidence of cervical cancer has been decreasing since the introduction of the Pap smear in 1941. There are about 12,800 new cases of invasive disease diagnosed each year and 4,800 deaths in the United States. The disease is more common in low socioeconomic groups and in third world countries (e.g., Latin America). In the United States, the mortality for African American women is twice that for caucasians, primarily due to more advanced disease at diagnosis. There is a bimodal age distribution, with peaks at 35 to 39 years and 60 to 64 years.

Risk factors for cervical cancer are strongly related to sexual activity and include early age of first intercourse, intercourse with multiple partners, and intercourse with a "high-risk" male (multiple partners, penile condyloma). Women who use barrier contraception have a decreased risk. Oral contraceptives have been possibly linked to increased incidence of dysplasia and invasive cancer, as well as to adenocarcinoma of the cervix. Cigarette smoking is also associated with an increased risk.

ETIOLOGIC FACTORS

The epidemiologic profile of cervical cancer is that of a sexually transmitted disease, so that studies on the etiology have focused on infectious agents, in particular herpes simplex virus type 2 (HSV-2) and human papilloma virus (HPV). HPV DNA has been found in a high percentage of cervical dysplasias and invasive cancers, and genetic integration of the viral genome into the cervical cell has been demonstrated. HPV proteins have also been found to bind to and inhibit the protein product of both the retinoblastoma and P53 tumor suppressor genes. HSV-2 and other cervical infections are now thought to be cofactors with HPV in the development of cervical neoplasia.

PATHOGENESIS/PATHOPHYSIOLOGIC FACTORS

Invasive cervical cancer is felt to progress in an orderly fashion from dysplasia to carcinoma in situ over a period of 10 to 20 years. This long lead time is partially responsible for the effectiveness of Pap smear screening. Also, there appears to be an early or "microinvasive" stage wherein the risk of nodal metastasis is negligible. Once invasion occurs, there is progression to regional lymphatics and occasionally hematogenous spread. Pelvic lymph nodes are usually involved prior to para-aortic nodes. Patients who are immunosuppressed have a higher incidence of lower genital tract HPV infection and neoplasia, and patients with AIDS have been found to experience more rapid progression of disease.

TABLE 221.1.	CLINICAL STAGING PROCEDURES FOR CERVICAL CANCER

Examination under anesthesia
Intravenous urogram
Barium enema
Chest x-ray
Skeletal x-ray
Cystoscopy
Proctoscopy

CLINICAL FINDINGS

Preinvasive and early invasive cervical cancer is asymptomatic and is usually detected by Pap smear screening or colposcopy. As the cancer spreads more deeply to the cervical stroma, abnormal vaginal bleeding can occur, particularly postcoital bleeding. Progression of disease is often associated with a malodorous discharge, a gross cervical tumor, weight loss, and local pain.

Cervical cancer is the only gynecologic malignancy staged clinically by the International Federation of Obstetrics and Gynecology (FIGO). Allowable studies are listed in Table 221.1. More sophisticated studies, such as computed tomography and magnetic resonance imaging, or surgical findings are not allowed for staging purposes but may be used for treatment planning.

LABORATORY FINDINGS

Patients with cervical cancer are often anemic, and the serum creatinine may be elevated in the presence of ureteral obstruction. Serologic markers such as the cancer antigen (CA-125) and the squamous cell carcinoma antigen have been found to be elevated in some patients with cervical cancer but in general are not useful in screening or follow-up.

OPTIMAL MANAGEMENT

Microinvasive cervical cancer can only be diagnosed by cone biopsy. In very early lesions, if the margins are negative, conization itself may be adequate treatment. In the United States, if the depth of invasion is less than 3 mm and there is no lymphovascular invasion evident in the cervical stroma, simple hysterectomy is the most common treatment.

Disease limited to the cervix with deeper invasion (stage IB) or to the upper vagina (stage IIA) may be treated with radical hysterectomy and regional lymph node dissection, or radiation therapy. The ovaries may be preserved with radical hysterectomy, but they cease to function after radiation therapy. The 5-year survival for stage I disease is about 85% with either treatment modality. Patients found to have positive lymph nodes, deep stromal invasion, or positive margins at radical hysterectomy should be offered postoperative radiotherapy. Recent evidence also suggests that the addition of cisplatin and 5-fluorouracil chemotherapy to radiotherapy may prolong survival. In selected cases, patients who present with bulky (more than 4 cm) tumors confined to the cervix may also be considered for treatment with preoperative radiation and chemotherapy followed by simple

hysterectomy. When cancer invades the lower vagina, parametrium, or surrounding organs (stages IIB to IVA), radiation therapy combined with chemotherapy, either cisplatin alone or cisplatin plus 5-fluorouracil, is indicated. Pretreatment evaluation of the para-aortic lymph nodes by lymphangiography, computed tomography, or extra-peritoneal lymph node dissection may be performed to determine whether patients require extended-field radiation. Cisplatin and ifosfamide are the two most active chemotherapeutic agents for distant disease, although paclitaxel has recently also demonstrated activity in squamous and nonsquamous cervical cancer.

A central recurrence of cervical cancer after radiation therapy is potentially curable with exenterative surgery. This usually involves removal of the bladder, rectum, and vagina. Newer techniques of urinary diversion, vaginal reconstruction, and surgical critical care have made this a more acceptable procedure in terms of morbidity and mortality.

Current clinical trials are evaluating the role of new chemotherapeutic agents and combinations of agents in advanced disease. Neoadjuvant chemotherapy is also being tested to reduce tumor size in bulky disease confined to the cervix prior to radical hysterectomy. In addition, viral vaccines, using-HPV related antigens, are being actively investigated in disease treatment and prevention.

■ UTERINE CANCER

Cancer of the uterus usually refers to adenocarcinoma of the endometrium, although the term includes uterine sarcomas and, rarely, squamous cell cancers. Sarcomas account for only about 3% of uterine malignancies and are distinguished from benign mesenchymal growths by their high mitotic count and nuclear atypia. Mixed mesodermal tumors combine admixtures of malignant epithelial and stromal elements and account for about 40% of uterine sarcomas.

INCIDENCE AND EPIDEMIOLOGIC FACTORS

In 1999 there were an estimated 37,400 new cases of uterine cancer and 6,400 deaths in the United States. This makes uterine cancer the most common gynecologic malignancy. It is more common in caucasian women and occurs primarily in postmenopausal women.

Risk factors are related to prolonged unopposed exposure to estrogen, such as occurs with obesity, anovulation, estrogen therapy without progesterone, and estrogen-secreting tumors. Smoking and oral contraceptives decrease the risk. Recently, tamoxifen, probably because of its weak estrogen effect, has been associated with an increased risk of endometrial cancer. Endometrial cancer also may be seen as part of the Lynch II familial cancer syndrome in association with breast, colon, or ovarian cancer.

ETIOLOGIC FACTORS

Whether endometrial cancer progresses from endometrial hyperplasia has been debated for years. It appears that both can develop in response to unopposed estrogen; however, the likelihood of progression of hyperplasia to cancer is very low in the absence of cytologic atypia.

PATHOGENESIS/PATHOPHYSIOLOGIC FACTORS

Approximately 85% of endometrial cancers are stage I or II (limited to the uterus and cervix). Endometrial adenocarcinoma invades the myometrium and may spread by lymphatics, blood vessels, or local extension to other organs. It may also spread into the peritoneal cavity through the fallopian tubes. Pelvic lymph nodes are almost always involved when more distant para-aortic nodes are found to contain disease. Depth of invasion into the myometrium and histologic grade of the tumor are directly related to the probability of lymph node involvement and prognosis. The Gynecologic Oncology Group (GOG) has evaluated this in a large surgical staging study (Table 221.2). Patients with estrogen and/or progesterone receptors have a better prognosis than those without receptors. The papillary serous histologic type is notorious for early spread, especially to the upper abdomen (similar to the spread pattern of epithelial ovarian cancer).

CLINICAL FINDINGS

Postmenopausal bleeding is by far the most common symptom associated with endometrial cancer. However, abnormal uterine bleeding in premenopausal women with a history of anovulation may be a sign of endometrial cancer. Diagnosis may be made by an office endometrial biopsy, but if this is not diagnostic, then a dilation and curettage should be performed. Hysteroscopy is sometimes helpful as well. Currently, there is no ideal screening test for asymptomatic women.

The complete staging of endometrial cancer requires surgery to remove the uterus and ovaries, to sample retroperitoneal lymph nodes, and to obtain peritoneal cytologic specimens. Computed tomography and magnetic resonance imaging are not routinely recommended in the preoperative evaluation.

LABORATORY FINDINGS

There are no tumor markers specifically associated with endometrial cancer, although CA-125 may be elevated in patients with recurrent or metastatic disease, especially in the abdomen. Estrogen and progesterone receptors status may be useful in guiding future therapy. High levels of hormone receptors are more common in well-differentiated lesions.

OPTIMAL MANAGEMENT

Total abdominal hysterectomy and bilateral salpingo-oophorectomy should be performed whenever possible. Washings are obtained for pelvic and peritoneal cytologic study and the abdominal cavity is explored. Although complete staging requires sampling of pelvic and para-aortic lymph nodes, these procedures are often omitted when the tumor is confined to the endometrium, or the grade is low (G1) and invasion is superficial. These prognostic factors may be assessed during surgery by frozen section of the resected uterus. Vaginal hysterectomy, with laparoscopic evaluation of the abdomen and lymph nodes, is currently being studied. Radical hysterectomy is sometimes used when there is extension to the cervix (stage II). Some centers use preoperative radiotherapy in patients with stage II disease or high-grade (G3) disease. If disease has spread beyond the pelvis, hysterectomy may still be useful to palliate bleeding. The role of debulking surgery in advanced disease is uncertain, although it is probably beneficial if all gross disease can be removed.

Patients with positive pelvic lymph nodes are usually treated with postoperative external-beam pelvic radiation. Patients with high-risk factors in the uterus (e.g., deep invasion and histologic grade 2 or 3) and negative lymph nodes may benefit from radiation therapy, at least in terms of recurrence, but a survival benefit is not clear at this time. Some patients with positive para-aortic lymph nodes may be salvaged with extended field radiotherapy. The role of vaginal radiotherapy, alone or in combination with external-beam therapy, is controversial. Intraperitoneal phosphorus 32 or whole-abdominal radiotherapy has been advocated for patients with positive peritoneal cytology, although the significance of this finding and proper treatment for these patients is still being debated.

Patients with advanced or recurrent disease with well-differentiated tumors and high levels of progesterone receptors are much more likely to respond to progestin therapy, with response rates of 80% or higher being reported. Unfortunately, these patients tend to have more poorly differentiated lesions. This probably accounts for the response rate of only 18% reported in the GOG study of the use of progestins in endometrial cancer. In addition, the effect of progestins does not appear to be dose-related above a certain threshold. Responses to tamoxifen (an antiestrogen) have been reported, and the role of tamoxifen combined with sequential progestin is currently being explored.

Doxorubicin is the most active chemotherapeutic agent in endometrial cancer, with a response rate of about 40%. The addition of cisplatin to doxorubicin improves response rates, but an improvement in survival has not been demonstrated.

| TABLE 221.2. | PELVIC AND PARA-AORTIC NODAL INVOLVEMENT IN STAGE I ENDOMETRIAL CANCER BASED ON DEPTH OF MYOMETRIAL INVASION AND HISTOLOGIC GRADE (%) |

Depth of Myometrial Invasion	Histologic Grade			
	G1	G2	G3	Total
Endometrium	0 (0)	3 (3)	0 (0)	1 (1)
Inner third	3 (1)	5 (4)	9 (4)	5 (3)
Middle third	0 (5)	9 (0)	4 (0)	6 (1)
Outer third	11 (6)	19 (14)	34 (23)	25 (7)
Total	3 (2)	9 (5)	18 (11)	

Recently, paclitaxel has been found to be active against endometrial cancer and is being tested in combination with doxorubicin.

The mainstay of therapy for uterine sarcomas is total abdominal hysterectomy and bilateral salpingo-oophorectomy. Surgical excision of stage I tumors is the only known curative therapy. Adjuvant chemotherapy with doxorubicin has not proven beneficial. Radiation therapy appears to decrease pelvic recurrence after hysterectomy but does not improve survival. Doxorubicin is the most active single agent in advanced leiomyosarcoma, and cisplatin, paclitaxel, and ifosfamide have the highest response rates (30% to 40%) in mixed mesodermal tumors.

OVARIAN CANCER

DEFINITION

Epithelial cancers of the ovary, which account for about 90% of ovarian malignancies, derive from the coelomic epithelium of the ovarian surface. Approximately 75% of epithelial ovarian cancers are of the serous type, with mucinous, endometrioid, clear cell, Brenner, and undifferentiated lesions making up the rest. In addition, tumors of low malignant potential (borderline tumors) can occur, especially in young women. These tend to behave in a relatively benign fashion, although they can metastasize and be fatal.

INCIDENCE AND EPIDEMIOLOGIC FACTORS

There are about 25,200 new cases per year in the United States with 14,500 deaths, making ovarian cancer the most common cause of death from gynecologic malignancy. The incidence increases with age, and there is a lifetime risk of 1% to 2% in the United States.

The incidence of ovarian cancer decreases with increasing parity. It is unclear as to whether infertility by itself contributes to the risk, but there is some suggestion that ovulation-inducing drugs may increase a woman's risk. Oral contraceptives and tubal sterilization have consistently been associated with a decreased risk, although there appears to be no significant effect from postmenopausal hormone use. Perineal talc use has also been associated with increased risk, possibly due to contamination with asbestos. Dietary intake of fat is related to increased risk, but the effects of coffee, alcohol, and tobacco are unclear. Patients with ovarian cancer appear to be at a greater risk for breast cancer and vice versa.

A hereditary component has been suggested by well-described, familial cancer syndromes such as site-specific ovarian cancer, breast/ovarian cancer, and the Lynch II cancer family syndrome. Despite these well-publicized syndromes, familial ovarian cancer probably occurs in only 5% to 10% of patients. Nevertheless, a woman with one first-degree relative with ovarian cancer has about a threefold increased risk, and two first-degree relatives with the disease may confer up to a 50% chance of developing ovarian cancer. Mutations in the *BRCA1* or *BRCA2* gene play a role in many cases of familial ovarian cancer.

ETIOLOGIC FACTORS

Epidemiologic evidence suggests that women at highest risk for ovarian cancer have a reproductive history consistent with repetitive ovulation. This has led to the "incessant ovulation" theory whereby repetitive epithelial injury and regeneration leads to more frequent mutations and subsequent neoplasia. Elevated pituitary gonadotropins have also been postulated as an etiologic factor because of the association with infertility and "fertility drugs." Finally, carcinogens such as talc, radiation, or environmental toxins have been implicated.

PATHOGENESIS/PATHOPHYSIOLOGIC FACTORS

Epithelial cancers of the ovary probably grow within the substance of the ovary, in most cases before dissemination. Occasionally, however, they may arise on the surface of the ovary and spread intraperitoneally early in the disease process before recognizable ovarian enlargement has developed. It is possible that in some cases an ovarian-like cancer may develop simultaneously in areas of metaplasia in several sites in the peritoneal cavity.

Approximately 75% of ovarian cancers will have metastasized at the time of diagnosis. Spread from a primary ovarian cancer is predominantly by exfoliation into the peritoneal cavity, although lymphatic dissemination is common. Clockwise circulation of peritoneal fluid often spreads ovarian cancer to paracolic and subdiaphragmatic surfaces, especially on the right side. Pleural or parenchymal liver involvement tends to occur late in the course of disease.

CLINICAL FINDINGS

Early ovarian cancer rarely causes symptoms and is usually found fortuitously on pelvic examination or ultrasonography. As the disease progresses and spreads, pelvic pain and bowel dysfunction occur, and patients are frequently evaluated for gastrointestinal disease with inconclusive results. As ascites develop, the patient may complain of abdominal bloating. This is often attributed to weight gain following menopause.

A solid mass or nodularity in the cul-de-sac may be felt on pelvic exam. In advanced disease, an abdominal fluid wave may be detected or physical exam may detect a pleural effusion. Survival is highly correlated with stage. More than 80% of patients with stage I or II disease survive for 5 years, whereas fewer than 20% of stage III and IV patients survive for that long a time.

There is no proven effective screening method for ovarian cancer, although transvaginal ultrasound combined with serum tumor antigens and Doppler flow studies of ovarian circulation are currently being evaluated. Although these methods are unproven in the general population, transvaginal ultrasound and serum CA-125 studies are reasonable approaches at this time in high-risk women, such as those with a strong family history of ovarian cancer.

LABORATORY FINDINGS

Elevation of the serum CA-125 level, a glycoprotein detected by the ovarian cancer monoclonal antibody (OC-125), is the

TABLE 221.3.	NON–OVARIAN CANCER CAUSES OF ELEVATED CANCER ANTIGEN 125
Gynecologic	**Nongynecologic**
Uterine fibroids	Pancreatitis
Pregnancy	Cirrhosis
Endometriosis	Peritonitis
Pelvic inflammatory diseases	Pancreatic carcinoma
Fallopian tube carcinoma	Lung carcinoma
Endometrial carcinoma	Breast carcinoma
Cervical carcinoma	Colon carcinoma

most consistent laboratory abnormality in patients with epithelial ovarian cancer. Although only about 50% or patients with stage I disease have elevations, more than 90% of patients with stage III and IV disease will have elevated levels. Unfortunately, many other conditions, both benign and malignant, have been associated with increased levels, thereby limiting its usefulness as a screening test (Table 221.3). The most accepted use for CA-125 measurement is to follow the clinical course of the disease once diagnosed and to follow patients in clinical remission. Carcinoembryonic antigen (CEA), CA 19-9, lipid-associated sialic acid, and other antigens are sometimes elevated in patients with ovarian cancer, but their current role in management or screening is unclear. Although an elevated CA-125 is a reliable predictor of persistent disease, a normal CA-125 (less than 35 units per milliliter) cannot rule out the presence of disease in patients who otherwise appear to be in clinical remission.

OPTIMAL MANAGEMENT

Since ovarian cancer is a surgically staged disease, exploration of the abdomen and pelvis should be performed as initial management in almost every case. Although ultrasonography, magnetic resonance imaging, and computed tomography are often used in the evaluation of an adnexal mass, they are not accurate enough to reliably distinguish a benign from malignant tumor or to estimate the extent of intra-abdominal disease.

Surgical management of an apparent early stage should involve a vertical midline incision that extends above the umbilicus. Washings of the pelvis and upper abdominal surfaces should be obtained for cytologic purposes. The primary tumor (ovary) should be removed intact if possible, and in most cases a total abdominal hysterectomy and bilateral salpingo-oophorectomy should be performed. In select cases of young women desiring to bear children, a unilateral adnexectomy may be performed if there is no other evidence of disease spread. A meticulous exploration of the abdomen should be performed, including evaluation of the subdiaphragmatic surfaces, along with random biopsies. At least an infracolic omentectomy should be performed. Para-aortic and pelvic nodes should be sampled on the side of the tumor. The role of laparoscopic treatment and staging of early ovarian cancer is currently being evaluated at several centers.

Patients with stage I low-grade tumors are adequately treated with surgery alone, as this is curative in over 90% of patients.

Patients with higher grade cancers and positive peritoneal cytology are at higher risk for recurrence (20% to 40%) and are usually treated with adjuvant therapy. Early studies reported that intraperitoneal phosphorus 32 or melphalan were equivalent as adjuvant treatment; however, results from an Italian trial suggest that cisplatin is superior to phosphorus 32 or no therapy in prolonging disease-free survival in patients with stage I high-risk disease. The role of combination chemotherapy in early disease is being studied.

Advanced ovarian cancer currently requires an aggressive surgical approach to remove as much disease as possible since many clinical studies have documented the importance of the extent of residual disease as a prognostic factor. Optimal surgery has generally been defined as removal of all tumor nodules larger than 1 or 2 cm. Surgical cytoreduction or "debulking" usually involves a total abdominal hysterectomy with bilateral salpingo-oophorectomy, total omentectomy, retroperitoneal lymph node dissection, and, in select cases, bowel resection or splenectomy. A retroperitoneal approach is often used in the presence of massive pelvic tumor. Based on the results of a European trial, for patients who cannot be successfully debulked during initial surgery, a second attempt may be considered following several courses of chemotherapy. Patients who are debulked to residual tumor nodules less than 1 cm are good candidates for intraperitoneal chemotherapy.

The role of second-look laparotomy in ovarian cancer is controversial. Most evidence fails to suggest a survival benefit. However, second-look surgery is useful to define responses in patients without measurable disease, may provide some benefit by allowing secondary cytoreduction, and can define a group of patients suitable for aggressive second-line treatment protocols such as intraperitoneal chemotherapy or high-dose chemotherapy with autologous bone marrow or stem cell support. Surgery for resection of recurrent disease after primary chemotherapy may be beneficial if the time to recurrence is prolonged (6 to 12 months).

Currently, combination chemotherapy with platinum-based therapy is the standard treatment in patients with advanced ovarian cancer. A trial reported in 1996 by GOG has demonstrated superior response rates and survival with cisplatin and paclitaxel versus cisplatin and cyclophosphamide in patients with suboptimal disease. Carboplatin and paclitaxel seems to be as effective as cisplatin and paclitaxel, and can be given over a shorter duration as an outpatient. Although high response rates have been demonstrated with high-dose chemotherapy and stem cell support, a clear benefit in either primary or secondary treatment has yet to be demonstrated. This approach should be limited to carefully designed clinical trials at present. Promising new agents such as topotecan, liposomal doxorubicin, and gemcitabine have activity in the second-line setting and may eventually be incorporated into front-line therapy.

GESTATIONAL TROPHOBLASTIC DISEASE

Gestational trophoblastic disease encompasses a spectrum of disease from localized hydatidiform mole to metastatic choriocarci-

TABLE 221.4.	SCORING SYSTEM OF GESTATIONAL TROPHOBLASTIC DISEASE			
	Score[a]			
Prognostic Factor	0	1	2	4
Age (y)	<39	>39		
Antecedent pregnancy	Hydatidiform mole	Abortion	Term	
Interval[b]	<4	4–6	7–12	>12
hCG (IU/L)	10^3	10^3–10^4	10^4–10^5	>10^5
ABO groups (female × male)		O × A	B	
		A × O	AB	
Largest tumor, including uterine tumor		3–5 cm	>5 cm	
Site of metastases		Spleen, kidney	GI tract, liver	Brain
Number of metastases identified		1–4	4–8	>8
Prior chemotherapy			Single drug	2 or more drugs

[a] The total score for a patient is obtained by adding the individual scores for each prognostic factor. Total score: ≤4, low risk; 5–7, middle risk; ≥8, high risk.
[b] Interval months between end of antecedent pregnancy and start of chemotherapy.
hCG, human chorionic gonadotropin; GI, gastrointestinal.

noma. Although persistent and metastatic trophoblastic disease usually follows a molar pregnancy, it may occur after any kind of gestation, even a term pregnancy. Molar pregnancy occurs in about 1 in 1,500 to 1 in 2,000 gestations per year in the United States and malignant disease occurs in approximately 15% to 20% of these. Trophoblastic disease is almost always associated with the production of human chorionic gonadotropin, which serves as a sensitive tumor marker. Women with molar pregnancies are at increased risk for trophoblastic disease with subsequent pregnancies.

Molar pregnancy is successfully treated by evacuation of the uterus in over 80% of cases. In the remainder, persistent elevation of the human chorionic gonadotropin should provoke a search for metastatic disease. Lung metastases are most common, but disease may also be found in the vagina, liver, gastrointestinal tract, or central nervous system. In the absence of metastatic disease, hysterectomy may be offered as part of the primary treatment, although chemotherapy with methotrexate is curative in over 90% of cases. Patients with metastatic disease may be divided into high-, middle-, and low-risk (Table 221.4). Low-risk patients, even those with pulmonary metastasis, may be treated with single-agent methotrexate or actinomycin D with complete remission in close to 100% of patients. High- and middle-risk patients require multiagent chemotherapy. Using a combination of etoposide, methotrexate, actinomycin D, cyclophosphamide, and vincristine [Oncovin] (EMA-CO), a complete remission rate of 70% to 80% may be expected. Normal reproduction can be expected in most patients after treatment for persistent trophoblastic disease.

BIBLIOGRAPHY

Burghardt E, Winter R, Tamussno K, et al. Diagnosis and surgical treatment of cervical cancer. *Crit Rev Oncol Hematol* 1994;17:181–231.
Colombo N. Controversial issues in the management of early epithelial ovarian cancer: conservative surgery and role of adjuvant therapy. NIH Consensus Development Conference on Ovarian Cancer. Program and Abstracts, April 5–7, 1994:45–48.
Creasman WT, DiSaia PJ. Screening in ovarian cancer. *Am J Obstet Gynecol* 1991;165:7–10.
Heller PB, Malfetano JH, Bundy BN, et al. Clinical–pathologic study of stage IIB, III, and IVA carcinoma of the cervix: extended diagnostic evaluation for paraaortic node metastasis—a Gynecologic Oncology Group Study. *Gynecol Oncol* 1990;38:425–430.
McGuire WP, Hoskins WR, Brady MF, et al. Cyclophosphamide and cisplatin compared with paclitaxel and cisplatin in patients with stage III and stage IV ovarian cancer. *N Engl J Med* 1996;334(1):1–6.
Morrow CP, Bundy BN, Kurman R, et al. Relationship between surgical–pathological risk factors and outcome in clinical stage I and II carcinoma of the endometrium: a Gynecologic Oncology Group Study. *Gynecol Oncol* 1991;40:55–65.
Rubin SC. Surgery for ovarian cancer. *Hematol-Oncol Clin North Am* 1992; 6:851–865.
Soper JT. Management of gestational trophoblastic disease. *Oncology* 1993; 7:68–74.
Trimble EL, Kosary MA, Park RC. Lymph node sampling and survival in endometrial cancer. *Gynecol Oncol* 1998;71:340–343.

Kelley's Textbook of Internal Medicine, fourth edition. Edited by H. David Humes.
Lippincott Williams & Wilkins, Philadelphia © 2000.

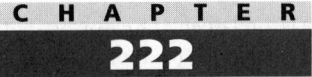

CHAPTER
222

GERM CELL MALIGNANCIES IN MEN

STEPHEN D. WILLIAMS

DEFINITION

Germ cell tumors are a heterogeneous group of diseases occurring in men and women. They are distinctly unusual tumors,

TABLE 222.1.	PATHOLOGIC CLASSIFICATION OF GERM CELL TUMORS

Seminoma
Nonseminoma
   Embryonal carcinoma
   Teratoma
   Endodermal sinus tumor
   Choriocarcinoma
   Mixed tumors

but their importance is increased by the fact that they typically occur in young persons in the prime of life. These malignancies arise in germinal epithelium, typically the testis or ovary. In men and women, pathologically and biologically similar malignancies can also originate in extragonadal sites, typically but not invariably the retroperitoneum or mediastinum. Occasionally, the origin of a germ cell tumor may be obscure. Laboratory investigations are beginning to increase the understanding of the fundamental biology of these neoplasms.

The pathologic classification of male germ cell tumors is outlined in Table 222.1. About 40% of germ cell tumors are pure seminomas. The remaining tumors may be a pure cell type, but they frequently are composed of more than one type. The major therapeutic implications of this classification is that seminomas are quite responsive to radiation therapy, but tumors other than seminomas are less so; surgery and chemotherapy are used in the treatment of nonseminomas.

The treatment of testicular cancer has improved dramatically in the past 20 years. Most men who develop this disease can be successfully treated and cured, with a low incidence of late adverse effects of treatment. This therapeutic triumph has occurred because of close collaboration among physicians of many different disciplines, and it represents one of the great therapeutic successes of our time.

INCIDENCE AND EPIDEMIOLOGY

Testicular cancer is a relatively rare disease, with an annual incidence in the United States of approximately 5.5 per 100,000 males. For reasons that are not clear, the incidence of this disease has increased somewhat. There are fairly marked geographic and racial differences in the frequency of this tumor. In Scandinavian countries, particularly Denmark, it is much more common, and in Asian countries it is less common. The incidence is significantly lower among blacks.

Testicular cancer is a disease of young men. Most affected patients are in their twenties or thirties. Testicular cancer does occur in pediatric patients and older men, but it is much less common in these age groups. Patients with pure seminomas tend to be a bit older than those with tumors other than seminomas. The most common cell type in childhood is sometimes referred to as infantile embryonal carcinoma, which is essentially

an endodermal sinus tumor. Pure endodermal sinus tumors in adults are rare.

Testicular cancer patients have a higher than expected incidence of congenital anomalies of the genitourinary tract. Testicular cancer patients also have a higher than expected incidence of dysplastic nevi and melanoma. Male relatives of these patients have a higher than expected incidence of testicular cancer, and about 1 of 100 testicular tumor patients develop a synchronous or metachronous tumor in the contralateral testis.

Extragonadal germ cell tumors are rare. They usually occur in young persons and share many common characteristics with their testicular counterparts, although there are some important differences. Extragonadal tumors, particularly mediastinal germ cell tumors, have a less favorable prognosis than testicular cancer. Mediastinal germ cell tumors are associated with Klinefelter's syndrome. Mediastinal tumors that contain elements of teratoma are associated with the synchronous or metachronous development of various hematologic malignancies, usually acute leukemia. The mechanism underlying this association is relevant to understanding the cause of these tumors.

ETIOLOGIC FACTORS

The cause of testicular germ cell tumors is unknown. It is much more likely to occur in individuals with a history of undescended testis. The involved testis and the contralateral testis are at increased risk. In patients with a history of unilateral cryptorchidism who develop testicular cancer, about 25% of the tumors occur in the opposite testis. It is likely that cryptorchidism and testicular cancer are related to some underlying disorder. There is presumptive evidence that early orchiopexy may lessen the risk of malignant degeneration. Absolute proof of this, however, is lacking. The relation between maternal diethylstilbestrol exposure and the subsequent development of testicular cancer is controversial.

Most patients with testicular cancer and extragonadal tumors have a characteristic cytogenetic abnormality located on chromosome 12. This finding can be helpful in classifying poorly differentiated neoplasms of obscure origin and will probably provide more information about the cause of these tumors.

PATHOGENESIS

Testicular cancer typically spreads in an orderly way to the retroperitoneal lymphatics and lung. Liver, bone, or brain involvement is sometimes found at diagnosis. Testicular cancer is a disease with a generally short natural history and early hematogenous dissemination; the diagnostic evaluation and initiation of therapy should be done in a timely fashion. Because of the pattern of spread, staging procedures should include a chest x-ray film and abdominal computed tomography (CT) scan. A chest

TABLE 222.2.	STAGING OF TESTICULAR GERM CELL TUMORS

Stage I: Tumor confined to the testis
Stage II: Involvement of testis plus retroperitoneal nodes
Stage III: Supradiaphragmatic or visceral involvement

CT scan should be done if the chest x-ray film is normal or equivocal. Serum markers and a lactate dehydrogenase (LDH) determination should be done. Other radiographic procedures should be done only as clinically indicated. With these standard procedures, most patients' disease is staged according to the staging system shown in Table 222.2.

CLINICAL FINDINGS

A patient with testicular cancer ordinarily presents with a scrotal mass. The mass may be painless or it may be associated with discomfort. Occasionally, patients may have acute onset of severe pain and be misdiagnosed as having testicular torsion. Another common symptom is back pain related to retroperitoneal lymphadenopathy. This pain may be severe and typically is worsened with recumbency. Patients with very high serum levels of human chorionic gonadotropin (hCG) may have gynecomastia. Pulmonary symptoms, such as dyspnea, cough, or hemoptysis, occur occasionally, but it is unusual for patients to have advanced pulmonary disease at the time of diagnosis. Symptoms related to other potential areas of involvement (e.g., liver, bone, brain) are rare because of the uncommon involvement of these areas at diagnosis.

The symptoms of extragonadal tumors are variable. Patients with mediastinal tumors ordinarily have chest pain, dyspnea, or cough at the time of diagnosis. Patients with retroperitoneal tumors usually have back pain as a prominent symptom.

Most patients with testicular cancer have abnormal scrotal examination findings. The key finding is a mass that is not clearly separable from the testis. Occasionally, it may be difficult to differentiate a testicular mass from a hydrocele. An important maneuver is transillumination. A scrotal mass that does not transilluminate should be considered to be a testis tumor until proven otherwise. Other potential physical findings include an abdominal or supraclavicular mass and gynecomastia.

LABORATORY FINDINGS

An important finding in the diagnosis and therapy of testicular cancer is the laboratory determination of tumor markers. α-Fetoprotein (AFP) and β-hCG levels are elevated in many patients, and these determinations are useful in the follow-up of such patients. However, most patients with seminomas and early-stage nonseminomas have normal markers. If elevated, they are useful in the diagnosis of a scrotal mass, but normal markers

do not imply that a scrotal mass found on physical examination is benign. Most patients with bulky stage II and stage III tumors have an elevation of one or both markers at the time of diagnosis. The rate of marker decline after chemotherapy or surgery provides important information. A rising hCG or AFP level during or after therapy indicates recurrence or progression. LDH is frequently elevated, but the relative lack of specificity of LDH elevation makes it less clinically useful.

Testicular ultrasonography is useful in defining the scrotal anatomy and differentiating testicular from epididymal lesions. A few patients present with signs or symptoms of metastatic tumor, and with careful evaluation using ultrasonography they are found to have primary sites within the gonads that were unsuspected clinically. Another use of ultrasonography is for patients with suspected extragonadal germ cell tumors. In such patients, it is important to exclude a testis primary tumor by careful examination and ultrasonography.

Other radiographic studies that should be done include a chest x-ray film and, if normal, a chest CT scan and an abdominal CT scan. Other radiographic studies are done only if indicated by clinical findings.

OPTIMAL MANAGEMENT

In the 1970s, the activity of a then-new chemotherapy agent, cisplatin, in patients with advanced testicular cancer was recognized. Several trials employing this agent in combination chemotherapy regimens were conducted. The most widely used regimen is cisplatin combined with etoposide and bleomycin (BEP regimen; Table 222.3). All three drugs are active as single agents and have different toxicities that allow them to be administered in full or nearly full doses in combination. Cisplatin and etoposide appear to be synergistic in vitro and in vivo. Most patients with metastatic tumors treated with a cisplatin-containing regimen survive their disease. The development of an effective chemotherapy regimen for advanced disease has had profound implications for the management of patients with early-stage tumors.

Patients with stage III or bulky stage II nonseminomas are treated initially with BEP after inguinal orchiectomy, which confirms diagnosis and initiates therapy. Patients can be grouped into those with limited metastatic disease and a resultant favorable prognosis (more than 90% cure) and those with high tumor volume and a lower likelihood of survival (50% to 60% cure). Patients in the former group are those with small-volume retro-

TABLE 222.3.	BEP CHEMOTHERAPY REGIMEN FOR TESTICULAR CANCER

Three to four courses given at 3-week intervals:
Cisplatin: 20 mg/m² on days 1–5
Etoposide: 100 mg/m² on days 1–5
Bleomycin: 30 U/week

BEP, bleomycin, etoposide, cisplatin.

peritoneal or pulmonary metastases and those with elevated markers as the only evidence of disease. Patients with high-volume tumors have large-volume pulmonary metastases, bulky retroperitoneal tumors plus supradiaphragmatic tumors, or liver, bone, or brain metastases. The relevant issues in the former group are cost and toxicity reduction; in the latter group, the important issue is improved therapeutic efficacy. A recent international collaborative study has noted the adverse prognostic impact of nonpulmonary visceral metastases and marked elevations of hCG, AFP, or LDH.

For good-prognosis patients, clinical trials have shown that three courses of BEP are equivalent to four courses; that if three courses of chemotherapy are given, the omission of bleomycin worsens the results; and that if bleomycin is not given, patients should receive four courses of treatment. Trials have also shown that carboplatin plus etoposide is less effective than etoposide plus cisplatin.

In patients with high tumor volumes, the use of high-dose cisplatin did not improve results, and there is no regimen that is known to be better than conventional dose BEP given for four courses.

Modern antiemetics (ondansetron, granisetron, and dolasetron) and other supportive-care aspects have allowed this form of chemotherapy to be relatively well tolerated. Although alopecia is universal, serious toxicities (e.g., cisplatin-induced renal damage, bleomycin-induced lung disease) are rare; however, continuous intravenous hydration must be given to avoid nephrotoxicity. About 25% of patients experience an episode of fever and neutropenia, which is rarely of major consequence when managed appropriately.

Treatment must be given on schedule in appropriate doses to be optimally effective. Chemotherapy courses should almost never be delayed. The cisplatin dose is not altered. The etoposide dose was ordinarily reduced 25% for previously irradiated patients and those with an intervening episode of neutropenic fever or severe thrombocytopenia. However, the availability of hematopoietic growth factors (granulocyte colony-stimulating factor and granulocyte–macrophage colony-stimulating factor) have altered this approach (see Chapter 256). The routine use of these agents is unnecessary, but patients who are very ill may benefit from one of these drugs. It probably is appropriate to add a growth factor rather than reduce the dose for patients with a prior episode of neutropenia and fever. Bleomycin is immediately discontinued if clinical or radiographic signs of pulmonary fibrosis are detected. Subtle clinical findings that warrant discontinuation of bleomycin include basilar rales or a lag or diminished expansion of a hemithorax.

The importance of surgery after chemotherapy for patients with a persistent mass is well recognized. As many as 25% to 40% of patients undergoing chemotherapy have a radiographically apparent mass at the conclusion of treatment; the most common location is the retroperitoneum. It is impossible to accurately predict the histology of these masses. It has become common practice to surgically remove the masses after suitable recovery from chemotherapy. About 45% of these masses contain only fibrosis and necrosis. Another 45% contain mature or immature teratomas. The mechanism by which this "benign"

tumor persists after treatment for a malignancy is unclear; presumably, it survives the chemotherapeutic eradication of the malignant elements. The remaining 10% to 15% of masses have microscopic evidence of persistent carcinoma. This latter group of patients have a high risk of recurrence and receive two courses of postoperative chemotherapy of the same type as given initially. Patients who are complete responders and those who undergo complete resection of teratomas following chemotherapy have a risk of relapse of about 10% and receive no further treatment. Patients with incompletely resected teratomas are at some risk of progressive local growth and cancer recurrence, and such individuals benefit from meticulous surgical resection.

Patients with *testicular nonseminoma* without pulmonary metastases and no or less than bulky retroperitoneal tumor undergo retroperitoneal lymph node dissection (RPLND) as a part of their initial therapy. After RPLND, patients with tumor-negative nodes do not receive adjuvant treatment; only about 10% of these tumors recur. However, the risk of recurrence in patients with completely resected tumor-positive nodes is much higher (about 50%), and these patients in former times routinely received adjuvant chemotherapy. The development of effective systemic treatment mandated reassessment of this concept.

The alternative approach involves observation, with treatment deferred until relapse occurs. This allows about 50% of patients destined to be cured by surgery to avoid chemotherapy. With careful follow-up, those who relapse can be treated promptly with chemotherapy if they have limited metastatic disease.

The alternative approaches were compared in an international randomized trial. About 50% of the observed patients had recurrences of their disease, but virtually all were successfully treated, and survival did not differ from that of patients who received two courses of immediate adjuvant chemotherapy, which prevented relapse. If observation is chosen, patients must be seen monthly for the first year and every other month for the second year, with a chest radiograph and hCG and AFP determinations done at each visit. Patients with pathologic stage I disease should be followed in the same fashion because 10% have recurrences; however, most of these patients can be cured with chemotherapy if treated when the tumor volume is small.

The concept of routine RPLND for patients with clinical stage I nonseminoma tumors has been challenged. If these patients undergo routine RPLND, about 15% to 30% are found to have tumor-positive nodes. Following a line of reasoning similar to that for pathologic stage II tumors, it seems possible that these patients could be followed with regular determinations of marker levels, chest x-ray films, and abdominal CT scans and avoid RPLND, with further treatment given only at the time of relapse. Although no randomized trials have been done for this situation, there are several studies with reasonably long follow-up of patients who have been observed after orchiectomy. Results of such management are excellent and seem to rival the almost universal cure rate of such patients treated with RPLND. The issues regarding choice of initial therapy are complex. For patients willing to submit to careful follow-up, either surveillance or RPLND is appropriate, with the choice based on patient preference and physician expertise.

The advantages of retroperitoneal lymph node dissection include the following:

1. Precise pathologic staging and a more certain natural history are available.
2. If desired, brief adjuvant chemotherapy can be given to node-positive patients.
3. There is less reliance on patient and physician compliance during follow-up.
4. The risk of recurrence is limited to 2 years; 3- and 4-year recurrences are rare but have been seen in some observed patients.
5. Fewer tests are required; observed patients should have an abdominal CT scan every 2 months during the first year and less frequently in subsequent years.
6. The cure rate approaches 100%.
7. As some stage II patients are cured with surgery alone, fewer patients require chemotherapy.

The advantages of observation include the following:

1. Surgery can be avoided.
2. Less urologic expertise is required.

The potential effects of treatment on subsequent fertility must also be considered. In earlier times, RPLND invariably disrupted the autonomic system responsible for ejaculation and produced infertility. A newer surgical procedure—nerve-sparing RPLND—preserves ejaculatory function in most patients. The impact of RPLND on fertility may be less than that of observation because fewer patients need chemotherapy.

The diagnosis of *seminoma* requires that the tumor be pathologically composed of seminoma only and that the serum AFP level be normal. Seminomas are extremely sensitive to radiation. Most seminoma patients have tumors limited to the testis at the time of diagnosis. These patients generally receive radiotherapy to their retroperitoneal lymphatics; the required dosage is low. Almost all remain free of cancer. Most patients with clinical stage II seminoma are also treated with radiation therapy. Of those with limited stage II tumor (IIA, less than 5 cm), 80% to 90% remain free of cancer after therapy.

Large-volume stage II disease fortunately is a rare occurrence. Reasonable therapeutic alternatives are irradiation or initial chemotherapy. The latter therapy cures most patients, and about 60% remain tumor-free after irradiation. However, most failing patients are successfully treated with chemotherapy at the time of relapse. Chemotherapy is also the choice for the rare patients with supradiaphragmatic involvement at diagnosis.

Most patients with early-stage seminomas and nonseminomas survive their disease with modern management. Fully 80% of patients with metastatic tumors are cured with chemotherapy. Only a small group of patients with extensive visceral metastases is at significant risk of death. Overall, about 95% of patients with nonseminomas survive their disease, as do a similar or higher number of patients with seminomas. The natural history of testicular cancer is short, and virtually all patients, regardless of stage and treatment, who are continuously disease-free for 2 years after initiation of treatment remain cancer-free.

For surviving patients, the late effects of treatment are an important issue. Anecdotal reports suggested that cisplatin-based chemotherapy might be associated with an increased risk of cardiovascular disease. The likelihood of adverse events was investigated in patients who were entered into a study of the therapeutic alternatives and outcomes for early-stage tumors other than seminomas. This study registered and observed patients with pathologic stage I tumors; some patients ultimately relapsed and required chemotherapy. Patients with stage II tumors randomly received two courses of adjuvant chemotherapy or were observed. Relapsing patients received four courses of therapy. A prospectively defined patient population received no chemotherapy or received two or four courses of treatment. There were no differences in the groups in terms of the incidence of cardiovascular disease or hypertension. The only differences noted were the frequencies of distal extremity paresthesias or Raynaud's phenomenon, primarily due to cisplatin, which were more likely to occur in patients who received longer courses of chemotherapy.

Etoposide is associated with the late development of a distinctive type of leukemia. This event appears to be dose-related and is rare in germ cell tumor patients who receive less than a total dose of etoposide of 2,000 mg per square meter. This total dose is exceeded only in testicular cancer patients who fail to achieve durable complete remissions with initial therapy.

The impact of chemotherapy on fertility is less severe than originally thought, although it is likely that at least some patients have chemotherapy-induced oligospermia or azoospermia. However, many men resume normal or nearly normal spermatogenesis, and a significant number have fathered children.

BIBLIOGRAPHY

Bokemeyer C, Schmoll H-J. Treatment of testicular cancer and the development of secondary malignancies. *J Clin Oncol* 1995;13:283–292.

Bosl GJ, Motzer RJ. Testicular germ-cell cancer. *N Engl J Med* 1997;337:242–253.

Group IGCCC. International germ cell consensus classification: a prognostic factor–based staging system for metastatic germ cell cancers. *J Clin Oncol* 1997;15:594–603.

Hainsworth JD, Johnson DH, Greco FA. Cisplatin-based combination chemotherapy in the treatment of poorly differentiated carcinoma and poorly differentiated adenocarcinoma of unknown primary site: results of a 12-year experience. *J Clin Oncol* 1992;10:912–922.

Nichols C, Roth B, Heerema N, et al. Hematologic neoplasia associated with primary mediastinal germ cell tumors—an update. *N Engl J Med* 1990;322:1425–1429.

Nichols CR, Roth BJ, Williams SD, et al. No evidence of acute cardiovascular complications of chemotherapy for testicular cancer: an analysis of the Testicular Cancer Intergroup Study. *J Clin Oncol* 1992;10:760–765.

Read G, Stenning SP, Cullen MH, et al. Medical Research Council prospective study of surveillance for stage I testicular teratoma. *J Clin Oncol* 1992;10:1762–1768.

Smith MA, Rubinstein L, Anderson JR, et al. Secondary leukemia or myelodysplastic syndrome after treatment with epipodophyllotoxins. *J Clin Oncol* 1999;17:569–577.

Williams SD, Stablein DM, Einhorn LH, et al. Immediate adjuvant chemotherapy versus observation with treatment at relapse in pathological stage II testicular cancer. *N Engl J Med* 1987;317:1433–1438.

Kelley's Textbook of Internal Medicine, fourth edition. Edited by H. David Humes. Lippincott Williams & Wilkins, Philadelphia © 2000.

PROSTATE CANCER

KENNETH J. PIENTA
DAVID C. SMITH

DEFINITION

Prostate cancer generally refers to adenocarcinoma of the prostate, which accounts for more than 98% of all prostate cancers. Seventy percent of these cancers occur in the peripheral zone, 20% in the transitional zone, and 10% in the central zone. Less common prostatic malignancies include neuroendocrine tumors, squamous tumors, sarcomas, and transitional cell carcinomas.

INCIDENCE AND EPIDEMIOLOGY

Prostate cancer is the most common cancer in men (excluding skin cancers) and the second leading cause of cancer-related deaths in men. In 1998, an estimated 184,500 new cases of prostate cancer were diagnosed, and 39,200 prostate cancer–related deaths occurred. Currently, the incidence rates for prostate cancer are 82 per 100,000 for men aged 50 to 54; 518 for men aged 60 to 64; and 1,326 for men aged 70 to 74. The age-adjusted death rate due to prostate cancer in 1995 was 17.3 per 100,000 population. In 1994, prostate cancer accounted for 6.2% of white male cancer deaths and 9.4% of African American male cancer deaths. Deaths attributed to prostate cancer have demonstrated a slight decrease of 1% to 2% per year over the last 2 years, which may in part reflect the increased use of prostate-specific antigen (PSA) as a screening tool starting in the early 1990s.

The prevalence of both histologic and clinical prostate cancer increases with age. The presence of histologic cancer increases so that by age 80 approximately 70% to 80% of men have evidence of this latent cancer at autopsy. Most studies suggest that the baseline prevalence of latent disease is similar around the world, but the rate of clinically evident cancer varies tremendously from country to country. Only about 10% of these histologic cancers appear to develop into clinically significant disease, and the factors that influence disease promotion remain undefined.

ETIOLOGIC FACTORS

After age 50, the incidence rates of prostate cancer increase nearly exponentially with age. Risk continues to increase with age and, unlike other cancers, does not demonstrate a peak at any age. If the incidence of prostate cancer is reviewed by region, it is highest in Scandinavia and lowest in Asia. However, the highest incidence of prostate cancer in the world is found in African American men, who have a 9.8% lifetime risk of developing clinically recognized prostate cancer. The genetic and/or cultural factors contributing to this increased risk remain undefined. Interestingly, Japanese immigrants to the United States demonstrate an incidence rate intermediate between men living in Japan and white men in North America, suggesting that environmental factors contribute to the risk of developing clinically significant prostate cancer.

A hereditary risk of developing prostate cancer has been demonstrated, and early analysis suggests that an autosomal dominant pattern of inheritance may be responsible for a small percentage of the prostate cancer seen in men younger than 55 years and for slightly less than 9% of prostate cancer patients overall. If a first-degree family member has the disease, a male relative has a relative risk of approximately 2, which rises with each additional affected family member.

Several studies have demonstrated that socioeconomic factors, prostatitis, occupational exposures, smoking, infectious agents, and level of sexual activity are not linked to prostate cancer risk. Prostate cancer is an androgen-sensitive disease, and it has been hypothesized that a higher level of circulating androgens over time may increase prostate cancer risk; however, a clear link between endogenous testosterone levels and prostate cancer development has not been demonstrated. The role of vasectomy in the development of prostate cancer has been controversial, with several studies suggesting that a link, if it exists, is very weak. Currently, vasectomy is not considered a risk factor for prostate cancer.

Dietary fat and high red meat consumption may increase prostate cancer risk. A native Asian diet low in red meat intake is also rich in soy products and vegetables, which may confer a chemopreventive effect. Recent studies suggest that the antioxidants vitamin E and selenium may also lower the risk of developing prostate cancer if taken on a regular basis. The effect of vitamin A, carotenes, and vitamin D on the development or prevention of prostate cancer is not clear.

PATHOGENESIS AND PATHOPHYSIOLOGIC FACTORS

The prostate gland is a walnut-shaped organ situated at the base of the bladder. Most tumors arise in the peripheral zone of the prostate and are potentially palpable by digital rectal examination (DRE). The transitional zone is the area of the prostate that classically enlarges with age (benign prostatic hyperplasia).

The most prominent grading system for prostate cancer was defined by Gleason and reflects aberrations in glandular architecture. Tumors are graded on a scale of 1 to 5, from the most to the least well differentiated (Table 223.1). Tumor specimens are assigned a Gleason score that represents the sum of the most common and second most common patterns of tumor (e.g., 4 + 3 = 7). The Gleason score (2 to 10) has predictive power for clinical outcome. Stage for stage, patients with higher Gleason scores have shorter survivals.

Another common histologic finding on needle biopsy is high-

TABLE 223.1.		THE UPDATED GLEASON GRADING SYSTEM
Old Gleason System	**New Gleason System**	**Description**
2–4	2–4	Well-differentiated cancer that looks a lot like normal prostate cells and is minimally aggressive
5–7	5–6	Moderately differentiated cancer that looks somewhat like normal cells and is moderately aggressive
—	7	Moderately to poorly differentiated cancer that slightly resembles normal cells and is aggressive
8–10	8–10	Poorly differentiated cancer that does not look anything like normal cells and is very aggressive

or low-grade prostatic intraepithelial neoplasia (PIN). Data suggest that high-grade PIN is a precursor lesion for prostate carcinoma. Subsequent biopsies detect cancer in 35% to 50% of patients with high-grade PIN.

The most commonly employed staging paradigms are the American (ABCD) and tumor–node–metastasis (TNM) systems (Table 223.2). The American system is less accurate than the TNM but is still commonly used. The TNM system is more representative of the manner in which the diagnosis is made as well as providing a more accurate pathologic staging system.

Specifically, many tumors are diagnosed based on an elevated PSA, negative DRE, but positive biopsy. These are classified as T1c tumors in the TNM system but cannot be classified by the American system.

In men who are not treated, average survival is approximately 8 to 10 years for stage A and B disease, 3 to 6 years for stage C, and 2 to 3 years for stage D disease. Men with higher Gleason grade tumors have shorter survival in each stage group. The most common site for distant metastasis is bone, with more than 90% of patients with metastatic disease developing bony lesions. The

TABLE 223.2.		THE NEW ABCD AND TNM CLINICAL STAGING SYSTEMS FOR LOCALIZED PROSTATE CANCER AND WHAT THEY REALLY MEAN
ABCD	**TNM**	**Description**
—	TX	Cancer cannot be staged at this time
	T0	There is no evidence of a cancer
A	T1	Cancer not palpable on DRE
A1	T1a	Cancer found at TURP occupying <5% of prostate tissue removed
A2	T1b	Cancer found at TURP occupying >5% of prostate tissue removed
B0	T1c	Cancer not palpable on DRE but detected by biopsy of one or both prostate lobes because of an initial high PSA level
B1 or B2	T2	Cancer confined within prostate and/or apex of the prostate but not beyond the prostate capsule
B1	T2a	Cancer involves only one lobe of the prostate
B2	T2b	Cancer involves both lobes of the prostate
C1–C2	T3	Cancer goes through the prostate capsule
C1	T3a	Cancer with unilateral or bilateral extracapsular extension
C2	T3b	Cancer with invasion of one or both seminal vesicles
C2	T4	Cancer with invasion of nearby structures (other than the seminal vesicles), including bladder neck, external sphincter, rectum, muscles, and/or pelvic wall
—	NX	Lymph nodes cannot be staged
—	N0	No cancer in regional (pelvic) lymph nodes
D1	N1	Cancer in regional (pelvic) lymph nodes
—	MX	Metastases cannot be assessed
—	M0	No evidence of metastasis
D2	M1	Cancer has metastasized
D2	M1a	Cancer has metastasized to a nonregional node or nodes
D2	M1b	Cancer has metastasized to bone
D2	M1c	Cancer has metastasized to viscera

DRE, digital rectal examination; TURP, transurethral prostatic resection; PSA, prostate-specific antigen.

spine is most commonly affected, and the metastases are generally osteoblastic in nature. Among patients with metastases who develop symptomatic hormone-refractory disease, the mean survival time is 6 to 9 months.

CLINICAL FINDINGS

Localized prostate cancer is an asymptomatic disease. Urinary symptoms, such as frequency, dysuria, or decreased force, can be seen with prostate cancer but are much more common findings with benign prostatic hyperplasia. Microscopic hematuria, gross hematuria, or blood in the ejaculate may be associated with prostate cancer but are more representative of a urinary tract infection, urinary tract stones, or a bladder or kidney tumor. Patients with metastatic disease may present with bone pain, weight loss, or fatigue. Currently, approximately 75% of patients are diagnosed with clinically localized disease, mainly due to the use of PSA as a screening tool.

Just as there are few symptoms of localized prostate cancer, there are few clinical signs. The most obvious sign for prostate cancer is an abnormal DRE finding. DRE alone is not a sufficiently sensitive or specific test for the detection of prostate cancer, and as many as 50% of patients diagnosed by a DRE have tumor beyond the prostate capsule. Localized bone pain or urinary retention may be evident in more advanced cases but is neither sensitive nor specific for prostate cancer.

LABORATORY FINDINGS

Serum PSA determination has had a profound effect on the diagnosis and management of prostate cancer. It has taken a central role in prostate cancer screening and this is more fully described in Chapter 207. PSA is a 34-kd glycoprotein serine protease that is a member of the kallikrein family of proteins. Normal epithelium, infected normal tissue, benign prostatic hyperplasia, and prostate cancer all produce PSA with a normal value that has been established as less than 4.0 ng per milliliter. Unfortunately, a value less than 4.0 ng per milliliter does not guarantee the absence of cancer (20% to 35% of clinically detectable prostate tumors display a PSA of less than 4.0 ng per milliliter), nor does a value above 4.0 ng per milliliter confirm the presence of cancer. As the PSA value increases, the chance of being diagnosed with cancer increases. A PSA value of 4 to 10 ng per milliliter has approximately a 20% chance of being associated with prostate cancer, and a PSA level above 10 ng per milliliter increases this association to over 50%. The combination of DRE and serum PSA is more sensitive and specific for detecting prostate cancer than either of these methods alone. It remains to be determined if this higher detection rate can decrease the death rate of this disease, but early indications suggest that this is true.

Serum PSA measurements are an excellent method to monitor patients after radical prostatectomy or radiation therapy, and they often provide the earliest data about treatment failure. In the post-surgical period, serum PSA levels should be in the undetectable range; following radiation therapy, serum PSA levels should remain stable. Persistent elevation of PSA postoperatively denotes surgical failure, as does the reappearance of detectable PSA levels after surgery. The interpretation of serum PSA measurements in patients treated with radiation therapy patients is less clear, but a favorable response usually occurs in those whose nadir values fall below 4.0 ng per milliliter or into the undetectable range and remain there. A rise in PSA level on three consecutive measurements is considered evidence of disease progression in this setting.

The diagnosis of prostate cancer is almost always made by transrectal ultrasound–guided needle biopsy of the prostate using a standard sextant biopsy technique in which samples are taken from the base, midportion, and apex of the prostate on each side. Additional biopsies may be obtained, depending on the level of clinical suspicion of disease and the presence of palpable lesions or visualized disease on transrectal ultrasound.

The skeletal system is the primary site of metastatic disease and a bone scan is the most sensitive method to detect osseous metastases. Bone scans must be interpreted with caution, however, because (1) they are not specific and (2) they demonstrate bony disease secondary to arthritis or injury. Patients with a PSA below 10 ng per milliliter have an extremely low chance of demonstrating bone metastasis, and for such patients, a bone scan may be eliminated as part of the metastatic workup. Computed tomography is also not routinely indicated in patients with PSA below 10 ng per milliliter.

OPTIMAL MANAGEMENT

The optimal treatment of any prostate cancer must take into account the age and health of the patient, the nature of the tumor (stage and grade), and the intent of treatment (cure or palliation). Treatment decisions with the intent to cure must be based on the probability of enhancing the 10-year and 15-year survival of any given patient.

LOCALIZED DISEASE

Standard treatment options for patients with clinically localized disease include watchful waiting, radical prostatectomy, and external-beam radiotherapy. Active observation, with androgen ablation reserved for palliative use at the time of progressive disease, may be a reasonable option for patients with a low-grade tumor and/or less than a 10-year expected survival. This must be assessed on a patient by patient basis.

For patients with an expected survival greater than 10 years, radical retropubic prostatectomy is considered a standard of care for men younger than 70 years. This procedure includes removal of the prostate and seminal vesicles in conjunction with a limited pelvic lymph node dissection. The surgical mortality rate is less than 0.5% and hospitalization is generally less than 4 days with newer methods of postoperative care. The principal morbidities from this surgery are permanent urinary incontinence, occurring in less than 5% of patients, and impotence, which occurs in over 50% of patients, depending on age, weight, and sexual function before surgery. Many patients display some degree of stress urinary incontinence. Patients with localized disease have an overall 5-year, PSA-negative, disease-free survival rate of 95%.

External-beam radiation therapy is another standard form of therapy for localized prostate cancer and is the preferred form of treatment for clinical stage C or T3 disease. Patients over the age of 70 are also commonly referred for radiotherapy. Treatment is provided in a fractionated manner for a total of 6,000 to 7,800 cGy. During therapy, patients may experience transient, non-debilitating bowel or bladder irritation. Long-term complications include a 2% to 5% rate of painless rectal bleeding or diarrhea, less than 1% incidence of incontinence, and a 20% to 80% incidence of erectile dysfunction. Studies suggest that androgen ablation by luteinizing hormone–releasing hormone (LHRH) agonists given through the course of radiation therapy increases the time to clinical recurrence of the disease. A recent study suggests that androgen ablation should continue for 3 years after completion of radiation therapy.

Retrospective comparisons of external-beam radiation therapy and radical prostatectomy do not demonstrate any significant differences in survival at 10-year follow-up assessments and these modalities are considered to be equivalent modes of therapy for localized disease. Patients often benefit from a multidisciplinary clinic approach where they are offered joint consultation from the departments of urology and radiation oncology so that they can develop an appreciation of the risks and benefits of each procedure.

Recently, the implantation of radioactive seeds (interstitial radiation or brachytherapy) has gained popularity as an experimental treatment for localized prostate cancer. Seeds consist of radioactive iodine or palladium and are placed through a transperineal approach using ultrasonographic guidance. Cryosurgical ablation of prostate tissue via transperineal probes is another investigational technique being performed at a few centers. Both of these techniques should be considered investigational, and long-term results with these techniques are not yet available.

RECURRENCE FOLLOWING PRIMARY THERAPY

Prostate-specific antigen provides an early indicator of disease recurrence in patients following definitive primary therapy. Typically, these patients will have no evidence of metastatic disease on bone and CT scan, and recurrence is only documented by a rising PSA. Postprostatectomy patients should have an undetectable PSA, and any elevation is an indication of disease recurrence. The time to recurrence has been shown to be an important prognostic indicator, with those patients whose PSA never becomes undetectable or whose PSA begins to rise within a year of prostatectomy having a high likelihood of diffuse metastatic disease. In contrast, patients developing a rising PSA after a year may be manifesting local recurrence. Treatment in this situation is controversial, but some studies have suggested that a significant proportion of these patients may be cured by salvage radiotherapy. This is also the situation in which newer imaging modalities may prove useful. Unfortunately, currently available tests lack sufficient sensitivity and specificity to be useful.

Defining PSA recurrence following radiotherapy is more difficult. Patients receiving radiation do not have complete ablation of the gland; thus, persistence of some level of PSA is frequent. PSA failure after radiotherapy has been defined as three consecutive rising PSA values. This definition has faced wide criticism but is a reasonable approach if applied appropriately. Patients meeting this definition who were reasonable candidates for prostatectomy initially may be considered for salvage prostatectomy. This procedure is associated with a high probability of incontinence due to the cumulative effects of radiation and surgery.

Patients with a rising PSA who are not candidates for radiotherapy or salvage prostatectomy present a difficult management problem. Some will not develop significant evidence of disease progression for prolonged periods. Others will rapidly develop diffuse metastatic disease. Initiation of hormonal therapy in this setting is controversial in that individual patients may be committed to a prolonged period of therapy without evidence that early hormonal therapy is of benefit. Decisions in this setting are often based on individual patient preference since definitive data to guide therapy are lacking. These patients may be excellent candidates for clinical trials designed to test new approaches to the therapy of prostate cancer since they presumably have a minimal tumor burden. Trials conducted in this setting must have a low probability of toxicity since this population is generally otherwise healthy; trials must also have appropriately defined biologic end points since measurement of overall benefit is difficult.

METASTATIC DISEASE

Patients with positive lymph nodes but negative osseous disease are generally treated with some form of androgen ablation. The use of pelvic irradiation in these patients remains controversial but is often used in younger patients. The 5-year overall survival rate is 70% to 85%.

Patients with distant metastatic disease (osseous or bone disease) are classically treated with androgen deprivation, which results in tumor regression in at least 80% of patients. The typical duration of response is approximately 2 years. Androgen deprivation is accomplished either through surgical castration or through the administration of depot-injectable LHRH agonists such as leuprolide and goserelin. The principal side effects of androgen deprivation are diminished libido, erectile dysfunction, hot flashes, sweats, and weight gain. When severe, hot flashes may be controlled by megesterol acetate (10 to 40 mg daily), bellargal, or low doses of the newer generation of serotonin antagonist antidepressants. Upon initiation of treatment with an LHRH agonist, the pituitary releases an initial surge of follicle-stimulating hormone and luteinizing hormone, followed by cessation of excretion. In the first month of therapy this surge should be blocked by administration of an antiandrogen, such as flutamide, bicalutamide, or nilutamide.

Administration of LHRH agonists or orchiectomy will result in castrate levels of circulating androgens, but 5% to 10% of circulating androgens from adrenal and peripheral adipose sources remain. The continued use of antiandrogens after the first month has been termed "complete or total androgen blockade." It remains a controversial strategy, with mixed results from studies that have attempted to determine whether this approach results in improved survival.

Classically, chemotherapy has been unsuccessful in the treatment of hormone-refractory prostate cancer. Recent studies have begun to show some promise for chemotherapy in the setting of advanced metastatic prostate cancer. The regimen of mitoxantrone and prednisone has been demonstrated to improve quality of life in patients with hormone-refractory prostate cancer but not to improve survival. These studies led to the approval of mitoxantrone for the treatment of hormone-refractory prostate cancer by the Food and Drug Administration. Other promising chemotherapeutic approaches include estramustine-based regimens and other chemohormonal therapy combinations. Response rates as high as 60% have been reported for combinations of estramustine with either paclitaxel or docetaxel, and estramustine has also been combined with vinblastine, oral etoposide, and vinorelbine. Ketoconazole has been given in combination with doxorubicin, and more recently this combination was studied in an alternating schedule with estramustine and vinblastine with good results. Cyclophosphamide with prednisone has also been shown to have some activity in this disease. Each of these combinations must be given in a setting in which a full assessment of the individual patient's comorbidities has been performed. Although none of these combinations has yet proven to improve overall survival, the activity is promising and continued evaluation is under way.

BIBLIOGRAPHY

Beck RJ, Kattan MW, Miles BJ. A critique of the decision analysis for clinically localized prostate cancer. *J Urol* 1994;152:1894–1899.

Bolla M, Gonzalez D, Warde P, et al. Improved survival in patients with locally advanced prostate cancer treated with radiotherapy and goserelin. *N Engl J Med* 1997;337:295–300.

Catalona WJ. Management of cancer of the prostate. *N Engl J Med* 1994;331:996–1004.

Hanks GE, Krall JM, Hanlon AL, et al. Patterns of care and RTOG studies in prostate cancer. Long term survival, hazard rate observations, and possibilities of cure. *Int J Radiat Oncol Biol Phys* 1994;28:39–45.

Johansson JE, Holmberg L, Johansson S, et al. Fifteen year survival in prostate cancer: a prospective, population based study in Sweden. *JAMA* 1997;277:467–471.

Oesterling JE. Prostate specific antigen: a critical assessment of the most useful tumor marker for adenocarcinoma of the prostate. *J Urol* 1991;139:907–923.

Oh WK, Kantoff PW. Management of hormone refractory prostate cancer: current standards and future prospects. *J Urol* 1998;160:1220–1229.

Partin AW, Yoo J, Carter HB, et al. The use of prostate specific antigen, clinical stage and Gleason score to predict pathological stage in men with localized prostate cancer. *J Urol* 1993;150:110–114.

Pilepich MV, Krall JM, Al-Sarraf M, et al. Androgen deprivation with radiation therapy compared with radiation therapy alone for localized prostate carcinoma: a randomized comparative trial of the Radiation Therapy Oncology Group. *Urology* 1995;45:616–623.

Walsh PC. Radical prostatectomy: a procedure in evolution. *Semin Oncol* 1994;21:662–671.

Kelley's Textbook of Internal Medicine, fourth edition. Edited by H. David Humes. Lippincott Williams & Wilkins, Philadelphia © 2000.

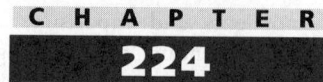

CHAPTER 224

SARCOMAS OF SOFT TISSUE AND BONE

J. SYBIL BIERMANN
LAURENCE H. BAKER

DEFINITION

Most cancers are epithelial and are called carcinomas. Common carcinomas include cancer of the lung, breast, prostate, and colon. Sarcomas usually arise in structures that derive from the mesoderm (i.e., bone, cartilage, fat, muscle, tendon, and fibrous tissue). Bone and soft-tissue sarcomas are among the least common malignancies. By convention, sarcomas also include malignant tumors that arise in peripheral nerves and are derived from neuroectoderm. Sarcomas may also arise in blood and lymphatic vessels. Sarcomas are malignant tumors that are locally aggressive and capable of invasive growth, recurrence, and distant metastasis. In the past two decades, there have been dramatic improvements in the management of osteogenic sarcomas, whereas progress in the management of soft-tissue sarcomas has lagged.

INCIDENCE AND EPIDEMIOLOGY

Only 1% of all cancers diagnosed in the United States this year will be sarcomas. In total, there will be approximately 8,000 new cases of which 2,000 will be bone sarcomas. Though uncommon, sarcomas occur in all age groups, even infants and newborns. Soft-tissue and bone sarcomas are second only to leukemias in incidence in the pediatric population. Evidence suggests there is an increase in the incidence of sarcomas, although most of this is related to HIV-associated Kaposi's sarcoma. The incidence and distribution of soft-tissue sarcomas seem to be similar in different regions of the world, and the incidence of osteosarcoma is also nearly identical from nation to nation. There are no known racial factors, with the exception that Ewing's sarcoma is rare in African Americans and Asians.

Sarcomas present in a wide variety of anatomical locations. Soft-tissue sarcomas occur most frequently in the extremities, chest wall, mediastinum, retroperitoneum, head and neck region, and within viscera (leiomyosarcoma of the uterus, gastrointestinal stromal sarcomas). Osteosarcomas have a predilection for the long-bone metaphyses and have been reported in nearly every bone. Occurring primarily in adolescents or young adults, osteosarcomas most often arise near the larger more active physes (distal femur, proximal tibia, proximal humerus), but may also arise in flat bones of the pelvis, skull, ribs, and scapula. The single most common site for sarcomas is the thigh, which is the region of the body with the most connective tissues.

Both soft-tissue and bone sarcomas are slightly more common in males. The gender and age incidences vary among the different histologic types. For example, embryonal rhabdomyosarcomas occur exclusively in the very young. Peak incidence for synovial sarcomas is in the third decade, and malignant fibrous histiocytoma is predominantly a tumor of older age with a peak incidence around 60 years.

ETIOLOGIC FACTORS

The pathogenesis of most soft-tissue or bone sarcomas remains unclear. Recognized causes include various environmental factors such as environmental carcinogens, radiation, and viruses, as well as inherited effects. Trauma is frequently implicated in sarcomas, but usually because trauma calls attention to a mass not previously recognized. The controversy on the role of pesticide exposure as a carcinogen continues. Evidence now exists for an increased incidence following exposure to phenoxacetic acids and the related chlorophenols. In recent years, there has been an increased concern over the long-term health risks associated with artificial breast implants. Thus far, all analyses have failed to show an increased risk for sarcoma after breast implantation.

There is a small but definite long-term risk for soft-tissue and bone sarcoma after therapeutic radiation. The mean latency period is 16 years; the median latency period is 10 years with a range of 4 to 31 years. The prognosis of these radiation-induced sarcomas is not worse than that of the sporadic sarcomas. Sarcomas have occurred following radiation to patients with Hodgkin's disease, breast cancer, and retinoblastoma. The most common postirradiation sarcoma is malignant fibrous histiocytoma; second is osteosarcoma, followed by fibrosarcoma.

Viruses play a role in the etiology of Kaposi's sarcoma. Virus particles have been found repeatedly in a variety of sarcomas, but no specific etiologic relationship has been identified. Immunologic deficiency may be the underlying mechanism in the development of angiosarcoma or lymphangiosarcoma that arises in an edematous extremity following modified radical mastectomy and external radiation (Stewart–Treves syndrome).

Several genetic diseases are associated with the development of sarcomas. Neurofibromatosis type I, an autosomal dominant disease, manifests early in life with large multiple café-au-lait spots, and later with the development of numerous neurofibromas. Malignant peripheral nerve sheath tumors will occasionally develop from malignant degeneration of a neurofibroma. This is the only example of a benign soft-tissue tumor becoming malignant.

The inherited bilateral form of retinoblastoma is frequently associated with the development of osteosarcoma, usually within the irradiated field, or with the development of a soft-tissue sarcoma well outside of any field of radiation. Further, the retinoblastoma gene *(Rb)* is frequently mutated in patients with sarcoma. Li–Fraumeni syndrome is a familial cancer syndrome in which there is a germ line mutation of the *p53* gene that results in familial rhabdomyosarcoma and other soft-tissue sarcomas or osteosarcomas, as well as early onset of bilateral breast cancer and several other neoplasms.

PATHOLOGIC FACTORS

Both bone and soft-tissue sarcomas are heterogeneous with regard to tumor grade, clonality, and morphologic subtypes. Most classifications are principally based on the line of differentiation of the tumor (i.e., the tissue being formed by the cancer rather than the tissue from which the cancer arose). Malignant fibrous histiocytoma and liposarcomas are the most common soft-tissue sarcomas in adults and together constitute about 40% of all sarcomas. Grading characteristics include the number of mitotic figures, the extent of tumor cell necrosis, and the degree of differentiation of the cancer. Some sarcomas including osteogenic sarcoma, Ewing's family of cancers, mesenchymal chondrosarcoma, and rhabdomyosarcoma are almost always high grade. Others, such as chondrosarcomas, liposarcomas, fibrosarcomas, and leiomyosarcomas, occur in low- and high-grade forms. High-grade lesions are potentially lethal and their clinical behavior is different from that of low-grade lesions. Once grade and tumor sizes are accounted for, the clinical behaviors of most types of soft-tissue sarcomas are similar.

Various chromosomal abnormalities have been detected in sarcomas. While the current classification of sarcomas continues to be based on morphologic resemblance between tumor cells and specific immunohistochemical staining patterns, the importance of cytogenetic criteria continually increases. Table 224.1 characterizes cytogenetic abnormalities in sarcomas.

CLINICAL FINDINGS

SOFT-TISSUE SARCOMAS

The clinical management of soft-tissue sarcomas begins with suspicion based on the clinical presentation and the imaging studies. In patients with an extremity sarcoma, a painless mass is the most common presenting symptom, with pain present only in about 25% of cases. Often patients give a history of trauma to the area that can lead to delay in the ultimate diagnosis. Delay in diagnosis is still quite common, with the common differential diagnosis often being hematoma or muscle strain/sprain. In general, any soft-tissue mass in an adult that is symptomatic or enlarging, greater than 5 cm in diameter, or any new mass that persists for more than 6 weeks should be considered for biopsy. Patients with intra-abdominal or retroperitoneal sarcomas often experience nonspecific abdominal discomfort.

Most retroperitoneal sarcomas are either liposarcoma or leiomyosarcoma. These patients usually present with very large masses and lower back pain. Rarely, these retroperitoneal sarcomas produce an insulin-like protein and the patient may present with hypoglycemia. Gastrointestinal stromal sarcomas (GISTs) are an uncommon GI malignancy (compared to epithelial cancers) and can occur in the stomach, small intestine, or colon. In the past these cancers were called leiomyosarcomas because of morphologic similarity. These patients present with a GI bleed and, less often, with symptoms of an intra-abdominal mass. Patients with sarcomas of the uterus usually present with abnormal vaginal bleeding. Uterine sarcomas can arise from an admixture of mesodermal and endometrial adenocarcinomatous

TABLE 224.1.	CHARACTERISTIC CYTOGENETIC ABNORMALITIES IN SARCOMAS	
Tumor	**Cytogenetic Abnormality**	**Frequency (%)**
Clear cell sarcoma	t(12;22)(q13;q12)	>75
Dermatofibrosarcoma protuberans	Ring chromosome 17	>75
Ewing's sarcoma	t(11;22)(q24;q12)	95
Intra-abdominal desmoplastic small round cell tumor	t(11;22)(p13;q12)	>50
Primitive neuroectodermal tumor	t(11;22)(q24;q12)	95
Extraskeletal myxoid chondrosarcoma	t(9,22)(q31;q12)	50
Hemangiopericytoma	Translocation at 12q13	>25
Leiomyosarcoma	Deletion of 1p	75
Liposarcoma		
Myxoid	t(12;16)(q13;p11)	75
Pleomorphic	Complex	90
Well-differentiated	Ring chromosome 12	80
Malignant fibrous histiocytoma		
High-grade	Complex	90
Myxoid	Ring chromosomes	>50
Malignant peripheral nerve sheath	Complex	90
Rhabdomyosarcoma		
Alveolar	t(2;13)(q35;q14)	80
Embryonal	+2q, +8, +20	80
Synovial sarcoma	t(X;18)(p11;q11)	95

elements (mixed mesodermal tumors), or from myometrium (leiomyosarcomas) or endometrial stroma (endometrial stromal sarcoma). In older men the genitourinary tract can be a site of sarcoma, usually in the paratesticular region, prostate, or bladder. Leiomyosarcoma and liposarcoma are the most common types of sarcoma.

Metastasis of soft-tissue sarcomas is usually hematogenous; lymphatic metastasis is uncommon. In more than 70% of patients, the first site of metastasis is the lung. These pulmonary lesions are characteristically multiple, in the lung periphery, and round (Fig. 224.1). Gastrointestinal stromal sarcomas and occasionally retroperitoneal sarcomas will most often metastasize to the liver.

EWING'S FAMILY OF TUMORS

Ewing's family of tumors comprises bone and soft-tissue, small round cell neoplasms of neuroectodermal origin defined by the chromosomal aberration t(11;22)(q24;q12), and closely related variants. Tumors of the soft tissues are sometimes called extraskeletal Ewing's or primitive neuroectodermal tumors (PNETs). Molecular and cytogenetic analysis of Ewing's sarcoma and PNETs has resulted in the identification of genetic mutations that can distinguish these tumors from other small round cell tumors such as rhabdomyosarcoma or lymphomas. Typically, Ewing's sarcoma occurs in adolescents and young adults; it usually arises in the diaphyseal portion of the bone. The most common primary sites are the femur and pelvis, although any bone may be affected. On imaging the bone appears as mottled. Periosteal reaction is classic and is due to a periosteal reaction; it is referred to as "onion skin" by radiologists. Fever, weight loss, and fatigue sometimes are constitutional symptoms. Abnormal laboratory studies may include elevated lactate dehydrogenase and leukocytosis. The lungs, bones, and bone marrow are the most common sites of metastasis. Nearly one-quarter of these patients present with signs and/or symptoms of disseminated disease.

OSTEOGENIC SARCOMA

The most common primary malignant tumor of bone is osteogenic sarcoma. Classic osteosarcoma composes nearly 80% of osteogenic sarcomas; it is a high-grade, spindle cell tumor that by definition manufactures osteoid (immature bone). It is intramedullary in location. The most common site for this cancer is the distal femur or proximal tibia. Pain followed by swelling is an early symptom. Because the pain in the beginning is often intermittent, confusing it with "growing pains" is common. Osteogenic sarcomas spread hematogenously, and lung is the most common metastatic site. Sometimes patients present with evidence of metastasis at the time of diagnosis. Several other variants of osteosarcomas occurring in an older population include osteo-

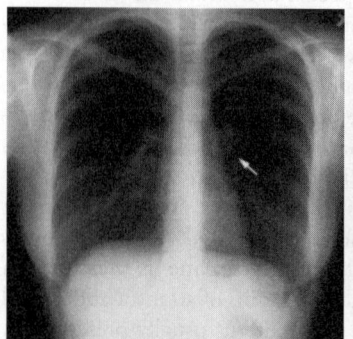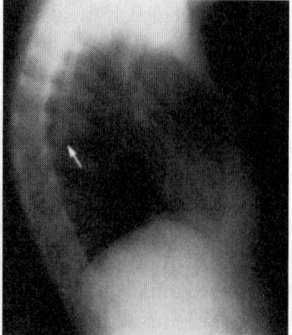

FIGURE 224.1. A small, round, peripheral metastasis in the lung fields characterizes metastatic sarcoma on this posteroanterior chest radiograph.

sarcomas secondary to Paget's disease or prior irradiation (bilateral retinoblastoma). The median age for all osteosarcoma patients is 20 years.

While most osteosarcomas are medullary, parosteal osteosarcoma is a low-grade variant occurring in a juxtacortical location, most often in the posterior distal femur. This variant tends to metastasize later than the classic form. Another juxtacortical variant is periosteal osteosarcoma, which most often involves the tibia and is intermediate in its behavior, falling somewhere between the parosteal and classic lesions.

The imaging of osteosarcomas includes plain films, which may show loss of trabeculation and new-tumor mineralization (Fig. 224.2). Computed tomography scan can show cortical disruption and extent of mineralization (Fig. 224.3). Magnetic resonance imaging (MRI) is the best multiplane imaging study because it shows intramedullary extent of the lesion as well as localization of any associated soft-tissue mass (Fig. 224.4). Alkaline phosphatase is frequently elevated in patients with osteosarcoma.

CHONDROSARCOMAS

Chondrosarcomas characteristically produce cartilage matrix devoid of osteoid from neoplastic tissue. These tumors are divided into primary lesions arising de novo from previously normal-appearing bone preformed from cartilage, and secondary tumors that arise or develop from preexisting benign cartilage lesions

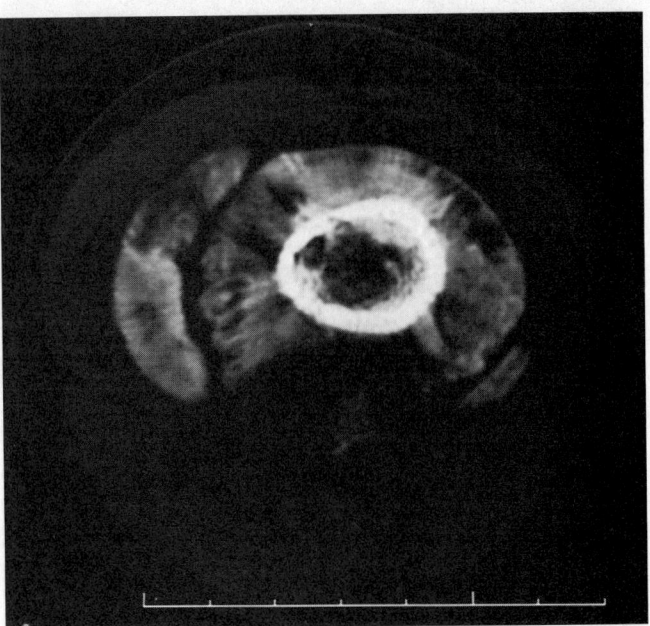

FIGURE 224.3. Computed tomographic scan of the femur with osteogenic sarcoma illustrates permeative destruction of the cortex and extensive extraosseous new-bone formation. Bones with osteosarcoma are often weakened despite their sclerotic appearance on plain films.

such as enchondromas or cartilaginous portions of osteochondromas. Malignant transformation has been reported in lesions of Ollier's disease (enchondromatosis). These sarcomas may occur at any age but usually begin 15 to 20 years after skeletal maturity. Whether the lesions are primary or secondary, the anatomical location and histologic grade are the important prognostic features. Primary chondrosarcomas constitute nearly two-thirds of all chondrosarcomas and can be high-grade lesions capable of distant metastasis as well as local invasiveness. Secondary tumors are usually low-grade with infrequent metastasis. Symptoms from chondrosarcoma are usually mild and depend on tumor size and location. Low-grade chondrosarcomas may become sizable without causing symptoms. Patients with pelvic lesions can present with severe pain and develop neurologic impairment, often because lesions arising in the pelvis are not recognized until late. Chondrosarcomas radiographically demonstrate cortical destruction and loss of medullary bone trabeculations with evidence of calcification. MRI will usually show the intramedullary extent as well as extraosseous extension of tumor.

▌ LABORATORY FINDINGS

There are no specific marker studies of blood or urine to diagnose a sarcoma. Lactate dehydrogenase is sometimes elevated, especially in Ewing's family of sarcomas. Alkaline phosphatase is often elevated in patients with osteosarcoma. Unfortunately, sarcomas are often presumed to be benign lesions until biopsy or removal. Some genetic conditions can predispose the diagnosis of sarcoma. Patients with neurofibromatosis (*NF1* gene) have a 10% incidence of a neurofibroma becoming malignant (neurofibrosarcoma). Similarly, patients with Ollier's disease or Maffucci's syndrome (enchondromatosis with hemangioma) are pre-

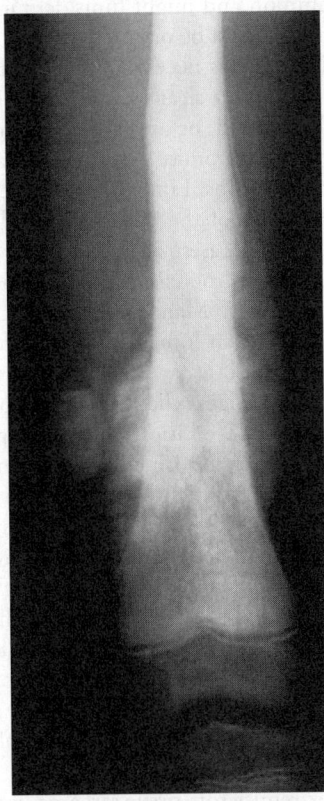

FIGURE 224.2. Anteroposterior view of a conventional osteoblastic osteosarcoma shows a poorly marginated sclerotic lesion with extensive soft-tissue mass and mineralization, as well as aggressive periosteal reaction.

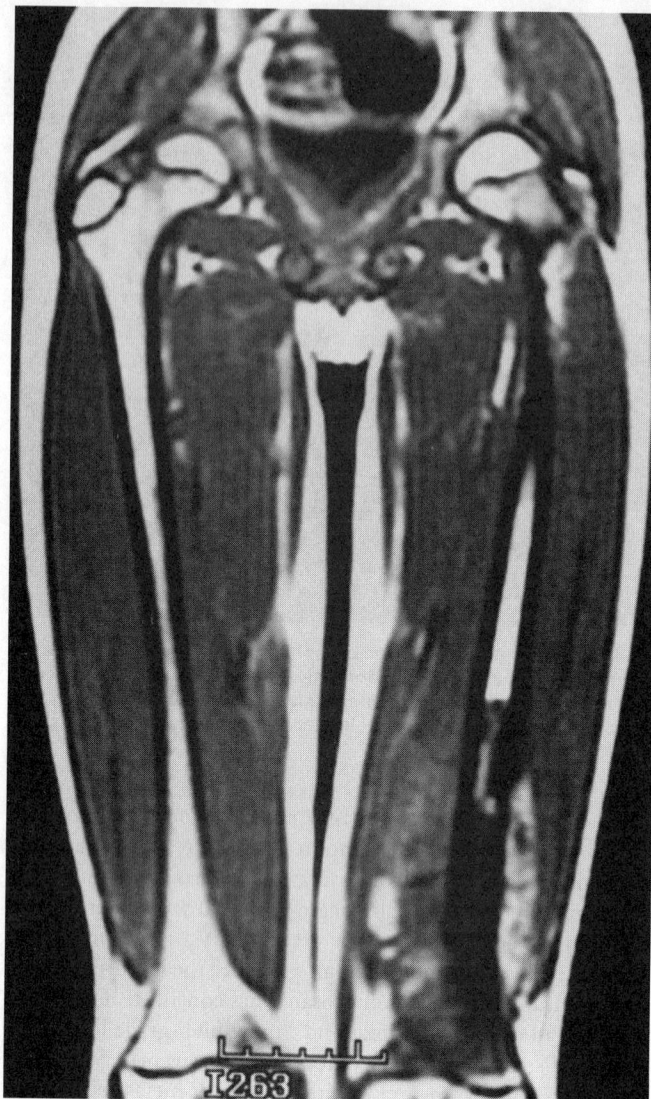

FIGURE 224.4. A T1-weighted coronal magnetic resonance image clearly defines the marrow extent of this tumor in the distal femoral diaphysis and metaphysis, extending into the epiphysis. The knee joint is uninvolved.

disposed to chondrosarcoma. The Li–Fraumeni syndrome is a rare hereditary disease characterized by the youthful occurrence of soft-tissue sarcomas, osteosarcomas, adrenocortical cancers, brain tumors, and bilateral breast cancer. The syndrome is inherited as an autosomal dominant trait with a high degree of penetrance. Within kindreds, the probability of an individual developing invasive cancer reaches 50% by age 30 and is 90% by age 70. Other predisposing conditions include prior exposure to radiation therapy and chronic lymphedema.

GENERAL MANAGEMENT PRINCIPLES

The relative small number of cases of soft-tissue and bone sarcomas and their significant diversity in anatomical location, his-

tologic appearance, and biologic behavior renders diagnostic and treatment decisions best served in a setting of multidisciplinary medicine with expertise in the management of these tumors. Team members should include an orthopedic oncologist, a pathologist, an interventional radiologist, a medical or pediatric oncologist, a radiation oncologist, and a physiatrist. Many patients consult a physician regarding a mass that is often painless or is intermittently painful.

Patients with intra-abdominal or retroperitoneal sarcomas often experience nonspecific abdominal discomfort and/or GI symptoms prior to diagnosis. Delays in diagnosis are common, with the most common incorrect diagnosis being hematoma or pulled muscle for an extremity or truncal lesion. Localized pain and swelling are the hallmark clinical features. Pain is often initially insidious and/or transient but becomes progressively more severe. Local soft-tissue swelling is often present.

Clinical management begins with suspicion based on the clinical presentation and the imaging studies. Locoregional staging should ideally be performed before the biopsy procedure. This implies that the T staging should be known prior to the procedure. MRI with and without contrast is the procedure of choice as it can determine tumor size, compartmental boundaries, neurovascular involvement, and presence of necrosis. Computed tomographic scanning may be indicated to evaluate possible cortical bone destruction and the presence or extent of mineralization.

After local tumor staging has been completed, the next step is to perform either a needle biopsy or an incisional biopsy. Biopsy should be done by an experienced surgeon because complications are common and might limit definitive limb-sparing surgery. Biopsy tracts must be oriented appropriately, usually in a vertical direction. This is necessary because the entire wound must be excised to obtain a clear margin in all directions. Transverse incisions, hematoma, or exposure of neurovascular structures may result in compromise of future surgical care and the loss of limb-sparing options. Limb salvage is the preferred surgical option for sarcomas of the extremities and can be accomplished in 95% of adult cases.

An important area in the clinical management of sarcomas is the follow-up strategy. Management of local recurrence is crucial since an increase in local failure leads to an increase in the rate of distant metastasis.

Surgical resection remains the cornerstone of primary treatment of sarcomas. Wide excision with limb preservation has supplanted amputation as the principal surgical method for eradication of local disease in patients with primary sarcomas of the limb and limb-girdle regardless of histologic type or tumor grade. Patient survival has not been compromised by this operative strategy. Development of soft-tissue and skeletal reconstruction techniques has expanded the capability of the limb reconstruction surgeon. Patients with metastatic disease to the lungs should be evaluated for surgical resection (metastasectomy). In one series, 72% of patients with isolated pulmonary metastases were rendered disease-free with surgery. The actuarial 3-year survival rate was 38%.

Radiation of extremity soft-tissue sarcomas is used as an adjuvant therapy after surgery. The routine use of radiation therapy in treatment of soft-tissue sarcomas is relatively recent. Only

TABLE 224.2.	FIVE-YEAR SURVIVAL BY TUMOR SIZE FOR INTERMEDIATE-GRADE AND HIGH-GRADE SARCOMAS TREATED WITH SURGERY AND REHABILITATION

Tumor Size	% Disease-Free
<2.5	94
2.6–4.9	77
5–10	62
10–15	51
15–20	42
>20	17

(Adapted from Brennan MF, Cosper ES, Harrison LB, et al. The role of multimodality therapy in soft tissue sarcoma. *Ann Surg* 1991; 214:328.)

patients with small, superficial tumors are spared adjuvant radiation therapy.

In patients with an extremity sarcoma who relapse, the site of failure is usually pulmonary (70%) and locally (10%). The 5-year disease-free survival rate by tumor size for patients with intermediate-grade and high-grade sarcomas treated with surgery and radiation is shown in Table 224.2. The treatment of retroperitoneal sarcomas and the role of radiation therapy remain a challenge. In no other location is the need for an adjunct modality after resection as high as in these patients.

The chemotherapeutic sensitivity of the soft-tissue sarcomas and osteogenic sarcomas is quite similar. The single most active drug in both disease categories is doxorubicin; the response rate is 26% in both tumor types. High-dose methotrexate therapy with folinic acid rescue appears to be more effective in patients with osteosarcoma (25% response) than the reported series of patients with soft-tissue sarcomas in which the response rate is 13%. Ifosfamide, like doxorubicin, has remarkably similar data in the two groups: 24% response in osteogenic sarcoma and 27% is soft-tissue sarcomas. Cyclophosphamide is also similar between the two groups (14% and 12%) and approximately half as effective as its analogue, ifosfamide. Cisplatin seems more effective in osteogenic sarcomas (18% versus 12%) than in soft-tissue sarcomas, and this is probably the reason for this drug to be included in adjuvant studies of osteogenic sarcomas, whereas adjuvant cisplatin therapy was only studied in patients with uterine sarcoma. The duration of response, frequency of complete remission, and overall survival all appear to be quite similar.

The data regarding the treatment of patients with disseminated soft-tissue sarcoma or osteogenic sarcomas with combination chemotherapy are again remarkably similar between the two groups. The combinations of doxorubicin and ifosfamide, or doxorubicin, ifosfamide, and dacarbazine, have reported response rates of 36% to 47%.

BIBLIOGRAPHY

Abeloff MA, Armitage JO, Lichter AS, et al. *Clinical oncology.* New York: Churchill Livingstone, 1995.

Antman KH, Crowley J, Balcerzak SP, et al. An intergroup phase III randomized study of doxorubicin and dacarbazine with or without ifosfamide and mesna in advanced soft-tissue sarcomas. *J Clin Oncol* 1993;11: 1276–1285.

Biermann JS, Baker LH. The future treatment of sarcoma. *Semin Oncol* 1997;24:592–597.

Biermann JS, Baker LH. NCCN practice guidelines: bone cancers. *Oncology* 1999;13(11A):365–390.

Brennan MF, Casper ES, Harrison LB, et al. The role of multimodality therapy in soft tissue sarcoma. *Ann Surg* 1991;214:328–338.

Denny CT. Gene rearrangements in Ewing's sarcoma. *Cancer Invest* 1996; 14:83–88.

Enzinger FM, Weiss SW. *Soft tissue sarcomas.* St. Louis: Mosby, 1995.

Kruzelock RP, Hansen MF. Molecular genetics and cytogenetics of sarcomas. *Hematol–Oncol Clin North Am* 1995;9:513–540.

Sarcoma Meta-Analysis Collaboration. Adjuvant chemotherapy for localized resectable soft tissue sarcoma of adults—meta-analysis of individual data. *Lancet* 1997;350:1647–1654.

Zalupski M, Baker LH. Ifosfamide. *JNCI* 1988;80:556–566.

Kelley's Textbook of Internal Medicine, fourth edition. Edited by H. David Humes. Lippincott Williams & Wilkins, Philadelphia © 2000.

CHAPTER

225

EPITHELIAL MALIGNANCIES OF THE HEAD AND NECK

GEORGE J. BOSL
DAVID G. PFISTER

Malignancies of the epithelial surface of the upper aerodigestive tract, often referred to as *head and neck cancer,* represent approximately 3.5% of all new cases of cancer in the United States. Worldwide, over 500,000 cases are diagnosed annually. In this chapter, head and neck cancer collectively refers to the squamous cell carcinomas and undifferentiated carcinomas of mucosal origin, as well as the adenocarcinomas of major and minor salivary gland origin. Control of the primary site and cervical lymph node metastases (i.e., locoregional control) dictate patient management, because two-thirds of patients die of advanced locoregional disease without distant metastases. Proper initial treatment of the primary site and, when appropriate, the cervical lymph nodes is crucial.

EPIDEMIOLOGY

Squamous cell carcinoma or one of its variants is the histologic type of 90% to 95% of head and neck cancers. With the exception of tumors of the nasopharynx, paranasal sinuses, and salivary glands, squamous cell carcinoma is usually associated with tobacco or ethanol abuse. The increased use and popularity of smokeless tobacco among adolescents and young adults are especially troublesome in this regard. The median age at diagnosis is in the sixth decade, and men predominate. Patients often present with concomitant pulmonary, hepatic, and general physiologic impairment, and they are at risk for second primary tumors because of prior tobacco and alcohol exposures. Neglect of symptoms often leads to presentation with advanced locoregional disease and debilitation due to pain and malnutrition.

The cause of salivary gland cancers is largely unknown, although an increased incidence in salivary gland tumors has been reported after radiation exposure, similar to that of thyroid cancer. Most malignant salivary gland tumors are subtypes of adenocarcinoma rather than squamous cell carcinoma. Nasopharynx and salivary gland cancers occur in younger patients than do squamous cancers of the other head and neck sites. Nasopharynx cancers are associated with Epstein–Barr virus exposure and an Asian ethnic background. Various occupational exposures have been associated with the development of sinonasal tract cancers.

CLINICAL PRESENTATION AND DIFFERENTIAL DIAGNOSIS

Squamous cell carcinoma usually presents as an ulceration in the mucosal surface. Although infection may mimic the symptoms of malignancy, any persistent lesion should be considered possibly malignant. Because much of the mucosal surface is not visualized through the open mouth, symptoms often occur that are not pursued. Hoarseness, odynophagia, dysphagia, dentalgia (particularly upper teeth from maxillary sinus cancer), and otalgia may precede obvious disease by months. Posterior neck pain is often associated with involvement of the retropharyngeal lymph nodes or prevertebral fascia. Otalgia may imply an obstructed eustachian tube in the nasopharynx, and otitis media in an adult, especially when unilateral, is a common presenting scenario for nasopharynx cancer. Laryngeal and pharyngeal cancers can also cause pain that radiates into the ear, misleading the examiner. Base of skull extension may cause a skull vertex headache or palsies of cranial nerves IX, X, or XII. Diplopia is associated with intraorbital tumor or palsies of cranial nerves III, IV, or VI due to cavernous sinus invasion.

Trismus implies involvement of the pterygoid musculature. Maxillary antrum cancers may cause facial dysesthesias resulting from involvement of branches of the fifth cranial nerve. A persistent submucosal mass or mass in the parotid or submandibular region suggests a salivary gland tumor. Asymptomatic cervical lymphadenopathy can be the presenting complaint of a malignancy of upper aerodigestive tract origin. The patient's age and risk factors are important to consider. If the initial head and neck examination does not reveal a cause, a trial of antibiotic therapy for presumed infection is warranted for 7 to 10 days, with careful follow-up to ensure resolution. Persistent symptoms, ulceration, or adenopathy, especially in the older patient with a history of tobacco or alcohol use, must be pursued, generally by referral to an otorhinolaryngologist or head and neck surgeon.

CLINICAL EVALUATION AND STAGING

Precise knowledge of tumor extent dictates proper management and maximizes the likelihood of locoregional control. A thorough physical examination must be done by an experienced examiner, with careful attention to mucosal surfaces and the cervical lymph nodes. A digital examination of the accessible oral mucosa occasionally reveals lesions not otherwise visualized. Besides direct palpation of a mass, local bleeding precipitated by gentle palpation may indicate the location of a subtle primary lesion. Indirect mirror and rigid or flexible endoscopic examination facilitates evaluation of all head and neck mucosal surfaces. Direct examination under anesthesia is necessary for tumors that cannot be visualized through the open mouth. The routine use of "triple endoscopy" (laryngoscopy, esophagoscopy, and bronchoscopy) is controversial. It appears to be of greatest usefulness in two groups: patients with diffuse mucosal abnormalities suggesting a higher risk of synchronous cancers and patients with cervical adenopathy and no clear primary lesion.

CT is required to evaluate the base of the skull; the superior and inferior extent of the tumor; the parapharyngeal, retropharyngeal, and cervical lymph nodes; possible encroachment on the carotid artery; and direct brain extension. It is the principal imaging technique used to evaluate the locoregional tumor extent in these patients. MRI is superior to CT for evaluating intracranial tumor extent and is also helpful in evaluating submucosal disease spread with tongue cancers. Some centers use ultrasonography to facilitate assessment of the neck. Routine use of all these studies is costly and is, in most cases, not indicated. Positron emission tomography (PET) is being investigated, but the data are currently limited for these diseases. PET can be useful in identifying an occult primary lesion.

Systemic metastases are uncommonly present at diagnosis in patients with head and neck cancers (except those with nasopharynx or hypopharynx cancer) and generally occur when cervical lymph nodes are involved. The most common metastatic sites are the lungs and bones. A routine chest radiograph is required for each patient, as much to detect a secondary primary tumor in the lung as to find a distant metastasis. A routine biochemical screen is indicated, with follow-up imaging of the liver or a bone scan only when appropriate biochemical abnormalities are identified. A complete blood count may suggest vitamin B_{12}, folate, or other nutritional deficiencies.

As with all malignancies, histologic proof of cancer is necessary, preferably of the primary site. Patients with an enlarged, suspicious lymph node or nodes without a clear primary lesion present a special challenge. An excisional lymph node biopsy should not be the first diagnostic step, because alteration of lymphatic drainage may occur. Fine-needle aspiration is the procedure of choice. Random directed biopsies of the more common sites for occult primary lesions, such as the nasopharynx, oropharynx (tonsillar fossa, base of tongue, vallecula), and hypopharynx (piriform sinus) are generally done when no mucosal abnormality is seen on routine examination.

The process of determining the site and extent of a malignancy is called *staging*. Each primary site lesion is staged clinically in terms of the tumor (T) stage, the nodal involvement (N) stage, and the metastatic (M) stage (Table 225.1). Prognosis broadly follows the stage for each primary site, but the prognosis for a patient with a stage III glottic larynx cancer is different from the prognosis for a patient with a stage III oral tongue cancer. Accordingly, the prognosis depends on the overall stage

TABLE 225.1.	STAGING OF SQUAMOUS CELL CARCINOMAS OF THE HEAD AND NECK FOR SELECTED SITES				
	Oral Cavity	**Oropharynx**	**Hypopharynx**	**Paranasal Sinus (Ethmoid)**	**Larynx**
T Stage					
Tis	Carcinoma in situ	Carcinoma in situ	Carcinoma in situ	Carcinoma in situ	Carcinoma in situ
T1	0–2 cm	0–2 cm	One site and 0–2 cm	Confined to ethmoid; bone erosion allowed	Limited to one site or to vocal cords
T2	2.1–4 cm	2.1–4 cm	>1 subsite or 2.1–4 cm; no vocal cord fixation	Nasal cavity extension	>1 site, or local impaired vocal cord mobility
T3	>4 cm	>4 cm	>4 cm or vocal cord paralysis	Anterior orbit or maxillary sinus extension	Vocal cord paralysis; postcricoid or preepiglottic space extension
T4	>4 cm with massive invasion	>4 cm with massive invasion	Massive soft-tissue invasion	Massive invasion	Massive invasion through soft-tissue or cartilage
N Stage (same for all primary sites)					
N0	No clinically apparent cervical lymph nodes				
N1	Clinically apparent solitary ipsilateral lymph node ≤3 cm				
N2	Clinically apparent ipsilateral lymph nodes, either solitary 3–6 cm (N_{2a}), multiple of size ≤6 cm (N_{2b}); bilateral or contralateral only ≤6 cm (N_{2c})				
N3	Clinically apparent nodes >6 cm				
M Stage					
M0	No distant metastases				
M1	Distant metastases present				
Stage Grouping					
Stage I	T1, N0, M0				
Stage II	T2, N0, M0				
Stage III	T1–3, N1, M0				
	T3, N0, M0				
Stage IV	T4, N0–1, M0 (IVA)				
	All Tx, N2, M0 (IVA)[a]				
	All Tx, N3, M0 (IVB)				
	All Tx, Nx, M1 (IVC)				

[a] For paranasal sinus cancer, TxN2M0 is stage IVB, not stage IVA.

and the primary site. Inspection of the T stages shows that staging of the primary site is complicated by the inability to measure accurately the size of most primary head and neck cancers, further complicating comparisons between primary sites. Although general rules with regard to staging the neck and the creation of overall stages apply to selected sites as highlighted in Table 225.1, the outlined paradigm does not uniformly apply to all primary sites. For example, staging of salivary gland tumors follows a different overall staging scheme; nasopharynx cancers have different neck and overall staging criteria.

OPTIMAL MANAGEMENT

GENERAL PRINCIPLES

Control of the primary tumor and draining lymph nodes is the principal goal of all head and neck cancer treatment. Surgery, radiation therapy, and chemotherapy play roles in various circumstances. In many situations, a patient can be treated in more than one way with survival results that are equivalent. Accordingly, other factors such as anticipated functional or cosmetic outcome may influence choice of therapy.

Tumors begin as mucosal lesions, sometimes progressing from leukoplakia or erythroplasia. The whitish plaques of leukoplakia usually progress slowly and rarely develop invasive cancer. Erythroplasia is less common than leukoplakia but more likely to harbor in situ or invasive cancer, mandating more aggressive evaluation and intervention. Progression of the primary lesion occurs by superficial extension and deep infiltration. The depth of invasion (deeper than 2 mm) is associated with a greater potential for regional lymph node metastases. As a tumor grows, natural barriers such as fascial planes, cartilage, and bone are traversed. The diffuse mucosal abnormalities—field cancerization or condemned mucosa—often found are compatible with prior tobacco and alcohol exposure, multiple sites of premalignant change, and increased risks of synchronous and metachronous cancers. Indeed, even normal-appearing mucosa surrounding a tumor may harbor premalignant changes on genetic analysis.

The larger the primary tumor, the greater is the likelihood of regional lymphadenopathy. The lymph nodes at risk are determined by the primary site and are generally ipsilateral to the primary tumor. The nodes are often classified by *levels*. Level I is the submental triangle; levels II, III, and IV are the upper, middle, and lower thirds of the jugular lymph node chain; and level V is the posterior cervical triangle. The location of involved lymph nodes in patients without a clear primary site is often helpful in directing further evaluation. For example, a level I lymph node should prompt careful scrutiny of the oral cavity; an isolated level IV node should raise the possibility of a primary site below the clavicles.

SURGERY

Surgery for head and neck cancer is multidisciplinary. An adequate surgical resection requires margins free of tumor. This may result in considerable cosmetic or functional alterations for large tumors. Conservation procedures that preserve vital structures while completely removing the tumor exist, but they should not be confused with a conservative resection that violates surgical oncologic principles and incompletely excises a tumor. Because diffuse mucosal abnormalities are common, a negative margin by immunohistochemical criteria can be falsely reassuring. Other factors at the molecular biologic level (e.g., p53 mutations) are being investigated as a means to ensure a more complete resection.

Total laryngectomy or glossectomy is sometimes required. Mandibular mobilization may be necessary to expose large primary tumors, such as those of the tonsil and base of the tongue. Resection of bone (i.e., hard palate or mandible) may be required to resect all disease with adequate margins. A maxillofacial prosthodontist is often required to create obturators to close defects and restore speech and swallowing.

Radical neck dissection is required in patients with bulky or multiple affected nodes. The contents of the ipsilateral neck are frequently resected en bloc with the primary tumor. A classic radical neck dissection includes resection of the spinal accessory nerve, the internal jugular vein, and the sternocleidomastoid muscle. Various less morbid modified neck dissections are available for specific indications. The need for neck dissection in patients with a high likelihood of cervical metastases but without clinical incidence of disease is controversial. Postoperative irradiation provides equivalent control in these patients. However, a neck dissection that does not find involved nodes may prevent the need for radiation therapy, depending on how the primary site is managed.

Relative or absolute contraindications to surgery include nasopharynx cancer, fixed lymphadenopathy, base of skull extension, trismus, and fixation to the prevertebral fascia. In these circumstances, clear margins are rarely achieved. The plastic surgeon, prosthodontist, and others involved in the reconstruction and repair of the surgical defect should evaluate the patient preoperatively to facilitate treatment planning. Reconstructive procedures appropriate for repair of the surgical defect are optimally done at the time of the definitive ablative procedure.

RADIATION THERAPY

Radiation therapy alone may be administered by itself as definitive treatment for less advanced squamous cell head and neck cancers, or it may be delivered preoperatively or postoperatively. Although at least one large study showed that preoperative radiation therapy of 5,000 cGy did not increase the morbidity of surgery, most patients are treated postoperatively, because locoregional control appears to be better with this approach.

The treatment volume and primary site dictate the radiation technique to be used. Total dose depends on the setting (definitive management or preoperative/postoperative) and fraction size. Treatment may require external-beam therapy and a temporary or permanent implant (*brachytherapy*). The treatment plan must be carefully designed to maximize effect and minimize treatment toxicity. Primary tumors treated with radiation alone generally require 6,500 to 7,000 cGy delivered over 6½ to 8 weeks in fractions of 180 to 200 cGy per day. Interstitial boosts with iridium Ir 192 by an afterloading technique (*temporary implant*) or iodine I 125 (*permanent implant*) may be required to boost the radiation dose in small volumes at high risk for recurrence. Altered fractionation (e.g., twice-daily radiation) is under study for treating large-volume tumors and appears to improve local tumor control. Conformal radiation therapy and intensity-modulated radiation therapy are being investigated as ways to optimally deliver treatment to the tumor while sparing more of the normal tissues and thus potentially facilitating dose escalation. Neutron-beam therapy has been suggested for certain salivary tumors, but it is not widely available.

Acute radiation injury impairs alimentation, and the maintenance of food intake is vital. A feeding tube or percutaneous gastrostomy may be required. Altered fractionation schemes or the concomitant use of chemotherapy with radiation can exacerbate acute toxicity. Evaluating ways to ameliorate or prevent local acute mucosal damage (e.g., chemoprotectants such as amifostine, growth factors, topical measures) are an important research priority. Long-term radiation injury includes xerostomia, accelerated caries formation, and weight loss. The results of a placebo-controlled randomized trial suggest that pilocarpine may help to ameliorate the salivary gland dysfunction and dry mouth associated with radiation therapy. Osteonecrosis is less common because of the advances in treatment planning and proper dental care. A dental consultation before radiation therapy is mandatory. Diseased teeth must be extracted, infected gingiva treated, and prophylactic fluoride treatment initiated.

CHEMOTHERAPY

By itself, chemotherapy cannot cure squamous cell head and neck cancers. The most active and commonly used single agents include cisplatin, carboplatin, methotrexate, bleomycin, 5-fluorouracil, paclitaxel, docetaxel, ifosfamide, and gemcitabine. Response rates depend on tumor bulk, degree of pretreatment, and drugs used. With cisplatin-based combination chemotherapy such as cisplatin plus continuous-infusion 5-fluorouracil, complete responses have been reported in 15% to 50% of previously untreated patients with stage III and IV disease and complete plus partial responses in 50% to 90%. Potential toxic effects such as nausea, vomiting, ototoxicity, nephrotoxicity, mucositis, and severe pancytopenia must be taken into account when considering chemotherapy in these sometimes debilitated patients.

The use of combination chemotherapy in patients with stage III and IV squamous cell head and neck cancer has been widely studied in the hope of improving survival or decreasing the extent of required resection. Chemotherapy can be administered before surgery or radiation (by induction or neoadjuvant therapy), after this treatment (by adjuvant or maintenance therapy), concomitantly with radiation (typically for unresectable tumors), or with some combination of these approaches. Unfortunately, randomized trials have failed to demonstrate a survival advantage for the addition of neoadjuvant or adjuvant chemotherapy to planned surgery and radiation therapy in patients with locally advanced, resectable disease.

For example, one study allocated more than 460 patients with stage III and IV disease to three treatment arms. The survival distribution of patients receiving chemotherapy (i.e., one cycle of preoperative with or without 6 months of adjuvant chemotherapy) was equivalent to that of the standard surgery plus postoperative radiation therapy arm, although there was a decrease in distant metastases among patients receiving adjuvant chemotherapy. This and other similar studies have several methodologic limitations. Studies have frequently not been site-specific, combining patients with different prognostic and management issues. Most studies have focused on improved overall survival, which is difficult to prove for a disease with a relatively low proportion of distant metastases, high proportion of locoregional relapses, and competing causes of mortality (e.g., medical comorbidities, second primary cancers, and neoadjuvant or adjuvant therapy-related deaths). Other important outcomes, such as quality of speech and swallowing, often are poorly or not formally quantitated. Nonetheless, based on available data, the use of chemotherapy with planned surgery and radiation therapy in patients with resectable, advanced locoregional disease should be viewed as investigational.

Chemotherapy has evolved significantly in two settings in the last 10 years. The first setting is as part of a larynx-preservation strategy. In general, the response to radiation therapy parallels the response to chemotherapy. A major response to neoadjuvant chemotherapy at the primary site implies a high likelihood of further response with radiation therapy. Applying these concepts, pilot studies have shown that preservation of larynx function is feasible with neoadjuvant chemotherapy, followed by radiation therapy, with surgery reserved for nonresponse or relapse. These studies suggested that survival was similar to survival after standard total laryngectomy plus postoperative radiation therapy, and the larynx can be preserved in approximately two-thirds of these patients. Tumors of the larynx itself have been most extensively studied, but some oropharynx and hypopharynx tumors that require total laryngectomy as part of the planned initial therapy have also been evaluated. Major randomized trials by the Veterans Administration Laryngeal Cancer Study Group and the European Organization for Research and Treatment of Cancer (EORTC) evaluating this approach in patients with advanced larynx and hypopharynx cancers confirmed that larynx preservation can be achieved in a significant proportion of such patients. Survival was not compromised compared with standard management with surgery, including total laryngectomy, and postoperative radiation therapy. Preservation of function continues to be an important end point in studies of combining chemotherapy and radiation. The data for other primary sites are more preliminary.

The second promising area of chemotherapy with radiation therapy is the management of patients with unresectable disease. Evolving data from randomized trials and meta-analyses suggest that concomitant chemotherapy and irradiation is superior to irradiation alone in the management of these patient with most advanced disease. The optimal combination of chemotherapy and radiation therapy has yet to be defined. As noted earlier, novel radiation fractionation schedules are also being pursued in treating these patients with locally advanced disease. Two recent randomized trials report an improvement in disease control with the concomitant addition of cisplatin, 5-fluorouracil ($\pm$leucovorin) to an altered fractionation radiation program compared with the same radiation scheme alone. Toxicity, however, was greater with the addition of the systemic therapy.

SPECIFIC TUMOR MANAGEMENT

Oral Cavity

The oral cavity extends anteriorly from the vermilion border posteriorly to a plane joining the line of the circumvallate papillae of the tongue with the junction of the hard and soft palate. Primary sites within the oral cavity include the lip, hard palate, buccal mucosa, the alveolar ridges, the floor of the mouth, the oral tongue, and the retromolar trigone. Tumors are generally easy to visualize, but oral tongue and floor of mouth tumors have high local relapse rates because of unrecognized invasion of the root of the tongue and the tissues of the anterior neck. Cervical node metastases occur first in levels I or II.

Initial surgical resection or radiation therapy are probably equally effective for most stage I and II disease, but surgical excision is sometimes preferred to avoid the potential risk of osteoradionecrosis of the mandible and xerostomia. Surgery with postoperative radiation therapy is required for all resectable stage III and IV cancers. Systemic chemotherapy has no proven role in resectable oral cavity cancers.

Oropharynx

The oropharynx extends from the plane joining the circumvallate papillae and the junction between the hard and soft palate posteriorly to the posterior pharyngeal wall, superiorly to the superior border of the soft palate, and inferiorly to the level of the epiglottis. Primary tumor sites include the soft palate, pharyngeal wall, base of the tongue, and tonsil. Because of their location, the tumors tend to be larger at presentation than oral cavity tumors. The base of tongue tumors particularly may escape detection and be found only after months of symptoms.

Most early tonsil and soft palate tumors are treated with radiation therapy alone. More advanced tumors require surgery and postoperative radiation therapy. Prophylactic radiation therapy or radical neck dissection is needed for stage III or IV tumors, because the likelihood of microscopic disease is high. Based on nonrandomized data, interstitial radiation therapy by the afterloading technique with Ir 192 may reduce the likelihood of recurrence at the primary site from base of tongue tumors when it is added to standard external beam therapy. Cervical node metastases generally first involve levels II and III, and they may be bilateral for base of tongue tumors because of unrecognized spread across the midline. The management of stage III and IV tumors of the base of tongue occasionally requires total laryngectomy to prevent the sequelae of chronic severe aspiration. The role of chemotherapy in the advanced, resectable setting is in evolution, especially as part of an organ-preservation strategy. Preliminary data suggest that similar management principles can be successfully applied to this primary site in the organ-preservation setting.

Larynx

The larynx extends superiorly from the epiglottis and inferiorly to the level of the cricoid, where it meets the trachea. A tumor may be of supraglottic, glottic, or subglottic origin, depending on its relation to the true vocal cords. Larynx cancer is the most common of all head and neck cancers. Supraglottic and glottic tumors constitute about 99% of larynx cancers. Supraglottic tumors often have lymph node metastases, but glottic tumors only uncommonly metastasize.

Radiation therapy is equivalent to surgery for stage I and II tumors. Treatment with radiation therapy or surgery is individualized. Advanced laryngeal cancers typically require total laryngectomy, although function-preserving procedures such as supraglottic laryngotomy and hemilaryngectomy can be applied in selected patients, and rehabilitative options to facilitate speech such as a tracheoesophageal puncture (TEP) can be performed. Subglottic larynx cancers require special management because of their propensity to spread to paratracheal lymph nodes. Embryologically, the subglottis arises from the lung bud and meets the upper aerodigestive tract at the glottis, thus explaining the propensity to involve inferiorly draining lymphatics that is characteristic of these tumors. Because total laryngectomy is among the head and neck operations most feared by patients, the use of chemotherapy with radiation as part of an organ preservation approach has received considerable attention. Randomized and nonrandomized studies indicate that laryngectomy can be potentially avoided in patients with stage III and IV larynx cancer by the chemotherapy plus irradiation approach outlined previously, without compromising survival.

Hypopharynx

The hypopharynx extends superiorly from the level of the epiglottis and inferiorly to the level of the cricoid, where it meets the cervical esophagus. Primary tumor sites include the posterior pharyngeal wall, the postcricoid mucosa, and the piriform si-

nuses. Patients often present with long histories of odynophagia and level III or IV cervical lymph node metastases.

Aggressive surgery and radiation therapy are usually indicated, including total laryngectomy. Even early-stage lesions can have deceptively bulky disease, compromising the efficacy of radiation therapy as a single modality. As noted previously, results from a randomized trial suggest that chemotherapy plus radiation treatment with the intent of larynx preservation, similar to that studied in patients with advanced larynx cancer, can be applied to these patients as well.

Nasopharynx

The nasopharynx begins with the superior border of the soft palate and extends to the roof of the pharynx. The eustachian tubes enter the nasopharynx laterally. Tumors are often asymptomatic until nasal obstruction, unilateral or bilateral level II or V cervical node metastases, otitis media, or cranial nerve palsies occur. The incidence of distant metastases is especially high among patients with undifferentiated carcinomas—the type more common in Asia and the Mediterranean basin.

Historically, radiation therapy has been the cornerstone of standard management. Surgery to the primary site is rarely used, except in highly selected cases in the recurrent disease setting, because the resection of even small primary lesions poses substantial technical challenges and can be associated with significant morbidity. Until recently, chemotherapy's role was primarily limited to the palliative setting. However, a recently reported study favored concomitant chemotherapy-radiation in stage III and IV disease.

Paranasal Sinuses

Tumors of the paranasal sinuses are rare, and those of the maxillary sinus are the most common. Presenting symptoms are often obscure and nonspecific, mimicking the much more common inflammatory symptoms. Patients with maxillary sinus tumors often present with proptosis due to orbital invasion, facial swelling, or dysesthesia, upper gingivobuccal sulcus ulceration, or trismus. Primary tumors of the ethmoid are uncommon, and tumors of the frontal and sphenoid sinuses are rare.

The widest spectrum of pathologic entities in the head and neck arise in the sinuses or nasal cavity. Surgery and radiation therapy are standard, but recurrence rates for all paranasal sinus malignancies are high. Integrated chemotherapy radiation is increasingly used for patients with unresectable disease.

Recurrent and Metastatic Disease

Recurrent or metastatic disease usually occurs within 2 years of initial treatment. Once a patient is beyond surgical or radiotherapeutic management, there is no cure. With the best available therapies, the median survival of these patients is approximately 6 months. Palliation is the goal. The same combinations of chemotherapy used in the neoadjuvant setting have been applied to patients with recurrent and metastatic disease. Response rates are significantly lower for recurrent than for previously untreated epidermoid cancer, and durable complete responses are very uncommon. Response proportions are somewhat higher with combination chemotherapy compared with treatment with single agents, but toxicity is also increased, and randomized trials fail to document a significant survival advantage for combinations over weekly single-agent methotrexate or single-agent cisplatin. Referral for clinical trials of new agents should be considered.

Salivary Gland Cancer

Cancers of the major and minor salivary glands are rare, constituting less than 10% of all head and neck malignancies. Histologic types include mucoepidermoid carcinoma, solid adenocarcinoma, and adenoid cystic carcinoma. The most common salivary tumor is the benign mixed tumor. Facial nerve paralysis generally implies a malignant primary parotid tumor.

Radical surgery and postoperative radiation therapy are indicated in the management of anything but the smallest malignant tumor. Unlike cases of squamous cell head and neck cancer for which surgery and irradiation are typically interchangeable for early-stage disease, surgery is the preferred treatment for early-stage salivary gland tumors. There is no standard chemotherapy.

The most common minor salivary gland tumor is adenoid cystic carcinoma. These tumors have a long natural history and high incidence of local recurrence. Surgery and radiation therapy are standard management. Pulmonary metastases may develop years later and are generally slowly progressive. No treatment is the standard approach in patients with only pulmonary metastases, because the disease progresses so slowly. There is no standard chemotherapy, but doxorubicin, cisplatin, and 5-fluorouracil have some activity against this tumor.

Second Malignancies

Second primary tumors occur at a rate of 3% to 5% per year in patients with squamous cell carcinomas of the head and neck. These are related to the tobacco and ethanol abuse that led to the first tumor. The risk persists for years, even if the patient abstains from subsequent tobacco and alcohol use. The second malignancies are generally of the mouth and throat, lung, and esophagus. The site of the index primary tumor can predict the likely site of the second primary tumor. For example, patients with laryngeal cancer, a site at which tobacco is a key risk factor, often have lung cancer as their second primary tumor. If a patient is free of disease from the first tumor for at least 2 years, a new tumor is more likely to be a second primary cancer than a recurrence. A solitary lung nodule should always be considered a new primary tumor unless proven to the contrary. Patients with head and neck cancer, particularly those who continue alcohol and tobacco abuse, must be kept under close and competent observation for the rest of their lives, seeking second and subsequent primary cancers.

Strategies to curb or eliminate tobacco and alcohol use by these patients are crucial. Accumulating evidence suggests that certain vitamin A analogues, called retinoids, may be able to interrupt or reverse premalignant changes. A randomized, placebo-controlled trial suggested that treatment with 13-*cis*-retinoic acid (50 mg per square meter daily) decreased the rate of second primaries, although overall survival was not improved. A confirmatory trial is in progress. Until these results become available, the use of chemopreventive agents remains investigational in the adjuvant setting.

BIBLIOGRAPHY

Al-Sarraf M, LeBlanc M, Giri PGS, et al. Chemoradiotherapy versus radiotherapy in patients with advanced nasopharyngeal cancer: phase III randomized intergroup study 0099. *J Clin Oncol* 1998;16:1310–1317.

Brizel DM, Albers ME, Fisher SR, et al. Hyperfractionated irradiation with or without concurrent chemotherapy for locally advanced head and neck cancer. *N Engl J Med* 1998;338:1798–1804.

Department of Veterans Affairs Laryngeal Cancer Study Group. Induction chemotherapy plus radiation compared with surgery plus radiation in patients with advanced laryngeal cancer. *N Engl J Med* 1991;324: 1685–1690.

El-Sayed S, Nelson N. Adjuvant and adjunctive chemotherapy in the management of squamous cell carcinoma of the head and neck region: a meta-analysis of prospective randomized trials. *J Clin Oncol* 14;1996: 838–847.

Hong WK, Lippman SM, Itri L, et al. Prevention of second primary tumors with isotretinoin in squamous cell carcinoma of the head and neck. *N Engl J Med* 1990;323:795–801.

Kramer S, Gelber RD, Snow JB, et al. Combined radiation therapy and surgery in the management of advanced head and neck cancer: final report of study 73-03 of the Radiation Therapy Oncology Group. *Head Neck Surg* 1987;10:19–30.

Laramore GE, Scott CB, Al-Sarraf M, et al. Adjuvant chemotherapy for resectable squamous cell carcinomas of the head and neck: report on intergroup study 0034. *Int J Radiat Oncol Biol Phys* 1992;23:705–713.

Lefebvre JL, Chevalier D, Luboinski B, et al. Larynx preservation in pyriform sinus cancer: preliminary results of a European Organization for Research and Treatment of Cancer phase III trial. *J Natl Cancer Inst* 1996;88:890–899.

Pfister DG, Shaha AR, Harrison LB. The role of chemotherapy in the curative treatment of head and neck cancer. *Surg Clin North Am* 1997; 6(4):749–768.

Sidransky D, Schantz SP, Harrison LB, et al. Cancer of the head and neck. In: DeVita VT Jr, Hellman S, Rosenberg SA, eds. *Cancer: principles and practice of oncology*, fifth ed. Philadelphia: JB Lippincott, 1998: 735–847.

Kelley's Textbook of Internal Medicine, fourth edition. Edited by H. David Humes.
Lippincott Williams & Wilkins, Philadelphia © 2000.

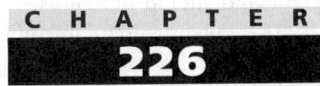

CHAPTER 226

CANCER OF UNKNOWN PRIMARY ORIGIN

JOHN D. HAINSWORTH
F. ANTHONY GRECO

Metastatic cancer with no obvious primary site accounts for about 5% of all cancers. Until recently, affected patients attracted little attention, because prognosis was believed to be uniformly poor, regardless of treatment. Effective therapy is now available for many types of advanced cancer, and it is not surprising that some carcinomas of unknown primary site are sensitive to chemotherapeutic agents. The clinician must approach each patient with two objectives: to identify treatable neoplasms using clinical and pathologic criteria and to avoid superfluous diagnostic procedures and inappropriate treatment.

The typical patient has symptoms at a metastatic site, but the history, physical examination, chest radiograph, and laboratory studies fail to identify the primary site. Light microscopic study of the biopsy sample usually reveals adenocarcinoma, squamous cell carcinoma, or poorly differentiated carcinoma. Occasionally, the less specific diagnosis of poorly differentiated neoplasm is made; this means the pathologist cannot differentiate carcinoma from lymphoma, sarcoma, and melanoma. These four groups identified by light microscopy differ with respect to clinical characteristics, recommended diagnostic evaluation, treatment, and prognosis.

POORLY DIFFERENTIATED NEOPLASMS

The diagnosis of poorly differentiated neoplasm can describe several neoplasms, many of which are responsive to systemic therapy. Further pathologic evaluation is always necessary and usually results in a more precise diagnosis, often with specific therapeutic implications. The most common cause of a nonspecific pathologic diagnosis is a small, inadequate biopsy. Fine-needle aspiration biopsy is often the initial diagnostic procedure in patients with suspected cancer; however, this biopsy technique is usually inadequate in the evaluation of poorly differentiated neoplasms, because histologic characteristics are poorly preserved and adequate material is not available for special studies. Often, a definitive diagnosis can be made by obtaining a larger biopsy. Close communication between the surgeon and pathologist is important if repeat biopsy is performed.

In some patients, light microscopic examination alone fails to provide a diagnosis more specific than poorly differentiated neoplasm or poorly differentiated carcinoma, even with a large, adequately preserved biopsy specimen. Further evaluation with immunoperoxidase staining is indicated. Immunoperoxidase stains are not specific and should not be used alone to make a diagnosis, but they are frequently useful in conjunction with the light microscopy and clinical features. Staining for leukocyte common antigen provides strong evidence for the diagnosis of lymphoma; other diagnoses that can be suggested by immunoperoxidase staining include melanoma, neuroendocrine carcinoma, and sarcoma. Some neoplasms can only be called carcinomas, and inconclusive results are obtained for about 30% of neoplasms.

Electron microscopy can provide important information in the differential diagnosis of poorly differentiated neoplasms. Because this diagnostic technique is less widely available than immunoperoxidase staining and requires special tissue preparation, electron microscopy is usually reserved for the examination of tumors for which immunoperoxidase staining provides inconclusive results. The detection of specific ultrastructural features

makes electron microscopy more specific than immunoperoxidase staining in the diagnosis of neuroendocrine carcinoma (i.e., in identifying neurosecretory granules) and melanoma (i.e., in identifying premelanosomes).

Two specific chromosomal changes associated with solid tumors have been identified and occasionally aid in the diagnosis of neoplasms. A large percentage of germ cell tumors have an isochromosome of the short arm of chromosome 12 (i12p). Peripheral neuroepithelioma and Ewing's tumor share a chromosomal translocation (11:22). Chromosomal analysis should be considered for young men with poorly differentiated mediastinal or retroperitoneal tumors and no specific diagnosis after other pathologic studies.

ADENOCARCINOMA OF UNKNOWN PRIMARY SITE

CLINICAL FEATURES AND NATURAL HISTORY

About 70% of all carcinomas of unknown primary site are adenocarcinomas. Although many patients are elderly and have multiple sites of metastases, the clinical features of this patient group are variable. Common metastatic sites include liver, bones, and lungs.

The clinical course is usually dominated by symptoms related to the sites of metastases. The primary site becomes evident during life in only 15% of patients. Autopsy series performed before the routine use of CT scanning detected primary sites in almost 70% of patients, often in the pancreas, lung, or other gastrointestinal sites. Improved diagnostic methods currently available undoubtedly result in the detection of many of these primary sites at initial evaluation, so the results from previous autopsy series are probably misleading. Adenocarcinomas of the breast and prostate, which are common in the general population, are rarely found in these patients.

PATHOLOGY

The diagnosis of adenocarcinoma is based on the formation of glandular structures and is usually made easily by light microscopy. The morphologic characteristics of the biopsy usually are not specific for the site of origin. Specialized pathologic evaluation rarely is useful. Immunoperoxidase stains for prostate-specific antigen (PSA) or estrogen receptors should be considered when a patient has clinical findings suggesting prostate or breast cancer, respectively.

The diagnosis of poorly differentiated adenocarcinoma should be viewed with caution, because patients may differ in tumor biology and responsiveness to systemic therapy. This diagnosis is often made when only minimal glandular formation is seen by light microscopy or sometimes is based on a positive mucin stain alone in a tumor that would otherwise be called poorly differentiated carcinoma. Additional pathologic study with immunoperoxidase stains or electron microscopy should be considered. Evaluation and treatment should be the same as for patients with poorly differentiated carcinomas.

TABLE 226.1.	EVALUATION OF CANCERS OF UNKNOWN PRIMARY SITES			
Histology	**Clinical Evaluation**[a]	**Special Pathologic Studies**	**Subgroups Effectively Treated**	**Prognosis**
Adenocarcinoma	CT scan of abdomen Men: prostate-specific antigen Women: mammograms Additional radiologic studies to evaluate abnormal symptoms, signs, laboratory values	Men: prostate-specific antigen (immunoperoxidase) Women: estrogen receptor, progesterone receptor	Women with axillary node metastasis Women with peritoneal carcinomatosis Men with blastic bone metastasis	Poor for entire group (median survival, 4 to 8 months) Better for treatable subgroups
Poorly differentiated carcinoma	CT scan of abdomen and chest Serum human chorionic gonadotropin, α-fetoprotein Additional radiologic studies to evaluate abnormal symptoms, signs, laboratory values	Immunoperoxidase staining Electron microscopy	Neuroendocrine tumors Predominant tumor location in mediastinum, retroperitoneum, lymph nodes	Variable—some curable with cisplatin-based chemotherapy
Squamous carcinoma (cervical lymph nodes)	Direct laryngoscopy with visualization of nasopharynx Fiberoptic bronchoscopy		Nodes located in high or midcervical region	30–50% Long-term survival with radical surgery or radiation therapy

[a] In addition to a history, physical examination, blood cell counts, serum chemistries, and a chest radiograph.
CT, computed tomography.

DIAGNOSTIC EVALUATION

A summary of the recommended evaluation is outlined in Table 226.1. CT scans of the abdomen can identify the primary site in 20% to 35% of patients and should probably be included. Additional evaluation should address findings identified by the history, physical examination, or routine laboratory studies; radiologic or endoscopic evaluation of asymptomatic areas is rarely useful.

TREATMENT AND PROGNOSIS

Optimal therapy depends on the recognition of certain treatable patient subgroups. Women who have adenocarcinoma involving axillary lymph nodes should be considered as possibly having breast cancer. About 50% of these women have primary tumors found at mastectomy, even when physical examination and mammographic results are normal. Estrogen receptors in the tumor strongly suggest breast cancer. Women who have no evidence of other metastatic sites should be treated by following guidelines for stage II breast cancer and are frequently cured with therapy. Initial treatment should include either a mastectomy or an axillary node dissection plus radiation therapy to the breast. Systemic therapy should be based on estrogen receptor status and the number of nodes involved. Women with metastatic sites in addition to axillary lymph nodes may have metastatic breast cancer; hormonal therapy or chemotherapy often provides palliation.

Some women who have peritoneal involvement with adenocarcinoma can be treated effectively using the guidelines established for ovarian cancer. The histology in these women often suggests ovarian cancer, even when the ovaries are pathologically uninvolved or in cases of previous bilateral oophorectomy. Therapy should include laparotomy with maximal surgical cytoreduction, followed by combination chemotherapy effective against ovarian carcinoma (e.g., paclitaxel plus platinum). Median survival in this group of patients is 18 to 24 months, with 10% to 15% achieving long-term, disease-free survival.

Male patients with blastic bone metastases, elevated serum PSA levels, or tumor staining with PSA should be suspected of having adenocarcinoma of the prostate and should receive a trial of hormonal therapy as used in advanced prostate cancer.

Occasional patients have only a single detectable metastasis after complete evaluation. These single lesions can occur in a wide variety of sites, including bone, lymph nodes, lung, adrenal gland, and brain. Definitive local treatment is recommended, either with surgical resection or radiation therapy, depending on the site of involvement. Such treatment affords substantial palliation, and many patients have significant intervals before further metastases appear.

Most patients with adenocarcinoma of unknown primary site do not fit into any of these clinical subsets. If such patients have good performance status, a trial of empiric chemotherapy should be considered. A recently developed regimen containing paclitaxel, carboplatin, and etoposide produced a 47% response rate and a 13-month median survival in these patients; 20% of patients lived more than 3 years. For patients who are debilitated, symptomatic care remains the most appropriate management.

SQUAMOUS CELL CARCINOMA OF UNKNOWN PRIMARY SITE

Squamous cell carcinoma of unknown primary site is unusual. Because effective treatment is available for some patients, appropriate evaluation is important.

The most common metastatic site is in the cervical lymph nodes. Most patients are middle-aged or elderly and have a history of tobacco use. Patients with involvement in upper or mid-cervical lymph nodes should be suspected of having a primary lesion in the head and neck region. These patients need a thorough examination of the oropharynx, nasopharynx, hypopharynx, larynx, and upper esophagus by direct laryngoscopy, with biopsy of any suspicious areas. Patients with tumor involving the lower cervical or supraclavicular lymph nodes are more likely to have lung cancer and should be evaluated with bronchoscopy if the head and neck examination and chest radiograph are unrevealing.

In patients with no identified primary site, treatment should follow guidelines for regionally metastatic head and neck cancer. Similar treatment results have been obtained with radical neck dissection, high-dose radiation therapy, or a combination. However, approximately 40% of patients treated with radical neck dissection alone eventually develop an obvious primary site in the head and neck region; for this reason, radiation therapy is usually included as part of initial therapy. In patients with high or midcervical adenopathy, 3-year survival rates range from 35% to 60%; patients with smaller adenopathy have a better prognosis. The chance of long-term survival is relatively poor for patients with lower cervical or supraclavicular adenopathy, probably because most have lung cancer. A minority (less than 15%) achieve long-term survival after local treatment to the cervical area, as described previously.

Patients with squamous cell carcinoma involving the inguinal lymph nodes usually have identifiable primary lesions in the genital or anorectal area. Women should undergo careful examination of the vulva, vagina, and cervix, with biopsy of any suspicious areas. Uncircumcised men should have careful inspection of the penis. The anorectal area should also be examined digitally and by anoscope in both sexes, with biopsy of suspicious areas. Therapy for carcinomas of the vulva, vagina, cervix, and anus can be curative in some patients even after spread to regional lymph nodes. When no primary site is identified, long-term survival has been reported after inguinal node dissection.

Patients with metastatic squamous cell carcinoma in other visceral sites almost always have lung cancer. If clinical features suggest the possibility of lung cancer, CT scans of the chest and bronchoscopy are appropriate. As described for patients with adenocarcinoma, the clinician should be suspicious of the diagnosis of poorly differentiated squamous cell carcinoma, particularly if other clinical features are unusual for lung cancer (e.g., young patient, nonsmoker, unusual metastatic site). Additional pathologic evaluation and a trial of therapy as described for patients with poorly differentiated carcinoma should be considered.

POORLY DIFFERENTIATED CARCINOMA OF UNKNOWN PRIMARY SITE

About 20% of carcinomas of unknown primary site have a poorly differentiated histologic pattern. Until recently, patients with this diagnosis were not considered separately from the larger group with adenocarcinoma of unknown primary site. However, a minority of these patients has tumors that are highly sensitive to platinum-based chemotherapy; therefore, a trial of systemic therapy is recommended in all of these patients.

PATHOLOGY

Additional pathologic study is indicated with immunoperoxidase staining and electron microscopy, as described for patients with poorly differentiated neoplasms. These studies can suggest unsuspected diagnoses in up to 25% of these patients, including some malignancies, such as lymphoma, germ cell tumor, and neuroendocrine tumors, for which specific therapy is available.

DIAGNOSTIC EVALUATION

The initial evaluation should be similar to that described for patients with adenocarcinoma of unknown primary site (Table 226.1). CT scanning of the chest and abdomen should be performed because these tumors frequently involve the mediastinum and retroperitoneum. Measurement of the serum tumor markers, human chorionic gonadotropin and α-fetoprotein, is essential, because markedly elevated levels suggest the diagnosis of a germ cell tumor.

TREATMENT

When specialized pathologic studies result in a specific diagnosis (e.g., lymphoma, melanoma), patients should be treated appropriately. Young men who have clinical features of extragonadal germ cell tumor (location in mediastinum or retroperitoneum; elevated human chorionic gonadotropin or α-fetoprotein) should be treated using the guidelines for poor prognosis germ cell tumors, even if the diagnosis of germ cell tumor cannot be confirmed pathologically.

Another subset of patients with poorly differentiated carcinoma have high-grade neuroendocrine tumors identified by immunoperoxidase staining or electron microscopy or both. Although the nature of these tumors is unclear, the response rate to platinum-based chemotherapy is approximately 75%, and a minority of patients (10% to 15%) have long-term survival. Paclitaxel-containing regimens may further improve treatment results and are under active investigation.

Most patients with poorly differentiated carcinoma of unknown primary site do not have a more specific diagnosis made after complete pathologic evaluation. An empiric trial of platinum/etoposide-based chemotherapy should be given to all patients in this group except those who are very debilitated. Those who will benefit from chemotherapy can be identified after a brief trial (3 to 6 weeks). Clinical features predicting chemotherapy responsiveness include location of tumor in the mediastinum, retroperitoneum, or lymph nodes (instead of other visceral sites); tumor limited to one or two metastatic sites; no previous cigarette use; and younger age.

BIBLIOGRAPHY

Abbruzzese JL, Abbruzzese MC, Hess KR, et al. Unknown primary carcinoma: natural history and prognostic factors in 657 consecutive patients. *J Clin Oncol* 1994;12:1272–1280.

Ellerbroek N, Holmes F, Singletary E, et al. Treatment of patients with isolated axillary nodal metastases from an occult primary carcinoma consistent with breast origin. *Cancer* 1990;66:1461–1472.

Hainsworth JD, Erland JB, Kalman LA, et al. Carcinoma of unknown primary site: treatment with 1-hour paclitaxel, carboplatin, and extended-schedule etoposide. *J Clin Oncol* 1997;15:2385–2393.

Hainsworth JD, Greco FA. Treatment of patients with cancer of an unknown primary site. *N Engl J Med* 1993;329:257–263.

Hainsworth JD, Johnson DH, Greco FA. Poorly differentiated neuroendocrine carcinoma of unknown primary site: a newly recognized clinicopathologic entity. *Ann Intern Med* 1988;109:364–371.

Hainsworth JD, Johnson DH, Greco FA. Cisplatin-based combination chemotherapy in the treatment of poorly differentiated carcinoma and poorly differentiated adenocarcinoma of unknown primary site: results of a 12-year experience. *J Clin Oncol* 1992;10:912–922.

Jones AS, Cook JA, Phillips DE, et al. Squamous carcinoma presenting as an enlarged cervical lymph node. *Cancer* 1993;72:1756–1765.

Menzin AW, Aikens JK, Wheeler JE, et al. Surgically documented responses to paclitaxel and cisplatin in patients with primary peritoneal carcinoma. *Gynecol Oncol* 1996;62:55–58.

Motzer RJ, Rodriguez E, Reuter VE, et al. Molecular and cytogenetic studies in the diagnosis of patients with midline carcinomas of unknown primary site. *J Clin Oncol* 1995;13:274–283.

Nystrom JS, Weiner JM, Hoffelfinger-Juttner J, et al. Metastatic and histologic presentations in unknown primary cancer. *Semin Oncol* 1977;4:53–58.

Ransom DT, Patel SR, Keeney GL, et al. Papillary serous carcinoma of the peritoneum: a review of 33 cases treated with platin-based chemotherapy. *Cancer* 1990;66:1091–1094.

Kelley's Textbook of Internal Medicine, fourth edition. Edited by H. David Humes. Lippincott Williams & Wilkins, Philadelphia © 2000.

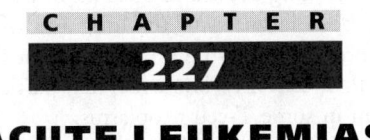

ACUTE LEUKEMIAS

PETER H. WIERNIK

Acute leukemias result from the uncontrolled proliferation of a malignant clone of hematopoietic cells. The abnormal clone has

survival advantages over normal progenitor cells and becomes dominant. Dominance is achieved because the malignant clone responds poorly or not at all to regulatory factors that control normal hematopoietic cell growth. The abnormal clone does not differentiate and mature normally and may suppress the growth and differentiation of normal hematopoietic cells. The result is an expanding clone of functionless cells together with a progressive decrease in the number of normal blood cells. Anemia, thrombocytopenia, and granulocytopenia, rather than abnormal cell production, cause most of the serious problems that beset the patient.

Acute lymphocytic leukemia (ALL) is characterized by the presence of an abnormal clone of cells with morphologic, biochemical, and immunologic characteristics of lymphoid cells. The term *acute myeloid leukemia* (AML) is used for all other types of acute leukemia. Subgroups of AML are defined by morphologic and other characteristics of the abnormal cells that predominate in the blood and marrow, and terms such as erythroleukemia or acute myelocytic, promyelocytic, monocytic, myelomonocytic, and megakaryocytic leukemia more precisely characterize AML in a given patient.

INCIDENCE AND EPIDEMIOLOGY

About 10,000 new cases of acute leukemia are diagnosed in the United States each year, and the rates have remained constant during the past 25 years. Of all neoplastic diseases, acute leukemia is associated with the least variation in incidence worldwide. Acute leukemias are more common in male adults and children than female adults and children, and in the United States, they are more common in whites than blacks. Acute leukemia is especially more common in elderly whites than in elderly blacks and is more common in Jews than in non-Jews. The unifying factor may be socioeconomics rather than genetics, because acute leukemia is more common in higher socioeconomic groups. There is an increased incidence of acute leukemia among patients with diseases associated with chromosomal nondisjunction, such as Down's syndrome, or increased chromosomal fragility, such as Bloom's syndrome and Fanconi's anemia. Although spatial, time, and familial clusters of acute leukemia are occasionally observed, no incontrovertible evidence exists that human acute leukemia is a transmissible disease.

Only about 25% of patients with ALL are older than 15 years. The incidence of the disease is roughly equal in all decades of adult life, and the median age of patients with the adult disease is about 42 years. Most adults respond well to initial therapy, but unlike children with ALL, most ultimately die of the disease. Although the initial treatment results for adult ALL may be better than those for adult AML, the long-term results are not and may actually be worse.

The average patient with AML is older than 55 years at diagnosis. Most AML patients are adults, and the incidence of AML increases steadily in successive decades of life. Most patients ultimately die of leukemia, but an increasing percentage—perhaps

30% to 40% or more—is apparently cured with current therapy. The likelihood of cure is greater for younger patients.

ETIOLOGY

The cause of human acute leukemia is obscure, but certain facts are known. Ionizing radiation is leukemogenic in humans, and radiation dose is directly correlated with the incidence of AML. Chemicals, including certain drugs that may cause bone marrow hypoplasia, are also associated with an appreciable incidence of AML. Most notable among such agents are benzene, chloramphenicol, and phenylbutazone.

Some cancer chemotherapeutic agents, especially alkylating agents and topoisomerase II inhibitors, are associated with an increased incidence of AML in surviving cancer patients. The incidence of secondary AML in such patients may be as high as 2% to 3% and is highest in patients who were treated with alkylating agents and radiation therapy, especially when such treatments were given sequentially for recurrent cancer. In some diseases, such as multiple myeloma, the incidence of secondary AML is higher in patients treated continuously with alkylating agents than in those treated with the same total dose of drug using an intermittent high-dose schedule. However, patients with chronic lymphocytic leukemia may receive alkylating agents for many years without an increased incidence of acute leukemia. The implication of this observation is that interaction of alkylating agents with another unknown (possibly genetic) factor may be leukemogenic, but either factor alone may not be. Alternatively, the agent responsible for the underlying neoplasm may also be important in the cause of what is recognized as secondary leukemia, and secondary leukemia may be a late manifestation of the primary disease experienced by some long-term survivors.

Certain viruses are known to be leukemogenic in rodents, birds, cats, and other species, and a specific RNA tumor virus (i.e., human T-cell lymphotrophic virus type I [HTLV-I]) is the causative agent of the adult T-cell leukemia-lymphoma syndrome, a rare form of leukemia endemic in certain areas of Japan and the Caribbean and seen in immigrants from those areas in the United States as well.

Oncogenes are genes found in normal human cells that are homologues of viral genes that are leukemogenic or carcinogenic in certain animals. They may provide a link between putative leukemogenic agents such as ionizing radiation and chemicals. Oncogenes may play a role in the regulation of normal cellular growth and differentiation. Oncogenes can be activated by a chromosomal translocation that physically separates a given gene from the promoter–enhancer region that normally controls it. By this mechanism, an oncogene is moved to a location on another chromosome, where it comes under the influence of a promoter–enhancer region normally associated with a transcriptionally active gene, and the second gene is removed to another location by the same event. Such translocations may be of great significance in human leukemogenesis. In such cases, increased oncogene product results from increased transcriptional activity, and the total amount of oncogene DNA remains normal. This situation has been demonstrated in Burkitt's lymphoma-leuke-mia in which it is associated with increased *MYC* gene transcriptional activity and product.

PATHOGENESIS AND PATHOPHYSIOLOGY

The leukemic cell has a relatively normal generation time of 15 to 16 hours and a low growth rate of about 5%. Normal blood cell precursors undergo a series of sequential developmental events that ultimately yield a differentiated, specialized cell that circulates and eventually dies. The capacity for cell division is lost in the process of differentiation. Leukemic cells do not have the capacity to differentiate completely. Although most leukemic cells are in the G0 phase of the cell cycle at any one time, they retain the capacity for cell division and may be induced to divide by a variety of events at random. The result is an expanding mass of immature immortal cells. Leukemic cells are randomly introduced into the blood from the bone marrow. They may divide in the blood or infiltrate an organ such as the spleen, liver, or lymph nodes, in which they may also divide and then reenter the blood.

The marrow precursor of normal circulating blood cells is a pluripotent, self-generating stem cell that forms progenitor cells irreversibly committed to a certain hematopoietic cell lineage. It is unclear whether these cells become committed to restricted differentiation pathways by an intrinsically determined mechanism or by the influence of microenvironmental factors. The commitment of their progeny to mature along one of the various hematopoietic lineages depends on the expression of receptors for certain factors that regulate cell proliferation, maturation, and mortality.

Starting at band 5q22-35 and extending to the terminus of human chromosome 5, the genes for granulocyte-macrophage colony-stimulating factor (GM-CSF), multi-CSF, β_2-adrenergic receptor, platelet-derived growth factor receptor, endothelial cell growth factor, macrophage colony-stimulating factor (CSF1) and its receptor (encoded by the *CSF1R* gene, formerly designated *FMS*), interleukin-3, -4, and -5 are sequentially located. Deletions often involve this region of the long arm of chromosome 5 in AML, which may result in homozygosity for the *CSF1R* locus, truncation of the GM-CSF gene (*CSF2*), or deletion of the gene for *CSF1*. Whether loss or mutation of any of these genes important for normal hematopoiesis is a crucial event in leukemogenesis is still unclear.

The genes encoding the α and δ chains of the human T-cell receptor have been localized to the long arm of chromosome 14, near the breakpoint for t(11;14), a pattern found in 25% of children with T-cell ALL. Those loci may participate in oncogene activation in some T-cell neoplasms.

Adult T-cell leukemia-lymphoma syndrome associated with HTLV-I may rely on a different mechanism. The viral genome encodes a protein that stimulates viral replication and mediates cellular transformation. This protein may activate cellular genes capable of immortalizing and transforming T cells. It is unknown whether such transformation is limited to the spectrum of T-cell diseases associated with the HTLV group or whether it has greater significance.

CLINICAL FINDINGS

ACUTE LYMPHOCYTIC LEUKEMIA

Adults with ALL usually present with subacute onset of nonspecific signs and symptoms, such as fatigue, lethargy, malaise, anorexia, pallor, and occasionally weight loss. Symptoms of anemia may be dominant. Evidence of thrombocytopenia, such as petechiae, easy bruising, prolonged or heavy menstruation, or other bleeding may cause the patient to seek medical attention. Young adults may have bone pain or arthralgias as evidence of an expanding bone marrow mass. Most patients have palpable lymphadenopathy, especially cervical, and the spleen is palpable in 50% of patients, but the liver is infrequently palpable. An abdominal radiograph may reveal kidneys enlarged by leukemic infiltration.

Signs of increased intracranial pressure or cranial nerve dysfunction secondary to leukemic infiltration of the central nervous system (CNS) may be evident at diagnosis, although such findings are more common in childhood ALL. The long cranial nerves (VI and VII) are the most frequently infiltrated with leukemic cells. Funduscopic evidence of increased intracranial pressure or leukemic infiltration of the retina appearing as Roth-like spots, both of which may be silent clinically, may be found.

About 15% of patients present with fever due to infection, which may be occult. Classic signs may be absent on the chest radiograph of a patient with pneumonia, and fluctuance and inflammation may be minimal at the site of a soft-tissue infection because of severe granulocytopenia.

The diagnosis of ALL can be made by examining the peripheral blood in most cases. In about 15% of adult patients, peripheral blood studies reveal serious abnormalities but no characteristic lymphoblasts necessary for the diagnosis. Bone marrow examination establishes the diagnosis. Bone marrow examination is necessary in all patients to assess marrow cellularity, the status of normal blood cell production, cytogenetic abnormalities, immunophenotype, and histochemical reactions to classify the leukemia properly and to obtain important prognostic information.

Anemia, granulocytopenia, and thrombocytopenia are almost always present at the time of diagnosis of ALL. Anemia is usually moderate, and granulocytopenia is often severe but rarely absolute. The platelet count is usually less than 100,000 per microliter and frequently less than 40,000 per microliter. Patients rarely sustain serious hemorrhage if the platelet count is more than 20,000 per microliter or maintained above that level with transfusion. The white blood cell (WBC) count is normal or elevated in more than 90% of patients and reduced in the rest. The WBC count usually is between 10,000 and 30,000 cells per microliter at diagnosis, but extreme hyperleukocytosis (more than 100,000 cells per microliter) occasionally occurs. The peripheral blood smear is consistent with the blood counts. For 85% of patients, examination of the blood smear reveals characteristic lymphoblasts, usually in large numbers. They usually have small nucleoli and agranular cytoplasm. Unlike typical lymphoblasts of childhood ALL, these cells have more than a scant rim of cytoplasm, and morphologic variation from cell to cell is much greater in adults.

The bone marrow biopsy specimen is almost always hypercellular. Lymphoblasts predominate, and normal hematopoietic elements are reduced in number. The normal marrow fat spaces are partially or completely obliterated by the leukemic infiltrate.

It is especially important to examine the cerebrospinal fluid (CSF) in patients with ALL, but only after successful platelet transfusion if the patient is thrombocytopenic. This procedure is done to determine whether CNS leukemia is present, which may occur without signs or symptoms. Meningeal leukemic infiltration is usually associated with CSF pleocytosis, which is readily detected by examining the fluid with methods that concentrate cells on a glass slide or millipore filter. The diagnosis of CNS leukemia is important because most antileukemic agents are denied access to the leukemic cells by the blood–brain barrier.

Two mechanisms have been suggested for meningeal infiltration. One is that leukemic cells are deposited in the pia-arachnoid by petechial hemorrhage. This is supported by the inverse relation between the incidence of meningeal leukemia and the blood platelet count. Another postulation after study of an experimental mouse model suggests that an expanding skull bone marrow mass causes leukemic infiltration of the dura and eventual infiltration of the adventitia of vessels that traverse the potential space between the dura and the pia-arachnoid. Recently, differentiation of human neural stem cells into early hematopoietic cells has been demonstrated. This fact and the fact that tissues lining the third ventricle in certain lower species function as a hematopoietic organ suggest that CNS leukemia may arise in situ under some circumstances.

Lumbar puncture in a patient with meningeal leukemia reveals a normal or elevated opening pressure. The CSF is usually clear and colorless and has a normal glucose concentration, but the protein concentration is usually elevated. The cell count by routine methods is normal or high. When normal, leukemic cells are demonstrable in more than 50% of patients with meningeal leukemia by cell-concentrating techniques. When cranial nerves alone are infiltrated with leukemic cells, the CSF is devoid of leukemic cells. However, the CSF protein concentration is almost always elevated, and the β2-microglobulin concentration may be elevated, as in overt meningeal leukemia. Determination of the latter may provide a sensitive and relatively specific indicator of meningeal leukemia in the absence of other suggestive CSF findings.

Independent factors in ALL patients that negatively influence the likelihood of a complete response to therapy are advanced age and mature B-cell immunophenotype. Factors that shorten response duration and survival are a hyperleukocytosis at diagnosis, a complex abnormal karyotype, and CNS leukemia at diagnosis or shortly thereafter.

ACUTE MYELOID LEUKEMIA

Adults with AML usually present with a vague history of chronic, progressive lethargy. However, as many as one third may present acutely ill with significant infection, usually of the respiratory tract, with or without septicemia. The patients usually have petechiae. More serious bleeding such as ecchymoses or orificial hemorrhage secondary to a combination of clotting factor deficiency and fibrinogenolysis may be evident in some patients, especially those with the *acute promyelocytic* (APL) *subtype of AML.*

Lymphadenopathy is unusual, splenomegaly is found in less than 20% of patients with de novo AML, and hepatomegaly is even less common. Gingival hypertrophy from leukemic infiltration occurs in about 50% of patients with the acute myelomonocytic or monocytic variants. Patients with these subtypes are more likely to have extramedullary leukemic infiltrations of all sorts and are the AML patients most likely to present with or subsequently develop meningeal leukemia, retinal infiltrates, and leukemia cutis.

Granulocytic sarcomas are tumors of leukemic cells that may be palpable, especially around the ribs or orbits, to which they are usually firmly attached. They have rarely been observed in organs such as the dura, ovary, and small intestine. Granulocytic sarcomas may appear before other diagnostic evidence of AML, soon after diagnosis, or as the first evidence of relapse. When biopsied, the lesions often have a dull green color, which fades rapidly on exposure to air because of the high peroxidase content of the leukemic cells. In some studies, granulocytic sarcomas, especially paraspinal tumors, were more common in patients with the t(8;21) cytogenetic translocation.

WBC count is normal, elevated, or depressed with equal frequencies at diagnosis of AML. Leukopenia is somewhat more common in AML than in ALL patients, and among the AML subtypes, it is most common in acute promyelocytic leukemia (APL), a subtype that accounts for approximately 10% of AML patients. Roughly 5% of patients with AML present with a WBC count of more than 100,000 cells per microliter. The rare patient who presents with extreme hyperleukocytosis ($\geq$200,000 cells per microliter) has a substantial risk of dying of sudden intracerebral hemorrhage. Unlike mature cells, myeloid blast cells have great intrinsic viscosity, and in such numbers, they cause sludging at the low-pressure venous side of the capillary bed. As the cell mass enlarges, the capillary may rupture. If this happens in the brain, sudden death may occur.

Blast cells are initially absent from the peripheral blood in about 15% of patients with AML. Such patients require bone marrow examination to make the correct diagnosis. Granulocytopenia is essentially universal in patients with AML, and 50% of patients have a serious risk of infection because of severe granulocytopenia of 500 cells per microliter or less. The platelet count is usually lower than in ALL, and platelet counts of less than 20,000 per microliter are common. Electronic platelet counts may be falsely elevated in acute monocytic leukemia, because cytoplasmic fragments the size of platelets are frequently broken off of monoblasts and may be counted as platelets. Phase-contrast microscopy is necessary to estimate the true platelet count in these patients. The hematocrit is almost always low in AML, but severe anemia is uncommon.

The bone marrow is usually markedly hypercellular but may be hypocellular in secondary AML that developed after treatment for another neoplastic disease. It may also be hypocellular in elderly patients, especially those with an antecedent preleukemic phase. At least 50% to 75% of the marrow nucleated elements are leukemic cells in the typical patient with AML. Megakaryocytes are reduced in number, as are red blood cell precursors in most patients. However, some patients with acute

myelomonocytic leukemia have a relative increase in red cell precursors involved in ineffective erythropoiesis. There is little evidence of maturation in marrow granulocytes in most patients. In addition to a routine morphologic examination, the special studies required by patients with ALL are also required for those with AML.

Patients with end-stage acute leukemia may rarely manifest special problems caused by leukemic infiltration of various organs. Heart conduction defects and pericarditis have been reported, and an acute asthma-like syndrome resulting from pulmonary capillary plugging by leukemic cells occasionally occurs.

Patients with secondary acute leukemia, which is almost always myeloid, may be difficult to diagnose accurately. Such patients are often severely pancytopenic and may have only an occasional blast cell in the peripheral blood smear. The marrow may be hypocellular and relatively devoid of frank blast cells. The predominant marrow cell may be a dysmyelopoietic promyelocyte or myelocyte with megaloblastoid features. An increased number of sideroblasts, including ringed sideroblasts, may be observed in the marrow. It may be difficult to differentiate secondary leukemia from refractory anemia with excess blasts or from other myelodysplastic or myeloproliferative disorders. Cytogenetic studies may be helpful in such cases.

Other hematologic disorders may mimic acute leukemia. Severe folate deficiency may be misdiagnosed as acute leukemia. Such patients are severely pancytopenic and have an extremely hypocellular bone marrow with many bizarre blastlike cells. The patient almost always gives a history of more than one cause of folate deficiency, such as alcoholism and pregnancy. Red cell folate levels are usually extremely low, if measurable at all, which is never the case in uncomplicated acute leukemia. Idiopathic or drug-induced aplastic anemia may superficially mimic acute leukemia, because pancytopenia can be a feature of both. Adults with aplastic anemia rarely have organomegaly or blasts in the marrow or blood. Acute leukemia may be preceded by aplastic anemia, however, and increasing marrow cellularity with a predominance of immature forms may be a harbinger of that transition rather than marrow recovery.

Patients with disseminated tuberculosis may present with a leukemoid reaction characterized by infiltration of the blood and marrow with cells indistinguishable from those of AML. Patients with blasts containing Auer rods have been reported whose hematologic disorder resolved with antituberculous therapy alone.

LABORATORY FINDINGS

Morphology, histochemical reactions, cytogenetics, enzymology, and cell surface antigen identification are the principal laboratory tools used to differentiate ALL from AML and to identify clinically important subtypes of both.

Serum lactate dehydrogenase levels are usually elevated in patients with ALL because of intramedullary destruction of lymphoid cells. The serum uric acid concentration is often elevated in ALL and AML patients, and renal tubular urate deposition may cause renal failure, especially in those with ALL. The serum and urinary lysozyme (muramidase) concentration is usually markedly elevated in acute myelomonocytic or monocytic leukemia. Excretion of lysozyme may cause renal tubular damage, resulting in hypokalemia. Patients with APL may have decreased plasma fibrinogen concentrations and increased serum fibrin degradation products. In such cases, factor-dependent coagulation tests give abnormal results.

Leukemic cell morphology is usually examined with Wright's stain or a similar stain of a peripheral blood and bone marrow aspirate smear. The blast cells of AML are generally larger and have more cytoplasm than those of ALL. Also, greater variation in the size and shape of blasts and of their nuclei and nucleoli is seen in AML than in ALL, but adults with ALL usually have more cell-to-cell variation in morphology than do children. Most patients with AML have some cytoplasmic granularity in most blast cells, but ALL blast cells are agranular. Cytoplasmic granules (lysosomes) in about 10% of patients with AML may appear as large, elongated, pink or red structures (Auer rods), especially in patients with t(8;21). Occasionally, cytoplasmic granules may be too small to be observed by light microscopy, even with specific histochemical stains, but they are detectable by electron microscopy or by a monoclonal antibody to myeloperoxidase. Lymphoblasts have negative reactions to histochemical stains that identify the granules of myeloid cells but frequently have a strong reaction to periodic acid–Schiff (PAS) reagent. The blasts of some patients with AML may also be PAS-positive because of fine, punctate cytoplasmic staining rather than the chunky cytoplasmic positivity of ALL.

The study of leukemic cell surface antigens with monoclonal antibodies results in more precise definition of the lineage from which a given leukemic cell population is derived. Many antibodies are available, and those with reactivity against the same antigen are given a common cluster of differentiation (CD) designation. More than 160 clusters have been created, based on antibody specificity determined at several international workshops.

Most patients with ALL have terminal transferase (TdT) activity in the blast cell nucleus, which may be detected immunologically. Usually, 90% or more of blasts are TdT$^+$. In adult ALL patients, B-lineage leukemias are more common than those of T lineage. Among B-lineage ALL patients, the CALLA$^+$, CD10$^+$ early pre-B subtype is the most common one. Philadelphia chromosome–positive ALL is characterized by CD10 and CD34 expression. TdT$^+$ blast cells are found in 5% to 50% of patients with AML. Often, no other lymphoid antigens are found in such cases. T-cell antigens, especially CD7, are more commonly expressed on leukemic myeloblasts than are B-cell antigens. Myeloid antigens can be detected on the surface of leukemic lymphoblasts in 50% to 80% of cases. However, intracytoplasmic antigens, such as intracytoplasmic CD3, intracytoplasmic CD22, and myeloperoxidase may be considered lineage-specific for T-ALL, B-ALL and myeloid leukemia, respectively, in such cases.

Cytogenetic studies yield important information about classification and prognosis in acute leukemia. Aneuploidy resulting from the addition or deletion of specific chromosomes, or part of them, affects prognosis positively (e.g., trisomy 21 in patients without Down's syndrome) or negatively (e.g., −5, −7), depending on the chromosome involved. Balanced translocations usually involving two chromosomes are often associated with significant disease characteristics. Specific karyotypic abnormalities are identified in 80% or more of acute leukemia patients, more frequently in AML than in ALL. ALL chromosomes frequently appear fuzzy, with indistinct delineation of bands, and they are usually shorter than those of AML. This makes the observation of subtle translocations difficult in ALL. Cytogenetic analyses are best performed on bone marrow cells, because mitoses are more frequently found in them than in blood blasts. Specimens for immonophenotyping and cytogenetic analysis must be collected in heparin, acid citrate dextrose, or EDTA (ethylenediaminetetraacetic acid).

Cytogenetic information is not usually available when initial treatment decisions are made because of limitations of current technology. Such information is used primarily to define prognosis rather than to dictate initial therapy. However, cytogenetic information may be helpful in formulating postremission therapy for patients with AML. Some new molecular techniques can provide results rapidly and may be useful in diagnosis and treatment planning in some cases. For instance, the PML-RARα fusion transcript, pathognomonic of APL, can be detected by such techniques within 24 hours. Therefore, patients suspected of having APL can be identified by the detection of that transcript long before the classic t(15;17) is revealed by standard cytogenetic studies. This is important, because relatively specific therapy has been developed for APL, as discussed in a subsequent section.

SUBTYPES OF ACUTE LYMPHOCYTIC LEUKEMIA

The French–American–British (FAB) morphologic classification system is used to define subtypes of acute leukemia. Three subtypes of ALL have been designated: L1, L2, and L3. Features of these subtypes are detailed in Table 227.1. At least 80% of children with ALL have the L1 subtype, and the L2 subtype is at least twice as common as L1 in adults. The rare L3 subtype, identical with the cells of Burkitt's lymphoma, occurs equally as frequently in ALL patients of all ages and accounts for less than 2% to 3% of all ALL.

The L1 and L2 subtypes in children other than infants are usually CD10$^+$ and other early B antigen-positive, as well as TdT$^+$. In infants, there is a preponderance of undifferentiated ALL or pre–pre-B (CD10$^-$, TdT$^+$) ALL. In adults, CD10$^+$, or early pre-B ALL is the major immunophenotypic subtype. A minority of children and adults with L1 or L2 morphology have pre-B ALL, which has intracytoplasmic μ heavy immunoglobulin chains and is CD10$^+$. A small number of patients have immature (TdT$^+$, early T antigen$^+$) or mature T-lineage ALL (TdT$^-$). The L3 subtype almost always consists of relatively mature B cells (CD10$^{+/-}$ and TdT$^-$) with surface immunoglobulins, usually IgM. Except for mature B-ALL, there appears to be little prognostic significance of B-lineage ALL subtypes. T-lineage ALL seems to have a better prognosis than B-lineage ALL in some studies. ALL surface immunologic features are detailed in Table 227.2.

The Philadelphia chromosome is found in approximately 15% of adult patients with ALL. These patients usually have L1 or L2 morphology and CD10$^+$, CD34$^+$, and TdT$^+$ blasts.

TABLE 227.1.	FAB CLASSIFICATION OF ACUTE LYMPHOCYTIC LEUKEMIA		

FAB Type	Morphology	Histochemistry	Cytogenetics
L1	Small blasts with scant cytoplasm; little variation; round nucleus with single, small nucleolus	PAS+, POX−, acid ptase and naphthyl esterase+ if T-cell ALL	t(1;19) t(9;22) 11q23 14q11
L2[a]	Larger cells with more abundant cytoplasm; variation from cell to cell; irregularly shaped nucleus, often with multiple nucleoli	Same as L1	t(9;22) 11q23
L3	Large cells with basophilic cytoplasm that may be vacuolated; fine chromatin in a round nucleus; multiple nucleoli, often basophilic	PAS−, POX−; vacuoles usually oil red O-positive	t(8;14) t(8;22)

ALL, acute lymphocytic leukemia; PAS, periodic acid–Schiff reaction; POX, myeloperoxidase.
[a] The most common morphology in adult ALL.

This finding raises the question whether de novo ALL or lymphoid blast crisis of chronic myelocytic leukemia is the correct diagnosis. Molecular studies can be helpful, because the breakpoints that result in t(9;22), recognized cytogenetically as the Philadelphia chromosome, are usually but not always different in the two leukemias. Translocations between chromosome 8 and 2, 14, or 22 are common in B-cell ALL and involve genes encoding immunoglobulin heavy chains (chromosome 14) and light chains (chromosomes 2 and 22). Translocations involving chromosome 14 also occur in T-cell ALL at a chromosomal breakpoint different from that found in B-lymphoid malignancies and involve the T-cell receptor α- or δ-chain locus.

SUBTYPES OF ACUTE MYELOID LEUKEMIA

The FAB system describes nine subtypes of AML, characteristics of which are given in Table 227.3. FAB types M1, M2, and M4 each account for approximately 20% of adult AML patients. Subtypes M2, M3, and M4 generally have the best prognoses for complete remission, remission duration, and survival. FAB subtypes M5A and M6 have variable prognoses, and patients with the rare M0 and M7 subtypes have a dismal prognosis. The leukemic cells in subtypes M0, M1, and M2 express early myeloid antigens on the surface and are positive for a major histocompatibility complex class II antigen, HLA-DR (HLA-DR+), and often for the hematopoietic precursor antigen CD34. FAB subtype M3 expresses most of the myeloid antigens expressed by subtypes M0 through M2, but it is HLA-DR− and CD34−. FAB subtypes M4 and M5 express antigens specific for monocytoid cells. Myeloid antigens found in M0 through M3 may also be found in M4. M6 expresses glycophorin A, blood group H antigen, or both. Antibodies to specific megakaryocytic antigens allow identification of subtype M7, which cannot be identified by morphology alone.

Cytogenetic abnormalities correlate with FAB subtype, immunophenotype, or both. For instance, t(15;17) is pathognomonic of APL, or FAB M3. The translocation t(8;21), which occurs primarily in FAB subtype M2, and inversion (inv)16, which occurs primarily in FAB subtype M4E, confer a good

TABLE 227.2.	IMMUNOLOGIC CHARACTERISTICS OF ACUTE LYMPHOCYTIC LEUKEMIA			

Immunologic Type[a]	TdT	CD10	HLA-DR	Other
Undifferentiated ALL	+	−	+	None
Pre–pre-B ALL	+	−	+	Cytoplasmic CD22, CD19
Early pre-B ALL	+	+	+	None
Pre-B ALL	+	+	+	Cytoplasmic μ, CD20
B-cell ALL	±	±	+	Surface immunoglobulins
Prothymocyte ALL	+	−	±	Cytoplasmic CD3, CD7
Early thymocyte ALL	+	±	±	CD2, CD5
Common thymocyte ALL	+	−	−	CD1, CD4 + CD8
Mature thymocyte ALL	+	−	−	CD4 or CD8, membrane CD3
T-cell ALL	−	−	−	Surface T-cell receptor proteins

ALL, acute lymphocytic leukemia; TdT, terminal transferase.
[a] These immunologic types of ALL are independent of FAB morphologic types, except for B-cell ALL, which is almost always FAB type L3. In adults, ALL is most commonly FAB type L2 and immunologically more often positive for CD10 than negative. Ph-chromosome–positive adult ALL is always CD10 positive.

| TABLE 227.3. | FAB CLASSIFICATION OF ACUTE MYELOID LEUKEMIA |

FAB Type	Morphology	Histochemistry	Cytogenetics	Immunophenotype
M0	Acute myelocytic leukemia No cytoplasmic granules by light microscopy	Sudan black, POX$^-$	Abnormal (variable)	POX$^+$ by antibody, stem cell antigens (CD34, HLA-DR, CD7); CD33$^+$ and/or CD13$^+$
M1	Acute myelocytic leukemia Undifferentiated cells with occasional cytoplasmic granules; some promyelocytes seen	Occasional POX$^+$ cell	t(9;22), −7 inv(3) del(12p)	CD33$^+$CD13$^+$CD65s$^\pm$
M2	Acute myelocytic leukemia Granulated blasts predominate; few monocytoid cells present; differentiation beyond the promyelocyte stage is evident; Auer rods may be seen	Strongly POX$^+$	t(8;21) t(6;9)baso^a del(12p)baso^a	CD33$^+$CD13$^+$CD65s$^+$CD15$^+$
M3	Acute promyelocytic leukemia Hypergranular promyelocytes predominate; large basophilic and eosinophilic granules	Strongly POX$^+$	t(15;17)	CD34$^-$HLA-DR$^-$ CD11b$^-$CD117$^+$
M4	Acute myelomonocytic leukemia Both monocytic and granulocytic precursors are found; serum lysozyme elevated	Strongly POX$^+$; may have punctate PAS$^+$ cells	11q23 trisomy 4	CD11b$^+$CD14$^\pm$
M4eo	Acute myelomonocytic leukemia Same as M4 but young eosinophils with small eosinophilic granules and large basophilic primary granules constitute up to 30% or more of marrow cells; serum lysozyme elevated	Same as M4	inv(16)	Same as M4
M5A	Acute monoblastic leukemia Large monoblasts with abundant, relatively agranular cytoplasm that may be vacuolated and basophilic; more common in children; serum lysozyme elevated	May be POX$^+$ and PAS$^+$; nonspecific esterase$^+$	11q23	CD34$^-$MPO$^-$CD11b$^+$CD14$^-$
M5B	Acute monocytic leukemia The predominant cell has a characteristic twisted, indented, or folded nucleus, more common in adults; serum lysozyme elevated	Same as M5A	t(8;16)ery^b	CD14$^+$
M6	Erythroleukemia Megaloblastoid red cell precursors predominate, but myeloid blasts also seen; multinucleated red cell precursors are common	Red cell precursors PAS$^+$; ringed sideroblasts seen	Complex	CD34$^-$HLA-DR$^-$ Blood group H antigen$^+$ Glycophorin A$^\pm$ CD36$^\pm$
M7	Megakaryocytic leukemia Variable morphology; megakaryocytic features may not be seen by light microscopy	Variable; platelet peroxidase demonstrated by electron microscopy	t(1;22)	CD41$^+$ CD42$^+$ (more mature) CD36$^\pm$

PAS, periodic acid–Schiff; *POX*, myeloperoxidase.
^{a} Associated with abnormal basophilia.
^{b} Associated with erythrophagocytosis.

prognosis. Patients with secondary acute leukemia often have a loss of all or part of chromosome 5, chromosome 7, or both, or they have a translocation involving 11q23. In other cases, very complex cytogenetic abnormalities involving many chromosomes may be found. All these cytogenetic abnormalities confer a poor prognosis for response to therapy and response duration in secondary acute leukemia.

OPTIMAL MANAGEMENT

ACUTE LYMPHOCYTIC LEUKEMIA

Therapy for acute leukemia should be offered only in a facility with adequate supportive care resources and conducted only by an experienced team of physicians, nurses, and other health care professionals. The difference between success and failure often is experience and adequacy of supportive care rather than leukemic cell drug resistance.

Before instituting chemotherapy, active infection must be brought under control with intravenous antibiotics, and hyperuricemia must be resolved with hydration and administration of allopurinol. The latter should be given at least 24 hours before starting chemotherapy, even if the serum uric acid level is normal and continued until the blood WBC count is in the low-normal range. Other presenting medical problems should be addressed and resolved, if possible, before antileukemic therapy is given.

Standard induction therapy regimens for adult ALL include drugs such as vincristine, prednisone, daunorubicin, and L-asparaginase. Vincristine (2 mg) is given intravenously weekly, and oral prednisone (60 mg per square meter per day) is given for 4 weeks. Daunorubicin (45 mg per square meter per day) is given intravenously daily for the first 3 days of treatment, and L-asparaginase (6000 U per square meter per day) is given intramuscularly daily on days 17 to 28 of this 4-week program. A complete response rate of at least 75% can be expected in unselected adults with ALL so treated, and good-risk patients, such as those younger than 50 years who do not have the Philadelphia chromosome or a B-cell ALL phenotype have an 85% or greater complete response rate.

Daunorubicin is myelosuppressive, and treatment with it results in profound marrow hypoplasia and severe pancytopenia for 2 to 3 weeks or longer. During that time, the patient has a significant risk of infection and hemorrhage. Empiric broad-spectrum antibiotic therapy is required for fever with granulocytopenia (less than 500 granulocytes per liter) in at least 75% of treatment courses, and prophylactic platelet transfusion is almost always required for severe thrombocytopenia (less than 20,000 platelets per liter). Daunorubicin is relatively contraindicated in patients with underlying heart disease because it is cardiotoxic. Cardiotoxicity is manifested clinically in only about 1% of patients with normal pretreatment cardiac function who receive a cumulative total dose of 450 mg per square meter or less of daunorubicin. Nevertheless, the drug can be dangerous in patients with an impaired cardiac ejection fraction, especially if cardiomyopathy is the underlying cause. In such patients and certain others, moderately large doses of intravenous methotrexate may be substituted for daunorubicin in the regimen described previously, without significant change in overall results.

After the patient has achieved complete remission and recovered from induction therapy, some form of intensive postremission therapy is necessary to maximize the duration of response. If no such therapy is given, relapse occurs in at least 95% of patients within months. Usually, drugs not used during induction therapy are used here, with or without allogeneic or autologous bone marrow transplantation. There is no consensus on the best therapy for ALL, but randomized, prospective trials are addressing this question. The purpose of this phase of treatment is to kill subclinical leukemia, which, if not eradicated, will almost certainly lead to recurrent and relatively resistant disease. If chemotherapy alone is used during this phase it is usually delivered repetitively over many months and is often followed by less intensive therapy given for years. Intensive

chemotherapy followed by bone marrow transplantation is fraught with greater toxicity, but the treatment requires less time than chemotherapy alone.

Complete responders to treatment for ALL have a 25% to 40% chance of developing CNS leukemia during remission. This complication is more common in patients who present with leukocytosis, have L3 morphology, or T-cell ALL. Incidence of CNS leukemia is also inversely related to age at diagnosis. Prophylactic CNS leukemia therapy greatly reduces its incidence. The standard approach is to give cranial irradiation and multiple intrathecal methotrexate (12 mg per dose) injections as soon as complete hematologic remission is documented. This reduces the incidence of CNS leukemia to 5% or less among patients who remain in long-term complete remission. Cytarabine is sometimes substituted for methotrexate for intrathecal therapy, but there is a greater chance of adhesive arachnoiditis (perhaps 1%) with it.

The median duration of complete remission in adult ALL treated as outlined is approximately 1 to 2 years. Approximately 30% to 40% of patients are 5-year disease-free survivors, and most appear to be cured. Long-term results are best in patients younger than 40 years. Although late relapses do occur, they are infrequent, and most relapses occur within 3 years of obtaining complete remissions.

Patients who relapse generally achieve a second complete remission, especially if the relapse occurs more than 1 year after complete remission was diagnosed initially. Virtually no relapsed patient is subsequently cured, except for some younger patients who have successfully undergone allogeneic marrow transplantation for early relapse or while in second complete remission. About 25% to 40% of such patients have second remissions substantially longer than the first, which is uncommon when second remission is achieved without transplantation.

Relapse may first occur in the CNS and may be manifested by signs and symptoms of increased intracranial pressure. Lumbar puncture typically discloses increased opening pressure, CSF pleocytosis, increased CSF protein concentration, and normal glucose concentration. Examination of a concentrated CSF specimen shows blast cells, which in most cases are TdT^+. Intrathecal methotrexate given every 3 days usually results in complete resolution of this complication after treatment for 1 to 2 weeks. The treatment must be given monthly thereafter to maintain a leukemia-free CSF for as long as possible. An intraventricular reservoir (Ommaya) placed under the scalp may be used to avoid repeated lumbar puncture. If CNS relapse has occurred within 1 year of the initial diagnosis of ALL, bone marrow relapse is likely. Isolated late CNS relapse may occur, however, and not influence the patient's chance for cure.

ADULT ACUTE MYELOID LEUKEMIA

Remission induction therapy for adult AML usually consists of only two drugs, cytarabine and daunorubicin or idarubicin. Idarubicin, an analogue of daunorubicin, was found in three prospective, randomized studies to be a more effective remission induction agent in treating adult AML. Idarubicin is given as an intravenous bolus injection of 12 mg per square meter per day for 3 consecutive days. Cytarabine is given as a continuous intravenous infusion for 7 days at the rate of 100 mg per square meter per day. Both drugs are started on the same day. The treatment leads to severe bone marrow hypoplasia and pancytopenia, from which the patient does not recover for 3 to 4 weeks after treatment. There is considerable risk of infection and hemorrhage after treatment, and almost all patients require prophylactic platelet transfusions periodically, and at least 90% of patients require empiric broad-spectrum antibiotic therapy for fever while they are granulocytopenic.

Complete remission is achieved in 70% or more of adults with this regimen, and about 90% of patients who completely respond do so after only one treatment course. Some complete responders require an additional treatment course, as evidenced by only partial improvement in the marrow after the first treatment. It is imperative in those patients to document that complete remission has not been achieved with two bone marrow examinations performed with an intervening interval of several days or more before embarking on a second course of therapy. The platelet count usually rises steadily once normal marrow regeneration has begun and may reach 100,000 per microliter or more before granulocytes reappear in the blood. It is tempting to deliver a second course of induction therapy to a patient whose platelet count has risen to that level or higher when the granulocyte count remains low. In such cases, a bone marrow examination usually demonstrates a cellular marrow without a significant number of leukemic cells. Time alone usually demonstrates that no further treatment is necessary. Occasionally, these patients may more quickly achieve normal blood and marrow parameters with the administration of folate or with the withdrawal of other myelosuppressive drugs such as amphotericin B and allopurinol.

Some patients, especially some with APL, achieve complete remission after treatment without enduring major marrow hypoplasia. Leukemic cell differentiation and maturation may have been induced by chemotherapy in such cases. The facility with which APL cells can be induced to mature and differentiate in vitro when exposed to a multitude of agents led to the discovery that all-*trans* retinoic acid (ATRA) induces remission of APL by induction of maturation and differentiation rather than by cytotoxicity. Most patients respond completely to ATRA with less toxicity than expected from standard chemotherapy. ATRA rapidly corrects the coagulopathy associated with APL, and, in some studies, more patients survive induction therapy with ATRA than with standard chemotherapy. ATRA therapy is not entirely safe, however. The WBC count must be kept low during its initial administration to avoid a potentially fatal pulmonary syndrome that may occur secondary to engorgement of pulmonary capillaries and alveoli with maturing granulocytes. This is most commonly done by administering chemotherapy immediately after ATRA has resolved the coagulopathy.

Complete remissions induced with ATRA alone are frequently short for reasons that are not entirely understood but may be related to the fact that the agent induces its own catabolism through a mechanism involving cytochrome P450. There is little evidence that cytarabine has significant activity against APL but abundant evidence that anthracyclines do. Some investigators have recommended immediate therapy with idarubicin alone after ATRA. Complete response rates approaching 90%

have been reported with this approach, and remissions have been of substantial duration for most patients so treated.

Because only a few AML patients develop CNS leukemia while in remission, prophylactic therapy is not usually given. CNS leukemia may rarely be present at diagnosis, especially in patients with the M4E subtype. Most such patients have no CNS signs or symptoms. It is probably not necessary to perform a lumbar puncture to discover CNS leukemia in asymptomatic AML patients with no signs of increased intracranial pressure because therapeutic levels of cytarabine will be achieved in the CSF with doses parenterally administered during induction therapy.

Intensive postremission therapy prolongs the complete remission duration in AML. The four options usually considered are high-dose cytarabine (3 g per square meter given as an intravenous bolus injection every 12 hours every other day for 12 doses), allogeneic bone marrow transplantation, autologous bone marrow transplantation, and prolonged maintenance therapy. It is unclear which method is more effective in yielding cures, but each can cure 30% to 40% of selected complete responders. Various factors must be considered when choosing a postremission therapy. Allogeneic bone marrow transplantation is available to only a few patients with AML, because an HLA-compatible and related donor is required for optimal results. There are age limitations to both types of marrow transplantation because of the significant toxicity associated with each. Age greater than 45 years usually is a contraindication to high-dose cytarabine therapy because of toxicity, and some evidence exist that this therapy may be effective only in patients with favorable karyotypes such as inv(16) and t(8;21).

Only long-term, relatively tolerable maintenance therapy may be available to most AML patients in complete remission who are older than 50 years. A successful maintenance regimen consists of the administration of cytarabine (100 mg per square meter) given intravenously every 12 hours together with oral 6-thioguanine given on the same schedule and at the same dose. The regimen is given every 3 months for 5 to 10 days, until significant marrow hypoplasia is achieved. Cycles are repeated for 2 to 3 years. This regimen has been well tolerated and has been given safely to patients up to 75 years of age, with results that are comparable to the more intensive treatments described previously.

The median duration of complete remission in adults with AML is 12 to 24 months in most studies in which some form of intensive postremission therapy is given. About 30% to 50% of complete responders survive disease-free for at least 5 years after discontinuing all therapy. Late relapses occur but, as in ALL, they are rare. Results with all methods of induction and postremission therapy are best in young patients. Elderly patients are particularly vulnerable to serious toxic effects from treatment, but less intensive treatment of the elderly reduces their opportunity for successful outcomes without reducing the overall toxicity. The safety of standard treatment for the elderly may be enhanced by administering a hematopoietic growth factor, such as GM-CSF, after marrow hypoplasia has been achieved with induction therapy and until the granulocyte count has recovered.

Most AML patients who experience relapse after complete remission of at least 1 year's duration achieve a second complete remission, often with the same drugs that were initially successful. Most second remissions are shorter than first remissions, except when allogeneic bone marrow transplantation is performed early in second remission, in which case 15% to 20% of patients appear to be long-term disease-free survivors. Some evidence exists that maintenance chemotherapy prolongs the second remission and that biologicals such as interleukin-2 may be useful in this setting.

BIBLIOGRAPHY

Berman E, Little C, Gee T, et al. Reasons that patients with acute myelogenous leukemia do not undergo allogeneic bone marrow transplantation. *N Engl J Med* 1992;326:156–160.

Bjornson CRR, Rietze RL, Reynolds BA, et al. Turning brain into blood: a hematopoietic fate adopted by adult neural stem cells in vivo. *Science* 1999;283:534–537.

Cassileth PA, Harrington DP, Appelbaum FR, et al. Chemotherapy compared with autologous or allogeneic bone marrow transplantation in the management of acute myeloid leukemia in first remission. *N Engl J Med* 1998;339:1649–1656.

Copelan EA, McGuire EA. The biology and treatment of acute lymphoblastic leukemia in adults. *Blood* 1995;85:1151–1168.

Mayer RJ, Davis RB, Schiffer CA, et al. Intensive postremission chemotherapy in adults with acute myeloid leukemia. *N Engl J Med* 1994;331:896–903.

Scheinberg DA, Maslak P, Weiss M. Acute leukemias. In: DeVita Jr VT, Hellman S, Rosenberg SA, eds. *Cancer: principles and practice of oncology,* fifth ed. Philadelphia: JB Lippincott, 1997:2293–2316.

Tallman MS, Andersen JW, Schiffer CA, et al. All-*trans* retinoic acid in acute promyelocytic leukemia. *N Engl J Med* 1997;337:1021–1028.

Wiernik PH. Diagnosis and treatment of acute myeloid leukemia. In: Wiernik PH, Canellos GP, Dutcher JP, et al. eds. *Neoplastic diseases of the blood,* third ed. New York: Churchill Livingstone, 1996:331–352.

Wiernik PH, Dutcher JP, Paietta E, et al. Long-term follow-up of treatment and potential cure of adult acute lymphocytic leukemia with MOAD: a non-anthracycline containing regimen. *Leukemia* 1993;7:1236–1241.

Kelley's Textbook of Internal Medicine, fourth edition. Edited by H. David Humes. Lippincott Williams & Wilkins, Philadelphia © 2000.

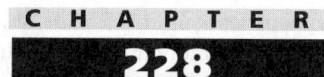

CHAPTER 228

CHRONIC LEUKEMIAS

GEORGE P. CANELLOS

The chronic leukemias are a group of heterogeneous proliferative disorders derived from lymphoid or myeloid precursor cells that retain some capacity for differentiation to recognizable mature elements. The natural history of the chronic leukemias tends to be longer than untreated acute leukemia, but successful therapy of the latter has narrowed the differences. Depending on the aggressiveness of the chronic leukemia, the natural history may be abbreviated.

The symptoms and signs of the chronic leukemias result from the continuous proliferation and eventual replacement of the normal hemopoietic components of the bone marrow. Although intensive therapy is required to survive the acute leukemias, most chronic leukemias are still treated palliatively with less intense treatments. Perhaps because of the availability of malignant cells for study, the molecular biology and pathogenesis of the chronic leukemias have become much better understood during the past 5 years.

CHRONIC LYMPHOCYTIC LEUKEMIA

CLINICAL FEATURES

The chronic lymphocytic leukemias (CLLs) represent a group of disorders in which the malignant cell is a recognizable mature lymphocyte of varied structure. The subtypes can be divided according to immunophenotypic origin. Most patients have a disease of cells originating in the bone (B) marrow. B-cell CLL is primarily a disease of Western (European) populations. CLL with thymic (T) markers is more common in Japan but can occur in Western countries, where it is usually associated with a generally worse prognosis. The immunophenotype of B-cell and T-cell CLL tends to favor a more differentiated pattern, which is readily defined by appropriate antibodies. Immunofluorescence for cell surface immunoglobulins is usually less intense than normal. The immunophenotype of the CLL lymphocyte includes the presence of CD5, a mature T-cell marker in addition to the usual pan–B-cell markers, CD19 and CD20. Flow cytometry also reveals a clonal preponderance of immunoglobulin light chain. CLL also has CD23 present in 70% of cases and is associated with a more favorable prognosis.

CLL occurs at the median age of 60 years at diagnosis and is equally distributed among men and women. The diagnosis tends to be made earlier because of the use of automated blood counts. The clinical features and extent of involvement determine the prognostic state of the CLL. About 50% of the patients present with *lymphadenopathy* in addition to a lymphocytosis that is usually greater than 15,000 per microliter. Splenomegaly may also be observed at presentation.

Patients may give a history of infections and even exaggerated responses to insect bites. Anemia and thrombocytopenia are usually late features unless an early autoimmune hemolytic anemia or thrombocytopenia has supervened. About 10% of patients have a small monoclonal M spike on serum electrophoresis, but in most cases absolute hypogammaglobulinemia occurs, worsening with progression of the CLL. Fever and painful lymphadenopathy are not features of the disease and usually suggest infection. In the absence of peripheral lymphocytosis, a variant low-grade lymphoma (small lymphocytic) has the same histologic picture on lymph node biopsy.

The bone marrow is usually diffusely replaced by small mature lymphocytes, but a nodular involvement may occur and be a more favorable sign. The peripheral blood usually reveals a monotonous lymphocytosis, but some patients may show an admixture of large transformed lymphoid cells (prolymphocytes). Hyperuricemia occurs only in patients with marked lymphocytosis and organomegaly. The median survival of patients can be prolonged to more than 10 to 15 years if only lymphocytosis and minimal lymphadenopathy are present at diagnosis; anemia and thrombocytopenia reduce the median survival to 2 to 4 years.

Cytogenetic abnormalities in B-cell CLL occur in 55% to 65% patients, with trisomy 12 being the most common anomaly. Abnormalities in the long arm of chromosome 13 or 14 also occur. The prognosis is usually more favorable with no cytogenetic abnormalities present.

The clinical course of CLL is determined by the initial presenting stage, but in time, it may accelerate, exhibiting an increased peripheral prolymphocyte count, anemia or thrombocytopenia, progressive lymphadenopathy, and marked splenomegaly. Prolymphocytes are usually recognized with prominent nucleoli that are absent from mature or CLL lymphocytes. In a few patients, the course of CLL may be complicated by abdominal tumors (e.g., gastric, small bowel, retroperitoneal), which has a histologic picture of large cell lymphoma (Richter's syndrome) with constitutional symptoms, fever, weight loss, and rapid deterioration. Associated autoimmune phenomena, such as hemolytic anemia, thrombocytopenia, and pure red blood cell aplasia can occur at any time in the natural history of the disease but usually do not influence the prognosis.

T-cell CLL is usually a more aggressive lymphoproliferative disorder than B-cell CLL, with anemia, thrombocytopenia, splenomegaly, and lymphadenopathy. A relatively unique feature of T-cell CLL is skin infiltration. The T-cell leukemia tends to respond less well to therapy than does the B-cell variety. The malignant cell may have a more convoluted nucleus and manifest the helper (CD4) T-cell immunophenotype. Suppressor (CD8) T-cell CLL is rare and usually presents as marked anemia or neutropenia out of proportion to the extent of marrow and organ involvement. The latter may also be defined as large granular cell leukemia. Death is usually related to infection because of granulocytopenia and hypogammaglobulinemia.

THERAPY

CLL usually has an indolent course with a natural history measurable in years and usually predicted by initial presenting features. Asymptomatic lymphocytosis with minimal lymphadenopathy with no anemia or thrombocytopenia does not require therapy. As a general rule, therapy is palliative and may not influence the overall survival.

In time, progressive lymphadenopathy and hepatosplenomegaly with or without anemia or thrombocytopenia require therapy. The reduction of the leukemic burden is achieved with oral alkylating agents such as chlorambucil (0.1 mg per kilogram) on a daily oral basis or intermittent monthly courses (0.8 mg per kilogram). Other oral alkylating agents, such as cyclophosphamide or melphalan, are also effective. Prednisone adds to the lymphocytolytic effect and can be added for short courses as a daily oral medication. Chronic prednisone therapy can produce other steroid-related problems and is best reserved for cases with anemia, thrombocytopenia, or autoimmune complications such as autoimmune hemolytic anemia. Patients refractory to alkylating agents may respond to parenteral fludarabine. Fludar-

abine is also an effective initial therapy but is more immunosuppressive because of its marked T-lymphocytotoxic effect and is associated with a relatively high rate of infection. In randomized comparisons of fludarabine with chlorambucil or combination chemotherapy, the former demonstrated a significantly higher overall and complete response rate but, as yet, no survival advantage.

Other therapeutic approaches to CLL are usually dictated by the clinical circumstances. Hypersplenism may respond to low doses of fractionated radiation therapy, but hypersplenic cytopenias are more directly benefited by splenectomy. Autoimmune complications may require a variety of immunosuppressive agents, such as corticosteroids, cyclosporine, and azathioprine (Imuran).

An aggressive turn in the natural history, such as a lymphomatous transformation (Richter's syndrome) or prolymphocytic leukemia, requires parenteral combination chemotherapy such as that used for large cell lymphoma, including vincristine and doxorubicin, which are not used for the chronic lymphoproliferative disorders.

The median survival, varying according to presenting stage, is 3 years to more than 10 years. In select circumstances, younger patients with advanced CLL have received allogeneic bone marrow transplants with about 50% surviving in remission at 3 years. The role of autologous transplantation is under investigation and may be a consideration in younger patients.

■ CHRONIC MYELOCYTIC LEUKEMIA

Chronic myelocytic leukemia (CML) is one of the myeloproliferative disorders that results from a clonal proliferation of cells of bone marrow stem cell origin with a predominance of mature granulocytic precursors, although abnormalities of red blood cell and platelet production are also present. Studies to date indicate that CML is a disorder of the stem cell common to bone marrow cells and B lymphocytes. It is unclear, except through indirect evidence, that the T lymphocytes may be involved. Nonclonal reactive bone marrow–derived fibroblasts can result in myelofibrosis, especially with heavy deposition of reticulum. This is especially a feature of an advanced or accelerated phase.

Precursors of the cells previously mentioned, except fibroblasts, have the Philadelphia (Ph^1) chromosome. This represents a reciprocal translocation of chromosomal material between chromosomes 22 and 9, with translocation and activation of the protooncogene, *ABL,* from chromosome 9 at band 34 to chromosome 22 t(9;22)(q34;q11). This occurs in over 90% of patients with CML. The *ABL* gene is translocated close to a site of chromosomal breakage on chromosome 22, known as the breakpoint cluster region (*BCR*). The chimeric *ABL/BCR* gene codes for a new transcript of 8.2-kb mRNA, producing a unique oncoprotein of 210 kd, which has greater tyrosine–kinase activity than the normal *ABL*-encoded protein (145 kd). Translocation of *ABL* appears to be a critical abnormality. It is considered a crucial component but perhaps not the sole event in CML leukemogenesis. Ph^1 chromosome-positive acute lymphocytic leukemia (ALL) in adults, for example, is associated with a different structural *BCR/ABL* chimeric protein of 180 kd, reflecting a different breakpoint in *BCR*. The oncogenic mechanism of the *BCR/ABL* protein is suggested by its capacity for multiple protein–protein interactions linked to signal transduction pathways. New agents have been designed to inhibit the tyrosine kinase activity of *BCR/ABL*. Molecular probes for *BCR* rearrangement can increase the sensitivity for detection of leukemic cells. The Ph[1] and the *BCR/ABL* abnormality remain through the natural history of the disease. Additional new cytogenetic abnormalities may occur during evolution of the disease to a more aggressive phase, such as duplication of the Ph[1] chromosome, trisomy 8, and isochromosome 17.

PATHOLOGY AND CLINICAL CHARACTERISTICS

The basic hematologic abnormality of CML involves an excess production of mature-appearing granulocytes and intermediate mature cells, such as myelocytes and metamyelocytes. CML is usually diagnosed in midlife or later. Initially, patients are essentially asymptomatic, although complaints referable to a bulky spleen may be noted. The peripheral blood white blood cell (WBC) count is characteristically two to four times the upper limit of normal, and the WBC differential count discloses some immaturity of the granulocyte series, represented by myelocytes and metamyelocytes. The platelet count is usually normal or elevated, and anemia may not be present. Leukocyte alkaline phosphatase activity is low or absent in uncomplicated patients. Although the test is rarely done, it is normal or elevated in most other benign or myeloproliferative disorders such as polycythemia vera and agnogenic myeloid metaplasia.

The bone marrow is hypercellular—primarily because of an expanded, immature (but not blastic) granulocyte compartment—and the numbers of megakaryocytes and red cell precursors are often increased. This results in progressive granulocytic leukocytosis, with the appearance of bands, myelocytes, and metamyelocytes in the blood in increased numbers. Eosinophilia and basophilia may occur. Marrow or blood karyotypes demonstrate the Ph[1] chromosome in almost all patients, although it may not be present in every metaphase examined. In some patients with otherwise typical CML, no Ph[1] chromosome can be identified by cytogenetics, although the rearranged *BCR/ABL* gene can be detected with molecular biologic techniques. As the disease progresses, the accumulation of granulocytes is expanded in other reticuloendothelial sites such as spleen and the portal areas of the liver. Biochemical abnormalities, such as hyperuricemia and an elevated B_{12}-binding protein (derived from granulocytes) in CML are related to the extent of granulocytosis.

The initial prognosis can be correlated with the extent of leukocytosis, presence of blasts in the peripheral blood, extent of splenomegaly, and thrombocytosis. All these features are associated with a poor prognosis. Profound anemia and thrombocytopenia are almost unknown initially but can occur as the disease progresses, usually in 2 to 4 years after diagnosis. The latter stage, known as the accelerated phase, may be associated with marked basophilia, anemia, myelofibrosis, progressive splenomegaly, and the emergence of new cytogenetic abnormalities in addition to the Ph[1] chromosome.

In a median of 36 to 50 months (later for patients with disease diagnosed early), there is a transformation of the CML to a more blastic leukemia, referred to as *blastic phase* or *blast crisis*. This usually represents a terminal phase of the disease, with all of the features of the accelerated phase possible in addition to thrombocytopenia, anemia, and an increase in the number of blast cells in the marrow and blood to over 30%.

Rarely, myeloblastomas develop in lymph nodes, skin, bone, and other sites. The rapid rise in blast cell count to more than 100,000 per cubic millimeter can result in leukostasis in the cerebral and pulmonary vasculature.

The morphologic characteristics of the blastic phase can vary; 60% to 70% of patients retain the myeloblastic features, but a significant minority have lymphoid or mixed myeloid–lymphoid features in their blast cells. Megakaryocytic and erythroblastic transformation rarely occurs. The lymphoblasts of CML in lymphoid transformation are usually of pre-B-cell phenotype, consistent with the cell of common childhood ALL. Rarely, T-cell transformation with a mixed T-cell–myeloid phenotype has occurred. The median survival of the blastic phase is from 2 to 4 months.

DIFFERENTIAL DIAGNOSIS

Juvenile CML is a distinct disorder of children younger than 14 years of age. The accelerated course of this CML variant usually manifests with thrombocytopenia, monocytosis, and elevation of fetal hemoglobin. The Ph[1] chromosome is absent.

Ph[1]-negative CML, erroneously described in older textbooks, probably does not exist. Patients whose illness has been categorized by this term usually had an elevated WBC count (secondary to an immature granulocytosis) in common with Ph[1]-positive CML but were commonly anemic, thrombocytopenic, elderly, and ill when diagnosed, unlike most patients with Ph[1]-positive CML. They may have an increased number of monocytic cells. The response to therapy and survival rates are inferior to Ph[1]-positive CML. Careful evaluation of patients with apparent Ph[1]-negative CML usually leads to a diagnosis of myelodysplastic syndrome or acute or chronic myelomonocytic leukemia (Chapters 227 and 229).

Although bone marrow specimens from patients with polycythemia vera or primary thrombocytosis (essential thrombocythemia) may occasionally be confused with the marrow of patients with CML, numerous clinical and laboratory features of the three entities clearly segregate them (Chapters 217 and 231).

Primary myelofibrosis with myeloid metaplasia may be confused clinically with CML, but the Ph[1] chromosome is absent and leukocyte alkaline phosphatase activity is normal or elevated. Myelofibrosis and extramedullary hematopoiesis may occur late in CML, but they rarely dominate the clinical picture. Initial massive splenomegaly, anemia, thrombocytopenia, and hepatomegaly occur more frequently in myelofibrosis than CML, and bone marrow in the former condition characteristically cannot be aspirated. A marrow core biopsy in patients with myelofibrosis usually discloses abundant, diffuse fibrosis and marked hypocellularity, rather than the hypercellularity characteristic of those with CML.

Leukemoid reactions to infection or neoplastic disease may

suggest CML. Leukemoid reactions secondary to both underlying conditions are characterized by a mature granulocytosis without abnormalities or platelet or red cell production and without splenomegaly. Leukocyte alkaline phosphatase activity is often elevated and never low.

THERAPY

Treatment of those in the chronic phase of CML is directed toward control proliferation of the granulocyte mass. The principal chemotherapeutic agent is hydroxyurea given by mouth at 1 to 3 gm per day as initial therapy with reduction of dose when the WBC count approaches 50% of the initial value. The drug is short-acting so that continuous maintenance is needed. Excessive dosage can result in macrocytic anemia. The myelosuppressive effects are short-lived when the drug is stopped. There do not appear to be any long-term toxic effects to other organs. Allopurinol should be used initially but may be discontinued when the WBC count approaches the normal range.

Recombinant interferon-α is a very effective agent in the therapy of the chronic phase. A percentage of patients (about 20%) can be treated chronically to a relatively low granulocyte count and achieve a transient disappearance of the Ph[1] chromosome. Interferon requires frequent injections and has more side effects than oral chemotherapy. Some randomized trials from Europe suggested the superiority of interferon over hydroxyurea, but conversely two others showed no significant difference. These treatments are palliative and it is uncertain whether the blastic phase is delayed. The cytotoxic action requires continuous therapy but lacks the myeloablative action of the cytotoxic drugs.

The achievement of cytogenetic remission may require prolonged therapy over 6 to 8 months at up to 5 million units per square meter per day. If the higher doses are tolerated, then 80% will achieve a hematologic remission, including a cytogenetic response. In a recent randomized trial comparing hydroxyurea with interferon, the latter showed a 16% complete or partial (less than 35%) cytogenetic response rate compared with 2% (only partial) with hydroxyurea. The overall survival was similar. Complete responders have a longer survival. The toxic effects of interferon include flulike symptoms and long-term fatigue. The combination of interferon and cytotoxic agents, such as cytosine arabinoside, can increase the hematologic and cytogenetic remission rate, but the impact on survival is to be defined. Accelerated proliferation of granulocyte precursors in the accelerated or blastic phase may respond to increased doses of hydroxyurea or otherwise require more intensive antileukemic therapy. Lymphoid morphology and phenotype occur in about 20% of patients entering the blastic phase. In this circumstance, anti–ALL-type therapy may achieve a hematologic remission with persistence of the Ph[1] chromosome. The median survival remains less than 1 year but is better than the 1 to 2 months for cases of myeloblastic transformation.

Allogeneic bone marrow transplantation in the chronic phase of CML from a matched sibling donor can cure about 50% of patients. Younger patients have a better prognosis. Patients in relapse from allogeneic transplantation can be treated with peripheral WBCs from the original marrow donor and achieve a second immune cell–mediated remission, but not without the risk of graft-versus-host disease. Autologous bone marrow transplantation is transiently beneficial in the blastic phase and may alter the percentage of Ph[1]-positive cells when done in the chronic phase. Splenectomy can palliate hypersplenic symptoms but does not affect the natural history of the disease. Recent data suggest that matched unrelated donor transplants are feasible with a 50% 5-year survival rate, with even better results with early transplantation of patients younger than 50 years.

HAIRY CELL LEUKEMIA

CLINICAL FEATURES

Hairy cell leukemia (HCL) is a rare form of a B-cell chronic lymphoproliferative disorder, whose malignant lymphoid cells have unique filamentous cytoplasmic projections and are nondividing. Unique cytochemical and immunologic characteristics of the abnormal lymphoid cells in HCL readily differentiate this disorder from CLL. They are of B-cell lineage according to surface markers and immunoglobulin gene rearrangement. Tartrate-resistant acid phosphatase is commonly found in HCL cells. Some surface antigens are uniquely expressed in HCL, and antibody studies may be diagnostic. The antigens that differentiate HCL from CLL include CD11c (myelomonocytic marker) and CD25 (interleukin-2 receptors).

The median age for presentation is in the sixth decade with a male predominance. Patients usually present with pancytopenia and impaired marrow function due to infiltration by leukemic cells. Splenomegaly is common. The course is indolent, with a tendency toward more profound marrow suppression and splenomegaly. On occasion, the cellular projections require electron microscopy for demonstration. Hairy cells are usually found readily in the blood, although in some patients they may be present in small numbers. The bone marrow is characteristically hypercellular, and aspiration is difficult or impossible.

THERAPY

The therapy for HCL has improved considerably over the last decade. Splenectomy was the only treatment for the associated cytopenias until the introduction of systemic agents, such as interferon-α and the purine analogues 2′-deoxycoformycin and 2-chlorodeoxyadenosine (2-CDA). The latter two agents can produce lasting complete remissions that were rarely achieved with interferon-α. 2-CDA has been used extensively. This agent is capable of inducing the long-lasting remission with a single course of parenteral treatment at 0.1 mg per kilogram by continuous infusion for 7 days. Patients refractory to interferon-α can also be successfully treated with the purine analogues. The major toxic effects of the purines are myelosuppression and lymphocytopenia. The overall response rate, however, is more than 90%, with almost 75% of patients achieving durable complete remissions. Relapse can be successfully retreated with the same drug.

BIBLIOGRAPHY

The Benelux CML Study Group. Randomized study on hydroxyurea alone versus hydroxyurea combined with low-dose interferon-alpha 2b for chronic myeloid leukemia. *Blood* 1998;91:2713–2721.

Carella AM, Frassoni F, Melo J, et al. New insights in biology and current therapeutic options for patients with chronic myelogenous leukemia. *Haematologica* 1997;82:478–495.

Cheson BD. Therapy for previously untreated chronic lymphocytic leukemia: a reevaluation. *Semin Hematol* 1998;35(Suppl 3):14–21.

Clift RA, Buckner CD, Thomas ED, et al. Marrow transplantation for chronic myeloid leukemia: a randomized study comparing cyclophosphamide and total body irradiation with busulfan and cyclophosphamide. *Blood* 1994;84:2036–2043.

Gale RP, Hehlmann R, Zhang M-J, et al. Survival with bone marrow transplantation versus hydroxyurea or interferon for chronic myelogenous leukemia. *Blood* 1998;91:1810–1819.

Hansen JA, Gooley TA, Martin PJ, et al. Bone marrow transplants from unrelated donors for patients with chronic myeloid leukemia. *N Engl J Med* 1998;338:962–968.

Keating MJ, O'Brien S, Lerner S, et al. Long-term follow-up of patients with chronic lymphocytic leukemia (CLL) receiving fludarabine regimens as initial therapy. *Blood* 1998;92:1165–1171.

Khouri IF, Przepiorka D, van Besien K, et al. Allogeneic blood or marrow transplantation for chronic lymphocytic leukaemia: timing of transplantation and potential effect of fludarabine on acute graft-verus-host disease. *Br J Haematol* 1997;97:466–473.

Montserrat E, Bosch F, Rozman C. B-cell chronic lymphocytic leukemia: recent progress in biology, diagnosis, and therapy. *Ann Oncol* 1997; 8(Suppl 1):93–101.

Saven A, Burian C, Koziol JA, et al. Long-term follow-up of patients with hairy cell leukemia after cladribine treatment. *Blood* 1998;92: 1918–1926.

Kelley's Textbook of Internal Medicine, fourth edition. Edited by H. David Humes. Lippincott Williams & Wilkins, Philadelphia © 2000.

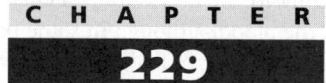

CHAPTER 229

MYELODYSPLASTIC SYNDROME

FREDERICK R. APPELBAUM

The myelodysplastic syndrome (MDS) describes a group of clonal hematopoietic disorders characterized by impaired maturation of blood cells and the development of peripheral cytopenias. MDS is the result of neoplastic transformation of a cell at a level of differentiation close to that of the hematopoietic stem cell. Unlike acute leukemia, the transformed cell and its progeny retain the ability to differentiate, although not entirely normally, for a period of months to years. With time, the abnormal clone suppresses normal hematopoiesis and becomes increasingly abnormal, ultimately resulting in fatal pancytopenia or progression to an acute leukemia-like syndrome.

To aid in categorizing patients with MDS, the French–American–British (FAB) Morphology Cooperative Group recognizes five distinct forms of MDS based on marrow and peripheral blood morphology (Table 229.1): refractory anemia (RA), refractory anemia with ringed sideroblasts (RARS), refractory anemia with excess blasts (RAEB), refractory anemia with excess blasts in transition (RAEB-t), and chronic myelomonocytic leukemia (CMMoL). This classification system is used widely but includes a syndrome (CMMoL) thought by many to more appropriately be considered a myeloproliferative disorder and ignores the generally recognized syndromes of hypoplastic myelodysplasia and myelodysplasia with marrow fibrosis.

INCIDENCE

Earlier reports characterized MDS as being relatively rare, with an annual incidence of approximately 1 case per 100,000 persons. Later studies suggested a much higher incidence, particularly if mild forms of the disease are included. Although sometimes seen in young patients, the disorder is much more common in the elderly, with a median age of onset of over 60 years. Beyond the age of 70, the incidence of MDS is greater than 1 case per 1,000 persons, making it among the most common hematologic malignancies of the aged.

ETIOLOGY

The cause of the defect leading to MDS in most cases is unknown. Some cases of MDS are seen in children with DNA repair deficiency syndromes (e.g., Bloom's syndrome, Fanconi's anemia, ataxia-telangiectasia), Down's syndrome, and the Li–Fraumeni syndrome, and MDS occurs in siblings of patients with familial monosomy 7 syndrome. Secondary (therapy-related) MDS is increasingly recognized as a major complication of irradiation and chemotherapy. A number of cases of MDS involving chromosome 5 or 7 develop 3 to 5 years after patients have been exposed to alkylating agents. Other patients develop MDS involving chromosome locus 11q23 after exposure to the topoisomerase II inhibitors etoposide and teniposide.

PATHOGENESIS AND PATHOPHYSIOLOGY

The exact pathogenesis of MDS remains unclear, but studies of chromosomal morphology, glucose-6-phosphate dehydrogenase isoenzymes, and molecular markers suggest that the development of MDS is a multistep process involving the accumulation of genetic lesions. Early in the course of the disease, there appears to be a genetic event in an early hematopoietic progenitor, resulting in its expansion to a clonal population of hematopoietic stem cells, which, at least initially, maintains many normal characteristics. Evidence for early clonal hematopoiesis comes from studies of X-linked polymorphisms in patients with MDS with only very mildly disordered hematopoiesis that demonstrate that myeloid, erythroid, platelet, and, in some cases, lymphoid cells all arise from the same clone.

The reasons for expansion of the abnormal clone are not understood but appear to be related to independence from normal growth factor control, insensitivity to normal inhibitory

| TABLE 229.1. | FAB CLASSIFICATION OF MYELODYSPLASTIC SYNDROMES |

Classification	Marrow Blasts (%)	Peripheral Blood Blasts (%)	Ringed Sideroblasts >15% of Bone Marrow	Monocytes (>1,000/μL)
Refractory anemia	<5	≤1	–	–
Refractory anemia with ringed sideroblasts	<5	≤1	+	–
Refractory anemia with excess blasts	5–20	<5	–/+	–
Refractory anemia with excess blasts in transition	20–30	>5	–/+	–/+
Chronic myelomonocytic leukemia	≤20	<5	–/+	+

factors, and active suppression of normal hematopoiesis. The abnormal clone appears to be genetically unstable, and successive genetic changes occur, accompanied by increasingly disordered hematopoiesis. Pancytopenia develops in the face of a hypercellular marrow as a result of defective maturation and premature intramedullary death of cells, presumably by means of an apoptosis pathway. With further genetic changes, hematopoiesis becomes increasingly malignant, ultimately resulting in a picture similar to acute leukemia.

The nature of the initial genetic event leading to MDS is unknown. Some studies have examined the role of protooncogenes and tumor suppressor genes. Mutations in the RAS protooncogene family, particularly NRAS, are found in 20% to 50% of cases and appear to be more common in more aggressive forms of MDS. Whether RAS mutations cause MDS or are a result of earlier genetic events is unknown. Similarly, mutations in the FMS protooncogene are found in some cases of MDS; as many as 20% of CMMoL patients demonstrate FMS mutations. Mutations in P53, although common in other malignancies, are seen in only a small percentage of MDS cases.

Single or complex cytogenetic abnormalities are found in 50% to 65% of patients with primary MDS and up to 90% of cases of secondary MDS. Whether some of these abnormalities represent the primary genetic event or are secondary to underlying genetic instability is unknown. The possibility that some cytogenetic abnormalities at least contribute to the development of disordered hematopoiesis is raised by observations that interstitial deletions of the long arms of chromosomes 5 and 7 are extremely common in MDS and that a large number of normal genes involved in hematopoietic growth and development map to these regions, especially to the 5q23–5q31 region, where the genes for interleukin-3 (IL-3), IL-4, IL-5, colony-stimulating factor 1 (CSF-1), and interferon regulatory factor–1 (IRF-1) are located.

CLINICAL FINDINGS

Clinical findings associated with MDS are almost solely the consequence of bone marrow failure. Fatigue, pallor, infection, and bruising or bleeding are the most common presenting complaints. Most MDS patients are anemic at diagnosis, and approximately 50% are granulocytopenic or thrombocytopenic as well. Splenomegaly is found in about 10% of cases. Occasional patients present with rheumatic or immunologic abnormalities, including cutaneous vasculitis or lupus-like syndromes.

LABORATORY FINDINGS

Laboratory findings in patients with MDS vary according to the category of disease. In RA, anemia is invariably accompanied by a low reticulocyte count. The numbers of peripheral blood granulocytes and platelets are normal or diminished slightly, and leukemic blasts are usually absent from the periphery and account for less than 5% of marrow cells. RARS has findings essentially identical with those of RA except that ringed sideroblasts make up 15% or more of marrow cells.

In patients with RAEB, thrombocytopenia and granulocytopenia are common; blasts make up 5% to 20% of marrow cells and account for up to 5% of the circulating white cells. RAEB-t has laboratory features similar to those of RAEB, but blasts are more common, accounting for up to 30% of marrow or peripheral blood leukocytes. If more than 30% of marrow or peripheral blood cells are blasts, the diagnosis of acute myeloid leukemia (AML) can be made. CMMoL has features similar to those of RAEB, with the addition of a circulating monocyte count of more than 1,000 per microliter.

Clonal chromosomal abnormalities are found in up to 65% of patients with primary MDS and 90% of patients with secondary MDS. Abnormalities of chromosome 5 or 7 are found in 25% of patients with primary MDS and 55% of those with secondary MDS. Other common abnormalities include trisomy 8 and interstitial deletions of the long arm of chromosomes 11, 13, 17, or 20. These abnormalities are also seen in some patients with AML and in that setting are associated with a poor prognosis. The cytogenetic abnormalities associated with a good prognosis in patients with AML, including t(8;21), t(15;17), and inv(16), are rarely seen in patients with MDS. Several myelodysplasia syndromes are associated with particular cytogenetic abnormalities. Patients with an interstitial deletion of the long arm of chromosome 5 (5q−) as the sole abnormality are frequently elderly women with macrocytic anemia and normal or elevated platelet counts. The bone marrow of such patients shows erythroid hyperplasia with hypolobulated megakaryocytes. This syndrome has a relatively benign course. t(5;12) (q33;p13) is specifically associated with the CMMoL subtype of MDS. As noted in the following text, cytogenetics is useful in determining prognosis in MDS.

OPTIMAL MANAGEMENT

The course of untreated MDS is highly variable; some patients survive for more than a decade, and others die within a year of presentation. An essential element in determining appropriate therapy is an assessment of the patient's prognosis. The FAB classification is of some prognostic use in that patients with RA and RARS have a better prognosis than patients with RAEB, RAEB-t, or CMMoL.

Several scoring systems provide greater prognostic precision. An International Prognostic Scoring System (IPSS) has recently been developed based on an analysis of 816 patients. The system rates the risk of a patient's disease according to three criteria: number and degree of cytopenias, bone marrow blast percentage, and cytogenetic findings. Risk scores for each of these three variables are defined, and by combining the scores, patients can be categorized as belonging to one of four prognostic categories: low-risk (median survival 5.7 years), intermediate-risk 1 (median survival 3.5 years), intermediate-risk 2 (median survival 1.2 years) or high-risk (0.4 years) (Table 229.2 and Fig. 229.1). Death of patients with MDS usually results from complications of pancytopenia or disease progression to AML. Infection and hemorrhage associated with low blood counts are the cause of 35% to 50% of all deaths in MDS. Patients with RAEB or RAEB-t have a 40% to 65% probability of disease progression to AML within 2 years, but the risk is much smaller for patients with RA or RARS.

Because of the considerable variability in the aggressiveness of MDS, appropriate management also varies. Patients with RA or RARS with normal or near-normal granulocyte and platelet counts (low-risk according to the IPSS) may require no therapy or, at most, support with red blood cell transfusions. Patients with RAEB or RAEB-t (intermediate-risk 1, intermediate-risk 2, and high-risk by IPSS) have, on average, a predicted survival of 0.4 to 3.5 years, and more aggressive interventions should be considered.

The only form of therapy that can cure MDS is allogeneic marrow transplantation, which results in long-term disease-free survival of 40% to 60% of transplanted patients. Transplantation results are best in younger patients, those with human leukocyte antigen–matched siblings to serve as donors, and patients without excess blasts. Although many patients with MDS are not candidates for transplantation because of advanced age or lack of a donor, transplantation should be considered for any patient younger than 55 years with intermediate-risk 1 or higher-risk disease.

Although several therapeutic interventions have been explored in patients who are not transplantation candidates, the evidence that any of these approaches are superior to supportive care alone is scant. Although an occasional response to glucocorticoids has been reported, the likelihood of such a response is low and, because of the increased risk of infection with these agents, glucocorticoids are not recommended as routine therapy. A few responses to androgens have been reported, but in prospective, randomized trials, no benefit of androgen therapy was detected.

The demonstration that several compounds can induce myeloid differentiation in vitro led to testing similar agents in patients with MDS. Phase I and II trials suggested responses of 20% to 30% with one such agent, 13-*cis*-retinoic acid, but two prospective, randomized studies failed to detect any improvement in progression-free or overall survival rates.

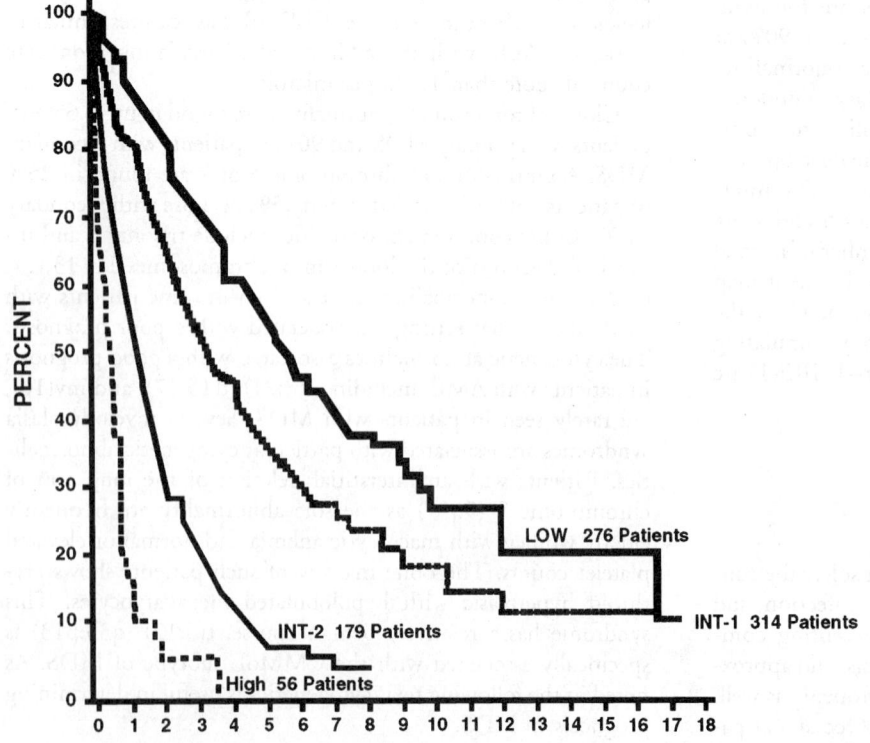

FIGURE 229.1. Survival according to IPSS risk classification. (From Greenberg P, et al. International scoring system for evaluating prognosis in myelodysplastic syndromes. *Blood* 1997;89:2079, with permission).

TABLE 229.2.	INTERNATIONAL PROGNOSTIC SCORING SYSTEM (IPSS) FOR MYELODYSPLASTIC SYNDROME

Characteristic	Individual Score
Cytogenetics	
Good (normal, del 5q, del 20q, and −y)	0
Intermediate	0.5
Poor (3 or more abnormalities or abnormalities of 7)	1.0
Blasts (% in marrow)	
<5	0
5–10	0.5
11–20	2.0
21–30	2.0
Cytopenias (Hb <10 g/dL, ANC <1800/mm³, platelets <100,000/mm³)	
0–1	0
2–3	0.5
Risk Groups	**Total Score**
Low	0
Intermediate risk-1	0.5–1.0
Intermediate risk-2	1.5–2.0
High	>2.0

ANC, absolute neutrophil count; Hb, hemoglobin.
The IPSS assigns each patient a score for each of three characteristics: cytogenetics, marrow blast percent, and peripheral cytopenias. An overall risk group is determined by adding the three scores.

The use of hematopoietic growth factors has been actively studied in MDS with the hope that these agents might reverse cytopenias by increasing production of normal cells or by inducing abnormal progenitors to differentiate more normally. The two most studied myeloid agents are granulocyte-macrophage colony-stimulating factor (GM-CSF) and granulocyte colony-stimulating factor (G-CSF). Use of either agent leads to an increase in granulocyte counts in approximately 75% of MDS patients and appears to do so by increasing the production of normal and abnormal cells. Improvements in platelet or red cell production are uncommon with the use of GM-CSF or G-CSF, occurring in only 10% to 15% of patients. Two large, randomized studies of the use of myeloid growth factors in treating MDS have been reported. In both studies, increases in granulocytes occurred, accompanied by a decrease in infectious complications. However, neither study demonstrated a survival advantage or a delay in time to progression to AML. There is no consistent evidence of clinical benefit associated with the chronic administration of GM-CSF or G-CSF in MDS, but it is appropriate to consider the use of such agents in neutropenic patients with infection.

Erythropoietin has been studied in MDS patients with anemia. Although most MDS patients have high endogenous levels of erythropoietin, high doses of exogenous drug improved red cell production in 20% of patients, with more frequent responses seen in patients with lower pretreatment endogenous erythropoietin levels. Combinations of erythropoietin and G-CSF may increase the frequency of an erythroid response.

Chemotherapeutic approaches to MDS have ranged from low-dose single-agent therapy to high-dose multiagent treatments similar to those used in AML. Use of low-dose cytarabine (20 mg per square meter per day) has been extensively studied, with the hope that this treatment could induce differentiation of myeloid cells. A summary of numerous phase II reports and the results of one randomized study indicated that low-dose cytarabine produced responses in approximately 15% of patients but did not increase overall survival. Like low-dose cytarabine, low-dose 5-azacitidine can result in hematologic responses in some patients. A recently completed randomized trial suggests 5-azacitidine may prolong the interval to leukemic transformation or death by as much as 10 months and thus merits consideration in patients with intermediate-risk 2 or high-risk disease. The topoisomerase inhibitor, topotecan, has been studied as a single agent in MDS and found to result in short-lived but complete responses in approximately 30% of patients. Intensive combination chemotherapy, including higher-dose cytarabine and daunomycin, can produce complete responses in 30% to 60% of patients. However, few complete responses last longer than 12 months, and only rare patients are cured, results distinctly inferior to those seen in patients with de novo AML. Children with MDS appear to respond somewhat better to intensive chemotherapy than adults.

ACKNOWLEDGMENT

This work was supported, in part, by grant number CA-18029 from the National Cancer Institute, and by grant number HL36444 from the National Heart, Lung, and Blood Institute, National Institutes of Health, DHHS.

BIBLIOGRAPHY

Appelbaum FR, Anderson J. Allogeneic bone marrow transplantation for myelodysplastic syndrome: outcomes analysis according to IPSS score. *Leukemia* 1998;12(Suppl 1):S25–S29.

Beran M, Kantarjian H, O'Brien S, et al. Topotecan, a topoisomerase I inhibitor, is active in the treatment of myelodysplastic syndrome and chronic myelomonocytic leukemia. *Blood* 1996;88:2473–2479.

Estey E, Thall P, Beran M, et al. Effect of diagnosis (refractory anemia with excess blasts, refractory anemia with excess blasts in transformation, or acute myeloid leukemia [AML]) on outcome of AML-type chemotherapy. *Blood* 1997;90(8):2969–2977.

Greenberg P, Cox C, LeBeau MM, et al. International scoring system for evaluating prognosis in myelodysplastic syndromes. *Blood* 1997;89:2079–2088.

Hellström-Lindberg E. Efficacy of erythropoietin in the myelodysplastic syndromes: a meta-analysis of 205 patients from 17 studies. *Br J Haematol* 1995;89:67–71.

Mecucci C. Molecular features of primary MDS with cytogenetic changes. *Leukemia Res* 1998;22(4):293–302.

Miller KB, Kyungmann K, Morrison FS, et al. The evaluation of low-dose cytarabine in the treatment of myelodysplastic syndromes: a phase-III intergroup study. *Ann Hematol* 1992;65:162–168.

Silverman LR, Demakos EP, Peterson B, et al. A randomized controlled trial of subcutaneous azacitidine (aza c) in patients with the myelodysplastic syndrome (MDS): a study of the Cancer and Leukemia Group B (CALGB) [Abstract]. *Proc Am Soc Clin Oncol* 1998;17:14a.

Willman CL. Molecular genetic features of myelodysplastic syndromes (MDS). *Leukemia* 1998;12(Suppl 1):S2–S6.

CHAPTER 230

APLASTIC ANEMIA AND BONE MARROW FAILURE SYNDROMES

JOEL RAPPEPORT

APLASTIC ANEMIA

Aplastic anemia is a bone marrow failure syndrome characterized by pancytopenia of the peripheral blood and a hypocellular bone marrow devoid of the progenitors of all three hematopoietic cell lines. This condition results from a quantitative decrease in pluripotential stem cells. Aplastic anemia, which must be differentiated from other causes of pancytopenias, affects patients of all ages, may be constitutional or acquired, and is variable in severity.

INCIDENCE AND EPIDEMIOLOGY

The incidence of aplastic anemia is estimated to be two to six new cases per 1 million persons annually in the United States. The incidence appears to vary worldwide, with an increased rate in Asia. Whether the variation reflects different rates of exposure to known causes or different genetic predispositions is unclear. Patients of all ages and both sexes are affected. Most cases appear to be acquired, but approximately 50% have no identifiable cause and are classified as idiopathic. Well-defined autosomal recessive constitutional syndromes such as Fanconi's anemia are uncommon causes of aplastic anemia.

ETIOLOGY

The causes of up to 50% of aplastic anemia cases are difficult to define, but several drugs, toxins, and infections have been associated with acquired aplastic anemia (Table 230.1). Other drugs are suspected as causal agents but have a less certain association with aplastic anemia.

The antibiotic chloramphenicol may cause both dose-related marrow suppression and idiosyncratic aplastic anemia. The dose-related suppression is usually reversible, and the idiosyncratic disorder is usually irreversible, severe, and frequently fatal. The idiosyncratic reaction is estimated to occur in approximately 1 of 50,000 patients, with aplasia developing weeks to months after treatment. Most cases have been associated with oral administration, but a few cases have occurred with intravenous chloramphenicol. Although used infrequently in the United States, chloramphenicol is commonly used in developing nations. Other, seemingly unrelated, drugs that result in an idiosyncratic reaction include other antibiotics, anti-inflammatory agents, and antiseizure medications. Whether an agent may re-

TABLE 230.1.	CAUSES OF APLASTIC ANEMIA

Idiopathic conditions
Genetic disorders (e.g., Fanconi's anemia, dyskeratosis congenita)
Drugs
  Dose-related reversible aplasia
    Cyclophosphamide
    Anthracyclines
    Antimetabolites (e.g., nucleotide analogues, folic acid antagonists)
    Antimitotics
    Epipodophyllotoxins
    Platinum-containing agents
    Chloramphenicol
  Dose-related irreversible aplasia
    Busulfan
    Nitrosureas
    Phenylalanine mustard
    Thiotepa
  Idiosyncratic
    Chloramphenicol
    Sulfonamides (e.g., antibiotic, antidiabetic, antithyroid)
    Anti-inflammatory agents (e.g., phenlybutazone, indomethacin)
    Gold
    Antiseizure agents (e.g., hydantoin derivatives, carbamazepine, felbamate)
    Penicillamine
    Allopurinol
Environmental toxins
  Benzene
  Toluene
  Insecticides
  Arsenic
Ionizing radiation
Infection
  Hepatitis (hepatitis A, B, and non-A, non-B, non-C)
  Epstein–Barr virus
Pregnancy
Paroxysmal nocturnal hemoglobinuria
Immunologically mediated conditions
  Systemic lupus erythematosus
  Diffuse eosinophilic fasciitis
  Rheumatoid arthritis

sult in dose-related aplasia or an idiosyncratic reaction is often unclear.

Most chemotherapeutic agents result in a severe pancytopenia and aplastic bone marrow, but with the exception of a few agents given in high doses, this process is reversible within a finite time. Chemotherapeutic drugs have a cumulative effect on hematopoiesis, and combination chemotherapy can have an additive effect.

Several viral infections have been associated with the development of aplastic anemia. The most common infection is non-A, non-B, non-C hepatitis, although some cases have been reported after hepatitis B and hepatitis A. A few severe cases have been reported after Epstein–Barr virus infections.

A variety of environmental toxins have been associated with aplastic anemia. These include benzenes, toluenes, arsenicals, and insecticides. Benzenes and other hydrocarbons are widely used in industrialized societies. Other hematologic effects develop secondary to benzenes. The development of aplastic anemia seems to be dose related, although there is individual susceptibility to these agents. Both industrial and home exposures should be sought.

PATHOPHYSIOLOGY

Aplastic anemia results from various pathophysiologic processes affecting the pluripotential stem cell. The primary defect is an absence of pluripotential hematopoietic stem cells. This concept is supported by the facts that all hematopoietic cell lines are affected, the bone marrow is morphologically empty, all committed progenitors are decreased, and the simple infusion of normal identical-twin bone marrow into unconditioned recipients results in hematopoietic reconstitution in 50% of patients.

"Damaged" pluripotential stem cells offer a second explanation. These cells are unable to differentiate and are functionally ineffective.

The third pathologic mechanism is a hostile microenvironment that may include structural defects of the marrow cavity stroma, decreased production of marrow-stimulating cytokines, or the development of an autoimmune antihematopoietic stem cell process. A defect in the supporting stroma probably occurs infrequently, given the high rate of engraftment of transplanted marrow. Most identified cytokines are present in aplastic anemia patients in physiologic amounts. An autoimmune process that is at least partially responsible for the development of aplastic anemia is detected in a significant number of patients. In addition to a large body of laboratory evidence, an autoimmune process is evidenced by partial responses to immunosuppression in approximately 40% of cases.

CLINICAL PRESENTATION

Two types of clinical presentation occur, depending on the severity of pancytopenia. Some patients experience a gradual onset of signs and symptoms of anemia, including gradually increasing fatigue, dyspnea, and pallor. Laboratory evaluation demonstrates a variable, but often mild pancytopenia and a hypoplastic bone marrow. Some patients present with signs and symptoms of thrombocytopenia and leukopenia in addition to anemia. These patients may have the sudden onset of high-spiking fevers and spontaneous petechiae and ecchymosis predominantly on the lower extremities and in areas of pressure. In a more fulminant emergent form of the disorder, patients may have epistaxis, retinal hemorrhages, and sustained oral mucosal bleeding. Fever may begin abruptly or be recurrent and persistent. Except for petechiae, ecchymosis, and other evidence of spontaneous hemorrhage, the physical examination reveals few pathologic findings. Lymphadenopathy and splenomegaly are not part of the clinical manifestations. In the absence of adequate granulocytes, sites of infection may include necrotic ulcerations, particularly in the oral cavity. The findings of pneumonia may be minimal and subtle.

Patients with Fanconi's aplastic anemia often have a variety of somatic abnormalities on physical examination, including absent radii, abnormalities of the thumbs, café au lait spots, and microcephaly. Dyskeratosis congenita, an ectodermal dysplasia, is associated with a reticular hyperpigmentation of the neck, face, and shoulders and with dystrophy of the nails and leukoplakia. Although both syndromes classically manifest in childhood, aplasia may begin in young adulthood. The diagnosis of these disorders is important, because the therapeutic options vary from those for acquired aplastic anemia.

LABORATORY FINDINGS

The laboratory findings in aplastic anemia include pancytopenia and a hypocellular bone marrow revealed by bone marrow biopsy. Aplastic anemia is classified as a normochromic, normocytic anemia, although some patients have macrocytosis. Residual leukocytes are morphologically normal, but the number and size of platelets are decreased. The reticulocyte count also is inappropriately decreased. The bone marrow reveals decreased hematopoiesis, and in its severe form, only a few lymphocytes, plasma cells, and mast cells may be evident. The bone marrow is replaced by fat, but without other apparent causes of pancytopenia. At examination, the different cell lines may be variably affected, and in some patients, a small amount of erythropoiesis may be evident. The iron-binding capacity is usually fully saturated, and an iron stain of the bone marrow reveals normal to increased iron stores.

Previously, the term *hypoplastic anemia* was differentiated from aplastic anemia and used to describe mild pancytopenia and hypocellularity of the marrow. Aplastic anemia is currently defined as mild or severe, based on the severity of the pancytopenia and the degree of cellularity of the bone marrow (Table 230.2). Patients with mild aplasia (not meeting the criteria in Table 230.2) may have a prolonged course or a complete spontaneous recovery. They may also degenerate into a severe aplastic anemia. Patients with severe aplastic anemia have only a 15% to 20% chance of spontaneous recovery and are likely to have a fulminate course with early death without successful treatment.

Laboratory evaluation should include studies that attempt to identify the possible cause of the aplasia, including tests for paroxysmal nocturnal hemoglobinuria, systemic lupus erythematosus, hepatitis, infectious mononucleosis, and pregnancy in females of childbearing age. Cytogenetic analysis should attempt

TABLE 230.2.	CHARACTERISTICS OF SEVERE APLASTIC ANEMIA

Peripheral Blood Values

All three of the following or two of three plus bone marrow criteria:
   Absolute neutrophil count of <500/mm³
   Untransfused platelet count of <20,000/mm³
   Reticulocyte count (corrected for hematocrit) of <1%

Bone Marrow

Markedly hypocellular bone marrow (<25% normal cellularity)
Moderately hypocellular bone marrow (25% to 50% normal cellularity) with <30 hematopoietic cells

Progressive Decline in Blood Counts During the First 3 Months

to identify patients with hypocellular myelodysplastic syndrome and those patients with underlying chromosomal fragility states such as Fanconi's aplastic anemia. Flow cytometry enhances identification of an underlying paroxysmal nocturnal hemoglobinuria and abnormal lymphocyte subsets. The evaluation of a congenital disorder should include x-ray films of the hands, wrists, and kidneys. Unfortunately, no reliable tests exist to determine the presence of environmental toxins.

Further laboratory testing is needed for patient treatment. Complete erythrocyte typing should be established before transfusion. The patient's cytomegalovirus history should be determined serologically to provide appropriate transfusion products and to determine an appropriate hematopoietic stem cell transplant donor. Immediate human leukocyte antigen (HLA) typing of the patient and family should be undertaken to determine the availability of a potential sibling transplant donor. On rare occasions, a parent may be a suitable donor. Typing should include serologic typing for HLA-A, HLA-B, and HLA-DR. If a search for an unrelated donor is to be pursued, molecular typing for HLA-DR should also be performed.

OPTIMAL MANAGEMENT

Treatment for aplastic anemia involves general supportive management and specific treatment, both of which are determined by the clinical scenario and the severity of the aplastic anemia. Exposure to possible causal agents should be eliminated. Drugs that interfere with platelet function should be avoided. Women of childbearing age should have their menses suppressed, and in cases of menorrhagia, control of menses may require platelet transfusion and aggressive pharmacologic therapy. Because of the need for frequent blood drawing and infusions, an assessment of vascular access may suggest the placement of indwelling lines. Patients with low neutrophil counts should avoid exposure to potential infectious pathogens. Fever and potential infection should be managed promptly and aggressively. For the patient with mild aplastic anemia, no further treatment may be required except for anticipatory clinical and laboratory observation. About 20% of patients with severe aplasia may have spontaneous recoveries within 3 to 6 weeks (Table 230.3).

Transfusions should be administered judiciously. Erythrocyte transfusions should be based on both the hematocrit and the clinical features. Young patients often tolerate hematocrit values that are in the low teens, but older patients may become symptomatic at higher levels. Platelets should also be transfused on the basis of the count and the clinical evaluation. Active bleeding, particularly in the region of the head, should be treated promptly with platelet transfusions, especially if the count is less than 20,000 per cubic millimeter. Prophylactic platelets need not be administered until the platelet count is less than 5,000 to 10,000 cubic millimeter. Transfusions should be leukocyte depleted, and family-derived transfusions should be avoided if a family-derived stem cell transplant is being considered. The cytomegalovirus antibody–negative patient should receive blood products from cytomegalovirus antibody–negative donors. In the event of a suboptimal response, nonimmunologic causes should be

TABLE 230.3.	TREATMENT OF APLASTIC ANEMIA

Initial Approach
Elimination of any potential causative agents
Assessment of severity of aplastic anemia
Rapid evaluation of potential therapeutic maneuvers
Careful and frequent serial medical and laboratory evaluation
Observation of mild aplasia

Supportive Care
Judicious transfusion support
Prevention of infection
Suppression of menses in females of childbearing age
Aggressive and prompt evaluation and treatment of fever and hemorrhage
Chelation therapy

Definitive Treatment
Hematopoietic stimulation
  Androgens
  Cytokines
Immunosuppression
  Antithymocyte globulin
  High-dose corticosteroids
  Cyclosporine
Bone marrow transplantation
  HLA-identical family member
  Matched unrelated donor

HLA, human leukocyte antigen.

evaluated. With alloimmunization, HLA-compatible transfusions should be attempted. Long-term transfusion-dependent patients may develop transfusional hemosiderosis, requiring iron chelation with desferrioxamine. Early transfusion therapy may influence the ultimate outcome of a subsequent hematopoietic stem cell transplantation.

Specific therapy for aplastic anemia includes marrow stimulation, immunosuppression, and hematopoietic stem cell transplantation. Although some patients with severe aplastic anemia respond to androgen therapy, studies have revealed no statistically significant response rate. However, patients with mild aplasia may often respond. Several cytokines have been tested in patients with severe aplastic anemia, and there is no evidence that patients have recovered with this therapy. However, some patients with neutropenia have a temporary response to the administration of granulocyte colony-stimulating factor or granulocyte-macrophage colony-stimulating factor, and these should be tried in cases of life-threatening infection and severe neutropenia. These agents do not affect erythroid or platelet production. Studies of other hematopoietic-stimulating cytokines singularly and in combination and concurrently being administered with immunosuppressive agents are under investigation.

Immunosuppressive therapy improves the hematologic status of approximately 40% to 50% of patients with severe aplastic anemia, although only a small percentage of patients appears to have a complete response. This therapy consists of antithymocyte globulin, high-dose corticosteroids, high-dose cyclophosphamide, and cyclosporine. More favorable and complete responses have been achieved in patients receiving a combination of immunosuppressive agents. Responses may take as long as 12 weeks, and the patient often requires interim transfusion support. Long-term follow-up reveals that a significant number of patients may develop recurrences, a myelodysplastic syndrome or acute leukemia, or paroxysmal nocturnal hemoglobinuria. These complications are probably not the result of the therapy; they result from the long-term persistence of damaged hematopoietic stem cells. It is not clear whether these patients normalize their survival.

Because the most common pathophysiologic defect is functionally absent hematopoietic stem cells, the most logical treatment of severe aplasia is hematopoietic stem cell transplantation. The factors limiting broad application of marrow grafting are identification of an appropriate donor and transplant-related complications. If typing identifies an HLA-identical sibling donor, the primary therapy for younger patients with severe aplasia should be hematopoietic stem cell transplantation. For previously untransfused patients 18 years of age and younger, the long-term survival rate is 80%. Although the cure rate decreases to approximately 30% for older patients, hematopoietic stem cell transplantation should be considered as primary therapy for patients younger than 40 to 45 years of age. Because of the poorer results of transplantation in older patients, a trial of immunosuppression should be considered as initial treatment. The choice of primary treatment is extremely important, because an adequate trial of immunosuppression places the patient at risk of requiring transfusion support and developing a life-threatening infection, and transplantation complications may result in death.

Frequent complications of hematopoietic stem cell transplantation for aplastic anemia are graft failure, with either failure to achieve primary engraftment or subsequent graft rejection. In an HLA-identical donor and recipient, this immunologic rejection results from minor non-HLA transplantation antigen differences. Adequate immunosuppression must be achieved with the preparative regimen. Patients of any age with a normal identical twin should undergo hematopoietic stem cell transplantation. However, even in this circumstance, immunosuppressive preparation may be necessary in 50% of patients. HLA-identical sibling donors are identified for 35% to 40% of patients. Although donors matching at five of six HLA antigens can serve as marrow donors for patients with malignant disorders, the success rate in those with aplastic anemia is less favorable. Similarly, hematopoietic stem cell transplantation with matched unrelated donors has been less successful in aplastic anemia patients than in those with malignant disorders. Umbilical cord blood transplantations have been successful. Without a matched family donor, consideration should be given to immunosuppression as the initial therapy.

Patients with genetic aplastic anemia have different therapeutic options. These patients often have primary responses to androgen treatment, but immunosuppressive therapy is unlikely to be successful. Transplantation in this setting has its own preparative regimens and features. The long-term course of these patients is complicated by the development of a variety of malignancies.

PURE RED CELL APLASIA

Pure red cell aplasia (PRCA) is a selective bone marrow failure syndrome uniquely involving erythroid production. The disorder involves a normocytic normochromic anemia, usually with normal leukocyte and platelet production. The patient has a severe reticulocytopenia, with virtual absence of erythroid precursors in the bone marrow. This disorder may be genetic or acquired, and acquired forms may be primary or secondary.

INCIDENCE AND EPIDEMIOLOGY

Congenital red cell aplasia (Diamond–Blackfan syndrome) is a rare disorder with autosomal dominant and recessive patterns of inheritance. Ninety-five percent of patients with this syndrome present by 2 years of age; some may present as late as 6 years of age. Diamond–Blackfan anemia may be associated with a variety of skeletal anomalies. This disorder must be differentiated from transient erythropenia of childhood.

PRCA is rare in adults, although transient red cell aplasia may be associated with a variety of infections, including B19 parvovirus, especially in the setting of stress erythropoiesis. PRCA of adults occurs equally in both sexes and most commonly in middle age.

PRCA may be a primary or secondary process. In adult PRCA, the major identifiable cause is thymoma, occurring in approximately 30% to 50% of patients. Approximately 5% of patients with thymoma develop PRCA. However, the disorder is also associated with a variety of lymphoproliferative disorders and autoimmune disorders such as systemic lupus erythematosus or rheumatoid arthritis. Approximately 5% of patients with chronic lymphocytic leukemia develop PRCA. Other associations include AIDS, viral hepatitis, nonhematologic solid tumors, and a variety of drugs, including α-methyldopa, chloramphenicol, diphenylhydantoin, isoniazid, and phenylbutazone.

PATHOGENESIS AND PATHOPHYSIOLOGY

The major pathophysiologic mechanism in PRCA involves a cellular or antibody autoimmune process directed against erythropoietin, erythropoietin-responsive cells, or erythroblasts. The cellular processes may be inhibitory or cytotoxic. In cases of thymoma, erythroid-suppressive thymic cells migrate to the marrow. Drug-associated PRCA may result from direct toxic effects of the drugs or from drug-associated immune suppression.

CLINICAL FINDINGS

The major clinical symptom of PRCA is progressive fatigue resulting from the anemia. The major physical finding is pallor. The disorder is not associated with organomegaly or lymphadenopathy unless it is associated with underlying precipitating conditions.

LABORATORY FINDINGS

The major findings in patients with PRCA are a normochromic, normocytic anemia and a reticulocyte count less than 1% and often zero. The platelet and leukocyte counts are usually normal. The serum iron is elevated, with saturation of the iron-binding capacity. The bone marrow is usually normocellular, with normal numbers of myeloid cells and megakaryocytes but lacking erythroid precursor cells. Occasionally, a small increase in lymphocytes occurs. A CT scan of the chest may demonstrate a thymoma. Laboratory investigations should include a search for underlying disorders, including immune system abnormalities, hepatitis, B19 parvovirus, AIDS, and myasthenia gravis.

OPTIMAL MANAGEMENT

The major supportive therapy for these patients is erythrocyte transfusions to remedy the absence of red cell production. In patients with refractory PRCA, long-term transfusions inevitably lead to transfusion siderosis, with damage primarily to the heart, liver, and pancreas. Patients should be periodically evaluated for their iron status, and, when appropriate, they should be considered for early chelation therapy before the development of organ dysfunction.

All possible offending drugs should be immediately eliminated; in such cases, resolution occurs within a few weeks. If thymoma is the underlying problem, thymectomy should be performed. In an inoperable situation, irradiation of the thymoma has also been effective. Thymectomy has not been effective in patients without thymomas. If an underlying malignancy is identified, therapy should be directed to this disorder. Persistent parvovirus infection often responds to intravenous γ-globulin infusions.

Immunosuppressive therapy should be carefully attempted in the patient with persistent PRCA, usually beginning with corticosteroids. If a response is not achieved, other immunosuppressive therapies, such as cyclophosphamide, azathioprine, antithymocyte globulin, and cyclosporine or combinations of these therapies, have induced responses. After the patient achieves adequate reticulocyte production and a sustained hematocrit, attempts should be made to decrease or discontinue therapy. Approximately 80% of patients have spontaneous or therapy-induced responses, although relapses occur.

BIBLIOGRAPHY

Brodsky RA, Sensenbrennen LL, Jones RJ. Complete remission in severe aplastic anemia after high-dose cyclophosphamide without bone marrow transplantation. *Blood* 1996;87:491–494.

Frickhofen N, Kaltwasser JP, Schrezenmeier H, et al. Treatment of aplastic anemia with antilymphocyte globulin and methylprednisolone with or without cyclosporine. *N Engl J Med* 1991;324:1297–1304.

Gluckman E, Esperou-Bourdeau H, Baruchel A, et al. Multicenter randomized study comparing cyclosporin A alone and antithymocyte globulin with prednisone for treatment of severe aplastic anemia. *Blood* 1992; 79:2540–2546.

Gluckman E, Horowitz MM, Champlin RE, et al. Bone marrow transplantation for severe aplastic anemia: influence of conditioning and graft-versus-host disease prophylaxis regimens on outcome. *Blood* 1992;79: 269–275.

Kohli-Kumar M, Morris C, DeLaat C, et al. Bone marrow transplantation in Fanconi anemia using matched sibling donors. *Blood* 1994;84: 2050–2054.

Krantz SB. Acquired pure red cell aplasia. In: Hoffman R, Benz EJ, Shattil SJ, et al, eds. *Hematology: basic principles and practice.* New York: Churchill Livingstone, 1995:350–361.

Young N. The pathogenesis and pathophysiology of aplastic anemia. In: Hoffman R, Benz EJ, Shattil SJ, et al, eds. *Hematology: basic principles and practice.* New York: Churchill Livingstone, 1995:299–336.

Young NS, Alter BP. *Aplastic anemia: acquired and inherited.* Philadelphia: WB Saunders, 1994.

Kelley's Textbook of Internal Medicine, fourth edition. Edited by H. David Humes. Lippincott Williams & Wilkins, Philadelphia © 2000.

CHAPTER

231

MYELOPROLIFERATIVE DISORDERS: POLYCYTHEMIA VERA, THROMBOCYTHEMIA, AND MYELOFIBROSIS

EUGENE P. FRENKEL

The term "myeloproliferative" encompasses a group of disorders linked by common clinical and laboratory features resulting from an autonomous clonal proliferation of a multipotential stem cell that produces a generalized expansion of all of the bone marrow elements. The clinical nomenclature delineates subtypes based on the predominant peripheral blood expression of the autonomous hyperplastic marrow response: polycythemia vera (PV) indicates a proliferation of red cells; chronic myelogenous leukemia, white cells; myelofibrosis, extramedullary hematopoiesis; and primary or essential thrombocythemia, platelets.

The generic term myeloproliferative disorder is clinically useful, although it denotes our lack of understanding of the mechanisms through which growth control is lost as well as the absence of absolute marrow histologic criteria. It is especially appropriately applied to some patients for whom the specific peripheral phenotypic expression of the panmyelosis has not yet become clear. The term also suggests that transition from one type to another may occur.

Neoplastic transformation of the pluripotential stem cell is a multistep process. Events confer a growth advantage for this clone over those normally regulated in the marrow, and subsequent events provide further selective proliferation and amplification of a cell lineage-specific population (e.g., red cells in polycythemia). Because the molecular biologic, cytogenetic, and signal mechanisms have been characterized for chronic myelogenous leukemia (Chapter 228), it is appropriate to separate it from the more generic group described in the subsequent sections.

POLYCYTHEMIA VERA

PV is an autonomous clonal proliferation of a multipotential stem cell that results in a generalized hyperplasia (panmyelosis)

TABLE 231.1.	CRITERIA FOR THE DIAGNOSIS OF POLYCYTHEMIA VERA PROPOSED BY THE POLYCYTHEMIA VERA STUDY GROUP (PVSG)[a]

A1	Raised red cell mass Male > 36 mL/kg Female > 32 mL/kg	B1	Thrombocytosis Platelet count > 400 × 10⁹/L
A2	Normal arterial oxygen saturation >92%	B2	Leukocytosis > 12 × 10⁹/L and no fever or infection
A3	Splenomegaly on palpation	B3	Raised neutrophil alkaline phosphatase score > 100 or raised B_{12} (>900 ng/L) or raised unsaturated B_{12} binding capacity (>2,200 ng/L)

Diagnosis of PV is acceptable if the following combinations are present: A1 + A2 + A3 or A1 + A2 + any two from category B

The Rotterdam Criteria of Polycythemia Vera Proposed by the Thrombocythemia Vera Study Group (TVSG)[b]

A1	Raised red cell mass Male >36 mL/kg Female >32 mL/kg	B1	Thrombocytosis Platelet count >400 × 10⁹/L
A2	Absence of any cause of secondary erythrocytosis by clinical and laboratory investigations	B2	Granulocytosis >10 × 10⁹/L and/or raised neutrophil alkaline phosphatase score of >100 in the absence of fever or infection
A3	Histopathology of bone marrow biopsy increase of: Cellularity, panmyelosis Enlarged megakaryocytes with hyperploid nuclei Reticulin fibers (optional)	B3	Splenomegaly on palpation or isotope/ultrasound
		B4	Erythroid colony formation in absence of EPO: spontaneous EEC

A1 + A2 + A3 is consistent with early stage PV ("idiopathic erythrocytosis")
A1 + A2 + A3 + any one from category B establishes overt polycythemia vera
A3 + B1 is consistent with essential thrombocythemia
A3 + B3 and/or B4 is consistent with a primary myeloproliferative disorder

EPO, erythropoietin; EEC, EPO-independent erythroid colonies.
[a] (Adapted from Berlin NI. Diagnosis and classification of the polycythemias. *Semin Hematol* 1975;12:338.)
[b] (Adapted from Michiels JJ, Juvonen E. Proposal for revised diagnostic criteria of essential thrombocythemia and polycythemia vera by the thrombocythemia vera study group. *Semin Thromb Hemat* 1997;23:339.)

of the bone marrow, increased production of red blood cells (RBCs), and an absolute increase in the numbers of circulating RBCs. The term *vera* implies that the erythron expansion occurs without an identifiable mechanism, separating it from nonautonomous causes of RBC production. The diagnostic criteria for PV developed by the Polycythemia Study Group are delineated in Table 231.1. The American criteria were affected by the belief that bone marrow examination was nonspecific. During recent years, a European consortium has reexamined these criteria and emphasized the bone marrow morphologic findings of megakaryocyte clustering and hyperploid nuclei. In addition, a classic finding in PV is spontaneous erythroid colony growth with no erythropoietin (EPO). Their diagnostic criteria are also shown in Table 231.1.

EPIDEMIOLOGY

The annual incidence of PV in the United States is about 5 cases per 1 million persons. It is diagnosed most often in persons between 50 and 70 years of age, although it occurs in all age groups. A slight male predominance (1.2: 1) exists, but a previously reported predilection for Jews of European extraction has not been confirmed. No other epidemiologic factors have been defined.

PATHOGENESIS

Neither the pathogenetic mechanisms nor the molecular biologic events in PV are known. The clonal origin of the acquired muta-

tion of the multipotential hematopoietic stem cell has been firmly established by isoenzyme characterization, clonogenic assays, and cytogenetic analysis. Cytogenetic abnormalities found in 12% of patients at diagnosis include trisomy 8, trisomy 9, and deletion of the long arm of chromosome 20 [del(20)(q12)]. The trisomy 8 is common in PV patients around the world, but the geographic distribution of the other genetic changes is not uniform. The molecular correlates of these pathogenic changes are unknown. Chromosomal evolution occurs during the course of the disease; but, the chromosomal abnormalities do not correlate with the clinical course, nor do they predict survival or leukemic transformation.

Clonal panmyelosis is a hallmark of all the myeloproliferative disorders. In PV, the process is exhibited through an unknown perturbation of the multipotential stem cell that results in selective proliferation and amplification of RBCs. Studies of cellular mosaicism and erythroid colony growth have shown the existence of normal and neoplastic multipotential stem cells and progenitors in the marrow early in the disease. Subsequent amplification of the neoplastic clone results in decreased production from the normal clones, especially beyond the erythroid burstforming stage. Their growth appears relatively independent of erythropoietin, and the receptor structure, binding, and internalization are normal. The thrombopoietin receptor (Mpl) is absent or markedly reduced in platelets and megakaryocytes in patients with PV. Because thrombopoietin inhibits apoptosis, its dysfunction may result in a defect in programmed cell death with resultant cellular accumulation providing a mechanism for expansion of the erythron.

CLINICAL FINDINGS

The early clinical findings in PV result from the expanded RBC mass; however, during the disease course, several clinical stages evolve and manifest different features.

The *preerythrocytic* or *inapparent phase* of PV is often unrecognized, and the signs and symptoms of this developmental stage are commonly insidious. During this phase, the circulating RBC mass has not yet increased, and only splenomegaly or pruritus after bathing may be noticed. Occasionally, mild thrombohemorrhagic symptoms or erythromelalgia (painful, burning erythematous palms and soles) occur. This phase lasts for a few months to 1 or 2 years. Portal vein thrombosis, particularly with isolated splenomegaly, is a significant clinical event. The diagnostic complex is normal hematocrit, a low serum EPO, and evidence of spontaneous erythroid colony growth with no EPO.

The classic picture of PV is seen in the *erythrocytic phase,* often first recognized because of an occlusive arterial or venous lesion, such as cerebral or myocardial infarction or ischemia, portal venous obstruction, or peripheral venous thrombosis. The expanded RBC mass produces symptoms of hyperviscosity, and the reduced cerebral blood flow can result in headaches, dizziness, and visual disturbances. Plethora and conjunctival or oral mucosal suffusion are common. Some patients present with hemorrhagic phenomena, usually affecting the mucosa or skin in the form of epistaxis, gastrointestinal or genitourinary bleeding, or ecchymosis. Bleeding sufficient to result in normal or low RBC values may obscure the underlying condition and confuse the diagnosis. Gastrointestinal symptoms and peptic ulcer disease also occur with increased frequency in this patient population.

Splenomegaly is the most common physical finding, identified in almost 90% of these patients; hepatomegaly occurs in about 50%. Episodes of acute gout associated with overproduction of urate may occur in 5%, and gout is occasionally the presenting complaint. With therapy, the erythrocytic phase may last 5 to 20 years.

In time, significant thrombocytosis occurs, frequently accompanied by renewed thrombohemorrhagic signs and symptoms; this change identifies the *proliferative phase* of PV. Asymptomatic leukocytosis is usually a feature of this phase, and increasing splenomegaly is common. The proliferative phase usually lasts a few years.

Subsequent evolution into the *postpolycythemic myeloid metaplasia phase* is gradual and occurs in 20% of patients. The median time to conversion is about 10 years. Asthenia is the most common symptom. Weight loss and generalized wasting, with clinical features of myelofibrosis, develop during this phase. Progressive splenomegaly occurs with increasing anemia and hemorrhagic findings. Extramedullary hematopoiesis in lymphoid sites may produce pressure symptoms in the gastrointestinal, respiratory, or central nervous system. Most patients in this phase have a shortened survival, dying of clinical complica-

tions, or the disease evolves to acute leukemia within 3 years, conferring an equally poor prognosis.

A small subset of patients undergo transition to a leukemic phase, producing the typical picture of acute nonlymphocytic leukemia. Such progression is most common (25% to 50%) in those who develop myeloid metaplasia. As in most secondary leukemias, therapy rarely produces durable remissions, and the survival is short.

LABORATORY FINDINGS

PV is usually recognized by an increase in the RBC count, hemoglobin concentration, and hematocrit. Early in the disease, the RBCs are of normal size. Because mucosal bleeding is common, iron deficiency frequently ensues, and RBC microcytosis develops. A low RBC mean corpuscular volume (less than 80 fL) with normal RBC values on presentation of a patient with recent blood loss is suggestive of PV.

Thrombocytosis (platelet count greater than 450,000 per microliter) is often seen at the time of the patient's initial diagnosis. Platelet size heterogeneity is common, as evidenced by the increased mean platelet volume, asymmetric histograms, or examination of the peripheral smear. Megakaryocytic hyperplasia, increased platelet production rate, and shortened platelet survival are found. Platelet functional abnormalities are common, and these correlate with an increased thrombohemorrhagic phenomena.

Leukocytosis, primarily granulocytosis with increased numbers of basophils, is seen in almost 50% of patients at diagnosis. There is increased granulocyte production, an increase in leukocyte alkaline phosphatase activity, and the production of cobalamin-binding proteins, which results in increased serum B_{12} levels.

An absolute increase in the measured RBC mass, corrected for age, sex, and body surface area, is required for the diagnosis of PV. Measurement of the RBC mass is performed with radiochromate-tagged RBCs. As a consequence of the increase in the RBC mass, the whole blood viscosity is elevated in patients, and the incidence of vascular occlusive events relates to this increase.

The bone marrow is diffusely hypercellular (almost 100%), with an increase in all hematopoietic elements (panmyelosis) and an increase in clustered enlarged megakaryocytes with hyperploid nuclei and usually absent iron stores. Marrow reticulin fibers increase during the course of the disease.

Some of the laboratory changes correlate with clinical manifestations of the disease. Increased numbers of basophils, producing histamine or histamine-like substances, probably explain the postbathing pruritus. Hyperuricemia and clinical gout result from the increased cell turnover. The "spurious hyperkalemia" resulting from potassium released from the increased numbers of qualitatively defective platelets is common and can confuse laboratory results.

Three other aspects of laboratory evaluation merit emphasis. First, although cytogenetic analysis has not identified any specific nonrandom change, trisomy 8, trisomy 9, or deletion of the long arm of chromosome 20 can be detected in about 12% of untreated cases. Second, serum erythropoietin levels are reduced

Third, the demonstration of erythropoietin-independent erythroid colonies in vitro is diagnostic.

As PV progresses to the later phases, other laboratory features become evident. Leukoerythroblastosis (abnormal-shaped and nucleated RBCs and immature white cells) occurs with progressive anemia and thrombocytopenia, and marrow fibrosis develops during the postpolycythemic myeloid metaplasia phase. Patients who enter the leukemic phase have laboratory and cytogenetic findings characteristic of a secondary type of acute leukemia.

DIAGNOSIS

The criteria for the diagnosis of PV are shown in Table 231.1. Established by the Polycythemia Study Group in 1967, these criteria have provided consistent parameters for the evaluation of the disease course and of responses in therapeutic trials. The recent modifications of these criteria by the European investigators are also shown.

OPTIMAL MANAGEMENT

The survival of patients with PV changed remarkably with the advent of treatment. Median survival without therapy was 18 months, but the median survival is 8.9 years for patients treated with an alkylating agent, 11.8 years with radiophosphorus therapy, and 13.9 years with phlebotomy alone. Appropriate therapy results in survival times approaching those expected for age-matched controls.

The changing clinical features that characterize the evolving phases of PV require different therapeutic approaches. In the preerythrocytic phase, when pruritus is a common symptom, histamine H_2 antagonists (e.g., 300 mg of cimetidine administered three times daily) in combination with an H_1 blocker (e.g., 4 mg of cyproheptadine three times daily or 10 mg of astemizole daily) are effective. Recombinant interferon-α (rIFN-α) has been effective at pruritus control where other measures have failed.

The excellent median survival rate accomplished with phlebotomy therapy alone had established this as the treatment of choice during the erythrocytic phase. Unfortunately, thrombotic events are common during the first 2 to 3 years of phlebotomy therapy. Alternate approaches now commonly instituted include hydroxyurea and, more recently, rIFN-α. These latter are particularly important in patients with a history of thrombotic events or in the elderly (particularly if obese or diabetic) in whom there is an enhanced risk of thrombosis with phlebotomy. Phlebotomy is still an important part of the maintenance program. Initially, antiplatelet agents, such as aspirin, were considered hazardous; recent results have led to the addition of low-dose aspirin. Clearly, however, the risk of thrombosis is best controlled by maintaining the hematocrit under 45.

Hyperuricemia should be managed with daily allopurinol. The iron deficiency secondary to phlebotomy does not merit therapy, because iron replacement encourages further expansion of the RBC mass.

For younger patients with a high phlebotomy requirement (more than 6 units per year) or for anyone with significant prolif-

erative features (e.g., thrombocytosis, splenomegaly), myelosuppressive therapy is indicated. Hydroxyurea, has been the drug of choice, although recent data have defined an emerging therapeutic role for rIFN-α. The typical dosage for hydroxyurea is 10 to 15 mg per kilogram per day, administered with the goal of maintaining the hematocrit below 50% and the platelet count below 650,000 per microliter. Dosage adjustments may be required—downward for the development of cytopenias or upward for inadequate control. Most patients achieve excellent control within 12 weeks of beginning therapy. Uncommonly, hydroxyurea has been associated with painful refractory leg ulcers requiring its cessation. In addition, it is now evident that hydroxyurea does not protect against the leukemic transformation prevalent in the era of radiophosphorus therapy nor does it delay emergence of myelofibrosis. It is associated with approximately a 10% leukemic conversion by the tenth year. For these reasons, rIFN-α (3 million U three times per week; increased to 6 million per dose at 3 months if suppression is inadequate) has been used. It has been successful at myelosuppression in controlling pruritus and reducing spleen size. Its long-term efficacy relative to transformation is uncertain.

For patients in whom persistent thrombocytosis is a major problem, anagrelide, an imidazoquinazolin compound, is effective in reducing platelet numbers by interference with megakaryocyte maturation. In clinical trials, it was effective at a daily dose of 0.5 to 3 mg and produced little toxicity; it appears to be nonmutagenic and nonleukemogenic.

Therapy during postpolycythemic myeloid metaplasia is supportive. Erythropoietin has reduced the transfusion requirement. Symptomatic extramedullary tumors respond well to radiation therapy. Recurrent painful splenic infarctions or symptomatic congestive splenomegaly may require splenectomy. Allogeneic HLA-matched bone marrow or peripheral stem cell transplantation has been successful for patients under the age of 55. The transition to leukemia, as with the development of other secondary leukemias, is associated with a poor response to therapy.

Surgery is a special problem in PV. Untreated patients have significant operative morbidity and mortality, but these risks decline to normal when the elevated RBC values are reduced to normal and remain stable before surgery.

■ PRIMARY THROMBOCYTHEMIA

Primary thrombocythemia, often called *essential thrombocythemia,* is an autonomous clonal proliferation of a multipotential stem cell that results in marrow panhyperplasia, increased platelet production, and an increased number of circulating platelets. The diagnostic criteria are shown in Table 231.2. By definition, all secondary causes of increased platelet numbers, such as infection, trauma, and splenectomy, are absent. The controversial issue focuses on the number of platelets that makes up the primary parameter. The Polycythemia Vera Study Group in the United States had used 650,000 per microliter and the European Thrombocythemia Vera Study Group has used 400,000 per microliter; the reasonable rationale of the latter has focused on counts that are above normal, where other mechanisms have been excluded. Because the clinical correlates of thrombohemor-

TABLE 231.2.	DIAGNOSTIC CRITERIA FOR PRIMARY (ESSENTIAL) THROMBOCYTHEMIA

Platelet count greater than 450 × 10⁹/L (confirmed on more than one occasion)
Absence of an identifiable cause for the increased platelet counts
Absence of a myelodysplastic syndrome or other myeloproliferative state
Bone marrow with:
  Megakaryocytic hyperplasia
  Fibrosis less than 1/3 of marrow cross-section
Ancillary supportive criteria:
1. Splenomegaly
2. In vitro: spontaneous megakaryocyte colony formation

rhagic manifestations only weakly relate to the absolute platelet numbers, the approach of the European groups appear appropriate.

EPIDEMIOLOGY

Incidence data and epidemiologic characterization do not exist for primary thrombocythemia. Most reported clinical series have a predominance of women.

PATHOGENESIS

Neither the pathogenic mechanisms nor the molecular biologic events are known. The clonal origin of the stem cell has been established by isoenzyme (glucose-6-phosphate dehydrogenase) distribution in heterozygotes. Using X-chromosome inactivation analysis of women with the appropriate diagnostic parameters, it is now evident that many patients are polyclonal. No consistent cytogenetic abnormalities have been identified. The net mass of megakaryocytes is increased, and the increased platelet production does not respond to the usual regulatory mechanisms. The autonomous proliferation of megakaryocytes increases the megakaryocytic volume, the reverse of reactive thrombocytosis, in which megakaryocytic volume decreases with increased platelet numbers. Unlike PV, the thrombopoietin receptor expression is normal.

CLINICAL FINDINGS

A significant but unknown percentage of patients with primary thrombocythemia are asymptomatic and are identified by an increased platelet count during a routine blood study. Thrombohemorrhagic symptoms and findings are the classic manifestations. It appears that the polyclonal patients may have fewer thrombotic events than the monoclonal ones. Mucosal bleeding is most common, followed by arterial and venous vascular thromboses that produce the variety of symptoms and signs expected with a vascular occlusion. Headaches and neurologic findings due to microvascular occlusions and Budd–Chiari syndrome are particularly prominent clinical problems. The only physical finding directly related to primary thrombocythemia is splenomegaly, which is detected in 20% of patients. Erythromel-

algia, a characteristic thrombotic complication that results in red, swollen, burning painful extremities, also occurs.

LABORATORY FINDINGS

The criteria for diagnosis are shown in Table 231.2. The primary diagnostic laboratory finding is a persistent elevation of the platelet count in the absence of a definable reactive cause, such as blood loss, splenectomy, cancer, chronic infectious or inflammatory states, or drugs. Large, atypical platelets and a measurable platelet functional defect are common. Pseudohyperkalemia and an elevated uric acid level are detected. Bone marrow examination reveals classic panmyelosis and clusters of mature megakaryocytes.

OPTIMAL MANAGEMENT

Therapy is directed toward reduction of platelet numbers. Hydroxyurea (approximately 10 to 15 mg per kilogram per day) has commonly been used. It can produce painful leg ulcers requiring its discontinuation. More complex and unsettled is its role in the uncommon leukemic transformation. An alternative is rIFN-α, which is successful in approximately 70% of patients, but durable control off therapy is uncommon. Control usually requires 5 million units per day, and maintenance requires 1 to 2 million units per day, making this therapy expensive and subject to the symptoms associated with interferon therapy.

Anagrelide is an alternative therapy. It is highly effective in reducing platelet numbers in patients with primary thrombocythemia and in other myeloproliferative disorders; the average daily oral dose is 0.5 to 3.0 mg. In acute or severe evolving thrombotic or hemorrhagic events, thrombocytopheresis can be used for crisis intervention; rapid reduction in platelet numbers can be achieved, but the effects are transient.

Pregnancy in patients with primary thrombocythemia is associated with frequent obstetric complications and fetal loss. The risks of the usual platelet suppressive measures have led to the use of aspirin, which has been effective and has allowed term delivery. This experience, as well as its remarkable efficacy in erythromelalgia, has led to the more general use of low-dose aspirin in patients with primary thrombocythemia.

■ MYELOFIBROSIS

Myelofibrosis is characterized by bone marrow fibrosis and extramedullary but ineffective hematopoiesis, which involves all cell lineages; the clinical signs and symptoms are the result of this extramedullary activity. This is a clonal stem cell disorder, typical of all myeloproliferative lesions.

The use of a variety of names, such as agnogenic myeloid metaplasia, myelosclerosis, and myeloid metaplasia, emphasizes our limited knowledge of the biology of this syndrome. No epidemiologic data exist for myelofibrosis.

ETIOLOGY AND PATHOGENESIS

Because a variety of mechanisms of marrow injury produce marrow fibrosis, the syndrome is generally considered to be the result of a defined or idiopathic injury. Two events, although not coordinated, appear to define myelofibrosis. Hematopoietic stem cells that are found in increased numbers in the circulation settle, develop, and proliferate in nonmarrow sites. The proliferation is clonal and has a "trilineage" of red and white cells and platelets. Fibroblastic proliferation in the marrow, the result of injury or the product of abnormal megakaryocytopoiesis, is reactive (nonclonal). It results in a decreased marrow mass, a disordered sinusoidal pattern with premature release of cells of all lineages, and an increased release of hematopoietic stem cells.

The known causes of myelofibrosis are chemicals (especially benzene), radiation, infections (especially granulomatosis disease), metastatic cancer, and immune complexes; nevertheless, most cases of myelofibrosis are idiopathic.

CLINICAL FINDINGS

All the clinical findings in patients with myelofibrosis are directly attributable to marrow fibrosis and extramedullary hematopoiesis. A presymptomatic phase may be indicated by splenomegaly or abnormal peripheral blood. Later, constitutional symptoms, such as fatigue, weakness, and fever, form the common presentation. These result from the anemia and ineffectual hematopoiesis. Focal pressure symptoms due to potentially massive sites of extramedullary hematopoiesis are the hallmark of myelofibrosis, especially secondary to splenomegaly. Later, the lymph nodes and liver become enlarged. In time, easy bruising and mucosal bleeding occur, often constituting a cosmetic more than clinical problem. Symptomatic gout occurs in 10% of patients. Late clinical complications include portal hypertension and Budd–Chiari syndrome, ascites, and endocardial fibrosis with right-sided heart failure.

LABORATORY FINDINGS

Peripheral blood findings of leukoerythroblastosis (anemia with anisocytosis, teardrop-shaped and nucleated RBCs, leukocytosis with a left shift of white cells and increased basophils, and large, atypical platelets) provide evidence of an altered sinusoidal marrow matrix and resultant premature release of cells. These findings of ineffective hematopoiesis are documented by increased levels of lactate dehydrogenase, uric acid, and muramidase. Bone marrow aspiration is usually ineffective, and a biopsy reveals increased reticulum fibers (and in time, increased collagen) enmeshing a panhyperplastic marrow with particular megakaryocytic entrapment. Examination of the spleen, liver, and nodes reveals trilineage hematopoiesis characteristic of extramedullary hematopoiesis. Bone x-ray films or MRI findings reveal osteosclerosis.

OPTIMAL MANAGEMENT

After specific causes for myelofibrosis have been eliminated, all therapy is directed toward the clinical symptoms and complications. The care is supportive. Erythropoietin has reduced the transfusion requirement, particularly when serum levels are lower than expected for the degree of anemia. Other cytokine support is being examined. Low-dose hydroxyurea (500 mg every day or every other day) has been associated with reduction

in spleen size, decreased marrow fibrosis, and improved peripheral blood findings; responses are very slow, usually requiring 12 to 18 months. Splenectomy has been used with success for specific indications: severe abdominal symptoms, especially suggesting splenic infarctions; severe unresponsive hemolysis or thrombocytopenia; and portal hypertension with bleeding varices. Allogeneic human leukocyte antigen (HLA)-matched bone marrow or peripheral stem cell transplantation has been used with success in patients younger than age 55.

BIBLIOGRAPHY

Frenkel EP. Myeloproliferative syndromes: polycythemia vera, primary (essential) thrombocythemia, and myelofibrosis. In: Calabresi P, Schein P, eds. *Medical oncology: basic principles and clinical management of cancer,* second ed. New York: McGraw-Hill, 1993:503–515.

Frenkel EP. The clinical spectrum of thrombocytosis and thrombocythemia. *Am J Med Sci* 1991;301:69–80.

Gruppo Italiano Studio Policitemia. Polycythemia vera: the natural history of 1213 patients followed for 20 years. *Ann Intern Med* 1995;123:656–664.

Harrison CN, Gale RE, Machin SJ, et al. A large proportion of patients with a diagnosis of essential thrombocythemia do not have a clonal disorder and may be at lower risk of thrombotic complications. *Blood* 1999;93:417–424.

Lamy T, Devillers A, Bernard M, et al. Inapparent polycythemia vera: an unrecognized diagnosis. *Am J Med* 1997;102:14–20.

Michiels JJ. Erythromelalgia and vascular complications in polycythemia vera. *Semin Thromb Hemost* 1997;23:441–454.

Moliterno AR, Hankins WD, Spivak JL. Impaired expression of the thrombopoietin receptor by platelets from patients with polycythemia vera. *N Engl J Med* 1998;338:572–580.

Murphy S, Peterson P, Iland H, et al. Experience of the polycythemia study group with essential thrombocythemia: a final report on diagnostic criteria, survival, and leukemic transition by treatment. *Semin Hematol* 1997;34:29–39.

Najean Y, Rain J-D (for the French Polycythemia Study Group). Treatment of polycythemia vera: use of 32P alone or in combination with maintenance therapy using hydroxyurea in 461 patients greater than 65 years of age. *Blood* 1997;89:2319–2327.

Silver RT. Interferon alfa: effects of long-term treatment for polycythemia vera. *Semin Hematol* 1997;34:40–50.

Kelley's Textbook of Internal Medicine, fourth edition. Edited by H. David Humes.
Lippincott Williams & Wilkins, Philadelphia © 2000.

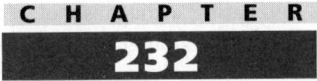

HODGKIN'S DISEASE

SANDRA J. HORNING

Hodgkin's disease is a B-cell lymphoid neoplasm originally described as a clinical entity in 1832 by Thomas Hodgkin and defined microscopically by pathologists Carl Sternberg and Dorothy Reed at the turn of the twentieth century. The diagnosis is based on the recognition of Reed–Sternberg (R-S) cells interspersed among a reactive mixed-cell population of lymphocytes, eosinophils, histiocytes, plasma cells, and neutrophils. Four histologic types (lymphocyte predominance, nodular sclerosis, mixed cellularity, and lymphocyte depletion) are distinguished on the basis of the morphology and immunohistochemistry. The anatomical extent of disease, associated symptoms and, to a lesser degree, the histologic subtype are the primary factors determining the presenting features, prognosis, and optimal therapy of Hodgkin's disease.

Although uncommon, Hodgkin's disease is significant because the systematic, multidisciplinary approach to diagnosis, staging, and treatment serves as a paradigm in oncology. As one of the most highly curable malignancies, therapy for Hodgkin's disease is approached with optimism; however, late effects of treatment continue to instruct and provide an impetus for new therapeutics.

INCIDENCE AND EPIDEMIOLOGY

The annual incidence of Hodgkin's disease, about 7,600 cases or 3.2 per 100,000, has been stable over the past decade in the United States. The incidence is higher in men than women and higher in whites than blacks. A bimodal age–incidence curve has been described in which rates rise through early life, peak in the third decade, decline until age 45, and thereafter rise steadily. The nodular sclerosis subtype is more common in young adults, whereas the mixed-cellularity subtype predominates in children and the elderly. In the young adult population, high socioeconomic status, high intelligence, small family size, single-family dwelling, and high educational attainment of patients and their immediate families all have been associated with increased risk of Hodgkin's disease.

The incidence of Hodgkin's disease varies by geographic patterns. In less developed countries, childhood and mixed-cellularity histology predominate. In developed countries, young adults with more favorable histologic subtypes are typical. These data have led to the hypothesis that one or more subtypes of Hodgkin's disease has an infectious cause. Several reports of clustering of Hodgkin's disease at the time of diagnosis suggested the possibility of infectious transmission but these studies have been sharply criticized. A large population study has demonstrated abnormally high titers of some anti-EBV (Epstein–Barr virus) antibodies antedating a diagnosis of Hodgkin's disease. The demonstration of EBV viral genomes in R-S cells supports a relation between EBV and Hodgkin's disease, and the epidemiologic features fit a polio model in which delayed age at infection leads to an increased risk of young adult disease. However, the association with EBV in tumor tissue is inconsistent with the model in that positive cases occur most often in children, especially in less developed countries and with mixed-cellularity histology.

ETIOLOGY

The fact that R-S cells account for only about 1% to 10% of the cellular composition in Hodgkin's tissues complicated their classification for more than 100 years. Recent studies involving isolation of single cells demonstrate that R-S cells are B cells with an excessive load of mutations within the variable region of the immunoglobulin heavy-chain gene, resulting in a loss of function. A second transforming event is postulated since these follicular center B cells fail to undergo apoptosis despite crippling mutations. EBV has been implicated as the transforming event based on multiple lines of evidence. With in situ hybridization methods, 18% to 50% of Hodgkin's cases are EBV-positive, and the viral genomes are present in a monoclonal population of cells. As already discussed, EBV in Hodgkin's tissues is associated with histology and demographic variables.

The histologic subtypes of Hodgkin's disease are defined by the relative amounts of collagen sclerosis, inflammatory cells, and the cytology of the malignant R-S cells. As observed on primary tissue and well-established cell lines, R-S cells secrete a variety of cytokines that may be responsible for the presence and activity of the nonmalignant cells surrounding them. These reactive cells, in turn, produce cytokines that can influence R-S cells in complex autocrine or paracrine interactions.

A genetic basis for increased susceptibility to Hodgkin's disease is supported by a marked risk in monozygous twins and increased risk among siblings and close relatives. It has been hypothesized that immunoregulatory genes within or near the major histocompatibility complex that may govern susceptibility to viral infections influence susceptibility to Hodgkin's disease. This theory is supported by data demonstrating specific human lymphocyte antigen (HLA) regions in the cause of Hodgkin's disease and increased HLA haplotype sharing among relatives in multiple-case families. Furthermore, Hodgkin's disease is associated with a variety of defects in cellular immunity, and successfully treated patients may continue to have suppressed responses to neoantigens for years.

PATHOLOGY

Nodular sclerosis accounts for 40% to 70% of all cases of Hodgkin's disease and is distinguished by distinctive fibrous bands that divide the lymphoid tissue into cellular nodules in addition to R-S cells and the appropriate cellular background. Mixed-cellularity histology is found in 30% to 50% of patients at diagnosis. Classic R-S cells are easily found amid a cellular background composed of lymphocytes, eosinophils, plasma cells, and histiocytes. Lymphocyte predominance (LP) is primarily composed of benign lymphocytes and relatively abundant multilobated "popcorn" cells.

LP Hodgkin's disease is uncommon, representing about 10% of cases. The pathologic diagnosis is based on the expression of surface markers as well as microscopic features. Classic Hodgkin's disease (nodular sclerosis and mixed cellularity) express the CD30 antigen, a marker of lymphocyte activation, and the CD15 antigen, which has been found on granulocytes, monocytes, activated T cells, and virus-infected cells. In contrast, the B-cell antigen CD20 is expressed by the multilobated cells of the LP subtype. Lymphocyte-depleted (LD) is a rare form of Hodgkin's disease in which two histologic variants have been described: a reticular type characterized by sheets of pleomorphic neoplastic cells and the diffuse fibrosis type, which has a prominent fibroblastic proliferation with few normal lymphocytes and sparse R-S cells. On retrospective review, many cases of LD Hodgkin's disease have been reclassified as non-Hodgkin's lymphoma.

CLINICAL FINDINGS

Constitutional symptoms, referred to as "B" symptoms, may accompany the diagnosis of Hodgkin's disease and influence prognosis. These include temperature higher than 38°C, drenching night sweats, and weight loss exceeding 10% of baseline body weight during the 6 months preceding diagnosis. Fevers, present in about one-third of patients, are usually low grade and irregular, although, rarely, a cyclic pattern of high fevers for 1 to 2 weeks is noted to alternate with afebrile periods of similar length. This classic Pel–Ebstein fever is virtually diagnostic of Hodgkin's disease. Internists should be alert to unexplained, generalized pruritus in young adults as symptomatic of Hodgkin's disease. Pain immediately after the ingestion of alcohol in involved lymph nodes is a curious complaint that is nearly pathognomonic for Hodgkin's disease. The cause of these symptoms, speculated to be related to cytokines, remains largely unexplained.

Detection of an unexplained mass or swelling in the superficial lymph nodes, especially the neck, is the most common presentation of patients with Hodgkin's disease. The lymph nodes are characteristically nontender and have a rubbery consistency. A diffuse, puffy swelling rather than a discrete mass may be apparent in the supraclavicular, infraclavicular, or anterior chest wall regions. Facial swelling and engorgement of the veins in the neck and upper chest may result from compression of the superior vena cava. Physical examination is relatively insensitive to the detection of intra-abdominal and pelvic adenopathy or organ enlargement, but examination should be oriented toward the liver, spleen, and iliac and inguinal nodal regions.

Clinical features are strongly correlated with histologic subtype in Hodgkin's disease patients. There is a 4:1 male predominance in LP Hodgkin's disease, and patients typically present with limited peripheral adenopathy. Involvement of the lower cervical, supraclavicular, and mediastinal lymph nodes in adolescents and young adults, particularly females, is characteristic of the nodular sclerosis subtype. Mixed-cellularity Hodgkin's disease is seen at both ends of the age spectrum, is more commonly associated with advanced, symptomatic disease, and is the predominant subtype found in patients infected with HIV. The rare LD subtype is overrepresented in older patients, who may present with fever of unknown origin, jaundice, and hepatosplenomegaly without palpable adenopathy. This subtype is also associated with AIDS.

LABORATORY FEATURES

The laboratory features of Hodgkin's disease are nonspecific. A routine complete blood count may reveal granulocytosis, eosino-

philia, lymphocytopenia, thrombocytosis, or anemia of chronic disease. Cytopenias may occur as a result of marrow involvement, hypersplenism, or an autoimmune mechanism. The degree of elevation of the erythrocyte sedimentation rate (ESR) has prognostic significance, correlating with advanced disease and constitutional symptoms. Serum alkaline phosphatase may be elevated in patients with Hodgkin's disease, nonspecifically in those with limited disease, or in association with involvement of liver, bone, or bone marrow in advanced disease. Hypercalcemia is unusual in Hodgkin's disease and appears to be secondary to synthesis of increased levels of 1,25-dihydroxyvitamin D by Hodgkin's tissues. Laboratory abnormalities may be prominent in rare presentations of Hodgkin's disease. These include abnormal liver function tests associated with marked enlargement of porta hepatis nodes and biliary obstruction or intrahepatic cholestasis. The nephrotic syndrome is a rare presentation of Hodgkin's disease.

OPTIMAL MANAGEMENT

Upon establishment of a histologic diagnosis of Hodgkin's disease by an expert pathologist, a diagnostic evaluation is undertaken. In addition to a complete history and physical examination, all patients should have computed tomographic (CT) scans of the chest, abdomen, and pelvis. Intrathoracic disease is present in two-thirds of patients at diagnosis and is particularly common in young women with nodular sclerosis. Chest CT scans may reveal hilar adenopathy, pulmonary parenchymal involvement, pleural effusions, pericardial effusions, and chest wall masses, especially with bulky mediastinal disease. CT of the abdomen and pelvis may detect celiac, portal, splenic hilar, retroperitoneal, and pelvic lymph nodes. Despite technologic advances, the correlation with histologic involvement of the spleen continues to be disappointing. Exploratory (staging) laparotomy has been phased out of routine staging owing to changes in treatment as described in the following text. Bone marrow biopsy is indicated in patients who are symptomatic or have extensive disease or cytopenias. Patients with bone pain should have bone scans and directed skeletal x-rays, which may demonstrate osteolytic, osteoblastic, or mixed lesions. Single positron-emission computed tomography (SPECT) gallium scanning may be useful in serial evaluation of extensive mediastinal disease before and after treatment.

The diagnostic evaluation of a person with Hodgkin's disease leads to the assignment of stage and directs the patient's therapy. The anatomical distribution of Hodgkin's disease in contiguous lymphatic structures is largely predictable and nonrandom. These patterns of association form the basis for the four-stage Ann Arbor classification, used to define the extent of Hodgkin's disease. Disease on one side of the diaphragm is considered stage I (one nodal site) or II (two or more sites), whereas stage III is disease confined to lymph nodes on both sides of the diaphragm. Extranodal disease, representing extracapsular extension of lymph node disease that can be treated with a curative dose of radiation therapy, is distinguished from disseminated, stage IV disease. Staging is further characterized by the presence (B) or absence (A) of constitutional symptoms. The correlation of this staging classification system with prognosis has been extensively verified, and, in a recent modification known as the *Cotswold classification,* additional prognostic information has been included.

In practice, as noted in Figure 232.1, patients are determined to have favorable stage I–II disease (asymptomatic, nonbulky), intermediate stage I–II disease (symptomatic, or bulky or contiguous extranodal disease), or advanced stage III–IV disease. Extended-field radiation therapy was the treatment of choice for favorable stage I–II Hodgkin's disease for more than three decades. However, late complications occurring 15 to 25 years after radiation therapy have created interest in combined-modality approaches using less toxic or abbreviated chemotherapy programs with involved-field radiation therapy. The combined-modality approach obviates the need for staging laparotomy and extended-field irradiation. Cure rates higher than 90% are regularly reported with this approach, which may require no more than 2 to 4 months of combination chemotherapy followed by 30 to 36 Gy of involved-field irradiation. Several chemotherapy combinations have been investigated in this setting. The ABVD (doxorubicin, bleomycin, vinblastine, dacarbazine) combination is favored by many practitioners because of its relatively favorable toxicity profile.

Combined-modality therapy is indicated for intermediate Hodgkin's disease presenting as a bulky mediastinal mass. Cure can be expected in 70% to 80% of such patients. Chemotherapy alone or chemotherapy plus involved-field radiation therapy are standard treatments for stage IIB Hodgkin's disease. ABVD chemotherapy is recommended based on a randomized clinical trial demonstrating the superiority of this combination compared with an alternate regimen, both delivered with radiation therapy, in intermediate Hodgkin's disease.

On the basis of a series of successive randomized trials, ABVD chemotherapy has emerged as the most effective and least toxic combination for advanced Hodgkin's disease. Treatment with six to ten cycles yields continuous disease-free survival in 65% to 70% of patients with stage III or IV disease 5 years after treatment. Although high rates of cure have been reported with consolidative radiation therapy given in low dose after chemotherapy, randomized trials have failed to establish definite benefit. Further improvement in these outcomes has been reported with newer chemotherapy programs, but assessment of these requires longer follow-up and confirmation in additional studies.

As demonstrated in Figure 232.2, the prognosis for patients with any stage of Hodgkin's disease is excellent with current approaches. This is due to advances in staging, identification of

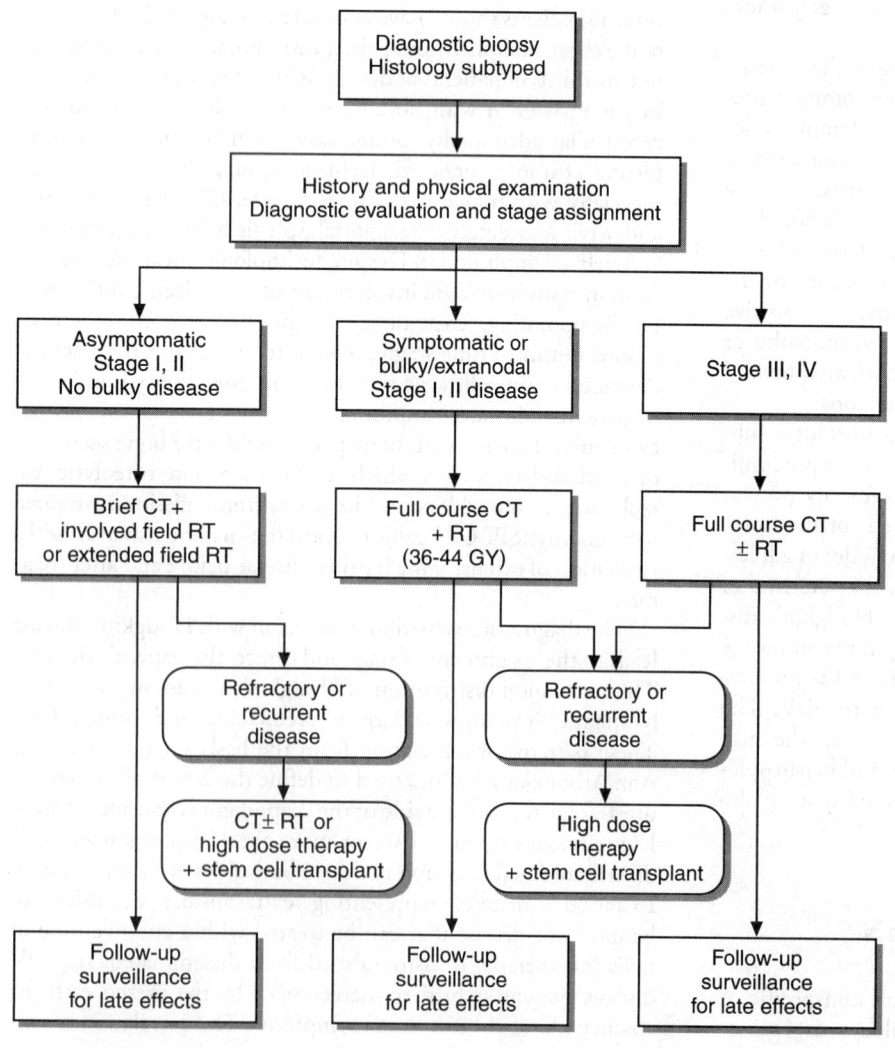

FIGURE 232.1. Optimal management of Hodgkin's disease. (*CT,* chemotherapy; *RT,* radiation therapy.)

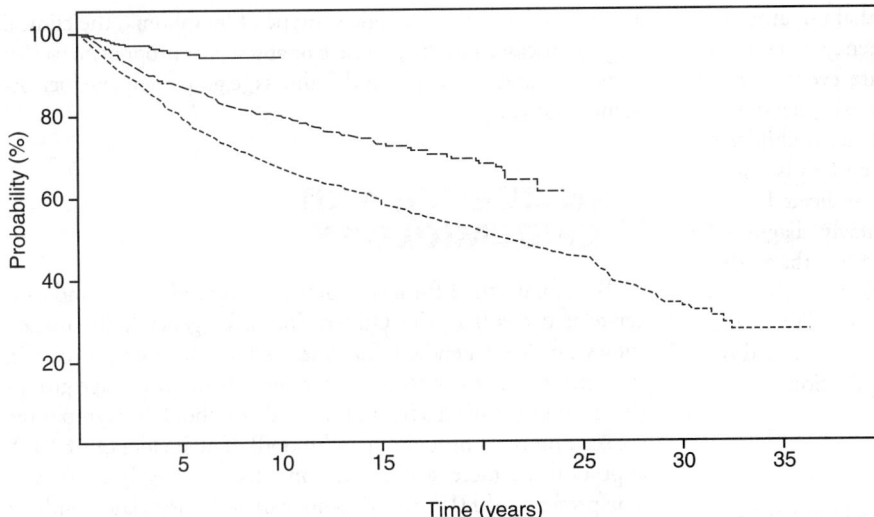

FIGURE 232.2. Overall survival in 2,789 patients with Hodgkin's disease treated at Stanford University from 1962 to 1999. Curves represent the eras 1962 to 1974 (*dotted line*), 1975 to 1988 (*dot and dash*), and 1989 to 1999 (*solid*). (Courtesy of SJ Horning, RT Hoppe, and SA Rosenberg, Stanford University.)

prognostic features that direct therapy, and the application of curative radiation therapy and chemotherapy. Nonetheless, a number of challenges remain. Older age, high tumor burden, and preexisting immunodeficiency have been recognized repeatedly as adverse prognostic factors in Hodgkin's disease. In 1998, an international group described seven adverse prognostic factors for advanced Hodgkin's disease: age over 45 years, stage IV disease, male gender, white blood count higher than 15,000 per microliter, lymphocyte count less than 600 per microliter or less than 8%, albumin less than 4 g per deciliter, and hemoglobin less than 10.5 g per deciliter. Disease-free survival at 5 years was 74% for patients with 0 to 2 factors compared with 55% for patients with more than three factors.

The prognosis for patients with Hodgkin's disease is significantly less favorable for those who fail primary chemotherapy alone or combined with radiation therapy. The initial duration of remission and sensitivity to chemotherapy has a significant effect on the ability of patients to respond to subsequent treatment and maintain their response. High-dose therapy and stem cell rescue constitute the current favored treatment for patients who fail primary induction or have a relapse. Approximately 50% of such patients are alive and disease-free at 5 years.

The high rates of cure anticipated with any presentation of Hodgkin's disease have led to more emphasis on treatment complications. Acute side effects are relatively easily managed, whereas late treatment effects including second malignancy and cardiopulmonary disease, constitute a major concern. Whereas the risk of acute leukemia and myelodysplasia was increased proportional to the cumulative dose of alkylating agents in early combination chemotherapy for Hodgkin's disease, this risk is significantly less after ABVD chemotherapy. Non-Hodgkin's lymphomas (NHLs) may occur either early or late after treatment for Hodgkin's disease. No clear relation to the type of primary treatment is known. These NHLs may be attributed to ongoing immunodeficiency or a common cell of origin.

Cancers of the lung, stomach, breast, bone, and soft tissue have been observed after treatment for Hodgkin's disease in a temporal pattern consistent with radiation-induced neoplasms.

An increased risk of solid cancers has been identified by several groups; the overall actuarial risk in the Stanford series was about 18% at 5 years. However, the latency for developing second cancers is an important consideration, because many are not noted with follow-up of less than 10 years and the risk appears to continue to increase beyond that time. Age at exposure may also be important. Breast cancer risk is increased in women treated before age 30 and is markedly increased in children and adolescents. The solid tumor risk has been related to radiation therapy, with tumors occurring infield or at the edges of the radiation therapy field. However, recent data indicate an increased risk of lung cancer in Hodgkin's patients treated with chemotherapy alone.

An increased risk of death from coronary artery disease and acute myocardial infarction has been identified in adults and children treated with mediastinal radiation therapy. Other types of cardiac disease that occur after chest radiation therapy are valvular disease, constrictive pericarditis, and cardiomyopathy. Theoretically, the use of ABVD might be associated with an increased risk of cardiac disease (doxorubicin-related cardiomyopathy) or pulmonary toxicity (bleomycin-related pneumonitis). In practice, cardiopulmonary complications have been infrequent.

The ABVD combination is associated with temporary amenorrhea and azoospermia, with full recovery noted in most patients. In contrast, sterility may follow the use of alkylating agents in high-dose regimens, in which the risk is related to cumulative dose, age at exposure, and gender. No increase in birth defects or complications of pregnancy has been seen after treatment for Hodgkin's disease.

The internist should be particularly aware of the late complications of treatment, many of which are related to radiation therapy. Screening programs for breast cancer should be initiated within 10 years of treatment in young women, and heightened surveillance for second malignancy and cardiovascular disease is indicated for all patients treated with radiation therapy. Furthermore, about 30% of patients develop hypothyroidism after neck irradiation, and the thyroid-stimulating hormone level should be monitored. Hyperthyroidism, Graves' ophthalmopathy, or thyroid neoplasms occur with increased frequency after neck radiation therapy. Overwhelming sepsis is a rare event among patients who have been splenectomized or received splenic irradiation in treatment for Hodgkin's disease, particularly children. Periodic vaccination for encapsulated bacteria and early intervention with antibiotics for febrile episodes are indicated.

It is anticipated that more than 80% of newly diagnosed patients will be cured of Hodgkin's disease, and less than 10% will die directly from the disease. However, serious morbidities and increased risks of life-threatening second neoplasms and cardiac disease are of concern. Current therapies are focused on maintaining high cure rates and reducing complications.

BIBLIOGRAPHY

Hancock SL, Hoppe RT. Long term complications of treatment and causes of mortality after Hodgkin's disease. *Semin Radiat Oncol* 1996;6: 225–242.

Hasenclever D, Diehl V. A prognostic score for advanced Hodgkin's disease. International Prognostic Factors Project on Advanced Hodgkin's Disease. *N Engl J Med* 1998;339:1506–1514.

Horning SJ, Yahalom J, Tesch H, et al. Treatment of Stage III-IV Hodgkin's disease. In: Mauch PM, Armitage JO, Diehl V, et al, eds. *Hodgkin's disease*. Philadelphia: Lippincott Williams & Wilkins, 1999:483–506.

Mauch PM. Controversies in the management of early stage Hodgkin's disease. *Blood* 1994;83:318–329.

Yuen AR, Rosenberg SA, Hoppe RT, et al. Comparison between conventional salvage therapy and high-dose therapy with autografting for recurrent or refractory Hodgkin's disease. *Blood* 1997;89:814–822.

Kelley's Textbook of Internal Medicine, fourth edition. Edited by H. David Humes. Lippincott Williams & Wilkins, Philadelphia © 2000.

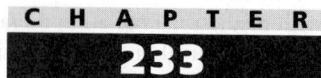

C H A P T E R

233

NON-HODGKIN'S LYMPHOMAS

R. GREGORY BOCIEK
JULIE M. VOSE
JAMES O. ARMITAGE

The term "lymphoma" comprises two clinically and biologically distinct groups of neoplasms—Hodgkin's disease and non-Hodgkin's lymphoma (NHL). NHLs are a heterogeneous group of malignancies that begin as a clonal malignant expansion of B or T lymphocytes. The clinical presentation of these illnesses is variable. Patients may give a history of chronic asymptomatic lymphadenopathy, which may have been present for months to years, or may present acutely with rapidly progressive lymphadenopathy, constitutional symptoms, and organ failure secondary to extranodal involvement from lymphoma. The choice of ther-

apy is based on the histologic subtype of lymphoma, the clinical stage of disease, and the presence or absence of prognostic factors known to affect outcome in this illness (e.g., patient age, performance status).

INCIDENCE AND EPIDEMIOLOGY

NHLs remain the fifth most common cause of cancer and cancer-related death in the United States. In general, the disease shows an age-dependent increase over time, although certain subtypes appear to be seen more frequently in certain age groups (for example, Burkitt's lymphoma and lymphoblastic lymphoma are seen more commonly in childhood). The incidence of NHL appears to be increasing for reasons that are largely unknown. The presence of HIV infection appears to be associated with an increased risk of developing NHL, and the increasing prevalence of HIV therefore likely accounts for some of the increase in incidence of the disease. However, the increasing prevalence of HIV is not solely responsible for the increase in NHL, as demonstrated by the observation that lymphomas in patients over the age of 60 are also on the increase, as are lymphomas not typically associated with HIV infection (e.g., indolent NHLs). Newer diagnostic studies such as immunophenotyping have led to the identification of certain subtypes of NHLs that may have been previously misclassified as Hodgkin's disease. The increasing use of solid organ and stem cell transplantation to treat various diseases may also be contributing to the increase in NHL as a result of the long-term effects of chronic immunosuppression.

Mortality rates from NHL appear to be higher for urban areas and for higher socioeconomic groups. Mortality and morbidity rates in the United States and Europe have risen gradually over the past several decades among older adults, although mortality rates among children and young people have fallen slightly. NHL occurs throughout the world at rates that range from a threefold to fourfold increase in recent years. The maximum rates are seen in Western developed countries.

ETIOLOGY

Factors that predispose to the development of NHL include congenital (e.g., ataxia-telangiectasia, Wiskott–Aldrich syndrome) or acquired (e.g., solid organ or stem cell transplantation, HIV infection) immunodeficiency states. Autoimmune diseases such as Hashimoto's thyroiditis (thyroid lymphomas) and Sjögren's syndrome (lacrimal/salivary gland lymphomas) are thought to be associated with an increased risk of lymphomas as a result of chronic inflammatory stimulation of the affected glands. Infectious agents such as human T-lymphotrophic virus type 1 (HTLV-1), Epstein–Barr virus, and *Helicobacter pylori* have also been associated with an increased risk of NHL. HTLV-1 appears to be the causative agent in T-cell leukemia/lymphoma endemic to southern Japan and some parts of the Caribbean. Epstein–Barr virus has been associated with African Burkitt's lymphoma and with post-transplantation lymphoproliferative disorders. Gastric infection with *H. pylori* has been associated with the development of mucosal associated lymphoid tissue (MALT) lymphomas.

Observational studies have demonstrated an increased risk of NHL in association with a variety of occupational and environmental exposures. Exposure to agents such as organophosphates and phenoxyacetic acid herbicides (e.g., in farm workers) has been associated with an increased risk of NHL. In some studies, the risk appears to correlate with increasing levels of exposure, particularly for those who handled or mixed substances directly. Exposure to organic solvents or chemicals (e.g., benzene, creosote, paint thinner) and hair dyes has also been linked to an increased risk of NHL. Finally, an increased risk of developing NHL has been observed in association with exposure to high nitrate levels in drinking water and in diets with a high intake of meat and fat from animal sources. Most lymphomas diagnosed in the United States, however, have no readily identifiable cause.

PATHOGENESIS AND PATHOPHYSIOLOGY

NHL results from the malignant transformation of normal lymphoid cells at various stages of differentiation. During normal development and differentiation, lymphocytes undergo genetic rearrangement of either immunoglobulin genes (B-cell development) or T-cell receptors (T-cell development). Specific chromosomal translocations involving these genes are seen in many NHLs. These translocations are useful markers for diagnosis and prognosis and in certain subtypes of lymphoma lend some understanding to the pathogenesis of the disease. For example, Burkitt's lymphoma uniformly involves translocation of the *MYC* oncogene on chromosome 8 into the immunoglobulin heavy-chain (chromosome 14) or light-chain (chromosomes 2 and 22) genes. The resulting chromosomal translocations t(8;14), t(2;8), or t(8;22) deregulate the *MYC* gene and result in the constitutive production of a DNA-binding protein that appears to control aspects of gene expression or DNA replication. Approximately 70% to 80% of follicular lymphomas are associated with the presence of the translocation t(14;18), which translocates the *bcl-2* gene on chromosome 18 into the immunoglobulin heavy-chain locus on chromosome 14. This dysregulation of *bcl-2*, normally a gene associated with cellular apoptotic control, may result in the formation of a malignant clone of cells that lose normal apoptotic control and achieve a functional form of immortality, resulting in the generation of a follicular lymphoma. Most mantle cell lymphomas bear the translocation t(11;14), which translocates the *PRAD* 1 (*CCND* 1) gene into the immunoglobulin heavy-chain locus on chromosome 14. This results in the overexpression of cyclin D1, which appears to cause disturbances in the regulation of the cell cycle. Exactly how this leads to lymphogenesis is not yet understood, but cyclin-D1 is known to regulate in some way movement of cells through G1 to S phase.

Several scenarios have been postulated to explain how Epstein–Barr virus infection and the observed chromosomal translocation interact to result in malignant transformation into a clinically recognized Burkitt's lymphoma. All these theories incorporate viral infection, spontaneous or virally induced mutation, environmental factors, and host factors including immune dysfunction. In the post-transplantation setting, the spectrum of Epstein–Barr virus–induced lymphoproliferation ranges from a predominance of polyclonal disease to true monoclonal aggressive NHL.

CLASSIFICATION OF NON-HODGKIN'S LYMPHOMAS

Classification of NHL has undergone a temporal evolution based on morphologic and biologic understanding of the illness at particular points in time. The Rappaport system developed in the 1950s classified lymphomas on the basis of appearance (nodular versus diffuse) and differentiation (well-differentiated versus poorly differentiated). In the 1970s, it became apparent that NHLs were derived from B or T lymphocytes. This knowledge became reflected in the staging system of Luke and Collins, in which lymphomas were classified primarily according to their presumed normal lymphoid counterparts. Confusion arising from the use of multiple classification schemes led to the development of the Working Formulation, which was proposed in 1982 (Table 233.1). This classification scheme identified specific histologic subtypes of NHL based largely on the appearance of the disease within the lymph node (i.e., a follicular versus diffuse pattern), as well as on the principal size of lymphoma cells within the node (small cleaved cells versus large noncleaved cells versus mixed populations). Although imperfect and subject to some degree of diagnostic interobserver variability, this classification scheme was able to divide NHLs into three reasonably distinct groups based on biology and prognosis: low-grade lymphomas, intermediate lymphomas, and high-grade lymphomas. Treatment patterns were based largely on these three subgroups, recognizing that within each group the illnesses were still to some degree, distinct entities.

Over the past 10 years, evolving knowledge and techniques

TABLE 233.1	**THE WORKING FORMULATION CLASSIFICATION OF NON-HODGKIN'S LYMPHOMAS**

Low Grade

A. Small lymphocytic lymphoma/chronic lymphocytic leukemia
B. Follicular, predominantly small cleaved-cell lymphoma
C. Follicular, mixed, small cleaved and large-cell lymphoma

Intermediate Grade

D. Follicular, large-cell lymphoma
E. Diffuse, small, cleaved-cell lymphoma
F. Diffuse, mixed, small cleaved and large-cell lymphoma
G. Diffuse, large-cell lymphoma

High Grade

H. Immunoblastic lymphoma
I. Lymphoblastic lymphoma
J. Small noncleaved-cell lymphoma
   Burkitt's
   Non-Burkitt's

TABLE 233.2.	MODIFIED WORLD HEALTH ORGANIZATION (WHO) CLASSIFICATION OF NON-HODGKIN'S LYMPHOMAS

Precursor cell lymphomas
  B-lymphoblastic leukemia/lymphoma
  T-lymphoblastic leukemia/lymphoma
Mature cell lymphomas
  B-cell lymphomas
    Follicular lymphoma
    B-cell chronic lymphocytic leukemia/prolymphocytic leukemia/small lymphocytic lymphoma
    Marginal zone lymphomas
      MALT (mucosa-associated lymphoid tissue) lymphoma
      Nodal marginal zone B-cell lymphoma
      Splenic marginal zone B-cell lymphoma
    Mantle cell lymphoma
    Diffuse large B-cell lymphoma
    Mediastinal diffuse large B-cell lymphoma
    Burkitt's lymphoma
  T-cell lymphomas
    Peripheral T-cell lymphoma, unspecified
    Anaplastic large T/null cell lymphoma
    Mycosis fungoides/Sézary syndrome
    Adult T-cell lymphoma/leukemia

for studying and understanding the biology of NHL led to the recognition that newer entities were being discovered that did not have a place in the Working Formulation (e.g., mantle cell lymphoma). In 1994, an international group of hematopathologists proposed a new classification scheme for both Hodgkin's disease and NHLs using morphologic, immunologic, and genetic techniques to more readily identify a list of easily definable disease entities. The proposed name was the "Revised European-American Classification of Lymphoid Neoplasms" or the "REAL" classification. Although some of the disease entities from the Working Formulation were essentially preserved (e.g., chronic lymphocytic leukemia, Burkitt's lymphoma) many new ones recognized by the REAL classification became quickly recognized as being clinically or biologically distinct entities (e.g., mantle cell lymphoma, primary mediastinal B-cell lymphoma). A recent retrospective study by the NHL Classification Project confirmed the clinical importance of these new disease entities. A revision of this classification was recently revealed by the World Health Organization. A modified version of this classification is presented in Table 233.2.

COMMON OR CHARACTERISTIC DISEASE ENTITIES

B-cell chronic lymphocytic leukemia and small lymphocytic lymphoma are clinical variations of the same biologic process. This disease most often occurs after the fifth decade and tends to be an indolent slowly progressive illness. Lymphadenopathy is commonly present, and patients may present with repeated infections or evidence of hypogammaglobulinemia. Pathologically, the illness is characterized by monomorphic small lympho-

cytes, usually involving the bone marrow, often with evidence of circulating lymphoma cells. By convention, patients with large numbers of circulating lymphocytes are considered to have chronic lymphocytic leukemia rather than small lymphocytic lymphoma. Larger cells, prolymphocytes may be present either at diagnosis, or as part of a process of transformation to a higher-grade illness. The malignant cells express B-cell antigens (e.g., CD19, CD20) and may generate a monoclonal gammopathy. The disease is incurable with standard treatment, and survival is not known to be improved by early or more aggressive therapy.

Follicular lymphomas account for approximately 30% to 40% of all NHLs. This group of lymphomas is common in older adults and often involves lymph nodes, bone marrow, and spleen at diagnosis. Occasionally, extranodal disease is seen, although certain extranodal sites (e.g., central nervous system [CNS]) are distinctly uncommon. Although the course is generally indolent, transformation to a higher-grade illness is seen at a rate of about 6% per year and is generally associated with a poorer prognosis. Histologic transformation is often associated with identification of another cytogenetic abnormality in addition to the original clone. In advanced stages, follicular lymphomas are incurable with standard therapy, although early-stage disease may be curable with radiation therapy in a percentage of patients.

Mantle cell lymphoma was not recognized within the Working Formulation. Pathologically, it most often consists of a diffuse lymphoma with small lymphocytes, although it can have a nodular histologic pattern also. Mantle cell lymphoma seems to incorporate the worst features of both indolent and aggressive lymphomas. Although often relatively slow growing, this lymphoma does not share the high degree of responsiveness so characteristic of other indolent lymphomas. The median survival of patients with mantle cell lymphoma is distinctly shorter than patients with other forms of indolent lymphoma (in particular, the diffuse subtype) and appears to be incurable with standard therapy.

Diffuse large B-cell lymphoma (representing diffuse large cell and immunoblastic lymphoma in the Working Formulation) is the most common NHL subtype and represents an aggressive intermediate-grade or high-grade form of lymphoma. Patients with diffuse large B-cell lymphoma most often present with disease in the lymph nodes and tend more often to have localized disease compared with those with indolent lymphomas. However, extranodal sites of disease (e.g., involvement of gastrointestinal tract, testes, thyroid, skin, breast, or central nervous system) are seen more frequently than in indolent lymphomas. Involvement of Waldeyer's ring is associated with approximately a 20% risk of simultaneous or subsequent involvement of the gastrointestinal tract in other sites. When patients present with involvement of Waldeyer's ring, a complete evaluation of the small and large bowel should be included in their initial evaluations. Bone marrow involvement is seen in only 10% of diffuse large B-cell lymphoma at diagnosis. Unlike indolent lymphomas, in which enlarging tumor masses tend to abut but not invade contiguous organs, diffuse aggressive lymphomas can result in compression or infiltration of organs, such as peripheral nerves, spinal cord, liver, great vessels, bronchi, and bone. These lymphomas are curable in a number of patients.

High-grade lymphomas such as lymphoblastic lymphoma occur most commonly in children or adolescents. Lymphoblastic lymphoma is histologically and clinically similar to acute lymphoblastic leukemia. The illness is more common in males, and approximately 50% of patients present with mediastinal lymphadenopathy. Although the disease may appear to be localized at the time of diagnosis, rapid dissemination usually occurs to the bone marrow, peripheral blood, and meninges. Although highly clinically aggressive, the disease is curable in a subset of patients (generally those without adverse prognostic features) with currently available therapy. Burkitt's lymphoma is another high-grade lymphoma originally described as an endemic disease in Africa. It is more common in men, and the endemic form usually presents with large extranodal tumors involving the maxilla, mandible, or other facial bones. In the non-African (nonendemic) form of Burkitt's lymphoma, patients most often present with disease in the abdomen and bowel, with subsequent bone marrow and CNS involvement as the disease progresses. Patients with endemic Burkitt's lymphoma have a median age at presentation of approximately 7 years, and the sporadic cases occur over a broader age range, up to the third decade, with a median age of 11 years. The initiation of therapy in high-grade lymphomas can lead to tumor lysis syndrome, and frequent monitoring of electrolytes, calcium, phosphate, and urate are important during the first few days of therapy, because rapid tumor lysis can lead to life-threatening complications, such as hyperkalemia and acute renal failure.

CLINICAL FINDINGS

Patients with NHL generally seek medical attention as a result of progressive lymphadenopathy. However, numerous other signs and symptoms may be seen as the presenting features of the illness. Patients may present with unexplained constitutional symptoms (so-called B symptoms, consisting of fever, drenching night sweats, and unexplained weight loss), fatigue, early satiety secondary to splenomegaly, abdominal pain from enlarging or infiltrating tumor masses, or chest pain or dyspnea resulting from a large mediastinal mass. Some patients present with atypical or recurrent infections resulting from immune dysregulation or with anemia or thrombocytopenia secondary to bone marrow involvement or as a result of autoimmune phenomena.

To some extent, specific histologic entities may reflect the presenting clinical features. Patients with follicular lymphomas may give a history of waxing and waning lymphadenopathy over a prolonged period of time, occasionally years. Patients with follicular lymphomas also commonly present with bone marrow involvement, and cytopenias may therefore be seen in these patients. Patients with intermediate-grade lymphomas generally present with a shorter history of enlarging nodes or constitutional symptoms that have been progressive over weeks or months. Finally, patients with high-grade lymphomas often present with tumor masses that have been enlarging rapidly over a short period of days or weeks, evidence of marrow failure, and circulating lymphoma cells in the peripheral blood and often have evidence of CNS (most commonly meningeal) involvement.

LABORATORY EVALUATION

The suspicion of a diagnosis of lymphoma should lead the clinician to notify the pathologist such that a series of special additional studies can be performed on the biopsy (cytogenetics, cell surface marker determinations, immunohistochemistry stains, and molecular biologic studies) in addition to the routine histology. These additional studies can add valuable information to help differentiate in particular some of the new NHL entities.

After confirmation of the diagnosis, various staging procedures are performed to assist in the determination of prognosis and to guide therapy. To some degree, the histologic subtype of NHL and the condition of the patient direct the type and speed of staging procedures performed. For example, a patient with a high-grade lymphoma that is rapidly progressing requires prompt, limited staging procedures to permit timely initiation of therapy. Indolent lymphomas in asymptomatic patients can be staged at the convenience of the patient and physician.

The various tests that are useful for staging NHLs are listed in Table 233.3. Baseline studies should include a complete history and physical examination; a complete blood count; liver chemistries; renal function studies; and lactate dehydrogenase (LDH), β_2-microglobulin, and calcium determinations. Imaging studies should include CT scans of the chest, abdomen, and pelvis as well as a bone marrow aspirate and biopsy. Additional studies that may be appropriate in certain circumstances are cytologic examination of effusions; a bone scan (with plain films of abnormal or symptomatic areas) if bony symptoms are present, and MRI of the brain or spinal cord if central or peripheral CNS symptoms are present. The presence of gastrointestinal symptoms or of lymphoma in Waldeyer's ring should prompt complete investigations of the gastrointestinal tract. Patients with high-grade lymphomas and patients with CNS symptoms compatible with meningeal involvement by lymphoma should receive a diagnostic lumbar puncture. Gallium Ga 67 scanning using single-photon emission CT sometimes can be useful in

TABLE 233.3.	DIAGNOSTIC AND STAGING INVESTIGATIONS FOR PATIENTS WITH NON-HODGKIN'S LYMPHOMAS

Lymph node biopsy with attention to additional studies as indicated
Complete blood and platelet counts
Serum chemistry panel (electrolytes, renal and hepatic function, serum calcium)
Lactate dehydrogenase level, β_2-microglobulin level
CT scan of chest, abdomen, and pelvis
Bone marrow biopsy
MRI of head and other locations[a]
Bone scan[a]
Lumbar puncture[a]
SPECT gallium scan[a]

CT, computed tomography; MRI, magnetic resonance imaging; SPECT, single photon-emission computed tomography.
[a] As indicated based on histologic subtype and presence of pertinent symptoms.

differentiating active lymphoma from fibrotic tissue, particularly when baseline scans reveal the presence of gallium-avid tumor, which can be reimaged at the completion of therapy.

Staging is classified according to the Ann Arbor staging system, which was originally developed for Hodgkin's disease (Chapter 232). The combination of stage and histologic subtype of lymphoma guides stratification of patients for appropriate treatment. Previously abnormal tests should be repeated part way through therapy, at the completion of therapy, and at regular intervals thereafter. Patients failing standard therapies at any point in time should be considered for clinical trials of newer therapies.

Several prognostic factors are associated with poor outcomes in patients with NHL. Histologic transformation of follicular NHL was one of the first unfavorable prognostic factors identified. In one study, the median survival of patients with follicular lymphoma and subsequent transformation to a diffuse large cell lymphoma was 12 months, compared with 40 months for patients with de novo diffuse large cell lymphoma. Other characteristics associated with a poor outcome in many studies include advanced age, advanced stage, poor performance status or the presence of B symptoms, the presence of CNS or bone marrow involvement, the presence of bulky sites of tumor, an elevated LDH or β_2-microglobulin level, cytogenetic abnormalities such as chromosome 17 abnormalities and slow tumor responsiveness to therapy.

The International Prognostic Index was developed in 1993 as a means to capture prognostic information in patients with intermediate-grade or high-grade NHL. A retrospective analysis was performed on patients who had been treated with anthracycline-based chemotherapy regimens. An index was derived that could stratify newly diagnosed patients into risk categories based on the number of independent risk factors present at diagnosis: age (≤ 60 years versus >60 years), stage (I or II versus III or IV), LDH concentration (normal versus $>$normal), Eastern Cooperative Oncology Group (ECOG) performance status (0 or 1 versus 2, 3, or 4) and the number of extranodal sites of disease (≤ 1 versus >1). The probability of survival was grouped according to the number of adverse prognostic factors (Fig. 233.1). The principal clinical use of the International Prognostic Index has been the identification of patients at diagnosis who are unlikely to be cured with standard anthracycline-based chemotherapy and in whom trials of novel therapies are warranted.

MANAGEMENT OF NON-HODGKIN'S LYMPHOMA

Treatment must be tailored to the individual patient and depends on the histologic subtype, stage, and other prognostic factors mentioned previously.

FOLLICULAR NON-HODGKIN'S LYMPHOMA

Localized (stage I or nonbulky stage II) follicular NHL is treated with radiation therapy, and approximately 40% to 50% of patients treated in this fashion remain disease-free at 10 years' follow-up. Patients with advanced disease (stage III or IV) are

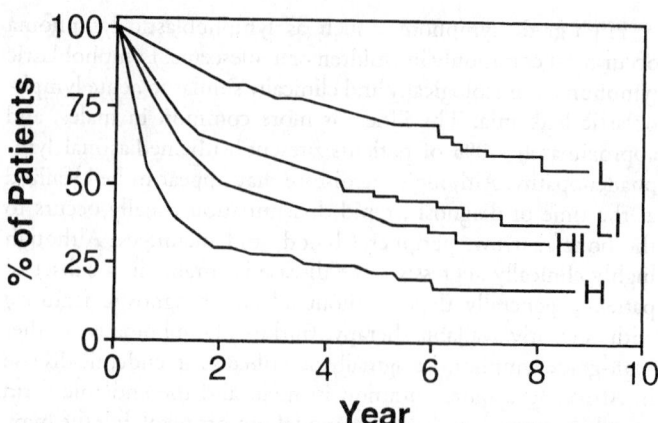

FIGURE 233.1. Survival according to risk groups defined by the International Prognostic Index. Patients are placed into four risk groups defined by the number of risk factors at diagnosis. *L,* low; *LI,* low intermediate; *HI,* high intermediate; *H,* high risk. (From Shipp MA, et al. A predictive model for aggressive non-Hodgkin's lymphoma: the International Non-Hodgkin's Lymphoma Prognostic Factors Project. *N Engl J Med* 1993;329:987, with permission.)

incurable with standard therapy but have a median survival of 8 years or more and generally have disease that is responsive to simple nontoxic chemotherapy regimens. However, overall survival is not known to be prolonged by the use of any form of standard chemotherapy. For this reason, a "watch and wait" approach is often offered to patients with advanced disease in whom no significant disease related symptoms or organ dysfunction are present. When symptoms or organ dysfunction lead to the decision to begin treatment, single-agent therapy with oral alkylating agents, such as chlorambucil (Leukeran) or cyclophosphamide (Cytoxan), is often used.

Another initial therapy frequently used in this clinical setting is the CVP regimen of **c**yclophosphamide, **v**incristine, and **p**rednisone. The use of aggressive combination chemotherapy regimens typically used for intermediate-grade and high-grade NHLs can lead to a more rapid therapeutic response in patients with low-grade lymphoma. Unfortunately, responses with any form of conventional chemotherapy are not durable, lasting a median of 2 years. Postchemotherapy maintenance interferon-α has been demonstrated to prolong disease-free and overall survival in randomized trials, but patients often find the associated flu-like symptoms difficult to endure. High-dose chemotherapy with autologous stem cell transplantation is now commonly used for the treatment of patients with refractory or relapsed follicular NHL. A lack of controlled trials in this area and the long natural history of the disease make it difficult to directly measure the magnitude of benefit associated with high-dose therapy. Extended follow-up of these patients is necessary to evaluate the curative potential of this approach.

Monoclonal antibodies directed against lymphocyte-specific antigens have been evaluated for the treatment of NHL and found to have potential especially for patients with relapsed low-grade or follicular lymphomas. These agents have been assessed both as isolated agents and as conjugates with toxins, chemotherapeutic agents, radioisotopes, or immunotherapeutic molecules. Rituximab, an unlabeled monoclonal antibody directed against the CD20 antigen has recently demonstrated response rates of approximately 50% (with a median duration of response of 10 to 12 months) in patients with relapsed low-grade or follicular lymphomas. Preliminary trials with radiolabeled antibodies for the treatment of low-grade NHL have also yielded promising results.

DIFFUSE LARGE B-CELL LYMPHOMA

The subtype of NHL, diffuse large B-cell lymphoma should be treated with curative intent. For the past two decades, combination chemotherapy has formed the basis of curative therapy for patients with this disease. First-generation chemotherapy regimens formulated in the early 1970s (e.g., CHOP, COMLA, and CHOP-Bleo; Table 233.4) were the first to produce long-term disease-free survival in a proportion of treated patients. Long-term follow-up from the original CHOP studies demonstrates that approximately one-third of patients are alive and disease-free a decade after treatment. Second- and third-generation regimens were developed by adding new agents to the original CHOP regimen, by taking advantage of alternative modes of administration, or by using alternating non–cross-resistant chemotherapeutic agents. These regimens include COP-BLAM, CAP-BOP, ProMACE-MOPP, m/M-BACOD, MACOP-B, and ProMACE-CytaBOM (Table 233.4).

Patients with localized (stage I or nonbulky stage II) disease are generally treated with short-course combination chemotherapy and involved-field irradiation. This results in long-term disease-free survival in approximately 70% to 80% of patients. Patients with bulky stage II, stage III, or stage IV disease have 5-year survival rates of 30% to 50% in most chemotherapy series. A definitive large, multicenter, randomized trial published in 1993 compared the four most popular combination chemotherapy regimens: CHOP, m-BACOD, MACOP-B, and ProMACE-CytaBOM. At 3 years' follow-up, the time to treatment failure and overall survival rates were no different for the four treatment arms. CHOP was associated with a trend toward less treatment mortality and, as such, has become the generally accepted standard combination chemotherapy regimen for these patients.

Lymphoma in certain anatomical locations necessitates additional therapy. For example, NHL in the testicle, paranasal sinuses, and epidural spaces can be associated with CNS relapse, and CNS prophylaxis should be used in these patients. Irradiation of the contralateral testicle is necessary for patients with primary testicular NHL.

Patients with recurrent diffuse large B-cell lymphoma have a poor prognosis with routine salvage chemotherapy. Multiagent chemotherapy regimens such as DHAP, MINE, IMVP-16, and ESAP (Table 232.4) have been evaluated in this setting. Despite a 20% to 30% complete response rate with most of these regimens, less than 5% of the patients are long-term disease-free survivors. A randomized trial (known as the Parma trial) comparing high-dose chemotherapy with autologous bone marrow transplantation was published in 1995. Patients with relapsed intermediate-grade or high-grade lymphoma were treated with two courses of conventional salvage chemotherapy. The patients responding to initial chemotherapy were then randomized to receive further conventional salvage chemotherapy or high-dose chemotherapy with autologous bone marrow transplantation. At 5 years' follow-up, patients randomized to high-dose chemotherapy/autologous bone marrow transplantation had a superior event-free (46% versus 12%) and overall (53% versus 32%) survival, and these differences have been sustained with further follow-up. This trial essentially established high-dose chemotherapy/autologous transplantation as the standard of care for patients with chemosensitive relapsed intermediate-grade or high-grade NHL.

In many transplantation centers, patients with poor prognostic features at diagnosis as established by the International Prognostic Index have been treated with high-dose chemotherapy/autologous stem cell transplantation in first partial or complete response to improve the long-term outlook. Some evidence suggests that outcomes are superior in patients who receive high-dose chemotherapy/autologous stem cell transplantation. For example the largest such study randomized poor-risk patients 55 years of age or younger to consolidative high-dose chemotherapy/autologous bone marrow transplantation in first complete remission. Patients with two or more adverse risk factors by the International Prognostic Index randomized to high-dose chemotherapy/autologous bone marrow transplantation

TABLE 233.4.	COMBINATION CHEMOTHERAPY REGIMENS FOR LYMPHOMA
Regimen	**Drugs Used**
CHOP	Cyclophosphamide, doxorubicin, vincristine, prednisone
CNOP	Cyclophosphamide, mitoxantrone, vincristine, prednisone
COP-BLAM	Cyclophosphamide, vincristine, prednisone, bleomycin, doxorubicin, procarbazine
CAP-BOP	Cyclophosphamide, vincristine, procarbazine, bleomycin, doxorubicin, prednisone
ProMACE-MOPP	Prednisone, methotrexate, doxorubicin, cyclophosphamide, etoposide, nitrogen mustard, vincristine, procarbazine
m/M-BACOD	Methotrexate, bleomycin, doxorubicin, cyclophosphamide, vincristine, dexamethasone
MACOP-B	Methotrexate, doxorubicin, cyclophosphamide, vincristine, prednisone, bleomycin
ProMACE-CytaBOM	Prednisone, methotrexate, doxorubicin, cyclophosphamide, etoposide, cytarabine, bleomycin, vincristine
VACOP-B	Etoposide, doxorubicin, cyclophosphamide, vincristine, prednisone, bleomycin
DHAP	Cisplatin, cytarabine, dexamethasone
MINE	Ifosfamide, mitoxantrone, etoposide
ESAP	Etoposide, cisplatin, cytarabine, methylprednisone
IMVP-16	Ifosfamide, methotrexate, etoposide

had a superior disease-free (59% versus 39%) and overall (65% versus 52%) survival at 5 years after transplantation.

Alternative therapies that are being evaluated for patients who are not transplantation candidates include infusional chemotherapy, modulation of the multidrug resistance gene (*PGY*), and monoclonal antibody therapy alone or with conjugated toxins, chemotherapy, or radiolabeled isotopes.

LYMPHOBLASTIC LYMPHOMA

Intensive chemotherapeutic regimens similar to those used in acute lymphoblastic leukemia patients produce the best long-term disease-free survival for patients with lymphoblastic lymphomas. Because of the propensity for CNS relapse, CNS prophylaxis (intrathecal chemotherapy and craniospinal irradiation) is a routine part of most treatment regimens. Particularly in adult patients, bone marrow involvement, CNS involvement, and elevated LDH levels at the time of diagnosis are poor prognostic signs. For patients with these poor prognostic features, many transplantation centers advocate high-dose chemotherapy with autologous stem cell transplantation as consolidative therapy. Some series have suggested that the use of a human leukocyte antigen (HLA)-identical sibling donor results in an increased chance of long-term disease-free survival in young patients.

■ CONCLUSION

The management strategy for patients with newly diagnosed or relapsed NHL is formulated on the basis of the histologic subtype of the disease, the results of staging investigations, and the presence or absence of the previously outlined prognostic factors. This approach for the selection of therapy ensures delivery of the best possible treatment for each patient.

BIBLIOGRAPHY

A predictive model for aggressive non-Hodgkin's lymphoma: the International Non-Hodgkin's Lymphoma Prognostic Factors Project. *N Engl J Med* 1993;329:987–994.

Bosch F, López-Guillermo A, Campo E, et al. Mantle cell lymphoma. *Cancer* 1998;82:567–575.

Bouabdallah R, Xerrsti L, Bardou VJ, et al. Role of induction chemotherapy and bone marrow transplantation in adult lymphoblastic lymphoma: a report on 62 patients from a single center. *Ann Oncol* 1998;9:619–625.

Cantor KP, Blair A, Everett G, et al. Pesticides and other agricultural risk factors for non-Hodgkin's lymphoma among men in Iowa and Minnesota. *Cancer Res* 1992;52:2447–2455.

Fisher RI, Gaynor ER, Dahlberg S, et al. Comparison of a standard regimen (CHOP) with three intensive chemotherapy regimens for advanced non-Hodgkin's lymphoma. *N Engl J Med* 1993;328:1002–1006.

Haioun C, Lepage E, Gisselbrecht C, et al. Benefit of autologous bone marrow transplantation over sequential chemotherapy in poor-risk aggressive non-Hodgkin's lymphoma: updated results of the prospective study LNH87-2. *J Clin Oncol* 1997;15:1131–1137.

Harris NL, Jaffe ES, Diebold J, et al. World Health Organization classification of neoplastic diseases of the hematopoietic and lymphoid tissues: report of the Clinical Advisory Committee meeting—Airlie House, Virginia, November 1997. *J Clin Oncol* 1999;17:3835–3849.

Landis SH, Murray T, Bolden S, et al. Cancer statistics 1998. *CA Cancer J Clin* 1998;48:6–29.

Lyons SF, Liebowitz DN. The roles of human viruses in the pathogenesis of lymphoma. *Semin Oncol* 1998;25:461–475.

McLaughlin P, Grillo-López AJ, Link BK, et al. Rituximab chimeric anti-CD20 monoclonal antibody therapy for relapsed indolent lymphoma: half of patients respond to a four-dose treatment program. *J Clin Oncol* 1998;16:2825–2833.

Kelley's Textbook of Internal Medicine, fourth edition. Edited by H. David Humes. Lippincott Williams & Wilkins, Philadelphia © 2000.

C H A P T E R

234

PLASMA CELL DISORDERS

PHILIP R. GREIPP

The principal plasma cell disorders are multiple myeloma (MM), monoclonal gammopathy of undetermined significance (MGUS), macroglobulinemia of Waldenström, and amyloidosis of the light-chain type. They arise when an abnormal clone of plasma cells produces a monoclonal immunoglobulin (M protein). The M protein is often first discovered on a screening serum electrophoresis. It assumes the shape of a monoclonal peak on a serum electrophoresis densitometric tracing and is often referred to as an *M spike*. Immunoelectrophoresis or immunofixation of the serum proves the suspected protein as monoclonal, having a single IgG, IgA, IgM, IgD, or IgE immunoglobulin heavy-chain class and a single kappa (κ) or lambda (λ) isotype immunoglobulin light chain.

In an asymptomatic patient with a small amount of IgG or IgA M protein (less than 2 g per deciliter), the most likely diagnosis is monoclonal gammopathy of undetermined significance (MGUS). This most often represents a "benign" condition, which remains stable during the patient's lifetime, but in 25% of patients it can also be a precursor to a serious disorder such as multiple myeloma (MM). Less commonly, amyloidosis of the light-chain type may develop (Chapter 235).

A small monoclonal protein of the IgM type in an asymptomatic person most often represents MGUS. It may also be a precursor to macroglobulinemia, malignant lymphoma, chronic lymphocytic leukemia, or a chronic lymphoproliferative disorder. These disorders are discussed in Chapters 228 and 236.

■ INCIDENCE AND EPIDEMIOLOGY

Twenty-five percent of MGUS patients eventually develop MM or another serious plasma cell disorder at the rate of 1% per year. In order of frequency, patients with MGUS have IgG, IgM, IgA, or IgD M protein in the serum and either a κ or λ light chain as part of the immunoglobulin molecule. Monoclonal gammopathy increases with age. It is uncommon in persons younger than 40 years of age. The annual incidence of MM is 3 to 4 cases per 100,000 persons with a 2 : 1 male predominance. As in other B-cell malignancies, the death rate from MM appears to be increasing. MM is projected to cause 14,000 deaths in the United States. It accounts for 1% of all malignancies and 2% of all cancer deaths. The median age is 60 to 65 years in referral populations and 75 years in the general population. MM is two times more common among blacks than whites, regardless of economic environment; this suggests a possible genetic or biologic predisposition.

TABLE 234.1.	PRINCIPAL DISORDERS ASSOCIATED WITH MONOCLONAL GAMMOPATHY

Monoclonal gammopathy of undetermined significance
Smoldering multiple myeloma
Multiple myeloma
Solitary plasmacytoma
Macroglobulinemia
Primary amyloidosis
Heavy-chain diseases (γ, α, and μ)
Cryoglobulinemia (types I and II)

ETIOLOGY

The causes of monoclonal gammopathy and myeloma are unknown. Although MGUS and MM have been reported in twins, family members, and spouses, no broad-based genetic predisposition or familial tendency is established. MGUS occurs more frequently among patients with HIV infection and those who have had bone marrow transplantation, suggesting that immune dysregulation can provide the milieu for the development of MGUS. Correlations with radiation or pesticide exposure have been challenged. Findings of herpes simplex virus HSV8 in dendritic cells and the detection of other viruses raise the possibility of viral oncogenesis.

PATHOGENESIS

In MM, cytokines mediate myeloma cell proliferation and bone destruction. Interleukin-1β (IL-1β) is produced by myeloma cells, and it can increase marrow stromal cell production of IL-6. In turn, IL-6 can stimulate proliferation of susceptible myeloma cells, block their apoptosis, and activate osteoclasts. Resulting pure "punched-out" lytic bone lesions are typical of MM. In about 15% of patients with MM, osteoporosis and compression fractures without radiographic bone lesions may develop. Hypercalcemia occurs in about 20% of patients owing to rapid loss of bone mineral. Renal failure in MM is associated with higher urinary excretion of monoclonal light chain (Bence Jones proteinuria), typically more than 1 g of protein in a 24-hour collection. Nephrotoxic light chains can concentrate in the renal medulla and form protein casts with Tamm–Horsfall mucoprotein. Flattened tubular epithelium, protein casts, and foreign-body giant cells characterize the myeloma kidney, which is especially susceptible to the effects of hypercalcemia, dehydration, x-ray contrast media, and nephrotoxic medications. Excess intake of vitamin C acidifies the urine and can cause Bence Jones protein casts and renal failure.

Myeloma plasma cells often have an immature appearance. Plasmablastic features suggest a poor prognosis. A high plasma cell proliferation rate, measured using the plasma cell labeling index (PCLI), defines MM as separate from MGUS and suggests a poor prognosis. A high level of IL-6 in the serum or plasma suggests more advanced MM. C-reactive protein is made by the liver in response to IL-6 and serves as a surrogate for IL-6

measurement. β_2-Microglobulin levels, which are elevated in patients with advanced myeloma, also convey a poor prognosis.

Myeloma cell surface adhesion molecules such as CD56 interact with marrow stromal cells, providing myeloma cells with a selective growth advantage by placing them close to the source of needed cytokines.

Because myeloma cells proliferate too slowly to produce metaphases for standard cytogenetic analysis, cytogenetic abnormalities, which contribute to MM progression, have been observed in only 20% of cases. Loss of chromosome 13 or a portion of it is associated with a poor prognosis. Fluorescence in situ hybridization (FISH) for interphase cells detects such abnormalities more sensitively than standard cytogenetics and in the near future will detect critical translocations. Molecular abnormalities contribute to myeloma progression by dysregulation of the *p53* and *bcl2* genes late in the disease. Like IL-6, these abnormalities decrease apoptosis, or programmed cell death. IL-1β upregulation is an important step between MGUS and overt MM. A combination of cytogenetic and molecular abnormalities leads to an expansion of the myeloma cell clone. *Ras* mutations can further increase the expansion of the myeloma cell clone. Abnormal gene expression causing glucocorticoid and multidrug resistance lead to a refractory, progressive, and terminal phase of the disease.

Infections are related to low levels of normal immunoglobulins and a defective primary antibody response to new antigen exposures. After chemotherapy, neutropenia and more deeply impaired T-cell immunity predispose to more infections.

The differential diagnosis of monoclonal gammopathies depends on the understanding of the disorders listed in Tables 234.1 and 234.2. The algorithm shown in Figure 234.1 can be used as a guide to evaluate the most common monoclonal gammopathies.

SPECIFIC PLASMA CELL DISORDERS
MONOCLONAL GAMMOPATHY OF UNDETERMINED SIGNIFICANCE

Clinical Findings

Patients with MGUS are asymptomatic. No associated abnormalities are seen on physical examination. MGUS is often coin-

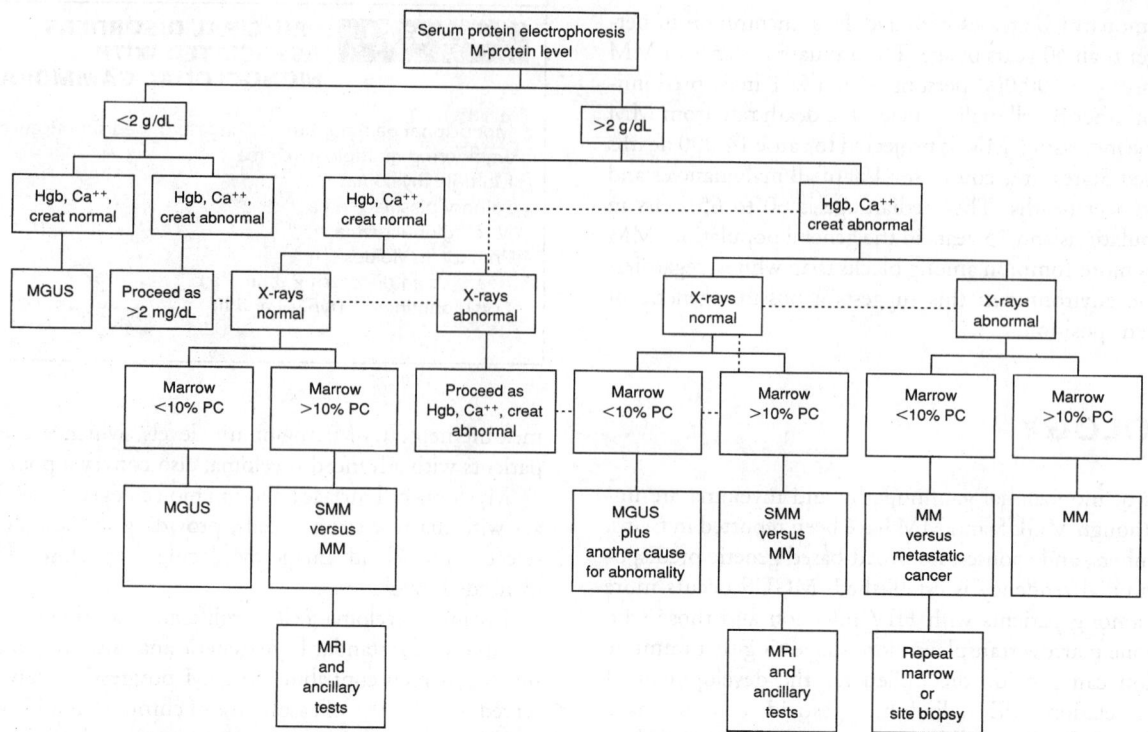

FIGURE 234.1. An algorithm for the differential diagnosis of monoclonal gammopathy (IgG, IgA types), including stepwise evaluation for patients with small (less than 2 g per deciliter) and larger (more than 2 g per deciliter) M-protein levels. Other ancillary tests refer to the C-reactive protein level, β_2-microglobulin level, plasma cell labeling index (PCLI), and test for circulating plasma cells. Patients with more than 2 g per deciliter of serum M protein should have a 24-hour urine protein electrophoresis. If Bence Jones protein is more than 5 g in 24 hours, proceed as if the Hgb, Ca^{++}, and Creat values are abnormal. Ca^{++}, serum calcium level; *Creat,* serum creatinine level; *Hgb,* hemoglobin level; *M protein,* monoclonal protein; *MGUS,* monoclonal gammopathy of undetermined significance; *MM,* multiple myeloma; *MRI,* magnetic resonance imaging; *PC,* plasma cells; *SMM,* smoldering multiple myeloma.

cidentally found with other diseases, including heart disease, cancer, and diabetes, which are common in older populations in whom MGUS is most prevalent. Symptoms such as bone pain, fatigue, and symptoms of hypercalcemia or renal insufficiency are absent in MGUS, and their unexplained presence suggests MM.

Laboratory Findings

A small monoclonal spike (less than 2 g per deciliter) on the serum protein electrophoresis of an asymptomatic patient supports a diagnosis of MGUS rather than MM. An M-protein concentration in the serum greater than 2 g per deciliter suggests the need to rule out MM. The urine should be examined by electrophoresis of a 24-hour collection for any patient with a serum M-protein concentration greater than 2 g per deciliter or whose urinalysis reveals proteinemia. A large spike on the urine protein electrophoretic tracing with a urine M-protein level greater than 300 mg per 24 hours suggests the need to rule out MM.

Serum special protein studies, including immunoelectrophoresis, immunofixation, and more recently developed capillary electrophoresis with immunosubtraction occasionally show free monoclonal light chain in the serum (Bence Jones proteinemia),

which is not apparent on the standard electrophoresis. This strongly suggests MM or amyloidosis. Such patients also have high levels of free κ or λ monoclonal light chain in the urine (Bence Jones proteinuria).

Anemia, hypercalcemia, and renal insufficiency are absent in the patient with MGUS. A bone survey shows no lytic lesions. Osteoporosis suggests the need to rule out MM, but it may be coincidental because of the age of the population involved. The bone marrow always shows less than 10% plasma cells. The PCLI of the marrow plasma cells is invariably very low, and circulating plasma cells are typically absent. Measurement of normal immunoglobulins is rarely helpful. They can be suppressed in MGUS or MM. C-reactive protein and β_2-microglobulin levels are rarely helpful in differentiating MGUS from early-stage MM.

Optimal Management

If no symptoms or laboratory findings suggest MM, amyloidosis, or another monoclonal gammopathy–associated condition, no further diagnostic studies are needed. Patients with MGUS should be followed up by serial electrophoresis at 3- to 6-month intervals until their M-protein level is stable, then at least annually thereafter. Quantitative immunoglobulin levels of IgG, IgA,

TABLE 234.2.	DISORDERS ASSOCIATED WITH MONOCLONAL GAMMOPATHY

Light-chain deposition disease
    Renal glomerular deposition of monoclonal light chain (usually λ)
Adult-acquired Fanconi's syndrome
    Renal tubular deposition of monoclonal light chain (usually κ)
Scleromyxedema (ie, papular mucinosis or lichen myxedematosis)
    Mucinous deposition in the skin (usualy IgG λ)
Peripheral neuropathy (usually IgM)
Osteosclerotic myeloma
    Single or multiple osteosclerotic bone lesions (usually λ)
    Associated POEMS of angiocentric follicular lymph node hyperplasia
Cold agglutinin disease
    IgM κ on erythrocytes
Systemic capillary leak syndrome
    Usually an IgG κ M protein with episodic hypotension and hemoconcentration
Acquired C_1-esterase inhibitor syndrome
    Often an IgM M protein with associated angioedema and episodic abdominal pain
Acquired von Willebrand disease
    Usually IgM, with typical platelet defect of von Willebrand

Ig, immunoglobulin; *κ*, kappa; *λ*, lambda; *POEMS*, polyneuropathy, organomegaly, endocrinopathy, M protein, and skin changes.

or IgM are helpful, especially if the spike is too small or difficult to measure on electrophoresis. An increase greater than 0.5 g in the serum electrophoretic spike or an increase in the quantitative immunoglobulin level during follow-up for the appropriate M protein suggests the need to rule out MM. A similar increase in an IgM-type protein suggests lymphoma, chronic lymphocytic leukemia, or macroglobulinemia, topics covered in other chapters.

Accurate differentiation of MGUS from MM can prevent unnecessary complications of treatment. If unexplained anemia, hypercalcemia, or renal insufficiency is present, x-ray films of the axial skeleton, skull, and proximal long bones should be obtained to search for lytic lesions. Bone marrow aspiration and biopsy are also indicated. Measurement of the PCLI and assessment of circulating plasma cells can be very useful in more difficult diagnostic situations.

SMOLDERING AND INDOLENT MULTIPLE MYELOMA

Clinical Findings

Smoldering and indolent multiple myeloma lie between MGUS and MM. Unlike MGUS, patients with smoldering multiple myeloma (SMM) have a higher level of M protein in the serum (often more than 3 g per deciliter) and a higher number of plasma cells in the marrow (higher than 10%). Patients are asymptomatic, and their disease is not progressive, so one can observe the patient without treatment for years. Affected patients may have mild nonprogressive anemia but no bone lesions, hypercalcemia, or renal failure. Disease of asymptomatic patients

who have scattered small bone lesions that are not progressive has been called stage I or indolent multiple myeloma (IMM). Most IMM patients progress to overt MM in less than 1 year. Eventual development of overt MM is to be expected in patients initially diagnosed with SMM or IMM, but the interval varies from months to many years.

SMM or IMM patients are asymptomatic. Physical examination reveals no abnormalities. Bone pain, fatigue, or symptoms of unexplained hypercalcemia or renal insufficiency suggests a diagnosis of MM.

Laboratory Findings

In addition to a higher serum M-protein spike and more than 10% plasma cells in the marrow with aggregates of plasma cells on the marrow biopsy, a 24-hour urine collection usually shows less than 500 mg of M protein. A higher level suggests overt MM. Some patients with less than 3 g per deciliter of M protein have more than 10% plasma cells in the marrow. These can also be classified as SMM. The PCLI is low, usually 0.0% to 0.2%, and circulating plasma cells are less than 3×10^6 per liter. The bone density is normal or borderline, and the MRI of the lumbar spine is normal. Mild anemia may exist and remain stable for years. Although bone fractures, hypercalcemia, and renal insufficiency constitute evidence of overt MM, idiopathic osteoporosis, hyperparathyroidism, and other occult renal disease must be considered in the differential diagnosis.

Optimal Management

Patients with SMM are followed up more closely than are patients with MGUS. A reasonable approach is to perform serum electrophoresis at 3-month intervals the first year and, if stable, at 6-month intervals thereafter. A second bone survey and marrow examination should be done if the M-protein level increases. A complete blood count and chemistry profile with serum calcium and creatinine should be done at least twice each year. Careful attention should be given to any symptoms that may indicate MM.

Early chemotherapy in asymptomatic MM does not improve survival, and the use of alkylating agent-based chemotherapy can cause pancytopenia, cytogenetic abnormalities, myelodysplastic syndrome, or acute leukemia. Although the overall risk of these problems is only 2% or 3%, the risk increases with time, reaching 10% at 10 years. Bisphosphonate therapy may prevent progression of bone disease. Observation is sometimes the best course.

The use of MRI of the lumbar spine is especially helpful when osteoporosis is evident on plain x-rays. If the diagnosis of idiopathic osteoporosis versus MM cannot be resolved, bisphosphonate therapy such as pamidronate and close follow-up is usually the best alternative.

MULTIPLE MYELOMA

Clinical Findings

Unlike MGUS and SMM, the plasma cell clone in MM expands progressively and produces one or more of the following: bone lesions, anemia, renal failure, or hypercalcemia. De novo plasma cell leukemia is a particularly malignant form of myeloma. Bone lesions are less common, and patients often have hepatosplenomegaly—findings uncommon in typical MM. Confirmation of a diagnosis of MM requires a finding of more than 10% plasma cells in the marrow aspirate or aggregates of monoclonal plasma cells on the marrow biopsy. If the malignant plasma cell proliferation cannot be found in the marrow, a site-directed biopsy of a plasmacytoma plus other lytic lesions satisfies diagnostic criteria.

The typical course of MM lasts 3 to 4 years. There is wide variation in survival, ranging from only a few weeks or months in 10% of patients to more than 10 years in 5% of patients. The cause of death is usually infection or bleeding associated with a chemotherapy resistant state.

Most patients with MM are anemic. They can present with pallor, fatigue, and shortness of breath. Most patients also have bone lesions, which manifest as movement-related bone pain. Bone tenderness or pathologic fractures of the vertebrae, ribs, or sternum may occur with little or no trauma. Bone pain can be dismissed as musculoskeletal pain for months before diagnosis. Hypercalcemia may develop, causing a loss of appetite, somnolence, nausea, vomiting, constipation, dehydration, or renal failure. Absence of significant anemia or bone lesions does not preclude the diagnosis of MM.

Recurrent infection with capsular organisms, including *Streptococcus pneumoniae, Staphylococcus epidermidis,* and *Haemophilus influenzae,* occur in less than 10% of patients. Patients with pneumonia may develop meningitis because of immune impairment. Standard immunization does not prevent *S. pneumoniae* infection. Gram-negative bacterial infections are common during the course of MM because of the effects of chemotherapy and neutropenia.

Bleeding in the initial months of MM is uncommon. A bleeding diathesis later in the course of the disease may result from interference of the M protein with coagulation factors, combined with thrombocytopenia due to chemotherapy superimposed on diminished marrow reserves.

Amyloidosis may occur in 10% of cases of myeloma, but usually the diagnosis is incidental with no symptoms or complications.

Laboratory Findings

Serum and urine immunoelectrophoresis and immunofixation are done in all cases. A serum monoclonal protein is present in 85% of patients with MM, and a urine monoclonal protein is found in 75%. Ten percent of these may lack the characteristic spike on electrophoresis of the serum and urine. For about 1% to 2% who have no M protein detected in the serum or urine by any method, the disease is called *nonsecretory* or, very rarely, *nonproducer myeloma* in which the malignant plasma cells are negative for cytoplasmic immunoglobulin by immunocytochemistry.

A bone survey including radiographs of the skull, axial skeleton, ribs, sternum, shoulder and hip girdles, and proximal long bones show characteristic lytic bone lesions in two-thirds of patients with MM. Osteoporosis and lytic lesions plus an M protein alone are insufficient criteria for the diagnosis of MM. MRI of the spine or CT scan of a suspected area may be needed to demonstrate bone lesions.

Accurate diagnosis depends on the demonstration of an M protein in the serum or urine, accompanied by more than 10% plasma cells in the marrow aspirate or aggregates of plasma cells in the biopsy sample, and demonstration of bone lesions, anemia, hypercalcemia, or renal failure. The average bone marrow examination demonstrates 30% plasma cells. Sheets of plasma cells replace the marrow in advanced disease. Rarely, fibrosis is present. Amyloidosis is found on the marrow biopsy in a small percentage of patients and is most often clinically inconsequential. About 2% of patients present with plasma cell leukemia, defined as more than 2,000 circulating plasma cells per cubic millimeter. In advanced disease, the blood smear may show a leukoerythroblastic reaction.

Hypercalcemia (calcium level higher than 12 g per deciliter) occurs in one of ten patients, and renal failure (creatinine greater than 2 mg per deciliter) in one of six patients. Fifty percent of patients have an elevated serum β_2-microglobulin level, which correlates with high tumor burden or renal insufficiency. Confirmatory tests include the PCLI and determination of circulating plasma cells.

Laboratory findings have yielded a staging system that reflects the tumor burden. Patients with stage I disease have a hemoglobin concentration greater than 10 g per deciliter, normal calcium, no bone lesions or a solitary lesion, an IgG level less than 5 g per deciliter, an IgA level less than 3 g per deciliter, and urine light-chain values less than 4 g per 24 hours. Patients with stage III disease have a hemoglobin concentration less than 8.5 g per deciliter, a calcium level greater than 12 g per deciliter, multiple lytic lesions, an IgG level greater than 7 g per deciliter, an IgA level greater than 5 g per deciliter, and a urine light-chain value greater than 12 g per 24 hours. Patients with intermediate values have stage II disease. Patients without and with renal insufficiency are classified, respectively, as A or B. An improved prognostic system relies on measurement of PCLI and β_2-microglobulin. The serum C-reactive protein level and soluble IL-6 receptor level also appear to be independent prognostic factors.

Optimal Management

Optimal management of a patient with MM depends on a prompt, accurate diagnosis and appropriate use of chemotherapy, radiation therapy, stem cell transplantation, management of bone disease, pain management, and psychologic support. Much of the improvement in survival observed during the last decade resulted from prompt recognition of complications and better supportive therapy. The patient and physician need to be aware of the symptoms of MM complications and their treatment.

Long-term disease control rather than cure is the goal of standard and even transplantation therapy regimens. Chemotherapy usually reduces the tumor burden, but most patients have residual disease. A plateau reached in most patients is marked by a stable decrease in the level of M protein. During this plateau, chemotherapy may be discontinued, and the M-protein level assayed regularly. The choice to use interferon in prolonging this phase should be weighed against the side effects it produces. Survival is not improved by maintenance interferon. Eventual relapse is the rule, and the chance for prolonged survival depends on whether the patient's myeloma is sensitive to second-line chemotherapy.

For patients over age 70 years who are not candidates for transplantation, simple melphalan (Alkeran) and prednisone chemotherapy produces an objective response in about 50% of patients. An objective response is defined as a reduction of the serum M-protein levels by more than 50% and a disappearance of the urine M protein. The dosage of melphalan is 0.15 mg per kilogram per day for 7 days, administered with 60 mg of prednisone daily for 7 days, cycled every 6 weeks. Although the objective response rate with combination chemotherapy may be higher than with melphalan and prednisone, there appears to be little survival advantage. However, combination chemotherapy may be advantageous for rapidly lowering the tumor burden. Disadvantages include side effects, expense, and more infections in older or infirm persons.

Precautions and prophylaxis against infection may improve outcome. Administration of trimethoprim-cotrimoxazole during the first 3 months of treatment, when the risk of infection is highest, is a reasonable approach, especially with combination chemotherapy regimens. Ciprofloxacin (500 mg twice daily) can be substituted. Granulocyte colony-stimulating factor may be used, but its comparative effectiveness is not proved, and it is costly. Penicillin VK (500 mg twice daily) taken orally prevents the recurrent *S. pneumoniae* infections that occur in less than 10% of patients.

Radiation therapy is used for locally threatening lesions. About 5% of MM patients develop spinal cord compression during the course of their disease. Prompt recognition of the symptoms and signs can prevent major disability. These include severe unremitting back pain, especially nerve root (radicular) pain, unilateral or bilateral numbness of the lower extremities, paresis or paralysis, urinary or bowel control problems, hyperreflexia, and pathologic reflexes. Myeloma is exquisitely sensitive to radiation therapy. Local recurrence is rare. Residual tumor mass, if any, is often dormant or caused by persistent amyloid in the mass. Fields and doses of radiation should be limited to control the locally threatening tumor and to avoid permanent effects on normal marrow. Radiation may be necessary for painful localized lesions in other bones, but it should be reserved for symptoms that pose threats to life or that might cause long-term disability.

Surgical internal fixation may be necessary in the case of impending fracture of a long bone. The most reliable sign of impending fracture is persistent pain. An orthopedist who has experience with MM should be consulted, and appropriate conservative measures, such as bracing for refractory pain or other support measures, or surgery should be chosen after considering the patient's long-term outlook and the degree of the threat posed by localized tumor growth. Oral calcium supplements, fluoride, and vitamin D do not adequately prevent fractures. Bisphosphonates, although costly, have been proved to prevent fractures and should be used for an indefinite period of time for any patients with myeloma bone disease.

Early recognition and treatment of hypercalcemia help to prevent renal insufficiency. Appropriate initial treatment includes high-dose corticosteroids and vigorous hydration to initi-ate a diuresis. Patients initially may have a large initial intravascular volume deficit that must be replaced. If saline diuresis has been initiated, natriuretic diuretics may be administered to enhance calcium excretion. Intravenous bisphosphonates are effective in treatment of hypercalcemia.

Renal insufficiency is a serious but often reversible complication of MM. Causes includes light-chain proteinuria, hypercalcemia, hyperuricemia, and hyperviscosity caused by very high levels of M protein. Aggravating factors include infections, dehydration, use of contrast dyes, nephrotoxic antibiotics, and excess doses of vitamin C. Prevention requires avoidance of these factors. Treatment includes vigorous intravenous hydration and discontinuation of nephrotoxic agents. Allopurinol, alkalinization of the urine, and plasmapheresis may be of benefit. Hydration and diuresis are the most important measures. Dialysis is rarely needed, and patients who require hemodialysis generally have more aggressive and resistant myelomas.

Patients younger than 70 years of age healthy enough to undergo the rigors of intensive therapy should be considered candidates for peripheral stem cell transplantation (PSCT) from the outset. After an initial period of cytoreductive chemotherapy with vincristine, doxorubicin (Adriamycin), and dexamethasone (VAD) or a similar regimen, stem cell harvest is carried out. Harvested cells are then cryopreserved in liquid nitrogen for immediate PSCT. Alternatively, standard chemotherapy can be given and PSCT reserved later for relapsed disease. MM treatment-related mortality in most centers is less than 5%. Intensive therapy and PSCT are attractive because they achieve a greater reduction in tumor burden and a higher complete response (CR) rate averaging 25% compared with the lower complete response rates obtained with standard chemotherapy. Patients who achieve CR live longer than other responding patients. Patients with primarily resistant disease on VAD chemotherapy may also respond particularly well to stem cell transplantation compared with the response from standard chemotherapy.

Allogeneic transplantation has a higher treatment-related mortality rate than autologous stem cell transplantation. In addition to a 30% to 40% mortality rate in the first 6 months, there is risk of developing severe chronic graft-versus-host disease. Allogeneic transplantation is restricted to centers where outcome is reported and special studies are conducted to reduce morbidity and mortality. Enthusiasm for potential cure by autologous and allogeneic transplantation is tempered by the reality that relapses occur in most cases. New agents and modalities holding promise are thalidomide, other antiangiogenic approaches, immunomodulation, and vaccination.

Pain management and psychologic support are important in patients with MM. A patient needs to know that response to treatment yields longer survival, often many years. Patients should know that other approaches are available in case of relapse. The availability of clinical trials should be stressed before treatment is started. Ideally, patients should assume a role in the choice of initial treatment. They should be guided toward developing an awareness of the importance of prompt treatment of complications. Patients should be told that they could live a normal life during the stable phase of the disease. With the support of analgesics, most patients afflicted with even the most severe bone pain can maintain activity levels that encourage better bone mineralization. They can increase fluid intake to prevent dehydration and reduce the risk of renal damage. Such patients can learn to promptly recognize and report fever or other evidence of infection.

SOLITARY PLASMACYTOMA

Most patients with solitary plasmacytoma have a single solitary plasmacytoma of bone (SPB), and some have an extramedullary plasmacytoma (EMP). Most have a monoclonal protein in the serum or urine. They do not fulfill criteria for MM, because they do not have anemia, disseminated bone lesions, hypercalcemia, or renal insufficiency and because they have less than 10% plasma cells in the marrow. Although most patients with SPB remain asymptomatic after initial treatment, about one-third develop MM an average of 4.5 years after initial diagnosis of SPB. About 40% are disease-free at 10 years. EMP can affect almost any organ. Some patients with EMP later develop local spread rather than overt MM.

Clinical Findings

The findings in SPB depend on the site of involvement. SPB most commonly affects the vertebrae but may also affect the ribs, scapulas, pelvis, and skull or any medullary site. Involvement of adjacent bone and tissue sites by direct extension does not constitute evidence of MM. Spinal cord compression and its attendant clinical symptoms and signs are potential complications that must be detected early and treated on an emergency basis.

Laboratory Findings

Evaluation of patients with suspected SPB should include serum and urine electrophoresis and immunofixation, bone radiographs, a complete blood count, a blood chemistry panel, and a marrow examination. Unlike patients who have MM, the spike in the serum of patients with SPB is small and usually disappears with treatment. Patients do not have major light-chain proteinuria. Hemoglobin, calcium, and creatinine levels are normal. Bone x-ray films fail to reveal additional bone lesions. The marrow examination usually detects no monoclonal plasma cells, but if they are present, the patient is likely to require chemotherapy for myeloma within only a few years.

Optimal Management

A patient with a SPB and an M protein does not satisfy criteria for MM, even with a small percentage of monoclonal plasma cells in the marrow. Chemotherapy should not be given as part of initial treatment for SPB. Many patients with SPB are given chemotherapy, but local irradiation alone may bring about long-term control without recurrence. Unlike the palliative irradiation used for controlling locally threatening disease in patients with MM, the goal in patients with SPB is cure. Radiation fields should generously encompass the known area of involvement, and full doses should be given.

The patient's prognosis depends on the biology of solitary plasmacytoma more than its size or extent. Morphologic immaturity of the plasmacytoma is not a negative prognostic factor

for progression to overt MM. The presence of monoclonal plasma cells in the marrow or persistent M protein in the serum or urine suggests that the patient will eventually develop MM. Patients remain at risk of MM for years. Local recurrence is extremely rare after local irradiation or complete surgical resection. These patients should be followed up in the same manner as those with SMM.

HEAVY-CHAIN DISEASES

Heavy-chain diseases are rare variants of monoclonal gammopathies that are characterized by the production by plasma cells of abnormal heavy chains of immunoglobulin. Immunoelectrophoresis and immunofixation may show that monoclonal heavy chains migrate differently from the migration of associated monoclonal light chains. This usually reflects critical deletions in coding the heavy chain to which the light chains are normally covalently linked. The underlying disorder varies.

Clinical Findings

The clinical spectrum of the heavy-chain diseases varies from that of a collagen vascular disorder to a lymphoma. Most common in the United States is γ heavy-chain disease, corresponding to IgG monoclonal gammopathy. Patients characteristically have hepatosplenomegaly or lymphadenopathy. Sometimes, they have pharyngeal involvement and uvular swelling (Franklin's disease). Usually, no free light chain is produced, and the course is extremely varied. The α heavy-chain disease, corresponding to IgA monoclonal gammopathy, is seen mainly in the Mediterranean area. Patients have abdominal nodal involvement, small-bowel involvement, and associated malabsorption. In μ heavy-chain disease, the presentation varies from lymphoma-like disease to that of chronic lymphocytic leukemia.

Laboratory Findings

A small, broad-based spike may be easily missed on electrophoresis. Lytic bone lesions are uncommon.

Optimal Management

Mediterranean lymphoma or α heavy-chain disease can cause malabsorption. Treatment varies from antibiotics for certain patients to cytotoxic therapy as for low-grade lymphoma. The response rate is high and the subsequent course highly variable. Cures are rare.

CRYOGLOBULINEMIA

Cryoglobulins precipitate from serum at reduced temperatures in vitro and may redissolve on rewarming. Type I cryoglobulinemia consists of a monoclonal protein, frequently IgM. The clinical picture varies from MGUS lymphoma or macroglobulinemia in the case of IgM M proteins to myeloma in the case of IgG or IgA M proteins. Type II cryoglobulinemia consists of a monoclonal immunoglobulin, usually IgM, which forms complexes with polyclonal immunoglobulin, usually IgG, and binds and removes complement causing low levels of C3 and C4. High rheumatoid factor levels are common. Type III cryoglobulins are characteristically polyclonal IgM immunoglobulin complexed with polyclonal IgG immunoglobulin.

Clinical Findings

Patients with type I cryoglobulinemia have acral cyanosis and even infarction if the cryoglobulin precipitates near body temperature. Most patients are asymptomatic. Cryocrits may be very high without any symptoms.

Patients with type II or mixed cryoglobulinemia develop vasculitides, with involvement of the skin, kidneys, and peripheral neuropathy. The clinical syndrome resembles immune complex disease, and complement levels may be low.

Type III cryoglobulins occur secondary to underlying infections, such as mononucleosis.

Laboratory Findings

Immunoelectrophoresis of redissolved cryoglobulin identifies the type of cryoglobulin. Thermal insolubility assays are useful in type I cryoglobulinemia to predict whether the patient will have symptoms.

Optimal Management

Patients with symptomatic type I cryoglobulinemia may require treatment for the underlying lymphoma or myeloma. Patients with type II or mixed cryoglobulinemia may benefit from corticosteroids and cytotoxic therapy. Interferon therapy may control disease without the long-term negative effects of cytotoxics and corticosteroids. Patients with type III cryoglobulinemia are rarely symptomatic and seldom require treatment.

▌ CONDITIONS ASSOCIATED WITH MONOCLONAL GAMMOPATHY

Table 234.2 lists other conditions associated with monoclonal gammopathy. Renal insufficiency in association with monoclonal gammopathy may be caused by amyloidosis of the light-chain type (Chapter 235), adult-acquired Fanconi's syndrome, or light-chain deposition disease. These disorders can overlap and mimic MM because of the finding of renal failure and increased plasma cells in the marrow associated with a monoclonal gammopathy, but most patients do not develop overt MM. They may live for years without requiring chemotherapy.

A full description of each of these syndromes is beyond the scope of this chapter. Most patients with one of these syndromes should be observed without treatment. Chemotherapy should be given only if the patient has overt systemic myeloma or if the risk of the disease outweighs the risk of chemotherapy-induced myelodysplasia and acute leukemia.

ACKNOWLEDGMENT

Supported by Grants CA62242 and CA21115 from the National Cancer Institute (National Institutes of Health).

BIBLIOGRAPHY

Alexanian R, Barlogie B, Dixon D. Renal failure in multiple myeloma: pathogenesis and prognostic implications. *Arch Intern Med* 1990;150: 1693–1695.

Donovan KA, Lacy MQ, Kline MP, et al. Contrast in cytokine expression between patients with monoclonal gammopathy of undetermined significance or multiple myeloma. *Leukemia* 1998;12:593–600.

Ellis PA, Colls BM. Solitary plasmacytoma of bone: clinical features, treatment and survival. *Hematol Oncol* 1992;10:207–211.

Gertz Ma, Kyle Ra. Amyloidosis—prognosis and treatment. *Semin Arthritis Rheum* 1994;24:124–138.

Greipp P, Lust J, O'Fallon W, et al. Plasma cell labeling index and beta 2-microglobulin predict survival independent of thymidine kinase and C-reactive protein in multiple myeloma. *Blood* 1993;81:3382–3387.

Greipp PR, Leong T, Bennett JM, et al. Plasmablastic morphology—an independent prognostic factor with clinical and laboratory correlates: Eastern Cooperative Oncology Group (ECOG) myeloma trial E9486 report by the ECOG Myeloma Laboratory Group. *Blood* 1998;91: 2501–2507.

Greipp PR, Witzig T. Biology and treatment of myeloma [see comments]. *Curr Opin Oncol* 1996;8:20–27.

Hawkins PN. Diagnosis and treatment of amyloidosis. *Ann Rheum Dis* 1997;56:631–633.

Kay NE, Leong T, Kyle RA, et al. Circulating blood B cells in multiple myeloma: analysis and relationship to circulating clonal cells and clinical parameters in a cohort of patients entered on the Eastern Cooperative Oncology Group phase III E9486 clinical trial. *Blood* 1997;90: 340–345.

Kyle RA, Greipp PR. Smoldering multiple myeloma. *N Engl J Med* 1980; 302:1347–1349.

Kyle RA, Rajkunnar SV. Monoclonal gammopathies of undetermined significance. *Hematol Oncol Clin North Am* 1999;13:1181–1202.

Mehta J, Tricot G, Jagannath S, et al. Salvage autologous or allogeneic transplantation for multiple myeloma refractory to or relapsing after a first-line autograft. *Bone Marrow Trans* 1998;21:887–892.

Noel P, Kyle RA. Plasma cell leukemia: an evaluation of response to therapy. *Am J Med* 1987;83:1062–1068.

Tricot G, Sawyer JR, Jagannath S, et al. Unique role of cytogenetics in the prognosis of patients with myeloma receiving high-dose therapy and autotransplants. *J Clin Oncol* 1997;15:2659–2666.

Witzig TE, Kyle RA, O'Fallon WM, et al. Detection of peripheral blood plasma cells as a predictor of disease course in patients with smouldering multiple myeloma. *Br J Haematol* 1994;87:266–272.

Kelley's Textbook of Internal Medicine, fourth edition. Edited by H. David Humes. Lippincott Williams & Wilkins, Philadelphia © 2000.

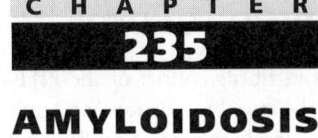

CHAPTER 235

AMYLOIDOSIS

ROBERT A. KYLE

▌ DEFINITION

Amyloid is a substance that consists of fibrils. It appears homogeneous and amorphous under a light microscope and stains pink with hematoxylin and eosin. With polarized light, amyloid

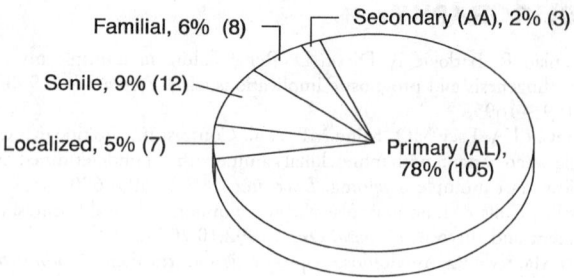

FIGURE 235.1. Types of amyloidosis among 135 cases diagnosed in 1997. (Modified from Kyle RA, Gertz MA. Primary systemic amyloidosis: clinical and laboratory features in 474 cases. *Semin Hematol* 1995;32: 45–59, with permission of W.B. Saunders Co.)

stained with Congo red produces apple-green birefringence. Linear, nonbranching, aggregated fibrils 7.5 to 10 nm wide and of indefinite length are seen with an electron microscope.

INCIDENCE AND EPIDEMIOLOGY

The types and distribution of amyloidosis are shown in Fig. 235.1. The age- and sex-adjusted annual rate of primary amyloidosis (AL) in Olmsted County, Minnesota, is 0.89 cases per 100,000 persons. Approximately 2,450 new cases occur annually in the United States. The median age at diagnosis is 64 years, but only 1% of patients are younger than 40 years.

ETIOLOGY

The cause of AL is unknown. Secondary amyloidosis (AA) is associated with an inflammatory process such as rheumatoid arthritis or its variants, inflammatory bowel disease (especially Crohn's disease), or bronchiectasis. In some parts of the world, tuberculosis and leprosy are major causes. Amyloidosis rarely is associated with hypernephroma, macroglobulinemia, Hodgkin's disease or other lymphomas, or heavy-chain diseases.

PATHOGENESIS AND PATHOPHYSIOLOGY

In AL, the amyloid fibrils consist of the NH_2-terminal amino acid residues of the variable portions of a monoclonal κ or λ light chain. AL is closely related to multiple myeloma, and it is difficult to differentiate AL from multiple myeloma with amyloidosis. Because the prognoses are similar, both should be considered AL. In AA, the main component of the amyloid fibril is protein A, which is derived from serum amyloid A protein and is not related to any known immunoglobulin. The amyloid fibrils in familial amyloidosis consist of transthyretin. More than 50 point mutations of transthyretin have been recognized. Fibrinogen, apolipoprotein A-I, gelsolin, lysozyme, cystatin-C, and β protein also may be associated with familial amyloidosis. The amyloid fibrils in senile amyloidosis consist of normal trans-

thyretin. Among patients undergoing long-term hemodialysis or peritoneal dialysis, periarticular or bony deposition of amyloid fibrils consisting of β_2-microglobulin often develops. Localized amyloid most often produces carpal tunnel syndrome. The catabolism or breakdown of amyloid fibrils is an important factor in pathogenesis, but little is known of this process. Amyloid P component, a glycoprotein, and glycosaminoglycans are present in amyloid deposits, but their functions are unknown.

CLINICAL FINDINGS

PRIMARY AMYLOIDOSIS

Weakness, fatigue, and weight loss are the most common features of AL. Purpura, particularly in the periorbital and facial areas, occurs among 15% of patients. Light-headedness, syncope, change in the tongue or voice, jaw or hip claudication, paresthesias, dyspnea, and edema are the most frequent symptoms. The liver is palpable in almost one-fourth of patients, but the spleen is palpable in only 5%. Macroglossia occurs in about 10%. Nephrotic syndrome or renal failure affects more than one-fourth of patients at diagnosis. Congestive heart failure, carpal tunnel syndrome, sensorimotor peripheral neuropathy, and orthostatic hypotension are other important features (Fig. 235.2). The presence of one of these syndromes and a monoclonal protein in the serum or urine are strong indications of AL, and appropriate biopsies are needed for diagnosis.

SECONDARY AMYLOIDOSIS

At diagnosis, more than 90% of patients with secondary amyloidosis have renal insufficiency or nephrotic syndrome. Gastrointestinal involvement often is manifested as a malabsorption syndrome. Nausea and vomiting from pseudoobstruction may occur. In contrast to AL, AA rarely involves the heart and peripheral nerves.

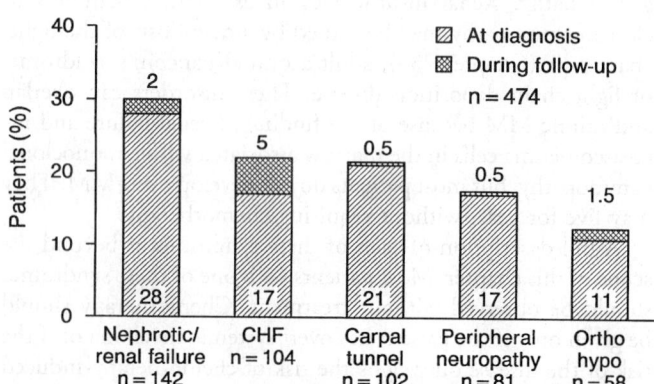

FIGURE 235.2. Frequency of amyloid syndromes at diagnosis of primary amyloidosis and during follow-up care. *CHF,* Congestive heart failure; *Ortho hypo,* orthostatic hypotension. (From Kyle RA, Gertz MA. Primary systemic amyloidosis: clinical and laboratory features in 474 cases. *Semin Hematol* 1995;32:45–59, with permission of W.B. Saunders Co.)

FAMILIAL AMYLOIDOSIS

For clinical purposes, familial amyloidosis can be classified most easily as neuropathic, cardiopathic, or nephropathic. The neuropathic type is characterized by sensorimotor peripheral neuropathy beginning in the lower extremities and by autonomic dysfunction, disturbances of bladder and gastrointestinal function, and vitreous opacities. Carpal tunnel syndrome may be a major feature. Some patients do not have symptoms until the sixth or seventh decade of life. Most patients described have been from Portugal, Sweden, and Japan. Familial Mediterranean fever is characterized by recurrent episodes of fever and abdominal pain and results in nephrotic syndrome or renal insufficiency. Hypertension and renal failure are the main features of amyloidosis in other families. The heart may be the main organ of amyloid deposition among families from Denmark, the Appalachian region of the United States, and many other parts of the world.

SENILE SYSTEMIC AMYLOIDOSIS

Patients with senile systemic amyloidosis usually have congestive heart failure. Atrial fibrillation is common. Echocardiography shows findings consistent with amyloidosis, and a biopsy reveals amyloid consisting of normal transthyretin. It is important to recognize these patients, because the survival period is much better than it is for AL (60 months versus 5 months) and because patients with senile systemic amyloidosis should not receive chemotherapy.

DIALYSIS-ASSOCIATED AMYLOIDOSIS

Patients undergoing long-term hemodialysis or peritoneal dialysis often have carpal tunnel syndrome and pain involving the shoulders, hands, wrists, hips, and knees. Deposition of amyloid in bones commonly produces radiolucencies.

■ LABORATORY FINDINGS

PRIMARY AMYLOIDOSIS

Anemia is not a prominent feature of AL, but when present, it is usually a result of multiple myeloma, renal insufficiency, or

gastrointestinal bleeding. Thrombocytosis occurs among 10% of patients. Serum creatinine level is higher than 2.0 mg per deciliter among 20% of patients. For one-half of patients, serum protein electrophoresis shows a modest localized band or spike (median, 1.4 g per deciliter). A monoclonal protein is found in the serum and the urine of more than 70% of patients. λ Light chains are twice as common as κ light chains. A monoclonal protein is found in the serum or urine in 90% of patients with AL. The bone marrow contains 5% or less plasma cells in almost one-half of patients.

Low voltage or characteristics of anteroseptal infarction, arrhythmia, and heart block are common electrocardiographic features. The echocardiogram is abnormal among two-thirds of patients. The main features are increased thickness of the left and right ventricular walls, abnormal myocardial texture (granular sparkling), atrial enlargement, valvular thickening and regurgitation, pericardial effusion, and abnormal diastolic and ultimately reduced systolic ventricular function.

The diagnosis depends on the demonstration of amyloid deposits (Fig. 235.3). Results of abdominal fat aspiration or bone marrow biopsy are positive among 90% of patients. If these sites are normal, tissue should be obtained from the rectum or a possibly involved organ such as the kidney, liver, heart, or sural nerve. A monoclonal population of bone marrow plasma cells or a monoclonal protein in serum or urine occurs among 98% of patients with AL.

SECONDARY AMYLOIDOSIS

Serum creatinine level is increased among two-thirds of patients with secondary amyloidosis. Eighty-seven percent of Mayo Clinic patients had more than 1 g of protein in 24-hour collections of urine. Serum albumin level was reduced among almost 90% of patients, but alkaline phosphatase level was increased among only 14%. Results of organ biopsy among patients with AA are similar to those among patients with AL.

FAMILIAL AMYLOIDOSIS

The laboratory findings among patients with neuropathic and cardiopathic amyloidosis are nondescript. Renal insufficiency

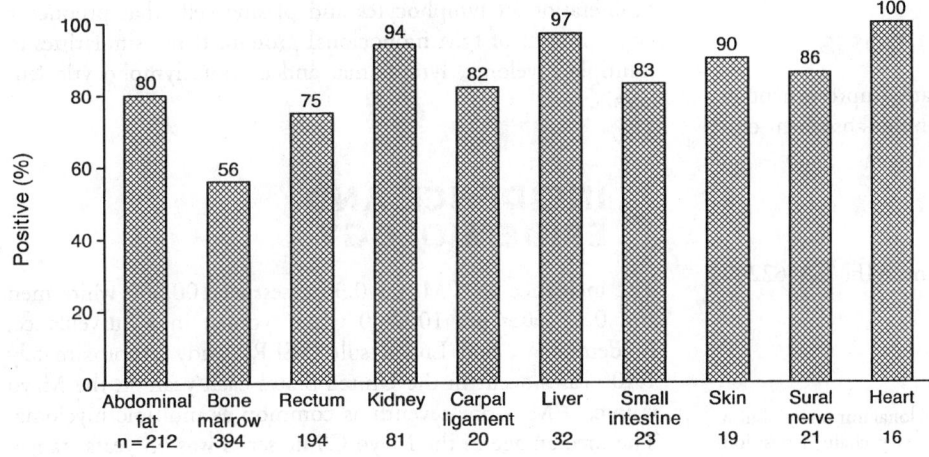

FIGURE 235.3. Results of biopsy among patients with primary amyloidosis. (From Kyle RA, Gertz MA. Primary systemic amyloidosis: clinical and laboratory features in 474 cases. *Semin Hematol* 1995;32:45–59, with permission of W.B. Saunders Co.)

and nephrotic syndrome frequently occur among persons with nephropathic amyloidosis. The diagnosis depends on the demonstration of amyloid. The incidence of positive biopsy results for bone marrow and rectum are similar to those in AL. The type of transthyretin mutation must be determined.

STRATEGIES FOR OPTIMAL CARE

PRIMARY AMYLOIDOSIS

In a series of 474 patients with AL seen within 1 month of diagnosis at the Mayo Clinic from 1981 to 1992, the median duration of survival was 13 months. The median survival period was 4 months for patients with congestive heart failure and 2 years for those with nephrotic syndrome or renal failure. Therapy for AL is unsatisfactory. Treatment should be attempted with alkylating agents known to be effective against plasma cell proliferative processes, because the amyloid fibrils consist of the variable portion of a monoclonal light chain. My colleagues and I demonstrated that melphalan and prednisone produce a significantly longer survival period than does colchicine (18 versus 9 months). We found no difference in survival time in a prospective study comparing melphalan and prednisone with a combination of alkylating agents. Intensive therapy consisting of high-dose chemotherapy followed by rescue with peripheral stem cells shows some promise. A useful treatment option may be 4'-iodo-4'-deoxyrubicin (I-DOX), which has an affinity for amyloid fibrils.

SECONDARY AMYLOIDOSIS

The median duration of survival is approximately 2 years for AA. Treatment depends on the underlying disease. Resorption of amyloid after therapy for osteomyelitis, tuberculosis, or empyema has been reported. Renal transplantation is helpful.

FAMILIAL AMYLOIDOSIS

The median actuarial survival period for familial amyloidosis was 5.8 years in the Mayo series. Liver transplantation produces a dramatic reduction in variant transthyretin serum level. In theory this should stop further deposition of amyloid.

DIALYSIS-ASSOCIATED AMYLOIDOSIS

Renal transplantation often leads to dramatic improvement in joint symptoms. The use of a β2-microglobulin-absorbent column may be helpful.

ACKNOWLEDGMENT

This work was supported by research grant NIH CA 62242 from the National Cancer Institute.

BIBLIOGRAPHY

Buxbaum JN, Chuba JV, Hellman GC, et al. Monoclonal immunoglobulin deposition disease: light chain and light and heavy chain deposition diseases and their relation to light chain amyloidosis: clinical features, immunopathology, and molecular analysis. *Ann Intern Med* 1990;112: 455–464.

Dubrey SW, Cha K, Anderson J, et al. The clinical features of immunoglobulin light-chain (AL) amyloidosis with heart involvement. *Q J Med* 1998;91:141–157.

Gertz MA, Kyle RA. Secondary systemic amyloidosis: response and survival in 64 patients. *Medicine (Baltimore)* 1991;70:246–256.

Gertz MA, Kyle RA, Thibodeau SN. Familial amyloidosis: a study of 52 North American-born patients examined during a 30-year period. *Mayo Clin Proc* 1992;67:428–440.

Gertz MA, Lacy MQ, Lust JA, et al. Prospective randomized trial of melphalan and prednisone versus vincristine, carmustine, melphalan, cyclophosphamide, and prednisone in the treatment of primary systemic amyloidosis. *J Clin Oncol* 1999;17:262–267.

Kyle RA, Gertz MA. Systemic amyloidosis. *Crit Rev Oncol Hematol* 1990; 10:49–87.

Kyle RA, Gertz MA. Primary systemic amyloidosis: clinical and laboratory features in 474 cases. *Semin Hematol* 1995;32:45–59.

Kyle RA, Gertz MA, Greipp PR, et al. A trial of three regimens for primary amyloidosis: colchicine alone, melphalan and prednisone, and melphalan, prednisone, and colchicine. *N Engl J Med* 1997;336:1202–1207.

Kyle RA, Spittell PC, Gertz MA, et al. The premortem recognition of systemic senile amyloidosis with cardiac involvement. *Am J Med* 1996; 101:395–400.

Sipe JD. Amyloidosis. *Annu Rev Biochem* 1992;61:947–975.

Kelley's Textbook of Internal Medicine, fourth edition. Edited by H. David Humes. Lippincott Williams & Wilkins, Philadelphia © 2000.

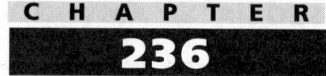

C H A P T E R
236

WALDENSTRÖM'S MACROGLOBULINEMIA

ROBERT A. KYLE

DEFINITION

Waldenström's macroglobulinemia (WM) is characterized by proliferation of lymphocytes and plasma cells that produce a large amount of IgM monoclonal protein. It has similarities to multiple myeloma, lymphoma, and chronic lymphocytic leukemia.

INCIDENCE AND EPIDEMIOLOGY

The incidence of WM was 0.34 cases per 100,000 white men and 0.17 cases per 100,000 white women in a Surveillance, Epidemiology, and End-Result (SEER) study. Approximately 1,400 cases occur in the United States each year. At the Mayo Clinic, WM is one-seventh as common as multiple myeloma. The median age in the Mayo Clinic series was 63 years (range,

30 to 89 years). The disorder rarely occurs before 40 years of age. About 60% of patients are male.

ETIOLOGY

The cause of WM is unknown. The condition has been recognized among first-degree relatives of several families and among monozygotic twins. In a case-control study, patients with WM were slightly better educated than controls, but there were no differences in sociodemographic factors, history of prior medical conditions, medication use, cigarette or alcohol consumption, specific occupational exposures, or employment in any particular industries or occupations. First-degree relatives appeared to have more diverse immunologic abnormalities than did controls.

PATHOGENESIS AND PATHOPHYSIOLOGY

WM is a monoclonal B-cell proliferative process in which lymphocytes or plasma cells produce an IgM monoclonal protein. WM is part of a spectrum that includes monoclonal gammopathy of undetermined significance of the IgM type, lymphocytic lymphoma or other malignant lymphoproliferative disorders, chronic lymphocytic leukemia, and primary amyloidosis. The monoclonal B cells always express monoclonal IgM of the same light-chain type as in the serum. Clonal chromosomal changes may be found, but no specific abnormality has been defined.

CLINICAL FINDINGS

Weakness and fatigue are the most common features of WM. Chronic nasal bleeding or oozing from the gums is characteristic, but postsurgical or gastrointestinal bleeding may occur. Blurring or loss of vision may be prominent. Dizziness, headache, vertigo, nystagmus, sudden deafness, ataxia, or diplopia may be present. Dyspnea and congestive heart failure may develop. Fever, night sweats, loss of weight, and recurrent infections may occur. Retinal vein engorgement and flame-shaped hemorrhages are common. Papilledema, somnolence, coma, and cerebral hemorrhage may develop in some cases. Although most patients have symptoms when the relative viscosity is more than 4 centipoises (cP), the correlation between serum viscosity and clinical manifestations is imprecise. Symptoms rarely are attributable to hyperviscosity if the relative viscosity is less than 4 cP. Bone pain is rare. About one-fourth of patients have hepatomegaly when WM is diagnosed. Splenomegaly and lymphadenopathy are slightly less common.

Diffuse pulmonary infiltrates, isolated masses, or pleural effusion may be a major manifestation. Diarrhea and steatorrhea from infiltration of monoclonal IgM rarely occur. Obstructive jaundice and portal hypertension have been reported. Although retroperitoneal and mesenteric lymphadenopathy often occur, they usually are asymptomatic. Renal insufficiency is uncommon. Nephrotic syndrome is rare in WM, but when present, it usually is caused by amyloidosis. Sensorimotor peripheral neuropathy is the most common neurologic manifestation. This may be caused by deposition of IgM or amyloid. Infiltration of the meninges rarely occurs.

LABORATORY FINDINGS

Most patients with symptomatic WM have anemia. Increased plasma volume is a frequent finding and is responsible for spuriously low hemoglobin and hematocrit levels. Rouleaux formation is prominent, and erythrocyte sedimentation rate usually is greatly increased. Lymphocytosis or monocytosis is a routine finding. Serum creatinine value almost always is normal.

Serum protein electrophoresis shows a sharp, narrow spike or dense band usually migrating in the γ area. About 75% of the IgM proteins are κ. The IgM level obtained by means of nephelometry often is 1,000 to 3,000 mg per deciliter more than that found with serum protein electrophoresis. The reduction in uninvolved IgG and IgA immunoglobulins is less striking than in multiple myeloma. About 10% of macroglobulins precipitate in the cold (cryoglobulinemia). A urinary monoclonal light chain is detected by means of immunofixation among 70% to 80% of patients. Fewer than 5% have lytic bone lesions.

A bone marrow aspirate often is hypocellular, but the biopsy specimen usually is hypercellular and extensively infiltrated with lymphoid or plasmacytoid cells. The presence of mast cells may help differentiate macroglobulinemia from myeloma or lymphoma.

STRATEGIES FOR OPTIMAL CARE

The diagnosis of WM depends on the presence of an IgM monoclonal protein and lymphocyte–plasma cell infiltration of the bone marrow that produces symptoms and physical findings of WM. The level of IgM protein is not helpful in predicting survival and is of importance only in producing the hyperviscosity syndrome. Patients with WM should not be treated unless they have symptoms. The median survival period is 5 years. Older age, loss of weight and other constitutional symptoms, low hemoglobin level, and the presence of cryoglobulinemia or cytopenia indicate shorter survival.

Plasmapheresis with a cell separator quickly alleviates the symptoms of hyperviscosity. Specific therapy should be directed against the proliferating lymphocytes and plasma cells. Chlorambucil given in a daily or intermittent course has been the usual treatment for more than three decades and produces an objective response among 70% of patients. Therapy should be continued until the IgM protein reaches a plateau level and constitutional symptoms have resolved. Because the response is slow, patients should be treated for at least 6 months before chlorambucil therapy is abandoned. The combination of vincristine, BCNU (carmustine), melphalan, cyclophosphamide, and prednisone is an alternative regimen. Interferon alfa-2 has produced benefit for some patients.

The nucleoside analogs fludarabine and 2-chlorodeoxyadenosine are reported to produce a response among as many as 80% of previously untreated patients. However, a large study involving 117 patients showed a response to fludarabine among only 34% of the patients. Only one-third of patients resistant to alkylating agents respond to the nucleoside analogs. Rituximab (Rituxan) produces a response among approximately one-half of patients.

ACKNOWLEDGMENT

This work was supported by research grant NIH CA 62242 from the National Cancer Institute.

BIBLIOGRAPHY

Dimopoulos MA, Alexanian R. Waldenström's macroglobulinemia. *Blood* 1994;83:1452–1459.

Dimopoulos MA, Kantarjian H, Weber D, et al. Primary therapy of Waldenström's macroglobulinemia with 2-chlorodeoxyadenosine. *J Clin Oncol* 1994;12:2694–2698.

Dimopoulos MA, O'Brien S, Kantarjian H, et al. Treatment of Waldenström's macroglobulinemia with nucleoside analogues. *Leuk Lymphoma* 1993;11[Suppl 2]:105–108.

Facon T, Brouillard M, Duhamel A, et al. Prognostic factors in Waldenström's macroglobulinemia: a report of 167 cases. *J Clin Oncol* 1993;11:1553–1558.

Gertz MA, Kyle RA, Noel P. Primary systemic amyloidosis: a rare complication of immunoglobulin M monoclonal gammopathy and Waldenström's macroglobulinemia. *J Clin Oncol* 1993;11:914–920.

Gobbi PG, Bettini R, Montecucco C, et al. Study of prognosis in Waldenström's macroglobulinemia: a proposal for a simple binary classification with clinical and investigational utility. *Blood* 1994;83:2939–2945.

Groves FD, Travis LB, Devesa SS, et al. Waldenström's macroglobulinemia: incidence patterns in the United States, 1988–1994. *Cancer* 1998;82:1078–1081.

Kyle RA. Waldenström's macroglobulinemia. In: Malpas JS, Bergsagel DE, Kyle RA, et al., eds. *Myeloma: biology and management,* 2nd ed. Oxford, UK: Oxford University Press, 1998:639–662.

Kyle RA, Garton JP. The spectrum of IgM monoclonal gammopathy in 430 cases. *Mayo Clin Proc* 1987;62:719–731.

Linet MS, Humphrey RL, Mehl ES, et al. A case-control and family study of Waldenström's macroglobulinemia. *Leukemia* 1993;7:1363–1369.

Kelley's Textbook of Internal Medicine, fourth edition. Edited by H. David Humes. Lippincott Williams & Wilkins, Philadelphia © 2000.

CHAPTER

237

INHERITED DISORDERS OF BLOOD COAGULATION

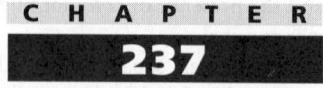

DAVID GINSBURG

DEFINITION

Hemostasis depends on a finely tuned balance among a large number of cellular and protein components of blood. The initial response to vascular injury is mediated by the interaction of platelets with specific plasma proteins and the vessel wall. Activation of the coagulation cascade leads to the deposition of fibrin, the principal structural component of the clot, and the fibrinolytic system coordinates subsequent dissolution of the clot. Inherited functional abnormalities at many points in this complex circuit can cause pathologic bleeding or thrombosis. Inherited disorders that lead to pathologic thrombosis (thrombophilia) are reviewed in Chapter 240 and inherited abnormalities in platelet function in Chapter 239. This chapter discusses inherited bleeding disorders caused by genetic deficiencies in coagulation factor function (Table 237.1). Although generally mild, the most common inherited bleeding disorder is von Willebrand disease (VWD), whereas hemophilia is the most frequent cause of a clinically severe hemorrhagic diathesis. Deficiencies of other clotting factors are considerably less common and can cause bleeding of varying severity.

HEMOPHILIA

Coagulation factors VIII and IX form a complex that activates factor X, leading to thrombin formation and deposition of a fibrin blood clot. Deficiency of factor VIII results in hemophilia A (classic hemophilia) and deficiency of factor IX in hemophilia B (Christmas disease). The factor VIII and factor IX genes both are located on the X chromosome, accounting for the typical X-linked inheritance of these two disorders.

INCIDENCE AND EPIDEMIOLOGY

Hemophilia A is the most common form. The prevalence is estimated at 1:5,000 to 1:10,000 male births. Approximately 80% to 90% of cases of hemophilia are classified as hemophilia A; the others are hemophilia B. Because of the X-linked inheritance, homozygous females (inheritance of two mutated copies of the *FVIII* or *FIX* gene) are exceedingly rare. Heterozygous female carriers should have approximately one-half of the normal factor level and generally have no symptoms. However, mild bleeding sometimes may be encountered, particularly in settings of unequal X chromosome inactivation.

Hemophilia occurs with similar prevalence in all populations. Approximately one-third of patients with hemophilia A or hemophilia B have "new mutations," and thus there is no family history of hemophilia. Observation of marked bleeding among females or male-to-male transmission of factor VIII deficiency should raise the suspicion of another disorder, particularly the type 2N variant of VWD (see later).

ETIOLOGY AND PATHOGENESIS

Hemophilia A and hemophilia B are caused by mutations in the genes for factor VIII and factor IX, respectively. Deficiency of the corresponding protein causes decreased clot formation and abnormal bleeding, particularly after trauma, although spontaneous hemorrhage may also occur.

The severity of bleeding in both hemophilia A and hemophilia B can be correlated directly with the level of residual clotting factor activity (Table 237.2). Most patients have unde-

TABLE 237.1.	INHERITED DISORDERS OF BLOOD COAGULATION		
Disorder	**Inheritance**	**Prevalence**	**Clinical Features**
Hemophilia A	X-linked recessive	1:5,000–10,000	Mild to severe hemorrhage, soft tissues and joints
Hemophilia B	X-linked recessive	~1:50,000	Mild to severe hemorrhage, soft tissues and joints
von Willebrand disease (VWD)			
Type 1	Autosomal dominant	1:100–1,000	Mild bleeding: skin, mucosa, menorrhagia; incomplete penetrance
Type 3	Autosomal recessive	~1:1,000,000	Severe bleeding, resembling both type 1 VWD and hemophilia A
Type 2A, Type 2B	Autosomal dominant	~1:5,000	Similar to type 1 but penetrance more complete; thrombocytopenia in type 2B
Type 2N	Autosomal recessive	?	Resembles mild to moderate hemophilia A, but autosomal inheritance
Other variants	Variable	Rare	Variable
Factor XI	Autosomal recessive	Common among Ashkenazi Jews	Similar to hemophilia; poor correlation with factor level
Factor XII, prekallikrein, high-molecular-weight kininogen	Autosomal recessive	Rare; factor XII most common	No hemorrhage, isolated laboratory abnormality (markedly prolonged aPTT)
Isolated deficiency of factor II, V, VII, or X	Autosomal recessive	Rare	Similar to hemophilia
Combined factor V and factor VIII deficiency	Autosomal recessive	Rare	Similar to mild-moderate hemophilia
Factor XIII	Autosomal recessive	Rare	Delayed bleeding, variable severity
Afibrinogenemia	Autosomal recessive	Rare	Variable, can be severe
Hypofibrinogenemia	Autosomal recessive	Rare	Generally mild bleeding or asymptomatic
Dysfibrinogenemia	Autosomal dominant	Rare (more common than fibrinogen deficiency)	Thrombosis more common than hemorrhage
α_2-Antiplasmin, plasminogen activator inhibitor–1 deficiencies	Autosomal recessive	Rare	Mild to moderate, particularly after trauma

aPTT, activated partial thromboplastin time.

tectable levels of factor activity (< 1%), and the hemophilia is classified as severe. Residual activity in the 1% to 5% range is classified as moderate hemophilia and in the 5% to 25% range as mild hemophilia. Severe hemophilia generally is recognized soon after birth or as soon as the child becomes active. Mild hemophilia may go undiagnosed until later in adult life or at the time of major surgery or trauma. The remarkable moderating effect of even small levels of residual factor VIII or factor IX activity on clinical severity forms the rationale for prophylaxis with intermittent factor replacement. This approach is becoming common practice in the management of newly diagnosed pediatric cases of severe hemophilia A.

Severe hemophilia is caused by genetic defects that disrupt the factor VIII or factor IX gene. These include deletions of part

TABLE 237.2.	CLINICAL CLASSIFICATION OF HEMOPHILIA A AND B	
Classification	**Factor IX or Factor VIII Activity**	**Clinical Manifestation**
Severe	<1%	Spontaneous hemorrhage beginning in early infancy; frequent hemarthroses and other serious hemorrhage
Moderate	1–5%	Hemorrhage after trauma; occasional spontaneous hemorrhage
Mild	5–25%	Bleeding generally only after severe trauma or surgery
	>25%	No substantial bleeding

or all of the gene and point mutations that disrupt the protein coding sequence. Moderate and mild forms of hemophilia generally are associated with single amino acid substitutions that only partly compromise protein function.

CLINICAL FINDINGS

The clinical presentations of hemophilia A and hemophilia B are essentially indistinguishable, and the differential diagnosis is based entirely on the results of clotting factor activity assays. The diagnosis of hemophilia should be suspected in any boy with a severe congenital bleeding disorder and in older males with mild bleeding. Patients with mild hemophilia may have easy bruising and excessive bleeding after trauma or surgery. In contrast to the bleeding of VWD or primary disorders of platelet function, which is predominantly cutaneous or from mucosal surfaces, the bleeding of hemophilia is primarily localized to soft tissues or joints.

The most serious life-threatening complication is central nervous system bleeding, which can follow even minor trauma and may lead to death or severe disability. Central nervous system bleeding accounted for about 25% of deaths among patients with hemophilia before the AIDS era. Joint bleeding (hemarthrosis) occurs predominantly into the large joints. Though usually first recognized as mild pain and some limitation of motion, symptoms often increase over several hours and can cause severe pain with continued bleeding. Repeated injury can lead to chronic degenerative arthritis, frequently necessitating joint replacement in later adulthood. Large intramuscular bleeds can lead to compartment syndromes. Pharyngeal bleeding causing airway obstruction is a particularly serious complication. Large bleeds into soft tissues can be walled off to form large masses with a liquefied center, referred to as *pseudocysts*. Hematuria is a common problem among many patients with hemophilia at some time during their lives and may lead to ureteral obstruction due to clots. Median life expectancy for patients with hemophilia expanded dramatically from 11 or 12 years in the early 1900s to close to normal in the late 1990s.

The bleeding manifestations of hemophilia have been overshadowed by the profound infectious complications related to therapy. Most patients who received blood products for hemophilia before 1984 were exposed to HIV, and approximately 90% of the patients heavily exposed during that time have positive test results for the virus. Nearly two-thirds of this cohort have died. The prevalence of hepatitis also was nearly uniform among this patient population. Although over the past 15 years hemophilia care has been dominated by management of HIV complications, this trend is shifting gradually because the younger population, who began treatment after 1984, is generally virus free.

Another important complication of hemophilia treatment is the development of antibody inhibitors to the infused missing clotting factor (factor VIII or factor IX). These inhibitors, which develop in 10% to 20% of patients with hemophilia A and 5% to 6% of those with hemophilia B, can dramatically complicate therapy. Antibodies can reach extremely high titers, which can be difficult or impossible to overwhelm with high doses of factor replacement.

LABORATORY FINDINGS

Bleeding time, which is thought primarily to represent a measure of platelet plug formation, is normal in hemophilia A and hemophilia B. Prothrombin time is normal in both disorders, and activated partial thromboplastin time (aPTT) is moderately prolonged in the severe form of these disorders and at least mildly prolonged among patients with factor VIII or IX levels less than 30%. The critical diagnostic tests for both disorders are specific assays for factor VIII and factor IX procoagulation activity. Patients with severe hemophilia have less than 1% factor activity, levels in the range of 1% to 5% being classified as moderate and 5% to 25% as mild (Table 237.2). Levels in excess of 25% generally are associated with normal hemostasis. VWF activity and protein level (the latter sometimes mistakenly referred to as factor VIII–related antigen or factor VIIIR:Ag) are normal in hemophilia. The inhibitory antibodies that develop in some patients are quantified in Bethesda units. One unit corresponds to the amount of antibody needed to neutralize the clotting factor activity contained in 1 mL of normal blood.

DNA testing can be performed for mutations in both the factor VIII and the factor IX gene. However, the clinical diagnosis of hemophilia, prediction of severity, and therapy all are based on the factor VIII or factor IX clotting activity measurement. Approximately one-half of severe hemophilia A is caused by the same recurrent DNA inversion event, referred to as the *factor VIII gene inversion*. It usually is most effective to begin testing with a screen for this abnormality. In the one-half of patients with severe hemophilia who do not have the inversion, direct DNA sequencing of the 26 factor VIII gene exons identifies the responsible mutation in most instances.

Identification of the gene mutation can facilitate precise carrier determination and facilitate prenatal diagnosis when a pregnancy is at risk. In the few cases in which the actual mutation cannot be identified, prenatal diagnosis often is still possible with genetic linkage analysis. In the past, hemophilia A carrier status among at-risk female patients often was determined by means of measurement of factor VIII activity in comparison with levels of VWF, although the sensitivity and specificity of this determination were low. Carrier status now can be resolved much more accurately in most cases by means of DNA diagnosis.

STRATEGIES FOR OPTIMAL CARE

The foundation of management of severe hemophilia A and hemophilia B is replacement of the missing clotting factor. The products for replacement are rapidly changing and the best choice of product is generally left to a hemophilia specialist. In the past, factor VIII and factor IX concentrates were prepared by means of pooling blood from large numbers of donors followed by limited biochemical purification. It is these products that carried the tragic infectious risk for HIV infection and hepatitis. Since the mid 1980s, heat and detergent treatment appear to have eliminated the hepatitis and HIV risk, but the potential for infection with other as yet unidentified agents remains a serious concern. For this reason, most patients found to have hemophilia are treated with recombinant factor VIII or factor

IX. However, the high cost and limited availability of these products restricts use to the acute management of profuse hemorrhage or prophylactic treatment before surgical procedures or after trauma.

Continuous prophylaxis among children with newly diagnosed hemophilia has become a more widespread approach. A factor VIII dose of 50 units per kilogram generally raises the factor VIII level from 0 to 100%. A level of factor VIII that is 50% or higher should be adequate for normal hemostasis, even under extreme circumstances. The half-life of factor VIII is approximately 8 hours, necessitating treatments several times per day or continuous infusion. Mild or moderate hemophilia A can sometimes be successfully managed with desmopressin (DDAVP), which can produce a two- to fivefold increase in factor VIII that lasts for several hours. Desmopressin is generally not effective in severe hemophilia. ϵ-Aminocaproic acid can be effective in the management of dental or superficial bleeding.

Management of the inhibitory factor VIII antibodies that develop in 10% to 20% of cases is a challenge that generally requires the expertise of a specialist. Treatment approaches include immunosuppression, infusion of porcine factor VIII, and various tolerance-inducing regimens. Both hemophilia A and hemophilia B are primary targets of a variety of gene therapy approaches, and several clinical trials have been initiated. Comprehensive care of patients with hemophilia also requires the cooperative input of many specialists, including orthopedists and geneticists. Care often is coordinated through a comprehensive hemophilia center.

■ VON WILLEBRAND DISEASE

DEFINITION

von Willebrand disease (VWD) is closely related to hemophilia A; von Willebrand originally called it *pseudohemophilia*. VWD is caused by a deficiency of von Willebrand factor (VWF) a large, multimeric plasma glycoprotein that serves as a carrier for factor VIII and as an adhesive bridge between blood platelets and the vessel wall. Bleeding ranges from mild in the most common form (type 1) to potentially life threatening (with hemorrhagic complications that resemble those of severe hemophilia) in the rare severe form of VWD (type 3). The large number of identified variants of VWD has led to a confusing and complex nomenclature.

INCIDENCE AND EPIDEMIOLOGY

The mild form of VWD, type 1, is the most common inherited bleeding disorder. Results of several epidemiologic studies have suggested that as many as 1% to 3% of the general population may be affected. In many of these studies, the diagnosis was based on minimal reductions in laboratory values not necessarily associated with major bleeding. The prevalence of clinically significant VWD is probably closer 1:1,000. The situation is clearly complicated by the incomplete penetrance of VWD—that is, not all persons who inherit the genetic defect actually express clinically significant bleeding. The number of

patients with symptoms is probably less than 60% of persons carrying a VWD genetic defect. Penetrance is greater among women because of the hemostatic stresses of pregnancy and menstruation; VWD is an important cause of menorrhagia. Type 1 VWD is autosomal dominant in inheritance, though because of reduced penetrance, less than 50% of offspring of an affected parent have appreciable bleeding. Accurate estimates of the frequency of VWD also are compounded by the extremely common and nonspecific nature of mild bleeding symptoms among the general population. For example, in some studies as much as 20% of the population reports symptoms such as easy bruising.

Type 3 VWD is associated with severe, life-threatening bleeding, similar to that observed in severe hemophilia. Type 3 VWD is estimated to occur with a frequency of approximately 1:1,000,000 and may be more common in Scandinavia, where it was first described. Parents of patients with type 3 VWD generally have no symptoms, leading to the classic description of the inheritance pattern as autosomal recessive. However, a subset of type 3 parents is found to have typical type 1 VWD. The type 2 variants of VWD account for 20% to 30% of cases and are probably more highly penetrant. The inheritance of most type 2 VWD variants is autosomal dominant.

ETIOLOGY AND PATHOGENESIS

VWF is one of the largest proteins circulating in blood. It is formed from multimers of up to 100 identical subunits, ranging up to 20 million dalton in molecular mass. VWF serves as the adhesive link between blood platelets and the injured vessel wall and is critical for efficient formation of the initial platelet plug at sites of vascular injury. VWF also carries factor VIII and localizes it to sites of initial clot formation. VWF is produced by endothelial cells and platelets. Plasma VWF is derived exclusively from endothelial cells. Platelet VWF is stored in the platelet α-granule and is released during platelet activation.

VWD is generally the result of mutations within the VWF gene on chromosome 12. Type 1 and type 3 VWD are produced by mutations that completely disrupt the function of VWF, whereas the type 2 variants usually are caused by single-amino-acid substitutions that lead to mildly decreased or altered function. Patients with type 3 VWD generally have inactivating mutations in both copies of the VWF gene that cause production of very low or undetectable levels of VWF. Factor VIII is very unstable without VWF, and patients with severe VWD also have very low levels of factor VIII, contributing to the severe bleeding diathesis. Patients with type 1 VWD generally have VWF levels in the range of 20% to 50% of normal, associated with mild bleeding, and are generally presumed to carry an inactivating mutation in one copy of the VWF gene. The remaining VWF, though reduced in quantity, is qualitatively normal, accounting for the mild symptoms.

The type 2 VWD variants result from qualitative dysfunction of the VWF protein. Types 2A and 2B VWD are associated with loss of the largest and functionally most active VWF multimers. In type 2B this occurs because increased spontaneous affinity for the platelet surface leads to clearance of both platelets and VWF from plasma and loss of the large VWF multimers as well as thrombocytopenia.

Type 2N VWD is caused by mutations within the factor

VIII binding domain of VWF, resulting in loss of factor VIII binding, although VWF platelet binding function is normal. Patients who are homozygous for a type 2N VWD mutation may resemble those with mild to moderate hemophilia A with normal VWF platelet binding function but a mild to moderately reduced factor VIII level. It is important to differentiate type 2N VWD from hemophilia A. This diagnosis should be suspected when a female patient has reduced factor VIII levels or when other aspects of inheritance are not consistent with an X-linked pattern.

In addition to mutations within the VWF gene, a variety of other genetic and environmental factors are known to affect levels of plasma VWF, including estrogen level, stress, and most notably ABO blood group. Patients with type O blood have average VWF levels 20% to 30% lower than those with type A, B, or AB blood. A number of other genetic factors undoubtedly modify the severity of VWD, but these remain to be identified.

Among patients with mild type 1 VWD, the modest reduction in factor VIII level probably only minimally contributes to bleeding and the primary pathologic finding relates to the corresponding quantitative decrease in platelet adhesion. This pathophysiologic mechanism explains why patients with VWD have bleeding different from that of patients with hemophilia.

CLINICAL FINDINGS

Unlike that of hemophilia, the bleeding of VWD is immediate and most prominent from mucosal surfaces. Bleeding generally is mild, except in type 3 disease. Nosebleeds are common, as are easy bruising, gastrointestinal bleeding, and excessive menstrual bleeding. Postpartum bleeding may occur, as may bleeding after trauma or surgery. Bleeding into joints or deep tissue as in hemophilia generally does occur in VWD, except among patients with type 3 VWD, who also have markedly reduced levels of factor VIII.

LABORATORY FINDINGS

The laboratory diagnosis of VWD is considerably more complex and less reliable than the simple factor assays that are the hallmark of hemophilia diagnosis. As a result of the limitations of laboratory testing, along with the incomplete penetrance and variable expression of VWD, many instances of mild VWD are incorrectly diagnosed or not diagnosed at all. Because of the frequency of VWD, many patients with mild or questionable bleeding histories are incorrectly given this diagnosis. Nonetheless, VWD is the most likely diagnosis for any patient with a mild congenital bleeding disorder, particularly when the disorder is associated with a family history that indicates autosomal dominant inheritance.

Prothrombin time and aPTT are generally normal, except among patients with type 3 VWD, among whom a marked reduction in factor VIII can lead to prolongation of aPTT. The bleeding time is expected to be prolonged in VWD but is a notoriously unreliable screening test with frequent false-positive and false-negative findings. For this reason, many experts discourage the use of bleeding time as a routine screening test. The standard evaluation for VWF consists of a battery of three laboratory tests: VWF activity (also called *ristocetin cofactor activity*, because it is based on the platelet aggregation induced by the antibody ristocetin in the presence of VWF), factor VIII coagulation activity, and VWF antigen level (previously called factor VIII–related antigen). As for all other clotting factors, these activities are expressed as a percentage of a pooled normal control (normal defined as 100%) or units (one unit is defined as the activity in 1 mL of control plasma).

Among patients with typical type 1 VWD, all three assays (factor VIII activity, VWF activity, and VWF antigen) generally are similarly decreased to the range of 20% to 50% of normal. Unfortunately, there is extensive overlap in observed values between patients and healthy persons, because the normal range for all of these factors is approximately 50% to 150%. For this reason, repeated testing often is necessary, and the diagnosis should generally not be made or excluded on the basis of a single measurement.

Specialized testing is needed to identify the type 2 variants of VWD. Analysis of VWF multimers generally is performed only in a reference laboratory. A normal distribution of multimer size is expected with type 1 VWD whereas selective loss of large multimers occurs in type 2A and type 2B. Diagnosis of type 2N VWD requires measurement of factor VIII VWF binding and again is performed only in a few reference laboratories. Diagnosis of type 2B VWD requires a specialized ristocetin-induced platelet aggregation study (RIPA) and must be differentiated from a closely related disorder, pseudo-VWD. The latter disorder is caused by mutations in the platelet receptor for VWF (GPIb).

Although DNA analysis of mutations within the VWF gene has the potential to be of great diagnostic value, this study is currently only available in research laboratories. The mutations responsible for most common type 2 VWD variants are known, although only a few type 1 mutations have been identified. Though not currently available outside research laboratories, prenatal diagnosis can be performed by means of mutation detection or linkage analysis, but is generally only indicated for type 3 VWD.

STRATEGIES FOR OPTIMAL CARE

Desmopressin can produce a two- to threefold increase in plasma levels of VWF and factor VIII that can last for 4 to 12 hours. Because the toxicity of this drug is modest, desmopressin has become a mainstay for the management of mild VWD. Desmopressin can be administered by means of intravenous bolus injection and is now available in a nasal spray. The increase in VWF occurs promptly, and adequate levels often can be maintained with repeated dosing once or twice per day, although tachyphylaxis can occur. Accurate diagnosis is essential, because desmopressin may be relatively contraindicated in the management of type 2B VWD. In type 2B disease, increased release of abnormally reactive VWF may exacerbate thrombocytopenia and clinical bleeding. However, this view is controversial, and some patients with type 2B VWD have been successfully treated with desmopressin. Desmopressin is generally not effective therapy for type 2A or type 3 VWD.

Patients with severe VWD (type 3) often need treatment with factor replacement. Unfortunately, a recombinant VWF product is not available. Treatment is limited to selected factor VIII concentrates prepared from pooled plasma that contain large amounts of VWF, such as humate P. Patients also can be treated with fresh frozen plasma or cryoprecipitate, although efforts should be made to minimize exposure to these plasma products, which may still carry high risk for viral infection. The fibrinolytic inhibitor ϵ-aminocaproic acid may be useful in reducing mucosal bleeding among VWD patients, particularly after dental extractions. Estrogens and oral contraceptives increase VWF levels and can be useful for treatment of women, particularly for menorrhagia. This effect also decreases the risk for profuse bleeding during pregnancy, though postpartum bleeding is common.

INHERITED DEFECTS OF OTHER COAGULATION FACTORS

Other coagulation factor deficiencies are considerably less common than hemophilia or VWD. However, they have a wide range of clinical manifestations, from asymptomatic laboratory abnormality to severe, life-threatening hemorrhage. For most of these disorders, a purified or dedicated factor concentrate is not available and treatment is thus limited to replacement with fresh frozen plasma or other general measures.

DISORDERS OF FIBRINOGEN

A variety of disorders of fibrinogen caused by mutations within the α, β, or γ chain genes have been reported. Because balanced synthesis of all three chains is needed for functional fibrinogen, an abnormality in any one chain can cause reduced or absent fibrinogen synthesis or synthesis of dysfunctional fibrinogen. These disorders are called *hypofibrinogenemia, afibrinogenemia,* and *dysfibrinogenemia,* respectively. The inheritance of afibrinogenemia is autosomal recessive, and, although rare, life-threatening hemorrhage similar to that associated with hemophilia can occur. Despite the absence of any detectable fibrinogen, bleeding severity is surprisingly variable. Some patients have only mild to moderate symptoms. Bleeding in hypofibrinogenemia is uncommon, unless the fibrinogen level is less than 50 mg per deciliter. Treatment is with cryoprecipitate, which contains large amounts of fibrinogen.

Dysfibrinogenemia is caused by single-amino-acid substitutions within one of the three fibrinogen chains; the substitutions lead to abnormal fibrinogen function. These disorders can be associated with pathologic bleeding or thrombosis, more often the latter. Inheritance usually is autosomal dominant, and the diagnosis should be suspected when assays of fibrinogen function give markedly lower levels than those obtained with chemical or immunologic methods.

FACTOR XI DEFICIENCY

Factor XI deficiency is autosomal recessive in inheritance and is particularly common for Ashkenazi Jews, among whom the prevalence has been estimated to be as high as 1:190. One-half of all patients are in this population, two mutations accounting for most instances. Unlike the situation for hemophilia, plasma factor XI level is a poor predictor of bleeding severity; marked bleeding occasionally occurs among heterozygotes. Most patients are only mildly or moderately affected; bleeding is most common after surgical procedures and dental extractions. This diagnosis often is detected with a prolonged screening aPTT and confirmed with a factor XI clotting activity assay.

DEFICIENCY OF FACTOR XII, PREKALLIKREIN, AND HIGH-MOLECULAR-WEIGHT KININOGEN

All three of these disorders are associated with marked prolongation of aPTT but no clinically significant bleeding. They are primarily identified through routine screening with aPTT before a surgical procedure. Factor XII deficiency may be associated with increased risk for thrombosis, although this has not been confirmed. Factor XII is the most common of these three disorders; the others represent rare case reports. No specific therapy is necessary.

DEFICIENCY OF OTHER COAGULATION CASCADE FACTORS

Deficiency of factor X, factor VII, factor V, and factor II (prothrombin) are all very rare, but they cause bleeding similar to that of hemophilia. The genes for all these factors are located on autosomes, and inheritance is autosomal recessive. Factors II, VII, and X (along with factor IX) are all vitamin K–dependent proteins the levels of which are reduced by vitamin K deficiency or treatment with warfarin. Rare cases of patients with combined deficiency of all of the vitamin K–dependent factors have been reported and are caused by defects in vitamin K metabolism or in the γ-carboxylase enzyme itself. Accurate diagnosis of all these conditions depends on specific activity assays for each of the coagulation factors.

Autosomal dominant inheritance of factor V deficiency restricted to the platelet (factor V Quebec) is known to be caused by a generalized enhancement of proteolysis within the platelet rather than a specific mutation within factor V. Combined deficiency of both factors V and VIII has been identified in a number of families, particularly of Middle East origin. The levels of both factors are reduced to the 5% to 25% range. This autosomal recessive disorder is now known to be caused by, in most instances, mutations in the *ERGIC-53* gene, a component of the endoplasmic reticulum to Golgi transport pathway.

FACTOR XIII DEFICIENCY

Factor XIII deficiency is autosomal recessive in inheritance and is caused by mutations in either the A or B subunits, each encoded by a different gene. Factor XIII cross links fibrin and stabilizes the blood clot. Because initial clot formation is normal, bleeding generally does not occur until late, when the less stable clot is prematurely lysed. This delayed pattern of bleeding is characteristic. Serious bleeding can occur, and the diagnosis often is made on the basis of prolonged umbilical cord bleeding.

Results of routine coagulation tests are normal, although a specific clot solubility test can be used to identify this defect. Treatment is with fresh frozen plasma or cryoprecipitate.

DEFECTS IN THE FIBRINOLYTIC SYSTEM

The fibrinolytic system acts through an independent series of steps to activate the proteolytic enzyme plasmin, which degrades the fibrin blood clot to counterbalance the coagulation cascade. Abnormalities of two regulatory inhibitors in this pathway have been associated with inherited bleeding, although both conditions are rare. α_2-Antiplasmin is the specific inhibitor of plasmin itself. Autosomal recessive deficiency has been reported in several families, and it causes a mild to moderate bleeding disorder. Genetic deficiency of plasminogen activator inhibitor 1 (PAI-1), the primary inhibitors of the plasminogen activators tissue plasminogen activator (tPA) and urokinase (uPA), has also been reported. PAI-1 deficiency has been identified primarily among the Amish population, where it may be a fairly common mutation. Homozygous patients with the deficiency have mild to moderate bleeding, particularly after trauma. Both PAI-1 and α_2-antiplasmin deficiency often can be effectively managed with inhibitors of the fibrinolytic system such as ϵ-aminocaproic acid.

BIBLIOGRAPHY

Colman RW, Hirsh J, Marder VJ, et al., eds. *Hemostasis and thrombosis basic principles and clinical practice.* Philadelphia: JB Lippincott, 1994: 3–18.

Furie B, Limentani SA, Rosenfield CG. A practical guide to the evaluation and treatment of hemophilia. *Blood* 1994;84:3–9.

Ginsburg D. Hemophilia and other inherited disorders of hemostasis and thrombosis. In: Rimoin DL, Connor JM, Pyeritz RE, et al., eds. *Emery and Rimoin's principles and practice of medical genetics.* New York: Churchill Livingstone, 1997:1651–1676.

Hoyer LW. Hemophilia A. *N Engl J Med* 1994;330:38–47.

Loscalzo J, Schafer AI, eds. *Thrombosis and hemorrhage.* Baltimore: Williams & Wilkins, 1998:729–755.

Nichols WC, Ginsburg D. von Willebrand disease. *Medicine (Baltimore)* 1997;76:1–20.

Kelley's Textbook of Internal Medicine, fourth edition. Edited by H. David Humes. Lippincott Williams & Wilkins, Philadelphia © 2000.

C H A P T E R

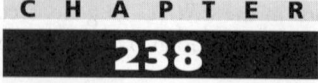

ACQUIRED DISORDERS OF BLOOD COAGULATION

ALVIN H. SCHMAIER

The most common forms of bleeding that physicians encounter are acquired disorders of blood coagulation. These entities occur frequently and often are encountered in the hospital practice of the internist. They commonly arise not as primary disorders themselves but as secondary manifestations of a primary disease or as result of therapy for an underlying disorder. Thus they often are iatrogenic, and the physician must be vigilant to prevent them. The diagnostic approach to acquired disorders of blood coagulation follows from the same method that one would use for all bleeding states. Careful analysis of results of screening tests for bleeding disorders (prothrombin time, activated partial thromboplastin time, platelet count, bleeding time, and fibrinogen level) and an understanding of the patient's underlying illness often point to the nature of the acquired disorder of blood coagulation. The bleeding associated with these entities can be profuse or mild, or there may be no bleeding at all. Recognition of the cause of an acquired bleeding disorder should lead to prompt therapy.

A physical examination for bleeding disorders is useful but seldom provides enough information for a diagnosis. In general, defects in plasma proteins become manifest as intramuscular hematomas, retroperitoneal hematomas, and intraarticular hemorrhage. Defects in number and quality of platelets can cause petechiae on the conjunctiva, soft and hard palate, and anterior portions of the arms and legs. Hemorrhagic bullae of the soft palate are characteristic of severe thrombocytopenia. Easy bruising on the skin of the upper arms and chest without recognition of recent trauma and ecchymosis around venipuncture sites also characterize disorders of platelet and von Willebrand's factor. Often only evaluation of routine coagulation screening tests alerts the physician to an acquired bleeding disorder. Activated partial thromboplastin time (aPTT) and prothrombin time (PT) together or alone help detect all known bleeding disorders caused by plasma proteins except for factor XIII deficiency and defects or deficiencies in α_2-antiplasmin, plasminogen activator inhibitor 1, and α_1-antitrypsin Pittsburgh. Platelet count and bleeding time are used to detect quantitative or qualitative defects in platelets and von Willebrand's factor. Thus with the results of a few inexpensive laboratory studies, the physician gains great diagnostic insight.

DISORDERS ASSOCIATED WITH A PROLONGED ACTIVATED PARTIAL THROMBOPLASTIN TIME AND PROTHROMBIN TIME

The most common acquired disorders of blood coagulation become manifest with a prolonged PT and aPTT (Table 238.1). These entities include anticoagulation, disseminated intravascular coagulation (DIC), liver disease, vitamin K deficiency, massive transfusion, and a number of rare disorders caused by acquired inhibition or deficiency of various coagulation proteins.

ANTICOAGULATION

By far the most common defects in the coagulation system among patients in hospitals is related to therapeutic anticoagulation. Anticoagulants are widely pervasive in the treatment of

TABLE 238.1.	APPROACH TO ACQUIRED BLEEDING DISORDERS

Prolonged PT and aPTT

Use of anticoagulants
Disseminated intravascular coagulation
Liver disease
Vitamin K deficiency
Massive transfusion
Rare acquired inhibition of coagulation proteins
   Paraproteinemia
   Dysfibrinogenemia
   Systemic amyloidosis
   Inhibitors of factors V, II, X
   Antiphospholipid syndrome

Prolonged aPTT, Normal or Prolonged PT, Normal aPTT

Acquired inhibition of factor VIII-c
Acquired inhibition of factor IX:c or factor XI:c
Acquired inhibition of factor VII-c

Abnormal Bleeding Time but Normal PT and aPTT

Acquired von Willebrand's disease
Uremia
Use of medications

Abnormal Bleeding but Normal Bleeding Time, PT, and aPTT

Inhibitors to factor XIII
α-Antiplasmin deficiency

PT, prothrombin time; aPTT, activated partial thromboplastin time.

patients with thrombotic disorders and those undergoing interventional procedures. Use of these agents is growing in the practice of medicine, and the number of agents also is increasing. Standard heparin functions as an anticoagulant by potentiating the naturally occurring plasma protease inhibitor antithrombin to inhibit coagulation factors IIa (thrombin), Xa, IXa, VIIa, XIa, XIIa, and kallikrein. The protection against thrombosis provided by heparin is mostly caused by the ability of the drug to inhibit factors IIa and Xa. Heparin mostly prolongs aPTT but in high enough concentrations also prolongs PT.

Low-molecular-weight forms of heparin mostly inhibit factor Xa. They cannot be monitored with PT or aPTT, but if the plasma level is sufficiently high, they prolong both times. Hirudin (an active site thrombin inhibitor) and danaparoid sodium (a heparinoid factor Xa inhibitor) also prolong both the aPTT and PT.

The oral anticoagulant warfarin inhibits two enzymes in vitamin K metabolism. The inhibition decreases the amount and uncarboxylated forms of coagulation factors II, VII, IX, X, protein C, and protein S. Decarboxylated vitamin K–dependent proteins are unable to bind to cell membranes to be activated. Warfarin anticoagulation mostly prolongs the PT, but because it inhibits factor IX synthesis and activity, it also prolongs aPTT at therapeutic concentrations when stable levels are achieved.

Bleeding during anticoagulant therapy occurs when there is a site for bleeding. Bleeding occurs most commonly among elderly patients and may be associated with cerebral amyloid angiopa-

thy. It also can occur within 2 weeks after a surgical procedure. The addition of drugs that interfere with hemostasis increases risk for bleeding. Acquisition of blood through anticoagulated indwelling lines and catheters is a common cause of abnormal results of coagulation screening tests among hospitalized patients.

Treatment of patients with bleeding caused by use of anticoagulants can be a serious problem. Standard heparin has a short half-life of 1 hour; therefore stopping the drug usually corrects the problem within 4 hours. If need be, heparin can be neutralized with protamine sulfate, but excess protamine sulfate can function as an anticoagulant itself. Warfarin anticoagulation is more difficult. It takes 5 days to bring about anticoagulation with warfarin because of the long half-lives of factors X and prothrombin. It also takes 5 days to correct the effect of warfarin in a nutritionally replete person with normal liver function. For asymptomatic prolongation of PT or an increase in international normalized ratio, merely withholding the drug is sufficient. Vitamin K infusion (5 to 10 mg) shortens or corrects an abnormal PT within 4 to 12 hours if liver function is normal.

Serious bleeding can be corrected with fresh frozen plasma infusion. Life-threatening bleeding or intracranial bleeding can be corrected with infusion of vitamin K–dependent concentrates with a goal of 50% normal levels of factors. Low-molecular-weight forms of heparin have much longer half-lives, 3 to 18 hours depending on the preparation. Excessive anticoagulation with these agents theoretically can be corrected with protamine sulfate. Low-molecular-weight forms of heparin are eliminated through renal excretion and therefore the doses should be reduced in the treatment of patients with kidney disease. Danaparoid sodium, a heparinoid, has an 18-hour half-life. It is not corrected with protamine sulfate. Patients with serious bleeding associated with this agent need supportive care until the drug is metabolized. Hirudin has a short half-life (2 hours) and is eliminated renally. Doses of this drug have to be markedly reduced in the care of patients with renal dysfunction. Patients with abnormal bleeding can only be given supportive care. It is important to remember that some of these patients may be taking platelet inhibitors (aspirin, thienopyridines) which also contribute to abnormal bleeding. Platelet transfusion sometimes can be helpful to control abnormal bleeding in the care of these patients.

DISSEMINATED INTRAVASCULAR COAGULATION

DIC is a clinicopathologic syndrome that is not a specific disease but is a manifestation of an underlying disorder. Recognition that a patient has DIC obligates the physician to search for an underlying medical disorder. In simplest terms, DIC can be described as a loss of balance between procoagulant (clot forming) and fibrinolytic (clot lysing) capacities. In biochemical terms, DIC is the loss of balance between the main clotting enzyme, thrombin, and the main enzyme of fibrinolysis, plasmin. The clinical and laboratory manifestations of DIC reflect the multiple actions of thrombin and plasmin. The degree to which thrombin or plasmin is formed depends on the inciting etiologic factor, the acuteness of the initiating event, and the clearance of activated products of coagulation and fibrinolysis.

The clinical manifestations of DIC follow from the inciting etiologic factor and the degree to which thrombin or plasmin is formed. DIC can become manifest as an acute hemorrhagic event as result of excessive fibrinolysis from plasmin formation. It also can manifest itself as a subacute or chronic illness that becomes manifest as venous thrombosis caused by a procoagulant state due to excessive thrombin formation. In the acute, hemorrhagic variety of DIC, patients have mucosal bleeding, skin ecchymosis especially around venipuncture sites, and petechiae. What is seen on the skin mirrors what is found diffusely in the body—multiple punctate hemorrhage in all tissues, including the brain. In the subacute or chronic form of DIC, evidence of venous or arterial thrombosis may be the only manifestation of the disorder.

DIC results from tissue injury of any cause. The many and varied causes of DIC can be classified according to the appearance of an acute, hemorrhagic disorder or a subacute, thrombotic disorder (Table 238.2). In acute, hemorrhagic DIC, the clinical and laboratory features develop rapidly over a period of time ranging from a few hours to days. The inciting etiologic factors usually are infection, obstetric complications, malignant disease, or gross tissue injury. Unlike acutely ill patients with complicating DIC, other patients may have a mild or protracted clinical course of consumption of coagulation factors or even subclinical disease with signs and symptoms that can be referred to thrombosis. These illnesses often are associated with malignant disease or vasculitis. They manifest themselves with fibrin deposition in the intravascular compartment that causes venous thrombosis, marantic endocarditis, and arterial embolism.

The laboratory diagnosis of DIC follows from the screening

TABLE 238.3.	DIAGNOSIS OF DISSEMINATED INTRAVASCULAR COAGULATION

Screening Assays
Prothrombin time
Activated partial thromboplastin time
Platelet count
Fibrinogen

Confirmatory Tests
D-dimer
Fibrin degradation products
Fibrin monomer

---

assays used in hemostasis (Table 238.3). If results of two of these tests are abnormal, the diagnosis of DIC is possible. If results of three of these tests are abnormal, the diagnosis of DIC is probable; if results of all screening tests are abnormal (PT, aPTT, platelet count, fibrinogen), the diagnosis is likely. In rare instances, such as after a timber rattlesnake bite or therapeutic thrombolysis, results all of these tests can be abnormal without DIC. The diagnosis of DIC is confirmed with a test that specifically shows plasmin and thrombin formation. Measurement of D-dimer is the confirmatory test for DIC. D-dimer is plasmin-liberated, insoluble cross-linked fibrin produced by prior thrombin cleavage of fibrinogen that has formed a neoantigen between the two D domains of fibrin. A positive D-dimer result a priori indicates DIC because it demonstrates the simultaneous formation of thrombin and plasmin. Measurement of fibrin degradation (split) products (FDPs) shows only plasmin-cleaved insoluble cross-linked fibrin, soluble fibrin, or fibrinogen. It does not indicate prior thrombin formation. In most instances a positive FDP result indicates DIC, but the FDP result can be positive from thrombolytic therapy, liver disease, and resolving hematoma without DIC. Measurement of soluble fibrin monomer is another confirmatory test. A positive result indicates that thrombin has been formed and fibrinogen has been cleaved. In acute DIC, fibrin monomer may be very transient and completely proteolyzed and thus not detected.

The first principle in therapy for DIC is to manage the underlying cause. Infections are managed with the appropriate antibiotics; obstetric complications are managed with the appropriate surgical treatment, and recognized cancer is managed with chemotherapy. Once treatment has been directed at the primary illness, therapy can be directed at the DIC itself. Before embarking on additional treatment, the physician always must carefully weigh the expected outcome with the possible benefits of therapy. The first principle is to replace the missing factor or factors. If a patient is depleted in fibrinogen, administration of cryoprecipitate is appropriate. If the patient has thrombocytopenia, platelet replacement is indicated; fresh-frozen plasma also may be helpful. Infusion of fresh frozen plasma may allay the illness because there are excess plasma protease inhibitors in plasma to "cool" the active proteases of DIC. If a patient with self-limited DIC has acral cyanosis and digital ischemia, standard heparin therapy may be instituted once the patient has received replacement therapy. In these cases, full-dose anticoagulation is not the

---

TABLE 238.2.	DIFFERENTIAL DIAGNOSIS AND CLINICAL CLASSIFICATION OF DISSEMINATED INTRAVASCULAR COAGULATION

Acute DIC

Infection: gram-positive and gram-negative septicemia, typhoid fever, Rocky Mountain spotted fever, viremia, infestation with parasites
Obstetric complications: abruptio placentae, amniotic fluid embolism, hypertonic saline abortion, eclampsia
Malignant disease: acute promyelocytic leukemia
Tissue injury: snake bite, necrotizing enterocolitis, freshwater drowning, heat stroke, brain and crush injury, renal homograft rejection, dissecting aortic aneurysm, hemolytic transfusion reaction
Other causes: homozygous protein C and S deficiency, factor V Leiden, severe liver disease, heparin-induced thrombocytopenia and thrombosis syndrome

Subacute or Chronic DIC

Malignant disease: mucin-producing adenocarcinoma
Obstetric complications: retained dead fetus
Vascular disorders: connective tissue disorders, giant cavernous hemangioma, chronic renal disease, venous thrombosis, pulmonary embolus, marantic endocarditis, arterial embolization

goal. Standard heparin usually is given at one-fourth the usual dose (4 to 5 units per kilogram per hour as a constant infusion) without a large intravenous loading dose. This lowered amount of heparin is sufficient to inhibit factor X activation and thus block further thrombin formation.

LIVER DISEASE

Liver disease can manifest a variety of coagulation protein disorders. All coagulation proteins (II, VII, IX, X, fibrinogen, prekallikrein, high-molecular-weight kininogen, XI, XII, XIII), anticoagulants (protein C, protein S), fibrinolytic protein (plasminogen), and plasma protease inhibitors (antithrombin, C_1 inhibitor, $\alpha_2$antiplasmin) are synthesized in the liver. Prekallikrein is the first protein in the liver whose synthesis is decreased in liver disease. Fibrinogen usually is the last protein the synthesis of which is lost in liver disease. Dysfibrinogenemia frequently is associated with liver disease. Patients with liver disease have reduced clearance of activated coagulation proteins. Patients with liver disease and cirrhosis experience hypersplenism, which manifests itself with thrombocytopenia. Some patients with liver disease have increased bleeding because of reductions in the amounts of hemostatic proteins and platelets and from anatomic lesions (gastritis, esophageal varices, peptic ulcer, hemorrhoids) related in part to portal hypertension and abuse of alcohol.

The earliest stages of liver disease are associated with a prolonged PT and later a prolonged aPTT. With disease progression and the appearance of dysfibrinogenemia, thrombin time lengthens and fibrinogen level decreases. FDP levels may rise because of reduced clearance, and platelet count may fall. Hemostatic abnormalities may be treated with vitamin K and fresh frozen plasma. If surgery is planned and a patient has thrombocytopenia, massive platelet transfusion may be necessary, although platelet transfusion usually is not helpful because the enlarged spleen serves as a reservoir for the transfused platelets. Cryoprecipitate therapy is useful to manage severe fibrinogen deficient states. Successful liver transplantation ameliorates these problems.

VITAMIN K DEFICIENCY

Vitamin K has a critical role in amino terminal carboxylation reactions (the addition of carboxy groups on the γ-carbon of glutamic acid residues, γ-carboxyglutamic acid) of the so-called vitamin K–dependent proteins. This reaction is essential for these proteins to interact with lipid surfaces and cell membranes to participate normally in hemostatic reactions. Vitamin K, a lipid-soluble vitamin, is provided by dietary intake of leafy green vegetables and by synthesis of intestinal flora. The body has a 1-month store of this vitamin. Deficiency of vitamin K can be caused by anatomic lesions that cause the small intestine to be bypassed, malabsorption, biliary tract obstruction, and rarely by a reduction in dietary intake. The last cause usually occurs among nutritionally depleted persons with alcoholism or patients in hospitals who have received intravenous nutrition for more than 1 month without vitamin K replacement. Antibiotics also interfere with the growth of intestinal bacteria and impair

vitamin K synthesis and oral absorption. The oral anticoagulant warfarin also interferes with the metabolism and function of vitamin K. Bleeding associated with vitamin K deficiency, which includes warfarin treatment, indicates that there is a bleeding site. It is incumbent on the physician to search for that site rather than to fully ascribe the bleeding to the vitamin K deficiency.

MASSIVE TRANSFUSION

Massive blood transfusion associated with trauma or surgery can lead to an acquired bleeding state. Infusion of a volume of fluid greater than 1.5 times the patient's blood volume in 24 hours can cause coagulopathy as the result of plasma dilution and increased concentration of the anticoagulant sodium citrate dextrose circulating in the patient's blood. Increased numbers of packed red cells and crystalloid infusion can dilute circulating platelets, and the dilution contributes to the problem. Plasmapheresis and extracorporeal circulation for cardiac surgery and respiratory failure without adequate fresh frozen plasma replacement also can decrease the level of plasma coagulation factors. In general it is useful to give one unit of fresh frozen plasma and one ampule of calcium gluconate for every 4 to 5 units of packed red cells given to patients in a short period of time.

RARE ACQUIRED INHIBITORS OF COAGULATION PROTEINS

Patients with hypergammaglobulinemic states (multiple myeloma, Waldenström's macroglobulinemia) acquire bleeding disorders. Immunoglobulin binds to fibrinogen and other coagulation proteins to interfere with their function. The presence of functionally abnormal fibrinogen (dysfibrinogenemia) is common in these patients, as is other nonspecific evidence of coagulation protein inhibitors. Primary therapy is management of the underlying disease. Plasmapheresis is useful for rapid correction of the hypergammaglobulin defect and for cessation of abnormal bleeding.

The presence of antibodies to fibrinogen that interfere with its function is not infrequent. Antibodies that interfere with fibrinopeptide A release can be associated with bleeding. These patients have prolonged thrombin and reptilase times. Antibodies to fibrinopeptide B release can cause strikingly long PT and aPTT but no bleeding history. Patients have abnormal thrombin times but normal reptilase times.

Systemic primary amyloidosis or amyloidosis associated with multiple myeloma has been associated with isolated deficiencies of factor X. Combined deficiencies of factors IX and X occasionally have been seen among patients with amyloidosis. The cause of this phenomenon is not completely known. Some patients have responded to splenectomy; others have responded to melphalan and prednisone therapy. The presence of antibodies to factor X has been reported. Bleeding is controlled with prothrombin complex concentrates.

Heparin-like or heparinoid-like anticoagulants have developed spontaneously in patients as a manifestation of underlying hematologic malignant disease (plasma cell dyscrasia, lymphoma, leukemia). Management of the underlying disease may ameliorate the condition. Isolated coagulation factor inhibitors of factor V are rare but serious and often lethal disorders. These inhibitors usually are present in older patients. Some cases may be iatrogenic as a result of the use in surgery of topical bovine thrombin contaminated with bovine factor V. Factor V deficiency also has been reported to occur with chronic myelogenous leukemia. Isolated hypoprothrombinemia can occur among patients with antiphospholipid antibody syndrome.

Antiphospholipid syndrome frequently becomes manifest as a prolonged aPTT and PT, especially if the reagent for the latter study has a lower international sensitivity index. The most common sign of the presence of antiphospholipid antibodies is an isolated prolonged aPTT. Antiphospholipid antibodies are heterogenous, being directed to acidic and neutral phospholipids, phospholipids in complex with various proteins (prothrombin, kininogen, prekallikrein, factor XI), or β_2-glycoprotein I. Antiphospholipid antibodies may prevent annexin V, a membrane anticoagulant, from binding to endothelial cells and thus indirectly promoting prothrombinase activity. In general, the presence of antiphospholipid antibodies is not associated with bleeding unless there is associated hypoprothrombinemia and thrombocytopenia. They also are associated with various degrees of severity of thrombosis.

DISORDERS ASSOCIATED WITH A PROLONGED ACTIVATED THROMBOPLASTIN TIME OR PROTHROMBIN TIME

Acquired disorders of coagulation with bleeding associated with a prolonged aPTT but a normal PT usually are spontaneous inhibitors of factor VIII:c. Each of us apparently has the potential to produce inhibitors to factor VIII:c. Spontaneous factor VIII:c inhibitors develop in immunosuppressed persons—patients with B-cell malignant disease, those with systemic lupus erythematosus or another connective tissue disorder, pregnant women, elderly patients, persons who take certain medications (penicillins, sulfa drugs, phenytoin), and patients with hemophilia A. A patient without hemophilia who has acute bleeding and a high titer (more than 5 Bethesda units) can be treated with activated prothrombin complex concentrates or porcine factor VIII:c. Among patients with an inhibitor but no evidence of acute hemorrhage, immunosuppressive therapy with cyclophosphamide (Cytoxan), vincristine, and prednisone is successful in 80% of cases.

Inhibitors to factor IX are present in only about 5% of patients with hemophilia B. They are quite rare among healthy persons. Large gene deletions have been reported to occur among patients with hemophilia B who have spontaneous inhibitors. Isolated deficiency of factor IX has been reported with Gaucher's disease. Specific inhibitors to factor XI have been recognized most commonly among patients with lupus anticoagulants. Three patients with factor XI deficiency were found to have inhibitors to factor XI; two of the inhibitors were against the high-molecular-weight kininogen-binding site on factor XI. Spontaneous inhibitors to factor VII have been found in a patient with lung cancer. The only initial sign was isolated prolongation of PT.

DISORDERS ASSOCIATED WITH AN ABNORMAL BLEEDING TIME ONLY

Acquired bleeding disorders with prolonged bleeding times but normal PT and aPTT usually arise from inhibitors to von Willebrand factor or result from uremia. Acquired von Willebrand disease has been associated with use of medications (procainamide, valproic acid), connective tissue disorders, lymphoproliferative disorders, and a variety of tumors. Antibodies can be directed to von Willebrand factor itself or platelet glycoprotein Ib/IX/V complex. Patients with acute and chronic renal failure can have multiple causes of bleeding. No one mechanism can explain all causes of bleeding. Patients with uremia often have ecchymosis, muscular hematomas, gastrointestinal bleeding, and oozing on the mucosal surfaces. For many of these patients severe anemia contributes to the bleeding tendency.

Medications are common causes of abnormal bleeding. Aspirin is widely used as primary and secondary prevention of acute coronary syndromes and stroke. Some persons are quite sensitive to the antiplatelet effect of aspirin and have spontaneous bleeding. The thienopyridines (ticlopidine, clopidogrel) are antiplatelet agents that inhibit the expression of the adenosine diphosphate (ADP) receptor on platelets. With the wide use of these medications in cardiovascular medicine, increased bleeding will occur when these patients receive additional anticoagulants. Abnormal bleeding among patients taking the irreversible platelet inhibitors aspirin and the thienopyridines is best managed by means of platelet transfusions.

DISORDERS ASSOCIATED WITH ABNORMAL BLEEDING BUT NORMAL SCREENING TESTS

Inhibitors to factor XIII have occurred among patients with factor XIII deficiency who have received multiple transfusions. Many of these patients were receiving isoniazid when the inhibitor developed. α_2-Antiplasmin is a serine protease inhibitor of plasmin. In acute promyelocytic leukemia primary fibrinolysis develops as a result of membrane expression of annexin II on the membrane of acute leukemic cells. An increase in annexin II on leukemic cell membranes increases plasminogen activation and causes acquired deficiency of α_2-antiplasmin. The congenital form of α_2-antiplasmin deficiency is associated with bleeding that does not cause abnormal results of screening tests. Thrombocytopenia often occurs with acute promyelocytic leukemia, and evidence of DIC frequently also is present. The bleeding in acute promyelocytic leukemia is best controlled with transfusion support and heparin. Data suggest that *all-trans*-retinoic acid actually down-regulates tissue factor and annexin II on leukemic cells to control bleeding independently of replacement therapy and heparin.

BIBLIOGRAPHY

Alving BM. Antiphospholipid syndrome, lupus anticoagulants, and anticardiolipin antibodies. In: Loscalzo J, Schafer AI, eds. *Thrombosis and hemorrhage.* Baltimore: Williams & Wilkins, 1998:817–833.

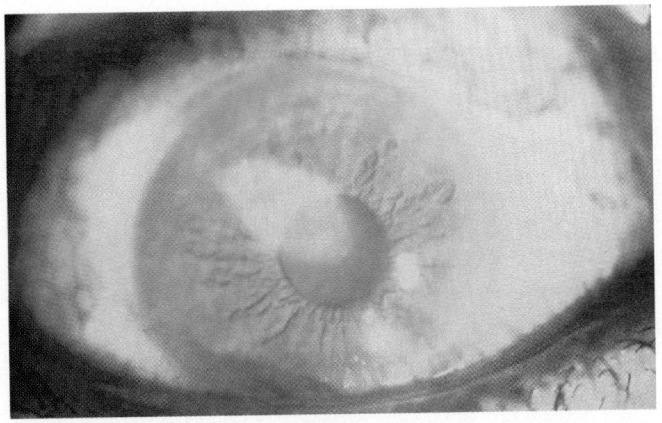

FIGURE 50.2. Neovascularization of the disc and retina.

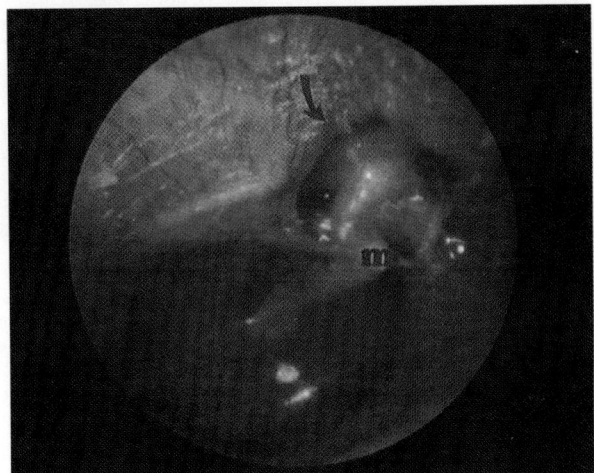

FIGURE 51.1. Otoscopic photograph of right tympanic membrane with large attic retraction pocket causing erosion of the bony external auditory canal. A serous effusion is also present. *m*, malleus short process.

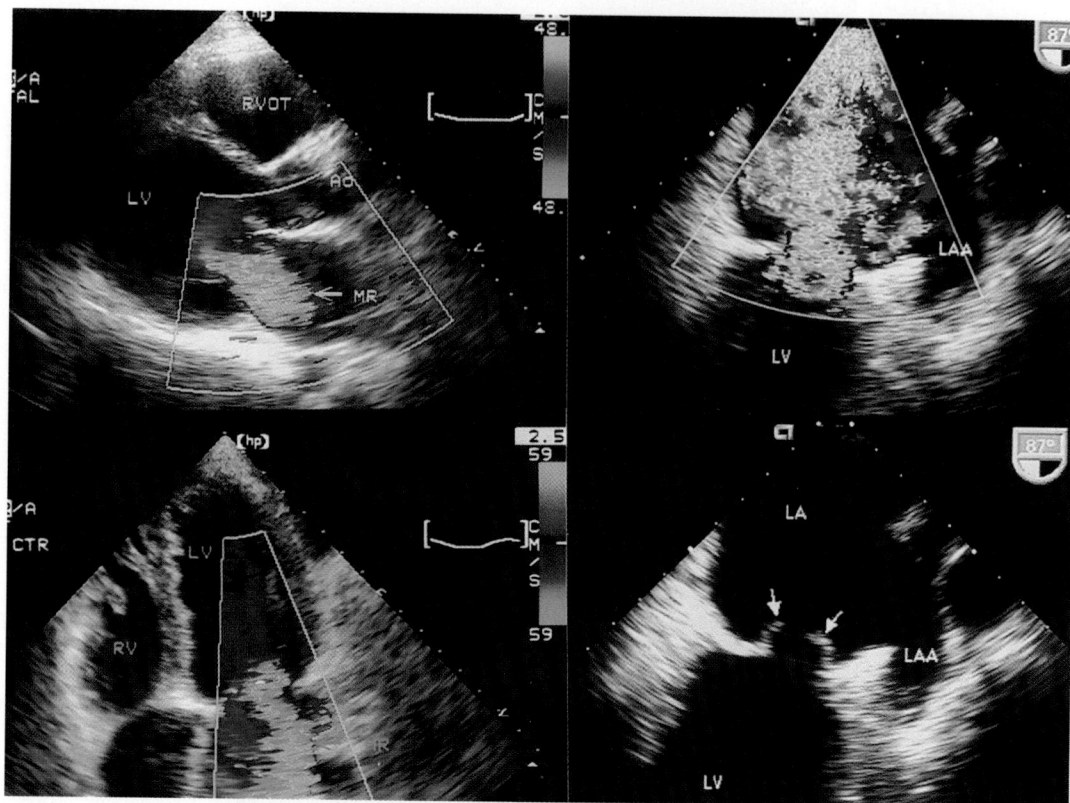

FIGURE 85.5. Four-panel view of patients with mitral regurgitation. The two panels on the left are transthoracic echocardiograms. The upper panel was recorded in a parasternal long-axis view and reveals moderate mitral regurgitation filling approximately 50% of the left atrium. The lower panel reveals a more eccentric mitral regurgitation jet along the lateral wall of the left atrium. The upper right panel is a transesophageal echocardiogram revealing severe mitral regurgitation and the lower panel the same view with the color signal suppressed. In this view, a flail anterior and posterior mitral valve leaflets *(arrows)* can be visualized as the mechanism for severe mitral regurgitation. LAA, left atrial appendage.

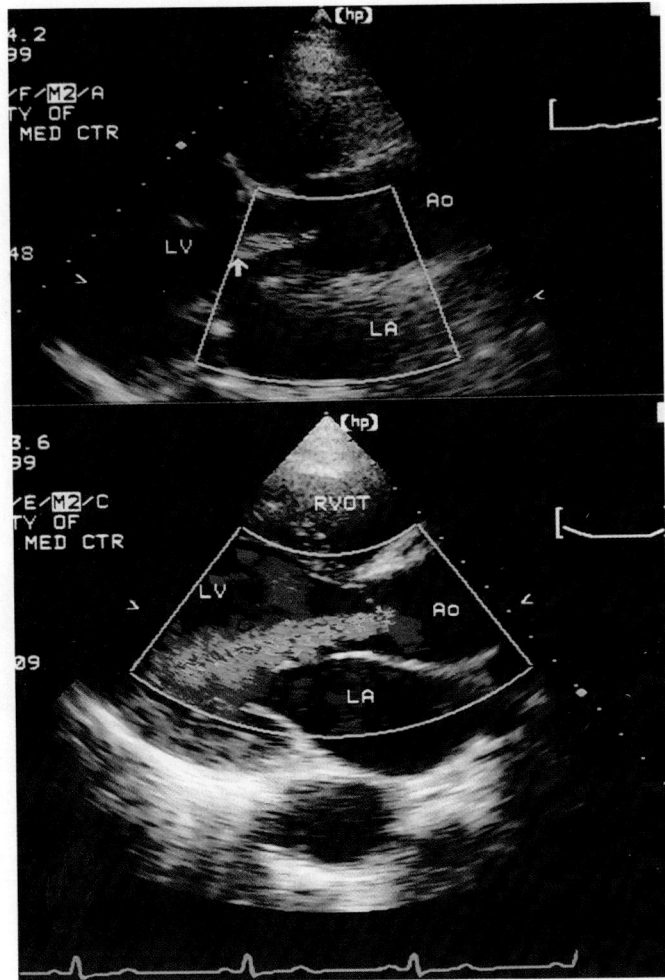

FIGURE 85.7. Parasternal long-axis views of two patients with aortic insufficiency. In each case the images were recorded in diastole. In the upper panel mild aortic insufficiency with a relatively small, narrow jet is seen (arrow). The lower panel demonstrates a greater degree of aortic insufficiency with a wide jet that penetrates down past the tips of the mitral valve leaflets.

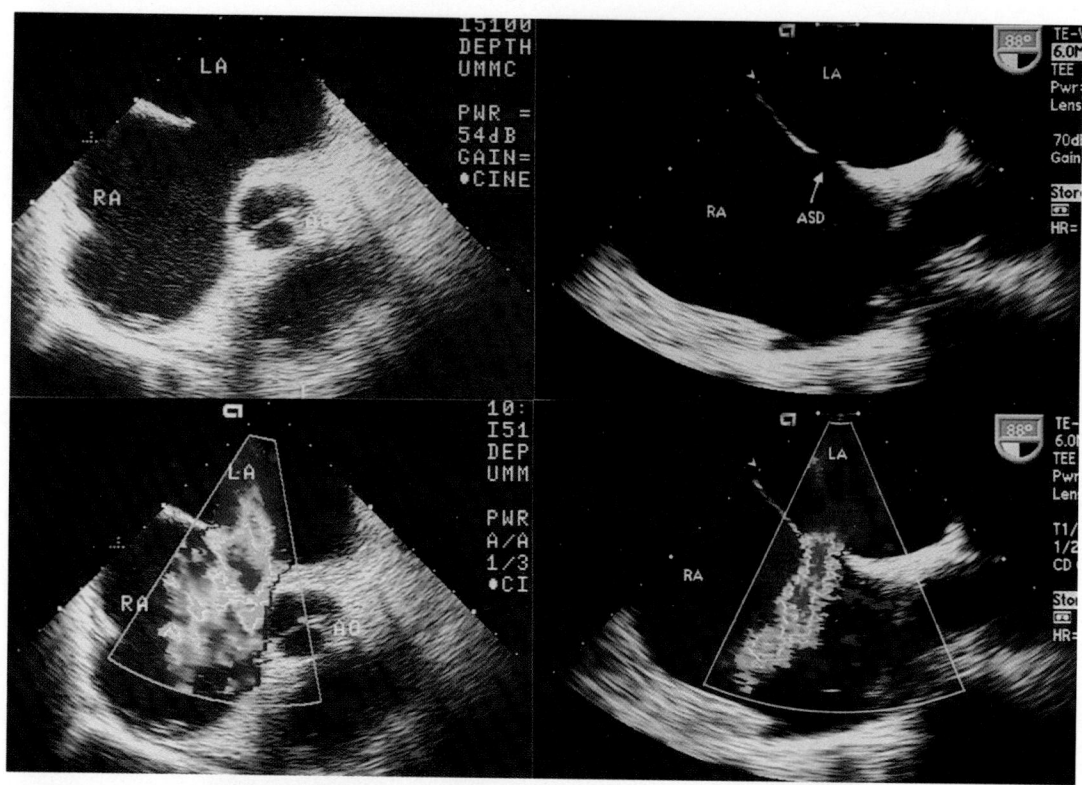

FIGURE 85.8. Transesophageal echocardiograms recorded in two patients with ASDs. On the left is a large ASD seen as echo dropout in the atrial septum on the two-dimensional image. The lower left panel shows the color flow image representing flow from the left atrium to the right atrium. The two right panels represent standard two-dimensional imaging and color flow imaging of a patient with a smaller ASD and predominant left-to-right shunting. ASD, atrial septal defect.

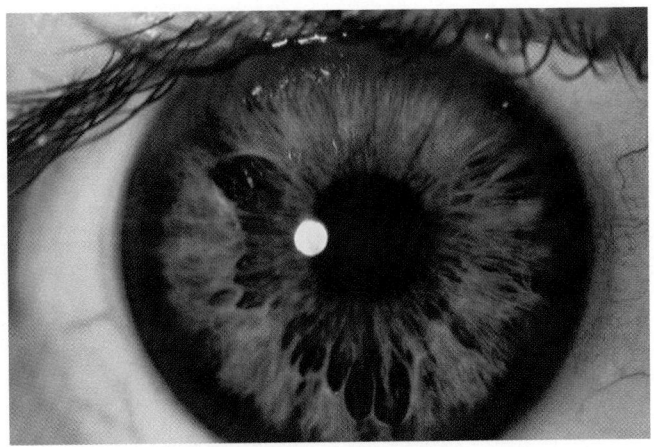

FIGURE 105.4. Kayser–Fleischer ring.

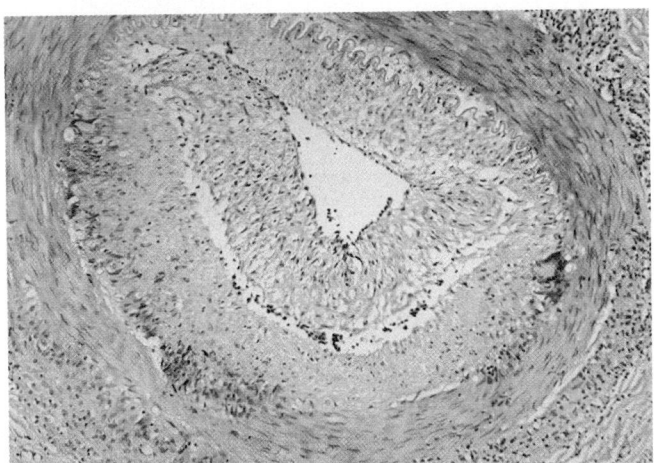

FIGURE 181.2. Temporal artery biopsy in a 64-year-old woman with new onset severe headaches, scalp tenderness, and polymyalgia rheumatica. Note the intense inflammatory changes in the adventitia and media, where giant cells are present. Intimal proliferation has caused luminal narrowing.

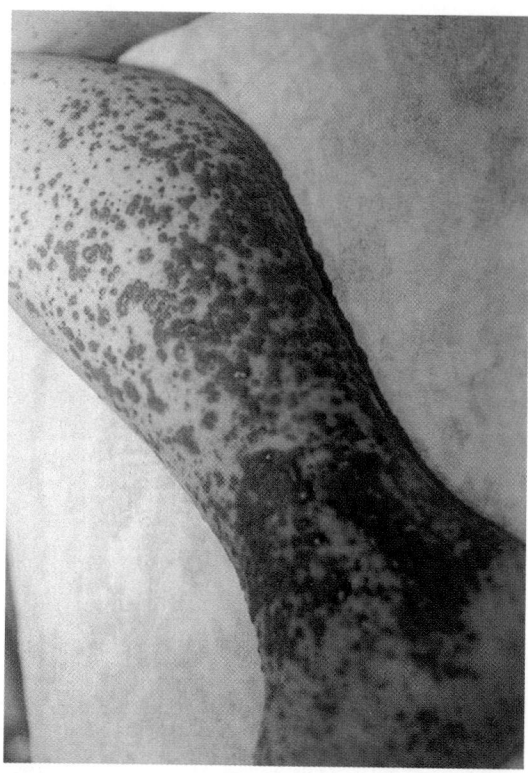

FIGURE 181.5. Henoch–Schönlein purpura. Skin lesions in this 14-year-old girl are particularly striking. Fever, polyarthralgias, and purpura cleared without glucocorticoid therapy. However, several recurrences followed a period of wellness.

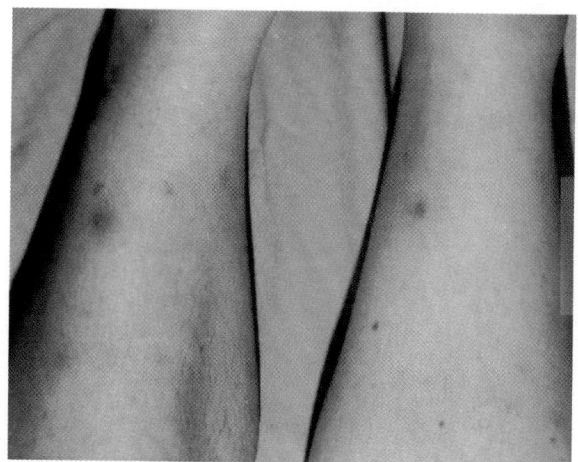

A

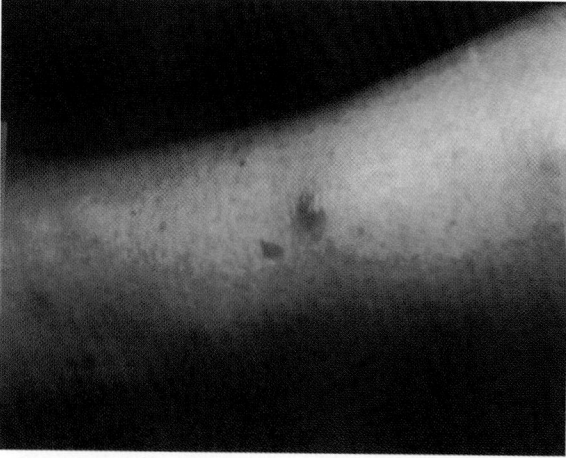

B

FIGURE 182.1. Disseminated gonococcal infection. **A:** Multiple skin lesions on lower extremities. **B:** Papule on hemorrhagic base. (Courtesy of Thomas H. Rae, MD.)

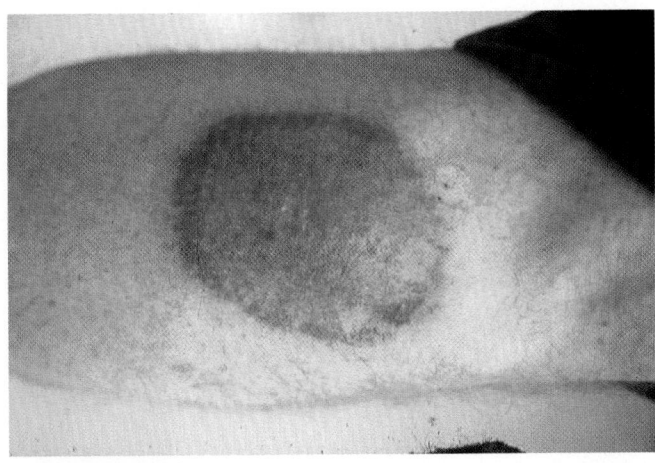

FIGURE 183.1. Lyme disease, erythema chronicum migrans. (Courtesy of Pfizer Central Research.)

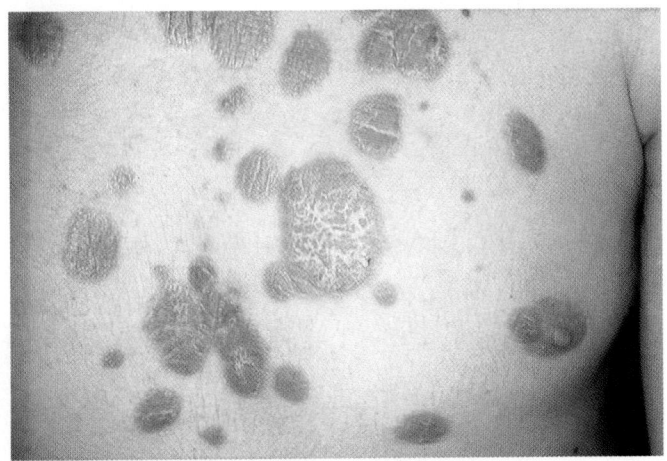

FIGURE 193.1. Chronic plaque-type psoriasis.

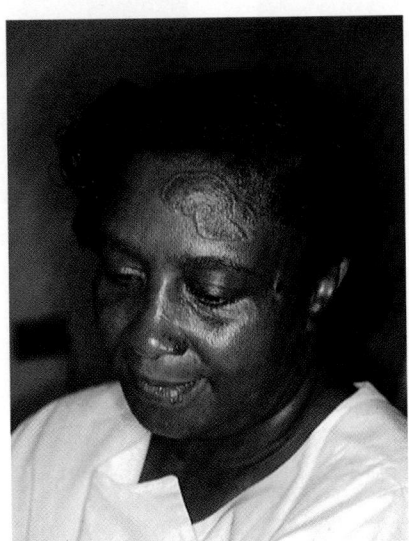

FIGURE 200.1. Annular: sarcoidosis.

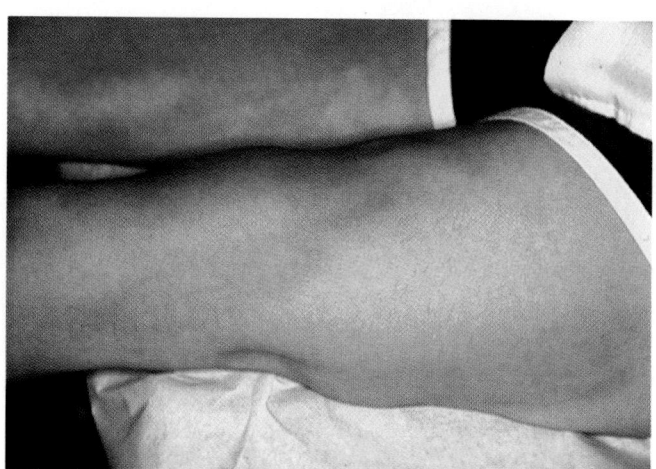

FIGURE 200.2. Atrophy: lipoatrophy.

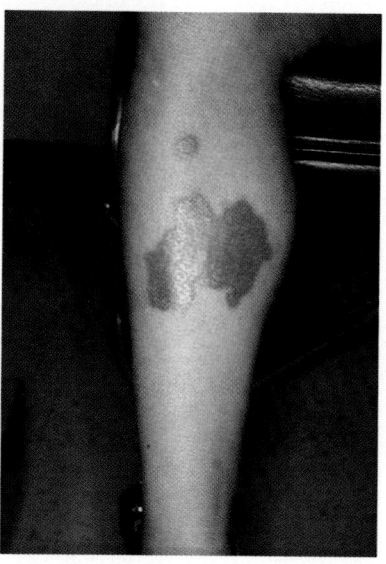

FIGURE 200.3. Atrophy: necrobiosis lipoidica diabeticorum.

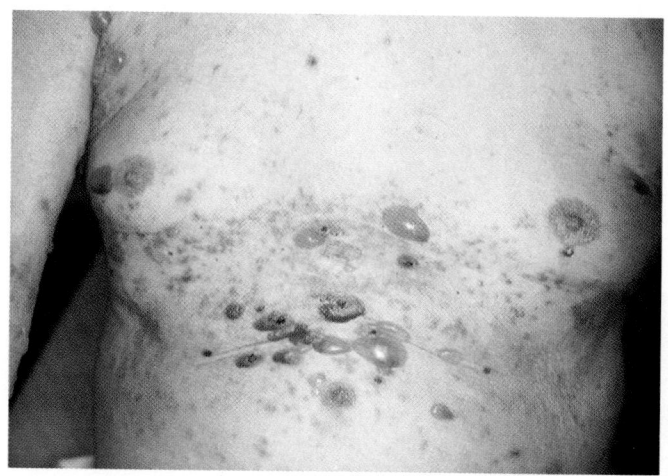

FIGURE 200.4. Vesicle and bulla: bullous pemphigoid.

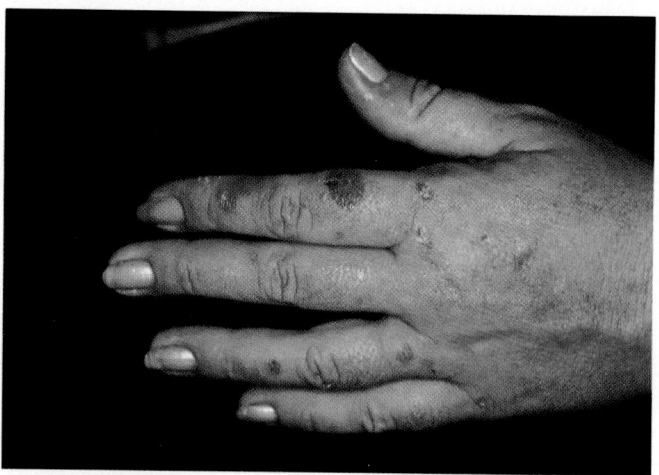

FIGURE 200.5. Erosion: porphyria cutanea tarda.

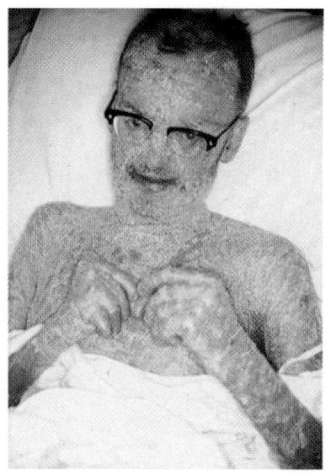

FIGURE 200.6. Exfoliation: psoriasis.

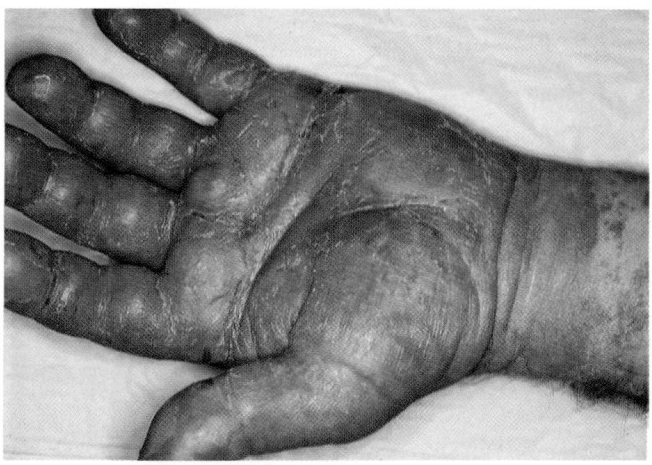

FIGURE 200.7. Fissure: hand eczema with erythema.

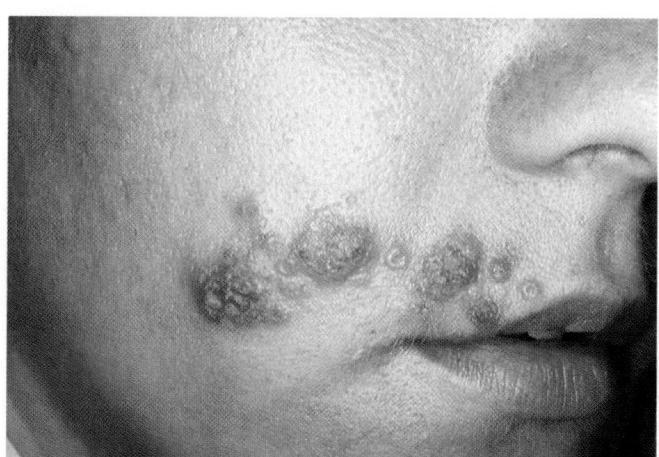

FIGURE 200.8. Herpetiform: herpes simplex with umbilicated vesicles.

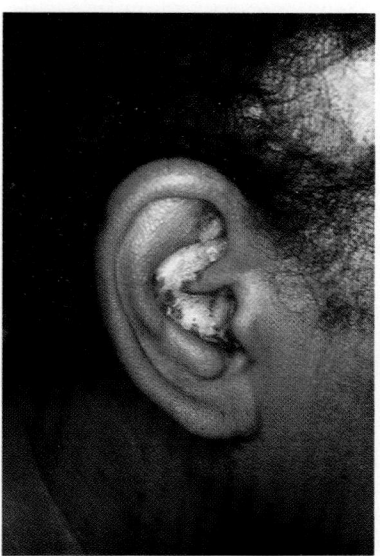

FIGURE 200.9. Hyperpigmentation/hypopigmentation: discoid lupus erythematosus with atrophic, hypopigmented center and hyperpigmented border.

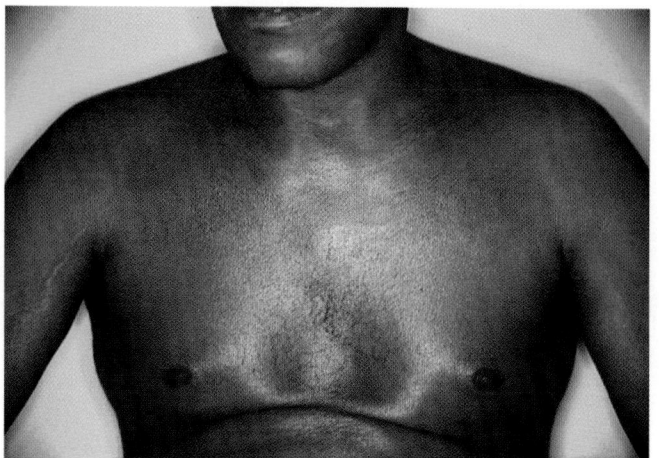

FIGURE 200.10. Indurated: scleroderma with diffusely shiny, taut skin.

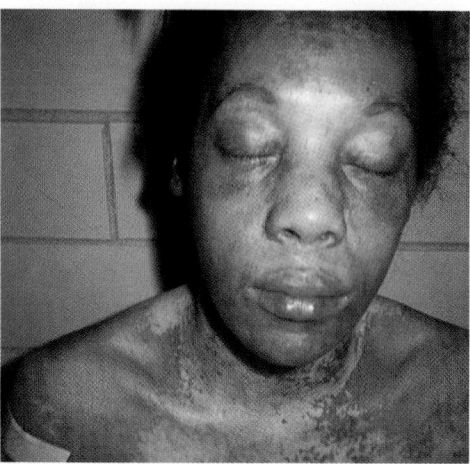

FIGURE 200.11. Lichenification: chronic eczematous dermatitis with hyperpigmentation.

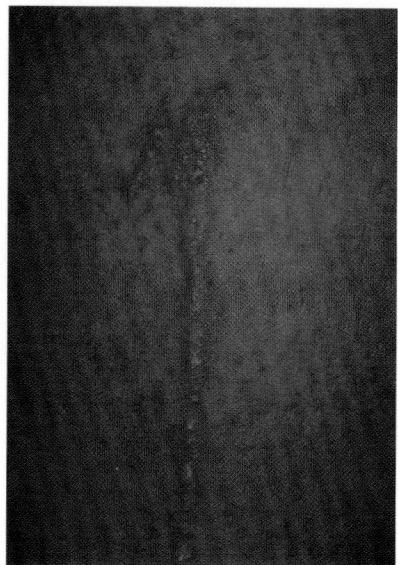

FIGURE 200.12. Linear: poison ivy contact dermatitis.

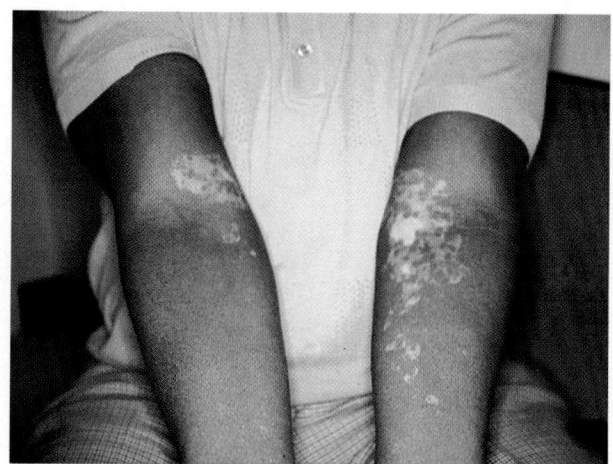

FIGURE 200.13. Macule: vitiligo.

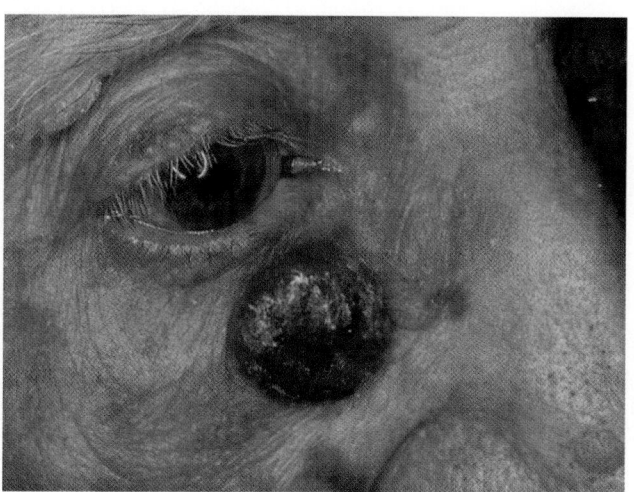

FIGURE 200.14. Nodule: squamous cell carcinoma.

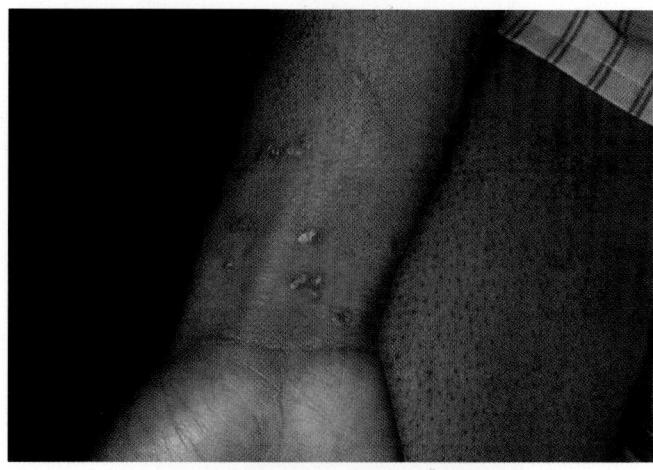

FIGURE 200.15. Papule: lichen planus.

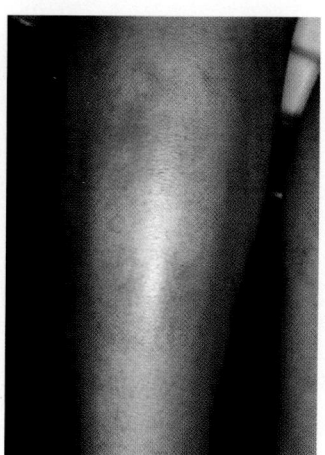

FIGURE 200.16. Plaque: erythema nodosum.

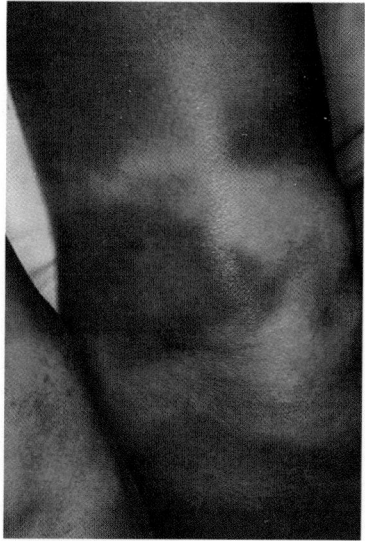

FIGURE 200.17. Purpura/ecchymosis: autoerythrocyte sensitization.

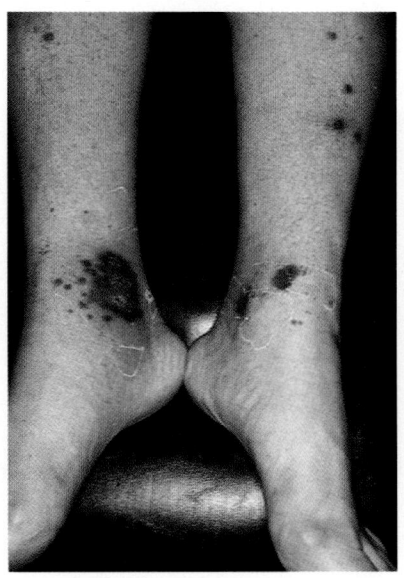

FIGURE 200.18. Purpura/petechiae: leukocytoclastic vasculitis.

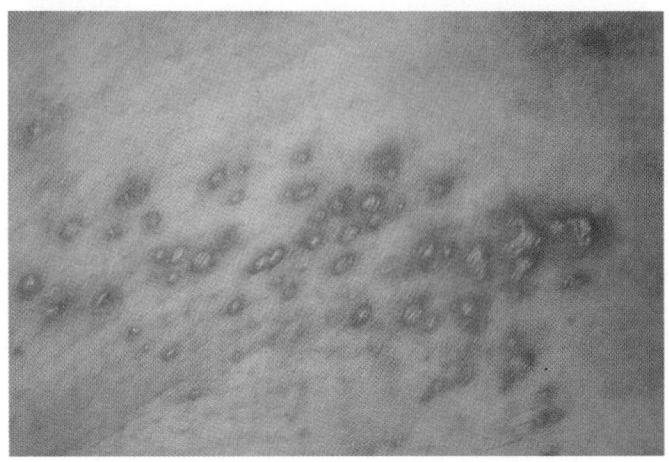

FIGURE 200.19. Pustule: pustular psoriasis.

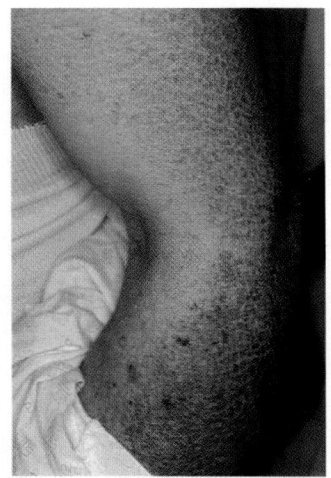

FIGURE 200.20. Scale: X-linked ichthyosis.

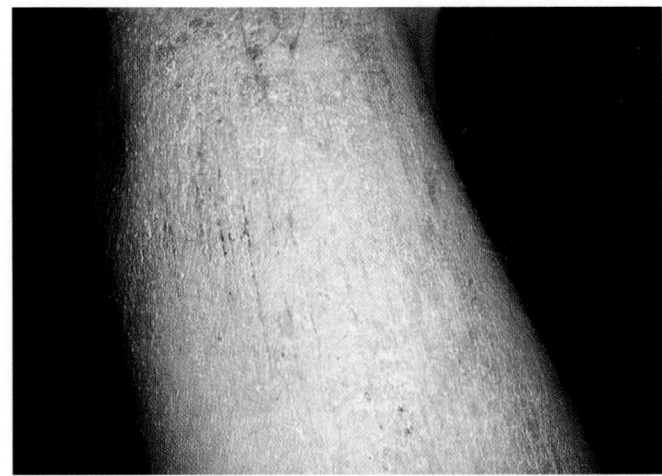

FIGURE 200.21. Excoriation: atopic dermatitis.

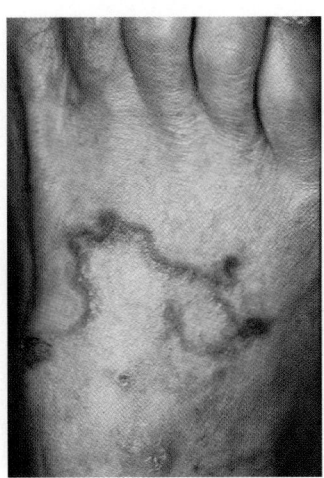

FIGURE 200.22. Serpiginous: cutaneous larva migrans.

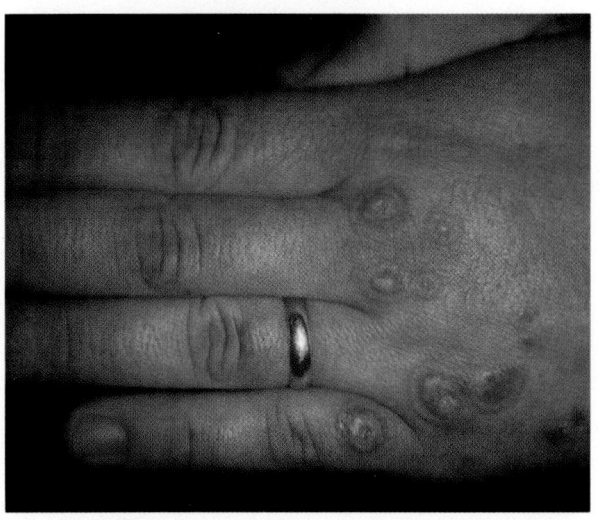

FIGURE 200.23. Target/iris: erythema multiforme.

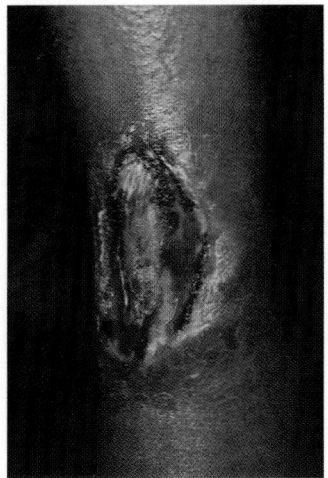

FIGURE 200.24. Ulcer: stasis ulcer with crusts.

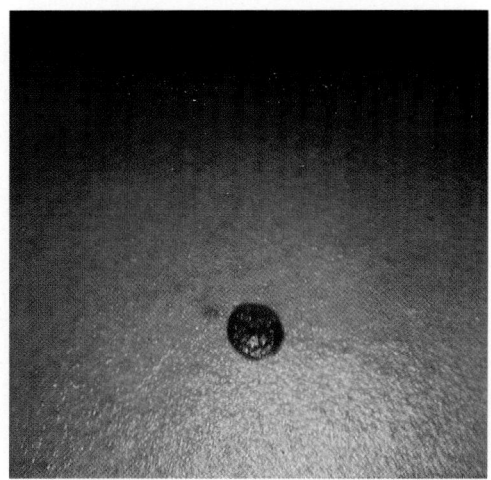

FIGURE 200.25. Verrucous: seborrheic keratosis.

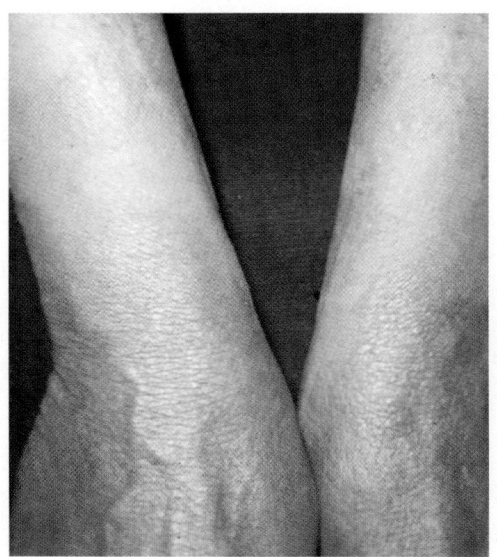

FIGURE 200.26. Violaceous: heliotrope discoloration of dermato-myositis.

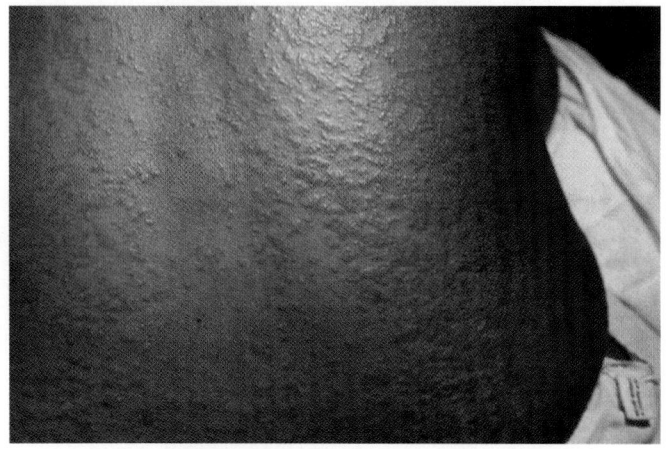

FIGURE 200.28. Case 1—Drug allergy secondary to ampicillin.

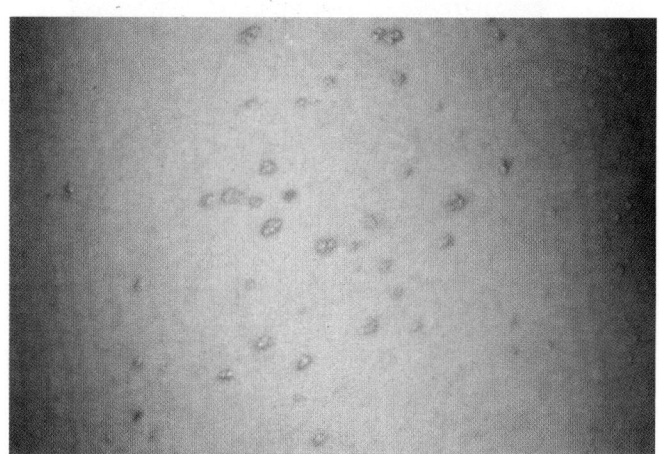

FIGURE 200.29. Case 2—Eruptive xanthomas secondary to diabetes mellitus.

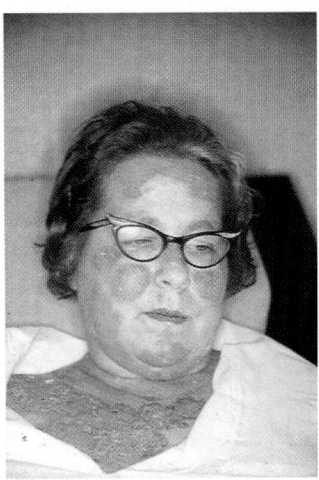

FIGURE 200.30. Case 3—Systemic lupus erythematosus.

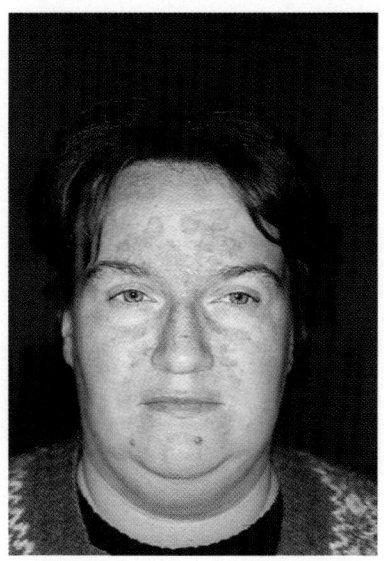

FIGURE 200.31. Case 4—Seborrheic dermatitis.

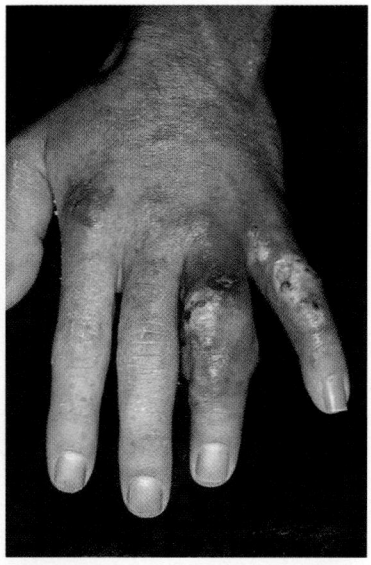

FIGURE 200.32. Case 5—Multicentric reticulohistiocytosis.

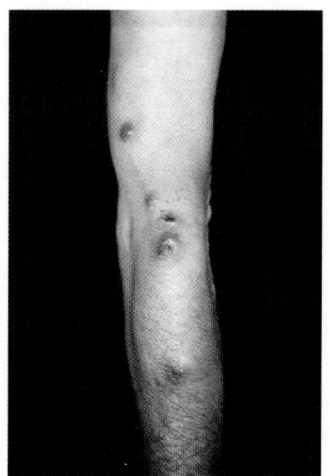

FIGURE 200.33. Case 6—Sporotrichosis.

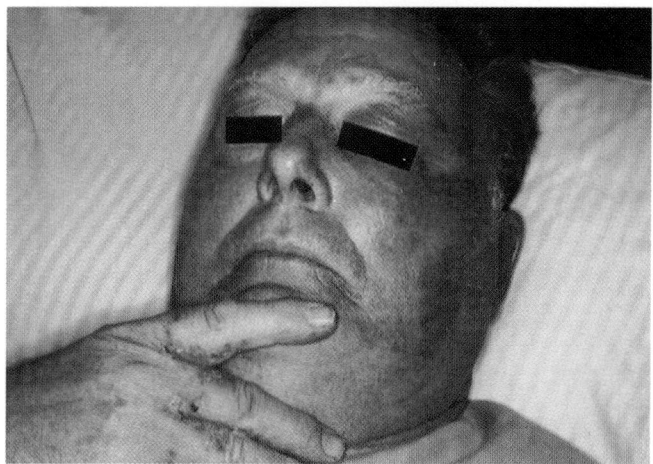

FIGURE 275.1. Erysipelas involving the left malar and preauricular areas of the face. The borders of the infection are clearly demarcated, and the lesions are elevated. Note the impetiginous lesions on the fingers.

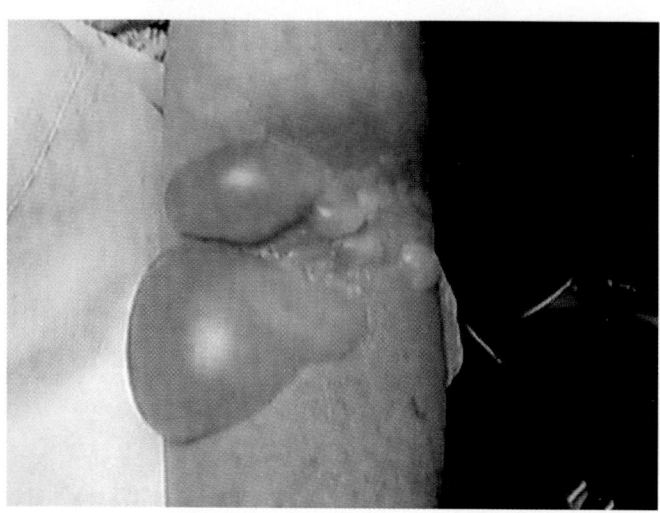

FIGURE 275.2. Group A streptococcal necrotizing fasciitis in a child with preceding varicella infection. Note the large bullous lesions with surrounding violaceous discoloration of skin. (Courtesy of Dr. Larry Slack, Vanderbilt University.)

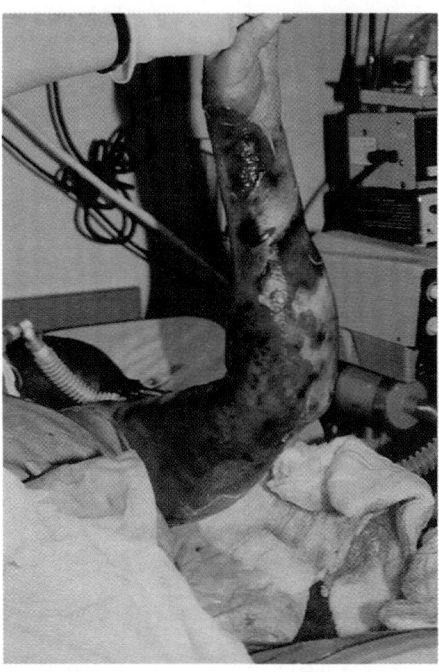

FIGURE 275.3. Group A streptococcal necrotizing fasciitis.

Colman RW, Robboy SJ, Minna JD. Disseminated intravascular coagulation (DIC): an approach. *Am J Med* 1972;52:679–689.

Green D. Factor VIII and other coagulation factor inhibitors. In: Loscalzo J, Schafer AI, eds. *Thrombosis and hemorrhage.* Baltimore: Williams & Wilkins, 1998:803–815.

Grosset ABM, Rodgers GM. Acquired coagulation disorders. In: Lee GR, Foerster J, Lukens J, et al., eds. *Wintrobe's clinical hematology,* 10th ed. Baltimore: Williams & Wilkins, 1999:1733–1780.

Schmaier AH. Disseminated intravascular coagulation: pathogenesis and management. *J Intensive Care Med* 1991;6:209–228.

Kelley's Textbook of Internal Medicine, fourth edition. Edited by H. David Humes. Lippincott Williams & Wilkins, Philadelphia © 2000.

CHAPTER 239

DISORDERS OF PLATELET FUNCTION

KEITH R. MCCRAE
SANFORD J. SHATTIL

Platelets arrest hemorrhage by adhering to the wall of damaged blood vessels and aggregating to form the primary hemostatic plug. Activated platelets, damaged endothelial cells, and other cells within the vessel wall participate in secondary hemostasis by providing a membrane surface on which coagulation proteins can assemble, interact, and produce a fibrin plug. Even in the absence of overt vessel damage, platelets are involved in maintaining the integrity of the vascular endothelial lining. Each of these functions may become inadequate in the presence of thrombocytopenia or a qualitative disorder of platelet function.

The clinical hallmarks of platelet dysfunction are bleeding from the skin and mucous membranes (epistaxis, gingival bleeding, menorrhagia), excessive posttraumatic or postoperative hemorrhage, and a prolonged bleeding time. All of these events reflect inadequate formation of the primary hemostatic plug. Disturbances of the role of platelets in maintaining vascular integrity may account for the development of petechiae, which are pinpoint hemorrhages in the skin or mucous membranes. These occur most commonly on the distal lower extremities or other dependent areas under increased hydrostatic pressure. Although hemorrhage involving larger and deeper areas of the skin (purpura and ecchymoses) may occur, these lesions are less specific than are petechiae as an indicator of platelet-type bleeding. Spontaneous hemorrhage into muscles or joints is not a feature of platelet dysfunction and suggests a defect in the formation or stability of the fibrin plug.

A bleeding time test is used clinically as a measurement of platelet plug formation. With a blood pressure cuff on the arm set at 40 mm Hg, a 1-mm deep incision is made on the volar surface of the forearm with a disposable, spring-triggered device, and the duration of bleeding is assessed. Bleeding time, which normally ranges from 2 to 9 minutes, usually is prolonged when there is a disorder of platelet function. However, the results of this test have not been shown to be a predictor of surgical bleeding and do not replace the need for meticulous history taking in screening for hemostatic defects.

The bleeding history is the most important screening test for platelet function defects. In the history interview one should attempt to obtain qualitative and quantitative information about earlier bleeding episodes. For example, reports of easy bruising are common and subjective and may or may not indicate an underlying problem. Oral bleeding can continue for as long as 24 hours after molar extraction even among persons with normal bleeding profiles. In contrast, bleeding that necessitates transfusion after minimal trauma or surgery is abnormal. Whereas bleeding of recent onset generally suggests an acquired defect in platelet function, a family history of bleeding suggests an inherited disorder, the diagnosis of which may be facilitated by pedigree analysis. Patients always must be questioned about the use of prescription and nonprescription drugs, because many such medications markedly alter platelet function. If a disorder of platelet function is suspected on the basis of the history and a prolonged bleeding time, additional laboratory studies are warranted to make a specific diagnosis and plan therapy.

NORMAL PLATELET FUNCTION

A discussion of platelet dysfunction is facilitated by an understanding of platelet anatomy and biochemistry. A platelet is enveloped by a plasma membrane that invaginates extensively into the cytoplasm to form a surface-connected open canalicular system. This membrane consists predominantly of a bilayer of phospholipid and cholesterol and contains numerous integral and peripheral membrane glycoproteins. Some of these glycoproteins mediate the interaction of the platelet with its environment and have been assigned Roman numerals on the basis of molecular weight. Several cytoskeletal proteins are closely associated with the cytoplasmic surface of the membrane, and these may be involved in a number of membrane functions, including control of cell shape. Platelets also contain a calcium-sequestering vesicular organelle called the *dense tubular system,* mitochondria, and four distinct types of storage granules. Electron-dense granules (δ granules) contain serotonin and metabolically inactive adenosine diphosphate (ADP). α Granules contain several proteins, including fibrinogen, von Willebrand factor (VWF), thrombospondin, platelet-derived growth factors, vascular endothelial cell growth factor, and platelet factor 4. The membrane of the α granule also contains a glycoprotein, P-selectin, which is expressed on the cell surface after platelet secretion and may be involved in the interaction of activated platelets with other cells in a vascular wound. Finally, λ-granules contain lysosomal enzymes, and microperoxisomes contain catalase.

Platelet adhesion refers to the contact and spreading of platelets on the wall of a damaged blood vessel. Adhesion is promoted by red blood cells, in part through rheologic effects, and is mediated by interactions of platelets with substances in the subendothelial matrix. Platelets contain binding sites for a number of matrix proteins, including collagen, fibronectin, vitronectin,

VWF, and laminin. In the capillary microcirculation, where blood shear rates are high, interactions between VWF and the platelet glycoprotein Ib/IX/V complex promotes initial platelet adhesion. VWF is a 225-kD protein synthesized by endothelial cells and megakaryocytes, where it undergoes a series of post-translational modifications, including formation of large multimers with molecular weights ranging from 0.8 to 20×10^6 kD. VWF multimers are released constitutively from endothelial cells into the vessel lumen and are deposited abluminally into the subendothelial matrix. The multimers also are stored within endothelial cells and may be released in response to certain stimuli. Although the VWF molecule contains distinct binding domains for platelets and collagen, it normally circulates in plasma in a conformational state that does not interact with circulating platelets. However, subendothelial VWF remains in an active conformation, perhaps through conformational changes induced after its binding to collagen. After vessel damage, exposed VWF within the subendothelial matrix binds to platelets; the larger VWF multimers are more effective in this regard.

Interactions between VWF and platelets occur largely through platelet GpIb, a 170-kD integral membrane protein composed of a 143-kD α subunit disulfide-linked to a 23-kD β subunit, the subunits arising from separate genes. GpIb normally forms a complex with a smaller, 17-kD membrane protein, GpIX, and an additional surface glycoprotein, GpV. Approximately 25,000 molecules of GpIbα, GpIbβ, and GpIX are expressed on the surface of each platelet with one-half as many molecules of GpV, for a putative overall stoichiometry for the GpIbα-Ibβ-IX-V complex of 2:2:2:1. In vitro, compounds such as ristocetin and botrocetin stimulate the binding of VWF to the complex, causing platelet agglutination; this property is used diagnostically to assess the function of VWF and platelet GpIb.

Binding of platelets to VWF leads to rolling adhesion to the vessel wall, and induces signaling events that lead to inside-out activation of integrin αIIbβ3, also called platelet GpIIb-IIIa, the platelet fibrinogen receptor (see later). αIIbβ3 may then mediate stronger, stationary adhesion through interactions with VWF and perhaps other matrix proteins containing Arg-Gly-Asp sequences. Adhesion of platelets to exposed collagen also occurs through interactions with platelet collagen receptors, including the integrin α2 (GpIa, molecular weight 168 kD) β1 (GpIIa, molecular weight, 130 kD) complex and glycoprotein VI (61 kD).

After adhering to the wall of a damaged vessel, platelets must aggregate to form the primary hemostatic plug. *Platelet aggregation* requires the binding of extracellular fibrinogen to αIIbβ3 (molecular weights 142 and 99 kD, respectively, for the αIIb and β3 chains). Although approximately 80,000 αIIbβ3 molecules are on the surface of each platelet, the fibrinogen receptor function is not expressed until the platelet is activated by an agonist, an event that occurs through several interrelated pathways. Activation of αIIbβ3 after binding of an agonist to platelets involves specific conformational changes in the integrin complex. Each activated αIIbβ3 complex binds a single fibrinogen molecule in a calcium-dependent manner. Because the fibrinogen molecule is dimeric, fibrinogen may bind to receptors on adjacent activated platelets, resulting in receptor bridging and

platelet-to-platelet aggregation. In addition to binding fibrinogen, activated αIIbβ3 can bind VWF, which may play an accessory role in platelet adhesion. VWF also may bind to activated αIIbβ3 and support platelet aggregation when fibrinogen is lacking.

Platelet activation and inside-out signaling are initiated by the binding of agonists such as thrombin, collagen, ADP, and epinephrine to specific receptors on the platelet surface membrane. When platelets are stirred in an aggregometer, weak agonists such as epinephrine and ADP can stimulate activation of αIIbβ3 and promote fibrinogen binding and the formation of small, or first-wave, platelet aggregates that may undergo disaggregation. If the concentration of a weak agonist is sufficiently high, the aggregating platelets produce and release thromboxane A_2. This endogenously formed agonist in concert with ADP secreted from δ granules promotes further αIIbβ3 activation, platelet secretion, and formation of large, irreversible, second-wave aggregates. These aggregates are stabilized by thrombospondin secreted from α granules. Exposure of functional αIIbβ3 also is stimulated by strong agonists such as thrombin, which directly stimulates thromboxane A_2 synthesis and granule secretion without the need for initial aggregation. Although collagen does not directly stimulate aggregation, it induces production of endogenous platelet thromboxane A_2, induces granule secretion, and therefore induces a delayed aggregation response.

Platelet secretion requires a contractile response involving actin and myosin and the fusion of granule membranes with the plasma membrane. These processes are initiated by the agonist-induced activation of two phospholipid-cleaving enzymes, phospholipase C and phospholipase A_2. One or more heterotrimeric guanine nucleotide binding proteins (G proteins) are interposed between agonist receptors and the phospholipases. G_q appears particularly important in this regard. Phospholipase C converts phosphatidylinositol 4,5-bisphosphate to diacylglycerol and inositol 1,4,5-triphosphate, and each of these reaction products stimulates platelet secretion. Diacylglycerol activates protein kinase C, which phosphorylates proteins involved in the secretory response. Inositol-1,4,5-triphosphate stimulates calcium release from the dense tubular system, causing a rise in cytoplasmic free calcium and activation of calcium-dependent enzymes such as phospholipase A_2 and myosin light-chain kinase. Phospholipase A_2 releases arachidonic acid from phospholipids, promoting the synthesis of prostaglandins and thromboxane A_2. These reactions stimulate platelet activation, but the overall activation state of the platelet depends on the balance between stimulatory and inhibitory influences. The latter include prostacyclin from endothelial cells and prostaglandin D_2 (PGD2) from platelets, which bind to their platelet membrane receptors and stimulate adenylate cyclase. That process increases intracellular concentrations of cyclic adenosine monophosphate (cAMP), which maintains platelets in the resting state. Endothelial cells may regulate platelet activation through the release of an ecto-ADPase.

Platelet procoagulant activity refers to the capability of platelets to support several key coagulation reactions, especially intrinsic pathway–mediated activation of factor X, and the conversion of prothrombin to thrombin. The platelet facilitates these reactions by providing a surface on which coagulation enzymes, substrates, and cofactors interact. Platelet procoagulant activity is markedly increased on activation by thrombin or collagen and is accounted for, at least in part, by exposure of acidic phospholipids on the surface of activated platelets and small membrane vesicles released from these cells.

CLASSIFICATION OF DISORDERS OF PLATELET FUNCTION

Defects in platelet adhesion, aggregation, and procoagulant activity may be inherited or acquired. Inherited defects (Table 239.1) usually have a predominant effect on only one of these functions, so classification is based on the underlying functional defect. Of the inherited platelet function disorders, von Willebrand disease and platelet activation defects are most prevalent, whereas storage pool disorders are less common, and membrane glycoprotein deficiencies are rare. In contrast, acquired conditions that impair platelet function often affect adhesion, aggregation, and procoagulant activity simultaneously, and in many such cases the precise underlying pathophysiologic mechanism is difficult to discern. It is most useful at present to classify acquired platelet function defects in the context of their associated clinical setting (Table 239.2). Ingestion of aspirin and other nonsteroidal anti-inflammatory drugs is the most common cause of acquired platelet dysfunction and of platelet dysfunction overall.

TABLE 239.1.	INHERITED DISORDERS OF PLATELET FUNCTION
Pathophysiologic Mechanism	**Specific Disorder**
Disorders of Platelet Adhesion	
Defects of adhesive proteins	von Willebrand disease
Defects of adhesion receptors	Bernard–Soulier syndrome
	Platelet-type von Willebrand disease
	Glycoprotein (Gp) Ia or Gp VI (deficiency)
Disorders of Platelet Aggregation	
Deficiency of the ligand (fibrinogen)	Afibrinogenemia
Defects of the receptor (Gp IIb–IIIa)	
Defects of Gp IIb–IIIa quantity or quality	Glanzmann thrombasthenia and variants
Defects of Gp IIb–IIIa activation	Platelet activation defects; Bartter's syndrome
Storage pool defects	Storage pool disease (δ and αδ storage pool diseases); gray platelet syndrome
Disorders of Platelet Procoagulant Activity	Scott syndrome

TABLE 239.2.	ACQUIRED DISORDERS OF PLATELET FUNCTION

Drugs That Affect Platelet Function

Nonsteroidal anti-inflammatory drugs
β-Lactam antibiotics
ADP-receptor antagonists
  Ticlopidine
  Clopidogrel
Glycoprotein IIb/IIIa receptor antagonists
  Abciximab (ReoPro)
  Eptifibatide (Integrilin)
  Tirofiban (Aggrastat)
  Others
Miscellaneous drugs

Systemic Conditions That Affect Platelet Dysfunction

Chronic renal disease
Cardiopulmonary bypass
Antiplatelet antibodies
Disseminated intravascular coagulation

Hematologic Diseases That Affect Platelet Dysfunction

Acute myelogenous leukemia, myelodysplastic syndromes, myeloproliferative disorders
Multiple myeloma and other B-cell neoplasms
Antiplatelet antibodies

INHERITED DISORDERS OF PLATELET FUNCTION

Disorders of Platelet Adhesion

von Willebrand Disease

von Willebrand disease and platelet-type von Willebrand disease are discussed in Chapter 237.

Bernard–Soulier Syndrome

Bernard–Soulier syndrome is a rare disorder transmitted in an autosomal recessive manner. Consanguinity is frequent in affected families. Homozygotes or compound heterozygotes experience menorrhagia and recurrent mucocutaneous, posttraumatic, or postoperative bleeding, which may be variable in severity but can be life threatening. The first bleeding episode occurs in infancy or childhood, sometimes after circumcision. In addition to a prolonged bleeding time, patients with this disorder have giant platelets on a peripheral blood film (many as large or larger than red blood cells). These persons also have mild to moderate thrombocytopenia, which in some cases is caused by shortened platelet survival. Heterozygotes do not have a bleeding tendency or thrombocytopenia, although their platelets may be larger than normal.

The main functional abnormality in Bernard–Soulier syndrome is impaired adhesion of platelets to the subendothelial matrix. This defect is the result of a marked deficiency or absence of the GpIb-IX-V complex, and the deficiency causes impaired interaction of platelets with subendothelial VWF. Bernard–Soulier syndrome should be suspected when there are giant platelets on a blood smear and when ristocetin does not induce platelet agglutination in the presence of normal VWF. The diagnosis is confirmed by means of measurement of GpIb and GpIX electrophoretic and immunologic techniques. Heterozygotes have about one-half the normal levels of GpIb-IX-V.

Several molecular defects that underlie the platelet phenotype in Bernard–Soulier syndrome have been characterized. Most of these are point mutations in GpIbα that lead to specific amino acid substitutions, although in one case a point mutation leading to premature chain termination has been described. In some cases, deletions in the GpIb coding sequence have led to frameshift mutations. Similar mutations have affected the genes for GpIbα and GpIX, although Bernard–Soulier syndrome caused by mutations in the gene for GpV has not been reported. The expression of unaffected subunits of the GpIb-IX-V complex (for example, GpIbα and GpIbβ in the case of a GpIX mutation) and GpV also is markedly reduced in platelets from patients with Bernard–Soulier syndrome. Although this observation remains unexplained, efficient expression of GpIbα, GpIbβ, or GpIX in vitro occurs only in the presence of a gene that encodes at least one other member of the complex. Though GpV is not needed for expression of the other proteins, its expression is enhanced in their presence. These studies suggest that association of the GpIbα, GpIbβ, and GpIX subunits during or soon their after synthesis and insertion into the endoplasmic reticulum facilitates their transport to the cell surface. The abnormal morphologic features of Bernard–Soulier platelets also suggest that the proper assembly of this complex plays a role in platelet and megakaryocyte development. Bernard–Soulier platelets also display delayed aggregation in response to thrombin, perhaps because GpIb-IX-V may mediate platelet activation by low concentrations of thrombin, and are resistant to damage by quinine- or quinidine-dependent antiplatelet antibodies, which are specific for an epitope consisting of the drug bound to the GpIb-IX-V complex.

Integrin α1 (Glycoprotein Ia) or Glycoprotein VI Deficiency

Studies have begun to define the role of integrin α2β1 (GpIa-IIa) and GpVI in adhesion to and activation of platelets by collagen. Binding of collagen to each of these sites may induce platelet activation, although different pathways appear to be involved. For a patient whose platelets contained only 10% of the normal levels of GpVI, platelet adhesion and spreading was reduced only modestly, although platelet aggregation and ATP release after exposure to collagen were absent. These observations suggest that platelet α2β1 is primarily involved in adhesion and arrest of platelets under flow conditions, whereas GpVI may largely function as a signaling receptor. GpVI is physically associated with the platelet Fc receptor γ chain, a signal-generating subunit of the Fc receptor. *Src* family kinases are associated with the GpVI-FcR-γ complex and may be involved in platelet activation occurring through this pathway.

Patients with deficient collagen receptor expression have a mild bleeding tendency and prolonged bleeding time consistent with that of a platelet adhesion disorder. Platelets from such persons display diminished adhesion to or spreading on subendothelial collagen but are fully responsive to other agonists. Little information is available concerning the molecular defects that underlie diminished expression or function of these receptors. However, a linked polymorphism in the coding regions of the α_2 integrin gene at nucleotides 807 (C or T) and 873 (G or A) has been described in which carriers of the $C_{807}G_{873}$ allele express higher levels of α2β1 and may be at greater risk for the development of myocardial infarction at a young age. In vitro platelets from these persons adhere more rapidly to type I collagen at high shear rates.

Disorders of Platelet Aggregation

Decreased platelet aggregation may be caused by (a) quantitative or qualitative abnormalities of platelets αIIbβ3 (thrombasthenia) or (b) decreased activation of αIIbβ3 caused by a platelet biochemical defect or storage pool deficiency.

Glanzmann Thrombasthenia

Glanzmann thrombasthenia is an autosomal recessive disorder characterized by a prolonged bleeding time, absent platelet aggregation, and mucocutaneous or posttraumatic bleeding. The bleeding diathesis is severe in many patients, although some patients have no excessive bleeding throughout their lives. For most patients, hemorrhage is sporadic and unpredictable; however, childhood epistaxis and vaginal bleeding at menarche or parturition represent serious risks. Glanzmann thrombasthenia usually is diagnosed before the age of 5 years, and although some authorities believe that its severity tends to decrease in later life, this opinion may simply represent a decreased incidence of minor trauma among adults. The disease is rare in most areas of the world (for example, 1 case per million in Scandinavia), but some populations have a high incidence, such as Jordanian Arabs and Jewish emigres from Iraq.

In the classic form of Glanzmann thrombasthenia there is a marked deficiency or absence of platelet αIIbβ3. Many patients have an associated decrease in the content of α granule fibrinogen, although plasma fibrinogen is normal. As a result of the deficiency of αIIbβ3, activated platelets are not capable of binding fibrinogen and cannot aggregate to form the platelet plug. Thrombasthenic platelets, however, can undergo a normal secretory response and can adhere to the vessel wall, although defects in platelet spreading have been described. The diagnosis is established with detection of a near absence of agonist-induced platelet aggregation and of αIIbβ3 by means of electrophoretic and immunologic techniques. The platelets of persons heterozygous for this disorder contain about one-half the normal amount of αIIbβ3, and these persons generally do not have a bleeding diathesis. Thrombasthenic platelets are deficient in the Bak (Lek) antigen, normally found on integrin αIIb, and the PL^A and YUK antigens, normally found on integrin β3.

Integrins αIIb and β3 are the products of separate genes on chromosome 17. Numerous studies have identified several molecular defects leading to the development of Glanzmann thrombasthenia. These lesions may involve the genes that encode either integrin αIIb or integrin β3 and at this point appear to involve each of these genes with approximately equal frequency. Most reported lesions have been either small deletions or substitutions of one base pair, which in some cases have involved splice donor sites, although larger deletions of up to 4.5 kb have been characterized. Most patients with Glanzmann thrombasthenia appear to be compound heterozygotes, although some persons with homozygous defects have been identified. These defects may be particularly common among Iraqi Jews with thrombasthenia, who often display a characteristic 11 base pair deletion in exon 12 of integrin β3.

As observed with mutations in proteins composing the GpIb-IX-V complex, platelets from patients with thrombasthenia who have mutations that affect only one member of the αIIbβ3 complex contain smaller amounts of the other member as well. The reduction in cell surface expression of integrin αIIb or β3 often is markedly greater than the total platelet content of these proteins. These findings suggest that proper complex formation between the two integrin chains must occur in the endoplasmic reticulum for the intact complex to be properly processed and transported to the cell surface. Proper complex formation may depend on each protein's assuming a particular folding pattern, which depends on the ability of the protein to bind specific chaperone proteins.

A mutation instructive with respect to the mechanisms of fibrinogen receptor activation has been a single base pair substitution in the cytoplasmic domain of integrin β3. Platelets from this patient exhibited variant thrombasthenia in that they contained immunologically reactive αIIb and β3 chains but did not bind fibrinogen or aggregate after platelet activation. Expression of this mutated receptor in stable cell lines has confirmed the importance of the cytoplasmic domain of integrin β3 in mediating inside-out signaling and activating αIIbβ3 receptor. Additional rare patients with variant thrombasthenia caused by other mutations or deletions in αIIbβ3 have been described.

Prolonged bleeding time and decreased platelet aggregation also may occur in congenital afibrinogenemia. The aggregation defect is generally mild, in part because VWF can bind to integrin αIIbβ3 after platelet activation and support aggregation.

Platelet Activation Defects

This group of inherited disorders is characterized by diminished platelet aggregation and secretion in response to one or more agonists. Unlike αIIbβ3 in Glanzmann thrombasthenia and its variants, αIIbβ3 in these defects is quantitatively and qualitatively normal. Some clinical platelet activation defects can be subtle. Bleeding time may be normal or only slightly prolonged, and the bleeding history may be mild or intermittent. If these patients ingest aspirin, however, their bleeding times may become inordinately prolonged, and they may also bleed excessively after surgical procedures.

Activation defects often are referred to as aspirin-like and represent a number of poorly defined abnormalities in the metabolic pathways responsible for stimulus-response coupling. In theory, the functional defect can be caused by an abnormality

of agonist receptors, transducing elements (G proteins), enzymes, or intracellular second messengers necessary for optimal αIIbβ3 activation, cell aggregation, and secretion. In some families, specific deficiencies of or mutations in agonist receptors (e.g., thromboxane A_2 receptors) or enzymes (e.g., cyclooxygenase or thromboxane synthetase) have been found. Other patients have been described whose platelets were unable to elevate intracellular ionized calcium levels after exposure to thrombin. These defects were not caused by deficiencies of thromboxane production or insensitivity to inositol 1,4,5-triphosphate but were postulated to be caused by deficiency or dysfunction of phospholipase C. In type I glycogen storage disease, a platelet activation defect is presumed to be related to chronic hypoglycemia and a decrease in the amount of metabolic adenosine triphosphate (ATP) available to support cell activation.

Bartter's syndrome is a rare disorder associated with renal juxtaglomerular hyperplasia, hypokalemia, hypertension, and increased blood levels of renin, angiotensin II, and aldosterone. Patients do not have a great deal of bleeding, but they may have a slightly prolonged bleeding time and decreased platelet aggregation in response to ADP and epinephrine. The platelets are intrinsically normal, but activation appears to be partially inhibited by a plasma factor the identity and mechanism of action remain to be determined.

Storage Pool Diseases

Storage pool diseases are a heterogeneous group of disorders characterized by a decrease in the number or content of platelet storage granules. It is presumed that these disorders are caused by a defect in megakaryocyte granule formation or in the synthesis or uptake of substances by the granules. The associated bleeding diathesis may be minimal to moderate in severity. An isolated deficiency of dense granules (δ storage pool disease) and a combined deficiency of α granules and dense granules (αδ storage pool disease) are transmitted in an autosomal dominant manner. δ Storage pool disease also may be associated with other congenital anomalies, such as Hermansky–Pudlak syndrome (tyrosine-positive oculocutaneous albinism, ceroidlike pigment in macrophages, autosomal recessive inheritance); Chediak–Higashi syndrome (oculocutaneous albinism, abnormally large granules in many cell types, recurrent pyogenic infections, autosomal recessive inheritance); Wiscott–Aldrich syndrome (eczema, thrombocytopenia, recurrent infections, X-linked recessive inheritance); and TAR syndrome (thrombocytopenia and absent radii, either inherited or acquired in utero).

In δ or αδ storage pool diseases, hemostasis is impaired because the secretory response is inadequate, leading to formation of a smaller than normal platelet aggregate in the hemostatic plug. In vitro there is an absence of the second wave of platelet aggregation. This is largely caused by a reduction in the amount of ADP released from δ granules. The diagnosis is confirmed with detection of a reduction in the amount of platelet δ granule substances (ADP) or α granule substances (platelet factor 4, VWF, multimerin, or β-thromboglobulin). Pure α granule deficiency is a rare autosomal recessive trait associated with the presence of large platelets, mild thrombocytopenia, diminished second-wave platelet aggregation, and mild reticulin fibrosis in the marrow. It is called *gray platelet syndrome* because of the characteristic lack of blue granularity of the platelets on Romanovsky-stained blood smears. Although gray platelets are deficient in many α granule substances, they do appear to contain the membranes of α granules. The defect in intracellular membrane structure and function present in gray platelets appears to be specific for megakaryocytes, because the endothelial homologues of platelet α granules, Weibel–Palade bodies, are present in the endothelial cells of these patients in normal amounts and have a normal content of VWF and P-selectin. Isolated microsomes from platelets of patients with the gray platelet syndrome display abnormalities in ionized calcium transport, which may be associated with deficiencies in the phosphorylation of specific proteins that regulate this process.

Disorders of Platelet Procoagulant Activity

Only a few patients with a primary deficiency of platelet procoagulant activity have been described. This disorder has been called *Scott syndrome.* Because such an abnormality primarily affects formation of fibrin rather than of the platelet plug, bleeding time is normal. Persons with this disorder may have spontaneous intramuscular hematomas and episodic but severe bleeding after tooth extractions, surgical procedures, and parturition. Serum prothrombin time is used as a screening test. In this test, when the patient's blood is allowed to clot in a test tube, prothrombin is converted to thrombin inefficiently, leaving residual amounts of the prothrombin in the serum. As a result, a prothrombin time subsequently performed on the patient's serum is shorter than that of control serum. Pedigree analysis of a single family with this disorder suggests that Scott syndrome may be inherited in an autosomal recessive manner.

When studied in vitro, platelets from patients with Scott syndrome do not express a procoagulant surface after activation. This is the result of failure of exposure of acidic phospholipid on the surface of activated platelets and platelet-derived microvesicles. Normal amounts and activity of a phospholipid scramblase protein that accelerates transbilayer migration of phospholipid have been found in platelets, red blood cells, and lymphocytes from patients with Scott syndrome. Thus the pathogenesis of this disorder remains uncertain. Because platelet procoagulant activity is normally increased after platelet activation by thrombin or collagen, many other inherited and acquired disorders of platelet function may be associated with a secondary deficiency of platelet procoagulant activity.

ACQUIRED DISORDERS OF PLATELET FUNCTION

Drugs That Affect Platelet Function

Aspirin and Other Nonsteroidal Anti-inflammatory Drugs

Aspirin acetylates and irreversibly inhibits cyclooxygenase, the enzyme that converts arachidonic acid to prostaglandin endoperoxides. As a result, platelets cannot undergo a secretory response or second wave of aggregation in response to the presence of ADP and epinephrine. The cyclooxygenase in circulating plate-

lets is inhibited almost completely after ingestion of a single 300 to 600 mg dose of aspirin or after ingestion of only 30 mg of aspirin per day for several days. Because platelets circulate for 7 to 10 days, aspirin may affect platelet function for as long as a week after it is discontinued. Although aspirin usually prolongs the bleeding times of healthy persons to about twice baseline value, this change usually is of little clinical consequence. Among persons with other hemostatic defects, however, aspirin may drastically prolong bleeding time and exacerbate the bleeding diathesis. Nonsteroidal anti-inflammatory agents such as indomethacin, ibuprofen, and phenylbutazone inhibit cyclooxygenase reversibly. Unlike those of aspirin, the effects of these drugs subside once the drugs are eliminated from the circulation. Acetaminophen does not affect platelet function in conventional doses.

Ticlopidine and Clopidogrel

Other drugs that inhibit platelet aggregation include the thienopyridines ticlopidine and clopidogrel. The mechanism of action of these drugs, although incompletely understood, appears to involve inhibition of the binding of ADP to the low-affinity type 2 platelet purinergic receptor. As a result, the drugs inhibit ADP-induced platelet aggregation. Aggregation in response to other platelet agonists such as collagen, thromboxane, thrombin, and platelet-activating factor also is inhibited at submaximal agonist concentrations. These drugs prolong bleeding time in a dose- and time-dependent manner, generally to a greater extent than does aspirin. Maximal prolongation of the bleeding time takes 4 to 7 days, although some investigators have suggested that clinical responses may occur more rapidly. Bleeding times take as long as 10 days to normalize after discontinuation of ticlopidine or clopidogrel. This finding suggests that the effects of these agents on platelet aggregation are irreversible. Administration of these agents in combination with aspirin may cause synergistic inhibition of platelet aggregation.

Inhibition of platelet aggregation by ticlopidine is responsible for the ability of this agent to reduce the incidence of (a) recurrent stroke, transient ischemic attacks, or primary cerebrovascular events among patients with peripheral arterial atherosclerotic disease, (b) vascular death or myocardial infarction among patients with unstable angina or peripheral arterial atherosclerosis, (c) coronary and peripheral arterial stent thrombosis, and (d) saphenous vein graft occlusion after coronary artery bypass surgery. Although ticlopidine may be a marginally more effective inhibitor of in vivo platelet function than is aspirin, toxicity has limited its applicability. Ticlopidine is associated with a 1% incidence of severe neutropenia, a 0.02% incidence of thrombotic thrombocytopenic purpura, rare cases of aplastic anemia, and frequent dermatologic and gastrointestinal side effects. The results of the CAPRIE trial (Clopidogrel versus Aspirin in Patients at Risk of Ischaemic Events) suggest that clopidogrel may have similar efficacy as ticlopidine and have led to the recent U.S. Food and Drug Administration approval of this agent for secondary prevention of vascular events among patients with symptomatic atherosclerosis (recent ischemic stroke, myocardial infarction within 35 days, or documented peripheral arterial disease). To date use of clopidogrel has not been associated with an increased incidence of neutropenia, though rare cases of thrombotic thrombocytopenic purpura have been reported.

Integrin αIIbβ3 Inhibitors

A diverse family of drugs is emerging that directly inhibits platelet aggregation by means of interfering with the binding of fibrinogen to αIIbβ3. The prototype of this family is abciximab (ReoPro), a human–murine chimeric Fab fragment derived from a monoclonal antibody that inhibits fibrinogen binding to αIIbβ3 and inhibits platelet aggregation. Abciximab cross-reacts with a related integrin, $\alpha_v\beta_3$, which also is expressed at low levels in platelets and at higher levels in vascular smooth muscle and endothelial cells. In several studies, abciximab has significantly reduced the incidence of death, myocardial infarction, and the need for subsequent revascularization procedures among patients undergoing coronary angioplasty. A significant reduction in mortality was found after follow-up periods that exceeded 3 years among patients who received abciximab in the EPIC trial (Evaluation of 7E3 for the Prevention of Ischemic Complications) (Fig. 239.1). These observations confirm the role of platelet aggregation in the morbidity and mortality associated with angioplasty. Results of other studies suggest that abciximab may be a promising agent in therapy for acute stroke.

Eptifibatide (Integrilin) is a cyclic heptapeptide containing a Lys-Gly-Asp sequence based on that in the snake venom disintegrin barbourin. The sequence of eptifibatide resembles that of a region within the carboxy terminus of the fibrinogen γ chain that mediates binding of fibrinogen to αIIbβ3. Eptifibatide rapidly inhibits platelet aggregation and causes mild prolongation of bleeding time after infusion into humans. Tirofiban (Aggrastat) is a small-molecule peptidomimetic, the structure of which was designed to mimic that of the Arg-Gly-Asp sequence within fibrinogen, VWF, and other αIIbβ3 ligands. Tirofiban inhibits the binding of fibrinogen to αIIbβ3 and reversibly inhibits platelet aggregation. Eptifibatide and tirofiban markedly decrease the incidence of death, myocardial infarction, and the need for additional coronary intervention among patients with unstable angina or non-Q-wave myocardial infarction, effects that have persisted in follow-up periods of 6 months (Fig. 239.1). An orally available peptidomimetic αIIbβ3 antagonist, lamifiban, has shown promise in phase III clinical studies (Fig. 239.1), and other oral agents have entered earlier phases of development.

In early studies, parenteral αIIbβ3 inhibitors appeared to be responsible for a high incidence of bleeding complications. Results of subsequent studies showed that these complications were primarily attributable to excessive doses of heparin administered concurrently. The rate of bleeding complications decreased significantly in later trials of weight-adjusted heparin dosing. No increased incidence of intracerebral hemorrhage has been observed with these drugs, and emergency coronary artery bypass grafting has been performed without excessive bleeding complications. Thrombocytopenia develops among 0.5% to 1.0% of treated patients, possibly because of the exposure of ordinarily

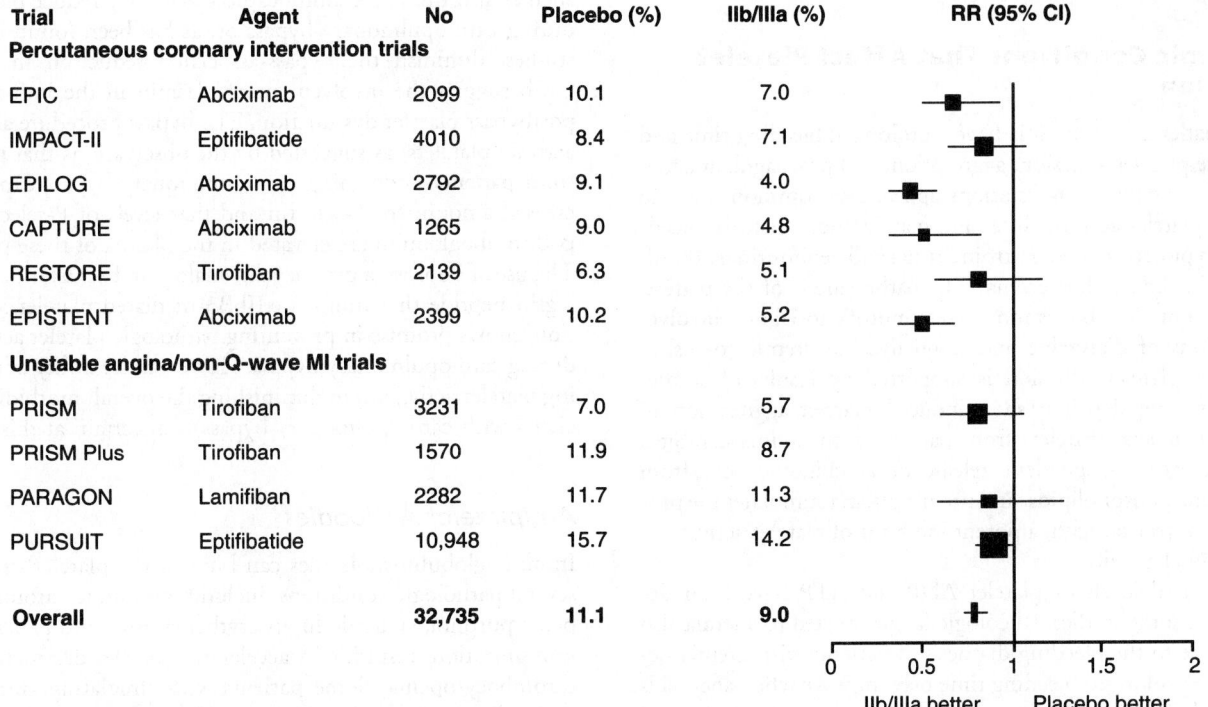

Trial	Agent	No	Placebo (%)	IIb/IIIa (%)	RR (95% CI)
Percutaneous coronary intervention trials					
EPIC	Abciximab	2099	10.1	7.0	
IMPACT-II	Eptifibatide	4010	8.4	7.1	
EPILOG	Abciximab	2792	9.1	4.0	
CAPTURE	Abciximab	1265	9.0	4.8	
RESTORE	Tirofiban	2139	6.3	5.1	
EPISTENT	Abciximab	2399	10.2	5.2	
Unstable angina/non-Q-wave MI trials					
PRISM	Tirofiban	3231	7.0	5.7	
PRISM Plus	Tirofiban	1570	11.9	8.7	
PARAGON	Lamifiban	2282	11.7	11.3	
PURSUIT	Eptifibatide	10,948	15.7	14.2	
Overall		32,735	11.1	9.0	

IIb/IIIa better   Placebo better

FIGURE 239.1. Death or nonfatal myocardial infarction outcomes at 30 days in 10 randomized, placebo-controlled trials of glycoprotein (Gp) IIb/IIIa blockers. Risk ratio (RR) with 95% confidence interval (CI), size of RR box being proportional to total sample size. Frequency of death of nonfatal myocardial infarction in columns 4 and 5. Overall (all 10 trials) benefit of GpIIb-IIIa blockade is highly significant (RR = 0.79; 95% CI, 0.73 to 0.85; $p < 10^9$). (From Topol EJ, Byzova TV, Plow EF. Platelet GpIIb-IIIa blockers. *Lancet* 1999;353:227–231, with permission.)

cryptic epitopes on αIIbβ3 after binding of the drug. The safety of long-term αIIbβ3 inhibition has not yet been fully assessed.

Miscellaneous Drugs

Many drugs can affect platelet function in vitro, although relatively few prolong bleeding time. Large doses of carbenicillin, other penicillins, and the cephalosporin moxalactam prolong bleeding time and affect platelet aggregation in a dose-dependent way. This effect begins within hours of drug administration and may last for several days after the drug is discontinued. Severe bleeding caused solely by this effect is uncommon, however. In vitro, high concentrations of penicillins impair the interaction of agonists with the platelet surface membrane, but the mechanism of the effects in vivo is not clear. Bleeding time also may be prolonged among some persons receiving conventional doses of heparin, presumably because this drug reduces the component of platelet activation normally mediated by thrombin. Dextran and large doses of the plasma expander hydroxyethyl starch may prolong bleeding time among some patients, but bleeding is uncommon unless other hemostatic defects are present. Fibrinolytic agents, such as streptokinase or tissue plasminogen activator, may affect platelets by stimulating the production of plasmin. Under some conditions in vitro, plasmin may impair platelet function by causing an increase in fibrin degradation products and by cleaving platelet GpIb and αIIbβ3, although the contribution of platelet dysfunction to the efficacy or the hemorrhagic side effects of fibrinolytic therapy has not been determined.

Systemic Conditions That Affect Platelet Function

Many patients with uremia have a prolonged bleeding time and defective platelet adhesion, aggregation, and procoagulant activity. Hemorrhagic manifestations appear less common than do in vitro platelet abnormalities and may include epistaxis, bleeding from puncture sites, gastrointestinal and genitourinary bleeding, and subdural hematoma. The pathogenesis of the platelet defect is not clear but is most likely multifactorial and involves the actions of dialyzable and nondialyzable uremic toxins. A defect in platelet adhesion is supported by results of studies demonstrating deficient shear-induced platelet aggregation of uremic platelets. Platelets from patients with uremia exhibit a reduced agonist-dependent release of arachidonic acid from membrane phospholipids, and uremic plasma stimulates the production of prostacyclin, a potent inhibitor of platelet activation, by endothelial cells.

Decreased levels of platelet ADP and ATP have been described in some studies. Rheologic factors related to anemia also contribute to the bleeding diathesis of patients with uremia because the prolonged bleeding time may improve when anemia is corrected. The plasma of patients with uremia contains elevated levels of L-arginine, the precursor of the potent vasodilator and inhibitor of platelet adhesion and aggregation, nitric oxide (NO). Uremic platelets generate more NO and contain higher levels of cyclic guanosine monophosphate (GMP), a second messenger of NO, than do control platelets, and uremic plasma stimulates the production of NO from cultured endothelial cells. The potential role of NO in uremia-induced platelet dysfunction is supported by the observation that the bleeding time of uremic rats normalizes after treatment with N-monomethyl-L-arginine, a potent inhibitor of NO synthesis. In addition to platelet dysfunction, factors such as uremic serositis or heparin anticoagulation during dialysis may be a predisposing factor for bleeding among patients with renal disease. The prolonged bleeding time and bleeding diathesis associated with uremia often improve with dialysis.

Cardiopulmonary Bypass

A prolonged bleeding time develops among almost all patients during cardiopulmonary bypass but usually reverses within 4 hours of the procedure. For some patients, the prolonged bleeding time may persist and be associated with substantial postoperative bleeding. The platelet defect in these patients is multifactorial and not adequately explained by the moderate thrombocytopenia that frequently occurs or the heparin administered during the procedure. Results of some studies suggest that during cardiopulmonary bypass, a percentage of both GpIb and αIIbβ3 may be lost from the platelet surface. The potential mechanisms accounting for this loss are uncertain and may reflect the effects of either mechanical trauma from turbulence and shear stress within the extracorporeal oxygenator or those of proteolytic enzymes, such as plasmin, activated during the bypass procedure. With respect to the latter, observations that protease inhibitors such as aprotinin or ε-aminocaproic acid may reduce blood loss during cardiopulmonary bypass or, as has been found in some studies, diminish the bypass-associated reduction in platelet GpIb suggest the involvement of plasmin in the induction of postbypass platelet dysfunction. The bypass procedure also may activate platelets, as suggested by the observations that platelets from patients undergoing cardiopulmonary bypass express increased amounts of P-selectin and that levels of P-selectin and β-thromboglobulin are elevated in the plasma of these patients. The use of iloprost, a prostacyclin analog, and echistatin, a disintegrin peptide that inhibits αIIbβ3-mediated platelet aggregation, shows promise in preventing pathologic platelet activation during cardiopulmonary bypass. However, the utility of inhibiting platelet activation in diminishing the overall morbidity associated with cardiopulmonary bypass is uncertain at this time.

Antiplatelet Antibodies

Immunoglobulin molecules can bind to the platelet surface in several pathologic conditions, including immune thrombocytopenic purpura, systemic lupus erythematosus, and platelet alloimmunization, resulting in accelerated platelet destruction and thrombocytopenia. Some patients with circulating antiplatelet antibodies also may have impaired platelet aggregation and a prolonged bleeding time, even when thrombocytopenia is modest or absent. In a few cases, the IgG purified from the patient's plasma or eluted from the platelets inhibited aggregation of normal platelets. Abnormal aggregation may be related to an acquired form of storage pool disease caused by antibody-mediated platelet activation and secretion occurring in vivo. In one report, platelets in immune thrombocytopenic purpura exhibited an activation defect manifested by diminished conversion of arachidonic acid to thromboxane A_2. Results of experiments with an ex vivo perfusion system have indicated that some antiplatelet antibodies also may inhibit adhesion of platelets to the subendothelial matrix. Several patients have been described who had autoantibodies with specificity for GpIb-IX-V or αIIbβ3 or that caused an acquired form of Bernard–Soulier syndrome or thrombasthenia

After repeated platelet transfusions, alloantibodies to GpIb or αIIbβ3 develop in some patients with the inherited forms of Bernard–Soulier syndrome or Glanzmann thrombasthenia, respectively. Such antibodies may limit the efficacy of subsequent transfusions by reducing the function or survival of donor platelets. In one case of a woman with Bernard–Soulier syndrome, an alloantibody with specificity for the GpIb-IX complex was able to cross the placenta during pregnancy and cause neonatal alloimmune thrombocytopenia.

Disseminated Intravascular Coagulation

Diminished platelet aggregation is but one of several hemostatic defects in disseminated intravascular coagulation (DIC) and may be caused by a combination of severe fibrinogen depletion and inhibition of fibrinogen binding by high concentrations of fibrin degradation products. The hemorrhagic diathesis in this disorder usually is dominated by abnormalities in coagulation and fibrinolytic proteins, as well as thrombocytopenia, rather than platelet dysfunction per se.

Hematologic Diseases That Affect Platelet Function

Acute Myelogenous Leukemia, Myelodysplastic Syndromes, and Chronic Myeloproliferative Disorders

Platelet dysfunction occurs among some patients with acute myelogenous leukemia, myelodysplastic syndromes, and chronic myeloproliferative disorders, particularly essential thrombocythemia, myelofibrosis with myeloid metaplasia, and polycythemia vera. A number of intracellular and membrane defects have been reported that are presumed to be caused by platelets arising from a neoplastic clone. The pattern of abnormality varies from patient to patient, however, and none of the functional defects is a reliable predictor of hemorrhage. In rare instances acquired forms of von Willebrand disease or Bernard–Soulier syndrome have occurred. In most of these disorders, thrombocytopenia usually is a more important cause of bleeding than is platelet dysfunction. An exception is essential thrombocythemia, in which bleeding may occur in association with an elevated platelet count (>400,000 per milliliter), even in the presence of a normal bleeding time. Patients with essential thrombocythemia also may have digital ischemia (erythromelalgia) or other vascular ischemic syndromes caused by microvascular platelet occlusion.

Bleeding and thrombotic complications may improve when the platelet count is lowered by means of plateletpheresis or

chemotherapy. Aspirin may be useful in the management of digital ischemia but should be avoided in the care of bleeding patients or those with active peptic ulcer disease. Results of some studies suggest that low doses of aspirin (75 to 100 mg per day) may be as effective as larger doses in reducing thrombotic complications and are accompanied by a lower incidence of bleeding. Essential thrombocythemia must be differentiated from secondary thrombocytosis, because elevated platelet counts in the latter are not associated with platelet dysfunction. Secondary thrombocytosis may occur in several settings, including hemolysis, iron deficiency anemia, aftermath of splenectomy, carcinoma, chronic inflammatory disorders, and transient rebound thrombocytosis after marrow suppression. The presence of other features of a myeloproliferative syndrome in essential thrombocythemia can be helpful in the differential diagnosis. These include splenomegaly, leukocytosis, and histologic features of bone marrow that demonstrate reticulin fibrosis and large clusters of megakaryocytes. When these clues are not present, documentation of decreased platelet aggregation in response to agonists such as epinephrine support a diagnosis of essential thrombocythemia.

Multiple Myeloma and Other B-cell Neoplasms

Prolonged bleeding time occurs among some patients with plasma cell neoplasms, such as multiple myeloma and Waldenstrom's macroglobulinemia. Platelet dysfunction may cause serious bleeding for some patients with these disorders. In these situations, the paraprotein appears to be responsible. Although a direct effect on one or more membrane proteins is suspected, the mechanism has not been characterized in most patients. As do rare patients with autoimmune thrombocytopenia, some patients with multiple myeloma may have acquired thrombasthenia caused by to a paraprotein that specifically reacts with αIIbβ3 and inhibits fibrinogen binding. Acquired von Willebrand disease has been reported among a small number of patients with multiple myeloma and other B-cell neoplasms. Rare patients with monoclonal antithrombin antibodies also have been described.

Bleeding among patients with monoclonal gammopath, particularly those with Waldenstrom's macroglobulinemia and IgM paraproteins, is more often a manifestation of the hyperviscosity syndrome than of platelet dysfunction per se. In either case, bleeding resolves after reduction of the paraprotein through plasmapheresis or chemotherapy.

THERAPY FOR PLATELET FUNCTION DISORDERS

GENERAL PRINCIPLES

Once the diagnosis of platelet dysfunction is made and the underlying defect established, an appropriate therapeutic strategy must be formulated to deal with a bleeding episode or to prevent hemostatic failure during surgery. Treatment must be individualized on the basis of variables such as the severity of the underlying platelet defect, the degree of stress that will be placed on the hemostatic system, and the efficacy and risks of a particular form of treatment. The physician must educate the patient to avoid aspirin and other platelet-inhibiting drugs, particularly before surgery.

Although the bleeding time is a useful test for evaluating patients for disorders of platelet function, it is affected by a number of technical variables that influence its sensitivity. Studies have shown that bleeding time is not clinically useful in finding individuals in unselected populations who are at greatest risk for surgical bleeding. Although a normal bleeding time, properly measured, gives reasonable assurance that the patient's ability to form a platelet plug is clinically sufficient, the significance of a prolonged bleeding time is far less certain and depends on whether the patient has a history that suggests a bleeding disorder. It is reasonable to use bleeding time as an indicator of the effect of therapy on patients with an inherited platelet function defect or to evaluate patients with a history of bleeding who may have a congenital or acquired disorder of platelet dysfunction. Results of studies suggest that automated platelet analyzers such as the PFA-100 device may have equal and perhaps better sensitivity and specificity than bleeding time for the detection of clinically significant platelet dysfunction. However, the utility of this technology awaits additional testing in expanded clinical settings.

Many defects of platelet function are mild, and clinical judgment must be brought to bear on therapeutic decisions. For example, when a patient with a clinically mild platelet defect is to undergo a minor surgical procedure or when meticulous hemostasis can be obtained with local measures, attempts to normalize bleeding time with platelet transfusions or other potentially toxic therapy are unwarranted.

MANAGEMENT OF THE UNDERLYING DISEASE

The most rational therapeutic approach to platelet dysfunction is to treat the patient for the underlying disease. The platelet dysfunction associated with systemic lupus erythematosus, lymphoma, plasma cell neoplasia, DIC, myeloproliferative disorders, or the presence of antiplatelet antibodies usually improves with successful therapy for the underlying disorder. Potentially life-threatening bleeding associated with multiple myeloma can be controlled successfully with plasmapheresis to remove the offending paraprotein. Acute episodes of bleeding in essential thrombocythemia may respond to plateletpheresis and pharmacologic suppression of platelet production. In afibrinogenemia or von Willebrand disease, replacement therapy with cryoprecipitate or factor VIII preparations rich in multimeric VWF may be warranted. Management of von Willebrand disease is discussed in Chapter 237.

In uremia, a prolonged bleeding time per se is not an indication for treatment. If the patient has clinically significant bleeding, intensive dialysis may be useful. Desmopressin (DDAVP) has been reported to shorten bleeding time for 50% to 75% of patients. Some of these patients have subsequently undergone surgical procedures without undue hemorrhage, although no results of controlled trials of this therapy have been reported. The drug has been well tolerated in a dose of 0.3 μg per kilogram

given intravenously over 15 to 30 minutes and has been successfully administered through the subcutaneous and intranasal routes, although absorption may be erratic with intranasal administration. Facial flushing, mild tachycardia, water retention, and hyponatremia are potential side effects. Caution in the use of this drug in the care of elderly patients with symptomatic atherosclerotic cardiovascular disease is warranted. The drug has been reported to precipitate myocardial ischemic episodes. The efficacy of desmopressin in therapy for uremia may reflect its ability to induce the release of VWF and factor VIII from tissue stores; however, it is unlikely that this is the only mechanism involved since levels of these proteins in patients with uremia are generally normal or elevated. The shortening of the bleeding time induced by desmopressin generally lasts for several hours after the infusion, and the drug has sometimes been administered repeatedly at 12- to 24-hour intervals, although tachyphylaxis may develop after several doses. Furthermore, because desmopressin is not efficacious for all patients, a therapeutic trial before surgery is indicated.

An additional treatment that may shorten bleeding time among adult patients with uremia who are undergoing dialysis is conjugated estrogens (0.6 mg per kilogram per day for 5 days intravenously or 50 mg per day by mouth). Although the mechanism of action of these agents is obscure, bleeding time may improve after the first dose, and the effect may persist for several days. The bleeding times of many patients with uremia also may improve after the hematocrit rises to greater than 30% with administration of red blood cell transfusions or recombinant erythropoietin. This improvement may reflect rheologic effects, although elevation in the hematocrit also has been reported to enhance platelet adhesion in δ storage pool disease, perhaps because of shear-induced release of red cell ADP.

ADJUNCTIVE THERAPIES

Platelet transfusion is indicated for severe bleeding due to intrinsic platelet defects such as Glanzmann thrombasthenia, Bernard–Soulier syndrome, storage pool disease, and cardiopulmonary bypass. The increased use of platelet function inhibitors, particularly αIIbβ3 blockers, in the care of patients with cardiovascular disease will likely lead to increased bleeding among some patients. Because specific antagonists of these agents are not available, treatment of such persons once alternative causes of bleeding are excluded should include platelet transfusion. The number of transfused platelets needed to secure hemostasis must be determined empirically and depends variables such as the patient's blood volume, the severity of the underlying defect, the functional integrity and life span of the donor platelets, and the presence of alloantibodies. Because of the inherent dangers associated with blood transfusion and the development of refractoriness after multiple transfusions, platelet transfusions should be reserved for situations in which they are clearly indicated.

In a number of uncontrolled and placebo-controlled studies, use of desmopressin successfully shortened the bleeding time for at least one-half of patients with inherited or acquired disorders of platelet function, including storage pool disease, platelet activation defects, and aspirin ingestion. The drug has not been efficacious in the treatment of patients with Glanzmann thrombasthenia, although bleeding time is shortened transiently among some patients with Bernard–Soulier syndrome. The mechanisms by which these effects are mediated are not clearly defined, and additional experience is needed to determine the precise mechanisms of action and overall efficacy of desmopressin to manage bleeding among patients with platelet function disorders. Prednisone, 20 to 50 mg per day for 3 days, has been reported to improve bleeding time among some patients with platelet activation defects. The mechanism is equally obscure.

Women with menorrhagia associated with defects of platelet function may benefit from hormonal therapy. Local hemostatic agents, such as topical thrombin, adsorbable collagen hemostat, or mouth rinses with tranexamic acid may alleviate bleeding during dental extractions. Prophylactic oral administration of antifibrinolytic agents such as ∈-aminocaproic acid or tranexamic acid may be useful in the treatment of patients with von Willebrand disease or hemophilia who are undergoing dental extractions. These agents may precipitate thrombosis among patients with DIC and should not be used in their care.

BIBLIOGRAPHY

George JN, Caen JP, Nurden AT. Glanzmann's thrombasthenia: the spectrum of clinical disease. *Blood* 1990;75:1383–1395.

George JN, Shattil SJ. The clinical importance of acquired disorders of platelet dysfunction. *N Engl J Med* 1991;324:27–39.

López JA, Andrews RK, Afshar-Kharghan V, et al. Bernard–Soulier syndrome. *Blood* 1998;91:4397–4418.

Mannucci PM. Desmopressin (DDAVP) in the treatment of bleeding disorders: the first 20 years. *Blood* 1997;90:2515–2521.

Rao AK. Congenital disorders of platelet function: disorders of signal transduction and secretion. *Am J Med Sci* 1998;316:69–76.

Rodgers RPC, Levin J. A critical reappraisal of the bleeding time. *Semin Thromb Hemost* 1990;16:1–20.

Santoso S, Kunicki TJ, Kroll H, et al. Association of the platelet glycoprotein Ia C807T gene polymorphism with nonfatal myocardial infarction in younger patients. *Blood* 1999;93:2449–2453.

Sharis PJ, Cannon CP, Loscalzo J. The antiplatelet effects of ticlopidine and clopidogrel. *Ann Intern Med* 1998;129:394–405.

Shattil, SJ, Kashiwagi H, Pampori N. Integrin signaling: the platelet paradigm. *Blood* 1998;91:2645–2657.

Topol EJ, Byzova TV, Plow EF. Platelet GpIIb-IIIa blockers. *Lancet* 1999;353:227–231.

Weigert AL, Schafer AI. Uremic bleeding: pathogenesis and therapy. *Am J Med Sci* 1998;316:94–104.

Kelley's Textbook of Internal Medicine, fourth edition. Edited by H. David Humes. Lippincott Williams & Wilkins, Philadelphia © 2000.

CHAPTER

240

THROMBOTIC DISORDERS

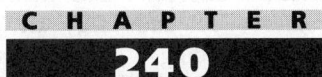

JOEL S. BENNETT

DEFINITION

Thrombotic disorders, the most common causes of morbidity and mortality in Western civilization, result from the formation of fibrin or platelet thrombi. Thrombi form when the normal hemostatic balance that maintains the fluidity of blood shifts to favor their formation. The composition of thrombi reflects the nature of the blood flow conditions in which they form. Under the high shear conditions found on the arterial side of the circulation, thrombi are composed primarily of platelets (white thrombi). Under the low shear conditions found in the venous circulation, thrombi are composed primarily of fibrin and entrapped erythrocytes (red thrombi).

INCIDENCE AND EPIDEMIOLOGY

Arterial thrombosis is most often a complication of atherosclerotic vascular disease and, as such, the most common cause of death in the United States. Coronary artery thrombosis results in approximately 800,000 new and 450,000 recurrent myocardial infarctions per year and resulted in 498,000 deaths in 1989. The prevalence of cerebrovascular disease in 1989 was 10 per 1,000 population, leading to 147,000 deaths. Venous thromboembolism affects 1 per 1,000 people annually. Pulmonary embolism is the most serious complication of this disorder, but because the diagnosis of pulmonary embolism may be difficult to establish and its occurrence frequently is overlooked, accurate data regarding its incidence are difficult to obtain. It has been estimated that there are 50,000 deaths from pulmonary embolism annually. Moreover, because only 10% of episodes of pulmonary embolism are fatal, the annual incidence of pulmonary embolism is probably close to 500,000. Evidence of pulmonary embolism is found in 25% to 30% of routine autopsies, which suggests that even this figure is an underestimate. Pulmonary embolism is also a major cause of postpartum and postoperative deaths. It accounts for 4,000 to 8,000 such deaths annually and in 1 to 2 deaths per 1,000 patients over age 40 undergoing major surgery.

ETIOLOGY

Thrombotic disorders are the result of inherited disorders of the hemostatic system (Table 240.1) or stem from other disorders

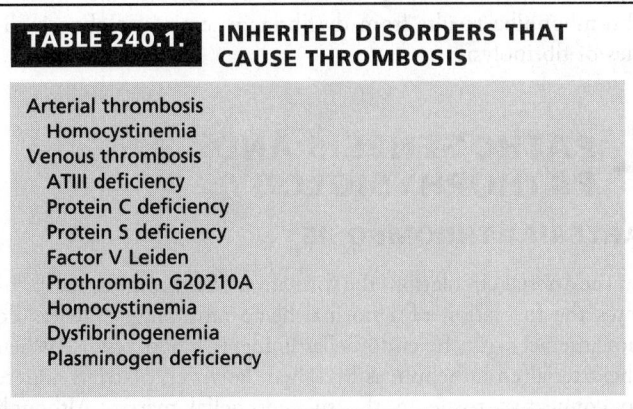

TABLE 240.1.	INHERITED DISORDERS THAT CAUSE THROMBOSIS

Arterial thrombosis
  Homocystinemia
Venous thrombosis
  ATIII deficiency
  Protein C deficiency
  Protein S deficiency
  Factor V Leiden
  Prothrombin G20210A
  Homocystinemia
  Dysfibrinogenemia
  Plasminogen deficiency

TABLE 240.2.	ACQUIRED DISORDERS THAT CAUSE THROMBOSIS

Arterial thrombosis
  Atherosclerosis
  Antiphospholipid antibody syndrome
  Myeloproliferative disorders
  Arteritis
  Thrombotic thrombocytopenic purpura
  Heparin-induced thrombocytopenia
Venous thrombosis
  Malignant disease
  Immobilization during medical and surgical illness
  Pregnancy
  Oral contraceptive and estrogen use
  Nephrotic syndrome
  Antiphospholipid antibody syndrome
  Paroxysmal nocturnal hemoglobinuria

(Table 240.2). Although arterial thrombosis most often derives from atherosclerosis, it also can be a complication of homozygous and heterozygous homocystinemia, arteritis, myeloproliferative disorders, thrombotic thrombocytopenic purpura (TTP), heparin-induced thrombocytopenia (HIT), and the antiphospholipid antibody syndrome.

The predilection to venous thrombosis is termed *thrombophilia* and occurs most often in patients with malignancy, in immobilized medical and surgical patients, in women who are pregnant or taking oral contraceptives, and in patients with the nephrotic syndrome, the antiphospholipid antibody syndrome, and paroxysmal nocturnal hemoglobinuria. In many patients, especially those who experience venous thrombosis at a young age, thrombophilia may be familial in origin. In 5% to 10% of these patients, there are abnormalities in proteins that control coagulation, including deficiencies of antithrombin (AT), protein C (PC), or protein S (PS). Approximately 40% of patients with venous thrombosis, 50% to 60% of patients with a family history of venous thrombosis, and 2% to 5% of normal individuals are resistant to the anticoagulant effect of activated PC (APC), most often owing to a polymorphism of the factor V (FV) molecule termed *factor V Leiden*. A relatively common genetic variation in the 3′ untranslated region of the prothrombin gene, prothrombin G20210A, is also associated with a moderate risk of venous thrombosis, as is an increased plasma concentration of the sulfur-containing amino acid homocysteine. Rarely, thrombophilia results from dysfibrinogenemia and abnormalities of fibrinolysis.

PATHOGENESIS AND PATHOPHYSIOLOGY

ARTERIAL THROMBOSIS

In the arterial circulation, the formation of a thrombus recapitulates the formation of a normal hemostatic plug. Platelets do not interact with the endothelial lining of blood vessels. When the arterial endothelium is breached, however, platelets adhere to connective tissue in the subendothelial matrix. Although platelets can adhere to collagen, fibronectin, and laminin in the matrix when the shear stress is high, adherence requires the presence of von Willebrand factor. Concurrently, platelets in the vicinity of the wound are stimulated by agonists, such as thrombin and ADP. This results in the binding of fibrinogen or von Willebrand factor to glycoprotein IIb/IIIa (GpIIb-IIIa) complexes on the surface of these platelets. The GpIIb-IIIa-bound protein then cross-links these platelets into aggregates that bind to the layer of adherent platelets, forming a hemostatic plug or an occlusive thrombus. Stimulated platelets also secrete ADP stored in their dense granules to amplify the aggregation process and convert arachidonic acid released from membrane phospholipid to thromboxane A_2, a potent platelet agonist and vasoconstrictor.

Platelet thrombi form on the surface of atherosclerotic plaques when there is extensive endothelial cell denudation. More often, thrombi result from disruption of the plaque and exposure of blood to highly thrombogenic material in the plaque interior. Plaque disruption occurs most often at the junction of the fibrous cap of the plaque and normal intima. This permits blood to enter the lipid pool in the plaque interior and leads to the formation of a platelet-rich thrombus. An extension of the thrombus composed of densely packed fibrin may reenter the vessel lumen and partially or totally occlude the flow of blood. A partially occlusive thrombus can embolize to produce vascular occlusion downstream or organize to increase arterial narrowing. An occlusive thrombus produces tissue infarction unless adequate collateral blood flow has developed.

Many patients homozygous for cystathionine β-synthase (CBS) deficiency die of vascular disease before the age of 30. The basis for their predisposition to premature atherosclerosis and arterial thrombosis is unknown. Approximately one-third of some cohorts of patients with premature atherosclerosis also have lesser degrees of hyperhomocystinemia after methionine loading, suggesting that hyperhomocystinemia is an independent risk factor for vascular disease. Arteritis due to collagenvascular diseases, such as systemic lupus erythematosus (SLE), can produce widespread recurrent arterial thrombi. The arterial and venous thromboses associated with the myeloproliferative disease polycythemia vera result from the increased blood viscosity and thrombocytosis that accompany this disease. Arterial and venous thromboses are also a feature of essential thrombocythemia and result from the increased number of abnormal platelets that characterize this disorder. Paradoxically, two thrombocytopenic syndromes (TTP and HIT) are associated with thrombosis rather than bleeding. TTP is characterized by widespread arteriolar platelet thrombi that cause evanescent symptoms of ischemia. Arterial and, occasionally, venous thrombosis develops in a minority of patients with HIT and can lead to stroke, myocardial infarction, or the need for amputation of an extremity. The antiphospholipid antibody syndrome is associated with both arterial and venous thrombosis and is discussed in the next section.

VENOUS THROMBOSIS

Venous thrombi are composed primarily of fibrin and entrapped erythrocytes and result from a series of biochemical reactions that begin with the exposure of tissue factor in a damaged vessel and lead to the sequential activation of coagulation factor X (FXa), cleavage of prothrombin by FXa to liberate thrombin, and cleavage of fibrinogen by thrombin to produce fibrin monomers. Fibrin monomers spontaneously polymerize into strands of fibrin that are irreversibly cross-linked by thrombin-activated factor XIII to produce an insoluble clot. Fibrin clots eventually are removed by the enzyme plasmin or organized by connective tissue. Because thrombin is directly responsible for the conversion of fibrinogen to fibrin, its generation from prothrombin and its activity in plasma are carefully regulated. The predominant inhibitor of thrombin and FXa activity in plasma is AT, the protein that mediates the anticoagulant effect of heparin and a member of the serpin family of protease inhibitors.

Two other proteins that limit the generation of thrombin from prothrombin are present in plasma. The production of sufficient FXa by activated factor IX (FIXa) to cleave prothrombin at a physiologically relevant rate and the cleavage of prothrombin itself require activated factor VIII (FVIIIa) and activated factor V (FVa), respectively. A complex formed by APC and PS acts as a brake on thrombin production by enzymatically cleaving both FVIIIa and FVa. Sensitive assays have shown that small amounts of FXa and thrombin are generated continuously in normal individuals, but their activities are controlled by AT and the APC-PS complex to prevent the formation of fibrin thrombi. Consequently, thrombosis can occur either when the production of FXa and thrombin is enhanced or when the activity of the control proteins is diminished.

Antithrombin Deficiency

AT irreversibly inhibits thrombin and FXa (as well as FIXa and factors XI and XII) by forming a covalent complex at the active site of each coagulation factor. Heparin binds to AT and accelerates its function approximately 1,000-fold by inducing a conformational change in the molecule. Abnormalities of AT are inherited in an autosomal dominant fashion and have been detected in about 5% of individuals with venous thrombosis who are less than 45 years old. There are two types of inherited AT deficiency. Type I deficiency is characterized by an equivalent decrease in the concentration and activity of AT in plasma, indicating reduced protein synthesis from one or both AT genes. In type II deficiency, however, AT activity is reduced out of proportion to its plasma concentration, reflecting synthesis of a defective protein. Although thrombosis due to AT deficiency affects one in 2,000 to 5,000 individuals, the prevalence of AT deficiency in the general population approaches 0.2% to 0.4%. Thus, additional factors appear to be required to induce thrombophilia in AT-deficient individuals.

The AT activity in the plasma of individuals heterozygous for AT deficiency is generally 50% of normal. The incidence of venous thrombosis in these individuals is about 50%. Thrombosis develops spontaneously in half of these individuals and is associated with other predisposing factors in the remainder. In two-thirds of patients, thrombosis is recurrent and is associated with pulmonary embolism in 40%. There is a single case report of two homozygous neonates with type I deficiency, suggesting that homozygous type I deficiency is incompatible with survival

beyond the neonatal period. The predisposition to thrombosis in patients with type II deficiency varies with the type of AT mutation. Mutations involving the protease binding site predispose to thrombosis, whereas mutations affecting the heparin binding sites, at least in heterozygous individuals, do not. However, individuals who are homozygous for the latter mutations have thrombophilia.

AT deficiency can be acquired. The concentration of AT occasionally declines after acute thrombosis but frequently decreases during the course of disseminated intravascular coagulation (DIC). Diminished AT concentrations also can result from liver disease because of decreased synthesis, from the nephrotic syndrome because of urinary loss, and with the use of oral contraceptives or other estrogen-containing drugs. The concentration of AT does not change substantially during pregnancy.

Protein C Deficiency

PC is a vitamin K–dependent zymogen that is converted to an active enzyme by thrombin bound to the endothelial cell membrane protein thrombomodulin (TM). When thrombin is generated from prothrombin, a portion of it binds to TM. Thrombin bound to TM is no longer able to cleave fibrinogen but converts PC to APC. APC, in turn, forms a complex with PS and intact FV to suppress further thrombin generation by inactivating FVIIIa and FVa. Thus, PC-deficient individuals are prone to thrombosis because they are unable to suppress thrombin generation adequately. PC deficiency is inherited as an autosomal dominant disorder, and heterozygotes with 50% levels of PC are at risk for thrombosis. Heterozygous individuals are usually asymptomatic until the third decade of life, when they begin to experience thrombosis, most often involving the veins in the legs. There is also a reported association between thrombotic stroke in young adults and PC deficiency.

Although heterozygous PC deficiency has a prevalence of one in 200, penetrance of the disorder varies. While up to 75% of individuals in some affected families have experienced thrombosis, members of other affected families are asymptomatic. Obligate heterozygous family members of infants with homozygous PC deficiency and purpura fulminans also have been asymptomatic. Like AT deficiency, additional factors may be required to induce thrombophilia in PC-deficient kindreds. Two types of PC mutations have been described. The more common type I mutation leads to a decline in PC synthesis, whereas type II mutations result in the synthesis of a functionally defective protein. Homozygous or doubly heterozygous PC deficiency with PC concentrations of less than 1% has been described in newborns and results in fatal purpura fulminans unless PC replacement is promptly initiated.

Acquired PC deficiency develops in the context of liver disease because of decreased synthesis. DIC and the adult respiratory distress syndrome result in PC deficiency by increasing consumption. Vitamin K antagonists, such as warfarin, lower the concentration of functional PC in plasma by inhibiting its γ-carboxylation in the liver. The administration of warfarin to patients heterozygous for PC deficiency has been associated infrequently with the development of skin necrosis. This occurs because the half-life of PC, like that of factor VII (FVII), is short (about 6 to 12 hours), while the half-life of the other vitamin K–dependent clotting factors is considerably longer. Thus, the administration of warfarin, especially in high loading doses, produces a transient hypercoagulable state, an effect exaggerated in individuals who are PC deficient.

Protein S Deficiency

PS is a vitamin K–dependent cofactor for the APC-mediated cleavage of FVIIIa and FVa. Normally, 60% of the PS in plasma is bound to C4b-binding protein (C4bBP). Because the unbound fraction is the cofactor for APC, PS measurements must differentiate between free and C4bBP-bound PS. C4bBP is an acute-phase reactant; changes in its concentration alter the concentration of free PS. Hereditary deficiency of PS predisposes to thrombosis and is inherited in an autosomal dominant fashion with an estimated prevalence of one in 20,000. The clinical manifestations of heterozygous PS deficiency are similar to those of PC deficiency, including an association with arterial thrombosis in young individuals. The total PS concentration of heterozygotes is approximately 50% of normal (type I), but deficiency states have been described in which the total PS concentration is normal while the free fraction is diminished (type II). Type III PS deficiency is due to the synthesis of a dysfunctional protein. Severe homozygous PS deficiency can result in neonatal purpura fulminans.

Acquired PS deficiency results from liver disease, DIC, pregnancy, and oral contraceptive use. The reduced concentrations of free PS that arise after acute thromboembolic disease, in part due to increases in C4bBP, make a diagnosis of PS deficiency difficult to establish at this stage of the disease. The concentration of functional PS declines with warfarin therapy, with a half-life of about 42 hours. Nevertheless, a case of warfarin-induced skin necrosis in a PS-deficient patient has been reported.

Factor V Leiden

Approximately 40% of patients with venous thromboembolism who are not AT, PC, or PS deficient are resistant to the ability of purified APC to prolong the activated partial thromboplastin time (aPTT). In thrombophilic families, the prevalence of this abnormality can reach 50% to 60%. In more than 90% of cases, APC resistance is due to an Arg506→Gln polymorphism in the FV molecule (FV Leiden). Because Arg506 is one of the APC cleavage sites in FV, FV Leiden is less sensitive than normal FV to inactivation by APC. The thrombophilia in families with FV Leiden is inherited as an autosomal dominant disorder: 30% of the heterozygotes and 44% of the homozygotes in these families have experienced one or more thromboembolic episodes. Looked at another way, heterozygosity for FV Leiden increases the risk of venous thrombosis five- to tenfold, while homozygosity raises this risk by a factor of 50 to 100. Furthermore, the relative risk of venous thromboembolism in relatives of patients heterozygous for FV Leiden has been reported to be 4.2, with the annual incidence increasing from 0.25% at ages 15 to 30 to 1.1% in individuals older than 60. Because the prevalence of FV Leiden in white populations may be as high as 2% to 5%, it is likely to be a significant second risk factor for thrombosis

in individuals otherwise prone to thrombosis. For example, the risk of venous thromboembolism in women taking oral contraceptives is magnified about eightfold by the presence of FV Leiden. On the other hand, the polymorphism is rare or absent in African, Chinese, Japanese, and Native American populations.

Prothrombin G20210A

Because prothrombin is the precursor for thrombin, an analysis of the prothrombin gene as a candidate gene for venous thrombosis revealed that a G to A polymorphism at the last position (20210) of its 3′ untranslated region was associated with an increase of about 25% in the plasma concentration of prothrombin and a 2.8- to 4.8-fold rise in the relative risk of venous thrombosis. In white populations, heterozygosity for prothrombin G20210A is present in 1% to 2% of healthy individuals and in 4.6% to 7.9% of patients with venous thrombosis. Like FV Leiden, prothrombin G20210A is rare in individuals of African, Asian, or Native American origin. Prothrombin G20210A also has been reported to be a risk factor for cerebral venous thrombosis, more frequently in women using oral contraceptives; for myocardial infarction in young women, especially those with other risk factors for coronary artery disease; and for cerebrovascular ischemic disease in younger patients.

Homocystinemia

An increased plasma concentration of the sulfur-containing, potentially toxic amino acid homocysteine, a product of methionine metabolism, is a risk factor for both premature atherosclerosis and deep venous thrombosis. It has been estimated that 10% of the risk for coronary artery disease may be attributable to homocysteine and that homocysteine concentrations in patients with symptomatic vascular disease are 31% greater than in normal controls. The homocysteine concentration in cells and plasma is controlled by two biochemical reactions: remethylation of homocysteine to methionine by sequential reactions involving the enzymes N^5, N^{10}-methylenetetrahydrofolate reductase (MTHFR) and methionine synthase (the latter requiring vitamin B_{12} as a cofactor) and transsulfuration, in which homocysteine condenses with serine to form cystathionine in a reaction catalyzed by the vitamin B6-dependent enzyme CBS. Homozygous deficiency of CBS or MTHFR leads to congenital homocystinuria with plasma homocysteine concentrations as high as 400 μmol/L.

Approximately 50% of patients with congenital homocystinuria have a thromboembolic event before the age of 30, with a mortality rate of 20%. Smaller increases in plasma homocysteine are present in individuals who are either heterozygous for CBS deficiency or homozygous for the common thermolabile MTHFR C667T variant when their plasma folate concentrations are low. In these individuals, there is a graded relationship between plasma homocysteine concentration and the risk of coronary artery disease, stroke, and death. Homocysteine concentrations above the 95th percentile for normal controls also have been reported to raise the risk for deep venous thrombosis by a factor of 2.5. Supplementing the diet of MTHFR C667T homozygotes with folate decreases their plasma concentration of homocysteine. Whether fortification of cereal grain products with folate to prevent congenital neural tube defects will have a beneficial effect on the overall incidence of thrombotic disorders remains to be determined.

The Antiphospholipid Antibody Syndrome

This refers to the association of lupus anticoagulants (LACs) and anticardiolipin antibodies (ACAs) with venous and arterial thrombosis. LACs are IgG and IgM antibodies directed against the anionic phospholipid component of the aPTT and prothrombin time (PT) clotting assays and prolong these assays. Although these antibodies were described first in patients with SLE, in whom they can be detected in 30% to 50% of cases, they also are found in patients with other chronic autoimmune disorders; patients taking such drugs as procainamide, phenothiazines, hydralazine, and quinidine; patients recovering from acute viral infections; patients infected with HIV; women with histories of several spontaneous abortions; and patients with prolonged aPTTs (as an incidental finding). While LACs prolong the aPTT, and occasionally the PT, they are not associated with bleeding unless they are accompanied by significant prothrombin deficiency or thrombocytopenia.

ACAs react with cardiolipin, the phospholipid antigen for the serologic testing for syphilis, but ACAs differ from reagin, the antiphospholipid antibody found in syphilis. Purified ACAs do not interact with phospholipid unless the lipid is complexed with the plasma protein β_2-glycoprotein I, suggesting that the antigens they recognize reside on a lipoprotein complex. ACAs are detectable in about 40% of patients with SLE and in patients with many of the same conditions in which LACs are found. There is as yet no satisfactory explanation for the association of LACs and ACAs with thrombosis, however. It remains to be determined whether LACs and ACAs are actually pathogenic or are simply markers of a hypercoagulable state.

A history of thrombosis can be established for 30% to 40% of patients with SLE and LACs and/or ACAs and in 15% to 30% of patients with LACs and/or ACAs but without SLE. LACs and ACAs that arise after acute infection or drug ingestion usually are not associated with thrombosis. Venous thrombosis typically affects the lower extremities but may involve unusual sites, such as the hepatic veins, cerebral venous sinuses, or the axillary veins. Arterial thrombosis can result in strokes, transient ischemic attacks, or gangrene of the extremities or digits. Thromboembolic disease associated with nonbacterial aortic and mitral valve vegetations has been reported, as has the concurrence of livedo reticularis and cerebrovascular disease (Sneddon syndrome). Patients with histories of venous thrombosis tend to have recurrent venous thrombi, while patients with histories of arterial thrombosis tend have recurrent arterial thrombi. There is also an association between persistently positive results on tests for LACs and ACAs in women with SLE and recurrent fetal loss, presumably owing to thrombosis of placental vessels and placental infarction. It is not clear whether such an association exists for women without SLE.

Rare Causes of Thrombophilia

A minority of the reported cases of congenital dysfibrinogenemia are associated with thrombosis. There is no ready explanation for thrombosis in most of these cases, but in several, defective thrombin binding to the abnormal fibrinogen was thought to increase the concentration of free thrombin; in others, defective plasminogen activation or fibrinolysis has been detected. Although thrombophilia has been associated with abnormalities of plasminogen and abnormal fibrinolysis, the contribution of the abnormalities to thrombosis remains to be established.

◼ OPTIMAL MANAGEMENT

The clinical and laboratory findings and strategy for treating patients with thrombosis are discussed in Chapter 219. Drugs that are useful for treating patients with thrombosis are discussed in the next sections. The goal of medical management of arterial thrombosis is to prevent recurrence using drugs that inhibit platelet function. In specific circumstances, fibrinolytic agents have been administered to directly lyse arterial thrombi.

ANTIPLATELET AGENTS

Aspirin remains the antiplatelet agent of choice, and there is substantial evidence for its benefit in lowering the incidence of arterial occlusion. Aspirin inhibits platelet function by irreversibly inactivating the enzyme cyclooxygenase. Because platelets are unable to synthesize new cyclooxygenase, the effect of aspirin persists for the life of the platelet. Inactivation of platelet cyclooxygenase prevents synthesis of prostaglandin endoperoxides and thromboxane A_2 and inhibits platelet responses requiring these substances. A single 100-mg dose of aspirin almost completely inhibits platelet thromboxane synthesis. The effect of lower aspirin doses is cumulative, and 30 to 50 mg daily will completely inhibit thromboxane synthesis by 7 to 10 days. Side effects of aspirin are primarily gastrointestinal irritation and bleeding. A small increased incidence of hemorrhagic strokes was observed in one clinical trial.

Alternatives to aspirin are the thienopyridines ticlopidine and clopidogrel, drugs that primarily inhibit ADP-induced platelet aggregation. In contrast to aspirin, the onset of action of these drugs is delayed, limiting their usefulness in acute situations. Their effect also persists for 4 to 10 days after they are stopped. Ticlopidine has a number of serious side effects, including neutropenia in 2% to 3% of patients and rare cases of aplastic anemia; moreover, a number of reports have associated its use with the development of TTP. These side effects have not been attributed to clopidogrel, but it has been used for a shorter period of time. Drugs that inhibit platelet aggregation directly by antagonizing GpIIb-IIIa are beneficial in improving the outcome of angioplasty in patients with acute coronary syndromes. Their utility and safety in other syndromes associated with arterial thrombosis and when given over the long term remain to be determined.

THROMBOLYTIC AGENTS

Thrombolytic agents, such as streptokinase, urokinase, recombinant tissue plasminogen activator (rtPA), and anisoylated plasminogen streptokinase activator complex, catalyze the conversion of the zymogen plasminogen to the fibrinolytic enzyme plasmin and have been used to lyse arterial and venous thrombi. Because tPA converts fibrin-bound plasminogen to plasmin, it was hoped that rtPA would be clot specific, but this is not the case; at clinically effective doses, each drug cleaves fibrinogen as well as fibrin. The use of a thrombolytic agent within 4 to 6 hours of the onset of a myocardial infarction results in coronary artery reperfusion in 50% to 80% of cases and reduces mortality rates by 30% to 55%. Local thrombolytic therapy is an alternative to surgery in selected cases of peripheral artery occlusion. Thrombolytic therapy is the treatment of choice for massive pulmonary embolism and submassive embolism superimposed on chronic cardiopulmonary disease, with an overall success rate of 80% to 90%. The role of thrombolytic therapy in the management of deep venous thrombosis of the lower extremities is unclear, because the risk of hemorrhage is greater with the use of these agents than with conventional anticoagulants and because it has not been shown to prevent the postphlebitic syndrome. It is an option for treatment of subclavian or axillary vein thrombosis.

The major hazard of thrombolytic therapy is hemorrhage due to lysis of physiologic as well as pathologic blood clots. The reported incidence of bleeding ranges from 5% to 40%, including a 0% to 2% incidence of intracranial bleeding. Absolute contraindications for thrombolytic therapy include active bleeding and damage and disturbances of the central nervous system. Relative contraindications include surgery or trauma within 10 days, arterial punctures, gastrointestinal ulcer disease, known coagulation or platelet disorders, severe hypertension, hepatorenal insufficiency, pregnancy, and subacute bacterial endocarditis.

Venous thrombosis is treated by anticoagulation. Anticoagulation also has been used to prevent recurrence or extension of arterial thrombi. Acute venous thrombosis is treated initially with heparin. Heparin also is used as prophylaxis against venous thrombosis in hospitalized patients at risk for thrombosis. The oral anticoagulant warfarin is administered for prophylaxis against venous thrombosis in outpatients.

HEPARIN

Heparin is a highly sulfated glycosaminoglycan that is extracted from tissues rich in mast cells. Commercial heparin is extracted from bovine lung or pork intestine and is a heterogeneous preparation of sugar fragments whose molecular weights range from 3,000 to 30,000. The anticoagulant function of heparin stems from its ability to potentiate the function of AT. Heparin binding to AT is mediated by a specific sequence of five sugar residues that is found in only 30% of heparin molecules.

Heparin is not absorbed orally and must be administered intravenously or subcutaneously. Both its anticoagulant activity and duration of action increase disproportionately with dose: the half-life of an i.v. dose of 100 U per kilogram is approximately 60 minutes, while the half-life of an i.v. dose of 400 U per kilogram is about 150 minutes. Heparin is cleared primarily by the reticuloendothelial system, though a small amount is excreted in the urine. Heparin is not transported across the placenta and can be used safely in pregnant women. When heparin is used to treat acute venous thrombosis, it generally is administered by continuous i.v. infusion at a dose sufficient to prolong the mean control aPTT by 1.5 to 2.5 times. This usually requires a dose of about 30,000 U per 24 hours, preceded by a bolus dose of 5000 U. Heparin also can be given by subcutaneous injection at 12-hour intervals. When heparin is used as prophylaxis against venous thrombosis and pulmonary embolism, it is given at a fixed dose of 5,000 U subcutaneously every 8 to 12 hours and generally does not prolong the aPTT. Although this regimen is effective in most instances, it is not effective after orthopedic procedures and hip fractures; a regimen adjusted to keep the aPTT at the upper limit of normal is required.

Heparin that is depolymerized or fractionated into fragments of 4,000 to 6,500 MW (low-molecular-weight heparin, or LMWH) preferentially catalyzes the inactivation of FXa instead of thrombin by AT. LMWH has a number of potential therapeutic advantages over unfractionated heparin: greater and predictable bioavailability, a half-life of 2 to 4 hours after i.v. injection and 3 to 6 hours after subcutaneous injection, and dose-dependent clearance. Thus, it has been used frequently without laboratory monitoring. LMWH has been administered in fixed daily or twice-daily subcutaneous doses to prevent venous thrombosis in general surgery patients, in patients undergoing hip surgery, and in patients with stroke and spinal injury. It also has been used to treat venous thrombosis and has been given to patients with unstable angina and ischemic stroke. In each of these circumstances, it has proved to be at least as effective and safe as unfractionated heparin. Moreover, LMWH may be useful for the outpatient management of venous thrombosis, bypassing the considerable costs of hospitalization.

The principal side effect of therapy with unfractionated heparin and LMWH is hemorrhage, which occurs in 2% to 7% patients. When bleeding is mild, it is usually sufficient to simply stop the drug. If bleeding is severe, the anticoagulant effect of unfractionated heparin can be reversed by an i.v. infusion of protamine sulfate in a ratio of 1 mg protamine per 100 U of heparin. Protamine sulfate also neutralizes the anti-thrombin activity of LMWH, but it is less effective in reversing its anti-FX activity. Thus, the reliability of protamine sulfate in reversing the anticoagulant effect of LMWH is less certain. HIT due to anti-heparin antibodies develops in approximately 1% of patients receiving heparin by any route, usually within 5 to 10 days of the initial dose. HIT generally is not associated with hemorrhage, but because a small number of patients with HIT experience thrombi, it is an indication for discontinuing heparin. The incidence of HIT is thought to be lower in patients receiving LMWH. Long-term heparin administration to pregnant women can cause osteoporosis and spontaneous vertebral fractures, but this complication may also be less frequent in women given LMWH.

ORAL ANTICOAGULANTS

Oral anticoagulants are vitamin K antagonists and lessen the plasma concentration of the functional forms of FVII, FIX, and FX and prothrombin (factor II). They also decrease the plasma concentration of functional PS and PC. Vitamin K is an essential cofactor for the γ-carboxylation of a number of amino-terminal glutamic acids of these coagulation factors. The γ-carboxylated glutamic acids interact with calcium, and, in their absence, the coagulation factors are biochemically inactive. During γ-carboxylation, vitamin K is oxidized from a hydroquinone to an epoxide and must be regenerated to a hydroquinone for further γ-carboxylation to occur. The two enzymes involved in regenerating vitamin K hydroquinone (vitamin K epoxidase and vitamin K reductase) are inhibited by vitamin K antagonists.

Warfarin, a 4-hydroxycoumarin, is the most commonly used oral vitamin K antagonist. Warfarin is absorbed almost completely from the gastrointestinal tract, and 97% is bound to albumin. Only the free fraction of warfarin is biochemically active. Warfarin is metabolized in the liver by enzymes of the cytochrome P450 system, and its plasma half-life is 36 to 42 hours. After warfarin ingestion, the levels of functional prothrombin, FVII, FIX, and FX decline according to their half-lives in plasma. FVII declines first (half-life of 6 hours), FIX and FX decline next (half-lives of 24 hours), and prothrombin declines last (half-life of 72 hours). The decline of functional PC (half-life of 6 to 12 hours) is similar to that of FVII, while the decline in PS is considerably slower (half-life of 42 hours).

Warfarin usage is complicated by the effect of exogenous factors on its metabolism (Table 240.3). Fat malabsorption enhances the anticoagulant effect of warfarin by impairing vitamin K absorption, while increased intake of foods rich in vitamin K is inhibitory. The resin cholestyramine binds warfarin in the gastrointestinal tract, preventing its absorption. Drugs that induce the synthesis of cytochrome P450 enzymes in the liver lessen the effect of warfarin by increasing its metabolism. Conversely, the effect of warfarin is enhanced by drugs that displace it from albumin and temporarily increase its free concentration or directly interfere with its metabolic clearance by the liver.

Warfarin is given to patients with venous thrombosis, after treatment with heparin, to prevent recurrence of the thrombosis and to patients with chronic atrial fibrillation and prosthetic heart valves to prevent embolization. It has been used to prevent stroke and pulmonary embolism in patients with myocardial infarction, but its efficacy in preventing reinfarction is not clear. The warfarin dosage is regulated by measuring the PT. Because PT measurements depend on the potency of the thromboplastin used for the test, the PT has been standardized by comparing the potency of various thromboplastins with a thromboplastin standard. This comparison is termed the International Sensitivity Index, or ISI. PT values are now reported as the International Standardized Ratio, or INR [INR = (measured PT/control PT)^{ISI}]. This represents the PT ratio that would have been obtained if the standard thromboplastin had been used. INRs recommended to prevent recurrent venous thromboembolism and embolization in patients with chronic atrial fibrillation are 2.0 to 3.0, while INRs of 3.0 to 4.0 have been recommended to prevent embolization from mechanical heart valves. Small doses of warfarin, on the order of 1 mg daily, have been reported to be effective in preventing thrombosis in subclavian vein catheters and as prophylaxis after gynecologic surgery.

Bleeding occurs in 5% to 10% of patients treated with warfarin when the INR is within the therapeutic range and in a higher percentage when the INR is excessive. When bleeding develops in a patient whose INR is in the therapeutic range, the presence of a structural lesion should be considered. When mild bleeding is associated with an excessive INR, it may be necessary only to withhold warfarin until the INR declines into the therapeutic range. When bleeding is severe, defective coagulation can be corrected immediately by the transfusion of fresh frozen plasma. In the most severe cases, the warfarin effect also should be reversed by administering vitamin K. It should be remembered that vitamin K may make the patient resistant if warfarin therapy is reinstituted. Rarely, the initiation of warfarin therapy causes severe skin necrosis. Some, but not all, patients with skin necrosis are heterozygous for PC or PS deficiency. In patients with known PC deficiency, skin necrosis has been prevented by heparin administration during the initiation of warfarin therapy. Warfarin crosses the placenta and can lead to fetal bleeding. It also can cause a form of embryopathy characterized by nasal hypoplasia and stippled epiphyses when it is administered during the first trimester and possibly central nervous system abnormalities when it is administered during any trimester. Consequently, heparin is the preferred anticoagulant during pregnancy. Warfarin does not have an anticoagulant effect on breast-fed infants.

TABLE 240.3.	DRUGS THAT INFLUENCE THE ANTICOAGULANT ACTIVITY OF WARFARIN

Drugs That Increase Warfarin Activity and Prolong Prothrombin Time

Acetohexamide	Metronidazole
Allopurinol	Nalidixic acid
Amiodarone	Omeprazole
Anabolic steroids	Phenylbutazone
Antibiotics that depress the intestinal flora	Phenytoin
Chloramphenicol	Piroxicam
Chlorpropamide	Quinidine
Cimetidine	Sulfinpyrazone
Clofibrate	Sulfonamides
Disulfiram	Tamoxifen
Erythromycin	Thyroid hormone
Fluconazole	Tolbutamide
Isoniazid	Trimethoprim-sulfamethoxazole
Ketoconazole	Vitamin E (megadose)

Drugs That Decrease Warfarin Activity and Shorten Prothrombin Time

Barbiturates	Griseofulvin
Carbamazepine	Haloperidol
Chlorthalidone	Oral contraceptives
Cholesytramine	Vitamin K

BIBLIOGRAPHY

Collen D, Lijnen HR. Basic and clinical aspects of fibrinolysis and thrombolysis. *Blood* 1991;78:3114–3124.

Hirsh J. Heparin. *N Engl J Med* 1991;324:1565–1574.

Hirsh J. Oral anticoagulants. *N Engl J Med* 1991;324:1865–1875.

Love PE, Santoro SA. Antiphospholipid antibodies: anticardiolipin and lupus anticoagulant in systemic lupus erythematosus (SLE) and in non-SLE disorders. *Ann Intern Med* 1990;112:682–698.

Middeldorp S, Henkens CMA, Koopman MWM, et al. The incidence of venous thromboembolism in family members of patients with Factor V Leiden mutation and venous thrombosis. *Ann Intern Med* 1998;128: 15–20.

Patrono C. Aspirin as an antiplatelet agent. *N Engl J Med* 1994;330: 1287–1294.

Poort SR, Rosendaal FR, Reitsma PH, et al. A common genetic variation in the 3′-untranslated region of the prothrombin gene is associated with elevated prothrombin levels and an increase in venous thrombosis. *Blood* 1996;88:3698–3703.

Simioni P, Prandoni P, Lensing AWA, et al. The risk of recurrent venous thromboembolism in patients with an Arg506→Gln mutation in the gene for factor V (Factor V Leiden). *N Engl J Med* 1997;336:399–403.

Weitz JI. Low-molecular weight heparins. *N Engl J Med* 1997;337: 688–698.

Welch GN, Loscalzo J. Homocysteine and atherothrombosis. *N Engl J Med* 1998;338:1042–1050.

Kelley's Textbook of Internal Medicine, fourth edition. Edited by H. David Humes. Lippincott Williams & Wilkins, Philadelphia © 2000.

TABLE 241.1. COMPOSITION OF NORMAL HUMAN HEMOGLOBINS

Name of Hemoglobin	Subunit Structure	Time of Expression
Hemoglobin Portland	$\zeta_2\gamma_2$	Embryonic life
Hemoglobin Gower I	$\zeta_2\epsilon_2$	Embryonic life
Hemoglobin Gower II	$\alpha_2\epsilon_2$	Embryonic life
Hemoglobin F	$\alpha_2{}^G\gamma_2$	Fetal life[a]
	$\alpha_2{}^A\gamma_2$	
Hemoglobin A$_2$	$\alpha_2\delta_2$	Minor adult hemoglobin
Hemoglobin A	$\alpha_2\beta_2$	Major adult hemoglobin

[a] Produced in small amounts in a limited subpopulation of cells (F cells) in adults.

C H A P T E R 241

HEMOGLOBINOPATHIES

GEORGE F. ATWEH
EDWARD J. BENZ, JR.

Disorders that affect the structure, function, or production of hemoglobin are called *hemoglobinopathies*. Hemoglobinopathies usually are inherited as mutations within the globin gene clusters, but rare acquired hemoglobinopathies can be caused by toxic exposures or hematologic neoplasms. These conditions range in severity from asymptomatic laboratory abnormalities to death in utero. In many geographic areas, these disorders represent serious public health problems. Because the pathophysiologic mechanism is uniquely well understood at the molecular level, hemoglobinopathies serve as the paradigm for understanding the physiologic consequences of deranged gene function. In this chapter, the molecular basis, pathophysiologic mechanism, and clinical features of selected hemoglobinopathies are considered.

■ ESSENTIAL BIOLOGIC FEATURES OF HUMAN HEMOGLOBINS

HEMOGLOBIN STRUCTURE

Several different hemoglobins are produced during embryonic, fetal, and adult life (Table 241.1). Each consists of a tetramer of globin polypeptide chains: a pair of α-like chains and a pair of non-α chains. The main adult hemoglobin, HbA, has the

structure $\alpha_2\beta_2$. Within each chain is a single heme moiety consisting of a protoporphyrin IX ring that forms a complex with a single iron atom in the ferrous state (Fe^{2+}). The heme moiety is situated within each globular polypeptide chain in a manner optimal for reversible binding of oxygen. Each heme moiety can bind a single oxygen molecule, and every molecule of hemoglobin can transport up to four oxygen molecules.

The *primary structures* (amino acid sequences) of the various globins are highly homologous to one another, suggesting that all of the proteins arose from a common ancestral gene. Each globin has a largely helical *secondary structure*. About 80% of each polypeptide exists in the form of an α helix. The non-α chains contain eight helical segments, designated A through H, as shown in Fig. 241.1. The helices fold into three-dimensional globular *tertiary structures* that are remarkably similar for the α and non-α globins (Fig. 241.1).

The exterior surface of the globin polypeptide chains are enriched in polar (hydrophilic) amino acids that enhance solubility. The interior is composed almost exclusively of nonpolar groups that form a cleft between the E and F helices into which the heme ring is deeply buried. This heme pocket is lined with hydrophobic groups that exclude water from the vicinity of the heme, allowing numerous noncovalent, hydrophobic, weak bonds to form and stabilize the interaction between heme and globin chains. A histidine in the F helix, called histidine F8, forms a strong covalent bond with the heme iron as a result of this configuration. These features are important for normal solubility and oxygen-binding properties of the hemoglobin molecule.

The *quaternary structure* of normal adult HbA has been characterized in considerable detail. The tetramer actually consists of two αβ dimers. The two α chains in the complete tetramer do not interact directly with each other. Rather there are numerous tight interactions ($\alpha_1\beta_1$ contacts) between the α and β chains within each dimer. The two chains within each dimer interact at points that remain relatively fixed during the complex conformational changes that accompany binding and release of oxygen. The complete tetramer is held together by interfaces ($\alpha_1\beta_2$ contacts) between the α-like chain of one dimer and the

OXY

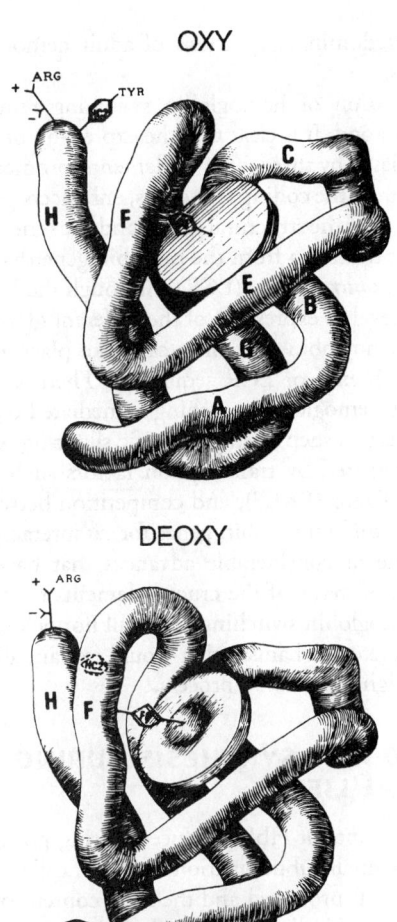

DEOXY

FIGURE 241.1. The helical and globular structure of the α-globin chain. Schematic shows the ways in which the folding of globin-chain amino acid sequences produces a hydrophobic pocket into which heme can be inserted. Iron atoms are maintained in an optimal configuration for reversible oxygen binding.

non-α chain of the other dimer. These contact points undergo large shifts during binding and release of oxygen.

The conformational changes that occur during binding and release of oxygen have been studied extensively. It is sufficient to understand that the hydrophilic surface amino acids, the hydrophobic amino acids lining the heme pocket, the F8 histidine, and the amino acids that form the $\alpha_1\beta_1$ and $\alpha_1\beta_2$ contact points represent critical positions. Mutations in these strategic regions tend to be the ones that alter clinical behavior.

FUNCTION OF HEMOGLOBIN

Hemoglobin functions effectively as an oxygen carrier in humans because it can bind efficiently to oxygen at the P_{O_2} of the alveolar capillary bed, retain the bound oxygen as the red blood cells (RBCs) traverse the circulation, and unload this oxygen to the tissues at the modestly lower oxygen tensions of tissue capillary beds. The ability of hemoglobin to fulfill the body's requirements for oxygen acquisition and delivery over a relatively narrow range of oxygen tensions results from a property inherent

in the tetrameric arrangement of heme and globin subunits within the hemoglobin molecule. This property has been called *cooperativity* or *heme–heme interaction.*

The importance of heme–heme interaction in generating the normal oxygen dissociation curve of HbA is shown in Fig. 241.2. Monomeric globin-like peptides, such as individual globin subunits or myoglobin, are useless as oxygen carriers. These proteins acquire oxygen readily but can release it only at low oxygen pressures that are incompatible with life. In contrast, the hemoglobin tetramer exhibits an S-shaped oxygen dissociation curve. At low oxygen tensions, the hemoglobin is fully deoxygenated. As the oxygen tension rises, increases in oxygen binding occur slowly at first. As soon as some oxygen has been bound by the hemoglobin molecule, there is an abrupt increase in the slope of the curve. This cooperative or autocatalytic mechanism causes hemoglobin molecules that have bound some oxygen to develop a higher oxygen affinity, greatly accelerating their ability to combine with more oxygen.

The cooperative nature of oxygen binding has been extensively studied with x-ray crystallography. The complete deoxy form is stabilized by several strong salt bonds (electrostatic bonds), which must be broken before the first oxygen molecule can bind to heme. Because the transition to the oxyhemoglobin

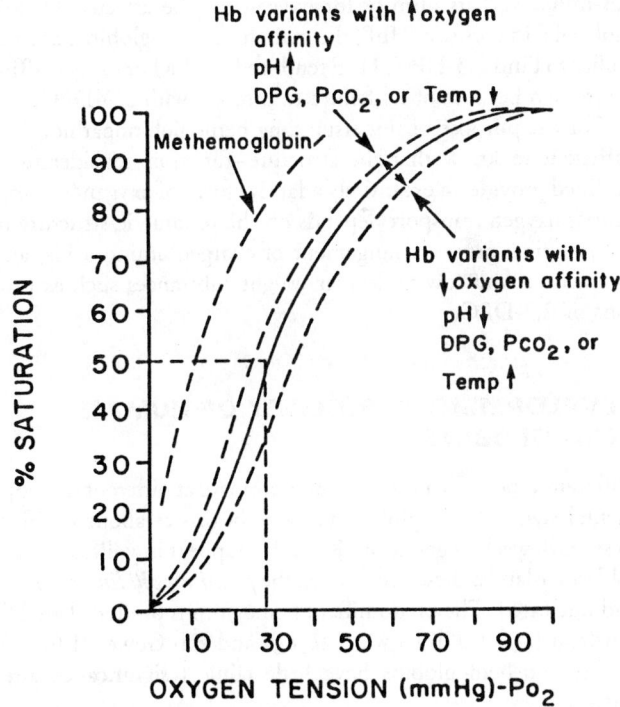

FIGURE 241.2. The oxygen dissociation curve of hemoglobin. Drawing shows the sigmoidal oxygen-binding curve of normal hemoglobin (*solid line*) and changes in dissociation that cause a shift to the left (increased oxygen affinity) or a shift to the right (decreased oxygen affinity), as indicated by the *dashed lines*. The far left shift, caused when hemoglobin is converted to methemoglobin, is indicated by an additional *dashed line*. The P_{50} value of the hemoglobin dissociation curve is used as an indication of oxygen affinity. The *right-angled dashed lines* indicate that the P_{50} value is measured as the partial pressure of oxygen at which a particular hemoglobin preparation is 50% saturated with oxygen.

state requires breaking of these bonds, the first oxygen to bind to the hemoglobin molecule must overcome much resistance. After one oxygen molecule has bound, however, the bonds are broken. Oxygen affinity then approaches that of the individual subunits and causes a marked increase in the slope of the oxygen-binding curve. This results in the physiologically more useful S-shaped oxygen equilibrium curve, along which substantial amounts of oxygen loading and unloading can occur over a narrow range of oxygen tensions.

The oxygen affinity of normal hemoglobin is affected by several factors. The classic effect of pH on oxygen affinity is known as the Bohr effect. It is caused by the stabilizing action of protons on the deoxy confirmation. Deoxyhemoglobin binds protons more readily than does oxyhemoglobin because it is a weaker acid. At low pH, hemoglobin has a lower oxygen affinity, facilitating delivery of oxygen to tissues.

Small molecules, called *allosteric effectors,* alter oxygen affinity of hemoglobin. The most important physiologic regulator of hemoglobin function in humans is 2,3-diphosphoglycerate (2,3-DPG). 2,3-DPG is generated as an intermediate of glycolysis in RBCs. Formation and destruction of this substance are enzymatically regulated and can be adjusted to changing physiologic conditions. Binding stabilizes the deoxy state. High levels of 2,3-DPG or other conditions that increase affinity for 2,3-DPG lower oxygen affinity. HbA has a reasonably high affinity for 2,3-DPG, and its affinity for oxygen can be affected by this molecule. In contrast, HbF, the main fetal hemoglobin, has little ability to bind 2,3-DPG. HbF tends to have higher oxygen affinity in vivo because of its failure to interact with 2,3-DPG.

For the purpose of understanding hemoglobinopathies, it is sufficient to know that the structure–function considerations outlined provide an exquisitely adaptive form of oxygen binding. Proper oxygen transport depends on the tetrameric structure of the proteins, proper arrangement of charged amino acids, and interaction with low-molecular-weight substances such as protons or 2,3-DPG.

DEVELOPMENTAL BIOLOGY OF HUMAN HEMOGLOBINS

Different types of hemoglobin predominate at different developmental stages. Hemoglobin synthesis begins at about the fifth to seventh week of gestation. RBCs first appear in yolk sac erythroblastic islands; these cells, called the *primitive cell line,* are large and nucleated. The predominant hemoglobins produced are Hb Portland ($\zeta_2\gamma_2$), Hb Gower I ($\zeta_2\epsilon_2$), and Hb Gower II ($\alpha_2\epsilon_2$). Embryonic hemoglobins have little clinical significance after birth.

Erythropoiesis shifts to the liver at 10 to 11 weeks of gestation, coincident with a transition from predominance of embryonic hemoglobins to predominance of fetal hemoglobin (HbF: $\alpha_2\gamma_2$). HbF is a heterogeneous mixture of two hemoglobins; they differ in the composition of the γ-chain component. The $^A\gamma$ chains have alanine, and $^G\gamma$ chains have glycine at position 136. Production shifts to bone marrow during the sixth to seventh month of gestation, but HbF continues to predominate until about 38 weeks of gestation, when a switch (HbF→HbA

switch) to predominant synthesis of adult hemoglobin (HbA: $\alpha_2\beta_2$) occurs.

The regulation of hemoglobin switching remains incompletely understood. It is clear that the expression of the β-globin genes is regulated by three types of elements: promoters immediately upstream of the coding sequences, enhancers present within or downstream of the structural genes, and the series of hypersensitive sites far upstream from the β-globin gene that are referred to as the *locus control region* (LCR). Although the LCR is critical for the high level of expression of the different globin genes, the process of hemoglobin switching can take place in transgenic mice in the absence of LCR sequences. There is considerable evidence that hemoglobin switching is mediated by a variety of different processes such as stage-specific silencing, stage-specific activation mediated by transcription factors such as erythroid Kruppel-like factor (EKLF), and competition between the promoters of the different globin genes for *cis* interaction with the LCR. In spite of considerable advances that have led to the identification of many of the crucial elements necessary for appropriate hemoglobin switching, it is still not possible to reconstruct a complete mechanism that would explain all the intricacies of this highly regulated process.

HEMOGLOBIN F SYNTHESIS DURING POSTNATAL LIFE

The small amounts of HbF produced during postnatal life are confined to a small subpopulation of RBCs called F cells. The number of F cells produced and the HbF content of each F cell appear to be genetically determined. Although F cells express few other features of fetal cells, they seem to be distinct from true fetal RBCs.

F cells are produced by the complex kinetics of the erythroid pool of progenitor cells. Results from a number of laboratories have suggested that the most immature committed erythroid precursors (BFU-e) undergo a series of proliferative and differentiating cell divisions before they enter the pool of the more differentiated progenitors poised to become proerythroblasts. To a first approximation, the most immature or undifferentiated BFU-e retain the highest potential to express fetal hemoglobin in adults. Under normal conditions of erythropoiesis, these cells continue to proliferate slowly and to differentiate into more mature BFU-e before being recruited into the pool of maturing progenitors (CFU-e and proerythroblasts). By this time, they have largely lost their ability to produce fetal hemoglobin. Only a small number of early BFU-e are recruited into the maturing pool, accounting for the small number of F cells produced under normal conditions.

Under conditions of marked erythroid stress, such as chronic congenital hemolytic anemia or recovery from bone marrow transplantation or chemotherapy, many BFU-e are recruited into the maturing pool of progenitors before they have had the chance to undergo the differentiating cell divisions. These cells retain considerable potential to produce fetal hemoglobin, resulting in higher than normal levels of HbF in clinical conditions characterized by marked erythroid stress. The molecular mechanisms mediating these complex events remain obscure. Nonetheless, it is believed that this phenomenon may explain, at least in

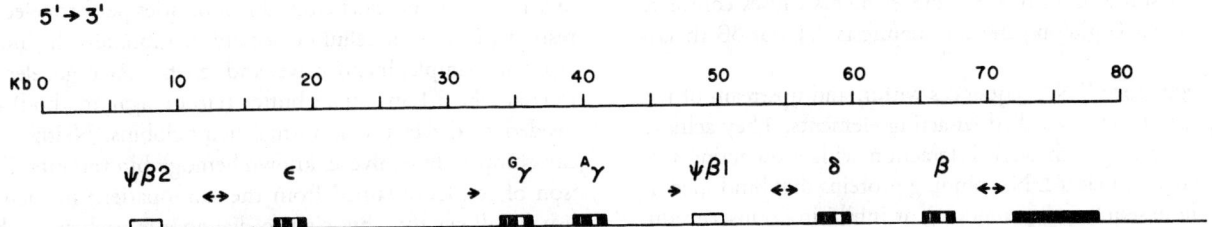

FIGURE 241.3. Structural organization of the non–α-globin gene cluster. Diagram shows the approximate topography of non–α-globin genes as they are arrayed along chromosome 11. The entire cluster is about 80 kb long. The gene loci are diagrammed as alternating patterns of introns and exons. *Open boxes* represent two pseudogenes, labeled ψβ1 and ψβ2. These are inactive remnants of globin genes that have become nonfunctional during evolution. The *arrows* pointing in the forward and reverse directions indicate repetitive sequence elements that are scattered throughout both globin gene clusters. The *large solid box* indicates a distinctive repetitive element downstream of the globin gene clusters. A strong enhancer that controls tissue-specific expression of the gene cluster is located within this region. The α-globin gene cluster has similar topography. A region about 10 kb upstream of the ε gene has been shown to promote maximal rates of globin gene expression.

part, the increased levels of HbF among patients with sickle cell disease treated with hydroxyurea. The same is true of the activation of HbF production with injections of high doses of recombinant erythropoietin. The expression of the fetal globin genes can be increased in postnatal life by treatment with agents such as butyrate, which can inhibit histone deacetylase and modify the structure of chromatin.

GENETICS AND BIOSYNTHESIS OF HUMAN HEMOGLOBIN

Production of the various human hemoglobins is controlled by two tightly linked gene clusters (Fig. 241.3). The α-like globin genes are clustered on chromosome 16 and the non-α genes on chromosome 11. The α-like cluster consists of two α-globin genes and a single copy of the ζ gene. The non-α gene cluster consists of a single ε gene, the ^{G}γ and ^{A}γ fetal globin genes, and the adult δ and β genes. Interspersed among the globin genes are pseudogenes that have been inactivated by mutations that prevent their expression.

In most respects, the functional anatomy of globin genes is typical of eukaryotic genes (Fig. 241.4). Each globin gene contains two intervening sequences (introns) interspersed among three blocks of sequence (exons) that ultimately code for messenger RNA. The non-α globin genes contain a small (130 bases) and a large (900 to 1,100 bases) intervening sequence. Both of the intervening sequences in the α- and ζ-globin genes are small (100 to 200 bases).

Flanking sequences at each end of the genes are important for regulating function of the genes. Immediately upstream (39 to 70 bp) are typical eukaryotic promoter elements necessary for the assembly of the transcription initiation complex, which includes RNA polymerase. Regions 100 to 300 bases upstream are important for proper developmental expression. The sequences in these regions are moderately well conserved among the globin gene clusters of several species. Sequences in the 5′ flanking region of the γ genes and the β genes appear to be crucial for the correct developmental regulation of these genes.

Important elements that function as classic enhancers have been identified in the 3′ flanking regions of the β-globin gene. All these regulatory regions exist in erythroid cells in a relatively open chromatin configuration that is characterized by increased DNAse sensitivity. The LCR more than 50 kilobases upstream of the β-globin gene consists of five sites characterized by a higher level of sensitivity to DNAse and is called *HS1 to HS5*.

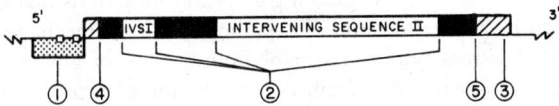

A. TRANSCRIPTION SIGNALS

① Region of relatively high homology required for faithful transcription

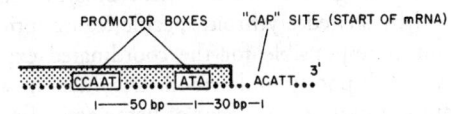

B. mRNA PROCESSING SIGNALS

② Splice sites: 5′GU...IVS...AG 3′

③ Polyadenylation signal: 5′..AAUAAA...GC 3′

C. mRNA TRANSLATION SIGNALS

④ Initiator codon (AUG in mRNA) (Start of translation)

⑤ Terminator codon (UAA in mRNA) (End of translation)

⑥ "Open" reading frame – no "in-phase" translation termination signals between initiation codon and termination codon

FIGURE 241.4. Anatomic features of the β-globin gene. Bar diagram shows the position of the anatomic features listed below each type of signal.

Deletion of some or all of these HS elements causes complete silencing of the β-globin gene and manifests as β- or δβ-thalassemia.

The regulatory DNA sequences within and upstream of the globin gene cluster are called *cis*-acting elements. They achieve their biologic effects through interaction with *trans*-acting factors, which are nuclear DNA binding proteins that bind specifically to these sequences, promoting or inhibiting transcription. Several transcription factors that bind to sequences in the globin gene promoters and enhancers have been identified. Some of these are ubiquitous transcription factors that are present both in erythroid and nonerythroid cells (e.g., Sp1 and YY1), whereas others are more or less limited to erythroid cells (e.g., GATA-1, NFE-2, and EKLF). These erythroid-specific factors appear to be involved in regulating the expression of other erythroid genes such as the genes that encode the enzymes of the heme biosynthetic pathway.

It is especially relevant to the discussion of the thalassemia syndromes to emphasize that the final product of the process, the hemoglobin tetramer, is highly soluble, whereas the individual globin chains are insoluble. To avoid precipitation and denaturation of monomeric globin chains, it is essential that α and non-α globins be synthesized in equal amounts. When globin chain synthesis is balanced, each newly synthesized α- or non–α-globin chain has an available mate with which to pair. The mechanisms responsible for maintaining the delicate balance between the expression of the α- and non–α-globin genes in normal RBCs is poorly understood. This delicate balance is disturbed when the α- or non–α-globin genes carry mutations that interfere with their expression. The pathophysiologic mechanism of the thalassemia syndromes involves imbalance of globin chain synthesis. The imbalance causes precipitation of unpaired chains and premature destruction of the RBCs.

The production of normal RBCs requires the coordinated expression of the globin genes and of all the genes responsible for heme and iron metabolism. Although it is clear that the genes that encode globin and the heme biosynthesis enzymes are regulated by shared erythroid-specific transcription factors, the mechanism responsible for the coordinated expression of these genes is still poorly understood. Disorders in which iron or the protoporphyrin component of heme are deficient generally cause secondary reduction in the level of globin synthesis. For complex reasons, a mild imbalance in globin chain synthesis also occurs; α-chain synthesis is more impaired by heme or iron deficiency than is β-chain synthesis. In other words, anemia characterized by deficiency of iron or heme tends to be mildly α-thalassemic. Because imbalances in this regulatory scheme occur frequently in a variety of conditions such as thalassemia, iron deficiency anemia, and disorders of heme biosynthesis, it can be inferred that the normal regulatory mechanisms are rather easily disrupted.

DETECTION AND CHARACTERIZATION OF HEMOGLOBINOPATHIES

Of the many methods available for hemoglobin analysis, two electrophoretic techniques are in routine clinical use. For routine or screening tests, most clinical laboratories perform electrophoresis at pH 8.6 on cellulose acetate membranes; this method is especially simple, inexpensive, and reliable. Agar gel electrophoresis at pH 6.1 in citrate buffer (citrate agar method) often is needed to detect the abnormal hemoglobins. Neither method can completely resolve all known hemoglobin variants. Comparison of results obtained from the same patient in each system usually allows the physician to diagnose most hemoglobinopathies unambiguously. The two electrophoretic methods should be regarded as complementary. In each case, the hemoglobins migrate toward the cathode. Cellulose acetate separations clearly resolve HbA, F, S, and A_2, but hemoglobins D and Lepore comigrate with HbS, and HbE and C migrate with HbA_2. Citrate agar gels resolve HbS and E from each other and allow identification of Hb Lepore and HbC as bands comigrating with HbS on cellulose acetate but with HbA on citrate agar. Most common variants can be defined through similar reasoning.

Quantitative assessment of the hemoglobin profile often is desirable. HbA_2 frequently is elevated in association with β-thalassemia trait and depressed with iron deficiency. HbF is elevated in conditions referred to as *hereditary persistence of fetal hemoglobins,* some β-thalassemia syndromes, and occasional periods of erythroid stress or marrow dysplasia. For characterization of sickle cell trait, sickle thalassemia syndromes, or HbSC disease and for monitoring the progress of exchange transfusion therapy to lower the percentage of circulating HbS, measurement of individual hemoglobins is needed. In most laboratories, measurement is performed only if the test is specifically ordered.

Many clinically important hemoglobin variants are not detected with electrophoresis. They cannot be differentiated from HbA with either of the previously described techniques. Most of these mutant hemoglobins can be detected with more specialized techniques, such as isoelectric focusing or high-pressure liquid chromatography, that are not widely available in clinical laboratories. Conversely, some nonsickling hemoglobins, such as HbO Arab and HbD, can comigrate with HbS on cellulose acetate. Electrophoretic assessment always should be regarded as incomplete unless functional assays for hemoglobin sickling, solubility, or oxygen affinity also are performed, as dictated by the clinical signs and symptoms.

The best assays for hemoglobin sickling involve measurement of the degree to which the hemoglobin sample becomes insoluble, or gelated, as it is deoxygenated (sickle solubility test). Some centers still offer an older test (the Sickledex test) in which a drop of blood is suspended in a reducing (deoxygenating) agent such as sodium metabisulfite and sealed under a coverslip. The cell suspension is examined with a microscope for formation of sickled cells.

Unstable hemoglobins are best detected with tests for solubility in isopropanol or after heating to 50°C. Unstable hemoglobins precipitate under these conditions; normal hemoglobins do not. High-affinity and low-affinity variants can be detected through measurement of P_{50}, the partial pressure of oxygen at which the hemoglobin sample becomes 50% saturated (in the oxy form) with oxygen. Direct tests for percentage carbonmonoxy-hemoglobin and methemoglobin in which spectrophotometric techniques are used can readily be performed in most clinical laboratories, even on an urgent basis.

For complete characterization of abnormal hemoglobin or thalassemia, including amino acid sequencing or gene cloning and sequencing, several investigational laboratories around the world are available for referral. Whereas such characterization used to take months, with the polymerase chain reaction (PCR), allele-specific oligonucleotide hybridization, and automated DNA sequencing, it is possible to identify globin gene mutations in a few days. Most hematologists are familiar with these resources.

Despite the plethora of sophisticated methods to characterize and confirm the diagnosis of hemoglobinopathy, the primary diagnosis is still most frequently established through recognition of a characteristic history, physical findings, morphologic findings on a peripheral blood smear, and abnormalities of the complete blood cell count, such as profound microcytosis with minimal anemia in thalassemia trait. Laboratory evaluation is still mostly an adjunct rather than the sole diagnostic method for most of the clinically important forms of hemoglobinopathy.

TYPES AND DISTRIBUTION OF HEMOGLOBINOPATHIES

CLASSIFICATION

There are five major classes of hemoglobinopathy. *Structural hemoglobinopathies* (Table 241.2) are disorders in which mutations alter the amino acid sequence of the globin polypeptide chains. The altered properties of the variant hemoglobins generate the characteristic clinical syndromes. Some hemoglobins polymerize abnormally, as in sickle cell anemia; others exhibit abnormal solubility or oxygen affinity. The *thalassemia syndromes* are characterized by defective synthesis of globin chains. Thalassemia syndromes are caused by mutations that impair production or translation of globin messenger RNA. Clinical abnormalities are attributable to an inadequate supply of hemoglobin and resulting anemia, imbalances in the production of individual globin chains and resulting premature destruction of RBCs, and the consequences of iron overload caused by a combination of increased absorption of dietary iron and transfusional iron load.

Thalassemic hemoglobin variants have features of thalassemia (abnormal globin biosynthesis) and of structural hemoglobinopathies (abnormal amino acid sequence). In *hereditary persistence of fetal hemoglobin,* there is continued synthesis of fetal hemoglobins beyond the perinatal period. *Acquired hemoglobinopathies* are derangements of hemoglobin structure or synthesis resulting from acquired conditions. A common example is modification of the hemoglobin molecule by toxins (acquired methemoglobinemia). Abnormal hemoglobin synthesis, such as high levels of HbF production in preleukemia and α-thalassemia in myeloproliferative disorders also occur sporadically. More than 400 structural variants and 100 thalassemia mutations have been identified. Only a few selected forms of hemoglobinopathy that are especially important clinically or theoretically are considered here.

TABLE 241.2.	**CLASSIFICATION OF HEMOGLOBINOPATHIES**

Structural hemoglobinopathies—hemoglobins with altered amino acid sequences that result in deranged function or altered physical or chemical properties
  Abnormal hemoglobin polymerization—hemoglobin S
  Altered O$_2$ affinity
    High affinity—polycythemia
    Low affinity—cyanosis, pseudoanemia
Hemoglobins that oxidize readily
  Unstable hemoglobins, hemolytic anemia, jaundice
  M hemoglobins—methemogobinemia, cyanosis
Thalassemia—defective production of globin chains
  α-Thalassemia
  β-Thalassemia
  δβ-, γδβ-, αβ-Thalassemia
Thalassemic hemoglobin variants—structurally abnormal hemoglobin associated with coinherited thalassemia phenotype
  Hemoglobin E
  Hemoglobin Constant Spring
  Hemoglobin Lepore
Hereditary persistence of fetal hemoglobin—persistence of high levels of hemoglobin F into adult life
  Pancellular—all red blood cells contain elevated hemoglobin F levels
    Nondeletion forms
    Deletion forms
    Hemoglobin Kenya
  Heterocellular—only specific subpopulations of red blood cells contain elevated levels of hemoglobin F
Acquired hemoglobinopathy
  Methemoglobin due to toxic exposures
  Sulfhemoglobin due to toxic exposures
  Carboxyhemoglobin
  Hemoglobin H in erythroleukemia
  Elevated hemoglobin F in states of erythroid stress and bone marrow dysplasia, usually heterocellular

EPIDEMIOLOGY

Hemoglobinopathy is especially common in areas in which malaria is endemic. It has been assumed that the clustering of hemoglobinopathies in the malaria belt is a reflection of a selective survival advantage for the thalassemic RBCs after infection with the malaria parasite. The RBCs are presumed to provide a less hospitable environment during the obligate intraerythrocytic stages of the parasitic life cycle. This hypothesis has been challenged after the observation that very young children with α-thalassemia are susceptible to infection with nonlethal *Plasmodium vivax,* which can act as a natural vaccine to protect them against infection with the more lethal *Plasmodium falciparum* later in life.

INHERITANCE

Hemoglobinopathies are inherited either as autosomal recessive or autosomal codominant traits; compound heterozygotes who inherit a different abnormal globin allele from each parent have composite features of each abnormal allele. For example, patients who inherit a β-thalassemia gene from one parent and a β^s (sickle) allele form the other have sickle β-thalassemia, a condition with features of β-thalassemia and sickle cell anemia. Each hemoglobinopathy is transmitted as a tightly linked allele of the β-globin gene.

The α-chain hemoglobinopathies cause abnormalities of HbA, HbA$_2$, and HbF, because the α chain is present in all of these hemoglobins. The α-globin hemoglobinopathies are manifested in utero and after birth because normal function of the α-globin gene is required throughout gestation and adult life. In contrast, β-globin gene expression is not abundant until after birth. Infants with β-globin hemoglobinopathies tend to have no symptoms until 3 to 9 months of age, when HbA has largely replaced HbF.

■ STRUCTURALLY ABNORMAL HEMOGLOBINS

SICKLE CELL SYNDROMES

The sickle cell syndromes are caused by a mutation in the β-globin gene that changes the sixth amino acid from glutamic acid to valine. HbS ($\alpha_2\beta_2^{6Glu\rightarrow Val}$) exhibits normal behavior when oxygenated, but deoxy HbS polymerizes reversibly to form a gelatinous network of fibrous polymers called *tactoids.* These tactoids exert deleterious effects on the circulating RBCs, including stiffening of the membrane, increased viscosity, dehydration due to potassium leakage and calcium influx, and distortion of morphologic features that produces the sickle shape that characterizes these syndromes (Fig. 241.5). Sickle cells lose pliability and cannot traverse small capillaries. The altered membrane of sickled RBCs is sticky and adheres to endothelial cell walls with a tenacity that further impedes flow through the microvasculature.

Sickling has two main pathophysiologic consequences. First, the abnormal sickle cells are destroyed by the spleen, and hemolytic anemia occurs. The presence of anemia can be beneficial in sickle cell disease because it reduces total blood viscosity and improves blood flow to the periphery. Therefore the mere presence of anemia in sickle cell disease is not an indication for

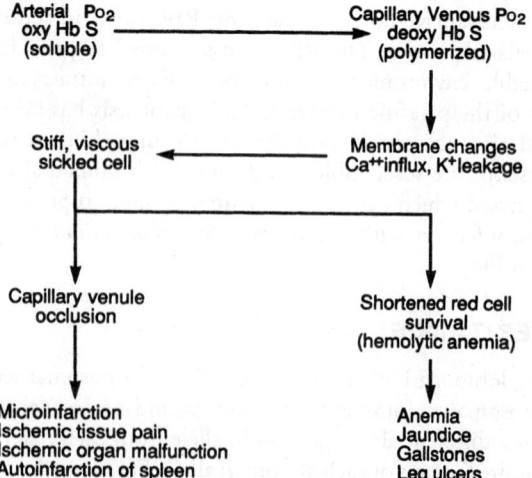

FIGURE 241.5. Pathophysiologic mechanism of sickle cell anemia. Diagram summarizes the pathogenesis of the two features of sickle cell disease—hemolytic anemia and vaso-occlusive crises.

transfusion therapy. Second, the sickle cells clog small capillaries and venules. Tissue supplied by the occluded vessels becomes ischemic, provoking symptoms ranging from pain to end-organ damage. This veno-occlusive component of the disease usually dominates the clinical signs and symptoms. Prominent manifestations include ischemic pain (painful crises) and ischemic malfunction or frank infarction in the spleen, central nervous system, bones, liver, kidneys, and lungs. The finding that sickle RBCs adhere to the endothelium, particularly in acute vaso-occlusive crises, suggests that the adhesive mechanisms themselves may be targets for new therapies. Several sickle syndromes occur as the result of inheritance of HbS from one parent and another hemoglobinopathy, such as β-thalassemia or HbC ($\alpha_2\beta_2^{6Glu\rightarrow Lys}$) from the other parent. The prototype disease, sickle cell anemia, is the homozygous state for HbS. The sickling syndromes are considered in Chapter 245 and are not discussed further here.

UNSTABLE HEMOGLOBINS

Unstable hemoglobins are produced by an amino acid substitution that renders the hemoglobin less soluble or more susceptible to oxidation. Both α- and β-globin variants can cause this condition. The mutations that produce insoluble hemoglobins tend to alter the helical segments, such as Hb Genova ($\beta^{28Leu\rightarrow Pro}$), to interfere with contact points between the α and β subunits, such as Hb Philly ($\beta^{35Tyr\rightarrow Phe}$), or to disrupt interactions of the hydrophobic pockets of the globin subunits with heme, such as Hb Koln ($\beta^{98Val\rightarrow Met}$).

Precipitation of hemoglobin in circulating RBCs produces intracellular inclusions called *Heinz bodies,* which are readily detectable with supravital dyes such as crystal violet. This method is the basis of a diagnostic test for Heinz body hemolytic anemia. The spleen attempts to remove these inclusions, and pitted, rigid cells form that eventually become sequestered and produce hemolytic anemia. Patients with severe forms of this anemia need long-term transfusion support. Splenectomy often is effective for relief of anemia. Leg ulcers and premature gallbladder disease occur frequently.

Unstable hemoglobins are rare compared with sickle cell anemia and thalassemia. They occur sporadically in many ethnic groups, often by means of spontaneous new mutations. The heterozygous state often is symptomatic, because large numbers of Heinz bodies form even when the unstable variant accounts for only one-half of the total hemoglobin. Most of the symptomatic unstable hemoglobins are β-globin variants, because sporadic mutations affecting the α-globin loci would usually involve only one of the four alleles, generating only 20% to 30% abnormal hemoglobin. The propensity of unstable hemoglobins to precipitate is exaggerated with oxidative stress, such as infection or exposure to oxidizing drugs such as quinine.

HEMOGLOBINS WITH ALTERED OXYGEN AFFINITY

High-affinity hemoglobins, such as Hb Zurich ($\beta^{His\rightarrow Arg}$), have high avidity for oxygen, causing the oxygen dissociation curve to shift to the left. These hemoglobins bind oxygen readily but are not likely to deliver the oxygen to tissues at normal capillary oxygen pressures. The resultant mild tissue hypoxia leads to inappropriately high RBC production and polycythemia. In extreme cases, hematocrits of 60% to 65% can occur. High-affinity variants are caused by several forms of mutations that alter interactions within the heme pocket, disrupt the Bohr effect or salt-bond site, or impair the interaction of HbA with 2,3-DPG. Because 2,3-DPG lowers the oxygen affinity of HbA, reduced 2,3 DPG-binding causes an effective increase in oxygen affinity. The presence of high-affinity hemoglobins should be considered in the case of patients with unexplained erythrocytosis. In some cases, the elevated hematocrit can increase blood viscosity and produce hyperviscosity symptoms. Phlebotomy is then needed.

Low-affinity hemoglobins, such as Hb Kansas ($\beta^{102Asn \rightarrow Thr}$), usually produce misleading laboratory abnormalities and physical findings but no symptoms. These hemoglobin variants bind sufficient oxygen in the lungs despite their lower oxygen affinity to achieve full saturation; however, at capillary oxygen tensions, they release excessive amounts of oxygen. These patients can deliver normal amounts of oxygen at hematocrits that indicate anemia and can have pseudoanemia. Capillary hemoglobin desaturation can be sufficiently dramatic that more than 5 g per deciliter of unsaturated hemoglobin is present in the vascular beds, producing clinically apparent cyanosis. Despite these findings, patients usually need no specific treatment.

METHEMOGLOBINEMIA

Methemoglobin is generated by oxidation of the iron moieties to the ferric state. Methemoglobin has such high oxygen affinity that almost no oxygen is delivered to tissues. Methemoglobin levels greater than 50% to 60% of total hemoglobin produce fatal tissue hypoxia. Methemoglobin also has a characteristic bluish-brown muddy color that causes patients to appear cyanotic.

Congenital methemoglobinemia is caused by mutations that interact with the heme pocket to favor stabilization of iron in the ferric state, such as HbM Iwate ($\alpha^{87His \rightarrow Tyr}$), or by inherited deficiency of the enzyme that reduces methemoglobin to hemoglobin, such as methemoglobin reductase, nicotinamide adenine dinucleotide phosphate (NADP), or diaphorase. Acquired methemoglobinemia is caused by exposure to toxins that oxidize heme iron, notably nitrate and nitrite-containing compounds. Patients with congenital methemoglobinemia rarely need treatment. Patients with nitrate or nitrite poisoning, if sufficiently severe, need therapy with ascorbic acid and methylene blue.

TREATMENT OF PATIENTS WITH UNSTABLE HEMOGLOBINS, HIGH-AFFINITY HEMOGLOBINS, AND METHEMOGLOBINEMIA

Diagnosis of the presence of an *unstable hemoglobin variant* should be suspected when a patient has nonimmune hemolytic anemia, jaundice, splenomegaly, or premature biliary tract disease. Unstable hemoglobins, like other congenital hemolytic

states, are part of the differential diagnosis of neonatal jaundice. Most cases of hemolytic anemia due to the presence of unstable hemoglobins are detected during infancy. Some mildly unstable variants may become manifest in adult life with mild to moderate anemia or only with unexplained reticulocytosis, hepatosplenomegaly, premature biliary tract disease, or leg ulcers. Because these variants frequently are caused by spontaneous mutation, a family history of anemia may not exist. A peripheral blood smear often shows anisocytosis, abundant cells with punctate inclusions, and irregular shapes (poikilocytosis).

The two best tests for diagnosing unstable hemoglobins are the Heinz body preparation and the isopropanol or heat stability test. The latter test is used to assess the ability of hemoglobin to remain in solution when heated or exposed to a mildly nonpolar solvent. Many unstable Hb variants are not detected with electrophoresis; they migrate in a position indistinguishable from that of HbA. The result of electrophoresis often is normal. The test is useful for confirmation but not as a ruling-out strategy.

Young children with severe hemolytic anemia caused by the presence of unstable hemoglobins may need transfusions for the first 3 years of life, because splenectomy before 3 to 4 years of age is associated with immune deficit. Splenectomy is the therapy of choice thereafter. Most patients have marked improvement. Rare patients may need lifelong transfusion support. Even after splenectomy, patients should be observed for signs of cholelithiasis and leg ulcers. Splenectomy should be considered in the care of patients with the secondary complications of chronic hemolysis, even if anemia is absent.

Many unstable hemoglobins precipitate more rapidly when subjected to oxidative stress. Principles of management that apply to glucose-6-phosphate dehydrogenases deficiency are applicable to the care of patients with unstable hemoglobins, even after splenectomy.

The presence of *high-affinity hemoglobin variants* should be suspected when a patient has unexplained erythrocytosis. The best test for confirmation is measurement of P_{50}. A significant left shift (lower numeric value of the P_{50}) suggests the possibility of the presence of high-affinity hemoglobin. The most important confounding variable is tobacco smoking. Carbonmonoxy-hemoglobin level frequently is elevated in heavy smokers and causes the P_{50} to fall.

Many high-affinity hemoglobins produce no symptoms, but rubor or plethora may be apparent. When the hematocrit exceeds 55% to 60%, headache or other symptoms of high blood viscosity and sluggish flow may occur. These patients may benefit from judicious phlebotomy. The guiding principle of phlebotomy should be to improve oxygen delivery by reducing blood viscosity and increasing blood flow. Erythrocytosis represents an appropriate attempt to compensate for the impaired oxygen delivery of the abnormal variant. Overzealous phlebotomy may stimulate increased erythropoiesis or aggravate symptoms by thwarting this compensatory mechanism. Phlebotomy should be directed at improvement of symptoms and viscosity, not at restoration of a normal hematocrit.

The presence of *low-affinity hemoglobins* should be suspected when a patient has cyanosis or a low hematocrit for no reason that is apparent after thorough evaluation. The P_{50} test can confirm the diagnosis. Awareness of the diagnosis, counseling, and reassurance are the interventions of choice.

The presence of *methemoglobin* should be suspected when a patient appears cyanotic but has a PaO$_2$ sufficiently high that hemoglobin should be fully saturated with oxygen. It may not be possible to ascertain whether a patient has ingested nitrite or another oxidant; some exposures may be inapparent to the patient, and others may be caused by suicide attempts. Methemoglobin gives a characteristic muddy appearance when blood is drawn. The test of choice to establish the diagnosis is measurement of methemoglobin content, which can readily be performed on an emergency basis in most clinical laboratories.

Congenital methemoglobinemia almost never necessitates therapy. Acquired methemoglobinemia may be associated with symptoms of cerebral ischemia if levels exceed 15% to 20%. Levels greater than 60% usually are lethal. Emergency therapy for methemoglobinemia involves intravenous injection of 1 mg per kilogram of methylene blue. Management of milder cases and follow-up therapy for severe cases can be achieved with oral methylene blue (60 mg three to four times a day) or ascorbic acid (300 to 600 mg a day). Methylene blue can induce hemolysis in patients with glucose-6-phosphate dehydrogenase deficiency.

THALASSEMIA SYNDROMES

The thalassemia syndromes are inherited disorders of α- or β-globin chain biosynthesis. There are two major consequences of reduced synthesis of a specific globin chain. First, the reduced supply of globin diminishes production of hemoglobin tetramers, causing hypochromia and microcytosis. Second, unbalanced synthesis of α and β subunits occurs because impaired synthesis of one chain is not associated with comparable reductions in synthesis of the other globin. Unpaired globin chains accumulate: α chains in β-thalassemia and β chains in α-thalassemia. The pathophysiologic process of thalassemia is dominated by the behavior of these unpaired chains. Clinical severity varies widely depending on the degree to which the synthesis of the affected globin is impaired and on modifying factors, such as altered synthesis of other globin chains or coinheritance of other abnormal globin alleles.

β-THALASSEMIA SYNDROMES

β-Thalassemia may be caused by mutations that affect every step in the pathway of globin gene expression: transcription, processing of the mRNA precursor, translation, and posttranslational integrity of the β-polypeptide chain (Fig. 241.6). Complete deletion of the β-globin gene alone has not been encountered, but complex deletions removing two or more non-α genes and partial deletion of the β-globin gene do account for rare cases. Other mutations alter promoter regions, polyadenylation signals, the translation initiator codon, and other steps in the synthetic pathway. The most common forms of β-thalassemia are caused by mutations that impair splicing of the mRNA pre-

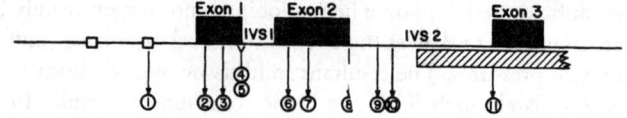

FIGURE 241.6. β-Thalassemia may be caused by mutations that affect every step in the pathway of β-globin gene expression: transcription, processing of the mRNA precursor, translation, and posttranslational integrity of the β-polypeptide chain. *Circled numerals* at various positions of the gene diagram at the top indicate the positions within the gene at which structural lesions are located. The lesions, numbered *1* through *11* down the left side, show the fine structure of these mutations.

cursor into mature mRNA in the nucleus or prevent translation of the mRNA in the cytoplasm.

Other less common but informative thalassemia mutations have been described. The patient may have a severe β-thalassemia phenotype, but the β-globin gene and its promoters are present and have entirely normal nucleotide sequences. This thalassemia phenotype may be caused by deletion of the LCR sequences needed for high levels of expression in developing RBCs. These LCR sequences are located thousands of bases upstream from the ε-globin gene of the β-globin gene cluster.

In each β-thalassemia syndrome, inadequate amounts of hemoglobin tetramers are produced because the supply of β globin is reduced. Hypochromia and microcytosis result. Among heterozygotes (β-thalassemia trait), this is the only abnormality, and the anemia is minimal. Unbalanced α- and β-globin accumulation also occurs. Excess α-globin chains accumulate because the α-globin genes continue to be expressed at a normal level. These α-globin chains are highly insoluble. They precipitate in early erythroblast precursors of homozygotes, forming inclusion bodies that exert toxic effects, killing most erythroblast precursors in the marrow. Massive ineffective erythropoiesis results. Few of the proerythroblasts beginning erythroid maturation in the bone marrow survive. The occasional RBC that survives and makes it out of the bone marrow bears a burden of inclusion bodies. These cells are sequestered in the spleen. The RBC life span is shortened, producing severe hemolytic anemia.

These factors combined produce profound deficits in the oxygen-carrying capacity of the blood. Erythropoietin is produced in an attempt to stimulate compensatory erythroid hyperplasia, but the marrow response is sabotaged by the inclusion body–mediated ineffective erythropoiesis. Profound anemia persists despite massive bone marrow expansion, driving erythroid hyperplasia to still higher levels and becoming so exuberant in some cases that masses of extramedullary erythropoietic tissue form in the abdomen or pelvis.

Massive bone marrow expansion has adverse effects on growth and development. Children with thalassemia have characteristic chipmunk facies owing to maxillary marrow hyperplasia and frontal bossing. Thinning and pathologic fracture of the long bones and vertebrae caused by cortical invasion by erythroid elements and profound growth retardation and endocrine deficiencies are common. Hemolytic anemia causes hepatosplenomegaly and high-output congestive heart failure. The metabolic drain caused by the conscription of so many caloric resources for erythroid hyperplasia leads to inanition, susceptibility to infection, and in the most severe cases, death during the first 20 years of life. Treatment with RBC transfusions sufficient to maintain a hematocrit of more than 30% improves oxygen delivery, suppresses the excessive ineffective erythropoiesis, and prolongs life. Without aggressive iron chelation therapy, complications of chronic transfusion therapy, notably iron overload, usually prove fatal before the age of 30 years.

The severity of β-thalassemia varies markedly among patients. Many factors contribute to this clinical heterogeneity. Individual alleles vary with respect to severity of the biosynthetic lesion. Other modulating factors ameliorate the burden of unpaired α-globin inclusion bodies. Coinheritance of the α-thalassemia trait reduces clinical severity by restricting production of excess α globin. High levels of fetal hemoglobin expression persist to various degrees in β-thalassemia. γ-Globin gene expression supplies γ chains as a substitute for β chains, simultaneously generating more functional hemoglobin and reducing the α-globin inclusion burden. This marked clinical heterogeneity has led to adoption of the terms *β-thalassemia major* and *β-thalassemia intermedia*. Patients with β-thalassemia major need intensive transfusion support to survive. Patients with β-thalassemia intermedia have somewhat milder clinical complications and can survive without transfusion. *β-Thalassemia minor* is the term sometimes used to describe asymptomatic β-thalassemia among heterozygotes (β-thalassemia trait).

α-THALASSEMIA SYNDROMES

The four classic types of α-thalassemia are α-thalassemia-2 trait, in which one of the four α-globin genes fails to function; α-thalassemia-1 trait, with two dysfunctional genes; HbH disease, with three genes affected; and hydrops fetalis with Hb Bart's with all four genes defective. These syndromes usually are caused by deletion, respectively, of one, two, three, or all four of the α genes (Fig. 241.7). Deletions of α-globin genes are much more common than deletions of β-globin genes because duplication of the α-globin genes on chromosome 16 causes a marked increase in the risk of homologous recombination. Nondeletion forms of α-thalassemia have been described. They are caused by mutations similar to those described for β-thalassemia.

α-Thalassemia-2 trait is an asymptomatic, silent carrier state produced through deletion or dysfunction of a single α-globin gene. α-Thalassemia-1 trait is caused by deletion or dysfunction of two α-globin genes. Offspring from one person with α-thalassemia-2 trait and another with α-thalassemia-1 trait can have a form of thalassemia more severe than that caused by either trait alone, called *HbH disease*. In Asian and Mediterranean populations, a deletion that removes both genes from the same chromosome (*cis*-deletion) is common, as is homozygosity for α-thalassemia-2 (*trans*-deletion). Both produce asymptomatic hypochromia and microcytosis.

HbH disease usually is caused by coinheritance of the *cis*-α-thalassemia-1 deletion and α-thalassemia-2 trait. HbA production is only 25% to 30% of normal; unpaired γ chains accumulate during gestation, and unpaired β chains accumulate during adult life. The unpaired β-globin chains are somewhat more soluble than the α-globin chains that accumulate in β-thalassemia, forming recognizable $β_4$-tetramers called HbH. HbH forms very few inclusions in erythroblasts; rather, it precipitates from circulating RBCs. Patients with HbH disease usually have the clinical signs and symptoms of thalassemia intermedia characterized by a moderately severe hemolytic anemia with relatively mild ineffective erythropoiesis. Patients with HbH disease often survive into adult life and usually are not dependent on blood transfusions.

Hydrops fetalis with HB Bart's is caused by total absence of α-globin synthesis caused by the homozygous state for the α-thalassemia-1 *cis*-deletion. No physiologically useful hemoglobin is produced beyond the embryonic stage. Free γ globin accumulates, forming tetramers called *Hb Bart's*. Hb Bart's has an extraordinarily high oxygen affinity, comparable with that of myoglobin. It binds oxygen delivered to the placenta but delivers almost none of it to fetal tissues. Severe anemia and asphyxia occur at the tissue level, causing profound edema (hydrops), congestive heart failure, and death in utero. Advances in prenatal diagnosis and the early institution of intrauterine blood transfusions have allowed a small number of live births. Unfortunately, most of the infants have permanent damage to the central nervous system.

α-Thalassemia-2 trait is common among people of African descent, with a gene frequency of 15% to 30% in some populations. The *cis*-α-thalassemia-1 deletion almost never occurs, however. Although α-thalassemia-2 and the *trans* form of α-thalassemia-1 are common, HbH disease and hydrops fetalis are almost never encountered among blacks.

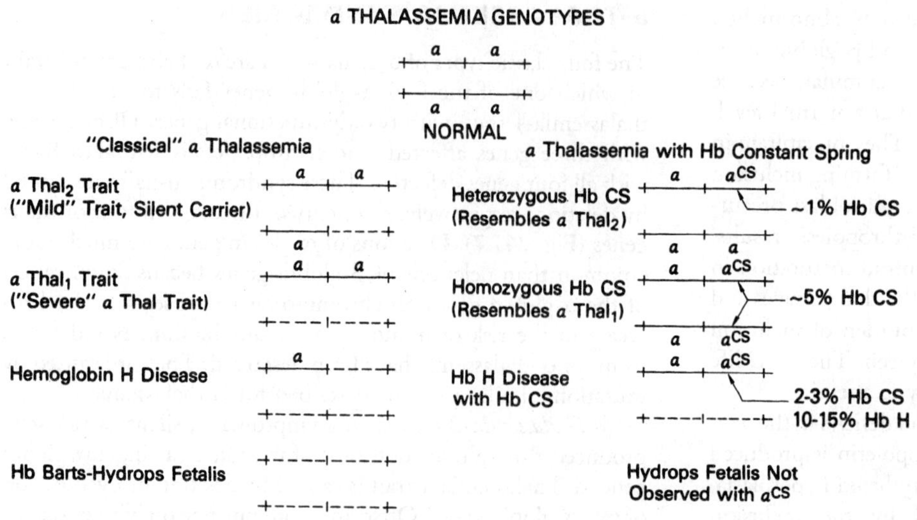

FIGURE 241.7. Classic forms of α-thalassemia with and without the Hb Constant Spring type of hemoglobin. *Top,* Normal duplicated α-globin genes (four gene loci per diploid cell). *Left,* The four classic forms of α-thalassemia that produced through deletion of one, two, three, or all four loci. *Right,* α-Thalassemia syndromes caused by Hb Constant Spring.

THALASSEMIC STRUCTURAL VARIANTS

Thalassemic structural variants are abnormal hemoglobins characterized by a biosynthetic defect and abnormal structure. The few examples considered herein are either particularly instructive examples or are clinically relevant because they are common.

Hemoglobin Lepore

Hb Lepore—$\alpha_2(\delta\beta)_2$—is the prototype of a group of hemoglobinopathies characterized by fused globin chains. These hemoglobinopathies are caused by unequal crossover and recombination events that fuse the proximal end of one gene with the distal end of a closely linked gene downstream. During meiosis, mispairing and crossover of the highly homologous δ and β genes can occur, resulting in a Lepore chromosome that contains only the fused δβ gene and an anti-Lepore chromosome that contains the reciprocal fusion product (βδ) and intact β- and δ-globin genes.

Lepore globin is synthesized in small amounts because the fusion gene is under the control of the δ-globin promoter, which normally sustains transcription at only 2% to 5% the level of the β-globin promoter. Because there are no other β-like globin genes on this chromosome, patients with Hb Lepore have the phenotype of β-thalassemia, differentiated by the added presence of 2% to 10% Hb Lepore and slightly increased levels of HbF in the 3% to 5% range. Anti-Lepore globin is not associated with thalassemia because of the presence of an intact β-globin gene on the same chromosome. Heterozygotes for Hb Lepore have the clinical phenotype of β-thalassemia trait; homozygotes behave as patients with homozygous β-thalassemia. Compound heterozygotes for Hb Lepore and a classic β-thalassemia allele also can have severe thalassemia. The presence of Hb Lepore should be suspected when a person with hypochromic microcytic RBCs also produces an abnormal hemoglobin that migrates in the position of HbS on routine electrophoretic gels.

Hemoglobin E

HbE ($\alpha_2\beta_2^{26Glu\rightarrow Lys}$) is extremely common in Cambodia, Thailand, and Vietnam. Heterozygotes resemble persons with mild β-thalassemia trait. Homozygotes have somewhat more marked abnormalities but no symptoms. Compound heterozygotes for HbE and a β-thalassemia gene can have β-thalassemia intermedia or β-thalassemia major, depending on the severity of the coinherited thalassemic gene. HbE is mildly unstable, but this instability by itself is insufficient to greatly affect the life span of RBCs. The high frequency of the presence of HbE gene may be a result of the thalassemia phenotype associated with its inheritance.

The only nucleotide sequence abnormality found in the β^E gene is the base change in codon 26 that causes the amino acid substitution. This mutation occurs at a cryptic RNA splice site. It alters the consensus sequence surrounding a potential GT donor splice site, activating the site. Alternate splicing at this position occurs 40% to 50% of the time, generating a structurally abnormal globin mRNA that cannot be translated. The 40% to 50% of mRNA precursors spliced at the normal sites generate functional mRNA that is translated into β^E globin because the mature mRNA carries the base change that alters codon 26.

HbE is important because it is so common in Southeast Asian populations. However, the prevalence of this gene in some parts of the United States has increased markedly with the increase in migration of Asians to the United States. For example, HbE has become the most common mutant hemoglobin detected in California. Genetic counseling of persons at risk should be directed at avoidance of the interaction between HbE and β-thalassemia, rather than HbE homozygosity. HbE is an instructive example of the pleiotropic mechanisms by which single mutations can give rise to a genetic disease.

HEREDITARY PERSISTENCE OF FETAL HEMOGLOBIN

The term *hereditary persistence of fetal hemoglobin* (HPFH) refers to a group of rare disorders characterized by continued synthesis of high levels of HbF in adult life. Patients have no deleterious effects, even when all the hemoglobin produced is HbF. These patients demonstrate convincingly that prevention or reversal of the fetal to adult hemoglobin switch would provide efficacious therapy for sickle cell anemia and β-thalassemia. Two main types of HPFH have been described. *Pancellular HPFH* is characterized by high levels of fetal hemoglobin synthesis and uniform distribution of HbF among all RBCs. *Heterocellular HPFH* is caused by inherited increases in the number of F cells.

Pancellular HPFH is divisible into two classes. The *deletion* forms are caused by large (80- to 100-kb) deletions within the β-globin gene cluster that appear to bring potent enhancer sequences into the proximity of the γ-globin genes, promoting their high expression. In *nondeletion* HPFH, single-base changes occur in the proximal promoter regions of the affected γ-globin gene, resulting in overexpression in adult life.

Most cases of heterocellular HPFH appear to be caused by mutations outside the β-globin gene cluster on chromosome 11. In some families, HbF is elevated only when factors that produce erythroid stress, such as sickle cell anemia, are present. The latter mechanism appears to account for the high levels of fetal hemoglobin in areas such as the eastern provinces of Saudi Arabia, where sickle cell disease is phenotypically very mild.

ACQUIRED HEMOGLOBINOPATHIES

The two most important acquired hemoglobinopathies are carbon monoxide poisoning and methemoglobinemia. Abnormalities of hemoglobin biosynthesis have been described in blood dyscrasias. An elevated HbF occasionally accompanies proliferation of an abnormal clone in myelodysplastic syndromes. Some patients with erythroleukemia and myeloproliferative disorders may have a mild form of HbH disease. The abnormalities frequently are restricted to one or a few clones of abnormal RBCs and are not severe enough to alter the course of the underlying disease.

MANAGEMENT OF THALASSEMIA

The diagnosis of β-thalassemia major usually is apparent during infancy and childhood. Severe anemia is accompanied by the characteristic signs of massive ineffective erythropoiesis with hepatosplenomegaly, profound microcytosis, characteristic results of a blood smear, and elevated levels of HbF, HbA_2, or both. These children should be cared for in consultation with a hematologist. Most need long-term transfusion therapy. Hypertransfusion should be directed at maintenance of a hematocrit greater than 27% to 30% so that erythropoiesis is suppressed. Splenectomy often is needed; it usually is performed if the annual transfusion requirement, expressed as volume of RBCs per kilogram of body weight, increases more than 50%. In most other respects, management is largely supportive. Folic acid supplements may be useful. Vaccination with Pneumovax in anticipation of eventual splenectomy is advised, as is close monitoring for infection, leg ulcers, and biliary tract disease. Early endocrine evaluation for glucose intolerance, thyroid dysfunction, and delayed onset of puberty or secondary sexual characteristics is indicated. Many patients have endocrine deficiencies as a result of iron overload.

Patients with β-thalassemia intermedia have the same signs and symptoms as those with β-thalassemia major but can survive without long-term transfusion. Management is particularly challenging because a number of factors can aggravate the anemia, including infection, onset of puberty, and development of splenomegaly and hypersplenism. Some patients benefit from splenectomy. The expanded erythron can cause absorption of excessive dietary iron and hemosiderosis, even without transfusion.

β-Thalassemia minor (thalassemia trait) usually is asymptomatic. The hallmark is profound microcytosis with only minimal or mild anemia. Mean corpuscular volume is rarely greater than 75 fL; hematocrit rarely is less than 30% to 33%. Hemoglobin electrophoresis classically reveals an elevated HbA_2 level (3.5% to 7.5%), but HbF, rather than HbA_2, may be elevated if the patient has δβ-thalassemia. The peripheral blood smear shows hypochromia and microcytic RBCs with many target cells. Reassurance, genetic counseling, and patient education usually are all that is needed. Patients with β-thalassemia trait should be alerted to the fact that their blood profile resembles that of iron deficiency and can be misdiagnosed. They should eschew routine use of iron. Iron deficiency can develop as among other persons, however, such as during pregnancy or from chronic bleeding. These patients should not be given the impression that iron is never appropriate.

The RBCs of persons with α-thalassemia trait are hypochromic, but the patients usually do not have anemia. HbA_2 and HbF levels are normal. The patients usually need only genetic counseling. Hydrops fetalis rarely is associated with survival beyond the perinatal period. HbH disease resembles β-thalassemia intermedia with the added complication that the HbH molecule behaves as a moderately unstable hemoglobin. Patients with HbH disease should undergo splenectomy if excessive anemia or a transfusion requirement develops. Oxidative drugs should be avoided. In severe cases of HbH disease, iron overload and death may happen in early adulthood.

Antenatal diagnosis of thalassemia syndromes is readily available, even though the techniques are used in clinical practice at only a few centers throughout the world. The best tests involve direct analysis of genes for specific mutations that predominate in a given area. Molecular epidemiologic studies have allowed investigators to identify the five to seven mutations that usually account for 90% to 99% of patients at risk in a given geographic area. These methods have dramatically reduced the incidence of homozygous thalassemia births in Greece, Sardinia, Cyprus, and parts of Italy. DNA diagnosis is based on polymerase chain reaction amplification of fetal DNA obtained through amniocentesis or chorionic villus biopsy followed by hybridization to allele-specific oligonucleotides probes. The probes can be designed to detect simultaneously the subset of mutations that account for 95% to 99% of the instances of β-thalassemia that occur in a particular ethnic group.

■ STRATEGIES FOR OPTIMAL CARE

The management of specific hemoglobinopathies is described earlier. A few important situations or new approaches to these disorders are as follows.

MANAGEMENT OF TRANSFUSIONAL HEMOSIDEROSIS

Long-term blood transfusion is associated with many untoward complications: blood-borne infection, alloimmunization, and iron overload. Iron overload can be lethal to patients undergoing long-term transfusion. Thalassemia and other forms of anemia associated with accelerated erythropoiesis predispose patients to more rapid development of iron overload than situations in which the erythron is not expanded, such as aplastic anemia and pure RBC aplasia. The expanded erythron provokes excessive absorption of dietary iron, exacerbating the hemosiderosis.

Healthy persons need 1 to 2 mg elemental iron each day, an amount readily delivered in most diets. A unit of packed RBCs contains 250 to 300 mg iron (1 mg per milliliter), and a single transfusion of two units of packed RBCs is about equal to a 1- to 2-year intake of iron. There are no mechanisms for increasing the excretion of iron beyond normal daily losses. Iron rapidly accumulates in patients undergoing long-term transfusion therapy.

Transfused iron is at first safely sequestered in the form of ferritin and hemosiderin, but patients who receive more than 100 units of packed RBCs usually have symptoms of iron overload, such as endocrine dysfunction, glucose intolerance, delayed puberty, cirrhosis of the liver, and cardiomyopathy. The diagnosis is made by means of assessment of ferritin level or liver biopsy, which shows parenchymal and reticuloendothelial iron. There are other accurate and noninvasive methods for assessing iron in the liver, such as use of a superconducting quantum-interference device (SQUID). However, such instruments are not widely available around the world. Cardiac toxicity includes early development of pericarditis and later dysrhythmia and pump failure. The onset of clinically apparent pump failure is an ominous finding, often presaging death within a year.

Therapy for iron overload is largely ineffective after symptoms have become apparent. It is essential to anticipate the need for long-term transfusion support and to institute therapy with iron-chelating agents relatively early in life. The only approved and available iron chelator is deferoxamine mesylate (Desferal). This drug is extremely expensive, however, and poorly absorbed from the gastrointestinal tract. Its iron-binding kinetics are such that chronic, slow, subcutaneous infusion of the drug is necessary. In effect, patients benefit most from iron chelation therapy if a chelator is present most of the time in the bloodstream. The constant presence of the drug improves the efficiency of chelation and protects tissues from occasional releases of the most toxic fraction of iron—low-molecular-weight iron—which may not be sequestered by protective proteins.

Oral iron-chelating agents such as deferiprone have shown considerable promise in early clinical trials. However, long-term trials have raised some doubts about the efficacy and safety of these drugs. Thus the role of these new agents in the management of iron overload in thalassemia remains to be determined. The only currently established method for iron chelation, however, is long-term subcutaneous infusion of desferoxamine mesylate through a metered pump. Patients vary greatly in their ability to excrete iron when treated with deferoxamine mesylate. Candi-

dates should first be given a test dose, and iron excretion in the urine should be monitored for 24 hours. Long-term therapy varies greatly with respect to dose and scheduling of pumping time among different medical centers. Specific recommendations cannot be provided herein. Patients should be treated in consultation with a center that has expertise in this area.

Long-term use of high doses of deferoxamine mesylate is occasionally associated with the development of cataracts and deafness. Local skin reactions, including urticaria, are common, but there are few other acute side effects. Skin reactions usually can be managed with antihistamines. Intensive iron chelation therapy is effective in the sense that negative iron balance can be achieved, even in the face of a high transfusion requirement. However, restoration of iron balance does not ensure prevention of long-term morbidity and mortality among patients undergoing long-term transfusion therapy. Patients with β-thalassemia major appear to have a significant survival advantage when therapy is started before 5 to 8 years of age. Irreversible end-organ damage may start at relatively modest levels of iron overload, even if symptoms do not appear for many years thereafter. Most experts recommend institution of therapy early in the course of a long-term transfusion regimen because it seems clear that iron toxicity can begin even at early stages.

EXPERIMENTAL THERAPIES FOR HEMOGLOBINOPATHY

Several new approaches to definitive treatment of hemoglobinopathy are being actively investigated. These include bone marrow transplantation, gene therapy, and pharmacologic induction of HbF synthesis. Bone marrow transplantation has been used to treat a large number of patients with β-thalassemia and a small number of patients with sickle cell anemia. Bone marrow transplantation replaces the patient's stem cells with cells capable of producing adequate amounts of normal hemoglobin. The outcome is excellent when the procedure is performed early in the course of disease before end-organ damage occurs. Cure is achieved among more than 90% of patients. When the procedure is performed in centers with considerable experience in bone marrow transplantation, the mortality is less than 10%. Even a low mortality such as this is difficult to accept, however, in the care of patients with nonmalignant disorders when survival into adult life is possible with conventional therapy.

Gene therapy in which a normal β- or γ-globin gene is inserted into the genome of the patient's own hematopoietic stem cells is another therapeutic modality that might provide cures for patients with hemoglobin disorders. Although the human β-globin gene was one of the first human genes used in retroviral gene transfer experiments, application of this new technology to gene therapy for thalassemia and sickle cell disease has been exceptionally difficult. The earlier generations of globin retroviral vectors suffered from genetic instability and low titers and gave rise to low-level expression of the transferred β-globin gene in transduced erythroid cells. The efficiency of gene transfer into nondividing hematopoietic stem cells was disappointingly low. Several groups of investigators have solved the problems of genetic instability, low titers, and low-level expression in transduced cells. However, the problem of low efficiency of retrovirus-mediated gene transfer into nondividing hematopoietic stem cells has remained intractable. The development of lentivirus-type vectors that can transduce nondividing cells offers considerable hope for solving the problem of low efficiency of gene transfer into hematopoietic stem cells. Once this is achieved, gene therapy should become a therapeutic option for patients with hemoglobin disorders.

Patients with β-chain hemoglobinopathy could be effectively treated by means of reestablishment of high levels of fetal hemoglobin synthesis. The clinical well-being of patients with hereditary persistence of fetal hemoglobin validates this strategy. Initial attempts to stimulate HbF synthesis were based on the fact that the γ-globin genes were found to be heavily methylated in adult erythroid cells. Methylation of the GC base pairs in 5' regions of genes has been known for some time to correlate with inactivation of expression of many genes. In experimental systems and in laboratory animals, administration of 5'-azacitidine, a drug that inhibits methylation of genes, was shown to markedly stimulate HbF synthesis. A short-term clinical trial with this agent to treat patients with thalassemia had the same effect. One patient needed no transfusions during the short course of the study. Unfortunately, 5'-azacitidine is too toxic and carcinogenic for wide use, especially in the care of children.

The augmentation of fetal hemoglobin synthesis obtained with 5'-azacitidine could be replicated by other chemotherapeutic agents such as hydroxyurea, which does not have any DNA-hypomethylating activity. Cytotoxic agents such as hydroxyurea and cytarabine promote high levels of HbF synthesis by means of stimulating proliferation of the primitive HbF-potent progenitor cell population (F-cell progenitors), accounting for increased levels of fetal hemoglobin. The mechanisms by which these events occur remain mysterious. In a randomized, placebo-controlled, multicenter clinical trial, the use of hydroxyurea led to a decrease in the incidence of the two most common complications of sickle cell disease (vaso-occlusive crises and acute chest syndrome). Although hydroxyurea has also shown some HbF-inducing activity in patients with β-thalassemia, no dose regimen has been identified yet that corrects the anemia and ameliorates the clinical manifestations of the disease. In spite of encouraging results of therapy for sickle cell disease with hydroxyurea, there are some lingering concerns about long-term toxicity of a DNA-damaging agent such as hydroxyurea. Butyrate belongs to a group of short-chain fatty acids that are also capable of stimulating HbF production in tissue culture cells and in several animal species. Results of the initial short-term human study with butyrate were encouraging. Results of a longer study showed loss of the initial HbF response after extended therapy with continuous high doses of arginine butyrate. The use of newer therapeutic regimens based on pulse or intermittent administration of butyrate caused sustained induction of HbF among most patients with sickle cell disease. It is still not clear whether butyrate will have similar activity in patients with β-thalassemia.

APLASTIC CRISIS AMONG PATIENTS WITH HEMOGLOBINOPATHY

Patients with chronic hemolytic anemia rely on high levels of erythropoiesis. Because of the shortened life span of their circulating RBCs, even transient depression of erythropoiesis can profoundly aggravate anemia. Healthy persons can tolerate suppression of erythropoiesis for several days without serious effects, because less than 1% of the circulating RBCs are replaced every day. Patients with hemolytic anemia sometimes have an alarming decline in hematocrit during and immediately after acute illnesses. These hypoplastic crises usually are transient and self-correcting before intervention is needed. These events probably represent an exaggerated manifestation of the suppression of bone marrow function that occurs in almost everyone during acute inflammatory illnesses. They can occur repeatedly during adult and childhood years.

Aplastic crisis refers to a profound cessation of erythroid activity among patients with chronic hemolytic anemia. It is associated with a rapidly falling hematocrit. Episodes usually are self-limited. Aplastic crises are caused by infection with a particular strain of parvovirus, B19A. Children with this viral infection usually develop permanent immunity. Aplastic crises do not often reoccur and are rare among adults. Management requires close monitoring of hematocrit and reticulocyte count. If anemia becomes symptomatic, transfusion support is indicated. Most crises resolve within 7 to 14 days.

Kelley's Textbook of Internal Medicine, fourth edition. Edited by H. David Humes. Lippincott Williams & Wilkins, Philadelphia © 2000.

C H A P T E R

242

IRON DEFICIENCY AND IRON LOADING ANEMIAS

KENNETH R. BRIDGES

IRON DEFICIENCY

Iron deficiency is a leading cause of anemia, affecting more than one-half billion people worldwide. Among adults, blood loss nearly invariably is the culprit. The high demand for iron that accompanies neonatal and adolescent growth spurts occasionally produces iron deficiency among children. Nevertheless, blood loss is the most frequent cause of iron deficiency for this group as well. Body iron stores for women normally vary between 1 and 2 g, whereas men average 3 to 4 g. The liver is the site of most stored iron. Depletion of iron stores precedes impaired production of iron-containing proteins, the most prominent of which is hemoglobin. The two important stages of iron deficiency are (a) depletion of iron stores without anemia and (b) depletion of iron stores with anemia. Therapy for iron deficiency cannot be comfortably undertaken until the cause of the iron deficit is ascertained.

ETIOLOGY

Abnormal Iron Uptake from the Gastrointestinal Tract

Although iron is the second most abundant metal in the earth's crust, its low solubility makes acquisition for metabolic use a challenge. Iron is not maintained in an easily absorbed form in the absence of gastric acid. Surgical interventions, such as vagotomy or hemigastrectomy for peptic ulcer disease, formerly were the major causes of impaired gastric acidification with secondary iron deficiency. Today the use of histamine H_2 blockers and acid pump blockers to manage peptic ulcer disease and acid reflux is among the most common causes of defective iron absorption. Although this complication is infrequent, use of these medications is widespread. Consequently, the likelihood of physicians' encountering secondary iron deficiency with use of these medications is rising.

The impaired function of the gastric parietal cells associated with pernicious anemia not only reduces production of intrinsic factor but also lessens gastric acidity. Impaired iron absorption can result. In addition, the megaloblastic enterocytes absorb iron poorly. Frank iron deficiency can accompany the anemia produced by cobalamin deficiency.

Disruption of the Enteric Mucosa

Some disorders, such as Crohn's disease, disrupt the integrity of the enteric mucosa and hamper iron absorption. Occult gastrointestinal bleeding exacerbates the problem of iron balance. Sprue, both the tropical and the nontropical variety (celiac disease), also can interfere with iron absorption. The disease can be mild to the point that it produces few or no symptoms. A gluten-free diet improves bowel function for many such patients, and anemia is corrected.

Blood Loss

Blood loss is the world's leading cause of iron deficiency. Menstrual blood loss is the primary physiologic cause of blood loss. Bleeding into the gastrointestinal tract is the most common cause of pathologic blood loss. Structural defects that bleed into the gastrointestinal tract can be malignant, such as adenocarcinoma of the colon, or benign, such as duodenal peptic ulcer. The rate of blood loss frequently is so low that symptoms of severe anemia are the first indication of bleeding.

The world's leading cause of gastrointestinal blood loss is parasitic infestation. Hookworm infection, caused primarily by *Necator americanus* or *Ancylostoma duodenale,* affects more than one billion people, most in tropical or subtropical areas. Daily blood loss exceeds 11 million liters. *Trichuris trichiura,* or whipworm, is believed to infest the colons of 600 to 700 million persons, about 10% to 15% of whom have iron deficiency. Urinary blood loss usually is sufficiently alarming that patients seek medical attention before substantial iron deficiency develops. Although pulmonary blood loss sufficiently severe to produce iron deficiency occurs, the phenomenon is distinctly rare, (as in chronic infection that causes bronchiectasis).

Chronic intravascular hemolysis occasionally produces iron deficiency due to loss of iron into the urine. Paroxysmal nocturnal hemoglobinuria is a classic but uncommon culprit in this regard. Two proteins in the circulation, haptoglobin and hemopexin, guard against such losses. The former complexes tightly with any hemoglobin in the plasma and is cleared by the liver. The latter binds free heme in the circulation to form a complex that also is cleared by the liver. The binding capacity of these two proteins is relatively low, however. Chronic intravascular hemolysis can overwhelm these two systems, allowing renal filtration of hemoglobin dimers (molecular weight 32 kd). The renal tubule cells absorb the hemoglobin dimers, digest the protein, and retain the iron as hemosiderin. When the tubule cells slough into the urine, the hemosiderin can be detected by means of Perls' Prussian blue staining. Intravascular hemolysis can be documented long after the event because renal tubule cells are not shed completely for weeks.

CONSEQUENCES OF IRON DEFICIENCY

Although anemia is the problem most prominently linked to iron deficiency, the condition produces a wide range of abnormalities, depending on its severity and duration. Some of these abnormalities, such as cognitive dysfunction among children, have been recognized only recently.

Anemia

Microcytic, hypochromic anemia impairs tissue oxygen delivery and produces weakness, fatigue, palpitations, and light-headedness. The rate at which anemia develops greatly influences the severity of the symptoms. Very severe anemias, for example, a hemoglobin level of 4 or 5 g per deciliter, occurs among some patients who have iron deficiency caused by slow, chronic bleeding. Often these patients report only mild fatigue. Among older patients, angina from cardiac ischemia can be the first symptom of iron deficiency.

Thalassemia trait is sometimes confused with iron deficiency. Iron deficiency unevenly alters the size of red blood cell. Electronic blood analyzers are used to determine mean corpuscular volume and the range of variation in red cell size (expressed as red blood cell distribution width, RDW). RDW, which is measured with every electronically processed complete blood cell count, is normal among patients with thalassemia trait but is high among those with iron deficiency. Other common features of thalassemia trait are basophilic stippling and the presence of target cells. These characteristics are not sufficiently unique, however, to differentiate thalassemia trait from iron deficiency.

Growth and Developmental Retardation

Iron deficiency with or without concomitant anemia commonly impairs growth and intellectual development among children. Current data indicate that some of the injury is irreversible. Concomitant lead exposure can further hamper the psychological development of these children. The mechanism by which iron deficiency impairs neurologic function is unknown. Many enzymes in neural tissue require iron for normal function. The cytochromes involved in energy production, for example, predominantly are heme proteins. Iron deficiency may impair cytochrome synthesis and produce an energy deficit during the formative years of neural cell growth and development.

The effect of iron deficiency on childhood growth is difficult to separate from overall nutritional deficiency. The high prevalence of childhood iron deficiency among less affluent people has yoked deficiencies of iron and general nutrients. When the two factors are separated, correction of iron deficiency improves growth independently of nutritional status.

Epithelial Changes

Iron deficiency alters the gastrointestinal tract, reflecting the enormous proliferative capacity of this organ. Some patients have angular stomatitis and glossitis with painful swelling of the tongue. The flattened, atrophic lingual papillae make the tongue smooth and shiny. A rare complication of iron deficiency is Plummer–Vinson syndrome with formation of a postcrycoid esophageal web. Long-standing, severe iron deficiency affects the cells that generate the fingernails and produces koilonychia, or spooning. The nail substance is so soft, that ordinary pressure on the fingertips, as occurs with writing, produces a concave deformity. Most of these abnormalities are now uncommon among industrialized nations.

Miscellaneous

Pica occurs variably among patients with iron deficiency. The precise pathophysiologic mechanism of the syndrome is unknown. Patients consume unusual items, such as laundry starch, ice, and soil clay. Both clay and starch can bind iron in the gastrointestinal tract, exacerbating the deficiency.

Unexplained thrombocytosis occurs frequently with platelet counts of 500,000 to 700,000 cells per femtoliter. Megakaryocytes and normoblasts are derived from a common committed progenitor cell, the colony-forming unit–granulocytic, erythroid, myelomonocytic. Thrombopoietin, the molecule that stimulates megakaryocyte growth and platelet production, is structurally homologous to erythropoietin, the molecule that promotes red blood cell development. Some investigators have speculated that elevated levels of erythropoietin among patients with iron deficiency anemia might modestly increase platelet production by cross-reacting with the thrombopoietic receptor. Results of investigations with recombinant human erythropoietin and thrombopoietin, however, indicate little cross-reactivity.

DIAGNOSIS OF IRON DEFICIENCY ANEMIA

Iron deficiency anemia lowers the number of circulating red blood cells, a feature of all types of anemia. The red blood cells are microcytic (usually less than 80 fL) and hypochromic. The quantity of the iron-carrying protein, transferrin, in the circula-

tion increases 50% to 100% over baseline. The quantity of iron on transferrin can decrease by as much as 90%. Consequently transferrin saturation frequently declines from its usual 30% to less than 10%. The most useful single laboratory value for the diagnosis of iron deficiency may be plasma ferritin level. Plasma ferritin level often falls to less than 10% of baseline level with substantial iron deficiency.

Other phenomena, such as chronic inflammation with rheumatoid arthritis, perturb the plasma values of iron, transferrin, and ferritin and complicate the diagnosis of iron deficiency among these patients. The situation is further obscured by the fact that chronic inflammation per se can produce anemia. Newer tests, such as assay of circulating transferring receptors, sometimes can help with the diagnosis of iron deficiency. If all else fails, bone marrow biopsy with Prussian blue staining for iron is the touchstone for the diagnosis.

THERAPY FOR IRON DEFICIENCY

The most important steps in the evaluation and management of iron deficiency are identifying the cause of the deficiency and correcting the abnormality. Malignant disease of the gastrointestinal tract is the haunting specter among adults with iron deficiency. After the cause of the iron deficiency has been ascertained, oral iron supplementation replaces stores most efficiently.

Oral Iron Supplementation

Oral iron supplementation is the ideal way to replace iron stores because the body's normal mechanisms are used. The shortcoming is the limited capacity of the gastrointestinal tract for iron absorption. Only about 5 to 10 mg of elemental iron is absorbed, even when 50 or 100 mg is presented to the gastrointestinal lumen. Most orally consumed iron flows untouched through the alimentary tract. Replenishing a 2,000 mg iron deficit can take most of a year. With ongoing blood loss, replacement of stores with oral iron becomes a Herculean task. Many if not most patients do not comply with such a prolonged medical regimen (Table 242.1).

TABLE 242.1.	CAUSES OF POOR RESPONSE TO ORAL IRON

Noncompliance
Ongoing blood loss
Insufficient duration of therapy
High gastric pH
    Antacids
    Histamine H_2 blockers
    Gastric acid pump inhibitors
Inhibition of iron absorption and utilization
    Lead
    Aluminum intoxication (hemodialysis patients)
    Chronic inflammation
    Neoplasia
Incorrect diagnosis
    Thalassemia
    Sideroblastic anemia

Parenteral Iron Replacement

Parenteral iron is available either as iron dextran or iron saccharide (commonly ferric polymaltose). Only iron dextran is available in the United States, whereas both forms are available throughout most of the rest of the world. Iron saccharide complexes are superior to iron dextran because they produce fewer side effects. Parenteral administration of iron is indicated when (a) oral iron is poorly tolerated, (b) rapid replacement of iron stores is needed, or (c) gastrointestinal iron absorption is compromised. Iron dextran can be administered by means of intramuscular or intravenous injection. A test dose of 10 mg iron should be given and the patient observed by a physician for 30 minutes to rule out an anaphylactic reaction to the medication (such reactions are infrequent). About 10% to 15% of patients experience transient mild to moderate arthralgia the day after intramuscular or intravenous administration of iron-dextran. Acetaminophen usually effectively relieves the discomfort. In uncomplicated cases of iron deficiency, intravenous replacement produces subjective improvement in a few days. Peak reticulocytosis occurs after about 10 days, and complete correction of the anemia can take 3 to 4 weeks.

FUNCTIONAL IRON DEFICIENCY

With steady-state erythropoiesis, iron and erythropoietin flow to the bone marrow at constant, low rates. Among patients with end-stage renal disease, recombinant human erythropoietin (rHepo) is administered in intermittent surges, most commonly as intravenous boluses. The resulting kinetics of erythropoiesis are markedly unphysiologic and strain the production process. Erythropoietin, the accelerator of erythroid proliferation is not coordinated with the supply of iron, the fuel for erythroid proliferation. This imbalance almost never occurs naturally. The rHepo jars previously quiescent cells to proliferate and produce hemoglobin. The requirement for iron jumps dramatically and outstrips the rate of delivery by transferrin. The late arrival of newly mobilized storage iron does not prevent production of hypochromic cells. This is functional iron deficiency or iron-erythropoietin kinetic imbalance. Functional iron deficiency is a major cause of erythropoietin resistance among patients with end-stage renal disease.

▌ IRON OVERLOAD

ETIOLOGY

Transfusional Iron Overload

A unit of blood (250 mL) contains about 225 mg iron. The iron is an integral component of the heme in hemoglobin and cannot be removed from the blood. Senescent red blood cells are destroyed by reticuloendothelial cells, primarily in the liver and spleen. The iron from the hemoglobin is not excreted. The elements either is used to make new red blood cells or is placed in storage (primarily in the liver). Among patients with transfusion-dependent anemia, nearly all of the iron from the transfused red blood cells goes into storage and eventually produces severe iron overload.

Erythroid Hyperplasia

The connection between hematopoiesis and iron absorption is most strikingly apparent among patients with ineffective erythropoiesis. Disorders such as β^+ thalassemia (thalassemia intermedia) or sideroblastic anemia increase the fractional absorption of ingested iron. Patients often have iron overload without transfusion. The mechanism by which bone marrow activity modulates gastrointestinal iron absorption is unclear. Without some compounding variable, such as hereditary hemochromatosis trait, iron loading without transfusion is uncommon in conditions such as sickle cell disease or hereditary spherocytosis, in which the increase in erythroid activity is less dramatic.

CONSEQUENCES OF IRON OVERLOAD

The effect of iron overload on some organs, such as the skin, is trivial, whereas hemosiderotic harm to other organs, such as the liver, can be fatal. Few unique symptoms precede advanced injury. Abdominal discomfort, lethargy, and fatigue are common but nonspecific characteristics. Dyspnea with exertion and peripheral edema indicate cardiac compromise and advanced iron loading.

Liver

As the main site of iron storage, the liver is a conspicuous victim of iron overload. Mild to moderate hepatomegaly develops early and is followed by shrinkage caused by fibrosis and cirrhosis. Hepatic tenderness occurs inconsistently. Hematoxylin and eosin staining reveals a sepia pigment in the hepatocytes that Perls' Prussian blue staining unmasks as iron. Large deposits of iron develop in the Kupfer cells of patients with transfusional iron overload, reflecting the destruction of senescent erythrocytes by these cells. This iron redistributes to the tissues, producing organ injury that is almost identical to that in hereditary hemochromatosis. Long-standing iron overload frequently fosters micronodular cirrhosis. Hemosiderotic liver damage produces very little inflammation. Hepatic iron deposition and even fibrosis can develop with very little increase in serum transaminase levels. Disturbances in liver synthetic function indicate advanced disease.

Heart

Congestive cardiomyopathy is the most common cardiac defect that occurs with iron overload, but other problems have been described, including pericarditis, restrictive cardiomyopathy, and angina without coronary artery disease. The cumulative number of blood transfusions correlates strongly with functional cardiac derangements among children with thalassemia.

The findings at physical examination are surprisingly benign even among patients with heavy cardiac iron deposition. Once evidence of cardiac failure appears, however, heart function rapidly deteriorates, often without response to medical intervention. Biventricular failure produces pulmonary congestion, peripheral edema, and hepatic engorgement. Vigorous iron extrication has occasionally reversed this potentially lethal cardiac complication.

The most useful noninvasive procedures are echocardiography for children and radionuclide ventriculography for adults. The echocardiographic abnormalities correlate roughly with the number of transfusions. Exercise radionuclide ventriculography is particularly sensitive in the detection of cardiac dysfunction among patients with iron overload.

Endocrine

Dysfunction of the endocrine pancreas is common among patients with iron overload. Some patients incur overt diabetes mellitus that necessitates insulin therapy. Disturbances in carbohydrate metabolism often are more subtle, however. An oral glucose tolerance test frequently unmasks abnormal insulin production in the absence of frank diabetes mellitus. Vigorous removal of the excess iron occasionally reverses the islet cell dysfunction. Exocrine pancreatic function, in contrast, usually is well preserved.

Pituitary dysfunction produces a plethora of endocrine abnormalities. Reduced gonadotropin levels are common. When the decrease in gonadotropin level is coupled with a primary reduction in gonadal synthesis of sex steroids, patients can suffer decreased libido or impotence. Although Addison's syndrome is uncommon with iron overload, production of corticotropin can be deficient. A metapyrone stimulation test shows delayed or diminished pituitary secretion of corticotropin.

Miscellaneous Abnormalities with Iron Overload

Hyperpigmentation is a nonspecific skin response to a variety of insults, including excessive exposure to ultraviolet light (tanning), thermal injury, and drug eruptions. Cutaneous iron deposition damages the skin and enhances melanin production by melanocytes. With particularly heavy iron overload, visible iron deposits sometimes appear in the skin as a grayish discoloration. Defective bone mineralization is a problem for patients with thalassemia. Osteoporosis weakens the bones, making the patients subject to fractures, both traumatic and pathologic. Arthropathy, a common feature of hereditary hemochromatosis, is rare among patients with transfusional iron overload due to acquired anemias. Other troubling musculoskeletal problems include severe, recurrent cramps and disabling myalgia. Muscle biopsy shows iron deposits in the myocytes, but the pathophysiologic connection between the pain and the cramps is unclear.

Iron Overload and Opportunistic Infections

Withholding iron from potential pathogens is one strategy used in host defense. The extremely high affinity of transferrin for iron coupled with the fact that two-thirds of the iron binding sites of the protein normally are unoccupied essentially eliminates free iron from plasma and extracellular tissues. Both trans-

TABLE 242.2. INFECTIONS ASSOCIATED WITH IRON OVERLOAD

Bacterial
  Listeria monocytogenes
  Yersinia enterocolitica
  Salmonella typhimurium
  Klebsiella pneumoniae
  Vibrio sputorum
  Escherichia coli
Fungal
  Cunninghamella bertholathae
  Rhizopus oryzae
  Mucor species

ferrin and the structurally related protein lactoferrin are bacteriostatic in vitro for many bacteria. The very high transferrin saturations that occur among patients with iron overload compromise the bacteriostatic properties of the protein. Iron sequestration is not a frontline defense against microbes. Therefore iron overload does not produce the susceptibility to infection that occurs with defects in more central systems (chronic granulomatous disease, for example.) Nevertheless, a number of infections, often with unusual organisms, have been reported among patients with iron overload (Table 242.2).

THERAPY FOR IRON OVERLOAD

Phlebotomy is the most effective means of removing excess iron. This option is not available to transfusion-dependent patients and is available to few patients with ineffective erythrophoresis. For patients with transfusional iron overload, chelation is the only available treatment.

Parenteral Chelation Therapy

Desferrioxamine (desferoxamine mesylate) is the most widely used chelator in the management of transfusional iron overload. Several characteristics of the drug place severe constraints on its use. First, absorption from the gastrointestinal tract is limited, dictating parenteral administration. Second, a bolus of the compound is excreted from the circulation with a half-life of only about 10 to 15 minutes. The chelator binds little or no iron during this time. Therefore slow, continuous parenteral administration is required. Third, desferrioxamine irritates tissues, meaning that only a small amount can be administered at a given site.

The practical translation is a drug given by means of continuous subcutaneous infusion with a rate-controlled pump. Skin irritation, manifested as raised, painful, erythematous welts, is less severe among children than among adults but is troublesome nevertheless. Patients can minimize but not eliminate the problem by rotating the infusion site daily. The infusion is given over 12 to 16 hours, allowing freedom from the pump for part of the day. Iron mobilization often falls to unacceptable levels when the infusion time is less than 12 hours. Desferrioxamine therapy is most effective when the pump is used daily. Few patients can conform to such a rigid schedule. The infusion should be conducted at least 5 days a week, however.

Otovestibular toxicity occurred in one group of children treated with doses of desferrioxamine that exceeded 150 μg per kilogram in some instances. Full recovery followed cessation of treatment. The drug produced no problems when reinitiated at a level of 25 to 50 μg per kilogram per day. Long-term chelation therapy with desferrioxamine sometimes produces bone disease. Chelation of minerals needed to form hydroxyapatite in developing bone is the presumed cause of this complication.

Oral Chelation Therapy

An orally effective iron chelator would be nirvana for patients with transfusional iron overload. None of the many agents advanced to date has met the exacting requirements for effective treatment. Only one drug occupies the field of competition, 1,2-dimethyl-3-hydroxypyrid-4-one, also called L1 or deferiprone. After early initial promise, L1 became embroiled in controversy. The issue at the center of the storm is whether L1 prevents progression of hepatic damage. Different groups of investigators have reached diametrically opposed conclusions with essentially the same data. This controversy, along with the infrequent but serious granulocytopenia that occurs with administration of the drug clouds the future of L1.

BIBLIOGRAPHY

Bini EJ, Micale PL, Weinshel EH. Evaluation of the gastrointestinal tract in premenopausal women with iron deficiency anemia. *Am J Med* 1988; 105:281–286.

Bonkovsky HL. Iron and the liver. *Am J Med Sci* 1991;301:32–43.

Bridges KR, Seligman PA. Disorders of iron metabolism. In: Handin R, et al., eds. *Blood*. Philadelphia: JB Lippincott, 1995:1433–1472.

Pippard MJ. Iron overload and iron chelation therapy in thalassaemia and sickle cell haemoglobinopathies. *Acta Haematol* 1987;78:206–211.

Pollitt E, Saco-Pollitt C, Ceibel RC, et al. Iron deficiency and behavioral development in infants and preschool children. *Am J Clin Nutr* 1986; 43:555–565.

Stoltzfus RJ, Dreyfuss ML, Chwaya HM, et al. Hookworm control as a strategy to prevent iron deficiency. *Nutr Rev* 1997;55:223–232.

Kelley's Textbook of Internal Medicine, fourth edition. Edited by H. David Humes.
Lippincott Williams & Wilkins, Philadelphia © 2000.

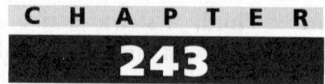

CHAPTER 243

MEGALOBLASTIC ANEMIAS

RALPH CARMEL

Megaloblastic anemia is a very characteristic disturbance of hematopoiesis that gives rise to large cells (macrocytosis) combined with nuclear abnormalities. All blood cell lines are affected—indeed, all dividing cells, such as skin and intestinal cells, show the same defect.

Several pathologic processes can produce megaloblastic anemia, but the most common by far are deficiencies of folate or cobalamin (vitamin B_{12}). These vitamin deficiencies are being identified with increasing frequency in patients who have little or no anemia, due, in part, to more sophisticated diagnostic approaches and earlier recognition.

■ NORMAL BIOCHEMISTRY AND PHYSIOLOGY

FOLATE

Biochemistry

Folic (pteroylglutamic) acid becomes metabolically active only upon reduction to tetrahydrofolic acid (THF) by dihydrofolate reductase (Fig. 243.1, reaction 1). Moreover, active folates have up to seven γ-carboxyl-linked glutamic acid side chains. This polyglutamated state enhances folate binding to enzymes and thus folate's coenzyme activity. It also is the usual intracellular form of folate because the highly polar polyglutamate side chain promotes cellular retention of the folate. Folates in the plasma are largely monoglutamates.

The main metabolic function of folate involves one-carbon unit transfers. Several amino acid conversions require folate; an important one is the methylation of homocysteine to methionine, with 5-methyl THF as a cosubstrate for methionine synthase (Fig. 243.1, reaction 4). Folate is also involved in purine synthesis. The clinically most apparent role, however, is in the methylation of deoxyuridine monophosphate to thymidine monophosphate by thymidylate synthase, which requires 5,10-methylene THF (Fig. 243.1, reaction 5). It is the compromise of this reaction in folate deficiency that leads to megaloblastic anemia. Precisely how the compromised reaction does so is unclear, because the diminished thymidylate synthesis appears to be compensated by the salvage pathway (Fig. 243.1, reaction 6), but there may be different thymidylate pools. Moreover, the deoxyuridine excess, along with the thymidylate insufficiency, promotes misincorporation of uracil in place of thymidine into DNA.

Nutrition, Absorption, and Metabolism

Folate derives its name from the leafy vegetables that are rich in it; many other foods, such as meat, dairy products, cereals, and flour, are also good sources. To avoid deficiency, adults normally require about 0.2 mg of folate daily. Total body stores vary but are about 10 mg. Thus, daily turnover is 1% to 2% of stores.

Food folate, largely reduced and usually methylated, is labile. For example, cooking fish, frying meat, or boiling vegetables can decrease the folate content of these foods by 50% to 90%. Even simple storage can diminish the folate content of some foods. Such information must be considered in assessing the adequacy of a patient's dietary intake. Moderate fortification

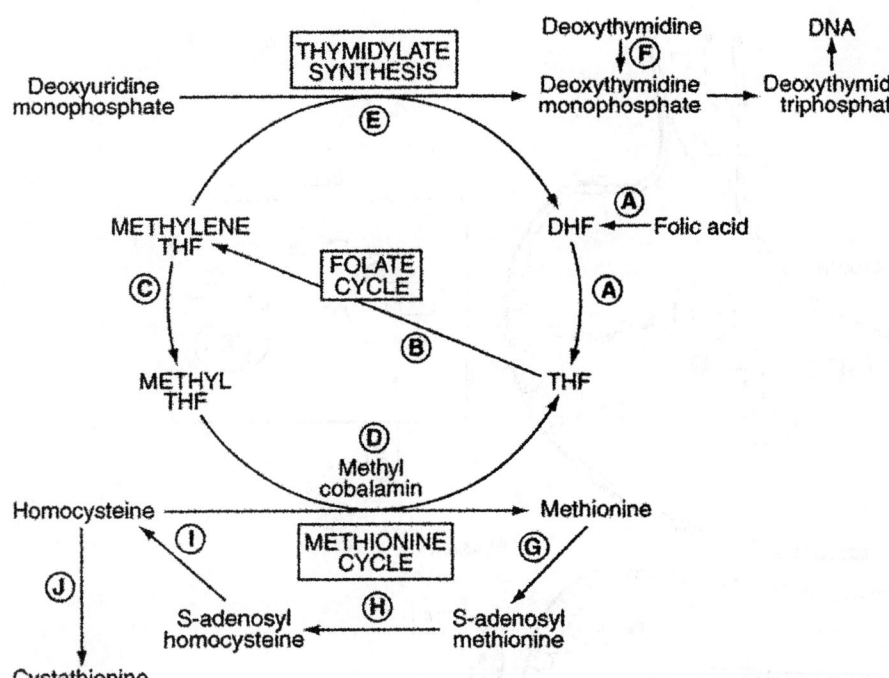

FIGURE 243.1. Folate metabolism and its interrelations with DNA synthesis (*top*) and cobalamin and homocysteine (*bottom*). This diagram includes only selected folate pathways in human beings. *1*, Two steps in the reduction of folic acid and dihydrofolate to tetrahydrofolate (THF), mediated by dihydrofolate reductase. *2*, The generation of 5, 10-methylene THF, coupled to serine-glycine metabolism. *3*, Reaction mediated by 5, 10-methylene THF reductase; this reaction is augmented when methionine and S-adenosylmethionine production falls, as might occur in cobalamin deficiency, and thus potentiates the "methyl THF trap." *4*, Reaction mediated by methionine synthase (homocysteine:methionine methyltransferase); it requires methylcobalamin and is the focal point of the methyl THF trap hypothesis. *5*, *De novo* synthesis of thymidine, mediated by thymidylate synthase. *6*, Salvage pathway of thymidylate synthesis, mediated by thymidine kinase. *7*, In addition to its remethylation to methionine (reaction 4), homocysteine is also metabolized to cystathionine; the initial reaction in the transsulfuration pathway is mediated by cystathionine β-synthase and pyridoxal phospate.

with folate of all cereal-grain products was mandated by the Food and Drug Administration in 1998.

Dietary folate is absorbed after its polyglutamate side chain is converted by folate conjugase to the monoglutamate form, which more readily crosses membranes. Most nonmethylated folate is also converted to methyl THF during absorption. Medicinal folic acid is absorbed to a large extent by a different process than is food folate. The efficiency of absorption depends on the form of folate, but usually more than 60% is absorbed; the process is an active, saturable one, and it is most efficient in the jejunum.

Absorbed methyl THF enters cells for use or is recycled to the liver for storage or enterohepatic recirculation by way of bile. Most folate in the blood at any time, therefore, represents recently absorbed folate and is largely methyl THF.

Two folate-binding protein activities exist in plasma. One involves low-affinity, nonspecific binding promoted by various proteins. The second is a specific protein with a high affinity for mostly oxidized rather than reduced folates and a low binding capacity. The physiologic roles of these proteins are uncertain. The nonspecific binder may prevent renal loss of folate.

Folate is ultimately degraded, and some of it may be lost through the urine. Biliary loss appears to be relatively minor.

COBALAMIN

Biochemistry

Cobalamins are corrinoids (compounds that contain a porphyrin-like corrin ring with a central cobalt atom) that have a 5,6-dimethyl benzimidazole side chain. The major physiologic cobalamins are hydroxocobalamin, methylcobalamin, and 5′-deoxyadenosyl cobalamin. By International Union of Pure and Applied Chemistry-International Union of Biochemistry nomenclature,

vitamin B_{12} refers specifically to cyanocobalamin, a cobalamin with a cyanide moiety attached to its central cobalt, a form found only in medicinal preparations.

Cobalamins are known to take part in only two reactions in humans. First, 5′-deoxyadenosyl cobalamin is the coenzyme for methylmalonyl CoA mutase in the isomerization of methylmalonyl CoA to succinyl CoA, as part of mitochondrial propionate metabolism. Methylmalonic acidemia is a useful indicator of cobalamin deficiency.

The second reaction involves methylcobalamin as a cofactor in the methylation of homocysteine to methionine, in which methyl THF is converted to THF (Fig. 243.1, reaction 4). This key role has many important ramifications. Cobalamin deficiency impairs the demethylation of methyl THF, thus inducing a block in folate metabolism. This forms the basis of the "methyl THF trap" hypothesis. The resulting depletion of 5,10-methylene THF, needed for reaction 5 in Fig. 243.1, explains why cobalamin deficiency leads to megaloblastic anemia. It also explains why therapy with folic acid, by temporarily bypassing the block, can transiently correct the megaloblastic anemia of cobalamin deficiency (Fig. 243.1, reactions 1, 2 and 5). Probably related to the increase of the largely monoglutamated methyl THF, cellular accumulation of folates also becomes impaired in cobalamin deficiency; tissue folate levels, including red cell folate, fall while serum levels rise. Another ramification of the trap is that hyperhomocysteinemia and partial methionine deficiency can result, along with impaired generation of S-adenosylmethionine, a universal methyl donor; these changes are now thought to have many important consequences.

Nutrition, Absorption, and Metabolism

Cobalamin is synthesized by bacteria. Humans usually acquire it secondhand from animals that have ingested these bacteria

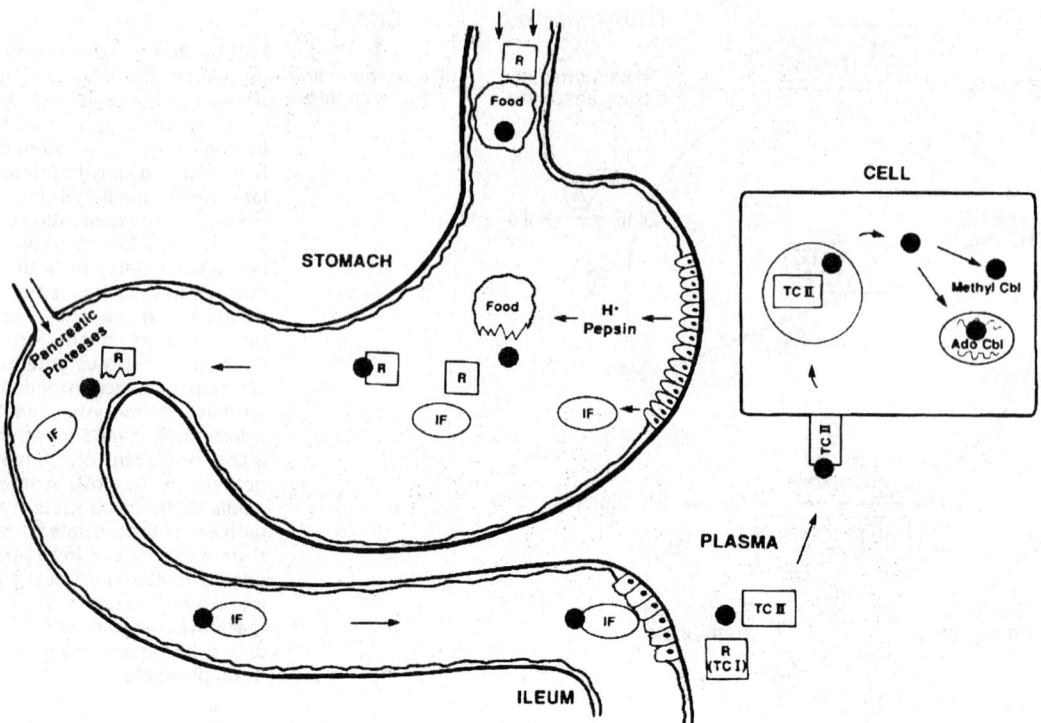

FIGURE 243.2. Sequence of events in cobalamin assimilation and use. *Filled circles,* cobalamin; *R,* salivary R binder; *IF,* intrinsic factor; *TC II,* transcobalamin II; *R(TC I),* plasma R binder (transcobalamin I); *Methyl Cbl,* methylcobalamin; *Ado Cbl,* 5'-deoxyadenosylcobalamin. (Modified from Carmel R. Clinical and laboratory features of the diagnosis of megaloblastic anemia. In: Lindenbaum J, ed. *Nutrition in hematology.* New York: Churchill Livingstone, 1983, with permission.)

and stored the cobalamin. The best food sources are meats, seafood, and products of animals, such as dairy products and eggs. Vegetables and fruits are poor sources, as are cereals, rice, flour, and nuts. The daily cobalamin requirement is thought to be 1 to 5 μg, and the usual North American diet provides more than that. Because of cobalamin's specific, saturable absorption, no more than 1 to 2 μg is absorbed in any one meal. Total body stores are estimated at 2 to 10 mg. Thus, daily turnover is only about 0.1% of stores.

Cobalamin assimilation follows the sequence of events in Figure 243.2. Ingested vitamin is split from its food binding by pepsin at a low pH. It is then bound by one of two binding proteins. The ultimately important binder is intrinsic factor. This glycoprotein is secreted by the gastric parietal cell in great excess over requirements. The other binding protein, R binder or haptocorrin, is secreted by glandular epithelial cells, such as those in the salivary gland. This glycoprotein is a less specific binder than intrinsic factor in that it also binds nonfunctional corrinoids. R binder binds cobalamin preferentially in the stomach at low pH but is then degraded in the jejunum by pancreatic proteases. Its cobalamin, thus released, is then bound by intrinsic factor.

Considerable enterohepatic recirculation of cobalamin occurs by way of biliary R binder, whose cobalamin is presumably released by pancreatic protease activity and transferred to intrinsic factor.

The intrinsic factor–cobalamin complex attaches to specific receptors for intrinsic factor on ileal epithelial cell membranes. These receptors are particularly numerous in the distal ileum. The complex is internalized, after which the cobalamin is exported from the ileal cell into the circulation.

In the bloodstream, cobalamin is bound by either of two binding proteins. Transcobalamin II binds cobalamin as it exits from the ileal cell and very quickly delivers it to all cells by way of specific receptors for transcobalamin II on their membranes. Without this binder, cellular uptake of cobalamin is inadequate. After internalization, the cobalamin becomes available as a coenzyme in the cytoplasm or mitochondria. On the other hand, transcobalamin I, the plasma representative of the R binder family, carries circulating cobalamin with a half-life of 9 to 10 days, without delivering it to cells. As a result, most measurable cobalamin in the plasma is normally attached to it, but its function is unknown; desialylated transcobalamin I may ultimately be involved nonspecifically in the hepatobiliary clearance of the vitamin.

The binding proteins are of additional interest in their own right. Plasma levels of transcobalamin I and its bound cobalamin are consistently elevated in chronic myelogenous and acute promyelocytic leukemias and sometimes in other conditions. Plasma transcobalamin II behaves like an acute phase reactant.

Various nonfunctional corrinoid analogues are found in the blood. Their source is unknown, but intestinal bacteria synthesize them and some multivitamin preparations are rich in them. Their role, deleterious or otherwise, is also uncertain.

ETIOLOGY

COBALAMIN (VITAMIN B12) DEFICIENCY STATES

The disorders presented here follow the assimilation sequence for cobalamin in Figure 243.2. Because of the large body reserves of cobalamin, virtually all disorders take several years to produce clinically obvious deficiency. Increasingly often now, they are diagnosed before the symptoms of deficiency appear.

Dietary Insufficiency

The great margin of safety provided by the 1,000 : 1 ratio of body stores to daily requirements, combined with unimpaired reabsorption of biliary cobalamin, explains why dietary insufficiency rarely causes cobalamin deficiency in the United States. Cobalamin deficiency does not occur in general malnutrition such as among homeless persons with alcoholism or malnourished patients with renal failure or cancer. For a deficiency to develop, one must be a particularly strict vegetarian for many years, usually avoiding eggs and dairy products not to mention cobalamin supplements. Even patients who meet all the criteria for dietary insufficiency usually have coexisting malabsorptive disorders that explain their deficiency on closer examination.

Nevertheless, marginal cobalamin status may well be common in vegetarians. Even if megaloblastic anemia is rare, low serum cobalamin levels have been described in several surveys. The one type of patient who often exhibits overt signs of deficiency, especially neurological signs, is the infant born to and nursed by a vegan mother; interestingly, the mother usually has no symptoms.

Disorders of the Stomach

Pernicious Anemia

Pernicious anemia is the most common cause of clinically overt cobalamin deficiency. Despite its hematologic name, it is really a gastroenterologic entity defined by malabsorption of cobalamin due to failure of the stomach to secrete intrinsic factor. One can have pernicious anemia without being anemic.

Classical, or addisonian, pernicious anemia features severe atrophic gastritis in which autoimmune phenomena are prominent. The gastritis often spares the antrum (type A gastritis) and gastrin levels usually are elevated. Achlorhydria is universal, but the crucial defect is loss of intrinsic factor secretion by the parietal cell. Although there is still no evidence that they are pathogenic, circulating antibodies to the H+,K+-ATPase of parietal cells (55% to 90% of cases) and the cobalamin-binding site of intrinsic factor (55% to 75% of cases) are often present.

Pernicious anemia is typically a disease of the elderly person of northern European ancestry but is found in all races. Moreover, pernicious anemia can occur in younger people; occurence in the third or fourth decade of life is especially common among black women. When the disease occurs in children or teenagers, it is called *juvenile pernicious anemia* (not to be confused with congenital pernicious anemia, a hereditary disorder without atrophic gastritis). Pernicious anemia shows a slight female preponderance.

The gastric defect is irreversible. The vitamin deficiency that it produces, however, is easily reversed and does not recur as long as maintenance therapy with cobalamin is given. A small source of risk for increased mortality is the predisposition to gastric cancer, estimated at two to five times that of the general population. An initial endoscopy is generally favored but the value of aggressive screening programs with periodic endoscopic examination is not established. Gastric carcinoids may be even more common but usually have a benign course. Other diseases that coexist with pernicious anemia more often than expected include autoimmune endocrinopathies (hypothyroidism, hyperthyroidism, diabetes mellitus, hypoparathyroidism, Addison's disease) and various immunologic disorders (hypogammaglobulinemia, [in which gastric cancer occurs particularly often], myasthenia gravis, vitiligo, autoimmune hemolytic anemia, and immune thrombocytopenic purpura). Of these, thyroid disease is by far the most common and may precede, follow, or coexist with pernicious anemia. Iron deficiency also is common in patients with pernicious anemia.

Postgastrectomy State

Cobalamin deficiency develops in 15% to 30% of patients who undergo subtotal gastrectomy. Loss of intrinsic factor can occur as a result of atrophic gastritis in the remnant stump. Bacterial overgrowth in the upper intestine may also contribute to the malabsorption. However, malabsorption limited to food-bound cobalamin is much more common and is discussed in the following section. Iron deficiency occurs frequently and can mask the hematological changes of cobalamin deficiency; folate deficiency may also coexist.

Other Gastric Diseases

Cobalamin deficiency can result from extensive infiltrative disease of the stomach and the attendant loss of intrinsic factor. Deficiency has also been described after gastric stapling or bypass for obesity.

The concept that atrophic gastritis leads to cobalamin malabsorption and deficiency only if intrinsic factor secretion is lost (pernicious anemia) is no longer tenable. Patients who have lost only acid and pepsin secretion absorb free cobalamin adequately. However, they may not always be able to liberate, and thus absorb, cobalamin from food or attached to protein, a defect identified only by modifications of the standard absorption test. This form of malabsorption has been described in patients with achlorhydria associated with gastritis, patients who have undergone subtotal gastrectomy or vagotomy, and patients taking acid-suppressive drugs. Food-cobalamin malabsorption accounts for 25% to 40% of cases of low cobalamin levels where the Schilling test result, which measures only absorption of free cobalamin, is normal.

Hereditary Disorders

Congenital pernicious anemia produces cobalamin deficiency because of a selective failure to secrete intrinsic factor or the secretion of an abnormal intrinsic factor. The stomach is otherwise morphologically and functionally intact. No autoimmune phenomena are seen, and the patient is not at increased risk for gastric cancer. Although the patients usually come to medical attention in the first few years of life, some are first diagnosed in adolescence or even adulthood.

Disorders of the Intestinal Lumen

Bacterial Contamination of the Intestine

The small intestine can become overgrown with bacteria that take up cobalamin. This bacterial overgrowth can result from blind loops, large diverticula, strictures, or disorders of bowel motility. Increased bacterial counts in the upper intestine may be seen in patients with gastric achlorhydria but are of uncertain significance. Bacterial contamination can produce cobalamin deficiency before any other intestinal symptoms or signs are apparent. Treatment includes antibiotic therapy, but unless the underlying cause of the bacterial overgrowth can be reversed, recurrence is common.

Tapeworm Infestation

Diphyllobothrium latum avidly takes up cobalamin. The greater the number of parasites, the more likely there is to be cobalamin deficiency. The major source of the tapeworm is poorly cooked fish from infested lakes. The disorder is rare in the United States.

Pancreatic Insufficiency

Pancreatic insufficiency produces an abnormal cobalamin absorption test result in about half of patients. The cause is the unavailability of pancreatic proteases to degrade the R binder to which cobalamin initially binds in the stomach. As a result, less vitamin becomes available for binding to intrinsic factor. Nevertheless, deficiency rarely develops, perhaps because pancreatic replacement therapy usually is given before cobalamin deficiency supervenes.

Gastrinoma

The Zollinger–Ellison syndrome can produce cobalamin malabsorption. The low intestinal pH inhibits intrinsic factor attachment to ileal receptors.

Disorders of the Ileum

Acquired Diseases Involving the Ileum

Nearly any disease involving enough of the ileum, especially the distal ileum, can produce cobalamin malabsorption. Cobalamin deficiency can be the first manifestation of tropical sprue, which may appear long after emigration from the endemic area and is often combined with folate deficiency. Loss of ileum due to surgical resection or diversion (e.g., the Kock pouch) or due to damage after pelvic radiotherapy can also produce malabsorption. Low serum cobalamin levels occur in 15% to 25% of patients with AIDS, and ileal malabsorption can be demonstrated in some of these cases.

Drugs, Toxins, and Nutritional Deficiency

Alcohol and many drugs (e.g., neomycin, biguanides, colchicine, slow-release potassium chloride, cholestyramine, and para-aminosalicylic acid) can impair cobalamin absorption. Absorption tests can become abnormal within a week or two of beginning drug therapy. Actual cobalamin deficiency is uncommon, however, because the drugs are rarely taken long enough to deplete stores.

Cobalamin deficiency itself sometimes produces megaloblastic changes in intestinal epithelial cells. The transient ileal malabsorption of cobalamin (i.e., even when exogenous intrinsic factor is supplied in the Schilling test), seen in 40% to 75% of patients with pernicious anemia, has been attributed to this phenomenon. The malabsorption normally reverses with cobalamin therapy after a few days or weeks. When the ileal malabsorption takes several months to reverse, it seems more plausible to implicate coexisting small bowel disorders.

Hereditary Disorders

In congenital malabsorption of cobalamin (Imerslund–Gräsbeck syndrome), malabsorption is limited to cobalamin only. The genetic defect is thought to involve the ileal receptor for intrinsic factor, cubilin, which is also found in kidney tubular cells. Mild proteinuria occurs in nearly all cases. Deficiency of the vitamin usually appears in the first few years of life but is sometimes delayed until the second decade. Malabsorption also accompanies hereditary transcobalamin II deficiency. This seems to be due to the inability of absorbed cobalamin to leave the ileal cell.

Disorders of Transport, Metabolism, and Utilization

Nitrous Oxide Exposure

Nitrous oxide inactivates cobalamin by oxidizing cob(I)alamin and inactivates methionine synthase (Fig. 243.1, reaction 4). Repeated exposure produces megaloblastic anemia and neurologic symptoms, with the latter often predominating. Cobalamin levels are usually normal and methylmalonic acidemia cannot always be demonstrated, so that the diagnosis of cobalamin abnormality can be difficult to make unless a history of exposure is elicited. Transient exposure during routine anesthesia produces no clinical sequelae unless a coexisting cobalamin deficiency has been overlooked.

Transcobalamin II Deficiency

Congenital deficiency of this crucial transport protein produces a life-threatening cellular depletion of cobalamin early in life. Serum cobalamin levels are usually, but not invariably, normal.

Occasional cases may not be diagnosed until the second decade of life, but these usually are patients who had been misdiagnosed and inadequately treated earlier. Curiously, neurologic disturbances are not initially prominent in most patients. However, some patients have developed such deficits, perhaps as a result of inappropriate folate therapy.

R Binder (Transcobalamin I) Deficiency

Because most cobalamin circulates in the blood attached to transcobalamin I, absence of the binder produces low serum levels of the vitamin even though cellular levels are adequate. The binder appears to have no other role in cobalamin metabolism, and these patients are nondeficient and asymptomatic (although one patient had unexplained, progressive myelopathy and dysarthria). The patients usually are discovered by accident because of an unexplained low serum cobalamin level. Absence of R binder in both blood and secretions such as saliva establishes the diagnosis. Deficiency of lactoferrin, which, like transcobalamin I, originates in neutrophil specific granules, coexists in some cases.

Inborn Errors of Metabolism

Recognition of abnormalities that interfere with cellular cobalamin activity begins with the demonstration of methylmalonic acidemia, homocysteinemia, or both, but the biochemical and clinical defects vary. Some disorders with abnormality limited to the 5′-deoxyadenosyl cobalamin-mediated reaction feature only acidosis, methylmalonic acidemia, and perhaps developmental problems (as in *cblA* and *B* mutations). Others have defective methylcobalamin activity as well (*cblC, D,* and *F* mutations); these patients usually have homocysteinemia in addition to methylmalonic acidemia. Their clinical pictures have ranged from mild neurologic symptoms appearing in adolescence to severe hematologic and neurologic abnormalities terminating in death in infancy. Thrombotic complications sometimes occur. In the *cblE* and *G* mutations, only methylcobalamin activity is impaired; homocysteinemia occurs without methylmalonic acidemia, and patients have hematologic and neurologic manifestations. The inborn errors should be considered in children who have developmental or neurologic problems as well as in children who have megaloblastic anemia. Some of the disorders may first be detected in adolescence or young adulthood.

Miscellaneous

Aging and mild cobalamin deficiency

Although the causes vary, low cobalamin levels occur in about 10% of the healthy elderly population. Most of the low levels are not accompanied by clinical symptoms or anemia but metabolic testing has shown evidence of cobalamin deficiency in 50% to 70% of cases. Food-cobalamin malabsorption explains 30% to 40% of these and pernicious anemia or ileal disease only about 10%; dietary insufficiency is rare.

FOLATE DEFICIENCY STATES

Deficiency of folate often is multifactorial in origin. In part this stems from the relative ease with which nutritional insufficiency can supervene in any illness. Alcohol and various drugs also have multiple effects on folate status that often are complicated by poor diet, coexisting disease, or the underlying illness for which the drugs are used. The disorders are presented here in the sequence of folate intake, absorption, and utilization.

Dietary Insufficiency

Poor dietary intake is the most common cause of folate deficiency. Because body stores are only about 100 times the daily requirement and because food folate is labile, significant tissue depletion can occur within a few months.

Certain factors potentiate the problem of poor or marginal intake. Chief among these is ingestion of alcohol. When combined with poor diet, alcohol use often has been implicated as the major cause of folate deficiency. Another potentiating factor can be an increased requirement for folate, which may strain body stores if the diet is marginal.

Disorders of Absorption

Diseases of the Small Intestine

Almost any condition involving enough of the upper small intestine can produce folate malabsorption. This includes sprue, infiltrative diseases, Whipple's disease, and resection of the small intestine. Bacterial contamination of the small intestine, however, does not produce folate deficiency, although it can produce cobalamin deficiency.

Drugs, Toxins, and Nutritional Deficiency

Several drugs and toxins have been associated with folate malabsorption. The chief one is alcohol (discussed in a later section). Sulfasalazine and para-aminosalicylic acid have been implicated in folate malabsorption. Malnutrition and its effects on the intestine also have been postulated to impair folate absorption.

Hereditary Disorders

The nature of the defect in congenital folate malabsorption is unknown, but it affects monoglutamate as well as polyglutamate absorption. A concurrent transport block into the cerebrospinal fluid has been implicated, perhaps explaining the frequent cerebral abnormalities these patients have in addition to their anemia.

Disorders of Transport, Metabolism, and Utilization

Alcohol

Alcohol has multiple effects on folate economy. Serum folate levels drop sharply with alcohol ingestion. Suggested mechanisms include impaired ability to form methyl THF in the liver, curtailed enterohepatic recirculation of folate, and increased urinary losses of folate. These putative defects are superimposed on the previously mentioned dietary insufficiency and on the possible absorptive defect. However, alcohol also can directly induce red cell macrocytosis that is not related to altered folate status and does not respond to folate therapy.

Drugs

Folate metabolism is a major target in antineoplastic therapy. Methotrexate inhibits dihydrofolate reductase (Fig. 243.1, reaction 1), thus inhibiting the generation of metabolically active THF.

Several antibiotics, such as trimethoprim, sulfamethoxazole, and pyrimethamine, inhibit dihydrofolate reductase in microorganisms, but the human enzyme is much less susceptible. Triamterene, a pteridine derivative, and sulfasalazine, which also affects two other folate-related enzymes, inhibit dihydrofolate reductase. All these drugs can, on rare occasions, directly induce folate deficiency. Nevertheless, whenever deficiency occurs, the initial focus should be to find coexisting disorders such as malnutrition or other diseases that compromise folate status.

Patients receiving anticonvulsant therapy often become folate-deficient. The mechanism is unclear, and a poor diet often contributes to the deficiency. In addition to possibly impairing absorption, hydantoins may impair cellular folate metabolism.

Acute Folate Deficiency

Acute folate deficiency has been found among some patients in intensive care units. These patients develop cytopenia and megaloblastic bone-marrow changes, but the peripheral blood appearance is often unaltered and vitamin levels are normal. The cause of this syndrome of cellular folate depletion is unknown.

Hereditary Disorders

Hereditary folate metabolic disorders are often associated with cerebral abnormalities, such as retardation or seizures; megaloblastic anemia is not always present. Methylene THF reductase deficiency may be the most common disorder (Fig. 243.1, reaction 3). It is associated with low serum folate levels due to impaired generation of methyl THF. Neurological symptoms are common, but megaloblastic anemia does not occur because methylene THF remains available for thymidine synthesis (Fig. 243.1, reaction 5). The disorder has been found among teenagers as well as among younger children.

A milder genetic mutation producing a thermolabile methylene THF reductase is very common. It produces no symptoms but can contribute to mild hyperhomocysteinemia and perhaps an increased thrombotic risk.

Increased Requirements and Losses

Low folate levels are common in pregnancy. Megaloblastic anemia sometimes ensues, especially in the last trimester. Routine prenatal folate supplementation has decreased its incidence.

Folate requirements are increased in chronic hemolytic anemias and other chronic states of increased cell turnover. However, clinical deficiency from the increased demand alone is unusual, and it is wise to search for contributing problems. Controlled studies have not demonstrated any clinical benefit from the common practice of routinely giving folate prophylactically to patients with chronic hemolysis, such as those with sickle-cell anemia. Cobalamin levels should be checked first if folate supplementation is planned.

Increased folate losses have been described in patients undergoing dialysis for renal failure, and supplementation is routinely given.

OTHER CAUSES OF MEGALOBLASTIC ANEMIA

Megaloblastic changes are sometimes caused by mechanisms unrelated to either folate or cobalamin deficiency and do not respond to therapy with either vitamin.

Drugs and Toxins

Drugs that impair nucleoprotein synthesis directly, for example, antineoplastic drugs like 5-fluorouracil, cytosine arabinoside, and hydroxyurea, often produce megaloblastic changes and macrocytosis. Hypersegmentation of neutrophil nuclei occurs with steroid therapy and reverses with its discontinuation; the mechanism is unknown. Arsenic poisoning does not produce truly megaloblastic changes, but the nuclear fragmentation and increased mitoses that result can be confused with megaloblastic anemia.

Primary Disorders of the Hematopoietic Stem Cells

Many primary disorders of the hematopoietic stem cells are associated with macrocytosis (Table 243.1). Some, like the myelodysplastic syndrome, may also feature erythroid maturation changes that resemble those of megaloblastic anemia. Neutrophils may have hypersegmented nuclei in some myeloproliferative diseases.

Hereditary Disorders Unrelated to Cobalamin or Folate

Orotic aciduria affects two enzymes in orotic acid metabolism. Among other features, severe megaloblastic anemia appears in the first year of life. The Lesch–Nyhan syndrome, a disorder of purine metabolism, sometimes produces megaloblastic anemia. Thiamine-responsive megaloblastic anemia, whose mechanism is unknown, may not produce anemia until late in childhood. Diabetes mellitus and sensorineural deafness are regular findings.

▓ CLINICAL FINDINGS

The clinical expressions of cobalamin or folate deficiency are the same no matter what the underlying cause of the respective deficiency. Sometimes, however, especially in cobalamin deficiency, the only recognizable abnormality is simply a low vitamin level in the blood or metabolic evidence of insufficiency.

MEGALOBLASTIC ANEMIA

The severity of morphologic changes tends to correspond with the severity of anemia. All cells, whether precursors or mature cells, tend to be larger than normal. A nuclear–cytoplasmic asynchrony appears in the precursor cells. Erythrocytes are often oval in addition to being macrocytic, and there may be considerable poikilocytosis. Mature granulocytes have hypersegmented nuclei, and metamyelocytes and bands tend to be large with large, bizarrely shaped nuclei and abnormally fine chromatin. Hypersegmentation in granulocytes can be defined in several ways: the presence of at least one neutrophil with six or more nuclear lobes; the presence of more than 3% to 4% five-lobed neutrophils; or an increased neutrophil lobe average. Granulocytic changes occur early in deficiency and are found in nearly all cases, whereas erythroid abnormalities are sometimes partially masked (e.g., by coexisting iron deficiency) and macrocytosis may be absent.

Functionally, the anemia is primarily one of ineffective hematopoiesis. Up to 90% of the cells may die within the bone marrow. The resulting indirect hyperbilirubinemia and increased serum lactate dehydrogenase are often striking, unless the anemia is mild. Evidence of hemolysis, including low serum haptoglobin levels and hemosiderinuria, is sometimes seen but reticulocytosis does not occur.

Leukopoiesis and thrombopoiesis are also ineffective, and pancytopenia may occur. Granulocyte and platelet dysfunctions are sometimes demonstrable but rarely produce clinical manifestations.

NEUROLOGIC ABNORMALITIES

Cobalamin deficiency often produces characteristic and usually symmetric myelopathy and neuropathy. Pathologic examination shows axonal degeneration with loss of myelin. This predominates in the posterior and lateral columns in the upper thoracic spinal cord. Patchy changes may also be found in the brain. How the deficiency produces the neurologic lesions is unknown. Current evidence favors impaired homocysteine–methionine conversion with an altered S-adenosylmethionine/S-adenosylhomocysteine equilibrium as the key to the defect. Some patients have severe neurologic deficits with little or no evidence of hematologic abnormality, whereas in others the reverse is true.

The earliest symptom is usually paresthesia in the feet. Vibration and position sense become impaired. Deep tendon reflexes may be diminished. Later, ataxia and a positive Romberg's sign may appear. As the lesion progresses, the deficits ascend. Spasticity, increased deep tendon reflexes, and weakness appear as the lateral columns are involved. Ultimately, paraplegia, bladder atony, poor control of sphincters, and impotence may result.

Mild cerebral manifestations such as depression, memory impairment, and irritability are common. Electroencephalographic abnormalities are frequently demonstrable. Psychiatric symptoms, confusion, or dementia may appear. Rarely, the disturbances can include ophthalmoplegia and optic atrophy.

Folate deficiency does not produce the neurologic abnormalities that cobalamin deficiency does. Minor cerebral symptoms, such as irritability, memory loss and personality changes, may occur, however, and neuropathy has been described by some observers. The nature of these changes is unclear. Cerebral disturbances such as mental retardation, seizures, and psychosis are prominent in children with inborn errors of folate metabolism.

The neurologic deficits of cobalamin deficiency, unlike the hematologic ones, do not respond to folate therapy. Indeed, the risk is that they may progress unchecked while hematologic improvement occurs.

MISCELLANEOUS ABNORMALITIES

Some patients, especially those with cobalamin deficiency, may have glossitis and atrophy of the tongue papillae. Oral symptoms even predominate in some cases. Infertility has also been attributed to cobalamin deficiency. Other abnormalities that reverse with cobalamin therapy include unexplained weight loss, pigment changes in skin, hair, and nails, and low serum levels of bone alkaline phosphatase and osteocalcin.

Folate deficiency has been implicated in damage to fragile sites on chromosomes. Some studies have also described protection by folate supplementation against progression of cellular atypia to neoplasia, but the phenomenon is unclear. Periconceptional folate supplementation of the mother partially protects her fetus against neural tube defects. This effect, whose mechanism is unknown, prompted the recent fortification of all cereal-grain products with folate.

HYPERHOMOCYSTEINEMIA

Although asymptomatic per se, acquired as well as hereditary hyperhomocysteinemia may be clinically important. Epidemiologic evidence shows it to be, even when mild, a risk factor for thrombotic and arteriosclerotic disease. Studies are underway to determine if reducing homocysteine levels by vitamin therapy reduces the vascular risk. Hyperhomocysteinemia, which predominates in men and in the elderly, can be caused by folate, cobalamin, or pyridoxine deficiency (Fig. 243.1), by several enzyme deficiencies or by renal failure.

■ LABORATORY FINDINGS

DIAGNOSIS OF MEGALOBLASTIC ANEMIA

Classic megaloblastic anemia is easy to diagnose. The advent of electronic cell sizing has made macrocytosis instantly obvious in the routine blood cell count. Alertness to details optimizes diagnosis in the early phases of deficiency and in mild anemias, atypical presentations, and the presence of findings altered by coexisting problems. Macrocytosis typically precedes the anemia and can be invaluable in making an early diagnosis. Even a red blood cell mean corpuscular volume in the upper range of normal should be viewed with suspicion. Macrocytosis is not invari-

TABLE 243.1.	CAUSES OF MACROCYTOSIS

Megaloblastic Anemia

Cobalamin or folate deficiency

Drugs

Alcohol

Agents that interfere with nucleoprotein synthesis
  Chemotherapeutic and immunosuppressive drugs
  Zidovudine

Hematologic Disorders

Aplastic anemia
Pure red blood cell aplasia
Myelodysplastic syndrome
Myeloproliferative disease
Leukemia
Multiple myeloma
Refractory anemia
5q− syndrome
Hemolytic anemia

Nonhematologic Disease

Liver disease (usually, but not invariably, alcoholic)
Hypothyroidism

Physiologic Process

Red blood cells are normally enlarged in the first 4 wk of life

Idiopathic Factors[a]

Pregnancy
Chronic lung disease, smoking
Cancer

Artifact of Electronic Cell Sizing

Cold agglutinins
Severe hyperglycemia
Hyponatremia
Stored blood
Warm antibody to red blood cells

[a] Higher mean corpuscular volumes than usual (although not necessarily above normal range) have been observed in these conditions, but the mechanism is unknown and the possibility of subtle megaloblastosis exists in some cases.

able, however; more than 25% of patients with pernicious anemia have normal or even low mean corpuscular volumes when first seen. Coexisting iron deficiency or thalassemia minor often is responsible for this, or the patient may simply have early deficiency or, for other, unknown reasons, may have only minimal hematologic abnormality. On the other hand, many nonmegaloblastic processes can also cause a high mean corpuscular volume (Table 243.1).

Neutrophil hypersegmentation is a sensitive index of the megaloblastic process. Hypersegmentation can also be found in nonmegaloblastic conditions, however, examples of which include myeloproliferative disease, corticosteroid therapy, and congenital hypersegmentation; it is nevertheless always advisable to demonstrate that vitamin deficiency does not coexist. The bone marrow aspirate is the court of last resort and should be examined before initiating therapy whenever the diagnosis is in doubt. However, megaloblastic changes may be subtle in mild or early deficiency,

and megaloblastic erythroid changes may be blunted by coexisting iron deficiency.

Various features of the anemia can mimic other disorders. Pancytopenia is sometimes severe enough to be confused with aplastic anemia. The maturation abnormalities, particularly if accompanied by exuberant myeloid proliferation or transient red blood cell hypoplasia, have been mistaken for leukemia. Increased iron levels and abnormal sideroblasts can mimic sideroblastic anemia. The frequent hyperbilirubinemia, elevated lactate dehydrogenase, decreased haptoglobin, and hemosiderinuria may resemble primary hemolytic anemia.

DIAGNOSIS OF THE VITAMIN DEFICIENCY

For all practical purposes, megaloblastic anemia in adults is secondary to deficiency of folate, cobalamin, or both (Table 243.2). Cobalamin deficiency should also be considered in any patient with neuropathy, myelopathy, or cerebral disturbances, whether or not megaloblastic anemia is present.

Serum vitamin levels, even though they reflect body stores indirectly, are the mainstay of diagnosis. Indeed, low serum levels are sometimes the only evidence of deficiency. However, they are sometimes too sensitive (especially serum folate, which falls with poor intake within days) and at other times are falsely low (Tables 243.3 and 243.4). Although the lower the serum level, the more likely it is that a deficiency exists, even mildly decreased values require investigation. The burden of proof is always on the physician to demonstrate that deficiency is not present, given its treatability and the potentially serious consequences of failure to treat it. Serum cobalamin levels also tend to fall in folate deficiency, whereas serum folate tends to rise in cobalamin deficiency. Low levels of both vitamins may indicate combined deficiencies, especially in malabsorption syndromes.

Measuring tissue levels is an ideal goal but is impractical, aside from determining red cell folate levels. Red cell levels are truer indices of folate status than serum levels and are not immediately affected by vitamin therapy. Their chief shortcomings are laboratory performance problems and the fact that low levels often occur in cobalamin deficiency as well.

TABLE 243.2.	LABORATORY DIAGNOSIS OF COBALAMIN AND FOLATE DEFICIENCY

	In Deficiency of		
	Cobalamin	Folate	Cobalamin and Folate
Serum cobalamin	↓	N–↓	↓
Serum folate	N–↑	↓	↓
Red blood cell folate	N–↓	↓	↓
Methylmalonic acid[a]	↑	N	↑
Homocysteine[b]	↑	↑	↑

N, normal level; ↓, decreased level; ↑, increased level.
[a] Can be assayed in serum or urine.
[b] Should be assayed in EDTA-anticoagulated plasma.

TABLE 243.3.	CAUSES OF LOW SERUM COBALAMIN LEVELS

Cobalamin Deficiency

Overt deficiency
Mild or preclinical deficiency
   Latent pernicious anemia or other malabsorptive state, including food-cobalamin malabsorption
   Old age[a,b]
   Vegetarianism[a]

Unexplained but Sometimes Associated with Compromised Cobalamin Status

Long-term dialysis for renal failure
Hydantoin therapy
Cancer
AIDS

Presumed not to Represent Cobalamin Deficit[b]

Pregnancy (last trimester)
Folate deficiency
Transcobalamin I deficiency
Multiple myeloma and Waldenström's macroglobulinemia
Aplastic anemia
Hairy cell leukemia
Oral contraceptive use
Severe iron deficiency

Artifact

Radioactive serum (e.g., after isotopic scanning procedures)
High-dose ascorbic acid ingestion

[a] Only a few patients will display clinically overt evidence of cobalamin deficiency.
[b] Some patients in these categories can have coexisting cobalamin malabsorption and either clinically overt or mild, preclinical deficiency.

Metabolic tests are becoming increasingly useful. Elevated homocysteine levels are a helpful marker for folate or cobalamin deficiency but occur in other conditions too. High methylmalonic acid levels are relatively specific for cobalamin deficiency. Serum levels of both metabolites also rise in renal insufficiency,

TABLE 243.4.	CONDITIONS ASSOCIATED WITH LOW SERUM FOLATE LEVELS

Folate deficiency
Low serum levels apparently not reflecting overt folate deficiency
   Transiently poor dietary intake without actual folate deficiency
   Sickle-cell anemia and other chronic hemolytic states
   Drug use (e.g., oral contraceptives, acetylsalicylic acid, alcohol)
   Idiopathic factors
Artifact
   Improper handling of specimen (e.g., long storage)
   Radioactive blood[a]
   Folate-binding protein abnormality in renal failure[a]
   Drugs that inhibit microbial growth (e.g., antibiotics)[b]

[a] Source of artifact only in radioisotopic assay.
[b] Source of artifact only in microbiologic assay.

however. Some patients with cobalamin deficiency have abnormal metabolite levels even when their serum cobalamin levels are normal. Testing for these two metabolites is occasionally helpful in acquired vitamin deficiencies and is mandatory when considering hereditary disorders. Perhaps an even more sensitive test for both vitamin deficiencies, the deoxyuridine suppression test in bone marrow cells, which tests reactions 5 and 6 in Fig. 243.1, is still a research tool.

DIAGNOSIS OF THE UNDERLYING DISEASE

Each of the two deficiencies has a distinct differential diagnosis. In cobalamin deficiency, the most common cause is pernicious anemia; for folic acid, it is dietary insufficiency, often combined with alcohol abuse. The temptation to automatically assume the most common diagnosis must be resisted, however.

Testing of cobalamin absorption is central to the diagnostic evaluation because nearly all cobalamin deficiency in the Western Hemisphere is either of gastric or intestinal origin. This is done by measuring the absorption of a small oral dose of radioactive cyanocobalamin. Radioactivity can be measured in urine (Schilling test), plasma, or feces, or whole-body retention can be measured. Each method has its advantages. The Schilling test is the most commonly used, but it requires a complete 24-hour urine collection and normal renal function. Pernicious anemia is diagnosed by an abnormal absorption test that is corrected by retesting with an oral dose of intrinsic factor. A popular version of the Schilling test combines both of the above steps but gives falsely normal results in 30% to 40% of cases due to isotope exchange.

The presence of anti-intrinsic factor antibody in the blood is diagnostically useful; it is rarely positive in patients without pernicious anemia, but an artifact can be produced if blood is sampled within 48 hours after a cobalamin injection is given. Antibody to parietal cells, on the other hand, is specific for atrophic gastritis, not pernicious anemia. High serum gastrin and low pepsinogen I levels occur in 80% to 90% of patients with pernicious anemia.

Malabsorption of food-bound cobalamin cannot be detected by standard absorption tests that use free cobalamin, such as the Schilling test. Absorption tests using cobalamin in scrambled egg yolk or bound to chicken serum have been devised but are still not widely available.

Diagnosing the cause of folate deficiency requires a good dietary history, evaluation for possible alcoholism, and a careful drug history. Malabsorption is responsible for 10% to 20% of cases. Because tests of folate absorption are not widely available, folate malabsorption is usually diagnosed indirectly by documenting other malabsorptive phenomena.

◼ OPTIMAL MANAGEMENT

TREATING THE SYMPTOMS

Megaloblastic anemia responds rapidly to small doses of the appropriate vitamin. A single injection of cobalamin or one folic acid pill reverses megaloblastic erythropoiesis. A feeling of well-being often precedes hematologic response by days. Reticulocytosis begins within a day or two and peaks at 5 to 7 days, at which time the hemoglobin level begins rising noticeably, although hypersegmented neutrophils may persist for several weeks. With adequate treatment, the blood count should always become completely normal within 8 weeks.

Transfusion is rarely indicated, given its hazards, the well-compensated state of even severely anemic patients, and the responsiveness to vitamin therapy. If clinical findings necessitate transfusion, a unit of packed red blood cells should be given slowly and the patient reevaluated before proceeding.

Vitamin therapy can be safely deferred in most patients until the specific vitamin deficiency has been identified, but it can be started in an emergency as soon as the necessary diagnostic specimens have been obtained. The neurologic symptoms of cobalamin deficiency call for more urgent therapy, but there is no evidence that higher doses or more frequent injections are necessary. The completeness of the neurologic response is not as predictable as the hematologic response. The more extensive the neurologic involvement and the longer the symptoms have been present, the less likely it is that complete reversal will occur. Nevertheless, some degree of neurologic improvement is possible even in longstanding cases, although it may take 6 to 12 months to occur. In any case, neurologic dysfunction never progresses when therapy is given. Patients with spasticity, gait disturbances or bladder problems require early rehabilitative efforts.

TREATING THE VITAMIN DEFICIENCY

Before therapy is begun, it is essential to be sure of the diagnosis. Treatment of cobalamin deficiency with folic acid must be avoided. If both vitamins are given, proper diagnosis may become difficult if the initial test results are inconclusive. Giving both vitamins can also blur the specificity of the diagnosis in the patient's mind, if therapy is continued for long. The two main goals are to reverse the abnormalities produced by the deficiency and to prevent relapse. A third goal is to replete tissue stores and provide a reserve, although there is no evidence that fully repleted stores are essential to the patient's well-being.

Because cobalamin deficiency is usually due to malabsorption, therapy should be parenteral. Lifelong maintenance is required when the underlying disease is irreversible, as in pernicious anemia. Usual doses are 100 to 1000 μg; a smaller fraction of the 1000-μg dose, but a larger absolute amount, is retained. Cyanocobalamin is the common form of cobalamin used, but hydroxocobalamin is better retained and requires less frequent injections. Once repletion has been achieved, monthly maintenance injections can be given. However, individual requirements vary: some patients may need more frequent injections, whereas others can do with less frequent ones. Metabolic and transport blocks require very frequent injections. Oral cobalamin suffices in dietary insufficiency. It can be used even in malabsorption because a small fixed proportion is absorbed by mass action, but at least 100 μg must be taken daily, and its effectiveness must be continuously monitored.

Folate therapy can usually be given orally because most deficiencies are dietary in origin. Daily doses of 1 mg are sufficient

and stores can be repleted within a few weeks. Long-term maintenance is necessary only when the underlying disorder cannot be reversed. Oral folic acid can often be absorbed normally even in malabsorption syndromes, but higher doses should be used.

TREATING THE UNDERLYING DISEASE

The underlying disease must always be identified. Several causes have their own specific therapy, such as antibiotics for bacterial contamination of the gut and gluten-free diets for sprue, and others have specific complications and prognostic implications. Vitamin therapy can be discontinued if the underlying disease has been reversed and does not recur.

COMPLICATIONS

Vitamin therapy itself has no complications (allergic reactions are rare), unless the wrong vitamin is given. Because a transient hematologic response can be obtained with folate in cobalamin deficiency while neurologic abnormalities continue to progress, this can be a serious problem. A more common occurrence is an incomplete hematologic response despite appropriate vitamin therapy. This is indicated by a blunted reticulocyte response during the first week or by failure of the blood count to become completely normal within 2 months and is almost always due to coexisting disorders. Iron deficiency often coexists and may initially be masked in untreated megaloblastic anemia, with completely normal blood and marrow tests of iron status.

Transfusion should be avoided whenever possible; volume overload is only one of the many risks involved.

Long-term complications are those related to the underlying disease itself. For example, in pernicious anemia, there are the increased risks of gastric cancer, carcinoid tumors, and immune endocrine disorders, particularly hypothyroidism.

PATIENT EDUCATION

Because cobalamin therapy usually becomes a lifelong concern, patient education is essential. Too many patients discontinue therapy once their symptoms disappear. Reinforcement and careful explanation of the nature of the underlying disease may help. Some patients can be taught to inject themselves, which saves costs and often improves compliance as well. Dietary education is essential in most cases of folate deficiency. Addressing alcohol problems is also important.

BIBLIOGRAPHY

Bailey LB, ed. *Folate in health and disease.* New York: Marcel Dekker, 1995.
Carmel R. Prevalence of undiagnosed pernicious anemia in the elderly. *Arch Intern Med* 1996;156:1097.
Carmel R. Cobalamin, the stomach and aging. *Am J Clin Nutr* 1997;66:750.
Carmel R, ed. Beyond megaloblastic anemia: new paradigms of cobalamin and folate deficiency. *Semin Hematol* 1999;36:1.

Chanarin I. *The megaloblastic anaemias,* 2d ed. Oxford: Blackwell Scientific, 1979.

Graham SM, Arvela OM, Wise GA. Long-term neurologic consequences of nutritional vitamin B$_{12}$ deficiency in infants. *J Pediatr* 1992;121:710.

Healton ER, Savage DG, Brust JCM, Garrett TJ, Lindenbaum J. Neurologic aspects of cobalamin deficiency. *Medicine* 1991;70:229.

Kokkola A, Sjöblom S-M, Haapiainen R, et al. The risk of gastric carcinoma and carcinoid tumors in patients with pernicious anaemia. A prospective follow-up study. *Scand J Gastroenterol* 1998;33:88.

Nilsson K, Gustafson L, Fäldt R, et al. Plasma homocysteine in relation to serum cobalamin and blood folate in a psychogeriatric population. *Eur J Clin Invest* 1994;24:600.

Wickramasinghe SN, ed. Megaloblastic anaemia. *Bailliére's Clin Haematol* 1995;8:441.

Kelley's Textbook of Internal Medicine, fourth edition. Edited by H. David Humes. Lippincott Williams & Wilkins, Philadelphia © 2000.

CHAPTER 244

HEMOLYTIC ANEMIAS

JOSEPH P. CATLETT

APPROACH TO THE PATIENT

PRESENTATION

Hemolytic anemia may be defined as the premature destruction of erythrocytes occurring by a number of mechanisms. For this reason, the presenting signs and symptoms of hemolysis may vary from patient to patient, depending, in large part, on the mechanism of erythrocyte destruction and the acuteness of the process. Patients with chronic hemolytic anemias may be asymptomatic despite severe depression of the hematocrit, whereas patients with acute anemia may be at risk for circulatory failure. It is therefore important to obtain accurate clinical and laboratory information before proceeding to potentially inappropriate or unnecessary therapeutic interventions.

PATHOPHYSIOLOGY

Normal erythrocytes have a life span in the circulation of 100 to 120 days. The oldest 1% of the erythrocyte mass is destroyed in the spleen and replaced each day by the bone marrow. Newly released erythrocytes, known as *reticulocytes,* normally constitute about 1% of circulating erythrocytes and can be recognized in a blood film as large, bluish gray cells. Through progressive loss of membrane and intracellular organelles, reticulocytes are gradually "remodeled" in the spleen and microcirculation into a biconcave disk. The erythrocyte depends on the biochemical integrity of its membrane, the stability of its proteins and metabolic processes, and the fluidity of its cytoplasm to maintain a critical ability to deform itself to negotiate passages less than one-tenth its diameter. The biconcave disk shape of the resting erythrocyte confers optimal surface-to-volume ratio facilitating both gas exchange and deformation in the microcirculation. During flow, these cells transiently assume "teardrop" and "parachute" shapes. As the erythrocyte ages, it acquires a more spherical shape through gradual loss of metabolic activity, deformability, and membrane surface, and accumulates surface immunoglobulin.

The erythropoietic capacity of the bone marrow normally is capable of a sixfold increase in erythrocyte production to compensate for a proportional acceleration of hemolytic rate. Anemia results when the rate of erythrocyte destruction exceeds the erythropoietic capacity of the bone marrow.

Intrinsic hemolytic disorders primarily are inherited alterations of erythrocyte membrane, hemoglobin structure or synthesis, or enzyme activity. *Extrinsic* hemolytic states are largely acquired and include erythrocyte injury caused by antibody to erythrocyte antigens, complement, bacterial toxins, parasites, or physical injury within the circulation. Hemolysis may take place within the circulatory system (*intravascular* hemolysis) such as that due to a defective prosthetic heart valve or thrombotic thrombocytopenic purpura (TTP), or within the reticuloendothelial system, e.g., the spleen (*extravascular* hemolysis), such as is seen with hereditary spherocytosis (HS). In some hemolytic anemias, e.g., certain forms of immune hemolysis, both mechanisms are operative. A mechanistic classification of hemolytic anemias is shown in Table 244.1.

TABLE 244.1. CLASSIFICATION OF HEMOLYTIC ANEMIAS BY MECHANISM OF ERYTHROCYTE INJURY

Abnormalities of the erythrocyte membrane
  Hereditary
    Spherocytosis
    Elliptocytosis
    Acanthocytosis
    Stomatocytosis
  Acquired
    Acanthocytosis, stomatocytes, target cells (liver disease)
    Echinocytosis (uremia)
    Paroxysmal nocturnal hemoglobinuria
Metabolic deficiencies of the erythrocyte
  Hexose-monophosphate shunt enzyme deficiencies
  Glycolytic pathway enzyme deficiencies
  Purine and pyrimidine metabolic abnormalities
Immune-mediated hemolytic anemia
  Warm antibody–mediated
  Cold agglutinin syndrome
  Paroxysmal cold hemoglobinuria
  Combined warm and cold antibody
  DAT-negative autoimmune hemolysis
  Drug-induced
Hemoglobinopathies and thalassemias
Physical erythrocyte injury
  Fragmentation hemolysis
  Microangiopathic
  Cardiac and large-vessel disease
  Thermal and chemical injury
  Erythrocyte parasitization (malaria, bartonellosis, babesiosis)

HISTORY AND PHYSICAL EXAMINATION

Historical data may be helpful in directing further evaluation and can include recurrent leg ulceration, pigmented gallstones requiring cholecystectomy at an early age, intermittent or chronic jaundice, intermittent dark urine, fevers, chills, fatigue, malaise, drenching night sweats, or weight loss. Acute hemolysis may follow self-administered or prescribed drug ingestion indicating the presence of an immune-mediated process or enzyme deficiency. Physical findings indicative of a hemolytic process may include jaundice, splenomegaly, hepatomegaly, petechial hemorrhages and purpuric lesions, or lymphadenopathy.

LABORATORY STUDIES AND DIAGNOSTIC TESTS

The presence of hemolytic anemia should be determined first on the basis of simple laboratory tests. Unless an underlying deficiency is present, reticulocytosis is present on the blood film (termed *polychromasia)* with the absolute count usually in excess of 100,000 per microliter. In many cases of hemolysis, the lactic dehydrogenase (LDH) levels will be elevated along with varying degrees of indirect hyperbilirubinemia. Haptoglobin levels are depressed in intravascular and some cases of extravascular hemolysis, and free hemoglobin may be demonstrated in the plasma and urine. A direct antiglobulin (Coomb's) test (DAT) is positive for immunoglobulin, complement, or both in most instances of immune-mediated hemolysis. Review of the peripheral blood smear may also demonstrate the presence of *spherocytes*, or fragmented cells, termed *schistocytes*, which are seen in certain types of hemolysis (described later).

DIFFERENTIAL DIAGNOSIS

When hemolytic anemia is present, the differential diagnosis, as noted in Table 244.1, should be reviewed and the necessary investigations performed to arrive at a precise diagnosis. The workup of each disorder will be described throughout this chapter.

STRATEGIES FOR OPTIMAL CARE MANAGEMENT

Establishing an accurate diagnosis is the key to the proper management of hemolytic anemia, regardless of the underlying cause. The optimal care of these patients depends on the underlying etiologic factors in the hemolytic process. However, certain therapies may be applicable to patients with hemolysis irrespective of its origin.

Management, Complications, and Pitfalls

Red blood cell transfusion often is indicated in patients with severe anemia. The decision to transfuse packed red cells in patients with hemolytic anemia has to be made in light of the known risks of transfusion, including febrile or allergic reactions, acute and delayed hemolytic transfusion reactions, and the transmission of infectious diseases. Long-term erythrocyte transfu-

sion, more commonly necessary in congenital hemolytic anemias, may lead to iron overload (*transfusional hemosiderosis)* requiring iron chelation therapy. For patients with extrinsic hemolysis (e.g., microangiopathy, autoimmune hemolysis), the transfused cells can be expected to have the same short survival suffered by the patient's own red cells. The presence of autoantibodies may render compatibility testing difficult (see later).

Oral folic acid in a dose of 1 mg per day is recommended initially since hemolysis increases the daily folic acid requirement and may deplete folic acid stores.

In patients with congenital hemolysis, gallstones may appear during adolescence and become symptomatic in early adulthood. Asymptomatic gallstones are often documented by ultrasound or other noninvasive testing. It is generally recommended that cholecystectomy be reserved for patients with symptomatic disease. Unfortunately, calcium bilirubinate gallstones, common in patients with chronic hemolysis, are not dissolved by chenodeoxycholic acid.

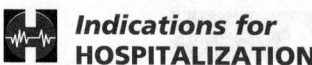

Indications for HOSPITALIZATION

Patients with severe symptomatic anemia, evidenced by dyspnea at rest, tachycardia, and hypotension, should be hospitalized for transfusion on an emergency basis. Those with high-output cardiac failure or impending circulatory collapse should be monitored in an intensive care setting. Most nonemergency transfusions can be done on an outpatient basis without undue complication.

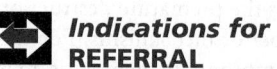

Indications for REFERRAL

A patient with anemia unexplained by routine lab workup should be referred to a hematologist for further evaluation and management. For many patients, one or two visits will suffice to establish a diagnosis for which follow-up and management can be done by the primary care physician. The same can be said for stable or asymptomatic congenital disorders. For more acute disorders, such as active immune-mediated hemolysis or TTP, a hematologist should assume total care of these complex problems.

Cost-Effectiveness

It is difficult to gauge the cost-effectiveness of the many therapies used to treat hemolytic anemia. Certainly, in asymptomatic or minimally symptomatic patients who may have immune-mediated hemolysis, prednisone is more cost-effective than transfusion, when possible. Asymptomatic patients with chronic hemolytic processes usually do not require admission, despite a low hematocrit, and can safely be evaluated and treated on an outpatient basis. Many therapies that were once considered inpatient procedures, such as plasma exchange for relapsing TTP, can be safely done in a properly appointed ambulatory facility, thus avoiding hospital costs.

 ## SPECIFIC DISORDERS

ABNORMALITIES OF THE ERYTHROCYTE MEMBRANE

Inherited Hemolytic Anemias Resulting from Membrane Protein Abnormalities

The erythrocyte membrane is formed by a lipid bilayer intercalated by membrane proteins. The bilayer is fluid in nature but is stabilized by its interaction with the membrane skeleton, a scaffold of proteins consisting mainly of spectrin, actin, and protein 4.1. This cytoskeleton is a major determinant of erythrocyte shape, strength, and flexibility. Numerous inherited and acquired alterations in erythrocyte membrane structure or intracellular content result in diminished deformability of the red cell with consequent accelerated hemolysis.

The molecular basis of erythrocyte membrane abnormalities can be divided into vertical and horizontal interactions. Vertical interactions are perpendicular to the plane of the membrane and stabilize the lipid bilayer. They involve interactions between spectrin, ankyrin (band 2.1; binds the lipid bilayer to the membrane skeleton), and ion transport channel (band 3); protein 4.1 and glycophorin C; and skeletal proteins with negatively charged lipids of the inner bilayer. Horizontal interactions are parallel to the plane of the membrane and support the structural integrity of the cells after their exposure to shear stress. These interactions involve the assembly of spectrin heterodimers into tetramers, the principal building blocks of the skeleton, and the binding of the distal ends of spectrin heterodimers with actin and protein 4.1.

Hereditary Spherocytosis

Definition
Hereditary spherocytosis (HS) is a common inherited hemolytic disorder of varying severity, characterized by spherocytosis on the blood smear, increased erythrocyte osmotic fragility, and a favorable clinical response to splenectomy.

Prevalence and Epidemiology
Reported in persons of most races, HS is the most common inherited anemia in patients of European descent, with an incidence of 1 in 2,000 among individuals in the United States and England. Despite the fact that the clinical severity of HS is highly variable among different kindreds, it is relatively uniform within a given family, where it is inherited in an autosomal dominant fashion. Recessively inherited HS has also been described, in some cases presenting with severe hemolytic anemia.

Etiologic Factors
Hereditary spherocytosis occurs as a result of a multistep process caused by an inherited deficiency or dysfunction of one of the skeletal proteins of the erythrocyte membrane including ankyrin, band 3, α-spectrin, β-spectrin, and protein 4.2 (pallidin) (Table 244.2). Accelerated erythrocyte destruction occurs in the spleen, where these intrinsically abnormal cells are retained and "conditioned." A combined deficiency of spectrin and ankyrin is found in most cases of HS, followed by deficiencies of band 3, spectrin only, and protein 4.2 (seen in the Japanese). Ankyrin "anchors" the spectrin-based skeleton to the intracellular portion of band 3. Multiple genetic defects are responsible for the array of protein abnormalities seen in HS; however, with few exceptions, mutations are private (unique for a given kindred).

Pathogenesis
The pathophysiology of HS is thought to involve aberrant vertical interactions occurring between the spectrin-based cytoskeleton and the lipid bilayer. Because of the decrease in spectrin content, the density of the membrane skeletal monolayer is reduced, leading to a destabilization of the lipid bilayer and a release of lipids from the membrane. This decrease in cell surface-to-volume ratio accounts for the spheroidal shape and decrease in deformability, which is diminished further by a high internal viscosity resulting from mild cellular dehydration. The red cells that are "conditioned" in the splenic pulp are considerably more osmotically fragile and more spherical. Some of the conditioned cells reappear in the peripheral circulation; their presence is suggested by a tail in the osmotic fragility curve, representing a subpopulation of the most fragile cells (Fig. 244.1). The primary cause of hemolysis is postulated to be entrapment of spherocytes in the splenic microcirculation and ingestion by splenic macrophages. Low pH, low glucose, and

TABLE 244.2.	**CLINICAL AND MOLECULAR HETEROGENEITY OF HEREDITARY SPHEROCYTOSIS**		
Inheritance	**Clinical Presentation**	**Reported Molecular Defect**	**Prevalence**
Autosomal dominant	HS with minimal, mild to moderate hemolysis	Ankyrin	Probably common
		β-Spectrin	About 10% of all patients
Autosomal recessive	HS with severe hemolysis	α-Spectrin	Probably rare
	HS with mild to moderate hemolysis	4.2	Rare in whites, may be more common in Japan
		? Anion transport protein	

HS, hereditary spherocytosis.

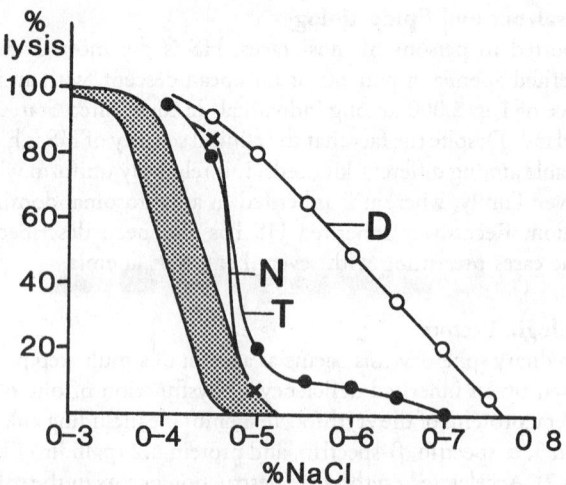

FIGURE 244.1. Different types of osmotic fragility curves in hereditary spherocytosis (HS). *N*, Normal-type curve, revealing an overall increase of osmotic fragility. Shaded area represents the normal range. *T*, Tailed curve, revealing a second population (a tail) of very fragile cells. *D*, Diagonal curve, in patients with severe HS, in whom the two cell populations are not easily separable. (Adapted from Dacie J. The haemolytic anaemias. In: *The hereditary haemolytic anaemias, vol 1. 3rd ed.* Edinburgh: Churchill Livingstone, 1985:114, with permission.)

toxic free radicals released by macrophages have been postulated to contribute to the early demise of these red cells. Recent murine studies suggest that a membrane permeability defect may also exist.

Clinical Findings

The clinical manifestations of HS are highly variable and correlate with the severity of spectrin deficiency, ranging from an asymptomatic condition to severe, life-threatening hemolysis (Table 244.2). In its more common form, the clinical features include a mild, often compensated hemolytic anemia, acholuric jaundice, splenomegaly, and the presence of similar findings in one or more siblings, children, or parents of the patient. In some, the clinical expression is mild, with normal or slightly elevated serum bilirubin and reticulocyte counts, and only subtle changes in erythrocyte morphology. The disease may be discovered during evaluation of asymptomatic splenomegaly, a family study of a patient with more typical symptoms of the disease, or exacerbation of hemolysis secondary to infection. Rarely, the diagnosis may first be made in old age. There is evidence to support the presence of an asymptomatic carrier state.

HS should be distinguished from other spherocytic hemolytic anemias, such as autoimmune hemolytic anemia (AIHA), unstable hemoglobins, and the rare Rh deficiency syndrome. Spherocytes in HS usually can be distinguished from those in immunohemolytic anemia by their relatively uniform shape and increased hemoglobin concentration. Occasional spherocytes are also seen in patients with large spleens (i.e., cirrhosis, myelofibrosis) or in patients with microangiopathic anemias, but it is usually not difficult to distinguish these conditions from HS.

Aplastic crisis may occur in association with infection by parvovirus, which inhibits erythropoiesis in vitro and in vivo. The infection is asymptomatic or manifests as a flulike syndrome

with fever, chills, mild respiratory symptoms, and a maculopapular rash on the face (slapped cheek syndrome), trunk, and extremities. Aplastic crisis should be differentiated from acute megaloblastic changes resulting from folate deficiency, such as during pregnancy, when the increased folate requirements of hyperplastic erythropoiesis are compounded by the high folate demands of the developing fetus. Bilirubin gallstones occur in more than half of all patients, including those with a relatively mild form of the disease. Other complications may include leg ulcerations or dermatitis, which heal quickly after splenectomy. Occasionally, extramedullary hemopoiesis, manifesting as a single mass or multiple masses, has been detected. Iron overload has been reported in several patients with HS who were heterozygous for human leukocyte antigen–linked hemochromatosis.

Laboratory Findings

Elevated unconjugated bilirubin, low haptoglobin, and reticulocytosis indicate hemolysis. The mean corpuscular hemoglobin concentration is increased, occasionally reaching 40 g per deciliter, which reflects mild cellular dehydration, and the erythrocyte volume is often inappropriately low considering the increase in reticulocytes, which have a larger volume than mature erythrocytes. Spherocytes are readily apparent only in more severe forms of the disease, whereas they can be missed in mild HS. In patients with severe or atypical forms of HS, additional morphologic abnormalities include surface spicules, irregular contour, and "pincered" erythrocytes with a mushroom-like appearance (Fig. 244.2).

The principal diagnostic test, erythrocyte osmotic fragility, measures the surface-to-volume ratio of the cells. Because their membranes are virtually unstretchable and impermeable to cations, erythrocytes act as nearly perfect osmometers—swelling in hypotonic solutions, then undergoing hemolysis after reaching a spheroidal shape. Because of a diminished surface-to-volume ratio, HS cells hemolyze more in hypotonic salt solutions than normal cells do (Fig. 244.1).

Deficiencies of one or more membrane proteins can be demonstrated in about 80% of cases by sodium dodecyl sulfate/polyacrylamide gel electrophoresis (SDS-PAGE) of erythrocyte membrane proteins or by radioimmunoassay.

Optimal Management

Patients with mild clinical features may require no specific therapy beyond folic acid supplementation. Splenectomy corrects the hemolytic anemia, but erythrocyte survival may remain slightly shortened in some patients. Spherocytosis becomes less prominent and osmotic fragility improves. Indications for splenectomy are somewhat controversial, but unequivocal criteria include severe symptomatic hemolytic anemia or its complications, particularly gallstones; mild hemolytic anemia in association with gallstones; and a history of gallstones in similarly affected family members. Splenectomy is not recommended in patients with mild HS who do not have family histories of gallbladder disease because these patients tend to have relatively uneventful courses. Splenectomy failures may be due to an accessory spleen, which can occur in up to one-third of patients; accidental autotransplantation of splenic tissue into the peritoneal cavity at the time of splenectomy followed by the develop-

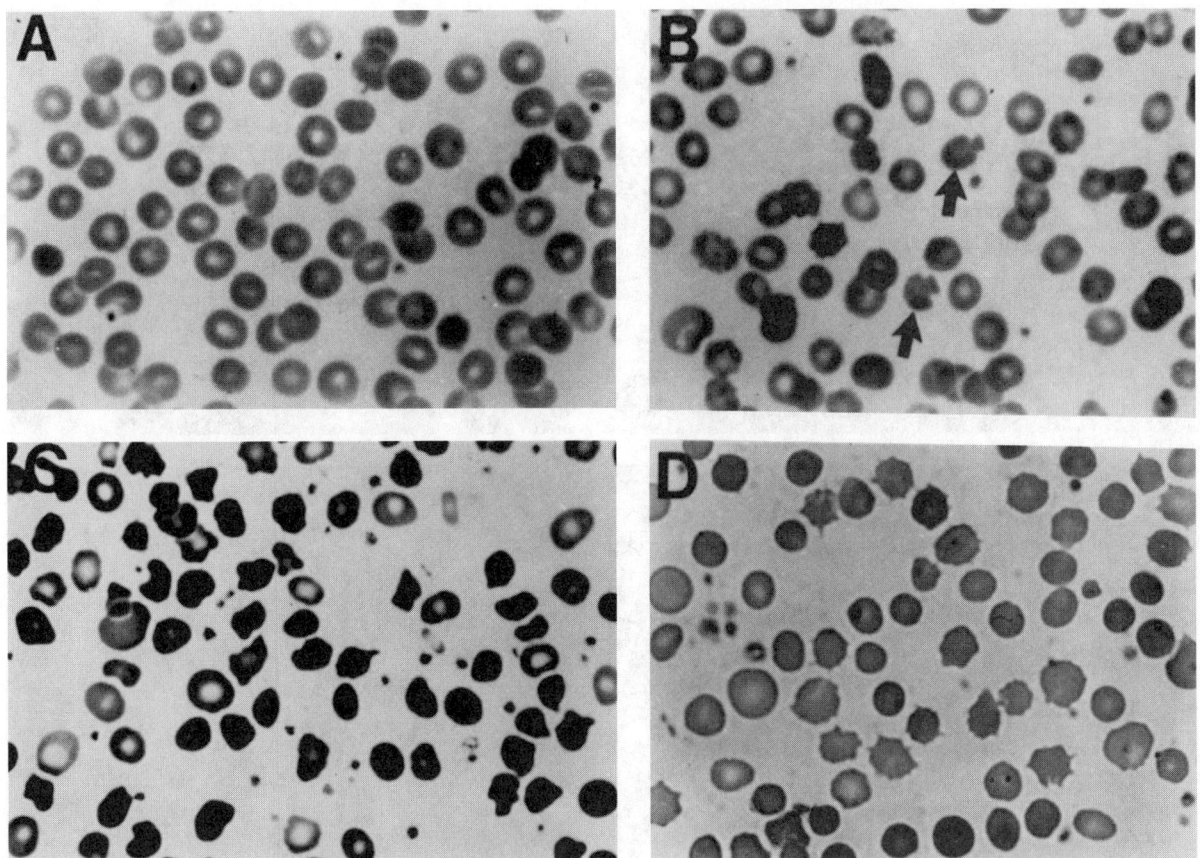

FIGURE 244.2. Blood films from patients with HS of varying severity. **A:** Typical HS. Although many cells have a spheroidal shape, some of them retain a central concavity. **B:** HS with pincered red blood cells (*arrows*). Occasional spiculated red blood cells also are present. **C:** Severe atypical HS due to a severe combined spectrin and ankyrin deficiency. In addition to spherocytes, many cells have an irregular contour. **D:** HS associated with abnormal β-spectrin that binds defectively to protein 4.1 (Spβ-4.1). Some of the spherocytes have prominent surface projections, and resemble spheroacanthocytes. (From Palek J. Anemias due to increased destruction of erythrocytes with abnormal shape and membrane defects. In: Williams WS, Beutler E, Ersler AJ, et al., eds. *Hematology.* New York: McGraw-Hill, 1989:558, with permission.)

ment (7 to 15 years later) of new splenic tissue (splenosis); or another concomitant hemolytic disorder.

Partial splenectomy (removal of 80% to 90% of splenic tissue), has been effective in decreasing the hemolytic rate while maintaining splenic phagocytic function and has been recommended in children, particularly transfusion-dependent infants. Prior to splenectomy, all patients should receive polyvalent vaccines against *Pneumococcus, Haemophilus influenzae,* and *Meningococcus.*

Because of a high prevalence of gallstones, all patients with HS should undergo periodic ultrasonographic examinations of the gallbladder. Patients in aplastic crisis from parvovirus or other infection should be supported with red cell transfusions until the crisis resolves.

Hereditary Elliptocytosis and Related Disorders

Definition

Hereditary elliptocytosis (HE) is a clinically, genetically, and biochemically heterogenous group of inherited disorders, having

in common elliptical erythrocytes. Three distinct subtypes have been described based on erythrocyte morphology. *Common HE,* the most prevalent form, is characterized by biconcave elliptocytes and, occasionally, rod-shaped cells, and, in its more severe form, designated hereditary pyropoikilocytosis (HPP), by poikilocytes, microspherocytes, and fragmented erythrocytes. *Spherocytic HE* is a phenotypic hybrid of HE and HS. *Stomatocytic HE,* also known as *Southeast Asian ovalocytosis* or *Melanesian ovalocytosis,* is characterized by "spoon-shaped" erythrocytes and other red cells that are more round and have a longitudinal or transverse slit (Fig. 244.3).

Incidence and Epidemiology

The true incidence of HE is unknown since many individuals are asymptomatic, but it is estimated at 1 in 2,000 to 1 in 4,000 worldwide. It is considerably higher (1.2 in 2,000 to 2.4 in 4,000) in equatorial Africa. In Southeast Asia, the incidence of Southeast Asian ovalocytosis is as high as 30%. The inheritance characteristically is autosomal dominant, but occasional patients inherit HE from an asymptomatic carrier who has the same

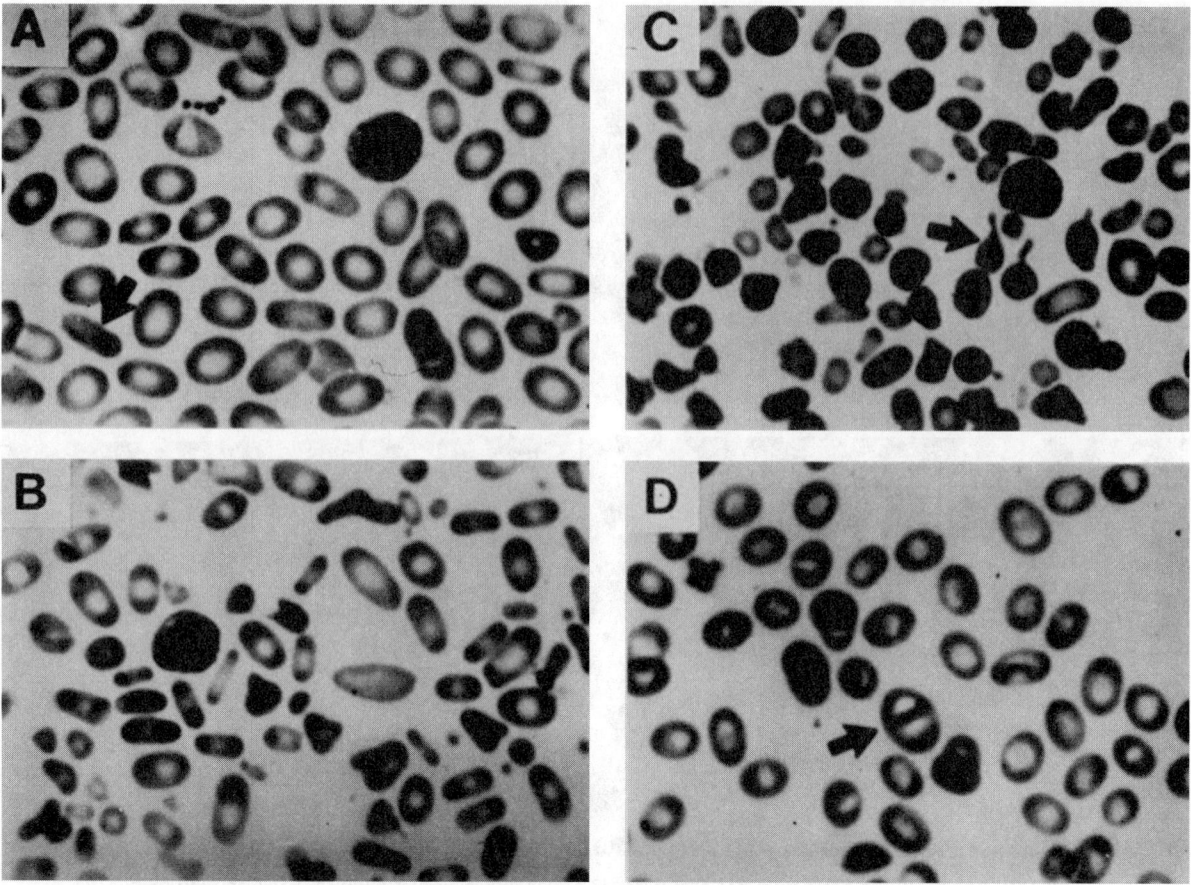

FIGURE 244.3. Blood films of patients with various forms of hemolytic elliptocytosis (HE). **A:** Dominantly inherited, mild, common HE. Note the predominant elliptocytosis with some rod-shaped cells (*arrows*) and the virtual absence of poikilocytes. **B:** Dominantly inherited severe HE. In addition to elliptocytosis, there are numerous small fragments and poikilocytes. **C:** Hereditary pyropoikilocytosis. The patient is a double heterozygote for mutant α-spectrin and a presumed synthetic defect of this protein. Note prominent microspherocytosis, micropoikilocytosis, and fragmentation. Only a few elliptocytes are present. Some poikilocytes are in the process of budding (*arrow*). **D:** Southeast Asian ovalocytosis. Most of the cells are oval, some of them containing a longitudinal slit or a transverse ridge (*arrow*). All blood smears were photographed at the same magnification (×1000).

membrane protein mutation. The clinical severity is highly variable, reflecting heterogeneous molecular causes. HPP is inherited as an autosomal recessive disorder. Typically, one of the parents of the offspring with HPP carries an identifiable molecular defect (e.g., mutation of spectrin) and is asymptomatic or has mild HE, whereas the other asymptomatic parent does not have an identifiable molecular defect or carries an asymptomatic spectrin mutation. Genetic studies have linked HE to blood group antigens Rh and Duffy, the genes of which reside on the short arm of chromosome 1. The gene for Duffy blood group is close to that of α-spectrin, and the Rh gene is close to the region containing the gene for protein 4.1.

Etiologic Factors

The underlying defect involves dysfunction or a deficiency of one of the major skeletal proteins. The clinical expression of these defects is shown in Table 244.3. The most common defects in HE are mutations of α- or β-spectrin. At the level of protein function, these abnormal spectrins are characterized by the ina-

bility of spectrin heterodimers to self-associate into tetramers. The second group consists of defects of protein 4.1. A total absence of protein 4.1 (homozygous condition) is associated with severe hemolytic HE, whereas a partial deficiency is associated with mild dominantly inherited HE. Several abnormal isoforms (increase or decrease in the size of the protein) have been reported. In a few patients with minimal HE, deficiency of glycophorin C has been detected.

Pathogenesis

In most patients with HE and HPP, the principal lesion involves horizontal membrane protein associations, namely, the spectrin dimer–dimer contact. This protein interaction, which is parallel to the plane of the membrane, maintains the structural integrity of the skeleton. The formation of elliptocytes is most likely a result of a permanent plastic deformation of the membrane skeleton. The elliptocytic shape is acquired in the circulation (Fig. 244.3), but the pathobiologic processes involved in this shape change are unclear. The clinical expression of HE is correlated

| TABLE 244.3. | CLINICAL AND MOLECULAR HETEROGENEITY OF HEREDITARY ELLIPTOCYTOSIS |

Clinical Presentation	Hemolysis	Red Blood Cell Morphology	Reported Molecular Defects	Inheritance
Common HE				
Asymptomatic carrier state	Absent	Normal	α- or β-spectrin mutations affecting SpD-SpD self-association	Offspring may have HE or HPP
Mild HE	Minimal or absent	Biconcave elliptocytes, some rod-shaped cells	α- or β-spectrin mutations affecting SpD-SpD self-association 4.1 Deficiency or abnormal 4.1 protein Glycophorin C deficiency	Autosomal dominant
HE with sporadic hemolysis	Moderate	Biconcave elliptocytes, rod-shaped cells, some poikilocytes	Probably the same spectrin defects as in mild HE	Other family members may have mild HE
HE with neonatal poikilocytosis	Moderate	Micropoikilocytes, fragments, elliptocytes	Probably the same spectrin defects as in mild HE	One parent has mild HE
HE with chronic hemolysis	Moderate	Biconcave elliptocytes, rod-shaped cells, some poikilocytes	Simple heterozygotes for some spectrin mutations; occasionally, homozygotes for α-spectrin mutants causing mild defects in SpD–SpD self-association	Autosomal dominant, occasionally homozygous or doubly heterozygous HE
Severe hemolytic HE	Severe	Elliptocytes, poikilocytes, fragments, occasional microspherocytes	Homozygotes or double heterozygotes for α- or β-spectrin mutations	HE homozygotes or double heterozygotes
HPP[a]	Severe, occasionally moderate	Poikilocytes, fragments, microspherocytes, occasional elliptocytes	Spectrin mutations causing SpD–SpD defect and spectrin deficiency	Autosomal recessive; usualy both parents are asymptomatic, occasionally one of them has mild HE
Spherocytic HE (Hereditary Ovalocytosis)				
Heterozygous state	Mild	Round elliptocytes, variable percentage of spherocytes	Partial 4.1 deficiency in some patients	Dominant
Homozygous state	Severe	Poikilocytes, microspherocytes, fragments, round elliptocytes	Complete deficiency of the 4.1 protein	Homozygous HE
Stomatocytic HE (Southeast Asian Ovalocytosis)				
	Mild or absent	Stomatocytic elliptocytes	Anion transporter	Autosomal dominant

[a] Most patients with HPP are double heterozygotes for an α-spectrin mutant and another defect (presumably a synthetic defect of this protein). Occasionally, the HPP phenotype is seen in patients who are doubly heterozygous for two α-spectrin mutations.
HE, hereditary elliptocytosis; HPP, hereditary pyropoikilocytosis; SpD, spectrin heterodimer.

directly with the severity of the spectrin dimer self-association defect as evidenced by the increase in the spectrin dimer percentage in the erythrocyte. Data suggest that the critical threshold of unassembled spectrin in the cell is 40% to 50%, above which patients exhibit severe hemolysis.

Clinical Findings

Common HE can be divided into several subgroups based on clinical severity. The most common is mild HE, an asymptomatic condition discovered during routine blood film evaluation.

Some of these patients do not have clinical evidence of hemolysis, and their erythrocyte survival may even be normal. Others, although clinically asymptomatic, have laboratory evidence of mild compensated hemolysis. Transient hemolysis develops in some patients with mild HE when the "minimal" HE defect is augmented by superimposed events such as viral, bacterial, or protozoal infection; renal transplant rejection; splenomegaly; B_{12} deficiency; or even normal pregnancy. In addition to elliptocytes and rod-shaped cells, blood films of such patients show considerable poikilocytosis. The underlying cause of increased hemolysis is not known. The prevailing hypothesis proposes that the marginally unstable erythrocytes of HE are damaged by the excessive shear stress of an altered microcirculation. There are several reports of HE with moderate to severe chronic hemolytic anemia requiring splenectomy. Some of these patients have a homozygous form of the disease, whereas in others, hemolytic HE is inherited through several generations. Asymptomatic carriers, with α-spectrin mutations involving the spectrin heterodimer association site, also have been reported. Typically, such patients are the parents (or siblings) of patients with HPP or, occasionally, HE.

HPP is an autosomal recessive disorder characterized by a severe hemolytic anemia with striking micropoikilocytosis and microspherocytosis with a mean corpuscular volume as low as 50 μm³. Patients with HPP are heterozygous for an α- or β-spectrin mutation associated with defective spectrin self-association and another defect possibly involving spectrin synthesis, which leads to a superimposed partial deficiency of spectrin. The same phenotype has been described in patients who are compound heterozygotes or homozygotes for one or two α-spectrin mutations; the concomitant spectrin deficiency presumably results from instability of one of these spectrin mutants. HPP is predominantly a disease of the black race, but it also has been seen in nonblacks. HPP represents a subset of HE: some of the relatives of HPP probands may have mild HE and carry identical α-spectrin mutations; however, the defect is more severe in HPP, where it is present in conjunction with a partial spectrin deficiency.

Spherocytic HE, also known as HE with spherocytosis or hemolytic hereditary ovalocytosis, is characterized by the presence of occasional spherocytes on the blood film and an increased osmotic fragility. These patients often have a clinically apparent hemolytic anemia in spite of relatively subtle changes in erythrocyte morphology.

Southeast Asian ovalocytosis is common (15% to 30%) among aboriginal populations of Malaysia, Melanesia, and possibly Indonesia. The condition is asymptomatic and appears to confer resistance to invasion by several strains of malarial parasites.

These disorders should be distinguished from other conditions in which elliptocytes and poikilocytes are commonly encountered, including iron deficiency, thalassemias, megaloblastic anemias, myelofibrosis, myelophthisic anemias, myelodysplastic syndromes, and pyruvate kinase deficiency. However, in these conditions, the quantity of elliptocytes in the peripheral smear seldom exceeds 60%.

Laboratory Findings

The percentage of elliptocytes on the blood film of a patient with a biochemically defined molecular defect of skeletal proteins is highly variable, ranging from 15% to 100%. A positive family history is more important for the diagnosis of HE than is any precise percentage of elliptocytes; therefore, evaluation of the peripheral blood smear, together with study of other family members, represents an essential step in diagnosis. Osmotic fragility is normal in mild forms of common HE but is increased in spherocytic HE, common HE with severe hemolysis, and HPP, reflecting the presence of spheroelliptocytes, microspherocytes, and fragments. In HPP, erythrocytes fragment and their

mutant spectrin denatures at temperatures of 45°C to 46°C, whereas this same process occurs in normal cells at 49°C to 50°C. Thermal instability also has been detected in heterozygous patients with HE who carry spectrin mutations.

Techniques for diagnosing these conditions involve the separation of membrane proteins by SDS-PAGE, which can detect deficiencies or defects based on migration patterns. In patients with common HE, mutations of the spectrin protein are present in roughly 60%, and most can be detected readily by this method. An increased fraction of unassembled, dimeric spectrin also typically is present in erythrocyte extracts.

Optimal Management

For patients who manifest hemolytic disease, treatment with splenectomy in a fashion similar to that used for HS reverses the anemia. HPP and hereditary stomatocytosis may also respond partially to splenectomy.

Acanthocytosis

Definition

Spur cells, or acanthocytes (from the Greek *acantha*, or thorn), are erythrocytes with multiple irregular projections that vary in width, length, and surface distribution (Fig. 244.4). They were first described in a patient with atypical retinitis pigmentosa, a progressive ataxic neuropathy, and fat malabsorption in whom subsequent studies showed congenital absence of β-lipoproteins. Acanthocytes also are seen in certain inherited neurologic disorders without abetalipoproteinemia (chorea–acanthocytosis syndrome), in association with the McLeod phenotype, and as an acquired disorder (see later).

Etiologic Factors

Both *abetalipoproteinemia* and *chorea–acanthocytosis syndrome* are inherited as autosomal recessive disorders. Acanthocytes have been described in association with markedly reduced red cell expression of Kell antigens, referred to as the *McLeod phenotype*, which is inherited in an X-linked fashion.

Pathogenesis

The primary molecular defect in abetalipoproteinemia involves a congenital absence of apolipoprotein-β in plasma. Consequently, all plasma lipoproteins containing this apoprotein and plasma triglycerides are nearly absent, and plasma cholesterol and phospholipid levels are markedly reduced. Plasma sphingomyelin is relatively increased at the expense of phosphatidylethanolamine. Bone marrow erythrocyte precursors have normal morphologic characteristics. The acanthocytic shape becomes progressively more apparent as the red cells mature and age in the circulation. The most striking abnormality of the acanthocyte membrane in abetalipoproteinemia is an increase in membrane sphingomyelin. This phospholipid is located predominantly in the outer hemileaflet of the membrane bilayer, and the excess sphingomyelin causes an expansion of its surface area that probably is responsible for the surface irregularities.

In the McLeod phenotype, the acanthocytic lesion is directly related to the absence of the Kx antigenic substance, a precursor

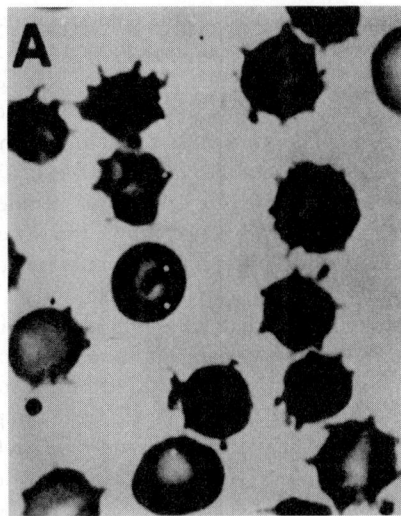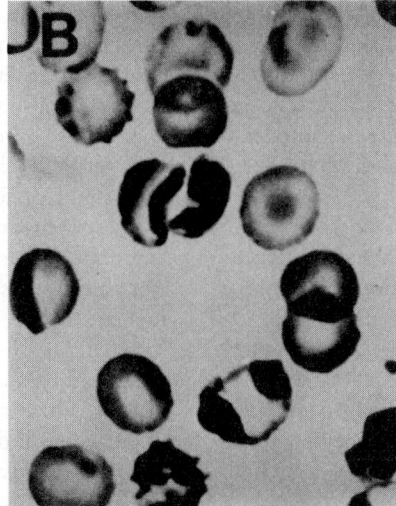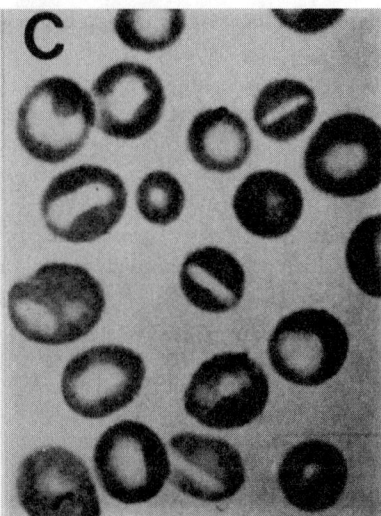

FIGURE 244.4. Blood films of patients with liver cirrhosis and spur cell anemia (A), hereditary xerocytosis (dessicocytosis; B), and stomatocytosis (hydrocytosis; C). (Adapted from Cooper RA, Kimball DB, Durocher JR. The role of the spleen in membrane conditioning and hemolysis of spur cells in liver disease. *N Engl J Med* 1974;290:1279; and Lande WM, Mentzer WC. Haemolytic anaemia associated with increased cation permeability. *Clin Haematol* 1985;14:89, with permission.)

molecule necessary for Kell antigen expression. However, the molecular basis of acanthocytosis in the McLeod syndrome is unknown.

The mechanism of acanthocytosis in chorea–acanthocytosis syndrome is unknown, but a recent report suggested an abnormality of the anion transport protein (band 3).

Clinical and Laboratory Findings

Abetalipoproteinemia manifests in the first month of life by steatorrhea. Retinitis pigmentosa (often resulting in blindness) and progressive neurologic abnormalities, characterized by ataxia and intention tremors, develop between ages 5 and 10 years, with death occurring in the second or third decade. Hematologic manifestations include mild normocytic anemia with acanthocytosis (50% to 90%) and normal to slightly elevated reticulocyte counts. Patients may have nutritional deficiencies (iron, folate) from fat malabsorption, resulting in more severe anemia.

Chorea–acanthocytosis syndrome is a disease of adult onset characterized by progressive neurologic dysfunction with orofacial dyskinesis, limb chorea, neurogenic muscle hypotonia and atrophy. Hematologic manifestations are minimal and include a variable percentage of acanthocytes on the peripheral smear without anemia.

In some cases, the McLeod phenotype coexists with chronic granulomatous disease of childhood, retinitis pigmentosa, and Duchenne's muscular dystrophy. The genetic loci of these disorders are in proximity of the p21 region of the X chromosome. Therefore, males are affected, and carrier females can be identified by flow cytometric analysis for Kell blood group antigen expression.

Optimal Management

In abetalipoproteinemia, treatment involves dietary restriction of triglycerides and supplementation of lipid soluble vitamins

A, D, E, and K. Vitamin E supplementation may stabilize or improve the retinal and neuromuscular abnormalities. Because the hematologic manifestations are minimal in the chorea–acanthocytosis and McLeod syndromes, no specific therapy has been described.

Stomatocytosis

Definition

Stomatocytes contain a wide transverse slit or stoma. On three-dimensional views, these cells have the shape of a cup or bowl. The slitlike appearance on blood films is an artifact, resulting from folding of the cells during blood smear preparation. Few stomatocytes (3% to 5%) commonly are found on blood films of normal persons. Several inherited and acquired disorders are associated with stomatocytosis; these include *hereditary stomatocytosis, hereditary xerocytosis,* and *Rh deficiency syndrome.*

Etiologic Factors and Pathogenesis

Inherited disorders are associated with abnormalities in erythrocyte cation permeability and volume, which is increased (hence the designation hydrocytosis), decreased (desiccocytosis or xerocytosis), or near normal. Although the mechanism behind this morphologic abnormality is unknown, stomatocytosis can be produced in vitro by certain drugs that intercalate into the inner half of the asymmetrical lipid bilayer, resulting in surface area expansion relative to that of the outer half of the bilayer.

In hereditary stomatocytosis, overhydration and swelling of cells occurs as a result of a membrane permeability defect, which leads to marked sodium influx into the cells, producing an increase in intracellular sodium and water content. The underlying molecular lesion is unknown.

Hereditary xerocytosis is characterized by erythrocyte dehydration and decreased osmotic fragility. The underlying defect in hereditary xerocytosis is complex and involves a net loss of potassium from the erythrocytes that is not accompanied by a proportional gain of sodium, resulting in a reduced net intracellular cation and cell water content. Except for an increase in membrane-associated glyceraldehyde-3-phosphate dehydrogenase, which binds to band 3, no other abnormalities have been detected.

The term *Rh deficiency syndrome* is used to designate those rare individuals who have absent (Rh_{null}) or markedly reduced (Rh_{mod}) expression of the Rh antigen in association with hemolytic anemia and the presence of stomatocytes and occasional spherocytes on the blood film. The erythrocytes of this disorder are also dehydrated as evidenced by decreased cell cation and water content and increased cell density. However, the relation between the absence of the Rh antigen and erythrocyte alterations leading to hemolysis is unknown.

Clinical/Laboratory Findings and Disease Management

Hereditary stomatocytosis is an uncommon dominantly inherited hemolytic anemia that also has been designated hereditary hydrocytosis to indicate an overhydration and swelling of cells. The disorder manifests as moderate to severe hemolysis with 10% to 30% stomatocytes on the blood film, an increased mean corpuscular volume, and a reduced mean corpuscular hemoglobin concentration. Osmotic fragility is markedly increased. The hemolytic anemia is improved, although often not fully corrected, by splenectomy.

Hereditary xerocytosis presents as an autosomal dominant hemolytic anemia. Sporadic cases have been described that share features of hereditary stomatocytosis and xerocytosis. Both stomatocytes and some target cells are seen on the blood film. Splenectomy may ameliorate hemolysis in some, whereas in others it is ineffective.

Osmotic fragility is increased in Rh deficiency syndrome, reflecting a marked reduction of the membrane surface area. Splenectomy results in a marked improvement of hemolytic anemia.

Acquired Abnormalities of the Erythrocyte Membrane

Numerous acquired hemolytic states are caused primarily by alteration of the balance among the membrane lipid moieties. Increased membrane cholesterol causes the membrane surface to expand, producing *target cells*. Substances that localize in the outer membrane lamina cause *echinocytic* (burr cell) shape change; those that bind to the inner lamina produce *stomatocytic* (slitlike or bowl-shaped) alterations.

Acquired Acanthocytosis, Target Cells, Stomatocytosis, and Echinocytosis

Definition, Etiologic Factors, and Pathogenesis

Acquired acanthocytosis is found most commonly in patients with severe alcoholic hepatocellular disease. It may be associated with a rapidly progressive hemolytic anemia, termed *spur cell anemia*, which is a rare but ominous complication of severe

liver disease. In the usual state, plasma free cholesterol readily equilibrates with the erythrocyte membrane cholesterol pool, in contrast to esterified cholesterol, which cannot be transferred from plasma to the erythrocyte membrane. Patients with severe liver disease have abnormal lipoproteins that contain a high free (unesterified) cholesterol/phospholipid ratio. The excess free cholesterol preferentially partitions into the outer hemileaflet of the erythrocyte membrane, which normally contains equal amounts of free cholesterol and phospholipids, and leads to an expansion of its surface relative to the inner hemileaflet. This increase in free cholesterol together with remodeling in the spleen results in acanthocyte formation. Phospholipid biosynthesis and repair may also be impaired, thus contributing to this process. These cells enter the circulation but are readily trapped in the spleen and destroyed. A similar clinical syndrome has been described in advanced metastatic liver disease, cardiac cirrhosis, Wilson's disease, and fulminant hepatitis. A few acanthocytes are seen in malnutrition, hypothyroidism, post-splenectomy states, and AIDS, possibly because of a superimposed nutritional deficiency. Acanthocytes should be differentiated from echinocytes (see later).

Target cells (codocytes) seen in patients with cirrhosis, hepatitis, acute (alcoholic) fatty liver, or obstructive jaundice have expanded membrane surface area because of symmetrically increased membrane cholesterol and phospholipid. In contrast, target cells occurring in hemoglobinopathies and iron deficiency have a high membrane surface area relative to the decreased hemoglobin content.

Acquired stomatocytosis is associated most commonly with ethanol abuse and obstructive hepatocellular liver diseases in which asymmetrical expansion of the inner lipid layer of the erythrocyte membrane occurs. Stomatocytosis can also be produced in vitro by procaine, phenothiazines, and calcium channel blockers, and may be seen in malignant neoplasms.

Echinocytes (burr cells) differ from acanthocytes in that they have uniform, fine surface spicules. The most common cause of echinocytosis is a laboratory artifact related to blood storage, contact with glass, or increased pH. Echinocytes are also seen in uremia, in pyruvate kinase deficiency, and following red cell transfusion. The mechanism of echinocytosis in uremia is unknown, but in pyruvate kinase and post-transfusional states, it may be associated with depletion of adenosine triphosphate (ATP), a state known to produce echinocytes in vitro. Hemolytic anemia with echinocytosis has been described in athletes after strenuous physical exertion, and in patients with hypomagnesemia and hypophosphatemia, presumably due to decreased intracellular ATP stores.

Clinical and Laboratory Findings

The anemia of chronic liver disease is multifactorial (gastrointestinal blood loss, iron and folic acid deficiencies, hemodilution, and alcohol effects on erythrocyte precursors). In patients with end-stage liver disease, development of spur cell anemia is associated with a grim prognosis.

Optimal Management

In patients with end-stage liver disease, treatment is largely supportive, with nutritional replacement and transfusions as needed.

Although the spleen plays a major role in the remodeling and sequestration of acanthocytes, its removal is not advisable.

Paroxysmal Nocturnal Hemoglobinuria

Definition
In its classic form, paroxysmal nocturnal hemoglobinuria (PNH) is characterized by hemolysis accompanied by nocturnal hemoglobinuria. It is unique among hemolytic anemias in being an acquired intrinsic abnormality of the erythrocyte, but it is also a clonal hematopoietic disorder affecting all hematopoietic elements.

Etiologic Factors and Pathogenesis
PNH appears to be caused by the acquisition of a mutation in the *pig-A* gene in a totipotent hematopoietic stem cell. This results in the inability of the affected stem cell and its progeny to synthesize the glycosylphosphatidylinositol (GPI) anchor that is used to attach numerous integral membrane proteins to the cell surface. One such protein, membrane inhibitor of reactive lysis (MIRL; CD59), protects cells from lysis by the complement membrane attack complex. Decay-accelerating factor (DAF; CD55) controls C3 convertase. The combined deficiency of DAF and MIRL accounts for the increased susceptibility to lysis by complement. Lack of these proteins may be responsible for the underlying hypercoagulability and may also account for the increased incidence of infections and deficient hematopoiesis.

Clinical Findings
Patients with PNH manifest all of the clinical and laboratory signs of chronic hemolytic anemia. Nocturnal hemoglobinuria occurs in a minority of patients. More commonly, hemoglobinuria is irregular in its occurrence and may be infrequent or even absent. Other symptoms are recurrent abdominal pain, vomiting, severe headaches, and ocular pain. Iron loss occurs in the urine, and hemosiderinuria is a constant feature of the disease, frequently leading to iron deficiency.

One of the most serious manifestations of PNH is the formation of venous thromboses at several unusual sites. Budd–Chiari syndrome, resulting from hepatic vein thrombosis, is a particularly common development that has an ominous prognosis. Clots in the cerebral veins, the splenic vein, and the veins of the dermis have occurred, the last resulting in necrotic skin lesions.

Laboratory Findings
Anemia is accompanied by reticulocytosis. If iron deficiency is present, the red cells may be microcytic and hypochromic. The bone marrow usually is hypercellular as a result of increased erythropoiesis, and the myeloid-to-erythroid ratio may be reversed. Hypoplasia of the marrow is not unusual. PNH commonly is associated with aplastic anemia. Aplasia may be the presenting disorder or, less commonly, develop during the course of PNH. Both erythrocyte membrane acetylcholinesterase and leukocyte alkaline phosphatase activities are decreased.

The most convenient screening test for PNH is the sucrose hemolysis test. If the results of this test are positive, the diagnosis may be confirmed using the acidified serum lysis test (Ham test) in which the red cells have an increased susceptibility to lysis by complement. Hemosiderin is usually found in the urine. Flow cytometry is used to demonstrate the lack of CD59 and CD55.

Optimal Management
The course of PNH is highly variable, with some patients dying within months of the onset of symptoms and others surviving for decades. Although the long-term outlook is good for many patients, the disease can be fatal, particularly as a result of the thrombotic manifestations or complications of pancytopenia.

Acute hemolysis may be treated with glucocorticoids, which inhibit the activation of complement. Iron deficiency due to chronic urinary loss is corrected with supplementation. If iron is given, the apparent rate of hemolysis rises as a result of increased marrow production of complement-sensitive red cells. To maintain an adequate hematocrit, transfusion may be necessary.

Acute thrombotic events are managed with anticoagulation. In some instances, such as hepatic vein thrombosis, thrombolytic therapy has been recommended. Bone marrow aplasia has responded to infusions of antithymocyte globulin. PNH may be cured by allogeneic or syngeneic bone marrow transplantation.

HEMOLYTIC ANEMIAS RESULTING FROM METABOLIC DEFICIENCIES

The metabolism of the mature erythrocyte depends on glucose catabolism by the glycolytic pathway and the hexose monophosphate (HMP) shunt. These metabolic pathways depend on the function of more than 20 enzymes and the availability of five major substrates: glucose, glutathione, nicotinamide adenine dinucleotide (NAD), nicotinamide adenine dinucleotide phosphate (NADP), and adenosine diphosphate (ADP). Glucose catabolism maintains the integrity of protein constituents, cell shape, and deformability; maintains hemoglobin iron in the ferrous form; and modulates the oxygen affinity of hemoglobin. These functions are achieved by the generation of sufficient levels of ATP, reduced glutathione, reduced NAD, reduced NADP, and 2,3-bisphosphoglycerate (2,3-BPG; formerly known as 2,3-diphosphoglycerate, or 2,3-DPG).

The principal role of the glycolytic pathway is the generation of ATP, which is required for ATP-linked sodium–potassium and calcium membrane pumps and is essential for cation homeostasis and erythrocyte deformability. The production of 2,3-BPG is regulated by the Rapoport–Luebering shunt. 2,3-BPG lowers hemoglobin–oxygen affinity and facilitates oxygen unloading at the partial pressure of oxygen levels found in the tissues. The major function of the HMP shunt is the production of reduced glutathione for the protection of hemoglobin and other cellular and membrane proteins against oxidant damage.

Hemolytic Anemias Resulting from Erythrocyte Glycolytic Enzyme Defects

Pyruvate Kinase Deficiency and Related Disorders

Definition and Pathogenesis
The principal consequences of glycolytic pathway defects are a decrease in the production of ATP and a decrease or increase

in the level of 2,3-BPG. Deficiencies of erythrocyte hexokinase (HK), glucose phosphate isomerase, phosphofructokinase (PFK), and pyruvate kinase (PK) all lead to a decrease in the ATP concentration. Although inherited deficiencies of nearly all of the glycolytic enzymes have been described, PK deficiency accounts for more than 95% of the hemolytic anemias resulting from glycolytic abnormalities. Glucose phosphate isomerase, HK, and PFK deficiencies are rare but next most common. All glycolytic enzyme defects are autosomal recessive in inheritance except for phosphoglycerate kinase, which is X-linked.

Clinical/Laboratory Findings and Optimal Management

Glucose phosphate isomerase and HK deficiencies are rare non-spherocytic hemolytic anemias that result in decreased ATP and 2,3-BPG concentrations with reduced exercise tolerance; these anemias show improvement after splenectomy. A form of acquired HK deficiency occurs in Wilson's disease, in which hypercupricemia inhibits the enzyme and may lead to episodes of brisk hemolytic anemia. PFK deficiency (Tarui's disease) combines hemolytic anemia with muscle glycogen storage disease. A low red cell ATP level leads to low-grade hemolysis, but muscle pain and weakness on exertion usually are the limiting symptoms. PK deficiency usually is manifested in early childhood as moderate hemolytic anemia with jaundice, splenomegaly, and failure to thrive. Echinocytes, spherocytes, and acanthocytes are observed in the peripheral blood. These cells (called xerocytes) are markedly dehydrated because of low levels of ATP resulting in potassium and water loss and have an increased mean corpuscular hemoglobin concentration. They are poorly deformable, which results in splenic entrapment and destruction. Splenectomy in PK-deficient patients results in significant improvement in the hemolytic anemia, but usually is reserved for patients with poor quality of life, chronic transfusion requirements, and persistent anemia.

Hemolytic Anemia Caused by Disorders of the Hexose Monophosphate Shunt

Glucose-6-Phosphate Dehydrogenase Deficiency

Definition

Glucose-6-phosphate dehydrogenase (G6PD) deficiency is the most common inherited abnormality of erythrocyte metabolism and by far the most clinically important defect of the HMP shunt. Defects of other HMP shunt enzymes are rare but should be considered in cases of oxidant-induced hemolysis when G6PD levels are normal.

Incidence and Epidemiology

In blacks, the predominant form of the enzyme is designated GdA, the faster migrating isozyme; GdA − is the designation for the usual African type of deficiency, which is estimated to occur in about 12% of African American males. In regions of West Africa, its gene frequency is even higher, perhaps because it confers a survival advantage against *Plasmodium falciparum* malaria. The gene is carried on the X chromosome and exhibits extensive polymorphism. Heterozygous carrier females have two erythrocyte populations, one normal (GdA or GdB) and one

deficient (GdA −). Female carriers possess varying degrees of erythrocyte enzyme deficiency depending on the extent of inactivation ("lyonization") of the affected X chromosome bearing the abnormal gene.

A second form of G6PD deficiency, seen in 3% to 5% of persons of Mediterranean ancestry, Ashkenazi Jews, and Asians, is exemplified by the deficient variant G6PD–Mediterranean, designated GdB −.

Etiologic Factors and Pathogenesis

Nearly 300 genetic variants of G6PD have been described and are grouped into categories depending on whether they possess normal, moderately deficient, or severely deficient activity, or are associated with chronic hemolytic anemia. GdA − is a moderately deficient variant that is unstable and has a shortened duration of activity; enzyme levels are normal in young red cells and deficient in older cells, which are susceptible to oxidant-induced hemolysis. GdB − is extremely unstable and remains active in the red cell for only a few hours; therefore, both reticulocytes and older cells are extremely susceptible to oxidant hemolysis.

The hemolytic mechanism in G6PD deficiency results from a failure to produce sufficient quantities of reduced NADP to maintain adequate levels of reduced glutathione. Oxidant drugs generate hydrogen peroxide and other peroxides on interaction with oxyhemoglobin. These and other oxidant radicals oxidize reduced glutathione, which complexes with hemoglobin to form a mixed disulfide, resulting in alteration of globin chain configuration, loss of heme, and further mixed disulfide formation. The resultant denatured hemoglobin aggregates into *Heinz bodies*, which bind to membrane cytoskeletal proteins. Cells containing Heinz bodies have decreased deformability and are entrapped primarily in the spleen, where membrane is lost by "pitting" of Heinz bodies. The severity of hemolysis in G6PD-deficient persons depends on the level of enzyme in the erythrocytes and the severity of the oxidative stress.

Clinical and Laboratory Findings

Patients with GdA − do not manifest anemia until an oxidant challenge, in the form of an oxidant drug, diabetic ketoacidosis, severe liver injury, or bacteremia, provokes brisk hemolysis with hemoglobinemia, hemoglobinuria, and a fall in the hematocrit. The oxidant drugs that most commonly cause hemolysis in G6PD-deficient persons are listed in Table 244.4, and those drugs that are probably safe in therapeutic dosages are listed in Table 244.5.

Drug-induced hemolysis in G6PD-deficient persons usually is mild and self-limited. Between 1 and 3 days after the ingestion of a oxidant compound, hemolysis becomes evident, with a fall in the hematocrit and, possibly, hemoglobinuria. The peripheral blood film shows bite cells, spherocytes, and polychromatophilia. Heinz bodies can be demonstrated on incubation of red cells with supravital dyes such as cresyl violet. The hematocrit reaches its nadir at 7 to 10 days, and the reticulocyte response, which begins at about day 3, peaks at 7 to 14 days. Because young cells are resistant to hemolysis, recovery of the hematocrit occurs despite continuation of the offending agent. Hemolysis

TABLE 244.4.	DRUGS AND CHEMICALS THAT CAUSE CLINICALLY SIGNIFICANT HEMOLYTIC ANEMIA IN PERSONS WITH GLUCOSE-6-PHOSPHATE DEHYDROGENASE DEFICIENCY

Acetanilid	Phenylhydrazine
Dapsone	Primaquine
Furazolidone (Furoxone)	Sulfacetamide
Isobutyl nitrite	Sulfamethoxazole
Methylene blue	Sulfanilamide
Nalidixic acid	Sulfapyridine
Naphthalene	Thiazolesulfone
Niridazole	Toluidine blue
Nitrofurantoin (Furadantin)	Trinitrotoluene (TNT)
Phenazopyridine (Pyridium)	Urate oxidase

may occur in women but is milder because G6PD levels are higher.

Patients with GdB— may have chronic nonspherocytic hemolytic anemia, with persistent splenomegaly. They manifest favism (hemolysis after the ingestion of fava beans), which can be severe or fatal, particularly in children. Newborns often have hemolytic anemia with neonatal icterus.

The clinical findings should make the diagnosis highly suspect. In the presence of increased reticulocytes, which possess normal enzyme levels, screening tests may fail to detect G6PD deficiency. Establishment of the diagnosis in a patient with he-

TABLE 244.5.	DRUGS THAT ARE PROBABLY SAFE WHEN GIVEN IN NORMAL THERAPEUTIC DOSES TO PERSONS WITH GLUCOSE-6-PHOSPHATE DEHYDROGENASE DEFICIENCY

Acetaminophen	Phenytoin
Aspirin (acetylsalicylic acid)	Phytomenadione (vitamin K)
p-Aminobenzoic acid	Probenecid
Aminopyrine	Procainamide hydrochloride
Antazoline	Pyrimethamine
Antipyrine	Quinidine
Ascorbic acid (vitamin C)	Quinine
Chloramphenicol	Streptomycin
Chlorguanidine	Sulfacytine
Chloroquine	Sulfadiazine
Colchicine	Sulfaguanidine
Diphenhydramine	Sulfamerazine
Isoniazid	Sulfamethoxypyridazine
Levodopa	Sulfisoxazole
Menadione (menaphthone)	Trihexyphenidyl (benzhexol)
Menadione sodium bisulfite	Trimethoprim
Phenacetin (acetophenetidin)	Tripelennamine
Phenylbutazone	

(From Beutler E. Glucose-c-phosphate dehydrogenase deficiency. In Stanbury JB, Wynpaarden JB, Fredrickson DS, et al., eds. *The metabolic bases of inherited disease,* fifth ed. New York: McGraw-Hill, 1983;29, with permission.)

molytic anemia requires the use of quantitative spectrophotometric measurement of G6PD enzyme activity, with adjustment for the reticulocyte count.

Optimal Management
Treatment involves patient education and the avoidance of oxidant drugs and chemicals. Patients deemed at risk, such as those about to start an oxidant drug, should be screened for the defect and the information clearly documented in the medical record. If an implicated drug is continued, hemolysis may be self-limited, chronic, and low grade.

In other forms of G6PD deficiency, erythrocytes of all ages are deficient, producing chronic hemolysis and more severe hemolytic reactions on exposure to an oxidant stress.

Hemolytic Anemia Due to Disorders of Erythrocyte Purine and Pyrimidine Metabolism

Adenylate Kinase Deficiency and Related Disorders

Definition and Pathogenesis
Adenylate kinase deficiency is the most common of the rare hemolytic disorders of erythrocyte purine and pyrimidine metabolism that produce hemolytic anemia, and leads to decreased adenosine production by the normal salvage pathway. Lack of ATP within the red cell leads to the same metabolic consequences described for glycolytic defects.

In another rare disorder, hemolysis is caused by *adenosine deaminase hyperactivity*, which precludes normal salvage of adenosine from plasma and its subsequent phosphorylation of ATP. Decreased red cell ATP is believed to be the cause of hemolysis.

Pyrimidine 5'-nucleotidase deficiency is a defect in pyrimidine metabolism associated with hemolysis.

Clinical/Laboratory Findings and Optimal Management
Person with adenylate kinase deficiency have a chronic nonspherocytic hemolytic anemia and splenomegaly. Splenectomy is of questionable value.

In its congenital form, the hemolytic anemia of pyrimidine 5'-nucleotidase deficiency is often associated with mental retardation. Hemolysis is associated with prominent coarse basophilic stippling identical to that seen in the anemia of lead intoxication, in which the same enzyme deficiency is induced.

IMMUNE-MEDIATED HEMOLYTIC ANEMIAS

Autoimmune hemolytic anemias (AIHAs) are a diverse group of disorders in which red cell destruction is caused by an autoantibody. A classification of AIHAs is given in Table 244.6.

Warm Antibody Autoimmune Hemolytic Anemias

Definition

About 70% of AIHAs are associated with warm autoantibodies (i.e., antibodies that are optimally reactive at 37°C).

TABLE 244.6.	CLASSIFICATION OF AUTOIMMUNE HEMOLYTIC ANEMIAS

Warm-antibody autoimmune hemolytic anemia
  Idiopathic
  Secondary (e.g., chronic lymphocytic leukemia, lymphomas systemic lupus erythematosus)
Cold-agglutinin syndrome
  Idiopathic
  Secondary: *Mycoplasma pneumoniae* infection or infectious mononucleosis (polyclonal cold agglutinin); malignancies, such as chronic lymphocytic leukemia or lymphomas (monoclonal cold agglutinin)
Combined cold- and warm-antibody autoimmune hemolytic anemia
Paroxysmal cold hemoglobinuria
  Idiopathic
  Secondary to viral infection (common) or syphilis (rare)
Hemolytic anemia with a negative direct antiglobulin test
Drug-induced autoimmune hemolytic anemia
  Caused by methyldopa, procainamide, levodopa, phenacetin, chlorpromazine, mefenamic acid[a]

---

[a] Other nonsteroidal anti-inflammatory drugs (e.g., ibuprofen, naproxen, tolmetin, sulindac, fenoprofen) have caused hemolysis, but the mechanism is not clearly attributable to red blood cell autoantibodies.

Etiologic Factors

Nearly 50% of warm antibody AIHAs are associated with autoimmune, infectious, or neoplastic diseases (chronic lymphocytic leukemia, systemic lupus erythematosus, ovarian tumors, ulcerative colitis), whereas others are related to drug-induced phenomenon or are idiopathic.

Pathogenesis

In warm antibody AIHA, the patient's erythrocytes almost always are coated with IgG, complement (C3d), or both. Macrophages in the reticuloendothelial system recognize either the Fc portion of the immunoglobulin or the complement component coating the erythrocyte and then phagocytize these cells. Partial phagocytosis results in loss of erythrocyte membrane, with a decrease in surface area/volume ratio, and is the pathogenic mechanism for the formation of the spherocyte (a common finding in the blood film).

Clinical Findings

In some patients, the onset of AIHA is insidious, with the gradual emergence of symptoms of anemia, often associated with fever and jaundice. In others, the onset is sudden, with pain in the abdomen and back, malaise, and manifestations of rapidly increasing anemia. The anemia may be severe and progress before therapy becomes effective. A history of dark urine results from the presence of bile pigments or hemoglobinuria. The latter is a prominent finding in the most seriously ill patients. Jaundice is present in about 40% of patients. In idiopathic AIHA, spleno-

megaly occurs in 50% to 60%, hepatomegaly in 30%, and lymphadenopathy in about 25%. Splenomegaly, hepatomegaly, and lymphadenopathy are absent in about 25% of patients.

Laboratory Findings

The cardinal feature of AIHA is a positive DAT. Antiglobulin serum contains antibodies to IgG or C3d, and, when reacted with erythrocytes coated with the appropriate globulin, causes their agglutination. Warm antibodies are found in the serum or can be eluted from the red cells. They typically are of the IgG class and react with normal red cells. Platelet and leukocyte counts usually are normal but are elevated in some patients, often with the presence of occasional metamyelocytes and myelocytes. However, platelet and leukocyte antibodies have been documented, resulting in thrombocytopenia or leukopenia. As in other types of hemolytic anemia, a persistently raised reticulocyte count is a characteristic, although not invariable, finding. The peripheral blood film often reveals spherocytosis and mild to moderate poikilocytosis. Polychromatophilia is present except in patients with reticulocytopenia. Erythroid hyperplasia or, less commonly, hyperplasia of all cell lines is seen in the bone marrow.

Optimal Management

Warm reactive IgG autoimmune antibodies produce hemolytic anemia predominantly through the interaction of antibody-coated red cells with macrophage Fc receptors. In most patients, this process can be altered rapidly with corticosteroids. Initial treatment with prednisone, 1 to 1.5 mg per kilogram per day orally, usually decreases the rate of hemolysis in 3 to 7 days and produces stable erythrocyte counts in 4 to 6 weeks. The initial effect of corticosteroids is to reduce the destruction of antibody-coated red cells, without changing antibody production or the strength of antiglobulin testing. Long-term corticosteroid therapy for several weeks to several months usually leads to a reduction in autoantibody concentration.

After the hematocrit has stabilized, prednisone is gradually tapered by 10 to 20 mg per day increments each week. As the dosage is reduced below 20 mg per day to 10 mg per day, slower tapering is required. Hematocrit and reticulocyte counts should be obtained frequently during this tapering process. Alternate-day therapy with prednisone may be used with dosages below 30 mg per day. Some patients can be treated successfully by reducing the prednisone dosage below 10 to 15 mg per day, but many patients experience relapse as the dosage is decreased. Warm reactive IgG AIHA is a chronic relapsing disease, and repeated courses of treatment may be necessary. If the prednisone dosage cannot be reduced to an acceptable level, alternative forms of treatment should be used. A prednisone dosage above 20 mg per day for more than 3 to 6 months produces iatrogenic Cushing's syndrome, which increases the perioperative morbidity and mortality of splenectomy.

Splenectomy is the next appropriate therapeutic procedure for most patients with warm reactive IgG AIHA who do not respond adequately to prednisone. The major effect of splenectomy is to reduce the destruction of antibody-coated red cells, but some patients also benefit by a reduction in antibody production. Unfortunately, isotopic red cell survival or sequestration studies do not predict the response to this therapy. Patients who are to undergo splenectomy should receive pneumococcal *H. influenzae* type b and meningococcal vaccines and be warned of the susceptibility to acute overwhelming sepsis. About two-thirds of patients have sustained hematologic improvement after splenectomy, and most maintain hematologic remission after corticosteroid therapy has been discontinued. In a smaller subset of post-splenectomy patients, lower dosages of corticosteroids may be necessary to control hemolysis. Because of the chronic relapsing nature of this disease, patients need long-term follow-up.

Other types of immunosuppressive therapy are useful in patients who cannot be treated by or do not respond to splenectomy. Cyclophosphamide or azathioprine may be useful at initial dosages of 50 to 100 mg per day and 50 to 150 mg per day, respectively, with subsequent maintenance dosages designed to prevent the absolute granulocyte count from falling below 1,000 per microliter or the platelet count from falling below 100,000 per microliter. At least 3 to 6 months of such therapy usually is necessary to decrease antibody production. Because long-term cytotoxic therapy carries an increased risk of secondary malignancy, such as acute leukemia, it should be considered only in older patients. Patients with refractory AIHA also have been treated successfully with high doses of intravenous δ-globulin, plasmapheresis, or the androgen danazol. However, experience is limited and reports of favorable responses are anecdotal.

Transfusion is indicated in patients with hemodynamic compromise. Antierythrocyte autoantibodies may make compatibility testing difficult to perform by masking the presence of erythrocyte alloantibodies. In these cases, the autoantibody from the serum should be adsorbed using autologous erythrocytes or carefully selected allogeneic erythrocytes to detect the presence of alloantibodies. Even though the autoantibody may react with all normal erythrocytes, so that it is impossible to find compatible blood, transfusion must never be regarded as contraindicated. In such patients, transfusion with the "least incompatible" blood is warranted and necessary.

Cold Agglutinin Disease

Definition

Cold agglutinin disorders are caused by autoantibodies that react at cooler temperatures (4°C to 18°C). Depending on the underlying disease process, cold agglutinins can be either monoclonal or polyclonal.

Incidence and Epidemiology

About 15% of patients with AIHA have cold agglutinin syndrome. This syndrome typically affects the middle-aged or elderly, with a peak incidence of onset from 51 to 60 years of age.

Etiologic Factors

Typically, cold agglutinin syndrome is idiopathic, but it may be associated with several infectious diseases, particularly *Myco-plasma pneumoniae* pneumonia and infectious mononucleosis. Although unusual, some patients have cold agglutinin syndrome in association with hematologic malignancies, particularly chronic lymphocytic leukemia, Hodgkin's disease, and the lymphocytic lymphomas.

Pathogenesis

The pathogenic antibody in the cold agglutinin diseases is IgM, which is highly effective in activating the complement cascade on the erythrocyte membrane. These antibodies are active in the peripheral circulation and dissociate from the erythrocyte as it enters the warmer visceral circulation. However, this time is sufficient to activate the complement cascade to the stage of C3b, which remains on the surface of the erythrocyte. Those erythrocytes that are not cleared by the C3b receptor, expressing hepatic macrophages, enter the circulation where C3b is degraded to C3dg or C3d, or both. Since opsonization with C3d is even less effective than that with C3b, these cells usually escape destruction and are responsible for the findings on the DAT.

Clinical Findings

Symptoms often are those of a chronic anemia. Some patients experience hemoglobinuria, particularly in cold temperatures, and many complain of acrocyanosis of the ears, tip of the nose, fingers, and toes—a condition that vanishes quickly with warming. Physical findings include pallor, jaundice, and, in most cases, splenomegaly. Hepatomegaly and lymphadenopathy are not prominent findings.

Laboratory Findings

In classic cases, the degree of anemia varies with the degree of cold exposure. However, a fairly stable anemia that is mild or moderate in severity is much more common. Autoagglutination of blood samples is characteristic and creates problems in making satisfactory blood films and performing blood counts. Erythrocyte morphology is less abnormal than in warm antibody AIHA, with lesser degrees of spherocytosis, anisocytosis, and poikilocytosis. Reticulocytopenia is rare, as are abnormalities of leukocytes and platelets.

The DAT is positive in cold agglutinin syndrome as a result of C3d on the red cells. The causative IgM antibody usually is not demonstrated on the erythrocytes in vitro by the DAT because antiglobulin serum does not readily detect IgM antibodies. The autoantibodies in the patient's serum cause the agglutination of normal erythrocytes to a higher titer than normal (greater than 1:50) at 4°C and react to a lesser titer up to a temperature of at least 30°C. In classic cases, the cold agglutinin titer at 4°C is greater than 1,000, and it may be as high as 256,000. In about 40% of cases, however, the cold agglutinin titer is less than 1,000. The antibody usually has specificity within the Ii blood group system, most commonly anti-I.

Optimal Management

Most patients with cold reactive IgM antibodies do not have severe hemolysis, and those with overt intravascular hemolysis may respond to cold avoidance. Patients must be educated about the importance of maintaining skin temperature at or as close to body temperature as possible. They may experience overt hemolysis with reduction in temperature of exposed skin that is not perceived as unacceptably cold.

For the unusual patient with severe cold agglutinin immune hemolytic anemia who does not respond to cold avoidance, immune manipulations may be attempted. Prednisone is usually not helpful but has been used in doses similar to those for warm reactive hemolytic anemias. It may benefit a subset of patients by decreasing antibody production or the interaction of complement-coated red cells with phagocytic cells. Splenectomy usually is not helpful since most red cell destruction occurs in the liver. Other immune manipulations, such as cytotoxic chemotherapy, have been used. Plasmapheresis, although theoretically effective in removing an IgM antibody, must be undertaken with extreme caution because inadvertent cooling of blood in the tubing or the pheresis apparatus can lead to severe hemolysis.

Most cold agglutin diseases are chronic, with intermittent exacerbations. Simply avoiding exposure to cold temperatures may suffice to ameliorate the hemolysis and avoid exacerbations. In patients with secondary causes, treatment of the underlying process is indicated.

The prognosis of patients with idiopathic cold agglutin syndrome is significantly better than that of patients with warm antibody AIHA. Many patients have a chronic course and tolerate their mild or moderate anemia well. Death may result from complications of slowly progressive anemia or long-term blood transfusion therapy.

Paroxysmal Cold Hemoglobinuria

Definition, Etiologic Factors, and Pathogenesis

Paroxysmal cold hemoglobinuria (PCH) is a rare disorder that composes about 1% of AIHAs. Historically, PCH occurred after cold exposure in patients who had congenital syphilis or who were in the quiescent stage of late syphilis. The causative agent is an IgG antibody, usually with anti-P specificity, which fixes to normal red cells in the cold and subsequently causes hemolysis of the cells when they are warmed to 37°C in the presence of complement (the Donath–Landsteiner test).

Clinical and Laboratory Findings

Paroxysmal cold hemoglobinuria is most common in children, and most patients have histories of a recent viral disorder or flulike illness. However, a history of cold exposure may not be elicited. Hemolysis is acute in onset and causes severe and rapidly progressive anemia. Patients may have symptoms of chills, fever, malaise, abdominal distress, aching in the back or legs, and nausea. Manifestations of intravascular hemolysis are present, such as hemoglobinemia and hemoglobinuria. The blood film may reveal spherocytosis, anisocytosis, poikilocytosis, erythrophagocytosis, and nucleated erythrocytes.

The diagnosis of PCH is established by demonstrating the presence of the erythrocyte autoantibody. The so-called Donath–Landsteiner antibody fixes the first two components of complement in the cold and completes the cascade on warming to 37°C. The DAT is usually negative but occasionally complement can be demonstrated. Since the Donath–Landsteiner test is not routinely available, diagnosis of the disorder rests on recognition of the clinical manifestations.

Optimal Management

Since the acute illness characteristically resolves spontaneously after several weeks, usually no specific treatment is indicated, save for transfusional support as needed. Corticosteroids are not effective.

Combined Cold and Warm Antibody Autoimmune Hemolytic Anemias

Definition, Etiologic Factors, and Pathogenesis

About 8% of patients with AIHA have serologic findings that satisfy the criteria for both warm antibody AIHA and cold agglutinin syndrome. The cold antibody in such cases is normal or only modestly elevated in titer at 4°C but reacts up to at least 30°C. There appears to be an association between combined cold and warm antibody AIHA and systemic lupus erythematosus because this disorder is present in more than 25% of patients.

Clinical Course

Most patients have severe hemolysis and, although the initial response to therapy (see above) usually is excellent, many have a chronic course.

Autoimmune Hemolytic Anemias With Negative Direct Antiglobulin Tests

Definition and Clinical/Laboratory Findings

Some patients who ultimately are diagnosed as having AIHA have negative DAT results. These patients have findings suggestive of AIHA; that is, they have an acquired hemolytic anemia, spherocytes are present on the peripheral smear, no other diagnosis is apparent after exhaustive evaluation, and the response to therapy is similar to that in patients with AIHA who have characteristic immunohematologic findings. Small concentrations of autoantibodies usually can be demonstrated on red cells or in an eluate from the red cells using techniques that are more sensitive than the routine DAT, such as tests using radiolabeled antiglobulin sera or agglutinating potentiators.

Drug-Induced Immune Hemolytic Anemias

Definition and Etiologic Factors

Drugs have been identified as the cause of acquired immune hemolytic anemia in about 10% of cases. In most instances, a drug-specific antibody can be shown in vitro to react with erythrocytes in the presence of the drug or one of its metabolites. In other cases, the antibody has specificity for intrinsic red cell antigens and is similar to autoantibodies found in warm antibody AIHA.

Pathogenesis

Because drugs have relatively low molecular weight, they may function as haptens by combining with red cell membrane proteins to become immunogenic. The resulting antibody may react with drug absorbed to the cell surface or with a compound antigen consisting of the drug and erythrocyte membrane proteins. Because the binding of most drugs to cellular proteins seems too labile to be immunogenic, however, an alternative proposal suggests that a more probable immunogen might be a drug–plasma protein compound. The resulting antibody may react with the drug to form an immune complex that in turn reacts with erythrocytes by an unknown mechanism. Some drugs, such as penicillins, do bind tightly to red cells, and hemolysis may result from the reaction of antidrug antibody with the cell-bound drug. In some patients, the antibodies responsible for immune hemolysis cannot be shown to react with drug-specific antigens but instead have specificity for intrinsic red cell antigens, and the resultant disorder is classified as drug-induced AIHA. The causative drugs may alter erythrocyte antigens, causing them to be recognized by the immune system as nonself. Alternatively, the primary effect of the drugs may be on cells of the immune system, causing unregulated production of erythrocyte autoantibodies.

Clinical and Laboratory Findings

More than 75 drugs have caused the development of drug-specific antibodies and immune hemolytic anemia. These include acetaminophen, cephalosporins, chlorpromazine, chlorpropamide, erythromycin, hydralazine, hydrochlorothiazide, penicillins, phenacetin, quinidine, quinine, rifampicin, tetracycline, tolbutamide, and triamterene. The DAT result is usually positive with polyspecific antiserum, an anticomplement reagent, or both. The causative antibody is detected by the incubation of drug-coated red cells with the patient's serum or by the incubation of a mixture of the patient's serum, a solution of the drug, and erythrocytes, followed by observation for in vitro hemolysis, agglutination, or the development of a positive indirect antiglobulin test.

Prototype drugs responsible for causing AIHA are methyldopa and procainamide, with rare cases also associated with levodopa, mefenamic acid, phenacetin, and chlorpromazine. Therapy with methyldopa for at least 3 months is required before hemolysis develops; anemia usually develops gradually. The DAT is strongly positive using anti-IgG antiserum and is negative using anticomplement. The antibodies in the serum and in a red cell eluate react with normal red cells and have serologic characteristics similar to those found in idiopathic warm antibody AIHA. Because no serologic evidence of a relation between the antibodies and the drug has been demonstrated, proof that methyldopa causes AIHA has come from clinical observations.

Optimal Management

When clinical findings lend strong support to a diagnosis of drug-induced immune hemolytic anemia, the possible offending drug should be discontinued while confirmatory laboratory tests are carried out. This is particularly important because many drug-induced immune hemolytic anemias lead to the development of renal failure, especially when signs of intravascular hemolysis, such as hemoglobinemia and hemoglobinuria, are present. Such brisk hemolysis commonly occurs when drug-specific antibodies are present against drugs that are loosely bound to the erythrocyte. Hemolysis usually resolves within a matter of days after cessation of the causative drug. Drug-induced AIHA usually is less acute in onset but can become life threatening if the diagnosis is not recognized. A short course of corticosteroids may be indicated when the hemolysis is severe. Blood transfusion may be necessary and, in patients with drug-specific antibodies, compatibility testing is not affected.

HEMOLYTIC ANEMIAS DUE TO TRAUMATIC RED CELL FRAGMENTATION

Erythrocyte fragmentation is caused by the interaction of red cells with altered intravascular surfaces or by direct physical trauma to the cells resulting from excessive shear forces within the circulation. The resultant fragmentation hemolytic anemia is characterized by intravascular hemolysis with elevated plasma hemoglobin levels, decreased haptoglobin levels, hemoglobinuria, hemosiderinuria (becomes evident after a week or more), and the diagnostic fragmented erythrocyte known as a *schistocyte*. Table 244.7 lists the laboratory findings in fragmentation hemolysis, and Table 244.8 indicates the disorders associated with this condition.

Microangiopathic Disease

Definition and Etiologic Factors

Intrinsic microvascular disease is the most common cause of fragmentation hemolytic anemia and has led to the term *microangiopathic hemolytic anemia* (MAHA). This type of hemolysis may accompany acute vasculitides such as occur in polyarteritis nodosa, lupus, rheumatoid arthritis, and allergic vasculitis, which primarily involve small arteries and arterioles. Fragmentation hemolysis has also been observed in diabetic microvascular disease, although the association has not been proved, and disseminated intravascular coagulation (DIC). DIC is associated most commonly with sepsis, shock, placental abruption, intrauterine fetal death, and malignancy. Evidence for fragmentation hemo-

TABLE 244.7.	**LABORATORY FINDINGS IN FRAGMENTATION HEMOLYSIS**

Normocytic or microcytic anemia with elevated absolute reticulocyte count and increased red blood cell distribution width
Schistocytes and polychromatophilia
Elevated indirect bilirubin value
Elevated serum lactic dehydrogenase value
Elevated plasma hemoglobin value
Decreased serum haptoglobin value
Hemoglobinuria
Hemosiderinuria

TABLE 244.8.	DISORDERS ASSOCIATED WITH FRAGMENTATION HEMOLYTIC ANEMIA

Microangiopathic Disorders
  Vasculitis, collagen vascular disorders
  Disseminated intravascular coagulation
  Disseminated malignancy
  Thrombohemolytic microangiopathy
    Thrombotic thrombocytopenic purpura
    Hemolytic-uremic syndrome
  Cavernous hemangiomas
  Homograft rejection (renal, hepatic, cardiac)
  Footstrike hemolysis (and related disorders)
Cardiac and Large-Vessel Diseases
  Cardiac valvular disease: aortic stenosis, calcific mitral stenosis
  Defective cardiac valvular prostheses
  Patch repairs of intracardiac defects
  Aortic and large-vessel prostheses and grafts

lysis is found in about 40% of cases of DIC, regardless of cause, and correlates with the severity of the coagulopathy. Disseminated malignancy usually leads to fragmentation hemolysis through associated DIC, which often is of low grade. Local intravascular coagulation leading to fragmentation hemolysis can occur in giant cavernous hemangiomas (Kasabach–Merritt syndrome) and during organ homograft rejection reactions, particularly of the kidney, but also of the liver and heart.

Pathogenesis

In the acute vasculitides, endothelial injury by immune complexes is accompanied by perivascular inflammation and fibrin deposition in the vessel lumen. In syndromes associated with DIC, coagulation is activated and leads to the generation of excessive thrombin, which results in deposition of fibrin strands and thrombi in arterioles and capillaries. In tumor-associated hemolysis, abnormal tortuous tumor vessels and tumor-released thromboplastins contribute to the associated DIC. Mucin-producing adenocarcinomatosis has a particular association with DIC and fragmentation hemolysis, often presenting before treatment and temporarily worsening with effective chemotherapy of the tumor as more mucin thromboplastin is released into the circulation. A similar phenomenon may be seen with acute promyelocytic leukemia and other acute leukemias.

Optimal Management

The clinical and laboratory findings of vasculitis can be found elsewhere in this book. Successful therapy results in resolution of the hemolytic process, although an element of anemia of chronic disease may persist. In DIC, treatment of the underlying disorder, if possible, is the key to controlling the hemolytic process. The fragmentation hemolysis seen in organ rejection will abate when rejection is abrogated.

Thrombohemolytic Microangiopathy
Definition

Thrombohemolytic microangiopathy includes TTP and hemolytic-uremic syndrome (HUS).

Etiologic Factors

Thrombotic thrombocytopenic purpura has been associated with drugs, hypersensitivity reactions, bone marrow and solid organ transplantation, viral and bacterial infections, pregnancy, and other causes. However, no clear etiologic process has emerged. Most cases of HUS are preceded by viral or bacterial infections, particularly of the gastrointestinal tract. The rare adult form of HUS is observed in peripartum women with complications of pregnancy and delivery, and in untreated patients with disseminated cancer. Both HUS and TTP have been caused by numerous chemotherapeutic agents. Mitomycin C is the most commonly implicated drug, but others include bleomycin, cisplatin, vinca alkaloids, the combination of mitomycin and 5-fluorouracil, cyclosporine, and FK-506. Quinine sensitivity is a relatively newly recognized cause of HUS where an immune mechanism has been well documented.

Pathogenesis

Intravascular fibrin and platelet thrombus formation characterizes the arteriolar lesion. Fibrin thrombi entrap erythrocytes during flow. The increased shear forces within these pathologic microvessels physically disrupt the red cells by tearing them away from points of attachment or fracturing them across fibrin strands. This direct physical hemolysis leads to the production of schistocytes with markedly reduced circulatory survival. Inhibitory antibodies against von Willebrand's factor–cleaving protease have also recently been described in patients with acute TTP and may have a role in the pathogenesis of this disorder.

Clinical Findings

Thrombotic thrombocytopenic purpura is a clinical syndrome comprising the pentad of fragmentation hemolysis, thrombocytopenia, fluctuating neurologic signs, renal dysfunction, and fever. It occurs primarily in young and middle-aged adults and is more common in women. TTP manifests as two clinical forms: (a) a chronic relapsing variety that extends from weeks to years and (b) the more common acute fulminant type that represents a medical emergency. Although formerly associated with an 80% mortality rate, TTP can be cured in most cases if it is recognized and treated before irreversible neurologic and renal injury has occurred.

HUS is primarily a disease of infants and children that presents as renal failure, fragmentation hemolytic anemia, thrombocytopenia (less marked than in TTP), and fever. In its less common adult form it is difficult to distinguish from TTP, except that the central nervous system is spared and renal dysfunction is more severe.

Laboratory Findings

Laboratory findings of DIC are absent. The peripheral blood film shows striking erythrocyte fragmentation with thrombocytopenia accompanied by polychromasia, and elevation of the LDH (more than 500 IU per deciliter) and indirect bilirubin.

Varying degrees of renal dysfunction are present, the severity of which depends on whether TTP or HUS is present.

Optimal Management

High-volume plasma exchange is the treatment of choice in TTP. Plasma infusions may be given until plasma exchange can be arranged. Recovery is marked by a fall in serum LDH, as well as improvement of anemia, thrombocytopenia, and the neurologic and renal parameters of the disease. Adjuncts to treatment include corticosteroids, antiplatelet agents, and vincristine. Platelet transfusions are contraindicated, except in suspected or documented central nervous system or other severe bleeds, as they can exacerbate the underlying process. Splenectomy may have some efficacy in prevention of relapses in the chronic form of the disease, although this is based on anecdotal data.

Management of both the childhood and adult forms of HUS relies on the combination of plasma exchange and, with severe renal dysfunction, dialysis. Additional measures have included vincristine, high-dose intravenous immunoglobulin, and splenectomy. Corticosteroids and antiplatelet drugs have been of limited value. With effective therapy, more than 85% of children recover, but a subset have persistent impairment of renal function and are subject to relapse. Adult HUS has higher mortality and propensity for residual renal dysfunction.

Footstrike Hemolysis

Definition, Etiologic Factors, and Pathogenesis

Footstrike hemolysis originally was recognized as *march hemoglobinuria* in German soldiers subjected to strenuous marches. Related forms of hemolysis caused by physical injury to the feet and hands have been recognized in long-distance runners, conga drummers, and pneumatic hammer operators.

Optimal Management

Cessation of the cause of injury always leads to resolution of the anemia.

Heart Valve Hemolysis

Definition

Heart valve hemolysis is the term applied to fragmentation states caused by pathologic heart valves or defective cardiac valvular prostheses. The most common associated valvular abnormality is severe aortic stenosis, with calcific mitral stenosis or septal defects implicated less often.

Etiologic Factors and Pathogenesis

Surgically implanted prosthetic valves, especially artificial aortic valve prostheses, tend to cause frequent and severe heart valve hemolysis. Several intracardiac or vascular surface and flow alterations contribute to hemolysis. Increased turbulence and jet effects produce high shear forces that may disrupt red cells directly or tear them across fibrin strands. Prosthetic valvular, vascular, or patch surfaces that are not endothelialized may become covered with a fibrin–platelet meshwork that entraps and fragments the erythrocytes.

Clinical and Laboratory Findings

Hemolytic anemia usually is mild, characterized by red cell fragmentation and hemoglobinuria that worsens with increased cardiac output, tachycardia, and heart failure. Hemolysis often is greater during activity in the daytime and decreases during rest at night. Chronic hemoglobinuria and hemosiderin loss in the urine lead to iron deficiency. Iron-deficient red cells have greater mechanical fragility. Worsening anemia leads to further hemodynamic deterioration, which increases the hemolytic rate.

Optimal Management

Successful therapy for this disorder requires breaking the cycle by correcting the iron deficiency and optimizing the patient's hemodynamic state. When severe hemolysis is present, it often is necessary to replace the defective valve or prosthesis.

HEMOLYTIC ANEMIAS RESULTING FROM PARASITISM OF RED BLOOD CELLS

Malaria

Definition

Malaria is the most common cause of hemolytic anemia worldwide. The following description is confined to changes that occur with *Plasmodium falciparum* infections, since the consequences of *P. malariae*, *P. ovale*, and *P. vivax* infections usually are much milder.

Etiologic Factors and Pathogenesis

Merozoites emerging at first from the tissues and later from previously parasitized red cells enter the erythrocyte and grow intracellularly. The intracellular development of the parasites leads to intravascular rupture of the red cells, but the degree of hemolysis and anemia always is in excess of what could be accounted for by this one mechanism. An immune mechanism may also be present since a positive DAT is present in some patients, the erythrocytes being sensitized by IgG with or without complement. The antibody eluted from the red cells has been shown to have activity against *P. falciparum* schizont antigen. The destruction of parasitized red cells appears to be a largely splenic phenomenon whereby pitting of the parasites from the red cells occurs (i.e., the parasite surrounded by a small ring of red cell and membrane is retained in the pulp and phagocytosed, whereas the remaining unparasitized part of the red cell emerges into the splenic sinus and returns to the circulation). The circulating fragment is spherocytic, has increased osmotic fragility (as do cells containing plasmodium), is more rigid, and is prone to sequestration when it next reaches the spleen.

Clinical and Laboratory Findings

Splenomegaly is usually present in chronic infections. *P. falciparum* malaria occasionally is associated with particularly severe hemolysis that may result in dark, almost black, urine, known as *blackwater fever*. It was common among Europeans in Africa and India, usually after treatment with quinine. Free and intraerythrocytic malarial parasites can be seen on thick-film preparations of the peripheral blood.

Optimal Management

When acute and unusually severe hemolysis occurs in the course of *P. falciparum* malaria, the physician should be certain that a hemolytic drug is not being administered to a G6PD-deficient person. Transfusions may be needed in blackwater fever; if renal failure occurs, extracorporeal dialysis may be required.

Bartonellosis

Definition

Human bartonellosis is transmitted by the sandfly, and the red cells become infected with *Bartonella bacilliformis*.

Pathogenesis and Clinical Findings

The organism does not appear to grow within the red cell but adheres to its exterior surface. During the first stage of the disease, most patients manifest no clinical symptoms whereas some have an acute, severe hemolytic anemia known as *Oroya fever*. The second stage of *Bartonella* infection, verruca peruviana, is a nonhematologic disorder characterized by an eruption of warty, bleeding tumors over the face and extremities.

Optimal Management

The mortality rate among untreated patients is high, but Oroya fever responds well to antibiotics and supportive care.

Babesiosis

Definition

Babesiosis is an intraerythrocytic protozoan infection that is transmitted by ticks and is characterized by malaria-like symptoms and hemolytic anemia.

Etiologic Factors and Pathogenesis

Most cases in the United States have been attributed to infection with *Babesia microti*, a rodent parasite maintained by *Ixodes dammini* ticks, the primary vector of the agent of Lyme disease (*Borrelia burgdorferi*). The parasite also may be transmitted by blood transfusion.

Clinical and Laboratory Findings

Asplenic, immunocompromised, and elderly persons are at greatest risk for severe illness, whereas other infected persons commonly are asymptomatic or mildly symptomatic. The disease usually has a gradual onset, with malaise, anorexia, fatigue, fever, sweats, and muscle and joint pains. Intraerythrocytic parasites can be seen on thin blood films, and serologic tests for antibodies to *Babesia* have been described.

Optimal Management

The disorder has responded well to treatment with clindamycin and quinine.

BIBLIOGRAPHY

Coppel Rl, Cooke Bm, Magowan C, et al. Malaria and the erythrocyte. *Curr Opin Hematol* 1998;5:132–138.

Gallagher PG, Ferriera JDS. Molecular basis of erythrocyte membrane disorders. *Curr Opin Hematol* 1997;4:128–135.

Jacob H, Telen M. Hyperdestructive anemias and other erythrocyte disorders. In: Jacob H, ed. *Hematology medical knowledge self-assessment program*, second ed. Philadelphia: American College of Physicians–American Society of Internal Medicine, 1999:114–134.

Joiner CH, Franco RS, Jiany M, et al. Increased cation permeability in mutant mouse red blood cells with defective membrane skeleton. *Blood* 1995;86:4307–4314.

Luzzatto L, Bessler M. The dual pathogenesis of paroxysmal nocturnal hemoglobinuria. *Curr Opin Hematol* 1996;3:101–110.

Palek J, Jarolim P. Red cell membrane disorders. In: Hoffman R, ed. *Hematology: basic principles and practice*, second ed. New York: Churchill Livingstone, 1995:667–709.

Schwartz RS, Silberstein LE, Berkman EM. Autoimmune hemolytic anemias. In: Hoffman R, ed. *Hematology: basic principles and practice*, second ed. New York: Churchill Livingstone, 1995:710–729.

Tasai HM, Chun-Yet Lian E. Antibodies to von Willebrand factor–cleaving protease in acute thrombotic thrombocytopenic purpura. *N Engl J Med* 1998;339:1585–1594.

Tchernia G, Ganthier F, Mielot R, et al. Initial assessment of the beneficial effect of partial splenectomy in hereditary spherocytosis. *Blood* 1993;81:2014–2020.

Telen MJ, Neeraja R. Recent advances in immunohematology. *Curr Opin Hematol* 1994;1:143–150.

Kelley's Textbook of Internal Medicine, fourth edition. Edited by H. David Humes. Lippincott Williams & Wilkins, Philadelphia © 2000.

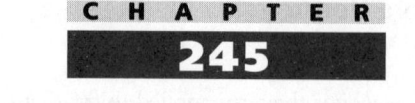

C H A P T E R
245

SICKLE CELL ANEMIA

BERTRAM H. LUBIN

Sickle cell disease is a hereditary hemoglobin disorder that results in sickling of the red cell, leading to chronic hemolytic anemia, vascular occlusion, and progressive organ damage. Sickle cell anemia (SS disease), sickle hemoglobin C disease (SC disease), and sickle β-thalassemia are the most common forms of the disease. For detailed information concerning each of these diseases, the reader is referred to several recent books listed in the bibliography.

INCIDENCE AND EPIDEMIOLOGY

The estimated incidence of sickle cell anemia in newborn African Americans is 1 in 600, for SC disease 1 per 800, and for sickle β-thalassemia 1 per 1,700. About 8% of African Americans have sickle cell trait. The distribution of the sickle cell gene throughout the world parallels that of *Plasmodium falciparum.* Persons with sickle cell trait who are infected with this parasite have a selective advantage over those who do not have sickle cell trait. Given this fact, it is not surprising that newborn screening programs for hemoglobinopathies have identified sickle cell hemoglobin in a substantial number of nonblacks.

ETIOLOGIC FACTORS

Sickle cell disease is a hereditary hemoglobin disorder due to a mutation in the β-globin gene. It is inherited in an autosomal codominant manner. In sickle cell anemia, both of the β-globin chains have a substitution of valine for glutamic acid in their sixth position, and all β-globin in the red cell is sickle. In SC disease, one β-globin gene codes for sickle globin and the other for hemoglobin C, which has lysine substituted for glutamic acid, also in the sixth position of the β-globin chain. In sickle β-thalassemia, one β-globin gene has the sickle cell mutation and the other has a thalassemia mutation. Depending on the type of thalassemia mutation, the synthesis of the normal β-globin chain is completely (β^0) or partially (β^+) suppressed. Sickle cell trait occurs when one β-globin gene codes for sickle hemoglobin and the other for hemoglobin A.

PATHOGENESIS AND PATHOPHYSIOLOGIC FACTORS

Adult hemoglobin (hemoglobin A) is a tetrameric protein containing two α-globin and two β-globin chains. Sickle hemoglobin (hemoglobin S) contains two normal α-globin chains and two sickle β-globin chains. The substitution of the neutral amino acid valine for an acidic amino acid (glutamic acid) changes the charge on the surface of the deoxygenated hemoglobin molecule and causes it to polymerize into a 14-stranded structure. Polymerized sickle hemoglobin is relatively insoluble, rigid, and unstable, and it causes the abnormal red cell properties resulting in sickle cell disease. Hemoglobin C can form polymers with hemoglobin S, resulting in SC disease. Hemoglobin A ($\alpha_2\beta_2$) and hemoglobin F (fetal hemoglobin, $\alpha_2\gamma_2$) prevent polymer formation, explaining the lack of clinical symptoms in persons with sickle cell trait, the mild clinical course of sickle β^+-thalassemia, and the therapeutic benefit of elevated fetal hemoglobin.

The generation of hemoglobin polymers within the cell depends on several factors. Hypoxia and acidosis promote sickling by lowering the oxygen saturation of hemoglobin. In the arterial circulation, where the P_{O_2} is about 95 mm Hg and hemoglobin is at least 90% saturated with oxygen, about 10% of the cells are sickled. In mixed venous blood, where the P_{O_2} is about 40 mm Hg, hemoglobin is approximately 60% saturated with oxygen, and as many as 70% of the cells may be sickled. Systemic hypoxemia secondary to pulmonary insufficiency is likely to increase the number of sickled cells in the peripheral blood. Conditions within the kidney, spleen, retina, and bone marrow are sufficiently hypoxic and acidotic to induce polymer formation and sickling, and are likely to explain why these organs are often affected.

Studies of the kinetics of polymerization of sickle hemoglobin have demonstrated that after complete deoxygenation of the molecule, a delay time of about 11 milliseconds occurs before polymer formation. This delay time is dramatically shortened when the mean corpuscular hemoglobin concentration (MCHC) is increased. Under normal circumstances, where the transit time of blood through capillaries is about 1 second, hemoglobin is reoxygenated before sufficient numbers of polymers can form inside the cell to cause it to sickle. However, if the transit time is prolonged (an event that could occur as a consequence of adhesive interactions between the red cell and the endothelial cell, abnormal deformability of the red cell, or increased plasma viscosity) or if the MCHC is elevated, polymer formation is favored. When significant amounts of polymer are formed within a red cell, the morphology of the cell transforms from a biconcave disk into a sickle shape. This process is reversible in most red cells by reoxygenation. In a subpopulation of red cells, called irreversibly sickled cells, abnormal morphology persists in the completely oxygenated state.

Although the hemoglobin defect is the primary cause of sickle cell disease, several acquired red cell membrane alterations occur as a consequence of sickling. These include increased calcium permeability and elevated intracellular calcium, decreased intracellular potassium and water, oxidation of membrane proteins and lipids, membrane phospholipid abnormalities, and abnormal expression of adhesive receptors, particularly in reticulocytes. These secondary membrane effects probably contribute to the hemolytic anemia and vaso-occlusive events characteristic of sickle cell disease, and they may be important factors in determining clinical severity.

In addition to the red cell, a number of other factors may contribute to the clinical severity of sickle cell disease. These include an elevated white blood cell count, a hypercoagulable coagulation profile, and upregulation of endothelial cell receptors in the large and small microvascular system. The search for genetic polymorphisms in addition to the sickle cell gene is likely to uncover multiple genes that contribute to clinical severity and help to explain the extreme variability in clinical manifestations that characterize this disease.

CLINICAL FINDINGS

The clinical manifestations of sickle cell disease can be classified into two categories: anemic and vaso-occlusive. The anemic category includes chronic hemolytic anemia, aplastic crisis, splenic

TABLE 245.1.	CLINICAL MANIFESTATIONS OF SICKLE CELL DISEASE

Ocular: Proliferative retinopathy, tortuous conjunctival vessels
Cardiac: Cardiomegaly, high-output failure, transfusion-related hemosiderosis, hypertension
Pulmonary: Acute chest syndrome, infection (pneumococcal, mycoplasmal), chronic hypoxemic lung disease
Gastrointestinal and Hepatic: Gallbladder disease, splenic sequestration, splenic infarction, hepatic crises
Musculoskeletal: Infarction (painful crises), aseptic necrosis, pain, infection (*Salmonella* osteomyelitis), arthritis (collagen vascular, gout)
Genitourinary: Renal concentration defects, hematuria, nephrosis, chronic renal failure, priapism
Immune: Susceptibility to infection, defect in the alternative complement pathway, functional asplenia, phagocytic defects
Skin: Leg ulcers
Hematopoietic: Chronic hemolytic anemia, aplastic crises, hyperhemolysis
Neurologic: Stroke, transient ischemic attacks, silent infarctions

sequestration, and hyperhemolysis. The vaso-occlusive category includes painful crisis and organ impairment, such as splenic infarction, stroke, aseptic necrosis of the hip, and acute chest syndrome. Although the term "crisis" is used in sickle cell disease to indicate a change in the patient's clinical course, it has no particular medical significance. Almost every organ system in the body can be significantly affected by sickle cell disease (Table 245.1).

ANEMIC COMPLICATIONS

The life span of the red cell in sickle cell anemia may be only 15 to 20 days, compared to the normal 120 days. Increased production of bilirubin due to hemoglobin catabolism is reflected by the frequent occurrence of bilirubin-containing gallstones and, in patients with compromised liver function, an elevated serum bilirubin level. Gilbert's disease should be ruled out in patients who have persistent or extreme elevations in bilirubin. This can now be accomplished using molecular diagnostic techniques. The spleen may be enlarged in young children but is rarely palpable in adults. If dietary folic acid intake is limited, megaloblastic changes can occur. Low dietary folate can also affect the hypercoagulable profile due to its effects on homocysteine metabolism. Factors that lower intracellular polymer formation, such as α-thalassemia trait (low MCHC), elevated fetal hemoglobin (β-globin haplotype), small amounts of hemoglobin A (sickle β+-thalassemia), and hemoglobin C (SC disease), decrease the rate of hemolysis and cause an increase in the hemoglobin. Variations among patients exist, but a given patient's hemoglobin value and reticulocyte count are relatively stable.

Patients with sickle cell anemia are very susceptible to infectious or inflammatory processes that suppress erythropoiesis. A common infection is due to parvovirus B19. This virus, previously thought to be restricted to veterinary medicine, is a common cause of red cell hypoplasia or aplasia in sickle cell anemia. Specific receptors for the virus are found on erythroid progeni-

tors. Infected patients have a rapid fall in the reticulocyte count and hemoglobin level, called an aplastic crisis. If not promptly treated, congestive heart failure can result. Within 7 to 10 days, bone marrow recovery is heralded by an increase in the reticulocyte count, followed by a rise in hemoglobin. Currently, trials of a vaccine to prevent parvoviral infections are in progress. A hyperhemolytic crisis has been reported in patients with sickle cell anemia that is characterized by anemia and a marked increase in the reticulocyte count over baseline values. This event may be secondary to glucose-6-phosphate dehydrogenase (G6PD) deficiency or Gilbert's disease, or it may be a sign of recovery after an aplastic crisis.

Acute splenic sequestration is a hematologic complication that primarily occurs in infants and young children. Within hours, the spleen rapidly enlarges and sequesters most of the circulating red cells. Although rarely documented, it is thought that a splenic sequestration crisis is preceded by a viral infection. Massive splenomegaly and a fall in the hemoglobin concentration to as low as 1 g per deciliter can rapidly occur and cause death. Parents should be taught to palpate the spleen and to bring the child to the physician if they feel the spleen is enlarged. In some children, chronic splenic sequestration associated with pancytopenia occurs.

VASO-OCCLUSIVE COMPLICATIONS

Vaso-occlusive and pain crises are the clinical manifestations that distinguish sickle cell disease from other hemolytic anemias. Pain crises occur sporadically and are unpredictable. They may last for a few days or up to several weeks. The frequency of painful crises varies over time and between patients, with an average of one to one and a half crises per year. Although a few patients appear to be particularly prone to these complications, the mechanisms responsible for this unique susceptibility are unknown. An inverse correlation exists between the fetal hemoglobin level and the frequency of painful crises. Patients with frequent vaso-occlusive crises have a shorter life span than those with infrequent ones.

Almost every organ system in the body can be affected by sickle cell disease. A proliferative retinopathy, similar to that in diabetes, can result in loss of vision if not treated promptly. Several cardiovascular abnormalities can occur. Cardiomegaly may result as a consequence of the chronic high-output state due to anemia, or cardiac dysfunction may occur secondary to transfusion-related hemosiderosis. Hypertension has been observed in association with painful crises, after an exchange transfusion, or in patients with progressive renal disease.

Acute pulmonary disease is responsible for 20% of deaths in sickle cell disease. Although patients can develop focal pulmonary infections with limited severity, in others a rapidly progressive disease, acute chest syndrome, is noted. The clinical manifestations are similar to those noted in adult respiratory distress syndrome. Patients typically present with symptoms consistent with a vaso-occlusive crisis, but within hours pulmonary disease develops and spreads to both lungs, resulting in pulmonary failure. The cause of acute chest syndrome is often not established since bronchoscopy, although safe in sickle cell patients, is rarely used to obtain the tissue required for a diagnosis. Infection or bone marrow fat embolism should be considered in the differential diagnosis. Elevated plasma levels of phospholipase A_2 predict embolism derived from bone marrow fat as a cause of acute chest syndrome. Changes in nitric oxide levels may also be predictive. Chronic restrictive pulmonary disease resulting in persistent hypoxemia may occur after recurrent episodes of acute chest syndrome.

The most common gastrointestinal complication in sickle cell anemia is gallbladder disease. Ultrasonograms have detected bilirubin stones as early as the first decade of life. Biliary problems can include common duct stones, biliary sludge, cholelithiasis, and cholestasis. The decision to perform a cholecystectomy should be based on the patient's symptoms, not the presence of stones. Intense hyperbilirubinemia (up to 60 to 80 mg per deciliter) can occur when the common bile duct is obstructed. This hepatic crisis is associated with hepatic enlargement and abnormal liver function. Liver biopsy shows bile stasis, hepatitis, hemosiderin, and sickled cells. The course of this complication may be as long as 14 days. In rare cases, hepatic failure occurs.

Musculoskeletal manifestations of sickle cell anemia include bone and muscle pain, aseptic necrosis of the bone, and osteomyelitis. Bone pain occurs in the hands and feet in young children. In adults, it usually involves the long bones and lower back. The hip and shoulder joints are often sites of aseptic necrosis. The microcirculatory blood flow in the head of the femur or humerus lends itself to permanent vascular obstruction by sickled cells. Although aseptic necrosis in the humerus has limited morbidity, aseptic necrosis of the head of the femur, due to the weight-bearing role of this bone, can result in permanent disability. When clinical symptoms suggest a hip problem, conventional radiography or magnetic resonance imaging should be used to establish a diagnosis. Conservative management should initially be attempted, but if necrosis progresses, a decompression coring procedure or total hip replacement should be considered. Although osteomyelitis can occur secondary to infection with *Staphylococcus aureus,* it is not unusual to find *Salmonella* in aspirates obtained from inflammatory bone sites. The mechanisms responsible for the susceptibility to *Salmonella* osteomyelitis are unknown, but biliary disease and bone infarction probably contribute.

The kidney is particularly prone to complications in sickle cell anemia due to its hypoxic, acidotic, and hypertonic environment. Renal concentration defects, silent hematuria, nephrosis, and chronic renal failure occur. Even in people with sickle cell trait, renal infarction, hematuria, and hyposthenuria occur. Urinary specific gravity cannot be used as an index of hydration in sickle cell anemia. In adults with hematuria, causes in addition to sickle cell anemia, such as malignancy, must be considered in the differential diagnosis. Hyperuricemia resulting in gouty arthritis is usually related to renal pathologic processes. Chronic renal failure is common in older patients. Since it can be associated with a fall in the baseline hemoglobin value, patients may have fewer vaso-occlusive crises due to decreased blood viscosity. Renal transplantation has been successful in patients with renal failure.

Acute priapism may occur during or shortly after a penile erection due to sluggish blood flow and sickling within the glans of the penis. It is associated with significant pain. Although transfusions may help, surgical intervention is often required. Intermittent episodes of priapism can also occur; these may be remedied by chronic transfusion therapy. Clinical trials using nitric oxide are currently being considered for this complication.

Patients with sickle cell anemia have a marked increase in susceptibility to bacterial infections, including *Streptococcus pneumoniae, Haemophilus influenzae,* and, less commonly, *Staphylococcus aureus* and *Mycoplasma pneumoniae.* The absence of splenic function is a primary factor in regard to infections due to polysaccharide-encapsulated organisms. Other immune defects may be secondary to transfusion-related hemosiderosis, defects in the alternate complement pathway, and phagocytic defects.

Skin ulcerations result from sluggish blood flow in superficial capillaries. These ulcerations, which often occur over the lateral malleoli of the tibia, often become infected and require systemic and local therapy. Transfusion therapy should be considered for patients who are severely disabled by skin ulcers.

Neurologic events occur in 15% to 25% of patients with sickle cell anemia. Stroke, convulsions, transient ischemic attacks, and behavioral disturbances have been reported. Hemorrhagic strokes are more common in adults, infarctive strokes more common in children. After transfusion to lower the percentage of hemoglobin S, dramatic clinical improvement is often observed. Early identification of cerebrovascular changes, followed by transfusion therapy, may prevent major central nervous system complications. Noninvasive techniques such as transcutaneous Doppler ultrasonography may be a useful way to detect patients at risk. Computed tomography scans have shown evidence of infarction in children who do not have overt strokes. Transfusion therapy for at least 5 years is recommended for patients who have had a stroke, but the appropriate treatment for "silent" cerebral infarcts remains to be established. Hydroxyurea administration and bone marrow transplantation are alternative therapies that are now being evaluated in patients who require long-term intervention for stroke.

The frequency and severity of anemic and vaso-occlusive complications among patients with sickle cell disease are highest in patients with sickle cell anemia, followed by sickle β^0-thalassemia, sickle β^+-thalassemia, and sickle hemoglobin C disease. However, the individual complications may be as severe in any type of sickle cell disease.

LABORATORY EVALUATION

Laboratory evaluation of a patient with suspected sickle cell disease should include examination of the peripheral blood smear; a complete blood count with red cell indexes; a reticulocyte count; hemoglobin electrophoresis on cellulose acetate (pH 8.6) and citrate agar (pH 6.2); and quantitative determinations of hemoglobins A, S, A_2, and F, or other variant hemoglobins. A solubility test (Sickledex) can be performed to confirm that a hemoglobin migrating in the S position on electrophoresis is S and not D or G. In many programs, molecular techniques are being used to confirm the hemoglobin diagnosis.

The peripheral blood smear in sickle cell anemia may show irreversibly sickled cells, polychromatophilic macrocytes, and occasional cell fragments. The mean corpuscular volume is high due to the presence of young red cells. Granulocytes are increased in number and a slight shift to the left may occur. Platelets are increased in number and size. The presence of nuclear remnants (Howell–Jolly bodies) within the red cell indicates functional asplenia. In sickle β^+-thalassemia or sickle β^0-thalassemia, hypochromic microcytic cells, target cells, and occasional sickle cells are noted. The hemoglobin A_2 level is increased as a consequence of the β-thalassemia gene. Iron deficiency must also be excluded if sickle β^+-thalassemia is being considered. The mean cell volume is below normal for age. Although patients with sickle β^+-thalassemia have both hemoglobin A and S, like people with sickle cell trait, the quantitative measurement of hemoglobins S and A can distinguish these two. Patients with sickle cell trait have more hemoglobin A than S; patients with sickle β^+-thalassemia have more hemoglobin S than A. In sickle hemoglobin C, target cells and rare sickle forms are seen. The mean cell volume is normal or slightly decreased and the reticulocyte count is slightly elevated. Molecular techniques can be used to definitively establish the diagnosis of sickle cell trait versus sickle cell–thalassemia.

Table 245.2 lists the clinical and laboratory findings characteristic of these common forms of sickle cell disease.

Several laboratory parameters have been evaluated in an attempt to predict clinical severity. Among these, the coinheritance of α-thalassemia trait (which lowers the mean corpuscular volume and MCHC) and an increase in fetal hemoglobin are two that have shown beneficial effects. Analysis of the β-globin haplotype is a good predictor of the fetal hemoglobin level and as such has some predictive value. However, there are no specific measurements for predicting clinical severity that can be used to direct experimental therapy in newly diagnosed patients.

Cord blood screening, which is mandatory in an increasing number of states, can identify all forms of sickle cell disease during the newborn period. Detection of sickle cell disease by analysis of fetal DNA makes prenatal diagnosis by amniocentesis or chorionic villus sampling safe and reliable for couples at risk. Collection of cord blood for potential use in transplantation should be encouraged in families that have a child with sickle cell disease. Discussions regarding this should be initiated during consultation for prenatal diagnosis.

OPTIMAL MANAGEMENT

Although bone marrow transplantation offers the only cure for sickle cell disease at the present time, comprehensive care can minimize many of the associated complications. Data from the

| TABLE 245.2. | CLINICAL AND HEMATOLOGIC FINDINGS IN SICKLE CELL DISEASE |

Disease	Clinical Severity	Hemoglobin Electrophoresis				Hematologic			
		S (%)	F (%)	A2 (%)	A (%)	Hb g/dL	Retic (%)	MCV (fl)	RBC Morphology
SS	Usually marked	>90	<10	<3.5	0	6–10	5–20	>80	Sickle cells Nrbc Normochromic Anisocytosis Polkilocytosis Target cells Howell-Jolly bodies
Sβ⁰ Thal	Marked to moderate	>80	<20	>3.5	0	6–10	5–20	<80	Sickle cells Nrbc Hypochromic Microcytosis Anisocytosis Poikilocytosis Target cells
Sβ⁺ Thal	Mild to moderate	>60	<20	>3.5	20 (A)	9–12	5–10	<75	No sickle cells Hyperchromic Microcytosis Anisocytosis Polkilocytosis Target cells
SC	Mild to moderate	50	<5	—	50 (C)	10–15	5–10	75–95	"Fat" sickle cells Anisocytosis Polkilocytosis Target cells

Nrbc, nucleated red blood cells; *Sβ⁺ Thal,* sickle beta no thalassemia; *Sβ⁺ Thal,* sickle beta plus thalassemia; *SC,* hemoglobin SC disease; *SS,* sickle cell anemia.

National Cooperative Study of Sickle Cell Disease demonstrate that among patients with sickle cell anemia receiving care in designated sickle cell programs, 50% are alive at age 45 years. A comprehensive manual distributed by the Sickle Cell Program at the U.S. National Institutes of Health (NIH) provides detailed information on current management and treatment guidelines.

There is an unfortunate tendency among health care providers to emphasize episodic treatment and to underestimate the importance of comprehensive health care. In addition to providing health care maintenance, the patient's primary physician, psychosocial services, and nursing and rehabilitation personnel are responsible for helping patients to cope with the chronicity of their illness, to deal with pain, to continue their education, to adjust to adolescence, and to plan for the future. Clinical examination should focus on early identification of problems by establishing standardized evaluations of various organ systems. Therapy should be directed at prevention, eliminating factors such as hypertonicity, acidosis, or hypoxia. Even mild dehydration must be corrected by the oral or intravenous route, recognizing that the inability to concentrate urine requires one and a half to two times the usual volume of fluids. Also, limited cardiac function may predispose the patient who is aggressively treated with intravenous fluids to pulmonary edema. Acidemia and hypoxia should be corrected, but routine oxygen therapy should be avoided, as it can suppress erythropoiesis. Managed care organizations must be educated as to the importance of comprehensive care and the data that demonstrate its cost-effectiveness.

Painful crises should be treated with adequate analgesia once surgical causes of pain have been excluded. Physicians should be familiar with the pharmacology of narcotic analgesics and should use doses sufficient to block painful symptoms quickly. Severe pain requires the parenteral administration of morphine, preferably by patient-controlled methods. Patients may benefit from the addition of nonsteroidal anti-inflammatory agents, provided the effects on renal function are considered. Pulmonary exercises should be added to the treatment plan to prevent atelectasis and hypoxia. As pain abates, the dose of analgesic can be reduced, but the dosing interval should not be changed. With continued improvement, a switch to oral analgesics can be considered. Although addiction is a concern in any patient who requires narcotic analgesics, the factors that predispose to addiction are usually based on social rather than medical issues.

Because of the frequency and serious consequences of septicemia, the sudden appearance of unexplained fever should be considered a medical emergency. A careful medical history should be taken and a complete physical examination performed. Blood and urine cultures and prompt therapy with intravenous antibiotics are required. Signs of neurologic involvement should determine if a lumbar puncture is required. The white cell count and differential should be compared to baseline values. Chest x-ray should be considered to exclude pneumonia. If an infiltrate is noted, the choice of antibiotics should include coverage for *M. pneumoniae.* Although most patients have been immunized with polyvalent purified pneumococcal polysaccharide antigen, this vaccine has not provided sufficient protection against the most virulent forms of *S. pneumoniae,* and newer vaccines are under development. Because all therapy must cover *S. pneumoniae,* the possibility of penicillin resistance must be considered. Improved

TABLE 245.3.	TRANSFUSIONS IN SICKLE CELL DISEASE

Definite:
  Cardiac decompensation
  Severe acute anemia during an acute splenic sequestration or hepatic crisis
  Erythroid hypoplasia or aplasia with a hemoglobin <5.0 g/dL
  Cerebrovascular accidents and transient ischemic attacks
  Multiorgan failure syndrome
  Acute chest syndrome
  Acute priapism unresponsive to fluid and analgesic therapy
  Preoperative preparation for major surgery
Equivocal:
  Intractable or frequent painful events
  Before injection of hypertonic contrast material
  Leg ulcers
  Complicated pregnancy
  Chronic organ failure
  Extreme diminution in performance status due to recurrent complications of sickle cell disease
  Growth failure
Nonindications and Contraindications:
  Chronic steady-state anemia
  Acute painful episodes
  Infections
  Minor surgery not requiring prolonged general anesthesia
  Aseptic necrosis of the hip or shoulder (except when surgery is required)
  Uncomplicated pregnancy

vaccines, such as the new conjugated pneumococcal vaccines, may be of benefit in patients with sickle cell anemia.

Early recognition of an aplastic crisis is facilitated by obtaining a reticulocyte count during the initial evaluation of an acutely ill patient and comparing it to baseline values. Identification of a splenic sequestration crisis can be facilitated by teaching the caregivers how to palpate the spleen. In both of these complications, transfusion therapy is often required.

Red cell transfusions are the mainstay of interventional therapy in sickle cell anemia. Table 245.3 lists the indications for transfusion, according to the recent NIH guidelines. As a consequence of transfusion requirements, iron overload has now become a problem for many patients and iron chelation therapy is often required. Use of techniques such as erythrophoresis may decrease the extent of iron overload in the patient who requires a chronic transfusion program.

For aplastic crisis, splenic sequestration crisis, acute stroke, or acute chest syndrome, partial exchange transfusion may be indicated. Preoperative transfusions minimize the risk of major surgery and should be administered to provide a hemoglobin level of 10 g per deciliter. Chronic blood replacement therapy in patients who have had a stroke or who are being treated for organ failure can be given at 3- to 4-week intervals. The posttransfusion hemoglobin level should never exceed 13 g per deciliter; at this level, the whole-blood viscosity approaches a range likely to cause vascular obstruction. Alloimmunization is a common problem in transfused patients due to the lack of African American blood donors. Providing phenotypically matched blood (especially for C, E, and Kell antigens) decreases this risk. Transfusion reactions can be confused with painful crises, and such reactions might be life threatening.

During the past decade, new therapeutic agents have been evaluated in patients with sickle cell anemia. Treatment with hydroxyurea, although not curative, can increase the red cell volume, increase the fetal hemoglobin level, decrease the frequency of painful crises, and increase the hemoglobin level. The incidence of acute chest syndrome is lower in patients treated with hydroxyurea. This drug must be carefully titrated to prevent toxicity. Its use during pregnancy has not been associated with toxicity. Patients with hemoglobin SC disease have also benefited from treatment with hydroxyurea. Short-chain fatty acids also reportedly elevate fetal hemoglobin levels but not to the extent noted with hydroxyurea. Among these, butyric acid appears to be the most promising. Treatment with clotrimazole and with magnesium has been shown to hydrate red cells by preventing potassium loss during sickling. Clinical trials with magnesium salts are currently under way. Allogeneic bone marrow transplantation has effected a cure in more than 80 patients with sickle cell anemia. A 10% risk of death following this procedure was reported. Alterations in pretransplantation conditioning regimes and use of cord blood as a source of stem cells are being evaluated. Criteria for consideration of transplantation are stringent and may be modified due to its success. Identification of risk factors for clinical severity should assist in the early selection of patients who should be considered for transplantation. Other therapies likely to be developed in the future are those that modify the adhesive receptors on red cells and endothelial cells. Progress in gene therapy has been slow, although use of improved vectors to deliver genes to hematopoietic stem cells has increased the chance that this approach will be successful.

BIBLIOGRAPHY

Beuzard Y, Lubin B, Rosa J, eds. *Sickle cell disease and thalassaemias: new trends in therapy.* London: John Libbey, 1995.
Brugnara C, Gee B, Armsby C, et al. Therapy with oral clotrimazole induces inhibition of the Gardos channel and reduction of erythrocyte dehydration in patients with sickle cell disease. *J Clin Invest* 1996;97:1227–1234.
Charache S, Lubin BH, Reid CD, eds. *Management and therapy of sickle cell disease,* second ed. Washington DC: US Department of Health and Human Services, 1995.
Charache S, Terrin M, Moore R. Effect of hydroxyurea on the frequency of painful crises in sickle cell anemia. *N Engl J Med* 1995;332:1317–1322.
De Franceschi L, Bachir D, Galacteros F, et al. Oral magnesium supplements reduce erythrocyte dehydration in patients with sickle cell disease. *J Clin Invest* 1997;100:1847–1852.
Embury SH, Hebbel RP, Mohandas N, et al. *Sickle cell disease: basic principles and clinical practice.* New York: Raven Press, 1994.
Platt O. The sickle syndromes. In: Handin R, Lux S, Stossel T, eds. *Blood: principles and practice of hematology.* Philadelphia: JB Lippincott, 1995.
Platt O, Thorington B, Brambilla D. Pain in sickle cell disease: rates and risk factors. *N Engl J Med* 1991;325:11–16.
Serjeant G. *Sickle cell disease,* second ed. Oxford: Oxford University Press, 1992.
Vichinsky E, Earles A, Johnson R, et al. Alloimmunization in sickle cell anemia and transfusion of racially unmatched blood. *N Engl J Med* 1990;322:1617–1621.
Walters MC, Patience M, Leisenring W, et al. Bone marrow transplantation for sickle cell disease. *N Engl J Med* 1996;335:369–376.

Kelley's Textbook of Internal Medicine, fourth edition. Edited by H. David Humes. Lippincott Williams & Wilkins, Philadelphia © 2000.

C H A P T E R
246
ANEMIA OF CHRONIC DISEASE

ROBERT T. MEANS, JR.

The anemia of chronic disease (ACD) is the anemia associated with chronic infectious, inflammatory, and neoplastic diseases. It is defined by the demonstration of a hypoproliferative anemia with low serum iron but adequate marrow iron stores. The syndrome does not include anemias associated with chronic renal or liver failure, with endocrine deficiencies, or with chronic bleeding. Many authors also include anemia associated with acute infections in the category of ACD. For these reasons, the term "anemia of chronic disease" is often criticized, and alternatives, such as "anemia of inflammation" or "anemia of defective iron reutilization," have been proposed. However, the disorders associated with ACD are united by the involvement of cytokines in their pathogenesis; these cytokines, in turn, are responsible for the resultant anemia (discussed below).

INCIDENCE

Anemia of chronic disease is generally considered to be the second most common anemia syndrome encountered in clinical practice. Blood loss, with consequent iron deficiency, is usually the cause of anemia. ACD can be identified in up to 27% of outpatients with rheumatoid arthritis and in 58% of patients admitted to the hospital with new rheumatologic diagnoses. In 1985/86, Cash and Sears performed iron studies on all anemic persons admitted to the medical service of a busy metropolitan public hospital during two 2-month periods. After patients with bleeding, hemolysis, or known hematologic malignancies were excluded, 52% of the remaining anemic patients met clinical laboratory criteria for ACD.

PATHOGENESIS

Three processes contribute to the development of ACD (Table 246.1). There is first a modest shortening of red cell survival,

TABLE 246.1.	PATHOGENETIC MECHANISMS IN THE ANEMIA OF CHRONIC DISEASE

Shortened red cell survival in vivo
Impaired marrow erythropoietic response to increased red cell requirements
Blunted erythropoietin response to anemia
Inhibited marrow progenitor response to erythropoietin
Impaired mobilization and utilization of reticuloendothelial iron stores

creating an increased demand for red cell production. The marrow cannot fully respond to this increased red cell requirement, and anemia develops. The marrow cannot increase red cell production because of abnormalities in the mobilization and utilization of reticuloendothelial iron stores and because of impaired erythroid progenitor response. The impaired erythroid progenitor response, in turn, results from two processes.

The production of erythropoietin (EPO), the renal hormone that is the principal regulator of erythropoiesis in vivo, is blunted in ACD; that is, at any given hemoglobin or hematocrit, an ACD patient has a lower EPO level than does a patient with iron deficiency anemia. However, this blunting of the EPO response to anemia cannot fully explain the poor erythropoietic response of these patients. The EPO level in an ACD patient is still higher than the level found in a normal person who is not anemic, indicating that erythroid progenitors are also defective in their ability to respond to EPO.

The observation that the severity of anemia was correlated with the activity of the associated infectious or inflammatory disease led investigators to consider the possibility that the cytokines that mediate inflammation and the response to infection or to tumor invasion, such as tumor necrosis factor (TNF), interleukin-1 (IL-1), and the interferons (IFN), may be responsible for ACD. Evidence accumulated over the last several years indicates that the three pathogenetic mechanisms implicated in the development of ACD (Table 246.1) can be attributed to the actions of these cytokines. The shortened red cell survival ob-

served in anemic patients with rheumatoid arthritis (a model for ACD) correlates with plasma IL-1 levels. Production of EPO in vitro by hepatoma cell lines is inhibited by TNF and IL-1, mimicking the blunted EPO response observed in ACD. The impaired response of erythroid progenitors to EPO can be produced in vitro by IL-1 and TNF acting through IFN-γ and IFN-β, respectively.

Interleukin-1 increases translation of ferritin messenger RNA, implying a shift of transferrin-bound iron immediately available for erythropoiesis to the storage form, ferritin. Acute-phase reactants such as α_1-antitrypsin also impair the binding of iron-bearing transferrin to erythroid precursors and the internalization of occupied transferrin receptors. Thus, cytokines and other mediators of the acute-phase reaction impair mobilization of iron and its use by erythroid precursors.

CLINICAL AND LABORATORY FINDINGS

Anemia of chronic disease is typically a moderate anemia, although 20% to 30% of patients have a hemoglobin level of 8 g per deciliter or less. Clinical findings are essentially those of the associated disease and of anemia. Early studies described ACD as a microcytic anemia; in more recent series, 70% to 80% of patients with ACD are normocytic. The reticulocyte response is typically low for the degree of anemia.

The hallmark of ACD is the demonstration of a low serum iron level with adequate reticuloendothelial iron stores. The major syndrome with which ACD is confused is iron deficiency anemia. This is an important distinction: a diagnosis of iron deficiency typically implies the need to identify a site of blood loss, usually by endoscopic investigation of the gastrointestinal tract. Typical laboratory results for ACD and iron deficiency are compared in Table 246.2.

Evaluation of suspected ACD begins with the determination of the serum iron level, serum total iron-binding capacity (TIBC), and the serum ferritin level. In ACD, the serum iron level is low, with a low serum TIBC, a TIBC saturation greater than 16%, and a normal or elevated serum ferritin level. Iron

| TABLE 246.2. | IRON DEFICIENCY VS. ANEMIA OF CHRONIC DISEASE[a] |

Factor	Iron Deficiency	Anemia of Chronic Disease
Serum iron	Low	Low
Serum TIBC	Typically increased	Decreased
TIBC saturation	<10%	>16%
Serum ferritin	Low	Normal or elevated
Mean corpuscular volume	Decreased	Typically normal
Serum transferrin receptor concentration	Increased	Normal
Marrow iron stores	Absent	Present

[a] These are typical findings; exceptions are discussed in text.
TIBC, total iron-binding capacity.

deficiency is typically associated with a low serum iron level, an elevated TIBC, a TIBC saturation less than 10%, and a low serum ferritin level. However, in some circumstances these observations may not hold true. A patient with concomitant inflammation may fail to show an increase in serum TIBC in response to iron deficiency. Conversely, if the serum TIBC is less than 200 μg per deciliter, a TIBC saturation of less than 16% may be observed in ACD. A low serum ferritin level always indicates iron deficiency; however, the serum ferritin may be elevated to as high as 200 ng per milliliter by inflammation in the absence of marrow iron stores.

Other tests may help distinguish iron deficiency from ACD. The mean corpuscular volume is low in iron deficiency anemia and normal in most cases of ACD. The red cell distribution width is elevated in iron deficiency and typically (but not always) normal in ACD. The serum soluble transferrin receptor level (sTfR) was initially reported to be elevated in iron deficiency and normal in ACD. In other studies, the distinction is less absolute, but it appears that an elevated serum sTfR identifies iron deficient patients with increased serum ferritin concentrations due to inflammation.

If iron deficiency cannot be ruled out, bone marrow examination should be performed. The evaluation of a Prussian blue–stained marrow aspirate or particle section should provide a definitive determination of the presence or absence of marrow iron stores. The evaluation of iron status is the principal indication for marrow examination in suspected ACD. The morphologic features of the bone marrow in ACD are nonspecific, and the diagnosis remains a clinical one.

TREATMENT

There is no specific treatment for ACD; therapy should be directed at the associated disease. The use of iron supplementation and of recombinant human (rh) EPO deserve special mention.

There is no role for iron therapy in the treatment of ACD. Reports in which iron therapy has partially corrected this anemia probably represent cases in which patients with ACD subsequently developed iron deficiency, as when patients with ACD due to rheumatoid arthritis have gastrointestinal blood loss provoked by nonsteroidal anti-inflammatory drugs. In these cases, only the component of anemia due to iron deficiency is corrected; the ACD component of the anemia is not corrected.

Recombinant human EPO can correct the anemia of patients with ACD. Results from the study of erythroid progenitors in vitro and in animal models suggest that this effect results from the ability of high rhEPO concentrations to oppose the inhibitory effects of cytokines. However, most patients with ACD are only moderately anemic and lack symptoms attributable to anemia. rhEPO therapy would not be indicated in these patients, but it should be considered in patients sufficiently anemic on a chronic basis to be symptomatic or to require transfusion, in patients who wish to donate blood to be stored for autologous transfusion at elective surgery, in patients who are anemic from cancer chemotherapy, and in significantly anemic patients with

HIV infection. Patients who have anemia due to cancer chemotherapy or who have severe ACD requiring transfusions may be treated with subcutaneous rhEPO 150 units per kilogram 3 times weekly or 50 units per kilogram 5 times weekly. The practice of using a once-weekly rhEPO dose at 40,000 units, shown to be effective in cancer patients, is also likely to be effective in ACD. HIV patients may be treated with subcutaneous rhEPO 100 to 150 units per kilogram 3 times weekly or 4000 units 6 times weekly.

Responses are typically seen by 6 weeks. Failure to respond suggests iron deficiency (which may develop in association with the response to rhEPO in a patient not previously iron-deficient), blood loss, or active inflammation suppressing erythropoiesis. It is generally good practice to treat a patient with ferrous sulfate 325 mg 3 times a day during rhEPO therapy; the alternative, monitoring the serum ferritin every other week to ensure that it is 100 ng per milliliter or more, is much more costly. Patients with clinically significant iron overload would be an exception to this practice. If iron deficiency, blood loss, or active inflammation is not present, a dose increment (usually 50% to 100%) can be tried. Failure to respond to the increased dose after an additional 6 weeks indicates that the patient is unlikely to respond to further therapy with rhEPO. The rhEPO doses of responding patients should be adjusted to maintain a hematocrit of 36% or a hemoglobin level of 12 g per deciliter. Patients donating blood for autologous transfusion may be treated with subcutaneous rhEPO 150 units per kilogram 3 times weekly or 300 units per kilogram twice weekly (and ferrous sulfate 325 mg 3 times a day) during the 3 to 4 weeks before surgery. Autologous blood for storage can then be collected according to the local blood center's protocol.

BIBLIOGRAPHY

Baer AN, Dessypris EN, Goldwasser E, et al. Blunted erythropoietin response to anaemia in rheumatoid arthritis. *Br J Haematol* 1987;66: 559–564.

Baer AN, Dessypris EN, Krantz SB. The pathogenesis of anemia in rheumatoid arthritis: a clinical and laboratory analysis. *Semin Arthritis Rheum* 1990;14:209–223.

Cash JM, Sears DA. The spectrum of diseases associated with the anemia of chronic disease: a study of 90 cases. *Am J Med* 1990;87:638–644.

Ferguson BJ, Skikine BS, Simpson KM, et al. Serum transferrin receptor distinguishes the anemia of chronic disease from iron-deficiency anemia. *J Lab Clin Med* 1992;19:385–390.

Means RT. Clinical application of recombinant human erythropoietin in the anemia of chronic disease. *Hematol Oncol Clin North Am* 1994;8: 933–944.

Means RT. Erythropoietin in the treatment of anemia in chronic infectious, inflammatory, and malignant diseases. *Curr Opin Hematol* 1995;2: 210–213.

Means RT, Krantz SB. Progress in understanding the pathogenesis of the anemia of chronic disease. *Blood* 1992;80:1639–1647.

North M, Dallalio G, Donath AS, et al. Correlation of serum transferrin receptor levels with other parameters in patients undergoing evaluation of iron status: observed vs. predicted results. *Clin Lab Haematol* 1997; 19:93–97.

Schilling RF. Anemia of chronic disease: a misnomer. *Ann Intern Med* 1991; 115:572–573.

C H A P T E R
247

PARANEOPLASTIC SYNDROMES

GREGORY P. KALEMKERIAN

■ DEFINITION AND INCIDENCE

The paraneoplastic syndromes are a heterogeneous group of clinical disorders with signs and symptoms affecting sites distant from both the primary tumor and metastatic foci. Although paraneoplastic syndromes occur, by definition, in patients with cancer, nearly all of them have also been reported in the absence of underlying malignancy. Indeed, many of these syndromes occur more frequently in patients without cancer, whereas only a few have been reported solely in the paraneoplastic setting. For instance, less than 10% of patients with dermatomyositis are found to have cancer, whereas necrolytic migratory erythema is considered pathognomonic for glucagonoma. Paraneoplastic syndromes are most frequently associated with carcinomas of the lung, stomach, and breast, or with hematologic malignancies, especially Hodgkin's disease and non-Hodgkin's lymphoma. A few paraneoplastic syndromes, such as cancer-related anemia and anorexia–cachexia, occur frequently in patients with a variety of malignancies, while most others are associated with specific histologic types of cancer. Despite the high frequency of nonspecific symptoms in cancer patients, most of the organ-specific paraneoplastic syndromes are rare, with an estimated overall incidence of 5% to 10%. As an example, although many patients with lung cancer exhibit gross neuromuscular or autonomic deficits, less than 2% of them are found to have definable neurologic syndromes. However, the high incidence of constitutional symptoms and laboratory abnormalities in cancer patients has recently led investigators to suggest that paraneoplastic syndromes may affect over 50% of these patients. It is important for the primary care physician to be familiar with the myriad manifestations of paraneoplastic syndromes because these disorders are frequently the earliest indication of cancer and their prompt recognition may allow for the diagnosis of the disease at an earlier, more treatable stage. In addition, the timely initiation of appropriate treatment for a specific paraneoplastic syndrome can have a tremendous impact on quality of life, even in the setting of advanced disease.

■ PATHOGENESIS

Although the cause of most paraneoplastic syndromes remains unknown, several mechanisms by which tumors can induce these syndromes have been described, including (a) ectopic production and secretion of peptide hormones or hormone precursors; (b) metabolic conversion of steroid hormones; (c) production and secretion of cytokines; and (d) stimulation of autoimmune antibody production. The endocrine syndromes, such as humoral hypercalcemia and the syndrome of inappropriate secretion of antidiuretic hormone (SIADH), are generally caused by the ectopic production of peptide hormones by tumor cells. Many normal and malignant nonendocrine cells produce small quantities of protein hormones that serve autocrine or paracrine functions. However, some cancers produce large quantities of these hormones or have greater potential for converting precursor molecules to the active form, resulting in a clinically apparent systemic syndrome. Paraneoplastic syndromes caused by the overproduction of steroid hormones are exceedingly rare due to the complexity of the steroid synthetic pathways. However, sarcomas and hepatocellular carcinomas can express increased aromatase activity that enhances the conversion of androgens to estradiol, resulting in gynecomastia. In addition, some hematologic malignancies express increased vitamin D hydrolase activity leading to elevated levels of calcitriol and systemic hypercalcemia. Although the production of a wide variety of cytokines by tumor cells has been well documented, the direct causal relationship between these substances and specific syndromes remains unproven. Nevertheless, available data suggest that the secretion of cytokines may be responsible for some of the more common paraneoplastic syndromes, including leukocytosis, tumor fever, and anorexia–cachexia. A variety of paraneoplastic syndromes, especially those with neurologic manifestations, are associated with the generation of autoantibodies directed against tumor-expressed antigens that are not normally accessible for immune recognition. These autoantibodies can cross-react with antigens on normal cells, such as neurons, resulting in tissue-specific cytotoxicity, or they can form complexes with circulating antigen to induce end-organ damage through immune complex deposition. In a few syndromes with an apparent autoimmune mechanism, specific causative antibodies have been identified, such as the anti-Yo and anti-Hu antibodies in subacute cerebellar degeneration, but in most the etiologic antigen and antibody remain unknown. The ability to establish a causal link between specific antibody production and a clinical syndrome has been confounded by the findings that many cancer patients without neurologic symptoms express low levels of autoantibodies and that some afflicted patients lack expression of the putative antibody.

■ CLINICAL FINDINGS

The signs and symptoms of paraneoplastic syndromes can precede the diagnosis of cancer by months or years, or can arise at any time during the course of known malignant disease. Paraneoplastic syndromes are usually associated with a relatively rapid onset of symptoms, which should heighten the clinician's suspicion of an underlying malignancy. The constellation of symptoms can also be affected by this rapid course and can help establish a cancer-associated etiology. For instance, paraneoplastic Cushing's syndrome differs from Cushing's disease in that it is rarely associated with truncal obesity, cutaneous striations, and hyperpigmentation. Although the clinical course of a paraneoplastic syndrome can be notoriously unpredictable, in most cases it closely parallels that of the underlying malignancy.

As noted in Table 247.1, nearly every organ system and anatomical site can be affected by paraneoplastic syndromes. Patients with neurologic syndromes typically display worsening of symptoms over weeks to months prior to stabilization of disease at a level of moderate to severe disability. The dermatologic

syndromes can cause significant cosmetic and functional morbidity that is usually underestimated by health care providers; in rare cases, severe desquamation, such as that associated with paraneoplastic pemphigus, can be fatal. Among the endocrine syndromes, SIADH and humoral hypercalcemia can induce severe, even lethal, metabolic disturbances. Similarly, anemia is a major contributing factor in cancer-related fatigue and cardiopulmonary morbidity, while thromboembolic phenomena are

TABLE 247.1.	SELECTED PARANEOPLASTIC SYNDROMES		
Syndrome	**Major Features**	**Cause**	**Common Malignancies**
Endocrine			
Cushing's syndrome	Weakness, alkalosis, ↓ K$^+$, hypertension	ACTH	SCLC, carcinoid, thymoma, medullary thyroid
Inappropriate antidiuretic hormone secretion	↓ Serum Na$^+$, relative urine hypertonicity, confusion	Arginine vasopressin, ANF	SCLC, GI, esophageal
Hypercalcemia	↑ Serum Ca^{2+}, confusion, polyuria/polydipsia	PTHrP	NSCLC, H&N, breast
		Osteoclast activating factors	Myeloma, breast, lymphoma
		↑ Vitamin D hydroxylation	T-Cell leukemia/lymphoma
Hypoglycemia	↓ Serum glucose, confusion	IGF-II	Sarcoma, HCC
Oncogenic osteomalacia	↓ Serum phosphate, ↓ 1,25-OH vitamin D, osteopenia, bone pain	↑ Renal phosphate loss	Sarcoma, prostate, SCLC
Acromegaly	Coarsened facial features, increased hand/foot size	Growth hormone	Lung, stomach, breast
		GHRH	Carcinoid, islet cell
Gynecomastia	Enlarged male breasts	hCG	NSCLC, GI, sarcoma
		↑ Aromatase activity	HCC, sarcoma
Neuromuscular			
Encephalomyelitis	Altered affect, dementia	ANNA-1 (anti-Hu)	SCLC
Subacute cerebellar degeneration	Ataxia, dysarthria, vertigo	Anti–Purkinje cell antibody (anti-Yo, anti-Hu)	SCLC, breast, ovarian
Cancer-associated retinopathy	Visual loss, photosensitivity	Antirecoverin antibody	SCLC
Opsoclonus-myoclonus	Involuntary motions	ANNA-2 (anti-Ri)	Breast, SCLC, neuroblastoma
Subacute motor neuropathy	Lower motor neuropathy	Anterior horn cell loss	Hodgkin's disease, NHL
Subacute myelopathy	Ascending weakness and sensory loss	Unknown	Lung, Hodgkin's disease
Subacute sensory neuropathy	Pain, sensory loss	Dorsal root ganglion degeneration/demyelination	SCLC, breast
Acute polyneuropathy (Guillain–Barré syndrome)	Ascending paralysis	Inflammation, demyelination	Hodgkin's disease
Intestinal pseudo-obstruction	Paralytic ileus	Anti–myenteric plexus neuron antibody	SCLC
Myasthenia gravis	Weakness, blurred vision	Anti–acetylcholine receptor antibody	Thymoma
Eaton–Lambert syndrome	Weakness, autonomic dysfunction	Anti–voltage-gated calcium channel antibody	SCLC
Hematologic			
Anemia	↓ Hgb/Hct, nl MCV	Relative ↓ erythropoietin	All
	Schistocytosis	Autoimmune hemolysis	Lymphoma, CLL
	↓ Erythroid precursors	Pure red cell aplasia	Thymoma
Erythrocytosis	↑ Hgb/Hct	Erythropoietin	Renal cell, HCC
Leukemoid reaction	WBC >20,000/mm^3	Cytokines	All
Thrombocytopenia	↓ platelet count	Antiplatelet antibody (ITP)	Lymphoma
Thrombocytosis	↑ platelet count	(?) Thrombopoietin	Hodgkin's disease, NHL, solid tumors
Thromboembolism (Trousseau's syndrome, marantic endocarditis)	Migratory thrombosis, sterile valvular vegetations, systemic emboli, CVA	Unknown	Mucinous adenocarcinomas (NSCLC, GI)
Disseminated intravascular coagulopathy	Anemia, ↑ PT/PTT, thrombocytopenia	Unknown	AML-M3, solid tumors

TABLE 247.1. *Continued*

Syndrome	Major Features	Cause	Common Malignancies
Dermatologic			
Acanthosis nigricans	Intertriginous brown, velvety plaques	Unknown	GI (stomach)
Tripe palms	Hyperpigmented, thickened, velvety palms	Unknown	Stomach, lung
Bazex's disease	Acral hyperkeratosis, nail dystrophy	Unknown	Esophageal, H&N, squamous lung
Sign of Leser-Trelat	Eruptive seborrheic keratoses	Unknown	GI, adenocarcinomas
Paget's disease	Eczematous plaques	Unknown	Breast
Erythema gyratum repens	Scaling erythema	Immune complex deposition	Lung, breast
Necrolytic migratory erythema	Gyrate blistering erythema	Glucagon (? metabolite)	Glucagonoma
Flushing	Episodic erythema of face/neck	Serotonin, other vasoactive peptides	Carcinoid, medullary thyroid
Erythroderma	Diffuse macular erythema	Unknown	Hodgkin's disease, NHL
Paraneoplastic pemphigus	Mucocutaneous bullae	(?) Antidesmoplakin antibody	Sarcoma, NHL
Acquired icthyosis	Diffuse dry, cracking, hyperkeratotic skin	Unknown	Hodgkin's disease, NHL
Hypertrichosis lanuginosa	Rapid growth of long, fine hair (lanugo)	Unknown	Lung, breast, GI, gynecologic
Pruritis	Diffuse itching	Unknown	Hodgkin's disease, NHL
Sweet's syndrome	Painful plaques, fever, neutrophilia	Unknown	Hematologic malignancies
Rheumatologic			
Dermatomyositis/polymyositis	Muscle weakness/inflammation, rash	(?) Antimyosin or antimyoglobin antibody	Lung, ovarian, breast, stomach
Vasculitis	All forms	Immune complex deposition	Hematologic malignancies
Pulmonary hypertrophic osteoarthropathy	Clubbing, bone pain, synovitis, periostitis	Unknown	Lung, mesothelioma, pulmonary metastases
Renal			
Glomerulonephritis	Membranous GN	Immune complex deposition	Lung, GI, breast, lymphoma
Nephrotic syndrome	Minimal GN (lipoid nephrosis)	Unknown	Hodgkin's disease
Hepatic			
Stauffer's syndrome	Hepatic dysfunction, fever, weight loss	(?) Antihepatocyte antibody	Renal cell
Systemic			
Anorexia-cachexia	Involuntary weight loss	(?) TNF-α (cachexin)	All
Fever	Absence of infection	(?) Pyrexins	Renal cell, Hodgkin's disease, hepatic metastases

ACTH, adrenocorticotropic hormone; AML-M3, acute promyelocytic leukemia; ANF, atrial natriuretic factor; ANNA, anti–neuronal nuclear antibody; CLL, chronic lymphocytic leukemia; CVA, cerebrovascular accident; GHRH, growth hormone–releasing hormone; GI, gastrointestinal adenocarcinomas; GN, glomerulonephropathy; H&N, head and neck squamous cell carcinoma; HCC, hepatocellular carcinoma; hCG, human chorionic gonadotropin; Hgb/Hct, hemoglobin/hematocrit; IGF-II, insulin-like growth factor II; ITP, idiopathic thrombocytopenic purpura; MCV, mean corpuscular volume; NHL, non-Hodgkin's lymphoma; NSCLC, non–small-cell lung cancer; PTHrP, parathyroid hormone–related peptide; PT/PTT, prothrombin time/partial thromboplastin time; SCLC, small-cell lung cancer; TNF-α, tumor necrosis factor–α; WBC, white blood cell count.

not an uncommon cause of death in patients with advanced cancer.

DISEASE MANAGEMENT

The appropriate management of paraneoplastic syndromes is dependent on the specific nature of the syndrome, the severity of symptoms, the therapeutic responsiveness of the underlying malignancy, and the overall prognosis of the patient. Usually, the dual goals of treatment are to alleviate the symptoms of the paraneoplastic syndrome and to control the associated cancer. In patients with mild paraneoplastic symptoms and surgically resectable or chemosensitive tumors, such as small-cell lung cancer or lymphomas, anticancer treatment alone may be sufficient. However, specific therapy directed at the paraneoplastic syndrome is usually required in patients with significant symptoms and/or advanced or poorly responsive tumors. Frequently, it is appropriate to forego specific therapy in favor of comfort measures in patients in the terminal phases of disease.

Paraneoplastic syndromes resulting from hormone or cytokine overproduction usually improve with successful anticancer therapy and recur upon relapse of disease. Ancillary therapies, such as the inhibition of cortisol production with aminoglutethimide or ketoconazole in Cushing's syndrome, hydration and bisphosphonates in humoral hypercalcemia, fluid restriction and demeclocycline in SIADH, and phosphate and vitamin D replacement in oncogenic osteomalacia, are frequently useful for symptom palliation. In contrast, the symptoms associated with autoimmune neurologic syndromes are often due to specific neuronal damage that is usually irreversible at diagnosis. Although clinical improvement is noted in less than 10% of these patients after cytotoxic or immunosuppressive therapy, such as plasmapheresis and corticosteroid administration, these measures frequently prevent further neurologic deterioration. Topical and systemic immunosuppressive approaches have also been tried with varying degrees of success in a wide variety of the dermatologic syndromes. Recent advances have led to substantial improvements in the quality of life of patients with some of the most common paraneoplastic syndromes. For example, appetite stimulants, such as medroxyprogesterone acetate, can reverse weight loss in up to 50% of patients with cancer-associated anorexia–cachexia, and erythropoietin can alleviate fatigue in a significant subset of patients with cancer-related anemia.

BIBLIOGRAPHY

Agarwala SS. Paraneoplastic syndromes. *Med Clin North Am* 1996;80: 173–184.

Bick RL, ed. Paraneoplastic syndromes. *Hematol Oncol Clin North Am* 1996;10.

Dropcho EJ. Principles of paraneoplastic syndromes. *Ann NY Acad Sci* 1998;841:246–261.

John WJ, Patchell RA, Foon KA. Paraneoplastic syndromes. In: DeVita VT, Hellman S, Rosenberg SA, eds. *Cancer: principles and practice of oncology*, fifth ed. Philadelphia: Lippincott-Raven Publishers, 1997: 2397–2422.

Kurzrock R, Cohen PR. Cutaneous paraneoplastic syndromes in solid tumors. *Am J Med* 1995;99:662–671.

Levin KH. Paraneoplastic neuromuscular syndromes. *Neurol Clin North Am* 1997;15:597–614.

Nathanson L, Hall TC, eds. Paraneoplastic syndromes. *Semin Oncol* 1997; 24:265–268.

Nelson KA, Walsh D, Sheehan FA. The cancer anorexia–cachexia syndrome. *J Clin Oncol* 1994;12:213–225.

Kelley's Textbook of Internal Medicine, fourth edition. Edited by H. David Humes. Lippincott Williams & Wilkins, Philadelphia © 2000.

DIAGNOSTIC AND THERAPEUTIC MODALITIES IN ONCOLOGIC AND HEMATOLOGIC DISORDERS

CHAPTER

248

IMAGING IN ONCOLOGY

STEPHEN I. MARGLIN
RONALD A. CASTELLINO

Perhaps more so than for the majority of other medical specialties, oncology relies on the quality of information uniquely provided by radiologic imaging. Because of the rapidity with which radiology has evolved and the consequent increase in the number of examinations from which to choose, selecting the most appropriate examination has become an increasingly difficult and daunting challenge. As a result, and in the belief that technologic advances are likely to continue, this chapter emphasizes what we believe to be the principles of oncologic imaging rather than the specific examinations that should be used in a given clinical setting. The indications for oncologic imaging and the manner in which one might attempt to evaluate these modalities are also emphasized. The technologies currently most applicable to oncology are also reviewed.

PRINCIPLES OF ONCOLOGIC IMAGING

The choice of an examination for a patient with a known or suspected malignancy depends primarily on the questions being posed. Put somewhat differently, the decision depends on the reason the information is being sought and on how the information will be used. Unless "the question" is carefully considered, an inappropriate test might be chosen—one that would waste valuable time, unnecessarily burden the patient, and produce little if any useful information. Table 248.1 lists some common reasons for obtaining an imaging examination.

Imaging is often used, before a diagnosis of cancer has been established, as a way to elucidate the etiology of symptoms or to better understand a palpable or biochemical abnormality.

During these examinations, it is not uncommon to encounter unexpected abnormalities. However, these aberrations do not invariably represent cancer. An important contribution that radiologists can render is the ability and experience to discriminate between benign and malignant lesions (i.e., between abnormalities that require histologic confirmation and those that do not). As an example, a lung nodule should, as a rule, be considered potentially malignant, particularly in a smoker or in someone over age 50. However, if the nodule is homogeneously or concentrically calcified, the lesion is almost certainly benign (i.e., it represents the residuum of an earlier granulomatous infection). Similarly, a hypodense liver lesion discovered on a contrast-enhanced computed tomography (CT) examination also should be viewed with concern. However, if scans obtained after the administration of intravenous contrast demonstrate that the lesion equilibrates in attenuation or "fills in," and particularly if the lesion avidly accumulates radiotracer on a tagged red cell scan, a radiologist can provide a high degree of reassurance that the abnormality is a benign hemangioma.

Although the radiographic appearance of an abnormality is an important component in the decision as to whether to perform additional tests, rarely can the appearance be relied on to provide a histologically specific diagnosis. Few findings are sufficiently pathognomonic (e.g., the CT appearance of a meningioma) to permit an unequivocal pronouncement regarding treatment or prognosis. This limitation must be borne in mind. Major decisions, especially those relating to the choice of initial therapy, generally require pathologic verification of the nature of the abnormality.

Having said this, accurate depiction of a lesion, especially when presented in cross-sectional format, is often exceedingly helpful in deciding how best to obtain tissue. Sometimes a conventional (open surgical) biopsy may be necessary. On other occasions, an image-guided, percutaneous aspiration or biopsy may provide the information needed to guide management.

Because most forms of imaging provide anatomical rather than histologic or metabolic information, the test's specificity must be well understood. It is essential that the predictive accuracy of a positive diagnosis not be overstated or misinterpreted. This is particularly important when staging a newly diagnosed cancer (i.e., when decisions regarding initial therapy are being made). CT or magnetic resonance imaging (MRI) examinations

TABLE 248.1.	COMMON INDICATIONS FOR IMAGING IN ONCOLOGY

To aid in establishing a diagnosis (i.e., establishing how best to obtain tissue)
Staging
Evaluating extent of disease
Establishing a baseline
Formulating prognosis
Planning treatment
Assessing response to therapy
Detecting relapse
Evaluating possible complications of disease or therapy
Detecting infections
Detecting second neoplasms
Evaluating cardiac dysfunction
Clinical research

of patients with newly diagnosed lung cancer commonly reveal enlarged mediastinal lymph nodes. It might be tempting to declare such patients inoperable. However, extensive experience has shown that an appreciable number of these enlarged nodes are reactive (i.e., do not contain tumor). Excessive reliance on the size and appearance of such nodes might therefore contribute inadvertently to the loss of a unique opportunity to treat, and possibly to cure, such patients.

Staging and defining the anatomical extent of disease are not necessarily synonymous, nor do these tasks necessarily require the same type or intensity of imaging. As an example, in non-Hodgkin's lymphoma, a bone marrow biopsy may be all that is required to categorize a patient as having advanced (stage IV) disease. This is quite different from the information that would be necessary to describe the degree of involvement in all nodal and extranodal sites. Thus, for certain diseases, if all that is required is "staging," little or no imaging may be required. To visualize the actual extent of disease, however, multiple examinations (e.g., CT or MRI) may be necessary. As always, the decision about which imaging tests to use depends on understanding what information is required and how that information is going to be used.

If appropriate management requires identification of all major sites of disease, the selection of examinations requires substantial knowledge of the anticipated biologic behavior of the tumor. Sites that are suggested by the results of biochemical tests or symptoms should of course be evaluated. But what about sites that are clinically silent? If a tumor is known to have a low propensity to metastasize to a given location, radiologic interrogation of that site is probably not warranted. For instance, in Hodgkin's disease, neither bone scans nor contrast examinations of the gastrointestinal (GI) tract are routinely performed in newly diagnosed patients because the yield is low to nonexistent, respectively.

There is one important caveat to this approach. If the consequences of missing metastatic disease in a particular location are serious enough (i.e., if they pose an unacceptable risk to the patient), a given test may still be warranted, even when the yield from that examination is known to be low.

Earlier we noted that the selection of a radiologic examination depends in part on a tumor's anticipated biologic behavior. This information is also essential for the accurate interpretation of a radiologic examination. In Hodgkin's disease, clinical research has demonstrated that the tumor spreads in a remarkably predictable manner. Thus, disease in the neck or mediastinum is known to place the upper abdominal lymph nodes and the spleen at risk. If CT or lymphography fails to demonstrate abnormalities in these sites but instead reveals enlargement of pelvic lymph nodes, radiologists and clinicians should interpret these findings with caution; something other than Hodgkin's is more likely responsible for the pelvic adenopathy.

When treatment is to consist of or include irradiation, the precision and accuracy of the information needed may be extraordinarily high. However, if the patient is going to receive chemotherapy, much can be accomplished without this same degree of anatomical precision; chemotherapeutic agents can accomplish their task without precise road maps.

If imaging is being performed to evaluate response to treatment or to detect relapse, it is useful to ask whether it is necessary to visualize all known sites of disease. Many tumors behave in a synchronous fashion; sites of disease wax or wane synchronously as they respond to variations in therapy. For these tumors, it may be possible to limit examinations to so-called index sites (sites of original bulk disease). Other sites, barring evidence to the contrary, can be assumed to behave in concert with the sites being imaged.

In reviewing the literature, it is sometimes difficult to decipher the significance of reports describing new therapeutic interventions, largely because of differences in the way in which the patients were evaluated. If the results of a patient's treatment are likely to be of interest to others, and particularly if the patient has been enrolled in an investigation that compares the efficacy of differing forms of therapy, some thought should be given to using the same imaging studies, in the same way, as other investigators.

EVALUATING DIAGNOSTIC MODALITIES

Having decided that some form of imaging is indicated, the clinician must then decide which examinations to obtain. Other things, such as cost and invasiveness, being equal, it might appear that the choice would come down to a straightforward comparison of the accuracy of the competing tests. Unfortunately, the task is not nearly so simple.

For any test, the term *accuracy* means the number of correct diagnoses divided by the number of examinations performed. Although this definition describes one facet of a test's performance, it provides no explicit information concerning its actual ability to detect disease. Consider the example of a tumor with a low likelihood of distant spread. If we assume that the tumor metastasizes between 1% and 10% of the time, and if the test in question were to be uniformly reported as "negative," the overall accuracy would be 99% and 90%, respectively. This test might therefore be considered respectable despite the fact that not a single incident of disease spreading beyond the confines of the original site was detected. Although the overall accuracy of this test is high, such a test is unlikely to be particularly helpful.

Thus, because the "accuracy" of a test provides limited information, it has become customary to report the results of tests in terms of their sensitivity and specificity (Fig. 248.1). These parameters provide much more information concerning the test's ability to detect disease. Useful information is also provided concerning the test's propensity to produce false-positive diagnoses. If the prevalence of the abnormality being studied is known, knowledge of a test's sensitivity and specificity permits one to calculate the probability of a false-positive or a false-negative diagnosis.

Although these amplifications and modifications represent significant improvements, they are still not entirely satisfactory. First, published results often represent the best that can be achieved by dedicated specialists under the best possible circumstances. Other well-trained, highly motivated physicians may not be able to replicate these results. More importantly, the results are significantly influenced by the prevalence of disease in the population originally studied. If that population differs greatly from the population in the "real world," results such as the "accuracy of positive diagnoses" or the "accuracy of negative diagnoses" will not be the same. If, however, the prevalence (the pretest probability of disease in the real world) is known, it is possible to recalculate the new and locally applicable values.

It is perhaps of greatest importance that simply providing a list of the relevant parameters of accuracy (sensitivity, specificity, predictive accuracy of positive and negative diagnoses, and overall accuracy) does not easily or inexorably lead to the selection of one examination over another. Which is better: a test with high sensitivity (one that can detect more cancers) or one with high specificity (one that has fewer false-positive diagnoses)? Even the conventional five parameters of accuracy only serve to describe a single point on a continuous curve, a curve that plots the sensitivity of the test against its false-positive fraction (the inverse of specificity). This curve, known as a receiver operating characteristics (ROC) curve (Fig. 248.2), is a better descriptor of the performance of a given examination and of the people who use it. If all other things are equal, comparing the areas

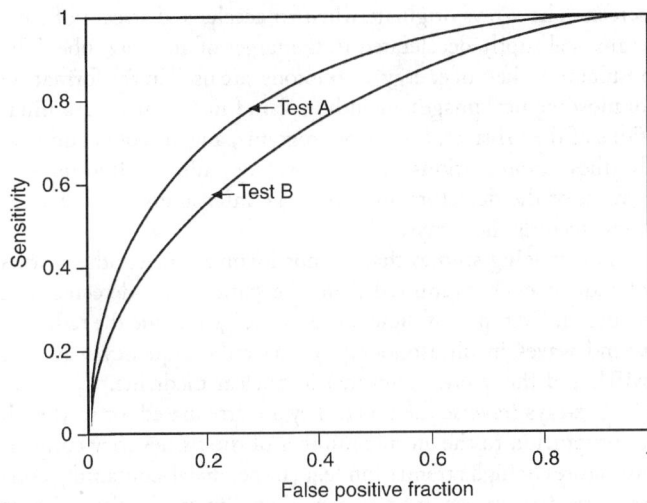

FIGURE 248.2. Receiver operating characteristic (ROC) curves of two hypothetical imaging examinations. Test A is theoretically the more accurate; that is, for each sensitivity or true-positive fraction, it has a lower false-positive fraction.

under the ROC curves of different tests permits one to identify the test that is theoretically the best.

However, the generation of an ROC curve is an artificial and somewhat labored process. The curve describes what *might* occur, given certain conditions—not all of which are likely. The single point described by the parameters of accuracy actually describes how the test performed in a given clinical setting. In other words, although the area under test A's ROC curve may exceed that for test B, the single point of practice for test B may still be judged as producing better results than the site that users have adopted for test A.

Finally, published reports of the prowess and accuracy of a given modality often describe what specialists under optimal conditions can achieve. It is unrealistic to assume that similar results will be obtained in every hospital and in every clinic. Thus, the preferences, skills, and talents of the radiologists performing the examinations must be considered and integrated into the decision.

SPECIFIC MODALITIES

Plain radiographs are usually the first imaging examinations that are obtained. Although they are less sensitive and less specific than the more sophisticated and expensive examinations, they are probably a reasonable compromise. If an abnormality is detected (which is certainly not uncommon) and/or if the signs and symptoms are sufficiently compelling, further evaluation invariably proceeds. Because plain radiographs, particularly those that examine the chest, are readily available and low in cost, they are also important in the periodic surveillance of patients with cancer.

Plain radiographs are produced when x-rays pass through the human body, interact with structures in their path, and contact and become recorded by a detector such as film or a luminescent

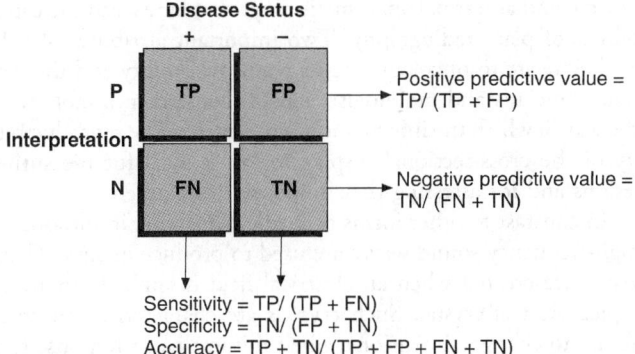

FIGURE 248.1. A classification table of test results compared with a gold standard. D, disease status; FN, false-negative; FP, false-positive; N, negative interpretation; P, positive interpretation; TN, true negative; TP, true positive.

screen. The x-rays originate when an accelerated stream of electrons is abruptly decelerated in the target of an x-ray tube. The resultant packets of energy, or photons, are used in the formation of most medical images, including plain films, contrast examinations of the GI tract, excretory urograms, angiography, and CT. In these examinations, a detector (e.g., film, a fluoroscopic screen, or the detectors used in image intensifiers and CT gantries) records the x-rays.

For imaging studies that do not involve x-rays, other forms of radiant energy, emitted from the patient, are detected and analyzed. Examples of these forms of energy include the reflected sound waves in ultrasonography, the radiofrequency waves in MRI, and the γ-rays (photons) in nuclear medicine.

As x-rays traverse the body, they are attenuated, or scattered, in proportion to the atomic number of the tissues they contact. Structures of high attenuation (e.g., bone, metal-containing contrast media) absorb more x-rays than "water-density" tissues (e.g., organs, blood), which absorb more than fat-containing and finally air-containing structures. The packets of energy that emanate from the body represent the summation of the atomic composition of the objects in the path of the beam. In most plain film examinations, the x-rays interact with a luminescent screen that produces light in direct proportion to the number of x-rays that reach it. The light exposes a film, which when developed results in the formation of an image. This projection image (e.g., a chest or abdominal radiograph) superimposes or compresses the patient's three-dimensional anatomy onto a two-dimensional sheet of film.

In addition to plain radiographs obtained without contrast, examinations performed after contrast administration (e.g., upper GI series, barium enemas, and intravenous urograms) are important means of interrogating specific organ systems. These examinations permit excellent definition of anatomical abnormalities that arise from the mucosa, as well as from the walls of a hollow viscus. A limitation of these examinations is their relative insensitivity to the presence of enlarged lymph nodes and/or nearby masses, even when such masses are quite large.

Angiography is a unique form of plain film radiography. In this increasingly important and technically demanding subspecialty, a contrast agent is injected into a vessel, enabling visualization of segments of anatomy that would otherwise be hidden from view. Angiography actually embraces a number of different examinations (e.g., arteriograms, venograms, and lymphangiograms). When the task involves establishing a diagnosis of cancer, CT and MRI have largely supplanted arteriography. However, if resection of part of the liver is being considered (e.g., for a hepatoma or for a small number of apparently localized metastases), performing a hepatic or superior mesenteric arteriogram can significantly increases CT's sensitivity to the presence of lesions.

In many radiology departments, angiography is combined with interventional radiology, reflecting the fact that what was formerly a purely diagnostic specialty has evolved into one that has become increasingly therapeutic. In addition to depicting normal and abnormal vascular anatomy, angiograms are now used to deliver cytotoxic agents and to embolize a tumor's blood supply. Sometimes this is done for palliation; on other occasions, it may be used as an adjunct to surgery (e.g., to diminish blood loss). Interventional radiology has proved particularly effective as a means of obtaining diagnostic material and as a way of percutaneously draining infected fluid collections.

Lymphography is a form of imaging in which an oily, iodinated contrast agent is directly infused into tiny lymphatic channels that course beneath the skin on the dorsum of the feet. Part of the contrast becomes trapped in the sinusoids of abdominal and pelvic lymph nodes, thereby permitting remarkably detailed visualization of the nodes' internal architecture. Lymphography was once a mainstay in the armamentarium of diagnostic oncology. Today CT has largely supplanted it. However, in certain diseases, such as Hodgkin's disease, lymphography has a small statistical advantage over CT. Despite this, the technical demands of the procedure, combined with the relatively infrequency with which it is performed, have led many radiologists to abandon it. In centers that specialize in cancer and in many large urban hospitals, lymphography is still performed. If the information provided by lymphography is considered important and if expertise in performing and interpreting lymphograms is unavailable locally, consideration should be given to referring the patient to a center that specializes in this examination.

Unlike conventional radiography, in which x-rays traverse a patient and directly produce a transmission image on film, in CT the images are actually rendered by a computer. The fundamental principle of CT is that an object's structure can be elicited and depicted on the basis of information obtained from sequentially passing x-rays through the object from multiple, different directions. In practice, a narrow slice of anatomy is interrogated with a series of thin, tightly collimated x-ray beams. The transmitted radiation is measured with several sensitive radiation detectors. In contrast to conventional radiography, the detectors in CT do not actually capture or form the image; rather, they tally or record the energy of the transmitted photons. The numerical data are then computer-processed to reconstruct the image.

Plain radiography transcends virtually all other forms of medical imaging in the ability to distinguish two or more closely positioned objects, a property known as *spatial resolution*. CT's spatial resolution is far below that of plain films. However, CT has a remarkable capacity to distinguish the densities of objects, or regions within an object, that differ only minimally in their electron density. This prowess enables CT to graphically depict normal and abnormal anatomy in ways that far exceed the capabilities of plain radiography. Two important attributes of CT, as they relate to oncology, are its ready availability and the fact that clinicians and radiologists have become comfortable with the way in which the information is presented. The reproducibility of the cross-sectional display makes it ideal for measuring lesions and for assessing their response to treatment.

In contrast to other forms of medical imaging, in ultrasound high-frequency sound waves are used to produce images. These waves are created when an electrical field is applied rapidly to a piezoelectric crystal. Such crystals are characterized by their ability to change dimensions, albeit minimally, in response to a change in electrical voltage. The deformation of the crystal and its subsequent return to normal produce sound waves that are directed to, and focused on, segments of a patient's anatomy. These waves travel at speeds determined by the densities and elasticities of the tissues. When sound waves encounter a tissue of different acoustic impedance, a sound wave (echo) is reflected back in the direction of the transducer. These returning echoes are processed by ultrasound computers to generate images. The location of various interfaces, deep within the body, are determined from the length of time it takes for the echoes to return; the longer the time, the farther an interface is from the transducer.

Ultrasound is an appealing examination, in part because it is less expensive than CT or MRI, but also because it is portable, and because it does not use ionizing radiation. Since images are obtained in real time, ultrasound is extremely valuable for guiding biopsies and other interventional procedures, such as drainage. The quality of an ultrasound image, somewhat analogously to the images obtained at GI fluoroscopy, depends very much on the skills of the person who performs the examination. This relative lack of reproducibility, coupled with the vagaries in visualization that occur as a result of changes in the position and amount of bowel gas, make ultrasonography less successful than CT for periodic surveys. Ultrasonography, however, is a very helpful adjunct to other examinations and an exceptional tool for solving specific problems.

Magnetic resonance imaging uses perturbations in the energy states of objects within a strong, externally applied magnetic field to create two- and three-dimensional images that are notable for their clarity and detail. The strength of the magnetic field can vary both within and between the products of different manufacturers, usually between 0.5 and 2.0 tesla (1 tesla is about 10,000 times the strength of the earth's magnetic field, measured at the surface). In CT, image contrast is related to differences in the electron density of tissues. In MRI, however, contrast is determined by differences in the concentration of mobile hydrogen protons. Without embarking on a treatise in physics, the single most important virtue of MRI, compared to CT and other forms of imaging, is its extraordinary contrast resolution.

The examinations that have been discussed above, as excellent as they are, all suffer from one common limitation. The information that they provide is primarily morphologic. While they are generally excellent at delineating both normal and abnormal anatomy, they sporadically fail to resolve clinically important questions. As an example, when a mass is seen, particularly in a patient who has previously been treated, it can be difficult to know whether the mass represents viable tumor or merely the extinct residuum of earlier disease. It is nuclear medicine's unique ability to provide physiologic information that has resulted in its recent resurgence as an oncologic imaging tool.

In nuclear medicine, radioisotopes are used to interrogate the function or biologic activity of a particular organ or a region of the body. Areas of increased activity are produced by tissues that concentrate the administered isotope (e.g., when a lymphoma concentrates gallium 67). Areas of diminished activity occur when a tumor displaces cells that are normally imaged, e.g., when hepatocytes are displaced by liver metastasis on a technetium Tc-99m sulfur colloid liver scan. Photopenic areas can also arise when a biologic activity such as bone repair is impaired. In the past, nuclear medicine examinations were occasionally derided because of their perceived poor image quality. Today, improvements in detection, recording electronics, and imaging processing have greatly improved the clarity of the images and the sensitivity of the examinations.

Of the radionuclide examinations currently employed, bone scanning is the most common. This test is based on the observation that bone metastases tend to elicit the formation of new bone. Consequently, when a bone-seeking agent (e.g., a ^{99m}Tc-phosphonate compound) is administered, the radionuclide is incorporated into hydroxyapatite crystal near the site of metastasis. Regrettably, however, bone scanning cannot distinguish between tumors, arthritis, or the residuum of prior trauma. Because of this, unless the results are viewed as unequivocally positive, i.e., related to a malignancy, consideration should be given to obtaining corroborative plain films. Like all tests, bone scans are not perfect; sometimes they fail to detect metastases. If a patient's pain is severe and if a planar bone scan is normal or equivocal, consideration should be given to further evaluation with a tomographic scan (e.g., CT, MRI, or single photon emission CT).

The most recent addition to nuclear medicine's arsenal is positron emission tomography (PET). In contradistinction to other nuclear medicine examinations that primarily provide semiquantitative physiologic information, PET provides truly quantitative metabolic information. As such, PET has shown remarkable proficiency in tumor detection and in characterizing potentially abnormal areas depicted on other examinations. Of similar significance, PET offers the potential to rapidly assess a tumor's response to therapy. Without question, PET promises to be one of the most powerful and important modalities for cancer imaging.

■ CONCLUSION

Given the high cost of health care and the public's skepticism over whether all of the health care services being purchased are worth their cost, the practice of oncology has come under considerable scrutiny. Because imaging is an important component of the costs associated with treating cancer, these costs and their associated benefits will continue to be carefully analyzed.

With this in mind, it is important to carefully consider whether the information obtained from a given examination is worth the cost, defined in both physical and economic terms. If the information being sought is not likely to alter a patient's stage or treatment, the examination probably should not be performed. A second tenet, only a little less axiomatic than the first, is that a test of limited accuracy probably should not be obtained, even if the prevalence of disease in a given location is high. Third, although the "accuracy" of a test may be high, if the prevalence of disease in the location interrogated is low, the test should probably not be performed. An important caveat concerning the second and third recommendations concerns situations in which the discovery of an abnormality would greatly influence therapy. If the "cost" of missing the presence of disease in a given location is regarded as sufficiently high, the test may still be warranted.

BIBLIOGRAPHY

Begg CB, McNeil BJ. Assessment of radiologic tests: control of bias and other design considerations. *Radiology* 1988;167(2):565–569.

Conti PS, Lilien DL, Hawley K, et al. PET and [18F]-FDG in oncology: a clinical update. *Nucl Med Biol* 1996;23(6):717–735.

Goldenberg DM. Perspectives on oncologic imaging with radiolabeled antibodies. *Cancer* 1997;80(12 Suppl):2431–2435.

Heiken JP, Weyman PJ, Lee JK, et al. Detection of focal hepatic masses: prospective evaluation with CT, delayed CT, CT during arterial portography, and MR imaging. *Radiology* 1989;171(1):47–51.

Kaplan WD. Residual mass and negative gallium scintigraphy in treated lymphoma: when is the gallium scan really negative? [editorial; comment]. *J Nucl Med* 1990;31(3):369–371.

McNeil BJ, Keller E, Adelstein SJ. Primer on certain elements of medical decision making. *N Engl J Med* 1975;293(5):211–215.

Rummeny EJ, Wernecke K, Saini S, et al. Comparison between high-field-strength MR imaging and CT for screening of hepatic metastases: a receiver operating characteristic analysis. *Radiology* 1992;182(3):879–886.

Schiepers C, Hoh CK. Positron emission tomography as a diagnostic tool in oncology. *Eur Radiol* 1998;8(8):1481–1494.

Scott WJ, Shepherd J, Gambhir SS. Cost-effectiveness of FDG-PET for staging non-small cell lung cancer: a decision analysis. *Ann Thorac Surg* 1998;66(6):1876–1883; discussion 83.

Valk PE, Pounds TR, Tesar RD, et al. Cost-effectiveness of PET imaging in clinical oncology. *Nucl Med Biol* 1996;23(6):737–743.

Kelley's Textbook of Internal Medicine, fourth edition. Edited by H. David Humes. Lippincott Williams & Wilkins, Philadelphia © 2000.

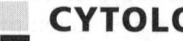

C H A P T E R

249

PATHOLOGY AND CYTOLOGY

VIRGINIA A. LIVOLSI
JOHN E. TOMASZEWSKI

The morphologic examination of tissue is a powerful diagnostic modality. Human disease is highly polymorphic in its biology and clinical characteristics. Imaging at the light microscopic and ultrastructural levels captures data-dense packages of information that are efficient representations of illness in the majority of circumstances. In each image there is an enormous wealth of integrated information. The pictures created in the morphologic examination of tissue are really summary statements as to which genes are present and active and how they are related to one another. For a particular disease process the entire interplay of genetics, biochemistry, and physiology is often retold in microscopic imaging studies, if only the observer is astute enough to deduce the tale!

Because of this robust nature, microscopic imaging can be an efficient and cost-effective means of arriving at a diagnosis. Biopsy early in the course of a patient's workup can significantly accelerate the establishment of a diagnosis and the design of a therapeutic program. Modern biopsy techniques offer the opportunity of obtaining image-based data at the microscopic level with a minimal risk of morbidity. Biopsy material may also be used for antigenic phenotyping, flow cytometry, and molecular

diagnosis. Clinicians should see the biopsy as a powerful tool to be considered early in many diagnostic algorithms and not as a procedure of last resort.

CYTOLOGY

The specialty of cytopathology (the evaluation of cellular changes) has developed over the past 50 years. Sampling for cytology can be viewed in two discrete manners, one as a screening technique and the other as a diagnostic modality.

SCREENING

The origin of cytopathology as a subspecialty of anatomical pathology began in the late 1940s with the work of Dr. Papanicolaou who discovered, while screening vaginal pool aspirates for hormonal abnormalities, cases of dysplastic and malignant cells. Doctor Papanicolaou recognized the possible use of this technique as a screening test for cervical carcinoma. Hence, the "Pap" smear was born. Since then, by the wide application of this screening test, pathologists have been able to define and diagnose preclinical, pre-invasive lesions of both the squamous epithelium and glandular epithelium of the cervix. This has lead to a decrease in the incidence of the mortality from invasive cervical squamous carcinoma.

Other areas in which cytologic screening of high-risk groups have been shown to be of use include screening for urothelial abnormalities in individuals who are exposed to work-related chemicals that are known transitional cell carcinogens. Individuals working in the aniline dye industry are an example. The screening of sputa for pre-clinical and dysplastic bronchial lesions in individuals who are heavy smokers or who have associated with asbestos is another example. However, the cost-effectiveness of these screening programs has not yet been proven.

DIAGNOSTIC CYTOPATHOLOGY

The screening tests described above are noninvasive or minimally invasive procedures. Diagnostic cytopathology usually involves evaluation of specimens obtained by at least minimally invasive procedures. Hence, cytologic evaluation of effusions (pleural, pericardial or peritoneal) can be very useful in diagnosing the spread of carcinomas to these sites. It has been shown by numerous studies that adenocarcinomas are much more commonly identified in fluids than are squamous cell carcinomas. When one assesses the likelihood of a primary site based on the cytologic findings, the following "clinical pearl" is of use regarding adenocarcinoma:

In pleural fluid in a woman, the primary site is usually breast.

In peritoneal fluid in a woman, the primary site is usually ovary.

In pleural fluid in a man, the primary site is usually lung.

In pericardial fluid, the primary sites are: lung in a man, and breast in a woman.

In addition to effusion cytology, assessment of endoscopically obtained samples, such as from the bronchus (bronchial wash-

TABLE 249.1.	UTILITY OF FINE-NEEDLE ASPIRATION

Site	Specificity (%)
Thyroid	90
Breast	77–99
Lymph nodes	
Metastases	90–96
Lymphoma	80
Salivary glands	96–98
Kidney	89
Liver, pancreas	61–91

ings and bronchial brushings), gastrointestinal tract (esophageal and gastric brushings), and other sites, has proven useful. If one uses biopsy techniques, the sampling from these various endoscopically available sites is relatively limited, whereas if one uses washings and brushings, one can obtain cells from a broader area allowing for a greater chance of obtaining diagnostic material.

The statistics of success rates in the evaluation of such specimens obtained by minimally invasive procedures are excellent with specificities of 95% to 97%. During evaluation of effusions, the chance of a diagnostic sampling obviously increases when there is a history of a known carcinoma in the patient; the diagnostic accuracy increases in endoscopically obtained samples when an endoscopically visible lesion is present.

FINE-NEEDLE ASPIRATION CYTOLOGY

In the past 10 to 15 years, the technique of fine-needle aspiration (FNA) cytology has been utilized in virtually every organ. This involves placing a small-bore needle, usually 23 to 25 gauge, into a clinically visible, palpable, or radiologically accessible lesion and obtaining a small aspirate sample. In the latter case, direct visualization under ultrasonographic or computed tomographic guidance can be most helpful in actually obtaining an adequate and diagnostic sample.

The successes with FNA cytology have been most notable in the thyroid gland, the breast, and superficial nodules including lymph nodes (in the latter instance especially for the diagnosis of metastatic carcinoma). For deep-seated lesions, especially those evaluated and sampled under radiologic control, the diagnostic sensitivity is about 90% (Table 249.1). A variety of special techniques can be applied to these samples including immunohistochemistry, in situ hybridization, special stains, flow cytometry, and molecular diagnosis methods.

When the FNA sample contains adequate material, a histologic preparation of residual material not used for smears can be obtained. This is known as a *cell block*. This is a histologic preparation of tissue fragments and can be a diagnostic supplement to the smeared aspiration slides.

■ BIOPSY

Biopsy pathology, as opposed to cytopathology, involves the evaluation of tissue. The advantage of biopsy sampling over cyto-

logic examination is that the pathologist can identify structures, as well as the relationships between cells and between cells and stroma. This is extremely useful in making diagnoses, especially in the realm of oncologic specimens. In certain areas, biopsy samples have replaced cytology sampling and FNA. These include prostatic biopsies with the utilization of the small biopsy needle, leading to histologic preparations and breast core biopsies (especially under stereotactic radiologic control).

Biopsies may be excisional or incisional. The latter is more commonly encountered in the modern surgical pathology practice. The biopsy should be handled properly with all pieces of the biopsy sent to the pathology laboratory for analysis. Care should be taken especially in endoscopically obtained samples not to crush the tissue since this can interfere with diagnostic interpretation. The tissue should be placed in fixative immediately because drying artifact will also hamper correct interpretation.

Another problem with biopsies involves sampling error. Since the biopsy surveys an area that is less broad than the endoscopic brush technique, the possibility of false-negative results due to sampling error must be recognized. One must be careful in evaluating specimens that are excessively inflamed or contain extensive areas of necrosis. In very large lesions, biopsies may encounter only the superficial aspects of the lesion and therefore may not be representative. For example, a superficial biopsy of an ulcerated gastric mass may show only granulation tissue and necrotic debris, whereas the neoplasm is present beneath the ulcer.

It is important to recognize that the biopsy of a visualized lesion is usually more productive than a random biopsy of an organ in which no lesion is identified. Biopsies obtained under direct visualization such as endoscopic procedures have excellent diagnostic yields (greater than 95%).

■ FROZEN SECTION

The utilization of frozen sections as an intraoperative technique for diagnosis has declined over the past decade for several reasons. Many patients now have preoperative testing, biopsies under endoscopic control, FNA cytology sampling, and so forth, at which time the diagnosis is made and surgery is the definitive procedure.

Frozen section should be utilized for three purposes only: (a) to define the nature of the pathologic process (often this has already been done preoperatively); (b) to determine adequacy of margins of resection; and (c) to ascertain if appropriate and sufficient diagnostic tissue has been obtained. Hence, frozen section should be performed only to guide the surgeon in the immediately subsequent surgical procedure being performed on the patient. In many institutions, intraoperative cytology is used to offer a diagnosis using a minimal amount of the lesion and avoiding compromise of the sample.

As lesions are detected by more effective radiologic techniques, they are identified when very small and therefore not clinically palpable. Frozen sections are inappropriate on such samples. This has become a problem most recently in breast biopsies that are directed by mammographic abnormalities without palpable lesions. Often there is no gross lesion and many of the lesions that are malignant are in situ, noninvasive cancers. It is inappropriate to ask for frozen sections on these lesions because with the availability of techniques to perform flow cytometric ploidy analysis and immunohistochemistry for steroid receptor and oncogenes on paraffin-embedded material, the most important function that a pathologist can serve in these cases is to ensure adequate material for diagnosis. Frozen section, by the nature of the technique, wastes precious diagnostic material. This can impede diagnostic accuracy and may so distort the tissue as to make definitive diagnosis impossible.

The technique of frozen section in experienced hands can be diagnostically accurate. Depending on the organ or system sampled, accuracy rates of 99% should be expected. False-positive results are very unusual. In some organs, however (e.g., thyroid, lymph nodes, spleen for lymphoproliferative diseases), a high deferral rate should be expected.

GROSS EXAMINATION OF TISSUE

The gross examination of tissue is a simple and cost-effective way to obtain important data. Resected specimens are best examined in the fresh state after rapid transport from the operating rooms to the anatomical pathology laboratories. In our institution, a pneumatic tube device is used to facilitate this delivery. Specimen orientation is critical so that a tumor's relationship to the margins of resection or other vital structures can be determined. Orientation can be communicated by marker sutures or direct consultation between the surgeon and the pathologist. The latter method is preferable since areas of particular concern can be immediately chosen for sampling. Multicolored inks can be used by the pathology staff to maintain orientation and allow microscopic visualization of the margins throughout the entire sectioning and embedding process.

Standardized approaches to gross description are fast becoming the norm in anatomical pathology. The most progressive labs embed gross description templates into their laboratory information systems. Tumor size, shape, color, texture, scarring pattern, anatomical location, and relationship to margins are all generic features that should be mentioned with each neoplasm.

TISSUE PREPARATION

The way in which tissue is prepared determines which types of tests can be performed on the sample. Certain methodologies are better suited for the evaluation of selected tissue types and require special handling. If the clinician is uncertain as to the best method of tissue handling, a prebiopsy consultation with the pathologist is encouraged. Following are discussed several preparative methods and their utility.

10% NEUTRAL BUFFERED FORMALIN FIXATION

Immediate fixation in 10% formalin is the standard protocol for the majority of tissues in most labs. Neutral buffered formalin (NBF) penetrates tissue slowly. Small biopsies may fix in a few hours, whereas large specimens with a high lipid content may take days for adequate penetration and thorough fixation. Partially fixed tissue will not process adequately and this can jeopardize a diagnosis. A 20:1 ratio of fixative to specimen volume is recommended. Immunohistochemistry, in situ hybridization, flow cytometry, and molecular diagnosis can all be performed on NBF-fixed tissue, although the sensitivity of these studies may be affected by time of fixation.

BOUIN'S FIXATIVE

Bouin's fixative is a combination of formalin, acetic acid, and picric acid that imparts a yellow color. Bouin's has the advantage of penetrating tissue relatively rapidly. It is an excellent nuclear fixative, and for this reason it is well suited for small biopsies where nuclear detail may be critical. Immunohistochemistry works well in Bouin's-fixed tissue. Nucleic acids are more rapidly degraded and molecular diagnosis in situ hybridization is problematic. Bouin's is contraindicated for flow cytometry.

MERCURY-BASED FIXATIVES

Fixatives containing heavy metals such as mercury may also produce superior nuclear cytology. This is particularly advantageous in certain material such as hematopoietic tissue. Zenker's fixative and Helly's fluid are examples of mercury-based fixatives. Hazardous waste disposal issues may limit the use of these fixatives.

NON–CROSS-LINKING AND WEAKLY CROSS-LINKING FIXATIVES

Alcohols and proprietary fixatives such as Omnifix or Histochoice are non–cross-linking, whereas paraformaldehyde is a weakly cross-linking fixative. Non–cross-linking fixatives denature by precipitation. Antigens and nucleic acids in tissue section are more easily recognized by antibodies and probes, and most immunohistochemical and in situ hybridization studies can be performed with these fixatives. The disadvantage is the poorer morphologic preservation.

DECALCIFICATION

Decalcification is best performed using a strong acid such as nitric or sulfuric acid. Decalcification of small biopsy specimens can be accomplished in 24 hours. Larger specimens or specimens with very dense bone may take several days. Residual acid must be neutralized after decalcification and before processing to allow nuclear visualization with basophilic dyes. Nucleic acids are fragmented by decalcification, making in situ hybridization and flow cytometry problematic. Tissue antigens are variable in their resistance to acid fixation.

FRESH TISSUE

Fresh tissue is the most flexible form with which to conduct analysis. It can be divided in the pathology laboratory to provide specimens that are optimally preserved for a variety of studies. Certain studies, such as cryostat sections for intraoperative consultation or classic karyotypic analysis, can only be performed on fresh tissue. The interval between harvest and processing is critical. Certain labile antigens may degrade within minutes. Morphologic preservation varies depending on the tissue type. Rapid delivery to the laboratory for immediate processing is recommended.

TISSUE PROCESSING, EMBEDDING, AND SECTIONING

Fixed tissue must be cleared with a series of organic solvents, impregnated with paraffin, embedded in a wax block, sectioned on a rotary microtome, and stained before slides are available for review. Even with discrete-mode processing this procedure takes a minimum of 6 hours. Cost-efficient labs must utilize batch processing with next-day turnaround.

ANCILLARY TESTS

SPECIAL HISTOCHEMISTRY

These tests represent the classic "special stains." Various dyes and reagents will bind to cell and matrix components in a differential manner. The advantages of these tests are that there is a large body of knowledge as to their operating characteristics, most labs are conversant with the methodologies, and many tests can be done in a rapid fashion. Enzyme histochemistry tests tissues for the presence of endogenous enzymes by providing the appropriate substrates coupled to a visual reporter system. Table 249.2 is a small partial listing of biologic components that can be highlighted with special histochemistry tests.

IMMUNOHISTOCHEMISTRY

Immunohistochemistry has been used heavily in the practice of diagnostic pathology for the past dozen years. Testing relies on the binding of preserved antigenic epitopes to an antibody reagent and the visualization of this reaction by some reporter signal that allows localization to a tissue substructure. Antibodies may be either polyclonal or monoclonal. Monoclonal antibodies offer the advantage of reproducibility; however, their sensitivity may be limited by the narrowness of their antigen target. Polyclonal antibodies see a broader range of specificities and in general are more sensitive. The problem of reagent standardization for polyclonal antibodies has been addressed with the newer methods of peptide immunization.

The original immunohistochemical methodologies employed antibodies directly labeled with fluorochromes. This "immunofluorescence" technique has been used to great advantage in nephropathology to stratify the glomerulonephritides. The disadvantage of direct immunofluorescence is the relatively poor sensitivity of the method and thus the requirement for large amounts of target before useful visualization. Over the years a

TABLE 249.2.	COMMON HISTOCHEMICAL TESTS
Basement membranes	Silver stains, PAS
Cell wall	PAS, Gram, silver stains
Collagen	Trichrome
Amyloid	Congo red, crystal violet
Mucins	Mucicarmine, PAS, Alcian blue
Myeloid granules	Giemsa
Lipids	Oil red O, Sudan black

PAS, periodic acid–Schiff.

number of multistep procedures have been linked with histochemical amplification systems to markedly enhance the sensitivity of immunohistochemistry. Current methodologies often employ variations of the avidin–biotin complex technique of Hsu wherein the primary antibody is reacted with a biotin-conjugated secondary antibody and then the signal is amplified using enzyme-linked avidin–biotin complexes. The sensitivity of modern multilayer techniques exceeds that of direct immunofluorescence by several logs.

Since differential diagnostic questions are most often raised after review of the standard light microscopic sections, formalin-fixed, paraffin-embedded tissue is often the starting point for any special studies. Immunohistochemistry has been hampered by the limited availability of antibody reagents that see formalin-resistant epitopes. An alternative approach has been to "unmask" antigens that are hidden by the cross-linking process. "Antigen retrieval" refers to the use of enzymes, microwave irradiation, or steam heat to break some of the steric hindrance that prevents antigen–antibody recognition in tissue section. The diagnostic effect of antigen retrieval methods has been to improve the sensitivity of immunohistochemical testing.

IN SITU HYBRIDIZATION

Nucleic acid probes may be applied to tissue sections for the localization of either genomic elements or transcripts. In situ hybridization offers the opportunity for the pathologist to (a) distinguish antigen uptake from cellular production by the simultaneous localization of transcripts and antigen in the same cell; (b) identify infectious genomic elements; and (c) perform interphase cytogenetics on tissue. The first and second uses are established in the literature and their application is rapidly expanding in many diagnostic labs. To date, interphase cytogenetics on smears or tissue section has mostly been confined to the analysis of microsatellite distribution and the evaluation of chromosomal deletions, translocations, or amplifications. The sensitivity of in situ hybridization as performed in our diagnostic labs is about ten copies. Point mutations cannot be seen with this method. New amplification techniques such as in situ polymerase chain reaction may allow the tissue localization of known mutations as this technology matures.

TABLE 249.3.	TISSUE MARKERS IN IMMUNOHISTOCHEMISTRY AND/ OR IN SITU HYBRIDIZATION

Marker	Utility
Prognostic	
Estrogen receptor protein	Certain
Progesterone receptor protein	Certain
Oncogenes (*Ras, Neu, Myc,* etc.)	Investigational
Tumor suppressor genes (*p53, WT1, Rh*)	Investigational
Proliferation markers (PCNA, Ki-67, Cyclins)	Investigational
Histogenetic Assignment	
Prostatic (PSA)	Certain
Thyroid (Thyroglobulin)	Certain
Hematopoeitic markers (LCA, T-cell, B-cell, myeloid)	Certain
Epithelial differentiation (cytokeratins, EMA)	Certain
Neural and Melanocytic (S-100, HMB45)	Certain
Vascular endothelium (Factor VIII, CD31)	Certain
Muscle differentiation (Desmin, HHF35, myoglobin)	Certain
Neuroendocrine differentiation (chromogranin, neuron-specific enolase, cell-specific hormones)	Certain
Infectious Agents	
Hepatitis B, Herpes, EBV, HPV chlamydia, and many others	Certain

PCNA, proliferative cell nuclear antigen; PSA, prostate-specific antigen; LCA, leukocyte common antigen; EMA, epithelial membrane antigen.
HMB45, melanoma marker; HHF35, muscle action marker.

UTILITY OF IMMUNOHISTOCHEMISTRY AND IN SITU HYBRIDIZATION

Immunohistochemical analysis may be used in tumors for the assignment of histogenetic origin, as a prognostic marker, or in the identification of infectious elements. Table 249.3 lists some of the tests which can be performed in each of these three categories. The exact classification of poorly differentiated tumors can be quite difficult based only on standard light microscopic examination. Since the determination of histogenetic origin may significantly impact on therapy, employing immunohistochemistry can be very helpful. Table 249.4 shows a short panel of five antibodies that can help in the separation of poorly differentiated carcinoma, sarcoma, high-grade lymphoma, and melanoma.

FLOW CYTOMETRY

Flow cytometry can be used either as a tool for ploidy analysis or as a method for immunophenotyping. In the former instance, nuclei are stained with a fluorochrome (propridium iodide or acridine orange) that stoichiometrically binds to nucleic acid and provides a quantitative measure of DNA content. Aneuploid populations can be identified and S phase calculated. The DNA Consensus Conference has reviewed the literature on the clinical utility of flow cytometry in several settings. The Conference recommends ploidy analysis as a significant prognostic feature in transitional cell carcinoma of the bladder, with less defined roles for breast and prostate cancer. S-phase analysis is recommended as a prognostic variable in breast cancer and non-Hodgkin's lymphoma.

MOLECULAR DIAGNOSIS

The reader is referred to Dr. Sklar's excellent chapter on molecular diagnosis in oncology (Chapter 251). Expert selection of the target tissue is critical for obtaining informative results. Fresh tissue that is to be used for molecular diagnosis should be collected rapidly, snap-frozen in liquid nitrogen, and a scout frozen section of the block performed. Areas of tumor should be subdivided as directed by the pathologist's review of the frozen section. Microdissection techniques can be performed if finer discrimination of the target is required. RNAase protection should be used if Northern analysis or reverse transcriptase polymerase chain reaction is considered, although we have not found RNAase protection necessary for in situ hybridization in paraffin-embedded tissue.

BIBLIOGRAPHY

Bibbo M, ed. *Comprehensive cytopathology,* second ed. Philadelphia: WB Saunders, 1997.
Elias JM. *Immunohistochemistry: a practical approach to diagnosis.* Chicago: ASCP Press, 1990.

TABLE 249.4.	IMMUNOHISTOCHEMISTRY IN THE EVALUATION OF ANAPLASTIC TUMORS

Antibody	Carcinoma	Lymphoma	Sarcoma	Melanoma
LCA (CD45)	—	+	—	—
Cytokeratin	+	—	—	—
EMA	+	—	—	—
S-100	+/−	—	—	+
HMB45	—	—	—	+

LCA, leukocyte common antigen; EMA, epithelial membrane antigen; HMB45, melanoma marker.

Fechner R. Practice parameter: frozen section and the mammographically detected breast lesion. *Am J Clin Pathol* 1995;103:6–7.

Gown A, de Weber N, Battifora H. Microwave-based antigenic unmasking. A revolutionary new technique for routine immunohistochemistry. *Appl Immunohistochem* 1993;1:256–266.

Hedley DW, Shankey TV, Wheeless LL. DNA cytometry consensus conference. *Cytometry* 1993;14:471–500.

Hsu SM, Raine L, Fanger H. Use of avidin–biotin peroxidase complex (ABC) in immunoperoxidase techniques: a comparison of ABC and unlabeled antibody (PAP) procedure. *J Histochem Cytogenet* 1981;29:577.

Hutchinson ML, Cassin C, Ball HI. The efficacy of an automated preparation device for cervical cytology. *Am J Clin Pathol* 1991;96:300–305.

Rosai J. *Ackerman's surgical pathology.* St. Louis: CV Mosby, 1996.

Silverberg SG. ADASP recommendations on tumor reporting. *Pathol Case Rev* 1998;3:215–270.

Spicer SS. *Histochemistry in pathologic diagnosis.* New York: Marcel Dekker, 1987.

Kelley's Textbook of Internal Medicine, fourth edition. Edited by H. David Humes. Lippincott Williams & Wilkins, Philadelphia © 2000.

CHAPTER 250

TUMOR MARKERS

DANIEL F. HAYES

Tumor markers provide an indication of the risk, presence, status, or future behavior of malignancy; they are genetic or biochemical changes that can be identified in association with one of these states. Detection or monitoring of these changes is useful in several clinical situations (Table 250.1): to identify otherwise healthy persons who are predisposed to develop cancer (i.e., are at higher risk than persons without the marker), to detect cancer at a very early stage, to determine a differential diagnosis, to predict the future behavior of an established malignancy, to monitor a patient who is free of clinically detectable disease for signs of early relapse, and to follow a patient with widespread disease to determine the effects of therapy.

Tumor markers can be detected using various assay technologies. Two fields of technological progress have revolutionized the ability to detect biochemical and genetic molecular changes. The development of tumor immunology—in particular, the emergence of hybridoma/monoclonal antibody technology—has permitted the detection of specific tumor-associated antigens and the capacity to map individual epitopic sites present on distinct molecular structures. The second advance is the ability to identify specific genetic changes at the DNA or RNA level, or both. Indeed, before the 1980s tumor markers were limited to visual observations of histopathology and crude assays using polyclonal antisera. With the development of these technologies, there are examples of clinically useful markers in nearly all, if not all, of the clinical categories listed above.

Identifiable genetic or biochemical changes that represent markers of malignancy may be detected in various tissues. In this regard, germ line genetic markers in all cells of the body might predict an inherited susceptibility to the development of cancer. Markers of early malignant transformation, tumor burden, or tumor biology might be assayed within the target organ tissue itself, either through biopsy or needle aspirate, or by collection of excreted/secreted contents, either directly (in aspirates, urine, stool, sputum, effusions) or indirectly (circulating in blood, serum, or plasma).

Circulating tumor markers are of particular interest because blood, plasma, and serum can be so easily obtained for assay with only minor inconvenience and cost to the patient. Circulating tumor markers have been most widely applied with respect to carcinomas (in contrast to malignancies of hematologic or mesenchymal origin). Examples of these markers include carcinoembryonic antigen (CEA), prostate-specific antigen (PSA), α-fetoprotein (AFP), and beta human chorionic gonadotropin (βhCG). A series of newer markers identified using monoclonal antibody–based assays include CA 125, CA 15-3, CA 549, CA 27.29, CA 19-9, and squamous cell antigen (SCA). Although each of these was originally purported to be associated with a specific malignancy, subsequent studies have usually demonstrated that elevated levels can be detected in patients with carcinomas originating from other sites.

Appropriate use of tumor markers requires an understanding of the biology underlying the premise that the marker might be useful and of the technology used for the assay. For example, several different monoclonal antibodies might be used to assay a single molecular structure, such as an oncogene product. These might detect different epitopes that might be differentially expressed on the oncogene under different circumstances, and they might have varying affinities and avidities for that epitope. Furthermore, distinct changes in the expression of the oncogene might be related to various alterations, such as mutations, deletions, or amplifications of the gene, or over- or underexpression of the product. Therefore, seemingly similar assays for the same marker, such as an assay for "HER-2/neu," might result in very different correlations with clinical outcome. Moreover, simply identifying a possible future outcome does not imply clinical utility. Therefore, clinicians should not automatically alter therapeutic decisions based on marker data if it has not been proven that such a change results in a more favorable clinical outcome, such as cure, improved survival, or enhanced quality of life. For example, a marker may reliably predict a poorer prognosis and therefore the clinician may be inclined to treat the patient more aggressively. However, if the application of more aggressive therapy is not beneficial, the patient may actually suffer from inappropriate interpretation of the marker results.

TABLE 250.1. POTENTIAL UTILITIES OF TUMOR MARKERS

Determine risk
Screen for early diagnosis
Determine differential diagnosis
Predict prognosis or response to therapy
Detect early relapse
Monitor course of metastatic disease

Finally, marker results may duplicate information already known. The clinician may not need or want marker results if they will repeat the information already ascertained by an equally reliable but less expensive or more easily performed test, such as the history and physical examination.

In summary, tumor markers are valuable only if they provide information that cannot be obtained by other means, or if they are either less expensive (in terms of financial or morbidity factors) or more reliable than other sources of information. The clinician must take into account the available biologic, technological, and clinical data to use tumor markers wisely.

DETERMINATION OF RISK AND SCREENING

DETERMINATION OF SUSCEPTIBILITY TO CANCER

Identifying patients who are at a higher risk to develop cancer might permit more efficient application of prevention or screening strategies, if they exist. Recently, several candidate "cancer" genes have been identified and cloned. In their normal state, these "tumor suppressor" genes appear to be responsible for maintaining the nonmalignant state. If a person inherits one abnormal copy of one of these genes (a germ line mutation), he or she is at an extraordinarily high risk of developing one or more malignancies in his or her lifetime. Although the abnormal gene is carried in every cell in the person's body (and can therefore be identified in DNA that is easily obtained from circulating white blood cells or scraped buccal smears), most of these genes appear to be associated with malignancies of specific organ types. These scientific discoveries are very exciting. However, screening of the normal population for genetic susceptibility to cancer is fraught with ethical, social, economic, cultural, and medical problems that have not been resolved. At present, routine screening for genetic susceptibility is recommended only in the context of a well-designed genetic counseling program. The patient can then obtain the pros and cons of being tested as well as appropriate support and advice once the results are available.

SCREENING FOR EARLY MALIGNANCY

Screening for signs of malignancy might provide an opportunity for early treatment. Indeed, screening and early treatment reduce the mortality rate for several malignancies, including breast, colon, cervical, and perhaps prostate carcinomas. Genetic or biochemical markers of early malignancy might be an inexpensive, low-risk means of monitoring for early malignant changes.

Monitoring circulating tumor markers (those found in serum or plasma) is a particularly convenient and appealing method of screening. Unfortunately, no currently available circulating marker has been proven to be sufficiently sensitive or tumor-specific for this application. PSA has received the widest publicity because in men it is almost absolutely tissue-specific, and rising levels are reasonably predictive for the presence of a histologically identifiable prostate carcinoma (see Chapter 207). However, PSA levels are also elevated at low levels in men with

benign prostatic hypertrophy. Furthermore, considerable controversy exists regarding whether early diagnosis and treatment of prostate cancer universally improves survival. Some patients may have only "occult" cancer that never becomes clinically relevant, and others may already have incurable, advanced disease by the time PSA levels are high enough to warrant further evaluation. Randomized trials are ongoing to determine whether circulating PSA levels, alone or in combination with other diagnostic tests, offer an advantage over currently used clinical methods.

New markers may become available for screening blood or urine and or sputum for the presence of early malignancies, especially of the uroepithelial and/or aerodigestive tracts. Acceptance of such markers requires demonstration of survival benefit in large-scale, well-designed, prospective trials with long follow-up to avoid the pitfalls of lead and length time biases.

DIFFERENTIAL DIAGNOSIS

Tumor markers would be of great value in helping to distinguish benign from malignant tumor symptoms, clinical findings, or radiographic changes. In patients with established tumors of unknown origin, tissue immunophenotyping may be helpful in distinguishing epithelial from hematopoietic or mesenchymal malignancies (Table 250.2). Highly specific and sensitive markers are available that distinguish hematopoietic malignancies from other neoplasms. Furthermore, markers of myeloid, T-cell, and B-cell origin allow classification into separate categories of hematopoietic malignancies and should be performed routinely on tissue or circulating neoplastic cells from patients with lymphomas and leukemias. The Philadelphia chromosome (t9;22) is nearly pathognomonic for chronic myelogenous leukemia. Certain markers of epithelial or mesenchymal origin, such as cytokeratins, epithelial membrane antigen (EMA), and S-100, can be helpful in separating carcinomas from sarcomas. Germ cell neoplasms, if not identifiable by routine histopathology, can occasionally be diagnosed on the basis of immunoperoxidase staining for AFP or βhCG. Likewise, staining for AFP may also be helpful in confirming the diagnosis of hepatocellular carcinoma.

Unfortunately, few other markers separate the common epithelial carcinomas from one another. Estrogen and progesterone receptor (ER, PgR) content is principally associated with breast cancer and should be assayed in all newly diagnosed breast cancers (see below). However, ER and PgR have been identified in many other malignancies, including lung, uterine, and ovarian carcinomas and in melanomas. CEA, keratin, and mucin (epithelial mucin antigen, CA 125, and others) expression is commonly observed in most types of epithelial malignancy and cannot be used to determine the tissue of origin.

Circulating tumor markers are only occasionally helpful in differential diagnosis. Elevated AFP or βhCG levels are nearly pathognomonic for germ cell malignancy in male patients who have a testicular mass or other evidence of germ cell cancers. However, AFP may also be elevated in hepatocellular carcinoma, and βhCG is occasionally elevated in gastric and other malignancies. These markers may also be of value in female patients with

TABLE 250.2.	POTENTIAL MARKERS TO DETERMINE DIFFERENTIAL DIAGNOSIS	
Differential	**Candidate Marker**	**Utility**[a]
Cancer vs. Benign	P53, ras, HER-2, other	±
Epithelial	EMA, cytokeratins	+ +
Sarcoma	Vimentin, desmin, smooth-muscle actin, S-100, neurofilament markers	+ + +
Melanoma	Melanin, HMB45, S-100	+ + +
Hematologic	LCA T, B, and myeloid antigens	+ + +
	T-cell receptor and other gene rearrangements	
CML	Philadelphia chromosome	+ + +
Germ cell	AFP, βhCG	+ + +
Breast	ER, PgR	+ +
	GCDP	+ +
	Mucin-like (DF3, HMFG)	−
Colon	CEA	−
Lung	SCA	−
Ovarian	CA 125	+/−
Prostate	PSA	+ + +
Thyroid	Thyroglobulin	+ + +

[a] + + +, Marker can be used independently to make clinical decisions; + +, Marker is helpful, adds to other clinical information to make clinical decision; +, Data are available suggesting possible clinical utility, but still investigational; ±, Preliminary data promising, but highly investigational; −, Marker results of no clinical utility.
EMA, epithelial membrane antigen; HMB, human melanoma; LCA, leukocyte common antigen; CML, chronic myelogenous leukemia; SCA, squamous cell antigen; AFP, α-fetoprotein; βhCG, β–human chorionic gonadotropin; ER, estrogen receptor; PgR, progesterone receptor; GCDP, gross cystic disease protein; HMFG, human milk fat globule; CEA, carcinoembryonic antigen; CA 125, cancer antigen 125; PSA, prostate-specific antigen.

germ cell malignancies, although such markers are less specific due to reproductive considerations.

As noted, circulating CEA, CA 125, and mucin markers, such as CA 15-3 and CA 27.29, do not reliably distinguish one type of epithelial cancer from another. Of course, an "M spike" detected by serum protein electrophoresis is highly suggestive of multiple myeloma.

PROGNOSIS

DETERMINATION OF PROGNOSIS IN PATIENTS WITH NEWLY DIAGNOSED CANCER

After the general diagnosis for a patient has been established, tumor markers can be used to place the patient into a subcategory based on the expected outcome. It is helpful to divide these types of factors into two groups. The first category, prognostic factors, contains factors associated with natural malignant features, such as invasive, metastatic, and growth potentials. The second category, predictive factors, includes factors that foretell

that a given tumor is likely to respond to a specific type of therapy. Prognostic factors can be used to determine whether a patient is likely to do well with no or minimal therapy, or whether the patient is very likely to suffer from the effects of the malignancy over time. Such patients might be candidates for subsequent therapy, if such therapy is known to be beneficial. If therapy is indicated, predictive factors can be used to select the most appropriate regimen. These categories may be related; indeed, one factor may fall into both. For example, high ER levels in primary breast cancer tissue are associated with more slowly growing tumors and better outcomes for untreated patients, but they are also highly predictive of potential benefit from adjuvant endocrine treatment.

Prognostic and predictive factors have the potential to be very helpful in the evaluation and treatment of patients with solid malignancies. This is particularly true in such malignancies as breast and colorectal cancers, in which adjuvant systemic therapy is known to be beneficial. Specific molecules that have been intensively studied in solid tumors include the oncogenes *p53*, *her-2*/c-*neu*, c-*myc*, and c-*ras*. Abnormalities in each of these (mutations, deletions, amplification, over- or underexpression) have been reported to be associated with a worse prognosis in breast, colon, lung, ovarian, bladder, prostate, cervical, and other carcinomas, as well as several types of sarcomas (see Chapter 251). Biologic behavior may also be predicted by measuring specific processes, such as enzyme activity potentially related to invasion and metastasis, and angiogenic activity. However, none of these has been adopted for routine evaluation and care for any solid malignancy.

Few markers truly predict response to specific therapies. Perhaps the best example of a clinically useful predictive factor is the correlation of the ER content of a primary breast cancer with the odds of responding to hormone therapy, in either the metastatic or the adjuvant setting. Patients with ER-rich tumors are very likely to benefit from hormone therapies such as tamoxifen, but those with ER-negative tumors are very unlikely to benefit from endocrine manipulation and are better treated with chemotherapy.

Few if any circulating markers are of prognostic or predictive value, independently of stage, because levels usually reflect tumor burden and not necessarily biology. In lymphomas, pretreatment lactate dehydrogenase (LDH) levels are associated with a worse prognosis, but in general treatment planning is not based on LDH alone. In patients with a history of germ cell malignancies, postoperative βhCG or AFP levels should be determined after a sufficiently long period to account for the clearance of preoperative marker from the circulation (10 to 14 postoperative days). Elevated levels beyond these times are absolute indications to begin systemic treatment. Pre- and postoperative levels of PSA, CA 125, and CEA may provide some prognostic information for prostate, ovarian, and colon cancer, but a decision to treat a patient with an elevated marker in the absence of other findings is controversial for all of these diseases.

DETECTION OF MICROMETASTASIS/MINIMAL RESIDUAL DISEASE

Patients with leukemia and lymphoma almost always have systemic disease at the time of diagnosis. Therefore, they are usually treated with systemic therapy to induce remission. Once these patients are free of clinically detectable disease (history, physical examination, radiographic evaluation), residual clones of malignant cells can be detected in the bone marrow by polymerase chain reaction (PCR) assays that detect genetic changes such as translocations or mutations specific to the malignancy (see Chapter 251). Patients who harbor these clones may have a significantly worse outcome than those who have been rendered completely disease-free. Patients with such findings might be candidates for more aggressive or alternative treatment approaches, but these findings are not absolute. For example, t(8; 21) translocations have been detected in bone marrow from patients who are otherwise free of any evidence of recurrent leukemia for as long as 14 years after treatment.

Most patients with newly diagnosed solid tumors present without evidence of distant disease and can be rendered disease-free by local treatment (surgical excision, radiation therapy). Carcinoma tissue–associated prognostic markers may be used to estimate the presence of distant micrometastatic disease. Indeed, as discussed previously, histopathologic identification of regional lymph node metastasis is essentially an in vivo assay for tumor metastatic potential. Other ways of detecting occult metastasis in regional lymph nodes could indicate a long-term risk of recurrence in patients who have histopathologically negative lymph nodes. However, it is unclear that the long-term prognosis of patients with occult regional lymph node metastases, detectable only by immunologic or genetic assays, is substantially different from that of patients who do not have such detectable lymph node metastases.

In addition to the evaluation of regional lymph nodes, immunocytochemical staining for tumor-associated antigens can demonstrate whether micrometastases are present in distant organs as well. Up to 25% of patients with stage I and II breast cancer have bone marrow metastases at the time of their primary surgery. Similarly, for patients who receive high-dose chemotherapy and subsequent autologous hematopoietic progenitor cell support (bone marrow or peripheral progenitor cells), these techniques may be used to identify microscopic contamination by tumor cells. In small studies with short follow-up, occult bone marrow micrometastases have been associated with a significantly worse disease-free and overall survival. Other investigators have urged caution regarding these methods, as the specificity of these assays is not absolute and the treatment implications are uncertain.

■ EVALUATION AND MONITORING FOR RECURRENT DISEASE

MONITORING PATIENTS WHO ARE FREE OF DETECTABLE DISEASE FOR EARLY RELAPSE

Patients with a history of invasive cancers are at risk for relapse for variable time periods after initial therapy. Therefore, patients with a history of malignancy might be screened for impending relapse throughout their course. Such screening would require time-dependent marker changes, as opposed to static marker changes such as those measured in primary tissue. For patients with a history of leukemia, serial bone marrow evaluations are easily performed, which are reasonably reliable predictors of recurrence. However, with routine histopathology, leukemic cells can be detected only at a sensitivity of 1 per 20 normal cells. Using even more sensitive techniques, the detection limit may only be as high as 1 per 50 for cytogenetics and 1 per 100,000 for PCR assays. When these relatively poor sensitivities are coupled with the ambiguity over the clinical significance of such findings, the value of routine serial bone marrow monitoring over a prolonged time is limited.

For solid malignancies (including lymphomas, sarcomas, and carcinomas), soluble/circulating tumor markers found in serum (or plasma) and urine would be ideal for such monitoring. The best example of this strategy is the use of serial βhCG and AFP to detect impending relapse in men with a history of germ cell malignancy. Rising marker levels after treatment (surgery or chemotherapy) in these patients are an absolute indication to begin "salvage" chemotherapy, which can be curative. Several circulating tumor markers associated with epithelial cancers, such as CEA (colon and other gastrointestinal, lung, breast, and ovarian cancers), CA 125 (ovarian cancer), PSA (prostate cancer), CA 15-3, CA 27.29, CA 549, breast cancer mucin, mammary serum antigen, and mucinous carcinoma antigen (breast cancer), and AFP (hepatocellular carcinoma), may permit detection of occult recurrence. However, these markers usually provide lead times of only a few months before the metastases would have been made evident by symptoms. As for any screening test, the positive and negative predictive values (i.e., that a positive test accurately predicts subsequent relapse and that a negative test reliably predicts that the patient will remain disease-free) depend on the likelihood of relapse in the first place and the sensitivity and specificity of the test (which require careful delineation of cutoff levels).

Detecting impending relapse may not be associated with any clinical benefit. In many malignancies, the treatment of asymptomatic metastases with potentially toxic systemic therapy has not been demonstrated to result in either increased cure or survival rate, and treatment of patients with asymptomatic metastasis is unlikely to provide improved palliation. However, for certain types of leukemias and lymphomas, detection of early relapse might provide an increased opportunity to establish higher cure rates through the use of high-dose chemotherapy and bone marrow transplantation. The advantage of early detection of recurrence for germ cell malignancies is established, and these patients should be routinely followed with periodic βhCG and AFP levels.

Resection of isolated colorectal carcinoma liver metastases renders a small percentage of patients disease-free for prolonged periods of time. Although it has never been tested in a randomized trial, monitoring patients after initial colectomy with serial CEA levels provides an indication of early and occasionally isolated hepatic relapse, and a few such patients may be cured as a result of this approach. Likewise, monitoring ovarian cancer patients after initial treatment with serial CA 125 levels may provide an indication of microscopic peritoneal recurrence. In this case, rising CA 125 levels are an indication for further evaluation, and early treatment with chemotherapy may result in modest prolongation of survival and even cure. Such advantages have not been demonstrated for patients with other malignancies, including breast or lung cancer.

MONITORING PATIENTS WITH METASTATIC DISEASE

Palliation of patients with recurrent or metastatic malignancy may be accomplished with a series of treatment modalities, including surgery, radiation, hormone therapy, and chemotherapy, depending on the tumor type. Although each may provide benefit, the risks and toxicities of the separate therapies differ widely. Therefore, accurate knowledge of the status of a patient's disease is essential in deciding whether to continue the current therapy or proceed to an alternate regimen.

Circulating and bone marrow levels of leukemic blasts provide rough estimates of the effects of chemotherapy during induction and consolidation. For most leukemias, patients who do not clear their marrows of blasts have a very poor prognosis. In patients with myeloma, quantitative analysis of serum globulin levels provides an indication of the relative success or failure of treatment. For lymphomas, serial LDH is a reliable indicator of clinical course, although usually the tumor itself is relatively easily followed by physical or radiographic examination. In patients with germ cell malignancies, βhCG and AFP are exquisite indicators of the response to chemotherapy, and they should be monitored with each treatment cycle. For epithelial malignancies, serial levels of CEA (gastrointestinal, breast, lung, and others), CA 125 (ovarian, lung, breast), and CA 15-3 or CA 27.29 (breast, ovarian) can supplement clinical estimates of the disease course. In general, rising levels suggest progression, decreasing levels suggest response to therapy, and stable levels suggest stable disease. These marker trends are not always perfectly associated with the expected clinical changes; for example, all three may transiently rise and then decrease (so-called tumor spikes) in relation to early tumor response, presumably a result of the release of stored marker protein during tumor lysis. Moreover, the production of CEA levels is related to tumor differentiation in colon cancer, and serial levels may decrease during a time of tumor dedifferentiation and progression. Finally, several benign conditions, especially benign inflammatory diseases of the bowel, lung, and especially liver, can elevate levels of these glycoproteins.

■ SUMMARY

Many tumor-associated antigenic and genetic markers have been proposed for identification, screening, prognosis, detection, or monitoring of patients with suspected or established malignancies. The precise clinical utilities of these markers must be carefully evaluated to avoid inappropriate changes in clinical care based on false-positive or false-negative results. Even if the marker results correlate reliably with the underlying biologic process or status of the disease, the clinician must decide on a therapeutic change only if such a change is known to provide clinical benefit. The relative independence of the marker in relation to other available markers must be determined to avoid the

unnecessary cost and expense of redundancy. With these caveats in mind, judicious application of germ line, tissue, and soluble tumor markers can improve the clinical care of patients at risk for and with cancer.

ACKNOWLEDGMENT

Supported in part by NIH Grant CA64057.

BIBLIOGRAPHY

ASCO Expert Panel. Clinical practice guidelines for the use of tumor markers in breast and colorectal cancer: report of the American Society of Clinical Oncology expert panel. *J Clin Oncol* 1998;16:793–795.

ASCO Sub-committee on Genetic Testing for Cancer Susceptibility. Statement of the American Society of Clinical Oncology. Genetic testing for cancer susceptibility. *J Clin Oncol* 1998;14:1730–1736.

ASCO Expert Panel. Recommended breast cancer surveillance guidelines. American Society of Clinical Oncology. *J Clin Oncol* 1997;15:2149–2156.

Bennett JM, Catovsky D, Daniel M, et al. Proposed revised criteria for the classification of acute myeloid leukemia. *Ann Intern Med* 1985;103:620–625.

Chen Z-X, Xue Y-Q, Zhang R. A clinical and experimental study on all-trans retinoic acid-treated promyelocytic leukemia patients. *Blood* 1991;78:1413–1419.

Droz J-P, Kramar A, Rey A. Prognostic factors in metastatic disease (germ cell). *Semin Oncol* 1992;19:181–189.

Hayes DF, ed. Tumor markers in adult solid malignancies. *Hematol Oncol Clin North Am* 1994.

Hayes DF, Trock B, Harris A. Assessing the clinical impact of prognostic factors: When is "statistically significant" clinically useful? *Breast Cancer Res Treat* 1998;52:305–319.

International Non-Hodgkin's Lymphoma Prognostic Factors Project. A predictive model for aggressive non-Hodgkin's lymphoma. *N Engl J Med* 1993;329:987–994.

Sell S, ed. *Serologic cancer markers.* Totowa, NJ: Humana Press, 1992.

Kelley's Textbook of Internal Medicine, fourth edition. Edited by H. David Humes. Lippincott Williams & Wilkins, Philadelphia © 2000.

CHAPTER
251

MOLECULAR DIAGNOSIS OF CANCER

JEFFREY SKLAR
NEAL LINDEMAN

The field of molecular diagnosis can be defined as the detection of diseases and conditions by the analysis of specific nucleotide sequences within DNA and RNA. Application of molecular diagnosis to cancer grew out of two major developments of the late 1970s: the demonstration that certain inherited diseases, such as hemoglobinopathies, could be diagnosed by the direct detection of mutations in DNA for specific genes, and the understanding that cancers arise from clonal proliferations of cells derived from single progenitor cells that acquire critical mutations that render those cells neoplastic. Inspired by these developments, researchers shortly thereafter set out to devise methods for diagnosing and monitoring cancer through the identification of changes in nucleic acids that distinguish malignant from normal tissues.

Interest in the molecular diagnosis of cancer has increased over the ensuing years because this approach to diagnosis has several advantages over conventional histopathology. These advantages include the relative objectivity of the results of molecular tests compared to the more subjective, morphologic criteria on which histopathologic diagnosis is based. Molecular diagnosis also is potentially far more sensitive for detecting small numbers of cancer cells, a feature that is particularly relevant to monitoring the effects of therapy. Additionally, molecular methods can be used for the presymptomatic determination of inherited predispositions to various types of cancer—a form of diagnosis not generally possible by other means. Finally, certain molecular methods lend themselves to efficient, simultaneous screening of numerous diagnostic markers—a feature that has generated enormous recent enthusiasm, especially for improved systems of tumor subclassification and for the determination of prognosis.

BASIC PRINCIPLES

At their core, all methods currently utilized in the molecular diagnosis of cancer rely on the principle of molecular hybridization, i.e., the ability of two strands of DNA or RNA to bind to each other through formation of hydrogen bonds between adenosine (A) and thymidine (T) or guanosine (G) and cytosine (C) nucleotides in the two strands. Strands of nucleic acid that are capable of forming high numbers of consecutive A:T and G:C nucleotide pairs over their lengths are said to be complementary. The presence of greater numbers of such A:T and G:C nucleotide pairs between the strands leads to tighter binding and higher stability with respect to factors such as increased temperature, high pH, low ionic strength, and elevated concentrations of various chemicals, all of which tend to disrupt hydrogen bonds and separate, or denature, nucleic acid duplexes. DNA in most situations is made up of complementary strands of nucleotides, so that two fragments of DNA containing identical or similar nucleotide sequences may exchange strands if first denatured and renatured together. Based on this property, the hybridization of strands from a labeled or tagged DNA fragment, often referred to as a *probe,* with strands of an unlabeled DNA is a common step in many procedures used in molecular diagnosis. DNA may be labeled with radioactivity, fluorescent adducts, or antigenic substituents that can be detected by the subsequent binding of an antibody tagged in one of a variety of ways. Probe fragments of DNA are routinely prepared by molecular cloning procedures in bacterial hosts. Relatively short, single-stranded DNA fragments, termed *oligonucleotides,* can also be synthesized in the test tube by chemical methods to contain specific nucleotide sequences complementary to defined regions of DNA.

RNA usually exists as single strands of ribonucleotides rather than the deoxyribonucleotides found in DNA; however, the small structural difference between ribo- and deoxynucleotides (the substitution of a hydroxyl group for a hydrogen in the pentose sugar moiety of the nucleotide) does not appreciably affect hybridization, and complementary strands of DNA and RNA will pair with each other, as will two complementary strands of RNA. The RNA normally transcribed from the DNA of a gene as the first step in protein synthesis is complementary in nucleotide sequence to the template strand of the DNA and can therefore be detected by hybridization with a probe derived from the DNA of that gene.

TECHNOLOGY OF CANCER DIAGNOSIS

SOUTHERN BLOT HYBRIDIZATION

Four techniques have played prominently in the molecular diagnosis of cancer. The first of these is Southern blot hybridization. In this technique, DNA extracted from tissue is digested by one or more bacterial restriction enzymes, which cleave DNA at specific short sequences (usually six nucleotides long) recognized by the particular restriction enzyme or mixture of restriction enzymes used. The resulting collection of fragments are separated according to size by electrophoresis through an agarose gel. The DNA within the gel is denatured to single strands by soaking in alkali and then is transferred to a nylon membrane, where the DNA fragments bind irreversibly, forming an invisible ladder of bands on the membrane with each band containing fragments of different size. DNA of interest is identified by hybridization with a radiolabeled probe containing complementary nucleotide sequence. After sufficient time has elapsed for binding of complementary sequences within the probe to target sequences of the membrane, the membrane is dried and placed in the dark against x-ray film for autoradiography. Following exposure of the membrane to the film (usually lasting hours to days), the film is developed and the position of the DNA on the membrane complementary to the probe sequence is revealed as a band or bands in the film, or autoradiogram. From start to finish, Southern blot analysis of DNA requires at least 4 or 5 days.

POLYMERASE CHAIN REACTION

The second technique, which is an integral part of methods that have largely superseded Southern blot hybridization for many purposes, is the polymerase chain reaction (PCR). This technique permits enormous amplification of any nucleotide sequences contained in DNA or RNA through repetitive cycles of brief in vitro DNA synthesis, provided the sequences of the nucleic acid flanking the region to be amplified are known. In the past, the size of the region amplified could not exceed 1 or 2 kb; more recently, methods have been described for amplifying regions up to 20 kb or greater. To perform PCR, short, single-stranded oligonucleotides (usually 15 or more nucleotides long and termed *primers*) are constructed to be complementary to these known sequences on both sides of the region to be amplified. A small amount of DNA template, such as total tissue

DNA, is added to a reaction tube containing a great molar excess of the two primers, along with nucleoside triphosphates (the form of nucleotide monomers that are joined together by DNA synthetic enzymes referred to as DNA polymerases) and heat-resistant DNA polymerase purified from thermophilic species of bacteria. The reaction mixture is heated to denature the template DNA to single strands, cooled to allow primers to hybridize to their complementary sequences, and brought to the proper temperature for polymerization of nucleotides. The DNA polymerase then processively adds nucleotides to the 3′ end of the primers according to the sequence specified by the template strand downstream of the two primers (heat-resistant DNA polymerases used in this reaction, like most DNA polymerases, cannot begin synthesis de novo but can only extend preexisting 3′ ends within DNA).

The steps of template denaturation, primer hybridization, and primer extension are repeated about 20 to 60 times during a standard PCR amplification. In each cycle, DNA synthesized in the previous cycle becomes a template for the subsequent cycle, thereby doubling the amount of template DNA and leading in theory to the accumulation, after 20 cycles, of about one million copies of the target sequence for each copy of the template provided at the beginning of the reaction. The products of PCR consist of fragments containing the amplified sequences and having a length precisely determined by the distance between the two sequences complementary to the primers in the template DNA. The success and specificity of the reaction is usually assessed by formation of a discrete band within a gel after electrophoresis. Sufficient product is often generated so that a band representing the product fragments can be viewed directly in the gel by staining with the fluorescent dye ethidium bromide and illuminating the gel with an ultraviolet lamp. PCR analysis can easily be completed in 1 or 2 days. Unlike Southern blot analysis, PCR can be performed on the short fragments of DNA that are recoverable from formalin-fixed and paraffin-embedded tissue (still the predominant form in which tissue is preserved in most pathology departments).

To detect sequences in RNA, the usual PCR procedure has been modified by the addition of an initial step in which a complementary copy, or cDNA, of the RNA is generated in vitro by a reverse transcription reaction using an DNA-dependent RNA polymerase, termed *reverse transcriptase*, which is produced by one of several retroviruses. Thereafter, the sequences within the cDNA are amplified by standard PCR. PCR carried out in this manner is commonly referred to as RT-PCR.

Two major problems are associated with PCR used for diagnostic purposes. One problem concerns false-positive results arising from spurious amplification of sequences due to contamination of the initial reaction mixture with small amounts of product from previous reactions. Another problem is that PCR generally does not provide quantitative information regarding the number of template molecules present at the start of the reaction. This deficiency is related to the fact that the accumulation of product in PCR plateaus after some number of cycles, so that the amount of product that results from the amplification of only one template can be almost as great as that amplified from abundant template. Several solutions have been employed to counteract this problem. For example, the template present

in a sample may be calculated by assuming that a single template molecule will give rise to product and performing multiple amplication reactions on successively higher dilutions of the template material until no further product is generated. As an alternative to numerous reactions required in this method of limiting dilution, quantitation of PCR has been attempted by adding known concentrations of an internal standard in the form of template that gives a product distinct from that produced from the real template but can also be amplified using the same primers. However, this approach presupposes that the sequences in the standard template will be amplified with same kinetics as those in the real template, and this assumption is not always justified. The most effective solution for quantitating PCR is real-time measurement of amplification as the reaction progresses. This is achieved by using fluorescent oligonucleotide probes that bind to adjacent sequences within the template and are released as DNA synthesis moves through that portion of the template, thereby disrupting the transfer of energy between the probes and quenching a fluorescent signal. The amount of template in the reaction can be accurately determined by comparing the results with template standards containing the same sequence. The procedure has additional advantages, such as completion of the entire process within a sealed tube (reducing the chances of contamination in subsequent reactions) and elimination of gel electrophoresis in many cases to check the specificity of the reaction. Unfortunately, the instruments that have the capability for real-time PCR measurement are expensive.

ANALYSIS OF NUCLEOTIDE SEQUENCE

The third technique fundamental to molecular diagnosis is direct analysis of nucleotide sequence. As most widely practiced, sequence analysis is performed using single-stranded DNA to be sequenced as a template for in vitro DNA synthesis directed by a bacterial or bacteriophage DNA polymerase. Four separate synthetic reactions are carried out, each beginning at the same oligonucleotide primer complementary to DNA immediately flanking the region to be sequenced. The reactions are performed in the presence of the four nucleoside triphosphates, one of which is labeled with sulfur 35 to permit detection of the products. The four reactions differ from each other by the inclusion of a chain-terminating nucleotide analogue (2′,3′-dideoxynucleoside triphosphate) for one or the other of the four bases in DNA, so that some portion of the primer-extension reaction stops whenever the nucleotide complementary to the dideoxy analogue appears in the template. The result of each reaction is a series of radioactive, single-stranded products having the same 5′ end but varying in length by the distance between the positions of the nucleotides in the template complementary to the nucleotide analogue in the reaction. The products of the four reactions are analyzed by electrophoresis in adjacent lanes of a polyacrylamide gel, followed by autoradiography of the gel. The sequence for the template is deduced by reading up the autoradiogram, moving back and forth from lane to lane, noting which lane contains the next band nearest the bottom. A nucleotide corresponding to the nucleotide analogue used in the reaction to generate the lane is added to the sequence for each band that appears in that lane. Up to about 700 nucleotides can be ascertained by performing sequence analysis with a single primer. Sequence analysis in recent years has increasingly relied on nucleoside triphosphates tagged with fluorescent chromophores rather than radioactivity. Using this modification, each of the primer extension reactions can be separately labeled with a different chromophore, run together in one lane of the electrophoretic gel, and analyzed with gel readers that scan the same lane at the four different wavelengths corresponding to the various chromophores that distinguish the products of the four reactions.

FLUORESCENCE IN SITU HYBRIDIZATION

The fourth important technique in molecular diagnosis of cancer is fluorescence in situ hybridization (FISH). In this procedure, DNA probes usually containing many thousands of nucleotide pairs of DNA are hybridized to metaphase chromosomes or interphase nuclei deposited on glass microscope slides. The probe is labeled either directly with a fluorescent chromophore or with an antigenic tag that can be detected immunochemically, and the hybridized material is viewed through a fluorescence microscope. The hybridized probes appear as dots within the nuclei or on the metaphase chromosomes at the site of the DNA contained in the probe.

■ MOLECULAR MARKERS OF CANCER DIAGNOSIS

A wide variety of different nucleic acid markers have been applied in some form of cancer diagnosis, at least on an experimental basis. Among the purposes for which these markers have been applied are primary determination of malignancy in biopsy specimens, tumor classification, staging of disease extent, assessment of prognosis, detection of residual disease, screening of patients for cancer in body fluids, and evaluation of patients for hereditary predisposition to cancer. Table 251.1 lists the more commonly used markers, along with the cancers, methods, and diagnostic purpose associated with their use.

ANTIGEN RECEPTOR GENE REARRANGEMENTS

Among those markers that have most clearly already established a role for themselves in cancer diagnosis are rearrangements of antigen receptor genes (i.e., genes that direct synthesis of the polypeptide subunits that make up immunoglobulins and T-cell receptors). Rearrangements of these genes are not markers for cancer per se but rather for clonality of lymphocytes in non-Hodgkin's lymphoma and lymphocytic leukemias. These rearrangements are created by a series of genetic recombination events that occur normally in the process of assembling functional antigen receptor genes during early stages of lymphocyte development. As inherited in the germ line and retained in all nonhematopoietic cells, each of these genes is encoded over relatively large stretches of DNA as discontinuous segments belonging to three or four multimember sets, termed V, D, J, and C. During gene rearrangement, one D segment becomes joined to one J, and one V segment becomes joined to the previously

linked DJ segments. Some antigen receptor genes lack D segments, in which case a V segment is joined directly to a J segment. The joined VDJ or VJ segments are transcribed into RNA along with a downstream C segment, and the resulting transcript is spliced to produce a mature V(D)JC transcript that can then be translated into an antigen receptor polypeptide. In normal B-cell precursors, this process takes place in two or three immunoglobulin genes (the heavy-chain gene and one or both of the light-chain genes, κ and λ), and rearrangement may occur in one or both alleles for each gene. In normal T-cell precursors, two of the four T-cell receptor genes (α and β or γ and δ) are rearranged. In general, once rearrangement is completed within a gene, that configuration of V, D, and J segments is fixed in the cell and any descendants that it may produce.

From a biologic perspective, the joining of various V, D, and J segments serves as a mechanism to generate structural diversity that is the basis of the specificity of immunoglobulins and T-cell receptors for binding individual antigens; from a diagnostic perspective, joining of V, D, and J segments provides a marker for a given cell or any clone derived from that cell. These rearrangements of segments in antigen receptor genes among cells within a lymphocytic population can be assessed by Southern blot analysis using a probe containing genomic DNA sequences lying downstream of the last J segment. To be visible as a band in the autoradiogram, the same rearrangement must be present within at least 5,000 to 10,000 cells (or about 1% of the 5 to 10×10^5 total cells routinely assayed in one analysis). In non-neoplastic processes in lymphoid tissues, such as inflammatory lesions, or in normal blood or bone marrow, clonal populations constituting as many as 1% of the cells within a tissue are very rare; consequently, non–germ line bands are not seen in Southern blot autoradiograms prepared from such tissues. In contrast, in analyses of tissues containing lymphocytic cancers, one or two non–germ line bands (depending on whether one or both alleles are rearranged within the tumor) are usually detected, provided the clonal population of neoplastic lymphocytes exceeds the 1% threshold.

In most cases, when sufficient material is available, several antigen receptor genes are ordinarily screened, often by analyzing two or three separate restriction enzyme digests of DNA with the same probe. This procedure yields a rearranged band in one or more immunoglobulin genes in B-cell tumors or T-cell receptor genes in T-cell tumors. A small fraction of lymphoid tumors show no detectable bands in the Southern blot autoradiogram, probably due in some cases to technical reasons that are not fully understood or to the origin of these tumors from natural killer cells or other lymphoid cells that do not normally rearrange their antigen receptor genes. In other cases, tumors may arise from lymphocyte precursors that have not yet rearranged their antigen receptor genes. A version of this situation is seen among acute lymphoblastic leukemias, in which many rearranged bands may be detected, presumably because malignant transformation occurs in a pre–pre-B cell precursor that generates descendants capable of rearranging their antigen receptor genes in diverse ways. The converse problem—detection of antigen receptor gene rearrangements in certain disorders traditionally regarded as clinically benign—is also encountered. Such disorders, which include lymphomatoid papulosis, lymphoepi-

TABLE 251.1. EXAMPLES OF MORE COMMONLY USED MOLECULAR MARKERS IN CANCER DIAGNOSIS

Disease	Molecular Marker	Means of Detection	Principal Application(s)
Hematologic Cancers			
Leukemias			
CML	t(9;22)(q34;q11) [BCR/ABL]	SB, RT-PCR, FISH	Primary diagnosis, residual disease
CLL	AGRs	SB, PCR	Primary diagnosis
	Trisomy 12	FISH	"
ALL			
B-lymphoid	AGRs	SB, PCR	Primary diagnosis, residual disease
	t(9;22)(q34;q11) [BCR/ABL]	RT-PCR, FISH	Primary diagnosis, residual disease
	t(1;19)(q23;p13) [E2A/PBX]	"	"
	t(8;14)(q24;q32)		
	t(2;8)(p11;q24), t(8;22)(q24;q11) [MYC;IGH,IGK,IGL]	SB, FISH	Primary diagnosis
	t(4;11)(q21;q23) [MLL/AF2]	RT-PCR, FISH	Primary diagnosis, residual disease
	t(12;21)(p13;q22) [TEL/AMLI]		
T-lymphoid	AGRs	SB, PCR	Primary diagnosis, residual disease
	t(1;14)(p32;q11) del(1p32) [TALI; TCRA]	SB, PCR, FISH	"
AML			
M2	t(8;21)(q22;q22) [AMLI/ETO]	SB, RT-PCR, FISH	Primary diagnosis, residual disease
M3	t(15;17)(q21;q11) [PML/RARA]	"	"
M4	t(6;9)(p23;q34) [DEK/CAN]	SB, FISH	Primary diagnosis
M4Eo	inv (16(p13q22) t(16;16)(p13; q22) [MYHI/CBFβ]	SB, RT-PCR, FISH	Primary diagnosis, residual disease
Non-Hodgkin's Lymphomas			
All subtypes	AGRs	SB, PCR	Primary diagnosis, residual diseases
Follicular	t(14;18)(q32;q21) [BCL2/IGH]	SB, PCR	"
Burkitt's	t(8;14)(q24;q32)	SB	"
	t(2;8)(p11;q24), t(8;22)(q24;q11) [MYC;IGH,IGK,IGL]	SB, FISH	Primary diagnosis
	EBV DNA	SB, PCR	"
Mantle cell	t(11;14)(q13;q32) [BCL1;IGH]	SB	"
Large-cell	t(3;14)(q27;q32) [BCL6/IGH]	SB	"
Anaplastic large-cell	t(2;5)(p23; of 35) [NPM/ALK]	SB, PCR	
Lymphomas associated with immunosuppression	EBV DNA	SB, PCR	"
Adult T-cell leukemia/lymphoma	HTLVI DNA	"	"
Primary body cavity lymphoma	HHV8 DNA	PCR	"
Solid Cancers			
Sarcomas			
Ewing's sarcoma, PNET	t(11;22)(q24;q12) [FLI1/EWS]	SB, RT-PCR	Primary diagnosis, residual disease
Desmoplastic small round cell tumor	t(11;22)(p13;q12) [EWS/WT1]	"	Primary diagnosis
Clear cell sarcoma of soft tissue	t(12;22)(q13–14;q12) [EWS/ATF1]	"	"
Alveolar rhabdomyosarcoma	t(2;13)(q35;q14) [PAX3/FKHR]	"	"
	t(1;13)(p36;q14) [PAX7/FKHR]	"	"
Myxoid liposarcoma	t(12;16)(q13–15;p11) [TLS/CHOP]	"	"
Synovial sarcoma	t(X;18)(p11.2;q11.2) [SYT/SSX]	"	Primary diagnosis, prognosis
Kaposi's sarcoma	HHV8 DNA	PCR	Primary diagnosis

TABLE 251.1.   Continued

Disease	Molecular Marker	Means of Detection	Principal Application(s)
Carcinomas			
Breast Ca	*HER2/NEU/ERBB2* amplification	SB, FISH	Prognosis, response to therapy
Prostate Ca	PSA mRNA	RT-PCR	Staging
Bladder Ca,	*P53* mutation	PCR/oligonucleotide hybridization	Staging, monitoring for relapse
Squamous Ca of head and neck	''	''	''
Colonic Ca	*KRAS* mutation	PCR/oligonucleotide hybridization	Monitoring for relapse
Esophageal Ca	*TP53*	PCR/SSCP PCR/ sequence analysis	Prognosis risk of progression to Ca in Barrett's esophagus)
Pancreatic Ca	*KRAS* mutation	PCR/oligonucleotide hybridization	Primary diagnosis
Cervical Ca	HPV16, 18 DNA	PCR	Primary diagnosis, risk of progression
Other cancers			
Neuroblastoma	*MYCN*	SB, FISH Amplification	Prognosis
Melanoma	Tyrosinase mRNA	RT-PCR	Staging
Familial Cancers and Cancer Syndromes			
Breast Ca, ovarian Ca	*BRCA1, BRCA2* mutations	PCR/SSCP PCR/BRC PCR/DGGE PCR/sequence analysis	Diagnosis of hereditary predisposition
Colonic Ca	*APC, MSH2, MLH1, PMS1, PMS2* mutations	''	''
Retinoblastoma, various sarcomas	*RB* mutations	''	''
Wilms' tumor	*WT1, WT2* mutations	''	''
Li–Fraumeni syndrome	*TP53* mutations	''	''
MEN 2	*RET* mutation	''	''
Kidney Ca (von Hippel–Lindau)	*VHL* mutation	''	''
Pheochromocytoma (neurofibromatosis)	*NF1, NF2* mutation	''	''
Melanoma	*MTS1* mutation	''	''
Astrocytoma (tuberous sclerosis)	*TSC1, TSC2* mutation	''	''
Basal cell Ca	*PTCH* mutation	''	''
Cowden's syndrome	*PTEN* mutation	''	''
Non-Hodgkin's lymphoma (ataxia telangiectasia)	*ATM* mutation	''	''
Acute lymphoblastic leukemia (Bloom's syndrome)	*BLM* mutation	''	''
Acute lymphoblastic leukemia (Fanconi's anemia)	*FACA, FACC* mutation	''	''

CML, chronic myeloid leukemia; CLL, chronic lymphoid leukemia; AML; acute myeloid leukemia; ALL, acute lymphoid leukemia; AGR antigen receptor gene rearrangement; SB, Southern blot hybridization; genes are indicated by italicized capital letters; genes involved in translocations are shown in brackets below the translocation; FISH, fluorescence in situ hybridization; RT-PCR reverse transcriptase polymerase chain reaction; HPV, human papillomavirus; PNET, peripheral neuroepithelioma; MEN, multiple endocrine neoplasia; SSCP, single-strand conformational polymorphism; BRC, bacteriophage resolvase cleavage; DGGE, denaturing gradient gel electrophoresis. Familial cancer syndromes are listed in place of a specific cancer when the condition is associated with multiple forms of cancer.

thelial lesions of the salivary gland, and so-called pseudolymphomas, tend to be chronic and are associated with relatively high risk of subsequent lymphoma or leukemia. Increasingly, these disorders are considered to be either benign neoplasms with a propensity for progression to malignancy, or very low-grade cancers.

Rearrangements of antigen receptor genes can also be analyzed as clonal markers using PCR. Whereas Southern blot analysis of antigen receptor gene rearrangements examines the configuration of specific rearranged V, D, and J gene segments, PCR focuses on the nucleotide sequences at the junctions between rearranged segments. During the rearrangement process, prior to fusion of the segments, novel sequences are created at these sites by the combined effects of two events: deletion of variable numbers of nucleotide pairs at the ends of the gene segments and insertion of variably sized short stretches of random nucleotide pairs between the segments. The sequences at the VDJ and VJ junctions can be amplified using primers complementary to sequences in the V and J segments flanking these junctions. Uniform junctional sequences indicative of clonal populations of lymphocytes can be identified as discrete bands in electrophoretic gels. Resolution of these bands may be based solely on the size of the PCR products (using standard agarose or polyacrylamide gels) or on the size plus the sequence of the products (using gradient denaturing gels). Either approach has about the same sensitivity for detecting clonal populations of lymphocytes as Southern blot analysis. However, as a practical prerequisite for PCR amplification of a given antigen receptor gene, sufficiently similar sequences must exist in the various V and J segments to permit amplification with a limited set of primers complementary to these sequences. For this reason, immunoglobulin heavy-chain and γ T-cell receptor genes are the only genes routinely analyzed for rearrangements by PCR. Furthermore, clonal rearrangements in only about 75% to 80% of B-cell neoplasms can be detected by PCR with multiple sets of primers for immunoglobulin heavy-chain genes. Nevertheless, the speed and convenience of PCR analysis (significantly, the avoidance of radioactive chemicals) relative to Southern blot analysis makes PCR a useful technique to assess gene rearrangements, at least as a preliminary screen before having to resort to Southern blot analysis. Additionally, because of the power of PCR to amplify very small amounts of DNA, it can be the only means to evaluate the clonality specimens having few lymphocytes, such as in skin biopsy specimens containing possible early cutaneous T-cell lymphoma.

Junctional sequences between segments of rearranged antigen receptor genes have also been utilized to search for residual disease after therapy. In this application, the V(D)J junction is amplified by PCR from the DNA of a diagnostic biopsy sample. Nucleotide sequence analysis is performed on the amplified fragment, and the tumor-specific junctional sequence is used to prepare an oligonucleotide primer or probe. Specimens obtained after administration of therapy can be then analyzed for residual disease by attempting amplification of DNA with the tumor-specific primer and a second nonspecific primer complementary to V or J sequences. Alternatively, V(D)J sequences can be amplified in aggregate from the DNA of a posttherapy specimen and the products tested for the tumor-specific junctional sequence by hybridization with an oligonucleotide probe constructed from the sequence determined from the original diagnostic specimen. These strategies have the ability to detect one malignant cell from a total of about 10^5 total cells.

The greatest interest in applying PCR of antigen receptor genes for monitoring of residual disease has centered on acute lymphoblastic leukemia because of the potential curability of the disease and the theoretical option of intensifying therapy or performing bone marrow transplantation if leukemic cells are found to persist in patients undergoing treatment. Studies attempting to correlate residual disease detected by these techniques with clinical outcomes have yielded somewhat contradictory results. Overall, a rapid decline in the detection of a clonal junctional sequence and continued absence of this sequence throughout the course of therapy predicts a better chance of survival. However, large fluctuations in the level of the clonotypic sequence can be found during therapy, and some patients lacking detectable clonotypic sequences at the end of therapy will ultimately relapse. Relapses among these patients are likely due to residual disease below the threshold detectable by testing for junctional sequences and in some cases to origin of the leukemia from pre–pre-B cells, which can give rise to subclones having different V(D)J sequences. Perhaps most surprising is evidence that some patients in clinical remission for years following cessation of all therapy continue to harbor viable cells bearing the junctional sequence found in their leukemic clone at diagnosis.

CHROMOSOMAL REARRANGEMENTS

Chromosomal rearrangements represent a large category of marker for the molecular diagnosis of certain cancers, especially hematopoietic neoplasms and sarcomas. Many of these rearrangements can also be detected by conventional cytogenetic analysis of metaphase chromosomes obtained from cancer cells. However, when molecular methods are applicable, they usually provide test results faster than cytogenetics and with much greater sensitivity for detecting small numbers of abnormal cells. Interpretation of these results does not require the degree of technical expertise needed for cytogenetics. Furthermore, biopsy specimens that fail to yield adequate metaphases for standard cytogenetic analysis or produce overgrowth of normal fibroblasts in culture do not affect molecular analysis. Molecular analysis can also detect diagnostically relevant submicroscopic chromosomal alterations that cannot be resolved by standard cytogenetics and disease-specific chromosomal rearrangements that are obscured in cytogenetic preparations by complex nonspecific karyotypic changes.

Chromosomal translocations have received particular attention as diagnostic markers, compared to other chromosomal abnormalities such as deletions or inversions, both because translocations are relatively common in cancer and because they are especially favorable markers for detection by molecular means. The most important technical consideration in detecting translocations within biopsy specimens is the variability of the positions of breakpoints in the DNA. Usually these breakpoints on the two participating chromosomes join portions of two genes, creating a chimeric gene with novel functions or properties that contribute to the malignant transformation of the cells that contain them. Sometimes the positions of the breakpoints for a specific translocation cluster closely over short lengths of DNA, in which case the translocation can be detected by Southern blot analysis using a probe complementary to DNA near one of the breakpoints, or by PCR using two primers that flank the point of fusion between the two chromosomes. Detection of a translocation is indicated by the presence of a band in a non–germ line position in the Southern blot autoradiogram or by a band produced by gel electrophoresis of the PCR products. The threshold for detecting neoplastic cells by these methods is about 1% (Southern blot analysis) and $1/10^5$ (PCR).

Rather than being tightly clustered within DNA, the positions of the chromosomal breakpoints more often vary considerably among cases with a specific translocation, particularly over the sizable stretches of DNA that constitute introns within the affected genes. Detection of translocations in this situation requires the use of multiple probes for Southern blot analysis and frequently precludes PCR of DNA for most practical purposes. To circumvent this problem, RT-PCR of RNA from biopsy tissues is commonly performed. Primers are constructed to complement sequences within exons lying on both sides of the site of breakpoint fusion. For most translocations, this approach permits detection of neoplastic cells using a few sets of primers and with a sensitivity at least as high as that obtained by PCR of DNA.

Because of the great sensitivity of PCR-based detection of chromosomal translocations, amplification across sites of chromosomal fusion has been extensively employed for monitoring residual disease after therapy or for identifying small numbers of neoplastic cells in autologous bone marrow transplantation. To date, most experience with these methods has been obtained in chronic granulocytic leukemia using the t(9;22)(q34;q11), the Philadelphia chromosome (Ph), as a marker. In general, the findings have paralleled those described above with PCR of V(D)J junctional sequences in acute lymphoblastic leukemias; levels of Ph may vary widely over the course of therapy and detectable numbers of it may persist for years in patients who remain in complete clinical remission. Even longer disease-free intervals have been seen in patients with M2 acute myelogenous leukemia carrying numbers of the t(8;21)(q22;q22) detectable by RT-PCR. On the other hand, early treatment of patients in whom detectable levels of the t(15;17)(q21;q11) have reappeared after therapy seems to prolong survival in M3 acute myelogenous leukemia.

In addition to Southern blot analysis and PCR, FISH has been applied for detecting translocations and other forms of chromosomal rearrangement. To test for chromosomal translocations, two probes are utilized, each distinguished by a different color of fluorescence and each complementary to DNA near one or the other breakpoints on the two participating chromosomes. If the appropriate translocation is present, three dots are seen—one with the color of the labeled probe for each of the normal chromosomal homologues and one with the combined colors corresponding to a product of the translocation. The principal virtue of FISH for diagnostic testing is its speed; analysis can be completed within hours when interphase cells are used. Furthermore, it can be used to detect chromosomal translocations, such as those involving the *MYC* gene in Burkitt's lymphoma, in which the breakpoints are so widely scattered in the DNA of chromosome 8 that neither Southern blot analysis, PCR, nor RT-PCR is applicable. A drawback to FISH is that cells must be examined individually, and therefore the method does not lend itself to the monitoring of residual disease. The sensitivity of FISH is further reduced by the fact that in any individual cell there is a significant risk of missing a dot because of failure of hybridization to DNA within the largely intact nuclei on the slide. Inconsistent hybridization within intact nuclei also complicates the use of FISH to detection of small deletions by probes to the deleted region; consequently, the method has not been widely employed for this purpose beyond experimental situations. On the other hand, detection of addi-

tions or deletions of whole chromosomes is generally less problematic in this way since strongly hybridizing probes to highly repetitive sequences surrounding chromosomal centromeres can be used.

Amplification of genes is another type of chromosomal rearrangement that has a potential role in the molecular diagnosis of certain cancers, particularly for assessment of prognosis. In one cancer, neuroblastoma, both the presence and degree of amplification of the N-*myc* oncogene is a well-recognized prognostic indicator. For other genes and cancers, such as the *her2/neu/c-erbB-2* oncogene in breast cancer, the significance of amplification as an independent prognostic variable is more controversial (although *HER2* amplification appears to be a valuable indicator of responsiveness to the therapy with recombinant monoclonal antibodies directed against the HER2 protein). In the past, increased copy number of these genes has been detected by Southern blot, but FISH on interphase nuclei has lately been increasingly used for this purpose. However, in some instances immunohistochemistry for the protein product of these genes may be more convenient than molecular diagnostic methods or may provide results more directly correlated with subsequent tumor behavior than copy number of the gene.

Efforts have also been made to exploit amplifications and deletions of much smaller regions of DNA for cancer diagnosis. These regions of DNA contain so-called microsatellite sequences made up of short stretches of tandem di- or trinucleotide repeats (most commonly CA dinucleotides) located at thousands of sites throughout the genome, predominantly outside of coding sequences. Microsatellite sequences are prone to replicative errors that occasionally add or subtract repeat units as cells proliferate, making most normal body tissues cellular mosaics with respect to the number of microsatellite repeats at certain loci. Additionally, mechanisms of mismatch DNA repair that work to prevent errors in DNA replication that occur in microsatellite sequences may be relaxed in cells early during tumorigenesis. The nonrepeated sequences surrounding many microsatellite repeats are known, and primers complementary to these sequences can be used to amplify individual microsatellite regions to search for changes in the number of repeats by noting alterations in the size of the resulting PCR product. The frequency of variation at any one microsatellite site is usually very low, so that a change in the size of the microsatellite region cannot be detected by amplification of total DNA from normal tissue. However, if clonal expansion has occurred, as happens during tumor development, alterations in size of the microsatellite region may become apparent. This type of clonal analysis has been used to assay for tumor cells in body fluids and even for free DNA released from tumors into blood. Unfortunately, many microsatellite regions may have to be examined before a polymorphism in repeat number can be identified, greatly reducing the utility of this approach to diagnosis.

VIRUS-DERIVED GENES

Viruses have been implicated as an etiologic factor in several forms of cancer, and the nucleic acids of these pathogens may serve as diagnostic markers in certain settings. Included within this group of viruses are Epstein–Barr virus (EBV), human T-cell leukemia/lymphoma virus type 1 (HTLV-1), human papillomavirus (mostly types 16 and 18), and human herpesvirus 8

(HHV-8). Detection of viral DNA in tissue biopsies can be carried out either by PCR or by Southern blot hybridization using primers or probes specific for the viral genome. However, both PCR and Southern blot analysis (although to a lesser extent with Southern blot analysis because of its lower sensitivity) run the risk of detecting infections by the above viruses unassociated with neoplasia. For example, neither method discriminates between the EBV DNA found in EBV-associated lymphomas and the EBV DNA in acute infections of patients with mononucleosis or in latently infected lymphoblasts found in most normal individuals. In the example of EBV, this problem has been overcome by performing Southern blot hybridization for the region of the DNA spanning the site where the termini of the linear genome present in the viral capsids are fused to form the circular episome found in infected cells. The termini differ from virion to virion due to varying numbers of tandemly repeated sequences 500 nucleotides long at the ends of the linear genome. Additionally, some repeat units may be discarded as the termini become joined through a process of homologous recombination. Consequently, the length of the restriction fragment containing the fused termini of the genome is likely to vary from one infected cell to another. The presence of an infected clone of lymphocytes, each member of which carries a uniform EBV episome with identical fused termini, is indicated by a predominant band in the Southern blot autoradiogram, in contrast to the ladder of bands that appear in autoradiograms produced from polyclonal cells infected by EBV.

ECTOPIC RNA

Structurally normal RNA molecules transcribed from cellular genes have been utilized as markers for cancer diagnosis in two contexts. One context involves the detection of metastatic tumor cells from non-hematopoietic tumors using as markers RNA transcribed from genes expressed primarily in the normal tissue from which that tumor arose. This approach to diagnosis takes advantage of the sensitivity of RT-PCR to detect specific RNA sequences and is based on the rationale that the finding of RNA at an inappropriate site must be due to metastasis. RT-PCR of such ectopic RNAs has the attractive feature of requiring no preliminary characterization of the primary tumor (e.g., identification of a specific chromosomal translocation or mutation). The chief limitation of the method has so far been the difficulty in discovering usable RNAs due to the phenomenon of so-called illegitimate transcription (the physiologically insignificant transcription of low levels of many or most genes in a wide variety of tissues). Low levels of nonspecific transcription in large numbers of normal cells at a site of possible metastasis is indistinguishable by RT-PCR from high levels of transcription in small numbers of metastatic cells at that site.

The original paradigm for application of RT-PCR of ectopic RNA for detecting metastatic cells was in testing for bloodborne tumor cells in melanoma patients using tyrosinase RNA as a marker for circulating malignant melanocytes. More recently, extensive study has been directed at the detection of metastatic tumor cells in blood, bone marrow, or pelvic lymph nodes of patients with prostate cancer by RT-PCR of RNA for prostate-specific antigen (PSA). Preliminary studies suggesting that detection of PSA RNA at ectopic sites predicts a shortened course await confirmation in larger prospective studies now underway.

TRANSCRIPTIONAL PROFILING

A second context in which RNA has been regarded as having great potential in cancer diagnosis is in the characterization of tumors through comprehensive surveys of gene transcription in cancer cells. These surveys are often called *transcriptional profiles* and have become feasible as a result of international efforts, now in progress, to determine the nucleotide sequence of all human genes. Another development critical for this work has been the creation of instruments and technologies that permit the construction on glass slides, often referred to as "chips" in this field, of microarrays composed of thousands of very small spots, each containing a different specific gene sequence. Two technologies have been used to construct microarrays: the deposition by robots of DNA fragments onto the chip and the photochemical synthesis of oligonucleotides directly on the chip surface. Additionally, chip-reading devices have been produced to rapidly collect signals generated from each individual spot.

The general procedure in transcriptional profiling is that pools of fluorescently labeled complementary DNAs (cDNAs) are synthesized from total-gene RNA in a tissue and hybridized to the chip. Hybridization of the test cDNA pool is usually performed together with a differently labeled cDNA pool prepared from a second source, and the chip reader compares the relative hybridization of the two cDNA pools at each spot. For example, cDNAs of an individual tumor can be compared in this way to the cDNAs of its normal tissue counterpart to determine those genes that are more or less active in the malignant versus the normal cells, or transcription in individual tumors can be compared pairwise to identify differences in the activities of certain genes. The diagnostic value of transcriptional profiling in cancer diagnosis rests on the concept that the clinical behavior of a tumor is largely determined by the activity of genes within it and that differences in gene activity will better define subclasses of tumors, predict responses to therapies, and dictate overall prognosis.

At present, transcriptional profiling of tumors is only beginning and there are difficulties to be overcome in the analysis and management of data from arrays containing as many as 10^5 spots (corresponding to the 10^5 unique genes in the human cell) and in problems posed by the cellular heterogeneity of many tumors. However, the latter difficulty may be mitigated by laser microdissection apparatuses that have been devised to excise homogeneous regions of pure tumor from tissue sections. It also remains to be seen as to whether transcriptional profiling will become a diagnostic method in itself or, perhaps more likely, a vehicle for the discovery of a set of critical markers that may be assessed by other methods, such as RT-PCR or immunohistochemistry.

POINT MUTATIONS

Point mutations—the substitution of one nucleotide pair for another within the DNA of genes—are a type of diagnostic marker with ramifications for many types of diagnostic applications in cancer. Such mutations are responsible for the conversion of some proto-oncogenes to oncogenes and often for the inactivation of tumor suppressor genes. In aggregate, these alterations probably represent the most common type of acquired genetic lesion present in human cancers. Furthermore, point mutations passed through the germ line, frequently in one allele of a tumor suppressor gene, account for most hereditary cancer syndromes. It is also widely anticipated that differences in single nucleotide pairs may affect gene products that interact with drugs and therefore could influence the response to therapy. Some of these differences will probably be acquired somatically, in the tumor itself. Other differences may be inherited, in which case they are usually referred to as polymorphisms rather than mutations because they are more common in the population than mutations and do not inactivate a gene or its product, although they may alter its function. The search for such genetic variations and their correlation with toxicities or therapeutic efficacy of drugs has engendered a new field of pharmacogenomics, which may significantly affect the practice of oncology in coming years.

Two considerations qualify the use of point mutations as diagnostic markers in cancer. One consideration relates to the essential multistep process of tumor development. Mutations in individual genes appear to be insufficient for full transformation to malignancy. Most cancers derive from progenitor cells that have accumulated a series of mutations, which may include nucleotide substitutions, deletions, amplifications, and chromosomal rearrangements, in addition to possible epigenetic changes (such as altered methylation of particular regions of DNA) that govern the activities of various genes. Therefore, mutations in a given oncogene or tumor suppressor gene may be present in dysplasias, in other premalignant conditions, or even in benign conditions, and these changes by themselves cannot be regarded as absolutely diagnostic of cancer. For example, mutations of the K-*ras* oncogene, found in about 90% of pancreatic adenocarcinomas, have also been detected in epithelial cells from the pancreatic ducts of a minority of patients with chronic pancreatitis. Moreover, point mutations present in the cells of primary tumors may also occasionally disappear in recurrences, underscoring the need for caution in applying these changes as markers for detection residual disease.

Nevertheless, if found in follow-up samples, point mutations that match those detected in an earlier specimen diagnosed by conventional morphologic and other criteria may be useful for staging of tumors or for monitoring of recurrent disease. For purposes of monitoring cancer, there are effective and relatively straightforward methods for "redetecting" such mutations. These methods usually depend on PCR of DNA for a particular gene, followed by molecular hybridization with oligonucleotides complementary to a sequence containing the specific mutation previously determined in the reference sample. Examples of these types of studies have been carried out using mutations of the *P53* tumor suppressor gene to screen for recurrences of bladder carcinoma in urinary sediments and to stage the extent of local spread in squamous carcinoma of the oropharynx. The maximal sensitivity of this method is on the order of detecting one malignant cell in 10^4 or 10^5 total cells, but working out the precise conditions for this level of detection can be challenging.

The second consideration in the attempt to use point muta-

tions as diagnostic markers pertains to technical difficulties in their de novo detection in primary diagnostic samples, as opposed to redetection in follow-up samples. Although mutations tend to occur repeatedly in certain positions of some cancer-related genes (notably genes of the *RAS* family, in which mutations occur predominantly in codons 12, 13, and 61), the sites of mutations are generally widely scattered throughout the sequence of most tumor suppressor genes among different cases and within those genes involved in hereditary cancers among different pedigrees. These mutations can be definitively determined by nucleotide sequence analysis of PCR products, but this process is generally considered to be too labor-intensive to be employed as a routine diagnostic procedure. In addition, nucleotide sequence analysis for cancer diagnosis is frequently complicated by the need to identify nucleotide changes in heterozygous tissues or in impure samples in which the malignant cells represent a minor component. Various methods have been devised to expedite detection of mutations. Most of these methods depend on the altered mobility of mutant DNA fragments in electrophoretic gels [single-strand conformational polymorphism analysis (SSCP) and denaturing gradient gel electrophoresis (DGGE)] or on the enzymatic cleavage at the position of mismatched bases within heteroduplexes of nucleic acids containing one normal strand and one mutant strand (enzyme mismatch scanning). These methods also have their disadvantages, including significant effort required to optimize the procedure in a given case and frequent false-negative results. Another potential solution to the problem of detecting point mutations is hybridization of DNA probes generated from tissue DNA to commercially prepared oligonucleotide microarrays containing all possible nucleotide substitutions for a given region of sequence. Although currently these microarrays are expensive, this approach has succeeded for detecting many mutations in certain genes and greatly reduces the labor needed to screen large segments of DNA for mutations at many possible sites.

BIBLIOGRAPHY

Ahrendt SA, Sidransky D. The potential of molecular screening. *Surg Onc Clin North America* 1999;8(4)641–656.

Rowley JD, Aster JC, Sklar JL. The impact of new DNA diagnostic technology on the management of cancer patients. *Arch Pathol Lab Med* 1993; 117:1104–1109.

Rowley JD, Aster JC, Sklar JL. The clinical applications of new DNA diagnostic technology on the management of cancer patients. *JAMA* 1993;270:2331–2337.

Schena M, Shalon D, Davis RW, Brown PO. Quantitative monitoring of gene expression patterns with a complementary DNA microarray. *Science* 1995;270(5235):467–470.

Sidransky D. Molecular markers in cancer: can we make better predictions? *Int J Cancer* 1995;64:1–2.

Sklar J. The molecular diagnosis of lymphoma and related disorders. In: Canellos G, Lister A, Sklar J, eds. *The lymphomas*. Philadelphia: WB Saunders, 1998:129–150.

Sklar J, Costa JC. Principles of cancer management: molecular pathology. In: DeVita VT Jr, Hellman S, Rosenberg SA, eds. *Cancer: principles and practice of oncology*. Philadelphia: JB Lippincott, 1997:259–284.

Vogelstein B, Kinzler KW, eds. *The genetic basis of human cancer*. New York: McGraw-Hill, 1998.

Kelley's Textbook of Internal Medicine, fourth edition. Edited by H. David Humes.
Lippincott Williams & Wilkins, Philadelphia © 2000.

CHAPTER
252

PRINCIPLES OF SURGICAL ONCOLOGY

JOHN M. DALY
MICHAEL D. LIEBERMAN

The surgical oncologist occupies a unique position in the management of the patient with cancer. Most cancer patients undergo some form of operative therapy for the diagnosis, primary treatment, or management of complications during the course of treatment for their neoplastic disease. Survival statistics of patients with cancer treated surgically have reached a plateau; earlier detection through selective screening and multimodal therapy should further improve cure rates. Inclusion of radiation therapy or chemotherapy or both may also preserve a comparable survival rate while permitting less extensive operative resection, thus enhancing cosmesis and function.

The surgical oncologist is responsible for the initial diagnosis and management of many types of cancer. Knowledge of tumor staging and the natural history of the disease should be integrated into a multimodal approach to treatment in concert with the medical oncologist and the radiation therapist. The guiding principles of the surgical oncologist should be the accurate diagnosis and staging of the cancer with adequate operative removal of locoregional disease.

The surgical oncologist's role varies with the type of cancer. For example, curative operations may be performed on patients with primary breast, head and neck, gastrointestinal, gynecologic, lung, skin, and urinary tract malignancies. In other forms of cancer, such as lymphoma, the surgeon may provide diagnostic and staging information. In patients with hematologic malignancies, the surgeon may provide vascular access or manage complications related to chemotherapy or radiation therapy.

PREOPERATIVE ASSESSMENT: CLINICAL DIAGNOSIS AND STAGING

On the first examination of the patient with cancer, a complete history and physical examination are indispensable before further judgments can be made regarding laboratory testing and treatment. Common symptoms range from anorexia, nausea, vomiting, hematemesis, abdominal pain, melena, and hematochezia in patients with gastrointestinal cancer to anorexia, productive cough, and hemoptysis in lung cancer, to an enlarging mass in breast and soft-tissue tumors. Symptoms generally correspond to the sites involved, but nonspecific symptoms such as night sweats and weight loss may be the initial manifestations of an underlying neoplastic tumor. The duration of symptoms may indicate the aggressiveness of the cancer. The degree of

impairment should be noted, as this will influence treatment decisions regarding palliation.

The patient's past medical history often provides clues to the diagnosis. The medical history also reveals environmental factors such as smoking, alcohol ingestion, or exposure to asbestos or aniline dyes that can be related to organ-specific sites of tumor development. Finally, a thorough medical history provides an important index of operative risk for the patient.

Physical examination should begin with an overall assessment, proceed through a systemic examination, and then focus on the specific sites suggested by the medical history. Simple screening examinations, such as a complete pelvic examination with uterine cervical Pap smear and fecal occult blood testing, should be performed routinely.

In addition to routine laboratory tests such as complete blood count, coagulation profile, multichannel serum biochemistry profile, and chest roentgenography, other studies are useful in determining the primary tumor site and extent of disease. The oncologist frequently requires assays for tumor markers in the blood or urine as well as radiologic studies.

Serum tumor markers have been most useful in following the patient's response to therapy (see Chapter 250). Serum markers such as carcinoembryonic antigen (CEA), β-human chorionic gonadotropin, CA 125, thyroglobulin, and α-fetoprotein (AFP) are useful in the management of patients with specific tumors.

The surgical oncologist relies heavily on preoperative imaging for diagnosis, staging, and planning the operation. Most commonly, a dynamic helical computed tomography (CT) scan is the first and only radiologic test required to assess an intra-abdominal process. Magnetic resonance imaging (MRI) is helpful for extremity sarcomas, retroperitoneal tumors, and the assessment of bowel wall penetration of rectal tumors. Endoscopic ultrasonography has a major role in the preoperative assessment of esophageal, gastric, and some pancreatic tumors. External ultrasonography is user-dependent but in experienced centers is a superb modality for evaluating tumors involving the hepatobiliary system. The use of preoperative angiography has been drastically reduced with the advent of Duplex ultrasound, magnetic resonance angiography, and contrast-enhanced helical CT scanning. However, preoperative arteriography can be useful in patients under consideration for hepatic artery infusional therapy. Mammography is useful for detecting occult breast masses and areas of suspicious microcalcifications, for stereotactic needle biopsies, and for providing needle localization of occult mammographic abnormalities for excisional biopsy. Radionuclide scans are useful for evaluating the presence of bone metastases in patients with symptomatic musculoskeletal complaints. Radiolabeled octreotide, cholesterol, and CEA scans have utility in staging patients with carcinoid, adrenal, and colorectal tumors, respectively. Positron emission tomography (PET) scanning complements other diagnostic modalities for lung, melanoma, and gastrointestinal cancers and may prove to be more cost-effective. Diagnostic sensitivity, specificity, and accuracy are 85% to 90% or better when assessing for primaries, metastases, or recurrence. The use of PET scanning altered patient manage-

TABLE 252.1.	ALTERED PATIENT TREATMENT WITH PET SCANNING

Disease	No. of Patients	Change in Treatment (%)
Recurrent colorectal cancer	93	38
Lung cancer	159	41
Lymphoma	74	15
Melanoma	50	44

(From Conti PS, Lilien DL, Hawley K, et al. PET and 18F-FDG in oncology: a clinical update. *Nucl Med Biol* 1996;23:717, with permission.)

ment in 15% to 44% of patients with recurrent colorectal cancer, lung cancer, lymphoma, and melanoma (Table 252.1).

PATHOLOGIC DIAGNOSIS AND STAGING

The importance of accurate pathologic diagnosis in the proper surgical treatment of cancer patients cannot be overstated. The determinations of histologic grade, primary site, and surgical resection margins provide critical information.

Diagnosis can frequently be made by the use of fine-needle aspiration cytology (FNA). Diagnosis using FNA (22- to 25-gauge needle) techniques concurs with the surgical pathologic diagnosis in 97% of tested lymph nodes in patients with metastatic solid tumors and 77% of primary breast tumors examined. This technique is rapid, minimally traumatic, and highly accurate for diagnosis of a clearly palpable mass or a radiographically visible lesion. False-positive results are rare; false-negative results may occur because of the small sample size and the site of the lesion. With the use of FNA techniques in combination with helical CT scans and ultrasonography, deep nonpalpable lesions have become amenable to diagnosis with minimal morbidity. Tumor cell implantation of the aspiration site is rare. FNA cytology is particularly useful in diagnosing palpable masses in the breast or thyroid or palpable suspected nodes in the neck, axilla, or groin. However, aspiration cytology cannot be relied on for grading solid tumors, for subdividing types of lymphoma, or for making an accurate diagnosis after radiation treatment, but a positive diagnosis of malignancy greatly facilitates diagnostic and treatment planning.

When an accurate diagnosis of tumor type and grade is necessary and cannot be accomplished by FNA, an incisional or excisional biopsy is required. Care should be taken in the planning of a surgical biopsy so as not to jeopardize later surgical extirpation or the use of skin flaps. In general, large soft-tissue lesions (5 to 7 cm) that are deeper than the superficial fascia are best sampled by incisional biopsy to provide a diagnosis and allow planning for a definitive procedure. Small (less than 2 cm) superficial lesions should be managed by excisional biopsy with a view to further treatment depending on tumor type, grade, and depth of invasion. Frozen section diagnosis should not be relied on to

provide accurate histologic grade and information about invasion depth. Surgical margins of resection should be evaluated by frozen section or permanent section examination of a properly marked and oriented specimen.

The surgical staging of intra-abdominal tumors with a concomitant decrease in morbidity has improved with minimal access surgery. Utilizing small incisions and ports with one-way valves, surgical instruments, and cameras can be introduced into the gas, CO_2, distended abdomen for exploration, direct organ ultrasonography, tissue biopsy, peritoneal cytology, and, sometimes, curative resection. Many surgical oncologists utilize laparoscopic techniques to rule out carcinomatosis prior to laparotomy for pancreatic, gastric, and hepatic malignancies. Limiting laparotomy to patients who may benefit from resection reduces patient morbidity, time to definitive therapy, duration of hospitalization, and cost.

PREOPERATIVE PREPARATION

Appropriate preoperative preparation includes knowledge of the natural history of the disease, evaluation of operative risk, decisions relevant to the need for and timing of operative intervention, estimation of the physiologic stress potentially imposed by the operation, and quantitative assessment of the patient's physiologic status. Comprehensive preparation of a patient for operative therapy requires physiologic and psychological support. The physician should consider potential abnormalities such as acid–base disorders, malnutrition, infection, respiratory insufficiency, hepatic and renal dysfunction, anemia, and clotting abnormalities.

The two aims of all treatment during the preoperative period should be to prepare the patient to withstand the stresses of operative therapy and to minimize the risks of the surgical procedure. The appropriate duration of the preoperative period depends on the urgency of the operative procedure. Determining this urgency requires knowledge of the operative risk and the natural history of the disease without immediate operative intervention. Included in this evaluation are factors such as age (chronologic and physiologic), degree of physiologic derangements and nutritional deficits, presence of organ system failure or insufficiency, and stage of the primary disease. Although the urgency of operative intervention may limit both the length of preoperative preparation and the methods available for correcting preexisting abnormalities, partial repair of deficiencies should be initiated promptly, with plans made for more complete correction during and after operative therapy. Months of chronic undernutrition cannot be corrected in a matter of hours, but anemia, dehydration, and electrolyte abnormalities can be ameliorated by early initiation of intensive intravenous support, guided by appropriate laboratory monitoring. Preoperative assessment of high-risk patients, in particular looking at reversible factors such as malnutrition, is essential for optimal outcome. Nutritional assessment techniques include a detailed history, noting the degree of weight change as well as dietary and alcohol intake, and physical examination. Other parameters studied are serum albumin and transferrin levels.

TABLE 252.2.	PROSPECTIVE RANDOMIZED TRIALS OF PREOPERATIVE TOTAL PARENTERAL NUTRITION IN SURGICAL PATIENTS				
Author	No. Patients	Preoperative TPN Duration (Days)	Nutrition Criteria Defined	Complication Rate (%) TPN vs. Control	Mortality Rate (%) TPN vs. Control
Holter	56	3	Wt. loss (≥10 lb)	13 vs. 19	7 vs. 8
Heatley et al.	74	7–10	N.D.	28 vs. 25	15 vs. 22
Hotler	26	2	Wt. loss (>10 lb)	16 vs. 18	N.D.
Moghissi	15	5–7	Severe dysphagia	30 vs. 50	N.D.
Preshaw	47	1	N.D.	33 vs. 17	N.D.
Simms	40	7–10	N.D.	N.D.	0 vs. 10
Lim	19	21–28	Severe dysphagia	30 vs. 50	10 vs. 20
Schildt	15	14	N.D.	38 vs. 50	0 vs. 0
Thompson	41	5–14	≥10 lb wt: loss	17 vs. 11 vs. 10	0 vs. 0 vs. 10
Sako	69	8–32	Nutrition status	50 vs. 56	50 vs. 25
Mueller	125	10	N.D.	11 vs. 19	3 vs. 11
Burt	18	14	≥20T wt. loss, unable to swallow liquids	N.D.	N.D.
Jensen	20	2	Wt. loss	Sig. in TPN group	N.D.
Starker	59	5–42	>10% wt. loss	12.5 vs. 45[a]	0 vs. 10[a]
Foshi	64	20	N.D.	18 vs. 47	3.5 vs. 12.5
Bellantone et al.	100	7	N.D.	5.3 vs. 22	5.3 vs. 6.6

[a] In those patients who received prolonged TPN.
TPN, Total parenteral nutrition; ND, not determined.
(Modified from Redmond HP, Daly JM. Preoperative nutritional therapy in cancer patients is beneficial. In: Simmons R, ed. *Debates in clinical surgery*. Chicago: Mosby–Year Book, 1991.)

The feeding regimen selected depends on the patient's nutritional status, the integrity of gastrointestinal function, and the type and magnitude of proposed treatment. If the patient cannot meet his or her daily nutritional requirements by voluntary oral ingestion of food, the first step in nutritional support should be oral nutrient supplementation and intensive dietary counseling. The patient who exhibits a moderate to severe degree of protein-calorie malnutrition by definition has failed to maintain himself or herself with spontaneous oral nutrient intake and must receive supplementation by an additional route and regimen of nutrition. A functional gastrointestinal tract is the best means to ensure normal digestion and assimilation of food, but the enteral route may be contraindicated by malabsorption, intestinal obstruction, upper gastrointestinal bleeding, or intractable vomiting or diarrhea. If the gastrointestinal tract is unavailable for use, intravenous nutritional support should be initiated. However, routine preoperative nutritional intervention has not been shown to diminish postoperative complications and may increase infectious complications. Thus, it should be reserved for the severely malnourished patient (Table 252.2).

After major elective operations, wound infection rates have varied from 0.5% to 40%, depending on whether the procedure was clean or contaminated (Table 252.3). Besides the added morbidity and potential mortality, surgical infection increases the average duration of hospitalization, resulting in a large increase in hospital costs. Resistance to infection (immune function), the quantity and virulence of invading bacteria, obesity, steroid usage, and the duration of the operation are major factors determining the probability of wound infection. Local wound resistance is aided by good surgical technique: gentle tissue handling, adequate hemostasis, debridement of dead tissue, good blood supply, avoidance of hematoma, and closure of the wound without tension.

The use of perioperative antibiotics to reduce infectious complications after surgery requires an understanding of the potential for encountering a contaminated viscus, the bacteriology of the contaminant, and the patient's immunity. When antibiotics are selected, the following guidelines are applied: antibiotics should be administered to allow adequate antibiotic levels in the wound before contamination; they should be administered for only a short time during the perioperative period; they should be specific for the most likely infecting organism; and they should be safe (Table 252.3).

GOALS IN SURGICAL INTERVENTION

The intent of operative intervention is to resect the tumor, to provide tissue for diagnosis and complete staging, or to palliate symptoms. A decision for curative operation presupposes that the tumor is localized or confined regionally, that the area of the tumor can be encompassed by regional excision, that distant metastases cannot be documented, and that the tumor is appropriately treated by operation. If a curative operation is selected, the extent of the surgical procedure must then be defined. In principle, an en bloc resection should be performed, encompassing the primary tumor, regional lymph nodes, and intervening

TABLE 252.3.	OPERATIVE SITES: INCIDENCE OF POSTOPERATIVE INFECTIONS AT THE OPERATIVE AREAS		
Operation	**Incidence (%)**	**Type of Infection**	**Major Pathogens**
Intradural craniotomy	4–8	Wound	*Staphylococcus aureus*
	0.5–1	Meningitis/abscess	Gram-negative
Head and neck	15–40	Wound	*S. aureus*, gram-negative anaerobes
Pulmonary	0.5–6	Wound	*S. aureus*
	1–2	Empyema	Gram-negative aerobes
Laparotomy	2–4	Wound	Anaerobes, gram-negative
Gastric resection	5–10	Wound	*Streptococcus*, anaerobes
Biliary tract	3–10	Wound	Gram-negative enterococci, clostridia
Colon resection	8–40	Wound	Anaerobes
	2–10	Abdominal abscess	Gram-negative aerobes
Mastectomy	1–3	Wound	*S. aureus*, gram-negative aerobes

From Bartlett JG. Choosing and using antibiotics. In: London RE, Decoste JJ, eds. *Surgical care.* Philadelphia: Lea & Febiger, 1980.

lymphatic channels. Perhaps this principle is best illustrated by operations for large bowel cancer, in which the regional lymphatics of the intra-abdominal colon course in one direction with the major arteries and veins.

Surgical resectability is determined by the tumor's relation to vital anatomical structures. Preoperative radiologic assessment is essential in defining the anatomy to guide the operative approach. For example, preoperative duplex ultrasonography and helical CT scanning have been invaluable in accurately defining the anatomical location, the number of tumors, and the relation of the tumor to the major vessels for resection of hepatic malignancies. Helical CT and endoscopic ultrasonography are highly accurate in defining the anatomy of pancreatic cancers. Intraoperative ultrasonography is now widely used to determine the resectability of hepatic and pancreatic tumors. PET scanning is quite sensitive for whole-body evaluation of the presence or absence of metastatic disease for many solid tumors. Laparoscopy has emerged as a powerful diagnostic as well as a therapeutic technique for the assessment of intra-abdominal solid tumors. These imaging techniques are extremely helpful in determining resectability or guiding resection, but often resectability is determined by careful surgical exploration.

The extent of resection is determined by the biology of the tumor, anatomy, and the patient's overall medical condition. Improved survival has been described for tumors of the esophagus, lung, and stomach with the addition of radical lymphadenectomy. Diminished local recurrence has been reported for rectal cancer after total mesorectal excision. However, a trend toward less radical surgical procedures is emerging. For example, wide local excision is preferred over limb amputation for extremity sarcomas. The technique of transanal excision or low anterior resection with coloanal anastomosis with or without chemoradiation for rectal cancer has increased sphincter preservation. Survival after segmental breast resection (lumpectomy) with axillary dissection and radiation therapy is comparable to that for modified radical mastectomy for stage I and II breast cancers. A recent prospective randomized trial from Denmark failed to demonstrate improved survival following extended lymphadenectomy

for stomach cancer. These results are in contrast to those reported in Japan.

Further attempts to limit patient morbidity by less radical surgical procedures have been incorporated in techniques to identify sentinel lymph nodes, the immediate draining nodes, with intraoperative radionuclide and dye lymphatic mapping. In 1990, Morton and colleagues first introduced the concept of lymphatic mapping and sentinel lymph node identification to select patients for radical lymphadenectomy for stage I malignant melanoma. Utilizing both dye and radionuclide, Morton was able to identify the sentinel lymph node in most patients (98%) with melanoma. Only patients with occult lymph node metastasis underwent complete lymph node dissection. Recent data from other investigators suggest that only patients with a positive sentinel lymph node or clinically palpable lymphadenopathy will benefit from a complete lymphadenectomy for malignant melanoma. The National Adjuvant Surgical Breast Project (NSABP) has recently initiated a large study evaluating the role of sentinel node sampling for patients with breast cancer (NSABP-B32). Other investigators are studying intraoperative lymph node mapping for squamous cell cancers of the head and neck, thyroid cancer, gastrointestinal and gynecologic malignancies. The role of intraoperative lymph node mapping for these diseases has not been defined.

The therapeutic value of regional node dissection has been questioned by some, but performed properly it may establish the data base for precise staging, which may require other adjuvant treatments. The extent of an operation may relate to the presence of additional precancerous lesions and genetics. For example, in a patient with familial polyposis coli or chronic and active ulcerative colitis (after 10 years), total proctocolectomy is recommended to prevent cancer of the colon. Finally, operability and treatment decisions must take into account the patient's medical status and ability to tolerate the proposed operation. Assessment of cardiopulmonary status, hepatic and renal function, and nutritional status is vital to proper determination of operative risk.

In various settings, operative intervention is used for palliative treatment. Bypasses are performed around obstructed viscera, e.g., gastrojejunostomy for obstructing carcinomas of the stomach, choledochoduodenostomy or choledochojejunostomy for a carcinoma of the pancreas obstructing the common bile duct, or nephrostomy for an obstructed ureter. Plastic Celestin tubes may be inserted through an obstructing esophageal carcinoma; colon diversion may be performed for obstructing large-bowel cancer. Transanal fulguration of an obstructing rectal tumor may provide adequate palliation for a debilitated patient.

The surgical oncologist must also be prepared to treat complications of radiation therapy or chemotherapy. Complications of radiation therapy, which occur infrequently, may include skin breakdown, intestinal fistulas, intestinal obstruction, and perforation. Radiation therapy as an adjunct in the management of gynecologic and urologic cancer may result in bladder and rectal injuries weeks to years after treatment. Ansline and associates reported 104 patients with radiation injury of the rectum; 50 patients required surgery for proctitis unresponsive to conservative measures ($n = 14$), rectal stricture or fistula ($n = 32$), or rectosigmoid perforation ($n = 4$). Diversion was considered the safest form of treatment for rectovaginal fistulas, rectal strictures, and proctitis; intestinal resection resulted in increased morbidity and mortality. Intestinal bypass or diversion is the safest approach to bowel obstruction or intestinal fistulas secondary to the late effects of pelvic irradiation. Diabetes mellitus, hypertension, and previous abdominal surgery predispose the bowel to radiation injury.

The surgeon is often called on to perform surgery on a patient who has been treated with radiation therapy or chemotherapy. Relatively small amounts of radiation therapy have no impact on the nature or extent of operation. More extensive amounts, such as 40 to 50 Gy over 5 weeks in the preoperative treatment of sarcomas or breast or rectal cancer, may require a delay of 4 to 6 weeks to allow resolution of skin erythema and tissue edema, and to obtain maximal tumoricidal effect. At the same time, operative risk is greater. Radiation may diminish local blood flow and tissue perfusion affecting subsequent wound healing. The risk of an anastomotic disruption may be sufficiently high in the setting of extensive preoperative radiation therapy to require a temporary proximal colostomy. It may also be necessary to apply reinforcement to a wound closure. The concurrent application of radiomimetic drugs, such as doxorubicin and actinomycin D, will augment the adverse side effects of radiation therapy to multiple tissues.

The surgeon may have to deal with the complications of chemotherapy. Patients with gastrointestinal lymphomas may perforate during radiation therapy or chemotherapy and thus require operative intervention. Patients undergoing chemotherapy may develop gastroenteritis or discrete ulcers leading to bowel perforation or bleeding, thus requiring surgical intervention. In the presence of perforation in a hematopoietically depressed patient, exclusion of the perforated intestine may provide a better chance for survival than resection and anastomosis.

Chemotherapy may inhibit wound healing, resulting in increased complications. Devereux and colleagues found significant impairment in wound healing when doxorubicin was given in the perioperative period (day 7 before surgery to day 3 after surgery). Corticosteroids, vincristine, methotrexate, actinomycin D, bleomycin, carmustine, and cyclophosphamide have also been shown to be deleterious in animal studies on wound healing.

The surgeon and the medical oncologist collaborate in regional chemotherapy in several areas. Cannulation of the gastroduodenal artery can be performed for chronic infusion of the hepatic artery with chemotherapeutic drugs for patients with hepatic metastases, particularly from large-bowel cancer. Hyperthermic limb perfusion in patients with melanoma or soft-tissue sarcoma has excellent results for patients with extensive tumors using combinations of cytokines (e.g., tumor necrosis factor) and chemotherapy.

Direct surgical interaction with radiation therapists includes the application of interstitial therapy (brachytherapy) by implanting radioactive isotopes or afterloading catheters in patients with lung and rectal cancer or after dissection for large, high-grade, soft-tissue sarcoma. Another area of growing interest is the application of intraoperative radiation therapy through the exposure of sites at operation, permitting direct contact of radiation at the desired tumor sites without the need for penetration of intervening skin, soft tissue, and viscera. Neuropathy remains the greatest morbidity factor associated with this method.

The surgical oncologist is responsible for the initial diagnosis and management of patients with various neoplasms. Accurate diagnosis and complete staging are coupled with adequate en bloc operative removal of localized disease. The surgical oncologist's role varies with the type of cancer (curative, palliative, staging) and should be integrated into a multimodal approach.

BIBLIOGRAPHY

Bilchik AJ, Giuliano A, Essner R, et al. Universal application of intraoperative lymphatic mapping and sentinel lymphadenectomy in solid neoplasms. *Cancer J Sci Am* 1998;4:351–358.

Botet JF, Lightdale CJ, Zauber AG, et al. Preoperative staging of gastric cancer: comparison of endoscopic ultrasonography and dynamic CT. *Radiology* 1991;181:426–432.

Conti PS, Lilien DL, Hawley K, et el. PET and 18F-FDG in oncology: A clinical update. *Nucl Med Biol* 1996;23:717–735.

Enker WE, Heilweil ML, Hertz REL, et al. En bloc pelvic lymphadenectomy and sphincter preservation in the surgical management of rectal cancer. *Ann Surg* 1986;203:426–433.

Fisher B, Redmond C, Poisson R, et al. Eight-year results of a randomized clinical trial comparing total mastectomy and lumpectomy with or without irradiation in the treatment of breast cancer. *N Engl J Med* 1989;320:822–828.

Kvols LK, Brown ML, O'Connor MK. Evaluation of a radiolabelled somatostatin analog (l-123 octreotide) in the detection and localization of carcinoid and islet cell tumors. *Radiology* 1993;187:129–133.

Martin EW Jr, Minto JP, Carey LC. CEA-directed second look surgery in the asymptomatic patient after primary resection of colorectal carcinoma. *Ann Surg* 1985;202:310–317.

Moertel CG, Fleming TR, Macdonald JS, et al. An evaluation of the carcinoembryonic antigen (CEA) test for monitoring colon cancer. *JAMA* 1993;270:943–947.

Redmond HP, Daly JM. Preoperative nutritional therapy in cancer patients is beneficial. In: Simmons R, ed. *Debates in clinical surgery*. Chicago: Mosby–Year Book, 1991.

Veronesi U, Adamus J, Bandiera DC. Inefficacy of immediate node dissection in stage I melanoma of the limbs. *N Engl J Med* 1997;279:627.

Kelley's Textbook of Internal Medicine, fourth edition. Edited by H. David Humes.
Lippincott Williams & Wilkins, Philadelphia © 2000.

PRINCIPLES OF RADIATION ONCOLOGY

ALLEN S. LICHTER

Radiation treatment is one of the most widely used forms of antineoplastic therapy. Radiation can be used as a sole modality to cure many types of malignant disease, such as Hodgkin's disease or carcinoma of the cervix. It is often used in combination with organ-preserving surgery to allow curative therapy without removing an important structure; examples include lumpectomy plus radiation instead of mastectomy for breast cancer, and wide local excision plus radiation instead of amputation for soft-tissue sarcomas of the extremities. Another important use of radiation is to provide increased local/regional control after definitive surgery. This therapy is frequently applied if positive regional lymph nodes are found at surgery, such as in most head and neck cancer sites or in node-positive lung cancer. Finally, radiation is probably the most important palliative therapy for malignant disease. Patients with metastasis to bone or to brain often achieve symptomatic relief for significant periods of time after a short course of radiation.

Since the discovery of the x-ray a century ago, there has been substantial progress in our understanding of the biologic and physical basis of radiation therapy and in the sophistication with which radiation can be applied in the treatment of malignant disease. This chapter will briefly summarize these areas.

■ PHYSICAL BASIS OF RADIATION THERAPY

X-rays are a short-wavelength, deeply penetrating form of energy. They are part of a continuum of waveform energy called the electromagnetic spectrum, which spans an extremely broad area from long-wavelength, low-energy waves, such as radio waves, to deeply penetrating, extremely short-wavelength energy such as cosmic rays. Therapeutic radiation can be derived from two sources: the decay of radioactive elements, called radionuclides, which can be naturally occurring or synthesized in nuclear reactors (these rays are often referred to as gamma rays); and x-ray generating equipment.

Radionuclides have played an important role in the treatment of cancer with radiation. Among the first therapeutic uses of radiation therapy was the direct application of the radioactive element radium directly onto superficial skin and lip cancers. Most of these radioactive materials are formed into small pellets or seeds that can be inserted directly into the tumor as part of an operative procedure. However, two radioactive materials are used in a somewhat different fashion.

Iodine 131 is commonly administered orally to patients with functioning thyroid malignancies. The malignant cells (as well as the normal cells) take up the radioactive iodine and are destroyed. This renders the patient hypothyroid and necessitates permanent thyroid replacement, but it is extremely effective and relatively nontoxic in its ability to control thyroid malignancies permanently.

Cobalt 60 is a radionuclide that produces a very energetic γ-ray. Cobalt has been used since the mid-1950s in machines designed to treat the patient with externally administered radiation. Due to the high energy of the cobalt γ-ray, deep-seated tumors could be safely treated, a distinct advantage over the low-energy x-ray generators of the time. Cobalt machines became the dominant form of external radiation treatment in the 1960s and continue to play a role in radiation therapy today.

However, the cobalt machine has largely been replaced by a synthetic x-ray generating device, the linear accelerator. From the initial discovery of the x-ray, production of these rays has involved accelerating an electron to high speed and allowing it to strike a target. There it is rapidly stopped and its kinetic energy is rapidly dissipated, mostly as heat but partially as the waveform we call an x-ray. Linear accelerators produce very high-energy x-rays but are small enough to be housed in a limited space (Fig. 253.1).

A cobalt machine produces a γ-ray of about 1.25 MeV (1 eV is the energy acquired by an electron as it passes from a negatively charged to a positively charged plate across a potential of 1 V). Low-energy linear accelerators produce x-rays in the range of 4 to 6 MeV, and high-energy accelerators produce 10- to 25-MeV x-rays. Other advantages that linear accelerators have over the older cobalt machines include the following:

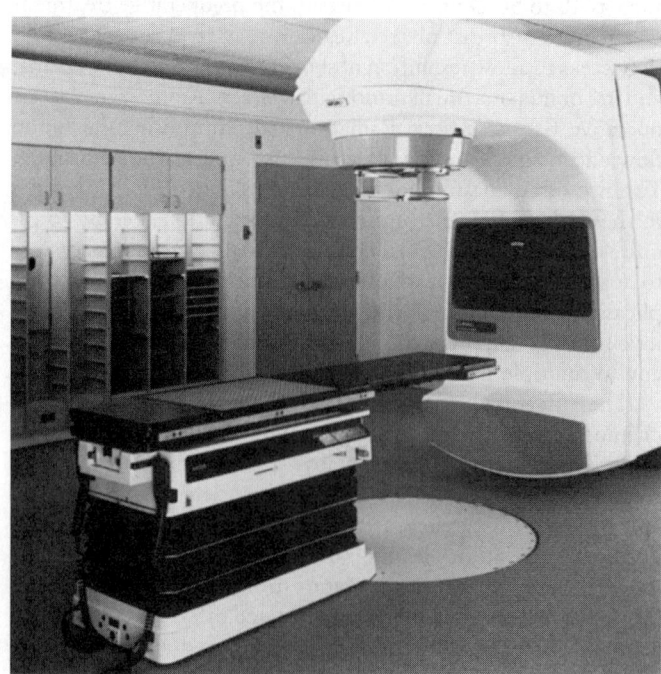

FIGURE 253.1. A modern linear accelerator. The patient lies on the rigid couch and the beam is directed precisely to treat the region of interest. The machine is capable of rotating 360 degrees around the patient so that treatment can be delivered from numerous cross-firing directions. (Photo courtesy of Varian Associates.)

1. The edges of the beam are much sharper than in a cobalt machine. This allows improved treatment precision, which is especially important when tumors lie very close to sensitive structures.
2. The target of a linear accelerator can be removed and the energetic electrons can be allowed to emerge from the machine directly. These charged particles can be used very effectively to treat superficial tumors, where a deeply penetrating beam is not necessary or desirable.
3. The amount of radiation emerging from the machine per unit of time can be varied, and extremely high dose rates can be produced. This allows effective treatment of large fields, such as those required for total body irradiation as part of bone marrow transplantation, where the patient must be a substantial distance from the machine to achieve the field size necessary. The dose rate of a cobalt machine is determined by the rate of nuclear decay of cobalt 60 (a fixed rate) and the physical amount of cobalt in the machine; there is no practical way to vary this dose rate.

For radiation to be useful in medical treatment, it must be measurable so that known amounts of radiation can be delivered from day to day, and so that one treatment center can communicate its treatment schema with another. The first unit of radiation measurement was the roentgen, abbreviated as "r." This was a unit of radiation exposure and was measured by quantifying the amount of ionization in the air produced by the radiation. The roentgen was a useful measurement unit several decades ago, but it had several major defects. It did not measure what was absorbed in the patient's tissues, only the amount of radiation present in the environment of the patient. For technical reasons, the roentgen can be measured only for relatively low energies, up to about 3 MeV. With the advent of high-energy linear accelerators, the roentgen became impractical. Finally, the roentgen is defined only for x-rays, not for particle irradiation. With the advent of electron beams and, later, many other particulate forms of radiation such as protons and neutrons, the roentgen could not be used.

In the early 1960s, a new unit that actually reflected the amount of radiation absorbed by tissue (the radiation absorbed dose) was defined and became known by its acronym, "rad." More recently, the rad has been replaced by the gray (named in honor of L. H. Gray, a British radiation biologist), which represents 100 rads. More commonly today, rads are converted to centigrays (cGy). A former prescription of 6,000 rad would now be written as 6,000 cGy, or 60 Gy.

◼ BIOLOGIC BASIS OF RADIATION THERAPY

X-rays are ionizing radiation; that is, they interact with atoms by striking an orbital electron and displacing it from the atom. The resulting atom lacks an electron for a short time and has thus been ionized. When radiation strikes biologic material, ionizations can occur anywhere within the cell, but it appears that the ionization and subsequent damage of DNA is the event that produces the biologic consequences of radiation that lead to cell death. DNA can be damaged directly by having an x-ray interact with atoms inside the DNA molecule itself. However, most of the damage to DNA appears to be indirectly mediated from the ionization of water. When a water molecule is irradiated, several highly reactive species, such as oxygen radicals, hydroxyl radicals, and aqueous electrons, are formed; these short-lived, highly reactive species can interact with the DNA molecule, damaging it.

Although DNA can be damaged in various ways (e.g., DNA/DNA cross-links, DNA–protein cross-links, base damage, single-strand DNA break), circumstantial evidence supports a specific lesion, the DNA double-strand break, as the biologically important lesion. For example, patients with ataxia telangiectasia have a very enhanced sensitivity to radiation and also have a defect in their ability to repair double-strand breaks. Radiation precisely near the nucleus of a cell results in cell death, whereas radiation to the cytoplasm has relatively little effect. The amount of DNA double-strand breaks appears to correlate very closely with cell lethality.

After DNA is damaged (by radiation or any other DNA-damaging agent, or simply by faulty replication of a DNA strand), repair enzymes in the nucleus repair the damage. Cells can efficiently, if not always faithfully, repair radiation damage. The rejoining of single-strand and double-strand breaks in DNA can be measured and appears to have a half-life of about 6 hours. If the cell has not sustained too much damage, and if the damage is repaired with acceptable fidelity, an irradiated cell can go on to function and divide, with relatively few effects from the radiation exposure. However, if the radiation damage is great and the repair is not sufficient to allow the cell to function normally, the cell generally dies. This cell death does not occur immediately but rather after one or more cell divisions (mitotic death); however, some cells die before mitosis, secondary to radiation-triggered apoptosis or programmed cell death. This latter form of radiation-induced cell death is gaining increasing attention: as the factors that influence the cells to die an apoptotic death are elucidated, experimental techniques to manipulate these factors to enhance cell death in target tissue and reduce cell death in normal structures will be applied.

When a dose of radiation is administered, both normal and malignant tissues are affected. There are few data to suggest that malignant tissue is preferentially more sensitive to radiation damage than normal tissue. The fact that radiation works to eradicate malignant populations while leaving normal tissues without permanent damage is well known but poorly understood. There may be subtle differences in the efficiency of radiation repair between normal and malignant cells that would be difficult to measure in the laboratory but clinically important over 25 or 30 daily treatment sessions. Clinically and experimentally, there are differences in radiation sensitivity among different types of malignancies. For example, melanoma and glioma cell lines appear to be much more radiation-tolerant than cell lines derived from breast or cervical cancers. The reasons for these differences are under intense radiobiologic investigation. Unraveling the factors that account for radiation resistance or sensitivity would open new avenues to improve the therapeutic gains from radiation. On the basis of our clinical experience, we have

TABLE 253.1.	RELATIVE SENSITIVITY OF CANCERS TO RADIATION TREATMENT

Sensitivity	Tumor Type
Very high	Lymphomas
	Small-cell cancers
	Seminoma
	Neuroblastoma
	Retinoblastoma
Medium	Head and neck cancer
	Breast cancer
	Lung cancer
	Gastrointestinal malignancy
	Gynecologic malignancy
	Prostate cancer
Low	Glioblastoma
	Sarcoma
	Renal cell cancer
	Melanoma

classified some tumors as relatively radiation-sensitive and others as much more difficult to cure with radiation (Table 253.1).

Along with histology, several other factors influence the effect of radiation on malignant cells. Tumor size is one of the most important factors. Microscopic disease, such as might be left behind in a surgical bed after gross total removal of a malignancy, can be controlled in 80% to 90% of cases with modest doses of radiation, typically 5,000 to 6,000 cGy. Small primary tumors can often be controlled with 6,500 to 7,000 cGy of radiation, whereas larger primary tumors are more difficult to control with doses in the 7,000-cGy region. For example, 80% to 90% of small lesions involving the true vocal cord can be cured with radiation, whereas large laryngeal cancers have only a 40% rate of local control with radiation. After wide excision of a soft-tissue sarcoma, local control can be obtained in 80% to 90% of patients with 6,000 cGy of radiation, but treating a bulky sarcoma of the same histology rarely produces local control. Thus, when possible, radiation treatment should be used with the smallest number of residual malignant cells. This can be done after surgical excision and more often is being done in combination with the cytotoxic effects of chemotherapy.

There are important effects on all normal tissues subjected to radiation exposure. Radiation effects are divided into acute effects (those occurring within 1 to 3 months after treatment) and late effects (which occur thereafter). In general, early effects are the direct result of parenchymal cell damage (e.g., loss of intestinal crypt cells in the small bowel, damage to type II pneumocytes in the lung); late effects are due to a combination of damage to parenchymal cells and longer term damage to the microvasculature, leading to late cell death and fibrosis.

Several important clinical observations can be explained by these facts. The first concerns the time course of clinical radiation effects. Because most cells die a mitotic death and many radiation effects are due to direct parenchymal cell damage, the speed at which tissues manifest clinical radiation damage should be in direct proportion to their rate of cell turnover; in fact, this is the case. Rapidly dividing tissues, such as the small intestine,

oral mucosa, and skin, show clinical radiation effects 2 to 3 weeks after the beginning of a course of radiation. Slowly dividing tissues, such as bone or brain, exhibit few if any acute effects and manifest their radiation damage months to years after a radiation exposure.

Another important clinical correlate is the potential dissociation between acute and late effects. Because parenchymal cell damage dominates the acute effects and vascular damage is a key component of late effects, there may be little correlation between early and late damage. Thus, a patient who has a very easy time getting through the treatment course may end up with severe radiation damage later, whereas a patient who has a very difficult time with acute symptoms may heal those injuries and never manifest further toxicity. The acute radiation effects to organs are listed in Table 253.2, and the long-term radiation tolerance of normal tissues is summarized in Table 253.3.

It would be ideal to manipulate the sensitivity of malignant and normal tissue to enhance the therapeutic benefit of radiation. Thus, over the past two decades, physical or chemical agents that purport to have radiation-sensitizing or protecting properties have been tested. Among these are radiation-sensitizing agents such as hypoxic cell sensitizers, DNA incorporation agents, and hyperthermia; the protective agent ethiofos has also been the subject of clinical trials. In general, these agents work extremely well in the laboratory, and the biologic basis for classifying them as radiation-sensitizing or protecting agents is incontrovertible. However, it has been extremely difficult to show that these agents improve the clinical outcome of a course of radiation. It is unknown as to whether the type of resistance or sensitivity that these cells overcome is not terribly important in the clinical environment, or whether these agents simply have not been applied in the proper dose or scheduling sequence with

TABLE 253.2.	ACUTE EFFECTS OF RADIATION[a]

Site	Symptom	Typical Onset[b]
Bladder	Dysuria frequency	2–4 wk
Bone marrow	Various cytopenias predominantly thrombocytopenia and leukopenia	1–3 wk
Esophagus	Dysphagia	2–3 wk
Heart	Acute pericarditis	3–6 mo
Liver	Radiation hepatitis	3–6 mo
Lung	Radiation pneumonitis	3–6 mo
Oral mucosa	Mucositis	2–3 wk
Rectum	Tenesmus	2–4 wk
Skin	Erythema desquamation	2–4 wk
Small intestine and stomach	Diarrhea	2–3 wk
	Nausea, vomiting	Hours/days
Systemic effects	Fatigue, lethargy	2–4 wk

[a] Effects are volume dependent: the greater the volume of an organ treated, the greater the chance that symptoms will be seen.
[b] After start of radiation.

| TABLE 253.3. | TOLERANCE OF NORMAL TISSUES TO RADIATION[a] (TREATMENT OF ENTIRE ORGAN) |

Organ	Dose-Limiting Toxicity	Radiation Dose (cGy)
Bladder	Contracture	6,500
Brain	Necrosis	6,000
Eye	Cataract	1,000
	Retinal injury	5,000
Esophagus	Stricture	6,000–6,500
Heart	Peri-paracarditis	4,500
Kidney	Nephritis	2,000
Liver	Hepatitis	3,000
Lung	Pneumonitis	2,000 (one lung)
Ovary	Menopause	500–1,000
Pituitary	Hypopituitarism	4,500
Rectum	Bleeding	6,500
Salivary gland	Xerostomia	3,000–4,000
Skin	Necrosis	6,000–6,500 (10 × 10 cm)
Stomach	Bleeding/ulceration	5,000
Spinal cord	Paralysis	5,000 (5-cm segment)
Testes	Azospermia	200–400
Thyroid	Hypothyroidism	4,500

[a] Approximately 5% chance of complication; treatment at 200 cGy/dose.

when applied along with radiation, the curability of various neoplasms has been enhanced. For example, radiation plus chemotherapy is much more effective in the curative treatment of esophageal carcinoma than radiation alone. Bladder cancers can be controlled more often with combined chemotherapy and radiation than with radiation alone. Anal carcinoma has effectively been cured with combinations of chemotherapy and radiation without the need for abdominoperineal resection. In randomized clinical trials, unresectable lung cancer and advanced cervical cancer have been more effectively treated with combined chemotherapy and radiation than with radiation alone.

The reason for the enhanced effectiveness of combined chemotherapy and radiation remains speculative. It could be simply a case of additive cell killing, with radiation destroying some of the cells and chemotherapy destroying others. There could be some measure of radiation sensitization involved; in other words, the chemotherapy could enhance the cytotoxicity of the radiation. Whatever the mechanism, it is increasingly common for radiation therapy to be combined with chemotherapy in the curative treatment of malignant disease.

CLINICAL APPLICATION OF RADIATION THERAPY

Radiation treatment for malignant disease begins with treatment planning. Once the decision to treat with radiation therapy is made, the patient usually begins the treatment planning process on a machine called a simulator. This machine has the exact geometry of a high-energy linear accelerator but produces diagnostic intensity x-rays and usually has fluoroscopy capabilities as well. The patient is positioned on the simulator table and the area that requires radiation is aligned in a simulated radiation field. One can then confirm immediately by fluoroscopy and

radiation. Much clinical research continues using these compounds, and further results can be expected in the next few years.

The cytotoxic chemotherapeutic agents have been successfully used to modify a course of radiation. Many of the commonly used drugs, especially cisplatin, 5-fluorouracil, and gemcitabine, are clearly radiation sensitizers in the laboratory, and

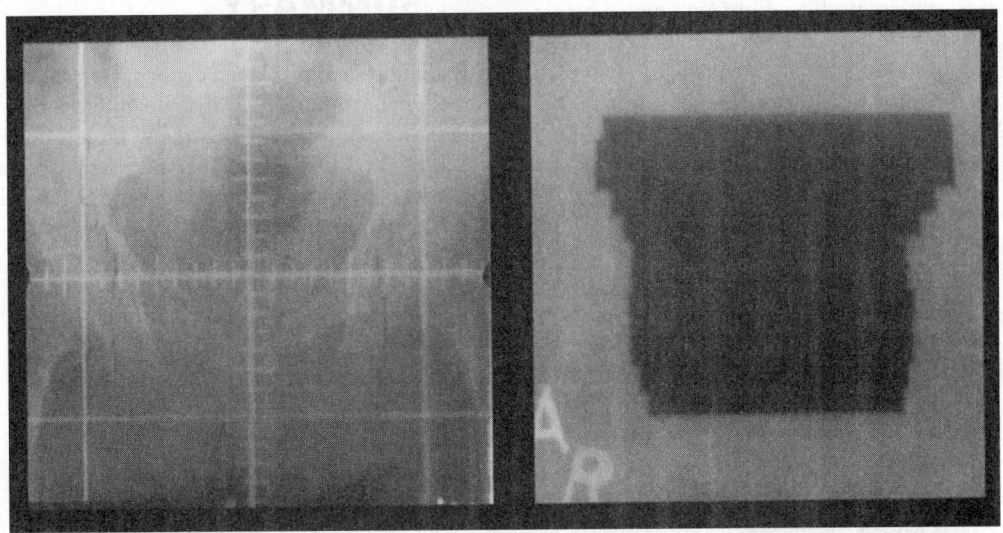

FIGURE 253.2. A simulation and port film for the treatment of a pelvic malignancy. The simulator film *(left)* shows the bony anatomy in detail. The small hash marks are a 1-cm scale. The hash marks cross at the center of the radiation field. The port film *(right)* shows less bony detail because it is taken with high-energy photons while the patient is on the linear accelerator table. However, the location of the field center *(dots)* and the field borders can be seen easily. The two films can be compared to ensure that the treatment is being carried out as desired.

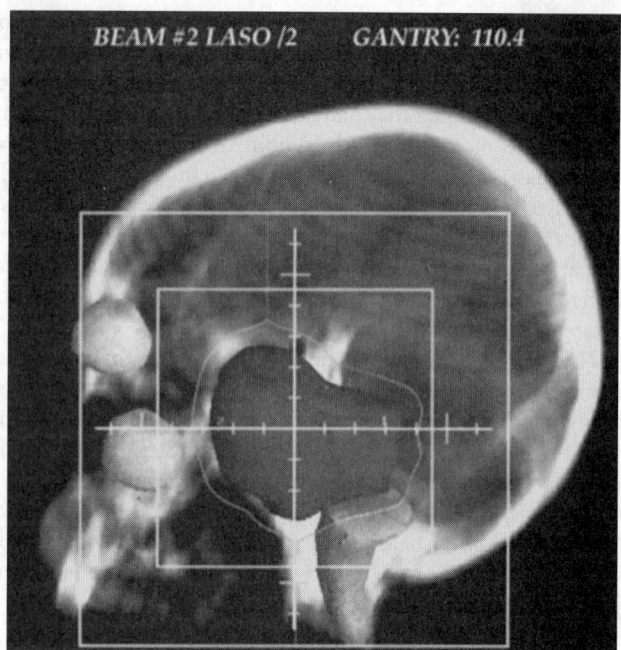

BEAM #2 LASO /2   GANTRY: 110.4

FIGURE 253.3. Computed tomographic scan information can be reformatted into useful three-dimensional images. In this case, a brain tumor is visualized lying directly superior to the brain stem. The eyes are on the left side of the figure. The target volume is represented by the large structure in the center of the cross-hairs. A shielding block has been drawn around the target to help protect the eyes and the brain stem from excessive radiation while exposing the target to full dose.

ultimately by simulator x-rays that the intended target region is within the radiation volume. Once the films of the treatment fields are taken, the radiation oncologist can further shape the field by indicating which areas of normal tissue should be further protected; these marks are then translated into custom-shaped lead blocks that can create the desired radiation aperture. Once the patient is on the treatment machine, films are exposed before the radiation treatment with the field-shaping blocks in place. This allows direct confirmation that the intended radiation plan is being delivered on the linear accelerator with appropriate precision (Fig. 253.2).

More sophisticated treatment planning is done with the aid of computed tomography (CT) and three-dimensional recon-

struction of the patient's anatomy. The process once again begins on the simulator, and the region to be treated is again marked out. The patient is then taken to the CT scanner, where multiple cross-sectional images are taken from several centimeters above to several centimeters below the intended region of treatment. These CT scans are then loaded into the treatment planning computer, and various normal tissues (e.g., external skin, lung, spinal cord, kidneys, liver) are outlined on a slice-by-slice basis. The area to be targeted with radiation is also indicated on each slice. Using relatively straightforward graphics techniques, three-dimensional renderings of the anatomical structures stacked one on another can be quickly made and viewed from any angle (Fig. 253.3). While the patient is comfortably at home, the appropriate beams can be placed onto the patient's anatomy and numerous combinations of fields can be tried until the appropriate plan has been created. In some respects, this is a simulation based on computer data rather than directly on the patient, and some have called it "virtual simulation." The fields to be treated are then verified on the simulator, and the accuracy of delivery is confirmed with films taken on the linear accelerator itself.

A typical course of radiation lasts 5 to 7 weeks, with treatment given daily, Monday through Friday. This fractionation of daily treatment is designed so that the normal tissues within the radiated volume can repair from one day to the next, allowing high doses of radiation to be safely administered with as few complications as possible. In some sites, especially in the head and neck, hyperfractionation (two fractions per day, ten fractions per week) has been used to spare normal tissue further, to allow higher doses of radiation to be given, and to shorten the overall time of treatment in some cases.

Radiation is used in the clinical treatment of virtually every type of tumor in the body. Table 253.4 summarizes the common types of malignancy treated with radiation.

■ SUMMARY

Radiation therapy plays a major role in the management of most malignant tumors. New insights into the biology and physics of radiation are making treatment more effective and less toxic, and hold promise for further advances. Used alone or in combination with local surgery or chemotherapy, radiation has allowed

TABLE 253.4.	**CLINICAL USES OF RADIATION IN CANCER MANAGEMENT**
Treatment	**Malignancy**
Definitive radiation	Hodgkin's, early-stage non-Hodgkin's lymphoma, gliomas, cervix, head and neck, lung, bladder, anal, esophagus, prostate, pancreas, skin, pituitary
Radiation follows organ-sparing (conservative) surgery	Breast, sarcoma, rectum
Radiation may follow radical surgery (to improve local control in selected cases)	Breast, rectum, lung, head and neck, endometrium, most margin-positive resections at many tumor sites (e.g., cervix, low-grade CNS tumors)
Palliation	All tumor types

more patients to survive their malignancy without the need for radical surgery and the removal of important structures. Progress in the use of combined-modality therapy in oncologic treatment can be anticipated.

BIBLIOGRAPHY

Baumann M, Bentzen SM, Ang KK. Hyperfractionated radiotherapy in head and neck cancer: a second look at the clinical data. *Radiother Oncol* 1998;46:127–130.

Coleman JN, Stevenson MA. Biologic basis for radiation oncology. *Oncology* 1996;10:399–411.

Lichter AS. Radiation therapy. In: Abeloff MA, Armitage JO, Lichter AS, et al., eds. *Clinical oncology*. Philadelphia: Churchill Livingstone, 2000: 423–470.

Lichter A, Lawrence T. Recent advances in radiation oncology. *N Engl J Med* 1995;332:371–379.

Mohan R, Mageras G, Wu Q. Computer-controlled delivery of 3D conformal radiation treatments. *Cancer Treat Res* 1998;93:49–67.

Schilsky RL. Biochemical pharmacology of chemotherapeutic drugs used as radiation enhancers. *Semin Oncol* 1992;19:2–7.

Stone HB, Dewey WC, Wallace SS, et al. Molecular biology to radiation oncology: a model for translational research? Opportunities in basic and translational research. From a workshop sponsored by the National Cancer Institute, Radiation Research Program, January 26–28, 1997, Bethesda MD. *Radiat Res* 1998;150:134–147.

Tannock IF. Treatment of cancer with radiation and drugs. *J Clin Oncol* 1996;14:3156–3174.

Weichselbaum RR, Hallahan DE, Sukhatme VP, et al. Gene therapy targeted by ionizing radiation. *Int J Radiat Oncol Biol Phys* 1992;24: 565–567.

Yarnold J. Molecular aspects of cellular responses to radiotherapy. *Radiother Oncol* 1997;44:1–7.

Kelley's Textbook of Internal Medicine, fourth edition. Edited by H. David Humes.
Lippincott Williams & Wilkins, Philadelphia © 2000.

C H A P T E R
254

PRINCIPLES OF CHEMOTHERAPY AND HORMONAL THERAPY

BRUCE A. CHABNER
MICHAEL SEIDEN
JEFFREY CLARK

Although it has been recognized as a disease entity for almost 200 years, cancer was not appreciated as a systemic illness until the last century, when careful pathologic examination of patients who had died of the disease disclosed the locally invasive and ultimately metastatic potential of a once-localized process. From this knowledge, surgical strategies evolved that attempted to encompass primary disease and regional lymph nodes, which were recognized as the initial site of spread. Radical surgery for colon, breast, genitourinary tumors, and soft-tissue tumors proved suc-cessful in establishing local control in most patients and cure in a smaller percentage of patients. Radiation therapy proved able to add to the cure rate for lymphomas and tumors of the head and neck and uterus. By the 1960s, about one-third of cancer patients could be rendered free of disease by these local treatment modalities. However, for the remaining two-thirds of patients with cancer, local therapies were unable to prevent or cure metastatic disease, and not until the first testing of chemotherapy in lymphomas at Yale in 1944 and in human leukemia at Harvard in 1948 did a truly systemic approach to cancer become a reality. Treatment for cancer was changed forever by these early experiments with drugs, as clinicians readily appreciated the logic of seeking systemic therapy for what is in most patients a disseminated process. At present, with these advances in treatment and with earlier diagnosis, 60% of newly diagnosed cancer patients live at least 5 years after initial disease recognition, mortality is decreasing for most solid tumors, and many more patients are cured.

This chapter describes the general process by which oncologists, including surgeons, radiation therapists, and medical oncologists, develop a treatment plan for the cancer patient. It considers in greater detail the role of drugs in cancer treatment. The reader should consult more specialized texts for an in-depth discussion of the pharmacology of cancer drugs and specific regimens used.

◼ INITIAL EVALUATION OF THE PATIENT WITH CANCER

The optimum care of the patient with cancer requires a multidisciplinary approach, including physicians of multiple specialties as well as nurses and social workers. This team approach helps ensure the close coordination of evaluation and treatment among the pertinent specialties of surgery, radiation therapy, and medical oncology and also aims to minimize treatment-related morbidity and the physical and emotional pain and suffering associated with malignancy.

The initial evaluation must be comprehensive, logical, expeditious, and ideally cost-effective. Obviously, development of a specific evaluation plan requires in-depth knowledge of the malignancy under consideration, in particular its typical presentation and patterns of dissemination. Nevertheless, general principles are applicable to all patients under evaluation and are reviewed in Table 254.1. Once in progress, evaluations should

TABLE 254.1.	EVALUATION OF THE PATIENT WITH A SUSPECTED MALIGNANCY

Unambiguous tissue diagnosis
Appropriate staging studies
Complete evaluation for significant comorbid diseases
Social and psychological history
Assessment of performance status
Design of appropriate treatment
Assessment of eligibility for clinical trial
Rehabilitation
Pain management, psychosocial support, end-of-life care

be thorough but rapid, because they often generate considerable anxiety for the patient and family, who want to know the extent of disease and the chances for cure, and anxiously anticipate the initiation of treatment.

The most important initial step is to establish an unambiguous tissue diagnosis. Essentially, every organ of the body may give rise to either benign or malignant tumors, and the treatment and prognosis of these tumors vary dramatically. Even patients with clinical findings suggestive of metastatic disease should have appropriate biopsies to establish the primary diagnosis and confirm suspicions of dissemination. Diseases such as sarcoidosis, histiocytosis, amyloid, multifocal osteomyelitis, neurofibromatosis, mononucleosis, vitamin deficiency, osteomalacia, Paget's disease, tuberculosis, and many others can mimic the presentation of metastatic malignant diseases.

Advances in minimally invasive techniques, including fine-needle aspiration, core biopsy, endoscope-guided biopsy, CT-guided stereotactic biopsy, laporoscopy, and thoracoscopy are available to diagnose and often stage most epithelial malignancies and can be performed safely and without significant risk of tumor dissemination. In some organs, such as the kidney and testis, most solid tumors are malignant, and tumor contamination through the biopsy site is a real concern. In these situations, primary surgical excision of the affected organ may be part of the appropriate initial evaluation. Patients with suspected lymphoma should have lymph node excision for a more complete histologic evaluation, including detailed evaluation of the pattern of lymph node replacement. Patients with suspected sarcomas of either soft tissue or bone should have biopsy sites carefully planned in conjunction with a surgeon so as not to cross and contaminate future resection planes.

Once tissue is available, standard histologic techniques usually generate an unambiguous diagnosis. Inability to make a diagnosis may result from tissue sampling errors, excessive tissue necrosis, crush artifact, or the presence of inflammatory cells with only rare malignant cells. In these cases, re-biopsy is indicated. Ideally, a second biopsy may collect a larger specimen or a specimen from a second lesion or may sample a more peripheral site in the primary tumor, where there is often less necrosis. Alternatively, some tumors are so poorly differentiated that identifiable histologic structures do not allow classification of the site or cell of origin. The differential diagnosis for these tumors often includes poorly differentiated carcinoma, lymphoma, melanoma, germ cell tumors, and rarely sarcoma. Because the drug sensitivities and potential curability of these various tumors are different, further evaluation should be undertaken. In these cases, immunohistochemistry, electron microscopy, tumor cytogenetics, serum tumor markers (such as human chorionic gonadotropin [HCG] or α-fetoprotein [AFP]), or molecular analysis of tumor DNA or RNA often allows unambiguous classification (Chapters 249 through 251).

Typically, tumor staging (TNM staging) is undertaken after the initial tumor biopsy. Staging of the neoplasm serves three important functions. First, it identifies the local and regional extension of tumor as well as the presence or absence of distant metastatic disease. Treatment plans for most cancers are based on clinical stage, which is determined by the size and local extension of the primary tumor, the involvement of regional lymph nodes, and the presence of distant metastasis. Second, staging often provides critical prognostic information for both the clinical care team and the patient. An understanding of the overall risk of disease progression and the impact of specific therapy provides information for clinical decision making by the physician and patient. Finally, staging is important in clinical research, because it allows accurate comparison of the outcome of different treatment modalities.

Appropriate staging requires knowledge of typical patterns of spread for a particular malignancy. In general, most carcinomas can spread hematogenously to organs such as bone, brain, liver, and lung as well as to regional lymph nodes via lymphatics. In contrast, some lymphomas (particularly Hodgkin's disease) often remain confined to lymphatic tissue, whereas others have a predilection for bone marrow spread (follicular lymphomas) and for organ invasion (large-cell lymphomas).

It is not mandatory or appropriate to perform whole-body radiologic evaluation in all patients with cancer. Techniques such as screening mammography and serum prostate-specific antigen have allowed early diagnosis of breast cancer and prostate cancer. Very few of these patients with small-volume primary carcinomas have evidence of metastatic disease. In breast cancer patients, assessment of regional lymph node involvement by surgical sampling is usually indicated, as is a chest x-ray and bone scan. But extensive evaluation for more distant disease by CT scans, bone marrow biopsies, or other invasive procedures is usually not rewarding when no symptoms are present. Alternatively, when very aggressive local therapies are considered, such as pelvic exenteration, pancreatoduodenectomy, partial hepatectomy, or extremity amputation, the presence of distant disease outside the operative field must be carefully excluded, because this finding may nullify the benefit of radical surgery.

After the histology and staging have been completed, a specific treatment plan should be established. Developing a treatment plan requires a careful review of the patient's medical history and current non-neoplastic illness. Significant cardiac, renal, pulmonary, neurologic, or hepatic dysfunction may absolutely preclude certain types of chemotherapy or immunotherapy, may predispose to toxicity, or may necessitate dose reductions. For example, patients with ventricular dysfunction are poor candidates for treatment with anthracyclines such as doxorubicin, daunorubicin, idarubicin, or mitoxantrone. Patients with renal dysfunction should not receive full doses of nephrotoxic chemotherapy drugs, such as cisplatin, or drugs that require extensive renal excretion, such as methotrexate. Patients with pulmonary dysfunction should not be treated with bleomycin because of the possibility of enhanced pulmonary damage. Neurologic impairment, particularly significant peripheral neuropathies, can be exacerbated by treatment with paclitaxel, vinca alkaloids (e.g., vincristine, navelbine), or cisplatin.

All patients with malignancy should have a careful evaluation of areas of pain, discomfort, and decreased mobility. Such symptoms may herald threatened fracture, skeletal instability, spinal cord compression, or visceral organ compromise. Early diagnosis of these complications may permit local therapeutic intervention that will minimize future complications and maximize symptom control. Multiple techniques and medications are available to

TABLE 254.2.	**KARNOFSKY PERFORMANCE STATUS SCALE**
Functional Capability	**Level of Activity**
Able to carry on normal activity; no special care needed	100%—normal; no complaints, no evidence of disease 90%—able to carry on normal activity; minor signs or symptoms of disease 80%—normal activity with effort; some signs or symptoms of disease
Unable to work; able to live at home; cares for most personal needs; varying amount of assistance needed	70%—cares for self; unable to carry on normal activity or to do active work 60%—requires occasional assistance but is able to care for most of own needs 50%—requires considerable assistance and frequent medical care
Unable to care for self; requires equivalent of institutional or hospital care	40%—disabled; requires special medical care and assistance 30%—severely disabled; hospitalization indicated, although death not imminent 20%—very sick; hospitalization necessary; active supportive treatment necessary 10%—moribund; fatal processes progressing rapidly 0%—dead

EASTERN COOPERATIVE ONCOLOGY GROUP PERFORMANCE STATUS SCALE

Grade	Level of Activity
0	Fully active, able to carry on all predisease performance without restriction (Karnofsky 90–100%)
1	Restricted in physically strenuous activity but ambulatory and able to carry out work of a light or sedentary nature, e.g., light house work, office work (Karnofsky 70–80%)
2	Ambulatory and capable of all self-care but unable to carry out any work activities; up and about more than 50% of waking hours (Karnofsky 50–60%)
3	Capable of only limited self-care, confined to bed or chair more than 50% of waking hours (Karnofsky 30–40%)
4	Completely disabled; cannot carry on any self-care; totally confined to bed or chair (Karnofsky 10–20%)

improve and often control pain from advanced malignancy (Chapter 260).

A patient's performance status is also important in the appropriate planning of cancer therapy and correlates directly with tolerance to therapy and outcome. Assessment of performance status is based on the patient's level of function and absence of symptoms. Patients who can care for their daily needs independently, have few or no symptoms, and carry on normal work and home activity are considered to have normal performance status. Patients who cannot care for themselves, have significant symptoms related to their malignancy, or spend part of the day in bed owing to fatigue, pain, or inanition have a poorer performance status, less tolerance for surgery, irradiation, or drugs, and a poorer prognosis. Several standardized but somewhat subjective scales of performance status are available (Table 254.2). More objective criteria such as the serum albumin level may be a better measure of prognosis.

Some cancer therapies are complex, requiring significant cooperation and participation by patients, and can be challenging or impossible in the mentally or physically impaired patient. Equally important is the patient's social and psychological background. Cancer therapy can be associated with significant morbidity, symptoms that can provoke anxiety and fear of loss of control. Patients with extensive social support systems generally cope better with the morbidity and fatigue associated with cancer therapy. Other patients can benefit from referral for psychosocial evaluation and support by professional staff.

Finally, cancer care can be very expensive, especially with some of the dose-intensive chemotherapy protocols in use, and

financial costs should be considered, particularly when the chance of benefit is minimal.

GENERAL THERAPEUTIC APPROACHES

After the diagnosis of cancer has been established and the staging completed, a specific plan of treatment must be established. The plan for a patient with newly diagnosed cancer usually requires the participation of more than a single specialist, in that both local control and systemic therapy must be addressed. In recent years, there has been increasing evidence for the early, up-front use of sequences or combinations of surgery, chemotherapy, and radiation to improve local disease control and to prevent distant recurrence, even in patients with apparently localized disease. The details of optimal sequence and optimal combination differ with each type and stage of cancer, but intelligent decision making requires participation of all three specialties in the planning stage. A number of factors influence the components of the plan of treatment. The most obvious of these is the stage, which is usually based on the size and extent of local, regional, and distant spread of the tumor. However, stage is not the only determinant of therapy. The histopathologic and molecular features of the tumor may provide information on likelihood of systemic spread and responsiveness to specific forms of therapy. Thus, apparently localized breast cancers that display lymphatic or blood vessel invasion, that lack hormone receptors, or that carry an amplified HER2/*neu* oncogene have a greater propensity for systemic spread and require aggressive adjuvant chemotherapy, usually with an anthracycline-containing regimen. In contrast, an elderly patient with a small tumor that is positive for estrogen receptor may best be treated with surgical excision and the estrogen antagonist, tamoxifen. Other tumors, such as well-differentiated prostate cancers may require only local therapy or, in older patients, observation, in that they have a minimal tendency to spread to distant sites and may not affect the patient's expected life span. For some malignancies, systemic therapy is required, regardless of stage, because of their aggressive pattern of growth and dissemination. These include large-cell lymphomas, small-cell lung cancers, and most cases of ovarian cancer.

When distant spread is detected, the treatment plan may have to accommodate special measures to prevent disability and restore function. Thus, brain metastases or spinal cord compression demand immediate treatment, and skeletal metastases that threaten to lead to fracture also require aggressive local therapy, usually radiation and possibly fixation. Superior vena cava obstruction by lymphoma or small-cell carcinoma may require immediate irradiation, with concomitant chemotherapy. Endobronchial, biliary, or ureteral obstruction similarly require restoration of flow, either through stenting, irradiation, or diversion by surgical intervention. Only in the case of a highly drug-responsive tumor such as a non-Hodgkin's lymphoma will drug therapy alone relieve obstruction in most cases.

Cancer treatments should be designed to accomplish specific goals beneficial to the patient. Optimally, therapy should be directed at the complete eradication of tumor cells both at the primary site, including the contiguous regional structures, and at systemic sites. Treatments should maximize effectiveness while minimizing morbidity, including disfigurement, pain, loss of function, and short- and long-term toxicity associated with the therapy. Local control is often best achieved through either complete surgical resection of the local (primary) tumor or a combination of surgery and irradiation. Very small breast cancers are often cured with lumpectomy alone, whereas larger tumors are often more difficult to resect completely, have a higher chance for microscopic dissemination, and require lumpectomy and chest wall irradiation. Such patients also have a higher risk of progressive metastatic disease. Locally advanced tumors not amenable to initial surgical resection may be resectable after radiation therapy, chemotherapy, or both. Such combined-modality approaches are often used in large locally advanced malignancies, such as cancers of the breast, lung, head and neck, rectum, esophagus, and bladder. Reducing the size of the primary tumor through the initial use of chemotherapy and radiation therapy shows promise of allowing preservation of the larynx, bladder, and anus in patients who formerly might have been treated by organ removal.

Adjuvant chemotherapy after a definitive local procedure reduces the burden of occult metastatic disease and thereby minimizes the risk of recurrence. The actual mechanisms whereby adjuvant therapy increases the cure rate of breast and colon cancer tumors is still uncertain. Reducing the amount of microscopic metastatic disease may permit normal host defenses to eradicate the residual disease. Even when complete eradication of the microscopic disease is not feasible, reducing the burden of microscopic metastatic disease may significantly prolong the period of time that the patient is clinically asymptomatic and may extend overall survival. Over the last several decades, randomized, controlled studies of adjuvant chemotherapy have demonstrated prolongation of survival in patients with apparently localized cancer of the breast, colon, or rectum. Adjuvant therapy also has a role in a number of solid tumors in children and young adults, including Ewing's sarcoma, Wilms' tumor, osteosarcoma, and neuroblastoma.

In patients with metastatic disease, local control remains an important goal, particularly if the primary tumor causes significant morbidity or loss of function (e.g., pain, obstruction). Even if curative therapy is unavailable, palliation is appropriate if the therapy prolongs survival, reduces pain or suffering, or delays a catastrophic complication of advancing malignancy (e.g., spinal cord compression, tracheoesophageal fistula, bowel obstruction).

Once a realistic goal is selected, the cancer care team must select the modalities most likely to achieve the desired outcome. When cure is impossible, the physician must weigh the likely benefit of therapy against its anticipated toxicity. For instance, very aggressive and toxic therapies may not be appropriate unless these measures are likely to provide symptomatic relief and alter the progression of disease in a positive manner.

Patients should be given the appropriate information to allow them to make an informed decision regarding their treatment options. This discussion should include information on prognosis and the benefits and toxicity associated with the recommended therapy. If other reasonable treatments are available, these should be discussed, too.

Special attention should be given to participation in clinical trials. Patients participating in studies designed to compare the relative efficacy of two therapies (phase III trials), the efficacy of new therapy (phase II trial), or the toxicity and efficacy of a new drug or biologic agent (phase I trial) should have a clear understanding of the purpose of the trial and the anticipated benefit and potential hazards of the proposed treatment.

■ PRINCIPLES OF CANCER CHEMOTHERAPY

Fundamental to the treatment of cancer is the understanding that qualitative and quantitative changes in the regulation of tumor growth cause malignancy. These changes occur as the result of genetic changes either inherited or resulting from environmental exposures, viruses, or more rarely chronic inflammation. Genetic damage may cause a loss of cell-cycle controls (*p53* mutation), a decreased ability to repair DNA damage (*BRCA-1* mutation), or a decreased ability to undergo apoptosis or programmed cell death (*bcl-2* activation). Cancer cells are distinguished by their ability for unrestrained growth, invasiveness, and metastasis. Initial attempts to treat cancer have been primarily directed at unrestrained growth and more specifically at the synthesis of DNA. However in recent years the biotechnology industry has targeted its efforts at the various factors that regulate proliferation, including growth factors and their receptors, and signal transduction pathways, as well as properties such as invasiveness, metastasis, and angiogenesis.

Cell growth and division in both normal and malignant cells

are accomplished by progression through the cell cycle. Cells in mature organs such as liver, brain, and pancreas spend most of their life cycle in the interphase or resting phase (also termed the G0 and G1 portions) of the cell cycle, which precedes DNA synthesis (S phase) and cell division (M phase). The precise signals that initiate cell division differ among different cells types, but both autocrine and paracrine growth factors are believed to initiate the transition from the resting phase into a phase of DNA synthesis and cell division. A cascade of biochemical changes is associated with progression through the cell cycle. These signals for proliferation may include autocrine growth factors, growth factors produced by neighboring cells (paracrine factors such as fibroblast growth factor or interleukins secreted by stromal cells or immune cells), or signals transmitted by cell-to-cell contact (adhesion molecules). Central to this progression is a collection of proteins named cell cycle–dependent kinases and their activators and inhibitors. Specific activators of these kinases, called cyclins, initiate cell movement through critical checkpoints at the G1/S and G2/M interface.

The best-known checkpoint is the p53 protein, which monitors the integrity of DNA and directs the process of DNA repair and, if DNA damage is too severe, promotes apoptosis or cell death. In normal cells, DNA synthesis is allowed to proceed only if the genome is intact and undamaged. Proteins that monitor DNA integrity and prevent the replication of damaged cells have been identified, and mutations of proteins such as p53 have been implicated as leading to genetic instability and cancer. Likewise, increased synthesis of cyclins and loss of the CDK4 inhibitor, p16, are common mutations associated with cancer.

Initial attempts to treat cancer have focused on the property of unrestrained proliferation. Through animal tumor screening, drugs capable of selectively killing tumor cells have been identified, although the basis for selectivity is incompletely understood. Drugs targeting DNA synthesis in general prove most effective against rapidly growing tumors, which logically spend more of their time in DNA synthesis. For many of these drugs, tumor cell kill is a function of the concentration of drug in plasma (C) and the duration of that cytotoxic concentration (T). For many DNA-interactive drugs, such as the anthracyclines, etoposide, antimetabolites, and carboplatin, C × T, the integral of the drug concentration versus time curve, correlates well with cytotoxicity, probably because for most cancer drugs the longer a cytotoxic concentration can be maintained, the greater the number of cells exposed to drug during their most vulnerable phase (S phase) of the cell cycle (Fig. 254.1). For others, including taxanes, toxicity is a direct function of duration of exposure above the threshold for cytotoxicity. For alkylating agents, which interact chemically with sites on DNA, drug dose and peak plasma concentration, and not duration of exposure, determine cell kill.

For drugs that cause DNA breaks or miscoding, cytotoxicity may result from either the initiation of the apoptotic pathway (programmed cell death) or, with more extensive cell damage, necrosis. Laboratory and clinical studies indicate that the presence of a functional p53 checkpoint is critical to the initiation of apoptosis in response to DNA damage due to irradiation, alkylating agents, and antimetabolites. Unfortunately, p53 is deleted or mutated in many human tumors, particularly during

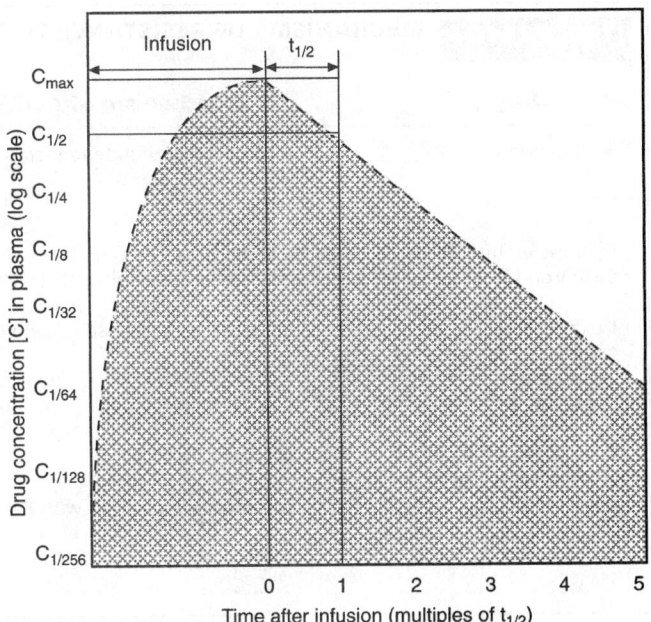

FIGURE 254.1. Hypothetical curve of logarithm of drug concentration versus time, where units of time are equal to the half-time ($t\frac{1}{2}$) for drug disappearance from plasma. Overall drug exposure, often expressed as the area under the C × T curve (AUC), equals the integral or space of the hatched area. C_{max}, the maximum concentration in plasma, is directly related to the infusion rate and inversely related to the $t\frac{1}{2}$ or rate of elimination of drug from plasma.

their late stages of growth, possibly contributing to treatment failure.

The growth characteristics of solid tumors change during tumor expansion. The most rapid growth occurs when tumors are relatively small and when the blood supply and nutrients are adequate. With further expansion, tumors must stimulate new blood vessel growth and often outgrow their existing blood supply, leading to a slowing of cell growth, tumor hypoxia, and even necrosis. Thus, the tumor cell growth characteristics vary with time and, at any instant in time, vary in different locations. In addition, tumors become increasingly heterogeneous as mutations occur over time; each metastasis, for example, represents a new clone of tumor cells, with altered growth characteristics, potential for survival, and drug sensitivity. Thus, it seems logical to initiate therapy as early as possible in the natural history of tumor development, as in the adjuvant setting to lessen the chance of encountering drug-resistant disease.

MECHANISMS OF DRUG RESISTANCE

The mutability of tumor cells, a central property of cancer, allows for diversity of phenotype and leads to the unique properties of these cells: invasiveness, metastasis, production of autocrine and paracrine growth factors, and the emergence of drug resistance. Indeed, the same biologic features that allow unrestrained growth and inhibit apoptosis—namely, loss of cell cycle checkpoints—also lead to drug resistance. Thus, biologic resistance

TABLE 254.3.	MECHANISMS OF RESISTANCE TO REPRESENTATIVE ANTICANCER DRUGS

Drug	Mechanism of Action	Mechanism of Resistance
Methotrexate (MTX)	Inhibits dihydrofolate reductase (DHFR)	Amplification of DHRF Mutation of DHFR Decreased transport of reduced folates Decreased polyglutamation (MTX)
Cytosine arabinoside	Inhibits DNA elongation	Decreased activation by deoxycytidine kinase
5-Fluorouracil	Inhibits thymidylate synthase (TS)	Decreased drug activation Increased TS activity
Doxorubicin	Inhibits topoisomerase II (topo II)	Decreased or mutated topo II Increased export due to *mdr* or *mrp* gene products
Topotecan	Inhibits topoisomerase I (topo I)	Decreased mutated topo I
Paclitaxel	Promotes polymerization of tubulin	Tubulin mutation decreases drug binding Increased export due to *mdr* gene product
Cyclophosphamide	Alkylates DNA	Increased DNA repair of alkylation Decreased apoptosis (p53 mutation)
Cisplatin	Forms covalent adduct with DNA	Increased repair of adduct Inactivation of drug by glutathione Decreased apoptosis (p53 mutation)

to drug therapy in many solid tumors and leukemias, is associated with mutation of the *p53* suppressor gene and with the overexpression of *bcl-2*, an antiapoptotic gene translocated in follicular cell lymphomas. In addition to these biologic resistance factors, other features of the tumor cell environment, such as increased interstitial fluid pressure, hypoxia, and poor perfusion, limit drug access and decrease response.

The high rate of spontaneous mutations also results in genetic changes that alter the specific target proteins against which cancer drugs act, thus providing a survival advantage for a particular tumor cell (Table 254.3). For example, methotrexate inhibits the enzyme dihydrofolate reductase, which is responsible for maintaining intracellular folic acid in its active and fully reduced form. If sensitive tumor cells are incubated with methotrexate over several generations, resistant sublines grow out, which contain alterations in the structure or levels of expression of dihydrofolate reductase. Resistant cells may also arise as the result of mutations that decrease the transmembrane uptake of the drug or its conversion to its long-lived polyglutamate form. Examples of these defects have been found in methotrexate-resistant tumor cells from patients treated with this drug.

Although the above alterations in methotrexate-resistant tumor cells have no impact on response to other agents, mutations induced by other drugs may confer broad patterns of drug resistance. For example, the multidrug-resistance gene (*mdr-1*) encodes a membrane glycoprotein, p170, which exports complex molecules across the cell membrane and increases resistance to various natural product drugs, including the vinca alkaloids, anthracyclines, and etoposide. Increased p170 expression is characteristic of many epithelial tumors, including lung, kidney, and colon cancers, and is also found in many patients with refractory forms of leukemia or lymphoma. Similar drug-exporting proteins encoded by the *mrp* gene and *bcrp* gene have been identified in human tumors and confer resistance to natural products such as anthracyclines. Patterns of drug cross-resistance and the likelihood of p170 expression in specific tumors are critical factors

in selecting new drugs for clinical development and in the design of combination chemotherapy regimens.

CHEMOTHERAPEUTICS

The drugs in use for cancer treatment, except for hormonal agents, have a narrow therapeutic index. The maximally effective conventional doses produce toxicity (primarily to gastrointestinal epithelium and bone marrow but also to other organs) and in some patients produce late toxic effects, such as secondary neoplasia, pulmonary fibrosis, peripheral neuropathy, and infertility. Despite the risks of toxicity, most clinical oncologists believe that the best results are obtained by regimens that use maximally tolerated doses. Results in drug treatment of breast cancer, ovarian cancer, lymphoma, and leukemia all support the notion that more intensive treatment, up to the limits of tolerance of normal tissues, increases the response rates and improves survival. Thus, the drugs should be used in a fashion that produces definite but readily controllable toxicity. In particular, regular monitoring of peripheral blood counts is essential after drug administration to detect periods of severe neutropenia and thrombocytopenia and to allow adjustments of subsequent doses of drug. The discovery of stimulating factors for granulocyte production (granulocyte colony-stimulating factor [G-CSF] and granulocyte-macrophage CSF [GM-CSF]) and more recently for platelet production (thrombopoietin) will undoubtedly allow further dose escalations, earlier recovery of blood counts, and fewer infectious complications and bleeding episodes from high-dose chemotherapy. Whether these products should be used as part of routine treatment has not been proved. Typically, drugs are delivered to maximal antitumor response as determined by physical examination, radiologic evaluation, and tumor marker measurement.

More than 50 chemotherapeutic drugs are currently available for the treatment of patients with malignancies (Table 254.4).

TABLE 254.4.	PROPERTIES OF ANTICANCER DRUGS

Drug	Site of Elimination[a]	Site of Action	Acute Toxicity (Immediate)	Delayed Toxicity (Days to Weeks)	Late Toxicity
Asparaginase (Elspar)	S	Destroys essential amino acid (L-asparagine)	*Nausea and vomiting;* fever; chills; headache; hypersensitivity, anaphylaxis, abdominal pain; hyperglycemia leading to coma; pancreatitis	CNS depression; thrombosis or hemorrhage	—
Azacitidine (Mylosar)	H, S	Inhibits DNA methylation	Nausea and vomiting; diarrhea; fever	*Leukopenia (may be prolonged):* thrombocytopenia; hepatic damage; muscle pain and weakness	—
Bleomycin (Blenoxane)	R	Free radical damage to DNA	*Nausea and vomiting;* fever; anaphylaxis and other allergic reactions	*Pneumonitis and pulmonary fibrosis;* rash; stomatitis; alopecia; Raynaud's phenomenon	Pulmonary fibrosis
Busulphan (Myleran)	S	Alkylates DNA	*Nausea and vomiting*	*Bone marrow depression;* hyperpigmentation; alopecia; gynecomastia; addisonian syndrome	Gonad failure, leukemia pulmonary infiltrates and fibrosis; bone marrow aplasia
Capecitabine (Xeloda)	H	Inhibits DNA, RNA synthesis	Nausea and vomiting, diarrhea, mucositis	Bone marrow suppression, palmar erythema	
Carboplatin (Paraplatin)	R	Crosslinks DNA	Nausea and vomiting	*Bone marrow depression,* esp. thrombocytopenia; peripheral neuropathy, anemia, renal toxicity in high-dose regimens	Leukemia
Carmustine (BCNU)	S	Alkylates DNA	*Nausea and vomiting;* local phlebitis	*Delayed leukopenia and thrombocytopenia (may be prolonged):* reversible liver damage	Pulmonary fibrosis, renal damage, leukemia
Chlorambucil (Leukeran)	S	Alkylates DNA	Minimal nausea at low doses	*Bone marrow depression;* hepatic toxicity	Pulmonary fibrosis, leukemia
Cisplatin (*cis*-diamine dichloroplatinum; *cis*-DDP	S, R	Crosslinks DNA	*Nausea and vomiting;* anaphylactic reactions; fever	*Renal damage;* ototoxicity; hemolysis; hypomagnesemia; hypocalcemia; hypokalemia; myelosuppression	Pulmonary fibrosis, leukemia, peripheral neuropathy
Cladribine (2-CdA, Leustatin)	R	Inhibits DNA synthesis	Nausea; headache	*Bone marrow depression;* fatigue; fever; rash; depressed CD4 lymphocyte counts	Opportunistic infection
Cyclophosphamide (Cytoxan, Neosar)	R	Alkylates DNA	*Nausea and vomiting;* hypersensitivity	*Bone marrow depression,* esp. neutropenia; hemorrhagic cystitis; hyponatremia; myocardial necrosis	Reproductive failure, pulmonary fibrosis, leukemia, bladder cancer

TABLE 254.4.   *Continued*

Drug	Site of Elimination[a]	Site of Action	Acute Toxicity (Immediate)	Delayed Toxicity (Days to Weeks)	Late Toxicity
Cytarabine HCl (Cytosine arabinoside, Cytosar-U)	H, S	Inhibits DNA synthesis	*Nausea and vomiting;* diarrhea; anaphylaxis, fever	*Bone marrow depression;* conjunctivitis; oral ulceration; hepatic damage; pulmonary edema and encephalopathy with high doses; gastrointestinal epithelial damage	—
Dacarbazine (DTIC; DIC; DTIC-)	H, S	Alkylates DNA	*Nausea and vomiting;* diarrhea; anaphylaxis; pain on administration; flulike syndrome	*Bone marrow depression;* alopecia; photosensitivity	—
Dactinomycin (actinomycin D: Cosmegen)	H	DNA intercalator[b]	*Nausea and vomiting;* diarrhea; local reaction and phlebitis; anaphylactoid reaction	*Stomatitis; oral ulceration; bone marrow depression;* alopecia; folliculitis; dermatitis in previously irradiated areas	—
Daunorubicin (daunomycin; Cerubidine)	H	DNA intercalator[b] Inhibits topoisomerase II	*Nausea and vomiting;* diarrhea; red urine (not hematuria); severe local tissue damage and necrosis on extravasation; transient ECG changes, esp. dysrhythmias; anaphylactoid reaction	*Bone marrow depression;* alopecia; stomatitis	Cardiotoxicity (congestive heart failure)
Deoxycoformycin (DCF)	R	Adenosine deaminase inhibitor	Nausea and vomiting, conjunctivitis	Nephrotoxicity; neurotoxicity; immune suppression, myelosuppression	—
Docetaxel (taxotere)	H	Prevents depolymerization of microtubules; blocks cells in mitosis	Hypersensitivity reactions; hypertension; bronchospasm; nausea; vomiting	*Bone marrow depression* (neutropenia); peripheral neuropathy; alopecia; peripheral edema; pleural effusion	—
Doxorubicin (Adriamycin)	H	DNA intercalator; generates free radicals; inhibits topoisomerase II	*Nausea and vomiting;* red urine (not hematuria); severe local tissue damage and necrosis on extravasation; diarrhea; transient ECG changes; ventricular dysrhythmia; anaphylactoid reaction	*Bone marrow depression;* alopecia; stomatitis; anorexia; conjunctivitis	*Cardiotoxicity* (may be irreversible, but may be decreased by weekly schedule) Leukemia
Estramustine	H	Inhibits microtubule formation	Nausea, vomiting, diarrhea, thrombocytopenia	Thrombosis, gynecomastia	
Etoposide (VP-16-213; Vespid)	H, R	Inhibits topoisomerase II	*Nausea and vomiting;* fever	*Bone marrow depression;* alopecia; peripheral neuropathy; allergic reactions; hepatic damage	Leukemia
Floxuridine (FUDR)	S, H	Inhibits thymidylate synthetase	*Nausea and vomiting;* diarrhea	*Oral and gastrointestinal ulceration; bone marrow depression;* alopecia; dermatitis	—

TABLE 254.4.   *Continued*

Drug	Site of Elimination[a]	Site of Action	Acute Toxicity (Immediate)	Delayed Toxicity (Days to Weeks)	Late Toxicity
Fludarabine (Fludara)	R	Inhibits ribonucleotide reductase and blocks DNA synthesis	Nausea and vomiting; diarrhea	*Bone marrow depression;* fatigue; fever; rash; edema; CNS toxicity at high doses	—
Fluorouracil (5-FU; Fluorouracil, Adrucil)	H, S	Inhibits thymidylate synthetase	*Nausea and vomiting;* diarrhea; hypersensitivity reaction	*Oral and gastrointestinal ulcers; bone marrow depression;* cerebellar toxicity; alopecia; chest pain indicating myocardial ischemia	—
Gemcitabine (Gemzar)	H, S	Inhibits DNA polymerase	Nausea and vomiting; flulike symptoms	*Bone marrow depression;* reversible increases in hepatic enzymes, proteinuria; rash	—
Hexamethylmelamine (HMM)	H	Alkylates DNA	Nausea and vomiting	*Bone marrow depression;* reversible increases in hepatic enzymes, proteinuria; rash	—
Hydroxyurea (Hydrea)	R	Inhibits ribonucleotide reductase	*Nausea and vomiting*	*Bone marrow depression;* CNS depression; peripheral neuritis, visual hallucinations	—
Ifosfamide (Ifex)	H	Alkylates DNA	Nausea and vomiting; CNS depression, seizures	*Bone marrow depression;* hemorrhagic cystitis; alopecia; sterility (may be temporary)	Leukemia, pulmonary fibrosis
Irinotecan (CPT-11)	H	Inhibits topoisomerase I	Diarrhea; myelosuppression	Diarrhea; bone marrow depression	—
Leucovorin calcium; folinic acid (Wellcovorin)	S	Reverses effects of methotrexate; potentiates binding of 5-FU nucleotide to thymidylate synthetase	—	—	—
Levamisole (Ergamisol)	?	Unknown (immune stimulant)	Nausea and vomiting; diarrhea	Bone marrow depression (rare); agranulocytosis	—
Lomustine (CCNU; CeeNu)	S	Alkylates DNA	*Nausea and vomiting*	*Delayed (4–6 weeks) leukopenia and thrombocytopenia (may be prolonged);* transient elevation of transaminase activity; neurologic reactions	Pulmonary fibrosis; leukemia
Mechlorethamine (nitrogen mustard; HN2; Mustargen)	S	Alkylates DNA	*Nausea and vomiting;* local tissue reaction to extravasation	*Bone marrow depression;* alopecia; diarrhea; oral ulcers	Pulmonary fibrosis; leukemia
Melphalan (Alkeran)	S	Alkylates DNA	Mild nausea; hypersensitivity reactions	*Bone marrow depression (esp. platelets)*	Pulmonary fibrosis; leukemia
Mercaptopurine (6-MP; Purinethol)	H, S	Inhibits purine synthesis	*Nausea and vomiting;* diarrhea	*Bone marrow depression; cholestasis and rarely hepatic necrosis;* oral and intestinal ulcers; pancreatitis; allopurinol may increase overall toxicity	—
Mesna (Mesnex)	R, S	Sulfhydryl group inactivates acrolein	Headache; nausea; vomiting; diarrhea	None reported	—

TABLE 254.4.   *Continued*

Drug	Site of Elimination[a]	Site of Action	Acute Toxicity (Immediate)	Delayed Toxicity (Days to Weeks)	Late Toxicity
Methotrexate (MTX; Methotrexate-Lederle; Mexate; Folex)	R	Inhibits dihydrofolate reductase	*Nausea and vomiting; diarrhea; fever; anaphylaxis*	*Oral and gastrointestinal ulceration; bone marrow depression;* hepatic necrosis; oral and intestinal ulcers; pancreatitis; allopurinol may increase overall toxicity; pulmonary infiltrates and fibrosis; alopecia; infertility; menstrual dysfunction; encephalopathy and anaphylactoid reactions (rare) and renal failure with high doses	Cirrhosis
Mitomycin (Mutamycin)	S	Crosslinks DNA	*Nausea and vomiting;* local reaction if extravasation; fever; hemolytic-uremic syndrome	*Bone marrow depression* (cumulative); stomatitis; alopecia; hepatotoxicity; renal toxicity	Pulmonary fibrosis; cardiac failure, esp. after anthracycline
Mitotane (o.p′-DDD; Lysodren)		Inhibits steroidogenesis	*Nausea and vomiting;* diarrhea	*CNS depression;* rash; visual disturbances; adrenal insufficiency; hematuria; hemorrhagic cystitis; albuminuria; hypertension; orthostatic hypotension	CNS dysfunction, cataracts
Mitoxantrone HCl (DHAD; Novantrone)	H	DNA intercalator[b] Inhibits topoisomerase II	Green pigment in urine, green sclerae; nausea	*Bone marrow depression;* white hair	Cardiac toxicity (congestive heart failure)
Paclitaxel (Taxol)	H	Prevents depolymerization microtubules	Hypersensitivity reaction; bradycardia, hypotension; nausea and vomiting	*Bone marrow depression;* myalgias and arthralgias; peripheral neuropathy; alopecia, mucositis	—
Plicamycin (Mithracin)	O	DNA intercalator[b]	*Nausea and vomiting; diarrhea; fever*	*Hemorrhagic diathesis;* bone marrow depression (thrombocytopenia); coagulation abnormalities, hepatic damage; hypocalcemia and hypokalemia; stomatitis; renal damage	—
Procarbazine HCl (Matulane)	H	Alkylates DNA	*Nausea and vomiting;* CNS depression; Antabuse-like effect with alcohol	*Bone marrow depression;* stomatitis; peripheral neuropathy; pneumonitis	Leukemia
Streptozocin (Streptozotocin; Zanosar)	S	Alkylates DNA	*Nausea and vomiting;* local pain; chills and fever	*Renal damage;* hypoglycemia; hyperglycemia; liver damage; diarrhea; bone marrow depression (uncommon), fever, eosinophilia	—
Teniposide (VM-26)	H, R	Inhibits topoisomerase II	Nausea and vomiting; phlebitis; anaphylactoid symptoms	*Bone marrow depression;* alopecia	Leukemia

TABLE 254.4. *Continued*

Drug	Site of Elimination[a]	Site of Action	Acute Toxicity (Immediate)	Delayed Toxicity (Days to Weeks)	Late Toxicity
6-Thioguanine (6-TG; Tabloid)	S, H	Guanine analogue, inhibits purine biosynthesis	*Occasional nausea and vomiting*	*Bone marrow depression;* hepatic damage; stomatitis	—
Thiotepa (triethylene thiophosphoramide)	S, H	Alkylates DNA	*Nausea and vomiting;* local pain	*Bone marrow depression*	Pulmonary fibrosis; leukemia
Topotecan	S	Topoisomerase I inhibitor	*Nausea and vomiting*	Bone marrow depression; diarrhea	—
Vinblastine sulfate (Velban)	H	Binds tubulin	*Nausea and vomiting;* local reaction and phlebitis with extravasation	*Bone marrow depression;* alopecia; stomatitis; peripheral neuropathy (mild)	—
Vincristine sulfate (Oncovin)	H	Binds tubulin	Local reaction with extravasation	*Peripheral neuropathy;* alopecia; mild bone marrow depression; constipation; paralytic ileus; inappropriate antidiuretic hormone secretion; hepatic damage; jaw pain	—
Vinorelbine tartrate (Navelbine)	H	Binds tubulin	Local reaction with extravasation	*Bone marrow depression;* granulocytopenia; mild alopecia; peripheral neuropathy; jaw pain	—

Dose-limiting effects are italicized.

[a] Site of elimination: R, renal excretion; H, hepatic metabolism; S, systemic metabolic breakdown.

[b] DNA intercalation: insertion of drug into DNA helix (either major or minor groove) with effects on DNA integrity, new DNA synthesis, and repair.

Physicians who use these drugs or who care for patients receiving such treatment must know the pharmacology and potential side effects of these toxic agents. However, treatment should not be individualized for each patient; protocol-based therapy is mandatory for the safe use of these drugs. The physician must consider whether the efficient elimination of the drug or drugs will be altered by abnormal renal or hepatic function; whether intercurrent neurologic, cardiac, or pulmonary disease presents special problems in drug tolerance; and whether past exposure to other drugs or radiation might predispose the patient to toxicity. The accompanying tables provide information on the mechanism of drug elimination for commonly used cancer drugs and suggest circumstances in which drug doses need to be altered. In general, doses of paclitaxel, docetaxel, and the vinca alkaloids must be reduced by at least 50% in patients with significant hepatic dysfunction (bilirubin higher than 3 mg per deciliter). Similarly, the doses of methotrexate, hydroxyurea, bleomycin, etoposide, carboplatin, fludarabine, cladribine, and deoxycoformycin should be reduced in proportion to decreases in creatinine clearance. The dose of carboplatin, a drug eliminated by renal excretion, should be calculated for the individual patient based on measurement of creatinine clearance.

Pharmacokinetic monitoring and dose adjustment is used infrequently in the routine practice of medical oncology, the only common example being the measurement of methotrexate levels 24 to 48 hours after high-dose administration. In this situation, abnormal drug levels in plasma prompt the institution of prolonged rescue with the antidote leucovorin (5-formyltetrahydrofolate).

Even when abnormal renal or hepatic function is taken into account in adjusting drug dosage, significant interindividual variability in drug clearance and tolerance remains among patients. In some cases, genetic defects in drug elimination or activation account for these findings. Examples include the absence of dihydropyrimidine dehydrogenase, the enzyme responsible for degradation of 5-fluorouracil. Persons lacking this enzyme have extreme sensitivity to 5-fluorouracil, even to topically administered drug for treatment of basal cell carcinomas, and may experience fatal toxicity from small doses. Low activity of thiopurine methyltransferase, the enzyme responsible for inactivating 6-mercaptopurine, is also associated with extreme drug toxicity. Both of these defects are found infrequently (less than 1 in 100 patients), but extreme toxic reactions should prompt testing for the mutation in question and caution in continuing drug treatment.

High-dose chemotherapy with rescue by bone marrow or peripheral blood stem cells allows dose escalation and curative responses in patients with leukemia or lymphoma refractory to standard chemotherapy, but introduces a unique set of toxicities. These include profound immunosuppression and opportunistic infection; vascular endothelial damage; severe damage to pulmonary and gastrointestinal epithelium; hepatocellular injury; myocardial necrosis; and secondary leukemia. The specific pattern of toxicity depends on the agents used, but alkylating agents remain the mainstay of high-dose therapy and are capable of producing any or all of the latter toxicities. In allogeneic marrow transplants, the immune response of the donor lymphocytes to the tumor (graft-versus-leukemia effect, for example) adds further benefit to the therapeutic response, but at the cost of graft-versus-host disease. Because of their linear dose-response relation extending into the high-dose range, alkylating agents are unlikely to be replaced in these regimens, although carboplatin, etoposide, and total body irradiation are often used in combination with the conventional alkylators.

Despite the disadvantages, high-dose chemotherapy with stem cell rescue has proved successful in producing long-term disease-free survival in acute and chronic myelocytic leukemia and other hematologic malignancies. However, the value of high-dose chemotherapy with bone marrow rescue remains unproven in most solid tumors, either for metastatic disease or in the adjuvant setting, and should be untaken only in the context of a clinical trial.

Cancer drugs can also cause late side effects (Table 254.4). The risk of secondary leukemias may reach 5% to 10% for regimens that use high doses of DNA-modifying agents, such as alkylating agents, procarbazine, and even certain natural products such as teniposide or etoposide. Often, these cases of leukemia occur 2 to 5 years after drug exposure, and most are refractory to treatment. Equally troublesome are the cardiac toxicity of anthracyclines; the pulmonary fibrosis that follows bleomycin, the nitrosoureas, and other high-dose alkylating agents; and the peripheral neurotoxicity of vincristine, paclitaxel, and cisplatin. Neurotoxicity usually develops within days or weeks of drug administration, but evidence of pulmonary fibrosis or cardiac failure may appear many months after drug treatment. The total dose limits for anthracyclines (550 mg per square meter for doxorubicin) should be respected to avoid cardiac failure.

PRINCIPLES OF COMBINATION CHEMOTHERAPY

In the treatment of malignant disease, as in the treatment of relatively resistant microbial infection, combinations of individually active agents can cure diseases that respond incompletely to single agents. This principle was first demonstrated in the successful treatment of acute lymphoblastic leukemia in children and later in the lymphomas and testicular cancer. With few exceptions, maximum benefit from chemotherapy requires the use of multiple drugs. The selection of the individual components of a regimen, as well as their scheduling and sequencing in combination, is usually based on pharmacologic and toxicologic considerations.

The basic principles of combination chemotherapy are reviewed in Table 254.5. These principles are useful but not rigid guidelines. Thus, although alkylating agents and anthracyclines are strongly myelosuppressive, their potent activity against lymphomas becomes the overriding factor in their common use in

TABLE 254.5.	**PRINCIPLES OF COMBINATION CHEMOTHERAPY**

Individual drugs should have antitumor activity
Toxicity of individual drugs should have minimal overlap
Combination regimens should avoid unfavorable drug interactions
Each drug should have different mechanism of action
Each drug should have different mechanism of drug resistance

combination against Hodgkin's disease and non-Hodgkin's lymphoma. In addition to the general consideration of toxicity and individual activity, drug interaction at the level of pharmacokinetics may lead to problems in regimen design (Table 254.6). Drugs may have organ toxicity that may affect the elimination of a second agent—for example, the renal toxicity of cisplatin can prolong the plasma half-life of methotrexate or bleomycin. Drug interactions at the biochemical level have guided the construction of many commonly used regimens (e.g., the use of leucovorin to enhance the binding of 5-fluorouracil nucleotide to its target enzyme [thymidylate synthase]). A thorough understanding of the pharmacology of the individual components of such regimens forms the underpinning of safe and effective combination chemotherapy.

PRINCIPLES OF HORMONAL THERAPY

Many neoplasms of the breast, prostatic, and uterine epithelium require corticosteroid hormones for rapid growth. Synthesis of these steroid hormones, namely estrogens, androgens, and pro-

TABLE 254.6.	**DRUG INTERACTIONS IN CANCER CHEMOTHERAPY**

Inhibition of Drug Elimination (Altered Pharmacokinetics)

Allopurinol blocks metabolism of 6-mercaptopurine by xanthine oxidase
Nonsteroidal analgesics block methotrexate excretion by kidneys
Cisplatin inhibits taxol metabolism by P-450 in liver

Biochemical Synergy

Leucovorin (5-formyltetrahydrofolate) enhances binding of 5-fluorouracil monophosphate to its target, thymidylate synthase.
Methotrexate enhances metabolic activation of 5-fluorouracil and 6-mercaptopurine through effects on phosphoribosylpyrophosphate pools.
l-asparaginase blocks protein synthesis and cell cycle progression, protects cells against methotrexate toxicity.
Repair of cisplatin/DNA crosslinks inhibited by antimetabolites (cytosine arabinoside, 5-fluorouracil).
Sulfhydril compounds (ethyol) protect kidney and bone marrow from cisplatin toxicity by intracellular inactivation of active platinum species and alkylating agents.

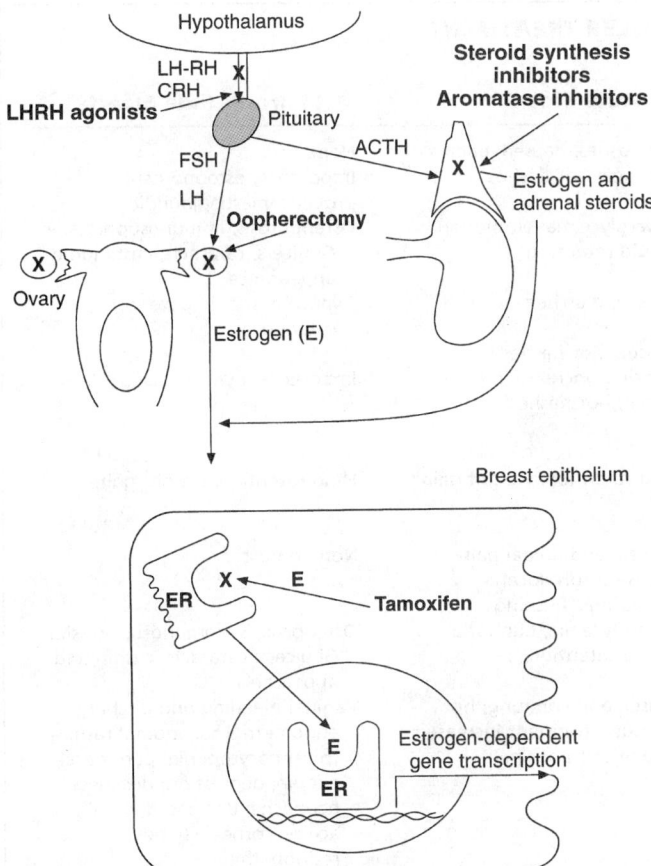

FIGURE 254.2. Endocrine-mediated growth of hormone-dependent breast cancer. X marks the sites of therapeutic pharmacologic or surgical interventions that interrupt the endocrine pathway.

gestins, depends on the action of hypothalamic hormones, such as luteinizing hormone-releasing hormone (LHRH) and pituitary hormones: follicle-stimulating hormone (FSH), luteinizing hormone (LH), and adrenocorticotropic hormone (ACTH). The latter hormones stimulate end organs such as the ovaries, testes, and adrenals to synthesize the appropriate steroid hormones that enter the circulation and bind to the intracellular receptors in tumor cells (Fig. 254.2). The ability of these hormones to stimulate growth is due to a complex interaction of these lipid-soluble hormones with their cytoplasmic receptors and the subsequent activation of gene transcription by the hormone–hormone receptor (ligand–receptor) complex. Structure and function studies of both the estrogen and androgen receptor demonstrate that these proteins contain hormone-binding, DNA-binding, and transactivating domains. Binding of the hormone to the receptor leads to a conformational change in the receptor, allowing the receptor–ligand complex to enter the nucleus and bind specific sites on DNA (estrogen- or androgen-responsive elements) through the DNA-binding portion of the receptor. Protein–protein interactions between the transactivating portion of the steroid receptor and other receptor-modulating proteins lead to unique patterns of expression of corticosteroid-dependent genes that determine the specific pattern of response in normal tissues and in tumors.

Tumors derived from hormonally sensitive tissues such as the breast, uterus, prostate, and thyroid retain responsiveness to hormonal manipulation. This manipulation can occur through either pharmacologic or surgical approaches that interrupt the axis between the hypothalamus and the pituitary gland, the pituitary gland and the end organ, or the end organ and the hormone receptor in tumor cells. For example, hormonal manipulation in breast cancer includes LHRH agonists to paradoxically decrease LH and FSH secretion, oophorectomy to reduce estrogen secretion, and the administration of tamoxifen, a competitive inhibitor of the estrogen–estrogen receptor interaction (Fig. 254.2). All three of these manipulations interrupt steroid-dependent tumor growth.

In some hormone-responsive tumors, such as breast and uterine cancer, the presence of hormone receptors (estrogen or progesterone receptors) marks the tumor as potentially hormone responsive; receptor levels should be measured on all primary breast tissue specimens and in metastases if hormonal therapy is a viable treatment option. Unfortunately, the presence of a hormone receptor does not guarantee that the tumor will respond to hormonal manipulation. Resistance to hormonal therapy, as with chemotherapy, can occur through many different mechanisms, including deletion of the hormone receptors or mutations that activate the receptor when bound to the antagonist. Androgen receptors in prostate cancer may undergo mutations such that androgen antagonists (which bind the receptors) act paradoxically as agonists and promote tumor growth. Alternatively, mutations may occur downstream from the site of hormone receptor action, allowing the constitutive expression of hormone-dependent genes even in the absence of hormone.

In many patients with metastatic breast or prostate cancer, hormonal manipulation is effective in prolonging survival. Randomized trials have also demonstrated the usefulness of hormonal manipulation in the adjuvant treatment of postmenopausal women with breast cancer and in the prevention of disease in high-risk women.

Although hormone receptors are present on various other tumor types, hormonal therapy has had its greatest impact on breast and prostate cancers, but not without toxic effects. Tamoxifen, for example, has both estrogen antagonist and agonist properties, depending on the tissue in question. In uterine tissue, tamoxifen acts as an estrogen-like agonist, increasing the long-term risk of endometrial cancer two- to threefold. This becomes an important consideration in the use of tamoxifen in the adjuvant setting and in cancer-prevention trials for patients at high risk for breast cancer. The drug has compensating beneficial effects on serum lipids and on bone mineralization in postmenopausal women and lowers the risk of osteoporotic fractures with long-term use. For prostate cancer patients, pharmacologic or surgical manipulations that result in a hypoandrogenic state also have side effects, including impotence and osteoporosis. Table 254.7 reviews many of the hormonal agents in use and their toxicities.

The interdigitation of hormonal and cytotoxic therapies is complex. Because hormonal antagonists place cancer cells in a quiescent, nondividing state, in experimental systems they tend to produce insensitivity to chemotherapy, which depends on active cell proliferation. In patients with breast cancer, hormonal

TABLE 254.7.	PROPERTIES OF HORMONES USED IN CANCER TREATMENT		
Agent	**Mechanism of Action**	**Acute Side Effects**	**Chronic Side Effects**
Anastrazole (Arimidex)	Selective aromatase inhibitor	Hot flashes; nausea; edema	None
Biculotamide (Casodex)	Nonsteroidal, antiandrogen	Diarrhea; hot flashes	Impotence; osteoporosis; gynecomastia; jaundice
Dexamethasone	Glucocorticoid, decreases cerebral edema	Hyperglycemia; euphoria; fluid retention	Osteoporosis; immunosuppression; GI ulcers; cataracts; cushingoid appearance
Flutamide (Eulexin-Schering)	Antiandrogen	Nausea, diarrhea	Gynecomastia; impotence; osteoporosis
Letrozole (Femara)2	Selective aromatase inhibitor	Nausea; hot flashes	
Lutenizing hormone (LH)-releasing hormone antagonist: Lupron-Abbott	Releases LH; "exhausts" pituitary	Transient increase in bone pain; hot flashes	Impotence; gynecomastia
Megestrol acetate (Megace-Bristol Myers)	Progestational agent	Fluid retention; weight gain	Fluid retention; weight gain
Octreotide acetate	Mimics somatostatin	Nausea; abdominal pain; loose stools, local reactions, flushing	None reported
Prednisone	Glucocorticoid; induces apoptosis, suppresses adrenal steroid production	Hyperglycemia; euphoria; fluid retention	Osteoporosis; immunosuppression; GI ulcers; cataracts; cushingoid appearance
Tamoxifen citrate (Nolvadex-Stuart)	Antiestrogen	Nausea and vomiting; hot flashes; transient increased bone or tumor pain	Vaginal bleeding and discharge; endometrial carcinoma; rash; thrombocytopenia; peripheral edema; depression; dizziness; headache; decreased visual acuity; corneal changes; retinopathy
Toremifene (Foreston)	Antiestrogen	Nausea; hot flashes; tumor flare; hypercalcemia	Thrombotic events

therapy is usually given before chemotherapy in metastatic disease and after chemotherapy in the adjuvant setting. A growing collection of new hormonal antagonists, including selective aromatase inhibitors and pure estrogen antagonists, LHRH antagonists, and alternative androgen antagonists, is now available. Their role in cancer treatment is now the focus of several cancer trials.

FUTURE ADVANCES IN CANCER THERAPEUTICS

The process of discovering effective drugs for treating cancer has proved difficult. More than 50 agents are in clinical use for this indication, but only a few have curative potential, and only in selected clinical settings. Most of these drugs were chosen for development because of their ability to inhibit rapidly dividing murine tumors, and most target aspects of DNA synthesis or interfere with its integrity. The difficulty of using such DNA-directed agents stems from the fact that, in most respects, cancers differ quantitatively but not qualitatively from normal proliferative tissue, such as bone marrow progenitors and epithelial cells; the enzymatic machinery that controls proliferation and that

serves as the target for these agents is common to both normal and malignant tissue. Greater specificity is provided by hormonal therapies, which slow the growth of breast cancer and prostate cancer but have no effect on proliferating normal tissues such as bone marrow or epithelium.

Advances in understanding the biology of cancer have led to the identification of cell surface antigens and intracellular proteins that are highly expressed on tumor cells. Many of these proteins confer a growth advantage to cancer cells, because they participate in signaling pathways that promote proliferation, inhibit apoptosis, or mediate angiogenesis or metastasis. Although most of these proteins are not truly tumor specific, many are expressed only in selected tissues and at specific stages in organogenesis. Thus, as drug targets, these proteins offer significant selectivity, compared with the anti-DNA–directed chemotherapy.

Among the most promising of these new targets are proteins such as the bcr-abl kinase, which is the unique product of the genetic translocation found in chronic myelocytic leukemia (CML). An inhibitor of the bcr-abl kinase has begun clinical trial, and initial reports indicate that it has striking activity in chronic-phase CML. The ras proteins are a second important molecular target. *H-ras* and *k-ras* genes are mutated (and thereby activated) in many human solid tumors, including pancreatic and colon cancer, and furnish continuous proliferative drive to the affected tumor cells. The ras proteins require modification with a lipid to insert in the cell membrane. Drugs designed to block this modification, called *farnesylation* inhibitors, have impressive activity against both *ras*-mutated and other tumor cells in experimental animals and have entered clinical trial. Similar molecules have been designed to inhibit alternative growth factor signaling pathways (inhibitors of protein kinase C, platelet derived growth factor receptor), as well as angiogenesis (inhibitor of vascular endothelial growth factor receptor), and metastasis (metalloproteinase inhibitors). The hope is that these molecules will offer greater specificity for tumors and fewer side effects than conventional chemotherapy.

BIBLIOGRAPHY

Boral AL, Dessain S, Chabner BA. Clinical evaluation of biologically targeted drugs: obstacles and opportunities. *Cancer Chemother Pharmacol* 1998;42(suppl):S3–S21.

Chabner B, Longo D. *Principles and practice of cancer chemotherapy and biological response modifiers*, 2nd ed. Philadelphia: JB Lippincott, 1996.

Chabner B, Boral AL, Multani P. Translational research: walking the bridge between idea and cure. Seventeenth Bruce F. Cain Memorial Award Lecture. *Cancer Res* 1998;58:4211–4216.

Fleming ID, Cooper JS, Henson DE, et al, eds. *AJCC cancer staging manual*, fifth ed. Philadelphia: Lippincott-Raven, 1997.

Kaelin WG. Taking aim at novel targets in cancer therapy. *J Clin Invest* 1999;104:1495–1496.

Kelley's Textbook of Internal Medicine, fourth edition. Edited by H. David Humes.
Lippincott Williams & Wilkins, Philadelphia © 2000.

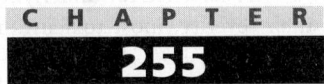

CHAPTER 255

PRINCIPLES OF BIOLOGIC THERAPY

JOHN W. SMITH II
WALTER J. URBA

Biologic therapy for the patient with cancer has changed substantially in recent years. These advances cross conventional treatment boundaries and provide a fourth treatment modality, in addition to surgery, radiation, and chemotherapy, which will increasingly influence the practice of medicine. The goal of biologic therapy is to achieve tumor regression through agents or approaches that modify the relation between tumor and host. Most biologic agents are found naturally in the body and have roles in the normal function of the immune system or another

physiologic process. They may act directly on the tumor to inhibit growth, to induce differentiation or death, or to block metastasis. Or, they may act indirectly on the host to augment an immune response or restore the activity of host defense mechanisms inhibited by the tumor itself or damaged by other cancer treatments.

Historically, biologic therapy has been synonymous with immunotherapy, but, despite some overlap, biologic therapy includes many strategies that do not necessarily have an immunologic rationale (e.g., differentiation and apoptosis-inducing agents). Furthermore, an historical classification of biologic approaches to cancer treatment ("active" for agents that stimulate the host, "passive" for agents that act directly against the tumor, and tumor-specific or tumor-nonspecific) has persisted but is inadequate for understanding biologic therapy. Many agents have several actions that defy such categorization. For example, tumor necrosis factor (TNF) has both active, or direct, cytotoxic effects on tumor cells and passive actions. It can kill tumor-associated vascular endothelial cells and activate monocytes that can kill tumor cells. Likewise, interferon can inhibit the growth of tumor cells, induce differentiation, and augment the activity of natural killer (NK) cells, and anti-CD20 antibodies can induce apoptosis or mediate tumor cell killing by complement fixation or antibody-dependent cellular cytotoxicity (ADCC).

Our limited understanding of in vivo tumor biology and tumor–host interactions and our inability to deliver agents to sites of tumors have presented significant barriers to the development of effective biologic therapy. A single cytokine, when isolated from the other mediators of a local inflammatory response and administered systemically at pharmacologic doses, probably does not act as it would as part of the finely orchestrated multicomponent physiologic process. Nevertheless, some significant clinical advances have emerged over the last decade. This chapter reviews the major biologic molecules of current use in clinical oncology.

NONSPECIFIC IMMUNE STIMULANTS

Bacteria and bacterial products are potent activators of the immune system. Some bacteria contain "superantigens," peptides capable of activating large populations of T cells. Bacteria and their products have been tested for their ability to act as immune "adjuvants" to stimulate the immune system in a nonspecific fashion in the hope that specific antitumor immunity would result. Bacillus Calmette–Guérin (BCG) is a strain of *Mycobacterium bovis* that has been used to elicit immune responses to vaccines. BCG has been tested in cancer patients, and the most impressive results have been observed when the inflammatory response was elicited at the site of tumor and the tumor cells were destroyed as bystanders of the inflammation. Direct injection of BCG causes regression of cutaneous melanoma and intravesical delivery is an approved, effective treatment for superficial bladder cancer.

CYTOKINES

Cytokines are polypeptides that control the function, growth, and differentiation of cells. Cytokines act by engaging a specific receptor on the surface of the target cell and transducing signals intracellularly that activate or repress particular genes. Several cytokines are approved for use in humans with cancer, and many more are undergoing clinical development.

INTERFERONS

Interferon-α (IFN-α) and IFN-β are class I interferons that share the same receptor, whereas interferon-γ is a class II interferon that binds to its own receptor and exhibits distinct biologic effects. Although IFN-β and IFN-γ are used in the treatment of multiple sclerosis and chronic granulomatous disease, respectively, neither is used in cancer therapy at this time. Two forms of recombinant IFN-α are available for clinical use: α2a and α2b. There are no important differences between them. The mechanism of action of IFN-α against tumor cells is unclear. It has the following diverse effects on tumor cells: induction of growth arrest or differentiation, inhibition of protein synthesis, up-regulation of major histocompatibility complex (MHC) class I expression and activation of NK cells. In addition, IFN-α can inhibit ornithine decarboxylase and thus block polyamine synthesis, an action that leads to growth arrest. Most of the clinical activity of interferon appears to be a direct antitumor effect.

IFN-α is active against chronic myelogenous leukemia (CML), cutaneous T-cell lymphoma, functional endocrine tumors, and AIDS-associated Kaposi's sarcoma. In patients with myeloma and follicular B-cell lymphoma, IFN-α appears to prolong the duration of a response to combination chemotherapy, and although active in hairy cell leukemia, it has been supplanted by the nucleoside, 2-chlorodeoxyadenosine, which produces more durable complete responses. IFN-α also induces tumor regression in patients with metastatic renal cell cancer and melanoma and may improve disease-free and overall survival of patients with high-risk melanoma (greater than 4-mm skin lesions or lymph node involvement) when given after surgery.

The dose of IFN-α required for antitumor activity varies (3 to 50 mU), and the usual route of administration is subcutaneous. The responses are usually partial and short-lived if treatment is discontinued, but they can be maintained, at times, for prolonged periods if therapy is continued. Dose-limiting toxicities are fatigue, muscle aches, headache, and anorexia (a flulike syndrome). Nausea, myelosuppression, proteinuria, elevated transaminase levels, and cardiac ischemia and dysrhythmias occur rarely. Resistance to IFN-α can be mediated by neutralizing antibodies. Alternate forms of IFN (e.g., lymphoblastoid IFN, a mixture of type I interferons) can be used to maintain the response. The antibodies are generally short-lived (median 8 months); when they disappear, IFNα can be reinstituted with restoration of efficacy.

INTERLEUKIN-2

Interleukin-2 (IL-2), originally named T-cell growth factor, is a 133-amino acid, 15-kD glycoprotein that plays a critical role in the activation and maintenance of an immune response to antigens. It is produced mainly by CD4 T cells after they encounter an immunogenic peptide presented by the human leukocyte antigen (HLA) class II molecule in combination with a second costimulatory signal. IL-2 promotes the proliferation, expansion, and activation to cytotoxicity of T cells, NK cells, and monocytes.

Early studies of recombinant human IL-2 (aldesleukin) also included the administration of peripheral blood leukocytes that had been cultured ex vivo with IL-2 for 3 to 5 days to generate lymphokine-activated killer (LAK) cells. The demonstration of dramatic tumor regressions (including complete regressions) in some patients with renal cell carcinoma and melanoma led to many confirmatory clinical trials. A randomized trial demonstrated that the LAK cells did not add to the benefit of IL-2 administered alone. IL-2 is the best example of a treatment for cancer that works purely by activating the immune system rather than by directly killing tumor cells. IL-2 is usually administered intravenously over 5 days by bolus or continuous infusion, but it can also be given subcutaneously at a much lower dose for a more protracted length of time. IL-2 toxicity is dose-related and can be substantial. In high doses, it induces a cytokine cascade that includes several other biologic mediators, such as IL-1, IFN, TNF, IL-6, and nitric oxide.

The clinical sequelae of IL-2 treatment are similar to that of septic shock except that the severity of symptoms may be controlled by skipping doses or discontinuing treatment. Patients experience chills, rigors, fever, decreased peripheral vascular resistance, hypotension, tachycardia, vascular leak of fluid into the tissues, fluid retention, prerenal azotemia, intrahepatic cholestasis, diarrhea, pruritic rash, and sometimes severe compromise of organ function such as pulmonary edema, cardiac arrhythmias, confusion, hallucinations, or seizures. Fatal complications occurred in up to 4% of patients in early studies, but have declined to less than 1%, because more experience with the agent was gained and patients were screened for underlying heart and lung disease. Despite their severity, most toxicities resolve within 3 to 5 days of discontinuing IL-2. Some IL-2–treated patients develop hypothyroidism, and some with melanoma develop patchy vitiligo, findings that have been reported to correlate with response rates.

The Food and Drug Administration (FDA) has approved IL-2 at high doses for the treatment of metastatic melanoma and renal cell carcinoma with which 15% to 20% of patients experience more than a 50% shrinkage of their tumor. The truly remarkable aspect of IL-2 treatment is that 7% to 8% of patients experience complete responses, 75% of whom continue without additional treatment in follow-up that ranges from 5 to 12 years. Similar response rates, including complete responses in patients with renal cell cancer treated with lower doses of IL-2, have been reported. Because the optimal regimen has not been determined, a variety of IL-2 doses are used in practice. The dose depends on the treating physician and on individual patient characteristics. IL-2 may represent the first curative systemic treatment for patients with metastatic melanoma or renal cell cancer. IL-2 has also been reported to improve remission duration for patients with acute myelogenous leukemia when given after allogeneic bone marrow transplantation and appears to produce sustained rises in the number of circulating CD4 cells in AIDS patients.

COLONY-STIMULATING FACTORS

Hematopoiesis is regulated by a complex network of cell interactions and positive and negative cytokine regulators of cell growth and differentiation. A single hematopoietic stem cell gives rise to all lymphocytes, erythrocytes, and myeloid cells (including granulocytes, eosinophils, basophils, mast cells, monocytes, macrophages, and platelets). Many of the factors that influence hematopoiesis have been cloned, and four (granulocyte colony-stimulating factor [G-CSF], granulocyte-macrophage colony-stimulating factor [GM-CSF], erythropoietin, and IL-11) are approved for clinical use in humans (Chapter 256).

OTHER CYTOKINES

TNF produced negligible antitumor effects when administered systemically to patients at its maximal tolerated dose, which was limited by toxicity to the cardiovascular system. However, when a tumor-bearing limb is isolated on the heart–lung machine and perfused with TNF, together with interferon, hyperthermia, and melphalan, dramatic antitumor effects have been observed in up to 90% of patients with sarcoma and melanoma.

IL-3, IL-4, IL-6, and IL-7 have been tested clinically for their hematopoietic, immunologic, and antitumor effects, but all have been abandoned because of their lack of efficacy or their toxicity. IL-12 demonstrated impressive antitumor activity in animal models of kidney cancer; however, phase II testing in patients with renal cell carcinoma failed to demonstrate significant responses. Its immunologic effects, the promotion of a Th1 T-cell response that promotes cytotoxic T-cell activity, are being investigated in many trials in which IL-12 is the adjuvant for a vaccine against an infectious disease or cancer.

ADOPTIVE CELLULAR THERAPY

Several different approaches have been used to activate cells ex vivo and administer them to cancer patients. LAK cell and IL-2 therapy was mentioned earlier. Macrophages cultured ex vivo with IFN-γ or lipopolysaccharide have also been used. Various routes of delivery have been used for both cell types: intravenous, intraperitoneal, intrapleural, and intra-arterial. Although occasional tumor regressions have been reported, neither cell type is used for the treatment of any malignancy.

In general, antigen-specific CD8 $^+$ T cells are thought to be the most potent killers of cancer cells. Accordingly, efforts have been made to activate T cells ex vivo for adoptive transfer. Rosenberg and colleagues have resected tumor masses, cultured the tumor-infiltrating lymphocytes with IL-2, and administered them back to patients along with intravenous IL-2. One-third of patients who received cells had regression of their tumors;

however, the advantage of this approach, compared with IL-2 without cells, is unclear.

T-cell therapy has been used to treat viral diseases. After adoptive transfer, CD8$^+$ T-cell clones specific for cytomegalovirus (CMV) and HIV have been shown to localize to sites of antigen and to lyse targets in vivo. These clones require CD4 $^+$ helper T cells to persist and replicate in vivo. In transplantation patients with a high risk of CMV, reconstitution of CMV-specific T-cell responses and protective immunity were observed after transfer of CD8 $^+$ CMV-specific cytotoxic T lymphocytes isolated from their HLA-matched sibling donor. In an important demonstration of the potency of the cellular immune response, adoptive transfer of Epstein–Barr virus (EBV)–specific, polyclonal, donor-derived CD4 $^+$ and CD8 $^+$ T cells prevented and also caused regression of established EBV-related lymphomas in allograft recipients. Thus, T-cell therapy may be useful against virus-associated malignancies, such as Hodgkin's disease, cervical carcinoma, and adult T-cell leukemia/lymphoma, which express EBV, human papillomavirus (HPV) and human T-cell leukemia/lymphoma virus (HTLV)-I–related antigens, respectively.

The most effective adoptive therapy is the graft-versus-tumor effect seen in patients undergoing allogeneic bone marrow transplantation. T cells from the donor graft mediate significant antitumor effects in acute leukemia, lymphoma, and Hodgkin's disease. Several strategies are being tested to exploit the graft-versus-tumor effect, including infusing recipients with donor lymphocytes, which induces sustained remissions in up to 80% of patients with relapsed CML. Unfortunately, the infusions are often accompanied by graft-versus-host disease (GVHD), which has led investigators to introduce suicide genes into donor lymphocytes, which can be eliminated if severe GVHD ensues.

ACTIVE IMMUNIZATION

The "Holy Grail" of tumor immunology is to prevent or treat cancer by active immunization (vaccination). An example of successful prevention is the reduction in hepatocellular cancer after vaccination for hepatitis B. This strategy is most easily understood in the context of viral-associated tumors, which may be eradicated by immune responses to viral-specific antigens. However, the molecular identification of nonviral antigens on cancer cells has provided the tools to develop strategies to immunize patients against other cancers as well. In some instances, true tumor-specific antigens have been described. For example, the immunoglobulin idiotype on a B-cell lymphoma, a mutated oncogene (*p53,Ras*) or a new hybrid protein created by the chromosomal translocation in promyelocytic leukemia (PML)(PML-RARα) or CML (*bcr-abl*). Under certain conditions, normal proteins may serve as tumor antigens. These antigens, often called *differentiation antigens,* are expressed by cancer cells and their normal counterparts. Examples include HER2/*neu* in breast cancer, and MAGE, MART-1, and gp100, among others, in malignant melanoma. These proteins may serve as tumor rejection antigens.

Experiments in mice and clinical trials in patients have demonstrated that immunity to a tissue autoantigen can induce antitumor effects without inducing evidence of autoimmune disease. A variety of clinical trials have been performed in which patients have been immunized with modified or unmodified whole tumor cells, DNA coding for the tumor antigen, viruses (adenovirus or vaccinia) carrying the tumor antigen, or peptide fragments of the tumor antigen. Major tumor responses have been observed in patients with metastatic melanoma vaccinated with whole cells (autologous or allogeneic) and with peptides given alone or with dendritic cells as antigen-presenting cells.

Similar results have been reported for patients with low-grade lymphoma vaccinated against the immunoglobulin idiotype. As vaccination strategies are demonstrated to be safe and effective in patients with advanced cancer, they are being used earlier in the course of disease. For example, a trial of melacine (a lysate of two allogeneic melanoma cell lines) versus observation has been completed in patients with completely resected melanoma. The results are pending. A recent European trial compared an autologous tumor cell vaccine given with BCG to observation in patients with stage II and III colon cancer. Researchers reported a 44% reduction in recurrence in vaccinated patients, but no significant differences in overall survival. These promising results indicate that vaccine strategies are likely to play a major role in the management of patients with cancer in the near future.

MONOCLONAL ANTIBODIES

The concept of generating antitumor antibodies to treat cancer has been around for many years but has been hampered by a number of largely technical difficulties. The ability to humanize murine antibodies has enhanced their circulating half-life and allowed repeated administration without the induction of anti-antibody immune responses. Antibodies have the theoretical attribute of tumor specificity and therefore reduced toxicity. Several mechanisms of action have been postulated for antitumor antibodies: Fc-mediated immune activation (complement fixation, antibody-dependent cellular toxicity [ADCC]), blockade or activation of a critical receptor molecule (e.g., growth factor receptor), induction of apoptosis after engagement of a cell surface receptor, and the delivery of lethal drugs, toxins, or radionuclides.

A variety of antibodies have been approved for use in patients with cancer. Arcitumomab and capromab, monoclonal antibodies to carcinoembryonic antigen (CEA) and prostate-specific membrane antigen, respectively, are approved as radiolabeled agents for diagnostic imaging; two humanized monoclonal antibodies, rituximab (Rituxan) and trastuzumab (Herceptin) have been approved for treatment of non-Hodgkin's lymphoma and breast cancer, respectively.

Rituximab, which binds to the B-cell marker, CD20, causes tumor regression in approximately 50% of patients with previously treated low-grade lymphomas. Recent studies show that it is also effective in patients with aggressive non-Hodgkin's lymphomas and is particularly effective if administered in combination with chemotherapy. Rituximab may mediate antitumor effects by traditional antibody mechanisms, such as complement fixation and ADCC, or by inhibiting B-cell proliferation directly and inducing apoptosis. Radionuclide-conjugated anti-CD20 antibody has had significant antitumor effects at doses that ablate bone marrow and even at moderate doses (not requiring stem cell support).

In September 1998, the FDA approved the first antibody for the treatment of breast cancer, trastuzumab, an antibody to HER2/*neu*, a cell surface protein of the epidermal growth factor receptor family that is overexpressed in 25% to 30% of breast cancer patients. Approval was based on its activity by itself in heavily pretreated women and in combination with paclitaxel chemotherapy as first-line treatment in women with metastatic breast cancer whose tumors overexpress HER2/*neu*. Weekly therapy with trastuzumab was well tolerated, and only one of 903 women developed an antibody response to trastuzumab. When given in combination with paclitaxel as first-line treatment of metastatic breast cancer, trastuzumab more than doubled the time to progression, the overall response rate, and the duration of response. The percentage of patients alive at 1 year increased from 61% to 73%. The mechanism of action of this antibody when used alone is thought to be due to the resultant down-regulation of HER2/*neu* expression and the disruption of HER2/HER3 and HER2/HER4 heterodimers, with both events leading to a decrease in cell proliferation. Upcoming clinical trials will test the value of trastuzumab in the adjuvant setting.

ALTERATION OF TUMOR CELL BIOLOGY

Agents have been identified that physically interfere with the interaction of a growth factor with its receptor (e.g., antibodies or peptides that block the receptor, and suramin, which binds to basic growth factors) or with one or more steps in the receptor's signal transduction pathway (e.g., antagonists of protein kinase C, phospholipase C, tyrosine kinase, and phosphoinositol-3 kinase). A protein kinase C antagonist, bryostatin, is in clinical development, as are various inhibitors of tyrosine kinases. Prospects for the development of agents to target the expression of particular genes include antisense oligonucleotides, which block gene expression, and ribozymes, which cleave specific RNAs. Although there are many barriers to overcome before these molecules become drugs, clinical testing of some of these agents has begun (Table 255.1). Tumor growth beyond a small avascular solid tumor requires the induction of new blood vessels (angiogenesis) to meet the growing tumor's need for oxygen and nutrients. For tumor cells to become invasive and metastatic, they must penetrate the epithelial basement membrane and migrate through the extracellular matrix (ECM) to the lymphatics and blood vessels and adhere to stromal proteins through specific attachment sites (integrins and laminin). The metastatic process may be blocked by interfering with several steps: the inhibition of laminin binding to its receptor, the inhibition of metalloprotease activity to prevent digestion of basement membrane and interstitial matrix, the inhibition of angiogenesis and the blockade of factors that promote tumor motility.

Matrix metalloproteases (MMPs) are a family of enzymes that are responsible for the turnover and remodeling of extracellular

TABLE 255.1.	NEW BIOLOGIC AGENTS IN CLINICAL TRIALS	
Type	**Strategy**	**Comments/Tumor Types**
Antibody	Block EGF receptor	Head and neck, breast
	Selective toxicity: anti-B4–blocked-ricin	B-cell lymphoma
	Selective radiation:^{131}I anti–CD20	B-cell lymphoma
Fusion protein	Selective toxicity: IL-2/diphtheria toxin (Denileukin Diftitox)	IL-2R + cutaneous T-cell lymphoma
Tyrosine kinase Inhibitors	Inhibit PDGF receptor	Small molecules act inside cell to block ATP-binding site and prevent signal transduction; gliomas, CML
	Inhibit EGF receptor	
	Inhibit *abl*	
Farnesyltransferase inhibitor	Prevent *Ras* activity	Useful for a variety of tumors; after activation by a tyrosine kinase, *Ras* draws other kinases to the cell membrane to transmit the growth signal in the cell
CDK inhibitors (cyclin-dependent kinase)	Block cell cycle	Flavopiridol is in clinical trial
Antisense		
bcl-2	Restore apoptosis	Non-Hodgkin's lymphoma
bcr-abl	Inhibit proliferation and survival of bcr-abl–expressing cells	CML
Gene therapy		
p53 retrovirus or adenovirus	Restore p53 tumor-suppressive activity	Head and neck; lung
p53 adenovirus	Selectively kill p53-deficient cells	Head and neck
Antiangiogenesis	Block new blood vessel function	TNP-470; vitaxin; thalidomide, anti-VEGF, marimastat, angiostatin, endostatin
MMP inhibitors	Inhibit tumor growth and metastasis by blocking proteases	Batimastat and other numbered compounds

ATP, adenosine triphosphate; CML, chronic myelogenous lymphoma; EGF, epidermal growth factor; VEGF, vascular endothelial growth factor.

matrix proteins. The ECM consists of a network of fibrous proteins including collagens, laminin, fibronectin, proteoglycans, and gelatins. MMPs are zinc and calcium-dependent enzymes that are subclassified according to their substrate specificity. Inhibitors of MMPs have the potential of slowing or preventing tumor growth, local invasion, and metastasis. Because MMPs are involved in angiogenesis, MMP inhibitors also have antiangiogenic effects. Clinical trials of several MMP inhibitors are underway and some have reached phase III testing.

The discovery of positive and negative regulators of angiogenesis has led to the development of exciting new strategies to inhibit angiogenesis in cancer. There are more than ten compounds in clinical trial that attempt to target angiogenesis. Approaches include antagonizing angiogenesis factors, such as vascular endothelial growth factor (VEGF) or angiopoietin 1 with antibodies or soluble receptors, or developing agents that act directly on endothelial cells to block their migration or proliferation or induce apoptosis. Angiostatin and endostatin belong to the latter group of compounds. The MMP inhibitors and antiangiogenic agents offer a different paradigm of treating cancer; instead of killing cancer cells, these agents prevent growth and metastasis—a strategy that may complement surgery, radiation, and chemotherapy.

Differentiating agents may alter the malignant phenotype. Retinoids already have a useful role in cancer prevention and treatment. Retinoids bind to specific nuclear receptors that influence gene expression. Isotretinoin (13-*cis*-retinoic acid) is therapeutic for the premalignant condition, oral leukoplakia, and prevents second cancers of the aerodigestive tract in patients with head and neck cancer. Toxic effects include dry skin, phlebitis, hypertriglyceridemia, and conjunctivitis; dose reductions are required in many patients. Tretinoin (all-*trans*-retinoic acid—ATRA) induces remission in most patients with acute promyelocytic leukemia (APL), which contains a t(15:17) translocation that causes abnormal distribution of the retinoic acid receptor. With tretinoin, the chimeric receptor localizes normally and the malignant cells undergo terminal differentiation. Tretinoin works best when used together with chemotherapy. In addition to the usual retinoid toxicities, tretinoin-treated APL patients may experience the "retinoic acid syndrome" (fever and respiratory distress related to hyperleukocytosis).

GENE THERAPY

Human gene therapy has progressed from the bench to the bedside in a very short time. In 1990, a 4-year-old girl with severe combined immunodeficiency received an infusion of her own gene-modified T cells, which helped correct her underlying adenosine deaminase deficiency. Gene-marked tumor-infiltrating lymphocytes and bone marrow cells have been used to monitor the trafficking of lymphocytes and to determine the origin of relapsed leukemia or neuroblastoma, respectively. Gene therapy has many applications for cancer, and clinical trials are already in progress. Inactivation of oncogenes and gene replacement for lost or mutated tumor suppressor genes have been attempted. In vivo delivery of normal p53 to "correct" p53-deficient tumor cells using retroviral or adenoviral vectors has been attempted with occasional tumor regressions observed. In a particularly novel approach, investigators removed the gene in a normal adenovirus that disables the cellular p53 gene. This creates an adenovirus that can only grow in and kill p53-deficient (i.e., cancer) cells only after infection. Intratumoral injection of virus kills tumors in mice and has elicited significant tumor regressions in patients with head and neck cancer. Gene transfer has been used to deliver drug sensitivity genes (e.g., the herpes simplex thymidine kinase gene, HSV-TK) to tumor cells or normal T cells. Gene-modified cells can be exposed to gancyclovir, and only those cells expressing TK metabolize the drug and die. This cellular suicide strategy has been used against brain tumors and is being used to eliminate T cells causing GVHD after infusion of donor lymphocytes in patients with CML. The transfer of drug resistance genes to bone marrow cells has been performed to increase the dose of chemotherapy that can be administered safely. The most common application of gene therapy at present is to enhance the immune response to tumor antigens. Specific tumor antigens have been cloned into viral vectors for immunization. Tumor immunogenicity has been enhanced by in vitro or in vivo insertion of foreign HLA antigens, cytokines, and costimulatory molecules, alone or in combination.

Despite an occasional promising response, many challenges to the successful application of gene therapy remain. Many obstacles associated with vector design, gene delivery, and tissue-specific expression, as well as immunogenicity of many of the components must be overcome. However, as technology and our understanding of the basic physiologic processes improve, gene therapy approaches will become part and parcel of our daily treatment plans for patients with cancer.

BIBLIOGRAPHY

Boon T, Coulie P, Marchand M, et al. Genes coding for tumor rejection agents: perspectives for specific immunotherapy. *Biol Ther Cancer Updates* 1994;4(1):1.

Ferrari AC, Waxman S. Differentiation agents in cancer therapy. *Cancer Chemother Biol Resp Modif Annu* 1994;15:337–366.

Greenberg PD, Finch RJ, Garvin MA, et al. Genetic modification of T-cell clones for therapy of human viral and malignant diseases. *Cancer J Sci Am* 1998;4 [Suppl 1]:S100–S105.

Hsu FJ, Benike C, Fagnoni F, et al. Vaccination of patients with B-cell lymphoma using autologous antigen-pulsed dendritic cells. *Nature Med* 1996;2:52–58.

Klagsbran M. Angiogenesis and cancer. AACR special conference in cancer research. *Cancer Res* 1999;59:487–490.

Multani PS and Grossbard ML. Monoclonal antibody-based therapies for hematologic malignancies. *J Clin Oncol* 1998;16:3691–3710.

Pfeffer LM, Dinarello CA, Herberman, RB, et al. Biological properties of recombinant alpha-interferons: 40th anniversary of the discovery of interferons. *Cancer Res* 1998;58(12):2489–2499.

Rooney CM, Smith CA, Ny CYC, et al. Infusion of cytotoxic T cells for the prevention and treatment of Epstein-Barr virus-induced lymphoma in allogeneic transplant recipients. *Blood* 1998;92:1549–1555.

Rosenberg SA, Yang JC, Topalian SL, et al. Treatment of 283 consecutive patients with metastatic melanoma or renal cell cancer using high-dose bolus interleukin 2. *JAMA* 1994;271(12):97–113.

Roth JA, Christiano RJ. Gene therapy for cancer: What have we done and where are we going? *J Natl Cancer Inst* 1997;89:21–39.

Kelley's Textbook of Internal Medicine, fourth edition. Edited by H. David Humes. Lippincott Williams & Wilkins, Philadelphia © 2000.

CHAPTER 256

HEMATOPOIETIC GROWTH FACTORS

MALCOLM A.S. MOORE

Hematopoietic growth factors (HGFs) make up a family of cytokines with pleiotropic and frequently overlapping activities that regulate steady-state lymphohematopoiesis and also mediate acute responses involving specific cell lineages. HGFs are named (a) after the lineage they regulate (e.g., erythropoietin [EPO], thrombopoietin [TPO]), (b) after an assay that permitted their detection (e.g., colony-stimulating factors [CSFs]), (c) by the cell populations from which they are produced and with which they interact (e.g., interleukins), or (d) by the receptors with which they interact (e.g., c-*kit* and Flk-2/Flt-3 ligands). There are currently 18 interleukins (IL-1–18), and three CSF species (granulocyte, macrophage, and granulocyte-macrophage [G-, M-, GM-CSF]). The factors are not thought to be instructive but rather to act permissively to support the expression of a differentiation program that may, in large part, be stochastically determined. In certain cases, biologic activity is observed only when an HGF is combined with another factor or factors, resulting in synergy or antagonism.

GROWTH FACTOR RECEPTORS

HGFs signal through either of two large classes of receptor: the family of type III tyrosine kinase receptors (c-*kit*, Flk-2/Flt-3, fms/M-CSF, αβPDGFR [platelet-derived growth factor receptor]) or a large family of structurally related hematopoietin receptors. The conserved extracellular motifs of this latter family are derived from the fibronectin type III module. Different family members contain one to three chains. All such receptors are associated with one or more members of a family of Janus kinases (JAKs). These kinases couple ligand binding to tyrosine phosphorylation, both of known signaling proteins and of a unique family of transcription factors termed the signal transducers and activators of transcription (STATs).

The receptors for IL-3, IL-5, and GM-CSF each consist of a ligand-binding α chain associated with a common β chain whose membrane proximal domain associates with JAK2, leading to signal transduction. The receptors for a number of cytokines, including IL-6, IL-11, and leukemia inhibitory factor (LIF), all use ligand-specific binding chains that associate with gp130, which, in turn, associates with and activates JAK1 and JAK2. A third category is that of receptors consisting of single chains, which associate with JAK2 through a receptor membrane–proximal domain (EPO, TPO, G-CSF, growth hormone, prolactin). The IL-2 receptor family (IL-2, IL-4, IL-7, IL-9, IL-15) and the interferon receptor family (IFN-α/IFN-β, IFN-γ_c, IL-10) represent an association pattern in which two chains are required for signaling. The IL-2 receptor contains α, β, and γ_c chains, the cytoplasmic domains of the latter two being required for signal transduction. The receptors for IL-4, -7, -9, and -15 each contain a ligand-specific α chain and a γ_c chain. The sharing of receptor subunits among different cytokine receptors accounts partly for the redundancy that is characteristic of the cytokine family.

GRANULOCYTE COLONY-STIMULATING FACTOR

The purification and molecular cloning of G-CSF were performed between 1984 and 1986, and clinical development commenced in 1986 with approval for clinical use in cancer patients treated with chemotherapy. Human G-CSF is a glycoprotein of 19,600 D, encoded by a single gene on chromosome 17q21-22. It is produced constitutively by many tissues, particularly by monocytes and macrophages, endothelial cells, and fibroblasts, and high serum levels are induced by a variety of inflammatory stimuli, including bacterial lipopolysaccharides. G-CSF receptors are expressed on mature neutrophils (500 to 3,000 per cell) as well as on the myeloblast-promyelocytes and pluripotent stem cells. In vitro, G-CSF stimulates committed progenitors to form neutrophil granulocyte colonies, but in synergy with other factors such as Kit ligand (KL), it enhances proliferation of pluripotent progenitors, including stem cells.

In vivo administration of G-CSF causes an increase in neutrophil granulocyte production, owing to a ~threefold increase in amplification divisions and a 3- to 4-day reduction in transit time to mature granulocyte. Unlike with GM-CSF, there is no effect on leukocyte half-life or margination. G-CSF is a potent activator of neutrophils (PMN), mobilizing secretory vesicles (leukocyte alkaline phosphatase, CD11b) and inducing the release of specific granules (lactoferrin, CD11b, and CD66b) and azurophil granules (elastase, α_1-antitrypsin complexes). G-CSF enhances PMN superoxide release, and this enhances respiratory burst metabolism. Administration of G-CSF causes a significant increase in circulating CD34$^+$ cells, including primitive subsets (CD34$^+$Thy-1$^+$, CD38$^-$), with levels of circulating CD34$^+$ progenitors of up to 35 times what is usually normally achieved by the fifth day. Extensive clinical application of G-CSF–mobilized, peripheral blood stem cells in autologous and, recently, allogeneic transplantation has resulted because of the ease with which large numbers of CD34$^+$ cells can be obtained by apheresis and the more rapid platelet and neutrophil recovery observed, compared with results obtained with conventional marrow transplantation.

G-CSF (Filgrastim) was initially used as an adjunct to chemotherapy for ameliorating neutropenia, one of the major side effects of cancer chemotherapy. Its use led to reduced infections and hospital admissions. G-CSF has been approved for treatment of myelosuppression after bone marrow transplantation and for treatment of aplastic anemia and severe chronic neutropenia (idiopathic and congenital). Patients with Kostmann's syndrome are characterized by severe neutropenia, maturation arrest of the neutrophil lineage, and onset of severe, recurrent bacterial infections in early childhood. Most of these patients show sustained neutrophil recovery upon continuous G-CSF treatment (5 to 20 μg per kilogram per day).

The use of G-CSF for treatment of acute myeloid leukemia (AML) and myelodysplastic syndrome (MDS) was initially contraindicated because of concern that it might lead to stimulation of leukemic clones. However, in several large randomized trials, G-CSF has proved effective in stimulating neutrophil recovery and reducing infectious episodes without promoting leukemic growth. It has also proved effective for reversing the neutropenia associated with AIDS. G-CSF also prevents progression of systemic nonresponsiveness in systemic inflammatory response syndrome and sepsis. It has been shown to stimulate host immunity by increasing leukocyte numbers and up-regulating neutrophil function in postoperative/post-traumatic patients at risk for sepsis.

MACROPHAGE COLONY-STIMULATING FACTOR

Over 30 years ago, a CSF was identified in serum, urine, and fibroblast cell line–conditioned medium that had a restricted ability to stimulate the development of colonies containing only macrophages. As a result of alternative splicing, three spliced variants of biologically active M-CSF are produced, a short or α form of 256 amino acids, a long or β form of 554 amino acids, and a γ form of 438 amino acids. The COOH terminus anchors some forms of M-CSF in an active cell-associated form, with the native secreted form of M-CSFα being generated by proteolytic cleavage. M-CSF is present in normal plasma at levels of 100 to 200 units per milliliter. That M-CSF is ubiquitously expressed may reflect production by cells common to many organs, such as macrophages, endothelial cells, fibroblasts, and mesothelial cells. Fluctuations in levels of circulating M-CSF reflect a balance between production and excretion, with M-CSF receptors on tissue macrophages responsible for significant clearance by specific binding of M-CSF, with subsequent endocytosis and intracellular destruction. Adherence and bacterial lipopolysaccharides are potent inducing stimuli for monocyte and macrophage M-CSF production. High-affinity (kd = 10^{-13}M) M-CSF binding sites (cfms) are expressed at levels of $1 \times 10^4 - 1 \times 10^5$ per cell on mature monocytes, macrophages, and osteoclasts. M-CSF is involved in survival, proliferation, and differentiation of monocyte-macrophage populations, and functions as a macrophage activator as part of an inflammatory host defense response. Acute events after M-CSF interaction with monocytes include increased cell spreading, membrane ruffling, receptor turnover, enhanced macrophage phagocytosis, enhanced bactericidal and amebicidal capacity, up-regulation of Fc receptor (FcR)γ, antibody-dependent cell-mediated cytotoxicity (ADCC), and induction of a variety of cytokines (IL-1, G-CSF, tumor necrosis factor [TNF], IL-6). At the progenitor level, highly purified populations are stimulated by M-CSF alone, as well as by GM-CSF and IL-3, with a frequency indicating that many progenitors have receptors for all three growth factors. Osteopetrotic (op/op) mice have an autosomal recessive, inactivating mutation of the M-CSF gene, resulting in absence of M-CSF. They have quantitative macrophage defects, are toothless, and marrow cavities occluded by bone overgrowth due to an osteoclast deficit, thus indicating a critical role of M-CSF in osteoclast development or function. Clinical trials of recombinant human (rh)M-CSF revealed that treatment leads to expansion of circulating mononuclear phagocytes, enhanced macrophage ADCC and phagocytosis, reduced platelet levels, and reduction in serum cholesterol. The cholesterol-lowering effect may be attributed to enhanced macrophage activities of neutral and acidic cholesterol ester hydrolases, enhancing net hydrolysis of acidic cholesterol ester.

GRANULOCYTE-MACROPHAGE COLONY-STIMULATING FACTOR

GM-CSF has a molecular weight of 23 kD, with glycosylation at two N-linked glycosylation sites, and is encoded by a gene located on chromosome 5q23-31 in very close proximity to the IL-3 gene. The long arm of chromosome 5 contains a clustering of hematopoietic regulatory genes that includes GM-CSF, IL-3, IL-4, IL-5, M-CSF, and the receptors for PDGF and M-CSF (c-fms). GM-CSF is an inducible product of a variety of cell types, including activated T and B lymphocytes and activated macrophages.

The biologic effects of GM-CSF were initially related to its ability to stimulate proliferation and differentiation of myeloid-committed progenitors (colony-forming unit–granulocyte-macrophage [CFU-GM]) into neutrophilic granulocytes and monocyte-macrophages. GM-CSF can promote proliferation and differentiation of eosinophils, basophils, megakaryocytes, erythroid and dendritic cells, in synergy with other factors (e.g., with EPO for erythropoiesis, with TNF or IL-4 for dendritic differentiation). In synergy with KL or Flt-3 ligand (FL), it stimulates multipotent progenitors and stem cells. GM-CSF promotes survival of myeloid cells, including mature neutrophils, by suppressing apoptosis. The pleiotropic functions of GM-CSF extend to enhancement of innate as well as specific immune responses, which can be initiated alone or in synergy with other cytokines, such as TNF. GM-CSF enhances antibody-dependent cell killing and phagocytosis by neutrophils and macrophages and acts as a neutrophil migration (and adhesion-)-inhibitory factor. It also enhances Fc γ-receptor RII and class II major histocompatibility complex expression on monocytes and neutrophils and stimulates monocyte/macrophage cytokine, leukotriene, and prostaglandin release.

Excess levels of GM-CSF, achieved by intravenous or subcutaneous injections of glycosylated or nonglycosylated recombinant human GM-CSF, in primates and humans results in a leukocytosis involving elevation of neutrophils, eosinophils, monocytes, and, to a lesser extent, lymphocytes. The therapeutic applications of GM-CSF were initially restricted to amelioration of chemotherapy-induced myelotoxicity, allowing dose intensification. GM-CSF may also promote wound healing and has been used topically as a treatment for nonhealing wounds and ulcers. It has proved effective in radioprotection. Sustained administration of GM-CSF alone or in combination with cytoxan induces mobilization of CD34$^+$ cells, including both stem and progenitor populations, into the circulation. The apheresis product can then be used for both autologous or allogeneic transplantation. GM-CSF has proved effective as adjuvant therapy for bacterial and fungal infections in cancer patients and for adjuvant treatment of opportunistic fungal infections in AIDS patients. GM-CSF has also been shown to be a potent stimulator of sustained, specific, antitumor immunity and is used in various cancer vaccine strategies.

ERYTHROPOIETIN

Human EPO is a glycoprotein of molecular weight 34,000 to 39,000 D, with a polypeptide backbone of 166 amino acids and N-linked carbohydrate side chains that are essential for full activity in vivo, owing to rapid clearance of the desialated hormone from the circulation. EPO is produced mainly in the kidney, with less than 10% produced by the liver. The cellular action of EPO begins at the erythroid progenitor (erythroid burst-forming unit [BFU-E]) stage, where, together with KL, IL-3, or GM-CSF, it promotes erythroid differentiation. EPO alone at low concentrations prevents apoptosis of CFU-E, and at higher concentrations, is mitogenic, stimulating the formation of colonies of 64 to 128 orthochromatic erythroblasts within 7 days. In vivo treatment with EPO induces polycythemia in healthy persons. Recombinant EPO has been approved for treatment of patients with anemia associated with renal failure and for treatment of anephric patients. It has also been shown to reduce blood transfusion requirements in cancer patients receiving myelosuppressive chemotherapy and to counteract the anemia frequently seen in AIDS patients treated with zidovudine (AZT).

PLATELET-STIMULATING FACTORS

INTERLEUKIN-11

IL-11 consists of 199 amino acids, including a 21–amino acid leader sequence, with a molecular weight of 19,154 D, encoded by a gene mapping to chromosome 19q13.3–19q13.4. The cytokine is expressed by a wide range of normal tissues, and expression is modulated by several proinflammatory cytokines (IL-1α, IL-1β, TGFβ), and agonists. IL-11 has pleiotropic effects on hematopoietic cells, osteogenic cells, intestinal epithelium, and neural tissue. It is also a potent stimulator of acute-phase reactants, an inhibitor of adipogenesis, and an inducer of febrile response. It is a potent synergistic factor, acting with a variety of cytokines (IL-3, IL-4, IL-7, IL-12, IL-13, KL, FL, GM-CSF) to stimulate proliferation of primitive stem cells and progenitors. In vitro, IL-11 acts synergistically with IL-3 and TPO or KL to stimulate production, differentiation, and maturation of megakaryocytes, and in vivo it results in marked stimulation of megakaryopoiesis, with modest platelet elevation. A number of multicenter, randomized, placebo-controlled trials of IL-11 have been undertaken in cancer patients and have shown significant reduction in platelet transfusion requirements after high-dose chemotherapy, resulting in Food and Drug Administration approval of the cytokine for treatment of chemotherapy-associated thrombocytopenia.

THROMBOPOIETIN

The existence of a lineage-specific factor regulating platelet production was doubted until the discovery of an orphan cytokine receptor, c-*Mpl*, expressed on progenitor cells, megakaryocytes, and platelets, and the subsequent isolation of its ligand, TPO. Human TPO comprises an amino-terminal domain of 153 amino acids, showing 50% similarity to EPO, and a unique 181–amino acid C-terminal domain that is highly glycosylated. TPO is expressed constitutively in various tissues, and serum levels appear to be regulated by platelet and megakaryocyte mass, with TPO sequestered via high-affinity (kD ~100 to 400 pmol) binding to c-*Mpl* receptors. In vitro, TPO stimulates development of colonies of polyploid megakaryoctes from committed progenitors (CFU-Meg). TPO also acts synergistically (KL, FL) or additively (IL-6, IL-3) with other HGFs to stimulate megakaryocyte production.

Evidence for action of TPO on stem cells has been obtained in studies showing that TPO directly promotes survival and suppresses apoptosis of human primitive CD34$^+$CD38$^-$ bone marrow cells and by demonstration of c-*Mpl* on populations of highly enriched stem cells. In combination with the Flk-2/Flt-3 ligand, TPO produces prolonged (24 weeks) and extensive expansion of cord blood stem cells. Two forms of the protein have been clinically evaluated, one (recombinant hTPO) is a full-length polypeptide; the other is a recombinant, truncated form of TPO, consisting only of the EPO-like domain chemically modified by addition of polyethylene glycol (PEG-conjugated megakaryocyte growth and differentiation factor [PEG-MGDF]). Both are fully functional in vitro and have been evaluated in vivo in primates and in clinical trials.

In cancer patients, the platelet count begins to rise after 3 to 5 days, with up to a tenfold increase in platelets, using doses of 1.0 μg per kilogram per day for 12 days, and no alteration in platelet activation status. TPO also mobilizes stem and progenitor cells into the circulation, an activity of value in peripheral blood stem cell transplantation. Platelet counts returned to baseline faster, and nadir counts were higher in cancer patients receiving myelosuppressive chemotherapy and PEG-MGDF.

The greatest potential for TPO in the near future may be in transfusion medicine, in collection and storage of platelets from healthy donors, or in autologous settings. A single dose of 3 μg per kilogram of PEG-MGDF increased the yield of platelets by a factor of 4 and was associated with a quadrupling of platelet counts in recipients of the apheresed platelets. Clinical trials of

MGDF have been terminated because some recipients developed thrombocytopenia due to development of cross-reacting antibodies to endogenous TPO. This serious side effect is not expected to be seen with full-length, glycosylated TPO.

INTERLEUKIN-3

IL-3 is a glycoprotein of 25 to 30 kD, with a core protein of 14.6 kD consisting of 152 amino acids with a 19–amino acid signal peptide. IL-3 is produced by activated T cells, natural killer (NK) cells, and mast cells after transient increase in gene transcription and messenger RNA (mRNA) stabilization. It is probably a locally acting factor, because it does not normally circulate at detectable levels in the blood.

IL-3 directly stimulates colony formation by a spectrum of progenitors, including pluripotent and neutrophil-, eosinophil, basophil-, and macrophage-restricted progenitors. In synergy with other factors, it stimulates megakaryocyte and erythroid progenitors and pluripotent stem cells. In addition to growth stimulation and shortening of doubling time of early hematopoietic cells, IL-3 also has an antiapoptotic action on progenitor populations at concentrations lower than necessary to initiate proliferation. IL-3 alters the function of mature phagocytes, acting as a survival factor for monocytes and inducing macrophage secretion of TNF-α IL-1β, and IL-6. In preclinical studies in primates, IL-3 administration after intensive myelosuppressive chemotherapy dramatically enhanced myeloid recovery and reduced the duration of neutropenia. Numerous clinical trials have shown the beneficial effect of IL-3 after cytotoxic therapy, in the post-transplantation period after bone marrow transplantation, and in a variety of neutropenic settings.

KIT-LIGAND

Mutations at both the *Steel* and *white spotting* loci in mice cause macrocytic anemia, absence of mast cells, infertility, and depigmentation. The S1 and W loci encode a ligand–receptor pair—the kit receptor tyrosine kinase, the gene product of the protooncogene c-*Kit*, and its ligand. Mice bearing the S1 mutant have normal stem cells but a defective hematopoietic environment, due to absent or truncated ligand production, whereas W mutants have intrinsic stem cell defects due to c-*kit* receptor mutations.

Two alternatively spliced KL RNA transcripts encode two cell-associated KL proteins, KL-1 and KL-2, of 248 and 220 amino acids, respectively. The presence of a major proteolytic cleavage site on KL-1 provides a mechanism for production of a biologically active, soluble form of KL, whereas KL-2 provides a differentially more stable, cell-associated form of the ligand. Soluble KL is a potent mast cell growth factor on its own and is a potent synergistic factor when combined with a variety of cytokines (Il-3, GM-CSF, G-CSF, EPO, TPO), stimulating both early and late progenitor populations of myeloid, erythroid, and megakaryocyte lineage. KL has an antiapoptotic action, promoting survival of primitive hematopoietic cells. KL also has important effects on cell–extracellular matrix and cell–cell interactions.

Potential clinical uses of KL have been limited by adverse

events involving dermal mast cell activation, with pruritic wheal formation and 10% to 20% of patients developing allergy-like reactions characterized by urticaria and, in some cases, laryngeal edema. Lower doses of KL (stem cell factor) have been used in conjunction with G-CSF for mobilization of CD34$^+$ cells, resulting in significant improvement in the quantity of CD34 cells harvested and in their quality, as measured by ex vivo expansion potential and stem cell content.

FLK-2/FLT-3 LIGAND

The Flk-2/Flt-3 receptor is activated by a cognate molecule termed the Flt-3 ligand (FL). The ligand exists in both a transmembrane and soluble form. FL promotes the survival and stimulates proliferation, differentiation, and mobilization of early hematopoietic progenitors, differing from KL in that it does not potentiate erythropoiesis nor stimulate mast cells, but it does potentiate the growth of pro-B cells in synergy with IL-6 and IL-7. It primarily acts as a synergistic factor, maximally stimulating CD34$^+$ stem and progenitor cell proliferation when combined with IL-3, IL-6, KL, GM-GCF, or TPO. FL enhances the rate of growth of IL-3–dependent colonies by shortening the duration of the G1 phase. Of all the cytokines, FL appears to be the most effective synergistic factor in promoting stem cell self-renewal, resulting in expansion of stem cell numbers.

In vivo treatment of mice and primates with FL demonstrated that it is a potent mobilizer of hematopoietic progenitors and, when combined with G-CSF, gives much higher mobilization levels than does either cytokine alone. Dramatic increases in dendritic cells of both T-lymphocyte and myeloid derivation are seen, in blood and lymphohematopoietic tissues, after FL treatment, and this response can promote an antitumor effect.

BIBLIOGRAPHY

Armitage JO. Emerging applications of recombinant granulocyte-macrophage colony-stimulating factor. *Blood* 1998;92:4491–4508.

Burdach S, Nishinakamura R, Dirksen U, et al. The physiologic role of interleukin-3, interleukin-5, granulocyte-macrophage colony-stimulating factor, and the beta c receptor system. *Curr Opin Hematol* 1998;5: 177–180.

Flanagan AM, Lader CS. Update on the biologic effects of macrophage colony-stimulating factor. *Curr Opin Hematol* 1998;5:181–185.

Garland JM, Quesenberry PJ, Hilton DJ, eds. *Colony stimulating factors: molecular and cellular biology*, second ed. New York: Marcel Dekker, 1997:1–566.

Hartung T, von Aulock S, Wendel A. Role of granulocyte colony-stimulating factor in infection and inflammation. *Med Microbiol Immunol* 1998; 187:61–69.

Johnston EM, Crawford J. Hematopoietic growth factors in the reduction of chemotherapeutic toxicity. *Semin Oncol* 1998;25:552–561.

Kaushansky K. Thrombopoietin. *N Engl J Med* 1998;339:746–754.

Lacombe C, Mayeus P. Biology of erythropoietin. *Haematologica* 1998;83: 724–732.

Lyman SD, Jacobsen SE. C-Kit ligand and Flt3 ligand: stem/progenitor cell factors with overlapping yet distinct activities. *Blood* 1998;91: 1101–1134.

Shpall EL, Wheeler CA, Turner SA, et al. A randomized phase 3 study of peripheral blood progenitor cell mobilization with stem cell factor and filgrastim in high-risk breast cancer patients. *Blood* 1999;93: 2491–2501.

Welte K, Gabrilove J, Bronchud MH, et al. Filgrastim (r-metHuG-CSF): the first 10 years. *Blood* 1996;88:1907–1929.

Kelley's Textbook of Internal Medicine, fourth edition. Edited by H. David Humes.
Lippincott Williams & Wilkins, Philadelphia © 2000.

CHAPTER 257

BLOOD TYPES, TISSUE TYPING, AND TRANSFUSION OF BLOOD PRODUCTS

FRANK T. HSIEH
STEVEN A. MECHANIC
EDWARD SNYDER
ALBERT DEISSEROTH

ABO BLOOD TYPES

Red blood cells (RBCs) contain numerous antigenic structures on their surfaces. The most important of these are the ABO antigens. The A and B genes of the ABO system code for glycosyl transferases that add *N*-acetyl galactosamine or galactose, respectively, to a common precursor H antigen. The O gene produces an enzyme with no activity, so only H antigen is present. These antigens form the basis for the ABO blood group system. ABO is the most important blood group system because most persons have naturally occurring IgM and IgG antibodies directed against non–self antigens of this system. These IgM antibodies can fix complement and cause rapid intravascular hemolysis. Major hemolytic transfusion reactions may cause hypotension, shock, disseminated intravascular coagulation (DIC), renal failure, and death. ABO antibodies directed against the antigens not present on an individual's own RBCs are normally present without prior exposure and are referred to as *naturally occurring antibodies.* Thus, in those with type A blood, anti-B antibodies are present, with type B blood, anti-A antibodies are present. Similarly, patients with type O blood recognize the A or B antigens as foreign and have naturally occurring anti-A and anti-B antibodies. Conversely, type O RBCs are not agglutinated by (do not react with) anti-A or anti-B antibodies. Therefore, transfused type O RBCs are compatible with any recipient blood type. Individuals of blood type AB, have neither anti-A or anti-B in their plasma.

The other major blood group system of clinical significance is the Rh system with five major antigens designated C, D, E, c, e (no "d" gene is expressed). Of the Rh antigens, the D antigen is the most important clinically. Fifteen percent of whites do not produce the D antigen; they are said to be Rh-negative. The D antigen is highly immunogenic. If an Rh-negative woman is transfused with Rh-positive RBCs, delivers an Rh-positive infant, or miscarries or aborts an Rh-positive fetus, resulting in fetomaternal hemorrhage with D antigen positive RBCs, she has a 70% chance of developing anti-D IgG antibodies. Because IgG can cross the placenta, any future Rh-positive infants will be at high risk for a potentially fatal intrauterine hemolytic anemia, also called *hemolytic disease of the newborn,* or erythroblastosis fetalis. For this reason, Rh-negative patients, particularly women with childbearing potential, should always be given Rh-negative blood. Furthermore, Rh-negative women who undergo abortion or delivery of an Rh-positive fetus are routinely treated with Rh Ig, a commercial hyperimmune globulin with anti-D specificity, which binds to the D antigen on the fetal Rh-positive blood cells that have entered the maternal circulation. Use of passive hyperimmune anti-D, Rh Ig prevents active D antibody formation in the mother by an as-yet undefined mechanism.

Because most fatal hemolytic transfusion reactions result from mistakes in patient identification made at the bedside rather than mistakes made in the laboratory, great care must be taken to draw the blood from the correct patient and to label the tube properly. When a physician orders a typing and cross-match, the blood bank requests a sample of blood from the recipient. The blood bank types the recipient's RBC using commercial reagent anti-A and anti-B antibodies. Then, the recipient's serum is tested for the presence of naturally occurring antibodies usually with commercial A and B reagent RBCs. An antibody screen is then routinely performed to reveal the presence of any "unexpected" RBC antibodies.

For the antibody screen, the recipient's serum is mixed with a set of two type O reagent RBCs that contain the antigens to which alloantibodies commonly develop. Agglutination in any reaction phase, that is, immediate spin, 37° C, or antihuman globulin, also known as *Coombs' phase,* would indicate the presence of an antibody. If a positive result is found with the antibody screening, then the recipient's serum is further studied by evaluating a panel of 10 or more type O reagent red cells whose antigen expressions are also known. Systematic elimination of nonreactive red cell antigens yields a pattern that can identify an antibody specificity. Antibodies that react with all panel cells are called panagglutinins; panagglutinins are seen in autoimmune hemolytic anemia. For transfusion, the recipient's serum is mixed in vitro (cross-matched) with an aliquot of RBCs from the units intended for transfusion. If compatible, the RBC unit is provided for transfusion.

▪ TISSUE TYPING

Just as RBCs contain antigenic structures on their surface membranes, some of which are highly immunogenic and limit transfusion, so do other cells contain immunogenic antigen structures. One specific family of antigens present on almost all cells other than RBCs is the human leukocyte antigen (HLA) system. This is another system of genetic polymorphisms for which multiple alleles are present in the population. HLA antigens are encoded by a closely linked cluster of genes on the short arm of chromosome 6. From the point of view of tissue typing, two types of surface antigens are encoded by the genes of the HLA locus. Class I molecules, which are present on virtually all cell

surfaces except RBCs and trophoblastic cells, are composed of two noncovalently linked polypeptide chains. The smaller chain is called β_2-microglobulin, with a molecular weight of 11.5 kD. The larger 44-kD glycosylated heavy chain carries the antigenic specificity and is inserted into the cell membrane. The heavy chains of the class I molecules are encoded for by three loci on chromosome 6: HLA-A, HLA-B, and HLA-C. Each locus has several possible alleles, so a given person has a specific set of class I molecule heavy chains, depending on the HLA-ABC set or haplotype inherited from each parent. β_2-microglobulin is encoded for by a gene on chromosome 15, and the same structure is shared by all three class I molecules. Class II antigens are composed of a 34-kD α chain and a 29-kD β chain. Both are inserted into the cell membrane and are noncovalently linked. Class II antigens are present on B lymphocytes, monocytes, and activated T lymphocytes. They are encoded by several loci (HLA-DP, HLA-DQ, HLA-DR) within the D region of the HLA complex on chromosome 6.

The antigens HLA-A, HLA-B, HLA-C, and HLA-DR can be determined serologically with specific antibody testing, just as performed in RBC blood group testing. In addition, some of the HLA-D antigens, particularly the HLA-DR antigens, can be defined by mixed lymphocyte culture. In mixed lymphocyte culture, the patient's lymphocytes are incubated with a panel of irradiated or mitomycin-treated lymphocytes of known HLA-D type. The patient's lymphocytes transform when exposed to lymphocytes of a different D type. The irradiated or mitomycin-treated lymphocytes, however, cannot transform because of the damage to their DNA. Lymphocytes to which the patient does not respond are considered to be of the same HLA-D type. Transfusion of non–leukocyte-reduced random-donor platelets results in HLA alloimmunization in up to 80% of patients with aplastic anemia who have an intact immune system. Clinically significant HLA alloantibodies occur in a smaller percentage of transfused patients with acute leukemia and in transfused bone marrow transplantation recipients, presumably because of the immunosuppressive effects of the patient's disease and treatment.

There is increasing evidence that since platelets carry only HLA class I antigens, "pure" concentrations of platelets (i.e., those units of platelet concentrates that are leukocyte-reduced) are minimally immunogenic. The development of antibodies to platelet class I HLA antigens appears to require the concurrent presence of foreign HLA class II antigens, which are present on lymphocytes and monocytes. Exclusive use of leukocyte-depleted blood products using third-generation absorption filters markedly delays or totally prevents the development of platelet HLA alloimmunization. In addition, by markedly decreasing the number of white blood cells (WBCs) in RBC or platelet transfusions, these filters can reduce chills or fever related to blood product infusion and likely prevent the transmission of cytomegalovirus (CMV) as well.

COMPONENT THERAPY

The standard blood donation is up to 500 mL (± 10%) of whole blood with addition of about 63 mL of an anticoagulant preservative solution containing citrate, phosphate, and dextrose

(CPD), or CPD and adenine (CPDA-1). Citrate binds calcium, which is essential for the coagulation cascade, and thus serves as an in vitro anticoagulant. Dextrose is added to serve as a substrate for glycolysis. Phosphate serves as a buffer, and adenine can be added to promote the generation of adenosine triphosphate (ATP), necessary for normal RBC sodium-potassium pump function. In addition to CPD, an additive solution containing saline, dextrose, and adenine (Adsol) may be added to further extend the storage life of RBCs. Despite addition of these substrates and 1 to 6° C refrigeration of the blood unit to slow metabolism, progressive RBC glycolysis results in lactic acid accumulation. Because mature RBCs lack mitochondria, they do not have a Krebs cycle to remove pyruvate and prevent lactate accumulation. This slow lactic acid accumulation lowers the pH and eventually results in loss of viability of the stored cells.

The shelf life of RBCs stored in liquid phase at 1 to 6 ° C, is 21 days in CPD and 35 days in CPDA-1. With the addition of an additive solution, the shelf life extends to 42 days, because the additive solution contains more adenine and can produce more ATP. Blood may also be frozen at −80° C for a maximum of 10 years using glycerol as a cryoprotective agent to prevent freeze–thaw damage. This technique is generally reserved for rare blood types.

Most collected whole blood can be separated into blood components such as RBCs, platelets, plasma, and cryoprecipitate. The plasma may be further fractionated to produce albumin, immune globulin, or specific clotting factor preparations. The major advantages of component therapy are that a patient's specific needs can be met and that each element of the donated unit of blood is optimally used (Table 257.1).

TABLE 257.1.	BLOOD COMPONENT THERAPY: INDICATIONS AND COMPLICATIONS	
Component	**Indications**	**Complications**
Red blood cells (RBCs)	Anemia	Fever Volume overload Hepatitis and other infections Urticaria Hemolytic transfusion reaction Increased viscosity
Leukocyte-poor RBCs	Prior febrile reactions to RBCs May delay or prevent human leukocyte antigen (HLA) alloimmunization	
Washed or plasma-poor RBCs	Prior urticarial reactions IgA deficiency Need to avoid complement transfusion (e.g., paroxysmal nocturnal hemoglobinuria)	
Frozen RBCs	Rare blood types Autologous donations Process also removes leukocytes and plasma	
Whole blood	None	
Random-donor platelets	Bleeding with platelet count <50,000/μL Bleeding and qualitative platelet dysfunction Elective surgery and thrombocytopenia Prophylactic for platelet <10,000–15,000/μL	Fever Urticaria Hepatitis Bacterial contamination
Single-donor platelets	Transplant of HLA alloimmunized recipients	
Leukocyte-poor platelets	Prior febrile reactions to RBCs or platelets May delay HLA alloimmunization	
HLA-matched single-donor platelets	Poor response to platelet transfusion due to HLA alloimmunization	
Granulocytes	Documented bacterial infection not responding to appropriate antibiotics with severe neutropenia; not expected to recover for several days	Fever, chills Respiratory distress Alloimmunization
Fresh frozen plasma	Coagulation factor deficiency, rapid warfarin reversal, with plasmapheresis for thrombotic thrombocytopenic purpura	Volume overload Hepatitis and other infections Hypocalcemia
Cryoprecipitate	Hypofibrinogenemia Uremic bleeding	Hepatitis and other infections
Humate-P or AlphaNine	Severe von Willebrand disease	
Intravenous immune globulin	Hypogammaglobulinemia Idiopathic thrombocytopenic purpura	Systemic reactions Local venous reaction Anaphylaxis
Recombinant lyophilized factor VIII	Hemophilia A	
Recombinant factor IX	Hemophilia B Factor VIII inhibitor	
Albumin	Volume expansion	

RED BLOOD CELLS

The main goal of RBC transfusion is to increase oxygen carrying capacity. The life span of the RBC is 120 days. In general, anemia is fairly well tolerated down to a hemoglobin level of 8 g per deciliter. Below this level, cardiac output increases to compensate for the decreased oxygen carrying capacity. Young patients without cardiopulmonary, hepatic, renal, or cerebrovascular disease may tolerate a hemoglobin level as low as 6 to 7 g per deciliter. In most adult patients, each unit of transfused RBCs raises the hemoglobin level by 1 g per deciliter or the hematocrit by 3%. Cancer patients who are anemic due to chemotherapy often are transfused at a hemoglobin of 7 to 8 g per deciliter unless a condition such as angina exists that may require transfusion to a higher hemoglobin. Transfusion of 1 to 2 units of RBCs is not an uncommon therapeutic intervention for a hemoglobin of 8 g per deciliter in a symptomatic cancer patient. In immunosuppressed persons, RBCs are irradiated to avoid the occurrence of life-threatening post-transfusion graft-versus-host disease (GVHD).

A unit of RBCs (non–leukocyte-reduced) has 100% of the RBCs, 100% of the WBCs, and 20% of the plasma originally present in the donated unit of whole blood. There is an increasing worldwide trend toward using blood products leukocyte-reduced by filtration. The leukocytes present in donated blood have been implicated in many transfusion complications, including febrile transfusion reactions, HLA alloimmunization, immunosuppression and immunomodulation, transmission of CMV, development of post-transfusion GVHD, and viral activation (see also Complications of Transfusion).

If the desired outcome is an increase in hemoglobin or hematocrit, the physician should order 1 to 2 units of RBCs. Whole blood is generally no longer available and has been replaced by infusion of additive-solution RBCs or RBCs plus crystalloid. Because of changes during storage, whole blood contains insufficient amounts of viable platelets and factors V and VIII. If a patient needs factor replacement, the following blood components are indicated: fresh frozen plasma for clotting factor deficiencies, cryoprecipitate for fibrinogen replacement, and platelets for thrombocytopenia or thrombocytopathy.

Occasionally, a physician may wish to avoid transfusing plasma to a patient, such as a patient who has had a prior allergic or anaphylactic reaction to plasma. Patients with a congenital IgA deficiency may develop an IgG anti-IgA antibody and may have severe anaphylactic reactions after exposure to plasma. The physician dealing with this problem should contact the blood bank to inform them that the recipient is IgA deficient and has an anti-IgA antibody. The blood bank can provide washed cellular components or obtain special-order IgA-negative components, including fresh frozen plasma.

Because of high costs and potential complications associated with RBC transfusions, attempts have been made to find an alternative method of increasing a patient's hematocrit. Erythropoietin is a glycoprotein that stimulates RBC production. It is produced in the kidney and stimulates the division and differentiation of committed erythroid progenitors in the bone marrow. Recombinant erythropoietin has been available for clinical use since 1989 and has become increasingly popular. Remarkably

well tolerated, one of the most important uses of recombinant erythropoietin therapy has been the correction of anemia associated with renal failure. Over 300,000 renal patients worldwide are now receiving this treatment.

Chronic renal failure is the prototypic erythropoietin-deficient state. More than 95% of patients with renal failure have a positive response to recombinant erythropoietin treatment. Moreover, with the commonly used weekly maintenance dose, this treatment can be cost-effective compared with RBC transfusions. Several studies have also demonstrated an improvement in quality of life in dialysis patients receiving erythropoietin and whose hemoglobin concentration increases from 6 to 7 g per deciliter to 9 to 10 g per deciliter. Besides its usage in renal failure patients, recombinant erythropoietin therapy can be used in other clinical settings as well, although with varying degrees of effectiveness.

Three other indications for use of recombinant erythropoietin therapy are approved by the Food and Drug Administration. They are, in decreasing order of evidence for their effectiveness, HIV-related anemia induced by zidovudine treatments with an erythropoietin level less than 500 mU per milliliter; chemotherapy-induced anemia in nonmyeloid malignancies; and reduction of perioperative allogeneic blood transfusions, limited to noncardiac and nonvascular elective surgeries in patients with hemoglobin higher than 10 and lower than 13 g per deciliter. Although only approximately 50% of unselected anemic cancer patients respond sufficiently to recombinant erythropoietin treatments, studies have shown that those who do respond have a significant increase in their energy level, functional status, and overall quality of life. Further studies are needed to define the optimum dose and schedule of recombinant erythropoietin administration and also to identify better predictors of response.

Other clinical settings in which the use of recombinant erythropoietin may provide benefit include the following: autologous blood collection, multiple myeloma, non-Hodgkin's lymphoma, myelodysplastic syndrome, rheumatoid arthritis, inflammatory bowel disease, acceleration of erythroid repopulation after allogeneic bone marrow transplantation, hyporegenerative anemia in patients undergoing organ transplantation and receiving cyclosporin A, and sickle cell anemia or thalassemia. Further studies are needed, however, to establish firm guidelines for the use of recombinant erythropoietin under these varied clinical circumstances.

PLATELETS

Platelet transfusions are indicated for treating patients with bleeding associated with thrombocytopenia or with a thrombocytopathy. For treating qualitative defects of platelet function, the indications for transfusion are complex. Often, because there is an excess of nonfunctional platelets, platelet transfusion may not correct the bleeding time to a measurable extent. Since the life span of platelets is about 8 days, this may mean that repeated platelet transfusions may be required if the clinical situation is life threatening. In general, the bleeding time begins to prolong as the platelet count falls below 100,000/μL and increases linearly down to a platelet count of 10,000 platelets/μL. In general, at a platelet count of 75,000/μL, the bleeding time is about 10 minutes; at 50,000/μL, it is about 15 minutes; and at 25,000/μL, it is about 20 minutes. At any given platelet level, patients with thrombocytopenia due to decreased production have a greater tendency to bleed than do patients with thrombocytopenia due to increased destruction, such as with idiopathic thrombocytopenic purpura. Circulating platelets in conditions with decreased production are older and physiologically less active, whereas in conditions associated with increased destruction, the marrow responds by markedly increasing its production of platelets. These circulating platelets generally are younger and more hemostatically effective.

In certain special clinical circumstances, such as life-threatening surgical bleeding or intracranial hemorrhage, a patient with 50,000 to 75,000 platelets/μL may benefit from a platelet transfusion. Patients who are actively bleeding after a major surgical procedure at a platelet count below 50,000/μL) might benefit from a platelet transfusion as well. Patients who are severely thrombocytopenic (less than 10,000 to 15,000 platelets/μL), particularly when the condition is due to decreased production, are often given prophylactic platelet transfusions to prevent intracranial or other serious bleeding. This practice must be balanced against the risk that frequent prophylactic platelet transfusions may result in alloimmunization, which limits the efficacy of further platelet transfusion (refractoriness). In non-neoplastic conditions such as aplastic anemia, 80% of patients given non–leukocyte-reduced random-donor platelets will develop HLA alloantibodies. In contrast, in cancer patients undergoing chemotherapy, the incidence of HLA alloimmunization is less than 30% (13% in some series). Single-donor platelets, either cross-matched or HLA-matched, are usually sufficient to improve low post-transfusion increments in HLA-alloimmunized patients. Use of leukocyte reduction filters for all blood transfusions will substantially reduce or eliminate the risk of HLA alloimmunization in these patients.

In immunosuppressed patients, including patients on chemotherapy, irradiation of blood products including platelets is recommended to avoid post-transfusion GVHD, which is associated with life-threatening bone marrow aplasia in addition to the usual skin, liver, and gastrointestinal tract manifestations of GVHD disease. Platelet sensitization also leads to febrile and allergic reactions. Platelet transfusions pose a risk of bacterial infections. About 1 in 1,500 to 1 in 2,500 units of platelets are believed to be contaminated with some type of bacteria.

Prophylactic platelet transfusions are designed to prevent serious bleeding episodes in persons with a platelet count below 10,000 to 15,000/μL. A pool of 4 to 6 units of random-donor platelets or a unit of single-donor platelets given once each day when the platelet count is below 10,000 to 15,000/μL is a reasonable clinical plan. If the patient is bleeding, repeated platelet transfusions may be indicated until the platelet count is above 50,000/μL or until the bleeding stops.

Platelet concentrates are prepared by centrifugation of whole blood or by platelet apheresis. One platelet concentrate contains 60% to 80% of the platelets originally present in the unit of whole blood and raises the post-transfusion platelet count by 5,000 to 10,000/μL. Apheresis platelets are collected by automated blood cell separators and contain the equivalent of 6 to 8 units of random-donor concentrates. There are several disease-related and other reasons why a patient may show poor post-transfusion platelet count increments, including HLA alloimmunization, splenomegaly, poor-quality platelets, use of ABO-incompatible platelets, rapid platelet consumption due to bleeding, sepsis, DIC, mucositis, antibiotics and other drugs, and antiplatelet antibodies. These causes all should be considered and the blood bank medical director consulted before committing a patient to a course of single-donor cross-matched platelets.

In patients suspected of having poor post-transfusion platelet count increments, platelet counts should be checked before, 1 hour after, and 24 hours after transfusion to ensure that an adequate increment has been attained. Patients who become alloimmunized (as evidenced by a less-than-expected increment in platelet count at 1 hour) can be treated with cross-matched, compatible, single-donor or HLA-matched platelets. The increment in platelet count achieved after transfusion can be calculated with the formula known as the corrected count increment (CCI):

$$CCI = (\text{Post-tx plt ct}) - (\text{pre-tx plt ct})$$
$$\times BSA/(\text{Platelets transfused} \times 10^{-11})$$

where pre-tx plt ct = pretransfusion platelet count, post-tx plt ct = post-transfusion platelet count, and BSA = body surface area in square meters. A CCI higher than 7,500 is considered an acceptable outcome. Each unit of random-donor platelet concentrate is estimated to contain 6×10^{10} platelets and a unit of apheresis platelets 3×10^{11} platelets. In individuals with qualitative defects of platelet function, a single transfusion of 4 to 6 units of random-donor platelets or a unit of single-donor platelets may have no significant clinical effect if a large excess of nonfunctional platelets is circulating at that time. Therefore, in patients who are being prepared for surgery, more frequent transfusion or pheresis of nonfunctional platelets from the recipient coupled with platelet transfusion from a normal donor may be required to correct the prolonged bleeding time associated with severe defects of platelet function.

Platelets lack Rh antigens. However, platelets from Rh-positive donors still should not be transfused to Rh-negative women of childbearing potential because Rh-positive RBCs are present in platelet concentrates and may immunize the mother. If there is no alternative to an Rh-incompatible platelet transfusion, the patient could receive intravenous or intramuscular Rh immune globulin to prevent formation of an active D antibody.

GRANULOCYTES

Over 200 billion granulocytes are circulating in the intravascular volume of a 70-kg person and another equal number of granulocytes is adherent to the endothelial surface. Since the life span of granulocytes is only 6 hours, the marrow usually has a reserve of nearly mature granulocytes that is six times the circulating granulocytes mass in the marrow ready for release. Granulocytes in stored whole blood are not viable. If granulocytes are needed, they must be freshly collected by apheresis technology. The efficacy of granulocyte transfusions is further limited by the following: the small number of neutrophils that can be collected from untreated normal volunteer donors, only 1 to 1.5×10^{10}/

collection; their short transfused half-life (6 hours); their short (24-hour) shelf-life; and the reactions encountered with their use, including acute respiratory distress. Higher doses of granulocytes can be collected from donors who are treated with granulocyte-colony stimulating factor (G-CSF) or granulocyte macrophage-colony stimulating factor (GM-CSF) (6 to 8 $\times$ 10^{10} PMN/collection). Transfusion of these granulocytes from G- or GM-CSF mobilized donors produces greater measurable post-transfusion neutrophil increments of 1 to 3,000/μL, even in adults.

Clinical trials of prophylactic granulocyte transfusions, however, conducted before G-CSF was available for donor mobilization did not show an impact on survival for the septic patient with leukemia. Studies using G-CSF–stimulated donors who are able to provide much larger numbers of neutrophils have not been reported. At this time, the indication for the use of granulocyte transfusions is restricted to the clinical settings of progressive local infection that is life threatening in patients who have been temporarily rendered neutropenic ($\leq$ 500 PMN per microliter) for a period of several days in response to their chemotherapy. Such patients should have a reversible clinical condition, and should exhibit progression of local infection despite appropriate antibiotics. Some clinicians have reported a negative interaction between the concomitant administration of amphotericin B and granulocyte transfusions. These two therapeutic interventions are best administered separately.

■ COMPLICATIONS OF TRANSFUSION

Transfusion of ABO-incompatible blood (e.g., type A blood given to a patient with type O blood) can generate a dangerous acute intravascular hemolytic transfusion reaction. Biologic response modifiers released during such a reaction in association with the fixation of complement, such as inflammatory cytokines interleukin-1 (IL-1), interleukin 6 (IL-6), and tumor necrosis factor-α (TNF-α), cause rapid intravascular hemolysis and may result in DIC, acute renal failure, bronchospasm, hypotension, shock, and death. Symptoms suggestive of evolving intravascular hemolysis include low back pain, chest pain, restlessness, shortness of breath, and pain at the site of transfusion. Physical signs may include fever, chills, tachypnea, wheezing, rash, hypotension, arrhythmia, tachycardia, oliguria or anuria, diaphoresis, hemoglobinuria, and generalized bleeding due to DIC. If a major hemolytic transfusion reaction is suspected, the clinician should do the following:

1. Stop the blood transfusion immediately.
2. Take measures designed to reverse potentially life-threatening conditions generated by the transfusion reactions: administer intravenous fluids and vasopressors as needed to support the blood pressure, including possibly renal-dose dopamine ($\leq$5 μg per kilogram per minute); ensure an adequate airway, provide oxygen and administer diphenhydramine, steroids, and epinephrine to reverse the bronchospasm. Use of diuretics should be considered after establishing adequate intravascular volume replacement. Diuretics, such as mannitol or furosemide will help to ensure adequate urine output to prevent oliguric renal failure and acute tubular necrosis. Mannitol should be avoided if renal failure has already begun.

3. Notify the blood bank.
4. Check the identification of the blood unit and patient.
5. Send the remaining blood to the blood bank.
6. Draw blood samples from another vein to check for hemoglobinemia and to repeat the typing and cross-match.
7. Obtain a urine sample to check for hemoglobinuria.

If the patient develops DIC and is bleeding with an increased prothrombin and partial thromboplastin time, replacement clotting factor therapy should be initiated using fresh frozen plasma. Cryoprecipitate should be given if the fibrinogen level is less than 50 to 80 mg per deciliter; platelet transfusion should be considered if the platelet count is less than 50,000 platelets/μL and the patient is bleeding. The patient's fluid intake and output, serum electrolytes, blood urea nitrogen, and creatinine should be monitored.

Patients exposed to blood transfusions may form antibodies against RBC antigens other than ABO. A transfusion reaction due to infusion of incompatible RBC antigens other than those antigens in the ABO system rarely results in acute intravascular hemolysis. Such patients, however, may have an acute or delayed extravascular reaction. Indeed, most non-ABO alloantibodies are IgG and are not present in high enough titers, or the antigen density on the RBC is not high enough, to activate the full C1–C9 complement sequence. If a patient has preexisting alloantibody from previous transfusions or pregnancies and blood containing the implicated blood group antigen is given, the patient usually does not have an acute intravascular hemolytic reaction. Instead, the transfused RBCs become coated with IgG and are removed by the spleen and the reticulendothelial system, resulting in a shortened life span. Associated with this extravascular reaction, the transfused blood undergoes relatively rapid destruction, with an increase seen in the recipient's level of indirect and total bilirubin and lactic dehydrogenase, but without signs of hemoglobinemia or hemoglobinuria. Also absent with an extravascular hemolytic reaction is the life-threatening clinical scenario seen with acute intravascular hemolysis as previously discussed.

RBC alloantibody actually may be present in a recipient at such low titer that it is not detected by the routine antibody screen or cross-match. This phenomenon is sometimes seen with alloantibody against antigens in the Kidd system (Jk^a or Jk^b). After transfusion with Jk^a antigen-positive RBCs, such a patient may have an anamnestic rise in antibody titer to high levels—usually in 5 to 7 days—and experience a rapid fall in hemoglobin and increases in the levels of bilirubin and lactic dehydrogenase. This is due to hemolysis of the previously transfused and still circulating Jk^a-positive RBCs, now hemolyzing because of the increased titer of Jk^a antibody in the recipient. This is termed a *delayed hemolytic transfusion reaction*. If the antibody binds complement to C9, the reaction produces hemoglobinemia and is considered a delayed intravascular hemolytic transfusion reaction; if complement is not fixed or is fixed only to C3, it produces an extravascular transfusion reaction. Similar reactions can be seen in patients with antibodies to antigens of the Rh, Kell, Duffy, and other blood group systems.

The most common transfusion reactions are febrile and allergic reactions. Febrile reactions are due to the reaction of the recipient to the foreign HLA and the leukocyte antigens present on transfused WBCs and to cytokines in non–leukocyte-reduced products (Table 257.2). HLA alloantibodies to transfused leukocytes occur in at least 20% of previously pregnant women and in up to 60% of multiply transfused patients. Since fever may be the presenting sign of a major hemolytic or septic transfusion reaction, when a patient develops a fever during transfusion the physician must stop the transfusion and send a blood sample to the blood bank for workup.

Although a serious concern, most post-transfusion chills and fever are rarely due to infusion of blood contaminated with bacteria. Normally, aseptic technique, cold storage, and the natural antibacterial effects of the neutrophils and plasma prevent bacterial growth in stored RBCs. Occasionally, however, gram-negative bacteria that can grow in the cold, such as *Yersinia*

enterocolitica, contaminate a unit of blood and produce endotoxin, both of which can cause DIC and shock after transfusion. Rarely, these contaminated units can be detected by visual inspection of the blood before transfusion. Any units with an unusual color, blood clots, or hemolysis must be quarantined or returned to the blood bank if the problem is not detected before arrival at the bedside. Platelets are also at risk of bacterial contamination since they are stored at 20° to 24° C. They can become contaminated with a variety of skin flora as well with enteric organisms. Infusion of such contaminated units can also produce septic shock.

Urticaria or hives may occur in 3% to 5% of transfusions and is thought to be due to reaction to plasma protein constituents. The transfusion must be stopped when these reactions are first noted. The transfusion may be resumed *only* if there are no signs of respiratory involvement or cardiovascular instability. If severe allergic signs are encountered or if wheezing, hypotension, or fever is noted, the transfusion must be stopped and the blood bank contacted. For serious allergic reactions, laryngeal edema, wheezing, dyspnea, or hypotension and tachycardia can occur, and a major hemolytic transfusion reaction should be ruled out. Diphenhydramine, hydrocortisone, and possibly epinephrine should be given as needed for treatment of other anaphylactic reactions.

The most severe post-transfusion anaphylactic reactions are occasionally fatal. They are usually due to IgA deficiency in a recipient who has developed anti-IgA antibodies. IgA deficiency is common (1:1000 persons), but antibody formation is rare. Patients with known IgA deficiency and an IgA antibody should receive washed RBCs and washed platelets; if these patients require plasma or plasma constituents, they should be derived from IgA-deficient donors.

Immunocompetent donor lymphocytes in donated blood can result in transfusion-associated GVHD in a susceptible recipient. Post-transfusion GVHD usually results in bone marrow aplasia and a minor rash, rather than conjugated serum hyperbilirubinemia or diarrhea, as usually seen in post-transplant engraftment syndromes. Post-transfusion GVHD is primarily restricted to severely immunosuppressed patients, such as those with congenital immunodeficiency syndromes, those with recent bone marrow or organ transplantation, and those with Hodgkin's disease or non-Hodgkin's lymphoma who are receiving intensive radiation and chemotherapy. Post-transfusion GVHD may also occur if immunocompetent patients receive blood from haplo-identical first-degree relatives. As a precaution, all such recipients should receive only irradiated cellular blood products.

With progressive storage, RBCs accumulate lactic acid and slowly leak potassium into the extracellular fluid. The increase in potassium rarely causes problems in adults. However, when transfusing patients in anuric renal failure or premature infants, blood less than 2 weeks old or washed RBCs have a lower extracellular potassium and may be preferred; the blood bank director should be consulted in such cases. In adults, major clinical problems associated with massive transfusion (more than 7 to 10 units within 24 hours) are thrombocytopenia and, if administration is too rapid, hypothermia. Hyperkalemia and acidosis after massive transfusion are problems primarily in newborns. Citrate toxicity resulting in hypocalcemia is primarily restricted to massively

TABLE 257.2.	DIFFERENTIAL DIAGNOSIS OF ACUTE TRANSFUSION REACTIONS
Clinical Feature	**Possible Diagnosis**
Fever and chills	Major hemolytic transfusion reaction
	Reaction to foreign human leukocyte antigens on transfused WBCs and platelets
	Contaminated blood
Dyspnea	Fluid overload
	Major hemolytic transfusion reaction
	Contaminated blood
	Air embolism
	Anaphylactic reaction due to transfusion of IgA-containing plasma to IgA-deficient recipient with anti-IgA
	Pulmonary leukoagglutinin
Bleeding	Disseminated intravascular coagulation due to major hemolytic transfusion reaction or contaminated blood
	Thrombocytopenia due to massive transfusion of RBCs
	Dilution of coagulation factors due to massive transfusion of RBCs
Dysrhythmia	Circulatory overload
	Hyperkalemia
	Hypothermia
	Hypocalcemia
	Major hemolytic transfusion reaction
	Contaminated blood
	Air embolism
Hypotension	Major hemolytic transfusion reaction
	Contaminated blood
	Anaphylaxis due to IgA deficiency
Hemoglobinuria	Major hemolytic transfusion reaction
	Excessive infusion pressure through small-bore needle
	Overheating with blood warmer
	Contaminated blood

RBCs, red blood cells; WBCs, white blood cells.

transfused patients with severe liver dysfunction who cannot metabolize the citrate in the anticoagulant/preservative solution. The routine administration of calcium to massively transfused patients is rarely necessary, however, because of the rapid metabolism of citrate in most patients.

Another important adverse event associated with transfusion is the transmission of infectious disease. Currently, blood donors are tested for hepatitis B surface antigen (HbsAg), hepatitis B core antibody (anti-HBc), human T-cell lymphotropic virus antibody (anti-HTLV-I/-II), anti–hepatitis C virus antibody (anti-HCV), HIV antibody-1/ -2, HIV-1 p24 antigen (Ag), and syphilis. Blood components can also transmit diseases caused by bacteria and parasites, mainly malaria, babesiosis, and trypanosomiasis. Changes to ensure the safety of the blood supply include addition of new-donor screening tests, elimination of paid donors, and the routine screening of blood donors using updated donor history questionnaires. Risks of disease transmission are presented in (Table 257.3). It is known that virus can be transmitted from a blood donor who has recently acquired a viral infection and who is infectious but whose donor screening tests are still negative. This is known as the "window period." The length of the window period of infection has been substantially shortened even further by inception of nucleic acid testing (NAT) to screen donors for HIV and HCV. NAT testing is basically PCR testing for HIV and HCV. Eventually, all donor blood testing for infectious diseases will be performed by NAT (PCR) testing. Such testing can shorten the window period for HCV from the current 70 days to 11 days, and HIV from 16 days to 10 days.

CMV infection causes a mononucleosis-like syndrome in normal hosts and can cause severe pneumonia, bone marrow failure, colitis, retinitis, and hepatitis in immunocompromised or bone marrow transplant patients. CMV disease can be largely prevented by the use of CMV-seronegative blood products or by the use of third-generation leukocyte depletion filters. Because CMV is a virus that resides in leukocytes, many medical centers are now using prestorage or in-laboratory leukocyte-depleted blood as an equivalent product to CMV-seronegative blood.

Each unit of blood contains 250 mg of iron, whereas the daily excretion of iron from the body is about 1 mg. Patients with a chronic hemolytic anemia and an ongoing transfusion requirement, such as patients with thalassemia major, may receive more than 80 to 100 units of blood over many years. These patients have a significant risk of transfusion hemosiderosis, which can lead to congestive heart failure, diabetes, liver dysfunction, and impotence. Patients with a reasonable life expectancy who are expected to receive large numbers of transfusions should be considered to be candidates for prophylactic iron chelation therapy such as desferroxamine infusion.

BIBLIOGRAPHY

Alter HJ, Purcell RH, Shih JW, et al. Detection of antibody to hepatitis C virus in prospectively followed transfusion recipients with acute and chronic non-A, non-B hepatitis. *N Engl J Med* 1989;321:1494–1500.

Bordin JO, Heddle NM, Blajchman MA. Biologic effects of leukocytes present in transfused cellular blood products. *Blood* 1994;84: 1703–1721.

Cazzola M, Mercuriali F, Brugnara C. Use of recombinant human erythropoietin outside the setting of uremia. *Blood* 1997;89:4248–4267.

DeChristopher PJ, Anderson RR. Risks of transfusion and organ and tissue transplantation: practical concerns that drive policies. *Am J Clin Pathol* 1997;107(suppl 1):S2–S11.

Goodnough LT, Brecher ME, Kanter MH, AuBuchon JP. Transfusion medicine. *N Engl J Med* 1999;340:438–533.

Heddle NM, Klama L, Singer J, et al. The role of the plasma from platelet concentrations in transfusion reactions. *N Engl J Med* 1994;331: 625–628.

Kelton JG, Heddle NM, Blajchman MA. *Blood transfusion: a conceptual approach.* New York: Churchill Livingstone, 1984.

Mollison PL. *Blood transfusion in clinical medicine,* eighth ed. Oxford: Blackwell Scientific Publications, 1987.

Triulzi DJ, ed. *Blood transfusion therapy,* sixth ed. American Association of Blood Banks, 1999.

Kelley's Textbook of Internal Medicine, fourth edition. Edited by H. David Humes.
Lippincott Williams & Wilkins, Philadelphia © 2000.

TABLE 257.3.	INFECTIOUS RISKS OF BLOOD TRANSFUSION

Infectious Cause	Estimated Frequency (per unit)
Viral	
HIV	1:760,000
Hepatitis A	1:1,000,000
Hepatitis B	1:80,000
Hepatitis C	1:100,000
Parvovirus B19	1:10,000
HTLV types I and II	1:800,000
Bacterial (Contamination)	
Platelets	1:2,500
Red cells	1:500,000

HTLV, human T-cell leukemia virus. (Adapted from Goodnough LT, Brecher ME, Kanter MH, AuBuchon JP. Transfusion medicine. *N Engl J Med* 1999;340:438.)

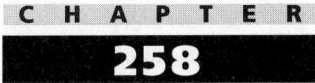

CHAPTER 258

HEMATOPOIETIC STEM CELL TRANSPLANTATION

STEPHANIE J. LEE
JOSEPH H. ANTIN

Hematopoietic stem cell transplantation refers to the use of marrow-derived or circulating totipotent cells to reestablish normal marrow and immune function that has been compromised. This advanced form of hematologic support is necessary when malignancies are treated with high-dose chemotherapy or radiation (or both) or when there are congenital or acquired deficiencies in hematopoiesis or immunity as in severe combined immunodeficiency syndrome, thalassemia, or aplastic anemia. Two fundamentally different types of hematopoietic transplantations are performed: autologous procedures (in which the patient serves as his or her own stem cell donor) and allogeneic procedures (in which another person donates the stem cells). For the most part, the goal of hematopoietic stem cell transplantation has been cure of the underlying disease; given the risks of the procedure and short- and long-term side effects, hematopoietic stem cell transplantation is not usually considered appropriate for palliation. Table 258.1 shows the current indications for stem cell transplantation.

The use of high-dose therapy with stem cell transplantation is becoming more common. Worldwide, 30,000 to 40,000 transplantations are performed annually, and this rate is increasing by 10% to 20% per year. Improved supportive care, advances in the understanding of immunology and tissue typing, and greater availability of unrelated donors has expanded the role of stem cell transplantation to a wider spectrum of patients and indications. It is increasingly likely that physicians of varied specialties will encounter patients who are appropriate candidates for stem cell transplantation or who have been treated with this modality.

 # HISTORICAL PERSPECTIVE

The first reported (although unsuccessful) attempt to infuse allogeneic bone marrow into another human for therapeutic purposes was in 1939. A patient with aplastic anemia was given sibling bone marrow intravenously but died 5 days later. In 1940, another patient with aplastic anemia received sibling bone marrow by direct injection into his sternum. No prior chemotherapy or radiation was given. Although the patient's blood counts improved, methods for confirming engraftment were not available, and it is likely that spontaneously autologous recovery rather than allogeneic engraftment occurred. In 1957, Dr. E. Donnell Thomas reported six patients with malignancies treated unsuccessfully with infusions of allogeneic bone marrow. All these early attempts took place before an understanding of human leukocyte antigen (HLA) typing. It was 11 years before advances in HLA typing, transfusion medicine, and treatment of infectious diseases allowed the first documented successful human allogeneic transplantations. In 1968, three children with immunodeficiency diseases were engrafted using bone marrow from siblings. These patients are alive and well today.

Other discoveries integral to the modern practice of stem cell transplantation soon followed. One of the greatest barriers to allogeneic transplantation is an immunologic reaction of mature competent donor lymphocytes against host tissues, a phenomenon known as *graft-versus-host disease* (GVHD). The ability to minimize this complication with the use of fully matched donors and prophylactic administration of cyclosporine (approved by the Food and Drug Administration in 1983) has expanded stem cell sources beyond sibling bone marrow. The first successful umbilical cord blood transplantation was in 1988, and the number of these procedures is growing rapidly. The dramatic increase in the use of compatible unrelated donors and improving results observed during the 1990s is partly due to the ability to identify better HLA matches using molecular techniques. Finally, use of allogeneic peripheral blood rather than marrow as a stem cell source is growing rapidly.

Although early efforts focused more on allogeneic than on autologous transplantation, the number of autologous procedures performed annually exceeded allogeneic ones in 1990, and the gap continues to widen. The first two human autologous transplantations were reported in 1960 for patients with non-Hodgkin's lymphoma and mycosis fungoides. However, the procedure did not gain popularity until the late 1980s. Granulocyte colony-stimulating factor (G-CSF) and granulocyte-macrophage colony-stimulating factor (GM-CSF) were approved in 1991 and have probably contributed the most to the diffusion of this technology. These drugs facilitate collection of adequate circulating progenitors and speed engraftment. Most autologous procedures are now performed using peripheral blood stem cells and not marrow.

General trends are recognizable owing to work by the International Bone Marrow Transplant Registry (IBMTR) and other

TABLE 258.1.	MAJOR INDICATIONS FOR STEM CELL TRANSPLANTATION

Acute and Chronic Leukemias
Acute myelogenous leukemia (AML)
Acute lymphoblastic leukemia (ALL)
Chronic myelogenous leukemia (CML)
Chronic lymphocytic leukemia (CLL)

Lymphomas
Non-Hodgkin's lymphoma
Hodgkin's disease

Plasma Cell Disorders
Multiple myeloma
Amyloidosis

Solid Tumors
Breast cancer
Ovarian cancer
Testicular
Non–small-cell lung cancer
Neuroblastoma

Immunodeficiencies/Metabolic Disorders
Severe combined immunodeficiency disorders
Wiskott–Aldrich syndrome
Chédiak–Higashi syndrome
Hunter's/Hurler's syndrome
Adrenoleukodystrophy

Nonmalignant Hematologic Disorders
Aplastic anemia
Myelodysplastic disorder
Paroxysmal nocturnal hemoglobinuria
Sickle cell disease
Diamond–Blackfan anemia
Fanconi's anemia
Thalassemia
Amegakaryocytic thrombocytopenia

large organizations that track transplant activity worldwide. Statistics collected over the last 20 years show that transplantation has evolved from a therapy used primarily in a young population with nonmalignant disease to a modality most often applied to older patients with malignancies. Physicians used to wait until patients were quite ill before proceeding with aggressive therapy. Now, as the procedure has become safer and prognostic factors predicting poor results with nontransplantation therapy are better recognized, transplantation is being offered earlier in the disease course. Seventy-five percent of allogeneic procedures are now performed for leukemia while 75% of autologous transplants are done for breast cancer or lymphoma.

SOURCES OF STEM CELLS

Cells capable of reconstituting hematopoiesis and lymphopoiesis reside primarily in the bone marrow, but also circulate and may be isolated from other sites. Sources of stem cells include bone marrow, peripheral blood, and umbilical cord blood. Potential donors include the patient themselves (autologous procedures), identical twins (syngeneic donors), and other related or unrelated individuals (allogeneic donors). In recognition of the different sources of stem cells, the common acronym BMT (for bone marrow transplantation) is changing to hematopoietic stem cell transplantation.

Under current technology and donor selection criteria, stem cell donation is very safe. Peripheral stem cell collection is similar to platelet donation and is often carried out in outpatient blood donor centers. Hematopoietic colony-stimulating factors are used to increase the numbers of circulating progenitor cells, which are then collected by leukapheresis. These stem cells are either cryopreserved for later use or infused directly into the patient.

Bone marrow is harvested in the operating room with patients under general or spinal anesthesia. Approximately 10 to 15 mg per kilogram recipient weight of marrow is removed using multiple (5 to 10 mL) bilateral aspirations of the posterior iliac crest. This represents about 5% of the donor's marrow volume, which will quickly regenerate. Most patients recover without difficulty and require only oral analgesia upon discharge home. However, some do suffer from pain at the harvest sites and prolonged fatigue, and 0.1% to 0.3% have major or life-threatening complications. The risk of death from marrow donation has been estimated at 1 in 15,000 to 1 in 20,000, approximately one-third to one-half the yearly risk of driving an automobile.

Umbilical cord blood is another source of allogeneic stem cells. Blood is collected from the umbilical cord and placenta at the time of delivery, samples are taken from the mother and baby for infectious disease testing and tissue typing, and the units are cryopreserved for later use. Because of the limited number of stem cells available in the small volume of cord blood, concerns about the ability to engraft adults have restricted this procedure primarily to pediatric patients. Several central repositories are now banking cord blood for transplantation. Data suggest that the risk of acute GVHD is less than with stem cells obtained from older donors, but platelet engraftment is delayed. The reduction in GVHD risk may allow the use of products with higher degrees of incompatibility than is otherwise tolerable.

The normal dose of nucleated cells infused is 1 to 5×10^8 per kilogram of recipient weight. All available evidence suggests that this inoculum is sufficient for regeneration of adequate hematopoiesis to last the patient's lifetime. When bone marrow, peripheral blood, or cord blood is infused into the patient, still undefined adhesion molecules allow the stem cells to infiltrate into marrow cavities, where expansion occurs. No detectable recovery of peripheral counts is visible until 8 to 21 days later. In fully engrafted allogeneic recipients, all hematopoietically derived elements including blood components, tissue macrophages, Kupffer's cells in the liver, dermal Langerhans' cells, and probably some microglial cells are donor derived. However, the bone marrow stroma and any remaining thymic tissue remain host-derived. Although not common, allergies, immunities, and autoimmune diseases and predispositions may also be transplanted with an allogeneic stem cell graft. Unfortunately, little donor immunity against infectious agents is transferred, necessitating substantial immune reconstitution and reimmunization against common pathogens.

PREPARATION FOR TRANSPLANTATION

Unlike the situation facing solid organ recipients where a limited, nonregenerable supply of organs exists, no triage system in stem cell transplantation determines priority. However, the procedure is rigorous, and patients must be carefully screened. The high doses of chemotherapy and radiation, need for extensive polypharmacy, and inevitable complications of transplantation place significant strains on the cardiac, pulmonary, hepatic, and renal systems, which will be exacerbated by underlying dysfunction. Patients typically undergo a full battery of tests to determine suitability for transplantation and to detect any correctable deficits before the procedure. Echocardiograms or MUGA (multigated angiogram) scans and pulmonary function tests are performed. Patients are tested for evidence of exposure to herpes simplex virus, cytomegalovirus, Epstein–Barr virus, varicella zoster, hepatitis B and C, human T-cell lymphotrophic virus 1 (HTLV-1), HIV, *Treponema pallidum* infection, *Toxoplasma* infection, and tuberculosis. Detection of HIV has generally been an absolute contraindication to transplantation. Before admission, patients must be made aware of the real possibility of serious and fatal side effects of the therapy. In most hospitals, full informed consent is required.

Patients are conditioned for transplantation using a variety of chemotherapy- and irradiation-based regimens. The goal of conditioning, which usually takes place in the 7 to 10 days before infusion of the stem cells, is to provide antitumor effects, to create "space" in the marrow by depletion of host hematopoiesis, and, in the case of allogeneic transplants, to immunosuppress patients enough to allow engraftment of the donor stem cells. Commonly used chemotherapy agents are cyclophosphamide, etoposide, busulfan, melphalan, carmustine, and thiotepa, often in combination. Fractionated total body irradiation is given in doses of 1200 to 1400 cGy. For the most part, no established conditioning regimen is clearly superior to the others.

After conditioning is accomplished, reinfusion of stem cells is by simple transfusion. It is not currently known how the cells home to the marrow. Evidence of engraftment occurs approximately 8 to 21 days after stem cell infusion and is influenced by the stem cell source, cell count, use of hematopoietic growth factors, and the type of GVHD prophylaxis (in allogeneic transplantation). Engraftment is defined as the day that the absolute neutrophil count is greater than 500 per milliliter. Platelet and red cell engraftment usually occurs after neutrophil engraftment.

SUPPORTIVE CARE

Most centers have dedicated teams of physicians, nurses, social workers, nutritionists, and other support personnel who care for transplantation patients. Early after transplantation, the acute toxicities of the conditioning regimen and the complications of neutropenia dominate. During the time period waiting for engraftment, patients require transfusions of red cells and platelets, broad-spectrum antibiotics and often antifungal agents if fevers develop, and pain medication and parenteral nutrition if mucositis is severe. Central venous catheters allow intravenous access, given the extensive infusion needs. Patients remain in sterile environments, typically in specialized units where they are cared for by specially trained nurses. Some centers are now performing outpatient transplantations for low-risk patients, but even these centers must have access to adequate inpatient facilities to manage any emergency complications.

ISSUES IN AUTOLOGOUS TRANSPLANTATION

Autologous transplantation is used primarily for patients with non-Hodgkin's and Hodgkin's lymphomas, multiple myeloma, and solid tumors including breast, ovarian, testicular, non–small-cell lung cancer, and neuroblastoma. These tumors are thought to have a dose response to chemotherapy. Thus, administering high doses of conditioning may increase the response rate while marrow toxicity is ameliorated with the stem cell infusion. Patients with chemotherapy-responsive disease in a minimal disease state are the best candidates for autologous transplantation.

The advantages of autologous over allogeneic stem cell sources are the immediate availability of a donor, relative lack of toxicity, and faster lymphohematopoietic recovery. The duration of neutropenia is often briefer, and since the reconstituting graft is genotypically identical to the patient, there is no risk of GVHD. However, the overwhelming cause of treatment failure after an autologous transplantation is relapse of the original disease. Tumor cells contaminate both peripheral blood and bone marrow collections. Investigators have tried to reduce the number of tumor cells infused back to the patient with the graft by either negative selection (purging using tumor-specific antigens or in vitro chemotherapy agents) or positive selection (retaining only cells with markers for early progenitor cells). None of these techniques has proved to reduce relapse rates. Indeed, it is unlikely that most of the infused cells are biologically capable of causing disease. Most patients recur in original tumor sites, sug-

gesting that it is residual disease and not reinfused cells that is responsible for most relapses. The lack of a graft-versus-tumor effect (see below) probably also contributes to the high relapse rates. If the conditioning regimen is not sufficient to eliminate the tumor, there is no immunologic barrier to eventual relapse.

ISSUES IN ALLOGENEIC TRANSPLANTATION

The theoretical advantages of allogeneic transplantation include (a) replacement of the hematopoietic system in patients in whom stem cell damage or disease preclude autologous transplantation, (b) no risk of relapse from the stem cell source, and (c) the new immune system offers the possibility of a graft-versus-tumor effect and lower relapse rates. However, it is acknowledged that these advantages come with a variety of disadvantages, including higher treatment-related mortality and risk of acute and chronic GVHD. Although relapse is the single most likely cause of treatment failure after allogeneic transplantation, most deaths are due to transplant-related mortality such as infection, GVHD, and organ failure. More people die from the procedure itself than from relapse of their original disease.

One problem with allogeneic transplantation is that most patients do not have suitable family member donors. Since both maternal and paternal HLA alleles are expressed and a child inherits one allele from each parent, full siblings have a 25% chance of matching each other. Given the average family size in the United States, only 30% of patients have sibling donors. For a patient with multiple siblings, the chance of having an HLA-identical sibling donor is equal to $1 - (0.75)^n$, where n is the number of siblings. The chances of finding a nonsibling family member who would be an appropriate donor is approximately 5% and makes typing of the extended family reasonable in certain circumstances. Nevertheless, two-thirds of patients need to look beyond their families for their donors.

For those unable to find a related donor, identification of a matched unrelated donor is a possibility. Almost 3 million volunteers are in the National Marrow Donor Registry, the major registry in the United States. Many other registries exist around the world. Cooperation among them through an organization called Bone Marrow Donors Worldwide allows transplantation centers to search the world for the most appropriate donors. Approximately 85% of white patients, 59% of African American, 62% of Asian American, and 76% of Hispanic patients initiating unrelated donor searches eventually find donors. Allogeneic donors are selected on the basis of the degree of match with the patient, their relationship to the patient (sibling, other family member, unrelated individual), age, gender, prior history of pregnancy or transfusion, and infectious disease status.

The human major histocompatibility complex (MHC) is located on the short arm of chromosome 6 and codes for the HLAs. These highly polymorphic glycoproteins are found on almost all cells and are critical to the immune response. Class I (HLA-A, -B, -C) and class II antigens (HLA-DR, -DP, -DQ) may be identified by either serologic or molecular methods. Although the traditional "perfect" match is 6/6 (HLA-A, -B, -DR), more refined HLA typing is changing this definition so that people now speak of 10/10 or even 12/12 matches. Failure to be completely matched at known loci is associated with greater degrees of GVHD, graft rejection, and poorer immune reconstitution, resulting in higher morbidity and mortality. Efforts to cross HLA barriers using 5/6 matched or other alternative donors have met with difficulty in overcoming these complications. Even when completely matched allogeneic donors are used, differences in minor histocompatibility antigens can result in serious GVHD.

GVHD occurs when a cascade of events, triggered by immunologic differences between patient and donor, cause tissue damage. Alloreactive T cells play a critical role in this complication, and allogeneic recipients require either chemoprophylaxis (cyclosporine and methotrexate) or T-cell removal to prevent severe acute GVHD. In contrast to solid-organ transplantation, immune tolerance eventually occurs in most allogeneic recipients, allowing discontinuation of all immunosuppressive therapy. Either clonal deletion of alloreactive cells or induction of anergy may be the mechanism for this tolerance.

Patients undergoing allogeneic transplantation do not recover substantial immune function until at least 1 year after transplantation, whereas those receiving stem cells from an unrelated donor are considered severely compromised for at least 2 years. Before immune recovery, patients have defects in both cellular and humoral immunity. They are often hypogammaglobulinemic, do not respond to immunizations appropriately, and have a risk of overwhelming infections. In patients with chronic GVHD, which is also associated with ongoing need for immunosuppression, the immune defects may last indefinitely.

SPECIFIC COMPLICATIONS OF HEMATOPOIETIC STEM CELL TRANSPLANTATION

By definition, high-dose therapy carries a much higher risk of mortality and toxicity than conventional-dose chemotherapy. Estimated treatment-related mortality rates vary from 1% to 5% for autologous procedures to 10% to 50% for allogeneic procedures. Table 258.2 summarizes the most common complications of hematopoietic stem cell transplantation.

EARLY COMPLICATIONS

Early complications account for most treatment-related deaths. Most conditioning regimens, by virtue of their effects on actively dividing cells, result in mucositis and alopecia. Nausea and vomiting are common despite use of serotonin antagonists. During the period of neutropenia, patients have a significant risk of developing gram-positive, gram-negative, and fungal infections, and antibiotics and antifungal agents are used frequently. The herpesviruses tend to reactivate during and after transplantation and require prophylactic treatment or careful observation and prompt treatment of infection.

Failure to engraft is a rare but dire complication. In autologous transplantation patients, this is usually due to a poor harvest or to progenitor damage when multiple chemotherapy regimens deplete stem cells before collection. In allogeneic transplantation

TABLE 258.2.	COMPLICATIONS OF HEMATOPOIETIC STEM CELL TRANSPLANTATION

Early

Nausea, vomiting
Mucositis
Diarrhea
Pancytopenia
Failure to engraft, graft rejection
Deep venous thrombosis—catheter-related
Pericarditis, cardiomyopathy
Hemorrhagic cystitis
Acral dermatitis
Alopecia
Infections: bacterial, viral, fungal
Interstitial pneumonitis
Venoocclusive disease
Acute graft-versus-host disease (allogeneic)

Late

Infections: bacterial, viral, fungal, protozoal
Chronic graft-versus-host disease (allogeneic)
Graft failure
Myelodysplasia
Secondary malignancies
Cataracts
Avascular necrosis
Infertility
Hypothyroidism

patients, failure to engraft may be due either to an inadequate dose of stem cells or to graft rejection by residual host T lymphocytes. Additional infusions of stem cells, with or without further conditioning of the patient, is required in these situations. Because of the intensity of the conditioning regimen, graft rejection occurs in less than 1% of matched sibling transplants when cyclosporine and methotrexate are used for GVHD prophylaxis. The use of T-cell–depleted grafts has been associated with a higher rate of graft rejection.

Veno-occlusive disease (VOD) occurs in 5% to 50% of patients and is a syndrome characterized by elevation in bilirubin, hepatomegaly, right upper quadrant pain, weight gain, and ascites. Pathophysiologically, endothelial damage from the conditioning regimen results in microthromboses in hepatic venules and sinusoids. Patients develop jaundice and have a capillary leak syndrome with third spacing of fluids. They are intravascularly volume-depleted despite total body fluid overload. Treatment is supportive and usually resolves without sequelae, although VOD may be fatal if severe. Predictive factors include a history of hepatic insults, hepatitis, and hepatotoxic medications (including estrogens and busulfan).

Pulmonary complications are common and often serious. Pulmonary edema may occur even in those with normal cardiac function because of the aggressive fluids administered during transplantation and capillary leak from the conditioning regimen. Bacterial and fungal pneumonias may occur. Interstitial infiltrates and hypoxia not due to fluid or bacterial or fungal infection is known as *interstitial pneumonitis*. One type of interstitial pneumonitis is caused by reactivation of cytomegalovirus, which may also be associated with hepatitis and myelosuppression. Although cytomegalovirus was a major cause of death in the past, better antiviral agents and strategies for detecting early reactivation have dramatically decreased the incidence of this complication. Another type of interstitial pneumonitis is *diffuse alveolar hemorrhage*, a syndrome characterized by bleeding into the alveoli with resultant respiratory distress. The cause is unknown, and the syndrome is associate with high mortality. Treatment is largely supportive, but high-dose corticosteroids are often used to reduce any damage from immunologic injury or cytokines.

Acute GVHD occurs in 30% to 70% of sibling donor recipients and 40% to 90% of unrelated donor recipients despite prophylaxis. Incidence depends on many patient and donor factors, such as source of stem cells, degree of HLA match, type of prophylaxis, patient and donor age, gender, cytomegalovirus status, and donor parity and transfusion history. GVHD is thought to be due to donor T cells that are triggered by contact with minor histocompatibility antigens. These cells interact with host tissues, either through direct cellular attack or cytokine-mediated changes (tumor necrosis factor-α [TNF-α] and γ-interferon) affecting the skin, liver, and gastrointestinal tract. Patients exhibit rashes, nausea, diarrhea, or liver abnormalities. The severity of acute GVHD is expressed as individual organ stages (0 to 4) combined to render an overall grade (0 to IV). Treatment is with increased immunosuppression (usually corticosteroids), and most cases respond. Nevertheless, severe GVHD may be refractory to treatment and can be fatal, either from direct organ damage or from infection related to the intensified immunosuppression.

LATE COMPLICATIONS

The chemotherapy and radiation delivered in the conditioning regimen and rigors of transplantation may have long-term effects. Children may suffer stunted growth and intellectual deficits, especially patients receiving cranial and total body irradiation. Many of the conditioning regimens are sterilizing for both men and women and result in infertility. Patients receiving extended corticosteroid therapy may suffer from avascular necrosis, osteoporosis, hypertension, and diabetes in addition to ongoing risk for infection.

Chronic GVHD is a complication of allogeneic transplantation occurring in 30% to 70% of survivors and is a major cause of late morbidity and mortality. Prior acute GVHD, older patient age, use of a mismatched donor, and peripheral blood as a stem cell source all have been associated with higher rates of this complication. Chronic GVHD can affect almost any organ and is largely treated with increased immunosuppression and supportive care. Some examples of chronic GVHD manifestations are skin rashes, joint contractures, mouth ulcers, fatigue, myalgias, gastrointestinal symptoms, bronchiolitis obliterans, and interstitial pneumonitis. Laboratory evaluation may show thrombocytopenia and evidence of cholestasis and transaminitis. Onset is usually between 100 days and 6 months after transplantation, although earlier and later development is possible. Patients with chronic GVHD are severely immunosuppressed, and infection is the major cause of death in this population. How-

ever, in most patients with chronic GVHD, organ involvement eventually resolves after 1 to 2 years, allowing discontinuation of immunosuppression.

Myelodysplasia is a late complication of autologous transplantation, particularly after cyclic pretransplantation chemotherapy and in patients who have evidence of clonal hematopoiesis before transplantation. Prognosis is grim, and affected patients often do poorly even with subsequent allogeneic transplantation.

Late malignancies are increased after transplantation compared with the normal population, but adequate studies using patients treated with nontransplant chemotherapy as controls have not been conducted. The quoted late malignancy rates (primarily cutaneous malignancies, brain tumors, and head and neck cancers) for allogeneic recipients are up to 2.2% at 10 years and 6.7% at 15 years. Patients treated with autologous transplants for Hodgkin's disease have a 5% rate of secondary malignancies at 5 years.

■ LONG-TERM ISSUES

Most studies document reasonable quality of life after autologous and allogeneic transplantation, although many patients continue to report significant side effects. Most autologous and allogeneic patients return to work, resume their pretransplantation social relationships, and report good health. However, many continue to notice fatigue, sexual difficulties, skin changes, susceptibility to colds, and sleep disturbances. Autologous patients probably recover faster than allogeneic or unrelated-donor patients. In allogeneic transplantation, chronic GVHD is a major impediment to return to normal function.

Patients have ongoing risk of infection long after transplantation. They receive prophylaxis against *Pneumocystis carinii* pneumonia for at least 1 year after transplantation and longer if they remain on corticosteroids. Herpes simplex and varicella zoster virus may reactivate, and many centers continue antiviral therapy for a prolonged period. Varicella virus may present clinically in unusual patterns, including visceral reactivation (causing severe abdominal pain), viral meningitis, or early dissemination. Patients with chronic GVHD have a particularly high risk of infections due to hypogammaglobulinemia and immune dysfunction. These patients are often given daily penicillin prophylaxis against pneumococcus and immunoglobulin replacement if found to be deficient in IgG_2 and IgG_4 subclasses.

After transplantation, patients lose their immunity to prior vaccinations and must be reimmunized at 1 and 2 years for tetanus, diphtheria, polio, pneumococcus, meningococcus, and *Haemophilus influenzae* type B. Immunizations earlier than 1 year after transplantation are not likely to be effective because of inadequate immune recovery. Influenza A vaccinations may begin 6 months after transplantation and should be given annually. At 2 years after transplantation, patients receive immunizations for measles, mumps, and rubella if they are off immunosuppression and free of chronic GVHD (since this is a live virus vaccine). If patients are returning to work in occupations in which they may be exposed to hepatitis B, immunity should be confirmed and reimmunization undertaken, if necessary.

Patients must continue to be monitored for primary disease relapse, secondary malignancies, chronic GVHD, and long-term effects of chemotherapy and radiation, such as cataracts and hypothyroidism. Patients with chronic GVHD on prolonged immunosuppression have a higher incidence of cutaneous and mucosal malignancies. They should avoid excessive sun exposure, given their predisposition to skin cancers and risk of exacerbating chronic GVHD. All survivors should have routine eye examinations, dental checkups, mammograms, Papanicolaou (Pap) smears, sigmoidoscopies, and prostate examinations at recommended intervals. Aggressive treatment for hypertension, osteoporosis, and hyperlipidemia should not be neglected. Most women treated with total body irradiation undergo premature menopause, and hormone replacement therapy should be addressed. However, rare patients retain fertility, and appropriate family planning should be offered to these individuals.

■ SPECIFIC APPLICATIONS

Since transplantation results vary considerably, depending on the stage of disease, type of transplant, and other clinical factors, broad ranges of statistics are available in the literature. Care must be taken in interpreting these numbers because significant selection bias confounds comparison with conventional therapy and among institutions. For specific details regarding these diseases, see individual chapters. General concepts for the major indications are presented in the following sections.

ACUTE MYELOGENOUS LEUKEMIA AND ACUTE LYMPHOBLASTIC LEUKEMIA

Despite encouraging remission rates, most adult patients with acute myelogenous leukemia (AML) and acute lymphoblastic leukemia (ALL) treated with conventional chemotherapy still suffer relapse and eventually die of their disease. This observation has provided the impetus to intervene with stem cell transplantation before refractory disease develops. Transplantation statistics for disease-free survival (DFS) at 3 to 5 years include the following:

Autologous transplantation (AML or ALL)—first complete remission (CR1) 30% to 50% (AML or ALL, greater than CR1, 10% to 30%).

Allogeneic transplantation (AML or ALL), CR1 40% to 70%; AML, first relapse or greater than CR1, 30% to 40%; ALL, greater than CR1, 20% to 40%.

It is notable that as the ability to give higher-dose consolidation chemotherapy has improved, transplantation has been reserved for patients with high-risk disease in the first complete remission and for those who relapse. Results for patients with AML in first relapse are about the same as when the procedure is performed in those in second remission, so patients in early relapse often proceed straight to transplantation without reinduction. In contrast, ALL patients in relapse have a much poorer outcome, and every effort is made to get patients back into remission before performing the transplantation procedure.

Transplantation physicians consider a patient's age, physical status, disease characteristics (subtype, cytogenetic abnormalities, response to therapy, duration of remission), donor availability, and preferences when evaluating appropriateness for transplantation.

CHRONIC MYELOGENOUS LEUKEMIA

Chronic myelogenous leukemia (CML) is a major indication for stem cell transplantation because it is incurable by any other means. The best results are obtained when the procedure is performed within the first year after diagnosis for patients in the early phase of the disease. Ten-year DFS is approximately 40% to 80% using sibling donors, and results of unrelated donor transplantation are approaching these figures. Patients in accelerated phase have an approximately 20% to 40% DFS, whereas the success rate drops to 0% to 20% for patients in blast crisis. CML seems to be exquisitely sensitive to graft-versus-leukemia effects, and relapses after stem cell transplantation may be salvaged with donor lymphocyte infusions.

APLASTIC ANEMIA

Although aplastic anemia was a common indication for transplantation early in the development of the field, it is actually a rare disease with multiple causes. Survival rates with allogeneic transplantation approach 60% to 90% with little toxicity in young (under 30 years) persons. Early difficulties with higher rates of graft rejection, presumably due to the immunologic activity associated with the disease, have been largely overcome. Although most patients present with profound pancytopenia, transfusions before transplantation may sensitize patients and increase mortality, so they should be avoided in transplantation candidates. Patients who develop aplastic anemia in the setting of Fanconi's anemia must be recognized before the transplantation procedure. Impaired DNA repair mechanisms makes these patients much more susceptible to alkylator therapy, and they will suffer fatal organ toxicity if given standard doses of cyclophosphamide during conditioning.

MYELODYSPLASTIC SYNDROME

Patients with a diagnosis of myelodysplastic syndrome constitute a growing percentage of the transplant population, since other options are largely supportive. Patients with less biologically aggressive disease (refractory anemia or refractory anemia with ringed sideroblasts) do much better (50% to 70% DFS) than patients transplanted with more advanced disease (refractory anemia with excess blasts, refractory anemia with excess blasts in transformation), who tend to have much higher rates of transplant-related mortality and relapse (20% to 30% DFS). Patients with secondary AML do poorly with any therapy. The new international prognostic scoring system (which uses number of cytopenias, cytogenetic abnormalities, and blast count) was developed in patients treated with nontransplantation therapies. However, this system also has prognostic importance after allogeneic transplantation.

CONGENITAL DISORDERS

Allogeneic transplantation has been successfully performed in patients with inherited disorders of hematopoiesis, immune function, and metabolism. In most of these disorders, the timing of transplantation is complicated because many patients can survive with reasonable quality of life for prolonged periods. Transplantation should be performed once the poor trajectory of the disease is established, but before irreversible deficits occur and significant organ damage substantially increases the risks. Recurrent infections, iron overload from transfusions, and neurologic damage all decrease the success of the procedure.

MULTIPLE MYELOMA

Both autologous and allogeneic transplantations have been performed for multiple myeloma. Studies thus far have not shown a plateau on the survival curve, although transplantation does seem to delay progression of disease and prolong survival, but with high transplantation-related mortality. However, most patients undergoing allogeneic transplantation eventually suffer relapse, with only 5% to 20% remaining alive and disease-free more than 4 years after the procedure. Results are somewhat better in patients undergoing autologous transplantation with a 6-year DFS of approximately 25%.

NON-HODGKIN'S LYMPHOMAS AND HODGKIN'S DISEASE

Non-Hodgkin's lymphomas and Hodgkin's disease are usually approached by autologous transplantation unless extensive bone marrow involvement or other mitigating circumstances are present. Randomized studies have shown that transplantation results in better DFS in patients who relapse after a short duration. Estimates of DFS are approximately 10% to 50%, depending on stage, prior therapy, chemotherapy responsiveness, and histology. The role of autologous transplantation in patients with slowly responding disease or high-risk disease in first complete remission is being studied.

SOLID TUMORS

Autologous transplantation has been used for a variety of solid tumors, including breast cancer, testicular cancer, small-cell lung cancer, ovarian cancer, neuroblastoma, and brain tumors. Breast cancer constitutes the most rapidly growing indication for autologous transplantation and has been the reason for several highly publicized lawsuits against health maintenance organizations and insurance companies who have denied women coverage for the procedure. Ongoing randomized national trials will help define the role of hematopoietic cell transplantation in the management of high-risk primary and metastatic solid tumors. Nonrandomized trials report a DFS of 10% to 20% in patients with metastatic breast cancer after limited follow-up.

BIBLIOGRAPHY

Antin JH, Smith Br. Bone marrow transplantation. In: Handin RI, Lux SE, Stossel TP, eds. *Blood: principles and practice of hematology.* Philadelphia: JB Lippincott, 1995:2055–2103.

Atkinson K. Chronic graft-versus-host disease. *Bone Marrow Transplant* 1990;5:69–82.

Deeg HJ, Leisenring W, Storb R, et al. Long-term outcome after marrow transplantation for severe aplastic anemia. *Blood* 1998;91:3637–3645.

Deeg HJ, Socie G. Malignancies after hematopoietic stem cell transplantation: many questions, some answers. *Blood* 1998;6:1833–1844.

Duell T, van Lint MT, Ljungman P, et al. Health and functional status of long-term survivors of bone marrow transplantation. *Ann Intern Med* 1997;126:184–192.

Ferrara JLM, Deeg HJ, Burakoff HJ, eds. *Graft-versus-host disease,* second ed. New York: Marcel Dekker, 1997.

Hansen JA, Gooley TA, Martin PJ et al. Bone marrow transplants from unrelated donors for patients with chronic myeloid leukemia. *N Engl J Med* 1998;338;14:962–968.

Philip T, Guglielmi C, Hagenbeek A, et al. Autologous bone marrow transplantation as compared with salvage chemotherapy in relapses of chemotherapy-sensitive non-Hodgkin's lymphoma. *N Engl J Med* 1995;333: 1540–1545.

Rubinsteizn P, Carrier C, Scaradavou A, et al. Outcomes among 562 recipients of placental-blood transplants from unrelated donors. *N Engl J Med* 1998;339:1565–1577.

Thomas ED, Blume KG, Forman SJ, eds. *Hematopoietic cell transplantation.* Malden: Blackwell Science, 1999.

Kelley's Textbook of Internal Medicine, fourth edition. Edited by H. David Humes. Lippincott Williams & Wilkins, Philadelphia © 2000.

C H A P T E R

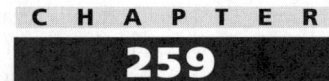

259

ANTICOAGULANT AND FIBRINOLYTIC THERAPY

BRUCE FURIE

Three pharmacologic agents predominate in the treatment or prevention of thromboembolic disease. Warfarin is unique in that it is administered by the oral route and thus can be taken long term by outpatients. Because it inhibits the synthesis of biologically active blood-clotting proteins, it does not work instantaneously nor does it act on existing thrombi. Heparin, administered by the intravenous or subcutaneous route, acts immediately to inhibit the active enzyme forms of the blood-clotting proteins. However, it does not cause existing clots to dissolve but prevents their enlargement. Fibrinolytic therapy using streptokinase, urokinase, or tissue plasminogen activator is administered parenterally. Because these enzymes digest fresh existing thrombi, such therapies rapidly accelerate the clearance of the vessel blockage that thrombi cause. The indications, complications, advantages, and disadvantages of these drugs dictate their proper use.

Anticoagulant therapy is used for two distinct indications. In one application, anticoagulants are used to prevent the development of thromboembolic disease in patients predisposed to such problems. This includes patients with an hereditary tendency to hypercoagulability due to protein C deficiency, proteins S deficiency, antithrombin III deficiency, or resistance to activated protein C. In addition, atrial fibrillation, prosthetic heart valves, and heart failure are among the medical problems that can lead to thrombus formation and subsequent embolization. These patients require *prophylactic* anticoagulant therapy to prevent the development of thromboembolic disease. Other patients with *active* thromboembolic disease, including deep venous thrombosis and pulmonary embolism, require anticoagulant therapy to prevent extension of existing thrombi and to allow reversal of vessel occlusion by physiologic fibrinolytic mechanisms.

ORAL ANTICOAGULANTS

The coumarin anticoagulants, specifically warfarin, are popular antithrombotic agents, which function as antagonists of the action of vitamin K in the synthesis of the vitamin K–dependent blood coagulation proteins (prothrombin, factor VII, factor IX, and factor X), proteins that contain γ-carboxyglutamic acid. After synthesis, these proteins undergo post-translational processing in a vitamin K–dependent reaction in which glutamic acid residues on the protein are modified to γ-carboxyglutamic acid. Warfarin inhibits enzymes in the vitamin K cycle, thus inhibiting γ-carboxylation and leading to the synthesis of inert forms of the blood-clotting proteins (Fig. 259.1). Because warfarin inhibits the biosynthesis of the vitamin K–dependent pro-

TABLE 259.1.	INTENSITY OF ANTICOAGULANT THERAPY: RECOMMENDED INR VALUES
Prevention of	
Deep venous thrombosis	2.0–3.0
Subclavian venous thrombosis	2.0–3.0
Pulmonary embolism	?
Prophylaxis Against Systemic Thromboembolic Disease	
Atrial fibrillation	2.0–3.0
Cardiac valve replacement	
Mechanical valves	2.5–3.5
Tissue valves	2.0–3.0

INR, international normalized ratio.

teins but not the activity of already synthesized protein, the effect of warfarin is delayed until the fully active blood-clotting proteins are cleared from the blood. Warfarin must be administered for 4 to 5 days before the antithrombotic action is therapeutic.

Warfarin sodium, administered orally, is completely absorbed, although there remains variation in the rate of absorption. In the blood, 97% of warfarin circulates bound to albumin; the unbound fraction is biologically active. The prothrombin time, which measures the extrinsic pathway, is used to monitor therapy with warfarin. Decreases in the activities of factor VII, factor X, and prothrombin prolong the prothrombin time. Warfarin is administered to prolong the prothrombin time into the therapeutic range. The international normalized ratio (INR) corrects for the variation in potency of different thromboplastins. The recommended therapeutic range varies with the indication for warfarin anticoagulation (Table 259.1).

Warfarin is contraindicated in patients who will not take the drug reliably or will not obtain regular laboratory measurement of the prothrombin time. In addition, patients with either hereditary or acquired bleeding disorders or with anatomical lesions that predispose them to serious bleeding should not be given warfarin. This drug should not be used in pregnancy because it is teratogenic and is associated with the fetal warfarin syndrome.

Bleeding complications occur in 10% to 20% of warfarin-treated patients. Bleeding includes epistaxis, purpura, hematuria, retroperitoneal bleeding, large hematomas, or gastrointestinal bleeding. Intracranial bleeding can be life-threatening. Overdosage of warfarin is a common cause of excessive bleeding. Proper action varies from the withholding of warfarin, administration of vitamin K, or the administration of fresh frozen plasma, depending on the seriousness of the bleeding complication.

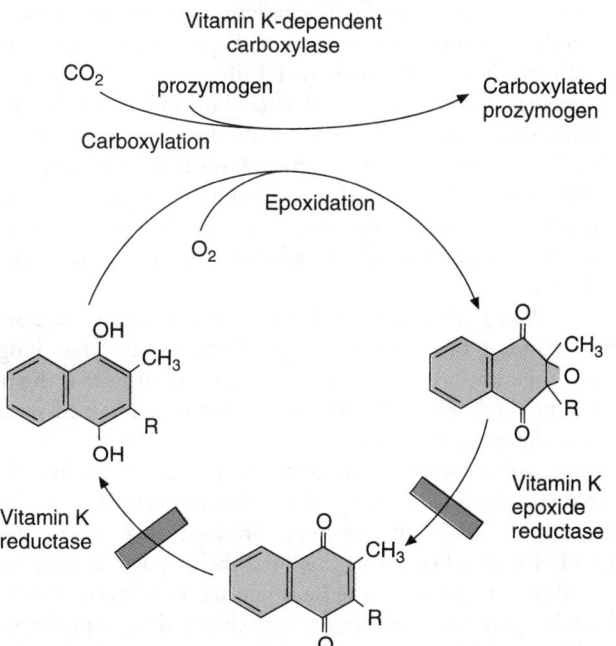

FIGURE 259.1. Vitamin K cycle and its inhibition by warfarin. Vitamin K is reduced to the vitamin K hydroquinone by a vitamin K reductase inhibited by warfarin. The vitamin K hydroquinone is a cofactor for the vitamin K–dependent carboxylase. In this reaction, the hydroquinone is oxidized to the vitamin K epoxide, and glutamic acid is converted to γ-carboxyglutamic acid. The carboxylase is not inhibited by warfarin. The vitamin K epoxide is salvaged by a vitamin K epoxide reductase, an enzyme sensitive to warfarin inhibition, and is recycled back to vitamin K.

HEPARIN

Heparin is a widely used anticoagulant that inhibits the active enzyme forms of most of the blood clotting proteins. A high-molecular-weight sulfated glycosaminoglycan (mean molecular weight 12,000) isolated from porcine intestinal mucosa or bovine lung, heparin accelerates the binding of antithrombin III, a plasma protease inhibitor, to factor Xa, thrombin, and other proteases in the blood coagulation pathways.

Heparin, most frequently used to treat thromboembolic disease, is administered by either the intravenous or subcutaneous route. Intravenous heparin by bolus injection or by continuous infusion leads to immediate anticoagulation. This results in a prolongation of the partial thromboplastin time, the prothrombin time, and the thrombin time. By convention, the adjustment of therapeutic heparin doses are titrated against the partial thromboplastin time, which is maintained at about 1.5- to 2 times the control value. Heparin prevents the extension of existing thrombi but does not dissolve these thrombi.

Heparin is also used prophylactically to decrease the risk of the development of thromboembolic disease. Patients at risk of thromboembolic disease who are undergoing intra-abdominal surgery benefit from mini-dose heparin prophylaxis. Some patients requiring chronic anticoagulation in whom warfarin is either not satisfactory or not indicated receive chronic subcutaneous heparin. Prophylactic low-dose heparin need not be monitored with the partial thromboplastin time, but adjusted-dose subcutaneous heparin therapy depends on the regular monitoring of the partial thromboplastin time.

The most common complication of heparin therapy is bleeding. This may occur when excessive heparin therapy has been used but can also be associated with therapeutic heparin doses. Bleeding may be limited to ecchymoses and purpura or may be more serious gastrointestinal, retroperitoneal, or intracranial bleeding. In about 5% of patients, thrombocytopenia complicates heparin therapy. Heparin-induced thrombosis is a rare but serious complication. Osteoporosis is a complication of long-term heparin therapy. Heparin may be used in pregnancy when an anticoagulant is required. With a half-life of about 2 hours, heparin is cleared by the reticuloendothelial system. When heparin therapy is discontinued because of mild bleeding complications, the anticoagulant effect is reversed over a course of hours. For serious bleeding complications, the heparin effect can be reversed with protamine.

Low-molecular-weight heparins, such as enoxaparin, are fractionated from heparin and enriched for their anticoagulant activity. Low-molecular-weight heparin is administered subcutaneously. Enoxaparin is given every 12 hours at a dose of 30 mg for prophylactic therapy and at 60 mg for treatment of thromboembolic disease. Another low-molecular-weight heparin, dalteparin (Fragmin), is given on a daily schedule. No monitoring of either the prothrombin time or the partial thromboplastin time is required with low-molecular-weight heparins, since neither is affected.

HIRUDIN

Hirudin, the anticoagulant component of the saliva of the medicinal leech, is a polypeptide that inhibits the action of thrombin. Prepared by recombinant DNA techniques, it is now available for clinical use as an alternative to heparin. Because hirudin is structurally unrelated to heparin, it can be used in patients requiring anticoagulant therapy who have heparin-induced thrombocytopenia or heparin-induced immune responses. Hiru-

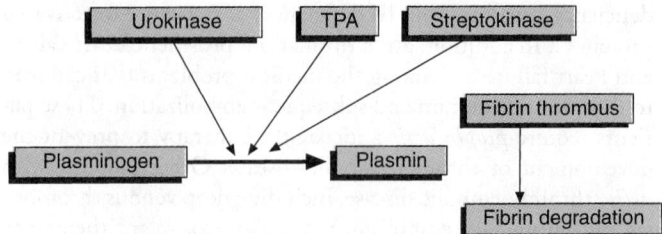

FIGURE 259.2. Mechanism of fibrinolytic therapy. Urokinase, tissue plasminogen activator (*TPA*), or streptokinase catalyze the conversion of plasminogen to plasmin. Plasmin digests the fibrin thrombus.

din is given intravenously and is used only for short-term anticoagulation.

FIBRINOLYTIC THERAPY

In contrast to warfarin and heparin, fibrinolytic therapy involves the infusion of enzymes into the blood to digest arterial and venous thrombi. Flow, blocked by thrombi, is rapidly restored when fibrinolytic therapy is effective. Urokinase, streptokinase, and tissue plasminogen activator are three agents used for fibrinolytic therapy (Fig. 259.2). Streptokinase is derived from β-hemolytic streptococci, urokinase is purified from human urine, and recombinant tissue plasminogen activator is expressed in heterologous mammalian cells based on the gene for human tissue plasminogen activator. These enzymes convert plasminogen to plasmin, and plasmin digests fibrin within the clot. Although the indications for fibrinolytic therapy vary, hemodynamically compromised patients with pulmonary emboli may benefit greatly from this therapy. Fibrinolytic therapy with acute myocardial infarction and acute arterial thrombosis or thromboembolic occlusion has been well established. The use of fibrinolytic therapy for deep venous thrombosis is controversial.

Fibrinolytic therapy is administered by the intravenous route. Therapy can be administered systemically through a peripheral vein or instilled through a catheter adjacent to the site of thrombus.

The dosage of fibrinolytic therapy is monitored by measuring the thrombin time, the fibrinogen level, or the plasminogen level. In general, measurement of the thrombin time is the preferred method, where the thrombin time is maintained at two- to five times the control level.

The major complication of fibrinolytic therapy is bleeding. Urokinase, streptokinase, and tissue plasminogen activator digest fibrinogen, thus leading to hypofibrinogenemia and increased risk of bleeding. Because of this risk, fibrinolytic therapy is contraindicated in patients who have had recent surgery, who have thrombocytopenia, and who are actively bleeding or predisposed to bleeding. Patients with central nervous system abnormalities should not receive fibrinolytic therapy. Streptokinase, derived from bacteria, may be associated with allergic reactions.

BIBLIOGRAPHY

Furie B. Oral anticoagulant therapy. In: Hoffman R, Benz EJ, Shattil SJ, et al, eds. *Hematology: basic principles and practice,* third ed. Philadelphia: WB Saunders, 2000:2040–2046.

Furie B, Bouchard B, Furie BC. Vitamin K-dependent biosynthesis of γ-carboxyglutamic acid. *Blood* 1999;93:1798–1808.

Furie B, Furie BC. The molecular and cellular biology of blood coagulation. *N Engl J Med* 1992;326:800–806.

Ginsberg J: Heparin. In: Hoffman R, Benz EJ, Shattil SJ, et al, eds. *Hematology: basic principles and practice,* third ed. Philadelphia: WB Saunders, 2000;2046–2056.

Greinacher A, Volpel H, Janssens U, et al: Recombinant hirudin provides safe and effective anticoagulation in patients with heparin-induced thrombocytopenia. *Circulation* 1999;99:73–80.

Marder V. Fibrinolytic therapy: indications and management. In: Hoffman R, Benz EJ, Shattil SJ, et al, eds. *Hematology: basic principles and practice,* third ed. Philadelphia: WB Saunders, 2000:2056–2074.

Kelley's Textbook of Internal Medicine, fourth edition. Edited by H. David Humes. Lippincott Williams & Wilkins, Philadelphia © 2000.

C H A P T E R
260

CANCER PAIN MANAGEMENT

JANET L. ABRAHM

Pain is often the first thing that comes to mind when patients are told they have cancer; families want to know if the patient will suffer. In fact, the fear of prolonged, unrelieved suffering may prevent patients from accepting potentially curative therapies. It is therefore reassuring to know that with current techniques, pain can be relieved in 90% of cancer patients, even when the cause of the pain cannot be eliminated. To accomplish this, the clinician must perform a thorough evaluation and assessment of the pain complaint, select the correct combination of therapies, and prevent and treat side effects caused by pain-relieving medications.

TRANSMISSION OF THE PAIN SIGNAL

For a patient to feel "pain," a signal arising from a noxious stimulus in the periphery must be transmitted to the centers in the brain that create the experience of pain. Histamine, serotonin, and bradykinin released at the site of tissue injury initiate the transmission of the signal, and prostaglandins, which do not themselves activate these fibers, sensitize them to lower levels of mechanical and chemical stimulants.

After activation of peripheral receptors, the signal passes along myelinated A_δ or unmyelinated C fibers and enters the spinal cord through the dorsal root. Substance P and the excitatory neurotransmitters glutamate, aspartate, and adenosine diphosphate mediate and enhance the transmission of this signal. The pain signal next usually crosses over and ascends in one of the two contralateral spinothalamic tracts to the hypothalamus and the somatosensory cortex.

Transmission of the pain signal can be inhibited at several places along this course. The dorsal longitudinal fasciculus is the descending pathway that inhibits transmission of the pain signal as it enters and ascends the spinothalamic tracts. Endogenous and exogenous opiates inhibit transmission and provide pain relief by binding to opiate receptors in the dorsal horn of the spinal cord, the ventromedial thalamic nuclei, and the periaqueductal gray.

EVALUATION OF THE COMPLAINT OF PAIN

Every effort should be made to detect, treat, and, if possible, eliminate the cause of the pain. Some of these causes, however, are not anatomical. The pain complaint may be the only manner in which the patient can express to the physician nonspecific feelings of distress. In patients with cancer, for example, Chapman has recognized three categories of such distress: anxiety, arising from fear of disfigurement, uncontrollable pain, loss of social position, loss of self-control, or fear of death; anger at the failure of physicians to provide a cure; and depression from loss of physical ability, a sense of helplessness, and the impact of financial problems. Because these concerns may exacerbate any concomitant painful sensations, alleviating them can significantly reduce distress and decrease the need for pain therapies.

Effective pain management requires repeated comprehensive assessment of the patient's pain. Pain reports by patients should be believed. Health care providers may not know that the clinical presentation of a patient suffering from chronic pain is very different from that of a patient in acute pain. If a patient does not manifest the common autonomic manifestations of acute pain (e.g., tachycardia, sweating, elevated blood pressure) or facial grimacing, the health care provider may not believe the patient is suffering from severe pain. A patient with severe but chronic pain does not manifest these autonomic findings, but is often withdrawn, quiet, and depressed or irritable. He or she moves very little spontaneously and complains of discomfort when moved. When the pain is relieved, such patients often exhibit completely different behaviors, becoming mobile, engaged, and involved with other people. Therefore, the first component in the assessment is to believe the patient's complaint.

Patient reports of pain are valid, reliable, and reproducible. They should be used, much as a blood sugar measurement is used in diabetes, to monitor the efficacy of therapy. Various assessment tools that generate results can be completed in 5 to 10 minutes. These should be used to determine several aspects of the pain: its location, intensity, quality, onset, and duration; what relieves or exacerbates it; and its functional consequences, including how it affects the patient's ability to sleep or eat and how it affects physical activity, relationships with others, emotions, and concentration.

The goal is to lower the pain to a level acceptable to the patient. For instance, in the Visual Analog Scale, 0 represents "no pain" and 10 is "the worst pain I can imagine" (Fig. 260.1) The change in the rating an hour after pain medication indicates what needs to be done next. Communication between nurse and physician is greatly improved by using these tools rather than

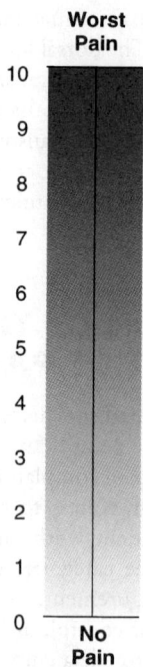

FIGURE 260.1. Visual analogue scale can be used to assess the effectiveness of pain interventions. The patient is asked to indicate on the scale the number that best corresponds to the intensity of his or her pain before and after the intervention and whether the degree of relief is satisfactory. Further adjustments in the regimen are then made, if needed.

qualitative descriptors such as "the pain is better" to guide pain management.

THERAPY FOR PAIN

A major component of any pain therapy is the attempt to reverse the underlying cause of the pain. Recurrent cancer may be discovered that is still responsive to surgery, chemotherapy, or radiation therapy. However, during diagnostic testing to define the cause, during specific therapy, or after all disease-related therapies are exhausted, pain still can be treated effectively.

The goal is to relieve patients' pain while preserving their ability to perform normal activities. The treatment regimen often includes nonpharmacologic approaches, the correct use of various medications that relieve pain with a minimum of side effects, and patient and family education throughout to foster communication and cooperation with the therapeutic plan. In addition, neurosurgical and anesthetic techniques are often useful.

NONPHARMACOLOGIC METHODS OF PAIN MANAGEMENT

Education and Reassurance

Patients with cancer often must undergo extensive diagnostic testing, which may include painful procedures. A rehearsal of the planned test or procedure, including the appearance of the

room, the length of time to be spent in the test apparatus, and so forth, can minimize the patient's anxiety. Such explanations given preoperatively lessen the need for postoperative medication and shorten the patient's hospital stay. For procedures such as venipuncture, lumbar puncture, thoracentesis, or paracentesis, which occur in the physician's office or in the patient's room, distraction procedures can be very helpful. The physician can encourage the patient to bring a portable tape player with earphones to listen to music or a book on tape during the procedure. Alternatively, the physician might play the television or radio in the patient's room and encourage him or her to pay attention to that rather than to the procedure. Patients with a good imagination can pretend to be someplace they have previously enjoyed, such as a beach or the mountains. They can dissociate themselves by concentrating on those pleasant memories, thereby diminishing the painfulness of the procedure.

Hypnosis

Practitioners with formal hypnotic training can use more elaborate hypnotic techniques to help their patients deal with painful procedures or conditions. Hypnosis takes advantage of the natural ability to enter a trancelike state, such as an athlete does when "playing through the pain." Patients who are trained to enter a trance at will can modify their perception of pain and diminish sleeplessness, anxiety, and anticipation of discomfort.

DRUG THERAPY

Drugs useful for pain relief include the non-opioid analgesics, opioid, and adjuvant drugs that either potentiate the actions of opioid analgesics or prevent or treat their side effects. A combination of medications is usually needed to provide optimal pain relief (Fig. 260.2).

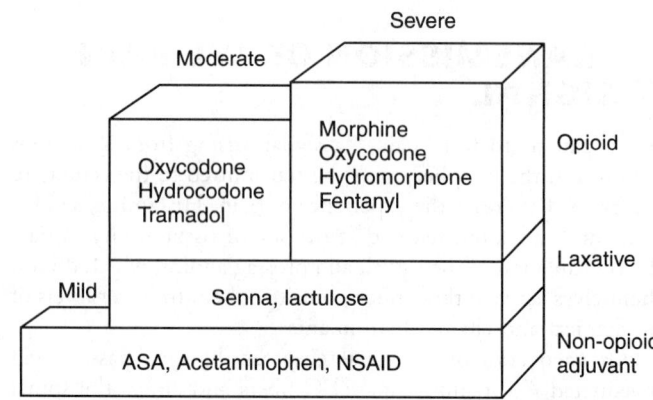

FIGURE 260.2. Mild pain should be treated with nonsteroidal anti-inflammatory drugs, acetylsalicylic acid (ASA), or acetaminophen. Moderate or severe pain requires the addition of a laxative and an opioid. For moderate pain, low-dose oxycodone (5 mg per tablet) is available in fixed-drug combinations that include ASA or acetaminophen. For severe pain, one of the other opioids listed, or higher doses of pure oxycodone, can be used.

Bone Pain

Non-opioid Analgesics

Non-opioid analgesics should be given to patients with mild pain of any cause. Aspirin, acetaminophen, and nonsteroidal anti-inflammatory drugs (NSAIDs), however, are especially useful in patients with bone pain, because they decrease local prostaglandin release and may thereby reduce the sensitization of pain receptors. Because NSAIDs cause renal insufficiency in some patients, renal function should be assessed 1 or 2 weeks after initiation of any of these agents. Ketorolac tromethamine (Toradol) is a particularly useful NSAID in relieving moderate to severe acute pain. An intramuscular dose of 30 mg ketorolac equals the pain-relieving potency of 12 mg intramuscular morphine; however, ketorolac has all the side effects of the NSAIDs and is not recommended for long-term use. If that degree of pain relief is needed chronically, an opioid agent should be substituted.

The non-opioid analgesics should be continued in appropriate patients when opioid analgesics are added, because they potentiate the pain-relieving effects of the opioids (Fig. 260.2).

Other Agents

Several effective new agents have recently become available, including the bisphosphonates (e.g., pamidronate), which reverse hypercalcemia from bony metastases and also relieve bone pain, and the injectable radionuclides (e.g., strontium 89, samarium-153-EDTMP).

Neuropathic Pain

Tricyclic antidepressants (amitriptyline), gabapentin, phenytoin, carbamazepine, and corticosteroids are non-opioid adjuvants with particular efficacy in relieving pain from nerve injuries. Corticosteroids can provide relief for patients with cord compression or plexus infiltrations. Doses of 16 to 100 mg of dexamethasone are needed to reduce vasogenic edema in spinal cord compression, but lesser doses (6 to 20 mg per day) can be helpful in patients with plexus injuries.

Opioid Analgesics

Narcotic analgesics are the mainstay of therapy for patients with moderate to severe pain of malignant or nonmalignant origin. To ensure compliance with an opioid prescription, however, education of other members of the health care team, the patient, and the family is often required to dispel the many misconceptions associated with opioid therapy. Even physicians who are cancer specialists hesitate to prescribe opioids as needed for patients with severe pain.

The fear of addiction is a common cause of inadequate dispensing of opioids and a barrier to their acceptance by patients. The physician can increase compliance by providing a full explanation of the differences between addiction and physical dependence, along with reassurance that research has repeatedly indicated that patients with malignancies who take opioids do not become addicts. Patients may also fear that if they allow themselves to take opioid medications for moderate pain, such medications will no longer be effective if more severe pain occurs. Because this fear can lead to undertreatment, the topic should be addressed whether or not the patient raises the question. A functional goal of therapy, such as returning to a favorite hobby or reinstituting normal activities of everyday life, may enable the patient and the family to accept the opioid.

Misconceptions about religious teachings may prevent health care personnel, patients, and their families from giving or accepting adequate pain medication. Roman Catholics, for example, may not be aware of the Church's position, as stated in the 1994 catechism, that opioids may be used at the approach of death, even if their use results in a shortening of life. The Church does not consider this use of pain medication to be suicide or euthanasia.

■ CHOICE OF MEDICATION

Because a wide variety of medications are available, pharmacokinetic considerations and side-effect profiles should be considered when choosing opioid agents (Table 260.1). Intermittent moderate to severe pain lasting hours to several days responds to oral analgesics with short half-lives (3 to 4 hours) with appropriate potency. Severe pain of relatively constant intensity should be treated with oral sustained-release opioid (taken every 8 to 12 hours) or transdermal fentanyl (renewed every 48 to 72 hours).

TABLE 260.1.	RELATIVE POTENCIES OF COMMONLY USED OPIOIDS	
Drug	**Parenteral (mg)**	**PO/PR (mg)**
Morphine	10	30
Oxycodone		20
Hydromorphone	1.5	7.5
Levorphanol	2	4
Methadone	10	20
Meperidine[a]	75	300

	Morphine (mg)	
Fentanyl (μg/h)	**IV/IM**	**PO**
25	10–30	30–90
50	31–50	91–150
75	51–70	151–210
100	71–90	211–270
125	91–110	271–330
150	111–130	331–390

IM, by intramuscular route; IV, by intravenous route; PO, by mouth; PR, by rectum.
[a] Not recommended for long-term use.
Adapted from Foley KM. Management of cancer pain. In: DeVita VT, Hellman S, Rosenberg SA, eds. *Cancer: principles and practice of oncology.* Philadelphia: JB Lippincott.
Donner B, Zenz M, Tryba M, et al. Direct conversion from oral morphine to transdermal fentanyl: a multicenter study in patients with cancer pain. *Pain* 1996;64:527–34.

Drugs with short half-lives should also be used for "rescue doses" given for breakthrough pain and for pain exacerbations between doses. The dose of the rescue medication should be 10% of the total 24-hour dose. For example, if a patient is receiving 300 mg of oral sustained-release morphine twice a day, the rescue dose should be 10% of 600 mg, or 60 mg of short-acting morphine. Agents with short half-lives such as morphine, hydromorphone, and oxycodone should also be used in the elderly and in patients with impaired renal or hepatic function. In patients with a previous history of drug abuse, agents with longer half-lives, such as methadone or levorphanol, are preferred.

The side-effect profiles of the opioid agents differ widely. It is often useful, therefore, to switch to another agent if a patient is experiencing dose-limiting side effects with the initial opioid chosen. For example, if a patient receiving morphine experiences disabling nausea, the physician may consider substituting hydromorphone (Dilaudid) at an equianalgesic dose (Table 260.1). Because of incomplete cross-tolerance, the initial dose for patients on higher doses of opioids should be only two-thirds to one-half of the calculated equianalgesic dose. For example, in the patient who takes 600 mg oral morphine a day, hydromorphone is begun at 75 or 100 mg a day (one-half or two-thirds of the 150-mg dose that would be equianalgesic).

Meperidine (Demerol) is the least useful opioid for patients with long-lasting moderate to severe pain. It provides pain relief for only about 1 to 2 hours and gives rise to an active metabolite, normeperidine, which induces dysphoria, excites the central nervous system, and can cause seizures. Normeperidine has a half-life of 13 to 24 hours, which can lengthen with renal failure. Thus, with the frequent administration of meperidine needed for pain control, normeperidine levels rise and the likelihood of seizures increases. The seizure incidence is further increased if the opioid antagonist naloxone (Narcan) must be given. If hyperirritability or a seizure occurs in a patient receiving meperidine, intravenous diazepam (Valium) rather than phenytoin should be used to control the seizure, and a new opioid should replace the meperidine for pain control.

ROUTES OF DELIVERY

Opioids can be delivered noninvasively (orally, rectally, or transdermally) or invasively (subcutaneously, intravenously, or by spinal infusion). Those interested in spinal delivery techniques are referred to the review by Hogan and associates, noted in the bibliography. Patients switched from oral or rectal to parenteral medication or vice versa must have the dose altered accordingly to avoid overdose or undertreatment (Table 260.1). No matter which route is chosen, patients who have continuous pain should receive the analgesics regularly, being awakened if necessary, to prevent pain recurrence.

The oral route is preferred for analgesic medications. Most patients can achieve excellent pain relief with either short-acting or sustained-release oral opioid preparations. Rectal opioids (morphine, oxymorphone, and hydromorphone) have about the same potency and half-life as oral agents and therefore must be given frequently.

For patients who cannot take oral medication and whose

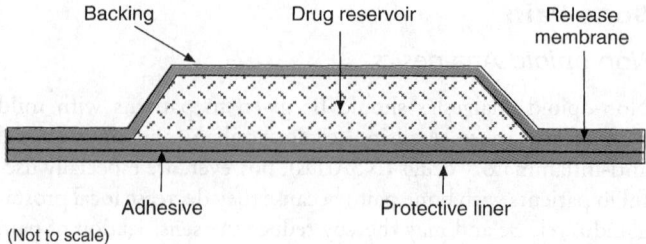

(Not to scale)

FIGURE 260.3. Duragesic patch. After the unit is placed on the chest wall, fentanyl, contained in the drug reservoir, diffuses through the release membrane into the skin. The drug is absorbed from the skin reservoir into the bloodstream. By 14 to 24 hours after the first patch is applied, fentanyl blood levels are sufficient to provide pain relief. New patches are usually applied every 72 hours.

opioid requirement precludes rectal delivery, the transdermal route is preferred to intravenous or subcutaneous drug delivery. The clinical usefulness of fentanyl in a transdermal delivery system (Duragesic) is well established. The transdermal system is a patch that adheres to the skin; fentanyl, a very lipophilic opioid, is rapidly absorbed from the contact adhesive into the skin. The drug then continuously diffuses from the patch reservoir into the skin through a rate-controlling membrane and is absorbed from the skin depot into the bloodstream (Fig. 260.3). There is, therefore, a significant delay (about 12 hours) before the drug begins to provide pain relief. A relatively constant plasma concentration of fentanyl is reached an average of 14 to 20 hours after the initial patch is placed. Rescue medication must therefore be provided during the first 48 hours of patch use.

Converting patients from an oral or parenteral opioid to the patch is easily accomplished using the information provided in Table 260.1. Most patients will require dose escalations, because the conversion is a conservative one. A new patch is applied every 72 hours, although a few patients require changes every 48 hours. Side effects include those due to the contact adhesive along with those commonly associated with other opioids.

The transdermal delivery system is not efficacious for patients with acute pain or for those with markedly fluctuating narcotic requirements. Lower doses may be required in elderly patients or those with respiratory insufficiency. Opioid overdoses can occur in patients using the system who develop fever or who have unstable hepatic function, because the drug's absorption or metabolism may be affected. Because the fentanyl continues to be absorbed from the skin, serum fentanyl levels remain at 50% as long as 14 to 25 hours after patch removal. In overdose, a naloxone infusion may be required until drug is eliminated from the skin depot.

For patients with severe or uncontrolled pain, continuous subcutaneous or intravenous administration of opioids should be used to provide pain relief in the shortest amount of time with the minimum amount of oversedation (see Management of Severe Pain). The drugs can be delivered by a portable infusion pump, initiated or continued at home. Patient-controlled analgesia systems for subcutaneous or intravenous drug delivery respond to the patient's pain threshold and eliminate the delays involved when nurses must administer supplemental medication.

ADJUVANT MEDICATIONS

Adjuvant medications are used to add to the analgesic effect of opioids and to prevent the complications opioids induce.

ADJUVANT ANALGESICS

The tricyclic antidepressants are among the most effective psychotropic analgesics. It has been suggested that they produce these effects by raising the concentration of the endogenous pain inhibitors, serotonin and norepinephrine, and increase the bioavailability of morphine. As opioid adjuvants, they act more promptly and at lower doses than those required for their antidepressant actions (e.g., amitriptyline is effective within 2 to 3 days at 50 to 100 mg per day).

The addition of dextroamphetamine (2.5 to 7.5 mg orally or 10 mg intramuscularly, twice daily) permits lowering the opioid dose by one-third to one-half while maintaining equivalent analgesia and less sedation. Methylphenidate (10 mg orally with breakfast and 5 mg orally with lunch) also can increase the analgesic effect and reduce sedation in patients receiving opioids. Pemoline, a chewable psychostimulant, is chemically unrelated to amphetamines but may be as useful in reversing opioid-induced sedation. Patients are started on one tablet (18.75 mg) in the morning and at noon, and the daily dose is gradually increased to a maximum of 75 mg. These combinations are very useful for patients who need to be more alert for a short period of time without interrupting their pain relief—for example, to attend a wedding.

LAXATIVES

Constipation is the most common opioid-induced side effect. Laxatives should be given routinely, not only on an as-needed basis, to patients treated with any of the drugs listed in Table 260.1. Detailed bowel preparation recommendations can be found, but none has been studied in a controlled fashion.

SLEEP MEDICATIONS

Sleep medications that themselves produce sedation (benzodiazepines, barbiturates, chloral hydrate) are not good choices for patients receiving opioids, because they produce excessive daytime sedation. Tricyclic antidepressants (e.g., 10 to 50 mg amitriptyline) are preferred, because they produce only night-time sedation and act as opioid adjuvants.

NALOXONE

Respiratory depression can occur in patients with mild to moderate pain during the initial use of opioids, although it is rare in patients with severe pain or in patients receiving long-term opioids. Caution should be used before giving naloxone to a patient receiving long-term opioids, because severe withdrawal may be precipitated. In such patients, rather than giving the usual dose of 0.4 mg per milliliter, the 0.4 mg of naloxone should be diluted with 10 mL of saline, and the minimum amount should be given that reverses respiratory depression. In a comatose patient, endotracheal tube placement is recommended to prevent aspiration from the salivation and bronchial spasm that will be induced.

SPECIFIC CLINICAL PROBLEMS

COAGULATION DISORDERS

Patients with coagulation disorders, whether inherited or acquired, have excessive bleeding risk if aspirin-containing pain relievers are used. If acetaminophen is ineffective, such patients may obtain significant relief from ibuprofen or the nonacetylated salicylates such as salsalate (Disalcid) or choline magnesium trisalicylate (Trilisate), which do not prolong the bleeding time.

PROBLEMS OF THE ELDERLY

Pain management in the elderly is complicated by difficulties in pain assessment, as well as the altered pharmacokinetics of opioids and psychotropic adjuvant medications. Elderly patients may underreport pain. Physicians may ascribe observed limitations in social contact and physical activity to age-related changes, when in fact they are pain-induced limitations.

Elderly patients are particularly susceptible to the side effects of NSAIDs, and patients taking them should be monitored closely. In general, in elderly patients (age 70 to 89), the volume of distribution for opioids is smaller, the drugs have a longer plasma half-life, and clearance is decreased, all of which lead to a prolonged duration of effect. Therefore, the effective doses for these patients are one-half to one-fourth of those needed in younger patients. Drugs without active metabolites are used (e.g., oxycodone or hydromorphone), and the initial doses should be low. Patients should be monitored carefully for the development of sedation or confusion, especially if they are receiving antihistaminic agents (e.g., cimetidine, diphenhydramine) or drugs with anticholinergic activity.

The acute urinary retention due to opioids (especially in patients with prostatic hypertrophy) and hypotension and tachycardia caused by tricyclic agents can be more frequent and of more clinical severity in the elderly population. The starting dose of the tricyclic should be low (for amitriptyline, usually 10 mg at bedtime), and the dose should be slowly increased as tolerated. Doxepin, which does not share these side effects, may be a better-tolerated opioid adjuvant.

PATIENTS WITH OPIOID ADDICTION

Drug requirements may be significantly higher and dosing intervals shorter in the addict. In patients on methadone maintenance, therapeutic dosing must be provided over and above their baseline dose. In all cases, the goal should be to deliver adequate medication to relieve the pain. The physician should always work from a written treatment plan. One physician should prescribe all psychotropic medication, and information about the patient's drug use should be obtained from sources in addition to the patient. When the question of "addiction" first arises, consultation should be obtained from an addiction medicine specialist. If opioids are needed, patients should be given limited quantities of long-acting medications on a scheduled basis.

MANAGEMENT OF SEVERE PAIN

Opioid therapy is the cornerstone of managing the patient with severe pain. We begin by reassuring patients and their families and explain that to relieve the pain as quickly as possible, intravenous narcotic medications will be started immediately, but oral pain medication will begin as soon as the pain is well controlled. Without this explanation, patients may misinterpret the morphine drip as an indication that they were thought to be terminal. The starting dose is calculated from the patient's baseline opioid requirement or weight (e.g., morphine, 0.05 mg kilogram per hour). A bolus is given, the drip is begun, and every 20 to 30 minutes the degree of pain relief is reassessed. If the relief is inadequate, another bolus is given, and in patients without severe underlying chronic obstructive pulmonary disease, the drip is increased in increments of 2 to 3 mg per hour. There is no maximal dose; we give whatever is required to relieve the pain. If the patient falls asleep, this usually indicates that pain relief has been achieved, not that the dose should be lowered. The dose is lowered if the respiratory rate falls below 10 to 12 breaths per minute.

Adjuvant agents are begun along with the opioid (Fig. 260.2). All patients are given one or two pills of senna concentrate (Senokot) orally each day, or one for every 30 mg morphine, to a maximum of eight pills daily. If more laxative effect is needed, lactulose is added; the starting dose is 15 to 30 mL orally at bedtime, repeated, if necessary, in the morning. Lactulose is effective and, unlike other agents, does not produce cramping or a feeling of fullness. Amitriptyline (10 to 50 mg orally) is usually ordered as a "patient may refuse" sleep medication. In opioid-naive patients, prochlorperazine (Compazine), 10 mg orally twice or three times daily, is offered for the first 48 hours to prevent the otherwise common development of nausea. In patients with bone or nerve pain, appropriate adjuvants are added.

When pain relief is adequate, the patient medication is converted to an equivalent dose of oral opioid (Table 260.1). For example, a patient who required 5 mg of intravenous morphine per hour (120 mg in 24 hours) will need 360 mg per day of the oral long-acting agent (120 mg × 3). This can be given as 180 mg orally every 12 hours or 120 mg orally every 8 hours. Two hours after the oral opioid is begun, the drip is discontinued. Short-acting, immediate-release morphine should be available for rescue dosing. If the amount of opioid taken as a rescue dose is significant, the daily dose of long-acting agent is increased accordingly.

BIBLIOGRAPHY

Chapman CR. Psychologic and behavioral aspects of cancer pain. In: Bonica JJ, Ventafridda J, eds. *Advances in pain research and therapy. Vol. II.* New York: Raven Press, 1979:44–56.
Doyle D, Hanks GWC, MacDonald N, eds. *Oxford textbook of palliative medicine,* second edition. Oxford: Oxford Medical Publications, 1998.
Foley KM. Management of cancer pain. In: DeVita VT, Hellman S, Rosen-
berg SA, eds. *Cancer: principles and practice of oncology,* fifth edition. Philadelphia: JB Lippincott, 1997.
Hogan Q, Haddox JD, Abran S, et al. Epidural opiates and local anesthetics for the management of cancer pain. *Pain* 1991;46:271–279.
Monks R. Psychotropic drugs. In: Bonica JJ, ed. *The management of pain,* second ed. Philadelphia: Lea & Febiger, 1990.
Payne R. Anatomy, physiology, and neuropharmacology of cancer pain. *Med Clin North Am* 1987;71:153–167.
Payne R. Transdermal fentanyl: suggested recommendations for clinical use. *J Pain Symptom Manage* 1992;7:S40–S44.
Portenoy RK. Constipation in the cancer patient: causes and management. *Med Clin North Am* 1987;71:303–311.
Wall PD, Melzack R, eds. *Textbook of pain,* third ed. Edinburgh: Churchill Livingstone, 1994.
White PF. Use of patient-controlled analgesia for management of acute pain. *JAMA* 1988;259:243–247.

C H A P T E R

261

ANTIEMETIC TREATMENT

RICHARD J. GRALLA

Many of the recent advances in oncology have occurred in supportive care. Although debate continues concerning the value of some supportive care agents, all agree that available antiemetics contribute markedly to the quality of life of patients with cancer and allow outpatient treatment that was not previously possible. Most patients given chemotherapy now need not experience vomiting. These improvements have been the result of a better understanding of the role of antiemetic drugs, the availability of a new class of antiemetic agents, and an increased knowledge of the neuropharmacology of emesis.

COMMON EMETIC PROBLEMS

As the control of emesis in patients receiving chemotherapy has improved, several different problems have become apparent. These include acute chemotherapy-induced emesis, delayed emesis, conditioned or anticipatory emesis, and emesis not related to chemotherapy. The most common problem is acute emesis.

Acute chemotherapy-induced emesis typically occurs 1 to 2 hours after chemotherapy in previously untreated patients not given effective antiemetics and can persist for several hours. Several schemes for assessing the potential of a chemotherapeutic agent for causing emesis have been devised. It is practical to divide the emetic risk into the following four categories: (a) severe, occurring in at least 99% of untreated patients (as seen with cisplatin); (b) moderate to high, occurring in 30% to 90%

(as seen with dacarbazine, nitrogen mustard, carboplatin, cyclophosphamide, and doxorubicin); (c) low, occurring in 10% to 30% (as seen with agents such as the taxanes, irinotecan, etoposide, and gemcitabine); and (d) very low, occurring in 0% to 10% (as seen with 5-fluorouracil, vincristine, bleomycin, vinblastine, and methotrexate). The most progress has been evident in the control of acute emesis, which must be treated prophylactically in all patients receiving chemotherapy with more than a very low risk of emesis.

Both delayed and acute emesis begin after the administration of chemotherapy. *Delayed emesis* is often defined as that beginning 24 hours after chemotherapy. The potential of chemotherapeutic agents to cause delayed emesis parallels that seen with the acute problem, occurring in 60% to 80% of patients treated with cisplatin and in 20% to 30% of those receiving carboplatin or doxorubicin. *Conditioned* or *anticipatory emesis* is the result of poor control of acute or delayed emesis. It is typically associated with anxiety before the next chemotherapy treatment, followed by nausea or vomiting before or during chemotherapy administration.

Commonly, all nausea or vomiting is attributed to chemotherapy. When the pattern of emesis is not typical of the chemotherapy administered, other causes should be considered. Medications (opiates, bronchodilators, antibiotics), tumor-related complications (intestinal obstruction, brain metastases), or other problems such as gastritis are often the cause of the emesis and require proper evaluation and a different approach.

Central to controlling chemotherapy-induced emesis is an understanding of how emesis is initiated and the mechanism of action of antiemetics.

THE NEUROPHARMACOLOGY OF EMESIS

Several neurotransmitters and their receptors are involved with this phenomenon in the brain and in the gut. Recently, interest has focused on serotonin and the type 3 serotonin receptor, (or 5-hydroxytryptamine [5-HT3] receptor). Agents that block this receptor are potent antiemetics and generally have few side effects (Table 261.1). The 5-HT3 receptors are found adjacent to enterochromaffin cells in the small intestine, in vagal nerve fibers, and in the medulla. Controversy exists concerning which site is the most important for stopping emesis. In addition, the duodenum contains a large amount of serotonin, which is liberated after cisplatin administration (but apparently not after cyclophosphamide). It is not clear whether the serotonin itself is important in causing emesis. Other receptors or mechanisms are also involved. This conclusion is reached because agents that do not affect 5-HT3 receptors (corticosteroids and dopamine-blocking agents) can be useful antiemetics and because emesis is not controlled in all patients.

PREVENTING EMESIS

The principles involved in the prevention of emesis include (a) selection of the most active antiemetics, (b) combination anti-emetic therapy of a 5-HT3 antagonist with a corticosteroid in appropriate settings, and (c) use of the most effective doses and schedules with minimization of side effects. Metoclopramide provided the first serotonin receptor antagonist antiemetic. Although metoclopramide also affects dopamine receptors, in high doses its efficacy is mediated by blocking 5-HT3 receptors. With the development of the selective 5-HT3 receptor antagonists, more specific treatment with fewer side effects and greater convenience became the standard.

Are there differences among the selective serotonin antagonists? In structure, potency per milligram, and pharmacokinetic profile, differences exist. In efficacy and side effects, the agents appear similar. Large, multicenter, randomized studies reveal equivalence among the three approved 5-HT3 receptor antagonists in the United States, ondansetron, granisetron, and dolasetron. Tropisetron, another serotonin antagonist, is not available in the United States, but with a therapeutic profile similar to the three latter agents. Trials report a low incidence of side effects shared by these drugs, such as mild headache, constipation, and a transient rise in transaminases.

Controversy persists concerning the ideal doses for the serotonin antagonists. The most practical and cost-effective approach is the single-dose regimen, as outlined in Table 261.1. The drugs are not schedule-dependent, and treatment can begin immediately before chemotherapy. Trials have repeatedly indicated that a single administration of an antiemetic regimen is as effective as multiple dosing in preventing acute chemotherapy-induced emesis. Evidence indicates that there is a "threshold" effect for these agents. After the relevant receptors are blocked, there is no value in increasing the dose, and lower doses are less effective. This threshold is in the range indicated in Table 261.1. In addition, the dose and regimen should be the same for chemotherapy with a severe, high, or moderate potential for causing emesis.

Location of relevant receptors in the gut may also be of importance. Large trials with serotonin antagonists in patients receiving either cisplatin or agents of moderate to high risk demonstrated that these agents given orally are as effective as the same agents given intravenously. Oral administration of a single dose of an antiemetic regimen provides the greatest flexibility for use in any chemotherapy setting. It also saves both pharmacy and nursing time. These considerations, together with lower acquisition costs for the oral agents, provide the background for making these equally efficacious combinations the regimens of choice for patients receiving most chemotherapy.

In those instances in which an antiemetic is needed with chemotherapy of a low emesis potential, a single dose of an oral or intravenous antiemetic is usually sufficient (generally a corticosteroid). Corticosteroids are active parenterally and orally and are active in various settings. Although the mechanism of action is not defined, it is different from that of other antiemetics. Thus, corticosteroids are easy to use in combination antiemetic regimens and enhance the activity of other active antiemetics. Side effects are generally mild and are well described for these agents. A recent trial indicates that a single dose of dexamethasone at 20 mg as a total dose is more effective than lower doses when added to a serotonin antagonist in patients receiving cisplatin.

In the past, many agents other than those just discussed have

| TABLE 261.1. | ANTIEMETIC AGENTS, DOSES, AND ADMINISTRATION SCHEDULES FOR PREVENTION OF ACUTE CHEMOTHERAPY-INDUCED EMESIS |

Antiemetic Agent	Dose Range	Schedule (for Acute Chemotherapy-Induced Emesis)
Serotonin Receptor Antagonists		
Dolasetron	100 mg or 1.8 mg/kg intravenously	One time, before chemotherapy
Dolasetron	100 mg orally	One time, before chemotherapy
Granisetron	1 mg or 0.010 mg/kg intravenously	One time, before chemotherapy
Granisetron	1 mg or 2 mg orally	One time, before chemotherapy
Ondansetron	8 mg or 0.15 mg/kg intravenously	One time, before chemotherapy
Ondansetron	Oral doses not well studied for acute emesis (usually 8 mg doses in delayed or radiation therapy [RT] emesis)	(Two to three times daily in delayed or RT emesis)
Tropisetron	5 mg intravenously	One time, before chemotherapy
Tropisetron	5 mg orally	One time, before chemotherapy
Corticosteroids		
Dexamethasone	8 mg to 20 mg[a] intravenously	One time, before chemotherapy
Dexamethasone	4 mg to 20 mg orally[a]	One time, before chemotherapy
Methylprednisolone	40 mg to 100 mg intravenously	One time, before chemotherapy

[a] The 20-mg dexamethasone dose is preferred for emetic situations of moderate or greater risk; the 4 mg dose is generally sufficient in settings of low emetic risk.

been used for chemotherapy-induced emesis. The phenothiazines, such as prochlorperazine, are commonly used in general medicine. High intravenous doses are better than the oral and intramuscular phenothiazines; however, orthostatic hypotension is a common toxicity. Other side effects include sedation and dystonic effects.

Lorazepam has only modest antiemetic effects, but with its antianxiety and amnestic properties has high subjective acceptance. It is also effective in reducing akathisia and is useful in decreasing dystonic reactions. The major side effect of lorazepam is sedation. It is recommended as an addition to effective antiemetics and not as a single agent.

Cannabinoids such as dronabinol (δ-9-tetrahydrocannabinol [THC]) have activity similar to oral phenothiazines but are markedly less effective than metoclopramide or the 5-HT3 receptor antagonists. Side effects are greater with cannabinoids than with serotonin antagonists or metoclopramide. The cannabinoid toxicities include sedation, dizziness, ataxia, orthostatic hypotension, dry mouth, and dysphoria. Although these agents have some antiemetic properties, other available agents have more activity and fewer side effects; thus, the role of cannabinoids in antiemetic treatment has not been well defined. Cannabinoids have great popularity in the lay press, aside from their tested properties. In addition, one well-conducted (random assignment, double-blind, crossover) study compared oral THC with inhaled marijuana. Both agents had similar but low activity, with a trend toward patient preference for the oral THC.

COMBINATION REGIMENS WITH CORTICOSTEROIDS

Antiemetic regimens combining a single dose of dexamethasone with either a serotonin antagonist (Table 261.1) or with met-oclopramide are more effective than a single agent. This has been demonstrated in at least a dozen studies and for emesis induced by cisplatin and other chemotherapeutic agents. Typically, antiemetic efficacy with cisplatin rises from the 40% to 50% range of complete control to 70% to 80% when dexamethasone is added to a 5-HT3 antagonist. With moderately emetogenic agents (e.g., cyclophosphamide, anthracyclines, or carboplatin), the complete control rate rises to over 90% with the combination regimen when compared with either a 5-HT3 antagonist or dexamethasone alone.

After more than a decade of use of combination regimens, few negative factors have emerged for the use of dexamethasone in this single-dose setting. Specifically, no evidence exists of impaired therapeutic response from chemotherapeutic agents, and there are only minor side-effects. Combination antiemetic regimens with corticosteroids should be considered treatments of choice for moderately emetogenic chemotherapy and cisplatin-containing regimens.

Treatment of delayed emesis differs from the approach to acute emesis (Table 261.2). The key agents for this problem are corticosteroids. Adding oral metoclopramide can enhance this activity. Serotonin antagonists are no more effective than metoclopramide when added to dexamethasone for preventing delayed emesis. The markedly greater cost of the serotonin antagonists without improved efficacy argues against their routine usage in the delayed emesis setting.

Anticipatory emesis is best approached by preventing this problem through the use of the most effective antiemetics with each course of chemotherapy. If, however, the problem occurs, treatment can be helpful. Behavior therapy techniques with desensitization can be useful. The usefulness of antianxiety agents has not been well studied.

TABLE 261.2.	RECOMMENDATIONS FOR THE PREVENTION OF DELAYED EMESIS

Indication

For patients who receive chemotherapy of moderate to severe risk

Antiemetic for Day of Chemotherapy

Use an effective combination antiemetic regimen of a serotonin antagonist plus a corticosteroid, as outlined in Table 261.1

Delayed Emesis Regimen

Beginning the morning after chemotherapy (approximately 12–24 hours after treatment)
Dexamethasone 8 mg orally BID for 2–3 days (2 days for moderate to high risk; 3 days for severe risk)
PLUS
Metoclopramide 30–40 mg BID orally for 2 days

CONCLUSION

Future directions of antiemetic treatment and research are taking many different paths. Better understanding of the roles and interactions of neurotransmitter receptors in emesis will allow for different approaches to this problem. Serotonin or dopamine pathways appear unlikely to be the only ones involved in chemotherapy-induced emesis. With 25% or more of patients not having complete control despite the use of active antiemetics, investigation of antiemetics with different mechanisms of action is a logical approach. Recent clinical studies indicate that the neurokinin antagonists are effective for both acute and delayed emesis. These trials have enlisted only a small number of patients, but, to date, the data are encouraging and indicate that these drugs will be useful additions to the serotonin antagonist plus corticosteroid combination regimens.

BIBLIOGRAPHY

Andrews PL, Naylor RJ, Joss RA. Neuropharmacology of emesis and its relevance to antiemetic therapy: consensus and controversies. *Support Care Cancer* 1998;6:197–203.

Gralla RJ, Clark RA, Kris MG, et al. Methodology in anti-emetic trials. *Eur J Cancer* 1991;27:S5–S8.

Gralla RJ, Itri LM, Pisko SE, et al. Antiemetic efficacy of high-dose metoclopramide: randomized trials with placebo and prochlorperazine in patients with chemotherapy-induced nausea and vomiting. *N Engl J Med* 1981;305:905–909.

Gralla RJ, Navari RM, Hesketh PJ, et al. Single-dose oral granisetron has equivalent antiemetic efficacy to intravenous ondansetron for highly emetogenic cisplatin-based chemotherapy. *J Clin Oncol* 1998;16:1568–1573.

Hesketh PJ, Kris MG, Grunberg SM, et al. Proposal for classifying the acute emetogenic of cancer chemotherapy. *J Clin Oncol* 1997;15:103–109.

Italian Group for Antiemetic Research. Dexamethasone, granisetron, or both for the prevention of nausea and vomiting during chemotherapy for cancer. *N Engl J Med* 1995;332:1–5.

Kris MG, Gralla RJ, Tyson LB, et al. Controlling delayed vomiting: double-blind, randomized trial comparing placebo, dexamethasone alone, and metoclopramide plus dexamethasone in patients receiving cisplatin. *J Clin Oncol* 1989;7:108–114.

Kris MG, Radford JE, Pizzo BA, et al. Use of an NK-1 receptor antagonist to prevent delayed emesis following cisplatin. *J Natl Cancer Inst* 1997;89:817–818.

Levitt M, Faiman C, Hawks R, et al. Randomized double blind comparison of delta-09-tetrahydrocannabinol (THC) and marijuana as chemotherapy antiemetics. *Proc Am Soc Clin Oncol* 1984;3:91.

Morrow GR, Roscoe JA, Kirshner JJ, et al. Anticipatory nausea and vomiting in the era of 5-HT3 antiemetics. *Support Care Cancer* 1998;6:244–247.

Navari R, Gandara D, Hesketh P, et al. Comparative clinical trial of granisetron and ondansetron in the prophylaxis of cisplatin-induced emesis. *J Clin Oncol* 1995;5:1242–1248.

Navari RM, Reinhardt RR, Gralla RJ, et al. Reduction of cisplatin-induced emesis by a selective neurokinin-1-receptor antagonist. *N Engl J Med* 1999;340:190–195.

Perez EA, Hesketh P, Sandbach J, et al. Comparison of single-dose oral granisetron versus intravenous ondansetron in the prevention of nausea and vomiting induced by moderately emetogenic chemotherapy: a multicenter, double-blind, randomized parallel study. *J Clin Oncol* 1998;16:754–760.

Phillips KA, Tannock IF. Design and interpretation of clinical trials that evaluate agents that may offer protection from toxic effects. *J Clin Oncol* 1998;16:3179–3190.

Roila F, Ballatori E, Contu A, et al. Optimal dose of intravenous (iv) dexamethasone (Dex) in the prevention of cisplatin (CDDP)-induced acute emesis: a double-blind randomized study. *Proc Am Soc Clin Oncol* 1998;17:50,195A.

Kelley's Textbook of Internal Medicine, fourth edition. Edited by H. David Humes. Lippincott Williams & Wilkins, Philadelphia © 2000.

C H A P T E R

262

DESIGN AND CONDUCT OF CANCER CLINICAL TRIALS

MICHAEL A. FRIEDMAN
RICHARD SIMON

Cancer clinical trials involve at least two broad objectives. The first is to identify promising new interventions; this objective is addressed by phase I and II trials. The second is to determine whether a promising treatment actually provides patient benefit; this is the objective of phase III trials. The design considerations for these two categories of trials are vastly different but are often confused.

Physicians play too limited a role in critically evaluating the treatments they dispense. Logically, the physician's responsibility to patients should demand discriminating analyses of all intentions, both old and new, but the traditional impediments to obtaining proper evaluation remain. These include the lack of recognition that treatments that "should work" often do not and in fact may be harmful; the desire to offer the patient a new treatment; the desire to shield the patient from uncertainties; and the desire to appear knowledgeable.

HUMAN PROTECTION ISSUES

The participation of a subject in a formal clinical trial is defined by an agreement embodying the highest medical, legal, and ethical principles. By enrolling a person in a study, the researcher assumes a set of obligations that transcend the conventional responsibility to provide proper medical attention. Participation in research is an active, voluntary choice; it is a commitment that may be withdrawn at any time without prejudicing ongoing care. The research subject has relatively complete autonomy. He or she can exercise choice limited only by access to services, the financial ability to pay for such services (private means or insurance), and a medical staff willing to provide these services. This active choice may be influenced by patient preference for one of the competing therapeutic options with similar efficacy (e.g., the choice of mastectomy or lumpectomy and irradiation for stage I breast cancer), or there may be no recognized effective option (e.g., in advanced pancreatic cancer). No matter what the clinical situation, the subject should be given relevant information by the medical staff to assist in the choice.

The informed consent process is an initial and fundamental interaction. The goal is to provide information in a clear, understandable, noncoercive manner. The essential elements of this process are defined by federal regulations and include a complete description of the therapy being offered, both standard care and investigational. The known, suspected, and potential risks and benefits should be fairly presented, as well as other reasonable alternatives worth considering by the subject. A pledge is made to preserve the subject's confidentiality, and a description is given of the circumstances under which access to medical records is permitted. Information describing compensation (if any) for toxicities encountered is also given, as well as specific means by which further information may be obtained.

DESIGN PRINCIPLES FOR PHASE I TRIALS

Historically, phase I studies define the distribution and metabolism (pharmacokinetics) and the toxicity (pharmacodynamics) characteristics of a new treatment to identify a safe but biologically active dosage and schedule of administration. Such studies of antitumor therapeutics are conducted in patients with refractory or resistant malignancies who lack any more efficacious option. The chance of patient benefit is less and the risk of toxicity greater than would be anticipated in later clinical trials.

Many new agents entering phase I trials are being selected more rationally to affect specific biologic (molecular) targets. Consequently, patients who have the targeted tumor or physiologic characteristics are the most appropriate candidates for early clinical trials. Such patients are more likely to benefit, and they also provide the opportunity to conduct relevant correlative laboratory studies.

To provide the most complete information for subsequent clinical trials, the pharmacologic characteristics of the new agent should be explored in populations of special interest; studies should be performed in both genders, in the young and the old, in those with coexisting organ dysfunction, and in specific racial or ethnic groups if relevant. These important clinical issues should be explored more thoroughly in phase II and III studies, but initial clues should be sought in the phase I setting.

DESIGN PRINCIPLES FOR PHASE II TRIALS

The primary purpose of a phase II study is to determine whether a treatment exhibits promising antitumor activity; the secondary purpose is to provide a more complete toxicity experience. Using a dose and schedule considered tolerable in phase I studies, relatively homogeneous populations of patients are entered into phase II studies. Phase II trials are generally conducted with patients for whom no curative therapy exists, so it is likely that the agent being tested will temporarily benefit only some of the patients. Moreover, there are no a priori means of identifying the responsive patients. Therefore, phase II trials are designed to detect specified rates of objective tumor shrinkage (or surrogate thereof). Although the assessment of transient, incomplete tumor regression (so-called partial response) is subject to observer misinterpretation, it is typically used.

The major methodologic problem for phase II studies is the reliable identification of antitumor activity (although incomplete) in the fewest number of patients. Typically, better-risk patients are more likely to benefit from any intervention, especially those who are younger, are more fit, or have been exposed to little prior antitumor therapy. Such patients are considered ideal candidates for phase II studies, as long as they are not being denied some other curative or highly effective therapy. The sort of biologic targeting described in the design of modern phase I trials should be carefully considered for phase II as well.

Before initiating the trial, a response rate representing an activity level of interest should be defined, because this will influence the study sample size and the interim monitoring procedure. This targeted response rate is determined by such factors as the inherent sensitivity of the disease to other therapies, the number of standard treatment options available, and the perceived benefits of these standard approaches. For example, a new agent with a 20% partial-response rate in patients with pancreatic cancer (for which no reasonable alternatives exist) would probably be of interest, but that level of activity might be of little benefit in lymphoma patients.

Two-stage designs provide simple, reasonably efficient frameworks for phase II trials. An initial cohort of patients is treated. If the response rate observed is inconsistent with the activity level of interest, then accrual is terminated. Otherwise, an additional cohort of patients is accrued. For an activity level of interest of 25% and a high probability of rejecting a drug with an activity level of 5%, a maximum sample size of 25 to 30 patients is needed. Such designs limit the chance that a study will be terminated prematurely (mistakenly assuming lack of antitumor activity) and also limit the chance that inappropriately large number of patients will be needlessly exposed to an ineffective regimen.

Phase II trials can provide only a general impression of activity; confidence intervals for the true response rate are generally wide. This level of specificity is acceptable because identifying phase II activity is not an end in itself but more properly is a means toward achieving survival or improvement in quality of life. Rather than expanding the size of phase II trials, efforts should be directed to moving smoothly and rapidly to definitive phase III trials, which hold the promise of providing information that improves medical practice.

DESIGN PRINCIPLES FOR PHASE III TRIALS

The key principle for the design of phase III clinical trials is to ask an important question and obtain a reliable answer. Asking an important question generally means identifying a hypothesis that may influence medical practice; using an experimental treatment that is promising, widely applicable, and substantially different from the control treatment; using a control treatment as a reference standard that is widely accepted; using an endpoint that is a direct measure of patient benefit; and studying patients who are broadly representative of the patients seen in practice by community physicians.

Survival is generally the endpoint most directly related to patient welfare. Tumor response may be appropriate for phase II trials as a measure of promising biologic activity, but it is only an indirect measure of patient benefit and therefore is generally unsuitable for phase III trials. Symptomatic relief or preservation of organ function can represent meaningful patient benefit, but direct measures of such effects are best used as endpoints rather than attempting to validate partial response as a valid surrogate.

Formerly, it was common in reports of uncontrolled phase II trials to see comparisons of the survivals of responders to the survivals of nonresponders. The fact that responders had longer survivals than nonresponders was inappropriately assumed to imply that the treatment extended survival. This analysis is invalid. To make valid inferences about the effect of a treatment on survival, the survivals of all the treated patients (not just the responders) must be compared with the survivals of a comparable control group receiving some control treatment.

If a clinical trial is to influence medical practice, the patients included in the trial must be representative of the population of patients to whom the results will be applied. Consequently, unduly narrow selection criteria for phase III clinical trials are generally inappropriate.

Getting a reliable answer also has several important components. Probably most important is the use of randomized treatment assignment. Most treatment improvements achieved for patients with solid tumors are relatively small compared with the natural variations in prognosis among patients. Many oncologists believe that nonrandomized trials are appropriate for determining what treatments are sufficiently promising to warrant evaluation in randomized clinical trials, but that we should not base major public health policies or patterns of care on methodologies that have led us astray so often.

A second important component of getting a reliable answer is an adequate sample size. Many clinical trials that are reported as negative are really just noninformative because they did not include enough patients to detect a medically important treatment effect. The use of confidence intervals to describe the magnitude of treatment differences that are consistent with the observed results are helpful in avoiding the common misinterpretation of "not statistically significant."

Intent-to-treat analysis is also an important component of getting a reliable answer. In this type of analysis, all eligible randomized patients are included in the group to which they were randomized, with no exclusions for noncompliance with treatment. Exclusions permit the results to be biased, because the excluded patients are usually prognostically different than the nonexcluded patients. A classic example of such bias occurred in the Coronary Drug Project in which placebo patients who were good compliers had much lower cardiovascular mortality than placebo patients who were poor compliers.

Performing numerous subset analyses is a cause of erroneous conclusions in many clinical trials. If the chance of a false-positive conclusion for a single question in a single analysis is 5%, then the chance that at least one false-positive conclusion will be obtained in 10 independent comparisons is about 40%. Many clinical trial reports describe more than 10 comparisons, considering the multiple endpoints and multiple subsets often considered. Such analyses should be viewed as exploratory, generating hypotheses that require independent testing in a focused clinical trial.

If a clinical trial of two equivalent treatments is analyzed repeatedly over the course of accrual and follow-up, then the probability that a $p < 0.05$ will be found in at least one interim or final analysis may exceed 25%, rather than the 5% expected. A powerful body of statistical methodology has been developed for interpreting interim data while keeping the type I error rate below 5%. Major multicenter clinical trials should also use data-monitoring committees to review accumulating data and to make recommendations about whether the trial should be changed, terminated, or reported. During the trial, interim efficacy results are withheld from physicians entering patients in the study (except possibly for the study chair) to protect both the patients and the study. The patients are protected because decisions on whether to continue, change, or terminate the trial are made by persons with no vested professional or financial interest in the trial. The study is protected from inappropriate early termination, which might occur if participating physicians were to become nervous about unreliable interim trends. Because physicians entering patients do not see the interim efficacy results, they remain free to interact with their patients honestly and to encourage their patients and colleagues to participate in the trial.

BIBLIOGRAPHY

Anderson JR, Cain KC, Gelber RD. Analysis of survival by tumor response. *J Clin Oncol* 1983;1:710–719.

Korn EL, Simon R. Using the tolerable-dose diagram in the design of phase I combination chemotherapy trials. *J Clin Oncol* 1993;11:794–801.

Simon R. Confidence intervals for reporting clinical trial results. *Ann Intern Med* 1986;105:429–435.

Simon R. Design and conduct of clinical trials. In: DeVita VT, Hellman S, Rosenberg SA, eds. *Principles and practice of oncology,* fourth ed. Philadelphia: JB Lippincott, 1993.

Simon R. Optimal two-stage designs for phase II clinical trials. *Control Clin Trials* 1989;10:1–10.

Simon R. Randomized clinical trials in oncology: principles and obstacles. *Cancer* 1994;74:2614–2619.

Simon R, Freidlin B, Rubinstein L, et al. Accelerated titration designs for phase I clinical trials in oncology. *J Natl Cancer Inst* 1997;89: 1138–1147.

Simon R, Wittes RE. Methodologic guidelines for clinical trial reports. *Cancer Treat Rep* 1985;69:1–3.

Smith MA, Ungerleider RS, Korn EL, et al. The role of independent data monitoring committees in randomized clinical trials sponsored by the National Cancer Institute. *J Clin Oncol* 1997;15:2736–2743.

Wittes RE, Marsoni S, Simon R, et al. The phase II trial. *Cancer Treat Rep* 1985;69:1235–1239.

Kelley's Textbook of Internal Medicine, fourth edition. Edited by H. David Humes. Lippincott Williams & Wilkins, Philadelphia © 2000.

7

INFECTIOUS DISEASES AND AIDS

Herbert L. DuPont, Editor

APPROACH TO THE PATIENT WITH INFECTIOUS DISEASES

APPROACH TO THE PATIENT WITH CELLULITIS AND OTHER SOFT-TISSUE INFECTIONS

RONALD T. LEWIS

Focal or diffuse soft-tissue infections are usually recognized easily, and they are well treated by local debridement and antibiotic therapy. However, infections may appear in many forms (Fig. 263.1). Those secondary to defined anatomical skin lesions, wounds, or dermatitis are usually obvious. But most infections are primary, and because they usually start with a break in the skin associated with minor trauma, they may be confused with inflammation without infection caused by trauma and other conditions. More important are severe, life-threatening, necrotizing soft-tissue infections, which may simulate nonoperative cellulitis. The astute clinician must be familiar with the usual modes of presentation of soft-tissue infections and should know and recognize the more serious conditions requiring aggressive management.

PRESENTATION

FOCAL CUTANEOUS INFECTIONS

The common focal lesions are readily diagnosed. Most lesions are seen as pyodermas without systemic signs, localized to the skin or to skin structures (Fig. 263.2).

Impetigo contagiosa is a highly communicable skin infection that occurs mainly on the face and legs of children. It begins as small vesicles with inflammatory halos that pustulate and dry out within 4 to 6 days, forming itchy but painless "stuck-on"

crusts. Most lesions are streptococcal in origin; the 10% caused by *Staphylococcus aureus* are bullous rather than vesicular at onset.

Folliculitis manifests as a pyoderma centered in one or more hair follicles, with mild surrounding inflammation, which culminates in a superficial pustule. A furuncle forms by deep extension of the perifollicular infection. A carbuncle results from coalescence of furuncles and still deeper extension of inflammation into the subcutaneous tissues. Fever and malaise are usually associated.

FOCAL INFECTIONS WITH TOXIC EFFECTS

Focal conditions include the staphylococcal scalded skin syndrome (SSSS) and toxic shock syndrome (TSS) and are characterized by remote staphylococcal infections associated with severe toxicity.

SSSS is usually found in young children; it is rare in adults and may occur in epidemic form in neonates (pemphigus neonatorum). A few days after a staphylococcal infection, fever develops, and an erythematous rash appears on the face 2 to 3 days later. Soon, the entire body is covered with a weeping rash that develops into large bullae. When the bullae break and slough, they leave denuded, wet, raw areas that heal within 10 days.

In TSS, vaginitis and vaginal discharge are associated with

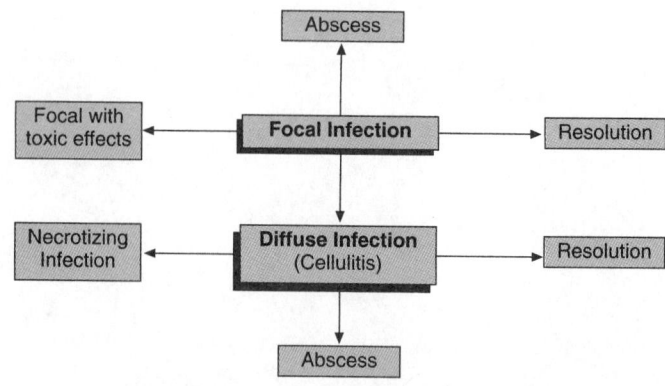

FIGURE 263.1. Presentation of soft-tissue infection.

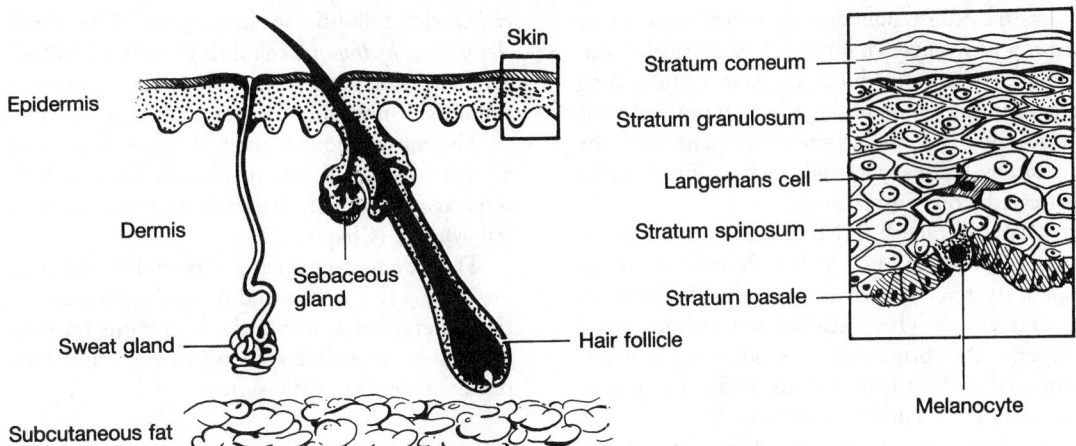

FIGURE 263.2. Anatomy of skin, skin structures, and subcutaneous fat. Soft-tissue infections are localized as follows: impetigo–epidermis; folliculitis, furunculosis, and carbuncle–hair follicle; focal infections with toxic effects–stratum granulosum; cellulitis–skin and subcutaneous fat; erysipelas–dermis. (Modified from Lookingbill DP, Marks JG. *Principles of dermatology*. Philadelphia: WB Saunders, 1993:4.

fever and a generalized macular erythematous rash that eventually desquamates. Hypotension occurs, and three or more organ systems may fail (Table 263.1). Rarely, TSS may follow other soft-tissue infections.

DIFFUSE INFECTIONS—CELLULITIS

Cellulitis is a spreading acute infection of the skin and subcutaneous tissues characterized by erythema, warmth, swelling, and tenderness. It may be primary or may be secondary to a local lesion or, uncommonly, to hematogenous spread of infection from a remote area. Cellulitis may be classified as mild and uncomplicated, severe, high risk, or necrotizing.

Most cellulitis is mild and uncomplicated and is caused by group A streptococci or by *S. aureus*. Diffuse erythema, swelling, and tenderness develop over 2 to 4 days. In an extremity, a red line along the course of the lymphatics indicates accompanying lymphangitis; enlarged, tender regional lymph nodes are common. Fever, malaise, and chills are often present. Cellulitis is potentially dangerous because of the rapidity with which infection spreads to the bloodstream.

Severe infections must be recognized, and patients must be admitted to the hospital for intravenous antibiotic therapy. The key signs are systemic: fever, chills, toxicity, and leukocytosis. Underlying disease (e.g., diabetes) and ischemia worsen the risk and should be sought specifically. Severity may also be graded in units by the intensity of each of its four elements (fever, erythema, swelling, and tenderness). Each element is rated as absent (0), mild (1), moderate (2), or severe (3), and the total score in severity units is the sum of scores for each element.

Some infections are designated as high risk because the sites at which they occur predispose to serious complications. These infections include orbital cellulitis, erysipelas, and other facial cellulitis; postadenectomy cellulitis and postvenectomy cellulitis in the extremities; and erysipeloid and infected human and animal bites on the hands.

Facial cellulitis is especially common in infants and children and is classified as odontogenic or nonodontogenic. Eighty percent occurs in the upper face. Odontogenic cellulitis refers to orofacial lesions originating from the teeth and periodontal structures. It accounts for 50% of all facial cellulitis, but 80% of lower facial cellulitis, and it occurs typically in older children

TABLE 263.1.	CRITERIA FOR DIAGNOSIS OF TOXIC SHOCK SYNDROME
Fever >38.8°C	Three or more of the following:
Rash	Gastrointestinal—vomit, diarrhea
Hypotension (BP <90 mm Hg)	Muscle—myalgias, CPK >2 × ULN
Negative	Renal—BUN, serum CR >2 × ULN
Culture of blood, throat, CSF	Liver—bilirubin ALT >2 × ULN
serology for leptospirosis, Rocky	Blood—platelets <100,000 mL^{-3}
Mountain spotted fever, measles	Neurologic—disorientation without focal signs

ALT, alanine aminotransferase; BP, systolic blood pressure; BUN, blood urea nitrogen; CPK, creatine phosphokinase; Cr, creatinine; CSF, cerebrospinal fluid; ULN, upper limit of normal.

of mean age 9 years. In contrast, nonodontogenic cellulitis occurs especially in infants and younger children. Thus, erysipelas usually follows a streptococcal sore throat in infants and young children. The anatomical location of the infection in the dermis and lymphatics accounts for the characteristic pain and the bright-red *peau d'orange* lesions whose advancing raised borders are sharply demarcated from normal skin.

Haemophilus influenzae type B (HIB) cellulitis occurs in the face and extremities of small children with fever and bacteremia from upper respiratory tract infections; recently, similar cases have been reported in adults. The typical lesion is painful, swollen, and purplish-red—the "bruised-cheek syndrome." It is unilateral when associated with ipsilateral otitis media, but it may be bilateral. Secondary meningitis may develop.

Orbital and periorbital cellulitis are marked by pain, redness, and swelling of the eyelids. Periorbital infections associated with minor trauma are common in childhood. Orbital cellulitis is a rare complication of acute sinusitis. The Chandler classification defines five stages: stage I, preseptal characterized by eyelid swelling only; stage II, postseptal orbital cellulitis in which infection has crossed the anterior orbital septum; stage III, subperiosteal abscess; stage IV, in which rupture of the periosteum allows extension of the abscess into the orbital cavity producing proptosis, chemosis, reduced eye motion, and a risk of blindness and of progression to stage V; and stage V, in which further complications such as meningitis and brain abscess occur. *S. aureus*, streptococci, and occasionally gram-negative aerobic bacteria are found.

Postadenectomy and postvenectomy cellulitis manifest as recurrent cellulitis in the lymphedematous extremity. Most patients with postadenectomy cellulitis have had a remote lymph node dissection for carcinoma of the breast, malignant melanoma, or gynecologic cancer. Postvenectomy cellulitis occurs in the legs of patients whose saphenous veins have been harvested for coronary artery bypass surgery. In both conditions, systemic signs such as fever, chills, and toxicity are prominent. Non–group A streptococci, particularly groups C and G, are usually implicated.

Erysipeloid is a form of cellulitis that occurs in workers handling fish, meat, and poultry. It is caused by the gram-positive bacillus *Erysipelothrix rhusiopathiae*. About 1 week after a minor injury to the hand, a violaceous painful area appears. As the central area clears, the lesion spreads outward with distinct raised borders. A more insidious marine infection caused by *Mycobacterium marinum* follows abrasions or puncture wounds in aquatic environments. Its presentation is a flat, macular, red area that disappears spontaneously or progresses to nodular and ulcerated lesions, which may extend along lymphatics or tendon sheaths and even to bone.

Animal and human bites are potentially dangerous because of tissue damage and secondary infection. Deep infections such as tenosynovitis are particularly common after human bites.

In some patients, cellulitis poses a high risk because of concurrent impaired host defense. This form of cellulitis is unusual, and the bacteria involved are unusual causes of primary soft-tissue infection. Pneumococcal cellulitis is associated with bacteremia and may resemble erysipelas. Cellulitis caused by Enterobacteriaceae is more insidious in onset. Examples include *Esche-* *richia coli* cellulitis in immunodeficient children or adults, *Aeromonas hydrophila* cellulitis (which follows minor lacerations acquired while swimming in fresh water), and *Serratia marcescens* cellulitis in immunocompromised patients with organ failure.

The most serious variant of cellulitis is *necrotizing cellulitis*, a term used for a variety of gangrenous soft-tissue infections often associated with anaerobic bacteria, tissue toxins, and bacterial synergy (Chapter 273).

The key to recognizing these infections is an awareness of underlying risk factors and of local signs: edema out of proportion to erythema, skin vesicles, crepitus on palpation or air in the tissues on radiologic examination, and local anesthesia or patchy gangrene of the skin.

PATHOPHYSIOLOGY

The pathophysiology of soft-tissue infections depends on anatomical localization (Fig. 263.2) and on the interaction of factors related to the invasiveness of the microorganism and to host defenses. Of the focal infections, impetigo is caused in 80% of cases by *Streptococcus pyogenes*, in 10% by *S. aureus*, or by both. Skin colonization favored by poor hygiene is followed by inoculation through minor abrasions, leading to clinical illness. Upper respiratory tract colonization occurs in the next 2 to 3 weeks but does not cause pharyngitis; in fact, the M-serotype skin strains are different from the throat strains that cause pharyngitis and tonsillitis.

The focal nature of the skin lesions is in keeping with poor lytic enzyme activity of the bacteria. In contrast, the large flaccid bullae typical of impetigo caused by group II phage-type *S. aureus* are a response to the exfoliative toxin (ET) produced by the organism. ET, also produced by *S. aureus* in SSSS, splits the epidermis in the stratum granulosum, resulting in large bullae and separation of sheets of skin (Nikolsky's sign). In TSS, group I phage *S. aureus* strains produce enterotoxin F (EF), which is responsible for the fever, skin rash, hypotension, and diarrhea. Most cases of TSS are associated with menstruation and with the use of superabsorbent tampons. A similar clinical picture has been described recently in extremity infections caused by group A streptococci, which produce a pyrogenic toxin similar to EF.

In diffuse cellulitis hyaluronidase, α and β toxins produced by *S. aureus* and DNase, hyaluronidase, streptokinase, and streptolysins produced by group A streptococci facilitate the spread of infection through tissue planes. A disparity exists between the intensity of the inflammatory response and the low density of bacteria found on culture or direct immunofluorescence techniques. These findings were previously attributed to lymphatic overload or failure, impaired protein clearance, and an exaggerated inflammatory response to the excess denatured protein. A better explanation has been found recently in a unique set of lymphoid and reticular cells in the skin (dendritic cells of Langerhans; Fig. 263.2) and keratinocytes. When exposed to bacterial cell components, these cells release cytokines such as interleukin-1 and tumor necrosis factor. In turn, these cytokines increase phagocytosis and cytotoxicity, causing rapid bacterial clearance, and they evoke an enhanced inflammatory response in the tissues.

In the severe cellulitis of diabetic foot infections, neuropathy, vascular insufficiency, and hyperglycemia combine to promote synergistic spreading infections, tissue necrosis, and delayed wound healing. Motor and sensory neuropathy causes altered weight-bearing and impaired sensation and proprioception. Vascular insufficiency impairs the healing of fissures and breaks in the skin, and hyperglycemia is associated with decreased neutrophil migration and phagocytosis, reduced fibroblast replication, and decreased collagen formation and strength.

The pathogenesis of HIB buccal cellulitis is unclear. Because the condition usually follows otitis media, lymphatic spread of HIB to buccal nodes has been suggested. Hematogenous spread has also been suggested because bacteremia is common in children with HIB cellulitis. However, bacteremia is uncommon in HIB cellulitis in the lower extremities of adults. In periorbital and orbital cellulitis, spread of infection occurs directly from the sinuses or by retrograde thrombophlebitis along valveless facial veins.

In postadenectomy and postvenectomy cellulitis, stagnated lymph fluid favors bacterial growth. This may explain why local infection and toxicity are more common in limbs with lymphedema than in normal limbs.

High-risk hand infections owe their severity to the depth of invasion of specific bacteria. These bacteria include the gram-negative coccobacillus *E. rhusiopathiae* in fish and meat handlers, *Pasteurella multocida*, and occasionally the gram-negative bacillus dysgonic fermenter-2 (DF-2) in dog and cat bites and the gram-negative bacillus *Eikenella corrodens* in human bites. DF-2 can produce fulminant bacteremia and disseminated intravascular coagulation in patients who have had splenectomy.

High-risk cellulitis in immunosuppressed patients is important for several reasons. First, in HIV-positive patients, the edema of Kaposi's sarcoma may simulate cellulitis, particularly in dark-skinned persons, in whom the neoplasm may not be noticeable. Second, gram-negative bacterial cellulitis and necrotizing infections occur with increased frequency in HIV-positive and other immunocompromised patients. Third, a recently described syndrome in the immunocompromised patient can cause lesions similar to those of Kaposi's sarcoma. The causative agent, *Rochalimaea henselae*, may be isolated from the cutaneous lesions and blood of patients with the syndrome.

In necrotizing cellulitis, impaired host resistance, anaerobic wound conditions, bacterial synergy, and lytic enzymes and toxins produced by the microbes involved are responsible for the rapidity of onset or progression. More recently, the streptococcal toxic shock syndrome has gained notoriety as a life-threatening "flesh-eating disease" in young adults. The pathogenesis is related to specific streptococcal pyrogenic exotoxins, which stimulate mononuclear cells and lymphocytes to produce cytokines that promote fever, shock, and tissue injury. The effect on the lymphocytes is greatly amplified because the exotoxins serve as "superantigens," interact with T lymphocytes in ways that are swifter and more universal than occur with conventional antigens, resulting in massive activation of lymphocytes and profuse release of damaging lymphokines.

INVESTIGATION

In all but the simplest cases of uncomplicated cellulitis, the physician should follow the ABCs of investigation of soft-tissue infection: **a**spiration of pus or deep tissue fluid for culture, **b**lood tests for risk evaluation, **c**ulture of deep tissue specimens and blood, and **d**iagnostic imaging.

ASPIRATION

Although superficial cultures are positive for pathogenic bacteria in two-thirds of cases, they are of little value in management because most are found in open lesions that respond to blind therapy with semisynthetic penicillins. Deep tissue culture is preferable, and needle aspiration is the best method of obtaining a satisfactory specimen of tissue fluid or pus. In patients without an obvious collection of pus, a fine-needle aspiration technique should be used.

BLOOD TESTS

Blood tests for risk evaluation should include a complete blood count and random blood sugar. In febrile or toxic patients, the blood urea nitrogen and serum creatinine levels should be determined; blood tests of liver function may be performed, if indicated. Blood cultures are usually negative and should therefore be done selectively. Leukocytosis is common. Organ dysfunction may be found in TSS and in necrotizing infections.

CULTURE

After deep tissue fine-needle aspiration, 0.5 mL thioglycolate broth is aspirated into the syringe and a few drops are inoculated

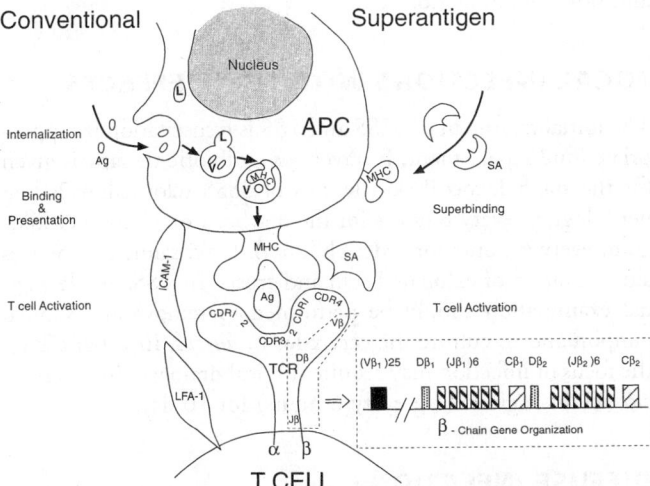

FIGURE 263.3. Activation of T lymphocytes by superantigens compared with that by conventional antigens. Ag, antigen; APC, antigen-presenting (mononuclear) cell; L, lysosome; V, vesicle; MHC, major histocompatibility class II molecule; SA, superantigen; ICAM, intracellular adhesion molecule; LFA, lymphocyte functional associated molecule; CDR, complementarity determining region; TCR, T cell receptor. Inset: Gene organization on β-chain of the T cell receptor. V, variable region; C, constant region; D, diversity segment; J, junctional zone. (From Lewis RT. Soft tissue infections. *World J Surg* 1998;22:146–151.)

onto plates of sheep blood agar, chocolate agar, and MacConkey agar and into a glass tube containing a semisolid thioglycolate medium. The agar plates and tube are then incubated for 48 hours at 35° C in 5% carbon dioxide, and a separate sheep blood agar plate is incubated in an anaerobic jar. Only 20% to 30% of cultures are positive in cellulitis; blood cultures are positive still less often.

DIAGNOSTIC IMAGING

Methods used include plain x-ray films, isotope and ultrasound imaging, and occasionally CT and MRI.

Plain films show air in the tissues in 90% of patients with necrotizing soft-tissue infection, so they are of great value in identifying these infections. Furthermore, when x-rays show medullary lysis, endosteal scalloping, or cortical erosion, they resolve immediately the issue of bony involvement. However, plain x-rays may be normal within the first 7 to 10 days of bony infection; therefore, bone scans are often obtained. In practice, it is best to delay scanning until soft-tissue infection has been controlled by intravenous antibiotics.

Isotope imaging may be performed with technetium (^{99m}Tc) pyrophosphate or gallium-indium. ^{99m}Tc pyrophosphate accumulates in areas of increased blood flow or new bone formation and may be positive within 48 hours of bone infection. Gallium citrate and indium chloride become fixed to sequestered polymorphs and macrophages, and to transferrin, which leaks from the bloodstream into areas of inflammation. Neither gallium nor indium accumulates specifically in areas of reactive bone. A 3-minute ^{99m}Tc scan is therefore preferable to the use of gallium-indium for differentiating clearly between soft-tissue and bone inflammation. When scans using both isotopes are available in a patient with osteomyelitis, ^{99m}Tc pyrophosphate shows a disproportionate concentration in bone, best seen when the studies are delayed until soft-tissue infection has subsided. In fact, when it it available MRI offers the greatest accuracy in diagnosing osteomyelitis. Secondary signs of bone involvement—ulcer, sinus, or cortical interruption—augment diagnostic confidence when an abnormal marrow signal is present.

Duplex scanning is the best method for identifying superficial and deep venous thrombosis. The study should be performed in patients with severe extremity inflammation to rule out venous thrombosis simulating or complicating cellulitis. MRI with gadolinium differentiates necrotizing from non-necrotizing soft-tissue infections by the absence of gadolinium contrast enhancement in T1-weighted CT imaging is mandatory in managing orbital infection. In particular, it identifies Chandler stage III disease and shows the details of stage V involvement.

▃ STRATEGIES FOR OPTIMAL MANAGEMENT

In managing soft-tissue infections, the first priority is to identify necrotizing infection. Figure 263.4 emphasizes the central role of risk factor analysis and clinical markers of necrotizing infection in the management scheme. A second priority is to rule out noninfectious conditions that may simulate or complicate

cellulitis. A third priority is to identify complications such as bone or joint infection in extremity cellulitis and orbital and intracranial infection in facial cellulitis. These priorities are met by attention to clinical presentation and to the ABCs of investigation. Treatment itself should include antibiotic therapy, local care, and resuscitation of some patients.

FOCAL NONTOXIC INFECTIONS

Impetigo is treated either by a single intramuscular injection of penicillin (300,000 to 600,000 units) or by oral penicillin V (15,000 units per kilogram) every 6 hours for 10 days. In penicillin allergy, oral erythromycin (10 mg per kilogram every 6 hours) should be given for 10 days. Local care is important and includes washing with soap and water to soften and remove crusts. In bullous impetigo, oral cloxacillin (15 mg per kilogram every 6 hours) is given for 10 days.

Folliculitis and furuncles are generally treated satisfactorily by local measures only; saline compresses speed regression or spontaneous drainage. Topical antibiotics may be helpful. Oral cloxacillin (500 mg every 6 hours) for 7 to 10 days is indicated for recurrent or facial furunculosis and for surrounding cellulitis or associated fever. In the penicillin-allergic patient, oral erythromycin (250 to 500 mg every 6 hours) for 7 to 10 days is a suitable alternative. Surgical drainage is required for large and fluctuant furuncles or carbuncles. In patients with recurrent disease, additional measures are recommended:

Shower daily with hexachlorophene soap to reduce skin colonization and autoinfection.

Cover draining lesions with sterile dressings to reduce the spread of contamination.

Discard dressings promptly after removing them.

Apply nasal bacitracin to decrease nasal carriage, shedding, and skin contamination.

FOCAL INFECTIONS WITH TOXIC EFFECTS

The initial treatment of SSSS and TSS is resuscitation by appropriate fluid replacement. Intravenous antibiotic therapy is given for the staphylococcal skin lesions of SSSS (cloxacillin 20 mg per kilogram every 6 hours for the newborn or 50 mg per kilogram every 6 hours for older children). Cold saline compresses aid separation of exfoliated skin and crusts. In TSS, gentle vaginal examination should be performed to remove any vaginal tampon and to culture the cervix for *S. aureus*. In variant TSS, the focus of infection may require surgical drainage. Intravenous cloxacillin is given (2 g every 6 hours) for 10 days.

DIFFUSE INFECTIONS

Most cases of cellulitis can be managed simply on an outpatient basis. However, severe infections, high-risk infections, and complicated infections usually require aggressive inpatient antibiotic therapy and often surgery. Patients with necrotizing infections must be admitted for surgery.

Uncomplicated mild cellulitis, commonly caused by *S. pyogenes* or *S. aureus*, responds well to oral cloxacillin or cephalexin

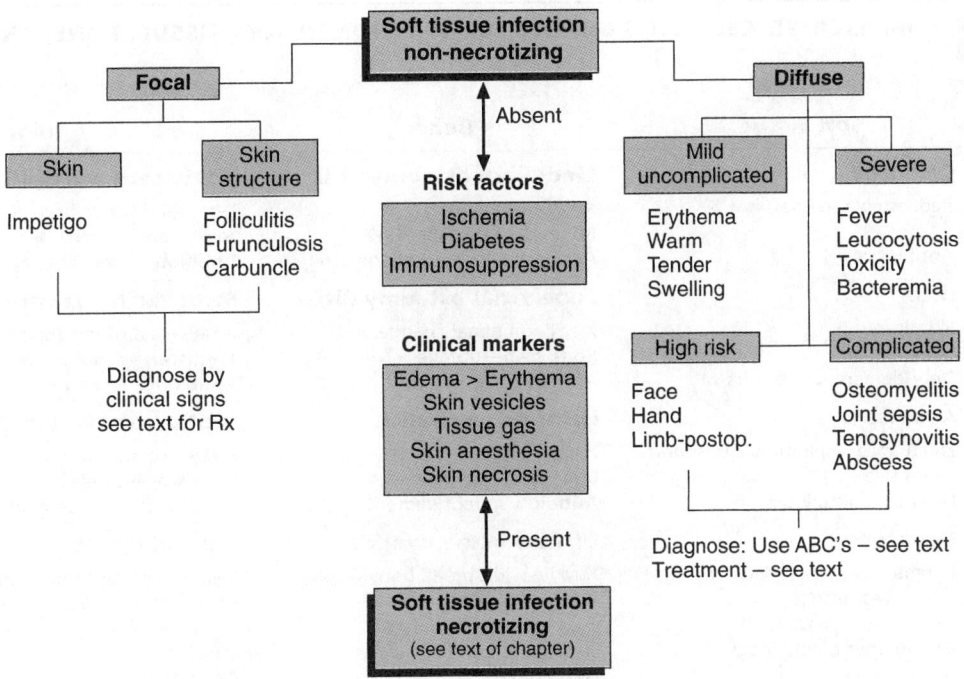

FIGURE 263.4. Management of soft-tissue infection.

(500 mg every 6 hours for 7 to 10 days). In patients allergic to penicillin, oral erythromycin (500 mg every 6 hours) is an alternative. Although various quinolones have been investigated for treating uncomplicated cellulitis, no advantage over less expensive antibiotics has been found. Local therapy includes cleansing the area and resting the extremity.

In severe cellulitis, treatment should start with intravenous cloxacillin (1 g every 6 hours). Intravenous vancomycin (500 mg every 8 hours) or the related glycopeptide antibiotic teicoplanin (1 g daily) are alternatives for the penicillin-allergic patient. An aminoglycoside such as gentamicin may be added when the clinical setting suggests that a gram-negative bacillus may play a role, for instance, in patients with failed oral cloxacillin therapy, in those with cellulitis after injury and exposure to contaminated fresh water, in those with perianal cellulitis, and in those who have risk factors for gram-negative bacterial infection (neutropenia, diabetes mellitus, organ failure, and corticosteroid treatment). However, many physicians now avoid aminoglycosides, particularly in diabetic and other patients who may have renal impairment. Second-generation cephalosporins such as cefoxitin (1 to 2 g every 6 hours) or cefotetan (1 to 2 g every 12 hours) have been used successfully and are particularly attractive in patients in whom anaerobic bacteria may play a role. Others prefer third-generation cephalosporins, particularly ceftazidime (2 g every 6 hours) or ceftriaxone (1 to 2 g daily), or the combination antibiotics piperacillin-tazobactam (3.375 g every 6 hours), ticarcillin-clavulanate (3.1 g every 8 hours), or ampicillin-sulbactam (3 g every 6 hours).

Some authors have suggested the use of nonsteroidal antiinflammatory drugs in cellulitis, based on the role of cytokines in the pathophysiology of soft-tissue infections. However, benefit is unproved, and caution has been suggested because of the risk

of promoting bacterial multiplication and because of an observed association with necrotizing skin infection. Local measures include elevation and immobilization of the part. Surgical drainage of focal lesions may be required.

Among high-risk facial infections, erysipelas usually responds to intravenous penicillin G (1 million units every 6 hours). Traditionally, HIB cellulitis is treated initially with intravenous ampicillin, but most institutions now favor intravenous cefuroxime (125 mg twice daily). Orbital cellulitis is also treated with broad-spectrum antibiotics. CT evidence of abscess or intracranial involvement and failure to respond to antibiotics within 48 hours are indications for prompt exploration and decompression of the orbit. Postadenectomy and postvenectomy cellulitis are treated as severe cellulitis. Of the high-risk hand infections, erysipeloid responds to amoxicillin-clavulanate or erythromycin. Animal and human bites require oral cloxacillin and local debridement. Neither *P. multocida* nor *E. corrodens* responds to erythromycin. Debridement is particularly important in human bites and clenched-fist injuries because of the major role of anaerobic bacteria in these states.

The treatment of complicated cellulitis is discussed in the following text, and necrotizing soft-tissue infection is considered in Chapter 273. In streptococccal toxic shock syndrome, evidence now favors use of intravenous high-dose penicillin and clindamycin, and human immunoglobulin is given to neutralize exotoxin.

COMPLICATIONS

Soft-tissue infection may be complicated by deep abscesses, tendon sheath infection, osteomyelitis, and other site-specific deep infections. In severe cellulitis, a deep abscess may be

TABLE 263.2.	COMPLICATED CELLULITIS GRADES OF INFECTION IN SOFT TISSUE, BONE, AND JOINT		
Anatomical Type	**Soft Tissue**	**Bone**	**Joint**
Simple	**Cellulitis**	**Medullary osteomyelitis**	**Acute septic arthritis**
Diagnosis	Red, edema, tender, hot	X-ray—bone lysis Bone scan—uptake + +	X-ray—joint swelling Joint scan—uptake + +
Treatment	Antibiotics	Antibiotics +/− drainage	Antibiotics +/− drainage
Superficial	**Ulcer**	**Superficial osteomyelitis**	**Septic arthritis with chondrolysis**
Diagnosis	Skin loss	X-ray—minimal changes Bone scan—uptake +	X-ray—loss of joint space Joint scan—uptake + +
Treatment	Debridement, antibiotics	Antibiotics +/− debridement	Antibiotics + drainage
Localized	**Abscess**	**Local osteomyelitis**	**Septic arthritis with osteomyelitis**
Diagnosis	Fluctuance, aspiration/ultrasound positive	X-ray—cortical erosion Bone scan—uptake + +	X-ray—cortical erosion, loss of joint space Bone scan—uptake + + in bone & joint
Treatment	Drainage, antibiotics	Antibiotics, debridement	Antibiotics, debridement
Diffuse	**Gangrene**	**Diffuse osteomyelitis**	**Unstable joint**
Diagnosis	Edema + +, gas in tissue, skin loss, vesicles	X-ray—widespread bony erosion Bone scan—uptake + + +	X-ray—cortical erosion, loss of joint space Bone scan—uptake + + + Unstable joint
Treatment	Debridement, antibiotics	Debride/amputate Antibiotics	Debride/fuse joint Antibiotics

Adapted from Calhoun JH, Mader JT. Infection in the diabetic foot. *Hosp Pract* 1992;27:81.

suggested by failure to respond to intravenous antibiotics or by clinical signs and results of investigation. A foreign body may serve as a nidus for abscess formation. The history may suggest it, and an x-ray film of the part or an ultrasound examination may confirm the diagnosis. Treatment includes removal of the foreign body, surgical drainage, and continued antibiotic therapy.

Tenosynovitis should be sought in all hand infections but is particularly likely after human bites of the hand. Kanavel's four signs suggest the diagnosis: uniform swelling of the digit, tenderness along the line of the tendon sheath, flexion of the resting digit, and worsening of the pain on extension. In early cases, intravenous antibiotics such as cloxacillin (1 g) or cefoxitin (2 g) every 6 hours may permit resolution, but surgical drainage is required if this fails and in advanced cases.

A classification of soft-tissue, bone, and joint infections has been suggested to aid in the diagnosis and management of infections of bone and joint complications (Table 263.2).

COST-EFFECTIVENESS

In an era of cost containment and managed health care, outpatient antibiotic therapy is playing an increasing role in the management of soft-tissue infection (Table 263.3). Evidence is increasing that parenteral antibiotics can be given effectively and safely to patients at home or in an ambulatory setting at substantially lower cost than inpatient care. Such therapy is made possible by antibiotics of prolonged half-life, which provide tissue

drug levels higher than the minimal inhibitory levels required for most pathogens that cause cellulitis. In addition, some new antibiotics are equally effective when given by mouth or by the intravenous route. More studies are required to define the best strategies for dealing with disease of varying grades of severity; particularly in diabetic foot infections where therapy for 3 or 4 weeks is recommended, it is convenient to start with intravenous therapy and continue with oral therapy. MRI is cost-effective in diagnosing osteomyelitis in providing the anatomical localization necessary for the aggressive surgical intervention that minimizes above-ankle amputation.

Other strategies suggested for reducing costs but are as yet unproven include the use of granulocyte colony-stimulating factor or hyperbaric oxygen therapy in diabetic foot infection and the use of platelet-derived growth factor to hasten healing of diabetic foot ulcers.

TABLE 263.3.	STRATEGIES FOR COST-EFFECTIVE OUTPATIENT ANTIBIOTIC THERAPY IN SEVERE CELLULITIS

Antibiotic therapy by mouth only
Single-dose parenteral antibiotic, followed by oral therapy
Daily parenteral antibiotic therapy until favorable response, followed by oral therapy

BIBLIOGRAPHY

Calhoun JH, Mader JT. Infection in the diabetic foot. *Hosp Pract* 1992; 27:81–90,99.

Castanet J, Lacour JPH, Perrin C, et al. *Escherichia coli* cellulitis: two cases. *Acta Dermatol Venereol (Stockh)* 1992;72:310–311.

Chandler JR, Langenbrunner DJ, Stevens ER. The pathogenesis of orbital complications in acute sinusitis. *Laryngoscope* 1970;80:1414–1428.

Chosidow O, Saiag P, Pinquier L, et al. Nonsteroidal antiinflammatory drugs in cellulitis: a cautionary note. *Arch Dermatol* 1991;127: 1845–1846.

Eron LJ, Park CH, Dixon DL, et al. Ceftriaxone therapy of bone and soft-tissue infections in hospital and outpatient settings. *Antimicrob Agents Chemother* 1983;23:731–737.

Fisher JR, Conway MJ, Takashita RT, et al. Necrotizing fasciitis: importance of roentgenographic studies for soft-tissue gas. *JAMA* 1979;241: 803–806.

Hook EW, Hooton TM, Horton CA, et al. Microbiologic evaluation of cutaneous cellulitis in adults. *Arch Intern Med* 1986;146:295–297.

Sachs MK. Cutaneous cellulitis. *Arch Dermatol* 1991;127:493–496.

Simpson GT, McGill TIJ, Healy GB. *Haemophilus influenzae* type B soft-tissue infections of the head and neck. *Laryngoscope* 1981;91:1200.

Stevens DL, Tanner MH, Winship J, et al. Severe group A streptococcal infections associated with a toxic shock-like syndrome and scarlet fever toxin A. *N Engl J Med* 1989;321:1–7.

Streilein JW. Skin-associated lymphoid tissue (SALT): origins and functions. *J Invest Dermatol* 1983;80(suppl):12S–16S.

Kelley's Textbook of Internal Medicine, fourth edition. Edited by H. David Humes. Lippincott Williams & Wilkins, Philadelphia © 2000.

C H A P T E R
264

INTRA-ABDOMINAL ABSCESS: DIAGNOSIS AND MANAGEMENT

MARIANNE CINAT
SAMUEL E. WILSON

An intra-abdominal abscess develops when infection within the greater or lesser peritoneal spaces becomes localized by a pyogenic membrane containing leukocytes, cellular debris, fibrin, and bacteria or fungi. This walling-off process represents temporary control of a potentially overwhelming peritonitis. Intraperitoneal abscesses often stem from perforation of a hollow viscus. Examples of enterogenous sources of intra-abdominal abscess are appendicitis, diverticulitis, and Crohn's disease. Intra-abdominal abscesses may develop as a result of invasive procedures, most commonly after gastrointestinal or biliary surgery (Figs. 264.1 and 264.2).

PATHOGENESIS

Secondary peritonitis results from loss of integrity from the gastrointestinal tract. It is usually due to a perforation of the intestine, is polymicrobial in nature, and may take the form of an intra-abdominal abscess or generalized peritonitis. Three forms of host defense occur after initial peritoneal contamination. Within minutes of bacterial contamination, microorganisms are cleared by lymphatics and are exposed to systemic defenses. Peritoneal macrophages become activated and act as phagocytic cells. If the invading microorganisms prevail, polymorphonuclear leukocytes migrate toward the area of infection. In addition, there is an increase in splanchnic blood flow and capillary permeability, leading to an exudation of 300 to 500 milliliters of fluid per hour, massive third-space fluid losses, and resultant hypovolemia. Fibrin produced from inflammatory cells entraps bacteria and limits their spread. These events help control generalized peritonitis, but they also promote the development of intra-abdominal abscesses.

MICROBIOLOGY

Pathogens isolated from intra-abdominal abscesses are derived from the flora of the gastrointestinal tract. Bacterial cultures are usually polymicrobial, commonly containing *Escherichia coli,* *Enterococcus,* anaerobes, and *Klebsiella* species. Anaerobic bacteria are found in up to 80% of intra-abdominal abscess cultures, with *Bacteroides fragilis* and *Clostridium* species identified most often. Initial antimicrobial therapy is usually presumptive, but subsequent modification is based on culture results. Pathogens other than bacteria may be involved, such as *Candida* or *Aspergillus* species, or parasites, such as *Pneumocystis carinii* or *Cryptosporidium.*

SITE

An abscess within the peritoneal cavity is not always located adjacent to the source of infection. Diaphragmatic movement draws peritoneal fluid upward, whereas gravity acts to pull peritoneal fluid into the pelvis. Accordingly, the subphrenic and pelvic areas are the most common sites of intra-abdominal abscess formation (Fig. 264.3). Twenty percent of patients have several sites of involvement, which is important to remember when deciding between image-guided and open treatment.

DIAGNOSIS

By means of a thorough history and physical examination and the appropriate noninvasive studies, the physician can localize intra-abdominal abscess with a high degree of accuracy. Enterogenous intraperitoneal abscess should be suspected when the patient has a history of diverticulitis, inflammatory bowel disease, peptic ulcers, pancreatitis, cancer, or long-term steroid use. The patient usually reports fever, anorexia, nausea, vomiting, and abdominal pain. Physical examination, estimated to be helpful or diagnostic in up to 75% of intra-abdominal abscesses, may pinpoint decreased or absent bowel sounds, indicating an

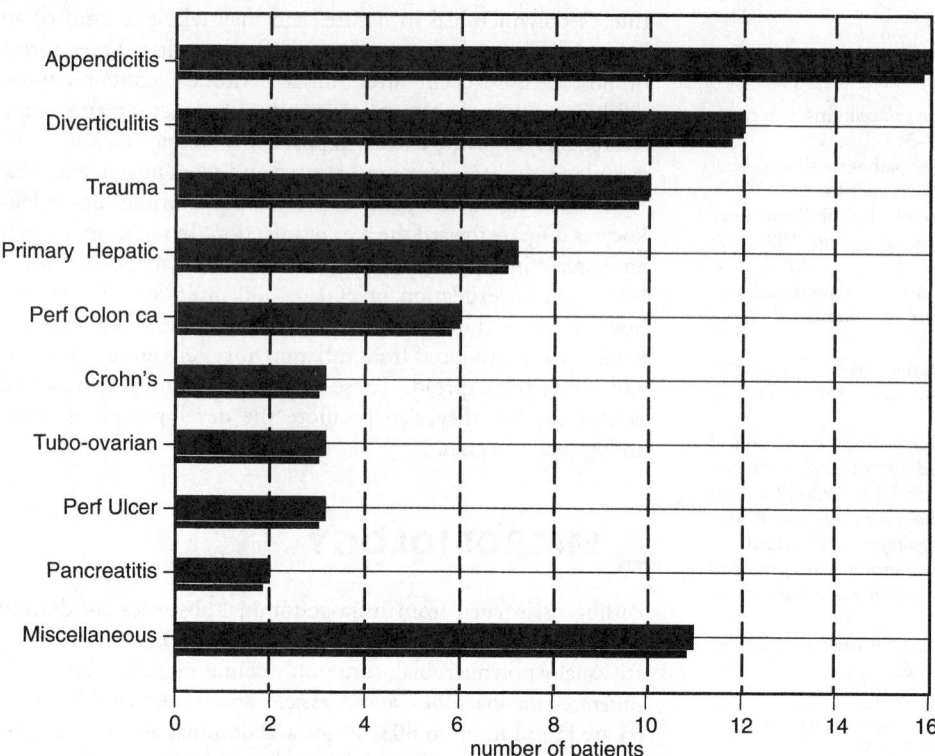

FIGURE 264.1. Origin of intra-abdominal abscesses arising from enterogenous disease or trauma. (From Saini S, Kellum JM, O'Leary MP, et al. Improved localization and survival in patients with intra-abdominal abscesses. *Am J Surg* 1983;145: 136–142, with permission.)

ileus, distention, and a mass with localized or diffuse tenderness. Peritoneal signs, such as rebound tenderness, may not be present, especially in those patients who are immunocompromised. Signs of peritonitis may have resolved by the time an abscess associated with a perforated viscus develops. Rectal and pelvic examinations are always carried out and can aid in localizing a pelvic or paracolic abscess. Abdominal tenderness is not to be expected with subphrenic abscesses; pulmonary symptoms, such as cough, dyspnea, and basilar rales, may be the only diagnostic clues. Diagnosis of a postoperative intra-abdominal abscess also represents a challenge, because these patients are receiving narcotics, have

peri-incisional tenderness and postoperative ileus, and may have low-grade fever unrelated to infection. Postoperative intraperitoneal abscess should be suspected when ileus, fever, and elevated leukocyte count are present beyond the fifth to seventh postoperative day in a patient who has had an intraperitoneal operation.

Imaging techniques have improved both diagnosis and treatment of intra-abdominal abscess. Plain film radiography will at best make visible only 50% of the abscesses that are present. Plain film findings suggestive of intra-abdominal abscess include displacement of bowel or other organs, extraluminal fluid collection with air-fluid level, or extraluminal air indicative of perforation. An elevated hemidiaphragm and pleural effusion seen on a chest radiograph may be the only findings suggestive of subphrenic abscess.

Computed tomography (CT) is the study of choice in imaging intra-abdominal abscesses, yielding up to 97% sensitivity and specificity in localizing intra-abdominal abscesses, with the added benefit of potentially identifying the primary disease process leading to abscess formation, such as appendicitis or diverticulitis. CT is superior to ultrasonography in making visible pelvic abscesses or several abscesses. CT findings of abscess include a well-defined fluid collection with a peripheral enhancing rim ("rind sign"), displacement of surrounding organs, and extraluminal air (Figs. 264.4 and 264.5).

When it is target directed, ultrasonography is useful in imaging intraperitoneal abscesses. Ultrasonography is less sensitive than CT, however, when used as a survey test and has a higher incidence of false-positive results. Saini and colleagues found no benefit from combined CT and ultrasonography when compared with CT alone in diagnosing intra-abdominal abscesses; they recommend CT as the sole imaging study whenever feasible.

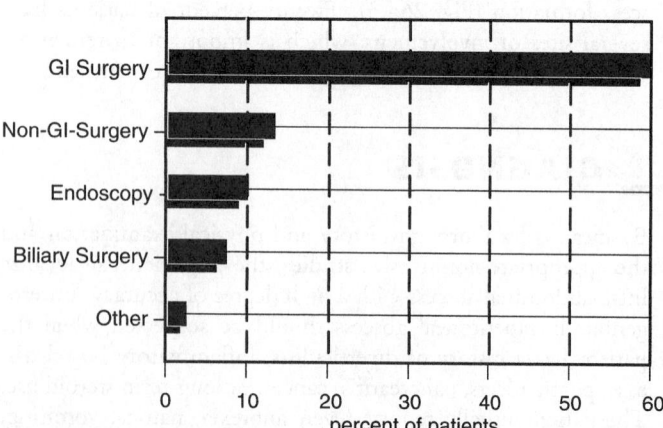

FIGURE 264.2. Origin of intra-abdominal abscess arising as a complication of surgical procedures. (From Saini S, Kellum JM, O'Leary MP, et al. Improved localization and survival in patients with intra-abdominal abscesses. *Am J Surg* 1983;145:136–142, with permission.)

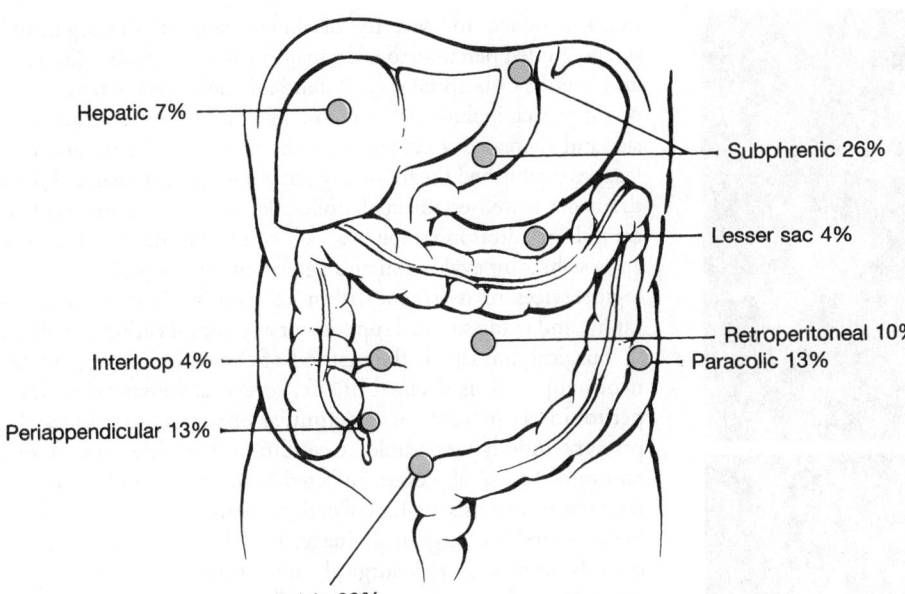

Hepatic 7%

Subphrenic 26%

Lesser sac 4%

Retroperitoneal 10%
Paracolic 13%

Interloop 4%

Periappendicular 13%

Pelvic 20%

FIGURE 264.3. Distribution of 130 abscesses in 100 patients (3% were in other locations) (From Saini S, Kellum JM, O'Leary MP, et al. Improved localization and survival in patients with intra-abdominal abscesses. *Am J Surg* 1983;145:136–142, with permission.)

Intraluminal gas, subcutaneous fat, and postoperative inflammation pose limitations to the use of ultrasonography. Nevertheless, with reported sensitivities greater than 82%, portability of equipment, and lack of radiation exposure, ultrasonography does have clinical utility, especially in pregnant patients and in patients too critically ill to be transported to a CT scanner.

Several radionuclides have been used to image intra-abdominal abscesses with some success. Both gallium 67 and indium 111 bind to leukocytes, localizing inflammation and abscesses as areas of focal uptake on scanning images. The great disadvantage of radioisotope scans is the high false-positive rates that occur because of localization of isotope in normal bowel, liver, and kidneys as well as in recent surgical sites and in neoplasms. On the other hand, a negative study result usually rules out significant intra-abdominal sepsis. With more rapid, accurate

diagnosis using CT and ultrasonography, radionuclide localization of intra-abdominal abscesses is not routinely performed today.

TREATMENT

Drainage of the infected fluid collection is the definitive step in treatment of an intra-abdominal abscess, but initial resuscitation with intravenous fluids and antimicrobial therapy must first be instituted without delay. Before the widespread use of CT and ultrasound technology, surgical drainage was the sole treatment of intra-abdominal abscesses. Since the mid-1970s, CT- or ultrasound-guided percutaneous drainage has been preferred to operative therapy in selected patients (Figs. 264.4 and 264.5). Pa-

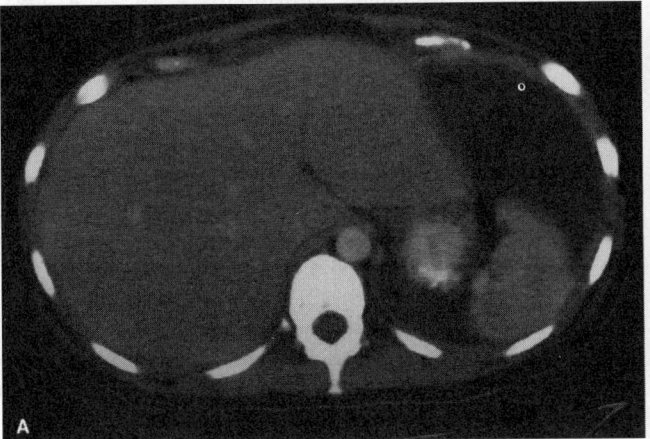
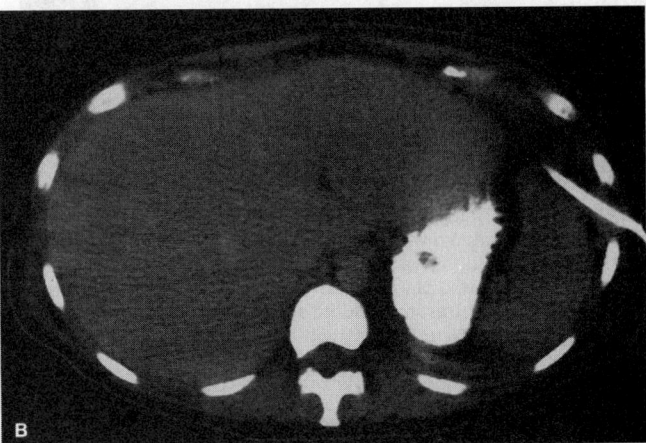

FIGURE 264.4. **A:** Computed tomographic (CT) scan of a 52-year-old woman, showing a large left subphrenic abscess caused by a perforated gastric ulcer. Note the extraluminal air within the fluid-filled abscess cavity. **B:** Follow-up CT scan 72 hours after CT-guided placement of a percutaneous drainage catheter into the left subphrenic abscess. The catheter is in a good position, and the abscess is almost completely resolved.

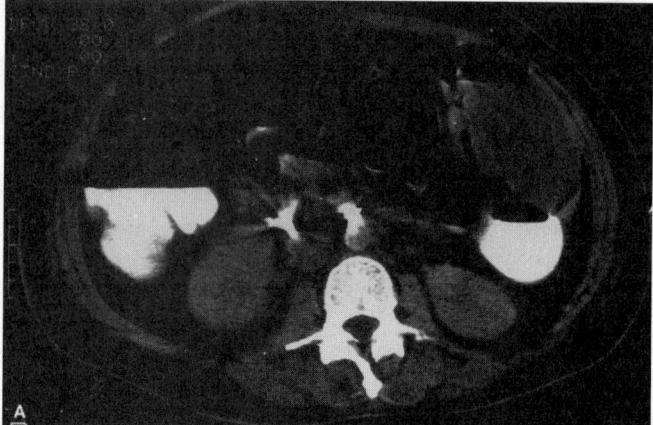

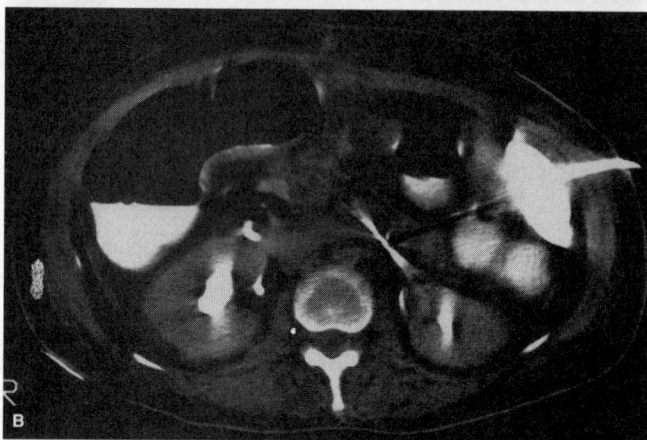

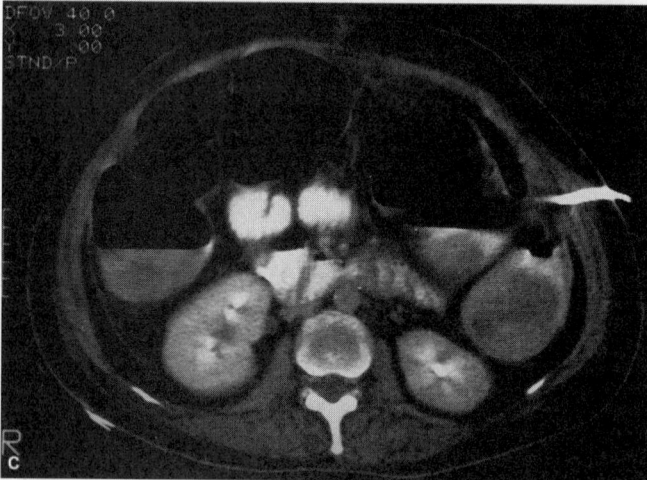

FIGURE 264.5. **A:** Computed tomographic (CT) scan of a 68-year-old woman with perforated diverticulitis, showing a left pelvic abscess. The abscess is well defined, with an enhancing rim, or "rind sign." **B:** Thirty-six hours after CT-guided placement of a drainage catheter, the catheter is injected with contrast to evaluate accurately the abscess response to drainage. With a 50% reduction in abscess size, drainage was continued for several more days. **C:** CT scan 72 hours after drain placement shows complete resolution of the left pelvic abscess.

tients matched for severity of illness, surgical drainage, and image-guided percutaneous drainage have similar mortality rates and lengths of hospital stay. Potential benefits of the percutaneous approach include reduced cost, avoidance of general anesthesia, and increased acceptance by the patient. Johnson and colleagues established the following criteria for percutaneous abscess drainage: a well-established unilocular fluid collection evident on CT or ultrasonography, a safe route for the percutaneous approach, joint evaluation and agreement by surgical and radiologic services, reassessment within 72 hours by CT or ultrasonography, and ready surgical support for any complication or failure.

Surgical drainage is the method of choice when the percutaneous approach is deemed unsafe, several abscesses exist, frank peritonitis is present, or a definitive operation to correct the primary underlying pathologic condition is feasible. The viscous nature of fungal abscesses, infected hematomas, and concomitant tissue necrosis make collections with these characteristics better suited for surgical drainage. Initial drainage is more frequently successful with surgical intervention, especially in centers where routine percutaneous abscess drainage is not performed.

Percutaneous and surgical abscess drainage can lead to similar complications, including fistulas, sepsis, bleeding, and recurrent abscesses. Olak found a 48% incidence of fistula formation associated with percutaneous drainage catheter placement, compared with 18.5% in the surgical group. Johnson and colleagues reported a 4% complication rate for percutaneous drainage and a 16% rate of complication for surgical drainage, mostly related to erosion caused by the indwelling catheter.

MANAGEMENT OF SPECIFIC ABSCESSES

PANCREATIC ABSCESS

At onset pancreatitis is a noninfectious, inflammatory process. Infection is the result of translocation of bacteria across ischemic bowel and secondary hematogenous or lymphatic spread of pathogens to pancreatic pseudocysts or to necrotic pancreatic parenchyma, with ultimate formation of a pancreatic abscess. The additional burden of a pancreatic abscess in a patient with fulminant pancreatitis can be devastating, as reflected in reported mortality rates of 14% to 57%. Malangoni and colleagues have found CT to be the most sensitive diagnostic test for pancreatic abscess; findings of peripancreatic fluid collections and gas in the area of the pancreatic bed are predictive of the presence of a pancreatic abscess. Use of CT-guided diagnosis, broad-spectrum antibiotics, and early surgical debridement and drainage has led to a decline in mortality rates from 38% to 18% since 1980. Freeny and colleagues had a 91% success rate in treating pancreatic abscess with percutaneous catheter drainage under CT guidance in well-selected patients. They concluded that in those patients with pancreatic abscesses but no extensive pancreatic necrosis, percutaneous drainage is an appropriate management choice. They recommend predrainage endoscopic retrograde cholangiopancreatography in all stable patients, to further delineate abscess location before choosing between percutaneous and surgical drainage. Pancreatic abscesses that have accompanying soft-tissue necrosis require open drainage and debridement.

PERIAPPENDICEAL ABSCESS

Chronic periappendiceal abscess is a complication of acute appendicitis in 2% to 3% of cases. Whereas acute appendicitis and its complications of perforation, peritonitis, or abscess mandate appendectomy, the presence of a subacute or chronic periappendiceal abscess indicates that perforation has already occurred and has been successfully walled off. Operation for periappendiceal abscess is effective in resolving the abscess, and appendectomy can usually be accomplished provided the ruptured appendix can be located. Percutaneous drainage under CT or ultrasonography guidance in carefully selected patients has proved effective in resolving periappendiceal abscesses. Interval appendectomy can then be safely performed approximately 6 weeks later.

DIVERTICULAR ABSCESS

Abscess resulting from diverticulitis and perforation has traditionally been surgically treated. Patients with small abscesses confined to the colonic wall or mesentery can undergo a one-stage procedure to remove the diseased segment and restore bowel continuity. If more extensive infection is present, it may be necessary to undertake a two-stage procedure involving resection of the diseased colon with temporary colostomy, followed by colostomy reversal at a later operation. Large, simple diverticular abscesses previously treated with a two-stage procedure are now successfully managed by initial percutaneous drainage, followed by an elective one-stage operation. Stabile and colleagues found percutaneous drainage followed by elective single-stage surgery to be successful in 75% of patients with contained diverticular abscesses. Percutaneous drainage followed by a one-stage operation is not appropriate when percutaneous catheter output is grossly feculent, which is associated with poor outcome.

SUBPHRENIC ABSCESS

The subphrenic spaces are common sites for development of intra-abdominal abscess; 40% are located on the left side. Subphrenic abscess typically arises as a complication of gastric or biliary tract surgery, which was the source in 52% of abscesses in one series. Less common causes include pancreatitis, colon surgery, trauma, and appendicitis. The clinical picture is often subtle, and findings on plain films may be confined to the chest radiograph, which may show pleural effusion, elevated hemidiaphragm, and atelectasis, thus prompting erroneous treatment of pneumonia. Abscess drainage can be carried out surgically via the transperitoneal or extraperitoneal approach or by image-guided percutaneous placement of drainage catheters. Percutaneous drainage is successful for 85% of unilocular subphrenic abscesses that are safely accessible. Surgical drainage is advocated if several abscesses or persistent infection is present and if no safe percutaneous route exists. Although there has been improvement in mortality rates from 40% in the 1960s to 30% in the 1990s, the mortality rate from subphrenic abscess remains high, probably because of the difficulty of establishing an early diagnosis.

PELVIC ABSCESS

Symptoms of pelvic abscess may include changes in bowel function, urinary urgency, and pelvic pain. Pelvic anatomy has necessitated more unusual routes of percutaneous drainage, such as the anterior, transgluteal, transrectal, and transvaginal methods, when intervening bowel, bladder, and pelvic vasculature complicate the anterior approach. The transgluteal route accesses the pelvis via the sciatic foramen, through which the sciatic nerve and superior gluteal artery travel. Because the gluteal musculature must be traversed, this approach is associated with increased discomfort for the patient. Gazelle and colleagues, who reported successful treatment of ten patients using CT-guided transrectal drainage of pelvic abscesses, contend that the transrectal approach avoids contamination of the peritoneum or the gluteal musculature and is tolerated well by patients. VanSonnenberg and colleagues reported superior visibility and cannulation of pelvic abscesses when using transvaginal ultrasonography.

POSTOPERATIVE INTRA-ABDOMINAL ABSCESS

A postoperative abscess typically develops about 7 days after contaminated intraperitoneal surgery, but it may not be diagnosed until some time later, owing in part to postoperative pain and fever, administration of pain medications, and inflammation that prevents detection on diagnostic studies. Operation for trauma is the most common antecedent, but 10% of postoperative abscesses follow elective operations. Certain risk factors identified at initial operation increase the likelihood of postoperative intra-abdominal sepsis and abscess formation, including emergency operation for peritonitis, abdominal operation for trauma, surgical procedures performed on elderly or unstable patients, and undue delay in original diagnosis. Increased vigilance through early use of CT for suspected abscess and prompt drainage by surgical or percutaneous means may result in improved outcomes.

■ MORTALITY RATE AND RISK FACTORS

Formation of an intra-abdominal abscess can be regarded as a host defense mechanism, confining potentially overwhelming or lethal peritonitis within a fibrinous capsule. Thus, the mortality rate from peritonitis is significantly lessened when intraperitoneal infection can be contained within an abscess. Nevertheless, an untreated intra-abdominal abscess will almost always eventually lead to death. Studies before the mid-1970s reported 30% to 50% mortality rates for intra-abdominal abscess. Since then, widespread application of CT and ultrasonography has afforded earlier diagnosis by rapid, accurate localization of abscesses and has led to a major decline in mortality rates for intraperitoneal abscess. Advances in microbial transport and culture have permitted more rapid identification of pathogens, including anaerobic bacteria, and broad-spectrum, low-toxicity antimicrobial therapy is highly effective. Through early diagnosis, resuscitation, and treatment, reported mortality rates for intra-abdominal abscess have decreased by half—from 12% to 30%.

The prognosis is predicted more by host-related factors than by the type and source of infection. A large retrospective review identified the APACHE II score, the Mannheim Peritonitis Index, hypoalbuminemia, hypocholesterolemia, and preoperative organ impairment as independent predictors of death. In another study, the preoperative serum albumin level was a good predictor of surgical outcome; mortality rates increased from 1% to 29% as the preoperative serum albumin level declined from 4.6 to 2.1 g per deciliter.

ANTIMICROBIAL THERAPY

Definitive treatment for intra-abdominal abscess is drainage of the infected fluid collection, either surgically or percutaneously. Appropriate adjuvant antimicrobial therapy directed at the suspected pathogens is also important. Both monotherapy and combination regimens have been shown to be effective and should be directed at the most prevalent organisms in intra-abdominal infections: gram-negative bacilli (*E. coli, Klebsiella, Enterobacter, Proteus* species), gram-positive cocci (*Enterococcus, Staphylococcus, Streptococcus*), and obligate anaerobes (*Bacteroides* and *Clostridium*). A large review of 480 patients with secondary bacterial peritonitis evaluated patients' outcomes as a function of intraoperative culture and sensitivity data and antibiotics used. Inadequate empiric antibiotic therapy was associated with increased rates of wound infection, deep abscess formation, need for reoperation, and prolonged length of hospital stay. Thus, adjuvant treatment with appropriate antimicrobials is of the utmost importance. Duration of therapy for complicated intra-abdominal infections with abscess should be 5 to 14 days and should continue until the patient is afebrile for 24°, the white blood count is less than 12.5, and bowel function has returned.

SUMMARY

Intra-abdominal abscess represents a broad spectrum of disease processes and locations. Early recognition based on clinical suspicion and imaging studies facilitates prompt treatment. Regardless of the underlying source or location of the abscess, antimicrobial therapy in conjunction with timely drainage constitute the essentials of management. Image-guided percutaneous drainage is often as effective as surgical evacuation in stable patients whose abscesses are well localized and accessible by the percutaneous route. Intra-abdominal abscess continues to be associated with significant morbidity and mortality but has declined by about half because of imaging technology and effective antimicrobials.

BIBLIOGRAPHY

Bohnen JMA, Solomkin JS, Dellinger P, et al. Guidelines for clinical care: anti-infective agents for intra-abdominal infection. A Surgical Infection Society Policy Statement. *Arch Surg* 1992;127:83–89.

Chang D, Wilson SE. Meta-analysis of the clinical outcome of carbapenem therapy in the adjunctive treatment of intra-abdominal infections. *Am J Surg* 1997;174:284–290.

Gibbs J, Cull W, Khuri S, et al. Serum albumin as a predictor of surgical mortality and morbidity: results from the National VA Surgical Risk Study. *Arch Surg* 1999;134:36–42.

Mclean KL, Sheehan GJ, Harding GKM. Intraabdominal infection: a review. *Clin Infect Dis* 1994;19:100–116.

Mosdell DM, Morris DM, Voltura A, et al. Antibiotic treatment for surgical peritonitis. *Ann Surg* 1991;214:543–549.

Pacelli F, Doglietto GB, Alfieri S, et al. Prognosis in intra-abdominal infections: a multivariate analysis. *Arch Surg* 1996;131:641–645.

Saini S, Kellum JM, O'Leary MP, et al. Improved localization and survival in patients with intra-abdominal abscesses. *Am J Surg* 1983;145:136–142.

Solomkin JS, Hemsell DL, Sweet R, et al. General guidelines for the evaluation of new anti-infective drugs for the treatment of intra-abdominal and pelvic infections. *Clin Infect Dis* 1992;15:S33–S42.

Wilson SE, Nord C. Clinical trials of extended spectrum penicillin/beta-lactamase inhibitors in the treatment of intra-abdominal infections: European and North American experience. *Am J Surg* 1995;169(suppl 5A):21S–26S.

Kelley's Textbook of Internal Medicine, fourth edition. Edited by H. David Humes. Lippincott Williams & Wilkins, Philadelphia © 2000.

CHAPTER

265

APPROACH TO THE PATIENT WITH OSTEOMYELITIS

LAYNE O. GENTRY

In the past 20 years, we have witnessed remarkable changes in the causes and antibiotic therapy of osteomyelitis. In the 1970s, most cases of osteomyelitis were caused by susceptible strains of *Staphylococcus aureus* and were cured with surgical debridement and a 4- to 6-week course of parenteral therapy with a β-lactamase-resistant penicillin, such as methicillin. In the 1990s, gramnegative organisms, frequently from nosocomial sources, often have been found, especially in cases of posttraumatic osteomyelitis. Polymicrobial infections are also common. In addition, coagulase-negative staphylococci, once considered saprophytic contaminants in bone, are now identified as virulent, persistent pathogens that require aggressive surgical debridement and parenteral therapy. Because many of these staphylococcal strains are resistant to methicillin, vancomycin may be the only effective antibiotic available to treat these infections. Furthermore, in the past, most cases of osteomyelitis were associated with severe bone trauma; the increase in the number of total joint replacements, however, has made osteomyelitis a dreaded complication of elective placement of orthopedic prostheses. These changes in causes and epidemiologic characteristics, combined with the introduction of safer and more effective antimicrobial agents, require us to reexamine the traditional treatment of patients with osteomyelitis.

CLASSIFICATION

Osteomyelitis, defined as inflammation of the bone marrow, the surrounding cortical bone, and the periosteum, has been

TABLE 265.1.	CIERNY AND MADER CLASSIFICATION SYSTEM FOR OSTEOMYELITIS

Anatomic Type	Description
I Simple	Medullary osteomyelitis
II Superficial	Superficial osteomyelitis
III Localized	Local osteomyelitis
IV Diffuse	Diffuse osteomyelitis
Physiologic class	
A	Normal immune response in host
B	Systemic compromise (Bs)
	Local compromise (Bl)
C	Minimal disability, treatment worse than disease; not a surgical candidate

(From Levine SE, Esterhai JL, Heppenstall RB, et al. Diagnosis and staging: osteomyelitis and prosthetic joint infections. *Clin Orthop Rel Res* 1993; 295:77, with permission.)

classified on the basis of pathogenesis, duration of disease, extent or type of bone involvement, anatomy of bone infection, and host characteristics. In the pathogenesis scheme, most infections either are hematogenous (predominantly in children) or result from spread from a contiguous focus of infection. The latter type of infection usually results from direct infection of the bone from an external source, such as surgery or open fracture, or from the progressive and continuous spread of infection from an adjacent focus, such as a soft-tissue abscess, a septic joint, or a bursa.

Many methodologies have been used to differentiate acute and chronic osteomyelitis. At our institution, we use a simple definition to distinguish the two. Acute osteomyelitis is defined as the first clinical episode, complete with the signs, symptoms, and radiographic, histologic, and microbiologic confirmation of bone infection. Chronic osteomyelitis is the diagnosis for all bone infections, based on these same criteria, that have failed one or more treatment attempts. Cierny and Mader have proposed a universal clinical staging system based on four anatomic types of bone infection and three physiologic conditions, where the clinical stage is defined by the combination of type and class (Table 265.1). This system permits the development of comprehensive treatment guidelines for each stage and allows for comparison of patients from different institutions.

PATHOPHYSIOLOGY

Pathogens gain access to bone in three ways: by hematogenous dissemination, by direct inoculation, or by extension from contiguous sites. Bone infections in children and in intravenous drug users are usually hematogenous and not associated with open fractures or a significant injury. In contrast, direct inoculation of microbes at the site of fracture or injury is a common initiating event in osteomyelitis in adults. Direct inoculation may also occur after human bites and orthopedic surgery. Finally, osteomyelitis extending from contiguous infected sites is

often seen in diabetic patients with foot infections or in patients with decubitus ulcers.

Regardless of the route of entry, the initial bone infection causes inflammation, vascular compromise, local hypoxia, and eventually the death of bone tissue. Infection may result in the formation of avascular tissue, or bone sequestrum, which forms a nidus for persistent infection and often prevents effective penetration of antibiotic into the area. If the periosteum is involved, soft tissue usually becomes infected, and localized abscesses result in a sinus tract that drains fluid and necrotic tissue from the deep focus of infection.

ETIOLOGY

S. aureus is the most common infecting organism causing hematogenous osteomyelitis in children and intravenous drug users. Other organisms that cause hematogenous osteomyelitis include gram-negative bacilli, coagulase-negative staphylococci, and pneumococci. In newborns, group B streptococci and gram-negative bacilli are common. The incidence of *Haemophilus influenzae* type B has declined as a result of *H. influenzae* vaccination.

In adults, the most common pathogens causing osteomyelitis are listed in Table 265.2. As in children, *S. aureus* is the most common single pathogen in adults, accounting for 50% to 70% of cases of osteomyelitis. The number of infections with gram-negative bacilli, either as a single infectious agent or as part of a polymicrobial infection, has increased recently; these organisms have been cultured in up to 50% of infections in some studies. Gram-negative pathogens are more likely to cause osteomyelitis in patients with open fractures and a history of prolonged hospitalization, in patients who have undergone several hospital procedures, and in those who have had a prolonged stay in the

TABLE 265.2.	COMMON PATHOGENS CAUSING OSTEOMYELITIS IN ADULTS[a]

Posttraumatic osteomyelitis
  Staphylococcus aureus
  Staphylococcus epidermidis
  Gram-negative bacilli
  Mixed infections
  Anaerobes
  Mycobacterium species
Postsurgical osteomyelitis
  Staphylococcus epidermidis
  Staphylococcus aureus
  Enterococcus faecalis
  Nosocomial gram-negative bacilli
  Mixed infections
  Candida species
Prosthetic joint infections
  Staphylococcus epidermidis
  Staphylococcus aureus
  Enterococcus faecalis

[a] Pathogens are listed in order of frequency of occurrence.

intensive care unit. Nosocomial gram-negative bacilli are a problem in osteomyelitis stemming from postsurgical wounds.

Osteomyelitis caused by methicillin-resistant *Staphylococcus epidermidis* and *S. aureus* is a growing concern. Infection with *S. epidermidis* is common after implantation of an orthopedic prosthesis. At our institution it is the most common cause of poststernotomy osteomyelitis in cardiovascular patients because of persistent infection around wired sutures of the sternal bone. Anaerobic bacteria should be considered when infection follows a human bite or is contiguous to a dental, intra-abdominal, foot, or ear-nose-throat infection. Polymicrobial aerobic and anaerobic infections are common in diabetic patients and in patients with decubitus ulcers.

HISTORY AND PHYSICAL EXAMINATION

A thorough history and physical examination are essential for diagnosing osteomyelitis. Most patients are adults who often have localized pain unresponsive to nonsteroidal drugs, heat, or rest. Swelling and redness may also be present at the site. Patients with vertebral osteomyelitis often have back pain; however, patients with infection of the larger cortical bones or patients with peripheral neuropathy, such as those with severe diabetes, may not experience pain. The extremity involved should be examined for local signs of venous stasis, acrocyanosis, edema, draining sinus tracts, erythema, induration, tenderness, range of motion, and sensory perception.

Children with osteomyelitis may have similar initial symptoms, but drainage is not usually present. Typical clinical findings in a child with hematogenous osteomyelitis include tenderness over the involved bone and decreased range of motion. The long bones, such as the femoral and tibial metaphyses, are typically involved. Systemic sepsis and fever may be present. Often, children with osteomyelitis have an associated infection; therefore, the history and physical examination should focus on evidence of both osteomyelitis and another focus of infection.

DIAGNOSIS

Diagnosis of osteomyelitis calls for a combination of clinical awareness, appropriate laboratory tests, and radiographic and radionuclide scanning studies. Diagnosis should be confirmed by histologic examination and microbiologic culture of bone specimens obtained either by surgery or percutaneous needle biopsy. Laboratory examinations should include a complete blood cell count with differential, erythrocyte sedimentation rate (ESR), urinalysis, and serum chemistries, including albumin and total protein. Although they are important in assessing health status, none of these tests specifically indicates the diagnosis of osteomyelitis. The white blood cell count is usually elevated only in the early stages of osteomyelitis. The ESR is usually elevated, but this finding is nonspecific and the ESR often returns to normal levels with successful therapy. The ESR is less reliable in newborns and in children with sickle cell anemia. In the early stages of osteomyelitis, specific findings on conventional radiography may be absent, since radiographic changes do not

manifest for at least 2 weeks. Within 4 weeks of infection, one or more of the following radiographic changes should be evident: periosteal elevation, lytic bone destruction, sclerosis, or the presence of sequestrum or overlying soft-tissue mass.

Computed tomography (CT) is a useful adjunct to conventional radiography in selected patients. CT studies have been effective in determining early periosteal proliferation in soft-tissue extension in patients who may have early injury or postoperative infection of bone and in whom conventional radiographic examination shows normal results. CT reliably detects destruction of cortical bone and the presence of sequestra. In addition, CT is helpful in evaluating bones, such as the spine, that are difficult to view.

Magnetic resonance imaging (MRI) is a highly sensitive tool for detecting and assessing the extent of infection of the musculoskeletal system. In addition to its sensitivity in detecting early infection, MRI has excellent specificity, especially in distinguishing bone tumor or infarction from osteomyelitis. The expense of this technique, however, precludes its use on a routine basis. Nevertheless, MRI is the technique of choice for detecting and assessing the site and extent of infection in the spine. In addition, MRI is the favored technique for staging the extent of infection in long cortical bones before definitive open debridement.

Bone scanning using technetium Tc 99m sulfur colloid, a readily available tool for radionuclide imaging, has excellent sensitivity for the diagnosis of osteomyelitis, especially within the first 2 weeks, but the specificity is relatively low. There may be false-positive results in patients with tumors or infarction or in patients with bone injury affecting the periosteum. Another disadvantage is that bone scan results remain positive for 6 weeks to 6 months after noninfectious bone injury or surgery.

In an attempt to increase the specificity of radionuclide imaging, gallium citrate Ga 67 scanning was introduced to detect osteomyelitis. Because the radiotracer binds to proteins associated with inflammation and infection, gallium uptake is nonspecific for infection. Thus, the specificity of this technique was enhanced by the combined interpretation of gallium and bone scans. Although initial results were promising, the accuracy rate of sequential scanning has approached only 70%. Advanced infections are more reliably detected with this method because of the increased numbers of white blood cells, whereas the number of white blood cells may be too few to detect in early stages of infection.

Indium In 111 altumomab pentetate white blood cell scanning, in which in vitro–labeled white blood cells are injected and imaging is performed 24 to 48 hours later, has been used to diagnose osteomyelitis. This technique may be useful in complicated cases or as an adjunct for detecting infections associated with orthopedic prostheses. The specificity of white blood cell scanning is higher than that of gallium imaging, and the sensitivity is moderate, even in the first 2 weeks. False-positive results may be seen in patients with infarction. The disadvantages of this technique include time- consuming ex vivo blood-handling techniques, special training of personnel, and the need for a large quantity of blood. In addition, white blood cell scanning is expensive. Immunoscintigraphy with technetium-99m-labeled monoclonal antigranulocyte antibodies (AGAb) has been used to image osteomyelitis; the sensitivity, specificity, and diagnostic accuracy compare favorably to those of white blood cell scanning. In a recent study, positron emission tomography with 2-18F-fluoro-2-deoxy-D-glucose was comparable to combined 99m-technetium-AGAb/99m-technetium-MDP in diagnosing chronic osteomyelitis in the peripheral skeleton and superior to AGAb imaging in the central skeleton.

There has been much debate on the diagnostic accuracy of specimens obtained for culture from various sites of infection and with various techniques. The gold standard for diagnosis of osteomyelitis is aerobic and anaerobic culture of a biopsy specimen taken under direct vision during surgery. Alternatively, at our center, culture of several specimens obtained by needle biopsy with a bone biopsy needle under fluoroscopic or CT guidance has been the most reliable, cost-effective means of diagnosing osteomyelitis. Combining surgical debridement and removal of sequestra with culture specimen acquisition is even more cost-effective. Specimens for culture should be obtained before beginning antibiotic therapy or at least 96 hours after ending therapy.

Blood cultures may show positive results during the acute phase of the disease, when bacteremia is present, and results usually indicate the etiologic agent in these cases. Bacteremia is rare in adults. Swab cultures of sinus tracts are not usually accurate because organisms not present in the bone may colonize the sinus tract. However, swab cultures may be more accurate in the diagnosis of osteomyelitis caused by a single pathogen than in osteomyelitis caused by several pathogens. In fact, some investigators have suggested that a presumptive diagnosis of *S. aureus* osteomyelitis may be justified when this organism is grown from culture of material from a sinus tract. At our center, however, experience has shown there is no substitute for a biopsy specimen.

OPTIMAL MANAGEMENT

Treatment of either acute or chronic osteomyelitis requires prolonged antibiotic therapy and complete surgical debridement of necrotic bone and soft tissue where there is evidence of residual sequestrum or foreign material. Even with appropriate therapy, relapses may occur. Broader-spectrum agents are frequently necessary for treatment of chronic osteomyelitis because polymicrobial infection is more common in such cases. These agents must be able to penetrate bone and must have limited toxicity over the course of administration.

The most effective strategy for the patient with osteomyelitis is the institution of appropriate antimicrobial therapy (Table 265.3) based on culture and sensitivity results, after complete surgical debridement of necrotic bone and soft tissue and after confirmation of the microbiologic diagnosis by biopsy. Typically, therapy fails if this routine is not strictly followed, regardless of the antimicrobial regimen. Empiric therapy for suspected organisms or for those grown from a sinus tract culture, however, may be necessary if the patient is acutely ill.

The type of surgical therapy depends on the extent of infection. In true cases of acute osteomyelitis, especially in children, antibiotic therapy alone may be sufficient. In most cases, however, complete surgical debridement is of paramount importance. Sequestered dead bone may serve as a focus for persistent infection. In our experience, inadequate surgical debridement is

the most common cause of treatment failure. Removal of foreign bodies is essential for successful treatment. If the bone is unstable after debridement, external fixation devices may be necessary. If the remaining bone is inadequate and debridement is extensive, reconstructive surgery with bone grafts and muscle flaps may be required. In cases of unrelenting osteomyelitis, amputation must be considered.

Although the cornerstone of therapy for osteomyelitis has been the intravenous administration of antibiotics through an indwelling catheter for 4 to 6 weeks, the oral fluoroquinolones, which are relatively nontoxic and are active against many of the typical pathogens that cause osteomyelitis, may be effective when susceptible organisms are isolated. Ciprofloxacin, the most actively studied fluoroquinolone, has been approved by the Federal Drug Administration as monotherapy for osteomyelitis. Particularly active against gram-negative pathogens, oral ciprofloxacin should be the antibiotic of choice when treating osteomyelitis caused by Enterobacteriaceae. Reports of resistance in some strains of *S. aureus* and *S. epidermidis* raise justifiable concerns about the use of ciprofloxacin in treating staphylococcal osteomyelitis. Recent studies have suggested that ofloxacin and lomefloxacin may be effective in treating osteomyelitis; however, neither agent has been approved for use in osteomyelitis. The combined administration of quinolones or fusidic acid and rifampin for prosthesis-related infections is promising.

In addition to the obvious economic benefits of reducing pharmacy and supply costs, the use of oral antibiotics eliminates the need for surgical insertion of a catheter and decreases catheter-associated complications. In children with acute hematogenous osteomyelitis, short-term parenteral therapy followed by long-term oral therapy is successful. Sequential intravenous–oral antibiotic therapy usually involves about 2 weeks of intravenous treatment followed by 3 to 6 weeks of oral treatment.

If parenteral therapy is necessary, outpatient home health nursing services can administer antibiotics at a significant savings over inpatient stays. In these cases, patients should be educated in the care, use, and administration of antibiotics via the catheter while they are still in the hospital. Outpatient care should include laboratory tests performed at 7- to 10-day intervals; a reduction in the ESR may be the only early indicator of improvement. Radiographs or radionuclide scans need to be performed only at the 4- to 6-month follow-up examination.

Newer, more powerful agents for treating serious gram-positive infections, including those resistant to methicillin, are under study. Teicoplanin, a glycopeptide, has been efficacious in treating osteomyelitis caused by resistant gram-positive organisms; however, teicoplanin has not been approved for any indication. In addition to the introduction of new antibiotics, novel approaches to medical therapy also have become available. Home intravenous therapy programs with belt-mounted, computer-controlled pumps for the intravenous delivery of antibiotics shorten hospital stays. In addition, this method allows the patient to resume daily activities during the long therapy period. Local antimicrobial therapy with antibiotic-impregnated acrylic beads has been effective in sterilizing local areas of infection. Used in open fracture wounds and in the management of dead space in resection of infected joint implants, antibiotic-impregnated beads may lessen some of the untoward side effects associ-

TABLE 265.3.   **ANTIMICROBIAL THERAPY FOR OSTEOMYELITIS IN ADULTS**

Organism	Therapy of Choice (Adult Dosage)
Gram-positive	
Staphylococcus aureus (methicillin susceptible)	β-lactamase-resistant penicillin Nafcillin (2 g i.v. q 6 hr) Oxacillin (2 g i.v. q 6 hr) or First-generation cephalosporin[a] Cefazolin (2 g i.v. q 8 hr) or Ciprofloxacin (750 mg p.o. q 12 hr)[b]
Staphylococcus aureus (methicillin resistant) or coagulase-negative *Staphylococcus*	Vancomycin (1 g i.v. q 12 hr)[c]
Streptococcus species	Ampicillin (2 g i.v. q 6 hr)
Enterococcus species	Ampicillin (2 g i.v. q 6 hr) + gentamicin (1 mg/kg q 8 hr)[d]
Gram-negative	
Pseudomonas aeruginosa	Third-generation cephalosporin Ceftazidime (2 g i.v. q 12 hr) Ceftriaxopne (2 g i.v. q 24 hr) or Ciprofloxacin (750 mg p.o. q 12 hr) or Semisynthetic penicillin[e] Piperacillin (3 g i.v. q 6 hr) Mezlocillin (3 g i.v. q 6 hr) and Aminoglycoside[e] Amikacin (15 mg/kg/d) Gentamicin or tobramycin (5 mg/kg/d)
Enterobacteriaceae and other gram-negative organisms	Ciprofloxacin (750 mg p.o. q 12 hr) or β-lactamase inhibitor Ticarcillin-clavulanic acid (3.1 g i.v. q 6 hr)[f] Imipenem-cilastatin (1 g i.v. q 6 hr)
Anaerobes	Clindamycin (0.9 g i.v. q 8 hr)[c] Metronidazole (0.5 g i.v. q 8 hr)

[a] Possible cross-reaction in penicillin-hypersensitive patients.
[b] Questionable efficacy of *Staphylococcus aureus* and rapid emergence of resistance are concerns.
[c] Possible combination with rifampin.
[d] Use combination for the first 2 weeks, followed by ampicillin alone.
[e] Use semisynthetic penicillin in combination with aminoglycoside
[f] Effective in mixed infections.
[g] Also active against staphylococci.

ated with the intravenous use of certain antibiotics, such as the aminoglycosides. Although antibiotic beads are not approved as a therapeutic treatment, orthopedic services often use homemade gentamicin beads. Japanese investigators have used porous pieces of calcium hydroxyapatite impregnated with antibiotics to treat patients with chronic osteomyelitis successfully.

SPECIAL CIRCUMSTANCES

PATIENTS WITH DIABETES MELLITUS

Osteomyelitis of the foot, common in patients with diabetes, often arises from extension of an infected soft-tissue ulceration. Bacteremia is rare in these patients. The infection, often polymicrobial, may include such pathogens as staphylococci, enterococci, anaerobes, and gram-negative bacilli and can be complicated by impaired wound healing and immune responses. Distinguishing bone infection from noninfectious neuropathic bony lesions is a diagnostic challenge. The most useful diagnostic tests in diabetic patients are the indium In 111–labeled leukocyte scan and MRI. In our center, the presence of diabetes does not affect outcome in patients with acute osteomyelitis; however, in patients with chronic osteomyelitis, diabetes significantly reduces long-term success rates for antimicrobial and surgical therapy (Table 265.4).

IMMUNOCOMPROMISED PATIENTS

The number of cases of osteomyelitis caused by unusual pathogens, such as fungi and mycobacteria, is increasing because of the rise in prevalence of immunocompromised patients. For fungal osteomyelitis, newer agents, such as fluconazole and itraconzol, should provide successful treatment with less toxicity than amphotericin B; however, these agents have not been approved for this indication. The resurgence in the incidence of tuberculosis has been accompanied by the development of resistant organisms. The most common skeletal sites for tuberculous infection are the hips, sacroiliac joints, and sternocostal joints. Tuberculous osteomyelitis, accompanied by pulmonary symptoms only half the time, may be difficult to diagnose, especially without vigilance and awareness on the part of the clinician. DNA

TABLE 265.4.	EFFECT OF DIABETES MELLITUS ON PROGNOSIS IN 124 PATIENTS WITH OSTEOMYELITIS (24-MONTH FOLLOW-UP)	
Clinical Success	Acute Osteomyelitis (%)	Chronic Osteomyelitis (%)
With diabetes	83	46
Without diabetes	84	67[a]

[a] $p < 0.01$.
(From Gentry LO. Antibiotic therapy for osteomyelitis. *Infect Dis Clin North Am* 1990;4:485, with permission.)

TABLE 265.5.	ECONOMIC SAVINGS FOR OUTPATIENT AND ORAL THERAPY IN TREATING OSTEOMYELITIS[a]
Outpatient therapy	
Inpatient room charge	
Four weeks at $250/day	$7,000
Outpatient clinic fees	
Eight visits at $60 each	480
Savings for outpatient therapy	$7,480
Oral Therapy	
Cost differential of using oral quinolone vs. third-generation cephalosporin	$1,640
Credit for four fewer clinic visits at $60 each	240
Credit for no insertion of Broviac catheter	1,500
Further savings for oral therapy	$3,380

Assume 2 weeks initial hospital stay completed and 4 additional weeks of therapy required. Prices are from St. Luke's, Episcopal Hospital Houston.
(From Gentry LO. Antibiotic therapy for osteomyelitis. *Infect. Dis Clin North Am* 1990;4:485, with permission.)

probes, when used as a complementary tool to culture, may enhance the laboratory's chances of identifying the organism.

In AIDS patients with osteomyelitis, suppressed clinical manifestations and compromised host defenses may result in dramatic and unusual radiographic findings. Usually, these infections are detected late and respond poorly to therapy. In addition, a wider array of sites and pathogens may be involved. Needle or surgical bone biopsies are essential to establishing the exact source in AIDS patients.

ECONOMIC CONSIDERATIONS

Long-term intravenous antibiotic regimens and the many surgeries associated with osteomyelitis therapy can be expensive. In this era of prospective reimbursement of providers, the goal should be to reduce health-care costs. Obviously, to hospitalize a patient with osteomyelitis who is afebrile and clinically stable for the sole purpose of administering parenteral antibiotics is not economical. Outpatient antibiotic therapy, by either clinic visits or a home health agency, can substantially minimize costs (Table 265.5). Because of the trend toward outpatient therapy, antibiotics that can be given every 8, 12, or 24 hours are preferred for treating osteomyelitis. Further economic benefits can be gained by using an orally administered agent, such as one of the fluoroquinolones.

BIBLIOGRAPHY

Boutin RD, Brossmann J, Sartoris DJ, et al. Update on imaging of orthopedic infections. *Orthop Clin North Am* 1998;29:41–66.

Gentry LO. Antibiotic therapy for osteomyelitis. *Infect Dis Clin North Am* 1990;4:485–499.

Gentry LO. Management of osteomyelitis. *Int J Antimicrob Agents* 1997; 951:37.

Gentry LO. Osteomyelitis. In: Rakel R, ed. *Conn's current therapy*. Philadelphia: WB Saunders, 1998.

Karwowska A, Davies HD, Jadavji T. Epidemiology and outcome of osteo-myelitis in the era of sequential intravenous–oral therapy. *Pediatr Infect Dis J* 1998;17:1021–1026.

Levine SE, Esterhai JL, Heppenstall B, et al. Diagnoses and staging: osteo-myelitis and prosthetic joint infections. *Clin Orthop Rel Res* 1993;295: 77–86.

Lew DP, Waldvogel FA. Osteomyelitis. *New Engl J Med* 1997;336: 999–1007.

Lipsky BA. Osteomyelitis of the foot in diabetic patients. *Clin Infect Dis* 1997;25:1318–1326.

Mader JT, Shertliff M, Calhoun JH. Staging and staging application in osteomyelitis. *Clin Infect Dis* 1997;25:1303–1309.

Magid D, Fishman EK. Musculoskeletal infections in patients with AIDS: CT findings. *Am J Roentgenol* 1992;158:603–607.

Rissing JP. Antimicrobial therapy for chronic osteomyelitis in adults: role of the quinolones. *Clin Infect Dis* 1997;25:1327–1333.

Tice AD. Outpatient parenteral administration of antimicrobial therapy for osteomyelitis. *Infect Dis Clin North Am* 1998;12:903–919.

Kelley's Textbook of Internal Medicine, fourth edition. Edited by H. David Humes. Lippincott Williams & Wilkins, Philadelphia © 2000.

CHAPTER
266

APPROACH TO THE FEBRILE PATIENT

PHILIP A. MACKOWIAK

NORMAL BODY TEMPERATURE

Although fever is a complex physiologic process involving numerous metabolic and immunologic reactions, it is recognized and characterized clinically predominantly by its thermal qualities. Implicit in such characterizations is the concept that the temperature of higher animals is tightly controlled within a narrow, species-specific range during the disease-free state. In healthy, young, human adults, this oral temperature range extends from 36.5°C (96°F) to 37.7°C (99.9°F).

Body temperature has a circadian rhythm, reaching its apogee during the evening and its nadir during the early morning. The circadian temperature rhythm is established during the first months after birth and retained throughout life. For as yet unclear reasons, children display exaggerated diurnal swings in temperature. Additional variability in the normal temperature may be seen as a result of transient elevations in temperature in response to meals, ovulation, or strenuous exertion. Generally, core temperature continues to exhibit diurnal variability during fever, although the median daily temperature is higher. Furthermore, circadian variations in temperature persist even during the course of such infections as bacterial endocarditis, in which levels of circulating exogenous pyrogens (i.e., bacteria) are constant throughout the day.

Clinicians typically regard temperature readings obtained at various anatomic sites as equivalent approximations of "body temperature," ignoring the fact that no one temperature provides a complete picture of the thermal status of the human body. This is because body temperature is actually a pastiche of many different temperatures, each representing a particular body part. Of the three sites most commonly used to estimate core temperature, none is universally accepted as the best. The mouth is generally preferred, because it is accessible, responds promptly to changes in core temperature, and has a long tradition of use in monitoring temperature in clinical practice. Nevertheless, there is also a general perception that rectal temperature provides a better approximation of core temperature, because the rectum is better insulated from the external environment. Unfortunately, rectal measurements are inconvenient, socially awkward, and associated with a higher risk of injury and cross-infection than oral determinations.

In theory, the tympanic membrane is the ideal site for measuring core temperature, because it is perfused by a tributary of the artery that supplies the body's thermoregulatory center. Unfortunately, numerous studies of many different tympanic membrane thermometers have shown that while they are convenient to use, such instruments give highly variable readings that correlate poorly with simultaneously obtained oral or rectal measurements. Because the temperature of the rectum, mouth, and tympanic membrane are related but not identical, it would be useful to have a reliable formula for converting data obtained at one site to those from another. On average, rectal readings of healthy young adults exceed concurrent oral readings by 0.4°C (0.7°F) and tympanic membrane readings by 0.8°C (1.4°F). Considerable individual variability exists in these relationships, however, especially in frail elderly patients.

THERMOREGULATION

Core temperature in higher animals is regulated by physiologic and behavioral means. In non-fur-bearing animals, the physiologic mechanisms that distinguish homeotherms (warm-blooded animals) from poikilotherms (cold-blooded animals) are concerned primarily with regulating heat loss by altering the amount of blood brought into contact with the skin surface. When excess thermal energy must be released during the thermoregulatory process, circulation to the skin and subcutaneous tissues is increased so that heat exchange with the external environment is potentiated. Sweating increases heat loss by providing water for vaporization. In fur-bearing animals, heat exchange by evaporation from the respiratory tract is the primary physiologic mechanism for effectuating heat loss. When thermal energy must be conserved to maintain normal core temperature, circulation to surface structures is reduced. When the demand for heat is great, either because the ambient temperature is low or because internal requirements are high (e.g., during sepsis), shivering may accompany peripheral vasoconstriction as a means of augmenting heat production. In higher animals, behavioral responses (moving to warmer or cooler environments) are also important features of the thermoregulatory response.

The neural mechanisms involved in thermoregulation are only partially understood. Although the spinal cord can initiate thermoregulatory responses, the preoptic area of the hypothalamus appears to be the primary site of integration of thermal stimuli and, through its input into the autonomic nervous system, initiation of thermal homeostatic mechanisms. As such, the anterior hypothalamus is generally regarded as the control center responsible for establishing a thermal set point for the body and for coordinating physiologic and behavioral responses that bring core temperature in line with that set point. Nevertheless, at least some thermophysiologists contend that the concept of a single, central set-point temperature oversimplifies the actual process of thermoregulation. They propose instead that core temperature is regulated within its narrow range by a composite set point of several thermosensitive neural networks, each controlling its own thermoregulatory response.

PYROGENIC CYTOKINES

Exogenous pyrogens, such as bacteria, viruses, or bacterial lipopolysaccharide, do not appear to cause fever by a direct action on the hypothalamic thermoregulatory center. Indeed, most exogenous materials enter brain tissue only with difficulty (the blood–brain barrier phenomenon). Rather, the weight of available evidence favors an indirect effect of exogenous pyrogens on the hypothalamus that is mediated by endogenous pyrogens (pyrogenic cytokines) produced by phagocytic leukocytes (Fig. 266.1). The most important cytokines in this regard are interleukin-1, tumor necrosis factor α, interferon, interleukin-6, and interleukin-2.

Production of pyrogenic cytokines by phagocytes appears to involve de-repression of specific genomes. After synthesis, molecules, such as interleukin-1, are released without significant storage and appear to act in specialized vascular areas of the hypothalamus as calcium ionophores, stimulating arachidonic acid release and thereby synthesis of prostaglandin E_2. Although prostaglandin E_2 exerts a direct pyrogenic effect on the hypothalamic thermoregulatory center, it is not yet clear whether this effect is essential for the febrile response or whether endogenous pyrogens act through some other process requiring protein synthesis. Early investigations focused on the capacity of endogenous pyrogens to increase core temperature. More recently, it has become apparent that pyrogenic polypeptides, such as interleukin-1, have a wide array of biologic (Table 266.1) and immunologic activities (Table 266.2).

TABLE 266.1.	BIOLOGIC ACTIVITIES ATTRIBUTED TO ENDOGENOUS PYROGENS

Fever	Hypercupremia
Muscle proteolysis	↓ Hepatic albumin synthesis
Hypoferremia	Leukocytosis
Fibroblast proliferation	↑ Lipoprotein lipase activity
Hypozincemia	↑ Hepatic acute-phase
↑ PGE$_2$ production	proteins

PGE$_2$, prostaglandin E$_2$.

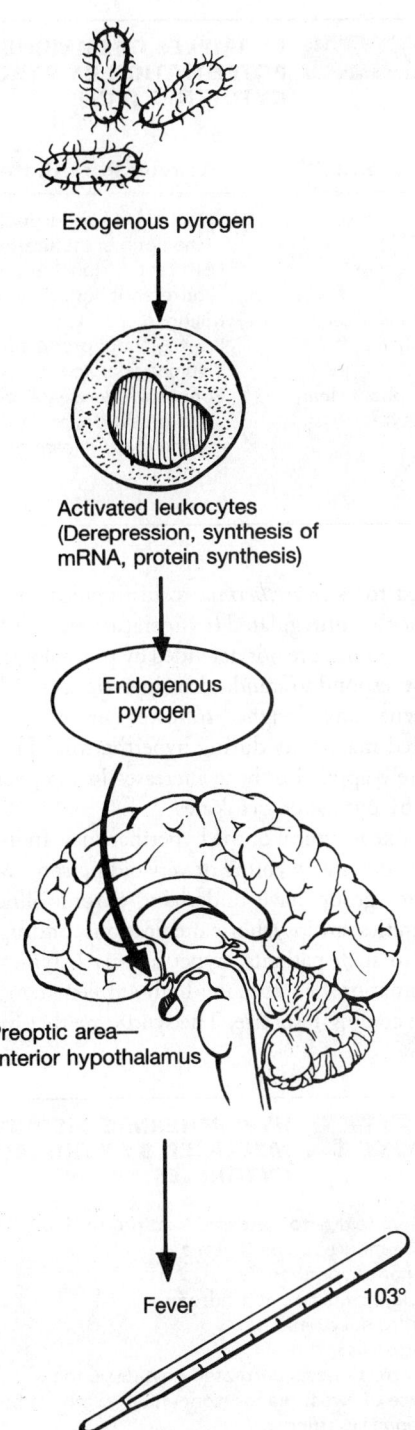

FIGURE 266.1. Postulated physiologic pathway for fever.

HYPERTHERMIA

Fever is a complex physiologic process mediated by the action of various pyrogenic cytokines on the anterior hypothalamus and characterized by a regulated rise in core temperature. There are also a number of disorders involving marked increases in core temperature, in which pyrogenic cytokines do not appear to play a major role (Table 266.3). Such increases in temperature

TABLE 266.2. EXAMPLES OF IMMUNE POTENTIATION BY PYROGENIC CYTOKINES (PCs)

Immune Cell	Activity Potentiated by PCs
T lymphocyte	Lymphokine production, chemotaxis, maturation
B lymphocyte	Maturation, clonal expansion, differentiation, chemotaxis
Natural killer cell	Killing
Macrophage	Prostaglandin production, tumoricidal activity
Polymorphonuclear leukocyte	Bone marrow release, margination, extravasation, chemotaxis, adherence, release of lysosomal enzymes

are referred to as *hyperthermia* to distinguish them from *fever*, because they are unregulated (temperature exceeds the thermoregulatory set point), are not defended by physiologic mechanisms, and do not respond to standard antipyretic agents. In fact, physiologic mechanisms designed to lower core temperature usually are activated maximally during hyperthermia. The term *fever* is appropriately applied only to increases in temperature that are mediated by pyrogenic cytokines.

Heatstroke is typical of the hyperthermias. In its classic form, heatstroke affects very young or very old persons. Many of those in the latter group have underlying chronic illnesses and are taking diuretics, antipsychotic medications, or drugs that inhibit sweating. In such patients, hyperthermia is typically the result of a combination of unusually high ambient temperatures and a defective cooling response. The syndrome that follows is characterized by a prodrome of chills and cutis anserina (goose bumps), hyperthermia, absence of sweating, and respiratory alkalosis. Lactic acidosis, if present, is not usually severe, and acute renal failure and rhabdomyolysis are either absent or mild. Confusion, delirium, seizures, and coma are common and reflect the special susceptibility of the central nervous system to hyperthermia-induced dysfunction.

The exertional form of heatstroke most commonly affects young to middle-aged men during episodes of unusually heavy exercise. Patients with exertional heatstroke are generally otherwise healthy, though many are using amphetamines at the time of the attack of heatstroke. Unlike patients with classic heatstroke, those with exertional hyperthermia rarely give histories of prodromal chills or goose bumps. They have only mild respiratory alkalosis but often have marked lactic acidosis, hypocalcemia, prominent rhabdomyolysis, and a 30% incidence of acute renal failure. Because the pathogenesis of both forms of heatstroke involves thermoregulatory failure, the core temperature can be lowered only by physical means. This may be accomplished either while briskly rubbing the body surface or by wetting body surfaces and then placing the patient in the wake of a powerful fan. The latter method is preferred by some authorities because it is less likely to cause shivering or frank seizures. In either case, vital signs should be monitored closely along with appropriate fluid and electrolyte replacement and continued until core temperature is reduced to 38.3°C (101°F).

ANTIPYRETIC THERAPY

In most clinical contexts, antipyretic drugs alone are sufficient to reduce fever. Of the many such agents available, aspirin and acetaminophen have the most extensive clinical history. Numerous studies comparing the antipyretic efficacy of these two agents have not found substantial differences. Moreover, both are probably equally effective in alleviating accompanying symptoms, such as malaise, headache, and myalgias. Neither drug lowers core temperature in the afebrile state. Thus, from a therapeutic standpoint, there is no compelling reason to choose one over the other. This decision is more often made on the basis of toxicity. Because of its adverse effects on the gastric mucosa and platelet function and its role in Reye's syndrome, aspirin should be avoided by patients with peptic ulcer disease and bleeding disorders and by children. Likewise, because of its potential for causing hepatotoxicity, acetaminophen should be avoided by patients with underlying liver disease.

During extreme pyrexia, physical methods are sometimes combined with antipyretic drugs to lower temperature. In hyperthermia, such measures may be the only therapy that is effective in lowering core temperature. When sponging is used to promote heat dissipation during fever, tepid water is preferred over ice water, because it is less likely to cause intense vasoconstriction, which acts to conserve body heat. In treating fever (as opposed to hyperthermia), lowering the hypothalamic thermal set point with antipyretic agents should be combined with physical measures to minimize physiologic reactions (shivering and peripheral vasoconstriction) that are working to maintain the elevated core temperature. Because external cooling measures

TABLE 266.3. HYPERTHERMIC DISORDERS NOT MEDIATED BY PYROGENIC CYTOKINES

Hyperthermia due to increased heat production
  Exercise-induced hyperthermia
  Malignant hyperthermia
  Neuroleptic malignant syndrome
  Pheochromocytoma
  Thyrotoxicosis
Hyperthermia due to decreased heat dissipation
  Absence of sweat glands (congenital, extensive burns)
  Autonomic dysfunction
  Dehydration
  Drug-induced (atropine)
  Heart failure (low-grade hyperthermia)
  Heatstroke (also ↑ heat production)
  Occlusive dressings
  Severe anemia (low-grade hyperthermia)
Hypothalamic disorders (rare)
  Drug-induced (phenothiazines)
  Infections (granulomas)
  Tumors
  Trauma
  Vascular accidents

have the capacity to induce coronary vasoconstriction as part of a cold pressor response, some investigators have questioned whether this form of antipyretic therapy should ever be used to treat fever (much less to treat patients hospitalized in intensive care units, for whom it is most commonly prescribed). If external cooling is used to treat fever, care must be taken to prevent shivering, which causes an increase in oxygen consumption. Unfortunately, even if shivering is prevented, there is no guarantee that a cold pressor response will be averted. Indomethacin likewise has been reported to cause coronary vasoconstriction in patients with coronary artery disease. For this reason, nonsteroidal anti-inflammatory drugs should be administered with caution to suppress fever in such patients.

FEBRILE CONVULSIONS

In experimental animals, fever has been shown to enhance survival in the context of a variety of infections. When fever is extreme, however, this beneficial effect is reversed. Although the former observation suggests that fever is a natural defense against infection and should not be suppressed pro forma, the latter observation argues for more liberal use of antipyretic therapy. Likewise, concern about febrile convulsions has led many clinicians to regard fever more as a liability than an asset in the infected patient. Approximately 3% of children experience febrile convulsions; as many as 11% of those who have febrile illnesses between the ages of 6 months and 5 years have such convulsions. Febrile seizures tend to run in families and are most often generalized. Simple febrile convulsions are characteristically brief, require no special treatment, and do not appear to cause brain damage.

Prophylactic anticonvulsant medication in general is not recommended for children with simple febrile convulsions. Epilepsy precipitated by fever, however, does require therapy with antiepileptic drugs and is distinguished from simple febrile convulsions by one or more of the following symptoms: prolonged seizures, focal convulsions of any duration, convulsions associated with fever in a child older than age 5 years, or electroencephalographic abnormalities suggestive of overt epilepsy.

FEVER OF UNKNOWN ORIGIN

Initially, all febrile illnesses are fevers of unknown origin (FUOs). To the internist, however, FUOs are an unusual and heterogeneous group of prolonged febrile disorders that elude diagnosis even after intensive investigation. Most published series of FUOs have considered only patients with temperatures above 38.3°C (more than 101°F). In general, a febrile illness is not designated a FUO unless fever is a dominant feature of the illness, has persisted for at least 2 to 3 weeks, and has defied diagnosis despite intensive investigation.

Most fevers either resolve spontaneously or are diagnosed quickly. Surprisingly, fevers that persist and defy intensive diagnostic scrutiny are more often the result of common diseases

TABLE 266.4.	CAUSES OF FEVER OF UNKNOWN ORIGIN IN 154 PEDIATRIC AND 234 ADULT PATIENTS IN FIVE PUBLISHED SERIES		
Source		**No.**	**%**
Infections		153	39
Endocarditis		18	5
Abdominal abscess		17	4
Hepatobiliary		17	4
Urinary		14	4
Mycobacterial		20	5
Brucellosis		2	1
Bone/joint		7	2
Meningitis (bacterial)		5	1
Viral		23	6
Other		30	8
Neoplastic		66	17
Lymphoma/leukemia		46	12
Carcinoma		13	2
Other		7	2
Collagen/vascular		68	18
Systemic lupus erythematosus		11	3
Rheumatoid arthritis		21	5
Other		36	9
Miscellaneous		101	26
Pulmonary emboli		6	2
Sarcoidosis		2	1
Hypersensitivity		9	2
Factitious		6	2
Other		36	9
No diagnosis		42	11

with unusual manifestations than exotic disorders (Table 266.4). Causes of FUO in children are similar to those in adults, except that in pediatric series, juvenile rheumatoid arthritis and chronic viral infections have been seen more often than in adult series. The three most common causes of the syndrome are infections (which account for more than a third of the cases reported in most series), malignant neoplasms (which account for about a fifth of such cases), and connective tissue disorders (which account for 8% of cases).

Familial Mediterranean fever is one of the few exotic diseases that must be considered in patients with FUO. This hereditary disorder is characterized by recurrent episodes of unexplained fever, frequently accompanied by peritonitis, pleuritis, or arthritis (generally monoarticular). It is a syndrome of unknown origin seen predominantly in Armenians, Sephardic Jews, and Arabs, in whom it affects males three times as often as females. Symptoms usually begin at puberty. Late complications include spontaneous abdominal adhesions and amyloidosis. During acute attacks, leukocytosis, an elevated erythrocyte sedimentation rate, and increases in various acute-phase reactants are characteristic. Laboratory test abnormalities are not seen between attacks. Long-term colchicine therapy reportedly lessens the incidence of such attacks and minimizes the likelihood of long-term complications.

The evaluation of the patient with FUO must be systematic. A detailed history and careful physical examination are its cornerstones. The epidemiologic history is especially important;

knowledge of communicable diseases among contacts, recent travel, animal exposure, food consumption, and occupation may provide important insight into the origin of the illness. When conducting the physical examination, close attention must be paid to the funduscopic findings (which may show choroid tubercles suggestive of miliary tuberculosis), the less prominent chains of lymph nodes (such as those along the inner aspect of the iliac crest), and the prostate, epididymis, and testicles (which may exhibit abnormalities signifying the presence of a prostate abscess, extrapulmonary tuberculosis or polyarteritis nodosa).

Laboratory evaluation must also be undertaken in a methodical fashion. Initial studies should include a complete blood count; urinalysis; biochemical tests; serologic studies for fungal infections and for connective tissue disorders; examination of the stool for the presence of occult blood; bacterial cultures of urine, sputum, and blood; testing of thyroid function; chest radiography; electrocardiography, and lumbar puncture. A tuberculin skin test should also be carried out.

The source of abnormalities detected in one or more of the initial studies should be pursued with more specific investigations. If these tests do not give conclusive results, empiric examinations, such as oral cholecystography and gastrointestinal endoscopy, should be considered. Biopsy of the liver, bone marrow, or skin may be indicated for some patients. Computed tomography scans of the brain, chest, and abdomen also may be helpful in such evaluations. Occasionally, lymphangiography or gallium scintigraphy identifies important abnormalities not apparent in other examinations. If these studies fail to yield a diagnosis, the physician has three options. The entire evaluation may be repeated in anticipation of the development of abnormalities on tests that previously showed normal results; a therapeutic trial directed against a probable but unproved diagnosis (e.g., a therapeutic trial of isoniazid and rifampin for suspected occult tuberculosis) may be initiated; or the patient may be observed for new signs or symptoms meriting further assessment.

DRUG FEVER

Many drugs—perhaps all—have the capacity to induce fever as an adverse reaction. Such fever may be the result of a pharmacologic effect of the drug, an idiosyncratic reaction, or a complication related to drug administration (phlebitis, chemical meningitis, sterile abscess). If fevers due to complications of drug administration are excluded, it is apparent that certain drugs, such as α-methyldopa, quinidine, and the penicillins, are more likely causes of the disorder than others, such as the aminoglycoside antibiotics and cardiac glycosides (Table 266.5). Although the list of drugs capable of inducing fever is long, the list of agents that actually cause the disorder is considerably shorter. Important former causes of drug fever, such as laxatives, bromides, arsenical agents, and vancomycin, are now rarely incriminated in the disorder, either because they are no longer used or because new preparations of the drugs are less pyrogenic (e.g., vancomycin).

Although patients with drug fever often have high, hectic fevers with chills and myalgias, suggesting sepsis, their course and general appearance generally reflect a less severe disorder.

TABLE 266.5.	AGENTS REPORTED AS CAUSES OF DRUG FEVER
Cardiovascular	**Antineoplastic**
Methyldopa	Bleomycin
Quinidine	Daunorubicin
Procainamide	Procarbazine
Hydralazine	Cytarabine
Nifedipine	Streptozocin
Oxprenolol	6-Mercaptopurine
Antimicrobial	L-asparaginase
Penicillin G	Chlorambucil
Ampicillin	Hydroxyurea
Methicillin	**CNS**
Cloxacillin	Diphenlhydantoin
Cephalothin	Carbamazepine
Cephapirin	Chlorpromazine
Cephamandole	Nomifensine
Tetracycline	Haloperidol
Lincomycin	Benztropine[a]
Sulfonamide	Theoidazine
Sulfa-trimethroprim	Trifluoperazine[a]
Streptomycin	Amphetamine
Vancomycin	LSD[a]
Colistin	**Anti-inflammatory**
Isoniazid	Ibuprofen
PAS	Tolmetin
Nitrofurantoin	Aspirin
Mebendazole	
Other	
Iodide	
Cimetidine	
Levamisole	
Metoclopramide	
Clofibrate	
Allopurinol	
Folate	
PGE$_2$	
Ritodrine	
Interferon	
Propylthiouracil	
Triamterene	

PAS, para-aminosalicylic; PGE$_2$, prostaglandin E$_2$; CNS, central nervous system; LSD, lysergic acid diethylamide.
[a] Fever observed during drug overdose.
(From Mackowick PA, LeMaistre CF. Drug fever. *Ann Intern Med* 1987;X:106–728, with permission.)

There is considerable variability in the length of time between the initiation of specific agents and the onset of drug-induced fever. In general, antineoplastic drugs are associated with the shortest lag times and cardiac drugs with the longest. The median lag time between the initiation of antibiotics causing drug fever and the onset of antibiotic-induced fever is 6 days.

Generally, drug fever is a diagnosis of exclusion, made in febrile patients whose fever abates within 48 to 72 hours of discontinuing the suspected pyrogenic drug. Even though some authors have emphasized the potential danger of rechallenging with the offending agent to confirm the diagnosis, the actual risk of such rechallenges is probably low. The uniformly rapid resolution of fever after discontinuation of the offending drug argues strongly against the need for other measures in treating the condition.

Two forms of drug-induced pyrexia are sufficiently distinctive to warrant separate consideration. The first, malignant hyperthermia, is a rare hereditary disorder characterized by rapidly evolving hyperthermia, muscular rigidity, and acidosis in patients undergoing general anesthesia. Although various inhalational anesthetic agents have been incriminated in the disorder, halothane (alone or in conjunction with succinylcholine) is the most common offender. The condition is often presaged by sudden ventricular ectopic activity, tachycardia, circulatory instability, and a sharp rise in core temperature. Metabolic acidosis and rhabdomyolysis are typical and often severe symptoms. The mortality rate in acute cases varies between 28% and 70%. Although the specific mechanisms of action responsible for the disorder are uncertain, a defect in the regulation of intracellular calcium appears to be involved. In susceptible patients, the sarcolemmic reticulum of skeletal muscle seems to be unstable and releases calcium inappropriately in response to certain anesthetic agents.

The other drug-induced pyrexia not generally included among the classic examples of drug fever is the neuroleptic malignant syndrome. The syndrome is characterized by hyperthermia (values more than 106°F have been observed and have been confused with heatstroke), diffuse muscular rigidity, autonomic instability, and altered consciousness. It most often develops as a side effect of haloperidol but also has been reported in association with other antipsychotic drugs, such as the phenothiazines and thioxanthenes. The primary defect responsible for the disorder appears to be inhibition of central dopamine receptor blockade, which causes sustained muscle contraction, excessive heat production, and inappropriate cutaneous vasoconstriction. Hyperthermia, dehydration, and exhaustion ensue and, if uncontrolled, may be fatal.

Treatment of neuroleptic malignant syndrome and malignant hyperthermia is the subject of controversy. Most authorities recommend administration of the peripheral muscle relaxant dantrolene for both conditions, in conjunction with external cooling and other supportive measures. Bromocriptine reportedly is effective in some cases of neuroleptic malignant syndrome.

BIBLIOGRAPHY

Atkins E. Fever: its history, cause and function. *Yale J Biol Med* 1982;55: 283–289.

Hirtz DG, Nelson KB. The natural history of febrile seizures. *Annu Rev Med* 1983;34:453–471.

Livingston S, Berman W, Pauli L. Febrile convulsions. *Lancet* 1973;2: 1441–1442.

Mackowiak PA. Concepts of fever. *Arch Intern Med* 1998;158:1870–1881.

Mackowiak PA. *Fever: basic mechanisms and management*, second ed. New York: Lippincott–Raven Publishers, 1997.

Mackowiak PA, LeMaistre CF. Drug fever: a critical appraisal of conventional concepts through an analysis of 51 episodes diagnosed in two Dallas hospitals and 92 episodes reported in the English literature. *Ann Intern Med* 1987;106:728–733.

Mackowiak PA, Plaisance KI. Benefits and risks of antipyretic therapy. *Ann NY Acad Sci* 1998;856:214–223.

Mackowiak PA, Wasserman SS, Levine MM. A critical appraisal of 98.6°F, the upper limit of the normal body temperature, and other legacies of Carl Reinhold August Wunderlich. *JAMA* 1992;268:1578–1580.

Moore-Ede MC, Czeicsler CA, Richardson GS. Circadian timekeeping in health and disease, parts 1 and 2. *N Engl J Med* 1983;309:469–536.

Petersdorf RG, Beeson PB. Fever of unexplained origin: report on 100 cases. *Medicine* 1961;40:1–30.

Pizzo PA, Lovejoy FH, Smith DH. Prolonged fever in children: review of 100 cases. *Pediatrics* 1975;55:468–473.

Kelley's Textbook of Internal Medicine, fourth edition. Edited by H. David Humes. Lippincott Williams & Wilkins, Philadelphia © 2000.

CHAPTER
267

APPROACH TO INFECTION IN THE IMMUNOCOMPROMISED HOST

KENNETH V. I. ROLSTON
GERALD P. BODEY

Immunocompromised patients pose special challenges because of the wide spectrum of infections encountered, the difficulties in establishing a diagnosis, and the limited efficacy of therapeutic regimens. Management strategies may differ based upon the underlying immunologic deficit. In patients with severe neutropenia, the risk of fulminant fatal infection is so great that the overriding factor in management is the prompt administration of empiric antibiotic therapy. In contrast, the spectrum of potential pathogens is so wide in patients with impaired cellular immunity (lymphoma, AIDS) that establishing a specific diagnosis is of paramount importance. Table 267.1 lists many of the important factors that predispose patients to infection and the specific infections frequently associated with them.

■ SPECIFIC IMMUNOLOGIC DEFICITS

DEFICIENCIES IN HUMORAL FACTORS

Humoral immunity includes protection afforded by such substances as immunoglobulins, opsonins, and complement, which attach to pathogens and/or facilitate phagocytosis by macrophages, monocytes, or neutrophils. Deficiencies in humoral immunity (multiple myeloma, Waldenström's macroglobulinemia) increase the likelihood of infections caused by encapsulated bacteria, such as pneumococci, meningococci, and *Haemophilus influenzae* organisms.

DEFICIENCIES IN CELLULAR FUNCTION

Specific defects in neutrophil function have been identified in some patients, including chemotaxis (Job syndrome) and bactericidal activity (chronic granulomatous disease, Chédiak–Higashi syndrome). These patients are especially susceptible to pyo-

TABLE 267.1.	DEFICIENCIES IN HOST-DEFENSE MECHANISMS AND ASSOCIATED INFECTIONS

Disease	Deficiency	Common Infections
Hereditary complement deficiency	Complement	*Neisseria* species
Multiple myeloma	Hypogammaglobulinemia	Pneumococcus, meningococcus; *Haemophilus influenzae*
Hodgkin's disease	Increased suppressor monocytes	*Cryptococcus, Listeria, Mycobacterium, Toxoplasma* species
Mucocutaneous candidiasis	T-lymphocyte function	*Candida albicans*
Bone marrow transplant	Increased suppressor T-lymphocyte activity	Gram-positive cocci, pneumocystis, cytomegalovirus
Acute leukemia	Neutropenia	Gram-positive cocci, gram-negative bacilli, *Candida* or *Aspergillus* species
Chronic granulomatous disease	Neutrophil bactericidal activity	*Staphylococcus, Serratta, Nocardia* species
Job syndrome	Impaired neutrophil chemotaxis	*Staphylococcus* species, *Aspergillus* species
AIDS	Decreased CD4$^+$ lymphocytes	Pneumocystis, cytomegalovirus; superficial *Candida*

genic bacterial infections, which are often chronic or relapsing. Patients with Hodgkin's disease have impaired monocyte function and are susceptible to infections caused by intracellular pathogens, among them, mycobacteria, *Listeria monocytogenes,* and *Cryptococcus neoformans.* Some patients with chronic mucocutaneous candidiasis have defects in T-lymphocyte function, including failure to mount a blastogenic response to multiple antigens or specifically to *Candida* antigens. Patients undergoing long-term adrenal corticosteroid therapy are especially susceptible to *Aspergillus* infections because steroids interfere with the ability of macrophages to kill *Aspergillus* spores.

DEFICIENCIES IN CELL NUMBERS

Although some diseases cause neutropenia, it is most often a consequence of myelosuppressive antineoplastic chemotherapy. The risk of infection is inversely related to the degree of neutropenia and directly related to its duration. Although the risk of infection begins to rise when the absolute neutrophil count falls below 1,000 per cubic millimeter of blood, most severe infections, including bacteremias, occur when the absolute neutrophil count is below 100 per cubic millimeter. Because the neutrophil is the primary defense against bacteria, *Candida* and *Aspergillus* infections caused by these organisms develop most often in neutropenic patients.

■ MANAGEMENT OF FEVER IN THE IMMUNOCOMPROMISED HOST

Immunocompromised patients with fever can be divided into two groups, each requiring different treatment strategies. The first group comprises patients with neutropenia, splenectomy, and other underlying deficiencies. In these patients, infection is usually acute in onset, bacteria are the predominant cause, and delaying therapy can result in fulminant infection and death. The second group includes patients with impaired lymphocyte or macrophage–monocyte function. In this group, infections are generally chronic in nature, the possible pathogens are myr-

iad and diverse, and establishing the correct diagnosis is critical to selecting appropriate antimicrobial therapy. It is important to establish the diagnosis expeditiously in these patients because infection can progress rapidly if left untreated. This is especially true for AIDS patients, who are susceptible to many infectious agents that have atypical signs and symptoms.

TREATMENT OF THE NEUTROPENIC PATIENT

When a neutropenic patient has fever, it should be considered indicative of infection unless it is associated with another obvious cause. A practical definition of fever is a temperature of at least 38.3°C (101°F) persisting for 2 hours. Appropriate cultures should be collected at the onset of fever, and a careful physical examination should be carried out. If the patient is acutely ill or has signs of infection, broad-spectrum antibiotic therapy should be initiated immediately (Fig. 267.1). Neutropenic patients cannot mount an adequate inflammatory response and can have extensive infection without characteristic signs and symptoms. Hence, patients who have fever that persists for 2 hours without other signs of infection should receive antibiotic therapy at that time, after the collection of a second blood culture specimen. This approach prevents the administration of antibiotics to patients who have a single temperature elevation for unknown reasons but avoids inappropriate delays in therapy for most infected patients. Prompt administration of therapy is critical: patients may die quickly if untreated, and delays diminish the efficacy of antibiotic therapy.

Selection of empiric antibiotics requires a knowledge of the usual organisms that cause infection in neutropenic patients. These infections are listed in Table 267.1. Although the most common bacterial pathogens are *Staphylococcus epidermidis, Staphylococcus aureus,* viridans streptococci, *Escherichia coli, Klebsiella pneumoniae,* and *Pseudomonas aeruginosa,* there are local institutional differences in the spectrum of infection. Antibiotic selection therefore should be guided by knowledge of the pathogens prevalent in the hospital as well as local susceptibility/resistance patterns. Extensive use of some antibiotics has resulted in the emergence of vancomycin-resistant enterococci, *Stenotro-*

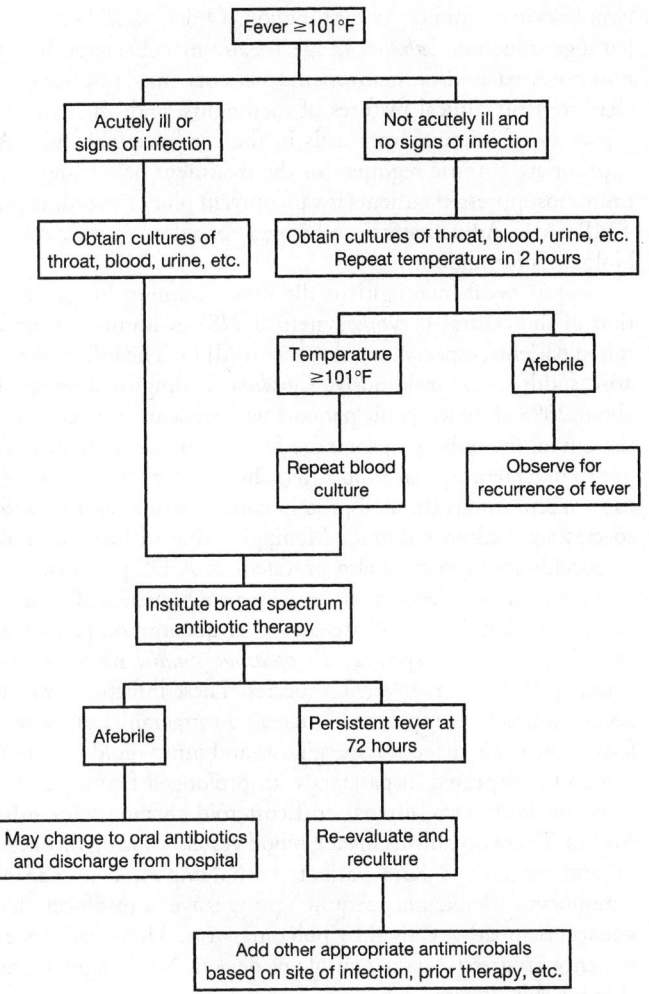

FIGURE 267.1. Approach to fever in neutropenic patients.

phomonas maltophilia, Candida krusei, and other multi-drug-resistant pathogens.

Various antibacterial regimens can be used for the empiric treatment of neutropenic patients, and no single regimen can be considered optimal. The current choices include combination regimens either with (vancomycin plus ceftazidime) or without (an aminoglycoside plus a broad-spectrum β-lactam) vancomycin or therapy with certain broad-spectrum agents (cefepime, imipenem, meropenem) used alone. Aminoglycosides are unreliable in the treatment of neutropenic patients even when the infecting organism is susceptible in vitro, and they are associated with substantial ototoxicity and nephrotoxicity. Suitable alternatives include the quinolones (ciprofloxacin, trovafloxacin) and trimethoprim-sulfamethoxazole (TMP-SMX). The current predominance of gram-positive pathogens has led to increased use of vancomycin-containing regimens. Vancomycin should be discontinued promptly if it is not needed, to reduce the selection of organisms (VRE, GISA) resistant to this agent.

If the patient responds to initial antibiotic therapy within a few days and never shows signs of local infection, therapy can be changed to oral medications, and the patient can be discharged from the hospital. Therapy should be continued for a week or until 4 days after the patient becomes afebrile, whichever is longer. The duration of therapy may be shorter if the neutrophil count recovers. If the patient is likely to remain neutropenic for a prolonged period, antibiotic prophylaxis should be considered, but therapeutic antibiotics need not be continued until the neutrophil count recovers. If the patient has signs of localized infection, the duration of therapy depends on the rapidity of response.

Treatment of the neutropenic patient who has no evidence of infection but remains febrile despite taking broad-spectrum antibacterial antibiotics is difficult. Potential sources of fever in these patients include drug, transfusion, tumor, or infection caused by antibiotic-resistant bacteria, viruses, mycobacteria, protozoa, or fungi. The most common cause of persistent fever in neutropenic patients is fungal infection. Because fungal infection may have no characteristic clinical findings and culture specimens often are not diagnostic, a therapeutic trial of antifungal therapy is appropriate. At least 30% of these patients respond, and therapy should be continued in such patients until their neutrophil counts recover or they remain afebrile for at least 10 days. Obviously, all patients with persistent fevers should be carefully evaluated for obscure infections, such as cytomegalovirus, tuberculosis, or toxoplasmosis. Judicious use of computed tomography and ultrasonography may pinpoint unsuspected sites of infection.

Risk-prediction models have enabled clinicians to classify febrile neutropenic patients into high-, moderate-, and low-risk categories at the onset of a febrile episode. High-risk patients (with hematologic malignancy with prolonged neutropenia or those with allogeneic bone marrow transplants) are treated in the standard manner with hospital-based, broad-spectrum parenteral, empiric antibiotic therapy. Moderate-risk patients (those who have solid tumors and have undergone intensive chemotherapy followed by autologous bone marrow transplantation or PBSCT) can be stabilized in the hospital over a 48- to 72-hour period and then discharged to complete therapy at home. Low-risk patients can be treated with broad-spectrum parenteral, sequential, or oral regimens without admission to the hospital at all. This risk-based therapy is becoming the new standard of care for febrile neutropenic patients: it is cost effective, is associated with fewer multi-drug-resistant superinfections, and results in more appropriate resource utilization (Table 267.2).

TABLE 267.2.	**RISK-BASED THERAPY FOR FEBRILE NEUTROPENIC PATIENTS**
Risk Group	**Therapy**
High risk	Standard, hospital-based, parenteral, broad-spectrum antibiotic therapy for duration of febrile episode
Moderate risk	Initial stabilization in hospital (48–72 hr) with standard therapy, followed by early discharge on outpatient regimens
Low risk	Outpatient (clinic/home) parenteral, sequential, or oral antibiotic therapy

TABLE 267.3.	CONSIDERATIONS IN THE MANAGEMENT OF INFECTION IN NON-NEUTROPENIC IMMUNOCOMPROMISED PATIENTS

Knowledge of specific deficiency and likely associated infections
Careful history, including travel and exposure to potential pathogens
Complete physical examination
Collection of appropriate culture specimens, with attention to special procedures
Attention to indicated serologic tests, skin tests, roentgenographic examination
Expeditious tissue biopsy for histologic examination and appropriate cultures
Correction of deficient host responses, if possible

TREATMENT OF OTHER IMMUNOSUPPRESSED PATIENTS

Although patients with impaired lymphocyte and monocyte function may experience fulminant infection, usually the infections are more indolent. Because of the variety of infectious processes that can arise in these patients, it is not usually advisable to treat them empirically. Table 267.3 lists important aspects in the evaluation of these febrile patients. The specific deficiency in host-defense mechanisms and the infections associated with this deficiency are critical to the selection of the proper diagnostic procedures. Often the pathogens are not ubiquitous, nor are they usually acquired in the hospital. Hence, it is important to obtain a careful history, paying attention to potential exposures. Special stains and culture procedures are often needed for patients' specimens, serologic tests, or skin tests. For example, *Nocardia* species may not be detected without special stains and processing of cultures, and cryptococcal meningitis occasionally is diagnosed only if the cerebrospinal fluid is tested for the presence of antigen. Biopsy of infected tissue is the most rapid and reliable diagnostic procedure and should be performed expeditiously when necessary. Routine dosages and schedules of antimicrobial agents for normal hosts may be inappropriate for immunocompromised patients. The duration of therapy is determined by the patient's response and not by predetermined schedules derived from experience in normal hosts.

MANAGEMENT OF INFECTION AT SPECIFIC SITES

CENTRAL NERVOUS SYSTEM

Acute bacterial meningitis is rare and occurs most often in asplenic or neutropenic patients. In the former case, pneumococci (20% to 60% of which are now penicillin resistant), meningococci, and *H. influenzae* are the most likely pathogens. In neutropenic patients, gram-negative bacilli, especially *P. aeruginosa*, predominate. Staphylococci are isolated most often from patients with shunt or other foreign-body-related meningitis. *L. monocytogenes* is a typical cause of meningitis in patients with

lymphocyte or monocyte dysfunction. Other possible bacterial pathogens include *Salmonella* species and mycobacteria. Immunosuppressed and/or neutropenic patients may not have the characteristic clinical features of meningitis, and often there is a paucity of inflammatory cells in the cerebrospinal fluid. An appropriate empiric regimen for the treatment of meningitis in immunosuppressed patients is vancomycin plus ceftazidime plus TMP-SMX. Adjustments can be made based on specific microbiologic information.

Cryptococcal meningitis is the most common fungal infection of the central nervous system (CNS) in immunocompromised patients, especially in those with AIDS. The infection may arise suddenly or insidiously. *Candida* meningitis develops in about 20% of neutropenic patients with disseminated candidiasis. Often, the only symptoms are fever, disorientation, and stupor. The cerebrospinal fluid often shows no characteristic feature, except for an elevated protein concentration, and *Candida* species are seldom cultured. Meningitis due to histoplasmosis or coccidioidomycosis is also prevalent in AIDS patients.

Intracerebral infections are usually a consequence of disseminated infection. Nearly all are caused by uncommon pathogens, including *Nocardia* species, *Toxoplasma gondii*, mycobacteria, cytomegalovirus, or *Aspergillus* species. These infections may be accompanied by symptoms of increased intracranial pressure or focal neurologic defects. Aspergillosis and other mold infections should be suspected in patients with prolonged neutropenia or those on long-term adrenal corticosteroid therapy who suffer strokes. These organisms invade blood vessels, causing thrombosis and infarction. Rare patients with lymphoma or chronic lymphocytic leukemia acquire progressive multifocal leukoencephalopathy, caused by polyoma virus. These patients experience progressive, fatal neurologic defects. No therapy is available for this disease.

SINUS INFECTIONS

Neutropenic patients occasionally have acute bacterial sinus infections, but these infections may be overlooked because of the diminished inflammatory response in such patients. *P. aeruginosa* is an infrequent cause of chronic sinusitis, otitis externa, otitis media, and mastoiditis. The most commonly recognized causes of sinus infection are molds (*Aspergillus, Fusarium, Mucorales*), seen primarily in neutropenic patients. These organisms can penetrate fascial planes, cartilage, and bone. Often the infected patient shows signs of a black necrotic ulcer on the exterior or interior of the nose or on the palate. Infection may erode through the base of the skull into the brain. The orbit often is affected in the process, and endophthalmitis may be a late complication. Amphotericin B therapy is indicated, and surgical debridement or excision should be performed if possible, though control of the infection depends on recovery of host defenses. Control may be effected in part with the use of hematopoietic growth factors and/or granulocyte transfusions.

OROPHARYNGEAL INFECTION

Most oropharyngeal infections arise in neutropenic and AIDS patients, though local factors can precipitate infections in other immunocompromised patients. Other susceptible patients are those who receive antitumor agents or radiation therapy that damages the epithelial cells, causing ulceration and infection. About 10% of leukemic patients experience bacterial infections in the oropharynx, many caused by gram-negative bacilli. Gingivitis, dental abscess, pericoronitis, pharyngitis, and, occasionally, gangrenous stomatitis may develop. *Capnocytophaga*, an anaerobic gram-negative bacillus that inhabits the oropharynx, causes bacteremia in neutropenic patients with mouth ulcers. Infections caused by *Stomatococcus mucilaginosus* are also common in this context. Severe mucositis may result in α-hemolytic streptococcal septicemia with shock, renal failure, or acute respiratory distress syndrome.

Thrush is the most prevalent oral infection in immunocompromised patients; it is seen in neutropenic patients (acute leukemia, marrow transplantation) and in patients with deficiencies in T-lymphocyte numbers or function (AIDS, mucocutaneous candidiasis). Thrush can be treated with topical antifungal agents (clotrimazole troches, nystatin suspension) or oral absorbable agents (fluconazole, itraconazole). Chronic and recurrent infection is the rule in patients with T-lymphocyte deficiencies (especially AIDS patients, who ultimately often require prolonged fluconazole prophylaxis). The emergence of resistant *Candida* species in this situation is a significant problem.

Serious herpes simplex infections occur in transplant recipients, AIDS patients, and neutropenic patients. They take the form of localized vesicular lesions but may progress to large hemorrhagic and necrotic lesions involving the oropharynx, lips, and surrounding facial tissues. Rarely, herpes simplex infection disseminates to internal organs, including the trachea, lungs, liver, and CNS. Another potentially serious complication of orocutaneous herpetic infection is bacterial superinfection, often caused by *S. aureus*. Intravenous acyclovir is an effective therapeutic agent, but some severely immunocompromised patients, such as bone marrow transplant recipients, may suffer from prolonged infection that responds slowly. Localized infections can be treated with oral agents, such as valaciclovir or famciclovir.

PNEUMONITIS

Pneumonitis is the most common infection in the immunocompromised host and has one of the highest mortality rates. Its management is challenging and difficult because of the diversity of causative organisms (Table 267.4). Bronchoalveolar lavage is often a useful diagnostic procedure, except in neutropenic patients, in whom even open lung biopsy often fails to establish a diagnosis. Infection may arise locally by inhalation of respiratory pathogens, such as *Aspergillus* organisms; by aspiration; or as a consequence of hematogenous dissemination, as in most cases of candidiasis. Some infections (*Pneumocystis* pneumonia, cytomegalovirus) may represent reactivation of latent infections.

Clues to the cause of pneumonitis can be derived from determination of the deficiency in host defenses, history of exposure, presenting signs and symptoms, extrapulmonary findings, and appearance of the chest roentgenogram. Neutropenic patients are most likely to have pneumonitis caused by gram-negative bacilli, *Candida* organisms, or *Aspergillus* species, whereas patients with impaired T-lymphocyte or monocyte function are

TABLE 267.4.	PNEUMONITIS IN THE IMMUNOCOMPROMISED PATIENT
Infection	**Agent**
Bacterial	Gram-positive cocci, gram-negative bacilli, and *Legionella, Nocardia,* and *Mycobacterium* species
Fungal	*Candida* species, *Aspergillus* species, and *Phycomycetes, Cryptococcus, Histoplasma, Coccidioides* organisms
Viral	Cytomegalovirus, herpes simplex, varicella zoster, respiratory syncytial virus, community respiratory viruses
Protozoal	*Toxoplasma Pneumocystis* species
Parasitic	*Strongyloides*
Noninfectious	Drug toxicity, hemorrhage, malignancy, nonspecific interstitial pneumonitis

susceptible to cryptococcosis, histoplasmosis, toxoplasmosis, pneumocystosis, mycobacteriosis, and cytomegalovirus. Community respiratory viruses, such as respiratory syncytial virus, influenza viruses, parainfluenza viruses, and adenoviruses, have been recognized as important sources of respiratory disease in immunocompromised patients.

Because *Aspergillus* species and other molds invade blood vessels, causing thrombosis and infarction, infected patients may show signs and symptoms of acute pulmonary embolism, including pleuritic chest pain and a pleural friction rub. Candidiasis usually occurs in patients with progressive debilitation who show signs of first-time or progressive pneumonitis while receiving antibacterial antibiotics. Patients with pneumonitis caused by cytomegalovirus or *Pneumocystis carinii* often experience severe tachypnea and cyanosis, with few abnormalities on chest auscultation. Pneumonia associated with CNS symptoms suggests infections such as cryptococcosis, listeriosis, or toxoplasmosis. Pneumonitis associated with myocarditis or hepatitis suggests the possibility of cytomegalic inclusion disease or toxoplasmosis. Pneumonitis caused by *Candida* or *Aspergillus* species or *P. aeruginosa* may be associated with characteristic skin lesions.

The chest roentgenogram also can provide clues to the cause of pneumonitis. Hilar or mediastinal lymphadenopathy would suggest such infections as histoplasmosis, coccidioidomycosis, or mycobacteriosis. Evidence of preexisting granuloma also indicates these infections. The earliest manifestation of pulmonary aspergillosis or other mold infection is the appearance of a single or several nodules that may progress to cavitation and formation of fungus balls. The presence of necrotizing pneumonia reflects infection by gram-negative bacilli. Abscess formation occurs in various infections, including those caused by *S. aureus*, gram-negative bacilli, or *Nocardia* species. Bilateral, diffuse pneumonitis in the neutropenic patient can be produced by bacteria, fungi, viruses, or protozoa. AIDS patients may have atypical initial roentgenographic manifestations. Empiric therapy is appropriate in neutropenic patients, but in most other immunocompromised patients, a vigorous approach to establishing the diagnosis is critical. Diagnosis should be expeditious, because apparently indolent infections can become fulminant.

ESOPHAGEAL INFECTION

Esophagitis has become a relatively common infection in recent years as a consequence of intensive myelosuppressive chemotherapy and AIDS. Esophageal candidiasis can develop in the absence of oral thrush. Initial signs are pain on swallowing and retrosternal discomfort. Barium contrast radiographic examination shows ulceration, spasm, and a cobblestone appearance to the esophageal mucosa. White patches and hemorrhagic ulcers can be seen on esophagoscopy. Esophagitis is usually caused by *Candida albicans* or herpes simplex virus; other causes include cytomegalovirus, bacteria, and peptic esophagitis. The diagnosis can be confirmed only by scrapings or a biopsy sample obtained during esophagoscopy. Fluconazole is the preferred therapy for *Candida* esophagitis and may be used empirically in susceptible patients, reserving esophagoscopy for patients who fail to respond after several days of therapy.

GASTROINTESTINAL INFECTIONS

A few infections of the gastrointestinal tract represent special problems for the immunocompromised patient. Colitis stemming from *Clostridium difficile* occasionally develops in patients receiving cancer chemotherapy who have not been exposed to antibiotics. Although it is not certain that *Salmonella* infections occur more frequently in patients with hematologic diseases, they affect extragastrointestinal sites in 50% of these patients. They arise primarily in patients with lymphoma, hemolytic anemia, autoimmune disorders, or AIDS. The common predisposing factor is impaired function of lymphocytes or the reticuloendothelial system. Most of the infections are caused by *S. typhimurium* and *S. enteritidis*. Chronic and relapsing infection is not uncommon, despite appropriate therapy.

At autopsy, signs of gastrointestinal candidiasis are often found in neutropenic patients, but it is seldom recognized clinically because most patients remain asymptomatic. Gastrointestinal infection often serves as the source of disseminated candidiasis. Cytomegalovirus can cause severe and even fatal infection of the gastrointestinal tract, especially in children. Occasionally, patients have died of protracted severe diarrhea that resulted in an uncontrollable electrolyte imbalance. Other patients have had ulcerations with severe hemorrhage or perforation. Strongyloidiasis is a rare problem in lymphoma and transplant patients, causing recurrent septicemia due to enteric organisms or hyperacute strongyloidiasis with pulmonary involvement.

Typhlitis is a unique and potentially serious infection in neutropenic patients. It is a patchy inflammatory disease characterized by well-demarcated ulcers, hemorrhage, and masses of organisms in the bowel wall, with a paucity of inflammatory cells. Usually, it is limited to the cecum, but it may affect the entire intestine. The typical presenting signs and symptoms are fever, abdominal pain, watery or bloody diarrhea, stomatitis, abdominal distention, tenderness (often in the right-lower quadrant), and diminished or absent bowel sounds. More than 70% of patients have septicemia caused by gram-negative bacilli or *Clostridium septicum*. Therapy consists of nasogastric suction, intravenous fluids, analgesics, and broad-spectrum antibiotic regimens that provide coverage against gram-negative bacteria, including *P. aeruginosa* and anaerobes. Surgical intervention may be necessary. The mortality rate is high unless the neutrophil count recovers.

Perirectal infections resulting in neutropenia develop in 5% to 10% of patients with hematologic diseases, but they are especially common in patients with acute monocytic and acute myelomonocytic leukemia. Perirectal infections and proctitis are prevalent infections in AIDS patients. The initial symptoms are pain aggravated by defecation, local tenderness, and septic or hectic fever. Infection often arises at the site of a hemorrhoid or fissure and may extend into the rectum, with extensive necrosis. Most of these infections are caused by aerobic gram-negative bacilli, especially *P. aeruginosa* and *E. coli*. In most cases, therapy consists of sitz baths or warm compresses, stool softeners, analgesics, and broad-spectrum antibiotics.

CUTANEOUS INFECTION

Infections of the skin and soft tissues may be localized or a manifestation of disseminated disease. Because many immunocompromised patients require frequent intravenous medications and blood tests, they often experience cellulitis. Some cancer chemotherapeutic agents are vesicants and lead to extensive tissue necrosis if they extravasate. Most local infections are caused by *S. aureus*, *S. epidermidis*, and gram-negative bacilli. Among the gram-negative bacilli that have a special propensity for generating localized infections are *P. aeruginosa*, *Aeromonas hydrophila*, and *S. maltophilia*. Occasionally, infections are caused by gram-positive organisms, such as *Bacillus* species and *Corynebacterium jeikeium*. Aspiration and biopsy of infected areas should be undertaken, but despite these procedures the pathogen often cannot be determined. Fungi that sometimes prompt local infections are *Candida*, *Aspergillus*, *Fusarium*, and *Mucorales* species. From time to time, genital herpes is seen in immunocompromised patients. Women may suffer extensive vulvovaginal infection that is disfiguring and painful. Genital condylomas may also develop in immunocompromised women, including renal transplant recipients and patients with hematologic malignancies. These lesions in immunocompromised patients are often difficult to eradicate by conventional methods.

Herpes zoster occurs in up to 25% of patients undergoing therapy for Hodgkin's disease. Most cases develop within a year after completion of therapy. Although zoster is considered a reactivation of latent infection, there have been outbreaks of infection in susceptible populations, suggesting exogenous acquisition of the virus. Infection tends to manifest where tumor is in close proximity to the nerve trunk or at sites of previous radiation therapy. Cutaneous dissemination takes place in 20% to 40% of patients; visceral dissemination is rare. Intravenous acyclovir should be given to patients with disseminated infection; it is also appropriate for patients with localized infections, to facilitate healing, minimize scarring, and prevent postherpetic neuralgia, which is more common in these patients than in normal hosts. Combination therapy (acyclovir plus foscarnet) may be beneficial in patients who fail to respond to acyclovir alone.

DISSEMINATED FUNGAL INFECTIONS

Disseminated candidiasis is especially common in neutropenic patients because the neutrophil is the primary defense against *Candida* organisms. Other factors predisposing to this infection include indwelling catheters, parenteral alimentation, broad-spectrum antibiotics, and adrenal corticosteroid therapy. There is nothing characteristic about the clinical picture of disseminated candidiasis in most patients. They often have fever as the only sign of infection, but some show symptoms suggestive of endotoxic shock, including shaking chills, tachycardia, tachypnea, and hypotension. *Candida* species is one of the more common sources of hematogenous pneumonia in neutropenic patients. A chronic form of candidiasis primarily involving the liver and spleen develops in some patients who achieve remission of leukemia or lymphoma. The infection arises when they are neutropenic but persists as a chronic, debilitating infection for prolonged periods after hematologic remission, despite the administration of antifungal therapy.

Diagnosing candidiasis is often difficult. The organism can be cultured from blood specimens of only 40% of patients with disseminated infection. Serologic tests of antibody or antigen have not been reliable for establishing the diagnosis. Because *C. albicans* is ubiquitous in patients receiving antibiotics, its recovery from several body sites often represents colonization rather than infection; recovery of *Candida tropicalis* from body sites appears to be more indicative of infection. Other *Candida* species, such as *C. glabrata*, *C. parapsilosis*, and *C. krusei*, have emerged as prevalent pathogens, especially among neutropenic patients. Computed tomography of the abdomen may pinpoint abscesses in the liver, spleen, or kidney. A definitive diagnosis often can be established only by tissue biopsy.

Aspergillus infection disseminates in about 30% of cases and mucormycosis less frequently. *Fusarium* species have emerged as a significant source of disseminated fungal infection in neutropenic patients. Because *Aspergillus* organisms invade blood vessel walls, causing thrombosis and infarction, symptoms of acute vascular events are typical. Conditions that are associated with disseminated infection include Budd–Chiari syndrome, myocardial infarction, cerebral infarction, gastrointestinal hemorrhage, and necrotic skin lesions. Although the diagnosis may be suspected from the clinical symptoms, it usually cannot be confirmed without tissue biopsy.

Although cryptococcosis usually appears as meningitis, it can also lead to disseminated infection of the lung, lymph nodes, skin, bone, liver, kidney, spleen, and adrenal glands. Skin lesions are acneiform, nodular, plaque-like, or ulcerated. Pneumonia may take the form of miliary, nodular, or cavitary lesions on chest roentgenograms. Reactivation of pulmonary granulomas caused by histoplasmosis or coccidioidomycosis may result in disseminated infection.

Amphotericin B has been the standard therapy for most fungal infections, but infusion-related toxicity and nephrotoxicity are significant limitations. The newer lipid formulations of amphotericin B are at least as effective and much less toxic, but they also are much more expensive than standard amphotericin B. The azole compounds (fluconazole, itraconazole) are alternative therapies for some fungal infections, but the appearance of resistant organisms (*C. krusei*) is a concern. Unfortunately, antifungal therapy may be ineffective unless the underlying immunologic defects can be corrected. The use of hematopoietic growth factors (granulocyte colony-stimulating factor and granulocyte–macrophage colony-stimulating factor) and granulocyte transfusions in addition to antifungal therapy may be of benefit in patients with disseminated fungal infections.

TRANSFUSION- AND TRANSPLANTATION-RELATED INFECTIONS

Organ transplantation has been associated with the acquisition of various chronic infections, including hepatitis B, cytomegalic inclusion disease, rabies, Creutzfeldt–Jakob disease, AIDS, and herpes simplex infection. Some immunocompromised patients require extraordinary numbers of transfusions; hence, they are susceptible to acquiring infections via this route. Herpes simplex, Epstein–Barr virus, and cytomegalovirus can be acquired from infected donor leukocytes. Babesiosis, malaria, leishmaniasis, and toxoplasmosis have been transmitted via blood products.

■ INFECTION PREVENTION

Programs to prevent infection have been developed for highly susceptible patients, such as organ transplant recipients and patients undergoing chemotherapy for acute leukemia. These programs include laminar air-flow rooms, special food preparation, skin-cleansing products, and antimicrobial agents. Conventional isolation is of little benefit and interferes with optimal patient care. Laminar air-flow rooms are expensive but effective in preventing exposure to respiratory pathogens, such as molds. Simple HEPA filtration units may be as effective and less costly. Foods may be contaminated with potential pathogens (gram-negative bacilli, *Candida* species). Special cooked diets can minimize this exposure, but they may be unnecessary for patients who are receiving antimicrobial prophylaxis.

Antimicrobial agents have been effective for prophylaxis in prospective, randomized trials. Fluoroquinolones and TMP-SMX are useful for antibacterial prophylaxis, but the former drugs are more effective where resistance to TMP-SMX is prevalent. Fluconazole is effective prophylaxis for *Candida* infections, though the emergence of resistant species is a concern. Ganciclovir can prevent cytomegalovirus infection, and acyclovir can prevent herpes simplex infection. The major worry with the use of prophylactic regimens is the potential for colonization and infection with resistant organisms. No regimen can provide protection against all potential pathogens or eliminate the risk of antimicrobial resistance.

Immunizations are a valuable measure for the prevention of some infections in immunocompromised patients. Because bone marrow transplant recipients and patients who have undergone splenectomy are susceptible to overwhelming pneumococcal infection, they should be given the pneumococcal vaccine. It should be administered before splenectomy for optimal benefit. The antibody response in patients receiving chemotherapy and in patients with impaired antibody synthesis is blunted, so vaccines are of limited value for them. Influenza vaccine is probably useful for patients taking immunosuppressive drugs, provided there is an interval between administration of the vaccine and the immunosuppressive therapy, to permit an adequate antibody response. The colony-stimulating factors (granulocyte colony-stimulating factor and granulocyte–macrophage colony-stimulating factor) may prevent infection during myelosuppressive chemotherapy by shortening the duration of neutropenia. Their role in infection prophylaxis remains the subject of controversy, primarily because of their expense.

BIBLIOGRAPHY

Bodey GP. Dermatologic manifestations of infections in neutropenic patients. *Infect Dis Clin North Am* 1994;8:655–675.

Bodey GP, Buckley M, Sathe YS, et al. Quantitative relationships between circulating leukocytes and infection in patients with acute leukemia. *Ann Intern Med* 1966;64:328–340.

Gomez L, Martino R, Rolston KV. Neutropenic enterocolitis: spectrum of the disease and comparison of definite and possible cases. *Clin Infect Dis* 1998;27:695–699.

Hughes WT, Armstrong D, Bodey GP, et al. 1997 Guidelines for the use of antimicrobial agents in neutropenic patients with unexplained fever. *Clin Infect Dis* 1997;25:551–573.

Koll BS, Brown AE. The changing epidemiology of infections at cancer hospitals. *Clin Infect Dis* 1993;17(suppl 2):S322–S328.

Ozer H, et al., and the ASCO Ad Hoc Colony-Stimulating Factor Guidelines Expert Panel. American Society of Clinical Oncology recommendations for the use of hematopoietic colony-stimulating factors: evidence-based, clinical practice guidelines. *J Clin Oncol* 1994;12:2471.

Pizzo PA. Management of fever in patients with cancer and treatment induced neutropenia. *N Engl J Med* 1993;328:1323–1332.

Rolston KVI, Rubenstein EB, Freifeld A. Early empiric antibiotic therapy for febrile neutropenia patients at "low-risk." In: Greene JN, Hiemenz JW, eds. *Infectious Disease Clinics of North America.* Philadelphia: WB Saunders, 1996:223.

Whimbey E, Englund JA, Couch RB. Community respiratory virus infections in immunocompromised patients with cancer. *Am J Med* 1997; 102(suppl 3A):10.

Wong-Beringer A, Jacobs RA, Guglielmo BJ. Lipid formulations of amphotericin B: clinical efficacy and toxicities. *Clin Infect Dis* 1998;27: 603–618.

Kelley's Textbook of Internal Medicine, fourth edition. Edited by H. David Humes. Lippincott Williams & Wilkins, Philadelphia © 2000.

C H A P T E R
268

APPROACH TO THE PATIENT WITH BACTEREMIA AND SEPSIS

GARY A. NOSKIN
JOHN P. PHAIR

More than 400,000 cases of bacteremia and sepsis occur each year in the United States, and they are associated with significant morbidity and mortality. In recent years, there has been a dramatic increase in the number of bacteremic infections due to gram-positive bacteria and fungi compared with infections due to gram-negative bacteria. This alteration in microbiology reflects, to a large extent, the widespread use of intravascular devices and extended-spectrum antimicrobial agents.

In some patients, bacteremia leads to a widespread inflammatory response now termed the systemic inflammatory response syndrome (SIRS). Only when SIRS stems from infection is it called sepsis. This distinction is crucial: many other conditions, such as trauma, severe burns, and pancreatitis, can result in SIRS and mimic sepsis, but they are unrelated to infection. Patients who become hypotensive as a result of sepsis are considered to have septic shock. The term multiple organ dysfunction syndrome has been coined for patients in septic shock who require intervention to maintain hemodynamic stability.

■ EPIDEMIOLOGY

Bacteremia occurs in both community- and hospital-acquired infections. Community infections commonly associated with bloodstream invasion include pneumonia, pyelonephritis, meningitis, and infections associated with perforating injuries of abdominal and thoracic viscera and lesions that obstruct the gastrointestinal or genitourinary tract. Patients with skin or soft-tissue infections, especially in association with diabetes mellitus, malnutrition, and HIV-1 infection, and those on corticosteroid therapy or other immunosuppressive agents (cyclosporine, azathioprine) are also at increased risk.

Nosocomial infections are those that develop in patients after admission to the hospital that were not present or were incubating at the time of admission, though this distinction is becoming blurred as more seriously ill patients are treated in the ambulatory setting. About 5% of patients admitted to hospitals experience an infection while hospitalized. These infections typically involve the urinary tract or are related to surgical wounds or pneumonia; at present, nosocomial bloodstream infections account for 14% of hospital-acquired infections. Manipulation of the genitourinary tract and the use of indwelling bladder catheters are associated with an increased risk of infection. Among catheterized patients, the most important risk factor is the duration of catheterization. Few of these infections result in bacteremia. Although women are infected most often, elderly men are the most likely to experience bloodstream infection.

Most surgical wound infections occur 3 to 7 days after surgery and are caused by bacteria introduced during the operation; however, decreasing lengths of hospital stay often make it difficult to identify these infections. Antibiotic prophylaxis administered in the perioperative period has had a significant effect on minimizing these infections. Less than 1% of surgical wound infections are complicated by bacteremia. Elderly men are at greatest risk after prolonged hospitalization, especially for surgery of the gastrointestinal or genitourinary tract.

Although nosocomial pneumonias occur less frequently than urinary tract infections or surgical wound infections, this form of pneumonia is the most lethal of the hospital-acquired infections, with a 30% to 50% mortality rate. Bacteremia is a consequence of nosocomial pneumonia more often than other nosocomial infections and is the reason for the higher mortality rate associated with this infection. The overall risk of dying from pneumonia is greatest for patients older than 60 years and those with multilobe involvement, respiratory failure, or severe underlying illness.

Primary bloodstream infection most often develops in patients with intravascular catheters, especially central venous access devices. Infection generally arises at the entry site, and the risk rises with frequent manipulation or prolonged duration of catheterization. Intravenous, arterial, and central venous catheters should be changed according to institutional infection-control guidelines. The introduction of antimicrobial impregnated catheters has been shown to lower this risk. Nosocomial bloodstream infection is associated with significant mortality rates, prolongs hospitalization, and increases costs. It is estimated that each nosocomial bloodstream infection increases the length of hospital stay by an average of 7.4 days and costs in excess of $5,000.

ETIOLOGY

The microbiology of bacteremia is evolving constantly. In the era before antibiotics, the pyogenic gram-positive cocci, *Streptococcus pneumoniae*, *Staphylococcus aureus*, and group A streptococci were common causes of bacteremia. In the late 1950s, nosocomial bacteremia due to gram-negative bacilli became more prevalent. The organisms most frequently isolated from blood cultures were *Escherichia coli*, *Serratia marcescens*, *Pseudomonas aeruginosa*, and *Proteus*, *Klebsiella*, and *Enterobacter* species. In the 1970s, renewed interest in anaerobic bacteriology resulted in the recognition of bacteremia due to *Bacteroides* species. Since the late 1980s, the gram-positive organisms, including *S. aureus* (especially methicillin-resistant species) and *Staphylococcus epidermidis*, as well as other coagulase-negative staphylococci, are being identified more frequently. The coagulase-negative staphylococci, many of which are methicillin-resistant, are a growing problem in patients with intravenous catheters, arteriovenous shunts or fistulas, prosthetic grafts, or cardiac valves. Enterococci, both *Enterococcus faecalis* and *Enterococcus faecium*, have emerged as important nosocomial pathogens with intensifying resistance to antimicrobial agents. The percentage of enterococci that are vancomycin resistant continues to rise in medical centers throughout the United States. It is of some concern that vancomycin resistance has occurred as enterococci have developed increasing resistance to penicillins and aminoglycosides. Even more of a problem is the recent identification of *S. aureus* with decreased susceptibility to vancomycin.

The site of the infection and the underlying disease often predict the organism that will be isolated from the blood. Examples include *S. epidermidis* in association with intravascular devices, *P. aeruginosa* with severe burns, aerobic enteric bacteria or *S. aureus* with neutropenia, anaerobic organisms with intra-abdominal disease, and encapsulated bacteria with defective humoral immunity. Bacteremia due to *Streptococcus bovis* is associated with carcinoma of the colon or inflammatory bowel disease;

thus, radiologic or endoscopic examination is necessary in patients with *S. bovis* bacteremia.

In patients with sustained gram-positive bacteremia, infective endocarditis or another intravascular site of infection must be considered. The organisms that most commonly cause endocarditis include viridans streptococci, enterococci, staphylococci, and *S. bovis*. Because bacteremia is continuous in patients with endocarditis, all or nearly all blood cultures show positive results. In the absence of previous antibiotic treatment, more than 95% of patients with endocarditis have positive results on blood cultures. Aerobic gram-negative bacilli, though they are a frequent cause of bacteremia, rarely infect heart valves. Persistent bacteremia due to these organisms suggests an intra-abdominal focus of infection, a perinephric abscess, septic phlebitis, or "pseudobacteremia" from a contaminated intravenous infusion or blood culture system. Patients with HIV-1 infection are predisposed to recurrent nontyphoid *Salmonella* species bacteremia. Bacteremia and sepsis due to *S. pneumoniae*, *Haemophilus influenzae*, and *Neisseria meningitidis* are associated with asplenia.

CLINICAL MANIFESTATIONS

It is impossible to identify patients with bacteremia exclusively on clinical grounds. It is necessary for the clinician to be vigilant and acutely aware to detect bloodstream infection, especially in the elderly, in patients who have low-grade fever, and in those who do not appear to be particularly ill. The initial symptoms in patients with bacteremia are nonspecific and may include fever, lethargy, fatigue, nausea, and mental status changes. Although fever is nonspecific, rigors suggest bacteremia. In the elderly, confusion, incontinence, or falls can provide subtle evidence of bacteremia. Blood cultures should be obtained from patients suspected of having bacteremia, even in the absence of fever. In fact, hypothermia (<36°C) can occur in the context of bacteremia (though it is more common in sepsis) and indicates a poor prognosis.

In some patients, a focal site of infection is evident because of symptoms, physical findings, or laboratory results. Examples include dysuria and pyuria in patients with urosepsis, productive cough and radiographic abnormalities in patients with bacteremic pneumonia, and rebound and guarding in patients with an intra-abdominal source of bacteremia. The skin of patients suspected of having bacteremia should be carefully examined, since some systemic infections manifest with cutaneous lesions. Many purpuric lesions can be seen in patients with meningococcemia or other gram-negative bacteremias. Ecthyma gangrenosum is associated with *P. aeruginosa*, and scattered maculopapular (or pustular) lesions suggest disseminated gonococcal infection. Multiple petechiae, Osler nodes, or Janeway lesions suggest infective endocarditis.

There may be many laboratory test abnormalities in patients with bacteremia, and they often reflect the source of bloodstream invasion. Like the clinical findings, they are nonspecific and should not be used to gauge the need for obtaining cultures. An elevated white blood cell count with an increase in immature forms suggests infection, though leukocytosis may be absent in elderly or immunocompromised patients. Furthermore, leukopenia can occur with overwhelming infection and portends a poor prognosis.

DIAGNOSIS

Blood cultures must be carried out when bacteremia is suspected (Table 268.1), because isolation of bacteria from the blood is the only way to confirm the diagnosis. The volume of blood is the most important factor in the accurate detection of bacteremia. Because bacteremia in adults is generally low grade (1 to 10 colony-forming units per milliliter), 10 to 20 mL of blood should be drawn. The yield of blood cultures is directly proportional to the volume of blood; results may be false-negative if the volume of blood is less than 10 mL.

Appropriate techniques for conducting blood culture are important, to avoid contamination with cutaneous flora. The skin should be prepared initially with an alcohol swab, followed by iodophor or tincture of iodine. Once applied, the iodine should be allowed to dry and should not be removed. The venipuncture should be made with sterile gloves; if nonsterile gloves are used, the site must not be palpated. It is unnecessary to change needles between venipuncture and inoculation into blood culture tubes, but a new needle must be used for each successive attempt. A separate venipuncture site should be used for each set of cultures. All blood collected from a single venipuncture represents one set, regardless of the number of tubes or the volume inoculated. Ideally, blood cultures should be taken 15 to 30 minutes apart, though there is little evidence that this increases the chance of a positive culture. In patients suspected of having infective endocarditis, three sets of cultures taken during a 24-hour period are sufficient.

One of the most difficult challenges facing clinicians is determining whether a positive blood culture result represents clinically significant bacteremia or contamination. Depending on the technique used and the experience of the person obtaining the culture, contamination occurs in up to 3% of all blood cultures.

TABLE 268.1.	INDICATIONS FOR BLOOD CULTURES

Patients with signs/symptoms of bacteremia
Patients with fever or hypotension not explained by noninfectious causes
In the absence of fever
   Patients with focal infection (pneumonia, meningitis, osteomyelitis)
   Children or elderly with failure to thrive
   Elderly patients with change in mental status from baseline
   Patients with renal insufficiency and unexplained leukocytosis or altered mental status
   Immunocompromised patients looking ill or with unexplained pulmonary, renal, or hepatic dysfunction
Patients receiving antibiotic therapy for documented bacteremia to confirm clearance of microorganisms from the blood

(From Chandrasekar PH, Brown WJ. Clinical issues of blood cultures. *Arch Intern Med* 1994;154:841, with permission.)

In general, contamination is suspected when only one culture is positive with normal skin flora (coagulase-negative staphylococci, *Corynebacterium* species, or *Propionibacterium acnes*) and isolation occurs after prolonged incubation. This is particularly important for patients whose clinical course is inconsistent with bacteremia associated with one of these organisms. For example, in an alcoholic patient with community-acquired pneumonia and a sputum Gram's stain with abundant gram-positive diplococci, isolation of *S. epidermidis* from blood probably represents contamination. On the other hand, a positive culture for *S. pneumoniae* would confirm the diagnosis of bacteremic pneumonia. In immunocompromised patients or those with prosthetic devices, the identification of coagulase-negative staphylococci may represent true infection and should alert the physician to the possibility of intravascular infection. Obviously, if several sets of blood cultures show positive results, there is a greater likelihood that bacteremia is present. Certain bacteria rarely represent contamination, including *S. pneumoniae*, *Streptococcus pyogenes*, *S. aureus*, *P. aeruginosa*, and the Enterobacteriaceae (enteric gram-negative bacilli).

Repeated cultures of blood are generally unnecessary in patients with stable clinical symptoms. Nevertheless, in immunocompromised patients, especially febrile persons with neutropenia, several cultures may be useful in detecting bacteremia or fungemia. If a patient with bacteremia is improving and receiving appropriate antimicrobial therapy, follow-up cultures are rarely indicated. On the other hand, if the patient does not respond to treatment, repeatedly positive cultures may indicate an undrained focus or an intravascular infection.

The diagnosis of sepsis is based on the early recognition of the systemic inflammatory response to infection—fever, tachycardia, tachypnea, and hypotension. As this syndrome progresses, there may be evidence of organ hypoperfusion, manifested by change in mental status, decreased urine output, hepatic dysfunction, and myocardial depression. If this inflammatory response continues, septic shock may develop, characterized by hypotension requiring vasopressors to maintain adequate organ perfusion, lactic acidosis, and worsening abnormalities of renal, hepatic, and central nervous system function. Insertion of a pulmonary artery catheter in such patients demonstrates a markedly increased cardiac index and low systemic vascular resistance and is useful to guide therapy.

PATHOGENESIS OF SEPSIS

The most serious complication of bacteremia, especially in association with gram-negative infections, is the development of sepsis and septic shock. It is estimated that sepsis is the thirteenth leading cause of death in the United States and accounts for at least $10 billion in annual health care costs. Despite advances in medical technology and the introduction of new antimicrobial therapy, the sepsis-related mortality rate has increased 83% in the past 15 years. Sepsis is defined as clinical evidence of infection associated with tachypnea, tachycardia, and fever or hypo-

TABLE 268.2.	AMERICAN COLLEGE OF CHEST PHYSICIANS AND THE SOCIETY OF CRITICAL CARE MEDICINE CONSENSUS CONFERENCE DEFINITIONS

Infection Microbial phemonenon characterized by an inflammatory response to the presence of microorganisms or the invasion of normally sterile host tissue by those organisms

Bacteremia The presence of viable bacteria in the blood

Systemic inflammatory response syndrome The systemic inflammatory response to a variety of severe clinical insults, manifested by two or more of the following conditions
Temperature >38°C or <36°C
Heart rate >90 beats/min
Respiratory rate >20 breaths/min or $Paco_2$ <32 mm Hg
White blood cell count >12,000/mm^3, <4,000/mm^3, or >10% immature (band) forms

Sepsis The systemic response to infection, manifested by two or more of the following conditions as a result of infection
Temperature >38°C or <36°C
Heart rate >90 beats/min
Respiratory rate >20 breaths/min or $Paco_2$ <32 mm Hg
White blood cell count >12,000/mm^3, <4,000/mm^3, or >10% immature (band) forms

Severe sepsis Sepsis-induced hypotension despite adequate fluid resuscitation, along with perfusion abnormalities that may include, but are not limited to, lactic acidosis, oliguria, or an acute alteration in mental status. Patients receiving inotropic or vasopressor agents may not be hypotensive at the time that perfusion abnormalities are measured.

Sepsis-induced hypotension A systolic blood pressure <90 mm Hg or a reduction of ≥40 mm Hg from baseline in the absence of other causes for hypotension

Multiple organ dysfunction syndrome Altered organ function in an acutely ill patient such that homeostasis cannot be maintained without intervention.

(From Bone RC, Balk RA, Cerra FB, et al. Definitions for sepsis and organ failure and guidelines for the use of innovative therapies in sepsis. *Chest* 1992;101:1646, with permission.)

thermia (Table 268.2). Septic shock occurs when sepsis results in hypotension associated with organ hypoperfusion.

The initial event in the sepsis cascade is the release of mediator or mediators from infecting bacteria at the site of infection or after invasion of the bloodstream (Fig. 268.1). These exogenous mediators initiate the inflammatory process that results in sepsis. The lipopolysaccharide (LPS) of the cell wall of gram-negative bacteria, or endotoxin, has been implicated as the primary exogenous mediator in the pathogenesis of gram-negative sepsis. Other bacterial components or products that may play a significant role in the pathogenesis of sepsis include peptidoglycan, muramyl dipeptide, lipoteichoic acid, staphylococcal enterotoxin B, toxic shock toxin 1, and *Pseudomonas* exotoxin A. Infusion of endotoxin in primates mimics much of the clinical picture of gram-negative shock seen in humans. The fact that symptoms in patients with gram-negative bacteremia initially worsen when antimicrobial agents are started suggests that endotoxin is released as bacterial cell walls are lysed as a result of therapy.

In the pathogenesis of sepsis, endotoxin activates monocytes and macrophages to secrete inflammatory cytokines and other mediators. These endogenous mediators of sepsis act on various target cells, leading to shock and multiorgan system failure. Two lipid A binding proteins have been identified that play an important role in sepsis—LPS binding protein (LBP) and bactericidal/permeability-increasing protein (BPI). Although LBP and BPI share similar DNA homology, they have different chemical properties. LBP potentiates the binding of endotoxin to CD14 receptors on monocytes, neutrophils, and endothelial cells necessary for the release of cytokines that mediate the sepsis syndrome. In contrast, BPI is a protein with bactericidal, endotoxin-neutralizing properties and blocks binding of LPS and LBP and hence the LPS/CD14 interaction. BPI is considered essential for polymorphonuclear cells to destroy gram-negative bacteria.

A series of observations have significantly advanced our knowledge of the pathophysiology of this syndrome. It appears that the signaling unit of the LPS receptor is a member of the Toll-like receptor (TLR) family. Expression of a member of the human TLR family, TLR2, confers LPS responsiveness. This responsiveness is dependent on LBP and CD14. Mutation or deletion of murine TLR results in a phenotype with markedly reduced or absent responses to LPS.

There are many potentially important endogenous mediators of sepsis in humans, such as tumor necrosis factor (TNF), interleukin-1 (IL-1), IL-6, IL-8, and platelet-activating factor. Secreted by mononuclear cells, TNF may be the most important endogenous mediator. In animal models, injection of TNF results in hypotension, neutropenia, and enhanced capillary permeability. Administration of TNF to healthy human volunteers produces signs of sepsis. Recent evidence, however, suggests that endotoxemia may produce the manifestations of sepsis independently of TNF. Therefore, the exact role of TNF in sepsis has not been elucidated completely. To complicate matters, despite the high circulating levels of TNF found in sepsis, increased levels also occur in the context of congestive heart failure, rheumatoid arthritis, and HIV wasting syndrome.

Other endogenous mediators of sepsis released after macrophage activation are IL-1, IL-6, and IL-8. In addition, arachidonic acid is metabolized to release leukotrienes, prostaglandins, and thromboxane A_2, which result in endothelial damage leading to hemodynamic instability in patients with septic shock. Another endogenous mediator, platelet-activating factor, exacerbates the generalized inflammatory response. These endogenous mediators have complex interactions and contribute to the end-organ damage that increases the mortality rate in patients with multiple organ dysfunction syndrome.

Nitric oxide (NO) has been investigated for its role in the pathophysiologic course of sepsis. In inflammatory conditions, NO production is catalyzed by the enzyme-inducible nitric oxide synthetase (iNOS). In animal models of infection, pneumococci induce NO, iNOS, and TNF production. Further studies are necessary to elucidate better the role of NO in the pathogenesis of sepsis.

FACTORS PREDISPOSING TO BACTEREMIA AND SEPSIS

Invasive bacterial infections occur more frequently in patients with a defect in a natural protective barrier to infection or a

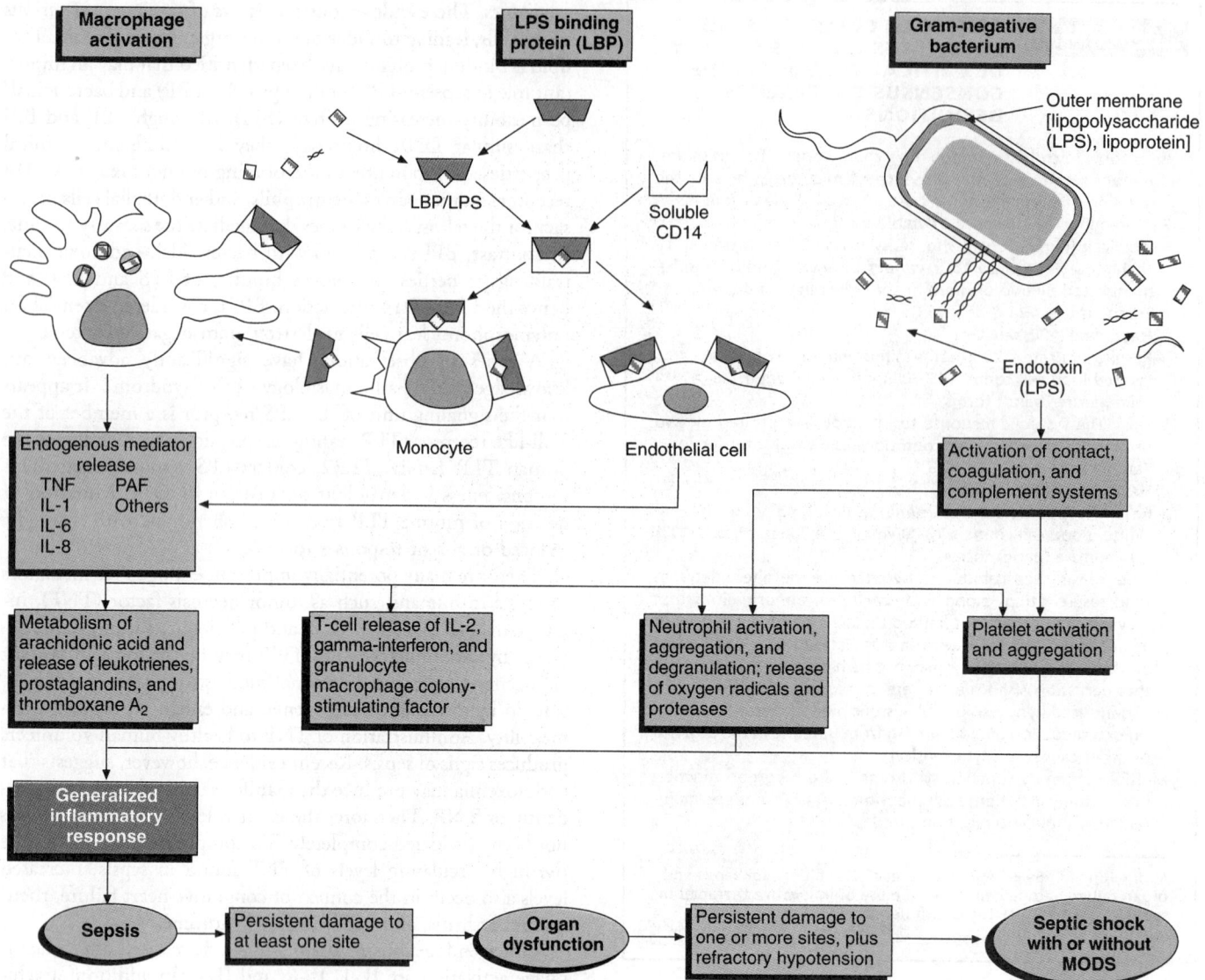

FIGURE 268.1. Schematic representation of the sepsis cascade. (From Bone RC. The pathogenesis of sepsis. *Ann Intern Med* 1991;115:457–469, with permission.)

deficiency in the inflammatory response or in the cellular or humoral immune system relevant to these infections. With most bacteria, control of infection depends on normal numbers and function of polymorphonuclear leukocytes (PMNs) and the serum opsonins, complement components, or specific antibody. Various conditions and therapies alter the normal functioning of these components of the host inflammatory response. Furthermore, serious underlying illnesses are also a major determinant of prognosis. The classification system of McCabe and Jackson, published in 1962, documented that patients with a rapidly fatal illness (acute leukemia) and an ultimately fatal illness (uremia) have a progressively worse prognosis than patients with bacteremia without underlying disease. Although there has been a marked improvement in the results of therapy for bacteremia over the past 30 years, this principle remains valid.

The most serious condition predisposing patients to bacteremia is neutropenia. The incidence and the lethality of bacteremia due to gram-negative bacilli and, to a lesser extent, gram-positive cocci, are directly proportional to the absolute neutrophil count. Although neutropenia is defined as an absolute neutrophil count less than 500 per microliter, the risk is greatest when the count is below 100 per microliter. Ultimate survival in all series correlates most directly with bone marrow recovery and restoration of normal white blood cell counts. The introduction of granulocyte colony-stimulating factors has lessened the duration of neutropenia in many patients after chemotherapy and bone marrow transplantation; however, their use has not been accompanied by a decreased risk of infection.

Age is another important determinant of bacterial invasion. This association has been most clearly documented in the case of nosocomial infections. The deficiency in older adults has not been delineated completely; although deterioration of the immune system has been postulated, the most plausible explanation is the increased incidence of cardiac, pulmonary, cerebrovascular, and neoplastic diseases and diabetes that occurs with advancing age. Catheterization of the urinary tract has also been shown to be a significant risk factor for bacteremia in the elderly.

Other conditions frequently associated with bacteremia include alcoholism with or without cirrhosis and diabetes. Acute alcohol intoxication impairs PMN function, as does hepatic disease. Diabetes mellitus is also associated with defective PMN responses to chemotactic stimuli, even if glucose metabolism is well controlled. In addition, phagocytosis and bacterial killing are defective in some patients with diabetes and in all patients with acidosis. Although *Candida* infections or staphylococcal skin infections develop with increased frequency, there is little evidence that infections are more prevalent in persons with well-controlled diabetes. Increased morbidity with infection has been documented in these patients, however.

In addition to the neutropenia due to malignant hematologic disease or cytotoxic chemotherapy, patients with neoplasms are at higher risk of serious infection. The hypogammaglobulinemia of lymphoproliferative diseases is associated with bacteremia due to encapsulated organisms. Obstruction of the gastrointestinal or genitourinary tract by tumors is a major cause of sepsis, and alteration in PMN function is also observed with certain solid tumors. Inhibitors of PMN chemotaxis have been described in patients with bronchogenic carcinoma and Hodgkin's disease. Malnutrition as a consequence of carcinoma also results in alteration in white cell function and serum opsonic capacity.

Treatment with medications other than cytotoxic chemotherapy also can be associated with an increased risk of sepsis due to abnormalities in white cell function. Corticosteroids have many effects on host defenses but clearly interfere with PMN function. Administration of glucocorticoids is associated with the release of cells from marrow reserves, but these agents also inhibit adhesion of PMNs to endothelial cells. Therefore, PMNs cannot leave the vascular compartment to reach the site of infection. Initial studies advocated the use of steroids as adjunctive therapy in patients with gram-negative bacteremia, especially those with septic shock. Subsequently, large, well-controlled, multicenter investigations clearly have shown no beneficial effect from the use of steroids in the treatment of sepsis.

Asplenic patients are particularly susceptible to bacteremic infections with encapsulated organisms, such as *S. pneumoniae* and *N. meningitidis*. These patients often have high-grade bacteremia, and organisms are identified frequently by examination of the peripheral blood smear. The exact mechanism of action responsible for this deficiency, which is also found in patients with sickle cell disease, is unclear. It is believed to be due to a deficiency of the alternate complement pathway, failure of antibody production, or failure of clearance mechanisms by the remaining reticuloendothelial system. For this reason, patients undergoing splenectomy should receive vaccination against *S. pneumoniae* before the procedure.

Deficiency of the terminal complement pathway is associated with an increased risk of bacteremic infections due to *Neisseria* species. This is a consequence of a defective lytic capacity of serum in the absence of the complement components 5 through 9. Deficiency of C3, the primary component in opsonization of *S. aureus* and gram-negative bacilli, results in a clinical picture resembling that seen in patients with neutropenia.

Patients with HIV-1 infection are also at increased risk of bacteremia, primarily due to encapsulated organisms. Although bacteremia traditionally has been considered a T-cell deficiency, HIV-1-infected persons also have defects in B-cell function. With disease progression, these patients often show signs of neutrophil dysfunction as well as abnormalities in cytokine production. These altered host defenses raise AIDS patients' risk of bacteremia due to encapsulated organisms, *S. aureus*, gram-negative bacilli, *Listeria monocytogenes*, and *Salmonella* species. In addition, infection due to *Rochalimaea henselae* and *Rochalimaea quintana*, the recently identified sources of bacillary angiomatosis and peliosis hepatis, are more common in HIV-1-infected persons.

Another predisposing factor for bacteremia is previous antibiotic therapy. Bloodstream infections due to enteric gram-negative bacilli, enterococci, and fungi are more common in patients with previous antimicrobial exposure. Examples include the association of second- and third-generation cephalosporins with enterococcal bacteremia and the relationship of vancomycin and vancomycin-resistant enterococci. *Klebsiella* sepsis has been noted in neurosurgical patients receiving antibiotic prophylaxis, *Enterobacter* sepsis has been associated with broad-spectrum antibiotic use, and *Stenotrophomonas* (*Xanthomonas*) *maltophilia* bacteremia can result from administration of imipenem.

The increased use of medical devices, such as intravenous and bladder catheters, is a major cause of nosocomial bacteremia, sepsis, and fungemia. It is estimated that 0.3% of all patients with an indwelling bladder catheter experience urosepsis. Devices that breach the natural protective barrier of the skin predispose patients to bloodstream infections with normal cutaneous flora, especially staphylococci. Although it rarely happens, intravenous fluids contaminated with bacteria also have been implicated as a source of bacteremia. Finally, prolonged survival of seriously ill patients, invasive diagnostic and therapeutic procedures, and increased use of immunosuppressive medications are all important risk factors for sepsis.

OPTIMAL MANAGEMENT

Diagnosis of bacteremia requires extreme vigilance and awareness, especially in patients who are afebrile or have low-grade fever. Therefore, blood cultures should be undertaken for all patients admitted to the hospital with an infectious disease. Prompt initiation of antimicrobial therapy is important in preventing death in patients with gram-negative sepsis and the complications that may result from bacteremia, such as endocarditis, osteomyelitis, or abscesses. In acutely ill patients, especially those in shock, a multidisciplinary approach is appropriate, often calling on clinicians with expertise in infectious disease and critical care medicine and, in some instances, surgeons.

After obtaining appropriate cultures, initial antimicrobial therapy should be directed at the most likely etiologic agent that results in the specific infection. No single antibiotic or combination of agents is effective for all patients with bacteremic infections. Ultimately, empiric therapy should be guided by the organisms most likely responsible for each infection and susceptibility patterns within each institution. When final identification and susceptibility are determined, however, therapy should be adjusted to provide the most narrow-spectrum, cost-effective antibiotic.

For patients in shock, a rapid assessment to determine the probable site of infection or portal of entry is critical. Careful attention should be paid to the respiratory and urinary tracts as possible foci of infection. To this end, examination of the urine for pyuria and bacteriuria and a chest radiograph are useful adjuncts to Gram's stain and cultures of blood, urine, and sputum. Empiric antibiotics and intravenous fluids should be administered cocomitantly with the initial assessment. If the patient is hypotensive and does not respond to fluid resuscitation, vasopressors should be initiated.

For suspected intravenous device infections, a penicillinase-resistant penicillin (oxacillin or nafcillin) or vancomycin is appropriate. Oxacillin is preferred if the infection is community acquired and vancomycin for nosocomial infections or for penicillin-allergic patients. For patients with an intra-abdominal focus of infection, antibiotics that provide coverage against enteric gram-negative bacilli, enterococci, and anaerobes are necessary. In the febrile patient with neutropenia, an antipseudomonal β-lactam antibiotic in combination with an aminoglycoside is preferred, but monotherapy with ceftazidime is effective. Empiric antifungal therapy is often required for patients with neutropenia who remain febrile on broad-spectrum antibiotics. Owing to delays in the diagnosis of fungemia, empiric antifungal therapy also may be warranted in patients with severe intra-abdominal infections, those on prolonged courses of antibiotics, and those receiving parenteral nutrition or corticosteroids.

Antibiotics should be administered at the highest dose consistent with the patient's physiologic condition. In general, the maintenance dose and interval should be based on the half-life of the agent and the expected clearance. With antibiotics that have narrow therapeutic windows, such as the aminoglycosides, serum concentrations should be monitored to prevent toxicity. The duration of antibiotic therapy in patients with bacteremia varies with the host and the specific organism. Guidelines have been developed through experience or clinical trials, but the duration of parenteral therapy requires clinical judgment. An exception is *S. aureus* bacteremia, for which 2 weeks of parenteral antistaphylococcal therapy is recommended in a normal host with a removable focus of infection. The greatest risk of inadequate therapy for staphylococcal bacteremia is the development of endocarditis or osteomyelitis. With bacteremic pyelonephritis, parenteral antibiotics can be discontinued when the patient is afebrile and clinically stable. In the febrile patient with neutropenia, parenteral antibiotics should be continued until the neutropenia resolves. If blood culture gives positive results, the duration of antibiotic therapy should be 14 days, even if neutropenia resolves. Patients with bacteremic pneumonia can be switched from parenteral to oral therapy when fever and toxicity abate. Patients with bacteremia should be monitored carefully for evidence of metastatic foci of infection, such as meningitis, endocarditis, osteomyelitis, and arthritis.

In addition to appropriate antibiotics, the management of bacteremia complicated by shock requires supportive care to alter the physiologic effects of sepsis. Initially, aggressive fluid replacement is necessary to reverse the cardiovascular collapse that can accompany shock. Saline is as effective as colloid solutions. Adequate volume replacement can best be determined by monitoring the pulmonary arterial wedge pressure with a pulmonary artery (Swan-Ganz) catheter in a critical care unit. Pulmonary artery wedge pressures should be maintained between 12 and 18 mm Hg.

Failure of adequate fluid administration to reverse hypotension is an indication for the use of vasopressors, such as dopamine. In doses below 5 μ per kilogram per minute, dopamine increases renal artery and mesenteric blood flow. At higher infusion rates (5 to 10 μ per kilogram per minute), dopamine exerts β-adrenergic effects; at rates above 10 μ per kilogram per minute, α-adrenergic effects predominate. If dopamine fails to raise blood pressure, norepinephrine should be administered. Dobutamine and isoproterenol can be used to increase cardiac output, but they should not be given alone because they diminish peripheral vascular resistance.

Many patients with septic shock require intubation and mechanical ventilation to correct hypoxia. Intubation should be considered for patients with a PaO_2 below 50 to 60 mm Hg despite supplemental oxygen or increasing respiratory muscle fatigue. A careful balance must be maintained between excessive positive end-expiratory pressure, causing barotrauma, and a high fraction of inspired oxygen, leading to oxygen toxicity.

Improvement in disseminated intravascular coagulation and the acidosis stemming from hypoperfusion results from control of infection and restoration of hemodynamic status. For this reason, only rarely is sodium bicarbonate or heparin indicated. In patients with severe depletion of clotting factors or platelets, infusion of fresh frozen plasma or platelets can be used to stop serious bleeding until the underlying infection is controlled.

One of the most exciting but controversial issues in the treatment of sepsis is the use of therapies aimed at blocking the deleterious effects of exogenous and endogenous mediators of sepsis (endotoxin, TNF, IL-1). Despite initial optimism, none of the controlled clinical trials using such agents provided a therapeutic benefit to all enrolled patients. With subgroup analysis, however, the evidence suggests that blocking mediators of sepsis might be of therapeutic value.

Monoclonal antibodies directed at the lipid A component of endotoxin have been the most rigorously investigated. E5 is a murine antibody and HA-1A is of human origin. Initially, HA-1A appeared to be effective in limiting mortality rates, and E5 seemed to be effective in minimizing organ dysfunction in patients with gram-negative bacteremia, but subsequent studies could not reproduce these initial results. The most recent large, multicenter, placebo-controlled trial with HA-1A failed to show improvement in the 14-day mortality rate in patients with gram-negative bacteremia and septic shock. There was a trend toward increased mortality rates among patients treated with HA-1A who had gram-positive bacteremia or fungemia.

Despite impressive results in animals, anti-TNF monoclonal antibodies have shown mixed results in humans. In a large multicenter study, anti-TNF antibodies were of no benefit in patients without circulatory (hemodynamic) collapse, but there was a reduction in mortality rates among patients with septic shock. Because of the different doses used, a statistically significant difference was not established, and another trial evaluating this agent is under way.

An IL-1 receptor antagonist (IL-1RA) has been shown to improve mortality rates in animal models of infection. In one large, multicenter, placebo-controlled trial, there was no benefit to IL-1RA in all patients enrolled or in the subgroup with shock. A retrospective review of this study found that IL-1RA lowered mortality rates in patients whose predicted mortality rate by APACHE III exceeded 24%. A prospective trial will be needed to confirm the usefulness of this agent in this subset of patients.

A recombinant protein has been developed that corresponds to the amino-terminal 23-kd fragment of BPI ($rBPI_{23}$). This protein has established antibacterial properties and has neutralized LPS activity in vitro. In animal models of sepsis, $rBPI_{23}$ has prevented binding of LPS to monocytes, thereby inhibiting the release of inflammatory cytokines. Experimental studies suggest that monoclonal antibodies directed at CD14 protect rabbits against organ injury and death after exposure to LPS. Additional animal studies and, ultimately, human trials will be necessary to evaluate the efficacy of these proteins in sepsis.

■ PREVENTION OF BACTEREMIA

The physician can do little to prevent bacteremia in community-acquired infections other than to administer prophylactic antibiotics to patients with valvular heart disease undergoing elective procedures associated with bacteremia. It is not as clear that patients with prosthetic joints should be treated in a similar fashion. There is increasing evidence that patients receiving chemotherapy who show signs of neutropenia are protected in part by prophylactic antibiotics; however, this benefit is counterbalanced by the increased risk of selection of resistant organisms. Widespread use of quinolones for prophylaxis has been associated with intensifying resistance to this class of antibiotics in *E. coli* and coagulase-negative staphylococci. In addition, the use of these agents predisposes patients with neutropenia to streptococcal bacteremia. More worrisome is the indiscriminate use of these and other antibiotics, which may lead to the dissemination of multidrug-resistant bacteria among the general population.

Nosocomial bacteremias can be limited by the recognition of known risk factors and adherence to proper infection-control procedures. An important vector for the transmission of nosocomial pathogens is the hands of hospital personnel: vancomycin-resistant enterococci can survive at least 1 hour on the hands of healthy adults and up to 1 week on environmental surfaces within the hospital. Therefore, major educational efforts and room design to facilitate hand washing can lessen the nosocomial spread of gram-negative bacilli, enterococci, and staphylococci.

The indiscriminate use of antibiotics also contributes to infection. The administration of second- or third-generation cephalosporins to hospitalized patients may predispose them to enterococcal bacteremia. In addition, pharyngeal colonization by gram-negative bacilli increases with prolonged antibiotic use; these organisms often are highly resistant to antimicrobial agents. The efficacy of antimicrobial prophylaxis before a surgical procedure is well established, but prolonged postoperative use of antibiotics should be discouraged.

Another determinant of bacteremia is the widespread use of intravenous and intra-arterial catheters. The incidence of local infection associated with vascular catheters varies from 4% to 57%, and the rate of bacteremia ranges from 4% to 14%. Infection rates increase with the length of time catheters are left in place. Guidelines regarding the proper use and maintenance of these devices have been published.

Various therapeutic methods used in the care of critically ill patients have been implicated as risk factors for bacteremia. Ventilatory equipment, nebulizers, pressure transducers, hyperalimentation fluids, blood, disinfectants, and irrigation fluids all have been associated with nosocomial infection. The advent of disposable equipment, appropriate sterilization, and single-use bottles and vials have helped control this problem. Patients infected or colonized with resistant organisms should be isolated according to standard infection-control procedures. Patients with enteric infections, draining wounds, and respiratory tract infections also require isolation. Standard guidelines outlining the proper methods of isolation and cohorting of patients during an outbreak have been published.

A surveillance program led by a knowledgeable physician is necessary for optimal infection control. Ongoing monitoring of bacterial flora causing nosocomial infections, their antimicrobial susceptibility, and the location of such infections can detect an early outbreak and prevent large or prolonged problems. The infection-control department must be committed to education, have authority, and be actively supported by hospital staff and administration. Prevention of infection and bacteremia in the hospital is difficult but necessary. Patients admitted to the hospital are increasingly ill, have more complex problems, and require aggressive support. Not all infections and bacteremias can be prevented, but careful attention to proper infection-control procedures can help manage this major problem.

BIBLIOGRAPHY

Bone RC. Toward an epidemiology and natural history of SIRS. *JAMA* 1992;268:3452–3455.

Bone RC, Balk RA, Cerra FB, et al. Definitions for sepsis and organ failure and guidelines for the use of innovative therapies in sepsis. The ACCP/SCCM Consensus Conference Committee. American College of Chest Physicians/Society of Critical Care Medicine. *Chest* 1992;101:1644–1655.

Chandrasekar PH, Brown WJ. Clinical issues of blood cultures. *Arch Intern Med* 1994;154:841–849.

Dajani AS, Taubert KA, Wilson W, et al. Prevention of bacterial endocarditis: recommendations by the American Heart Association. *JAMA* 1997;277:1794–1801.

DuPont HL, Spink WM. Infections due to gram-negative organisms: an analysis of 860 patients with bacteremia at the University of Minnesota Medical Center, 1958–1966. *Medicine (Baltimore)* 1969;48:307–332.

Gazzano-Santoro H, Meszaros K, Birr C, et al. Competition between $rBPI_{23}$, a recombinant fragment of bactericidal/permeability-increasing protein, and lipopolysaccharide (LPS)–binding protein for binding to LPS and gram-negative bacteria. *Infect Immunol* 1994;62:1185–1191.

Kirschning CJ, Wesche H, Ayres TM, et al. Human toll-like receptor 2 confers responsiveness to bacterial lipopolysaccharide. *J Exp Med* 1998;188:2091–2097.

Kohn FR, Ammons WS, Horwitz A, et al. Protective effect of a recombinant amino-terminal fragment of bactericidal/permeability-increasing protein in experimental endotoxemia. *J Infect Dis* 1993;168:1307–1310.

Linden PK. Clinical implications of nosocomial gram-positive bacteremia and superimposed antimicrobial resistance. *Am J Med* 1998;104(5A): 24S–33S.

Martin MA. Epidemiology and clinical impact of gram-negative sepsis. *Infect Dis Clin North Am* 1991;5:739–752.

McCabe WR, Jackson GC. Gram-negative bacteremia. *Arch Intern Med* 1962;110:847.

McCloskey RV, Straube RC, Sanders C, et al. Treatment of septic shock with human monoclonal antibody HA-1A: a randomized, double-blind, placebo-controlled trial. CHESS Trial Study Group. *Ann Intern Med* 1994;121:1–5.

Rackow EC, Astiz ME. Pathophysiology and treatment of septic shock. *JAMA* 1991;266:548–554.

Schimke J, Mathison J, Morgiewcz J, et al. Anti-CD14 mAb treatment provides therapeutic benefit after in vivo exposure to endotoxin. *Proc Natl Acad Sci USA* 1998;95:13875–13880.

Talan DA. Recent developments in our understanding of sepsis: evaluation of anti-endotoxin antibodies and biological response modifiers. *Ann Emerg Med* 1993;22:1871–1890.

Ziegler EJ, Fisher CJ Jr, Sprung CL, et al. Treatment of gram-negative bacteremia and septic shock with HA-1A human monoclonal antibody against endotoxin: a randomized, double-blind, placebo-controlled trial. *N Engl J Med* 1991;324:429–436.

Kelley's Textbook of Internal Medicine, fourth edition. Edited by H. David Humes. Lippincott Williams & Wilkins, Philadelphia © 2000.

C H A P T E R
269

APPROACH TO THE PATIENT WITH RECURRENT INFECTIONS

BURKE A. CUNHA

Recurrent infections are defined as repeated infections due to the same or different microorganisms, which may be immunologically or nonimmunologically related. Recurrent infections may be due to reinfection or relapse. Relapse refers to recurrent infection by the same organism, whereas reinfection refers to repeated infections caused by different microorganisms. Recurrent infections must be differentiated from coincidental recurrences that appear to have a recurrent pattern, for example, viral upper-respiratory tract infections. Furthermore, many multisystem disorders are characterized by exacerbations and remissions that mimic recurrent infections, among them, sarcoidosis and systemic lupus erythematosus. Noninfectious conditions that mimic recurrent infections are very common. Most recurrent infections are not immunologically mediated.

GENERAL CONCEPTS

Immunologically based recurrent infections are uncommon. Immunodeficiency disorders causing recurrent infections may be congenital or acquired. Acquired immunodeficiency syndromes are encountered more often in clinical practice (e.g., HIV-, drug-induced, malignancy-associated conditions), whereas congenital primary immunodeficiencies are very rare. Historical clues to immune-mediated, recurrent infections include repeated infections by encapsulated organisms or unusually severe, persistent infections by low-virulence hallmark organisms that are always associated with impaired host defenses, among them, invasive aspergillosis, *Pneumocystis carinii* pneumonia (PCP), and *Toxoplasma* meningoencephalitis. Immune-deficiency screening tests should not be undertaken for patients with coincidental or clustered recurrences of infection, especially those with repeated upper-respiratory viral illnesses. Immunologically mediated recurrent infections have characteristic histories and patterns of infection due to specific microorganisms. Screening for immune defects should be obtained only if there is an appropriate antecedent history of infectious pathogens associated with immunodeficiencies.

CLINICAL APPROACH

The most common recurrent infections are meningitis, otitis, pharyngitis, pneumonia, urinary tract infection, cellulitis, device-related infections, and chronic osteomyelitis. Recurrent meningitis may have an immune or nonimmune source. Most recurrent infections encountered by the internist are associated with structural defects, foreign bodies, inadequately drained abscesses, inadequate antimicrobial therapy (inadequate spectrum, dose/duration, or tissue penetration).

After coincidental recurrences have been eliminated from diagnostic consideration, noninfectious conditions that resemble recurrent infections should be ruled out. The differential diagnosis of noninfectious mimics of recurrent infection is best approached from a regional or organ system perspective. In multisystem disorders (e.g., systemic lupus erythematosus), with predominant findings in one organ system, there will be evidence of disease elsewhere, which should provide clues to the origin of the primary disease process. After eliminating recurrent infectious sources that are not immunologically mediated, the diagnostic approach should be directed toward immunologically based disorders. Either the pattern of organ involvement or the type of microorganism should suggest a defect in humoral (HI) or cell-mediated immunity (CMI).

NONIMMUNE-MEDIATED RECURRENT INFECTIONS

Urinary tract infections are a common cause of recurrent infection. Recurrent cystitis is usually due to repeated reinfection, but chronic prostatitis/pyelonephritis, genitourinary anatomical defects, and stones are prone to relapse. Recurrent pharyngitis is usually viral in origin and not due to group A streptococci (GAS). GAS frequently colonize patients with viral pharyngitis. The finding of GAS by rapid antibody testing or culture does not distinguish colonization from infection. Recurrent GAS colonization is a common problem among teachers and caretakers of children. Look for a viral source underlying *Mycoplasma pneumoniae*, *Chlamydia pneumoniae*, or recurrent pharyngitis with/without GAS colonization. Chronic osteomyelitis in the context of diabetes is one of the most common recurrent infections in adults. Chronic, deeply penetrating ulcers or draining sinus tracts are indicative of chronic osteomyelitis, which can be cured only by adequate surgical debridement. Infections associated with foreign bodies or prosthetic materials usually cannot be relieved by antimicrobial therapy—surgical removal is necessary.

IMMUNE-MEDIATED RECURRENT INFECTIONS

The medical history is important in establishing the pattern of recurrent infections due to immunity defects. Children with CMI problems often have initial signs of severe varicella, invasive fungal infections, or acute reactions to live vaccines. Older children and adults have histories of anergy or several malignancies. Children and adults with conditions related to CMI typically have recurrent infections due to intracellular organisms (herpes simplex, PCP, *Listeria*, *Aspergillus*).

Children with humoral defects often have a long history of recurrent sinopulmonary infections, meningitis, bacteremias, diarrhea, or cellulitis. Adults frequently give a family history of severe or recurrent infections, autoimmune diseases, or B-cell malignancies. Children and adults with HI defects have unusually severe infections due to common organisms (*Giardia*, enteroviruses, *Mycoplasma pneumoniae*) or repeated infection due to encapsulated organisms (*Neisseria meningitidis*, *Streptococcus pneumoniae*, or *Hemophilus influenzae*). The history together with the type of organism determine whether the recurrent infection is based on an HI or a CMI defect (Table 269.1).

IMMUNODEFICIENCY SCREENING TESTS

Tests for HI deficiencies should identify antibody, complement, or phagocytic defects. Antibody defects are the most common and are identified by quantitative serum immunoglobulins. Serum IgA levels are the single most important determination, because they are depressed in all immunodeficiency disorders with significant antibody defects. HI may also be assessed by measuring IgG antibody titers to protein/polysaccharide vaccines. Patients with defective or inadequate antibody responses will have low titers (or none at all) after common immunizations (diphtheria, tetanus, *Hemophilus*, *Streptococcus pneumoniae*). IgG subclass determinations should not be part of the antibody defects workup. Since IgG subclass deficiencies are associated with autoimmune diseases, not infectious diseases, complement defects can be screened by the serum CH 50 level. If the CH 50 level is low, the individual complement components (C2, C3 and C4) can be measured.

Terminal components of the complement cascade (C6-7) are associated with recurrent *Neisseria* infections. Phagocytic defects in HI can be detected by the white blood cell and differential count, which provides a quantitative measurement of circulating phagocytes. The nitroblue tetrazolium reduction test is used to assess phagocyte function. A serum IgE level is also helpful in identifying hyperimmunoglobulin E syndrome (Job's syndrome). CMI requires intact T-lymphocyte and macrophage function and can be assessed by total lymphocyte count and T-lymphocyte subsets. Anergy testing for impaired delayed-type hypersensitivity with PPD or *Candida* should be undertaken for patients with suspected CMI defects. HIV serologic studies should be carried out for patients who might have HIV. The focus of the diagnostic approach is to arrive at a definitive diagnosis of the immunodeficiency disorder responsible for recurrent infections after other causes have been excluded. The diagnosis of immunodeficiency disorders is syndromic (Table 269.2).

TREATMENT

The treatment for nonimmune recurrent infections is appropriate antibiotic therapy. Consideration should be given to the location of the infection and to whether the infection is intracellular, extracellular, or in a protected location. Pharmacokinetic considerations regarding intracellular tissue penetration are important in selecting optimal antimicrobial therapy. The duration of treatment is also important; it is prudent to treat patients with congenital or acquired immunodeficiency disorders for longer periods of time than usually are recommended.

Patients with some antibody deficiencies can be treated with intravenous gamma globulin therapy. Immunoglobulin replacement therapy is most useful in patients with agammaglobulinemia, antibody deficiencies with near normal immunoglobulin concentrations, Wiskott-Aldrich syndrome, severe combined immunodeficiency, and X-linked immunodeficiency with increased levels of IgM. Intravenous immunoglobulin preparations contain primarily IgG, and 400 mg per kilogram per month should be administered to approximate physiologic IgG levels. It is not possible to replace defects in secretory IgA with immunoglobulin therapy. Serum immunoglobulin contains very little IgA, and immunoglobulin therapy is contraindicated for IgA deficiency because of the high incidence of anti-IgA antibodies in intravenous immunoglobulin.

Primary immunodeficiency syndromes with CMI defects can be treated by bone marrow transplantation. The main concern of prolonged immunosuppression or treatment with chemotherapy is the development of subsequent malignancies. Patients with HIV have relapsing, recurrent infections. The infecting microorganisms are predictable by the degree of impaired CMI, as measured by the CD4 count. Prophylaxis or early treatment of infections in HIV/AIDS patients minimizes further T helper lymphocyte loss. Antigenic-induced stimulation of the immune system should be avoided in HIV patients. Purified protein derivative (PPD) testing also should not be undertaken in HIV patients, since it results in rapid destruction of T helper cells, hastening the patient's demise. Since most HIV patients are anergic, there is no point to PPD testing; tuberculosis should be diagnosed in other ways (sputum, blood, bone marrow, AF smears/culture).

TABLE 269.1   CLINICAL APPROACH TO THE PATIENT WITH RECURRENT INFECTIONS

Determine the recurrence problem.
  Distinguish coincidental recurrences (reinfection UTIs, repeated viral URIs) from true recurrent infections (more than one pneumonia/year or ≥3 episodes of pneumonia).
  In patients with recurrent infections, differentiate reinfection from relapse.
Eliminate noninfectious mimics of recurrent infections (very common).
  Recurrent systemic diseases that can resemble recurrent infections
    Sarcoidosis
    SLE
  Periodic drug reactions that can resemble recurrent infections
Recurrent nonimmunologically based infections (most common)
  Differentiate intermittent colonization from recurrent infection.
  Periodic reinfections
    Exacerbations of chronic bronchitis
    Recurrent group A streptococcal pharyngitis
    Recurrent lower-extremity group A streptococcal cellulitis
    Reinfection (cystitis)
    Recurrent aspiration pneumonia
  Congenital/structural abnormalities
    Recurrent meningitis/myelomeningocele
    Dural sinus leak
    Genitourinary structural abnormalities
    Right-middle-lobe syndrome/pneumonias
  Acquired abnormalities
    Foreign-body infections (removal required for cure)
      PVE
      CNS shunt infections
      Central i.v. line infections
      AV shunt infections
      Artificial joint replacements
      Infected prosthetic materials
  Antibiotic treatment failures (inadequate/inappropriate therapy)
    Intracellular pathogens, Salmonella, Chlamydia, Legionella
    Chronic prostatitis/pyelonephritis
    Endocarditis due to fastidious resistant organisms
  Protected/infected foci (surgical drainage required for cure)
    Undrained abscesses
    Biliary/renal stones
    Obstruction of CSF, bile, or urine
    Postobstructive pneumonias
    Chronic osteomyelitis

Recurrent immunologically based infections (rare)
  Diagnosis of immunologically based recurrent infections
    Rule out noninfectious mimics of recurrent infections.
    Rule out nonimmunologically mediated recurrent infections.
  Characteristics suggesting an immunologically based recurrent infection
    Characteristic patterns of organ involvement
      Recurrent sinopulmonary infections
      Recurrent skin abscesses (pyodermas)
      Bacteremias with metastatic focal infections
    Unusually severe/recurrent infections with common organisms
      Mycoplasma
      Giardiasis
    Persistent/chronic infection with common organisms
      Progressive Epstein–Barr virus
      Severe enteroviral meningoencephalitis
    Unusual host response to antigens/vaccines
      Absent DTH (anergy)
      Failure to develop immunity to protein/polysaccharide vaccines
      GVH response to blood transfusions
      Disease after live vaccines, e.g., vaccinia following smallpox vaccination
    Infections with hallmark organisms
      Severe infections with encapsulated organisms
        Streptococcus pneumoniae
        Hemophilus influenzae
        Neisseria meningitidis
      Severe infections with intracellular organisms
        Pneumocystis carinii pneumonia
        Invasive aspergillosis
        Toxoplasma
        Mycobacterium avium-intracellulare
Screening tests for suspected immunodeficiency syndromes

Suspected Immunodeficiency Problems

Humoral immunity
  (antibody/phagocyte/complement)
  Antibody defects
  Complement defects

  Phagocyte defects

Cell-mediated immunity (T lymphocyte/macrophage)

Screening Tests

Quantitative immunoglobulins (serum IgG, IgM, IgA levels)
Low/absent vaccine antibody IgG titers (diphtheria, tetanus, pneumococcus, *Hemophilus influenzae* type b)
CH 50
Serum C2, C3, C4, C5–9
WBC/differential count
NBT test
Serum IgE level
Total lymphocyte count
T-lymphocyte subsets
Anergy testing (PPD, *Candida*)
HIV serology

UTI, urinary tract infection; URI, upper-respiratory infection; SLE, systemic lupus erythematosus; CNS, central nervous system; AV, atrioventricular; CSF, cerebrospinal fluid; DTH, delayed-type hypersensitivity; GVH, graft versus host; WBC, white blood cell; NBT, nitroblue tetrazolium reduction test; PPD, purified protein derivative

TABLE 269.2	SYNOPSIS OF IMMUNODEFICIENCY SYNDROMES CAUSING RECURRENT INFECTIONS AND ASSOCIATIONS		
Clinical Onset	**Immunodeficiency Syndrome**	**Clinical Features**	**Comments/Clues**
Childhood	SCID (HI/CMI defect)	Recurrent oral candidiasis, recurrent diarrhea, recurrent otitis/sinopulmonary infections, anergy, 75% measles, childhood neonatal viral infections often fatal (HSV, CMV, RSV)	Eosinophilia, hypogammaglobulinemia, lymphopenia
Childhood	SCID with ADA deficiency (HI/CMI defect)	Recurrent oral candidiasis, recurrent diarrhea but no thymus, rib/scapular deformities, anergy	Eosinophilia, hypogammaglobulinemia, lymphopenia
Childhood	Ataxia-telangectasia (HI/CMI defect)	Recurrent oral candidiasis, recurrent diarrhea, recurrent pneumonia, progressive bronchiectasis, lymphoreticular malignancies, death from pulmonary infection/malignancy onset 2–3 years	↑ alpha fetoprotein, ↓ IgA (↓ IgG)
Infancy	Wiskott-Aldrich syndrome (HI/CMI defect)	Severe eczema; bleeding problems; recurrent otitis/sinopulmonary infections; bacteremias; lymphoreticular malignancies; anergy (late); death in childhood from infections or malignancies, neonatal bleeding; infection begins first year, death in childhood	↓ IgM (↑ IgA, ↑ IgE), thrombocytopenia (small platelets)
Childhood	Chronic granulomatous disease (HI/CMI defect)	Seborrheic dermatitis; gingivitis; aphthous ulcers; hepatosplenomegaly; draining lymph nodes with sinus tracts; recurrent abscesses of lungs, skin; osteomyelitis due to catalase (+) organisms; associated with discoid lupus 75% lupus	Eosinophilia
Childhood	Chediak–Higashi syndrome (CMI problem)	Partial oculocutaneous albinism; nystagmus; mental retardation; periodontal disease; peripheral neuropathy; lymphoma-like syndrome in young adults (hepatosplenomegaly)	Neutropenia; characteristic giant lysosomal granules in WBCs
Childhood	Hyperimmunoglobulinemia E (Job's syndrome) HI problem	Coarse facies; severe eczema; aphthous ulcers; periodontal disease; deep "cold" *Staphylococcus aureus* skin abscesses; associated with chronic mucocutaneous candidiasis	↑ IgE with mild eosinophilia
Infancy	X-linked (Bruton's) agammaglobulinemia (congenital), agammaglobulinemia (HI defect)	Aphthous ulcers; recurrent otiti/sinopulmonary infections; recurrent bacteremias; recurrent chronic enteroviral meningitis; associated with dermatomyositis, rheumatoid arthritis; no tonsils/nodes; asplenic men only; infections after first year, and 15% die of infection before adulthood	Hypogammaglobulinemia (↓ IgA, IgG, IgM), Howell-Jolly bodies
Infancy	Immunodeficiency with ↑ IgM (HI defect)	Resembles X-linked agammaglobulinemia	↑ IgM (↓ IgG, ↓ IgA)
Infancy	Selective IgA deficiency (HI defect)	Recurrent otitis/sinopulmonary infections; recurrent diarrhea (*Giardia*); bronchiectasis; anaphylactic reactions to blood, transfusions/gamma globulin; associated with rheumatoid arthritis, SLE	↓ IgA (normal IgG, IgM)
Childhood	Common variable immune deficiency, acquired hypogammaglobulinemia (HI problem)	Resembles X-linked agammaglobulinemia but normal tonsils, splenomegaly (25%), recurrent pneumonias, bronchiectasis; lymphoma-like presentation with fever, weight loss, generalized	Lymphocytosis (↓/N IgA, ↓ IgG, ↓/N IgM)
Childhood	X-linked lymphoproliferative disease (HI problem)	Males with EBV infection–complicated disease, acquired hypogammaglobulinemia, aplastic anemia, overwhelming infection/death, B-cell lymphomas	+ EBV serologies, hypogammaglobulinemia
Childhood	Selective IgM deficiency (HI problem)	Atopic, recurrent pneumococcal pneumonia/meningitis, splenomegaly, can live to adulthood if infections treated	↓ IgM
Adult	Hypogammaglobulinemia with thymoma (HI problem)	Severe diarrhea; RBC aplasia	Eosinopenia anemia
Infancy	DiGeorge syndrome (CMI problem)	Congenital heart disease (ASD/VSD), dysmorphic ears/facies, and neonatal hypocalcemic seizures; fatal reactions to live vaccines; antibody responses, not levels, impaired; may die in infancy of congenital heart disease; patients with mild cases may live to adulthood	Hypocalcemia ↓ IgA (↑ IgE)
Infancy	Nezelof syndrome (CMI problem)	Same as DiGeorge syndrome, but no facial abnormalities; small thymus	Lymphopenia
Childhood	Chronic mucocutaneous candidiasis (CMI problem)	Superficial, not invasive/disseminated candidiasis; anergic; associated with endocrinopathies	Polyclonal gammopathy

SCID, severe combined immunodeficiency; HI, humoral immunity; CMI, cell-mediated immunity; HSV, herpes simplex virus; CMV, cytomegalovirus; RSV, respiratory syncytial virus; WBC, white blood cell; SLE, systemic lupus erythematosus; EBV, Epstein–Barr virus; RBC, red blood cell; ASD, atrial septal defect; VSD, ventricular septal defect.

BIBLIOGRAPHY

Berger M, Sorensen RU. Immune defects associated with recurrent infections. *Adv Pediatr Infect Dis* 1989;4:111–138.

Buckley RH. Abnormal development of the immune system. In: Joklik WK, Willet HP, Amos DB, et al., eds. *Zinsser microbiology.* Norwalk, Connecticut: Appleton and Lange, 1992.

Fischer A. Severe combined immunodeficiencies. *Immunodef Rev* 1992;3: 83–100.

Grieco MH. *Infections in the abnormal host.* New York: Yorke Medical Books, 1980.

Puck JM. Primary immunodeficiency diseases. *JAMA* 1997;278: 1835–1841.

Wood RA, Sampson HA. The child with frequent infections. In: *Current problems in pediatrics.* New York: Year Book Medical Publishers, 1989.

Kelley's Textbook of Internal Medicine, fourth edition. Edited by H. David Humes.
Lippincott Williams & Wilkins, Philadelphia © 2000.

C H A P T E R

270

ENDOCARDITIS, INTRAVASCULAR INFECTIONS, PERICARDITIS, AND MYOCARDITIS

C. GLENN COBBS
MICHAEL SACCENTE

INFECTIVE ENDOCARDITIS

DEFINITION

Infective endocarditis (IE) refers to microbial invasion of the endocardium, including both valvular and nonvalvular surfaces. The term *infective endocarditis* is preferred to the older term *bacterial endocarditis* because the latter ignores microbial pathogens, such as rickettsiae, mycoplasma, chlamydiae, and fungi. Previously, the terms *acute bacterial endocarditis* and *subacute bacterial endocarditis* were used to distinguish varieties of the disorder with different clinical courses. Acute bacterial endocarditis referred to a clinical entity that was rapid in onset, was associated with toxicity and early complications, and typically was caused by *Staphylococcus aureus*, *Streptococcus pneumoniae*, *Streptococcus pyogenes*, or *Neisseria gonorrhoeae*. Subacute bacterial endocarditis described an illness with a more indolent and protracted course that was caused most often by viridans streptococci. These terms are no longer particularly useful, because there is a great deal of overlap, particularly with certain microorganisms. IE is also categorized as native valve endocarditis (NVE) or prosthetic valve endocarditis (PVE).

INCIDENCE AND EPIDEMIOLOGY

At present, the incidence of IE is approximately one case per 1,000 hospital admissions. The epidemiologic picture of IE is a function of the frequency of bloodstream invasion by pathogens and the prevalence of predisposing endocardial diseases. In developed countries during the past 50 years, there have been important changes in the sources of bacteremia and the prevalence of underlying endocardial lesions. The average age of patients with IE has increased from 35 in the era before antibiotics to the current mean age of about 55. This trend reflects the declining prevalence of rheumatic heart disease, the growing prevalence of degenerative valvular lesions, and the increased use of procedures in older patients that predispose to bacteremia. Mitral valve prolapse has been recognized more frequently as a predisposing lesion, especially in older men. Patients with the murmur of mitral regurgitation and/or valvular redundancy and thickening on echocardiography appear to be at highest risk.

Other factors that have resulted in changes in the epidemiologic characteristics of IE include the increased use of intravascular or intracardiac devices, such as prosthetic valves, pacemaker wires, pulmonary artery catheters, hemodialysis shunts, and intravenous catheters. Nosocomially acquired IE is becoming more prevalent. Parenteral drug use continues to be a significant problem in our society, and approximately 25% of patients with IE have injected illicit drugs. One episode of IE predisposes to a subsequent episode, and as increasing numbers of patients survive first episodes of IE, more cases of recurrent IE are being seen.

ETIOLOGY AND BACTERIOLOGY

Before 1960, *S. viridans* caused 60% to 70% of episodes of NVE, and staphylococci were responsible for 15% to 20% of cases; other microorganisms were less common. Since the 1970s, the percentage of cases caused by viridans streptococci has declined to about 35% (Table 270.1). The incidence of cases of staphylococcal and enterococcal IE has risen to account for 25% and 10% of cases, respectively.

Streptococci

Overall, streptococci are still the most commonly reported cause of NVE, with viridans streptococci predominating. About 80% of patients have underlying cardiac disease. Viridans streptococci are normal oral flora that gain access to the bloodstream through breaches in the oral mucosa. *Streptococcus bovis* IE is associated with bowel lesions, including colon cancer, and isolation of this organism from the blood should prompt an evaluation of the

| TABLE 270.1. | MICROBIAL ORIGIN OF NATIVE AND PROSTHETIC VALVE INFECTIVE ENDOCARDITIS[a] |

Microorganism	Incidence (%)		
	NVE	Early PVE	Late PVE
Streptococci	50	10[b]	30
Viridans	35	—	25
S. bovis	15	—	5
Enterococci	10	—	5
Staphylococci	25	50	40
S. aureus	23	15	10
Coagulase negative	2	35	30
Gram-negative bacilli	6	15	10
Diphtheroids	—	10	5
Fungi	1	10	5
Other and culture negative	8	5	5

NVE, native valve endocarditis; PVE, prosthetic valve endocarditis.
[a] Incidences are approximate; local experience will vary.
[b] Includes all streptococci and enterococci.

gastrointestinal tract. Ninety percent of patients with streptococcal IE are cured with appropriate therapy.

Enterococci

Enterococci are reported more and more often as the cause of IE. Older men undergoing genitourinary procedures, women undergoing gynecologic procedures, and parenteral drug users are at particular risk. The course is usually subacute but can be aggressive. Forty percent of patients have no known underlying heart disease.

Staphylococci

Overall, staphylococci cause 25% of cases of NVE; 90% are due to *S. aureus*. In some community hospitals, *S. aureus* is the most common microbe associated with IE. No previous valvular abnormality is found in about one-third of patients. The clinical course is often acute, and the mortality rate is 25% to 40% in non-addicts with mitral or aortic valve disease. In parenteral drug users with right-sided valvular infection, the clinical course is often less fulminant, and the prognosis is quite good. Complications more typically accompany *S. aureus* endocarditis than IE provoked by other bacteria; they include myocardial abscess, valve ring abscess, conduction defects, purulent pericarditis, and peripheral emboli. Metastatic suppuration in the brain, kidney, or spleen is seen in up to 40% of patients with left-sided *S. aureus* IE. Coagulase-negative staphylococci are the most prevalent source of PVE. They are unusual in the context of NVE.

Aerobic Gram-negative Bacteria

Aerobic gram-negative bacteria cause 5% to 10% of cases of IE. Intravenous drug abusers and patients with prosthetic valves are at greatest risk. When Enterobacteriaceae or *Pseudomonas aeruginosa* infect left-sided valves, the clinical course is frequently acute, and the mortality rate is high. The acronym HACEK is used to designate a special group of fastidious, aerobic, gram-negative bacteria that produce a characteristic clinical variety of NVE. This group includes *Haemophilus* species, *Actinobacillus actinomycetemcomitans*, *Cardiobacterium hominis*, *Eikenella corrodens*, and *Kingella* species. Clinical features include previous valvular disease, a subacute clinical course, embolic complications, large vegetations, and the frequent need for valve replacement.

Culture-negative Endocarditis

In 5% to 10% of patients with presumed IE, no etiologic microorganism is isolated from blood. The usual reason for this inability to identify the responsible microorganism is previous antimicrobial therapy. Fastidious microorganisms, such as HACEK group bacteria, nutritionally deficient streptococci, anaerobic bacteria, bartonellae, rickettsiae (*Coxiella burnetii*), and fungi, may not be detected with routine culture methods. When culture-negative IE is suspected, the clinician should discuss the case with clinical microbiology laboratory personnel. Appropriate use of special culture media and techniques and serologic studies can help identify the source of IE in some patients with negative results on blood culture. For example, the lysis centrifugation technique increases the yield of blood cultures in IE caused by intracellular fungi.

PATHOGENESIS

The initiating event in the pathogenesis of IE is disruption of the endocardial surface; this leads to exposure of underlying collagen, to which platelets and fibrin adhere to form a sterile platelet/fibrin complex. The endocardial surface is disrupted by turbulent blood flow caused by acquired (rheumatic heart disease, degenerative valvular disease) or congenital valvular lesions. Direct endocardial injury can occur with central intravenous catheters, pacemaker wires, or other intravenous devices that reside in the heart. IE results when circulating microorganisms colonize the endocardial surface.

Microorganisms (usually bacteria) can invade the blood in several ways. In some instances, bloodstream invasion results from microbial extension past local anatomic barriers (skin, mucous membrane, and subcutaneous tissues) to lymphatics and the thoracic duct. A second mechanism of invasion is direct inoculation into capillaries and venules, as happens during dental or periodontal surgery. Bacterial adherence to a platelet/fibrin complex depends on the interaction between bacterial surface components and tissue receptors and may vary considerably for different bacteria. Staphylococci and streptococci possess the virulence factors necessary for adherence (the FimA surface protein of oral streptococci) more often than enteric gram-negative bacilli.

CLINICAL FEATURES

Clinical features of IE reflect host responses to acute or subacute heart valve inflammation, complicated by microbial invasion of the bloodstream, altered cardiac physiology due to valve damage, and remote tissue injury caused by immune complex disease, emboli, ischemia, and infarction.

History

There may be a history of underlying heart disease and a preceding bacteremic event, such as dental work, instrumentation of the gastrointestinal or genitourinary tract, or parenteral drug use. Fever is present in more than 90% of patients. Most patients with subacute disease have other nonspecific symptoms, such as malaise, arthralgias, myalgias, and fatigue. Symptoms of heart failure are present in about 50% of patients with NVE. Emboli to the lungs or abdominal organs may provoke chest or abdominal pain.

Physical Examination

Most patients with left-sided valvular disease have heart murmurs at some point in their illness, but they may not be evident initially. Classic peripheral signs of IE include petechiae, Roth's spots (oval retinal hemorrhages), splenomegaly, clubbing, Osler's nodes (painful, purple to red nodules found on the pads of the fingers or toes), linear splinter hemorrhages beneath the fingernails or toenails, and red, macular Janeway lesions on the palms or soles.

LABORATORY FINDINGS

Blood Cultures

Blood culture is the most important laboratory test for the diagnosis of IE. Bacteremia associated with IE is typically low grade and constant. One of the first two sets of blood cultures yields the etiologic bacteria in 90% of patients. At least three sets of blood cultures should be obtained within the first 24 hours from patients suspected of having IE.

Other Laboratory Tests

Several nonspecific laboratory test abnormalities can be found in patients with IE; they generally reflect inflammation and/or immune injury. Anemia of chronic disease occurs in about 80% of patients with IE and is more likely to be present in patients with subacute disease. Leukocytosis, unusual in the context of subacute IE, is more likely to develop in acute endocarditis due to staphylococci, pneumococci, or gonococci. The sedimentation rate is generally elevated. IgM antibody against IgG (rheumatoid factor) has been confirmed in almost half of patients with subacute IE. Concentrations of C-reactive protein and circulating immune complexes have been used in monitoring response to therapy. Patients with IE may have abnormal results of urinalysis, including hematuria in about 40% and proteinuria in 50%. These abnormalities reflect immune complex injury and infarction.

Echocardiography

Echocardiography has proved very useful in the diagnosis of IE. Transthoracic echocardiography shows vegetations in about 50% to 60% of patients with IE diagnosed clinically. Transesophageal echocardiography (TEE) is more accurate, with a sensitivity approaching 90%. TEE more readily identifies small vegetations and vegetations on pulmonary and prosthetic valves. A single negative TEE result does not exclude IE, but more than one negative result has a high negative predictive value. Echocardiography is also useful for defining the severity of valvular destruction, detecting complications (fistula, myocardial abscess, and proximal aortic mycotic aneurysm), and assessing the hemodynamic effects of IE. TEE is more sensitive than transthoracic echocardiography for identifying myocardial abscess. Some investigators have found that the presence, size, and mobility of vegetations correlate with adverse events, including arterial emboli, heart failure, valve destruction, and death.

DIAGNOSIS

The gold standard for diagnosis of IE is histopathologic and/or microbiologic analysis of a vegetation obtained surgically or at autopsy. Because the majority of patients with IE do not undergo surgery, the antemortem diagnosis of IE typically depends upon clinical features, especially evidence of endocardial involvement, immunologic and vascular phenomena, and blood culture positivity. In 1981, von Reyn and colleagues proposed criteria for the diagnosis of IE based upon strict case definitions. These criteria do not include a category for definitive IE based solely on clinical data. Apparent shortcomings of the von Reyn criteria include the failure to consider parenteral drug use as an underlying condition, failure to use echocardiographic findings in diagnosis, difficulty classifying acute cases, and lack of prospective validation.

In 1994, Durack and colleagues at Duke University proposed diagnostic criteria that include a category of definitive IE based solely on clinical findings (Table 270.2). The von Reyn and Duke criteria have been directly compared in several large studies. The Duke criteria consistently classify more cases as definite and are more sensitive for the diagnosis of pathologically proven IE. The Duke system also appears to be highly specific in diagnosing IE.

SPECIAL SITUATIONS

Infective Endocarditis Associated with Parenteral Drug Use

The microbiologic and anatomic features of IE in intravenous drug users are shown in Table 270.3. Most cases occur in patients with no previously recognized valvular abnormality. *S. aureus* is the most common causative agent and most often infects the tricuspid valve. The microbiologic picture of IE provoked by gram-negative bacilli in intravenous drug users has shown geographical and temporal variation. For example, outbreaks of IE due to *P. aeruginosa* have occurred in Detroit and Chicago, while IE caused by *Serratia marcescens* seems to be unique to San Francisco.

Patients with tricuspid IE due to *S. aureus* typically experience acute onset of fever, pleuritic chest pain, dyspnea, and cough. A systolic murmur is usually heard, but classic signs of tricuspid regurgitation are present in at most 50% of patients at the time of admission. The initial chest radiograph shows abnormal re-

TABLE 270.2. **DUKE CRITERIA FOR THE CLINICAL DIAGNOSIS OF INFECTIVE ENDOCARDITIS**[a]

Major criteria
 Positive blood culture results for infective endocarditis
  Typical microorganism from two separate blood cultures
   Viridans streptococci, S. bovis, HACEK group, or community-acquired S. aureus or enterococci without a primary focus
 or
  Persistently positive blood culture results for a microorganism suggestive of infective endocarditis
   Blood cultures drawn more than 12 hours apart
 or
  All three or a majority of four or more separate blood cultures, with the first and last drawn at least 1 hour apart
 Evidence of endocardial involvement
  Echocardiogram showing an oscillating intracardiac mass in the absence of alternative anatomic explanation, abscess, or new partial dehiscence of a prosthetic valve
 or
  New valvular regurgitation (increase or change in preexisting murmur not sufficient)
Minor criteria
 Predisposing heart disease or intravenous drug use
 Fever >38.0°C (100.4°F)
 Vascular phenomena
 Immunologic phenomena
 Microbiologic evidence not meeting a major criterion or serologic evidence of active infection
 Consistent echocardiogram not meeting a major criterion

[a] IE is classified as definite if two major, one major and three minor, or five minor clinical criteria are met or if surgical or autopsy specimens meet pathologic criteria (not shown in this table).
(From Durack DT, Lukes AS, Bright DK. New criteria for diagnosis of infective endocarditis: utilization of specific echocardiographic findings. Am J Med 1994;96:200, with permission.)

sults in about two-thirds of cases and may show nodular opacities, abscesses with cavitation, patchy areas of pneumonitis, or pleural effusions. Left-sided IE takes much the same form as IE in other populations. Infection of valves on both sides of the heart by P. aeruginosa is associated with severe illness and high mortality rates. The overall mortality rate associated with IE in intravenous drug users is less than 10%. This observation is best explained by the relatively good prognosis of tricuspid IE compared with left-sided IE and the relatively young age of these patients compared with other patients with IE.

Prosthetic Valve Endocarditis

PVE develops in about 2% of patients after valve replacement. About one-third become ill within the first 2 months after surgery (early PVE) and two-thirds after this time (late PVE). The pathogenesis of early-stage PVE involves microbial colonization of the prosthesis at the time of surgery. Late-stage PVE more closely resembles NVE with regard to pathogenesis and origin (Table 270.1). Overall, staphylococci are the most common cause. Streptococci are an uncommon source of early PVE; they more often cause late disease. Gram-negative bacilli and fungi are relatively more common in PVE than in NVE.

Patients with PVE have many of the same clinical features as patients with NVE. A new or changing murmur is present initially more often in PVE, reflecting the higher incidence of local suppurative complications, such as valve ring abscess. A valve ring abscess may extend to form a myocardial abscess, septal abscess with perforation, or pericarditis. Most important, it may cause valve dehiscence. Overall, the mortality rate in PVE is 25% to 30%. The mortality rate is higher in patients with early-stage PVE and in PVE caused by gram-negative bacilli, staphylococci, or fungi.

COMPLICATIONS
Cardiac

Valvular damage resulting in hemodynamically important valvular dysfunction is the most critical cardiac complication of IE.

TABLE 270.3. **ETIOLOGY AND ANATOMY OF INFECTIVE ENDOCARDITIS ASSOCIATED WITH INTRAVENOUS DRUG ABUSE IN THE UNITED STATES**[a]

Bacteria	Number of Cases (% of Total)	Valve Involved		
		Right	Left	Mixed
Staphylococcus aureus	45 (61)	40	3	2
Oxacillin susceptible	27 (36)	25	1	1
Oxacillin resistant	18 (24)	15	2	1
Streptococci	10 (13.5)	3	7	0
Enterococci	2 (2.7)	2	0	0
P. aeruginosa	10 (13.5)	3	2	5
Corynebacterium JK	1 (1.4)	1	0	0
Polymicrobial	6 (8)	4	1	1

[a] Based on 74 cases from 1982 to 1983.
(From Levine DP, Crane LR, Zerror MJ. Bacteremia in narcotic addicts at the Detroit Medical Center. II. Infectious endocarditis: a prospective comparative study. Rev Infect Dis 1986;8:374, with permission.)

Valvular insufficiency is most common, but in the context of large vegetations, such as those seen in fungal endocarditis and in PVE, obstruction may occur. The mechanism of valvular insufficiency in NVE is destruction of the valve itself or disruption of the valve annulus by a valve ring abscess. With aortic IE and aortic insufficiency, the stream of regurgitant flow can lead to damage, infection, and rupture of the mitral valve chordae tendineae or papillary muscles.

The most serious consequence of valvular dysfunction in patients with IE is heart failure, which is the predominant cause of death in patients with IE. The rapidity of the development of valvular insufficiency as well as the valve involved determine hemodynamic consequences. Acute IE, especially if it is associated with acute aortic insufficiency, is more likely to be hemodynamically significant than subacute disease or IE complicating chronic aortic regurgitation. Mechanisms of congestive heart failure not involving valvular dysfunction include embolic myocardial infarction, myocarditis, and conduction disturbances. Extension of a paravalvular abscess into the conduction system may produce varying degrees of atrioventricular block and bundle-branch block. These complications are prevalent in aortic valve IE because of the proximity of the aortic valve ring to the conduction system. Pericarditis is found at autopsy in 15% to 20% of patients with IE. This condition is especially common in the context of staphylococcal disease.

Extracardiac

Emboli, which arise during the course of IE in about one-third of patients, may be bland (uninfected) or septic. In left-sided IE, symptomatic emboli most often involve the spleen, kidney, brain, and heart. Emboli appear to be more prevalent in IE caused by *S. aureus*, HACEK bacteria (especially *Haemophilus parainfluenzae*), anaerobes, and fungi. In fungal endocarditis, peripheral emboli may provide the only source of diagnostic material because of the difficulty of recovering certain fungi from routine blood cultures.

Neurologic abnormalities are seen in about 30% of patients with IE, and such patients experience higher mortality rates than those without neurologic complications. Neurologic complications most frequently accompany IE due to pyogenic organisms, such as *S. aureus*, enterococci, gram-negative bacilli, and anaerobes. Clinical syndromes include embolic stroke, subarachnoid hemorrhage, brain abscess, meningitis, encephalopathy, seizure, and psychiatric disturbance. Strokes represent 10% to 15% of neurologic complications and most often occur in the middle cerebral artery distribution. Brain abscess develops infrequently, and meningitis, due to bacteremic localization in the subarachnoid space or rupture of a parameningeal focus, is unusual. Encephalitic symptoms may be due to emboli, bleeding, or vasculitis.

A mycotic aneurysm is a pathologic dilatation of a vessel due to local infection and complicates the course of IE in 15% to 25% of patients. The pathogenesis of aneurysm formation is believed to involve invasion of a vessel wall after embolization of infectious vegetation material. Mycotic aneurysms develop most frequently in the central nervous system, the sinus of Valsalva, the abdominal aorta and its branches, and the coronary and pulmonary arteries. The main risk associated with a mycotic aneurysm is rupture with bleeding. Many are clinically silent

and may not be recognized for months to years after infection has resolved. The clinical signs and symptoms depend on the location of the aneurysm and whether there is attendant bleeding. Central nervous system mycotic aneurysms usually appear in the form of subarachnoid or intracerebral hemorrhage. Renal failure, a relatively typical finding before the advent of antibiotics, occurs in only 10% of patients today. Focal or diffuse glomerulonephritis is the most common feature, though membranoproliferative glomerulonephritis due to immune complex deposition has been seen in IE due to *S. epidermidis*. Macro- and microinfarcts are also frequently seen but only rarely cause renal failure.

OPTIMAL MANAGEMENT

There are certain general principles of antimicrobial therapy for patients with IE. Host defenses on the relatively avascular endocardium are inadequate to sterilize the site. Consequently, therapy must include bactericidal drugs given parenterally for a prolonged period of time. In vitro testing of the microorganism's susceptibility to antimicrobial agents is helpful in predicting cure. The minimum inhibitory and bactericidal concentrations of antimicrobial agents necessary to repress and kill the microorganism, respectively, are important in choosing treatment regimens. In the past, the serum bactericidal (Schlichter) test was used in an attempt to confirm the adequacy of a regimen in use.

When the diagnosis of IE is under consideration, two important questions arise: when to treat and how to treat. Antimicrobial therapy for IE should be started without delay in four situations: when the clinical diagnosis of IE seems certain even though blood culture results are not yet available, when the diagnosis seems likely and the patient is seriously ill or cardiac surgery is planned in the immediate future, when antimicrobial therapy for another condition is necessary, and when the patient may have IE and blood cultures show positive results. In the first three situations, the physician should obtain blood cultures and begin antimicrobial therapy directed against the most likely microorganisms (Fig. 270.1). If these criteria are not satisfied and the diagnosis is uncertain, antibiotics should be withheld until more data are available.

When therapy for IE is initiated without knowledge of the microorganism responsible, empiric therapy must include agents likely to be effective against enterococci. Antistaphylococcal agents should also be considered for patients with PVE, patients with rapidly progressive illness suggestive of acute endocarditis, patients with aortic valve symptoms who have no previous evidence of valvular abnormality, patients with a history of parenteral drug use, patients with a previously infected intravenous catheter, and patients on long-term hemodialysis. Once the infecting pathogen is identified and antimicrobial susceptibilities are determined, a more specific antibiotic regimen is administered. Recommended regimens for the most common causes of IE are shown in Table 270.4.

Recent studies concerning the therapy of IE have focused on evaluation of shorter courses of antibiotics and once-daily dosing regimens, which may, in some cases, allow for outpatient treatment. Uncomplicated IE caused by highly susceptible streptococci (minimal inhibitory concentration of penicillin ≤ 0.1 μg per milliliter) can be successfully treated with 4 weeks of once-

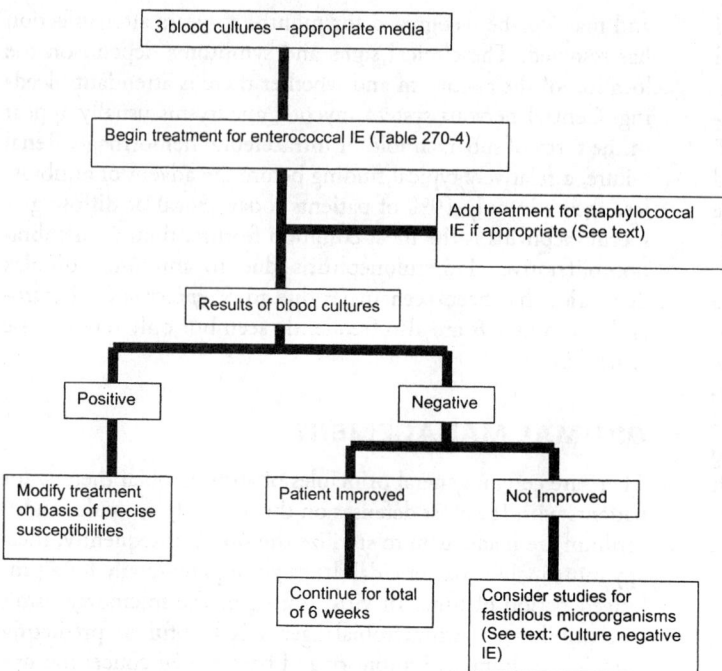

FIGURE 270.1. Strategy for diagnosing presumed infective endocarditis before identification of infecting microorganism.

daily ceftriaxone. Recent data suggest that 2 weeks of ceftriaxone plus an aminoglycoside given once daily is also effective for this disease. Parenteral drug users with uncomplicated tricuspid IE caused by oxacillin-susceptible *S. aureus* are usually cured with 2 weeks of a penicillinase-resistant penicillin (nafcillin) plus an aminoglycoside. Two-week therapy with a penicillinase-resistant penicillin alone may be equally effective.

Surgical Therapy

Valve replacement during active IE may be lifesaving. Indications for urgent surgery include severe or refractory heart failure, valvular obstruction, fungal endocarditis, ineffective antimicrobial therapy, and an unstable prosthetic valve. Relative indications for surgery in NVE include nonstreptococcal IE, recurrent IE, intracardiac extension of infection, two or more emboli, and vegetations or mitral valve preclosure seen by echocardiography. In PVE, additional relative indications include early-stage PVE, nonstreptococcal late-stage PVE, and periprosthetic leak.

Left-sided congestive heart failure complicating aortic valvular regurgitation is an indication for immediate valvular replacement. The mortality rate in this situation approaches 100% when heart failure does not respond to medical therapy. In contrast, the mortality rate after surgery in such patients is about 25%. The hemodynamic status, not the microbial activity of the disease, determines the need for surgery in patients with left-sided IE. Because life-threatening hemodynamic complications are rare in patients with tricuspid valve IE, persistent infection with resistant bacteria or fungi is the predominant indication for surgery. Tricuspid valvulectomy or repair with autologous pericardium is generally preferred over valve replacement.

A point system has been proposed to aid in determining the need for surgical intervention in IE (Table 270.5). Complications that develop during IE are assigned a point value according

to their importance as indicators of surgical therapy. If a patient's clinical status indicates five or more points, emergency surgery should be considered. Severe heart failure (heart failure that does not respond to maximum medical therapy) is an absolute indication for surgery and therefore is assigned five points. Other complications, such as conduction abnormalities, systemic emboli, and persistent bacteremia, are also given a point rating proportional to the importance of each as indicators of the need for surgery.

Treatment of Complications

Heart failure is treated in the usual manner, with afterload reduction, diuretics, and inotropic support and with surgical intervention if necessary (see later discussion). In patients with abnormal results on neurologic examination, the initial evaluation should include a thorough assessment for such systemic disorders as acidosis, hypoxia, and uremia. In most instances, computed tomography (CT) should be the initial diagnostic procedure. If no bleeding or mass lesion is noted, a lumbar puncture should be done to exclude meningitis. Angiography is indicated if cerebrospinal fluid analysis or the CT scan suggests subarachnoid hemorrhage or mycotic aneurysm.

Medical therapy alone is adequate for the treatment of mycotic aneurysms in about 30% of cases. Peripheral aneurysms, aneurysms that continue to enlarge on medical therapy, and ones that have bled should be debrided and clipped or resected if possible. This is not always feasible with aneurysms deep in the brain. An asymptomatic mycotic aneurysm in a difficult position for resection (e.g., the circle of Willis) and multiple mycotic aneurysms should be followed with another angiographic study after 1 to 2 weeks.

TABLE 270.4. ANTIMICROBIAL THERAPY FOR INFECTIVE ENDOCARDITIS[a]		
Microorganism	**Suggested Regimen**[b]	**Comments**
Penicillin-susceptible streptococci (viridans streptococci and *S. bovis* with MIC ≤0.1 µg/mL)	Aqueous crystalline penicillin G, 12–18 million U/24 hr for 4 weeks or Ceftriaxone, 2 g i.m./i.v. q day for 4 weeks or Aqueous crystalline penicillin G, 12–18 million U/24 hr, plus gentamicin, 1 mg/kg i.m./i.v. q 8 hr—both for 2 weeks[c]	Avoid aminoglycosides in patients older than 65 years and in those with impaired renal or eighth cranial nerve function. Substitute vancomycin, 30 mg/kg i.v. per 24 hr in two equally divided doses for 4 weeks, for penicillin in patients with immediate hypersensitivity to penicillin.[d]
Streptococci relatively resistant to penicillin G (MIC >0.1 µg/mL and <0.5 µg/mL)	Aqueous crystalline penicillin G, 18 million U/24 hr for 4 weeks, plus gentamicin, 1 mg/kg i.m./i.v. q 8 hr, for first 2 weeks[c]	Substitute cefazolin (or other first-generation cephalosporin) for penicillin in patients with non-life-threatening penicillin allergy. Substitute vancomycin, 30 mg/kg i.v. per 24 hr in two equally divided doses, for penicillin in patients with immediate hypersensitivity to penicillin[d]
Enterococci, nutritionally variant streptococci, and streptococci with penicillin MIC >0.5 µg/mL[e]	Aqueous crystalline penicillin G, 18–30 million U/24 hr (or ampicillin, 12 g/24 hr), plus gentamicin, 1 mg/kg i.m./i.v. q 8 hr—both for 4–6 weeks[c]	Substitute vancomycin, 30 mg/kg i.v. per 24 hr, in two equally divided doses for penicillin or ampicillin in patients with immediate hypersensitivity to penicillin. Cephalosporins are not acceptable alternatives.[d]
Penicillin-susceptible staphylococci (confirm with negative assay for β-lactamase production)	Aqueous crystalline penicillin G, 12–18 million U/24 hr for 4–6 weeks	Substitute cefazolin (or other first generation cephalosporin) for penicillin in patients with non-life-threatening penicillin allergy. Substitute vancomycin, 30 mg/kg i.v. per 24 hr, in two equally divided doses in patients with immediate hypersensitivity to penicillin.[d]
β-lactamase-producing, oxacillin-susceptible staphylococci	Nafcillin or oxacillin, 2 g i.v. q 4 hr for 4–6 weeks, with optional gentamicin, 1 mg/kg i.m./i.v. q 8 hr for first 3–5 days[c, f]	Substitute cefazolin (or other first-generation cephalosporin) for penicillin in patients with non-life-threatening penicillin allergy. Substitute vancomycin, 30 mg/kg i.v. per 24 hr in two equally divided doses, for nafcillin of oxacillin in patients with immediate hypersensitivity to penicillin.[d]
Oxacillin-resistant staphylococci	Vancomycin, 30 mg/kg i.v. q 24 hr in two equally divided doses for 4–6 weeks[d]	
HACEK group	Ceftriaxone, 2 g i.m./i.v. q day for 4 weeks or Ampicillin, 12 g/24 hr, plus gentamicin, 1 mg/kg i.m./i.v. q 8 hr—both for 4 weeks[c]	Do not use ampicillin if isolate produces β-lactamase
Culture-negative	Aqueous crystalline penicillin G, 18–30 million U/24 hr (or ampicillin, 12 g/24 hr) for 6 weeks, plus gentamicin, 1 mg/kg i.m./i.v. q 8 hr for 2 weeks	

MIC, minimal inhibitory concentration; HACEK group, *Haemophilus* species, *Actinobacillus actinomycetemcomitans, Cardiobacterium hominis, Eikenella corrodens,* and *Kingella* species.
[a] Suggested dosages are for patients with normal renal function. Table applies to native valve endocarditis. For patients with streptococcal endocarditis in the context of a prosthetic valve or other prosthetic material, use the regimen for enterococci and treat for 6 weeks. For staphylococcal prosthetic valve endocarditis, treat for at least 6 weeks with nafcillin, oxacillin, or vancomycin (depending on susceptibility) plus rifampin, 300 mg orally 1 8 hr, and include gentamicin as dosed above for the first 2 weeks.
[b] Aqueous crystalline penicillin G and ampicillin can be given either by continuous infusion or in six equally divided doses over 24 hr.
[c] Gentamicin dose is based on ideal body weight and should not exceed 80 mg. During therapy, further adjustments should be based on serum drug levels. Peak level of approximately 3 µg/mL is desirable.
[d] Vancomycin dose is based on ideal body weight. Vancomycin dosage should not exceed 2 g/24 hr unless serum drug levels are monitored. Peak serum level of 30–45 µg/mL is desirable.
[e] All enterococci causing endocarditis must be tested for antimicrobial susceptibility. Regimens suggested for enterococci in this table assume the isolate does not possess high-level resistance to penicillin, vancomycin, or gentamicin.
[f] Intravenous drug users who have uncomplicated tricuspid infective endocarditis due to oxacillin-susceptible *S. aureus* and no evidence of left-sided disease can be treated with nafcillin or oxacillin, 2 g i.v. q 4 hr, plus gentamicin, 1 mg/kg i.m./i.v. q 8 hr, both for 2 weeks. Vancomycin is not recommended as an alternative to nafcillin or oxacillin in 2-week regimens.

EVIDENCE LEVEL: A. Reference: Wilson WR, Karchmer AW, Dajani AS, et al. Antibiotic treatment of adults with infective endocarditis due to streptococci, enterococci, staphylococci, and HACEK microorganisms. *JAMA* 1995;274:1706–1713.

TABLE 270.5. POINT SYSTEM FOR ASSESSING THE NEED FOR CARDIAC SURGERY IN INFECTIVE ENDOCARDITIS[a]		
	Point Rating	
Complication	**Native Valve Infection**	**Prosthetic Valve Infection**
Heart failure		
Severe	5	5
Moderate	3	5
Mild	1	2
Fungal source	5	5
Persistent bacteremia	5	5
Source other than susceptible *Streptococcus*	1	2
Relapse after medical therapy	2	3
Single major embolus	2	2
Two or more systemic emboli	4	4
Vegetations seen on echocardiography	1	1
Evidence of early closure of mitral valve on echocardiography	2	NA
Ruptured chordae tendineae or papillary muscle	3	NA
Heart block	3	3
Ruptured sinus of Valsalva or ventricular septum	4	4
Unstable prosthesis	NA	5
Early PVE	NA	2
Periprosthetic leak	NA	2

NA, not applicable; PVE, prosthetic valve infection.
[a] Accumulation of five or more points implies the need for valve replacement.
(From Alsip SG, Blackstone EH, Kirklin JW, et al. Indications for cardiac surgery in patients with active infective endocarditis. *Am J Med* 1985;78:138, with permission.)

PROPHYLAXIS

Because of the significant morbidity and mortality associated with IE, prevention of this infection in susceptible persons has been emphasized for many years. Prophylactic antimicrobial therapy is based on two principles: bacteremia is common after certain invasive procedures, and particular patients appear to be at risk of IE after an episode of bacteremia. Although the use of prophylactic antibiotics to prevent IE is recommended in specific situations, it should be noted that no randomized, controlled trials addressing this issue have been performed among humans and that most cases of IE do not occur in association with an invasive procedure.

Prophylactic antibiotics should not be given if the risk of acquiring IE is lower than the risk of an adverse reaction to the antibiotic. The risk of bacteremia is highest for some dental and oral procedures, intermediate for genitourinary procedures, and lowest for most gastrointestinal procedures, including those that involve biopsy. Exceptions to the last generalization are esophageal dilatation and variceal sclerotherapy, both of which are associated with bacteremia rates of 30% to 40%. According to the American Heart Association, high-risk cardiac conditions include prosthetic valves, previous IE, complex cyanotic congenital defects, and surgically constructed systemic pulmonary shunts and conduits. Rheumatic heart disease and mitral valve prolapse with regurgitation are classified as moderate risk.

Antibiotic selection is directed against viridans streptococci for dental, oral, respiratory, and esophageal procedures and against enterococci for other gastrointestinal and genitourinary

procedures. Amoxicillin or ampicillin is the preferred antibiotic for most patients undergoing procedures in the former category. For genitourinary or nonesophageal gastrointestinal procedures, ampicillin or amoxicillin with or without gentamicin (depending on risk) is preferred.

■ SUPPURATIVE THROMBOPHLEBITIS

Inflammation, clot, and microbial infection within a vein characterize suppurative thrombophlebitis. Thrombophlebitis may develop in a previously normal vein or in association with an indwelling device, usually an intravenous catheter. It is more likely to occur the longer the intravenous device is left in place. Symptoms and signs associated with suppurative thrombophlebitis vary. In a few instances, there is no observable abnormality at the intravenous site; in others, there is mild erythema, pain, edema, and tenderness. Some patients may have frank pus at the intravenous site, which can be expressed from the vein after removal of the device. Because most intravenous catheters are placed in an upper extremity, this is the most common site of disease, and 90% of such patients have evidence of inflammation at the catheter site. In patients with severe burns, suppurative thrombophlebitis is frequently not apparent, even though there may be extensive clot and infection. Patients with suppurative thrombophlebitis involving a central venous catheter often show initial signs of sepsis.

Pelvic vein thrombophlebitis may develop in a previously normal vein as a complication of septic abortion, pelvic inflammatory disease, or the process of giving birth. The usual symptoms include fever accompanied by nausea and abdominal pain (usually the right-lower quadrant). Eighty percent of cases involve right-sided veins alone, and in about 15% of patients thrombophlebitis is bilateral. Only 5% of cases involve left-sided vessels alone.

Staphylococci (including coagulase-negative species) are the most common microorganisms responsible for catheter-related suppurative thrombophlebitis; gram-negative bacilli, enterococci, and *Candida* are also encountered. The incidence of suppurative thrombophlebitis due to *Candida* seems to be on the rise. Aerobic gram-negative bacilli and enterococci are more often responsible in patients with intra-abdominal venous thrombosis. In pelvic suppurative thrombophlebitis, anaerobic organisms, aerobic gram-negative bacilli, and streptococci predominate.

Bacteremia and inflammation or suppuration at an intravenous site support the diagnosis of suppurative thrombophlebitis. The diagnosis is substantiated if the same microorganism is isolated from the blood and catheter site exudate or if differential quantitative blood cultures or semiquantitative catheter cultures implicate the catheter as the source of bacteremia. Bacteremia is documented in 80% to 90% of patients, except in pelvic suppurative thrombophlebitis, where blood cultures show positive results in 20% to 30% of cases. For large central veins (abdominal or pelvic veins or the superior vena cava), venography or CT is useful for diagnosis.

Treatment of suppurative thrombophlebitis associated with an intravenous catheter begins with removal of the device. Further therapy almost always requires a combination of surgical and medical management. The surgical procedure of choice is venotomy and exploration plus removal of the affected segment. Excision is generally followed by defervescence within 24 hours. Initial antimicrobial therapy should include vancomycin plus an antibiotic likely to be active against nosocomial gram-negative bacilli, such as an aminoglycoside or ceftazidime. For central vein or pelvic vein suppurative thrombophlebitis, medical therapy alone is often effective. In the latter case, high doses of penicillin G plus an additional antianaerobic agent (metronidazole) or a β-lactam/β-lactamase inhibitor combination is usually effective. Heparin is often used in patients with pelvic or central vein suppurative thrombophlebitis. When *Candida* is the causative microorganism, excision plus amphotericin B (about 500 mg total) or intravenous fluconazole is recommended.

MYOCARDITIS AND PERICARDITIS

Infective myocarditis and infective pericarditis may be caused by a wide variety of microorganisms (Table 270.6). Many agents produce both myocarditis and pericarditis, but often only one of the syndromes predominates in terms of clinical symptoms. The most commonly identified cause of myocarditis in immunocompetent hosts is coxsackievirus B, an enterovirus. Several lines

TABLE 270.6.	INFECTIOUS CAUSES OF MYOCARDITIS AND PERICARDITIS

Viral
  Coxsackievirus
  Echovirus
  Influenza virus
  Poliovirus
  Herpes simplex virus
  Varicella zoster virus
  Cytomegalovirus
  Epstein–Barr virus
  Mumps virus
  Rubella virus
  Rubeola virus
  Hepatitis B virus
  Human immunodeficiency virus
  Adenovirus
Bacterial and Rickettsial
  Corynebacterium diphtheriae
  Streptococci
  Staphylococci
  Haemophilus influenzae
  Salmonella typhi and other gram-negative bacilli
  Neisseria meningitidis
  Listeria monocytogenes
  Campylobacter jejuni
  Brucella
  Clostridium perfringens and other anaerobic bacteria
  Legionella pneumophilia
  Mycoplasma pneumoniae
  Chlamydia psittaci
  Rickettsia rickettsii
  Coxiella burnetii
  Borrelia burgdorferi
  Mycobacterium tuberculosis
Fungi
  Aspergillus
  Histoplasma
  Candida
  Coccidioides
  Cryptococcus
  Blastomyces
Parasites
  Trypanosoma
  Toxoplasma
  Entamoeba
  Schistosomes
  Trichinella

of circumstantial evidence link viral myocarditis with the later development of idiopathic dilated cardiomyopathy.

The pathogenesis underlying enteroviral myocarditis is not completely understood, but evidence from animal models suggests that direct myocardial damage by the pathogen is followed by a host inflammatory response that persists after the virus is eliminated. Using techniques such as the polymerase chain reaction and in situ hybridization, enteroviral genomic sequences have been identified in myocardial tissue from patients with myocarditis. HIV-1 sequences have been detected in myocardial tissue from patients with HIV-1 infection and left ventricular dysfunction. In patients with Chagas' disease, *Trypanosoma cruzi* causes direct myocardial injury. Other mechanisms include damage by a toxin, as in diphtheria, and damage due to immunologic injury, as in acute rheumatic fever.

Symptoms of viral myocarditis include fever, fatigue, malaise, dyspnea, palpitations, and chest pain. Patients often report symptoms suggestive of antecedent viral illness. Physical examination typically finds nonspecific symptoms, such as fever and tachycardia and, in severe cases, congestive heart failure. Atrial and ventricular dysrhythmias and conduction defects are common electrocardiographic abnormalities in patients with viral myocarditis. Cardiac troponin I levels are more likely to be elevated in patients with biopsy-proven myocarditis than creatine kinase-MB levels. Magnetic resonance imaging and nuclear scanning with gallium 67 or indium-labeled antimyocyte antibodies are potentially useful diagnostic methods.

Only endomyocardial biopsy can confirm active myocarditis, but this procedure is subject to sampling error because myocardial involvement may be patchy. Viruses rarely have been isolated from biopsy specimens, and molecular diagnostic tests generally are not available for clinical use. In practice, the diagnosis of viral myocarditis is made when the clinical course is consistent, the virus is isolated from another site (oropharynx or stool), and there is a fourfold or greater rise in specific antiviral IgG antibody titers. Extracardiac manifestations of infection may implicate the causative agent in cases of nonviral myocarditis.

Antiviral agents as a rule are ineffective in the treatment of viral myocarditis. Because vigorous physical activity has been shown to worsen myocyte damage in animal models, supportive care of patients with myocarditis includes bed rest. Angiotensin-converting enzyme inhibitors and diuretics are the mainstays of therapy for those with congestive heart failure. Immunosuppression with prednisone and azathioprine or cyclosporine has not been shown to be beneficial. Immunosuppression should be reserved for patients with disease that is refractory to conventional measures. Cardiac transplantation can be considered for patients who fail all other therapies. Nevertheless, 1-year survival rates among patients who have undergone transplantation for myocarditis are lower than those among patients who have had the procedure for other reasons. Overall, 56% of patients enrolled in the Myocarditis Treatment Trial either died or had undergone transplantation when assessed at 5-year follow-up. For myocarditis caused by nonviral agents, effective antimicrobial agents are usually available.

Many patients with myocarditis also have pericarditis, especially with viral disease. Pericarditis results from hematogenous spread of the microorganism to the pericardium or contiguous spread to the pericardium from a site in the heart or within the chest. Formerly, bacterial pericarditis developed as a complication of pleuropulmonary disease, and pneumococci, other streptococci, staphylococci, and *H. influenzae* were the most common causative organisms. Since the advent of effective antibacterial therapy, bacterial pericarditis has become less common and is now primarily a nosocomial disorder. Bacteremia, postoperative wound infections, and endocarditis each account for about 25% of cases today. Antecedent noninfectious pericardial effusions predispose patients to bacterial pericarditis. Tuberculous pericarditis is seen in about 1% of patients with tuberculosis and is usually the result of spread from disease in a mediastinal lymph node. Fungal pericarditis, except for cases due to *Histoplasma*, is usually seen only in severely immunocompromised patients.

Chest pain may be absent, and clinical deterioration may be rapid in acute bacterial pericarditis, but in tuberculous pericarditis the onset is insidious, chest pain is usually present, and weight loss, fever, night sweats, and cough are typical. A pleural effusion is more common in tuberculous disease, but it is seen in at least one-third of patients with bacterial and viral sources of infection. Parenchymal pulmonary disease is most suggestive of acute bacterial pericarditis and least suggestive of a viral origin. A pericardial rub is found in half of patients with pericarditis. Jugular venous distention and muffled heart sounds suggest pericardial effusion. A paradoxical pulse and hypotension suggest cardiac tamponade. Initial electrocardiographic changes in patients with pericarditis are PR-interval depression and diffuse ST-segment elevation. T-wave inversion is usually a late finding, after ST-segment normalization. An enlarged cardiac silhouette on chest radiography is suggestive of pericardial effusion. Echocardiography is extremely useful for the detection of pericardial effusions and for the assessment of their hemodynamic significance.

Identification of the specific source of pericarditis depends on isolation of the causative microorganism. In viral pericarditis, isolation is unusual, and pericardiocentesis or pericardiectomy is unwarranted in the absence of hemodynamic compromise. Hemodynamic compromise is more often seen in bacterial and tuberculous pericarditis, and pericardiocentesis or pericardiectomy is often indicated to diagnose and treat these disorders.

Most cases of viral pericarditis are treated with bed rest and nonsteroidal anti-inflammatory drugs. Corticosteroids are indicated only for recurrences. Bacterial pericarditis is treated with antimicrobial agents directed at the causative organism plus surgical drainage. Antibiotics should be continued for 4 to 6 weeks after surgery. Patients with tuberculous pericarditis should receive standard antituberculous medications for 6 months plus corticosteroids for the first 6 weeks. Surgery is indicated for tuberculous pericarditis if there is evidence of hemodynamic compromise (tamponade or constriction). The prognosis for viral pericarditis is good—almost all patients experience spontaneous resolution. The mortality rate with bacterial pericarditis remains high, even with appropriate therapy.

BIBLIOGRAPHY

Alsip SG, Blackstone EH, Kirklin JW, et al. Indications for cardiac surgery in patients with active infective endocarditis. *Am J Med* 1985;78:138.

Baker CC, Petersen SR, Sheldon GF. Septic phlebitis: a neglected disease. *Am J Surg* 1979;138:97.

Brown CA, O'Connell JB. Myocarditis and idiopathic dilated cardiomyopathy. *Am J Med* 1995;99:309.

Dajani AS, Taubert KA, Wilson W, et al. Prevention of bacterial endocarditis: recommendations of the American Heart Association. *JAMA* 1997; 277:1794.

Durack DT, Lukes AS, Bright DK, et al. New criteria for the diagnosis of infective endocarditis: utilization of specific echocardiographic findings. *Am J Med* 1994;96:200.

Pelletier LL, Petersdorf RG. Infective endocarditis: a review of 125 cases from the University of Washington Hospitals, 1963–1972. *Medicine* 1977;56:287.

Tunkel AR, Kaye D. Neurologic complications of infective endocarditis. *Neurol Clin* 1993;11:419.

Watanakunakorn C, Burkert T. Infective endocarditis at a large community teaching hospital, 1980–1990. *Medicine* 1993;72:90.

Weinstein L. Life-threatening complications of infective endocarditis and their management. *Arch Intern Med* 1986;146:953.

Wilson WR, Karchmer AW, Dajani AS, et al. Antibiotic treatment of adults with infective endocarditis due to streptococci, enterococci, staphylococci, and HACEK microorganisms. *JAMA* 1995;274:1706.

Kelley's Textbook of Internal Medicine, fourth edition. Edited by H. David Humes. Lippincott Williams & Wilkins, Philadelphia © 2000.

CHAPTER

271

GENITOURINARY TRACT INFECTIONS, INCLUDING PERINEPHRIC ABSCESS AND PROSTATITIS

BALDWIN TOYE
ALLAN R. RONALD

■ URINARY TRACT INFECTIONS

Infections of the urinary tract are among the most often encountered of all bacterial infections; they account for up to 10 million ambulatory care visits and 1.5 million discharge diagnoses yearly in the United States. These infections are experienced by at least 35% of women; many have repeated infections, resulting in substantial morbidity and use of health care services. Urinary tract infections (UTIs) are also the most frequently reported nosocomial infection and the most common source of gram-negative bacteremia.

DEFINITIONS AND PRESENTATIONS

Bacteriuria refers to the presence of bacteria in urine. The term *significant bacteriuria* was introduced to differentiate contaminated from infected urine. The distinguishing criterion has been more than 10^5 colony-forming units per milliliter in a voided urine sample, but urine from patients with symptomatic UTIs may have lower colony counts. *Acute cystitis* is a clinical illness caused by inflammation of the bladder epithelium or urethra as a result of bacterial infection, though other sources produce similar symptoms (the dysuria/frequency syndrome—see Chapter 136). *Acute pyelonephritis* is a clinical syndrome of flank pain, fever, and chills due to the inflammatory response to bacterial invasion of the renal parenchyma. *Asymptomatic (covert) bacteriuria* is the presence of significant bacteriuria in the absence of any symptoms attributable to infection. *Complicated UTIs* are those that develop in patients with abnormal urinary tracts.

The terms *chronic cystitis* and *chronic UTI* are used to describe recurring infections. Recurrent infections may be categorized as relapse or reinfection. Relapse is the recurrence of bacteriuria with the original infecting organism because of its persistence within the urinary tract. Reinfection is recurrence of bacteriuria caused by entry of bacteria into the bladder from the fecal–perineal reservoir. The term *chronic pyelonephritis* should be restricted to calyceal dilatation with overlying cortical scarring.

MICROBIOLOGY AND EPIDEMIOLOGY

Urine is normally sterile. Most UTIs are caused by Enterobacteriaceae, with about 80% of community-acquired infections caused by *Escherichia coli* (Table 271.1). Other gram-negative organisms, including *Klebsiella* species, *Proteus mirabilis*, and *Enterobacter* species, together constitute 10% of community-acquired infections. *P. mirabilis* is of particular significance because it predisposes to the formation of struvite calculi. *Staphylococcus saprophyticus*, a novobiocin-resistant, coagulase-negative organism, is the second most common cause of acute cystitis in young, sexually active women. *Enterococcus faecalis* is an important gram-positive pathogen in the elderly and in patients who have had genitourinary tract instrumentation. *Staphylococcus aureus* bacteriuria is frequently the result of bacteremic seeding of the kidneys during the course of hematogenous infection.

The origin of hospital-acquired UTIs is substantially different. Patients often have indwelling urethral catheters or are receiving antimicrobial agents and thus are at greater risk of acquiring multiply resistant bacteria, often owing to cross-infection from other patients with UTIs. Infections of less susceptible strains of Enterobacteriaceae, *Pseudomonas aeruginosa*, and yeasts are common. Infection due to *E. faecalis* has become prevalent, especially in patients being treated with cephalosporins. Diphtheroids, α-hemolytic streptococci, lactobacilli, and anaerobes are rarely true urinary pathogens, although they are often present if searched for in voided urine.

The prevalence of bacteriuria has been defined in various population groups. In adult women, the prevalence is 3% to 7%, but it rises to 10% to 25% in women older than 60. In adult men, the prevalence is much lower (less than 0.1%) but increases in later years to 2% to 15%. The prevalence of bacteri-

TABLE 271.1.	MICROBIOLOGY OF URINARY TRACT INFECTIONS
Community acquired, uncomplicated (%)	
Escherichia coli	80
Staphylococcus saprophyticus	10
Klebsiella pneumoniae	5
Other	5
Hospital acquired, complicated (%)	
Escherichia coli	30
Enterococcus species	15
Pseudomonas aeruginosa	10
Other *Enterobacteriaceae*	20–25
Staphylococcus species	5–10
Yeasts	5–10
Other	10–20

uria in the elderly depends on the level of functional and anatomic impairment and may exceed 50% in nonambulatory persons. Various risk groups have been found to have an increased incidence of UTI. The association of UTI with sexual intercourse in women is reflected in the term *honeymoon cystitis*. Women who use spermicides have a greater risk of UTI than women who use other contraceptive methods. Infections in men are often related to anatomic abnormalities. The incidence of UTI is higher in uncircumcised men and in men who engage in penetrative anal intercourse. Patients with diabetes mellitus are at a higher than normal risk of asymptomatic and symptomatic UTIs. Does recurrent UTI with onset in adult life lead to renal failure? Although progressive renal scarring occurs in children as a result of infection, the damage takes place mostly before age 5. In adults, renal failure rarely results from recurrent or asymptomatic UTIs unless obstruction, diabetes mellitus, reflux, or analgesic abuse is also present.

PATHOPHYSIOLOGY

Although infection can arise by the hematogenous route (usually due to *S. aureus* or *Candida albicans*), the ascending route is the most important. Migration of uropathogens from the rectum to the vagina with introital and distal urethral colonization precedes the development of bladder infection. Antecedent antimicrobial use and diaphragm/spermicide use facilitate vaginal colonization with UTI pathogens. Bacterial entry into the bladder is enhanced by sexual intercourse. Upper tract involvement ensues when organisms ascend the ureters to reach the kidneys. The interaction between host defenses and the organism determines whether infection takes place. A major host defense is normal urinary flow, especially the flushing effect of micturition. The inherent antibacterial and antiadherent properties of bladder mucin and normal functioning of the ureterovesical junction aid in preventing infection.

The P fimbriae of *E. coli* are a virulence determinant and permit adherence to epithelial cells. Women with the P^1 blood group have increased susceptibility to pyelonephritis when they experience a UTI. Cytokines, specifically interleukin-6 (IL-6) and IL-8, are produced locally by epithelial cells in response to infection with virulent bacteria. These cytokines produce acute-phase proteins, and IL-8 acts as a chemoattractant for neutrophils. Most women with recurrent infection have normal urinary tracts. Any interruption of the normal flow of urine, such as obstruction, a neurogenic bladder, or calculi, results in residual urine and instrumentation, which increases the incidence of infection. Calculi also serve as a nidus for persistent infection. Vesicoureteral reflux contributes to upper UTI. The usual cause of reflux is an abnormality of the insertion of the ureter into the bladder, which often disappears during adolescence. Infection also causes reflux. Reflux alone may lead to renal damage, presumably from retrograde pressure, but most renal scarring is a complication of infection in patients with reflux.

HISTORY AND PHYSICAL EXAMINATION

Patients with acute cystitis show initial signs of dysuria, urgency, and frequency, sometimes accompanied by suprapubic discom-

fort or gross hematuria. Fever rarely exceeds 38°C (100.4°F) if infection is confined to the lower tract. The absence of upper tract symptoms is an unreliable marker in excluding renal infection; up to 30% of patients with so-called cystitis have subclinical pyelonephritis, as documented by localization studies.

The classic clinical picture of acute pyelonephritis in adults consists of fever (usually more than 38.5°C [more than 101°F]), chills, and flank pain. Only 60% of patients with this classic triad are subsequently confirmed to have pyelonephritis. Flank pain may radiate to the epigastrium or to the lower abdominal quadrants, but radiation to the groin suggests ureteral obstruction. Constitutional symptoms include malaise, anorexia, nausea, vomiting, diarrhea, myalgias, and headache. Up to 30% of patients have concomitant lower tract symptoms, often antedating upper tract symptoms. Physical features vary, ranging from none to the clinical features of septic shock. There is often percussion tenderness in the costovertebral angle.

The clinical picture of acute pyelonephritis can be confused with many other conditions, including bacterial pneumonia, myocardial infarction, acute hepatitis, cholecystitis, and acute pelvic inflammatory disease. Zoster, in the appropriate dermatome before the onset of vesicles, may also mimic renal pain. Patients with diabetes mellitus may not have flank pain, and loss of blood glucose control may be the sole feature of acute pyelonephritis. These patients are at risk for complications due to renal papillary necrosis and emphysematous pyelonephritis. Although classic features of pyelonephritis are seen in the elderly, flank tenderness is less common, and confusion and bacteremia are more common. Genitourinary sepsis leads to metastatic infection at other sites in 1% to 3% of patients, and patients can have initial symptoms localized to these sites rather than to the urinary tract. Examples of metastatic infection include endocarditis, meningitis, endophthalmitis, and vertebral osteomyelitis.

LABORATORY STUDIES AND DIAGNOSTIC TESTS

The exact diagnosis of UTI requires a culture of urine. The simplest method is to obtain a clean-voided midstream urine specimen. If patients are unable to give a clean-voided specimen, urine may be obtained by catheterization. The urine should be planted on culture media within 1 hour or refrigerated until it can be cultured, to avoid erroneously high colony counts.

Quantification of bacteriuria distinguishes infection from contamination. With voided urine, more than 10^5 bacteria per milliliter has been the traditional criterion that indicates infection. More than 90% of patients with acute pyelonephritis have bacteriuria of more than 10^5 per milliliter. A diagnosis of asymptomatic bacteriuria in women requires two voided specimens with more than 10^5 per milliliter of the same bacterium, to ensure 95% confidence of "true" bacteriuria. In men, a single specimen growing more than 10^4 per milliliter of a single organism is specific for bacteriuria. In women with symptomatic lower UTI, however, 30% have fewer than 10^5 per milliliter. The best diagnostic criterion for symptomatic infection with gram-negative aerobes is at least 10^2 per milliliter with pyuria. Pretherapy cultures do not improve therapeutic outcomes in women with acute cystitis.

Pyuria is the presence of more than five white blood cells (WBCs) per high-power field in centrifuged urine sediment or more than 10 cells per cubic millimeter of unspun urine. Counts of more than 10 cells per cubic millimeter are found in fewer than 1% of asymptomatic patients without bacteriuria, whereas they are present in 96% of symptomatic patients with bacteriuria, including low-count bacteriuria, and in more than 90% of symptom-free patients with bacteriuria (more than 10^5 per milliliter). The leukocyte esterase dipstick, a widely available office test, is less sensitive but is an acceptable alternative to microscopic diagnosis of pyuria. Microscopic hematuria is present in 50% of patients with acute cystitis.

Urine microscopy for bacteriuria can provide important information before culture results are available. The finding of any organism per oil-immersion field in a Gram's stain of unspun urine correlates with bacteriuria of more than 10^5 per milliliter with a sensitivity of 93%. Centrifuging urine prior to Gram staining increases the sensitivity to 98%.

Differentiating upper from lower UTIs predicts the response to treatment. Unfortunately, clinical criteria (absence or presence of upper tract signs) are imperfect and unreliable in localizing the site of infection. The Stamey test (ureteral catheterization) and Fairley test (bladder washout) both require instrumentation and are impractical in routine clinical practice. Noninvasive tests, such as measurement of antibody-coated bacteria, maximal urinary-concentrating ability, C-reactive protein or urinary proteins (β_2-microglobulin), or imaging with gallium scans, have limited use in the treatment of individual patients.

More than 90% of women with lower UTIs can be cured by a 3-day course of an antimicrobial agent; 90% of women with only lower tract symptoms who experience relapse (3-day failure) have upper UTIs. Failure to be cured with a short course of therapy may be the most practical measure to diagnose upper UTIs in women with only lower tract symptoms or asymptomatic bacteriuria. Bacteremia is shown to be present in about 20% of patients with acute pyelonephritis. WBC casts are present in two-thirds of patients with pyelonephritis and, when present, they suggest acute renal infection.

Diagnostic imaging is not required in many patients with urinary infection. Both sonography and intravenous pyelography are relatively insensitive, but they can be useful to exclude obstruction, calculi, or anatomic abnormalities in the urinary tract. Repeated evaluation after an initial normal examination result should be discouraged. Computed tomography (CT), specifically helical scanning enhanced with contrast, has become the most important study in patients who require imaging. Pelvic or ureteral calculi, renal parenchymal abnormalities, and perinephric collections of fluid all can be diagnosed readily in this way. Moreover, a proportion of patients with presumed acute renal infection do not have acute pyelonephritis. CT scanning often will confirm the primary diagnosis and substantially alter management. Specific diagnoses, including renal tuberculosis and xanthogranulomatous pyelonephritis, also can be made with sensitivity and specificity with CT scanning. In general, imaging studies are more often obtained in men with UTIs, owing to the higher incidence of anatomic abnormalities among men. Radiographic and cystoscopic examination of women with acute cystitis who have no clinical evidence of urologic disorders or upper tract involvement rarely identifies abnormalities that alter treatment.

DIFFERENTIAL DIAGNOSIS

Acute cystitis must be distinguished from sexually transmitted infections with *Neisseria gonorrhoeae*, *C. trachomatis*, and herpes simplex virus. Patients may confuse the symptoms of urinary infection with those of vulvovaginal monoliasis and other vaginal pathologic conditions. During the first episode of infection, laboratory tests, including urinalysis and urine culture, and a sexual risk assessment, are necessary; if the latter study shows positive results, sexually transmitted diseases should be excluded. Recurring episodes of acute bacterial cystitis are often confused with the diagnosis of interstitial cystitis. This term is a "wastebasket" diagnosis for patients with recurring symptoms that can be severe and are usually accompanied by negative results on urine culture, an absence of pyuria, and no response to treatment. Cystoscopy may show evidence of petechiae after bladder dilatation, but the sensitivity and specificity of cystoscopic diagnosis are still undetermined.

The diagnosis of acute pyelonephritis should always be made with supporting laboratory findings. About one-fifth of patients with an initial diagnosis of pyelonephritis will prove to have other conditions, including acute surgical conditions, acute pelvic inflammatory disease, ectopic pregnancy, diverticulitis, renal calculi, pneumonia, or acute cholecystitis. Because acute pyelonephritis can progress rapidly to the sepsis syndrome with hypotension and multiple organ failure, all patients with this diagnosis must be regarded as representing a medical emergency and should be examined and treated promptly and observed until improvement is confirmed.

STRATEGIES FOR OPTIMAL CARE

The mainstay of treatment is antimicrobial therapy with supportive measures, including hydration and analgesia. The goal of treatment is clinical resolution and bacteriologic cure. In patients with acute invasive renal infections, the antibiotic selected should achieve inhibitory blood and tissue levels. The initial choice of agent depends on local resistance patterns of uropathogens. Optimal treatment regimens and duration of administration for most UTIs remain the subject of controversy. Conventional therapy for UTIs has consisted of 7- to 14-day regimens (Table 271.2), but most studies have failed to differentiate upper and lower UTIs.

In women with acute cystitis, 3-day treatment courses cure 95% of infections (Table 271.3), a rate equivalent to more prolonged regimens. Therapy with trimethoprim-sulfamethoxazole (TMP-SMX) or ciprofloxacin is preferred because of the increasing prevalence of amoxicillin resistance. In some areas, TMP-SMX resistance is also at a level that may make the choice of one of the quinolones preferable. Advantages of short-course treatment include lower cost, improved compliance, and fewer and less severe side effects. There is also minimal effect on the fecal flora, so that repeated short courses can be used without emergence of resistant organisms. Self-diagnosis and initiation of short-course therapy is a cost-effective alternative to urine

TABLE 271.2.	**CONVENTIONAL REGIMENS FOR URINARY TRACT INFECTION IN ADULTS**

Drug	Dose[a]
Trimethoprim-sulfamethoxazole	160/800 mg p.o. b.i.d.
Trimethoprim	200 mg p.o. b.i.d.
Amoxicillin	500 mg p.o. t.i.d.
Cephalexin	500 mg p.o. q.i.d.
Ofloxacin	400 mg p.o. b.i.d.
Ciprofloxacin	500 mg p.o. b.i.d.
Nitrofurantoin	100 mg p.o. q.i.d.

[a] See text for duration depending on site of infection.

TABLE 271.4.	**INITIAL EMPIRIC PARENTERAL REGIMENS FOR ACUTE PYELONEPHRITIS IN ADULTS**

Drug	Dose[a]
Ampicillin	1 g q 6 hr
and	
Gentamicin[b]	4.5 mg/kg q 24 hr
Cefotaxime	1 g q 8–12 hr
Ceftazidime	1 g q 8–12 hr
Ceftriaxone	1–2 g q 24 hr
Imipenem	500 mg q 6–8 hr
Aztreonam	1 g q 8 hr
Ciprofloxacin	400 mg q 12 hr
Trimethoprim-sulfamethoxazole	160/800 mg q 12 hr
Piperacillin-tazobactam	3/0.375 g 6 hr

[a] Doses assume normal renal function.
[b] Other aminoglycosides can be used.

culture and diagnosis and treatment by a physician. Woman with symptoms suggestive of upper tract involvement should be treated with a 7- to 14-day course of an appropriate antimicrobial agent. Furthermore, women at risk of subclinical pyelonephritis (those with a history of genitourinary abnormalities, diabetes mellitus, duration of symptoms more than 7 days, documented relapse) should be treated for 7 to 14 days, as should women whose infections recur within 2 weeks of short-course therapy.

Patients with acute pyelonephritis are now more often being treated as outpatients. Frequently, an initial parenteral antibiotic is prescribed in the office or emergency room and followed with an oral regimen. Although ampicillin together with gentamicin has been the traditional parenteral treatment, monotherapy with various agents is as effective and may be preferred for patients with renal impairment or resistant pathogens (Table 271.4). The complications of acute pyelonephritis and indications for hospitalization are summarized in Table 271.5.

Most patients become afebrile with symptom resolution within 48 to 72 hours. Patients with complications or a delayed response to treatment should be investigated to exclude obstruction or other lesions that require urologic consultation. Once the patient is afebrile for 24 hours, therapy can be switched to oral medication and continued to complete the course. About two-thirds of nonpregnant adult patients with acute pyelonephritis are only moderately ill and may be treated initially with oral antibacterial agents, particularly the fluoroquinolone ciprofloxacin.

Asymptomatic infection usually should not be searched for and treated in nonpregnant patients. Treatment may be indicated, however, in selected subgroups of patients at increased risk of morbidity, including patients undergoing urinary tract manipulation, immunosuppressed patients, and patients with diabetes mellitus. Elderly patients and those confined to bed should not be treated, because of the futility of maintaining sterile urine, the probable emergence of resistant organisms, and the lack of evidence that any benefits are associated with treatment. Men with UTIs require treatment regimens similar to those women receive. A proportion of men have a prostatic focus, which may require much more prolonged treatment in order to eradicate a focus of infection.

RECURRENT INFECTIONS

Infections recur in 50% of patients within 1 year of treatment. Relapse results from failure to eradicate the organism from renal

TABLE 271.3.	**EFFECTIVE SHORT-COURSE REGIMENS FOR WOMEN WITH ACUTE CYSTITIS**

Drug	Dose[a]
Trimethoprim-sulfamethoxazole	160/800 mg b.i.d.
Trimethoprim	200 mg b.i.d.
Ciprofloxacin	500 mg b.i.d.

[a] Daily for 3 days.

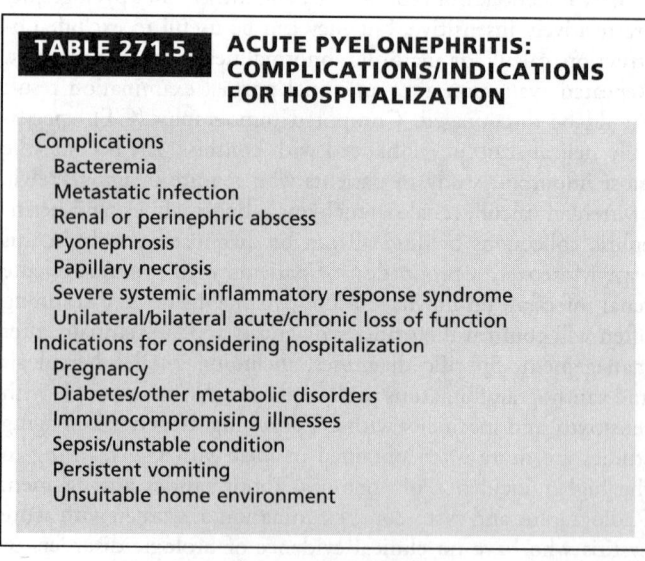

TABLE 271.5.	**ACUTE PYELONEPHRITIS: COMPLICATIONS/INDICATIONS FOR HOSPITALIZATION**

Complications
  Bacteremia
  Metastatic infection
  Renal or perinephric abscess
  Pyonephrosis
  Papillary necrosis
  Severe systemic inflammatory response syndrome
  Unilateral/bilateral acute/chronic loss of function
Indications for considering hospitalization
  Pregnancy
  Diabetes/other metabolic disorders
  Immunocompromising illnesses
  Sepsis/unstable condition
  Persistent vomiting
  Unsuitable home environment

TABLE 271.6.	REGIMENS FOR PREVENTION OF REINFECTION IN WOMEN
Drug	**Dose**
Trimethoprim-sulfamethoxazole	40/200; mg p.o. daily[a]
Trimethoprim	100 mg p.o. daily
Nitrofurantoin	50 mg p.o. daily
Norfloxacin	400 mg p.o. daily
Ciprofloxacin	250 mg p.o. daily

[a] Same dose taken thrice weekly is also effective.

or prostatic tissue. The treatment of patients who suffer a relapse after short-course therapy has been discussed. Relapse after a 2-week course of therapy typically can be cured with a 6-week course of therapy. Continuous long-term suppressive therapy should be considered for patients who have relapses after prolonged courses of treatment. Half the usual daily dose of TMP-SMX, amoxicillin, cephalexin, or a fluoroquinolone is often an effective suppressive regimen.

Most recurrent infections are reinfections that result from new organisms entering the bladder from the fecal–perineal reservoir. Prophylaxis or prevention of reinfection is cost effective in women who experience more than two infections per year (Table 271.6). Although resistant organisms replace the fecal flora of patients treated with β-lactams or sulfonamides, selection of highly resistant fecal flora is less common with TMP, nitrofurantoin, and the quinolones. A 6-month trial of prophylaxis is begun after existing infections are eradicated. Taking the medication at the time of intercourse is an alternative strategy. Women with sporadic infections may choose to self-diagnose and self-treat infections (Fig. 271.1). For postmenopausal women, the use of intravaginal estriol cream prevents recurrent UTIs, presumably by minimizing vaginal carriage of Enterobacteriaceae.

CATHETER-ASSOCIATED URINARY TRACT INFECTION

About 40% of nosocomial infections involve the urinary tract, and most are associated with indwelling urethral catheters. They are the most common source of gram-negative bacteremia in hospitalized patients and are associated with longer durations and higher costs of hospitalization. Major risk factors are female sex, advanced age, and severe general debility. The risk of infection after a single in-and-out catheterization is as low as 1% in young, healthy women. Closed sterile drainage significantly lowers the infection rate, but the risk with indwelling catheterization is still about 5% per day. Infection may result from contamination at catheter-collection junctions, with intraluminal proximal migration of bacteria into the bladder, or by periurethral migration of bacteria around the catheter.

Most patients are asymptomatic; lower tract symptoms can be obscured by the presence of the catheter. Although upper tract symptoms or even septic shock may develop, fever may be the only clinical indicator of a catheter-associated UTI. Other sources of fever must be considered, however, before assuming that the source of elevated temperature is an infected urinary tract. Diagnosis is obtained by catheter puncture using a sterile needle and syringe. Any bacterial count after urine is collected by needle aspiration and cultured is generally considered significant in patients with indwelling catheters.

Bacteriuria usually persists after catheter removal and should be treated. If the catheter cannot be removed, asymptomatic bacteriuria should not be treated, because treatment only selects for more resistant organisms. When symptoms develop, they should be treated initially with broad-spectrum agents, since more resistant organisms are often responsible; the spectrum should be narrowed once the antimicrobial susceptibility is known (Fig. 271.2). The most effective method of prevention

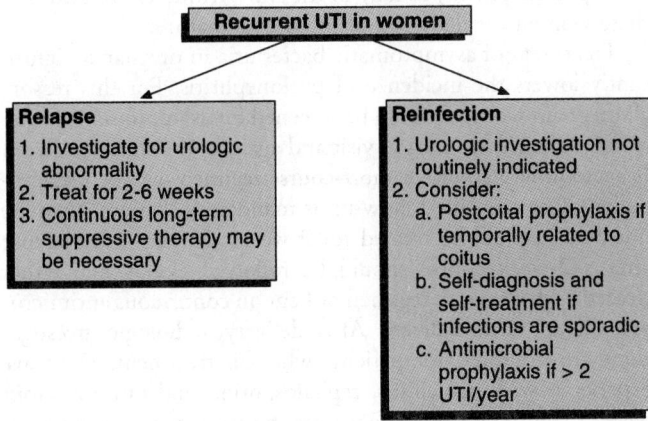

FIGURE 271.1. Recurrent urinary tract infections in women.

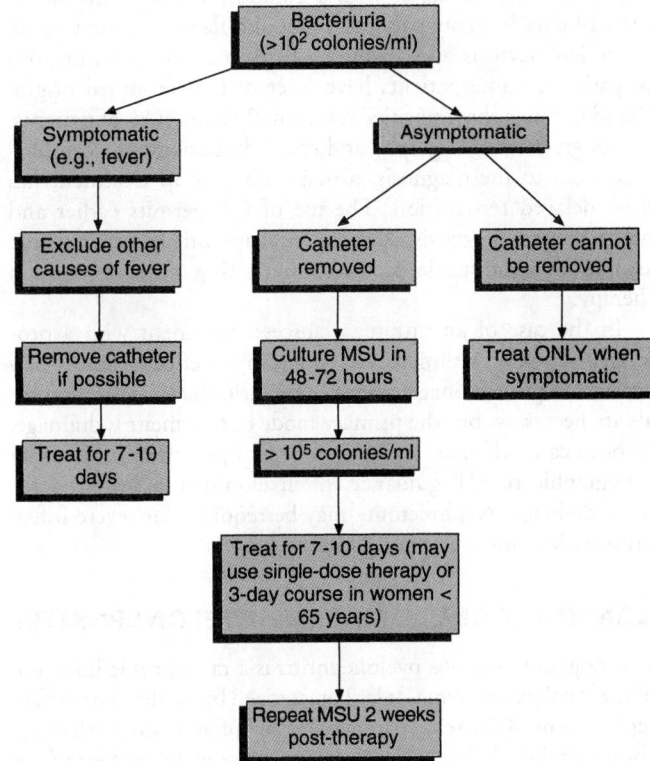

FIGURE 271.2. Approach to indwelling catheter–associated bacteriuria.

is to avoid catheterization and to remove the catheter as soon as possible. For management of the neurogenic bladder, intermittent catheterization is preferred over indwelling catheterization. The instillation of antiseptic solutions in drainage bags and meticulous periurethral care with antibacterial ointment have had limited success in lessening the incidence of infection.

PERINEPHRIC AND INTRARENAL ABSCESS

A perinephric abscess is suppuration in the perirenal fascia; an intrarenal abscess is suppuration within the renal parenchyma. The abscesses may coexist, and diagnosis can be difficult and is often delayed. The mortality rate is substantial—up to one-third of cases of perinephric and intrarenal abscess are diagnosed at autopsy. Patients with calculi, obstruction, or diabetes mellitus are predisposed to abscess formation. Intrarenal abscesses may be caused by hematogenous seeding (especially by *S. aureus*) of the renal cortex, but many develop as complications of acute pyelonephritis. In the latter case, gram-negative uropathogens are most common, with a predilection for the corticomedullary regions. The patient often has initial symptoms of fever and flank pain of acute onset associated with leukocytosis. Normal findings on urinalysis do not exclude the diagnosis, since pyuria is present only when there is communication of the abscess with the collecting system. A slow response to appropriate treatment in a patient with presumed pyelonephritis should suggest the diagnosis.

Most perinephric abscesses result from rupture of an intrarenal abscess into the perirenal space. Hematogenous seeding and direct extension from a nearby focus are less common. The onset is usually more insidious, with a duration of symptoms longer than 14 days in many patients. Fever and flank pain are typical, as are leukocytosis and anemia; a flank mass is found in 50% of patients. Some patients have fever of undetermined origin. Blood cultures show positive results in 20% to 40% of patients. Although chest radiography and renal ultrasonography can provide clues to the diagnosis, a major obstacle to treatment has been delayed recognition. The use of CT permits earlier and more accurate diagnosis, allowing for diagnostic and therapeutic aspiration. Serial studies facilitate monitoring of the response to therapy.

In the case of an intrarenal abscess, treatment with a prolonged course of antimicrobials alone may be effective, but many patients require drainage. For a perinephric abscess, antimicrobials are necessary, but the primary mode of treatment is drainage. In both cases, drainage can be performed percutaneously under sonographic or CT guidance, often eliminating the need for open drainage. Nephrectomy may be required for severe infections with a nonfunctioning kidney.

XANTHOGRANULOMATOUS PYELONEPHRITIS

Xanthogranulomatous pyelonephritis is a rare chronic infection of the renal parenchyma. It is characterized by localized or diffuse replacement of the renal parenchyma by inflammatory cells with abundant lipid-laden macrophages. A lysosomal defect interferes with digestion of bacterial products. It is most common in the fifth to sixth decades of life, with a predominance among

women. Chronic obstruction and recurrent UTIs are typical; malaise, flank pain, fever, weight loss, pyuria, and nephrolithiasis are common features. Cultures of urine and renal tissue often show positive results for *P. mirabilis*. Xanthogranulomatous pyelonephritis can mimic renal cell carcinoma, renal tuberculosis, renal abscess, or hydronephrosis. CT establishes the diagnosis through the finding of abnormal fatty tissue in the renal mass. Surgical resection of the affected material (total or partial nephrectomy) is curative. Accurate preoperative diagnosis may aid the surgeon in limiting the amount of tissue resection. A more conservative approach using long-term antibacterial therapy also may be successful.

MALACOPLAKIA

Malacoplakia is a rare granulomatous disease that develops in the same clinical context as xanthogranulomatous pyelonephritis, but infection is usually with *E. coli*. Lesions are found in the bladder or kidney and may involve the prostate and ureters. Gross examination shows yellow-brown plaques that form aggregates of large histiocytes (von Hanseman cells) containing intracytoplasmic inclusions (Michaelis–Gutmann bodies) that are believed to be calcified, incompletely digested organisms. Bladder involvement is characterized by irritative symptoms, and cystoscopy may show typical plaques. A patient with upper tract disease has fever, flank pain, or a mass in association with UTI. CT may show unifocal or multifocal masses. The pathogenesis of malacoplakia is incompletely understood, but it is believed to be due to a defect in intracellular killing of ingested microorganisms by macrophages. Bethanechol can reverse this defect in vitro, and treatment with bethanechol combined with TMP-SMX or a fluoroquinolone has been successful. Surgery is required for patients with progressive disease.

URINARY TRACT INFECTION IN PREGNANCY

The prevalence of asymptomatic bacteriuria in pregnancy is similar to the rate of bacteriuria in sexually active non-pregnant women (3% to 8%). Only 1% to 2% of women acquire bacteriuria during pregnancy. About one third of these infections involve the upper tract. If the infection is left untreated, 20% to 30% of bacteriuric pregnant patients experience symptomatic acute pyelonephritis, usually in the third trimester, and 20% of these women are delivered of infants prematurely.

Treatment of asymptomatic bacteriuria in pregnancy significantly lowers the incidence of pyelonephritis. For this reason, all pregnant women should be screened for asymptomatic bacteriuria at their first prenatal visit and again in the third trimester. If bacteriuria is found, a short-course regimen may be used initially. Close monthly follow-up is mandatory. Patients who are not cured should be treated for 2 weeks. Patients who relapse after a 2-week course should be followed closely and either treated with a 6-week regimen or kept on continuous antimicrobial therapy until delivery. After delivery, radiologic investigations are indicated for patients who fail treatment. Extensive experience with penicillins, cephalosporins, and nitrofurantoin have shown them to be safe for use in pregnancy. Sulfonamides may be used except during late pregnancy. Patients with pyelonephritis are frequently hospitalized to allow careful monitoring of mother and fetus. The response to therapy is often slow. If the patient is still febrile and ill after 72 hours of appropriate therapy, ultrasonography may be needed to delineate underlying abnormalities.

PROSTATITIS

Prostatitis is inflammation of the prostate gland. The diagnosis of prostatitis is often made without objective evidence. It is usually classified as bacterial prostatitis (acute and chronic), nonbacterial prostatitis (prostatosis), and prostatodynia. Except for acute prostatitis, it is often difficult to distinguish these categories on clinical criteria; diagnosis depends on microscopic and bacteriologic examination of prostatic fluid. Lower tract localization studies remain the gold standard for the diagnosis of bacterial infection of the prostate. The first-voided 10 mL of urine (VB_1), 10 mL midstream urine (VB_2), expressed prostatic secretions (EPS) obtained by prostatic massage, and the first 5 mL of urine voided immediately after prostatic massage (VB_3) are collected for quantitative culture and microscopic examination. Normal prostatic fluid contains fewer than 10 WBCs per high-power field. Most cases of bacterial prostatitis are caused by Enterobacteriaceae—*E. coli* is the most common pathogen. The most common gram-positive pathogen is *E. faecalis*, which is responsible for up to 10% of infections. A zinc-containing antibacterial factor present in normal prostatic fluid aids in resisting infection, and abnormally low levels of this factor have been found in men with bacterial prostatitis.

ACUTE PROSTATITIS

The typical picture of acute prostatitis consists of fever, chills, malaise, and irritative and obstructive voiding symptoms associated with lower back and perineal discomfort. On physical examination, the prostate is found to be exquisitely tender, warm, and swollen. Prostatic massage should not be performed, because of the risk of bacteremia. Most patients have bacteriuria caused by the same organism, and diagnosis of the source is thus possible.

Although some patients can be treated with oral antibiotic therapy, the acutely ill patient should be hospitalized and treated empirically (Table 271.4). After clinical response, therapy can be changed to an oral agent, usually TMP-SMX or a fluoroquinolone, depending on the susceptibility of the isolated organism. Therapy should be continued for 6 weeks. Most antimicrobial agents penetrate poorly into prostate tissue, but penetration is satisfactory in the acutely inflamed prostate. Supportive therapy with sitz baths, analgesics, and stool softeners is helpful. Urinary retention should be managed with suprapubic drainage. Other complications include prostatic abscess, pyelonephritis, bacteremia, epididymitis, and seminal vesiculitis.

CHRONIC PROSTATITIS

Patients with chronic prostatitis have irritative voiding symptoms often associated with perineal and lower back pain. This is an important cause of relapsing UTI in men. There are no specific physical features. Diagnosis is based on lower tract localization studies. The EPS has more than 10 WBCs per high-power field, with a few lipid-laden macrophages. Bacterial counts of EPS and VB_3 exceed that of VB_1 by at least tenfold. If the VB_2 shows bacteriuria (more than 10^5 per milliliter), the site of infection cannot be localized.

Treatment has proved unsatisfactory. A major problem is the inability of many antimicrobial agents to diffuse into the prostatic fluid. Prostatic calculi also may serve as a persistent focus of infection. TMP-SMX and fluoroquinolones penetrate into the prostatic tissue and have the best cure rates (32% to 71%). Treatment must be prolonged (8 to 12 weeks), but relapse is typical. Long-term suppressive therapy is often more successful than cure. Suppressive therapy often consists of a single nightly dose of TMP-SMX or a fluoroquinolone, and relapse can occur after years of successful suppression.

NONBACTERIAL PROSTATITIS

The clinical features of nonbacterial prostatitis (prostatosis) are identical to those of chronic bacterial prostatitis, including microscopic evidence of inflammation in the EPS. Bacterial pathogens are not isolated from EPS and urine cultures, however. Many pathogens, including *Ureaplasma urealyticum* and *C. trachomatis*, have been isolated from EPS, but an etiologic role is unproved. Nonetheless, some physicians recommend a course of therapy with tetracycline or erythromycin, to which some patients respond. Repeated and prolonged courses of therapy are not indicated. Treatment is mainly symptomatic, with a combination of sitz baths, prostatic massage, and analgesics.

PROSTATODYNIA

Patients with prostatodynia have symptoms that mimic chronic prostatitis, but they lack evidence of prostatic inflammation. Localization cultures show negative results for bacterial pathogens. Some patients have an element of associated emotional stress. The origin of these symptoms is unknown, but evidence suggests that it may be a primary voiding dysfunction due to overactivity of pelvic sympathetic nerves acting at the level of the external urethral sphincter. Antimicrobials are not indicated, and treatment is largely symptomatic, along with reassurance. Some patients obtain relief with α-adrenergic blockers, such as phenoxybenzamine or prazosin.

EPIDIDYMITIS

Epididymitis is the clinical syndrome resulting from inflammation of the epididymis. In men younger than age 35, it is usually sexually transmitted and is often associated with urethritis. The most common etiologic agents are *Neisseria gonorrhoeae* and *C. trachomatis*. In men 35 and older, there is typically underlying structural urologic abnormalities, bacterial prostatitis, or a history of recent genitourinary tract manipulation. Most cases are found to be bacteriuric. *E. coli*, other Enterobacteriaceae, and

Pseudomonas organisms account for most cases, though there are reports of streptococcal and anaerobic epididymitis.

Clinical symptoms include painful swelling of the scrotum, which usually arises acutely over 1 to 2 days, often in association with irritative lower tract symptoms. Early on, tender swelling is localized to the epididymis alone, but with time inflammation spreads to the ipsilateral testis, making the testes indistinguishable on palpation. A urethral discharge or evidence of inflammation should be sought because asymptomatic urethritis may be present, especially in patients younger than age 35. Urethral discharge should be submitted for culture or nucleic acid amplification, and midstream urine culture should be carried out. Cultures of epididymal aspirates are useful for patients who fail medical therapy or those who experience recurrences without confirmation of the source of disease.

The most important differential diagnosis to be considered is testicular torsion. Doppler ultrasonography, radionuclide scanning, CT, and emergency urologic consultation may be necessary to make the diagnosis. Other diagnostic considerations include testicular tumor, abscess, spermatocele, hydrocele, varicocele, hernia, and trauma. Treatment consists of nonspecific measures: bed rest, scrotal elevation, analgesics, and local ice packs. Specific treatment should be directed against etiologic agents suspected on initial evaluation. If sexually transmitted epididymitis is suspected, an appropriate course of treatment should be prescribed. When urethral Gram's stain or culture shows *N. gonorrhoeae*, one of the recommended treatment regimens (such as ceftriaxone followed by tetracycline) should be administered. Sexual partners should also be evaluated and treated.

Acutely ill men with nonsexually transmitted epididymitis can be treated initially with any of the empiric regimens used in the treatment of renal infections (Table 271.4). After clinical response, an oral agent is chosen based on the susceptibility of the organism isolated from urine. Men with epididymitis and bacteriuria should receive a 6-week course to minimize the risk of relapse. Surgery is reserved for those with no response to medical therapy or for those in whom testicular torsion is a very real possibility. Complications of epididymitis include abscess formation, testicular infarction, chronic pain, infertility, and bacteremia. Systemic infections that can involve the epididymis include tuberculosis, deep mycoses (blastomycosis, cryptococcosis, histoplasmosis, coccidioidomycosis), brucellosis, and schistosomiasis.

BIBLIOGRAPHY

Abrutyn E, Mossey J, Berlin JA, et al. Does asymptomatic bacteriuria predict mortality and does antimicrobial treatment reduce mortality in elderly ambulatory women? *Ann Intern Med* 1994;120:827–833.

Agace W, Hedges S, Ceska M, et al. Interleukin-8 and the neutrophil response to mucosa gram-negative infection. *J Clin Invest* 1993;92:780–785.

Harding GK, Nicolle LE, Ronald AR, et al. How long should catheter-acquired urinary tract infection in women be treated? A randomized controlled study. *Ann Intern Med* 1991;114:713–719.

Hooton TM, Scholes D, Hughes JP, et al. A prospective study of risk factors for symptomatic urinary tract infection in young women. *New Engl J Med* 1996;335:468–474.

Kunin CM. Does kidney infection cause renal failure? *Annu Rev Med* 1985;36:165–176.

Mushlin AI, Thornbury JR. Intravenous pyelography: the case against its routine use. *Ann Intern Med* 1989;111:58–70.

Nicolle LE, Harding GKM, Thompson M, et al. Efficacy of 5 years of continuous TMP-SMX prophylaxis for urinary tract infection. *J Infect Dis* 1988;157:1239–1242.

Raz R, Stamm WE. A controlled trial of intravaginal estriol in postmenopausal women with recurrent urinary tract infections. *N Engl J Med* 1993;329:753–756.

Sheinfeld J, Schaeffer AJ, Cordon-Cardo C, et al. Association of the Lewis blood-group phenotype with recurrent urinary tract infections in women. *N Engl J Med* 1989;320:773–777.

Smith HS, Hughes JP, Hooton TM, et al. Antecedent antimicrobial use increases the risk of uncomplicated cystitis in young women. *Clin Infect Dis* 1997;25:63–68.

Stamm WE, Hooton TM. Management of urinary tract infections in adults. *N Engl J Med* 1993;329:1328–1334.

Kelley's Textbook of Internal Medicine, fourth edition. Edited by H. David Humes. Lippincott Williams & Wilkins, Philadelphia © 2000.

C H A P T E R
272

SEXUALLY TRANSMITTED DISEASES AND GENITAL TRACT INFECTIONS

WILLIAM C. LEVINE

Sexually transmitted diseases (STDs) are those conditions caused by pathogens transmitted mainly through sexual contact (Table 272.1). Depending on the characteristics and natural history of each disease, the principal goals of treatment of patients with STDs and related genital tract infections are microbiologic cure of infection, relief of signs and symptoms, prevention of adverse effects, and prevention of horizontal and vertical transmission. Even as our knowledge of the organisms that cause STDs continues to grow, diagnostic methods improve, and new treatments become available, we continue to face therapeutic and epidemiologic challenges in the management of these diseases. For example, the optimal management of patients with syphilis and HIV co-infection remains the subject of controversy; the possibility exists that antiviral therapy prevents transmission of asymptomatic genital herpes simplex virus infection, but it has not been evaluated adequately; and emerging resistance is a growing problem for certain bacterial and viral sexually transmitted pathogens. In all cases, the approach to the patient with an STD should be guided by the knowledge that transmission of STDs can be prevented if the therapeutic encounter can be linked to education and counseling that will minimize an individual's risk of acquiring or transmitting infection.

Curable bacterial and persistent viral STDs are extremely common in the United States (Table 272.2), as they are in many

TABLE 272.1.	MAJOR SEXUALLY TRANSMITTED PATHOGENS

Bacteria
  Neisseria gonorrhoeae
  Chlamydia trachomatis
  Treponema pallidum
  Mycoplasma genitalium
  Mycoplasma hominis
  Ureaplasma urealyticum
  Haemopyhilus ducreyi
  Shigella species
  Calymmatobacterium granulomatis
  Campylobacter species
  Mobiluncus species (?)
  Group B streptococci (?)
Viruses
  Human immunodeficiency virus
  Herpes simplex virus
  Hepatitis A and B
  Hepatitis C (?)
  Cytomegalovirus
  Human papillomavirus
  Molluscum contagiosum virus
  Human T-cell lymphotropic virus, type 1
  Human herpesvirus 8
Protozoa
  Trichomonas vaginalis
  Giardia lamblia
  Entomoeba histolytica
Ectoparasites
  Phthirus pubis (crab louse)
  Sarcoptes scabei (scabies mite)

other countries. In the United States, the incidence of gonococcal infections has been declining since the 1970s, and rates of primary and secondary syphilis have dropped to their lowest level in many years. Nonetheless, outbreaks of these diseases continue to occur among heterosexual and gay populations. Rates of infection with bacterial STDs remain higher in the United States than in all other industrialized nations, except for Russia and some of the countries of eastern Europe, which have recently seen enormous epidemics of syphilis and gonorrhea. In

TABLE 272.2.	ESTIMATED INCIDENCE OF SELECTED SEXUALLY TRANSMITTED DISEASES IN THE UNITED STATES, 1996

STD	Number of Cases/Year
Chlamydia	3,000,000
Gonorrhea	650,000
Syphilis	70,000
Human papillomavirus	5.5 million
Genital herpes	1 million
Trichomoniasis	5 million
Hepatitis B	77,000
HIV	20,000

Source: American Social Health Association.

the United States, chlamydia is the most prevalent bacterial STD; the 1998 report by health departments to the Centers for Disease Control of approximately 600,000 cases is a gross underestimate, because efforts to screen routinely for this infection have missed many sexually active adolescents and young adults.

Chancroid, the STD most strongly associated with increased HIV transmission risk, remains endemic in certain parts of the United States, but it is underreported because of the difficulty in establishing the diagnosis by laboratory tests. Viral STDs also have a continuing high prevalence in the United States; an estimated 20 million persons are infected with human papilloma virus (HPV) and 45 million are infected with herpes simplex virus (HSV). Hepatitis B virus infects an estimated 240,000 persons annually in the United States; sexual transmission accounts for a substantial proportion of new infections. Whereas gonorrhea, syphilis, and chancroid tend to be concentrated in inner-city communities and associated with low socioeconomic status, chlamydia, HSV, and HPV are distributed more broadly throughout the general population.

■ CLINICAL SIGNS AND SYMPTOMS

Men with STDs usually appear for treatment because they have a prominent symptom or sign, such as urethral discharge, genital ulcers, genital warts, or proctitis. Women typically experience vaginal discharge, lower abdominal pain, or a genital lesion. STDs in both sexes may be asymptomatic, but asymptomatic infection is generally more common in women; infections in women are identified more frequently through screening tests. Gonorrhea or chlamydia may be detected through testing during a routine pelvic examination or screening of urine and syphilis during routine prenatal serologic screening. Patients may also have symptoms for which an STD is only one possible consideration in a differential diagnosis (arthritis, enteritis). Men and women also may be seen for treatment if they have been referred by a sex partner with a diagnosis of STD or if they believe that they have had a high-risk sexual encounter. STD-related syndromes and other reasons for which patients may seek medical care are listed in Table 272.3.

■ HISTORY AND PHYSICAL EXAMINATION

An assessment of a patient's STD risks is an essential component of the medical history. This assessment assists in the interpretation of physical findings and laboratory tests and provides information that may be helpful for treatment of the patient and his or her partner. The assessment of risk should be conducted in a sensitive, nonjudgmental manner within the usual context and flow of taking the medical history. Any anxiety or partiality on the part of the clinician toward a patient's sexual practices is likely to be detected and may make the patient reluctant to discuss aspects of his or her sexual behavior and thus impede optimal medical care.

TABLE 272.3.	CLINICAL SYNDROMES ATTRIBUTABLE TO SEXUALLY ACQUIRED INFECTION

AIDS
Urethritis
Cervicitis
Vaginitis
Pelvic inflammatory disease
Infertility and ectopic pregnancy
Fetal and neonatal infection (conjunctivitis, pneumonia, TORCH, etc.)
Adverse outcomes of pregnancy
Genital tract neoplasia
Genital ulceration
Proctitis and enteric infections
Hepatitis syndromes
Epididymitis
Arthritis (disseminated gonococcal syndrome, Reiter's syndrome)
Late syphilis
Molluscum contagiosum
Ectoparasite infestation (scabies, pubic lice)
Tropical spastic paraparesis
Kaposi's sarcoma

Essential information obtained from the sexual history includes the gender of the patient's sex partners; whether the patient engaged in sexual intercourse with new or several partners in the past 4 weeks (this timeframe includes the usual incubation period for many STDs); whether the patient had vaginal, oral, or anal sex with these partners (and if anal, whether the male patient who had male partners was the insertive or receptive partner); condom use during sex; and past history of STDs, including HIV infection. The patient's history of drug and alcohol use is also relevant, because substance abuse is often associated with sexual risk-taking behaviors and STDs.

For patients who have no symptoms and are being evaluated as part of a routine examination, an assessment of risk is helpful in deciding whether to screen for STDs. All sexually active women under the age of 25 years should be tested annually for chlamydial infections (per the recommendations included in the Health Employer Data Information Set), and women aged 25 years and older should be tested if they have one or more risk factors for infection (new partner or several partners in the past 2 to 3 months, clinical signs or symptoms suggestive of infection, or a sex partner with suspected or documented infection). Adolescent girls tend to have a high prevalence of infection (often 5% to 10%) and may benefit from testing at more frequent intervals, particularly if they have already been found to have infection. The increasing availability and declining cost of urine testing with nucleic acid amplification assays have made more frequent screening feasible and convenient. Men who are considered to be at risk of chlamydial infection also should be screened using urine tests, although specific recommendations for screening men have not yet been established.

Recognition of a patient's risks of STDs is important in considering the differential diagnosis of clinical syndromes for which STD is only one of several possible diagnoses. Sexually transmitted infections should be considered in the differential diagnosis

of dysuria in women (which may be caused by chlamydial or gonococcal infection), rashes (secondary syphilis or scabies), arthritis (disseminated gonococcal infection or Reiter's syndrome), and enteritis (*Shigella* or *Giardia* species). Persons who report recent oral or anal intercourse should undergo laboratory testing for gonococcal infection that includes specimens from oral and anal sites. Persons who have had oral–fecal contact are at increased risk of contracting sexually transmitted enteric infections, and those who have had receptive anal intercourse are at increased risk of proctitis.

The decision of whether to provide immediate treatment based on clinical findings or preliminary laboratory results may also depend on the risk assessment. A patient with a high risk of STD is more likely to be infected given a presumptive positive test or clinical findings that suggest the presence of an STD and may be less likely to be adversely affected by a false-positive result. Once a determination has been made that a patient has an STD, information obtained through the sexual history is necessary to begin the process of counseling about risk reduction and assisting in notifying and counseling sex partners.

The physical examination of the patient being evaluated for an STD includes components of the general physical examination: inspection of the skin, including an examination of the palms and soles for lesions that are typical of secondary syphilis; of the mouth for oral lesions; and of the lymph nodes not only for inguinal adenopathy but also for generalized lymphadenopathy that may develop in patients with syphilis or HIV. In women, the lower abdomen is examined for tenderness or an adnexal mass that suggests the diagnosis of pelvic inflammatory disease (PID). The gynecologic examination begins with inspection of the skin of the pubic area for genital warts, ulcerative lesions, and evidence of lice or scabies. With the speculum inserted in the vagina, the quantity and color of vaginal secretions are noted, and the cervix is closely examined for the presence of inflammation or lesions. After specimens are collected, the speculum is withdrawn slowly so that the vaginal epithelium can be seen.

The bimanual examination includes palpation of the Bartholin's glands, examination for cervical motion tenderness, and palpation of the uterus and adnexa for masses or tenderness. The urethra is gently stripped to search for the presence of purulent discharge. The pH of the vaginal secretions is measured using narrow-range pH paper, to assist in the diagnosis of vaginitis. In men, the skin of the inguinal area is examined for lesions. The penis also is examined for lesions, and if no urethral discharge is apparent, the shaft of the penis is stripped lengthwise to look for any discharge. The scrotum is scrutinized and the testicles and epididymis palpated for mass or tenderness. In both men and women, the anus should be inspected for warts, discharge, or ulcers; if proctitis is suspected in light of the patient's history, anoscopy should be performed.

LABORATORY STUDIES AND DIAGNOSTIC TESTS

Until rapid office-based tests are available that are highly sensitive and specific for STDs, gaps will continue to exist between treatment based on results of rapid tests with relatively low sensitivity or specificity and treatment based on results of more reliable tests not available until several days after the patient's visit. Clinicians must rely on an assessment of a patient's risks for STDs and the potential implications of either notifying the patient of false-positive test results when making decisions concerning immediate treatment based on tests with relatively low specificity or accepting the delay and expense involved in performing confirmatory tests. Because most screening tests are imperfect, an estimate of pretest probabilities of disease based on the prevalence of disease in the population and an individual patient's risks is important in evaluating the certainty of infection in view of a positive test result. The nonculture tests for gonococcal and chlamydial infection especially raise this concern; although specificities for most nonculture tests that are used for widespread screening are probably 99.5% or greater, lack of well-defined gold standards has made the true specificity of these tests uncertain.

Even a specificity of 99.5% raises potential problems unless the disease prevalence in the population is high. If a test for chlamydia with a specificity of 99.5% and a sensitivity of 80% is used to screen women with a chlamydia prevalence of 15%, the positive predictive value is 97%. The same test in a population with a 2% prevalence, however, has a positive predictive value of only 77%; nearly one-fourth of patients with a positive test result do not have infection. For this reason, in low-prevalence populations, positive results should be confirmed routinely before notifying the patient or administering therapy, especially if adverse consequences can result from notification of a false-positive result. For chlamydia, enzyme immunoassay results can be verified with a blocking antibody, and nucleic acid probe assays can be verified with a competitive probe. Verification can also be effected by repeating the test; optimally, a second test should be cell culture or a second nonculture test based on a different principle or on a different antigen or nucleic acid sequence from the one used in the initial test.

The Papanicolaou smear (cervical smear) is not a sensitive test for STDs. The finding of a pathogen (*Trichomonas vaginalis*) or cytologic changes suggestive of infection (*T. vaginalis, Chlamydia trachomatis*, HSV, HPV), however, can be useful in directing the choice of more specific tests. Diagnostic tests specific for HPV subtypes that have been associated with cervical cancer are commercially available. They are being evaluated for use in cervical cancer screening, triage of women with abnormalities on the Papanicolaou smear, and follow-up of women who have been treated for cervical cancer.

DIFFERENTIAL DIAGNOSIS

Details of the clinical course, pathophysiologic characteristics, and treatment of several STDs are presented elsewhere in this textbook. The treatment of common causes of vaginal discharge and the approach to several of the major STD syndromes and their differential diagnoses are discussed in the following sections. The major syndromes include genital ulcer disease, urethritis, vaginal discharge, cervicitis, and PID.

GENITAL ULCER DISEASE

In the United States, genital ulcers most often are caused by genital HSV infection, *Treponema pallidum* (primary syphilis), and *Haemophilus ducreyi* (chancroid). Lymphogranuloma venereum (caused by *C. trachomatis* serovars L$_1$, L$_2$, and L$_3$) and donovanosis (also called granuloma inguinale, caused by *Calymmatobacterium granulomatis*) are seen rarely in the United States; they are more common in developing countries. In some instances, genital ulcers are caused by trauma or by generalized or localized dermatologic conditions that are not STDs. The distribution of diseases causing genital ulcers varies widely according to the population of patients, the practice setting, and the patterns of local morbidity. Although in most U.S. cities chancroid is rare, in some cities it may be an endemic disease, found most often in association with prostitution and crack cocaine use. Genital ulcers of syphilis and chancroid are detected less often among women than among men, possibly because in some women the lesions manifest only in the vagina or on the cervix and therefore go unnoticed.

Syphilitic ulcers are typically painless and have smooth margins, indurated borders, and a clean, indurated base with serous exudate (Table 272.4). Bilateral, nonpainful inguinal lymphadenopathy is present in 60% to 70% of cases. Ulcers of chancroid usually are painful, deep, and irregular and have rough margins and a purulent exudate. Lymphadenopathy accompanying chancroid is often unilateral, painful, and tender and can become fluctuant, resulting in buboes that drain through the skin in severe cases. Fluctuant nodes should be aspirated, drained, and cultured. Whereas syphilis and chancroid lesions often begin as small papules or macules, ulcers of HSV infection take the initial form of vesicles that lead to superficial ulcers. First clinical episodes of HSV are often accompanied by fever, myalgia, and malaise. Patients who have a first clinical episode of HSV infection with HSV-1 or HSV-2 frequently experience less severe symptoms when they have previously had primary infection with the other subtype.

These symptoms and signs are characteristic of the different genital ulcer diseases, but atypical cases are common, and it is often not possible to distinguish one from another on clinical grounds. Clinical diagnosis of genital ulcers is incorrect in up to 40% of cases. Depending on the local epidemiologic characteristics of these diseases, persons infected with one disease may be co-infected with another. Conventional diagnostic tests identify no etiologic source in 25% to 50% of genital ulcers. For both syphilis and chancroid, diagnostic tests are relatively insensitive with a single examination. New diagnostic tests using DNA amplification for the three main organisms responsible for genital ulcers have been used experimentally, with substantial increases in sensitivity, but they are not yet commercially available. The sensitivity of a single dark-field examination of an ulcer for *T. pallidum* is probably quite low, depending on the quality of the specimen and the experience of the laboratory staff.

The nontreponemal RPR (rapid plasma reagin) card or VDRL (Venereal Disease Research Laboratory) tests have estimated sensitivities of 70% to 80%. If a patient with primary syphilis who has a nonreactive syphilis serologic test result returns for another test in 2 to 4 weeks, the test may be reactive;

TABLE 272.4.   CHARACTERIZATION AND DIFFERENTIATION OF GENITAL ULCERATION

Characteristic	Syphilis	Genital Herpes	Chancroid	Lymphogranuloma Venereum	Granuloma Inguinale
Causative agent	*Treponema pallidum*	Herpes simplex virus	*Haemophilus ducreyi*	*Chlamydia trachomatis*	*Calymmatobacterium granulomatis*
Initial lesion	Papule	Vesicle	Erythematous papule or pustule	Papule, pustule, or vesicle	Papule
Number of lesions	Single (multiple in 30–40% of patients)	Multiple	1–3	Single	Variable
Appearance of ulcer	Indurated, painless, clean-based ulcer with sharply demarcated, firm, raised borders	Multiple, small, nonindurated, painful, superficial, clean-based ulcers; in primary disease ulcerations tend to coalesce	Nonindurated, painful, erythematous ulcers with yellow-gray inflammatory exudate at the base; borders tend to be erythematous and undermined	Inconspicuous and quickly healing; demonstrable in less than 60% of patients; superficial, sometimes painful, erosionlike ulcer; may be associated with dorsal penile lymphangitis	Painless, gradually progressive, chronic genital ulcerations with a beefy, granulomatous heaped up appearance, tendency for prominent lesions to coalesce and local spread by autoinoculation
Associated inguinal lymphadenopathy	Firm, nontender Bilateral in 60–70%	In initial herpes: usually mildly tender and bilateral In recurrent herpes: rare, most often unilateral if present	Unilateral, tender lymphadenopathy in 50–60% of patients; may become fluctuant and spontaneously drain	Unilateral, tender, marked lymphadenopathy, often out of proportion to degree of ulceration, overlying skin may become brawny and adherent	Rare; however, pseudolymphadenopathy because of direct involvement of groin tissue in granulomatous process
Diagnostic approach	Dark-field (or immunofluorescence microscopy of material from ulcer) Serologic testing (negative in 20–30% of primary syphilis) No culture test available	Culture of vesicular lesion material, if possible Immunofluorescent antibody staining of lesion material Acute and convalescent serologic testing in nonresearch laboratories of highly variable usefulness	Culture of lesion or lymph node aspirate on selective chancroid media (consultation with clinical microbiologist recommended)	Culture of lymph node aspirate for *C. trachomatis* Serologic testing in consultation with an expert	No culture or serologic test available Diagnosis based on demonstration of bipolar staining bacilli within monocytes; best diagnostic specimen is biopsy of ulcer base at its margin

(From Hook EW III. Approach to sexually transmitted diseases and genital tract infections. In Kelly WN, *Textbook of Internal Medicine*, Second ed. Philadelphia: JB Lippincott, 1992:1608, with permission.)

however, it is possible that the test will remain nonreactive if treatment is instituted very early. The sensitivity of the fluorescent treponemal antibody-absorption test is somewhat higher than that of nontreponemal tests, but it cannot distinguish recent from past infection or exclude the possibility that the lesion is due to HSV or chancroid if the patient has a history of syphilis. The sensitivity of *H. ducreyi* culture (which is difficult and often not available) ranges widely, from about 35% to 80%, depending on the experience of the laboratory team. Tests for HSV have the highest sensitivity when vesicles are present.

In communities where both syphilis and chancroid occur, it is reasonable to presumptively treat a patient with genital ulcers for both diseases if diagnostic testing is not optimal and compliance with a request for a return visit is uncertain. Because chancroid, syphilis, and HSV have been associated with a higher than normal risk of HIV infection, and because HIV infection can result in the need for treatment with higher doses or longer courses of therapy, patients with genital ulcers due to any of these agents should be tested for HIV.

URETHRITIS

Symptomatic men with a visible urethral discharge or asymptomatic men with ≥5 leukocytes per oil-immersion field (1,000×) on a urethral smear have urethritis. Urethritis is classified as gonococcal urethritis (if it is caused by *Neisseria gonorrhoeae*) or nongonococcal urethritis (NGU). The most common cause of NGU in men 15 to 40 years of age is *C. trachomatis*; this organism is found in 15% to 40% of patients, with *Ureaplasma urealyticum* (10% to 40%) and *T. vaginalis* (2% to 10%) being the next most common organisms. Occasionally, HSV leads to urethritis, but in many cases, the cause is unknown. In men with gonococcal urethritis, 5% to 30% are co-infected with *C. trachomatis*. *Mycoplasma hominis* and *Mycoplasma genitalium* have also been associated with urethritis, but these organisms also can be found in patients without clinical evidence of urethral inflammation.

In symptomatic men a purulent discharge suggests gonococcal infection, and a serous discharge indicates NGU, but this distinction is not highly reliable. In men with a visible discharge, secretions at the tip of the penis are collected with a cotton or Dacron swab and evaluated by Gram's stain for the presence of leukocytes and intracellular gram-negative diplococci. If intracellular diplococci are seen, gonococcal urethritis is indicated; if not, the condition is considered to be NGU. The sensitivity and specificity of Gram's stain for gonococcal infection in symptomatic men are each more than 95% (compared with about 50% in infected men who have no symptoms).

In men without a visible discharge (even after stripping the urethra), a thin urethral swab should be inserted 2 to 3 cm to obtain secretions; this technique is particularly helpful in evaluating patients who report symptoms but who have no apparent sign of discharge at the time of examination. If urethritis is not confirmed at the initial visit of a patient who reports symptoms, the patient should return for another examination the following morning, before urinating. Although the urethral smear is useful for distinguishing men who have gonococcal urethritis from those who do not, men with a smear suggestive of gonococcal

infection should also be tested by culture for *N. gonorrhoeae*, in part for medicolegal reasons. Symptomatic men with NGU should be tested for *C. trachomatis*, because finding *C. trachomatis* is important for appropriate treatment of sexual partners.

For screening asymptomatic men for gonococcal and chlamydial infection, polymerase chain reaction and ligase chain reaction tests, which can be performed on urine, have higher sensitivities than other nonculture tests. An inexpensive option for detecting urethritis in asymptomatic individuals is the leukocyte esterase test, which can be performed on the initial 15 to 20 mL of voided urine. This technique has been best evaluated in adolescent boys, in whom the sensitivity of detecting *N. gonorrhoeae* and *C. trachomatis* ranges from 50% to 100%, and the specificity ranges from 80% to 100%.

Initial treatment of patients with urethritis should be based on the results of Gram's stain. (In the symptomatic patient, if a Gram's stain of urethral secretions is not immediately available, treatment for both gonococcal and nongonococcal urethritis is advised.) Tetracycline-resistant *U. urealyticum* and other sources of NGU should be considered in patients with persistent NGU who have completed therapy and have not been reexposed to an untreated sex partner.

VAGINAL DISCHARGE

Vaginal discharge is most often the result of bacterial vaginosis, vulvovaginal candidiasis, or trichomoniasis. The prevalence of these conditions varies according to the population of patients; bacterial vaginosis is usually the most common. Severe cervicitis caused by *N. gonorrhoeae*, *C. trachomatis*, or HSV infrequently results in vaginal discharge. Abundant vaginal secretions are occasionally physiologic and do not necessarily indicate the presence of infection. Treatment regimens for common causes of vaginal discharge are listed in Table 272.5.

The typical discharge of bacterial vaginosis is white or gray, homogeneous, and adherent to the walls of the vagina. Vulvovaginal candidiasis is characterized by a white, often curdlike discharge sometimes accompanied by vulvitis. Trichomoniasis produces a profuse yellowish discharge, and the vaginal walls may appear inflamed; a *strawberry cervix* with petechial lesions may be seen. It is often difficult to distinguish these conditions based on history and physical examination alone; the conditions may exist without symptoms, and co-infections are common. Frequent douching may also affect the appearance of vaginal secretions that are normally associated with these pathogens. It is important not only to perform diagnostic testing on the vaginal discharge but also to examine every patient with vaginal discharge for cervicitis and to test for gonorrhea and chlamydia, especially women with an STD risk factor.

In evaluating the possibility of vaginitis, a specimen of vaginal secretions should be collected from the posterior fornix of the vagina using a cotton or Dacron swab. Apply the swab to two microscope slides. One or two drops of 0.9% saline may be added to one slide for wet-mount examination for motile trichomonads and for the clue cells typical of bacterial vaginosis. A 10% potassium hydroxide (KOH) solution added to the second slide improves the examination for yeast or pseudohyphae.

Bacterial vaginosis results from an alteration in vaginal flora

TABLE 272.5.	TREATMENT REGIMENS FOR COMMON CAUSES OF VAGINAL DISCHARGE	
Disease	**Recommended Regimens**	**Alternative Regimens**
Bacterial vaginosis	Metronidazole, 500 mg orally two times a day for 7 days[a]; Clindamycin cream, 2%, one full applicator (5 g) intravaginally at bedtime for 7 days; or Metronidazole gel, 0.75%, one full applicator (5 g) intravaginally two times a day for 5 days	Metronidazole, 2 g orally in a single dose; Clindamycin, 300 mg orally two times a day for 7 days
Vulvovaginal candidiasis	Butoconazole, 2% cream, 5 g intravaginally for 3 days; Clotrimazole, 1% cream, 5 g for 7–14 days; Clotrimazole, 100-mg vaginal tablets for 7 days; Clotrimazole, 100-mg vaginal tablets, two for 3 days; Clotrimazole, 500-mg vaginal tablet, one tablet in a single application; Miconazole, 2% cream, 5 g intravaginally for 7 days; Miconazole, 200-mg vaginal suppository, one for 3 days; Miconazole, 100-mg vaginal suppository, one for 7 days; Nystatin, 100,000-unit vaginal tablet, one for 14 days; Tioconazole, 6.5% ointment, 5 g intravaginally in a single application; Terconazole, 0.4% cream, 5 g intravaginally for 7 days; Terconazole, 0.8% cream, 5 g intravaginally for 3 days; Terconazole, 80-mg suppository, one suppository for 3 days; or Fluconazole, 150 mg orally in a single dose[b]	
Trichomoniasis	Metronidazole, 2 g orally in a single dose[a]	Metronidazole, 500 mg twice daily for 7 days

[a] During pregnancy, the recommended regimen for bacterial vaginosis is metronidazole, 250 mg orally three times a day for 7 days. Trichomoniasis may be treated during pregnancy with metronidazole, 2 g orally in a single dose.
[b] Contraindicated during pregnancy.

that is characterized by replacement of the normally dominant *Lactobacillus* species with an overgrowth of *Gardnerella vaginalis*, *Mycoplasma hominis*, and anaerobic bacteria, including *Bacteroides* and *Mobiluncus* species. The typical clue cells seen in the 0.9% saline preparation are vaginal epithelial cells with a granular appearance and indistinct margins caused by adherent bacteria. The Amsel criteria for diagnosis of bacterial vaginosis require that the vaginal discharge have at least three of these four characteristics: typical vaginal discharge, clue cells present on wet mount, a typical fishy amine odor (often produced or enhanced when mixed with 10% KOH), or a vaginal pH of more than 4.5. New tests for bacterial vaginosis include a rapid test of vaginal secretions for elevated pH and amines and a nucleic acid probe assay for *G. vaginalis* antigens. Tests for *G. vaginalis* are not specific for bacterial vaginosis, however, because this organism is found in a high proportion of women with no signs or symptoms. In the absence of symptoms in nonpregnant women, a finding of bacterial vaginosis is not sufficient indication for treatment. Some experts recommend screening and treatment of asymptomatic pregnant women (particularly those with a history of premature delivery) or asymptomatic women about to undergo invasive gynecologic surgery, in light of evidence that treatment may help prevent premature births and postoperative infections. Bacterial vaginosis is associated with sexual intercourse, but no counterpart of this disease is found in men; treatment of men does not prevent recurrence of this syndrome in their sex partners.

Vulvovaginal candidiasis most often is caused by *Candida albicans* and less frequently by *Torulopsis* species and other *Candida* species. Diagnosis usually is made on clinical grounds and by examining the KOH preparation by microscopy. Vulvovaginal candidiasis is not sexually transmitted. The primary goal of therapy is alleviation of symptoms; *Candida* species often can be detected in vaginal secretions by culture, even in the absence of vaginal discharge. Patients with acute or recurrent vulvovaginal candidiasis (usually defined as three or more episodes annually) may have predisposing risk factors, such as antibiotic or glucocorticoid use, diabetes, immunosuppression, or HIV infection, though such factors are identified in a minority of cases. Many topical azole preparations are available for treatment of vulvovaginal candidiasis. Oral azole therapy is another option, but it should not be used during pregnancy. Over-the-counter topical preparations are available, but they should be used only by women in whom vulvovaginal candidiasis has been diagnosed previously and who experience symptoms similar to their previous episode; recurrences within 2 months of treatment should be reevaluated thoroughly.

Trichomonas vaginalis infection is a sexually transmitted protozoal infection that should be treated even when it is detected in patients with minimal or no symptoms. In patients with a typical vaginal discharge, the sensitivity of wet-mount examination is high, but in patients with milder symptoms, wet mount is less sensitive; culture or nucleic acid probe assay may assist in making the diagnosis. Sex partners of patients with *T. vaginalis* should be treated. Infections can be resistant to the standard doses of metronidazole; such infections may respond to re-treatment or to treatment with higher doses of the same drug (2 g of metronidazole taken orally in a single dose for 3 to 5 days). Infections that persist even after treatment with this higher dose should be evaluated for susceptibility to metronidazole and referred to an expert.

CERVICITIS

Mucopurulent cervicitis (MPC) is characterized by the presence of a yellowish, mucopurulent, endocervical secretion present at the cervical os or on a white endocervical swab. MPC is often associated with cervical friability (bleeding that occurs with insertion of the first endocervical swab used for specimen collection) and with an edematous zone of cervical ectopy. The presence of increased numbers of white blood cells (more than 30) on an endocervical Gram's stain also supports the diagnosis, but this sign is too nonspecific to be diagnostically useful. Although the source of MPC is identified in a minority of cases, it is typically found in association with chlamydial infection, sometimes with gonococcal infection, and occasionally with HSV.

All patients with MPC should be tested for *C. trachomatis* and *N. gonorrhoeae*. To assess the possibility of MPC and endocervical infection, first wipe away with a swab any vaginal secretions obscuring the cervical ostium. If endocervical specimens are to be collected, a swab for the gonorrhea test should be inserted 1 to 2 cm into the endocervix and left in place for 10 to 15 seconds to absorb secretions. When using an endocervical swab to collect a specimen for examination for *C. trachomatis*, at least one full rotation of the swab or Cytobrush should be made; in sampling for chlamydia, it is optimal to obtain columnar epithelial cells present on the endocervix, because chlamydia preferentially infect these cells. Urine tests for gonococcal and chlamydial infections using nucleic acid amplification methods can be performed in lieu of tests on endocervical specimens.

An endocervical Gram's stain for gram-negative intracellular diplococci has a sensitivity of no more than about 60% for *N. gonorrhoeae*, even in experienced laboratories, and is therefore not an adequate test. In patients with MPC who have a high likelihood of having both gonorrhea and chlamydia, the clinician should treat empirically for both diseases. If the likelihood of infection with *N. gonorrhoeae* is low but that of *C. trachomatis* is appreciable, the clinician should treat for chlamydial infection and await the gonorrhea test results. If neither infection is considered likely, the clinician should await the results of both diagnostic tests before prescribing therapy.

PELVIC INFLAMMATORY DISEASE

PID, a syndrome that includes endometritis, salpingitis, tuboovarian abscess, and, in severe cases, peritonitis and pelvic abscess, can be initiated by gonococcal or chlamydial infection and possibly by bacterial vaginosis. In many instances, however, none of these sources can be confirmed. In a substantial proportion of

TABLE 272.6.	CIRCUMSTANCES UNDER WHICH HOSPITALIZATION FOR TREATMENT OF PID IS ESPECIALLY RECOMMENDED

Surgical emergencies, such as appendicitis, cannot be excluded.
The patient is pregnant.
The patient does not respond clinically to oral antimicrobial therapy.
The patient is unable to follow or tolerate an outpatient oral regimen.
The patient has severe illness, nausea and vomiting, or high fever.
Patient has a tuboovarian abscess.
The patient is immunodeficient (i.e., has HIV infection with low CD4 count, is taking immunosuppressive therapy, or has another disease).

cases of PID, there is anaerobic infection of the upper genital tract, and some experts recommend providing all women with PID with comprehensive treatment for anaerobic infection in addition to therapy for gonorrhea and chlamydial infection. Because many patients with acute PID have no symptoms or only mild symptoms, it is difficult to make a clinical diagnosis of acute PID, and many cases go unrecognized. Severity of symptoms has not been shown to correlate with severity of tubal damage or related effects of PID; for this reason, the physician should have a low threshold for instituting therapy. PID should be suspected and treatment initiated when lower abdominal tenderness, adnexal tenderness, and cervical motion tenderness are present, if other causes have been excluded. More comprehensive evaluation should be undertaken if the symptoms and signs are more severe (a discussion is beyond the scope of this chapter). Hospitalization for PID is often indicated (Table 272.6).

STRATEGIES FOR OPTIMAL CARE

MANAGEMENT

In deciding on STD diagnostic and treatment services for a particular practice setting, consideration should be given to the risk profile of the patients served, the disease prevalence rates in the clinic population, and the likelihood that patients will comply with requests for a return visit. In settings providing services to many adolescents and young adults, it is essential to make available screening examinations for gonorrhea and chlamydia. Nucleic acid amplification assays for these agents, using urine specimens, can facilitate testing in places where gynecologic examinations are not routinely performed. In facilities where patients with urethritis and cervicitis are seen relatively often, on-site availability of medications for treatment of chlamydial infection and gonorrhea is important. In those primary care settings where patients with bacterial STDs are seen comparatively infrequently, emphasis may be placed on ensuring the availability of confirmatory or repeated testing, to exclude false-positive test results. Clinicians providing prenatal services to a population of patients with a notable prevalence of syphilis morbidity but uncertain follow-up should have on-site RPR card testing and benzathine penicillin G.

When follow-up of patients is uncertain or when continued disease transmission is a concern, immediate treatment (and possibly overtreatment) of curable STDs is preferred to delayed treatment pending the results of laboratory tests. For reasons of acceptability, adherence to treatment, and prevention of disease transmission, single-dose therapy is generally preferable to multidose therapy, and immediate dispensing of medications is preferable to requesting that a patient obtain medications at another site.

Patients diagnosed with one STD should be evaluated for others, including HIV. Practitioners serving populations with STDs should be prepared to perform HIV counseling and testing or to refer for this test. Practitioners serving populations with HIV infection also should be ready to evaluate HIV-infected patients for other STDs. Screening for STDs in HIV-infected patients should include a serologic test for syphilis and, in women, a complete gynecologic examination and tests for endocervical gonococcal and chlamydial infection. Patients with sexually acquired HIV are at increased risk of other STDs, and untreated STDs in these patients raise their risk of transmitting HIV to others.

Patients should be counseled about how to lessen their risk of acquiring STDs; such counseling should include guidance in the consistent and correct use of condoms. Identification, treatment, and counseling of sex partners are essential to prevent reinfection of the patient and further transmission of disease. The physician should assist with this process. In many cases, patients can be encouraged to bring or refer their sex partners for treatment. If patients are unwilling to notify partners, the

local health department should be asked to provide confidential partner notification.

COMPLICATIONS AND PITFALLS

The likelihood of surgical emergencies should be considered in persons with possible epididymitis (testicular torsion is part of the differential diagnosis) or PID (ectopic pregnancy and acute abdomen need to be excluded). There are many pitfalls in the treatment of patients with STDs; several are noted in Table 272.7.

➡️ ## Indications for REFERRAL

Persons who should be referred for further evaluation and treatment may include patients in need of specialized counseling or drug treatment services; patients with nonhealing lesions that may require biopsy; patients with persistent epididymitis, which, in the context of HIV, may be due to fungal or tuberculous infection; and patients with persistent vaginitis, which may be due to metronidazole-resistant trichomoniasis or recurrent vulvovaginal candidiasis.

COST-EFFECTIVENESS

The adverse effects of sexually transmitted infections are responsible for the high human and economic costs associated with these diseases. The annual medical cost of curing STDs (chlamydia, gonorrhea, syphilis, and trichomoniasis) is estimated to be approximately two billion dollars annually; over half of this cost is associated with PID and its effects—infertility, chronic pelvic pain, and ectopic pregnancy. Untreated syphilis during pregnancy results in fetal death in 40% of cases, and the average lifetime cost of care of an infant born with congenital syphilis is more than $130,000. The costs of non-HIV viral STDs (genital herpes, HPV, hepatitis B) and their side effects also have been estimated to be about two billion dollars annually. Several HPV types, mainly 16, 18, 31, 33, and 35, are associated with the development of cervical dysplasia and carcinoma, and hepatitis B is associated with hepatocellular carcinoma. There is strong evidence that both ulcerative and nonulcerative STDs enhance transmission of HIV, though the extent to which transmission of HIV infection is attributable to other STDs varies locally according to disease prevalence and transmission modes.

Because the economic consequences of STDs place a large burden on the health care system, primary prevention and early detection and treatment of STDs are highly cost-effective measures. The expense and preventability of congenital syphilis have made universal syphilis screening of women during pregnancy a standard preventive measure. Hepatitis A and B are the only STDs for which there are vaccines; the first trials of an HSV

TABLE 272.7.	COMMON PITFALLS IN THE MANAGEMENT OF PATIENTS WITH STDs

Incomplete assessment of a patient's STD risks
Incomplete physical examination
Improper specimen collection
Failure to consider the lack of sensitivity of certain diagnostic tests, leading to possible undertreatment
Failure to consider the lack of specificity of certain diagnostic tests and the possibility of false-positive results in low-prevalence populations
Lack of optimal on-site, immediate treatment of high-risk patients
Underrecognition and undertreatment of PID
Failure to consider HIV co-infection in patients with STDs and STDs in patients with HIV
Failure to provide education and counseling in risk reduction
Failure to prevent transmission or reinfection through identification, notification, and counseling of sex partners

STD, sexually transmitted disease.

vaccine were unsuccessful, and further efforts at vaccine development are under way. When tests are expensive and funds for testing are scarce, selective screening of populations at high risk for STDs may be wise, as described earlier for chlamydial infection. Preventive efforts, including counseling, also should be focused on patients at high risk; a careful risk assessment is a useful cost-effective tool.

BIBLIOGRAPHY

Alexander LL, Cates JR, Herndon N, et al., eds. *Sexually transmitted diseases in America: how many cases and at what cost?* Research Triangle Park, N.C.: American Social Health Association, 1998.

Brunham RC, Paavonen J, Stevens CE, et al. Mucopurulent cervicitis: the ignored counterpart in women of urethritis. *N Engl J Med* 1984;311: 1–6.

Centers for Disease Control and Prevention. Recommendations for the prevention and management of *Chlamydia trachomatis* infections, 1993. *MMWR* 1993;42(RR-12):1–39.

Centers for Disease Control and Prevention. 1998 recommendations for treatment of sexually transmitted diseases. *MMWR* 1998;47(RR-1): 1–111.

Centers for Disease Control and Prevention. HIV prevention through early detection and treatment of other sexually transmitted diseases—United States. *MMWR* 1998;47(RR-12):i–24.

Eng TR, Butler WT, eds. *The hidden epidemic: confronting sexually transmitted diseases.* Washington, D.C.: National Academy Press, 1997.

Holmes KK, Sparling PF, Mardh P-A, et al., eds. *Sexually transmitted diseases,* third ed. New York: McGraw-Hill, 1999.

Mertz KJ, Trees D, Levine WC, et al. Etiology of genital ulcers and prevalence of human immunodeficiency virus coinfection in 10 US cities. The Genital Ulcer Disease Surveillance Group. *J Infect Dis* 1998;178: 1795–1798.

Morse SA, Moreland AA, Holmes KK, eds. *Atlas of sexually transmitted diseases and AIDS,* second ed. St. Louis: Mosby, 1996.

Quinn TC. The polymicrobial origin of intestinal infections in homosexual men. *N Engl J Med* 1983;309:576–582.

Workowski KA, St Louis ME. 1998 guidelines for the treatment of sexually transmitted diseases. *Clin Infect Dis* 1999;28:S1–S3.

Kelley's Textbook of Internal Medicine, fourth edition. Edited by H. David Humes. Lippincott Williams & Wilkins, Philadelphia © 2000.

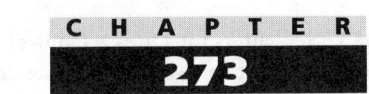

CHAPTER
273

SURGICAL INFECTIONS

E. PATCHEN DELLINGER

PATHOPHYSIOLOGY

Surgical infections are different from most medical infections because a mechanical or anatomical barrier to resolution of infection exists. Although the specific pathogens present are susceptible to antimicrobial agents, administration of these agents will

not resolve the infection unless the mechanical problem is corrected. Some examples include drainage of an abscess, either superficial or deep; removal of an obstructed and infected appendix; and repair or diversion of an intestinal perforation. Some procedures may not be thought of as "operations" but achieve the same purpose. Thus, opening an infected wound, placing a percutaneous catheter into an intra-abdominal abscess, or draining an obstructed, infected biliary duct system with an endoscopic stent all fulfill this purpose. The key to successful management of a surgical infection is to recognize the "surgical" nature of the infection and to perform the required procedure promptly, in coordination with appropriate antimicrobial administration and other treatment factors.

Infections that follow a surgical procedure are classically considered surgical infections because they occur as a consequence of the procedure; in addition, many of them also require surgical intervention such as opening of the wound, draining of an intra-abdominal abscess, or repair of a leaking anastomosis.

Postoperative fever raises the question of postoperative infection and in many cases serves as the stimulus for the administration of antibiotics. However, most febrile postoperative patients do not have an identifiable infection, and many infected patients do not have a fever in the early stages of infection. Depending on the definition of fever, 20% to 75% of postoperative patients have a fever in the first 5 days after the procedure. More than 75% of fevers noted in the first 2 days are never associated with an identifiable infection. By the fifth postoperative day, the likelihood that a new fever represents a wound infection is about 40% (Fig. 273.1). Thus, giving empirical antibiotics to a postoperative patient with fever is not a good strategy unless there is a clear presumptive diagnosis of an infection that is expected to respond to antibiotic administration (e.g., pneumonia or urinary tract infection). Other postoperative infections will not respond to antibiotic administration without the appropriate surgical management, and giving antibiotics before the

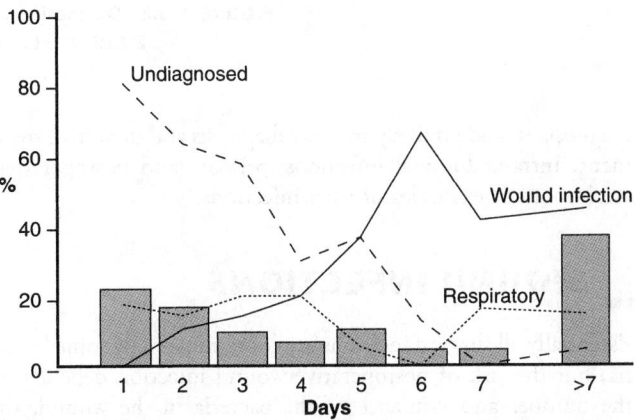

FIGURE 273.1. Bars indicate the percentage of all fevers that appear on each respective day. Lines indicate the percentage of new fevers on each day that are due to wound infection (------) or respiratory infection (. . .) or are unexplained (- - -). (Data from Garibaldi RA, Brodine S, Matsumiya S, et al. *Infect Control* 1985;6:273; and Gorbach SL, Bartlett JG, Blacklow NR. *Infectious diseases.* Philadelphia: WB Saunders, 1992: 754.

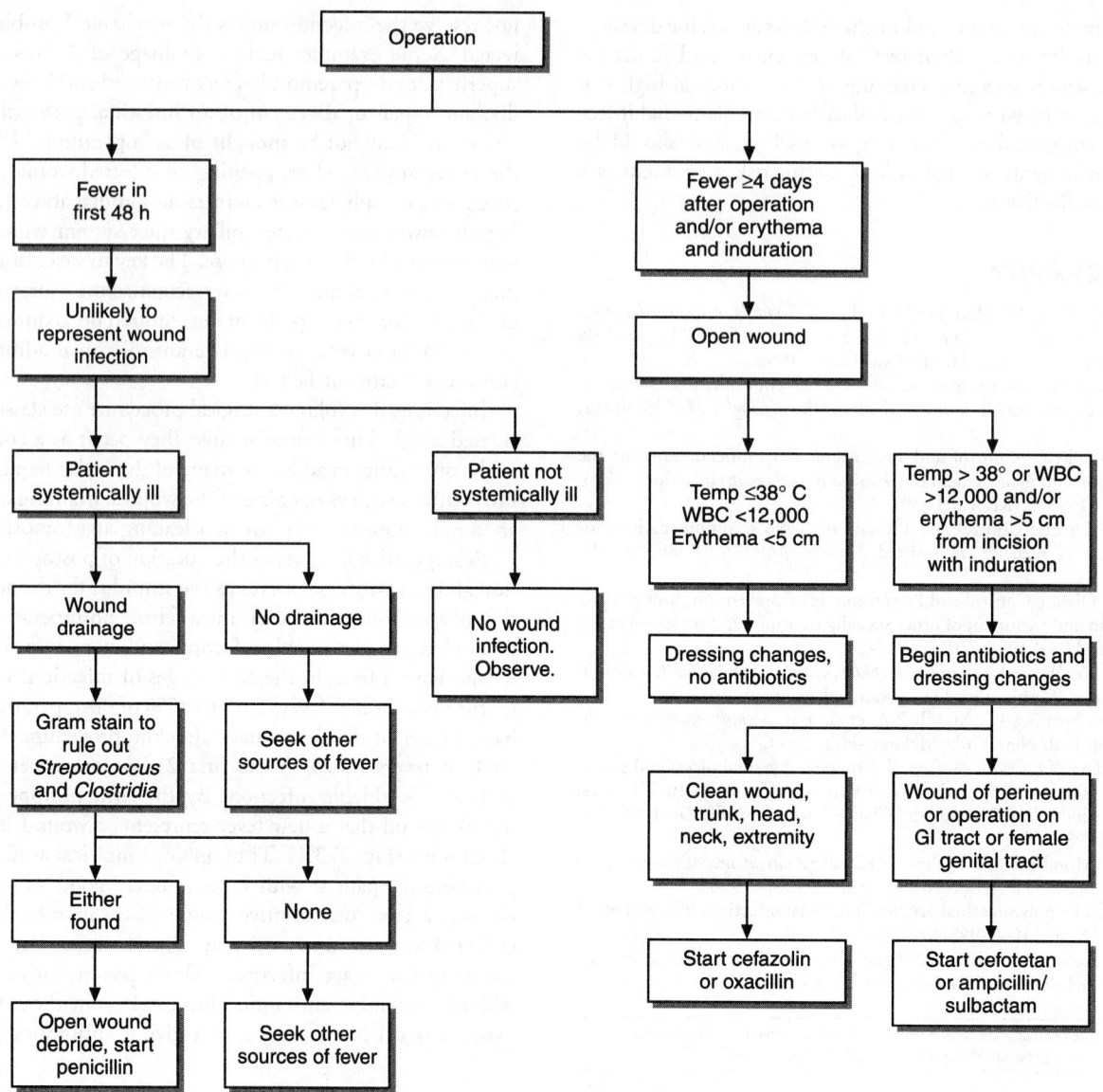

FIGURE 273.2. Diagnosis and treatment of postoperative infection.
EVIDENCE LEVEL: C. Expert Opinion.

diagnosis is made is likely to delay diagnosis and definitive treatment. Intra-abdominal infections, primary and postoperative, are important examples of such infections.

WOUND INFECTIONS

Essentially all surgical incisions are contaminated by some bacteria, but the risk of postoperative wound infection depends on the number and virulence of the bacteria in the wound, the state of underlying host defenses, and the extent to which the operation impairs local and systemic host defenses. Historically, wounds were classified solely by the risk of bacterial contamination during the procedure, as determined largely by entry into the gastrointestinal tract or an area of preexisting inflammation or infection. Currently, the most widely used scoring system,

developed by the U.S. Centers for Disease Control and Prevention (CDC), assigns a point for wounds that are contaminated or dirty, a point for an operation that lasts longer than the 75th percentile for that procedure, and a point if the patient is classified as physical status 3 or 4 according to the American Society of Anesthesiology. Using this score, CDC data show a risk of infection of 1.5% for a score of 0, 2.9% for a score of 1, 6.8% for a score of 2, and 13.0% for a score of 3. These data reflect modern surgical and anesthetic practices and current standards for use of perioperative prophylactic antibiotics.

Most wound infections are not evident clinically until after the fifth postoperative day, so with modern practice resulting in shorter hospital stays for most procedures, over half of all wound infections are diagnosed after hospital discharge. The only types of wound infection likely to be diagnosed in the first 48 hours after a procedure are those due either to β-hemolytic streptococci or to *Clostridium* species. They are rare, but when they occur they can move rapidly and have devastating consequences. Clostridial infections are noted for the absence of signs of local inflammation due to the leukocidal exotoxins released into the wound. The exudate typically contains gram-positive rods without spores and few or no white blood cells (WBCs). Streptococcal infections do show signs of inflammation, and the Gram smear shows both WBCs and gram-positive cocci. Both streptococcal and clostridial early wound infections are typically accompanied by signs of severe systemic response. Any suspicion of such an infection should cause direct inspection of the wound and a Gram smear of any exudate. If the diagnosis is made, the wound must be opened and debrided, high-dose penicillin should be administered, and vigorous cardiorespiratory stabilization and support should be instituted. Recent in vitro and animal data suggest a helpful role for clindamycin administration in such patients due to its action of suppressing toxin production by streptococcal and clostridial species.

The most important treatment for a wound infection is to open the wound. Most wound infections respond promptly and nicely to drainage alone without antibiotics (Fig. 273.2). Antibiotics are needed for wound infections only if there is evidence of invasive soft-tissue infection beyond the limits of the wound or if there is a systemic response to the infection indicated by elevated temperature (higher than 38°C) and WBC count (more than 12,000 per microliter). If an antibiotic is given, the choice should be guided by the Gram smear of the wound exudate and the type of wound. Antibiotic treatment should be continued only until local signs of inflammation or the systemic response have resolved (usually 2 or 3 days).

Infections following clean operations on the trunk or extremities are most likely to be caused by *Staphylococcus aureus*. Infections that follow operations in the axilla are more likely to involve gram-negative rods, and infections that follow operations on the perineum, the female genital tract, or the large intestine commonly involve a mixture of gram-positive cocci, gram-negative rods, and anaerobes.

PREVENTING WOUND INFECTIONS

Many think first of prophylactic antibiotic administration for preventing postoperative wound infections. However, many elements are important in preventing wound infections (Table 273.1), and unless these are considered, the use of prophylactic antibiotics will not achieve an acceptable result. In addition, several factors that are not under the surgeon's control increase the risk of infection (Table 273.2). Knowledge of these can increase the surgeon's awareness of risk and perhaps stimulate additional precautions, including the appropriate use of prophylactic antibiotics for cases that might otherwise not warrant them.

Principles for the effective use of prophylactic antibiotics have been refined over many years (Table 273.3). The three most common errors in the use of prophylactic antibiotics are failure to use them at all when indicated; initiating antibiotic administration more than 2 hours before the beginning of the procedure

---

TABLE 273.1.	IMPORTANT ELEMENTS IN PREVENTION OF WOUND INFECTIONS

- Do not perform an elective clean operation if there is a distant-site infection (urinary tract, sinusitis, subcutaneous abscess) or an adjacent open wound.
- Do not shave the operative site until just before the time of operation, or at all if possible.
- Perform complete mechanical bowel preparation before an elective colon operation.
- Use good sterile operative technique.
- Avoid tissue trauma during the operation.
- Avoid operative blood loss and minimize operative time.

---

or after the beginning of the procedure; and continuing prophylactic antibiotics for more than 12 hours after the completion of the procedure. Surgeons commonly wish to continue antibiotics for a longer time in high-risk patients or in the presence of a postoperative fever (see above), but there is no evidence that antibiotics administered after the completion of the procedure prevent postoperative infections. Even in trauma patients, where administration of prophylactic antibiotics before the injury is impossible, prospective trials of patients with penetrating intestinal injuries or open fractures have demonstrated that a 12-hour course of antibiotics is not inferior to prolonged administration of the same agents over 5 to 7 days.

Knowledge regarding the specific procedures that benefit from administration of prophylactic antibiotics has evolved over the past 20 years. Table 273.4 lists procedures for which prophylactic antibiotics are effective in reducing the rate of postoperative surgical site infections, and for which the benefit of this reduction is thought to outweigh any complications or costs of the antibiotics used. Prophylactic antibiotics are, however, commonly used in many other situations that have not been proven effective, or where reduction of infection has been demonstrated but the baseline infection rate is low or the consequences of infection are small. In the latter situation, some argue that the costs of the prophylactic use outweigh the benefits. However, there are data indicating that practicing surgeons can recognize patients who are at higher risk and tend to use prophylactic antibiotics in those settings. Factors such as those listed in Table 273.2 and found in the CDC index may justify the addition of a brief course of perioperative prophylactic antibiotics for procedures that do not have an official recommendation.

TABLE 273.2.	FACTORS THAT INCREASE THE RISK OF WOUND INFECTION

- Increased age
- Diabetes mellitus
- Obesity
- Malnutrition
- Steroid administration
- Smoking

TABLE 273.3.	PRINCIPLES OF PERIOPERATIVE PROPHYLACTIC ANTIBIOTIC USE

- Choose an appropriate agent (see text)
- Use a dose equal to or greater than the usual therapeutic dose for the agent chosen.
- Initiate antibiotic administration intravenously during the 60 min before the surgical incision.
- Discontinue antibiotic prophylaxis preferably at the end of the procedure, but certainly within 12 h.
- During a prolonged operative procedure, repeat doses of antibiotic at intervals of 1–2 times the half-life of the drug.

Many individual antibiotics have been tested and found effective in one or more settings for perioperative prophylaxis. In practical terms, the choice can be determined by whether the planned operation will involve the distal ileum, appendix, or colon. In this case, an agent with activity against enteric facultative and obligate anaerobic bacteria should be chosen. Cefotetan is recommended; cefoxitin is an alternative. For procedures where anaerobic bacteria are unlikely to be involved, the recommended agent is cefazolin. Vancomycin can be used for patients who are allergic to cephalosporins or in settings where methicillin-resistant *S. aureus* are common. However, vancomycin should not be used for prophylaxis unless the indications for it are strong because of its tendency to promote the emergence of vancomycin-resistant enterococci (VRE). Because vancomycin provides no activity against gram-negative rods, an agent such as aztreonam or an aminoglycoside can be added for upper intestinal operations, and metronidazole or clindamycin should be

TABLE 273.4.	PROCEDURES THAT BENEFIT FROM PROPHYLACTIC PERIOPERATIVE ANTIBIOTICS

- High-risk gastroduodenal procedures (operations for cancer, gastric ulcer, bleeding, or obstruction, and when the patient has received effective acid-reducing therapy or is morbidly obese)
- High-risk biliary tract procedures (age >60, common duct stones present, bile duct obstruction, recent acute cholecystitis, prior biliary tract operation or instrumentation)
- Any operation on the colon or distal ileum, including appendectomies
- Head and neck cancer operations
- Vascular procedures on the lower extremities or abdominal aorta
- Hysterectomy
- Primary cesarean section
- Joint replacement
- Placement of other prosthetic devices
- Cardiac procedures
- Craniotomy

Procedures for Which Prophylactic Antibiotic Indications Are Controversial

- Groin hernia repair without prosthetic mesh
- Breast mass excision and mastectomy
- Other clean procedures without prosthetic insertion

added if anaerobic bacteria will be encountered. For elective colonic procedures, current practice in the United States is to give an oral antibiotic regimen before the operation in addition to parenteral antibiotics at the time of the procedure. The most common regimen with firm support from prospective trials is neomycin 1 g and erythromycin base 1 g orally, given at 19, 18, and 9 hours before the planned procedure.

NECROTIZING SOFT-TISSUE INFECTIONS

These serious infections can be divided into those involving muscle (of which the most severe is clostridial myonecrosis, or gas gangrene) and those not involving muscle. Clostridial myonecrosis is noted for the rapid pace of its spread and the severe systemic reaction associated with it. Signs of inflammation are minimal (as noted in the section on postoperative infections) and the external evidence of infection is less than the underlying tissue involvement. Treatment requires aggressive resuscitation, large doses of penicillin, and aggressive operative debridement, often including extremity amputation. Hyperbaric oxygen probably helps if it is readily available, but the primary treatment must not be delayed by efforts to transfer the patient for its administration. Mortality and morbidity from this infection is high.

The serious nonclostridial infections have been given many names over the years, but the most common label is necrotizing fasciitis. This infection is much more common than serious clostridial infections. The fascia referred to is the superficial fascia, which consists of all tissue between the dermis and the underlying muscle. The difficulty with these infections is that the initial presentation is often misleading, resembling a simple cellulitis that would be expected to resolve with antibiotics alone. The following signs in association with an apparent cellulitis indicate that a necrotizing process is involved and that surgical exploration with probable debridement will be required: skin gangrene, ecchymoses, bullae, crepitus, edema in excess of other local signs of infection and inflammation, and failure to respond to apparently adequate antibiotic therapy. Necrotizing fasciitis can be caused by a synergistic combination of gram-negative rods, gram-positive cocci, and anaerobes, and can also be caused by β-hemolytic streptococci alone. Mixed infections tend to follow traumatic lacerations and operations on the perineum or in the abdomen involving bowel, or to complicate decubitus ulcers. Necrotizing infections that arise in trivial injuries such as varicella lesions, mosquito bites, or superficial scratches or occur with no known injury are almost always due to group A streptococci.

INFECTIONS IN BURN PATIENTS

Infection continues to be one of the primary mechanisms of morbidity and mortality in burn patients. The burn injury itself imposes major trauma with profound metabolic and immune consequences simultaneously with the destruction of the most important bacterial host defense organ, the skin. Bacteria gain access to the devitalized burn wound and previously sterile tissues beneath it at a time of profound depression of systemic host defenses. Therapeutic interventions create the risk of additional nosocomial infections, including pneumonia, urinary tract infection, and intravenous line–associated infection.

Efforts to prevent infection must begin with the initial evaluation of the patient. Tetanus toxoid should be administered. Burn wounds are washed and protected with a topical antimicrobial substance. The ideal agent should penetrate the burn wound, have broad-spectrum antibacterial activity, have little toxicity, and be both easy to apply and painless. Silver sulfadiazine is easy to apply, painless, and effective against most common burn wound pathogens, but it does not penetrate the burn wound. This makes it quite effective in preventing infection but not very effective if infection has already occurred. Mafenide acetate is also broad-spectrum and easy to apply, but it is somewhat painful on application. It penetrates the burn wound and is thus useful for reducing burn wound colonization, but this penetration can also lead to systemic absorption with resulting metabolic acidosis caused by one of the metabolites, which functions as a carbonic anhydrase inhibitor.

A burn wound is rarely sterile, but low levels of bacteria (fewer than 10^3 organisms per gram of tissue) do not cause clinical disease and are referred to as *colonization*. Infection occurs when bacterial overgrowth in the burn wound leads to invasion of adjacent viable tissue. Bacterial numbers associated with burn wound infection are usually more than 10^5 organisms per gram of tissue. Histologic sections of burn wound infection also show bacteria invading beyond the burn wound into viable tissue. Any acute change in the appearance of a burn wound or the surrounding tissues should lead to biopsy for culture and histology to make the diagnosis of invasive infection. Some signs that should stimulate biopsy include an increase in the depth of the burn wound injury, discoloration of adjacent tissue, hemorrhage beneath the burn wound, and greenish discoloration of the burn wound. Typical pathogens in burn wound infections include *S. aureus,* streptococci, *Pseudomonas aeruginosa, Proteus* species, *Escherichia coli,* and *Klebsiella* species. Use of parenteral antibiotics should be limited to documented infections, but they are needed for burn wound infection. The best way to prevent infection is through early closure of the burn wound, usually through a combination of excision and grafting.

BIBLIOGRAPHY

Burke JF. Identification of the source of staphylococci contaminating the surgical wound during operation. *Ann Surg* 1963;158:898.

Culver DH, Horan TC, Gaynes RP, et al. Surgical wound infection rates by wound class, operative procedure, and patient risk index. *Am J Med* 1991;91(Suppl 3B):152S–157S.

Dellinger EP. Antibiotic prophylaxis in trauma: penetrating abdominal injuries and open fractures. *Rev Infect Dis* 1991;13(Suppl 10):S847–S857.

Dellinger EP. Approach to the patient with postoperative fever. In: Gorbach SL, Bartlett JG, Blacklow NR, eds. *Infectious diseases in medicine and surgery.* Philadelphia: WB Saunders, 1991.

Dellinger EP, Gross PA, Barrett TL, et al. Quality standard for antimicrobial prophylaxis in surgical procedures. Infectious Diseases Society of America. *Clin Infect Dis* 1994;18:422–427.

Gilpin DA, Rutan RL, Herndon DN. Burn wound infection. In: Fry DE, ed. *Surgical infections.* Boston: Little, Brown and Company, 1995.

Howard RJ, Simmons RL, ed. *Surgical infectious diseases,* second ed. Norwalk, CT: Appleton & Lange, 1988.

Lewis RT. Necrotizing soft-tissue infections. *Infect Dis Clin North Am* 1992;6:693–703.

Platt R, Zaleznik DF, Hopkins CC, et al. Perioperative antibiotic prophylaxis for herniorrhaphy and breast surgery. *N Engl J Med* 1990;322:153–160.

Platt R, Zucker JR, Zaleznik DF, et al. Prophylaxis against wound infection following herniorrhaphy or breast surgery. *J Infect Dis* 1992;166:556–560.

U.S. Centers for Disease Control and Prevention. Recommendations for preventing the spread of vancomycin resistance. Recommendations of the Hospital Infection Control Practices Advisory Committee (HICPAC). *MMWR* 1995;44:1–13.

Kelley's Textbook of Internal Medicine, fourth edition. Edited by H. David Humes. Lippincott Williams & Wilkins, Philadelphia © 2000.

ORGANISM-SPECIFIC DISORDERS

BACTERIAL INFECTIONS

CHAPTER

274

STAPHYLOCOCCAL INFECTIONS

DENNIS R. SCHABERG

Infection due to staphylococci is one of the most common problems confronting clinicians in both ambulatory and hospital settings. Staphylococci are conveniently categorized by their ability to coagulate plasma and are referred to as coagulase-positive *(Staphylococcus aureus)* or coagulase-negative. *S. aureus* is a pluripotential pathogen causing a host of clinical syndromes in normal or compromised patients, whereas coagulase-negative staphylococci generally require major host compromise, in particular indwelling devices, in order to produce disease. Other coagulase-negative isolates are limited to selected infections, as is the case for *Staphylococcus saprophyticus,* which usually is restricted to the urinary tract. Despite the availability of very active antimicrobial therapy, staphylococcal infection appears to be on the increase with persistent significant morbidity and mortality.

EPIDEMIOLOGIC FACTORS

Humans are the primary reservoir for staphylococci. Neonates frequently become colonized soon after birth with *S. aureus* at the umbilical stump, perineum, and skin. Later in life, 20% to 40% of the general population become carriers of *S. aureus* with the anterior nasal vestibule as the usual site. Patients who share in common breaks in their skin such as insulin-dependent diabetics, intravenous drug users, hemodialysis patients, and patients receiving allergy injections can have markedly higher rates of carriage. AIDS patients also have very high carriage rates, perhaps related to alteration in integument, as do patients with eczema or psoriasis. Rarely, perineal carriage persists in adults, and approximately 10% of premenopausal women will carry *S. aureus* vaginally with the density of colonization increasing during menses. Coagulase-negative staphylococci are considered to be normal flora of human skin although the particular strains carried can be dynamic.

For *S. aureus,* organisms are transferred from time to time from the site of carriage to intact skin. Normal skin resists persistent colonization, but breaks in the integument provide an opportunity for persistence and further proliferation. This translocation process makes the carrier state very important clinically in that patients with higher carrier rates are at increased risk of infection and the opportunity to eradicate the carrier state presents an opportunity for prevention in high-risk populations. Development of coagulase-negative staphylococcal infection is usually traced to contamination of an implantable prosthetic device or catheter occurring at the time of placement.

Special attention must be made of the growing problem of β-lactam-resistant strains of *S. aureus,* often referred to as methicillin-resistant (MRSA). These organisms have become prominent hospital-acquired pathogens with transmission often occurring via the hands of health care personnel. Outbreaks have also been described in chronic care settings and chronic carriers often serve as reservoirs for the organism in institutional settings. In several urban centers, community-acquired MRSA has been described with major sources of infection arising from intravenous drug users.

Control and interruption of spread of *S. aureus,* especially in institutional environments, is an effective strategy to minimize the impact of this pathogen. Timely identification of isolates, surveillance cultures of potential patient reservoirs, barrier precautions for infected patients, and reinforcement of hand washing are helpful measures in interrupting transmission. Clear identification of patients carrying the organism is also helpful if only to heighten awareness of routine infection control precautions.

ETIOLOGY AND MICROBIOLOGY

Staphylococci are gram-positive cocci that appear as grapelike clusters on Gram stain. These organisms are distinguished by their growth characteristics, colonial morphology, and virulence characteristics. *S. aureus* typically forms yellow colonies, 2 to 3 mm in diameter, with β-hemolysis in blood agar plates.

Staphylococcus epidermidis and *S. saprophyticus* are white and nonhemolytic. The major laboratory feature distinguishing *S. aureus* from the other staphylococci is the ability to produce coagulase. Other tests that may be used include mannitol fermentation and the deoxyribonuclease test, both of which are positive for *S. aureus,* as opposed to coagulase-negative staphylococci. *S. saprophyticus* is further identified by its resistance to novobiocin.

PATHOGENESIS

Infections due to staphylococci are often initiated when a break in the normal barrier of the intact skin or mucosa allows staphylococci access to underlying tissues or to the bloodstream. Multiplication ensues, and whether the infection remains localized or spreads is dependent on the interaction of the virulence determinants of the organism and host defense factors. Risk for infection and dissemination is enhanced by the presence of foreign bodies and devices such as suture material and plastic catheters. A variety of serum and tissue constituents such as fibrinogen, fibronectin, and collagen rapidly coat these materials following implantation. Many *S. aureus* strains produce surface proteins (e.g., fibronectin-binding protein, collagen-binding protein, and elastin-binding protein), which bind to these extracellular matrix molecules enabling the organism to adhere and persist. Opsonophagocytosis is also impaired in the presence of foreign devices tilting the balance against the host.

The specific adherence interactions may help explain the propensity for *S. aureus* to cause endovascular infection and to disseminate widely from a minor skin or soft-tissue focus. The organism binds avidly to endothelial cells and is actually taken up by these cells. This intracellular location protects the organism from more traditional phagocytic cells and from certain classes of antimicrobials with poor cell penetration.

Polymorphonuclear leukocytes (PMNs) are the major defense against *S. aureus*. Anticapsular antibody and C3b complement deposition enhance PMN function. Traditional cellular immunity has a small role. Defects in PMN function or number are often complicated by *S. aureus* infection. The cell wall peptidoglycan of *S. aureus* evokes a brisk inflammatory response mediated via cytokines such as interleukin-1 (IL-1), IL-6, and tumor necrosis factor–α (TNF-α). While markedly increasing the migration of PMNs to the site of inflammation, paradoxically the presence of the cytokines enhances the growth of *S. aureus*.

Staphylococcus aureus is also armed with a variety of exotoxins that affect cell function and host defense. Some of the toxins, such as toxic shock syndrome toxin 1, are pyrogenic toxin superantigens and cause life-threatening disease. They bind directly as superantigens to the invariant region of major histocompatibility complex (MHC) class II molecules, causing an expansion of T cells and a massive release of cytokines. This in turn leads to endothelial injury and shock that is clinically indistinguishable from endotoxic shock. Other toxins are enterotoxins associated with a food poisoning syndrome characterized by sudden onset of nausea and vomiting. These are preformed in the food ingested, odorless, tasteless, and heat-stable. Other secreted toxins, such as α-toxin, probably contribute to pathogenesis mainly by enhancing tissue injury.

CLINICAL FINDINGS

SKIN AND SOFT-TISSUE INFECTIONS

Folliculitis is a pyoderma localized to hair follicles that responds to local care. A furuncle or boil is a more deep-seated infection presenting as a warm, painful, swollen, and indurated area that drains purulent material on excision. If these infections extend into the subcutaneous area, they may form a carbuncle and may be accompanied by systemic findings of fever and chills.

Impetigo is a soft-tissue infection, unrelated to hair follicles, that involves a superficial area of the skin. This disease afflicts mainly children and manifests by an erythematous macule that forms a vesicle of purulent material that ruptures and crusts. Although most cases of impetigo are caused by *S. aureus,* up to 20% are due to *Streptococcus pyogenes* or a mixed streptococcal and staphylococcal infection.

Staphylococcus aureus is the most common cause of postoperative wound infections; such infections typically occur more than 2 days after surgery and are associated with purulent or hemorrhagic drainage. Antibiotics are only secondary to the adequacy of surgical drainage and assist in local healing and preventing hematogenous spread.

In soft-tissue infections with systemic signs or symptoms, Gram stain, culture of drainage material, and blood cultures should be obtained. In mild cases of infection in the ambulatory setting where systemic symptoms are absent, empiric antistaphylococcal therapy may be prescribed for 7 to 10 days.

OSTEOMYELITIS AND SEPTIC ARTHRITIS

In adults, osteomyelitis most commonly arises from adjacent infections rather than the hematogenous spread common in children. In posttraumatic osteomyelitis, *S. aureus* is the most common organism recovered; in ischemic disease, *S. aureus* is the most common gram-positive organism recovered. The diagnosis of postoperative or traumatic osteomyelitis may be delayed or obscured by changes in plain radiographs and radionuclide scanning attributable to the underlying injury. Postoperative high fever after 2 days and objective evidence of inflammation should lead to the consideration of underlying infection. If drainage occurs, culture and recovery of *S. aureus* suggest a deep-seated infection. If mixed flora are identified, a deep aspirate should be performed for microbiologic confirmation. Adequate surgical drainage of abscesses and removal of devitalized bone and foreign material are important. Adults with *S. aureus* osteomyelitis should receive parenteral antimicrobial therapy for 4 to 6 weeks.

Staphylococcus aureus is the most common cause of septic arthritis in the elderly population and second only to gonococcal disease in persons aged 20 to 40. The patient with septic arthritis presents with a painful, swollen, warm joint; an aspirate yields high bacterial counts (usually more than 50,000 per cubic millimeter) and gram-positive cocci on Gram stain. Therapy for septic arthritis may be confounded by the inability to exclude adjacent osteomyelitis; therefore, parenteral therapy for 4 weeks with an effective antistaphylococcal agent is warranted.

Staphylococcus epidermidis is the most common cause of prosthetic joint infections, which usually occur within 3 months of surgical insertion of the prosthesis. Infections are most often accompanied by pain, joint instability, loosening of the prosthesis, and low-grade fever. Antimicrobial therapy and device removal are required for cure.

ENDOCARDITIS

Staphylococcus aureus is the most common cause of endocarditis associated with intravenous drug use and the second most common organism causing endocarditis not associated with addiction. The diagnosis is clear when the patient has fever, murmur, embolic disease, and persistent bacteremia. In an effort to include cases that have been previously excluded, proposed new criteria include two major criteria, or one major and three minor criteria, or five minor criteria for diagnosing infective endocarditis. Major criteria include positive blood cultures with organisms typical of endocarditis, all positive when drawn 12 hours apart or positive in more than three blood cultures, and evidence of endocardial involvement by echocardiography (oscillating intracardiac mass, abscess, or dehiscence of a prosthetic valve) or clinical evidence of regurgitation. Minor criteria include fever (higher than 38°C), vascular phenomenon, immunologic phenomenon, positive blood cultures not meeting the major criteria, or echocardiogram consistent with endocarditis but not meeting the major criteria.

Careful physical examination is necessary to differentiate endocarditis from nonendocarditis *S. aureus* bacteremia by detecting a new or increasing murmur or new embolic lesions. There are compelling reasons for careful clinical monitoring in the inpatient setting and avoidance of outpatient management of staphylococcal endocarditis with home infusion programs.

Laboratory evidence is generally supportive but not absolute in excluding a diagnosis of staphylococcal endocarditis. Echocardiography can be a useful adjunct, especially transesophageal echocardiography, which can approach sensitivities of 90%.

The diagnostic value of echocardiography in drug users appears to be less because visualization of the tricuspid valve, the most common site for drug use–associated endocarditis, is not significantly improved by an esophageal study over the transthoracic echocardiogram. In one series, 13% of endocarditis in intravenous drug users could not be predicted by clinical or laboratory criteria at presentation.

The mortality of endocarditis varies. The young drug user with right-sided disease has the most favorable outcome, with mortality of about 5%; the elderly hospitalized patient with heart failure or embolic disease has a mortality in excess of 70%.

Patients with *S. aureus* endovascular infection are given a parenteral bactericidal agent for 4 to 6 weeks. The duration of therapy for bacteremia without endocarditis should be 2 weeks. Although some recommend short-course therapy (2 weeks) for right-sided disease, there is limited experience with this approach to support its use on a widespread basis. Short-course therapy must be performed selectively to avoid relapses due to hematogenous seeding from extracardial sites.

The need for cardiac surgery is based on the presence of systemic emboli, cardiac compromise, or microbiologic failure manifest by prolonged persistently positive blood cultures. When a patient has *S. aureus* aortic valve endocarditis, cardiac decompensation should be expected and early surgical intervention considered. Cardiac surgery is seldom justified for right-sided disease.

PNEUMONIA

Staphylococcus aureus as a cause of nosocomial pneumonia is second only to *Pseudomonas aeruginosa*. Risk factors related to *S. aureus* pneumonia in adults include neurosurgical intervention, coma, extremes of age, prior influenza, underlying pulmonary disease, and bacteremic extrapulmonary sites of infection.

Staphylococcus aureus pneumonia also occurs in the community and is especially seen following antecedent viral infection, particularly influenza virus. Radiographs are nonspecific in distinguishing this form of pneumonia from that caused by other pathogens.

Cavities are common in children but relatively rare in adults. The criteria for diagnosis should include pulmonary infiltrate, fever, leukocytosis, and purulent tracheobronchial secretions. Gram stain and culture of the sputum should be obtained to help guide antimicrobial therapy, which usually lasts 2 weeks.

MENINGITIS

Meningitis rarely occurs by itself. Rick factors include central nervous system (CNS) trauma or surgery, intravenous drug use, extra-CNS sites of *S. aureus* infection, and diabetes mellitus. Lumbar puncture shows features typical of bacterial meningitis.

Cerebritis is the presence of microabscesses in the cerebral cortex associated with *S. aureus* bacteremia and usually endocarditis. These patients typically have a predominantly polymorphonuclear pleocytosis with counts lower than those of patients with meningitis and an elevated protein level. Gram stains are usually negative, but occasionally cultures are positive if a microabscess has recently ruptured.

TOXIN-MEDIATED SYNDROMES

Toxic shock syndrome (TSS) is usually but not always caused by *S. aureus*. Menstrual TSS was previously most common, but recently nonmenstrual TSS has become more common. Nonmenstrual TSS may be associated with vaginal colonization by toxin-secreting strains of *S. aureus* involving vaginal infections, contraceptive devices, abortion, childbirth, and the postpartum period. Other TSS-associated conditions include surgical wounds, nasal packing, osteomyelitis, skin and soft-tissue infections, and influenza-associated pneumonia.

The clinical manifestations include multiorgan dysfunction. The criteria established by the U.S. Centers for Disease Control and Prevention include fever (more than 38.9°C), systolic blood pressure below 90 mm Hg, and rash with desquamation on the palms and soles, plus involvement of three or more major organ systems: gastrointestinal (vomiting, diarrhea), muscular (myalgia, increased level of creatine phosphokinase), mucous membranes (hyperemia), renal (elevated creatinine level with pyuria without infection), hepatic (elevated levels of aspartate transaminase and alanine aminotransferase, bilirubin), blood (thrombocytopenia), and CNS (disorientation without focal neurologic signs). Hypocalcemia without other explanation can be a helpful clue. The patient should have a negative workup for Rocky Mountain spotted fever, leptospirosis, and measles.

Disease management requires aggressive fluid replacement, followed by a careful assessment to define the origin of the toxin-producing strains of *S. aureus*. An antistaphylococcal agent should be administered for 10 to 14 days. Culture of the vaginal flora should be obtained even in the absence of a focus of infection. Once a focus is identified, eradication of the carriage should be documented.

Food poisoning is another disease caused by toxin-producing *S. aureus*. The source is the contamination of food by a carrier. The onset of illness is acute (2 to 6 hours after ingesting the contaminated food), with nausea and vomiting followed by abdominal cramps and diarrhea. The patient with *S. aureus* food poisoning is afebrile. The illness resolves within a day, and antimicrobials are not required.

FOREIGN BODY DEVICES

Staphylococcus epidermidis is the major pathogen of prosthetic devices, leading to dysfunction of the device and often a subacute presentation of infection. For prosthetic heart valves, management usually but not always requires valve replacement; for other prosthetic devices, such as prosthetic joints, shunts, and dialysis access devices, device removal is required for cure of the infection.

LABORATORY FINDINGS

The diagnosis of staphylococcal infection requires confirmation by the microbiology laboratory by culturing material from the suspected site and blood cultures if there are systemic signs and symptoms. Three sets of blood cultures drawn from different sites should be obtained if endocarditis is suspected or possible. Separating collections of each blood culture by 15 to 60 minutes will help in identifying an endovascular infection. *Staphylococcus aureus* grows rapidly in the absence of antibiotics and is usually identified in 1 to 2 days. Obtaining blood cultures 48 hours after the first set can also be helpful in suggesting a possible endovascular focus of origin.

TREATMENT

Therapy for *S. aureus* and *S. epidermidis* depends on antimicrobial susceptibility testing, host tolerance or allergies, and the site of infection. Penicillin is no longer a first-line therapy, as resistance occurs with over 90% of *S. aureus* and *S. epidermidis* pathogens by production of β-lactamase. Since the 1970s, *S. aureus* has demonstrated a gradual increase in resistance to the antistaphylococcal penicillins. These isolates are referred to as methicillin-resistant or β-lactam-resistant, reflecting the cross-resistance to all β-lactams (antistaphylococcal penicillins, cephalosporins, and imipenem). Currently, 5% to 50% of *S. aureus* pathogens are β-lactam-resistant, and up to 65% of cases of *S. epidermidis* are methicillin-resistant.

Familiarity with local susceptibility patterns is critical to selecting empirical therapy. The mechanism for resistance to β-lactams is the production of penicillin-binding protein (PBP-2a), which has a lowered affinity for penicillin binding, thus permitting the peptidoglycan production necessary for cell wall formation to occur uninterrupted.

If the organism is susceptible to oxacillin, an antistaphylococcal penicillin should be considered such as methicillin, oxacillin, or nafcillin (100 to 200 mg per kilogram per day in six divided doses). Cefazolin, a first-generation agent, is more active than the third-generation cephalosporins (cefotaxime, ceftriaxone, ceftizoxime). Other agents with activity against *S. aureus* include clindamycin, fluoroquinolones, and imipenem cilastatin. With β-lactam-resistant staphylococci, the therapy of choice is vancomycin (15 mg per kilogram every 12 hours). For patients who cannot take vancomycin, sulfamethoxazole–trimethoprim has been shown to be effective against susceptible strains. The report of strains of *S. aureus* requiring markedly increased concentrations of vancomycin for inhibition is a disturbing new development. How widespread these isolates will become and what their clinical significance will be is unclear at present. Currently, it is prudent in particular to perform detailed antimicrobial susceptibilities on isolates from patients failing to improve clinically on vancomycin therapy or patients with end-stage renal disease who may have received vancomycin frequently in the past.

Combination therapy with aminoglycosides (gentamicin or tobramycin) added to the antistaphylococcal penicillin or vancomycin leads to a shortening of the duration of bacteremia. In prosthetic infections, especially cardiac valve prostheses, three-drug combinations (vancomycin, gentamicin, and rifampin) are associated with a more favorable outcome than two-drug regimens.

Treatment of nasal carriage may be considered if a carrier is responsible for recurrent disease or an outbreak of *S. aureus* infections. Successful eradication may occur with topical therapy to the anterior nares with mupirocin twice daily for 5 to 7 days; this agent decreases nasal and hand carriage. As with most other antistaphylococcal agents, resistance to mupirocin has occurred; consequently, indiscriminate use of this agent should be avoided.

BIBLIOGRAPHY

al-Ujayki B, Nafziger D, Saravolatz L. Pneumonia due to *Staphylococcus aureus. Clin Chest Med* 1995;16:111–120.

Crossley KB, Archer GL, eds. *The staphylococci in human disease.* New York: Churchill-Livingstone, 1997.

Lowy FD. *Staphylococcus aureus* infections. *N Engl J Med* 1998;339: 520–532.

Moreno F, Crisp C, Jorgensen JH, et al. Methicillin-resistant *Staphylococcus aureus* as a community organism. *Clin Infect Dis* 1995;21:1308–1312.

Wenzel RP, Perl TM. The significance of nasal carriage of *Staphylococcus aureus* and the incidence of postoperative wound infection. *J Hosp Infect* 1995;31:13–24.

Kelley's Textbook of Internal Medicine, fourth edition. Edited by H. David Humes. Lippincott Williams & Wilkins, Philadelphia © 2000.

C H A P T E R
275
STREPTOCOCCAL INFECTIONS

MONICA M. FARLEY
BENJAMIN SCHWARTZ

Streptococci are a diverse group of bacteria, including the major human pathogens *Streptococcus pyogenes* (group A streptococci), *Streptococcus agalactiae* (group B streptococci), and *Streptococcus pneumoniae* (pneumococci), that cause a wide range of clinical infections. Streptococci are important pathogens because of their diversity, their significance as common causes of infection in all age groups, and recent developments in the epidemiology and treatment of certain streptococcal infections. These developments include the emergence of antimicrobial resistance in several species, particularly *S. pneumoniae*; the increased awareness of severe infections caused by group A streptococci, including streptococcal toxic shock syndrome (STSS) and necrotizing fasciitis; and the occurrence of clusters of rheumatic fever cases in the United States. The emergence of vancomycin resistance in enterococci (until recently considered to be group D streptococci but now given their own genus designation) poses complicated treatment challenges and creates the potential for spread of vancomycin resistance to more virulent organisms.

Streptococci are gram-positive cocci that form chains in broth media. Most species are facultative anaerobes, although some are strictly anaerobic. Absence of catalase production and the formation of chains distinguish streptococci from most other gram-positive cocci, including staphylococcal species.

A number of classification schemes have been used to differentiate streptococci, and they often must be used in combination to accurately characterize organisms. The Lancefield serogroup is determined based on precipitin reactions of specific antisera to the cell wall carbohydrate antigen. Although over 20 Lancefield groups have been described, groups A, B, C, D, F, or G are the ones most often associated with human disease. The type of hemolysis that occurs when cultured on blood agar can classify strains: α-hemolytic strains partially hemolyze erythrocytes, producing a greenish zone of hemolysis, whereas β-hemolytic strains cause complete hemolysis, leaving a clear zone around a colony. Other strains are nonhemolytic (occasionally referred to as γ-

TABLE 275.1.	CLASSIFICATION OF CLINICALLY IMPORTANT STREPTOCOCCI		
Lancefield Group	**Species**	**Hemolysis**	**Clinical Illnesses**
A	S. pyogenes	β	Pharyngitis, pyoderma, bacteremia, streptococcal shock syndrome, necrotizing fasciitis, acute rheumatic fever, acute glomerulonephritis
B	S. agalactiae	β	Neonatal sepsis, endometritis, bacteremia, skin/soft tissue infection, pneumonia, urinary tract infection, meningitis, endocarditis
C	S. equisimilis, S. zooepidemicus	β	Cellulitis, bacteremia, pharyngitis
D (nonenterococcal)	S. bovis	None	Bacteremia, endocarditis
F or variable	S. intermedius, S. constellatus, S. anginosus (Intermedius or Milleri group)	Variable	Invasive pyogenic infections—abdominal cavity, brain, dental abscesses
G		β	Cellulitis, bacteremia, arthritis, pharyngitis
Nongrouped	S. pneumoniae	α	Pneumonia, otitis media, sinusitis, bacteremia, meningitis
Nongrouped	Viridans streptococci (Intermedius/Milleri group discussed above); S. mutans, S. sanguis, S. gordonii, S. crista, S. salivarius, S. mitis, S. oralis	α or none	Endocarditis, bacteremia in neutropenic patients

hemolytic). Streptococci are assigned to a species group based on metabolic characteristics and molecular techniques, including DNA homology and 16S ribosomal RNA (rRNA) sequencing. Table 275.1 shows the classification of clinically important streptococci based on these three schemas.

GROUP A STREPTOCOCCUS

DEFINITION

Group A *Streptococcus* includes a single species (*S. pyogenes*) and causes a wide array of pyogenic infections including pharyngitis, scarlet fever, skin and soft-tissue infections (e.g., impetigo, cellulitis, necrotizing fasciitis), infection of normally sterile sites (e.g., bacteremia, pneumonia), postpartum infection (puerperal sepsis), and STSS. Nonsuppurative sequelae of group A streptococcal infection include acute rheumatic fever (ARF) and acute glomerulonephritis (AGN).

PATHOGENESIS AND VIRULENCE

Group A streptococcal pathogenicity and virulence are mediated by a variety of cell-associated and extracellular factors (Table 275.2) and by the host immune response to them. The major virulence factor of group A streptococci is the M protein, which is antigenic and inhibits phagocytosis. More than 80 M protein serotypes and over 100 M protein gene sequence types (*emm* types) have been described. M protein expression is required for invasive infection. Long-term type-specific immunity follows infection, but reinfection with another M serotype is common.

In addition, in a susceptible host, cross-reactive antibodies to certain M-protein epitopes may result in the development of nonsuppurative sequelae such as rheumatic fever.

Streptococcal pyrogenic exotoxins have been implicated in the pathogenesis of serious streptococcal infections. These exotoxins, an extracellular protein known as streptococcal superantigen, and some M-protein fragments act as superantigens, inducing polyclonal T-cell activation and the massive release of inflammatory mediators. The hyaluronic acid capsule of the group A streptococci contributes to virulence by inhibiting phagocytosis, and heavy capsule production has been epidemiologically linked with rheumatic fever–associated isolates.

PHARYNGITIS

EPIDEMIOLOGIC FACTORS

Pharyngitis is the most common clinical manifestation of group A streptococcal infection. Pharyngitis is the fourth leading reason for acute-illness visits to a physician's office in the United States. Although group A streptococci are the most common bacterial cause of pharyngitis, they account for less than half of all pharyngitis episodes. Disease occurs most often in school-age children, but persons of all ages may be affected. Most infections occur during winter and spring. Infection spreads person to person by large respiratory droplets; thus, close contact, such as that in child care settings, crowded households, schools, and military barracks, enhances the spread of infection. In families where a child is infected, 20% of siblings and 5% of adults also develop infection. Asymptomatic pharyngeal carriage is common, affect-

TABLE 275.2.	VIRULENCE FACTORS AND EXTRACELLULAR TOXINS OF GROUP A STREPTOCOCCI

Factor	Activity
Cell-Associated Factors	
M Protein	Antiphagocytic, superantigenic in some cases
Hyaluronic acid capsule	Antiphagocytic
Streptolysin S	Leukocyte and erythrocyte cytotoxin, promotes spreading
C5a peptidase	Cleaves C5a, decreases neutrophil chemotaxis
Protein F	Mediates attachment to pharyngeal cells
Extracellular Factors	
Streptococcal pyrogenic exotoxins (SpeA, SpeB, SpeC, SpeF)	Superantigenic, responsible for scarlet fever rash, SpeB–cysteine protease precursor
Streptococcal superantigen	Superantigenic
Hyaluronidase	Cleaves hyaluronic acid in connective tissue, promotes spreading
Streptokinase	Cleaves plasminogen, promotes spreading
Streptolysin O	Leukocyte and erythrocyte cytotoxin, promotes spreading
DNase	Cleaves DNA and RNA, promotes spreading

ing 10% to 20% of school-age children during disease outbreaks. However, carriers are less likely to transmit infection, probably due to reduced numbers of organisms and loss of M-protein production in isolates associated with asymptomatic carriage. Foodborne outbreaks of streptococcal pharyngitis have been reported. Fomites and household animals have not been shown to play a role in transmission.

CLINICAL FEATURES

Characteristic symptoms include the acute onset of fever and sore throat; headache, abdominal pain, vomiting, and malaise may also occur, particularly in children. Physical examination typically reveals pharyngeal erythema and edema. Tonsils are enlarged and may have a gray–white exudate. Tender anterior cervical adenopathy is frequently present. Palatal petechiae, while less common, are consistent with a group A streptococcal etiologic process. Signs of upper respiratory infection, such as rhinorrhea, cough, and hoarseness, suggest a nonstreptococcal cause. Despite suggestive clinical findings, overlap with nonstreptococcal pharyngitis is common; thus, accurate diagnosis of group A streptococcal pharyngitis cannot be made with consistency based on clinical findings.

Several other pathogens may cause pharyngitis and can sometimes be differentiated from streptococcal infections, based on clinical and epidemiologic findings (Table 275.3). Respiratory viruses cause most pharyngitis; infection frequently is present in multiple family members and the community, and typical symptoms of upper respiratory congestion and cough are prominent. *Mycoplasma* infections also usually manifest signs of upper

TABLE 275.3.	ETIOLOGIES OF PHARYNGITIS AND DISTINGUISHING CLINICAL AND EPIDEMIOLOGIC FEATURES

Etiology	Clinical/Epidemiologic Characteristics
Group A streptococci	Tonsillar exudate, cervical adenopathy, absence of URI signs
Other β-hemolytic streptococci	Tonsillar exudate, cervical adenopathy, absence of URI signs
Arcanobacterium haemolyticum	Scarlatiniform rash, adolescent age group
Corynebacterium diphtheriae	Gray pseudomembrane, systemic toxicity, nonvaccination
Neisseria gonorrhoeae	History of sexual activity
Epstein–Barr virus	Generalized lymphadenopathy, splenomegaly, atypical lymphocytes
Adenovirus	Signs of URI, conjunctivitis (pharyngoconjunctival fever)
Influenza virus	Signs of URI, occurrence during influenza epidemic
Mycoplasma	Signs of URI, bullous myringitis
Enterovirus	Stomatitis (usually posterior), systemic signs
Herpes simplex virus	Stomatitis (usually anterior)

URI, upper respiratory infection.

respiratory infection, and bullous myringitis may be present. Infections caused by enterovirus and herpes simplex virus are more often stomatitis than pharyngitis. Culture of a throat swab specimen on sheep blood agar remains the gold standard for diagnosis of group A streptococcal pharyngitis. Rapid antigen detection tests, which identify the carbohydrate grouping antigen, offer a highly specific alternative method that allows for immediate diagnosis and initiation of appropriate early therapy. However, because of lower sensitivity, a negative rapid antigen test should be confirmed by conventional culture. Newer tests with greater sensitivity may eliminate the need for backup culture in the future.

OPTIMAL MANAGEMENT AND PROGNOSIS

Treatment of group A streptococcal pharyngitis reduces spread, prevents suppurative and nonsuppurative complications, and may shorten the duration of illness. Treatment with oral penicillin V (250 mg 3 times a day for 10 days) or intramuscular benzathine penicillin (600,000 units in patients weighing less than 27 kg and 1,200,000 units in patients weighing more than 27 kg) remains the treatment of choice for persons with group A streptococcal pharyngitis. Therapy can be initiated up to 9 days after onset of symptoms and still prevent the occurrence of rheumatic fever. Penicillin resistance among clinical isolates of group A streptococci has not been documented. Erythromycin is recommended for treatment of penicillin-allergic persons; in some countries, resistance to erythromycin may exceed 20%, but in the United States resistance is uncommon. Other β-lactam antibiotics also are effective as therapy when given in a 10-day course. Shorter course treatment options have been proposed (e.g., cefadroxil, cefuroxime, cefpodoxime, azithromycin), but data are limited and must be weighed against the increased cost and broader spectrum of activity of these agents.

Repeat throat culture after therapy to document cure is not recommended in asymptomatic persons. Notable exceptions include when a patient or household member has a history of rheumatic fever; during outbreaks of rheumatic fever or poststreptococcal glomerulonephritis; or during outbreaks of pharyngitis in closed communities. Although some persons will continue to carry group A streptococci, the risk both of disease spread and of developing rheumatic fever are low. Repeat therapy of asymptomatic carriers is not recommended except in special circumstances (e.g., patient or household member with history of rheumatic fever; efforts to terminate large outbreak in closed setting). Clindamycin (children: 20 to 30 mg per kilogram per day for 10 days; adults: 600 mg per day in 2 to 4 equally divided doses for 10 days) or amoxicillin/clavulanate (40 mg per kilogram per day in 3 equal doses for 10 days) have been recommended for symptomatic patients with multiple repeated culture-positive episodes of pharyngitis.

COMPLICATIONS

Suppurative complications of streptococcal pharyngitis include direct extension of infection resulting in peritonsillar or retropharyngeal abscess, sinusitis, otitis media, mastoiditis, or cervical lymphadenitis. Rarely, meningitis, brain abscess, intracranial venous thrombosis, and pneumonia may occur through this mech-anism. Bacteremic spread may result in metastatic foci of infection.

ACUTE RHEUMATIC FEVER

Nonsuppurative sequelae of infection include ARF and AGN. ARF occurs after pharyngeal group A streptococcal infection, whereas AGN most often follows cutaneous infection but may also occur after pharyngitis (see Chapter 150 for a discussion of acute glomerulonephritis). The incidence of ARF in the United States is estimated at 0.5 to 1 per 100,000 population. In developing countries, rates several hundred times higher may be observed, and rheumatic heart disease accounts for 25% to 40% of all cardiovascular disease. Although the incidence of rheumatic fever in the United States has declined steadily during the past century, outbreaks in the late 1980s occurred in several communities and military settings, reemphasizing the importance of diagnosing and treating streptococcal pharyngitis. ARF is most common in school-age children and is rare in those under 3 years. Attack rates vary from less than 1% to 3% in persons with untreated streptococcal pharyngitis. In general, ARF has been a disease of lower socioeconomic, minority populations in the United States, probably related to crowded living conditions. However, several outbreaks in the 1980s involved predominantly white, middle-class families in suburban and rural settings.

Although the pathogenesis of ARF is not entirely understood, the importance of tissue cross-reactive epitopes of the group A streptococcal M protein is clear. Antibodies to specific M-protein epitopes may cross-react with myocardial proteins, antigens in the basal ganglia of the human brain, and antigens in articular cartilage. Host factors, including class II HLA antigens (HLA-DR2 in blacks and HLA-DR4 in whites) may contribute to the pathogenesis of rheumatic fever. Certain M-protein types (types 1, 3, 5, 6, 18, and 24) and the mucoid or heavily encapsulated phenotype have been associated with "rheumatogenicity."

Acute rheumatic fever is defined by a combination of clinical and laboratory findings, occurring in the context of a preceding streptococcal pharyngitis (Table 275.4). In some cases, a history of clinical pharyngitis is absent. Major manifestations include carditis, arthritis, chorea, subcutaneous nodules, and erythema marginatum (a serpiginous, evanescent, erythematous, nontender rash on the trunk or extremities). Minor manifestations include fever, arthralgia, heart block manifested by a prolonged PR interval, and elevated acute-phase reactants (erythrocyte sedimentation rate or C-reactive protein). Preceding group A streptococcal infection can be ascertained by serologic tests and, less commonly, by culture.

Onset of ARF generally occurs 2 to 3 weeks after a preceding streptococcal pharyngitis; however, cases presenting with "pure" chorea may occur several months after a preceding infection. Arthritis is the most common manifestation of disease (47% to 100% of ARF). The ankles, knees, wrists, and elbows are most frequently affected by this migratory polyarthritis. Resolution occurs in several weeks without articular damage. Carditis occurs in 40% to 50% of cases and may vary in severity from pancarditis, resulting in heart failure and death, to subtle myocardial involvement, which can be detected only by echocardiogram.

TABLE 275.4.	THE MODIFIED JONES CRITERIA: 1992 UPDATE OF GUIDELINES FOR THE DIAGNOSIS OF AN INITIAL ATTACK OF ACUTE RHEUMATIC FEVER[a]

Evidence of Preceding Group A Streptococcal Infection[b]
Positive throat culture
Positive rapid antigen detection test
Elevated or rising streptococcal antibody titer (anti-streptolysin O [ASO], antihyaluronidase, anti-DNase B, or streptozyme)
Major Manifestations[c]
Carditis
Polyarthritis
Chorea
Erythema marginatum
Subcutaneous nodules
Minor Manifestations[d]
Clinical
   Arthralgia
   Fever
Laboratory
   Prolonged PR interval
   Elevated acute phase reactants

[a] In the face of a preceding group A streptococcal infection, two major manifestations or one major and two minor manifestations strongly support the diagnosis of acute rheumatic fever.
[b] Laboratory evidence of preceding group A streptococcal infection is necessary for the diagnosis of acute rheumatic fever, except when Sydenham's chorea or indolent rheumatic carditis is the presenting major criterion.
[c] Echocardiographic findings cannot be used as the sole criterion to define carditis; auscultatory findings must be present.
[d] Arthralgias cannot be counted as a minor criterion if arthritis is a major criterion.

Endocarditis primarily involves the mitral valve and, less commonly, the aortic valve. Although most valvular damage resolves, mitral and aortic valve stenosis may occur. Specific manifestations of ARF vary with age; carditis is more common in children and arthritis more common in adults.

The differential diagnosis of ARF includes other causes of arthritis, carditis, and chorea. Treatment is aimed at reducing inflammation. In less severe disease, high-dose aspirin to achieve a blood level of 20 mg per deciliter is adequate therapy; more severe illness is treated with corticosteroids. Bed rest is recommended, particularly for persons with carditis. Rheumatic heart disease is the only long-term consequence of infection. Patients without carditis during their acute episode are unlikely to develop cardiac disease later.

Recurrences of rheumatic fever may ensue with subsequent group A streptococcal infections. Such recurrences are prevented by continuous antimicrobial prophylaxis. Intramuscular benzathine penicillin given every 4 weeks is recommended and avoids problems with compliance. In settings where the risk of streptococcal infection is high, benzathine penicillin can be given every 3 weeks. Oral sulfadiazine, penicillin, and erythromycin for penicillin-allergic persons are all acceptable alternatives, although none of the oral regimens are as effective as intramuscular penicillin. Prophylaxis should continue until the risk of acquiring group A streptococcal pharyngitis is reduced and at least 5 years after acute illness. In persons with rheumatic carditis, some experts recommend lifelong prophylaxis.

SCARLET FEVER

Scarlet fever presents as a group A streptococcal infection in the presence of a characteristic *scarlatina* rash. It occurs most often in association with pharyngitis but may also present with pyoderma or wound infection (surgical scarlet fever). The epidemiology of infection is similar to that of group A streptococcal pharyngitis, with the exception that scarlet fever is rare in very young children. The cutaneous manifestations of scarlet fever are a result of delayed-type hypersensitivity to streptococcal pyrogenic exotoxins, requiring prior exposure for expression of disease. This probably explains the age distribution in that most infants have not had previous exposure or generated antibodies to the exotoxins.

The hallmark of scarlet fever is a generalized erythematous rash that is noted within 2 days of the onset of pharyngitis symptoms. The rash begins on the upper body and spreads distally, sparing the palms and soles; it is blanching and is composed of fine papules that give the skin the texture of sandpaper. Linear petechial streaks in skin folds are known as Pastia's lines. On the face, the area around the lips is spared, yielding a circumoral pallor. Enlarged papillae on a coated tongue may occur (strawberry tongue), with the tongue later becoming denuded. Nausea and vomiting are common and may be the initial clinical finding. Desquamation may occur during convalescence. The differential diagnosis of scarlet fever includes viral exanthems, Kawasaki's syndrome, and infection with *Arcanobacterium haemolyticus*. Treatment is the same as that for streptococcal pharyngitis.

STREPTOCOCCAL INFECTIONS OF THE SKIN AND SOFT TISSUES
DEFINITION

Group A streptococcal skin and soft-tissue infections differ in their clinical presentation and reflect varying degrees of invasiveness. Impetigo, often referred to as pyoderma, is the most common group A streptococcal skin infection, recognized by shallow ulcers with a honey-colored crust. Cellulitis is a deeper infection involving the subcutaneous tissues and is characterized by erythema, edema, and tenderness, with mild to moderate systemic toxicity. Erysipelas, a characteristic form of group A streptococcal cellulitis, produces lesions that are erythematous and sharply demarcated by a raised edge; the rash is very tender, may involve the face or lower extremities, and is usually accompanied by fever, chills, and leukocytosis (Fig. 275.1). Deep-tissue infections include necrotizing fasciitis and myositis.

EPIDEMIOLOGIC FACTORS

Impetigo is the second most common manifestation of group A streptococcal infection. It occurs primarily in pre-school-age and school-age children in late summer or fall. Group A strepto-

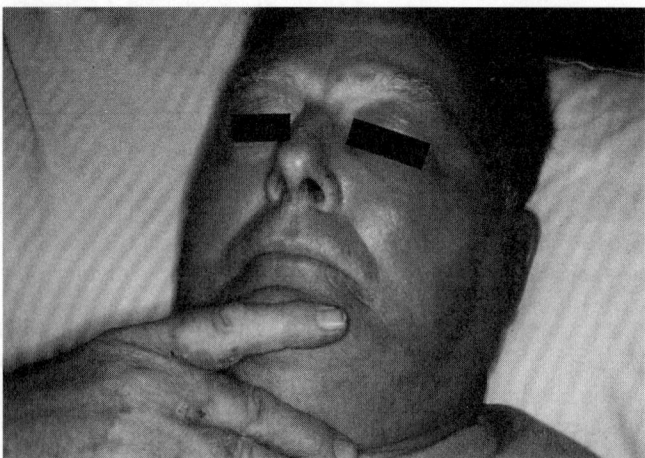

FIGURE 275.1. Erysipelas involving the left malar and preauricular areas of the face. The borders of the infection are clearly demarcated, and the lesions are elevated. Note the impetiginous lesions on the fingers. See color figure 275.1.

coccal colonization of intact skin may lead to impetigo following minor trauma or insect bites. Crowded conditions and poor sanitation enhance spread of streptococci from skin sites. As with pharyngitis, fomites are unlikely to have a major role in transmission.

Other group A streptococcal skin and soft-tissue infections, such as cellulitis, erysipelas, and necrotizing fasciitis, occur more frequently in adults. Infection may be associated with local trauma, surgical wounds, or chronic skin disorders such as eczema and psoriasis. Individuals with impaired lymphatic drainage may have recurrent episodes of cellulitis in the affected area. Intravenous drug use has been associated with acute cellulitis, at times associated with bacteremia, due to groups A, B, C, or G streptococci. Varicella infection can predispose to severe streptococcal skin and soft-tissue infection, including necrotizing fasciitis. Anecdotal reports and small case series have linked development of necrotizing fasciitis to the use of nonsteroidal anti-inflammatory drugs; however, an association has not been proved in a controlled study. Most cases of streptococcal necrotizing fasciitis occur in older adults, and the rates increase with age.

ETIOLOGIC FACTORS

In addition to group A streptococci, *Staphylococcus aureus* can frequently be isolated from impetigo lesions, but its relative clinical importance is not entirely clear. Streptococcal strains associated with impetigo differ in M-protein types from those associated with pharyngitis and include some highly nephritogenic M types that have been linked to community outbreaks of post-streptococcal glomerulonephritis.

Erysipelas is almost always caused by group A streptococci, occasionally by group C or G streptococci. In contrast, acute cellulitis may be associated with a number of organisms, most often β-hemolytic streptococci and *S. aureus. Streptococcus pneumoniae,* gram-negative organisms such as aeromonads and pseudomonads, vibrios, and clostridia may also be considered in cer-

tain epidemiologic settings. Many forms of necrotizing soft-tissue infections have been described and associated with a variety of etiologic agents including *Clostridium perfringens* and other clostridial species, *S. aureus,* mixed aerobes and anaerobes, and group A and rarely group B streptococci. Group A streptococcal necrotizing fasciitis may be distinguished from other forms of necrotizing fasciitis by the severity of pain and systemic toxicity, the rapid progression of necrosis, and association with multiorgan failure.

CLINICAL FEATURES

Impetigo lesions usually begin as papules that evolve to vesicles and pustules, which over several days break down, leaving shallow ulcerated lesions with a honey-colored crust. Regional lymphadenopathy may occur, and systemic signs are rare. In contrast to these lesions, staphylococcal pyoderma (bullous impetigo) presents with large bullae that rupture, leaving a nonpurulent, thin, shiny crust. Impetigo lesions occur most commonly on the face and extremities.

Streptococcal cellulitis occurs most often at the site of skin disruption, trauma, or in an area of impaired lymphatic drainage. Lesions are tender, erythematous, and edematous; lymphangitis is common. Systemic manifestations such as fever and leukocytosis often accompany the local findings. Differentiating streptococcal cellulitis from other causes, such as *S. aureus,* is not usually possible on clinical grounds. In contrast, the clinical appearance of erysipelas is characteristic. Lesions generally occur on the face or extremities and are characterized by a well-demarcated, raised, advancing edge. The affected area is tender and there is marked systemic toxicity. Blood cultures are usually negative in both erysipelas and streptococcal cellulitis.

Initial clinical signs of necrotizing fasciitis are similar to those of cellulitis, except that the degree of pain is severe and, at least at first, appears disproportionate to the appearance of the lesion. Skin lesions may become bullous, turning violaceous in color and then necrotic (Fig. 275.2). Infection advances rapidly with

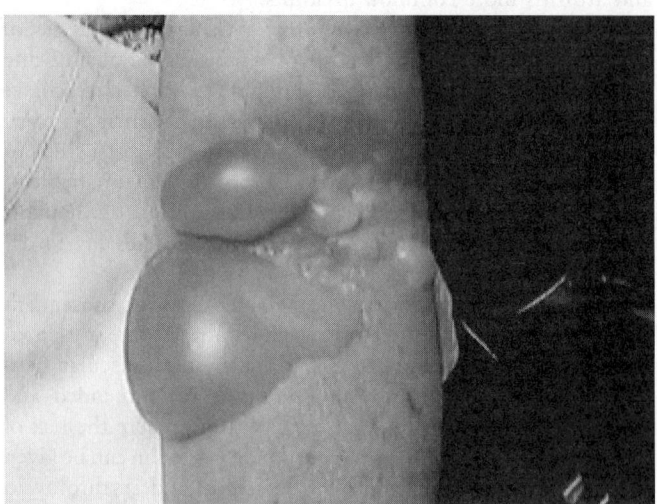

FIGURE 275.2. Group A streptococcal necrotizing fasciitis in a child with preceding varicella infection. Note the large bullous lesions with surrounding violaceous discoloration of skin. (Courtesy of Dr. Larry Slack, Vanderbilt University.) See color figure 275.2.

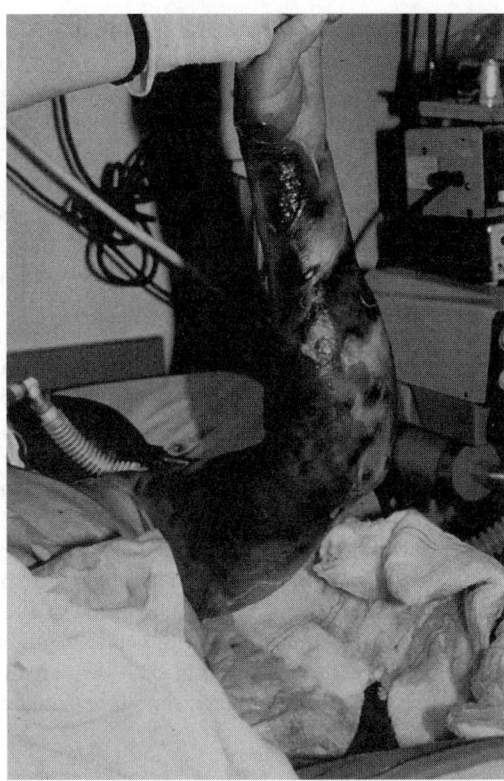

FIGURE 275.3. Group A streptococcal necrotizing fasciitis. See color figure 275.3.

progressive necrosis of subcutaneous fascia and fat, prompting the lay press to refer to it as the "flesh-eating" infection (Fig. 275.3). When the diagnosis is in question, magnetic resonance imaging and examination of frozen section biopsies may be useful in determining the extent of tissue involvement. Fever and systemic toxicity, at times progressing to multiorgan failure, are common. Approximately 50% of patients with necrotizing fasciitis are also diagnosed with STSS.

OPTIMAL MANAGEMENT

Penicillinase-resistant oral antibiotics are effective therapy for impetigo. Erythromycin therapy has proven effective in the past, but erythromycin resistance among *S. aureus* may compromise use of this agent in the future. Topical therapy with mupirocin also is very effective.

Cellulitis and erysipelas may require parenteral antibiotics. If the cause of the cellulitis is unknown, a semisynthetic, penicillinase-resistant penicillin or first-generation cephalosporin should be used. In necrotizing fasciitis, surgery is required to remove necrotic tissue or to relieve increased compartment pressure. The large inoculum of organisms with the propensity to be in a phase of growth during which expression of penicillin-binding proteins (PBPs) may be reduced results in reduced efficacy of penicillin in streptococcal necrotizing fasciitis (the Eagle effect). Clindamycin therapy has been shown to be superior to penicillin and unaffected by the inoculum size in experimental streptococcal myositis. Most experts currently recommend the

administration of clindamycin and penicillin. Intravenous immune globulin (IVIG) has been used when necrotizing fasciitis occurs in association with streptococcal toxic shock (see discussion of management of STSS below).

INVASIVE GROUP A STREPTOCOCCAL INFECTIONS

DEFINITION

Invasive group A streptococcal infections can be defined by the isolation of the organism from normally sterile sites and may be associated with skin and soft-tissue infections, respiratory tract infections, or, in some cases, bacteremia with no identified septic focus. STSS, which was first recognized in 1987, is characterized by hypotension and multiorgan failure (Table 275.5).

INCIDENCE AND EPIDEMIOLOGIC FACTORS

The incidence and severity of invasive group A streptococcal infections have increased since the mid-1980s. Incidence of disease ranges from 1.5 to 5 cases per 100,000 population. Rates of disease are highest among infants, the elderly, African Americans, and Native Americans. Rates of invasive group A streptococcal infection also are significantly increased in persons with chronic illness, malignancy, diabetes mellitus, varicella infection, HIV infection, and alcohol abuse. A number of outbreaks of invasive group A streptococcal disease in nursing homes have been reported.

More than 10% of invasive group A streptococcal infections occur in a nosocomial setting. Most common syndromes include

---

TABLE 275.5.	**DEFINITION OF STSS**[a]

I. Laboratory isolation of group A streptococci
  A. From a normally sterile site
  B. From a non-sterile site
II. Clinical findings occurring within 48 h of hospitalization or 48 h of illness for a nosocomial case
  A. Hypotension
  B. Multiorgan involvement defined by two or more of the following:
    1. Renal impairment
    2. Coagulopathy (thrombocytopenia or disseminated)
    3. Liver involvement
    4. Adult respiratory distress syndrome or evidence of diffuse capillary leak
    5. Generalized erythematous macular rash that may desquamate
    6. Soft-tissue necrosis, including necrotizing fasciitis or myositis, or gangrene

---

[a] An illness that meets criteria IA and II (both A and B) is defined as a *definite* case. An illness that meets criteria IB and II is defined as a *probable* case if no other etiology is identified.
Adapted from Working Group on Severe Streptococcal Infections. Defining the group A streptococcal toxic shock syndrome. *JAMA* 1993;269:390.

postpartum endometritis and sepsis, surgical wound infections, and catheter-related sepsis. Health care workers with asymptomatic skin, pharyngeal, vaginal, and anal carriage have been implicated in nosocomial outbreaks.

Streptococcal toxic shock syndrome accounts for 15% of invasive infections. Although younger, previously healthy individuals are emphasized in case reports of this syndrome, population-based surveillance reveals that the elderly and those with underlying illness are at greatest risk.

ETIOLOGIC FACTORS

Changes in the epidemiologic factors associated with invasive group A streptococcal infection and the emergence of STSS correspond to an increase in infections caused by M types 1 and 3 and an increase in the proportion of strains producing pyrogenic exotoxin A (SpeA). In the United States, statistically significant associations have been shown between these serotypes and SpeA production and STSS, whereas European investigators have associated pyrogenic exotoxin B (SpeB) production with disease severity. Although M types 1 and 3 are most common, many other M types have been associated with invasive disease, and geographic variation has been observed. M-protein genotyping (*emm* typing), based on sequencing of the variable region of the M-protein gene, is now available and will be useful in monitoring trends in M-protein prevalence.

CLINICAL FEATURES

Half of invasive group A streptococcal infections occur in association with skin and soft-tissue infection, followed by bacteremia without a defined source and respiratory tract infection. Clinical presentations and severity vary with the site of infection and the health status of the host. Overall mortality is 15% and it increases with advancing age.

Streptococcal toxic shock syndrome frequently begins with nonspecific, flulike symptoms, including fever, malaise, and myalgia. Although diagnosis at this early stage may be difficult, one should maintain an increased index of suspicion when evaluating patients in high-risk groups, particularly outside of the flu season, and in the setting of ongoing community outbreaks. Within 24 to 48 hours of onset, however, hypotension occurs accompanied by organ system impairment or acute respiratory distress syndrome. A generalized erythematous rash occurs in 10% to 20% of patients, and necrotizing fasciitis is observed in a similar proportion. Desquamation may occur during convalescence. Mortality ranges from 30% to 65%.

OPTIMAL MANAGEMENT

Parenteral therapy with a β-lactam agent or clindamycin is appropriate for invasive group A streptococcal infections. As with necrotizing fasciitis, a combination of clindamycin and penicillin is recommended for severe infections such as STSS. Inhibition of synthesis of streptococcal proteins such as M protein and pyrogenic exotoxins is an added benefit of clindamycin therapy. Supportive care and surgical intervention in the case of associated tissue necrosis or endometritis are also important. There is increasing evidence to suggest that high-dose IVIG may improve survival in persons with STSS. IVIG has been shown to contain neutralizing activity against streptococcal superantigens, although significant variation has been noted between IVIG preparations. Given the extremely high case fatality rates for STSS, the available data, though not based on randomized trials, support the use of IVIG in treatment of STSS. The recommended dosage is 1 to 2 g per kilogram given once and repeated if needed.

When an episode of postoperative or postpartum group A streptococcal infection is identified, health care workers involved in direct patient care during delivery, operative procedure, or wound care should be screened for asymptomatic carriage. Screening should include nares, throat, vagina, rectum, and skin. Medical and laboratory records should be reviewed to identify additional cases and efforts made to retrieve and subtype isolates to determine relatedness. Secondary cases of invasive group A streptococcal disease have been reported among household contacts of an index case. However, the magnitude of the risk of subsequent cases and optimal chemoprophylaxis regimens have not been adequately determined. Until such data are available, decisions regarding chemoprophylaxis should be based on individual assessment of risk in each case.

GROUP B STREPTOCOCCAL INFECTIONS

INCIDENCE AND EPIDEMIOLOGIC FACTORS

Group B streptococci (*S. agalactiae*) cause infection primarily in newborns, pregnant women, and adults with underlying medical conditions. Over the past several decades, group B streptococci (GBS) have emerged as the leading cause of sepsis, meningitis, and pneumonia in newborn infants in the United States; the incidence of invasive neonatal disease is about 1.0 case per 1,000 live births (approximately 3,900 cases in the United States per year). This represents a substantial recent decline likely related to implementation of new prevention guidelines. Epidemiologic risk factors for neonatal infection include African American background, low socioeconomic status, teenage pregnancy, and previous delivery of a GBS-infected infant. Risk is also increased in preterm delivery and in the presence of intrapartum risk factors such as maternal fever (38°C or above), prolonged rupture of membranes (18 hours or longer), and maternal colonization with GBS. The GBS are estimated to account for 15% to 25% of maternal infections.

In nonpregnant adults, the risk of invasive GBS infections increases with age and is higher among African Americans. The incidence of invasive GBS infections in adults is approximately 5 cases per 100,000 persons and has been noted to be increasing in recent years. Conditions that predispose nonpregnant adults to serious GBS infections include diabetes mellitus, malignancies in young and middle-aged adults, cirrhosis, presence of decubitus ulcers, and a neurogenic bladder. Nosocomial infection is relatively common (20% of invasive cases) and has been associated with placement of central venous catheters.

ETIOLOGIC FACTORS AND PATHOGENESIS

At least ten GBS serotypes have been identified; types Ia, Ib/c, Ia/c, II, III, and V are most common in the United States. Immunity is mediated by antibody to the capsular polysaccharide and is serotype-specific. Several studies have shown that susceptibility to neonatal infection is increased in infants born to mothers with low levels of anticapsular antibody. GBS are a common inhabitant of the gastrointestinal tract and lower genital tract. Rectal and vaginal carriage can be identified in 25% to 30% of pregnant women. Newborns may become infected from ascending infection after rupture of membranes while still in utero or during vaginal delivery.

Little is known about immunity to GBS infections in adults. The diverse group of underlying conditions among nonpregnant adults with GBS disease suggests that susceptibility to infection may be complex and include waning antibody levels, impaired immune response, and local factors such as skin breakdown, aspiration, and structural abnormalities in the urinary tract.

CLINICAL FEATURES

Pneumonia and bacteremia are the most common presentation of early-onset neonatal GBS disease. Meningitis is the most common presentation of late-onset infection in neonates; bacteremia, pneumonia, and bone and joint infection may also occur. The case fatality rate of neonatal infection is approximately 5%. Neurologic sequelae occur in up to one-third of infants who survive GBS meningitis.

Postpartum endometritis, wound infections (often associated with cesarean section), and bacteriuria are the most common presentations of maternal GBS infection. Signs of endometritis generally begin within 48 hours of delivery and include fever and uterine tenderness. Polymicrobial infection is common. The severity of GBS urinary tract infection ranges from asymptomatic bacteriuria to pyelonephritis.

In nonpregnant adults, the most common clinical diagnoses are skin, soft-tissue, or bone infection; bacteremia with no identified source; urosepsis; and pneumonia. Typical skin or soft-tissue infections include cellulitis, wound infection, and infection of foot ulcers or decubitus ulcers. More than half of patients with such infections have diabetes mellitus. Endocarditis and meningitis are uncommon manifestations of invasive GBS disease. There are rare reports of GBS associated with STSS and necrotizing fasciitis. Clinical findings vary with the site of infection. Overall mortality for invasive GBS in adults is approximately 25%; risk of death is higher in the elderly and in those with pneumonia.

The gold standard for diagnosis of GBS infection is culture. Optimal sensitivity of vaginal and rectal cultures from pregnant women requires inoculation of a selective broth medium rather than direct plating of the specimen. GBS antigen detection tests are thus far insufficiently sensitive to be used for prenatal or intrapartum screening. Invasive GBS disease may present as a polymicrobial bacteremia in nonpregnant adults, most often involving mixed infection with staphylococci.

OPTIMAL MANAGEMENT

Parenteral antibiotic therapy and supportive care are the mainstays of therapy. All GBS strains are susceptible to penicillin.

The combination of a β-lactam and aminoglycoside is recommended for severe neonatal infections. Erythromycin resistance is increasing and compromises the use of this agent in penicillin-allergic individuals. Use of clindamycin is preferred in this setting. Surgical debridement may also be important in the treatment of certain skin and soft-tissue infections.

PREVENTION

Many neonatal GBS infections can be prevented by intrapartum antimicrobial prophylaxis. Chemoprophylaxis with penicillin or ampicillin significantly reduces the incidence of neonatal infection and of postpartum maternal febrile illness. The approach recommended by the U.S. Centers for Disease Control and Prevention (CDC) includes prenatal screening cultures at 35 to 37 weeks' gestation; and intrapartum antibiotics for preterm deliveries (less than 37 weeks' gestation), GBS carriers, and mothers with intrapartum risk factors and unknown colonization status. Vaccines for the prevention of GBS infection in newborns are in development.

OTHER β-HEMOLYTIC STREPTOCOCCAL INFECTIONS

INCIDENCE AND EPIDEMIOLOGIC FACTORS

Group C and G streptococci have been implicated as causes of endemic and epidemic pharyngitis and of invasive infection. Because many group C streptococci are also bacitracin-sensitive, they may be misidentified as group A streptococci when this technique is used to identify positive throat cultures.

In one hospital-based case series, group G and C streptococci accounted for 11% and 5% of all bacteremic β-hemolytic streptococcal infections. Group G streptococcal infection, however, represented only 0.3% of all positive blood cultures. Populations at high risk for invasive group C and G streptococcal infections are similar to those populations at high risk for group B streptococci.

ETIOLOGIC FACTORS AND PATHOGENESIS

Most group C streptococcal infections in humans are caused by *Streptococcus equisimilis*. *Streptococcus zooepidemicus* is primarily an animal pathogen and rarely infects humans; outbreaks associated with unpasteurized dairy products have been reported. Only one case of bacteremic infection with *Streptococcus equi* has been reported. Group G streptococci generally are not characterized by species.

Both group C and G streptococci make streptolysin O, and *S. equisimilis* produces the streptokinase that is used for human thrombolytic therapy. Group G streptococci have M proteins that are antiphagocytic. Pyrogenic exotoxins have not been documented in either group C or G.

CLINICAL FEATURES

The clinical presentation of group C and G pharyngitis is similar to that of group A streptococcal infection. Both endemic disease and epidemics of foodborne infection can occur. A variety of suppurative infections due to group C and G streptococci have been reported. Bacteremic group C and G streptococcal infection presents most commonly with skin and soft-tissue infection, pulmonary infection (pneumonia and empyema), or with no defined focus. Endocarditis, puerperal sepsis, bone and joint infection, and peritonitis have also been reported.

TREATMENT

Penicillin is the treatment of choice for these infections. For severe infections (e.g., endocarditis), an aminoglycoside may be added for synergy. Similar to GBS infections, 26% of invasive group G streptococcal infections were polymicrobial, *S. aureus* being identified in half of the infections; thus, broader spectrum antimicrobial coverage may be indicated until culture results are known.

▪ STREPTOCOCCUS PNEUMONIAE

INCIDENCE AND EPIDEMIOLOGIC FACTORS

Streptococcus pneumoniae (pneumococcus), an α-hemolytic streptococcus, is the leading cause of bacterial meningitis, community-acquired bacteremia, and bacterial pneumonia in the United States. The annual incidence of pneumococcal bacteremia is 23 cases per 100,000 persons. Rates are highest at the extremes of age. The pneumococcus also accounts for 30% to 40% of otitis media cases—approximately 7 million cases per year in the United States. Risk factors for pneumococcal infection include chronic and immunosuppressive illness, particularly hematologic malignancies, HIV infection, anatomical and functional asplenia, cerebrospinal fluid leaks, and very young or older age. Rates of pneumococcal disease are increased in African Americans and certain Native American populations in the southwestern United States. Cigarette smoking and passive exposure to cigarette smoke have both been shown to increase the risk of invasive pneumococcal disease in nonelderly adults. Children with underlying diseases and those who attend day care are at increased risk for invasive pneumococcal disease.

Pneumococcal infection is transmitted person to person by direct contact with respiratory secretions. Although outbreaks of pneumococcal disease are uncommon, recent occurrences of clusters in an overcrowded jail, among military trainees, and in day care and nursing home settings emphasize the role of crowding as a risk factor for transmission. Pneumococcal infections usually occur during the winter and early spring, and may complicate infections caused by influenza and respiratory syncytial virus.

ETIOLOGIC FACTORS AND PATHOGENESIS

More than 80 capsular types of *S. pneumoniae* have been identified. Most infections are caused by relatively few of these types: the seven most common serotypes account for over 70% of infections in the United States. As with other streptococcal species, the capsule inhibits phagocytosis, and anticapsular antibody provides type-specific protection. The immune response to infection and to nasopharyngeal carriage varies with serotype and age.

Although several pneumococcal toxins have been identified, their pathogenic role remains unclear. Pneumolysin activity may be important in the development of pneumococcal pneumonia. Cell wall teichoic acid of *S. pneumoniae* elicits a potent inflammatory response. Peroxide production by the organism may also contribute to pathogenesis.

Pneumococcal upper respiratory infections, otitis media, and sinusitis occur following direct extension from the nasopharynx, and pneumonia occurs following aspiration of the organism. Host factors that promote aspiration or inhibit mechanical or immunologic defense mechanisms, such as alcohol abuse or smoking, increase the risk of pneumonia.

CLINICAL FEATURES

Pneumococcal otitis media and sinusitis present with findings typical of infection at those sites and cannot be distinguished clinically from other etiologies of infection. Pneumococcal pneumonia often presents with abrupt onset of fever and chills. Cough is productive of purulent to blood-tinged sputum. Pleuritic chest pain, tachypnea, and tachycardia are common. Hypoxemia and cyanosis may occur. On examination, the patient appears acutely ill. Rales and signs of consolidation are usually present. A pleural rub or signs of an effusion may occur. The abdomen may be distended and abdominal pain may occur with lower lobe pneumonia. Laboratory evaluation reveals leukocytosis with an increased proportion of neutrophils and band forms. The most common radiographic finding is lobar consolidation, usually involving a single lobe; however, multilobar disease or bronchopneumonia may also occur. Blood culture may be positive in 20% of patients. Examination of sputum specimens often reveals gram-positive, intracellular, lancet-shaped diplococci.

Pneumococcal bacteremia may occur in association with pneumonia or with no evidence of a primary focus. Up to half of all pneumococcal bacteremia in children occurs in those presenting to the emergency department with fever and no localizing signs; most children are clinically well and culture-negative on reevaluation at 24 to 48 hours, regardless of whether antimicrobial therapy was begun. In contrast, pneumococcal bacteremia in adults is generally associated with significant systemic toxicity and most patients are hospitalized for treatment of their disease. Metastatic focal infections including meningitis, osteomyelitis, septic arthritis, and peritonitis may occur following bacteremia in children and adults.

OPTIMAL MANAGEMENT

The emergence of antimicrobial resistance among pneumococci has had a major impact on therapy for these infections. Resistance to penicillin and other β-lactam antibiotics occurs through changes in the PBPs, which decrease their affinity for these agents. Resistance occurs along a continuum that depends on the number of changes within the PBPs. These changes occur following exchange of genetic material with other pneumococci or other streptococcal species. Resistance is unrelated to β-lactamase production and thus inhibitors of β-lactamase add nothing to the treatment of penicillin-resistant pneumococcal infections. Penicillin-resistant strains frequently have decreased susceptibility or resistance to the cephalosporins, including third-generation cephalosporins, which also rely on binding to PBPs for their activity. Penicillin-resistant pneumococci are also more likely to be resistant to erythromycin and trimethoprim–sulfamethoxazole, although by completely different mechanisms. Currently, most resistance is clustered within several serotypes, including 6A and B, 9V, 14, 19A, and 23F. Rates of resistance vary widely among geographic areas but have now reached significant levels in most areas of the United States.

Although penicillin resistance is defined by a minimum inhibitory concentration (MIC) of greater than 1 μg per milliliter and intermediate susceptibility by an MIC between 0.1 and 1 μg per milliliter, the clinical response to therapy depends on the antibiotic concentration that can be achieved at the site of infection. Pneumonia and bacteremia caused by intermediate strains may be successfully treated with high-dose penicillin. Fully resistant infections at these sites may still respond to penicillin or can usually be treated with a parenteral third-generation cephalosporin because achievable blood levels of the antibiotic are many times higher than the MIC. Recent trends toward ever higher MIC levels among pneumococci may compromise treatment with β-lactams in the future. Expanded spectrum fluoroquinolones have good activity against β-lactam-resistant pneumococci at this writing. However, use of such agents is not currently approved in children, and judicious use in adults is recommended to avoid rapid emergence of resistance.

Because of decreased penetration of penicillin across the blood–brain barrier and decreased opsonophagocytosis in the central nervous system, pneumococcal meningitis caused by intermediate or resistant strains cannot be treated with penicillin. In addition, the increasing prevalence of third-generation cephalosporin resistance makes reliance on these agents for empirical treatment of pneumococcal meningitis no longer acceptable. Treatment with a parenteral third-generation cephalosporin (cefotaxime or ceftriaxone) *in combination with* vancomycin is now recommended. The addition of rifampin has been advocated by some in difficult cases. All pneumococci remain susceptible to vancomycin. Amoxicillin remains the drug of choice as first-line empirical therapy for children with otitis media, although an increase in the dosage to 80 or 90 mg per kilogram per day is recommended.

PREVENTION

A 23-valent pneumococcal polysaccharide vaccine is recommended for persons over 2 years of age in high-risk groups and for all persons over 65. Approximately 90% of invasive pneumococcal infections are caused by a type included in the vaccine or a related type with cross-protection. Vaccine efficacy for bacteremic disease is about 70% and varies with underlying disease and age. Efficacy has not been demonstrated in persons with sickle cell anemia, Hodgkin's disease, and other hematologic malignancies. Penicillin prophylaxis has been effective in decreasing invasive pneumococcal infections in patients with sickle cell disease. Seven-, nine-, and eleven-valent polysaccharide/

protein conjugate vaccines will soon be available for use in infants and young children. Indications for use of the conjugate vaccines in adults have yet to be determined.

VIRIDANS STREPTOCOCCUS

DEFINITION

Viridans streptococci are a heterogeneous group of organisms that are not uniformly classified by either blood agar hemolysis or Lancefield serogroup classification systems. The Latin word *viridans*, meaning "green," was chosen because many of the species in this group are α-hemolytic; however, other species in this group are nonhemolytic and a few are β-hemolytic. The viridans streptococcal species do not have predictable, characteristic Lancefield serotypes, although an individual isolate may react with one or more Lancefield sera. In general, then, the viridans streptococci are a group defined more by exclusion than inclusion; they must be distinguished from pneumococci, enterococci, group D streptococci, and other groupable streptococci.

The nomenclature and number of species in the viridans streptococci group have changed several times over the past two decades. Clinically significant viridans streptococci include *S. mitis, S. oralis, S. sanguis, S. gordonii, S. cristi, S. salivarius, S. mutans,* and the Intermedius or Milleri group that includes *S. intermedius, S. constellatus,* and *S. anginosus.* Nutritionally variant streptococci were formerly classified as viridans streptococci and now form a separate group. They require pyridoxal or vitamin B_6 for growth. Although they will grow in broth blood culture media, which contains the necessary nutrients, they will not grow when subcultured onto agar unless the media is supplemented. Two nutritionally variant streptococcal species are proposed: *S. adjacens* and *S. defectivus.* Because the clinical features of nutritionally variant streptococcal disease are similar to those of the viridans streptococci, they are included in this section.

INCIDENCE AND EPIDEMIOLOGIC FACTORS

Because of changes in patient populations and underlying cardiac diseases, viridans streptococci are now responsible for about 35% of all cases of native valve endocarditis, whereas in the past they constituted a much greater proportion of cases. Most patients with endocarditis due to viridans streptococci have congenital or acquired valvular heart disease (rheumatic disease, congenital disease, mitral valve prolapse, and degenerative valve disease) or prosthetic valves. Although many species of viridans streptococci produce endocarditis, they are not distinguishable by clinical manifestations.

PATHOGENESIS AND CLINICAL FEATURES

Viridans streptococci are common commensals of the oral pharynx, gastrointestinal tract, and female genital tract. Viridans streptococci are organisms of low virulence, in part because they lack the usual repertoire of pathogenic mechanisms such as production of endotoxins, exotoxins, or pyogenic factors. The important characteristic that they do possess is the ability to adhere to and propagate on endocardial surfaces. This characteristic is mediated in part by production of extracellular dextran, a compound produced unpredictably by certain isolates, and by the production of lipoteichoic acid, which mediates binding to fibronectin on cardiac valves. Dextran not only mediates adherence to valvular surfaces but also decreases the ability of penicillin to kill organisms, resulting in enhanced vegetation size in dextran-producing strains.

Endocarditis is the major clinical disease caused by the viridans streptococci. The course of endocarditis caused by viridans streptococci is typically indolent, resulting in delayed diagnosis, often 2 to 5 weeks following the onset of symptoms (see Chapter 270).

The clinical significance of the growth of viridans streptococci from blood cultures is frequently questioned. However, viridans streptococci are well-established causes of significant bacteremia without endocarditis in immunocompromised hosts, particularly patients undergoing bone marrow transplant or chemotherapy for malignancy. In some centers, it is the most common cause of bacteremia in such patients. Bacteremia has been associated with neutropenia, the presence of mucositis, and prophylactic use of trimethoprim–sulfamethoxazole. *S. mitis* is the most frequently reported species. It typically occurs within 15 days of bone marrow transplant and is more common in children than adults. While the majority of patients have an uncomplicated febrile illness, up to one-fourth develop a fulminant shock syndrome characterized by vascular collapse, rash, adult respiratory distress syndrome, and subsequent desquamation.

Viridans streptococci can also cause meningitis, albeit rarely. Isolation of viridans streptococci from the cerebrospinal fluid poses a challenge of interpretation because only a single preantibiotic specimen is usually available. In the face of signs, symptoms, or other laboratory data indicating true meningitis, viridans streptococci must be considered in the list of causative agents and not summarily disregarded as a contaminant. Viridans streptococcal meningitis and bacteremia have been described among all age groups, including neonates. The Intermedius or Milleri group is well known for the propensity to cause pyogenic infections such as intra-abdominal and visceral abscesses, brain abscesses, and endocarditis complicated by myocardial or perivalvular abscesses.

OPTIMAL MANAGEMENT AND PROGNOSIS

Most but not all viridans streptococci remain very sensitive to penicillin G. Resistance to penicillin is mediated by alteration of the PBPs and not by β-lactamase production, similar to pneumococci. Strains with an MIC between 0.1 and 0.5 μg per milliliter are defined as relatively resistant or intermediate, and those with an MIC of 0.5 μg per milliliter or more are defined as resistant. The American Heart Association recommends treatment with a combination of high-dose parenteral penicillin (20 to 30 million units per day) with gentamicin or vancomycin with gentamicin for resistant (MIC 0.5 μg per milliliter or greater) infections. Cephalosporins should be used with caution in penicillin-resistant viridans streptococcal infections; because cephalosporins also bind to PBPs, alterations may cause some

degree of cephalosporin resistance in addition to penicillin resistance.

No vancomycin resistance among viridans streptococci has been reported; however, this drug should be considered only in cases in which no other therapy can be used, such as serious β-lactam allergy. A variety of other antibiotics may have activity against penicillin-resistant infections. These include chloramphenicol, imipenem, and teicoplanin. Sensitivity to these antibiotics is not uniformly predictable; therefore, MIC testing of the isolate should be done.

■ ENTEROCOCCUS AND GROUP D STREPTOCOCCI

DEFINITION

Enterococci are gram-positive, variably hemolytic cocci that usually react with Lancefield group D antisera but now form a separate genus. Two species, *Enterococcus faecalis* and *Enterococcus faecium*, account for 80% to 90% and 5% to 10% of human enterococcal disease, respectively. Enterococci are ubiquitous, hardy organisms, which are part of the normal human gastrointestinal flora and sometimes are found as part of the genital and skin flora. They are also found in the gastrointestinal tracts of other animals and in environmental sources such as soil and water. The remarkable capacity of enterococci to manifest antimicrobial resistance, most notably vancomycin resistance, makes this otherwise low-level pathogen a major clinical challenge.

INCIDENCE AND EPIDEMIOLOGIC FACTORS

Enterococci now rank as the second or third most prevalent cause of hospital-acquired infection. Although *E. faecalis* and *E. faecium* are responsible for the majority of human enterococcal disease, other *Enterococcus* species that are rarely encountered as human pathogens include *E. gallinarum*, *E. casseliflavus*, *E. durans*, *E. hirae*, *E. avium*, and *E. raffinosus*. Colonization with *Enterococcus* organisms is far more common than clinically relevant disease. The enterococcus is of low virulence in humans and most patients with serious enterococcal infection have significant underlying diseases.

Although enterococci are normal inhabitants of the gastrointestinal tract, studies have demonstrated that disease-causing isolates are frequently acquired exogenously. Such acquisition highlights the potential preventability of nosocomial infections and the importance of limiting the spread of resistant organisms from one patient to another. Health care workers whose hands become contaminated with vancomycin-resistant enterococci (VRE) may contribute to nosocomial transmission. Risk factors for nosocomial enterococcal disease include prolonged hospitalization, intensive care unit location, antibiotic therapy (particularly with cephalosporins or aminoglycosides), and use of vascular or urinary catheters. Critically ill patients in intensive care, oncology, and transplant units are at greatest risk of acquiring multidrug-resistant enterococci, particularly VRE.

CLINICAL FEATURES

The most common enterococcal infections involve the urinary tract and are often associated with structural abnormalities or recent instrumentation. Enterococci cause a variety of other clinical diseases, including wound and tissue infections, bacteremia, meningitis, endocarditis, intra-abdominal infections, and pelvic infections. Enterococci account for 5% to 10% of bacterial endocarditis cases. Underlying valvular damage or heart disease is not a prerequisite for infection. Enterococcal bacteremia is more common than endocarditis and is often identified in the setting of polymicrobial disease. A source of bacteremia may be identified in the abdomen, pelvis, biliary tract, urinary tract, or a wound. Patients with enterococcal bacteremia have a mortality rate in the range of 30% to 50%; host underlying illness and immunocompromised states contribute to this high case fatality rate.

Enterococcus is an unusual but well-known cause of meningitis, particularly among neonates. As with other enterococcal infections, meningitis occurs among patients with underlying disease, including structural abnormalities or trauma, previous procedures to the central nervous system, or previous antibiotic use or immunocompromised state. Enterococci are frequently isolated from polymicrobial intra-abdominal and pelvic abscesses; however, their role may be more synergistic than directly pathogenic. The need for specific antienterococcal therapy in this setting is not fully defined because resolution of many mixed infections is achieved through combinations of antibiotics that are not effective therapy for *Enterococcus*. Pure enterococcal pelvic and abdominal infections are described most notably among peritoneal dialysis patients, cirrhosis patients, and women following cesarean section. Mixed aerobic and anaerobic wound and tissue infections may include *Enterococcus;* however, as with abdominal infections, the precise pathogenic role of this organism is difficult to establish.

OPTIMAL MANAGEMENT

All enterococci exhibit low-level intrinsic antibiotic resistance to a variety of agents, including penicillin, cephalosporins, clindamycin, and aminoglycosides. Most enterococci have also acquired "tolerance" to cell wall–active agents such as β-lactams and vancomycin. High-level β-lactam resistance is most often seen in *E. faecium*. Penicillin resistance is generally due to decreased PBP affinity but β-lactamase production is occasionally detected. Synergistic activity occurs between cell wall–active agents, such as ampicillin, and aminoglycosides; combination therapy is standard for serious enterococcal infections. Unfortunately, high-level aminoglycoside resistance, now seen with increasing frequency, eliminates the synergistic benefit.

A striking increase in the prevalence of VRE has occurred in the last decade. VRE account for almost 15% of enterococcal infections in intensive care units, and their prevalence in other hospital locations is increasing. The vanA, vanB, vanC, or vanD resistance phenotypes that result in variably decreased glycopeptide antibiotic binding affinity mediate resistance to vancomycin. The vanA phenotype, inducible high-level vancomycin and teicoplanin resistance, is present in approximately 70% of VRE in the United States; the vanB phenotype, variable vancomycin

resistance and teicoplanin susceptibility, is present in about 25% of VRE.

The treatment of choice for susceptible infections that do not require bactericidal activity, such as urinary tract infections, remains ampicillin or penicillin. Use of vancomycin should be reserved for penicillin-allergic patients or in patients with *E. faecium* infections that show high-level penicillin resistance. For infections that require bactericidal therapy such as endocarditis, meningitis, and life-threatening bacteremia, a combination of a cell wall–active agent (e.g., penicillin, ampicillin, or vancomycin) and an aminoglycoside (e.g., gentamicin or streptomycin) is recommended. Clinical failures and relapses occur more often in persons infected with strains with high-level aminoglycoside resistance, when synergy cannot be achieved. Isolates with high-level gentamicin resistance should also be tested for streptomycin resistance, as streptomycin may occasionally remain active in this setting. Treatment options for high-level gentamicin- and streptomycin-resistant enterococci include therapy with higher doses or prolonged courses of ampicillin or vancomycin (e.g., ampicillin 12 to 16 g per day for 8 to 12 weeks for endocarditis).

Optimal treatment for VRE infections has not been established. VRE urinary tract infections can be successfully treated with nitrofurantoin. In many *E. faecalis* VRE infections, penicillin or ampicillin remains active and can be used for treatment. Teicoplanin may be useful in the subgroup of VRE infections with the vanB resistance phenotype, but emergence of teicoplanin resistance on therapy has been noted. VRE infections due to *E. faecium* are particularly problematic due to the common association with high-level penicillin resistance and resistance to most other available agents. Combinations of agents, including some fluoroquinolones, doxycycline, rifampin, novobiocin, and chloramphenicol, have been proposed; the bacteriostatic nature of these agents limits their use in endocarditis and meningitis. Quinupristin/dalfopristin offers another option for treatment of *E. faecium* VRE infections but it is not active against *E. faecalis*. The investigational drug linezolid, the first synthetic oxazolidinone, has shown good in vitro activity against both *E. faecalis* and *E. faecium* VRE.

Because most resistant enterococcal infections are hospital-acquired, strategies to prevent the spread of these strains are vital. These include prudent vancomycin use by clinicians and appropriate infection control measures to prevent person-to-person transmission.

GROUP D STREPTOCOCCI

Streptococcus bovis, a group D streptococcus, is a common colonizer of the gastrointestinal tract and relatively uncommon cause of endocarditis and bacteremia. *S. bovis* is responsible for approximately 15% of cases of infective endocarditis and the presentation is clinically indistinguishable from that caused by viridans streptococci. Invasive disease due to *S. bovis* has been associated with underlying gastrointestinal pathology, particularly colon cancer. As a result, most experts recommend that patients who have *S. bovis* isolated from blood be evaluated for colonic malignancies. Penicillin is the drug of choice for treatment of *S. bovis* infections; other antibiotics active against these bacteria include cephalothin, vancomycin, erythromycin, and clindamycin.

BIBLIOGRAPHY

Auckenthaler R, Hermans PE, Washington JA II. Group G streptococcal bacteremia: clinical study and review of the literature. *Rev Infect Dis* 1983;5:196–204.

Bisno AL, Gerber MA, Gwaltney RH, et al. Diagnosis and management of group A streptococcal pharyngitis: a practice guideline. *Clin Infect Dis* 1997;25:574–583.

Bisno AL, Stevens DL. Streptococcal infections of skin and soft tissues. *N Engl J Med* 1996:334:240–245.

Bronze MS, Dale JB. The reemergence of serious group A streptococcal infections and acute rheumatic fever. *Am J Med Sci* 1996;311:41–54.

Butler JC, Breiman RF, Campbell JC, et al. Pneumococcal polysaccharide vaccine efficacy: an evaluation of current recommendations. *JAMA* 1993;270:1826–1831.

Davies HD, McGeer A, Schwartz B, et al. A population-based assessment of the epidemiology of invasive group A streptococcal infections, including streptococcal toxic shock. *N Engl J Med* 1996;335:547–554.

Farley MM, Harvey RC, Stull T, et al. A population-based assessment of invasive disease due to group B streptococcus in nonpregnant adults. *N Engl J Med* 1993;328:1807–1811.

Hofmann J, Cetron MS, Farley MM, et al. The prevalence of drug-resistant *Streptococcus pneumoniae* in Atlanta. *N Engl J Med* 1995;333:481–486.

Moellering RC Jr. Vancomycin-resistant enterococci. *Clin Infect Dis* 1998; 26:1196–1199.

Murray BE. The life and times of the enterococcus. *Clin Microbiol Rev* 1990;3:46–65.

Salata RA, Lerner PI, Shlaes DM, et al. Infections due to Lancefield group C streptococci. *Medicine* 1989;68:225–239.

Schuchat A. Epidemiology of group B streptococcal disease in the United States: shifting paradigms. *Clin Microbiol Rev* 1998;11:497–513.

Villablanca JG, Steiner M, Kersey J, et al. The clinical spectrum of infections with viridans streptococci in bone marrow transplant patients. *Bone Marrow Transplant* 1990;6:387–393.

Wilson WR, Karchmer AW, Dajani AS, et al. Antibiotic treatment of adults with infective endocarditis due to streptococci, enterococci, staphylococci, and HACEK microorganisms. *JAMA* 1995;274:1706–1713.

Working Group on Severe Streptococcal Infections. Defining the group A streptococcal toxic shock syndrome. *JAMA* 1993;269:390.

Kelley's Textbook of Internal Medicine, fourth edition. Edited by H. David Humes. Lippincott Williams & Wilkins, Philadelphia © 2000.

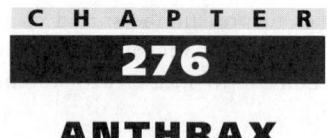

CHAPTER 276

ANTHRAX

RAYMOND A. SMEGO, Jr.

Anthrax is a zoonotic infection, affecting domestic livestock that acquire infection by grazing on spore-contaminated fields. It causes human disease by way of direct animal contact or through exposure to contaminated animal hides, meat, or other products. No human-to-human transmission has been demonstrated. *Bacillus anthracis*, the causative organism of anthrax, is an aerobic, nonmotile, gram-positive bacillus that can exist as a spore, thus allowing the organism to withstand adverse environmental conditions and persist in the soil for up to 60 years. The disease is the result of a virulence capsule and necrotizing toxin that are produced by the organism once it has invaded the host and reverted to its vegetative form.

INCIDENCE AND EPIDEMIOLOGIC FACTORS

With its name derived from the Greek derivative for "coal," anthrax has had an important place in human history. The disease was one of the plagues of the Middle Ages. Known as the "Black Bane," it swept through Europe during the seventeenth century. Rayor in 1850 described filiform bodies in the blood of dying livestock, and in 1863 Davaine transmitted anthrax to experimental animals by subcutaneous injection of infected blood. Robert Koch later recognized the sporulation of *B. anthracis* and its importance in the life cycle and environmental perpetuation of the organism. Anthrax has a place of importance in early immunization history as well; in 1881 Pasteur successfully administered a heat-attenuated anthrax vaccine to sheep.

Anthrax is rarely seen in industrialized countries, with sporadic cases occurring in individuals exposed to contaminated animal hides, hair, wool, bone, or other animal products. Cases of oropharyngeal and gastrointestinal anthrax are associated with ingestion of contaminated meat. The disease is endemic in parts of the Middle East, Africa, Asia, and Haiti. Recent large-scale outbreaks occurred during the 1970s to 1990s in Zimbabwe, Tanzania, and Haiti. In 1979, in Sverdlovsk in the former Soviet Union, the largest known epidemic of inhalational anthrax occurred; it was later found to have been the result of an accidental release of anthrax spores from a military research facility. This outbreak demonstrated the potential suitability of *B. anthracis* as a weapon of biologic warfare.

MICROBIOLOGY

Bacillus anthracis grows aerobically on 5% sheep blood agar without hemolysis. This gram-positive rod-shaped bacterium produces oval spores that are centrally or paracentrally located and produce no swelling of the bacillus. In tissues or discharges, the organisms appear in short chains (less than three bacilli). Lysis of specific γ-bacteriophage confirms identification.

PATHOGENESIS

The virulence of *B. anthracis* is due to an antiphagocytic poly-D-glutamic acid capsule and a three-component exotoxin consisting of protective antigen, edema factor, and lethal factor. After inoculation through the skin or mucous membranes, spores germinate in macrophages and grow at the local side to produce capsule and toxin, resulting in characteristic extensive tissue edema and a paucity of neutrophils. Edema factor has adenyl cyclase activity and raises cyclic adenosine monophosphate (cAMP) levels up to 200-fold, and is responsible for the edema and impaired neutrophil function. Spread of bacilli to regional nodes with further production of toxin gives rise to the hemorrhagic, necrotic, and edematous lymphademitis characteristic of anthrax.

CLINICAL FEATURES

Clinical forms of anthrax include cutaneous (more than 90% to 95% of cases), inhalational, oropharyngeal, gastrointestinal, sepsis, and meningeal disease. Typical cutaneous anthrax evolves through a range of local changes, even after initiation of antimicrobial therapy, beginning as a nonspecific, erythematous, painless, pruritic papule or macule that appears after an incubation period of 3 to 4 days. The lesion subsequently develops into a vesicle from which the organism can be isolated. The formation of the vesicle is accompanied by a mild to moderate ring of gelatinous edema that is usually more severe on the neck or face than on the trunk or extremities. The vesicle subsequently ulcerates and forms a characteristic centrally depressed black chancre (or malignant pustule) (Fig. 276.1). Other features of cutaneous anthrax include edema out of proportion to the size of the lesion, typical lack of pain, location on the face or extremities (Fig. 276.2), regional lymphadenitis, and rarity of neutrophils of Gram stain of lesion specimens. Approximately 80% of cutaneous lesions contain localized and resolve spontaneously within a few weeks. Cutaneous lesions that may mimic the early stages of anthrax include staphylococcal infections, plague, and tularemia. However, these diseases seldom lead to the severe skin necrosis seen in patients with anthrax.

Inhalational anthrax (or wool sorter's disease) begins with an influenza-like prodrome that lasts for 1 to 6 days, followed by sudden deterioration with dyspnea, strider, cyanosis, and hypoxemia. The key diagnostic feature is widening of the mediastinum due to hilar adenopathy; pleural effusions may be seen but pneumonia in uncommon. Inhalational disease is usually diagnosed late in its course and, like the extremely rare oropharyngeal and gastrointestinal forms, is usually fatal despite antibiotic therapy, often the result of sepsis or meningitis.

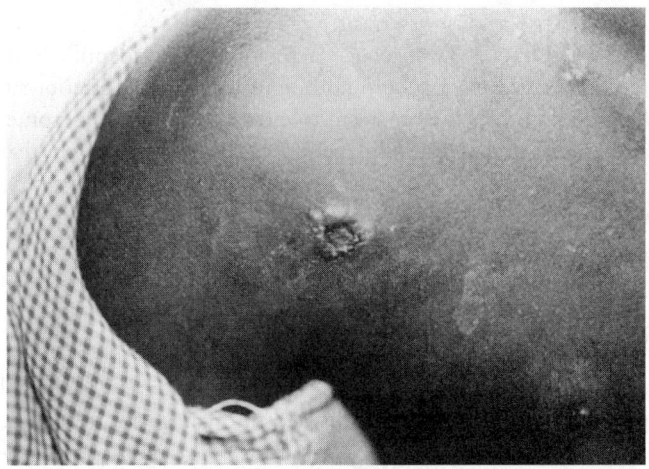

FIGURE 276.1. Typical anthrax eschar on the right shoulder of a 12-year-old boy.

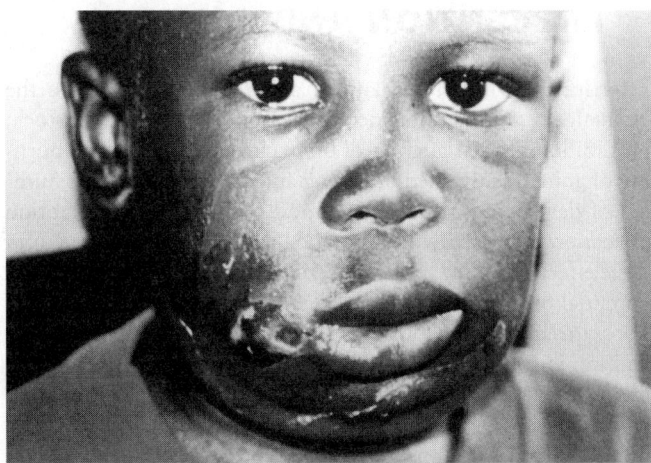

FIGURE 276.2. Cutaneous anthrax with eschar on the lip commissure and facial edema (day 3).

DIAGNOSIS

Worldwide most cases of animal and human anthrax are diagnosed on clinical and epidemiologic grounds, especially in developing countries where laboratory facilities and personnel are not readily accessible or available. Laboratory confirmation can be made by demonstration of the causative organism in blood, tissue fluids, and exudates by direct microscopic examination and culture, or by animal inoculation. Enzyme-linked immunosorbent assay (ELISA) or fluorescent antibody serologies are available but are rarely used or helpful ante mortem, especially in fulminant systemic disease. Polymerase chain reaction techniques can detect as few as three spores per clinical specimen, and a rapid hand-held immunochromatographic assay has recently been developed and made suitable for field use.

TREATMENT

Penicillin is the drug of choice for all clinical forms of disease. A daily dose of 1.2 to 8 million units of penicillin G (or V) for 7 to 10 days virtually eliminates the spread of cutaneous anthrax and essentially reduces the mortality rate to zero. Antibiotic therapy, however, will not prevent or retard the natural progression of the anthrax lesion. Penicillin has no effect on necrotizing toxin already secreted in the host tissue. It is also ineffective against *B. anthracis* spores but will stop further multiplication of the vegetative form of the organism, consequently preventing further spread of the disease. For serious systemic disease, high-dose penicillin (24 million units per day) is recommended. Tetracycline, erythromycin, chloramphenicol, and ciprofloxacin are suitable alternatives for penicillin-allergic patients. One uncontrolled study suggested a benefit of corticosteroids for serious systemic infection. Specific anthrax antiserum seems to be of value in toxic patients but it is not commercially available in most countries.

PREVENTION AND CONTROL

Effective agricultural regulations that reduce or eliminate the incidence of anthrax include vaccination of domestic livestock, prohibition of the slaughter of unvaccinated animals, and burning of animals suspected of having anthrax. Recently, in a number of developing countries, political instability and disruption of economic infrastructures have led to a lack of enforcement of these effective public health measures, thus creating a significant potential for an increase in the number of outbreaks of anthrax as occurred in Zimbabwe following the 1978–1980 civil war, and in Haiti in 1994 after the ousting of the dictatorial government. Newer human anthrax vaccines are under development. Clinicians and public health officials must be capable of recognizing this uncommon but epidemic-prone disease.

BIBLIOGRAPHY

Anthrax vaccine. *Med Lett Drug Ther* 1998;40:52–53.
Farrar EW. Anthrax: virulence and vaccines. *Ann Intern Med* 1994;121: 379–380.
File JC, Malone JD, Eitzen EM, et al. Anthrax as a potential biologic warfare agent. *Arch Intern Med* 1998;158:429–434.
LaForce FM. Anthrax. *Clin Infect Dis* 1994;19:1009–1013.
Meselson M, Guillemin J, Hugh-Jones M, et al. The Sverdlovsk anthrax outbreak of 1979. *Science* 1974;266:1202–1208.
Patra G, Vaissaire J, Weber-Levy M, et al. Molecular characterization of *Bacillus* strains involved in outbreaks of anthrax in France in 1997. *J Clin Microbiol* 1998;36:3412–3414.
Smego RA Jr, Gebrian B, Desmangels G. Cutaneous manifestations of anthrax in rural Haiti. *Clin Infect Dis* 1998;26:97–102.
World Health Organization. Anthrax control and research, with special references to national programme development in Africa: memorandum from a WHO meeting. *Bull WHO* 1994;72:13–22.
World Health Organization. Anthrax: memorandum from a WHO meeting. *Bull WHO* 1996;74:465–470.

Kelley's Textbook of Internal Medicine, fourth edition. Edited by H. David Humes. Lippincott Williams & Wilkins, Philadelphia © 2000.

C H A P T E R

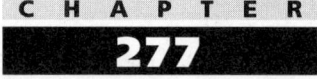

LISTERIA AND ERYSIPELOID INFECTIONS

BARRY ZELUFF
MARCIA KIELHOFNER
SUSAN J. BURGERT

LISTERIOSIS

INCIDENCE AND EPIDEMIOLOGY

Listeria monocytogenes is a β-hemolytic, facultative intracellular, gram-positive coccobacillus with a characteristic tumbling motil-

ity. This organism may be mistaken for a contaminant in the laboratory due to its similar appearance to diphtheroids. *Listeria* strains may be readily recovered from soil, water, and decaying vegetation, and have been isolated from sheep and cattle (where epizootics have been described) as well as other wild and domestic mammals and avian species. Despite this widespread distribution, invasive disease occurs in only 3.6 to 7.1 per million population in the United States, accounting for approximately 1,700 cases annually. The disease has an increasing incidence with age, and a slight male predominance (1.4:1) has been noted. The vast majority of patients with invasive listeriosis are immunocompromised; the disease has been associated with solid and hematologic malignancies, liver disease, systemic lupus erythematosus, steroid and other immunosuppressive therapies, renal failure, alcoholism, pregnancy, and transplantation (often in the context of treatment for allograft rejection). Although an uncommon infection in patients with AIDS, the frequency is reportedly up to 300 times that seen in the general population, most commonly occurring in patients with CD4 counts of less than 100.

The importance of foodborne transmission has been underscored by several outbreaks over the past two decades. Implicated vehicles include raw vegetables, processed undercooked meats, unpasteurized milk and soft cheeses. Other reported methods of transmission include transplacental spread, direct transmission to veterinarians delivering infected calves, and nosocomial outbreaks involving contaminated rectal thermometers and resuscitation equipment.

PATHOGENESIS

The development of invasive listeriosis is dependent on host susceptibility, bacterial virulence, and inoculum. The importance of T-cell-mediated immunity against this pathogen is exemplified by the populations at highest risk for disease. There may also be a role for humoral immunity, as low levels of IgM and decreased classic complement pathway activity have been correlated with neonatal disease. Gastric acidity is an important local defense against listeriosis.

Several important virulence factors have been identified: internalin, a protein that promotes entry into cells; listeriolysin O, which enables the organism to escape from phagolysosomes and evade intracellular killing; and Act A, a surface protein that induces actin filament assembly and facilitates cell-to-cell spread of the organism.

CLINICAL FEATURES

Listeria monocytogenes infections can exhibit a myriad of clinical presentations. These can be divided into categories to include central nervous system (CNS) infections, sepsis of unknown origin, focal infections, infections associated with pregnancy, and neonatal infections.

CENTRAL NERVOUS SYSTEM INFECTIONS

Two-thirds of adult infections involve the CNS, as either meningitis or meningoencephalitis. Unlike other common causes of bacterial meningitis, *L. monocytogenes* has a tropism for the brain (particularly the brain stem) as well as the meninges, and many patients present with altered levels of consciousness, movement disorders, or seizures that are more suggestive of a meningoencephalitis than pure meningitis. In a recent review of community-acquired bacterial meningitis at a large referral hospital, *L. monocytogenes* was the third most frequent cause of meningitis. It is second only to *Pneumococcus* as the leading cause of bacterial meningitis in adults older than 50 years. It is the leading cause of bacterial meningitis in organ transplantation patients, lymphoma patients, and any patient receiving corticosteroid therapy.

Meningitis due to *L. monocytogenes* usually resembles other forms of bacterial meningitis but may have a more subacute presentation akin to tuberculous meningitis. Nuchal rigidity is uncommon, with less than 50% of patients displaying meningismus on presentation. Movement disorders (ataxia, tremors, myoclonus) and seizures are common. Two-thirds of patients present with an altered sensorium, and a fluctuating mental status is common. The cerebral spinal fluid (CSF) findings are generally indistinguishable from other causes of bacterial meningitis. The white blood cell count is usually between 100 and 5,000 cells, and the majority of cells are neutrophils. Mononuclear cells predominate in one-third of patients. The CSF glucose is typically normal in two-thirds of patients. The CSF Gram stain is negative in two-thirds of patients and may be misleading as it is often misread as a "diphtheroid."

An unusual form of CNS infection involves primarily the brain stem and is termed *rhombencephalitis*. This syndrome is distinct from other forms of *Listeria* CNS infections in that the normal host appears more susceptible to this form of infection. The typical illness presents with a prodrome of fever, headache, nausea, and vomiting that lasts for approximately 4 days. This is followed by the abrupt onset of cerebellar signs, cranial nerve defects, and long-tract motor and/or sensory signs. Asymmetry of neurologic signs is characteristic of this syndrome. Nuchal rigidity is present in only 50% of the cases. Respiratory failure or arrest occurs in 40% of patients. The CSF findings are typically minimally abnormal, with the Gram stain positive in less than 10% of patients. The CSF cultures are positive in 40% whereas the blood cultures are positive in 60% of patients. Overall mortality is high, and serious neurologic sequelae are common in the survivors.

Brain abscesses are an unusual presentation of *Listeria* CNS infections occurring in less than 10% of cases. One-fourth of patients will have associated meningoencephalitis as manifested by positive CSF cultures. Bacteremia is present in the majority of cases, distinguishing *L. monocytogenes* from other causes of brain abscesses. Brain abscesses occur most commonly in persons at high risk for listerial infections. Unlike other causes of brain abscesses, involvement in the thalamus, pons, and medulla is common with *Listeria*. With appropriate antibiotic therapy,

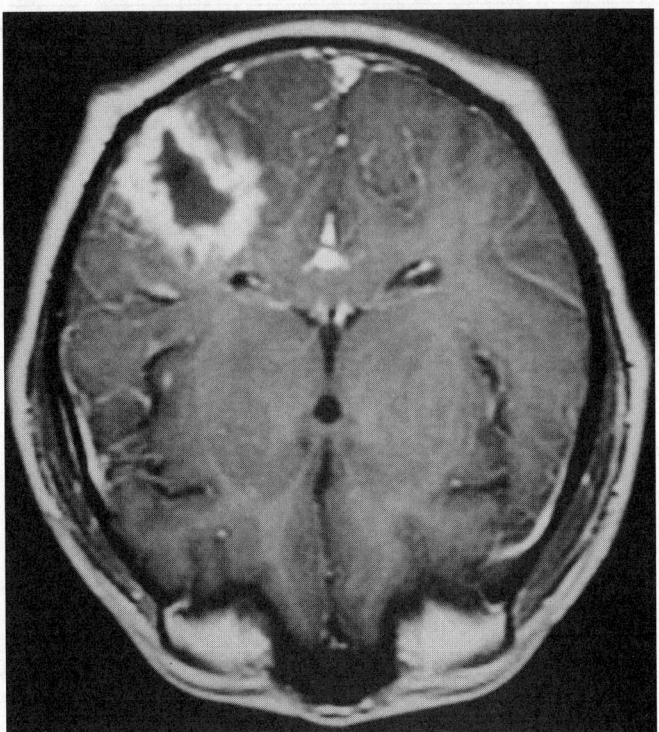

FIGURE 277.1. *Listeria* brain abscess in a patient taking corticosteroids.

prognosis is generally favorable, although residual neurologic sequelae are not uncommon (Fig. 277.1).

SEPSIS OF UNKNOWN ORIGIN

The second most common clinical presentation of *L. monocytogenes* infections is sepsis of unknown origin. The clinical picture may vary from a mild febrile illness to complicated septic shock. The pregnant woman often has a mild flulike illness with *Listeria* bacteremia, whereas her infant may develop overwhelming sepsis. The majority of adults with sepsis of unknown origin are immunosuppressed. The clinical presentation is indistinguishable from other causes of sepsis due to both gram-positive and gram-negative bacteremia.

Listeria monocytogenes endocarditis has been reported on both native and prosthetic valves. It usually presents as a subacute form of endocarditis that is indistinguishable from other causes of endocarditis, such as viridans streptococci. Multiple blood cultures are usually positive. Mortality with *Listeria* infection is high in both forms of endocarditis.

FOCAL INFECTIONS

Focal infections can be the result of hematogenous seeding or direct inoculation of *Listeria*-infected material. Veterinarians in direct contact with infected animals have reported a pustular rash. Purulent conjunctivitis has also been reported due to direct

TABLE 277.1.	MANAGEMENT OF LISTERIOSIS IN THE ADULT[a]			
Site of Infection	**First-Line Therapy**		**Second-Line Therapy**	**Duration**
Primary bacteremia	Ampicillin 6–10 g/d		TMP-SMX 20 mg/kg/d	2 wk
Meningitis	Ampicillin 6–10 g/d + Gentamicin 6 mg/kg/d[b]		TMP-SMX 20 mg/kg/d	3 wk
Brain abscess	Ampicillin 14 g/d + Gentamicin 6 mg/kg/d[b]		TMP-SMX 20 mg/kg/d	4–6 wk
Endocarditis	Ampicillin 6–10 g/d + Gentamicin 6 mg/kg/d[b]		TMP-SMX 20 mg/kg/d	4–6 wk
Bacteremia in pregnancy	Ampicillin 6–10 g/d		Erythromycin 4 g/d	2 wk

[a] Dosing based on trimethoprim component.
[b] No data regarding once-a-day vs. conventional dosing.
TMP-SMX, trimethoprim–sulfamethoxazole.

inoculation. *Listeria* pneumonia may be seen in neonates who aspirate infected amniotic fluid or adults who aspirate contaminated food. The pneumonia is lobar and is usually diagnosed by positive blood cultures for *Listeria*. Other focal infections reported include peritonitis, hepatitis and hepatic abscesses, cholecystitis, arteritis of both native and synthetic grafts, osteomyelitis, septic arthritis, and endophthalmitis.

LISTERIOSIS IN PREGNANCY

The cell-mediated immune defect that occurs during pregnancy places the pregnant woman at risk for listerial infection. In addition, the placenta appears to provide a protected site for proliferation of the organism. Bacteremia is the most common manifestation of infection and is seen most often in the third trimester. Symptoms are of a nonspecific, febrile, flulike illness. Perinatal infection is rarely life threatening to the mother; however, amnionitis may result, and premature labor is common with stillbirth or neonatal death in 22% of cases. Mortality is highest when infection occurs early in gestation. Early diagnosis and treatment improve outcome. For unclear reasons, listerial meningitis is uncommon in the pregnant woman.

LISTERIOSIS IN THE NEONATE

Infection in utero can result in spontaneous abortion, stillbirth, early disseminated disease known as granulomatosis infantiseptica, or early-onset sepsis. The most serious of these illnesses is granulomatosis infantiseptica, the hallmark of which is abscess and granuloma formation in multiple organs. The infant may have respiratory or hemodynamic compromise, pharyngitis, conjunctivitis, or meningitis. A rash may be present, with ulcerating papules on the trunk and extremities. The mortality in this syndrome may approach 100%. When infection occurs during vaginal delivery, the neonate more commonly presents with a late-onset meningitis 2 weeks post partum. This form of late infection may also be acquired by horizontal or nosocomial acquisition.

DIAGNOSTIC MODALITIES

Listerial infection is diagnosed by the isolation of the organism from a normally sterile site and identification by microbiological techniques. Routine culture methods are typically adequate to identify *Listeria* species, although cold enrichment techniques and the use of selective media may be employed when suspicion of listeriosis is high. Serologic tests are not useful in establishing this diagnosis.

OPTIMAL MANAGEMENT

Recommendations for antibiotic management of listeriosis are based on in vitro susceptibility data, animal studies, and clinical experience (Table 277.1). Large comparative trials evaluating antibiotic efficacy are lacking. Ampicillin is regarded as the drug of choice for *Listeria* species, although the data that support ampicillin use over penicillin use are controversial. Both drugs appear very active, while other β-lactam antibiotics are less active. Penicillin and ampicillin are, however, considered bacteriostatic for *Listeria* species. Although there are no comparative clinical data that clearly support combination therapy, the aminoglycosides demonstrate synergy with penicillin and ampicillin, and the addition of an aminoglycoside is thus recommended in some circumstances (i.e., in the treatment of meningitis, brain abscess, endocarditis, and in the immunocompromised host). Whether intrathecal aminoglycoside administration is necessary in the treatment of meningitis is unclear.

In penicillin-allergic patients, trimethoprim–sulfamethoxazole (TMP-SMX) is the preferred alternative. It is suitable for the treatment of both meningeal and nonmeningeal infection as it has excellent CNS penetration. In the pregnant patient, in whom sulfa drugs may be contraindicated, erythromycin appears to be effective for nonmeningeal infection if allergy precludes ampicillin use. There is limited clinical information regarding the newer macrolides in the treatment of listeriosis, although clarithromycin may show promise. Imipenem and meropenem also show good in vitro activity versus *Listeria* species, but supportive clinical data are awaited.

Drugs thought to have insufficient activity for reliable use in listeriosis include chloramphenicol, rifampin, tetracycline, currently available quinolones, and the cephalosporins. Variable success has been reported with vancomycin, but considering its poor CSF penetration, vancomycin likewise may not be a reliable agent—especially when CNS involvement is suspected. The inadequate activity of the cephalosporins is notable as these agents are frequently used in the initial empirical coverage for meningitis. In any patient with meningitis and a risk factor for listerial infection, ampicillin or TMP-SMX should be included in initial coverage unless there is Gram stain evidence supporting another bacterial etiologic process. The role of steroids in the treatment of listerial meningitis is unknown.

PREVENTION

Both isolated cases and outbreak cases of listeriosis have been associated with ingestion of contaminated foods. Persons at risk for infection with this organism should be counseled to avoid dietary habits associated with listeriosis. Recommendations are to avoid soft cheeses, unheated leftover foods, ready-to-eat foods (hot dogs), and unheated delicatessen foods. All persons should be mindful of ways to decrease acquisition of foodborne organisms: by cooking animal products thoroughly, washing raw vegetables, keeping uncooked meats separate from other foods, avoiding raw milk and milk products, and washing hands and utensils carefully after handling uncooked foods.

ERYSIPELOTHRIX RHUSIOPATHIAE

EPIDEMIOLOGY

Erysipelothrix rhusiopathiae is a nonsporulating, nonmotile, α-hemolytic, pleomorphic, gram-positive bacillus that was first established as a human pathogen by Rosenbach in 1909. The organism is known to produce both neuraminidase and hyaluronidase, the activity of which may correlate with virulence. The organism is distributed worldwide in decaying organic matter, where it can survive for weeks to months. Domestic swine, which are susceptible to infection with this organism, are the major reservoir of human infection. Sheep, horses, fowl, fish, shellfish, and many other wild and domestic animals may also be reservoirs of disease. Infection with *Erysipelothrix* is most commonly related to occupational exposure, particularly among veterinarians, butchers, fish handlers, and other persons in occupations involving possible trauma (typically puncture wounds) coupled with animal exposure. No human-to-human transmission has been documented.

CLINICAL FINDINGS

The most common manifestation of infection with *Erysipelothrix* is a nonsuppurative cellulitis of the upper extremity. Patients typically present 2 to 7 days following a cut or abrasion with severe pain and pruritus, swelling, and violaceous, well-defined areas of cellulitis. The central area often fades as the cellulitis spreads peripherally. Adenopathy and lymphangitis are seen in approximately one-third of patients, and low-grade fever and arthralgias in only 10%. This so-called "erysipeloid of Rosenbach" is typically self-limited over 3 to 4 weeks.

Occasionally, the cellulitis progresses proximally from the area of inoculation or appears at remote areas. In this setting, fever and arthralgias are common. Blood cultures are invariably negative with this form of disease. Recurrence of this more severe form of cellulitis is common and the course more protracted.

Bacteremic infection with *Erysipelothrix* is associated with infective endocarditis in 90% of cases. History of cutaneous lesions is elicited from more than one-third of these patients. The disease is more prevalent in males (likely reflecting occupational exposure to the pathogen). Underlying structural cardiac valve disease is noted in over 40% of cases of *Erysipelothrix* endocarditis, and the aortic valve is most commonly affected. Although a subacute presentation is common, the organism is often highly virulent, resulting in marked valve destruction with a high need for valve replacement (more than 33%) and high mortality (38%). Bacteremia without associated endocarditis may be more common in immunocompromised patients. Brain abscess, osteomyelitis, and chronic arthritis have also been caused by this agent.

OPTIMAL MANAGEMENT

Most strains of *Erysipelothrix* are susceptible to penicillins, cephalosporins, carbapenems, clindamycin, and ciprofloxacin. The in vitro activity of chloramphenicol, erythromycin, and tetracycline is variable. Notably, the organism is uniformly resistant to sulfonamides, aminoglycosides, and vancomycin (an agent commonly used empirically for the treatment of infective endocarditis). The regimen of choice for infective endocarditis is 12 to 18 million units of aqueous penicillin G daily for 2 to 4 weeks. While cutaneous disease may be self-limiting, antibiotic therapy may shorten the duration of symptoms.

Preventive measures against *Erysipelothrix* infection include the wearing of protective gloves among persons involved in occupations associated with this disease. A live attenuated vaccine is available for veterinary use.

BIBLIOGRAPHY

Cherubin CE, Appleman MD, Heseltine PNR, et al. Epidemiological spectrum and current treatment of listeriosis. *Rev Infect Dis* 1991;13:1108–1114.

Decker CF, Simon GL, DiGioia RA, et al. *Listeria monocytogenes* infections in patients with AIDS: report of five cases and review. *Rev Infect Dis* 1991;13:413–417.

Gorby GL, Peacock JE Jr. *Erysipelothrix rhusiopathiae* endocarditis: microbiologic, epidemiologic, and clinical features of an occupational disease. *Rev Infect Dis* 1988;10:317–325.

Hof H, Nichterlein T, Kretschmar M. Management of listeriosis. *Clin Microbiol Rev* 1997;10:345–357.

Jones EM, MacGowan AP. Antimicrobial chemotherapy of human infection due to *Listeria monocytogenes*. *Eur J Clin Microbiol Infect Dis* 1995;14:165–175.

Khayr WF, Cherubin CE, Bleck TP. Listeriosis: review of a protean disease. *Infect Dis Clin Pract* 1992;1:291.

Lorber B. Listeriosis. *Clin Infect Dis* 1997;24:1–11.

Reboli AC, Farrar WE. *Erysipelothrix rhusiopathiae*: an occupational pathogen. *Clin Microbiol Rev* 1989;2:354–359.

Schuchat A, Swaminathan B, Broome CV. Epidemiology of human listeriosis. *Clin Microbiol Rev* 1991;4:169–183.

Southwick FS, Purich DL. Review Articles: Mechanisms of Disease: Intra-cellular pathogenesis of listeriosis. *N Engl J Med* 1996;334:770–776.
U.S. Centers for Disease Control and Prevention. Update: food-borne liste-riosis—United States, 1989–1990. *MMWR* 1992;41:251.

Kelley's Textbook of Internal Medicine, fourth edition. Edited by H. David Humes.
Lippincott Williams & Wilkins, Philadelphia © 2000.

CHAPTER

278

CORYNEBACTERIAL INFECTIONS

ROBERT T. CHEN
CHARLES R. VITEK

DIPHTHERIA

The genus *Corynebacterium* contains pleomorphic gram-positive rods, of which *Corynebacterium diphtheriae* is the most important human pathogen. Other corynebacterial species (diphtheroids) are ubiquitous and generally innocuous except in immunocompromised hosts. Diphtheria is an acute communicable disease of humans caused by infection with *C. diphtheriae*. The respiratory form of diphtheria is classically characterized by an adherent pseudomembrane covering the tonsils or pharynx, whereas cutaneous diphtheria is classically characterized by the presence of nonhealing skin ulcers. Complications of diphtheria, such as myocarditis, neuritis, shock, and death, may occur due to an exotoxin elaborated by toxigenic strains. Immunization with diphtheria toxoid is highly effective in preventing diphtheria. Boosters throughout adulthood are needed to maintain immunity.

INCIDENCE AND EPIDEMIOLIC FACTORS

Humans are the only natural host of *C. diphtheriae*. Transmission is generally person to person through close respiratory and physical contact (important in cutaneous diphtheria). Because the vaccine protects against the toxin and not the bacterial infection, immune persons can become asymptomatic carriers of toxigenic *C. diphtheriae*. Patients are usually infectious for 2 to 4 weeks if untreated, less if treated with antibiotics. Chronic nasal carriage for more than 6 months may occur despite treatment.

Despite modest declines in incidence associated with improved living conditions, respiratory diphtheria was a leading cause of child mortality in the first decades of the twentieth century, with a marked winter seasonality in temperate zones. The introduction of diphtheria toxoid vaccine in the 1920s and routine childhood vaccination in the 1940s led to rapid declines in incidence and eventually to virtual elimination of indigenous respiratory diphtheria in most developed countries. Five or fewer cases have been reported annually in the United States since 1980, mostly among adults. The last large outbreak—1,100 cases, 86% of which involved cutaneous diphtheria—occurred in 1972 to 1982 among Seattle's "skid row" population. In tropical countries, cutaneous diphtheria is the most common form of the disease and is an important mechanism of natural immunity.

Due to the decline in the circulation of toxigenic strains of *C. diphtheriae* and the waning of vaccine-induced immunity in the absence of regular booster immunizations, a substantial proportion of adults in most developed countries have become susceptible to diphtheria. Diphtheria outbreaks can recur when toxigenic strains are reintroduced into a susceptible population, especially if hygienic and social conditions facilitate spread. Adult susceptibility, reintroduction of toxigenic strains, and poor socioeconomic conditions have led to a massive epidemic of diphtheria in the former Soviet Union, with more than 150,000 reported cases and over 5,000 deaths from diphtheria from 1990 through 1997. Most reported patients in this outbreak have been 15 to 50 years old. Although this outbreak is coming under control, travelers to these and other countries where diphtheria remains endemic may import the organism.

ETIOLOGIC FACTORS

Corynbacterium diphtheriae is an aerobic, unencapsulated, non-motile, nonsporulatin, gram-positive rod. It is destroyed by heat, light, and most disinfectants, but survives freezing and prolonged desiccation. In nutritionally deficient Löffler's medium, it develops a characteristic club shape arranged like Chinese characters. Recovery is selective on tellurite-containing media, on which corynebacteria form distinctive grayish black colonies. The three biotypes of *C. diphtheriae* (*gravis, mitis,* and *intermedius*) are distinguished by colonial morphology and fermentation reactions. The severity of disease is not correlated with biotype but depends on whether the strain produces toxin (toxigenic) or not (nontoxigenic).

The gene coding for toxin production, *tox*, resides in several closely related B phages that can lysogenize nontoxigenic diphtheria organisms, converting them to toxigenic strains. Diphtheria toxin is an extremely potent inhibitor of protein synthesis. Toxin expression requires low-iron conditions in vitro, but the clinical significance of this is unknown.

PATHOGENESIS

The upper respiratory tract is the most common portal of entry for *C. diphtheriae*. The organism remains localized on the mucosal epithelium. After an incubation period of 2 to 5 days, toxigenic strains elaborate toxin, killing local epithelial cellsand eliciting a severe inflammatory response. The resultant enmeshed fibrin, necrotic epithelium, leukocytes, and bacterial organisms form a 1- to 3-mm-thick pseudomembrane, which is adherent to the underlying tissue and becomes a fertile site for further bacterial growth and toxin production. Extension of the pseudomembrane is associated with greater toxin absorption and a grave prognosis. Mechanical obstruction of the bronchi may occur.

Absorbed toxin is disseminated by the circulation. All tissues are vulnerable, especially the heart, peripheral nerves, and kidneys.

In addition to the toxin, the pathogenesis of diphtheria is also mediated by its cell wall antigens and other enzymes. Nontoxigenic strains can produce mild localized disease without systemic complications.

CLINICAL FINDINGS

The clinical course is determined by the patient's preexisting immunity against diphtheria toxin, the virulence and toxigenicity of the infecting organism, other coexisting disease, and the anatomical location of the infection.

In the most common form, pharyngotonsillar diphtheria, onset occurs insidiously over several days (versus the acute course of streptococcal pharyngitis). Early symptoms are nonspecific. Fever is low (under 102°F) throughout the illness. The pharynx appears injected. The membrane begins as small, white patches on the tonsil(s); as it coalesces, it may spread to cover the pharynx, uvula, palate, and larynx. The membrane may become thicker and gray, with green or black necrotic patches. It is adherent to underlying tissue, and removal causes bleeding. Some patients may complain of sore throat, dysphagia, nausea, vomiting, and headache. Older membrane may become necrotic and odorous. Anterior cervical nodes are usually soft, swollen, and tender. In severe cases, marked edema of adjacent tissue results in a "bull's neck" appearance. In the laryngeal form, there may be difficult and noisy breathing, hoarseness, stridor, and cough. Anterior nasal diphtheria is mild. A membrane may form on the nasal septum, but toxins are poorly absorbed from this site.

In mild cases, the membrane generally sloughs off in about a week with a proportional decrease in systemic symptoms. Patients with severe disease appear toxic, with a racing pulse; they may develop stupor, coma, and death from circulatory or respiratory failure within 10 days. Myocarditis is detectable in half of patients, beginning 1 to 6 weeks after the onset of illness, with the mortality rate proportional to the rapidity of appearance. Clinical findings may include tachycardia, muffled S_1, dysrhythmias, and failure. Peripheral neuropathy, mainly bilateral, motor, and reversible, appears 3 to 7 weeks after onset in 20% of cases, resulting in paralysis of the soft palate, posterior pharynx, cranial nerves, and respiratory muscles. The effects may range from mild debilitation to sudden death. Other internal organs may suffer nonspecific damage from the toxin.

Cutaneous diphtheria classically manifests as punched-out ulcers; however, any skin lesion can be superinfected with *C. diphtheriae*. The clinical course tends to be mild, but skin lesions may be an important source of infection to others. Rarely, the eye, genitalia, and middle ear can be infected.

The death-to-case ratio for respiratory diphtheria was 35% before the availability of antitoxin therapy and as high as 90% for laryngeal diphtheria. The fatality rate with antitoxin therapy has remained around 5% to 10% and is associated with delays in the initiation of antitoxin therapy.

Antitoxin should be given if diphtheria is clinically suspected, as therapy cannot await culture confirmation. Diphtheria should be considered whenever a patient presents with a membrane in the throat. The differential diagnosis includes group A streptococcal or viral tonsillopharyngitis, infectious mononucleosis, candidiasis, and Vincent's angina. Diagnosis based on smears of lesions alone is unreliable.

Cultures should be obtained from the nose and throat and from any other lesions. Part of the membrane or the material underneath should be obtained using a swab. The laboratory should be alerted to the possibility of diphtheria so that they can inoculate the specimen onto a Löffler or Pai slant, a tellurite-containing medium, and a blood agar plate. Silica gel is recommended if transport requires more than 24 hours. Rapid presumptive diagnosis may be obtained after incubation of the slant overnight and examination for characteristic morphology under methylene blue staining. Cultures may be negative if obtained after the initiation of antibiotic therapy. Culturing of close contacts may also be helpful. All isolates of *C. diphtheriae* should be tested for toxigenicity using the in vivo guinea pig lethality test or the in vitro Elek immunodiffusion test. Toxigenic and nontoxigenic strains can coexist, so that multiple colonies should be tested. In addition to culture, a polymerase chain reaction assay for diphtheria toxin is available through the U.S. Centers for Disease Control and Prevention (CDC). Serology can occasionally be useful; a low pretreatment antitoxin titer is consistent with but does not prove the diagnosis, whereas a high titer makes diphtheria unlikely.

LABORATORY FINDINGS

Laboratory findings are nonspecific and may include moderate leukocytosis and transient albuminuria and thrombocytopenia. Serial electrocardiograms and cardiac enzyme assays are needed for early detection of myocarditis; when present, patients should be transferred to units with adequate monitoring and therapy for serious dysrhythmias and conduction defects.

OPTIMAL MANAGEMENT

After ensuring airway patency, the only specific therapy is diphtheria antitoxin. Equine antitoxin should be administered after conjunctival or intradermal testing for hypersensitivity. Antitoxin should be administered as early as possible, as it can neutralize only toxin not already bound to cells. The recommended antitoxin dosage varies from 20,000 to 120,000 units (see package insert), depending on the anatomical site and the severity and duration of illness. Antitoxin is available from the CDC at (404)639-2888.

Antibiotics do not alter the course or outcome of disease or the incidence of complications but are used to eliminate the organism from the patient. This prevents further toxin production and transmission of the organism. Erythromycin (1 to 2 g per day orally for adults, 40 to 50 mg per kilogram orally for children) or penicillin (intramuscularly or intravenously in age-appropriate doses) should be administered for 14 days. Patients should be isolated until two successive cultures, taken at 24-hour intervals after completion of therapy, are negative. General supportive care includes strict bed rest and observation and treatment for cardiac and respiratory complications. Intubation to maintain the airway or bronchoscopy to remove obstructing membrane may be necessary. Steroids do not appear to prevent myocarditis or neuritis. Age-appropriate doses of diphtheria toxoid should be administered during convalescence, as disease may not induce immunity. Without antitoxin therapy, mortality may reach 30% to 50%. Even with antitoxin therapy, mortality of 5% to 10% may be observed, probably due to delays in diagnosis and therapy. The rapid onset of cardiac complications portends a poor prognosis.

For children less than 7 years old, active immunization is with diphtheria toxoid [6.7 to 12.5 Lf (limits flocculation units)/dose] combined with tetanus toxoid (DT), or also with acellular pertussis vaccine (DTaP). A primary series of three doses at 2, 4, and 6 months of age, followed by boosters at 12 to 18 months of age and 4 to 6 years of age, is recommended in the United States. Older persons should receive adult tetanus and diphtheria (2 Lf) toxoids (Td) to complete their primary series. A Td booster every 10 years is recommended to prevent waning immunity.

Control efforts after the diagnosis of an index case should be directed to the early diagnosis, isolation, and treatment of patients. The health department should be notified. Close contacts (e.g., household, school) should receive an age-appropriate booster dose of diphtheria-containing vaccine if they have not completed a primary series or received a booster dose within 5 years. All such contacts should also be cultured, started on antibiotic prophylaxis with either erythromycin or penicillin, and observed for symptoms for 7 days.

OTHER CORYNEBACTERIA

Corynebacteria are ubiquitous and are frequent contaminants of cultures. Many are known pathogens of animals; some may also produce an exotoxin and infect humans. *Corynebacterium ulcerans*, *C. haemolyticum*, and *C. pyogenes* organisms can cause pharyngitis. *C. ovis* organisms cause a granulomatous lymphadenitis in sheep handlers. Opportunistic pathogens in severely compromised hosts, frequently related to indwelling catheters and prosthetic heart valves, have been reported with *C. xerosis*, *C. pseudodiphtheriticum*, *C. equi*, *C. matruchotii*, and a group called JK. The organisms can be differentiated based on their morphologic, biochemical, and genetic features. Erythromycin is the drug of choice for all except group JK, for which vancomycin is preferred.

BIBLIOGRAPHY

Bisgard K, Hardy I, Popovic T, et al. Respiratory diphtheria in the United States, 1980–1995. *Am J Publ Hlth* 1998;88:787–791.

Farizo KM, Strebel PM, Chen RT, et al. Fatal respiratory disease due to *C. diphtheriae*: case report and review of guidelines for management, investigation, and control. *Clin Infect Dis* 1993;16:59–68.

Galazka AM, Robertson SE. Diphtheria: changing patterns in the developing world and the industrialized world. *Eur J Epidemiol* 1995;11: 107–117.

Galazka AM, Robertson SE. Immunization against diphtheria with special emphasis on immunization of adults. *Vaccine* 1996;14:845–857.

Immunization Practices Advisory Committee. Diphtheria, tetanus and pertussis: recommendations for vaccine use and other preventive measures. *MMWR* 1991;40(RR-10):1–28.

Kleinman LC. To end an epidemic: lessons from the history of diphtheria. *N Engl J Med* 1992;326:773–777.

Lipsky BA, Goldberger AC, Tompkins LS, et al. Infections caused by non-diphtheria corynebacteria. *Rev Infect Dis* 1982;4:1220–1235.

Naiditch MJ, Bower AG. Diphtheria: a study of 1433 cases observed during a 10-year period at the Los Angeles County Hospital. *Am J Med* 1954; 17:229.

Pappenheimer AM. Diphtheria: studies on the biology of an infectious disease. *Harvey Lectures* 1982;76:45.

Vitek C, Wharton M. Diphtheria in the former Soviet Union: re-emergence of a pandemic disease. *Emerging Infect Dis* 1998;4:539–550.

Kelley's Textbook of Internal Medicine, fourth edition. Edited by H. David Humes. Lippincott Williams & Wilkins, Philadelphia © 2000.

CHAPTER 279

MENINGOCOCCAL INFECTIONS

PETER DENSEN

Meningococcal disease takes the form of several well-described syndromes, ranging from chronic relapsing bacteremia to focal meningitis to full-blown sepsis and shock. But it is the epidemic potential of this organism combined with its ability to strike suddenly, causing rapidly fatal disease that imparts a healthy respect, if not dread, in physicians and lay persons alike. Recent excellent clinical investigations have clarified fundamental epidemiologic and immunologic details, and in so doing have served to elucidate the pathogenesis of endotoxic shock in general.

INCIDENCE AND EPIDEMIOLOGIC FACTORS

Globally, the incidence of meningococcal disease (cases per 100,000 population) varies over several orders of magnitude: from about 0.1 case in Japan (hypoendemic), to one in the United States (endemic), to approximately 10 in recent group B epidemics in South America and Norway, to approximately 100 in the group A and C hyperepidemics in Africa and China. Crowding, low socioeconomic status, poor public hygiene, and the level of immunity in a population clearly constitute major risk factors for meningococcal disease in general, but they provide an incomplete understanding of the epidemic potential of this organism.

The incidence of meningococcal disease also varies with age, being highest (10 to 15 cases per 100,000 population, i.e., epidemic levels) between 2 months and 2 years of age. About 70% of U.S. cases occur before 10 years of age. For unknown reasons, perhaps related to intimate socialization, epidemic disease is associated with a shift in the median age of infected individuals from childhood to the mid-teens.

Although 13 meningococcal serogroups have been described, serogroup A, B, C, Y, and W135 strains cause over 99% of all meningococcal infections. Group A meningococci are responsible for epidemic disease in Africa, the Middle East, and China, whereas group B, C, W135, and Y disease predominates in the United States, Europe, and South America. Epidemic disease has not occurred in the United States since the late 1940s. Rather, clusters of disease activity are reported yearly, group B disease predominating in children less than 2 years of age and group C disease in older individuals, especially college students in association with dormitory living and alcohol-related socialization.

BACTERIOLOGIC STUDIES

In clinical specimens, *Neisseria meningitidis* appear as asymmetrical gram-negative cocci that resemble kidney beans. They tend to occur in pairs, with the poles of paired cocci touching one another. They typically engender a polymorphonuclear inflammatory response and are often seen extracellularly because of the antiphagocytic properties of their capsule. On primary isolation they grow best when incubated at $37°C$ in a 5% CO_2 atmosphere on chocolate agar. Meningococci are oxidase-positive and metabolize both glucose and maltose.

Like other gram-negative bacteria, meningococci have a trilaminar cell wall consisting of an inner cytoplasmic membrane, a periplasmic space, and an outer membrane composed of a lipid bilayer containing lipopolysaccharide and outer membrane proteins. External to the cell wall lies a polysaccharide capsule, which is pierced by hairlike protein filaments called pili.

Classically, meningococci are serogrouped according to their capsular polysaccharides and subdivided further into serotypes on the basis of 5 classes of major outer membrane proteins and 12 different lipoligosaccharides (LOSs). As a consequence, meningococci differing in their serogroup may nevertheless share the same serotype or partial serotype.

Genetic mechanisms enable the meningococcus to rapidly and independently shift its display of outer membrane molecules. Organisms expressing a "new" protein or LOS molecule appear with a frequency of 10^{-3} to 10^{-5}. The factors that promote the emergence of these new strains are poorly understood but are clearly important clinically and epidemiologically.

Since genetic shifts also occur rapidly upon subculture, the accuracy of serologic techniques in tracking the relatedness of disease strains becomes a limitation. Consequently, new techniques have been developed that classify meningococci on the basis of either several "housekeeping" gene products [multilocus enzyme electrophoresis (MEE)] or the pattern of genomic DNA generated by cutting with splicing enzymes [pulsed-field gel electrophoresis (PFGE)]. The electrophoretic types (ET) generated by MEE can be grouped into electrophoretic complexes that have proven particularly useful in tracking meningococcal disease both locally and globally. The ET-5 complex has been responsible for the group B epidemics in Norway and Cuba, whereas the clusters of group C disease that have occurred in recent years in the United States and Canada are caused by meningococci belonging to the ET-37 complex.

PATHOGENESIS

Humans are the unique reservoir for *Meningococcus*. Organisms are spread via large respiratory droplets during close contact between the 2% to 15% of the population who carry them in the oropharynx and noninfected persons. On inhalation, meningococci attach to respiratory epithelial cells, but only in a tiny proportion of infected individuals (less than 1%) does this acquisition progress to invasive disease. The ratio of carriage to cases of invasive disease varies among the serogroups, ranging from around 400:1 for ET-37 complex C strains to more than 12,000:1 for group Y strains, respectively. Invasion, when it does occur, appears to do so shortly (2 to 10 days) after acquisition. Viral respiratory infections, by altering ciliary function, mucus secretion, exposure of respiratory epithelium, or the expression of glycoproteins and lipids on these cells, are well-described antecedent events that can affect whether an encounter with the meningococci results in invasive disease rather than carriage of the organism.

A current model of the acquisition event proposes that pili are the primary meningococcal structures mediating initial adhesion to host cells. Attachment is promoted further by the class 5 outer-membrane proteins interacting with the glycose moiety on host cell glycoproteins and lipids, and by host cell proteins binding to the oligosaccharide moiety of meningococcal LOSs. On the other side of the coin, the meningococcal capsule and/or LOS sialylation inhibit attachment. Thus, intimate contact and internalization of meningococci by respiratory mucosal epithelial cells is favored by the acquisition of acapsulate, unsialylated strains—precisely those commonly identified in culture surveys.

Genetic shifts in the expression of meningococcal class 5 and LOS allotypes select for those mutations within an infecting strain that are best matched with the corresponding ligands on host epithelial cells to promote optimal attachment between the two entities. Following internalization, some meningococci remain within intracellular vacuoles, whereas others are discharged into the submucosal space. Subsequent uptake by vascular endothelial cells and breach of this barrier leads to bloodstream invasion by a single meningococcal clone that is heavily piliated and possesses a capsule and sialylated LOSs. These structural differences compared to those on the initially acquired strain speak to the critical role of dynamic genetic plasticity of these surface molecules in the pathogenesis of meningococcal disease.

In most instances, bloodstream invasion results in low-level bacteremia. Most circulating meningococci are cleared by the spleen, but a few adhere to and migrate through endothelial cells at other sites, most typically the choroid plexus, where they cause local infection. Low concentrations of antibody, complement, and neutrophils in cerebrospinal fluid contribute to the predilection of meningococci to cause meningitis. As local infection progresses, meningococci may reinvade the bloodstream, causing secondary bacteremia in addition to local infection.

During multiplication, either locally or within the vascular tree, the meningococcus releases outer membrane blebs that elicit local and systemic inflammatory responses. LOSs within blebs stimulate the release of various mediators, e.g., tumor necrosis factor (TNF), interleukins, interferon-γ, platelet-activating factor, from professional and nonprofessional immune cells, as well as the activation of various cascade systems (e.g., complement, clotting, fibrinolysis arachidonate). The interaction of blebs or intact meningococci with microvascular endothelial cells and the activation of the cascade systems at the blood–endothelial cell interface impair vascular integrity throughout the body, producing the petechial–purpuric rash that typifies clinical meningococcal disease. Thus the distribution and concentration of LOSs is the major organism-based determinant of the extent and compartmentalization of the inflammatory response, clinical findings, and outcome in meningococcal disease.

From the standpoint of the host, the outcome of its interaction with the meningococcus is affected primarily by the presence and concentration of specific antibodies, as well as the complement system. The fact that the highest age-specific incidence of meningococcal disease (2 months to 5 years) is inversely related to the presence of serum bactericidal activity for the meningococcus underscores the extreme importance of specific antibody in determining the outcome of the encounter of the host with the meningococcus in the general population. Antibody to capsular polysaccharide, which is protective by virtue of its ability to promote bactericidal and opsonophagocytic activity, is particularly important. Antibodies to subcapsular antigens are also bactericidal, and because they cross-react with epitopes shared across distinct serogroups, they play a significant role in natural immunity to meningococcal disease. This is especially true for group B disease because humans have limited capacity to synthesize antibody to the homopolymeric sialic acid that constitutes its capsule. Antibodies to subcapsular antigens are generated during the carrier state, during colonization with related organisms (e.g., *Neisseria lactamica*), and as a result of exposure to epitopes shared with enteric organisms.

Serum bactericidal activity arises from the ability of specific antibody to activate the complement cascade. Thus, persons with either acquired (e.g., systemic lupus erythematosus, C3 nephritic factor) or inherited complement deficiencies who are unable to generate complement-dependent bactericidal activity experience about a 1,000-fold increased risk of acquiring meningococcal disease. The probability that a given person with meningococcal disease has a complement deficiency is inversely proportional to the incidence of the disease in the general population (or age group); it is between 5% and 10% in countries with endemic disease and even higher in countries with hypoendemic disease.

Acquired or genetic antibody or complement deficiencies increase the risk of invasive meningococcal disease. In contrast, the severity and prognosis of the disease are modulated by genetic polymorphisms that affect the intensity of the inflammatory response. For example, a polymorphism (B2) in the promotor region of the TNF-α gene results in higher concentrations of TNF-α, more severe disease and a worse prognosis in patients with meningococcal disease. Similarly, the FcγR IIa R131 polymorphism, which results in impaired phagocytic efficiency, is associated with more severe meningococcal disease. In contrast, complement deficiencies, though they increase the probability of invasive disease, are associated with less severe disease, presumably because complement-dependent amplification of the inflammatory response is blunted.

■ CLINICAL FEATURES AND LABORATORY FINDINGS

Meningococcal disease occurs year-round, but most cases occur between November and March, coincident with the peak in respiratory viral illnesses; about 50% of diseased patients have a several-day history of antecedent upper respiratory illness. There are four distinct patterns of meningococcal disease. Meningitis and meningococcemia account for 65% to 80% and 20% to 35%, respectively, of the total burden of meningococcal infections. Chronic meningococcemia and focal infection (e.g., pneumonia, suppurative arthritis, urethritis) are uncommon and account for less than 5% of all meningococcal disease.

Meningococcal meningitis is the second most common cause of acute bacterial meningitis in most developed countries. Most incidents (70%) occur in children between ages 2 months and 10 years. Patients typically appear quite ill and describe the relatively sudden onset of fever, headache, and stiff neck. The illness progresses rapidly: the median time from the onset of symptoms until presentation is 26 hours. A rash is present in 75% of patients when they are first seen. In most cases, it consists of petechiae or 2- to 5-mm purpuric lesions. Lesions may develop rapidly and involve the mucosal membranes, a consideration that necessitates repeated careful examination. The cerebrospinal fluid typically demonstrates an elevated white count (more than 1,000 neutrophils per microliter), a markedly depressed glucose level, and an elevated protein level (more than 150 mg %). Gram stain of the cerebrospinal fluid is positive in 50% to 70% of patients, and the culture is positive 80% to 90% of the time. Blood cultures are positive in 20% to 35% of infected patients. With prompt recognition and institution of appropriate antibiotic therapy, the prognosis is good, with a mortality of 5% to 10% in most developed countries.

The clinical syndrome of meningococcemia represents bacteremia without evidence of infection elsewhere. It reflects primary invasion of the bloodstream and uncontrolled, often explosive organism growth within the vascular tree, and a clinical picture that ranges from simple bacteremia to fulminant sepsis and shock. The disease progresses extremely rapidly, with the median time from the onset of illness to presentation being just 12 hours. Patients are typically restless or extremely anxious, have a very high temperature, and complain of severe myalgia. The absence of a rash in 25% of patients and the absence of meningeal symptoms or signs makes the specific diagnosis difficult. However, orthostatic changes in the blood pressure and pulse, or frank hypotension, are present in most patients and should point to a diagnosis of sepsis. The presence of a petechial or purpuric rash strongly supports a clinical diagnosis of meningococcemia. Laboratory data reveal an elevated white blood cell count with a neutrophilic predominance, but some patients exhibit leukopenia; in either setting, a marked left shift is usually present. The patient frequently exhibits some degree of thrombocytopenia. Elevated prothrombin and partial thromboplastin times are often observed, and frank disseminated intravascular coagulopathy occurs about 10% of the time. In this setting, consideration should be given to the possibility of accompanying adrenal hemorrhage (Waterhouse–Friderichsen syndrome), and appropriate diagnostic and therapeutic intervention instituted. Patients with meningococcemia usually have very high levels of bacteremia; consequently, blood cultures are positive in 90% of infected patients. In contrast, the cerebrospinal fluid usually contains few or no cells, and most cerebrospinal fluid cultures fail to grow meningococci. Prompt institution of antibiotic therapy and appropriate supportive care have reduced mortality to 15% to 20%. Acute renal failure, myocarditis, extensive dermal infarction, and autoamputation of distal digits result in significant morbidity in an additional 10% to 15% of survivors.

As discussed above, the outcome in meningococcal infections is directly related to the number of meningococci, the concentration of meningococcal endotoxin, and the resulting high levels of inflammatory cytokines at the site of infection. In meningococcal meningitis, with or without accompanying bacteremia, the primary infection is largely contained within the subarachnoid space, and the concentration of both microbial and host inflammatory mediators is high within the cerebrospinal fluid but low or undetectable in the systemic circulation. Consequently, organ damage is largely confined to the brain, and most patients survive. In contrast, in patients with meningococcemia, the concentration of these mediators is low or undetectable in the cerebrospinal fluid but high in the systemic circulation. The highest levels of these mediators are seen in fulminant meningococcemia (LOS concentration greater than 700 ng per milliliter); as such, this form of the disease represents an extreme example of the systemic inflammatory response syndrome, and resultant mortality is high.

Several prognostic scores have been developed to predict patient outcome. The simplest, the Glasgow Meningococcal Septicemia Prognostic Score, assigns points for hypotension (3), skin/rectal temperature difference more than 3 (3), coma score less than 8 (3), lack of meningismus (2), deterioration in past hour (2), base deficit more than 8 mmol per liter (1), and extending or widespread ecchymoses (1). Scores greater than 8 to 10 progressively predict mortality exceeding 36% to 45%. Chronic meningococcemia is an uncommon infection characterized by recurrent episodes of low-grade fever, scattered petechial lesions, arthritis, and low-grade intermittent bacteremia. Often patients do not appear acutely ill and recover spontaneously only to experience a recurrence days to weeks later. Blood cultures are often negative, and the diagnosis is often missed or mistaken for the gonococcal dermatitis/arthritis syndrome.

Focal meningococcal infection is also uncommon, but pneumonia, arthritis, and urethritis are well described. Given the frequency with which the organism colonizes the upper respiratory tract, the diagnosis of meningococcal pneumonia requires both a compatible clinical picture and a positive blood culture. Genital meningococcal infection has been reported in persons practicing oral sex.

Complement deficiency should be suspected in persons who have a family history of meningococcal disease, who have recurrent meningococcal infection, whose first infection occurs at 15 to 17 years of age or older, and whose infection is caused by serogroup Y, W135, or X.

TREATMENT

Meningococcal disease is a medical emergency. Outcome is directly related to the interval from presentation to diagnosis and institution of therapy. Delays in treatment are due to the failure of parents, referring doctors, and hospital physicians to recognize specific aspects of the disease. Treatment should be initiated in the emergency department or before transfer, even if diagnostic cultures have not been completed. Because the disease can progress extremely rapidly, patients should be admitted to an intensive care unit for appropriate treatment and supportive therapy. Intravenous penicillin (10 to 20 million units per day) remains the standard treatment for meningococcal disease. However, the desirability of achieving antibiotic concentrations 10-fold greater than the minimal inhibitory concentration for the organism and cost considerations have prompted regular use of third-generation cephalosporins, particularly ceftriaxone (1 to 2 g per day intravenously). Chloramphenicol (50 mg per kilogram to a maximum of 4 g per day in divided doses every 6 to 8 hours) is used in penicillin-allergic patients and for treatment of penicillin-resistant strains. Therapy is administered for 2 weeks, contingent on the clinical response, although small case series support 5 days of treatment.

Patients should be placed in respiratory isolation and the disease reported to public health officials. Family members living with the patient have a ≥500-fold increase in the risk of developing meningococcal disease. This degree of risk also applies to dormitory roommates or medical personnel involved in the resuscitation, but not routine care, of infected patients. These close personal contacts should receive chemoprophylaxis. Oral rifampin (10 mg per kilogram, to a maximum of 600 mg, every 12 hours for 2 days) remains the standard antibiotic treatment for the elimination of the carrier state in exposed persons. However, single-dose therapy with intramuscular ceftriaxone (250 mg) or oral ciprofloxacin (500 mg) appears even more effective. Administration of the tetravalent meningococcal capsular polysaccharide vaccine (serogroups A, C, Y, and W135) is recommended when the respective serogroups have caused disease because up to 50% of secondary infections occur 2 to 4 weeks after the index case—a period sufficient to permit a protective immune response. Policy decisions regarding administration of the vaccine and/or chemoprophylaxis to control cluster outbreaks in schools are best made in conjunction with public health authorities.

A number of additional therapeutic interventions have been tried in patients with severe meningococcal disease; however, controlled trials supporting their utility are generally lacking. Clearly, corticosteroid administration is essential in documented adrenal failure. Dexamethasone is commonly administered for the first 2 days of treatment for meningococcal meningitis. Heparin can be useful in the treatment of disseminated intravascular coagulopathy but is clearly secondary to treatment of the infection itself. Infusion of fresh frozen plasma to replace protein C may improve outcome. The utility of plasmapheresis and treatment with monoclonal antibody to lipid A remain uncertain but probably are not beneficial.

BIBLIOGRAPHY

Brandtzaeg P, Halstensen A, Kierulf P, et al. Molecular mechanisms in the compartmentalized inflammatory response presenting as meningococcal meningitis or septic shock. *Microb Pathogen* 1992;13:423–431.

Duncan A. New therapies for severe meningococcal disease but better outcomes? *Lancet* 1997;350:1565–1566.

Figueroa JE, Densen P. Infectious diseases associated with complement deficiencies. *Clin Microbiol Rev* 1991;4:359–395.

Nadel S, Newport MJ, Booy R, et al. Variation in the tumor necrosis factor–α gene promoter region may be associated with death from meningococcal disease. *J Infect Dis* 1996;174:878–880.

Nadel S, Britto J, Maconochie I, et al. Avoidable deficiencies in the delivery of health care to children with meningococcal disease. *J Accid Emerg Med* 1998;15:298–303.

Powars D, Larsen R, Johnson J, et al. Epidemic meningococcemia and purpura fulminans with induced protein C deficiency. *Clin Infect Dis* 1993;17:254–261.

Raymond NJ, Reeves M, Ajello G, et al. Molecular epidemiology of serogroup C meningococcal disease. *J Infect Dis* 1997;176:1277–1284.

Schwartz B, Al-Ruwais A, A'ashi J, et al. Comparative efficacy of ceftriaxone and rifampicin in eradicating pharyngeal carriage of group A *Neisseria meningitidis*. *Lancet* 1988;1:1239–1242.

Virji M. Meningococcal disease: epidemiology and pathogenesis. *Trends Microbiol* 1996;4:466–470.

Kelley's Textbook of Internal Medicine, fourth edition. Edited by H. David Humes. Lippincott Williams & Wilkins, Philadelphia © 2000.

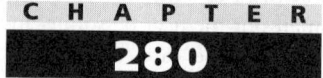

CHAPTER 280

GONOCOCCAL INFECTIONS

GEORGE F. BROOKS

Gonococcal infections are caused by the gram-negative diplococcal bacteria *Neisseria gonorrhoeae*. The most common form of gonococcal infection in men is urethritis. In women, endocervicitis is most common, but the complication of uterine tube infection [pelvic inflammatory disease (PID)] is most important.

■ INCIDENCE AND EPIDEMIOLOGIC FACTORS

Gonorrhea remains a major public health problem worldwide. In the United States, the incidence of gonorrhea began to increase in the mid-1950s, and by 1975 nearly 500 cases per 100,000 population or about 1 million cases were reported; the actual incidence may have been twice that because of unreported cases. In recent years, the incidence of reported gonorrhea has declined significantly to less than 125 cases per 100,000 popula-

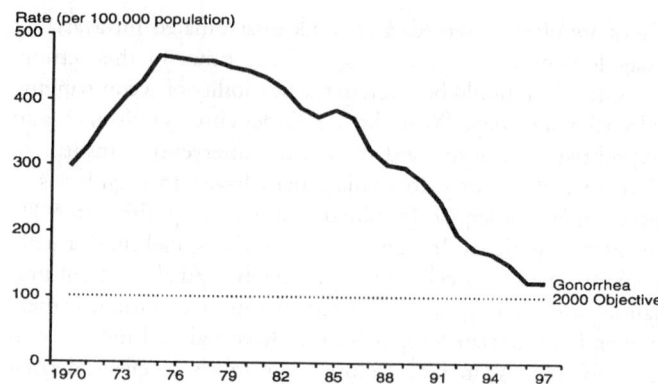

FIGURE 280.1. Reported rates of gonorrhea for the United States, 1970–1997. The incidence of gonococcal infections in the United States peaked at nearly 500 cases per 100,000 population in 1975. By 1996 the rate had fallen below 125 cases per 100,000 population. (From Division of STD Prevention. *Sexually Transmitted Disease Surveillance, 1997*. U.S. Department of Health and Human Services. Atlanta: Centers for Disease Control and Prevention, September 1998; http://www.cdc.gov.

tion (Fig. 280.1). This decline reflects changes in sexual behavior and safe-sex practices in response to AIDS.

In the United States, the incidence of gonorrhea is highest in adolescents and young adults (15 to 24 years old), particularly the urban poor and minority ethnic groups. In developing countries and in the military, where male contact with prostitutes is more common, the male/female ratio approaches 10:1. In civilian populations of Western countries, the ratio is about 1.5:1. Gonococcal infection in a child often indicates sexual abuse of the child.

Neisseria gonorrhoeae is transmitted by sexual contact. Inoculation of infected genital secretions by hand sometimes occurs, yielding secondary sites of infection and, rarely, infection of another person.

■ ETIOLOGY

Neisseria gonorrhoeae is a member of the genus *Neisseria*. *Neisseria meningitidis* is the other important pathogen in the genus and is closely related to *N. gonorrhoeae*. Gonococci ferment glucose but not maltose, lactose, or other sugars, which differentiates them from other *Neisseria* species. Fluorescence microscopy, coagglutination tests, enzyme immunoassays, and DNA probes can also be used to separate the species. All gonococci require cysteine for growth. Gonococcal strains can be typed by determining nutritional requirements (auxotyping) and by determining the porin protein serovar.

GROWTH CONDITIONS

Gonococci grow on agar containing hemin and additional supplements, and do not routinely grow on standard nutrient or sheep blood agar. Modified Thayer–Martin medium with hemin, IsoVitaleX, and antibiotics is the selective medium used in the United States for clinical cultures to diagnose gonococcal infections. Gonococci grow best at 35°C to 37°C in a humid environment with 5% to 10% CO_2; often a candle extinction jar is used to grow them. Gonococci do not grow in ambient air. Cultures of clinical specimens on selective medium should be examined after overnight incubation and again after 48 hours before discarding. Typical colonies are small (0.5 to 2 mm), grayish, convex, and shiny. When grown on translucent agar, large and small colonies that are opaque or transparent can be seen, depending on the expression or nonexpression of pili and opacity-associated proteins.

STRUCTURE

Knowledge of the surface or outer-membrane structures has been the key to understanding the pathogenesis of and immunologic factors involved in gonococcal infection, as well as infections by other mucosal pathogens.

PILI

Pili (fimbriae) are the hairlike appendages that extend from the gonococcal cell surface. Piliation is required to yield infection in human volunteers. Pili are made of repeating units of pilin protein. Pili function in the adherence of gonococci to host cells on the mucosal surface. Pilin antigenic variation aids the gonococci in evading the immune system. Each strain of *N. gonorrhoeae* has a series of genes that code for antigenically different pilin, and these are variably expressed during growth. Also, nearly every strain of gonococci expresses pilin molecules that are antigenically different from every other strain. Thus, there are hundreds or thousands of antigenically different gonococcal pili.

PORIN PROTEIN

The porin protein (Por) occurs in trimers and extends through the gonococcal outer membrane to form channels through which some nutrients enter the cell. Only one antigenic type of Por is expressed by each strain of gonococci, but different strains have distinct Por types. There are two major Por types, A and B, and more than 40 subtypes, based on monoclonal antibody typing systems. Serotyping of Por is a major tool used in epidemiologic studies but is not available for routine clinical use. Monoclonal antibodies against Por are routinely used to identify gonococci in fluorescent antibody tests.

OPACITY-ASSOCIATED PROTEIN

Opacity-associated proteins (Opas) are named because gonococci in opaque colonies on agar have an Opa in the outer membrane. Opas are variably expressed outer-membrane proteins that function in gonococcal attachment to and invasion of host cells, and in evasion of the immune system. Each strain of gonococcus has 10 to 12 *opa* genes that code for six to eight antigenically different Opas. Clinical isolates of *N. gonorrhoeae* typically have one to four Opas on their surface. There are hundreds of antigenically different Opas.

LIPOLIGOSACCHARIDE

Lipoligosaccharide (LOS) is the toxic substance of the outer membrane. Gonococci can simultaneously and variably express several antigenically different forms of the LOS carbohydrate chains. Gonococci make LOS molecules that structurally resemble human glycosphingolipids, a form of molecular mimicry. The gonococcal LOS and the human glycosphingolipid of the same class react with the same monoclonal antibodies, indicating their structural similarities. One conserved LOS structure has the same lacto-*N*-neotetraose glycose moiety as the human glycosphingolipid paraglobaside series. Other LOS glycose structures are shared with those of the globoside, ganglioside, and lactoside series. This molecular mimicry helps the gonococci evade the immune system.

ANTIGENIC VARIATION

Clinical isolates of *N. gonorrhoeae* have pili and Opa. In the laboratory, these proteins show phase variation—expression or nonexpression. Pili, Opa, and LOS each have a high frequency of antigenic variation: they switch expression from one antigenic form to another at a frequency of about 1 in every 10^3 gonococci (mutation rates for bacteria are one in 10^8 or 10^9). The variation for each of these antigens is independent of the others. Thus, every strain of *Gonococcus* may have different surface antigens from other strains, and each strain changes its surface antigens at a high frequency.

Gonococci also have several outer-membrane proteins that are antigenically similar in all strains, including Rmp (reduction-modifiable protein), Lip, and iron-regulated proteins.

GENETICS

Gonococci take up and integrate naked DNA (transformation); piliated gonococci do this much better than nonpiliated gonococci. Gonococci in contact can mate (conjugation) and exchange genetic information. Transduction does not occur in gonococci.

Gonococci have three types of plasmids (circular nonchromosomal DNA). The smallest plasmid is about 2.5 MD in size, occurs in 95% of gonococci, and has no known function. The second type of plasmid is 3.4 to 4.7 Md, carries the genes for penicillinase (β-lactamase) and other antibiotic resistance, and is found in 10% to 50% or more of gonococci, with geographic variation. The 24.5-Md plasmid controls gonococcal conjugation; this plasmid occurs with high frequency in areas where the 3.4- to 4.7-Md plasmids and resistance to penicillin G are common. The conjugative plasmid promotes the transfer of the plasmids that code for antibiotic resistance.

■ PATHOGENESIS

ADHERENCE, MUCOSAL COLONIZATION, AND INVASION

Pili appear to mediate the initial adherence of gonococci to mucosal epithelial cells; Opa is a secondary adherence effector. Por has been shown to insert and translocate across plasma membranes and, during the adherence process, may be inserted into the host cell membrane.

In over 95% of newly infected men, attachment and colonization of the urethra by gonococci results in an inflammatory response, predominantly of polymorphonuclear leukocytes. Asymptomatic infection occurs in 3% to 5% of new infections but may be of high prevalence because it is of long duration and not treated. About 25% of female patients have endocervical inflammation or urethral infection with sufficient signs and symptoms for them to seek medical care. Other women have asymptomatic infection of the endocervix or urethra. Asymptomatic endocervical infection is, then, an important reservoir of *N. gonorrhoeae*, leading to transmission during sexual intercourse. Pharyngeal carriage and rectal carriage also are often asymptomatic or only mildly symptomatic.

A few gonococci survive within polymorphonuclear leukocytes, which may also provide a reservoir for transmission of infection. In the female genital tract, gonococci may gain access to the fallopian tube by attaching to spermatozoa, by propulsion by coital contractions, or by migration during menses.

Gonococcal invasion of mucosal cells has been studied in in vitro human genital epithelial cell and fallopian tube models of infection. Once inoculated onto the genital epithelial cell surface, the gonococci adhere to the microvilli; pili and Opa may both be required for this process. In the fallopian tube model, the gonococci adhere primarily to the microvilli of nonciliated epithelial cells. The gonococcal LOS destroys the ciliated cells, causing them to slough. The gonococci enter the nonciliated epithelial cells by a poorly understood engulfment mechanism, multiply in the cells, pass through and destroy them, and enter the submucosal space. The result is major damage to the epithelial surface, which can yield ectopic pregnancy or infertility.

Gonococci enter the bloodstream from sites of active inflammation or, more commonly, from sites of asymptomatic infection (e.g., the endocervix at menstruation). Gonococci isolated from the blood are resistant to killing by antibodies and complement in normal human serum; gonococci isolated from uncomplicated mucosal infections are often serum-sensitive. Resistance to antibody- and complement-mediated killing is an important virulence factor for dissemination in patients with normal complement systems.

IMMUNITY

Humans infected with gonococci often have high levels of serum IgG and IgM that are reactive with outer-membrane structures; serum IgA is less important. The primary genital antibodies are IgA and IgG, which react predominantly with pili, Opa, and LOS.

Gonococci and other pathogens that reside on human mucosa (e.g., *N. meningitidis, Haemophilus influenzae, Streptococcus pneumoniae*) make the enzyme IgA$_1$ protease. IgA1 is the major IgA subclass present on mucosal surfaces. The enzyme splits IgA1, inactivating it.

There is no known protective immunity for uncomplicated gonococcal infection; a person can have repeated infections. The highly variable surface antigens help gonococci to evade antibod-

ies and repeatedly infect humans. Longitudinal studies in high-risk women have shown that antibodies against Rmp correlate with increased risk for infection, especially PID. Antibodies against Opa correlate with decreased risk for PID but do not change the risk for uncomplicated infection.

Persons with congenital deficiency of one of the late-acting components of complement (C5, C6, C7, or C8) are at high risk for systemic gonococcal or meningococcal infection because the circulating antibody- and complement-mediated bactericidal system will not kill the *Neisseria* organisms. As many as 20% of patients with meningococcal bacteremia or meningitis have one of these complement deficiencies. The incidence of complement deficiency is lower in gonococcal bacteremia because gonococci that cause bacteremia are commonly resistant to killing by antibody and complement.

Pili, Por, and whole-killed gonococci have been studied as vaccines for gonorrhea, but all have failed.

■ CLINICAL FEATURES

INFECTIONS OF WOMEN

Lower Genital Tract

Symptoms of endocervical infection are recognized by only 20% to 25% of infected women. Typically, they have an unusual or purulent vaginal discharge, and may have irregular or abnormal periods. Infection of Bartholin's or Skene's glands can yield swelling and formation of pus. Gonococcal urethritis is not routinely diagnosed in women, but dysuria and a urethral discharge are often present. Positive urethral cultures can often be obtained from women with acute uncomplicated gonorrhea. Gonococci are one of the causes of the acute urethral syndrome, in which a woman presents with acute dysuria suggestive of a bladder infection.

Pelvic Inflammatory Disease

In about 20% of women with endocervical gonorrhea, the infection spreads to involve the endometrium, fallopian tubes, and peritoneum, causing PID. This is the most important consequence of gonococcal infection. In the United States, gonococci cause 30% to 50% of cases of PID; *Chlamydia trachomatis* and mixed infections with anaerobes and aerobes are the other major causes. Mixed infections with anaerobes and aerobes cause the most severe symptoms in acute PID, including fever, adnexal masses, and pyosalpinx. Gonococcal PID is intermediate in clinical symptoms. *C. trachomatis* PID often has relatively few symptoms, but it may have the worst prognosis in terms of subsequent infertility and ectopic pregnancy.

Patients with PID present with lower abdominal pain, increased vaginal discharge, and fever, usually around the time of menstruation. Physical findings are limited to the lower abdomen and pelvis; the most common findings are adnexal tenderness, pain on cervical motion, and a palpable adnexal mass. A wide range of symptoms and physical findings in patients with PID make clinical diagnosis imprecise, short of laparoscopy. The differential diagnosis of PID includes ectopic pregnancy, appendicitis, and other intra-abdominal conditions.

Gonococcal PID predisposes to recurrent episodes of PID, which may be nongonococcal. The probability of sterility or ectopic pregnancy increases with each recurrence.

Perihepatitis (Fitz-Hugh–Curtis Syndrome)

Perihepatitis in women can occur with gonococcal or *C. trachomatis* infection after retrograde spread of infection from a pelvic focus. It rarely follows bacteremia. Right upper quadrant tenderness is common, and there may be an associated friction rub and elevated liver enzyme levels. If laparoscopy is done, adhesions between the hepatic capsule and the parietal peritoneum are evident. Response to antibiotic therapy is rapid.

INFECTIONS OF MEN

Urethritis

The likelihood of a man acquiring urethral gonococcal infection after a single exposure to an infected woman is about 25%. The incubation period is 3 to 5 days to the development of symptoms, typically consisting of urethral discharge, dysuria, or both. Between 5% and 40% of men have asymptomatic infection, and this can last for months. Asymptomatic infection is most likely to be found in men whose female consorts have disseminated gonococcal infection, PID, or positive screening cultures.

Epididymitis

Neisseria gonorrhoeae and *C. trachomatis* are the common causes of epididymitis in men under age 35. Acute epididymitis develops in men with untreated gonococcal infection. Pain and swelling of the epididymis occur. The diagnosis is made clinically and by culturing *N. gonorrhoeae* from an epididymal aspirate; a presumptive diagnosis is made by culturing the bacteria from a urethral swab specimen.

INFECTIONS OF WOMEN AND MEN

Conjunctivitis

Ophthalmia Neonatorum

Gonococcal ophthalmia neonatorum is an important cause of blindness in children in developing countries. It is uncommon in the United States because of antenatal screening and the widespread use of prophylaxis with antibiotic eye drops. Ophthalmia neonatorum usually presents after an incubation period of 2 to 3 days. Signs are bilateral conjunctival inflammation and chemosis, followed by purulent discharge. Dissemination can occur from the conjunctivae, leading to septic arthritis.

Adult Gonococcal Conjunctivitis

Gonococci can be inoculated into the conjunctivae on fingers contaminated with infected genital secretions and, rarely, by

bacteremia. The infection presents as an acute purulent conjunctivitis, often unilateral.

Pharynx

Pharyngeal gonococcal infection is acquired by oral–genital sex, most commonly fellatio. Transmission by kissing or oral secretions is rare. Disseminated gonococcal infection may result from pharyngeal carriage. Symptomatic infection with a mild to severe sore throat occurs in only about 5% of persons with pharyngeal infection. A purulent exudate may be present. The differential diagnosis of severe gonococcal pharyngitis includes group A β-hemolytic streptococcal disease, infectious mononucleosis, diphtheria (very rare in the United States), and various viruses that occasionally cause severe sore throats. Gonococcal pharyngitis is diagnosed by culture. The indication for a pharyngeal culture for gonococci is a history of oral sex.

Rectum

Isolation of *N. gonorrhoeae* from the anal canal is common in women who have endocervical gonococcal infection and may be due to contamination by vaginal secretions or anal intercourse. Anorectal gonococcal infection in men occurs in those who engage in receptive anal intercourse with an infected partner. Symptomatic rectal infection (gonococcal proctitis) occurs in a few infected persons; symptoms include pruritus, tenesmus, purulent discharge, and bloody diarrhea. On proctoscopy, a mucopurulent discharge or a friable mucosa is noted. The differential diagnosis of such findings in a male homosexual includes proctitis due to *C. trachomatis* or herpes simplex virus. Rectal cultures for gonococci should be done routinely for persons who practice rectal intercourse and are suggested for routine cultures of women, where anatomical proximity leads to rectal infection.

Disseminated Gonococcal Infection

Probably less than 1% of genital gonococcal infections lead to disseminated gonococcal infection (DGI). The rate appears to decreasing because the auxotype associated with DGI is less common in the United States. About 75% of cases of DGI occur in women, often in association with menstruation. The symptoms variably include fever, skin rash, joint or tendon pain, and a migratory polyarthritis. The skin rash occurs on the distal parts of the arms and legs, including the hands and feet. It starts as small red papules and evolves into pustules a few millimeters in diameter (Fig. 280.2). Other infectious diseases can yield similar rashes (e.g., meningococcemia, staphylococcal endocarditis). The arthritis usually stops with one joint, often a major joint such as the knee, with swelling and redness. The gonococcus is the most common cause of septic arthritis in young adults. Pus can be aspirated from the joint. When promptly treated, gonococcal arthritis rarely yields joint damage.

A presumptive diagnosis of DGI can be made in a young adult with typical clinical findings who has *N. gonorrhoeae* isolated from a mucosal surface and responds rapidly to antibiotic therapy directed at the gonococcus.

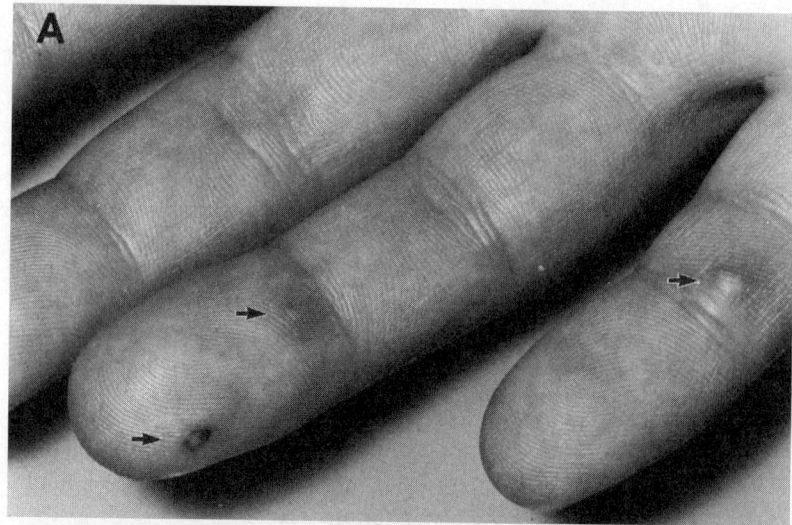

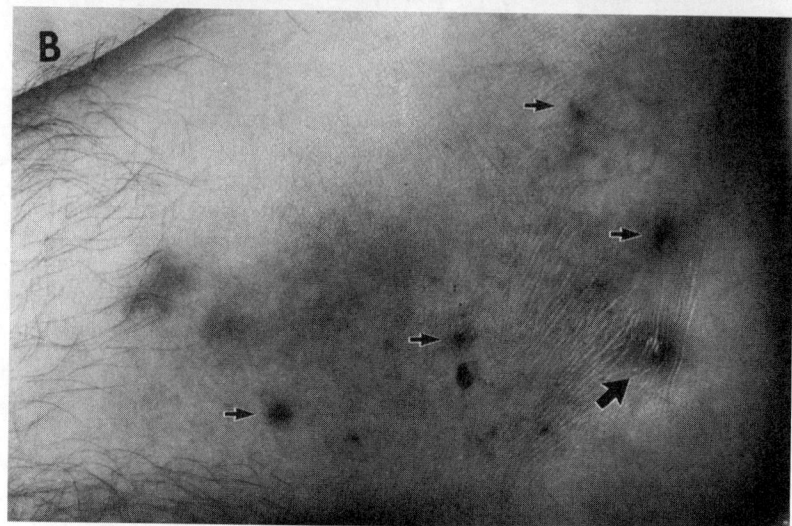

FIGURE 280.2. Petechial and small pustular lesions *(small arrows)* on the fingers **(A)** and foot **(B)** of a patient with disseminated gonococcal infection. The large arrow indicates a hemorrhagic bullous lesion on the foot.

Gonococcal endocarditis is rare in the antibiotic era but can result in rapid valve destruction. Gonococcal meningitis cannot be distinguished clinically from meningococcal meningitis.

LABORATORY FINDINGS

GRAM STAIN AND OTHER RAPID DIAGNOSTIC TECHNIQUES

In men with symptomatic urethritis, the diagnosis of gonorrhea can be made by a Gram stain of the urethral discharge and the finding of polymorphonuclear cell–associated (intracellular) gram-negative diplococci (Fig. 280.3). The sensitivity of the Gram stain for symptomatic men exceeds 90%, and the specificity is 98% to 99%. The predictive value of a positive Gram stain is very high and cultures for gonococci are not indicated if the stain is positive. Gram stain of the exudate from the endocervical canal in women is less sensitive (about 50%). In women (and at nongenital anatomical sites), the normal mucosal bacterial

flora can obscure or mimic gonococci, and the stain is not a sensitive diagnostic tool. Gram stain may be helpful in the initial diagnosis of conjunctivitis but does not indicate the species of bacteria.

CULTURE AND OTHER DIRECT DIAGNOSTIC LABORATORY METHODS

The diagnosis of gonococcal infection in women and at all anatomical sites except the male urethra is best made by culture. Modified Thayer–Martin or other selective medium should be used for culture of specimens from mucosal sites. Enriched chocolate agar without antibiotics can be used for joint fluid specimens.

Urethral cultures are obtained by inserting a small sterile swab about 0.50 in. into the anterior urethra. Anal cultures are obtained by inserting a swab 1 in. into the anal canal, avoiding contact with feces. In women, a swab is inserted in the endocervical canal and rotated. The specimen should be placed directly

tion in the form of the polymerase chain reaction also can be used to diagnose gonococcal infection.

OPTIMAL MANAGEMENT

ANTIBIOTIC RESISTANCE

Neisseria gonorrhoeae strains that are resistant to penicillin, tetracycline, or both are common in the United States (Fig. 280.4) and worldwide. Gonococci resistant to ciprofloxacin also have been isolated but are relatively uncommon; spectinomycin resistance has been reported as well. All gonococci are susceptible to the third-generation cephalosporins; they are the mainstay of therapy in developed countries but may be too costly for use in developing areas.

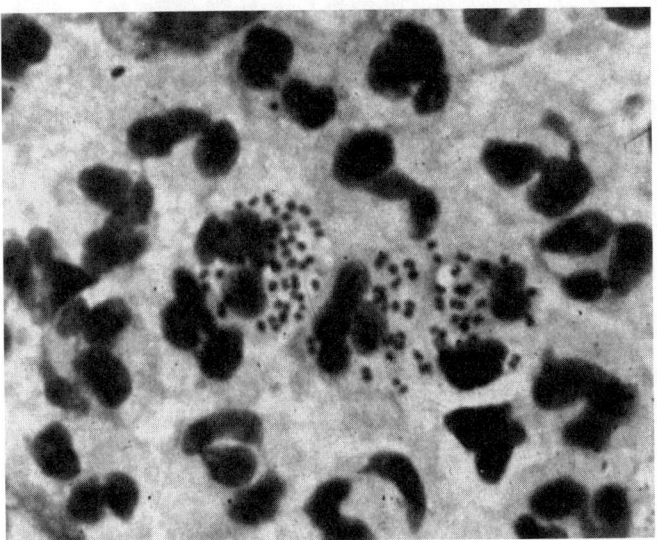

FIGURE 280.3. Gram stain of urethral exudate from a male patient with gonococcal urethritis showing gram-negative intracellular diplococci. (Courtesy of U.S. Centers for Disease Control and Prevention.)

onto the culture medium when possible, or put in transport medium and sent directly to the laboratory.

In DGI, blood cultures are positive in only 25% of cases and joint fluid cultures in about 10% of cases. Gonococci do not grow well in liquid media and are often susceptible to sodium polyanethol sulfonate, an anticoagulant and antiphagocytic factor commonly included in blood culture media. Early subculturing of blood cultures or the use of the lysis–centrifugation system may increase the yield for gonococci.

When genital Thayer–Martin medium cultures of sexually transmitted disease clinic patients are positive, a simple and inexpensive laboratory identification (e.g., fluorescent antibody test) is sufficient. Positive cultures of any other patients or from any anatomical site outside the genital tract require more extensive laboratory confirmation tests, preferably by two separate methods, because other *Neisseria* or other gram-negative cocci that do not cause gonorrhea can be isolated. Careful laboratory confirmation of gonococcal infection is especially important if the patient is a child and there is a possibility of sexual abuse.

An enzyme immunoassay is available to diagnose genital gonococcal infections in men and women. The assay is equivalent to the Gram stain for men but is much more expensive, and it is less sensitive and specific than culture to diagnose endocervical infections.

Another direct method to detect gonococci in genital tract specimens uses a nonisotopic probe to hybridize with gonococcal ribosomal RNA in a 2-hour test. The sensitivity of the test is 90% to 95% compared with culture. The specificity after discrepant analysis is 97% to 100%.

Nucleic acid amplification in the form of the ligase chain reaction can be used to diagnose gonococcal infection. In this test a sequence in the *N. gonorrhoeae opa1* gene is amplified. The sensitivity of this test is 90% to 100% and the specificity after discrepant analysis is 99% to 100%. Nucleic acid amplifica-

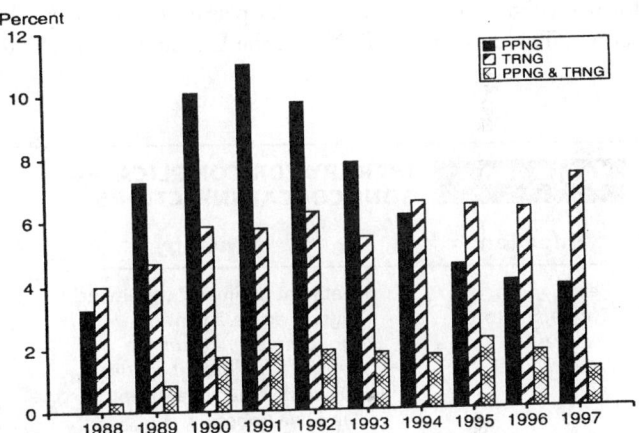

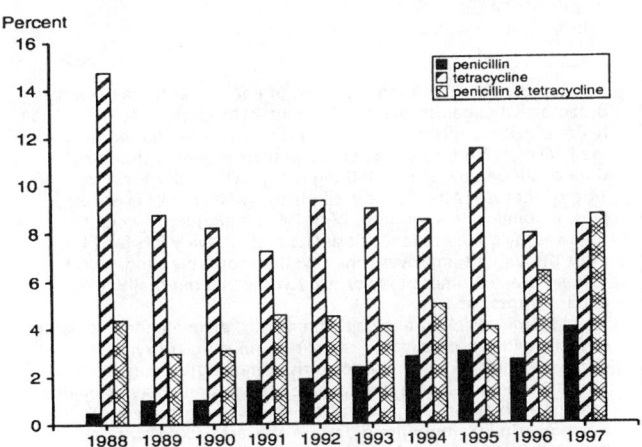

FIGURE 280.4. Trends in gonococcal resistance to penicillin and tetracycline, 1988–1997, from the Gonococcal Isolate Surveillance Project. **A:** Plasmid-mediated resistance. PPNG, penicillinase-producing *Neisseria gonorrhoeae*; TRNG, tetracycline-resistant *N. gonorrhoeae*. **B:** Chromosomally mediated resistance; resistant is a minimum inhibitory concentration of penicillin (β-lactamase-negative) or tetracycline of ≤2 μg/mL. (From Division of STD Prevention. *Sexually Transmitted Disease Surveillance, 1997.* U.S. Department of Health and Human Services. Atlanta: Centers for Disease Control and Prevention, September 1998; http://www.cdc.gov)

TABLE 280.1.	THERAPY FOR UNCOMPLICATED GONOCOCCAL INFECTIONS
Site	**Therapy**
Cervix, urethra, and rectum	Cefixime 400 mg orally in a single dose, *or* ceftriaxone 125 mg IM in a single dose, *or* ciprofloxacin 500 mg orally in a single dose, *or* ofloxacin 400 mg orally in a single dose, *plus* a regimen effective against possible coinfection with *Chlamydia trachomatis* such as azithromycin 1 g orally in a single dose, *or* doxycycline 100 mg orally b.i.d. for 7 d
Pharynx	Ceftriaxone, *or* ciprofloxacin, *or* ofloxacin, *plus* azithromycin, *or* doxycycline as above

Penicillinase-producing *N. gonorrhoeae* (PPNG) are resistant to penicillin G because they produce a *TEM-1* β-lactamase that inactivates penicillin. The plasmids of *N. gonorrhoeae* that code for penicillinase are related to similar plasmids in *Haemophilus* species. The incidence of PPNG in the United States is 6% to

TABLE 280.2.	THERAPY FOR COMPLICATED GONOCOCCAL INFECTIONS
Infection	**Therapy**
Pelvic inflammatory disease	Treatment regimens[a] should include agents active against *N. gonorrhoeae*, *Chlamydia trachomatis*, gram-negative facultative bacteria, streptococci, and anaerobes
Disseminated gonococcal infection[b]	Ceftriaxone[c], 1 g IM or IV every 24 h

[a] Examples of combination regimens of parenteral therapy with broad activity against major pathogens: cefotetan 2 g IV every 12 h, or cefoxitin 2 g IV every q 6 h, plus doxycycline 100 mg IV or orally every 12 h for 24 h after the patient improves clinically; then continue doxycycline 100 mg orally twice a day for a total of 14 d of therapy. Alternatively, clindamycin 900 mg IV every 8 h plus gentamicin loading dose IV or IM (2 mg/kg body weight) followed by a maintenance dose (1.5 mg/kg) every 8 h for 24 h after the patient improves clinically; then continue clindamycin 450 mg orally 4 times a day or doxycycline 100 mg orally twice a day for a total of 14 d.
[b] A total of 1 week of antibiotic therapy is recommended. Reliable patients with uncomplicated cases (e.g., no purulent synovial effusions or evidence of endocarditis or meningitis) may be discharged 24–48 h after improvement begins and may complete therapy with an oral regimen of cefixime 400 mg twice a day, or ciprofloxacin 500 mg twice a day, or ofloxacin 400 g twice a day. Parenteral therapy may be continued longer in patients with gonococcal arthritis and large purulent effusions. With the possible exception of the hip, drainage is not usually indicated. Gonococcal meningitis and endocarditis require high-dose IV therapy (e.g., ceftriaxone 1–2 g IV every 12 h) for 10–14 days and 4 wk, respectively.
[c] Ceftizoxime, 1 g IV every 8 h, or cefotaxime, 1 g IV every 8 h, is an alternative. For persons allergic to β-lactam drugs the options include ciprofloxacin 500 mg IV every 12 h, or ofloxacin 400 mg IV every 12 h, or spectinomycin 2 g IM every 12 h.

10% of all *N. gonorrhoeae* strains with some year-to-year variation (Fig. 280.4). PPNG are common in many other places in the world. PPNG also are often resistant to tetracycline.

Tetracycline resistance in gonococci may also be plasmid-mediated. Insertion of the streptococcal *tet-M* gene into the gonococcal conjugative plasmid (25.2 Md) yields the high-level tetracycline resistance (minimal inhibitory concentration 16 μg per milliliter or more).

A second type of resistance to penicillin is mediated by gene(s) on the chromosome and is not related to penicillinase production. Gonococci with chromosomally mediated penicillin resistance are increasingly common worldwide. Chromosomally mediated resistance to tetracycline also is common.

ANTIBIOTIC THERAPY

Guidelines for treatment of uncomplicated and complicated gonococcal infections reflect the emergence of antibiotic-resistant *N. gonorrhoeae*, the high frequency of coexisting chlamydial infections in patients with gonorrhea, and the potential serious complications of these infections (Tables 280.1 and 280.2). Cephalosporins (e.g., ceftriaxone, cefixime), quinolones (e.g., ciprofloxacin, ofloxacin), and spectinomycin are active against antibiotic-resistant gonococci. A complete set of recommended therapies and options are presented in the *Guidelines for Treatment of Sexually Transmitted Diseases* published by the U.S. Centers for Disease Control and Prevention.

All gonorrhea patients should have serologic tests for syphilis and should be offered counseling and testing for HIV infection. Ceftriaxone therapy for gonorrhea cures incubating syphilis, but spectinomycin and quinolones may not.

◼ PROGNOSIS

Untreated gonococcal urethritis may cure spontaneously, or a less purulent urethral discharge or asymptomatic carriage may result. Effective antibiotic therapy eradicates gonococcal infection, and resolution of symptoms indicates cure. Follow-up cultures are not needed. Gonococcal salpingitis may lead to infertility, ectopic pregnancy, or recurrent PID. Treated gonococcal arthritis usually has no sequelae.

BIBLIOGRAPHY

Britigan BE, Cohen MS, Sparling PF. Gonococcal infection: a model of molecular pathogenesis. *N Engl J Med* 1985;312:1683–1694.
Hook EW, Holmes KK. Gonococcal infections. *Ann Intern Med* 1985;312:229–243.
Koumans EH, Johnson RE, Knapp JS, et al. Laboratory testing for *Neisseria gonorrhoeae* by recently introduced nonculture tests: a performance review with clinical and public health considerations. *Clin Infect Dis* 1998;27:1171–1180.
U.S. Centers for Disease Control and Prevention. 1998 Guidelines for treatment of sexually transmitted diseases. *MMWR* 1998;47(No. RR-1):59–69.

Kelley's Textbook of Internal Medicine, fourth edition. Edited by H. David Humes. Lippincott Williams & Wilkins, Philadelphia © 2000.

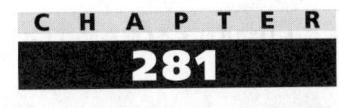

CHAPTER 281

SALMONELLOSIS

SONJA J. OLSEN
ROBERT V. TAUXE

■ DEFINITION

Salmonellosis is one of the most common bacterial infections in the United States. The various types of the *Salmonella* bacteria cause a variety of clinical syndromes, including enterocolitis, bacteremia, enteric fever, and severe focal infections. Persons with AIDS are particularly susceptible to invasive infections.

■ INCIDENCE AND EPIDEMIOLOGIC FACTORS

Between 1970 and 1985, the incidence of reported *Salmonella* infections in the United States increased from 11 per 100,000 to 28 per 100,000, after which it declined slightly (Fig. 282.1). Because of marked underdiagnosis and underreporting, it is likely that the true number of incidents is approximately 1.4 million each year. The emergence of nontyphoidal salmonellosis is related to changes in food animal production and slaughter practices that make contamination of fresh meat likely, and to the increasing number of highly susceptible persons in the population.

The incidence of salmonellosis is highest among children under 1 year of age and is particularly likely if the infant is bottle-fed. Incidence is also higher among the elderly. Infections can occur year-round but are more likely to occur in the summer and early fall. About 10% of cases are linked to recognized outbreaks, but most occur sporadically.

With the exception of *S. typhi*, which is found almost exclusively in humans, most nontyphoidal *Salmonella* infections in humans are related directly or indirectly to infected animals, including birds, mammals, and reptiles. Most human infections result from the ingestion of contaminated food, particularly foods of animal origin contaminated by *Salmonella* from the animals themselves. More recently, fresh fruits and vegetables have been implicated in an increasing number of outbreaks. Waterborne transmission has occasionally occurred, and direct person-to-person transmission has been demonstrated in newborn nurseries. *Salmonella* organisms can also be easily transmitted from pet reptile to child. Pet iguanas are an increasingly common source. Most typhoid fever cases are associated with travel to the developing world and consumption of contaminated food or water there.

Nontyphoid *Salmonella* organisms are commonly isolated from raw foods of animal origin, including unpasteurized milk, raw eggs, and raw meat. They are readily killed by heating to 74°C (165°F), but multiply rapidly on food held at ambient temperature. Most outbreaks and sporadic infections result from food handling practices that allow the organisms to survive and multiply in food. Common food vehicles include beef, chicken, and turkey, and grade A shell eggs, which have emerged as a particularly common source of *S. enteritidis* in most of the industrialized world. Large outbreaks occur when salmonellae contaminate a mass-produced food; in 1985, one outbreak caused by *S. typhimurium* in pasteurized milk produced more than 200,000 cases. Salmonellosis outbreaks have also been traced to many other vehicles, including raw milk, precooked roast beef, homemade and commercial ice cream, marijuana, sprouts, orange juice, tomatoes, cantaloupe, and pharmaceutical agents such as carmine dye and pooled platelets.

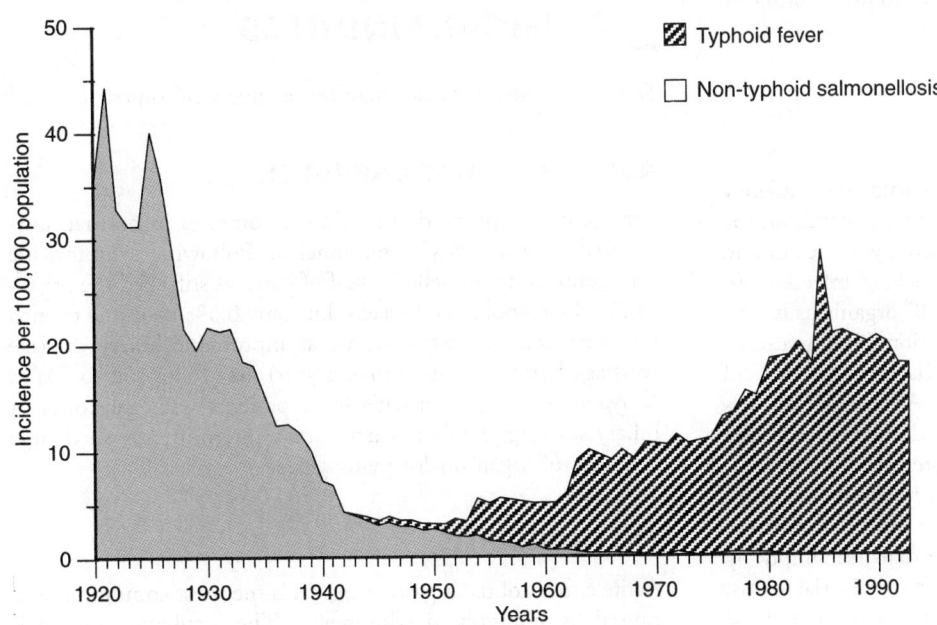

FIGURE 281.1. The annual incidence of reported typhoid fever and nontyphoidal salmonellosis in the United States, 1920–1997.

TABLE 281.1.	THE 10 MOST COMMON SEROTYPES IDENTIFIED AMONG HUMAN *SALMONELLA* INFECTIONS IN 1980, 1990, AND 1997[a]							
	1980			**1990**			**1997**	
Serotype	**No. of Isolates**	**Percentage**	**Serotype**	**No. of Isolates**	**Percentage**	**Serotype**	**No. of Isolates**	**Percentage**
Typhimurium	10,248	34.9	Typhimurium	8,817	20.8	Typhimurium	9,116	26.3
Heidelberg	1,940	6.6	Enteritidis	8,734	20.6	Enteritidis	7,924	22.9
Enteritidis	1,884	6.4	Heidelberg	3,955	9.3	Heidelberg	2,104	6.1
Newport	1,594	5.4	Hadar	1,837	4.3	Newport	1,584	4.6
Infantis	1,390	4.7	Newport	1,802	4.3	Agona	740	2.1
Agona	1,374	4.7	Agona	980	2.3	Montevideo	718	2.1
Saint-Paul	753	2.6	Montevideo	928	2.2	Thompson	695	2.0
Montevideo	658	2.2	Braenderup	758	1.8	Javiana	675	2.0
Typhi	588	2.0	Infantis	753	1.8	Infantis	651	1.9
Oranienberg	483	1.6	Thompson	750	1.8	Hadar	643	1.9
Other	8,427	28.7	Other	13,024	30.8	Other	9,758	28.2
Total	29,339		Total	42,338		Total	34,608	

[a] National Salmonella Surveillance System, CDC.

ETIOLOGIC FACTORS

Salmonellae are gram-negative, flagellated, nonsporulating aerobic bacilli. They are serotyped using the schema developed by Kauffman and White using somatic (O) and flagellar (H) antigens; more than 2,000 serotypes have been identified. Current convention refers to the serotype as a serovar of the species *S. enterica*, for example: *Salmonella* serotype *typhimurium, S. dublin*, or *S. enteritidis*. Most clinical laboratories use only the O antigen to group salmonellae into broad serogroups A through G. Complete serotyping is available through state public health laboratories and can be clinically and epidemiologically useful. Ten serotypes account for the majority of infections (Table 281.1). Many serotypes have specific animal reservoirs and exhibit unique patterns of age specificity, invasiveness, antibiotic resistance, and geographic distribution.

PATHOGENESIS

The pathogenesis of *Salmonella* infections remains incompletely understood. The clinical expression of infection depends on the serotype and strain of the organism, the underlying health and gut flora of the host, and the dose and vehicle of infection. In normal volunteers, the presence of 10^5 to 10^9 organisms is usually necessary to produce symptomatic infection. Highly susceptible hosts or foods that protect the bacteria from gastric acid may lead to infection at much lower doses. After ingestion, salmonellae must survive gastric acid and successfully colonize the small intestine. Disruption of the normal intestinal flora by antimicrobial agents decreases the dose needed to produce illness.

The bacteria attach to and penetrate the intestinal mucosa. In most infections, salmonellae may cause diarrhea simply by direct damage to the mucosa or by local action of bacterial toxins. However, salmonellae can invade the gut-associated lymphoid tissues, multiply within macrophages, and reach the bloodstream. Some serotypes are particularly invasive and more likely to result in bacteremia, enteric fever, and distant focal infections.

Persons at the extremes of age, those with reduced gastric acidity, and those who have recently taken an antibiotic are more susceptible to *Salmonella* infection following exposure. Persons silently infected with a resistant strain of *Salmonella* may develop clinical illness if they take an antibiotic to which the infecting strain is resistant. Disorders of reticuloendothelial cell function, such as sickle cell anemia, and defects in cellular immunity, such as those associated with AIDS, lymphoma, leukemia, or antineoplastic therapy, predispose to bacteremia and invasive disease.

CLINICAL FINDINGS

Salmonella infections can manifest as five syndromes.

ASYMPTOMATIC CARRIAGE

Transient asymptomatic infection is common in normal hosts exposed to low doses of salmonellae. Following symptomatic nontyphoidal salmonellosis, half of patients still shed the organism in their stool after 4 weeks, but only 0.5% continue to shed for more than a year. Chronic asymptomatic biliary carriage (carriage lasting for more than a year) may follow up to 3% of *S. typhi* infections, particularly in patients with gallstones or biliary scarring. Typhoid carriers may intermittently shed large numbers of organism for many years.

ENTEROCOLITIS

Acute enterocolitis or gastroenteritis is the most common illness caused by nontyphoid salmonellae. The incubation period is typically 8 to 48 hours. The initial symptoms include nausea and vomiting, followed by abdominal cramps and diarrhea, which is occasionally bloody. About half of patients have fever and headache. The severity of diarrhea may vary from a few loose stools per day to profuse watery or bloody diarrhea. Diarrhea typically subsides in 3 to 5 days but may persist for 2 weeks. Acute infection with nontyphoidal salmonellae can trigger the reactive postinfectious syndrome of Reiter's arthropathy in persons with a susceptible genotype.

ENTERIC FEVER

The enteric fever syndrome is typically seen with *S. typhi* infection but may occur with other strains, particularly *S. paratyphi* type A and B. The incubation period is usually 1 to 3 weeks, depending on the dose ingested. Early symptoms are nonspecific and include cough, sore throat, myalgia, and abdominal pain. The patient may experience constipation or mild diarrhea. Within a week, a pronounced and sustained fever develops, and headache, anorexia, lethargy, and a characteristically clouded mental state become prominent. Physical examination often reveals relative bradycardia, hepatosplenomegaly, and abdominal tenderness. Rose spots (clusters of delicate pink, irregular macules 2 to 4 mm in diameter that blanch with pressure) may be seen on the trunk. Complications of enteric fever include myocarditis, bone marrow depression, and intestinal perforation and hemorrhage.

BACTEREMIA

Sustained bacteremia, characterized by high fevers and leukocytosis but without other clinical features of enteric fever or diarrhea, can occur with a variety of serotypes, but is most typical for *S. choleraesuis.* Recurrent *Salmonella* bacteremia, usually with *S. typhimurium* or *S. enteritidis,* is an important problem among patients with AIDS; relapse may follow prolonged courses of antibiotics.

FOCAL INFECTIONS

Focal *Salmonella* infections have been reported in many sites, including the brain, meninges, lung, pleural space, pericardium, kidney, bone, liver, spleen, bladder, heart valve, and endarterial lesions. Such infections follow an initial bacteremia, which may be silent. *Salmonella* meningitis occurs almost exclusively in young infants. Salmonellae appear to have a predilection for infecting atherosclerotic lesions, particularly atherosclerotic aortic aneurysms.

◼ LABORATORY FINDINGS

Definitive diagnosis depends on identification of *Salmonella* organisms. Unless antibiotic treatment has already been given, routine bacteriologic techniques will readily yield salmonellae from stool, blood, cerebrospinal fluid, or other clinical specimen. No specific serologic tests are available. Typhoid fever can present

a particular diagnostic challenge, as stool cultures are often negative early in the illness and blood cultures may be negative in some patients, particularly those who have been partially treated. Cultures of bone marrow, bile obtained by duodenal string test, and, in the future, polymerase chain reaction–based diagnostic tools may be helpful in such cases. The Widal serologic test is fraught with problems. False-positive test results may be caused by other infections or previous vaccine administration, and some typhoid fever patients may never mount an antibody response.

ANTIMICROBIAL RESISTANCE

Salmonellae have become increasingly resistant to antimicrobial agents. Although treatment is not indicated for uncomplicated gastroenteritis, resistance can lead to treatment failure in severe infections. To monitor trends in resistance, a national surveillance system was recently implemented. In 1997, more than 1,300 nontyphoidal *Salmonella* isolates from 15 states and local health departments were tested for antimicrobial resistance to 17 agents; 34% of strains were resistant to at least one antimicrobial agent and 27% were resistant to multiple agents—a substantial increase from earlier surveys. Similar resistance is found in salmonellae isolated from meats and is a direct consequence of the use of antimicrobial agents in animal husbandry. Multiply-resistant *S. typhi* and nontyphoidal salmonellae are now being identified in many developing countries.

◼ OPTIMAL MANAGEMENT

The treatment of salmonellosis depends on the type of infection. Antimicrobial agents are not indicated for uncomplicated enterocolitis since they do not shorten the illness and actually prolong bacterial shedding. Fluid and electrolyte losses should be replaced and antimotility agents avoided. Convalescent carriage of nontyphoidal salmonellae is not shortened by antimicrobial therapy, and treatment of convalescent carriers is not indicated. Because chronic carriers of *S. typhi* represent a major reservoir for that organism and are excluded from some jobs, elimination of carriage is desirable. Prolonged high doses are required, with the most encouraging results reported for either norfloxacin 400 mg twice a day or ciprofloxacin 750 mg twice a day for 4 weeks.

Chloramphenicol, ampicillin or amoxicillin, or trimethoprim–sulfamethoxazole have long been the treatments of choice for enteric fever. However, increasing antimicrobial resistance limits the current usefulness of these agents. Third-generation cephalosporins, including ceftriaxone, cefotaxime, and cefoperazone, and fluoroquinolones, including norfloxacin and ciprofloxacin, have demonstrated efficacy in treating typhoid fever. Although in vitro sensitivity may be reported, tetracyclines and first- and second-generation cephalosporins are not effective for *Salmonella* infections, including typhoid fever.

Bacteremia and focal infections have also traditionally been treated with chloramphenicol, ampicillin, and trimethoprim–sulfamethoxazole, and more recently with fluoroquinolones. For meningitis and osteomyelitis, ceftriaxone and cefotaxime offer excellent in vitro activity, achieve good levels in tissue, and are bactericidal. Prolonged therapy of 2 to 4 weeks should be given. Localized abscesses, infected aneurysms, and infected heart valves usually require surgical management. Because of the frequency of recurrence, long-term suppressive therapy with an oral antimicrobial agent should be considered for AIDS patients with *Salmonella* bacteremia.

PREVENTION

Salmonellosis can be prevented by simple measures that care-givers can encourage. Particular care is warranted to avoid salmo-nellosis in infants, the elderly, and the immunocompromised, among whom severe outcomes are most likely. Breast-feeding is strongly protective against this and other diarrheal diseases in infants. Unpasteurized milk and raw eggs should be avoided. Care in handling meat, eggs, and other foods of animal origin will prevent many cases, if the foods are cooked thoroughly, and if hands, knives, and work surfaces are immediately washed with soap. Most reptiles carry salmonellae and are not appropriate pets for households with infants or HIV-infected persons. The risk of salmonellosis in institutions such as hospitals and nursing homes can be further decreased by use of pasteurized eggs rather than shell eggs, and by standard food safety measures. Salmo-nellosis outbreaks in hospital nurseries have been curtailed by infection control, hand washing, and cohorting. The risk of ac-quiring salmonellosis from fresh fruits and vegetables can be reduced by the use of chlorinated water in all postharvest product handling.

New measures to reduce the risk of *Salmonella* infection through foodborne transmission include cleaner slaughter prac-tices on the farm and, in the future, irradiation of meat and poultry products. Judicious use of antibiotics in all arenas, espe-cially animal husbandry, will help to prevent the development of antibiotic-resistant strains of *Salmonella*. It is important for clinicians to culture all specimens from persons suspected of having *Salmonella* infection and for laboratories to serotype all isolates; all suspected outbreaks should be reported to local or state health departments.

Typhoid fever in the United States has been controlled by improvements in water and sewage treatment. Travelers to devel-oping countries can lower their risk by careful selection of food and drink. Vaccination is recommended for people living in or visiting areas of endemic disease for extended periods or under conditions of poor hygiene, for family members of chronic ty-phoid carriers, and for microbiology personnel who are likely to be exposed to *S. typhi*. Three licensed typhoid vaccines are available in the United States. One is a heat- and phenol-inacti-vated preparation that has been shown to provide 65% to 70% protective efficacy after two initial doses one month apart. Ad-verse reactions are common (25% to 45%) and include local pain, fever, myalgia, and headache. The second vaccine is a live attenuated oral one made from the Ty21a strain, taken in four oral doses at 48-hour intervals. In field trials, efficacy of a three-dose regimen was 66%, and the vaccine was virtually free of side effects. Finally, a parenteral vaccine containing purified Vi polysaccharide antigen from *S. typhi* provides 55% to 74% effi-cacy after a single dose and is associated with only mild local reactions. All require boosting at intervals. In the future, Vi polysaccharide conjugated to carrier proteins may increase im-munogenicity in young children.

BIBLIOGRAPHY

Aserkoff B, Bennett JV. Effect of antibiotic therapy in acute salmonellosis on the fecal excretion of salmonellae. *N Engl J Med* 1969;281:3–7.

Chalker RB, Blaser MJ. A review of human salmonellosis: III. Magnitude of *Salmonella* infections in the United States. *Rev Infect Dis* 1988;10:111–124.

Cohen JI, Bartlett JA, Corey GR. Extra-intestinal manifestations of *Salmo-nella* infections. *Medicine (Baltimore)* 1987;66:349–388.

Cohen ML, Tauxe RV. Drug-resistant *Salmonella* in the United States: an epidemiologic perspective. *Science* 1986;234:964–969.

Griffin PG, Tauxe RV. Food counseling for patients with AIDS [Letter]. *J Infect Dis* 1988;158:668.

Hornick RB, Greisman SE, Woodward TE, et al. Typhoid fever: pathogene-sis and immunologic control. *N Engl J Med* 1970;283:686–691, 739–746.

Lee LA, Puhr ND, Maloney K, et al. Increase in antimicrobial-resistant *Salmonella* infections in the United States, 1989–1990. *J Infect Dis* 1994;170:128–134.

Levine WC, Buehler JW, Bean NH, et al. Epidemiology of nontyphoidal *Salmonella* bacteremia during the human immunodeficiency virus epi-demic. *J Infect Dis* 1991;164:81–87.

Neill MA, Opal SM, Heelan J, et al. Failure of ciprofloxacin to eradicate convalescent fecal excretion after acute salmonellosis: experience during an outbreak in health care workers. *Ann Intern Med* 1991;114:195–199.

U.S. Centers for Disease Control and Prevention. Typhoid immunization. Recommendations of the Advisory Committee on Immunization Prac-tices (ACIP). *MMWR* 1994;43(RR-14):1–6.

Kelley's Textbook of Internal Medicine, fourth edition. Edited by H. David Humes. Lippincott Williams & Wilkins, Philadelphia © 2000.

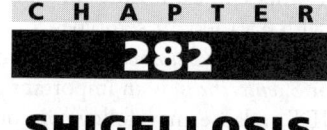

282

SHIGELLOSIS

KAREN KOTLOFF
MYRON M. LEVINE

DEFINITION

Shigellosis is the clinical syndrome that occurs when bacteria of the genus *Shigella* invade the human terminal ileum and colon. The spectrum of symptoms may include asymptomatic infec-tion, mild watery diarrhea, or severe dysentery characterized by high fever, toxemia, cramps, and tenesmus. The term *shigellosis* is commonly used to describe prototypic bacillary dysentery (the passage of frequent scanty stools containing blood and mucus).

ETIOLOGY

Shigella are gram-negative, non-lactose-fermenting, nonmotile bacilli of the family Enterobacteriaceae. Four species or groups of *Shigella* are recognized: *S. dysenteriae* (group A), *S. flexneri* (group B), *S. boydii* (group C), and *S. sonnei* (group D). Groups A, B, and C have multiple serotypes and subtypes, whereas group D has only a single serotype.

There is geographic variation in the predominant serogroup of *Shigella* that appears to be related to the local standard of sanitation and hygiene. *S. sonnei* is by far the most common type found in industrialized countries, accounting for more than 70% of isolates reported in the United States. *S. flexneri* predominates in developing countries but constitutes only about 20% of isolates in the United States. *S. dysenteriae* occurs in the least developed areas of the world where it causes a small proportion (about 6%) of endemic disease. In addition, the *S. dysenteriae* type 1 serotype, also known as the Shiga bacillus, elaborates Shiga toxin and is uniquely capable of forming pandemics of severe disease that spread in waves from country to country. In the United States, *S. dysenteriae* type 1 has been eliminated except when introduced by travelers. *S. boydii* is an uncommon serogroup in both developing and industrialized countries.

INCIDENCE AND EPIDEMIOLOGIC FACTORS

The predominant mode of transmission is by fecal–oral contact, and a low infectious inoculum (as few as 10 organisms can cause illness) renders *Shigella* highly contagious for humans, the only natural host. Sustained person-to-person transmission from symptomatic individuals is largely responsible for persistence of this pathogen. Spread by ingestion of fecally contaminated food or water is less common (*Shigella* causes about 3% of bacterial foodborne outbreaks in the United States) since the organism survives poorly in the environment, but individual outbreaks can be extensive. Salad is the most common vehicle; contamination is usually related to a breech in hygienic practices by an infected food handler. Transmission subsequent to swimming in fecally contaminated water occasionally occurs. In certain settings where disposal of human feces is inadequate, houseflies may transmit infection. Among homosexuals, transmission via anal–oral contact has been reported.

Shigella infections occur worldwide but are most prevalent in settings where crowding, poor sanitation, inadequate water supplies, and primitive personal hygiene coexist. Seasonal peaks appear in the late summer and fall in temperate climates. Throughout the world, the incidence of shigellosis is highest among children 1 to 4 years of age. Infants and young children who are breast-fed have fewer episodes of shigellosis, and when an episode occurs, it is less severe compared to that in children who are not breast-fed.

In the United States, endemic foci of shigellosis persist among poor, urban children belonging to ethnic minorities, and in some Native American communities. An elevated risk of shigellosis is also found among young children in day care centers, residents of custodial institutions, travelers to less developed countries, and soldiers in field conditions. The incidence of shigellosis in the United States has been estimated based on national laboratory surveillance data collected by the U.S. Centers for Disease Control and Prevention (CDC). Since the 1960s, periodic peaks

and troughs have been observed, ranging from 5.4 to 10.1 isolations per 100,000 population. Since only about 15% of cases are reported, this figure is believed to markedly underestimate the actual rate of *Shigella* infection in the United States. Nonetheless, *Shigella* remains a relatively uncommon enteropathogen in the United States, causing fewer than 5% of diarrheal episodes among children younger than 5 years. Data on case fatality are limited, but it has been estimated at about 0.4%, resulting in approximately 60 deaths per year in the United States.

Two notable demographic trends were reported in the United States in recent years. Since the late 1970s, marked increases have been observed in the rate of infection reported among women of childbearing age. Presumed to reflect transmission from infected children to their mothers (rates of secondary transmission of *S. sonnei* in households with small children often exceeds 50%), this trend could be explained by a steady increase in the use of day care facilities whose role in disseminating shigellosis in the community is well recognized. Increases in isolation of *S. flexneri* from adult men in the 1980s were attributed to transmission among homosexual men.

The burden of disease from *Shigella* infection is greatest in developing countries, where endemic *Shigella* (mainly *S. flexneri* serotypes) is responsible for about 1% to 15% of diarrheal episodes among young children. Overall it is estimated that *Shigella* causes 163 million cases of diarrhea in developing countries and 1.1 million deaths annually. In addition, pandemic Shiga dysentery has appeared in Central America, South and Southeast Asia, and sub-Saharan Africa since the late 1960s, primarily affecting populations in areas of political upheaval and natural disaster. The pandemic strains are notoriously multiply antibiotic-resistant and cause high attack rates and mortality in all age groups. The ravaging effects of *S. dysenteriae* among refugee populations in pandemic areas was observed when approximately 800,000 Rwandans fled to Democratic Republic of Congo in 1994. During the first month of the crisis alone, approximately 20,000 persons died from dysentery caused by a multiply antibiotic–resistant strain of *S. dysenteriae* type 1.

PATHOGENESIS

In response to certain environmental signals, shigellae can exhibit remarkable acid resistance. This apparently enables the bacteria to survive transit through the gastric acid defense barrier following oral ingestion. Ultimately, shigellae reach the terminal ileum and colon, where they invade and proliferate within enterocytes, produce cell death, and incite an intense inflammatory reaction.

The cardinal pathogenic feature is invasion of intestinal epithelial cells that involves a bacteria–host cell interaction wherein shigellae secrete invasins that induce ruffling of the enterocyte membrane. Fusion of these flowerlike membrane projections leads to bacterial internalization via macropinocytosis. Within minutes of entry, the bacteria escape the membrane-bound pinocytotic vacuole to reach nutrients within the cytosol that are required for the next phase of intense bacterial replication. These nonmotile bacteria then acquire the ability to undergo directed intracellular movements, navigating via reorganization of the host cell cytoskeleton to form a unipolar actin comet tail. Some bacteria are propelled toward the cell surface, leading to the development of long protrusions that penetrate adjacent epithelial cells. As contiguous enterocytes become infected and die, areas of ulceration and hemorrhage are formed.

Invasion of the intestine by shigellae elicits a potent inflammatory response characterized by polymorphonuclear leukocyte (PMN) chemotaxis, edema, infiltration of the lamina propria with PMNs and mononuclear cells, and formation of mucosal microabscesses. Shigellae induce apoptotic death of macrophages, their own front-line predator in subepithelial tissues. Apoptotic killing of macrophages confers two distinct advantages: it allows bacterial survival, and it releases cytokines that trigger inflammation and render the epithelial barrier more permeable to *Shigella* invasion. Integrity of the epithelial lining is disrupted as PMNs migrate through the intercellular space to reach luminal organisms, opening additional pathways for invasive organisms to access enterocytes.

Until recently, the pathogenesis of the watery diarrhea that typically precedes dysentery and that is often the sole clinical manifestation of mild infection remained enigmatic. Then two novel *Shigella* enterotoxins, designated ShET1 and ShET2, were incriminated as the likely mediators of the watery diarrhea seen early in the clinical course. Transudation and decreased absorption of water by an inflamed colon may also play a role.

The *S. dysenteriae* type 1 serotype uniquely produces a highly potent exotoxin called Shiga toxin. Shiga toxin is a powerful inhibitor of protein synthesis; however, its precise role in the pathogenesis of Shiga dysentery is still not entirely clear. Mutants of *S. dysenteriae* type 1 that are invasive but do not express Shiga toxin nevertheless have caused typical Shiga diarrhea and dysentery when fed to monkeys and volunteers, although less endothelial damage to intestinal microvasculature was evident.

Hemolytic–uremic syndrome is a well-recognized, life-endangering complication of *S. dysenteriae* type 1 infection in children, which manifests as thrombotic thrombocytopenic purpura in adults. The central pathophysiologic process is believed to be vascular endothelial cell death induced by systemically absorbed Shiga toxin. Whereas the inciting agent is usually *S. dysenteriae*

type 1 in developing countries, most cases in the United States and other industrialized countries follow infection with enterohemorrhagic *Escherichia coli*, a category of diarrheagenic *E. coli* (most commonly serotypes O157:H7 and O26:H11) that elaborates Shiga toxin (or the related Shiga toxin 2).

CLINICAL FINDINGS

The incubation period is usually 1 to 4 days but may be as long as 8 days with *S. dysenteriae* type 1. Shigellosis often progresses through several phases. Typically the illness begins with fever and other constitutional symptoms such as headache, malaise, anorexia, and, occasionally vomiting, followed by several hours of watery diarrhea (Table 282.1). Most cases in the United States are limited to these milder manifestations. However, progression to frank dysentery may occur with frequent scanty stools containing blood and mucus, accompanied by lower abdominal cramps and tenesmus. Disease is most severe in young children and in the elderly, whereas many adults have asymptomatic or mild illness.

Most cases of shigellosis in otherwise healthy individuals are self-limited and resolve within 5 to 7 days. Acute, life-threatening complications occur most frequently among infants and young children living in developing countries, and among people infected with *S. dysenteriae* type 1, although in endemic areas any species of *Shigella* can cause severe illness or death. Intestinal complications include toxic megacolon, rectal prolapse from tenesmus, and intestinal perforation (Table 282.1). Extensive damage to the intestinal mucosa of young children can cause marked exudation of proteins, leading to hypoproteinemia and acute kwashiorkor. Dehydration, hyponatremia, hyperkalemia, and hypoglycemia are acute metabolic derangements requiring immediate therapeutic intervention. *Shigella* sepsis, seen most often in young, malnourished children, occurs uncommonly but is a leading cause of death during shigellosis. In the United States, bacteremia has occasionally been reported among HIV-infected and other immunocompromised patients. Rarely, *Shi-*

TABLE 282.1.	CLINICAL MANIFESTATIONS OF SHIGELLOSIS	
Acute Manifestations	**Complications**	
	Intestinal	**Extraintestinal**
Fever	Toxic megacolon	Dehydration
Headache	Rectal prolapse	Electrolyte abnormalities
Malaise	Intestinal perforation	Hypoglycemia
Anorexia	Persistent diarrhea	Hypoproteinemia
Vomiting	Protein-losing enteropathy	Malnutrition
Watery diarrhea		Bacteremia
Dysentery		Extraintestinal infection
Abdominal cramps		Hemolytic–uremic syndrome
Rectal tenesmus		Thrombotic thrombocytopenia purpura
		Reactive arthritis
		Reiter's syndrome

gella organisms cause focal infections such as meningitis, osteomyelitis, arthritis, and splenic abscess.

A variety of unusual extraintestinal manifestations can occur (Table 282.1). The most common is seizures, which are reported in 5% to 45% of children hospitalized with shigellosis. They usually occur in children younger than 5 years who have fever or metabolic derangements known to precipitate seizures. Rarely encephalopathy is encountered. Hemolytic–uremic syndrome, manifesting as microangiopathic hemolytic anemia in association with thrombocytopenia and renal insufficiency, can follow infection with Shiga toxin–producing organisms. Another hematologic complication encountered with *S. dysenteriae* type 1 infection is a leukemoid reaction with PMN counts exceeding 50,000 to 100,000 per cubic millimeter.

An uncommon late sequela seen primarily in adults is reactive arthritis, alone or as part of a constellation of arthritis, conjunctivitis, and urethritis known as Reiter's syndrome. Arthritis has an acute onset usually 2 to 4 weeks after the intestinal illness and most often follows infection with *S. flexneri* serotypes. Joint symptoms can range from mild arthralgia to severe polyarthritis, which becomes chronic in about 10% of cases. Individuals with the HLA–B27 histocompatibility antigen are predisposed, accounting for approximately half of cases. It has been suggested that there are "arthritogenic" *Shigella* strains that carry a small plasmid encoding a cross-reactive peptide.

APPROACH TO LABORATORY DIAGNOSIS

There is no commercially available serologic assay indicating acute infection. Leukocytosis is often present, sometimes with marked bandemia in the peripheral blood smear. Measurement of serum electrolytes, glucose, blood urea nitrogen, creatinine, and protein is indicated in patients who appear dehydrated, malnourished, or have changes in mental status.

STOOL MICROSCOPY

If *Shigella* infection is suspected, fresh stool should be examined for the presence of fecal leukocytes. The observation of large numbers of fecal leukocytes in a patient with acute diarrheal illness provides evidence that a bacterial pathogen has invaded the colonic mucosa and produced inflammation. *Campylobacter jejuni*, enteroinvasive *E. coli*, *Yersinia enterocolitica*, and nontyphoidal *Salmonella* species are bacterial pathogens aside from *Shigella* that cause dysentery accompanied by abundant fecal leukocytes. Stool microscopy also differentiates other infectious causes of bloody diarrhea from enteroinvasive bacterial infection. Notably, amebic dysentery and enterohemorrhagic *E. coli* do not induce abundant fecal leukocytes.

STOOL CULTURE

A specific diagnosis can usually be made within 48 hours by bacteriologic culture. When feces are acidic, bacteria remain viable for only a few hours; therefore, culture of a fresh stool is optimal. If this is not feasible, buffered glycerol saline makes the best transport medium. Differential, moderately selective media such as xylose–lysine deoxycholate (XLD) agar and *Salmonella–Shigella* (SS) should be used. Culture of two or more stool specimens increases the likelihood of isolating *Shigella* organisms. If *S. dysenteriae* is suspected, Tergitol-7 agar is particularly useful, but XLD agar can also isolate this fastidious bacterium. Susceptibility testing of isolates should be performed.

OPTIMAL MANAGEMENT

Hygienic behavior such as hand washing is effective in interrupting transmission. Segregation of ill persons is important in controlling infection in settings where hygienic practices are difficult to enforce, such as outbreaks occurring in institutions for the mentally handicapped. Antibiotics should not be given to prevent infection.

Correction of fluid and electrolyte deficits and replacement of ongoing losses is a central feature of management. The clinician should be alerted to other possible complications of shigellosis that may require specific therapy, such as seizures and intestinal perforation.

No evidence suggests that common antidiarrheal preparations, such as kaolin–pectin formulas, lactobacilli, or bismuth salicylate, have a significant beneficial effect, nor does evidence suggest that these agents are deleterious and therefore contraindicated. Agents that suppress intestinal motility, such as diphenoxylate, loperamide, and tincture of opium, have generally been avoided in known or suspected shigellosis because they may prolong or exacerbate the clinical and bacteriologic course of the disease, particularly in young children. Nonetheless, a randomized, double-blind, placebo-controlled trial demonstrated that adults with dysentery due to *Shigella* (predominantly *S. flexneri*), or the closely related enteroinvasive *E. coli*, who were treated with loperamide plus ciprofloxacin had significantly fewer diarrheal stools (median 2.0 stools) than subjects who were treated with ciprofloxacin alone (median 6.5 stools), and a significantly shorter duration of diarrhea (19 hours versus 42 hours, respectively). Adverse effects from loperamide were not detected. These findings suggest that loperamide may offer additional benefit to ciprofloxacin in adults with *Shigella* dysentery. However, loperamide should not be given to children, to debilitated or immunocompromised patients, to patients who may be infected with ciprofloxacin-resistant strains, or to those infected with *S. dysenteriae*.

Many controlled clinical trials have shown that appropriate antibiotics significantly decrease the duration of fever, diarrhea, and excretion of the pathogen in shigellosis. Most patients in these studies were infected with either *S. flexneri* or *S. dysenteriae*. The advantages of treating *S. sonnei*, which is usually self-limited, are less clear; benefit is likely to be greatest when therapy is initiated early in the course of illness. Nonetheless, this cumulative experience, in conjunction with the fact that treatment of ill persons may interrupt transmission, provides the rationale for treating patients with shigellosis with antibiotics.

The decision to treat must be reconciled with the reality that only a few antibiotics have proven to be clinically efficacious and that resistant *Shigella* strains eventually emerge from wide-

TABLE 282.2.	TREATMENT OF SHIGELLOSIS		
Antibiotic	**Route**	**Adult Dose**	**Pediatric Dose**[a]
Ampicillin	PO, IV	500 mg q.i.d. for 5 days	25 mg/kg q.i.d. for 5 days
TMP-SMX	PO, IV	160 mg TMP/800 mg SMX b.i.d. for 5 days	5 mg/kg TMP/25 mg/kg SMX b.i.d. for 5 days
Quinolones			
Ciprofloxacin	PO, IV	500 mg b.i.d. for 5 days[b]	10 mg/kg b.i.d. for 5 days[c]
Norfloxacin	PO	400 mg b.i.d. for 5 days[b]	See note[c]
Nalidixic acid	PO	1.0 g q.i.d. for 5 days	15 mg/kg q.i.d. for 5 days
Azithromycin	PO	500 mg on day 1, followed by 250 mg q.d. on days 2–5	Efficacy not evaluated in children

[a] Maximum dose not to exceed adult dose.
[b] In settings such as developing countries where the expense and practicality of a 5-day course of therapy are problematic, shigellosis caused by serotypes other than *S. dysenteriae* type 1 can be successfully treated with a 1–3 day regimen.
[c] These quinolones have not yet been approved for use in children younger than 18 years. However, there is growing evidence that they are safe and effective for use in multiply resistant childhood shigellosis.
TMP-SMX, trimethoprim–sulfamethoxazole.

spread use of these antibiotics. In 1997, nearly 20% of *Shigella* isolates reported to the CDC were resistant to both ampicillin and trimethoprim–sulfamethoxazole (TMP-SMX). *Shigella* isolates in Oregon between 1993 and 1998 demonstrated high-level (greater than 60%) resistance to either ampicillin or TMP-SMX. Resistance is more likely to be encountered if there is a history of recent foreign travel in the patient or in a household member with diarrhea. In Asia and Africa, nearly all *S. dysenteriae* type 1 strains are now resistant to tetracycline, ampicillin, TMP-SMX, and nalidixic acid (the drugs previously used to treat this infection), and other *Shigella* species are commonly resistant to these agents.

If the strain is susceptible, then inexpensive and highly effective antibiotics for adults include ampicillin (but not amoxicillin), tetracycline, TMP-SMX, and nalidixic acid (Table 282.2). Fluoroquinolones (e.g., ciprofloxacin, norfloxacin) are a highly effective albeit more expensive choice. A recent trial demonstrated that azithromycin was therapeutically equivalent to ciprofloxacin and may be considered as a second-line agent. Infections with strains having unknown susceptibility can be empirically treated with a fluoroquinolone; the increasing levels of TMP-SMX resistance suggest that this is no longer appropriate empiric therapy for shigellosis in many areas. Some antibiotics should be avoided because they lack clinical efficacy even though shigellae appear to be susceptible in vitro; these include nitrofurans, aminoglycosides, and first- and second-generation cephalosporins.

Therapy for children is similar to that for adults, with the following four exceptions. For one, despite growing evidence that they are safe and effective, fluoroquinolones have been used cautiously in children younger than 18 years because they cause arthropathy in young animals. Nonetheless, limited use of fluoroquinolones in children has shown that standard doses do not cause arthropathy. Similar experimental toxicity is observed with the quinolone nalidixic acid, but it was approved for use in children before this toxic effect was known and it has been used extensively without associated joint damage. Second, tetracycline should be avoided in children younger than 9 years because it may cause tooth enamel hypoplasia and discoloration. Third,

data on the efficacy of azithromycin in treating children with shigellosis are insufficient to formulate recommendations. Finally, whereas oral cefixime was not efficacious in adults, both oral cefixime and parenteral ceftriaxone have appeared to be beneficial in children.

Antibiotics are usually given for 3 to 5 days. In developing countries where costs of therapy constitute a critical consideration, short (1- to 3-day) courses of oral quinolones have been shown to be effective for milder illness caused by serotypes other than *S. dysenteriae* type 1; however, a 5-day course of therapy should be administered for severe illness or for suspected Shiga dysentery. With the exception of severely ill patients, therapy can be administered orally.

There is a pressing need for more effective control measures, such as improved hygiene and sanitation, and vaccination. In the 1960s, attenuated mutant strains of *Shigella* (in particular streptomycin–dependent mutants) were shown to be safe and protective when used as live oral vaccines. However, these vaccines had drawbacks and never gained widespread popularity. Research in this area has continued and has resulted in newer candidate vaccines, some of which have entered clinical trial. The objective is safe vaccines that provide broad-spectrum, long-lived immunity after administration of only one or two oral doses.

BIBLIOGRAPHY

Bennish ML, Salam MA, Khan WA, et al. Treatment of shigellosis: III. Comparison of one or two dose ciprofloxacin with standard 5 day therapy. A randomized, blinded trial. *Ann Intern Med* 1992;117:727–734.

Khan MU, Shahidulla M. Interruption of shigellosis by handwashing. *Trans R Soc Trop Med Hyg* 1982;76:164–168.

Kotloff KL, Winickoff JP, Ivanoff B, et al. Global burden of *Shigella* infections: implications for vaccine development and implementation. *Bull WHO* 1999;77:651–656.

Murphy GS, Bodhidatta L, Echeverria P, et al. Ciprofloxacin and loperamide in the treatment of bacillary dysentery. *Ann Intern Med* 1993;118:582–586.

Lee LA, Shapiro CN, Hargrett-Bean N, et al. Hyperendemic shigellosis is the United States: a review of surveillance data for 1967–1988. *J Infect Dis* 1991;164:894–900.

Sansonetti PJ, Tran Van Nhieu G, Egile C. Rupture of the intestinal epithelial barrier and mucosal invasion by *Shigella flexneri*. *Clin Infect Dis* 1999;28:466–475.

Tauxe RV, Puhr ND, Wells JG, et al. Antimicrobial resistance of *Shigella* isolates in the USA: the importance of international travelers. *J Infect Dis* 1990;162:1107–1111.

Kelley's Textbook of Internal Medicine, fourth edition. Edited by H. David Humes. Lippincott Williams & Wilkins, Philadelphia © 2000.

CHAPTER 283

INFECTIONS CAUSED BY *VIBRIO* AND *CAMPYLOBACTER* SPECIES

J. GLENN MORRIS, JR.
MARTIN J. BLASER

The pathogenic genera *Vibrio, Aeromonas, Plesiomonas,* and *Campylobacter* represent a diverse collection of gram-negative bacteria. *Vibrio cholerae* strains in O groups 1 and 139 cause cholera; patients with cholera have profuse, watery diarrhea that in the absence of treatment can rapidly lead to dehydration, shock, and death. Diarrhea is the most common clinical manifestation seen in association with other *V. cholerae* serogroups and other disease-causing species and strains in these genera. Some species also cause wound infections or septicemia. Septicemia, when it occurs, is usually limited to impaired hosts. Table 283.1 summarizes the principal features of the agents reviewed.

MICROBIOLOGY

Essentially all thin, curved, motile, gram-negative bacteria were originally considered to be vibrios, but closer examination has indicated that several distinct genera can be justified, including *Vibrio, Aeromonas, Plesiomonas, Campylobacter,* and *Helicobacter*. *Campylobacter* species were segregated because they are microaerophilic, whereas the true *Vibrio* species are facultative aerobes. All pathogenic *Vibrio* species other than *V. cholerae* require salt for growth. Isolation of *Vibrio* species from a stool specimen may be done by direct plating on thiosulfate citrate bile salt sucrose (TCBS) medium. After overnight incubation, suspect colonies can be identified; pre-enrichment in alkaline peptone water may increase the yield of culture. For *V. cholerae,* a reference microbiology laboratory (such as a state health department laboratory) can differentiate between cholera-associated strains (strains in O groups 1 and 139), and strains in other O groups, which may or may not be pathogenic. *V. cholerae* in O group 1 (*V. cholerae* O1) may be further classified by biotype (El Tor or classical) and serotype (Inaba or Ogawa).

Aeromonas and *Plesiomonas* species are rod-shaped bacteria of the family Vibrionaceae. Species considered to be pathogenic for human beings include *Aeromonas hydrophila, Aeromonas caviae, Aeromonas sobria,* and *Plesiomonas shigelloides*. These organisms may be differentiated from the Enterobacteriaceae because most are oxidase-positive, non–lactose fermenters. Blood agar that contains ampicillin is a selective medium for fecal isolation.

Campylobacter species were not isolated from fecal specimens until selective methods were used; these include a microaerobic atmosphere (5% oxygen) and use of either an antibiotic-containing plate medium or filtration for selective enrichment. A wide variety of *Campylobacter* and closely related *Helicobacter* species have been associated with human diarrheal illnesses. These include *Campylobacter coli, Campylobacter fetus, Campylobacter lari, Helicobacter cinaedi, Helicobacter fennelliae, Campylobacter upsaliensis,* and *Campylobacter hyointestinalis*; however, *Campylobacter jejuni* remains the most important and the prototype for the other organisms. A related organism, *Helicobacter pylori,* has been isolated from the gastric mucosa from patients with gastritis. Several diagnostic methods are based on its highly conserved urease enzyme.

CHOLERA

EPIDEMIOLOGIC FACTORS

Cholera has been recognized in the Indian subcontinent for hundreds of years. Seven cholera pandemics have occurred since 1817, involving spread of cholera from endemic areas in India and Asia through much of the rest of the world. The seventh pandemic (caused by *V. cholerae* O1 strains with an El Tor biotype) started in Indonesia in the early 1960s and, in the intervening three decades, has spread through Asia, parts of southern Europe, Africa, Oceania, and, beginning in 1991, South America. In the fall of 1992, a new cholera strain, *V. cholerae* O139 Bengal, was identified as the cause of epidemic cholera in Madras, India. This new strain subsequently spread through much of Asia, and in the Indian subcontinent is now as common, if not more common, than seventh-pandemic *V. cholerae* O1 El Tor strains.

Vibrio cholerae is a free-living organism in estuarine and other aquatic environments. Strains in this environmental reservoir may proliferate with seasonal increases in water temperature or other stimuli, and may be introduced into human populations though contaminated seafood, food, or water. In areas with poor sanitation, fecal material from ill persons further contaminates water or food sources, leading to additional cases and initiating cycles of epidemic disease. In areas in which the disease has become established, epidemics of this type usually occur once or twice a year, at very predictable times ("cholera season"). In such areas, illness is most common among children; adults are thought to have some degree of immunity because of prior exposure to the organism. In contrast, when *V. cholerae* is introduced into populations without prior exposure to cholera (or when there are major modifications in the antigenic structure of the strain, as occurred with the emergence of *V. cholerae* O139 Bengal strains), attack rates are equal in all age groups.

TABLE 283.1. CLINICAL AND EPIDEMIOLOGIC FEATURES OF INFECTIONS CAUSED BY *VIBRIO* AND *CAMPYLOBACTER* SPECIES

Feature	V. cholerae (O1/O139)	V. cholerae (non-O1/non-O139)	V. parahaemolyticus	V. vulnificus	Aeromonas	Plesiomonas shigelloides	C. jejuni	C. fetus
Major reservoir	Fresh or brackish water	Fresh or brackish water	Brackish water	Brackish water	Fresh or brackish water		Intestinal tract of most mammalian and avian species	Cattle and sheep intestinal tract
Major vehicles	Water, food	Shellfish	Seafood	Shellfish	Untreated potable water	Shellfish	Poultry, raw milk, untreated water	Raw milk
Risk groups	In endemic areas; persons consuming fecally contaminated water or food, or raw or undercooked shellfish	Travelers, raw shellfish consumers, exposure to seawater	Seafood consumers	Raw shellfish consumers with liver disease, iron overload, immunosuppression	Raw water drinkers, swimmers	Travelers, raw seafood consumers	Children, young adults	Immunosuppression, debilitation
Pathogenetic mechanism	Cholera toxin	NAG-ST, other toxins; capsule (for bacteremia)	Hemolysin-associated	Capsule	Unknown	Unknown	Cytotoxin or invasion	Protein capsule
Ability to cause illness in previously healthy host	High	High (low for bacteremia)	High	Low	Unknown	Unknown	High	Low
Major syndrome	Massive watery diarrhea	Watery or bloody diarrhea	Watery or bloody diarrhea	Bacteremia	Watery or bloody diarrhea	Bloody, mucoid diarrhea with severe cramps	Febrile, bloody diarrhea	Bacteremia and systemic infections
Minor syndrome	Mild watery diarrhea	Bacteremia, extraintestinal infections	Wound infection	Wound infection, diarrhea	Wound infection, bacteremia, extraintestinal infection	Bacteremia	Bacteremia	Diarrhea
Usual diagnostic tests	Fecal culture on TCBS agar	Fecal culture on TCBS agar; blood culture	Fecal culture on TCBS agar; blood culture	Blood culture	Fecal culture on MacConkey agar; oxidase-positive colonies	Fecal culture on MacConkey agar; oxidase-positive colonies	Fecal culture on Campylobacter-specific agar, direct stool examination	Blood culture
Fecal leukocytes	No	Variable	No	NA	Usually absent	Yes	Yes	NA

TCBS, thiosulfate citrate bile salts sucrose; NA, not generally applicable; NAG-ST, heat-stable enterotoxin of nonagglutinating (non-O1) *Vibrio cholerae*.

PATHOGENESIS

The primary mechanism for disease is the production of a potent enterotoxin, *cholera toxin*, that, through stimulation of adenyl cyclase on the membrane of small intestinal crypt cells, results in a net secretion of salt and water into the intestinal lumen. This augmentation of normal physiologic mechanisms, not actual damage to tissue, produces the often severe diarrhea for which cholera is known.

Recent studies indicate that the cholera toxin gene is carried by a filamentous phage, which is capable of integration into the bacterial chromosome. The receptor for this phage appears to be encoded by a gene in the *Vibrio* pathogenicity island (VPI), which is carried by a second phage. Genes responsible for expression of critical surface antigens also appear to be capable of transfer among strains. These findings underscore the genetic plasticity of cholera strains, a plasticity that may have contributed to the ability of the microorganism to "reinvent" itself in a series of pandemics.

CLINICAL FINDINGS

The manifestations of infection with O1 *V. cholerae* range from asymptomatic carriage to a rapidly fatal, fulminating illness. In severe cases, the sequence is massive diarrhea, volume depletion, hypotension, shock, and death. Without fluid replacement, death can occur within hours of onset of symptoms. Initially, stools may be loose, but the classic "rice-water" appearance then develops. Because the manifestations of disease result from a noncytolytic intoxication, fever and abdominal cramping are uncommon. The most common other symptoms—thirst, anxiety, muscle cramps, and light-headedness—are related to the rate and extent of fluid and electrolyte loss. Vomiting may contribute to fluid loss and impair the use of oral rehydration regimens. Dulled sensorium or convulsions, especially in children, may be caused by hypoglycemia. Hypokalemia may result in ileus that disguises the extent of fluid loss (cholera sicca), weakness, or arrhythmia.

DIAGNOSIS

Clinical diagnosis depends on the presence of massive watery stools, the absence of fever or abdominal cramping, and, usually, an exposure history. Volume replacement therapy for depleted patients should be begun before information on the specific etiologic agent is available. Dark-field or phase contrast microscopic examination of stools may show the typical *Vibrio* forms with darting motility. Definitive diagnosis is based on isolation of the organism on plate media. Isolation is facilitated by use of TCBS, although the organism will grow on MacConkey agar.

OPTIMAL MANAGEMENT

Cholera is a medical emergency. The treatment of all diarrheal diseases, and especially cholera, is the adequate replacement of fluid and electrolyte losses. In most cases, oral rehydration is sufficient, and the most favorable outcome is associated with its early institution. Oral rehydration packets of electrolytes and sugar to be mixed with water are available in most areas of the world in which cholera is endemic. If they are unavailable, the following should be added to each liter of boiled drinking water: NaCl, 3.5 g; NaHCO$_3$, 2.5 g; KCl, 1.5 g; glucose, 20 g. In an emergency, only NaCl and glucose are necessary. For patients already in shock or unable to take oral fluids, intravenous therapy is necessary and should be begun immediately. Lactated Ringer's solution or normal saline containing NaHCO$_3$, 4 g per liter, and KCl, 1 g per liter, in volumes to replace stool losses should be given. After initial stabilization by either intravenous or oral fluids, ongoing fluid loss in adults should be counterbalanced by oral rehydration solution at a ratio of 1.5:1 (150 mL of oral rehydration solution for every 100 mL of diarrheal stool). For children, losses should be replaced at a ratio of 1.1:1.

Antibiotics can shorten the duration of cholera diarrhea and the period of excretion of *V. cholerae*. However, antimicrobial therapy is clearly secondary in importance to fluid replacement: patients recover without difficulty in the absence of antimicrobial therapy but die without volume repletion. Tetracycline is the drug of choice, administered as 500 mg 4 times a day for 3 days; a single dose of 300 mg of doxycycline is also effective. Resistance to tetracycline is becoming increasingly widespread, particularly in sub-Saharan Africa. For tetracycline-resistant strains, alternative agents include ciprofloxacin, erythromycin, trimethoprim–sulfamethoxazole, and furazolidone.

PREVENTION

In endemic areas, prevention ultimately must be based on improving the quality of the water supply for drinking and cooking as well as for bathing and washing. The simple expedient of hand washing during outbreaks may diminish intrafamilial transmission. In epidemic situations, the widespread availability of oral hydration solutions is life saving. The use of older, parenteral, killed, whole-cell cholera vaccines is currently not recommended; protection with these vaccines was minimal, and they were associated with substantial side effects. Live attenuated and killed oral vaccines are currently undergoing evaluation and should become commercially available in the near future.

■ *VIBRIO CHOLERAE* IN O GROUPS OTHER THAN O1 AND O139

EPIDEMIOLOGIC FACTORS

As noted earlier, *V. cholerae* is common in estuarine and other aquatic environments. Non-O1/non-O139 strains of *V. cholerae* are particularly common environmental isolates, and are often present in shellfish, such as oysters, which are filter feeders. In the United States, cases of gastroenteritis caused by these strains are almost always associated with eating raw oysters. Outside of the United States, non-O1/non-O139 *V. cholerae* strains are recognized as a cause of travelers' diarrhea.

PATHOGENESIS

Most non-O1/non-O139 *V. cholerae* strains do not produce cholera toxin. Diarrheal illness has been reported in association

TABLE 283.2.	RECOMMENDED AGENTS FOR ANTIMICROBIAL TREATMENT OF INFECTIONS WITH *VIBRIO* AND *CAMPYLOBACTER* SPECIES	
Infection	**Agent of Choice**	**Alternative**
V. cholerae	Tetracycline, 500 mg PO q6h for 3 d or single 300-mg dose of doxycycline (g ciprofloxacin for bacteremia)	Furazolidone, 100 mg PO t.i.d.
V. parahaemolyticus	Tetracycline, 500 mg PO q.i.d. for 3 d	Ciprofloxacin, 500 mg PO b.i.d.
V. vulnificus	Minocycline 100 mg q12h PO, and cefotaxime 2.0 g q8h IV	Ciprofloxacin, 500 mg PO b.i.d.
		Tetracycline, ciprofloxacin, chloramphenicol
Aeromonas species	Trimethoprim–sulfamethoxazole	Ciprofloxacin
Plesiomonas shigelloides	Trimethoprim–sulfamethoxazole	Tetracycline
C. jejuni	Erythromycin, 250 mg PO q.i.d. for 5 d	Tetracycline, 500 mg PO q.i.d. for 5 d; furazolidone, 100 mg PO t.i.d. for 5 d; or ciprofloxacin, 500 mg b.i.d. for 5 d
C. fetus	Gentamicin for systemic infection; erythromycin, 250 mg PO q.i.d. for 5 d for diarrhea	Chloramphenicol for systemic infection

with a subset of strains that produce a heat-stable enterotoxin called NAG-ST; the association between other enterotoxins and cytotoxins and illness remains unclear. Strains which are heavily encapsulated are more likely to cause septicemia.

CLINICAL FINDINGS

Gastrointestinal infections manifest with diarrhea and abdominal cramps in most cases. In contrast to O1/O139 *V. cholerae*, infections with non-O1/non-O139 strains frequently result in fever or bloody diarrhea. The incubation period is usually less than a day, and illness lasts less than a week and often for 48 hours or less. Non-O1/non-O139 *V. cholerae* strains can cause otitis externa and wound infections in people bathing in estuarine or other water containing the organism. People who have liver disease or who are immunosuppressed are at risk for bacteremia. Mortality rates for patients with bacteremia exceed 60%.

DIAGNOSIS

Diagnosis is based on isolation of the organism from stool, wound, or blood cultures. Isolation from stool is facilitated by use of TCBS medium.

OPTIMAL MANAGEMENT

Therapy of diarrhea should focus on appropriate fluid replacement. Although no data on efficacy are available, it would appear reasonable to treat patients with severe or prolonged gastroenteritis with tetracycline or ciprofloxacin. Patients with bacteremia require aggressive antimicrobial therapy (with tetracycline or ciprofloxacin) and good supportive care (Table 283.2).

VIBRIO PARAHAEMOLYTICUS

EPIDEMIOLOGIC FACTORS

Vibrio parahaemolyticus may frequently be isolated from seawater, sediment, fish, and shellfish; however, only a minority of

these environmental strains are pathogenic for human beings. Illness is usually associated with the eating of raw or undercooked seafood, or the cross-contamination of cooked food by raw seafood. In Japan, *V. parahaemolyticus* is the most commonly reported bacterial cause of acute enteritis. Illness occurs year round in tropical areas, but in temperate areas it occurs mostly in the summer. The largest North American outbreak of *V. parahaemolyticus* infection reported to date occurred in July–August 1997, in the Pacific Northwest, in association with the eating of raw oysters; increases in seawater temperatures above historic levels were felt to be one factor contributing to occurrence of the outbreak.

PATHOGENESIS

Traditionally, virtually all *V. parahaemolyticus* strains isolated from human beings were β-hemolytic on blood agar (Kanagawa-positive), whereas most environmental isolates were negative. Studies suggest that the thermostable direct hemolysin (TDH), the primary hemolysin responsible for this effect, has a direct role in production of diarrhea; the possible contributions of other factors to pathogenesis remain to be determined. More recently, a subset of isolates that are urease-positive but Kanagawa-negative have been linked with case clusters along the Pacific coast of the United States and in Asia.

CLINICAL FINDINGS

Vibrio parahaemolyticus usually produces a brief, explosive gastroenteritis with watery diarrhea, nausea, vomiting, headache, and low-grade fever. Stools generally are not bloody, although a subset of patients with dysentery-like illness has been reported. The incubation period ranges from 4 to 96 hours. Although diarrhea may occasionally be massive, illness is self-limited to 3 to 5 days in most cases. Wound infections and septicemia may also occur.

DIAGNOSIS

Diagnosis is based on isolation of the organism from culture. As with other *Vibrio* species, isolation from stool is facilitated by use of TCBS medium.

OPTIMAL MANAGEMENT

Specific antimicrobial treatment is not needed in most cases. In severe illness, tetracycline appears to be the treatment of choice (Table 283.2).

VIBRIO VULNIFICUS

EPIDEMIOLOGIC FACTORS

Vibrio vulnificus is ubiquitous in coastal waters, particularly during the warm summer months when water temperatures exceed 20°C. Oysters harvested from these waters commonly carry *V. vulnificus*. Injuries from shellfish or direct contamination of preexisting wounds with coastal waters may cause wound infections. *V. vulnificus* septicemia may result from a wound infection or follow ingestion of the organism in raw shellfish. Severe illness tends to be restricted to persons with underlying liver disease, hemochromatosis, chronic renal insufficiency, use of immunosuppressive agents, or heavy alcohol consumption.

PATHOGENESIS

Ability to cause either local or systemic infection is associated with the resistance of encapsulated *V. vulnificus* to complement-mediated serum lysis and to phagocytosis. The microorganism also produces a potent cytolysin and protease, which may contribute to the observed clinical syndrome.

CLINICAL FINDINGS

Wound infections may remain localized or, in persons in the risk groups noted above, may spread rapidly, with formation of bulli. In the most severe cases, the clinical appearance may be similar to that seen with necrotizing fasciitis.

Septicemia may result from a wound infection or follow ingestion of shellfish containing the bacterium. Patients with septicemia usually have the abrupt onset of fever, chills, and hypotension. Characteristic bullous skin lesions develop within the first 24 hours of infection in a majority of cases. Mortality rates for patients with *V. vulnificus* septicemia exceed 50%; mortality is greater than 90% for patients who present in shock or become hypotensive within 24 hours of hospital admission. Even if patients survive the first few days, multiorgan system failure is a common sequela to septicemia, resulting in weeks of hospitalization in an intensive care unit and necessitating prolonged rehabilitation.

DIAGNOSIS

Diagnosis is based on a high index of suspicion among people with seawater or raw shellfish exposure, especially in high-risk patients. The presence of bullous skin lesions in a person with an appropriate history is a sensitive indicator of *V. vulnificus* sepsis. Definitive diagnosis is based on isolation of the causative organism from wound or blood culture.

OPTIMAL MANAGEMENT

Wound infections require rapid surgical debridement and aggressive antibiotic therapy; tetracycline and ciprofloxacin are the drugs of choice. Recent in vitro and animal studies from Taiwan indicate that there is synergism between minocycline and cefotaxime in treatment of serious *V. vulnificus* infections. In light of these latter studies, therapy with minocycline (100 mg q12h PO) and cefotaxime (2.0 g q8h IV), with doses appropriately adjusted for underlying renal or hepatic disease, is recommended for patients with septicemia or serious wound infections. Early initiation of antibiotic therapy has been associated with increased survival for patients with septicemia, and consequently therapy should be started immediately if there is any suspicion of the diagnosis. Patients who are hypotensive require aggressive supportive care in an intensive care unit.

OTHER VIBRIOS

EPIDEMIOLOGIC FACTORS

Other vibrios of medical significance include *V. mimicus*, *V. alginolyticus*, *V. damsela*, *V. hollisae*, *V. fluvialis*, and *V. furnissii*. These organisms have been isolated from estuarine environments, and in some cases illnesses have been associated with consumption of raw or undercooked seafood.

PATHOGENESIS

Although these vibrios have been isolated from patients with diarrheal illnesses or wound infections, their roles as pathogens are not well defined.

CLINICAL FINDINGS

Patients infected with *V. fluvialis* frequently have diarrhea, vomiting, and fever, as well as fecal leukocytes and blood. *V. mimicus* infection has also been associated with bloody diarrhea. *V. damsela* and *V. alginolyticus* are primarily associated with wound or ear infections rather than gastroenteritis.

DIAGNOSIS

Diagnosis of these infections is based on their isolation from stool cultures using selective media or isolation from wound or blood cultures.

OPTIMAL MANAGEMENT

For all diarrheal illnesses, treatment is based on repletion of volume lost in the stools. The role of specific antimicrobial therapy for diarrheal illnesses associated with these agents has not been determined. Wound infections and bacteremia should be treated with tetracycline or ciprofloxacin.

AEROMONAS

EPIDEMIOLOGIC FACTORS

Aeromonas species are widely found in environmental water sources, in highest concentrations in warm water and during the summer months. Potable water, especially if untreated, is usually considered the most important vehicle for this organism. Swimming in fresh or estuarine brackish water is a risk factor for wound infection. People of all ages may be affected with diarrheal disease. Rates of asymptomatic stool excretion of *Aeromonas* are also high in both adults and children, suggesting that not all strains are able to cause diarrhea. Extraintestinal infection occurs chiefly in compromised hosts.

PATHOGENESIS

Although several enterotoxins and cytotoxins have been described, their biologic role is uncertain and it is not known which environmental strains are pathogenic for humans.

CLINICAL FINDINGS

Infection may cause acute, watery diarrhea, dysentery, or a syndrome of chronic diarrhea. Acute, watery diarrhea is most common among children. Illness in these cases is usually self-limited, with a duration of less than 7 days. The dysenteric syndrome resembles shigellosis, with blood and mucus in feces, abdominal cramps, and fever. Chronic or intermittent diarrhea may persist for months to 2 years or more. *Aeromonas* species are associated with wound infections in people with exposure to estuarine and aquatic environments. Extraintestinal infections, including bacteremia, meningitis, endocarditis, and soft tissue, muscle, and bone infections, are also reported; these latter infections usually are limited to compromised hosts.

DIAGNOSIS

Aeromonas infection should be suspected in people who become ill after drinking or swimming in untreated water. Diagnosis is based on isolating organisms from a fecal culture using a selective medium or on isolating organisms from wound or blood cultures.

OPTIMAL MANAGEMENT

For those intestinal infections requiring treatment (those with fever, bloody diarrhea, or chronicity beyond 1 week), trimethoprim-sulfamethoxazole, a quinolone, or tetracycline are the agents of choice (see Table 283.2). For extraintestinal illness, trimethoprim-sulfamethoxazole is the treatment of choice, with ciprofloxacin a possible alternative.

PLESIOMONAS SHIGELLOIDES

EPIDEMIOLOGIC FACTORS

Water and seafood, especially raw oysters, appear to be the main environmental sources for *Plesiomonas* infection of human beings. Both environmental and human isolates occur more frequently in the summer months. Diarrheal illness occurs chiefly in immunocompetent hosts, whereas extraintestinal infection is most common in compromised hosts. *Plesiomonas* appears to be a cause of traveler's diarrhea.

PATHOGENESIS

The pathogenic mechanisms of *Plesiomonas* are not known, nor has it been determined as to which environmental and fecal isolates are virulent.

CLINICAL FINDINGS

Most patients infected with *Plesiomonas* organisms have bloody, mucus-containing stools with fecal leukocytes. Other patients may have severe abdominal cramps, vomiting, and dehydration. Acute colitis also may be present. Extraintestinal manifestations include cellulitis, meningitis, and septicemia.

DIAGNOSIS

Because the pathogenic potential of *Plesiomonas* strains is not known, by convention, isolation is considered clinically significant when these organisms are found in large numbers from stools using relatively nonselective media, such as MacConkey agar.

OPTIMAL MANAGEMENT

Antimicrobial therapy (Table 283.2) is indicated for patients with acute toxicity, bloody diarrhea, or long-standing infection; trimethoprim-sulfamethoxazole or tetracycline is considered to be the treatment of choice. Chloramphenicol should be used for septicemia, but self-limited bacteremia also occurs.

CAMPYLOBACTER JEJUNI

EPIDEMIOLOGIC FACTORS

Campylobacter jejuni and closely related organisms in the genera *Campylobacter*, *Helicobacter*, and *Arcobacter* are carried in the intestinal flora of a wide variety of avian and mammalian species, especially those used for food production. Transmission to human beings occurs primarily from undercooked chicken, unpasteurized milk, untreated water, and exposure to infected pets; occasionally, transmission also occurs from young children who are infected. Although infections occur year round, incidence peaks during the summer. In the United States, highest attack rates are in children younger than 1 year of age, but most cases occur in persons 15 to 29 years of age. Persons of any age may be affected, and asymptomatic excretion is uncommon. In developing countries, infection is hyperendemic, but immunity appears to be acquired at a young age; asymptomatic excretion is common.

PATHOGENESIS

The ileum, colon, or both is the usual target of infection, which is manifested as an acute inflammation with neutrophilic infiltration of the lamina propria and destruction of mucous glands. Fecal leukocytes and gross or occult blood are common, but the pathogenic mechanism is unknown. Although both enterotoxins and cytotoxins have been described, whether they are of biologic significance is unknown.

CLINICAL FINDINGS

Most patients infected with *C. jejuni* in the United States have an acute febrile gastroenteritis. Common symptoms are a prodrome lasting for 12 to 48 hours, with fever, myalgia, and other constitutional complaints before the onset of gastrointestinal symptoms. Diarrhea is the most common symptom, and stools may be watery, mucoid, or bloody. At the peak of illness, which usually occurs in the first 48 hours, most patients have 10 or more bowel movements per day. Abdominal cramping is common and may be sufficiently severe to mimic an acute abdomen or acute appendicitis. On occasion, fever and constitutional symptoms may predominate, producing an enteric fever syndrome. Gastrointestinal involvement also may include toxic megacolon or frank lower gastrointestinal hemorrhage, sometimes necessitating colectomy. Extraintestinal manifestations are uncommon but may include bacteremia, cholecystitis, pancreatitis, and pneumonia. Late complications include nonsuppurative arthritis, especially in human leukocyte antigen B27–positive hosts, and the Guillain–Barré syndrome. Altogether, 20% to 50% of all Guillain–Barré syndrome cases follow *Campylobacter* infections.

DIAGNOSIS

The epidemiologic setting may suggest the diagnosis, and it should be remembered that *C. jejuni* is implicated as the cause for acute diarrheal illnesses more frequently than *Salmonella* and *Shigella* species combined. In patients with febrile or bloody diarrhea, microscopic examination of stools may show leukocytes; their presence is an indication for fecal culture and may help identify invasive or cytotoxigenic diarrheal pathogens. Examination of fecal preparations by Gram stain or dark-field microscopy is a rapid technique for diagnosing *Campylobacter* infection; although specificity is close to 100%, sensitivity is about 60%. Definitive identification is made by fecal culture onto *Campylobacter*-specific selective plate media. Most diarrheal illnesses are caused by *C. jejuni*, and less often by *C. coli*, *C. lari*, *C. fetus*, *C. hyointestinalis*, or *C. upsaliensis*, *Helicobacter* species such as *H. cinaedi* and *H. fennelliae*, or *Arcobacter* species. Differentiation must be made by biochemical testing. On occasion, febrile diarrheal disease due to infection with *Campylobacter* species may be diagnosed by blood culture.

OPTIMAL MANAGEMENT

Most gastrointestinal infections due to *Campylobacter* species are self-limited to 5 to 7 days, and specific antimicrobial therapy is not necessary. Treatment (Table 283.2) is recommended, however, for people with more severe illness that includes bloody diarrhea, continued fever, 10 or more bowel movements a day,

persistence of symptoms beyond a week, or underlying immunocompromise.

The agent of choice is erythromycin, 250 mg by mouth 4 times daily for 5 days. Ciprofloxacin also has excellent activity against *Campylobacter* and is an attractive agent for use in patients before culture results are known because of its broad-spectrum activity against a number of bacterial enteric pathogens. However, resistance of *Campylobacter* to ciprofloxacin and other quinolones is increasing globally, with recent rapid increases in resistance in parts of the United States. For resistant organisms, the alternatives are tetracycline, 250 mg orally 4 times daily for 5 days, or furazolidone.

■ *CAMPYLOBACTER FETUS*

EPIDEMIOLOGIC FACTORS

Campylobacter fetus is contained in the intestinal flora of cattle, sheep, swine, and reptiles. Transmission to human beings through unpasteurized milk or uncooked meat has been documented, but the source for the organism in most human infections has not been established. Diarrheal illnesses due to *C. fetus* infection may develop in persons of any age, but pregnant women, individuals at the extremes of age, or those debilitated by preexisting illnesses, such as malignancy, liver disease, diabetes, HIV infection, or advanced atherosclerosis, are at risk for development of systemic infection.

PATHOGENESIS

Campylobacter fetus can cause systemic disease because of its resistance to complement-mediated serum lysis and to phagocytosis—properties conferred by a protein capsule. Host defects in reticuloendothelial function or in providing a locus for the organism to multiply also seem important.

CLINICAL FINDINGS

Campylobacter fetus may cause acute diarrheal illnesses with onset and symptoms indistinguishable from those due to *C. jejuni*. For the systemic infections, there may be a prodrome of constitutional symptoms. Fever is the cardinal manifestation; it may be intermittent or continuous, and it may be low grade or part of a syndrome of sepsis. The major types of infection are bacteremia, meningitis, arthritis, abscesses, and endovascular infections, including endocarditis, infected aortic aneurysms, and septic thrombophlebitis. The manifestations of these infections are typical for pyogenic processes at these sites but may persist. Prognosis depends in part on the site of infection, the rapidity with which therapy is begun, and the underlying host status; however, fatal infections are common. Gastrointestinal symptoms may or may not be present.

DIAGNOSIS

Diagnosis is made by isolation of *C. fetus* from cultures of blood or fluid from affected areas. These organisms are fastidious and slow growing, and microbiologic identification may be difficult.

OPTIMAL MANAGEMENT

Diarrheal illnesses, when severe or prolonged, may be treated with erythromycin. Although self-limited bacteremia may occur, extraintestinal *C. fetus* infections usually are severe. Antimicrobial therapy is required in such infections (Table 283.2); the initial agent of choice is chloramphenicol or an aminoglycoside. Definitive therapy depends on susceptibility of the organism as well as location (e.g., meninges), and the necessity for surgical debridement or drainage of abscesses or other foci of necrosis.

BIBLIOGRAPHY

Allos BM, Blaser MJ. *Campylobacter jejuni* and the expanding spectrum of related agents: state of the art. *Clin Infect Dis* 1995;20:1092–1101.

Blaser MJ. *Campylobacter fetus*: emerging infection and model system for bacterial pathogenesis at mucosal surfaces. *Clin Infect Dis* 1998;27:256–258.

Blaser MJ, Wells JG, Feldman RA, et al. *Campylobacter* enteritis in the United States: a multicenter study. *Ann Intern Med* 1983;98:360–365.

Chuang, YC, Ko WC, Wang ST, et al. Minocycline and cefotaxime in the treatment of experimental murine *Vibrio vulnificus* infection. *Antimicrob Agents Chemother* 1998;42:1319–1322.

Guerrant R, Lahita RG, Winn WC, et al. Campylobacteriosis in man: pathogenic mechanisms and review of 91 bloodstream infections. *Am J Med* 1978;65:584–592.

Hlady WG, Klontz KC. The epidemiology of vibrio infections in Florida, 1981–1993. *J Infect Dis* 1996;173:1176–1183.

Holmberg SD, Schell WL, Fanning GR, et al. *Aeromonas* intestinal infections in the United States. *Ann Intern Med* 1986;105:683–689.

Kaper JB, Morris JG Jr, Levine MM. Cholera. *Clin Microbiol Rev* 1995;8:48–86.

Karaolis DKR, Somara S, Maneval DR Jr, et al. A bacteriophage encoding a pathogenicity island, a type-IV pilus and a phage receptor in cholera bacteria. *Nature* 1999;399:375–379.

Klontz KC, Lieb S, Schreiber M, et al. Syndromes of *Vibrio vulnificus*: clinical and epidemiologic features in Florida cases, 1981–1987. *Ann Intern Med* 1988;109:318–323.

Smith KE, Besser JM, Hedberg CW, et al. Quinolone-resistant *Campylobacter jejuni* infections in Minnesota, 1992–1998. *N Engl J Med* 1999;340:1525–1532.

U.S. Centers for Disease Control and Prevention. Outbreak of *Vibrio parahaemolyticus* infections associated with eating raw oysters—Pacific Northwest, 1997. *MMWR* 1998;47:457–462.

Kelley's Textbook of Internal Medicine, fourth edition. Edited by H. David Humes.
Lippincott Williams & Wilkins, Philadelphia © 2000.

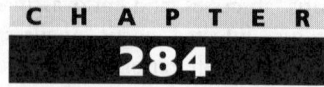

C H A P T E R
284

INFECTION BY HELICOBACTER PYLORI

DAVID Y. GRAHAM

Prior to the isolation of *Helicobacter pylori*, a number of diseases were known to be tightly linked to gastritis, including peptic ulcer disease, gastric cancer, and primary gastric lymphoma. The proof that *H. pylori* infection was the major cause of gastritis resulted in a reappraisal of many concepts in gastroenterology and allowed many disparate facts to be linked through the common pathway of a bacterial infection. The identification of a major cause of gastritis also suggested that it might be possible to prevent and to cure the gastritis-associated diseases.

MICROBIOLOGY

Helicobacter pylori bacilli are small (0.5 × 2.5 (m), flagellated, spiral, gram-negative organisms with sheathed unipolar flagella. *H. pylori* are slow growing in vitro, microaerophilic, and require complex media. Three enzymes are uniformly present and useful for laboratory identification: oxidase, catalase, and urease. Urease activity is especially intense in comparison with other urease-producing bacteria and forms the basis of a number of different diagnostic tests.

EPIDEMIOLOGIC FACTORS

Members of the genus *Helicobacter* are widespread in the animal kingdom. *H. pylori* infects humans, although animals, notably other primates, may become infected because of contact with infected humans. *H. pylori* has worldwide distribution. Current evidence is consistent with humans as the major and probably the only important reservoir. The most common mode of transmission is the fecal–oral route but gastro–oral (e.g., exposure to contaminated nasogastric tubes or endoscopes) has also been documented. Risk factors for acquiring *H. pylori* infection include birth in a developing country, low socioeconomic status, crowded living conditions, large family size, unsanitary living conditions, unclean food or water, presence of infants in the home, and exposure to gastric contents of infected individuals.

Current data suggest that, once acquired, *H. pylori* infection is often life-long. The increasing prevalence of infection with age is thought to be the consequence of a birth cohort phenomenon and reflects the fact that older individuals were born in a time when sanitation and standards of living were lower than they are today. *H. pylori* infection is typically acquired in childhood, and the prevalence of the infection at age 20 provides a reasonable estimate of the frequency of symptoms for that birth cohort throughout the remainder of their lives. In adults, the likelihood of acquiring the infection is about 0.5% per year. The natural tendency of the infection is to disappear, and in developed countries the prevalence is falling in every age group probably as a result of the widespread use of antibiotics or other reasons.

PATHOGENESIS

Both urease activity and motility are important for *H. pylori* colonization of the human stomach. *H. pylori* is uniquely adapted to gastric-type epithelium and may colonize the stomach, duodenum, esophagus, or wherever gastric type epithelium is found. The bacteria attach to the epithelium, and there is also evidence for limited invasion of epithelial cells. Attachment is associated with a marked inflammatory response, affecting neutrophils as well as mononuclear cells.

The search for factors that predict virulent versus nonvirulent *H. pylori* has not been rewarding. Nevertheless, strains that contain the *cag* pathogenicity island are associated with more intense acute inflammation and a higher likelihood of symptomatic disease than those that lack that characteristic. This increase in risk is of a low order of magnitude and testing for the presence of any putative virulence has not proven useful.

CLINICAL FINDINGS

The outcome of any infection is closely related to the pattern of gastritis. Although the bacteria are scattered throughout the gastric mucosal surface, the severity of gastritis differs within the stomach. The corpus of the stomach is relatively resistant to developing more than mild gastritis. This resistance can be overcome by any mechanism that reduces acid secretion such as vagotomy or the use of proton pump inhibitors or higher doses of H_2 receptor antagonists, suggesting that it is acid that "protects" this portion of the stomach. Inflammation is typically worse in the non-acid-secreting portions of the stomach, (antrum and cardia). Antral predominant gastritis is typical of duodenal ulcer and is consistent with the old notions and observations that unimpeded acid secretion was a perquisite of development of duodenal ulcer disease. Corpus gastritis causes a reversible reduction in gastric acid secretion and is associated with a lower frequency of duodenal ulcer disease and also gastroesophageal reflux disease. The pattern of multifocal pangastritis with atrophy and intestinal metaplasia is the phenotype with the highest risk of gastric ulcer and gastric cancer. The fact that *H. pylori* infection may appear to "protect" against gastroesophageal reflux disease is a reflection of the prevalence of multifocal atrophic pangastritis. This has been misinterpreted by some as evidence for the presence of less harmful *H. pylori* organisms.

One outcome of *H. pylori* infection is for there to be a progression from superficial gastritis to pangastritis with atrophy, metaplasia, dysplasia, and, finally, gastric adenocarcinoma. It is currently unknown at which point the cure of *H. pylori* infection halts the progression. Epidemiologic evidence has also linked *H. pylori* infection with low-grade B-cell lymphoma of mucosa-associated lymphoid tissue (MALToma). This lymphoma is of special interest because it appears to be stimulated by the presence of *H. pylori* antigens and regresses when *H. pylori* is treated.

DIAGNOSIS

Diagnostic tests for *H. pylori* can be divided into those performed on gastric biopsy specimens (and therefore requiring upper gas-

TABLE 284.1.	DIAGNOSTIC TESTS FOR *HELICOBACTER PYLORI* INFECTION

Invasive (performed on endoscopic biopsy specimen)
   Histology with special stains
   Bacterial culture
   Biopsy urease test
Noninvasive
   Serology
   Urea breath test (carbon 13 or 14)

trointestinal endoscopy) and noninvasive tests (Table 284.1). Noninvasive testing is preferred and should be the approach of choice unless there is another indication for endoscopy such as the presence of features suggesting cancer (e.g., a mass) or an ulcer complication (e.g., bleeding).

The two main noninvasive tests for *H. pylori* are serology and the urea breath test. The urea breath test is the test of choice, especially after treatment. Urea breath testing is inexpensive compared to endoscopy; it is also simple and reliable. The patient ingests isotopically labeled urea, and if *H. pylori* urease is present the urea is hydrolyzed and labeled carbon dioxide produced can be measured in breath samples. The two isotopes commonly used in the test are carbon 13 and carbon 14, the latter of which is radioactive. As with all tests that require active *H. pylori* infection, false-negative results may occur if the patient had recently taken drugs that reduce the bacterial load such as antibiotics, proton pump inhibitors, or bismuth compounds. H_2 receptor antagonists may also lead to false-negative results with the carbon 14 urea breath test but is not a problem with the carbon 13 urea breath test; this probably relates to the quantity of substrate used in each.

Serologic testing is rapid, convenient, and inexpensive and may be the test of choice for those with active ulcer disease. Unfortunately, serology cannot be used to check early treatment success because reliable falls in antibody levels from the pretreatment baseline may take more than a year. Only IgG-based tests have proven to be clinically useful. There are no IgM or IgA anti–*H. pylori* tests currently approved by the Food and Drug Administration, and those that are available commercially "for research only" are in our experience unreliable and should not be used.

TABLE 284.2.	RECOMMENDED ANTIBIOTIC REGIMENS FOR TREATMENT OF *H. PYLORI* INFECTION

1. Proton pump inhibitor (b.i.d.) or ranitidine bismuth citrate (b.i.d.) plus two of the following:
   Amoxicillin 1 g b.i.d.
   Clarithromycin 500 mg b.i.d.
   Metronidazole 500 mg b.i.d.
2. Bismuth citrate or subsalicylate (2 tablets q.i.d.) plus tetracycline (500 mg q.i.d.) plus one of either
   Metronidazole 500 mg t.i.d.
   Clarithromycin 500 mg t.i.d.

Endoscopy has an advantage in that it can also establish the diagnosis of peptic ulcer or gastric cancer. Histologic examination of stained gastric biopsy specimen gives information regarding *H. pylori* status as well as the type and severity of gastritis. Hematoxylin and eosin staining alone has repeatedly proven to be unreliable for detection of *H. pylori*, and the clinician should demand that the pathologist examine the tissue with a special stain. We recommend the triple stains of Genta, El-Zimaity, or the combination of a slide stained with hematoxylin and eosin and another stained with Diff-Quik. Bacterial culture is not widely available but is required if antibiotic susceptibility testing is needed (an increasingly common indication). The third commonly used biopsy-based test, the rapid urease test, involves placing a biopsy specimen in a medium containing urea and a pH indicator. A color change occurs if urease is present. These tests are cheap and reliable, and they serve as a good check on the pathologist. Many endoscopists use rapid urease testing as a method to decide which biopsy specimens to send for histologic examination (specimens from patients with negative rapid urease tests are submitted for histologic examination).

OPTIMAL MANAGEMENT

Because of the risks associated with *H. pylori* infection (e.g., one in six patients develop peptic ulcer; lifetime risk for gastric cancer of 1% to 3%) and because the infection is always transmissible, there is general agreement that diagnosis should be followed by treatment. Current discussions concerned whom to test. There is no disagreement about peptic ulcer because cure of *H. pylori* infection cures that disease. Most would test and treat infected patients with dyspepsia based on the premise that the population of otherwise uninvestigated dyspeptics will be enriched for those with peptic ulcer. Most patients with proven nonulcer dyspepsia do not appear to benefit symptomatically from *H. pylori* treatment, but, as there is no method of distinguishing which patients will benefit, many clinicians will test and treat. Other groups that are potential candidates for testing are first-degree relatives of patients with peptic ulcer or with gastric cancer as both groups have markedly increased risk of developing symptomatic *H. pylori* disease. The question about when to refer is addressed in Fig. 284.1.

The principle of therapy is to test, treat, and then confirm cure. No patient who does not have an *H. pylori* infection should receive triple antibiotic therapy because they will experience side effects without any possibility of benefit. The actual therapy consists of at least two antibiotics plus a proton pump inhibitor (or a bismuth compound) prescribed in divided doses (Table 284.1). Which antibiotics? The first question in choosing a specific regimen is, what is the likelihood that resistant organisms are present? For example, resistance to metronidazole or clarithromycin is expected if either of those antibiotics has been used in earlier attempts to cure the infection. Clarithromycin resistance predicts failure with the results of triple antibiotic combinations being reduced to what would be expected with a dual therapy of the remaining drugs (the combination of a pro-

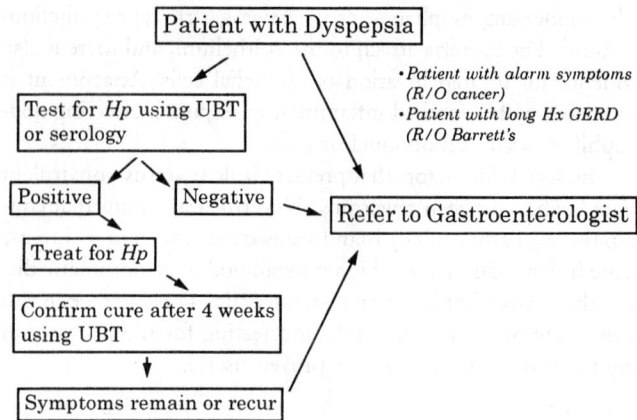

FIGURE 284.1. Clinical pathway for the treatment of patients with suspected peptic ulcer (dyspepsia) to assist in decision making regarding when to refer the patient to a gastroenterologist.
EVIDENCE LEVEL: C. Expert Opinion.

ton pump inhibitor, clarithromycin, and amoxicillin would be equivalent to the proton pump inhibitor plus amoxicillin in the face of clarithromycin resistance). In contrast, the deleterious effects of metronidazole resistance can be partially or completely overcome by increasing the dosage of metronidazole and possibly the duration of therapy. Although there has been a tendency to reduce the duration of therapy from 14 days to 10 days or even 7 days, head-to-head comparisons have generally shown that the best results are obtained with a 14-day duration. Four to six weeks after therapy, one should confirm that the therapy was successful. This can easily be done using a urea breath test or possibly an *H. pylori* stool antigen test. Follow-up endoscopy is indicated for those with suspicious histology (e.g., dysplasia) and possibly those with gastric ulcer.

BIBLIOGRAPHY

Breuer T, Malaty HM, Graham DY. The epidemiology of *H. pylori*-associated gastroduodenal diseases. In: Ernst P, Michetti P, Smith PD, eds. *The immunobiology of* H. pylori *from pathogenesis to prevention*. Philadelphia: Lippincott–Raven Publishers; 1997:1–14.

El-Zimaity HM, Ota H, Scott S, et al. A new triple stain for *Helicobacter pylori* suitable for the autostainer: carbol fuchsin/Alcian blue/hematoxylin–eosin. *Arch Pathol Lab Med* 1998;122:732–736.

El-Zimaity HM, Segura AM, Genta RM, et al. Histologic assessment of *Helicobacter pylori* status after therapy: comparison of Giemsa, Diff-Quik, and Genta stains. *Mod Pathol* 1998;11:288–291.

Graham DY, Yamaoka Y. *H. pylori* and cagA: relationships with gastric cancer, duodenal ulcer, and reflux esophagitis and its complications. *Helicobacter* 1998;3:145–151.

Graham DY. Antibiotic resistance in *Helicobacter pylori*: implications for therapy. *Gastroenterology* 1998;115:1272–1277.

Graham DY. Can therapy ever be denied for *Helicobacter pylori* infection? *Gastroenterology* 1997;113:S113–117.

Graham DY. *Helicobacter pylori* infection in the pathogenesis of duodenal ulcer and gastric cancer: a model. *Gastroenterology* 1997;113:1983–1991.

Howden CW, Hunt RH. Guidelines for the management of *Helicobacter pylori* infection. Ad Hoc Committee on Practice Parameters of the American College of Gastroenterology. *Am J Gastroenterol* 1998;93:2330–2338.

Ota H, Genta RM. Morphological characterization of the gastric mucosa during infection with *H. pylori*. In: Ernst P, Michetti P, Smith PD, eds. *The immunobiology of* H. pylori *from pathogenesis to prevention.* Philadelphia: Lippincott–Raven Publishers; 1997:15–28.

Kelley's Textbook of Internal Medicine, fourth edition. Edited by H. David Humes. Lippincott Williams & Wilkins, Philadelphia © 2000.

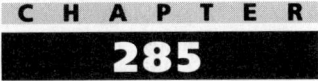

285

BRUCELLOSIS, TULAREMIA, PASTEURELLOSIS, AND YERSINIOSIS

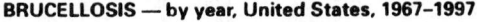

EDWARD J. YOUNG

The infections discussed in this chapter share a common feature: they are diseases of animals (zoonoses), and humans are accidental hosts who play no role in maintaining the disease in nature. Man's risk of contracting these infections is principally direct or indirect contact with diseased animals or their products.

■ BRUCELLOSIS

DEFINITION

Brucellosis is a systemic infection caused by species of the genus *Brucella.*

INCIDENCE AND EPIDEMIOLOGIC FACTORS

Brucellosis exists worldwide, especially in developing countries. As a result of the control and near-elimination of the disease in domestic animals, human brucellosis is now rare in the United States, with less than 0.05 case per 100,000 population being reported in recent years (see Fig. 285.1). Although occupational exposure (e.g., ranchers, veterinarians, abattoir workers) poses an increased risk of infection, most cases in the United States are now associated with the consumption of unpasteurized dairy products (e.g., milk, cheese) originating in areas where the disease is endemic. No animate vectors are known, and person-to-person transmission is rare.

ETIOLOGIC FACTORS

The brucellae are small, gram-negative coccobacilli that lack capsule, endospores, flagellae, or natural plasmids. Although closely related genetically, *Brucella* species are traditionally classified according to their usual animal hosts (nomen species): *B. abortus*

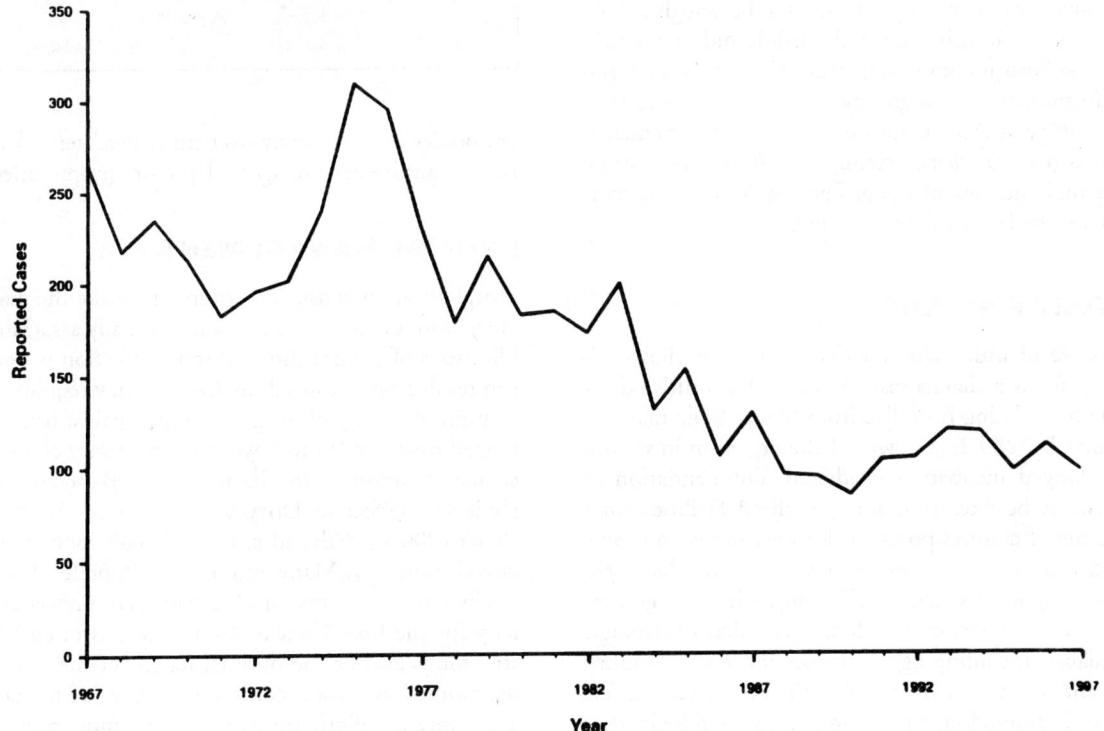

FIGURE 285.1. Number of reported cases of brucellosis by year, 1967–1997. (From U.S. Centers for Disease Control and Prevention. Summary of notifiable diseases, United States, 1997. *MMWR* 1997; 46(54):26.)

(cattle), *B. melitensis* (goats and sheep), *B. suis* (swine), *B. canis* (dogs), *B. ovis* (sheep), and *B. neotomae* (wood rats). Only the first four species are known to cause human infection. A new species (tentatively termed *B. maris*) has recently been isolated from marine mammals.

PATHOGENESIS

Brucellae are facultative intracellular pathogens that can survive and multiply within phagocytic cells of the host. The major virulence factor appears to be cell wall lipopolysaccharide. Among the nomen species, *B. melitensis* and *B. suis* are the most virulent. During infection the bacteria localize within mononuclear phagocytes of the reticuloendothelial system (e.g., lymph nodes, spleen, liver, and bone marrow), accounting for many of the clinical complications. Localization within cyetic products of some animals may explain their propensity for spontaneous abortions. The activation of macrophages by specifically committed T cells enhances their ability to kill intracellular brucellae. Although humoral antibodies play some role in resistance, recovery from infection depends on cell-mediated immunity.

CLINICAL FINDINGS

Brucellosis is characterized by a multitude of nonspecific complaints (e.g., fever, sweats, fatigue, joint pains, weight loss, and depression), with a paucity of abnormal physical findings other than occasional splenomegaly. The onset can be acute or insidious. Any organ system can be involved, but osteoarticular complications predominate (Table 285.1). A history of animal exposure or unusual food consumption should be sought. Life-threatening complications include endocarditis and meningitis. Childhood brucellosis is common in areas where *B. melitensis* is endemic. Infection during pregnancy can result in abortion if the disease is untreated. Accidental inoculation of live-attenuated animal vaccines (e.g., *B. abortus* strain 19 or *B. melitensis* strain Rev-1) can result in human infection. The new *B. abortus* vaccine RB51 appears to be less virulent for humans.

LABORATORY FINDINGS

Routine tests are of little value for diagnosing brucellosis, although leukopenia is a characteristic finding. A definitive diagnosis is made by isolating brucellae from blood, bone marrow, or other tissue (Fig. 285.2). Growth of the organism in vitro is slow and prolonged incubation is advised. Differentiation of *Brucella* species is best reserved for specialized facilities since routine handling of cultures poses a risk to personnel and some automated identification systems can result in a misdiagnosis. A presumptive diagnosis is made by showing high or rising titers of specific antibodies in serum (Fig. 285.2). A variety of serologic tests are available, including agglutination and enzyme-linked immunosorbent assay (ELISA). Smooth lipopolysaccharide (SLPS) is the immunodominant epitope, and serologic tests using this antigen can identify the three major nomen species. *Brucella canis* lacks SLPS and tests to diagnose this species require monospecific antigen. With treatment, levels of IgM and IgG

TABLE 285.1.	COMPLICATIONS OF HUMAN BRUCELLOSIS
Organ System	**Complications**
Osteoarticular	Sacroillitis
	Arthritis (large joints predominate)
	Spondylitis
	Osteomyelitis
	Reactive arthropathy
	Paravertebral abscess
Gastrointestinal	Peritonitis
	Ileitis
	Colitis
Hepatobiliary	Hepatitis
	Cholecystitis
	Pancreatitis
Genitourinary	Orchitis
	Epididymitis
	Pyelonephritis
Respiratory	Pneumonia/pneumonitis
	Empyema
	Lung abscess
Neurologic	Meningitis/encephalitis
	Brain abscess
	Radiculitis
	Peripheral neuritis
	Myelitis
Cardiovascular	Endocarditis
	Pericarditis
	Aneurysms
Ophthalmic	Uveitis
	Optic neuritis
	Optic atrophy
Cutaneous	Rashes
	Cellulitis
	Vasculitis
	Abscesses

antibodies decline slowly over time. Persistent elevation of IgG isotype antibodies presages relapse or chronic infection.

OPTIMAL MANAGEMENT

Hospitalization is usually required to make the diagnosis. Mortality from brucellosis is rare and is usually associated with complications of endocarditis. Chronic infection is uncommon but can result from localized disease that may require surgical intervention. A variety of drugs are active against brucellae, but prolonged treatment (4 to 6 weeks) is necessary owing to the intracellular location of the bacteria. The β-lactam antibiotics are clinically ineffective. Doxycycline (200 mg daily) plus rifampin (600 to 900 mg daily) administered orally for 6 weeks is generally effective therapy. Many authorities still prefer doxycycline for 6 weeks plus streptomycin (1 g daily) administered intramuscularly for the first 3 weeks. Gentamicin is often substituted for streptomycin, but the optimal length of therapy has not been determined. Relapse is common, usually due to inadequate therapy. Since antibiotic resistance is rare, most relapses are treated with a second course of the same agents. Treatment of pregnant women and children younger than 6 years, for whom tetracyclines are contraindicated, remains controversial. Drugs such as

TULAREMIA — counties reporting cases, United States, 1993

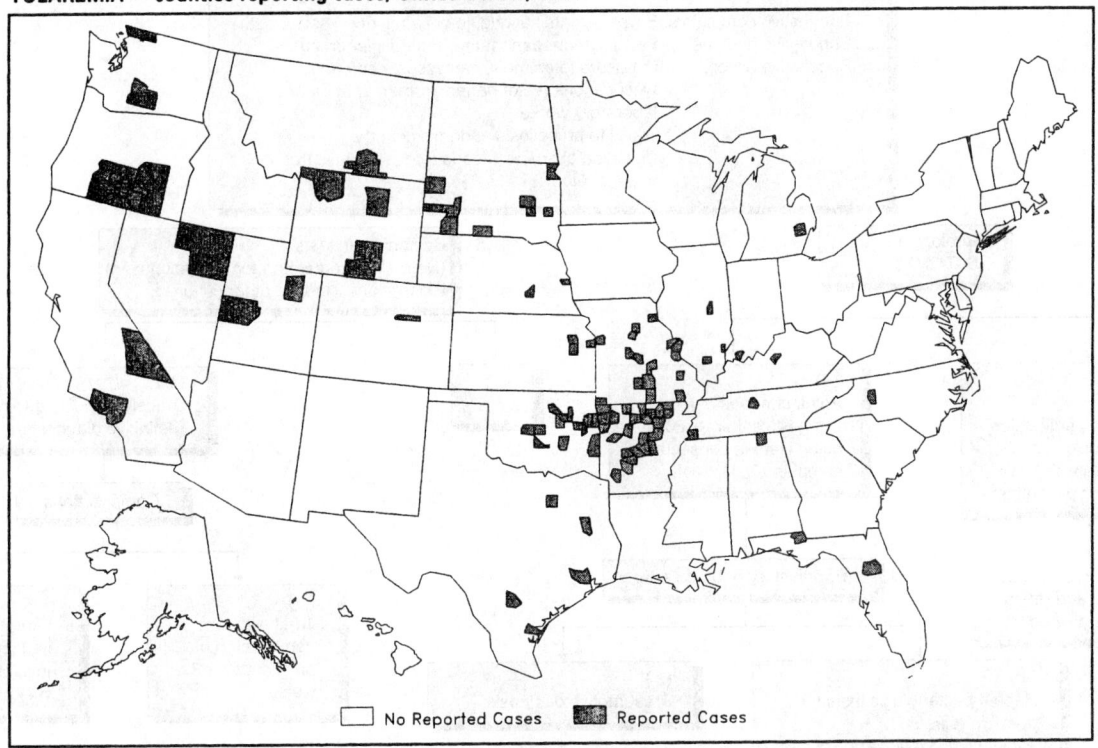

FIGURE 285.2. Number of reported cases of tularemia by year, United States, 1945–1993.

trimethoprim–sulfamethoxazole (TMP-SMX) (4 tablets in fixed dosage) for 6 weeks with or without rifampin have been used with some success. Fluoroquinolones administered orally for 6 weeks with rifampin or TMP-SMX have also been used, but monotherapy is never an option. Treatment of complications, such as meningitis or endocarditis, may require even longer courses of therapy, and valve replacement surgery is usually required.

◼ TULAREMIA

DEFINITION

Tularemia is an infection with variable clinical manifestations depending on the route of inoculation caused by *Francisella tularensis*.

INCIDENCE AND EPIDEMIOLOGIC FACTORS

Tularemia is endemic throughout the temperate zone of the Northern Hemisphere except in the British Isles. In the United States, the incidence of human infection is low (approximately 0.05 case per 100,000 population). Human tularemia has been reported from all states except Hawaii, but it is most prevalent in the western and midwestern regions (Fig. 285.3). Rodents and rabbits are the principal animal hosts, although more than 100 wild and domestic animals and birds are susceptible. Cases occurring during the summer are usually related to arthropod

bites, whereas direct contact with diseased animals accounts for most cases in the fall and winter. Contaminated water and undercooked meat are rare sources of infection.

ETIOLOGIC FACTORS

The genus *Francisella* contains three biovars: *tularensis*, which predominates in North America; *palaearctica*, which predominates in Europe and Asia; and *novicida*. *F. tularensis* is a small, nonmotile, nonsporulating, aerobic, gram-negative coccobacillus. It is nutritionally fastidious, requiring glucose–cysteine agar for isolation. It produces no exotoxins but is surrounded by a capsule-like material containing carbohydrate, protein, and large amounts of lipid. It is a hazard to laboratory personnel, and biohazard precautions are necessary when infectious material must be handled.

PATHOGENESIS

Traditionally, tularemia was classified into different types (ulceroglandular, glandular, oculoglandular, typhoidal) depending on the mode of inoculation. Routes of transmission include direct contact with diseased animals, bites of arthropod vectors (ticks, deerflies, mosquitoes), bites from domestic animals (cats) that have ingested infected rodents, inhalation of contaminated aerosols, and, rarely, ingestion of contaminated water or food.

As few as 10 to 50 *F. tularensis* organisms can cause infection when inoculated or inhaled, whereas 10^8 bacteria are required for oral infection. *F. tularensis* is a facultative intracellular patho-

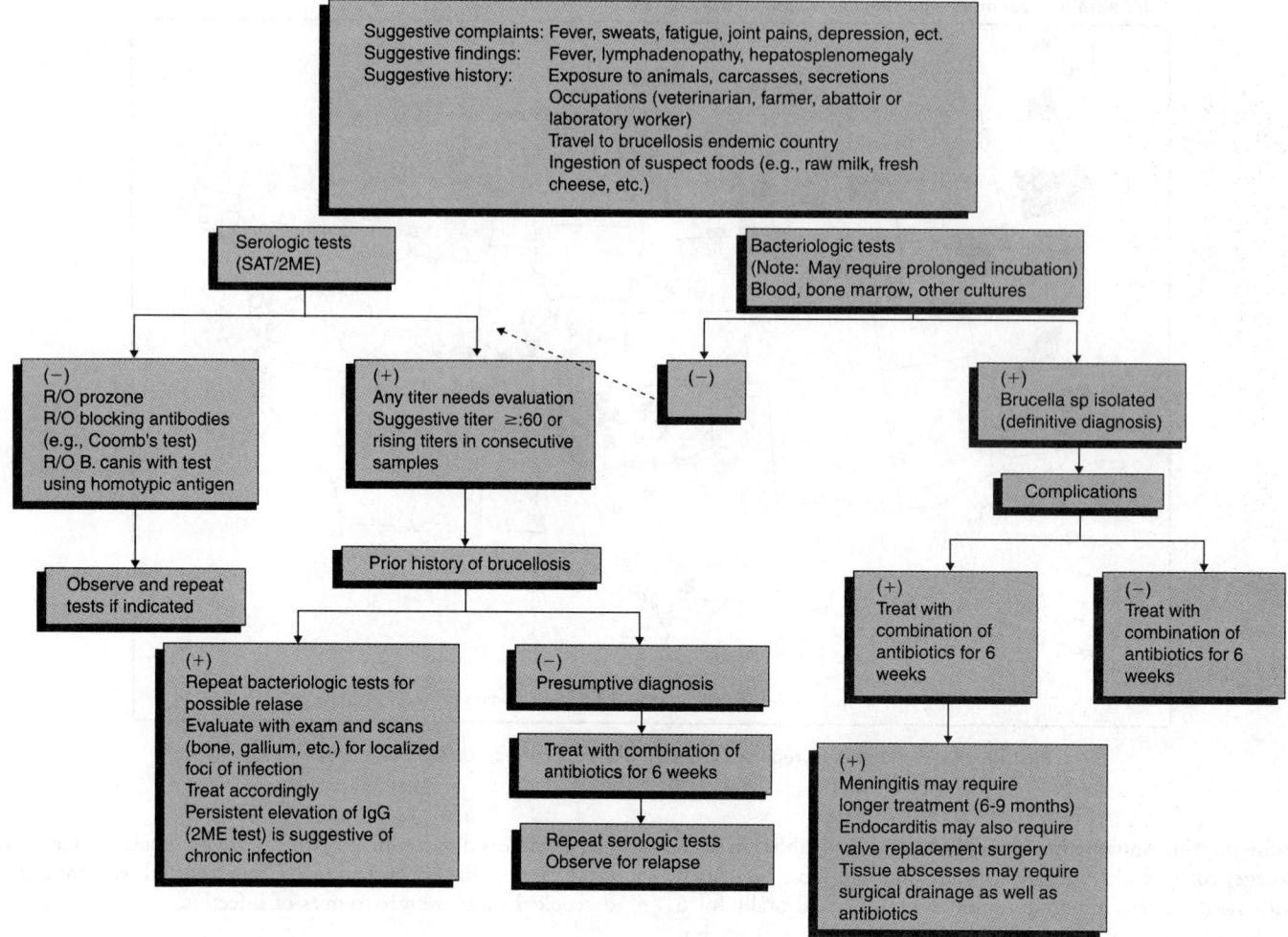

Suggestive complaints: Fever, sweats, fatigue, joint pains, depression, ect.
Suggestive findings: Fever, lymphadenopathy, hepatosplenomegaly
Suggestive history: Exposure to animals, carcasses, secretions
                         Occupations (veterinarian, farmer, abattoir or
                         laboratory worker)
                         Travel to brucellosis endemic country
                         Ingestion of suspect foods (e.g., raw milk, fresh
                         cheese, etc.)

Serologic tests (SAT/2ME)

(−)
R/O prozone
R/O blocking antibodies (e.g., Coomb's test)
R/O B. canis with test using homotypic antigen

(+)
Any titer needs evaluation
Suggestive titer ≥:60 or rising titers in consecutive samples

Bacteriologic tests
(Note: May require prolonged incubation)
Blood, bone marrow, other cultures

(−)

(+)
Brucella sp isolated (definitive diagnosis)

Complications

Observe and repeat tests if indicated

Prior history of brucellosis

(+)
Repeat bacteriologic tests for possible relase
Evaluate with exam and scans (bone, gallium, etc.) for localized foci of infection
Treat accordingly
Persistent elevation of IgG (2ME test) is suggestive of chronic infection

(−)
Presumptive diagnosis

Treat with combination of antibiotics for 6 weeks

Repeat serologic tests
Observe for relapse

(+)
Treat with combination of antibiotics for 6 weeks

(−)
Treat with combination of antibiotics for 6 weeks

(+)
Meningitis may require longer treatment (6-9 months)
Endocarditis may also require valve replacement surgery
Tissue abscesses may require surgical drainage as well as antibiotics

FIGURE 285.3. Approach to the patient with suspected brucellosis.

gen that survives within phagocytic cells of the host apparently by inhibiting phagosome–lysosome fusion. Before the development of immunity, granulocytes may inhibit the spread of tularemia in organs such as the liver by lysing parasitized hepatocytes. Immunospecific protection is afforded by natural infection or by vaccination with live attenuated strains of *F. tularensis*. Cellular immunity is the principal mechanism of recovery and resistance to tularemia.

CLINICAL FINDINGS

Fever, a cutaneous ulcer, and lymphadenopathy are the most commonly reported symptoms of tularemia (Table 285.2). Depending on the location of the tick bite, the most common areas of lymphadenopathy are inguinal, axillary, and cervical chains. Cutaneous ulcers are reported in about 85% of cases, involving the fingers, hands, legs, head, neck, and buttocks. Patients with pleuropulmonary tularemia present with fever, chest pain, cough, purulent sputum, and patchy alveolar infiltrates. Rarely, foodborne tularemia manifests as an exudative pharyngotonsillitis or mesenteric adenitis. Typhoidal tularemia results from hematogenous spread and can produce cutaneous, pulmonary,

and gastrointestinal symptoms. Patients experience fever, chills, confusion, meningismus, vomiting, and diarrhea; cutaneous lesions and lymphadenitis may be absent. Left untreated the typhoidal form is fatal in 30% to 40% of cases.

LABORATORY FINDINGS

Because *F. tularensis* is rarely seen in Gram-stained specimens and special medium is required for isolation, the diagnosis is usually made by serologic tests. Serum agglutinins are detectable within 10 to 14 days and a fourfold rise in titer is diagnostic. A single titer higher than 1 : 160 in a patient with compatible clinical findings is also considered diagnostic. Titers can remain elevated for years after an acute infection. Cross-reactions have been reported with other gram-negative bacteria, but usually in low titer. An ELISA and polymerase chain reaction have been used for diagnosis when the agglutination test yields equivocal results.

OPTIMAL MANAGEMENT

Before the introduction of antibiotics, tularemia was fatal in up to 15% of cases. The mortality has declined to about 1%, with

TABLE 285.2.	CLINICAL MANIFESTATIONS OF TULAREMIA			
Clinical Type	**Route of Transmission**	**Findings**	**Frequency**	**Mortality**
Ulceroglandular	Contact with infected animals Insect bites Animal bites	Fever Flulike symptoms Cutaneous papule (ulcerated) Lymphadenitis (generalized)	70%–80%	Low
Glandular	Same as for ulceroglandular	Same as for ulceroglandular, but lacking cutaneous lesion	10%–15%	Low
Oculoglandular	Inoculation into the conjunctival sac	Fever Conjunctivitis Periorbital inflammation Lymphangitis (regional)	1%–5%	Low
Pleuropulmonary	Inhalation of contaminated aerosol Hematogenous spread	Fever Pneumonia Pleural effusion	1%–5%	High
Oropharyngeal	Ingestion of contaminated food or water	Fever Tonsillitis (unilateral) Peritonsillar abscess Lymphangitis (regional)	Rare	Low
Typhoidal	Hematogenous spread	Fever Rigor Malaise Abdominal pain Nausea/vomiting Diarrhea Hepatitis Pneumonia Pericarditis Meningitis	Rare	High

typhoidal and pulmonary forms carrying the greatest risk. Streptomycin (7.5 to 10 mg per kilogram twice daily intramuscularly) has long been the recommended drug of choice, although gentamicin, tetracycline, and chloramphenicol are acceptable alternatives. An aminoglycoside is recommended as initial therapy for seriously ill patients, followed by tetracycline (2 g daily by mouth) for 3 to 4 weeks to prevent relapse. Fluoroquinolones have also been used, but their role as primary therapy awaits the results of larger trials. β-Lactam antibiotics including third-generation cephalosporins are not effective therapy.

PASTEURELLOSIS

DEFINITION

Pasteurellosis is an infection caused by members of the genus *Pasteurella*, most commonly *P. multocida*.

INCIDENCE AND EPIDEMIOLOGIC FACTORS

Pasteurella multocida, the species most often isolated from human specimens, is a normal inhabitant of the nasopharynx and intestines of a variety of animals and birds worldwide. Although a history of animal exposure is not always obtained, the majority of human infections are associated with bite or scratch wounds from animals (notably cats and dogs). Occasionally, the organism is recovered from respiratory secretions of healthy

persons who have close contact with animals. There is no evidence of foodborne or waterborne spread, nor is there person-to-person transmission. Cases have been reported after contact with inanimate objects soiled by animals.

ETIOLOGIC FACTORS

Pasteurellae are primarily animal pathogens causing diseases such as "shipping fever" in cattle or fowl cholera in birds. Once classified according to host species, in recent years, the taxonomy of pasteurellae has undergone changes based on DNA–DNA hybridization and 16S rRNA sequencing studies. The family *Pasteurellaceae* comprises *Pasteurella* species, *Haemophilus* species, and *Actinobacillus* species. Currently, *Pasteurella sensu stricto* includes 11 species and 3 subspecies of which *P. multocida* subspecies *multocida* and *septica*, *P. canis*, *P. stomatis*, and *P. dogmatis* account for the majority of human isolates. The organisms are small, encapsulated, aerobic, bipolar staining, gram-negative coccobacilli lacking flagella or endospores. They grow on blood, chocolate, and Mueller–Hinton media but not on MacConkey's agar.

PATHOGENESIS

After inoculation through cuts or abrasions in the skin, *P. multocida* multiplies rapidly in the extracellular space, invades the bloodstream, and localizes within the reticuloendothelial system. Little is known about virulence factors except for the capsule that inhibits phagocytosis and the cell wall that contains endotoxin and neuraminidase.

CLINICAL FINDINGS

Soft-tissue infection caused by *P. multocida* cannot be distinguished clinically from infections caused by more common pathogens such as streptococci. Wound infections usually respond to local care plus antibiotics, but patients with underlying liver disease, alcoholism, or immunosuppression are predisposed to hematogenous dissemination.

Infections of sinuses, pharynx, trachea, and lungs have been reported with a clear predilection for the compromised host. Cardiovascular complications include native and prosthetic valve endocarditis. Osteoarticular complications usually follow penetrating animal bites (notably cats) and septic arthritis is common in patients with preexisting inflammatory joint diseases. Central nervous system infections occur in less than 5% of cases, but meningitis, brain abscess, and subdural empyema are reported. Gastrointestinal complications include peritonitis, appendicitis, intra-abdominal abscess, and postoperative infections. Rare genitourinary infections are usually associated with preexisting cancer, ureterostomy, or ureteroileostomy. Ophthalmic manifestations are least common but can occur from direct trauma to the eyes involving animals.

OPTIMAL MANAGEMENT

Pasteurellae are almost universally sensitive to penicillin and ampicillin although rare penicillin-resistant strains are known. Alternative drugs include third-generation cephalosporins, tetracycline, chloramphenicol, and trimethoprim-sulfamethoxazole. Most strains are resistant to aminoglycosides. Experience with quinolones is limited, but ciprofloxacin is active in vitro. The duration of therapy depends on the primary disease process.

▉ YERSINIOSIS (INCLUDING PLAGUE)

Although the *Yersinia* species causing plague (*Y. pestis*) and the nonplague yersinioses (*Y. enterocolitica* and *Y. pseudotuberculosis*) are related, they are traditionally discussed separately because they differ in their epidemiologic factors and clinical manifestations.

DEFINITIONS

Plague is an acute, potentially lethal infection caused by *Yersinia pestis*. Yersiniosis is an infection caused by either of the enteropathogenic *Yersinia* species: *Y. enterocolitica* or *Y. pseudotuberculosis*.

ETIOLOGIC FACTORS

The *Yersinia* species are aerobic, gram-negative coccobacilli belonging to the family Enterobacteriaceae and are therefore lactose-negative. *Y. pestis* is nonmotile at all temperatures, whereas *Y. enterocolitica* and *Y. pseudotuberculosis* are motile at 25°C but not at 37°C. Differentiation of species is based on biochemical reactions, phage lysis patterns, and virulence for animals. A rapid identification of *Y. pestis* can be made using a specific fluorescent antibody.

PATHOGENESIS

The virulence of pathogenic *Yersinia* species appears to be related to a number of factors, some encoded by the bacterial genome, others by plasmids. A plasmid-mediated, capsule-like glycoprotein (fraction 1) of *Y. pestis* interferes with phagocytosis, and antibodies to this substance confer immunity. The ability to synthesize endogenous purines is a characteristic of virulent *Yersinia* species and appears to facilitate intracellular survival. The V and W antigens, closely linked to the expression of free calcium (Ca^{2+}) dependence, are encoded by a 75-kb plasmid and are important for intracellular survival. *Y. pestis*, *Y. enterocolitica* serotype 1B, and *Y. pseudotuberculosis* 0:1 strains possess a chromosomal determinant that is involved in iron uptake mediated by the siderophore yersiniabactin. This iron acquisition determinant (designated HPI for high-pathogenicity island) is necessary for virulence in mice. A plasmid-mediated bacteriocin (pestin), outer-membrane proteins, a heat-labile exotoxin, and endotoxin are additional virulence factors of *Y. pestis*. Genome-encoded proteins (invasins) of *Yersinia* species mediate endocytosis, which enhances their ability to invade intestinal mucosal cells.

LABORATORY FINDINGS

Yersinia pestis is readily isolated from clinical specimens, whereas special techniques are required for other *Yersinia* species. Bubonic plague can be diagnosed by smear and culture of bubo aspirate. *Y. enterocolitica* and *Y. pseudotuberculosis* can be readily isolated from otherwise sterile sites, such as blood, peritoneal fluid, or mesenteric lymph nodes. Recovery from feces requires selective media, such as cefsulodin–triclosan–novobiocin agar incubated at 25°C for 18 to 20 hours. Cold enrichment (4°C) of stool specimens in phosphate-buffered saline subcultured weekly for 4 weeks has been used to enhance recovery of small numbers of bacteria. Serologic tests can also be used for diagnosis; however, *Y. enterocolitica* O:9 is known to cross-react with *B. abortus* and *Escherichia coli*.

EPIDEMIOLOGY OF PLAGUE

Yersinia pestis exists worldwide, especially in developing countries. It is responsible for four great pandemics of human disease. Factors contributing to pandemic plague are epizootics in nature, poor sanitation, war, and famine. The most important *urban* reservoir of *Y. pestis* is rats. The principal *sylvatic* reservoir of plague in the United States is wild rodents such as ground squirrels and prairie dogs. Humans contract plague from the bite of fleas, from direct contact with diseased animals, or from contaminated aerosols.

Domestic cats and dogs can become infected and on occasion transmit plague to humans via bites, scratches, or aerosols. Person-to-person spread is rare except for cases of pneumonic plague.

CLINICAL FINDINGS IN PLAGUE

Bubonic plague accounts for 80% to 90% of cases of human infection with *Y. pestis*. The disease begins 2 to 8 days after the bite of an infected flea and is characterized by the rapid onset of fever and painful regional lymphadenopathy (buboes). Buboes, usually in the groin, axilla, or neck depending on the location of the bite, are exquisitely painful. Most patients experience transient (often asymptomatic) bacteremia. Bacteremia in the absence of buboes is termed *septicemic* plague, an illness with a grave prognosis. Although similar in presentation to sepsis caused by other bacteria, septicemic plague has a higher mortality, in part due to the high-grade bacteremia. Gastrointestinal symptoms are common, including vomiting, diarrhea, and abdominal pain. Another ominous finding is purpura, associated with disseminated intravascular coagulation. *Pneumonic* plague is a rare but greatly feared complication of hematogenous dissemination or direct inhalation of contaminated aerosols. The sputum usually contains organisms visible by Gram stain and the mortality is high despite antibiotic therapy. Plague *meningitis* is another rare but lethal complication that typically occurs more than a week after inadequately treated bubonic plague.

EPIDEMIOLOGY OF NONPLAGUE YERSINIOSES

Yersinia enterocolitica exists worldwide but appears to be more prevalent in cooler climates. Certain serotypes predominate in different geographic areas, with most human infections caused by types O:3, O:5, O:8, O:9, and O:27. The bacteria are found in the oropharynx and intestines of wild and domestic animals and in shellfish. They have also been recovered from water of lakes and streams and from unpasteurized animal milk. Person-to-person spread is rare, but cases have been traced to transfusions of refrigerated banked blood. *Y. pseudotuberculosis* resides in many of the same animals but is also found extensively in birds.

CLINICAL FINDINGS OF NONPLAGUE YERSINIOSES

The spectrum of disease caused by *Y. enterocolitica* ranges from self-limited infection to potentially fatal septicemia and post-infectious complications. The alimentary tract is the portal of entry in most cases, and enterocolitis is the presenting feature in two thirds of cases. After an incubation period of 4 to 7 days, patients present with fever, abdominal pain, and diarrhea lasting for 1 to 3 weeks. Most patients with enterocolitis are younger than 5 years, whereas older children and adults present with mesenteric adenitis that is indistinguishable from acute appendicitis. Focal extra-intestinal manifestations include pharyngitis; soft-tissue infection; osteomyelitis; and urinary, lung, and eye infections. Bacteremia, with and without seeding of other organs, is reported in patients with underlying diseases, such as alcoholism, cirrhosis, hemochromatosis, malnutrition, and malignancies. Septicemia has a mortality of 30% to 50%. Postinfectious complications include reactive polyarthritis, usually beginning days to a month after the onset of diarrhea and lasting for several months. Arthropathy is more common in patients who have the HLA allele B27 and molecular mimicry is postulated to be the mechanism for this association. The clinical features of *Y. pseudotuberculosis* infection resemble those of *Y. enterocolitica*, except that mesenteric adenitis is more common than enterocolitis.

OPTIMAL MANAGEMENT

The case fatality from untreated plague is at least 50%, especially with septicemic, pneumonic, and meningeal forms. Early diagnosis and treatment significantly reduces mortality. Streptomycin (30 mg per kilogram per day) intramuscularly in two divided doses for 10 days is the treatment of choice. No other drug has been shown to be more efficacious or less toxic. For patients with meningitis, chloramphenicol (75 mg per kilogram per day) intramuscularly in four divided doses for 10 days is recommended. Oral tetracycline (2 g per day) has been used for prophylaxis. A formalin-killed *Y. pestis* vaccine is recommended for laboratory personnel working with plague. The value of antimicrobial therapy for *Y. enterocolitica* and *Y. pseudotuberculosis* enterocolitis and mesenteric adenitis is unproven. Intestinal infections are usually self-limited. For patients with septicemia or other complications, intravenous gentamicin (5 mg per kilogram per day) alone or in combination with a third-generation cephalosporin (ceftriaxone or cefotaxime) has been suggested. Alternatively, TMP-SMX, doxycycline, and ciprofloxacin have been used. For serious infections with *Y. pseudotuberculosis*, intravenous ampicillin (100 to 200 mg per kilogram per day), streptomycin (20 to 30 mg per kilogram per day), or tetracycline (20 to 30 mg per kilogram per day) in divided doses has been used. The mortality from *Y. pseudotuberculosis* septicemia is 75% despite antibiotic therapy.

BIBLIOGRAPHY

Brucellosis

Solera J, Martinez-Alfaro E, Espinosa A. Recognition and optimum treatment of brucellosis. *Drugs* 1997;53:245–256.

Young EJ. Serologic diagnosis of human brucellosis: analysis of 214 cases by agglutination tests and review of the literature. *Rev Infect Dis* 1991; 13:359–372.

Young EJ. An overview of human brucellosis. *Clin Infect Dis* 1995;21: 283–290.

Tularemia

Cross JT, Jacobs RF. Tularemia: treatment failures with outpatient use of ceftriaxone. *Clin Infect Dis* 1993;17:976–980.

Evans ME, Gregory DW, Schaffner W, et al. Tularemia: a 30-year experience with 88 cases. *Medicine* 1985;64:251–269.

Tarnvik A, Eriksson M, Sandstrom G, et al. *Francisella tularesis*: a model for studies of the immune response to intracellular bacteria in man. *Immunology* 1992:76:349–354.

Pasteurellosis

Frederiksen W. Ecology and significance of pasteurellaceae in man-an update. *Int J Med Microbiol Virol Parisitol Infect Dis* 1993;279:27–34.

Kumar A, Devlin HR, Vellend H. *Pasteurella multocida* meningitis in an adult: case report and review. *Rev Infect Dis* 1990;12:440–448.

Weber DJ, Wolfson JS, Swartz MN, et al. *Pasteurella multocida* infections: report of 32 cases and review of the literature. *Medicine* 1984;63: 133–154.

Yersinioses

Brubaker RR. Factors promoting acute and chronic diseases caused by *Yersinia. Clin Microbiol Rev* 1991;4:309–324.

Butler T. *Yersinia* infections: centennial of the discovery of the plague bacillus. *Clin Infect Dis* 1994;19:655–663.

Crook LD, Tempest B. Plague: a clinical review of 27 cases. *Arch Intern Med* 1992;152:1253–1256.

Gayrand M, Scavizzi MR, Mollaret HH, et al. Antibiotic treatment of *Yersinia enterocolitica* septicemia: a retrospective review of 43 cases. *Clin Infect Dis* 1993;17:405–410.

Johnson RH: *Yersinia* infections. *Curr Opin Infect Dis* 1992;5: 654.

Verhaegen J, Charlier J, Lemmens P, et al. Surveillance of human *Yersinia enterocolitica* infections in Belgium: 1967–1996. *Clin Infect Dis* 1998; 27:59–64.

Kelley's Textbook of Internal Medicine, fourth edition. Edited by H. David Humes.
Lippincott Williams & Wilkins, Philadelphia © 2000.

CHAPTER
286

INFECTIONS CAUSED BY *HAEMOPHILUS* AND *BORDETELLA* SPECIES

**CHARLES J. SCHLEUPNER
KENNETH M. SOSNOWSKI**

◼ *HAEMOPHILUS* INFECTIONS

Haemophilus influenzae type B is the major invasive pathogen of this genus, especially in infants and children younger than 2 years of age. However, it also causes disease in adolescents and adults. The nontypable strains of *H. influenzae* are more commonly seen in patients with noninvasive disease and when host defenses are compromised. A biotype of *H. influenzae,* biogroup *aegyptius,* is the causative agent for Brazilian purpuric fever. *Haemophilus ducreyi* is a sexually transmissible pathogen that results in chancroid. The other *Haemophilus* species are less common causes of serious adult infections.

INCIDENCE AND EPIDEMIOLOGY

Haemophilus species are part of the normal flora of the pharynx and, to a lesser extent, the genital tract (excluding *H. ducreyi*).

The prevalence of nontypable *H. influenzae* colonization in the pharynx has been reported to be as high as 50% to 80% in healthy adults, whereas encapsulated (50% type B) strains are present in only 5% of healthy individuals. Carriers usually remain healthy. Table 286.1 lists the strains of *H. influenzae* that have been implicated as primary pathogens in both invasive and noninvasive diseases. Type B *H. influenzae* causes 95% of invasive disease in children and bacteremic infection in adults. Meningitis and epiglottitis have accounted for 68% to 80% of all bacteremic *H. influenzae* infections. *H. influenzae* type B was previously the leading cause of bacterial meningitis in children but has dramatically declined over the last 10 years—in some studies by as much as 86%.

In the past, about 8,000 cases occurred annually in the United States, but because invasive infections due to *H. influenzae* are not reportable to the public health departments in all states, infection rates are not accurate. Overall during 1998, only 1,023 cases of invasive *H. influenzae* disease were reported to the Centers for Disease Control and Prevention (CDC). Serious invasive infections occur more often in male children and adults, blacks, lower socioeconomic families, Alaskan Eskimos, and Navajo and Apache Indians, and during winter months. Children exposed by close contact to children with invasive *H. influenzae* type B disease have high colonization rates (up to 50%) and those younger than 2 years of age have up to a 500 times greater risk of secondary disease if not previously immunized.

The noninvasive diseases due to *H. influenzae* type B (bronchitis, otitis media, conjunctivitis) are more common but less serious overall; they tend to occur in all age groups. Invasive disease due to the nontypable strains of *H. influenzae* is uncommon and usually results from a compromise of the normal host defenses, such as occurs with chronic lung disease, AIDS, asplenia (anatomical or functional), chronic lymphocytic leukemia, multiple myeloma, a cerebrospinal fluid (CSF) leak, or prior head trauma, among other causes. The most common form of invasive infection is pneumonia in the elderly and in patients with chronic bronchitis. The most common forms of noninvasive infection due to the nontypable strains are sinusitis, otitis media, and conjunctivitis.

Other *Haemophilus* species less frequently cause disease and have a low pathogenicity. *Haemophilus parainfluenzae, Haemophilus parahaemolyticus, Haemophilus aphrophilus,* and others are part of the normal oral and pharyngeal flora of healthy people. Disease results from a lapse in host defenses leading to local or systemic infection. *H. ducreyi* infection is discussed in Chapter 288.

ETIOLOGY

Haemophilus species are small gram-negative, pleomorphic (cocco-) baccilli with specific growth requirements for X factor (hemin) or V factor (a coenzyme, nicotinamide adenine dinucleotide). *Haemophilus* species with the prefix "para" *(H. parainfluenzae, H. paraphrophilus,* and *H. parahaemolyticus)* require only the V factor for growth, whereas *H. aphrophilus* and H. ducreyi require only the X factor. The remaining clinically significant species, *H. influenzae* and *H. hemolyticus,* require both factors. *Haemophilus* (blood seeking) refers to the original source

TABLE 286.1.	**DISEASES ASSOCIATED WITH HAEMOPHILUS SPECIES**	
Haemophilus Species	**Classification**	**Type**
H. influenzae type b	Invasive, often with bacteremia	Meningitis, epiglottitis, endophthalmitis, cellulitis, osteomyelitis, septic arthritis, primary bacteremia, pneumonia
H. influenzae, biogroup *aegyptius*	Invasive, usually bacteremia	Brazilian purpuric fever
H. influenze, nontypable	Invasive, usually without bacteremia Noninvasive	Pneumonia, neonatal and maternal infections Otitis media, sinusitis, conjunctivitis, bronchitis
H. parainfluenzae, H. aphrophilus, H. paraphrophilus	Invasive and noninvasive (occasionally)	Endocarditis, sinusitis, otitis media, conjunctivitis, epiglottitis, pharyngitis, CNS infections, bone infections, genitourinary infections, hepatobiliary infections
H. ducreyi		Chancroid

of its required growth factors. However, *H. influenzae* cannot be grown on standard blood agar because the V factor is available only after being released from erythrocytes by heating the blood (chocolate agar). The phenomenon of "satelliting" refers to the growth of V factor requiring *Haemophilus* species on standard sheep blood agar only in the proximity of colonies of *Staphylococcus aureus*, which may secrete V factor or cause V factor to be released from erythrocytes by hemolysis. Isolation of these organisms is improved by prompt inoculation of clinical specimens and incubation in a humidified environment containing 5% to 10% carbon dioxide. When gram-stained, these organisms may be morphologically confusing, because although they appear coccobacillary in clinical specimens, they may appear filamentous in culture.

H. influenzae isolates can be differentiated into six serotypes (A through F) based on antigenically and biochemically distinct polysaccharide capsules, which are virulence factors. Type B encapsulated organisms are the most pathogenic, although all five other serotypes and nontypable organisms may also be pathogens.

PATHOGENESIS

The determinants of colonization with *H. influenzae* are not well understood. The organism potentially may express four types of fimbriae, one of which mediates epithelial adherence (and hemagglutination by way of the blood group antigen Anton). The role of fimbriae in virulence is unclear, because most nonencapsulated strains are fimbricated; however, this has not correlated with pathogenicity. Furthermore, fimbriae are lost during invasion, and this lack of fimbriae makes organisms less susceptible to phagocytosis. Some strains (encapsulated or unencapsulated) elaborate one or more cilioinhibitory factors that may impair clearance and thus enhance replication of the organism. These effects may ultimately lead to mucus penetration and binding to epithelial receptors. Nontypable *H. influenza* binds to human buccal and nasopharyngeal epithelial cells better than encapsulated strains.

H. influenzae secretes an IgA1 protease, but its role in virulence is unclear. Synthesis of histamine by *H. influenzae* may contribute to bronchoconstriction in pulmonary infection. The lipopolysaccharide of *H. influenzae* may play a role in damage

to the respiratory epithelium, thereby potentiating invasion. The peptidoglycan of *H. influenzae* type B plays a major role in the pathogenesis of meningitis by increasing blood–brain barrier permeability and CSF leukocytosis; the latter is also enhanced by the *H. influenzae* lipopolysaccharide.

The most important virulence factor for encapsulated *H. influenzae* is the polysaccharide capsule, a polymer of ribosyl ribitol phosphate (PRP). Type B capsule impedes phagocytosis in the absence of antibody (or other opsonic factors). Antibody to the PRP capsule enhances complement activation, opsonization, phagocytosis, and killing of the organism and is the major determinant of immunity in humans. The mechanism for acquisition of antibody to PRP by age 3 to 4 years in unimmunized persons is not well understood. The antibody response to initial type B *H. influenzae* infection in children 12 months of age or younger is poor owing to the limited antibody response of infants to T-cell–independent antigens, thereby allowing for recurrent infections.

The pathogenesis of infection with other *Haemophilus* species is primarily related to a lapse of a host defense. The roles of serum and secretory antibody against nontypable *H. influenzae* and the other *Haemophilus* species remain unclear. The role of mucosal immunity is also not well understood. The complement system plays a major role in the defense against both encapsulated and unencapsulated *Haemophilus* species in both immune and nonimmune hosts. Genetic deficiencies of selected complement components (e.g., C2, C3, C4) enhance the disease potential of *H. influenzae*.

CLINICAL FINDINGS

Meningitis

Meningitis due to type B *H. influenzae* is the most serious manifestation of invasive infection caused by this organism. In neonates, *H. influenzae* meningitis is rare. However, although it was previously the most common cause of meningitis in children from age 6 months to 5 years and was responsible for up to 20% of bacterial meningitis in adults, the incidence of *H. influenzae* meningitis has dramatically declined since 1985 in children older than 6 months. In children, an antecedent upper respiratory infection, commonly otitis media, is usual. In adults, antecedent head trauma, neurosurgery, sinusitis, otitis, or a CSF leak is found in two-thirds of cases. In adults, approximately 50% of cases are caused by nontypable organisms, whereas most episodes in children result from type B strains. The most common signs are fever and an altered mental status. In a child younger than 1 year of age, the disease may be fulminant with death occurring in a few hours; however, acute deterioration usually follows several days of mild upper respiratory illness. In adults, the pathogenesis involves contiguous spread from a primary site of infection, and the illness resembles other forms of acute bacterial meningitis. Associated bacteremia is more common in children than in adults. Coma and bacteremia in adults predict a worse outcome. Mortality rate may be up to 20% to 30% in adults, whereas less than 5% of childhood cases are fatal with therapy. Up to 50% of children even with appropriate antibiotic therapy are left with neurologic sequelae, including hearing and cognitive impairment and seizures. Subdural effusions are also a common complication. Data on the declining incidence of these sequelae are evolving.

Pneumonia and Tracheobronchitis

Primary lung infection due to nontypable *H. influenzae* occurs in adults and in children, especially in infants in developing countries, and has been associated with nosocomial spread resulting in both colonization and respiratory infection. In adults, *H. influenzae* is second only to *Streptococcus pneumoniae* as the most common cause of community-acquired pneumonia. The typical adult patient with invasive *H. influenzae* pneumonia is older than 60 years of age with evidence of chronic pulmonary disease, alcoholism, malignancy, use of steroids, diabetes mellitus, or a recent viral infection, especially influenza. Younger adults with *H. influenzae* pneumonia usually have evidence of alcohol abuse or AIDS, or have an invasive infection associated with other chronic immunocompromising diseases. Type B strains may be responsible only for up to 15% of pneumonia due to *H. influenzae* in adults, and are more frequently associated with bacteremia. Overall, up to 10% to 20% of pneumonias in adults are bacteremic.

The clinical and radiologic findings of *H. influenzae* pneumonia are indistinguishable from those of other bacterial pneumonias. Segmental lobar consolidation occurs frequently, but bronchopneumonia and diffuse interstitial disease have been observed. Cavitary disease and empyema occur; sterile parapneumonic effusions may occur in up to 50% of patients. A form of purulent, febrile tracheobronchitis due to nontypable *H. influenzae* has been reported. The clinical features of patients with a tracheobronchitis are indistinguishable from those with pneumonia; however, the two syndromes can be distinguished by chest radiography.

H. influenzae can be recovered from sputum of most patients with chronic bronchitis, often worsened by prior viral infection. Thus, the presence of the organism in sputum does not necessarily imply a pathogenic role in exacerbations of chronic bronchitis. However, nontypable *H. influenzae* is cultured more frequently during exacerbations of bronchitis than during symptom-free periods. The exact role of these organisms in exacerbations of chronic bronchitis remains controversial. Curiously,

tobacco and nicotine have been shown in vitro to stimulate growth of *H. influenzae*.

Other Respiratory Tract Infections

H. influenzae has been isolated from 20% of infants and children with acute otitis media, most commonly from children 6 months to 5 years old. Up to 90% of these strains are nontypable. *H. influenzae* has also been isolated from middle ear aspirates of adults with otitis media, but the prevalence of nontypable organisms in adults is unknown. Nontypable *H. influenzae* is also a common cause of sinusitis in children and adults. Acute epiglottitis (a cellulitis of supraglottic tissue) is a fulminant illness that occurs most often in children 2 to 7 years old, but also has been reported increasingly frequently in adults. In children, the disease typically has an explosive onset, with sore throat, fever, and dyspnea progressing rapidly to acute respiratory obstruction; *H. influenzae* type B is the usual pathogen and is associated with bacteremia in 65% to 90% of cases. Because of use of vaccines since 1985, current data support a declining incidence of epiglottitis in children, with a shift to older ages (from a peak incidence at 36 months to 55 to 80 months) and to nonwhite patients. Since 1985, the incidence of *H. influenzae* type B epiglottitis has not appreciably changed in the adult population. In adults, *H. influenzae* remains the most commonly identified cause of epiglottitis, but bacteremia is less common. The mortality rate in adult cases of epiglottitis has been greater than in pediatric cases, presumably resulting from failure to consider this diagnosis early.

Septic Arthritis

H. influenzae has been the most common cause of infectious arthritis in unimmunized children younger than 2 years. In children, infection usually involves a single, large weight-bearing joint. In adults, *H. influenzae* accounts for less than 1% of all cases of nongonococcal infectious arthritis. About 75% of adult patients with *H. influenzae* arthritis have predisposing conditions, including connective tissue disease, splenectomy, diabetes mellitus, alcoholism, hypogammaglobulinemia, multiple myeloma, lymphoma, or trauma. Up to 50% of affected adults have multiarticular and 65% have extra-articular sites of infection.

Other Infections

Nontypable *H. influenzae* is a cause of genitourinary tract infection, including tubo-ovarian abscess and chronic salpingitis. The association of fetal or neonatal infections with *H. influenzae* genital tract infections in women (endometritis, amnionitis) has been well described, especially after premature rupture of the membranes. Urinary tract infections usually occur in the setting of instrumentation or structural abnormalities of the urinary tract. Facial or neck cellulitis due to *H. influenzae* type B has previously occurred commonly in children between the ages of 6 months and 3 years. Classically, this infection involves one cheek or periorbital area. Immunization of children with conjugated *H. influenzae* type B vaccines has caused a decline of this syndrome. Neck cellulitis has been reported in adults older than 50 years, who present with pharyngitis, high fever, and rapidly progressive anterior neck swelling. The characteristic red-purple hue of the skin described in children with cellulitis may be absent in adults. A number of unusual infections have been attributed to *H. influenzae* in various case reports, including endocarditis, cholecystitis, peritonitis, and epididymo-orchitis.

H. aegyptius (identical with *H. influenzae* biotype 3, the Koch–Weeks bacillus) is associated with a conjunctivitis in children, which may occur in outbreaks. More recently, *H. aegyptius* has been implicated as the causative agent of Brazilian purpuric fever, a fulminant systemic illness first reported in children in Brazil in 1984. This organism has been shown to be toxic to endothelial cells in vitro. The illness has a peak incidence in children 1 to 4 years old, characteristically begins with purulent conjunctivitis, and progresses in a small percentage of patients to a febrile illness with petechial or purpuric skin lesions. If untreated, some patients have experienced overwhelming endotoxemia and fatal shock.

Other *Haemophilus* Species

H. parainfluenzae causes a spectrum of disease similar to *H. influenzae*, including respiratory tract infections, pneumonia, empyema, meningitis, endocarditis, septic arthritis, and hepatobiliary, central nervous system, urinary tract, and genital infections, among others. Over the last decade, *Haemophilus* species (*H. parainfluenzae*, *H. aphrophilus*, *H. paraphrophilus*, and *H. influenzae*) have been recognized as causative agents in about 5% of cases of endocarditis, probably associated with improved microbiologic techniques. These organisms colonize the upper respiratory tract; thus, endocarditis may result from periodontal disease, dental manipulation, or respiratory tract infections. *Haemophilus* species belong to the HACEK group of fastidious gram-negative bacteria associated with the previously termed "culture-negative" endocarditis. The organisms usually cause disease in the setting of previous valvular heart disease, prosthetic valve implants, or intravenous drug abuse in young to middle-aged adults.

Persons with *Haemophilus* endocarditis usually present with subacute onset indistinguishable from endocarditis due to viridans streptococci. The single major distinguishing feature of endocarditis due to *Haemophilus* species is the common occurrence of large valvular vegetations and major arterial embolization, which may occur in up to 60% of cases. Delay in diagnosis and difficulty in isolating and identifying these fastidious organisms may account for the significant morbidity and mortality associated with this form of endocarditis.

LABORATORY FINDINGS

Confirmation of the diagnosis of infection due to *Haemophilus* species should be based on Gram's stain and culture of specific body fluids (e.g., blood, middle ear, sinus, CSF, or aspirates of cellulitis or joint spaces). In the absence of bacteremia, demonstration of the organism by Gram's stain in a sputum screened microscopically for cellular content must be interpreted in the context of an appropriate clinical syndrome. Specimens obtained

by transthyrocricoid membrane aspiration or bronchoscopy yield more specific (and sensitive) diagnostic information. In addition, the pleomorphic nature of the organism may make Gram's stain interpretation difficult. In cases of meningitis, positive CSF Gram's stains have been reported in only 50% to 70% of cases. Detection of capsular antigen in serum or other body fluids using immunoelectrophoresis, latex agglutination, or enzyme-linked immunosorbent assays (ELISAs) may be an adjunct to diagnosis within the first 72 hours of illness. These methods for detection of capsular antigen may be positive in up to 90% of culture-positive fluids. Other laboratory data (complete blood count, serum electrolytes and chemistries) reflect only specific organ or body system dysfunction related to an ongoing bacterial process and may be nonspecifically abnormal.

A transthoracic or transesophageal echocardiogram may suggest the possibility of *Haemophilus* species as the cause of endocarditis because of the presence of large vegetations on the involved valve. Peripheral arterial embolization also suggests this cause.

OPTIMAL MANAGEMENT

Antibiotics

Without treatment, meningitis and epiglottitis due to *H. influenzae* may be rapidly fatal. Antimicrobial resistance among isolates of *H. influenzae*, and occasionally other *Haemophilus* species, has become an increasingly prevalent problem. Enzymatic resistance to ampicillin mediated by β-lactamases may be present in 24% to 32% of clinical isolates, whereas nonenzymatic resistance (altered outer membrane proteins or decreased affinity of penicillin-binding proteins) may occur in 2% to 4% of isolates. Type b strains are nearly twice as likely as strains other than type b to produce β-lactamase (about 30% and 15%, respectively), whereas the non–β-lactamase resistance to ampicillin is more commonly seen in nontypable strains. Since 1980, the emergence of strains resistant to chloramphenicol has also been described. Although less than 1% of isolates in the United States are chloramphenicol resistant, this phenomenon necessitates sensitivity testing and thoughtful antimicrobial selection. The third-generation cephalosporins, cefotaxime and ceftriaxone, are the preferred agents. They penetrate the CSF and have been shown to be effective in serious *H. influenzae* infections, including meningitis in children and adults.

Dexamethasone therapy to reduce cerebral edema and inflammation in children older than 2 months with meningitis is now accepted. Dexamethasone before or concomitant with the first dose of antibiotics and continued for the first 4 days of therapy of acute *H. influenzae* meningitis in children has been shown to decrease secondary deafness from 17% to 3%. The use of dexamethasone in adult meningitis remains controversial.

Less serious infections, such as otitis and sinusitis, due to β-lactamase–negative strains of *H. influenzae* usually can be managed with amoxicillin. Alternative oral agents for ampicillin-resistant disease include amoxicillin-clavulanic acid, trimethoprim-sulfamethoxazole, cefuroxime axetil, cefpodoxime proxetil, cefixime, ciprofloxacin, ofloxacin, azithromycin, and clarithro-

TABLE 286.2.	ANTIMICROBIAL SUSCEPTIBILITY OF 1,688 ISOLATES OF *HAEMOPHILUS INFLUENZAE* CANADA 1992–1993

Antibiotic	% Susceptible According to β-Lactamase Production	
	Positive (n = 479)	Negative (n = 1,209)
Ampicillin	0	99.6
Amoxicillin/cavulanate	100	99.6
Cefaclor	98.8	99.3
Loracarbef	97.9	100
Cefuroxime	100	100
Cefixime	100	100
Ciprofloxacin	100	100
Oflaoxacin	100	100
Erythromycin	6.8	3.7
Trimethoprim-sulfamethoxazole	93.7	94.7

(Adapted from Scriver SR, Walmsley SL, Kau CL. Determination of antimicrobial susceptibilities of Canadian isolates of *Haemophilus influenzae* and characterization of their β-lactamase. *Antimicrob Agents Chemother* 1994;38:1678–1680)

mycin (Table 286.2). Quinolones should be used with caution in children because of possible toxicities. The typical therapy for endocarditis due to infection with *Haemophilus* species is intravenous ampicillin with or without an aminoglycoside. Ceftriaxone monotherapy may be adequate management of endocarditis due to these organisms. The optimal duration of therapy for endocarditis due to *Haemophilus* organisms is unknown; a minimum of 4 weeks of treatment should be prescribed. Serum inhibitory and bactericidal assays may be used to monitor the potential effectiveness of therapy. Adequate therapy may reduce the previously documented 25% to 50% mortality rate to 10% to 15%.

Unimmunized young children younger than 2 years old in the same household as an infected person with serious invasive disease due to *H. influenzae* type b have a significantly increased risk of secondary invasive infections due to this organism. Secondary attack rates have been estimated at 2% to 4% in household contacts and 1.3% in day care centers. Rifampin prophylaxis, 20 mg per kilogram with a maximum dose of 600 mg per day given once daily for 4 days, is recommended for both children and adults in homes with children younger than 4 years old. To reduce nasopharyngeal carriage and potential spread, the index case should also be given prophylaxis if he or she is returning to the household of a child younger than 4 years of age.

PREVENTION

The possibility of active immunization against type b *H. influenzae* has become a reality during the 1980s. A vaccine composed of purified type b PRP was shown to give variable results in the United States. Several very effective PRP-conjugate vaccines are now available for children 2 months of age or older, given usually as a series of four injections at 2, 4, 6, and 15 to 18 months of age (Table 286.3). In the United States since 1987, the rate of disease due to *H. influenzae* in children younger than 5 years has decreased by 95%, whereas reported disease in people older than 5 years has remained stable. Conjugated *H. influenzae* vaccines combined with diphtheria–tetanus–acellular pertussis vaccine are now available for children 15 to 18 months. The use of conjugated *H. influenzae* vaccines in immunocompromised adults (i.e., with AIDS) is now being advocated.

For children who are receiving immunosuppressive chemicals, children with AIDS, or Native American infants, bacterial polysaccharide immune globulin (BPIG) may be of use in preventing *H. influenzae* disease before such children are able to respond to a PRP-conjugate vaccine. BPIG does not interfere with responses to vaccines (diphtheria–pertussis–tetanus or PRP-conjugate) given concurrently.

TABLE 286.3.	APPROVED *HAEMOPHILUS INFLEUNZAE* TYPE B VACCINES AND TARGETED POPULATIONS

FDA-Approved	Vaccine Type	Targeted Population
April 1985	Polyribosyl ribitol phosphate (PRP) polysaccharide	Children ≥18 months old
December 1987	PRP-diphtheria toxoid conjugate (PRP-D)[a]	Children ≥18 months old
December 1989	PRP-*Neisseria meningitidis* outer membrane protein conjugate (PRP-OMP)[b]	Children ≥18 months old
	PRP-oligosaccharide diphtheria toxoid conjugate (HbOO)[c]	
December 1990	PRP-OMP HbOC	Children ≥2 months old
March 1993	PRP-tetanus toxoid conjugate (PRP-T)[d]	Children ≥2 months old
September 1996	PRP-T reconstituted/mixed with DTaP	Children >15–18 months old (4th dose of DTaP)

DTaP, diphtheria and tetanus toxoid.
[a] Pro HIBIT (Connaught).
[b] Pedvax HIB (Merck).
[c] HibTITER (LEDERLE-PRAXIS).
[d] ActHIB (Pasteur Merieux); Omni HIB (SmithKline Beecham).
[e] Tri HIBit (Connaught-Pasteur Merieux).

■ *BORDETELLA* INFECTIONS

Of the seven species within the genus *Bordetella*, only *Bordetella pertussis* and *Bordetella parapertussis* routinely cause disease in humans. *B. pertussis* is the causative agent of whooping cough. Although a mild form of clinical disease has been attributed to *B. parapertussis* in the past, recent studies suggest a frequency of a classic pertussis syndrome due to this organism similar to that caused by *B. pertussis,* especially in children. *Bordetella bronchiseptica* rarely causes whooping cough–like illness in humans and opportunistic infections in compromised hosts. *Bordetella hirci, B. holmseii,* and *B. trematum* have rarely been isolated from human infection. *Bordetella avium* is not known to infect humans.

INCIDENCE AND EPIDEMIOLOGY

Pertussis is endemic worldwide, with epidemics occurring every 3 to 5 years. After the whole-cell vaccine (WCV) was introduced in the late 1940s, a marked decline occurred in the annual incidence of pertussis to a nadir of 1,010 cases in the United States in 1976. Because immunity after WCV is usually less than 12 years, most adults are susceptible and have little to no humoral immunity to provide through passive transfer to neonates. Since 1976, there has been a significant resurgence (82% increase) of cases in people 10 years of age or older. This has occurred because of the withholding of booster doses of WCV from adolescents and adults owing to the concern about systemic toxicity.

The attack rate among susceptible people after exposure to *B. pertussis* is 50% to 100%; infection is acquired by exposure to aerosol droplets from a coughing patient at a distance of 5 feet or less. The attack rate, as well as the morbidity and mortality, are higher in female children; the reason for this is unknown.

ETIOLOGY

The human pathogens (*B. pertussis* and *B. parapertussis*) are small, slowly growing, gram-negative, coccobacillary organisms that are nonmotile and require growth medium supplementation with nicotinamide (contained in synthetic medium or in the starch–blood agar medium described by Bordet and Gengou).

PATHOGENESIS

B. pertussis produces several biologically active virulence factors, including a dermonecrotic heat-labile toxin, a tracheal cytotoxin, adenylate cyclase toxin, agglutinogens, and a filamentous hemagglutinin, the last of which is involved in adherence to ciliated respiratory epithelium. The best-characterized virulence factor is pertussis toxin (pertussigen), which promotes epithelial adherence and, as a typical toxin with A and B binding sites, catalyzes the adenosine diphosphate ribosylation of guanine nucleotide-binding regulatory proteins in target cells. Pertussis toxin is also responsible for the lymphocytosis, the sensitization to histamine, and the enhancement of insulin secretion seen in experimental animals and human disease and is the likely cause of the systemic manifestations of disease. Tracheal cytotoxin, dermonecrotic toxin, and adenyl cyclase toxin cause damage to the respiratory epithelium, thereby potentiating infection. Phagocyte function is abrogated by pertussis toxin, adenyl cyclase toxin, and tracheal cytotoxin.

CLINICAL FINDINGS

Classic disease occurs primarily in children 1 to 5 years of age. The limited duration of vaccine immunity and the publicity generated by adverse reactions to the WCV have changed the epidemiology of the illness so that most cases now occur in infants younger than 1 year or adolescents and adults older than 15 years.

Clinical illness presents in three phases: the catarrhal phase, the paroxysmal phase, and the convalescent phase. After an incubation period of less than 1 to 3 weeks, the *catarrhal phase,* indistinguishable from other upper respiratory illnesses, may last for a few days to a week. This phase manifests as rhinorrhea, conjunctival injection, malaise, and low-level fever. The cough paroxysm ensues and consists of a series of short, staccato bursts followed by an inspiratory gasp, resulting in the classic "whoop." However, the whoop is uncommon among infants and adults with pertussis. The typical laboratory finding of lymphocytosis is noted in the late catarrhal and early paroxysmal phases. Lung consolidation is noted in 20% to 25% of infants and adults. Complications include otitis media, pneumonia, and the sequelae of the severe cough paroxysms, including petechiae, epistaxis, subconjunctival, scleral and central nervous system hemorrhages, and pneumothorax, among others. In children younger than 1 year old, seizures (3%), encephalopathy (0.9%), and death (0.6%) are seen. *B. pertussis* has been recognized as a cause of chronic infection in patients with HIV-1 infection.

LABORATORY FINDINGS

During the late catarrhal and early paroxysmal phases, leukocytosis may be as high as 50,000/mm^3, consisting primarily of a T- and B-cell lymphocytosis. The gold standard for diagnosis is culture of *B. pertussis* (or *B. parapertussis*), which may take up to 5 days for growth on specific medium. However, the overall sensitivity of nasopharyngeal culture for disease clinically consistent with pertussis may be a as low as 58%. Material for culture should be obtained by calcium alginate swab of nasopharyngeal secretions or by aspiration. Ability to diagnose by culture rapidly diminishes during the paroxysmal phase. Direct fluorescent antibody (DFA) stains of nasopharyngeal specimens or of cultured isolates may aid in more rapid diagnosis, although DFA on direct specimens is less sensitive and specific than culture.

DNA hybridization and polymerase chain reaction (PCR) techniques have been developed for detection of *B. pertussis* in secretions. PCR has been determined to be approximately 98% specific but often less than 50% sensitive when compared with serologic diagnosis. With further refinement, PCR may be a valuable complement to, if not replacement for, culture for the diagnosis of pertussis. Because of these diagnostic limitations, the diagnosis of pertussis in patients with a cough persisting for 2 weeks is often clinical. A retrospective serologic diagnosis of pertussis can be made with ELISA.

OPTIMAL MANAGEMENT

In addition to supportive measures, especially for infants who are at greatest risk for complications, azithromycin, clarithromycin, erythromycin, tetracycline, trimethoprim-sulfamethoxazole, and chloramphenicol eliminate *B. pertussis*. One isolate of *B. pertussis* resistant to erythromycin has been reported. These agents may act by affecting bacterial adherence through protein synthesis inhibition, thereby reducing the severity and duration of infection. However, clinical disease may not be altered by antimicrobial therapy.

PREVENTION

Isolation of cases is ineffective at preventing spread of pertussis because of the nonspecificity of symptoms during early illness. Macrolide prophylaxis may help to control transmission within households and during outbreaks.

Since the late 1940s, the WCV, combined with diphtheria and tetanus toxoids, has been more than 80% efficacious at preventing pertussis in children. The limited duration of immunoprotection is evidenced by the fact that 95% or more of disease occurs 12 or more years after immunization. However, disease is usually less severe in these patients. The WCV is usually given at age 2, 4, 6, and 15 months and at 4 to 6 years. The major limitation of a vaccine containing pertussis WCV is reactogenicity, both local and systemic, in the form of pain, swelling, fever, anorexia, and fretfulness. Encephalopathy and neurologic sequelae, previously associated with pertussis immunization, have been disproved as being caused by the vaccine. However, owing to these concerns, the WCV has been rarely used in older children and adults, except for outbreak control.

Declining immunity in adolescents and adults, despite vaccination levels of 93% in 1994, has led to the resurgence of this disease in many cities and countries since 1976. In 1993, there were 5,457 cases in the United States, representing an 82% increase compared with 1992 and a 540% increase since 1976, primarily in persons older than 5 years.

To avoid vaccine reactions and possibly to enhance the magnitude and duration of immunity, acellular pertussis vaccines combined with diphtheria and tetanus have now been licensed. The acellular pertussis components include from two to four purified or recombinant *B. pertussis* virulence antigens. These vaccines have demonstrated greater immunogenicity and fewer adverse effects. They have been incorporated into three licensed combined diphtheria–tetanus vaccines for administration at ages 2, 4, 6, and 15 to 18 months and at 4 to 6 years. Their potential usefulness for periodic booster immunizations during adult life is likely but not yet advocated.

BIBLIOGRAPHY

Bass JW, Wittler RR. Return of epidemic pertussis in the United States. *Pediatr Infect Dis J* 1994;13:343–345.
Centers for Disease Control and Prevention. Pertussis—United States, January 1992–June 1995. *MMWR* 1995;44:525–529.
Centers for Disease Control and Prevention. Recommendations of the Advisory Committee on Immunization Practices (ACIP). Pertussis vaccination: use of acellular pertussis vaccines among infants and young children. *MMWR* 1997;46(RR-7):1–25.
Centers for Disease Control and Prevention. Recommended childhood immunization schedule–United States, 1999. *MMWR* 1999;48(1):12–16.
Centers for Disease Control and Prevention. Recommended childhood immunization schedule–United States, 1998. *MMWR* 1998;47:8–12.
Cherry JD. Pertussis in adults. *Ann Intern Med* 1998;128:64–66.
Christie CDC, Marx ML, Marchant CD, et al. The 1993 epidemic of pertussis in Cincinnati: resurgence of disease in a highly immunized population of children. *N Engl J Med* 1994;331:16–21.
Edwards KM. Pertussis in older children and adults. *Adv Pediatr Infect Dis* 1998;13:49–77.
Farley MM, Stephens DS, Brachman PS, et al. Invasive *Haemophilus influenzae* disease in adults: a prospective, population-based surveillance. *Ann Intern Med* 1992;116:806–812.
Funkhouser A, Steinhoff MC, Ward J. *Haemophilus influenzae* disease and immunization in developing countries. *Rev Infect Dis* 1991;13(suppl 6):S542–S554.
He Q, Viljanen MK, Arvilommi H, et al. Whooping cough caused by *Bordetella* pertussis and *Bordetella* parapertussis in an immunized population. *JAMA* 1998;280:635–637.
Hoppe JE, Bryskier A. In vitro susceptibilities of *Bordetella* pertussis and *Bordetella* parapertussis to two ketolides (HMR 3004 and HMR 3647), four macrolides (azithromycin, clarithromycin, erythromycin A and roxithromycin), and two ansamycins (rifampin and rifapentine). *Antimicrob Agents Chemother* 1998;42:965–966.
Jorgensen JH. Update on mechanisms and prevalence of antimicrobial resistance in *Haemophilus influenzae*. *Clin Infect Dis* 1992;14:1119–1123.
Mink CM, Sirota NM, Nugent S. Outbreak of pertussis in a fully immunized adolescent and adult population. *Arch Pediatr Adolesc Med* 1994;148:153–157.
Muller FMC, Hoppe JE, von Konig CHW. Laboratory diagnosis of pertussis: state of the art in 1997. *J Clin Microbiol* 1997;35:2435–2443.
Schoendorf KC, Adams WG, Kiely JL, et al. National trends in *Haemophilus influenzae* meningitis mortality and hospitalization among children, 1980 through 1991. *Pediatrics* 1994;93:663–668.

Kelley's Textbook of Internal Medicine, fourth edition. Edited by H. David Humes.
Lippincott Williams & Wilkins, Philadelphia © 2000.

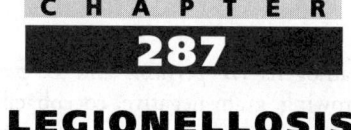

CHAPTER 287

LEGIONELLOSIS

**EMANUEL N. VERGIS
ROBERT R. MUDER**

DEFINITION AND ETIOLOGY

Legionnaires' disease was named after the outbreak of severe pneumonia at the 1976 American Legion Convention in Philadelphia during which over 180 people were afflicted and 34 died. The causative organism, *Legionella pneumophila*, was isolated from postmortem tissue by investigators from the Centers for Disease Control several months after the outbreak. *L. pneumophila* belongs to the family Legionellaceae, which includes a total of 34 described species. Furthermore, more than 50 serogroups are within the individual species of *Legionella*. *L. pneumophila* is the most common species encountered and accounts for approximately 90% of infections caused by the Legionellaceae. Of the 14 serogroups of *L. pneumophila*, serogroups 1, 4, and 6 are responsible for most of the infections among humans. Other *Legionella* species implicated with human infection (pneumonia) include *L. micdadei* (the Pittsburgh pneumonia agent), *L. bozemanii*, *L. dumoffii*, and *L. longbeachae*. These account for approximately 9% of pneumonia due to *Legionella*. Several other non-*pneumophila* species implicated in pneumonia are *L. jordanis*, *L. gormanii*, *L. feeleii*, *L. hackeliae*, *L. maceachernii*, *L. wadsworthii*, *L. birminghamensis*, *L. cincinnatiensis*, *L. oakridgensis*, *L. anisa*, *L. sainthelensi*, *L. tusconensis*, and *L. lansingensis*. Collectively, these less frequently encountered species are responsible for approximately 1% of cases of pneumonia. Another clinical syndrome caused by members of the Legionellaceae family is Pontiac fever, an acute febrile nonpneumonic illness that has been serologically linked to *L. pneumophila* and other *Legionella* species.

Legionellae are widely distributed in both natural and man-made aquatic environments, which include freshwater habitats such as lakes, rivers, streams, thermally polluted waters, cooling towers, evaporative condensers, whirlpool spas, and potable water systems. They are aerobic, gram-negative bacilli, with fastidious growth requirements rendering them incapable of growing on the usual microbiologic media. Their growth is supported by buffered charcoal yeast extract agar supplemented with cysteine, ketoacids, and iron. Legionellae are also considered facultative intracellular pathogens of mononuclear phagocytes, principally monocytes and alveolar macrophages.

INCIDENCE AND EPIDEMIOLOGY

The incidence of legionnaires' disease depends on the extent of contamination of the aquatic reservoir by the organism, the susceptibility of the population exposed to that water, and the intensity of the exposure. In addition, the discovery of this infection also depends on the expertise of the testing laboratory and on the availability of specialized laboratory tests. *L. pneumophila* has been consistently shown to be among the top three most common microbial causes of community-acquired pneumonia. The percentage of community-acquired pneumonia requiring hospitalization due to *L. pneumophila* ranges from 2% to 15% with a median incidence of 5%. Cigarette smoking, advanced age, chronic lung disease, and immunosuppressive therapy are major risk factors for acquisition of legionnaires' disease. Some studies have noted an increased risk among patients with alcoholism and renal failure. Persons with AIDS also appear to have a somewhat increased risk for *Legionella* infection.

Originally, nosocomial legionnaires' disease was believed to be epidemic in institutions. It is now believed that endemic infection is much more common. The incidence of nosocomial pneumonia due to *L. pneumophila* varies and depends largely on the degree of colonization of the hospital hot-water distribution system by the organism and the number of susceptible hosts. As with community-acquired disease, recognition requires availability of specialized testing for *Legionella* within the hospital. The percentage of nosocomial pneumonia due to *Legionella*

varies from less than 1% to 50%. The major predictor of nosocomial infection in susceptible persons is colonization of the hospital hot-water distribution system with *Legionella*. Persons at high risk for nosocomial legionnaires' disease include those who are highly immunocompromised, especially organ transplant recipients. Additional risk factors are recent surgery, endotracheal intubation, and the use of respiratory tract therapy equipment. In addition to *L. pneumophila*, *L. micdadei*, *L. dumoffii* and *L. bozemanii* can cause nosocomial legionnaires' disease provided that the water is colonized by these organisms.

There are many modes of transmission of *L. pneumophila* from a water source to humans. There is evidence of aerosolization, aspiration, and direct instillation into the lung during respiratory tract manipulation. Reports implicating cooling towers as point sources of transmission have gradually disappeared with the recognition that *Legionella* could be pervasive within water distribution systems. Colonization of potable water distribution systems in the home and in the workplace has been implicated in community-acquired cases of legionnaires' disease. Despite the initial isolation of *L. pneumophila* in a hospital from a showerhead, an epidemiologic link between showering and acquisition of disease has never been shown in prospective studies. Aerosols generated by humidifiers, nebulizers, and other respiratory care devices have been linked to infection. Tap water, which is frequently used to rinse respiratory equipment and tubing, may be contaminated by *Legionella*, resulting in infection by direct instillation of the organism into the lung. Aspiration of contaminated water or contaminated oropharyngeal secretions is probably the major mode of transmission. Nasogastric tube placement has been implicated as a risk factor in intubated patients in two prospective studies.

PATHOGENESIS

Legionellae enter the respiratory tract by aerosolization or aspiration of contaminated water. The development of disease subsequently depends on the inoculum and virulence of the organism and the immune competence of the host.

The initial barrier against infection is mechanical clearance of the organism effected by the mucociliary process of the respiratory epithelial cells. Mucociliary action is impaired in patients with chronic pulmonary disease, in cigarette smokers, and in alcoholics—patients in whom there is a consistent epidemiologic association of increased risk of legionnaires' disease. Upon reaching the alveoli, legionellae are phagocytized by alveolar macrophages, where they are capable of replication. The primary host defense mechanism against legionellae appears to be cell-mediated immunity. Evidence for this comes from observation that legionnaires' disease is more common and more severe for patients with cell-mediated immune dysfunction, including transplant recipients, patients receiving corticosteroid therapy, and patients with AIDS. Humoral immunity is a secondary host defense mechanism of limited effectiveness. Antibody does not promote the killing of *L. pneumophila* by complement and causes only a modest amount of killing of *L. pneumophila* by phagocytes. Virulence of *L. pneumophila* varies among different strains. Virulence may be associated with a particular surface epitope that is recognized by a monoclonal antibody (Mab-2). In vivo studies with guinea pigs have shown that a 24-kd protein referred to as *macrophage infectivity potentiator* (Mip) appears to be required for virulence.

CLINICAL FINDINGS

There are two clinical manifestations of *Legionella* infection: Pontiac fever and pneumonia (legionnaires' disease). No clear explanation exists regarding why there are two forms of clinical disease, but different inocula of the organism, different modes of transmission, and host factors are believed to be important. Pontiac fever is an acute, flulike illness without pneumonia, occurring after exposure to heavily contaminated aerosols. The attack rate is over 90%, and the incubation period is 1 to 2 days. Malaise, fatigue, and myalgias are frequently described in 97% of patients. Despite the presence of a nonproductive cough and chest pain, no radiographic evidence of pneumonia is seen. Fever with chills and headache are present in 80% to 90% of patients. Arthralgias, nausea, abdominal pain, and diarrhea are seen in less than 50% of patients. A modest leukocytosis with predominant neutrophils may be seen. The illness is self-limited with full recovery within 1 week without sequelae. *L. pneumophila* serogroups 1 and 6, *L. feeleii,* and *L. micdadei* have been implicated in several outbreaks of Pontiac fever.

Pneumonia is the predominant clinical finding in legionnaires' disease (Table 287.1). The disease can range from a mild cough and slight fever to bilateral pneumonia with multisystem failure. The incubation period ranges from 2 to 10 days. Nonspecific symptoms such as fever, malaise, myalgia, anorexia, and headache may be present early in the course of the illness.

Initially, the cough is nonproductive or minimally productive of nonpurulent sputum, which on occasion may be blood streaked. Gross hemoptysis is rare. Chest pain, either pleuritic or nonpleuritic, can be a prominent feature for some patients. An incorrect diagnosis of pulmonary embolus may be suggested by the combination of chest pain and hemoptysis. Gastrointestinal symptoms occur in up to 50% of patients. Watery, nonbloody diarrhea is most common. Other gastrointestinal complaints are nausea, vomiting, and abdominal pain. Neurologic symptoms ranging from headache and lethargy to encephalopathy are reported. However, change in mental status is the most common neurologic abnormality.

Examination of the patient with legionnaires' disease shows high fever, and chest findings are typical of bacterial pneumonia. Pulse–temperature dissociation has been unduly stressed as a useful clinical finding, but can occasionally be seen in elderly patients with severe legionnaires' disease. Hypotension and bradycardia are not unusual. However, pneumonia caused by *Legionella* cannot be distinguished from other pneumonias by clinical manifestations alone.

Extrapulmonary manifestations of *Legionella* infection are rare and presumably occur through hematogenous dissemination. Anecdotal reports of cellulitis, sinusitis, pericarditis, myocarditis, prosthetic valve endocarditis, peritonitis, pancreatitis, and acute pyelonephritis with renal abscesses have been reported. Wound infections have resulted from exposure to water containing *L. pneumophila.*

LABORATORY FINDINGS

ROUTINE STUDIES

Polymorphonuclear leukocytosis with immature forms is common in patients with legionellosis. Mild biochemical abnormalities are common, including azotemia, hepatic dysfunction, and hypophosphatemia. Hyponatremia (serum sodium less than 130 mEq per liter) occurs significantly more frequently in patients with legionnaires' disease than in those with pneumonias of other origin.

Gram's stain of sputum showing numerous neutrophils with few or no organisms is a typical finding when specimens are available and should raise clinical suspicion of *Legionella* infection. However, such a stain is also seen with *Mycoplasma, Chlamydia,* and viral pneumonia.

CHEST RADIOGRAPHY

The initial common finding on chest radiography is a unilateral alveolar infiltrate that may progress to consolidation. Radiographic evidence of pneumonia is seen by the third day of the illness. Pleural-based rounded opacities may resemble pulmonary infarction. Small to moderate pleural effusions are seen in one-third of patients. Progression of infiltrates may occur, involving multiple lobes even while the patient is on appropriate antibiotic therapy. With apparent clinical response, cavitation is a common feature in the immunocompromised patient receiving corticosteroids or immunosuppressive drugs for legionellosis. Radiographic improvement often lags behind clinical response, and several weeks to months may pass before infiltrates resolve completely.

SPECIALIZED LABORATORY TESTS

Specialized laboratory testing is required to make the diagnosis of legionnaires' disease because it lacks specific findings in its clinical and radiographic presentation. Growth on special media, direct fluorescent antibody (DFA), serologic antibody titers, and urinary antigen detection.

Recovery of *Legionella* from respiratory secretions on buffered charcoal-yeast extract media containing antimicrobial agents to

TABLE 287.1.	**CLINICAL CLUES FOR DIAGNOSIS OF LEGIONNAIRES' DISEASE**

Gram's stain of respiratory secretions showing numerous neutrophils, but few, if any, organisms
Hyponatremia
Failure to respond to β-lactam (penicillin or cephalosporin) and aminoglycoside antibiotics
Occurrence in a hospital or environment in which the water supply is known to be contaminated with *Legionella*

suppress competing microflora and dyes to enhance visibility is the gold standard test for diagnosis of legionnaires' disease. Acid-wash pretreatment of the sputum specimens reduces overgrowth of competing flora and improves sensitivity of the sputum culture. Specimens obtained by bronchoscopy have approximately the same yield as that for sputum samples; bronchoalveolar lavage gives higher yields than bronchial wash specimens. Pleural fluid obtained by thoracentesis should be evaluated by DFA stain and culture. The kit used for detection of *Legionella* antigen in urine has also detected *Legionella* in pleural fluid.

DFA staining is rapid and allows for direct visualization of *Legionella* in specimens. The sensitivity of the DFA stain of sputum ranges from 50% to 80%; organisms are more likely to be seen by DFA when multilobar infiltrates are present on chest radiography. The test is highly specific.

Serologic detection of antibodies is commonly made by either indirect fluorescent antibody or enzyme-linked immunosorbent assays. These techniques have become less useful owing to the availability of culture methods and specialized tests. Serologic diagnosis is made from acute and convalescent sera by documenting a fourfold rise in antibody titer to 1:128. A single titer of 1:256 in the setting of compatible clinical disease is considered presumptive evidence for legionnaires' disease. Maximal sensitivity requires both IgG and IgM tests. The sensitivity of serology is 40% to 60%. The specificity is estimated to be 95% and in cases of infection due to *L. pneumophila* serogroup 1. The usefulness of this test is therefore limited to epidemiologic studies. Specificity in diagnosing infection due to other serogroups or species is uncertain.

A rapid diagnosis of legionnaires' disease can be made by detecting *L. pneumophila* antigenuria. Urinary antigen testing is available only for *L. pneumophila* serogroup 1. The test is easy to perform and is not affected by antibiotics. The sensitivity for urinary antigen detection is 80%. The specificity approaches 100%.

OPTIMAL MANAGEMENT

The new macrolides, especially azithromycin, have replaced erythromycin as the drug of choice. Azithromycin, roxithromycin, clarithromycin, and josamycin have been therapeutically effective in anecdotal reports. These new macrolides have superior lung tissue penetration and more potent intracellular and in vitro activity than erythromycin. The quinolones also have greater intracellular and in vitro activity than the macrolides. There have been numerous anecdotal successes with the quinolones, especially ciprofloxacin and levofloxacin. Rifampin is highly active in vitro and in vivo against *Legionella*. Tetracycline proved efficacious in the 1976 Philadelphia outbreak, and doxycycline and minocycline have also been efficacious.

Parenteral therapy is preferred initially until there is an objective clinical response, usually within 3 to 5 days. Oral therapy can then be substituted and continued for a total duration of 10 to 14 days, although a 21-day course has been recommended for immunocompromised patients or those with extensive disease seen on chest radiograph. Five to 10 days of azithromycin therapy is sufficient.

We recommend therapy with a newer macrolide, especially for community-acquired pneumonia in the immunocompetent patient. For organ transplant recipients in whom *Legionella* is a possible pathogen, we recommend a quinolone, especially ciprofloxacin or levofloxacin, as the drug of choice. The macrolides (but not azithromycin) interact with tacrolimus and cyclosporine, which are used as immunosuppressive drugs after organ transplantation. Levels of tacrolimus and cyclosporine increase

TABLE 287.2.	ANTIBIOTIC THERAPY FOR *LEGIONELLA* INFECTION
Antimicrobial Agent	**Dosage**[a]
Azithromycin	500 mg[b] orally or intravenously every 24 h
Clarithromycin	500 mg orally or intravenously[c] every 12 h
Roxithromycin	500 mg orally every 12 h
Erythromycin	1000 mg intravenously every 6 h
	500 mg orally every 6 h
Dirithromycin	500 mg orally every 24 h
Levofloxacin	500 mg[b] orally or intravenously every 24 h
Ciprofloxacin	400 mg intravenously every 12 h
	750 mg orally every 12 h
Ofloxacin	400 mg orally or intravenously every 12 h
Doxycycline	100 mg[b] orally or intravenously every 12 h
Minocycline	100 mg[c] orally or intravenously every 12 h
Tetracycline	500 mg orally or intravenously every 6 h
Trimethoprim/sulfamethoxazole	160/800 mg intravenously every 8 h
	160/800 mg orally every 12 h
Rifampin	300–600 mg orally or intravenously every 12 h

[a] Dosages are based on clinical experience, not on controlled trials.
[b] We recommend doubling the first dose.
[c] Intravenous form not available in the United States.

considerably when macrolides are coadministered, resulting in renal toxicity. The quinolones lack significant interactions with tacrolimus and are therefore recommended in the transplant recipient. The addition of rifampin as adjunctive therapy for legionnaires' disease may be considered in the immunocompromised patient or in the patient with radiographic evidence of multilobar pneumonia. However, rifampin has significant interactions with both tacrolimus and cyclosporine. Coadministration of rifampin with tacrolimus or cyclosporine may result in marked reduction in the levels of the immunosuppressive drugs, which may increase the risk of acute rejection. The dosages of the various antibiotics are shown in Table 287.2.

Treatment of Pontiac fever is primarily symptomatic; no antibiotic therapy is required.

PROGNOSIS

Patients treated early with appropriate antibiotics usually have an objective clinical response within 3 to 5 days. Mortality rate from legionnaires' disease in the immunocompetent patient is about 10% and depends primarily on the severity of the underlying illnesses and the timing of initiation of appropriate antibiotics. Mortality may approach 50% in nosocomial *Legionella* infection and reflects the severity of the underlying illnesses. The chest radiograph is not useful for monitoring clinical response.

PREVENTION

Identification of the contaminated environmental water source and subsequent disinfection of the water supply is the ultimate preventive measure. Two methods for disinfection are feasible: superheating the water such that the distal outlet temperature is 70° to 80° C, with flushing of the distal sites (faucets, showerheads) for at least 30 minutes and installing copper–silver ionization systems. Superheating and flushing can be quickly implemented to stop an outbreak, but afford no residual protection for regrowth of *Legionella*. Hyperchlorination is no longer recommended. Copper–silver ionization provides residual protection throughout the water distribution system and has proved cost-effective in hospitals. Based on studies in animals, development of an effective vaccine is feasible, but none is currently available.

BIBLIOGRAPHY

Lowry PW, Tompkins LS. Nosocomial legionellosis: a review of pulmonary and extrapulmonary syndromes. *Am J Infect Control* 1993;21:21–27.
Muder RR, Yu VL. Other *Legionella* species. In: Mandel GL, Bennett JE, Dolin R, eds. *Principles and practice of infectious diseases,* fourth ed. New York: Churchill Livingstone, 1995:2097.
Potgeiter PD, Hammond JMJ. Etiology and diagnosis of pneumonia requiring ICU admission. *Chest* 1992;101:199.
Rello J, Quintana E, Ausina V, et al. A three-year study of severe community-acquired pneumonia with emphasis on outcome. *Chest* 1993;103: 232–235.
Stout JE, Yu VL. Legionellosis. *N Engl J Med* 1997;337:682–687.
Sopena N, Sabria-Leal M, Pedro-Botet ML, et al. Comparative study of the clinical presentation of *Legionella* pneumonia and other community-acquired pneumonias. *Chest* 1998;113:1195–1200.
Vergis EN, Yu VL. *Legionella* species. In: Yu VL, Merigan TC, Barriere SL, eds. *Antimicrobial therapy and vaccines.* Baltimore: William & Wilkins, 1999:257.
Woo AH, Goetz A, Yu VL. Transmission of *Legionella* by respiratory equipment aerosol generating devices. *Chest* 1992;102:1586–1590.
Yu VL, Vergis EN. Legionellosis. In: Fishman AP, Elias JA, Fishman JA, et al, eds. *Fishman's pulmonary diseases and disorders,* fourth ed. New York: McGraw-Hill, 1998:2234.

Kelley's Textbook of Internal Medicine, fourth edition. Edited by H. David Humes.
Lippincott Williams & Wilkins, Philadelphia © 2000.

CHAPTER
288

CHANCROID AND GRANULOMA INGUINALE

GEORGE P. SCHMID

CHANCROID

Chancroid is a sexually transmitted disease characterized by one or more painful genital ulcers, often accompanied by painful inguinal lymphadenopathy.

INCIDENCE AND EPIDEMIOLOGY

Chancroid occurs throughout the world but is most common in developing countries, where it is often the most common of the sexually transmitted diseases characterized by genital ulcers. In the United States, as a result of numerous outbreaks, the number of cases in 1989 (4,714) was the highest since World War II, but for unclear reasons the number of cases declined to 243 in 1997—the lowest since World War II.

The epidemiology of chancroid is characterized by prostitution (often associated with drug use in the United States), poverty, travel, and lack of circumcision. Most cases occur in men, commonly in male:female ratios of 5 to 10:1 in outbreaks. Such ratios have led researchers to look for colonization or asymptomatic infection in women. Colonization has uncommonly been found, although occasionally cervical or vaginal ulcers are found in women who have no symptoms. Most frequently, women have symptomatic vulvar ulcers but continue to have sexual intercourse as a result of need for money or lack of medical care. In locations where chancroid is rare, cases can often be traced to infected people arriving from endemic locations. Uncircumcised men are more likely to acquire chancroid than are circumcised men.

Chancroid, particularly in Africa, has been highly associated with infection by HIV. In one study, 43% of uncircumcised men in whom genital ulcers (most commonly caused by *Haemophilus ducreyi*) developed after intercourse with a prostitute (most, but not all, of whom had HIV) became HIV-infected.

H. ducreyi, first observed by Ducrey in smears of material from ulcers in 1889, is a small, gram-negative bacillus.

PATHOGENESIS AND CLINICAL FINDINGS

The typical incubation period of chancroid is less than 10 days. Many patients first notice a papule or pustule, which ulcerates in 1 or 2 days, leaving an excavated, painful, raw ulcer with irregular erythematous margins. Some ulcers appear to be superficial, but most are deep (Fig. 288.1). More than 50% of patients have multiple ulcers. The most common location of ulcers is the coronal sulcus in circumcised men and the prepuce in uncircumcised men; ulcers in uncircumcised men may be hidden by a painful phimosis. In women, ulcers occur most commonly on the vulva, but anal, vaginal, and cervical ulcers are also found. Painful inguinal lymphadenopathy, which may become a bubo, occurs in up to 50% of men but in a smaller proportion of women; lymphadenopathy may be bilateral.

LABORATORY FINDINGS

Definitive diagnosis of chancroid requires culture of *H. ducreyi*. Isolation is difficult, however, because the organism requires selective, enriched media and microbiologists experienced with the organism. Cultures taken from the cleaned ulcer should be placed directly onto culture media. Gram stains of ulcers, showing gram-negative coccobacilli in chains, suggest the diagnosis.

Other means of diagnosis, such as serologic testing or direct detection of organisms in lesions by immunofluorescence or polymerase chain reaction, are subjects of research.

OPTIMAL MANAGEMENT

Chancroid commonly must be differentiated from syphilis and genital herpes. Syphilis, a curable disease, should always be ex-

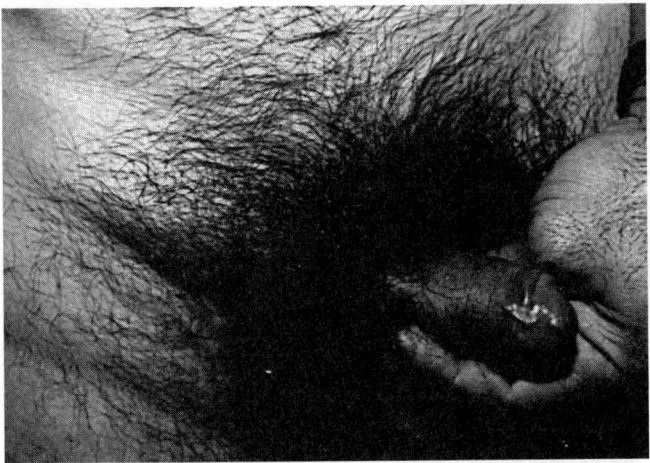

FIGURE 288.1. Single chancroid ulcer with unilateral lymphadenopathy.

cluded by serologic testing (and, when possible, by darkfield microscopy). Ideally, a subsequent serologic test for syphilis should be performed; about 10% of patients with chancroid simultaneously have syphilis or genital herpes.

Erythromycin base, 500 mg orally, four times a day for 7 days; ceftriaxone, one dose of 250 mg intramuscularly (IM); ciprofloxacin, 500 mg orally, twice a day for 3 to 5 days; or azithromycin, 1 g orally, are highly effective. Patients with HIV infection do not respond as well as patients without HIV infection; some experts prefer the erythromycin regimen for HIV-infected persons. For ulcers, a subjective response to eventually successful therapy is almost always present by 48 hours, but complete healing usually takes 10 to 11 days. Response of lymph nodes usually parallels that of ulcers, but some nodes progress to fluctuation despite successful therapy. Fluctuant nodes should be aspirated through normal skin or incised. If nodes are aspirated, aspiration may need to be repeated.

Patients should receive an HIV test at the time of diagnosis; if it or the syphilis serologic test is negative, follow-up serology at 3 months is advisable. Cases of chancroid should be reported to health authorities. Sex partners in the 10 days preceding onset should be examined and treated, regardless of the presence of lesions.

■ GRANULOMA INGUINALE (DONOVANOSIS)

Granuloma inguinale is an indolent disease, sexually transmitted in most cases, characterized by granulomatous ulcers that progressively cause extensive tissue destruction.

INCIDENCE AND EPIDEMIOLOGY

Granuloma inguinale is concentrated in Papua New Guinea, southern India, southern Africa, and the Caribbean; scattered cases are reported elsewhere. In the United States, fewer than 20 cases are reported annually. The disease is thought to be sexually transmitted because 90% of cases occur in the genital area, but it appears not to be highly contagious because many sex partners of infected persons have no symptoms. Slightly more cases occur in men than in women. Granuloma inguinale has been associated with increased risk of HIV infection.

Calymmatobacterium granulomatis, a gram-negative bacillus, was described by Donovan in 1905.

PATHOGENESIS AND CLINICAL FINDINGS

The typical incubation period is 7 to 30 days. The first manifestation is a papule or nodule, which, after several days, excavates into an ulcer with a beefy base that slowly enlarges over days to months (Fig. 288.2). The skin becomes infiltrated with plasma cells, neutrophils, and histiocytes. Several types of ulcers have been described, the most common being ulcerative (Fig. 288.2) and hypertrophic, with elevated and indurated lesions. Satellite lesions may occur on the genitalia or elsewhere from autoinoculation, and anal lesions are common in homosexual men. About

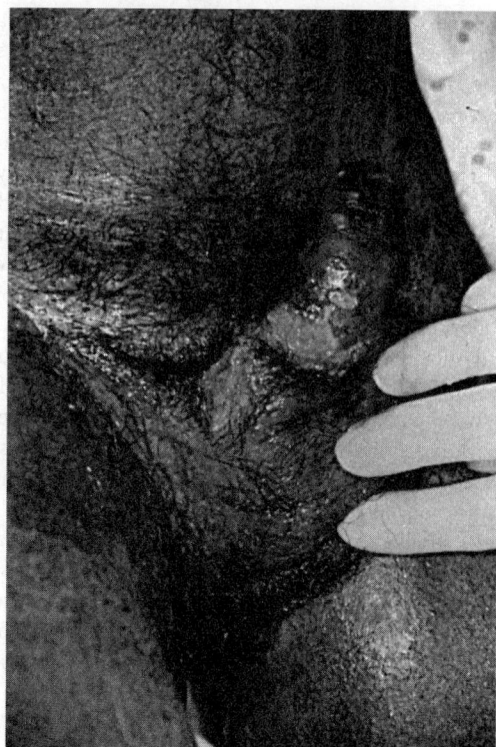

FIGURE 288.2. Granuloma inguinale causing erosion of the base of the penis and inguinal area. (Courtesy of Dr. F. Blais.)

10% of patients have extragenital lesions only, most commonly in the mouth.

LABORATORY FINDINGS

It is unclear whether *C. granulomatis* can be primarily isolated on artificial media; isolation in eggs and recently on culture using human mononuclear cells have been reported. Consequently, crush preparations of tissue looking for histiocytes with typical intracellular bacilli (Donovan bodies) are considered diagnostic. A small piece of tissue is placed on a slide, crushed with a second slide, air-dried or fixed on the slides with methanol, and stained. Giemsa or Wright stains are most commonly used. The Donovan bodies stain bipolarly, often with a capsule. Many crush preparations may be needed, and silver-stained biopsy specimens may provide an answer if crush preparations do not. Indirect immunofluorescence serology and polymerase chain reaction for detection of *C. granulomatis* in lesions are available on a research basis; skin tests are not available.

OPTIMAL MANAGEMENT

Extensive chancroid, carcinoma, secondary syphilis, and genital warts are the diseases that must usually be differentiated. No clearly preferred drug exists, and tetracycline, 500 mg orally four times a day, trimethoprim-sulfamethoxazole, two tablets orally twice a day, ceftriaxone, 1 g per day intramuscularly, chloramphenicol, 500 mg orally or intravenously three to four times a day, gentamicin, 1 mg per kilogram intramuscularly twice a day,

and streptomycin, 1 to 2 g per day intramuscularly, are variously recommended. Therapy should be continued a minimum of 21 days or until lesions have healed.

BIBLIOGRAPHY

DiCarlo RP, Armentor BS, Martin DH. Chancroid epidemiology in New Orleans men. *J Infect Dis* 1995;172:446–452.
Hart G. Donovanosis. *Clin Infect Dis* 1997;25:24–30.
Plummer FA, D'Costa LJ, Nsanze H, et al. Clinical and microbiologic studies of genital ulcers in Kenyan women. *Sex Transm Dis* 1985;12:193–197.
Schmid G. Treatment of chancroid, 1997. *Clin Infect Dis* 1999;28(suppl 1):S14–S20.

Kelley's Textbook of Internal Medicine, fourth edition. Edited by H. David Humes. Lippincott Williams & Wilkins, Philadelphia © 2000.

C H A P T E R

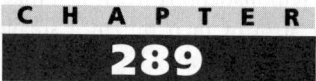

BARTONELLOSIS

NORBERT J. ROBERTS, JR

Cutaneous manifestations (verrugas) and the acute form (Oroya fever) of bartonellosis were shown to have a common bacterial cause by Daniel Carrión (hence, Carrión's disease) in 1885. Characteristics of the organism as well as the geographic restriction of infection differentiate bartonellosis from other hemotropic bacterial infections.

INCIDENCE AND EPIDEMIOLOGY

Classically, sandfly vectors transmit this infection in river valleys of the Andes Mountains at altitudes of 2,000 to 8,000 feet in Peru, Ecuador, and Colombia. In those areas, bartonellosis is endemic, and outbreaks of Oroya fever occur even in recent times. Recent studies have reported cases in lowland areas of Ecuador, and several lines of evidence have raised the possibility of a rodent or other reservoir in endemic areas. The absence of detectable organisms on human blood smears or in culture in post- or interepidemic surveys, the infection of humans in otherwise uninhabited areas, and correlations with disease in animals all support the existence of a natural animal reservoir or reservoirs.

ETIOLOGY

The cause of bartonellosis, *Bartonella bacilliformis*, is small, motile, aerobic, and pleomorphic (small bacillary or coccobacillary), with unipolar flagella. It grows best at 28° to 30° C in nutrient agar containing fresh rabbit serum and hemoglobin. The organism stains reddish-purple with Giemsa stain and is gram-negative, but counterstains poorly. Molecular analyses place the organism within the α-2 subgroup of *Proteobacteria*, within a proposed family Bartonellaceae. *B. bacilliformis* has the closest homology (97.9% to 98.8%) to the four *Bartonella* species formerly termed *Rochalimaea*.

PATHOGENESIS

In nonimmune people, infection with *B. bacilliformis* results in Oroya fever. Large numbers of bacteria adhere to erythrocytes and endothelial cells. The infection causes erythrocyte deformation, which is only slowly reversible even in the absence of bacterial internalization. Reticuloendothelial cells destroy infected erythrocytes, whose life span is markedly shortened, and the bone marrow response is acutely depressed. Thus, anemia develops, which can be rapid in onset and severe. Organisms in the blood disappear or decline markedly during recovery, and second episodes of Oroya fever are unusual. In some persons, however, the organism has been reported to persist for up to 1 year or more in the blood. After a variable period, a chronic benign form of infection called *verruga peruana*, hemangiomatous nodules commonly limited to the skin and subcutaneous tissues, usually develops.

CLINICAL FINDINGS

The incubation period of bartonellosis is about 3 weeks, but marked variability occurs. Blood cultures of apparently healthy people have been found to contain *B. bacilliformis*. In the nonimmune person, onset of the acute Oroya fever form of infection may be insidious or abrupt. Thus, the patient may have an insidious onset of anorexia, headache, malaise, and slight fever over several days. In this period, blood smears may be negative, but cultures may be positive. Alternately, the onset may be sudden with high fever, chills, diaphoresis, headache, and changes in mental function. A generalized, nontender lymphadenopathy may develop, but splenomegaly suggests the possibility of intercurrent infection. Jaundice, combined with an anemic pallor, may be present.

If the patient survives the acute episode, a convalescent phase begins with sudden disappearance of the organisms from the erythrocytes. Intercurrent infection is most common at this stage, with salmonellosis, tuberculosis, enteric bacterial infection, or parasitic infections most common (in more than 40% of cases) significantly affecting prognosis. Recurrence of fever or onset of marked leukocytosis suggests intercurrent infection.

Pain in the bones, joints, and muscles may persist after resolution of Oroya fever. The eruptive form of verruga may follow Oroya fever or may occur without a recent acute episode. The lesions usually appear on exposed parts of the body but may involve mucous membranes and internal organs. They appear in crops, and lesions in stages of growth and regression may coexist. The verrugas may be sessile, nodular, and pedunculated and can have a pustular or ulcerated form with secondary infection. Without complicating infection, they are nontender. The diversity of skin lesions, often appearing after the infected person leaves the endemic area, can make the diagnosis difficult. Epidemiologic data and other physical and microscopic observations aid in eliminating alternate diagnoses such as Kaposi's sarcoma and lymphoproliferative neoplasms. Onset of the cutaneous eruption usually is associated with a decrease in the joint pains and low-grade fever of the preeruptive stage, and anemia is not usually present.

The existence of mild clinical disease, leading to underreporting of bartonellosis has been suggested by serosurveys combined with clinical observations.

LABORATORY FINDINGS

The anemia of the Oroya fever form of bartonellosis is macrocytic, often hypochromic, with abnormal erythrocyte forms. A shift to the left in leukocyte differential, with variable absolute counts, is common. The erythrocyte count may fall rapidly, and numerous organisms can be seen on the blood smear. The most rapid diagnosis of Oroya fever patients, with the proper epidemiologic setting, may be obtained by eosin-thiazine stain (Diff-Quik) of blood smears. In a recently reported outbreak, approximately 60% of the cases had *B. bacilliformis* detectable on blood smears. IgM antibody may be present not only in patients with Oroya fever but in some healthy people, as well as those with verrugas. Crude *Bartonella* antigens, used in enzyme-linked immunosorbent assays, may cross-react with antibodies to other organisms, such as *Chlamydia psittaci*. Several purified *Bartonella* antigens, however, have been shown to be specific in immunoblot assays, and such assays can be used for confirmation when antibody is detected using crude *Bartonella* antigens.

The organism can be demonstrated histologically by electron microscopy and can be cultured from the cutaneous lesions and occasionally from the blood and bone marrow during the verruga peruana stage of the infection.

OPTIMAL MANAGEMENT

Prevention of bartonellosis requires control of the sandfly and insect repellents and bed netting for the individual. A dramatic clinical response in acute bartonellosis has been described with use of chloramphenicol, penicillin, and possibly other antibiotics. Organisms may persist beyond resolution of fever, which can occur within 24 hours. The presence of intercurrent infection may dictate the choice of antibiotics. Thus, chloramphenicol is often the drug of choice (2 g per day or more for 7 or more days) because of the frequency of complicating *Salmonella* infections. Newer antimicrobial agents with anti-*Salmonella* activity have not yet been reported to treat bartonellosis effectively. Severe anemia may require blood transfusions. The cutaneous lesions, if large or secondarily infected, may require surgical excision.

BIBLIOGRAPHY

Amano Y, Rumbea J, Knobloch J, et al. Bartonellosis in Ecuador: serosurvey and current status of cutaneous verrucous disease. *Am J Trop Med Hyg* 1997;57(2):174–179.

Arias-Stella J, Lieberman PH, Erlandson RA, et al. Histology, immunohistochemistry, and ultrastructure of the verruga in Carrión's disease. *Am J Surg Pathol* 1986;10:595–610.

Cooper P, Guderian R, Orellana P, et al. An outbreak of bartonellosis in Zamora Chinchipe Province in Ecuador. *Trans Royal Soc Trop Med Hyg* 1997;91,544–546.

Cuadra M. Salmonellosis complication in human bartonellosis. *Texas Rep Biol Med* 1956;19:47.

Dooley JR. Haemotropic bacteria in man. *Lancet* 1980;2:1237–1239.

Gray GC, Johnson AA, Thornton SA, et al. An epidemic of Oroya fever in the Peruvian Andes. *Am J Trop Med Hyg* 1990;42:215–221.

Howe C. Carrión's disease: immunologic studies. *Arch Intern Med* 1943; 72:147.

Knobloch J. Analysis and preparation of *Bartonella bacilliformis* antigens. *Am J Trop Med Hyg* 1988;39:173–178.

Ihler G. *Bartonella bacilliformis*: dangerous pathogen slowly emerging from deep background. *FEMS Microbiol Lett* 1996;144:1–11.

Matteelli A, Castelli F, Spinetti A, et al. Short report: verruga peruana in an Italian traveler from Peru. *Am J Trop Med Hyg* 1994;50:143–144.

Ricketts WE. Clinical manifestations of Carrión's disease. *Arch Intern Med* 1949;84:751.

Urteaga BO, Payne EH. Treatment of the acute febrile phase of Carrión's disease with chloramphenicol. *Am J Trop Med* 1955;4:507.

Kelley's Textbook of Internal Medicine, fourth edition. Edited by H. David Humes. Lippincott Williams & Wilkins, Philadelphia © 2000.

C H A P T E R

290

CLOSTRIDIAL INFECTIONS

W. LANCE GEORGE

Clostridia are gram-positive, spore-forming, obligate, anaerobic bacilli that are widely present in soil and the distal gastrointestinal tract of most animal species. They are in the feces of essentially all human beings. At least 40 to 50 different species of clostridia have been detected in studies of human normal fecal flora; these include all the species shown in Table 290.1 except *Clostridium botulinum*.

Certain clostridial diseases of human beings may present as distinctive clinical syndromes (e.g., botulism, tetanus, and gas gangrene), whereas others (e.g., clostridial wound infection and antimicrobial agent-associated diarrhea) may not be distinguishable clinically from processes that do not involve clostridia. Table 290.1 lists the clinical syndromes or diseases caused by clostridia and the species of *Clostridium* that are usually involved.

■ INCIDENCE AND EPIDEMIOLOGY

With the exception of mixed anaerobic–aerobic pyogenic infections and *Clostridium difficile*-associated (antimicrobial) diar-

TABLE 290.1.	CLOSTRIDIAL DISEASES OF HUMAN BEINGS
Clinical Syndrome	***Clostridium* Species Usually Involved**
Botulism	*C. botulinum*
Tetanus	*C. tetani*
Food poisoning	*C. perfringens*, type A
Enteritis necroticans	*C. perfringens*, type C
Antimicrobial agent–associated diarrhea and pseudomembranous colitis	*C. difficile*
Myonecrosis or gas gangrene	*C. perfringens*, *C. septicum*, *C. histolyticum*
Metastatic clostridial myonecrosis	*C. septicum*, *C. perfringens*
Neutropenic colitis	*C. tertium*, *C. septicum*, *C. perfringens*
Postabortal sepsis/uterine myonecrosis	*C. perfringens*
Emphysematous cholecystitis	*C. perfringens*
Suppurative or pyogenic infections (intra-abdominal abscess, fetid foot of the diabetic)[a]	*C. perfringens*, *C. ramosum*, *C. bifermentans*
Transient (uncomplicated) bacteremia[a]	*C. perfringens*, *C. septicum*

[a] Twenty-five to 30 other species have also been isolated in low frequency from these infections.

rhea, clostridial diseases of human beings are relatively rare; unfortunately, the potential for death from these rare processes is substantial. This potential is often exaggerated by the failure of medical personnel to make the correct diagnosis early.

Botulism is a rare disease, although appreciable underreporting probably occurs in all countries. Spores of *C. botulinum* can be found in soil and sediment throughout the world. Most cases are caused by contamination of home-canned food with type A or type B spores; type E disease is usually caused by contaminated canned fish products. Because commercially canned products may be distributed to a large number of people over a large geographical area, the detection of cases may be difficult.

The incidence of tetanus is inversely related to the extent to which the population has been immunized. The number of cases of tetanus reported in the United States is fewer than 100 per year. In other parts of the world, the incidence is much higher. Wound contamination with feces or soil containing *Clostridium tetani* spores is the usual predisposing event; unfortunately, the tetanus-causing wound sometimes appears trivial or even noninfected. Tetanus has also been reported in association with injection drug use, apparently as a consequence of inoculation of spores by needle puncture.

Clostridial food poisoning is a relatively common form of food poisoning and is typically related to preparation of large quantities of food as for banquets and to improper storage after preparation.

C. difficile diarrhea is almost always associated with antimicrobial therapy. Almost all antimicrobial agents that are secreted in bile after parenteral administration or incompletely absorbed after oral administration may reach the colon in appreciable concentrations. High concentrations of these agents produce major changes in the bacterial flora of the colon and thereby permit *C. difficile* (when present) to proliferate and produce its toxins. Nosocomial transmission of the disease has been demonstrated; the spores of *C. difficile* are hardy and may be transferred from one patient to another directly by hospital personnel or by fomites, or both. The most common offending antimicrobial agents are penicillins, cephalosporins, and clindamycin. The incidence of *C. difficile*-induced diarrhea with such agents is probably about 5% of all cases treated. Almost all antimicrobial agents appear capable of causing *C. difficile* diarrhea.

The incidence of clostridial myonecrosis is difficult to estimate. Historically, the disease has been a product of warfare in which traumatic wounds were grossly contaminated with dirt or fecal material and were not debrided promptly. In contrast, an appreciable proportion (perhaps one-third to one-half) of cases of civilian clostridial myonecrosis occur after surgery; the remainder are related to accidental trauma or fetal abortion performed by nonmedical personnel. The usual predisposition is contamination of devitalized tissue, particularly muscle, by *Clostridium perfringens* or other histotoxic clostridia. Although soil may be the source of the organism in some instances, it is becoming increasingly evident that an appreciable number of cases are derived from clostridia in the large bowel. Metastatic clostridial myonecrosis (rather than wound myonecrosis) is a rare disease.

PATHOGENESIS

The pathogenesis of clostridial diseases is varied and depends to a great extent on the specific clinical entity under consideration. In general, clostridial diseases can be divided into those in which production of a toxin is known to be important and those in which a role for toxins has not been shown. Of the clinical entities shown in Table 290.1, toxins are known to be important in all except emphysematous cholecystitis, transient (uncomplicated) bacteremia, and suppurative infections.

Botulism is a paralytic illness caused by *C. botulinum* types A, B, and E and occasionally type F. Each of these strains produces a potent neurotoxin that interferes with release of the neurotransmitter acetylcholine at peripheral cholinergic synapses; disease manifestations are related to this interference with neurotransmission. Minute quantities of the toxin (10^{-8} g) may be lethal. Disease in adults usually occurs as a consequence of ingestion of canned food contaminated with *C. botulinum*; after commercial or home canning, the heat-resistant spores germinate, multiply, and produce toxin. Unfortunately, canned foods that contain *C. botulinum* toxin may have a completely normal odor and appearance. Botulinal toxin is destroyed by boiling for 5 to 10 minutes or by heating to 80° C for 30 minutes. Rarely, an illness that resembles infant botulism occurs in adults; *C. botulinum* autointoxication, adult infectious botulism of unknown source, or "adult infant botulism" is caused by production of the toxin in the gut rather than toxin ingestion. Wound botulism is an uncommon entity that occurs when a traumatic wound is con-

taminated by soil and becomes infected by *C. botulinum*. Toxin is produced in situ and absorbed from the wound.

Tetanus, in contrast to botulism, is a spastic illness in which the cardinal manifestation is skeletal muscle tetany. The organism is usually introduced into the body through soil or fecal contamination of a traumatic wound; the wound occasionally may be so trivial as to not warrant medical attention. Toxin is elaborated in the soft tissues and in the nonimmune person is absorbed into the bloodstream and disseminated to tissues throughout the body. The toxin is thought to be taken up primarily by the peripheral endings of motor neurons and, to a lesser extent, by sensory and autonomic nerve endings. The toxin then travels along the neuron to the cell body in the central nervous system and then passes across the synapse into the presynaptic terminals of γ-aminobutyric acid–releasing spinal inhibitory neurons. The major activity of the toxin is prevention of neurotransmitter release by these inhibitory neurons; loss of this inhibitory effect leads initially to increased muscle tone and eventually to a sustained contraction (tetany) of both agonist and antagonist muscle groups.

Clostridial food poisoning is a relatively mild illness caused by enterotoxin-producing strains of *C. perfringens*. When foods, particularly meat or meat products, contaminated with *C. perfringens* are stored at ambient temperatures or are allowed to cool slowly after cooking, surviving organisms (usually spores) proliferate to extremely large numbers of vegetative cells. On ingestion, the vegetative cells begin sporulation and during sporulation produce an enterotoxin. In contrast to botulism, the toxin of *C. perfringens* is believed to be produced in vivo rather than being ingested.

Enteritis necroticans (pig-bel) is a severe necrotizing disease of the small intestine that is caused by the β toxin of *C. perfringens* type C. Although the pathophysiology of this disease is complex and unclear, essential factors appear to be reduced trypsin activity in the gut caused by poor nutrition and ingestion of protein-rich foods in conjunction with trypsin inhibitors (such as sweet potatoes). (Trypsin is thought to degrade the toxin.) The classic setting for enteritis necroticans is in the South Pacific islands when pigs are cooked in a manner that results in heavy contamination of the meat by *C. perfringens* type C. Clearly, however, other factors besides pig feasting predispose to enteritis necroticans, as indicated by outbreaks of disease in Europe in the 1940s and in other parts of the world in the 1980s and 1990s.

Antimicrobial agent–associated diarrhea and pseudomembranous colitis are caused by a toxin or toxins of *C. difficile*.

Clostridial myonecrosis (gas gangrene), uterine myonecrosis, and metastatic (or spontaneous) myonecrosis are entities that share the same pathophysiology. The first two processes involve accidental traumatic or surgical introduction of histotoxic clostridia (usually *C. perfringens*) into skeletal or uterine muscle. The process known as metastatic myonecrosis is initiated when a breach of the colonic or cecal mucosa permits *C. perfringens* or *Clostridium septicum* to gain access to the bloodstream. The most common bowel lesion is an unrecognized adenocarcinoma of the cecum, but other solid tumors of the bowel, leukemia, and neutropenia also have been implicated. By mechanisms that are not understood, the organism may lodge in a distant muscle and spontaneously cause myonecrosis. Myonecrosis is produced by local elaboration of α toxin, which is a lecithinase capable of hydrolyzing essential components of mammalian cell membranes. This toxin is therefore thought to be the principal cause of muscle necrosis and intravascular hemolysis.

Gangrenous or emphysematous cholecystitis is a particularly severe form of gallbladder disease that frequently yields *C. perfringens* on culture. Muscle invasion and clostridial toxemia are not features of this entity.

Suppurative or pyogenic infections involving clostridia are the most difficult for the clinician to interpret. Pyogenic infections caused by anaerobes are also likely to yield clostridia because anaerobic infections of the peritoneum, abdominal viscera, female genital tract, and lower extremities are usually derived from fecal flora. Such infections are often associated with soft-tissue (but not muscle) necrosis and may, on culture, yield several species of anaerobes (including clostridia) and several species of aerobic or facultative bacteria. Microscopic examination of infected tissue or exudate may reveal large gram-positive bacilli with square ends or spore-forming bacilli that resemble clostridia. Necrotizing clostridial toxins do not appear to be present in these infections, and many of the species of *Clostridium* that are recovered are not toxigenic.

Clostridial bacteremia in patients with skeletal or uterine myonecrosis is obviously a grave complication and may be associated with intravascular hemolysis. In other patients, however, bacteremia is often a benign clinical event. Frequently, the source of such bacteremia is not clinically evident, and the bacteremia is transient; the presumed source for such a process is the bacterial flora of the colon.

■ CLINICAL FINDINGS

BOTULISM

The typical incubation period for botulism is about 1 day, but it may range from several hours to 7 or 8 days. Early symptoms may be nausea, vomiting, and generalized lassitude. Extreme dryness of the mouth and throat may cause the patient to complain of sore throat. Ileus, constipation, urinary retention, and systemic hypotension may occur as a consequence of autonomic dysfunction. Neurologic symptoms are usually present early in disease. Symmetrical descending ocular and bulbar dysfunction manifest as diplopia, ptosis, blurred vision, dysphonia, dysarthria, and dysphagia occurs early and is followed by descending weakness of the muscles of respiration and of the extremities. The patient is afebrile, alert, and oriented. The presence of fixed or poorly reactive and dilated pupils in an alert patient is highly suggestive of botulism. The absence of ocular dysfunction does not exclude the disease. Neurologic examination may reveal generalized muscle weakness; sensation is intact; deep tendon reflexes may be present, absent, or depressed; and bowel and urinary bladder atony may be present. Wound botulism is similar clinically, except for the possible presence of fever due to wound infection.

Botulism has had a relatively poor prognosis. Because all aspects of the disease are reversible, the prognosis depends to a great extent on early diagnosis and institution of supportive care. The mortality rate now is 10% to 25%. The major problem in botulism is muscle weakness, which may progress after admission and be severe and protracted. Respiratory arrest has been the usual cause of death. Recovery from botulism is typically gradual over weeks to months.

TETANUS

Tetanus in adults has classically been described as having three clinical forms: cephalic tetanus, in which infection around the head leads to spasm of muscles supplied by the cranial nerves, particularly the facial nerve; local tetanus manifested by tetanic contractions of muscles at the site of infection; and generalized tetanus. Cephalic and local tetanus may progress to generalized tetanus; 75% or more of cases are of the generalized form. The incubation period varies from a few days to a few weeks and is roughly proportional to the distance of the wound from the central nervous system. Clinically, the first signs of tetanus are spasm of the jaw muscles (trismus), neck stiffness, and increased muscle tone and stiffness.

As the disease progresses, the muscle tone may increase to the point of rigidity. Rigidity of facial muscles leads to the facial sneer (*risus sardonicus*); the abdominal muscles and back muscles are tense; and rigidity of the extremity muscles holds the patient in a fixed position of extension. In severe disease, spasm of the powerful extensor muscles of the back may supervene over the spinal flexors to produce the backward arching of the back, termed *opisthotonos*. Muscle rigidity and spasm are extremely painful and can also readily produce bone fracture, particularly of the vertebrae. Spasm of pharyngeal muscles leads to difficulty in swallowing and may result in aspiration of oropharyngeal contents. Spasm of laryngeal muscles may cause airway obstruction, and diaphragmatic and intercostal muscle spasms may cause apnea. Autonomic dysfunction, manifested as fluctuating but sometimes severe hypertension and hypotension, tachycardia, cardiac arrhythmia, profuse diaphoresis, and fever (unrelated to infection) is common in severe cases. The patient's sensorium is not significantly impaired except in severe disease.

Tetanus is a reversible disease. The violent contractions of spasms may lead to respiratory insufficiency (the patient simply cannot ventilate) and to fractures, particularly of vertebrae. Complete recovery may require weeks or months.

OTHER DISEASE FORMS

The incubation period for *clostridial food poisoning* is usually 8 to 12 hours after ingestion of contaminated food. The prominent symptoms are watery diarrhea and moderately severe to severe midepigastric pain. Nausea may be present occasionally, but fever, chills, and emesis are rare, and the stools do not contain either blood or mucus. The disease resolves within 24 hours and is not associated with mortality or prolonged morbidity.

In contrast, *enteritis necroticans* is a serious, life-threatening disease. Illness usually occurs within 24 hours of ingestion of contaminated food and is characterized by vomiting, acute abdominal pain, diarrhea that is often bloody, and shock. Pathologically, inflammation and areas of necrosis are seen in the small intestine. Enteritis necroticans is a rapidly progressive disease. Because bowel necrosis is common, peritonitis may develop rather rapidly. Mortality with this illness has been about 40%.

C. difficile–associated diarrhea may develop during or up to 6 weeks after cessation of antimicrobial therapy. On occasion, it may occur as early as the second or third day of therapy. Occasionally, one or two doses of prophylactic antimicrobial therapy may cause *C. difficile* diarrhea. The course of *C. difficile*–associated diarrhea typically is that of a self-limited illness; resolution may occur in 80% to 90% of cases within 1 or 2 weeks after discontinuation of the offending antimicrobial agent. In a few patients, the illness may be protracted. Complications, including toxic megacolon, bowel perforation, and death, have been reported but are rare. Protein-losing enteropathy, with significant hypoalbuminemia, may be relatively common.

The incubation period of *clostridial myonecrosis* is variable but typically is 3 or 4 days; it may, however, be as short as 8 to 12 hours. The first sign of myonecrosis is often the sudden onset of severe, unremitting pain at the affected site. The severity of the pain is remarkable because it frequently seems inconsistent with the relatively benign clinical findings at the site of muscle involvement. Moderate fever is typically present. The pain becomes progressively more severe. There is prominent local swelling and blanching of the overlying skin; a thin, but sometimes copious, serous, serosanguineous, or hemorrhagic exudate develops. The wound typically has a sweet odor, but a foul, offensive odor has been noted on occasion. A purple or blue discoloration of the skin may develop, and bullae filled with serosanguineous fluid occur. The sensorium is clear, but the patient is apprehensive and often has a sense of impending doom; toxic delirium, if it occurs, develops late in the course of disease. Other late findings include renal failure and hypotension. Although gas may be present, it is often difficult to detect early in the illness and may become abundant only in the terminal stages of disease.

Uterine myonecrosis lacks the cutaneous features. Jaundice, renal failure, and hemoglobinuria are relatively prominent features of uterine myonecrosis.

Unfortunately, the diagnosis of clostridial myonecrosis can be made definitively only at surgery by inspection of the muscle. Early on, the muscle is pale and edematous; subsequently, contractility disappears, the blood supply is lost, and gas may be detectable. Progressive reddening and purple mottling of the muscle occur and then dark discoloration as the muscle becomes necrotic and liquefies. All these findings may be present simultaneously in various areas of the same muscle, because the changes occur rapidly and the process spreads outward from the initial site of infection.

Emphysematous cholecystitis is an uncommon but severe variant of cholecystitis in which gas is in the gallbladder lumen and later in the surrounding tissues; gangrene and perforation of the gallbladder may develop. Patients with this disease tend to be elderly and have diabetes mellitus.

Suppurative or *pyogenic infections* that involve clostridia as part of a mixed flora do not appear to be clinically distinct from such infections that do not yield clostridia on culture. These infections are reviewed in Chapter 291.

Bacteremia, which may occur with any of the myonecrosis syndromes, has also been associated with a form of neutropenic colitis; the organisms involved here are *C. septicum*, *C. perfringens*, and *Clostridium tertium*. Transient clostridial bacteremia, by definition, is a benign process that most frequently involves *C. perfringens*; a thorough history and physical examination are necessary and are usually sufficient to exclude potentially life-threatening infection. A second blood culture should be done as a precautionary measure. When *C. septicum* is the cause of transient bacteremia, however, investigation of the large bowel for occult malignancy is prudent.

Clostridial myonecrosis is an extremely rapidly progressive disease that may cause death within hours of onset; therefore, a clinical diagnosis must be established immediately and therapy instituted. The overall mortality rate is about 50%; mortality is lowest when an extremity (that can be amputated, if necessary) is involved and is highest when unresectable paravertebral or abdominal wall muscles are involved or when there is intravascular hemolysis.

■ LABORATORY FINDINGS

Laboratory findings, other than for selected tests, are not of clinical value and, for most of the important clostridial diseases, the diagnosis must be based on clinical criteria.

With regard to botulism, the cerebrospinal fluid examination is unremarkable. Electromyography, if done specifically as part of an evaluation for botulism, may yield findings consistent with that diagnosis; these findings include enhanced and prolonged post-tetanic facilitation, muscle fibrillation, and small-amplitude polyphasic motor unit potentials. Confirmation of disease by a reference laboratory is an important public health measure to help prevent additional cases. Hence, the suspect food item and the patient's serum, gastric contents, and feces should be tested for *C. botulinum*, toxin, or both, depending on the sample.

Although *C. tetani* may be recovered from the wound of patients with tetanus, it often is not. The diagnosis can be excluded (retrospectively) if protective levels of antitoxin from prior immunization are present in serum obtained before treatment with antitoxin.

Clostridial food poisoning is diagnosed by detecting high counts of enterotoxin-producing *C. perfringens* in the implicated food and by recovery of the same serotype from feces of affected patients.

C. difficile–induced diarrhea is most effectively diagnosed by detection in feces of either the enterotoxin or the cytotoxin, or both produced by the organism; the most sensitive and specific assay available is detection of a cytopathic effect in tissue culture.

Gram's stain of exudate in cases of suspected clostridial myonecrosis may reveal large, gram-positive bacilli with square ends and a paucity of intact leukocytes; culture of exudate or muscle fragments may help to establish the diagnosis retrospectively. For practical purposes, however, the diagnosis must be confirmed by inspection of the involved muscle.

■ OPTIMAL MANAGEMENT

The more severe clostridial diseases require extensive and aggressive supportive care because of a high incidence of complications, including secondary infection.

Specific therapy for food-borne botulism should include careful observation for signs of respiratory insufficiency and early institution of endotracheal intubation and ventilatory support. Purging of the bowel by gastric lavage, purgatives, and saline enemas is recommended. Trivalent antitoxin should be given as soon as the diagnosis has been established to neutralize toxin that may continue to circulate for prolonged periods. The antitoxin is available from state health departments and the US Centers for Disease Control and Prevention and is an equine preparation directed against *C. botulinum* types A, B, and E.

After hypersensitivity to horse serum has been excluded (or the patient has been desensitized), 2 ampules of the trivalent preparation should be administered and the dose repeated in 2 to 4 hours. Some experts recommend giving half of each dose intramuscularly and half intravenously, whereas others recommend giving the entire dose intravenously. Because the goal is to bind circulating toxin, it seems most appropriate to administer all of each dose intravenously. Hypersensitivity to horse serum occurs in about 20% of patients and anaphylaxis in 3% to 5%. The use of guanidine hydrochloride to promote acetylcholine release is not recommended because there is a lack of convincing scientific data regarding its efficacy. Treatment for wound botulism should also include aggressive debridement of the wound and therapy with penicillin G and other antibiotics as appropriate.

The most crucial aspect of tetanus management is ventilatory support. In full-blown tetanus, the spontaneous spasms prevent effective ventilation. Therefore, tracheostomy, assisted ventilation, and the liberal use of sedating agents, muscle relaxants,

and neuromuscular blockade are crucial. Agents that have been used successfully include the shorter-acting barbiturates, benzodiazepines, and, in the case of severe spasms, curare-like agents. The induction of spasms can be decreased by reducing external stimuli; thus, placing the patient in a quiet room and avoiding unnecessary physical stimuli are important. Feeding by means of gastrostomy and parenteral hyperalimentation are preferred to feeding through a nasogastric tube because of the risk of massive and fatal aspiration. Wound debridement and administration of penicillin G (and other antimicrobial agents as indicated) are important to prevent continued toxin production. Passive immunization should be given as soon as the diagnosis is suspected. Passive immunization can be effected by intravenous administration of 3,000 units of human tetanus immune globulin; horse antitoxin should be avoided because of the risk of hypersensitivity reactions. Active immunization should be given using the standard regimen for adsorbed tetanus toxoid, because clinical tetanus does not necessarily confer immunity.

Tetanus can be prevented by active immunization of children and by aggressive surgical management of traumatic wounds and the use of passive and active immunization in these patients (Table 290.2). Unimmunized adults should receive adsorbed tetanus (and diphtheria) toxoid using a three-dose schedule consisting of an initial dose, a second dose 1 month later, and the last dose 6 months later. Although immunization may be protective for many years, administration of a booster every 10 years is recommended.

The management of enteritis necroticans is basically surgical and involves resection of necrotic bowel along with antimicrobial treatment of peritonitis when present. Preliminary data suggest that immunization may be useful.

The management of *C. difficile*–induced diarrhea involves discontinuation of the offending antimicrobial agent (or, if further treatment is needed, a change to another agent that is unlikely to cause diarrhea) and consideration of treatment directed against *C. difficile*. If the disease is of mild to moderate severity, removal of the offending antimicrobial agent may suffice. If the disease is severe, if it develops after discontinuation of antimicro-

TABLE 290.2.	GUIDELINES FOR ACTIVE AND PASSIVE TETANUS PREVENTION	
Immunization Status	**Wound Status**	**Recommendation**
Unimmunized or incompletely immunized	Low-risk wound	Immunization (see text)
	Tetanus-prone wound[a] or any wound neglected for 24 hours	1 dose of TD[b] and administration of 250 U of HTIG[c]; complete immunization later
Fully immunized plus booster in past 10 years	Low-risk wound	None
	Tetanus-prone wound	1 dose of TD if no booster in past 5 years
	Any wound neglected for 24 hours	1 dose of TD plus 250 U HTIG
Fully immunized but no booster in past 10 years	Low-risk wound	1 dose of TD
	Tetanus-prone wound	1 dose of TD
	Any wound neglected for 24 hours	1 dose of TD plus 250 U HTIG

[a] A wound that is likely to have been contaminated with soil or feces (hence, *Clostridium tetani*).
[b] A combination of adsorbed tetanus and diphtheria toxoids for administration to adults; diphtheria–pertussis–tetanus vaccine should not be given to adults.
[c] Human tetanus immune globulin.

bial therapy, or it does not improve within 3 or 4 days after discontinuation of therapy, then treatment directed against *C. difficile* should be instituted. Orally administered vancomycin, metronidazole, and bacitracin have been shown to be effective, and all strains are susceptible to these agents. Based on low cost and worldwide availability, metronidazole, 500 mg orally three or four times per day, is considered to be the drug of choice. Vancomycin, 125 to 250 mg orally four times per day, is as effective as metronidazole but is appreciably more expensive. The dosage of bacitracin is 25,000 units four times per day. Because of recent concerns about the emergence of vancomycin-resistant enterococci, vancomycin is now recommended only in cases of life-threatening or refractory (to other agents) *C. difficile*–induced diarrhea. Therapy with any of these agents should be for 7 to 10 days, and oral administration should be used to ensure adequate gut levels of drug.

Cholestyramine and other binding resins are often used for treatment of *C. difficile*–induced diarrhea; the data, however, suggest that the resins probably do not contribute significantly to patient management. Antimotility agents may exacerbate rather than relieve symptoms in patients with infectious diarrhea and should not be used. A distressing problem in management of *C. difficile*–associated disease is the propensity for relapse of disease after apparent cure with metronidazole, vancomycin, or bacitracin therapy. Such relapse may occur from several days to 6 weeks after treatment. The relapse invariably responds to retreatment with the same drug and is not the result of antimicrobial resistance, but relapse may occur after cessation of treatment. Administration of cholestyramine (but not in association with vancomycin), reconstitution of the fecal flora, and ingestion of *Saccharomyces bourlardii* in capsular form have shown limited success in various reports. The most effective means of treating recurring relapsing disease is a prolonged tapering course of oral vancomycin over a 6- to 8-week period or longer.

The mainstay of treatment for clostridial myonecrosis is radical surgical debridement of affected tissues in an emergency setting; many operations are often needed to ensure that all devitalized tissue has been removed. High doses of penicillin G (about 20 million units daily for adults with normal renal function) is considered to be the antimicrobial therapy of choice; concomitant therapy may be indicated to cover resistant anaerobes such as *Bacteroides fragilis* and facultative gram-negative bacilli. Gas gangrene antitoxin has not been shown to be of value; because it is of equine origin, the potential benefit of such antitoxin is outweighed by the risk of adverse reactions. Similarly, hyperbaric oxygen therapy has been promoted for treatment of clostridial myonecrosis, but convincing data are not available. Definitive surgical debridement or amputation certainly should not be delayed to transport the patient to a facility that has a hyperbaric unit.

BIBLIOGRAPHY

Finegold SM. *Anaerobic bacteria in human disease.* New York: Academic Press, 1977.
Finegold SM, George WL, eds. *Anaerobic infections in humans.* San Diego: Academic Press, 1989.
Rolfe RD, Finegold SM, eds. *Clostridium difficile: its role in intestinal disease.* Orlando: Academic Press, 1988.
Smith LDS. *Botulism.* Springfield, IL: Charles C Thomas, 1977.
Smith LDS, Williams BL. *The pathogenic anaerobic bacteria,* third ed. Springfield, IL: Charles C Thomas, 1984.
Styrt B, Gorbach SL. Recent developments in the understanding of the pathogenesis and treatment of anaerobic infections. *N Engl J Med* 1989; 321:298–302.
Willis AT. *Clostridia of wound infection.* London: Butterworth & Co, 1969.

Kelley's Textbook of Internal Medicine, fourth edition. Edited by H. David Humes. Lippincott Williams & Wilkins, Philadelphia © 2000.

C H A P T E R

291

INFECTIONS CAUSED BY NONCLOSTRIDIAL ANAEROBES

SYDNEY M. FINEGOLD
W. LANCE GEORGE

Infections due to nonclostridial anaerobes include infections of all types anywhere in the body. The major types of anaerobic infections, in terms of frequency of occurrence, include oral and dental, pleuropulmonary, intra-abdominal, female genital tract, and skin and soft-tissue infections. Other infections in which anaerobic bacteria are commonly involved are brain abscess, chronic sinusitis, chronic otitis media, neck space infections, bite wound infections, and bone and joint infections. Some of these anaerobic infections, such as Vincent's angina and various forms of actinomycosis, are distinctive entities; most are not clinically distinguishable from similar infections not involving non–spore-forming anaerobes.

The clinically significant non–spore-forming anaerobic bacteria are found primarily in the genera *Bacteroides, Prevotella, Porphyromonas, Fusobacterium, Bilophila, Sutterella, Peptostreptococcus, Actinomyces, Propionibacterium,* and *Eubacterium.* The species most commonly encountered clinically are listed in Table 291.1. Microaerophilic streptococci are not true anaerobes but are included because they are commonly found in the same setting as true anaerobes and because anaerobic transport and culture techniques are usually necessary for their recovery from specimens. The non–spore-forming anaerobes are prevalent among the normal flora of the human body, particularly on mucosal surfaces. Infections with these organisms are of endogenous origin. They often involve many organisms, usually a mixture of both anaerobes and aerobic or facultative bacteria.

TABLE 291.1. MAJOR NONSPORING ANAEROBES ENCOUNTERED CLINICALLY

Gram-negative bacilli
  Bacteroides fragilis group
    Especially *B. fragilis, B. thetaiotaomicron, B. distasonis, B. ovatus, B. vulgatus*
  Other *Bacteroides*
    B. ureolyticus
    B. splanchnicus
  Campylobacter (*C. concisus, C. recta, C. curva, C. gracilis*)
  Porphyromonas species (*P. asaccharolytica, P. gingivalis, P. endodontalis*)
  Pigmented *Prevotella* species (*P. corporis, P. denticola, P. intermedia, P. loescheii, P. melaninogenica, P. nigrescens*)
  Other *Prevotella* species
    P. oris
    P. buccae
    P. oralis group
    P. bivia
    P. distens
  Fusobacterium species
    F. nucleatum
    F. necrophorum
    F. mortiferum
    F. varium
  Bilophila wadsworthia
  Sutterella wadsworthensis
Gram-positive cocci
  Peptostreptococcus
    Especially *P. anaerobius, P. micros, P. magnus, P. asaccharolyticus, P. prevotii*
  Microaerophilic streptococci[a] (especially *S. anginosus, S. constellatus, S. intermedius; Gemella morbillorum*)[a]
Gram-positive non–spore-forming bacilli
  Actinomyces (*A. israelii, A. meyerii, A. naeslundii, A. odontolyticus, A. viscosus, A. neuii, A. radingae, A. turicensis*)
  Propionibacterium propionicum (*Arachnia propionica*)
  Propionibacterium acnes
  Bifidobacterium dentium (*B. eriksonii*)
  Eubacterium (*E. lentum, E. nodatum*)

[a] Not true anaerobes

TABLE 291.2. CONDITIONS PREDISPOSING TO ANAEROBIC INFECTION

General

Diabetes mellitus
Corticosteroids
Neutropenia
Hypogammaglobulinemia
Malignancy
Immunosuppression
Cytotoxic drugs
Splenectomy
Collagen vascular diseases

Decreased Redox Potential

Obstruction and stasis
Tissue anoxia
Tissue destruction
Aerobic infection
Foreign body
Calcium salts
Burns
Vascular insufficiency

PATHOGENESIS

Infection with non–spore-forming anaerobes occurs primarily in an anaerobic environment, which usually results from impaired circulation, surgery, trauma, or malignant or other disease. A defect in the mucosal surface of the oral, intestinal, or female genital tract permits endogenous anaerobes to penetrate to the deeper tissues to set up infection. Previous or concurrent infection with nonanaerobic organisms may reduce the oxidation-reduction potential at the site. Other factors involved in synergy (common in mixed infections) include production of nutrients essential for growth of fastidious anaerobes and production of toxins or other virulence factors. Putative virulence factors produced by non–spore-forming anaerobes include the ability to adhere to various surfaces; production of capsular material (by *Bacteroides fragilis* in particular—the capsule inhibits macro-phage migration, is antiphagocytic for aerobes and anaerobes, interferes with T-cell function, and promotes abscess formation); production of catalase and superoxide dismutase (conferring oxygen tolerance); production of immunoglobulin proteases; production of hyaluronidase, collagenase, chondroitin sulfatase, neuraminidase, fibrinolysin, heparinase, and other coagulation-promoting factors; and production of lipopolysaccharide, leukotoxin, butyrate, and soluble inhibitors of chemotaxis and succinate, which inhibit neutrophil respiratory burst by reducing intracellular pH. Important pathogenetic factors and conditions predisposing to anaerobic infection are summarized in Table 291.2.

In aspiration pneumonia and other pleuropulmonary infections involving anaerobes, the pathogenesis is usually different, with aspiration of oropharyngeal or gastric contents the major background factor and periodontal disease or gingivitis also important in many patients. In the process of such aspiration, oral flora (in which anaerobes predominate) is carried down into the bronchial tree and alveoli.

The primary pathologic features of non–spore-forming anaerobic infection are a neutrophilic response, abscess formation, tissue invasion with necrosis and gas production, and, in the case of actinomycosis, granuloma formation and fibrosis.

EPIDEMIOLOGY

Even when non–spore-forming anaerobic infection is associated with surgical procedures and implantation of a foreign body (e.g., ventriculoatrial shunt, implanted intrauterine device), the infecting agents derive from the host's indigenous flora.

One non–spore-forming anaerobe that may spread from person to person and cause diarrhea is enterotoxin-producing *B. fragilis*.

CLINICAL FINDINGS

Non–spore-forming anaerobic bacteria are involved in a wide variety of infections; the clinical features vary with the site and type of infection. Specific clinical situations predisposing to anaerobic infection are given in Table 291.3. Table 291.4 lists infections in which anaerobes are commonly involved and others in which anaerobes seldom play a role.

Anaerobes have been recovered from 5% to 15% of all positive blood cultures in various series. The most common isolate, *Propionibacterium acnes*, usually represents a skin contaminant but may be involved in bacteremia in the setting of an implanted prosthetic or intravascular device. The *B. fragilis* group is the anaerobe most commonly encountered. The second most common blood culture isolates of clinical significance are various *Peptostreptococcus* species. Anaerobes are found with some frequency in polymicrobial bacteremia. Distinctive features that are occasionally found and may be suggestive of anaerobic bacteremia include suppurative thrombophlebitis, metastatic infection, and hyperbilirubinemia.

Obligate anaerobes are uncommon causes of endocarditis, but microaerophilic streptococci may be found in up to 5% to 10% of cases. The most common anaerobe encountered is *Peptostreptococcus*. There is a tendency for *Bacteroides*, and perhaps other anaerobes, to produce large vegetations and embolic phenomena in large vessels.

Anaerobic bacteria are the primary cause of brain abscess, accounting for over 90% of cases. Background factors are often sinus, ear, or mastoid infection, oral or dental infection, pulmonary infection, or hematogenous spread from other foci. The anaerobes most commonly involved are *B. fragilis* and other β-lactamase-producing organisms such as *Prevotella* and *Porphyromonas*, along with *Fusobacterium*, *Peptostreptococcus*, *Actinomyces*, and *Clostridium*. Other important organisms include microaerophilic and viridans group streptococci. Anaerobes are not uncommonly involved in subdural empyema and are found occasionally in epidural abscess. They are not at all common in

TABLE 291.3.	SPECIFIC CLINICAL SITUATIONS PREDISPOSING TO ANAEROBIC INFECTION

Malignancy
   Colon, uterus, lung
   Leukemia
Oral, gastrointestinal, female pelvic surgery
Oral, gastrointestinal, genital tract disease or trauma
Human and animal bites
Aspiration
Therapy with aminoglycosides, trimethoprim-sulfamethoxazole, earlier quinolones
Acatalasemia

TABLE 291.4.	ROLE OF ANAEROBES IN INFECTION

Infections in Which Anaerobes Are Commonly Involved

Brain abscess
Subdural empyema
Periodontal disease
Root canal infection
Odontogenic infections
Chronic sinusitis
Chronic otitis media, mastoiditis
Peritonsillar abscess
Neck space infections
Aspiration pneumonia
Lung abscess
Pleural empyema
Pyogenic liver abscess
Peritonitis
Intra-abdominal abscess
Appendicitis
Postoperative wound infection after bowel or female genital tract surgery
Endometritis
Salpingitis
Tuboovarian abscess
Human and animal bite infections
Infected foot ulcers, especially in diabetics
Decubitus ulcers
Anaerobic cellulitis
Synergistic nonclostridial anaerobic myonecrosis
Anaerobic streptococcal myonecrosis
Necrotizing fasciitis
Chronic osteomyelitis
Actinomycosis

Infections in Which Anaerobes Seldom Play a Role

Meningitis
Acute sinusitis
Acute otitis media
Pharyngitis
Bronchitis
Acute cholecystitis
Spontaneous peritonitis
Pyelonephritis
Cystitis
Acute osteomyelitis

meningitis that has no associated brain abscess or subdural empyema.

Evidence indicates that anaerobes are found in eye infections more frequently than had been appreciated in the past. Anaerobic eye infections are likely to occur in the settings of trauma, surgery, soft contact lens use, topical corticosteroid therapy, and antibacterial therapy. Peptostreptococci are among the most commonly encountered anaerobes in eye infection. *P. acnes* has been recovered a number of times from infection secondary to implantation of artificial lenses. One of the few distinctive clinical syndromes of anaerobic infection of the eye is lacrimal canaliculitis involving *Actinomyces* species, which leads to concretions in the lacrimal canal.

Infections in the head and neck region in which anaerobes may play a role include acute and, more commonly, chronic sinusitis and otitis media, mastoiditis, membranous tonsillitis (Vincent's angina), peritonsillar abscess, deep neck space infections, odontogenic infections, and infection after radical neck dissection or other head and neck surgery. The usual oral anaerobes are the anaerobes most often involved (peptostreptococci, *Prevotella, Porphyromonas,* [the *B fragilis* group may be found in 5% to 20% of certain infections in this area], and fusobacteria). *Fusobacterium necrophorum* is a key pathogen in Vincent's angina and its complications.

Anaerobic bacteria are commonly involved in root canal infection, periapical abscess, osteomyelitis of the jaw, periodontitis and abscess, stomatitis, noma, and other odontogenic infections.

Anaerobes are a major cause of pleuropulmonary infection but are often overlooked because of the difficulty in collecting appropriate specimens. Aspiration pneumonia and lung abscess involve anaerobes in over 90% of cases, and anaerobes are also found commonly in spontaneously occurring thoracic empyema. The most frequently encountered anaerobes are various species of pigmented and nonpigmented *Prevotella, Porphyromonas, Fusobacterium nucleatum,* and *Peptostreptococcus.* The *B. fragilis* group is found in about 5% of anaerobic pleuropulmonary infections. Viridans streptococci are also common. In hospitalized patients, colonization of the oropharynx with nosocomial pathogens such as staphylococci and various gram-negative bacilli may occur, and such organisms may then be involved in a subsequent aspiration pneumonia, along with the anaerobes.

Mediastinitis related to prior perforation of the esophagus, extension of a retropharyngeal abscess, or extension of cellulitis or abscess of dental origin from the neck commonly involves anaerobes.

In intra-abdominal infection, anaerobes play a prominent role, with the bowel as their point of origin. The *B. fragilis* group is found in most patients because it is the dominant member of the normal colonic flora. Other anaerobes encountered include *Bilophila wadsworthia, Peptostreptococcus, Sutterella,* and *Clostridium* species. *Escherichia coli* and streptococci, including enterococci, are also commonly found; in patients with prior hospitalization and antimicrobial therapy, more resistant gram-negative bacilli and staphylococci may be found. Wound and other postoperative infections have a similar infecting flora. In biliary tract infection, *Clostridium perfringens* and, less commonly, *B. fragilis* may be found, along with coliforms and enterococci. Anaerobes are probably the predominant pathogens in liver abscess; the most common anaerobic isolates are *Peptostreptococcus,* the *B. fragilis* group, *Prevotella, Porphyromonas, F. necrophorum,* other fusobacteria, clostridia, and *Actinomyces* species.

Anterior retroperitoneal abscess secondary to appendicitis or diverticulitis typically involves anaerobes. Colonic anaerobes, the *B. fragilis* group in particular, are commonly involved in perineal and perirectal infections.

Anaerobes are frequently involved in female genital tract infections of all types. Peptostreptococci, *Prevotella* (especially *Prevotella bivia* and *Prevotella disiens,* and pigmented species), and *Bacteroides,* including the *B. fragilis* group, are the most common anaerobic isolates, but clostridia, *Actinomyces,* and *Eubacterium* are also important.

Anaerobes are not involved in more than a small percentage of urinary tract infections; data indicate that at least 1.3% of cases of bacteriuria involve anaerobes. Anaerobic bacteremia after urethral dilatation and other manipulation of the urinary tract has been reported.

Non–spore-forming anaerobes are involved in a wide variety of infections of the skin and underlying soft tissues. Included are such processes as cellulitis, pyoderma, cutaneous and subcutaneous abscesses, hidradenitis suppurativa, infected diabetic and other foot ulcers, infected decubitus ulcers, bite wound infections, burn wound infections, bacterial synergistic gangrene, necrotizing fasciitis, anaerobic streptococcal myositis, muscle abscesses in narcotic addicts, and synergistic nonclostridial anaerobic myonecrosis (synergistic necrotizing cellulitis). Infected decubitus ulcers are an important portal of entry for anaerobic bacteremia.

Evidence exists that non–spore-forming anaerobic bacteria are an important cause of osteomyelitis, particularly chronic bone infection of the lower extremities and pelvis (especially in patients with diabetes mellitus, other causes of vascular insufficiency or neuropathy, or trauma). The anaerobes involved vary with the site of the infection, but peptostreptococci are by far the most common; *B. fragilis* group strains are found in 10% to 15% of cases. Other *Bacteroides* and pigmented *Prevotella* are also important. Purulent arthritis involving anaerobes is uncommon but not rare; the *B. fragilis* group is the most common organism when the source is hematogenous. *F. necrophorum* is much less frequently encountered in bone and joint infections than was true in the preantimicrobial era.

Subareolar and recurrent breast abscesses often involve anaerobic bacteria and, as a result, may present distressing problems, such as chronic draining sinuses with foul-smelling pus. The pathogenesis appears similar to that of hidradenitis suppurativa.

Actinomycosis is a chronic destructive process of soft tissue and bone, and sometimes viscera, caused by various species of *Actinomyces* or by *Propionibacterium propionicum.* Pathologically, there is suppuration or granuloma formation, and fibrosis is common, leading to the woody character that is typical of such lesions on palpation. This has led thoracic surgeons, on occasion, to resect a lung on the mistaken impression that carcinoma was present. Chronic draining sinuses are common. The three classic types of actinomycosis are cervicofacial, thoracic, and abdominal, but any part of the body may be involved. A number of cases have been described in connection with the use of intrauterine devices. Some of these cases, as well as cervicofacial actinomycosis, have yielded *Eubacterium nodatum,* an organism that resembles *Actinomyces* closely.

DIAGNOSIS

Clinical clues to anaerobic infection are noted in Table 291.5. The foul or putrid odor that may be evident is the only clue that is specific; no other organisms causing human infection aside from anaerobes (both clostridia and non–spore formers) lead to such an odor. The absence of such an odor, however, does not rule out the possibility of anaerobic infection. The other clues are nonspecific but are still useful in suggesting the

TABLE 291.5.   CLUES TO ANAEROBIC INFECTION

Foul odor of lesion or discharges

Location of infection in proximity to a mucosal surface

Classic clinical picture of anaerobic infection (e.g., actinomycosis, lung abscess)

Infections secondary to human or animal bite

Gas in tissues or discharges

Tissue necrosis, gangrene, abscess formation

Septic thrombophlebitis

Infection associated with malignancy (especially colon, uterus, lung)

Previous therapy with aminoglycoside antibiotics (such as neomycin, gentamicin, and amikacin), trimethoprim-sulfamethoxazole, most older quinolones, monobactams, cephalosporins with poor activity against anaerobes (e.g., ceftazidime)

Black discoloration of blood-containing exudates; these exudates may fluoresce red under ultraviolet light (pigmented *Prevotella* or *Porphyromonas* infections)

Presence of "sulfur granules" In discharges (actinomycosis)

Unique morphology on Gram's stain

No growth on routine culture—"sterile pus"

Failure to grow, aerobically, organisms seen on Gram's stain of original exudate

Growth in anaerobic zone of fluid media or of agar deeps

Growth anaerobically on media containing 75 to 100 μg/mL of kanamycin, neomycin, or paromomycin (or medium also containing vancomycin, in the case of gram-negative anaerobic bacilli)

Characteristic colonies on agar plates anaerobically (e.g., *Fusobacterium nucleatum*)

Young colonies of pigmented anaerobic gram-negative rods may fluoresce red under ultraviolet light (blood agar plate)

likelihood of infection with anaerobes. The combination of tissue necrosis and gas, along with abscess formation, is highly suggestive of the probability of anaerobic infection, although this may be encountered in other types of infection. The unique morphology on Gram's stain applies particularly to the anaerobic gram-negative bacilli (and certain clostridia); commonly noted are irregular staining and pleomorphism.

Two important considerations for the clinician to remember in documenting the presence of anaerobes in a specimen and in determining the specific cause of an infection are the need for proper specimen collection (to avoid picking up normal flora from a nearby mucosal surface because anaerobes are prevalent in such flora) and the need for transport of the specimen under anaerobic conditions (to avoid die-off related to oxygen exposure). In most situations, proper specimen collection is not difficult. In the case of suspected anaerobic pulmonary infection (e.g., aspiration pneumonia), however, it may be something of a problem.

If pleural fluid is present, it should be tapped. In a true anaerobic pulmonary infection, this is likely to be an empyema, and the microbiology of the empyema fluid will accurately reflect that of the lung parenchyma itself. For less serious degrees of suspected anaerobic pulmonary infection, empiric therapy is reasonable. In a seriously ill patient in whom accurate bacteriologic diagnosis is essential for optimal therapy, if empyema fluid is not available, bronchoalveolar lavage with quantitative culture

yields valuable information and may actually be life saving. Specimens obtained properly with a double-lumen, catheter-protected bronchial brush and cultured quantitatively are also satisfactory. A number of commercially available transport devices permit safe transport of delicate anaerobes as well as other organisms.

Results of anaerobic cultures are usually not available for at least a few days because anaerobes grow somewhat more slowly than nonanaerobes and because it may take some time to obtain in pure culture all the different organisms that may be present in a mixed infection. Accordingly, Gram's stain becomes a valuable diagnostic tool because, in a matter of minutes, the clinician may be able to suspect the presence of anaerobic bacteria of specific types and to determine the relative numbers of each of several organisms in a mixed infection.

OPTIMAL MANAGEMENT

The principles of treatment of non–spore-forming anaerobic bacterial infections are modifying the environment so that it is difficult for anaerobes to proliferate and checking the spread of anaerobes into healthy tissues. Measures to control the local environment include debridement of dead tissue, drainage of pus, elimination of obstruction, decompression of swollen tissues restricted by a tight fascia, release of trapped gas, improvement of circulation to the affected part, and improvement of tissue oxygenation. Antimicrobial agents play an important role in limiting the spread of anaerobes into healthy tissues.

The important role of surgical management should be evident from the previous discussion. There are some exceptions, however. Surgery is rarely indicated for lung abscess at present; it is actually contraindicated as a rule because of the hazard of spread of infection. In certain cases of abscess, especially intra-abdominal abscess, drainage may be effected by percutaneous aspiration, with or without catheter drainage, guided by ultrasonography or computed tomography. Hyperbaric oxygen is not beneficial in infection with non–spore-forming anaerobes.

Antimicrobial therapy is important in most anaerobic infections, whether or not surgical treatment has been carried out. Anaerobic bacteria have been manifesting increasing resistance to a number of antimicrobial drugs in recent years. The production of β-lactamases (by many species of anaerobic gram-negative rods and clostridia) is one of the major mechanisms of resistance. Others include plasmid-mediated transferable resistance, transposons, changes in the porin molecules of the outer membrane, and changes in the penicillin-binding proteins. The available agents are listed in Table 291.6 in terms of their in vitro activity against various non–spore-forming anaerobes. The table presents in vitro data, but there are generally comparable clinical data. In vitro results may vary with the test method used (especially with ceftizoxime), strain selection, and other factors. In choosing among several agents, considerations include bactericidal or bacteriostatic activity, penetration of the central nervous system, toxicity, impact on the normal flora, severity of the infection, availability of an orally administered preparation, and cost as well as spectrum of activity against clostridia and nonanaerobes that may be present in a mixed infection.

TABLE 291.6. SUSCEPTIBILITY OF GRAM-NEGATIVE ANAEROBIC BACTERIA

% Susceptible[a]	B. fragilis	Other B. fragilis Group[c]	C. gracilis	Other Bacteroides	Prevotella
>95	Piperacillin Amoxicillin + clavulanate Ampicillin + sulbactam Cefoperazone + sulbactam Piperacillin + tazobactam Ticarcillin + clavulanate Cefoxitin Biapenem Imipenem Meropenem Chloramphenicol Clinafloxacin Satifloxacin Levofloxacin Ofloxacin Trovalfloxacin Metronidazole	Ampicillin + sulbactam Cefoperazone + sulbactam Pipeacillin + tazobactam Ticarcillin + clavulanate Biapenem Imipenem Meropenem Chloramphenicol Clinafloxacin Satifloxacin Trovafloxacin Metronidazole Minocycline	Piperacillin Amoxicillin + clavulanate Piperacillin + tazobactam Ticarcillin + clavulanate Cefoxitin Ceftizoxime Ceftriaxone Biapenem Imipenem Meropenem Chloramphenicol Ciprofloxacin Clinafloxacin Satifloxacin Fleroxacin Lomefloxacin Sparfloxacin Trovafloxacin Metronidazole Azithromycin Clindamycin Erythromycin Roxithromycin Minocycline Tetracycline	Piperacillin Amoxicillin + clavulanate Ampicillin + sulbactam Ticarcillin + clavulanate Cefoperazone Cefoperazone + sulbactam Cefotaxime Cefoxitin Ceftizoximne Biapenem Imipenem Chloramphenicol Clinafloxacin Satifloxacin Levofloxacin Trovafloxacin Metronidazole Clindamycin	Piperacillin Amoxicillin + clavulanate Ampicillin + sulbactam Piperacillin + tazobactam Ticarcillin + clavulanate Cefoxitin Ceftizoxime Biapenem Imipenem Meropenem Chloramphenicol Clinafloxacin Satifloxacin Trovafloxacin Metronidazole Clindamycin
85–95	Cefotetan Ceftizoxime Clindamycin Minocycline	Amoxicillin + clavulanate Piperacillin Cefoxitin Ceftizoxime		Cefotetan Ceflazidime Ceftriaxone Clarithromycin Erythromycin Roxithromycin Minocycline	Ceftriaxone Azithromycin Clarithromycin Erythromycin Roxithromycin
70–84	Moxalactam Ceftriaxone Clarithromycin	Levofloxacin Clarithromycin Clindamycin		Penicillin G Moxalactam Ofloxacin Sparfloxacin Azithromycin	Ciprofloxacin Oflaxacin Sparfloxacin Minocycline
50–69	Cefoperazone Cefotaxime Ceftazidime Sparfloxacin	Cefoperazone Cefotetan Moxalactam Ofloxacin Sparfloxacin		Ciprofloxacin Tetracycline	Tetracycline
<50	Penicillin G[b] Ciprofloxacin Fleroxacin Lomefloxacin Azithromycin Erythromycin Roxithromycin Tetracycline	Penicillin G Cefotaxime Ceftazidime Ceftriaxone Ciprofloxacin Fleroxacin Lomefloxacin Azithromycin Erythromycin Roxithromycin		Fleroxacin Lomefloxacin	Fleroxacin Lomefloxacin

TABLE 291.6.   SUSCEPTIBILITY OF GRAM-NEGATIVE ANAEROBIC BACTERIA

Porphyromonas	Sutterella wadsworthensis	F. nucleatum	F. mortiferum and F. varium	Other Fusobacterium	B. wadsworthia
Piperacillin	Amoxicillin + clavulanate	Piperacillin	Piperacillin	Penicillin G	Piperacillin
Amoxicillin + clavulanate	Ticarcillin + clavulanate	Amoxicillin + clavulanate		Ampicillin + sulbactam	
Cefoxitin	Cefoxitin	Piperacillin + tazobactam	Piperacillin + tazobactam	Piperacillin + tazobactam	Ticarcillin
Ceftizoxime	Ceftriaxone	Ticarcilline + clavulanate	Ticarcillin + clavulanate		Amoxicillin + clavulanate
Ceftriaxone		Cefoxitin	Cefoxitin	Cefoxitin	Ampicillin + sulbactam
Biapenem	Imipenem	Ceftrizoxime	Biapenem	Biapenem	Cefotetan
	Meropenem		Imipenem	Imipenem	
Imipenem	Ciprofloxacin	Ceftriaxone	Meropenem	Meropenem	Cefoxitin
	Fleroxacin	Biapenem			Ceftizoxime
Meropenem		Imipenem	Chloramphenicol	Chloramphenicol	Imipenem
Chloramphenicol		Meropenem	Clinafloxacin		
Clinafloxacin		Chloramphenicol	Satifloxacin	Clinafloxacin	Chloramphenicol
Satifloxacin			Trovafloxacin	Satifloxacin	Ciprofloxacin
		Clinafloxacin		Metronidazole	
Sparfloxacin		Satifloxacin	Metronidazolne	Clindamycin	Satifloxacin
Trovafloxacin		Levofloxacin	Minocycline	Minocycline	Fleroxacin
Metronidazole		Ofloxacin		Tetracycline	Lomefloxacin
Azithromycin		Sparfloxacin			Sparfloxacin
Minocycline		Trovafloxacin			Trovafloxacin
		Clindamycin			Metronidazole
		Metronidazole			Minocycline
		Minocycline			Tetracycline
		Tetracycline			
Ciprofloxacin	Piperacillin		Amoxicillin + clavulanate	Piperacillin	Clindamycin
Clarithromycin	Piperacillin + tazobactam	Azithromycin	Ceftizoxime	Amoxicillin + clavulanate	
Clindamycin	Ceftizoxine		Ceftriaxone	Ticarcillin + clavulanate	
Erythromycin				Cefoperazone + sulbactam	
Roxithromycin	Trovafloxacin			Cefotaxime	
				Cefotetan	
				Ceftizoxime	
				Ceftriaxone	
	Metronidazole	Ciprofloxacin	Clindamycin	Ceftazidime	
			Tetracycline	Moxalactam	
				Ciprofloxacin	
				Sparfloxacin	
				Azithromycin	
Tetracycline	Clindamycin		Ciprofloxacin		
			Sparfloxacin		
Fleroxacin		Fleroxacin	Fleroxacin	Fleroxacin	Amoxicillin
Lomefloxacin		Lomefloxacin	Lomefloxacin	Lomefloxacin	Ampicillin
		Clarithromycin	Azithromycin	Clarithromycin	Penicillin G
		Erythromycin	Clarithromycin	Erythromycin	
		Roxithromycin	Erythromycin	Roxithromycin	
			Roxithromycin		

TABLE 291.6. SUSCEPTIBILITY OF GRAM-POSITIVE ANAEROBIC BACTERIA

% Susceptible	Peptostreptococcus	C. difficile[d]	C. ramosum
>95	Penicillin G Piperacillin Amoxicillin + clavulanate Ampicillin + sulbactam Piperacillin + tazobactam Ticarcillin + clavulanate Cefoperazone Cefoperazone + sulbactam Cefotetan Cefoxitin Ceftazidime Ceftizoxime Ceftriaxone Biapenem Imipenem Meropenem Chloramphenicol Clinafloxacin Satifloxacin Sparfloxacin Trovafloxacin Metronidazole	Ampicillin Piperacillin Ticarcillin Amoxicillin + clavulanate Ampicillin + sulbactam Piperacillin + tazobactam Ticarcillin + clavulanate Cefotetan Imipenem Meropenem Clinafloxacin Satifloxacin Trovafloxacin Metronidazole	Amoxicillin + clavulanate Piperacillin + tazobactam Ticarcillin + clavulanate Ceftizoxime Imipenem Clinafloxacin Satifloxacin Metronidazole
85–95	Levofloxacin Clindamycin Minocycline	Ceftriaxone Biapenem Chloramphenicol	Ampicillin Piperacillin Ampicillin + sulbactam Chloramphenicol Trovafloxacin Clindamycin
70–84	Ciprofloxacin Ofloxacin Azithromycin Clarithromycin Erythromycin		Cefoxitin Clindamycin
50–69	Fleroxacin Tetracycline Roxithromycin	Clindamycin Minocycline Tetracycline Azithromycin Clarithromycin Erythromycin Roxithromycin	Sparfloxacin Minocycline Tetracycline
<50	Lomefloxacin	Cefoxitin Ceftizoxime Ciprofloxacin Fleroxacin Lomefloxacin Sparfloxacin	Ciprofloxacin Fleroxacin Lomefloxacin Azithromycin Clarithromycin Erythromycin Roxithromycin

NSF-GPR, non–spore-forming gram-positive rod.
[a] According to the NCCLS-approved breakpoints (M11-A3), using the intermediate category as susceptible.
[b] NCCLS-approved breakpoint is 4 μg/mL. However, the breakpoint should probably be lowered to 1 μg/mL, which will considerably lower the values for % susceptible. For example, at 1 μg/mL, no strains of the B. fragilis group were susceptible.
[c] Excluding B. fragilis.
[d] Breakpoint is used only as a reference point. C. difficile is primarily of interest in relation to antimicrobial-induced pseudomembranous colitis. These data must be interpreted in the context of level of drug achieved in the colon and impact of agent on indigenous colonic flora.
[e] The order of listing of drugs within percent-susceptible categories is not significant.

TABLE 291.6. SUSCEPTIBILITY OF GRAM-POSITIVE ANAEROBIC BACTERIA

C. perfringens	Other Clostridium sp	NSF-GPR
Ampicillin	Amoxicillin	Penicillin G
Piperacillin	Ampicillin	Piperacillin
Ticarcillin	Carbenicillin	Amoxicillin + clavulanate
Ampicillin + sulbactam	Penicillin G	Ampicillin + sulbactam
Amoxicillin + clavulanate	Piperacillin	Piperacillin + tazobactam
Piperacillin + tazobactam	Ticarcillin	Ticarcillin + clavulanate
Ticarcillin + clavulanate	Ampicillin + sulbactam	Cefotaxime
Cefotetan	Amoxicillin + clavulanate	Ceftizoxime
Ceftizoxime	Biapenem	Biapenem
Biapenem	Imipenem	Imipenem
Imipenem	Chloramphenicol	Meropenem
Chloramphenicol	Clinafloxacin	Chloramphenicol
Ciprofloxacin	Satifloxacin	Clindamycin
Clinafloxacin	Trovafloxacin	Clinafloxacin
Satifloxacin	Metronidazole	Satifloxacin
Fleroxacin	Minocycline	Levofloxacin
Sparfloxacin		Minocycline
Trovafloxacin		
Metronidazole		
Azithromycin		
Clarithromycin		
Erythromycin		
Roxithromycin		
Lomefloxacin	Moxalactam	Cefotetan
Clindamycin		Cefoxitin
		Ceftriaxone
		Cefoperazone + sulbactam
		Trovafloxacin
		Azithromycin
		Clarithromycin
		Erythromycin
		Roxithromycin
Minocycline	Levofloxacin	Cefoperazone
	Ofloxacin	Moxalactam
	Sparfloxacin	Sparfloxacin
	Clindamycin	Tetracycline
	Tetracycline	
Tetracycline	Cefoperazone	Ciprofloxacin
	Cefotaxime	Ofloxacin
	Cefoxitin	Metronidazole
	Ceftizoxime	
	Ceftriaxone	
	Ciprofloxacin	
	Azithromycin	
	Clarithromycin	
	Erythromycin	
	Roxithromycin	
	Ceftazidime	Fleroxacin
	Fleroxacin	Lomefloxacin
	Lomefloxacin	

Aminoglycosides, such as gentamicin and amikacin, have little activity against anaerobes; this is true as well for trimethoprim-sulfamethoxazole, most older quinolones, monobactams, and ceftazidime. Penicillin V and ampicillin (as well as amoxicillin) are comparable to penicillin G in activity. Isoxazolyl penicillins (e.g., dicloxacillin) and nafcillin have rather poor activity against many anaerobes, as do first- and most second-generation cephalosporins.

Duration of therapy should ordinarily be prolonged for anaerobic infections. For example, lung abscess should generally be treated for not less than 3 weeks and often requires much more extended treatment. Metronidazole has had a favorable impact on the prognosis in brain abscess; the high levels achieved in the brain and the excellent bactericidal activity are responsible for its effectiveness. Ordinarily, penicillin G should be used with metronidazole in the treatment of brain abscess. Some failures have been reported with penicillin G in anaerobic pulmonary and head and neck infections because of the production of β-lactamases by the infecting flora. Penicillin can no longer be recommended for such infections.

PREVENTION AND CONTROL

A limited number of useful measures are available for control of infections caused by nonclostridial anaerobes. Good surgical technique is certainly important. Good oxygenation of tissues must be maintained, when possible. Patients who are not fully conscious must be watched because of the possibility of aspirating material into the respiratory tract. Appropriate antimicrobial prophylaxis should be used for dental and selected other procedures such as transurethral resection.

BIBLIOGRAPHY

Borriello SP, ed. *Clinical and molecular aspects of anaerobes.* Petersfield, Great Britain: Wrightson Biomedical, 1990.
Brook I. *Pediatric anaerobic infection: diagnosis and management,* second ed. St. Louis: CV Mosby, 1989.
Duerden BI, Drasar BS, eds. *Anaerobes in human disease.* New York: Wiley-Liss, 1991.
Finegold SM. *Anaerobic bacteria in human disease.* New York: Academic Press, 1977.
Finegold SM, George WL, eds. Anaerobic infections in humans. San Diego: Academic Press, 1989.
Finegold SM, Jousimies-Somer H. Recently described clinically important anaerobic bacteria: medical aspects. *Clin Infect Dis* 1997;25(suppl 2): S88–S93.
Kasper DL, Onderdonk AB, eds. International Symposium on Anaerobic Bacteria and Bacterial Infections. *Rev Infect Dis* 1990;12(suppl 2): S121–261.
Styrt B, Gorbach SL. Recent developments in the understanding of the pathogenesis and treatment of anaerobic infections. *N Engl J Med* 1989; 321:298–302.
Summanen P, Baron EJ, Citron DM, et al. *Wadsworth anaerobic bacteriology manual,* fifth ed. Belmont, CA: Star Publishing Co., 1993.
Wexler HM, Finegold SM. Current susceptibility patterns of anaerobic bacteria. *Yonsei Med J* 1998;39:495–501.

Kelley's Textbook of Internal Medicine, fourth edition. Edited by H. David Humes. Lippincott Williams & Wilkins, Philadelphia © 2000.

CAT-SCRATCH DISEASE, BACILLARY ANGIOMATOSIS, AND PELIOSIS HEPATIS

THOMAS H. BELHORN

Cat-scratch disease (CSD) is a common clinical entity initially described in 1950. The classic disease presentation involves a persistent regional lymphadenopathy in the area of lymphatic drainage from a recent cutaneous cat-scratch lesion. Many subsequent case series have further defined and broadened the clinical presentation and diverse complications associated with CSD.

Since the 1980s, significant advances have been made in defining the causative agent of CSD, *Bartonella henselae.* In addition, several diseases seen primarily in HIV-positive patients, namely, bacillary angiomatosis, bacillary peliosis hepatis, and relapsing febrile bacteremia, are associated with this etiologic agent or closely related *Bartonella* species. Serologic and molecular studies are clarifying the pathogenesis of and relations between these diverse diseases.

INCIDENCE AND EPIDEMIOLOGY

CSD occurs throughout the United States and is estimated to affect approximately 22,000 people and result in 2,000 hospitalizations each year. Most cases are reported in patients 18 years of age or younger, with a slight predominance in boys. However, the disease is seen in all age groups. The increasing number of cases occurring from September through January is thought to reflect either the seasonal variation in acquisition of new family pets or breeding patterns of the reservoir or vector for the pathogen.

In up to 99% of CSD cases, exposure to a cat, usually a kitten, is documented. Symptomatic CSD patients were found to be more likely than a control group to have a pet kitten younger than 12 months of age, to have been scratched or bitten by a kitten, and to have had a kitten with fleas. The domestic cat has been shown to be a major persistent reservoir for the etiologic agent of CSD, with some cats exhibiting prolonged asymptomatic bacteremia. Bites and scratches by other animals, including dogs, may also expose a person to the infectious agent.

Bacillary angiomatosis and peliosis hepatis are most frequently diagnosed in patients with AIDS but are also reported in organ transplantation and cancer patients and rarely in immunocompetent people. Although a recent cat scratch or bite was originally reported in less than 20% of cases of bacillary angiomatosis, further studies have found a strong relation with cat exposure, especially in *B. henselae*-associated disease.

ETIOLOGY

B. henselae (formerly *Rochalimaea henselae*) is the predominant causative agent of CSD as well as of many cases of bacillary angiomatosis and peliosis hepatis. Serologic, epidemiologic, molecular (polymerase chain reaction [PCR]), and culture data have established a convincing link between this organism and the aforementioned diseases. *Afipia felis*, a small, pleomorphic bacillus originally isolated from CSD nodes, may rarely be involved in the pathogenesis of CSD. *Bartonella quintana* (formerly *Rochalimaea quintana*), the causal agent of trench fever, also plays a role in the development of bacillary angiomatosis and peliosis hepatis in HIV-positive patients. Other species of *Bartonella, B. clarridgeiae* and *B. elizabethae*, are less commonly associated with these diseases.

CLINICAL FINDINGS

The patient's age, status of the immune system, and mode of transmission influence the clinical presentation. Table 292.1 lists the major characteristics of CSD and selected other diseases associated with *Bartonella* species.

The initial manifestation of CSD is the appearance of a papule at the site of inoculation, often within the line of a previous cat scratch. This skin lesion, which is noted in 50% to 90% of cases, appears 1 to 2 weeks after contact with the animal. The lesion may evolve from a macule and eventually appear vesicular.

Between 7 to 50 days after the appearance of the cutaneous lesion, the characteristic regional lymphadenopathy ensues. The involved node is enlarged and usually tender. A single node is involved in approximately 50% of the cases, rarely more than three nodes are involved, and the nodes are usually in the distribution of lymphatic drainage from the initial lesion. The nodes affected, in decreasing order of frequency, are axillary, cervical, submandibular, inguinal, preauricular, femoral, and epitrochlear; rarely, postauricular and clavicular nodes and nodes in the chest wall may be involved. Associated fever and mild constitutional symptoms are present in less than one-third of cases, and fever over 39° C is rarely seen. The total duration of symptoms varies from several weeks to several months; suppuration of the node occurs in only 12% of cases.

Unusual manifestations involving different body systems are reported in 10% of CSD cases. Oculoglandular syndrome of Parinaud, first described in the previous century, is a granulomatous conjunctivitis with preauricular adenopathy secondary to inoculation of the agent in the periocular area. Neurologic complications of CSD are reported in more than 2% of patients and include peripheral neuropathy, myelitis, radiculitis, encephalopathy, and retinitis. Patients with encephalopathy can present with headache, seizures, combative behavior, or lethargy; permanent neurologic sequelae are infrequent. A granulomatous hepatitis, occasionally asymptomatic and visualized as hypoechogenic lesions in imaging studies, as well as a granulomatous splenitis, may occur. Immunocompromised patients with CSD may have severe and disseminated disease; renal and liver transplant recipients may present with shock, seizures, and granulomatous hepatitis. Other conditions associated with CSD have included osteomyelitis, pleural effusion, erythema nodosum, erythema annulare, and maculopapular rashes. Prolonged fever without focus has been occasionally described secondary to CSD; enteric acquisition of the agent has been postulated to be responsible for disease without obvious lymphadenopathy.

Bacillary angiomatosis and bacillary peliosis hepatis are distinct pathologic entities occurring almost exclusively in immunocompromised hosts. Cutaneous bacillary angiomatosis presents as single or multiple, red or purple, nodular/papular lesions on the skin or mucosa. These lesions, often described as having a cranberry appearance with occasional crusting or scaling, can reach several centimeters in diameter and ulcerate. Lesions may resemble and must be differentiated from Kaposi's sarcoma. Fever, chills, malaise, headache, weight loss, and other associated constitutional signs and symptoms are not unusual. Extracutaneous manifestations have been described in such diverse organ systems as the central nervous system, muscles, soft tissue, bone marrow, liver and spleen, heart, and mucosal surfaces of the respiratory and gastrointestinal tract.

Bacillary peliosis hepatis is a vasoproliferative condition involving the liver of HIV-infected patients, presenting as multiple cystic, blood-filled spaces in the liver. The usual symptoms and signs include fever, abdominal distention, diarrhea, and hepato-

TABLE 292.1.	CHARACTERISTICS OF SELECTED DISEASES ASSOCIATED WITH *BARTONELLA* SPECIES	
	Cat-Scratch Disease	**Bacillary Angiomatosis/Bacillary Peliosis Hepatis**
Peak age	Children	Young adult
Host immune status	Immunocompetent	Immunosuppressed (HIV, cancer, other), rarely immunocompetent
Predominant clinical manifestation	Lymphadenitis	Cutaneous/visceral lesions, liver lesions
Bartonella species	*B. henselae*	*B. henselae* or *B. quintana*
Antibiotics with possible efficacy	Ciprofloxacin, rifampin, gentamicin, trimethoprim-sulfamethoxazole, azithromycin	Erythromycin, doxycycline, rifampin, azithromycin

splenomegaly. The diagnosis can be made concomitantly with bacillary angiomatosis or bacteremia due to *Bartonella* species. Recurrent bacteremia and endocarditis, including the development of valvular vegetations, may also complicate *Bartonella* infection in the immunocompromised host.

LABORATORY FINDINGS

The diagnosis of CSD has traditionally been based on clinical criteria, mainly the presence of a dermal or conjunctival lesion, regional lymphadenopathy with negative studies for alternative causes, and the history of cat contact. Historically, delayed-type hypersensitivity skin testing with material made from heated purulent lymph node aspirates from CSD patients could be used for confirmation of the diagnosis. However, this test was not standardized or licensed for routine use; serologic testing and alternate methodologies are currently used for confirmation of the diagnosis.

Histopathologic study of CSD lymph nodes characteristically demonstrates granulomas, nonspecific inflammatory infiltrates, and stellate abscesses with central suppurative necrosis and surrounding rims of epithelioid histiocytes. Silver stain impregnation can demonstrate bacilli, especially in nodes examined early in the disease process.

Serologic methods such as an indirect fluorescent antibody assay and an enzyme immunoassay are used for confirmation of *B. henselae* infection and epidemiologic studies. In preliminary studies, the indirect fluorescent antibody assay has shown that 88% of patients with suspected CSD had serum titers of 1:64 or higher to *B. henselae* antigen, whereas healthy control subjects exhibited a low prevalence (3%) of significant titers. A positive serologic test should be interpreted within the clinical context.

Culture of clinical specimens is not routinely performed, because *Bartonella* species are extremely fastidious and require special culture conditions. Varying methods exist for culture of the organisms, but prolonged incubation of lysis centrifugation blood cultures plated onto freshly prepared blood agar plates can be used. PCR has been a useful technique for demonstrating *Bartonella* DNA in clinical specimens and, if available, is considered superior to routine culture for diagnosis.

For diagnosis of bacillary angiomatosis and peliosis hepatis, lesion biopsy for staining and histologic examination, techniques using immunofluorescent antibody, culture, and PCR may be used. Histologic examination of bacillary angiomatosis lesions shows vascular proliferations with cuboidal "plump" endothelial cells protruding into the lumen. Bacillary forms on Warthin–Starry silver impregnation stain are seen in eosinophilic or basophilic granular material present in the interstitium. Infiltration of polymorphonuclear leukocytes is seen frequently. In addition to blood culture techniques described earlier, the agent can be cultured from tissues by incubation over bovine endothelial cell monolayers with subsequent transfer of supernatants to blood agar. Further optimization of culture and PCR methodologies are likely to enhance the sensitivity of these diagnostic techniques.

OPTIMAL MANAGEMENT

CSD is nonfatal and typically a self-limited disease, usually resolving in 2 to 4 months without specific therapy. Surgical biopsy or excision is not required unless malignancy cannot be excluded as a diagnosis. Routine incision of nodes should be avoided because chronic drainage may occur from the incision site. However, large-needle aspiration or incision and drainage of suppurative, painful nodes is indicated to relieve discomfort and to enhance recovery.

Although antibiotic therapy is unnecessary in patients with mild clinical presentations, patients with significant adenopathy or moderate to severe systemic manifestations may benefit from a course of antibiotics. Few controlled studies on the effectiveness of antibiotics in CSD exist, but various reports have indicated relief of systemic symptoms and a shorter duration of adenopathy with antibiotic therapy. In one prospective study, a 5-day course of azithromycin was found beneficial in decreasing CSD lymph node volume during the first month of observation. Uncontrolled studies have shown that treatment with rifampin, ciprofloxacin, intravenous gentamicin, trimethoprim-sulfamethoxazole, or doxycycline appears to yield the most beneficial results, whereas other antibiotics commonly fail to change the natural course of the disease or effect a decline in the sedimentation rate. The optimum duration of antibiotic therapy is likewise unclear, with courses ranging from 5 days up to 2 months. Some practitioners consider a 10- to 14-day course of ciprofloxacin the treatment of choice for adult CSD patients, although many other therapeutic regimens exist and alternate drugs are mandated in the young pediatric population.

Bacillary angiomatosis, bacillary peliosis hepatis, and febrile bacteremia associated with *B. henselae* are associated with significant morbidity and mortality if untreated. These diseases often respond relatively well to antibiotic therapy, however, and the response may differ from that seen in typical CSD. Erythromycin or doxycycline have been used with success to resolve systemic symptoms or lesions in these diseases; rifampin may be used in combination with either drug in severely ill patients. Tetracycline, azithromycin, and minocycline have also been used successfully for therapy. The optimum duration of therapy with these agents is unclear, but a minimum course of 2 to 4 months is recommended for immunocompromised patients, depending on the type and extent of disease. Relapses are not infrequent, and lifelong therapy in HIV-infected patients may be necessary to prevent recurrences.

BIBLIOGRAPHY

Adal, KA, Cockerell CJ, Petri WA. Cat-scratch disease, bacillary angiomatosis, and other infections due to *Rochalimaea*. *N Engl J Med* 1994; 330:1509–1515.

Armengol, CE, Hendley, JO. Cat-scratch disease encephalopathy: a cause of status epilepticus in school-aged children. *J Pediatr* 1999;134:635–638.

Bass, JW, Freitas, BC, Freitas, AD, et al. Prospective randomized double blind placebo-controlled evaluation of azithromycin for treatment of cat-scratch disease. *Pediatr Infect Dis J* 1998;17:447–452.

Carithers HA. Cat-scratch disease: an overview based on a study of 1200 patients. *Am J Dis Child* 1985;139:1124–1133.

Margileth AM. Antibiotic therapy for cat scratch disease: clinical study of therapeutic outcome in 268 patients and a review of the literature. *Pediatr Infect Dis J* 1992;11:474–478.

Sander A, Posselt M, Bohm N, et al. Detection of *Bartonella henselae* DNA by two different PCR assays and determination of the genotypes of strains involved in histologically defined cat scratch disease. *J Clin Microbiol* 1999;37:993–997.

Spach DH, Koehler JE. *Bartonella*-associated infections. *Infect Dis Clin North Am* 1998;12:137–155.

Kelley's Textbook of Internal Medicine, fourth edition. Edited by H. David Humes. Lippincott Williams & Wilkins, Philadelphia © 2000.

C H A P T E R
293
RAT-BITE FEVER

RONALD G. WASHBURN

Rat-bite fever is a rare febrile systemic illness typically transmitted by the bite of a rat or other small rodent. The infection can be caused either by *Streptobacillus moniliformis* or *Spirillum minus*, bacteria commonly found in the oropharynx of rodents. Streptobacillary disease accounts for the majority of cases in the United States, whereas *S. minus* infections occur mainly in Asia. In Japan, the infection caused by *S. minus* is called *sodoku* (*so*, rat; *doku*, poison). Table 293.1 compares the two different forms of rat-bite fever.

INCIDENCE AND EPIDEMIOLOGY

In the United States, persons at risk for percutaneous inoculation with *S. moniliformis* include animal laboratory workers and persons inhabiting crowded urban dwellings or rural areas infested with wild rats. Rat-bite fever is typically transmitted by the bite or scratch of rats, mice, squirrels, or carnivores that prey on those rodents, including cats, dogs, pigs, ferrets, and weasels. The infection may also be acquired by handling dead rats, with no apparent breach of intact skin. Between 10% and 100% of both wild and laboratory rats harbor *S. moniliformis* in their nasopharyngeal flora. Although healthy laboratory mice generally are not colonized with the organism, they do share with rats the susceptibility to epizootic infection characterized by pneumonia, otitis media, polyarthritis, and septicemia.

Oral ingestion of *S. moniliformis* has caused epidemics of Haverhill fever (erythema arthriticum epidemicum), an illness resembling rat-bite fever. Potential sources of such outbreaks include water or milk contaminated with rat excrement.

In the case of *S. minus*, the major route of transmission is through rat bites. In contrast to *S. moniliformis*, oral ingestion has never been shown to transmit *S. minus* infection. In endemic areas of Asia, approximately 25% of tested rats are positive for *S. minus* in nasopharyngeal and conjunctival secretions, pulmonary lesions, and blood.

ETIOLOGY

S. moniliformis is a pleomorphic, nonmotile, nonsporulating, nonencapsulated gram-negative bacillus. Filaments and beadlike chains may contain fusiform swellings. The organism is microaerophilic, requiring a partial pressure of CO_2 between 8% and 10%. On blood agar small cottonlike colonies appear after approximately 3 days of incubation at 37° C. In broth media, flocculent puffballs are seen at the bottom of the broth after 2 to 10 days. Fatty acid analysis by gas liquid chromatography is useful for rapid identification of *S. moniliformis*.

In contrast, the other agent of rat-bite fever, *S. minus*, is a short, thick, gram-negative, tightly coiled spiral rod. Terminal flagella confer darting motility, visible on darkfield examination. The organism cannot be cultured on artificial media, but can be recovered through xenodiagnosis (see Laboratory Findings).

TABLE 293.1.	COMPARISON OF TWO TYPES OF RAT-BITE FEVER	
	Streptobacillus moniliformis	*Spirillum minus*
Organism	Gram-negative bacillus	Gram-negative coiled rod
Geographical distribution	North America, Europe	Asia
Mode of transmission	Rat bite, ingestion	Rate bite
Clinical syndrome		
Relapsing fever	Yes	Yes
Rash	Yes	Yes
Arthritis	Yes	No
Ulceration of initial bite wound	No	Yes
Regional lymphadenopathy	No	Yes
Diagnosis	Culture	Direct visualization, xenodiagnosis
Therapy	Penicillin G	Penicillin G

PATHOGENESIS AND PATHOLOGY

Streptobacillary rat-bite fever is probably the consequence of failed local cutaneous defenses followed by bacterial dissemination. Autopsy reports describe focal mononuclear infiltrates. For the ingestion-induced form of the infection, Haverhill fever, organisms probably gain access to peripheral blood by penetrating gastrointestinal mucosa.

Relapsing spirillary rat-bite fever is postulated to be due to seeding of blood and distant foci during periodic reactivation of the primary bite lesion. Autopsy specimens show granulomatous inflammation at the original site of inoculation, accompanied by epithelial necrosis and mononuclear infiltration of the dermis. Regional lymph nodes are hyperplastic. Distant skin rash lesions contain dilated blood vessels and round cell infiltrates, whereas liver and kidney show hemorrhage and necrosis.

CLINICAL FINDINGS

The two forms of rat-bite fever share certain common clinical features but also possess their own distinctive signatures (Table 293.1). In streptobacillary infection, a brief incubation period follows the bite of the rat (usually less than 10 days; range 1 to 22 days). Abrupt onset of fever, chills, headache, vomiting, and migratory arthralgias and myalgias marks the onset of clinical disease. By that time, the wound itself has typically already healed. Indeed, the diagnosis is often initially missed because the patient may be unaware of a bite that occurred during sleep. Regional lymphadenopathy is minimal or absent. Within 2 to 4 days after the onset of fever, a nonpruritic maculopapular, morbilliform, petechial, or pustular rash erupts over the palms, soles, and extremities. Approximately 50% of patients develop asymmetric large-joint polyarthritis or true septic arthritis simultaneously with the rash or within a few days thereafter.

Haverhill fever differs from percutaneously acquired disease in the high incidence of pharyngitis and heightened severity of vomiting. The peripheral white blood cell count may range as high as 30,000/mm³ with left shift. Fever typically subsides spontaneously after 3 to 5 days without specific antibiotic therapy, and the remaining symptoms gradually resolve within 2 weeks. However, fever may occasionally relapse in an irregular pattern for weeks or months, producing a picture of fever of undetermined origin. Arthritis may persist for as long as 2 years.

Complications of *S. moniliformis* infection include endocarditis, myocarditis, pericarditis, meningitis, pneumonia, and amnionitis. Mortality of untreated cases ranges as high as 13%, and endocarditis in the preantibiotic era was uniformly fatal. Most of those intravascular infections occurred on valves with underlying lesions such as rheumatic valvulitis or calcification.

In *S. minus* infection, the initial bite wound promptly heals but then becomes painful, swollen, and purple approximately 1 to 4 weeks later. In contrast to streptobacillary disease, the bite wound is associated with prominent regional lymphangitis and lymphadenitis. The local inflammatory response heralds a systemic illness characterized by fever, chills, headache, and malaise. In contrast to streptobacillary rat-bite fever, arthritis and myalgias are rare in *S. minus* infection.

Next, the bite wound of *S. minus* infection commonly progresses to chancre-like ulceration and induration with eschar formation. During the first week of fever, a diffuse violaceous or reddish-brown macular rash erupts. Leukocytosis is common, with peripheral white blood cell counts of 10,000 to 20,000/mm³. Without specific antimicrobial therapy, fever lasts 3 to 4 days and recurs at regular intervals between afebrile periods of 3 to 9 days. Spontaneous resolution usually occurs within 1 to 2 months, but rarely leads to relapsing fever for years. Complications are similar to those of streptobacillary rat-bite fever, and mortality of untreated *S. minus* infection in the preantibiotic era was 6% to 10%.

LABORATORY FINDINGS

For *S. moniliformis* infection, direct visualization of pleomorphic bacillary organisms in Giemsa-, Wayson-, or gram-stained smears of blood, joint fluid, or pus may provide an early clue to diagnosis. However, laboratory diagnosis ultimately is based on culturing *S. moniliformis* using enriched media. The slide agglutination test is no longer available, but an enzyme-linked immunosorbent assay (ELISA) has recently been developed for detection of specific antibody against *S. moniliformis*.

S. minus cannot be grown on synthetic media, so initial diagnosis relies on direct visualization of spirochetes in blood, exudate, or lymph node tissue using Giemsa or Wright's stain or darkfield microscopy. Organisms can also be recovered from mice or guinea pigs 1 to 3 weeks after intraperitoneal inoculation, with the precaution that the animals must be prescreened to exclude preexisting spirochete infection. No specific serologic test is available for *S. minus* infection. Given the similarities between rat-bite fever and secondary syphilis, the clinician needs to be mindful of false-positive serologies for syphilis among those with rat-bite fever (25% to 50%).

OPTIMAL MANAGEMENT

Both agents of rat-bite fever are susceptible to penicillin. In the past, procaine penicillin G was given as 600,000 units intramuscularly every 12 hours for 10 to 14 days. Currently, intravenous penicillin G appears more appropriate. The Jarisch–Herxheimer reaction may complicate initial therapy of *S. minus* infection. Oral tetracycline, 500 mg every 6 hours, is preferred for penicillin-allergic patients.

Most patients respond promptly to therapy. For persons who appear well after 5 to 7 days of intravenous penicillin, therapy can be completed with an additional week of oral penicillin V or ampicillin, 500 mg every 6 hours. Patients with mild disease can probably be treated orally for the entire course. Endocarditis is so rare that optimal therapy is uncertain, but 4 weeks of intravenous penicillin, with or without streptomycin, is probably adequate.

After a rodent bite, the wound should be thoroughly cleaned, and tetanus prophylaxis should be administered if warranted by the patient's immunization history. A 3-day course of oral penicillin, 2 g per day, seems reasonable. However, the prophylactic efficacy of penicillin in this setting is unknown, and the patient should be advised to report any subsequent symptoms. Measures to limit the incidence of rat-bite fever include eradication of rats, avoidance of nonpasteurized milk and potentially contaminated water, and the use of gloves by laboratory workers when handling rodents.

BIBLIOGRAPHY

Anderson LC, Leary SL, Manning PJ. Rat-bite fever in animal research laboratory personnel. *Lab Anim Sci* 1983;33:292–294.

Baron EJ, Weissfeld AS, Fuselier PA, et al. Classification and identification of bacteria. In: Murray PR, Baron EJ, Pfaller MA, et al, eds. *Manual of clinical microbiology,* sixth ed. Washington, DC: American Society for Microbiology, 1995:249.

Boot R, Bakker RH, Thuis H, et al. An enzyme-linked immunosorbent assay (ELISA) for monitoring rodent colonies for *Streptobacillus moniliformis* antibodies. *Lab Anim* 1993;27:350–357.

Edwards R, Finch RG. Characterisation and antibiotic susceptibilities of *Streptobacillus moniliformis. J Med Microbiol* 1986;21:39–42.

Holmes B, Pickett MJ, Hollis DG. Unusual Gram-negative bacteria. In: Murray PR, Baron EJ, Pfaller MA, et al, eds. *Manual of clinical microbiology,* sixth ed. Washington, DC: American Society for Microbiology, 1995:499.

Leads from the Morbidity and Mortality Weekly Report. Rat-bite fever—New Mexico, 1996. *JAMA* 1998;279:740–741.

Raffin BJ, Freemark M. Streptobacillary rat-bite fever: a pediatric problem. *Pediatrics* 1979;64:214–217.

Rat-bite fever—New Mexico, 1996. *MMWR* 1998;47:89–91.

Rupp ME. *Streptobacillus moniliformis* endocarditis: case report and review. *Clin Infect Dis* 1992;14:769–772.

Kelley's Textbook of Internal Medicine, fourth edition. Edited by H. David Humes. Lippincott Williams & Wilkins, Philadelphia © 2000.

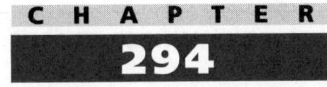

MYCOBACTERIAL INFECTIONS

CHAPTER
294

TUBERCULOSIS

LISA K. FITZPATRICK
CHRISTOPHER BRADEN

DEFINITION

Tuberculosis (TB) has been recognized in its various forms for thousands of years. Descriptions of TB date back to the first millennium B.C. in medical texts from Greece to India. The Greeks named the malady *phthisis,* which means "to waste." In the English-speaking world, *consumption* was the common name given the disease. It was during the Middle Ages, when TB became common in Europe, that it became known as the *white plague.* Other manifestations were described, including the rapid lung destruction of galloping consumption and the skin manifestations of lupus vulgaris. Percival Pott's description of TB of the spine resulted in the application of his name to this form of TB. With its varied manifestations, TB was considered to represent many different diseases. It was not until 1804 that Rene Laennec proposed his theory of a unified view of the various manifestations of this disease. In 1839, Schönlein proposed that the pathologic entity known as the *tubercle* was the fundamental basis of the disease and suggested that the word *tuberculosis* be used as a generic name for all its varied manifestations. In 1882, Robert Koch discovered that the causative agents of TB were the organisms of the *Mycobacterium tuberculosis* complex.

INCIDENCE AND EPIDEMIOLOGY

Two billion people (one-third of the world population) are infected with *M. tuberculosis.* In 1997, nearly 6 million cases of active TB worldwide were reported to the World Health Organization. Twenty-two countries in Asia and Africa account for more than 70% of these reported cases of TB. The number of reported cases of TB probably is an underestimate of the true number of cases in the world because many developing countries lack resources for TB control and public health programs. One of the highest estimated case rates (467 per 100,000 population) worldwide occurs in Africa, where TB is the most common opportunistic infection among persons with HIV infection.

In the United States, TB case rates steadily declined from the beginning of national TB surveillance in 1953 until 1985. During this time, national case rates decreased from 53.0 to 9.3 per 100,000 population. From 1985 to 1992, a resurgence of TB occurred, resulting in a 20% increase in cases nationwide (Fig. 294.1). This increase was attributable to the following factors: (a) the emergence of both drug resistance and the HIV

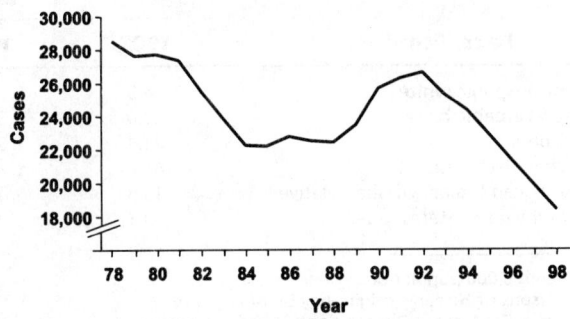

FIGURE 294.1. Reported cases of tuberculosis in the United States, 1978–1998.

epidemic, (b) increased immigration of persons from countries with a high prevalence of TB, (c) increased transmission in congregate settings, and (d) decreases in resources available to TB control programs. The development of complacency about TB during the previous period of decline in national case rates in conjunction with a lack of clinical expertise in management of the disease resulted in a deterioration in TB control programs and diagnostic suspicion of the disease.

In 1993 the number of cases of TB in the United States began to decline and has continued to decrease approximately 7% per year. This decline was attributable to three major changes, as follows: (a) decreased transmission in hospitals and correctional facilities, (b) implementation of directly observed therapy (DOT) nationwide, and (c) improvement in TB control efforts such as case finding, contact investigation, and administration of preventive therapy. In 1998 there were 18,361 cases (case rate 6.8 per 100,000) which represented a decrease of 1,480 (7%) cases compared from the previous year.

Six states of the United States share a disproportionate burden of cases of TB. More than 56% of cases are reported from California, Florida, Illinois, New Jersey, New York, and Texas. National surveillance of TB morbidity has consistently demonstrated that the burden of TB in the United States exists disproportionately among members of racial and ethnic minorities and tends to cluster in urban areas. Since 1985, case rates for persons of Asian and Pacific Island descent, blacks, and Hispanics have been as high as 15, 7, and 6 times higher, respectively, than case rates among whites born in the United States (Table 294.1). Although case rates for these racial and ethnic groups have declined simultaneously with national case rates, this trend of disproportionately higher case rates has remained undisturbed. TB among persons born outside the United States accounted for 42% of U.S. reported cases in 1998. Overall, the steady and appreciable decreases in TB case rates in other ethnic groups since 1993 are not parallelled among persons born outside the United States. Case rates for this group have remained two to three times higher than those for all persons born in the United States.

The HIV epidemic had considerable bearing on the resurgence of TB. Reporting of HIV status for persons with TB has been sporadic and incomplete since 1993, when TB was first included as an AIDS-defining illness. Attempts to cross-match TB and HIV registries have shown that less than 15% of persons with reported cases of TB also have HIV infection. The incomplete reporting of HIV test results limits the evaluation of temporal trends in HIV-related TB, and current data likely represent a gross underestimation of the number of persons with both TB and HIV disease. It is clear that the timing of the increase in cases of TB in the United States (1983–1992) coincided with the onset of the AIDS epidemic. Epidemiologic similarities between the two epidemics suggest that the number of coinfected persons is much higher. For instance, the largest increase in cases of TB between 1985 and 1992 occurred among persons 25 to 44 years of age, the same group who had the largest number of AIDS cases in the same years. Overlapping demographic data suggest a link among the two diseases. The geographic distributions of the two epidemics were similar; most cases of both diseases were reported from large urban areas in New York, California, Florida, and Texas.

The resurgence of TB in the United States was accompanied by an increase in the number of cases of multidrug-resistant tuberculosis (MDRTB). Primary drug-resistant TB is disease caused by infection with a drug-resistant strain of *M. tuberculosis*. Secondary, or acquired, drug resistance results from the development of resistance during therapy for disease. MDRTB has no standard definition. Some clinicians define multidrug resistance as resistance to any two or more of the five first-line antibiotics used for TB treatment (isoniazid, rifampin, ethambutol, streptomycin, and pyrazinamide). Others have defined it as resistance to at least isoniazid and rifampin because these two antibiotics have been shown to be the most potent anti-TB agents. Resistance to these two drugs greatly complicates the treatment of patients with TB and their contacts.

The increase in cases of MDRTB in the United States was caused in part by inappropriate, incomplete, or erratic management of active disease and several outbreaks of MDRTB related to poor infection control measures in health care settings and transmission in congregate settings, such as shelters for the homeless and prisons. In 1998, however, only 1.1% of all reported culture-positive cases of TB were resistant to isoniazid

| TABLE 294.1. | REPORTED RATES OF TUBERCULOSIS BY RACE AND ETHNICITY—UNITED STATES, 1985, 1992, 1997 |

	Rate[a]			Percentage Change	
Race, Ethnicity	1985	1992	1997	1985 vs 1992	1992 vs 1997
Non-Hispanic white	4.5	4.0	2.5	−11.1	−37.5
Non-Hispanic black	23.0	31.7	20.5	+37.8	−35.3
Hispanic[b]	21.4	22.4	14.4	+4.7	−35.7
Asian, Pacific Islander	41.6	46.6	40.6	+12.0	−12.8
American Indian, Alaskan Native	18.9	16.3	13.4	−13.8	−17.8
Total United States	9.3	10.5	7.4	+12.9	−29.5

[a] Per 100,000 population.
[b] Persons of Hispanic origin may be of any race.
Source: Centers for Disease Control and Prevention.

and rifampin. Approximately 50% of these cases were reported in California and New York.

ETIOLOGY

The *M. tuberculosis* complex belongs to the family Mycobacteriaceae and includes the subspecies *M. tuberculosis*, *M. africanum*, *M. bovis*, *M. canettii*, and *M. microti*. These bacilli are genetically similar but can be differentiated through biochemical analysis. *M. bovis* is primarily a pathogen of ruminants and may cause disease among humans that is clinically indistinguishable from TB. *M. africanum* is most commonly found in Africa, *M. microti* is a pathogen of rodents, and *M. canettii* is a newly described variant of *M. tuberculosis* that has been isolated from several patients who acquired infection in Africa.

The diagnosis of TB begins with stains performed on clinical specimens to find acid-fast bacilli (AFB). Detection of AFB requires approximately 10^4 colony-forming units (CFU) per milliliter of specimen with both the classic carbolfuchsin stains (Kinyoun and Ziehl–Neelsen) and the fluorochrome stains (auramine or auramine–rhodamine). AFB staining is not particularly sensitive or species specific, but it is rapid and inexpensive. Fluorochrome stains are more sensitive because they are easier to read. In many parts of the world the laboratory diagnosis of TB relies solely on AFB microscopic examination.

M. tuberculosis may be grown on specialized solid or liquid media. Solid media components include an egg base, such as Löwenstein–Jensen or agar base, such as Middlebrook 7H10 or 7H11. Use of liquid media systems has been shown to decrease the time to the detection of growth. It is recommended that liquid media systems be used for routine mycobacterial cultures. Compared with other bacteria, mycobacteria grow slowly; it usually takes 2 to 8 weeks to detect them.

DNA probes can be used to detect four species of mycobacteria (*M. tuberculosis* complex, *M. avium* complex, *M. kansasii*, and *M. gordonae*). When these DNA probes are used, subspecies may be identified in isolates within hours through the detection of species-specific messenger RNA. Nucleic acid amplification tests can be used to identify *M. tuberculosis* organisms directly from smear-positive sputum specimens. Because of the high cost and lack of sensitivity of smear- negative specimens, the practical applications of nucleic acid amplification tests are unclear. High-performance liquid chromatography (HPLC) also can be used for rapid identification. An advantage of this method over DNA probes and nucleic acid amplification tests is that many subspecies of mycobacteria can be identified with HPLC, whereas molecular diagnostics are limited to the small number of species for which DNA probes and primers have been identified and included in commercial kits.

Susceptibility testing against the primary anti-TB drugs is recommended for the initial isolate from all culture-positive cases of TB in the United States. Susceptibility testing should be repeated when clinical response to treatment is delayed or if patients have a relapse. Drug resistance is tested in the United States with the liquid medium BACTEC and the modified agar proportion method. In the modified agar proportion method, suspensions of *M. tuberculosis* bacilli are inoculated onto drug-containing solid media plates and a drug-free control plate. The number of colonies is counted for all plates, and the proportion of resistant bacilli are calculated by means of comparing the growth on the drug-containing media with the growth on the drug-free control media. Susceptibility testing takes 1 to 4 weeks.

Despite laboratory advances, complete testing, including detection, isolation, identification, and drug susceptibility, for *M. tuberculosis* is long process, requiring weeks and sometimes months. In any of these tests, new or old, contamination from environmental mycobacteria or direct contamination from other specimens in the laboratory may lead to false-positive results. The diagnosis of TB must be must be made carefully with both clinical and laboratory information.

PATHOGENESIS

TRANSMISSION

M. tuberculosis is transmitted through the air in the form of very small (1 to 3 mm) infectious particles, called *droplet nuclei*, which are expelled in the cough of a person with pulmonary or laryngeal TB. Two reported exceptions are prosector's wart caused by skin inoculation from contaminated sharp instruments and person-to-person transmission through contaminated bronchoscopes. The risk of transmission from an infected source person to a susceptible host is associated with the potential concentration of viable bacilli in an airspace. The risk of transmission from an infected source patient is low outdoors, where there is much exchange and essentially infinite dilution, or in spaces fitted and maintained with specialized ultraviolet light fixtures. The risk of transmission is greater in spaces lacking air volume, fresh air, and natural or ultraviolet light.

INFECTION AND DISEASE

Droplet nuclei are small enough to remain suspended in air currents and are able to bypass the natural filtering of larger particles in the upper respiratory tract. Once inhaled, the droplet nuclei may lodge in the alveoli of the lung to establish infection. Among approximately 5% of persons infected, bacilli may multiply locally over weeks to months to cause hilar or peritracheal lymph node enlargement or lobar pneumonia (usually in the middle or lower lobes) or incite a serosal reaction and pleural effusion. These events constitute primary TB. Most patients show no signs of infection other than development of delayed-type hypersensitivity to tuberculin proteins. The infection includes invasion of alveolar macrophages within which *M. tuberculosis* can survive and disseminate throughout the body. In response, macrophages containing bacilli may combine to form swirls of multinucleated giant cells in a stroma of fibrous inflammatory tissue, the hallmark of a tuberculous granuloma, or tubercle. Over a period of years, granulomas may become relatively large and calcified and become manifest on chest radiographs as small densities in the upper lung fields, apical pleura, and hilar lymph nodes.

If disease does not develop soon after infection, a relative equilibrium is established between host and pathogen. With the

TABLE 294.2.	HIGH-RISK CATEGORIES FOR TUBERCULOSIS

HIV infection
Diabetes mellitus
Prolonged corticosteroid use
Chronic renal failure
Bone marrow transplantation, organ transplantation
Malnutrition
Hematologic disorders (leukemia, lymphoma)
Silicosis
Gastrectomy
Jejunoileal bypass
Old, healed tuberculosis lesions on chest radiograph without history of appropriate therapy
Some forms of cancer chemotherapy

exception of immunocompromised persons, those who have been infected with *M. tuberculosis* are thought to be protected from reinfection. However, infection may progress to active disease over time. Factors that influence progression from infection to disease usually are host related and include extremes of age and immunocompromising medical conditions such as HIV infection (Table 294.2). Among immunocompetent persons, the risk of development of active disease after infection with *M. tuberculosis* is thought to be 10% over a lifetime. In contrast, three prospective studies in the United States showed that the rate of development of active disease among persons with HIV infection and *M. tuberculosis* infection ranged from 1.7% to 7.9% per year.

For a small portion of patients with latent infection, the infection reactivates after any number of years. Because lymphohematogenous dissemination takes place around the time of initial infection, reactivation can take place in almost any tissue. Certain locations are much more prone to reactivation, primarily the lung parenchyma (Fig. 294.2). Reactivation occurs in a granulomatous focus in the lung, often in the apical regions, in which caseation and local spread produce pneumonia. Large caseous foci may produce visible cavities in the lung parenchyma. Over several years, these foci may destroy lung tissue to such an extent as to induce pulmonary failure. Reactivation disease manifests much more commonly than primary disease.

INFECTIOUSNESS OF TUBERCULOSIS

Latent *M. tuberculosis* infection is not contagious. Pulmonary and laryngeal TB are the only active forms of TB considered contagious. The best predictors of infectiousness are the number of bacilli in the pulmonary secretions and the presence and frequency of coughing. The extent of pulmonary disease is based on the presence on a chest radiograph of signs of tuberculous infiltrates and cavities in the lung parenchyma. The number of bacilli in the pulmonary secretions is most easily determined by means of microscopic examination of sputum for AFB. Most clinical laboratories quantify the AFB in sputum specimens in three or four categories, such as rare, few, or many. This system may be used to ascertain whether a patient with pulmonary TB has contagious disease. At least 10^4 AFB per milliliter of sputum

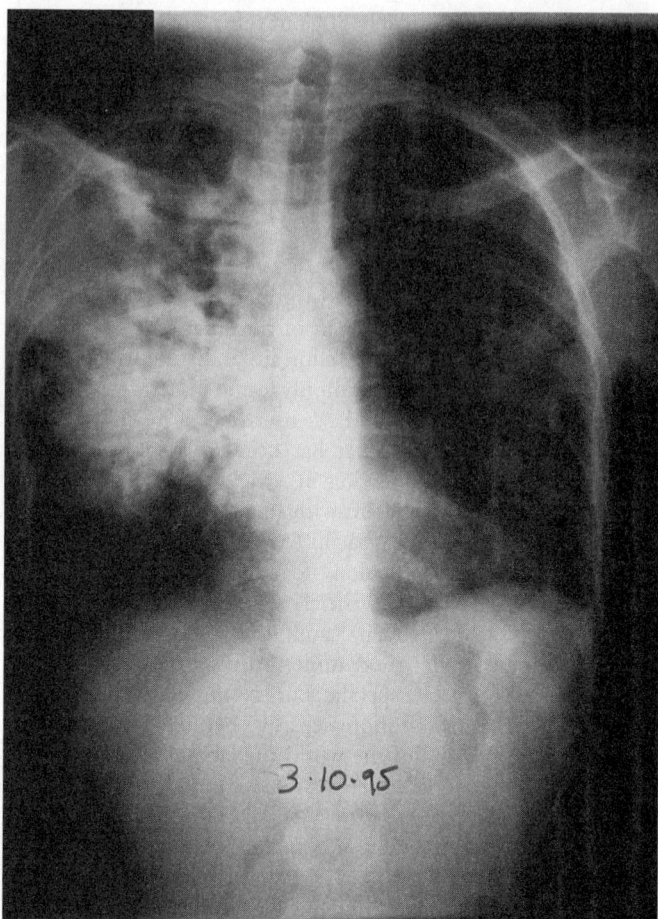

FIGURE 294.2. Radiograph of the chest shows signs of reactivation tuberculosis.

must be present for detection of AFB by means of microscopic examination. However, patients with fewer bacilli in their sputum may still have contagious disease even though they have negative smear results.

Current clinical dogma is that 2 weeks of appropriate anti-TB therapy renders patients noncontagious. However, the time needed to eliminate AFB from sputum, as determined with microscopic examination, varies greatly. For patients with extensive cavitary disease and a heavy burden of bacilli in the sputum or for patients with drug-resistant disease, conversion of sputum from AFB-positive to AFB-negative may take several months. For a patient with extensive cavitary disease and a florid positive smear result, it is possible that subsequent positive smears may contain nonviable organisms. Whether a patient undergoing therapy for TB has contagious disease has to be individually assessed on the basis of symptoms, especially coughing, AFB microscopic findings, and culture results.

CLINICAL FINDINGS

Tuberculosis can become manifest as pulmonary or extrapulmonary disease. Pulmonary TB constitutes 80% to 85% of active cases; the other 15% to 20% of cases are extrapulmonary. Concomitant pulmonary and extrapulmonary disease occurs in approximately 7% of cases, and miliary TB accounts for about 0.2% of cases. The diagnosis of TB can be elusive because TB can masquerade as many pulmonary illnesses, including bacterial or viral pneumonia, interstitial lung disease, and neoplasia. A thorough medical history and physical examination are essential to obtain pertinent information regarding the likelihood of infection and disease. Other important elements of an evaluation for for TB include a Mantoux tuberculin skin test (TST), the result of which is positive among 85% to 90% of immunocompetent patients with pulmonary TB, chest radiography, and AFB smears and cultures. It is important to obtain accurate information about past medical illnesses and about immunocompromising medications, which may place persons in high risk categories (Table 294.2). Information about exposure to persons with active cases of TB or past treatment of infection and disease assists in determining risk of active TB.

PULMONARY DISEASE

Patients with pulmonary TB exhibit a wide range of signs and symptoms, including cough with or without sputum production, fever, night sweats, and weight loss. Other symptoms include pleuritic chest pain, dyspnea, hemoptysis, fatigue, and anorexia. Ten percent to 20% of persons with active TB, particularly persons with early cases and elderly persons, may have no symptoms. TB often is an indolent illness, and symptoms may take several weeks to appear; therefore it is not uncommon for patients to come to medical attention with advanced disease.

Cough is the most prominent symptom of TB, particularly for the immunocompetent patients, although it may go unrecognized by patients with a history of chronic lung disease such as bronchitis or chronic obstructive pulmonary disease. Fever and night sweats occur among as many as 50% of patients. Considerable weight loss accompanies chronic illness and is a late manifestation of disease. Hemoptysis also is a prominent feature of pulmonary disease and usually accompanies advanced disease. Rasmussen's aneurysm is an uncommon source of massive hemoptysis and is caused by erosion of the pulmonary artery by intrusion of an expanding tuberculous cavity.

Physical examination findings are nonspecific and vary with stage of disease. In early disease the physical examination findings may be normal. Later notable symptoms include rales, rhonchi, or signs of consolidation, such as tubular breath sounds or vocal and tactile fremitus. In considerably advanced disease, wasting may be present.

EXTRAPULMONARY DISEASE

Extrapulmonary TB generally is a consequence of lymphohematogenous dissemination of M. tuberculosis during primary infection. Persons with immunosuppressive illnesses are more likely to have extrapulmonary TB. The most common forms of extrapulmonary TB are lymphatic (41%), pleural (21%), bone and joint (11%), genitourinary (7%), meningeal (5%), and peritoneal (4%). Other sites account for 11% of cases. Manifestations

in extrapulmonary disease vary according to the presence of local (lymphatic) versus systemic (miliary) disease. Symptoms of local disease generally are limited to the affected site. Symptoms of systemic disease are nonspecific and often are only constitutional symptoms such as fever, anorexia, and weight loss.

Lymphadenitis associated with TB (scrofula) is the most common form of extrapulmonary disease. Any node may be involved, but cervical and supraclavicular chains are most frequently affected. Patients come to medical attention with painless adenopathy, which often drains spontaneously. In early disease, nodes may be firm and discrete. In late disease, nodes may become soft and fluctuant. With the exception of fever, there usually are no systemic symptoms unless disease is present elsewhere. Diagnosis is by means of fine-needle aspiration or incisional biopsy of the affected node. AFB smears and cultures of nodal tissue usually show AFB and M. tuberculosis organisms.

Pleural disease usually becomes manifest with mild to severe pleuritic chest pain, which may be accompanied by dyspnea. Other constitutional symptoms include fever, night sweats, and weight loss. Disease may be acute or chronic and often causes a subtle effusion. Effusions generally are unilateral and accompany active parenchymal disease in 70% of patients. Pleural TB may develop at any stage of disease but frequently occurs as a primary disease manifestation and may occur as long as 6 months after infection with M. tuberculosis.

Vertebral TB (Pott's disease) accounts for 50% to 70% of skeletal TB. It is characterized by kyphosis and spinal-cord compression, so patients may have neurologic or motor symptoms. The lower thoracic and upper lumber vertebrae are the most common sites of disease. Patients typically have a history of 2 weeks to 3 months of back pain, fever, and weight loss. Paravertebral abscesses occur among 50% of patients. Patients with Pott's disease usually have radiographic evidence of spinal involvement, and 50% of patients have radiographic evidence of either active or old pulmonary TB. Diagnosis requires biopsy and culture of infected bone. Tuberculous arthritis characteristically manifests as an indolent monoarticular arthritis of weight-bearing joints (knees, hips, ankles). Pain is the most common symptom, and swelling with decreased range of motion in the involved joint may be present. Infection is preceded by trauma in 25% of cases. Biopsy of synovial tissue may contain granuloma, and culture results are positive for M. tuberculosis 60% to 75% of the time.

Genitourinary TB is indolent. It can produce signs and symptoms of local infection with few systemic manifestations, or disease may be completely asymptomatic. Urinary tract involvement typically causes dysuria, urinary frequency, and gross hematuria with or without flank pain. Disease among women may cause pelvic pain, menstrual irregularities, and infertility. Men may have a painless scrotal mass. One-fifth of patients with pyuria may have no symptoms. Disease is suspected when urinalysis shows white blood cells and hematuria without bacteria. The diagnosis is confirmed with a urine culture. Urine culture results are negative for the usual bacteria (sterile pyuria) and positive for M. tuberculosis. The diagnostic yield is greatest from early morning specimens. Three specimens should be submitted for culture. Findings at intravenous pyelography usually are nonspecific and often are unhelpful. Given the paucity of symptoms and its indolence, renal TB often is advanced at the time of diagnosis. Two-thirds of patients with genitourinary TB have abnormal chest radiographs that show signs of active or old pulmonary disease.

Tuberculous meningitis is caused by hematogenous spread of mycobacterial organisms into the meningeal space. This process may occur weeks to years after infection, and the presentation of central nervous system (CNS) TB may be acute or subacute. Disease may manifest clinically as bacterial meningitis. Acute symptoms may include headache, fever, or change in mental status. Other symptoms may last for weeks to months; these include fever, weight loss, anorexia, night sweats, malaise, and cranial nerve palsies. Sixth-nerve nerve palsy is the hallmark of CNS TB, but cranial nerves II, III, IV, and VII also may be affected. Examination may reveal meningism and papilledema. CNS TB may progress in three distinct stages. Stage 1 is characterized by nonspecific symptoms with few or no clinical signs of meningitis. Stage 2 denotes the development of signs of meningitis such as meningism, lethargy, and cranial nerve palsies. Stage 3 portends coma and neurologic sequelae such as paralysis. The diagnosis often is made on clinical grounds and is based on the presence of risk factors of TB, TST results, and chest radiography. Patients with CNS TB often have a gratifying response to TB treatment if therapy is initiated expeditiously (before stage 3). This alone may be adequate for diagnosis when clinical suspicion is high and results of laboratory studies are not enough to provide a diagnosis.

Miliary TB, an insidious and clinically elusive form of disease, develops after hematogenous dissemination of tubercle bacilli. This dissemination produces a miliary pattern (so named because it resembles millet seeds 2 mm in diameter) on chest radiographs or in biopsy specimens from the bone marrow, liver, or spleen. Miliary disease usually occurs among high-risk groups, including persons with HIV infection or other immunosuppressive illnesses, connective tissue disease, or hematologic neoplasms, persons who abuse alcohol, and those taking immunosuppressive medications, including high doses of steroids. Patients may have a mild illness for several weeks or months before seeking medical attention. Fever is the most prominent symptom of miliary disease, but many patients report nonspecific symptoms such as weakness, anorexia, weight loss, and night sweats. The physical examination is nonfocal. The diagnosis of miliary TB is made on the basis of clinical history, presence of a miliary pattern on a chest radiograph, and a positive culture results for *M. tuberculosis* from blood or a biopsy site such as the liver or bone marrow. The TST is an insensitive indicator of prior *M. tuberculosis* infection among persons with miliary disease; results have been reported to be positive in 25% to 75% of cases. In cases in which a laboratory diagnosis is difficult, monitoring the clinical response to anti-TB therapy may be helpful. Fever abates among 30% of patients within 2 weeks and among 60% to 70% of patients within 4 weeks.

Peritoneal TB is uncommon and often presents a diagnostic dilemma. The pathogenesis is not clearly understood, but the disease is thought to develop after hematogenous seeding, as in other forms of extrapulmonary disease. Symptoms vary from patient to patient but most commonly include abdominal pain and distention, fever, weight loss, and malaise. Symptoms may become chronic, and disease may progress to ascites or abdominal masses, which are probably amassed omentum, mesentery,

and bowel, which are responsible for the classic doughy abdomen found at physical examination. As many as 30% of patients may have pleural effusions.

Pericardial TB is an uncommon form of disease and carries considerable morbidity and mortality. The diagnosis may be extremely difficult because patients may have no evidence of disease at other sites. Localization of disease is caused by erosion of a mediastinal lymph node, which spreads directly into the pericardial sac. Symptoms include chest pain, cough, weight loss, dyspnea, orthopnea, ankle edema, and night sweats. Patients often seek medical attention because of symptoms of pericarditis such as relief of pain when they lean forward. Signs of disease include fever, cardiomegaly, hepatomegaly, jugular venous distention, and muffled heart tones. Electrocardiographic findings may be those of pericardial effusion or early tamponade (tachycardia, ST depression, low voltage). Management generally consists of anti-TB therapy with or without drainage in conjunction with parenteral administration of steroids, which may decrease the risk of long-term sequelae such as constrictive pericarditis.

LABORATORY FINDINGS

A posterior-anterior radiograph of the chest is imperative for evaluation of pulmonary TB. TB may have various manifestations on a chest radiograph, but the hallmark of pulmonary disease is an infiltrate with cavitation, mainly in the apical region (Fig. 294.2). Cavitation has been reported to occur in 19% to 50% of cases of reactivation of TB. Other findings include lymphadenopathy, lobar infiltrates, and interstitial infiltrates. The diagnosis of TB should not be eliminated on the basis of the radiographic location or appearance of infiltrates, because patients, especially those with HIV infection, may have atypical infiltrates or minimal radiographic findings. Computed tomography may be used to evaluate the extent of disease, but in general, unless occult disease is suspected, it is not helpful in the initial evaluation for TB. Chest radiography also is useful for identifying effusions in pleural disease. In pericardial disease, chest radiography usually shows cardiomegaly with or without a left-sided pleural effusion.

Laboratory abnormalities in pulmonary disease may include leukocytosis or leukopenia (either lymphocytic or neutrophilic), normochromic, normocytic anemia (usually with disseminated infection or long-term disease), or in rare instances hyponatremia due to extensive lung disease or concomitant CNS involvement. These laboratory abnormalities may be present in extrapulmonary disease but are much less common than in pulmonary disease.

Fluid chemical analysis is useful for some extrapulmonary sites such as the peritoneum, pleura, and pericardium. Effusions from these sites may be bloody or nonbloody lymphocytic exudates. Fluid glucose level usually is decreased but may be normal, and the protein is elevated. Smears, cultures, and biopsy specimens from peritoneal, pleural, and pericardial sites are necessary for diagnosis. The diagnostic yield of collective AFB smear, culture, and biopsy for these sites is 65%, 75% and 85%, respectively.

In CNS disease, laboratory findings in subacute and acute disease may reveal neutrophilic or lymphocytic predominance in the CSF with normal or low glucose and elevated protein. The diagnostic yield from CSF smear and culture is disappointingly low (15% and 50%, respectively). Polymerase chain reaction may be useful for detecting *M. tuberculosis* in the cerebrospinal fluid; however, this technique is expensive and is not standardized. Although imaging studies may reveal areas of enhancement, infarction, or hydrocephalus in CNS TB, these findings are not specific for TB and offer little diagnostic utility.

In miliary disease, blood cultures obtained with lysis centrifugation techniques often have been the initial means of diagnosis among persons with HIV infection. Such cultures also may be helpful in the diagnosis of miliary disease among immunocompetent persons. Yield from sputum specimens is less gratifying than in pulmonary TB; the results may be positive in only 50% to 60% of cases. Given this, biopsy specimens from alternative sites such as bone marrow, liver, lymph nodes, or lung should be examined for evidence of granuloma formation. Liver biopsy has been the most successful procedure in yielding a diagnosis. Classic chest radiographic findings may lag 2 to 3 weeks behind early clinical presentation.

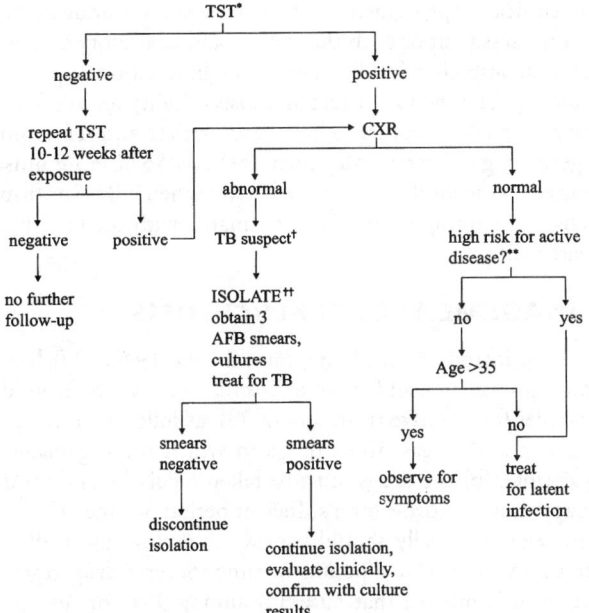

FIGURE 294.3. Initial treatment of patients exposed to tuberculosis. *TST, tuberculin skin test; CXR, chest radiograph. **See Table 294.2. †Report to local health department. ‡Isolation necessary only if hospitalized. Outpatients may have to restrict activity. Discharge conducted with local health department.

■ STRATEGIES FOR OPTIMAL CARE

TREATMENT OF A PATIENT BELIEVED TO HAVE TUBERCULOSIS

Some cases of TB are identified when a patient comes to medical attention with symptoms of TB. Other cases are found through screening after a TST result is read as positive (Table 294.3). It is important to determine the persons's degree of infectiousness when making decisions regarding disposition and restrictions in activity. Patients believed to have TB may be hospitalized or treated as outpatients depending on the severity of illness and the living situation (Fig. 294.3). In many cases, patients with TB have previously exposed household members, and there is minimal risk of continued transmission of infection in the home. If, however, the household includes children younger than 5 years or persons who are immunocompromised, it is prudent to minimize continued exposure from the persons with suspected TB. If patients are hospitalized, prompt isolation in a negative-

pressure room is critical for interrupting transmission and preventing transmission in the health care setting. For all patients believed to have TB, sputum specimens should be obtained on three consecutive mornings and subjected to AFB smear and culture. Anti-TB therapy should be initiated as soon as the presence of TB is suspected. If three smears do not contain AFB, the patient is considered not contagious and should have no restrictions placed on activity.

Patients in the hospital who have positive smear results should remain in isolation. Persons being treated as outpatients should remain at home until they have three consecutive negative smear results for AFB and have demonstrated a clinical response to anti-TB therapy (decrease in frequency of cough, defervescence, or decreasing bacterial burden on smear). Patients who do not

TABLE 294.3.	**CRITERIA FOR TUBERCULIN POSITIVITY BY RISK GROUP**[a]	
≥5 mm	**≥10 mm**	**≥15 mm**
Persons with HIV infection	Persons from high-prevalence countries	Persons with no risk factors
Injection drug users of unknown HIV status		
Persons with recent exposure to TB	Low-income populations	
Persons with chest radiographs that suggest old TB	HIV negative injection drug users	
	Residents of nursing homes or correctional facilities	
	Health care workers	
	Persons with certain medical conditions: diabetes, corticosteroid therapy, gastrectomy, silicosis, chronic malabsorption	

[a] Induration in millimeters.

have clinical improvement with therapy should undergo thorough reassessment of both the clinical and laboratory diagnoses. If clinical suspicion for TB remains high, additional specimens should be obtained for culture and susceptibility testing. Lack of response to what appears to be an appropriate anti-TB regimen suggests drug resistance. All patients believed to have TB must be reported to the local health department. When TB is confirmed, discharge planning should be coordinated with the local health department.

MANAGEMENT OF TUBERCULOSIS

Since the introduction of streptomycin the 1940s, TB has become a preventable and curable disease. There are three guiding principles for effective treatment of TB, as follows: (a) regimens must contain at least three drugs to which the organisms are susceptible, (b) the drugs must be taken regularly, and (c) drug therapy must continue for a sufficient period of time. The treatment regimen ideally should provide the safest, most effective therapy in the shortest period of time. Several drug regimens have been identified that cure TB among 95% of susceptible cases. For patients believed to have drug-susceptible disease, the regimens are based on the use of combinations of five first-line anti-TB drugs—isoniazid, rifampin, ethambutol, pyrazinamide, and streptomycin. Options for regimens are shown in Table 294.4.

The course of therapy is divided into two main components,

the initial intensive phase and the continuation phase. The intensive phase (which generally is 2 weeks to 2 months in duration depending on the chosen regimen) is designed to accomplish rapid killing of most of the bacilli causing disease. The continuation phase is 4 months or longer and is aimed at killing the few bacilli harbored in intracellular compartments that make disease eradication difficult.

For any patient, especially those with HIV coinfection, treatment should be extended beyond 6 months if the clinical or bacteriologic response is slow or otherwise suboptimal. Therapy for extrapulmonary TB follows the same principles as for pulmonary TB; the drug regimens and durations are the same. The exceptions are miliary TB, TB of bones and joints, and TB meningitis. Patients with these conditions should receive 12 months of therapy. For patients with TB pericarditis or meningitis, adjunctive therapy with corticosteroids has been shown to help prevent constrictive pericarditis and neurologic sequelae, respectively, especially when administered early in the course of disease.

There is a dearth of information concerning regimens for the management of MDRTB. The number of potential resistant patterns make randomized prospective trials almost impossible, and the drug regimens use for treatment are individualized on the basis of results of drug susceptibility testing and other factors. Regimens for drug-resistant TB always should be prescribed by an experienced health care provider.

TABLE 294.4.	TIME LINE: REGIMEN OPTIONS

Regimen Option	Time (Weeks of Treatment)										
	0	2	4	8	12	16	20	24	28	32	36
1	INH, RIF, and PZA taken daily (weeks 0–8)			INH, RIF taken daily or 2–3 times/week (DOT) (weeks 8–24)							
	with EMB or SM until susceptibilities known											
2	INH, RIF, PZA, and EMB or SM taken daily	INH, RIF, PZA and EMB or SM taken 2 times/week (DOT) (weeks 2–8)		INH and RIF taken 2 times/week (DOT) with EMB or SM until susceptibilities known (weeks 8–24)							
3	INH, RIF, PZA, and EMB or SM taken 3 times/week (DOT) (weeks 0–24)											
	For adults with sputum- and culture-negative pulmonary TB:											
4	INH, RIF, PZA, and EMB or SM taken daily as in options 1, 2, or 3 (weeks 0–8)			INH, RIF, PZA, and EMB or SM taken daily or 2–3 times/week (DOT) (weeks 8–16)							
5	When PZA is contraindicated: INH and RIF taken daily (weeks 0–8)			INH and RIF taken 2 times/week (DOT) (weeks 8–36)							
	with EMB or SM until susceptibilities known											

For patients who have no individual risk factors for drug resistance and who live in areas where primary INH resistance is <4%, EMB or SM may not be necessary in options 1, 4, 5, or after 8 weeks in option 2; and PZA may be discontinued after 2 months in option.
INH, isoniazid; RIF, rifampin; DOT, directly observed therapy; EMB, ethambutol; SM, streptomycin; PZA, pyrazinamide; AFB, acid-fast bacilli.

Drug-resistant TB may be suspected when the source of infection is known to have had drug-resistant disease or when a patient does not respond to an adequate therapy. Drug resistance may be identified with drug susceptibility testing of isolates. When a patient is believed to have disease that is resistant to at least isoniazid and rifampin, the initial treatment regimen should contain at least three drugs to which susceptibility is considered likely and to which the patient is naive. First- and second-line agents should be combined to achieve the optimal regimen. Second-line anti-TB drugs include quinolones, capreomycin, cycloserine, kanamycin, ethionamide, and para-aminosalicylic acid. Drug therapy ultimately should be guided by a complete panel of in vitro susceptibility results, and the medications should be administered under directly observed therapy. In the event of treatment failure, a single drug should never be added to a failing regimen. The correct procedure is to add to the regimen at least two new drugs not previously taken by the patient. Therapy for MDRTB should extend for at least 12 months after culture-negative status is achieved.

MANAGEMENT OF ACTIVE TUBERCULOSIS AMONG PERSONS WITH HIV INFECTION

It is estimated that more than 5 million people worldwide are coinfected with HIV and TB. TB is now an AIDS-defining illness. Given this, it is imperative to consider the diagnosis of TB when a person with HIV infection reports pulmonary symptoms. The reduction of cellular immunity is the greatest known risk factor for progression from *M. tuberculosis* infection to active disease.

Early diagnosis and management of TB among persons with HIV infection is critical for interrupting TB transmission, prompt initiation of therapy, and cure. In early HIV infection (CD4 count >300), TB becomes manifest in the same way it does among persons without HIV infection. In late HIV infection, symptoms generally are subtle, and chest radiographic findings may be atypical for TB. Lymphadenopathy or small lobar infiltrate may be the only radiographic manifestation, or the chest radiograph may be entirely normal. Immunosuppressed persons often are incapable of mounting an immune response sufficient for cavity formation or formation of dense lobar infiltrates. Disease then may present as fever, wasting, nonproductive cough, or night sweats.

Although persons with HIV infection are at increased risk of reactivation TB, cases of exogenous reinfection with a different strain of *M. tuberculosis* have been reported. Extrapulmonary disease, particularly miliary disease, is more common among persons with HIV infection than among those without HIV infection. All persons with HIV infection should undergo tuberculin skin testing at initial evaluation of the HIV infection to determine the need for preventive therapy. For persons with HIV infection, greater than or equal to 5 mm is considered a positive reaction (Table 294.3). Persons with advanced immunosuppression who are believed to be anergic should undergo periodic, thorough TB symptom reviews. Persons with known exposure to a person with an active case of TB (regardless of TST status) or who have a positive skin test result but no signs and symptoms of active disease should undergo treatment of latent infection as soon as possible regardless of age.

In cases of active TB, some clinicians choose to interrupt antiretroviral therapy during therapy for active TB. Others continue both medication regimens simultaneously. It is now recommended that rifampin be avoided by patients taking protease inhibitors as part of the antiretroviral regimen. In these cases, rifabutin should be substituted for rifampin because this drug is a less potent inducer of the cytochrome P450 system and has less interaction with protease inhibitors. When protease inhibitors and rifabutin are used concomitantly, it may be necessary to increase the dosages of the protease inhibitor, especially for patients taking nelfinavir and indinavir. Ritonavir should not be used with either form of rifamycin. Therapy for of active TB among persons with HIV infection should be undertaken only by care providers who are very familiar with both the side effects and pharmacologic interactions of anti-TB and antiretroviral medications.

SCREENING

Tuberculin skin test screening is performed to identify persons at high risk of infection with *M. tuberculosis* would benefit from preventive therapy (Table 294.5). Although cases of clinical disease often are identified with screening, this method should not be used to find new cases of active TB.

The Mantoux TST performed with 5 tuberculin units of purified protein derivative (PPD) is the standard method for detecting of *M. tuberculosis* infection. The PPD is placed subcutaneously into the volar surface of the forearm. Induration (palpable swelling) at the site of antigen placement is the hallmark of TB infection. Tests to detect induration are read 48 to 72 hours after PPD placement. Erythema often occurs, but this alone does not constitute a positive skin test reaction and should not be measured. A positive reaction is determined by the width of the induration in millimeters, which varies according to risk category (Table 294.3).

Persons with a positive TST reaction should undergo chest radiography and clinical evaluation to rule out active disease (Fig. 294.3). Contacts of a person with an active case of TB

TABLE 294.5.	**GROUPS AT RISK OF *M. TUBERCULOSIS* INFECTION AND FOR WHOM SKIN TESTING IS INDICATED**

Persons with HIV infection
Close contacts of persons with infectious tuberculosis
Persons with immunocompromising medical conditions[a]
Injection drug users
Persons from areas where tuberculosis is common
Homeless persons
Medically underserved, low-income population, including high-risk racial and ethnic groups (Asians, Pacific Islanders, blacks, Hispanics, Native Americans)
Residents or workers in congregate settings (e.g., correctional institutions, nursing homes, mental institutions, long-term care facilities, shelters)

---

[a] See Table 294.2.

should undergo skin testing as soon as possible after exposure. If the results of initial testing are negative, the TST should be repeated 10 to 12 weeks after the last time of exposure to the person with the infectious case, because delayed-type hypersensitivity (DTH) may take several weeks to become manifest. A false-negative reaction does not exclude the possibility of infection or disease. False-negative skin test reactions may occur among 15% to 20% of persons tested. False-positive reactions also may occur with administration of the TST. False-positive reactions are most often caused by the presence of antigens in tuberculin that are shared with nontuberculous mycobacteria such as *Mycobacterium avium* complex. Nontuberculous mycobacteria are ubiquitous in the environment; exposure to these may produce hypersensitivity responses to PPD.

Some persons may have incurred *M. tuberculosis* infection many years in the past. In these cases delayed-type hypersensitivity may wane over time, and the initial TST result may be negative. If waning sensitivity is suspected, two-step skin testing may be used to elicit the booster phenomenon. The booster phenomenon represents restimulation of the delayed-type hypersensitivity response among persons whose immunologic reaction to *M. tuberculosis* has waned. In two-step testing, the initial skin test is read 72 hours after placement of PPD. If the reaction is negative, the skin test should be repeated in 1 to 3 weeks. A positive result at repeat testing generally reflects a boosted reaction. A negative result of the repeated test is likely a true-negative reaction. Two-step testing is used to establish a baseline TST result for persons who undergo skin testing periodically and for persons who are at risk of exposure to *M. tuberculosis*, such as health care workers. Two-step testing in the health care setting also reduces the likelihood of misclassifying persons with boosted reactions as recent converters.

For persons born outside the United States who have a remote history of vaccination with bacille Calmette–Guérin, a positive TST reaction should be interpreted as infection with *M. tuberculosis*. Repeated intradermal injections of PPD do not sensitize uninfected persons to tuberculin.

MANAGEMENT OF LATENT TUBERCULOSIS INFECTION

Therapy for latent TB infection is recommended for certain groups of persons who have a positive TST reaction, many of whom are felt to be at increased risk of active disease (Table 294.6). The decision to treat a patient for latent infection should also be based on tuberculin positivity for risk groups (Table 294.5). For example, a close contact of a person with an active case of TB who has a TST reaction that shows 5 mm induration should undergo treatment of latent infection. However, a person younger than 35 years with no identifiable risk factors for progression to disease should undergo therapy for latent infection if the tuberculin induration is 15 mm or more. Children and adolescents with negative TST reactions (<5 mm induration) who have been close contacts of contagious persons within the 3 months before tuberculin testing are candidates for therapy for latent TB infection until a second test is performed 10 to 12 weeks after last exposure. If the second test reaction is positive, therapy is continued to completion; if it is negative, therapy

TABLE 294.6.	HIGH-PRIORITY GROUPS FOR THERAPY FOR TUBERCULOSIS INFECTION

Treat Regardless of Age

Persons known to have or likely to have HIV infection
Close contacts of a person with infectious tuberculosis
Persons who have a chest radiograph that suggests previous tuberculosis and who have received inadequate treatment
Persons who inject drugs
Persons with certain medical conditions[a]
Recent converters[b]
Children younger than 5 years

Treat Persons Who Are Younger Than 35 Years

Persons from areas where tuberculosis is common
Medically underserved, low-income populations, including high-risk racial and ethnic groups and residents of long-term care facilities
Locally identified high-prevalence groups (e.g., homeless, migrant farm workers)

---

[a] See Table 294.2.
[b] Persons whose tuberculin skin test reaction converted from negative to positive within the past 2 years (≥10 mm increase if younger than 35 years; ≥15 mm increase if 35 years or older).

may be discontinued unless there is continuing exposure to the contagious person.

A 6-month course of isoniazid once was the recommended and standard therapy for latent infection. Revised recommendations emphasize the greater efficacy of longer durations of therapy for latent infection. A 9-month course of daily isoniazid is now thought to be the most effective regimen. Other options for management of latent TB infection include intermittent isoniazid therapy given twice a week for 6 or 9 months or the previous standard of isoniazid given daily for 6 months. For persons with conditions in which neuropathy is common, such as diabetes, uremia, alcoholism, HIV infection, pyridoxine should be coadministered with isoniazid. Regimens with rifampin alone or rifampin plus pyrazinamide are being studied in clinical trials and are promising. Rifampin and pyrazinamide given for 2 months to persons with dual infection (HIV and *M. tuberculosis*) was as effective as 12 months of isoniazid therapy in a prospective, randomized trial. This regimen is thought to be equally efficacious in the care of persons without HIV infection. Although the cost is higher than that of regimens with isoniazid alone, a 2-month regimen may increase the acceptability of therapy for latent TB infection.

■ COST-EFFECTIVENESS

Regardless of patients' need for treatment of active TB disease or treatment of latent infection, TB control programs in most nations offer drugs and care at no charge. Many health departments offer directly observed therapy programs to help patients complete the full course of therapy. In a directly observed therapy program a health care provider watches patients swallow all doses of anti-TB drugs. The programs often provide food, transportation, and even housing if needed. This and many other strategies are necessary to achieve the national health goal of TB elimination by the year 2010. A multipronged approach that includes early recognition and timely therapy for active disease, effective contact investigations to find infected persons, and administration of therapy for latent infection are pivotal for successful elimination.

BIBLIOGRAPHY

American Thoracic Society. Diagnostic standards and classification of tuberculosis. *Am Rev Respir Dis* 1990;142:725–735.
American Thoracic Society. Control of tuberculosis in the United States. *Am Rev Respir Dis* 1992;146:1623–1633.
American Thoracic Society. Treatment of tuberculosis and tuberculosis infection in adults and children. *Am J Respir Crit Care Med* 1994;149: 1359–1374.
Cantwell MF, Snider D. Epidemiology of tuberculosis in the United States. *JAMA* 1994;272:535–539.
Centers for Disease Control and Prevention. Guidelines for preventing the transmissions of *M. tuberculosis* in health-care facilities. *MMWR Morb Mortal Wkly Rep* 1994;43:27–58.
Centers for Disease Control and Prevention. tuberculosis morbidity—United States, 1997. *MMWR Morb Mortal Wkly Rep* 1998;47: 253–257.
Centers for Disease Control and Prevention. Prevention and treatment of tuberculosis among patients infected with human immunodeficiency virus: principles of therapy and revised recommendations. *MMWR Morb Mortal Wkly Rep* 1998;47:11–40.
Huebner R, Schein M. The tuberculin skin test. *Clin Infect Dis* 1993;17: 968–975.
McCray E, Weinbaum C. Epidemiology of tuberculosis in the United States. *Clin Chest Med* 1997;18:99–113.

Kelley's Textbook of Internal Medicine, fourth edition. Edited by H. David Humes. Lippincott Williams & Wilkins, Philadelphia © 2000.

CHAPTER

295

NONTUBERCULOUS MYCOBACTERIAL DISEASES

DAVID E. GRIFFITH
RICHARD J. WALLACE, JR.

Although most human mycobacterial disease is still caused by *Mycobacterium tuberculosis* and *M. leprae,* a rapidly increasing number of other mycobacterial species are capable of producing disease. These organisms are especially important pathogens in the southeastern and central United States and in association with some immunocompromising conditions, especially AIDS. There are currently more than 50 recognized species of mycobacteria other than *M. tuberculosis* and *M. leprae.* Skin test data suggest that as many as 40 million persons in the Untied States

have been infected with these organisms, but development of disease remains infrequent despite widespread exposure. The main environmental sources, portal of entry, and mode of transmission have not been firmly established for many species of nontuberculous mycobacteria.

The best-known classification system of mycobacterial organisms was introduced by Ernest Runyon in the early 1960s. The system is based on colony pigmentation and rate growth. This classification system was intended to promote rapid identification of nontuberculous mycobacterial species by microbiologists, but unfortunately it was of little value to clinicians. With the advent of rapid diagnostic systems, this system is generally no longer used. In the classification recommended by the American Thoracic Society, patterns of disease, such as lung disease and lymph node disease, are related to the mycobacterial species most likely to be responsible for each type of disease (Table 295.1).

■ MICROBIOLOGY

Unlike *M. tuberculosis,* which is an obligate human pathogen, the nontuberculous mycobacteria are widely distributed in the environment. They differ from *M. tuberculosis* in rate of growth, morphologic features of the colony, frequent presence of yellow or orange colony pigment formation, biochemical reactivity, DNA and RNA composition, and pathogenicity. They are readily seen with routine acid-fast staining techniques, and most species grow well on standard tuberculosis culture media such as Lowenstein–Jensen medium or Middlebrook 7H10 agar at 35°C. *M. marinum, M. chelonei,* and *M. haemophilum* often require lower incubation temperatures (28°C to 30°C) for primary isolation. *M. haemophilum* requires the addition of iron-containing compounds for growth at any temperature. Current emphasis in the diagnosis of tuberculosis is on development of rapid diagnostic techniques. The result is greater emphasis on growing nontuberculous mycobacteria on broth media and on genetic and chromatographic methods. The nontuberculous mycobacteria also grow well in Middlebrook 7H12 broth that contains ^{14}C-labeled substrates. The BACTEC system (Becton-Dickinson, Cockeysville, MD) is used to measure production of radiolabeled carbon dioxide. With this technique growth of *M. avium* complex can be detected in an average of 5 days as opposed to the usual 2 to 3 weeks when solid medium is used.

Commercial DNA probes that allow species identification of pure cultures on solid or broth culture media in 1 day (Gen-Probe, San Diego, CA) are available for *M. tuberculosis, M. avium, M. intracellulare, M. kansasii,* and *M. gordonae.* For other species of mycobacteria, identification relies on techniques such as high-performance liquid chromatography or biochemical testing. Studies have emphasized the potential of molecular techniques, such as the polymerase chain reaction, for rapid species identification. The nontuberculous species of mycobacteria most commonly isolated in the presence of disease is *M. avium* complex (MAC) followed by *M. kansasii, M. abscessus, M. fortuitum,* and *M. marinum.*

TABLE 295.1.	COMMON CLINICAL DISEASES CAUSED BY NONTUBERCULOUS MYCOBACTERIA AND THE MOST FREQUENTLY RECOVERED SPECIES

Pulmonary Disease

M. avium complex
M. kansasii
M. abscessus
M. xenopi
M. szulgai
M. malmoense
M. simiae
M. fortuitum
M. celatum
M. smegmatis group[a]

Disseminated Disease

M. avium complex
M. kansasii
M. abscessus
M. chelonei
M. xenopi
M. genavense
M. haemophilum
M. gordonae

Lymphadenitis

M. avium complex
M. scrofulaceum
M. fortuitum
M. chelonei
M. abscessus
M. kansasii

Skin and Soft-Tissue Infection

M. marinum
M. fortuitum[b]
M. chelonei
M. abscessus
M. ulcerans
M. avium complex
M. kansasii
M. terrae nonchromogenicum complex
M. smegmatis group[a]

Catheter-Related Infection

M. fortuitum
M. chelonei
M. abscessus
M. mucogenicum

---

[a] M. smegmatis, M. goodii, M. wolinskyi.
[b] M. fortuitum, M. peregrinum, M. fortuitum third biovariant complex.

DIAGNOSIS

Isolation of a nontuberculous mycobacterial species does not necessarily indicate that it is responsible for a patient's disease, particularly if a single culture result from a sputum sample is positive but the acid-fast stain result is negative. This is especially true for species such as *M. gordonae, M. scrofulaceum, M. terrae* complex, and *M. phlei,* which are rarely, if ever, a cause of disease

among humans but can contaminate laboratory specimens. Recovery of organisms obtained under sterile conditions such as blood cultures and percutaneous aspiration or surgical biopsy is almost always indicative of infection. Some organisms (*M. marinum, M. kansasii*) are so rarely recovered from the environment and are so commonly associated with disease that recovery or these organisms from any source is almost always indicative of human disease. Other species are relatively common in the environment; recovery of those organisms is not absolute proof of the presence of disease.

Evaluating the significance of culture of a nontuberculous mycobacterial species from a sputum sample necessitates careful and sometimes protracted consideration to determine whether the organism is of clinical significance and causing disease. The American Thoracic Society criteria, most recently revised in 1997, are the diagnostic criteria used most often. The criteria are guidelines and must be interpreted in the context of a specific patient and the specific nontuberculous mycobacteria isolated from that patient. For instance, *M. kansasii* usually is not a contaminant or saprophyte; therefore a single culture of this organism may be important in a compatible clinical setting. For other nontuberculous mycobacterial isolates, it may take many months or years of clinical follow-up care to ascertain the clinical significance of the isolate.

Skin testing is not useful in the diagnosis of nontuberculous mycobacterial disease. Persons may react weakly or not at all to intermediate-strength purified protein derivative (PPD) tuberculin, and U.S. Food and Drug Administration–approved skin tests prepared from antigen extracts of nontuberculous mycobacterial species are not commercially available.

PULMONARY DISEASE

Chronic pulmonary disease is the most important clinical problem associated with infection by nontuberculous mycobacteria. MAC and *M. kansasii* are the most important pulmonary pathogens in the United States. Whether nontuberculous mycobacterial pulmonary disease represents a primary infection as a result of inhalation of an infected aerosol or reactivation of a previously acquired infection is unknown. The portal of entry is generally agreed to be the respiratory tract. As with pulmonary tuberculosis, there may be great variability in clinical presentation—asymptomatic disease found through routine chest radiography, the presence of nodular and interstitial infiltrates on chest radiographs associated with chronic coughing, or far-advanced disease with cavitation associated with weight loss, coughing, and hemoptysis. One clinical finding that usually is absent is fever. Fewer than 10% of patients with nontuberculous mycobacterial lung disease but 60% to 80% of patients with disease due to *M. tuberculosis* infection have a fever. The diagnostic criteria for nontuberculous mycobacterial disease among persons with and those without HIV infection are presented in Table 295.2.

Some radiographic findings suggest nontuberculous mycobacterial disease, especially the presence of large, thin-walled cavities (Fig. 295.1). No radiographic finding, however, provides enough information to confirm a diagnosis or can be used relia-

TABLE 295.2.	DIAGNOSTIC CRITERIA OF NONTUBERCULOUS MYCOBACTERIAL LUNG DISEASE AMONG HIV-SEROPOSITIVE AND -SERONEGATIVE HOSTS

A. If three sputum or bronchial wash results are available from the previous 12 months
  1. Three positive culture results with negative acid-fast bacillis (AFB) smear results
    or
  2. Two positive culture results and one positive AFB smear
B. If only one bronchial wash is available:
  1. Positive culture with a 2+, 3+, or 4+ AFB smear or 2+, 3+, or 4+ growth on solid medium
C. If sputum or bronchial wash evaluations do not provide enough information for diagnosis or another disease cannot be excluded:
  1. Transbronchial or lung biopsy yielding nontuberculous mycobacteria (NTM)
    or
  2. Biopsy showing mycobacterial histopathologic features (granulomatous inflammation, AFB, or both) and one or more sputum or bronchial washings positive for NTM even in low numbers

bly to differentiate tuberculosis from nontuberculous mycobacterial disease. Cavitary nontuberculous mycobacterial disease frequently accompanies chronic pulmonary disease related to pneumoconiosis, previous tuberculosis, smoking-related chronic obstructive lung disease, bronchiectasis, cystic fibrosis, and chronic aspiration.

MYCOBACTERIUM AVIUM COMPLEX

M. avium and *M. intracellulare* are separate species that resemble each other so closely they are indistinguishable with routine microbiologic methods and for practical purposes are referred to as the *M. avium* complex (MAC). MAC can be isolated from water and soil throughout the United States but is present in greatest concentration in the Southeast, especially in coastal waters and estuaries. In a study involving 275,000 Navy recruits who had never lived outside the counties in which they were born, reaction to MAC skin test antigen (PPD-B) was found among more than 70% of those who had resided in the coastal states from Virginia to Texas. Although the pathogenesis of chronic lung disease due to MAC infection is unknown, evidence strongly supports aerosol spread to humans from infected water sources as the principal mode of infection. There is no evidence of animal-to-human or human-to-human transmission. Whether this infection is contained and then reactivates, as does tuberculosis, is unknown but seems likely among patients with upper lobe predominance of MAC lung disease.

Patients with the first form of pulmonary MAC disease typically are middle-aged or older men from the rural southeastern United States who smoke and have preexisting chronic obstructive lung disease. Symptoms include coughing, sputum production, weight loss, and hemoptysis. Fever is infrequent, but if it does occur, it is less severe than with tuberculosis. A chest radiograph typically shows upper lobe cavitary infiltrates (Fig. 295.2).

A second form of MAC lung disease, often called *nodular bronchiectasis,* has been recognized since the late 1980s. Most of the patients are older women who do not smoke but who have coexistent bronchiectasis. The radiographic abnormalities are best defined with computed tomography. They include evidence of cylindrical bronchiectasis and fibronodular and interstitial infiltrates predominant in the middle and lower portions of the

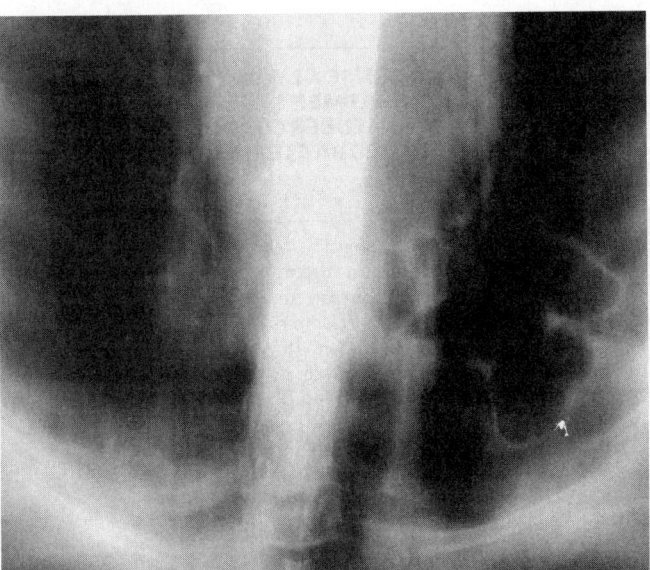

FIGURE 295.1. Multiple, large, thin-walled cavities in a young woman with infection with *Mycobacterium kansasii.* Although not enough information for diagnosis, cavities of this type with minimal surrounding infiltrate often are seen with infection by organisms of this species.

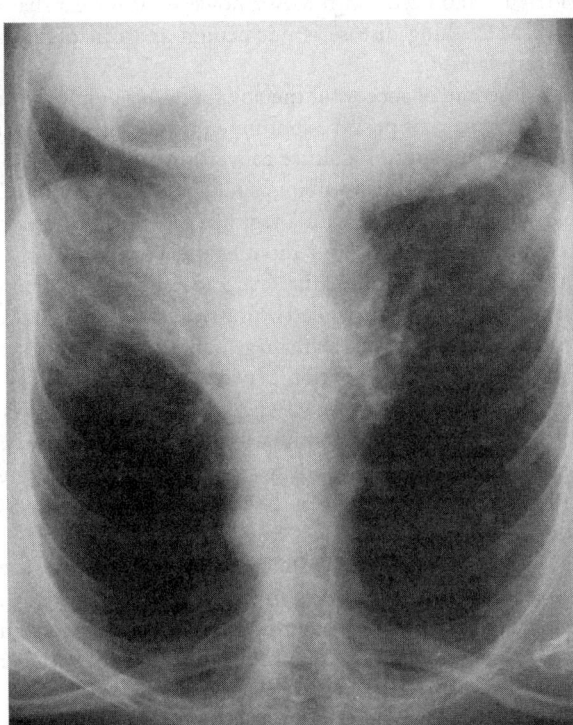

FIGURE 295.2. Upper lobe cavitary disease caused by *Mycobacterium avium* complex in a middle-aged male smoker.

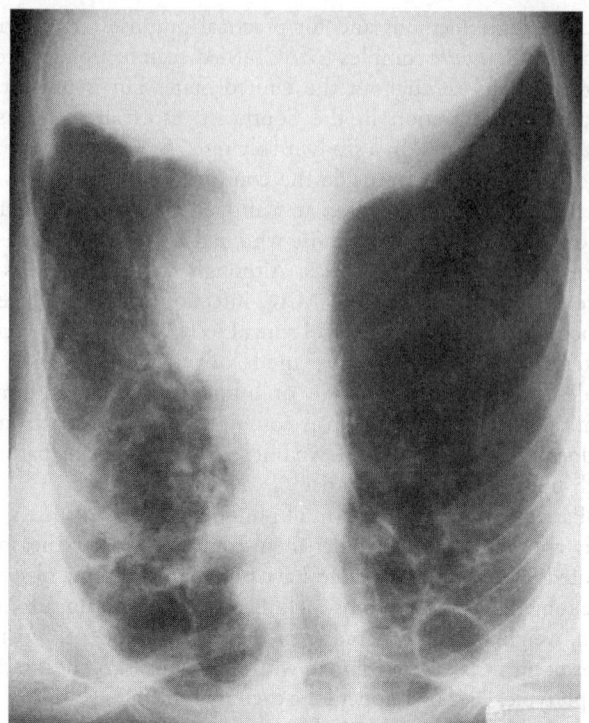

FIGURE 295.3. Nodular and interstitial infiltrates caused by *Mycobacterium avium* complex in an elderly female nonsmoker.

lung (Fig. 295.3). Initial symptoms usually are only cough and progressive fatigue but with progression may mimic those of classically described MAC lung disease. These patients once were considered "colonized" with MAC; however, it is clear that this form of MAC lung disease is not benign and can progress to respiratory failure.

The outcome of successful therapy for MAC pulmonary disease is conversion of positive sputum culture results to negative results. The best sputum culture conversion rates before the introduction of macrolide antibiotics ranged from 60% to 80%. Conversion was achieved with a regimen of isoniazid, rifampin, and ethambutol for 18 to 24 months and intramuscularly administered streptomycin for the first 3 to 6 months of therapy. This regimen was recommended by the American Thoracic Society in 1990. A problem in the management of MAC lung disease has been the lack of correlation between the results of in vitro drug susceptibility tests of the standard antituberculous drugs for *M. tuberculosis* infection and clinical or bacteriologic outcome. Relapse with antituberculous drug regimens has been common; long-term negative culture results have occurred in only 50% of cases.

An important development in therapy for MAC lung disease was the direct result of efforts to manage disseminated MAC disease among patients with AIDS. The AIDS epidemic stimulated the development and use of three new therapeutic agents: clarithromycin, azithromycin, and rifabutin. The macrolide antibiotics (clarithromycin and azithromycin), perhaps because of high tissue and macrophage concentrations, have rapidly evolved into the cornerstone of therapy for MAC lung disease. Studies

involving patients with MAC lung disease have demonstrated the superiority of macrolide-based regimens for MAC lung disease over previously used antituberculous regimens. The principal limitation of these new treatment regimens is side effects, especially of rifabutin. Studies are being conducted to determine the optimal drug combination for successful management of MAC lung disease (Table 295.3).

The regimen recommended by the American Thoracic Society in 1997 is clarithromycin 1,000 mg per day (or azithromycin 250 mg per day), rifabutin 150 to 300 mg per day, and ethambutol 25 mg per kilogram daily for the first 2 months then 15 mg per kilogram per day. Streptomycin 500 to 1,000 mg twice a week should be added in the first 3 months for patients with extensive disease. Intermittent treatment (three times a week with macrolide-containing regimens) has proved to be effective against MAC lung disease. For this regimen the drug doses remain the same, except that the dose of ethambutol is 25 mg per kilogram for the duration of treatment. Monthly sputum cultures must be obtained if possible, and patients are treated until they have negative culture results with therapy for 12 months. An initial study showed sputum conversion rates of 80% to 90% among patients able to tolerate all three drugs in the regimen. The success was more than 90% among patients not previously treated but was much lower among patients who had undergone an unsuccessful course of therapy.

Combined medical and surgical therapy has had excellent results for selected patients with localized cavitary disease and adequate pulmonary reserve. It generally has been restricted to patients with upper lobe fibrocavitary disease who do not have improvement after a minimum of 6 months of drug therapy or whose MAC isolate becomes macrolide resistant. Surgical resection is not an option for most patients who have extensive or bilateral disease. Other drugs such as clofazimine and the

TABLE 295.3.	**COMMONLY USED DRUGS FOR TREATMENT OF NONTUBERCULOUS MYCOBACTERIAL INFECTIONS**
Species	**Drugs**
M. avium complex	Clarithromycin (Azithromycin), ethambutol, rifabutin (rifampin), with or without streptomycin (amikacin)
M. kansasii	Isoniazid, rifampin, ethambutol
M. fortuitum group	Amikacin, cefoxitin, imipenem, clarithromycin (80%), newer quinolones, sulfonamides, doxycycline or minocycline (50%)
M. abscessus	Amikacin, cefoxitin, imipenem, clarithromycin
M. chelonei	Tobramycin, imipenem, clarithromycin, doxycycline or minocycline (25%), ciprofloxacin (20%)
M. marinum	Trimethoprim—sulfamethoxazole, doxycycline or minocycline, clarithromycin, rifampin, rifampin plus ethambutol

newer fluorinated quinolones have added little if anything to these treatment regimens.

MAC lung disease is a diagnostic and therapeutic challenge. Before the introduction of improved antibiotic therapy against MAC, nihilism about an aggressive approach to the care of these patients was understandable. With the availability of improved medical approaches, however, care must be taken in determining the importance of a MAC isolate in a sputum specimen. Some patients with indolent disease may need follow-up care for an indefinite period to determine whether a respiratory isolate of MAC is clinically significant and whether therapy against MAC is indicated.

MYCOBACTERIUM KANSASII INFECTION

The presence of *M. kansasii* organisms in the piped water systems of cities that have pulmonary disease caused by this species has led to the concept that infected aerosols from local tap water are the source of *M. kansasii* lung disease. Pulmonary *M. kansasii* disease is clinically and radiographically indistinguishable from tuberculosis. The typical patient is a middle-aged man from the Southwest or Midwest who is likely to have chronic obstructive pulmonary disease and resides in a major metropolitan area. The course of disease usually is slow progression over a number of years that may lead to extensive lung destruction, although more rapid disease progression can occur.

Untreated isolates of *M. kansasii* are susceptible to achievable serum concentrations of isoniazid (5 μg per milliliter), rifampin (1 μg per milliliter), and ethambutol (5 μg per milliliter), and sputum conversion rates with rifampin-containing regimens approach 100%. This differs from the standard regimen used to treat patients with tuberculosis. The tuberculosis regimen includes pyrazinamide, a drug that has no activity against *M. kansasii*. The American Thoracic Society recommends isoniazid 300 mg per day, rifampin 600 mg per day, and ethambutol 15 mg per kilogram per day for 18 months for disease management. Patients with HIV infection who take protease inhibitors should receive rifabutin at 150 mg daily in place of rifampin. Shorter regimens such as a 12-month regimen with these three drugs plus intramuscular streptomycin twice a week for the first 3 months also have proved successful. However, long-term results with short-course regimens are not known to be as good as those obtained with the American Thoracic Society recommended regimen.

Localized lung disease among patients with AIDS usually responds well to therapy. Lung disease associated with disseminated infection carries a less favorable prognosis. The key to successful therapy for *M. kansasii* infection is in vitro sensitivity to rifampin, because susceptibility to other drugs with tuberculosis test concentrations (0.2 or 1 μg per milliliter isoniazid) does not influence the outcome. Extensive disease and coexistence of other diseases also does not influence outcome of therapy. In rare instances rifampin resistance may emerge during drug therapy. Multidrug treatment regimens that contain clarithromycin may be beneficial in the treatment of these patients. With the availability of rifampin there is no proven role for surgical resection.

MYCOBACTERIUM ABSCESSUS INFECTION

M. abscessus is a rapidly growing species of mycobacteria and is ubiquitous. It is responsible for approximately 85% of cases of lung disease due to rapidly growing mycobacteria. Most *M. abscessus* lung disease occurs among women older than 60 years who do not smoke and have no underlying lung disease. Approximately 15% of patients have coinfection with MAC. Achalasia, previous granulomatous disease, bronchiectasis, cystic fibrosis, and chronic vomiting, but not HIV disease, are risk factors evident among a small percentage of patients, primarily those younger than 50 years. The disease is slowly progressive, and the symptoms usually are mild.

Radiographic examination shows that *M. abscessus* lung disease is primarily interstitial (reticulonodular) and that cavitation is infrequent. Medical therapy for this disease has had generally disappointing results. Antituberculous drugs are uniformly ineffective. Antibiotics such as amikacin, cefoxitin, and the newer macrolides provide temporary clinical improvement. Cure usually is effected only when surgical resection is possible. Clustered outbreaks of pseudoinfection have been caused by sampling with a bronchoscope contaminated in an automated washer.

INFECTION WITH OTHER MYCOBACTERIUM SPECIES

In rare instances, other nontuberculous mycobacteria can cause pulmonary disease. *M. xenopi* grows best at 45°C and is found in hot-water generators and storage tanks. It has been responsible for false outbreaks related to contamination of hot water systems in hospitals and for sporadic true outbreaks of disease. *M. xenopi* is especially common in England and Canada and appears to be increasing in frequency in the United States. The infection can be managed with the macrolide-containing regimen for MAC infection, but relapses appear to be common during periods when the patient is not taking the drugs. Other rare organisms that cause nontuberculous mycobacterial lung disease are *M. szulgai*, *M. fortuitum*, *M. smegmatis* group, *M. celatum*, and *M. simiae*.

◼ LYMPHADENITIS

Lymphadenitis caused by nontuberculous mycobacteria is more common today than tuberculous lymphadenitis. Since the mid 1980s, MAC has become the most commonly recovered pathogen and is responsible for almost 80% of cases of nontuberculous mycobacterial lymphadenitis. Before that time *M. scrofulaceum* was the most common pathogen. More than 95% of cases of disease involve only the cervical lymph nodes, are unilateral, and become manifest as a mass of matted, enlarged nodes, often with associated skin changes. The patients have no evidence of mycobacterial disease elsewhere, and their chest radiographs are normal. Children 1 to 5 years of age are most commonly affected and usually have no constitutional symptoms. The involved nodes may regress spontaneously or progress to softening, rupture, sinus formation, and drainage.

The diagnosis usually is established with the surgical finding of caseating granulomatous disease with or without acid-fast bacilli and (in only 50% of cases) a positive node culture result. The presence of disease is suspected on the basis of signs and symptoms, especially if a child with no tuberculosis contacts has a PPD test result that is weakly or strongly positive. Because of the threat of a chronically draining sinus, incision and drainage are contraindicated, and the treatment is excision of the major involved nodes. Antituberculous drugs usually are not helpful. Clarithromycin with rifabutin or ethambutol may be useful to patients with a poor response to surgical excision or patients who cannot undergo complete surgical excision of involved lymph nodes. No clinical trial has been conducted of this regimen in this setting.

SKIN AND SOFT-TISSUE INFECTION

RAPIDLY GROWING MYCOBACTERIA

The three major pathogenic species of rapidly growing mycobacteria, *M. abscessus*, *M. chelonei*, and *M. fortuitum*, produce a wide spectrum of diseases but are primarily responsible for skin and soft-tissue infections. Most infections occur among otherwise healthy hosts and follow surgery or accidental environmental wound contamination. Most are caused by *M. fortuitum*. The most common nosocomial infections include wound infection after median sternotomy or augmentation mammaplasty, abscesses at injection sites, and infection caused by long-term use of catheters. Outbreaks of pseudoinfection have occurred from contamination of automated bronchoscope washers in which tap water is used for rinsing. Disseminated cutaneous disease due to *M. chelonei* and occasionally *M. abscessus* infection occurs almost exclusively among patients undergoing long-term corticosteroid therapy who have multiple, nodular, draining skin lesions usually on the extensor surfaces of the lower legs with minimal systemic symptoms. HIV disease appears to be associated with no special risk of infection with these organisms.

The pathogenic, rapidly growing mycobacteria are highly resistant to antituberculous drugs but are susceptible to a number of traditional antibacterial agents. Because drug susceptibility is variable, susceptibility testing should be performed. The *M. fortuitum* group (*M. fortuitum*, *M. peregrinum*, *M. fortuitum* third biovariant complex) is uniformly susceptible to ciprofloxacin and ofloxacin, amikacin, imipenem, cefoxitin, and sulfonamides. About 80% of organisms are susceptible to clarithromycin and cefoxitin and about 40% to doxycycline. In *M. chelonei* disease, clarithromycin is effective against all untreated strains, but there is an approximately 10% risk with monotherapy of development of mutational resistance with therapy for disseminated disease. The best additional agents are tobramycin, which is better than amikacin against organisms of this species, and imipenem. For *M. abscessus* infection, amikacin, imipenem, cefoxitin, and clarithromycin are the most active agents (Table 295.3). In general, serious or invasive disease due to infection with *M. fortuitum* group or *M. abscessus* is managed with amikacin plus cefoxitin for 4 to 8 weeks followed by the best available oral agent to complete 6 months of therapy. Drugs used

to manage infection caused by gram-positive bacteria, including everninomicins and linezolid, are under investigation as therapy for infection with mycobacteria.

MYCOBACTERIUM MARINUM INFECTION

M. marinum is responsible for fish-tank granuloma. Fanciers of tropical fish and persons with saltwater injuries are the main populations at risk of disease. *M. marinum* skin lesions first appear as small papular or nodular lesions with central ulcerations at the site of inoculation (usually the hands or arms). The lesions characteristically appear weeks to months after exposure. The disease usually is self-limited, but in the absence of therapy may persist for 1 to 3 years. Some patients have proximal secondary lesions similar to those of sporotrichosis. Disseminated skin disease is rare but can occur among immunosuppressed patients, including patients with AIDS.

The key to diagnosis is a careful history interview. The diagnostic procedure of choice is skin biopsy for culture. Organisms of this species can be readily grown, but initial or primary isolation requires incubation at lower temperatures (28°C to 32°C) than the standard 35°C. Histopathologic study of biopsy specimens shows granulomatous inflammation, but only 5% to 10% specimens have demonstrable acid-fast bacilli. The PPD skin test result often is positive. There is no one drug treatment of choice, and trimethoprim-sulfamethoxazole, doxycycline, clarithromycin, and rifampin with or without ethambutol all have proved effective when given for a minimum of 3 months (Table 295.3). Surgery may be needed to manage extensive or rapidly progressive disease, especially when it involves the hand.

INFECTION WITH MISCELLANEOUS SPECIES

A number of other nontuberculous mycobacterial species may occasionally cause primary skin and soft-tissue disease, usually after trauma to an otherwise healthy host. This group includes MAC, *M. kansasii*, *M. smegmatis*, *M. goodii*, *M. wolinskyi* (the latter two closely related to *M. smegmatis*), and *M. terrae* complex (almost always infection of the hand). *M. ulcerans* infection is a relatively common cause of large necrotizing ulcers of the extremities in localized areas of Australia (Bairnsdale ulcer) and Africa (Buruli ulcer) but is not endemic in the United States.

DISSEMINATED DISEASE AND DISEASE ASSOCIATED WITH AIDS

INFECTION WITH MYCOBACTERIUM AVIUM COMPLEX

Disseminated disease caused by nontuberculous mycobacteria was rare before the 1980s. It occurred among immunocompromised patients, particularly those who had undergone renal transplantation. Disease was usually manifested by multiple subcutaneous nodules. *M. chelonei* and *M. kansasii* were the most commonly recovered agents.

With the advent of AIDS, however, disseminated nontuberculous mycobacterial disease, usually disseminated MAC disease, became relatively common. At one time, as many as 50% of persons with AIDS had evidence of disseminated *M. avium* disease at autopsy. The risk is closely related to CD4 count, risk by year reaching as high as 40% among patients with CD4 counts less than 10 cells per cubic millimeter. More than 95% of isolates are *M. avium* rather than *M. intracellulare*, and most belong to serotypes 4, 6, and 8.

The initial symptoms are nonspecific and include fever. With early disease the fever often is the only finding. With advanced disease, hepatosplenomegaly often is present, as are anemia and elevated levels of alkaline phosphatase. The organism can be isolated from numerous sites, including blood, bone marrow, liver, spleen, lymph nodes, and the gastrointestinal tract. Persistent bacteremia is present and provides the easiest and most accurate method of diagnosis (blood cultures). The lungs often are culture positive at autopsy, but histopathologic changes are rare. Chest radiographic abnormalities and respiratory symptoms usually are not a prominent feature. At bone marrow biopsy, well-formed granulomas are absent, so the histologic appearance of advanced disease is similar to that of lepromatous leprosy with large clumps of acid-fast bacilli. Isolation of the organism from the lower respiratory tracts of persons with AIDS does not necessarily confirm the presence of disease but can be a harbinger of dissemination.

Both clarithromycin (500 mg twice a day) and azithromycin (500 mg per day) have been shown to be effective therapy for disseminated *M. avium* disease. One of these agents should be used in a multidrug regimen that includes ethambutol. Clarithromycin appears to be more effective in sterilizing the bloodstream but has more drug interactions than does azithromycin. Results of one study showed that rifabutin did not increase bacteriologic clearing of the bloodstream but significantly reduced the risk of clarithromycin resistance, compared with a placebo, when included with ethambutol and clarithromycin. Other agents used are rifabutin and occasionally amikacin. Monotherapy for disseminated *M. avium* infection with clarithromycin or azithromycin results in emergence of a macrolide-resistant *M. avium* strain. Treatment is presumably lifelong. Disseminated *M. avium* disease clearly hastens death, and treatment seems to enhance short-term survival. In randomized prophylaxis treatment trials, clarithromycin (500 mg twice a day), azithromycin (1,200 mg once a week), and rifabutin (300 mg per day) reduced the incidence of disseminated *M. avium* infection. All three are approved for prophylaxis.

The most recent recommendations suggest that adults and adolescents with HIV infection who have a CD4 T-lymphocyte count of fewer than 50 cells per microgram per milliliter should undergo chemoprophylaxis against MAC. Most physicians appear to prefer the azithromycin regimen, because it requires fewer drug doses and has fewer drug interactions. Relapse isolates also are less likely to be macrolide resistant than with clarithromycin therapy. In the era of highly active anti-retroviral therapy, CD4 cell counts in many patients may increase above the threshold for instituting MAC prophylaxis. This recovery in CD4 cell counts appears to reduce but not abolish the risk of disseminated *M. avium* disease. Pending results of further studies, patients continue with MAC prophylaxis regimens even if their CD4

count exceeds 50 cells per milliliter. With improved AIDS treatment and with effective prophylaxis regimens, the threat of disseminated *M. avium* disease among patients with AIDS has dramatically abated.

Other nontuberculous mycobacteria, including *M. kansasii*, *M. genavense*, *M. haemophilum*, and *M. gordonae*, may cause localized or disseminated disease among patients with AIDS, although much less frequently than does *M. avium*. The isolation of any nontuberculous mycobacterium from a patient with AIDS necessitates careful evaluation. The profound immunosuppression associated with AIDS has allowed some mycobacterial species that are rarely encountered as pathogens, such as *M. haemophilum*, *M. genavense*, and *M. gordonae*, to emerge as pathogens.

BIBLIOGRAPHY

Bamberger DM, Driks MR, Gupta MR, et al. *Mycobacterium kansasii* among patients infected with human immunodeficiency virus in Kansas City. *Clin Infect Dis* 1994;18:395–400.

Chow SP, Ip FK, Lau JHK, et al. *Mycobacterium marinum* infection of the hand and wrist. *J Bone Joint Surg Am* 1987;69:1161–1168.

Fry KL, Meissner PS,. Falkinham JO III. Epidemiology of infection by nontuberculous mycobacteria: VI, Identification and use of epidemiologic markers for studies of *Mycobacterium avium*, *M. intracellulare*, and *M. scrofulaceum*. *Am Rev Respir Dis* 1986;134:39–43.

Griffith DE, Brown BA, Murphy DT, et al. Initial (6-month) results of three-times-a week azithromycin in treatment regimens for *Mycobacterium avium* complex lung disease in human immunodeficiency virus–negative patients. *J Infect Dis* 1998;178:121–126.

Griffith DE, Girard WM, Wallace RJ Jr. Clinical features of pulmonary disease caused by rapidly growing mycobacteria: an analysis of 154 patients. *Am Rev Respir Dis* 1993;147:1271–1278.

Horsburgh CR Jr, Selik RM. The epidemiology of disseminated nontuberculous mycobacterial infection in the acquired immunodeficiency syndrome (AIDS). *Am Rev Respir Dis* 1989;139:4–7.

Nelson KG, Griffith DE, Brown BA, et al. Results of operation in *Mycobacterium avium-intracellulare* lung disease. *Ann Thorac Surg* 1998;66:325–330.

Nightingale SD, Cameron DW, Gordin FM, et al. Two controlled trials of rifabutin prophylaxis against *Mycobacterium avium* complex infection in AIDS. *N Engl J Med* 1993;329:828–833.

Schaad UB, Votteler TP, McCracken GH Jr, et al. Management of atypical mycobacterial lymphadenitis in childhood: a review based on 380 cases. *J Pediatr* 1979;95:356–360.

USPHS/IDSA Prevention of Opportunistic Infections Working Group. Preface to the 1997 USPHS/IDSA guidelines for the prevention of opportunistic infections in persons infected with human immunodeficiency virus. *Clin Infect Dis* 1997;25:S299–S235.

Wallace RJ Jr, Brown BA, Griffith DE. Clarithromycin regimens for pulmonary *Mycobacterium avium* complex: the first 50 patients. *Am J Respir Crit Care Med* 1996;153:1766–1772.

Wallace RJ Jr, Cook JL, Glassroth J, et al. Diagnosis and treatment of disease caused by nontuberculous mycobacteria. *Am J Respir Crit Care Med* 1997;156:S1–S25.

Wallace RJ Jr, O'Brien R, Glassroth J, et al. Diagnosis and treatment of disease caused by nontuberculous mycobacteria: ATS statement. *Am Rev Respir Dis* 1990;142:940–953.

Wallace RJ Jr., Swenson JM, Silcox VA, et al. Spectrum of disease due to rapidly growing mycobacteria. *Rev Infect Dis* 1983;5:657–679.

Wolinsky E. Nontuberculous mycobacteria and associated diseases. *Am Rev Respir Dis* 1979;119:107–159.

Kelley's Textbook of Internal Medicine, fourth edition. Edited by H. David Humes. Lippincott Williams & Wilkins, Philadelphia © 2000.

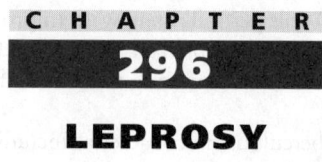

CHAPTER 296

LEPROSY

ROBERT R. JACOBSON

DEFINITION

Leprosy is a chronic infectious disease primarily involving skin and peripheral nerves. The more advanced types also may affect the eyes and mucous membranes of the upper respiratory tract.

INCIDENCE AND EPIDEMIOLOGY

Intensified control efforts worldwide have reduced the registered case load of leprosy to fewer than 900,000. About 150 new cases occur yearly in the United States, 20% of them among native-born citizens. The spread of the infection is believed to be mainly respiratory with a 3- to 5-year incubation period. Household contacts are at greatest risk.

ETIOLOGY

Leprosy is caused by *Mycobacterium leprae*, a slow-growing, obligate, intracellular parasite. It has never been grown in artificial media and divides only every 12.5 days in animal models.

PATHOGENESIS

Leprosy is believed to occur as a result of a relatively specific defect in the patient's cell-mediated immune response to *M. leprae*. More than 95% of a given population are apparently not susceptible to infection. The earliest manifestation may be indeterminate leprosy, which may self-heal or progress to another type. Persons with the most intact immune response keep the infection localized as tuberculoid leprosy, and few bacilli are evident. At the other extreme, among persons with a poor response the infection becomes generalized as lepromatous leprosy with large numbers of bacilli. Between these two extremes is the broad borderline group, which is usually subdivided into those with borderline-tuberculoid, mid-borderline, and borderline-lepromatous leprosy. The bacilli have a predilection for nerves, and the nerves involved may be damaged or destroyed.

CLINICAL FINDINGS

Leprosy should always be suspected when any patient has skin lesions and sensory loss. Physical examination includes inspec-

tion of the skin with documentation of the extent and types of lesions; sensory and motor testing; palpation of peripheral nerves for enlargement or tenderness; and examination of the eyes. The skin manifestations are protean and may include macules, plaques, papules, and nodules. Indeterminate disease commonly appears as a single, hypopigmented, occasionally erythematous macule, which may be hypoesthetic.

Tuberculoid disease typically becomes manifest with a single, large, scaly, anesthetic, hypopigmented macule that has a raised, well-defined margin. The sensory loss is confined to the lesion, but peripheral nerves in the vicinity of the lesion may be involved, leading to distal loss or to motor loss.

Lepromatous leprosy usually is generalized at diagnosis. It may appear as diffuse disease with no distinct lesions, as faint erythematous macules, or, most commonly, as papules and nodules. Early in the course of disease, there may be little or no sensory loss, but later the loss may be extensive, particularly over the distal extremities. Multiple peripheral nerves may be involved, but motor loss occurs late. Partial or complete loss of eyebrows and eyelashes, upper respiratory tract involvement, and eye involvement may occur. The lesions in borderline disease (Fig. 296.1) range from tuberculoid-like to lepromatous in character.

The borderline portion of the leprosy spectrum is characterized by immunologic instability and may shift toward lepromatous disease before treatment and toward tuberculoid disease with treatment. The latter may produce reactive episodes called *type 1* or *reversal reactions*. Nerve involvement often is extensive in borderline cases, and sensory and motor loss frequently occurs.

Reactive episodes vary markedly in severity and are more common after treatment is initiated. Type 1 reactions are characterized by the sudden onset of neuritis and edema and erythema of preexisting lesions and other skin areas that rarely may progress to ulceration. The neuritis may produce extensive loss of motor and sensory function if the patient is not properly treated. Erythema nodosum leprosum (type 2; ENL) reactions

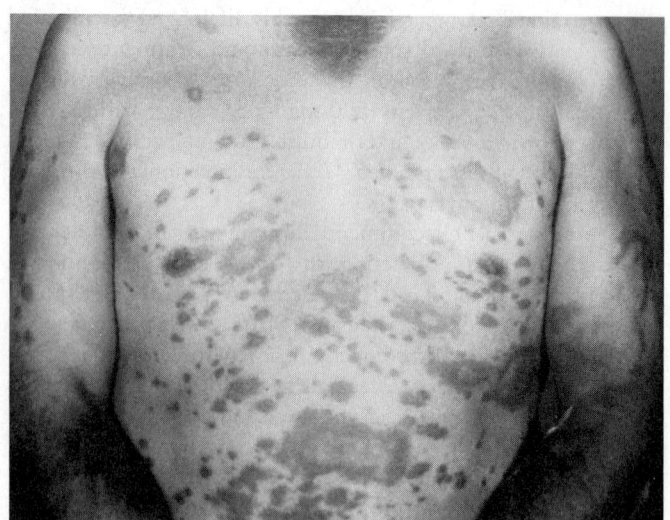

FIGURE 296.1. Borderline lepromatous leprosy. The multiple papules and nodules are typical of lepromatous disease, but the larger lesions, some of which are tuberculoid-like, indicate a borderline component.

cause fever and erythematous, frequently painful nodules. Erythema multiforme–like, pustular, and ulcerating forms also may be found. Neuritis, arthralgia, leukocytosis, lymphadenitis, iridocyclitis, orchitis, and nephritis may accompany ENL. Patients with lepromatous disease may have ENL, patients with borderline lepromatous disease may have either, and patients with other classifications may have only type 1 reactions. Neuritis, orchitis, and occasionally other components of reactive episodes may occur independently. The ulnar and median nerves are the most commonly involved.

LABORATORY FINDINGS

Diagnosis is based on the physical findings, the results of examination of skin scrapings, and biopsy findings. Some biopsy sections are stained for histopathologic study, and classification is based on the type of cellular infiltrate and the involvement of dermal nerves. Other biopsy sections and skin scrapings are stained for acid-fast bacilli. Bacilli are counted by means of a semilogarithmic scale to obtain the bacterial index (BI). This index ranges from 0 (no bacilli in 100 oil-immersion fields) to 6+ (more than 1,000 bacilli per oil-immersion field).

STRATEGIES FOR OPTIMAL CARE

Every patient should be given multidrug therapy to avoid drug resistance. Patients with paucibacillary disease (indeterminate, tuberculoid, and borderline tuberculoid with a BI of 0 at all sites on skin scrapings) are given dapsone 100 mg per day plus rifampin either 600 mg per day (U.S. recommendation) or once a month (World Health Organization [WHO] recommendation) for 12 months (U.S.) or 6 months (WHO). Therapy is then discontinued. Patients with multibacillary disease (midborderline, borderline lepromatous, and lepromatous or any patient with a BI of 1+ or greater at any site) are treated with dapsone 100 mg per day plus clofazimine 50 mg per day plus rifampin either 600 mg per day (U.S.) or per month (WHO). Therapy is given for 2 years (U.S.) or 1 year (WHO) and then discontinued, although patients in the United States often have been continued with dapsone indefinitely to prevent relapse.

Relapses apparently are uncommon even when therapy is stopped after 2 years. However, a relapse can occur 5 or more years after the original illness, so patients should undergo follow-up examinations at least once a year for 10 years. The *M. leprae* organisms in these patients usually remain fully sensitive to the drugs used, so treatment involves repeating the same regimen. Most skin lesions clear within 6 to 12 months, and the BI usually falls at a rate of 0.5 to 1 unit per year. Ofloxacin (400 mg per day), clarithromycin (500 mg per day), and minocycline (100 mg per day) are highly bactericidal for *M. leprae,* although less so than rifampin, and a number of regimens with one or more of them together with rifampin are under study to determine whether therapy can be further shortened.

Complications during therapy are most commonly reactions and neuritis. These respond to prednisone in a daily dose of 60 mg or more. This is the only approach that may reverse or prevent nerve damage. The time during which prednisone is needed varies from several weeks to years. Clofazimine in high doses is useful for the management of ENL. Thalidomide usually can control ENL, but it is teratogenic and must be used with caution. Assistance in the management of all cases can be obtained at any time from the Gillis W. Long Hansen's Disease Center in Louisiana.

PROGNOSIS

Treatment rapidly renders leprosy noninfectious, and the overall results are excellent. When they come to medical attention, however, some patients have disabilities caused by the disease. These disabilities are not reversed with treatment.

BIBLIOGRAPHY

Hastings RC, ed. *Leprosy,* 2nd ed. Edinburgh: Churchill Livingstone, 1994.

Jacobson RR, Yoder LJ. Leprosy. In: Evans AS, Brachman PS, eds. Bacterial *Infections of Humans, Epidemiology and Control,* 3rd ed. New York: Plenum, 1998:377–393.

World Health Organization Expert Committee on Leprosy. Seventh report (WHO technical report series no. 874). Geneva, Switzerland: WHO, 1998.

Kelley's Textbook of Internal Medicine, fourth edition. Edited by H. David Humes. Lippincott Williams & Wilkins, Philadelphia © 2000.

SPIROCHETAL INFECTIONS

CHAPTER
297

SYPHILIS

NAIEL N. NASSAR
JUSTIN DAVID RADOLF

DEFINITION

Syphilis is a chronic, systemic, sexually transmitted disease caused by the spirochete *Treponema pallidum* subspecies *pallidum.* After a variable incubation period (mean 21 days), classic untreated syphilis progresses through stages with highly variable clinical manifestations. Syphilis is capable of causing a wide spectrum of clinical disease that can affect almost all organ systems. The disease can cause manifestations over a tremendous length of time, varying from a genital ulcer weeks after the initial infection to a form of dementia 15 to 20 years later.

INCIDENCE AND EPIDEMIOLOGY

Humans are the only known natural hosts of *T. pallidum*. Most cases of newly acquired syphilis are caused by direct contact during sexual intercourse with the mucocutaneous lesions that occur during the primary or secondary stages of syphilis. Late syphilis is considered noninfectious. Other forms of sexual activity such as kissing, oral-genital, and oral-anal contact also may cause infection. An untreated pregnant woman can transmit syphilis to the fetus regardless of the stage of disease. Syphilis is rarely transmitted through nonsexual contact, accidental inoculation, or blood transfusion from a donor with syphilis .

By some estimates, the prevalence of syphilis in the late 1800s was as high as 10% of the population. Over the past 50 years, the incidence of syphilis in the United States has shown great variation. Reported cases of primary and secondary syphilis, which had been increasing steadily during the 1940s, peaked in 1947. From 1947 to 1957 a rapid diminution in reported cases appeared to be related to both the end of World War II and the introduction of penicillin as therapy for syphilis. Between 1955 and 1960, however, the number of new cases of syphilis rebounded substantially, and there were nearly steady annual increases through 1982. At the same time, a striking increase in the incidence of infectious syphilis among homosexual white men paralleled the newly recognized HIV epidemic.

Between 1986 and 1990, there was a surge in reported cases of syphilis in the United States. The highest rates of primary and secondary syphilis were in the southern states, where the rate was two to five times higher than in other regions of the United States. Higher levels of poverty and less access to health care services are postulated to be responsible for this regional variation. Throughout the 1990s, the rates of primary and secondary syphilis have declined 84% in the United States in all regions. Syphilis rates also have declined for all racial and ethnic groups; the largest decline occurred among Hispanics (90%) followed by blacks (85%) and non-Hispanic whites (81%). Rates of primary and secondary syphilis, however, remain high among blacks and among women of all races. Although syphilis remains an endemic disease in parts of the South, rates in this region have declined 80% since 1990. Factors that may have contributed to the decline in syphilis include increased state and federal resources allocated to syphilis control programs, implementation of HIV prevention activities, a decline in use of crack cocaine, and the presence of acquired immunity in the population at risk after the epidemic.

ETIOLOGY

The genus *Treponema*, which belongs to the family Spirochaetaceae, contains two species pathogenic for humans, *T. pallidum* and *T. carateum*, and a number of genetically unrelated nonpathogenic species. The causative organism of venereal syphilis is *T. pallidum* subspecies *pallidum*. Yaws and endemic syphilis are caused by *T. pallidum* subspecies *pertenue* and *T. pallidum* subspecies *endemicum*, respectively, whereas *T. carateum* is the agent of pinta. Although limited replication has been achieved in tissue culture systems, the pathogenic treponemes cannot be cultivated continuously in vitro. Experimental strains of *T. pallidum* subspecies *pallidum* are most commonly maintained by means of repeated intratesticular inoculation of rabbits. All four treponemes are morphologically and antigenically indistinguishable. Speciation traditionally has depended on differences in host range, mode of transmission, geographic distribution, and the clinical features of the respective diseases. More recently, however, investigators have identified genetic differences that should prove useful for differentiating these organisms.

T. pallidum subspecies *pallidum* is a fragile, helical bacterium 5 to 20 μm long and 0.1 to 0.2 μm wide. It divides by means of longitudinal binary fission with a dividing time of 30 to 33 hours. Although *T. pallidum* frequently is referred to as gramnegative, this is a misnomer inasmuch as the organism poorly takes up aniline dyes and contains no lipopolysaccharide. Electron micrographs demonstrate that the organism possesses both outer and cytoplasmic membranes separated by a periplasmic space. Ultrastructural studies reveal that *T. pallidum* organisms have an outer membrane that is unique among prokaryotes in that the membrane contains an extraordinarily low content of integral membrane proteins. The organelles of motility, the endoflagella, are located within the periplasmic space. Three endoflagella insert near each end of the organism. As in other spirochetes, peptidoglycan is thought to be associated with the cytoplasmic membrane. The approximately one megabase circular chromosome of the bacterium has been completely sequenced. This information confirms that *T. pallidum* lacks much of the metabolic and biosynthetic machinery typically found in cultivated bacterial pathogens.

PATHOGENESIS

The specific mechanisms and determinants of treponemal virulence are still being elucidated. The genomic sequence surprisingly revealed that *T. pallidum* appears to lack virulence factors previously characterized among other bacterial pathogens. Pathogenic, but not nonpathogenic, treponemes readily attach to and penetrate a variety of cultured cell monolayers. Attachment may be mediated by treponemal receptors for components of the extracellular matrix. Motility is thought to play an important role in cell penetration and host dissemination. Although evasion of host cellular and humoral immune responses is presumably prerequisite to establishment of latent infection, the mechanisms responsible for this phenomenon are poorly understood. It is known, however, that the surface of the organism reacts poorly with specific antibodies. The paucity of surface-exposed proteins is believed to explain this phenomenon. The tissue damage caused by syphilitic infection appears to be more a result of the host immune response rather than a direct toxic effect of *T. pallidum*.

Much of our knowledge of the course of untreated syphilis derives from three clinical studies. From 1910 onward, Boeck and successors at the University of Oslo followed the cases of approximately 2,000 patients with untreated early syphilis for almost 40 years (the Oslo Study). In 1932, the United States Public Health Service began a 30-year study of untreated syphilis among 431 black men with latent syphilis (the Tuskegee study) that provided insights into the incidence and nature of cardiovascular syphilis among black men. A study by Magnuson et al. in the 1950s with human volunteers in the Sing Sing Correctional Facility helped to clarify the time course of incubation of human syphilis and documented the development of immunity to reinfection among persons with untreated late latent syphilis.

Endogenous resistance to treponemal infection has been inferred from epidemiologic studies showing that syphilis develops among only one-third of persons exposed. Nevertheless, experiments with both human subjects and rabbits in which standardized inocula were used indicated that fewer than 10 organisms are capable of producing infection. In natural infection, organisms rapidly penetrate intact mucous membranes and microscopically abraded skin and disseminate hematogenously soon thereafter. Blood from a patient with incubating syphilis is infectious long before the appearance of a chancre. Transfusion of blood from such patients has transmitted the infection. Although neurologic symptoms may not become apparent until years after infection, treponemal invasion of the central nervous system occurs early. A high proportion of patients with early syphilis (syphilis of less than 1 year's duration) have cerebrospinal fluid (CSF) abnormalities despite a lack of neurologic symptoms. Treponemes often can be recovered by means of inoculation of rabbits with normal or abnormal spinal fluid during this period. Conversely, normal findings at spinal fluid examination 2 or more years after infection indicate low risk of subsequent development of neurosyphilis.

Syphilitic lesions at all stages of disease have two histopathologic characteristics. The first is obliterative endarteritis in which hyperplasia and swelling of endothelial cells cause narrowing and complete occlusion of blood vessels. The second is a loose perivascular infiltrate consisting of lymphocytes, macrophages, and, most characteristically, plasma cells. Granuloma formation in both secondary and, particularly, tertiary syphilitic lesions also is common. Circulating immune complexes containing treponemal antigens are regularly present in secondary syphilis and may contribute to clinical manifestations.

CLINICAL FINDINGS

Classic syphilis is divided into stages. It is important to emphasize at the outset, however, that staging of syphilis is imprecise because of the considerable temporal, clinical, and histopathologic overlap among stages.

A chancre, the primary lesion of syphilis, appears after an incubation period of 10 to 90 days (average 3 weeks) at the site of inoculation. It begins as an erythematous papule that ulcerates

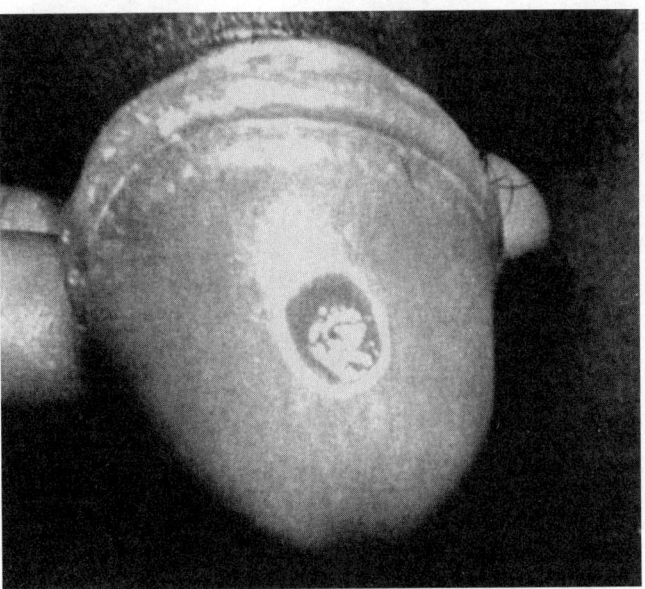

FIGURE 297.1. Typical syphilitic chancre.

before healing within 2 to 4 weeks (Fig. 297.1), even without treatment, and leaves a thin, atrophic scar. The typical chancre is painless, solitary, rounded, and has a raised, discrete border with a rubbery or cartilaginous consistency. The individual lesions vary in size from a few millimeters to 1 to 2 cm. Among heterosexual men, chancres are most commonly found on the glans, the coronal sulcus, and the foreskin. Among women clinically evident lesions usually are found on the external genitalia, particularly the labia majora and minora, the fourchette, and the perineum. Perianal, anal, and rectal lesions are common among homosexual men. Most chancres outside the anogenital region occur in or about the mouth, particularly the lips, where they tend to be somewhat painful, although any area of the body may become infected. Approximately 50% of patients with primary syphilis have painless, nonsuppurative, bilateral regional adenopathy.

Because many chancres are atypical in appearance, it is important to suspect that any genital lesion may be syphilitic. Papular lesions may occur among patients who seek treatment before the onset of ulceration. Multiple lesions occur among as many as 30% of patients. Tender, even exquisitely painful, primary lesions sometimes occur. Among homosexual men, chancres may be mistaken for trauma-induced anal fissures. Primary syphilis must be differentiated from the multiple other causes of genital ulceration, including venereal infection (e.g., chancroid, herpes genitalis, lymphogranuloma venereum, granuloma inguinale), nonvenereal infection (e.g., cat-scratch fever, rat-bite fever, sporotrichosis), and noninfectious lesions (e.g., traumatic wounds, malignant tumors).

Approximately 6 to 24 weeks after infection, usually when the chancre is either healing or has disappeared entirely, the secondary, or disseminated, stage of syphilis begins. Although characterized by widespread, sometimes florid, mucocutaneous lesions, secondary syphilis is a systemic infection that can affect almost every organ system. The ability of secondary syphilis to

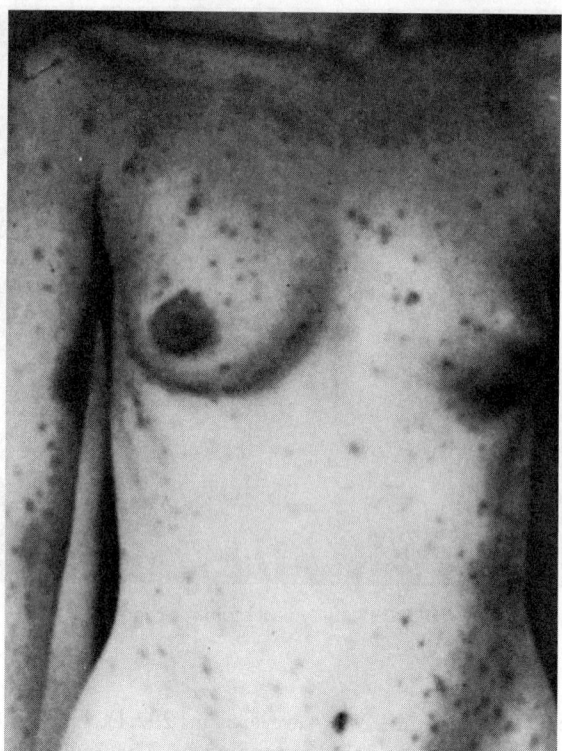

FIGURE 297.2. Typical rash of secondary syphilis.

mimic many other clinical conditions is largely responsible for its reputation as the "great imitator."

The cutaneous lesions of secondary syphilis (syphilids) usually are described as macular, maculopapular, papular, papulosquamous, and pustular. More than 95% of the skin lesions are of the first four varieties, macular and maculopapular lesions predominating in most series. The lesions usually are symmetrical and widespread, varying from several millimeters to several centimeters in diameter (Fig. 297.2). Pruritic eruptions can occur. Successive eruptions may evolve from macular to papular or papulosquamous; the different forms may be present simultaneously. Among some patients, lesions are characteristically confined to the distal extremities, especially the palms and soles. Syphilids with a squamous component may resemble psoriasis, lichen planus, or pityriasis rosea. A rare, unusually severe type of secondary syphilis formerly called *lues maligna* sometimes occurs. It appears as nodular-pustular lesions on the torso, the extremities, and sometimes the oral mucosa that evolve over the course of months into large, necrotic ulcerations. In the AIDS era, lues maligna has been linked with HIV infection; however, it is important to know that this rare but severe form of secondary syphilis was well recognized in the preantibiotic era. Other common mucocutaneous manifestations of secondary syphilis include patchy ("moth-eaten") alopecia and thinning of the eyebrows and beard; diffuse redness of the tonsils and pharynx; superficial ulcers of the oral and genital mucosa (mucous patches); and moist, papular excrescences in the intertriginous areas (condyloma lata) that teem with treponemes and are highly infectious.

Generalized lymphadenopathy often is present, and spleno-megaly often is evident in florid presentations. Other organ systems that may be involved in secondary syphilis include the gastrointestinal tract, the central nervous system, the eyes, the kidneys, and the bones. A markedly elevated alkaline phosphatase level, with or without other liver function abnormalities, usually indicates granulomatous hepatitis and occur in about 10% of patients with early syphilis. Renal involvement caused by immune complex deposition in secondary syphilis is rare. It usually manifests with isolated proteinuria, nephrotic syndrome, or acute glomerulonephritis. Symptomatic central nervous system involvement, usually headache and meningism (syphilitic meningitis), occurs among a small percentage of patients. In rare instances patients may have more severe neurologic disorders, such as a basilar meningitis with cranial nerve abnormalities (most commonly involving the third, sixth, seventh, and eighth cranial nerves), acute syphilitic hydrocephalus, optic neuritis, or cerebrovascular syndromes.

Anterior uveitis is relatively common in secondary syphilis and should be ruled out for all young adults with iritis. Less common is posterior uveitis, which can cause blindness through vitritis or destruction of the macula, and optic neuritis. There is a general impression that posterior syphilitic uveitis has become more prevalent, particularly among homosexual men, and it should be included among the causes of chorioretinitis in examinations of patients with HIV coinfection. Clinically significant osteitis and arthritis are rare; in contrast, mild forms of osteitis associated with bone pain are frequent.

After the manifestations of secondary syphilis subside, untreated patients enter the asymptomatic stage, called *latency*. An important finding of the Oslo Study was that approximately 25% of patients have one or more infectious relapses during the first 4 years of latency, primarily in the first year, and that infectious relapses thereafter are rare. This is the basis for the traditional distinction between early and late latency, whereas the period of greatest infectiousness is designated *early syphilis*. Relapses may be indistinguishable from the patient's previous secondary episode. Cutaneous lesions tend to be less florid than those in secondary disease, whereas mucosal lesions, such as mucous patches and condyloma lata, may predominate. Isolated visceral relapses, such as hepatitis, osteitis, and uveitis, also occur. Pregnant women with early latent syphilis are at great risk of infecting the fetus in utero.

According to the Oslo Study, approximately 30% of untreated patients with late latent disease have one or more forms of tertiary syphilis years, even decades, after infection. Tertiary syphilis is traditionally divided into the following three categories: benign tertiary (gummatous) syphilis, cardiovascular syphilis, and neurosyphilis. At present in the United States, all categories of tertiary syphilis are rare.

Gummatous syphilis is characterized by the development of one or more granulomatous lesions (gummas) 7 to 10 years after initial infection. Although most common on mucocutaneous surfaces and in bone, the lesions can occur in almost any location. Gummas begin as one or more small nodules that slowly enlarge through inflammatory changes, and central necrosis develops. They may vary from large, ulcerative skin lesions to space-occupying lesions within the central nervous system. Gummas of the facial structures and upper respiratory tract can produce marked disfigurement. Bone gummas can produce bone pain and give rise to pathologic fractures.

Cardiovascular syphilis is more common among men than among women and is a major cause of death among all patients with late syphilis. It is caused by obliterative endarteritis of the vasa vasorum of the large arteries, particularly the proximal ascending thoracic aorta. Medial necrosis develops and leads to progressive fusiform or saccular aneurysmal dilatation. In addition to extensive adventitial fibrosis, degeneration of the intima results in atherosclerotic plaque formation with calcification, evident as "tree barking" on chest radiographs. Syphilitic thoracic aortic aneurysms frequently remain asymptomatic until they rupture or encroach on neighboring mediastinal structures. Aortic root dilatation may give rise to aortic regurgitation and congestive heart failure. Some patients have symptoms of ischemic heart disease due to coronary artery ostial stenosis.

Syphilis of the central nervous system (neurosyphilis) constitutes a group of neurologic syndromes that occur mainly but not exclusively as a late manifestation of infection. Four categories of neurosyphilis usually occur in late syphilis: asymptomatic, meningovascular, parenchymatous, and gummatous. Asymptomatic neurosyphilis is the presence of one or more CSF abnormalities in a patient with late syphilis, usually defined as 1 or more years after infection. Meningovascular syphilis, manifesting as stroke, usually occurs 5 to 10 years after infection and can involve all parts of the central nervous system. The parenchymatous neurosyphilitic syndromes are tabes dorsalis and generalized paresis. Tabes dorsalis is caused by demyelinization of the posterior columns of the spinal cord, dorsal roots, and dorsal root ganglia. Patients have lancinating pain, pupillary abnormalities (most characteristically Argyll Robertson pupils), impotence, bladder incontinence, truncal ataxia, lower extremity areflexia, and a profound loss of position and vibratory sensation in the legs that gives rise to chronic traumatic arthritis (Charcot joints). Generalized paresis is an insidious dementia that may include seizures, dramatic and bizarre changes in personality, and intellectual deterioration. Gummas of the central nervous system are rare and manifest as mass lesions with or without CSF abnormalities consistent with chronic inflammation.

Congenital syphilis, a consequence of intrauterine infection, usually at 18 weeks or later during gestation, is divided into early and late stages. Early infection occurs within the first 2 years of life and is analogous to the secondary stage of acquired syphilis among adults. It can be fulminant, causing stillbirth and neonatal death. Other disorders include rhinitis (snuffles); highly infectious mucocutaneous lesions, such as bullae, maculopapules, mucous patches, and condyloma lata; and periostitis, hepatosplenomegaly, thrombocytopenia, leukopenia, anemia, and nephrosis. After a period of latency, manifestations of late congenital syphilis develop that include interstitial keratitis, dental anomalies (mulberry molars and Hutchinson's teeth), eighth nerve deafness, osteitis, gummas, facial deformities (saddle nose), and neurosyphilis. For unclear reasons, cardiovascular syphilis is a rare complication of congenital infection.

◼ LABORATORY FINDINGS

Because *T. pallidum* cannot be cultivated in vitro, diagnosis relies on either identification of the treponeme in clinical specimens

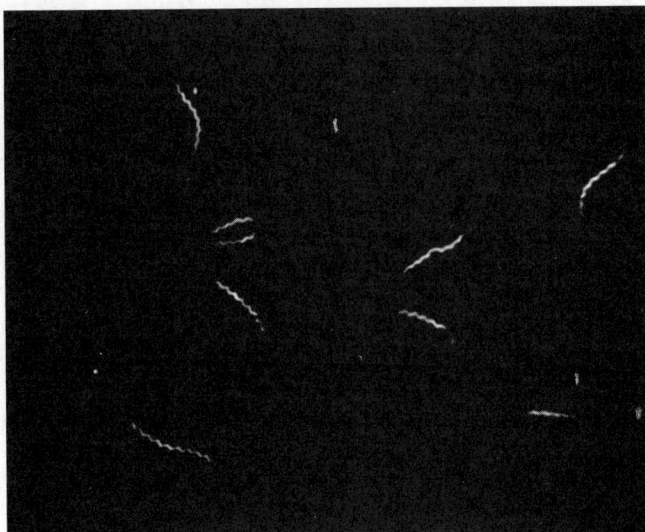

FIGURE 297.3. Photograph from dark-field microscopic examination depicts *Treponema pallidum* organisms.

or reactive serologic tests. Misdiagnosis or failure to diagnose the disease expeditiously is more frequently a consequence of the physician's unfamiliarity with the diverse manifestations of syphilitic infection than a lack of precision of diagnostic tests. Nevertheless, the limitations of syphilis diagnostics are such that a final diagnosis must at times be based on empiricism and mature clinical judgment.

The most rapid and direct means of identification of treponemes in clinical material is dark-field microscopic examination (Fig. 297.3). Exudates from chancres and moist secondary lesions such as condyloma lata are most amenable to this procedure. A slide should be examined for a minimum of 10 minutes before it is considered to be normal. Because visualization of treponemes with a dark-field microscope requires between 104 and 105 organisms per milliliter of fluid, normal findings do not eliminate the diagnosis of syphilis. Dark-field examination of material from mucosal surfaces is not recommended because these surfaces are colonized with nonpathogenic treponemes that may be confused with *T. pallidum*. Characteristic histopathologic findings may raise the suspicion of syphilis. Demonstration of treponemes in tissue may be accomplished by means of silver stain or the more sensitive and specific immunologic techniques in which anti–*T. pallidum* antibodies are used.

Serologic tests for syphilis are the mainstay of diagnosis. The fact that the assays can be used to measure two distinctly different kinds of antibodies, nontreponemal and treponemal, is a perpetual source of confusion to practicing physicians. *Nontreponemal tests,* such as the Venereal Disease Research Laboratory test (VDRL) and the rapid plasma reagin test (RPR), are used to measure flocculating antibodies to a mixture of cardiolipin, cholesterol, and lecithin. These antibodies are presumed to arise from the interaction of virulent treponemes with host tissue. Titers of nontreponemal antibodies tend to be highest in secondary disease and decline gradually thereafter. Approximately 30% of patients with primary, late latent, and tertiary disease have nonreactive results of nontreponemal tests. Some patients with extremely elevated levels of nontreponemal antibodies, as in secondary syphilis, have nonreactive nontreponemal results when the tests are performed at low serum dilutions but have reactive test results after the sera are diluted (prozone phenomenon). This phenomenon can be detected by means of performing nontreponemal tests on diluted and undiluted sera.

The *treponemal tests,* which are used to measure antibodies specific for the pathogenic treponemes, are needed to confirm that reactive nontreponemal serologic results are caused treponemal infection. The most commonly used treponemal tests are the fluorescent treponemal antibody absorption test and the microhemagglutination assay–*T. pallidum.* In the fluorescent treponemal antibody absorption test indirect immunofluorescence is used to detect serum antibody bound to treponemes dried on microscope slides. The microhemagglutination assay is used to measure the ability of serum antibodies to agglutinate red blood cells coated with *T. pallidum* antigens. The specificity of both assays is enhanced by the absorption of sera with material derived from a nonpathogenic commensal treponeme to remove cross-reacting antibodies. Inability completely to remove such antibodies is the most frequent cause of the falsely reactive treponemal tests that occur among as much as 2% of the general population.

A third treponemal test, called the *T. pallidum immobilization test,* is used to measure the ability of *T. pallidum*–specific antibody to immobilize virulent treponemes in the presence of complement. This highly specific test is not generally available. The sensitivities of the nontreponemal and treponemal tests for the different stages of syphilis are presented in Table 297.1. Newer tests such as the Captia Syph G and Capita Syph M, which are used to detect *T. pallidum*–specific IgG and IgM, appear to be helpful in the diagnosis of early primary and congenital syphilis and in differentiating biologic false-positive reactions and true syphilis. Although not commercially available, immunoblot assays facilitate differentiation of false- and true-positive treponemal tests. Polymerase chain reaction amplification of *T. pallidum* DNA appears to be of limited value because treponemes often are not present in the clinical specimens, such as serum, most easily obtained from persons with syphilis.

TABLE 297.1.	**SENSITIVITY (%) OF SEROLOGIC TESTS IN DIFFERENT STAGES OF SYPHILIS**

Stage	RPR	FTA-ABS	MHATP	TPI Test
Primary	75	85	80	40
Secondary and early latent	>99	100	100	98
Late latent and tertiary	70[a]	>99	98	95

Note: Values represent approximate means based on data from several clinical studies.
RPR, rapid plasma reagin; FTA-ABS, fluorescent treponemal antibody absorption test; MHATP, microhemagglutination assay–*Treponema pallidum;* TPI, treponemal immobilization.
[a] Reactivity of nontreponemal tests in tertiary syphilis varies greatly according to the specific syndrome.

Many diseases may give rise to either acute or chronic falsely reactive nontreponemal tests ("biologic" false positives). Some causes of the former include *Mycoplasma pneumoniae* infection, various viral illnesses (especially Epstein–Barr virus infections), and malaria. Chronic falsely reactive nontreponemal tests are produced most often by autoimmune disorders, such as systemic lupus erythematosus but also occur in conditions such as narcotic addiction, leprosy, and pregnancy and as an accompaniment of aging. A nonreactive treponemal test excludes syphilis for a patient with a reactive nontreponemal test.

For the diagnosis of neurosyphilis, CSF examination should be performed on any patient with reactive syphilis serologic findings and neurologic abnormalities. In the absence of a traumatic lumbar puncture, a reactive CSF-VDRL result is almost always specific for neurosyphilis. However, the CSF-VDRL may be reactive among only 50% to 70% of patients with neurosyphilis, ranging from nearly 100% in meningovascular syphilis to as little as 50% among patients with tabes dorsalis. Active neurosyphilis usually is accompanied by CSF pleocytosis, usually lymphocytic, and often by an elevated protein level. A decrease in CSF glucose level also can occur. Cases of neurosyphilis have been reported among patients with normal spinal fluid. A presumptive diagnosis of neurosyphilis can be made when a patient is believed to have neurosyphilis and has a nonreactive CSF-VDRL. Empiric therapy usually is indicated in this situation, and response to therapy may help confirm the diagnosis.

All patients with late syphilis ideally should undergo lumbar puncture to identify asymptomatic neurosyphilis. The Centers for Disease Control and Prevention (CDC), however, recommends that these efforts concentrate on patients with clinical signs or symptoms of neurologic or ophthalmic syphilis; serum nontreponemal antibody titers greater than 1:32 (unless duration of infection is less than 1 year); treatment failure (see later); other evidence of tertiary syphilis (aortitis, gummas, iritis); and penicillin allergy for whom nonpenicillin therapy for late latent syphilis is planned.

Physicians frequently encounter patients whose nontreponemal serologic results, usually obtained as screening tests, are unexpectedly reactive. A treponemal test should be obtained because a nonreactive treponemal test excludes the diagnosis of syphilis. A reactive treponemal test requires the physician to perform a complete evaluation, including consideration of lumbar puncture, and to treat the patient accordingly. In appropriate circumstances, the physician should ask about residence in areas endemic for nonvenereal treponematosis that is serologically indistinguishable from venereal syphilis.

For infants with relatively high treponemal burdens, the presence of congenital infection can be confirmed with detection of spirochetes in suspicious lesions, body fluids, or tissues by means of dark-field microscopic examination, silver staining or immunofluorescence, or polymerase chain reaction for *T. pallidum* DNA. Otherwise, serologic tests are the mainstay of diagnosis, as in acquired infection. A triad of enlarged hypercellular villi, proliferative fetal vascular changes, and acute or chronic villitis can be evident at microscopic examination of the placenta and can be helpful in establishing a diagnosis of congenital syphilis. Prenatal diagnosis of fetal syphilis is possible with ultrasonography, which can help identify hydrops fetalis, hepatosplenomegaly, and placentomegaly in the presence of maternal syphilis. Any infant born to a seropositive mother should undergo a complete examination to rule out evidence of congenital syphilis. In addition to the serologic testing, a lumbar puncture is necessary to evaluate the CSF for cell count, protein, and VDRL result. Immunoblot studies have demonstrated the feasibility of using *T. pallidum*–specific IgM antibodies in neonatal sera as unequivocal evidence of intrapartum infection.

STRATEGIES FOR OPTIMAL CARE

Penicillin is the drug of choice for therapy for all stages of syphilis. *T. pallidum* is exquisitely sensitive to this agent, and results with the drug have been excellent. Although regimens with benzathine penicillin G have come under considerable scrutiny, these agents are the preferred formulations for uncomplicated forms of syphilis because they provide prolonged treponemicidal levels. Despite reports of treatment failures with penicillin, there is no evidence that the sensitivity of *T. pallidum* to penicillin has diminished since the introduction of this antibiotic. Alternative antibiotics, such as tetracycline, erythromycin, and chloramphenicol, are believed to be less efficacious. There is much less clinical experience with these agents than there is with penicillin, particularly in therapy of complicated forms of disease such as neurosyphilis. The 1998 therapeutic recommendations of the CDC are shown in Table 297.2.

More than 95% of HIV-negative patients with syphilis of less than 1 year's duration are cured with intramuscular administration of 2.4 million units of benzathine penicillin G. Patients with complicated forms of early syphilis, such as posterior uveitis or meningeal infection with cranial nerve involvement, should receive high doses of intravenous penicillin, as for neurosyphilis. Nonpregnant patients with early syphilis who are allergic to penicillin can be treated effectively with tetracycline. Pregnant patients who are allergic to penicillin should undergo skin tests to confirm penicillin hypersensitivity. If skin tests are reactive, desensitization should be performed. Erythromycin should not be used to treat pregnant patients with penicillin allergies because of an unacceptable frequency of treatment failures among neonates.

Patients who seek treatment of gonorrhea are often presumed to be coinfected with syphilis. All treatment regimens for gonorrhea in which β-lactam antimicrobial agents are used probably are effective in the management of early, incubating syphilis. Quinolones, such as ciprofloxacin, levofloxacin, and grepafloxacin, and spectinomycin are not effective against incubating syphilis. Persons who have had sexual contact within 90 days with an untreated patient with early syphilis are also presumed to be infected and need the treatment given for early syphilis.

Patients who are not allergic to penicillin who have late latent, cardiovascular, and benign tertiary syphilis are treated with benzathine penicillin G. Symptomatic cardiovascular lesions may not improve with therapy, but progression of asymptomatic lesions usually is arrested. Tetracycline is recommended to treat patients who are -allergic to penicillin who have late latent syphilis. Intravenous penicillin G is recommended therapy for both

TABLE 297.2.	THERAPY FOR THE DIFFERENT STAGES OF SYPHILIS

Primary and secondary syphilis
  Benzathine penicillin G 2.4 million units IM in a single dose
Penicillin allergy
  Doxycycline 100 mg orally twice a day for 2 weeks *or* tetracycline 500 mg orally four times a day for 2 weeks
Early latent syphilis
  Benzathine penicillin G 2.4 million units IM in a single dose
Late latent syphilis or latent syphilis of unknown duration
  Benzathine penicillin G 7.2 million units total administered as three doses of 2.4 million units IM each at 1-week intervals
Penicillin allergy
  Doxycycline 100 mg orally twice a day *or* tetracycline 500 mg orally four times a day
Tertiary syphilis
  Benzathine penicillin G 7.2 million units total administered as three doses of 2.4 million units IM at 1-week intervals
Neurosyphilis
  Aqueous crystalline penicillin G 18–24 million units/day, administered as 3–4 million units IV every 4 hours for 10–14 days
  If compliance with therapy can be ensured, patients may be treated with the following alternative regimen: procaine penicillin 2.4 million units IM a day *plus* probenecid 500 mg orally four times a day, both for 10–14 days
Syphilis in pregnancy
  Treatment during pregnancy should be the penicillin regimen appropriate for the stage of syphilis
Congenital syphilis
  Aqueous crystalline penicillin G 100,000–150,000 units/kg a day, administered as 50,000 units/kg per dose IV every 12 hours during the first 7 days of life and every 8 hours thereafter for a total of 10 days *or* procaine penicillin G 50,000 units/kg per dose IM a day in a single dose for 10 days
  Infants and children who need treatment of syphilis but who have a history of penicillin allergy or have an allergic reaction presumed to be caused by penicillin should be desensitized, if necessary, and treated with penicillin

asymptomatic and symptomatic neurosyphilis. Because of numerous reports of treatment failures, the CDC has eliminated regimens in which only benzathine penicillin G is used to manage neurosyphilis. It is highly desirable that patients with neurosyphilis who are allergic to penicillin undergo skin tests to confirm penicillin hypersensitivity and that desensitization be attempted if skin test results are reactive. If desensitization fails or is not attempted, the patient should be treated in consultation with an expert in syphilis treatment.

Ceftriaxone, a third-generation cephalosporin with a relatively long half-life, has been used experimentally in the management of primary and secondary syphilis. Treatment is multiple once-daily intramuscular injections. Although initial reports appear promising, further studies need to be conducted before ceftriaxone therapy can be recommended. One small retrospective study evaluated ceftriaxone in the treatment of HIV-positive patients with late latent and asymptomatic neurosyphilis. There was a disappointing 23% failure rate with 10- to 14-day treatment with ceftriaxone. The failure rate was very similar for another group treated with the standard therapy of injection of benzathine penicillin G once a week for 3 weeks.

The azalide antibiotic, azithromycin has many properties that suggest it might be useful as therapy for early syphilis. It is active against *T. pallidum* in vitro and has been effective in experimental models of syphilis. Although plasma concentration of azithromycin may be nearly immeasurable, high levels can be achieved in tissue. The half-life of azithromycin is 68 hours, which makes it ideal for therapy against *T. pallidum*, an organism with a prolonged doubling time. Ongoing studies suggest that azithromycin may be useful for early syphilis and may be efficacious in a single-dose to prevent incubating syphilis among patients treated for gonococcal and chlamydial urethritis.

Patients who have initially reactive nontreponemal serologic results should be examined at regular intervals, ideally beginning 3 months after therapy, to determine that a cure has been achieved. Patients should be reexamined clinically and serologically 6 and 12 months after treatment ends. More frequent evaluation may be prudent if the likelihood of follow-up care is uncertain. It once was believed that 95% of patients with primary syphilis will have nonreactive nontreponemal test results within 1 year of therapy and that at least 75% of patients with secondary and early latent syphilis will have nonreactive nontreponemal test results within 2 years of therapy. However, a carefully performed retrospective study conducted in Canada demonstrated that the rate of serologic decline after successful therapy for early syphilis was slower than previously thought. The investigators found fourfold and eightfold decreases in rapid plasma reagin titers 6 and 12 months, respectively, after treatment among patients with primary and secondary syphilis and fourfold decreases 12 months later among patients with early latent syphilis. Serologic test titers may decline more slowly for patients who previously had syphilis.

Seroreversion is definitive evidence of cure. Patients with early syphilis whose nontreponemal test results remain reactive at a low, stable titer also may be considered cured. If a patient has signs or symptoms that persist or recur or has a sustained fourfold rise in nontreponemal test titer, treatment probably has failed or the patient has been reinfected. These patients should be treated after reevaluation for HIV infection. Unless reinfection with *T. pallidum* is certain, lumbar puncture also should be performed. Failure of nontreponemal test titers to decline fourfold within 6 months after therapy for primary or secondary syphilis indicates that a patient is at risk of treatment failure. Such patients should undergo reevaluation for HIV infection. Optimal treatment of such patients is unclear. At a minimum, they should undergo additional clinical and serologic follow-up studies. Patients with HIV infection should be examined more frequently (every 3 months rather than every 6 months). If additional follow-up care cannot be ensured, repetition of treatment is recommended. Some experts recommend CSF examination in such situations. When patients undergo repetition of treatment, most experts recommend intramuscular injection of 2.4 million units benzathine penicillin G once a week for 3 weeks unless CSF examination indicates that neurosyphilis is present.

Patients with late latent syphilis should have nontreponemal serologic tests repeated 6, 12, and 24 months after treatment. Serologic response to therapy for late latent syphilis is difficult to judge because there are limited data. Titers should decrease fourfold (two dilutions) if pretreatment titers are high (1 : 32 or more). Patients with late syphilis frequently have low (1 : 8 or more) nontreponemal titers that do not decline appreciably after therapy. Such results are considered "serofast," and treatment has not necessarily failed. Patients who have a fourfold rise titer or whose titers do not decline fourfold within 12 to 24 months and those who have symptoms and signs of syphilis should undergo reevaluation for neurosyphilis and be treated accordingly.

Patients with neurosyphilis should undergo spinal fluid examinations at 6-month intervals for a minimum of 3 years or until the cell count is normal. Pleocytosis should improve considerably within 6 months of therapy. Failure to normalize within 2 years suggests a need for repetition of treatment. Protein and CSF-VDRL values decline slowly after therapy and may take years to normalize. A serofast CSF-VDRL result is common and is not by itself an indication for repetition of treatment. Meningeal and meningovascular forms of neurosyphilis usually show good clinical response to therapy. Improvement in the presence of a parenchymatous syndromes is highly variable; the conditions of some patients may continue to deteriorate even after appropriate therapy.

Several hours after receiving therapy some patients experience sudden onset of symptoms that include chills, fever, tachycardia, headache, flushing, and mild headache. Patients with neurosyphilis may have exacerbations of their neurologic symptoms, and further transient visual deterioration may occur among patients with ophthalmologic involvement. This response, called the Jarisch–Herxheimer reaction, is especially common among patients with secondary syphilis, although it has been described in all stages of syphilis and with therapies other than penicillin. Symptoms of the reaction usually abate within 24 hours and can be managed with aspirin. Severe localized forms of the reaction may necessitate short courses of glucocorticoids. The mechanism of this reaction has not been identified.

SYPHILIS AND HUMAN IMMUNODEFICIENCY VIRUS INFECTION

Epidemiologic data have suggested that genital ulcers, including those caused by syphilis, are cofactors for HIV infection. Syphilitic lesions disrupt the normal epithelial and mucosal barriers and provide portals of entry for HIV. Moreover, the bases of chancres also contain large numbers of activated HIV target cells (activated lymphocytes and macrophages).

Because the cellular arm of the immune system is thought to be important in the containment of syphilitic infection, there is widespread concern that current recommendations regarding the diagnosis and management of syphilis may be inadequate in the care of patients with immunosuppression due to HIV infection. Numerous case reports document unusual presentations of syphilis, treatment failures, and accelerated development of neurosyphilis among patients with HIV infection. There also is concern that serologic tests for syphilis may not be reliable among patients with HIV infection. There have been three case reports in which both treponemal and nontreponemal test results were negative in the presence of biopsy-proven secondary syphilis.

Results of four controlled studies examining whether syphilis infection behaves differently among patients with HIV infection have been published. In a prospective study, neither neurologic manifestations nor central nervous system invasion by *T. pallidum* (detected by means of intratesticular inoculation of rabbits with CSF) were more common among patients with HIV infection. Another study compared results among users of injected drugs, 31 of whom had HIV infection and 19 of whom did not. No differences in stage of disease, serologic manifestations, or response to treatment were found in a median follow-up period of 11 months.

A case-control study involved 309 patients with early syphilis, of whom 70 (23%) had HIV infection. The clinical signs and symptoms of syphilis were different among the group with HIV infection in that they were more likely to come to medical attention with secondary syphilis and to have coexistent chancres with the secondary syphilis. However, no unusual dermatologic manifestations, no increased incidence of neurologic complications, and no increased rate of treatment failure with conventional regimens were found among the patients with HIV infection.

A recent CDC-sponsored, multicenter study compared use of the standard benzathine penicillin G regimen with use of the same regimen plus 2 g amoxicillin and 500 mg probenecid (orally three times a day for 10 days) for 553 HIV-seropositive and HIV-seronegative patients with primary, secondary, or early latent syphilis. There was only one reported clinical failure, which involved an HIV-seropositive patient who received standard therapy. Approximately 15% of patients who received treatment with either regimen did not meet the standard criterion for serologic success (a two-dilution decrease in nontreponemal serological titer) as late as 12 months after treatment. This occurrence was statistically more likely among HIV-seropositive participants than among their HIV-seronegative counterparts, although the clinical importance for both patient groups was uncertain. In the relatively short follow-up period of that study, none of the HIV-seropositive patients experienced the type of dramatic treatment failure that has been reported anecdotally over the past 10 years.

Despite the reports of unusual serologic responses among patients with HIV infection, the 1998 recommendations of the CDC state that treponemal and nontreponemal tests for syphilis are accurate for most persons with HIV coinfection. If there is suspicion of syphilis in the face of negative serologic results, other tests, such as dark-field microscopic examination, biopsy, and direct fluorescent staining of lesion material, should be performed.

Expert opinion based on available data is that patients with HIV coinfection may be at increased risk of treatment failure and neurologic complications, but the amount of increased risk appears to be small. In its 1998 treatment guidelines, the CDC recommended that patients with HIV infection and early syphilis receive the same treatment as patients without HIV infection and that they undergo follow-up evaluation 3, 6, 9, and 12 months after therapy to establish the adequacy of treatment. Patients with HIV infection who have particularly florid second-

ary syphilis may benefit from large intravenous doses of penicillin. Although the practice is of unproven benefit, some experts advocate examining the CSF of all HIV-positive patients who have early syphilis. Routine lumbar puncture is not endorsed by the CDC.

PREVENTION AND CONTROL

Major strides in the prevention and control of syphilis were made with the institution of routine premarital and prenatal screening by means of nontreponemal tests. In view of the far lower incidence of syphilis in the postantibiotic era, it has been argued that routine screening is no longer cost-effective. However, increases in the incidence of syphilis among lower socioeconomic groups has demonstrated the importance of continued targeted surveillance. Aggressive epidemiologic tracing and treatment of contacts remains the most effective means available to public health workers for curtailment of syphilis transmission by patients with active infection.

The marked decline in the incidence of syphilis during the past several years has encouraged the CDC to make complete eradication of syphilis within the United States a public health objective. The emerging strategy to reach this lofty but potentially achievable objective involves a series of epidemiologic, public health, and behavioral initiatives. The development of a syphilis vaccine, a long-standing goal of researchers into treponemal disease, should be viewed as a complementary approach. Efforts at identifying specific treponemal molecules that might function as vaccinogens have been hampered by the inability to cultivate pathogenic treponemes in vitro and a poor understanding of *T. pallidum* proteins capable of inducing a protective immune response. Although prospects for a syphilis vaccine have improved with the advent of recombinant DNA methods and the availability of the *T. pallidum* genomic sequence, it is unclear whether a vaccine will be available in the near future.

BIBLIOGRAPHY

Centers for Disease Control and Prevention. Primary and secondary syphilis—United States, 1997. *JAMA* 1998;280:1218–1219.

Centers for Disease Control and Prevention. Primary and secondary syphilis—United States, 1997. *MMWR Morb Mortal Wkly Rep* 1998;47:493–497.

Glaser JH. Centers for Disease Control and Prevention guidelines for congenital syphilis [Editorial]. *J Pediatr* 1996;129:488–490.

Harris DE, Enterline DS, Tien RD. Neurosyphilis in patients with AIDS. *Neuroimaging Clin North Am* 1997;7:215–221.

Hook EW III. Is elimination of endemic syphilis transmission a realistic goal for the USA? *Lancet* 1998;351:19–21.

Mashkilleyson AL, Gomberg MA, Mashkilleyson N, et al. Treatment of syphilis with azithromycin. *Int J STD AIDS* 1996;7:13–15.

Meyer JC. Laboratory diagnosis of syphilis. *Curr Probl Dermatol* 1996;24:1–11.

Rolfs RT, Joesoef MR, Hendershot, et al. A randomized trial of enhanced therapy for early syphilis in patients with and without human immunodeficiency virus infection. The Syphilis and HIV Study Group. *N Engl J Med* 1997;337:307–314.

Sanchez PJ. Laboratory tests for congenital syphilis. *Pediatr Infect Dis J* 1998;17:70–71.

Sanchez PJ, Wendel GD. Syphilis in pregnancy. *Clin Perinatol* 1997;24:71–90.

Kelley's Textbook of Internal Medicine, fourth edition. Edited by H. David Humes. Lippincott Williams & Wilkins, Philadelphia © 2000.

C H A P T E R

298

NONVENEREAL TREPONEMATOSES: YAWS, PINTA, AND ENDEMIC SYPHILIS

NAIEL N. NASSAR
JUSTIN DAVID RADOLF

■ DEFINITION

The nonvenereal or endemic forms of treponematosis—yaws, pinta, and endemic syphilis—constitute a group of chronic, granulomatous diseases in tropical and subtropical countries. They are caused by treponemes morphologically and serologically indistinguishable from *Treponema pallidum* subspecies pallidum, the agent of venereal syphilis. These diseases are transmitted by means of nonvenereal inoculation of mucocutaneous surfaces. They progress, as does venereal syphilis, through more or less defined clinical stages.

■ INCIDENCE AND EPIDEMIOLOGY

At the beginning of the twentieth century endemic treponematosis was rampant in almost all areas of the tropical belt but also occurred in some communities in the temperate zones. Endemic treponematosis typically is confined to remote, rural areas with poor sanitation and overcrowding. Economically disadvantaged peoples with frequent skin trauma, scanty clothing, and little or no access to health care are particularly at risk. Infection with the organisms that cause yaws and endemic syphilis occurs primarily during childhood, whereas infection with the pinta organism occurs during late childhood or adolescence.

YAWS

Yaws is known by a number of other names, including *frambesia*, *pian* (French), *parangi* (Malay), *paru* (Malay), and *bubas*. It is prevalent in rural, warm, tropical regions and initially affects children and adolescents, with a peak incidence between 6 and 10 years of age. Almost all new cases are diagnosed among children younger than 15 years. It is estimated that in the preantibiotic era 50 to 100 million active cases of yaws affected the 400 million people living in Africa, Asia, Latin America, and the Caribbean region. Yaws eradication programs launched in endemic areas by the World Health Organization in the 1950s brought about dramatic decreases in the prevalence of yaws in endemic areas. Unfortunately, there has been a mild resurgence of yaws because of inadequate facilities for treatment and inadequate surveillance methods. The main reservoirs of yaws are West and Central Africa, Southeast Asia, the Pacific islands, and Central and South America.

PINTA

Pinta is also known as *mal de pinto* (Mexico), *carate* (Colombia and Venezuela, and *azul* (Chile and Peru). Countries with high prevalence are Brazil, Venezuela, Colombia, Peru, Ecuador, Central America, and Mexico. In Brazil, some parts of the Amazonas state are an endemic focus of pinta. A few cases also have been reported from Southeast Asia, Central Africa, and the Pacific regions. However, the presence of pinta outside the Americas is the subject of controversy. Most patients acquire the disease in childhood or young adulthood. Like yaws and endemic syphilis, the primary foci of pinta are in remote rural regions. Precise data about the prevalence of pinta are scanty. A serosurvey taken in 1982 and 1983 in Panama revealed a 20% seropositivity rate. In this same survey, 2% to 3% of the population, primarily children younger than 5 years, were found to have active pinta.

ENDEMIC SYPHILIS

Also known as *bejel* (Bedouin Arabs in Syria and Iraq), *firjal* or *loath* (elsewhere in the Middle East), and *njovera* or *dichuchwa* (Zimbabwe), endemic syphilis continues to be a serious problem, particularly in dry, hot climates. Disease transmission occurs by means of direct contact with infectious lesions and by sharing drinking and eating utensils. Children between the ages of 2 and 15 years who live in isolated, closed communities with unhygienic and crowded conditions are the primary reservoir. Once highly prevalent among the nomadic and seminomadic rural populations of North Africa and the Middle East, endemic syphilis today is confined primarily to the Arabian peninsula and the Sahel, the southern border of the Sahara. The most recent data reveal that 15% to 40% of children in the Sahel have serologic evidence of treponemal infection and 2% to 20% have evidence of active infection. A prevalence of 27% has been documented among the Bedouin tribes of the Middle East.

■ ETIOLOGY

The agents of venereal syphilis, yaws, and endemic syphilis are *T. pallidum* subspecies *pallidum*, *pertenue*, and *endemicum*, respectively. *T. carateum* is the agent of pinta. The pathogenic treponemes are delicate, actively motile, helical bacteria 5 to 20 μm long and 0.1 to 0.2 μm wide. They stain poorly with aniline dyes, cannot be cultivated on artificial media, and can be seen only with a dark-field microscope or by means of histopathologic study. Differentiating these four treponemes is difficult. Speciation depends primarily on differences in host range in experimental animals, modes of transmission, geographic distribution, and clinical features of the respective diseases (Table 298.1). Differences identified at the genetic level may help in this regard. All four pathogenic treponemes stimulate the production of antibodies that are reactive in both nontreponemal and treponemal serodiagnostic tests.

■ PATHOGENESIS

All three nonvenereal forms of treponematosis are transmitted by close, person-to-person, nonsexual contact that allows inocu-

TABLE 298.1.	NONVENEREAL TREPONEMAL INFECTIONS				
Disease	Organism	Endemic Area	Primary Lesion	Secondary Lesion	Tertiary Lesion
Yaws	*T. pallidum* subspecies *pertenue*	Rural areas of Africa, Central and South America, the Caribbean, equatorial islands of Southeast Asia, and remote parts of India and Thailand	Papule Papilloma Ulcer	Diffuse papules, papillomas, or ulcers Osteitis Dactylitis	Destructive gummas of skin and bone
Pinta	*T. carateum*	Underdeveloped rural areas of Mexico and northern South America	Erythematous papule	Scaly papules Areas of altered skin pigmentation	Areas of altered skin pigmentation, hyperkeratosis
Bejel	*T. pallidum* subspecies *endemicum*	West Africa, small foci in Zimbabwe, Botswana, Arabian peninsula, and central Australia	Oral mucosal ulcer	Oral and pharyngeal ulcers Mucous patches Condyloma lata Perisostitis	Gummas of skin, bone, and joints

lation of skin and mucosal surfaces with virulent organisms from infectious lesions. Pinta is the least contagious of the three diseases and *T. carateum* the least virulent of the pathogenic treponemes. Soon after inoculation, treponemes invade local lymphatic vessels and the bloodstream to disseminate systemically. With the exception of endemic syphilis, in which primary lesions rarely are seen, a primary lesion develops at the site of inoculation after an incubation period of 3 to 4 weeks. Weeks to months later, highly infectious secondary lesions appear on skin or mucosal surfaces. In both untreated yaws and pinta, recurrences of secondary lesions may occur for months to years. With all three infections, after the secondary manifestations fade, the infection enters a highly variable latency period that is followed by late or tertiary disease. Patients with tertiary yaws and endemic syphilis have highly destructive, necrotizing granulomas of skin, mucous membranes, cartilage, and bone that histologically and clinically resemble the gummas of tertiary venereal syphilis. Lesions of late pinta, however, are nonnecrotizing cutaneous granulomas characterized by hyperkeratosis and depigmentation. Unlike venereal syphilis, endemic syphilis rarely involves the cardiovascular or central nervous system.

CLINICAL FINDINGS

YAWS

Primary yaws (frambesia) is characterized by a raised papule at the site of inoculation that enlarges to form a hyperkeratotic papilloma (mother yaw) before eventually forming a shallow ulcer that can persist for a few months to several years (Fig. 298.1). It often is accompanied by regional lymphadenopathy. The lesions of yaws tend not to be painful, except in cases of secondary bacterial infection. Yellow crust on the surface of a papilloma and a raised lesion are the best clues that a lesion is that of yaws. Crops of highly infectious, papular, lobulated, and

verrucous secondary lesions appear weeks to months after infection and frequently are accompanied by painful periostitis. Goundou is a rare form of hypertrophic osteitis of the nasal process of the maxilla that may occur in early yaws and produces a characteristic facies. After multiple infectious relapses, the disease enters an asymptomatic latent period.

Approximately 10% of untreated patients eventually have tertiary disease, which generally consists of solitary destructive

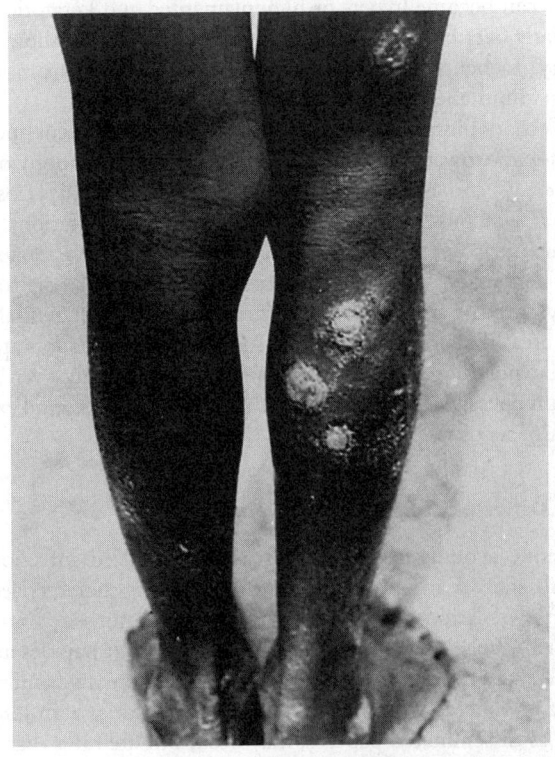

FIGURE 298.1. Shallow ulcers of yaws.

lesions of bone or mucocutaneous surfaces. Chronic osteitis of the tibia may lead to curvature, producing saber shins. Rhinopharyngitis mutilans (gangosa), highly destructive ulceration of facial structures, is a particularly severe form of tertiary yaws. Although yaws was classically described as sparing the nervous and cardiovascular systems (unlike venereal syphilis), some reports suggest the possibility of late ophthalmologic and neurologic involvement in yaws. The difficulty in definitively differentiating previous yaws infections from venereal syphilis makes conclusions in this regard difficult.

It is rare to see lesions of late yaws now. Patients usually have papilloma, lesions of early yaws. The classic yaws appearance of a person covered in papillomas is rare. There is a some consensus that an attenuated form of yaws with less florid skin manifestations may have developed as a result of mass treatment campaigns in the 1950s.

PINTA

Pinta is unique among the spirochetal diseases in having only skin manifestations. The initial lesion of primary pinta appears after an incubation period of 1 week to 4 months. The initial lesions are small squamous papules, which may be single or multiple, never ulcerate, and cause no lymphadenopathy. The papular lesion frequently is localized on exposed areas of the lower limbs, face, arms, and torso. The primary papule can resemble a lichenoid, eczematoid, or psoriasiform lesion. It may resolve spontaneously or continue its evolution, becoming indistinguishable from a secondary lesion. Secondary lesions (pintids) usually appear 2 to 6 months after the initial lesion. They are usually few. Pintids are usually smaller, nonpruritic, dyschromic, and more morphologically consistent than the primary lesions. They can become hyper- or hypopigmented and keratotic, particularly over bony prominences. The pintids do not show symmetry. Lichenoid, eczematoid, or psoriasiform lesions may develop simultaneously in the same patient.

Tertiary pinta (late pinta) takes 2 to 5 years to occur and has a tendency toward generalization and symmetry. Atrophy of the epidermis and epidermal appendages occurs mainly close to joints. Mucous membrane involvement (pigmentation) may occur but is not frequent. Tertiary lesions are characterized by well-defined patches of hyperchromic, hypochromic, achromic, or dyschromic areas. Hyperchromic spots occur preferentially in skin areas that are exposed to the sun; hypochromic spots appear in unexposed areas. Achromic lesions appear mainly over bony prominences; preferred areas are the hands, feet, face, and extensor aspects of the extremities.

ENDEMIC SYPHILIS

Endemic syphilis usually begins as a generalized infection in the absence of an obvious primary lesion. It is characterized by ulcerative lesions of the oropharyngeal mucosa (mucous patches), hoarseness, angular stomatitis and split papules at the corners of the mouth, intertriginous condylomata (similar to those of venereal syphilis), and painful periostitis. Skin lesions, such as disseminated papules, may occur but are rarer than secondary venereal syphilis. Tertiary gummas develop among most

untreated patients after a latency period of several years. These occur most commonly on the skin, in the nasopharynx, and in bone and may cause severe destruction and disfigurement.

DIAGNOSIS AND LABORATORY FINDINGS

Presumptive diagnosis of all three types of nonvenereal treponematosis can be based largely on the clinical presentation of the disease and its occurrence in an endemic area. Both the ulcerated primary lesion and the tertiary gummas of yaws have to be differentiated from other causes of skin ulceration common in tropical countries, including Buruli ulcer, sporotrichosis, pyoderma, leishmaniasis, and mycetoma. The skin lesions in all three stages of pinta may resemble conditions such as leprosy, psoriasis, and lichen planus.

Early lesions of all three infections contain large numbers of treponemes. A definitive diagnosis can be reached with darkfield microscopic or histopathologic analysis. As with venereal syphilis, treponemes usually are difficult to find in tertiary lesions. Reactivity in both nontreponemal (Venereal Disease Research Laboratory and rapid plasma reagin) and treponemal (fluorescent treponemal antibody absorption and microhemagglutination assay—*T. pallidum*) tests occurs with both nonvenereal treponematosis and syphilis and cannot, by itself, be used to differentiate these infections. In pinta, serologic tests may not become reactive until several months after infection, whereas nearly all patients with endemic syphilis have reactive serologic results when they come to medical attention.

STRATEGIES FOR OPTIMAL CARE

Intramuscular benzathine penicillin G is the therapy of choice for all three types of nonvenereal treponematosis. Adults and children older than 10 years with disease in the incubatory stage, with symptomatic disease, or with latent disease or those who are close contacts of infectious patients should receive 1.2 million units. Younger children should be given 600,000 units. Patients allergic to penicillin may be given 500 mg tetracycline by mouth four times a day for 15 days (total of 30 g). Children between 8 and 15 years of age should be given one-half the adult dose. Although erythromycin frequently is used as an alternative drug to treat young children, results of studies to determine its effectiveness have not been reported for any of the forms of nonvenereal treponematosis.

The lesions of patients with yaws become noninfectious within several days of therapy. The rate of decline of antibody titers is inversely proportional to the length of time the patient had been infected. Patients with endemic syphilis also become noninfectious within several days of therapy. If these patients are treated early, nontreponemal test results revert to nonreactivity. Pinta responds slowly to therapy. Early lesions take months to heal and frequently leave discolored residua. The serologic response to therapy for pinta likewise is absent or slow.

Therapy for all three diseases in the tertiary stages may arrest disease progression but does not always bring about healing of the destroyed tissues. As is true of venereal syphilis, serologic reactivity of treponemal tests usually lasts for life, regardless of therapy. Failure of penicillin therapy for yaws has been reported in Papua, New Guinea. The implications of this observation, if confirmed, for mass treatment programs in remaining yaws-endemic areas are very serious.

CONTROL AND PREVENTION

Earlier global eradication programs have demonstrated that mass treatment in conjunction with improved living standards can dramatically reduce the prevalence of nonvenereal treponematosis in endemic areas. Failure to continue surveillance and treatment programs in many endemic areas has led to resurgence of these diseases, particularly yaws. Improving overall health care access and integrating surveillance and treatment into the existing health care system in endemic areas may be the best method to control and eradicate nonvenereal treponematosis.

BIBLIOGRAPHY

Antal GM, Causse G. The control of endemic treponematoses. *Rev Infect Dis* 1985;7[Suppl 2]:S220–226.

Backhouse JL, Hudson BJ, Hamilton PA, et al. Failure of penicillin treatment of yaws on Karkar Island, New Guinea. *Am J Trop Med Hyg* 1998;59:388–392.

Engelkens HJ, Judanarso J, Oranje AP, et al. Endemic treponematoses, part 1: yaws. *Int J Dermatol* 1991;30:77–83.

Engelkens HJ, Niemel PL, ven der Sluis, et al. Endemic treponematoses, part 2: pinta and endemic syphilis. *Int J Dermatol* 1991;30:231–238.

Fuchs J, Milbradt R, Pecher SA. Tertiary pinta: case reports and overview. *Cutis* 1993;51:425–430.

Koff AB, Rosen T. forms of nonvenereal treponematosis: yaws, endemic syphilis, and pinta. *J Am Acad Dermatol* 1993;29:519–535.

Mecheus A, Antal GM. The endemic treponematoses: not yet eradicated. *World Health Stat Q* 1992;45:228–237.

Vorst FA. Clinical diagnosis and changing manifestation of treponemal infection. *Rev Infect Dis* 1985;7[Suppl 2]:S327–S331.

Kelley's Textbook of Internal Medicine, fourth edition. Edited by H. David Humes. Lippincott Williams & Wilkins, Philadelphia © 2000.

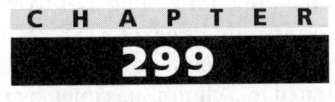

CHAPTER 299

LEPTOSPIROSIS

GEORGE J. ALANGADEN

DEFINITION

Leptospirosis is zoonosis of worldwide distribution caused by the pathogenic spirochetal species *Leptospira interrogans*. Human infection occurs through exposure to water or soil contaminated with infected animal urine. The clinical spectrum of illness can range from subclinical infection to life-threatening multisystem illness.

INCIDENCE AND EPIDEMIOLOGY

Leptospirosis affects most species of wild and domestic mammals. Humans are affected through exposure to infected animal urine. In the United States leptospirosis is currently not a reportable disease except in a few states. Thus the exact incidence and prevalence are not known. Until 1993 about 40 to 100 cases were identified each year, about one-half being reported from Hawaii. In the United States leptospirosis generally occurs sporadically; however, outbreaks have been reported in occupational or recreational settings. Persons at risk of leptospirosis are those likely to have contact with infected animals or contaminated water, such as farmers, veterinarians, abattoir workers, sewer workers, and military personnel. Sporadic cases of leptospirosis in urban settings have been reported.

The incidence of leptospirosis due to exposure during recreational activities such as swimming, canoeing, and hunting has been increasing. In 1996 an outbreak was identified among five persons who had returned from a whitewater rafting expedition on flooded rivers in Costa Rica. River water contaminated with leptospires was implicated as the probable cause of the disease. Leptospirosis also was the likely cause of an acute febrile illness among about 24 athletes who participated in a triathlon in Illinois and Wisconsin in 1998. The participants probably were exposed to the organism while swimming in a contaminated lake.

Although leptospirosis is uncommon in the United States, it is one of the most widespread zoonotic diseases in the world, especially in temperate or tropical climates. It is being increasingly recognized in some Latin American, Caribbean, and Asian countries, and temporal associations between heavy rainfall and flooding and leptospirosis among humans have been observed.

The pathogenic species is *L. interrogans*. Specific serotypes have been associated with infection among at least 160 different mammalian species. Human disease can be caused by different serovars (serologic variants) the prevalence of which varies worldwide. Human disease is generally caused by serotypes Canicola (found in dogs), Pomona, Hardjo and Hebdomidis (all found in livestock), Icterohaemorrhagiae (rodents), and Autumnalis and Grippotyphosa (found in wildlife).

ETIOLOGY

Leptospires are aerobic, mobile, thin (0.1 mm in diameter), helicoid, bacteria about 6 to 20 mm long with semicircular hooked ends. The genus *Leptospira* consists of two species *L. interrogans* (pathogenic) and *L. biflexa* (saprophytic). On the basis of agglutinogenic characteristics these species have been classified into 300 serovars, which have been grouped into about 23 serogroups. Seven species of pathogenic leptospires have been identified on the basis of DNA homology. They can be grown on artificial media (10% rabbit serum or 1% bovine broth and long-chain fatty acids) at pH of 6.8 to 7.4 and incubation at 30°C for 1 to 4 weeks. They can be seen with a dark-field or phase-contrast microscope.

PATHOGENESIS

Infection of humans occurs when the leptospires gain access to the bloodstream through abraded skin, mucosa, or conjunctiva. They then rapidly disseminate throughout the body including the central nervous system. The clinical manifestations are thought to result from generalized vasculitis. Leptospiral products such as sphingomyelinase C and possibly other leptospiral cytotoxins may be responsible for the vasculitis. In severe cases of leptospirosis hemorrhagic diathesis and hepatic and renal dysfunction can be caused by endothelial damage from the vasculitis. Hepatic dysfunction is associated with minimal hepatocellular necrosis. Renal ischemia and hypoxia causing tubular damage without appreciable interstitial inflammation is thought to be the primary cause of renal insufficiency. Complete resolution of the hepatic and renal dysfunction occurs with clinical recovery. Myalgia is common and is associated with transient nonspecific inflammatory changes within the myofibrils. Central nervous system involvement occurs during the leptospiremic phase, but signs of meningeal inflammation occur during the second week of illness. The vasculitis can lead to hemorrhagic pneumonitis or myocarditis. In severe cases multisystem involvement can cause shock. Recovery occurs when an immune response develops in the production of specific antibodies and elimination of leptospiremia although leptospiruria can persist for weeks.

CLINICAL FINDINGS

The incubation period of leptospirosis is about 5 to 14 days. Leptospirosis is typically a biphasic illness. The first phase is a septicemic phase characterized by leptospires in the blood and cerebrospinal fluid (CSF). The second phase is an immune period in which IgM antibodies develop and leptospires are present in the urine. The clinical manifestations are highly variable. This is an acute, systemic febrile illness without any specific features. In general two clinical syndromes have been described—anicteric leptospirosis, which accounts for as many as 90% of cases, and icteric leptospirosis (Weil's syndrome). Subclinical infections are rare.

Anicteric leptospirosis is a generally an acute, self-limited illness with abrupt onset of fever, chills, headache, myalgia (calf and back), anorexia, nausea, vomiting, and an occasional rash. Fevers (38°C to 39°C), conjunctival suffusion (without discharge), and muscle tenderness often are found at examination. Transient rashes, lymphadenopathy, and hepatosplenomegaly are found less commonly. The acute symptoms subside after a week when the leptospires clear from the blood and CSF and specific IgM antibodies develop. Aseptic meningitis with mild pleocytosis or low-grade fever can occur during the second week

(immune phase). Leptospiruria develops and can persist for as long as 3 weeks. Anicteric leptospirosis can become manifest with pulmonary hemorrhage, respiratory failure, and death, as occurred in Nicaragua.

Icteric disease is more severe than anicteric disease. The patient has varying degrees of hepatic, renal, hematologic, and other systemic dysfunction. The mortality is 5% to 10%. Jaundice and azotemia occur during the first week. Hyperbilirubinemia occurs but without appreciable hepatocellular dysfunction, as evidenced by relatively mild elevations in liver transaminase levels. Acute tubular necrosis manifested by oliguria, anuria, proteinuria, and hematuria can occur during the second week of the disease. Hemorrhagic manifestations such as epistaxis, gastrointestinal bleeding, hemorrhagic pneumonitis, hypotension, and myocarditis occur less commonly. It can take several weeks for patients with severe disease to recover completely.

LABORATORY FINDINGS

Mild leukocytosis with neutrophilia generally is present. Fivefold elevations in creatine kinase level occur in about one-half of cases. In the icteric form of leptospirosis bilirubin levels (predominantly conjugated) are generally less than 20 mg per deciliter and are associated with only mild elevations in liver transaminase levels (100 to 200 U per liter). Elevation in blood urea nitrogen level seldom exceeds 100 mg per deciliter and in creatinine level seldom exceeds 8 mg per deciliter. For an acutely ill and jaundiced patient the combination of marked increases in creatine kinase level with modest elevation in liver transaminase levels differentiates leptospirosis from viral hepatitis.

Most patients have CSF pleocytosis with cell counts generally less than 500 per cubic millimeter, normal glucose level, and mild elevations in protein level. About half of these patients may have meningeal signs. Nonspecific infiltrates from small nodular densities, or a diffuse ground-glass pattern, to areas of consolidation may be found on a chest radiograph. An electrocardiogram may show nonspecific transient changes.

The definitive diagnosis of leptospirosis requires demonstration or isolation of leptospires in clinical specimens, seroconversion, or a fourfold or greater rise in antibody titer. Leptospires can be isolated from blood and CSF during the first 10 days of illness and from the urine for as long as 4 weeks. Direct examination for leptospires in urine or CSF by means of dark-field microscopy often shows no abnormalities. Leptospires may be demonstrated in a clinical specimen by means of immunofluorescence. Isolation of the organisms requires inoculation of clinical specimens onto semisolid media, such as Fletcher medium or Ellinghausen–McCullough–Johnson–Harris and incubation at 28°C to 30°C for up to 6 weeks. Selective agent 5-fluorouracil may be added to the medium when it is believed the specimen might have been contaminated. A dark-field microscope is used to examine the cultures periodically for leptospires.

The microscopic agglutination test with live or formalin-fixed antigens is the standard confirmatory serologic procedure. Antigens representing the serovars in a geographic area must be used because of the serovar specificity of this test. A fourfold or greater increase in *Leptospira* agglutination between acute- and convalescent-phase serum obtained at least 2 weeks apart is needed. This test is labor intensive and usually is performed at leptospirosis reference centers. Thus a variety of easier screening tests to detect leptospiral IgM antibodies with enzyme-linked immunosorbent assay (ELISA) or dot-ELISA have been developed. Polymerase chain reaction (PCR) assays have been used to detect leptospiral DNA in blood, serum, CSF, urine, and aqueous humor. Rapid DNA-based typing of serovars using PCR assays, DNA probes, and pulse–field–gel electrophoresis techniques have been reported.

STRATEGIES FOR OPTIMAL CARE

Patients with severe disease are given supportive therapy to correct dehydration, hypotension, hemorrhagic diathesis, and hepatic and renal dysfunction. Although antimicrobial therapy is efficacious when initiated during the first 4 days, it can still be effective later in the course of the illness. Antimicrobial therapy can shorten the duration of the fevers, ameliorate the disease, prevent leptospiruria, and decrease hospital stay. Patients with moderate to severe disease need high doses of intravenously administered penicillin G (80,000 to 100,000 U per kilogram) or intravenous ampicillin (0.5 to 1.0 g every 6 hours). Patients with milder disease can be treated with oral amoxicillin or ampicillin (500 mg every 6 hours) or doxycycline (100 mg twice a day). A Jarisch–Herxheimer reaction may occur after treatment with penicillin. Most cases of leptospirosis are anicteric and self-limited with an uneventful recovery. The prognosis generally correlates with severity of the illness and the condition of the patient. Death is caused by hemorrhagic complications or renal failure.

Effective control and prevention are difficult because of the ubiquitous nature of the organism and the persistence of infection among animals. Control measures for leptospirosis include vaccination of domestic animals, rodent control, use of protective clothing, and avoidance of swimming in contaminated water. Doxycycline (200 mg a week) has been used as effective short-term chemoprophylaxis among military personnel. Vaccination of humans has been used in Europe and Asia.

BIBLIOGRAPHY

Centers for Disease Control and Prevention. Outbreak of leptospirosis among white-water rafters—Costa Rica, 1996. *MMWR Morb Mortal Wkly Rept* 1997;46:577–579.
Centers for Disease Control and Prevention. Update: leptospirosis and unexplained acute febrile illness among athletes participating in triathlons—Illinois and Wisconsin, 1998. *MMWR Morb Mortal Wkly Report* 1998;47:673–676.
Faine S. *Guidelines for the control of leptospirosis.* WHO offset publication no. 67. Geneva, Switzerland: World Health Organization, 1982.
Faine S. Leptospirosis. In: Collier L, Balows A, Sussman M, eds. *Topley and Wilson's microbiology and microbial infections,* 9th ed. Vol. 3, Hausler WJ Jr, Sussman M, eds. *Bacterial infections.* London, England: 1998: 849–869.
Farr RW. Leptospirosis. *Clin Infect Dis* 1995;21:1–8.
Friedland JS, Warrell DA. The Jarisch-Herxheimer reaction in leptospirosis: possible pathogenesis and review. *Rev Infect Dis* 1991;13:207–210.

Kaufmann AF, Weyant RS. Leptospiraceae. In: Murray PR, Baron EJ, Pfaller MA, et al., eds. *Manual of clinical microbiology,* 6th ed. Washington, DC: American Society for Microbiology, 1995:621–625.
Takafuji ET, Kirkpatrick JW, Miller RN, et al. An efficacy trial of doxycycline chemoprophylaxis against leptospirosis. *N Engl J Med* 1984;310: 497–500.
Trevejo RT, Rigau–Pérez JG, Ashford DA, et al. Epidemic leptospirosis associated with pulmonary hemorrhage—Nicaragua, 1995. *J Infect Dis* 1998;178:1457–1463.
Watt G, Padre MA, Tuazon L, et al. Placebo-controlled trial of intravenous penicillin for severe and late leptospirosis. *Lancet* 1988;1:433–435.

Kelley's Textbook of Internal Medicine, fourth edition. Edited by H. David Humes. Lippincott Williams & Wilkins, Philadelphia © 2000.

CHAPTER 300

RELAPSING FEVER

THOMAS BUTLER

DEFINITION

Relapsing fever is an acute febrile illness caused by blood spirochetes belonging to the *Borrelia* species. The two kinds are tick-borne relapsing fever, for which rodents are the reservoirs and ticks are the vectors, and louse-borne relapsing fever, for which humans are the reservoir and body lice are the vectors. The natural course consists of one or more phases of fever and spirochetemia, which last several days and are separated by afebrile intervals of several days without spirochetemia.

INCIDENCE AND EPIDEMIOLOGY

Tick-borne relapsing fever occurs in endemic foci in the western United States, southern British Columbia, Mexico, Central and South America, Africa, and the Middle East. Louse-borne relapsing fever occurs in parts of South America, Europe, Africa, and Asia. The disease often goes unrecognized because patients with febrile illnesses do not routinely have blood smears examined for spirochetes. Ethiopia appears to be the country with the highest incidence, estimated to be 10,000 or more cases per year.

The major reservoirs of the tick-borne relapsing fevers are wild rodents, including squirrels, deer mice, rats, and chipmunks. The vectors of these organisms are soft-bodied argasid ticks of the genus *Ornithodoros*. The infection is passed between the reservoir animals through tick bites. Humans become accidental hosts when they are bitten by infected ticks. Tick bites are painless and usually occur at night. Ticks are able to survive as long as 15 years between blood meals and to harbor viable spirochetes for years. Female ticks can pass *Borrelia* spirochetes through the ovaries to their offspring, allowing ticks to be infective without having bitten an infected host. Persons at greatest risk of infection are campers who sleep in log cabins. In tropical countries, people who live in dwellings that are not rodent proof are prone to infection.

For louse-borne relapsing fever, the human body louse *Pediculus humanus* is the vector, and the only known reservoir is humans. Lice acquire the infection by feeding on a person who has spirochetemia, and they remain infected for their entire life span, which is 10 to 61 days under laboratory conditions. Persons at risk are those living in crowded, unhygienic conditions that favor infestation with lice. Migrant workers and soldiers at war are particularly prone to this infection. Men are at much greater risk than women. In endemic areas of Ethiopia, the incidence increases during the cool winter season, when people wear heavier clothing that becomes infested with lice.

ETIOLOGY

The species of *Borrelia* that cause tick-borne relapsing fever are numerous and include *B. duttonii* in East Africa, *B. hispanica* in Spain, *B. persica* in Asia, and *B. hermsii* and *B. turicatae* in North America. *B. recurrentis* is the only species that causes louse-borne relapsing fever. *Borrelia* spirochetes are spiral organisms that measure 5 to 20 μm in length and about 0.5 μm in diameter. They are too thin to be seen in wet preparations with a light microscope, but they can be seen with a dark-field or phase-contrast microscope. The spirochetes have corkscrew-like motility. They can be stained with aniline dyes, such as Wright's and Giemsa stains, and can be seen well in tissue with application of silver stains, such as Dieterle's or Warthin–Starry stain.

Borrelia bacteria are microaerophilic and fermentative in their growth characteristics. They can be cultivated in a complex broth, Barbour–Stoenner–Kelly medium. The relapsing feature of *Borrelia* infection has been attributed to antigenic variation in the infecting population of spirochetes. In experimental infection of rats with *B. hermsii*, separate serotypes emerged sequentially during relapses, and specific antibody appeared in response to each of the antigenic variants. Each of 25 serotypes of *B. hermsii* expresses different variable major proteins that are encoded by genes located on linear plasmids of the spirochete. A specific antigen G1pQ is not present in the Lyme disease spirochete *B. burgdorferi* and promises improved serologic testing of patients.

PATHOGENESIS

After a person is exposed to an infected tick or louse, spirochetes enter the body through the skin and divide in the blood plasma during an incubation period, estimated to last from 4 to 18 days. When the spirochetes have built up to a concentration of 10^4 to 10^8 per milliliter of blood, symptoms begin suddenly. A small proportion of the spirochetes are within circulating polymorphonuclear phagocytes, and some spirochetes have been phagocytosed by fixed macrophages of the reticuloendothelial system of the spleen, liver, and bone marrow. Although occasionally pres-

ent in other tissues, such as brain, hepatic cells, kidneys, and subcutaneous tissues, spirochetes do not proliferate or elicit inflammatory reactions in these extravascular sites.

Borrelia spirochetes possess a heat-stable, nonendotoxic pyrogen that stimulates mononuclear phagocytic cells to elaborate the inflammatory cytokines tumor necrosis factor and interleukins 1, 6, and 8. Thrombocytopenia is caused by sequestration of platelets and disseminated intravascular coagulation and causes petechiae and sometimes other hemorrhagic phenomena. Levels of serum complement, Hageman factor, and prekallikrein are decreased, suggesting that activation of certain plasma proteins contributes to the pathogenesis. Before and during the Jarisch–Herxheimer reaction (a rigor elicited by antibiotic treatment), blood levels of the inflammatory cytokines rise. The reaction has been prevented in experiments by means of administration of antibodies against tumor necrosis factor. Patients develop antiborrelial antibodies. The antibodies kill and opsonize spirochetes and render patients immune to future infection with the same serotype of *Borrelia*. Patients who die of the disease have enlarged spleens with microabscesses, enlarged livers with necrosis and hemorrhage, hearts with myocarditis, and cerebral edema sometimes with cerebral hemorrhage.

CLINICAL FINDINGS

Relapsing fever begins abruptly with shaking chills, fever, headache, and fatigue. Most patients have these symptoms almost continuously throughout the day, whereas some patients report the intermittent appearance of symptoms several times a day. Patients frequently report myalgia, arthralgia, anorexia, dry coughing, and abdominal pain. Epistaxis occurs occasionally, and children may have seizures. These symptoms usually are mild on the first day of illness and increase in intensity over a few days, leading to prostration and a visit to a physician. The nonspecific nature of these symptoms leads patients or their physicians to believe they have a flulike illness. Patients may have seen ticks on their bodies, but the bites rarely leave a mark.

For pregnant women, severe disease is common and can induce labor, leading to abortion or preterm delivery with and high infant mortality. Neonates may acquire congenital infection from maternal blood, the illness being detected 4 to 12 days after delivery.

Temperature rises to 38.5°C to 40°C, and heart rate increases to about 115 beats per minute. Blood pressure decreases to about 105/70 mm Hg. Patients appear lethargic. Physical signs that are common but not regularly present are conjunctival injection, petechial skin rash that is more apparent on the torso than on the extremities, and palpable liver and spleen. Jaundice sometimes is present. Generalized muscle weakness is common. Some patients display mental confusion, delirium, or coma, and some have nuchal rigidity.

LABORATORY FINDINGS

Relapsing fever is readily diagnosed through microscopic examination of a thin film of peripheral blood obtained by means of

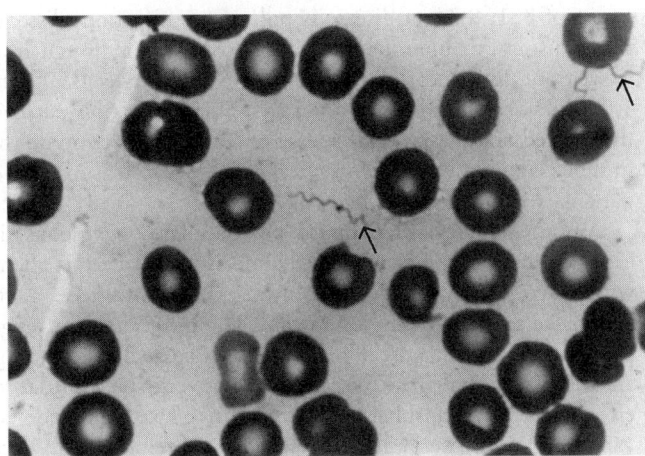 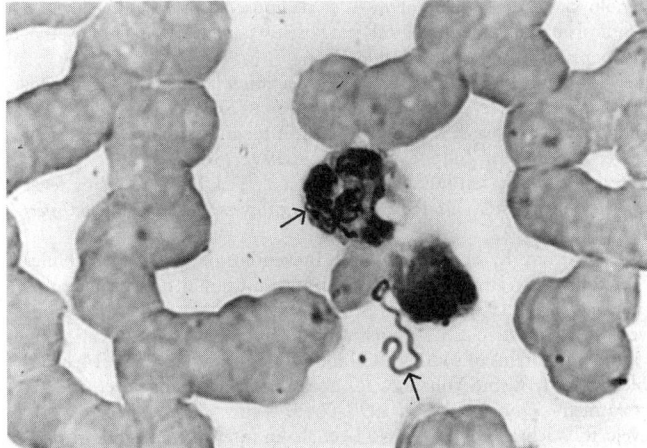

FIGURE 300.1. Blood smears of patients with relapsing fever show spirochetes (*arrows*) in plasma (*left,* Wright's stain) and within a polymorphonuclear leukocyte and in plasma (*right,* Warthin–Starry stain).

fingerstick or venipuncture. *Borrelia* spirochetes are stained blue in a routine blood smear treated with Wright's or Giemsa stain. The spirochetes are 5 to 20 μm long and lie in the plasma spaces between blood cells or overlie the blood cells (Fig. 300.1). Patients with relapsing fever who have an active fever typically have several spirochetes per high-power field. Patients who are in an afebrile interval between relapses have normal smear findings and undergo reexamination when the fever reoccurs. Serologic tests for relapsing fever are not generally available, and serologic tests for Lyme disease show false positive results caused by the presence of cross-reactive antigens.

The white blood cell count of patients with relapsing fever usually is normal, or there are with increased band forms and decreased eosinophils. Platelet counts often are less than 50,000 per cubic millimeter, and there may be prolongations of prothrombin time and partial thromboplastin time and increased titers of fibrinogen-fibrin degradation products. Results of liver function tests frequently are abnormal, and there are elevations in serum levels of alanine aminotransferase and bilirubin. Renal function tests often show mild abnormalities in the serum urea nitrogen and creatinine values, and patients may have proteinuria and microscopic hematuria.

■ STRATEGIES FOR OPTIMAL CARE

The relapsing fevers are effectively managed with tetracycline, erythromycin, or penicillin. Tetracycline is the treatment of choice except among children younger than 7 years and among pregnant women. A single 500-mg oral dose of tetracycline is as effective in clearing spirochetemia and preventing relapse as a longer course of treatment. Erythromycin, 500 mg by mouth in a single dose, is equally effective and is a satisfactory alternative to tetracycline. For patients unable to take oral medication, intravenous injection of 250 mg tetracycline or erythromycin is curative. Penicillin G has been used as therapy for relapsing fever, but it has been associated with slow clearance of spirochetes and relapses after treatment. Good results have been reported from

Africa with 400,000 or 600,000 units of procaine penicillin G given intramuscularly once or with the same dose repeated 12 hours later.

For most patients, antibiotic treatment provokes a distressing Jarisch–Herxheimer reaction. About 2 to 3 hours after antibiotic treatment is started, patients notice a chill that progresses to rigor. Temperature subsequently rises sharply, and blood pressure declines while spirochetes are cleared from the blood. Patients are extremely uncomfortable for several hours with shivering, intense body aches, and sometimes expressing a fear of impending death. Patients may need intravenous infusion of 0.9% saline solution to maintain adequate blood pressure on the day of treatment. Attempts to ameliorate the reaction by giving antipyretic or anti-inflammatory drugs have not been useful.

Complete recovery is expected among 95% or more of treated patients. Unfavorable prognostic signs are jaundice, coma, high spirochete counts in the blood, and hypotension. Death is caused by shock, liver failure, hemorrhage, or arrhythmia. Most neonates with relapsing fever die. During epidemics of louse-borne relapsing fever, untreated patients have mortality rates as high as 40%. Untreated patients also have relapses. In tick-borne relapsing fever, the first attack lasts about 3 days and is followed by an interval of about 7 days, after which an average of three relapses occur, each lasting about 2 days. In louse-borne relapsing fever, the first attack lasts about 6 days and is followed by an afebrile period of about 9 days. There usually is one relapse, which lasts only about 2 days.

Approaches to the control of relapsing fever include detection of disease among humans and treatment of the patients, vector control, rodent control, and public health education. Campers and hikers going into endemic areas should be advised to avoid staying in cabins that are inhabited by rodents and their ticks and to apply topical tick repellent (35% diethyltoluamide [DEET]) to their skin.

BIBLIOGRAPHY

Anda P, Sanchez-Yebra W, Vitutia MDM, et al. A new *Borrelia* species isolated from patients with relapsing fever in Spain. *Lancet* 1996;348: 162.

Borgnolo G, Hailu B, Ciancarelli A, et al. Louse-borne relapsing fever: a clinical and an epidemiological study of 389 patients in Asella Hospital, Ethiopia. *Trop Geogr Med* 1993;45:66.

Butler T, Hazen P, Wallace CK, et al. Infection with *Borrelia recurrentis*: pathogenesis of fever and petechiae. *J Infect Dis* 1979;140:665.

DuPont HT, La Scola B, Williams R, et al. A focus of tick-borne relapsing fever in Southern Zaire. *Clin Infect Dis* 1997;25:139.

Dworkin MS, Anderson DE, Schwan TG, et al. Tick-borne relapsing fever in the Northwestern United States and Southwestern Canada. *Clin Infect Dis* 1998;26:122.

Fekade D, Knox K, Hussein K, et al. Prevention of Jarisch-Herxheimer reactions by treatment with antibodies against tumor necrosis factor α. *N Engl J Med* 1996;335:311.

Lovett MA, Goldstein EJC, Fleischmann J. Fever in a couple vacationing in the mountains of southern California. *Clin Infect Dis* 1992;14:1254.

Rahlenbeck SI, Gebre-Yohannes A. Louse-borne relapsing fever and its treatment. *Trop Geogr Med* 1995;47:49.

Trevejo RT, Schriefer ME, Gage KL, et al. An interstate outbreak of tick-borne relapsing fever among vacationers at a Rocky Mountain cabin. *Am J Trop Med Hyg* 1998;58:743.

Kelley's Textbook of Internal Medicine, fourth edition. Edited by H. David Humes. Lippincott Williams & Wilkins, Philadelphia © 2000.

INFECTIONS CAUSED BY FUNGI AND HIGHER BACTERIA

C H A P T E R

301

ACTINOMYCETES: NOCARDIOSIS, ACTINOMYCETOMA, ACTINOMYCOSIS

RICHARD J. WALLACE

◼ NOCARDIOSIS

DEFINITION

Nocardiosis is the clinical disease produced by one of multiple species of the genus *Nocardia*. The spectrum of disease is extremely wide. It includes posttraumatic skin infections, brain abscess, pneumonia, and disseminated infection.

INCIDENCE AND EPIDEMIOLOGY

There does not appear to be a geographic predominance of nocardial infection in the United States. There is a male predomi-

nance of 3:1; 85% of disease is pulmonary infection, disseminated disease, or brain abscess. Published data (although from work done in the early 1970s) suggest that between 500 and 1,000 new cases of disease due to *Nocardia* infection occur in the United States each year. The effect of HIV infection on this number is unknown, but in several series, only 10% to 15% of patients with nocardiosis had AIDS.

Among patients with primary (posttraumatic) cutaneous disease, about 80% have no underlying disease. Among patients who have the more serious and invasive types of disease, about 80% have serious underlying disease. The most common single predisposing factor is use of high-dose corticosteroids to manage an underlying malignant disease, connective tissue disorder, or effects of organ transplantation. Other risk factors include advanced HIV disease, pulmonary alveolar proteinosis, and occasionally alcoholism. Among persons with HIV infection, nocardiosis occurs late. The mean CD4 lymphocyte count was 100 in one series of 30 patients.

ETIOLOGY

The causative agents of nocardiosis are aerobic members of the family Actinomycetaceae, genus *Nocardia*. *N. asteroides* complex is by far the most common clinical taxon and is responsible for 90% of cases of pulmonary disease, disseminated disease, or brain abscess. *N. asteroides* complex has long been recognized as containing multiple taxonomic groups. In the early 1990s two new species, *N. nova* and *N. farcinica*, were recognized as representing 20% each of isolates identified by means of routine methods as *N. asteroides* complex. The clinical disease appears comparable with that described in the past for *N. asteroides*, although *N. farcinica* appears to be the more virulent. The term *N. asteroides complex* has been introduced to describe the *N. asteroides* group in recognition of its taxonomic heterogeneity. *N. brasiliensis* is responsible for 60% to 80% of primary skin infections. Most pulmonary and extracutaneous disease caused by organisms that biochemically look like *N. brasiliensis* are caused by another new species, *N. pseudobrasiliensis*. Other species such as *N. transvalensis* and *N. otitidis-caviarum* are rare causes of any of these syndromes (Table 301.1).

PATHOGENESIS

Nocardia are environmental organisms but are rarely recovered from humans in the absence of disease. In primary cutaneous

TABLE 301.1.	CLINICALLY IMPORTANT PATHOGENIC SPECIES OF *NOCARDIA*	
Common		**Rare**
Nocardia nova		*Nocardia transvalensis*
Nocardia farcinica		*Nocardia otitidis-caviarum*
Nocardia asteroides complex		*Nocardia pseudobrasiliensis*
Nocardia brasiliensis		

disease, a history of trauma at the site of infection is almost always present. Most of these injuries occur outdoors and are associated with obvious potential soil contamination, such as a motorcycle accident or gardening accident. The point of entrance for other types of clinical disease (lung disease, disseminated disease, brain abscess) is assumed to be the lower respiratory tract, although the place and source where this inhalation occurs is rarely identified.

The nature of the immune response to *Nocardia* organisms is still under investigation. The basic tissue inflammatory response involves polymorphonuclear leukocytes. Microabscess and macroabscess formation is present with purulent drainage. Despite the polymorphonuclear leukocyte response, cell-mediated immunity and macrophage functions are considered to be extremely important in the pathogenesis of disease. Antibodies are measurable in most infections in an immunocompetent host, but they probably play no role in protection from disease.

CLINICAL FINDINGS

Table 301.2 lists the clinical diseases associated with *Nocardia* infection. Patients with primary cutaneous nocardiosis usually have a low-grade fever or no fever and have few or no systemic symptoms. Clinical disease is manifested as localized pyoderma with a central, ulcerated, draining lesion or an obvious abscess. These lesions are almost always on an extremity, but they frequently occur around the faces or necks of young children. Proximal lymphangitic spread with multiple subcutaneous nodules (abscesses) can exactly mimic sporotrichosis. This form of the disease is known as *sporotrichoid nocardiosis* and is almost always caused by *N. brasiliensis.*

Patients with pulmonary disease have the usual symptoms of pneumonia. Cough, usually productive of thick purulent sputum, is present. Chest pain of a pleuritic type occurs among some patients. Almost all patients have a fever, including those taking corticosteroids. The temperature may be as high as 39°C (103°F). In some instances the disease is detected at chest radiography before the onset of clinical symptoms.

Dissemination from a pulmonary focus (primarily to skin or brain) occurs among about 20% of patients. Symptoms of brain abscess may develop before or after the pulmonary symptoms or may occur without any apparent respiratory disease. The condition ranges from an asymptomatic state to the presence of fever, headache, lethargy, confusion, focal or grand mal seizures, or sudden development of a neurologic deficit.

LABORATORY FINDINGS

Nocardia organisms are not fastidious, but they grow more slowly than most bacterial species, taking 3 to 5 days to produce good growth. They grow well aerobically on blood and chocolate agar as well as on Löwenstein–Jensen medium. The presence of other mixed flora, especially in sputum, may obscure or even inhibit the growth of *Nocardia* organisms and is a major reason for failure to recover the organism. Despite the common misconception that these are fungi, nocardiae often grow poorly on Sabouraud's or antibiotic-containing media.

On Gram stain, the organism appears as beautiful, somewhat delicate, beaded, branched gram-positive filaments in tangled masses surrounded by acute inflammatory cells (Fig. 301.1). Only the anaerobic *Actinomyces* or *Propionibacterium* (formerly *Arachnia*) species such as *Actinomyces israeli*, have the same morphologic appearance. *Nocardia* organisms grow in blood cultures, usually from patients who are severely immunosuppressed, have overwhelming clinical disease, or have catheter-related sepsis.

The diagnosis of nocardial infection by means of Gram stain and culture is not difficult if the disease is considered and good laboratory assessment is available. Because purulent sputum is available from most patients with pulmonary disease and the organisms are easily identified with Gram stain, there should be little need for invasive procedures. Unfortunately, this often is not the case, and bronchoscopy, percutaneous needle aspiration, or in rare instances open lung biopsy is needed to make a definitive diagnosis.

Identification to species has traditionally involved hydrolysis of casein, tyrosine, and xanthine. This technique does not separate *N. nova* and *N. farcinica* from *N. asteroides* complex and *N. pseudobrasiliensis* from *N. brasiliensis.* The use of polymerase chain reaction restriction analysis of a heat-shock protein gene sequence, and antimicrobial susceptibility patterns have been suggested to allow more accurate species identification.

Radiographic studies of patients with pneumonia often show a dense, rounded infiltrate that goes on to cavitation with an

TABLE 301.2.	CLINICAL DISEASES ASSOCIATED WITH *NOCARDIA* INFECTION
Pneumonia	Brain abscess
Lung abscess	Bacteremia
Localized cutaneous infection	Disseminated disease
Sporotrichoid cutaneous infection	Meningitis
Osteomyelitis	Catheter sepsis
Septic arthritis	

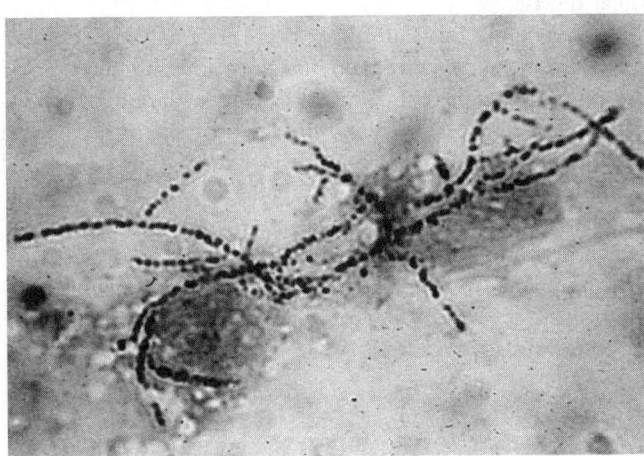

FIGURE 301.1. Gram stain of *Nocardia* organisms from the sputum of a patient with pulmonary nocardiosis. The organisms appear as a beaded, gram-positive, branching tangle adjacent to three necrotic white cells (original magnification ×1,000.)

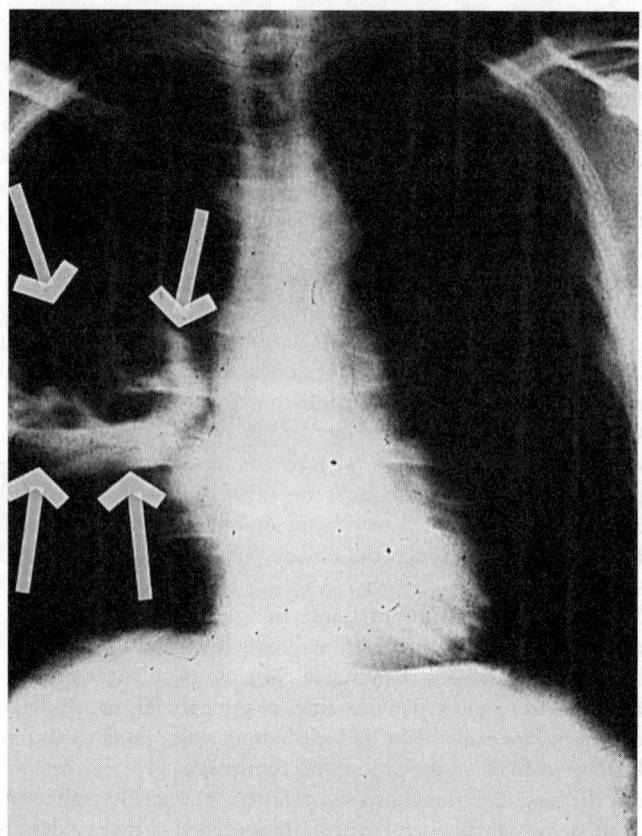

FIGURE 301.2. Chest radiograph of a patient with nocardial pneumonia (*arrows*) shows a large, rounded infiltrate that has undergone cavitation and has an air-fluid level.

air-fluid level (Fig. 301.2). Such a finding in an immunocompromised patient is almost enough evidence to confirm the diagnosis of nocardial infection. Unfortunately, nocardial infection has many other manifestations in the lung. They range from a nonspecific bronchopneumonic infiltrate to diffuse reticulonodular disease.

Because of the pyogenic nature of the nocardial disease, radionuclide scans or computed tomography of the abdomen should be considered in the evaluation of patients with pulmonary disease to find unsuspected sites of clinical involvement. Computed tomography or magnetic resonance imaging of the brain should be performed for all patients with pulmonary or presumed disseminated disease to exclude the presence of a brain abscess, which profoundly alters the patient's treatment and prognosis.

No serologic tests (antigen or antibody) are available. Leukocytosis of 15,000 to 25,000 cells per milliliter is present in most patients with serious disease.

COURSE AND PROGNOSIS

A number of factors have been associated with the poor prognosis of pulmonary nocardiosis, including the need for continued use of immunosuppressive drugs, disseminated disease, and central nervous system involvement. As recently as the early 1970s, these factors were said to be associated with a mortality of 80% or greater. Although exact numbers are not available, the current mortality of uncomplicated pneumonia is probably only about 10%. The presence of overwhelming disease, including diffuse pulmonary disease with respiratory failure, clearly carries a high mortality. Brain abscess is difficult to treat. It necessitates surgical drainage in most cases, and the mortality when only sulfonamides are used is 50%. The mortality appears to be much lower with the use of initial combination drug therapy (often sulfa, ceftriaxone, and amikacin). Patients with AIDS as the risk factor seem to respond as well to therapy as do patients at risk because of use of corticosteroids.

The course of primary cutaneous disease is not known but is probably self-limited. Cure with surgical debridement alone occurs in at least one-third of cases. Nevertheless, drug therapy is recommended for all patients.

■ STRATEGIES FOR OPTIMAL CARE

The therapy of choice for all forms of nocardiosis is a sulfonamide. The usual adult doses are sulfamethoxazole, 1 g three times a day, or sulfisoxazole, 2 g four times a day. Sulfadiazine is less desirable because of its high degree of insolubility in the urine. The optimal serum levels needed for clinical response have not been determined. An advantage of one sulfonamide preparation over another is not clinically evident.

Drugs in combinations with a sulfonamide are being used increasingly to manage nocardiosis. Trimethoprim has little in vitro activity against nocardiae, and a clinical advantage to using this drug in combination over using a sulfonamide alone has never been shown. Despite this, the combination of trimethoprim and sulfamethoxazole is commonly used to manage nocardiosis. Some practitioners consider it the treatment of choice.

In uncomplicated pulmonary or cutaneous nocardiosis, the response to sulfonamide therapy alone is so good that additional therapy is not routinely recommended, regardless of the risk factor. The need for additional agents comes with poor clinical response, overwhelming disease, disseminated disease, and brain abscess, for the mortality with sulfonamides alone is as high as 50%. Low-dose amikacin (peak serum levels approximately 20 μg per milliliter) and high-dose ceftriaxone (2 g twice a day for adults) are the usual choices to add to the sulfonamide until clinical improvement has occurred, which can take as long as 4 to 8 weeks. Amikacin is omitted first because of its greater toxicity. Other alternative agents include imipenem and cefotaxime.

The susceptibility of *N. asteroides* complex to antimicrobial agents other than the sulfonamides, is variable, so susceptibility testing should be performed if these agents are being considered. In vitro studies have shown that amikacin (95% susceptible to 2 μg per milliliter), imipenem (90% susceptible to 8 μg per milliliter), and cefotaxime or ceftriaxone (75% susceptible to 8 μg per milliliter) are the best alternative parenteral agents against *N. asteroides* complex. Minocycline (90% susceptible to 4 μg per milliliter) and amoxicillin-clavulanate (about 40% susceptible to 8/2 μg per milliliter) are the best oral agents. Specific drug susceptibility patterns are associated with other species or taxons of *Nocardia*. Isolates of *N. nova*, for example, are uniformly susceptible to erythromycin, clarithromycin, amikacin, and imipenem, whereas isolates of *N. farcinica* are resistant to all aminoglycosides except amikacin and the third-generation cephalosporins, including cefotaxime and ceftriaxone. Isolates of *N. brasiliensis* usually are susceptible to cefotaxime or ceftriaxone (less than 8 μg per milliliter), amoxicillin-clavulanate (less than 4/2 μg per milliliter), and amikacin (less than 2 μg per milliliter) but are resistant to imipenem (more than 8 μg per milliliter). Published experience with these agents is limited. Acquired drug resistance with therapy is rare but has occurred with amoxicillin-clavulanate and clarithromycin.

Because of the pyogenic and suppurative nature of nocardiosis, abscess formation is common. Drainage of these abscesses, especially in the brain and pleural space, is important.

The duration of therapy for nocardiosis varies with the type and extent of disease. The treatment period usually is 3 months for primary cutaneous disease, 6 months for pulmonary disease, and 8 to 12 months for a brain abscess. Relapses, if they occur, usually do so within 4 to 6 weeks of discontinuation of therapy.

ACTINOMYCETOMA

Actinomycetoma (Madura foot) is characterized by a large, swollen extremity with multiple draining sinuses and multifocal osteomyelitis. *Actinomadura madurae*, an aerobic, slow-growing species of actinomycetes, is the most common pathogen, but *Nocardia* species and true fungi also can produce this disease, which usually occurs among people from developing nations. Because of the extensive nature of this disease, the long-term prognosis is poor. *Actinomadurae* organisms grow aerobically on routine and fungal media and appear as a large clump of beaded gram-positive filaments. Some but not all isolates of *Actinomadura* produce β-lactamase. Penicillin or ampicillin is the therapy of choice for β-lactamase–negative strains, whereas erythromycin, sulfonamides, trimethoprim-sulfamethoxazole, and tetracycline are active against most but not all β-lactamase–producing isolates. Therapy for 12 to 24 months usually is needed. Surgery, including amputation, may be needed to control or cure the disease.

ACTINOMYCOSIS

Actinomycosis is the name for the group of diseases produced by six of the 14 currently recognized species of the genus *Actinomyces* and one species of the genus *Propionibacterium* (formerly *Arachnia*). Approximately 80% of cases of this disease are caused by the species *A. israeli*. These organisms are anaerobic bacteria. The usual reservoir is the gingival and tonsillar crypts, the gastrointestinal tract, and the female genital tract. Actinomyces are microaerophilic or obligate anaerobes and grow slowly. In disease they are almost always recovered with other anaerobic organisms.

Clinical disease is most commonly produced when oral anaer-

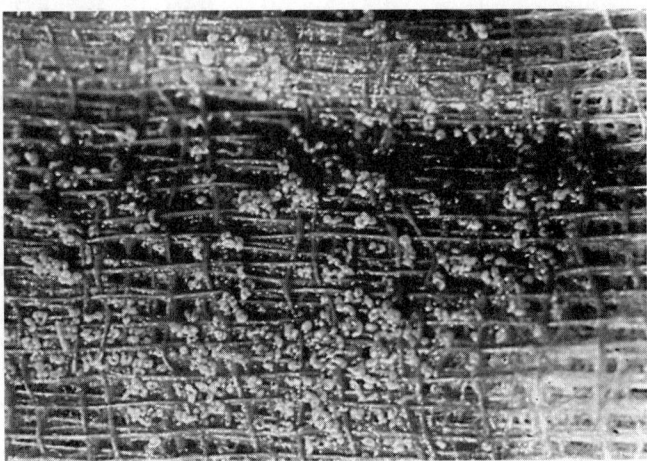

FIGURE 301.3. Sulfur granules of actinomycosis as they appear on a gauze bandage. They are light yellow and represent large clumps of organisms that have grown as a single mass.

obic flora can be pathogenic. Facial or cervical actinomycosis, so-called lumpy jaw (named for the hard, woody induration of the skin produced by the disease), usually is associated with periodontal disease. An intense fibrotic reaction, sinus track formation, and tendency to produce metastatic infections in other sites, especially the skin, are unique features of actinomycosis wherever it occurs and are not seen with infection by other anaerobes.

Pulmonary disease is rare and can be difficult to diagnose because the organisms rarely are seen on Gram stains of the sputum. It has the radiographic features of anaerobic lung disease, sometimes including cavitation. The actinomycotic nature of the disease usually is demonstrated when a draining chest wall abscess is found or when biopsy of a lesion shows typical sulfur granules (Fig. 301.3). Not uncommonly, the infiltrate can mimic carcinoma of the lung and ends up being resected, so-called pseudotumor. Because of difficulty in growing the organism, microbiologic diagnosis of more than 50% of cases is based on histopathologic findings. In rare instances actinomycosis can occur in sites other than the face or lung. Such conditions include perforation of the gastrointestinal tract, endometritis associated with the presence of an intrauterine device, brain abscess, and a disseminated form of the disease with multiple sites of visceral and cutaneous involvement.

Therapy for actinomycosis is penicillin. Cephalosporins, tetracycline, and clindamycin are good alternative agents for infections that do not include the central nervous system. Chloramphenicol is the alternative therapy for brain abscess. Penicillin usually is given in high intravenous doses (10 to 20 million units per day) until disease control is obtained. Then high-dose oral therapy (2 to 4 g per day) can be administered. The average duration of therapy is 3 months for cervical-facial disease and 6 to 12 months for pulmonary or disseminated disease. Surgical debridement is important, especially when an abscess forms.

BIBLIOGRAPHY

Beaman BL, Beaman L. *Nocardia* species: host-parasite relationships. *Clin Microbiol Rev* 1994;7:213.

Brown JR. Human actinomycosis: a study of 181 subjects. *Hum Pathol* 1973;4:319.

Lerner PI. Nocardiosis. *Clin Infect Dis* 1996;22:891.

McNeil MM, Brown J. The medically important aerobic actinomycetes: epidemiology and microbiology. *Clin Microbiol Rev* 1994;7:357.

Skoutelis A, Petrochilos J, Bassaris H. Successful treatment of thoracic actinomycosis with ceftriaxone. *Clin Infect Dis* 1994;19:161.

Smego RA Jr, Foglia G. Actinomycosis. *Clin Infect Dis* 1998;26:1255.

Tight RR, Bartlett MS. Actinomycetoma in the United States. *Rev Infect Dis* 1981;3:1139.

Uttamchandani RB, Daikos GL, Reyes RR, et al. Nocardiosis in 30 patients with advanced human immunodeficiency virus infection: clinical features and outcome. *Clin Infect Dis* 1994;18:348.

Wallace RJ Jr, Steele LC, Sumter G, et al. Antimicrobial susceptibility patterns of *Nocardia asteroides*. *Antimicrob Agents Chemother* 1988;32:1776.

Wallace RJ Jr, Tsukamura M, Brown BA, et al. Cefotaxime-resistant *Nocardia asteroides* strains are isolates of the controversial species *N. farcinica*. *J Clin Microbiol* 1990;28:2726.

Kelley's Textbook of Internal Medicine, fourth edition. Edited by H. David Humes. Lippincott Williams & Wilkins, Philadelphia © 2000.

C H A P T E R
302

INFECTIONS CAUSED BY DIMORPHIC FUNGI

THOMAS F. PATTERSON

The dimorphic fungi are soil-growing organisms that exist in a mycelial form in the environment but grow as a yeast or yeast-like form at body temperature (37°C). The major infections caused by these fungi are histoplasmosis, coccidioidomycosis, blastomycosis, paracoccidioidomycosis, sporotrichosis, and penicilliosis. All occur in distinct epidemiologic settings or in specific endemic regions (Fig. 302.1). Clinical manifestation of these infections depends on the immune status of the host. Among hosts with normal immune status, clinical infection may be minimal. Patients with altered host defenses, including patients with AIDS, may have overwhelming disseminated infection. The large number of persons with suppressed immune systems, including patients with HIV and patients undergoing immunosuppressive therapy, has increased the clinical relevance of dimorphic fungal infection. Although the use of highly active antiretroviral therapy has reduced the incidence of these mycoses among persons with HIV infection, patients not receiving or effectively responding to this therapy continue to be at high risk of infection with these organisms. An approach to antifungal therapy is discussed in Chapter 336.

■ HISTOPLASMOSIS

The dimorphic fungus *Histoplasma capsulatum* is the etiologic agent of histoplasmosis, a disease endemic to the Ohio River

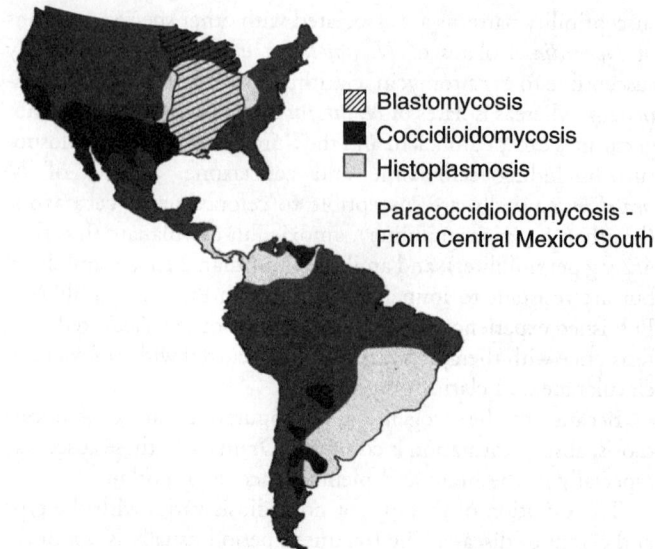

FIGURE 302.1. Endemic zones of dimorphic fungi in the Americas. (Adapted from Graybill JR. Opportunistic fungal infections in patients with AIDS. *Clin Courier* 1995:12:2, with permission.)

and Mississippi River valleys. The clinical manifestations range from asymptomatic infection to chronic pulmonary disease and disseminated infection.

INCIDENCE AND EPIDEMIOLOGY

Most cases of histoplasmosis occur in endemic regions in North America and Latin America (Fig. 302.1). The attack rate approaches 100% in certain areas, but most cases remain asymptomatic and are detected only with skin testing. The organism is found in soil contaminated with droppings from fowl, including pigeons, starlings, and chickens, and is associated with bird roosts, caves, and decaying buildings. Urban outbreaks of histoplasmosis have been linked to soil disturbances. Children have high attack rates in outbreaks because of lack of immunity, as do persons who live on the edges of the endemic regions. Reactivation of infection can occur among immunosuppressed patients, such as those undergoing chemotherapy and patients with AIDS.

PATHOGENESIS

The usual route of infection is inhalation of microconidia, which germinate into yeasts that can disseminate through the blood and lymphatic system. Host cells, including neutrophils, macrophages, and natural killer cells control the organism. Circulating yeasts are cleared by reticuloendothelial cells. Specific cell-mediated immunity to activate macrophages fungicidal to the organism develops within 2 to 3 weeks. Persons with deficient T-cell immunity cannot contain the organism, and severe infection is more likely. Risk factors for failure of cell-mediated immunity include AIDS, organ transplantation, malignant disease, and steroid use. Immunity is not complete, and reexposure may cause clinical infection, particularly if the inoculum is heavy. Host response to the organism results in a granulomatous inflammatory lesion associated with necrosis. The lesion can contain latent organisms that serve as a source of endogenous reactivation if host immunity is impaired.

CLINICAL FINDINGS

The clinical spectrum of histoplasmosis depends on underlying host defenses, the intensity of exposure, and previous immunity. After low-intensity exposure, symptomatic infection develops in only 1 in 100 people (Table 302.1). After a heavy inoculum, most infections are symptomatic. The acute self-limited illness of histoplasmosis is characterized by a flulike illness with fever, chills, headache, myalgia, anorexia, nonproductive cough, and chest pain. Chest radiographs may show enlarged hilar or mediastinal lymph nodes with patchy infiltrates. After a heavy inoculum, more extensive pulmonary disease may occur, including adult respiratory distress syndrome.

Inflammatory complications may accompany acute symptomatic infection in approximately 10% of patients and may include arthritis or severe arthralgia accompanied by erythema nodosum. These symptoms can last for months and are best managed with anti-inflammatory drugs. Viral-like pericarditis also may develop. Chest radiographs may show mediastinal lymphadenopathy as a clue to diagnosis of histoplasmosis. Most cases of acute histoplasmosis resolve without therapy, but residual calcified granulomas in the lung are commonly identified on chest radiographs of persons who reside in the endemic zones.

In approximately 1 in 2,000 cases, progressive pulmonary histoplasmosis follows acute infection. This condition is characterized by chronic pulmonary symptoms associated with apical lung cavities and fibrosis. Chronic pulmonary histoplasmosis is caused by the immune response to the inhaled organism and is more likely to develop in patients with preexisting lung disease, elderly patients, men, whites, and persons with suppressed immune systems. Clinical symptoms resemble those of other granulomatous infections. Fewer than one-third of the lesions heal spontaneously. More commonly, persistence of the organism leads to chronic infection and fibrosis; progressive infections occur among more than 50% of patients.

Disseminated histoplasmosis develops among approximately 1 in 2,000 patients with acute infection and also can be caused by reactivation of disease. Disseminated infection is more likely to occur among patients with advanced AIDS, organ transplant recipients, patients receiving steroids or chemotherapy, patients younger than 1 year, and patients with debilitating medical conditions. Severe disease is more likely to develop among the very young and among patients with suppressed immune systems, including patients with AIDS. Fever, pulmonary infiltrates (including adult respiratory distress syndrome), and a syndrome resembling septic shock are more likely to occur. Disseminated infection can include gastrointestinal ulcerations and bleeding, skin lesions, oropharyngeal ulcerations, adrenal insufficiency, meningitis, and endocarditis. Signs and symptoms of disseminated infection are nonspecific and can include fever, weight loss, hepatosplenomegaly, and lymphadenopathy. Chest radiographs usually depict a diffuse interstitial or reticulonodular infiltrate. Bone marrow involvement is common and can be suggested by leukopenia, thrombocytopenia, and anemia. A markedly elevated serum lactate dehydrogenase level can be an important clue to the disease.

LABORATORY FINDINGS

The diagnosis of histoplasmosis is established by means of culture, histopathologic examination, or serologic testing (Table 302.2). Skin tests for histoplasmosis are not useful to establish a diagnosis because most patients in endemic zones have skin test reactivity, and cross-reactions with other fungi are common. Patients with disseminated histoplasmosis may have a negative skin test reaction. Cultures are limited by the lack of positivity in self-limited disease and slow growth of the organism. Cultures are more rapidly positive among patients with a heavy organism burden, as occurs among patients with AIDS. More than 75% of patients with disseminated disease have positive cultures of blood, bone marrow, or urine. Identification of the organism requires conversion of the mold to a yeast and back to the mold, but exoantigen testing is used to establish the diagnosis. Almost two-thirds of patients with chronic pulmonary histoplasmosis have positive sputum culture results, although multiple samples may be needed. Histopathologic analysis of tissues, including bone marrow, skin lesions, and buffy coat smears of blood, is useful for a rapid diagnosis through demonstration of budding intracellular yeasts.

Detection of antibody to yeast- and mycelial-phase antigens is used to diagnose acute infection. Antibody is uncommonly detected among persons with remote exposures, but cross-reactions with other fungi can occur. Antibodies develop within 4 to 6 weeks after infection and gradually decrease over a 2- to 5-year period. Antibody develops in most people with acute symptomatic infection. A fourfold rise in complement fixation (CF) titers or a titer of at least 1:32 suggests active infection. In chronic pulmonary histoplasmosis, titers usually are lower.

TABLE 302.1.	CLINICAL MANIFESTATIONS OF HISTOPLASMOSIS		
Clinical Manifestation		Heavy Inoculum (%)	Light Inoculum (%)
Asymptomatic		50	99
Self-limited		50	1
Pulmonary (80% o symptomatic)			
Arthritis-erythema nodosum (10%)			
Pericarditis (10%)			
Mediastinal granuloma (unknown)			
Disseminated		Unknown	0.05
Chronic pulmonary		Unknown	0.05
Inflammatory manifestation			
Fibrosing mediastinitis		Unknown	0.02

Source: Adapted from Wheat LJ. *Histoplasma capsulatum.* In: Gorbach SL, Barlett JG, Blacklow NR, eds. *Infectious diseases.* Philadelphia: WB Saunders, 1992:1905–1912, with permission.

	Positive Results (%)		
TABLE 302.2. DIAGNOSTIC TESTS IN HISTOPLASMOSIS			
Test	**Self-Limited**	**Cavitary**	**Disseminated**
Antibody			
Immunodiffusion	75	100	63
Complement fixation	89	93	63
Either immunodiffusion or complement fixation	99	100	71
Antigen detection	40–75	21	92
Culture	15	85	85

Source: Adapted from Wheat LJ. *Histoplasma capsulatum.* In: Gorbach SL, Bartlett JG, Blacklow NR, eds. *Infectious diseases.* Philadelphia: WB Saunders, 1992:1905–1912, with permission.

The immunodiffusion (ID) test is used to measure H and M band antibody. Whereas the H band is more specific for the diagnosis, the M band is more sensitive. The diagnostic yield is increased with use of both the ID and the CF test.

A radioimmunoassay and an enzyme immunoassay were developed by Wheat et al. for detecting *Histoplasma* polysaccharide antigen in serum and urine. This method is particularly sensitive in detecting disseminated infection. Serial measurement of antigen provides a means for assessing the efficacy of therapy and for establishing relapse of disease. Therapy is discussed in Chapter 336.

COCCIDIOIDOMYCOSIS

Coccidioidomycosis is caused by the fungus *Coccidioides immitis*, a soil organism that is endemic in the southwestern United States, Mexico, and South America (Fig. 302.1).

INCIDENCE AND EPIDEMIOLOGY

In the United States, an estimated 100,000 cases of coccidioidomycosis occur annually. The clinical manifestations range from self-limited valley fever to disseminated disease. The number of cases increased in the 1980s and 1990s because of the epidemic of coccidioidomycosis in California and the occurrence of infection among patients with AIDS.

Infection occurs only in the Western hemisphere and primarily in the southwestern United States and Mexico. The semiarid conditions of the southwest United States are particularly favorable to growth of *C. immitis*. Epidemics of *C. immitis* infection in California have been associated with dust storms and soil disturbances from earthquakes. Cycles of drought and rain enhance dispersion of the organism because heavy rains facilitate growth of the organism in the nitrogenous soil wastes. Subsequent drought conditions favor aerosolization of arthroconidia.

PATHOGENESIS

The usual portal of entry for *C. immitis* is inhalation of arthroconidia. Pulmonary macrophages and neutrophils provide initial host defenses. Arthroconidia, endospores, and spherules are resistant to killing by these defenses, which may be related to the outer wall of the organism. Arthroconidia germinate to produce spherules filled with endospores, which is the characteristic tissue phase of the organism (Fig. 302.2). Spherules rupture to release vast numbers of endospores, which form additional spherules. These spherules are surrounded by neutrophils and macrophages, and this phenomenon leads to granuloma formation.

Cell-mediated defenses with T lymphocytes are central to the immune response. Deficient cellular immunity is associated with disseminated infection. It occurs among certain groups at high

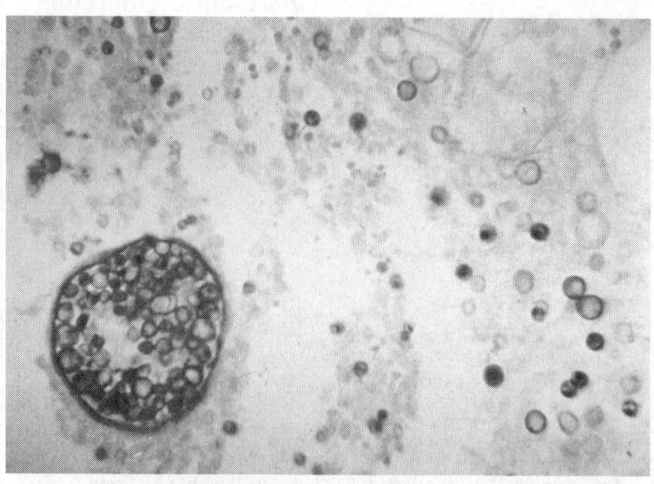

FIGURE 302.2. Periodic acid–Schiff stain of a thick-walled spherule of *Coccidioides immitis* filled with endospores in a tissue specimen.

risk of dissemination, particularly Filipinos and blacks, and immunosuppressed populations, such as organ transplant recipients, patients receiving steroid therapy or chemotherapy, and patients with AIDS. In certain endemic areas, 10% of patients with HIV infection contract coccidioidomycosis each year; the infection can be primary or reactivated. Male patients have higher rates of dissemination than do women, with the exception of pregnant women, among whom dissemination is common.

CLINICAL FINDINGS

Coccidioidomycosis is asymptomatic among 60% of persons with the infection. The presence of infection is indicated by a positive skin test reaction. The other 40% have a self-limited, influenza-like illness that develops 1 to 3 weeks after exposure. The illness is characterized by a dry cough, pleuritic chest pain, myalgia, arthralgia, fever, sweats, anorexia, and weakness. Patients with primary infection may have a variety of immune complex complications, including an erythematous macular rash, erythema multiforme, and erythema nodosum. Acute infection usually resolves without therapy, although symptoms may last for several weeks. Approximately 5% of patients have pulmonary residua, including nodules and cavities. Chronic progressive pulmonary infection is characterized, particularly among immunocompromised patients, by the development of extensive thin-walled cavities that may be complicated by cavity rupture, bronchopleural fistulas, and empyema.

Extrapulmonary disease develops in 1 in 200 patients and involves the skin and soft tissues, bone, and meninges. Among patients with meningitis, the mortality without therapy is greater than 90% after 1 year, and lifelong infection is common. Cerebrospinal fluid (CSF) findings include mononuclear pleocytosis associated with low glucose and elevated protein levels. CSF cultures frequently have negative results. The diagnosis is made through detection of complement-fixing antibodies in the CSF. Hydrocephalus is a common finding and may necessitate surgical intervention.

Dissemination to the skin is common. Lesions include verrucous, wart-like papules or plaques. Bone and joint dissemination also is common. The spine is the most frequent site of dissemination, but the typically lytic lesions also occur in the skull, hands, feet, and tibia. Joint involvement usually is monoarticular and occurs most commonly in the ankle and knee.

LABORATORY FINDINGS

Spherules are readily seen in histopathologic specimens and are diagnostic of coccidioidomycosis. *C. immitis* organisms are cultured within 3 to 4 days from clinical specimens. Large-volume CSF cultures may increase the yield from spinal fluid. The mycelial form of the organism grows as a white mold and is not distinctive. However, cultures are extremely infectious and should be handled with caution if the presence of *C. immitis* is suspected.

Serologic study is useful in establishing a diagnosis of coccidioidomycosis and in determining prognosis. IgM antibody may be detected within the first few weeks of infection with a tube precipitin test. IgG is detected after a few weeks of infection. One test combines ID and CF (IDCF). A positive IDCF result is highly suggestive of infection, and titers greater than 1 : 16 commonly indicate dissemination. Serum IDCF titers can be normal with single-site extrapulmonary infection. A positive CSF IDCF result is useful in the diagnosis of meningitis because results of culture of CSF rarely are positive. Serial titers can be used to assess the efficacy of therapy. Skin tests for coccidioidin are of limited utility. A positive result occurs with exposure, but the result may be negative in disseminated disease. Failure to develop a positive skin test reaction has been associated with poor response to therapy. Treatment is discussed in Chapter 336.

■ BLASTOMYCOSIS

Blastomyces dermatitidis, the etiologic agent of blastomycosis, is endemic in the central United States and causes disease that ranges from pulmonary to disseminated infection. The skin is especially susceptible to dissemination.

EPIDEMIOLOGY AND PATHOGENESIS

B. dermatitidis exists in nature as a mold. At body temperature it appears as a large, broad-based, budding yeast (8 to 30 μm) with a thick, refractory cell wall. The endemic zone for blastomycosis overlaps that of histoplasmosis. Most cases occur in the midwestern and southeastern United States, the Canadian provinces of Ontario, Quebec, and Alberta, and sporadically worldwide (Fig. 302.1). Dogs are also susceptible to infection with the organism.

Infection has been associated with soil exposure. The organism has been isolated from soil containing decayed vegetation or decomposed wood. Warm, humid temperatures and proximity to water or recent rains seem to facilitate growth of the organism. Occupational or recreational contact with soil has been associated with outbreaks of infection.

The usual route of infection is inhalation of conidia. In the alveoli, the organism transforms into yeasts and induces an acute inflammatory response that includes neutrophils and macrophages with granuloma formation. Once converted to a yeast, the organism is relatively resistant to phagocytosis and killing. Cell-mediated immunity is the principal acquired host defense against the organism and is critical in preventing dissemination. Blastomycosis is not a common opportunistic infection among immunocompromised hosts and is an uncommon late complication among patients with AIDS.

CLINICAL AND LABORATORY FINDINGS

An estimated 50% of persons with blastomycosis have symptoms, which are nonspecific and mimic influenza or bacterial infection with an abrupt onset of fever, chills, cough, myalgia, and arthralgia. Chest radiographs may show lobar or segmental consolidation, although a nodular pattern may be seen with chronic disease. The acute pulmonary symptoms may resolve but can cause progressive pulmonary disease or disseminated infection. The skin is the most frequent site of dissemination. Verrucous or ulcerative lesions appear on exposed areas of the body and may be mistaken for squamous cell carcinoma. Other extrapulmonary sites of infection include subcutaneous abscesses that may ulcerate, bones (particularly long bones, vertebrae, and ribs), genitourinary tract (prostate and epididymis), and central nervous system.

The diagnosis is established by means of demonstration of the organism on wet preparations or by means of histopathologic study. The organism can be differentiated on the basis of size and the presence of a refractile cell wall and broad-based buds. The organism is cultured, but the presence of the mycelial form is not evidence to confirm a diagnosis before conversion to a yeast. Serologic study is less reliable in establishing a diagnosis because of the lack of sensitive and specific antigens. Serum CF tests are less sensitive and specific than ID tests with A antigen. Positive test results occur among as many as 80% of patients and suggest the diagnosis. Negative test results, however, should not exclude the diagnosis, particularly if infection is disseminated. Klein et al. described specific antigens that may enhance serodiagnosis. Treatment is discussed in Chapter 336.

PARACOCCIDIOIDOMYCOSIS

Paracoccidioides brasiliensis, the etiologic agent of paracoccidioidomycosis (South American blastomycosis), is the principal dimorphic fungal infection in Latin America (Fig. 302.1).

EPIDEMIOLOGY AND PATHOGENESIS

P. brasiliensis produces a characteristic pilot-wheel appearance in tissues; 2- to 4-μm buds surround a central mother cell. Infection occurs only in Latin America but spares some areas, including the Caribbean region and Chile. Infection occurs among men older than 30 years and among patients with soil exposure, although the organism has only rarely been isolated in nature. The organism is inhaled and converts into yeasts. From the lung, the organism disseminates to regional lymph nodes.

CLINICAL AND LABORATORY FINDINGS

Infection ranges from self-limited acute infection to chronic pulmonary disease and dissemination. The lungs are the primary site of infection, and most patients never have symptoms. In those patients, however, the organism may remain dormant and later cause clinical disease if host defenses are impaired. Among patients younger than 30 years, a juvenile form of infection occurs that is subacute and has a severe prognosis. It also occurs

among patients with AIDS. These patients have minimal pulmonary symptoms. The major manifestations of infection involve the reticuloendothelial system. Among adult patients, symptoms can occur years after primary infection. They include a persistent cough, purulent sputum, chest pain, weight loss, weakness, malaise, dyspnea, and fever. The chest radiograph may show interstitial or alveolar infiltrates with nodules, cavitation, or hilar adenopathy. A paracoccidioidoma, a large cavitary mass, also can occur. Infection disseminates to skin and mucosa, including the oropharynx. Ulcerations contain characteristic hemorrhagic spots; oropharyngeal involvement may be associated with hoarseness or dysphagia. Other sites of dissemination are the lymph nodes, especially cervical nodes, adrenal glands, liver, spleen, central nervous system, and bones.

The diagnosis of paracoccidioidomycosis is established through examination of tissues or infected specimens for the characteristic pilot-wheel shape of the organism. Culture requires conversion to the yeast because the mycelial form is not distinctive. Detection of antibody by means of ID or CF testing is useful in suggesting the diagnosis and may be used to evaluate response to therapy. ID antibodies may remain positive for years, and cross-reactions with *Histoplasma* antigens are common with CF. Skin tests are not a reliable means to establish the diagnosis. Treatment is discussed in Chapter 336.

SPOROTRICHOSIS

Sporotrichosis is caused by the soil fungus *Sporothrix schenckii* and is characterized by skin lesions, although pulmonary and disseminated infection occurs.

EPIDEMIOLOGY, PATHOGENESIS, AND CLINICAL FINDINGS

Infections with *S. schenckii* occur by means of direct skin inoculation from contaminated soil or plants, especially thorned plants such as roses. Outbreaks of infection have been associated with exposure to contaminated plant material such as straw, wood, hay bales, and sphagnum moss. Most cases are associated with vocational or recreational exposures, and the disease occurs worldwide. Sporotrichosis is uncommonly associated with immunosuppression and is rare among patients with AIDS.

After an incubation period of 1 to 10 weeks or longer, reddish-purple, necrotic, nodular cutaneous lesions appear that follow the lymphatic vessels and commonly ulcerate. Involvement of distal extremities may be related to the intolerance of some strains to temperatures of 37°C. The organism sometimes spreads directly to joints or bones. Disseminated infection is uncommon, as is pulmonary infection, which occurs most often among patients with alcoholism.

LABORATORY FINDINGS

The diagnosis of sporotrichosis is established by means of culture of the organism from pus or cutaneous lesions. Growth of the organism may occur within 3 to 5 days. Histopathologic analysis demonstrates typical cigar-shaped yeasts that may be surrounded by a stellate material that is positive at periodic acid–Schiff staining and is known as an *asteroid body*. Serologic testing may be useful to detect extracutaneous infection such as meningitis, but antibodies may be present without the disease. Treatment is discussed in Chapter 336.

PENICILLIOSIS

Penicillium marneffei has emerged as an important dimorphic pathogen in Southeast Asia. It produces chronic disseminated infection in immunosuppressed hosts. The fungus is endemic to Southeast Asia and is associated with exposure to the bamboo rat. Infections have been reported in northern Asia, throughout China, and as imported cases in Europe and Texas. Most cases have occurred among patients infected with HIV.

The organism is acquired through inhalation, and disseminated infection develops. Signs and symptoms mimic those of disseminated histoplasmosis or coccidioidomycosis. They include fever, weight loss, cough, hepatosplenomegaly, lymphadenopathy, and skin lesions. Pulmonary infiltrates, anemia, and thrombocytopenia are common. The diagnosis is established with smears of bone marrow, ulcerative skin lesions, or buffy coat of blood. Examination of the smears show elliptic yeasts that resemble *H. capsulatum* organisms except that prominent cross-walls are present. The walls develop when the organism divides though fission. On culture, the mold colony produces a distinctive red pigment. Treatment is discussed in Chapter 336.

BIBLIOGRAPHY

Bradsher RW. Clinical features of blastomycosis. *Semin Respir Infect* 1997; 12:229–234.

Brummer E, Casteñeda E, Restrepo A. Paracoccidioidomycosis: an update. *Clin Microbiol Rev* 1993;6:89–117.

Corcoran GR, Al-Abdely H, Flanders C, et al. Markedly elevated serum lactate dehydrogenase levels are a clue to the diagnosis of disseminated histoplasmosis in AIDS. *Clin Infect Dis* 1997;24:942–944.

Dooley DP, Bostic PS, Beckius ML. Spook house sporotrichosis: a point-source outbreak of sporotrichosis associated with hay bale props in a Halloween haunted-house. *Arch Intern Med* 1997;157:1885–1887.

Hamilton AJ. Serodiagnosis of histoplasmosis, paracoccidioidomycosis and penicilliosis marneffei: current status and future trends. *Med Mycol* 1998;36:351–364.

Stevens DA. Coccidioidomycosis. *N Engl J Med* 1995;332:1077–1082.

Supparatpinyo K, Perriens J, Nelson KE, et al. A controlled trial of itraconazole to prevent relapse of *Penicillium marneffei* infection in patients infected with the human immunodeficiency virus. *N Engl J Med* 1998; 339:1739–1743.

Walsh TJ, Chanock SJ. Diagnosis of invasive fungal infections: advances in nonculture systems. *Curr Clin Top Infect Dis* 1998;18:101–153.

Wheat J. Histoplasmosis: experience during outbreaks in Indianapolis and review of the literature. *Medicine (Baltimore)* 1997;76:339–354.

Kelley's Textbook of Internal Medicine, fourth edition. Edited by H. David Humes.
Lippincott Williams & Wilkins, Philadelphia © 2000.

CHAPTER
303

OPPORTUNISTIC FUNGAL INFECTIONS

JOHN E. EDWARDS, JR.

CANDIDA SPECIES, INCLUDING CANDIDA GLABRATA

INCIDENCE, EPIDEMIOLOGY, AND ETIOLOGY

Although more than 150 species of *Candida* exist, only *Candida albicans, C. tropicalis, C. guilliermondii, C. parapsilosis, C. stellatoidea, C. pseudotropicalis, C. krusei,* and *C. glabrata* infect humans with frequency. The numbers of infections caused by *C. lusitaniae* is increasing. The importance of *C. lusitaniae* is its resistance to amphotericin B. The rate of infection with *C. dubliniensis* is increasing among patients with AIDS. *C. glabrata,* formerly called *Torulopsis glabrata,* is capable of infecting the urinary tract and disseminating to major organs in immunocompromised patients. The manifestations are similar to those associated with the other species. Recovery of *C. glabrata* organisms from the gastrointestinal tract, genitourinary tract of women, and blood has increased considerably.

Candida organisms are ubiquitous. They are normal commensals of humans and some animals, usually inhabiting mucous membranes or damaged skin. Evidence indicates that many health care workers carry the organisms on their hands. Most species exist in three forms in tissue: yeast, which can bud, hyphae, and pseudohyphae. The organisms are partially gram-positive and grow well in aerated blood culture bottles, lysis centrifugation isolators, and routine culture media.

PATHOGENESIS

Severe candidal infections usually are iatrogenic complications of modern therapeutics. The organism is emerging as a highly important nosocomial pathogen. The two most important predisposing factors are exposure to broad-spectrum antimicrobial agents and neutropenia. Neutropenia, however, is not requisite for disseminated candidiasis. About one-half of cases continue to occur among patients with complicated postoperative courses unrelated to underlying neoplastic diseases. *Candida* organisms are the fourth most commonly isolated microorganisms and the third most common pathogen in blood cultures of hospitalized patients. Several virulence factors of *Candida* have been studied, including the morphologic forms of the organism (especially germ tubes and hyphae), extracellular enzymes (e.g., protease and phospholipases), and its ability to interfere with host defense mechanisms.

CLINICAL FINDINGS

Skin and Mucous Membranes

Intertrigo on the warm, moist areas of the skin occurs among obese persons and those with diabetes. Infection of the hair follicles occurs among both healthy persons and addicts. Paronychia occurs among persons who immerse their hands in water for long periods. Candidal diaper rash is one of the most common cutaneous infections of infants. Chronic mucocutaneous candidiasis is a long-standing, severe mucocutaneous disease of patients with lymphocyte-mediated immune response deficiency. Among immunocompromised hosts, the macronodular lesions of disseminated candidiasis, which contain the organisms, are important in ascertaining the presence of widespread dissemination in the visceral organs. These lesions are raised and frequently have a hemorrhagic base. Results of biopsy with both culture and section for histopathologic study establish the cause.

Candidal infection of the mouth, or thrush, occurs among patients who have taken antibiotics or inhaled steroids, among neonates, among denture wearers, and among severely debilitated or immunocompromised patients. It is one of the most frequent manifestations of AIDS. Any person who has thrush without an identifiable predisposing factor should be evaluated for AIDS.

Candidal infections of the gastrointestinal tract have become common among immunocompromised patients. Candidal esophagitis occurs frequently among patients receiving cytotoxic chemotherapy and among patients with AIDS. Swallowing is painful, and white plaques on the esophageal mucosa can be identified with endoscopy. Because herpesvirus and cytomegalovirus infections are in the differential diagnosis, biopsy is necessary. Before a definitive diagnosis is made for selected patients, however, a therapeutic trial with antifungal agents is acceptable. Biopsy specimens of gastric ulcers have been found to contain *Candida* organisms. Therapy for the ulcer usually is successful without specific anti-*Candida* therapy. In refractory cases, however, antifungal therapy should be tried when *Candida* has infected the ulcer base. In severely neutropenic hosts, *Candida* may cause ulcers throughout the gastrointestinal tract and may disseminate from these sites.

Genitourinary Tract

Candida species are found in the urine of 8% of healthy male and 12% of healthy female subjects. Candiduria, however, may signify cystitis, pyelonephritis, papillary necrosis, perinephric abscess, fungus balls, and emphysematous cystitis. A common problem is prolonged colonization of the bladders of patients with indwelling Foley catheters. Among most patients, the candiduria is self-limited, but some patients may need an amphotericin B bladder washout or treatment with oral fluconazole. There is concern that urinary tract colonization can cause dissemination, so the threshold has lowered for treating hospital patients for urinary colonization and infection.

Blood Vessels

About 2% of cases of endocarditis are caused by *Candida* organisms, and 50% of these are complications of cardiac surgery.

Heroin addicts also are prone to the development of candidal endocarditis, usually with *C. parapsilosis*. The hallmarks of candidal endocarditis are large vegetations and occlusion of large vessels. Of particular importance is the increasingly common occurrence of candidal intravascular infection at sites of peripheral indwelling intravascular lines. Fungus balls in the right atrium have occurred as complications of the presence of indwelling central catheters. Persistent candidemia may be caused by these intravenous infections.

Central Nervous System

The most common candidal infection of the central nervous system (CNS) is microabscess of the brains of patients with widespread hematogenous candidiasis. A large percentage of biopsy specimens from such patients have shown brain involvement. The most common form of infection is multiple microabscesses and small macroabscesses. Larger parenchymal abscesses, granulomatous vasculitis, and meningitis also have been described. Other CNS conditions associated with cerebral candidiasis include complications of chronic otitis, cerebral trauma, neurosurgical procedures, and presence of indwelling intracranial devices, such as ventricular fluid shunts. A small number of patients have had candidal meningitis that occurred de novo. The leukocytosis in candidal meningitis may be predominantly polymorphonuclear or predominantly mononuclear. The most effective treatment is a combination of amphotericin B and 5-fluorocytosine.

Pulmonary System

Candidal pneumonia is uncommon. When it occurs, the most common form is diffuse miliary abscesses in the preterminal course of severe neutropenia. In rare instances *Candida* organisms may superinfect the lung parenchyma damaged by preceding bacterial pneumonia. Progressive, necrotizing, localized pneumonia may evolve. Because *Candida* organisms frequently are present in the sputum of ill patients previously treated with antibiotics, simple recovery of the organism does not prove pneumonia. Histopathologic demonstration of invasion of tissue is definitive.

Other Candidal Infections

Additional candidal infections are osteomyelitis, arthritis, pancreatitis, biliary infection with fungus ball formation in the gallbladder and biliary ducts, postoperative infection of sternotomy sites, infection of prosthetic implants, peritonsillar abscesses complicating thrush, sinus and otic infections, peritonitis, especially during long-term ambulatory dialysis, and infection of the skeletal muscle with severe pain. Candidal endophthalmitis is an important complication of hematogenous dissemination and an important clue to infection of other organs. Ocular candidal infection can occur as a complication of ophthalmic surgery. Numerous patients have had hepatosplenic candidiasis with focal abscesses in both organs. It usually requires prolonged antifungal therapy. The abscesses can be seen on computed tomographic scans, and percutaneous biopsy can be performed.

Syndrome of Disseminated Candidiasis

Widespread disseminated candidiasis occurs most frequently among patients with neutropenia and among patients with prolonged and medically complicated postoperative courses, not necessarily related to the presence of a neoplasm. Low-birth-weight neonates also are at risk. Predisposing factors include use of antibiotics, neutropenia, presence of indwelling intravascular catheters, hyperalimentation fluids, and steroids. *Candida* is one of the most common organisms recovered from blood cultures in major medical centers, usually within the top 5 to 10 organisms. A strong consensus has evolved to treat all patients who have candidemia with an antifungal agent.

Beginning in the 1980s, a syndrome called the *yeast connection* or *Candida-related complex* was described in the general press. The purported pathogenesis is overgrowth of *Candida* on mucous membranes, especially in the gastrointestinal tract. This overgrowth is said to be induced through use of antibacterial drugs and environmental toxins. The *Candida* organisms are said to be capable of producing toxins that inhibit the immune system. The publications claim that weakness of the immune system causes a diversity of general symptoms, including fatigue, irritability, poor memory, and many other similar nonspecific conditions. Treatment is supposedly antifungal agents and avoidance of yeast-containing foods. Because the reports appeared in the general press, many persons are convinced they have this condition. At least three medical societies have published position statements expressing skepticism about the syndrome and advising caution in the use of potentially toxic antifungal agents for treatment.

LABORATORY FINDINGS AND DIAGNOSIS

It is difficult to determine whether a positive blood culture result is related to the presence of an indwelling catheter and the infection may resolve with removal of the catheter or whether the result reflects underlying disseminated disease. The problem is compounded by the lack of any reliable serodiagnostic tests. A strong consensus has evolved that all patients with candidemia should be treated with an antifungal agent. Any patient prone to disseminated candidiasis because of exposure to the known predisposing factors needs serial blood cultures and a physical examination to detect evidence of renal, cardiac, or cerebral infection. The diagnosis of candidal infection of deep organs requires biopsy evidence of the organism that is invading the tissue. Determining whether macronodular skin lesions, candidal endophthalmitis, or candidal myositis is present is valuable because the presence of these infections is highly correlated with involvement in the brain, heart, or kidney. The diagnosis of candidal infection of the mucous membranes can be established on the basis of the clinical appearance of the lesions and recovery of the organism from scrapings of the infected area. There are no serodiagnostic tests for invasive candidiasis that are well accepted or widely used.

STRATEGIES FOR OPTIMAL CARE

Until further studies are completed, therapy for life-threatening candidal infection is amphotericin B. Studies have shown that fluconazole is acceptable for patients without neutropenia and patients with neutropenia and candidemia who do not have life-threatening infection. Mucocutaneous infections have been successfully controlled with azole antifungals, including fluconazole, itraconazole, and ketoconazole. Removal of as many predisposing factors as possible is critical. The consensus is that removal of a catheter and changing all intravenous lines is highly desirable whenever logistically feasible.

CRYPTOCOCCAL INFECTIONS

INCIDENCE, EPIDEMIOLOGY, AND ETIOLOGY

Within the genus *Cryptococcus, C. neoformans* is the dominant species; infection with non-*neoformans* species is rare. The organism is a ubiquitous, encapsulated yeast of worldwide distribution, found in soil, on fruit, in pigeon droppings, on eucalyptus trees, and in animals, including cats. It occurs predominantly in the yeast phase, and its capsule is easily seen in specimens of body fluids with the aid of india ink or nigrosin. Cryptococcosis is an aerosol-borne mycosis. Either overt or subclinical infection of the lungs occurs after inhalation of contaminated dust. Most patients with the infection do not give a history of unusual exposure to dust or pigeons. CNS infection is caused by hematogenous seeding. Direct human-to-human or animal-to-human infection is not known to occur.

PATHOGENESIS

Many patients with cryptococcosis have no known host defense defect or predisposing condition. Only limited clinical observations and data from experiments with mice suggest the possibility of a genetic predisposition to infection in these circumstances. Predisposing factors for cryptococcal infection include AIDS, lymphoma, use of corticosteroids, sarcoidosis, diabetes, cytotoxic antineoplastic therapy, and renal transplantation. The disease is substantially more frequent among men and more common among whites than other races.

CLINICAL FINDINGS

Central Nervous System

Involvement of the CNS is the most serious and frequent form of cryptococcosis. Certain host factors may be responsible for this common CNS localization, such as lack of an inflammatory response in the brain and meninges and the growth-supportive nature of the cerebrospinal fluid (CSF). Hematogenous seeding of the meninges usually causes subacute symptoms, including headache, meningism, and low-grade fever. However, approximately one-half of patients who do not have a recognizable immunocompromising condition do not have a fever when they come to medical attention. Some patients with AIDS may have almost no symptoms. Although uncommon, neuropathy and papilledema may occur. Because of the possibility of a brain abscess or other space-occupying lesion, computed tomography scan of the head is advisable before a spinal tap. Abnormal CSF values include elevated opening pressure, depressed CSF glucose levels, elevated protein levels, and pleocytosis with lymphocyte predominance. Many or all of these abnormalities can be absent among patients with AIDS. In about one-half of cases, cryptococci can be seen with a microscope in india ink or nigrosin preparations of the CSF. During the evolution of the AIDS epidemic, patients were in stable clinical condition at admission and had rapid herniation after therapy was begun. Whether therapy accelerated decompensation is related to initiation of antifungal therapy is speculative. In general, the prognosis among patients with AIDS has been poor, and the relapse rate has been high. Many patients have come to attention with only minimal or no neurologic signs or symptoms.

Pulmonary System

Healthy people may harbor cryptococci as part of the natural flora of the tracheobronchial system. Simple recovery of the organism does not define infection. Asymptomatic pulmonary nodules may occur. Cryptococcal pneumonia occurs most frequently among immunocompromised persons and is usually a subacute necrotizing process that tends to be lobar in distribution. Some patients with AIDS have radiographic findings indistinguishable from those of pneumocystic pneumonia.

Other Forms of Cryptococcal Infection

Subcutaneous, painless nodules have been associated with widespread hematogenous cryptococcal infection. Biopsy with visualization of the organism has established the presence of dissemination in some patients. Cellulitis, lesions resembling molluscum contagiosum (among patients with AIDS), and ulcerations have been described. Cryptococcal prostatitis has emerged as an important problem among patients with AIDS. Cryptococcemia is associated with a poor prognosis. Other sites of cryptococcal infection include the oral mucosa, kidney, bone, eye (chorioretinitis), heart, pericardium, mediastinum, liver, peritoneum, joints, and muscle. Myocardial involvement is an important complication among patients with AIDS and may be considerably underreported.

LABORATORY FINDINGS AND DIAGNOSIS

The definitive diagnosis of cryptococcal infection is made by means of detecting the organism in biopsy specimens. Finding the organism in india ink or nigrosin preparations is nearly enough information to confirm a diagnosis because of the small incidence of false-positive results when experienced personnel perform the test. Detection of cryptococcal polysaccharide antigen by means of latex agglutination is an important adjunct to diagnosis when controls are in place for the presence of rheumatoid factor. Sensitivity and specificity are high. The results of the test are not definitive, however, and finding the organism in a biopsy specimen or culture from the appropriate source remains the definitive diagnostic procedure. Antigen testing should be performed on both blood and CSF. Positive results are more frequent when the test is performed on CSF. Some patients with AIDS have extremely high antigen titers.

STRATEGIES FOR OPTIMAL CARE

The management of cryptococcal CNS infection is controversial and is under study. Amphotericin B in combination with 5-fluorocytosine or amphotericin B alone for 6 to 10 weeks (depending on clinical response) is considered standard therapy. Some patients who respond well to initial treatment can undergo a 2-week consolidation course with amphotericin B and 5-fluorocytosine followed by fluconazole for 10 weeks. Because of the improved prognosis for patients with AIDS in general, more aggressive therapy in now being used. The consensus is to treat patients with AIDS with a combination of amphotericin B and 5-fluorocytosine for 2 weeks followed by treatment with fluconazole for a minimum of 10 weeks at 400 mg per day. These patients then undergo maintenance therapy for 12 to 18 months taking fluconazole at 200 to 400 mg per day. If the patient is doing poorly, a 6- to 10-week course of combined amphotericin B and 5-fluorocytosine may be preferable. It has become popular to use fluconazole to control cryptococcal infection outside the CNS that is not life threatening. A consensus also has been established to remove CSF fluid to correct increased intracranial pressure.

Patients intolerant of fluconazole may be given itraconazole, but there is concern that itraconazole may be less effective than fluconazole. Data are accumulating that suggest the lipid formulations of amphotericin B may be alternatives for those patients who are especially intolerant of the standard preparation.

ASPERGILLOSIS

INCIDENCE, EPIDEMIOLOGY, AND ETIOLOGY

Aspergillus organisms are among the most ubiquitous microbes. Interpretation of positive culture results from clinical specimens must be critical because contamination by dust particles is common at collection and during the culture procedure. The ubiquitous nature of the organism also presents important considerations with regard to the hospital environment. Hospital air conditioning systems may be contaminated with *Aspergillus* organisms, which probably causes regional differences in infection rates. At least 10 species of *Aspergillus* are known to be pathogenic for humans. Of these, *A. fumigatus* and *A. niger* are the most common. The organism is readily grown on standard fungal culture media.

PATHOGENESIS

Neutrophils, monocytes, and macrophages are important host defense mechanisms, and functioning of these cells is enhanced through complement. Like the organisms that cause the zygomycoses, *Aspergillus* organisms are angiotropic. They invade vascular walls and cause thrombosis, vascular occlusion, and infarction.

CLINICAL FINDINGS

Disseminated Aspergillosis in an Immunocompromised Patient

Neutropenia and use of steroids are the most important predisposing factors for an immunocompromised host. *Aspergillus* organisms usually enters through the sinuses or lungs and seed hematogenously to almost any organ. Severe, necrotizing pneumonia may occur and can cause cavitation or infarction. The hallmark of aspergillosis among immunocompromised hosts is tissue infarction. Lung, liver, and brain are the most common examples, but skin, gastrointestinal tract, eye, and bone involvement also occur. *Aspergillus* infection can cause esophagitis or ulceration in other segments of the gastrointestinal tract. Sinus involvement may be extensive, and necrosis of the nasal septum can occur. Blood cultures rarely are positive in disseminated aspergillosis, and generalized meningitis is rare.

Pulmonary System

The syndrome of allergic bronchopulmonary aspergillosis occurs among persons with asthma who have an immediate-type skin response to *Aspergillus* antigens, anti-*Aspergillus* antibodies, elevated IgE, transient pulmonary infiltrates from bronchial plugging, and *Aspergillus* organisms in the bronchial tree that contribute to bronchial plugging. Invasion of the pulmonary parenchyma does not occur. A common form of aspergillar pulmonary involvement occurs among patients who have cavitary pulmonary disease from any cause and an *Aspergillus* fungus ball in the cavity. Symptoms may range from none to fatal hemoptysis. Chest radiographs show a superior crescent of air above the fungus ball that shifts with changes in position. Unless complications such as hemoptysis, bronchopulmonary fistula, or recurrent bacterial infection of the cavity occur, aspergilloma is left untreated.

A form of miliary pulmonary aspergillosis occurs among children with normal immune function after they inhale large numbers of *Aspergillus* spores. Deaths have occurred, but spontaneous resolution is the norm. Immunocompromised patients, including children with chronic granulomatous disease, may have severe, necrotizing, cavitating bronchopneumonia associated with pulmonary infarction. Widespread dissemination may result. Resolution of the neutropenia and aggressive amphotericin B therapy are associated with an improved prognosis. In rare instances this form of aspergillar pneumonia occurs among persons with normal immune function.

Other *Aspergillus* Infections

Aspergillus organisms may infect the sinuses of otherwise healthy persons. They also may be recovered from patients with allergic sinusitis. In rare instances fungus balls may form in the involved sinuses. When *Aspergillus* is considered to play a role in chronic sinus infection, extensive irrigation or surgical drainage is necessary. Postsurgical antifungal therapy usually is not needed. For unknown reasons, *A. flavus*, as opposed to *A. fumigatus*, is much more commonly recovered from sinus infections. In rare circumstances, aspergillar sinus infection may have features indistinguishable from those of rhinocerebral zygomycosis. *Aspergillus* may be one of several organisms recovered in culture from ears with chronic otitis externa. Although it rarely causes extensive disease, the organism usually is one of many recovered and does not necessitate specific treatment.

Aspergillus infection can cause endocarditis, but rarely does

so. The infection is most common among drug addicts and patients with prosthetic valves. Bone infection can be caused by contiguous extension, especially in the lung. Surgical contamination can occur, particularly in neurosurgical procedures. Infections of the mandible, larynx, tracheobronchial tree, external ear canal, pericardium, myocardium, eye, peritoneum, pericardium, urinary tract, and epiglottis have been reported.

LABORATORY FINDINGS AND DIAGNOSIS

The diagnosis of invasive aspergillosis is established by means of histopathologic and culture demonstration of the fungus invading tissues. Blood and CSF culture results rarely are positive in hematogenously disseminated aspergillosis in a patient with neutropenia. The infrequent recovery of *Aspergillus* organisms from body fluids (even from the blood of patients with endocarditis), coupled with difficulty in interpreting positive cultures results because of the ubiquitous nature of the organism, make the diagnosis of invasive aspergillosis one of the most difficult among the opportunistic mycoses. The serodiagnostic technology is still experimental; however, an enzyme-linked immunosorbent assay (ELISA) is used in Europe. Detection of anti-*Aspergillus* antibodies, however, is helpful in diagnosing allergic bronchopulmonary aspergillosis.

STRATEGIES FOR OPTIMAL CARE

Amphotericin B is considered standard therapy for *Aspergillus* infection. Itraconazole has been approved for management of aspergillosis, and successful treatment with this azole has been reported. The lipid formulations of amphotericin B are considered alternatives in the presence of amphotericin intolerance. An experimental triazole, voriconazole, is under evaluation. In selected circumstances, surgery combined with antimicrobial treatment is necessary, as in aspergilloma, enophthalmitis, sinus infection, endocarditis, and selected pulmonary infections that cause massive hemoptysis. A combination of corticosteroids and itraconazole is the preferred strategy to manage allergic bronchopulmonary aspergillosis. The use of inhaled amphotericin B is experimental.

■ ZYGOMYCOSIS (MUCORMYCOSIS)

EPIDEMIOLOGY, ETIOLOGY, AND PATHOGENESIS

The term *zygomycosis* will likely replace *mucormycosis* because the latter incorrectly implies infection by organisms of the genus *Mucor*. The term *zygomycosis* is derived from *Zygomycetes*, which is the subclass of fungi that produce zygospores. Within the order Mucorales, consisting of the four genera *Rhizopus, Absidia, Mucor,* and *Cunninghamella*, are most of the organisms that cause infection in an immunocompromised host. There has been increased reporting of infections caused by *Apophysomyces elegans*. Some of these infections have occurred in normal hosts.

Zygomycetes species are ubiquitous. Decaying organic material is their most frequent site. They occasionally are recovered from healthy persons. The spores can easily disseminate through the air, and in infected tissue, they form broad, thick-walled, nonseptate hyphae that branch at nearly right angles. The various species cannot be differentiated by means of histopathologic examination, nor can Zygomycetes species be reliably differentiated from other fungi on this basis.

The two most important factors of predisposition are any disease that causes systemic acidosis (not the hyperglycemia of diabetes) and neutropenia associated with cytotoxic chemotherapy. The use of deferoxamine in the care of dialysis patients has been a well-defined predisposing factor. The neutrophil is capable of damaging *Mucor* hyphae and probably is an important cell in host defense.

A hallmark of infection with Zygomycetes species is invasion of vascular walls. Black, necrotic debris frequently is present in pus from infected areas. The pertinent clinical signs and symptoms coupled with the finding of this black debris may facilitate diagnosis of zygomycosis.

CLINICAL FINDINGS

Rhinocerebral Zygomycosis

Rhinocerebral zygomycosis occurs most commonly among patients with diabetes who have ketoacidosis. The infection begins in the nasal sinuses and spreads through the ethmoid sinus into the retroorbital space. The first symptoms and clinical signs frequently are not detected until the retroorbital tissues become infected. Pain, loss of ocular movement, and proptosis usually are the initial manifestations. Headache, visual loss, and periorbital cellulitis may occur. Because of the propensity of the organism to invade vessel walls, direct extension through the apex of the orbit into the brain may occur. A surprising phenomenon is that computed tomographic scans of the orbit may be normal; only rarely is an organized retroorbital mass present. Involved ocular muscles also may appear normal at surgical exploration of the orbital area.

Thoracic Zygomycosis

The most common form of intrathoracic zygomycosis is infection of the lung parenchyma. The pulmonary form of zygomycosis occurs most commonly among immunocompromised patients, usually as a superinfection in an area of pneumonia caused by bacterial infection. Pulmonary infection also can occur from hematogenous seeding to the pulmonary artery with subsequent thrombosis and infarction. The pneumonia caused by Zygomycetes species generally is more indolent than most types of bacterial pneumonia. Bronchopneumonia infiltrates, consolidation, cavitation, and pleural effusions are present, as are fungus balls within cavities. Nonpulmonary intrathoracic forms of zygomycosis are much less common than pulmonary forms. Examples are hematogenous seeding of cardiac valves and of the coronary arteries accompanied by thrombosis and myocardial infarction.

Abdominopelvic Zygomycosis

In nearly all instances, zygomycosis of the gastrointestinal tract occurs in areas of underlying disease such as gastric ulcer, amebic colitis, pellagra, kwashiorkor, *Salmonella* infection, and local trauma from indwelling intragastric devices. Complications such as perforation, obstruction, and peritonitis may occur. Other sites of infection are the kidney, uterus, and bladder.

Cutaneous Zygomycosis

Among immunocompromised patients, cutaneous zygomycosis may occur as subcutaneous, nonspecific nodules or as hematogenous lesions that resemble ecthyma gangrenosum. Burn wounds can be infected with Zygomycetes species and contain black necrotic debris within the pus. The organisms also have infected needle tracks left after organ biopsies or steroid injections.

Widespread Dissemination

Widespread dissemination may occur from any cutaneous site. Most commonly, however, this dissemination occurs in a severely immunocompromised host treated with cytotoxic chemotherapy for leukemia or lymphoma. When hematogenous dissemination occurs, infarction of the infected organs may be a clinical clue to disseminated zygomycosis or aspergillosis if the patient has a fever and neutropenia. Patients with rhinocerebral zygomycosis associated with acidosis may have hematogenous dissemination to the lungs, coronary arteries, and other organs.

Miscellaneous Infections

Zygomycosis of the ear, venous grafts, bone (hematogenous osteomyelitis), renal cysts, heart valves, and prosthetic material used for breast implants has been described.

LABORATORY FINDINGS AND DIAGNOSIS

The diagnosis of disseminated zygomycosis frequently is difficult because patients usually have severe multisystem disease, drug toxicity, and almost never have positive results of blood cultures. There also is no satisfactory serodiagnostic test. The diagnosis is obtained when methenamine silver or periodic acid–Schiff staining of a biopsy specimen shows the organism invading tissue. Precise diagnosis depends on recovery of the organism from culture of the biopsy specimen, because the species cannot be identified on the basis of the appearance of histopathologic sections.

None of the signs or symptoms of zygomycosis is specific. Entities commonly included in the differential diagnosis are tumor, pyogenic retroorbital infection, Graves' ophthalmopathy, infection with non-Zygomycetes fungi, bacterial bronchopneumonia, or colonization with the organism without its causing infection. Laboratory contamination of specimens can occur because these organisms are ubiquitous. When a culture for zygomycoses is requested, alerting the laboratory is beneficial so that the technologist does not use media that contain cycloheximide. There are no useful serodiagnostic tests.

STRATEGIES FOR OPTIMAL CARE

Standard therapy for rhinocerebral zygomycosis is amphotericin B in combination with a surgical procedure. At one time, radical surgical intervention was routine. Today a more selective surgical procedure combined with amphotericin B therapy has become the standard approach. The importance of the operation cannot be overemphasized, because many strains of the organism are resistant to amphotericin B. The use of other antifungal agents in combination with amphotericin B is controversial. Although no systematic studies have been performed, the lipid formulations of amphotericin B may be important for management of zygomycosis, because many patients need large amounts of amphotericin B and relatively rapid acceleration of dosage schedules.

EMERGING OPPORTUNISTIC FUNGI

A large number of rare fungal organisms are emerging as an important group of pathogens in immunocompromised hosts. Reported fungi (incomplete list) include *Trichosporon beigelii, Malassezia furfur, Fusarium* species, *Geotrichum candidum, Curvularia* species, *Drechslera* species, *Pichia farinosa, Torulopsis pintolopesii, Saccharomyces cervisiae, Cunninghamella bertholletiae, Penicillium* species, *Rhodotorula rubra, Scedosporium inflatum (prolificans),* and *Alternaria* species. When these organisms are recovered from immunocompromised patients, the possibility of dissemination has to be carefully evaluated, rather than their being considered contaminants or inconsequential. Many of these species may be relatively resistant to amphotericin B. Some may be partially resistant to fluconazole. This list will continue to grow in parallel with the growth in the population of immunocompromised hosts.

BIBLIOGRAPHY

Aberg JA, Powderly WG. Cryptococcal disease: implications of recent clinical trials on treatment and management. *AIDS Clinical Review* 1997; 229.
Clemons KV, Stevens DA. Comparison of fungizone, Amphotec, AmBisome, and Abelcet for treatment of systemic murine cryptococcosis. *Antimicrob Agents Chemother* 1998;42:899.
Connolly JE Jr, McAdams HP, Erasmus JJ, et al. Opportunistic fungal pneumonia. *J Thorac Imaging* 1999;14:51.
Denning DW. Invasive aspergillosis. *Clin Infect Dis* 1998;26:781–803.
Edwards JE Jr, Bodey GP, Bowden RA, et al. International conference for the development of a consensus on the management and prevention of severe candidal infections. *Clin Infect Dis* 1997;25:43.
Hughes WT, Armstrong D, Bodey GP, et al. 197 guidelines for the use of antimicrobial agents in patients with neutropenia with unexplained fever. Infectious Diseases Society of America. *Clin Infect Dis* 1997;25:551.
Kauffman CA, Hedderwick S. Opportunistic fungal infections: filamentous fungi and cryptococcosis. *Geriatrics* 1997;52:40–42.
Kullberg BJ. Trends in immunotherapy of fungal infections. 1997;16:51.
Pfaller MA, Jones RN, Messer RA, et al. National surveillance of nosocomial blood stream infection due to species of *Candida* other than *Candida albicans*: frequency of occurrent and antifungal susceptibility in the SCOPE program. SCOPE Participant Group. Surveillance and Control of Pathogens of Epidemiologic. *Diagn Microbiol Infect Dis* 1998;30:121.
van der Horst CM, Saag MS, Cloud GA, et al. Treatment of cryptococcal meningitis associated with the acquired immunodeficiency syndrome. National Institute of Allergy and Infectious Diseases Mycoses Study Group and AIDS Clinical Trials Group. *N Engl J Med* 1997;337:15.

Kelley's Textbook of Internal Medicine, fourth edition. Edited by H. David Humes. Lippincott Williams & Wilkins, Philadelphia © 2000.

RICKETTSIAL INFECTIONS

CHAPTER 304

INFECTIONS CAUSED BY *RICKETTSIA, EHRLICHIA, ORIENTIA,* AND *COXIELLA*

DANIEL B. FISHBEIN

DEFINITION

The human pathogens in the genera *Rickettsia, Ehrlichia, Orientia,* and *Coxiella,* are fastidious, pleomorphic gram-negative bacteria that grow in association with eukaryotic cells. These organisms cause a number of different diseases and clinical syndromes (Table 304.1). All are zoonoses; the natural history requires an animal reservoir and, with the exception of Q fever, an arthropod vector. The epidemiology and geographic distribution of each disease are related to the distribution of these reservoirs, vectors, and humans who come into contact with them. The bacteria discussed in this chapter were formerly included the family Rickettsiaceae but have recently undergone substantial reclassification. They are considered together because of their historical, pathophysiologic, clinical, and therapeutic similarities.

SPOTTED FEVER GROUP *RICKETTSIA*

ROCKY MOUNTAIN SPOTTED FEVER, BOUTONNEUSE FEVER

Incidence and Epidemiology

Rocky Mountain spotted fever (*Rickettsia rickettsii*) was originally recognized in the early 1900s in the Bitteroot Valley of

TABLE 304.1. PATHOGENS IN THE GENERA *RICKETTSIA*, *EHRLICHIA*, *COXIELLA*, AND *ORIENTIA*

Genus and Group	Etiologic Agent	Disease
Rickettsia		
Spotted fever group	R. rickettsii	Rocky Mountain spotted fever
	R. conorii	Mediterranean spotted fever
	R. sibierica	Siberian tick typhus
	R. japonica	Japanese or Oriental spotted fever
	R. africae	African tick-bite fever
	R. australis	Queensland tick typus
	R. honei	Flinders Island spotted fever
	R. slovaca	Not named
	R. mongolotimonae	Not named
	Israeli tick typhus *Rickettsia*	Israeli spotted fever
	R. felis	California flea rickettsiosis
	R. akari	Rickettsial pox
	Not named	Astrakhan fever
Typhus group	R. typhi	Murine typhus
	R. prowazekii	Epidemic typhus, Brill–Zinser disease, flying squirrel–associated typhus
Orientia	O. tsutsugamushi	Scrub typhus
Coxiella	C. burnetii	Q fever
Ehrlichia	E. chaffeensis	Human monocytic ehrlichiosis
	E. phagocytophila or E. equi	Human granulocytic ehrlichiosis
	E. sennetsu	*Sennetsu* ehrlichiosis

Montana. Most of the approximately 500 cases reported each year in the United States occur in the south central states, especially Oklahoma, and along the Atlantic seaboard, especially North Carolina, but cases are reported from many other states (Table 304.2). Rocky Mountain spotted fever also occurs in other countries in the Western Hemisphere, from Canada to Brazil. Boutonneuse fever (*R. conorii*) follows exposure to infected *Rhipicephalus* ticks and is endemic throughout Africa, the Middle East, and southern Europe. These disease are most common among boys and men younger than 20 years. A history of tick bite, attachment, or exposure can be elicited from about 60% of patients. For Rocky Mountain spotted fever, tick exposure usually occurs in rural wooded or brushy areas but can also follow exposures in parks and other less-developed parts of large cities, New York, for example.

Clinical Findings

Rocky Mountain spotted fever and the Eastern Hemisphere spotted fever group infections are similar in most aspects. Illness begins 2 to 14 (usually 6 to 8) days after exposure. For most patients, the first symptoms are high fever, usually 39°C, severe headache, myalgia, and rash; about one-half of patients report nausea, abdominal pain, and vomiting. A macular rash, which often begins on the wrist and ankles, appears by day 5 among 75% of patients, spreads centripetally, and becomes petechial. About 50% of patients with spotted fever group infections other than Rocky Mountain spotted fever have a red papule appears at the bite site. The papule develops into a painless, punched-out ulcer covered by a dark crust (tache noire, eschar). Central nervous system signs, pulmonary and peripheral edema, hypotension, adult respiratory distress syndrome, hepatomegaly and jaundice, and renal failure indicate serious organ system involvement, occur in severe forms of the disease, and are poor prognostic signs. Some patients have permanent sequelae. If the patient is not treated, the disease lasts 2 to 3 weeks. About 3% to 5% of patients die. The risk of death increases with age and duration from onset of symptoms to initiation of treatment with tetracycline.

Laboratory Findings

Because no laboratory test has a consistently positive result during the first 2 weeks of illness, the initial diagnosis of spotted fever group infections must be based on epidemiologic and clinical features. Thrombocytopenia, anemia, leukopenia, abnormal hepatic aminotransferase levels, and hyponatremia are present toward the end of the first week of illness among about one-third of patients. A definitive diagnosis of most spotted fever group infections can sometimes be made early in the illness by means of polymerase chain reaction in a variety of specimens or immunologic detection of *Rickettsia* organisms in involved skin by means of direct fluorescent antibody technique. The diagnosis is best established with tests of both acute and convalescent phase sera. A fourfold rise in titer confirms the diagnosis; tests of single sera samples should be interpreted with caution. Indirect immunofluorescence assay is the standard serologic test, although a number of other detection systems are satisfactory. The Weil–Felix test lacks specificity.

STRATEGIES FOR OPTIMAL CARE AND PREVENTION

Early suspicion of spotted fever group infections is particularly important because delay in initiation of effective treatment increases the risk of complications and death. Infection with all *Rickettsia* species responds to doxycycline (100 mg every 12 hours) or tetracycline, 25 to 50 mg per kilogram per day for

TABLE 304.2.	**COMPARISON OF CLINICAL AND EPIDEMIOLOGIC FEATURES OF RICKETTSIAL DISEASES FOUND IN THE UNITED STATES**						
Feature	Rocky Mountain Spotted Fever	Rickettsial Pox	Murine Typhus	Flying Squirrel–Associated Typhus	Acute Q Fever	Human Monocytic Ehrlichiosis	Human Granulocytic Ehrlichiosis
Reported rate/ 100,000[a]	0.3–3.0	Unknown	Unknown	<1.0	Unknown	<1.0	0.4–2.9
Distribution	Along broad band from Texas, Oklahoma, and Kansas to and including the Piedmont plateau and parts of the Atlantic seaboard, including New York City seaboard	Primarily New York City	Seaboards in southern Texas, southern California, Hawaii	Primarily eastern states	Corresponds to the distribution of infected reservoirs	Southeastern and southcentral United States	Northeastern and upper midwestern United States
Habitat	Rural to suburban, occasionally urban parks	Urban	Urban areas	Rural, suburban	Abattoirs, farms, peridomestic (cats)	Rural	Rural, suburban
Seasonality	90% between April and September, 50% in May and June[a]	None	Warmer months	Late fall to early spring	Year round, peaks in the spring	66% May–July; 90% April–September	Year round; 75% May–September
Vector	Lone star tick, American dog tick, wood tick	Mites	Rat and cat fleas	Lice	Ticks (humans infected by aerosols)	Lone star tick	Black-legged tick
Reservoir	Same as vector	Mice	Rats, cats, opossums	Flying squirrel	Small wild rodents (ticks transmit the disease to sheep, goats, and domestic cats)	White-tailed deer	Deer
Case–fatality rate	3–5%	0	1%	0	<1%	2–5%	2–5%

[a] Reported statewide rates in states where the disease is endemic. Actual rates are higher because of unrecognized, unreported, unconfirmed, or subclinical cases.

10 to 14 days. Seriously ill patients should receive the drugs parenterally. Fever should begin to subside within 24 to 48 hours, and defervescence should be complete within 3 to 5 days. Although chloramphenicol has long been an alternative treatment, outcomes may be better with tetracycline or doxycycline. Avoiding tick-infested areas and animals, especially dogs, best prevents Rocky Mountain spotted fever and boutonneuse fever. When this is not practical, protective clothing should be worn, a tick repellent used, the body inspected for ticks twice a day, and ticks removed with a tweezers. No vaccine is available.

Rickettsial Pox

Rickettsial pox (*R. akari*) is transmitted to humans by mites of house mice. The first sign may be a painless red papule that forms 7 to 10 days after the bite, becomes vesicular and slowly

forms an eschar that lasts for weeks. About 1 week later, fever, chills, headache, myalgia, and 5 to 100 discrete papulovesicles develop. Therapy is the same as for Rocky Mountain spotted fever.

California Flea Rickettsiosis

California flea rickettsiosis (*R. felis*) is a spotted fever group rickettsial infection that resembles murine typhus clinically and epidemiologically.

TYPHUS GROUP *RICKETTSIA:* EPIDEMIC TYPHUS

INCIDENCE AND EPIDEMIOLOGY

Epidemic typhus (*R. prowazekii*) may have caused more deaths in the twentieth century than any other infectious disease. The disease occurs where war, famine, cold, poverty, poor hygiene, and crowding promote infestation and proliferation of body lice (the vector) on humans (the reservoir). Epidemic typhus became rare after the introduction of insecticides (especially DDT) effective against lice and antibiotics effective against the disease. The continued threat, however, is evidenced by outbreaks and endemic foci in Africa (Ethiopia, Uganda, Rwanda, and Burundi) and the highlands of the Americas (Peru). Brill–Zinsser disease, a recrudescent form, can occur decades after the primary infection. Acute infection has been found sporadically during the winter months in the eastern and southern United States. It appears to be associated with contact with the ectoparasites of flying squirrels, the sylvan reservoirs.

CLINICAL AND LABORATORY FINDINGS

In acute infection, an incubation period of 7 to 12 days is followed by an abrupt onset of symptoms. The patient appears seriously ill. Symptoms are similar to those of Rocky Mountain spotted fever, but the rash is an ill-defined macular one that appears on the fourth to seventh day in the axillae or sides of the torso, becomes hemorrhagic and generalized, but spares the face, palms, and soles. Untreated epidemic typhus is a serious infection. The case-fatality ratio reaches 50%. Patients with flying squirrel–associated typhus and Brill–Zinsser disease become quite ill but less so than patients with epidemic typhus. Thrombocytopenia, abnormal results of liver function tests, and microscopic hematuria and proteinuria are common laboratory abnormalities. Definitive diagnosis is best made by means of analyzing acute- and convalescent-phase sera in a test in which typhus group antigen is used.

STRATEGIES FOR OPTIMAL CARE AND PREVENTION

A single dose of doxycycline (100 to 200 mg) is as effective as the extended regimens used for Rocky Mountain spotted fever. Prevention efforts are directed at delousing the infested populations and improving living conditions that facilitate infestation.

TYPHUS GROUP *RICKETTSIA*: MURINE TYPHUS

Murine typhus (*R. typhi*) and California flea rickettsiosis (*R. felis*) are transmitted to humans by fleas. Murine typhus is endemic in many warm parts of the world where poor living conditions and flea-infested rats coexist. Although improved sanitation and rodent control programs have markedly reduced the incidence of this disease in the United States, recent cases in California and Texas have been associated with flea-infested free-ranging cats, dogs, and opossums.

Although milder than that of epidemic typhus, the onset of murine typhus can be abrupt. Fever more than 39°C, headache, chills, myalgia, and nausea are common. Only about 20% of patients have a rash when they seek medical attention. The rash usually is macular and appears on the torso, legs, or arms. Splenomegaly or hepatomegaly may be present. Laboratory abnor-

malities include mild depression of platelets, elevated hepatic aminotransferase levels, and hypoalbuminemia. Death (1% of cases) and complications are associated with delayed treatment and advanced age. Diagnosis requires a high index of suspicion because only a few patients report rodent contact or flea bites. Specific diagnostic tests are the same as those for suspected *R. prowazekii* infection. The therapeutic regimens are the same as those for spotted fever group infections. Relapses have occurred among patients treated with chloramphenicol. Infection can be prevented by means of avoiding flea-infested rats or using vector and rodent control measures. No vaccine is available.

ORIENTIA

SCRUB TYPHUS

Caused by *Orientia tsutsugamushi*, scrub typhus is found in Asia, Australia, and the South Pacific, where it can be a common cause of febrile illness. The reservoir and vector for humans are trombiculid mites (chiggers). Humans become infected when they intrude on the areas of transition (scrub) vegetation where the vectors thrive. Soldiers and agricultural workers are therefore especially likely to be infected. After a prodrome of headache, chilliness, and anorexia, almost all patients have a fever, headache, and chills. Most patients have generalized lymphadenopathy. About one-half of patients have an eschar, splenomegaly, and a maculopapular rash. Absolute lymphocytosis is often present, suggesting the diagnosis of mononucleosis. Without treatment, the fever lasts about 2 weeks. Complications include pneumonitis, meningoencephalitis, renal failure, and jaundice. About 10% of cases die. Unlike other rickettsial diseases, reinfection can occur with one of the multiple serotypes of this organism. The Weil–Felix test is of some diagnostic utility. The sensitivity and specificity are approximately those of the indirect immunofluorescence assay for this disease. Treatment with tetracycline results in rapid defervescence, but antibiotic resistance has been reported.

COXIELLA

Q FEVER

Incidence and Epidemiology

Q fever has been reported from at least 51 countries on 5 continents. Q fever is the only rickettsial infection transmitted in nature by aerosols. Because *Coxiella burnetii*, the etiologic agent, is extremely resistant to desiccation and physical and chemical agents and a single organism can cause infection, *C. burnetii* is a threat in a variety of natural settings and in health and research institutes. It also has been considered as an agent of bioterrorism. Although *C. burnetii* has been transmitted to humans from many species of domestic animals, most cases occur in association with exposure to livestock or livestock products and domestic cats. The disease usually is transmitted through aerosols from contaminated environments, but infection also can occur after direct contact with these animals, their birth products, milk, urine, and feces. Outbreaks of up to several hundred cases, sometimes of obscure origin, have occurred. Chronic Q fever occurs 1% to 10% of infections.

Clinical and Laboratory Findings

Asymptomatic infection is common. Acute Q fever can appear as pneumonia, a nonspecific febrile illness, as hepatitis, or as a combination of these diseases. *C. burnetii* infection has been associated with spontaneous abortion among humans. After an incubation period that ranges from 2 to 5 weeks, the onset usually is somewhat sudden with rigors and fever to 40°C or more. Other, nonspecific symptoms include fatigue, headache, myalgia, arthralgia, retrobulbar pain, chest pain, cough, nausea, and vomiting. Physical examination abnormalities are limited to evidence of pulmonary consolidation and, occasionally, hepatomegaly, splenomegaly, and generalized or focal neurologic signs. Liver function test results frequently are abnormal. As in other rickettsial diseases, diagnosis is best established by means of testing acute and convalescent serum specimens. In granulomatous hepatitis, liver biopsy reveals doughnut granulomas.

Chronic Q Fever

The chronic form of Q fever usually becomes manifest as culture-negative bacterial endocarditis in a patient with underlying rheumatic valvular disease or vascular aneurysms. About one-half the cases occur among persons with prosthetic aortic valves. The initial symptom also may be a fever of unknown origin.

▪ STRATEGIES FOR OPTIMAL CARE AND PREVENTION

Although acute Q fever almost always resolves without treatment, tetracycline reduces the duration of fever if administered during the first 3 days of illness. This drug is the treatment of choice. Quinolones, rifampin, and chloramphenicol may be effective. Effective control of Q fever endocarditis is extremely difficult. The antibiotics available are rickettsiostatic only in the face of a deep-seated infection and should be used in combination. Valve replacement is indicated if infection cannot be controlled or if there is hemodynamic instability. A vaccine is available in a number of countries and as an investigational new drug in the United States. Vaccination should be considered for persons at high risk of exposure and who have no demonstrated sensitivity to Q fever antigen.

▪ *EHRLICHIA*

HUMAN MONOCYTIC EHRLICHIOSIS AND HUMAN GRANULOCYTIC EHRLICHIOSIS

Ehrlichia species are members of the Rickettsiaceae family characterized by parasitism of macrophage-monocytes and the granulocytic cell line, which they invade by means of phagocytosis. Human monocytic ehrlichiosis (HME), a tick-borne infection

caused by *E. chaffeensis,* was first recognized in the United States in 1986. Human granulocytic ehrlichiosis (HGE), caused by organisms similar or identical to the veterinary pathogens *E. phagocytophila, E. equi,* and *E. ewingii,* was first reported in 1994. Clusters (morulae) of *Ehrlichia* organisms, sparse perivascular infiltrates, reticuloendothelial hyperplasia, and focal necrosis can be found in bone marrow, liver, spleen, and other organs.

Incidence and Epidemiology

E. chaffeensis infection has been recognized in the south central and southern United States as well as in Europe and Africa. Patients often are exposed to Lone Star ticks (*Amblyomma americanum*) during outdoor activities in brushy or woody areas. HGE, a clinically similar infection, is transmitted by black-legged ticks (*Ixodes scapularis*) in the upper midwestern and northeastern United States and *I. pacificus* in California. The disease also is found in western Europe and Slovenia. The incubation period usually is 1 to 2 weeks. Incidence rates of both forms of ehrlichiosis are higher among men and increase with age through 60 to 69 years.

Clinical and Laboratory Findings

The clinical spectrum varies from asymptomatic to life threatening. The onset usually is gradual, but it may be sudden. Early symptoms include malaise or myalgia. Fever often is higher than 39°C. Other common symptoms include headache, chills, and gastrointestinal symptoms. A rash occurs among only about one-third of patients and frequently is fleeting.

Both HME and HGE are suggested when leukopenia or thrombocytopenia is present during the first week of an otherwise unexplained febrile illness. Anemia and abnormalities in hepatic aminotransferase levels and renal function are common. Coagulopathy and cerebrospinal fluid pleocytosis also have occurred. Neutrophilic inclusions (morulae) occur among about 80% of patients with HGE and are a practical screening criterion, but inclusions are rare in HME. Serologic testing is performed with sera from the acute and convalescent periods. Indirect immunofluorescence assay is performed with the antigen of *E. chaffeensis* for HME and that of *E. equi* for HGE.

▪ STRATEGIES FOR OPTIMAL CARE AND PREVENTION

HME and HGE respond best to tetracycline and doxycycline. The dosages are the same as for infections with spotted fever group rickettsiae. Preventive measures are the same as for Rocky Mountain spotted fever.

BIBLIOGRAPHY

Bakken JS, Krueth J, Wilson-Nordskog C, et al. Clinical and laboratory characteristics of human granulocytic ehrlichiosis. *JAMA* 1996;275: 199–205.

Berman SJ, Kundin WD. Scrub typhus in South Vietnam: a study of 87 cases. *Ann Intern Med* 1973;79:26–30.

Buller RS, Arens M, Hmiel SP, et al. *Ehrlichia ewingii,* a newly recognized agent of human ehrlichiosis. *N Engl J Med* 1999;341:148–155.

Dalton MJ, Clarke M, Holman RC, et al. National surveillance for Rocky Mountain spotted fever: epidemiologic summary and evaluation of risk factors for a fatal outcome. *Am J Trop Med Hyg* 1995;52:405–413.

Duma RJ, Sonenshine DE, Boseman FM, et al. Epidemic typhus in the United States associated with flying squirrels. *JAMA* 1981;245:2318–2323.

Dumler JS, Taylor JP, Walker DS. Clinical and laboratory features of murine typhus in south Texas, 1980 through 1987. *JAMA* 1991;266:1365–1370.

DuPont HT, Raoult D, Broqui P, et al. Epidemiologic features and clinical presentation of acute Q fever in hospitalized patients: 323 French cases. *Am J Med* 1992;93:427–434.

Fishbein DB, Dawson JE, Robinson LE. Human ehrlichiosis in the United States, 1985–1990. *Ann Intern Med* 1994;120:736–743.

Kaplowitz LG, Fischer JJ, Sparling PF. Rocky Mountain spotted fever: a clinical dilemma. *Curr Clin Top Infect Dis* 1981;2:89.

Kass EM, Szaniawski W, Levy H, et al. Rickettsial pox in a New York City hospital, 1980–1989. *N Engl J Med* 1994;331:1612–1617.

Marrie TJ, ed. *Q fever: the disease.* Boca Raton, FL: CRC Press, 1990.

Perine PL, Chandler BP, Krause DK, et al. A clinico-epidemiological study of epidemic typhus in Africa. *Clin Infect Dis* 1992:14:1149–1158.

Raoult D, Ndihokubwayo JB, Tissot-DuPont H, et al. Outbreak of epidemic typhus associated with trench fever in Burundi. *Lancet* 1998;352:353–358.

Kelley's Textbook of Internal Medicine, fourth edition. Edited by H. David Humes. Lippincott Williams & Wilkins, Philadelphia © 2000.

MYCOPLASMAL AND CHLAMYDIAL INFECTIONS

C H A P T E R
305

INFECTIONS CAUSED BY MYCOPLASMA PNEUMONIAE AND THE GENITAL MYCOPLASMAS

CHARLES M. HELMS

DEFINITION

Mycoplasmas belong to the class Mollicutes, eubacteria that have evolved regressively from low G + C–containing gram-positive ancestors by means of genome reduction. Mycoplasmas are the smallest of the free-living organisms, about 200 nm in greatest dimension. They are pleomorphic and bounded by a single triple-layered membrane. The genome (500 to 1,000 kd) is only half that of the smallest bacterium. Unlike viruses, mycoplasmas are capable of cell-free growth in artificial media and are susceptible to some antibiotics. Unlike classic bacteria, mycoplasmas have no cell wall because they are genetically incapable of synthesizing cell wall precursors.

Several *Mycoplasma* species have been isolated from humans, but only three appear to be frequent human pathogens: *M. pneumoniae* is a respiratory pathogen, and *M. hominis* and *Ureaplasma urealyticum* are urogenital pathogens. *M. genitalium* is believed to be a genital pathogen. *M. fermentans, M. pirum,* and *M. penetrans* have been isolated from patients with HIV infection, but the pathogenic role of these organisms in association with AIDS is unclear. *M. salivarium, M. orale, M. buccale, M. faucium, M. lipophilum, M. primatum, M. spermatophilum, Acholeplasma laidlawii,* and *A. oculi* are isolated from humans but do not clearly or commonly cause disease.

INFECTIONS CAUSED BY MYCOPLASMA PNEUMONIAE

INCIDENCE AND EPIDEMIOLOGY

Infections with *M. pneumoniae* occur worldwide in all seasons. Pneumonia epidemics tend to occur at 4- to 8-year intervals, usually in the summer and fall. Infections are particularly troublesome among military recruits and college students, among whom the prevalence of *M. pneumoniae* pneumonia may be as high as 44%. In communities the overall prevalence is about 15%. Infection rates are highest among school-aged children and young adults. Illness tends to occur primarily among those 5 to 40 years of age. Thirty percent to 60% of cases of pneumonia that occur among these age groups are caused by *M. pneumoniae.* Although *M. pneumoniae* infections occur among the very young and in the elderly, serious illness appears to be uncommon. Humans are the only known reservoir of *M. pneumoniae.* Infection is spread in respiratory secretions, especially when contact is close. Infection among families usually is introduced by a school-aged child and spreads slowly but extensively.

ETIOLOGY, PATHOGENESIS, AND IMMUNITY

M. pneumoniae organisms are small (10×200 nm), filamentous, and motile. A key step in pathogenesis is binding of the organism to glycoprotein receptors on the luminal surface of ciliated respiratory epithelial cells. A specialized terminal attachment tip in the membrane binds the organism to the cell (Fig. 305.1). The tip contains a 170-kd cytadhesin (P1 protein) and accessory proteins that facilitate cytadherence. Antibodies directed against the P1 protein inhibit attachment and reduce histologic evidence of disease in hamsters. After attachment to host respiratory epithelium, ciliostasis occurs. This injury appears to be mediated through a complex array of virulence determinants, including hydrogen peroxide and superoxide radicals

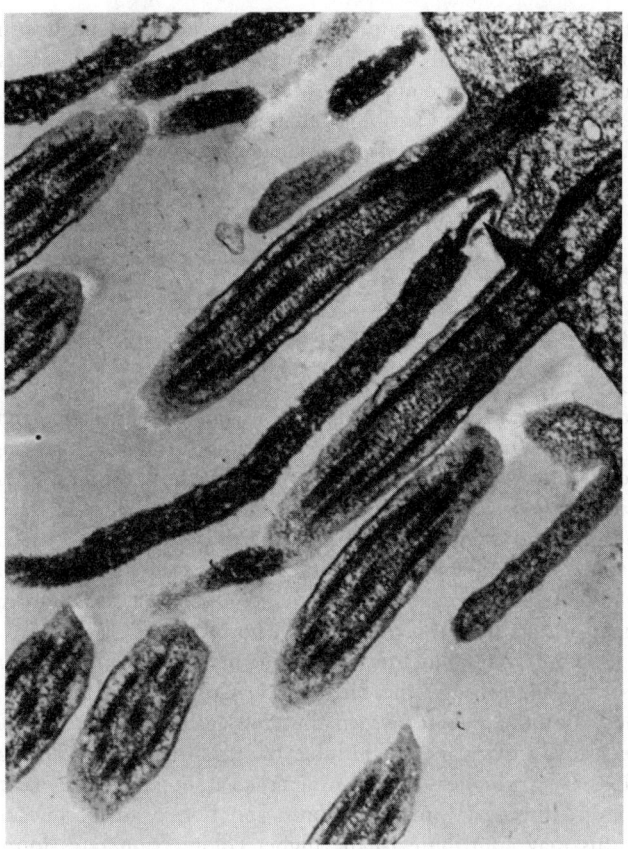

FIGURE 305.1. Electron photomicrograph shows *Mycoplasma pneumoniae* organisms attached to ciliated epithelial cells of a human fetal trachea organ culture. The specialized attachment tip of *M. pneumoniae* is indicated by an *arrow.* (From Collier AM. Pathogenesis of *Mycoplasma pneumoniae* infection as studied in the human foetal trachea in organ culture. *Ciba Found Symp* 1972:307, with permission.)

produced by the organism. Overt destruction of epithelial cells follows ciliostasis, and marked superficial disruption of the respiratory mucosa occurs.

The pathologic changes associated with *M. pneumoniae* infection likely involve host cellular immune processes and processes attributable directly to *M. pneumoniae.* The characteristic histopathologic host response involves peribronchial lymphocytes and plasma cells. Neutrophils and macrophages are present in the peribronchial area and within the bronchial lumen. Bronchitis, bronchiolitis, alveolitis, and interstitial infiltrates have been described. The organism induces a broad range of immunoregulatory events, among them T-cell and B-cell activation and cytokine production.

In recovering from respiratory infection with *M. pneumoniae,* the host produces specific local and systemic antibodies to the organism. Local antibodies may inhibit cytadherence, promote opsonization, or allow antibody-complement–mediated lysis. The presence of local and systemic antibodies has been related to resistance to infection. Immunity to *M. pneumoniae* infection increases with age but is not complete. There are well documented cases of second infection.

CLINICAL FINDINGS

Infections caused by *M. pneumoniae* are manifest most commonly as respiratory tract illnesses. Pneumonia, rhinitis, pharyngitis, otitis media, bullous myringitis, sinusitis, tracheobronchitis, bronchitis, and bronchiolitis are seen. Sometimes *M. pneumoniae* infection manifests itself primarily in extrarespiratory disease. A causal relation exists between *M. pneumoniae* infection and meningoencephalitis. Erythema multiforme (Stevens–Johnson syndrome), meningitis, mononeuritis and polyneuritis, myocarditis, pericarditis, arthritis, and pancreatitis have been reported in association with *M. pneumoniae* infection. The advent of DNA probes and polymerase chain reaction methods promises a better understanding of the etiologic relation between *M. pneumoniae* infection and many of these extrarespiratory manifestations.

For most cases of *M. pneumoniae* pneumonia, the incubation period ranges from 9 to 21 days. Onset is typically insidious with a prodrome of headache, malaise, fever, and upper respiratory tract symptoms. Cough is present in nearly all cases and is initially prominent and nonproductive. Temperature of at least 37.8°C (100°F) is present in 94% of cases and is at least 38.9°C (102°F) in 77% of cases. Chills occur in 58% of cases, but frank rigors are unusual. The patient usually is not toxic, and the physical examination except for rales often is not helpful. Bullous myringitis and rash occur in fewer than 20% of cases. Chest radiographic findings are nonspecific; the findings in as many as 25% of cases are those of segmental bronchopneumonia in the lower lobe or lobes and a small effusion. Leukocytosis is variable (more than 10,000 cells per microliter in only 27% of cases). An elevated cold agglutinin titer may be found in 50% of cases by the second week of illness. Sputum Gram stain does not show a predominant organism. The course of the typical case of *M. pneumoniae* pneumonia, even if untreated, is self-limited and rarely fatal. Nevertheless, uncontrolled illness often persists for 3 to 6 weeks or more and may cause considerable debilitation. Only about 2% of patients with pneumonia need admission to a hospital.

Although the usual case of *M. pneumoniae* pneumonia is mild and easily managed in the ambulatory setting, severe illness requiring hospitalization does occur. The hospitalized person may be previously healthy, have an underlying disease, such as sickle cell disease, or be immunocompromised. Complications occur among 2% to 10% of hospitalized patients. Respiratory complications include relapse, respiratory insufficiency, pneumatocele, lung abscess, bronchiectasis, and bronchiolitis obliterans organizing pneumonia. Extrarespiratory complications include erythema multiforme, meningoencephalitis, meningitis, mononeuritis and polyneuritis, myocarditis, pericarditis, and arthritis. Varied rashes, nephritis, hepatitis, intravascular hemolysis, disseminated intravascular coagulation, thrombocytopenic purpura, Raynaud's phenomenon, cerebellar ataxia, psychosis, transverse myelitis, postinfectious leukoencephalitis, optic neuritis, sudden deafness, and polymyositis have been reported.

Mechanisms underlying extrarespiratory findings in *M. pneumoniae* infection are not clear. Autoimmune mechanisms and toxins have long been postulated. Extrarespiratory spread and tissue invasion seem likely, however. Case reports of accumulate describing isolation of *M. pneumoniae* organisms from skin lesions, from cerebrospinal, pleural, pericardial, and synovial tissues and fluids, and from blood.

LABORATORY FINDINGS

The diagnosis of *M. pneumoniae* requires a careful history and physical examination. Elements of the epidemiologic and clinical history that may implicate the organism must be elucidated. Radiographic evidence of an infiltrate is critical to the diagnosis of pneumonia. The differential diagnosis of mycoplasmal pneumonia is extensive and includes infection with most bacterial and nonbacterial pathogens. The presence of cold agglutinins of the IgM class with anti-I specificity strengthens clinical suspicion, but is not sufficiently specific to confirm a clinical diagnosis of *M. pneumoniae* pneumonia. Infections caused by measles virus, Epstein–Barr virus, adenoviruses, and some tropical parasites have been associated with elevated cold agglutinin antibody titers. Likewise, the absence of cold agglutinins is not a sufficiently sensitive negative finding to exclude the diagnosis of *M. pneumoniae* pneumonia, because only about one-half of cases of *M. pneumoniae* pneumonia are associated with elevated titers of cold agglutinins.

Definitive diagnosis of mycoplasmal pneumonia involves isolation of *M. pneumoniae* on selective media from respiratory exudate. This usually takes 7 to 10 days. DNA probes and polymerase chain reaction methods can be sensitive, specific, and more timely. A fourfold or greater rise in specific antibody titer in convalescence also confirms the diagnosis. Antibodies usually are assayed with the complement fixation or enzyme-linked immunosorbent assay method with sera from the acute and convalescent phases, the latter obtained 4 to 6 weeks after onset of illness. None of the serologic approaches allows easy or rapid diagnosis of *M. pneumoniae* pneumonia.

STRATEGIES FOR OPTIMAL CARE

Because of diagnostic limitations, the decision to initiate therapy for most cases of *M. pneumoniae* pneumonia is empiric. Erythromycin, clarithromycin, azithromycin, ofloxacin, levofloxacin, sparfloxacin, and tetracycline are used for management of *M. pneumoniae* pneumonia. β-Lactam and other antibiotics active on cell wall synthesis are ineffective against *M. pneumoniae* infection because the organism lacks a cell wall.

Erythromycin and tetracycline have proved effective in controlled trials among military recruits and college students in shortening the morbidity of illness and the duration of hospitalization associated with *M. pneumoniae* pneumonia. Erythromycin or tetracycline in dosages of 0.25 to 0.5 g orally every 6 hours is recommended for treatment of selected patients. Intravenous therapy may be used if the patient has severe illness. Tetracycline should not be used to treat children younger than 8 years or pregnant women. Two or 3 weeks of erythromycin or tetracycline therapy is recommended to prevent relapse. Resistance to erythromycin and tetracycline has not emerged as a clinical problem.

Antibiotic therapy is not used for *M. pneumoniae* respiratory illnesses other than pneumonia unless the etiologic diagnosis is clear and the clinical course necessitates intervention. The course of extrarespiratory complications of *M. pneumoniae* infection seems unaffected by antibiotic therapy. There is no vaccine for the prevention of *M. pneumoniae* pneumonia.

■ INFECTIONS CAUSED BY GENITAL MYCOPLASMAS

INCIDENCE AND EPIDEMIOLOGY

U. urealyticum and *M. hominis* are the two species of *Mycoplasma* most frequently isolated from the human genitourinary tract. Both have been associated with a number of urogenital and reproductive diseases. Causal relations have been difficult to establish, however, because both agents may be isolated from healthy and from sick people. Nevertheless, a consensus has emerged that etiologically links these two species of genital *Mycoplasma* with selected urogenital infections and systemic infections among immunocompromised hosts.

Colonization of infants with genital mycoplasmas occurs during passage through the birth canal. Colonization rates then decrease until puberty, when they rise again in direct relation to sexual activity and the number of sexual partners. Colonization rates are higher among women than among men. Pregnancy may predispose a woman to colonization. Race or socioeconomic status may contribute to the higher colonization rates found among blacks than among whites and among patients attending municipal clinics rather than private clinics.

ETIOLOGY AND PATHOGENESIS

Results of inoculation studies with human and primate subjects have firmly established *U. urealyticum* as a cause of nongonococcal urethritis. At least 10% of cases of nongonococcal urethritis are caused by this organism. *M. genitalium* may also be a pathogen in this setting. Serologic examinations of some patients with pelvic inflammatory disease and its complications implicate *M. hominis* as an etiologic agent. In experiments in monkeys, isolates of *M. hominis* have produced salpingitis.

A causative role for *M. hominis* in postabortal and postpartum fever is supported by results of serologic studies and isolation of the organism from the blood. A probable role for *U. urealyticum* in chorioamnionitis is suggested by the results of serologic studies, isolation of the organism in pure culture from amnionic fluid, and isolation from the blood. Both *M. hominis* and *U. urealyticum* have been isolated from urine in cases of lower urinary tract disease, but only *M. hominis* has been implicated etiologically with culture and serologic data as an agent in in acute pyelonephritis.

There are well-documented reports of associations between *U. urealyticum* and *M. hominis* and septic arthritis in settings of hypogammaglobulinemia and immunosuppression. *M. hominis* and *U. urealyticum* organisms have been isolated from cultures of pericardial fluid and tissue in cases of pericarditis. *M. hominis* infection also has been associated with neonatal meningitis, meningoencephalitis, brain abscess, fever among burn and trauma patients, sternotomy infections, and extragenital infections among recipients of solid-organ transplants.

The pathogenetic mechanisms of the genital mycoplasmas are not well understood. Both *U. urealyticum* and *M. hominis* appear capable of adsorbing to the surface of mammalian cells and replicating. Subsequent structural and functional changes in sperm and fallopian ciliary cells have been found. The cytopathic effect induced by *U. urealyticum* has been related to its urealytic activity and subsequent release of ammonium ions. *M. genitalium* appears to have a specialized terminal attachment structure and a cytadhesin resembling the *M. pneumoniae* P1 protein.

CLINICAL AND LABORATORY FINDINGS

Genital mycoplasmal infection has been etiologically associated with nongonococcal urethritis, pelvic inflammatory disease and its complications, chorioamnionitis, postpartum and postabortal fever, and pyelonephritis. The clinical presentations of these infections are discussed in detail in Chapter 272. Exclusion of other, more common pathogens associated with a given urogenital clinical syndrome, such as *Neisseria gonorrhoeae* and *Chlamydia trachomatis* in urethritis, is a crucial part of diagnosis.

Definitive diagnosis requires laboratory isolation of the organism from the infection site in the absence of other pathogens. Culture techniques for isolation of genital mycoplasmas can be performed in many hospital microbiology laboratories. Isolation of genital mycoplasmas is optimized by immediate inoculation of the specimen into appropriate selective media and rapid transport to the laboratory for incubation. Unlike *M. pneumoniae* organisms, which have a long incubation time, genital mycoplasmas grow in culture within 1 to 3 days.

In interpreting culture results, it is important to remember that sexually active persons often are colonized with genital mycoplasmas. These colonize the urethral mucosa of men and may be found under the foreskin. In women, the organisms are found most frequently in the vagina but also are present in the endocervical canal and periurethral area.

STRATEGIES FOR OPTIMAL CARE

Even when diagnostic techniques to detect mycoplasmal urogenital infections are available, they may not be clinically useful because of the time inherent in culturing the organisms. Therapy for these infections therefore is almost inevitably empiric. It is in the clinical setting of antibiotic failure in the management of presumed bacterial urogenital infection that culturing of blood or the genital site for mycoplasmas may be most helpful in patient care.

Tetracycline and erythromycin continue to be the mainstays of therapy for presumed genital mycoplasmal infections. Azithromycin, other new macrolides, and fluoroquinolones are of increasing therapeutic value, however, because the prevalence of clinically significant tetracycline resistance is increasing among persons with *U. urealyticum* of *M. hominis* infection. Tetracycline should not be used to treat pregnant women or children younger than 8 years or in situations in which tetracycline resistance is suspected.

Erythromycin may be used as therapy for suspected or proven

U. urealyticum infections when tetracycline is contraindicated. Clindamycin may be used as alternative therapy for suspected or proven *M. hominis* infection. In vitro tests of antibiotic susceptibility may be used to guide therapy for genital mycoplasmal infections in which antibiotic resistance is a factor. The routine use of antimycoplasmal agents in empiric therapy for urogenital or other conditions in which a mycoplasmal cause has not been proved is not recommended.

BIBLIOGRAPHY

Baseman JB, Tully JG. Mycoplasmas: sophisticated, reemerging, and burdened by their notoriety. *Emerg Infect Dis* 1997;3:21–32.

Baum SG. *Mycoplasma pneumoniae* and atypical pneumonia. In: Mandell G, Bennett JE, Dolin R, eds. *Mandell, Douglas and Bennett's principles and practice of infectious diseases*, 4th ed. New York: Churchill Livingstone, 1995:1704.

Cassell GH, Waites KB, Watson HL, et al. *Ureaplasma urealyticum* intrauterine infection: role in prematurity and disease in newborns. *Clin Microbiol Rev* 1993;6:69–87.

Chanock RM, Hayflick L, Barile MF. Growth on artificial medium of an agent associated with atypical pneumonia and its identification as a PPLO. *Proc Natl Acad Sci USA* 1962;48:41.

Collier AM. Pathogenesis of *Mycoplasma pneumoniae* infection as studied in the human foetal trachea in organ culture. *Ciba Found Symp* 1972:307.

Kolski H, Ford-Jones EL, Richardson S, et al. Etiology of acute childhood encephalitis at the Hospital for Sick Children, Toronto, 1994–1995. *Clin Infect Dis* 1998;26:398–409.

Steingrimsson O, Olafsson JH, Thorarinsson H, et al. Single dose azithromycin treatment of gonorrhea and infections caused by *C. trachomatis* and *U. urealyticum* in men. *Sex Transm Dis* 1994;21:43–46.

Taylor-Robinson D. Infections due to species of *M.* and *Ureaplasma*: an update. *Clin Infect Dis* 1996;23:671.

Taylor-Robinson D, Bébéar C. Antibiotic susceptibilities of mycoplasmas and treatment of mycoplasmal infections. *J Antimicrob Chemother* 1997;40:622–630.

Valencia GB, Banzon F, Cummings M, et al. *Mycoplasma hominis* and *Ureaplasma urealyticum* in neonates with suspected infection. *Pediatr Infect Dis J* 1993;12:571–573.

Kelley's Textbook of Internal Medicine, fourth edition. Edited by H. David Humes.
Lippincott Williams & Wilkins, Philadelphia © 2000.

C H A P T E R
306

CHLAMYDIAL INFECTIONS

ROBERT B. JONES

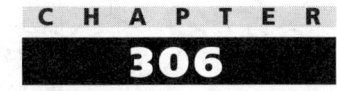 ## DEFINITION

The order Chlamydiales contains only a single genus, *Chlamydia,* and four species (Table 306.1) only three of which are associated with infection among humans—*C. psittaci, C. trachomatis,* and *C. pneumoniae.* Organisms in all three species are

TABLE 306.1.	CLASSIFICATION OF *CHLAMYDIA* SPECIES		
Species	**Biovar/Serovar**	**Primary Host**	**Associated Diseases in Humans**
C. psittaci	Many unclassified serovars	Tropical birds, domestic fowl, mammals	Atypical pneumonia, culture-negative endocarditis
C. pneumoniae	Single strain, TWAR	Humans	Pharyngitis, bronchitis, and atypical pneumonia
C. trachomatis	Lymphogranuloma venereum biovar Serovars: L₁, L₂, L₃ Trachoma biovar	Humans	Lymphogranuloma venereum, proctocolitis
	Serovars: A–C, Ba	Humans	Ocular trachoma
	Serovars: D–K	Humans	Inclusion conjunctivitis, urethritis, cervicitis, epididymitis, endometritis, salpingitis, proctitis, infant pneumonia
	Mouse pneumonitis biovar: single strain recognized	Mice	None
C. pecorum	Many unclassified serovars	Swine, ruminants, marsupials (koala)	None

obligate, intracellular parasites with a relatively complex life cycle (Fig. 306.1). The extracellular forms (elementary bodies) attach to susceptible cells and induce their own ingestion but are able to inhibit fusion of lysosomes with the endocytic vacuole. Thus they escape intracellular destruction and live in a protected environment inside the cell, where they reorganize into their replicative forms (reticulate bodies) and divide by means of binary fission. They are energy parasites in that high-energy phosphate compounds, as well as essential amino acids, are supplied by the host cell. Continuing replication results in an intracytoplasmic inclusion that ultimately fills the infected cell. The reticulate bodies then reorganize into elementary bodies, and the inclusion is either extruded from the cell or the cell is lysed to allow the cycle to continue. Despite many biologic similarities, there is less than 10% DNA homology among the three species.

Multiple strains of *C. psittaci* cause a wide variety of diseases among birds and other animals. TWAR is the only recognized strain of *C. pneumoniae*. *C. trachomatis* contains two biovars that infect humans. On the basis of degree of antigenic relatedness, these have been subdivided into 15 well-characterized serovars or strains (Table 306.1).

INCIDENCE AND EPIDEMIOLOGY

PSITTACOSIS

Most cases of psittacosis among humans are caused by contact with infected birds, especially members of the parrot family (psit-

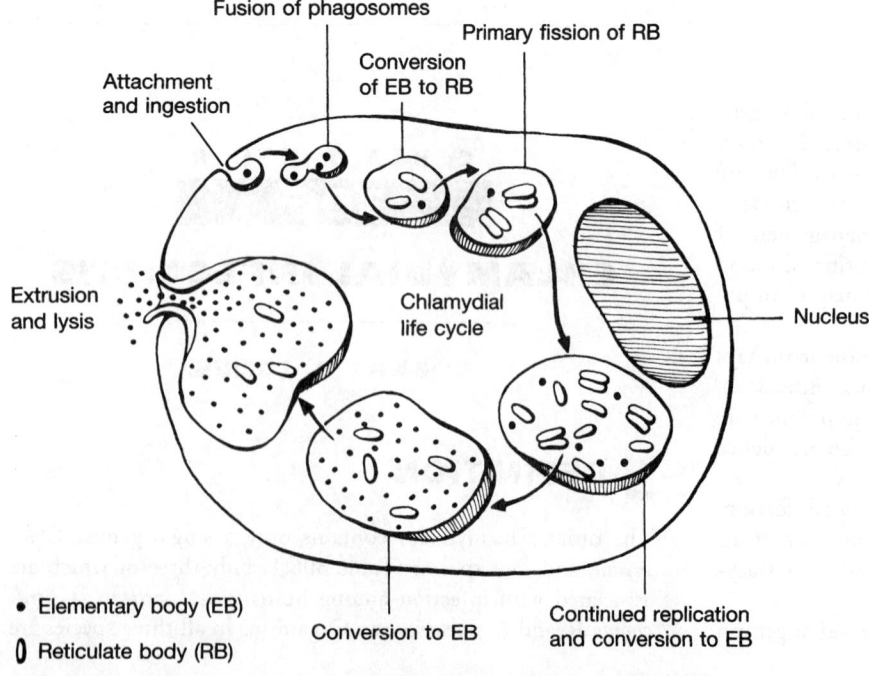

FIGURE 306.1. Schematic of life cycle of *Chlamydia trachomatis* organism. *C. psittaci* and *C. pneumoniae* organisms have similar life cycles but often have multiple cytoplasmic inclusions in each infected cell, unlike the one large inclusion of *C. trachomatis*.

tacine), such as parakeets or cockatiels. However, outbreaks also have been associated with exposure to turkeys in poultry-processing plants. *C. psittaci* can be recovered from the tissue, feathers, and droppings of infected birds. Humans are infected as a result of handling the sick birds or being exposed to aerosols of their excreta. Less than 500 cases per year are reported in the United States.

CHLAMYDIA PNEUMONIAE INFECTION

Clustering of cases suggests human-to-human transmission for what appears to be a fairly common cause of mild lower respiratory disease. Moreover, a growing body of evidence suggests that *C. pneumoniae* also may cause more severe disease, including pneumonia, either as a primary or a copathogen with other bacteria. Reinfection appears to be common. Epidemiologic and anatomic evidence suggests that chronic *C. pneumoniae* infection may play a role in the pathogenesis of atherosclerosis and coronary artery disease.

OCULOGENITAL INFECTIONS

C. trachomatis infection is among the most prevalent sexually transmitted diseases. In industrialized nations infection occurs among a substantial proportion of sexually active adults in both symptomatic and asymptomatic forms (Table 306.2). Infection is epidemiologically linked to younger age, nonwhite race, and level of sexual activity as determined by frequency of intercourse or number of partners. Transmission among adults is almost entirely a result of sexual activity, although ocular infection can occur as a result of autoinoculation with infected genital secretions. Untreated chlamydial urethritis or cervicitis resolves over

TABLE 306.2.	PRESENTATION AND APPROXIMATE PREVALENCE OF *CHLAMYDIA TRACHOMATIS* INFECTION IN SEXUALLY ACTIVE POPULATIONS

Presentation	Prevalence (%)
Men	
Nongonococcal urethritis	≈40
Gonococcal urethritis	≈20
No or ignored symptoms[a]	10–28
Women	
Gonorrhea	30–50
Sexual contact with partner with urethritis (gonococcal or nongonococcal)	33–66
Clinical diagnosis of pelvic inflammatory disease	20
Routine examination	
Family planning clinic	5.2–9
Adolescent clinic	9–28
College student health service	8–9

[a] Screening examination for condition not related to urogenital tract.

a few weeks in most instances, although the organism can persist for years in the absence of effective therapy. Identification of the organism does not always mean recent acquisition of infection. Presence of the organism alone should not be interpreted as prima facie evidence of recent sexual activity with a new partner. Among 20% to 30% of untreated women, the infection progresses to symptomatic salpingitis, and among an unknown proportion to asymptomatic endometritis or salpingitis. There is compelling evidence that urogenital infection with *C. trachomatis* is a risk factor for transmission or acquisition of HIV among both men and women. Serologic studies indicate that approximately 70% of infants born to infected women acquire the organism during passage through the infected birth canal. Ten percent to 30% contract inclusion conjunctivitis, pneumonia, or both.

PATHOGENESIS

PSITTACOSIS

Infection of human usually is a result of inhalation of infective elementary bodies. Progressive localized pneumonia can then occur. More frequently, however, the organism spreads hematogenously to the liver and spleen and, after additional growth at these sites, infects the lungs and other organs. Carditis, pericarditis, or endocarditis may occur. When pulmonary involvement is minimal, endocarditis may be the predominant manifestation.

OCULOGENITAL INFECTIONS

C. trachomatis is capable of infecting transitional and columnar epithelial cells of the conjunctiva, respiratory tract, and urogenital tract. Strains of the lymphogranuloma venereum (LGV) biovar are capable of infecting monocytes and macrophages. Primary infection with the trachoma biovar of *C. trachomatis* causes a polymorphonuclear leukocytic response of variable duration followed by infiltration of mononuclear cells and local lymphoid hypertrophy. Uncontrolled infection may resolve spontaneously or progress to low-grade persistent infection. In either case, it usually does not produce serious sequelae unless it is reactivated or reinfection occurs. In hyperendemic areas of ocular trachoma, reinfection is common. Reactivation also is a result of bacterial conjunctivitis. Flies play a major role in transmission. Findings characteristic of ocular trachoma include lymphoid follicular conjunctivitis with scarring, keratitis, and vascular pannus formation (pannus is a fibroid vascular infiltration across the limbus). Pannus formation and scarring cause distortion of the lid margins such that the eyelashes can turn in and scrape the bulbar conjunctiva, causing further scarring and blindness.

The urethra or endocervix usually is the initial site infected in the genital tract. The resulting degree of inflammation is variable, and the infection may resolve spontaneously, progress to more severe disease, especially in women, or evolve into a low-grade, persistent infection. In many if not all cases of endocervical infection, there is concurrent or subsequent involvement of the endometrium and fallopian tubes. The intensity of the inflammatory response is presumed to be a function of the host's earlier experience with the organism and the resulting immune status. Chlamydial endometritis is characterized by a plasma cell infiltrate with associated lymphoid hypertrophy. When the fallopian tubes are involved, clinically apparent or subclinical salpingitis may develop, and scarring, distortion, and blockage of the tubes occur. Such changes can lead to ectopic pregnancy or infertility.

The pathogenesis of adult or infant inclusion conjunctivitis is similar to that of initial infection in ocular trachoma. Repeated cycles of reinfection or reactivation of persistent infection do not occur, however, and serious sequelae are uncommon.

LYMPHOGRANULOMA VENEREUM

Although there frequently is a lesion at the site of initial inoculation, the primary manifestations of LGV infection are lymphangitis in the regional nodes draining the inoculation site. Among men, these usually are the inguinal nodes, and the enlarged, fluctuant nodes are called *buboes*. These may break down and drain spontaneously, producing cutaneous fistulas. Among women, the regional nodes frequently are sacral and perirectal. When these nodes suppurate and drain, they may produce rectal strictures and rectal or vaginal fistulas.

■ CLINICAL AND LABORATORY FINDINGS

PSITTACOSIS

Psittacosis usually begins suddenly with chills and a high fever 7 to 15 days after exposure. Severe headache, myalgia, and a persistent, dry cough are common. Physical findings usually are minimal and may consist only of rales in the lower lung fields. Nontender hepatomegaly is frequent, and palpable splenomegaly is present in 10% to 70% of patients. A pulse-temperature dissociation (a normal or slow heart rate at the time of a high temperature) is a frequent observation. Routine laboratory studies usually are not helpful. A chest radiograph usually reveals a patchy interstitial infiltrate, although lobar infiltrates also occur. The disease should be considered when there is a history of contact with pet birds or the patient is a poultry worker, has culture-negative endocarditis, or has non–hospital-acquired pneumonia not responsive to cell wall–active antibiotics, such as penicillin or cephalosporins.

CHLAMYDIA PNEUMONIAE INFECTION

Symptoms associated with *C. pneumoniae* infection of the respiratory tract include fever, cough, and sore throat (often with laryngitis). Clinical or laboratory evidence of pneumonia or bronchitis is common. However, it is difficult to differentiate pneumonia caused by *C. pneumoniae* from that caused by other bacterial pathogens, because the other pathogens frequently are recovered in association with serologic evidence of *C. pneumoniae* infection. Young people with *C. pneumoniae* infection usually have normal white blood cell and differential counts. Specific symptoms have not been associated with *C. pneumoniae* endo-

vascular infection, although such infections may be a precursor to the development of atherosclerosis.

OCULAR *CHLAMYDIA TRACHOMATIS* INFECTION

Ocular infection with *C. trachomatis* causes conjunctivitis. Signs and symptoms include a foreign body sensation, photophobia, erythema, and a mucopurulent discharge. Among infants who acquire the infection at birth, evidence of infection appears 2 to 25 days after birth. Without therapy, resolution occurs over several months, but chlamydiae may be recovered from the eye or nasopharynx for additional months thereafter. Specific therapy shortens the duration of disease and should be systemic. Adults usually have concurrent genital tract infection; infants have nasopharyngeal colonization.

UROGENITAL *CHLAMYDIA TRACHOMATIS* INFECTION

Urethral infection with *C. trachomatis* among men produces dysuria and a discharge that usually is scant and watery but occasionally is copious and purulent. Chlamydial urethritis among women usually is asymptomatic, but there may be associated dysuria and pyuria. Endocervical infection often produces a purulent discharge that is yellowish-green when viewed against the white background of a swab. The presence of a mucopurulent discharge and friability (bleeding after swabbing) of the endocervix is highly suggestive of chlamydial infection. *C. trachomatis* does not infect the squamous epithelial lining of the vagina of an adult but can infect the transitional epithelium of the prepubertal vagina and can cause vaginitis among prepubertal girls. Endometritis causes abdominal pain and changes in the pattern or volume of menstrual flow. Salpingitis produces abdominal pain. Salpingitis and endometritis may coexist. The intensity of pain varies considerably, but often it is fairly mild in spite of severe inflammatory disease that involves the fallopian tubes. Uncontrolled, the disease runs a protracted course with sequelae that include infertility, ectopic pregnancy, and chronic pelvic pain.

EPIDIDYMITIS, PROCTITIS, AND REITER'S SYNDROME

One percent to 3% of men with nongonococcal urethritis have chlamydial epididymitis. The usual initial symptoms are scrotal pain and swelling. Among heterosexual men younger than 35 years, *C. trachomatis* and *Neisseria gonorrhoeae* are the agents most frequently responsible for epididymitis. *C. trachomatis* infection also is associated with proctitis and proctocolitis, primarily among homosexual men. Symptoms include rectal discharge, pain, tenesmus, and constipation. Ulceration and bleeding of the rectal mucosa may be found at proctoscopy and granuloma formation at biopsy. Reiter's syndrome is characterized by urethritis, arthritis, uveitis, and lesions of the skin and mucous membranes. The cause is unknown, but it probably represents a disordered immune response to any of several infectious agents.

INFANT PNEUMONIA

The onset of *C. trachomatis* pneumonia among newborns usually is between 2 weeks and 3 months after birth. The infant has no fever but has a staccato cough and associated tachypnea, rales, and pulmonary hyperinfiltration. Signs of diffuse interstitial pneumonia are present on a chest radiograph, and there is often eosinophilia with elevated serum γ-globulin levels. If the patient is not treated, the clinical illness lasts several weeks. Rales and radiographic abnormalities may persist for months and pulmonary function abnormalities for years.

◼ DIAGNOSIS AND STRATEGIES FOR OPTIMAL CARE

CHLAMYDIA PSITTACOSIS INFECTION

Although *C. psittaci* organisms can be recovered relatively easily in tissue culture, they are hazardous organisms with which to work. Culture consequently is performed in only a few highly specialized laboratories. A fourfold rise in anti-chlamydial antibodies measured with the complement fixation test is considered diagnostic. Such increases usually occur by the end of the second week of illness. A single titer of at least 1:32 is considered presumptive evidence if a patient has a compatible illness. Early treatment with tetracycline, however, can delay the appearance of serum antibody for several weeks, and confirmation may necessitate repetition of serologic testing during an extended period of follow-up evaluation. *C. psittaci* organisms are not susceptible to the cell wall–active antibiotics that are most often used to treat patients with pneumonia. However, they are sensitive to tetracycline, doxycycline, erythromycin, and chloramphenicol, and the response to therapy usually is quite good.

CHLAMYDIA PNEUMONIAE INFECTION

Cultures for *C. pneumoniae* organisms and serologic testing for antibodies to them are performed in only a few research laboratories. Specific antibody can be measured by means of microimmunofluorescence with a *C. pneumoniae* elementary body antigen. Serologic criteria that have been proposed as diagnostic are (a) current infection (acute phase), fourfold or greater increase in antibody titer, IgM titer of at least 1:16, or IgG of at least 1:512 and (b) past infection and IgG titer of 1:16 to 1:512. Lower respiratory tract infections due to *C. pneumoniae* among young immunocompetent patients are relatively mild illnesses that respond to bed rest. Many patients, however, do not recover promptly and have a persistent cough for 1 to 2 months. Administration of tetracycline seems to shorten this duration considerably. Erythromycin is less effective. The course of *C. pneumoniae* infection among more seriously ill patients and the effectiveness of treatment are not known.

CHLAMYDIA TRACHOMATIS INFECTION

A presumptive diagnosis of LGV often can be made from the clinical presentation. Confirmation may be obtained through recovery of the organism from aspirated bubo material or by means of serologic testing. Serologic test results highly suggestive of LGV in an appropriate clinical setting are a single titer of at least 1:64, a fourfold increase in complement-fixing antibodies, or a microimmunofluorescent titer of at least 1:512 against an LGV serotype.

Except for LGV, serologic testing for chlamydia is not useful in the diagnosis of acute *C. trachomatis* infection, but *C. trachomatis* can be recovered in tissue culture from most persons with infection. Culture has been the standard against which other diagnostic tests have been measured. The sensitivity of culture in detection of oculogenital disease is approximately 70%, and the specificity is greater than 99%. Other tests include those used to detect chlamydiae by means of enzyme-linked immunosorbent assay, immunofluorescence, or nucleic acid hybridization. All these methods are less sensitive and specific than culture but are easily performed and relatively inexpensive. They may be of value for screening under some circumstances. Amplification tests based on detection of chlamydial DNA by means of polymerase (PCR) or ligase (LCR) chain reactions or specific chlamydial rRNA with transcription-mediated amplification (TMA) are available now (PCR and LCR) or soon will be (TMA). They are considerably more sensitive than culture and only slightly less specific. In some instances they can be used to detect *C. trachomatis* organisms in urine or on vaginal swabs, thereby obviating invasive sample collection. In the near future one or more of these techniques is likely to become the method of choice for the diagnosis of genitourinary *C. trachomatis* infection.

Early treatment appears to be effective. For approximately 95% of men and women with chlamydial infection, a 1-week course of doxycycline 100 mg orally twice a day or azithromycin 1 g orally as a single dose is sufficient to eradicate the infection. Most patients so treated who have infection after completion of therapy either did not complete the course of therapy or have

TABLE 306.3.	INDICATIONS FOR EMPIRIC THERAPY FOR POSSIBLE *CHLAMYDIA TRACHOMATIS* INFECTION
Men	**Women**
Sexual contact with partner with chlamydial infection or gonorrhea	Sexual contact with partner with chlamydial infection or gonorrhea
Urethritis (gonococcal or nongonococcal)	Sexual contact with partner with urethritis (gonococcal or nongonococcal)
Epididymitis (age <35 y)	Gonorrhea
	Clinical diagnosis of pelvic inflammatory disease
	?Mucopurulent cervicitis[a]

[a] Diagnosis imprecise. May either treat empirically or test for presence of *C. trachomatis* and *Neisseria gonorrhoeae* and base treatment on test results.

been reinfected. Notification and treatment of sexual partners is a critical component of care. Patients with complicated chlamydial infections such as salpingitis, epididymitis, and proctitis usually are treated for 2 weeks, but few data suggest that the longer course of therapy is more beneficial. No diagnostic test is 100% sensitive, and rapid diagnostic testing is not always feasible. Persons at high risk for infection should be treated empirically, regardless of test results (Table 306.3). Because a high proportion of persons with *C. trachomatis* infection have no symptoms, routine screening with an appropriate diagnostic test should be performed annually for all sexually active women 20 years of age or younger and for any woman with a history of multiple or new sexual partners since last test or a clinical diagnosis of mucopurulent cervicitis.

Oculogenital *C. trachomatis* infection can be prevented by means of education to avoid circumstances that may lead to transmission (to avoid "unsafe" sex) and by means of finding and treating persons with infection to reduce the pool of carriers. Where active control programs have been in place for some period of time, as in Seattle, Washington, and Indianapolis, Indiana, there have been declines in overall isolation rates of chlamydiae from patients attending sexually transmitted disease clinics.

BIBLIOGRAPHY

Black CM. Current methods of laboratory diagnosis of *Chlamydia trachomatis* infections. *Clin Microbiol Rev* 1997;10:160–184.

Centers for Disease Control and Prevention. Recommendations for the prevention and management of *Chlamydia trachomatis* infections. *MMWR Morb Mortal Wkly Rep* 1993;42:1–39.

Centers for Disease Control and Prevention. HIV prevention through early detection and treatment of other sexually transmitted diseases—United States. *MMWR Morb Mortal Wkly Rep* 1998;47:1–24.

Dawson CR, Schachter J. Strategies for treatment and control of blinding trachoma: cost-effectiveness of tropical or systemic antibiotics. *Rev Infect Dis* 1985;7:768–773.

Gaydos CA, Howell MR, Pare B, et al. *Chlamydia trachomatis* infections in female military recruits. *N Engl J Med* 1998;339:739–744.

Grayston JT. Infections caused by *Chlamydia pneumoniae* strain TWAR. *Clin Infect Dis* 1992;15:757–761.

Jones RB. *Chlamydia trachomatis* (trachoma, perinatal infections, lymphogranuloma venereum, and other genital infections). In: Mandell GL, Bennett JE, Dolin R, eds. *Principles and practice of infectious diseases,* 4th ed. New York: Churchill Livingstone, 1994:1679.

Perine PL, Osoba AO. Lymphogranuloma venereum. In: Holmes KK, Mardh PA, Sparling PF, et al., eds. *Sexually transmitted diseases,* 2nd ed. New York: McGraw-Hill, 1990:195.

Schachter J. Diagnosis of *Chlamydia trachomatis* infection. In: Orfila J, Byrne GI, Chernesky MA, et al., eds. *Chlamydial infections: proceedings of the Eighth International Symposium on Human Chlamydial Infections.* Bologna, Italy: Società Editrice Esculapio, 1994:293.

Schlossberg D. *Chlamydia psittaci* (psittacosis). In: Mandell GL, Bennett JE, Dolin R, eds. *Principles and practice of infectious diseases,* 4th ed. New York: Churchill Livingstone, 1994:1693.

Shepard MK, Jones RB. Recovery of *Chlamydia trachomatis* from endometrial and fallopian tube biopsies in women with infertility of tubal origin. *Fertil Steril* 1989;52:232–238.

C H A P T E R

307

INFECTIONS CAUSED BY ARBOVIRUSES

JAMES P. LUBY

Arboviruses are grouped by the three separate categories of disease they cause: encephalitis, hemorrhagic fever, and fever with or without a rash and arthralgias. Although this classification scheme is generally valid, some arboviruses cause disease in more than one category. For example, dengue viruses can elicit fever with a rash and arthralgias, but under certain circumstances they can also provoke hemorrhagic fever. Arboviruses also can be grouped by the geographic regions in which disease occurs. Although these geographic regions can be extensive, they are also restricted by the specific epidemiologic characteristics of the viruses. For example, St. Louis encephalitis (SLE) virus mostly causes disease in the western, midwestern, and southern United States. It exists in enzootic form in Central and South America, where it infrequently leads to disease. It does not exist outside the Western Hemisphere. Because arboviruses are geographically restricted, they may be named for the primary location where disease occurs or where they were first isolated. Sometimes arbovirus names are given by the affected native population and describe a disease manifestation, like chikungunya fever, literally meaning "that which bends up," which refers to the transient, severe joint pains that develop during the illness. Infections caused by arboviruses can be endemic, but one of the major reasons they incite fear is that they have the potential of producing epidemic disease. Epidemics can evolve with such intensity that they interrupt normal societal functioning.

◼ MICROBIOLOGY

Arboviruses causing human disease belong to four virus families: Togaviridae, Flaviviridae, Bunyaviridae, and Reoviridae. In the family Togaviridae, viruses in the *Alphavirus* genus include eastern equine encephalitis (EEE) and western equine encephalitis (WEE) viruses. Examples of flaviviruses include SLE virus and dengue virus. Members of the California encephalitis (CE) virus group belong to the Bunyaviridae family. Colorado tick fever virus, which belongs to the *Orbivirus* genus, is the most prominent member of the family Reoviridae. Alphaviruses are positive-sense, single-stranded RNA viruses 60 to 70 nm in diameter; the capsid with icosahedral symmetry becomes enveloped by primary budding through the plasma membrane. Flaviviruses are smaller positive-sense, single-stranded RNA viruses, 40 to 50 nm in diameter, with capsids of uncertain symmetry that become enveloped by budding into cytoplasmic vacuoles. Bunyaviridae family viruses are divided into several genera. They are about 100 nm in diameter and possess a negative-sense message that is coded in three distinct RNA segments. The virus of Colorado tick fever contains 12 genomic segments of double-stranded RNA.

ENCEPHALITIS

Arboviruses included in this category usually cause encephalitic illness, with fever, nuchal rigidity, and signs of deep-seated involvement of the central nervous system. Encephalitic illness is associated with cerebrospinal fluid (CSF) pleocytosis, a normal CSF glucose level, and a normal or elevated CSF protein concentration. Viruses in this group less commonly also produce aseptic meningitis (headache, stiff neck, and fever) or an afebrile headache (headache, fever without a stiff neck). All these viruses provoke asymptomatic infection, with variable ratios of asymptomatic infection to clinical cases. In the Western Hemisphere, the major arboviruses producing disease are EEE virus, WEE virus, Venezuelan equine encephalitis (VEE) virus, SLE virus, and the CE group of viruses (Table 307.1). Arboviruses of lesser importance that cause disease in localized areas include Powassan virus in North America, a flavivirus that is transmitted by ticks, and Rocio virus, a mosquito-borne flavivirus that has led to localized epidemics in Brazil.

The viruses of EEE, WEE, and SLE are maintained in nature by a mosquito-bird-mosquito transmission cycle, with humans being an end point in the cycle, because viremia of sufficient magnitude to infect mosquitoes does not develop in humans. CE and VEE viruses are maintained in nature by a mosquito–small mammal–mosquito cycle. When VEE virus becomes epizootic and epidemic, epidemiologically virulent subtypes of virus move into equine populations, where they can multiply to high titers in serum and serve as the virus source for mosquitoes. Powassan virus is maintained in a tick–small mammal–tick cycle, and Rocio virus most probably is maintained in a mosquito–bird–mosquito cycle. As far as is known, under natural circumstances SLE virus, the CE virus group, Rocio, and Powassan viruses cause disease only in humans. The arthropod vector remains infected for its lifetime and apparently is unharmed by the infection.

Cases of arthropod-borne encephalitis develop in the summer and early autumn months. Epidemics are often related to spring flooding or lack of spring rains and consequent stagnation of water and an excessive mosquito population. SLE is the most significant public health problem of the American arthropod-borne encephalitides, in terms of numbers of cases and its capacity to cause urban epidemics. Disease arises in urban and suburban Florida and in the midwestern and southern United States. Because of the mosquito vectors involved, SLE virus has the capacity to produce epidemics in cities (St. Louis, 1933; Tampa Bay, 1962; Houston, 1964; Dallas, 1966; Corpus Christi, 1966; Chicago, 1975). The CE virus group has member viruses that cause disease in various parts of North America. La Crosse virus is the major pathogen prompting disease. Rocio virus has caused disease in Brazil.

The ages of people infected by these viruses vary. EEE primarily affects infants, young children, and elderly people. In terms of severity, it is the most lethal arthropod-borne viral infection in the United States. WEE has a particular tendency to affect infants, whereas VEE usually causes disease in everyone infected. SLE principally affects older people in urban areas during epidemics. The reason for this predilection is not known, because

TABLE 307.1.	ARBOVIRUS ENCEPHALITIDES IN NORTH AMERICA			
Encephalitis	Virus	Vector	Geographic Distribution	Distinguishing Features
St. Louis	Flavivirus	Mosquito	Central, southern, western United States	Summer–fall epidemics in urban areas, especially involving elderly patients; endemic western rural spread
Eastern equine	Alphavirus	Mosquito	Eastern, southeastern United States; Caribbean	Disease in equines precedes human disease, most lethal arbovirus encephalitis in United States
Western equine	Alphavirus	Mosquito	Western, central United States; Canada	Disease in equines precedes human disease; case fatality rate in infants approximates 50%
Venezuelan equine	Alphavirus	Mosquito	Central, South America; Mexico; infrequent cases in Florida and Texas	Disease in equines precedes, human disease; all infected humans become ill; case fatality rate <1%
California	Bunyavirus, family Bunaviridae	Mosquito	Midwestern United States, West Virginia	Forest exposure in boys; case fatality rate <5%; sometimes mimics herpes simplex encephalitis
Powassan	Flavivirus	Tick	Canada; New York State	Encephalitis in people with forest exposure

infection rates during epidemics of this virus do not vary by age. CE particularly affects boys, since they go into the woods for recreational pursuits. Powassan virus causes disease related to intrusion into forested areas, and Rocio virus causes encephalitis most often in men working in forests.

Although the most common manifestation of infection is inapparent or asymptomatic, encephalitis is the usual clinical presentation of full-blown disease. The only exception is VEE, in which the typical feature is febrile headache. Patients with arthropod-borne encephalitis experience abrupt onset of illness with headache, fever, nausea and vomiting, and neck stiffness. They become somnolent, lethargic, and confused. Patients with SLE tend to have substantia nigra and extrapyramidal involvement—tremulousness is a prominent feature of the illness. Patients are usually seen by their physicians relatively early in the course of illness, with the aforementioned clinical history. On physical examination, the patient has fever, confusion, a stiff neck, possible seizure activity, and, occasionally, localizing neurologic abnormalities; tremulousness is evident in patients with SLE and in adults with WEE. The single most important laboratory examination is that of the CSF. The test almost always shows pleocytosis, a normal glucose level, and a normal or elevated protein concentration, particularly if a second lumbar puncture is performed. The case fatality rate in EEE at the extremes of life may approach 75%. WEE is particularly lethal in infancy. With SLE, the case fatality rate increases with age and can approach 30% in people older than 60 years of age. In CE, the case fatality rate usually is less than 5%, but localizing abnormalities may be found, and the differential diagnosis then includes infection with this virus and encephalitis due to herpes simplex virus.

It is critical for the physician to be aware that he or she will probably encounter one or more cases of arthropod-borne encephalitis at some time in their careers. In clinical terms, the disease cannot be distinguished with certainty from encephalitis caused by other agents, but if cases of encephalitis occur in close proximity in summer and autumn or if one or more of these patients die from encephalitis, diagnostic specimens should be sent immediately to an appropriate laboratory where tests can be performed. Two or three cases of encephalitis associated with tremulousness in elderly people during the summertime in a large city may be the harbingers of an SLE epidemic. Because there are potent means to bring these epidemics to a close—namely, the use of insecticide spraying—the diagnosis should be pursued vigorously. Diagnosis is usually made on the basis of a rise in titer between serial serum specimens by enzyme-linked immunosorbent assay (ELISA) or hemagglutination-inhibition, indirect immunofluorescence, or complement-fixation tests. A newer test, the IgM antibody capture test, promises early diagnosis and relies on detecting IgM antibody in CSF directed against the virus in question. This test is sensitive for the detection of specific IgM antibody; when results are positive, the diagnosis often can be made on the first sample of CSF obtained from the patient. Positive IgM indirect immunofluorescence antibody tests on serum also can be used to make the diagnosis early in the course of illness.

The differential diagnosis of arthropod-borne encephalitis includes a large number of illnesses, among them, herpes simplex encephalitis, encephalitis of other origins, and other infections of the central nervous system, such as tuberculous meningitis or cryptococcal meningitis. Sometimes patients with cerebrovascular accidents or partially treated bacterial meningitis show signs of disease similar to arthropod-borne encephalitis. Treatment of the patient with severe encephalitis can involve therapy for the syndrome of inappropriate secretion of antidiuretic hormone. Fluid administration should be curtailed under this circumstance, because the continued administration of intravenous saline or water in the elderly patient may lead to volume overload. Patients should be monitored closely for the development of seizure activity. Gastrointestinal bleeding stemming from gastric ulcerations is common. Nosocomial infections of the lung and the urinary tract must be diagnosed early and appropriately treated.

In the Eastern Hemisphere, the major viruses that cause encephalitis are Japanese encephalitis virus and tick-borne encephalitis virus, as it occurs in central Europe and in eastern Russia. Tick-borne encephalitis has been divided into the central European form of the infection and the eastern Russian and Siberian form, which is more severe and is associated with paralytic disease involving the lower brain stem and the upper cervical cord. Other viral encephalitides of lesser importance include Murray Valley encephalitis in Australia, louping ill in Great Britain, Tahyna virus encephalitis, a member of the CE virus group in central Europe, and other agents, such as West Nile virus and Rift Valley fever virus; the latter can cause encephalitis, though they usually provoke febrile illnesses.

Japanese encephalitis is a major problem in Japan, Southeast Asia, China, and India. A large outbreak affected five thousand people in India in 1978. The case fatality rate in the indigenous population approaches 25%. American servicemen not protected by vaccine who are serving in these regions can contract the disease and its severe adverse effects. The disease is characterized by abrupt onset of headache, confusion, ataxia, slurred speech, and tremulousness. Physical findings support these clinical features. The patients have abnormal CSF examination results, with pleocytosis, a normal glucose level, and a normal or high protein concentration. IgM antibody specific to Japanese encephalitis virus can be found in the CSF of most patients with Japanese encephalitis during the early phase of illness. An inactivated vaccine made in suckling mouse brain is available and has been shown to prevent illness in controlled trials.

Tick-borne encephalitis occurs in central Europe and in eastern Russia and Siberia. In the eastern Soviet Union and in Siberia, the disease has a case fatality rate approaching 20%, and some patients are left with paralysis of the shoulder girdle. Murray Valley encephalitis manifests in the northern part of Australia close to New Guinea and has precipitated epidemics in which the case fatality rate was at least 25%. It is caused by a flavivirus, as is louping ill, whose name is derived from the characteristic gait that sheep have when they are infected. Flavivirus is transmitted by ticks, but people who incur this viral infection are usually farmers, butchers, and store workers who handle carcasses of infected animals. Tahyna virus encephalitis is a minor complication of this viral infection in central Europe; the most common manifestation of infection is a febrile headache. West Nile virus, which is also a flavivirus, can cause encephalitis, but it more often produces fever with lymphadenopathy. In 1996, however, an epidemic of West Nile fever caused at least 350 central nervous system infections in Romania around Bucharest and in the lower Danube valley.

HEMORRHAGIC FEVERS

Worldwide the most important hemorrhagic fevers caused by arboviruses are dengue hemorrhagic fever, yellow fever, Congo-Crimean hemorrhagic fever, Omsk hemorrhagic fever, and Kayasanur Forest disease (Table 307.2). Dengue virus has four serotypes and exists throughout the tropical regions of the world. The vectors for dengue virus are *Aedes* species mosquitoes, particularly *Aedes aegypti*. After subcutaneous inoculation, the virus undergoes replication, with subsequent viremia. The incubation period usually is from 5 to 7 days. The illness may have a monophasic or biphasic febrile course. During the course of illness, the patient is acutely ill with fever and has a maculopapular skin rash and diffuse myalgias and arthralgias. In addition to fever and skin rash, the patient may have petechiae and generalized lymphadenopathy. Laboratory tests show features of leukopenia and thrombocytopenia. The illness lasts from 3 to 7 days, and the patient is a source of virus to mosquitoes during the viremic interval.

Epidemics of dengue can be extensive, and clinical symptoms of illness develop in most of the population that becomes infected. In the early 1950s, a new clinical syndrome became apparent. It occurred in children in Southeast Asian populations who had been exposed recurrently to different dengue virus serotypes. This new syndrome, the dengue hemorrhagic shock syndrome, was characterized by fever, shock, hemoconcentration, thrombocytopenia, and bleeding manifestations. In contrast to classic dengue, the leukocyte number often remained normal. Although hemorrhagic disease can develop in people with primary dengue infection, the body of evidence shows that dengue hemorrhagic shock syndrome manifested primarily in children who were experiencing a second infection, each with a different dengue serotype. In the context of partial immunity, there is thought to be an enhancement of dengue virus replication in peripheral blood monocytes. Shock and hemoconcentration have an immunopathologic basis, in that excessive cytokines are released and complement is activated, leading to diffuse capillary leak syndrome. Although the case fatality rate of dengue hemorrhagic shock syndrome initially was high, with good medical care it is usually less than 3% today. Because *A. aegypti* mosquitoes are common throughout the world and are closely associated with human habitation, the disease can be introduced from indigenous areas into countries free of infection, like the United States. Dengue has always been a problem for the military services, because epidemics can affect troops, immobilizing them. Diagnosis depends on serologic studies, such as ELISA, the hemagglutination-inhibition test, or the complement-fixation test, or on virus isolation. Attempts are under way to prepare a polyvalent vaccine, but none is currently available.

Yellow fever is a severe disease that used to occur along shipping routes, in ports where the infected mosquito vector or infected people could be introduced. In urban areas, the vectors are *A. aegypti* mosquitoes. The virus transmission cycle results from infected mosquitoes feeding on humans, who then become viremic, serving as a virus source for other mosquitoes. Control of *A. aegypti* mosquitoes paved the way for the control of yellow fever in urban areas of the world. It later was recognized that yellow fever could also exist in the jungle in a separate cycle involving nonhuman primates and forest canopy mosquitoes. Humans entering forested areas became infected sporadically, but there was always the potential of introduction of the virus into communities by way of such cases or through infected nonhuman primates or infected mosquitoes. The clinical illness consists of fever; jaundice related to hepatic involvement; hemorrhagic manifestations, including the cardinal sign of black vomitus; and diminished renal output associated with proteinuria. The case fatality rate can approximate 25%. The disease can be diagnosed by serologic studies or by virus isolation from

	TABLE 307.2.	ARBOVIRUS HEMORRHAGIC FEVERS			
Fever	**Virus**	**Vector**	**Geographic Distribution**	**Distinguishing Features**
Dengue hemorrhagic	Flavivirus	*Aedes* species mosquitoes	Worldwide	Hemorrhage, fever, hemoconcentration, thrombocytopenia; found predominantly in children experiencing secondary dengue infections
Yellow	Flavivirus	*Aedes aegyti* mosquitoes	Africa; Central and South America	Hepatic involvement, clotting factor disturbances, hematemesis
Congo-Crimean hemorrhagic	Nairovirus, family Bunyaviridae	Tick	South Africa to Crimean Peninsula	Decreased hepatic function, thrombocytopenia
Omsk hemorrhagic	Flavivirus	Tick, infected muskrat contact	Former Soviet Union	Exposure to forested areas, muskrat hunting
Kayasanur Forest disease	Flavivirus	Tick	India	Exposure to forested areas

TABLE 307.3.   ARBOVIRUS FEVERS

Fever	Virus	Vector	Geographic Distribution	Distinguishing Features
Dengue	Flavirus	*Aedes* species mosquitoes	Worldwide	Joint pains, rash, leukopenia, thrombocytopenia
Rift Valley	Phlebovirus, family Bunyviridae	Several mosquito species; contact with infected livestock, humans	Africa, Middle East	Fever; encephalitis in 5%; retinitis progressing to blindness
Chickagunya	Alphavirus	Mosquito	Africa; Asia	Fever, painful joint swelling
West Nile	Flavivirus	Mosquito	Africa; Middle East, southern Europe; Pakistan; India	Fever, headache, myalgias; encephalitis may develop
Colorado tick	Orbivirus	Tick	Western United States	Resembles Rocky Mountain spotted fever but rash is minimal; prolonged persistence of virus in erythrocytes

serum. An attenuated viral vaccine, 17D, is available and produces solid immunity for at least 10 years.

Congo-Crimean hemorrhagic fever is a new geographic entity, which may be an emerging disease of increasing importance. The disease is characterized by fever, headache and myalgia, vomiting, abdominal pain, hepatomegaly, and a hemorrhagic state with a petechial rash that becomes purpuric. The patient is viremic during the early stage of the illness. Hepatic dysfunction is present, along with leukopenia and thrombocytopenia. Some patients may become uremic at later stages of the illness. The basic pathologic process may result from an insult to endothelial cells, with subsequent activation of complement and the clotting process. The case fatality rate is close to 40%.

ARTHROPOD-BORNE VIRAL FEVERS

The most prominent arthropod-borne viral fever is dengue fever (Table 307.3), which is indigenous to the tropical areas of the world. Most of the other arboviruses provoking fever are localized to a distinct geographic region. Rift Valley fever virus is a growing concern as a source of disease. The disease caused by this virus was isolated to sub-Saharan Africa until 1977, when it crossed into Egypt and spread from Egypt into portions of the Sinai Peninsula. It is estimated that this epidemic caused as many as 200,000 human cases of disease and probably close to 600 deaths. The virus is transmitted to humans by contact with infected livestock and various mosquito species and possibly by nosocomial contact with other human cases. The clinical features consist of fever, headache, malaise, myalgias, anorexia, and vomiting. Encephalitis can develop during the course of illness in about 5% of patients. A hemorrhagic disease can eventuate in perhaps the same proportion of people suffering clinical illness. Retinitis, which can lead to blindness, also may develop. The tremendous capacity of this virus to spread from area to area and affect large populations of humans demonstrates its potential as a pathogen.

Chikungunya virus is also capable of causing widespread febrile disease and accompanying features, such as joint pains and skin rash. Ross River fever, an alphavirus infection, appears in Australia at irregular intervals and triggers a febrile disease with painful swelling of joints. Lymphadenopathy and leukopenia may be features of the illness. Although joint and muscle pains fade rapidly in most cases, some patients have recurrences of joint pain for up to a year. West Nile virus and phlebotomus fever viruses also provoke fever, headache, and myalgias. West Nile fever virus contributes significantly to undiagnosed fever among children in Egypt. Such viral diseases as O'Nyong-Nyong (Africa), Mayaro virus (South America), or Oropouche fever (South America) have appeared in circumscribed places at particular times in the past, causing large numbers of cases.

Colorado tick fever virus is an orbivirus transmitted in the western part of the United States by tick bite and associated with persistent parasitization of red blood cells by the virus. Symptoms are similar to those of Rocky Mountain spotted fever, except that the rash is relatively minimal and primarily affects the trunk. Although the disease usually runs a relatively circumscribed course, Colorado tick fever virus can be recovered from washed red cells of infected human beings for as long as 120 days after onset of symptoms. There are known instances of transmission of Colorado tick fever virus by transfusion of infected blood from patients.

BIBLIOGRAPHY

Calisher CH. Medically important arboviruses of the United States and Canada. *Clin Microbiol Rev* 1994;7(1):89–116.

Dickerson RB, Newton JR, Hansen JE. Diagnosis and immediate prognosis of Japanese B encephalitis. *Am J Med* 1952;12:277.

Gear JH. Clinical aspects of African viral hemorrhagic fevers. *Rev Infect Dis* 1989;(Suppl 4):S777–S782.

Halstead SB. Antibody, macrophages, dengue virus infection, shock, and hemorrhage: a pathogenetic cascade. *Rev Infect Dis* 1989;11(Suppl 4): S830–S839.

Luby JP. St. Louis encephalitis. In: Beran GW, Steele JH, eds. *Handbook of zoonoses*, second ed. Boca Raton, FL: CRC Press, 1994:47.

Monath TP, ed. *St. Louis encephalitis*. Washington, D.C.: American Public Health Association, 1980.

Tsai TF, Popovici F, Cernescu C, et al. West Nile encephalitis epidemic in southeastern Romania. *Lancet* 1998;352(9130):767–771.

Kelley's Textbook of Internal Medicine, fourth edition. Edited by H. David Humes.
Lippincott Williams & Wilkins, Philadelphia © 2000.

C H A P T E R

308

INFECTIONS CAUSED BY ARENAVIRUSES, HANTAVIRUSES, AND FILOVIRUSES

ALI S. KHAN
ANNE K. PFLIEGER

The term *viral hemorrhagic fever* describes a severe multisystem syndrome characterized by diffuse vascular damage and dysregulation. The etiologic agents of these diseases are zoonotic, lipid-enveloped RNA viruses, with dozens of members from four different viral families. This chapter discusses the arenavirus-, filovirus-, and hantavirus-associated diseases (Table 308.1). Most of these agents are localized geographically (Fig. 308.1), and associated with specific vector hosts in rural settings. The diseases they cause are episodic and arguably the most feared of the viral hemorrhagic fevers, given their high lethality and potential for transmission from person to person. Contributing to this perception is the paucity of information concerning their clinical manifestations, therapeutic options, pathogenesis, and ecologic factors. Except for the hantaviruses, these viruses do not cause disease in North America or Europe, but the occurrence of rare imported cases and infections caused by laboratory misadventure has heightened this concern. Additionally, the growing recognition that these agents can be employed for bioterrorism has highlighted the need for increased global surveillance and vigilance on the part of the individual clinician.

Correctly diagnosing a patient with a viral hemorrhagic fever presents an exercise in geographic medicine, after a thorough evaluation for more common treatable conditions of travelers, such as malaria, dysentery, and typhoid fever. Because of the availability of therapy for some hantaviral and arenaviral infections and the potential for nosocomial transmission, viral hemorrhagic fevers should always be considered in the differential diagnosis of a patient with the appropriate clinical symptoms. Although these fevers are somewhat nondescript in initial presentation, the subsequent development of hypotension, a flushed appearance suggesting early vascular injury, and, in particular, hemorrhage should trigger diagnostic suspicion. It is important to bear in mind that hemorrhage may be absent and, if present, is rarely life threatening in itself. Thrombocytopenia, except in Lassa fever, is the most characteristic laboratory feature. Virtually all arenaviral hemorrhagic fevers can be excluded, however, in the absence of proteinuria and/or hematuria. Given the vascular fragility of these patients, the only indication for transport should be to gain access to the closest intensive care services; this level of care is necessary because the condition of patients can deteriorate precipitously.

All filoviruses, most arenaviruses, and one hantavirus are asso-

TABLE 308.1.	SALIENT FEATURES OF SELECTED VIRAL HEMORRHAGIC FEVERS			
Family	**Virus**	**Disease**	**Geographic Region**	**Reservoir/Vector**
Arenaviridae	Junin	Argentine hemorrhagic fever	Argentina pampas	Rodent: *Calomys callosu*
	Machupo	Bolivian hemorrhagic fever	Beni Department, Bolivia	Rodent: *Calomys musculinus*
	Guanarito	Venezuelan hemorrhagic fever	Guanarito municipality of Portuguesa State and adjacent regions of Barinas State, Venezuela	Rodent: *Zygodontomy brevicauda*
	Sabiá	Unnamed	São Paulo State, Brazil	Unknown
	Lassa	Lassa fever	Nigeria, Sierra Leone, Liberia, Guinea, Ivory Coast	Rodent: *Matomys* species
Bunyaviridae	Hantaan and related viruses	Hemorrhagic fever with renal syndrome	Asia and Europe (rare in Africa and the Americas)	Rodents: Arvicoline and murine subfamilies
	Sin Nombre and related viruses	Hantavirus pulmonary syndrome	Americas	Rodents: Sigmodontine subfamilies
Filoviridae	Marburg	Marburg hemorrhagic fever	Sub-Saharan Africa	Unknown
	Ebola	Ebola hemorrhagic fever	Tropical forests, Africa (all strains except Ebola-Reston from Philippines)	Unknown

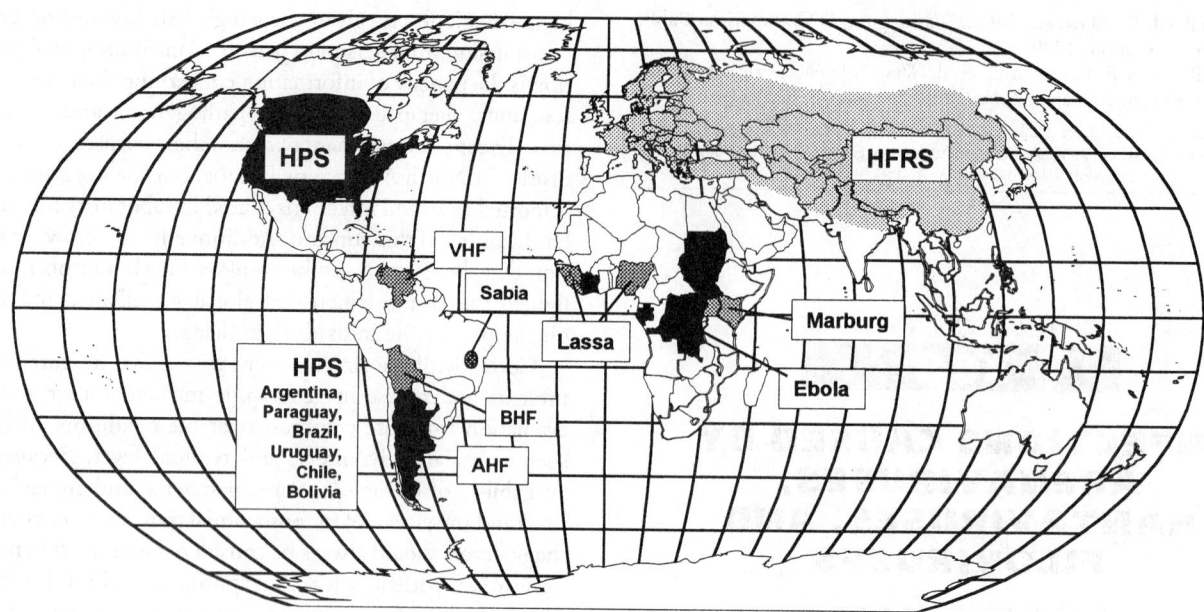

FIGURE 308.1. Geographic distribution of selected viral hemorrhagic fevers.

ciated with secondary transmission—often as the source of large nosocomial outbreaks. The potential mechanisms for person-to-person transmission include direct contact or direct projection (large-particle droplet spread) of droplets onto mucous membranes, indirect transmission via fomites and body fluids, and, rarely, airborne transmission via small-particle aerosols. Nonetheless, the absolute risk to family members and medical staff in U.S. hospitals is low, and these patients can be treated safely by adding precautionary guidelines for handling clinical samples. Enhanced safety measures for viral hemorrhagic fever include standard precautions in addition to transmission-based droplet and contact precautions; respiratory precautions are added for high-risk procedures likely to generate aerosols or if the patient is coughing. Minimizing human–rodent contact is the cornerstone of preventing natural infections with hantaviruses or arenaviruses. Although rodent abatement is readily accomplished in the peridomestic setting by eliminating rodent harborage, attempting to control rodent populations in rural occupational or recreational settings, where rodents are too abundant and geographically dispersed, is relatively futile. No recommendations can be made about eliminating natural infection by filoviruses, since the host is unknown. Nevertheless, the potential for infection from imported nonhuman primates has been minimized through new quarantine regulations and reliance on captive-bred animals for medical research.

Animal studies with hantaviruses and all laboratory studies with arenaviruses and filoviruses require biosafety level 4 containment, because these viruses are known to be infectious via small-particle aerosols in the laboratory, which generally mirrors the natural mode of transmission from their respective reservoirs. Except for hantaviruses, these viruses are readily isolated from acute or morbid patient samples. Enzyme-linked immunosorbent assays (ELISAs) have proved to be sensitive and specific for rapid antigen and/or antibody detection, though the older indirect fluorescent, neutralization, and complement fixation antibody techniques remain available. Diagnosis during acute phase of illness can be confirmed before antibody development by reverse transcription–polymerase chain reaction (RT-PCR) of blood or postmortem tissues. Immunohistochemical techniques are available for all of these agents for postmortem diagnosis. Specific diagnostic or treatment questions for patients suspected of harboring these viruses can be addressed to the Special Pathogens Branch, Centers for Disease Control and Prevention, Atlanta, Georgia.

ARENAVIRUSES

DEFINITION

The Arenaviridae family generally is divided into two complexes: those viruses associated with New World sigmodontine rodents and those associated with Old World murine rodents, including Lassa and lymphocytic choriomeningitis viruses. The New World arenaviral diseases tend to be more severe; these diseases include Argentine, Bolivian, Venezuelan, and a single, natural case of Brazilian, or Sabiá-associated, hemorrhagic fever caused by Junin, Machupo, Guanarito, and Sabiá viruses, respectively. Lassa fever, initially described in a series of nosocomial epidemics as a lethal hemorrhagic fever associated with a 50% case fatality, is now known to be a common, usually self-limited, febrile illness in West Africa with milder hemorrhagic manifestations. Lymphocytic choriomeningitis virus infection is ubiquitous within the distribution of its rodent reservoir, the cosmopolitan house mouse, and only rarely has been associated with a hemorrhagic diathesis. All arenaviruses that produce human disease are carried by chronically infected rodents. Person-to-person transmission is well documented for Lassa virus but also has been reported for Machupo and Junin viruses in *rare* instances.

INCIDENCE AND EPIDEMIOLOGY

Lassa Fever

Of the arenaviruses, Lassa virus is responsible for the greatest number of cases of human disease: an estimated 100,000 to 300,000 infections and approximately 5,000 deaths occur annually in disease-endemic areas of West Africa. Although the clinical features of Lassa fever were described in Sierra Leone in the 1950s, Lassa virus was first isolated in 1969, after causing the death of a missionary nurse who provided care for Lassa patients in the far northeastern region of Nigeria. In disease-endemic areas of Sierra Leone and Liberia, Lassa fever accounts for 10% to 16% of hospital admissions. Lassa fever is fatal for approximately 15% to 20% of those hospitalized, but it is a leading cause of fetal and maternal death in hospitalized patients. The overall mortality for Lassa virus infection is less than 1%.

The virus is transmitted to humans through direct contact with contaminated surfaces, ingestion of contaminated food, inhalation of aerosolized particles from rodent excreta, and rodent bites. Humans also may become infected when the *Mastomys species* rodents are caught and ingested. Prevention has focused on efforts to eliminate peridomestic rodents and to minimize handling of trapped rodents before thorough cooking. Human-to-human transmission takes place through contact with the blood, tissue, secretions, or excretions of an infected person or through inhalation of airborne particles contaminated by an infected person by such actions as coughing. Lax infection-control practices, such as the re-use of needles, can cause significant nosocomial transmission and contribute to explosive nosocomial epidemics. A serologic survey in 1992 identified previous infection in as many as one-sixth of ward aides in six health centers in Nigeria.

Lymphocytic Choriomeningitis

Lymphocytic choriomeningitis virus (LCMV) was the first arenavirus to be discovered and isolated (in 1933) and the first specific agent identified as causing nonfatal aseptic meningitis. The virus was shown to be responsible for 8% to 11% of central nervous syndromes in patients hospitalized at a medical center between 1941 and 1958. Serosurveys have documented a 2% to 5% prevalence of antibody to LCMV in individuals in the United States. Most infections occur during the fall, winter, and spring and generally affect young adults, though individuals of all ages are susceptible to infection. Unfortunately, the current incidence of the clinical syndromes associated with infection is not known, since diagnostic testing is rarely requested.

The epidemiologic features of the disease are congruent with the ecologic characteristics of the reservoir host, the common house mouse (*Mus musculus* and *Mus domesticus*). Peridomestic LCMV infections have been contracted by persons living in proximity to wild infected and pet mice, though there is also evidence that pet (Syrian) hamsters (*Mesocricetus aureus*) can be competent alternative reservoirs. Infections from house mice are associated with substandard housing, such as trailer parks and inner city dwellings. Outbreaks also have been documented among laboratory workers, especially those handling mice or hamsters or silently infected rodent cell lines. No cases of person-to-person transmission have been reported.

New World Hemorrhagic Fevers

Arenaviruses that cause New World hemorrhagic fevers are enzootic throughout South America, with intermittent periods of epizootic transmission. Most New World arenaviral diseases arise mainly in rural populations with peridomestic rodent contact and are focal in their distribution. In 1958 Junin virus, the causative agent of Argentine hemorrhagic fever (AHF), was the first of these viruses to be isolated, near the very circumscribed area of the town of Junin, in the province of West Buenos Aires. At present, AHF is reported to occur in the 150,000 km^2 agricultural areas of central and northwestern Argentina, specifically the Buenos Aires, Santa Fe, and the Cordoba states of the pampas region, which encompasses two million inhabitants. The majority of AHF cases develop during the harvest season, from February to May, when adult male agricultural workers have the greatest contact with infected rodents. With increased vaccination and changes in agricultural practices, disease case counts have declined from 4,000 to less than 100 per year. Sexual transmission during convalescence is well documented, and there has been one reported instance of nosocomial transmission; Junin virus also has been isolated from breast milk.

Similarly, Bolivian hemorrhagic fever (BHF), known as "black typhus" during the late 1950s, usually is associated with agricultural activity or peridomestic exposure to infected rodents. Its etiologic agent, Machupo virus, was first isolated in 1963 near the Machupo River in Bolivia. This virus was the source of large municipal outbreaks in 1963 and 1964, and accounted for more than 500 cases in the towns of the Beni Department in northeastern Bolivia. Cases of BHF acquired in a peridomestic setting affect both sexes and all ages. The peak incidence is in the fall and winter months, corresponding to the dry season. No cases were confirmed between 1971 and 1993, but sporadic cases have developed since 1993. Person-to-person transmission was reported during a small nosocomial outbreak that included two health care workers and a pathologist and a cluster of seven family members. Contact transmission was insufficient to explain disease transmission for some of these individuals.

Venezuelan hemorrhagic fever (VHF) has been recognized since 1989 in the ~9,000-km^2 rural areas of southern and southwestern Portuguesa State and the adjacent region of Barinas State in the central grassy plains of northwestern Venezuela. Guanarito virus, the etiologic agent of VHF, was determined to be genetically distinct from the other known South American arenaviruses in 1995. Between September 1988 and January 1997, 165 cases of VHF were reported, with a case fatality of 33%. This period included a 36-month interval from September 1992 to August 1996 when the disease virtually disappeared. VHF occurs predominantly in adult men (70% of cases) and peaks in November, December, and January, coinciding with intense harvesting and land clearing. As with BHF, disease often develops in an area where forest is cleared for smallhold agriculture and cattle ranching, providing opportunity for transmission from infected rodents. Rates of asymptomatic infection are low, and only one suspected case of person-to-person transmission has been documented—that of a female spouse who became ill 12 days after her husband's discharge from the hospital.

Brazilian, or Sabiá-associated, hemorrhagic fever was first recognized in 1990 after the death from what was thought to be yellow fever of a 25-year-old agronomist from São Paulo State, Brazil. In addition to the index case from Brazil, Sabiá virus has been documented in two laboratory-associated infections, including one in the United States.

ETIOLOGY AND ECOLOGY

The Arenaviridae comprise a family of enveloped, negative-stranded RNA viruses consisting of two single-stranded segments termed large (L) and small (S). Created as a new taxon in 1970, the family name describes the fine granules (*arena* meaning "sand" in Latin) seen within virions by electron microscopy. Arenaviruses infect a wide variety of cells in vitro, with little obvious cell damage or cytopathic effect. They are relatively unstable in vitro and rapidly inactivated at a pH of less than 5.5 and more than 8.5. Sensitive to ultraviolet and gamma irradiation, solvents, and detergents, these viruses are readily inactivated by the usual disinfectants.

Lassa virus is the only one of four African arenaviruses (Lassa, Mobala, Mopeia, and Ippy) that causes human disease. The virus persistently infects *Mastomys huberti* and *Mastomys erythroleucus,* the "multimammate rat" found in West, Central, and East Africa. LCMV, the only other Old World arenavirus that produces human illness, is distributed worldwide. Of the 14 New World arenaviruses, the agents known to cause human disease are Junin, Machupo, Guanarito, and Sabiá viruses, which are the etiologic agents, respectively, of Argentine, Bolivian, Venezuelan, and Sabiá-associated hemorrhagic fevers. These viruses are associated with specific sigmodontine rodents: Junin, Machupo, and Guanarito viruses are maintained by *Calomys musculinus, Calomys callosus,* and *Zygodontomys brevicauda,* respectively. The rodent reservoir of Sabiá virus has not yet been determined.

PATHOGENESIS

Lassa Fever

Hepatocellular necrosis is the most conspicuous pathologic finding, but splenic and adrenocortical necrosis, interstitial nephritis and pneumonia, and myocarditis often are found. High concentrations of virus are present in other organs that do not show distinct pathologic lesions. Circulatory collapse and death result from volume depletion through failed capillary endothelia. Generalized hemorrhaging from the gums, gastrointestinal tract, and vagina is not a result of disseminated intravascular coagulation (DIC) but may be related to circulating inhibitors of hemostasis and to platelet or endothelial dysfunction. Neutralizing antibodies may not be found in recovered patients, and the immunologic mechanisms related to recovery are undefined.

Lymphocytic Choriomeningitis

Arenavirus infections of cells in vivo and in vitro usually induce little or no obvious morphologic changes. Thus, their deleterious effects are mediated by more subtle alterations in cellular function. Classically, peripheral inoculation of adult mice produces no disease, whereas intracranial inoculation leads to a fatal convulsive disorder. The intracranial disease in mice results in acute choroid plexus damage and death, following a massive T-cell immune response with more than 50% of splenic CD8 cells specific for LCMV.

New World Hemorrhagic Fevers

Disease is characterized by single-cell necrosis of the epithelium of the gastrointestinal tract, interstitial pneumonia, lymphoid and hematopoietic cell necrosis, and the presence of platelet thrombi in a few blood vessels, associated with hemorrhage. Immunoelectron microscopy has identified intact virions and typical arenavirus inclusions in these tissues. The viruses replicate in mononuclear cells that seed the central nervous system (CNS) during viremia. A direct viral effect on megakaryocytes may explain thrombocytopenia; however, the suspected pathogenesis of arenavirus hemorrhagic fever is through effects on macrophages that induce cytokine activation. Interferon and tumor necrosis factor (TNF) are abundant in acute-phase serum samples, and their levels correlate with the severity of disease, supporting the idea that soluble mediators are important in the pathogenesis of these infections. Circulating antibodies coincide with clinical improvement.

CLINICAL FEATURES

Lassa Fever

Following an incubation period of 7 to 18 days, patients with Lassa fever experience a nonspecific constellation of symptoms, including fever, malaise, headache, and musculoskeletal pain. The illness evolves gradually and may lead to exudative pharyngitis, conjunctivitis, cough, substernal chest pain or epigastric pain, and complaints of abdominal cramping, diarrhea, and vomiting after 4 to 5 days. Neurologic symptoms, such as tremors, and encephalitis may occur. A maculopapular rash is frequently noted on light-skinned persons. Patients appear ill, are weak, and may be hypotensive. Fulminant disease is marked by shock, mucosal bleeding, facial and neck edema, and pulmonary edema; crepitant rales and pleural or pericardial effusions are evident on chest examination. The disease does not have characteristic petechiae, ecchymoses, or jaundice. Mild cases of Lassa fever resolve slowly, within 8 to 10 days. In severe cases, hospitalized patients appear toxic with profuse sweating and tachypnea and tachycardia commensurate to the degree of fever. The most common complications associated with Lassa fever include hemorrhage, spontaneous abortions, and pleural and pericardial effusions. Almost one-third of hospitalized Lassa fever patients experience acute hearing impairment at the beginning of convalescence, and approximately two-thirds of these patients are left with some degree of permanent hearing loss.

Malaria and typhoid fever can mimic Lassa fever, though gingival petechiae and purulent pharyngitis are unusual. Depending on the patient's travel history, diseases to exclude include the other locally endemic viral hemorrhagic fevers, such as dengue, yellow fever, and chikungunya; amebiasis; laryngeal diphtheria in a patient with stridor and facial and neck edema; streptococcal pharyngitis; leptospirosis; and bacterial pneumonia and sepsis.

Lymphocytic Choriomeningitis

After an incubation period of 6 to 13 days, the vast majority of patients suffer a nonspecific illness characterized by fever, headache, and severe myalgia that primarily affects the lumbar region. Patients may experience nausea, vomiting, pharyngitis, parotitis, lymphadenopathy, cough, chest pain, myocarditis, orchitis, and arthralgias. Biphasic fever occurs in one-fourth of cases, and after 4 to 7 days, blood dyscrasia may develop. Although studies indicate that a third of LCMV infections are asymptomatic, approximately half of all infected individuals show mild to moderate symptoms that usually resolve within a week of onset. Less than 10% of patients will have classic lymphocytic choriomeningitis with significant CNS manifestations, including meningism, altered mental state, generalized weakness, and abnormal reflexes; roughly a third of these patients develop encephalopathy or encephalitis. Although LCMV infections are rarely fatal, death has resulted from acute meningoencephalitis and after severe systemic illnesses complicated by pneumonia and generalized hemorrhages. The disease is associated with prolonged convalescence often marked by alopecia and arthritis. Pregnancy may produce a congenital syndrome in the fetus characterized by ocular abnormalities (usually chorioretinitis), micro- or macrocephaly with associated hydrocephalus, and long-term neurologic effects.

New World Hemorrhagic Fevers

After an incubation period of 5 to 19 days, all four diseases have similar clinical features: gradual onset of fever and malaise followed by headache, myalgia, arthralgias, and dizziness; gastrointestinal symptoms, such as nausea, vomiting, constipation, and diarrhea, also are present frequently. There may be retro-orbital pain, photophobia, and epigastric abdominal pain, but complaints of pharyngitis and other respiratory symptoms are uncommon. During the first week of illness, patients are usually acutely ill and irritable. Most have edematous and flushed facies, with nonexudative bulbar and palpebral conjunctival injection, generalized lymphadenopathy, and fine petechial eruptions in the oral pharynx, on the upper trunk, and especially in the axillae. After the first week, most patients enter a convalescent phase, but more than one-third experience neurologic or hemorrhagic complications. Severe cases are characterized by a hypotensive, hemorrhagic phase, reflecting a capillary leak syndrome that can lead to pulmonary edema and shock. Severely ill patients develop multiple hemorrhages in the gastrointestinal tract, uterus, and other mucosal surfaces. Acute renal failure and secondary bacterial infection are additional complications. In a significant number of patients, severe neurologic complications appear and may completely overshadow the vascular and homeostatic abnormalities. Fine intention tremors, hypo- or hyperreflexia, ataxia, and an altered state of consciousness are very common, but even among patients with severe neurologic involvement, the cerebro-spinal fluid (CSF) may be normal. CNS abnormalities, such as delirium, convulsions, and coma, are associated with an extremely poor outcome. The evolution of an individual infection toward a principally neurologic or hemorrhagic syndrome has been correlated with tropic properties of the infecting virus strain. Fatal outcomes occur in 15% to 30% of patients, usually within 2 to 14 days of hospitalization. There are no long-term effects, but convalescence may last up to several months, and diffuse hair loss, hearing loss, and transverse furrowing of the nail beds are common features of recovery.

The various hepatitides, including yellow fever and dengue, are important to consider in the differential diagnosis of the New World arenaviral hemorrhagic fevers. In the initial stages of illness, the clinical features of these potentially lethal diseases cannot be distinguished from those of other acute infections with hemorrhagic manifestations, such as meningococcemia, leptospirosis, yellow fever, dengue hemorrhagic fever, and thrombotic thrombocytic purpura.

LABORATORY FINDINGS

Lassa Fever

Common findings of Lassa fever include hemoconcentration and proteinuria. Leukopenia is usually noted except in severe cases, but thrombocytopenia is uncommon and mild if present. Amylase and creatine phosphokinase levels may be elevated; aspartate aminotransferase (ALT) levels of more than 150 U per milliliter suggest a poor prognosis. The diagnosis can be made on the basis of specific IgM or IgG antibody; however, a rise in IgM antibodies in the first 3 to 6 days rarely is seen in fatal cases, and only about half of patients evidence antibodies in the first week of illness. IgG antibody is not detected reliably until the second week of illness. Antigen-capture ELISA can be used in acute or fatal infection before the detection of IgM antibody. The virus can be cultured in 7 to 10 days, with high levels of circulating virus (median tissue culture infective dose, >103.6 per milliliter) predicting a poor outcome. RT-PCR also can be used to detect Lassa viral nucleic acid from blood or urine samples early in the course of illness or from postmortem tissues.

Lymphocytic Choriomeningitis

Patients with LCMV infection may have peripheral leukopenia. Pleocytosis may be evident on examination of the CSF, with up to 5,000 leukocytes per cubic millimeter. Lymphocytes predominate, but 25% of the cells may be polymorphs. Hypoglycorrhachia is found in 25% of patients. The acute diagnosis can be made by serologic testing or by IgM-capture ELISA of CSF, but LCMV can be recovered from the CSF, blood, or throat washings in as many as 50% of patients. If mice are used in virus-isolation attempts, the colony must be certified to be free of LCMV.

New World Hemorrhagic Fevers

Pronounced leukopenia, thrombocytopenia, and proteinuria are characteristic findings with New World hemorrhagic fevers, usually present in the first few days of illness. Transaminase levels may be elevated, and nonspecific electrocardiogram (ECG) changes have been reported in AHF. As in Lassa fever, IgM antibodies are detected late in the illness and may be absent in fatal cases; however, antigen-detection tests have been used recently with good success. Circulating antibodies appear 10 to 12 days after illness onset.

OPTIMAL MANAGEMENT

Lassa Fever

Intravenous ribavirin therapy in patients with an AST level ≥150 IU per liter lowers the case fatality from 55% to 5% if administered within 6 days but may have some benefit if administered later. Supportive therapy involves maintenance of fluid and electrolyte balance, with strict attention to the development of pulmonary or laryngeal edema, cyanosis, and hypotension. Acetaminophen should be used instead of aspirin for fever reduction.

Lymphocytic Choriomeningitis

Treatment is symptomatic; patients with CNS involvement are usually hospitalized and receive supportive therapy. Ribavirin has been effective in treating some severe cases.

New World Hemorrhagic Fevers

Specific therapy for AHF using passively administered immune plasma has proved effective in lowering the mortality to less than 1% when 2 units were given within 8 days of the onset of illness. Recovery is complete; however, in 10% of treated patients a neurologic syndrome of fever, ataxia, and tremor may develop 4 to 6 weeks after onset of serotherapy, which resolves without residual effects. Although convalescent-phase plasma has been used successfully to treat AHF, its efficacy in BHF and VHF is less well established. The similarities of these diseases, however, suggest that it may work. Supportive therapy for shock, hemorrhage, and secondary infection is critical in cases of hemorrhagic fever.

No clinical trials of intravenous ribavirin therapy for South American hemorrhagic fevers have been conducted, but work with animal models and early experience among humans with AHF, BHF, and Sabiá-associated infection suggest its usefulness. For AHF, intravenous ribavirin also should be considered if specific immune plasma is unavailable or if patients present after 8 days of disease onset. An experimental live-attenuated vaccine for AHF (Candid-1) was more than 95% effective in one large-scale human trial and may be effective for BHF.

HANTAVIRUSES

DEFINITION

The genus generally is divided into two groups: those associated with Old World murine and arvicoline rodents and those associ-

ated with New World sigmodontine rodents. In general, the so-called Old World hantaviruses are distributed more widely throughout areas of Europe, the Americas, and Asia. The illnesses caused by Old World hantaviruses, collectively known as hemorrhagic fever with renal syndrome (HFRS), share a clinical picture of renal compromise and bleeding diathesis. New World virus hosts inhabit specific regions of North and South America. Human infection with New World hantaviruses causes hantavirus pulmonary syndrome (HPS), associated with noncardiogenic pulmonary edema and shock. Primary renal dysfunction is reported in HPS, as is pulmonary edema in HFRS, which suggests more overlap between these syndromes than originally was recognized. Secondary person-to-person transmission, including nosocomial transmission, has been reported only with Andes virus infections in South America.

INCIDENCE AND EPIDEMIOLOGY

Hemorrhagic Fever with Renal Syndrome

Epidemic hemorrhagic fevers associated with renal failure and shock are ancient conditions with assorted regional names; they are major public health problems in such countries as China, where 40,000 to 100,000 cases are reported each year. Most cases are documented in Korea, China, Japan, Russia, Scandinavia, Holland, the United Kingdom, France, Belgium, and the Balkans, with broader serologic evidence of infection in Africa and Asia. Seoul virus has a worldwide distribution in persistently infected rats, but only three cases have been reported in the United States.

Infections from Seoul virus occur in sylvan and urban locations, with a fall and spring seasonality. Men, particularly agricultural and forestry workers, are at greatest risk of infection in sylvan locations. Laboratory outbreaks associated with rodent colonies have occurred frequently, and transmission has been documented after rodent bites. The exact mechanisms of human infection are unknown, but infective aerosols from urine or other excreta of chronically infected rodents are known to be dangerous and are likely the major route of transmission. Person-to-person transmission of HFRS has never been reported, though common point-source outbreaks from rodent exposure are documented.

Hantavirus Pulmonary Syndrome

HPS was first recognized after a high-profile investigation of a cluster of unexplained respiratory deaths in the southwestern United States during the spring of 1993. Retrospective identification of cases documented hantavirus infection in the United States as early as 1959. As of July 1999, more than 300 cases of HPS had been identified in seven other American countries: Argentina, Bolivia, Brazil, Canada, Chile, Paraguay, and Uruguay. Through July 15, 1999, the Centers for Disease Control and Prevention had confirmed 217 cases of HPS in the United States, with a case fatality in the past 2 years of approximately 25%. Unlike the initially recognized cases among Native Americans, HPS now is found mainly among whites. The mean age of these patients is 39 years (range, 10 to 69 years), and 60%

of them are male. The temporal distribution of cases since 1992 shows a major peak that corresponds to the outbreak in the summer of 1993 and another larger peak in 1999. With a spring through summer seasonality, cases have developed throughout the interim period in a pattern that appears to reflect the effects of El Niño on rodent populations (increased population density as a result of more abundant food sources). The temporal distribution of cases has oscillated between the southwestern United States during peak years and the Pacific Northwest during interim periods. Cases have been reported in 30 states, including most of the western half of the country and some eastern states as well.

The geographic distribution of HPS cases in the United States is related, at least in part, to the interaction of the rodent hosts with humans and their habitats. Rural residents have a 15-fold higher risk of HPS than do urban dwellers. Seventy percent of the patients with confirmed evidence of HPS for whom exposure information is available experienced exposure closely associated with peridomestic activities in homes that showed signs of rodent infestation. Possible cases of occupationally acquired Sin Nombre virus (SNV) infection have been recognized, but they are infrequent. Grain farmers, an extension livestock specialist, field biologists, and agricultural, mill, construction, utility, and feedlot workers have had documented hantavirus infections, but many of these individuals had concurrent peridomestic exposures.

No case of person-to-person transmission of New World hantaviruses has been reported in North America. Furthermore, a serologic survey among health care workers who took care of the initial cluster of HPS patients failed to show any sign of infection. Person-to-person and nosocomial transmission of Andes virus was identified in Argentina, however. Twenty cases in acquaintances, relatives, and five physicians, including three involved in direct patient care, were epidemiologically and genetically linked through direct contact with infected persons. Suspected cases of interperson transmission of Andes virus also have been reported in Chile, though no additional cases were identified among hospital staff attending these patients. Suspected transmission from breast milk also has been reported in Argentina.

ETIOLOGY AND ECOLOGY

Like other members of the family Bunyaviridae, hantaviruses are enveloped viruses with a genome that consists of three single-stranded RNA segments designated S (small), M (medium), and L (large). Hantavirus evolution is best understood as co-evolution within specific lineages in the rodent family Muridae. The apparent coupling between hantaviruses and their rodent hosts suggests that viruses of sigmodontine rodents share a common ancestor, as do viruses of the rodent subfamilies Arvicolinae and Murinae. This coupling also has a geographic and clinical correlate: viruses found in Old World murine rodents are associated with HFRS in Eurasia, whereas viruses carried by New World sigmodontine rodents are associated with HPS in the Americas. Transmission from rodent to rodent is believed to take place through contact—perhaps aggressive contact, with accompanying combat wounds. Hantaviruses are sensitive to heat, acid pH,

detergents, formalin, and lipid solvents and therefore can be inactivated with the use of commercially available cleaning products.

Hemorrhagic Fever with Renal Syndrome

Four genetically distinct hantaviruses are recognized and well characterized as etiologic agents of HFRS. Hantaan virus, the prototype member of the genus, is endemic to Asia and is associated with the striped field mouse (*Apodemus agrarius*). Seoul virus is found worldwide, reflecting the distribution of its rodent hosts, the black rat (*Rattus rattus*) and the Norway rat (*Rattus norvegicus*). Puumala virus is endemic in Western Europe, Scandinavia, and Russia to the west of the Ural Mountains and is carried by the European bank vole (*Clethrionomys glareolus*). Dobrava virus is known to be enzootic in the yellow-necked field mouse (*Apodemus flavicollis*) in the Balkans. Numerous other New World hantaviruses and their respective reservoir hosts have been identified but not implicated in human disease, including Prospect Hill virus, which is known to be enzootic in meadow voles (*Microtus pennsylvanicus*) in the United States.

Hantavirus Pulmonary Syndrome

The deer mouse, *Peromyscus maniculatus,* is the primary rodent reservoir in the contiguous United States, where it is widely distributed. Cases of HPS have been identified outside the range of *P. maniculatus,* however, and four additional hantaviruses with different rodent hosts have been identified. Black Creek Canal virus (BCCV) is associated with the cotton rat (*Sigmodon hispidus*) and a single case in Florida. Bayou virus of the rice rat (*Oryzomys palustris*) is linked to cases from Louisiana and Texas. Cases of HPS in the northeastern United States have been caused by an SNV variant (New York-1) from the white-footed mouse (*Peromyscus leucopus*), found in the eastern third of the United States. Another SNV variant, Monongahela virus, was identified in a patient from North Carolina and is associated with *Peromyscus maniculatus nubiterrae.* Cases of HPS can be expected to occur throughout the range of rodent distributions.

Viruses that cause HPS and their rodent hosts have been found in South America: Andes virus (*Oligoryzomys longicaudatus*) from Argentina, Chile, and Uruguay; Oran (*O. longicaudatus*) from Argentina; Lechiguanas (*Oligoryzomys flavescens*) from Argentina; Hu39694 (unknown host) from Argentina; Laguna Negra (*Calomys laucha*) from Paraguay and Bolivia; and Juquitiba, Castelo dos Sonhos, and Araraquara virus (all unknown hosts) from Brazil. Numerous other viruses and rodent reservoirs have been recognized but are not implicated in human disease.

PATHOGENESIS

Hemorrhagic Fever with Renal Syndrome

Severe HFRS causes widespread macroscopic and microscopic hemorrhages, capillary endothelial damage, and associated fluid transudation with retroperitoneal edema. The most striking ab-

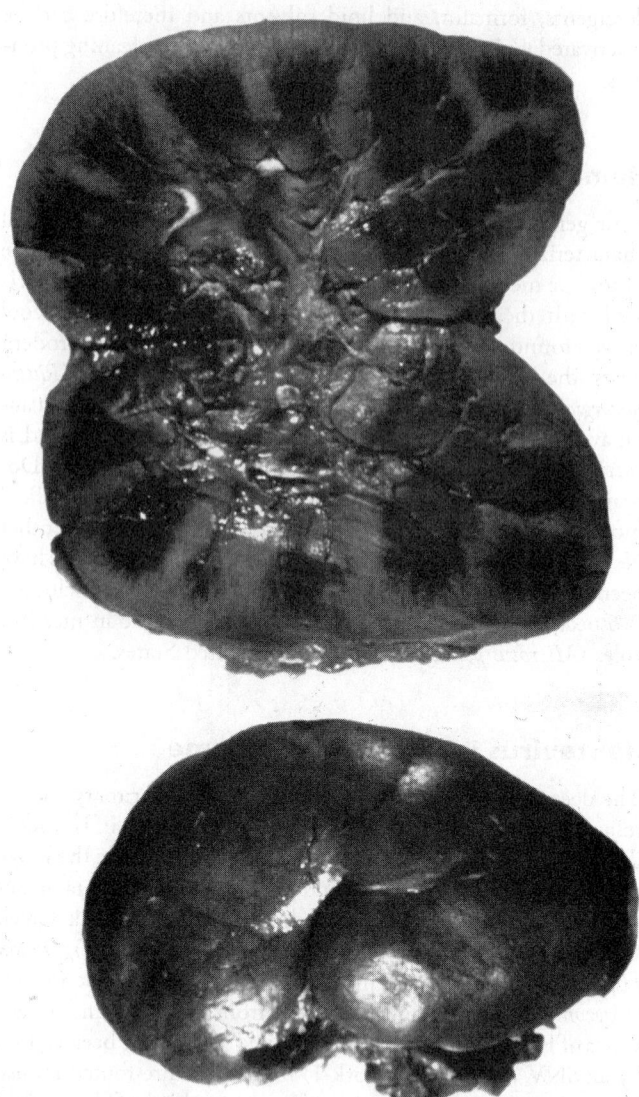

FIGURE 308.2. Kidney in hemorrhagic fever. The cortex is pale and swollen, and the medulla is congested and hemorrhagic, with submucosal hemorrhage in the pelvis.

normalities are in the kidneys (Fig 308.2), which show a pale, swollen cortex with a sharp demarcation from a varyingly hemorrhagic medulla, with similar findings in the right atrium and anterior pituitary. The most common histopathologic abnormality is acute tubulointerstitial nephritis with interstitial edema, extravasation of red blood cells, and inflammatory infiltrates. Although fibrin clots are absent, laboratory evidence suggests that the basis of hemorrhage involves a form of consumptive coagulopathy. Full clarification of the pathogenetic mechanisms of action will have to await development of an animal model.

Hantavirus Pulmonary Syndrome

The histopathologic lesions, mainly seen in the lung and spleen, are primarily vascular, with varying degrees of generalized capillary dilatation and edema. Morphologic changes of the endothe-

lium are uncommon. In most cases, the lungs evidence mild to moderate interstitial pneumonitis with different degrees of congestion, edema, and infiltration; on gross examination, they are dense, rubbery, and heavy. The cellular infiltrate is composed of a mixture of small and enlarged mononuclear cells, scanty neutrophils, and the appearance of immunoblasts. Focal hyaline membranes have been noted, as has diffuse alveolar damage. Other typical histopathologic findings include immunoblasts within the red pulp and periarteriolar sheaths of the spleen and paracortex, within sinuses of lymph nodes, and in the peripheral blood. Immunohistochemistry analysis has shown marked accumulations of hantaviral antigens in the pulmonary microvasculature and in follicular dendritic cells within the lymphoid follicles of the spleen and lymph nodes.

The timing of disease onset concurrent with development of antibody response, without evidence of cytopathologic viral changes, has suggested that the disorder is immunologically mediated. Functional impairment of vascular endothelium is central to the complex pathogenesis of HPS. Hypotension is often the source of the fatal outcome of infection, but it is unclear how the shock syndrome relates to such factors as viral distribution and immunologic and pharmacologic mediators of capillary permeability. There appears to be compartmentalization of a selective immune response in the lungs of HPS patients in combination with extremely high levels of viral antigens and cytokine production in the pulmonary vasculature; administration of TNF or interleukin-2 to animals causes syndromes that are similar to HPS.

CLINICAL FEATURES

Hemorrhagic Fever with Renal Syndrome

The most severe form of HFRS is caused by Hantaan virus and classically is associated with five consecutive phases, with a characteristic physiologic derangement and a 5% to 15% case fatality.

Febrile Phase

Onset is usually abrupt, with fever, chills, lethargy, and weakness after a 7- to 42-day incubation period. Other associated symptoms include frontal or retro-orbital headache that occasionally is associated with pain on eye movement, myalgia, lumbar aching, diffuse abdominal pain, blurred vision, and nausea and vomiting, which tends to develop a few days later. Within a few hours the patients are more or less prostrated and begin to experience marked thirst and anorexia.

Hypotensive Phase

Shock or hypotension of varying degrees sets in during the last 24 to 48 hours of the febrile phase, or about day 5 of illness. Tachycardia and bulbar conjunctival edema may be evident on physical examination.

Oliguric Phase

Blood pressure tends to normalize, with occasional episodes of brief hypertension, and oliguria is prominent. Most symptoms abate during this phase, although nausea and vomiting may continue. Approximately 15% of patients develop overt hemorrhagic manifestations, such as epistaxis, ecchymoses, and subconjunctival hemorrhage and, less often, gross hematuria, hemoptysis, and CNS and gastrointestinal bleeding. This phase reflects the overall severity of the illness and is associated with major electrolyte, fluid, and CNS abnormalities in addition to serious pulmonary complications.

Diuretic Phase

Progressive improvement is heralded by the onset of diuresis, usually within 2 weeks of onset of symptoms.

Convalescent Phase

Convalescence is marked by polyuria and loss of urine-concentrating ability. Rare reports have suggested long-term renal complications, such as renal tubular acidosis, renal hypertension, proteinuria, and end-stage renal disease. A residual inability to concentrate the urine may be permanent, and studies in the United States have suggested an association with hypertensive renal disease.

Patients with severe HFRS appear acutely ill; their symptoms include an erythematous flush of the face and upper torso, with blanching on pressure and dermatographia. Petechiae are present in axillary and waist folds and occasionally on the face and upper torso. Conjunctival injection is common; conjunctival petechiae and hemorrhage develop during days 3 to 5 in some patients. The soft palate also is intensely and diffusely reddened, with mild generalized lymphadenopathy noted on day 2. Splenomegaly, jaundice, and a maculopapular rash have not been reported.

The incidence and severity of clinical manifestations of hantavirus infection vary considerably, and the individual phases may overlap. This is most apparent in Puumala virus infections, in which shock does not develop and skipping of phases is common. The mildest form of this syndrome, known as nephropathia epidemica, is characterized by a mild degree of renal insufficiency without significant overt hemorrhage. Epistaxis, macroscopic hematuria, and mild gastrointestinal bleeding may occur in 5% of these patients in association with petechiae, but most patients experience only febrile grippe with proteinuria and an extremely low case fatality of 0.2%. Blurred vision and photophobia are typical findings, as is a myopic shift with narrowing of the anterior chamber and thickening of the crystalline lens. Puumala virus infection also has been associated with Guillian-Barré syndrome. Pulmonary edema is another classic feature, not just in the more severe Hantaan virus infections but in the much milder Puumula virus infections. Features of disease caused by Seoul virus infection are intermediate in nature between these two clinical pictures, whereas Dobrava virus infection appears to be more Hantaan-like. Hepatic involvement is more likely with Seoul virus.

Although it is difficult to mistake HFRS with classic polyphasic manifestation, this syndrome can be confused with Waterhouse–Friderichsen syndrome, acute glomerulonephritis, pyelonephritis, leptospirosis, scrub typhus, dengue fever, thrombocytopenic purpura, or acute renal vein thrombosis. Nephro-pathia epidemica cannot be distinguished clinically from other viral grippes. Consider these diseases in the differential diagnosis of all patients with unexplained febrile nephropathy with isosthenuria and proteinuria.

Hantavirus Pulmonary Syndrome

Hantaviral infection may be asymptomatic or mild or may cause severe disease (HPS). After a 1- to 5-week incubation period, patients usually experience a brief, 4-day prodrome characterized by malaise, diarrhea, and headache. Fever, chills, myalgia, nausea or vomiting, and cough develop one day later. Dizziness or light-headedness is also reported by approximately one-fourth of patients, whereas arthralgias, back pain, and abdominal pain are reported less frequently. Patients often are misdiagnosed during this early stage because differentiating characteristics, such as cough and tachypnea, generally do not develop until the end of the prodromal phase. Within 24 hours of initial evaluation, most patients abruptly enter the characteristic cardiopulmonary phase, with some degree of hypotension and progressive evidence of pulmonary edema and hypoxia, usually requiring mechanical ventilation. Patients who do not survive have severe hypotension frequently terminating with sinus bradycardia, electromechanical dissociation, or ventricular tachycardia or fibrillation. This terminal hemodynamic compromise can be independent of oxygenation status and occurs a median of five days after onset of symptoms. Multiorgan dysfunction syndrome is rarely seen. About 90% of patients are intubated by day 5 of illness. The disease resolves rapidly, usually preceded by or concurrent with a diuretic phase. Atypical clinical pictures of prominent renal insufficiency and myositis have been documented with Black Creek Canal, Bayou virus, and Andes virus. The typical length of stay in the hospital is 10 days, though patients may experience fatigue and exercise intolerance for several months. Occasional residual effects under investigation include cognitive impairments, sensorineural hearing loss, and modest small-airway obstruction, and a few patients have mild degrees of proteinuria and pulmonary hypertension.

Physical examination of the patient in the initial stage of infection shows normal results, except for fever, tachypnea, and tachycardia. Rashes, throat or conjunctival erythema, and peripheral or periorbital edema are absent. In South America, Andes virus may produce facial flushing (rubicundez), petechiae, and occasionally frank hemorrhage from the gastrointestinal or pulmonary tract. Rarely, there is overt hemorrhage in severe cases in North America, owing to DIC. Rapidly progressive respiratory and hemodynamic compromise reflects the evidence of increasing tachypnea, hypotension, and pulmonary edema and pleural effusions on serial examination.

Initial chest radiographs in almost all patients show abnormal results indicative of interstitial edema, specifically, Kerley B lines, hilar indistinctness, or peribronchial cuffing with normal cardiothoracic ratios. One-third of patients also have evidence of airspace disease on the initial radiograph. By 48 hours, all patients show evidence of interstitial edema, and two-thirds have extensive airspace disease that is initially bibasilar or perihilar in na-

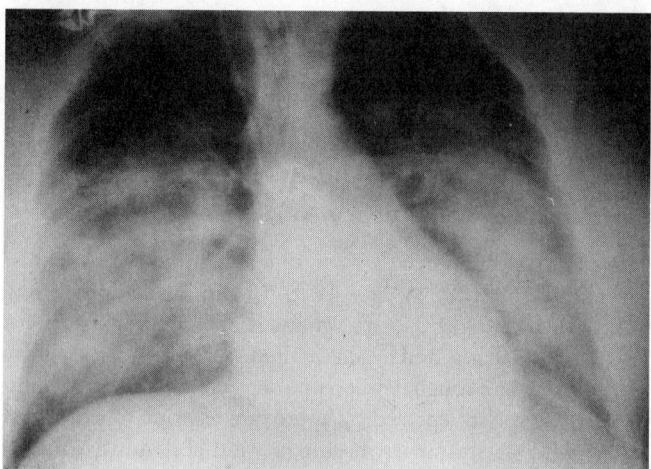

FIGURE 308.3. Chest radiograph of hantavirus pulmonary syndrome, taken 48 hours after admission, showing bilateral interstitial infiltrates.

ture, with some degree of pleural effusion (Fig. 308.3). Evidence of bilateral interstitial pulmonary infiltrates is required for a diagnosis of severe disease. The lack of peripheral distribution of initial airspace disease, the prominence of interstitial edema, and the presence of pleural effusions on radiography early in the disease process distinguish HPS from the acute respiratory distress syndrome (ARDS).

Diagnostic considerations include sepsis and severe pneumonia. The lack of sore throat and nasal symptoms facilitates differentiation of HPS from influenza, the lack of lobar infiltrates and chest pain distinguishes HPS from pneumococcal pneumonia, and certain laboratory test abnormalities help discriminate HPS from unexplained ARDS. Depending on the patient's history, other diagnoses to exclude are acute pulmonary edema due to myocardial infarction, septicemic plague, tularemia, leptospirosis, Q fever, ehrlichiosis, coccidioidomycosis, histoplasmosis, and diffuse pulmonary hemorrhage.

LABORATORY FINDINGS

Hemorrhagic Fever with Renal Syndrome

Laboratory findings are usually unremarkable at first, but progressive thrombocytopenia and leukocytosis develop during the course of the febrile phase and into the hypotensive phase. Abrupt onset of proteinuria is usually noted on about day 5 of illness, with isosthenuria (urine specific gravity of 1.010) and evidence of hemoconcentration. Renal insufficiency and electrolyte abnormalities are prominent during the oliguric phase.

Measurement of IgM-specific anti-hantaviral antibodies, using an IgM-capture ELISA or immunofluorescence assay, is the method of choice for the early diagnosis of HFRS. Specific antibodies are usually present on admission, and all patients should have measurable antibodies by day 7 of disease. Hemagglutination or neutralization tests are needed to distinguish hantaviruses serologically. RT-PCR also has been used in clinical diagnosis and to differentiate hantaviral strains. Recovery of virus from blood, various fluids, and tissues has rarely been done and has no diagnostic usefulness.

Hantavirus Pulmonary Syndrome

Notable hematologic findings include neutrophilic leukocytosis with increased mycloid precursors, circulating immunoblasts, thrombocytopenia, and hemoconcentration, especially at the onset of the cardiopulmonary phase. The triad of left-shifted neutrophils, thrombocytopenia, and immunoblasts may help make an early diagnosis. Hypoalbuminemia, proteinuria, and mild elevations of transaminases, creatinine phosphokinase, amylase, and creatinine also have been documented. Other abnormalities mirror hemodynamic and pulmonary involvement—the development of metabolic acidosis, rising serum lactate levels, and prolongation of the prothrombin time and partial thromboplastin time. Critical prognostic indicators include a plasma lactate level greater than 4.0 mmol per liter or a cardiac index of less than 2.2 L per minute per square meter. Elevated fibrin split products and decreased fibrinogen levels suggestive of DIC are uncommon.

Diagnosis can be confirmed rapidly by using ELISA to detect SNV-specific IgM and IgG antibodies in North America and Laguna Negra–specific antibodies in South America. A Western blot assay using recombinant antigens and isotype-specific conjugates for IgM–IgG differentiation is also available. Specific antibodies almost always are present on admission, and all patients should have measurable antibodies by day 7 of disease. Serologic confirmation of hantaviral infections traditionally has been done with neutralizing plaque assays; these assays have been described for SNV, though they are not readily available. IgG antibody is long lasting, but antibody reversions have been reported.

To date, no isolates of SNV-like viruses have been recovered from humans; therefore, virus isolation is not a diagnostic consideration. Detection of hantaviral RNA has been useful for diagnosis when fresh frozen lung tissue, blood clots, or nucleated blood cells are tested by RT-PCR. Serum does not appear to be as useful for amplification of viral RNA. Immunohistochemistry has an important role in the diagnosis of HPS in patients from whom serum samples and frozen tissues are not available for diagnostic testing.

OPTIMAL MANAGEMENT

Hemorrhagic Fever with Renal Syndrome

The principal therapeutic challenge is treatment of renal failure and shock, but pulmonary edema, stroke, primary encephalopathy, myocarditis, hepatitis, and pancreatitis may complicate the illness. The case fatality rate is less than 5% when good supportive care and access to dialysis and advanced intensive care are available. In a double-blind concurrent, placebo-controlled trial, intravenous ribavirin therapy has been shown to result in a sevenfold reduction in Hantaan-virus associated HFRS mortality, if it is administered within 6 days of fever onset to patients >14 years of age. It has been established that steroids ameliorate disease but do not affect fatality. Cyclophosphamide, which presumably inhibits immune-mediated damage, has been used in China outside any controlled trials, with conflicting results. Public health measures have focused on the control of rodents and building rodent-proof homes and grain storage facilities. A number of inactivated Hantaan virus vaccines are commercially available in Korea and China, but no effectiveness data are available. Preliminary human trials using a recombinant vaccine that expresses both the M and S segments for Hantaan virus are under way.

Hantavirus Pulmonary Syndrome

Treatment of patients with HPS also remains supportive in nature. Nevertheless, all patients should be placed on broad-spectrum antibiotics, including tetracycline, until the diagnosis of HPS is well established, since bacterial shock is far more common than hantaviral shock. Early intensive care is important, with prompt correction of electrolyte, pulmonary, and hemodynamic abnormalities. Flow-directed catheterization of the pulmonary artery is helpful not only in intensively monitoring and treating the patient but also in verifying the normal-to-low pulmonary wedge pressure, decreased cardiac index, and increased systemic vascular resistance in patients who progress to shock. This pattern of shock is in contrast to the typical hemodynamic profile for septic shock of increased cardiac index and low systemic vascular resistance. Fluid administration to correct hypotension should be limited, to prevent worsening pulmonary edema, and the early use of inotropic agents, such as dobutamine, is strongly encouraged. Early promising results with extracorporeal membrane oxygenation as salvage therapy for patients with poor prognostic indicators have not been reproduced. An open-label trial of treatment with intravenous ribavirin—which is effective in treating HFRS—failed to document a dramatic improvement in mortality. A single patient had a favorable outcome after inhaled nitric oxide therapy. Therapy with intravenous glucocorticoids has had positive results in South America and is to be tested in a controlled trial.

The thrust of the prevention effort regarding peridomestic rodents is to eliminate their access to domestic settings and to make domestic settings uninhabitable by rodents by properly storing or removing all sources of food and water. Standard precautions coupled with droplet precautions should be reinforced in South American countries, with an upgrade to aerosol precautions as indicated.

■ FILOVIRUSES

DEFINITION

Marburg and Ebola viruses are the prototypical emerging pathogens. They cause a hemorrhagic disease with a high case fatality associated with explosive outbreaks due to person-to-person transmission. Moreover, they occur unpredictably and have an unknown reservoir. There is no treatment at present. Since their initial discovery in 1967, there have been only a handful of filoviral outbreaks, mostly in remote locations. The documented occurrence of secondary cases in locations far from disease-endemic areas, however, raises the concern that filoviruses have the potential to generate unprecedented outbreaks in the future. This speculation has been validated by the identification of a fatal case of Marburg virus infection traced to the large-scale production of Marburg virus by Biopreparat, the biological weapons program of the former Soviet Union.

INCIDENCE AND EPIDEMIOLOGY

Marburg Viral Hemorrhagic Fever

In 1967, many cases of severe hemorrhagic fever with nosocomial transmission among European laboratory workers led to the identification of Marburg virus. The primary patients had all handled monkey blood, tissues, or cell cultures traced to a shipment of African green (vervet) monkeys (*Cercopithecus aethiops*) exported from Uganda. In 1975, a traveler became infected in Zimbabwe and transmitted the disease to a female companion and a nurse who attended the second victim. In 1980 and 1987, two episodes of Marburg VHF were identified among expatriates in southwestern Kenya, near the area in Uganda that produced the infected monkeys involved in the 1967 outbreak. Indigenous Marburg virus infection among native Africans in rural areas was confirmed during a large 1999 outbreak in Durba, in the northeastern region of the Democratic Republic of Congo, primarily affecting gold miners and with occasional secondary spread. This area had several similar small outbreaks that were termed "Durba syndrome," with retrospective confirmation of Marburg virus infection in a survivor from 1994.

Ebola Viral Hemorrhagic Fever

The first recognized outbreaks of Ebola VHF took place simultaneously in northern Zaire and southern Sudan in 1976 and were caused by two distinct subtypes. No index case was identified clearly in the Sudan outbreak, though early cases originating in Nzara, Sudan, arose among cotton factory workers. The disease initially spread through nosocomial transmission; the use of nonsterile needles and lack of barrier nursing practice fueled the epidemic. The case fatality in the Sudan outbreak was 53%. A small outbreak in southern Sudan in 1979 was linked to the same cotton factory.

The outbreak in Zaire centered around a Belgian mission hospital in Yambuku, Equateur region. During the 7-week period of the outbreak, 318 cases were confirmed, with a case fatality of 88%. A significant factor in the spread of infection in the hospital was the reuse of syringes and needles. The disease appeared to subside, except for an isolated case in northwestern Zaire in 1977. Then three separate outbreaks caused by an Ebola-Zaire subtype occurred in Gabon over a 3-year period. In 1994, an outbreak of Ebola VHF occurred north of the provincial capital of Ogooue-Ivindo, which was originally misdiagnosed as yellow fever. In January 1996, another outbreak, near the site of the 1994 outbreak, was linked to the butchering for consumption of a dead chimpanzee. In 1996–1997, there was a 7-month outbreak of 60 cases in Booue Province, Gabon (case fatality of 75%), associated with eight generations of secondary cases, some of which were found in the capital city. A noteworthy case of secondary transmission involved a nurse in Johannesburg who died from the disease after caring for a physician with Ebola VHF. In 1994, a new Ebola subtype was isolated from an infected ethologist in Côte d'Ivoire who had performed a necropsy on a chimpanzee from a group that had lost several members to an unidentified illness. This isolation extended the geographic distribution of known cases to include most of the African rain forest.

Ebola VHF dramatically reemerged in Zaire in 1995, when a total of 315 cases (81% case fatality) developed over 7 months, centered in Kikwit but taking in an additional 20 villages. The earliest documented patient was a charcoal worker, in whom the diagnosis was missed; for 3 months the disease spread from person to person in the community until it was amplified in the hospital setting and finally recognized. Owing to nosocomial transmission, one-fourth of the cases arose among health care workers. The application of basic barrier nursing methods rapidly terminated transmission in the hospital. Two individuals, designated "super-spreaders," may have been the source of infection for more than 50 cases; the mechanism of heightened transmission was not identified, though contact with a cadaver was implicated strongly.

In contrast to the three pathogenetic subtypes of Ebola virus from the African continent, a subtype of low or no pathogenicity for humans (Ebola-Reston) was recognized in November 1989 at a primate quarantine facility in Reston, Virginia. Unusually high mortality was noted in a shipment of cynomolgus monkeys (*Macaca fascicularis*) imported from the Philippines; the deceased monkeys subsequently were determined to have been infected with Ebola-Reston virus. Four cases of acute filovirus infection were confirmed among the human caretakers, none of whom experienced clinical illness.

The natural epidemiologic characteristics of these infections, besides those documented during internationally recognized outbreaks, are unknown. The latency between occurrence of index cases and the recognition of a subsequent outbreak suggests that sporadic cases of unrecognized filovirus infections are not uncommon. Serologic surveys have found an antibody prevalence of 9% to 10% among gold panners in Gabon and among rural villagers in the Democratic Republic of Congo. The explosive nature of these outbreaks belies the fact that the secondary attack rate is approximately 12% to 16% and close physical contact is necessary for disease transmission. Health care facilities have played a major role in amplifying the disease; the closure of or upgrade of infection control practices in these facilities, coupled with community education, has proved critical to the rapid cessation of these outbreaks.

ETIOLOGY AND ECOLOGY

Filoviruses are classified into a new family of RNA viruses, the Filoviridae, consisting of the single genus *Filovirus,* on the basis of their similarities in size, tubular morphologic features, and distinctive physicochemical properties. The genus contains four subtypes of Ebola virus (Zaire, Sudan, Ivory Coast, and Reston) and a single species of Marburg virus. Infectious virions can be inactivated when exposed to appropriate amounts of lipid solvents (such as detergents), formaldehyde, hypochlorite (bleach), b-propiolactone, quaternary ammonium and phenolic disinfectants, ultraviolet light, gamma irradiation, and prolonged heating at 60°C. Little is known of the geographic and natural distribution of Marburg or Ebola viruses or the circumstances leading to human infection in nature. The discovery of Reston viral infections in macaque monkeys from Asia suggests a wider, possibly global distribution of Ebola-related viruses. The best evidence for the putative host has come from experimental inocula-

tions that have demonstrated replication and circulation of high titers of virus in bats. The similarity of Ebola–Zaire subtypes from widely separated geographic and ecologic areas (northern Zaire, southern Zaire, and Gabon) and collections spanning 20 years suggest an extremely stable virus–host relationship.

PATHOGENESIS

Filoviral infection results in widespread cytopathic effects on parenchymal and endothelial cells and release of immune cell mediators. Several underlying mechanisms of damage have been postulated: suppression of the immune system through infection of fibroblastic reticular cells, the action of structural (spike) glycoproteins via a conserved immunosuppressive motif, and the binding of the secreted form of the Ebola virus glycoprotein to neutrophils. Disease has been characterized by widespread involvement of liver, lymphoid organs, and kidneys. The liver shows extensive eosinophilic degeneration with prominent vacuolar changes and intracytoplasmic viral inclusions. Interstitial pneumonia, interstitial nephritis, and follicular necrosis of the spleen are found frequently, but there is pathologic evidence of pantropic infection. The pathophysiologic features of bleeding and events leading to death are not understood fully. Platelet and endothelial cell dysfunction may be the primary causes of hemorrhage and shock. Tissue factor release from infected monocytes and fragmented tissue factor–rich cell membranes following viral budding and cell lysis have been hypothesized as mechanisms for DIC.

CLINICAL FEATURES

Marburg Viral Hemorrhagic Fever

After an incubation period of 5 to 9 days, the highly characteristic clinical syndrome begins with sudden onset of fever and headache accompanied by profuse vomiting and nonbloody diarrhea with varying evidence of conjunctivitis, myalgia, and lymphadenopathy. This picture is often accompanied by abdominal pain that may be intense enough to suggest a surgical abdomen. Patients frequently appear restless and anxious, and they later become disoriented, drowsy, and stuporous and exhibit other encephalopathic signs, such as lassitude. After 3 to 8 days, a morbilliform, usually confluent, nonpruritic rash starts on the upper trunk and spreads centrifugally to involve the entire body, sparing the face and neck; the rash fades in 48 hours, and desquamation occurs in 2 weeks. The oral cavity is usually dry, with small aphthous-like ulcers with slight posterior pharynx injection. The conjunctiva are only slightly injected and rarely icteric. Examination of the chest commonly shows bibasilar rales; there is no organomegaly on abdominal exam, but epigastric and right subcostal tenderness may be present. Severe hemorrhagic diathesis, with bleeding from the gums, the nose, and puncture sites as well as the gastrointestinal tract, is noted in approximately one-third of patients when the thrombocyte count is lowest, usually between day 6 and day 12. Multisystem failure from pneumonitis, hepatitis, pancreatitis, and tubulointerstitial nephritis combined with intractable hypotension usually leads to death.

Ebola Viral Hemorrhagic Fever

Beginning with a sudden onset of fever, asthenia, headache, and joint and muscle aches, the disease causes initially nonbloody diarrhea (81%), vomiting (59%), pain and dryness of the throat (63%), and abdominal pain. Chest pain (83%) is a characteristic feature of patients infected with Ebola-Sudan virus but uncommon in those infected with Marburg or Ebola-Zaire virus. Patients are usually hospitalized by the fifth day of illness with deep-set eyes, ghostlike expressionless facies, and extreme lethargy. A rubeola-like rash with later desquamation appears in approximately half of the patients at about the fifth day, though it may be difficult to evaluate in dark-skinned people. Hemorrhagic manifestations, usually gastrointestinal and rarely urogenital, are common and may be preceded by apparent improvement. Although hemorrhage is present in only half of all cases, almost all of the fatal cases showed some sign of hemorrhage, which typically is not life threatening in itself. During the 1995 Ebola-Zaire outbreak, 103 cases were studied prospectively and were characterized by a similar biphasic clinical syndrome with asthenia as an early sign and the later evolution of hemorrhagic manifestations, hiccups (15%), and, less frequently, neurologic symptoms. Terminally ill patients had obtundation, anuria, shock, tachypnea, and normothermia.

Convalescence after filoviral infection is prolonged—resolution of fatigue, anorexia, and cachexia takes as long as several weeks, and weight loss is very common. Tender livers and other hepatic abnormalities have been reported in the Marburg VHF patients, but these features may have been due to transfusion-associated hepatitis; relapse also has been described in Marburg patients. Patients infected with the Ebola-Zaire subtype continue to report myalgia and arthralgias 2 years after acute illness, which may be correlated with circulating antibody titers. The differential diagnosis depends on the initial stage of clinical illness and its evolution. Causes of VHFs in addition to those addressed in this chapter include dengue, yellow fever, Congo-Crimean hemorrhagic fever, and Rift Valley fever viruses. The travel and occupational histories of the patient are critical in narrowing the potential diagnoses, as are reports of clusters of illness or person-to-person transmission. Contact with severely ill humans or with sick or dead nonhuman primates and a history of injections in an African hospital are relevant (Fig. 308.4).

LABORATORY FINDINGS

Typical findings include thrombocytopenia, normal or depressed white blood cell counts, and the presence of "atypical" lymphocytes, plasma cells, plasmablasts, pyroninophil blast cells, or immunoblasts. Mild to severe elevations in liver transaminases and amylase levels, prothrombin time, partial thromboplastin time, and fibrin degradation products have been reported. Proteinuria and microscopic hematuria are also evident in some patients. Most of the initial Marburg VHF patients had high levels of aspartate aminotransferase (AST) and ALT (ALT greater than AST) and normal bilirubin, alkaline phosphatase, and creatine kinase levels. Elevated amylase also has been reported, and significant rises in blood urea nitrogen and proteinuria are characteristic of the most severe cases. Antibody is detected late (12

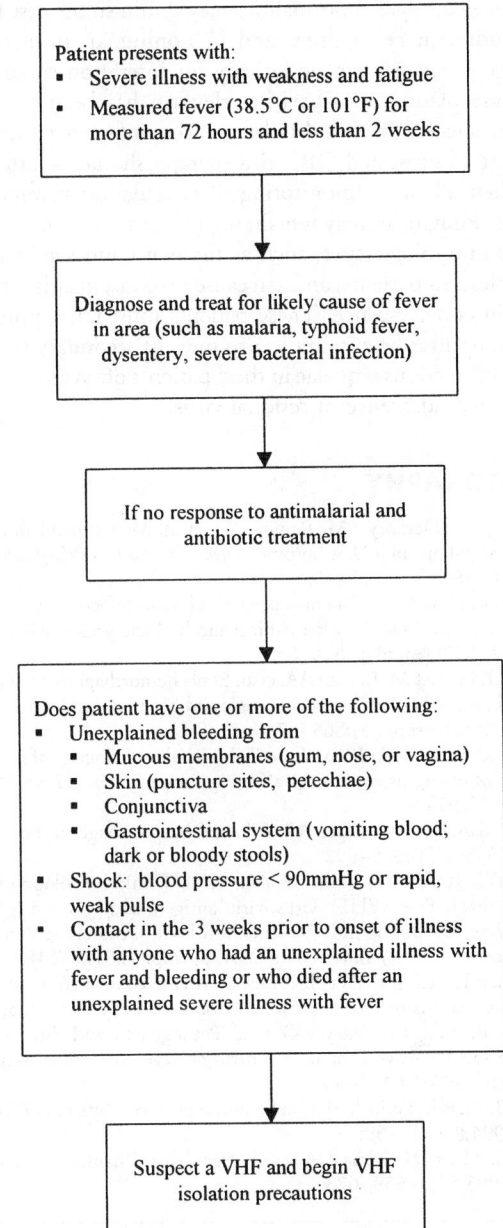

FIGURE 308.4. Approach to suspected cases of viral hemorrhagic fever (VHF).

to 13 days) among survivors by ELISA and indirect fluorescent antibody techniques; therefore, during the acute phase of illness, serum or blood should be tested for the presence of virus, viral antigen, or viral RNA. Fatal infections are best diagnosed from serum samples using antigen detection by ELISA, from liver touch preps using fluorescent antibodies, or from fixed solid tissue samples by immunohistochemistry and electron microscopy.

OPTIMAL MANAGEMENT

No specific therapy is available for filoviral infections. Extremely limited data suggest that utmost attention to correction of simple fluid and electrolyte abnormalities may diminish the case fatality rate. Studies in cell culture and in nonhuman primates and guinea pigs have shown no efficacy for interferon-α, convalescent-phase plasma, or ribavirin. Heparin has been used with apparent success in two Marburg virus–infected patients for treatment of suspected DIC; this therapy should be attempted only when adequate monitoring of coagulation parameters is available. Filoviruses may remain sequestered for months in protected immunologic sites, such as the uveal and seminal tracts of convalescent patients, and can cause myelitis, uveitis, or orchitis late in convalescence. These patients must take appropriate precautions after hospitalization to prevent secondary transmission. Postinfectious sequelae in these patients often are associated with the recrudescence of residual virus.

BIBLIOGRAPHY

Armstrong LR, Dembry LM, Rainey PM, et al. Management of a Sabiá-infected patient in a U.S. hospital. *Infect Control Hosp Epidemiol* 1999; 20:176–182.

Formenty P, Hatz C, Le Guenno B, et al. Human infection due to Ebola virus, subtype Cote d'Ivoire: clinical and biologic presentation. *J Infect Dis* 1999;179(suppl 1):S48–S53.

Georges AJ, Leroy EM, Renaut AA, et al. Ebola hemorrhagic fever outbreaks in Gabon, 1994–1997: epidemiologic and health control issues. *J Infect Dis* 1999;179(suppl 1):S65–S75.

Gonzalez JP, Sanchez A, Rico-Hesse R. Molecular phylogeny of Guanarito virus, an emerging arenavirus affecting humans. *Am J Trop Med Hyg* 1995;53(1):1–6.

Khan AS, Sanchez A, Pflieger AK. Filoviral haemorrhagic fevers. *Br Med Bull* 1998;54(3):675–692.

Ksiazek TG, Rollin PE, Williams AG, et al. Clinical virology of Ebola hemorrhagic fever (EHF): virus, virus antigen, and IgG and IgM antibody findings among EHF patients in Kikwit, Democratic Republic of the Congo, 1995. *J Infect Dis* 1999;179(suppl 1):S177–S187.

McCormick JB, King IJ, Webb PA, et al. A case-control study of clinical diagnosis and course of Lassa fever. *J Infect Dis* 1987;155:445.

Settergren B, Ahlm C, Alexeyev O, et al. Pathogenetic and clinical aspects of the renal involvement in hemorrhagic fever with renal syndrome. *Ren Fail* 1997;19(1):1–14.

Vainrub B, Salas R. Latin American hemorrhagic fever. *Infect Dis Clin North Am* 1994;8(1):47–59.

Young JC, Mills JN, Enria DA, et al. New World hantaviruses. *Br Med Bull* 1998;54(3):659–673.

Kelley's Textbook of Internal Medicine, fourth edition. Edited by H. David Humes. Lippincott Williams & Wilkins, Philadelphia © 2000.

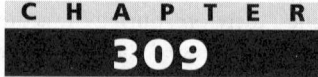

C H A P T E R

309

POXVIRUS INFECTIONS

BRIAN W. J. MAHY

There are nine poxviruses known to cause infection in humans. Six of them produce relatively rare zoonotic infections (cowpox,

milker's nodules, monkeypox, orf, tanapox, and yabapox), and two cause specifically human diseases (smallpox [variola] and molluscum contagiosum). The last, the most widely studied, is vaccinia virus (smallpox vaccine). Smallpox is the only infectious disease to have been eradicated globally; the last natural case occurred in Somalia in October 1977. The intensive worldwide campaign to eliminate smallpox began in 1966 and used vaccinia virus as a potent, stable vaccine. Eradication eliminated the need for smallpox vaccination, with enormous economic benefits; the entire cost to the World Health Organization of the 11-year campaign was recovered in 6 months once vaccination was no longer necessary.

■ DESCRIPTION

The poxviruses of medical importance belong to the subfamily Chordopoxvirinae of the family Poxviridae. Within this subfamily, viruses of four different genera affect humans: *Orthopoxvirus, Parapoxvirus, Yatapoxvirus,* and *Molluscipoxvirus.* Poxviruses consist of large brick-shaped or ovoid virions of complex structure, 220 to 450 nm by 140 to 260 nm in size (Fig. 309.1). There is an outer coat containing tubular lipoprotein subunits that encloses two "lateral bodies" and a core containing the double-stranded DNA genome, 130- to 220-kb pairs in length in different viruses. The genomes of vaccinia virus (191, 636 bp) and variola (smallpox) virus (186, 103 bp) have been sequenced completely and found to specify more than 180 polypeptides,

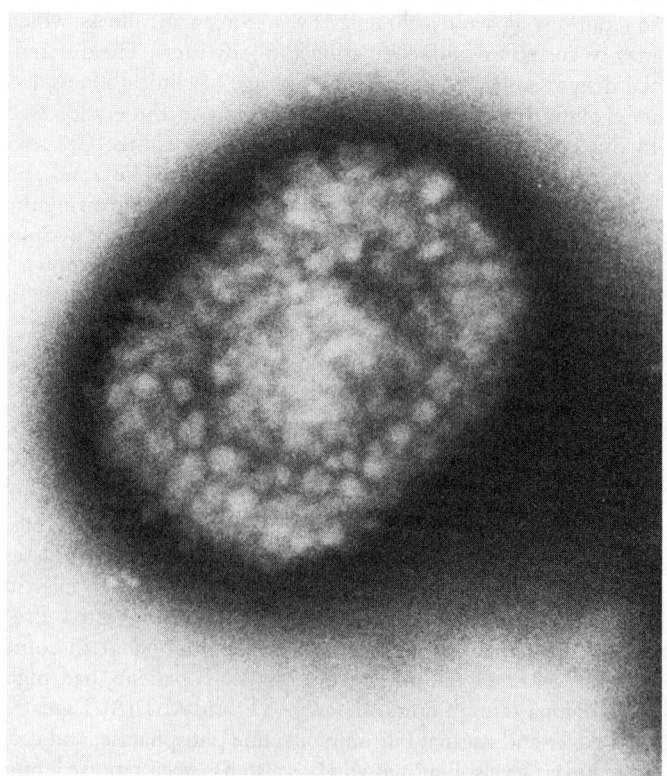

FIGURE 309.1. Smallpox (variola) virus. (Phosphotungstic acid, original magnification ×350,000. Courtesy of Frederick A. Murphy.)

151 of which are closely similar between the two viruses. In contrast to the other DNA viruses, poxviruses replicate in the cytoplasm, where they may form characteristic inclusions (Guarnieri bodies) detected on histologic examination.

Dozens of enzymes necessary for DNA transcription and replication are encoded in the virus genome, and after entry and uncoating of the virion, DNA transcription is initiated by enzymes contained within the virion itself. Transcription is controlled by the binding of certain viral proteins to promoter sequences on the DNA genome, and it takes place in three stages—early, intermediate, and late. Early genes encode almost 100 proteins needed for replication; once DNA replication begins, intermediate genes are expressed that encode several proteins secreted by infected cells that affect the host immune system. Finally, late genes are triggered that encode late enzymes and virion structural proteins. The entire replication cycle from virus entry to assembly and morphogenesis of progeny virions takes about 20 hours.

PATHOGENESIS

Poxviruses cause lesions on the skin that may be localized or, in more severe cases, generalized. The lesions normally form a pustular rash but can also be proliferative (in molluscum contagiosum). After infection, there is an incubation period of 10 to 14 days before fever, headache, and myalgia develop; the skin lesions appear 2 to 3 days later. In most infections, neutralizing antibodies emerge 4 to 6 days after the onset of clinical symptoms and protect against reinfection. In orthopoxvirus infections, other antibodies are directed against a virus-specific hemagglutinin produced in infected cells. Cell-mediated immune responses also play a critical role in recovery and protective immunity—agammaglobulinemic subjects were found to recover from smallpox provided their cell-mediated immunity was not impaired.

EPIDEMIOLOGY

Transmission of poxvirus infections usually requires close contact with an infected person or animal, although fomites can also disperse the virus. Smallpox was eradicated because (a) there was no animal reservoir for variola virus, (b) immunity after infection was long-lasting and infection did not lead to recurrence, (c) the vaccine (vaccinia virus) was extremely effective, and (d) antigenic variants of variola virus resistant to neutralization were not found. Smallpox was an extremely severe disease that spread worldwide and exacted a high toll in human morbidity and mortality over many centuries. Now that smallpox is extinct, the only human poxvirus disease of global importance is molluscum contagiosum, which is spread by contact with an infected person (or occasionally by fomites) but is quite benign. The zoonotic poxviruses that can be transmitted to humans in a variety of ways are not readily transmissible from human to human and are relatively rare.

CLINICAL FEATURES

HUMAN MONKEYPOX

Monkeypox virus was first recognized as the origin of a disease of captive nonhuman primates, but in 1970 cases of human infection were discovered in West and Central Africa, where smallpox had been eradicated. In the initial reports, six of 36 cases were fatal. The disease has features similar to smallpox—a generalized pustular rash, high fever, and toxemia—and could not be distinguished in clinical terms from smallpox. A mortality rate of about 11% has been recorded among unvaccinated children younger than 9 years of age, but not in adults; vaccination with vaccinia virus protects against monkeypox virus infection. Unlike smallpox, monkeypox is not readily transmissible between humans, and for this reason it is not a serious risk outside the limited disease-endemic area. The true reservoir of monkeypox virus appears to be species of squirrels of the genera *Funisciurus* or *Heliosciurus* that inhabit the tropical rain forest in Zaire and the surrounding regions. Monkeys as well as humans are secondary hosts.

COWPOX

Human infections with cowpox virus have been recorded only in Europe, mostly among farmworkers who have close contact with cattle. The cowpox virus is not enzootic in cattle, however, and it is believed to be maintained in a rodent reservoir, the species of which is not known. Cats frequently become infected with cowpox virus, and human infections from cats have been well documented. Infections in large feline species in zoos also have been reported. In humans, cowpox virus produces ulcerated, pustular lesions on the hands or face that are frequently hemorrhagic and most severe in young children.

PSEUDOCOWPOX (MILKER'S NODULES) AND ORF

Pseudocowpox (milker's nodules) and orf are occupational infections acquired from close contact with cattle or sheep, respectively, and caused by parapoxviruses. Both diseases manifest worldwide and are rare human zoonoses. Orf is the result of human infection with a virus causing contagious pustular dermatitis (scabby mouth) of sheep and goats. Human infections usually consist of a lesion on the finger that begins as an inflammatory papule; enlarges to a relatively painless, granulomatous lesion; and then crusts and regresses without vesicle formation. Many infections are mild, and reinfection is frequent during close contact with infected animals. Pseudocowpox, or milker's nodules, is primarily a disease of cattle, predominantly dairy herds, where it produces lesions on the teats and udder. Humans become infected by handling cattle, and small nodules on the hands are of little consequence and seldom require treatment.

MOLLUSCUM CONTAGIOSUM

The most serious parapoxvirus that affects humans is molluscum contagiosum virus, the only species in the genus *Molluscipox-*

virus. Molluscum contagiosum appears as many discrete, flesh-colored papules in the epidermal layer of the skin. It can arise on many parts of the body, probably as a result of mechanical contact spread; it does not appear to spread through viremia. The painless lesions are firm, usually 2 to 5 mm in diameter, and frequently umbilical with an opening at the top. After several months the lesions regress spontaneously, but they may persist for a year or more, particularly in immunocompromised people, such as patients with acquired immunodeficiency syndrome. The disease has a worldwide distribution and is spread by contact, usually in urban settings associated with public swimming baths, and perhaps through sexual contact. Although the cells in the papular lesions contain masses of virus particles in large cytoplasmic masses known as molluscum bodies, the virus cannot be grown in cell cultures. Confirmatory diagnosis consists of histologic examination for the presence of molluscum bodies; electron microscopic examination easily pinpoints the virus particles themselves.

TANAPOX AND YABAPOX

Tanapox and yabapox are two tropical zoonotic infections that occur mainly in Africa. The primary reservoir of these viruses is unknown, but monkeys become infected and may spread the disease to humans both in the wild and in captive primate colonies. Yabapox virus originally was discovered as the cause of benign fibrous tumors of the head and limbs of rhesus and cynomolgus monkeys in captivity in West Africa. Cases also have been found in primate colonies in other parts of the world. Although once considered a model tumor virus, yabapox virus induces lesions that are nonproliferative and regress as an immune response is mounted.

Tanapox virus was discovered 40 years ago in Kenya, where it is thought to be a zoonotic infection, though the reservoir host is not yet known. Mechanical transmission by arthropods is suspected. The disease frequently is acquired by humans through contact with monkeys, but they are not the primary host. Patients have fever and myalgia before a papule develops at the site of infection. There is thickening of the epidermis to produce a papule about 15 mm diameter that progresses to form an erythematous vesicle. Usually the lesion is solitary, though several lesions sometimes are seen, and healing takes place within a few weeks.

VACCINIA

Vaccinia virus is an attenuated smallpox (variola) virus, the origin of which is obscure. The virus shares 90% homology with smallpox virus and was directly responsible for the global eradication of smallpox. Vaccinia virus caused clinical disease during the smallpox eradication campaign when it was used to vaccinate children with eczema or with various forms of immunodeficiency. Since smallpox was eliminated in 1978, vaccination has ceased worldwide. Some countries (notably the United States) recommend vaccinations for laboratory workers who are conducting experiments using vaccinia virus, because it is preferable to experience primary infection with vaccinia virus after scarification and inoculation into the arm rather than as the result of

inadvertent infection at some other site, such as the eye, which may have serious consequences. Some European countries take a different view and prefer not to vaccinate unless exposure to vaccinia virus has been documented.

Vaccinia virus was such a successful vaccine against smallpox that it is being genetically engineered as a vector for other antigens, with a view to developing new vaccines. The US Department of Agriculture has approved a vaccinia-rabies glycoprotein recombinant virus for oral vaccination of wild animal species against rabies virus infection. For human use, much less virulent strains of vaccinia virus are being developed by attenuation using tissue culture passage or by genetically engineered deletion. Vaccinia virus is believed to be identical to buffalopox virus, which may induce lesions on the teats of buffaloes and infect humans in India who milk buffaloes. The virus is now endemic in the Indian buffalo population, but fortunately the human infections are not very serious.

BIBLIOGRAPHY

Baxby D. Indications for smallpox vaccination: policies still differ. *Vaccine* 1993;11:395–396.

Baxby D. Poxviruses. In: Mahy BWJ, Collier L, eds. *Virology.* London: Arnold, 1998:367. (*Topley and Wilson's microbiology and microbial infections,* ninth ed., vol. 1.)

Baxby D, Bennett M, Getty B. Human cowpox 1969–93: a review based on 54 cases. *Br J Dermatol* 1994;131:598–607.

Buller RM, Palumbo GJ. Poxvirus pathogenesis. *Microbiol Rev* 1991;55:80–122.

Dumbell K, Richardson M. Virological investigations of specimens from buffaloes affected by buffalopox in Maharashtra State, India, between 1985 and 1987. *Arch Virol* 1993;128:257–267.

Fenner F, Henderson DA, Arita I, et al. *Smallpox and its eradication.* Geneva: World Health Organization, 1988.

Jezek Z, Fenner F. *Human monkeypox.* Vienna: Karger, 1988. (*Virol Monogr,* vol 17.)

Moss B. Vaccinia virus: a tool for research and vaccine development. *Science* 1991;252:1662–1667.

Kelley's Textbook of Internal Medicine, fourth edition. Edited by H. David Humes. Lippincott Williams & Wilkins, Philadelphia © 2000.

C H A P T E R

310

RESPIRATORY VIRAL INFECTION

ROBERT L. ATMAR

Acute respiratory illnesses (ARIs) are among the most common diseases in humans, and respiratory viral infections are the principal cause of ARIs. Several community-based surveillance studies have shown that ARIs occur with the greatest frequency during the first 2 years of life and are common during the first decade

TABLE 310.1.	CHARACTERISTICS OF COMMON RESPIRATORY VIRUSES		
Virus	**Number of Types**	**Common Syndromes**	**Seasonal Occurrence**
Adenovirus	49	Febrile respiratory illness, pharyngoconjunctivitis	Year-round
Coronavirus	2	Common cold	Winter and spring
Influenza virus	3	Febrile respiratory illness with prominent systemic component (myalgias, headache)	Annual winter epidemics
Parainfluenza virus	4	Croup (children)	Fall (types 1 and 2) and year-round (type 3)
Respiratory syncytial virus	2	Bronchiolitis (children), pneumonia	Annual winter epidemics
Rhinovirus	>100	Common cold	Year-round, with increases in spring and fall

of life (five to nine ARIs per year). The frequency of ARIs declines to three to five illnesses per year thereafter. Somewhat higher rates are seen among adults with young children, owing to the introduction of infection into the family by the children.

Acute viral infections can be triggered by a number of different viruses, the most common of which are shown in Table 310.1. Respiratory viral infections are characterized by infection of the respiratory mucosa, though some viruses also can be isolated from tissues outside the respiratory tract. These viruses provoke a variety of clinical syndromes, including the common cold, pharyngitis, influenza-like illness, croup, tracheobronchitis, bronchiolitis, and pneumonia. The typical clinical syndromes associated with respiratory viruses also are listed in Table 310.1, but each of these viruses has been identified in association with most of the other clinical syndromes. Thus, the etiologic agent can be suspected based on the epidemiologic setting and clinical syndrome, but confirmation requires specific viral diagnostic studies. This chapter describes characteristics of the most common respiratory virus infections.

ADENOVIRUSES

DEFINITION

Adenoviruses are nonenveloped, icosahedral viruses 65 to 80 nm in size and containing a genome consisting of double-stranded DNA. The human adenoviruses belong to the genus *Mastadenovirus* and are divided into 49 distinct serotypes. The genus is divided into six subgroups (A to F) on the basis of DNA sequence homology and other characteristics. The adenovirus capsid consists of 240 capsomer called hexons and 12 pentons. The pentons are located at each of the vertices and have two structural components. The penton base anchors the penton to the capsid, and the fiber extends from the base and is the viral attachment protein. Type-specific and group-specific antigens are found on both the hexons and penton fibers. Adenoviruses can replicate in epithelial cells and lymphoid cells. In epithelial cells, infection results in lysis of the cell and release of infectious virus. Infection

of lymphoid cells can result in latent infection. Although some adenoviruses have been shown to cause tumors in rodents, these viruses have not been associated with tumors in humans.

INCIDENCE AND EPIDEMIOLOGY

Adenoviruses induce endemic and epidemic illness. The pattern of infection, mode of transmission, and clinical manifestations vary by serotype. For example, adenovirus types 1, 2, 5, and 6 are endemic, whereas types 4, 7, 14, and 21 more often cause small epidemics. The pattern of disease also can be affected by socioeconomic factors. In developing countries with poor hygienic conditions, adenovirus serotypes that cause conjunctivitis are frequently endemic; in contrast, epidemic illness with these serotypes is more common in developed countries.

Infection rates are highest in young children, in whom up to 5% of ARIs are associated with adenovirus infections. Less than 3% of ARIs in adults are related to adenovirus infection. The average incubation time is 6 to 10 days, but it may be as short as 2 days and as long as 3 weeks. Adenoviruses are transmitted in several ways. Fecal–oral transmission occurs in young children, within families, and with the enteric adenoviruses. Airborne (droplet) transmission is the primary route in outbreaks of acute febrile respiratory illness in closed settings (military barracks), and contact/fomite transmission is a major route for the spread of epidemic keratoconjunctivitis in the community and in nosocomial outbreaks. Infection usually results in the production of type-specific antibodies that are associated with protection against subsequent infection caused by the same serotype.

CLINICAL FEATURES

Adenoviruses prompt a variety of respiratory and nonrespiratory illnesses. In children, common respiratory syndromes associated with adenovirus infection include tonsillitis, otitis media, laryngitis, and pneumonia. These respiratory illnesses cannot be distinguished in clinical manifestations from those caused by other respiratory viruses, and exudative tonsillitis may be confused with tonsillitis caused by *Streptococcus pyogenes*. Pharyngoconjunctival fever, related most frequently to types 3 and 7, is characterized by conjunctivitis with follicular hypertrophy, pharyngitis, and fever. A pertussis-like syndrome, with prolonged cough, has been reported to be produced by several serotypes. Other clinical syndromes seen in children include nonspecific febrile illness, febrile convulsions, hemorrhagic cystitis (type 11), gastroenteritis (types 40 and 41), intussusception in infants, and encephalomeningitis.

In adults, epidemic febrile respiratory illness with symptoms of rhinorrhea, sore throat, and cough was first recognized in military recruits. This acute respiratory disease is associated most frequently with types 4 and 7; its other manifestations include hoarseness, tonsillitis, tracheobronchitis, and a patchy form of interstitial pneumonia. Epidemic keratoconjunctivitis (types 8, 19, and 37) is characterized by conjunctivitis with follicular hyperplasia, lacrimation, ocular pain, and photophobia. Pre-auricular adenopathy is common, and keratitis develops after a few days.

Adenovirus infection can be particularly severe in certain populations. Disseminated infection in neonates is often fatal and is associated with fever, lethargy, hepatomegaly, and pneumonia. Infection in immunocompromised patients, including bone marrow transplant recipients, solid organ transplant recipients, and AIDS patients, elicits a variety of syndromes, ranging from asymptomatic shedding to disseminated disease. Pneumonia, hepatitis, nephritis, colitis, hemorrhagic cystitis, and encephalitis are other complications seen in these patients. Disease may be caused by primary infection, by reactivation of latent infection in the immunocompromised patient, or by reactivation of infection transmitted from a transplanted organ.

LABORATORY FINDINGS

A variety of methods are used to identify adenovirus infections. The virus grows in a number of different cell culture systems, and a cytopathic effect is generally seen within 1 to 2 weeks of inoculation. Hemagglutination assays are used for initial classification into a subgroup, and serotype identification can be performed using neutralization assays or DNA restriction enzyme analysis. Virus can be detected by culture from a number of different clinical samples, including respiratory secretions, stool, urine, and conjunctival swabs. Viral shedding can be found in the stool for weeks or longer after recovery from respiratory illness, raising questions about the diagnostic usefulness (specificity) of such specimens.

Other diagnostic methods have been used to ascertain adenovirus infection. Enteric adenoviruses can be identified by rapid antigen detection assays (latex agglutination or enzyme immunoassay) and by electron microscopy. Immunofluorescence can pinpoint viral antigen in respiratory samples. Polymerase chain reaction assays have been applied successfully to the detection of adenovirus DNA in many different clinical specimens, but this methodology is not widely available, is not standardized from one laboratory to another, and must be considered investigational at this time. Serologic methods, including complement fixation, neutralization, hemagglutination inhibition, and enzyme immunoassays, are less useful in clinical practice because of the requirement for acute-phase and convalescent-phase serum samples. These methods have been useful in epidemiologic studies.

OPTIMAL MANAGEMENT

No specific treatment of adenovirus infection is available at this time. Supportive care is targeted toward symptom management.

PREVENTION

A vaccine for the prevention of the acute respiratory disease seen in military recruits has been developed and is used to control disease in the military (Table 310.2). The vaccine contains serotypes 4 and 7 and is administered as an enteric-coated capsule. The nonattenuated vaccine viruses cause asymptomatic infection of the gastrointestinal tract and induce both systemic and mucosal immune responses. Adenoviruses also are being evaluated as vectors for the delivery of foreign genes.

TABLE 310.2.	METHODS FOR SPECIFIC TREATMENT AND PREVENTION OF COMMON RESPIRATORY VIRAL INFECTIONS		
Virus	**Treatment**	**Prevention**	**Under Investigation**
Adenovirus	None	Live, enteric adenovirus vaccines (types 4 and 7)—military only	None
Coronavirus	None	None	None
Influenza virus	Amantadine, rimantadine	Trivalent, inactivated vaccines	Live, attenuated vaccines; neuraminidase inhibitors
Parainfluenza virus	None	None	Live, attenuated vaccines
Respiratory syncytial virus	Ribavirin	Respiratory syncytial virus immune globulin	Live, attenuated vaccines, subunit vaccines
Rhinovirus	None	None	Soluble receptor

CORONAVIRUSES

DEFINITION

Coronaviruses are pleomorphic, enveloped viruses ranging in size from 80 to 160 nm. The name of the virus is derived from the solar corona appearance produced by 20-nm-long, petal-shaped projections that extend from the viral envelope. The genome consists of single-stranded, positive-sense RNA, and it is surrounded by a viral nucleoprotein. Human coronaviruses are divided into two antigenic groups, represented by serotypes 229E and OC43. Two (229E) or three (OC43) envelope proteins are present on the viral surface. Other viral strains have been recognized, but difficulties in the cultivation of these viruses have made their characterization difficult. The cell receptor of the 229E virus is aminopeptidase N (CD13). The OC43 virus uses a different receptor that has not yet been identified.

INCIDENCE AND EPIDEMIOLOGY

Most of what is known about the epidemiologic characteristics of coronavirus infections is based on serologic studies. Infection is more common in the winter and spring, and cyclical epidemics of 229E and OC43 infections occur. There are few differences in infection rates in different age groups, and the annual incidence of infection ranges from 1% to more than 30% of the population, with a mean of 15% to 20%. Approximately 4% to 8% of respiratory illnesses are associated with coronavirus infection, and 15% to 20% of common colds are caused by these viruses. Spread of infection appears to be by the respiratory route; based on experimental human infection studies the incubation period is 1 to 5 days.

CLINICAL FEATURES

Coronaviruses provoke a common cold syndrome similar to that caused by rhinoviruses. Sore throat, malaise, headache, and cough are seen in approximately one-half of adults and low-grade fever in about 20%. Symptoms tend to be more severe in children, with low-grade fever occurring in up to 40%. Other respiratory illnesses associated with coronavirus infection include exacerbations of asthma and chronic obstructive lung disease and pneumonia. Coronavirus-like particles have been detected in the stools of persons with nonbacterial gastroenteritis, suggesting that viruses from this family also may cause diarrhea.

LABORATORY FINDINGS

Coronaviruses are difficult to grow in cell culture, and some strains have been isolated only in human embryonic tracheal organ cultures. Although serologic assays are the principal means of diagnosis, these assays are not readily available. Reverse transcription–polymerase chain reaction assays have been developed for virus detection and used successfully in epidemiologic studies, but the availability of these assays is limited to research laboratories.

OPTIMAL MANAGEMENT

No specific antiviral therapy is available, and treatment is targeted toward the relief of symptoms. The development of an effective vaccine is unlikely, owing to high reinfection rates, difficulties in propagating the virus in vitro, and the circulation of unidentified viral strains in humans.

INFLUENZA

DEFINITION

Influenza viruses are pleomorphic, enveloped viruses that form filamentous and spherical particles 80 to 120 nm in diameter. These viruses are members of the Orthomyxoviridae, and the genome is segmented and consists of single-stranded, negative-sense RNA. There are three types of influenza—A, B and C; influenza A and B viruses have eight gene segments, and influenza C viruses have only seven. Two glycoproteins, hemagglutinin and neuraminidase, extend as spikes from the surface of influenza A and B viruses, and variation in the antigenic composition of these proteins is responsible for recurring epidemics in humans. Influenza C viruses have a single surface glycoprotein (HE protein) that has both hemagglutination and esterase activity.

The replication cycle of influenza A and B viruses begins with the attachment of the viral hemagglutinin to sialic acid residues on the cell surface. The virus is taken into the cell by pinocytosis into endosomes. As the endosomes are acidified, protons pass through a transmembrane channel made of the viral M2 protein into the interior of the virus and trigger a conformational change in the hemagglutinin that results in the uncoating and release of the viral ribonucleoprotein complex into the cytoplasm. This complex is transported to the nucleus, where transcription and replication of viral RNA takes place. New virions are assembled at the surface of the infected cell and released by budding. The viral neuraminidase removes sialic acid residues on the cell surface to prevent aggregation of the virions being released from the cell.

INCIDENCE AND EPIDEMIOLOGY

Influenza A and B viruses are significant causes of morbidity and mortality. Influenza C viruses are a minor cause of respiratory disease. Epidemics of influenza A or B virus infection take place annually in temperate climates. These epidemics occur during the cold weather months, but they may begin in different months from year to year. Minor antigenic changes (antigenic drift) in hemagglutinin or neuraminidase lead to decreased reactivity with antibody acquired from previous influenza virus infection and result in enhanced susceptibility to the variant virus. New variant viruses emerge every few years as the immunity of the population to past variants increases. Viral strains are designated by their type, location of isolation, an identifying number from that location, year of isolation, and, for influenza A viruses, subtype of hemagglutinin and neuraminidase.

Major antigenic changes (antigenic shift) in hemagglutinin and neuraminidase also can occur with influenza A viruses and are due to reassortment of human strains with animal (principally avian) strains. Because of the significant changes in these proteins, the entire population is susceptible to infection and, if the virus can spread efficiently from person to person, a pandemic may result. There have been four pandemics during the 1900s.

Influenza is spread by contact with virus-containing respiratory secretions. This happens primarily from contact with respiratory droplets, but it also may occur following direct contact with secretions. The incubation period ranges from 1 to 5 days. Influenza is transmitted rapidly and efficiently within closed populations (nursing homes, military barracks). School-aged children facilitate the spread of influenza within the community. The proportion of infection is highest in this age group at the beginning of an epidemic and declines over time, while the proportion of infection in other age groups increases. Thus, the arrival of influenza in a community is heralded by appreciable increases in school absenteeism and a rise in the number of ARIs that come to medical attention. Influenza also sparks an increase in mortality rates attributed to pneumonia or influenza compared with historical rates. This excess mortality rate lags behind peak influenza activity in the community by about 2 weeks, and the majority of deaths are among the elderly and those with underlying cardiac or pulmonary disorders. The rise in mortality rates detected each year in association with influenza epidemics demonstrates the significant impact of these viruses on the population.

CLINICAL FEATURES

Influenza illness is characterized by systemic symptoms, such as fever, headache, myalgias, and malaise in association with respiratory symptoms, including sore throat and dry cough. This constellation of symptoms is seen in approximately one-half of infected subjects when related viruses have been circulating within the population. Approximately 30% of infected subjects have upper respiratory symptoms without fever, and in another 20% the infection is inapparent. With febrile influenza, the systemic symptoms are often more prominent at the onset of illness, and respiratory symptoms begin to dominate as systemic signs diminish. Fever and systemic symptoms typically last 3 to 5 days; cough may continue for several weeks. Alterations in pulmonary function are seen with acute influenza and may persist for months.

Both pulmonary and nonpulmonary complications develop during or after influenza virus infection. The two principal pulmonary complications are primary viral pneumonia and secondary bacterial pneumonia. Primary viral pneumonia is characterized by progressive symptoms of dyspnea, tachypnea, cough, and cyanosis beginning within days of the onset of symptomatic influenza. Rales are heard over both right and left lung fields, and signs of consolidation are absent. Chest radiography usually shows bilateral interstitial infiltrates. If sputum is produced, sputum Gram's stain fails to show a predominant bacterial organism. Histologic findings include diffuse epithelial damage and hemorrhagic pneumonia with lymphocytic infiltrate. This frequently fatal complication is usually seen in association with influenza A virus infection and occurs most frequently in persons

with underlying risk factors, including cardiovascular disease (especially rheumatic heart disease), pregnancy, organ transplants, and malignancy. There is also a milder and rarely fatal form of viral pneumonia, characterized by focal pulmonary features and the absence of progressive pulmonary symptoms.

Secondary bacterial pneumonia typically complicates influenza after a period of initial clinical improvement. Fever recurs, usually in association with increased cough and purulent sputum production; the symptoms and signs are the same as those seen with bacterial pneumonia in the absence of influenza. *Streptococcus pneumoniae*, *Staphylococcus aureus*, and *Haemophilus influenzae* are the most common bacterial pathogens. Unlike primary viral pneumonia, secondary bacterial pneumonia responds to pathogen-specific antibiotic therapy. Other pulmonary complications of influenza include bronchitis, exacerbations of asthma and other chronic obstructive pulmonary diseases, and croup.

Nonpulmonary complications also develop in association with influenza virus infection. Otitis media and sinusitis are secondary bacterial infections of the respiratory tract and are caused by the same organisms that give rise to secondary bacterial pneumonia. A toxic shock syndrome has been seen in association with colonization or secondary bacterial infection by toxin-producing *S. aureus*. Myositis is characterized by severe pain and muscle tenderness and has been associated most frequently with influenza B virus infection. Elevated serum creatine kinase levels and myoglobinuria are found on laboratory examination. Myocarditis, pericarditis, and several neurologic diseases, including transverse myelitis and Guillain-Barré syndrome, are rare complications of influenza virus infection.

Reye syndrome is a severe complication seen in pediatric patients. After the symptoms of influenza have abated, the affected child experiences nausea and vomiting followed by neurologic manifestations that may include lethargy, seizures, delirium, and coma. Hepatomegaly is typical, and liver biopsy shows fatty infiltration. Laboratory findings include hyperammonemia, hypoglycemia, and elevated serum transaminase levels with normal protein levels and cell counts in the cerebrospinal fluid. Death is common and is related to the mental status at admission. Supportive care should be given, with special emphasis placed on the management of hypoglycemia and cerebral edema. Because the use of salicylates has been associated with the development of Reye syndrome, salicylate-containing compounds should not be used during the treatment of influenza illness.

LABORATORY FINDINGS

A presumptive diagnosis of influenza virus infection can be made in the context of typical clinical features of febrile influenza when influenza is documented in the community. The diagnosis is confirmed by detection of the virus or a serologic response to the virus. Several rapid virus detection tests are now commercially available, allowing the identification of viral antigen in respiratory secretions in less than 1 hour. Although these tests have good specificity (more than 90%), their sensitivity is poorer in samples collected from adults (less than 60%) than in those collected from children (70% to 90%). Influenza virus can be isolated from respiratory secretions after inoculation into the amniotic and allantoic cavities of fertile chicken eggs or onto

TABLE 310.3.	**RECOMMENDATIONS FOR THE USE OF INFLUENZA VIRUS VACCINE (1998–1999)**

Target Groups for Special Vaccination Programs
　Groups at increased risk of influenza-related complications
　　Adults and children with chronic disorders of the pulmonary or cardiovascular systems, including asthma
　　Residents of nursing homes and other long-term-care facilities housing patients of any age with chronic medical conditions
　　Persons ≥65 yr of age
　　Adults and children who have required medical follow-up or hospitalization during the preceding year because of chronic metabolic diseases (including diabetes mellitus), renal dysfunction, hemoglobinopathies, or immunosuppression (including immunosuppression caused by medications)
　　Children and teenagers (aged 6 mo to 18 yr) who are receiving long-term aspirin therapy and therefore may be at risk of Reye syndrome after an influenza infection
　　Women who will be in the second or third trimester of pregnancy during the influenza season
　　Pregnant woman with high-risk conditions; vaccination before the influenza season regardless of the stage of pregnancy
　Groups potentially capable of transmitting influenza to high-risk persons
　　Persons caring for high-risk patients can transmit influenza infections to them while they themselves are experiencing subclinical infections or working despite the existence of symptoms. Some high-risk persons (the elderly, transplant recipients, or persons with acquired immunodeficiency syndrome) can have relatively low antibody responses to influenza vaccine. Efforts to protect them against influenza may be improved by limiting the chances that their care providers will expose them to influenza. Therefore, the following groups should be vaccinated:
　　　Physicians, nurses, and other personnel in both hospital and outpatient care settings
　　　Providers of home care to high-risk persons (visiting nurses, volunteer workers)
　　　Household members (including children) of high-risk persons
　　　Employees of nursing homes and chronic-care facilities who have contact with patients or residents
　Vaccination of other groups
　General population
　　Physicians administer influenza vaccine to any person who wishes to lower his or her chances of acquiring influenza infection. Persons who provide essential community services and students or other persons in institutional settings (schools and colleges) may be considered for vaccination, to minimize the disruption of routine activities during outbreaks.
　Persons infected with HIV
　　Limited information exists regarding the incidence and severity of influenza illness among HIV-infected persons. Nevertheless, because influenza can result in serious illness and complications in some HIV-infected persons, vaccination is a prudent precaution.
　Travelers to foreign countries
　　The risk of exposure to influenza during foreign travel varies depending on the season of greatest influenza activity, among other factors, —in the Southern Hemisphere, April–September. Because of the short incubation period for influenza, exposure to the virus during travel often results in clinical illness that begins during travel, which is an inconvenience or potential danger, especially for persons at high risk for complications. Persons preparing to travel to the tropics should review their vaccination histories. If they were not vaccinated the previous fall or winter, they should be considered for influenza vaccination before travel. Persons in high-risk categories should be encouraged to receive vaccine. The most-current available vaccine should be used. High-risk persons given the previous season's vaccine before travel should be revaccinated in the fall or winter with current vaccine.
Persons who should not be vaccinated
　Inactivated influenza vaccine should not be given to persons known to have an anaphylactic hypersensitivity to eggs (see next section).
　Persons with acute febrile illnesses usually should not be vaccinated until their symptoms have abated.
Side effects and adverse reactions
　Because influenza vaccine contains only noninfectious viruses, it cannot cause influenza. Occasional cases of respiratory disease after vaccination represent coincidental illnesses unrelated to influenza vaccination. The most common side effect of vaccination is soreness at the vaccination site for up to 2 d.
　In addition, the following two types of systemic reactions have occurred:
　　Fever, malaise, myalgia, and other systemic symtoms develop infrequently and most often affect persons who have had no exposure to the influenza virus antigens in the vaccine (young children). These reactions begin 6–12 hr after vaccination and can persist for 1 or 2 d. In adults, split-virus vaccine is not associated with higher rates of systemic symptoms than placebo.
　　Immediate, presumably allergic reactions (such as hives, angioedema, allergic asthma, or systemic anaphylaxis) occur extremely rarely after influenza vaccination. These reactions probably result from hypersensitivity to some vaccine component—most likely residual egg protein. Although current influenza vaccines contain only a small quantity of egg protein, this protein can induce immediate hypersensitivity reactions in persons with severe egg allergy. Persons who have experienced hives or have had swelling of the lips or tongue or acute respiratory distress or collapse after eating eggs should not be given influenza vaccine. Persons with a documented IgE-mediated hypersensitivity to eggs, including those who have had occupational asthma or other allergic responses from occupational exposure to egg protein, may also be at increased risk for reactions from influenza vaccine.
　　The 1976 swine influenza vaccine was associated with an increased incidence of GBS. Evidence for causal relationships with subsequent vaccines is less clear, though one study found a slightly higher relative risk of GBS associated with influenza vaccination in the 1992–1993 and 1993–1994 seasons. Even if GBS were a true side effect, the very low estimated risk for GBS (one to two per million population) is less than that of the severe influenza that could be prevented by vaccine. Although influenza vaccination can inhibit the clearance of warfarin and theophylline, clinical studies have consistently failed to show any adverse effects attributable to these drugs in patients receiving influenza vaccine.

HIV, human immunodeficiency virus; GBS, Guillain-Barré syndrome.
(From Advisory Committee on Immunization Practices. Prevention and control of influenza. *MMWR* 1988;47:1, with permission.)

cell culture monolayers. Virus isolation typically requires 3 to 7 days. Serologic assays necessitate the testing of acute-phase and convalescent-phase serum samples; the latter sample should be collected at least 2 weeks after the acute-phase sample.

OPTIMAL MANAGEMENT

Specific antiviral therapy is available for the treatment of influenza A virus infections. Amantadine and its α-methyl derivative, rimantadine, are effective in minimizing the duration of symptoms and viral shedding when administered within the first 48 hours of the onset of illness. These antivirals are not active against influenza B viruses. Resistance to these drugs develops frequently during the course of treatment, but in older children and adults such resistance has not been associated with diminished drug efficacy. Resistant virus can be transmitted, however, and causes a clinical syndrome indistinguishable from that caused by drug-sensitive virus. The major side effects stemming from the use of these antivirals are neurologic (insomnia, difficulty concentrating, lightheadedness, and irritability). These side effects are more common with amantadine and resolve after drug discontinuation. The daily dosage of amantadine must be adjusted in patients with renal insufficiency; both drugs are administered at lower dosages to patients over the age of 65 years.

Therapy also is directed toward the relief of symptoms. Antipyretics can be used for the reduction of fever, though salicylate-containing compounds should be avoided in children because of the risk of Reye syndrome. Newer antivirals that inhibit viral neuraminidase activity and that are active against both influenza A and B viruses are under development and may soon become available to the public.

PREVENTION

Inactivated influenza vaccines are the principal means used to minimize the impact of influenza virus infection. Vaccination in young, healthy adults is 70% to 90% effective in preventing clinical symptoms of influenza. Efficacy rates for disease prevention are lower in geriatric populations and in other risk groups, but the vaccine is still very successful in preventing hospitalization and death in these populations. The composition of the vaccine changes from year to year to reflect the antigenic changes seen in circulating influenza virus isolates. In recent years, the influenza vaccine has been trivalent, containing antigens from influenza A/H1N1, A/H3N2, and B virus strains. The specifics of vaccine composition and recommendations for use are made annually by the Advisory Committee on Immunization Practices; the recommendations for vaccine usage for the 1998 to 1999 vaccine are shown in Table 310.3.

The principal side effect of inactivated influenza virus vaccine is mild soreness at the injection site. Hypersensitivity reactions can occur and are usually due to allergy to residual egg protein contained in the vaccine; thus, persons with egg allergy should not be given inactivated vaccine. Guillain-Barré syndrome has been reported slightly more often in vaccinated individuals (one or two per million), but the influenza-related risks of hospitalization and death far outweigh the potential risk of Guillain-Barré syndrome.

TABLE 310.4. CHEMOPROPHYLAXIS FOR INFLUENZA A VIRUS INFECTION

Chemoprophylaxis is not a substitute for vaccination. In the context of a community outbreak, however, the use of rimantadine or amantadine prophylaxis should be considered for the following groups:
Persons at high risk who are vaccinated after influenza A virus activity has began (for up to 2 weeks after vaccination)
Persons providing care to those at high risk (especially if unvaccinated)
Persons who have immune deficiency (those unlikely to have an adequate immune response to vaccine)
Persons for whom influenza vaccine is contraindicated
Other persons who wish to avoid influenza A illness
All of these groups in situations in which the epidemic strain might not be controlled by the vaccine

Amantadine and rimantadine are approved for the prophylaxis of influenza A virus infections. These drugs are 70% to 90% effective in preventing disease due to influenza A viruses. Table 310.4 outlines circumstances in which amantadine or rimantadine can be considered in place of or in addition to vaccine for influenza prophylaxis. A live, attenuated, influenza virus vaccine is in clinical trials and may soon be available for use in children and others.

PARAINFLUENZA VIRUS AND RESPIRATORY SYNCYTIAL VIRUS

DEFINITION

Parainfluenza virus and respiratory syncytial virus (RSV) are pleomorphic, enveloped viruses 150 to 300 nm in diameter. These viruses are members of the family Paramyxoviridae and contain a single-stranded, negative-sense RNA. Two spikelike proteins are found on the viral surface: F (fusion) and HN (hemagglutinin–neuraminidase) for the parainfluenza viruses and F and G (attachment) for RSV. These viruses replicate in the cytoplasm of epithelial cells. Four types of parainfluenza virus and two types of RSV are recognized to cause human infection.

INCIDENCE AND EPIDEMIOLOGY

Parainfluenza viruses cause both epidemic and endemic disease, and RSV produces annual epidemics. Parainfluenza types 1 and 2 virus infections occur during autumn months, whereas parainfluenza type 3 has been noted to occur sporadically throughout the year and in epidemics during the spring. The epidemiologic characteristics of parainfluenza type 4 are still being defined. RSV infections are usually first seen beginning in the autumn, and epidemic disease continues through the winter months and sometimes into early spring. Approximately two-thirds of children are infected with RSV and parainfluenza type 3 during the first year of life, and reinfections with these viruses throughout life is common. The greatest impact of these viruses is seen with primary infection. It is estimated that 0.5% to 1% of children require hospitalization for management of RSV infection in their first year of life. Parainfluenza viruses and RSV are spread by direct contact with respiratory secretions or fomites and by large-droplet aerosol. Thus, they can be a significant cause of nosocomial viral respiratory disease. The average incubation period for these viruses is 3 to 6 days.

PATHOGENESIS

Several clinical observations have led to intense interest in the pathogenesis of RSV infections. As noted, the most severe disease manifestations develop with primary infection in infants less than 1 year of age, and many of these infections occur during the first 6 months of life, a time when maternal antibody provides infants with partial protection from other viral infections. When a formalin-inactivated, parenterally administered vaccine was given to infants, it potentiated disease resulting from natural exposure to virus rather than providing protection. These observations led to the suggestion that immunopathologic mechanisms play a role in disease development. Several additional observations, however, suggest that serum antibody protects against disease and infection: (a) the risk of lower respiratory disease in infants is inversely related to RSV antibody levels measured in umbilical cord serum; (b) the administration of RSV immune globulin to high-risk infants protects them from the development of lower respiratory tract disease due to RSV; (c) lower respiratory tract disease occurs in the absence of measurable serum anti-RSV antibodies; and (d) serum antibody levels to the F and G viral proteins are inversely correlated with risk of RSV infection. The roles of direct cytotoxicity caused by RSV infection, inflammatory mediators induced by infection, and RSV-specific IgE are other areas under active investigation to determine the pathogenesis of RSV-induced disease.

CLINICAL FEATURES

The prototypic illnesses related to parainfluenza viruses and RSV manifest in children. Croup, or laryngotracheobronchitis, is seen most often in association with parainfluenza type 1, but parainfluenza type 2 also causes epidemic disease, and type 3 is associated with sporadic cases of croup. Fever, hoarseness, and a barking cough are the principal signs of croup. This disease must be distinguished from epiglottitis, which has become less common with the use of vaccines for *H. influenzae* type b. Bronchiolitis and pneumonia are the prototypical illnesses seen in the context of RSV. Wheezing, air trapping, and cough are common signs; rhinitis and fever also occur in the majority of patients. A small percentage of cases of bronchiolitis and viral pneumonia are provoked by parainfluenza types 3 and 4. Acute otitis media is a complication that has been associated with infection with each of these viruses.

In healthy adults, infection with parainfluenza viruses and RSV cause mild upper respiratory illnesses and are uncommon causes of lower respiratory illness. Recent studies suggest that approximately 3% of community-acquired cases of pneumonia in adults during the RSV season are associated with RSV infection. These viruses can lead to exacerbations of asthma and

chronic obstructive pulmonary disease, but they do so less often than rhinoviruses and coronaviruses. In the geriatric population, RSV is the root of outbreaks of respiratory disease in nursing homes, and its clinical features are often indistinguishable from those of influenza. Severe, frequently fatal lower respiratory infections are seen in immunocompromised patients, especially bone marrow transplant recipients.

LABORATORY FINDINGS

The diagnosis of parainfluenza virus or RSV infection is made by detection of the virus or a serologic response to the virus. Rapid virus detection tests are commercially available for parainfluenza type 3 and RSV. All of these viruses can be isolated from respiratory secretions after inoculation onto cell culture monolayers. The preferred clinical sample for these studies is a nasal wash or aspirate. RSV is particularly labile, and there is rapid loss of viability if the specimen is not handled properly. Virus isolation typically requires 3 to 5 days for RSV and 5 to 14 days for the parainfluenza viruses. Serologic assays require the testing of acute-phase and convalescent-phase serum samples, so the results of such assays are delayed until a convalescent-phase sample can be collected (2 weeks or longer after the collection of the acute-phase sample).

OPTIMAL MANAGEMENT

Specific antiviral therapy for the treatment of parainfluenza virus infections is not yet available. Care of the patient with croup is supportive, and mist therapy has been reported to be of value. A single dose of systemic corticosteroids is used by many physicians to treat airway obstruction in severe croup. Ribavirin is licensed for the treatment of moderate to severe cases of bronchiolitis caused by RSV. There is still much debate about the usefulness of this antiviral agent in this syndrome. The high cost of the medication has led to its use being restricted in many hospitals. No treatment of RSV disease in adults is available, though anecdotal reports have suggested that ribavirin in combination with high-titered RSV immunoglobulin lowers mortality rates among bone marrow transplant patients.

PREVENTION

High-titered RSV immunoglobulin and a humanized RSV-specific monoclonal antibody preparation are both available for the prevention of RSV infection and disease in certain high-risk children (those with chronic lung diseases or premature infants). RSV immunoglobulin has the advantage of providing protection against other respiratory viruses, but it must be administered intravenously. The monoclonal antibody preparation is given intramuscularly. The use of subunit or live attenuated vaccines is another approach under evaluation for the prevention of RSV and parainfluenza virus infection. RSV can be a major cause of nosocomial respiratory virus infection. Nosocomial transmission has been prevented effectively by the simple infection-control measures of hand washing and the use of gloves. Cohorting of staff caring for infected patients and isolation of such patients are additional measures that have been effective in preventing spread within the hospital. Such measures are less practical within the community.

RHINOVIRUSES

DEFINITION

Rhinoviruses are small, nonenveloped, single-stranded, positive-sense RNA viruses in the family Picornaviridae. They are approximately 30 nm in size and are differentiated from enteroviruses by their loss of infectivity after exposure to a low pH. More than 100 serotypes of rhinovirus are recognized, and the cell receptor for the majority is intercellular adhesion molecule 1 (ICAM-1). Most of the rest of the rhinoviruses use the low-density lipoprotein receptor for cell attachment.

INCIDENCE AND EPIDEMIOLOGY

Rhinoviruses cause illness throughout the year, with peak periods during the fall and spring. All age groups are affected. Illness rates are higher in infants and small children, who experience an average of one rhinovirus illness per year. Older children and adults average approximately one rhinovirus illness every 2 years. Several serotypes can be found circulating in a community at any given time, and these serotypes tend to change over time. Transmission of virus occurs via aerosols and after direct contact with respiratory secretions or fomites. The average incubation period is 2 to 3 days.

CLINICAL FEATURES

The common cold is the usual clinical manifestation of rhinovirus infection, and at least 50% of common colds are precipitated by rhinoviruses. The major symptoms include sneezing, nasal discharge and congestion, and sore throat. Cough, malaise, and headache also may be significant features. The main complications of rhinovirus infection are sinusitis and otitis media. Rhinovirus infection also is present frequently in both pediatric and adult patients who have symptoms of wheezing. Recent studies suggest that rhinoviruses have an etiologic role in triggering exacerbations of asthma and other reactive airway diseases.

LABORATORY FINDINGS

Rhinovirus infection can be suspected based on clinical manifestations in the patient with a common cold. The principal means of confirming the diagnosis is by cell culture. Antigen detection assays have not been useful because of the large number of serotypes and the lack of a common group antigen. For similar reasons, serologic assays are not useful for most patients. The polymerase chain reaction has been evaluated by many research laboratories and has proved to be much more sensitive than cell culture, but this assay is not readily available to most clinicians.

OPTIMAL MANAGEMENT

Treatment of patients with rhinovirus infections is directed at symptomatic relief. Topical or systemically administered sympa-

thomimetics (pseudoephedrine, phenylpropanolamine) decrease nasal congestion and sneezing, whereas parasympatholytic agents (ipratropium bromide) diminish nasal mucus production. Acetaminophen, aspirin, and nonsteroidal anti-inflammatory agents provide relief from systemic symptoms without affecting local nasal symptoms. Dextromethorphan is a useful antitussive. The antihistamine chlorpheniramine also has been used to minimize sneezing and nasal mucous production. These medications often are used in combination to lessen local and systemic symptoms. There have been few studies of these medications in pediatric populations, and no studies have confirmed a clinical benefit of these medicines in the preschool child. The use of a decongestant plus an antihistamine has not limited the rate of development of secondary otitis media in preschool children.

Specific antiviral agents have not been effective in the treatment of rhinovirus-associated symptoms. Topical antiviral agents, including interferon-α and virus capsid binding agents have not shown consistent clinical benefits in the context of experimental human infection. Antibiotics have no role in the treatment of uncomplicated infection. Other treatments, such large doses of vitamin C, zinc lozenges, and warm humidified air, have failed to alter the clinical course of illness consistently.

PREVENTION

The large number of rhinovirus serotypes limits the likelihood of vaccine strategies for the prevention of rhinovirus infection. Interferon-α has been evaluated in studies of prophylaxis. When used topically in studies of natural transmission within the family, rhinovirus transmission was reduced by as much as 80%. The usefulness of this treatment strategy is limited by its lack of efficacy against other respiratory viruses, the unavailability of rapid diagnostic assays for rhinovirus infections, and the side effects associated with the use of topical interferon. Soluble ICAM-1 (the cellular receptor for the majority of human rhinoviruses) has been effective in the prevention of rhinovirus infections in a chimpanzee model; its efficacy in human beings remains to be determined. At present, the only available prevention strategies are nonspecific environmental controls, such as hand washing and measures to prevent autoinoculation.

BIBLIOGRAPHY

Advisory Committee on Immunization Practices. Prevention and control of influenza. *MMWR* 1988;47:1.

Arruda E, Pitkaranta A, Witek TJ Jr, et al. Frequency and natural history of rhinovirus infections in adults during autumn. *J Clin Microbiol* 1997; 35:2864–2868.

Baum SG. Adenovirus. In: Mandell GL, Bennett JE, Dolin R, eds. *Principles and practice of infectious diseases.* fourth ed. New York: Churchill Livingstone, 1995:1382.

Falsey AR, Cunningham CK, Barker WH, et al. Respiratory syncytial virus and influenza A infections in the hospitalized elderly. *J Infect Dis* 1995; 172:389–394.

Glezen WP, Couch RB. Influenza viruses. In: Evans AS, Kaslow RA, eds. *Viral infections of humans,* fourth ed. New York: Plenum Publishing Company, 1997:473.

Gwaltney JM. Rhinovirus. In: Mandell GL, Bennett JE, Dolin R, eds. *Principles and practice of infectious diseases,* fourth ed. New York: Churchill Livingstone, 1995:1656.

McIntosh K. Coronaviruses. In: Fields BN, Knipe DM, Howley PM, eds.

Fields virology, third ed. New York: Lippincott–Raven Publishers, 1996: 1095.

Nichol KL, Lind A, Margolis KL, et al. The effectiveness of vaccination against influenza in healthy, working adults. *N Engl J Med* 1995;333: 889–893.

Piedra PA, Englund JA, Glezen WP. Respiratory syncytial virus and parainfluenza viruses. In: Richman DD, Whitley RJ, Hayden FG, eds. *Clinical virology*. New York: Churchill Livingstone, 1997:787.

Whimbey E, Champlin RE, Couch RB, et al. Community respiratory virus infections among hospitalized adult bone marrow transplant recipients. *Clin Infect Dis* 1996:22:778–782.

Kelley's Textbook of Internal Medicine, fourth edition. Edited by H. David Humes.
Lippincott Williams & Wilkins, Philadelphia © 2000.

C H A P T E R
311

MEASLES, MUMPS, AND RUBELLA

WALTER A. ORENSTEIN
MELINDA WHARTON

■ MEASLES

DESCRIPTION AND PATHOGENESIS

Measles is an acute illness characterized by rash and fever and caused by a paramyxovirus. The virus is inhaled into the nasopharynx and upper respiratory tract, penetrates the mucosa, and probably establishes primary viremia within 2 days and a more extensive form of secondary viremia beginning about 5 days after initial infection. The organism can be found in many different tissues of the body but has a predilection for the respiratory tract. Three viral proteins have major roles in pathogenesis and in some of the complications seen with measles. The hemagglutinin that projects from the surface allows attachment to cells. The F (fusion) protein plays a part in cell-to-cell spread through membrane fusion, and the M protein is important in packaging of the final virion. Acute infection results in solid immunity, which is typically lifelong. Although second clinical attacks of measles have been cited, they have not been well documented; if they occur, they are rare.

EPIDEMIOLOGY

The disease is usually spread by respiratory contact, with the victim inhaling virus contained in droplets expelled by a patient. Airborne spread over greater distances has been documented, however, and instances of infection have occurred when the victim did not enter a room until at least 1 hour after the original patient had left. Laboratory studies have documented viral survival in small droplets for at least 2 hours. After an incubation period of 7 to 10 days, the first symptoms of illness appear; the patient becomes infectious at that time. Although virus can be recovered from several body fluids, including urine, the most important means of transmission is through respiratory secretions. The period of infectivity lasts through the prodromal symptoms and for 3 or 4 days after appearance of the rash in the normal host.

Measles is one of the most highly contagious illnesses; 90% or more of susceptible household contacts become infected in a single generation of spread. Because of its infectiousness, it is essentially a universal disease, except in isolated populations. In the developing world, where measles vaccine has not been used widely, transmission often occurs in very young children, and 95% of people have had measles by 10 years of age. In the United States, before measles vaccine became available, 95% of people had measles before reaching 15 years of age. Primary transmission occurred in elementary schools and day care centers. Since introduction of measles vaccine in 1963 and its subsequent widespread use, the overall incidence has declined dramatically.

Indigenous measles transmission appears to have been interrupted in this country many times since 1993. Genomic analysis of measles virus isolates shows that current strains are different from those that circulated before 1993. During the late 1990s several genotypes were detected, usually linked directly to international importations or to genotypes known to circulate in other counties. Only 100 cases were reported in 1998, down from more than 27,000 cases in 1990, the peak of a 3-year resurgence of measles at the beginning of the decade. A target has been set to eliminate indigenous measles from the Western Hemisphere by the end of the year 2000, and other regional measles elimination goals have been established for the European and eastern Mediterranean regions of the World Health Organization.

Transmission of measles has been reported in three major patterns: preschool; school age, including college; and mixed. Preschool cases of measles have developed primarily in inner city populations and predominantly affect unvaccinated children. In contrast, school-age measles infects people in junior and senior high school and college and is characterized by a high number of cases (often most cases) among people with a history of having been given one dose of vaccine. These vaccine failures are mainly the result of initial failure to seroconvert rather than waning immunity; with increasing implementation of the two-dose measles vaccination schedule, such cases are being seen less often. Mixed patterns often involve young adults, who usually are not enrolled in institutions, and young preschool children. Outbreaks have also been reported among health care personnel.

CLINICAL FEATURES

The typical pattern of measles symptoms is a 2- to 4-day prodrome of fever, malaise, cough, coryza, conjunctivitis, and photophobia. Koplik's spots, which are faint, white, 1- to 2-mm elevated lesions on an erythematous base, may be present for 1 or 2 days before and after onset of rash and are pathognomonic of measles. The prodrome is followed by the appearance of a characteristic rash beginning on the head, neck, and trunk and spreading centrifugally over the course of 2 or 3 days. The rash lasts 5 to 7 days and may be followed by a period of desquamation lasting up to 1 week. The usual pattern of illness is similar in children and adults, but complications are most likely to develop in infants and more likely to occur in adults than in school-age children.

Measles is usually an uncomplicated disease, but because of its universality, the overall burden of complications can be high. Otitis media is seen in 7% to 9% of children with measles; pneumonia (either primary viral or secondary bacterial) occurs in 1% to 6%; diarrhea is reported in about 6% of cases. In the past, about 1% to 3% of children with measles in the United States were hospitalized. Hospitalization rates may be higher now. Encephalitis develops in about one in 1,000 cases and is a greater risk after measles in adults. The reported ratio of deaths to cases in the United States is about one to two deaths per 1,000 cases. Measles virus is also capable of establishing long-term infection in the central nervous system, causing subacute sclerosing panencephalitis, a fatal degenerative central nervous system condition, about once in every 100,000 infections. The incubation period for subacute sclerosing panencephalitis is typically 7 years. In infants, adults, and people with malnutrition or other debilitating or immunocompromising conditions, complications and death are more common. Abnormalities of cell-mediated immunity predispose to measles complications. People with agammaglobulinemia appear to recover from measles in a fashion similar to that of normal hosts. Overall, it is estimated that about one million people die each year as a result of measles or its complications. Most of these deaths take place in developing countries.

Clinical primary infections are the rule. Exposure to measles virus can result in subclinical boosts in antibody titer in immune hosts. Circulating, passively acquired antibody to measles can prevent or modify the infection and make it subclinical or much less severe. Such situations commonly arise in infants (because of maternally derived antibody) and those who have received immune globulin. In fact, immune globulin is used after exposure to abort or minimize illness.

DIAGNOSIS

Laboratory confirmation can be accomplished most readily by detecting IgM antibodies in a single specimen. Alternatively, a significant rise in antibodies to measles virus between acute-phase and convalescent-phase serum samples is also an acceptable indicator. Hemagglutination inhibition largely has been replaced by enzyme-linked immunosorbent assay (ELISA). IgM antibodies can be verified beginning almost simultaneously with rash onset, peak at about 10 days after rash onset, and may persist for 1 month or longer; tests performed within 72 hours of rash onset may show negative results. ELISA tests using a capture format for IgM are preferred. Measles IgG antibodies peak 2 to 4 weeks after onset of rash and fall off slightly thereafter. After measles, most patients maintain demonstrable antibodies for life. In the absence of reexposure, however, a few patients lose antibody, as measured by standard tests. Such individuals appear to be immune, however, because antibody is detectable in special sensitive assays and because these individuals give a prompt sec-

ondary antibody response on vaccination. Subclinical reinfections are also associated with boosts in antibody titer.

Measles virus can be isolated from urine, respiratory secretions, or blood. Sequencing of the H and N genes of viral isolates allows tracking of measles transmission within the United States and internationally. Other illnesses that might be confused with measles in adults are rubella (usually a milder illness and of shorter duration), Rocky Mountain spotted fever, secondary syphilis, parvovirus infection, and adenoviral or enteroviral illnesses with rash.

OPTIMAL MANAGEMENT

There is no specific treatment. Antibiotics are typically used to treat pneumonia associated with measles, because it is often bacterial, commonly caused by infection with *Streptococcus pneumoniae* or *Staphylococcus aureus*.

PREVENTION AND CONTROL

In 1963, a killed virus vaccine and a live attenuated virus vaccine (Edmonston B strain) were introduced. The killed virus vaccine (which lacked the F protein) was soon shown to induce short-lived protection and to sensitize some recipients so that on subsequent exposure they contracted an unusual clinical illness with fever, atypical rash, and pneumonia (atypical measles syndrome). Consequently, this product was not distributed after 1967. The Edmonston B vaccine induced long-lasting immunity but also caused a mild measles-like illness in many recipients. As a result, it was usually given with immune globulin. In 1965, the further attenuated Schwarz strain vaccine, derived from Edmonston A virus, was introduced, followed in 1968 by the Moraten strain, which was similar to the Schwarz strain. These vaccines rapidly replaced the Edmonston B strain. The Moraten strain is the only vaccine strain used in the United States. Measles vaccine is available as a single antigen or combined with rubella (MR) or mumps and rubella (MMR).

More than 93% of susceptible people 12 to 15 months of age or older have antibodies after receipt of a single dose of the currently available measles vaccine. Seroconversion rates in infants are not as high because of interference from persisting maternally derived antibodies. Although antibody titers decline with time and may become undetectable (using standard tests), vaccine-induced immunity is long term, probably lifelong in almost all recipients. Although waning immunity has been reported, it appears to be rare. Measles transmission has been reported in highly vaccinated populations, primarily junior and senior high school and college students who received a single dose on or after their first birthday. These cases appear to represent mainly the 2% to 7% of vaccinees who initially fail to respond to vaccine.

To minimize measles vaccine failure, two doses of measles vaccine, given as MMR, began to be recommended for routine immunization starting in 1989. It is suggested that the first dose be administered at 12 to 15 months of age and the second dose at entry to school (kindergarten or first grade). A goal has been set to ensure that all children, in kindergarten through twelfth grade, receive a second dose of MMR by 2001. To prevent college outbreaks, all college entrants should have evidence of receipt of two doses of vaccine on or after the first birthday, previous physician-diagnosed measles, or laboratory evidence of immunity. All persons who work in health care facilities should be immune to measles as evidenced by the same criteria as for college students. Adults born before 1957 generally are considered to be immune as the result of early exposure to natural virus. Nonetheless, one dose of MMR should be considered for unvaccinated health care workers born before 1957, because cases of measles have been reported in this group.

During outbreaks, particularly in schools, all students and staff at risk should be vaccinated unless they have received two previous doses of vaccine on or after the first birthday, have evidence of previous physician-diagnosed measles, or have a positive serologic test for measles antibody. Reactions to measles vaccine are usually mild. Approximately 5% of recipients may have temperatures of 39.4°C (103°F) or more or rashes 5 to 12 days after vaccination. These features are usually mild and of short duration, though febrile convulsions have been reported. Encephalitis also has been reported within 30 days after vaccination at a rate of about one case per two million doses of vaccine distributed, but it is not clear that it is caused by the vaccine. Only nonimmune persons tend to have side effects attributable to vaccine virus complications, such as fever and rash. Reactions should be less common in people being revaccinated than in children receiving measles vaccine for the first time.

Measles vaccine virus is grown in chick embryo fibroblasts and may contain egg protein in picogram quantities. Most anaphylactic reactions are attributed to other vaccine components, however, and skin tests for egg hypersensitivity do not predict who will suffer anaphylactic reactions. Therefore, allergy to eggs, chickens, or feathers is not a contraindication to routine vaccination, though vaccination of those with anaphylactic hypersensitivity should be performed where epinephrine is available. Some cases of anaphylaxis may be related to sensitivity to gelatin. MMR also appears to cause thrombocytopenic purpura in one of 30,000 to 40,000 vaccinated children.

The only contraindications to receipt of measles vaccine are an immunocompromised state and, on theoretic grounds, pregnancy. Patients with human immunodeficiency virus (HIV) infection and no symptoms also should be vaccinated. Vaccine also should be considered for individuals with symptomatic HIV infection, but persons with HIV who are severely immunocompromised should not be vaccinated. In adults, this translates to CD4 counts of less than 200 per cubic millimeter or CD4 cells constituting less than 14% of total lymphocytes.

All people without contraindications who are not known to be immune to measles should be considered susceptible and should be vaccinated. Measles vaccine combined with other antigens should be used in anyone potentially susceptible to rubella or mumps. There is no harm in vaccinating someone who is already immune. People born before 1957 are likely to have been exposed to wild virus and can generally be considered immune. Women known to be pregnant should not be vaccinated. A practical way to deal with women of childbearing age is to ask them if they are pregnant or likely to become so in the next 3 months. If the answer is no, the potential risks are explained to them before they are vaccinated.

Immune globulin can be used to prevent or modify illness in people who have been exposed to measles. The usual dose is 0.25 mL per kilogram, up to a maximum of 15 mL. People with compromised immune systems should receive 0.5 mL per kilogram. Measles vaccine also can be used after exposure (≤72 hours) to prevent illness. The advantage of using vaccine is that if the exposure did not result in infection, the person is protected against subsequent exposure.

MUMPS

DESCRIPTION AND PATHOGENESIS

Mumps is an acute illness generally characterized by parotitis and caused by a paramyxovirus. The virus is typically inhaled, probably replicates in the respiratory epithelium or parotids, and disseminates through the bloodstream to localize in glandular or nervous tissue. Virus can be detected in saliva up to 7 days before onset and 7 days after clinical symptoms appear. Viruria can be confirmed up to 14 days after onset of illness. One infection confers long-lasting immunity; second attacks of clinical illness are rare.

EPIDEMIOLOGY

The incubation period typically is 16 to 18 days, with a range of 12 to 25 days. Infected people usually become contagious 1 or 2 days before symptom onset and can transmit virus for 5 to 9 days after parotid swelling. People with subclinical infection also can spread disease. Transmission is through inhalation of droplets of respiratory secretions containing virus and consequently involves face-to-face contact with an infected person. Mumps is highly infectious—more than 30% of susceptible household contacts are likely to be infected on exposure. Subclinical infection is common (20% to 40% of all infections) and also induces long-lasting immunity. Mumps traditionally has been a disease of school-age children, but cases have been documented in preschool children and adults. Widespread use of mumps vaccine has resulted in a dramatic decline in the incidence of mumps in the United States. Only 666 cases were reported in 1998, which represents less than 1% of prevaccine levels.

CLINICAL FEATURES

The illness typically begins with malaise and low fever. Within 1 or 2 days, parotitis (the most characteristic manifestation in 30% to 40% of cases) appears and lasts 4 to 6 days; it may be unilateral or bilateral. Fever usually persists 3 or 4 days. Recovery is complete and induces lifelong immunity. Complications are common, but they are generally mild. Aseptic meningitis develops in 4% to 6% of patients and, as a rule, it is mild, with no adverse effects. Mumps meningoencephalitis, a rare complication, can result in long-term side effects, including paralysis, cranial nerve palsies, and hydrocephalus. Many persons with mumps meningoencephalitis do not have parotitis. Orchitis is common in postpubertal men—it occurs in 20% to 40% of cases. Most cases are unilateral, and sterility is rare. Mastitis is seen frequently in postpubertal women. Other complications include oophoritis, thyroiditis, nephritis, arthritis, and myocarditis. Pancreatitis, usually mild, develops in about 4% of cases. In rare cases, diabetes has been associated temporally with mumps; however, the causal role of the virus, if any, has not been established clearly. The most common residual manifestation of mumps is nerve deafness, which seems to occur at a rate of about one case in 20,000 infections.

DIAGNOSIS

The diagnosis can be confirmed by a significant rise in mumps antibody levels using neutralization, complement fixation, ELISA, or hemagglutination inhibition tests. IgM ELISA antibody tests are highly sensitive and specific for mumps and allow diagnosis based on a single serum specimen. IgM antibodies usually are detectable during the first few days of illness and persist for weeks to several months. Immunity after infection appears to be lifelong, but antibody titers, particularly those measured by complement fixation, decline with time and frequently become nondetectable (thus negating the usefulness of the complement fixation test in serologic screening for immunity). Mumps virus can be isolated from the nasopharynx, saliva, urine, and cerebrospinal fluid; however, isolation is used infrequently for diagnosis. The serum amylase value is elevated in most cases. No other agents are known to cause epidemic parotitis, but sporadic cases may stem from a variety of infectious and noninfectious sources. Other viral agents associated with parotitis include parainfluenza, influenza, cytomegalovirus, and coxsackievirus.

OPTIMAL MANAGEMENT

There is no specific therapy.

PREVENTION AND CONTROL

Live attenuated mumps virus vaccine (Jeryl Lynn strain) was introduced in the United States in 1967; since 1971, it has been available in combination with measles and rubella vaccines (MMR). The vaccine induces seroconversion in more than 90% of susceptible people who are at least 12 months of age. Vaccine-induced immunity appears to be lifelong. Although most cases of mumps develop among unvaccinated people, vaccine failure has been noted in some outbreaks. During field evaluations of vaccine efficacy, protection levels of 75% to 95% have been reported after a single dose of mumps vaccine.

Reactions to mumps vaccine are few. Mild parotitis or orchitis have been reported, but these reactions are rare. The only contraindications are an immunocompromised state and, on theoretic grounds, pregnancy. Mumps vaccine is prepared in chick embryo cell culture. While rare and serious allergic reactions have been reported in recipients with histories of anaphylactic reactions to eggs, skin testing for egg sensitivity is not predictive of anaphylaxis, and most cases of anaphylaxis do not appear to be related to egg sensitivity. Therefore, persons with anaphylaxis to eggs may be vaccinated. In about one per 30,000 to 40,000 immunizations, thrombocytopenic purpura can follow mumps vaccination when it is administered as MMR.

Since 1989 a routine two-dose vaccination schedule with MMR has been recommended, and most children vaccinated since then will have received two doses of mumps vaccine as MMR. It is suggested that the first dose be administered at 12 to 15 months of age and the second dose at entry to school (kindergarten or first grade). All children in school (kindergarten through twelfth grade) should receive a second dose of MMR by 2001 if they have not received it previously. A single dose of mumps vaccine is acceptable evidence of mumps immunity for people not in the age group for two doses. Other acceptable evidence of mumps immunity includes documentation of physician-diagnosed disease or laboratory evidence of immunity. From a practical point of view, people born before 1957 are likely to have been exposed to wild virus and generally can be considered to be immune. Women of childbearing age should be vaccinated according to the guidelines presented earlier for measles vaccine. Immune globulin is not reliably effective in preventing or modifying the effects of mumps after exposure. No clear evidence suggests that mumps vaccine given after exposure prevents disease. If exposure did not result in infection, however, such vaccination prevents disease on subsequent exposure.

■ RUBELLA

DESCRIPTION AND PATHOGENESIS

Rubella (sometimes called German measles) is an acute illness caused by a togavirus. The virus typically is inhaled, penetrates the upper respiratory tract mucosa, and establishes viremia, which may be present from about 1 week before rash onset. The virus freely infects and crosses the placenta and damages fetal tissues that are undergoing rapid division and maturation. Immunity is thought to be lifelong.

EPIDEMIOLOGY

Transmission is usually through respiratory secretions and typically involves face-to-face contact with an infected person. Airborne spread also has been postulated. People with subclinical infections can transmit virus. The period of infectivity typically begins a few days before rash onset and lasts up to 5 to 7 days after onset of rash. Before rubella vaccine was introduced, primary transmission of rubella occurred in school-age children; antibodies developed in 80% to 85% of people in the United States by 15 years of age. Because of the level of susceptibility in the young adult population, however, outbreaks of disease did develop among adults, with tragic outcomes. As a result of the nationwide epidemic in 1964 to 1965, an estimated 20,000 infants were born with congenital defects stemming from congenital rubella infection, and an additional 12,000 pregnancies ended in spontaneous or induced abortion.

Widespread use of rubella vaccine has resulted in marked declines in the incidence of both rubella and congenital rubella syndrome. In 1998, a total of 364 cases of rubella and seven cases of congenital rubella syndrome (two of which were imported) were reported in the United States. This number represents less than 1% of prevaccine era levels. A target has been set to eliminate indigenous rubella and congenital rubella syndrome in the United States by the year 2000. In the 1990s rubella emerged as a disease seen predominantly among Hispanic adults who were not born in the United States and who grew up in countries without programs for routine rubella vaccination of children. The recent epidemiologic characteristics of congenital rubella syndrome (most cases now arise among infants born to Hispanic women) reflect the current epidemiologic features of rubella.

CLINICAL FEATURES

Rubella is usually a mild illness and may pass unnoticed. Subclinical infections are common (25% to 50%). The typical illness begins 16 to 18 days (range, 2 to 3 weeks) after exposure, with slight malaise and low-grade fever, followed in 1 or 2 days by the appearance of a maculopapular rash that typically is not as widespread as in measles and lasts only 2 or 3 days. Occipital and postauricular lymphadenopathy are common and indicate the diagnosis. Arthralgia is common in adults (particularly in women) and may be found in half or more of cases. All manifestations typically subside within 2 to 5 days, and the patient subsequently has lifelong immunity.

Complications are rare and include thrombocytopenia and encephalitis, both of which usually resolve without residual effects. The major burden of rubella is related to infection in a woman in the early stages of pregnancy. Overall, more than 20% of women infected during the first trimester give birth to infected infants. The virus infects the placenta and the fetus and affects rapidly dividing and developing tissue. The incidence of defects is highest during the first month of gestation. By the fifth month, essentially there is no serious risk. Consequently, the major manifestations of congenital rubella infection depend on the stage of pregnancy in which infection occurs.

The most common manifestations of congenital rubella are fetal death, deafness, cataracts, congenital heart lesions, and mental retardation. Infection early in the first trimester is associated with major congenital anomalies, such as congenital heart disease, whereas infection in the fourth month is more likely to result in deafness alone. Because deafness may not be detected for some time after birth, babies with congenital rubella syndrome may appear normal in the neonatal period. Congenital infection can lead to chronic infection, and infants with congenital rubella syndrome may excrete virus (and infect others) for periods as long as a year after birth. Chronic infection also can lead to diabetes or progressive rubella panencephalopathy, which is a rare condition that is similar to subacute sclerosing panencephalitis.

DIAGNOSIS

Diagnosis based on clinical symptoms is unreliable. Laboratory confirmation involves detection of IgM antibodies in any blood specimen or evidence of a significant increase in antibody titer (using a variety of tests, including hemagglutination inhibition, complement fixation, ELISA, indirect fluorescent antibody, and hemolysis-in-gel tests) or virus isolation. ELISA is the most common test. Diagnosis in infants with suspected congenital rubella infection can be confirmed by detection of rubella-specific IgM, persistence of antibodies beyond the expected rate of decay from transplacental passage, virus isolation, or detection of rubella virus by the polymerase chain reaction.

OPTIMAL MANAGEMENT

There is no specific therapy.

PREVENTION AND CONTROL

The only effective preventive technique is the use of rubella vaccine. Live attenuated rubella virus vaccines were first introduced in 1969. Their widespread use in the United States has led to the virtual disappearance of rubella and congenital rubella syndrome. Vaccines have been prepared in a variety of different cell lines; currently available vaccine (RA 27/3) is prepared in human diploid cells (WI-38) and is commonly combined with measles and mumps vaccines as MMR. More than 95% of susceptible people at least 1 year of age have antibodies after administration of rubella vaccine. Levels of antibody are lower than those after natural infection and may decline to undetectable levels over time. Nonetheless, vaccine-induced immunity is long term, probably lifelong, in almost all vaccine recipients who seroconvert.

Less than 5% of recipients of vaccine experience mild fever or rash 10 to 15 days after vaccination. The most prominent adverse effect, arthralgia, is seen primarily in women and may develop in about 25% of susceptible vaccinees. It typically lasts 1 day to 3 weeks, is only rarely responsible for work loss, and does not recur. Frank arthritis occurs in approximately 10% of susceptible adult female vaccinees. Joint symptoms manifest only in susceptible vaccinees. Recurrence or persistence of arthralgia and frank arthritis has been reported, though the incidence rate is similar to incidence rates in unvaccinated populations, implying that rubella vaccine does not cause chronic arthropathy. Comparative studies show that chronic or recurrent joint symptoms after rubella disease are considerably more common than after rubella vaccines. In rare instances, thrombocytopenic purpura has followed rubella vaccine when administered as MMR.

Because rubella virus damages fetuses, there has been concern that the vaccine virus might have the same effect. Between 1971 and 1989, the Centers for Disease Control and Prevention maintained a registry of women who received vaccine when they were unknowingly pregnant. There were reports of 321 women, known to be susceptible to rubella, who had received RA 27/3 rubella vaccine within the 3 months before or after conception and who carried their pregnancies to term. None delivered a child with congenital deformities suggestive of congenital rubella syndrome. Although the measured risk is 0, the maximum theoretic risk is 1.6%, which is considerably lower than the measured risk of 20% or more with wild rubella virus in the first trimester. Although five of the infants had serologic evidence of in utero infection by the vaccine virus, no clinical abnormalities were verified.

Fetal tissues obtained at abortion have also yielded vaccine virus on occasion. Consequently, the potential for fetal infection exists even though experience indicates no cases of congenital rubella syndrome caused by vaccine virus. Because of this theoretic risk, rubella vaccination is contraindicated in pregnancy. A reasonable approach to vaccinating women of childbearing age is to ask if they are pregnant or likely to become pregnant within the next 3 months. If they say no, the possible risks should be explained, and they should be vaccinated. The possibility of risks to the fetus of rubella vaccine virus have been evaluated by the Advisory Committee on Immunization Practices, which concluded that the risk, if any, is negligible. Therefore, vaccination of a woman later found to be pregnant within 3 months of vaccination should not in itself be considered an indication for abortion. A final decision must rest with the woman and her physician.

Although one dose of rubella vaccine appears to be adequate, many people receive two doses as part of MMR. The first dose usually is administered at 12 to 15 months of age and the second dose at entry to school (kindergarten or first grade). By 2001, all students, kindergarten through twelfth grade, should receive a second dose of MMR if they have not been given a second dose previously. Because the clinical diagnosis of rubella is unreliable, people should be considered immune to rubella only if they have documentation of having received rubella vaccine on or after the first birthday or if they have laboratory evidence of immunity. Most persons born before 1957 can be considered immune from exposure to natural infection. Women of childbearing age who might become pregnant should be vaccinated if they lack evidence of vaccination or serologic evidence of immunity. The only contraindications for vaccination are pregnancy and an immunocompromised state. Immune globulin given after exposure can modify the clinical manifestations of rubella, but it does not reliably prevent fetal infection or fetal damage. Consequently, it should be used only for a pregnant woman exposed to rubella who would not consider abortion under any circumstance.

BIBLIOGRAPHY

Bosma TJ, Corbett KM, Eckstein MB, et al. Use of PCR for prenatal and postnatal diagnosis of congenital rubella. *J Clin Microbiol* 1995; 33:2881–2887.

Centers for Disease Control and Prevention. Measles, mumps, and rubella: vaccine use and strategies for elimination of measles, rubella and congenital rubella syndrome and control of mumps. Recommendations of the Advisory Committee on Immunization Practices (ACIP). *MMWR* 1998;47(RR-8):1–57.

Centers for Disease Control and Prevention. Epidemiology of measles—United States, 1998. *MMWR* 1999;48:705–709.

Cooper LZ, Krugman S. Clinical manifestations of postnatal and congenital rubella. *Arch Ophthalmol* 1967;77:434–439.

Hefland RF, Heath JL, Anderson LJ, et al. Diagnosis of measles with an IgM capture EIA: the optimal timing of specimen collection after rash onset. *J Infect Dis* 1997;175:195–199.

James JM, Burks AW, Roberson PK, et al. Safe administration of the measles vaccine to children allergic to eggs. *N Engl J Med* 1995;332:1262–1266.

Philip RN, Reinhard KR, Lackman DB. Observations on a mumps epidemic in a "virgin" population. *Am J Hyg* 1959;69:91–111.

Plotkin SA. Rubella vaccine. In: Plotkin SA, Orenstein WA, eds. *Vaccines*, third ed. Philadelphia: WB Saunders, 1999:409–438.

Plotkin SA, Wharton M. Mumps vaccine. In: Plotkin SA, Orenstein WA, eds. *Vaccines*, third ed. Philadelphia: WB Saunders, 1999:267–292.

Ray P, Black S, Shinefield H, et al. Risk of chronic arthropathy among women after rubella vaccination. Vaccine Safety Datalink Team. *JAMA* 1997;278:551–556.

Redd SC, Markowitz LE, Katz SL. Measles vaccine. In: Plotkin SA, Orenstein WA, eds. *Vaccines*, third edition. Philadelphia: WB Saunders, 1999:222–266.

Rota JS, Rota PA, Redd SB, et al. Genetic analysis of measles viruses isolated in the United States, 1995–1996. *J Infect Dis* 1998;177:204–208.

Schluter WW, Reef SE, Redd SC, et al. Changing epidemiology of congenital rubella syndrome in the United States. *J Infect Dis* 1998;178:636–641.

Kelley's Textbook of Internal Medicine, fourth edition. Edited by H. David Humes. Lippincott Williams & Wilkins, Philadelphia © 2000.

C H A P T E R
312

HERPES SIMPLEX VIRUS INFECTIONS

MICHAEL N. OXMAN

Herpes simplex viruses (HSVs) are ubiquitous, remarkably host-adapted human pathogens. Initial (primary) HSV infection is usually asymptomatic or mild and self-limited, but instead of disappearing from the body during convalescence, the virus establishes a latent infection that persists for life. This latent infection is subject to intermittent reactivation, which results in recurrent disease or asymptomatic virus shedding and transforms each affected person into a lifelong reservoir of HSV infection. The prompt recognition of HSV infection is extremely important because of the potential for transmission and the availability of effective antiviral chemotherapy.

MICROBIOLOGY

There are two HSVs, type 1 (HSV-1) and type 2 (HSV-2), which are closely related but differ in their epidemiologic characteristics. They are classified as members of the herpesvirus family on the basis of virion architecture and genome structure. HSV-1 and HSV-2 are morphologically indistinguishable from each other and from other members of the herpesvirus family, including the six other human herpesviruses (HHV) discovered to date: varicella-zoster virus (HHV-3), Epstein–Barr virus (HHV-4), human cytomegalovirus (HHV-5), HHV-6 (the cause of roseola infantum), HHV-7, and HHV-8 (etiologically linked to Kaposi's sarcoma).

The HSV virion consists of a linear double-stranded DNA genome within an icosahedral protein shell, or capsid. This structure, the HSV nucleocapsid, is surrounded by a layer of viral protein (the tegument) and, finally, by a lipoprotein envelope containing viral glycoproteins that mediate virus attachment to and penetration into susceptible host cells. Because of the essential role of these envelope glycoproteins, only enveloped virions are infectious, and HSV infectivity is rapidly destroyed by organic solvents, detergents, proteolytic enzymes, heat, drying, and extremes of pH. The genomes of HSV-1 and HSV-2 share about 50% of their nucleotide sequences. Each encodes about 80 proteins, most of which are antigenically related and elicit cross-reactive immune responses. Replication of HSV is highly regulated. Viral genes are expressed in a sequentially ordered cascade controlled by viral regulatory proteins.

PATHOLOGY AND PATHOGENESIS

The pathologic changes that characterize HSV infections are the result of cytopathic effects induced by HSV in infected cells plus local inflammatory responses. Exogenous HSV infection is initiated when virus comes into contact with a mucosal surface (oropharynx, conjunctivae, vaginal mucosa, cervix) or penetrates the stratum corneum of the skin at a site where this barrier has been disrupted by small cracks, minor trauma, or disease. HSV replicates locally in cells of the stratum spinosum, producing papular lesions that rapidly evolve into intraepidermal vesicles. Inflammatory cells soon invade the vesicle, turning the fluid cloudy and transforming it into a pustule. The fluid is then absorbed, leaving a flat, adherent crust that is subsequently detached when subjacent epithelial cells grow back. The lesions heal without scars. Lesions in mucous membranes develop in the same way, but the thin roof of the vesicle quickly breaks down, leaving a shallow ulcer.

In most infected persons, even those who have a primary infection (the initial HSV infection of a host with no immunity to HSV-1 or HSV-2), virus replication and cell destruction are terminated quickly at the site of inoculation, and the infection remains asymptomatic or unrecognized. In some cases, however, virus replication and cell destruction are more extensive, resulting in clinically manifest disease at the portal of entry, spread of virus to regional lymph nodes, and some degree of viremia. In the normal host, nonspecific and specific defense mechanisms combine to localize infection, terminate virus replication, and eventually eliminate infectious virus from tissue at the portal of entry and at any sites of viremic spread.

HERPES SIMPLEX VIRUS LATENCY AND REACTIVATION

The most significant biologic property of the HSVs, which they share with other members of the herpesvirus family, is their ability to establish lifelong persistent infections that ensure their perpetuation in the human population. The key to this behavior is neuronal latency and reactivation. Early in the course of both symptomatic and asymptomatic infections, virus invades local sensory or autonomic nerve endings and is transported within axons to regional sensory or autonomic ganglia, where ongoing latent infections are established in neurons. Thereafter, despite the host's immunity, this latent virus is reactivated periodically,

either spontaneously or by various stimuli, such as trauma to the ganglion or nerve root, fever, menstruation, ultraviolet light, sexual intercourse, or emotional stress. The reactivated virus travels within axons back to the periphery and reinfects epithelial cells in the skin or mucous membranes at or near the original portal of entry. There, virus replication and cell-to-cell spread may produce intraepidermal vesicles like those produced during primary infection. When reactivation of latent HSV results in clinically manifest disease, it is called a recurrence or an episode of recurrent HSV infection. In the normal host, immune mechanisms rapidly limit local virus replication and spread so that recurrent HSV infections are generally less severe, less extensive, and of shorter duration than primary infections. In fact, in the majority of instances, the local infection is so circumscribed that no recognizable lesions are produced and reactivation results only in asymptomatic virus shedding.

Several important questions about HSV latency with implications for prevention and treatment remain to be answered. The first is the mechanism by which HSV latency is established in sensory neurons. Studies with a variety of HSV mutants, as well as the use of antiviral agents that block HSV DNA synthesis, have shown that latency can be established and maintained in the absence of detectable HSV replication and even in the absence of significant HSV gene expression. Thus, the establishment of HSV latency appears to be a passive process governed by neuronal factors rather than by any specific viral gene products.

The absence of detectable HSV gene expression in latently infected neurons and the ability of replication-negative HSV mutants to establish and maintain latency in animal models indicate that HSV DNA replication, at least that catalyzed by HSV-encoded DNA polymerase, is not required for the maintenance of HSV latency in neurons. Consistent with this conclusion is the clinical observation that prolonged suppression of recurrent genital herpes with acyclovir, which blocks HSV DNA synthesis catalyzed by the viral DNA polymerase, fails to abolish latent HSV infection in the sacral ganglia.

IMMUNITY

In the normal host, an array of overlapping local and systemic defense mechanisms limit HSV replication and spread, destroy HSV-infected cells, and eventually eliminate infectious virus. These defenses fall into two categories, nonspecific and specific, that are most clearly differentiated during primary HSV infections. Only nonspecific defenses are operative during the first several days of primary infection, that is, until specific immune responses develop, yet these are sufficient to prevent the development of clinically manifest disease in the majority of infected individuals.

The normal cornified epithelium is an important nonspecific barrier—the first line of defense against the initiation and spread of HSV infection. When it is defective (as in patients with atopic eczema or burns), HSV infections are frequently severe, widespread, and occasionally disseminated. Once primary HSV infection is initiated in the skin or mucous membranes, a number of nonspecific defense mechanisms are mobilized, actuating a local inflammatory response. These include complement activation; production of interferons and other lymphokines; and the activity of neutrophils, monocytes, macrophages, and natural killer cells. Together, they slow HSV replication and limit its spread.

Antibodies to HSV are first detected several days after the onset of infection; they are elicited by epitopes on most of the HSV-encoded proteins, but those that are protective are directed primarily at the envelope glycoproteins that are exposed on the surface of virions and virus-infected cells. Later, during the second week of infection, HSV immune T lymphocytes can be detected. In addition to lysing cells that express HSV glycoproteins, these T lymphocytes lyse cells that express the immediate early (alpha) HSV proteins ICP4 and ICP27. Consequently, they are able to destroy HSV-infected cells early in the virus replication cycle, before any progeny virus is produced.

Because of the multiplicity and overlap of these host defenses, it is difficult to determine the exact role and relative importance of each. Nevertheless, clinical and experimental observations indicate that the natural resistance of the normal epithelium and the virucidal and cytolytic capacities of macrophages and natural killer cells play a crucial role in localizing infection at the portal of entry and slowing virus replication during the first few days, before specific immune responses have developed. When these defenses are deficient, as they are in patients with eczema or extensive burns and in the newborn, there is risk of early virus dissemination and overwhelming systemic infection.

Antibody-dependent cellular cytotoxicity (ADCC), the appearance of which coincides with resolution of the systemic symptoms of primary HSV infections, also has an important role in limiting virus replication at the portal of entry and preventing visceral dissemination. Deficiencies in ADCC, due primarily to numerical or functional deficiencies in effector cells, are associated with a markedly increased risk of severe disseminated HSV infection in the newborn and in certain patients with leukemia; the presence of antibodies mediating ADCC is predictive of a better outcome in neonatal HSV infections. Finally, HSV-reactive T lymphocytes appear to be required for the eventual eradication of infectious virus from mucocutaneous sites of infection. Patients with deficient T-lymphocyte function, such as those infected with HIV, experience severe, persistent, locally progressive mucocutaneous HSV infections but rarely have hematogenous dissemination.

EPIDEMIOLOGY

The principal mode of transmission of HSV is close personal contact, which mediates the direct transfer of virus by infected secretions or from an infected mucocutaneous surface to the recipient's mucous membranes or skin. Because the intact stratum corneum is resistant to HSV infection, transmission to cutaneous sites generally requires some disruption of this barrier, either by trauma or disease. HSV is labile. Consequently, despite experimental evidence that it can survive for hours on a variety of contaminated surfaces, there is no documented transmission from inanimate objects (such as toilet seats) or from swimming pools or hot tubs, and there is no evidence of natural transmission by aerosols. There is no evidence of differing racial or sexual

susceptibility to HSV or of significant seasonal or sexual variation in the incidence of overt disease. Genital herpes is transmitted more efficiently from men to women than from women to men, however, and the prevalence of antibody to HSV-2 is higher in women, even after controlling for other risk factors.

Epidemiologic studies have been complicated by two characteristics of HSV: the prevalence of occult infections and the nature of the immune response. More than two-thirds of initial HSV infections are asymptomatic or unrecognized, and reactivation of latent HSV results in asymptomatic virus shedding far more often than overt disease. Thus, at any point in time, persons shedding HSV asymptomatically (many of whom are totally unaware of ever having been infected) far outnumber those with clinical disease. Consequently, clinical surveys greatly underestimate the incidence and prevalence of HSV infection. Furthermore, though the amount of virus in the lesions of overt disease is greater than that shed asymptomatically, most new HSV infections result from contact with persons who are shedding HSV in the absence of recognized symptoms or lesions. In addition, the immune response to HSV is largely to type-common antigenic determinants. Thus, most serologic assays do not distinguish reliably between antibody responses to the two HSV serotypes.

The epidemiologic characteristics of HSV-1 and HSV-2 infections differ because of differences in their modes of transmission. HSV-1 is transmitted principally by contact with infected oral secretions or lesions, and consequently the incidence and prevalence of HSV-1 infection are influenced by factors that affect the degree of exposure to these sources of infection, such as crowding, poor hygiene, and age. Thus, the rate of acquisition of HSV-1 infection is inversely related to socioeconomic status. This was shown by early serologic studies that found that the age-specific prevalence of antibodies to HSV-1 was lower in upper-income groups than in lower-income groups. In children of low-income families in developing countries, seroconversion (primary HSV-1 infection) takes place early in life; the majority acquire antibodies to HSV-1 by 5 years of age, and 95% are seropositive by age 15 years. Similar results were obtained in low-income families in the United States and Western Europe during the 1950s.

Predictably, the age-specific prevalence of antibodies to HSV-1 has been declining during the past 40 years in Western industrialized countries, especially in middle-class populations, as the standard of living has improved. The prevalence of antibodies to HSV-1 in white adults in the United States has decreased to 40% to 60%. It is only 25% in white 14-year-olds and 25% to 30% in white college students; the figures are much higher for blacks (70% in 14-year-olds and 50% to 60% in college students), undoubtedly reflecting lower socioeconomic status and crowded living conditions during childhood. In a study of college students, most of whom were initially seronegative for HSV-1, primary infections occurred in nearly 10% per year. Thus, whereas primary HSV-1 infections are confined largely to early childhood in developing countries and even in poor urban populations in the United States, the majority of middle- and upper-income children in Western societies escape HSV-1 infections during childhood and are infected as adolescents or adults. Because the clinical manifestations of primary oropharyngeal HSV infection differ in young children (gingivostomatitis) and adults (pharyngotonsillitis and a mononucleosis-like syndrome), this epidemiologic change has resulted in the appearance of a previously unrecognized disease in young adults: acute herpetic pharyngotonsillitis.

Clinical surveys indicate that 20% to 25% of adults in the United States suffer herpes labialis; the majority experience no more than one episode per year, but approximately one-third have two to six episodes per year, and about 5% have recurrences as often as once per month. The frequency and severity of episodes tend to decline with age, and many persons infected with HSV-1 (i.e., with antibodies to HSV-1) do not appear to experience herpes labialis. Nevertheless, seropositive children and adults, including those with no history of symptomatic primary or recurrent infections, periodically shed HSV asymptomatically in their saliva and are the major source of virus causing new HSV-1 infections. The proportion shedding virus at any given time appears to range from 1% to 10%, but it may be greater in children during the first year or two after primary infection and is markedly increased in immunosuppressed patients. Current data on seroprevalence indicate that approximately 130 million U.S. citizens of all ages (50%) are infected with HSV-1.

HSV-2, the predominant cause of genital herpes, is transmitted sexually by contact with infected genital secretions or mucocutaneous surfaces. Thus, HSV-2 infection is rare before puberty, and its acquisition thereafter is related to sexual activity. The highest rates of infection occur between ages 15 and 35 years: more than 80% of all primary HSV-2 infections develop in this age group. The prevalence of antibodies to HSV-2 varies from essentially zero in children younger than 14 years and celibate adults to more than 80% in prostitutes. Once an uncommon disease among members of the white middle class in Western industrialized countries, symptomatic genital herpes has increased dramatically in prevalence since the mid-1960s. Contributing factors include the increasing sexual activity of adolescents, the declining use of barrier contraceptives, and the lower proportion of white middle-class adolescents who have partial immunity to HSV induced by childhood HSV-1 infection.

HSV-2 antibody prevalence rates are 20% to 30% in middle-class women in the United States and more than 20% in the U.S. general population. Some 60% to 80% of these seropositive individuals have no history of symptomatic genital herpes. The incidence of initial HSV-2 infections is 1% to 2% per year in college students, 2% per year in middle-class women of child-bearing age, 5% to 10% per year in multipartner heterosexual sexually transmitted disease (STD) clinic patients, and 5% per year in sexually active homosexual men. There are now 40 to 60 million people in the United States infected with HSV-2, an increase of more then 30% since the late 1970s, and more than a million new infections occur each year.

Risk factors for HSV-2 infection include several sexual partners, early age at first intercourse, years of sexual activity, history of other STDs, low family income, race, and gender; the age-specific prevalence of antibodies to HSV-2 is two to three times higher in black than in white persons and is consistently higher in women than in men. In heterosexual women in the United States, the probability of being infected with HSV-2 rises markedly with the number of sexual partners. It is less than 10% in

women with one lifetime sexual partner, increasing to 40% with two to 10, 60% with 11 to 50, and more than 80% in women with more than 50 lifetime sexual partners. The corresponding probabilities of HSV-2 infection in heterosexual men are less than 1%, 20%, 35%, and 70%.

As in the case of HSV-1, latency and asymptomatic virus shedding play critical roles in maintaining HSV-2 in human populations. The majority of new HSV-2 infections are acquired from a sexual partner shedding virus in the absence of recognized signs or symptoms of disease. The decreasing prevalence of HSV-1 infections before puberty and the increasing popularity of orogenital sexual practices are changing the epidemiologic features of genital herpes. In the United States and Western Europe, 10% to 40% of initial episodes of genital herpes are now caused by HSV-1.

CLINICAL MANIFESTATIONS

The clinical manifestations of HSV infection are determined by the portal of entry of the virus; the previous experience of the host with HSV; the serotype and amount of virus initiating infection; and such host factors as age, immunocompetence, nutritional status, and the presence or absence of conditions like eczema or burns that compromise the normal resistance of the skin. Although HSV-1 is responsible for the majority of infections at anatomic sites above the waist and HSV-2 for the majority of infections at sites below the waist, both serotypes can cause infections at any site, and there is generally no discernible difference between the clinical presentation and course of a given syndrome caused by HSV-1 or by HSV-2. One exception appears to be the frequency of recurrences of oral–labial and genital HSV infections caused by the two viruses. The recurrence rate of genital herpes is at least five times greater when it is caused by HSV-2 than by HSV-1, whereas the recurrence rate of oral–labial herpes is 10 to 100 times greater when it is caused by HSV-1 than by HSV-2. Because transmission of HSV and thus its survival in human populations depend chiefly on recurrent infections, the greater recurrence rate of HSV-1 than of HSV-2 in oral–labial infections and of HSV-2 than HSV-1 in genital infections may reflect the adaptation of the two serotypes to their respective anatomic niches. These differences help explain why HSV-1 is isolated from lesions of recurrent genital herpes so much less frequently than from lesions of primary genital herpes and why HSV-2 is almost never isolated from lesions of herpes labialis.

OROPHARYNGEAL HERPES SIMPLEX VIRUS INFECTIONS

Acute Herpetic Gingivostomatitis

Acute herpetic gingivostomatitis is a manifestation of primary oropharyngeal HSV-1 infection. It develops most often in children between 6 months and 5 years of age, but it is being reported with increasing frequency in older children and adults. The source of infection is usually an adult who has herpes labialis or who is shedding HSV-1 asymptomatically in saliva, but it may be another infected child. The incubation period is usually 3 to 6 days (range, 2 days to 2 weeks). Onset is abrupt, with temperatures as high as 102°F to 104°F (38.9°C to 40.6°C), anorexia, and listlessness. The mouth becomes sore before oral lesions appear, and the child is restless, irritable, and unwilling to eat or drink. Gingivitis is the most striking manifestation of the disease. The gums are first hyperemic and then become markedly swollen, reddened, friable, and exquisitely tender. They bleed easily, and there is a bright red line along the dental margin. Vesicular lesions develop on the oral mucous membranes; they begin as tiny vesicles surrounded by narrow zones of erythema but quickly rupture, leaving tender, round, 1- to 3-mm, shallow, yellowish gray, indurated ulcers or plaques. These often coalesce and are surrounded by a thin red halo. They can manifest anywhere on the mucous membrane of the mouth or pharynx but are most common on the tongue, the inner surface of the lips, and the buccal and sublingual mucosa. Lesions develop less frequently on the soft palate and on the gums themselves, occasionally in the pharynx, and rarely in the larynx. Herpetic epiglottitis, esophagitis, and otitis media are unusual complications.

The submandibular and anterior cervical lymph nodes are enlarged and tender. Salivation and drooling are marked, and the breath is fetid owing to overgrowth of anaerobic oral bacteria. Herpetic lesions often develop in areas of skin contaminated with infected saliva, which contains large quantities of HSV. Thus, many children develop herpetic vesicles in the perioral skin, and herpetic whitlow is seen in finger suckers. Autoinoculation also can result in herpetic vulvovaginitis and HSV infections of the eye. The disease is self-limited and without adverse affects in normal children, but it varies considerably in severity and duration. Although viremia is rarely documented, it probably occurs in many cases of uncomplicated herpetic gingivostomatitis. Primary infection with HSV-1 causes acute herpetic gingivostomatitis in adults as well as in children, but the disease is generally less severe, and pharyngitis is much more prominent. Perioral skin lesions are uncommon, and lesions produced by autoinoculation are rare.

Acute Herpetic Pharyngotonsillitis

In adults, primary oropharyngeal HSV-1 infection causes pharyngitis and tonsillitis much more frequently than gingivostomatitis. The illness begins with fever, malaise, headache, and sore throat. Tiny vesicles appear on the tonsils and posterior pharynx, but they quickly break down to form shallow ulcers that run together. A grayish yellow exudate forms on the tonsils and posterior pharynx in more than half of patients, but lesions in the anterior mouth or lips are seen in fewer than 10%. In college and university students, about 70% of whom are HSV seronegative, HSV is a major cause of pharyngitis and tonsillitis. Although most cases appear to be caused by HSV-1, HSV-2 is being isolated with increasing frequency, especially when pharyngotonsillitis is associated with orogenital contact or occurs in the course of symptomatic genital herpes.

The disease is usually indistinguishable in clinical manifestations from pharyngotonsillitis caused by the group A β-hemolytic streptococcus, and it also may be confused with infectious mononucleosis caused by Epstein–Barr virus, primary HIV infection, herpangina, diphtheria, tularemia, and pharyngotonsillitis associated with adenovirus and enterovirus infections. Persons seropositive for HSV as a result of previous herpetic pharyngotonsillitis are latently infected. They experience periodic asymptomatic shedding of HSV in saliva and subsequently may show signs of herpes labialis. Recurrences of infection do not appear to result in recurrent pharyngotonsillitis.

Herpes Labialis

Herpes labialis (cold sore, fever blister) is the most common manifestation of recurrent HSV-1 infection. Most patients (50% to 80%) have a prodrome of pain, burning, tingling, or itching at the site of the subsequent eruption, which usually precedes its onset by 6 hours or fewer but occasionally last 24 to 48 hours. This is followed by the appearance of a small cluster of erythematous papules that rapidly develop into tiny, thin-walled, intraepidermal vesicles. These generally become pustular and then either burst, leaving shallow ulcers, or dry and form a scab. Left undisturbed, the scab is displaced by the regrowth of epithelium. The evolution of the lesions is generally rapid, the papular stage lasting only a few hours and the vesicles crusting within 2 days. Lesion area (usually less than 100 mm^2) and pain are maximal during the vesicular stage and decline rapidly thereafter. Healing is completed, with loss of scabs and without scarring, in 6 to 10 days. Patients sometimes have local lymphadenopathy but no constitutional symptoms.

The most common site of herpes labialis is the vermilion border of the lip (95%), usually the outer third and more often the lower lip than the upper. Other sites include the nose, the chin, the cheek, and, rarely, the oral mucosa. Although HSV occasionally provokes recurrent lesions of the oral mucosa, it is not the cause of recurrent aphthous ulcers, which afflict many persons with no history of HSV infection and no antibodies to HSV. Herpes labialis afflicts 20% to 25% of the adult population, but this figure varies with the prevalence of latent HSV-1 infection (i.e., of antibody to HSV-1) in the population surveyed. Most people subject to herpes labialis suffer fewer than two episodes per year, but a small minority have recurrences at intervals of a month or less. In a given person, the lesions generally recur at the same site, and the provoking factor (exposure to sunlight, menses, fever, stress) is often stereotypic.

The quantity of HSV present is highest during the first 24 hours, when the lesions are vesicular, and it declines steadily thereafter; rarely is virus recovered after 5 days. HSV is usually present in the saliva during episodes of herpes labialis, and it also can be recovered from 1% to 10% of saliva samples obtained when persons are free of disease, though the concentration of virus is considerably lower. Intraoral lesions are rarely present, and HSV is not recovered from parotid gland secretions. Thus, the source of virus in the saliva remains a mystery. Because of the very low rate of reactivation following primary oral–labial infections caused by HSV-2, HSV-2 is almost never isolated from cases of herpes labialis.

OCULAR HERPES SIMPLEX VIRUS INFECTIONS

Primary HSV infections of the eye are found most commonly in children, often as a result of autoinoculation during acute herpetic gingivostomatitis or asymptomatic primary oropharyngeal HSV infection. The conjunctiva also may be the portal of entry of HSV and infection of the eye the sole manifestation of primary HSV infection. Most infections are asymptomatic or unrecognized, but even when ocular disease is obvious, the causal role of HSV often is unappreciated. Except in newborns, HSV infection of the eye almost always is caused by HSV-1. When it is symptomatic, primary ocular HSV infection usually manifests as unilateral follicular conjunctivitis often accompanied by blepharitis and preauricular lymphadenopathy. There may be herpetic vesicles on the lid margins and periorbital skin. Symptoms typically include photophobia, excessive lacrimation, chemosis, and edema of the eyelids. Some primary infections involve the cornea, producing acute herpetic keratoconjunctivitis accompanied by pain and a foreign body sensation.

Primary infection results in the establishment of HSV latency in the trigeminal ganglion and is followed by periodic reactivation. Most reactivations are asymptomatic, with shedding of HSV in tears, but some result in symptomatic recurrences characterized by keratitis, blepharitis, or keratoconjunctivitis. Recurrences develop in at least 25% of patients who have symptomatic primary infection and in many persons who are seropositive with no history of disease. Recurrent infections tend to involve the underlying stroma; with repeated recurrences, there may be progressive corneal scarring and neovascularization, with eventual loss of vision. HSV is the leading infectious cause of blindness in the United States and other developed countries. Corneal transplantation is frequently performed for end-stage corneal scarring caused by HSV. Unfortunately, some recipients experience recurrent HSV infection of the graft, which is easily confused with allograft rejection. Corticosteroids exacerbate ocular HSV infections, and they are contraindicated unless accompanied by effective antiviral therapy. Acute retinal necrosis is a rare, rapidly progressive form of HSV retinitis that occurs in immunocompetent as well as in immunocompromised persons. It also can be caused by varicella-zoster virus.

HERPES SIMPLEX VIRUS INFECTIONS OF THE SKIN

Because of the resistance of the intact cornified epithelium, isolated exogenous HSV infections of the skin are uncommon in normal adults. When they do arise, they usually are associated with cutaneous trauma. Most primary cutaneous HSV infections develop in the course of acute herpetic gingivostomatitis or primary genital herpes. The skin lesions typically result from autoinoculation or zosteriform spread from an infected mucosal site in the same dermatome. Vesicles tend to be discrete, rather than grouped, and heal without scarring in 7 to 14 days. A normal person with acute herpetic gingivostomatitis or primary genital herpes occasionally experiences widespread cutaneous dissemination, resulting in a varicella-like rash. This rash is accompanied by malaise and fever, but rarely is there serious visceral infection.

Regardless of their location or pathogenesis, cutaneous HSV infections result in the establishment of latency in corresponding sensory ganglia, and the patient is subject to recurrences. Because the virus responsible for recurrent infections originates in sensory ganglia and is transported to the skin by sensory nerves, the lesions of recurrent cutaneous herpes appear as grouped vesicles rather than the discrete vesicles seen in primary infections, and they may assume a segmental or dermatomal distribution that resembles that of herpes zoster. In contrast to herpes zoster, recurrent zosteriform HSV infections recur repeatedly in the same dermatome.

A prodrome of pain, burning, itching, or tingling usually heralds the herpetic eruption, preceding it by 2 or 3 hours (occasionally by up to 2 or 3 days). Lesions begin as grouped, erythematous papules that progress to vesicles, pustules, and crusts and then heal without scarring in 6 to 10 days. There is often regional lymphadenopathy, but constitutional symptoms are rare. Recurrent cutaneous herpes sometimes is associated with severe local neuralgia. Recurrences on the extremities may be accompanied by local edema, erythema, lymphangitis, and tender axillary or inguinal lymphadenopathy. Thus, they may be misdiagnosed as streptococcal cellulitis.

Traumatic Herpes (Herpes Gladiatorum, Scrumpox)

Primary cutaneous HSV infections occasionally appear in normal persons in the absence of oropharyngeal or genital herpes. Such lesions generally result from direct exogenous infection of skin rendered susceptible by trauma. They may develop when an adult shedding HSV in saliva "kisses away" the pain of a child's abrasion or tends an infant with diaper rash. Primary cutaneous herpes also is seen in wrestlers and rugby players (herpes gladiatorum, scrumpox); presumably, traumatized skin is infected by contact with an adversary's cutaneous lesions or virus-bearing saliva. In addition to local vesicular lesions, which are generally confined to the area of traumatized skin (usually the head, trunk, or extremities), regional lymphadenopathy and often constitutional symptoms are present. Recurrences are common, often heralded by a prodrome of pain, burning, tingling, or itching. They frequently are accompanied by regional lymphadenopathy but almost never by symptoms of systemic illness. Herpes gladiatorum is endemic in many groups of high school and college wrestlers, with reported attack rates exceeding 50%. In this context, the primary mode of transmission appears to be direct skin-to-skin contact.

Herpetic Whitlow

Herpetic whitlow (herpetic paronychia) is a painful HSV infection of a terminal phalanx (Fig. 312.1). The thumb or index finger is most often affected, and the portal of entry is usually a damaged cuticle. Involvement of more than one finger is uncommon. In children, it is frequently caused by HSV-1 and occurs in the course of primary oropharyngeal infection as a result of finger sucking. The source of infection also may be an adult who kisses away the pain of an injured finger. In adults, herpetic whitlow is a preventable (by using gloves) occupational

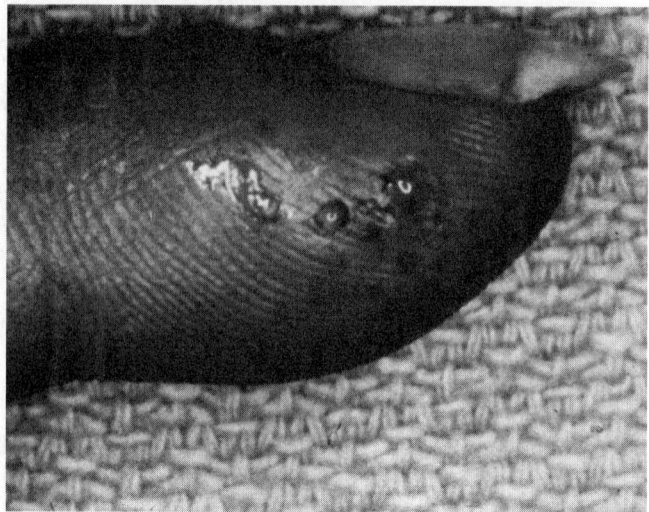

FIGURE 312.1. Herpetic whitlow. The terminal phalanx of the index finger of a respiratory therapist is exquisitely painful, swollen, and erythematous, with multiple deep and superficial vesicles. Herpes simplex virus type 1 was isolated from vesicle fluid. (From Oxman MN. Herpes stomatitis. In: Braude AI, Davis CE, Fierer J, eds. *Infectious diseases and medical microbiology*, second ed. Philadelphia: WB Saunders, 1986: 752–772, with permission.)

disease of medical and dental personnel exposed to oropharyngeal secretions containing HSV-1. The majority of adult cases are caused by HSV-2, acquired by autoinoculation during concurrent genital herpes. Although it can appear in persons with preexisting antibodies to HSV-1 or HSV-2, most initial episodes of herpetic whitlow are primary exogenous infections.

The whitlow begins 2 to 7 days after exposure, with intense itching, pain, and erythema in the infected finger. Within a day, a deep vesicle appears, soon followed by others, which tend to coalesce. The process continues, destroying considerable tissue. In many cases, there appears to be pus under the cuticle, but incision discloses only a little clear fluid or, at a later stage, thick, yellow necrotic debris. Intense local pain is always present. Systemic symptoms and epitrochlear or axillary lymphadenopathy are common, and lymphangitis and neuralgia may occur. The lesions tend to progress for about 10 days, during which time pain persists unabated. There is then abrupt improvement, and the lesions begin to dry. Resolution is usually complete in 18 to 20 days. If the lesion is incised, the period of disability is prolonged, and there is risk of secondary bacterial infection.

Recurrences at the same site are typical; they are often as painful as the primary infection but are shorter in duration and rarely accompanied by constitutional symptoms. The recurrent whitlow is frequently heralded and accompanied by severe neuralgic pain in the hand and arm, and it is often associated with swelling and edema of the hand, lymphangitis, and regional lymphadenopathy. Herpetic whitlow is often confused with bacterial paronychia. When it is associated with lymphangitis and lymphadenopathy, it can be confused with streptococcal cellulitis. Prompt diagnosis is essential to avoid transmission (herpetic whitlow is an important source of nosocomial HSV infection) and inappropriate attempts at surgical drainage.

Herpes Simplex Virus Infections of Abnormal Skin

Cutaneous HSV is often severe and life threatening in patients with disorders of the skin, such as eczema, Darier disease, pemphigus, or burns, which permit more extensive local virus replication and spread and facilitate visceral dissemination. Infection may be acquired nosocomially or by autoinoculation from symptomatic oropharyngeal or genital lesions or asymptomatic virus shedding. Innumerable vesicular lesions can spread throughout the affected skin—a syndrome known as eczema herpeticum or Kaposi varicelliform eruption. The lesions may be ulcerative and nonspecific in appearance, though careful examination may uncover vesicles, especially in adjacent normal skin. Thus, diagnosis requires careful examination and clinical vigilance, with prompt biopsy and culture for virus. Patients are febrile and toxic and, without antiviral therapy, can die from widespread visceral dissemination. Enormous amounts of virus are present in the lesions, and such patients are often a source of nosocomial infections. Recurrences are common; while they may be extensive, they are usually less severe than the primary infection.

CENTRAL NERVOUS SYSTEM HERPES SIMPLEX VIRUS INFECTIONS

In children and adults, central nervous system infections with HSV are relatively uncommon complications of primary or recurrent HSV infections at peripheral sites. In contrast, central nervous system infection is a major component of neonatal HSV infection, occurring in at least 50% of affected newborns.

Herpes Simplex Encephalitis

Herpes simplex encephalitis is an acute necrotizing viral encephalitis that, beyond the neonatal period, nearly always is caused by HSV-1. It has a higher mortality rate than most other forms of viral encephalitis—greater than 70% in the absence of specific therapy. Although it is rare, this form of encephalitis is the most common cause of sporadic acute necrotizing encephalitis in the United States, with an annual incidence estimated to be two to three per million. In contrast to most other forms of viral encephalitis, there are no seasonal epidemics, and cases manifest throughout the year. Serologic data indicate that herpes simplex encephalitis takes the form of a primary infection in about 30% of patients and a recurrent infection in the remainder, but there is no obvious difference between the two groups in initial symptoms, clinical course, or outcome.

The mode of manifestation, clinical features, and side effects are determined largely by the nature and distribution of the pathologic process—acute asymmetric necrotizing encephalitis that involves primarily the orbitofrontal and temporal cortex and the limbic system. Although the manifestations and rates of progression vary, most patients have two recognizable groups of findings: (a) nonspecific changes seen in most forms of encephalitis, which include fever (present in more than 90%), headache, signs of meningeal irritation, nausea, vomiting, global confusion, generalized seizures, and alteration of consciousness, and (b) changes referable to focal necrosis of the orbitofrontal and temporal cortex and the limbic system, which include anosmia, memory loss, peculiar behavior, defects of speech (especially expressive aphasia), hallucinations (particularly olfactory and gustatory hallucinations), and focal seizures. There is rapid progression in some cases, with the appearance of reflex asymmetry, focal paralysis, hemiparesis, and coma. Cerebral edema contributes to these manifestations and plays an important role in the outcome of the disease. Other patients have a more protracted course, with several days of mild, nonspecific illness punctuated by intermittent periods of bizarre behavior alternating with lethargy or sleep. These patients may present a picture of acute psychosis or delirium tremens and be admitted to the hospital for psychiatric care until the appearance of localizing neurologic signs, seizures, and coma alerts their physicians to the severe organic nature of their disease. Rarely, patients have initial symptoms of a brain stem encephalitis that bears little resemblance to the usual case of herpes simplex encephalitis.

Cerebrospinal fluid (CSF) examination usually shows mononuclear pleocytosis (50 to 500 cells per microliter); there are often 10% to 25% neutrophils, and neutrophils may predominate early in the disease. Red blood cells are present initially in 40% and at some time in more than 80% of cases. The protein concentration generally is elevated (50 to 200 mg per deciliter) and often increases markedly over time. Initially, the glucose concentration is often normal (5% of patients have hypoglycorrhachia), but it may be depressed later in the context of extensive cerebral necrosis. Some 5% to 10% of patients have normal CSF on first examination. Magnetic resonance imaging appears to be the most sensitive imaging procedure. The results of electroencephalography are almost always abnormal, and this method often localizes the area of maximum involvement; a pattern of periodic sharp wave or spike-and-wave complexes (periodic lateralized epileptiform discharges) on a background of arrhythmic slow wave activity is characteristic but not pathognomonic.

Detection of HSV DNA in CSF after polymerase chain reaction (PCR) amplification provides a rapid and definitive diagnosis. The sensitivity and specificity of this technique approach 100%, and it has replaced brain biopsy as the primary means of establishing the diagnosis of herpes simplex encephalitis. Antibodies to HSV generally appear in the CSF, but they are rarely detectable until 10 days or more after onset and are thus not helpful in establishing an early diagnosis. Mortality and morbidity rates can be minimized by early initiation of antiviral therapy, but 5% or more of patients suffer a clinical relapse after antiviral therapy has been discontinued. The efficacy of more prolonged antiviral therapy is under investigation. It has been proved on brain biopsy that more than half of patients thought to have herpes simplex encephalitis have another condition, including 9% with other treatable diseases. Thus, the diagnosis should be vigorously pursued, usually with brain biopsy, if PCR analysis of the CSF fails to identify HSV DNA.

Herpes Simplex Meningitis

Herpes simplex meningitis is an acute, generally benign lymphocytic meningitis that develops in otherwise normal adults, often in association with primary genital herpes. Most documented cases have been caused by HSV-2, which can often be isolated from the CSF. Symptoms, which include headache, fever, photophobia, nausea and vomiting, myalgia, and nuchal rigidity, usually resolve in about a week, but 15% to 25% of patients experience one or more recurrences, sometimes in association with an episode of recurrent genital herpes. Herpes simplex meningitis has been observed in children, from whose CSF HSV-1 has been isolated. The detection of HSV DNA in the CSF after PCR amplification has established HSV, predominantly HSV-2, as the principal cause of benign recurrent lymphocytic (Mollaret) meningitis.

Ganglionitis and Myelitis Associated with Herpes Simplex Virus Infections

Genital and anorectal HSV infections may be complicated by lumbosacral ganglionitis, radiculitis, and ascending myelitis. Clinical manifestations include urinary retention, obstipation, abdominal and lower extremity muscle weakness, paresthesia and anesthesia over sacral dermatomes, and severe sacral neuralgia. These symptoms usually resolve spontaneously after a week or two, but some, especially sacral neuralgia, recur in association with episodes of recurrent genital or anorectal herpes.

GENITAL HERPES SIMPLEX VIRUS INFECTIONS

Because of their extensive cross-reactivity, HSV-1 and HSV-2 both induce heterologous humoral and cell-mediated immune responses. Consequently, infection with one HSV serotype limits susceptibility to infection by the other and moderates the severity of those infections that do occur. The prevalence of antibodies to HSV-2 is lower in women with antibodies to HSV-1 than in HSV-1-seronegative women, indicating that HSV-1 infection, presumably acquired in childhood, provides partial protection against subsequent HSV-2 infection. Women with antibodies only to HSV-2 are more likely to have a history of symptomatic genital herpes than women with antibodies to both viruses, indicating that preexisting immunity to HSV-1 diminishes the severity of any HSV-2 infections, so that a higher proportion are subclinical. The protective effect of previous HSV-1 infection has been confirmed by prospective transmission studies in couples discordant for antibodies to HSV-2. The risk of acquiring HSV-2 infection is three to four times greater in women who lack antibodies to both HSV-1 and HSV-2 than in women with previously acquired antibodies to HSV-1.

Prospective clinical studies have shown that initial episodes of genital herpes caused by HSV-2 are less severe in patients with serologic evidence of previous HSV-1 infection than in those with no preexisting antibodies to HSV. In addition, initial episodes of genital herpes caused by HSV-1 are extremely rare in patients with preexisting antibodies to HSV-1, indicating that previous (presumably oropharyngeal) HSV-1 infection protects against genital herpes caused by the same HSV serotype. Finally, most initial HSV-2 infections are asymptomatic, but they still result in the establishment of latent infections that are subject to periodic reactivation. Consequently, many people experiencing their first recognized episode of symptomatic genital herpes are not, as they believe, experiencing an initial episode of exogenous infection. Instead, they are suffering their first symptomatic recurrence caused by reactivation of a latent infection established in the course of an earlier asymptomatic or unrecognized exogenous HSV infection. Such episodes frequently result in confusion and consternation, especially when they occur in one member of a monogamous couple, neither of whom has any history of recognized genital herpes. In this situation, imparting a clear understanding that the source of the virus responsible for the episode may be endogenous rather than exogenous is often more therapeutic than antiviral therapy.

These considerations, which are important in counseling patients and in evaluating any forms of treatment or prophylaxis, lead us to classify an initial episode of clinically manifest genital herpes as a primary infection if it arises in a person with no previous HSV infection at any site, as evidenced by the absence of antibodies to HSV-1 and HSV-2; as an initial nonprimary infection if it occurs in a person with preexisting antibodies to the heterologous HSV serotype (e.g., a first episode of symptomatic genital herpes caused by HSV-2 in a person with preexisting antibodies to HSV-1); and as a recurrent infection if it develops in a person with preexisting antibodies to the same HSV serotype. The average duration and severity of manifestations of clinical disease are greater in primary than in nonprimary first episodes of genital herpes, and episodes of recurrent genital herpes are usually the shortest and least severe. There is sufficient overlap, however, that distinctions are often difficult to make on clinical grounds in individual patients; even in referral clinics with experienced clinicians, almost 10% of persons judged to have a first episode of genital herpes prove to have a recurrent infection, and the proportion is substantially higher in pregnant women.

Acute Herpetic Vulvovaginitis in Infants and Children

In young infants and children, acute herpetic vulvovaginitis may result from autoinoculation during symptomatic or asymptomatic primary oropharyngeal HSV-1 infection or from contact with an adult shedding HSV (e.g., when diapers are changed). Because it also may result from sexual abuse (in which case, it may be caused by HSV-2), its occurrence warrants a thorough and sensitive appraisal of the child's social situation and possible contacts. Every attempt should be made to isolate and type the responsible virus, which then should be saved for comparison with isolates from suspected contacts. Symptoms include fever and malaise, and the perineal area is red, edematous, and studded with tiny vesicles that rapidly evolve into shallow, yellowish white ulcers 2 to 4 mm in diameter. The lesions are extremely painful and often coalesce to form large ulcers. HSV urethritis is generally present, and dysuria may lead to urinary retention. The inguinal lymph nodes are enlarged and tender. Fever and constitutional symptoms subside in a week, and healing is complete without scarring within 12 to 18 days.

Primary and Initial Nonprimary Genital Herpes

The incubation period after sexual contact is usually 3 to 7 days, with a range of 1 day to more than 2 weeks. Most infections in both sexes are asymptomatic, but symptomatic primary genital herpes is more severe in women than in men. Women have a larger total area of lesions, more intense and prolonged local symptoms, more frequent constitutional symptoms, more numerous extragenital lesions, and more complications. They have a higher rate than men of dysuria (83% versus 44%), urethritis (85% versus 27%), meningitis (93% versus 13%), and pharyngitis (13% versus 7%). Primary genital herpes in women often begins with the appearance of herpetic vesicles, but this may be preceded by a short period of local burning, tenderness, and erythema of the labia minora and vaginal introitus. Typical herpetic vesicles first appear on the external genitalia, typically involving the labia majora, labia minora, vaginal vestibule, and introitus. New lesions continue to appear bilaterally in the same areas, and the eruption often extends to the mons pubis, clitoris, urethral orifice, perianal skin, buttocks, and thighs. In most areas within the labia minora, vesicles quickly rupture, leaving shallow, exquisitely tender ulcers covered with a yellowish gray exudate and surrounded by a red areola (Fig. 312.2). In drier areas, such as the outer surface of the labia majora and the adjacent skin, vesicles may remain intact, evolve into pustules, and then crust in several days.

New lesions continue to appear for a week or more. They are often extensive and may coalesce, forming bullae and large areas of ulceration that resemble a second-degree burn. The vaginal mucosa and vulva are inflamed and edematous. The cervix is almost always involved, and there is usually a profuse watery vaginal discharge. Examination typically reveals diffuse friability

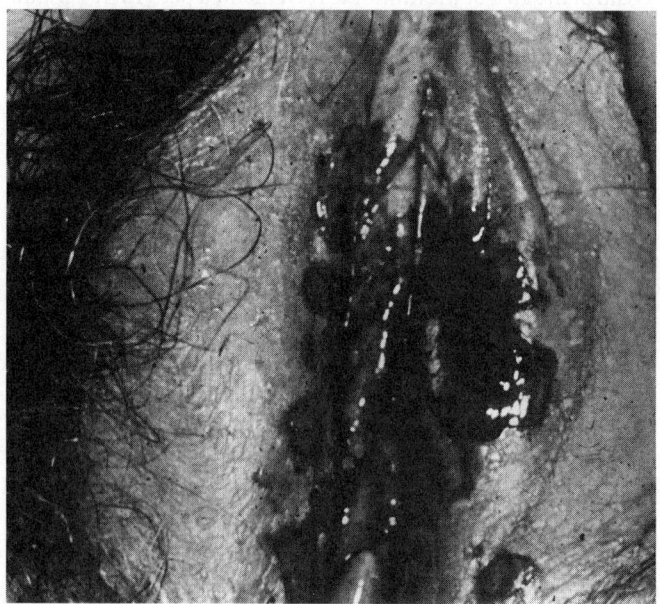

FIGURE 312.2. Primary genital herpes in a female patient. This young woman with primary herpetic vulvovaginitis has shallow, exquisitely tender ulcers on the inner surface of the labia majora, the labia minor, and the vaginal mucosa. The ulcers are covered with a yellowish gray exudate and surrounded by a narrow zone of erythema. Further examination shows herpetic cervicitis. (From Oxman MN. Genital herpes. In: Braude AI, Davis CE, Fierer J, eds. *Infectious diseases and medical microbiology*, second ed. Philadelphia: WB Saunders, 1986:1041–1054, with permission.)

of the cervical epithelium; sometimes there is extensive ulceration and, occasionally, severe necrotic cervicitis. Herpetic cervicitis is sometimes the only clinical manifestation of primary genital herpes. Most patients have severe vulvar pain, exquisite tenderness of the affected tissues, and dysuria, which is sometimes severe enough to cause urinary retention. Dysuria nearly always is associated with urethritis and the presence of HSV in the urine. HSV appears to be present in the urine in a higher proportion of patients with primary genital herpes caused by HSV-1 than by HSV-2.

Most infected women have constitutional symptoms, including fever, headache, malaise, and myalgias, which usually peak during the first 3 to 4 days and disappear by the end of the first week. They also experience bilateral painful inguinal and pelvic lymphadenopathy. The local symptoms generally worsen during the first week, reach a peak between days 8 and 10, and gradually subside. Even when it is severe, primary genital herpes is normally self-limited. Virus replication is maximal during the first 3 to 4 days and declines thereafter; the mean duration of virus shedding is 11 to 12 days, though a few patients shed virus for several weeks. Pain usually remits in 10 to 14 days, and healing takes place without scarring in 2 to 4 weeks. Mucosal lesions heal without crusting. The cervix appears to be the source of virus that may be shed for weeks after visible lesions have healed and symptoms have disappeared.

In men, the lesions of primary genital herpes usually appear bilaterally on the glans penis, the prepuce, and the shaft of the penis and less often on the scrotum, thighs, and buttocks. Their evolution is similar to that in women. In dry skin (on the shaft of the penis), they progress from papule to vesicle to pustule to crust and then heal, as a rule by the middle of the third week. In moist areas (under the prepuce), the vesicles are quickly macerated and evolve into ulcers identical to those described in women. New lesions continue to appear for a week or more, and there is local pain, tenderness, inflammation, and edema. Dysuria, usually associated with herpetic urethritis and accompanied by a small amount of clear mucoid urethral discharge, develops in 30% to 40% of men with primary genital herpes. It is generally more painful than the dysuria of gonococcal or nongonococcal urethritis, and HSV typically can be isolated from urethral swabs. There is bilateral tender inguinal and pelvic lymphadenopathy, but it is less severe and of shorter duration than in women. Less than half of men with primary genital herpes have significant constitutional symptoms. Virus is present in large amounts during the first 3 to 5 days, and the mean duration of virus shedding is 10 to 11 days. Pain usually resolves during the second week, and healing ensues without scarring in 2 to 3 weeks.

The clinical manifestations and course of primary genital herpes caused by HSV-1 and HSV-2 are indistinguishable, but the rate of subsequent recurrences is lower after primary genital herpes caused by HSV-1. The clinical manifestations of initial nonprimary genital herpes are similar to those of primary genital herpes, but the disease is less severe and of shorter duration. There is a marked decline in the incidence of constitutional symptoms, extragenital lesions, and complications, and a smaller proportion of women shed HSV from the cervix.

Recurrent Genital Herpes

In all, 60% to 90% of individuals with symptomatic primary or initial nonprimary genital herpes experience one or more episodes of recurrent genital herpes during the subsequent year. The recurrence rate is lower for HSV-1 than for HSV-2. The mean monthly rate of recurrence for genital herpes caused by HSV-1 is 0.08, compared with 0.34 for genital herpes caused by HSV-2, and approximately 40% of HSV-2-infected patients will have six or more recurrences per year. This is probably why HSV-1 is isolated from 10% to 40% of patients with primary genital herpes but from only 1% to 5% of patients with recurrent disease. A study of patients with concurrent genital and oropharyngeal infections with the same HSV serotype showed that the oropharyngeal recurrence rate is higher for HSV-1 (0.12 per month) than for HSV-2 (0.001 per month). These differences in site-specific recurrence rates may reflect the adaptation of HSV-1 and HSV-2 to different anatomic niches. The rate of symptomatic recurrence is approximately 20% higher in men than in women.

Recurrent genital herpes is generally less severe and of shorter duration than either primary or initial nonprimary genital herpes. Although the same sites tend to be affected, there are fewer lesions, the area involved is more circumscribed, and the lesions often are unilateral. Most patients have a prodrome of tenderness, pain, burning, tingling, or itching at the site of the impending eruption, beginning from a few hours to 1 or 2 days before the appearance of lesions. Some have a prodrome of ipsilateral sacral neuralgia, with severe burning, aching, or lancinating pain in the leg, buttock, or genital area. The lesions of recurrent genital herpes begin as clusters of tiny erythematous papules, which quickly develop into clusters of tiny vesicles on an erythematous base. They sometimes coalesce, and they evolve in the same manner as in primary genital herpes but more rapidly. There is less pain, fewer days of new lesion formation, and a much smaller total area of lesions.

The clinical manifestations of recurrent genital herpes are more severe in women than in men. In women, the lesions are almost always painful. Most often they are located on the labia minora, labia majora, or perineum, but they may manifest on the mons pubis, perianal skin, or buttocks. Some women have linear ulcerations in the fourchette, which resemble inflamed excoriations and often are not recognized as herpetic by patients or their physicians. Lymphadenopathy may be present, but fever and constitutional symptoms are uncommon; only about one-fourth of women with recurrent genital herpes have dysuria. Virus is present in much smaller amounts in recurrent than in primary herpetic lesions (mean peak titers of 103 plaque-forming units or fewer per swab versus 105 plaque-forming units or more per swab); virus is shed for an average of 5 days, and its recovery after the seventh day is uncommon. Pain disappears during the first week, and the lesions generally heal within 8 to 10 days. The rate of positive results on cervical culture (5% to 10%) is much lower during recurrent than during primary episodes of genital herpes. Furthermore, there are no visible cervical lesions, and the amount of virus present is at least 1,000-fold less than the amount present during primary infections.

In men, recurrent genital herpes most often manifests in the

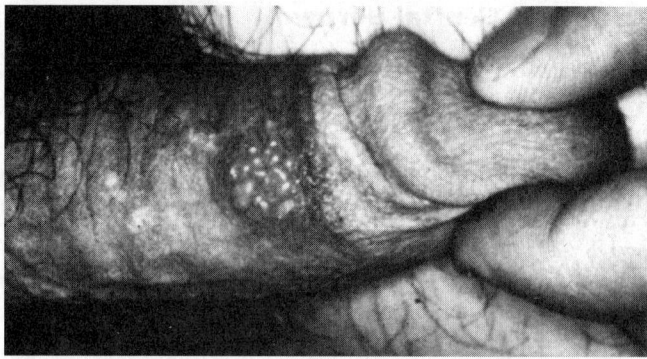

FIGURE 312.3. Recurrent genital herpes in a male patient. A typical patch of grouped vesicles on an erythematous base is seen on the shaft of the penis. (From Oxman MN. Genital herpes. In: Braude AI, Davis CE, Fierer J, eds. *Infectious diseases and medical microbiology,* second ed. Philadelphia: WB Saunders, 1986:1041–1054, with permission.)

form of one or more patches of grouped vesicles on the shaft of the penis, prepuce, or glans (Fig. 312.3). Lesions, which are usually unilateral, begin as papules and, on dry skin, evolve into vesicles, pustules, and crusts in the same manner as the lesions of herpes labialis. Under the prepuce, vesicles are quickly macerated, forming shallow, painful ulcers. There may be mild inguinal lymphadenopathy, but constitutional symptoms are rare, and urethritis is uncommon. Urethral cultures show positive results for HSV in less than 5% of men with recurrent genital herpes. The titer of virus is lower in recurrent than in primary lesions, and HSV rarely can be recovered after 4 to 5 days. Pain is present in about 60% of men with recurrent genital herpes. It is usually mild and disappears with the virus. Lesions heal in 7 to 10 days.

In approximately 5% of patients, recurrent herpes genitalis may appear initially as a single, large, shallow, minimally tender ulcer, up to 1 cm in diameter, that has a clean, granular base and a sharply demarcated border. This lesion, which has been called a *herpetic chancre,* can be mistaken for a syphilitic chancre. Because herpes genitalis and syphilis can coexist in the same patient, diagnosis on the basis of laboratory tests is essential. Symptomatic genital HSV infections are only the tip of an iceberg. The majority of initial primary and nonprimary genital HSV infections are asymptomatic or unrecognized, and 70% to 80% of people with antibodies to HSV-2 have no history of symptomatic genital herpes. Nevertheless, these seropositive individuals are infected latently and experience periodic virus reactivation, as evidenced by virus shedding. The majority of these reactivations also are asymptomatic or unrecognized. Consequently, episodes of asymptomatic virus shedding are far more frequent than episodes of symptomatic recurrent genital herpes.

The rate of asymptomatic virus shedding is generally 1% to 2% in immunocompetent persons with antibody to HSV-2, but it is substantially higher (6% or more) in the first few months after initial HSV-2 infection, in the days immediately before and after a symptomatic recurrence, and in individuals with a high rate of symptomatic recurrence. HSV DNA can be detected by PCR at a rate approximately eight times higher than that reported for infectious virus, but the biologic significance of low levels of HSV DNA in the absence of infectious virus remains to be determined. Asymptomatic shedding appears to be at least

as common from the usual lesion site on the vulva as from the cervix, and anal shedding is documented frequently.

The epidemiologic importance of asymptomatic genital HSV infection is underscored by the fact that most new cases of genital herpes are acquired from a partner shedding HSV asymptomatically who has no history of recognized HSV infection. It is also evidenced by the observation that the majority of mothers of infants with neonatal herpes have had no signs or symptoms of genital herpes during pregnancy and no history of symptomatic genital herpes.

Complications of Genital Herpes

Although genital herpes is often physically and mentally distressing, in the normal host it is almost always self-limited and usually resolves spontaneously without major complications or adverse effects. Complications can be divided into three categories: bacterial or fungal superinfection, extragenital infection or aberrant behavior by the virus in an apparently normal person, and HSV infections in compromised hosts.

Bacterial and fungal superinfections are surprisingly uncommon. Rarely, balanoposthitis develops on the prepuce of an uncircumcised male due to bacterial superinfection of herpetic ulcers, and candidal balanitis is seen occasionally. Ulcerative lesions in moist skin areas may become superinfected. *Candida* vaginitis occurs in about 10% of women with primary genital herpes and is more common in patients with diabetes. These complications typically respond to local therapy and rarely require systemic antibiotics.

Most complications of genital herpes result from infection of extragenital sites. Virus may reach these sites by direct extension, autoinoculation, viremia, or neural (zosteriform) spread. Extragenital sites also may be infected exogenously at the time of genital infection, for example, concurrent oral and genital HSV-1 infection may result from exposure to infected saliva. These complications are much more common in primary than in initial nonprimary infections, and they are also more common and generally more severe in women than in men. Once established, these extragenital HSV infections may recur, but they rarely are initiated during episodes of recurrent genital herpes.

The cervix is infected in almost every woman with symptomatic primary genital herpes and in many asymptomatic cases as well. On occasion, the cervical infection may be extremely severe, producing necrotic cervicitis. Symptoms include profuse vaginal discharge; dysuria; abdominal, pelvic, or genital pain; and constitutional symptoms. The cervix is extremely tender, bleeds easily, and exhibits extensive superficial necrosis with sloughing of necrotic epithelium. Healing takes place spontaneously in 2 to 3 weeks. Herpetic cervicitis may be seen in the absence of other genital lesions. Now and then, extensive herpetic infection of the glans penis can produce necrotizing balanitis. Misdiagnosis and inappropriate therapy are typical.

Herpetic urethritis frequently accompanies primary genital herpes, arising in 20% to 40% of men and more than 80% of women. Typical herpetic lesions may be visible near the urethral meatus, or they may be intraurethral. There is usually severe burning pain on micturition but minimal discharge. Typical intranuclear inclusion bodies and multinucleated giant cells may be found in urethral smears. The urethritis may recur, with or without recurrent genital lesions, and herpetic urethritis may sometimes be the only clinical manifestation of primary genital herpes. Herpetic cystitis also has been observed in patients with primary genital herpes and may account for some instances of dysuria and urinary retention. Virus can reach the bladder by direct extension from the urethra or by neural transmission from infected sacral ganglia. The presence of cystitis caused by HSV-1 in adults with oropharyngeal HSV infection suggests that the bladder also may be infected as a result of viremia.

During an episode of primary genital herpes, cutaneous lesions frequently appear on the buttocks, thighs, or other areas of skin below the waist. They can result from contiguous spread, zosteriform neural transmission from newly infected sacral ganglia, or autoinoculation. When these lesions recur (typically in the absence of genital lesions), they can resemble herpes zoster and often are associated with a prodrome of deep neuralgic or sciatic pain. Frequent recurrence distinguishes this syndrome of "zosteriform herpes simplex" from true herpes zoster caused by varicella-zoster virus, which rarely recurs in the same dermatome. Many patients with zosteriform herpes simplex have never had a recognized episode of genital herpes. Nevertheless, they still have asymptomatic genital shedding of HSV and require counseling regarding transmission of infection to sexual partners.

From 10% to 30% of patients with primary genital herpes caused by HSV-1 or HSV-2 experience symptomatic herpetic pharyngotonsillitis, often as the first manifestation of HSV infection. In most cases, virus probably is introduced directly by oral–oral or oral–genital contact, but it may reach the pharynx by viremia. Clinical manifestations range from mild erythema to severe exudative pharyngotonsillitis, which may even result in pharyngeal obstruction. Most patients have constitutional symptoms and anterior cervical lymphadenopathy. Many are misdiagnosed as having streptococcal pharyngitis or infectious mononucleosis, especially if genital signs and symptoms are absent or ignored.

Autoinoculation of the finger during an episode of primary genital herpes may result in a herpetic whitlow that is indistinguishable from the forms of whitlow that develop in hospital personnel as a result of contact with HSV-1 in saliva and respiratory secretions. Most cases of herpetic whitlow in adults now are associated with primary genital herpes and are caused by HSV-2. These troublesome lesions are seen primarily in women and tend to recur. Autoinoculation occasionally results in skin lesions at other sites and appears to be responsible for herpetic keratoconjunctivitis, which may be seen in as many as 1% of patients with primary genital herpes.

Anorectal herpes and herpetic proctitis may be complications of genital herpes in women, the virus traveling from the vulva to the perineum, anus, and anal canal directly or by zosteriform spread from infected sacral ganglia. Most cases, however, result from anal intercourse, and the disease is seen most frequently in homosexual men. Typical herpetic lesions arise on the perianal skin and in the anal canal, where they frequently coalesce, producing an ulcerative cryptitis. Pain is severe, frequently radiating to the groin, buttocks, and thighs. There is often a serous rectal discharge and bilateral inguinal adenopathy, and constitutional symptoms are common. Pain in the anal canal usually results in reflex inhibition of defecation and sometimes tenesmus. In spite of its severity, the disease is self-limited; symptoms resolve, and healing typically takes place without scarring in 2 to 4 weeks. Recurrent attacks of anorectal herpes are common after primary infections.

Primary genital or anal herpes sometimes is complicated by urinary retention, which may be accompanied by sacral neuralgia, impotence, and blunting of sensation over the sacral dermatomes. Patients with this syndrome have hypotonic bladders and CSF pleocytosis, indicating that urinary retention reflects acute herpetic ganglionitis or lumbosacral radiculomyelitis. This complication of genital herpes normally resolves spontaneously without residual effects in 7 to 10 days; the only report of prolonged dysfunction was in a patient treated with corticosteroids.

Recurrent genital herpes and recurrent zosteriform herpes simplex involving the skin below the waist may be associated with severe local neuralgia, usually in an L5-S1 dermatome distribution. When recurrent herpetic lesions and neuralgia affect the extremities, there may be local edema and lymphangitis, which can lead to a misdiagnosis of bacterial cellulitis. Neuralgia may precede the eruption by several days and usually resolves along with the cutaneous lesions. Although resolution is generally complete and multiple recurrences occur without permanent residual effects, repeated attacks over a period of years sometimes can result in chronic pain and permanent sensory and motor deficits. A similar syndrome occasionally is seen with recurrent herpetic whitlow.

Genital herpes sometimes disseminates in immunocompromised patients, producing widespread cutaneous lesions or fatal involvement of several visceral organs, especially the liver. This highly lethal complication of genital herpes, seen most often in organ allograft recipients in the first month after transplantation, is usually a consequence of reactivation of latent endogenous HSV infection, though it may result from exogenous infection introduced by the transplanted organ. It can be prevented by the use of acyclovir prophylaxis. Asymptomatic shedding of HSV-2 is markedly amplified in immunocompromised patients.

The diseases to be considered in the differential diagnosis of herpes genitalis and its complications include syphilis, chancroid, lymphogranuloma venereum, gonorrhea, nongonococcal urethritis, chlamydial urethritis, granuloma inguinale, herpes zoster, erythema multiforme, Behçet syndrome, mucocutaneous manifestations of inflammatory bowel disease, contact dermatitis, candidiasis, trichomoniasis, bacterial folliculitis, and impetigo. Multinucleated giant cells with eosinophilic intranuclear inclusion bodies indicate the presence of either HSV or varicella-zoster virus; direct detection and identification of HSV antigens or nucleic acids or virus isolation can give the specific diagnosis. PCR assays of the CSF can distinguish enteroviral from HSV aseptic meningitis. Because patients often have more than one STD, it is important to rule out other possibilities (e.g., syphilis) as well as HIV infection, even when an HSV infection is documented.

NEONATAL HERPES SIMPLEX VIRUS INFECTION

One of the most serious complications of genital herpes is the transmission of infection in a pregnant woman to her newborn infant. The infant usually is infected perinatally during passage through the birth canal of a mother with asymptomatic genital herpes. In some cases, ascending infection occurs shortly before birth, typically in a woman with prolonged rupture of membranes. Ascending infection can also be iatrogenic, introduced by a fetal monitor. The risk of neonatal infection is estimated to be 30% or more for infants born to mothers with an initial primary HSV infection acquired late in pregnancy who have not developed measurable levels of neutralizing antibody before the onset of labor, and the risk is greater from a primary than a nonprimary maternal infection. Conversely, the risk is much lower (probably less than 1%) when virus shedding at term results from recurrent infection or even from an initial primary or nonprimary HSV infection acquired early enough in gestation for complete seroconversion to take place before the onset of labor.

Congenital infection, a consequence of primary maternal HSV infection earlier in pregnancy, is responsible for 3% to 5% of cases among neonates. Some infants acquire infection postnatally from the mother, other family members, or nursery personnel with nongenital HSV infections or by nosocomial transmission from another infected infant. One-third of neonatal HSV infections are now caused by HSV-1. The overall rate of neonatal HSV infection in the United States is estimated to be 1 in 3,000 to 9,000 live births. Antiviral therapy has lowered the mortality rate and increased the proportion of survivors who function normally at 1 year of age. Early recognition of neonatal HSV infections is hampered by the absence of skin lesions in 30% or more of infected infants.

HERPES SIMPLEX VIRUS INFECTIONS AT OTHER SITES

Transient viremia is probably common during primary HSV infections in normal persons, but host defense mechanisms generally limit virus replication and spread so that foci of hematogenous infection in the skin and internal organs remain subclinical. These host defenses also limit the direct extension of HSV infection from the oropharynx to the trachea and esophagus. Nevertheless, clinically manifest disease due to hematogenous dissemination or direct extension of HSV infection does develop in normal hosts, though it is much more common in immunocompromised patients.

Disseminated Herpes Simplex Virus Infections

Primary oropharyngeal and genital HSV infections in apparently normal children and adults occasionally are complicated by clinically significant viremia, with cutaneous or visceral dissemination. This may even happen during otherwise asymptomatic primary infections, in the absence of signs or symptoms of disease at the portal of entry. In most cases, clinically significant dissemination is confined to the skin, producing an illness that is virtually indistinguishable from varicella (except when oropharyngeal or genital lesions are present). The illness is self-limited and resolves in 7 to 14 days, but skin lesions often recur.

Rarely, there is severe, often fatal visceral dissemination,

which may or may not be accompanied by vesicular lesions in the skin. Several organs are involved, but fulminant HSV hepatitis is usually predominant, and it is generally accompanied by leukopenia, thrombocytopenia, and disseminated intravascular coagulation. This syndrome, fatal in the majority of untreated cases, occurs with greatest frequency in pregnant women, typically during the third trimester. Some cases have been associated with primary oropharyngeal HSV-1 infections, but most have accompanied primary genital herpes caused by either HSV serotype. The disease in these pregnant women resembles that observed in renal transplant recipients and other immunosuppressed patients and in the neonate. HSV-specific cellular immunity is depressed during the third trimester of pregnancy, which may explain the susceptibility of pregnant women to disseminated HSV infection. Disseminated HSV-1 and HSV-2 infections in apparently normal children and adults have been associated with herpetic esophagitis, adrenal necrosis, interstitial HSV pneumonitis, HSV cystitis, monarticular HSV arthritis, HSV meningitis, and, now and then, HSV encephalitis.

Respiratory Tract and Gastrointestinal Tract Infections Caused by Herpes Simplex Virus

Herpetic tracheobronchitis due to aspiration of oropharyngeal secretions containing HSV-1 may develop in apparently normal persons. This happens most often in the elderly and in association with endotracheal intubation. Clinical manifestations range from asymptomatic infection to severe tracheobronchitis with widespread mucosal ulceration. Focal or multifocal HSV pneumonitis can result from further aspiration or contiguous spread of infection, and these patients often have concurrent HSV esophagitis. Viremic infection of the lungs, more common in immunosuppressed patients, is rare in immunocompetent persons; it results in bilateral interstitial pneumonia. Diagnosis is complicated by contamination of specimens with HSV shed asymptomatically in saliva.

HSV esophagitis, a commonplace manifestation of HSV infection in immunocompromised patients, also can develop in otherwise normal children and adults, especially in the presence of a nasogastric tube. Initial signs are fever, odynophagia, dysphagia, substernal pain, and, infrequently, hematemesis, but it is often asymptomatic. Endoscopy shows typical shallow herpetic ulcers of the esophageal mucosa. Herpetic esophagitis usually stems from direct extension of symptomatic oropharyngeal infection or from infection of traumatized esophageal mucosa by HSV shed in saliva, but it can be a recurrent infection resulting from reactivation of virus latent in the vagus ganglion. Symptoms usually resolve spontaneously within a day or two after removal of the nasogastric tube. HSV esophagitis may be difficult to distinguish from *Candida* esophagitis, and both organisms sometimes can participate in the pathogenetic process. HSV esophagitis usually responds to systemic antiviral chemotherapy.

HERPES SIMPLEX INFECTIONS IN IMMUNOCOMPROMISED HOSTS

The frequency and severity of HSV infections increase markedly in patients with hematologic and lymphoreticular malignancies, in patients with AIDS, and in organ and bone marrow allograft recipients, particularly during the first 4 to 6 weeks after transplantation, when immunosuppression is greatest. These infections develop mainly in patients with preexisting antibodies to HSV, reflecting reactivation of endogenous latent infection. Most seropositive transplant recipients shed HSV. Although these HSV infections are sometimes asymptomatic, they usually are associated with symptomatic mucocutaneous disease (herpes labialis, recurrent genital herpes). These recurrent infections often behave normally and resolve without complications. Sometimes, however, the local lesions do not resolve but slowly enlarge, ulcerate, become necrotic, and extend to deeper tissues.

Satellite lesions develop, and mucous membrane involvement is often extensive, with ulcerative, sometimes nodular, lesions on the lips, buccal mucosa, tongue, and palate. Pain and chronicity are hallmarks of the disease. These chronic, atypical mucocutaneous HSV infections, which involve the perioral or anogenital region, are a major cause of morbidity in profoundly immunosuppressed patients. They are common in patients with AIDS. They often heal spontaneously when cellular immunity improves on induced remission of lymphoreticular malignant neoplasms, reduction in iatrogenic immunosuppression in organ allograft recipients, or effective chemotherapy of HIV infection.

Latent HSV is also reactivated during postchemotherapy mucositis; the majority of patients who suffer stomatitis after cancer chemotherapy shed HSV in saliva, and it is difficult to assess the relative contribution of chemotherapy and HSV to the mucosal disease. HSV dissemination is rarely associated with any of these chronic mucocutaneous HSV infections in seropositive patients, but local extension can be a major problem. Virus can spread from the oropharynx to the esophagus and trachea, where infection is facilitated by mucosal damage caused by radiation, chemotherapy, or intubation. Herpetic esophagitis is a common, but often unrecognized complication of oropharyngeal HSV infection in immunocompromised and debilitated patients, especially in the presence of a nasogastric tube. There are typical herpetic ulcers of the esophageal mucosa that may become confluent in the lower third. Herpetic esophagitis can lead to viremia, with infection of the liver and other organs, and the mucosal lesions are often superinfected with *Candida* species, which further obscures the diagnosis.

The lungs also can be infected by HSV, either by direct extension of infection from the oropharynx or as a consequence of viremia. Direct extension is facilitated by injury to the respiratory epithelium (by endotracheal intubation, chemotherapy, radiation, or burn injury). This probably explains the high incidence of herpetic tracheobronchitis in hospitalized burn victims and the frequency of local HSV infection in patients intubated for adult respiratory distress syndrome. In these contexts, most patients have focal or multifocal pneumonitis, and concurrent HSV esophagitis is common. There is usually evidence of active oropharyngeal infection long before the onset of pneumonia. Diffuse bilateral interstitial pneumonia, a consequence of hematogenous HSV dissemination, is rare except in profoundly immunosuppressed patients and is much more likely to occur in the course of a primary rather than a recurrent HSV infection.

HERPES SIMPLEX VIRUS INFECTION AS A CAUSE OF ERYTHEMA MULTIFORME

Recurrent HSV infections may be associated with allergic cutaneous and mucocutaneous disorders, especially erythema multiforme. In 15% to 70% of patients with erythema multiforme, especially those with recurrent erythema multiforme, the onset of disease is regularly preceded by a symptomatic attack of recurrent HSV infection (Fig. 312.4). Furthermore, the disease has been induced by the intradermal inoculation of inactivated HSV antigens in patients who suffer erythema multiforme but not in persons who have a history of uncomplicated recurrent herpes simplex. Erythema multiforme usually begins 3 to 10 days after the appearance of the herpetic lesions. It can range in severity from mild disease with typical target (iris) lesions on the extremities (erythema multiforme minor) to severe and extensive disease with lesions over the entire body, including the palms and soles, and painful bullous, erosive lesions on the mucous membranes of the eyes, nose, oropharynx, genitalia, and anus (erythema multiforme major or Stevens–Johnson syndrome).

Although the mucosal lesions can be confused with lesions caused directly by HSV infection, their histopathologic appearance is different. The lesions of erythema multiforme result from vasculitis, and vesicles, when present, are subepidermal. They do not result from virus replication in the skin, and thus they do not contain inclusion bodies or multinucleated giant cells, and they almost never yield HSV on culture. Their formation represents an allergic response, presumably to circulating HSV

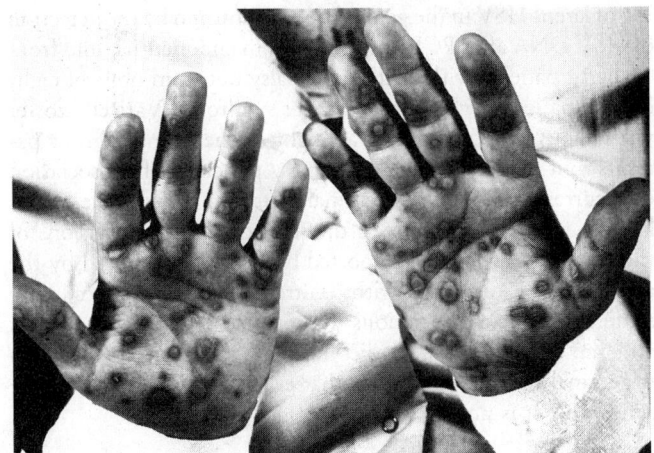

FIGURE 312.4. Recurrent erythema multiforme associated with recurrent cutaneous herpes simplex. Erythema multiforme regularly develops in a young man with recurrent herpes simplex involving a small area of skin over his left scapula (herpes gladiatorum), 3 to 5 days after the onset of each herpetic recurrence. The rash consists of characteristic target (iris) lesions primarily affecting the skin of the trunk and extremities, including the palms and soles, and there is oropharyngeal mucositis. Herpes simplex virus type 1 is isolated from the herpetic lesions over the scapula, but not from the target lesions or oral mucosa, and no multinucleated giant cells or intranuclear inclusion bodies have been detected in biopsy specimens of the erythema multiforme lesions. Suppression of the patient's recurrent bouts of cutaneous herpes simplex with acyclovir, 400 mg orally twice daily, has eliminated recurrences of erythema multiforme. (From Oxman MN. Herpes stomatitis. In: Braude AI, Davis CE, Fierer J, eds. *Infectious diseases and medical microbiology*, second ed. Philadelphia: WB Saunders, 1986:752–772, with permission.)

antigens or antigen–antibody complexes, and these complexes, as well as HSV DNA, have been detected in the skin lesions. Suppression of HSV recurrences with oral acyclovir can prevent the occurrence of erythema multiforme in the majority of patients.

HERPES SIMPLEX VIRUS AND IDIOPATHIC NEUROLOGIC SYNDROMES

The intimate association of HSV with neurons has aroused suspicion that the virus plays a part in the pathogenesis of a variety of neurologic syndromes of unknown cause, including trigeminal neuralgia (tic douloureux), atypical pain syndromes, idiopathic facial paralysis (Bell's palsy), temporal lobe epilepsy, recurrent psychosis, and multiple sclerosis. The ubiquity of HSV, its lifelong latent residence in seropositive persons, and its frequent reactivation in response to a variety of stimuli, however, minimize the etiologic significance of any temporal association between the occurrence or recurrence of HSV infection and the onset of another disease. Nevertheless, the association of HSV with atypical pain syndromes, including trigeminal neuralgia, enjoys a measure of clinical and serologic support. Recurrent cutaneous HSV infections sometimes are associated with a prodrome of severe neuralgic pain, and repeated attacks over a period of years occasionally have resulted in the development of chronic pain and permanent sensory loss.

HSV appears to be the principal cause of idiopathic facial palsy (Bell's palsy). Previously based primarily upon serologic data, this association has been strengthened greatly by the finding of latent HSV in the geniculate ganglion and by the detection of HSV DNA after PCR amplification in endoneurial fluid from 11 of 14 patients with acute Bell's palsy but from none of eight control patients with Ramsay Hunt's syndrome. Varicella-zoster virus DNA was detected in all eight of the Ramsay Hunt patients, but in none of the Bell's palsy patients. The association of recurrent HSV with trigeminal neuralgia, which, like herpes labialis, almost always affects the second and third divisions of the trigeminal nerve, is supported by serologic data and by the association of some cases with recurrent cutaneous herpes in the same area. These associations do not prove causality, however, and the absence of antibodies to HSV in some patients with trigeminal neuralgia indicates that even if HSV does cause the syndrome, it is not the only cause.

GENITAL HERPES AS A RISK FACTOR FOR HUMAN IMMUNODEFICIENCY VIRUS INFECTION

It has long been recognized that genital ulcer disease enhances the transmission of HIV infection among sexually active persons. HIV transmission is facilitated by disruption of the epithelial barrier and the presence of HIV-infected T lymphocytes and macrophages in the ulcer base. In North America and Europe, where HSV infection is the most common cause of genital ulcer disease, epidemiologic evidence indicates that orogenital HSV infection is an important risk factor for HIV infection. Thus, controlling symptomatic HSV infections with effective antiviral chemotherapy may contribute to AIDS prevention.

HERPES SIMPLEX VIRUS INFECTION AND CANCER

The capacity of HSV to induce cell transformation in vitro and the observation made in many (but not all) seroepidemiologic studies that the prevalence of antibodies to HSV-2 is higher in women with carcinoma of the cervix than in matched control subjects led to the suggestion that HSV-2 might play a causal role in cervical carcinoma. The epidemiologic studies indicate only that HSV-2 infection and cervical carcinoma are covariable: both are linked to sexual promiscuity and early age at first coitus. Convincing evidence of any more direct linkage is lacking. Furthermore, compelling data now indicate that human papillomavirus infections are responsible for most cases of cervical carcinoma.

DIAGNOSIS

The potential for transmission and the availability of specific antiviral agents now place a high premium on early and reliable diagnosis. A presumptive diagnosis of HSV infection often can be made on clinical and epidemiologic grounds (in patients with typical herpes labialis or recurrent genital herpes). Many other diseases can be confused with HSV infections, however, and lesions caused by HSV are often atypical, especially in immunocompromised patients. Even among very experienced physicians, the specificity of a clinical diagnosis of HSV infection is less than 80%. Thus, diagnosis based on laboratory testing is often required, and it is always desirable. There is, however, an important caveat. The high prevalence of unrecognized HSV infections and the frequency of asymptomatic virus shedding—which is markedly higher in the context of immunosuppression and the stress and fever of most illnesses—limit the etiologic significance of the presence of HSV in many clinical specimens (e.g., a specimen of lung obtained by transbronchial biopsy, which may be contaminated with saliva). In such situations, diagnosis requires histopathologic evidence of the direct involvement of HSV in the pathologic process.

VIRUS ISOLATION

Virus isolation in cell culture has been the gold standard for the diagnosis of HSV infections. It offers high sensitivity and unsurpassed specificity when specimens are obtained early in the course of HSV infection (at the vesicular stage) and handled properly to avoid loss of infectivity. It also yields virus for subsequent studies, such as measurement of sensitivity to antiviral drugs and restriction endonuclease fingerprinting, and it may detect pathogens other than HSV. HSV grows readily in a variety of human and nonhuman cells, and characteristic cytopathic effects typically are apparent in 1 to 3 days. Even with culture enhancement techniques (including early immunostaining for HSV antigens), however, results are generally not available for 24 hours or longer. Because many therapeutic decisions require diagnostic information in minutes to hours, much effort has been devoted to developing methods for rapid diagnosis.

RAPID DIAGNOSIS—HISTOPATHOLOGY

The histologic appearance of lesions caused by HSV provides a rapid and practical means of diagnosis. Multinucleated giant cells containing eosinophilic intranuclear inclusion bodies distinguish the lesions of HSV from those produced by almost all other pathogens. Other than HSV, only measles and varicella-zoster virus produce multinucleated giant cells with eosinophilic intranuclear inclusion bodies. Measles does not resemble HSV infection in clinical features or epidemiologic characteristics, the rash is normally not vesicular, and the skin lesions are distinct in histologic appearance from those caused by HSV. The characteristic cytologic changes induced by HSV can be seen easily in Tzanck smears prepared at the bedside. Cells are scraped from the base of an early vesicle, spread gently on a glass microscope slide, and stained with hematoxylin-eosin, Giemsa, Papanicolaou, or Paragon multiple stain. A punch biopsy taken at the edge of a lesion provides better tissue for cytologic and immunologic diagnosis, especially in atypical ulcerative lesions, such as those found in immunocompromised patients. Biopsy also facilitates diagnosis in the prevesicular stage. Specimens also can be examined for virus particles by electron microscopy. While these cytologic techniques are useful in rapidly differentiating HSV infection from most other vesicular diseases (contact dermatitis, hand-foot-and-mouth disease), they are relatively insensitive (50% to 80%), and they do not distinguish between HSV and VZV infections.

RAPID DIAGNOSIS—DIRECT DETECTION OF HERPES SIMPLEX VIRUS ANTIGENS OR NUCLEIC ACIDS IN CLINICAL SPECIMENS

Rapid direct detection and identification of HSV antigens and nucleic acids in clinical specimens are now a reality. Although they are often less sensitive than virus isolation, these techniques can detect viral proteins and nucleic acids late in the course of disease, when infectious virus may not be recovered. Immunofluorescent or immunoenzyme staining with monoclonal antibodies to HSV-1, HSV-2, and varicella-zoster virus can strengthen sensitivity and provide a specific diagnosis, distinguishing HSV from varicella-zoster virus and HSV-1 from HSV-2.

IDENTIFICATION OF HERPES SIMPLEX VIRUS DNA BY POLYMERASE CHAIN REACTION ASSAYS

The development of PCR assays for the detection of viral DNA and RNA has vastly improved the laboratory diagnosis of virus infections. The use of primers from DNA sequences that are common to HSV-1 and HSV-2 (e.g., DNA polymerase) permits detection of either HSV serotype, whereas primers from type-specific DNA sequences can be used to identify the HSV serotype. Because of their extraordinary sensitivity (substantially greater than virus isolation or direct detection of HSV antigens or nucleic acids), assays employing PCR amplification have revolutionized the diagnosis of HSV infections. In herpes simplex encephalitis, detection of HSV DNA in CSF now provides a noninvasive diagnostic technique that is at least as sensitive as brain biopsy. PCR assays also have established that HSV (usually HSV-2) is the principal cause of benign recurrent lymphocytic (Mollaret) meningitis and confirmed a strong association between HSV-1 infection and Bell's palsy. PCR assays are substantially more sensitive than virus isolation for detecting symptomatic and asymptomatic virus shedding in patients with genital herpes. Their use has led to a three- to eightfold increase in the estimated rate of HSV shedding by HSV-2 seropositive women. The clinical significance of small quantities of HSV DNA detected by PCR in the absence of infectious virus remains to be determined.

SEROLOGIC DIAGNOSIS

The usefulness of serologic assays for the diagnosis of HSV infections has been limited by the need to obtain a sample of convalescent-phase serum to establish seroconversion; by the fact that recurrent infections, which account for much of the morbidity of HSV, generally do not stimulate a significant increase in antibody titers; and by the antigenic cross-reactivity of HSV-1 and HSV-2. Commercially available enzyme immunoassays do not discriminate reliably between HSV-1 and HSV-2 infections despite claims to the contrary. These assays are useful only for confirming a diagnosis of primary HSV infection by documenting HSV seroconversion and for identifying persons not infected with either HSV serotype (who are HSV seronegative).

Type-specific serologic assays are now available in which serum samples are reacted with HSV proteins that have predominantly type-specific epitopes (e.g., gG1 from HSV-1 and gG2 from HSV-2) in solid-phase enzyme immunoassays or with electrophoretically separated HSV-1 and HSV-2 proteins in Western blot assays. The enzyme immunoassays are accurate and simple to perform on large numbers of serum samples, but antibodies to gG2 may not develop until 6 to 8 weeks after initial HSV-2 infections and may remain undetectable in some patients, especially immunosuppressed patients, with culture-proven recurrent HSV-2 infections. Western blot assays are more cumbersome, but they can ascertain early seroconversion, identify HSV-2 infections when antibodies to gG2 are not detectable, and detect seroconversion to HSV-2 in patients with previous HSV-1 infections despite their early anamnestic response to type-common epitopes. Type-specific assays can distinguish between initial primary and nonprimary HSV infections and identify persons previously infected with HSV-1, HSV-2, or both (e.g., when screening organ donors and recipients, pregnant women and their sexual partners, and potential vaccine recipients). The clinical application of these type-specific assays has revolutionized the serologic diagnosis of genital herpes and led to a clear delineation of the epidemiologic characteristics of HSV-1 and HSV-2 infections.

■ TREATMENT

No treatment is presently available that can eradicate latent HSV infections or prevent the establishment of HSV latency. Nevertheless, antiviral chemotherapy can limit the morbidity and mortality of HSV infections, and suppressive therapy can markedly lessen the rate of symptomatic recurrences and of asymptomatic virus shedding. Nine compounds that interfere with HSV DNA replication—idoxuridine, trifluorothymidine, vidarabine, acyclovir, penciclovir, foscarnet, cidofovir, famciclovir, and valacyclovir—have been proved effective and are licensed for use in the United States. Idoxuridine and trifluorothymidine are effective for topical treatment of HSV keratitis but are too toxic for systemic use. Vidarabine, acyclovir, penciclovir, foscarnet, and cidofovir are licensed for both topical and systemic use.

Acyclovir, the first truly selective inhibitor of HSV replication to be evaluated in clinical practice, is phosphorylated actively by HSV-encoded thymidine kinase (TK) but is a poor substrate for cellular TKs. Thus, it is concentrated in HSV-infected cells. Cellular enzymes then convert acyclovir monophosphate to acyclovir triphosphate, which is a selective inhibitor of HSV-encoded DNA polymerase. In addition, any acyclovir triphosphate that is incorporated into DNA causes chain termination. As a consequence of these properties, acyclovir is a highly effective and nontoxic inhibitor of HSV replication. It is available in intravenous, oral, and topical formulations, though topical acyclovir is rarely indicated.

Penciclovir is similar to acyclovir in mechanism of action and anti-HSV activity but differs in its pharmacologic properties (e.g., penciclovir triphosphate has a much longer intracellular half-life than acyclovir triphosphate). Penciclovir is available in intravenous and topical formulations. Two licensed prodrugs, famciclovir (prodrug of penciclovir) and valacyclovir (prodrug of acyclovir), provide much greater oral bioavailability than acyclovir, which permits less frequent dosing and results in blood levels of antiviral activity heretofore achievable only with intravenous acyclovir. Foscarnet and cidofovir are more toxic than acyclovir and penciclovir, and their use is limited to the treatment of acyclovir-resistant HSV infections. Additional compounds that target HSV-encoded DNA polymerase are being evaluated, and viral protease inhibitors offer another promising avenue for selective inhibition of HSV replication.

In normal persons infected with HSV, virus replication is terminated effectively by host defense mechanisms, and clinical manifestations, when present, resolve quickly without medical intervention. This is especially true of such recurrent HSV infections as herpes labialis. Consequently, antiviral therapy may have little clinical impact. In contrast, when HSV replication is prolonged, as it is in symptomatic primary infections and in immunocompromised patients, antiviral therapy can limit morbidity and mortality markedly.

TREATMENT OF PRIMARY AND INITIAL NONPRIMARY HERPES SIMPLEX VIRUS INFECTIONS

Symptomatic treatment should be directed toward prevention of autoinoculation and bacterial superinfection and minimization of local discomfort. Lesions should be kept clean and dry and nonspecific creams and ointments avoided. Burrow solution compresses or sitz baths are often helpful. Painful urination in women with genital herpes may be relieved by urinating in a sitz bath or bathtub. HSV infections of the eye respond to topical antiviral therapy—trifluridine appears to be the drug of choice.

Systemic therapy with oral acyclovir, famciclovir, or valacyclovir should be added if deeper tissues are affected. Eye infections should always be managed in collaboration with an experienced ophthalmologist.

In double-blind, placebo-controlled studies, both acyclovir and vidarabine have been shown to reduce the mortality and morbidity rates of neonatal HSV infections and herpes simplex encephalitis. Because of its lower toxicity, greater ease of administration, and superior efficacy in HSV encephalitis, intravenous acyclovir has replaced vidarabine for the treatment of these and other serious HSV infection. Suppression with oral acyclovir or valacyclovir after initial therapy with intravenous acyclovir is being evaluated for prevention of relapses of herpes simplex encephalitis and cutaneous recurrences in neonatal HSV infections.

Acyclovir is the drug of choice for the treatment of primary and nonprimary first episodes of genital herpes. Oral and intravenous therapy substantially shortens the duration of local symptoms and virus shedding; accelerates healing; and diminishes new lesion formation, dysuria, vaginal discharge, and extragenital manifestations. Oral acyclovir generally is recommended (Table 312.1). Intravenous therapy is reserved for disease severe enough to require hospitalization, especially if there are such extragenital manifestations as urinary retention or HSV meningitis. Topical acyclovir has no role in the therapy of initial genital HSV infections. Famciclovir and valacyclovir produce higher blood levels of antiviral activity and offer the possibility of less frequent administration. Their clinical efficacy does not appear to be superior to that of oral acyclovir, however, and they are generally more expensive. Unfortunately, no form of therapy appears to lessen the frequency or severity of subsequent recurrences.

Oral acyclovir is indicated for immunocompetent persons who have severe herpetic gingivostomatitis or pharyngotonsillitis; initial episodes of herpetic whitlow; HSV protitis; primary herpetic infections of the skin, such as herpes gladiatorum. Higher daily doses of oral acyclovir appear to be required for HSV infections at these sites. Intravenous therapy is suggested for patients hospitalized with severe infections or with visceral or neurologic complications. Famciclovir or valacyclovir may be preferable to oral acyclovir, but studies establishing their superiority are not available at present.

TREATMENT OF RECURRENT HERPES SIMPLEX VIRUS INFECTIONS

Recurrent HSV infections typically are limited in duration and extent and resolve spontaneously without complications. Nevertheless, they cause sufficient physical and emotional distress to prompt most afflicted persons to seek some form of relief. Oral acyclovir, even when administered during the prodrome, has only a modest effect on the course of herpes labialis and recurrent genital herpes, and it does not seem to alter the frequency or severity of subsequent recurrences. Oral acyclovir does provide meaningful relief to patients whose episodes are more extensive and prolonged and to most patients with recurrent herpetic whitlow. Topical acyclovir is ineffective for recurrent HSV infections in normal hosts, but topical penciclovir shows modest clinical efficacy in patients with herpes labialis. Because treatment of herpes labialis and recurrent herpetic whitlow require higher doses of acyclovir than treatment of recurrent genital herpes, famciclovir or valacyclovir may be preferred.

PROPHYLAXIS (SUPPRESSION) OF FREQUENTLY RECURRING HERPES SIMPLEX VIRUS INFECTIONS

Long-term prophylaxis with oral acyclovir markedly reduces the incidence and severity of repeated episodes of genital herpes in persons with frequent recurrences. Suppressive therapy can be continued safely for 10 years or longer, but even such prolonged suppression does not eliminate HSV shedding or abolish latency; recurrences resume when suppressive therapy is stopped. Although suppression with acyclovir does not eliminate asymptomatic shedding, it limits it markedly, and the effect of this reduction on HSV transmission is under investigation. Until these results are available, it seems reasonable to prescribe suppressive therapy for sexually active patients with recurrent genital herpes but to advise them that they still may be capable of transmitting the infection when they are asymptomatic. Famciclovir and valacyclovir administered twice daily are comparable in efficacy to acyclovir, but these prodrugs are generally more expensive.

Suppression with oral acyclovir is also effective for recurrent herpetic whitlow, HSV proctitis, and cutaneous HSV infections. Suppression with oral acyclovir is especially beneficial for patients whose recurrences are associated with severe complications, such as recurrent meningitis, erythema multiforme, or neuralgia, and for patients with recurrent ocular HSV infections associated with stromal keratitis or iritis. Placebo-controlled studies of natural sunlight–induced and experimental ultraviolet light–induced herpes labialis have shown that prophylaxis with oral acyclovir lessens the incidence of lesion formation and the severity of the lesions that do occur. Suppression of herpes labialis requires higher doses of acyclovir than suppression of recurrent genital herpes, however, and, in any case, is less effective (50% to 78% vs. 80% to 90%). Perhaps famciclovir or valacyclovir would be more effective, but results of comparative studies are not available.

TREATMENT AND PROPHYLAXIS OF HERPES SIMPLEX VIRUS INFECTIONS IN IMMUNOCOMPROMISED PATIENTS

Symptomatic initial and recurrent mucocutaneous HSV infections in immunocompromised patients respond to intravenous or oral acyclovir (Table 312.1). The addition of topical acyclovir or penciclovir may speed resolution of external lesions. Recurrent HSV infections are a major cause of illness in patients undergoing organ or bone marrow transplantation or remission-induction chemotherapy for acute leukemia; mucocutaneous HSV infections develop in 60% to 90% of seropositive patients during the early posttransplantation period, when immunosuppression is greatest. A number of placebo-controlled studies have shown that intravenous and oral acyclovir provide effective prophylaxis, lowering the rate of recurrences by 90% or more. Long-term suppression with oral acyclovir is often indicated, but immuno-

compromised patients require high doses of acyclovir, and famciclovir is a useful alternative.

DEVELOPMENT OF RESISTANCE TO ANTIVIRAL DRUGS

Because the selective antiviral activity of acyclovir involves two HSV-encoded enzymes, TK and DNA polymerase, mutations altering either one can lead to resistance. Resistant mutants, most of which are TK deficient, are readily selected in the laboratory and have been isolated sporadically from immunocompetent patients before, during, and after acyclovir therapy. These acyclovir-resistant isolates have been associated only in rare instances with treatment failure. Clinically significant acyclovir resistance is being encountered with increasing frequency, however, in severely immunocompromised patients, especially HIV-infected patients and bone marrow transplant recipients receiving acyclovir for persistent mucocutaneous HSV infection. Many of these viruses have caused locally invasive disease and even disseminated infections that were unresponsive to acyclovir. Most are TK deficient and thus also resistant to penciclovir and ganciclovir.

Although these mutants are susceptible to both foscarnet and vidarabine in vitro, only foscarnet is effective in vivo. Occasionally, acyclovir resistance is due to a mutant TK with altered substrate specificity; though resistant to acyclovir, such viruses may still be sensitive to penciclovir. DNA polymerase mutants resistant to both acyclovir and foscarnet have been isolated from immunocompromised patients with lesions unresponsive to these drugs. These mutants have been found to be sensitive to cidofovir and trifluridine. The emergence and potential spread of such drug-resistant mutants place at risk our recently acquired capacity to treat HSV infections.

◼ PREVENTION OF HERPES SIMPLEX VIRUS INFECTION

PREVENTION OF EXPOSURE

At present, avoidance of exposure is the only proven means of preventing HSV infection. Consistent condom use appears to be an effective means of curbing genital HSV transmission. The high incidence of asymptomatic virus shedding, however—usually by persons who have no history of symptomatic infection to alert them to their potential infectiousness—makes avoiding exposure impractical except in special circumstances. For example, health care workers who have herpetic whitlow should not engage in direct care of patients. Hospitalized patients with extensive HSV infections, such as eczema herpeticum, should be isolated. Persons with herpes labialis and recurrent genital herpes should avoid sexual contact when active lesions are present, and all sexually active persons should be aware that infection frequently is transmitted during episodes of asymptomatic virus shedding. Pregnant women who have active genital herpes at term should be delivered by caesarean section before membranes rupture, to lower the risk of neonatal HSV infections. Susceptible pregnant women with seropositive sexual partners should

TABLE 312.1. ANTIVIRAL THERAPY OF HSV INFECTIONS[a,b]

Disease	Treatment	Alternative Treatment	Suppression or Prophylaxis[c,d]	Comments
Oropharyngeal HSV Infections				
Acute herpetic gingivostomatitis or Acute herpetic pharyngotonsillitis	Acyclovir 400 mg orally (600 mg/m² in children <12 years of age), 4 times daily for 10 days or Famciclovir 250–500 mg orally, 3 times daily for 10 days, or Valacyclovir 1000 mg orally, 2 times daily for 10 days.	Acyclovir 5–10 mg/kg (250–500 mg/m² in children <12 years of age) intravenously over 1 hour every 8 hours for 7 days (or until clinical resolution) in patients with severe disease or complications necessitating hospitalization.[g]		Continue treatment longer if new lesion formation or symptoms continue.
Herpes labialis	Penciclovir 1% cream applied to lesions every 2 hours while awake for 4 days, or Acyclovir 400–800 mg orally, 3–4 times daily for 5 days, or Famciclovir 500 mg orally, 3 times daily for 5 days, or Valacyclovir 1000 mg orally, 2 times daily for 5 days.		Acyclovir 400 mg orally, 2–3 times daily for prevention of frequent and/or severe herpes labialis or HSV-associated erythema multiforme. or Acyclovir 400 mg orally, 3 times daily; or famciclovir 500 mg orally, 3 times daily; or valacyclovir 1000 mg orally, 2 times daily; beginning before sun exposure or surgical procedure and continuing until 3 days after sun exposure ceases or 7 days after the surgical procedure.	Long term suppression of recurrent herpes labialis should be considered for selected patients with frequent recurrences (>6 per year); or HSV-associated erythema multiforme. Short term prophylaxis should be considered for selected patients who are anticipating a period of intense sun exposure or stress; undergoing surgical procedures on the trigeminal ganglion or nerve; or undergoing facial surgery (including chemical peel or laser skin resurfacing).
Ocular HSV Infections				
First-clinical episode of ocular HSV infection	1% trifluridine (trifluoro thymidine) ophthalmic solution 1 drop every 2 hours while awake until reepithelialization of corneal ulcer, then 1 drop every 5 hours while awake for 7 more days, plus Acyclovir 400 mg orally, 3 times daily for 10–14 days (or until clinical resolution),	Vidarabine ophthalmic ointment and idoxuridine ophthalmic solution are less effective than trifluridine.		Treatment of ocular HSV infection should always be carried out in collaboration with an experienced ophthalmologist. The addition of oral acyclovir is always warranted when deeper tissues are involved (e.g., stromal keratitis, iritis).

Infection	Regimen	Comments
	or Famciclovir 500 mg orally, 3 times daily for 10–14 days, or Valacyclovir 1000 mg orally, 2 times daily for 10–14 days.	
Recurrent ocular HSV infection	1% trifluridine (trifluoro thymidine) ophthalmic solution 1 drop every 2 hours while awake until reepithelialization of corneal ulcer, then 1 drop every 5 hours while awake for 7 more days, plus Acyclovir 400 mg orally, 3 times daily for 7–10 days (or until clinical resolution) when deeper tissues are involved (e.g., stromal keratitis, iritis), or Famciclovir 500 mg orally, 3 times daily for 7–10 days, or Valacyclovir 1000 mg orally, 2 times daily for 7–10 days.	Vidarabine ophthalmic ointment and idoxuridine ophthalmic solution are less effective than trifluridine. Acyclovir 400 mg orally, 2–3 times daily. Suppression is of greatest benefit in patients with a history of stromal keratitis because they tend to have recurrences of stromal keratitis that result in corneal scarring and loss of vision. Patients with a history of only superficial forms of HSV eye disease (e.g., epithelial keratitis, conjunctivitis, blepharitis) tend to have similar recurrences that generally resolve with short term topical antiviral therapy without permanent damage.

HSV Infections of the Skin

Infection	Regimen	Comments
First clinical episode of traumatic herpes (herpes gladiatorum, scrumpox) or Herpetic whitlow	Acyclovir 400 mg orally, 4 times daily for 10 days, or Famciclovir 500 mg orally, 3 times daily for 7–10 days, or Valacyclovir 1000 mg orally, 2 times daily for 7–10 days.	Treatment should be continued until clinical resolution.
Recurrent cutaneous herpes or Recurrent herpetic whitlow	Acyclovir 400 mg orally, 3 times daily for 5 days, or Famciclovir 500 mg orally, 3 times daily for 5 days, or Valacyclovir 1000 mg orally, 2 times daily for 5 days.	Acyclovir 400 mg orally, 2 times daily. or Famciclovir 250 mg orally, 2 times daily. or Valacyclovir 500 mg orally, 2 times daily. Suppression of recurrent episodes is appropriate in patients with frequent recurrences (≥6 per year); recurrences associated with erythema multiforme; or recurrences with neurologic complications.

(continued)

TABLE 312.1. *Continued*

Nervous System HSV Infections

Disease	Treatment	Alternative Treatment	Suppression or Prophylaxis[c,d]	Comments
Herpes simplex encephalitis	Acyclovir 10 mg/kg intravenously over 1 hour every 8 hours for 14–21 days.[g]			Early initiation of therapy is crucial. Occurrence of relapse after cessation of therapy has prompted many physicians to prolong intravenous therapy to 21 days.
First clinical episode of aseptic meningitis caused by HSV	Acyclovir 10 mg/kg intravenously over 1 hour every 8 hours for 7–10 days.[g] or Valacyclovir 1000 mg orally, 3 times daily for 7–10 days. or Famciclovir 500 mg orally, 3 times daily for 7–10 days.			Suppression with oral valacyclovir following intravenous therapy is under investigation. Aseptic meningitis caused by HSV generally resolves spontaneously without sequelae.
First clinical episode of ganglionitis or myelitis associated with HSV infection	Acyclovir 10 mg/kg intravenously over 1 hours every 8 hours for 7–10 days.[g]	Valacyclovir 1000 mg orally, 3 times daily for 7–10 days. or Famciclovir 500 mg orally, 3 times daily for 7–10 days.		
Idiopathic facial paralysis (Bell's palsy)	Valacyclovir 1000 mg orally, 3 times daily for 5 days. or Famciclovir 500 mg orally, 3 times daily for 5 days.			Corticosteroids are frequently used in addition to antiviral therapy in an attempt to reduce inflammation.
Recurrent aseptic meningitis caused by HSV (benign recurrent lymphocytic [Mollaret] meningitis) or Recurrent ganglionitis or myelitis associated with HSV infection.	Acyclovir 10 mg/kg intravenously over 1 hour every 8 hours 7–10 days.[g]	Valacyclovir 1000 mg orally, 3 times daily for 7–10 days. or Famciclovir 500 mg orally, 3 times daily for 7–10 days.	Acyclovir 400 mg orally, 2–3 times daily. or Famciclovir 250 mg orally, 2 times daily. or Valacyclovir 500 mg orally, 2 times daily.	Consider suppressive therapy in patients with frequent recurrences (≥4 per year) or severe/prolonged recurrence with sequelae.
Trigeminal neuralgia (tic douloureux)			Acyclovir 400 mg orally, 2–3 times daily. or Famciclovir 250 mg orally, 2 times daily. or Valacyclovir 500 mg orally, 2 times daily.	Suppression of trigeminal neuralgia should be considered, especially when it is associated with recurrent labial or facial HSV infection.

Genital HSV Infections

Condition	Regimen	Severe disease	Comments
First clinical episode of genital herpes (i.e., initial primary and nonprimary genital herpes)	Acyclovir 400 mg orally, 3 times daily for 10 days. *or* Acyclovir 200 mg orally, 5 times daily for 10 days. *or* Famciclovir 250 mg orally, 3 times daily for 10 days. *or* Valacyclovir 1000 mg orally, 2 times daily for 10 days.	Acyclovir 5 mg/kg intravenously over 1 hour every 8 hours for 5–10 days (or until clinical resolution) for severe disease with neurologic complications, such as urinary retention or aseptic meningitis; cutaneous dissemination; or visceral complication, such as pneumonitis or hepatitis.[9]	Continue treatment longer if new lesion formation or symptoms continue. Treatment of first episode of genital herpes does not appear to affect the frequency or severity of subsequent recurrences.
Recurrent genital herpes	Acyclovir 400 mg orally, 3 times daily for 5 days. *or* Acyclovir 200 mg orally, 5 times daily for 5 days. *or* Acyclovir 800 mg orally, 2 times daily for 5 days. *or* Famciclovir 125 mg orally, 2 times daily for 5 days. *or* Valacyclovir 500 mg orally, 2 times daily for 5 days.	Acyclovir 400 mg orally, 2 times daily (safety and efficacy have been deomonstrated in patients taking daily suppressive therapy for as long as 10 years). *or* Acyclovir 400 mg orally, 3 times daily. *or* Acyclovir 200 mg orally, 3 times daily. *or* Famciclovir 250 mg orally, 2 times daily. *or* Valacyclovir 250 mg orally, 2 times daily.	Treatment of recurrent genital herpes is most effective when it is patient-initiated early (e.g., during the prodrome). Suppressive treatment reduces but does not eliminate asymptomatic HSV shedding. Its effect of HSV transmission is unknown. Poor response to suppression of frequently recurring genital herpes is usually because the diagnosis of genital herpes is incorrect. When breakthrough lesions proven to be HSV occur, the patient may not be receiving an adequate dose, either because of non-compliance or poor absorption. In this case, increase acyclovir dosage to 3 times daily or switch to famciclovir or valacyclovir.

HSV Proctitis (in Immunocompetent Patients)

Condition	Regimen	Severe disease / Suppression	Comments
First clinical episode of HSV proctitis	Acyclovir 400 mg orally, 4–5 times daily for 10 days. *or* Famciclovir 500 mg orally, 3 times daily for 10 days. *or* Valacyclovir 1000 mg orally, 2 times daily for 10 days	Acyclovir 5 mg/kg intravenously over 1 hour every 8 hours for 7 days for severe infections.[9]	Treatment should be continued until clinical resolution. Topical therapy (in addition to oral or intravenous therapy) may speed resolution of external lesions. Higher doses of oral acyclovir are preferred for treatment and suppression of HSV proctitis in male homosexuals who may be immunosuppressed as a result of HIV-1 infection.
Recurrent HSV proctitis	Acyclovir 400 mg orally, 4–5 times daily for 5 days. *or* Famciclovir 500 mg orally, 3 times daily for 5 days. *or* Valacyclovir 1000 mg orally, 2 times daily for 5 days.	Acyclovir 400 mg orally, 2 times daily. *or* Famciclovir 250 mg orally, 2 times daily. *or* Valacyclovir 500 mg orally, 2 times daily.	Suppression should be considered for patients with frequent recurrences (≥4–6 times per year); severe symptoms; or neurologic complications. Topical therapy (in addition to oral therapy) may speed resolution of external lesions.

(continued)

TABLE 312.1.   *Continued*

Disease	Treatment	Alternative Treatment	Suppression or Prophylaxis[c,d]	Comments
Neonatal HSV Infections				
	Acyclovir 15–20 mg/kg intravenously over 1 hour every 8 hours for 14–21 days.[g]			Suppression of cutaneous recurrences with prolonged oral administration of acyclovir or valacyclovir following initial intravenous therapy is being evaluated.[e,f]
Disseminated HSV Infections in Immunocompetent Patients				
	Acyclovir 5 mg/kg intravenously over 1 hour every 8 hours for 7–10 days.[g]	In immunocompetent patients with cutaneous dissemination and no evidence of visceral or neurologic involvement: Famciclovir 500 mg orally, 3 times daily for 7 days. or Valacyclovir 1000 mg orally, 2 times daily for 7 days.		Increase dose to 10 mg/kg every 8 hours when there is CNS involvement. Treatment should continue until clinical resolution.
Visceral HSV Infections in Immunocompetent Patients				
HSV esophagitis or HSV pneumonitis	Acyclovir 5 mg/kg intravenously over 1 hour every 8 hours for 7–10 days.[g]	In patients with less severe disease and little or no immunosuppression: Famciclovir 500 mg orally, 3 times daily for 7 days. or Valacyclovir 1000 mg orally, 2 times daily for 7 days.		
Erythema Multiforme Associated With HSV Infections				
	Acyclovir 400 mg orally, 3–4 times daily for 7–10 days. or Famciclovir 500 mg orally, 3 times daily for 7–10 days. or Valacyclovir 1000 mg orally, 2 times daily for 7–10 days.		Acyclovir 400 mg orally, 2–3 times daily. or Famciclovir 250 mg orally, 2 times daily. or Valacyclovir 500 mg orally, 2 times daily.	Episodic treatment is sometimes successful in preventing HSV-associated erythema multiforme, but long-term suppression of HSV recurrences is more reliable. The frequency with which erythema multiforme is associated with asymptomatic HSV infections warrants a trial of acyclovir suppression even when the recurrent erythema multiforme is not associated with clinically manifest recurrent HSV infection.

Mucocutaneous HSV Infections in Immunocompromised Patients

Acyclovir 5 mg/kg (250 mg/m²) intravenously over 1 hour every 8 hours for 7–10 days.[g]

Acyclovir 400 mg orally, 4–5 times daily for 10 days.

or

Famciclovir 500 mg orally, 3 times daily for 10 days.

or

Valacyclovir 1000 mg orally, 2 times daily for 10 days.

Acyclovir 5 mg/kg (250 mg/m²) intravenously over 1 hour every 8 hours prevents recurrences during periods of intense immunosuppression (e.g., the immediate post-transplantation period). Regimens of intravenous acyclovir followed by oral therapy for 3–6 months are well tolerated and highly effective in organ allograft recipients.[g]

or

For immunocompromised (e.g., HIV-1 infected) patients with recurrent mucocutaneous HSV infections:
Famciclovir 500 mg orally, 2 times daily.

Penciclovir 5 mg/kg intravenously every 12 hours appears to be equivalent in efficacy to acyclovir 5 mg/kg intravenously every 8 hours.[g]
Continue treatment longer if new lesion formation or symptoms continue. The addition of topical therapy may speed resolution of external lesions. Long-term suppression is often desirable, but requires larger doses of antiviral drugs than are recommended for immunocompetent persons.

Mucocutaneous HSV Infections Due to Acyclovir-Resistant HSV

Foscarnet 40 mg/kg intravenously every 8 hours for 7–21 days in patients with disease that is clinically resistant to acyclovir, valacyclovir, or famciclovir.

Topical treatment of external lesions with foscarnet 1% cream or cifofovir 1% gel is often effective.

Rare in immunocompetent patients, resistance to acyclovir is a significant problem in immunocompromised patients receiving multiple courses of therapy, especially in severely immunocompromised patients (e.g., bone marrow transplant recipients; patients with AIDS). Despite in vitro sensitivity to vidarabine, acyclovir-resistant HSV infections rarely respond to treatment with vidarabine *in vivo*.
Infections with HSV resistant to both acyclovir and foscarnet have responded to topical or intravenous cidofovir (HPMPC), or to a combination of topical trifluridine and interferon-α.

---

[a] Dosage reduction may be required in patients with renal insufficiency (see manufacturer's instructions)
[b] Treatment regimens in boldface type are preferred by the author. Treatment regimens currently approved by the Food and Drug Administration are indicated with a " ". All other treatment regimens are based upon the results of clinical trials or anecdotal experience.
[c] For long-term suppression, the antiviral drug should be titrated to the lowest effective dose.
[d] Suppression should be interrupted at 12–24 months interval to reassess the need for it.
[e] Suppression of symptomatic genital herpes in late pregnancy may be considered to prevent neonatal infection and avoid cesarean section.
[f] Prophylactic treatment of asymptomatic infants born to mothers who are culture (+) at term is also being evaluated.
[g] Intravenous acyclovir may produce reversible renal insufficiency due to crystallization of the drug in renal tubules. This is avoided by administering the drug slowly over 1 hour and insuring that the patient is well hydrated.

practice abstinence, including abstinence from oral–genital contact, during the 6 weeks before delivery, to avoid acquiring primary infection near term.

PREEXPOSURE PROPHYLAXIS

No means of prophylaxis has been proved to be effective in humans. In addition, the high proportion of HSV infections that follow unrecognized exposures suggests that even if effective, short-lived forms of prophylaxis, such as the administration of acyclovir or antibodies to HSV, would have little practical application. On the other hand, effective preexposure immunization could provide an ideal means of prophylaxis. Several experimental vaccines have entered clinical trials, but results obtained to date have been disappointing. Therapeutic immunization to reduce the rate of recurrent HSV infections has a long and colorful history. Placebo-controlled trials of vaccines containing recombinant HSV-2 glycoproteins D and B have shown only very modest clinical activity. Trials of additional vaccines are likely to follow.

POSTEXPOSURE PROPHYLAXIS

The short incubation period of symptomatic HSV infection, the early establishment of latency, and the ability of replication-negative HSV mutants to become latent all suggest that postexposure prophylaxis will be ineffective in preventing HSV infection or the establishment of latency. However, studies in animal models indicate that postexposure prophylaxis with antibodies to HSV, with antiviral agents, or with combinations of the two may lower the incidence and severity of disease in some circumstances. This approach is being evaluated in clinical trials of acyclovir prophylaxis in newborns exposed to HSV at delivery, in the hope of improving the results achieved with antiviral therapy initiated after the onset of the symptoms and signs of neonatal HSV infection.

BIBLIOGRAPHY

Balfour HH. Antiviral drugs. *N Engl J Med* 1999;340:1255–1268.

Belongia EA, Goodman JL, Holland EJ, et al. An outbreak of herpes gladiatorum at a high-school wrestling camp. *N Engl J Med* 1991;325:906–910.

Benedetti JK, Zeh J, Selke MA, et al. Frequency and reactivation of nongenital lesions among patients with genital herpes simplex virus. *Am J Med* 1995;98:237–242.

Bernstein DI, Stanberry LR. Herpes simplex virus vaccines. *Vaccine* 1999;17:1681–1689.

Brice SL, Krzemien D, Weston WL, et al. Detection of herpes simplex virus DNA in cutaneous lesions of erythema multiforme. *J Invest Dermatol* 1989;93:183–187.

Brown ZA, Selke S, Zeh J, et al. The acquisition of herpes simplex virus during pregnancy. *N Engl J Med* 1997;337:509–515.

Centers for Disease Control and Prevention. CDC 1998 guidelines for treatment of sexually transmitted diseases. *MMWR* 1998;47(RR-1):1–118.

Corey L, Langenberg AG, Ashley R, et al. Recombinant glycoprotein vaccine for the prevention of genital HSV-2 infection: two randomized controlled trials. *JAMA* 1999;282:331–340.

Diamond C, Selke S, Ashley R, et al. Clinical course of patients with serologic evidence of recurrent genital herpes presenting with signs and symptoms of first episode disease. *Sex Transm Dis* 1999;26:221–225.

Douglas JM, Critchlow C, Benedetti J, et al. A double-blind study of oral acyclovir for suppression of recurrences of genital herpes simplex virus infection. *N Engl J Med* 1984;310:1551–1556.

Erlich KS, Mills J, Shatis P, et al. Acyclovir-resistant herpes simplex virus infections in patients with acquired immunodeficiency syndrome. *N Engl J Med* 1989;320:293–296.

Fleming DT, McQuillan GM, Johnson RE, et al. Herpes simplex virus type 2 in the United States, 1976 to 1994. *N Engl J Med* 1997;337:1105–1111.

Gutierrez KM, Falkovitz Halpern MS, Maldonado Y, et al. The epidemiology of neonatal herpes simplex virus infections in California from 1985 to 1995. *J Infect Dis* 1999;801:199–202.

Hensleigh PA, Andrews WW, Brown Z, et al. Genital herpes during pregnancy: inability to distinguish primary and recurrent infections clinically. *Obstet Gynecol* 1997;89:891–895.

Hook EW III, Cannon RO, Nahmias AJ, et al. Herpes simplex virus infection as a risk factor for human immunodeficiency virus infection in heterosexuals. *J Infect Dis* 1992;165:251–255.

Jabs DA. Acyclovir for recurrent herpes simplex virus ocular disease. *N Engl J Med* 1998;339:340–341.

Lakeman FD, Whitley RJ. Diagnosis of herpes simplex encephalitis: application of polymerase chain reaction to cerebrospinal fluid from brain-biopsied patients and correlation with disease. *J Infect Dis* 1995;171:857–863.

Langenberg AGM, Corey L, Ashley RL, et al. A prospective study of new infection with the herpes simplex virus type 1 and type 2. *N Engl J Med* 1999;341:1432–1438.

Lazarus HM, Belanger R, Candoni A, et al. Intravenous penciclovir for treatment of herpes simplex infections in immunocompromised patients: results of a multicenter, acyclovir-controlled trial. *Antimicrob Agents Chemother* 1999;43:1192–1197.

McClements WL, Armstrong ME, Keys RD, et al. Immunization with DNA vaccines encoding glycoprotein D or glycoprotein B, alone or in combination, induces protective immunity in animal models of herpes simplex virus-2 disease. *Proc Natl Acad Sci USA* 1996;93:1141–1420.

Mertz GJ, Benedetti J, Ashley R, et al. Risk factors for the sexual transmission of genital herpes. *Ann Intern Med* 1992;116:197–202.

Oxman MN. Genital herpes. In: Gorbach SL, Bartlett JG, Blacklow NR, eds. *Infectious diseases*, second ed. Philadelphia: WB Saunders, 1997:986–1007.

Oxman MN. Herpes simplex viruses. In: Gorbach SL, Bartlett JG, Blacklow NR, eds. *Infectious diseases*, second ed. Philadelphia: WB Saunders, 1997:2022–2062.

Reichman RC, Badger GJ, Mertz GJ, et al. Treatment of recurrent genital herpes simplex infections with oral acyclovir: a controlled trial. *JAMA* 1984;251:2103–2107.

Safrin S, Crumpacker C, Chatis P, et al. A controlled trial comparing foscarnet with vidarabine for acyclovir-resistant mucocutaneous herpes simplex in the acquired immunodeficiency syndrome. *N Engl J Med* 1991;325:551–555.

Spruance SL, Rea TL, Thoming C, et al. Penciclovir cream for the treatment of herpes simplex labialis: a randomized, multicenter, double-blind, placebo-controlled trial. *JAMA* 1997;277:1374–1379.

Spruance SL, Rowe NH, Raborn GW, et al. Peroral famciclovir in the treatment of experimental ultraviolet radiation–induced herpes simplex labialis: a double-blind, dose-ranging, placebo-controlled, multicenter trial. *J Infect Dis* 1999;179:303–310.

Stamm WE, Handsfield HH, Rompalo AM, et al. The association between genital ulcer disease and acquisition of HIV infection in homosexual men. *JAMA* 1988;260:1429–1433.

Stanberry LR. Control of STDs: the role of prophylactic vaccines against herpes simplex virus. *Sex Transm Infect* 1999;74:391–394.

Stanberry L, Cunningham A, Mertz G, et al. New developments in the epidemiology, natural history and management of genital herpes. *Antiviral Res* 1999;42:1–14.

Straus SE, Wald A, Kost RG, et al. Immunotherapy of recurrent genital herpes with recombinant herpes simplex virus type 2 glycoproteins D and B: results of a placebo-controlled vaccine trial. *J Infect Dis* 1997;176:1129–1134.

Tatnall FM, Schofield JK, Leigh IM. A double-blind, placebo-controlled trial of continuous acyclovir therapy in recurrent erythema multiforme. *Br J Dermatol* 1995;132:267–270.

Tedder DG, Ashley R, Tyler KL, et al. Herpes simplex virus infection as a cause of benign recurrent lymphocytic meningitis. *Am Coll Phys* 1994; 121:334–338.

Wald A, Zeh J, Barnum G, et al. Suppression of subclinical shedding of herpes simplex virus type 2 with acyclovir. *Ann Intern Med* 1996;124: 8–15.

Whitley RJ, Cobbs CG, Alford CA Jr, et al. Diseases that mimic herpes simplex encephalitis: diagnosis, presentation, and outcome. NIAD Collaborative Antiviral Study Group. *JAMA* 1989;262:234–239.

Kelley's Textbook of Internal Medicine, fourth edition. Edited by H. David Humes. Lippincott Williams & Wilkins, Philadelphia © 2000.

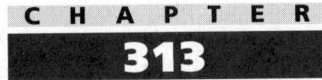

CYTOMEGALOVIRUS

SARAH H. CHEESEMAN

DEFINITION

Cytomegalovirus (CMV), a member of the herpesvirus family, derives its name from the characteristic enlargement of infected cells, or cytomegaly. The first human disease linked to this virus was a devastating congenital infection syndrome, called cytomegalic inclusion disease. CMV is a major cause of heterophile-negative infectious mononucleosis as well as significant disease in transplant recipients and patients with AIDS.

INCIDENCE AND EPIDEMIOLOGY

Most infection with CMV is asymptomatic, and seroprevalence studies show early acquisition, almost universal by age 2, in countries with poor socioeconomic conditions. In the United States, 0.4% to 2.5% of newborns excrete the virus at birth, and about 3,000 cases of cytomegalic inclusion disease are expected each year. A large number of children become infected in the first 2 months of life from exposure to maternal genital secretions at delivery and through subsequent breast-feeding. Despite the similarities to the epidemiologic characteristics of perinatal HIV or hepatitis B virus, CMV acquired postnatally by these routes is a benign infection without clinical manifestations or long-term effects. Infants and toddlers in close contact transmit infection to each other and to their caretakers, at home or day care, via excretion of virus in urine and saliva. Later in life, sexual transmission predominates, but acquisition by other routes also takes place, with a seroconversion rate of 1% to 2% per year for the general population, leading to seroprevalence rates in excess of 60% by age 60. Infection by CMV is lifelong, and fluctuations of serum antibody titer as well as culture evidence of shedding indicate that silent reactivation of the infection occurs. It is not surprising, therefore, that blood products and solid organ transplants can transmit CMV to their recipients.

In normal hosts, most symptomatic CMV disease is the result of primary acquisition, though even in adults, primary acquisition is often asymptomatic. In this respect, the pattern of CMV closely resembles that of Epstein–Barr virus (EBV), though the seroprevalence rate at any given age is lower. Most persons with AIDS who acquired their infections by routes other than transfusion of blood or clotting factors also have CMV, so the late-stage syndromes are assumed to be due to reactivation. In the context of solid organ transplantation, disease may result either from reactivation of the recipient's own previous CMV infection, reinfection with a different strain derived from the donor, or primary infection derived from the donor. Disease manifestations follow a gradient, with the most severe syndromes occurring in seronegative recipients of an organ from a seropositive donor [D(donor)+, R(recipient)−], followed by seropositive recipients of a seropositive organ (D+R+) and seropositive recipients of organs from seronegative donors (D+R−). The least severe disease manifests in seronegative recipients of seronegative organs, whose infections may come from blood products. By contrast, in allogeneic bone marrow transplantation, the recipient with pretransplant antibody to CMV is at highest risk of CMV disease after transplant, though the risk in autologous marrow transplantation is quite low.

The most feared consequence of CMV infection may well be the congenital infection syndrome. Overt symptomatic CMV disease at birth is the result of maternal primary infection during pregnancy, with only two or three well-documented exceptions; most cases derive from infection in early gestation. For a pregnant woman diagnosed with primary CMV infection, the risk that the baby will be infected congenitally is 40%. Among babies with congenital infection due to primary maternal infection during pregnancy, 18% have symptomatic CMV infection (fatal in 4% to 12% and leaving 90% of the survivors with neurologic impairment) and 25% have some adverse consequence (15% having sensorineural hearing loss). A woman with primary CMV infection in early pregnancy faces a 10% risk that her baby will have neurologic impairment as a result of this infection. Only 1% of infants born to mothers thought to have had primary CMV infection before pregnancy are congenitally infected, of whom 5% to 8% have any neurologic consequences.

PATHOGENESIS

Remarkably little is known about the pathogenesis of CMV infection beyond that which can be inferred from its epidemiologic characteristics. Although antibody is a useful marker of infection, the concentration of disease in patients with severe deficiency of cell-mediated immunity points to the importance of this mechanism of protection, as does protection of CMV-seropositive allogeneic bone marrow transplant recipients by infusion of donor-derived CMV-specific cytotoxic lymphocytes. Active CMV infection produces immunosuppression, measurable in both the normal host and in solid organ transplant recipients; in the latter group, an increased rate of other opportunistic infections, especially fungal infections, accompanies CMV disease. CMV can transactivate HIV in vitro; studies in hemophiliacs suggest that co-infection hastens the progression of immunodeficiency. Overt CMV disease does not develop in HIV-infected persons until there has been profound depletion of CD4 cells (median CD4 count of 25/μL).

CMV can be isolated from circulating leukocytes, principally neutrophils, in normal hosts with CMV mononucleosis, and detection of viremia by a variety of means accompanies and may precede clinical manifestations of CMV disease in immunosuppressed hosts. CMV disease has been reported in almost every organ, but the site of true viral persistence remains a mystery. Attempts to link various chronic diseases with CMV, based on seroprevalence studies or detection of viral antigens or polymerase chain reaction (PCR) fragments in tissues, have not yet defined any causal associations, but one has been disproved: Kaposi's sarcoma is now thought to be related to human herpesvirus 8.

CLINICAL FEATURES

Symptomatic primary infection, or CMV mononucleosis, is a febrile illness sharing many features with the classic infectious mononucleosis syndrome produced by EBV: malaise, fatigue, and atypical lymphocytes (generally not as numerous in CMV disease as in EBV). Pharyngitis and lymphadenopathy are not as common as in EBV; they are found in about one-third of patients with primary CMV. Elevated liver enzymes are present in at least 90%. Either leukocytosis or leukopenia may be present, and relative or absolute neutropenia is a useful clue. The illness may last for several weeks. Particularly in young people, this diagnosis should be sought before embarking on a costly workup for fever of unknown origin. Pope John Paul II contracted CMV mononucleosis as a consequence of blood transfusions after his attempted assassination. When acquired in this manner, CMV takes the form of a late postoperative fever, with an incubation period of 3 to 6 weeks. Specific organ involvement is rare in normal hosts, but case reports have described most of the syndromes seen in immunocompromised hosts in normal individuals as well. Slow but spontaneous resolution is the rule.

CMV disease is becoming less frequent in immunocompromised hosts, thanks to gentler immunosuppression and screening of blood products for transplant recipients and to the impact of more effective antiretroviral therapy in AIDS. Before the introduction of protease inhibitors, CMV retinitis afflicted more than a third of AIDS patients before they died; now it is unusual even among those with an inadequate response of HIV infection to protease inhibitor–containing regimens. Recent reports, however, suggest that protection may wane as the CD4 count drops below 50/μL.

Patients with CMV retinitis report spots or floaters before their eyes, a curtain or veil over a portion of the visual field, or blurred vision—not eye pain or conjunctival injection. Funduscopic examination shows exudates, often tracking along blood vessels and with hemorrhage, described as "cottage cheese and ketchup" or "cheese pizza"; these exudates represent retinal necrosis. Undilated funduscopy permits examination of only 25% of the retina, and many examiners see much less. Examination of visual fields by confrontation may define a more

peripheral area of visual loss, but the patient with suggestive symptoms should be referred to an ophthalmologist. Untreated CMV retinitis progresses over a few weeks and eventually results in blindness. Very rapid progression may occur when the patient with undiagnosed and untreated CMV retinitis begins highly active antiretroviral therapy. A new syndrome of vitritis in patients on these therapies whose CMV retinitis is in control is presumed to result from immune recovery and response to CMV antigens; the clinical symptoms are floaters and impaired visual acuity. Sudden visual loss in a patient treated for CMV retinitis most often indicates retinal detachment.

CMV can produce a form of necrotizing encephalitis difficult to distinguish from that due to HIV but frequently associated with preexisting CMV retinitis. It can also cause a distinctive syndrome characterized by periventricular enhancement on neuroimaging studies and neutrophilic pleocytosis and a low glucose level in the cerebrospinal fluid (CSF). The same CSF abnormalities occur in CMV polyradiculopathy or cauda equina syndrome, with initial signs of urinary retention and lower-extremity weakness often accompanied by pain. The other major target for CMV in AIDS is the gastrointestinal tract. CMV colitis results in abdominal pain and diarrhea, which is often bloody. CMV esophagitis causes odynophagia in bone marrow transplant recipients as well as AIDS patients. It is the third most frequent cause of esophagitis in HIV-infected persons, after candida and aphthous ulceration.

By far the most dreaded complication of CMV in transplant recipients is pneumonia. The highest fatality rates are seen among bone marrow transplant recipients with graft-versus-host disease and solid-organ recipients with accompanying neutropenia and liver enzyme abnormalities. Chest radiography shows an interstitial infiltrate early in the course of infection, but it may progress to confluent opacification ("white-out") with respiratory failure.

CMV also causes a febrile illness without specific organ manifestations in transplant recipients, characterized by leukopenia, elevated liver enzymes, and atypical lymphocytes (in small numbers, since the immunosuppressive medications tend to produce lymphopenia); this condition is often termed the "CMV syndrome." Another curious feature of CMV is its association with rejection and other disease of the transplanted organ: re-stenosis of coronary arteries in heart transplants, hepatitis in liver transplants, and glomerulonephritis in transplanted kidneys.

LABORATORY FINDINGS

Primary CMV infection can be diagnosed with assurance when a specimen of blood obtained early in the illness tests negative for CMV antibody and antibody is detected in specimens obtained 2 to 3 weeks later. More often, however, low levels of antibody are present by the time someone considers the diagnosis. Evidence of a fourfold rise in titer between acute and convalescnet specimens tested in the same assay, along with the presence of IgM antibody to CMV, constitutes strong evidence of primary CMV infection. Unfortunately, IgM antibody testing for CMV is not as reliable as one would like for the most critical situations (such as pregnancy)—27% false-negatives and 11% false-positives were found in a careful evaluation of one commercial assay. IgM testing is also not useful in immunosuppressed hosts, who may not make IgM even when they sustain primary infection, or in patients whose CMV disease is a result of reactivation.

With new methods of inoculation and detection of CMV early antigens by fluorescent antibody staining, isolation of CMV in cell culture has become a semirapid test, yielding results within 24 hours. A positive culture result is proof of infection, but it may not always establish that CMV is the cause of clinical symptoms: 7% of asymptomatic seropositive normal persons shed CMV in the urine, and the rate is much higher among immunocompromised patients. Isolation of virus from a person lacking serum antibody, however, can confirm primary infection, and isolation of virus from a newborn infant proves congenital infection.

Isolation of CMV from blood is strongly suggestive of the role of CMV in the clinical syndrome under investigation, but it is neither 100% specific nor 100% sensitive and may not be sufficiently rapid. The overnight method is not as successful with buffy coat as with urine. Detection of virus in blood by PCR or by examination of leukocytes for viral matrix antigen (leukocyte antigen detection) has become the mainstay of diagnosis in transplant patients, permitting early initiation of therapy, even before (and with the hope of forestalling) clinical symptoms. PCR of CSF can be helpful in the diagnosis of central nervous system disease due to CMV.

The gold standard for establishing infection of a target organ is histopathologic diagnosis of CMV by identification of the typical enlarged cell with a basophilic intranuclear inclusion with surrounding halo that resembles an owl's eye. This finding is particularly important in distinguishing CMV pneumonia or upper gastrointestinal tract disease from clinically insignificant viral shedding detected by culture of secretions—even those obtained at bronchoscopy or endoscopy, since both may be contaminated by saliva. To avoid false-negative histopathologic results, biopsy samples should be taken at ulcer edges and at several lesion sites and even apparently uninvolved areas in the colon. CMV retinitis diagnosed by an experienced ophthalmologist requires no laboratory test for confirmation.

OPTIMAL MANAGEMENT

Reassurance and counseling are all that are needed for the normal host. A diagnosis of primary CMV infection may be a welcome finding in a workup that included the possibility of newly acquired HIV infection and a useful opening to discuss prevention of other sexually transmitted diseases; care should be taken to recognize that CMV may have been acquired by other routes. Since the highest risk of symptomatic congenital CMV infection is associated with acquisition near the time of conception, attempts at pregnancy should be postponed.

Specific antiviral therapy is indicated for transplant recipients with evidence of CMV disease. The addition of immune globulin to antiviral therapy is lifesaving in bone marrow transplant recipients with CMV pneumonia. Many centers monitor patients prospectively for viremia and initiate preemptive antiviral therapy as soon as it is detected as well as at the first sign of any potential symptoms. Ganciclovir and foscarnet, administered by the intravenous route, are the two drugs currently approved for systemic therapy. Patients with AIDS and CMV retinitis can be treated systemically with these drugs or cidofovir or with an intravitreal implant that releases ganciclovir locally. In the absence of potent antiretroviral therapy, the risk of contralateral or disseminated CMV disease was very high for patients treated only with implants, and those on maintenance systemic therapy could expect periodic activation of retinitis. Patients whose CD4 counts rise substantially as a result of antiretroviral therapy seem to be at very low risk of progression even if they stop maintenance therapy once retinitis has healed (though recurrences are now being reported among patients whose CD4 counts drop below 50/μL). All patients requiring treatment for CMV infection should be referred to an expert.

BIBLIOGRAPHY

Falagas ME, Snydman DR, George MJ, et al. Incidence and predictors of cytomegalovirus pneumonia in orthotopic liver transplant recipients. *Transplantation* 1996;61:1716–1720.

Fowler KB, Stagno S, Pass RF, et al. The outcome of congenital cytomegalovirus infection in relation to maternal antibody status. *N Engl J Med* 1992;326:663–667.

Karavellas MP, Lowder CY, Macdonald JC, et al. Immune recovery vitritis associated with inactive cytomegalovirus retinitis: a new syndrome. *Arch Ophthalmol* 1998;116:169–175.

McCutchan JA. Cytomegalovirus infections of the nervous system in patients with AIDS. *Clin Infect Dis* 1995;20:747–754.

Meyers JD, Ljungman P, Fisher LD. Cytomegalovirus excretion as a predictor of cytomegalovirus disease after marrow transplantation: importance of cytomegalovirus viremia. *J Infect Dis* 1990;162:373–380.

Musch DC, Martin DF, Gordon JF, et al. Treatment of cytomegalovirus retinitis with a sustained-release ganciclovir implant. *N Engl J Med* 1997;337:83–90.

Rodriguez-Barradas MC, Stool E, Musher DM, et al. Diagnosing and treating cytomegalovirus pneumonia in patients with AIDS. *Clin Infect Dis* 1996;23:76–81.

Walter EA, Greenberg PD, Gilbert MJ, et al. Reconstitution of cellular immunity against cytomegalovirus in recipients of allogeneic bone marrow by transfer of T-cell clones from the donor. *N Engl J Med* 1995;333:1038–1044.

Wilcox CM, Straub RF, Schwartz DA. Cytomegalovirus esophagitis in AIDS: a prospective evaluation of clinical responses to ganciclovir therapy, relapse rate, and long-term outcome. *Am J Med* 1995;98:169–176.

Kelley's Textbook of Internal Medicine, fourth edition. Edited by H. David Humes. Lippincott Williams & Wilkins, Philadelphia © 2000.

CHAPTER

314

EPSTEIN–BARR VIRUS AND THE INFECTIOUS MONONUCLEOSIS SYNDROME

JOSEPH S. PAGANO

Best known in North America as the causative agent of infectious mononucleosis (IM), Epstein–Barr virus (EBV) infection is also associated with malignancy, especially Burkitt's lymphoma (BL) in Africa and nasopharyngeal carcinoma (NPC) in China. The question of how a single virus can play a part in these disparate diseases, one benign and two malignant, is long-standing and now complicated by more associations. In terms of the prevalence of EBV diseases, IM and NPC head the list, followed by lymphoproliferative disorders in immunodeficient states; other lymphomas, including Hodgkin's disease (HD); hairy leukoplakia of the tongue; and gastric carcinoma. These diseases have some common features at the molecular pathobiologic level.

The herpesvirus group, of which EBV is a member, has three hallmark phases of infection: primary, latent, and reactivated. The symptoms of primary and reactivated EBV infection differ strikingly; in general, the malignancies are associated with viral reactivation. EBV has many claims as a human tumor virus, but it acts as contributor rather than as sole cause, which is in agreement with the idea of the genesis of malignancy as a multifactorial, stepwise molecular process. Its disease associations are still emerging, influenced by such therapies as organ transplantation, the onslaught of acquired immunodeficiency syndrome (AIDS), and new molecular diagnostic techniques.

VIROLOGY

EBV, one of two human members of the Gammaherpesvirinae, looks like other herpesviruses. It is enveloped and has an icosahedral nucleocapsid containing a double-stranded piece of DNA consisting of about 172,000 nucleotide base pairs. This linear genome is replicated by virally encoded DNA polymerase, the target for most antiviral drugs. The genome itself is characterized by distinctive sequence reiterations. At the termini are ten to 20 copies of a 500-base-pair repeated sequence that is complementary and therefore permits circularization of the linear genome to form the EBV episome. The fused termini of episomes are useful for determining clonality of EBV conditions.

The EBV episome is the molecular basis for latent infection. It is a circular intracellular form of the genome not found in virus; instead it maintains a persistent relationship within the cell, like an autonomous piece of DNA situated in the chromatin. The episome is replicated by host DNA polymerase and thus is not susceptible to antiviral drugs specific to viral enzymes. Each copy of the EBV episome is replicated only once during the cell cycle, so that constant numbers are maintained from one cell generation to the next, which is part of the mechanism of persistence of the EBV genome in latency.

The EBV genome encodes about 100 genes, but only a few are expressed during latent infection and in tumor cells. These genes are keys to latency, and some are involved in immortalizing cells. Proteins encoded by these genes are found either in the nucleus or in the plasma membrane. One of the nuclear antigens, Epstein–Barr nuclear antigen 1 (EBNA-1), is the universal EBV protein needed to replicate and maintain the latent EBV episome in cells; EBNA-1 binds to the origin of replication, ori-P, used by episomes. Another nuclear protein, EBNA-2, is a transcription factor necessary for cell immortalization; it activates cellular proliferation genes as well as the other EBV latency and immortalization genes. Lymphocyte membrane-associated protein 1

(LMP-1), is the EBV oncoprotein. LMP-1 affects cellular processes that promote proliferation; it also counters apoptosis by inducing bcl-2, and it activates the epithelial growth factor receptor. LMP-1 uses the tumor necrosis factor receptor intracellular signaling pathway by engaging tumor necrosis factor receptor–associated factors, which are involved in cell transformation.

There are at least three forms of EBV latency, classified according to the pattern of viral protein expression. Type 1, in which chiefly EBNA-1 is expressed, is exemplified by BL. Type 2 latency, typified by NPC and HD, expresses EBNA-1 and the three latent membrane proteins, LMP-1, LMP-2a, and LMP-2b. In type 3 latency, represented by EBV lymphoproliferative diseases, the full range of latency antigens is expressed—all six nuclear antigens and the three membrane proteins. In all latently infected and immortalized cells, certain small nuclear RNAs called EBERS are also expressed. Although the function of these non–protein-coding RNAs is unknown, their abundance in EBV-immortalized cells makes them sensitive detectors of latent infection and EBV malignant cells. In most tumors, 100% of cells are latently infected. The fact that BL does not express either of the two principal EBV transforming proteins, LMP-1 or EBNA-2, underscores that the virus is not the etiologic agent for BL, as is discussed later. Finally, LMP-1 not only is itself an oncoprotein, it also can induce a cellular enzyme that is important for tumor invasion and metastasis, matrix metalloproteinase 9. LMP-1 is expressed in EBV-associated tumors with a proclivity for invasiveness, such as NPC and lymphoproliferative neoplasias. Thus, latency type also relates to disease phenotype.

In contrast, in productive infection, virtually all the EBV genes are expressed, starting with the immediate-early genes (R and Z), which encode transcriptional transactivator proteins that trigger the viral replicative cycle by inducing expression of early viral genes needed for viral replication. The early viral genes encode enzymes involved in viral replication, including early antigen-diffuse (EA-D), a DNA processivity factor required for DNA replication, and the virally encoded DNA polymerase, which is the target for most current antiherpetic drugs. Different origins of replication, ori-lyt, are used for replication of linear genomes. EA-D, which has served for years as a diagnostic antigen, is now a target for a new antiviral drug. The rest of the cytolytic cycle genes encode proteins that make up the virion structure. For the most part, none is activated in tumor cells, though antibodies to Z protein, the key activator of the cytolytic cycle, attain high titers during viral reactivation and are detected early in the genesis of NPC. The Z protein can dampen the growth-suppressor protein p53, while its immediate-early partner, the R protein, interacts with Rb; both may act in tandem to stimulate transiently the cell cycle and synthesis of cellular macromolecules needed for viral DNA replication.

EPIDEMIOLOGY

EBV is found worldwide, and infection is virtually universal. In underdeveloped countries, most infants are infected asymptomatically within the first year of life, but not in utero or in the first few months after birth, because maternal EBV antibodies are protective. In upper-socioeconomic classes, most people are infected within the first three decades of life; the infection is often asymptomatic or undiagnosed. Typically, IM occurs in adolescence and the early third decade of life and rarely in older people. The virus spreads from person to person by close contact and exchange of oral secretions. Although there are no epidemics of IM, the incidence is higher in college students in early fall and winter, when semesters begin, presumably because of new opportunities for virus exposure. The incubation period, variable and difficult to estimate because of the insidious onset, is about 4 to 6 weeks. Asymptomatic cervical infection with EBV has been detected in up to 20% of sexually active women, but its significance is unknown. Two types and many strains of EBV can be distinguished by polymorphisms in the *EBNA2* gene. Although these viral differences do not account for the different EBV diseases, there are patterns of geographic distribution of some of the intratypic variants, especially in NPC. The rich and often puzzling epidemiologic features of EBV-associated malignancies are presented with the specific diseases.

PATHOGENESIS

The virus infects the oropharynx, where it replicates in epithelial cells, the seat of productive infection. Virus replicates in pharyngeal lining cells, parotid ductal cells, and perhaps on the tongue, accompanied early by infection of B lymphocytes, where the virus becomes latent. The principal features, then, are superficial infection of epithelium and infection of lymphocytes. In lymphocytes (CD21 cells), attachment of virus is accomplished by means of a normal cellular complement receptor (C2R). In epithelial cells, replication of linear EBV genomes dominates, in a complete cycle leading to virus production and cytolysis. In contrast, in B lymphocytes there is production of EBV episomes with expression of latent EBV gene functions and cell proliferation. These infection events are often subclinical. The dual cell-stimulatory aspects of the primary infection, both of B lymphocytes and reactive T cells, are self-limiting except in rare people with specific inborn genetic defects or acquired defects that produce severe deficiency in cell-mediated immune systems. In such people, B-cell proliferation escapes, and lymphomas result.

The pharyngitis of IM arises from cytolysis of epithelial cells caused by virus replication, which diminishes to the point of being asymptomatic, though small amounts of virus are shed into the saliva for months or years. Most of the other manifestations of IM are caused by cytotoxic T-cell and natural killer cell responses to the EBV-infected B lymphocytes, which present new virally encoded antigens on their plasma membranes. The atypical lymphocytosis in the peripheral blood (up to 40%) that is so characteristic of EBV-caused IM represents a cytotoxic T-cell response in which both CD4 and CD8 lymphocytes participate. When infection is at its height, up to 10% of circulating B cells are latently infected. Rather than being lysed, these cells are stimulated to proliferate polyclonally, and, indeed, B cells explanted from the peripheral blood are immortalized and will form EBV-infected cell lines in vitro. The numbers of EBV-infected B lymphocytes subside gradually, but a low level persists in the circulation many years after infection. These cells contain EBV episomes.

The molecular and immunologic bases for IM thus fall into a still hypothetical but rational scheme that suggests the genesis of EBV-infected lymphomas in immunodeficient states. The role of EBV in BL and NPC follows different pathways, however, because clinical immune dysfunction precedes neither BL nor NPC and patients appear normal after treatment. From a molecular pathogenetic standpoint, NPC stands apart because it is an epithelial malignancy that must represent the exception to the cytolysis usually produced by EBV in epithelial cells, perhaps through a variance in viral gene expression.

CLINICAL FEATURES

INFECTIOUS MONONUCLEOSIS

While IM formerly was considered a constellation of symptoms of unknown origin, after the studies of Werner and Gertrude Henle in 1968, EBV now can be deemed the sole source of 90% of cases. The onset is insidious. Most symptoms are caused not by direct viral invasion but by secondary immunopathic responses that affect the brain, liver, and bone marrow; the virus does not infect the dominant cell types in these organs. IM is the result of primary, not reactivated infection. Acute pharyngitis often brings the patient to the physician. The classic features are fever lasting up to 3 weeks or more, lymphadenopathy, splenomegaly, and florid, atypical lymphocytosis along with malaise that may be slow to resolve, consistent with the subacute nature of the illness. Coupled with a positive heterophil antibody reaction or "monospot test," these features are enough for diagnosis in most cases. Heterophil antibodies are nonspecific IgM antibodies that react with surface antigens of sheep and horse but not guinea pig red blood cells. The diagnosis is verified by the presence of EBV antibodies. The symptom complex characterizing IM develops in postpubescent people in the second or early third decade of life. Infections earlier in life produce nondescript symptoms, such as fever and malaise alone.

IM can be complicated by neurologic syndromes, such as encephalitis, neuritis, transverse myelitis, and Guillain-Barré syndrome, and by hematologic abnormalities, such as agranulocytosis, aplastic anemia, and thrombocytopenia. Acute hepatitis is the most common complication, but it is usually short-lived and mild. Because the virus is not directly cytolytic in these organ tissues, the often alarming complications of IM tend to resolve without treatment. A rare complication is splenic rupture. Some patients with prominent lymphadenopathy, splenomegaly, and fever have a fluctuating course that mimics lymphoma. Sometimes acute IM seems to lapse into a chronic phase lasting a year or more, marked by persistent fatigue, low-grade fevers, malaise, and a labile emotional state.

Protracted virus excretion has raised the possibility that a subset of the so-called *chronic fatigue syndrome* (CFS) may be caused by EBV infection. CFS, which is ill defined, certainly has a variety of causes. CFS attributable to EBV begins with acute IM proven by EBV serologic testing and lasting a year beyond a subacute phase. Persistently high EA-D antibody levels, formerly thought to point to CFS, are not a reliable indicator, in that normal people may have such titers several years after primary infection. CFS is rarely caused by EBV. Mononucleosis caused by cytomegalovirus infection mimics EBV mononucleosis, though sore throat and atypical lymphocytosis may not be prominent features and the heterophil reaction is usually negative. Toxoplasmosis can be confused with IM because a rash may develop in IM, especially if ampicillin is given. When complications of IM dominate, the differential diagnosis is extended and complex.

BURKITT'S LYMPHOMA

In the 1950s, an Irish surgeon, Dennis Burkitt, working in Uganda wondered whether a common childhood malignancy that appeared in the form of a tumor of the jaw might be caused by a transmissible agent because of its pattern of incidence (Table 314.1). The tumor, BL, is endemic at lower elevations in a belt sweeping from east to west across equatorial Africa. It is a rapidly growing, multifocal B-cell lymphoma whose initial symptom is a tumor of the jaw that can impinge on the ocular orbit; it is usually multifocal, affecting parenchymatous organs, the ovaries, and the testes. Bone marrow involvement is rare, in contrast to the sporadic American form of the disease. The virus now called EBV was first isolated from explanted specimens of the tumor. Patients with BL in Africa often had high titers of EBV antibodies. A firm link of virus to disease was established only by molecular hybridization analyses, which showed that cryptic viral genome, but not virus itself, was present in African BL tissue, first linking a human malignancy with a virus. More than 98% of cases of African BL contain EBV DNA, present as the EBV episome, in contrast to about 15% of the American form of BL. EBV infection precedes by years the development of lymphoma.

The role of EBV in the genesis of BL appears to be as contributory cofactor.

In the endemic regions, the incidence of BL is estimated to be about ten per 100,000, with evidence of a downward trend. The sporadic form of BL that occurs in North America and western Europe is a much rarer disease. Although EBV is no longer thought to cause BL, it takes prime place because the virus was discovered in this neoplasm. The mean age for occurrence of BL in Africa is approximately 7 years. Because most children there are infected in the first few months of life, this figure establishes the average latency period of EBV infection in the development of BL. In the endemic areas, BL is more likely to develop in children with higher than average titers of EBV antibodies followed prospectively. Cofactors are postulated to explain the high incidence in the endemic regions. One is holoendemic malaria, the geographic distribution of which is similar to that of endemic BL. In recent years the incidence of authentic BL has risen in nonendemic regions because of AIDS, and in the United States it now exceeds the incidence in Africa.

Translocations involving the immunoglobulin loci on chromosomes 14, 22, and 2 and the c-*myc* locus on chromosome 8 are found in all cases of BL regardless of geographic origin or whether they are coincident with EBV infection, with the result that expression of the c-*myc* proto-oncogene is turned on by the immunoglobulin regulatory sequences. The role of EBV as a cofactor for BL arises from its stimulation of B lymphocytes to proliferate, which increases the likelihood of selection of cells with such a mutation, because overexpression of c-*myc* results in enhanced growth properties. This molecular lesion also accounts for the monoclonality of BL. BL cells are not recognized by the immune system, even though they express EBNA-1, an antigen. The EBNA-1 protein contains a distinctive Gly-Gly-Ala polymer, which inhibits its presentation as an antigen by major histocompatibility complex class I molecules and therefore protects BL cells from destruction by cytotoxic T lymphocytes.

B-CELL LYMPHOMAS

In contrast to BL, which arises in immunocompetent hosts (as well as in patients with AIDS), EBV lymphoproliferative syndromes (also called immunoblastic sarcomas) are complications of organ transplantation and AIDS. At first, lymphoproliferation (diffuse or localized) is polyclonal; monoclonal lymphomas are likely to evolve. None of these B-cell lymphomas has the chromosomal changes of BL, but the lymphomas are consistently infected with EBV, at least in transplant recipients. The virus is believed to be directly responsible for neoplastic growth, just as it can drive polyclonal growth of B cells in culture. Solitary lymphomas of the brain are striking examples—all are latently infected with EBV. Masses in the retroperitoneum are also common. These neoplasias almost certainly are triggered by EBV alone, without the necessity for cofactors. The tumors exhibit the type 3 latency phenotype, which is characterized by expression of all the EBV latency genes. In its early phases, lymphoproliferation in transplant recipients can be reversed by reduction of immunosuppression. With conversion to monoclonality, the proliferation is not reversible and is notoriously difficult to treat.

TABLE 314.1.	**DISEASES ASSOCIATED WITH EPSTEIN–BARR VIRUS INFECTION**
Tissues Affected and Diseases	**Role of Epstein–Barr Virus**
Lymphoid	
Burkitt's lymphoma	Cofactor, nonessential; clonal
B-cell immunoblastic lymphomas	Causal
T-cell lymphomas	Clonal association
Hodgkin's disease	Clonal association, Reed–Sternberg cells infected
Chronic interstitial lymphocytic peumonitis	Causal
Epithelial	
Nasopharyngeal carcinoma	Essential factor
Parotid carcinoma	Clonal association
Gastric carcinoma	Clonal association
Hairy leukoplakia of the tongue	Causal
Lymphoid and epithelial	
Infectious mononucleosis	Causal
Other	
Leiomyosarcoma	Clonal association; in AIDS

Even with successful anti-HIV therapy, such tumors may still progress, depending on stage.

HD was associated inconclusively with EBV in the past because of high EBV antibody titers in some patients and a somewhat higher incidence of HD after IM detected in epidemiologic surveys. Stronger direct evidence of a link with the virus emerged during the early 1990s. The EBV genome is detected in up to 70% of HD tissues, in some cases as monoclonal episomes in Reed–Sternberg cells. The profile of EBV gene expression includes EBNA-1, LMP-1, LMP-2, and EBER RNA, similar to the pattern in NPC. EBV infection may contribute to the genesis of HD. EBV is more likely to be expressed in the mixed cellularity form than in the nodular sclerosing form of the disease; expression of EBV in lymphocyte-depleted HD is inconsistent and probably rare. EBV-associated HD is more common in pediatric and middle age or older patients.

There is also developing evidence of EBV infection in T-cell lymphomas, which comes as a surprise because EBV is predominantly B-lymphotropic. The tumors appear as solitary or several neoplasms or sometimes as a diffuse T-cell proliferation; they also can be sited in the nasopharynx, sometimes as a midline lesion. All are reported as negative for human T-cell leukemia virus 1 infection. They are rare conditions (up to now found in Japan, Taiwan, and the United States), but they are significant because of the monoclonality of the EBV episomes found in them and the possible new perspective on the genesis of lymphomas. Finally, the human herpesvirus 8–associated primary effusion lymphomas of B cells in patients with AIDS are sometimes co-infected with EBV, raising the possibility of an interaction between these viruses, which contain several genes in common. Lesions of Kaposi's sarcoma are not infected with EBV.

NASOPHARYNGEAL CARCINOMA

An epithelial malignancy that arises in the posterior nasopharynx in the fossa of Rosenmüller in Waldeyer's ring, NPC is a fascinating malignancy in terms of etiologic and epidemiologic characteristics, early detection, and the prospects for novel therapeutic approaches. The most common histologic type (World Health Organization [WHO] type 1) is the anaplastic form. Often infiltrated with T lymphocytes (NPC is described as a lymphoepithelioma), the EBV episomes nonetheless are found in the transformed epithelial cells, not the lymphocytes, which are normal and may be a response to a lymphokine secreted by the carcinomatous cells. NPC exhibits type 2 latency with expression of EBNA-1 and the EBV oncoproteins LMP-1 and LMP-2. The association of EBV with this malignancy is consistent worldwide, regardless of whether the disease appears in regions of sporadic or endemic incidence. EBV genomes or gene products can be detected uniformly, though with more difficulty in the rarer differentiated form (WHO type 3), where genome copy numbers are low. EBV genomes are detected even in tissues with the earliest changes leading to NPC, namely, hyperplasia. Since hyperplastic and dysplastic lesions rarely are detected, even in the endemic regions where prophylactic instrumentation and biopsy are routine in high-risk persons and full-blown NPC is common, progression of this malignancy is probably rapid.

Although it is one of the major malignancies in the world, NPC is a sporadic disease in North America and western Europe. The incidence of NPC in southern China is about 100 times higher than in the United States. Cofactors proposed to explain this high incidence are diet (ingestion of salted fish in infancy); exposure to medicinal herbs containing phorbol esters, which can induce reactivation of EBV replication from the latent state; and genetic predisposition. Other regions of high incidence include Taiwan, Singapore, Hong Kong, Malaysia, and, to a lesser extent, the west coast of North America, where southern Chinese immigrate. The incidence is also high among the Inuits of North America. NPC has a moderately high incidence in whites in North Africa, where the disease affects younger persons as well as the characteristic middle age group. North African expatriates in France have a high incidence of NPC for at least a generation, much like the Chinese immigrants. Explanations for these extraordinary epidemiologic patterns are largely speculative.

The pathogenesis of NPC in the endemic region of southern China can be outlined tentatively. EBV infection occurs early in life in the whole population. A long period of latent infection, typical of EBV, ensues until middle age (40 to 60 years). There then appear circulating IgA antibodies to EBV replicative cycle antigens, which signal viral reactivation, presumably in the nasopharynx. The trigger of this viral replication is unknown, but activation may take place when the target epithelial cells are infected. The early neoplastic changes of NPC after viral infection probably develop in selected persons with somatic mutations acquired during the latency period from the suspected environmental or nutritional carcinogens or through genetic predisposition. Monoclonal episomes in the carcinomatous cells indicate that virus infection comes before cellular proliferation leading to malignancy. The p53 gene is not mutated in NPC, except occasionally late in the course of disease, as a secondary event. Thus, in this scheme, infection is not dormant in nasopharyngeal epithelial cells. Instead, the target cells for NPC in the fossa of Rosenmüller are newly infected, perhaps mediated by IgA antibodies as a consequence of viral reactivation elsewhere. In any case, the appearance of EBV IgA antibodies is a harbinger of NPC, either already present or in incipient stages; carcinoma is detected within 12 to 18 months.

Carcinomas of other portions of the upper aerodigestive tract, including supraglottal and laryngeal carcinomas, thymomas of epithelial origin, and some parotid carcinomas, also are suspected of having a link to EBV infection. The parotid gland is a site of EBV replication, and all these tissues have a common origin in the primitive oropharynx. Infection of the aerodigestive tract extends, unexpectedly, to the stomach. Some gastric carcinomas contain clonal EBV genomes and express an EBV latency gene (*EBNA2*) not detected in the other epithelial malignancies.

A distinctive EBV-associated disease is hairy leukoplakia of the tongue, which usually produces lesions on one side of the tongue; on histologic examination there is epithelial proliferation, followed by shedding of cells, which lyse. The disease was recognized first as a lesion in patients with AIDS, but it also occurs in some allograft recipients. The most remarkable feature is the enormous number of herpesvirus particles in the lesion, identified as EBV by molecular hybridization analyses; there is florid virus replication, often with several EBV strains, leading to viral recombination. Hairy leukoplakia responds promptly to treatment with acyclovir, though it may recur.

LABORATORY FINDINGS

The EBV-associated diseases are distinctive in their clinical features, but in each case diagnosis should be established by specific tests. For IM, evidence of antibodies to the EBV viral capsid antigen (VCA), both IgG and IgM in primary infection, and, ideally, EA-D antibodies but not EBNA antibodies confirms the diagnosis. Antibodies to EA-D are transient and indicate recent infection or reactivated infection; however, EA antibody titers may persist for several years, probably because of sporadic asymptomatic virus reactivation. Antibodies to EBNA-1 often are not detectable in primary infection, appearing up to 6 months later. The characteristic pattern of past infection would be a moderate titer of IgG VCA antibodies and a low titer of EBNA antibodies, both persisting for life.

Virus is detected in saliva by exposure of cord-blood lymphocytes to filtered throat washings, which results in proliferation of the cells within 4 to 6 weeks after infection. The cell lines that emerge are immortalized and bear EBNA-1 antigen and EBV episomes in low copy numbers. The usefulness of this test is limited by its difficulty and because of protracted virus shedding in saliva. Past infection is also confirmed by cultivation of peripheral blood lymphocytes; the EBV-infected fraction in 50% or more of infected people proliferates spontaneously, and the resulting polyclonal B-cell lines bear EBV antigens and genomes.

In BL, diagnosis is based on distinctive histopathologic characteristics and cytogenetic analysis for the characteristic chromosomal translocations. In the African endemic regions, all patients with BL have VCA, EA-R, and EBNA-1 antibodies, often in high titers. Molecular hybridization analyses of tumor tissue show EBV episomes and EBER RNA. In the sporadic form, EBV serologic and viral hybridization analyses are of little value.

EBV-induced lymphoproliferative syndromes result from primary or reactivated infection and arise in the context of immunodeficiency states, most usually acquired, as in allograft recipients (up to 10% of graft recipients, depending on the intensity of immunosuppressive therapy). Primary immunodeficiency states, though rare, are associated with a very high incidence of EBV-induced lymphomas; they include X-linked lymphoproliferative syndrome (Duncan's syndrome), Wiskott–Aldrich syndrome, ataxia–telangiectasia, and combined immunodeficiency disease. The proliferations, initially polyclonal, express B-cell surface markers and do not have distinctive chromosomal abnormalities. The tumor cells evidence EBNA-1 on touch preparations, EBV episomes by Southern blot hybridization, and EBER RNA by in situ cytohybridization. Except for the absence of EBNA-1 antibodies in some EBV-infected patients with primary immunodeficiency, the serologic pattern is not distinctive; both VCA and EA antibodies are present or elevated.

Patients with NPC have a highly distinctive EBV serologic profile marked by IgA antibodies to VCA and EA antigens as well as high titers of the usual IgG antibodies to these same antigens (VCA and EA-R or EA-D). The titers of IgG antibodies to viral products, such as DNAse and BZLF1 (Z), are useful as indexes of response to therapy and recurrence. The EBV IgA antibodies appear in the earliest stages of disease, including the period when premalignant hyperplastic changes are found in biopsy samples of the fossa of Rosenmüller. Evidence of EBV IgA antibodies therefore may be uniquely valuable for early detection of disease or even to predict onset in high-risk groups. In addition to EBER RNA, NPC tissues invariably contain EBV episomes, though the number of copies is low or not detectable in the differentiated WHO type 3 form. Hairy leukoplakia of the tongue is diagnosed by EBV replicative antigens and linear forms of the genome in tissue biopsy samples, which also show evidence of abundant virions on electron microscopy.

OPTIMAL MANAGEMENT

In EBV-infected cell cultures, replication of virus can be checked entirely by exposure to any of a number of nucleoside analogs and other antiviral drugs used experimentally. Latently infected cells in the cultures are unaffected. Controlled trials of acyclovir for treatment of IM have shown marginal benefit, in part because many of the symptoms of IM are caused by secondary immuno-pathologic processes unaffected by antiviral treatment. In theory, a nontoxic, nonmutagenic, orally administered drug that produces high blood and salivary levels plus an immunomodulator, such as a corticosteroid—coupled with early diagnosis—might be effective for the treatment of IM. An ideal antiviral pro-drug for such a regimen is valcyclovir. Another highly effective drug for use in vitro, an L-benzimadizole riboside that is thought to inhibit an EBV protein kinase, with the unique result of disabling a necessary replication cofactor—the EBV DNA processivity factor—is in development. Certain rare forms of chronic EBV infection of the lung in infants, called chronic interstitial lymphocytic pneumonitis, appear to respond transiently to acyclovir. There is no evidence that so-called chronic mononucleosis responds to antiviral drugs; the single placebo-controlled trial of acyclovir for CFS showed no benefit. The cases were heterogeneous, however, and the time after primary EBV infection uncertain.

Polyclonal B-cell lymphoproliferation may be reversed in its early phases by reducing the immunosuppressive regimen. Acyclovir may add some benefit by preventing infection of additional B lymphocytes. Other approaches are still theoretical. The concept of curing latent infection by disrupting episomal replication with the use of antisense deoxyribonucleotide oligomers to EBNA-1 in mRNA or analogous ribozymes is attractive but limited by difficulties in delivery. Such antisense oligomers should stop not only replication of EBV episomes but also proliferation of the EBV-immortalized lymphocytes. Their proliferation is also retarded by interferon-α.

Gene therapy of solitary brain lymphomas poses an interesting challenge. Approaches would be by direct inoculation of viral vectors with several objectives. One proposal is delivery of a vector carrying the herpes simplex virus thymidine kinase (tk) gene or other viral kinase, which will locally activate a systemically administered cytotoxic drug, such as ganciclovir. Similarly, the cytosine deaminase (CD) gene has been delivered to EBV lymphomas grown in SCID mice. When the pro-drug 5-fluorocytosine is given to the mice, it becomes activated by CD in the tumors, which regress. Another hypothetical approach would be to deliver by direct inoculation a viral vector containing the EBV activator gene Z. Expression of the Z protein will specifically convert latent EBV infection to active viral replication that is cytolytic. Moreover, expression of viral cytolytic cycle enzymes can activate cytotoxic pro-drugs. The difficulty is penetration into all the tumor cells; however, a bystander effect may expand cytotoxicity. Finally, systemic administration of a drug, such as a butyrate compound, might induce EBV reactivation in tumor cells (as well as in other latently EBV-infected cells), which in turn, would provide virally encoded enzymes that could activate a cytotoxic drug in the tumor cells. This strategy avoids direct inoculation but requires an effective, relatively nontoxic inducing agent.

Cell-mediated immunotherapy is no longer hypothetical for systemic treatment of EBV lymphomas. EBV-specific autologous T cells are selected and clonally expanded in vitro. Infusion of these cells has produced dramatic long-term remissions without graft-versus-host disease. The target cells in EBV lymphoproliferative disease have the type 3 latency phenotype, which responds best because all the latency proteins are expressed and only some are good antigens. A similar strategy for treatment of HD and NPC may not be as effective, because of the more restricted viral latency protein profile in these diseases. African BL, even in advanced stages, responds well to chemotherapy with cyclophosphamide. Protocols also include vincristine, methotrexate, and prednisolone. Complete, long-term remissions are expected in the EBV-associated form of the disease. The American form of BL, with dissemination to bone marrow, responds less well.

NPC is best approached in its earliest or incipient stages, which are heralded in endemic regions by the distinctive EBV IgA responses to replicative antigens. In theory, antiviral therapy with an acyclovir pro-drug might be beneficial if started early enough. Retinoids prevent second primary head and neck tumors (EBV negative) by favoring epithelial differentiation. In vitro retinoids interfere with the triggering effect of the EBV BZLF-1 (Z) protein in viral reactivation. Combination of a retinoid with a viral inhibitor at the earliest stages of pathogenesis of NPC might therefore be of benefit, but it has not been tested. Genetically engineered EBV vaccines, mainly using the GP350 membrane protein as antigen in several viral vectors, have been tested in animal models. The purified protein is not expected to prevent primary infection, but it may prevent disease.

BIBLIOGRAPHY

Cesarman E, Chang Y, Moore PS, et al. Kaposi's sarcoma–associated herpesvirus-like DNA sequences in AIDS-related body cavity–based lymphomas. *N Engl J Med* 1995;332:1186–1191.

Glemser B. *Mr. Burkitt and Africa.* New York: World Publishing Company, 1970.

Kenney S, Ge J-Q, Westphal E, et al. Gene therapy strategies for treating Epstein–Barr virus–associated lymphomas: comparison of two different Epstein–Barr virus–based vectors. *Hum Gene Ther* 1998;9:1131–1141.

Kieff E. Epstein–Barr virus and its replication. In: Fields BN, Knipe DM, Howley PM, eds. *Virology.* Philadelphia: Lippincott–Raven Publishers, 1996:2343–2396.

Miller G, Grogan E, Rowe D, et al. Selective lack of antibody to a compo-
nent of EB nuclear antigen in patients with chronic active Epstein–Barr virus infection. *J Infect Dis* 1987;156:26.

Pagano JS. Viral causation of malignant disease. In: Hoeprich PD, Jordan MC, Ronald AR, eds. *Infectious diseases: a modern treatise of infectious diseases,* fifth ed. Philadelphia: JB Lippincott, 1994:1473.

Pagano JS. Epstein–Barr virus: therapy of active and latent infection. In: Jeffries DJ, De Clercq E, eds. *Antiviral chemotherapy.* London: John Wiley & Sons, 1995:155.

Raab-Traub N. Epstein-Barr virus and nasopharyngeal carcinoma. *Semin Cancer Biol* 1992;3:297.

Raab-Traub N, Flynn K. The structure of the termini of the Epstein–Barr virus as a marker of clonal cellular proliferation. *Cell* 1986;47:883.

Rickinson AB, Kieff E. Epstein–Barr virus. In: Fields B, Knipe D, Howley P, et al., eds. *Virology,* third ed. Philadelphia: Lippincott–Raven Publishers, 1996:2343–2396.

Rooney CM, Smith CA, Brenner MK, et al. Prophylaxis and treatment of Epstein–Barr virus lymphoproliferative disease using genetically modified cytotoxic T lymphocytes. *Lancet* 1995;345:9–13.

Shibata D, Weiss L. Epstein–Barr virus associated gastric carcinoma. *Am J Pathol* 1992;140:769–774.

Webster-Cyriaque J, Edwards R, Quinlivan E, et al. Epstein–Barr virus and human herpesvirus 8 prevalence in human immunodeficiency virus–associated oral mucosal lesions. *J Infect Dis* 1997;175:1324–1332.

Kelley's Textbook of Internal Medicine, fourth edition. Edited by H. David Humes. Lippincott Williams & Wilkins, Philadelphia © 2000.

CHAPTER

315

VARICELLA-ZOSTER VIRUS INFECTION

ANNE A. GERSHON

Varicella and zoster are two diseases that are caused by the varicella-zoster virus (VZV). Varicella (chickenpox), the primary infection, is mainly a disease of young children, but about 5% of adults in the United States remain susceptible; varicella tends to have more severe effects in adults than in children. Zoster, the secondary infection, is caused by reactivation of latent VZV that was acquired during infection with varicella. Zoster is mainly a disease of adults; after the age of 50 years, the incidence begins to climb steeply. Zoster is also more common in immunocompromised people than in normal people of similar ages. It results when cell-mediated immunity to VZV wanes either with time or because of underlying illness.

■ DEFINITION

VZV is a member of the herpesvirus family, closely related to herpes simplex virus (HSV) types 1 and 2, cytomegalovirus, and Epstein–Barr virus. These agents are composed of a DNA core surrounded by a protein capsid, a tegument, and an outer envelope consisting of lipids and glycoproteins. Their diameter is about 200 nm. Herpesviruses become latent after primary infection and may later reemerge and provoke a second clinical illness. VZV causes latent infection in dorsal root ganglia; its DNA and RNA have been identified there in autopsy specimens.

EPIDEMIOLOGY

In temperate climates, varicella is largely a disease of children; most cases develop before the age of 10 years. In these areas, about 95% of adults are immune to chickenpox. Most adults who recall having had clinical symptoms of varicella are immune, but only about 25% with no recollection of varicella are actually susceptible. In countries with tropical climates, there is often less spread of VZV among children and consequently a greater percentage of adults who are susceptible. The basis of this phenomenon is unknown, but it may be related to lack of urbanization, a warm ambient temperature, or both. Varicella in temperate climates is mainly seen in cold weather seasons.

After varicella infection, specific antibodies and cell-mediated immune responses develop and persist for many years. They probably play a major role in prevention of second cases of varicella, which are unusual. Varicella is a highly contagious disease; in families, about 90% of susceptible people in the household become infected. Immune people who are reexposed to the virus often experience a boost in VZV antibody and cell-mediated immunity without symptoms. In contrast to varicella, zoster occurs with equal frequency throughout the year. It is unusual in young adults, including those frequently exposed to VZV. Zoster is rare in childhood, but its occurrence increases with age, especially during the fifth decade; its rate approaches 20% in the ninth decade. Immunocompromised patients are also at higher risk of zoster; the risk is proportional to the degree of compromise in immunity. For example, zoster has been reported in as many as half of patients with advanced Hodgkin's disease. Zoster usually develops despite residual humoral immunity to VZV; most people who have it have depressed cell-mediated immunity to VZV. Cell-mediated immunity to VZV decreases with advancing age, beginning at about 50 years of age.

PATHOGENESIS

Varicella is an exogenous, primary infection (Table 315.1). External sources of VZV are vesicular skin lesions and the respiratory tract. VZV, which is spread by the airborne route, presumably reaches the respiratory tract of a susceptible person and begins to multiply, invading the local lymph nodes and eventually causing primary viremia. The virus then reaches the viscera and multiplies further, causing secondary viremia that delivers VZV to the skin.

Zoster is caused by reactivation of latent VZV in sensory ganglia, with transport of the virus down the sensory nerve to the skin. Development of zoster has not been recognized as a sign of underlying malignancy. It has been noted, however, as an early clinical sign of acquired immunodeficiency syndrome (AIDS) in people at high risk for human immunodeficiency virus infection.

CLINICAL FEATURES

Varicella takes the form of a generalized rash, after an incubation period ranging from 10 to 21 days (mean, 14 days; Fig. 315.1). The rash, which usually is accompanied by fever, is most concentrated on the trunk and head, and it consists progressively of maculopapules, vesicles, pustules, and crusts. There often are several crops of lesions, so that all forms of the rash may be seen in any one area of skin. The rash is intensely pruritic, and skin vesicles are full of infectious virions. In healthy children, the disease is usually mild. A second case in a family is often more severe than the first case. All vesicles usually crust within 5 to 7 days, and the patient is no longer infectious to others. Complications in otherwise healthy children are unusual.

Varicella in pregnant women may be severe; they should be observed closely in case antiviral therapy is required. A rare constellation of congenital anomalies has been reported in roughly 2% of infants born to women who contract varicella during the first or second trimester of pregnancy. These anomalies include skin scarring; a hypoplastic limb; eye abnormalities, such as chorioretinitis; low birth weight; and mental retardation. There

---

TABLE 315.1. **CHARACTERISTICS OF DISEASES CAUSED BY VARICELLA-ZOSTER VIRUS**

Characteristics	Varicella	Zoster
Type of infection	Primary	Secondary
Distribution of rash	Generalized, especially trunk and face	Localized to one to three dermatomes, unilateral
Usual age at onset	Childhood	After age 50 years
Specific antibody at onset	Absent	Present
Cellular immunity to virus at onset	Absent	Low
Complications	Progressive, potentially fatal in untreated immunocompromised patients, including human immunodeficiency virus–positive patients Bacterial encephalitis superinfection	Generalized rash with viremia in immunocompromised patients May be first sign of acquired immunodeficiency syndrome Postherpetic pain in the elderly after healing of acute illness

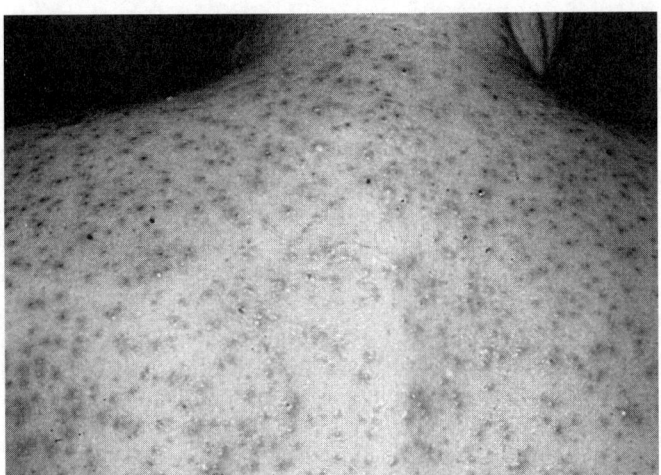

FIGURE 315.1. Skin eruption of chickenpox in an adult patient.

is no recognized means of prenatal diagnosis. Ultrasonography may be helpful in assessing limb formation in case abortion is being considered.

Varicella in immunocompromised patients, including patients being treated for underlying malignancy, those with immunodeficiency diseases, and patients treated with high doses of corticosteroids (more than the equivalent of 1 mg per kilogram per day of prednisone), may be severe or fatal. Patients with underlying leukemia or lymphoma are at greatest risk; untreated, their mortality rate approaches 10%. Severe varicella may be either fulminant—with hemorrhagic skin lesions, disseminated intravascular coagulation, and death—or more indolently fatal. In the latter case, the disease seems to progress normally for the first week. Fever continues, however, and many new, often large vesicles appear during the second week, when pneumonia often develops, which is usually the fatal event. According to the Centers for Disease Control and Prevention, estimated fatalities due to varicella are two per 100,000 in otherwise healthy children, 50 per 100,000 in adults, and 7,000 per 100,000 in children with an underlying malignancy. Newborns whose mothers have varicella at term are also at increased risk for severe chickenpox, which resembles varicella in immunocompromised patients and has a mortality rate of about 20%.

Adults may have extensive skin lesions, and they have a high incidence of varicella pneumonia. Pulmonary involvement occurs 1 to 6 days after the onset of rash. In studies of military recruits, the incidence of pulmonary disease (cough and shortness of breath) is 4% of adult cases, with abnormal chest radiographic features in 16%. The typical radiologic finding in varicella pneumonia is diffuse nodular infiltration. In contrast to children, adults tend to have a prodromal period before onset of rash, and their convalescent period may last several weeks. The severity of pneumonia appears to reflect directly the degree of cutaneous involvement. Adults with varicella should be observed closely so that antiviral therapy can be administered if necessary. It should be given, for example, to adults in the early stages of varicella pneumonia.

Zoster appears as a unilateral rash in a dermatomal distribution; from one to three dermatomes are usually involved. Fever

may be present. Zoster is seen most commonly in the thoracic region, followed by the facial–cervical area, trunk, and extremities. Pain is associated with the acute phase of zoster, and older patients may experience postherpetic neuralgia that may last for many months after the rash has healed. The incidence of postherpetic pain begins to increase sharply at about the age of 50 years. Zoster actually represents a spectrum of disease—some patients experience only dermatomal pain without rash, some have only a few vesicular lesions, and some show extensive dermatomal involvement. It is not uncommon for 10 to 15 scattered vesicular lesions to develop outside the dermatomal area.

Zoster of the face often involves the ophthalmic division of the trigeminal nerve; this is commonly associated with central nervous system symptoms, such as headache, aphasia, and seizures. Granulomatous angiitis, appearing as contralateral paralysis days to weeks after the onset of trigeminal zoster, may be caused by VZV infection of the cerebral blood vessels; it is seen most often in elderly patients. The time course of zoster varies and is often longer in immunocompromised people. Patients are no longer infectious to others after all lesions are dried. The mortality rate from disseminated zoster in immunocompromised patients is 1% to 2%.

DIAGNOSIS

Infections caused by VZV are usually distinctive in clinical features, and for this reason, laboratory confirmation often is not required (Table 315.2). The concentration of lesions on the face and trunk as well as the vesicular and pruritic character of the rash in varicella are most helpful diagnostically. Epidemiologic clues, such as exposure to VZV and the season of the year, also may be helpful. Zoster is less likely to be confused with other diseases, with the exception of HSV infection. About 10% of cases diagnosed as zoster actually are caused by HSV. Recurrent

---

TABLE 315.2.   DIAGNOSIS OF VARICELLA-ZOSTER VIRUS INFECTION

Differential for varicella
  Contact dermatitis, coxsackievirus infection, generalized herpes simplex virus infection, impetigo, insect bites, rickettsialpox, scabies, Stevens–Johnson syndrome
Laboratory testing
  Examine skin lesions for evidence of VZV
    Detect viral antigen by immunofluorescence (using commercial tagged monoclonal antibodies); detect viral DNA by polymerase chain reaction
    Culture moist lesions for virus (can take a week or longer)
    Tzanck smear (not specific for VZV)
  Detect fourfold or greater increase in specific antibody titer in acute- and convalescent-phase serum specimens (takes at least 10 days to collect specimens)
    Assays: immunofluorescence, enzyme-linked immunosorbent assay, radioimmunoassay, latex agglutination, complement fixation

VZV, varicella-zoster virus.

dermatomal rashes are almost always attributable to HSV rather than VZV. A specific diagnosis of VZV infection is best made by examination of skin scrapings of vesicular lesions. A fourfold or greater rise in VZV antibody is considered diagnostic of varicella. It is usually indicative of zoster as well, but patients with HSV who have had varicella at one time may also have a concomitant rise in VZV antibody titer. Therefore, zoster is best diagnosed by analysis of vesicular fluid. In VZV encephalitis, it is rare to isolate the virus from cerebrospinal fluid. High VZV antibody titers in cerebrospinal fluid may suggest this complication. Polymerase chain reaction assays for VZV DNA in cerebrospinal fluid may show positive results.

OPTIMAL MANAGEMENT

Local treatment measures, such as calamine lotion for varicella and Burow's solution for zoster, are often used. Aspirin should not be given to children and adolescents with varicella, because of the risk of Reye's syndrome; acetaminophen may be taken to control fever. Antihistamines may control itching. Acyclovir (ACV), a selective inhibitor of VZV DNA synthesis, is useful for therapy of VZV infections. Patients with severe or potentially severe infections should be treated with the intravenous formulation at a dose of 30 mg per kilogram per day for adults and adolescents and 1,500 mg per square meter per day for children (in both instances given in three divided doses), because only about 20% of the oral formulation is absorbed from the gastrointestinal tract. ACV is excreted by the kidneys; for this reason, patients with creatinine clearances of less than 50 mL/min/1.73 m^2 should receive one-half to one-third the normal dosage. ACV should be infused over at least 1 hour, with maintenance fluids given both before and during the infusion. Precipitation of the drug in the renal tubules, with reversible increases in serum creatinine levels, has been associated with bolus administration. Other side effects of ACV include phlebitis, rash, nausea, and neurologic manifestations, such as headache and tremor; however, the drug is remarkably well tolerated, in part because an enzyme induced by VZV is required for the antiviral effect of ACV.

Because ACV has little toxicity and therapy within 3 days of onset has been associated with the best outcomes, it is recommended that early treatment be instituted for patients at high risk of severe VZV infections, to prevent dissemination of the virus. This therapy should not be considered merely potentially lifesaving; in many cases, considerable morbidity can be prevented by antiviral treatment in immunosuppressed patients. In zoster patients, intravenous ACV is associated with more rapid healing of skin lesions and resolution of acute pain than if no specific treatment is given.

There has been considerable interest in the question of whether orally administered ACV is useful for treatment of varicella and zoster in patients who are not immunocompromised. Dosages used are 4 g per day (in five divided doses) for adults and 80 mg per kilogram per day (in four divided doses) for children. Therapy with oral ACV begun within 24 hours of rash onset shortens the course of varicella by about 1 day but does not prevent complications or spread of VZV. For zoster, drug efficacy has been established even if 3 days have elapsed since onset, but the earlier ACV is begun, the greater the effect is likely to be. Although it has not been verified conclusively, there is some indication that therapy minimizes the pain associated with zoster. It has therefore become customary to treat elderly patients with early zoster, because the older the patient with this disease, the more likely it is that pain (especially postherpetic neuralgia) will be a problem. A study conducted by Wood and colleagues found no difference in outcome in older patients with zoster whether they were treated with ACV for 7 days or 21 days. Moreover, healing was no more rapid, and postherpetic neuralgia was no less likely to occur, if a 3-week course of tapering prednisolone (beginning at 40 mg per day) was given in addition to ACV.

One concern about widespread use of ACV is that drug resistance may develop. Resistance is less of a problem with VZV than for HSV. In the case of HSV, VZV resistant to ACV has been reported, most often in patients with underlying AIDS. The antiviral drug foscarnet, which is more toxic than ACV and can be administered only intravenously, has proved useful for therapy of ACV-resistant VZV. The antiviral drug famciclovir has been approved by the Food and Drug Administration for oral therapy of zoster. This antiviral is the prodrug of the active compound penciclovir, to which it is rapidly converted in the body. Like ACV, penciclovir has no antiviral activity until it is phosphorylated by viral enzymes. Its main advantage over ACV is that it can be administered three times a day (1,500 mg per day) rather than five times daily, which may lead to better compliance. There are no data concerning whether varicella can be treated successfully with famciclovir, nor are there any published data on the use of famciclovir in immunocompromised patients. A drug analogous to famciclovir, valcyclovir, has also been approved for treatment of zoster.

PREVENTION AND CONTROL

Passive immunization against varicella may be achieved with varicella-zoster immune globulin (VZIG). VZIG is available through local blood centers and the American Red Cross. It is indicated for prevention or modification of severe varicella in high-risk people, including those with an underlying malignancy or immunodeficiency disease, patients receiving high doses of corticosteroids for any reason, and newborns whose mothers have had onset of varicella 5 days or less before or within 2 days after delivery. Recipients should also have had intimate exposure to varicella within the preceding 5 days, but preferably within 3 days. Intimate exposure is usually defined as that occurring in a household, as the result of indoor play in a closed area for more than 1 hour, or through having adjacent hospital beds. Exposure to either varicella or zoster is considered significant.

Immunocompromised adults as well as immunocompromised children with no history of varicella also should be passively immunized after an exposure. It is helpful to determine the immune status of such immunocompromised adults in advance. Because 95% of people older than the age of 30 years are immune to varicella, adults with detectable VZV antibodies measured by a reliable method do not require passive immunization should an exposure occur.

VZIG should not be used to try to control nosocomial varicella because it may not necessarily prevent clinical symptoms of chickenpox but rather modify them. In addition, it increases the possible time of risk, because the incubation period of varicella may be increased. VZIG should be given to otherwise healthy adults only if they have been proved by serologic testing to be susceptible to chickenpox. It should not be given to healthy children for modification of benign disease. Overuse of VZIG in populations not at high risk of severe varicella is unnecessarily expensive. VZIG has not been found to be useful for treatment of VZV infections or for prevention of zoster in high-risk patients. High-risk patients who have received VZIG may still experience a mild form of varicella. They need to be observed carefully, but only rarely do they require any specific antiviral chemotherapy. Nosocomial varicella typically can be controlled by a combination of testing of employees (in advance) for susceptibility to varicella, obtaining accurate histories for varicella in all patients admitted to the hospital, furloughing susceptible personnel during potential incubation periods, cohorting exposed susceptible children and those with active varicella, and discharging exposed susceptible patients early.

A live attenuated varicella vaccine was developed in Japan in the early 1970s. It is extremely effective in preventing severe varicella. Mild breakthrough cases of varicella have been noted in a few vaccinees. Thus far, these cases have required no specific therapy, even in highly immunocompromised children. Immunization has been associated with a decline in the incidence of zoster in leukemic children. In 1995, this vaccine was approved for routine use in healthy persons susceptible to the disease who are more than 1 year of age. Adults should be given two doses 1 month apart for optimal protection.

BIBLIOGRAPHY

Centers for Disease Control and Prevention. Varicella-zoster immune globulin for the prevention of chickenpox. *MMWR* 1984;33:84.

Committee on Infectious Diseases. Live attenuated varicella vaccine. *Pediatrics* 1995;xx:791.

Friedman SM, Margo CE, Connelly BL. Varicella-zoster virus retinitis as the initial manifestation of the acquired immunodeficiency syndrome. *Am J Ophthalmol* 1994;117:536.

Gershon A. Varicella-zoster virus: prospects for control. *Adv Pediatr Infect Dis* 1995;10:93.

Hope-Simpson RE. The nature of herpes zoster: a long-term study and a new hypothesis. *Proc R Soc Med* 1965;58:9.

Jacobson MA, Berger TG, Fikrig S. Acyclovir-resistant varicella-zoster virus infection after chronic oral acyclovir therapy in patients with the acquired immunodeficiency syndrome. *Ann Intern Med* 1990;112:187.

Leclair JM, Zaia J, Levin MJ, et al. Airborne transmission of chickenpox in a hospital. *N Engl J Med* 1980;302:450.

Pahwa S, Biron K, Lim W, et al. Continuous varicella-zoster infection associated with acyclovir resistance in a child with AIDS. *JAMA* 1988; 260:2879.

Takahashi M, Otsuka T, Okuno Y, et al. Live attenuated varicella vaccine used to prevent the spread of varicella in hospital. *Lancet* 1974;2: 1288.

Wood MF, Johnson RW, McKendrick MW, et al. A randomized trial of acyclovir for 7 days or 21 days with and without prednisolone for treatment of acute herpes zoster. *N Engl J Med* 1994;330:896.

Whitley RJ, Straus S. Therapy for varicella-zoster virus infections: Where do we stand? *Infect Dis Clin Pract* 1993;2:100.

Kelley's Textbook of Internal Medicine, fourth edition. Edited by H. David Humes.
Lippincott Williams & Wilkins, Philadelphia © 2000.

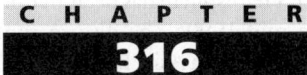

ENTEROVIRUS INFECTIONS

ROSS E. MCKINNEY, JR.

■ DEFINITION

The enteroviruses are small, nonenveloped, single-stranded RNA viruses. They are members of the family Picornaviridae (*pico* meaning "small"—hence, "small RNA viruses") and consist of a single RNA strand and a capsid made up of four virus-encoded proteins. The enteroviruses are divided into subtypes, shown in Table 316.1. The missing serotypes (for example, echovirus 10) are due to reclassification of early serotypes as further information became available. Hepatitis A previously was classified as one of the enteroviruses but was reclassified as a separate genus in 1991 (Hepatovirus). The classification of a given virus as an echovirus, coxsackievirus, or poliovirus is determined by the virus receptor (the cell protein to which the virus attaches before entry).

■ EPIDEMIOLOGY

The enteroviruses spread from person to person through the fecal–oral route. As nonenveloped viruses, they are physicochemically very stable and persist in the environment for long periods of time. The lack of an envelope and their dense protein capsid make the enteroviruses relatively resistant to inactivating agents, such as soaps and detergents. They are shed in the feces of infected people and may be excreted for as long as months. Sewage frequently contains enteroviruses and may be a source of contamination of water supplies. Young children, with their

TABLE 316.1.	MEMBERS OF THE GENUS *ENTEROVIRUS*
Poliovirus	Types 1–3
Coxsackievirus, group A	Types 1–22, 24
Coxsackievirus, group B	Types 1–6
Echovirus	Types 1–9, 11–27, 29–33
Enterovirus	Types 68–71

feces contained in diapers, are another important source of enteroviral exposures. Children also have the highest attack rates of enteroviral infection and disease. The enteroviruses are distributed worldwide and are affected by the seasons in temperate climates, occurring more frequently during the summer and early fall. In the tropics, they have a year-round incidence.

Poliovirus eradication has been an important international objective since the development of polio vaccines in the 1950s. While the Western Hemisphere has been free of wild-type poliomyelitis since the mid-1990s, the disease continues to be endemic in Africa and southern Asia. Because human beings are the only animal host for polio, there is still hope that with complete vaccination, wild-type polio eventually will be eliminated.

PATHOGENESIS

The enteroviruses are cytolytic. Once they infect a cell, they monopolize the cellular protein synthesis system so that the cell produces almost only viral proteins. These proteins are assembled into viral particles, and the cell ruptures. Virus particles are released into the extracellular milieu, and eventually the viruses attach to the receptor on another susceptible cell. The requirement for an extracellular step in the life cycle makes the enteroviruses vulnerable to neutralizing antibodies as a host defense.

The enteroviruses invade their human hosts through mucosal surfaces. Initial penetration and replication take place either in the oral mucosa and tonsillar tissues or in the lower gastrointestinal tract. The viruses are stable in an acid environment and thus are able to pass through the stomach into the intestines. The virus traverses the intestinal wall, and replication occurs in submucosal lymphatic tissue, particularly Peyer's patches. From the intestinal tract, some virus enters the circulation. This period is usually asymptomatic but can result in mild symptoms, primarily fever; this is referred to as the "minor viremia." During this phase the virus spreads to more distal lymphatic tissue. In some cases, the minor viremia produces a sufficient antigenic stimulus to trigger an immune response, and the virus is controlled, predominantly through the production of neutralizing antibodies (rather than cytolytic T cells). Tropism of the virus determines the sites where the virus is able to replicate as it is carried through the circulation. For example, poliovirus has tropism for the central nervous system, particularly the anterior horn cells of the spinal cord, and thus produces central nervous system disease.

CLINICAL FEATURES

The most common clinical result of an enterovirus infection is asymptomatic viremia and gastrointestinal shedding or a mild febrile illness of a few days' duration. Nonetheless, there are several important clinical syndromes associated with enteroviral infection.

POLIOMYELITIS

More than 90% of poliovirus infections are asymptomatic. Only one in 1,000 infected people show signs of paralytic disease.

Symptomatic poliomyelitis is often biphasic. The first phase, or "minor illness," develops in roughly 10% of poliovirus disease. It begins with fever and nonspecific symptoms, such as myalgias, headache, and sore throat. This phase resolves within 1 or 2 days. The major illness with polio infection is marked by the abrupt onset of aseptic meningitis. The symptoms include fever, headache, nuchal rigidity, and vomiting. The cerebrospinal fluid evidences pleocytosis, mildly elevated protein levels, and a normal glucose level. At this stage, aseptic meningitis cannot be distinguished from any other enteroviral meningitis.

The characteristic motor disease of poliomyelitis begins with severe myalgias. The pain is alleviated by exercise, such that patients may pace or perform other maneuvers in the early stages of disease to minimize myalgia. The pain and subsequent weakness are characteristically asymmetrical. Flaccid paralysis begins 1 to 2 days into the major phase of illness. Any combination of limbs can be afflicted, but the muscle groups are generally proximal more often than distal. The lower limbs tend to be affected more frequently than the upper limbs. Painful spasms can arise in nonparalyzed muscles. Deep tendon reflexes diminish or disappear, and sensory function remains normal. Bowel and bladder dysfunction can be an early symptom.

In general, paralysis peaks within 5 days, and recovery is slow; most recovery occurs within 6 months. Sixty percent of patients are left with residual weakness. Less than 10% of patients die; those that do commonly succumb to respiratory failure. Cranial nerve involvement (bulbar poliomyelitis) is noted in 5% to 35% of paralytic disease. It can strike any cranial nerve, but the ninth and tenth are the most often affected. The major concern with bulbar poliomyelitis is the effect on respiration. Other diseases can mimic polio. Several enteroviruses can produce a poliomyelitis syndrome, particularly coxsackie A7 and enterovirus 71. Guillain-Barré syndrome and neonatal botulism can mimic polio, but symptoms of these diseases are symmetrical, in contrast to polio. Moreover, Guillain-Barré syndrome often has sensory manifestations.

ASEPTIC MENINGITIS

Most of the enteroviruses can cause aseptic meningitis. The typical pattern is fever, malaise, headache, nuchal rigidity, and sometimes a petechial rash. The onset is typically acute, most often in the summer or early fall. Cerebrospinal fluid shows moderate pleocytosis with neutrophils predominating in the early stage; over the course of 24 hours this changes to lymphocyte predominance. The total leukocyte count is generally in the range of 30 to 400, the protein level is mildly elevated, and the glucose level is normal. The usual course of illness is 2 to 5 days. The disease can be more serious in young infants, though there are generally no significant residual effects at any age. A small number of infants experience disease-associated seizures, but these are usually easily controlled.

ENCEPHALITIS

Most cases of enteroviral encephalitis are truly a form of meningoencephalitis, involving both brain matter and the meninges. In the immunologically normal host, symptoms initially are those of aseptic meningitis. Progression to confusion, lethargy, and irritability occurs over days. Seizures, coma, or death are possible outcomes. At times, the syndrome can mimic the symptoms of herpes encephalitis. Children and adults with X-linked agammaglobulinemia are susceptible to an unusual chronic form of enteroviral meningoencephalitis. The disease takes the form of slowly diminishing cognitive function and cortical atrophy on computed tomographic or magnetic resonance imaging. Hypogammaglobulinemic children not treated prophylactically with intravenous immune globulin may show signs of a dermatomyositis-like syndrome.

MYOCARDITIS

The enteroviruses, particularly coxsackie B viruses, are the most common cause of acute viral myocarditis, producing 25% to 35% of the cases for which a source can be determined. Neonates are particularly susceptible, though the disease can affect persons of any age. Symptoms include signs of congestive heart failure, palpitations, and chest pain. The pain can mimic that of a myocardial infarction. Arrythmias as a result of myocardial inflammation can be life threatening. Blood levels of cardiac isoenzymes may be elevated. The pericardium is often involved; at times there may be significant pericardial fluid and tamponade. A small proportion of patients progress to chronic congestive heart failure, endocardial fibroelastosis, or dilated cardiomyopathy. In most patients (80% or more) the disease resolves completely.

PLEURODYNIA

Pleurodynia, also known as the Devil's grippe and Bornholm disease, is an inflammation of costal and abdominal muscles. It is produced most often by the coxsackie B viruses and is marked by sharp pain on cough or deep breathing. The illness begins with typical enteroviral symptoms of fever and malaise, before the onset of thoracic symptoms. The illness lasts 7 to 10 days, though the symptoms may recur for a period of weeks. Treatment is symptomatic.

PANCREATITIS AND DIABETES MELLITUS

Enteroviruses are one of the most common causes of acute viral pancreatitis, though the disease itself is relatively uncommon. There is also a long-standing suspicion that the enteroviruses, especially coxsackie B viruses, contribute to the pathogenesis of diabetes mellitus, perhaps through triggering an autoimmune process in a genetically susceptible host.

HAND, FOOT, AND MOUTH DISEASE

Outbreaks of hand, foot, and mouth disease often occur in the summer months. The most common source is coxsackie A16 virus, but enterovirus 71 and other coxsackie A serotypes also can induce the disease. Typically, the patient has fever, headache, a maculopapular rash on the palms and soles, and small oral ulcers. Both the palm/sole exanthem and the oral enanthem can be painful. The oral rash frequently involves the palate and

posterior pharynx, making it distinct from the more anterior lesions of herpes simplex stomatitis. Occasionally, hand, food, and mouth disease can be severe. During a 1998 outbreak in Taiwan, 90,000 cases of the disease were reported; 320 patients required hospitalization, and 55 died. The cause of death was most often shock beginning 2 to 7 days after a nonspecific febrile prodrome. Most of the victims were children less than 3 years old.

ACUTE HEMORRHAGIC CONJUNCTIVITIS

Acute hemorrhagic conjunctivitis is characterized by swelling of the eyelids, acute eye pain, photophobia, headache, and subconjunctival hemorrhages. Most hemorrhagic conjunctivitis is caused either by enterovirus type 70 or by a coxsackievirus A24 variant. The virus is spread primarily in tears, an unusual pattern for the enteroviruses. Paralytic disease similar to poliomyelitis has been reported in some enterovirus type 70 outbreaks.

OTHER

The enteroviruses are one of the most common causes of parotitis (inflammation of the parotid glands) and are part of the differential diagnosis of possible mumps infection. Herpangina, which is distinct from hand, foot, and mouth disease, appears as multiple papulovesicular lesions on the posterior palate and tonsils. The gums are rarely afflicted. Coxsackie A viruses are most often implicated, and treatment is symptomatic.

■ LABORATORY FINDINGS

The enteroviruses can be detected by either culture or polymerase chain reaction testing. Detection by tissue culture is relatively quick—typically less than a week—and is marked by a characteristic cytopathic effect. Nonetheless, not all enterovirus types grow well in tissue culture. Most coxsackie A viruses, for example, are cultured more effectively in the brains of suckling mice than in vitro. The echoviruses, polioviruses, and coxsackie B viruses can be detected fairly reliably in tissue culture. Culture also can be used to determine the serotype of a given enterovirus through the use of overlapping pools of neutralizing antibodies.

Virus detection by polymerase chain reaction is faster and more sensitive than culture, though it is not yet widely available. The method detects a conserved noncoding region of the virus and is able to recognize enteroviruses regardless of serotype. It is particularly useful in detecting low levels of virus in such conditions as chronic enteroviral meningoencephalitis in agammaglobulinemic patients. Antibody tests are of little general diagnostic benefit. If the serotype of virus is known, a rise in antibody titer can be used to confirm infection. In most cases, however, the specific serotype is uncertain, and screening batteries of antibodies are often inaccurate, because of both false-positives and false-negatives.

■ MANAGEMENT

The primary management strategy for poliovirus has been prevention through vaccination. The approach recommended at present is inactivated polio vaccine (Salk). This strategy limits the exposure of immunocompromised children to live virus like the Sabin attenuated poliovirus vaccine at a time when their immune problem may not be diagnosed. The major treatment for enteroviral infections is symptomatic care. Intravenous immunoglobulin is useful to prevent enteroviral disease in hypogammaglobulinemic patients and can be administered to treat chronic meningoencephalitis in agammaglobulinemic individuals. Pleconaril is an experimental antiviral that has shown early promise in the treatment of serious enteroviral disease. It acts at the level of virus uncoating and blocks the release of viral RNA once the virus has entered a cell. Its use in human disease is still at an early stage.

BIBLIOGRAPHY

Abzug MJ, Keyserling HL, Lee ML, et al. Neonatal enterovirus infection: virology, serology, and effects of intravenous immune globulin. *Clin Infect Dis* 1995;20:1201–1206.

Centers for Disease Control. Paralytic poliomyelitis—United States, 1980–1994. *MMWR* 1997;46:79–83.

Centers for Disease Control. Acute hemorrhagic conjunctivitis—St. Croix, U.S. Virgin Islands, September–October 1998. *MMWR* 1998;47: 899–901.

Centers for Disease Control. Deaths among children during an outbreak of hand, foot, and mouth disease—Taiwan, Republic of China, April–July 1998. *MMWR* 1998;47:629–632.

Grandien M, Forsgren M, Ehrnst A. Enteroviruses. In: Lennette EH, Lennette DA, Lennette ET, eds. *Diagnostic procedures for viral, rickettsial, and chlamydial infections*. Washington, D.C.: American Public Health Association, 1995:279–297.

McKinney RE. The enteroviruses. In: Joklik WK, Willett HP, Amos DB, et al., eds. *Zinsser microbiology*, twentieth ed. Norwalk, Conn.: Appleton & Lange, 1992:980–985.

McKinney RE, Katz SL, Wilfert CM. Chronic enteroviral meningoencephalitis in agammaglobulinemic patients. *Rev Infect Dis* 1987;9:334–356.

Rotbart H. Enterovirus. In: Katz SL, Gershon AA, Hotez PJ, eds. *Krugman's infectious diseases of children*, tenth ed. St. Louis: Mosby–Year Book, 1998:81–97.

Rotbart HA, ed. *Human enterovirus infections*. Washington, D.C.: American Society for Microbiology, 1995.

Kelley's Textbook of Internal Medicine, fourth edition. Edited by H. David Humes. Lippincott Williams & Wilkins, Philadelphia © 2000.

CHAPTER 317

VIRAL GASTROENTERITIS

ROGER I. GLASS

In the past, diarrhea often was attributed to viruses when a bacterium or parasite could not be pinpointed as the causative agent. In 1972, the Norwalk agent was the first virus to be identified as a source of diarrhea in humans; since then, rotaviruses, enteric adenoviruses, astroviruses, and other human caliciviruses, including both Sapporo-like viruses and Norwalk-like viruses, have been recognized to cause diarrhea in humans. Other viruses—among them, torovirus, picobirnavirus, coronavirus, enterovirus 22, pestivirus, and parvovirus—have been found in fecal specimens of patients with diarrhea but have not yet been proved to be causative agents of human disease. Viral gastroenteritis is generally mild and self-limited, but in some patients, particularly small infants, the elderly, and the immunocompromised, illness can be severe, leading to extreme dehydration and occasionally death. Viral gastroenteritis induces either diarrhea or vomiting, or both. Viruses are the recognized source of a syndrome previously described as *winter vomiting disease*.

EPIDEMIOLOGY

Viral diarrheas take two distinct forms—common childhood diarrheas that develop in all children during their first 5 years of life and epidemic disease that afflicts both children and adults in sporadic outbreaks. Childhood diarrhea is associated with rotavirus (group A), enteric adenovirus, astrovirus, and human caliciviruses, including both Sapporo-like viruses and Norwalk-like viruses. These viruses infect most children in their first few years of life. First infections usually are associated with disease, and their modes of transmission are generally unknown but may be by direct contact or through airborne droplets. For those agents whose epidemiologic characteristics have been better studied, the declining incidence of disease with increasing age and the low rate of subsequent infections suggest that immunity develops after early infections. In the United States, as well as in other developed countries, a majority of all diarrheal illness in children is provoked by viruses, whereas in developing countries, these agents also are present but complemented by many other bacterial and parasitic pathogens. In temperate climates, rotavirus, astrovirus, and Norwalk-like viruses have a distinct seasonality from late fall to early spring, whereas in tropical settings disease occurs year-round.

Epidemics are typically caused by the Norwalk-like viruses, whose many representatives (Snow Mountain, Hawaii, and Taunton agents) share a characteristic small, round-structured appearance seen on electron microscopy (EM); nonetheless, they are antigenically distinct. Epidemics associated with the Norwalk-like viruses are the most commonly identified and affect groups of all ages. Transmission often can be traced to fecally contaminated water or foods, especially oysters, and dissemination by direct contact, vomitus, or air-borne droplets has been suggested when no other route of transmission has been identified. Epidemics often can be aborted by distinguishing the mode of transmission—particularly contaminated food or water or an ill food handler—and implementing specific public health controls. Rotaviruses of group B have triggered epidemics of cholera-like diarrhea throughout China since 1982 and also have been identified in India. Rotaviruses of group C have been implicated in epidemics worldwide, mostly in infants and small children, but the epidemiologic features of disease caused by this virus are poorly understood, because detection methods are not commonly available. The observation that endemic childhood diarrhea (rotavirus, astrovirus) has been identified less frequently in outbreaks also suggests that their mode of transmission in these settings may be different. For example, rotavirus can cause outbreaks among children in day care centers or in hospital wards, where patients may have direct contact with contaminated food or other vehicles of transmission (toys, surfaces).

The disease burden of viral diarrheas is enormous. Globally, rotavirus alone accounts for an estimated 600,000 deaths per year in children under age 5 and about one-third of all hospitalizations for childhood diarrhea, making it the most severe cause of childhood diarrhea. In the United States, approximately 10% to 12% of all hospitalizations among children less than 5 years old are for diarrhea—160,000 hospitalizations per year, with a mean duration of 3.5 days. The majority of these illnesses are associated with viral agents. Among adults, 1.5% to 2% of all hospitalizations are for diarrhea, and a bacterial pathogen can rarely (less than 10%) be identified, suggesting that many of these episodes are due to viruses.

MICROBIOLOGY

All enteric viruses can be seen by EM and confirmed in reference or research laboratories, but in clinical settings simple diagnostics using commercially available assays are available only for rotavirus and adenovirus. The difficulty in detecting gastrointestinal viruses has precluded in-depth investigation of the epidemiologic characteristics of disease caused by these agents, particularly for sporadic cases requiring hospitalization. It also has made clinicians underestimate their importance.

Rotavirus (group A), a member of the the family Reoviridae and the most important source of severe diarrhea in children worldwide, is a 70-nm triple-shelled virus that contains 11 segments of double-stranded RNA and can be cultivated. Two outer capsid proteins are involved in neutralization activity and specify the four main serotypes commonly found in humans. The immune response to infection can be measured by antibodies in serum, though the mechanism of protection, believed to be mediated by local immunity, is not well understood. Rotaviruses with other group antigens—groups B and C—that cause epidemic diarrhea in humans are indistinguishable by EM from the more common group A strains of rotavirus. Diagnosis rests on their distinct profile on polyacrylamide gel electrophoresis (PAGE), their failure to be detected with common immunoassays to group A strains, and detection of their unique antigens by enzyme immunoassay and their distinct genetic sequences by reverse transcription–polymerase chain reaction (RT-PCR).

Norwalk-like viruses and Sapporo-like viruses are genetically distinct groups in the family Caliciviridae. They are 27 to 35 nm in size; contain positive-sense, single-stranded RNA; and cannot be grown in tissue culture or propagated in animal models. Sapporo-like viruses were previously called *classic human caliciviruses* because of the large calicis at their rim surrounding a distinct Star of David structure at the core. Until recently, the virus could be detected routinely only by EM, which is quite insensitive. Immunoassays for the Norwalk-like viruses in fecal specimens and antibodies in serum samples required non-replenishable virus and paired samples obtained from human volunteers. The recent cloning of these viruses has led to new

molecular methods to detect virus (RT-PCR, Southern blot hybridization) and characterize strains by sequence analysis, but these techniques are not yet suitable for routine use. Expression of the capsid protein of Norwalk virus in baculovirus has yielded viruslike particles that have been useful in immunoassays to detect seroconversion. Further advances in our understanding of the epidemiologic features and clinical importance of these agents will require improved diagnostic assays and further advances from research laboratories.

Enteric adenoviruses, particularly of serotypes 40, 41, and 31, are 80-nm icosohedral viruses with double-stranded DNA that grow fastidiously in cell culture. They can be detected by commercially available immunoassays to the adenovirus hexon and then serotyped using monoclonal antibodies to serotypes 40 and 41, the strains that most often provoke diarrhea. Astroviruses are rarely seen by EM and were thought to be an uncommon cause of diarrhea in children. The recent development and application of simple immunoassays to detect virus in fecal specimens and to confirm and serotype positive strains by culture and molecular methods have led to the recognition that this virus is a common pathogen in children. By EM, the 30-nm virus is often visible in large sheets and has a smooth outer surface that occasionally surrounds a star-shaped structure that gives it its name. The core contains single-stranded RNA, which has an unusual replication strategy and has been classified in its own family, Astroviridae. Simple diagnostic methods for astrovirus may be commercially available soon. Other viruses have been found by EM or PAGE in fecal specimens from patients with diarrhea, but their role as etiologic agents has not been established. They include the toroviruses, picobirnavirus, coronavirus, reovirus, pestivirus, and parvovirus.

PATHOGENESIS

Whereas the pathogenetic conduits of most viral agents of gastroenteritis have been well studied in animals, our understanding of their pathogenicity in humans is quite limited. Generally, infection occurs in the proximal portion of the small intestine and the pathologic agents, like the disease, are transitory. Rotavirus infects and damages the villous tips of mature epithelial cells, causing sluffing of the mucosa and secretory diarrhea. Norwalk infects epithelial cells as well, producing blunting of the villous tips, hypertrophy of crypt cells, and accumulation of inflammatory cells in the lamina propria. Infections with these viruses are localized to the intestine; extra-intestinal manifestations have been documented but are rare. For example, rotavirus has been found in the liver of patients who have died of severe combined immunodeficiency syndrome, and rotaviral RNA has been found by RT-PCR in cerebrospinal fluid of children with rotavirus diarrhea and seizures.

CLINICAL FEATURES

The clinical features of viral gastroenteritis can range from asymptomatic infection to overwhelming, dehydrating diarrheal illness. Vomiting is often prominent and precedes the onset of diarrhea. Rotavirus is associated with low-grade fever and dehydration that can last 3 to 7 days. In the United States, a majority of children less than 2 to 3 years of age who are hospitalized in the winter season have rotavirus. Rotavirus diarrhea is uncommon in the first 3 months of life, and the incidence declines rapidly after 2 years of age. Rotavirus also can develop in adults as a form of traveler's diarrhea, among parents and caretakers of infants with rotavirus, and among immunocompromised patients who experience prolonged shedding. Childhood diarrhea associated with other viruses is indistinguishable from that of rotavirus diarrhea.

Viral gastroenteritis in adults typically is provoked by Norwalk-like viruses and has symptoms of vomiting and diarrhea. Older patients suffer from low-grade fever, abdominal cramps, myalgias, malaise, and headaches. The incubation period is 18 to 36 hours, and the illness lasts for 18 to 48 hours and is self-limited. Fecal leukocytes and elevated white blood counts are absent. Viral agents have not been associated with dysentery, and chronic diarrhea in the context of infection with these viruses has been documented only in immunocompromised patients.

DIAGNOSIS

EM is the only method to detect the variety of agents causing diarrhea, and most diagnoses require help from a reference laboratory. Commercial assays for rotavirus and adenovirus are based on the detection of antigen in fecal specimens using enzyme-linked immunosorbent assays, latex agglutination, and PAGE. Molecular methods, including RT-PCR, are available in research laboratories to detect the caliciviruses (Norwalk-like viruses) and characterize Sapporo-like virus as well as astrovirus. Proper collection and handling of specimens are key to establishing a viral origin. Fecal specimens collected in large volume and maintained at 4°C are best suited for electron microscopy and can be used for both immune and molecular diagnostic assays. Paired acute- (0 to 5 days) and convalescent-phase (14 to 28 days) serum samples are useful to document an immune response to the virus and help establish that the virus was the causative agent of the disease and not a mere traveler in the intestinal tract.

TREATMENT

Treatment of viral diarrhea rests on the replacement of fluid and electrolyte losses with oral rehydration therapy in patients who are alert and on intravenous rehydration in patients with severe dehydration (more than 10%), recurrent vomiting, or inability to take an adequate volume of oral rehydration solution. Since most diarrheas in children are of viral origin, antibiotics are specifically contraindicated, and antimotility drugs have no established role. In immunocompromised patients, immune globulin has been suggested to treat gastroenteritis stemming from rotavirus infection; it may minimize symptoms of diarrhea caused by other viral agents.

PREVENTION AND CONTROL

At present, no specific measures are available for the control of the common childhood diarrheas caused by viral agents, except

for rotavirus. Rotavirus vaccine (Tetravalent Rhesus Rotavirus—RotaShieldR) has been licensed and recommended for the routine immunization of American children. Three oral doses of this vaccine provide more than 80% efficacy against severe rotavirus disease. This vaccine and others under development hold the prospect of preventing this specific cause of childhood diarrhea. In outbreaks, identification of the mode of transmission (water, food, shellfish, or an infected food handler) can lead to specific public health interventions. In the absence of specific control measures, nonspecific enteric precautions are recommended, particularly for outbreaks in day care centers, retirement homes, or hospital settings. These precautions include hand washing; the hygienic disposal of diapers, feces, and vomitus; and provision of clean food and water.

BIBLIOGRAPHY

American Academy of Pediatrics. Prevention of rotavirus disease: guidelines for use of rotavirus vaccine (RE9840). Policy statement. *Pediatrics* 1998; 102(6):1483–1491. Internet: www.aap.org/policy/re9840.

Blacklow NR, Greenberg HB. Viral gastroenteritis. *N Engl J Med* 1991; 325:252–264.

Centers for Disease Control and Prevention. Rotavirus vaccine for the prevention of rotavirus gastroenteritis among children. Recommendations of the Advisory Committee on Immunization Practices. *MMWR* 1999; 48(RR-2):xxx–xxx.

Duggan C, Santosham M, Glass RI. The management of acute diarrhea in children: oral rehydration, maintenance, and nutritional therapy. *MMWR* 1992;41(RR-16):1–20.

Fankhauser RL, Noel JS, Monroe SS, et al. Molecular epidemiology of small round structured viruses in outbreaks of gastroenteritis in the United States. *J Infect Dis* 1998;178:1571–1578.

Glass RI, Kilgore PE, Holman RC, et al. The epidemiology of rotavirus diarrhea in the United States: surveillance and estimates of disease burden. *J Infect Dis* 1996;174(suppl 1):S5–S11.

Glass RI, Noel JS, Mitchell D, et al. The changing epidemiology of astrovirus-associated gastroenteritis: a review. *Arch Virol* 1996;12(suppl): 287–300.

Grohmann GS, Glass RI, Pereira HG, et al. Enteric viruses and diarrhea in HIV-infected patients. *N Engl J Med* 1993;329:14–20.

Herrmann JE, Taylor DN, Echeverria P, et al. Astroviruses as a cause of gastroenteritis in children. *N Engl J Med* 1991;324:1757–1760.

Kapikian AZ, Estes MK, Chanock RM. Norwalk group of viruses. In: Fields BN, Knipe DM, Howley PM, et al., eds. *Fields Virology*, third ed., vol 1. Philadelphia: Lippincott–Raven Publishers, 1996:783–810.

Kelley's Textbook of Internal Medicine, fourth edition. Edited by H. David Humes. Lippincott Williams & Wilkins, Philadelphia © 2000.

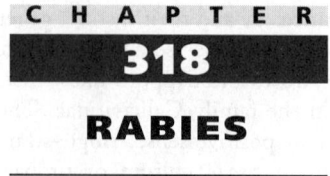

CHAPTER 318

RABIES

CHARLES E. RUPPRECHT

DEFINITION

Rabies is an acute, fatal encephalomyelitis due to infection with rabies and related lyssaviruses. It is widespread among mammals worldwide, with the exception of areas that have prevented its establishment (Oceania) or achieved secondary elimination (Great Britain). Humans almost always become infected from the bite of a rabid animal by way of virus-laden saliva. Human infection is also known as hydrophobia; unlike more recently recognized emerging conditions, such as acquired immunodeficiency syndrome and hantavirus pulmonary syndrome, rabies is one of the oldest known viral diseases.

INCIDENCE AND EPIDEMIOLOGY

Rabies is a zoonosis with diverse natural reservoirs; hence, its incidence is poorly quantified because of the variables related to the wild populations at risk. Predominant hosts are bats and mammalian carnivores. These animals include canids, such as the domestic dog as the principal global reservoir; foxes in the Arctic, eastern Canada, portions of New England, Central and Western Europe, the Middle East, and scattered foci throughout the western United States; coyotes in the western United States and Latin America; skunks, primarily in the central and western United States, Canada, and portions of Latin America; raccoons, in the eastern United States; and several species of viverrids, such as the mongoose in Asia, Africa, and several Caribbean islands. "Bat" rabies per se is a New World phenomenon, described primarily among the insectivorous species in the Western Hemisphere and the hematophagous vampires in Latin America. Related lyssaviruses have been diagnosed in African, European, and Australian bat species. Although the disease is naturally maintained by relatively few taxa, rabies can affect any mammal, such as ungulates, and result in a largely "dead-end" infection. Contrary to popular belief, cases of rabies in rodents (mice, rats), lagomorphs (rabbits, hares), and other small mammals are uniformly rare.

Rather than a global rabies pandemic, single or multispecies assemblages are apparent when disease surveillance is practiced systematically. Combined with historical temporal and geographic data, antigenic characterization and nucleotide sequence analysis can be used to understand and compartmentalize rabies virus with different reservoirs responsible for their perpetuation and thus attribute relative risks of human disease from differential animal exposure. For example, during 1997, only four human fatalities but 8,509 animal rabies cases (an increase of 19% over 1996) were reported in the United States (including the District of Columbia and Puerto Rico). In contrast to fulminant canine rabies before World War II, more than 90% of current animal rabies cases are in wildlife. Most of these cases resulted from continued spread of a predominant raccoon rabies virus variant, because of unrestricted progression of an outbreak initiated during the late 1970s by animal translocation to the Virginias from an infected nidus in the southeastern United States. By 1997, New York State (including New York City) alone reported 1,266 rabies cases (versus only 54 in 1989), primarily as a consequence of the raccoon outbreak; in contrast, Hawaii remains unique in never reporting a case of indigenously acquired rabies, the result, in part, of its isolation.

Rabies cases in other important wildlife were also reported, primarily skunks (2,040 cases) and foxes (448 cases), in the Midwest, Alaska, and the eastern and western United States, respectively, and 958 bat rabies cases were widely distributed over 46 states and the District of Columbia. Alarmingly, new wildlife rabies outbreaks continue to emerge: 83 cases of rabies in coyotes were diagnosed in 1995 (80 from southern Texas). By comparison, only seven rabid coyotes had been reported from that state during 1997, which put in place a large-scale oral vaccination program. Domestic animals most at risk include those with a lower probability of induced immunity from vaccination but higher potential for rabies exposure if poorly supervised, such as cats. Consequently, the 300 cases of rabies reported in cats during 1997, almost entirely from states also reporting raccoon rabies, constituted a 13% increase over 1996; rabies cases in cats often surpass its canine counterpart, owing in part to the increased popularity of cats as pets but also to lower rates of vaccination. By temporal comparison, 126 cases of rabies in dogs were reported in the United States during 1997, an increase of 14% from 1996.

Human rabies is rare in developed countries. Before the 1940s, human rabies cases numbered in the hundreds, but between 1981 and 1998, only 37 human deaths were reported in the United States, 12 of which were likely acquired abroad. Of the remaining cases suspected to have resulted from infection while in the United States, 22 were associated with bat rabies virus variants. Before 1960, most U.S. human rabies cases originated from the bite of rabid dogs and, more rarely, cats, whereas a definitive history of animal exposure often is difficult to elicit in the case of most of the current human fatalities. In contrast to North America and Europe, where wildlife rabies predominates, in Southeast Asia, Latin America, and Africa, dogs continue to be the principal causative vectors of rabies to humans, with a consequent high case load (estimated at more than 25,000 annual human fatalities in India alone).

ETIOLOGY

Rabies belongs to the RNA virus family Rhabdoviridae, genus *Lyssavirus*. On electron microscopy, rabies virus has a characteristic bullet-shaped morphologic picture (~75 × 180 nm), a nucleocapsid core composed of ribonucleoprotein, and a lipid envelope through which spikes of glycoprotein project. Lyssaviruses are inactivated readily by heat, ultraviolet radiation, and most detergents. Two antigens of rabies virus have diagnostic and clinical importance: antibodies to the nucleocapsid can identify intracytoplasmic viral inclusions (Negri bodies) in neurons, and the surface glycoprotein stimulates virus-neutralizing antibodies.

Viruses isolated from rabid animals previously were thought to be indistinguishable, regardless of species or geographic origin. Variants of rabies virus and other lyssaviruses now can be differentiated by monoclonal antibody typing and genetic sequencing. Although true rabies viruses are global in distribution, related lyssaviruses potentially capable of zoonotic transmission are restricted to the Old World (Duvenhage, Mokola, and Lagos bat; European bat; and Australian bat viruses).

PATHOGENESIS

Much of what is known concerning the dynamic events after rabies virus infection is based on experimental animal inoculation. Transmission in nature usually originates from the bite of an infected animal, with the introduction of virus-laden saliva deep into the wound. Virus gains direct access to the central nervous system (CNS) from severed or intact unmyelinated peripheral nerves, in the vicinity of motor end plates or a neuromuscular spindle apparatus. Virus may attach at acetylcholine-related receptors or a separate series of unrelated receptors. Rabies virus travels centripetally at approximately 2 to 3 mm per hour by retrograde axoplasmic flow to the CNS, where replication and assembly of mature virions ensue. Movement across neuronal synapses may involve budding from intracytoplasmic and plasma membranes, or spread may result from direct cell-to-cell passage by fusion mechanisms. Viremia has not been implicated to any significant extent. Successive cycles of replication and passive transport result in widespread dissemination throughout the brain, particularly the brain stem, hippocampus, subcortical nuclei, limbic cortex, and Purkinje cells in the cerebellum. Infection progresses from the CNS with the centrifugal migration of virus through the nerve terminals of a variety of organs, most notably the salivary glands, by way of neural innervation of secretory cells. At this portal of exit, additional viral replication may take place.

Variations on the generalized neurotropic pathogenesis scheme may include localization of virus in striated muscle at or near the bite site for long periods before neural transit and replication in dorsal root ganglia; direct infection of sensory neurons or olfactory neuroepithelia by aerosol transmission of virus under unique environmental conditions; viral entry through the gastrointestinal route; sequestration of virus in additional non-nervous tissue; and, very rarely, transplacental transmission. Traditionally, the bite route is regarded as the primary means of rabies virus transmission, but less is known about other lyssaviruses.

The final outcome of rabies virus–induced encephalitis usually is death from neurologic dysfunction of vital brain regions. Gross findings are lacking in most cases. The histopathologic lesions are nonspecific and include neuronal degeneration, neuronophagia, and monocytic cellular infiltration with perivascular cuffing, as expected from viral inflammation of the CNS. Cytoplasmic inclusion bodies of viral nucleocapsid aggregates, or Negri bodies, in CNS neurons formed the basis of postmortem laboratory examination in concert with the intracerebral inoculation of laboratory animals with suspect brain material, until replacement by the more sensitive fluorescent antibody technique as the preferred method of rabies diagnosis.

Rabies virus infection per se is not synonymous with death. Patients' outcomes can be predicated in part on the dose of virus, the route of infection, the particular virus variant, the biting animal species in question, as well as the age and physiologic status of the host. The incubation period is usually 1 to 3 months, but it is highly variable and ranges from days to years. The particular role played by humoral and cell-mediated immunity in the pathogenesis of rabies and viral evasion of host-derived responses until late in the course of infection are poorly understood.

CLINICAL FEATURES

Exposure to rabies is defined by transdermal or mucosal contact with potentially infectious virus-laden material, such as saliva or CNS tissue. The primary route of transmission is the bite of a rabid animal. Very rarely, rabies develops as the result of a few other nonbite conduits; four patients are believed to have acquired infection by the aerosol route (two from laboratory accidents and two from prolonged exposure to the highly humid air from caves inhabited by millions of bats). Human-to-human transmission is possible in theory, but it has not been readily documented, with the exception of eight cases resulting from corneal transplant; both the donors and the recipients succumbed to rabies.

The symptomless period between exposure and first sign of disease is usually 1 to 3 months, rarely less than 10 days or more than a year. During a prodromal phase of 4 to 7 days, the symptoms are initially nonspecific, with complaints including moderate fever, headache, chills, cough, sore throat, dyspnea, lack of appetite, weakness, nausea, vomiting, or general malaise. Thereafter, in the acute neurologic phase, there may be an array of signs and symptoms, including intermittent anxiety, confusion, excitation, agitation, insomnia, hallucinations, percussion myoedema, cranial nerve deficits, chorea, dysphagia, anorexia, hypersalivation, piloerection, priapism, paresis, paralysis, and sometimes maniacal behavior, interspersed with periods of calm. Classic symptoms include paresthesia at or near the site of bite exposure and hydrophobia (a synonymous term for the human disease) or aerophobia, manifesting as phobic pharyngeal or inspirational musculature spasms after provocative stimuli, such as anticipation of swallowing or air currents. One type of the disease, "dumb rabies," may spare central consciousness but take the form of ascending paralysis and progressive unresponsiveness as primary features of the clinical spectrum, gradually progressing to coma. Once the neurologic phase nears its termination in 2 to 10 days, the remaining clinical course is rapid and downhill, with death ensuing within days and usually attributable to respiratory or cardiac failure. Because human rabies is rare in developed countries and disease onset is nonspecific, diagnosis may be delayed until late in the course of disease or at postmortem examination.

LABORATORY FINDINGS

Rabies should be suspected in any case of unexplained viral encephalomyelitis, especially if there is a history of animal bite within the past 3 months. It is important to include arbovirus, enterovirus, and herpesvirus encephalitides in the differential diagnosis. In suspect animals, diagnosis is confirmed only at euthanasia by the fluorescent antibody test on brain tissue. In human cases, routine laboratory tests are nonspecific. Antemortem diagnosis can be confirmed by the finding of rabies antigen

00

with fluorescent antibody testing of a brain biopsy specimen or in highly innervated areas, such as a full-thickness nuchal skin biopsy sample. Virus may be isolated from saliva in cell culture or by animal inoculation. Rabies virus RNA can be detected by the reverse transcription–polymerase chain reaction technique from saliva or sometimes from other tissues. Evidence of rabies-specific antibodies in the serum of an unvaccinated person or at anytime in the cerebrospinal fluid of a suspect patient also confirms the diagnosis.

OPTIMAL MANAGEMENT

Rabies remains a significant global viral disease that almost inevitably results in death, without spontaneous recovery. With the institution of prompt and proper prophylaxis, its prevention is virtually ensured. In excess of 1,000,000 humans annually undergo antirabies postexposure prophylaxis, and an estimated 50,000 others or more succumb, primarily from the bite of an infected dog and inappropriate or no prophylaxis. Contact between humans and animals is frequent, but exposure to a rabid animal is a relatively rare event in most developed countries. Application of regional epidemiologic surveillance and knowledge of rabies pathogenesis can significantly minimize human morbidity and mortality through the identification of likely reservoirs, development of vaccination consideration charts, and estimation of occupational risk groups (Tables 318.1, 318.2, and 318.3). After a bite from an infected mammal, postexposure treatment of rabies in humans, as recommended by the United States Advisory Committee on Immunization Practices, includes proper wound care and the simultaneous administration of multiple doses of an efficacious rabies vaccine together with antirabies immune globulin of human origin (HRIG).

Modern inactivated rabies vaccines produced in cell culture are used throughout the developed world and are major improvements over the Pasteurian neural attenuated products of animal origin from the past century. The human diploid cell vaccine was the first of this new generation of biologics, one of only three vaccines now licensed in the United States. The other two are rabies vaccine, adsorbed, which is produced in fetal rhesus lung culture, and a purified chick embryo cell vaccine, grown in primary chicken fibroblast culture; both are used for either preexposure or postexposure treatment (Tables 318.2 and 318.4). Although the concept of potent cell culture vaccines and HRIG inclusion is not new, it is little practiced; the majority of prophylactic treatment in Africa, Asia, and Latin America is with nerve tissue vaccines only, because of the associated high cost of production of alternative products. It is unclear whether the lack of an even greater burden of human death due to rabies can be attributed to relative human insusceptibility, differences in regional genetics, variation in local virus virulence, wound severity factors, degree of surveillance, or other phenomena.

Preexposure rabies vaccination may be offered to certain risk groups whose activities often bring them into contact with rabies virus or rabid animals. Such immunization simplifies postexposure prophylaxis; benefits those exposed whose postexposure prophylaxis might be delayed, such as travelers to regions of enzootic dog rabies; and may protect people at risk of inapparent exposure. Although preexposure vaccination does not eliminate the need for local wound care and proper boosters, it does simplify such therapy by removal of the need for HRIG administration and minimization of the number of vaccine doses required.

PROGNOSIS

Once symptoms manifest in the naive patient, rabies is invariably fatal; recovery has been well documented in only four patients,

TABLE 318.1.	RABIES POSTEXPOSURE PROPHYLAXIS GUIDE, UNITED STATES	
Animal Type	**Evaluation and Disposition of Animal**	**Postexposure Prophylaxis Recommendations**
Dogs, cats, and ferrets	Healthy and available for 10 days' observation	Should not begin prophylaxis unless signs of rabies develop in the animal[a]
	Rabid or suspected rabid	Immediate vaccination
	Unknown (escaped)	Consult public health officials
Skunks, raccoons, foxes, and most other carnivores; bats	Regarded as rabid unless laboratory tests show negative results[b]	Immediate vaccination
Livestock, rodents, lagomorphs (rabbits and hares), and other mammals	Consider individually	Consult public health officials
		Bites of squirrels, hamsters, guinea pigs, gerbils, chipmunks, rats, mice, other small rodents, rabbits, and hares almost never require antirabies prophylaxis

[a] During the 10-day holding period, begin prophylaxis at the first sign of rabies in a dog, cat, or ferret that has bitten someone. The suspect animal should be euthanized immediately and tested.
[b] The animal should be euthanized and tested as soon as possible. Holding for observation is not recommended. Discontinue vaccine if immunofluorescence test results are negative.
(From Centers for Disease Control and Prevention. Human rabies prevention—United States, 1999. *MMWR* 1999;48(RR-1):1, with permission.)

TABLE 318.2.	RABIES POSTEXPOSURE PROPHYLAXIS SCHEDULE, UNITED STATES

Vaccination Status	Treatment	Regimen[a]
Not previously vaccinated	Wound cleansing	All postexposure prophylaxis should begin with immediate, thorough cleansing of all wounds with soap and water. If available, a virucidal agent, such as a povidone-iodine solution, should be used to irrigate the wounds.
	HRIG	Administer 20 IU/kg body weight. If anatomically feasible, the full dose should be infiltrated around the wound(s), and the rest should be administered i.m. at an anatomical site distant from vaccine. HRIG should not be administered in the same syringe as vaccine. Because HRIG may partially suppress active production of antibody, no more than the recommended dose should be given.
	Vaccine	HDCV, RVA, or PCEC, 1.0 mL i.m. (deltoid area), one each on days 0, 3, 7, 14, and 28[b]
Previously vaccinated[c]	Wound cleansing	All postexposure prophylaxis should begin with immediate, thorough cleansing of all wounds with soap and water. If available, a virucidal agent such as povidone-iodine solution should be used to irrigate the wounds.
	HRIG	HRIG should not be administered.
	Vaccine	HDCV, RVA, or PCEC, 1.0 mL i.m. (deltoid area), one each on days 0 and 3[b]

HRIG, human antirabies immune globulin; i.m., intramuscular; HDCV, human diploid cell vaccine; RVA, rabies vaccine, adsorbed; PCEC, purified chick embryo cell vaccine.
[a] These regimens are applicable for all age groups, including children.
[b] The deltoid area is the only acceptable site of vaccination for adults and older children. For younger children, the outer aspect of the thigh may be used. Vaccine should never be administered in the gluteal area.
[c] Any person with a history of preexposure vaccination or previous postexposure prophylaxis with HDCV, RVA, or PCEC or previous vaccination with any other type of rabies vaccine and a documented history of antibody response to the previous vaccination.
(From Centers for Disease Control and Prevention. Human rabies prevention—United States, 1999. *MMWR* 1999;48(RR-1):1, with permission.)

TABLE 318.3.	RABIES PREEXPOSURE PROPHYLAXIS GUIDE, UNITED STATES

Risk Category	Nature of Risk	Typical Populations	Preexposure Recommendations
Continuous	Virus present continuously, often in high concentrations; specific exposures likely to go unrecognized; bite, nonbite, or aerosal exposure	Rabies research laboratory worker, rabies biologics production workers[a]	Primary course, serologic testing every 6 months, booster vaccination if antibody level is below acceptable level[b]
Frequent	Exposure usually episodic, with source recognized, but exposure may also be unrecognized; bite, nonbite, or aerosal exposure	Rabies diagnostic laboratory workers, spelunkers, veterinarians and staff, and animal-control and wildlife workers in rabies enzootic areas[a]	Primary course, serologic testing every 2 years, booster vaccination if antibody titer is below acceptale level[b]
Infrequent (greater than population at large)	Exposure nearly always episodic with source recognized, bite or nonbite exposure	Veterinarians and animal-control and wildlife workers in areas with low rabies rates, veterinary students, travelers visting areas where rabies is enzootic and immediate access to appropriate medical care—including biologics—is limited	Primary course, no serologic testing or booster vaccination
Rare (population at large)	Exposures always episodic with source recognized, bite or nonbite exposure	U.S. population at large, including persons in rabies epizootic areas	No vaccination necessary

[a] Judgment of relative risk and extra monitoring of vaccination status of laboratory workers is the responsibility of the laboratory supervisor.
[b] Minimum acceptable antibody level is complete virus neutralization at a 1:5 serum dilution by the rapid fluorescent focus inhibition test. A booster dose should be administered if the titer is below this level.
(From Centers for Disease Control and Prevention. Human rabies prevention—United States, 1999. *MMWR* 1999;48(RR-1):1, with permission.)

TABLE 318.4.	RABIES PREEXPOSURE PROPHYLAXIS SCHEDULE, UNITED STATES

Type of Vaccination	Route	Regimen
Primary	i.m.	HDCV, RVA, or PCEC, 1.0 mL (deltoid area), one each on days 0, 7, and 21 or 28
	i.d.	HDCV, 0.1 mL, one each on days 0, 7, and 21 or 28
Booster[a]	i.m.	HDCV, RVA, or PCEC, 1.0 mL (deltoid area), day 0 only
	i.d.	HDCV, 0.1 mL, day 0 only

i.m., intramuscular; i.d., intradermal; *HDCV*, human diploid cell vaccine; *RVA*, rabies vaccine, adsorbed; PCEC, purified chick embryo cell vaccine.
[a] Administration of routine booster dose of vaccine depends on exposure risk category.
(From the Centers for Disease Control and Prevention. Human rabies prevention—United States, 1999. *MMWR* 1999;48(RR-1):1, with permission).

two with serious neurologic adverse effects. Cardiac dysrhythmias, respiratory failure, and systemic nosocomial infections may all occur. Specific antiviral treatment is currently unavailable. Despite the experimental use of parenteral or intrathecal application of rabies immunoglobulin, $F(ab')_2$ rabies immunoglobulin fragments, cytosine or adenine arabinoside, interferon, acyclovir, antithymocyte globulin, steroids, vidarabine, tribavirin, inosine pranobex, or ribavirin, no treatment of clinical human rabies has shown any proven benefit. The most effective means to protect humans against this zoonosis are preventive measures designed to lessen the opportunity of contact with the virus, including compulsory companion animal vaccination and reduction of the risk of wildlife exposure through targeted public education and sound animal control policies, and postexposure prophylaxis when these measures fail.

BIBLIOGRAPHY

Centers for Disease Control and Prevention. Compendium of animal rabies control, 1999. *MMWR* 1999;48(RR-3):1–9.

Centers for Disease Control and Prevention. Human rabies—Virginia, 1998. *MMWR* 1999;48:95–97.

Centers for Disease Control and Prevention. Human rabies prevention—United States, 1999. Recommendations of the Advisory Committee on Immunization Practices. *MMWR* 1999;48(RR-1):1–21.

Hanlon CA, Rupprecht CE. The reemergence of rabies. In: Scheld WM, Armstrong D, Hughes JM, eds. *Emerging infections*, vol 1. Washington, DC: ASM Press, 1998:59.

Krebs JW, Smith JS, Rupprecht CE, et al. Rabies surveillance in the United States during 1997. *J Am Vet Med Assoc* 1998;213:1713–1728.

Noah DL, Drenzek CL, Smith JS, et al. Epidemiology of human rabies in the United States, 1980 to 1996. *Ann Intern Med* 1998;128:922–930.

Rupprecht CE, Dietzschold B, Koprowski H. Lyssaviruses. *Curr Top Microbiol Immunol* 1994;187:1.

Rupprecht CE, Smith JS, Krebs J, et al. Current issues in rabies prevention in the United States. *Public Health Rep* 1996;111:400–407.

Smith JS. New aspects of rabies with emphasis on epidemiology, diagnosis, and prevention of the disease in the United States. *Clin Microbiol Rev* 1996;9:166–176.

World Health Organization. *Eighth report of the WHO expert committee on rabies*. Geneva: World Health Organization, 1992. (WHO technical report series 2824.)

Kelley's Textbook of Internal Medicine, fourth edition. Edited by H. David Humes. Lippincott Williams & Wilkins, Philadelphia © 2000.

C H A P T E R 319

HUMAN PAPILLOMAVIRUSES

WILLIAM BONNEZ

DEFINITION

Human papillomaviruses (HPVs) form a large, ubiquitous collection of more than 100 distinct DNA viruses that latently or actively infect the tegumental and mucosal epithelia. Active infections manifest in the form of tumors that range from benign (such as warts) to malignant (such as squamous cell carcinomas). HPVs can be divided into three broad groups according to the tissues they infect and their biologic characteristics (Table 319.1). The first group is represented by the cutaneous HPVs, which are distributed over the distal extremities of the body, where they occasion deep plantar warts, common warts, and flat warts. The anogenital HPVs constitute the second group. They are found not only over the external genitalia, vagina, cervix, anus, and anal canal but also in the upper respiratory mucosal surfaces. They produce such conditions as nasal or laryngeal papillomas but mostly anogenital warts, intraepithelial neoplasias, and cancers. HPVs of the third group are dispersed over

TABLE 319.1.	MAIN DISEASES AND HPV TYPES ASSOCIATIONS[a]

Diseases	HPV Types
Deep plantar warts	1, 2
Common warts	2, 1
Flat warts	3, 10
Anogenital warts (condylomata acuminata)	6, 11
Intraepithelial neoplasia	
Low grade	6, 11
High grade	**16, 18**[b]
Cervical carcinoma	**16, 18**[b]
Recurrent respiratory papillomatosis	6, 11
Epidermodysplasia verruciformis	2, 3, 10, **5, 8**, 9, 12, **14**, 15, **17**[b]

[a] HPV, human papillomavirus. Further information on HPV types can be found at http://hpv-web.lanl.gov.
[b] HPV types with high malignant potential are indicated in bold.

the trunk, proximal extremities, and face. They cause the rare disease epidermodysplasia verruciformis as well as skin lesions in allograft transplant recipients.

INCIDENCE AND EPIDEMIOLOGY

Cutaneous warts are most common in children and affect up to 20% of the population. More than two-thirds of affected patients have common warts, while one-third, usually older patients, have plantar warts. Flat warts make up less than 5% of cutaneous warts. The mode of acquisition is not well understood, but microtrauma and humidity can play a role.

It is estimated that in the United States 500,000 subjects acquire anogenital warts each year and 1% of the sexually active population is affected. The incidence seems to have risen over the past 30 years. In a study done in the United States, 8% of college women had cytologic evidence of HPV infection by Papanicolaou (Pap) smear of the uterine cervix. When the presence of cervical HPV infection was determined by using an HPV DNA polymerase chain reaction assay, the prevalence increased to 46%. Many cervical HPV infections are in fact transient, and it appears that the development of cytologic lesions is associated with persistence and high levels of HPV DNA.

Anogenital HPV infections are mostly sexually transmitted, as evidenced by their association with the onset of sexual activity and the number of sexual partners. In the case of rare recurrent respiratory papillomatosis, risk factors in the juvenile-onset form of the disease include the presence in the mother of genital warts at the time of delivery and oral sex in the adult-onset form. The smoke plume generated during wart ablation by laser or electrosurgery may be infectious, but the role of fomites in disease transmission remains to be established.

There is now very strong evidence that some of the HPV types associated with anogenital infection cause cancer of the uterine cervix. The DNA of these so-called high-risk types (e.g., HPV-16 and HPV-18) was found in 93% of cervical squamous cell carcinomas worldwide. In addition, the presence of high-risk HPV types in the cervix of women with normal cytologic features is a very strong predictor of the development of high-grade cervical intraepithelial neoplasia, the lesion precursor to cancer. Seroepidemiologic studies also have confirmed these relationships. Although HPV infection is a necessary factor for the vast majority of cervical cancers, it is not sufficient. The other co-factors are not well characterized but may include immunosuppression.

A strong epidemiologic association has been established between anal cancer and anal HPV infection or, to a lesser degree, anogenital warts. Co-infection with the human immunodeficiency virus (HIV) is an additional risk factor for anal cancer. Weaker links exist between HPV infection and cancers of the vulva, vagina, and penis. Lesions of epidermodysplasia verruciformis can degenerate into squamous cell carcinomas, and the role of HPV in nonmelanoma skin cancers is being investigated.

ETIOLOGY

HPVs belong to the *Papillomavirus* genus of the family Papovaviridae and are made of a naked, icosahedral, 55-nm capsid that encloses a circular, double-stranded, super-coiled DNA approximately 7,900 base pairs in length. These small viruses have the same genetic organization, which consists of three different functional regions. A noncoding stretch, called the upstream regulatory region, possesses numerous binding sites for cellular and viral proteins that are the main biologic switches for the virus. A second region is made up of several genes (E1, E2, E4, E5, E6, and E7) that code for nonstructural proteins. Among them, E1 and E2 are necessary for viral replication, whereas E6 and E7 are essential to the oncogenic properties of HPV by interfering with at least two key cellular tumor-suppressor proteins. The E6 protein binds to the p53 tumor-suppressor protein and leads to its accelerated degradation, while E7 binds to and inactivates the retinoblastoma protein, Rb. E7 is the major oncogene. Introduced alone or in concert with E6, it causes cell immortalization and malignant transformation in cell lines, and in transgenic mice it leads to the formation of skin squamous cell carcinomas. The third genomic region comprises the two structural genes L1 and L2 that encode the major and minor capsid proteins, respectively.

Because of the inability to propagate HPVs in vitro and, under most circumstances, to purify virions, the rich diversity of these viruses was recognized only in the past three decades using genetic methods rather than the more traditional serotyping. HPV genotypes differ from one another by more than 10% in DNA homology of the L1 gene. At least 75 distinct HPVs have been characterized fully, and more have been identified. HPV virions appear to be relatively resistant to physico-chemical factors and thus may persist in the environment.

PATHOGENESIS

HPVs infect the keratinized and nonkeratinized stratified epithelia only of human beings, but each HPV type has particular anatomic predilections that result in different diseases (Table 319.1). The typical incubation period of HPVs causing cutaneous and genital warts is 3 to 4 months. Incubation durations ranging from 6 weeks to as long as 2 years have been observed in experimental inoculation experiments. Susceptibility to infection appears to vary among individuals, and in the case of genital warts, only two-thirds of the asymptomatic sexual partners of patients show signs of warts within 2 years of follow-up.

The virus is presumed to infect the keratinocytes in the basal, dividing layer of the epithelium. As the keratinocytes differentiate while moving toward the epithelial surface, the different phases of the HPV life cycle are activated sequentially, resulting in the formation of viral particles that eventually are released with the desquamating epithelial cells. In benign infections, this process is associated with the proliferation of all the epithelial layers, except the basal layer, hence causing papillomatosis, acanthosis, parakeratosis, and hyperkeratosis. Another characteristic feature of the infection, seen often with some HPV types, is the development in the upper stratum spinosum of a large cell with a distinctive perinuclear vacuole, the koilocyte (from the Greek *koilos*, meaning "cavity").

Only a subset of HPV types also causes malignant lesions, typically squamous cell carcinomas (Table 319.1). In the anogenital epithelia, intraepithelial neoplasias (also improperly called dysplasias) are transitional lesions that may regress eventually or progress to invasive carcinoma. Intraepithelial neoplasia is characterized by a proliferation of basal cells and an abundance of abnormal mitoses (dyskaryosis). While HPV DNA remains episomal in benign lesions, in the highest grades of intraepithelial neoplasias (carcinoma in situ) copies of the viral genome become integrated into the host genome. This integration typically disrupts the E2 gene, which loses its negative regulatory properties on the expression of E6 and E7 oncogenes. The vast majority of HPV infections are neither active nor oncogenic, but latent. The factors that maintain latency are not known.

Immunosuppression and immunodeficiency are risk factors for more frequent and florid disease manifestations, a persistent course, and, when oncogenic HPVs are involved, malignant evolution. Genetic factors control the development of epidermodysplasia verruciformis. HPV infection elicits an inconsistent humoral response. The significance of neutralizing antibodies in human beings is unclear at present, but in animal papillomavirus infection-neutralizing antibodies are protective.

■ CLINICAL FEATURES

CUTANEOUS WARTS

The three main types of cutaneous warts are deep plantar warts, common warts, and plane or flat warts. Deep plantar warts (or myrmecia, from the Greek for "anthill") are typically few in number and range in size from 2 to 10 mm. Each lesion looks like a deep-seated, soft, multistranded bundle of keratin fibers, transected as it protrudes from the skin. Deep plantar warts are often present on pressure points, which makes them painful and sometimes confused with corns and calluses. Shaving of the wart surface, however, reveals the punctation of bleeding blood vessels, a distinctive sign. Myrmecia can be present on the palms as well.

Common warts are well-demarcated, hemispheric papules with a rough, hyperkeratotic surface. They can be found anywhere on the hand, but also on the soles of the feet, where they may coalesce and flatten to form mosaic warts. Occasionally, they can be found in the oral cavity. Plane warts are characteristically small, flat, slightly irregular papules found on the face, neck, and hands of children. Most cutaneous warts spontaneously disappear. In one study of children, the rates of resolution at 1 and 5 years follow-up were 50% and 90%, respectively. Malignant degeneration is extremely rare.

ANOGENITAL WARTS AND RELATED DISEASES

Anogenital or venereal warts (also called condylomata acuminata) take the form of flesh-colored or more pigmented papules that are sessile or attached by a broad and short peduncle. They offer great variation in size, but usually their diameters range from 2 to 8 mm. Their surface contour may look like a mulberry or a cauliflower, but they can be jagged or acuminate. In men, warts are mostly distributed over the penile shaft and in the preputial cavity of the uncircumcised penis. In women, the vulva, particularly the introitus, can be affected. Perianal lesions are more common in women than in men, but their prevalence is increased substantially by anal intercourse, which also is associated with extension of the disease to the anal canal. In a minority of women, vaginal and cervical involvement can occur in the form of condylomas.

HPV papillomas tend to turn white when exposed to acetic acid. Thus, previous soaking of the genitalia with 3% to 5% acetic acid (or white vinegar) for 1 to 3 minutes and examination with magnifying optics, like a loupe or a colposcope, facilitate the detection and identification of lesions, particularly on the cervix. The presence of acetowhite macules on the vulva alone is not diagnostic of HPV infection. Symptoms are absent in about three-fourths of patients with anogenital warts; when present, they typically consist of itching, burning, or tenderness. The greatest impact of the disease is psychosexual. Our knowledge of the natural history is very limited, but 10% to 20% of patients experience complete spontaneous resolution over a 3- to 4-month period.

Exophytic anogenital warts rarely transform into carcinomas, but large, bleeding, or darkly pigmented lesions merit expert attention and biopsy, because they may be intraepithelial neoplasias or early carcinomas. Intraepithelial neoplasias (IN) can involve the penis (PIN), vulva (VIN), vagina (VAIN), anus (AIN), and cervix (CIN). They all carry a risk of progression to cancer that has been defined best for CIN and increases from grade 1 through grade 3. For example, CIN-3, the highest grade, is associated with a 12% chance of progression to cancer. The presence of perianal warts and a history of passive anal intercourse should prompt an anoscopic exam, particularly in a patient infected with HIV, because of the increased risk of AIN and anal carcinoma.

Recurrent respiratory papillomatosis is uncommon and typically develops either in early childhood or young adulthood. It is heralded by voice hoarseness, stridor, or dyspnea, which reflect the proliferation of papillomas in the larynx. The course of the disease can be relentless, with obstruction of the airways, local extension, and, occasionally, malignant transformation after irradiation. Nasal papillomatosis is another rare condition, which, like recurrent respiratory papillomatosis, is caused by an infection with anogenital HPVs. Anogenital HPVs can produce oral condylomas (the mouth should be examined) and conjunctival papillomas.

EPIDERMODYSPLASIA VERRUCIFORMIS AND RELATED CONDITIONS

Epidermodysplasia verruciformis (EV) is a very rare condition characterized by flat papules or red macules distributed over the face, torso, and upper extremities, which transform into squamous cell carcinomas at high rates in sun-exposed areas. EV-associated viruses have been recovered in squamous cell carcinomas, EV-like lesions, and the healthy skin of immunosuppressed solid-organ-transplant recipients. HPV-5 has been implicated in the etiologic course of psoriasis.

LABORATORY FINDINGS

HISTOLOGY AND CYTOLOGY

Histologic examination is the gold standard used for the diagnosis of HPV disease. Biopsy is indicated when the clinical diagnosis is in question or when there is a risk of malignancy. Screening for cervical malignancy is done by cytology (Pap smear). Cytologic findings are usually reported according to the Bethesda classification, which distinguishes four types of squamous cell abnormalities: (a) atypical squamous cell of unknown significance (ASCUS), the single largest category of diagnoses; (b) low-grade squamous intraepithelial lesion (LSIL), which corresponds to CIN-1 by histology; (c) high-grade squamous intraepithelial lesion (HSIL), the correlate of CIN-2 and -3; and (d) squamous cell carcinoma. As a detection tool of cervical carcinoma in the general population, the Pap smear is 80% sensitive and more than 99% specific.

SEROLOGY

The best serologic assays of HPV infection use HPV viruslike particles (VLP), but they are not commercially available. VLPs are produced by expression in eukaryotic cells via the appropriate vector (baculovirus, vaccinia virus, and so on) of the gene (L1) that encodes the major capsid protein. The protein self-assembles into a capsid-like structure that bears the same antigenic properties as the virion. The antigenicity seems genotype-specific. Unfortunately, only half to two-thirds of infected patients have detectable antibodies, which limits the assays' usefulness for clinical diagnosis.

MOLECULAR DIAGNOSIS

The diagnosis of HPV infection, particularly in the absence of disease, rests on the detection of viral nucleic acids. The Hybrid Capture assay (Digene Diagnostics) is the only HPV detection kit approved by the Food and Drug Administration and currently on the market. In that assay, HPV DNA is extracted from the target tissue or cells and bound in liquid phase to an HPV type-specific RNA probe. The DNA–RNA complex is captured by an antibody coating the test tube and detected quantitatively by another antibody conjugated to alkaline phosphatase. The assay uses two pools of probes—one that detects anogenital HPVs with a low oncogenic risk and another that recognizes anogenital HPVs with a high oncogenic risk. A more sensitive hybrid capture that detects additional high-risk HPVs is likely to become commercially available. The Hybrid Capture assay appears to be helpful in the management of Pap smear with ASCUS, in the proper triage strategy to colposcopy, and in the screening of postmenopausal women. Polymerase chain reaction assays are the most sensitive tools for the detection and typing of HPV DNA, but they are reserved for research only. Consensus and degenerate primers have been designed to amplify known and new HPV types.

OPTIMAL MANAGEMENT

Three principles govern the management of HPVs. First, current treatments are directed at the diseases rather than at the infections caused by HPVs. Second, the often self-limited nature of benign HPV diseases should be kept in mind when considering the costs and limitations of the available treatment methods. Third, screening and detection of premalignant and malignant anogenital lesions is part of the optimal management of HPV diseases.

CUTANEOUS WARTS

Most cutaneous warts will spontaneously disappear; if treatment is desired for cosmetic reasons or to alleviate symptoms, it is important to consider carefully the risk of scarring and mutilation. Hand warts are best treated with a salicylic and lactic acid (SAL) paint (salicylic acid, lactic acid, collodion, 1:1:4). Numerous over-the-counter medications are available (Duofilm, Occlusal, Paplex, among others), and about two-thirds of patients respond to daily self-application for up to 12 weeks. Cryotherapy administered every 3 weeks gives the same response rate. This is the favored mode of treatment for eyelid, nasal, and periungual warts. Mosaic warts respond to topical SAL paint, 10% glutaraldehyde, or 5-fluorouracil. Deep plantar warts respond even better to treatment with SAL paint or 25% podophyllum resin, but preliminary paring may be necessary. Flat warts usually do not require treatment.

The cited treatment methods generally are well tolerated. Curettage to partially remove a deep plantar wart may be appropriate, but more extensive surgery is not needed as a rule. Electrosurgical techniques tend to cause scarring and are better reserved for small and well-localized lesions. Myriad other treatments, including suggestion, have been proposed for the treatment of cutaneous warts without being submitted to a rigorous evaluation.

ANOGENITAL WARTS

It is unclear whether the treatment of anogenital warts has any effect on the eradication of HPV, the risk of HPV transmission, or the extremely rare malignant transformation of the lesions. Consequently, the indications for therapy are the alleviation of physical and psychological symptoms and cosmesis. Because none of the treatment options are completely satisfactory, it is important to discuss with the patient the goals of therapy, the costs, the possible adverse reactions, and the alternatives, including the fact that spontaneous resolution is not uncommon. A great variety of therapies have been promoted for the treatment of anogenital warts. We focus on the most common and best studied and make comments regarding their application to related conditions. As with cutaneous warts, most of the treatments aim at the destruction of wart tissues by physico-chemical means.

TABLE 319.2.	MANAGEMENT STRATEGIES FOR ANOGENITAL WARTS	
Priority[a]	**Provider**	**Therapy**[b]
First line	Patient	Imiquimod
		Podofilox
First line	Practitioner	Cryotherapy
		Trichloracetic acid
		Podophyllin
		Cold-blade excision
		Electrosurgery
Second line	Practitioner	Laser surgery
		Intralesional interferon

[a] If the patient fails a given first-line treatment, it is not necessarily an indication for trying a second-line treatment. A different first-line treatment, or even the same one, may still prove effective.
[b] The determination of the cost/benefit ratios of the different treatments should include not only the cost of the medication but also that of the visits to the practitioner. Consequently, there will be substantial geographic variation in these ratios. Nevertheless, second-line therapies are markedly more expensive than any of the first-line choices.

PHYSICAL TREATMENTS

Cryotherapy usually is delivered weekly either with a cryoprobe or a liquid nitrogen spray. Severe pain is transient and, as with all the physical methods, can be controlled by the previous application of EMLA (lidocaine and prilocaine) cream. Reported complete response rates vary between 50% and 100%, and response may take six or more treatments. Long-term scarring is unusual.

Electrosurgical techniques (electrocautery, electrodesiccation, fulguration, electrocoagulation) can be quite efficacious, possibly more so than cryotherapy, but they require some expertise. Scarring may occur. The loop electrosurgical excision procedure is the most common tool for the treatment of HPV cervical diseases.

Cold-blade excision, which is done under local anesthesia with curved (iridectomy) scissors, is a prompt and very effective way of treating anogenital warts that are few in number. Hemostasis is achieved by the application of a chemical cauterizing agent (trichloracetic acid), and long-term scarring is rare.

Laser surgery is very costly and demands expert handling. The surgery also requires local or general anesthesia. The effectiveness of laser surgery is not necessarily superior to that of the other physical methods, but laser surgery is a useful tool for the treatment of cervical lesions and is ideally suited for the management of laryngeal papillomas.

CHEMICAL TREATMENTS

Podophyllin, a resin extract from the rhizome of *Podophyllum peltatum* (podophyllum resin, USP), has long been used, usually as a 25% solution in benzoin. It is a cytotoxic agent that acts on the microtubules. Because it causes skin necrosis, it should not be applied to healthy skin. Podophyllin ingestion or extensive application can lead to serious, sometimes fatal hematologic, neurologic, pulmonary, or renal complications. The product is cheap, but the efficacy is poor, ranging from 20% to 40%. Moreover, it needs to be applied by a health practitioner. Podofilox (podophyllotoxin) is the most active compound in podophyllin. It is a standardized product that is also less toxic and, for that reason, can be self-administered. Complete response rates typically vary from 45% to 60%, but recurrences are common. Podophyllin and podofilox are contraindicated during pregnancy.

Trichloracetic and bichloracetic acids in a 10% to 90% solution are favored by gynecologists. Topical application is painful and causes temporary ulcerations. Pregnancy is not a contraindication. This common and cheap treatment has not been well evaluated, but it may be as effective as cryotherapy. Interferons have been well studied for the treatment of genital warts, but the results have been disappointing in general. Intralesional, as opposed to systemic or topical, administration is the most effective route. The 35% to 60% response rates that are reported apply only to the usually few lesions that are injected. Systemic interferon administration is used to some advantage for the treatment of recurrent respiratory papillomatosis. Imiquimod, the newest addition to the therapeutic armamentarium against anogenital warts, is an inducer of interferon-α and other cytokines. In one pivotal study, the topical application by the patient of a 5% cream formulation for up to 16 weeks was associated with a 50% complete response rate, compared with 14% in the placebo group. Only about 10% of patients experienced recurrence in

TABLE 319.3.	GENERAL DOSING INFORMATION FOR ANOGENITAL WART MEDICAL THERAPIES	
Drug	**Commercial Name and Presentation**	**Dosing Regimen**
Imiquimod	Aldara: 5% cream, box of 12 single-use, 250-mg packets	Thrice-weekly, every-other-day applications, ≤16 weeks
Podofilox	Condylox: 0.5% solution, 3.5-mL bottle with cotton-tipped applicators	Every-other-day applications for 3 consecutive days per week, ≤4 cycles
Podophyllin	Podophyllum USP, Podocon: 25-, 15-mL bottle; Podofin: 15-mL bottle	Once-weekly application, ≤6 applications
Bi- or trichloracetic acid	Bichloracetic acid: 80%, 10-mL bottle; Tri-chlor: 80%, 15-mL bottle	Once-weekly application, ≤6 applications

the 12-week follow-up period. The treatment was more effective in women than men, 72% versus 33%. Side effects were local and well tolerated. They included itching, burning, erythema, erosions, and swelling.

Tables 319.2 and 319.3 summarize how the different treatment methods can be used to the benefit of patients. Self-applied treatments are usually preferred by patients and can be delivered easily by primary caregivers. Nonetheless, patients should be instructed in the proper use of the medication and show that they can apply it properly (women may find the use of a mirror helpful).

FOLLOW-UP AND REFERRAL

There are no guidelines for the follow-up of patients with anogenital warts, but periodic evaluations should be arranged at least for those patients with persistent or recalcitrant disease. Histologic verification of the clinical diagnosis is appropriate in instances of long duration, progressive growth, or pigmentation or if the patient is immunosuppressed or immunodeficient. Referral to an expert is recommended.

CERVICAL CANCER SCREENING

Cervical cancer screening should not be overlooked in women (Table 319.4). The Pap smear collection gives the opportunity to examine the vagina and cervix. Cytology reports of HSIL and squamous cell carcinoma are mandates for colposcopic examination and directed biopsies of the cervix. Different management strategies have been proposed for the more common diagnoses of ASCUS and LSIL. Compliance on the part of the patient and the pathologist's impression are important. Under the most favorable circumstances, the patient can be followed with repeated Pap smears every 4 to 6 months for 2 years until three consecutive Pap smears have shown negative results. The management of internal HPV disease is best left to the specialist.

RECURRENCE AND PREVENTION

HPV disease recurrence is caused mostly by relapse rather than reinfection; thus, barrier methods of contraception would be

chiefly of benefit to the asymptomatic sexual partner. Unfortunately, the evidence of their effectiveness is sparse and equivocal. Investigations of animal papillomaviruses have shown that HPV VLPs (see Laboratory Findings and Serology) can be used as effective vaccines. Anogenital HPV VLP-based vaccines are under development and hold great promise.

BIBLIOGRAPHY

Am J Med 1997;102(5A).
J Natl Cancer Inst Monogr 1996;(21).
Obstet Gynecol Clin North Am 1996;23(3,4).
Anonymous. 1998 Guidelines for the treatment of sexually transmitted diseases. *MMWR* 1998;47(RR-1):1–116. Internet: http://www.cdc.gov/epo/mmwr/preview/mmwrhtml/00050909.htm).
Beutner KR, Reitano MV, Richwald GA, et al. External genital warts: report of the American Medical Association Consensus Conference. *Clin Infect Dis* 1998;27:796–806.
Bonnez W. Papillomavirus. In: Richman DD, Whitley RJ, Hayden FG, eds. *Clinical virology*, first ed. New York: Churchill Livingstone, 1997.
Bonnez W, Reichman RC. Papillomaviruses. In: Mandell GL, Bennett JE, Dolin R, eds. *Principles and practice of infectious diseases*, fifth ed. Philadelphia: WB Saunders, 1999.
Chopra KF, Tyring SK. The impact of the human immunodeficiency virus on the human papillomavirus epidemic. *Arch Dermatol* 1997;133:629–633.
Miller DM, Brodell RT. Human papillomavirus infection: treatment options for warts. *Am Fam Phys* 1996;53:135–143, 148–150.
Walsh JM. Cervical cancer: developments in screening and evaluation of the abnormal Pap smear. *West J Med* 1998;169:304–310.

Kelley's Textbook of Internal Medicine, fourth edition. Edited by H. David Humes.
Lippincott Williams & Wilkins, Philadelphia © 2000.

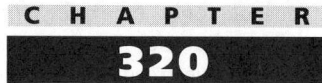

CHAPTER 320

HUMAN HERPESVIRUS 6

THOMAS H. BELHORN

DEFINITION

Human herpesvirus 6 (HHV-6), a herpesvirus first reported in 1986, not only is a common pathogen in young children but is capable of causing significant morbidity and mortality in immunocompromised patients. In addition, because HHV-6 and HIV can coinfect T lymphocytes, much speculation exists concerning the consequences of interactions between these two viruses.

INCIDENCE AND EPIDEMIOLOGIC FACTORS

Serologic studies have demonstrated that HHV-6 is a ubiquitous pathogen. The peak age of acquisition is from 6 months to 2

TABLE 319.4.   CERVICAL CANCER SCREENING GUIDELINES

1. Obtain the first Papanicolaou (Pap) smear when the patient becomes sexually active or reaches her eighteenth birthday. Follow-up with at least two other annual Pap smears.
2. The Pap smear should be obtained every 6 months in the year that follows the diagnosis of HIV infection and annually thereafter.
3. In the absence of HIV infection or other sexually transmitted diseases (including anogenital warts) in the previous year, Pap smears can be obtained every 3 to 5 years if three previous annual Pap smears have all shown negative results and if the patient is compliant with follow-up. Otherwise, Pap smears should be obtained annually.

years, with more than 90% of children having evidence of prior infection by age 2 to 3 years. Although the precise mechanism of infection is not documented, it is assumed that infection occurs by way of infected secretions, as saliva has been shown to contain HHV-6.

ETIOLOGIC FACTORS

Human herpesvirus 6 exhibits the general characteristics of a herpesvirus, including an enveloped icosahedral structure, a double-stranded DNA genome with a large coding capacity, and the apparent ability to establish a latent infection with reactivation after the initial primary infection in the human host. Unlike previously discovered herpesviruses, HHV-6 preferentially replicates in T lymphocytes. The genome of HHV-6 is most homologous with that of HHV-7 and human cytomegalovirus; cross-reacting monoclonal antibodies to these viruses have been documented. Restriction endonuclease profiles, nucleotide sequence comparisons, monoclonal antibody reactivity, and growth properties can be used to distinguish two distinct variants of HHV-6, termed variant A and variant B. HHV-6 variant B is isolated from children with acute febrile illness or roseola, whereas either variant may be isolated from immunocompromised patients.

CLINICAL FINDINGS

Primary infection with HHV-6 in young children can be asymptomatic, manifest as roseola, or present as an acute febrile illness without rash. Roseola (also called exanthem subitum or sixth disease), a disease presenting in late infancy or early childhood, has long been defined clinically by several days of high fever with few or no localized findings of infection, followed by defervescence concurrent with onset of a rose-colored rash. Both roseola and the acute febrile illness without the rash associated with HHV-6 primary infection may be associated with a febrile seizure. The rare primary infection occurring in an older child or adult may manifest as adenopathy or an acute mononucleosis-like illness. Kikuchi's disease, a necrotizing adenitis with a characteristic histologic pattern, may also be associated with HHV-6.

Human herpesvirus 6 persists after the primary infection and is capable of reactivation from a latent state. Although such reactivation is thought to be asymptomatic in most adults, the clinical consequence of HHV-6 reactivation in an immunocompromised host is variable. HHV-6 reactivation has been associated with fever, leukopenia, rash, encephalitis, pneumonitis, and graft rejection. In transplant recipients, HHV-6 may induce bone marrow suppression. The virus is clearly neurotropic, and the association between HHV-6 infection and multiple sclerosis as well as white matter demyelinization in AIDS dementia complex is under investigation. The association of HHV-6 with specific malignancies, specifically Hodgkin's disease and non-Hodgkin's lymphoma, has been reported but not proven. Ongoing research will hopefully elucidate the precise role HHV-6 plays in such disease processes in immunocompromised populations.

LABORATORY FINDINGS

The diagnosis of roseola has historically been made clinically, and laboratory findings are nonspecific. Serologic studies are available to aid in the confirmation of a primary HHV-6 infection by documenting seroconversion. Serologic testing is of little use in documenting reactivation disease. Virus can be isolated from blood, saliva, and, occasionally, tissue in primary infection as well as in reactivation disease; specimens are usually cultured in cord blood lymphocytes, which may not be available in many laboratories. Polymerase chain reaction and hybridization techniques are valuable for HHV-6 detection and are being used more frequently to document the presence of HHV-6 in immunocompromised patients.

OPTIMAL MANAGEMENT

Primary infection in children is a self-limiting disease that requires no specific antimicrobial therapy. The prognosis for primary disease with the usual manifestations of roseola or an acute febrile illness is excellent, with no long-term sequelae. Severe disease associated with HHV-6 infection or reactivation in an immunosuppressed host should be treated with an appropriate antiviral regimen and supportive measures. In vitro data support the efficacy of either foscarnet or ganciclovir in the therapy of HHV-6 infections, although the usefulness of these agents has not been well documented in vivo. No effective means of prophylaxis for HHV-6 infection or reactivation exists, and no vaccine is available.

BIBLIOGRAPHY

Braun DK, Dominguez G, Pellett PE. Human herpesvirus 6. *Clin Microbiol Rev* 1997;10:521–567.

Dockrell DH, Smith TF, Paya CV. Human herpesvirus 6. *Mayo Clin Proc* 1999;74:163–170.

Hall CB, Long CE, Schnabel KC, et al. Human herpesvirus-6 infection in children: a prospective study of complications and reactivation. *N Engl J Med* 1994;331:432–438.

Kimberlin DW, Whitley RJ. Human herpesvirus-6: neurologic implications of a newly-described viral pathogen. *J Neurovirol* 1998;4:474–485.

Lusso P, Ensoli B, Markham PD, et al. Productive dual infection of human CD+ T lymphocytes by HIV-1 and HHV-6. *Nature* 1989;337: 370–373.

Singh N, Carrigan DR. Human herpesvirus-6 in transplantation: an emerging pathogen. *Ann Intern Med* 1996;124:1065–1071.

Soldan SS, Berti R, Salem N, et al. Association of human herpesvirus 6 (HHV-6) with multiple sclerosis: increased IgM response to HHV-6 early antigen and detection of serum HHV-6 DNA. *Nature Med* 1997; 3:1394–1397.

Kelley's Textbook of Internal Medicine, fourth edition. Edited by H. David Humes. Lippincott Williams & Wilkins, Philadelphia © 2000.

CHAPTER
321

INTESTINAL PROTOZOA

PABLO C. OKHUYSEN
CYNTHIA L. CHAPPELL

■ CRYPTOSPORIDIOSIS

Cryptosporidium parvum inhabits the mucosal epithelium of the small bowel. The oocyst (3 to 5 μm; Fig. 321.1) sporulates within the parasitophorous vacuole prior to release into the intestinal lumen and when shed in feces are directly infectious to others. The incubation period ranges from 4 to 24 days post exposure.

C. parvum is a ubiquitous organism that can infect humans and is a common pathogen of many mammals. Two distinct transmission cycles occur in nature and are related to specific genotypes. Infections with genotype H demonstrate preference for causing infection in humans, whereas genotype C favors a zoonotic transmission. Oocysts are resistant to water chlorination and hospital disinfectant solutions. In the height of the AIDS epidemic in the United States, cryptosporidiosis was the AIDS-defining infection in 4% of patients reported to the U.S. Centers for Disease Control and Prevention, and prior to the advent of highly active antiretroviral therapy, up to 50% of HIV-infected patients experienced *Cryptosporidium* infection at some point of their disease. The incidence of AIDS-associated cryptosporidiosis has decreased significantly in recent years due to effec-

tive antiretroviral therapy and the prophylactic use of macrolides. Transmission via the fecal–oral route may occur by contact with an infected person, farm animals, or pets, or by drinking contaminated water. Those at increased risk of acquiring disease include travelers to developing countries, children in day care centers, immunosuppressed persons, the elderly, veterinarians, and dairy farmers. As few as ten oocysts can cause infection in healthy volunteers and presumably even fewer in immunocompromised individuals. Immunocompetent individuals may experience a self-limited illness that rarely lasts more than 14 days. Symptoms of cryptosporidial infection include watery stools, fatigue, abdominal pain, general malaise, and in 20% nausea and vomiting. Low-grade fever can also occur. In HIV-infected individuals, when CD4 counts are higher than 200 per cubic milliliter, *C. parvum* infection may resolve spontaneously; however, in the later stages of HIV disease (CD4 counts under 100), chronic infection can lead to dehydration, malnutrition, and wasting, frequently culminating in death. In profoundly immunosuppressed hosts, extraintestinal infections have been described. The invasion of the biliary tract may manifest as cholestasis, acalculous cholecystitis, or cholangitis with right upper quadrant pain, marked elevation of serum alkaline phosphatase, and slight or no elevation of serum bilirubin. Associated strictures may respond to ampullary dilatation with endoscopic retrograde cholangiopancreatography (ERCP). A diarrheagenic toxin has been suggested, but evidence to date is incomplete. Experimental data suggest that interferon-γ, intestinal intraepithelial lymphocytes, and CD4 and CD8 T-cell lymphocytes are important in clearing cryptosporidiosis.

Diagnosis is made by identifying oocysts with a modified acid-fast stain of a fresh fecal specimen. Leukocytes are usually absent. Recently, more sensitive, monoclonal-based, direct immunofluorescence assay and enzyme-linked immunosorbent assay (ELISA) have been introduced. Since oocyst excretion is variable, the analysis of several specimens may be necessary to confirm the diagnosis.

The treatment of cryptosporidoisis in an otherwise healthy individual is supportive. In AIDS-associated cryptosporidiosis,

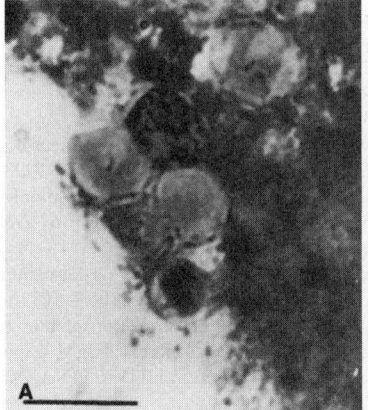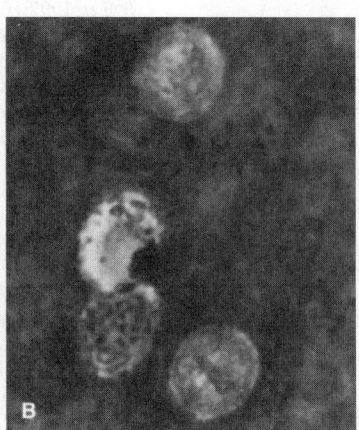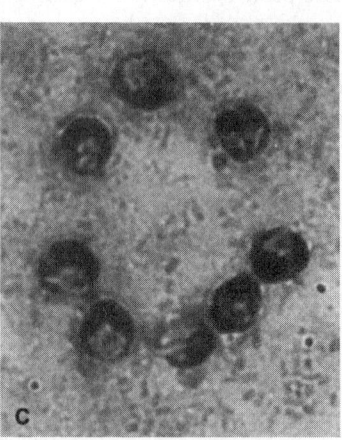

FIGURE 321.1. **A:** *Cyclospora;* **B:** *Cryptosporidium muris;* **C:** *Cryptosporidium parvum.* Bar represents 10 μm. (From Ortega Y, et al. *Cyclospora* species: a new protozoan pathogen of humans. *N Engl J Med* 1993;328:1308, with permission.)

the combination of paromomycin and azithromycin improves symptoms and decreased parasitic burden. Uncontrolled studies using hyperimmune bovine colostrum have shown some benefit in HIV-infected patients, and controlled, clinical trials have shown little effect.

ISOSPORIASIS

Isospora belli produces large (12 × 30 mm), oval-shaped oocysts that sporulate outside the body. This process takes 2 to 3 days before the oocysts become infectious. Isosporiasis was rarely diagnosed prior to the HIV epidemic, although healthy individuals can also become infected. The organism is endemic in tropical and subtropical environments, is associated with outbreaks of diarrheal disease, and has been implicated in traveler's diarrhea. *I. belli* infection is confined to humans and, perhaps, to dogs. No other animal reservoir has been identified. Transmission is associated with contaminated water, although that route is not proven.

Biopsies of severe cases reveal flattened villi and crypt hyperplasia of the small bowel with a cellular infiltrate of lymphocytes and eosinophils. The watery diarrhea caused by this organism suggests an enterotoxin, but no evidence for this molecule yet exists. The clinical features of *I. belli* infection in immunocompetent hosts are abdominal pain, cramping, nausea, and watery diarrhea, occasionally with eosinophilia. In immunodeficient hosts, prolonged diarrhea with malnutrition may occur. Several case reports have documented dissemination to the mesenteric lymph nodes or acalculous cholecystitis in advanced HIV infection.

Oocysts can be visualized with an acid-fast stain. Symptomatic infection responds to treatment with trimethoprim–sulfamethoxazole (TMP-SMX; Table 321.1). In AIDS patients with recurrent disease, secondary prophylaxis with TMP-SMX and pyrimethamine sulfadoxine prevents relapses. Nitazoxanide, a thiazolide compound, and its desacetyl derivative, tizoxanide, have antimicrobial properties against anaerobic bacteria, as well as against helminths and protozoa. Therefore, it is a promising agent in the treatment of this and other parasitoses.

CYCLOSPOROSIS

Cyclospora cayetanensis is excreted as an unsporulated oocyst. It has been found in developing countries and in the United States during outbreaks in children, travelers to developing nations, and AIDS patients. An initial study has found a prevalence rate of 10.9% in Peruvian children. Data regarding pathologic factors are absent, but the organism is suspected of infecting the proximal jejunum. After an incubation period of approximately 17 days, an explosive diarrhea occurs accompanied by cramping, abdominal pain, nausea, vomiting, fatigue, and, occasionally, fever. In one study, the median duration of diarrhea was 43 days, at which point symptoms resolved spontaneously in immunocompetent hosts. However, the immunocompromised may experience an unusually prolonged course.

Cyclospora and *Cryptosporidium* show staining similarity, but *Cyclospora* oocysts are slightly larger (8 to 10 mm) (Fig. 321.1). *Cyclospora* oocysts can also be identified in fecal samples by autofluorescence at 330 to 380 nm. Small-bowel biopsies reveal local erythema and villous atrophy. Open-label studies of TMP-SMX have demonstrated rapid improvement in the clinical symptoms and clearing of *Cyclospora* after 10 days (Table 321.1) and may thus be of use in the treatment and prevention of relapses.

MICROSPORIDIOSIS

Microsporidia are small, obligate, intracellular parasites that infect vertebrate and invertebrate hosts. Only a few of the more than 1,000 species known to belong in this phylum have been identified as pathogenic agents for humans. Two species are associated with enteric infection: *Enterocytozoon bieneusi* and *Encephalitozoon intestinalis* (formerly known as *Septata intestinalis*); the former is the more common. Microsporidia share several common characteristics, including specialized polar tubes that transfer the parasite to the host cell. Intracellular asexual reproduction leads to formation of small (0.5 to 0.9 × 1.5 μm), thick-walled spores that can survive for months in the environment. *E. bieneusi* and *E. intestinalis* can be distinguished morphologically by electron microscopy of small-bowel biopsies.

To date, *E. bieneusi* has only been reported in humans, but it is apparently found worldwide. The prevalence in selected groups of HIV-infected patients in different countries has indicated a range of 1.7% to 30%.

Both *E. bieneusi* and *E. intestinalis* infections are identified with diarrhea in individuals with CD4 counts lower than 100 and frequently also in asymptomatic carriers. *E. bieneusi* infects the enterocytes of the proximal jejunum and occasionally spreads to the biliary tract. In comparison, *E. intestinalis* is found in enterocytes, macrophages, and fibroblasts. In both infections, changes in the local cellular architecture may vary from a mild inflammatory, lymphocytic infiltrate to severe epithelial deterioration with decreased brush-border enzymes. *E. intestinalis* infects the intestinal tract but may also disseminate to the mesenteric nodes and kidney.

Free and intracytoplasmic spores can be stained with Giemsa or fluorochrome stains (Calcofluor, Uvitex 2B) that have affinity for chitin, but identification of the specific species requires electron microscopy. Preliminary data suggest that albendazole may be of use in the treatment of *E. intestinalis* (Table 321.1) and in *Encephalitozoon* infections.

AMEBIASIS

Entamoeba histolytica infection of the colonic mucosa is initiated by the ingestion of cysts (8.5 to 19.0 mm). After excystation, asexual division results in the formation of trophozoites (12 to 60 μm diameter), which bind to mucous secretions and intestinal cells via a galactose-specific lectin. A portion of the trophozoites develop into cysts and are excreted.

TABLE 321.1.   RECOMMENDED TREATMENTS FOR THE MAJOR HUMAN INTESTINAL PROTOZOAN PARASITES

Organism	Treatment	Dosage	Side Effects
Cryptosporidium parvum	Supportive. Paromomycin in combination with azithromycin partially effective in AIDS-associated cryptosporidiosis	Paromomycin 500 mg t.i.d. in combination with azithromycin 1,200 mg po b.i.d. × 1 d then 1,200 mg PO q.d. for 27 d then 600 mg/d for chronic suppression	Avoid when concomitant intestinal ulcerative lesions are present as inadvertent absorption may cause nephropathy or ototoxicity
Giardia lamblia	Metronidazole *or*	250 mg t.i.d. for 5 d	Metallic taste, disulfiram-like reaction when ingested with alcohol, peripheral neuropathy
	Albendazole *or*	400 mg PO b.i.d. for 5 d	
	Quinacrine *or*	100 mg t.i.d. for 5 d	May color the sclera, skin, urine; may cause dizziness, headache, toxic psychosis; contraindicated in psoriasis; avoid alcohol or primaquine
	Furazolidone	100 mg q.i.d. for 7–10 d	Disulfiram-like reaction with alcohol; hypersensitivity reactions
Enterococcus histiolytica			
Asymptomatic cyst passer	Diloxanide furoate *or*	500 mg t.i.d. for 10 d	Poorly absorbed; excessive flatulence
	Paromomycin	30 mg/kg/d in 3 doses for 5–10 d	As above
Invasive rectocolitis	Metronidazole *or*	750 mg t.i.d. 10 d, *plus* diloxanide or paromomycin	As above
	Tinidazole *or*	1 g PO q12 × 3 d	
	Ornidazole	500 mg PO q 12 × 3 d	
Liver abscess	Metronidazole *or*	750 mg tid 10 d *plus* diloxanide or paromomycin	As above
	Dehydroemetine	1–1.5 mg/kg/d (max 90 mg/d) IM for up to 5 d *plus* diloxanide or paromomycin	Cardiovascular toxicity
Cyclospora	Trimethroprim/ sulfamethoxazole	One DS tablet b.i.d. for 3 d, in AIDS-associated infection DS b.i.d. for 10 days then chronic suppression with DS t.i.w.	Rash, nausea, vomiting, chelitis, neutropenia; contains sulfites
Iosopora belli	Trimethroprim/ sulfamethoxazole	Two DS tablets b.i.d. for 2–4 weeks. In AIDS-associated diarrhea may need chronic suppression with daily DS dose	Rash, nausea, vomiting, chelitis, neutropenia; contains sulfites. In sulfa-allergic patients pyrimethamine 75 mg/d + folic acid
Microsporidia:			
Encephalitozoon intestinalis	Albendazole *or*	400 mg b.i.d.	Diarrhea, abdominal pain, leukopenia, alopecia, Increased ALT, AST. Chronic suppression needed in AIDS-associated microsporidiosis
Enterocytozoon bieneusi	Atovaquone	750 mg PO b.i.d.	Shown to have effect in a small trial
Balantidium coli	Tetracycline	500 mg q.i.d. 10 d	Skin rash, photosensitivity, staining of teeth, contraindicated in pregnancy
Dientamoeba fragilis	Iodoquinol	650 mg t.i.d. 20 d	Maximum dose is 2 g/d, longer courses may cause optic neuritis. Tetracycline and paramomycin are alternatives.

DS, double-strength; ALT, alanine aminotransferase; AST, aspartate aminotransferase.

E. histolytica infection is especially prevalent in Mexico, India, Africa, and Central and South America. Major routes of transmission are through contaminated water and food or by direct fecal–oral contact. Individuals at highest risk for infection include travelers to developing nations, immigrants or migrant workers, immunocompromised individuals, and individuals housed in psychiatric facilities.

Both pathogenic and nonpathogenic strains of *E. histolytica* occur in humans. The strains are morphologically indistinguishable but can be differentiated by zymodeme patterns, monoclonal antibodies, and DNA probes. Nonpathogenic strains are associated with asymptomatic infection and do not usually elicit a serologic response. In contrast, 10% of infections are with pathogenic strains, resulting in symptomatic illness (80% to 98%) or invasive disease (2% to 20%) and the production of serum antibodies. After invasive disease, there is development of immunity to subsequent invasion but not to colonization; immunity is thought to be mediated by cellular mechanisms. Pathogenic amebae release a pore-forming protein, soluble toxic molecules, and increased concentrations of a cysteine proteinase, which can degrade matrix proteins. Host leukocytes, neutrophils, and macrophages also play a role in cell damage when they are lysed and release their toxic products. Ulcerative lesions in the intestinal mucosa and liver abscesses are characterized by a moderate inflammatory response. Advanced lesions have necrotic centers with amebae concentrated at the outer zone of normal tissue.

Entamoeba histolytica can cause intestinal syndromes, including the following: (a) a dysenteric syndrome with production of small volumes of bloody, mucoid stools without fecal leukocytes; (b) colitis characterized by ulcerations of the colonic mucosa with typical flask-shaped abscesses; or (c) the formation of a fibrotic mass in the intestinal wall (ameboma). Chronic amebic colitis is clinically indistinguishable from inflammatory bowel disease, and those receiving corticosteroids are at risk for toxic megacolon and perforation. Infective trophozoites can migrate hematogenously to the right lobe of the liver, causing abscess formation, abdominal pain, jaundice, and fever. Adjacent anatomic structures, such as the pulmonary parenchyma, peritoneum, and pericardium, can become involved. Amebae can also disseminate to the brain. Immunosuppressed or malnourished individuals, those at the extremes of age, patients with malignancy, and women during pregnancy and postpartum stages are especially at risk for invasive amebiasis. Indications for surgical drainage of an amoebic abscess include large dimensions, impending rupture, left lobe location, or lack of therapeutic response.

Identification of *E. histolytica* cysts and trophozoites requires examination of a fresh stool and a trichrome stain. New fecal antigen detection methods (ELISA) may also prove useful. Periodic acid–Schiff-stained tissue obtained by colonoscopy may be required to confirm the diagnosis. An episode of dysentery may not necessarily precede abscess formation. In areas of low endemicity, a positive serologic response correlates with severe colitis or invasive disease. However, titers persist for prolonged periods of time and are of no use in determining acute versus remote infection in areas of high endemicity. The identification of cysts in an asymptomatic host should prompt treatment with diloxa-

nide or paromomycin (Table 321.1). Invasive disease, such as severe colitis or parenchymal abscess, should be treated with metronidazole followed by a luminal agent to prevent future invasion with any remaining cysts.

GIARDIASIS

Gardia lamblia can produce infection in humans and is also a zoononsis. *G. lamblia* cysts are ingested with contaminated water or food. In the environment this prozooan parasite is found in a cystic stage that is resistant to conventional concentrations of chlorine used to treat drinking water. Giardiasis is a common problem in day care centers and has also been associated with water-borne outbreaks. Brief exposure to temperatures higher than 50°C results in inactivation. Once cysts are ingested, trophozoites (10 to 20 mm) emerge in the duodenum and adhere to the upper small-bowel microvillar surface, crypts, and occasionally to the common bile duct epithelium. A ventral suction cup is thought to mediate the attachment. After an incubation period of 7 to 9 days, infectious cysts (8 × 12 mm) are excreted intermittently.

The clinical manifestations are variable and range from completely asymptomatic infections to watery diarrhea with abdominal cramping and distention. Urticaria and eosinophilia are rarely associated with giardiasis. During heavy infestations, microvillar blunting and malabsorption can ensue. Infection may resolve spontaneously or result in chronic diseases with steatorrhea, malabsorption, and weight loss. Chronic or recurrent giardiasis should prompt an evaluation for IgA deficiency because of its association with giardiasis.

Giardia can be visualized in trichrome iodine stains of fecal smears. Infection can be identified by sensitive ELISA. A direct immunofluorescence assay that can detect *Cryptosporidium* and *Giardia* simultaneously is available commercially. Staining a sampling of duodenal bile obtained by the Enterotest capsule method may improve the diagnostic yield. Treatment of asymptomatic cyst passers remains controversial since most individuals clear the infection spontaneously. However, for those in whom the likelihood of reinfection is low (e.g., an asymptomatic traveler returning to a developed nation who is found to pass cysts), eradication of *G. lamblia* may be indicated. For individuals with symptomatic disease the antiparasitic agent of choice is metronidazole administered as outlined in Table 321.1.

BIBLIOGRAPHY

Didier ES. Microsporidiosis. *Clin Infect Dis* 1998;27:1–8.
Peng MM, Xiao L, Freeman AR, et al. Genetic polymorphism among *Cryptosporidium parvum* isolates: evidence of two distinct human transmission cycles. *Emerg Infect Dis* 1997 Oct–Dec;3(4):567–573.
Soave R, Herwaldt BL, Relman DA. Cyclospora. *Infect Dis Clin North Am* 1998 Mar§(1):1–12.
Marshall MM, Naumovitz D, Ortega Y, et al. Waterborne protozoan pathogens. *Clin Microbiol Rev* 1997; Jan;10(1):67–85.

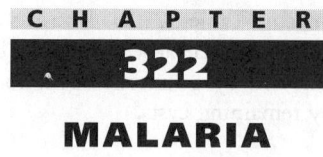

MALARIA

DONALD J. KROGSTAD

DEFINITION

Four species of plasmodia infect humans: *Plasmodium falciparum*, *Plasmodium vivax*, *Plasmodium ovale*, and *Plasmodium malariae*. Humans acquire malaria from the bite of infected female *Anopheles* mosquitoes (Fig. 322.1). After their injection under the skin by a mosquito, sporozoites travel through the circulation to enter the liver cell (hepatocyte). Within the hepatocyte, the parasite matures to a tissue schizont containing large numbers of infectious merozoites (2,000 to 30,000). The merozoites then invade red blood cells (RBCs) and mature through a series of asexual erythrocytic stages: ring, trophozoite, and schizont. After either 48 or 72 hours, the schizont stage of the parasite lyses its host RBC, freeing 6 to 32 merozoites, which then invade other RBCs and repeat the asexual erythrocytic cycle.

Some intraerythrocytic parasites develop into the sexual forms (male or female gametocytes) necessary to complete the life cycle.

In the mosquito, the gametocytes (which are haploid, like the asexual erythrocytic stages) transform to gametes and fuse to form a diploid oocyst. The oocyst then undergoes a reduction division (meiosis) to produce haploid sporozoites that migrate to the salivary gland, where they are infectious for humans.

Two malaria species (*P. vivax* and *P. ovale*) have persistent liver stages (hypnozoites) that may remain dormant in the liver for 6 to 11 months or more. When hypnozoites finally mature to tissue schizonts and release merozoites, they produce either a delayed primary attack (if the patient was taking antimalarial chemoprophylaxis and did not develop symptomatic parasitemia within 2 to 4 weeks of the initial infection) or a relapse (if symptomatic parasitemia developed at the time of initial infection).

Malaria may also be transmitted by the parenteral inoculation of infected blood (inadvertent transfusion of parasitized RBCs, sharing of needles among drug addicts). Because induced malaria is acquired from parasitized RBCs (rather than sporozoites), no hypnozoites form in the liver and relapses do not occur, even with *P. vivax* or *P. ovale* infection.

EPIDEMIOLOGIC FACTORS

Malaria is endemic in most of the developing tropical world. Because malaria transmission depends on the *Anopheles* mosquito, it usually does not occur at altitudes above 1,500 m. Because of their importance for both chemoprophylaxis and

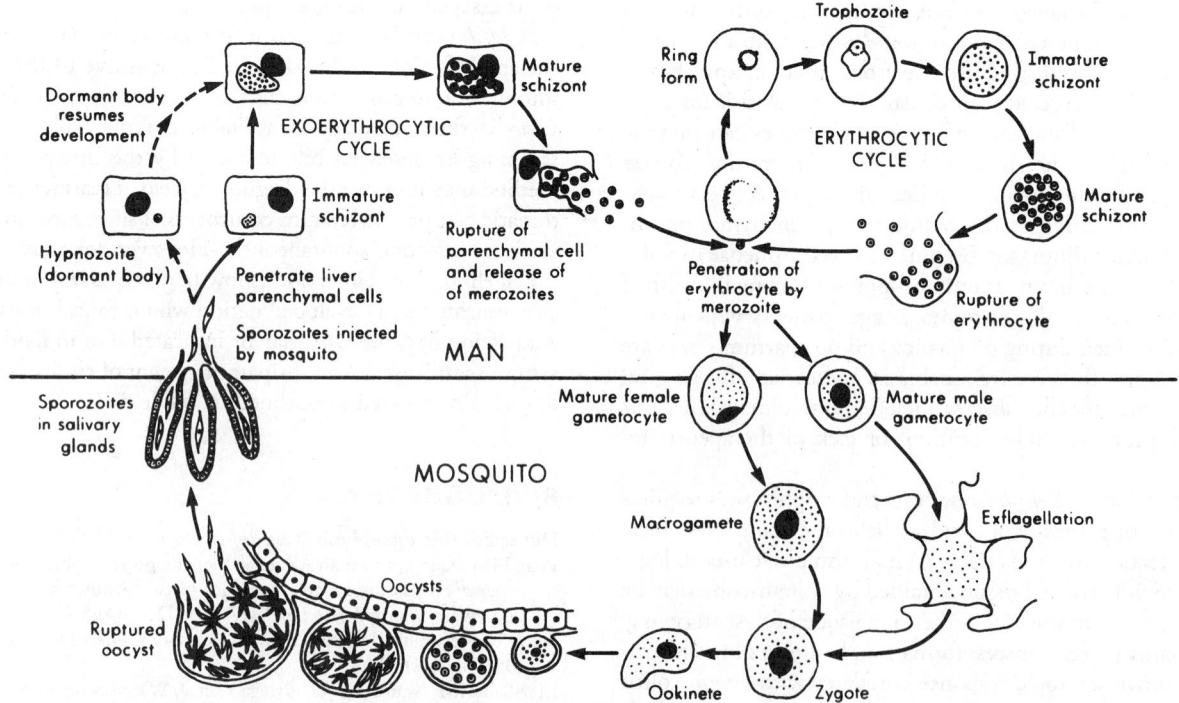

FIGURE 322.1. Malaria life cycle. Red cell infection (the asexual erythrocytic form of the parasite) is responsible for the morbidity and mortality associated with malaria. The hypnozoite is responsible for relapse in *Plasmodium vivax* and *Plasmodium ovale* infection. (From Remington, Swartz. *Curr Clin Top Infect Dis* 1982;3:56, with permission.)

| **TABLE 322.1.** | **COUNTRIES WITH CHLOROQUIINE-RESISTANT *PLASMODIUM FALCIPARUM* MALARIA**[a] |

Africa

Angola
Benin
Botswana
Burkina Faso
Burundi
Cameroon
Central African Republic
Chad
Comoros
Congo
Cote d'Ivoire
Democratic Republic of the Congo (formerly Zaire)
Djibouti
Equatorial Guinea
Eritrea
Ethiopia
Gabon
Gambia
Ghana
Guinea
Guinea-Bissau
Kenya
Liberia
Madagascar
Malawi
Mali
Mauritania
Mauritius (not in urban areas)
Mayotte
Mozambique
Namibia
Niger
Nigeria
Rwanda
Sao Tome and Principe
Senegal
Sierra Leone
Somalia
South Africa (not in urban areas)
Sudan
Swaziland
Tanzania
Togo
Uganda (now Democratic Republic of the Congo)
Zambia
Zimbabwe

Asia

Afghanistan
Bangladesh
Bhutan (not in urban areas)
Cambodia
China (not in urban areas)
India
Indonesia
Iran (not in urban areas)
Laos
Malaysia
Myanmar (not in urban areas)
Nepal (not in urban areas)
Oman
Pakistan
Philippines (not in urban areas)
Sri Lanka (not in urban areas)
Thailand (not in urban areas)
Vietnam
Yemen

Latin America

Bolivia (not in urban areas)
Brazil
Colombia (not in urban areas)
Ecuador
French Guiana
Guyana (not in urban areas)
Panama (east of Canal, including
   San Blas Islands) (not in urban areas)
Paraguay (not in urban areas)
Peru (not in urban areas)
Suriname (not in urban areas)
Venezuela (not in urban areas)

Australia and Oceania

Papua New Guinea
Solomon Islands
Vanuatu

[a] Based on information from the Medical Letter on Drugs and Therapeutics and the U.S. Centers for Disease Control and Prevention (CDC), which maintains a 24-hour phone line for malaria advice for travelers and physicians (888-232-3228) and a second phone line to help physicians in the treatment of severe and complicated malaria (404-639-2888). Similar information is available on the Internet at the CDC web site http://www.cdc.gov/.

treatment, the areas where chloroquine-resistant *P. falciparum* is present are outlined in Table 322.1. Note that this list is continually in flux as new data become available. In countries such as the United States, the lack of transmission results primarily from the lack of infected people. This is because competent mosquito vectors are present in many regions of the United States (*A. albimanus, A. quadrimaculatus,* and *A. freeborni*). Therefore, malaria transmission can (and does) occur in the United States when significant numbers of infected people are exposed to (and reinfect) the domestic anopheline mosquito pool. For this reason, malaria introductions occurred in the United States after World War II, after the Korean and Vietnam Wars, and after the entry of large numbers of refugees from Southeast Asia.

PATHOGENESIS

The morbidity and mortality of *P. falciparum* malaria are related in large measure to the cytoadherence of RBCs containing mature parasites to the microvascular endothelium. RBCs containing mature parasites cytoadhere because their surfaces contain parasite proteins that mediate adherence to ligands on endothelial cells such as CD36 and intercellular adhesion molecule 1. The clinical consequences of this microvascular disease may include ischemia (hypoxia), hypoglycemia, and acidosis in the affected tissues. Thus unresponsive coma or seizures (cerebral malaria) may be produced by metabolic factors, such as hypoglycemia, or physical factors, such as the presence of cytoadherent parasitized RBCs on the microvascular endothelium of the brain. Pulmonary edema in malaria is associated with a capillary leak syndrome, not with congestive heart failure, and may result from parasite-stimulated release of tumor necrosis factor-α (TNF-α), as it does in gram-negative bacterial septicemia. Acute renal failure may result from hemolysis and the microvascular disease associated with *P. falciparum* infection, particularly in the renal cortex.

The morbidity and mortality of malaria are also related to the magnitude of the parasitemia. Thus, *P. falciparum*, which is able to invade RBCs of any age, may produce parasitemias greater than 10^6 per microliter. In contrast, *P. vivax* and *P. ovale*, which are able to invade only younger RBCs such as reticulocytes, and *P. malariae*, which is restricted to older RBCs, produce more limited parasitemias ($\leq$25,000 per microliter and $\leq$10,000 per microliter, respectively), and therefore pose a lower risk of complications and death.

Complications observed with malaria caused by plasmodial species other than *P. falciparum* include an immune complex nephrotic syndrome associated with *P. malariae* infection. These immune complexes contain parasite antigens, complement, and host antibodies to parasite antigens, consistent with an immune complex glomerulonephritis.

CLINICAL FINDINGS

The cardinal clinical features of malaria are recurring fevers and chills (associated with the lysis of RBCs containing mature schizonts) in the absence of localizing signs. The periodicity of the fevers and chills is typically 48 hours with *P. vivax* or *P. ovale*, and 72 hours with *P. malariae*. In contrast, irregular, hectic fevers and chills are usually observed with *P. falciparum* infection, especially in nonimmune patients (those who have never been exposed to plasmodia), who are at the greatest risk of complications and death.

In severe *P. falciparum* infection ($\geq$$10^6$ parasites per microliter of blood), acute complications include coma (due to hypoglycemia, the microvascular disease produced by the parasite, or TNF-α), pulmonary edema, acute renal failure, thrombocytopenia, and gastroenteritis (predominantly diarrhea). Chronic *P. falciparum* infection may produce splenomegaly, which typically resolves after suppressive treatment with prophylactic doses of antimalarials for 6 to 12 months.

P. malariae infection is associated with an immune complex nephrotic syndrome (see previous discussion). *P. vivax* infection predisposes to late splenic rupture with trauma (1 to 3 months after the initial, or primary, infection).

LABORATORY FINDINGS

Malaria is diagnosed by the identification of parasites on a Giemsa-stained blood film. Wright's stain is less sensitive than Giemsa, especially for inexperienced observers. Correct identification of the infecting species is essential for treatment because many *P. falciparum* strains are resistant to chloroquine, pyrimethamine–sulfadoxine (Fansidar), and other antimalarials. In contrast, all *P. ovale* and *P. malariae* organisms are susceptible to chloroquine. Although most *P. vivax* organisms are susceptible to chloroquine, chloroquine-resistant *P. vivax* organisms have been reported.

With Giemsa stain, the parasite cytoplasm and nucleus are light and dark blue, respectively. In *P. falciparum* infections, the diagnostic crescent-shaped gametocytes may appear only after an additional 7 to 10 days. In addition, only ring-stage asexual parasites are visible initially on the peripheral smear. This is because *P. falciparum*-parasitized RBCs containing the more mature trophozoite- and schizont-infected RBCs are sequestered in the peripheral microvasculature and therefore do not circulate in the bloodstream. In contrast, in *P. vivax*, *P. ovale*, and *P. malariae* infections, all asexual erythrocytic stages circulate in the bloodstream and are therefore seen on the blood smear because they do not cytoadhere.

In acutely ill patients, the differential diagnosis can usually be simplified to *P. falciparum* versus *P. vivax*. This is because *P. ovale* is virtually identical to *P. vivax* (morphologically and clinically) and because *P. malariae* typically produces a more chronic infection. On a thin blood film (in which the morphologic characteristics of the RBCs are preserved), *P. vivax*–parasitized RBCs characteristically demonstrate both Schüffner's dots in the RBC cytoplasm (eosinophilic dots 0.2 μm in diameter) and RBC enlargement with parasite maturation. In contrast, neither Schüffner's dots nor RBC enlargement occur with *P. falciparum* infection. Potentially confusing factors include Maurer's dots in the cytoplasm of *P. falciparum*–parasitized RBCs and infections with more than one parasite species (in 5% to 7% of patients with malaria).

Thick blood films (in which the RBCs have been lysed) permit the examination of approximately ten times as much blood per unit time as thin films and are therefore often diagnostic in patients with low parasitemias. However, inexperienced observers are frequently confused by thick films because RBC lysis makes it impossible to determine the effect of parasite maturation on RBC size.

Although serologic (antibody) testing ultimately demonstrates increases in species-specific antibody titers in most patients with malaria, it is not useful for the management of acutely ill patients because 3 to 4 weeks or more is typically required to produce a diagnostic rise in antibody titer. Conversely, antigen detection (e.g., based on parasite lactate dehydrogenase) may be useful and is now available in kit form.

DNA probes have been developed for several plasmodia, especially *P. falciparum*. In combination with amplification using the polymerase chain reaction and nonradioactive probes, they provide sensitivities and specificities similar to those of the thick smear. Despite this progress, DNA probes are not used routinely

TABLE 322.2. TREATMENT OF MALARIA

Drug and Route	Dosage
All species except chloroquine-resistant *Plasmodium falciparum* and chloroquine-resistant *Plasmodium vivax*	
Oral regimens	
Chloroquine	600-mg base (1,000 mg chloroquine phosphate), followed by 300-mg base after 6 h and 300-mg base again on days 2 and 3
Parenteral regimens	
IM Chloroquine	2.5-mg base/kg q4h or 3.5-mg base/kg q6h (total not to exceed 25 mg base/kg)
IV Chloroquine	10-mg base/kg over 4 h, followed by 5-mg base/kg q12h given in a 2-h infusion (total dose not to exceed 25-mg base/kg)
Chloroquine-resistant *P. vivax*	
Oral regimens	
Mefloquine alone	1,250 mg mefloquine × 1
Quinine sulfate plus doxycycline or pyrimethamine–sulfadoxine	650 mg quinine sulfate q8h × 3–7 d *plus* 100 mg doxycycline q12h × 7 d, *or* 75/1,500 mg pyrimethamine-sulfadoxine (3 tablets) × as a single dose on the last day of quinine
Chloroquine-resistant *P. falciparum*	
Oral regimens	
Quinine sulfate plus doxycycline, pyrimethamine-sulfadoxine, or clindamycin	650 mg quinine sulfate salt (540-mg base) q8h for 3 d or until substantial improvement *plus* 100 mg doxycycline q12h × 7 d, *or* 3 tablets of pyrimethamine–sulfadoxine (75/1,500 mg Fansidar) in a single dose on the last day of quinine, *or* 900 mg clindamycin q8h × 5 d
Mefloquine alone	1,250 mg mefloquine (1,140-mg base) as a single dose, or 750 mg followed by an additional 500 mg 6–8 h later
Halofantrine[a]	500 mg halofantrine q6h × 3 doses, repeat in 1 week
Atovaquone plus proguanil or doxycycline	1,000 mg atovaquone q.d. × 3 d *plus* 400 mg proguanil q.d. × 3 d, *or* 100 mg doxycycline q12h × 3 d
Artesunate plus mefloquine	4 mg artesunate/kg q.d. × 3 d *plus* 1,250 mg mefloquine × 1 dose
Parenteral regimens	
IV Quinidine gluconate	6.25-mg base/kg (10 mg quinidine gluconate/kg, maximum of 600 mg) IV over 1–2 h, followed by a constant infusion of 0.0125-mg quinidine base/kg/min (0.02 mg quinidine gluconate/kg/min) IV until the parsitemia is <1% or oral treatment can be begun
IV Quinine dihydrochloride	16.7-mg base/kg (20 mg salt/kg) loading dose over 4 h, followed by 8.3-mg base/kg over 2–4 h q8h
IM Quinine dihydrochloride	8.3-mg base/kg (10 mg salt) q8h (maximum of 1,800 mg salt (1,500-mg base)/d

[a] Neither halofantrine nor the artemisinin derivatives are available in the United States. Halofantrine regimens in use in Southeast Asia reflect dose escalation for the treatment of multidrug-resistant *P. falciparum*: **oral halofantrine**—500 mg q8h × 72 h (total dose of 4,500 mg); **oral halofantrine**—500 mg q4h × 3 doses on day 1, followed by 500 mg/d × 6 d (total dose of 4,500 mg). Parenteral artemisinin regimens reported to be effective include 4 mg artemether per kg × 1 IM, followed by 2 mg/kg IM q8h × ≥72 h in adults; and 3.2 mg/kg × 1 IM, followed by 1.6 mg/kg IM q.d. × 3 days for a total of 4 days in children, followed by 750 mg mefloquine.
[b] Halofantrine may fail with mefloquine-resistant parasites, and there are risks of neuro- and fetotoxicity with artemisinin compounds.
IM, intramuscular; IV, intravenous.

because neither the necessary reagents nor the expertise to use them are readily available in most malaria-endemic areas.

OPTIMAL MANAGEMENT

CHOICE OF ANTIMALARIALS

Infection of the nonimmune patient with *P. falciparum* is considered a medical emergency, and treatment is based accordingly (Table 322.2). Chloroquine should be used if the patient has come from an area where there is no evidence of chloroquine resistance, such as Haiti. In contrast, nonimmune patients who have taken chloroquine chemoprophylaxis in areas with chloroquine resistance should be treated initially with other agents. Semi-immune persons exposed to chloroquine-resistant *P. falci-*

parum, who have not taken chemoprophylaxis, are not critically ill and have no more than 10^4 parasites per microliter, may be treated initially with chloroquine if they can be observed carefully. However, other antimalarials known to be effective against chloroquine-resistant *P. falciparum* should be given at the first sign of clinical deterioration or if the parasitemia rises above 10^4 per microliter.

The choice of antimalarials for persons who may be infected with chloroquine-resistant *P. falciparum* is controversial and difficult. Oral mefloquine is available in the United States and is effective in most chloroquine-resistant *P. falciparum* cases. However, persons who have been on mefloquine prophylaxis should not be treated with halofantrine because many mefloquine-resistant *P. falciparum* organisms are also halofantrine-resistant. Pyrimethamine–sulfadoxine (Fansidar) may be effective but should not be used for critically ill, nonimmune patients because resistance to the drug has occurred in many areas with chloroquine-resistant *P. falciparum*. Quinine and quinidine are usually effective and may be given orally or parenterally, although they have substantial toxicity (see following discussion), especially when begun with an intravenous loading dose in elderly patients. Qinghao and other artemisinin derivatives (artemether, arteether, artesunate) are used with increasing frequency in Southeast Asia and Africa because they are active in most cases involving chloroquine-resistant *P. falciparum* and typically produce rapid parasite clearance. Unresolved questions about these compounds that have impeded their acceptance in the United States include evidence for neurotoxicity in animal models, a question of cerebellar toxicity in humans, and uncertainty about their safety in pregnancy. Atovaquone plus proguanil is a recently available option for chloroquine-resistant *P. falciparum* infections. In summary, potentially chloroquine-resistant *P. falciparum* infections are usually treated with mefloquine or quinidine in countries such as the United States.

Chloroquine is the treatment of choice for *P. vivax*, *P. ovale*, and *P. malariae* infections. However, there are reports of resistance to chloroquine among *P. vivax* organisms from Indonesia, Papua New Guinea, and elsewhere. Thus far, these infections have responded to treatment with quinine (plus doxycycline or pyrimethamine–sulfadoxine) or single-dose mefloquine (1,250-mg salt; Table 322.2). The addition of primaquine is recommended for patients with *P. vivax* or *P. ovale* infections acquired by mosquito-borne transmission to prevent late relapse from persistent hypnozoites in the liver. Primaquine is usually given after the initial treatment with chloroquine has cleared the patient's parasitemia. This permits time for glucose-6-phosphate dehydrogenase (G6PD) testing of the patient's RBCs to avoid the hemolysis that may occur in patients with G6PD deficiency and obviates potential confusion between the side effects of primaquine and the patient's illness.

MODE OF ADMINISTRATION AND TOXICITY

Because of its cardiotoxicity (arrhythmogenic potential), chloroquine should not be given by rapid intravenous infusion. It may be given intramuscularly or by slow (carefully controlled) intravenous infusion (Table 322.2).

Quinine is often given intravenously for the treatment of chloroquine-resistant *P. falciparum* infection but may produce cinchonism (vertigo, nausea, tinnitus) at excessive serum concentrations (≥ 5 μg per milliliter). Hypoglycemia is an important side effect of both quinine and quinidine because they stimulate the release of insulin directly from the pancreatic β cell, regardless of the plasma glucose concentration. For this reason, and because hypoglycemia may also result from the parasite's consumption of glucose and there is decreased oral intake during the patient's illness, comatose patients infected with *P. falciparum* should be treated empirically with intravenous glucose if blood glucose measurements are not available on an emergency basis. Patients who are comatose because of hypoglycemia typically respond to treatment with one or two ampules of 50% dextrose intravenously. In countries such as the United States, intravenous quinidine is now preferred because it is two to three times more active than quinine against the parasite because quinidine

(but not quinine) drug levels can be measured in many hospitals (to identify dose level–related side effects) and because intravenous quinine is now available only through the U.S. Centers for Disease Control and Prevention.

For patients with *P. falciparum* infections that may be partially resistant to quinine, a quinine loading dose (16.7-mg base per kilogram intravenously over 4 hours) has been recommended to produce therapeutic serum levels more rapidly than maintenance doses alone (8.3-mg base per kilogram intravenously every 8 hours) because it clears the parasitemia more rapidly. Corticosteroids are not recommended for the treatment of coma in cerebral malaria because controlled studies have shown that patients who receive steroids take longer to recover from coma and clear their parasitemias more slowly than control patients who did not receive steroids.

◾ PREVENTION AND CONTROL

DEVELOPMENT OF A MALARIA VACCINE

Most investigators believe that an effective malaria vaccine will need at least three antigens—specifically, sporozoite, merozoite (asexual), and gametocyte (sexual) stage antigens—to simultaneously reduce infection of the liver by sporozoites, replication of asexual forms in the bloodstream, and infectivity for the anopheline mosquito vector. Although the genes responsible for the immunodominant epitopes on the sporozoite, merozoite, and gamete have been cloned and are now being used to produce candidate vaccines, it is not yet clear as to whether those candidate vaccines will be successful or when a safe and effective malaria vaccine will be available.

CHEMOPROPHYLAXIS

For the immediate future, chemoprophylaxis is the most important preventive measure for nonimmune travelers to malaria endemic areas (Table 322.3). Chloroquine remains the chemoprophylactic agent of choice for areas without chloroquine resistance because of its safety (even during pregnancy) and the lack of visual side effects (at doses used for malaria chemoprophylaxis). Alternative chemoprophylactic agents for areas with chloroquine resistance include mefloquine (which is probably safe during pregnancy) and doxycycline (which is not safe during pregnancy or for young children, and produces yeast vaginitis frequently and a photosensitive dermatitis infrequently).

ANCILLARY MEASURES

Especially in areas with chloroquine resistance, it is important to reduce vector exposure as much as possible with conventional measures such as mosquito netting and mosquito repellents (*N,N*-diethyl-*m*-toluamide, or DEET). Bed nets or curtains impregnated with pyrethroid insecticides (permethrin, deltamethrin) have been shown to reduce the frequency of biting by anophelines and the prevalence of infection. However, the impact of this strategy on the incidence of severe and complicated malaria is not yet clear.

TABLE 322.3.	CHEMOPROPHYLAXIS OF MALARIA

Drug	Dosage
All species except chloroquine-resistant *Plasmodium falciparum*	
Chloroquine phosphate (Aralen)	300-mg base (500 mg chloroquine phosphate) weekly, beginning 1 wk before exposure, and continuing for 4 wk after exposure
Chloroquine-resistant *P. falciparum*	
Mefloquine (Lariam)	250 mg mefloquine (228-mg base) weekly during exposure and continuing for 4 wk after exposure
Doxycycline (Vibramycin)	100 mg/d beginning 1 d before exposure, continuing during the period of exposure, and for 4 wk thereafter
Proguanil (Paludrine[a])	200 mg/d in combination with weekly chloroquine during the period of exposure and for 4 wk thereafter
Prevention of late relapse due to *Plasmodium vivax* or *Plasmodium ovale*	
Primaquine phosphate	15-mg primaquine base (26.3 mg primaquine phosphate) per day $\times$ 14 d after leaving the endemic area

[a] Not available in the United States.

BIBLIOGRAPHY

Anonymous. Drugs for parasitic infections. *Med Lett Drugs Ther* 1998;40: 1–12.

Gluzman IY, Krogstad DJ, Orjih AU, et al. A rapid in vitro test for chloroquine-resistant *Plasmodium falciparum*. *Am J Trop Med Hyg* 1990;42: 521–526.

Grau GE, Taylor TE, Molyneux ME, et al. Tumor necrosis factor and disease severity in children with falciparum malaria. *N Engl J Med* 1989; 320:1586–1591.

Krogstad DJ, Gluzman IY, Kyle DE, et al. Efflux of chloroquine from *Plasmodium falciparum*: mechanism of chloroquine resistance. *Science* 1987;238:1283–1285.

Krotoski WA. The hypnozoite and malarial relapse. *Prog Clin Parasitol* 1989;1:1–19.

Marsh K, Forster D, Waruiru C, et al. Indicators of life-threatening malaria in African children. *N Engl J Med* 1995;332:1399–1404.

Phillips-Howard PA, Wood D. The safety of antimalarial drugs in pregnancy. *Drug Safety* 1996;14:131–145.

Piper R, Lebras J, Wentworth L, et al. Immunocapture diagnostic assays for malaria using *Plasmodium* lactate dehydrogenase (pLDH). *Am J Trop Med Hyg* 1999;60:109–118.

Taylor TE, Molyneux ME, Wirima JJ, et al. Blood glucose levels in Malawian children before and during the administration of intravenous quinine for severe falciparum malaria. *N Engl J Med* 1988;310:1040–1047.

Schuurkamp GJ, Spicer PE, Kereu RK, et al. Chloroquine-resistant *Plasmodium vivax* in Papua New Guinea. *Trans R Soc Trop Med Hyg* 1992; 86:121–122.

Stoute JA, Slaoui M, Heppner DG, et al. A preliminary evaluation of a recombinant circumsporozoite protein vaccine against *Plasmodium falciparum* malaria. *N Engl J Med* 1997;336:86–91.

Su X, Heatwole VM, Wertheimer SP, et al. The large diverse gene family *var* encodes proteins involved in the cytoadherence and antigenic variation of *Plasmodium falciparum*–infected erythrocytes. *Cell* 1995;82: 89–100.

Su XZ, Kirkman LA, Fujioka H, et al. Complex polymorphisms in an approximately 330 kDa protein are linked to chloroquine-resistant *P. falciparum* in Southeast Asia and Africa. *Cell* 1997;91:593–603.

Tran TH, Day NP, Nguyen HP, et al. A controlled trial of artemether or quinine in Vietnamese adults with severe falciparum malaria. *N Engl J Med* 1996;335:76–83.

Van Hensbroek MB, Onyiorah E, Jaffar S, et al. A trial of artemether or quinine in children with cerebral malaria. *N Engl J Med* 1996;335: 69–75.

Wang R, Doolan DL, Le TP, et al. Induction of antigen-specific cytotoxic T lymphocytes in humans by a malaria DNA vaccine. *Science* 1998; 282:476–480.

Warrell DA, Looareesuwan S, Warrell MJ, et al. Dexamethasone proves deleterious in cerebral malaria: a double-blind trial in 100 comatose patients. *N Engl J Med* 1982;306:313–319.

Kelley's Textbook of Internal Medicine, fourth edition. Edited by H. David Humes. Lippincott Williams & Wilkins, Philadelphia © 2000.

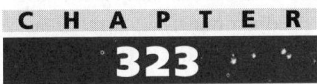

CHAPTER
323

LEISHMANIASIS

A. CLINTON WHITE, JR.
PETER C. MELBY

DEFINITION, INCIDENCE, AND EPIDEMIOLOGY

Leishmaniasis is a group of chronic cutaneous, mucosal, and visceral infections caused by protozoan parasites of the genus *Leishmania* (Table 323.1). Approximately 400,000 new cases are reported each year worldwide with an estimated 12 million persons infected. Over 15 different species of parasite cause human leishmaniasis, each with subtle differences in geographic distribution, host specificity, insect vectors, and disease manifestations. All, however, are transmitted by the bite of female blood-eating sandflies (genus *Phlebotomus* in the eastern hemisphere and *Lutzomyia* in the western hemisphere). In the natural life cycle, the parasites are transmitted between the sandflies and

TABLE 323.1.	MAJOR *LEISHMANIA* SPECIES THAT CAUSE HUMAN DISEASE

	Species	Main Presentation	Unusual Presentations	Main Geographic Location
L. donovani complex	*L. donovani*	VL	PKDL	India, Bangladesh, China, Africa
	L. infantum	VL	CL	Middle East, Mediterranean, North Africa, China
	L. chagasi	VL	CL	Central and South America
L. tropica complex	*L. tropica*	CL	VL, LR	Middle East, Mediterranean, West Asia
	L. major	CL	ML, SL	Middle East, Central Asia, Africa
	L. aethiopica	CL	DCL	East Africa
L. mexicana complex	*L. mexicana*	CL	DCL	From Texas and Mexico to northern South America, Dominican Republic
	L. amazonensis	CL	DCL	From Bolivia and Brazil north to Costa Rica
	L. venezuelensis	CL		Venezuela
L. braziliensis complex		(subgenus *Vianna*)		
	L. braziliensis	CL	ML, SL	South America, Central America from northern Argentina to Guatemala
	L. panamensis	CL	(ML), SL	Ecuador, Colombia, Venezuela, Central America
	L. guyanensis	CL	(ML), SL	Amazon basin, Guyana, Surinam, French Guiana

CL, cutaneous leishmaniasis; DCL, disseminated cutaneous leishmaniasis; LR, leishmaniasis recidivans (lupoid leishmaniasis); ML, mucosal leishmaniasis; PKDL, post–kala azar dermal leishmaniasis; SL, sporotrichoid or lymphatic leishmaniasis; VL, visceral leishmaniasis.
(Adapted from Evans TG. Leishmaniasis. *Infect Dis Clin North Am* 1993;7:527; Grimaldi G Jr, Tesh RB. Leishmaniasis of the new world: current concepts and implications for future research. *Clin Microbiol Rev* 1993;6:230.)

mammalian reservoir hosts. Human infection is a zoonosis that occurs when infected sandflies feed on humans as a substitute for the reservoir host. The diseases are usually chronic, lasting months to years. In the eastern hemisphere (Old World), cutaneous leishmaniasis is usually caused by parasites of the *Leishmania tropica* complex (*L. major, L. tropica, L. aethiopica*, and others). The reservoirs for *L. major* are rodents, and human infection occurs predominantly in rural areas. *L. tropica* is transmitted through a zoonotic cycle (the reservoirs have not been fully defined) in some rural areas, and through an anthroponotic cycle (humans are the reservoir) in some densely populated urban centers. The endemic regions for Old World cutaneous leishmaniasis include widespread areas in Asia, the Middle East, and Africa, but most cases are acquired in the Middle East and Central Asia. In the western hemisphere (New World), cutaneous leishmaniasis is usually caused by parasites of the *Leishmania mexicana* complex (subgenus *Leishmania; L. mexicana, L. amazonensis*, and others) or *Leishmania braziliensis* complex (subgenus *Viannia; L. braziliensis, L. guyanensis, L. panamensis*, and others). The reservoir hosts for *L. mexicana* complex parasites are primarily forest rodents. The reservoirs of *L. braziliensis* include forest rodents and domestic animals (e.g., dogs, equines). The other members of the *L. braziliensis* complex are primarily parasites of arboreal edentates of the rain forests. Thus, American cutaneous leishmaniasis occurs primarily among people who work or settle in or near neotropical forests. *L. braziliensis* complex parasites are also associated with mucosal disease in which patients develop potentially mutilating metastatic infections involving the nasal or oropharyngeal mucosa. Most cases are due to *L. braziliensis*, but rarely cases may be due to *L. braziliensis* complex parasites, *L. amazonensis, L. major*, or *L. donovani* complex parasites. With *L. braziliensis* infection, only 2% to 3% of infected patients

develop mucosal disease. Mucosal disease occurs more commonly in patients with multiple or large ulcers and in patients not adequately treated for cutaneous leishmaniasis.

Visceral leishmaniasis occurs when parasites disseminate from the site of cutaneous inoculation to infect the macrophages of the reticuloendothelial system (liver, spleen, bone marrow). It is present in both hemispheres and is associated with parasites of the *L. donovani* complex (*L. donovani, Leishmania infantum*, and *Leishmania chagasi*). Visceral leishmaniasis occurs in four major endemic foci, which differ in epidemiology and disease manifestation. In eastern India and Bangladesh, visceral leishmaniasis is primarily a disease of young adults and older children. Transmission occurs via peridomestic sandflies, which are anthropophilic. No animal reservoir host has been identified, and human-to-human transmission is presumed. In East Africa, visceral leishmaniasis occurs as sporadic cases and in epidemics, such as occurred among refugees in the Sudan beginning in the mid-1980s. Disease typically occurs in older children and adults. Rodents are thought to be the major reservoir host. Canines and humans may also be important reservoir hosts. Visceral leishmaniasis occurs as a sporadic disease in the Middle East, the Mediterranean littoral, and China. Scattered foci are also noted in Central and South America. In the Middle East and the Mediterranean region, and in Latin America, visceral leishmaniasis is primarily a disease of children younger than 5 years. Dogs and other canines are the major reservoir hosts.

ETIOLOGIC FACTORS

Leishmania parasites are dimorphic protozoans. In the sandfly, they take the form of promastigotes, with a body 10 to 15 μm long and an anterior flagellum. The promastigotes multiply in the midgut of the sandflies, then migrate anteriorly. During this migration, they undergo developmental changes, most notably in the structure of the surface lipophosphoglycan, into the infectious metacyclic stage. When an infected sandfly takes a blood meal, the promastigotes are deposited in the wound. In the mammalian host, the parasites are obligate intracellular pathogens found almost exclusively in macrophages. The parasites attach to tissue macrophages, using host cell complement and carbohydrate receptors, and are rapidly incorporated into phagolysosomes. Within the phagolysosome, the parasites transform into rounded or oval amastigote forms, which are 2 to 4 μm in diameter and lack a visible flagellum. The amastigotes replicate within the macrophage, eventually destroying it and spreading to other macrophages. The life cycle is completed when the sandflies are infected by ingesting amastigotes and infected macrophages along with a blood meal.

Leishmania species cannot be distinguished morphologically. Initially, parasite species were designated based on clinical manifestation, animal reservoirs, and geographic distribution. Current methods of parasite speciation include isoenzyme electrophoresis, monoclonal antibody typing, and a variety of DNA-based techniques. Using these techniques, investigators have shown that one species of parasite may give rise to a variety of clinical manifestations. For example, in parts of Central America, *L. chagasi* may cause either visceral or cutaneous disease. Likewise, visceral disease due to *L. tropica* has been described among veterans of the Persian Gulf war. Some investigators classify the parasites by subgenus. The subgenus *Viannia* denotes parasites that undergo part of their development in the sandfly hindgut and includes the parasites of the *L. braziliensis* complex. All other human species are included in the subgenus *Leishmania*.

PATHOGENESIS

After infection of macrophages in the skin, the promastigotes transform to amastigotes and multiply locally. An accompanying influx of host inflammatory cells is present, and some of these cells become infected. As more macrophages and lymphocytes are recruited locally, they may form a small erythematous papule. In localized cutaneous leishmaniasis, the cellular infiltration is associated with the development of a cell-mediated immune response accompanied by delayed-type cutaneous hypersensitivity (Montenegro, or leishmanin, skin test). The cellular infiltrate forms granulomas, which lead to ulceration and slow healing. Healing is accompanied by the production of T-helper type 1 cytokines (interleukin-2 and interferon-γ). Macrophages activated by these cytokines are then able to kill the parasites. A minority of patients fail to develop an effective immune response. They are anergic to the Montenegro skin test and develop the spreading nodular lesions of disseminated cutaneous leishmaniasis. In murine models, progressive disease is accompanied by production of T-helper type 2 cytokines (interleukin-4 and interleukin-10). In the case of visceral disease, the parasites spread to the macrophages of the liver, spleen, and bone marrow. Visceral leishmaniasis is also accompanied by the suppression of the cellular immune response to the parasite with negative skin

tests and suppression of the T-helper type 1 cytokines (interleukin-2 and interferon-γ). In contrast, there is augmented production of T-helper type 2 cytokines, particularly interleukin-10. In mucosal disease, the parasites metastasize from the site of infection in the skin to mucosa of the nose and mouth. An intense granulomatous infiltrate, with a mixed T-helper types 1 and 2 cytokine profile, is present in the mucosa. Few parasites can be detected, and it is thought that the tissue destruction is mediated by the intense host inflammatory response.

CLINICAL FEATURES AND MANAGEMENT OF VISCERAL LEISHMANIASIS (KALA AZAR)

Most infections with *L. donovani* complex parasites are either asymptomatic or oligosymptomatic. Only a minority of infections progress to classic visceral leishmaniasis. Oligosymptomatic infection may be characterized by intermittent fever, malaise, diarrhea, and cough. Nearly all patients will have hepatomegaly, but splenomegaly is less common. Most cases will resolve spontaneously over 3 years, but a minority will progress to classic visceral leishmaniasis.

The incubation period for classic visceral leishmaniasis (kala azar) is usually 2 to 8 months. Most patients will note gradual onset of fever. Rarely, there is an abrupt onset of high fever and chills. Other common symptoms include abdominal distention or pain (due to hepatosplenomegaly), weight loss, and lethargy. Complaints of pallor, cough, diarrhea, bleeding, and amenorrhea are less common. On examination, splenomegaly, which may be massive, is nearly always observed. Most patients will have abdominal distention, hepatomegaly, pallor, and wasting. Laboratory evaluation reveals normocytic anemia. Most patients also have leukopenia, thrombocytopenia, and elevated γ-globulins. Mild elevations of transaminases, prolonged prothrombin time, and depressed albumin are also common. Secondary bacterial infections are common in patients with visceral leishmaniasis, especially skin and respiratory tract infections. The primary cause of death is superinfection, including bacterial sepsis, pneumonia, tuberculosis, and dysentery.

Visceral leishmaniasis can present as an opportunistic infection in immunosuppressed patients (e.g., patients with AIDS or with solid organ transplants). In contrast to normal hosts, immunosuppressed patients are less likely to have splenomegaly, and fever is less prominent. Involvement of the lungs, pleura, gastrointestinal mucosa, and skin has also been reported. There are also reports of visceral infection due to parasites of other complexes, including visceral *L. tropica* infection in U.S. troops who served in Operation Desert Storm. The symptoms resembled those seen in visceral leishmaniasis (chronic low-grade fever, malaise, fatigue, and diarrhea) but tended to be milder.

Post–kala azar dermal leishmaniasis is seen in a minority of patients. The lesions vary from hyperpigmented macular to nodular skin lesions primarily on the face and trunk that usually develop months to years after an apparently successful treatment of visceral leishmaniasis. In contrast to cutaneous disease, these lesions will persist unless treated.

CUTANEOUS LEISHMANIASIS (OLD WORLD)

Cutaneous leishmaniasis in the eastern hemisphere is caused predominantly by *L. major, L. tropica,* or *L. aethiopica.* After a typical incubation period of several weeks to several months, an erythematous nodule develops at the site of the insect bite (usually in exposed areas). The center of the nodule begins to crust and then develops an ulcer with raised, inflamed borders containing amastigotes and granulomatous inflammation. The central ulcer gradually crusts. Ulcers will usually heal spontaneously, but healing may require months to years and may leave extensive scarring. *L. major* more frequently causes multiple lesions, is more likely to cause necrosis and ulceration (wet-type lesions), and always heals spontaneously (usually within a few months). *L. tropica* more frequently causes single lesions, often forms a crust rather than ulceration (dry-type lesions), and may heal slowly or not at all. *L. tropica* is associated with leishmaniasis recidivans, in which nodular granulomatous papules recur near the edge of a scar, resembling lupus vulgaris. In addition to localized cutaneous leishmaniasis, *L. aethiopica* is associated with disseminated cutaneous leishmaniasis, with chronic nodular skin lesions disseminated throughout the skin.

CUTANEOUS LEISHMANIASIS (NEW WORLD)

In the western hemisphere, cutaneous leishmaniasis can be caused by parasites of the *L. mexicana* and *L. braziliensis* (subgenus *Viannia*) complexes. The clinical presentation of cutaneous leishmaniasis is similar in eastern and western hemispheres, with papular lesions developing at the site of sandfly bites, followed by ulceration and eventual healing. In one study from Guatemala, lesions caused by *L. braziliensis* were likely to be more numerous, larger, and less likely to heal spontaneously than lesions caused by *L. mexicana* (Figure 323.1). Biopsy specimens also showed

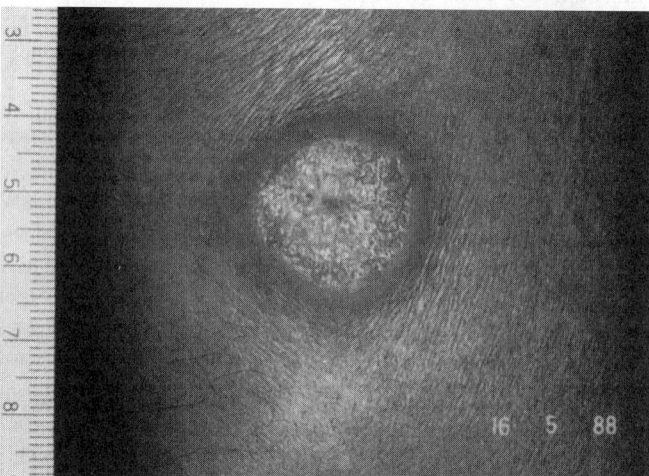

FIGURE 323.1. Typical lesion of cutaneous leishmaniasis showing a cutaneous ulcer with an indurated erythematous border. This patient was infected in Guatemala. (Photograph courtesy of Dr. Thomas R. Navin. From Herwaldt BL et al. American cutaneous leishmaniasis in U.S. travelers. *Ann Intern Med* 1993;118:779.)

fewer parasites in the lesions caused by *L. braziliensis.* Nodular or ulcerative lesions developing along the lymphatics, termed sporotrichoid leishmaniasis, have been associated with *L. braziliensis* complex parasites. *L. mexicana* complex parasites may result in disseminated cutaneous leishmaniasis. Disseminated cutaneous and visceral infections due to *L. braziliensis* have been reported in patients with AIDS. The diagnostic methods are the same for all cases of cutaneous leishmaniasis.

MUCOSAL LEISHMANIASIS

Mucosal leishmaniasis results from the spread of amastigotes from a cutaneous lesion to the mucosa of the nose, mouth, throat, and upper respiratory tract. Mucosal lesions may develop concurrently with a cutaneous lesion, but more commonly the primary lesion has healed before (in some cases decades before) the onset of mucosal disease. Patients initially develop epistaxis or nasal congestion. Untreated disease may progress to involve the nasal septum, palate, lips, oropharyngeal mucosa, larynx, and epiglottis. The appearance of the lesions may range from erythema, edema, or infiltration to frank ulceration. Severe disease may result in destruction of the nasal architecture. Aspiration pneumonia is a common complication of advanced disease and can be fatal.

DIAGNOSIS

The clinical presentation of visceral leishmaniasis is often indistinguishable from other coendemic diseases including malaria, typhoid fever, typhus, acute Chagas' disease, amebic liver abscess, brucellosis, schistosomiasis, lymphoma, or lymphocytic leukemias. Definitive diagnosis depends on demonstration of amastigotes in tissues or of promastigotes in cultures. Bone marrow aspirates are the most common source of diagnostic material. Giemsa- or Wright-stained smears are positive in two-thirds of cases. Splenic aspiration is more sensitive but is avoided because of the risk of potentially life-threatening bleeding. In patients with lymphadenopathy, it is often possible to demonstrate organisms in lymph node aspirates. Cultures of bone marrow or splenic aspirates are positive in 70% to 96% of cases. Serologic tests (indirect immunofluorescence antibody assay, ELISA, direct agglutination assay) show high titers of antileishmania antibodies in patients with active visceral leishmaniasis, providing presumptive evidence of infection. In some regions, cross-reactivity to other infectious agents (most notably *Trypanosoma cruzi*) may diminish the specificity. Recently, a serologic test using a recombinant *Leishmania* antigen (rK39) was shown to be highly sensitive and specific. The sensitivity of serologic tests in patients with AIDS is poor. Other techniques have been used to identify parasites, including immunofluorescence with monoclonal antibodies and polymerase chain reaction.

Diagnosis of cutaneous leishmaniasis is made by identifying organisms on biopsy specimens or on aspirates taken from the dermis of the nonulcerated edge of the lesion. Touch preparations are thought to be more sensitive than biopsies. The diagnostic yield can be improved by culturing the aspirate or ground biopsy material. Serologic tests have limited value in the diagnosis of cutaneous leishmaniasis. Montenegro skin tests are usually positive in localized cutaneous disease and mucocutaneous disease, but are negative in disseminated cutaneous and visceral leishmaniasis. A presumptive diagnosis of mucosal disease can be made in patients with typical lesions and exposure history. Biopsy specimens show granulomatous inflammation but few parasites. Cultures may also be negative.

To culture for *Leishmania* promastigotes, aspirates or tissue homogenates should be inoculated onto a biphasic medium consisting of blood agar [Nicolle–Novy–MacNeal (NNN) medium] overlayed with tissue culture medium (available from the Division of Parasitic Diseases, U.S. Centers for Disease Control and Prevention, Atlanta, GA). When cultured at 24°C to 26°C, the tissue amastigotes transform into motile, flagellated promastigotes that are visible within a few days to several weeks. The isolation of promastigotes enables species identification by a reference lab.

MANAGEMENT

The treatment of choice for visceral leishmaniasis is pentavalent antimony. Sodium stibogluconate (Pentostam, Burroughs Wellcome, London; available in the United States only through the Drug Service of the U.S. Centers for Disease Control and Prevention), containing 100 mg per milliliter of antimony, or meglumine antimonate (Glucantime, Rhône-Poulenc, Paris), containing 85 mg per milliliter, are given by either intramuscular or intravenous routes. Optimal response requires a dose of 20 mg per kilogram per day of antimony. In visceral disease, therapy should be continued for 28 days. Response rates are generally over 90%. Lower rates are seen in patients previously treated with antimonials, during epidemic transmission, and in immunosuppressed hosts. Common side effects include myalgias, arthralgias, mild elevation of liver enzymes, elevation of pancreatic enzymes, and nonspecific electrocardiographic changes. These necessitated interruption of treatment in 28% of cases in one large study, but there were no lasting sequellae. Severe side effects are rare but include cardiac arrhythmias, hematologic abnormalities, and pancreatitis. In patients who fail normal doses of antimonials, prolonging the duration of antimony therapy (e.g., 20 mg per kilogram per day for 40 days) appears to increase response rates. Amphotericin B is also highly effective, but complications are common. Recent studies using lipid formulations of amphotericin B (liposomal amphotericin, AmBisome, Vestar, San Dimas, CA; amphotericin lipid complex, Abelcet, Liposome Technology, Menlo Park, CA; or amphotericin cholesteryl sulfate complex, Amphotec, Sequus, Menlo Park, CA) demonstrated high response rates with few side effects. Pentamidine has been used as an alternative but is associated with higher failure rates as well as toxicity. Parenteral paromomycin (aminosidine) has been shown to be highly effective in Indian kala azar for which antimony treatment has a high failure rate. Aminosidine, interferon-γ, and allopurinol have all been reported to improve response rates when used in combination with pentavalent antimonials.

In immunosuppressed patients (e.g., AIDS patients), there is a poor initial response to antimonials and a high relapse rate. Better initial response rates have been reported using liposomal amphotericin or pentavalent antimonials combined with allopurinol or interferon-γ. Secondary prophylaxis to prevent relapses may be needed, but the optimal regimen has not been defined.

Specific antileishmanial therapy is not routinely indicated for uncomplicated cutaneous leishmaniasis caused by strains that usually self-heal (*L. major, L. mexicana*). Lesions that are extensive, located where a scar would result in disability or cosmetic disfigurement, or do not begin healing within 3 to 4 months should be treated. Cutaneous lesions suspected or known to be caused by members of the *Viannia* subgenus (New World) should be treated because of the low rate of spontaneous healing and the potential risk of developing into mucosal disease. All patients with mucosal disease should receive therapy.

Pentavalent antimonials are also the primary therapy for Old World cutaneous leishmaniasis and should be given at a dose of 20 mg per kilogram per day for 20 days. Topical treatment with heat, paromomycin, or intralesional antimony has been reported to be effective in some cases. Uncontrolled trials have described cures with oral allopurinol or ketoconazole.

The treatment of American cutaneous leishmaniasis has only recently been studied in carefully controlled trials. Pentavalent antimonials are the standard treatment and should be given at a dose of 20 mg per kilogram per day of antimony. The recommended duration of therapy is 20 days, but excellent response rates have been reported with 10 days of treatment. Oral allopurinol was superior to pentavalent antimony in a trial from Colombia for leishmaniasis due to antimony-resistant *L. panamensis* but was not effective in trials from Ecuador and Panama. Ketoconazole has some efficacy, but trials of itraconazole have been disappointing. Ketoconazole at 600 mg per day was superior to antimonials for *L. mexicana* in a trial from Guatemala. One study noted excellent response rates to pentamidine. Reports also exist of successful immunotherapy using a vaccine composed of bacille Calmette-Guérin and killed *Leishmania* promastigotes.

Mucocutaneous disease responds poorly to antiparasitic agents. The recommended therapy is pentavalent antimonials at 20 mg per kilogram per day for 28 days. Cure rates with isolated nasal disease approach 75%. With involvement of the oropharynx, cure rates range from 10% to 63%. Failures include patients who do not respond and others relapsing after initial improvement. Prolonging therapy does not improve the response rate. Amphotericin B or lipid preparations of amphotericin have most often been used in patients failing antimonials.

Cure of disseminated cutaneous leishmaniasis is difficult and relapses are the norm. Some efficacy has been reported with a combination of pentavalent antimony and interferon-γ. Disseminated cutaneous disease in the Old World responds poorly to antimonials but may respond to pentamidine.

BIBLIOGRAPHY

Alvar J, Canavate C, Gutierrez-Solar B, et al. *Leishmania* and human immunodeficiency virus coinfection: the first 10 years. *Clin Microbiol Rev* 1997;10:298–319.
Aronson NE, Wortmann GW, Johnson SC, et al. Safety and efficacy of

intravenous sodium stibogluconate in the treatment of leishmaniasis: recent U.S. military experience. *Clin Infect Dis* 1998;27:1457–1464.

Ashford RW, Desjeux P, deRaadt P. Estimation of population at risk and number of cases of leishmaniasis. *Parasitol Today* 1992;8:104.

Berman JD. Human leishmaniasis: clinical, diagnostic, and chemotherapeutic developments in the last 10 years. *Clin Infect Dis* 1997;24:684–703.

Berman J. Chemotherapy of leishmaniasis: recent advances in the treatment of visceral leishmaniasis. *Curr Opin Infect Dis* 1998;11:707.

Davidson RN, di Martino L, Gradoni L, et al. Short-course treatment of visceral leishmaniasis with liposomal amphotericin B (AmBisome). *Clin Infect Dis* 1996;22:938–943.

Franke ED, Llanos-Cuentas A, Echevarria J, et al. Efficacy of 28-day and 40-day regimens of sodium stibogluconate (Pentostam) in the treatment of mucosal leishmaniasis. *Am J Trop Med Hyg* 1994;51:77–82.

Herwaldt B, Berman JD. Recommendations for treating leishmaniasis with sodium stibogluconate (Pentostam) and review of pertinent clinical studies. *Am J Trop Med Hyg* 1992;46:296–306.

Jha TK, Thakur CPN, Kanyok TP, et al. Randomised controlled trial of aminosidine (paromomycin) v sodium stibogluconate for treating visceral leishmaniasis in North Bihar, India. *Br Med J* 1998;316:1200–1205.

Pearson RD, de Queiroz Sousa A. Clinical spectrum of leishmaniasis. *Clin Infect Dis* 1996;22:1–13.

Seaman J, Mercer AJ, Sondorp HE, et al. Epidemic visceral leishmaniasis in southern Sudan: treatment of severely debilitated patients under wartime conditions and with limited resources. *Ann Intern Med* 1996;124:664–672.

Kelley's Textbook of Internal Medicine, fourth edition. Edited by H. David Humes. Lippincott Williams & Wilkins, Philadelphia © 2000.

CHAPTER

324

AFRICAN AND AMERICAN TRYPANOSOMIASES

MARIO PAREDES-ESPINOZA
PATRICIA PAREDES-CASILLAS

DEFINITION

African and American trypanosomiases, also called sleeping sickness and Chagas' disease, respectively, are caused by protozoan parasites that belong to the genus *Trypanosoma*. The subspecies *Trypanosoma brucei gambiense* and *T. brucei rhodesiense* cause West African and East African trypanosomiases, respectively, and are transmitted by blood-sucking tsetse flies. *T. b. brucei* is a third African trypanosome subspecies that causes a usually fatal disease of cattle called nagana, which means "in low spirits" in Zulu. Chagas' disease is caused by the species *Trypanosoma cruzi,* which is transmitted by numerous species of hematophagous triatomine insects, also called kissing bugs.

ETIOLOGIC FACTORS

These organisms are fusiform hemoflagellate protozoans belonging to the family Trypanosomatidae, order Kinetoplastida. Their single mitochondrion contains a unique structure called the kinetoplast, which contains many thousands of interlocking circular DNAs. Most morphologic stages of these trypanosomes have a flagellum anchored by an undulating membrane that produces forward motion of the parasite resembling that of an auger (*trupanon* in Greek). The nucleus is large and oval with a central karyosome. Trypanosomes have complex life cycles involving mammals as well as insect vectors, and in passing from one group of hosts to the other undergo major morphologic and metabolic changes. In the case of *T. b. brucei,* discovered by David Bruce in Zululand in 1894, some of the longitudinally dividing slender bloodstream trypanosomes in mammals differentiate into relatively stumpy forms that are preadapted for infecting tsetse flies (Fig. 324.1). Carlos Chagas discovered *T. cruzi* in 1907. Infected triatomine insects transmit the disease while painlessly sucking blood for 20 or more minutes from mammals. Rising intra-abdominal pressure causes the bug, in many instances, to deposit parasite-containing feces on the skin at or near the puncture site. These organisms can enter the mammalian host through breaks in the skin, including the puncture site, as well as through normal mucosas or conjunctivas (Fig. 324.2).

AFRICAN TRYPANOSOMIASIS

INCIDENCE AND EPIDEMIOLOGIC FACTORS

The complex epidemiology of African (or Rhodesian) trypanosomiasis involves tsetse flies ("flies that destroy cattle" in Zulu), trypanosomes, humans, game animals, and the ecological circumstances within which they all coexist. The bite of riverine tsetse *Glossina palpalis* and open-savannah *Glossina morsitans* transmit the disease in sub-Saharan West, Central, and East Africa in an area approximately equal to the size of the United States.

Approximately 50 million people live in areas endemic for sleeping sickness, and 20,000 to 30,000 cases of acute and chronic sleeping sickness are reported annually. The actual number of cases probably is many times this figure, and as many as 55,000 persons may die annually due to sleeping sickness. In Angola, the Democratic Republic of Congo, the Sudan, and Uganda, the disease is considered epidemic, with a prevalence greater than 50% in many villages, a high transmission rate, and total deaths equal to or greater than those due to AIDS. Little is known about the epidemiology of sleeping sickness in countries such as Ethiopia, Liberia, or Senegal. Infected tsetse can transmit the disease to young babies who are being carried on their mothers' backs. Game wardens, hunters, poachers, honey gatherers, firewood collectors, and others who venture into areas

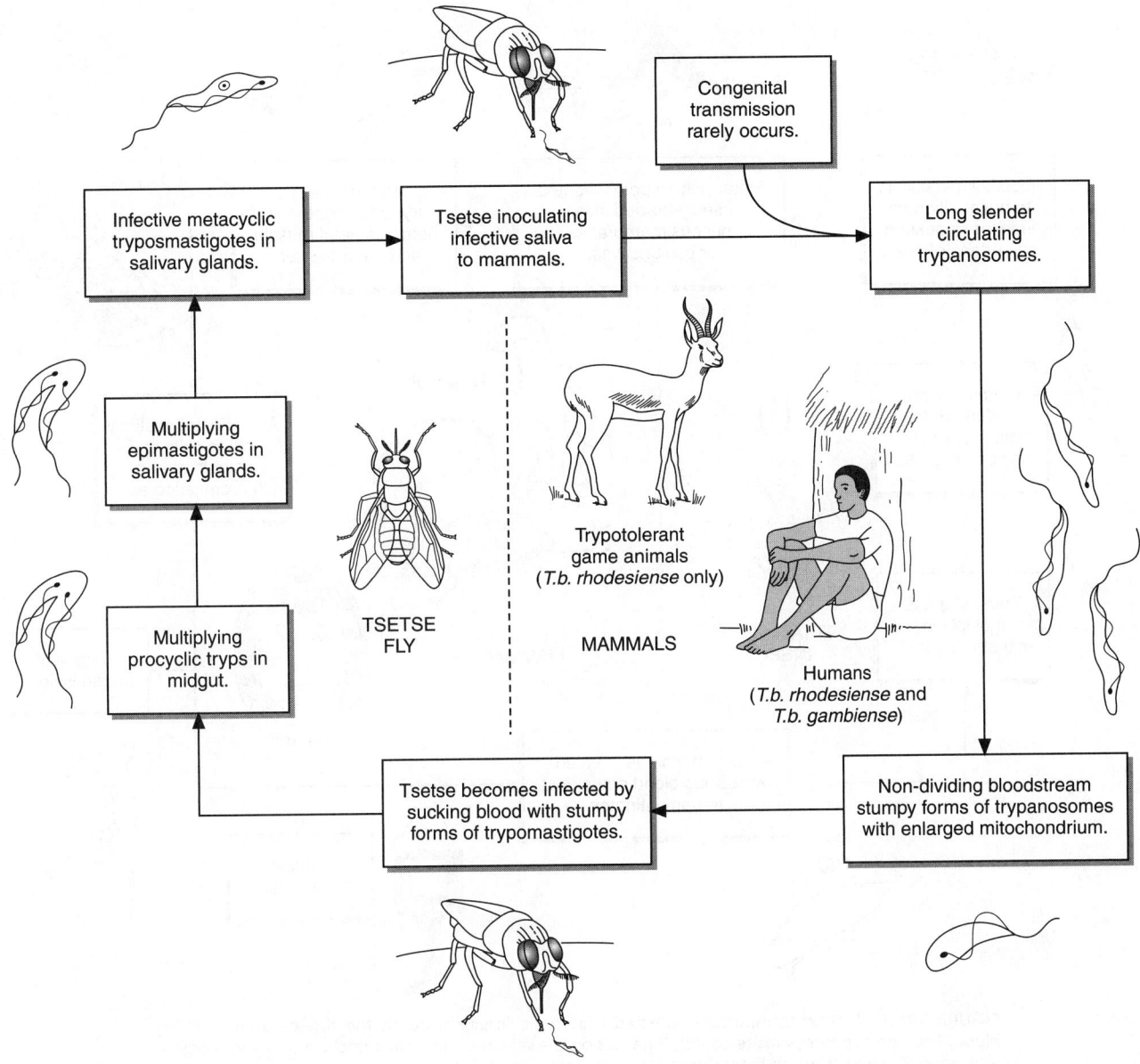

FIGURE 324.1. *T. b. brucei.* Differentiation in mammals of the longitudinally dividing slender bloodstream trypanosomes, preadapted for infecting tsetse flies.

populated by wild animal reservoirs are at risk for acquiring Rhodesian trypansomiasis in East Africa.

PATHOGENESIS

Once inoculated into a mammalian host with tsetse saliva, trypanosomes multiply locally and often invade the lymphatics. Parasitemia appears within a week or two but is initially controlled by antibody-mediated mechanisms of destruction. Symptomatic, periodic parasitemia occurs throughout the life of the host due to sequential antigenic variations of the surface glycoprotein of the parasite. No long-standing immunity develops. Direct parasite–macrophage interactions initiate a cascade of immunomod-

ulatory mechanisms that eventually lead to profound immunosuppression. A diffusible *T. b. rhodesiense* immunosuppressive factor has been shown to block interleukin-2R (IL-2R) expression by activated human lymphocytes in vitro. There is initial polyclonal activation of CD5$^+$ B-cell proliferation with consequent exhaustion of antigen B lymphocytes and arrest of T-cell proliferation.

CLINICAL FINDINGS

A trypanosomal chancre appears within days at the site of the infected tsetse bite. This is generally a tender and indurated inflammatory lesion several centimeters in diameter. Weeks or

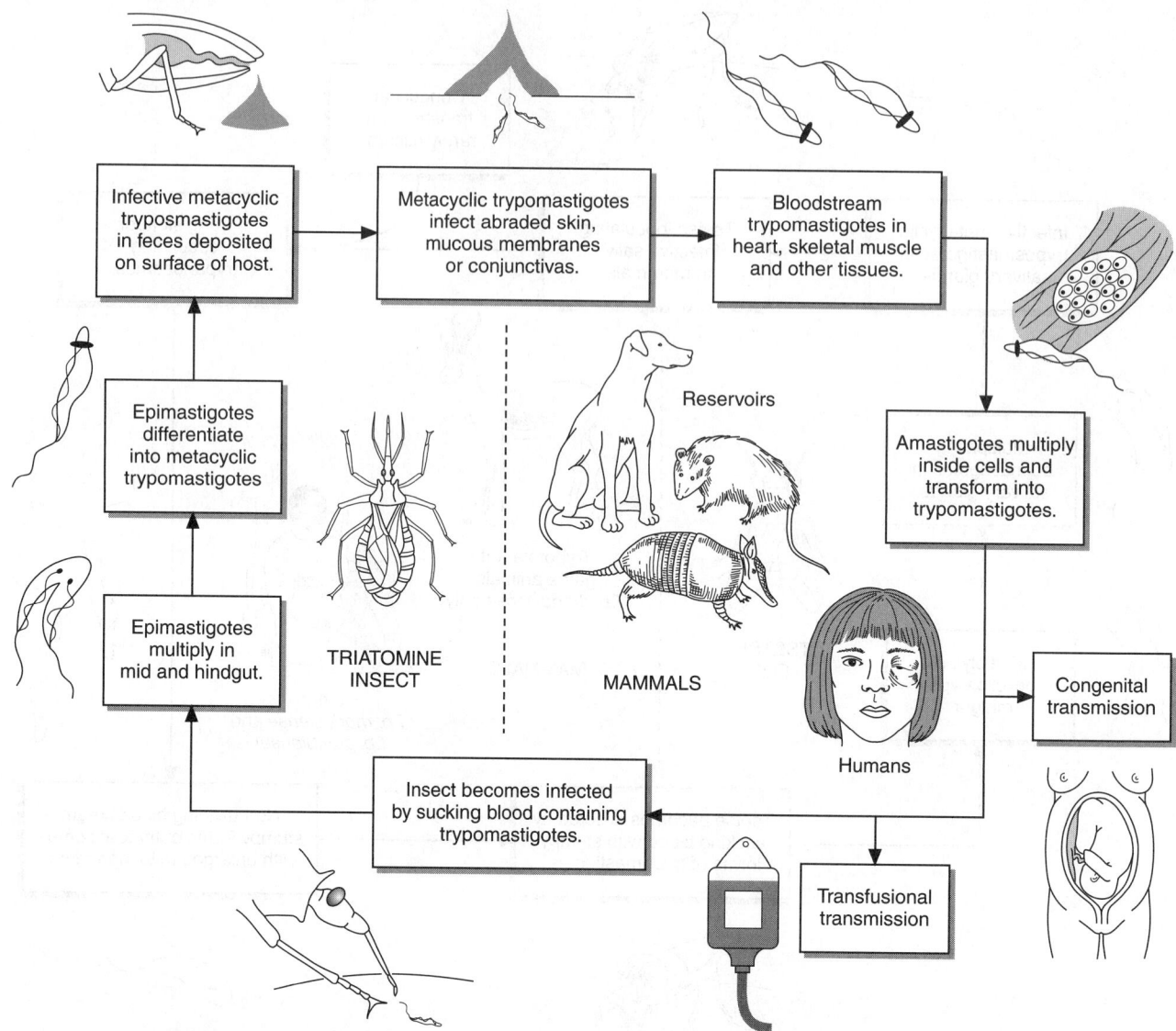

FIGURE 324.2. *T. cruzi* transmission. Infected triatomine insects transmit the disease while sucking blood. The bug deposits parasite-containing feces on the skin at or near the puncture site. These organisms enter the host through breaks in the skin, mucosas, or conjunctivas.

months later the hemolymphatic stage of the disease develops, which is notable for cyclic episodes of high fever, severe headaches, and malaise alternating with progressively shorter asymptomatic periods.

Areas of pruritic annular skin rash up to 10 cm in diameter (trypanids) may appear on the trunk and shoulders. Kerandel sign is an uncommon but nearly pathognomonic form of hyperesthesia that causes patients to become obsessed with a fear of hurting themselves. Hepatosplenomegaly and diarrhea (more marked in children), initial polyphagia, severe hemolytic anemia, wasting, recurrent pneumonia, spontaneous abortion, amenorrhea, impotence, and high abortion rate occur. Progressive myocarditis with heart failure and disseminated intravascular coagulation with or without severe central nervous system (CNS)

involvement may cause death within weeks to a few months in the East African form of the disease, whereas the course of West African trypanosomiasis is usually less aggressive.

Particularly in the case of infections with *T. b. gambiense*, months after the beginning of the hemolymphatic stage chronic progressive meningoencephalitis may develop, with profound somnolence and apathy. Prominent adenopathy in the posterior cervical triangle (Winterbottom's sign) may represent lymphatic drainage of trypanosomes from the ventricles and the base of the brain. Extrapyramidal and cerebellar damage, emotional lability, slurred speech, sad expression, facial edema, cachexia, and death occur over a course of 2 to 3 years. Sleeping sickness in children usually follows a rapid course. Reactivation of chronic gambiense infection has not been observed in HIV-infected patients.

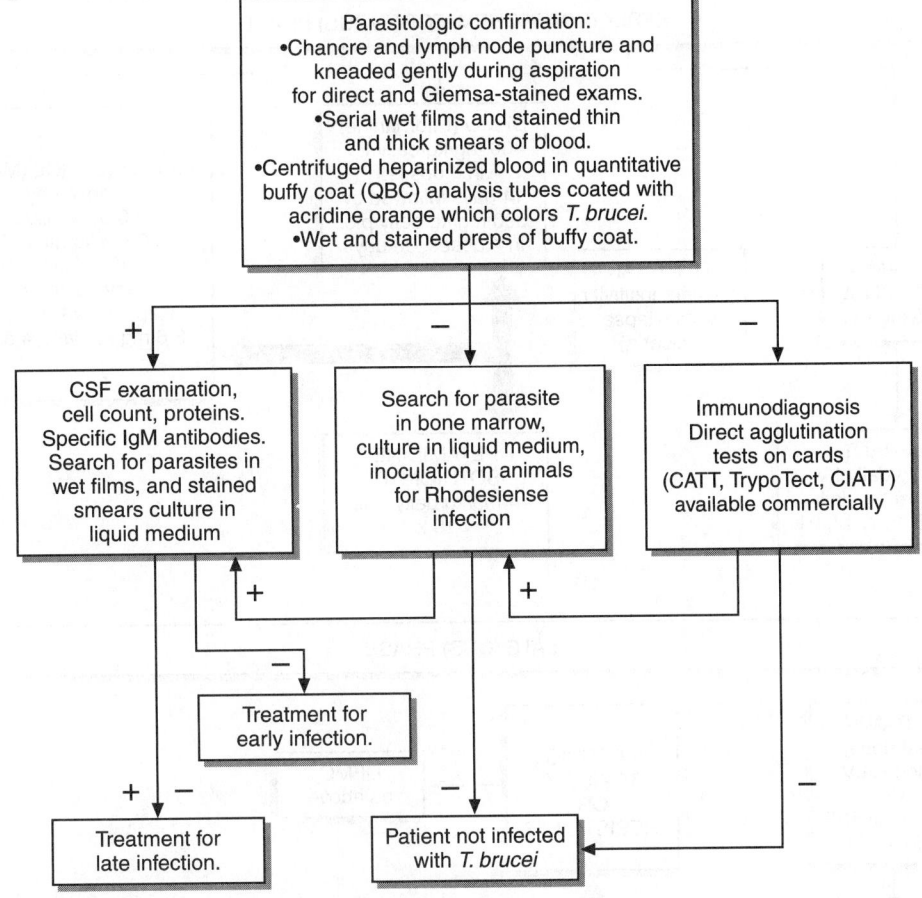

FIGURE 324.3. Lymph fluid, as well as cerebrospinal fluid, can be examined for a diagnosis of sleeping sickness.

LABORATORY FINDINGS

The diagnosis of sleeping sickness must be made by parasitologic methods. Therapy should never be started until parasites have been visualized because of the potential toxicity of the drugs used for treatment. Microscopic examination of wet preparations and Giemsa-stained thin and thick smears of peripheral blood or buffy coat is a sensitive method for detecting African trypanosomes. Fluid aspirated from a swollen lymph node or the bone marrow, as well as cerebrospinal fluid, can be examined similarly (Fig. 324.3). Implementation of even these simple approaches is limited in many endemic regions because of a lack of human and material resources.

OPTIMAL MANAGEMENT

Suramin, arsenicals, and eflornithine [2-(difluoromethyl)-DL-or-nithine; DFMO] achieve a parasitologic cure in over 90% of cases of early and late stage sleeping sickness (Fig. 324.4). Drug toxicity is high, especially with arsenicals, and related mortality may exceed 5%. Untreated sleeping sickness is usually fatal. Corticosteroids can be used as adjunctive treatment of late-stage sleeping sickness with CNS involvement or to prevent reactive

encephalopathy induced by arsenicals, which occurs in about 10% of patients and has a mortality of 50%. The signs and symptoms of reactive arsenical encephalopathy can include headache, fever, psychosis, seizures, and coma.

■ AMERICAN TRYPANOSOMIASIS

INCIDENCE AND EPIDEMIOLOGIC FACTORS

Insect-borne acquisition of *T. cruzi* by humans, which is the most common mode of transmission, depends on the interaction of a number of complex factors relating to vector density and feeding habits, biological characteristics of the parasites, host immune status, and a conducive physical environment (Table 324.1). Some 50 triatomine species are known to transmit *T. cruzi,* and over 100 species of mammals are reservoirs of the parasite. The wild mammals most commonly infected with *T. cruzi* are armadillos, raccoons, and opossums. *Triatoma infestans, Panstrongylus megistus, Rhodnius prolixus, T. dimidiata,* and *T. barberi* are vector species that are well adapted to living in rural dwellings in endemic regions. *T. cruzi* also can be transmitted by transfusion of contaminated blood, and many thousands of

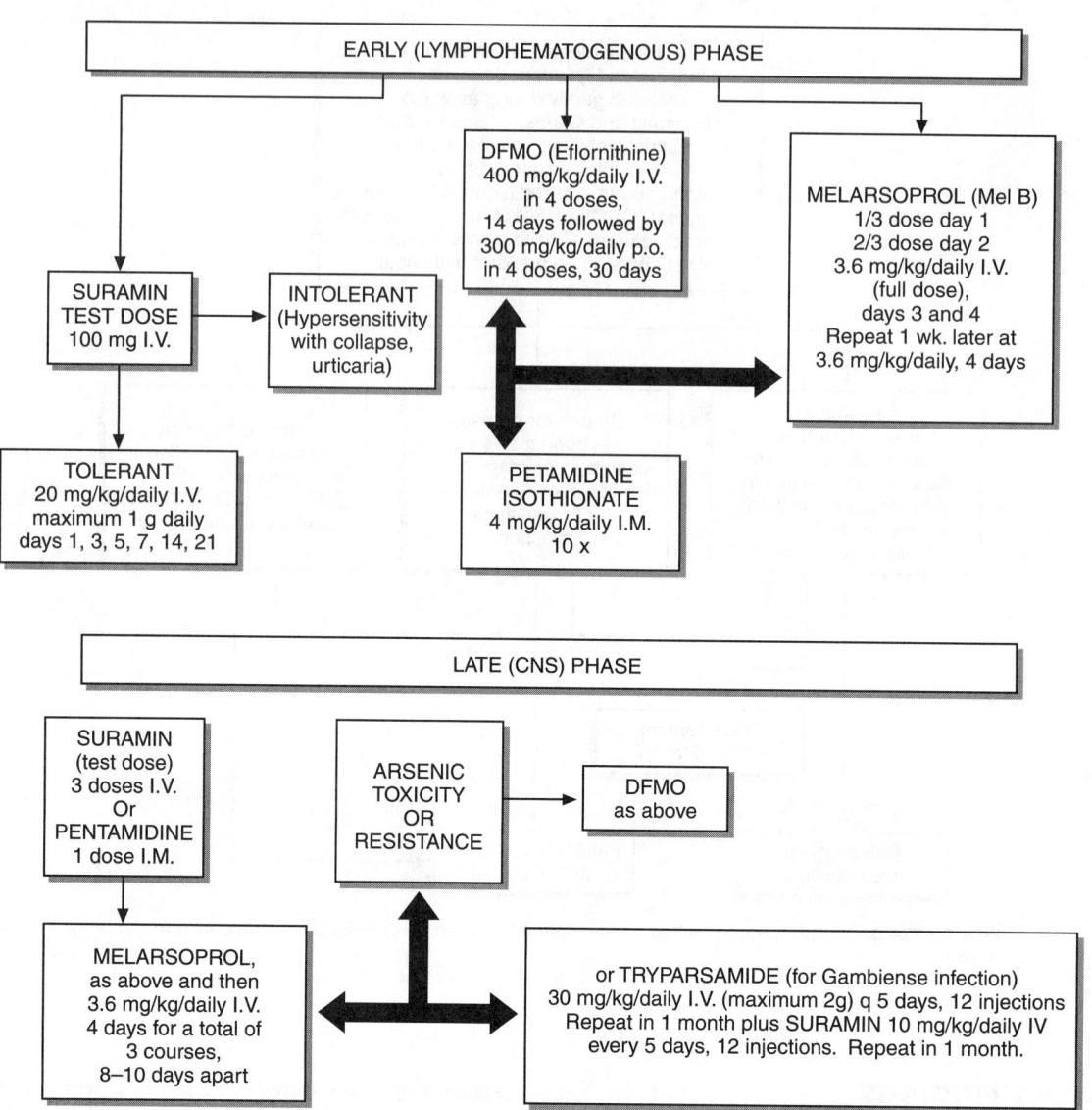

FIGURE 324.4. Effectiveness of treatment with Suramin, arsenicals, and eflornithine in cases of early and late stage sleeping sickness.

transfusion recipients become infected by this route each year in areas where effective donor-screening programs have not been implemented. Prevalence of *T. cruzi* among blood donors in many endemic regions is higher than that of HIV and hepatitis B and C viruses. Congenital *T. cruzi* infection is present in a small portion of babies born to infected mothers, but precise incidence data are not available.

Over 100 million Latin Americans are at risk of acquiring *T. cruzi* infection, and 16 to 18 million chronically harbor the parasite. Roughly 5 million persons have symptomatic disease and 45,000 die of the illness each year. One hundred eight acute cases of Chagas' disease have been reported on the west coast of Mexico. The annual economic loss resulting from disability and early mortality due to Chagas' disease, which frequently occurs in economically productive young adults, currently is estimated to be more than U.S. $8 billion.

It is estimated that 50,000 to 100,000 Latin American immigrants currently living in the United States are chronically infected with *T. cruzi*. No assay for detecting *T. cruzi* infection in donated blood has been cleared by the U.S. Food and Drug Administration. Currently, a questionnaire is being used in an

TABLE 324.1.	TRANSMISSION OF *TRYPANOSOMA CRUZI* TO HUMANS
Contact with triatomine feces	
Blood transfusions	
Congenital transmission	
Laboratory accidents	

effort to identify high-risk donors. Transfusions of *T. cruzi*–infected blood are particularly hazardous in immunosuppressed patients.

PATHOGENESIS

After contacting susceptible tissues of a mammalian host, infective forms of *T. cruzi* enter macrophages and other cells where they transform into amastigotes. The amastigotes then multiply and eventually differentiate into flagellated trypomastigotes. The latter are released when infected cells rupture and then spread via the lymphatics and the bloodstream to invade other cells, mainly in the heart, skeletal and smooth muscle, CNS, parasympathetic neurons, and reticuloendothelial system.

Most circulating parasites are destroyed by specific antibodies plus complement or in combination with Fc receptor–bearing leukocytes. In turn, trypanosomal immunosuppressor factor (TIF) inhibits the production of IL-2 and down-regulates the expression of IL-2R. Polyclonal activation is observed during *T. cruzi* infection, which triggers uncontrolled proliferation of autoreactive clones of B cells, leading to possible autoimmune reactions. The persistent presence of *T. cruzi* in the heart has been demonstrated with sensitive techniques such as immunohistochemistry and polymerase chain reaction (PCR)–based assays. *T. cruzi* is the first microorganism described to suppress the expression of T-cell receptor molecules, which is required for antigen recognition. Parasympathetic cardiac denervation occurs. Destruction of cells of the myenteric plexus can cause megaesophagus and megacolon.

CLINICAL FINDINGS

When the skin is the portal of entry of *T. cruzi*, an indurated, erythematous, and painless primary chagoma with regional adenopathy may develop. When the conjunctiva is the site of entry, unilateral, palpebral swelling, called the Romaña sign, can arise. After multiplication at the site of entry, spread of the organisms results in acute Chagas' disease. This may be asymptomatic, manifested by mild symptoms, or may cause life-threatening disease (Table 324.2). Congenital Chagas' disease is a form of

TABLE 324.2.	**MANIFESTATIONS OF ACUTE CHAGAS' DISEASE**

Portal of Entry:
  Primary chagoma or Romaña sign
Systemic Manifestations:
  Fever
  Malaise
  Adenopathy
  Edema
  Hepatosplenomegaly
  Myocarditis
  Meningoencephalitis
Skin Manifestations
  Schizotrypanids (skin rash)
  Secondary chagomas

TABLE 324.3.	**MANIFESTATIONS OF CHRONIC CHAGAS' CARDIOPATHY**

Ventricular extrasystoles
Atrioventricular block
Brady and tachyarrhythmias
Right bundle-branch block, left anterior hemiblock
Ventricular tachycardia
Ischemic chest pain
Dilated cardiomyopathy, ventricular aneurysms
Congestive heart failure, clot formation, embolization
Sudden death

acute Chagas' disease. Its manifestations can also be mild to severe, and occasionally may involve megaviscera, which is not seen acutely in patients infected by other mechanisms. Acute Chagas' disease resolves spontaneously in 4 to 8 weeks in almost all patients, who then enter the indeterminate form of the illness characterized by lifelong, subpatent parasitemias and easily detectable levels of specific anti–*T. cruzi* antibodies.

Years or even decades after resolution of the acute infection, up to a third of chronically infected patients develop symptomatic cardiac and/or gastrointestinal disease. Chagas' cardiopathy typically involves rhythm disturbances and progressive cardiomyopathy causing congestive heart failure (Table 324.3). Megadisease is usually manifested as megaesophagus and/or megacolon. Immunosuppressed patients, including persons with AIDS, who are chronically infected with *T. cruzi* are at risk for developing reactivated acute Chagas' disease that may be manifested in its typical form or atypically as ulcerating skin lesions or brain abscesses.

LABORATORY FINDINGS

The diagnosis of acute Chagas' disease must be made by parasitologic methods. Parasites sometimes can be seen in wet preparations of anticoagulated blood or buffy coat, or in Giemsa-stained smears of these same specimens. Bone marrow aspirates may be examined similarly. Hemocultures in a specialized media have a sensitivity of about 80% but have the disadvantage of taking several weeks before parasites are evident. Sensitive and specific PCR assays that amplify highly repetitive nuclear or kinetoplast DNA sequences of *T. cruzi* have been described, but their accuracy still needs further definition and they are not available commercially.

The diagnosis of chronic *T. cruzi* infection is made by serologic methods, and parasitologic approaches play a secondary role. The sensitivities of conventional serologic methods, such as indirect immunofluorescence assay, complement fixation test, and enzyme-linked immunosorbent assay, are high, but a lack of specificity has been a persistent problem historically. False-positive reactions typically occur with specimens from patients with other parasitic and infectious diseases, as well as with collagen vascular diseases, and because of this it is generally recommended that two or three tests be employed before a specimen is accepted as positive. Alternatively, confirmatory testing can be carried out using a radioimmune precipitation assay that has been shown to be highly sensitive and specific (L. V. Kirchhoff,

TABLE 324.4.	PREVENTION OF CHAGAS' DISEASE

Health education
Housing improvement
Vector control with insecticides
Serologic screening of donated blood

University of Iowa). A role for PCR assays in chronic Chagas' disease has not been defined.

OPTIMAL MANAGEMENT

A panel of experts that recently convened under the sponsorship of World Health Organization recommended that all patients infected with *T. cruzi* be treated with one of the two currently available drugs. This recommendation was based on recent laboratory and clinical data indicating that the progression of lesions is less in animals and humans who have been cured parasitologically. However, the two drugs used to treat *T. cruzi*, nifurtimox and benznidazole, lack efficacy, and the probability of parasitologic cure is approximately 70% in patients with acute Chagas' disease and 20% in persons with longstanding chronic infections. Benznidazole is the drug of choice for treatment of *T. cruzi*, and the recommended course is 5 mg per kilogram per day in two divided doses for 60 days. Leukopenia and skin eruptions are the most common side effects of benznidazole. The recommended dose of nifurtimox is 8 to 10 mg per kilogram per day for adults, 12.5 to 15 mg per kilogram per day for adolescents, and 15 to 20 mg per kilogram per day in children 10 years of age or less. In all patients the daily dose should be given orally in four divided doses and continued for 90 to 120 days. The most common side effects of nifurtimox are anorexia, nausea, and vomiting, and they are generally more bothersome than those of benznidazole.

Chagas' disease is an illness that primarily affects poor people living in rural settings. A major effort for eliminating vectorial and transfusional transmission of *T. cruzi* in the Southern Cone nations of South America was launched in 1992, and major successes have been achieved in several regions. Uruguay was certified as transmission-free in 1997, and the spread of the parasite in Chile is expected to be stopped by the end of this year. Brazil and Argentina are expected to follow this pattern within the next few years. The success of the Southern Cone initiative and the implementation of similar programs in the northern part of South America and Central America provide a basis for optimism regarding the eventual elimination of transmission (Table 324.4).

BIBLIOGRAPHY

Donelson JE, Hill KL, El-Sayed NMA. Multiple mechanisms of immune evasion by African trypanosomes. *Mol Biochem Parasitol* 1998;91: 51–66.

Kierszenbaum F, ed. *Parasitic infections and the immune system.* San Diego: Academic Press, 1994.

Kirchhoff LV. American trypanosomiasis (Chagas' disease): a tropical disease now in the United States. *N Engl J Med* 1993;329:639–644.

Kirchhoff LV. American trypanosomiasis (Chagas' disease). *Gastroenterol Clin North Am* 1996;25:517–533.

Kirchhoff LV, Gam AA, Gusmao RD, et al. Increased specificity of serodiagnosis of Chagas' disease by detection of antibody to the 72- and 90-kilodalton glycoproteins of *Trypanosoma cruzi. J Infect Dis* 1987;155: 561–564.

Moncayo A. Progress toward elimination of transmission of Chagas disease in Latin America. *World Health Stat Q* 1997;50:195–198.

Mulligan HW. *The African trypanosomiasis.* New York: Wiley-Interscience, 1970.

Pepin J, Milord F. The treatment of human African trypanosomiasis. *Adv Parasitol* 1995;33:1–47.

Schmunis GA. *Trypanosoma cruzi*, the etiologic agent of Chagas' disease: status in the blood supply in endemic and nonendemic countries. *Transfusion* 1991;31:547–557.

Truc P, Jamonneau V, N'Guessan P, et al. Parasitological diagnosis of human African trypanosomiasis: a comparison of the QBCR and miniature anion-exchange centrifugation techniques. *Trans R Soc Trop Med Hyg* 1998;92:288–289.

Kelley's Textbook of Internal Medicine, fourth edition. Edited by H. David Humes. Lippincott Williams & Wilkins, Philadelphia © 2000.

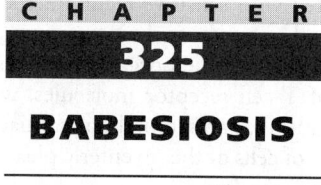

CHAPTER 325

BABESIOSIS

MURRAY WITTNER

DEFINITION

Babesiosis is a worldwide tick-borne hemolytic disease of wild and domestic animals that is caused by intraerythrocytic protozoan parasites of the genus *Babesia*. Human infection with several diverse species of *Babesia* may cause a broad spectrum of clinical features, from severe and occasionally fatal hemolytic anemia, with fever, jaundice, and splenomegaly, to a condition that is entirely asymptomatic.

EPIDEMIOLOGIC FACTORS

Since 1957, when the first human case of babesiosis was described in a Yugoslavian farmer who died of severe hemolytic anemia, sporadic cases have been reported with increasing frequency, especially along the northeastern coast of the United States. In the United States, infections have been reported from California, Missouri, Minnesota, Washington State, and Georgia; the most endemic areas, however, are the islands off the coast of Massachusetts, including Nantucket and Martha's Vineyard, and eastern and south central Long Island, including Shelter Island and Fire Island in New York. Foci in Connecticut that overlap with Lyme disease, as well as in Wisconsin and

Indiana, have been recorded. Sporadic cases have also been reported from France, Great Britain, Ireland, the Soviet Union, and Mexico. In the United States, with one possible exception, the murine species *Babesia microti* has been implicated. However, in the western United States those cases of babesiosis reported from California have been caused by a non–*B. microti* species, whereas those cases reported from Washington State, although morphologically indistinguishable from *B. microti,* were shown to be antigenically and genotypically distinct from *B. microti.* Most European and African cases have been caused by bovine and other nonmurine species of *Babesia.*

Recent reports have suggested an increased prevalence of babesiosis in such areas of New England as Connecticut, possibly because of the marked increase in the population of white-tailed deer, which are essential to the life cycle of the northern deer tick. In this regard, in a recent study of 1,000 *Borrelia burgdorferi*–seropositive patients from Connecticut, 10% were also seropositve for *B. microti.*

Babesia microti is transmitted through the bite of the northern deer tick, *Ixodes dammini* (= *scapularis*). Dissemination of *B. microti* to humans appears to be the result of indiscriminate feeding by infected larval and especially nymphal stages of *I. dammini* on a variety of hosts, including humans. Epidemiologic studies on Nantucket have shown that about 60% of the trapped white-footed or deer mice (*Peromyscus leucopus*) are infected with *B. microti.* Throughout its larval, nymphal, and adult stages, *I. dammini* feeds on three hosts, dropping off between each blood meal. In the larval and nymphal stages, it usually feeds on white-footed mice; the adults usually feed and mate on deer, who are naturally immune. Human infection usually occurs from late spring to early fall, when many nymphs are questing and when humans enter the tick-infested habitat. Evidence of transovarial transmission in *B. microti,* as there is in other species of *Babesia,* has been reported occasionally.

Seroepidemiologic studies carried out on residents of Nantucket and Shelter Islands have shown a 4% to 7% seroconversion. Similar results were obtained in studies on residents of a rural area along the Gulf Coast of Mexico that was a known focus of babesiosis of domestic animals, These studies imply that asymptomatic human infection seems to be common. In some of these symptom-free individuals, low numbers of circulating parasites have been found and have been a source of transfusion babesiosis. Despite the widespread prevalence of putative asymptomatic infection, clinical disease has not been reported from people immunodepressed during a course of corticosteroid or cyclophosphamide therapy. However, patients with AIDS are apparently unable to control their infection naturally or after usual treatment, and must be maintained on antibiotic therapy indefinitely.

The risk for transmission of *B. microti* infection via contaminated blood products has been recognized since the late 1970s. However, direct measures of risk are not available, and estimates of the likelihood of acquiring *Babesia* from a unit of blood are based on reported cases or seroepidemiologic studies. Although *B. microti* is the second most commonly reported cause of transfusion-transmitted parasitic infection, testing of all blood donors for evidence of *B. microti* infection has not been considered cost-effective. Despite the low overall incidence of transfusion-

transmitted babesiosis, it is likely that the risk of transmission of babesiosis by blood products depends on where the blood is collected. For example, a seroepidemiologic study from Connecticut estimated the risk to be 0.17% per unit of packed cells. Furthermore, since in the vast majority of immunocompetent individuals infection with *B. microti* is subclinical and therefore undiagnosed, the standard question "Have you ever had babesiosis?" is unlikely to be useful in excluding infected donors. Given the lack of effective screening strategies, the widening geographic range of *B. microti,* and the concomitant increase in human infections with this parasite, one may expect the incidence of transfusion-associated babesiosis to increase.

PATHOGENESIS

After an infectious tick bite, the organisms invade red blood cells and a trophozoite differentiates, replicating asexually by budding with the formation of two to four merozoites. A second type of undifferentiated trophozoite is also formed that does not replicate but rather enlarges and differentiates into gametocyte-like forms similar to that seen in *Plasmodium* species. Merozoites eventually disrupt infected erythrocytes and reinvade other red blood cells. These events cause a hemolytic anemia that, when severe, can bring about hemoglobinuria, renal insufficiency, or renal failure.

Although symptomatic infection with *B. microti* is seen regularly in otherwise immunocompetent people, the most severe cases have been recorded from patients splenectomized for a variety of reasons, including trauma.

Splenectomized animals have more severe infections than those with intact spleens, and they often die with an extraordinarily high parasitemia. In animal experiments, after recovery from a *B. microti* infection, splenectomy often provokes a severe and fatal relapse.

If untreated, clinically symptomatic *B. microti* infections in immunocompetent patients are usually self-limited; it has been shown that both humoral and cell-mediated immune mechanisms influence the outcome of the infection. Experimental studies have demonstrated that without T-helper cells specific humoral immunity cannot be established and the animals die. Similarly, athymic nude mice have been shown to have severe and fatal infections. Several studies have documented that in patients with acute babesiosis, in vitro lymphocyte mitogenic responses were profoundly depressed; on recovery, these T-cell changes returned to normal. It is not clear as to whether the age of the host influences the severity of a *Babesia* infection, except at the extremes of life, when these patients are probably immunocompromised.

CLINICAL FINDINGS

After a recognized tick bite, the incubation period varies from 5 to 33 days, whereas after an infected blood transfusion, the clinical incubation period has been 6 to 9 weeks. In a recent cluster of transfusion-derived babesiosis the clinical incubation period was 43 days. Frequently, however, infected people are unaware of being bitten because (a) *I. dammini* is 1 to 2 mm in overall diameter, (b) feeding is painless, and (c) soon after feeding the organisms drop off the host. In persons with intact spleens, the clinical onset can be gradual, beginning with a general feeling of malaise and myalgias, followed by fatigue, weakness, and chilliness, to frank shaking chills with fever and diaphoresis. This presentation is often mistaken for malaria, and the symptoms continue for weeks if untreated. Some patients have severe arthralgias. Occasionally, nausea and vomiting and severe headache, as well as mood and personality changes, are noted. As frequently found in malaria, splenomegaly is often evident but lymphadenopathy is not. A mild to severe hemolytic anemia and a normal to slightly depressed leukocyte count are usually found. In most patients, the serum bilirubin, aspartate aminotransaminase, and alkaline phosphatase values are mildly elevated, and the parasitemia can range from below 1% to more than 50%. Splenectomized patients usually have greater levels of parasitemia and more severe hemolytic anemia. Unless other clinical problems intervene, patients with *B. microti* infections usually recover. In patients with underlying heart disease, babesiosis may precipitate cardiac failure; elderly patients in particular have died after acute myocardial infarction.

Because *I. dammini* is also the vector of *B. burgdorferi* (the etiologic agent of Lyme disease) and *Ehrlichia chafaensis,* and because babesiosis, Lyme disease, and ehrlichiosis coexist in a number of localities in the northeastern United States, it is important to be alert for the coexistence of these diseases. This has been reported, and the spirochete has been demonstrated in the myocardium.

In Europe, human babesiosis with bovine species of *Babesia* is seen exclusively in splenectomized patents in whom the disease is fulminant and characterized by chills, fever, nausea, vomiting, and severe hemolytic anemia. These patients were often icteric, had acute renal insufficiency or failure, and died.

■ LABORATORY FINDINGS

The diagnosis of babesiosis should be entertained in anyone with a febrile hemolytic disorder, regardless of a history of tick bite, who has been to an endemic area or who has received a blood transfusion. The diagnosis can be firmly established with the finding of characteristic intraerythrocytic parasites on thick or thin blood smears stained with Giemsa or Wright's stain. *B. microti* is frequently mistaken for ring forms of *Plasmodium falciparum,* especially when multiple rings are present in a single erythrocyte. *Babesia* species do not produce residual hemozoin pigment, a by-product of hemoglobin digestion, as is usual with late-stage malarial schizonts. In some instances, cruciate, Maltese cross, or tetrad forms lacking pigment can be seen in a blood smear. These are characteristic and diagnostic (Fig. 325.1). It may be necessary to examine blood smears made at frequent intervals with low-level parasitemia. An indirect immunofluorescence test performed by the U.S. Centers for Disease Control and Prevention can be helpful, but low-titer cross-reactions between *Babesia* and P 1024 are present during acute disease and decline over the ensuing year to a ratio of 1:256 to 1:32 or

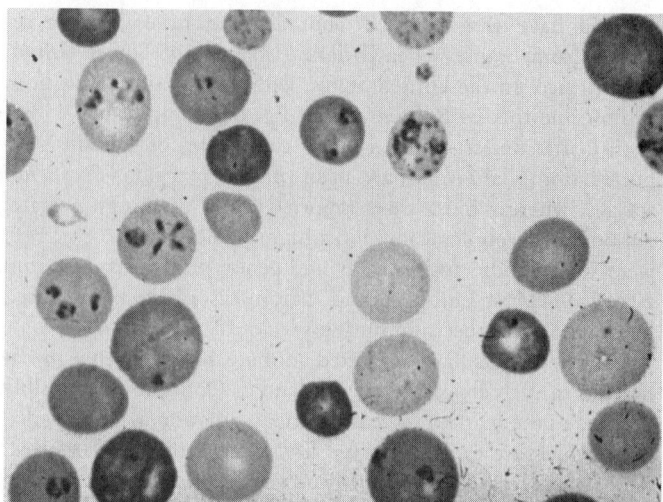

FIGURE 325.1. Blood smear showing intraerythrocytic parasites of *Babesia microti.* Many ring forms that resemble those of *Plasmodium falciparum* are evident, but the pathognomonic "tetrad" or "Maltese cross" form is also present. (Original magnification ×1,250.)

less. If 1 mL of the patient's blood is inoculated intraperitoneally into a golden hamster or gerbil, a parasitemia becomes evident. High *Babesia* antibody titers (1:12 to 14 days) should help to confirm the diagnosis. The use of polymerase chain reaction (PCR) is especially useful to assess whether infection has been eliminated. Recent studies suggest that this procedure is more sensitive than microscopic examination of thin blood smears. This has also been reported for other infectious agents including *P. vivax* and *B. burgdorferi.*

Babesiosis can be mistaken for rickettsial disease, especially when there is a history of tick bite, fever, myalgias, headache, hemolytic anemia, and thrombocytopenia. A blood smear should quickly eliminate this diagnosis. In case of *B. microti* infection, concurrent Lyme disease should also be considered, especially when arthralgias, rash, and cardiac symptoms are evident. The diagnosis of coexisting Lyme disease or erlichiosis can be made serologically. PCR for these is conditions also available.

■ OPTIMAL MANAGEMENT

In patients who are otherwise immunocompetent and who have normal, intact spleens, spontaneous recovery from *B. microti* infection seems to be the rule, although lingering symptoms with low-grade parasitemia can be evident for months.

In asplenic patients and those infected with *Babesia bovis* or *Babesia divergens,* symptoms are often too severe to temporize. Bovine babesiosis usually is severe with a fulminant downhill course and must be treated aggressively if the patient is to survive. Several patients who were placed on renal dialysis and transfused have survived. Diminazene aceturate (Berenil), an aromatic diamidine that is an effective babesiacide in animals, was unsuccessful in a fatal case of *B. divergens* infection. More recently, however, a human case of *B. divergens* infection was treated successfully with trimethoprim–sulfamethoxazole and pentamidine.

Treatment for human *B. microti* infection has been more successful. Initially, most patients received chloroquine, primarily because of the morphologic similarities of *B. microti* to *P. falciparum* in human blood smears. However, there is little evidence of its efficacy. Experimental babesiosis in hamsters was shown to be unaffected by chloroquine, as well as by sulfadiazine, primaquine, or metronidazole in combination with pyrimethamine. Minocycline and tetracycline, when used at high and toxic doses, had some effect in reducing parasitemia; at usual therapeutic levels, however, tetracycline had no effect. Pentamidine isethionate (Pentam 300), 4 mg per kilogram per day for 14 days by deep-muscle injection, has had limited success when used to treat human *B. microti* infection, lowering but not eliminating the parasitemia. Recrudescence occurred after completion of therapy. Significant side effects included the development of renal insufficiency, severe pain at the injection site, and formation of large sterile abscesses. Red blood cell or whole-blood exchange transfusion has been used with apparent success in several ill patients who had high parasitemias (40% to 60%).

Since the mid-1980s, clindamycin plus quinine has been regarded as the standard therapy for this infection on the basis of numerous clinical observations and experimental hamster studies. Clindamycin, 1,200 mg intravenously every 12 hours for 7 days, combined with quinine, 650 mg orally every 8 hours for 7 days, has been used successfully to treat in adults. The pediatric dose is clindamycin, 20 to 40 mg per kilogram per day in three doses for 7 days, and quinine, 2.5 mg per kilogram per day in three doses for 7 days. However, there have been several reports and unpublished observations that, in some immunocompromised and HIV-infected patients, babesiosis has been difficult to treat successfully with the standard therapy and as a result other modalities, such as exchange transfusion, have been required. In these patients, it was unclear as to whether this was because of relapse, persistence, or emergence of resistance. AIDS patients initially respond to quinine–clindamycin therapy but usually experience relapse after it is discontinued. They often become refractory to further repeated treatment with this regimen. Experimental animal studies have suggested that azithromycin and quinine may be an effective alternative for *B. microti* infections. Animal and human studies have suggested that the combination of atovaquone and azithromycin is effective in immunocompromised patients who have become resistant to the quinine–clindamycin regimen.

The use of atovaquone, an agent with antimalarial, anti-*Pneumocystis*, and anti-*Toxoplasma* activity, was prompted by two recent studies demonstrating the efficacy of atovaquone in the hamster model of *B. microti* infection. When used as monotherapy, atovaquone was reported to be effective for both treatment and prophylaxis. However, other studies have shown that with monotherapy, recrudescence and development of high-grade resistance appeared that was not encountered with the atovaquone–azithromycin combination. Rapid emergence of resistance with atovaquone monotherapy also has been reported in malaria chemotherapy.

In malaria, the combination therapy of atovaquone plus proguanil has been used successfully in a fixed combination. Studies in several species of *Plasmodium* have indicated that the site of action of atovaquone is at the mitochondrial cytochrome bc1 (complex III). This agent inhibited electron transport at the bc1 complex by collapsing the mitochondrial membrane potential. However, the role of proguanil is not clear since it did not appear to function as a dihydrofolic acid reductase inhibitor.

PREVENTION

Specific chemoprophylaxis is not available. Those who are immunocompromised, especially postsplenectomized patients, should avoid tick-infested areas. Because normal, immunocompetent people may acquire symptomatic and sometimes severe disease, they also should be wary when entering these areas. Because *I. dammini* is small and often feeds undetected for long periods (48 hours), patients should inspect themselves and their pets daily and remove ticks completely. Gentle traction with a forceps applied close to the capitulum (head) usually suffices to remove the entire tick. If the tick is deeply entrenched in the skin, mineral oil or even a hot needle can be applied and usually causes the tick to relax its hold. In tick-infested areas, repellents should be used on clothes, especially on the lower parts of trousers. It is advisable to wear long-sleeved garments, and shirts should be tucked under the belt. One of the most effective tick repellents is *N,N*-diethyl-*m*-toluamide, or DEET. It is commercially available in concentrations up to 100%. Care should be taken in its use because 10% to 15% of each application can be recovered in urine. Serious toxic and allergic reactions have been reported in those individuals who have used it frequently or in high concentrations. In young children, toxic encephalopathy has occurred. Use of nonabsorbable, long-acting formulations such as Ultrathon or DEET-Plus should obviate many of these adverse reactions. In any event, DEET products containing more than 38% DEET should be avaoided.

BIBLIOGRAPHY

Benezra D, Brown AE, Polsky B, et al. Babesiosis and infection with human immunodeficiency virus (HIV). *Ann Intern Med* 1987;107:944.

Dammin GJ, Spielman A, Benach JL, et al. The rising incidence of clinical *Babesia microti* infection. *Hum Pathol* 1982;12:398–400.

Dobroszycki J, Herwaldt B, Boctor F, et al. A cluster of transfusion-associated babesiosis cases traced to a single asymptomatic donor. *JAMA* 1999; 281:927–930.

Jacoby GA, Hunt JV, Kosinski KS, et al. Treatment of transfusion-transmitted babesiosis by exchange transfusion. *N Engl J Med* 1980;303: 1098–1100.

Persing DH, Mathieson D, Marshall WF, et al. Detection of *Babesia microti* by polymerase chain reaction. *J Clin Microbiol* 1992;30:2097–2103.

Raoult D, Soulayrol L, Toga B, et al. Babesiosis, pentamidine and cotrimazole. *Ann Intern Med* 1987;107:944.

Rowin KS, Tanowitz HB, Wittner M. Therapy of experimental babesiosis. *Ann Intern Med* 1982;97:556–558.

Smith T, Kilbourne FL. Investigation into the nature, causation, and prevention of Texas or south cattle fever. *USDA Industry Bull* 1893;1:1.

Spielman A. Human babesiosis on Nantucket Island: transmission by nymphal *Ixodes* ticks. *Am J Trop Med Hyg* 1976;25:784–787.

Spielman A, Wilson ML, Levine JF, et al. Ecology of *Ixodes dammini*-borne human babesiosis and Lyme disease. *Annu Rev Entomol* 1985; 30:439–460.

Srivastava IK, Rottenberg H, Vaidya AB. Atovaquone, a broad spectrum antiparasitic drug, collapses mitochondrial membrane potential in a malarial parasite. *J Biol Chem* 1997;272:3961–3966.

Vaidya AM. Mitochondrial physiology as target for atovaquone and other antimalarials. In: Sherman IW, ed. *Malaria: parasite biology, pathogenesis, prevention*. Washington, DC: American Society for Microbiology Press, 1998.

Weiss LM, Wittner M, Wasserman S, et al. Efficacy of azithromycin for treating *Babesia microti* infection in the hamster model. *J Infect Dis* 1993;168:1289–1292.

Wittner M, Lederman J, Tanowitz HB, et al. Efficacy of atovaquone for the treatment of *Babesia microti* infection: experimental studies and clinical experiences. *Am J Trop Med Hyg* 1996;54.

Wittner M, Rowin KS, Tanowitz HB, et al. Successful chemotherapy of transfusion babesiosis. *Ann Intern Med* 1982;96:601–604.

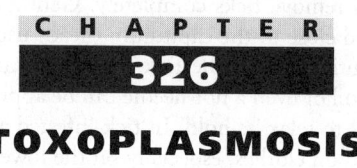

CHAPTER 326

TOXOPLASMOSIS

BENJAMIN J. LUFT

Toxoplasmosis, the disease caused by the obligate intracellular protozoan *Toxoplasma gondii*, is a ubiquitous zoonosis that is responsible for significant morbidity and mortality in both animals and humans throughout the world. Long recognized as a cause of serious disease in congenitally infected neonates and immunocompromised hosts, it is only with the advent of AIDS that toxoplasmosis has occurred in epidemic proportions. It is one of the most common causes of focal central nervous system (CNS) infection in patients with AIDS.

PATHOGENESIS

Toxoplasma gondii is a coccidian, classified among the Sporozoa in the suborder Eimeria. It exists in three life forms: oocysts, tachyzoites (trophozoites), and tissue cysts. The complete life cycle takes place only in felines. Humans become infected most commonly by ingesting raw or undercooked meat containing tissue cysts, or foods or beverages contaminated with oocysts, and by ingesting oocysts following exposure to excrement from an infected cat. After replicating in the intestinal mucosa, tachyzoites invade the lymphatics and blood and disseminate widely, infecting all organs and tissues. The intracellular proliferation of tachyzoites usually causes host cell death. Cell death may result in acute disease or asymptomatic infection, depending on the host's immune response. Both humoral and cell-mediated immunity are important, but cell-mediated immunity is of particular consequence. In the immunodeficient host, the acute infection may continue unabated and cause potentially fatal local or diffuse disease such as encephalitis, myocarditis, or pneumonitis. With the development of an adequate immune response, tachyzoites disappear and tissue cysts form.

Generally, infected individuals will remain seropositive for anti–*T. gondii* antibodies, and viable tissue cysts will remain in various organs for the remainder of the host's life. For AIDS patients, the predominant pathogenetic mechanism is recrudescence of a chronic, latent infection arising from tissue cysts. The spontaneous and simultaneous development of multifocal areas of encephalitis in these previously seropositive patients strongly supports this assumption. In contrast, there is often epidemiologic evidence that the toxoplasmosis was newly acquired in other immunocompromised patients.

EPIDEMIOLOGIC FACTORS

In humans, serologic surveys report an increasing prevalence of antibodies to *T. gondii* with increasing age, with no significant difference between the sexes. Lower prevalence is noted at higher altitudes, in cold regions, and in hot arid climates. In the United States, serologic evidence of prior infection has been demonstrated in 6% to 21% of children and in 10% to 67% of adults over the age of 50. The seroprevalence rate is much higher in other countries, particularly France, Central Africa, and El Salvador, often reaching 90% in the population 40 years of age or older. A number of factors affect the incidence of toxoplasmosis among different populations, including climactic conditions, cat population, methods of farming and animal husbandry, and hygienic and cultural habits with regard to food preparation and consumption. The two major routes of transmission in humans are oral and congenital. Other modes of transmission include blood or leukocyte transfusion as a result of persistent parasitemia in a normal asymptomatic donor, accidental self-inoculation of tachyzoites in laboratory workers, and organ transplantation.

Transplacental transmission deserves particular mention. In the immunocompetent host, the fetus is at risk of infection only when the mother is acutely infected for the first time during gestation. The incidence and severity of fetal infection are related to the trimester during which maternal infection takes place. If maternal infection during the first trimester is untreated, then transplacental infection occurs in about 25% of infants and the disease may be severe. Transplacental infection during the second and third trimesters occurs in 54% and 65% of infants, respectively, but disease tends to be less severe or asymptomatic during the neonatal period. In rare cases, maternofetal transmission has been reported in women of childbearing age who contract acute toxoplasmosis 6 to 8 weeks prior to conception. It is recommended that pregnancy be avoided for at least 6 months in these cases.

For women infected with HIV, the primary mode of transmission in congenital toxoplasmosis is from reactivation of chronic infection. This is a risk only for immunocompromised patients and has been reported for pregnant women with Hodgkin's disease, with systemic lupus erythematosus for which corticosteroids are being given, and with AIDS. Of the 29 cases of toxoplasmosis in HIV-infected children reported to date, 15 (51%) of infections were acquired in utero. Most of these infections occurred during reactivation of chronic maternal toxoplasmosis, which was either symptomatic and manifested as toxoplasmic encephalitis (TE), or asymptomatic. At the time of fetal infection, maternal CD4 lymphocytes counts have been as high as 459 per cubic millimeter. The initial manifestations of infection are similar to those observed in non–HIV-infected infants, but the disease seems to follow a more progressive course. The frequency of vertical transmission of *T. gondii* in chronically infected women with AIDS is under study.

CLINICAL MANIFESTATIONS

Clinical manifestations of toxoplasmosis vary with the timing of infection (acute, newly acquired, or reactivation of chronic latent disease), the particular type of host (immunocompetent versus immunocompromised), and the organs involved. In the immunocompetent host, it is convenient to consider toxoplasmosis as congenital, acquired, or ocular (either congenital or acquired), and in the immunocompromised host as acquired or reactivation of chronic infection.

CONGENITAL TOXOPLASMOSIS

The fetus is at risk of infection regardless of the severity of disease during pregnancy. Acute infection in the mother is most frequently asymptomatic; symptomatic disease (usually lymphadenopathy) is seen in only 10% to 20% of cases. No correlation exists between the severity of disease in the infant and that of the mother. Eighty percent of infected newborns are asymptomatic at birth. The incidence of chorioretinitis in untreated infants with subclinical infection has been found to be greater than 85% on follow-up in one series (Koppe et al.). Infants with clinically apparent disease at birth may have any combination of the following: a mild nonspecific illness, failure to thrive, fever or hypothermia, lymphadenopathy, hepatosplenomegaly, pneumonitis, myocarditis, CNS involvement, or ocular disease. Clinically apparent disease in the neonate is usually associated with severe sequelae, whereas asymptomatic disease at birth may be followed by either mild or severe sequelae, particularly retinochoroiditis, hydrocephalus, mental retardation, sensorineural hearing loss, blindness, and delayed psychomotor development. Congenital toxoplasmosis as a result of reactivation of latent infection in HIV-infected women has been described. The initial clinical manifestations are similar to those of non–HIV-infected infants at birth but may progress more rapidly.

ACQUIRED TOXOPLASMOSIS

The spectrum of disease in acquired toxoplasmosis in the immunocompetent host ranges from subclinical lymphadenopathy to fatal fulminant infection. The most common manifestation is asymptomatic lymphadenopathy, which may be generalized or localized to a single node or area. The cervical nodes are most frequently enlarged. Nodes are usually discrete and vary in firmness and tenderness; suppuration is not seen. Associated signs and symptoms include fever, headache, fatigue, and malaise. A few patients may have a *mononucleosis-like* syndrome consisting of fever, maculopapular rash, sore throat, myalgia, headache,

hepatosplenomegaly, and atypical lymphocytosis. The lymphadenopathic form is usually self-limited; symptoms resolve within several weeks but may recur for months. Routine laboratory studies are unremarkable other than a slight lymphocytosis, an increased sedimentation rate, and mildly elevated hepatic transaminases. The differential diagnosis usually includes lymphoma, infectious mononucleosis, and cytomegalovirus infection. Rarely, severe disease occurs with signs and symptoms referable to the specific organ involved: myocarditis, pneumonitis, hepatitis, polymyositis, or encephalitis. Fever of unknown origin has also been described. Prolonged parasitemia in asymptomatic, acquired toxoplasmosis has been observed and associated with transfusion-related infection (particularly whole blood). *T. gondii* was shown to survive in whole citrated blood stored at 4°C for up to 50 days.

OCULAR TOXOPLASMOSIS

Ocular toxoplasmosis is most frequently a late manifestation of congenital infection but is also seen in acute acquired disease (about 1% of cases) and in patients with AIDS. It is estimated that toxoplasmosis accounts for 35% of all cases of retinochoroiditis. Clinical manifestations include decreased visual acuity, scotomas, eye pain, photophobia, epiphora, loss of central vision (with macular involvement), nystagmus, and strabismus if the extraocular muscles are affected. Signs of systemic infection are uncommon except in AIDS patients in whom ocular toxoplasmosis is frequently associated with CNS disease. Ophthalmologic examination reveals single or, more frequently, multiple yellow–white patches with elevated indistinct margins surrounded by an area of hyperemia usually involving the posterior pole of the retina. If inflammation of the vitreous is present, the fundus may be obscured. Older lesions are atrophic, whitish gray plaques with distinct borders and black spots of retinal pigment. Lesions of varying age may be seen, indicating episodic flare-ups of activity. Multiple recurrences that progressively destroy the retina can lead to glaucoma. In patients with AIDS, toxoplasmic retinochoroiditis can be identified by the following: absence of hemorrhage, location at the posterior pole, presence of inflammation of the vitreous and anterior chamber, and fluorescein angiography. In addition, cytomegalovirus retinitis is virtually seen only when absolute CD4 counts are fewer than 50 per cubic millimeter.

INFECTION IN THE IMMUNOCOMPROMISED HOST

Severe infections with *T. gondii* are seen in epidemic proportions in patients with AIDS and are one of the most common causes of focal CNS infection in these patients. Other immunodeficient states associated with toxoplasmosis are malignancies of the reticuloendothelial system, especially Hodgkin's disease, leukemia, collagen vascular diseases, solid organ transplantation, and chronic corticosteroid use. The pathogenesis is usually reactivation of latent infection particularly in the overwhelming majority of cases of AIDS- associated toxoplasmosis. Signs and symptoms may include those noted in the immunocompetent host with acquired toxoplasmosis. However, the most common clinical manifestations reflect involvement of the CNS and, less frequently, the lungs, eyes, and heart.

Patients at risk for developing toxoplasmosis from reactivation of latent infection can easily be identified by measuring serum anti–*T. gondii* antibody titers. In this setting, toxoplasmosis is most frequently manifested by encephalitis, usually alone or, less frequently, as part of a multiorgan infection. Isolated organ involvement without CNS disease is uncommon. Toxoplasmosis becomes clinically apparent when CD4 counts fall below 200 per cubic millimeter with over 80 % of cases occurring in patients with less than 100 per cubic millimeter. The clinical characteristics are protean and depend on the number, size, and location of the lesions. Signs and symptoms of focal or generalized neurologic dysfunction or, more frequently, a mixture of both are seen. Cerebral edema and, on occasion, frank hemorrhage, which can occur concomitantly with active infection, also contribute to the disease process. Fifty percent to 89% of patients have a subacute onset with focal neurologic deficits, with or without evidence of generalized cerebral dysfunction. Seizures may be the initial manifestation of TE in 15% to 25% of cases. Occasionally, generalized cerebral dysfunction is the predominant initial manifestation; focal neurologic deficits develop as the infection progresses. The most common focal neurologic deficits are hemiparesis and speech disorders. Headache, when present, can be focal, generalized, and unremitting. Fever is not invariably present. TE is predominantly intra-axial, so that meningeal involvement is rare; thus, signs and symptoms of meningeal irritation are unusual.

A form of TE that appears to be unique to AIDS patients is a *diffuse encephalitis* manifested by rapidly progressive, fatal, generalized cerebral dysfunction without focal neurologic deficits or focal lesions on neuroradiographic study. Myelitis without TE can occur. *T. gondii* pneumonitis with or without associated TE is clinically indistinguishable from *Pneumocystis carinii* pneumonia. The diagnosis requires a high index of clinical suspicion and the demonstration of *T. gondii* in specimens obtained via bronchoalveolar lavage (BAL) or lung biopsy. Cardiac involvement may be asymptomatic or manifest with cardiac tamponade or biventricular failure. Clinical manifestations attributable to infection of other organs (testis, gut, liver, pancreas, kidney, bladder, adrenals, and skeletal muscle) occur infrequently.

■ DIAGNOSIS

The diagnosis of toxoplasmosis can be made by several means: isolation of *T. gondii* from blood or other body fluids; demonstration of tachyzoites or *T. gondii* antigens in tissue sections, smears, or body fluids; use of serologic tests; or detection of *T. gondii* DNA by polymerase chain reaction (PCR) in tissue or body fluids.

TOXOPLASMOSIS IN THE IMMUNOCOMPROMISED HOST

Clinically, serologic tests for the diagnosis of toxoplasmosis in AIDS patients are useful only to identify HIV-infected individuals at risk for developing TE and to support the diagnosis of TE

in AIDS patients with focal brain lesions. Many serologic tests are available that can detect different classes of antibodies. It is important to be aware that the results from these tests vary considerably in different laboratories.

The Sabin–Feldman dye test is the accepted standard for measurement of IgG antibodies, which have been shown to be higher in AIDS patients with TE than in those without TE. IgG titers usually appear 1 to 2 weeks after infection, reach levels of 1 : 1,000 by 6 to 8 weeks, then gradually decline over months and years. Low titers (1 : 65) may persist throughout life. The indirect fluorescence assay is used more commonly and measures the same IgG antibodies as the dye test. Commercially available kits are poorly standardized, and the results must be used within the context of the clinical setting. Almost 100% of AIDS patients with TE will have detectable IgG by dye test or indirect fluorescentce assay. The level of the titer can be variable, however, and is unimportant in diagnosis. Variable IgG levels also occur in patients with toxoplasmosis infections other than TE. Patients with TE rarely show a significant rise in antibody titer over time. Simply the presence of antibodies in the serum of an HIV-infected individual identifies a patient at risk for development of TE. The absence of these antibodies strongly suggests an alternative cause for a patient presenting with neurologic signs and symptoms.

The current standard of care allows the treatment of TE to be initiated on presumptive diagnosis in the presence of a characteristic neuroradiographic abnormality (e.g., multiple contrast enhancing mass lesions) on computed tomography (CT) or magnetic resonance imaging (MRI) and clinical manifestations that include signs and symptoms of focal or generalized neurologic dysfunction. MRI is a more sensitive neuroradiographic imaging study than CT for the demonstration of focal CNS lesions. If CT scanning is unremarkable in a clinical setting consistent with TE, multiple lesions may be detected on MRI. The presence of multiple lesions on CT or MRI greatly increases the probability of TE versus other causes of focal CNS disease. The probability of a CNS lymphoma is higher than or equal to that of TE in the presence of a solitary lesion on MRI. However, the clinical manifestations and radiographic findings are not specific for toxoplasmosis. The differential diagnosis includes other infections that cause space-occupying CNS lesions such as tuberculoma, cryptococcoma, and, most frequently in the United States, CNS lymphoma. A definitive diagnosis requires a brain biopsy, which should be reserved for the following settings: (a) patients whose baseline abnormalities (except headaches and seizures) do not improve within the first 10 to 14 days of therapy or whose condition deteriorates early in the course of therapy; (b) patients with solitary CNS lesions on CT or MRI; and (c) patients receiving trimethoprim–sulfamethoxazole (TMP-SMX) for *P. carinii* prophylaxis. The absence of a response to therapy does not always exclude TE because concurrent disease processes (e.g., other infections or lymphoma) may be present.

A presumptive diagnosis of TE may be confirmed by inoculation of tissue specimens into mice or tissue cultures. In addition, using histopathologic methods, definitive diagnosis is made possible by demonstration of the protozoa, usually the tachyzoite form, in tissue sections or smears (e.g., brain biopsy, bone marrow aspirate) or body fluids (e.g., cerebrospinal fluid and amniotic fluid). Direct or indirect fluorescent antibody methods and peroxidase–antiperoxidase methods have been used with success to identify the organism by Wright, Giemsa, immunoperoxidase, or eosin–methylene blue II staining. Since meningeal involvement is not prominent, examination of the CSF was usually unrewarding and was only used in excluding other diseases. However, detection of *T. gondii* DNA by poylmerase chain reaction (PCR) in CSF has proven a rapid and sensitive test that is especially useful in the diagnosis of TE in AIDS patients, avoiding the more invasive brain biopsy. However, variations in technique can affect results. Diagnostic sensitivity decreases when patients are receiving antiparasitic therapy.

TOXOPLASMOSIS IN THE PREGNANT WOMAN AND FETUS

Women who acquire toxoplasmosis during pregnancy expose their fetuses to the risk of infection. Infection of the fetus may result in stillbirth, spontaneous abortion, or birth of a symptomatic or an asymptomatic infant.

In 1994, Wong and Remington recommended a systematic, standardized screening program for all pregnant women. Accordingly, all pregnant women should be tested as early as possible for antibodies to *T. gondii* by dye test or an equivalent battery of serologic assays. Ideally, women should be tested no later than at 10 to 12 weeks of gestation. If results are seronegative, the pregnant woman should be tested again at 20 to 22 weeks. If seroconversion is substantiated, prenatal diagnostic testing should be performed, if feasible. For non–HIV-infected women, a definitive prenatal diagnosis of congenital infection may be accomplished by several methods: isolation of *T. gondii* from fetal blood (mouse inoculation) or amniotic fluid (mouse inoculation, cell culture), or detection of IgM *Toxoplasma* antibodies in fetal blood. The IgM enzyme-linked immunosorbent assay (ELISA) is based on the earlier appearance and disappearance of IgM antibodies. The presence of IgM antibodies in the fetus and neonate represents synthesis in utero because, unlike the IgG antibodies, IgM antibodies do not cross the placental barrier. If diagnostic tests are used in combination, a correct diagnosis could be achieved for the vast majority (more than 90%) of cases. The results of inoculation studies may not be available for 3 to 6 weeks, however, and this delay is of particular concern when pregnancy termination is being considered. The use of PCR assay for the detection of *T. gondii* DNA in amniotic samples has been shown to be of value in early diagnosis. It is a rapid (1 to 2 days) and highly sensitive (70% to 100%) diagnostic tool. Amniocentesis followed by both PCR and mouse inoculation may prevent the risk of fetal loss as a result of fetal blood sampling. It has been hypothesized that transmission of HIV may be more likely during fetal blood sampling as compared with amniocentesis, but no published studies support or refute this theory.

■ TREATMENT

Most episodes of toxoplasmosis in immunocompetent hosts are asymptomatic and do not require therapy. However, specific instances do occur when treatment is necessary based on the location of infection, its severity, mode of transmission (e.g., congenital disease), and host immune status. Therapeutic regimens are based on data from in vitro and in vivo experimental animal models (mostly murine) of infection, as well as a few large, well-controlled clinical trials, and the practice of physicians experienced in the treatment of toxoplasmosis. The ideal dosage, combination of drugs, and length of therapy are still under study.

TOXOPLASMOSIS IN THE IMMUNCOMPETENT HOST

The majority of infections in this setting are asymptomatic and do not require therapy. Lymphadenopathy, the most common manifestation, is self-limited and usually resolves within 1 to 3 weeks. Treatment in this setting should only be considered if systemic symptoms are severe or prolonged, or in the rare event that visceral involvement (encephalitis, pneumonitis, myocarditis) is present. Acute infection as a result of laboratory accident or transfusion may be severe and should be treated. The treatment regimen consists of a combination of pyrimethamine (Daraprim) and sulfadiazine or trisulfapyrimidine (a mixture of equal parts of sulfamethazine, sulfamerazine, and sulfadiazine) given for 2 to 4 weeks with folinic acid (leucovorin) (Table 326.1). Oral pyrimethamine is administered at a loading dose of 2 mg per kilogram per day, up to a maximum of 100 to 200 mg for 2 days, followed by 25 to 50 mg per day, along with 10 mg of folinic acid. Sulfadiazine or trisulfapyrimidine is administered orally at 100 mg per kilogram per day (maximum daily dose of 4 to 8 g) in four equally divided doses. In the event of pyrimethamine-induced hematologic toxicity (cytopenia), the dose of folinic acid may be increased. For patients allergic to sulfa, clindamycin (300 mg orally every 6 hours) in combination with pyrimethamine and folinic acid is successful.

OCULAR TOXOPLASMOSIS

Toxoplasmic retinochoroiditis is usually a manifestation of congenital infection but is also seen occasionally in acute acquired disease and in patients with AIDS. Signs of systemic involvement are uncommon except in patients with AIDS, in whom ocular disease can be a harbinger of CNS infection. Diagnosis is based on the ophthalmologic examination combined with serologic evidence of toxoplasmosis. Treatment is required to prevent relapse with the risk of progressive visual loss and other complications such as glaucoma. The drugs of choice are oral pyrimethamine and sulfadiazine or trisulfapyrimidine with folinic acid in the same dosages as described for the immunocompetent host. Therapy is given for 4 weeks and repeated as needed. Adjunctive therapy with systemic corticosteroids (prednisone, 80 to 120 mg per day, or an equivalent) is indicated if the macula, optic nerve or papillomacular bundle is involved. In particular cases, photocoagulation and vitrectomy may be necessary.

TOXOPLASMOSIS IN THE IMMUNOCOMPROMISED HOST

Therapy for TE in HIV-positive patients is generally started empirically based on the clinical and neuroradiographic evidence

TABLE 326.1.	OVERVIEW OF DRUGS CURRENTLY USED IN TREATMENT OF TOXOPLASMOSIS		
Antimicrobial	**Adverse Effects**	**Recommended Dose (Immunocompetent)**	**Recommended Dose (Immunocompromised)**
Pyrimethamine (Daraprim) Oral	Cytopenias, rash, GI intolerance	Loading dose = 2 mg/kg/d (max 100–200 mg) for 2 d; then 25–50 mg/d, 2–4 wk; with folinic acid oral, 10–20 mg/d	Acute: Loading dose = 100–200 mg; 50–75 mg/d, 3–6 wk; with oral folinic acid (leucovorin), 10–20 mg/d Maintenance: 25–50 mg/d; with folinic acid oral, 10–20 mg/d
Sulfadiazine or trisulfapyrimidine* Oral	GI intolerance, rash (Stevens-Johnson syndrome) cytopenias, nephrolithiasis, crystalluria, interstitial nephritis, encephalopathy	100 mg/kg/d (max 4–8 g/d) in 4 equally divided doses, 2–4 wk	Acute: 4–8 g/d, 3–6 wk Maintenance: 2–4 g/d in 4 equally divided doses
Clindamycin* Oral & IV	GI intolerance, rash, pseudomembranous colitis	300 mg every 6 h, 4 wk; repeat as needed	600 mg every 6 h, 3–6 wk Maintenance: same

* Used in combination with pyrimethamine.

in a patient with CD4 lymphocyte counts lower than 200 per cubic millimeter and seropositive for anti–*T. gondii* antibodies. The combination of pyrimethamine, an initial 100- to 200-mg loading dose in two divided doses followed by 50 to 75 mg per day orally, and sulfadiazine, 4 to 6 g per day orally in four divided doses, remains the mainstay of treatment. Oral folinic acid, 10 to 20 mg per day, is added to preclude the hematologic toxicities associated with antifolate agents. Acute therapy is given for at least 3 weeks; 6 weeks or more is indicated in severely ill patients and when a complete clinical and radiographic response has not been achieved. Patients with sulfa allergy can be given clindamycin, 600 mg orally or intravenously every 6 hours, in combination with pyrimethamine as described. Seventy percent of patients with TE have a quantifiable clinical improvement by day 7 of therapy. Conversely, patients not responding to empirical therapy usually have evidence of progressive disease within the first 10 days. Ninety percent of patients have improvement on neuroradiographic studies within 6 weeks of starting therapy.

Chronic suppressive therapy is indicated in all immunocompromised patients until an adequate cell-mediated immune response is restored. Pyrimethamine, 25 to 50 mg per day, and sulfadiazine, 2 to 4 g per day orally in four equally divided doses, with 10 mg per day of oral folinic acid, is recommended based on the low relapse rate associated with this combination. In sulfa-allergic patients, clindamycin is used. The combination of clindamycin and pyrimethamine has a higher relapse rate than pyrimethamine and sulfadiazine. Prophylactic use of anticonvulsants is not recommended. Corticosteroids should not be used routinely but are indicated if there is evidence of increased intracranial pressure. The use of corticosteroids may complicate the interpretation of the response to empirical therapy because clinical and radiographic involvements may be related to reduced cerebral edema or the size of a steroid-sensitive CNS lymphoma. The same chemotherapeutic regimens are used for extraneural toxoplasmosis; however, there are limited data available on the optimal length and outcome of treatment.

Primary chemoprophylaxis is a very attractive therapeutic op-

tion for patients known to be at risk of developing toxoplasmosis (e.g., HIV-infected patients with known CD4 counts less than 100 per cubic millimeter and seropositive for *T. gondii* antibodies). Based on retrospective data, oral TMP-SMX (1 double-strength tablet per day, 160 mg TMP–800 mg SMX) has been shown to be effective. Dapsone and pyrimethamine as single agents are not as efficacious; however, in combination, pyrimethamine (50 mg per week) and dapsone (50 mg per day) plus folinic acid provides a good alternative. In sulfa-allergic patients, desensitization is also an option.

Drug regimens currently being studied for their usefulness as initial and maintenance therapy include atovaquone (Mepron). A recent ACTG trial evaluating atovaquone-containing regimens (in combination with pyrimethamine or sulfadiazine) shows greater than 80% initial response to therapy (unpublished data). As salvage therapy, atovaquone alone induced initial clinical response in 50% of study patients. The response to atovaquone has been directly correlated with serum drug levels achieved. The newest formulation of atovaquone is administered as an oral suspension 1.5 g twice daily with food, preferably fatty foods, to increase its bioavailability. The new macrolide antibiotics clarithromycin (Biaxin) and azithromycin (Zithromax) in combination with pyrimethamine have limited utility as alternative agents.

TOXOPLASMOSIS IN THE PREGNANT WOMAN

It has been shown that early prenatal antibiotic therapy may reduce the incidence and severity of congenital infection. Pyrimethamine plus a sulfonamide or spiramycin (a macrolide antibiotic available in Western Europe, Mexico, Canada, and through the U.S. Food and Drug Administration) appear to decrease the incidence of infection and sequelae in the fetus when given to women who acquire *T. gondii* during pregnancy. Pyrimethamine is teratogenic and should not be used during the first trimester. The sulfonamides should be offered during the first trimester as they have been shown to be effective in animal

TABLE 326.2.	DRUGS USED IN TREATMENT TOXOPLASMOSIS IN PREGNANT WOMEN AND FOR CONGENITAL TOXOPLASMOSIS			
Antimicrobial	Adverse Effects	Recommended Dose (Pregnancy—1st Trimester)	Recommended Dose (Pregnancy—2nd & 3rd Trimester)	Recommended Dose (Congenital)
Spiramycin* Oral	Nausea, vomiting	30–50 mg/kg/d, in 3 divided doses	30–50 mg/kg/d, in 3 divided doses; if fetal infection confirmed or suspected, pyrimethamine and sulfadiazine may be superior for treatment of fetus	50–100 mg/kg/d in 2 equally divided doses; 4–6 wk course alternating with 3-wk course of pyrimethamine and sulfadiazine for up to age 1 y
Pyrimethamine (Daraprim) Oral	Cytopenias, rash, GI intolerance	Not recommended—teratogenic	Loading dose = 100 mg/d for 2 d; then 50 mg/d with folinic acid, 10 mg orally (with sulfadiazine or trisulfapyrimidine)	Loading dose = 2 mg/kg for 2 d, then 1 mg/kg with folinic acid, 10 mg orally, 3 times/wk up to 1 y (with sulfadiazine or trisulfapyrimidine)
Sulfadiazine or trisulfapyrimidine Oral	GI intolerance, rash (Stevens-Johnson syndrome) cytopenias, nephrolithiasis, crystalluria, interstitial, nephritis, encephalopathy	50–100 mg/kg/d in 2 equally divided doses (alone)	50–100 mg/kg/d (max 4 g/d) in 2 equally divided doses (with pyrimethamine)	50–100 mg/kg/d in 2 equally divided doses for up to 1 y (with pyrimethamine)

* Spiramycin is available on request from U.S. Food and Drug Administration.
Remington JS, McLeod R, Desmonts G. Toxoplasmosis. In: Remington JS, Klein JO, eds. *Infectious diseases of the fetus and newborn infant*. 4th ed. Philadelphia: WB Saunders, 1995; 140.

models. If spiramycin can be obtained, pregnant women acutely infected in the first trimester may be treated with 30 to 50 mg per kilograms per day orally in three divided doses until fetal infection is documented or excluded. Treatment with spiramycin alone decreases the incidence of transmission but not the severity of established congenital infection. Maternal treatment with pyrimethamine and sulfadiazine plus folinic acid appears to attenuate the clinical manifestations in the fetus. If fetal infection is suspected or confirmed after the first trimester, pyrimethamine, sulfadiazine, and folinic acid should be used to treat the maternal infection (Table 326.2).

CONGENITAL TOXOPLASMOSIS

Optimal treatment for congenital toxoplasmosis is not yet established. However, a National Institute of Allergy and Infectious Diseases Collaborative Treatment trial based in Chicago yielded a favorable preliminary outcome with the use of pyrimethamine, sulfadiazine, and folinic acid in infants with congenital infection. Medications were given to infants 2.5 months old and continued for 1 year. Two different doses of pyrimethamine were compared. The most significant adverse effect was transient neutropenia, which responded favorably to the withholding of increasing doses of folinic acid or pyrimethamine. Preliminary results indicate that this therapeutic regimen can be safely administered to children. Interestingly, the majority of the treated children had normal development on follow-up despite severe initial findings of CNS and ophthalmologic disease. Longitudinal follow-

up studies are still in progress. The current guidelines for treatment of congenital toxoplasmosis are oral pyrimethamine (loading dose of 2 mg per kilogram for 2 days, then 1 mg per kilogram per day) plus sulfadiazine or trisulfapyrimidine (50 to 100 mg per kilogram per day orally, in two equally divided doses) plus folinic acid (10 mg orally, 3 times a week) for up to 1 year. If the patient has evidence of an inflammatory process (chorioretinitis, high CSF protein content, generalized infection, jaundice), then corticosteroids (prednisone and methylprednisolone, 1 to 2 mg per kilogram per day orally, as two equal portions, 12 hourly) should be prescribed until the inflammation subsides.

PREVENTION

Humans are an incidental host in the life cycle of *T. gondii*. One can help to prevent infection by only eating meat that has been well cooked (more than 60°C; when no longer pink in the center) or frozen (less than −20°C for at least 24 hours) and thawed. It is important to be aware that home freezers do not achieve this temperature. Consistent hand washing after the handling of cats or their feces should help to decrease the ingestion of oocysts. Also, cat litter boxes should be emptied daily, before the oocysts can become infectious. Cat owners should keep their cats indoors, if possible, and feed them commercial cat food or well-cooked table food only. Pregnant women and immunocompromised hosts, especially HIV-infected individuals, should observe these prevention strategies.

BIBLIOGRAPHY

Cochereau-Massin I, LeHoang P, Lautier-Frau M, et al. Ocular toxoplasmosis in human immunodeficiency virus–infected patients. *Am J Ophthalmol* 1992;114:130–135.

Dannemann B, McCutchan A, Israelski D, et al. Treatment of toxoplasmic encephalitis in patients with AIDS. *Ann Intern Med* 1992;116:33–43.

Foulon W, Villena I, Stray-Pedersen B, et al. Treatment of toxoplasmosis during pregnancy: a multicenter study of impact on fetal transmission and children's sequelae at age 1 year. *Am J Obstet Gynecol* 1999;180:410–415.

Koppe JG, Loewer-Sieger DH, de Roerer-Bonnet H. Results of 20-year follow-up of congenital toxoplasmosis. *Lancet* 1986:101:254–256.

Luft BJ, Hafner R, Korzun AH, et al. Toxoplasmic encephalitis in patients with the acquired immunodeficiency syndrome. *N Engl J Med* 1993;329:995–1000.

Luft BJ, Remington JS. Toxoplasmic encephalitis in AIDS. *Clin Infect Dis* 1992;15:211–222.

Mariuz P, Luft BJ. New therapeutic approaches to toxoplasmic encephalitis. *Curr Opin Infect Dis* 1991;4(6):826–833.

McAuley J, Boyer KM, Patel D, et al. Early and longitudinal evaluation of treated infants and children and untreated historical patients with congenital toxoplasmosis: the Chicago Collaborative Treatment trial. *Clin Infect Dis* 1994;18:38–72.

Novati R, Castagna A, Morsica G, et al. Polymerase chain reaction for Toxoplasma gondii DNA in the cerebrospinal fluid of AIDS patients with focal brain lesions. *AIDS* 1994;8:1691–1694.

Pomeroy C, Felice GA. Pulmonary toxoplasmosis: a review. *Clin Infect Dis* 1992;14:863–870.

Porter SB, Sande M. Toxoplamosis of the central nervous system in the acquired immunodeficiency syndrome. *N Engl J Med* 1992;327:1643–1648.

Remington JS, McLeod R, Desmonts G. Toxoplasmosis. In: Remington JS, Klein JD, eds. *Infectious diseases of the fetus and newborn infants,* fourth ed. Philadelphia: WB Saunders, 1995:140–267.

Renold C, Sugar A, Chave JD, et al. Toxoplasma encephalitis in patients with the acquired immunodeficiency syndrome. *Medicine* 1992;71:224–239.

Wong SY, Remington JS. Biology of *Toxoplasma gondii. AIDS* 1993;7:299–316.

Wong SY, Remington JS. Toxoplasmosis in pregnancy. *Clin Infect Dis* 1994;18:853–861.

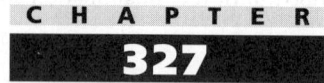

CHAPTER 327

PNEUMOCYSTOSIS

DONALD ARMSTRONG
EDWARD M. BERNARD

EPIDEMIOLOGIC FACTORS

Pneumocystis carinii, while long considered to be a protozoan parasite, is now recognized as a fungus that appears to be passed from person to person by the respiratory route. Animals other than humans harbor similar organisms in their lungs. Morpho-logically, the organisms that infect humans, rats, ferrets, and mice are indistinguishable, but there are genetic and antigenic differences. There is no evidence of transmission of the organism from other animals to humans. Reports of clusters of cases and of rises in antibody titers among health care workers exposed to heavily infected patients suggest that person-to-person transmission can occur.

Research findings based on ribosomal gene sequences and gene regulatory mechanisms provide strong evidence that *P. carinii* is a fungus rather than a protozoa. This raises the possibility that the organism may be found in soil or other environmental sources. Like the most common opportunistic fungus, *Candida albicans, P. carinii* may colonize or latently infect humans and cause infection from colonizing sites.

There is no convincing evidence of seasonal variation in the incidence of pneumocystosis. The infection appears to be less common among immunocompromised patients in nonindustrialized countries. This may be attributable to the higher incidence of other, more virulent infections, such as tuberculosis and cryptococcosis, and to different standards of medical care.

In summary, *Pneumocystis* is an unusual fungus that resides in the lower respiratory tract of humans and spreads by the respiratory aerosol route. It usually is not pathogenic until it has the opportunity to multiply and invade because of a T-helper cell defect.

PATHOGENESIS

The organisms are found in the alveolar space during both asymptomatic infection and disease. Multiplication is unleashed in the setting of T-helper cell depletion or dysfunction and induces a frothy alveolar exudate that is acellular or contains mononuclear cells. A plasma cell exudate has been described in epidemics of pneumocystosis among malnourished children. Extrapulmonary disease rarely was described in immunocompromised hosts before the advent of AIDS and now is recognized increasingly in patients with AIDS. Disseminated disease appears to be a rare complication of *Pneumocystis* pneumonia. However, its frequency is uncertain because most patients with pneumonia receive systemic agents that should be effective at both extrapulmonary and pulmonary sites of infection. Reports of the organisms causing granulomas in the external auditory canal suggest the possibility of contiguous spread from the upper respiratory tract. The finding of organisms in liver, spleen, brain, and other organs demonstrates that hematogenous dissemination can occur.

Granulomatous lesions occur in nonpulmonary sites and, rarely, in the lung. Pulmonary lesions range from the usual mononuclear infiltrate to a neutrophil infiltrate and even necrosis with cavity formation. Pneumothorax usually is the result of necrotizing lesions in the lung pleura. It should be assumed, unless proven otherwise, that a pneumothorax in a patient at risk for pneumocystosis is caused by active disease that requires immediate and appropriate treatment.

DIAGNOSIS

The symptoms and signs of pneumocystosis usually are those of an acute diffuse pneumonia. It has become apparent, with the increasing number of cases, that a variety of pulmonary presentations occur, including solitary lesions, patchy infiltrates, lobar pneumonias, and cavitary pneumonias (Fig. 327.1). Patients receiving aerosol pentamidine for prophylaxis tend to have apical pneumonias and fewer clinical symptoms and signs. The pulmonary disease can progress slowly or rapidly. In some cases, pulmonary symptoms are absent and the primary complaint is fever, night sweats, or diarrhea. Any persistent constitutional symptom in a patient at risk for the development of *P. carinii* pneumonia (PCP) should prompt consideration of the diagnosis of pneumocystosis. There are other infections that can mimic PCP, and these should be ruled out as the cause of the patient's illness (Table 327.1). Concurrent infections can complicate pneumocystosis, and investigation of clinical specimens should include appropriate tests for other organisms.

Unexplained anemia, adenopathy, hepatosplenomegaly, or external auditory canal lesions can be caused by extrapulmonary pneumocystosis; biopsy specimens or exudates should be stained with methenamine silver and immunohistochemical reagents to detect *P. carinii* as well as other opportunistic pathogens.

The diagnosis of PCP usually is made by bronchoalveolar lavage followed by examination of the lavage fluid using various stains. The methenamine silver, Gram–Weigert, and toluidine blue O stains are used to detect cyst-like forms, and the Giemsa stain is used to detect trophozoite-like forms. The direct fluorescence antibody test detects both forms of the organism. Application of the polymerase chain reaction to the diagnosis of pneumocystosis appears to offer improved sensitivity over

TABLE 327.1.	PATHOGENS AND CONDITIONS THAT MAY ACCOMPANY OR MIMIC *PNEUMOCYSTIS CARINII* INFECTIONS

Bacteria
    Streptococcus species
    Haemophilus influenzae
    Staphylococcus aureus
    Mycobacterium tuberculosis
Fungi
    Cryptococcus neoformans
    Histoplasma capsulatum
Parasites
    Toxoplasma gondii
    Strongyloides stercoralis
Viruses
    Cytomegalovirus
    Herpes simplex
    Adenovirus
Other
    Kaposi's sarcoma
    Lymphoma
    Drug toxicity
    Lymphoid interstitial pneumonia

conventional methods. All of these methods are highly sensitive and specific in the hands of an experienced laboratory. Our preference is to use several methods. Bronchoalveolar specimens are sent to the microbiology laboratory for toluidine blue O staining and to the cytology laboratory for Gram–Weigert staining; transbronchial biopsy specimens are sent to the pathology laboratory for Gram–Weigert and methenamine silver staining. Some laboratories have reported remarkable success using sputum induction to make a diagnosis of PCP. This should be attempted if there is sufficient time. Transbronchial biopsy can be helpful in detecting cytomegalovirus, drug toxicity, lymphocytic interstitial pneumonia, or neoplasms.

The diagnosis of extrapulmonary pneumocystosis usually is made by examining biopsy specimens of the tissue involved using appropriate stains such as methenamine silver. The organism cannot be recovered by culture of clinical specimens.

PREVENTION

Because prevention of PCP reduces mortality and morbidity and decreases costs, every effort should be made to identify patients who are at risk and to provide them with safe and effective chemoprophylaxis (Table 327.2).

Patients who are at risk for the development of PCP and who should receive prophylaxis include adults and adolescents with HIV infection and fewer than 200 CD4$^+$ T-helper cells per μL; children with HIV, regardless of their CD4$^+$ T-helper cell count; all newborns of HIV-infected mothers; patients with leukemia or lymphoma who are receiving cytotoxic therapy; patients with solid tumors or other conditions who are taking high doses of adrenocorticosteroids (see later); and organ or bone marrow transplant recipients. We recommend prophylaxis for

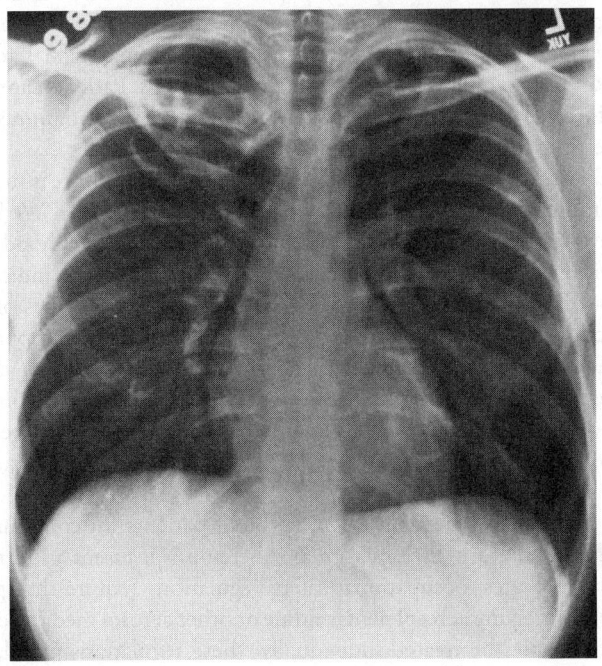

FIGURE 327.1. Chest radiograph of a patient with open-lung biopsy–proven pneumocystosis and large cavitary lesions.

TABLE 327.2.	PREVENTION OF PNEUMOCYSTOSIS	
Drug	**Dose**	**Utility**
Trimethoprim–sulfamethoxazole	Single- or double-strength tablet, daily or 3 times/wk	Highly effective, inexpensive, also prevents other infections
Dapsone	100 mg/d	Good to poor tolerance, moderately effective
Aerosol pentamidine	300 mg/mo, Respirgard nebulizer	Well tolerated, moderately effective
Atovaquone	1,500 mg/d	Good to poor tolerance, moderately effective

all patients being treated with adrenocorticosteroids at dosages of prednisone equivalents of 20 mg per day or higher for more than 2 weeks. Prophylaxis should be continued during tapering of corticosteroid therapy and for 1 month thereafter.

Trimethoprim–sulfamethoxazole (TMP-SMX) is almost always effective in preventing PCP. It can virtually eliminate the risk of PCP among patients with cancer or HIV infection. Several dosing regimens have been used successfully for this indication. One double-strength tablet given daily or 3 days per week has been shown to prevent PCP. A double-strength tablet contains 160 mg of TMP and 800 mg of SMX. Advantages of TMP-SMX include high efficacy, systemic action, activity against bacterial pathogens and against toxoplasmosis, and low cost. Use of folinic acid is not recommended because it raises costs and does not increase efficacy or significantly reduce toxicity.

The major limitation of TMP-SMX is that some patients cannot tolerate it. It can cause rash, nausea, fever, neutropenia, and other adverse reactions. Hypersensitivity to the sulfonamide component is the most common adverse reaction. Intolerance of TMP-SMX occurs more often among patients with HIV infection than among other patients. This reflects a higher rate of allergic reactions to medications and an increased opportunity to become sensitized because of the longer period for which prophylaxis is needed. In most cases, patients can be desensitized, and this should be attempted before considering alternative agents.

Aerosol pentamidine and dapsone are alternative methods for prophylaxis of PCP. Although not as reliably effective as TMP-SMX, they have been shown to reduce the risk of PCP among HIV-infected patients. Aerosol pentamidine also has been used successfully in bone marrow transplant recipients and in patients with cancer who cannot tolerate sulfonamides.

Dapsone has been administered for PCP prophylaxis at daily oral doses of 100 mg; some clinicians add pyrimethamine at 50 mg once a week. Patients should be tested for glucose-6-phosphate dehydrogenase deficiency before taking dapsone because this genetic deficiency increases the risk of dapsone-induced hemolysis. Methemoglobinemia occurs with dapsone therapy and may be clinically significant in patients with anemia or lung disease. The most common side effects of dapsone are rash, pruritus, nausea, and fever.

Dapsone, a sulfone, is chemically related to the sulfonamides, and many patients who are allergic to SMX experience hypersensitivity reactions to dapsone. There is reasonably good evidence

that dapsone plus pyrimethamine and TMP-SMX also provide some protection against toxoplasmosis. Dapsone is an inexpensive and effective alternative agent for PCP prophylaxis.

Aerosol pentamidine is tolerated better than TMP-SMX or dapsone. It is less effective than TMP-SMX but equal or superior to dapsone. Because pentamidine has a long half-life in tissue, protective levels can be maintained with low and infrequent dosing. Administration by the aerosol route delivers the drug to the desired site of action while limiting toxicity to other organs. Systemic side effects are rare, although rash, pancreatitis, and hypoglycemia have been reported.

The only regimen approved in the United States for aerosol pentamidine involves the administration, every 4 weeks, of 300 mg of pentamidine through the Respirgard II nebulizer. The jet nebulizer requires a compressor or source of compressed air or oxygen. Some practitioners recommend that this regimen be given every 2 weeks to patients at highest risk for PCP. We recommend that the monthly regimen of 300 mg be preceded by a loading regimen of five doses of 300 mg given over 2 weeks. The use of a loading regimen is particularly important in bone marrow transplant recipients and patients receiving cytotoxic therapies. If a loading regimen is not used, it may take 1 to 3 months to establish protective levels in the lungs. Patients cannot afford to wait for protection when they have a high and immediate risk for this life-threatening infection.

There is disagreement about whether pneumothorax is more common among patients receiving aerosol pentamidine. We believe that aerosol pentamidine, by increasing the likelihood of apical pneumonia and pleural involvement, can be an indirect contributory factor. Because aerosol pentamidine provides protection to the lung and not to other organs, extrapulmonary pneumocystosis is a rare but significant complication of this method of prophylaxis. The most common side effects are cough and bronchospasm; both usually can be prevented by pretreatment of susceptible patients with an inhaled bronchodilator such as albuterol.

Careful and frequent examination of patients for communicable respiratory diseases such as tuberculosis is essential. In the United States, occupational safety regulations require that patients receiving aerosol pentamidine or other aerosol medications or therapies be treated individually; these regulations mandate the use of barriers, filters, and masks that prevent exposure of health care workers and other patients to potentially infectious aerosols and to aerosol medications. These measures add to the expense and can cause anxiety and discomfort for patients.

Other potential agents for PCP prophylaxis are atovaquone or clindamycin–primaquine, and sulfadoxine–pyrimethamine (Fansidar). The long-acting sulfonamide sulfadoxine should not be used because adverse reactions can be severe. Atovoquone is less effective than TMP-SMX but appears to be similar in effectiveness to dapsone. Clinical studies have yet to provide evidence of a role for clindamycin–primaquine in prophylaxis against PCP.

It has been recommended that once prophylaxis is indicated, for an HIV-infected patient, it should be continued for life. The advent of highly active antiretroviral therapy (HAART) has prompted reexamination of the need for lifelong prophylaxis. There is mounting evidence that patients who experience immune reconstitution as a result of successful HAART therapy may be able to discontinue prophylaxis against PCP and other opportunistic infections. Additional studies are needed before the recommendation can be definitively changed. At this time, the decision to discontinue must be made on a case-by-case basis.

TREATMENT

The preferred therapy for pneumocystosis is TMP-SMX (Table 327.3). Although other agents have been shown to be effective in the treatment of PCP, most are less effective and none is superior to TMP-SMX. Except in mild cases, intravenous pentamidine is the treatment of choice for patients who cannot tolerate SMX. Several oral therapies provide alternatives to intravenous pentamidine: dapsone-TMP, atovaquone, or clindamycin–primaquine. These agents should be considered only for the treatment of patients with mild episodes of PCP (PaO_2 greater than 70 mm Hg or A-a gradient less than 35 mm Hg). Trimetrexate plus leucovorin can be used in moderate to severe cases of PCP in patients who cannot tolerate TMP-SMX

or pentamidine. Early treatment with adjunctive corticosteroids is recommended for patients with AIDS who have PCP and hypoxia (PaO_2 less than 70 mm Hg). On completion of therapy, patients should receive prophylaxis to prevent recurrence of pneumocystosis for as long as they remain immunocompromised.

For the treatment of acute PCP, TMP-SMX can be administered orally or intravenously. Unless the episode is exceedingly mild and there is no evidence or suspicion of gastrointestinal dysfunction, we prefer to use the intravenous route. Intravenous or oral treatment should be administered at dosages of 15 to 20 mg per kilogram per day of TMP and 75 to 100 mg per kilogram per day of SMX; it can be given in three to four divided doses. We recommend continuation of treatment for 21 days. Initial treatment with intravenous doses can be followed by oral dosing in responsive patients. Careful monitoring for clinical response and for adverse reactions is needed throughout the treatment period. Hospitalization is recommended during the induction phase of treatment; some patients with mild episodes can be treated as outpatients, and many patients can complete therapy successfully using oral medications at home.

The most common toxicities with TMP-SMX are rash, fever, hepatic dysfunction, and leukopenia. These reactions do not always require discontinuation of the drug. If the side effects are moderate or severe, or if symptoms are not improved after 5 to 7 days of treatment, alternative therapies must be considered. In most cases, the alternative therapy of choice is intravenous pentamidine. Many patients who have had allergic reactions to TMP-SMX can receive initial therapy with intravenous pentamidine while being desensitized to SMX over a 3- to 7-day period. This allows completion of therapy with oral TMP-SMX and its continuation as prophylaxis.

Intravenous pentamidine appears to be as effective as TMP-SMX in the treatment of PCP. It should be administered by intravenous infusion at 3 to 4 mg per kilogram per day over 1 to 2 hours. Response to pentamidine therapy often is slow; it

TABLE 327.3.	TREATMENT OF PNEUMOCYSTOSIS
Drug	**Dosage**
Initial Therapy	
Trimethoprim–sulfamethoxazole	15/75 mg/kg to 20/100 mg/kg, IV (preferred) or PO, in 4 divided doses, 14–21 d
Alternative Therapy for Mild to Severe Disease	
Pentamidine	3–4 mg/kg, IV, 14–21 d
Alternative Therapy for Mild to Moderate Disease	
Dapsone-trimethoprim	Dapsone at 100 mg/d, PO, plus trimethoprim at 20 mg/kg/d, PO in 3 divided doses, 14–21 d
Atovaquone	750 mg PO t.i.d. with food, 14–21 d
Clindamycin-primaquine	Primaquine 15 mg PO q.d. for 21 d, plus clindamycin 600 mg IV q6h for 10 d, followed by 450 mg PO q6h for 11 d
Alternative Therapy for Moderate to Severe Disease When Standard Therapies Cannot Be Used	
Trimetrexate-leucovorin	Trimetrexate 45 mg/m^2–leucovorin 20 mg/m^2 q6h

may take four or more doses to achieve effective pulmonary concentrations of the drug. Treatment should be continued for 2 to 3 weeks. Pentamidine is reserved for patients who cannot tolerate or fail to respond to TMP-SMX because pentamidine can cause hypotension, renal dysfunction, hypoglycemia, fever, or pancreatitis. Although these potential toxicities require careful monitoring, it is our experience that most patients who require intravenous pentamidine can be treated successfully with this alternative therapy. Pentamidine should not be administered by intramuscular injection because this route is associated with the formation of painful and debilitating sterile abscesses at the site of injection.

There are several proven alternatives to intravenous pentamidine that should be considered for the treatment of mild episodes of PCP in patients who cannot tolerate TMP-SMX. Oral dapsone (100 mg per day) with TMP (20 mg per kilogram per day) is effective for this indication. Although dapsone is chemically related to SMX, some patients who are allergic to SMX can tolerate dapsone. Patients receiving dapsone should be observed carefully for rash, fever, liver function abnormalities, and methemoglobinemia.

Atovaquone (750 mg orally 3 times a day) is a hydroxynaphthoquinone that is effective therapy for mild to moderate PCP. It usually is better tolerated than TMP-SMX or intravenous pentamidine, but therapeutic failures occur with greater frequency. The higher failure rate may be attributable to the fact that absorption of the drug is poor among some patients. Improved formulations have mitigated this significant problem.

Clindamycin plus primaquine is another option for the treatment of sulfa-intolerant patients with mild PCP. Controlled clinical trials with this combination have shown that it is effective but can cause adverse reactions, including rash, diarrhea, anemia, and neutropenia. Trimetrexate plus leucovorin is available as salvage therapy for patients with moderate to severe PCP. It is effective in some patients and should be considered if standard therapies fail or cannot be tolerated.

Aerosol pentamidine, although shown to be effective in the prevention of PCP, is markedly less effective than standard therapies for acute PCP. Aerosol pentamidine should not be used for the treatment of this life-threatening infection.

Adjunctive corticosteroids improve survival and decrease the likelihood of respiratory failure in patients with AIDS who have confirmed PCP and hypoxia (PaO_2 < 70 mm Hg). The recommended dosage of prednisone is 40 mg twice daily for 5 days, followed by 40 mg daily for 5 days, then 20 mg daily until completion of therapy for PCP. There was concern that corticosteroid therapy might increase the risk for developing other opportunistic infections or neoplasms, but this risk seems to be outweighed by the benefits of this adjunctive therapy.

BIBLIOGRAPHY

Cushion MT. Taxonomy, genetic organization, and life cycle of *Pneumocystis carinii*. *Semin Respir Infect* 1998;13(4):304–312.

Fishman JA. Treatment of infection due to *Pneumocystis carinii*. *Antimicrob Agents Chemother* 1998;42(6):1309–1314.

Furrer H, Egger M, Opravil M, et al. Discontinuation of primary prophylaxis against *Pneumocystis carinii* pneumonia in HIV-1–infected adults treated with combination antiretroviral therapy. Swiss HIV Cohort Study. *N Engl J Med* 1999;340(17):1301–1306.

Hughes WT. Use of dapsone in the prevention and treatment of *Pneumocystis carinii* pneumonia: a review. *Clin Infect Dis* 1998;27(1):191–204.

Masur H, Kaplan J. Does *Pneumocystis carinii* prophylaxis still need to be lifelong? [editorial; comment] *N Engl J Med* 1999;340(17):1356–1358.

Sepkowitz KA. Effect of prophylaxis on the clinical manifestations of AIDS-related opportunistic infections. *Clin Infect Dis* 1998;26(4):806–810.

Shelhamer JH, Gill VJ, Quinn TC, et al. The laboratory evaluation of opportunistic pulmonary infections. *Ann Intern Med* 1996 Mar 15; 124(6):585–599.

US Public Health Services/Infectious Diseases Society of America. 1997 USPHS/IDSA guidelines for the prevention of opportunistic infections in persons infected with human immunodeficiency virus: disease-specific recommendations. USPHS/IDSA Prevention of Opportunistic Infections Working Group. *Clin Infect Dis* 1997(Suppl 3):S313–S335.

Kelley's Textbook of Internal Medicine, fourth edition. Edited by H. David Humes. Lippincott Williams & Wilkins, Philadelphia © 2000.

C H A P T E R

328

TRICHOMONIASIS

JOSE A. PRIETO
JORGE D. BLANCO

DEFINITION AND EPIDEMIOLOGY

Trichomonas vaginalis, a unicellular, flagellated protozoan first described in 1836, is a major cause of infectious vulvovaginitis, occurring in 25% of symptomatic women. The organism also can be found in a significant percentage of asymptomatic, sexually active women. In men, *T. vaginalis* can colonize and invade the prostate, urethra, or seminal vesicles, but it rarely produces symptoms. About 5% of all episodes of nongonococcal urethritis in men are caused by this organism.

The prevalence of trichomoniasis ranges from 3% of patients attending student health clinics to 37% of patients attending sexually transmitted disease clinics. Because the only established mode of transmission is sexual intercourse, patients should be evaluated for other sexually transmitted diseases, such as gonorrhea, syphilis, chlamydial infection, and HIV infection.

CLINICAL FEATURES AND DIAGNOSIS

Among symptomatic women, common presenting complaints include vaginal discharge (white, yellow, or green), vulvar itching, dyspareunia, malodor, and dysuria. The supposedly classic frothy, yellow–green discharge associated with vaginal wall erythema and a "strawberry" cervix is seen in only 10% of cases.

Because the presentation can vary, the clinician should not rely on clinical symptoms alone in making the diagnosis.

Vaginal, prostatic, or urethral secretions should be examined for the presence of *Trichomonas* organisms. A positive wet mount prepared with fresh normal saline reveals the motile organisms. The sensitivity of this method varies from 22% to 76%, but it is highly specific when positive. Spence and colleagues found the sensitivity of cultures (Diamond's medium) to be greater than that of wet mounts. However, culture diagnosis is labor-intensive, expensive, and not commonly available.

TREATMENT

Metronidazole (Flagyl) is the effective therapy for trichomoniasis. Initially, the recommended dosage was 250 mg orally three times a day for 7 to 10 days. However, controversial studies suggesting possible carcinogenicity of metronidazole led to the development of other treatment regimens. In 1972, Csonka compared a single 2-g oral dose with prolonged multidose regimens and found similar effectiveness. Aubert and Sesta reported comparable adverse effects with the two regimens. Based on these and subsequent studies, the U.S. Centers for Disease Control and Prevention in 1985 began recommending a single 2-g oral dose as the treatment of choice. The cure rate with this regimen exceeds 90%.

Because *Trichomonas* is transmitted sexually, partners of infected patients should be treated concurrently. Preventive measures, such as the use of condoms, also should be prescribed.

Pregnant patients with trichomoniasis present a treatment challenge. Most authorities agree that metronidazole should not be used during the first trimester. However, investigations suggest that trichomoniasis may be associated with premature birth and premature rupture of the membranes. Therefore, most clinicians treat symptomatic patients during the second and third trimesters with a single 2-g dose or three 250-mg doses every day for 7 days.

Although rare, treatment failures can occur. However, repeated exposure is the most common cause for recurrent disease. In such cases, a prolonged oral regimen, intravaginal administration, or intravenous therapy may be necessary. A reasonable first step is a regimen of 500 mg to 1 g orally twice a day for 7 days. Alternatively, intravaginal therapy with two uncoated 500-mg tablets twice a day for 7 days may be useful.

TRICHOMONAS AND HUMAN IMMUNODEFICIENCY VIRUS INFECTION

Trichomonas and HIV are transmitted by sexual contact and share the same behavioral risk factors. In a prospective study by Laga and associates, incident gonorrhea, chlamydial infection, and trichomoniasis were associated with an increased risk of HIV seroconversion in women, even after the number of sexual partners and level of condom use were considered. Nonulcerative sexually transmitted diseases such as trichomoniasis may facili-

tate the acquisition of HIV infection by causing mucosal disruption of the genital tract.

Screening for HIV infection is justified in both symptomatic and asymptomatic patients with trichomoniasis. Likewise, early detection and treatment of trichomoniasis is essential in HIV-infected patients.

BIBLIOGRAPHY

Aubert JM, Sesta HJ. Treatment of vaginal trichomoniasis, single 2-gram dose of metronidazole as compared with a seven-day course. *J Reprod Med* 1982;27:743–745.

Csonka GW. Trichomonal vaginitis treated with one dose of metronidazole. *Br J Vener Dis* 1971;47:456–458.

Gardner H, Dukes CD. *Haemophilus vaginalis* vaginitis: a newly defined specific infection previously classified "nonspecific" vaginitis. *Am J Obstet Gynecol* 1955;69:962.

Hager WD. *Trichomonas vaginalis* infection. In: Pastorek J, ed. *Obstetric and gynecologic infectious disease.* New York: Raven Press, 1994:537.

Laga M, Maroka A, Kivuru M, et al. Non-ulcerative sexually transmitted diseases as risk factors for HIV-1 transmission in women. Results from a cohort study. *AIDS* 1993;7:95–102.

Latif AS, Mason PR, Marowa E. Urethral trichomoniasis in men. *Sex Transm Dis* 1987;14:9–11.

Minkoff H, Grunebaum AN, Schwarz RH, et al. Risk factors for prematurity and premature rupture of membranes: a prospective study of the vaginal flora in pregnancy. *Am J Obstet Gynecol* 1984;150:965–972.

Plummer FA, Simonsen JN, Cameron DW, et al. Co-factors in male–female sexual transmission of human immunodeficiency virus type I. *J Infect Dis* 1991;163:233–239.

Rein MF, Muller M. *Trichomonas vaginalis.* In: Holmes KK, Mardh PA, Sparling PF, et al., eds. *Sexually transmitted diseases.* New York: McGraw-Hill, 1984:525.

Spence MR, Hollander DH, Smith J. The clinical and laboratory diagnosis of *Trichomonas vaginalis* infection. *Sex Transm Dis* 1980;7:168–171.

U.S. Centers for Disease Control and Prevention. Sexually transmitted diseases treatment guidelines—1985. *MMWR* 1985;34:25.

Kelley's Textbook of Internal Medicine, fourth edition. Edited by H. David Humes. Lippincott Williams & Wilkins, Philadelphia © 2000.

CHAPTER

329

NAEGLERIA, ACANTHAMOEBA, AND LEPTOMYXID AMEBIC INFECTIONS

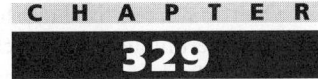

RICHARD J. DUMA

CENTRAL NERVOUS SYSTEM INFECTIONS

The most commonly recognized infection caused by free-lining amebae (FLA), in both humans and other animals, is meningoencephalitis. *Naegleria* organisms, and occasionally *Acanthamoeba* organisms, produce an acute, fulminating, almost always fatal infection, referred to as primary amebic meningoencephalitis (PAM), whereas *Acanthamoeba* species and leptomyxid amebae of the genus *Balamuthia mandrillaris* produce a subacute or chronic meningoencephalitis, referred to as granulomatous amebic meningoencephalitis (GAE).

MICROBIOLOGY, PATHOGENESIS, AND EPIDEMIOLOGIC FACTORS

Although *Naegleria* and *Acanthamoeba* belong to the order Amoebida, families Vahlkampfiidae and Acanthamoebidae, respectively, leptomyxid amebae belong to the order Leptomyxida, family Leptomyxidae. Pathogenic amebae in all three groups are biologically distinct but differ from *Entamoeba histolytica* in that they are highly aerobic, possess a large karyosome within a single nucleus, have no known intermediate hosts, are not considered parasites, are commonly found as trophozoites in soil and water, and are highly resistant to a wide array of chemotherapeutic agents, especially those used to treat *E. histolytica*.

Naegleria fowleri is the only species of *Naegleria* reported to infect humans. However, other potentially pathogenic species exist (e.g., *Naegleria australiensis*). Under light microscopy, trophozoites measure 10 to 20 μm, have a single contractile vacuole, and possess food vacuoles that may contain ingested red blood cells; they have blunt or lobose pseudopodia. Their movement is active and slug-like. Cysts are uninucleate and circular, and possess smooth, doubly contoured walls with pores for excystation. Most importantly, trophozoites can transform into characteristic flagellates, distinguishing them from *Acanthamoeba* and other FLA. However, only trophozoites are found in infected tissues.

At least five species of *Acanthamoeba* infect humans: *A. polyphaga*, *A. culbertsoni*, *A. rhysodes*, *A. astronyxis*, and *A. castellani*. Under light microscopy, trophozoites are 15 to 40 μm long, have a single contractile vacuole, may contain red blood cells, and possess pseudopodia that taper to finely rounded ends (acanthapodia). In addition, their nuclei are indistinguishable from those of *Naegleria*. Their movement is sluggish and, at times, barely perceptible. Cysts are uninucleate and characteristically appear stellate or wrinkled. Both trophozoites and cysts can be found in infected tissues.

Balamuthia mandrillaris is the only leptomyxid ameba reported to infect humans. Trophozoites are irregularly shaped, range in length from 12 to 60 μm, and are predominantly uninucleate. Although locomotion is generally sluggish, at times they exhibit a spider-like walking movement. Cysts are circular, 6 to 30 μm in diameter, and possess a very thick wall that on ultrastructual examination consists of three layers. Both trophozoites and cysts are found in infected tissues, but distinction from *Acanthamoeba* is difficult and is usually acomplished with immunologic staining techniques.

Naegleria and *Acanthamoeba* can be cultured axenically in artificial media, nonaxenically on plain agar seeded with Enterobacteriaceae as a food source, or in a variety of tissue culture cell lines. However, *B. mandrillaris* does not grow well with bacteria as a food source, and inoculation of tissue culture cell

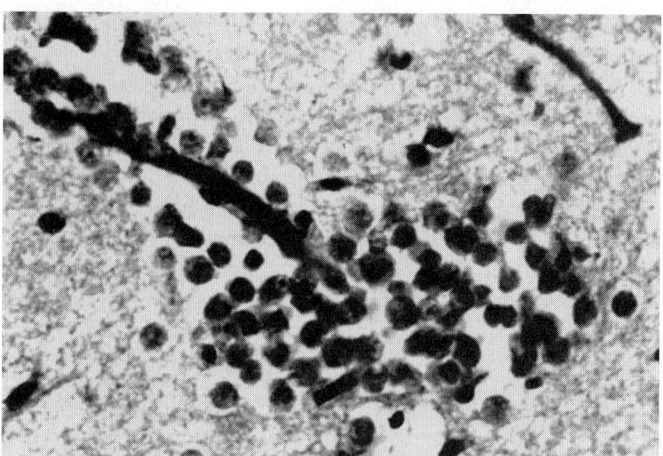

FIGURE 329.1. Perivascular collection of *Naegleria* in the frontal cortex of a patient with primary amebic meningoencephalitis (×500). Prominent, dark karyosomes and surrounding halos within the nuclei of the organisms are visible. (From Duma RJ, Ferrell HW, Nelson CE, et al. Primary amebic meningoencephalitis. *N Engl J Med* 1969;281:1315, with permission.)

lines, such as African green monkey kidney cells (E6), is needed. Pathogenic FLA are stable at room temperature (23°C), grow well at 33°C to 37°C, and may withstand 44°C. Most tolerate temperatures below 5°C poorly; hence, clinical specimens containing organisms should not be refrigerated if isolation is desired.

Naegleria fowleri organisms invade the central nervous system (CNS) of mammals directly through the olfactory nerve pathways after penetrating the nasal mucosa (Fig. 329.1). *Acanthamoeba* species invade the CNS directly by the nasal route or indirectly by hematogenous spread from a site outside the CNS (e.g., lung, skin, uterus, prostate, eye). The portal of entry for *B. mandrillaris* is unknown. The risk of infection from almost all FLA is related to the size of the inoculum and the site of instillation. In a variety of tissue culture cell lines, a cytopathogenic effect (CPE) is initiated by contact of amebae with cells (contact-dependent cytolysis), and portions of cell cytoplasm also appear to be removed by a "nibbling-out" process referred to as *trogocytosis*. In vitro, *N. fowleri* organisms migrate preferentially toward nervous tissue (tropism).

Examination of brain tissue from patients with GAE often reveals extensive demyelination associated with trophozoites of *Acanthamoeba*, suggesting the release of cytotoxic enzymes. Pathogenic *Acanthamoeba* species contain more phospholipase A than do nonpathogenic species. Brain infection due to *B. mandrillaris* is usually associated with considerable arteritis or angiitis, with perivascular cuffing and necrotizing granulomas.

The first line of host defense against invasion by *Naegleria* appears to be the polymorphonuclear leukocyte; against *A. culbertsoni*, however, polymorphonuclear leukocytes appear to be ineffective unless they are preexposed to activated macrophages. Fresh human serum lyses *N. fowleri* and *Acanthamoeba* organisms through activation of the alternate pathway for complement, and mice depleted of hemolytic complement are more susceptible to infection from *Naegleria* than are those with normal levels of complement. The roles of cell-mediated immunity and humoral antibodies against *Naegleria* are unclear, but humoral antibodies and complement activation appear to be primary mechanisms of defense against *Acanthamoeba*. Antibodies to *Acanthamoeba* are present in healthy individuals and in some patients with nonspecific respiratory tract infections. Host defense mechanisms against *B. mandrillaris* are as yet poorly defined, but they probably are similar to those involved with *Acanthamoeba*.

Infections caused by *Naegleria* species usually occur during the hottest times of the year, may be epidemic, and are acquired almost invariably from intimate contact with fresh or brackish water (swimming, diving, water skiing). The incubation period is predictably 5 to 7 days. Infections occur worldwide and often in epidemics (point source).

The epidemiology of infections caused by *Acanthamoeba* and *Balamuthia* species are unclear; however, immunocompromised individuals appear to be infected more often than normals. The incubation periods are unknown. Infections occur worldwide. CNS infections occur sporadically, although epidemics of ocular infections due to *Acanthamoeba* species related to contaminated contact lenses or their cleaning solutions have been reported.

CLINICAL FEATURES AND DIAGNOSIS

Naegleria fowleri produces an acute, fulminant meningoencephalitis (PAM) that in the early stages of infection resembles bacterial meningitis (Table 329.1). Male individuals are involved more often than female individuals (3:2), and healthy children or young adults are at greatest risk. Examination of the cerebrospinal fluid (CSF) reveals a preponderance of neutrophils, low glucose, and elevated protein; bacteria are absent. Because amebae soon invade the brain, causing hemorrhagic necrosis of CNS tissues, signs of encephalitis appear. Computed tomography (CT) scanning can be helpful if it demonstrates a hemorrhagic lesion of the brain in the presence of a purulent meningitis. Untreated infections last 24 to 72 hours. Death usually results from cerebral edema and brain stem herniation or from heart failure caused by unexplained myocarditis. The diagnosis can be established by finding characteristic amebae in unstained CSF; occasionally flagellate forms are seen, which is diagnostic. Fluorescein-tagged antibody directed against *Naegleria* can be applied directly to CSF or tissues, but serologic tests are of little value. At autopsy, the diagnosis is usually not difficult, since many rounded amebae without cyst forms are found throughout the brain.

Acanthamoeba organisms can produce a PAM that is clinically indistinguishable from that produced by *Naegleria* organisms, but they more often produce a picture of subacute or chronic meningoencephalitis (GAE). No patient age preference exists, but males predominate and about half of patients have underlying diseases or immunodeficiency problems. More than a dozen patients with AIDS are reported to have been infected, in which cases the clinical pictures resembled disseminated cutaneous fungal or algal diseases, or CNS toxoplasmosis. The portal of entry

TABLE 329.1.	**COMPARISON OF *NAEGLERIA* AND *ACANTHAMOEBA/BALAMUTHIA* MENINGOENCEPHALITIS**[a]	
Factor	**Naegleria**	**Acanthamoeba/Balamuthia**
Age	Child or young adult	Any age, but often extremes of life
Sex ratio	3:2 (males/females)	Males >females
Prior health	Excellent	May be normal, but often underlying disease or immunodeficiency present, e.g., AIDS
Epidemiology	History of recent intimate contact with freshwater	Unknown
Incubation period	5–7 d	Unknown, but highly variable; usually >20 days for GAE
Portal of entry	Olfactory mucosa	Skin, prostate, uterus, eye, lung, ear, olfactory mucosa for Acanthamoeba; may be skin for Balamuthia
Invasion route to CNS	Olfactory nerves	For Acanthamoeba usually hematogenous, but occasionally via the olfactory nerve; unknown for Balamuthia
Clinical picture	PAM; resembles acute pyogenic meningitis	Resembles brain abscess or space-occupying mass
Diagnosis	CSF light microscopy, clinical picture, and culture	Brain biopsy (with immunostaining), neuroimaging, clinical picture, occasionally serology and/or culture
Clinical course	Rapidly fatal (2–3 d)	Fatal, but usually subacute or chronic course
Treatment	Amphotericin B is mainstay, rifampin (adjunct)	Surgery in selected cases; sulfa, 5-fluorocytosine, imidazoles; rifampin and pentamidine for Acanthamoeba
Pathology	Hemorrhagic necrosis (acute neutrophilic) response with involvement principally of frontal and/or temporal lobes; only trophozoites present	Hemorrhagic necrosis (chronic inflammatory cells, reparative gliosis, and granulomas) occurs, midline structures usually spared; both trophozoites and cysts present. Necrotizing granulomas and angiitis with Balamuthia
Protozoology	Amebae seen in and isolated from CSF. Flagellato stage important to identify	No amebae usually seen in CSF, but occasionally can be isolated

[a] Leptomyxid amebic infections usually resemble chronic *Acanthamoeba* infections.
CNS, central nervous system; CSF, cerebrospinal fluid, GAE, granulomatous amebic meningoencephalitis; PAM, primary amebic meningoencephalitis.

varies. The nose, skin, sinuses, and respiratory tract are incriminated most commonly, and preceding or concomitant skin lesions, nasal ulcerations, sinusitis, or pneumonitis containing amebae may be present. In GAE, examination of the CSF reveals a preponderance of round cells, normal to low-normal glucose, and modestly elevated protein. The clinical picture is one of focal or localized CNS disease (resembling brain abscess); however, as the infection progresses, the involvement of multiple areas, usually in centrally located structures, becomes evident. Death usually results from brain stem herniation. Diagnosis may be difficult because amebae rarely are found in the CSF. CT scans may be useful for localization of lesions but are not diagnostically specific. Premortem brain biopsy may be necessary. The application of fluorescein-tagged antibody (directed against surface antigens of the amebae) to infected CSF fluid or tissues may be useful, but false-negative results occur if species not included in the diagnostic preparation are present. Serologic testing may be useful, but only if the infection is chronic.

Infections of the CNS caused by *B. mandrillaris* resemble GAE caused by *Acanthamoeba*, but the clinical course of infection ranges from 14 to 240 days. Patients at the extremes of life and who are immunocompromised appear to be most often infected; however, immunocompetent individuals, particularly children, are occasionally reported. Infants or children presenting with a strokelike picture of unknown cause should be considered as possibly infected by *Balamuthia*. CT scans and/or magnetic resonance imaging (MRI) may help to differentiate these entities, in which case hyperdense, nonenhancing, multiple- or single-space–occupying masses are seen. Examination of the CSF may also be useful but generally is not diagnostic. A variable pleocytosis (occasionally mononuclear) is present, associated with slightly low sugar, elevated protein, and an absence of bacteria. Amebae are not generally found in the CSF by light microscopy, but they may be isolated in tissue culture cell lines (vide supra). For definitive premortem diagnosis, brain biopsy is usually necessary.

OTHER INFECTIONS

Ocular infections caused by *Acanthamoeba* species are not uncommon and usually are chronic, refractory to therapy, and extremely painful. They first appear as shaggy, irregular corneal ulcers resembling those of herpes. *A. castellani* and *A. polyphaga* are the organisms most commonly involved. Almost always, a history of injury containing a foreign body (e.g., dirt or splinters) or the use of a contaminated contact lens is obtained. A characteristic 360-degree or partial paracentral stromal ring infiltrate with recurrent corneal epithelial breakdown typifies the lesion. The diagnosis usually is made from histologic studies of appropriate stains and cultures of ulcer scrapings. A variety of other anatomical sights may also be infected by *Acanthamoeba* (e.g., air sinuses, lungs, skin, uterus, and prostate); and occasionally by *B. mandrillaris* (e.g., lungs and skin), and for *Acanthamoeba* these infected sites are believed to represent the source of hematogenous seeding of the CNS.

TREATMENT AND PREVENTION

The treatment of choice for PAM caused by *Naegleria* is amphotericin B. A daily dose of 1 mg per kilogram is given intravenously over 1 to 2 hours. Because the drug diffuses poorly into the CSF, direct intraventricular instillation may be used, but not without risk. Rifampin may be added, but its value is not established. Standard antiamebae agents (those used against *E. histolytica*) are useless and may be toxic.

Medical therapies for infections caused by *Acanthamoeba* usually are unsatisfactory. Most CNS infections (PAM and GAE) are fatal, although an insufficient number of patients have been studied carefully before death to allow an accurate assessment of presumed mortality rates. For early localized disease, excision of the lesion may be useful, but surgical dissemination of amebae is a distinct risk. Sulfur, 5-fluorocytosine, and the imidazoles may be effective in preventing infections in animals, but their therapeutic usefulness in humans (once disease appears) is essentially unproved. Rifampin and pentamidine were used together in the successful treatment of one renal transplant recipient with disseminated *Acanthamoeba* infection, but more studies are needed to confirm the value of these drugs.

GAE due to *B. mandrillaris* is universally fatal, and to date no medical therapy is available to treat this disease. However, like infections due to *Acanthamoeba*, early surgery may be tried.

Similar problems exist for the treatment of ocular infections caused by *Acanthamoeba*. Some patients appear to benefit from imidazoles and propamidine isethionate. Hexamidine (0.1% hexamidine isethionate eyedrops) also appears to be effective. Surgery usually is necessary and may be curative, but often a penetrating keratoplasty or corneal transplantation is necessary.

Prevention of infections caused by FLA is difficult because the organisms are ubiquitous in nature. The risk of PAM from *Naegleria* may be reduced by wearing nose clips or avoiding swimming or bathing in warm (more than 30°C) freshwaters or brackish waters. Halogenation of natural bodies of water is difficult, but chlorination of enclosed swimming pools effectively kills *Naegleria* organisms. *Acanthamoeba* organisms, especially cysts, are highly resistant to chemical agents and survive chlorination.

After an ocular injury is sustained, the incidence of keratitis and infection from FLA can be reduced by ensuring that foreign bodies are removed immediately and that the injured eye, if washed out, not be rinsed with water containing FLA. Finally, soft contact lenses should always be cleansed in sterile, ameba-free water.

The epidemiology of *B. mandrillaris* or how it infects humans is unclear, but infections are believed to be more common than reported. Little is known about disinfectants for leptomyxid amebae.

BIBLIOGRAPHY

Carter RF. Primary amoebic meningo-encephalitis: clinical, pathological, and epidemiological features of six fatal cases. *J Pathol Bacteriol* 1968; 96:1–25.

Driebe WT, Groden LR, Genvert G, et al. *Acanthamoeba* keratitis associated with contact lenses—United States. *MMWR* 1986;35:405–408.

Duma RJ, Ferrell HW, Nelson CE, et al. Primary amebic meningoencephalitis. *N Engl J Med* 1969;281:1315–1323.

Griesemer DA, Barton LL, Reese CM, et al. Amebic meningoencephalitis caused by *Balamuthia mandrillaris*. *Pediatr Neurol* 1994;10(3): 249–254.

John DT. Opportunistically pathogenic free-living amebae. In: Kreier JP, Baker JR, eds. *Parasitic protozoa*, vol 3, second ed. San Diego: Academic Press, 1993:143.

Jones DB, Visvesvara GS, Robinson NM. *Acanthamoeba polyphaga* keratitis and *Acanthamoeba* uveitis associated with fatal meningoencephalitis. *Trans Ophthalmol Soc UK* 1975;95:221–232.

Niu MT, Duma RJ. Amebic infections of the nervous system. In: Harris AA, ed. *Handbook of clinical neurology,* vol 8. *Microbial disease.* Amsterdam: Elsevier, 1988.

Perrine D, Chenu JP, Georges P, et al. Amoebicidal efficiencies of various diamidines against two strains of *Acanthamoeba polyphaga*. *Antimicrob Agents Chemother* 1995;39:339–342.

Riestra-Castaneda JM, Riestra-Castaneda R, Gonzalez-Garrido AA, et al. Granulomatous amebic encephalitis due to *Balamuthia mandrillaris* (Leptomyxiidae): report of four cases from Mexico. *Am J Trop Med Hyg* 1997;56(6):603–607.

Seidel JS, Harmatz P, Visvesvara GS, et al. Successful treatment of primary amebic meningoencephalitis. *N Engl J Med* 1982;306:346–348.

Sison JP, Kemper CA, Loveless M, et al. Disseminated *Acanthamoeba* infection in patients with AIDS: case reports and review. *Clin Infect Dis* 1995;20:1207–1216.

Visvesvara GS, Martinez AJ, Schuster FL, et al. Leptomyxid ameba, a new agent of amebic meningoencephalitis in humans and animals. *J Clin Microbiol* 1990;28:2750–2756.

CHAPTER

330

INTRODUCTION TO HELMINTHIC DISEASES

ADEL A.F. MAHMOUD

Parasitic metazoa (worms) constitute an important group of infectious diseases worldwide. The unique biologic features of these agents result in significant epidemiologic and clinical characteristics. Worms are multicellular organisms that vary in size from a few millimeters to several meters. They are capable of parasitizing a restricted or wide range of mammalian hosts and may need more than one host to complete their life cycle. Infection is acquired by ingestion or by direct penetration of human skin. Except for *Strongyloides* and *Echinococcus*, worms do not multiply within the human host; increase of parasite population in a specific mammalian host occurs only upon reexposure to the infective stage of the helminth.

Because of the complexity of the antigenic structure of worms and the multiplicity of their stages within the host, the immunologic sequelae of these infections are considerable. The host immune response to worms may play a protective role in limiting infection or disease, or it may cause immunopathologic reactions. In addition, eosinophilia is a prominent feature of the clinical course of tissue-invading worm infections. Eosinophils have been shown to have a significant protective effect against the invasive or tissue-residing stages of worms.

Individuals with suspected worm infections usually have nonspecific complaints. Both a detailed geographic history and epidemiologic information are important. Specific organ system disease, such as hepatomegaly, splenomegaly, or the presence of peripheral blood or sputum eosinophilia, usually is suggestive of worm infection. Definitive diagnosis depends on the identification of a stage of infection in body fluids or tissues. In some situations, serologic evidence of infection is helpful.

BIBLIOGRAPHY

Mahmoud AAF, ed. *Tropical and geographical medicine companion handbook,* second ed. New York: McGraw-Hill, 1993:468.

Warren KS, Mahmoud AAF, eds. *Tropical and geographical medicine,* second ed. New York: McGraw-Hill, 1990:1159.

Drugs for parasitic infections. *Med Lett* 1999.

CHAPTER

331

TISSUE NEMATODE INFECTIONS

JAMES W. KAZURA

FILARIASIS AND TROPICAL EOSINOPHILIA

Filarial infection in humans can cause clinically significant pathology in the lymphatic system, lungs, skin, or eyes. The causative organisms are endemic only in tropical and subtropical areas of the world. They can be divided broadly into three groups based on the major anatomical sites of pathology in the parasitized human host (Table 331.1).

ETIOLOGIC FACTORS

Wuchereria bancrofti, Brugia malayi, and *Brugia timori* are commonly referred to as lymphatic-dwelling filariae because adult worms are localized primarily to the afferent lymphatic vessels and cause disease in these sites. Microfilariae of lymphatic-dwelling filariae circulate in the bloodstream. Adult worms of *Loa loa* are located in subcutaneous tissues and induce pathologic reactions there. Adult worms and microfilariae of *Onchocerca volvulus* dwell in subcutaneous tissue and the skin or eye, respectively. The major pathologic reactions in onchocerciasis result

TABLE 331.1.	FEATURES OF MAJOR HUMAN FILARIAL INFECTIONS			
Organism	**Vector**	**Geographic Distribution**	**Clinical Features**	**Treatment**
W. bancrofti, *B. malayi,* *B. timori*	Mosquito	Tropical Africa, Asia, South Pacific, South America	Mainly asymptomatic, lymphatic obstruction. Tropical Africa	Diethylcarbamazine, Ivermectin
O. volvulus	Blackfly (*Simulium* sp.)	West and Central Africa, Central and South America	Dermatitis, eye disease, hanging groin	Ivermectin
L. loa	Horsefly or deerfly (*Chrysops* sp.)	West and Central Africa	Calabar swelling renal disease, CNS disease	Diethylcarbamazine
M. ozzardi	Midges (*Culicoides* sp.)	Africa, Carribean, Central and South America	Usually asymptomatic, dermatitis	Diethylcarbamazine or no treatment required

from pathologic processes induced by microfilariae in the skin and eye.

The complex life cycle of these filarial nematodes includes an obligate intermediate insect vector that inoculates infective or third-stage larvae into humans during blood feeding. Infective larvae subsequently molt to fourth-stage larvae and develop over about 6 to 12 months into sexually mature adult male or female worms. The latter can live for more than 5 years and release microfilariae, which subsequently are taken up by the insect vector. Microfilariae molt and develop into infective larvae in the insect in 7 to 15 days.

WUCHERERIA BANCROFTI, BRUGIA MALAYI, AND BRUGIA TIMORI INFECTIONS

EPIDEMIOLOGIC FACTORS

Infections with *W. bancrofti*, *B. malayi*, and *B. timori* affect some 120 million people worldwide. *W. bancrofti* infection is endemic in focal areas of the Caribbean, such as Haiti; tropical areas of South America, Africa, and the South Pacific; and Southeast Asia, particularly India and Indonesia. Malayan filariasis is limited in its distribution to India, the Philippines, Malaysia, Indonesia, and China. *B. timori* occurs in the Indonesian islands of Timor and Flores.

Wuchereria bancrofti, the most widespread of these filariae, infects only humans and is transmitted predominantly by culicine mosquitoes. *Anopheles* and *Aedes* mosquitoes also transmit *W. bancrofti*, largely in rural areas. These mosquitoes feed at night, a behavior coincident with the nocturnal periodicity of *W. bancrofti* microfilaremia in many endemic areas. Usually, less than 1% to 2% of mosquitoes in an endemic area harbor infective larvae. Furthermore, less than 20% of such larvae develop into adult worms in the nonimmune host. Therefore, multiple mosquito bites are required for the successful development of a few adult worms. *B. malayi* may be a zoonotic infection because cats can act as a reservoir.

PATHOGENESIS AND CLINICAL MANIFESTATIONS

Infection with lymphatic filariae produces a wide spectrum of disease manifestations in residents of endemic areas. Most chil-

dren younger than 10 years of age and a smaller proportion of adults (20% to 80% in various endemic areas) have no symptoms. Filarial fevers usually are the initial manifestation of symptomatic infection in teenagers and young adults. Abrupt onset of fever greater than 38°C is associated with myalgia and a peculiar retrograde lymphangitis. Swelling proceeds distally from the inguinal area and produces inflamed cordlike lesions and lymphedema. Occasionally, regional lymph nodes enlarge to a diameter of several centimeters. These eventually may rupture and form abscesses. Symptoms persist for 5 to 10 days and may reappear several times per year. Filarial fevers commonly are misdiagnosed as acute attacks of malaria that fail to respond to antimalarial chemotherapy. After recurrent attacks of filarial fevers and acute lymphedema and lymphangitis, lymphedema may not regress and lymph flow from the affected site may become severely limited. The end stage of the process results in chronic obstructive pathology or classic elephantiasis of the upper or lower extremities. The skin is brawny and thickened, with a doughy consistency. Fissures may appear, with breakdown of the skin and secondary bacterial infections. In males with *W. bancrofti* infection, hydroceles and permanent scarring of the spermatic cords occur. Such hydroceles may reach immense size. Obstruction of lymphatic draining of the renal pelvis may produce intermittent chyluria with significant proteinuria.

The pathologic lesions in the lymphatics include intact or remnants of degenerating adult worms surrounded by plasma cells, eosinophils, and macrophages. Granulomas consisting of giant cells, macrophages, eosinophils, and collagen deposits obliterate the lumina of lymphatic vessels. Studies suggest that lymphatic obstruction results in part from these T-cell-mediated granulomatous reactions and from secondary bacterial infections of the extremities. At an epidemiologic level, transmission intensity correlates with the prevalence of lymphatic disease.

Nonresidents of endemic areas have a pattern of clinical manifestations that is different from that of residents. Based on observations of U.S. servicemen stationed in endemic areas during World War II and of migrant adults displaced from nonendemic to endemic areas of Indonesia, it appears that brief, intense exposure (6 months or more) to infective larvae can result in acute manifestations of infection. These include lymphangitis of the lower extremities or genitalia. Such individuals rarely have microfilaremia. Biopsy of affected lymph nodes reveals eosinophil-rich inflammatory lesions surrounding adult worms and sexually immature parasites. Signs and symptoms do not recur if these individuals leave the areas where infection is transmitted. These acute, allergic-type manifestations are thought to result from lack of neonatal immunologic tolerance conferred by maternal infection.

In the case of tropical eosinophilia, the major pathologic reactions are to microfilariae localized in the lung. For reasons that are unclear, microfilariae in such individuals are trapped in the small pulmonary blood vessels and elicit initially histiocyte-rich alveolar and interstitial responses. These evolve into eosinophilic abscesses and infiltrates surrounding degenerating microfilariae. Multiple eosinophil-rich granulomatous lesions eventually may develop in the lung and, in untreated individuals, progress to interstitial fibrosis. Similar lesions with eosinophilic precipitates may be present in lymph nodes and are referred to as *Meyers–Kouwenaar bodies.*

OPTIMAL MANAGEMENT

The definitive means of diagnosis is by demonstration of microfilariae in the blood. Because parasitemia often has a nocturnal periodicity, blood should be obtained between midnight and 4 a.m. to optimize the likelihood of detecting parasites. In the case of bancroftian filariasis, infection in the absence of microfilaremia can be detected by the presence of circulating parasite antigens.

The mainstay of therapy for lymphatic filariasis is the drug diethylcarbamazine (DEC). DEC is administered to a cumulative dosage of 72 mg per kilogram (orally twice a day for 10 to 14 days), beginning with dosages of 50 and 200 mg per day for the first 2 days in adults. The drug reduces the level of parasitemia by more than 90% within 1 or 2 days and also kills a proportion of adult-stage worms. The major side effects of DEC are fever and acute adenolymphangitis, most commonly in patients with high-intensity parasitemia. Microfilaremia may reappear within 12 to 24 months, especially in patients who continue to be exposed to mosquitoes containing infective larvae. It is not clear as to whether DEC given in conventional dosages reverses lymphatic obstruction, although single annual doses of DEC have been shown to reduce the prevalence of hydroceles in endemic communities. Physiotherapy of the affected extremities and treatment of secondary bacterial infections decreases the degree of limb swelling in patients with elephantiasis.

Ivermectin given as a single oral dose has been shown to be as effective as DEC in lowering the intensity of microfilaremia, although it does not kill adult worms. There are no differences between the two drugs in regard to the severity of side effects.

TROPICAL PULMONARY EOSINOPHILIA

Tropical pulmonary eosinophilia occurs primarily in young adult men who are lifelong residents of endemic areas of bancroftian or Malayan filariasis. The disease is especially common in areas of southern Asia. Patients often have asthmatic symptoms, especially at night. Sputum production is scant. The physi-

cal examination may be normal except for rhonchi, wheezing, and, particularly in children, lymphadenopathy and splenomegaly. Chest radiography shows transient pulmonary infiltrates in the early stages of the disease, which may progress to a mottled appearance (representing granulomatous reactions to trapped microfilariae) and eventually interstitial fibrosis in untreated individuals. The results of pulmonary function tests initially are consistent with mixed restrictive and obstructive airways disease, followed by a restrictive picture.

Other diagnostic criteria include absence of microfilaremia, elevated total and filarial-specific IgE (total IgE levels often greater than 3,000 units per milliliter), high titers of IgE antimicrofilarial antibodies, eosinophilia (usually more than 3,000 cells per microliter of blood), and a beneficial response to DEC given in a 2-week course. Pulmonary function test results and eosinophilia also return rapidly to normal and are sustained for at least 1 year after administration of the drug. Repeated treatment with DEC is necessary in some cases.

LOIASIS

Loa loa infection is limited to equatorial areas of Central and West Africa. The obligate insect vector is the deerfly *(Chrysops).* After deposition of infective larvae in the skin by the blood-feeding fly, adult worms develop over a period of several months and migrate throughout subcutaneous tissues, including the conjunctiva. *L. loa* microfilariae circulate in the blood with a diurnal periodicity, such that peak intensities occur at noon.

PATHOGENESIS AND CLINICAL MANIFESTATIONS

The most prominent clinical manifestations of loiasis are migratory angioedema and Calabar swellings. Calabar swellings are egg-like lesions that are 0.5 to 3 cm in diameter, red, and commonly located over bony prominences of the extremities such as the elbows or wrists. They are painful and believed to represent angioedematous reactions to antigens released from adult *L. loa* migrating through the subcutaneous tissues. The swellings resolve over 2 to 4 days but usually recur. Adult worms may be visible as the nematode passes through the bulbar conjunctiva. Immunologically "naive" individuals, such as recent immigrants to endemic areas, may have severe disease manifestations if their exposure is intense.

OPTIMAL MANAGEMENT

Definitive diagnosis is made by demonstration of microfilariae in blood obtained during the daytime. Microfilariae of *L. loa* can be readily distinguished from those of *W. bancrofti* on morphologic grounds. DEC (8 to 10 mg per kilogram per day in three divided doses for 21 days) is the appropriate treatment. The drug kills both microfilariae and adult worms of *L. loa.* Side effects such as fever, malaise, and subcutaneous nodules may develop. On initiation of DEC therapy, a neurologic syndrome characterized by changes in the level of consciousness and signs of meningitis may develop in patients with high intensities of microfilaremia (more than several thousand parasites per milliliter of blood). These patients should be treated with low doses of DEC (1 mg per kilogram over 1 to 2 days) in conjunction with corticosteroids (1 mg per kilogram per day of prednisone) for the first 3 days. DEC (300 mg once per week) has been shown to be an effective prophylactic agent in previously uninfected individuals who have moved to endemic areas.

MANSONELLA OZZARDI, MANSONELLA PERSTANS, AND MANSONELLA STREPTOCERCA INFECTIONS

Several filarial parasites uncommonly infect humans. *Mansonella ozzardi* infection occurs in the Caribbean and in Central and South America, and is transmitted by biting midges and black-flies. Adult-stage parasites inhabit the peritoneal cavity and microfilariae are present in the bloodstream. Infection usually is asymptomatic and associated with eosinophilia. Joint pain has been suggested as a disease manifestation in some individuals.

Mansonella perstans infection is endemic in tropical West and Central Africa and northeastern South America. It is transmitted by biting midges. Adult worms are found in the peritoneal and pleural cavities. Microfilariae circulate in the blood. Most infected individuals have no symptoms. There is clear documentation, however, that *M. perstans* infection may cause angioedematous lesions similar to Calabar swellings, fever, and headache. Treatment of *M. perstans* infection diagnosed on the basis of microfilaremia is by administration of DEC at the dosage described for lymphatic filariasis. Multiple courses of DEC may be necessary to eliminate microfilariae from the blood.

Mansonella streptocerca infection is transmitted in the rain forests of West and Central Africa by biting midges. Adult worms and microfilariae migrate in the skin and induce inflammatory reactions, consisting of many eosinophils and macrophages. Clinical diagnosis is made by identification of the parasites in biopsy specimens. Manifestations include macular eruptions, hypopigmentation, pruritus, and lymph node enlargement. DEC (6 mg per kilogram per day for 21 days) kills both adult worms and microfilariae.

ONCHOCERCIASIS

Onchocerciasis ("river blindness") is caused by chronic infection with the filarial parasite *O. volvulus*. It usually is manifested by skin or ocular disease, and is a leading cause of socioeconomic disruption in endemic areas.

ETIOLOGIC FACTORS

Onchocerca volvulus is transmitted from person to person by the bite of female blackflies of the *Simulium* species. The adult male and female worms, located in the subcutaneous tissues and deeper fascial planes, coil up into spherical bundles and repro-

duce sexually to yield millions of larvae, called microfilariae, which migrate through the skin and ocular tissues. Microfilariae are ingested by the fly and develop into infective larvae in 6 to 8 days. Infective larvae are transmitted to a new human host when the fly bites again. The larvae then take 9 to 18 months to develop into adult worms. Adult females measure 20 to 70 cm in length and males measure 3 to 5 cm. Microfilariae are unsheathed and measure 210 to 320 μm in length. Infective larvae are about 600 μm in length. The average life span of the adult worm in humans is about 6 to 10 years.

EPIDEMIOLOGIC FACTORS

Onchocerca volvulus infects an estimated 20 million individuals in endemic foci that are scattered across West, Central, and East Africa. The major focus in Latin America is in Guatemala, with additional foci in southern Mexico, Venezuela, northwestern Brazil, Colombia, and Ecuador. Small, scattered foci exist in Yemen and Saudi Arabia near the Red Sea.

Blackflies deposit eggs on objects in freely flowing streams and rivers, and these subsequently develop into larvae and pupae. Because of the dependency of the *Simulium* vector on waterways for reproduction, flies concentrate around streams and rivers and usually are found within a few kilometers of waterways. Humans are exposed to biting flies during daily activities such as farming, fishing, bathing and washing, and water collection.

Because blindness resulting from severe ocular disease or debility associated with severe skin disease often affects productive adults during the third and fourth decades of life, the effect of the disease on the economic viability of the community is particularly devastating. About 1% to 4% of infected individuals become blind, and onchocerciasis ranks as the fourth leading cause of blindness in humans. In some hyperendemic areas, more than half of all adults become blind, and a much higher percentage have skin disease or some ocular involvement.

PATHOGENESIS AND CLINICAL MANIFESTATIONS

The basis of most of the pathologic changes in onchocerciasis is believed to be the host reaction to microfilariae in dermal and ocular tissues. In involved tissues, the pathologic appearance of the lesions reflects a low-grade chronic inflammatory process.

Onchocerca dermatitis is recognized microscopically by the presence of increased numbers of fibroblasts throughout the dermal layer and a moderate infiltrate of lymphocytes, histiocytes, plasma cells, and eosinophils. Microfilariae are relatively difficult to find. The end stage of disease in the skin includes loss of elastic fibers, atrophy, and fibrosis. In the eye, neovascularization and scarring of the cornea lead to loss of transparency and blindness. The remainder of the eye often is involved by a chronic nongranulomatous inflammatory process. Onchocercoma, which are subcutaneous nodules containing live adult worms surrounded by a collagenous stroma, show chronic inflammation with fibrosis and extensive capillary infiltration.

Clinically, onchocercomas are firm, nontender, and freely movable if not attached to periosteum. Common locations of palpable nodules include the superior iliac crests, the coccyx, the greater trochanter of the femur, the bony thorax, and the scalp and head region.

Differences in the clinical manifestations of disease between individuals native to endemic areas and those newly arrived or only briefly resident in the areas result from the relatively light infections in the latter individuals. Nodules often are not palpable in lightly infected individuals. The earliest signs of infection include pruritus and an intermittent papular rash with some thickening of the skin, which may be localized in one area of the body. Transient episodes of localized rash, erythema, and edema are common.

In more chronic disease, permanent skin changes include loss of elasticity and a chronic, scaling, hyperkeratotic, maculopapular, pruritic rash with mottled hypopigmentation or hyperpigmentation. Atrophy may lead to areas of ulceration with the risk of superinfection. In Central America, the dermal manifestations are most prominent around the head and neck, whereas in Africa they more commonly involve the trunk, buttocks, and lower extremities. Enlargement of femoral and inguinal lymph nodes with secondary obstructive changes in the groin region or in an extremity is a common problem in Africa and Yemen.

Early ocular manifestations include conjunctivitis, punctate keratitis, and anterior uveitis. Chronic changes include sclerosing keratitis, chorioretinitis, optic atrophy, and complications resulting from persistent anterior uveitis, such as glaucoma. In general, the severity of disease correlates with the intensity and duration of infection.

OPTIMAL MANAGEMENT

The diagnosis is established by demonstration of microfilariae of *O. volvulus* in the skin. Skin snipping to the level of the tips of the dermal papillae is the optimal method of diagnosis. The technique for this type of skin biopsy involves the use of a corneoscleral biopsy instrument or a razor blade to yield 1 or 2 mg of skin in a bloodless manner. The skin snips are placed in tissue culture medium or saline solution in microplate wells and the microfilariae that emerge are counted after a 3-hour or overnight incubation. Skin snipping has the advantage of providing a measure of intensity of infection, with fewer than ten microfilariae per milligram of skin constituting a light infection and more than 100 constituting a heavy infection. For greatest reliability, four to six biopsies are done in different areas, including the hips, calves, and shoulders.

A presumptive diagnosis can be made clinically by the presence of onchocercoma, typical skin changes, or ocular findings of onchocerciasis, including microfilariae in the cornea or anterior chamber in otherwise normal-appearing eyes. Although elevated titers of antifilarial antibodies may support the diagnosis of onchocerciasis, a standardized immunodiagnostic technique has not been perfected.

Ivermectin has no effect on adult worms and has replaced DEC as the standard therapy. It is well tolerated and is given as a single oral dose of 150 μg per kilogram. It should be taken orally on an empty stomach and at least 2 hours before the next meal. Most patients have little or no reaction in response to dying microfilariae. One percent to 10% (up to one-third in some endemic areas) have mild cutaneous edema and pruritus.

A maculopapular rash develops in less than 5% of patients, and bullous lesions develop over the extremities or in the groin area in rare cases. Symptomatic hypotension develops in about 1 patient per 10,000, and ocular reactions are rare. The frequency and severity of reactions after ivermectin treatment probably are related to the intensity of infection. Contraindications to ivermectin treatment include breast-feeding within the first 3 months after birth and central nervous system disorders (particularly meningitis), and other conditions that may increase penetration of ivermectin into the central nervous system (e.g., age younger than 5 years). Special caution is warranted in patients with asthma because ivermectin therapy may precipitate bronchospasm.

Because ivermectin does not eradicate adult parasites and significant microfilariae production begins again about a year after treatment, skin snips should be taken yearly to document the effect and establish the need for retreatment. In lightly infected expatriates, who often remain symptomatic, treatment can be given every 6 months even in the absence of recurrent microfilariae in skin snips.

DRACUNCULIASIS

Dracunculus medinensis is a spiroid nematode with a wide distribution in West Africa from Mauritania to Cameroon, the Nile Valley and eastern equatorial Africa, India, and the Arabian Peninsula. Ten million cases of dracunculiasis are estimated to occur annually, although this number has diminished markedly with worldwide efforts to eradicate this infection.

Human infection results from the ingestion of drinking water contaminated with copepods (cyclops) containing third-stage larvae of the parasite. The prepatent period is about 12 months, during which larvae develop into adult worms in the peritoneal cavity. A fertilized adult female migrates superficially to form a blister; then a loop of uterus prolapses through the body wall or mouth, and first-stage larvae are released. These larvae are ingested by cyclops present in the water and develop into infective third-stage larvae over about 10 days. Adult females measure about 70 to 120 cm in length and males measure about 3 to 5 cm.

Symptoms relate to the local ulcer that develops when the adult female penetrates the skin and to associated infectious complications, including tetanus. Before the worm penetrates the skin, various systemic symptoms often occur, including vague dysphoria and urticaria. The local lesion initially is erythematous and pruritic. It subsequently becomes papular and then vesicular, measuring several centimeters in diameter. Rupture of the blister is followed by protrusion of the adult female. The healing process commonly takes several weeks or even months. The affected individual usually is disabled during this time. Chronic complications include contracture of the limbs. Common locations of lesions include the ankles, the soles of the feet, and peripherally in the upper extremities.

Treatment consists of manually extracting the worm by winding it onto a stick with gentle traction. The administration of metronidazole may facilitate the extraction. Local care should be used to prevent bacterial superinfection, and tetanus precautions are warranted. Simple preventive measures can be effective, including providing safe drinking water in bore holes, filtering water through a 100-μm or finer mesh fiber, and boiling water. Infected individuals should avoid sources of drinking water.

▊ TOXOCARIASIS

The ingestion of embryonated eggs of the dog roundworm *Toxocara canis* may lead to visceral larva migrans (VLM) or ocular larva migrans (OLM). VLM and OLM are cosmopolitan in their distribution and occur predominantly in children. The roundworms of cats *(Toxocara cati)* and raccoons *(Baylisascaris procyonis)* are rare causes of a syndrome similar to VLM.

ETIOLOGIC FACTORS

Toxocara canis is a roundworm of dogs and foxes. Adult worms inhabit the upper small intestine of these definitive hosts and release embryonated eggs, which are passed in feces. Humans are infected when they ingest soil or other materials contaminated with embryonated *T. canis* eggs. After ingestion, embryonated eggs hatch in the upper bowel and release larvae. These do not develop into adult roundworms but instead migrate to multiple sites, including muscle, liver, lung, eye, and, occasionally, brain.

EPIDEMIOLOGIC FACTORS

Several factors account for the observation that exposure to *T. canis* eggs is much greater in children than in adults. Pica and geophagia are particularly common in children. Proximity to areas where dogs defecate, such as playgrounds and sandboxes, also enhances the opportunity to ingest parasite eggs. Intimate contact and playing with puppies is important because they may be infected from dams by the transplacental route and by larvae contained in maternal milk, feces, and vomitus.

PATHOGENESIS AND CLINICAL MANIFESTATIONS

Most *T. canis* infections are asymptomatic. Surveys of healthy children between 1 and 11 years of age residing in several areas of the United States show that the seroprevalence of anti-*Toxocara* antibodies ranges from about 4% to 13%, with the highest values occurring in rural children of low socioeconomic status. Symptomatic infection presumably results from the ingestion of many *T. canis* eggs.

Tissue damage results from the necrotic and hemorrhagic tracts produced by migratory larvae. Eosinophil-rich granulomatous reactions also develop around trapped larvae and cause local organ damage. *T. canis* larvae eventually encyst in human tissue and do not undergo further development. Long-term follow-up of seropositive children suggests that there are no sequelae to asymptomatic infections.

Visceral larva migrans is the most common clinically detectable form of *T. canis* infection. The disease occurs predominantly in children younger than 8 years (mean age, 5 years) and is characterized by the gradual onset (1 to 2 weeks) of low-grade fever, wheezing, cough, and, occasionally, right upper quadrant pain. These symptoms may persist for several weeks. In exceptional cases, heart failure or seizures associated with the invasion of many larvae and eosinophils into the myocardium and brain occur. Physical examination of children with VLM reveals rhonchi and wheezes, with no signs of consolidation. The liver is slightly enlarged and tender to palpation in about 25% of cases.

Ocular larva migrans accounts for less than 10% of the reported cases of symptomatic *T. canis* infection of humans. Patients with OLM have changes in vision that are not clinically distinct from other, more common ocular diseases of children. Examination of the eye shows intraretinal and posterior pole granulomas, endophthalmitis, and leukokoria. In some patients, larvae periodically migrate in the retina over years and cause intermittent signs and symptoms of OLM. OLM usually occurs in children older than those with VLM. VLM and OLM rarely develop in the same individual.

OPTIMAL MANAGEMENT

Eosinophilia (more than 500 cells per microliter of blood), moderate leukocytosis, hypergammaglobulinemia, and transient infiltrates on chest radiography suggest the diagnosis of VLM. Elevated antibody titers to *Toxocara* larvae as determined by enzyme-linked immunosorbent assay is the most specific laboratory indicator available, but high titers persist after the resolution of acute disease. Definitive diagnosis can be made only by identification of larvae in tissue such as lung or liver. However, biopsy is not recommended.

The approach to management of VLM is controversial. In patients with acute symptoms of VLM and high-grade eosinophilia (more than 80% of the total leukocyte count), antihelminthics such as DEC (6 mg per kilogram per day in three doses over 7 to 10 days) or mebendazole (300 mg twice daily over 14 to 21 days) may more rapidly diminish eosinophilia and laboratory abnormalities relative to untreated patients; however, their effects on symptoms are not well established. Anti-inflammatory agents such as corticosteroids have no proven benefit but may be warranted in severely ill children with myocardial or central nervous system disease.

Ocular larva migrans represents a diagnostic challenge because the lesions can be confused with retinoblastomas, which require enucleation. Measurement of anti-*Toxocara* antibodies in aqueous fluids is warranted if the diagnosis cannot be made by clinical examination and other laboratory tests, such as fluorescein angiography and computed tomography. Antibody titers in the ocular fluids of patients with OLM are higher than the simultaneous values in sera.

Treatment of OLM requires ophthalmologic expertise. The utility and safety of antihelminthic drugs in the management of OLM have not been established. VLM and OLM may be prevented by deworming puppies within 6 weeks of birth and limiting contact between children and dogs.

CUTANEOUS LARVA MIGRANS

Cutaneous larva migrans, or creeping eruption, is caused by the larval stage of animal hookworms such as *Ancylostoma braziliense, Uncinaria stenocephala,* and *Bunostomum phlebotomum,* or by human nematodes, such as *Necator americanus, Ancylostoma duodenale,* and *Strongyloides stercoralis.* Infections occur most commonly in the setting of intimate skin contact with moist surfaces that contain fecal material from dogs, cats, or humans, such as under porches or in vegetation on beaches. Initial symptoms include the rapid onset of intense pruritus at the site of larval penetration. The larvae penetrate to the epidermal–dermal junction and migrate laterally, producing pruritic, serpiginous, red tracts that move 1 to 2 cm every few days. The diagnosis is made by obtaining a history of exposure (many patients recall the exact time of infection because pruritus can appear within hours) and observing the characteristic physical findings. Creeping eruption can be treated by the topical application of thiabendazole suspension or one oral dose of ivermectin (200 μg per kilogram).

TRICHINOSIS

Trichinosis is a helminthic infection with a worldwide distribution, including arctic, temperate, and tropical climates. The prevalence of trichinosis in the United States has decreased markedly over the past several decades, largely because of legislation prohibiting the practice of feeding garbage (contaminated with carcasses of *Trichinella spiralis*–infected rodents) to hogs.

ETIOLOGIC FACTORS

Trichinella spiralis is a nematode with an enteric and systemic phase of its life cycle in the mammalian host. Human infection is initiated by the ingestion of third-stage larvae encysted in striated muscle. The larvae escape from their cysts in the acid–pepsin environment of the stomach and develop into adult male and female worms that lie coiled in the small intestinal mucosa. Female worms then release many newborn larvae; these migrate through the intestinal wall to the systemic circulation and invade host myocytes. The helminths eventually encyst in these sites and can remain dormant for years.

Humans are infected most commonly by the ingestion of poorly cooked pork products (especially when purchased from a noncommercial source), bear, boar, and walrus. Undercooked horse meat has been documented as a source of infection in France and Italy. Encysted *Trichinella* larvae remain viable in flesh held at 4°C and at temperatures associated with the cooking of meat to rare. The practice of smoking uncooked meat or microwaving does not kill encysted third-stage larvae.

EPIDEMIOLOGIC FACTORS

Trichinosis usually occurs in common outbreaks associated with the ingestion of homemade and undercooked meat products, such as pork sausage and wild game.

PATHOGENESIS AND CLINICAL MANIFESTATIONS

The severity of illness resulting from *T. spiralis* infection is related to the number of parasites ingested and the associated inflammatory response to tissue-dwelling larvae. The mean interval from exposure to initial complaints is 8 days, with a range of 1 to 34 days. Gastrointestinal symptoms such as cramps and diarrhea often are the initial manifestation of trichinosis. These symptoms have been reported in 10% to 58% of cases and usually last 1 to 2 weeks, although a report of trichinosis in Arctic Inuits eating raw walrus meat indicates that prolonged diarrhea (13 to 98 days) can be the major and sole manifestation of *T. spiralis* infection. Two to eight weeks later, myalgia, periorbital edema, peripheral blood eosinophilia, and fever (higher than 38°C) appear. These signs and symptoms are coincident with invasion of muscle by newborn larvae and elicitation of eosinophil-rich inflammation reactions in these sites. These symptoms occur in 60% to 88% of cases confirmed by serologic or parasitologic testing. Heavily infected individuals may have myocardial involvement leading to heart failure and dysrhythmia, or central nervous system involvement causing seizures. In most cases, fever and myalgia resolve spontaneously over several weeks. Eosinophilia exceeding 500 cells per microliter of blood usually develops and can persist for several months after the resolution of myalgia and periorbital edema. Nonspecific elevations of the erythrocyte sedimentation rate and serum immunoglobulin level also occur, as in many other acute infections. Muscle damage is accompanied by elevations in creatine phosphokinase.

OPTIMAL MANAGEMENT

The diagnosis of trichinosis should be investigated when the described signs and symptoms occur in the setting of possible ingestion of *T. spiralis*–infected meat. In the United States, most cases, occurring in outbreaks, have been associated with the ingestion of smoked homemade pork sausage or wild game such as bear, boar, and cougar. Meat must reach a temperature of 81.2°C (177°F) to kill *T. spiralis* larvae.

Serologic tests for trichinosis are performed by the U.S. Centers for Disease Control and Prevention. The results of these antibody-based tests usually become positive within 2 to 4 weeks of infection. In situations in which a history of infected meat ingestion cannot be clearly documented and the results of serologic tests are negative or equivocal, muscle biopsy (e.g., from the gastrocnemius) to identify larvae may be useful.

The treatment of trichinosis depends on the phase of infection at which the diagnosis is made. If a patient is suspected of having ingested contaminated meat within the previous 1 to 3 weeks, the administration of mebendazole (200 to 400 mg 3 times daily for 3 days, then 400 to 500 mg 3 times daily for 10 days) may be useful because this drug kills gut-dwelling adult worms. Treatment of the larval phase of infection is primarily symptomatic and includes the administration of antipyretics and analgesics. In patients with myocarditis or central nervous system disease, corticosteroids may be administered with the intent of diminishing the local inflammatory response to larvae. However, the benefit of corticosteroids in this situation has not been established in controlled trials. Case reports suggest that benzimidazoles also may kill muscle-stage larvae.

 # ANGIOSTRONGYLIASIS

Angiostrongylus (more recent taxonomy: *Parastrongylus*) *cantonensis* is the most common cause of eosinophilic meningitis worldwide. Endemic areas of angiostrongyliasis include the South Pacific (American Samoa, Papua New Guinea, New Caledonia); southeast Asia; Egypt; and areas of West Africa, such as Côte d'Ivoire. Other helminths less commonly associated with eosinophilic meningitis include *T. spiralis*, *Taenia solium* (cysticercosis), *T. canis* (VLM), *Gnathostoma spinigerum*, and *Paragonimus westermani*.

ETIOLOGIC FACTORS

Infection of humans occurs through the ingestion of raw or poorly cooked slugs, snails, freshwater prawns, and mollusks, which are intermediate hosts of *A. cantonensis*. Vegetables and fomites contaminated with *A. cantonensis* larvae also may be sources of infection. Ingested larvae burrow through the intestinal wall and migrate through the systemic circulation to blood vessels in the brain, occasionally the spinal cord, and rarely the eye. Unlike infection in the definitive rat host, the nematodes do not complete their life cycle in humans.

PATHOGENESIS AND CLINICAL MANIFESTATIONS

Migrating *A. cantonensis* larvae elicit eosinophil-rich inflammatory reactions in the brain and leptomeninges. Necrotic tracks attributable to migrating parasites have been observed in specimens of brain and spinal cord. About a week after the ingestion of *A. cantonensis* larvae, headache, stiff neck, and fever appear. In one series, headache was a major presenting symptom in half of all cases, whereas fever exceeding 38°C occurred in less than half. Paresthesia, vomiting, extraocular muscle weakness, and papilledema are less common. Most patients recover from these symptoms in 1 to 2 weeks.

OPTIMAL MANAGEMENT

Angiostrongylus cantonensis infection of the central nervous system should be suspected in a patient who has a history of eating a potential carrier of parasite larvae, symptoms of angiostrongyliasis, and typical findings on examination of cerebrospinal fluid. The most important cerebrospinal fluid finding is eosinophilia (usually more than 20% of the differential cell count). Cerebrospinal fluid protein levels also may be slightly elevated (60 to 100 μg per deciliter). Glucose levels usually are normal relative to blood values. *A. cantonensis* larvae rarely are identified in cerebrospinal fluid. Serologic tests for antibodies to *A. cantonensis* have not been examined rigorously for sensitivity or specificity and are not widely available.

No specific antihelminthic drug is recommended for this self-limited disease. Corticosteroids have no proven benefit. Analgesics should be used to alleviate headache. Preventive measures include education regarding the possible hazards of eating raw or poorly cooked snails and mollusks from endemic areas.

BIBLIOGRAPHY

Bockarie MJ, Alexander ND, Hyun P, et al. Randomised community-based trial of annual single-dose diethylcarbamazine with or without ivermectin against *Wuchereria bancrofti* infection in human beings and mosquitoes. *Lancet* 1998;351:162–168.

Clausen MR, Meyer CN, Krantz T, et al. *Trichinella* infection and clinical disease. *Q J Med* 1996;89:631–636.

Drugs for parasitic infections. *Med Lett Drugs Ther* 1998;40:1–12.

Glickman LT, Magnaval J-F. Zoonotic roundworm infections. *Infect Dis Clin North Am* 1993;7:717–732.

Greene BM, Taylor HR, Cupp EW, et al. Studies on onchocerciasis in the United Cameroon Republic: II. Comparison of ivermectin and diethylcarbamazine in the treatment of onchocerciasis. *N Engl J Med* 1985;313:133–138.

MacLean JD, Viallet J, Law C, et al. Trichinosis in the Canadian Arctic: report of five outbreaks and a new clinical syndrome. *J Infect Dis* 1989;160:513–520.

Nutman TB, Miller KD, Mulligan M, et al. *Loa loa* infection in temporary residents of endemic areas: recognition of hyperresponsive syndrome with characteristic clinical manifestations. *J Infect Dis* 1986;154:10–18.

Nutman TB, Miller KD, Mulligan M, et al. Diethylcarbamazine provides effective prophylaxis for human loiasis: results of a double-blinded study. *N Engl J Med* 1988;319:752–756.

Ottesen EA, Nutman TB. Tropical pulmonary eosinophilia. *Annu Rev Med* 1992;43:417–424.

Punyagupta S, Juttijudata P, Bunnag T. Eosinophilic meningitis in Thailand: clinical studies of 484 cases probably caused by *Angiostrongylus cantonensis. Am J Trop Med Hyg* 1975;24:921–931.

Kelley's Textbook of Internal Medicine, fourth edition. Edited by H. David Humes. Lippincott Williams & Wilkins, Philadelphia © 2000.

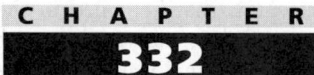

C H A P T E R

332

INTESTINAL NEMATODES

ROBERT A. SALATA

Nematodes, or roundworms, consists of over 500,000 species and are generally classified as those that infect primarily the gastrointestinal tract or those that infect deep tissue. In this chapter, the most frequently encountered intestinal nematode infections of humans including enterobiasis, trichuriasis, ascariasis, hookworm infection, and strongyloidiasis are described. The causative agents along with their geographical distribution, means of infection, and major clinical manifestations are summarized in Table 332.1.

TABLE 332.1.	**MAJOR INTESTINAL NEMATODE INFECTIONS OF HUMANS**			
Organism	Common Name	Geographic Distribution	Means of Infection	Major Clinical Manifestations
Enterobius vermicularis	Pinworm	Cosmopolitan, especially in temperate zones	Oral–fecal	Anal pruritus
Trichuris trichiura	Whipworm	Cosmopolitan, most common in poor, tropical, rural communities that lack sanitary facilities	Oral–fecal	Mild anemia, bloody diarrhea, growth retardation, rectal prolapse with heavy infection
Ascaris lumbricoides	Giant roundworm, ascariasis	Cosmopolitan, but most prevalent in tropics	Oral–fecal	Löffler's-likesyndrome, malnutrition, obstruction of biliary or intestinal tracts
Ancylostoma duodenale Necator americanus	Hookworm	Tropics, subtropics between 45°N and 30°S	Skin	Iron-deficiency anemia and hypoalbuminema
Strongyloides stercoralis	Strongyloidiasis	Tropics and subtropics	Skin	Abdominal pain, diarrhea, rash, eosinophilia, Löffler's-like syndrome, hyperinfection syndrome in immunocompromised hosts

ENTEROBIASIS

Etiology

Enterobius vermicularis (pinworm) is a small, white, threadlike worm that inhabits the cecum and adjacent colon in infected individuals. Gravid female worms detach from the colonic mucosa and migrate at night to the perianal and perineal areas and lay sticky eggs. The final developmental phase of *E. vermicularis* larvae within the egg shell occurs upon contact with an aerobic environment and is continued in temperatures of 30° to 40°C. Eggs containing fully developed larvae are infectious within 4 to 6 hours. The most common mode of transmission is through the hands of the individual by scratching or handling bed clothes and linen. On ingestion, eggs hatch into larvae, which develop into adult worms in 36 to 54 days.

Epidemiology

Enterobiasis is highly prevalent throughout the world, especially in temperate climates. It is the most common helminthic infection in the United States and Europe, with an estimated 42 million cases and infecting individuals at every socioeconomic level. Infection with *E. vermicularis* is most frequent in children between the ages of 5 and 14 years and is commonly seen in families, in overcrowded conditions, and institutionalized groups. Because the life-span of adult worms is relatively short, long-standing infection probably results from continuous reinfection.

Pathogenesis and Clinical Manifestations

Enterobius worms cause little mechanical injury to the colonic mucosa. No evidence suggests that infection with *E. vermicularis* is associated with a hypersensitivity reaction, as no eosinophilia or increased IgE levels have been observed. Most *Enterobius* infections are light and asymptomatic. The most common complaints in 25 percent of infected individuals include perianal and perineal pruritis and restless sleep. Occasionally, the migrating worms may produce appendicitis, salpingitis, and predispose to secondary bacterial perianal skin and urinary tract infections.

Management

Diagnosis of enterobias by detecting worms or/eggs is made by examination of an adhesive cellophane tape pressed to the perianal area early in the morning ("scotch tape test"). A single examination detects 50% of infections, and five examinations detect 99%. In contrast, *E. vermicularis* eggs are found in feces in only 10% to 15% of infected individuals. Occasionally, adult worms, mainly female, can be observed in the perianal area or during anoscopy, proctoscopy, on vaginal inspection, or in the feces during diarrhea or after antihelminthic therapy.

Drug therapy of enterobiasis with mebendazole (100 mg once) or pyrantel pamoate (11 mg/kg once) or albendazole (400 mg once) results in cure rates of 90% to 100% percent. For heavy and symptomatic infections, repeat treatment after 2 weeks may be necessary. Drug therapy is recommended for all infected members of families with intense or symptomatic infections.

TRICHURIASIS

Etiology

Adult *Trichuris trichiura* (whipworm) are located in the cecum of infected individuals. Female worms with a life expectancy of 1 year, shed 3,000–20,000 eggs per day. After excretion in the stool, embryonic development of eggs takes place under optimal moisture and shade conditions in 15 to 30 days. When humans ingest embryonated eggs through contaminated food or water, the larvae hatch and mature into ovipositing adults in 1 to 3 months.

Epidemiology

More than 800 million people are infected with *Trichuris trichiura* worldwide, most living in tropical or subtropical areas. In the rural southeastern part of the United States, over 2.2 million individuals have been estimated to be infected with whipworm. Children in the 5 to 15 year age group have the highest prevalence and probably have higher worm burdens than do adults.

Pathogenesis and Clinical Manifestations

Adult *Trichuris* worms are primarily found in the cecum and ascending colon but may be present from the terminal ileum down to the rectum in heavy infection. Colonic pathologic findings, which may be seen in heavily infected individuals, resembles that seen with inflammatory bowel disease.

The human immunologic response in *Trichuria* infection is not fully known. Infection induces a specific human antibody response, but no evidence indicates that this is effective in controlling or eliminating disease. Murine infection with *T. muris* stimulates both humoral and cellular immunity, which results in expulsion of the worms.

Infection with *T. trichiuria* is most commonly asymptomatic. A form of acute dysentery associated with malnutrition has been ascribed to heavy *Trichuris* infection. Clinically, this presentation may be indistinguishable from bacterial or amebic dysentery or inflammatory bowel disease. Children in the 2 to 10 year age group are most frequently affected. In addition, these children may have growth retardation. In cases of massive infantile trichuriasis, there is often mucosal or full-thickness prolapse of the rectum on defecation and worms may be visualized on the bloody, edemetous surface. Anemia may also complicate this presentation. Worm burden in this syndrome is usually greater than 500 and can reach 5,000 or more.

Chronic *Trichuris* colonic infection in children presents with growth retardation and failure to thrive. This presentation may continue for years and occasionally evolves into the classical acute dysentery syndrome.

Management

The presence of the characteristic lemon-shaped eggs in stool is diagnostic of *Trichuris* infection (Table 332.2). Given the correlation between worm burden and colonic abnormality, quantitation of infection can also be assessed most conveniently by the Kato method.

Mebendazole is the drug of choice in treating *Trichuris* infec-

TABLE 332.2.	DIAGNOSIS AND TREATMENT OF INTESTINAL NEMATODE INFECTIONS			
			Therapy	
Infection	**Diagnosis**	**Drug of Choice**	**Adult Dosage**	**Pediatric Dosage**
Enterobiasis (pinworm infection)	"Scotch tape test" in early morning	Mebendazole *or*	100 mg PO once	100 mg PO once for children >2 y
	Looking for worms (white threads)	Pyrantel pamoate *or* Albendazole	11 mg/kg (maximum 1 g) once 400 mg once; repeat in 2 weeks	11 mg/kg (maximum, 1 g) once 400 mg once; repeat in 2 weeks
Trichuriasis (whipworm infection)	Stool examination for characteristic lemon-shaped ova	Mebendazole *or* Albendazole	100 mg b.i.d. × 3 d 400 mg once	100 mg b.i.d. × 3 d for children >2 y 400 mg once
Ascariasis	Stool examination for eggs	Mebendazole *or* Albendazole Piperazine citrate for obstruction of intestinal/biliary tracts	100 mg b.i.d. × 3 d 400 mg once 75 mg/kg (maximum, 3.5 g)/d × 2 d	100 mg b.i.d. × 3 d for children >2 y 400 mg once 75 mg/kg (maximum, 3.5 g)/d × 2 d
Hookworm infection	Stool examination for eggs	Mebendazole *or* Pryantel pamoate *or* Albendazole	100 mg b.i.d. × 3 d 11 mg/kg (maximum, 1 g) × 3 d 400 mg once	100 mg bid × 3 d for children >2 y 11 mg/kg (maximum, 1 g) × 3 d 400 mg once
Strongyloidiasis	Larvae in feces or duodenal fluid	Thiebendazole *or* Ivermectin *or* Albendazole	25 mg/kg b.i.d. (maximum, 3 g/d) × 2 d[a] 200 µg/kg/d × 2 d 400 mg qd × 3 d	25 mg/kg b.i.d. (maximum 3 g/d) × 2 d† Not established 400 mg qd × 3 d

[a] For disseminated strongyloidiasis, therapy should be continued for 5–15 d.

tion with cure rates of 70% to 90% and reduction in egg output of 90% to 99%; (see Table 332.2). Although single-dose oral therapy with 100 mg of mebendazole is convenient for chemotherapeutic control programs and adequate for asymptomatic infection, therapy over 3 days increases the probability of complete cure in symptomatic cases. Albendazole and ivermectin are also well tolerated and effective drugs for this condition.

ASCARIASIS

Etiology

Ascaris lumbricoides (giant roundworm) adults reside in the lumen of the small bowel, most commonly the jejunum and middle ileum, and have a life span of 10 to 24 months. More than 200,000 ova per day are produced by mature female worms. The fertile egg is broadly oval and has a thick shell with an outer mammilated albuminous covering. After passage with feces, embryogenesis occurs in soil under favorable environmental conditions, and fully developed infective larvae dvelop within the eggs in 5 to 10 days. When these egges are ingested by humans, larvae hatch in the small intestine, penetrate through the intestinal mucosa, and migrate through the venous circulation to the heart and lungs. They then break into the alveolar spaces and pass up through the bronchi and trachea. After being swallowed, the larva mature into adult worms in the small intestine. The time required to produce a mature female has been estimated to be 2 months.

Epidemiology

Ascaris infection is the most common helminthic infection of humans, with an estimated prevalence of 1 billion. This parasitic infection is cosmopolitan in distribution but is most common in tropical and subtropical areas occurring most commonly in malnourished individuals. In the United States, it infects an estimated 4 million people mainly in the southeast. Schoolaged children are most commonly infected. Transmission of *A. lumbricoides* is through a fecal-oral route and usually hand to mouth. Infection is facilitated by the extremely high output of eggs by mature females and the ability of eggs to resist unfavorable environmental conditions. *Ascaris* ova can live for 2 years at 5° to 10°C, can survive anaerobic conditions for up to 3 months, and can resist desiccation for 2 to 3 weeks at 22°C. In loose, moist, sandy soil, ova can live 6 years and survive freezing winter temperature.

Pathogenesis and Clinical Manifestations

During the passage of larvae through the intestinal mucosa, some larvae are covered with eosinophils and may be enveloped in eosinophilic granulomas and destroyed. Hypersensitivity reactions are pronounced during pulmonary migration with alveolar sacs being filled with serous exudate and eosinophilic infiltration of peribronchial tissue. The intensity of this host reaction varies greatly, but is usually correlated with the number of larvae destroyed during migration. General hypersensitivity reaction observed during pulmonary larval migration include asthma, tran-

sient pulmonary infiltrates (Loeffler's syndrome), angioneurotic endema, and urticaria. The symptoms of asthma and urticaria have been associated with circulating IgE antibodies.

Overt disease in established *Ascaris* infection is infrequent. The most common clinical manifestations are pulmonary and nutritional disorders, and obstruction of the intestinal or biliary tracts. Pulmonary symptoms which occur during the stage of larval migration through the lungs include cough, wheezing, pulmonary infiltrates and peripheral eosinophilia. Children with heavy gastrointestinal infection may exhibit malabsorption. Most of these observations have occurred in the developing world, in which polyparasitism and multiple nutritional deficiencies cannot be excluded. Masses of *Ascaris* worms may occasionally obstruct the lumen of the small bowel. These children present with obstructive symptoms including abdominal pain, distention, and vomiting. Another complication that may be encountered is obstruction of the biliary tract, mostly the common bile duct, with a single worm. Clinically, these patients complain of abdominal pain (right upper quadrant or epigastric), nausea, and vomiting. Jaundice is uncommon.

Management

Ascariasis is diagnosed by finding adult worms, larvae, or eggs (Table 332.2). With pulmonary symptoms, larvae may be found in sputum or gastric washings between days 8 and 16 after exposure and are occasionally identified in lung biopsy material. Eggs appear in the feces 60 to 75 days after exposure. Because of the enormous output of eggs by gravid female ascarids, direct smear of fecal material is usually sufficient for diagnosis.

The drug of choice for treatment of ascariasis is mebendazole (100 mg twice daily for 3 days: see Table 332.2). Albendazole given 400 mg once is an effective alternative. In cases associated with intestinal or biliary obstruction, piperazine citrate has been recommended. This agent narcotizes the worms and helps relieve obstruction. Surgery is sometimes necessary in patients with complete obstruction, an acute surgical abdomen, or complications of perforation, peritonitis or volvulus.

HOOKWORM INFECTION

Etiology

Adult hookworms of two species, *Ancylostoma duodenale* (old world hookworm) and *Necator americanus* (new world hookworm), are small, grayish-white roundworms. These helminths live mainly in the upper small intestine, attached to the mucosa by their strong buccal capsules. Hookworms cause significant daily blood loss from the gut; 0.03 mL for *N. americanus* and 0.26 mL for *A. duodenale*. Adult hookworms have a mean lifespan of 2 to 5 years, and lay an average of 7,000 eggs daily. Under suitable conditions of soil, humidity, and temperature, the eggs hatch into infective larvae. Humans become infected through the skin by contact with larvae-infected soil. On penetration, these organisms circulate to the lungs, break through the alveolar walls and ascend the trachea. The larvae follow a pathway similar to *Ascaris* and are carried to their final place of habitat in the small intestine. Mature female worms begin to produce eggs 4 to 6 weeks after skin penetration.

Epidemiology

Hookworm infection is estimated to affect at least one quarter of the world's population and remains a significant problem in the developing world with 500 million to 1 billion estimated infections. In the United States, a low frequency of infection is still encountered in the southeast. Immigrants and foreign visitors often harbor hookworms and may be symptomatic. In the soil, larvae are found mainly in superficial layers facilitating penetration of human skin. Hookworm larvae will not develop at temperatures below 13° to 15°C. Larvae are destroyed by drying and direct sunlight. Other epidemiological factors associated with hookworm infection include methods of fecal waste disposal, and the habit of walking barefoot.

Pathogenesis and Clinical Manifestations

The most important pathophysiological features of hookworm infection are due to attachment of the worms to the intestinal mucosa. Blood is sucked by the worms as well as being spilled around. This leads to iron-deficiency anemia as the predominant clinical feature of hookworm infection. Associated symptoms may include fatigue, edema, heart failure, and palpitations. There is a strong association between anemia and the intensity of hookworm infection as well as the amount of absorbable dietary iron. The relationship between iron deficiency and hookworm infection may be complicated by severe malnutrition and hypoproteinemia and an enteropathy endemic to the tropics. Malabsorption has been described more frequently in infected children than in adults and can be associated with growth and developmental retardation.

During skin penetration, disease manifestations may include intense pruritis, erythema and a papular-vesicular rash ("ground itch") at the site of larval penetration. With pulmonary migration, cough, wheezing and transient pulmonary infiltrates associated with eosinophilia (Loffler's syndrome) may be observed; these pulmonary features are much less common than in other migrating nematode infections.

Management

Diagnosis depends upon identification of eggs in the stool (see Table 332.2). Direct fecal smears are usually adequate to diagnosis moderate to heavy infections; concentration techniques may be necessary for light infections.

Mebendazole, 100 mg twice daily for 3 days or albendazole 400 mg once are the drugs of choice for hookworm infection. This regimen has resulted in cure rates of 95%, with an egg count reduction by 99.9%. Iron therapy should also be given when anemia is present. In preliminary studies, ivermectin has been well tolerated and effective.

STRONGYLOIDIASIS
Etiology

Strongyloides stercoralis is unique among intestinal nematodes because of the ability to cause hyperinfection syndrome in the immunosuppressed host. Adult worms inhabit the upper small intestine, where the females burrow through the mucosa. Females deposit ova, which hatch into larvae. These organisms bore through the intestinal epithelium to the gut lumen and are passed with feces. Larvae in the outside environment can either molt and differentiate into free-living adult males and female worms or metamorphose into the infective filariform larvae. Free-living adults can either continue their cycle in the soil or produce filariform infective larvae.

The most common route of human infection is through skin contact with contaminated soil. Humans may also be infected through the mucosa of the lower gastrointestinal tract or in the perianal area from larvae that have transformed into the filariform infective form during their passage with feces. This capacity to replicate within the host is the basis for persistence of infection for many years and the hyperinfection that is seen in overwhelming strongyloidiasis in compromised hosts.

After penetration of skin or gut mucosa, larvae pass through the circulation to the lungs, break into the alveolar spaces, ascend the trachea and are then swallowed to their final residence in the small bowel. Deposition of eggs by gravid females begins about 28 days after initial infection.

Epidemiology

Strongyloidiasis, although uncommon in comparison to other major intestinal nematodes, is widely distributed in the tropics and subtropics. In the United States, transmission still occurs at a very low rate in the southern states. Infection is also seen among residents of institutions for the mentally retarded.

Infection is acquired most commonly when infective larvae in soil come in contact with skin. The patient's worm burden in strongyloidiasis is dependent on the size of the larval inoculum and the degree of autoinfection. Because this helminthic parasite can increase its numbers within the human host, all infected people are at risk for developing potentially fatal disseminated strongyloidiasis if suppression of their immune system occurs.

Pathogenesis and Clinical Manifestations

The factors mediating host susceptibility and pathogenesis in *Strongyloides* infection are not well understood. In chronic infection, a balance is reached whereby worms are restricted in number and confined principally to the gastrointestinal tract, but the organism is not eradicated. With depression of host defenses, worms may multiply rapidly and disseminate.

The cutaneous reactions seen with strongyloidiasis appear to be mediated by an immediate hypersensitivity skin reaction to migrating worms or their products. Enteritis that is observed may result from direct mechanical trauma as well as the host inflammatory response and secondary bacterial infection of ulcerated lesions. In mild infection, diarrhea may occur while abdominal pain and malabsorption are usually seen with heavy infection. In disseminated infection, migrating larvae may damage tissues directly, resulting in widespread secondary bacterial infections as bacteria are carried by migrating larvae or enter the circulation through ulcerative lesions in the gastrointestinal tract.

Over one-third of patients infected with *S. stercoralis* have no symptoms. Symptoms of acute infection probably reflect the intensity of infection. Local cutaneous manifestations include a pruritic, erythematous, papular rash at the site of larval penetration. With pulmonary migration of larvae, a Loeffler's syndrome with cough, wheezing, pulmonary infiltration and eosinophilia can be observed.

Chronic infections are usually asymptomatic, but gastrointestinal manifestations may be encountered. Burning or colicky abdominal pain, often epigastric in location, may be associated with diarrhea, vomiting, weight loss and evidence of malabsorption or a protein-losing enteropathy. Eosinophilia is typically prominent. Cutaneous manifestations may be seen in as many as two-thirds of chronically infected individuals. A localized or generalized urticarial rash perianally and extending to the buttocks, abdomen, and thighs is common.

Massive larvae invasion of the lungs and other organs may occur with autoinfection, especially in patients immunocompromised by hematological malignancies, therapy with corticosteroids and cytotoxic agents, as well as infection with the human immunodeficiency virus. In disseminated strongyloidiasis, high fever, severe generalized abdominal pain, diffuse pulmonary infiltrates, ileus or small bowel obstruction, jaundice, shock, and meningitis or sepsis from gram-negative enteric bacilli may be seen. Eosinophilia may not be present.

Management

A high clinical index of suspicion for strongyloidiasis should be maintained in patients presenting with abdominal pain, diarrhea, or urticaria particularly if they have lived at some time in their life in an endemic area. Diagnosis of strongyloidiasis depends on the demonstration of *S. stercoralis* larvae in the feces or duodenal fluid. Concentration techniques should be employed to improve diagnostic yield. Repeated examinations may be required to confirm the diagnosis. The presence of eosinophilia or an elevated IgE serum level can be useful indicators of strongyloidiases, but neither are constant features in chronic infection. Furthermore, the eosinophil count is frequently normal in patients with disseminated strongyloidiasis. Immunodiagnostic assays may occasionally be helpful for the diagnosis of chronic strongyloidiosis.

All individuals infected with *S. stercoralis* should be treated because of the threat of autoinfection and disseminated disease. Thiabendazole (25 mg/kg twice a day for 2 days) is a readily available effective agent. In disseminated strongyloidiasis, early diagnosis is critical. Therapy with thiabendazole should be continued for 2 to 3 weeks; mortality rates remain high despite treatment. Preliminary studies have suggested that ivermectin is extremely well tolerated and probably more effective than thiabendazole in disseminated disease. Supportive therapy as well as treatment of secondary gram-negative bacterial infections is essential in the hyperinfection syndrome. Individuals with a past history of exposure to *S. stercoralis* should be comprehensively examined and treated before undergoing immunosuppressive therapy.

BIBLIOGRAPHY

Celedon JC, Mathur-Wagh U, Fox J, et al. Systemic strongyloidiasis in patients infected with the human immunodeficiency virus. *Med* 1994; 73:256–263.

Cooper ES, White-Alleng CAM, Finzi-Smith JS, et al. Intestinal nematode infections in children: The pathophysiological price paid. *Parasitology* 1992;104:S91–S103.

DeVault GA, King JW, Rohr MS, et al. Opportunistic infections with *Strongyloides stercoralis* in renal transplantation. *Rev Infect Dis* 1990;12: 653–671.

Hotez PJ, Pritchard DI. Hookworm infection. *Sci Amer* 1995;272:68–78.

Liu LX, Weller PF. Strongyloidiasis and other intestinal nematode infections. *Infect Dis Clin No Am* 1993;7:655–682.

Russell LJ. The pinworm *Enterobius vermicularis*. *Primary Care* 1991;18: 13–24.

Tietze PE, Tietze PH. The roundworm, *Ascaris* lumbricoides. *Primary Care* 1991;18:25–41.

Walden J. Parasitic Diseases. Other roundworms. Trichuris, hookworm, and strongyloides. *Primary Care* 1991;18:53–74.

Kelley's Textbook of Internal Medicine, fourth edition. Edited by H. David Humes. Lippincott Williams & Wilkins, Philadelphia © 2000.

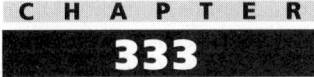

CHAPTER 333

CESTODE INFECTIONS

RONALD BLANTON

■ DEFINITION

Adult cestodes are descriptively referred to as tapeworms. They consist of 3 to 3,000 flattened segments *(proglottids),* each relatively independent and mainly dedicated to the production of eggs. The organism anchors itself to the intestinal mucosa by a set of specialized hooks and/or suckers attached to its first segment *(scolex).* While the adults cause little direct morbidity, the larval stages of these parasites are invasive and can produce severe, life-threatening disease. Humans can be infected with one or both stages, depending on the parasite species.

■ TAENIASIS (BEEF AND PORK TAPEWORM INFECTION)

INCIDENCE AND EPIDEMIOLOGIC FACTORS

The highest prevalence of *Taenia saginata* (beef tapeworm) occurs in Africa, Southwest Asia, and Eastern Europe. In Western countries, uncooked beef dishes, such as steak tartare, have resulted in tapeworm infections, particularly where inspection of beef is inadequate. *Taenia solium* (pork tapeworm) infection is most prevalent in Central America, South America, and Asia.

ETIOLOGIC FACTORS

Humans become infected when they consume parasite larvae embedded in raw or undercooked beef or pork. Adult *T. saginata* and *T. solium* develop in the small intestine and reach an average length of 4 to 6 m. The adults are long-lived, and spontaneous cure is unusual.

PATHOGENESIS AND CLINICAL FINDINGS

The adult worms are not usually pathogenic. Due to their size, however, *T. saginata* and *T. solium* may rarely obstruct the small bowel, the pancreatic duct, or the common duct. In contrast, larval forms of *T. solium* are a common and important cause of morbidity (see section "Cysticercosis").

LABORATORY FINDINGS

The laboratory findings in adult beef or pork tapeworm infection are not specific. The diagnosis depends on identification of the organisms or their eggs in stool, although the eggs will not permit distinction between these two species. It is important to identify the species for public health reasons since *T. solium* carriers may infect others and cause serious morbidity. Diagnostic characteristics of *T. saginata* are the presence of 15 to 30 uterine branches in proglottids and the absence of hooks on the scolex. In contrast, *T. solium* has 7 to 12 uterine branches and a scolex armed with hooks.

OPTIMAL MANAGEMENT

The treatment of choice for taeniasis is a single dose of praziquantel (10 mg per kilogram). A single dose of niclosamide is also effective given at 2 g for adults, 1.5 g for children weighing more than 34 kg, and 1 g for children weighing 11 to 34 kg. Niclosamide tablets should be chewed thoroughly and then swallowed. Since this drug is not absorbed, it will not affect the invasive intermediate form of *T. solium*, which may or may not be desirable (see section "Cysticercosis"). Infection can be prevented by improved inspection of beef and pork and by thorough cooking of meat. The side effects of both drugs are mild abdominal discomfort, nausea, headache, and dizziness.

■ CYSTICERCOSIS

INCIDENCE AND EPIDEMIOLOGIC FACTORS

Cysticercosis is the most common parasitic infection of the brain. Its distribution in the Americas, India, Southeast Asia, parts of Africa, and Eastern Europe follows that of *T. solium* infections, since cysticercosis is caused by the invasive intermediate form of this tapeworm. In areas of high prevalence, more than 2% of autopsies show evidence of infection. Serologic assays indicate that in highly endemic areas more than 10% of persons have been exposed. The number of cases is rising in the United States as a result of increased immigration from endemic areas and increased recognition.

ETIOLOGIC FACTORS

Pigs harbor only the tissue stage *(cysticercus)* of the parasite, whereas humans may be infected with either the intestinal or the tissue stages. Cysticerci develop in humans or pigs after they ingest food or water contaminated with parasite eggs. Invasive larvae hatch from eggs in the proximal small bowel, then penetrate the gut wall, and are carried in the bloodstream to multiple tissues (most notably brain and muscle). Individuals infected with adult worms can infect themselves with the larval stage by the fecal–oral route or by retrograde movement of eggs into the upper small bowel and stomach. Most studies have shown low rates of dual infection with both larval and adult stages, suggesting that autoinfection is uncommon.

PATHOGENESIS

The cysticercus is a 6- to 10-mm cystic structure containing a single (proto)scolex. Morbidity is caused by compression of adjacent tissues, obstruction of cerebrospinal fluid (CSF), or the immunopathologic response to dying parasites. Viable organisms induce only a mild reaction, whereas dying parasites produce marked inflammation and severe swelling. In muscles, cysticerci survive for months or years, then collapse and calcify within 4 to 5 years. Cysts in the brain also collapse and calcify, but more slowly. Cyst location, intensity of infection, and immune response are so varied that any neurologic, cognitive, or personality disorder in an individual from an endemic area may represent neurocysticercosis. All areas of the central nervous system can be affected, but parenchymal lesions predominate.

CLINICAL FINDINGS

Parenchymal Neurocysticercosis

Parenchymal neurocysticercosis accounts for 50% of cases of neurocysticercosis. This form most commonly presents with focal seizures or focal neurologic deficits. More diffuse symptoms of intellectual deterioration with dementia or parkinsonism may not suggest the diagnosis until focal signs appear. There is a fulminant encephalitis–like presentation most often seen in children, characterized by showers of cysticerci, an acute inflammatory response, and diffuse cerebral edema.

Subarachnoid Neurocysticercosis

Chronic basilar arachnoiditis due to cysts in the basal cisterns accompanies many forms of neurocysticercosis and makes up some 30% of cases. The lack of surrounding tissues allows the cysts at times to expand into a large mass of interconnected cysts without protoscolices *(racemose cysticercosis)*. Inflammation or external mechanical obstruction of ventricles by subarachnoid cysts produces hydrocephalus. Rarely, there is cerebral infarction from the obstruction of small terminal arteries or vasculitis.

Intraventricular Neurocysticercosis

Intraventricular neurocysticercosis composes 15% of cases of neurocysticercosis, and when cysts obstruct CSF it can be associated with hydrocephalus and acute or subacute signs of increased intracranial pressure including headache, nausea, vomiting, change in mental status, loss of balance. The symptoms may be positional, since cysts are free-floating in the CSF. The fourth ventricle is most often affected.

Spinal Cysticercosis

Spinal cysticercosis accounts for 3% to 15% of cases of neurocysticercosis and presents as cord compression, nerve root pain, transverse myelitis, or meningitis.

Ocular Cysticercosis

Ocular infection is seen in less than 1% of cases and causes decreased visual acuity as a result of cysticerci floating in the vitreous humor, retinal detachment, iridocyclitis, or muscle involvement.

LABORATORY FINDINGS

The most important diagnostic tools are a history that includes travel and personal contacts, neuroimaging, and blood serologic testing. Parenchymal cysts are easily seen by magnetic resonance imaging (MRI; Fig. 333.1) or head computed tomography (CT). MRI is more sensitive than CT for subarachnoid or intraventricular cysts, but less sensitive for calcifications. The serum enzyme-linked immunoelectrotransfer blot (EITB) is the most sensitive and specific serologic test available. The sensitivity of EITB decreases when there is no inflammation, when there is a single or few parenchymal cysts, and when all lesions are calcified. Examination of CSF is often less helpful, but the presence of eosinophils is highly suggestive.

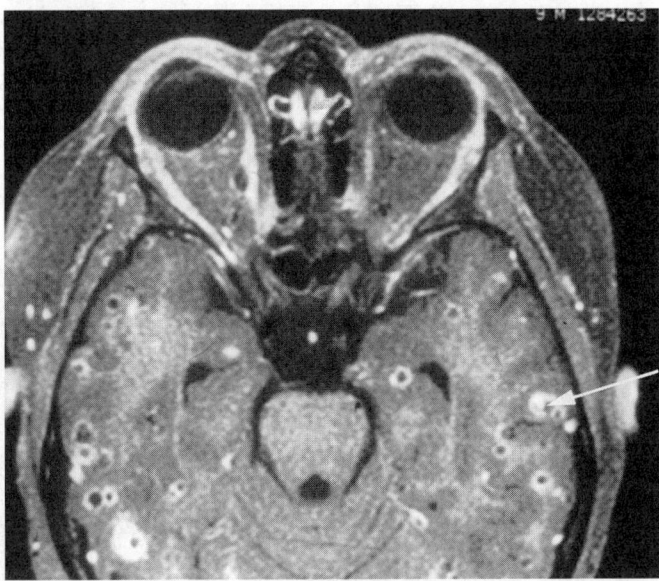

FIGURE 333.1. Magnetic resonance imaging T1-weighted image with gadolinium showing multiple cysticerci at various stages of development in the parenchyma and ocular muscle. Note presence of a protoscolex *(arrow)* within the left parenchymal cysticercus. (Courtesy of Nelson Ferreira, Hospital Beneficênce Portugesa, Med. Imagem, São Paulo, Brazil.)

OPTIMAL MANAGEMENT

Treatment decisions must be individualized with each patient and based on the viability and location of cysticerci. There is general agreement that when hydrocephalus is present, ventricular shunting should precede any antiparasitic therapy. Furthermore, the encephalitic form of disease should be treated with anticysticercal drugs after shunting if there is hydrocephalus. When imaging shows resolved or largely resolved lesions, no antiparasitic therapy is indicated. Beyond these points, management of parenchymal disease is controversial. A large prospective study indicated that the frequency of seizures and seizure control was better in those who received antiparasitic drugs. However, subjects in this study were largely self-selected and not randomized. In contrast, there are natural history studies that conclude that the outcome is unchanged by specific therapy.

Albendazole, the drug of choice, is administered at 15 mg per kilogram per day in two or three divided doses for 15 days. It has few undesirable interactions with other drugs, and there is some evidence that it has higher efficacy than praziquantel. Praziquantel is also effective at 50 mg per kilogram per day in three divided doses for 15 days. Transient worsening of inflammation occurs in 20% of cases after treatment, as a response to rapidly dying parasites. To prevent or blunt some of this effect, dexamethasone should be given at 10 to 20 mg intramuscularly once daily for the first 4 days of therapy. As a further benefit, steroids increase plasma levels of albendazole by as much as 50%. Corticosteroids and antiepileptics, however, reduce plasma concentrations of praziquantel. When using praziquantel, corticosteroids should either be withheld until symptoms develop or administered with cimetidine to reduce activity of the hepatic P-450 system. Imaging should be repeated 3 months after therapy to evaluate response. Patients who do not respond initially should be treated once more and observed for evidence of progression before another course is given.

There is growing use of medical therapy for extraparenchymal disease, although surgery is usually needed for disease that is intraventricular, ocular, or spinal. Ventricular cysts should be removed surgically or by neuroendoscopy, since they frequently become symptomatic or obstruct shunt function. Some cases are known to resolve with albendazole or praziquantel, but there is a risk of precipitating ependymitis and chronic obstruction. It is prudent in most cases to place a ventricular shunt prior to therapy for even asymptomatic ventricular cysticerci. Surgery is also the preferred therapy for spinal and ocular disease.

DIPHYLLOBOTHRIASIS (FISH TAPEWORM INFECTION)

INCIDENCE AND EPIDEMIOLOGIC FACTORS

Transmission occurs near freshwater lakes in northern climates, such as Scandinavia, Alaska, and the Great Lakes areas of the United States and Canada. The fish tapeworm has also become established in some temperate regions of Africa and South America. In this country, infection is usually associated with the ingestion of raw salmonid fish.

ETIOLOGIC FACTORS

Infection with the adult fish tapeworm, *Diphyllobothrium latum*, occurs after the consumption of raw or undercooked freshwater fish carrying the infectious stage of the parasite. Megaloblastic anemia is a notable but uncommon complication of infection.

PATHOGENESIS AND CLINICAL FINDINGS

Diphyllobothrium latum may produce megaloblastic anemia by competing with the host for the absorption of vitamin B_{12} and blocking absorption by dissociating the B_{12}–intrinsic factor complex in the gut. Complaints are relatively nonspecific even when anemia is present. Hematologic disorders may be masked in patients who have a good intake of vitamin B_{12} and folate, but deficiency may then present as glossitis or neurologic signs due to degeneration of the spinal cord dorsal and lateral columns.

LABORATORY FINDINGS

The presence of normal gastric acid and intrinsic factor combined with folate-resistant anemia is characteristic of the megaloblastic anemia caused by *D. latum* infection. Examination of the stool reveals abundant ovoid eggs with a distinctive cap structure *(operculum)* (Fig. 333.2) or worm segments.

OPTIMAL MANAGEMENT

Therapy for diphyllobothriasis is the same as for taeniasis. Cooking fish at temperatures higher than 50°C for at least 5 minutes or completely freezing at −18°C kills infective larvae. Proper sewage disposal decreases transmission because humans are the most important definitive host.

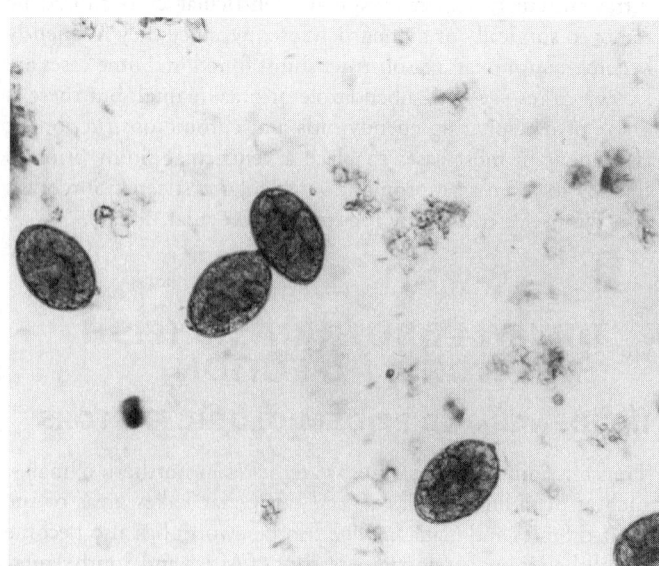

FIGURE 333.2. Fish tapeworm *(Diphyllobothrium latum)* eggs, 70 × 45 mm.

ECHINOCOCCOSIS (HYDATID DISEASE)

INCIDENCE AND EPIDEMIOLOGIC FACTORS

Echinococcus granulosus and *Echinococcus multilocularis* are responsible for unilocular and alveolar hydatidosis, respectively. Although both forms are serious, alveolar hydatidosis carries the worst prognosis. *E. granulosus* has a worldwide distribution concentrated in sheep herding regions of the world, such as North Africa, Southwest Asia, Southern Europe, and Australia. Some of the highest prevalences of disease, however, have been reported in Kenya and Western China. In highly endemic areas, more than 1% of all surgical admissions are for hydatidosis. In North America, transmission occurs in a sylvatic moose–wolf cycle in Alaska and Canada and between dogs and sheep in the western states. Transmission of *E. multilocularis* in a rodent–fox cycle is maintained primarily in the sub-Arctic regions of Alaska, Canada, and Northern and Eastern Europe and China.

ETIOLOGIC FACTORS

Dogs develop the adult stage after eating the viscera of slaughtered game or livestock. The adult parasite is a small tapeworm (3 to 6 mm) of three or four segments that develops in the intestine of canine hosts and is shed in their feces. Intermediate hosts for *E. granulosus* include most domestic and wild herd animals, pigs, and humans. These hosts become infected through the ingestion of pasture or food contaminated with eggs or through close contact with infected dogs. In unilocular disease, infecting larvae of *E. granulosus* invade the host's lung or liver and form solitary cysts with a tough fibrous capsule that sometimes will contain internal daughter cysts. Protoscolices, the infective form for the dog, can be found in the cyst fluid or attached to the cyst wall. They have a characteristic ring of hooklets when viewed from above (Fig. 333.3). Infection with *E. multilocularis* produces a larval form that multiplies by external budding from the primary cyst. The result is an expanding cluster of lobules instead of the single encapsulated mass produced by *E. granulosus*. Adult worms of *E. multilocularis* develop in foxes,

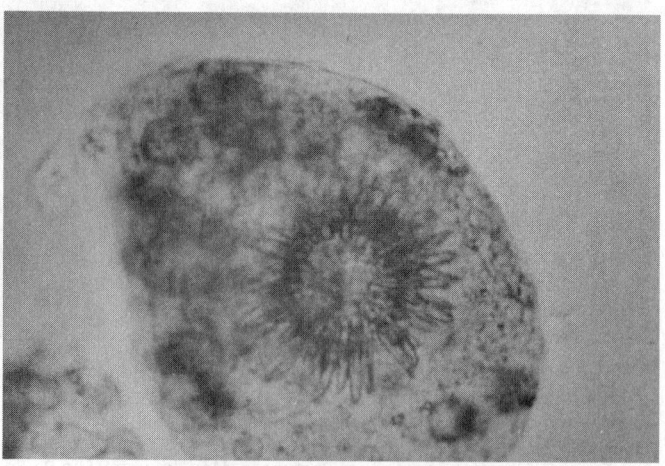

FIGURE 333.3. *Echinococcus granulosus* protoscolex.

wolves, and sled dogs, and are similar in appearance to those of *E. granulosus.*

PATHOGENESIS

The pathology associated with hydatid disease is a result of pressure effects, obstruction, or allergic responses to cyst fluid. Cysts can grow to enormous proportions but average 0.5 to 1 L. Pressure on adjacent tissues leads to pain, organ dysfunction, or obstruction. Spontaneous or traumatic rupture of a cyst or spillage of cyst fluid during surgery into the peritoneum disseminates daughter cysts. Cyst leakage or rupture can provoke minor urticarial reactions in the host, peritonitis, or anaphylaxis. The hydatid of *E. multilocularis* is a cluster of firm gelatinous cysts that invades adjacent tissue and produces distant metastases, similar to a malignant tumor. Enlargement occurs rapidly and most infections are fatal if untreated.

CLINICAL FINDINGS

Hydatid cysts are found in liver (50% to 70%), lung (20%), and, infrequently, other organs or the skin. As the cysts enlarge, the liver becomes palpable and obstruction of the biliary tree can occur. In the lung, the lack of surrounding tissue allows cysts to become much larger. Rupture of lung cysts induces cough and hemoptysis, and hydatid membranes are occasionally coughed up. A cyst in bone thins the cortex and can cause a pathologic fracture. In the kidney, cysts cause pain and hematuria. Spinal cord and brain hydatid cysts are very rare and result in clinical syndromes similar to cysticercosis. Cysts also become secondarily infected with bacteria and can present as abscesses. Untreated alveolar hydatid disease produces liver failure.

LABORATORY FINDINGS

The radiologic appearance of uncomplicated unilocular hydatid cysts on plain films, ultrasonography (Fig. 333.4), and CT is that of a smooth, well-circumscribed cystic mass that may be partially calcified and may have internal septae representing daughter cysts. In contrast, alveolar disease displays a loose collection of infiltrating lobules. The immunoblot assay is the most specific for *Echinococcus* species, except for cross-reactions with *T. solium* infections. The sensitivity is approximately 30%.

OPTIMAL MANAGEMENT

The World Health Organization has produced an excellent set of guidelines for the management of hydatid disease. Importantly, not all cysts require removal. Some are small, do not enlarge, and cause no symptoms unless secondarily infected. Surgery is recommended for large, complex cysts (involution or multiple daughter cysts present) or very superficial cysts that are apt to rupture. Surgical removal is also the treatment of choice for cysts that are symptomatic, enlarging, or infected. Albendazole prophylaxis is recommended, and during surgery scolecidal agents such as hypertonic saline are infused into the cyst cavity. However, scolicides should not be used in the presence of bile-

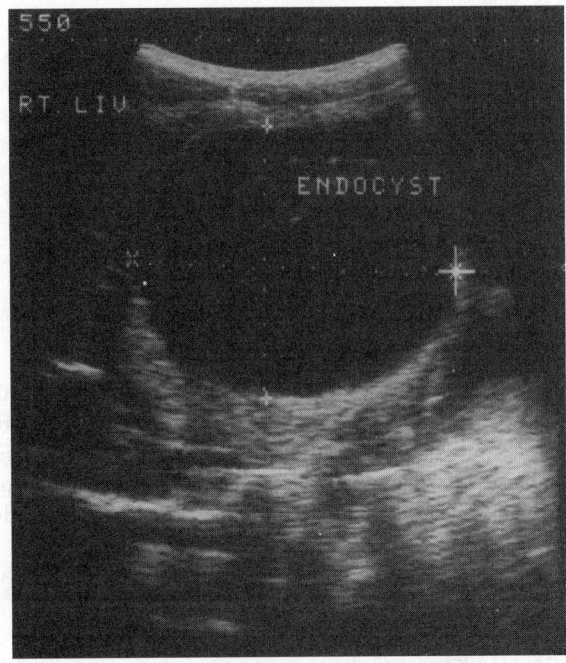

FIGURE 333.4. Ultrasound image of a hydatid cyst, 10.5 × 8.4 cm.

stained cyst fluid because of the risk of inducing sclerosing cholangitis. The mortality rate is 1% to 3% with the first operation for hydatid disease and increases dramatically with each subsequent operation.

A major complication is spillage of cyst contents, since each liberated protoscolex can form a secondary cyst. Morbidity and mortality are significantly lower in centers that are experienced with hydatid surgery. Some centers report a normal life span compared with matched control subjects for their patients who undergo surgery for unilocular cysts. Surgery rarely is successful for alveolar hydatid disease, except in early lesions that can be removed completely. Liver transplant may be an option if metastatic disease is not present.

*P*ercutaneous *a*spiration with *i*nstillation (of a scolicidal agent) and *r*epeat aspiration (PAIR) in experienced hands has little morbidity and excellent results when the cyst is without internal structures or daughter cyst and is not superficial. Ethanol, hypertonic saline, and cetrimide are acceptable scolicidal agents; however, formalin is contraindicated. The scolicide should remain in contact with the cyst for at least 15 minutes. Cyst fluid should be hypotonic and crystal clear, but it should contain protoscolices or free hooks. Liver cysts with bile-stained fluid and lung cysts should be managed with surgery or chemotherapy. The procedure can be complicated by bleeding, spillage of cyst fluid, ethanol toxicity, or hypernatremia.

Albendazole is the drug of choice where surgery or PAIR is contraindicated, refused, or the cysts have low potential for morbidity. A recommended drug regimen is three to six cycles of albendazole (10 to 15 mg per kilogram per day) twice daily for 28 days, followed by 14 days rest. There is some evidence that 3 to 6 months of continuous therapy is more efficacious without an increase in side effects (hepatotoxicity, neutropenia, thrombocytopenia, alopecia). For surgical prophylaxis, at least

4 days of therapy before and for 1 month afterward are recommended. The collective experience with albendazole indicates that 30% of patients are cured and 50% improve. Albendazole therapy can halt the progression of alveolar hydatid disease but does not appear capable of curing this condition.

OTHER CESTODE INFECTIONS

HYMENOLEPIASIS (DWARF TAPEWORM INFECTION)

Hymenolepis nana is a small tapeworm (30 mm) found throughout the world under conditions of poor hygiene. No symptoms can be attributed to light infections with *H. nana,* but heavy infections are associated with anorexia, diarrhea, and abdominal pain. Recommended therapy is a single dose of niclosamide or praziquantel.

MULTICEPS MULTICEPS (BLADDER WORM INFECTION)

Multiceps multiceps is a pathogen of sheep that rarely infects humans. In humans, it causes a disease similar to cysticercosis, with intermittent increased intracranial pressure or epilepsy. Praziquantel is thought to be useful, but surgery usually is impossible because of the organism's size, lobular morphology, and close association with host tissues.

SPARGANOSIS (SPIROMETRA SPECIES)

Spirometra species are tapeworms of dogs and cats whose intermediate stage *(sparganum)* is found in frogs, snakes, and rodents. Infection in humans occurs through the ingestion of contaminated water, the uncooked flesh of infected animals, or through the folk practice of applying crushed or split amphibians or reptiles to sites of inflammation. Although distributed worldwide, the majority of cases are from Asia. Infected individuals have painful inflammatory masses around the larvae. Treatment is by incision and removal of the parasite. Common sites are subcutaneous areas of the chest, abdomen, or thighs, and sometimes the brain. Praziquantel is used to treat inoperative infections.

BIBLIOGRAPHY

Amman R, Eckert J. Cestodes: *Echinococcus. Gastroenterol Clin North Am* 1996;25:655–689.
Anonymous. Guidelines for treatment of cystic and alveolar echinococcosis in humans. WHO Informal Working Group on Echinococcosis. *Bull WHO* 1996;74:231–242.
Caplan LR. How to manage patients with neurocysticercosis. *Eur Neurol* 1997;37:124.
Cuetter AC, Garcia-Bobadilla J, Guerra LG, et al. Neurocysticercosis: focus on intraventricular disease. *Clin Infect Dis* 1997;24:157–164.
Salgado P, Rojas R, Sotelo J. Cysticercosis: clinical classification based on imaging studies. *Arch Intern Med* 1997;157:1991–1997.
Sotelo J, Jung H. Pharmacokinetic optimisation of the treatment of neurocysticercosis. *Clin Pharmacokinet* 1998;34:503–515.

White AC Jr. Neurocysticercosis: a major cause of neurological disease worldwide. *Clin Infect Dis* 1997;24:101–113.

Kelley's Textbook of Internal Medicine, fourth edition. Edited by H. David Humes. Lippincott Williams & Wilkins, Philadelphia © 2000.

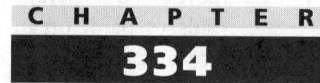

CHAPTER 334

TREMATODE INFECTIONS

CHARLES H. KING

BLOOD FLUKES: SCHISTOSOMIASIS

DEFINITION

Schistosomiasis, also known as bilharziasis, is caused by infection with parasitic trematodes (flukes) that colonize the venous circulation (Fig. 334.1). The five *Schistosoma* species that cause human infection are *S. mansoni, S. haematobium, S. japonicum, S. intercalatum,* and *S. mekongi.* Each parasite has a distinct geographic zone of transmission defined by the distribution of its snail vector, and each causes a specific clinical syndrome according to its preferred anatomical distribution in the human host. In some areas of the world, humans also may become infected transiently by the schistosomal parasites of other animals, especially birds (i.e., *Trichobilharzia* and *Bilharziella* species). These latter schistosomes do not mature into adult worms but may cause significant dermatitis.

EPIDEMIOLOGIC FACTORS

Mature schistosomal worms, like most other helminthic parasites, cannot multiply inside the human host. Therefore, envi-

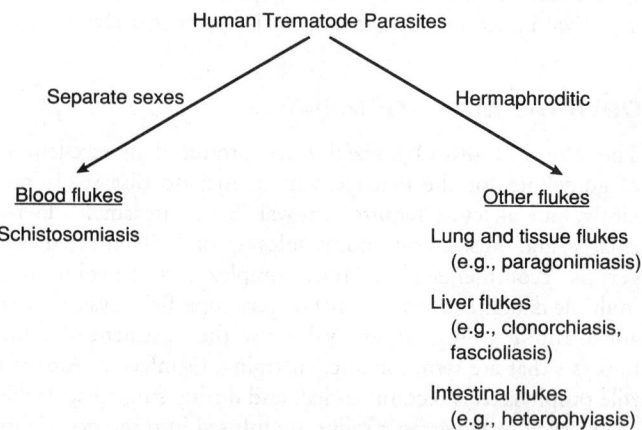

FIGURE 334.1. Human trematode parasites.

ronmental factors that promote continued patient exposure to infected water can help to determine the intensity of chronic infection. Areas endemic for schistosomiasis are characterized by three factors: the presence of a reservoir of human infection, the availability of suitable snail intermediate hosts, and socioeconomic conditions or breaks in sanitation that allow contamination of and exposure to local bodies of water. *Schistosoma* species are endemic within specific geographic regions: *S. mansoni* in Africa, the Middle East, the Caribbean (including Puerto Rico), and South America; *S. haematobium* in Africa and the Middle East; *S. japonicum* in the Far East; *S. mekongi* in scattered foci in Southeast Asia; and *S. intercalatum* in Central and West Africa.

Typical epidemiologic features of schistosomiasis include an increase in age-specific prevalence from birth to about 15 to 20 years. This is followed by a small but significant decline in prevalence in older age groups. In distinction, estimates of intensity of infection (based on standardized egg counts) indicate that worm burden increases progressively up to 15 to 20 years of age, after which there is a dramatic decline in intensity of infection among adults. This decrease has been taken as evidence that older individuals acquire immunity to infection with time, but it also may reflect changes in water use and duration of water contact in older age groups. The distribution of infection intensity in endemic populations is not uniform: most infected individuals (50% to 75%) carry light infections, and a small percentage (1% to 5%) carry extremely heavy infections and pass thousands of eggs daily. This is clinically significant in that morbidity from parasitic infection is correlated with infection intensity. Disease caused by schistosomal infection is more common in children and young adults, and is particularly common among those few individuals who have heavy infections.

ETIOLOGIC FACTORS

Schistosomal infection is acquired when humans enter bodies of fresh water that contain infected snails (Fig. 334.2). Free-swimming schistosome cercariae, released by these snails, seek

Schistosome Life Cycle

Adult worms in mestenteric or urinary tract veins pass eggs into host tissues
↓
Eggs reach feces or urine and are excreted
↓
Eggs hatch in fresh water to become miracidia
↓
Miracidia infect freshwater snails, multiplying to become cercariae
↓
Cercariae released into water penetrate human skin to become schistosomula
↓
Schistosomula develop in the body to become adult worms

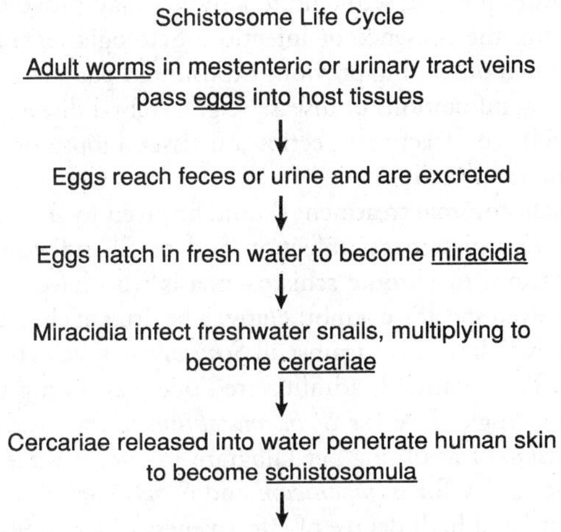

FIGURE 334.2. Schistosome life cycle.

human skin and penetrate through the epidermis to initiate infection. Cercarial transformation into schistosomula is completed in the dermis or capillary circulation. During the next 6 to 9 weeks, maturing schistosomula migrate through the lungs, liver, and other tissues to reach their final destination in the portal, periureteral, or perivesicular veins. Individual schistosomula mature into male or female worms. After mating, mature female worms deposit several hundred (*S. haematobium, S. mansoni*) to several thousand (*S. japonicum*) eggs each day into the host's venous circulation. About half of the deposited eggs are trapped permanently within host tissues. The remainder penetrate through the tissues to reach the lumina of the ureters or bowel. Eggs mixed with feces or urine then pass into the environment to reach bodies of freshwater. There the eggs hatch, releasing motile miracidia that in turn infect snail intermediate hosts to complete the parasite life cycle. Miracidia in the snail tissues undergo extensive (200- to 400-fold) asexual multiplication, then transform into cercariae (the parasite stage that is infective for humans).

PATHOGENESIS AND CLINICAL MANIFESTATIONS

Disease caused by schistosomal infection is the result of many factors, the most significant of which is the interaction of the host immune response with the parasite and its eggs. Clinical manifestations are related to the duration and intensity of previous exposure, the intensity of current infection, and the age, gender, and nutritional status of the infected host. The earliest form of disease, *cercarial dermatitis,* is seen most commonly after exposure to *S. haematobium, S. mansoni,* or the avian schistosomal species. Clinically, it is manifested by a maculopapular eruption in the areas of skin exposed to cercariae-infested water. The dermatitis is caused by an immediate or late cutaneous hypersensitivity reaction that begins 1 or 2 days after exposure and lasts for a few days. Symptoms are reported more commonly by newcomers to an endemic area than by local inhabitants. Cercarial dermatitis is self-limited and responds to local care.

The migratory period and the early phases of parasite egg deposition are associated, in some infected individuals, with *acute schistosomiasis* (also known as snail fever or Katayama fever). This syndrome is seen most commonly in travelers from temperate zones who visit areas in which schistosomiasis is endemic. In acute schistosomiasis, patients have fever, generalized lymphadenopathy, hepatosplenomegaly, and peripheral blood eosinophilia. The cause of the syndrome may be related to allergic hypersensitivity to the parasite and to the formation of soluble immune complexes that cause an illness resembling serum sickness. Although usually self-limited and rarely fatal, the disease manifestations can be severe and may be exacerbated by antiparasitic therapy. Symptomatic treatment with anti-inflammatory agents is recommended before treatment of the parasitic infection.

The next phase of disease, called *chronic schistosomiasis,* develops as parasite eggs remaining in host tissues become surrounded by a delayed-type hypersensitivity granulomatous inflammation formed by host lymphocytes, eosinophils, and macrophages. This response, regulated by acquired humoral and cellular immunity, kills and destroys the eggs. Subsequent resolution of the inflammation is, however, associated with the deposition of collagen scar. The accumulation of scar tissue within an organ, especially near vascular beds, can lead to significant venous hypertension or organ dysfunction. In addition, inflammation near the ureters and bowel wall can lead to ulceration and significant blood loss into the urine or feces, resulting in iron and protein malnutrition. In chronic schistosomiasis, the severity of disease is determined both by the intensity of parasite infection and by the intensity of host immunity; paradoxically, disease often is modulated by a spontaneous down-regulation of host cell–mediated immune response to parasite eggs.

The clinical syndromes associated with chronic schistosomiasis occur months to years after initial infection. They are species-dependent because different anatomical locations are preferred by different parasite species. Occasionally, unusual symptomatology is related to the aberrant migration of developing worms (e.g., in the central nervous system) or is a by-product of host immune response, as in glomerulonephritis related to the deposition of immune complexes in the kidney.

For *S. haematobium* infection, the main clinical symptoms are related to egg deposition in the bladder and lower ureters. More than half of those infected complain of dysuria, frequency, and terminal hematuria. Evidence of obstructive uropathy can be demonstrated by ultrasonographic or contrast radiographic examination. Findings include bladder wall thickening, granulomas, calcification, hydroureter, and hydronephrosis. In some endemic areas, there is an epidemiologic association between *S. haematobium* infection and squamous cell carcinoma of the bladder. During the course of chronic *S. haematobium* infection, repeated bacteremia, particularly with *Salmonella* species, also may be observed.

In individuals infected with *Schistosoma* species that localize to the intestinal circulation (*S. mansoni, S. japonicum, S. mekongi,* and *S. intercalatum*), two stages of disease can evolve. The more common and milder form of disease usually manifests as cramping abdominal pain and diarrhea, which may contain blood. The less common presentation of severe disease includes hepatosplenomegaly, portal hypertension, and hematemesis. Unlike postviral or alcoholic cirrhosis, liver disease caused by mesenteric schistosomes is a unique form of presinusoidal fibrosis that preserves liver function until late in the course of illness. Characteristic *Schistosoma*-associated organ damage is readily detected on ultrasonographic examination. Because hepatocyte nutrition and respiration are preserved (as a result of arterialization of the liver blood supply), most organ functions remain normal. Only late in *Schistosoma*-induced liver disease or when intercurrent insults such as viral hepatitis intervene is there evidence of widespread liver cell damage.

Other syndromes associated with chronic schistosomal infection include cor pulmonale and central nervous system (CNS) disorders. Cor pulmonale occurs in *S. mansoni* or *S. japonicum* infection after the onset of portosystemic shunting; because of retrograde venous flow, parasite eggs are swept into the pulmonary circulation, causing local pneumonitis and vascular hypertension. CNS disorders associated with schistosomiasis are caused by the inadvertent deposition of eggs into the brain,

spinal cord, meninges, or ventricles. Resulting syndromes include seizures, transverse myelitis, cord compression, and hydrocephalus. Other sites of schistosomal egg deposition (skin and genital tracts) have been described, along with associated inflammatory disorders, but these are rare.

OPTIMAL MANAGEMENT

The preferred method for diagnosing schistosomiasis is by identification of parasite eggs in urine or feces. Nucleopore filtration of urine or Kato thick smear of fecal samples provides an effective concentration of eggs and an appropriate measurement of egg output. In individuals with low worm loads or low egg excretion rates, examination of tissue biopsy material may be necessary to diagnose infection. Rectal snips are less invasive than bladder or liver biopsies and are obtained more easily in general practice. The identification of schistosomal eggs in tissue or excreta is based on their size and characteristic morphology. *S. haematobium* eggs measure 140 to 150 $\times$ 60 μm and have a terminal spine, whereas *S. mansoni* eggs measure 150 $\times$ 60 μm but have a lateral spine. *S. japonicum* eggs are 90 $\times$ 60 μm with a terminal knob that often is not seen. *S. mekongi* organisms resemble *S. japonicum* but are smaller (about 57 μm). *S. intercalatum* organisms are 170 $\times$ 58 μm in size, with a terminal spine similar to that of *S. haematobium*. *S. intercalatum* eggs can be distinguished from *S. haematobium* eggs by positive Ziehl–Neelsen staining after fixation in Bouin's fluid. In individuals who have been treated for infection or who have only remote exposure to infection, nonviable eggs may be passed in excreta or detected in biopsy specimens. This finding may or may not reflect active infection, and viability testing by vital staining or miracidial hatching may be necessary to establish the presence of active infection.

Serologic tests for *Schistosoma* infection are available. When used in schistosomiasis-endemic areas, serologic testing tends to be sensitive but not specific for active infection. In this setting, a negative serologic test result is useful to exclude exposure, but a positive result does not establish infection. In travelers from nonendemic zones who have had only brief, defined periods of exposure, positive serologic test results may prove useful in establishing the presence of infection. Serologic testing also is useful in demonstrating previous exposure in patients who have aberrant manifestations of disease (e.g., cerebral disease) and no other evidence of active infection on tissue biopsy or on stool and urine examination.

Antischistosomal treatment should be given to all individuals with active schistosomal infection and to all individuals with manifestations of chronic schistosomiasis who have not previously received specific chemotherapy. The drug of choice is praziquantel, which is active against all *Schistosoma* species that infect humans. Praziquantel is administered orally at 40 mg per kilogram as a single dose for *S. haematobium, S. mansoni,* and *S. intercalatum,* or at 60 mg per kilogram in two or three divided doses over a day for *S. japonicum* and *S. mekongi*. Praziquantel treatment has a high degree of effectiveness (70% to 90% cure) with limited side effects. Specific therapy results in the eradication of adult parasites and, if given early in the course of infection, can result in the reversal of infection-associated morbidity, including hepatosplenomegaly, bladder deformity, and hydrone-phrosis. In older individuals with established fibrotic or obstructive sequelae, reversal of pathologic changes may not be possible. Other supportive endoscopic or surgical interventions may be necessary, particularly for hematemesis, hepatic cell failure, or bladder carcinoma.

Travelers visiting areas in which *Schistosoma* is endemic can avoid infection by staying out of infected bodies of freshwater. For practical purposes, all bodies of freshwater in endemic areas, whether still (ponds, lakes) or flowing (rivers, streams), should be considered infected and should be avoided. No other prophylactic measures are available.

Control of schistosomal infection and infection-associated morbidity has proven an elusive goal in most endemic areas. Attempts at using chemicals to kill vector snails have not provided consistent or long-lasting results. In contrast, chemotherapy given selectively to those with heavy infection (e.g., school-age children) has resulted in significant reductions in transmission and in the prevalence of infection-associated morbidity. With the development of safe, orally administered, effective antischistosomal agents, this control modality assumes an important role.

LIVER, LUNG, AND INTESTINAL FLUKES

DEFINITION

The tissue and intestinal flukes that commonly cause human disease are listed in Table 334.1. These trematode parasites have a complex life cycle that involves the passage of parasite eggs (in sputum or feces) into freshwater or brackish water, the infection of an intermediate aquatic snail host, and the release of parasite larvae (cercariae) from infected snails. Cercariae of the tissue and intestinal flukes must encyst as metacercariae in a second intermediate host (water plants, fish, crabs, crayfish, or insects) and be consumed to produce human infection.

EPIDEMIOLOGIC FACTORS

Infection with tissue and intestinal flukes requires travel to or residence in an endemic region of the world (Table 334.1).

TABLE 334.1.	**CLINICALLY SIGNIFICANT TISSUE AND INTESTINAL FLUKES**				
Group and Species	**Geographic Distribution**	**Common Infective Foods**	**Diagnosis**	**Potential Complications**	
Liver Flukes					
Clonorchis sinensis	Asia	Cyprinid freshwater fish (carp, minnows)	Stool examination	Cholangitis, cirrhosis, cholangiocarcinoma	
Opisthorchis felineus	Asia, eastern Europe				
Opisthorchis viverrini	Asia				
Fasciola hepatica	Worldwide	Watercress		Fever, hepatomegaly, biliary/pharyngeal obstruction	
Fasciola gigantica	Africa, Asia	Water plants		Fever, hepatomegaly, biliary obstruction	
Dicrocoelium dendriticum	Europe, Asia, Africa	Ants		Hepatomegaly, biliary colic	
Tissue Flukes					
Paragonimus westermani	Asia, Africa, South and Central America	Crustaceans (crabs, crayfish from fresh or brackish water)	Sputum, stool examination	Lung abscess, seizures, gastrointestinal ulceration	
Other Paragonimus species			Sputum, stool examination and biopsy	Lung and cerebral lesions, tissue abscess	
Intestinal Flukes					
Fasciolopsis buski	India, Asia	Water plants	Stool examination	Intestinal ulceration, diarrhea, ascites	
Gastrodiscoides hominis	India, Russia and former Soviet republics, Asia	Water plants		Mucous diarrhea	
Echinostoma ilocanum	Asia, India, Philippines	Fish, tadpoles		Abdominal pain, diarrhea	
Heterophyes heterophyes	Egypt, Asia, India, Philippines	Fish		Diarrhea, central nervous system and cardiac lesions	
Metagonimus yokogawai	Asia, eastern Europe, Spain	Fish		Intestinal ulceration	
Metorchis conjunctus	Canada	Fish		Nausea, diarrhea, fatigue	
Nanophyetus salmincola	North America, Siberia	Salmonid fish			

Transmission depends on the dietary preferences and the sanitary practices of the local population. For these reasons, when evaluating a patient's risk for fluke infection, it is important to obtain a careful exposure history, including a complete travel and residence history and a detailed history of food consumption.

ETIOLOGIC FACTORS

Patients acquire parasite infection by eating raw, pickled, smoked, or undercooked foods containing viable metacercarial forms. Metacercariae hatch in the gut and, depending on the parasite species, maturing flukes penetrate the intestinal wall to migrate to preferred organ sites within the body (as tissue flukes) or to develop within the lumen of the intestine (as intestinal flukes). Because the tissue/intestinal flukes are hermaphroditic, infection with only a single mature fluke is sufficient for parasite egg production.

PATHOGENESIS

Disease produced by fluke infection is caused by local irritation of the biliary tree and intestinal tract, or by localized immune response in host tissues to antigens released by migrating parasites or their eggs. For intestinal fluke infections, symptoms usually are absent or mild, but may include cramping, diarrhea, and gastrointestinal bleeding. The early phases of tissue and liver fluke infection include a period of migration by immature parasites from the intestine to the definitive organ site. During this migration period, mild to severe inflammatory symptoms, including allergic-type reactions, may occur in any of several organ systems, depending on the current location of the parasite. The host response to migrating flukes involves both humoral and cell-mediated immunity to parasite antigens. Symptoms usually wane as the parasite reaches its mature form. In some cases, mature parasites or their eggs inadvertently reach critical organs, such as the spinal cord, brain, or pericardium, leading to severe local and distal symptoms caused by swelling, obstruction, inflammation, or fibrosis. Chronic fluke infection of the biliary system may predispose to the development of multicentric cholangiocarcinomas in the biliary tree.

LIVER FLUKES

Parasites specific to the liver include the Chinese liver fluke, *Clonorchis sinensis*, and *Opisthorchis felineus* and *Opisthorchis viverrini* species. Also included in this group are the species *Fasciola hepatica*, *Fasciola gigantica*, and *Dicrocoelium dendriticum*.

Clonorchis sinensis infection is acquired by the ingestion of metacercariae encysted under the scales of freshwater fish. The consumption of pickled, smoked, raw, or undercooked fish is responsible for infection. After hatching, developing larvae migrate from the intestine through the ampulla of Vater to reside in the distal branches of the biliary tree or in the pancreatic duct. Mature worms reach 15 × 3 mm, releasing light brown eggs of 30 × 14 μm into the bile that eventually pass out of the body with the feces. Symptoms associated with acute infection may include anorexia, epigastric pain, jaundice, hepatomeg-

aly, and diarrhea. Laboratory studies may show elevations of serum bilirubin, alkaline phosphatase, aspartate aminotransferase, alanine aminotransferase, and blood eosinophilia. Chronic clonorchiasis itself usually results in limited morbidity and commonly is asymptomatic. Individuals with chronic clonorchiasis may have symptoms of cholelithiasis, cholangitis, pancreatitis, or biliary stricture resulting from parasite-induced hyperplasia of the biliary ducts. Cholangiocarcinoma of the distal biliary radicals may be a late complication of infection.

Opisthorchiasis is caused by human infection with the species *O. felineus* and *O. viverrini*, which also infect cats and dogs. Like clonorchiasis, opisthorchiasis is acquired by the ingestion of raw or incompletely cooked freshwater fish. By contrast, the liver fluke *D. dendriticum* is acquired by the ingestion of metacercariae-infected ants. The course of *Opisthorchis* or *Dicrocoelium* infection resembles that of *Clonorchis* infection, with the same spectrum of symptoms and late complications.

Fascioliasis is caused by accidental human infection with the livestock parasites *F. hepatica* or *F. gigantica*. Sporadic infections have been described in most major sheep- and cattle-raising areas of the world. Infection is acquired by the ingestion of freshwater plants, particularly wild watercress, that contain encysted *Fasciola* metacercariae. After the metacercariae hatch, the *Fasciola* larvae penetrate the duodenal wall and undergo a prolonged (6- to 9-week) tissue migratory phase. This period can be associated with pronounced signs and symptoms, including fevers, hepatomegaly, right upper quadrant pain, jaundice, urticaria, and eosinophilia. Parasites eventually penetrate through the liver capsule to reside in the larger ducts of the biliary tree. Local inflammation may cause fibrosis and biliary cirrhosis with symptoms of chronic biliary obstruction. Occasionally, migrating parasites fail to reach the liver and become encysted within other intraperitoneal and extraperitoneal organs, including lung, skin, eye, brain, and muscles, resulting in atypical symptoms. Parasites encysting in the subdural space may cause eosinophilic meningitis, obstruction of the flow of cerebrospinal fluid, or destruction of the CNS. In the Middle East, an unusual form of secondary *Fasciola* infection has been described that is caused by the ingestion of raw meat from infected sheep or goats. Immature parasites from the meat stimulate or penetrate the upper alimentary tract to cause a severe, acute nasopharyngitis called *halzoun* or *marrara*, which may be associated with respiratory compromise.

LUNG/TISSUE FLUKES

The various *Paragonimus* species that cause tissue fluke infections are found around the world, including North and Central America. Human infection is acquired by the consumption of uncooked crustaceans, including crayfish and crabs, harvested from contaminated freshwater or brackish water. The lung fluke, *Paragonimus westermani*, is most common in China, Japan, Korea, Laos, the Philippines, Vietnam, Thailand, and Kampuchea, but also can be found in India, West Africa, and South and Central America. Other *Paragonimus* tissue flukes, such as *P. africanus*, *P. mexicanus*, and *P. kellicotti*, which encyst in organs other than the lung, are more common in Africa and the Americas. In *P. westermani* infection, metacercariae penetrate the gut wall to reach the peritoneal cavity, then spend weeks to months migrating through the diaphragm to reach the pleural space and lung parenchyma. During this migration, patients may have abdominal pain, diarrhea, fever, urticaria, chest pain, dyspnea, and night sweats. As the parasite matures in the lung, local inflammation may lead to mucoid hemoptysis or secondary bacterial infection, resulting ultimately in pulmonary fibrosis, bronchiectasis, atelectasis, or vasculitis of the lung. Extrapulmonary localization of *Paragonimus* flukes can result in inflammatory disease of the intestines, peritoneal cavity, lymph nodes, pleura, diaphragm, heart, skin, and CNS.

INTESTINAL FLUKES

Intestinal flukes cause infection limited to the lumen of the gastrointestinal tract. These species are transmitted by the consumption of freshwater plants (including water chestnuts, water bamboo, and caltrop, for *Fasciolopsis buski*), by the consumption of fish from freshwater or brackish water (for *Heterophyes heterophyes, Metagonimus yokogawai, Nanophyetus salmincola, Metorchis conjunctus,* and *Gastrodiscoides hominis*), or by the consumption of snails, tadpoles, and shellfish (for *Echinostoma ilocanum*). These fluke species are primarily endemic to Asia and Africa. Exceptions are the animal flukes *N. salmincola* and *Metorchis,* which are transmitted in uncooked salmon in northwestern North America. Light infection often is asymptomatic, but heavy infection with intestinal flukes is associated with local inflammation and abscess formation. This results in abdominal pain, diarrhea, malabsorption, and intestinal ulceration. In severe cases, there may be associated edema of the trunk, face, and extremities, with ascites.

OPTIMAL MANAGEMENT

The diagnosis of liver fluke infection should be considered in individuals with the triad of fever, hepatomegaly, and eosinophilia. For established intrabiliary infections, the diagnosis is made by examination of stool or duodenal aspirates for parasite eggs. Density separation and egg concentration techniques enhance the sensitivity of egg detection in light infections. In endemic areas, it is important to restrict the patient's diet before testing to exclude spurious recovery of eggs in the stool resulting from the consumption of meat (especially liver) from infected animals. Early or ectopic infection requires serologic testing (which is not completely sensitive or specific) or surgical biopsy to establish the diagnosis.

The diagnosis of lung fluke infection is suggested by a history of travel or residence in an endemic area and by the presence of a chest x-ray film containing patchy infiltrates or ringlike shadows (early disease), or pleural thickening and calcification (late disease). The diagnosis should be confirmed by sputum and stool examination for parasite eggs. Nonpulmonary infection may require serologic testing or biopsy to establish the diagnosis.

The diagnosis of intestinal fluke infection is made by parasitologic examination of stool or duodenal aspirates for parasite eggs, or by fluke recovery on endoscopy.

The recommended therapy for all active fluke infections (except *F. hepatica*) is praziquantel (25 mg per kilogram 3 times a day for 1 or 2 days). To ensure cure, follow-up stool or sputum examinations should be obtained 1, 6, and 12 months after therapy, and a second praziquantel regimen should be given if the first course is unsuccessful. Localized or generalized inflammatory lesions, particularly of the CNS, may require corticosteroid therapy or surgical removal to relieve symptoms. Although praziquantel therapy may prove successful in some cases of *F. hepatica* infection, the drug of choice for *F. hepatica* is bithionol (30 to 50 mg per kilogram given on alternate days, for a total of 10 to 15 doses). In the United States, bithionol is classified as an investigational drug and is obtained through the U.S. Centers for Disease Control and Prevention in Atlanta, Georgia. Successful therapy of *F. hepatica* and of paragonimiasis has also been reported with the investigational drug triclabendazole (see WHO Fact Sheet 191, April 1998; www.who.int/inffs/en/fact191.html).

BIBLIOGRAPHY

Anonymous. Drugs for parasitic infections. *Med Lett* 1998;40:1–12.

Cheever AW, Yap GS. Immunologic basis of disease and disease regulation in schistosomiasis. In: Freedman DO, ed. *Immunopathogenetic aspects of disease induced by helminth parasites: chemical immunology,* vol 66. Basel: Karger, 1997:159–176.

Gang CM. *Schistosoma japonicum* and *S. japonicum*–like infections: epidemiology, clinical and pathological aspects. In: Jordan P, Webbe G, Sturrock RF, eds. *Human schistosomiasis.* Wallingford, UK: CAB International, 1993:237–270.

Harinasuta T, Bunnag D. Liver, lung and intestinal trematodiasis. In: Warren KS, Mahmoud AAF, eds. *Tropical and geographical medicine,* second ed. New York: McGraw-Hill, 1990:473–489.

Kagawa FT. Pulmonary paragonimiasis. *Semin Respir Infect* 1997;12:149–158.

King CH. Disease in schistosomiasis haematobia. In: Mahmoud AAF, ed. *Schistosomiasis.* (Tropical medicine: science and practice series.) London: Imperial College Press, 2000 *(in press)*.

Kusner DJ, King CH. Paragonimiasis of the central nervous system. *Semin Neurol* 1993;13:201–208.

Liu LX, Harinasuta KT. Liver and intestinal flukes. *Gastroenterol Clin North Am* 1996;25:627–636.

Mahmoud AAF, Abdel Wahab MF. Schistosomiasis. In: Warren KS, Mahmoud AAF, eds. *Tropical and geographical medicine,* second ed. New York: McGraw-Hill, 1990:458–473.

Visser LG, Polderman AM, Stuiver PC. Outbreak of schistosomiasis among travelers returning from Mali, West Africa. *Clin Infect Dis* 1995;20:280–285.

World Health Organization. IARC Monographs on the evaluation of carcinogenic risks to humans. *Schistosomes, liver flukes and* Helicobacter pylori, vol 61. Geneva: 1994;45–100.

Kelley's Textbook of Internal Medicine, fourth edition. Edited by H. David Humes. Lippincott Williams & Wilkins, Philadelphia © 2000.

DIAGNOSTIC AND THERAPEUTIC MODALITIES IN INFECTIOUS DISEASES

ANTIMICROBIAL THERAPEUTIC AGENTS

WILLIAM A. CRAIG

In the 60 years since the beginning of the modern era of chemotherapy, a large variety of antimicrobial agents have become available for the treatment and prevention of infectious diseases. The introduction of sulfonamides in 1936 was followed by penicillin, the first β-lactam antibiotic, in the early 1940s. The "golden era" for antimicrobial agents during the 1950s saw the introduction of chloramphenicol, erythromycin, streptomycin, and tetracycline. The emergence of penicillin-resistant staphylococci led to the discovery of new agents, such as methicillin, cephalothin, lincomycin, and vancomycin. Similarly, the emergence of multiply resistant gram-negative bacilli stimulated the search for ampicillin, gentamicin, and nalidixic acid. During the past 25 years, most new antimicrobials have been modifications of older agents and provide enhanced antimicrobial activity or improved pharmacokinetic characteristics. This has led to antimicrobials with potent activity against *Pseudomonas aeruginosa* and other gram-negative bacilli, enhanced penetration into the cerebrospinal fluid (CSF), prolonged elimination half-lives, and excellent oral absorption. Despite the large number of available agents, the emergence of multiply resistant pneumococci, staphylococci, enterococci, and mycobacteria demonstrates a need for further antimicrobials, including those with new sites of action.

FACTORS THAT INFLUENCE ANTIMICROBIAL SELECTION AND OUTCOME OF THERAPY

INFECTING ORGANISM AND SUSCEPTIBILITY TESTING

Cultures obtained from appropriate sites of patients with suspected infection and the Gram's stains of these cultures usually identify the infecting pathogen. Because therapy often is required before culture and susceptibility test results are known, the clinician must formulate the probable pathogens for the site and severity of infection and the underlying diseases in the patient. Knowledge of the local susceptibility patterns helps the clinician decide whether initial therapy should address the possibility of special problem pathogens, such as penicillin-resistant *Streptococcus pneumoniae* and methicillin-resistant *Staphylococcus aureus*. Subsequent modifications in therapy are made after the culture and susceptibility findings are known.

The standard method for measuring antimicrobial activity in vitro is determination of the *minimal inhibitory concentration* (MIC) and the *minimal bactericidal concentration* (MBC). By definition, the MIC is the lowest concentration of drug that prevents visible bacterial growth over an 18- to 24-hour incubation period. The MBC is the lowest concentration that kills 99.9% of the organisms over the same period. In the past, these determinations were too complicated and time-consuming to be used routinely in clinical microbiology laboratories. Instead, qualitative methods, such as the disk diffusion test, were used to classify organisms as susceptible, intermediate, or resistant. Automated techniques now allow many laboratories to report MIC values routinely. MBC determinations also can be performed readily, but usually are reserved for infections in which bactericidal activity is necessary. In general, the MBC of a bactericidal agent is one to four times the MIC. An organism that is not killed by an antibiotic that usually kills that species is said to be tolerant; *tolerance* usually is defined as an MBC greater than 16 times the MIC.

ANTIMICROBIAL RESISTANCE

A major limitation to the continued success of almost all antimicrobial agents has been the emergence of resistance. The mechanisms of resistance are varied and include drug inactivation, alteration of the drug's site of action, decreased permeability of the outer cell membrane, and active drug efflux from the cell. The genes that account for these resistance mechanisms are acquired by the mutation of existing DNA or by the acquisition of new DNA. For example, the emergence of resistance in staphylococci and mycobacteria to rifampin is by mutation, whereas the resistance in gonococci and *Haemophilus influenzae* to penicillins is by the acquisition of genes encoding β-lactamases. New genes mediating resistance usually are spread from organism to organism by plasmids or *transposons,* the so-called jumping genes. The ability of different bacteria to share certain antibiotic resistance genes explains the remarkable speed at which some resistance mechanisms spread and increase.

SITE OF INFECTION AND HOST DEFENSES

Most tissues in the body are supplied by capillaries with pores that readily allow the passage of antimicrobials. If therapeutic drug concentrations can be obtained in serum, they usually can be obtained at most extracellular sites of infection. Even antimicrobial penetration into abscesses usually is adequate, although low pH and other factors may reduce drug efficacy when drainage is not performed. Foreign bodies such as prosthetic valves and prosthetic hips provide niduses where bacteria can be protected from antibiotics.

The penetration of antimicrobial agents into cells and into tissues that lack porous capillary beds, such as the central nervous system and ocular vitreous humor, depends much more on the lipid solubility of the drugs than on their pharmacokinetics in serum. Rifampin and the macrolides are examples of drugs with high intracellular penetration and activity against intracellular pathogens, such as mycobacteria and *Legionella pneumophila.* The most important factor for increasing antibacterial concentrations in the CSF is inflammation. For drugs such as penicillin G and ampicillin, inflammation enhances the influx of drug into the CSF and reduces the active transport of drug from the CSF. Rifampin, metronidazole, and chloramphenicol are examples of lipid-soluble drugs that have adequate CSF penetration in the absence of inflammation. The aminoglycosides, clindamycin, and the early cephalosporins are drugs that exhibit marginal or inadequate penetration even with inflamed meninges.

Whether a drug is bacteriostatic or bactericidal has little importance for many infections. The antimicrobial drug needs only to slow or inhibit the growth of the organism, because the body's host defenses (neutrophils, macrophages, antibodies) will kill and eliminate the infecting pathogen. However, endocarditis, meningitis, and osteomyelitis are infections that occur in areas of impaired host defenses. Bactericidal drugs are required for effective treatment of these infections. Patients with neutropenia or significant defects in neutrophil function also should receive bactericidal drugs.

PHARMACODYNAMICS AND DOSING REGIMEN

Although MIC and MBC values can reflect the potency of different antimicrobials against a pathogen, these parameters poorly describe the time course of antimicrobial activity. The MBC does not express the rate of bacterial killing and whether it can be enhanced by increasing concentrations. For some drugs, such as the aminoglycosides and the fluoroquinolones, bactericidal activity is concentration-dependent. The higher the drug level, the faster is the rate of killing. The ratios of the peak concentration or the area under the serum concentration-versus-time curve (AUC) to the MIC are important determinants of efficacy for these drugs. On the other hand, bacterial killing with β-lactams

usually is slower, with little dependence on the drug concentration. The duration of time that drug concentrations exceed the MIC is the major determinant of efficacy for the β-lactams.

Another potentially important parameter not assessed by MIC and MBC testing is the postantibiotic effect. This term refers to a persistent suppression of bacterial growth after limited drug exposure. The presence or absence of a postantibiotic effect may be an important determinant of the frequency of antimicrobial dosing. Some antimicrobials, such as the aminoglycosides exhibit prolonged postantibiotic effects with gram-negative bacilli, which provide a rationale for widely spaced dosing regimens. In contrast, β-lactams produce short or no postantibiotic effects with gram-negative bacilli. The frequency of dosing with these drugs depends largely on the speed at which they are eliminated from the body.

Parenteral administration is preferred in serious infections and those that require high dosages, such as endocarditis and meningitis. The high oral bioavailability of certain antimicrobials makes oral therapy an acceptable alternative to parenteral therapy for certain moderately severe infections. For example, the fluoroquinolones are effective orally for the treatment of osteomyelitis. In the setting of renal impairment, the dose or frequency of administration of an antimicrobial may need to be reduced. Any drug that is excreted primarily unchanged in the urine requires a downward adjustment in proportion to the decrease in renal function. Similar modifications are necessary in the setting of hepatic impairment for antimicrobials with major hepatic metabolism or biliary excretion. The usual dosage regimens for the various antimicrobial drugs and the need for dosage modification in patients with renal and hepatic impairment are shown in Table 335.1.

ANTIBIOTIC COMBINATIONS

The primary reason for using drugs in combination is to enhance antimicrobial activity. For example, the addition of an aminoglycoside to penicillin improves the killing effect against most enterococci. This combination also results in better efficacy for enterococcal endocarditis than is obtained with monotherapy. Antimicrobial combinations also are used to treat mixed infections, to broaden coverage in infections with unknown causes, and to prevent the emergence of resistant organisms. Tuberculosis is the primary infection for which drug combinations have been shown to prevent the emergence of resistant organisms.

The major disadvantages of antimicrobial combinations are the added cost and enhanced side effects. Furthermore, the combination of bacteriostatic and bactericidal drugs can exhibit antagonism, as has been shown with the use of penicillin plus tetracycline for pneumococcal meningitis.

▆ INDIVIDUAL AGENTS

β-LACTAMS

The β-lactam antibiotics are the most commonly used antimicrobial agents because of their high potency, low incidence of serious adverse reactions, and proven effectiveness. All members

TABLE 335.1.	PHARMACOLOGIC ASPECTS OF SELECTED ANTIMICROBIAL AGENTS

Class or Drug	Route	Average Adult Dosage	Dosage Adjustment — Hepatic Impairment	Dosage Adjustment — Renal Insufficiency
Aminoglycosides				
Amikacin	IM, IV	15 mg/kg q 24 h, 7.5 mg/kg q 12 h, or 5 mg/kg q 8 h	No	Major
Gentamicin, tobramycin	IM, IV	3–5 mg/kg q 24 h, 1.5–2.5 mg/kg q 12 h, or 1–1.7 mg/kg q 8 h	No	Major
Netilmicin	IM, IV	4–6.5 mg/kg q 24 h, 2–3.3 q 12 h, or 1.3–2.2 mg/kg q 8 h	No	Major
Cephalosporins				
FIRST-GENERATION				
Cephalothin, cephradine, cephapirin	IV	1–2 g q 4–6 h	No	Yes
Cefazolin	IM, IV	0.5–2 g q 8 h	No	Yes
Cefadroxil	PO	500–1000 mg q 12 h	No	Yes
Cephalexin, cephapirin	PO	250–500 mg q 6 h	No	No
SECOND-GENERATION				
Cefamandole	IM, IV	1–2 g q 4–6 h	No	Yes
Cefuroxime	IM, IV	1–1.5 g q 6 h	No	Yes
Ceforanide	IM, IV	0.5–1 g q 12 h	No	Yes
Cefonicid	IM, IV	1–2 g q 24 h	No	Yes
Cefoxitin	IM, IV	1–2 g q 4–6 h	No	Yes
Cefotetan	IM, IV	1–2 g q 12 h	No	Yes
Cefmetazole	IV	1–2 g q 6–8 h	No	Yes
Cefaclor	PO	250–500 mg q 8 h	No	Minor
Cefuroxime axetil	PO	250–500 mg q 12 h	No	Minor
Cefixime	PO	400 mg q 24 h	No	Minor
Cefpodoxime proxetil	PO	100–200 mg q 12 h	No	Minor
Cefprozil	PO	250–500 mg q 12 h	No	Minor
Cefdinir	PO	300 mg q 12 h	No	Minor
Ceftibuten	PO	400 mg q 24 h	No	minor
Loracarbel	PO	200–400 mg q 12 h	No	Minor
THIRD-GENERATION				
Ceftriaxone	IM, IV	1–2 g q 12–24 h	No[a]	No[a]
Cefotaxime	IM, IV	1–2 g q 4–8 h	No	Yes
Ceftizoxime	IM, IV	1–2 g q 8–12 h	No	Yes
Cefoperazone	IM, IV	1–2 g q 8–12 h	Yes	No
Ceftazidime	IM, IV	0.5–1 g q 8–12 h	No	Yes
FOURTH-GENERATION				
Cefepime	IM, IV	1–2 g q 8–12 h	No	Yes
Chloramphenicol	PO, IV	0.25–1 g q 6 h	Yes	No
Clindamycin	IM, IV	0.6 g q 6–8 h	Yes	No
	PO	150–300 mg q 6 h		
Fosfomycin	PO	3 g single dose	No	No
Macrolides				
Azithromycin	PO	500 mg load, then 250 mg q 24 h	No	No
Clarithromycin	PO	250–500 mg q 12 h	No	Minor
Dirithromycin	PO	500 mg q 24 h	No	No
Erythromycin	IV	0.5–1 g q 6 h	Yes	No
	PO	250–500 mg q 6 h	No[a]	No
Metronidazole	IV, PO	0.5 g q 6–8 h	Yes	No
Nitrofurantoin	PO	50–100 mg q 6 h	No	Avoid

[a] Use lower end of recommended dosage in severe impairment.

TABLE 335.1.   *Continued*

Class or Drug	Route	Average Adult Dosage	Dosage Adjustment Hepatic Impairment	Dosage Adjustment Renal Insufficiency
Other β-Lactams				
Aztreonam	IM, IV	1–2 g q 8–12 h	No	Yes
Imipenem (cilastatin)	IV	0.5–1 g q 6–8 h	No	Yes
Meropenem	IV	0.5–1 g q 8 h	No	Yes
Amoxicillin/clavulanic acid	PO	250/125–500/125 mg q 8 h or 875/125 mg q 12 h	No	Minor
Ampicillin/sulbactam	IV	1/0.5–2/1 g q 6 h	No	Yes
Piperacillin/tazobactam	IV	2/0.25–4/0.5 g q 6 h	No	Yes
Ticarcillin/clavulanic acid	IV	3/0.1 g q 4–6 h	No	Yes
Penicillins				
Penicillin G	IM, IV	0.4–4 million U q 4 h	No	Yes
Penicillin V	PO	250–500 mg q 6 h	No	No
Ampicillin	IM, IV	0.5–2 g q 4–6 h	No	Yes
	PO	250–500 mg q 6 h	No	Minor
Amoxicillin	PO	250–500 mg q 8 h	No	Minor
Oxacillin	IM, IV	1–2 g q 4 h	No[a]	No[a]
Nafcillin	IM, IV	1–2 g q 4 h	Yes	No
Cloxacillin, dicloxacillin	PO	500–1000 mg q 6 h	No[a]	No
Indanyl carbenicillin	PO	500–1000 mg q 6 h	No	Avoid
Ticarcillin	IM, IV	2–3 g q 4–6 h	No	Yes
Mezlocillin, piperacillin	IM, IV	2–3 g q 4–6 h	No	Yes
Quinolones				
Ciprofloxacin	IV	200–400 mg q 12 h	No	Yes
	PO	250–750 mg q 12 h	No	Yes
Enoxacin	PO	200–400 mg q 12 h	No	Yes
Gatifloxacin	IV, PO	400 mg q 24 h	No	Yes
Grepafloxacin	PO	400–600 mg q 24 h	Avoid	No
Levofloxacin	IV, PO	250–500 mg q 24 h	No	Yes
Lomefloxacin	PO	400 mg q 24 h	No	Yes
Moxifloxacin	PO	400 mg q 24 h	Avoid	No
Norfloxacin	PO	400 mg q 12 h	No	Yes
Ofloxacin	IV, PO	200–400 mg q 12 h	No	Yes
Sparfloxacin	IV, PO	400 mg first dose; then 200 mg q 24 h	No	Yes
Trovafloxacin	IV	200–300 mg q 24 h	Avoid	No
	PO	100–200 mg q 24 h		
Rifampin	IV, PO	600 mg q 24 h	Yes	No
Tetracyclines				
Tetracycline	IV, PO	0.25–0.5 g q 6 h	Avoid	Avoid
Doxycycline	IV, PO	100 mg q 12–24 h	No	No
Minocycline	IV, PO	100 mg q 12 h	No	No
Trimethoprim or Sulfonamide				
Sulfisoxazole, sulfadiazine	PO	1 g q 6 h	Yes	Yes
Trimethoprim-sulfamethoxazole	IV	5/25–20/100 mg/kg/d divided into 2, 3, or 4 equal doses	Minor	Yes
	PO	80/400–160/800 mg q 12 h	No	Yes
Trimethoprim	PO	100 mg q 12 h	No	Yes
Vancomycin	IV	1 g q 12 h	No	Major

[a] Use lower end of recommended dosage in severe impairment.

of the group contain the four-member β-lactam ring that must remain intact to express antimicrobial activity. Variation in the rings attached to the β-lactam ring divides the β-lactams into various subgroups (penicillins, cephalosporins, carbapenems, and monobactams). The further addition of different side chains to the basic nucleus generates analogues with altered in vitro activity and pharmacokinetic properties. The in vitro activities of selected β-lactams are shown in Table 335.2.

Penicillins

The penicillins can be divided into three main groups: the natural penicillins, the penicillinase-resistant penicillins, and the extended-spectrum penicillins.

Mechanisms of Action and Resistance

Penicillins inhibit growth by interfering with the synthesis of the cell wall. Penicillins bind covalently to various enzymes (also called penicillin-binding proteins) involved in cell wall synthesis. For most bacteria, inhibition of cell wall synthesis indirectly activates bacterial enzymes (murein hydrolases) that cause killing by cell lysis.

The primary mechanism for resistance to the penicillins is enzymatic cleavage of the β-lactam ring by β-lactamases. Most penicillins are susceptible to inactivation by the penicillinase produced by most strains of S. aureus. Penicillinase production in staphylococci is plasmid mediated and apparently has spread to enterococci. In gram-negative bacilli, β-lactamases are located in the periplasmic space between the outer and inner cell membranes. In general, the extended-spectrum penicillins have enhanced penetration across the outer membrane rather than a reduced rate of drug inactivation. The spread of β-lactamase genes among the Enterobacteriaceae and to H. influenzae and Neisseria gonorrhoeae has greatly altered susceptibility to the penicillins. The selection of stable clones that produce large amounts of a chromosomally mediated β-lactamase has increased resistance to penicillins in P. aeruginosa.

New or altered penicillin-binding proteins with decreased affinity for penicillin also can lead to the development of resistance. This mechanism accounts for methicillin resistance in staphylococci and penicillin resistance in pneumococci and other streptococci. Altered permeability of the outer membrane of gram-negative bacilli provides another mechanism for resistance to the penicillins. Organisms that exhibit tolerance to the killing activity of penicillins, such as the enterococci, appear to have reduced or altered autolytic activity with exposure to these drugs.

Activity and Clinical Use

Penicillin G is still the drug of choice for many streptococcal infections, meningococcal infections, actinomycosis, anthrax, rat-bite fever, erysipeloid, fusospirochetal infections, gas gangrene, tetanus, Pasteurella multocida infections, periodontal infections, leptospirosis, and treponemal infections, including all stages of syphilis. Penicillin V has a similar spectrum of activity against gram-positive organisms, but is less active than penicillin G against gram-negative bacteria.

The penicillinase-resistant penicillins include methicillin, nafcillin, oxacillin, cloxacillin, and dicloxacillin. These agents have bulky side chains that greatly reduce their susceptibility to inactivation by penicillinase. They are the drugs of choice for infections caused by S. aureus, except for methicillin-resistant strains. Penicillinase-resistant penicillins are slightly less potent than penicillin G against streptococci.

Ampicillin and amoxicillin have a spectrum of activity similar to that of penicillin G, except that they are more potent against certain gram-negative bacteria, including Escherichia coli, Proteus mirabilis, Shigella, Salmonella, and H. influenzae. Amoxicillin is also the most potent penicillin against penicillin-resistant pneumococci. These drugs provide effective therapy for otitis media, sinusitis, and exacerbations of chronic bronchitis. Their use for severe H. influenzae infections, Salmonella and Shigella infections, and urinary tract infections has been reduced by the appearance of resistant strains. Ampicillin is preferred over penicillin G for enterococcal and listerial infections.

Even greater activity against gram-negative bacteria is obtained with carbenicillin, ticarcillin, mezlocillin, and piperacillin. Carbenicillin is available only in an oral form used for urinary tract infections. Ticarcillin, mezlocillin, and piperacillin are used to treat serious gram-negative infections, including those caused by P. aeruginosa. Piperacillin is more potent than ticarcillin and mezlocillin against P. aeruginosa, but this has not resulted in any major increase in clinical efficacy.

Pharmacology

Penicillin G and several other penicillins are unstable in acid and largely restricted to parenteral administration. Penicillin V, amoxicillin, cloxacillin, and dicloxacillin are acid stable and are the major penicillins used orally. The indanyl ester of carbenicillin is also well absorbed.

The distribution of the penicillins within the body is governed to some degree by the extent of protein binding. Avidly bound drugs tend to exhibit high serum levels and low tissue concentrations. In general, the penicillins are confined to extracellular fluids. Concentrations of unbound drug in various tissues and inflammatory fluids are close to those in serum. In the absence of infection, penetration into the CSF is less than 3%; infection usually results in adequate CSF levels for the common organisms producing meningitis, except penicillin-resistant pneumococci.

Penicillins are eliminated primarily by glomerular filtration and tubular secretion. They also are excreted into bile, but only nafcillin, oxacillin, cloxacillin, dicloxacillin, mezlocillin, and piperacillin exhibit significant elimination by this route. Because the elimination half-life of the penicillins varies from only 30 to 60 minutes, the usual dosing intervals for these drugs are 4 to 6 hours.

Benzathine and procaine salts of penicillin G are relatively insoluble preparations that are absorbed slowly from intramuscular injection sites. These formulations result in lower, more sustained serum concentrations than those obtained with aqueous penicillin G. Serum concentrations of benzathine penicillin are so low that this preparation is used only for syphilis and

TABLE 335.2.   RELATIVE IN VITRO ACTIVITIES OF SELECTED β-LACTAMS

	Penicillin	Amoxicillin and Ampicillin	Nafcillin	Cephalosporins[a]			Piperacillin	Ticarcillin/ Clavulanate	Imipenem	Aztreonam
				First-Generation	Second-Generation	Third-Generation				
Staphylococcus aureus (methicillin-susceptible)	0–1+	0–1+	4+	3–4+	2–3+	2–3+	0–1+	3+	4+	0
Streptococci	4+[a]	4+[a]	3–4+	3–4+[a]	3+[a]	2–3+[a]	3–4+	3+	4+	0
Enterococci	3+[a]	3+[a]	1+	0–1+	0–1+	0–1+	3+[a]	2+	3+	0
Listeria monocytogenes	3+	3+	2+	2+	1–2+	0–1+	2–3+	2–3+	3–4+	0
Neisseria gonorrhoeae	4+[b]	4+[b]	1+	1–2+	2–4+	4+	4+	4+	4+	4+
Neisseria meningitidis	4+[b]	4+[a]	1+	1–2+	2–4+	4+	4+	4+	4+	4+
Haemophilus influenzae	3+[b]	3–4+[b]	0	1–2+	3+	4+	3+	3–4+	4+	4+
Escherichia coli, Proteus mirabilis	0–1+	1–3+[b]	0	2–3+	3+	4+	3+[b]	3+	4+	4+
Klebsiella, Enterobacter, Serratia	0	0–2+[b]	0	2+[c]	2–3+[c]	3–4+[c]	2–3+[b]	2–3+	3–4+	3–4+[ac]
Pseudomonas aeruginosa	0	0	0	0	0	1–3+[c]	2–3+[b]	2–3+	3+	2–3+[c]
Bacteroides fragilis	0–1+	0–1+	0	0–1+	0–3+[d]	1–2+	2–3+	3+	3–4+	0

[a] Plasmid-mediated resistance occurs occasionally.
[b] Plasmid-mediated resistance occurs commonly.
[c] Members of these species (except *Klebsiella pneumoniae*) produce a chromosomal β-lactamase that can inactive these drugs.
[d] Among the cephalosporins, cefoxitin, cefotetan, and cefmetazole have the best activity.
0, no activity at usual achievable levels; 1+, poor to fair activity; 2+, minimal inhibitory concentrations, for most strains are adequate but greater than in the higher categories; 3+, good activity; 4+, excellent activity against almost all strains.

streptococcal pharyngitis and for prophylaxis against rheumatic fever.

Adverse Reactions

Hypersensitivity reactions are the most common adverse effects of the penicillins. Immediate hypersensitivity reactions vary from mild urticaria to severe anaphylaxis. Morbilliform rashes also are common, especially with ampicillin and in patients with infectious mononucleosis or those receiving concomitant allopurinol. Erythema multiforme, vasculitis, serum sickness, drug fever, and Coombs'-positive hemolytic anemia are uncommon adverse effects of the penicillins. Adverse reactions with an increased incidence for specific drugs are hepatotoxicity with oxacillin, interstitial nephritis with methicillin, and neutropenia with nafcillin. Platelet dysfunction can result from high doses of ticarcillin, but clinical bleeding is rare. Neurotoxicity also can be seen with high-dose penicillin therapy, particularly in patients with renal impairment. Drug interactions with the penicillins are uncommon.

β-LACTAMASE INHIBITORS

Clavulanic acid, sulbactam, and tazobactam are β-lactams with weak antibacterial activity. However, they are potent, irreversible inhibitors of the β-lactamases of staphylococci, *Bacteroides fragilis, Klebsiella,* and most of the common plasmid-mediated enzymes found in *H. influenzae, E. coli,* and other gram-negative bacteria. They do not inhibit the chromosomal β-lactamases produced by *Enterobacter, Citrobacter, Serratia,* and *Pseudomonas.*

The combinations of amoxicillin with clavulanic acid and ampicillin with sulbactam have been useful for otitis media, sinusitis, and lower respiratory tract infections caused by *H. influenzae* and *Moraxella catarrhalis.* They are effective in staphylococcal and streptococcal skin infections and in bite wound infections. Ticarcillin with clavulanic acid and piperacillin with tazobactam have provided effective therapy in nosocomial pneumonia, intra-abdominal infections, and severe skin and soft-tissue infections. The half-lives of clavulanic acid, sulbactam, and tazobactam are similar to those of the penicillins with which they are combined. Their adverse reactions also are similar to those of the penicillins, except that amoxicillin with clavulanic acid produces more diarrhea than does amoxicillin alone.

Cephalosporins

The cephalosporins differ from the penicillins in that they have another site for the attachment of side chains that can alter the activity or pharmacology of the drug. The cephalosporins can be divided into four generations based on variations in antimicrobial activity.

Mechanisms of Action and Resistance

The cephalosporins inhibit cell wall synthesis and exhibit bactericidal activity by the same mechanisms as do the penicillins.

Resistance to the cephalosporins results from β-lactamase production, decreased permeability, and altered penicillin-binding proteins. β-Lactamases that hydrolyze the cephalosporins are encoded on the chromosomes of certain gram-negative bacilli, especially *Enterobacter* and *Pseudomonas* species. Mutation of the regulatory genes controlling the synthesis of these enzymes can lead to overproduction and resistance to the cephalosporins. Mutations of common plasmid-mediated β-lactamases that hydrolyze penicillins have extended their spectrum to include many cephalosporins. These enzymes, found primarily in *Klebsiella* species and *E. coli* are called *extended-spectrum β-lactamases* (ESBLs).

Activity and Clinical Use

The first-generation cephalosporins are active against staphylococci, most streptococci, *E. coli, Klebsiella pneumoniae,* and *P. mirabilis.* However, these drugs are used primarily as an alternative to penicillin for staphylococcal and streptococcal infections and for surgical prophylaxis. The second-generation cephalosporins can be divided into two groups. Cefoxitin, cefotetan, and cefmetazole have increased activity against *B. fragilis* and are used primarily for the prevention and treatment of mixed aerobic and anaerobic infections. The other group of drugs includes many oral and parenteral cephalosporins with increased activity against *H. influenzae,* including β-lactamase–producing strains. These drugs are used for upper and lower respiratory tract infections. The third-generation cephalosporins are 10 to 100 times more potent against enteric bacteria than are the earlier cephalosporins. Ceftazidime and cefoperazone also have activity against *P. aeruginosa.* These drugs are used for a variety of serious gram-negative bacillary infections. All the third-generation drugs are less active against gram-positive bacteria than are the first-generation cephalosporins. Cefepime, a fourth-generation cephalosporin, combines the activity of first- and third-generation cephalosporins, as well as being less susceptible to chromosomal β-lactamases in gram-negative bacilli. Enterococci and *Listeria* remain resistant to all the cephalosporins.

Pharmacology

The pharmacology of the cephalosporins is similar to that of the penicillins, with a few exceptions. The half-lives of most of the second-, third- and fourth-generation agents are longer than those of the penicillins. Ceftriaxone, cefonicid, cefotetan, ceforanide, and cefixime have half-lives ranging from 3 to 8 hours, which allows for once- or twice-daily dosing. Although most cephalosporins are eliminated by the kidney, cefoperazone and ceftriaxone are excreted extensively into bile. Cefuroxime and all the third-generation drugs, except cefoperazone, provide adequate CSF concentrations in the presence of inflamed meninges and are approved for bacterial meningitis. The third-generation drugs also are effective for gram-negative meningitis.

Adverse Reactions

The cephalosporins can produce the same adverse reactions as the penicillins. Allergic reactions are most common, and cephalosporins usually are avoided in patients with prior anaphylactic reactions to penicillins. Prolongation of the prothrombin time and a disulfiram-like reaction can occur with drugs that have a methylthiotetrazole side chain. This includes cefamandole, cefmetazole, cefoperazone, and cefotetan. Superinfection with enterococci, including vancomycin-resistant strains, has also been associated with use of the third-generation cephalosporins.

Carbapenems

Imipenem and meropenem have a broader spectrum of activity than other antimicrobial agents. Only a few organisms are characteristically resistant and include *S. maltophilia, Enterococcus faecium,* methicillin-resistant staphylococci, and *Corynebacterium jeikeium* diphtheroids. Resistance has emerged primarily in *Pseudomonas* and is associated with decreased permeability to the carbapenems, but not to penicillins or cephalosporins. When administered alone, imipenem is inactivated in the kidney by a dehydropeptidase enzyme found along renal tubular cells. Blocking the activity of this enzyme with cilastatin eliminates nephrotoxicity and produces high urine levels. The commercial preparation of imipenem contains both drugs. Meropenem is much less susceptible to inactivation in the kidney. These drugs have similar half-lives of 1 hour that allow for dosing every 6 to 8 hours. In general, the side effects of the carbapenems are similar to those of other β-lactams. Seizures have occurred occasionally with imipenem, primarily in patients with renal impairment being given high doses, but not with meropenem.

Monobactams

Monobactams consist of only a β-lactam ring and attached side chains. Aztreonam is the only monobactam available. Its activity is limited to facultative gram-negative bacteria; the drug has no activity against gram-positive bacteria or anaerobes. Its activity against gram-negative bacteria is similar to that of ceftazidime. Aztreonam is given parenterally, is well distributed into most body fluids, and is excreted unchanged in the urine. Its half-life of 2 hours allows for 8-hour dosing. An advantage of aztreonam is that it does not appear to cause cross-reactivity in patients with allergic reactions to other β-lactams.

Aminoglycosides and Aminocyclitols

Streptomycin, kanamycin, neomycin, gentamicin, and tobramycin are the naturally occurring aminoglycosides available in the United States. The emergence of resistance to these drugs has increased considerably, especially in hospital isolates. Two semisynthetic agents, amikacin and netilmicin, were developed for their activity against resistant strains. Spectinomycin has some similarity to these drugs in that they all have aminocyclitol rings, but it is not an aminoglycoside.

Mechanisms of Action and Resistance

The aminoglycosides inhibit protein synthesis by binding to bacterial ribosomes. The uptake of these drugs by bacteria depends on an oxygen-requiring active transport system, explaining the resistance of anaerobes. Aminoglycoside resistance is caused primarily by inactivating enzymes that phosphorylate, acetylate, or adenylate key portions of the molecules. The genes for these enzymes are carried on plasmids and transposons and can spread among many species. Changes in the outer membrane leading to decreased permeability also occur, especially with *P. aeruginosa.* Resistance to streptomycin commonly results from mutational change of the target ribosome.

Activity and Clinical Use

The aminoglycosides are active primarily against aerobic gram-negative bacilli (Table 335.3). Tobramycin is the most active agent against *P. aeruginosa,* whereas amikacin is the most resistant of all the aminoglycosides to the inactivating enzymes. Despite their potential for toxicity, the aminoglycosides are recommended for use in combination with broad-spectrum β-lactams in patients with serious gram-negative bacillary infections. Streptomycin is still a useful agent for tuberculosis, tularemia, plague, and brucellosis (in combination with a tetracycline). Neomycin is used orally (to reduce bowel organisms) or topically. Spectinomycin is used only to treat gonorrhea, especially β-lactamase–producing strains.

The aminoglycosides have poor activity against most gram-positive cocci. However, in combination with β-lactams, they exhibit synergism with staphylococci, streptococci, and enterococci unless the bacteria show high-level resistance because of inactivating enzymes. Such combinations have improved the efficacy or shortened the duration of therapy for endocarditis and bacteremia caused by gram-positive cocci.

Pharmacology

All the aminoglycosides have poor oral absorption and require parenteral administration for systemic infections. The drugs distribute primarily in extracellular fluid and penetrate poorly into the CSF. The aminoglycosides are eliminated almost entirely by glomerular filtration. Because their efficacy is improved by obtaining peak concentrations that are at least eight times higher than the MIC, many physicians give the drugs in single daily doses rather than two or three divided doses.

Adverse Reactions

The aminoglycosides produce significant nephrotoxicity and ototoxicity. The damage to renal tubules usually is reversible and can be reduced by monitoring renal function and adjusting dosages appropriately. Once-daily administration also has been shown to reduce nephrotoxicity in several studies. Ototoxicity, which may be auditory or vestibular, is increased by prolonged courses of therapy in elderly patients and those with renal impairment.

QUINOLONES

The quinolones are synthetic compounds consisting of nalidixic acid and its fluorinated derivatives. The early fluoroquinolones

TABLE 335.3.   RELATIVE IN VITRO ACTIVITIES OF SELECTED ANTIMICROBIALS

	Vancomycin	Clindamycin	Macrolides	Tetracyclines	Gentamicin and Tobramycin	Ofloxacin and Ciprofloxacin	Trimethoprim/ Sulfamethoxazole
Staphylococcus aureus (methicillin-susceptible)	3–4+	2–3+†	2+†	1–2+	0–2	2–3+	2–3+
Staphylococcus aureus (methicillin-resistant)	3–4+	0–1+	0–1+	1–2+	0–1+	1–2+	2+
Streptococci	4+	3+*	3+*	2+	0–1+‖	0–2+	2+
Enterococci	3+*	0–1+	0–1+	1–2+	0–1+‖	1–2+	1–2+
Listeria monocytogenes	2+	2+	2+	2+	0–1+‖	1–2+	3+
Neisseria gonorrhoeae	0	0	1+	3+†	0–1+	4+	0–1+
Neisseria meningitidis	0	0	1–3+‡	2–3+	0	4+	0–1+
Haemophilus influenzae	0	0	0	2–3+	2+	4+	3–4+
Escherichia coli, Proteus mirabilis	0	0	0	0–2+	3–4+†	4+*	3–4+*
Klebsiella, Enterobacter, Serratia	0	0	0	0–2+	3–4+†	3–4+*	2–3+
Pseudomonas aeruginosa	0	0	0	0	2–3+†‖§	3+†	0
Bacteroides fragilis	0	3–4+	0–1+	0–2+	0	0–1+	0

* Plasmid-mediated resistance occurs occasionally.
† Plasmid-mediated resistance occurs commonly.
‡ Among the macrolides, azithromycin and clarithromycin have the best activity.
§ Among the aminoglycosides, tobramycin has the best activity.
‖ Used in combination with a β-lactam antibiotic to enhance bactericidal activity.
0, no activity at usual achievable levels: 1+, poor to fair activity; 2+, minimal inhibitory concentrations, for most strains are adequate but greater than in the higher categories; 3+, good activity; 4+, excellent activity against almost all strains.

(ciprofloxacin, enoxacin, lomefloxacin, norfloxacin, and ofloxacin) were primarily active against gram-negative bacilli. The newer fluoroquinolones (gatifloxacin, grepafloxacin, levofloxacin, moxifloxacin, sparfloxacin, and trovafloxacin) have increased activity against gram-positive cocci.

Mechanisms of Action and Resistance

The quinolones inhibit the function of topoisomerase IV and DNA gyrase, which is involved in supercoiling strands of bacterial DNA. By inhibiting DNA synthesis, the drugs are rapidly bactericidal, even against nongrowing bacteria. The major mechanisms of resistance involves mutations in the topoisomerase IV and DNA gyrase, which reduce their affinity for the quinolones. Resistance also has developed as a result of alterations of outer membrane porins in gram-negative bacilli and of increased drug efflux in gram-positive cocci.

Activity and Clinical Use

The quinolones have excellent activity against aerobic gram-negative bacteria. Ciprofloxacin is the most potent agent against *P. aeruginosa* and several other gram-negative bacilli. The activity of quinolones against staphylococci, streptococci, and anaerobes varies among the different agents (Table 335.3). Quinolones have demonstrated efficacy in sinusitis, lower respiratory tract infections, urinary tract infections, skin and soft-tissue infections, osteomyelitis, and joint infections. Many quinolones are active against intracellular pathogens, such as mycobacteria, *Chlamydia,* and *Legionella.* Their efficacy also has been documented in a variety of gastrointestinal infections, including traveler's diarrhea and bacterial gastroenteritis.

Pharmacology

All the quinolones are well absorbed orally, and most are eliminated by urinary excretion. Grepafloxacin, moxifloxacin, sparfloxacin, and trovafloxacin have major hepatic clearance. The quinolones are distributed widely in tissues and body fluids, including the CSF. Intracellular concentrations are higher than serum levels, which accounts for their activity against intracellular pathogens. The elimination half-lives of the quinolones vary from 3 to 4 hours for norfloxacin and ciprofloxacin to 6 to 18 hours for other quinolones. This permits once- to twice-daily dosing of these drugs.

Adverse Reactions

The incidence of adverse effects to the quinolones is low, with gastrointestinal disturbances being most common. Central nervous system reactions such as dizziness, headache, and insomnia can occur, but seizures are rare. Nephrotoxic reactions caused by crystalluria and hepatotoxicity also are rare. Moderate to severe phototoxicity is observed infrequently, primarily with lomefloxacin and sparfloxacin. Enoxacin and, to a lesser extent, ciprofloxacin and grepafloxacin increase theophylline and caffeine levels. Because the quinolones have been reported to produce cartilage

damage in young animals, none of these drugs is approved for use in children.

OTHER AGENTS

VANCOMYCIN

Vancomycin is a glycopeptide antibiotic that inhibits cell wall synthesis at an earlier step than do the β-lactam drugs. Vancomycin is active against most gram-positive bacteria, including methicillin-resistant *S. aureus* and *Staphylococcus epidermidis,* penicillin-resistant pneumococci, *Clostridium difficile,* and enterococci; gram-negative organisms usually are resistant. The increased use of vancomycin over the past decade has contributed to the emergence of vancomycin-resistant enterococci. Resistance can occur by several mechanisms and may be transferred by plasmids and transposons.

Because of its poor absorption, vancomycin can be used orally for the treatment of *C. difficile* colitis. After intravenous administration, it distributes to most body fluids and has marginal to adequate penetration into the CSF in the presence of inflamed meninges. The drug is eliminated almost entirely by the kidney, with a half-life of 6 hours. In patients with normal renal function, dosing is every 12 hours. The dosing frequency in patients with renal impairment is determined by drug level monitoring,

Vancomycin use has been associated with nephrotoxicity and ototoxicity, but this problem has decreased with more recent and purer preparations. Rapid infusion can cause histamine release that produces a syndrome somewhat similar to anaphylaxis. Even with slower infusion, thrombophlebitis can occur.

MACROLIDES

Erythromycin, clarithromycin, dirithromycin, and azithromycin are bacteriostatic agents that inhibit protein synthesis. Resistance among gram-positive cocci usually results from methylation of the ribosomal site of action, which prevents the binding of all three macrolides. Resistance resulting from active efflux and drug inactivation also has been described. The macrolides are broad-spectrum agents with primary activity against gram-positive bacteria. The newer macrolides, clarithromycin and azithromycin, have increased activity against *H. influenzae* and nontuberculous mycobacteria. Erythromycin is used clinically for mild to moderate streptococcal and staphylococcal infections, *Legionella* infections, *Mycoplasma* and *Chlamydia* pneumonitis, *Campylobacter* enteritis, and pertussis. The broader spectrum of activity of the newer agents has fostered their use for a variety of upper and lower respiratory tract infections. These drugs also have become major agents in the treatment and prophylaxis of atypical mycobacterial infections.

The macrolides, especially the newer agents, are absorbed adequately after oral dosing. The drugs are well distributed to most tissues and body fluids; the high intracellular tissue concentrations account for their efficacy against intracellular pathogens. Most of the drug is excreted in the bile. The half-lives vary from 1.5 hours for erythromycin to more than 24 hours for azithromycin. As a result, erythromycin, clarithromycin, and azithromycin usually are given every 6, 12, and 24 hours, respectively. Erythromycin is an extremely safe drug, although gastrointestinal disturbances with oral use and thrombophlebitis with intravenous administration are common. The incidence of gastrointestinal symptoms is decreased markedly with the newer macrolides.

CLINDAMYCIN

The mechanism of action and resistance of clindamycin is similar to that of the macrolides. It is active against most staphylococci, streptococci, and anaerobes. The drug also has activity against *Pneumocystis carinii, Toxoplasma gondii,* and *Plasmodium falciparum.* It is used primarily in anaerobic infections, especially lung abscesses, and as an alternative agent in mild to moderate streptococcal and staphylococcal infections.

Clindamycin is well absorbed orally; it is widely distributed in most tissues, but penetrates poorly into the CSF. The drug is metabolized in the liver and excreted largely in the bile. The major complication of clindamycin therapy is the development of antibiotic-associated colitis resulting from the overgrowth of *C. difficile.* This problem is not unique to clindamycin and has been observed with many other antimicrobial agents.

TETRACYCLINES

The tetracyclines are bacteriostatic agents that inhibit protein synthesis. Resistance results primarily from the acquisition of genes that cause active efflux of the drug from the cell. The tetracyclines have a broad spectrum of antimicrobial activity. They are useful drugs for sexually transmitted diseases, such as nongonococcal urethritis, granuloma inguinale, and lymphogranuloma venereum. The drugs also are indicated for rickettsial infections, Lyme disease, brucellosis (with streptomycin or rifampin), *Mycoplasma* and *Chlamydia* pneumonitis, and chronic bronchitis. In addition, the tetracyclines are used as alternative agents for infections such as syphilis, plague, and malaria.

All the tetracyclines are well absorbed orally; doxycycline and minocycline are the least affected by food. These agents also have the longest half-lives, allowing for once- or twice-daily dosing. Although the older tetracyclines are excreted largely by the kidneys, doxycycline and minocycline are eliminated primarily in the bile. Because tetracycline can worsen azotemia by inhibiting protein synthesis, dosage modification is required even in patients with mild renal impairment. Doxycycline does not accumulate in patients with renal failure and can be used safely without dosage adjustment. High doses of tetracycline, especially in pregnant women, can induce hepatotoxicity. The tetracyclines should not be used in pregnant women or children because of discoloration of teeth and bones. All the tetracyclines have the potential for phototoxicity, diarrhea, and vaginal candidal overgrowth. Minocycline can cause vestibular toxicity.

CHLORAMPHENICOL

Chloramphenicol exerts a bacteriostatic effect by binding to the bacterial ribosome and inhibiting protein synthesis. Resistance results primarily from inactivating enzymes that acetylate the drug. The antimicrobial spectrum of chloramphenicol is similar to that of the tetracyclines. Because of its potential to produce bone marrow suppression, the use of chloramphenicol is restricted to specific situations in which alternative agents are unavailable. The main indications for chloramphenicol are for the treatment of typhoid fever, brain abscesses, meningitis caused by ampicillin-resistant strains of *H. influenzae,* and pneumococcal and meningococcal meningitis in penicillin-allergic patients.

Chloramphenicol is well absorbed orally, distributed widely into tissues and fluids (including the CSF), and metabolized in the liver. With prolonged use, reversible inhibition of bone marrow function develops in most patients. Irreversible aplastic anemia occurs rarely (about 1 per 40,000 patients).

METRONIDAZOLE

Metronidazole is used clinically for the treatment of giardiasis, amebiasis, trichomoniasis, and anaerobic infections. The drug is converted only in anaerobic bacteria to a series of compounds that damage DNA. Metronidazole must be used with other agents in mixed aerobic and anaerobic infections. Oral and parenteral dosing of metronidazole produce comparable serum concentrations; the drug also is metabolized by the liver. Its bactericidal activity and excellent penetration into the CSF and tissues make metronidazole an ideal choice for endocarditis and meningitis caused by anaerobic bacteria. Side effects include gastrointestinal intolerance, a disulfiram-like reaction, and peripheral neuropathy with prolonged use. Although metronidazole is carcinogenic in animals and mutagenic in bacteria, it has not been associated with carcinogenesis in humans.

SULFONAMIDES AND TRIMETHOPRIM

The sulfonamides and trimethoprim are synthetic compounds that inhibit different enzymes involved in the bacterial synthesis of folic acid. Resistance results from the acquisition of genes that encode for enzymes not inhibited by these drugs. Both agents are broad-spectrum drugs that inhibit many gram-positive and gram-negative bacteria, chlamydia, and certain protozoa. As monotherapy, the sulfonamides are used primarily for urinary tract infections and nocardiosis. The combination of sulfamethoxazole and trimethoprim is used for urinary tract infections, typhoid fever, traveler's diarrhea, and *P. carinii* infections. The trimethoprim analogue, pyrimethamine, is combined with the sulfonamides for the treatment of *T. gondii* and some *P. falciparum* infections.

The sulfonamides and trimethoprim are readily absorbed orally. These drugs penetrate well into the CSF and other fluids, are metabolized partially in the liver, and are excreted as intact drug and metabolites in the urine. Both the sulfonamides and trimethoprim can produce rash and drug fever; more severe skin reactions are observed in patients with HIV infection. Trimethoprim can produce bone marrow suppression, and the sulfonamides can cause hemolytic anemia in patients with glucose-6-phosphate dehydrogenase deficiency. Crystalluria can occur with high doses of sulfadiazine. The sulfonamides also can displace bilirubin from albumin and produce kernicterus in newborns.

RIFAMPIN

Rifampin interferes with protein synthesis by inhibiting DNA-dependent RNA polymerase. Resistant mutants, which occur commonly with most bacteria, have altered RNA polymerase that no longer binds the drug. Despite its broad-spectrum and bactericidal activity, rifampin's propensity for resistance keeps it from being used alone. It is given in combination with other drugs for mycobacterial, staphylococcal, *Brucella,* and *Legionella* infections. Short courses of rifampin alone are useful as prophylaxis for contacts of patients with severe meningococcal infections and for reducing carriage of *S. aureus.* A related drug, rifabutin, is used for the prophylaxis of mycobacterial infections in HIV-infected patients with low CD4 counts.

Rifampin is well absorbed orally; it also is distributed widely in tissues and body fluids, including the CSF. The drug is metabolized and excreted by the liver. Side effects include hepatitis, orange discoloration of the urine, interstitial nephritis, and a flulike syndrome with erratic use. Rifampin is a potent stimulator of the hepatic metabolism of other drugs, such as warfarin, oral hypoglycemics, and oral contraceptives.

URINARY ANTISEPTICS

Nitrofurantoin is a nitrofuran derivative used to treat and prevent urinary tract infections. It is active against most gram-positive and gram-negative urinary pathogens, except *Proteus* and *P. aeruginosa.* Adverse reactions include gastrointestinal disturbances, an acute hypersensitivity pneumonitis, and hemolysis in patients with glucose-6-phosphate dehydrogenase deficiency. A single, large oral dose of fosfomycin also provides similar efficacy to nitrofurantoin for uncomplicated urinary tract infections in females.

Methenamine breaks down at an acid pH to form formaldehyde, which is active against most bacterial species. The drug is used to suppress or prevent recurrent bacteriuria. Although methenamine is available in combination with mandelic or hippuric acids, urine acidification by ammonium chloride or ascorbic acid usually is required.

BIBLIOGRAPHY

Bartlett JG. Tables of antimicrobial agents. In: Gorbach SL, Bartlett JG, Blacklow NR, eds. *Infectious diseases,* second ed. Philadelphia: WB Saunders, 1998:428.

Craig WA. Pharmacokinetic/pharmacodynamic parameters: rationale for antibacterial dosing of mice and men. *Clin Infect Dis* 1998;26:1–12.

Davies J. Inactivation of antibiotics and the dissemination of resistance genes. *Science* 1994;264:375–382.

Nikaido H. Prevention of drug access to bacterial targets: permeability barriers and active efflux. *Science* 1994;264:382–388.

The choice of antibacterial drugs. *Med Lett Drugs Ther* 1998;40:33–42.

C H A P T E R

336

APPROACH TO THE TREATMENT OF SYSTEMIC FUNGAL INFECTIONS

JOHN H. REX

The frequency of serious fungal infections is rising as a result of the increasingly successful use of antineoplastic therapy, the growing number of patients infected with HIV type 1, and the widespread use of broad-spectrum antibacterial agents. The number of drugs available to treat such infections also has increased, and their use is reviewed in this chapter.

ANTIFUNGAL AGENTS

AMPHOTERICIN B

Long the mainstay of antifungal therapy, amphotericin B remains an important agent. Its antifungal effect results from its ability to bind to fungal membrane sterols, especially ergosterol, and alter membrane permeability. Although it is potent against almost all fungal infections, its use is limited by its toxicity. Because amphotericin B is otherwise insoluble in aqueous solutions, it is made soluble by the addition of deoxycholate. It is reconstituted in water or water-containing dextrose; any addition of sodium or potassium salts causes aggregation. Amphotericin B must be given intravenously, and phlebitis almost invariably develops unless it is administered through a central venous catheter. The addition of heparin (500 to 1000 units) to the infusion is thought to ameliorate the phlebitis. Single daily doses of 0.5 to 1.5 mg per kilogram are given, to total doses of 15 to 30 mg per kilogram, with the precise daily and total doses depending on the severity of infection, the infecting agent, and the patient's response to therapy.

Fever, chills, and hypotension are common during the initiation of therapy. Occasionally, the reaction is striking, and many clinicians begin therapy with a 1-mg test dose to identify patients who have severe reactions to the drug. Patients usually adjust to amphotericin B after a few doses, but acetaminophen (650 mg) or diphenhydramine (50 mg) can be administered before each dose to alleviate fever and nausea, and meperidine (25 to 50 mg) can be administered intravenously to interrupt profound rigors.

The addition of 25 to 50 mg of hydrocortisone to each infusion also may help prevent these symptoms. After the acute adverse effects resolve, many patients have persistent malaise, mild nausea, and weight loss. Later in the course of therapy, nephrotoxicity often develops. Elevation of the creatinine level to 2.5 to 3 mg per deciliter is common and does not warrant discontinuation of therapy. The azotemia is accompanied by renal tubular acidosis, hypokalemia, and hypomagnesemia. The electrolyte losses can be severe, but are predictable, and a regular program of electrolyte replacement is required. Salt loading with 500 to 1000 mL of normal saline before each dose of amphotericin B appears to reduce nephrotoxicity. Administering twice the daily dose every other day or three times a week also ameliorates nephrotoxicity somewhat. Concomitant with the renal dysfunction, a normochromic, normocytic anemia develops. The hemoglobin falls to 8 to 10 mg per deciliter and the erythropoietin level is low. Although amphotericin B causes irreversible renal damage in some patients (especially those with preexisting renal dysfunction or those receiving other nephrotoxic agents), the azotemia and anemia usually abate completely within a few months of the cessation of therapy.

LIPID-ASSOCIATED FORMULATIONS OF AMPHOTERICIN B

Three lipid-associated formulations of amphotericin B are now licensed for use in humans: amphotericin B lipid complex (ABLC), amphotericin B colloidal dispersion (ABCD), and liposomal amphotericin B (L-AmB). All are mixtures of amphotericin B with lipids, but only L-AmB has the molecular configuration of a spherical lipid bilayer. Regardless of configuration, all three preparations are associated with significantly reduced nephrotoxicity, and the licensed doses are significantly higher than for standard amphoterin B deoxycholate: 5 mg per kilogram per day (ABLC), 3 to 5 mg per kilogram per day (AmBisome), or 3 to 4 mg per kilogram per day (ABCD). These compounds are at least equipotent with 0.5 to 1 mg per kilogram amphotericin B deoxycholate. Although all three compounds cause less nephrotoxicity, creatinine elevation and electrolyte losses still develop and must be monitored. ABLC and L-AmB are also associated with reduced acute administration-related toxicity. The principal advantage of these compounds is that their reduced nephrotoxicity often permits extended usage, even in patients with preexisting renal dysfunction or in those receiving therapy with other nephrotoxic agents. These agents are, however, very costly and are in general most appropriate for patients who are refractory to or intolerant of therapy with standard amphotericin B deoxycholate.

AZOLE ANTIFUNGAL AGENTS

The development of azole antifungal agents has proceeded rapidly, and three agents now are used to treat systemic infections (Table 336.1). These agents have their effect by inhibiting an enzyme in the fungal sterol biosynthetic pathway. All the azole antifungal agents have oral formulations, which is one of their principal advantages over amphotericin B. All are given at dosages ranging from 100 to 400 mg per day, although data suggest that fluconazole can be given safely at dosages up to 800 mg per day. The principal adverse effect of the azoles is occasional hepatotoxicity, typically with a hepatocellular injury pattern. Slight elevation of transaminase levels (up to 1.5 times the upper limit of normal) is common, and progressive elevation associated with clinical symptoms of hepatitis and jaundice occurs occasionally. This hepatitis resolves with discontinuation of the drug, but continued azole therapy in the face of hepatitis or rechallenge

| TABLE 336.1. | GUIDELINES FOR ANTIFUNGAL AGENT SELECTION IN INVASIVE MYCOSES |

Disease	First-Line Agents[a]	Second-Line Agents[b]
Aspergillosis	AmB, LAFB[c]	Itra
Blastomycosis	AmB, Itra	Keto, Fluco
Candidiasis	AmB, Fluco	Itra
Coccidioidomycosis	AmB, Fluco	Keto, Itra
Cryptococcosis	AmB ± 5-FC, Fluco	Itra
Histoplasmosis	AmB, Itra, Keto	Fluco
Mucormycosis	AmB, LAFB[c]	
Paracoccidioidomycosis	Keto, Itra	AmB, Sulfadiazine
Sporotrichosis	AmB, Itra, Keto	Fluco

AmB, amphotericin B; LAFB, lipid-associated formulation of amphotericin B; Keto, ketoconazole; Itra, itraconazole; Fluco, fluconazole.
[a] Proved active in one or more clinical trials.
[b] May be active, but their efficacy has either not been fully established or appears inferior to the first-line agents.
[c] The lipid-associated formulations of amphotericin B may be especially useful for these diseases and should be considered promptly if standard therapy is not immediately effective.

after an episode of hepatitis can lead to substantial hepatic dysfunction or even death. Hepatitis most often manifests during early therapy and is not clearly dose related. Most clinicians recommend serial transaminase determinations during therapy, but these do not consistently predict late-onset hepatitis and should not be relied on exclusively. Patients receiving azoles should be instructed to report promptly any symptoms of hepatitis and to discontinue the drugs until they can see their physicians.

Nausea is another common adverse effect of the azoles, especially at higher doses of ketoconazole and itraconazole. Cutaneous reactions include pruritus, rash, and Stevens–Johnson syndrome. Ketoconazole can interfere significantly with corticosteroid hormone biosynthesis and produce decreased libido, gynecomastia, menstrual irregularities, and, rarely, symptomatic adrenal insufficiency. Itraconazole occasionally causes edema, hypokalemia, and hypertension.

The azoles have several notable pharmacologic properties. First, predictable absorption of ketoconazole and itraconazole requires attention. Ketoconazole absorption requires gastric acidity. Itraconazole is available both as a capsule and a solution. Absorption of the capsule form, although modestly sensitive to gastric acidity, is increased if taken with food. Itraconazole solution is best absorbed if taken on an empty stomach and has a bioavailability approximately 30% greater than the capsule form. Ketoconazole and itraconazole are cleared by hepatic metabolism and do not require dosage adjustment in the face of renal dysfunction. In contrast, fluconazole is predictably well absorbed when given orally, but is cleared by the kidneys and requires dosage adjustment for renal dysfunction. Unlike ketoconazole and itraconazole, fluconazole also has a parenteral form.

The azoles have the potential for pharmacokinetic interaction with many other agents. Particularly important interactions include decreased ketoconazole and itraconazole levels with the simultaneous use of antacids, H_2-blockers, or sucralfate; decrease in the levels of all azoles with concomitant rifampin therapy; and increased cyclosporine, phenytoin, and terfenadine levels with the use of any of the azoles.

FLUCYTOSINE

Flucytosine, also known as 5-fluorocytosine, is a fluorinated pyrimidine analogue that often is used in combination with amphotericin B. In susceptible fungi, it is deaminated to 5-fluorouracil, which subsequently is incorporated into DNA or RNA. Such incorporation interferes with DNA and RNA function and leads to cell death. Flucytosine can be given orally or parenterally, although the parenteral form is not available in the United States. The dosage is 25 to 37.5 mg per kilogram given four times per day. Flucytosine is cleared by the kidneys and may accumulate in patients with renal dysfunction. If blood levels exceed 50 to 100 (g per milliliter, leukopenia and thrombocytopenia may occur. Colitis and hepatitis also may be seen, particularly when blood levels of flucytosine rise.

CHOICE OF ANTIFUNGAL THERAPY

The choice of antifungal therapy for individual patients requires careful thought. In general, amphotericin B is preferred as initial therapy in profoundly ill patients. The azoles are used as primary therapy in less acutely ill patients and as long-term therapy after a brief course of amphotericin B. However, the application of these general rules is evolving rapidly as new studies continue to demonstrate that azoles can be used as first-line therapy for certain fungal infections (e.g., itraconazole for disseminated histoplasmosis and fluconazole for candidemia in nonneutropenic patients). Some guidelines for antifungal selection are given in Table 336.1, but expert advice should be obtained for all but the most straightforward systemic fungal infections.

BIBLIOGRAPHY

Como JA, Dismukes WE. Oral azole drugs as systemic antifungal therapy. *N Engl J Med* 1994;330:263–272.
Francis P, Walsh TJ. Evolving role of flucytosine in immunocompromised patients: new insights into safety, pharmacokinetics, and antifungal therapy. *Clin Infect Dis* 1992;15:1003–1018.
Gallis HA, Drew RH, Pickard WW. Amphotericin B: 30 years of clinical experience. *Rev Infect Dis* 1990;12:308–329.
Rex JH, Walsh TJ, Anaissie EA. Fungal infections in iatrogenically compromised hosts. *Adv Intern Med* 1997;43:321–371.
Wong-Beringer A, Jacobs RA, Guglielmo BJ. Lipid formulations of amphotericin B: Clinical efficacy and toxicities. *Clin Infect Dis* 1998;27:603–618.

Kelley's Textbook of Internal Medicine, fourth edition. Edited by H. David Humes.
Lippincott Williams & Wilkins, Philadelphia © 2000.

ANTIMICROBIAL CHEMOPROPHYLAXIS

F. MARC LAFORCE

GENERAL PRINCIPLES

In the early 1940s, it was noted that when sulfadiazine when was administered to closed populations with epidemic meningococcal disease, the result was an immediate cessation of cases of the disease and the virtual disappearance of carriers. This dramatic success stimulated interest in the concept of chemoprophylaxis. A half-century later, we have learned more about the limits of chemoprophylaxis. For example, the most successful prophylactic regimens are generally those that prevent infection from a single type of organism for a relatively brief period. Conversely, the least success is achieved when prophylaxis is aimed against multiple species for an extended period.

The strategy of prevention by chemoprophylaxis has important drawbacks that have been understated. Antibiotics and their administration are expensive, and some agents are inappropriately and extravagantly overused. Perhaps the most serious consequence of the widespread use of antibiotics as prophylactic agents is the emergence of resistant organisms. One common example of inappropriate chemoprophylaxis is the attempt to suppress bacteriuria in the patient with a chronic indwelling bladder catheter. All prophylactic regimens that use antibiotics fail in this setting, and organisms that finally colonize the urinary tract are invariably resistant to the prophylactic agent being used. In such circumstances, it is more prudent to ensure that there are no obstructions to urine flow and to treat acute infections as they occur.

Some medical indications for antimicrobial chemoprophylaxis are presented in this chapter. Other chapters in this text deal with specific infectious agents and should be consulted for more detailed information. Perioperative chemoprophylaxis is discussed in Chapter 273.

GROUP A STREPTOCOCCAL INFECTIONS AND RHEUMATIC FEVER

Patients with poststreptococcal rheumatic heart disease require continuous prophylaxis to prevent streptococcal infections (Chapter 275). The preferred regimen is monthly injections of 1.2 million units of benzathine penicillin G. Oral penicillin V also is an acceptable prophylactic regimen, but is less effective than monthly penicillin injections because of compliance problems. Patients who are allergic to penicillin can be treated with erythromycin. The optimum duration of continuous antibiotic prophylaxis is unclear. The risk of rheumatic fever recurrences decreases with age and the length of time since the last episode. Some experts suggest that prophylaxis should not be discontinued until a patient is in his or her 20s and until at least 5 years have elapsed since the last attack.

MENINGOCOCCAL INFECTIONS

Household contacts of patients with meningococcal infections are at risk for infection with *Neisseria meningitidis* (Chapter 279). Similar high-risk conditions occur in closed populations such as college dormitories and nursery schools. Hospital personnel do not have increased risk, except for those who have had intimate exposure, such as mouth-to-mouth resuscitation. Recommended therapy for meningococcal prophylaxis in adults is with rifampin (600 mg every 12 hours for 2 days).

RECURRENT URINARY TRACT INFECTIONS

Several studies have shown that nightly use of trimethoprim-sulfamethoxazole (½ tablet consisting of 40 mg of trimethoprim and 200 mg of sulfamethoxazole) or nitrofurantoin (50 mg) can decrease significantly the incidence of recurrent urinary tract infections in women (Chapter 271). In some women, recurrences are associated with sexual activity, and a single dose of trimethoprim-sulfamethoxazole or nitrofurantoin taken after sexual intercourse is effective.

INFLUENZA

Amantadine and rimantadine are effective chemoprophylactic agents against influenza A, but not influenza B (Chapter 310). During an influenza A epidemic, amantadine or rimantadine prophylaxis can be initiated at the same time that susceptible persons receive influenza vaccine. Prophylaxis can be discontinued 2 weeks later when antibody titers presumably are protective. Amantadine use in the elderly has been associated with central nervous system side effects, and the recommended prophylactic dosage is 100 mg per day. Rimantadine has fewer central nervous system side effects. Amantadine or rimantadine also can be used in patients who cannot receive influenza vaccine because of egg sensitivity or in high-risk persons when the vaccine does not contain a good antigenic match to the circulating influenza A virus.

PNEUMOCYSTIS INFECTIONS

Patients recovering from *Pneumocystis* pneumonia remain at high risk for the development of recurrent disease as long as the predisposing immunosuppression persists (Chapter 327). Trimethoprim-sulfamethoxazole has proved effective as chemoprophylaxis against *Pneumocystis* infection. In addition, this agent decreases the incidence of toxoplasmosis and may lower infection rates from *Streptococcus pneumoniae* and *Haemophilus influenzae*. Patients with AIDS have a high rate of reaction to trimethoprim-sulfamethoxazole, and many cannot tolerate it. Effective alternative agents include dapsone, dapsone plus pyrimethamine, and monthly aerosolized doses of pentamidine.

MALARIA

Malaria is an important health risk for travelers to tropical non-industrialized countries (Chapter 322). Chloroquine (300 mg once weekly) is the drug of choice in areas without chloroquine-resistant malaria. Chloroquine-resistant *Plasmodium falciparum* occurs in most of Africa, Southeast Asia, and the Amazon region of South America. Travelers to chloroquine-resistant areas should use mefloquine (250 mg per week). Travelers who cannot take mefloquine should take doxycycline (100 mg per day). Travelers should also carry a three-tablet treatment dose of pyrimethamine-sulfadoxine (Fansidar) to be taken in the event of a febrile illness. Prophylactic antimalarial regimens should be initiated 2 weeks before departure except for doxycycline, which can be begun at the time of entry into a malarious area. All prophylactic regimens should be continued for 4 weeks after the traveler has returned home.

TUBERCULOSIS

Isoniazid (300 mg per day for 1 year) is effective prophylactic therapy for most adults whose tuberculin skin test results have become positive (Chapter 294). Tuberculin skin reactors with

---

TABLE 337.1.	**CURRENT RECOMMENDATIONS FOR ENDOCARDITIS PROPHYLAXIS IN ADULTS**

- Prophylactic regimens for dental, oral, respiratory tract, or esophageal procedures
- Amoxicillin, 2 g PO 1 h before procedure
- Allergic to penicillin:
  Clindamycin, 600 mg PO 1 h before procedure
  or
  Azithromycin or clarithromycin, 500 mg PO 1 h before procedure
- Prophylactic regimens for genitourinary and gastrointestinal procedures
- High-risk patients: ampicillin 2 g intravenously (IV) or intramuscularly (IM) plus gentamicin 1.5 mg/kg within 30 minutes of starting procedure; 6 h later ampicillin 1 g IM/IV or amoxicillin 1 g orally
- High-risk patients allergic to ampicillin/amoxicillin: vancomycin 1 g IV over 1–2 h plus gentamicin 1.5 mg/kg (not to exceed 120 mg); complete infusion within 30 minutes of starting procedure

From Dajani AS, Taubert KA, Wilson W, et al. Prevention of bacterial endocarditis: recommendations of the American Heart Association. *JAMA* 1997;277:1794–1801.

radiographic changes suggestive of tuberculosis but with negative culture results, and those with special risk factors such as diabetes, gastrectomy, or immunosuppression also should receive isoniazid chemoprophylaxis. Exposure to isoniazid-resistant tuberculosis can be managed with rifampin (600 mg per day).

ENDOCARDITIS

Recommendations for prophylaxis against bacterial endocarditis have recently been changed and are summarized in Table 337.1 (see Chapter 270). Persons considered to be at high risk for bacterial endocarditis include those with prosthetic valves, histories of endocarditis, aortic or mitral valve lesions, congenital heart diseases (except atrial septal defects), and alimentation catheters or arteriovenous fistulas.

BIBLIOGRAPHY

Dajani AS, Taubert KA, Wilson W, et al. Prevention of bacterial endocarditis: recommendations of the American Heart Association. *JAMA* 1997; 277:1794–1801.
www.cdc.gov (This is a user friendly web site with accessible and useful current information on chemoprophylaxis.)

Kelley's Textbook of Internal Medicine, fourth edition. Edited by H. David Humes. Lippincott Williams & Wilkins, Philadelphia © 2000.

C H A P T E R

338

HOSPITAL EPIDEMIOLOGY AND INFECTION CONTROL

JAN EVANS PATTERSON

HISTORICAL PERSPECTIVE

Hospital epidemiology is rooted in the principles of infectious disease epidemiology and antisepsis developed by investigators such as Semmelweiss, Nightingale, Lister, and Holmes. The term *hospital epidemiologist* first appeared in the 1940s in relation to controlling institutional outbreaks of diarrhea, then disappeared during the initial successes of antibiotic therapy. The term and the practice of hospital epidemiology reappeared with the emergence of penicillinase-producing staphylococci and outbreaks of nosocomial staphylococcal infections during the late 1950s and 1960s. Eventually, the Hospital Infections branch of the Centers for Disease Control (CDC) was established to address the problem of nosocomial infections. The role of infection control nurses was recognized as critical to hospital programs and a professional organization of these practitioners, the Associ-

ation for Professionals in Infection Control (APIC; previously the Association for Practitioners in Infection Control), was established and is still thriving. The role of hospital epidemiologists, physicians with expertise in epidemiology and infection control, evolved more slowly, but now is recognized as essential to a successful infection control program. The Society for Healthcare Epidemiology of America (SHEA; previously the Society for Hospital Epidemiology of America) has grown rapidly with the increased demand for physicians with expertise in this field.

SURVEILLANCE, PREVENTION, AND CONTROL

The function of hospital epidemiology and infection control is the surveillance, prevention, and control of nosocomial infections. Several studies show an association between decreased nosocomial infection rates and effective infection control programs. The most notable is the Study on the Efficacy of Nosocomial Infection Control (SENIC), a nationwide controlled trial that was performed by the CDC in the late 1970s. The SENIC documented a 32% decrease in nosocomial infection rates associated with specific components of surveillance and infection control programs, including an infection control practitioner for every 250 beds and a physician with expertise in infection control. Routine surveillance components of infection control programs have evolved with institutional needs. Previously, whole-house (i.e., total) nosocomial infection surveillance was done in many hospitals, but this no longer is considered practical or necessary in many settings.

Hospitals may select high-risk areas for surveillance based on their specific needs. This often includes intensive care units (ICUs) and other high-risk units that house immunocompromised patients and those with specific infections such as surgical wounds. A form of whole-house surveillance may be used by the infection control staff, who review the clinical microbiology reports to detect clusters of multiply resistant or other epidemiologically significant organisms. To obtain national data on nosocomial infections, the CDC established the National Nosocomial Infections Surveillance System (NNIS), a collaborative system that includes about 150 hospitals in the United States. The NNIS provides data for comparison rates for hospitals in the United States (even those outside the system) and is useful for identifying nationwide trends. Four surveillance components are used in this system: hospital-wide, ICU, high-risk nursery, and surgical patient.

The NNIS has incorporated device-associated infection rates to control for exposure to the principal risk factor for infection, and reports these rates in device days to control for the duration of hospitalization. For example, catheter-associated bloodstream infections are reported per 1,000 central catheter days and ventilator-associated pneumonias are reported per 1,000 ventilator days. Many hospitals outside the NNIS have begun to report infection rates in device days so that NNIS data can be used to generate comparison rates.

NOSOCOMIAL INFECTIONS

A nosocomial infection is defined as an infection that is not present or incubating at the time of admission to a health care facility. Although many infections that are detected more than 48 hours after hospital admission are nosocomial, diseases with longer incubation periods (e.g., viral exanthems, legionellosis, aspergillosis, hepatitis) often are recognized only after hospitalization. Several nationwide studies document the universality of nosocomial infections in health care institutions and suggest that about 5% of hospitalized patients will have at least one nosocomial infection. These infections contribute significantly to extended hospital stays. Hospital-acquired infectious complications result in 1 to 7 extra days of hospitalization and in $1,000 to $7,000 in extra charges per patient per infection. Astute hospital administrators have become interested in improving infection control programs to improve quality of care, increase cost savings, and meet risk management incentives.

NOSOCOMIAL PATHOGENS

The overall pathogen distribution for major sites of nosocomial infection reported to the NNIS from 1986 to 1989 is shown in Table 338.1. *Escherichia coli* is the most common pathogen because of the predominance of urinary tract infections, but other organisms are increased significantly from previous comparison periods. Enterococci are the second most common nosocomial pathogens overall. *Pseudomonas aeruginosa* and *Staphylococcus aureus* are the next most prevalent, followed by coagulase-negative staphylococci. Coagulase-negative staphylococci increased from 4% in 1980 to 9% from 1986 to 1989, primarily as causative agents of bloodstream infection. *Candida albicans* also increased in all major sites of infection from 2% in 1980 to 5% from 1986 to 1989. *Enterobacter* and *Klebsiella* species are some of the next most prevalent gram-negative nosocomial pathogens.

Trends in the epidemiology and antimicrobial resistance of these nosocomial pathogens are troubling. Most hospital isolates and many community isolates of *E. coli* are resistant to ampicillin. The enterococci have acquired numerous new mechanisms of resistance in the past decade, including high-level aminoglycoside resistance and vancomycin resistance. Vancomycin-resistant enterococci have been deemed the nosocomial pathogens of the decade, because these organisms usually are multiply resistant to alternative antibiotics and cause infection in seriously ill hospitalized patients. In addition, vancomycin-resistant enterococci can persistently colonize the gastrointestinal tract and become prevalent on environmental surfaces, allowing for ready cross-transmission in the hospital setting.

Methicillin-resistant *S. aureus* (MRSA) has increased in prevalence among all hospital *S. aureus* isolates from 2.4% in 1975 to 47% in 1998. Recent studies document that a significant percentage of MRSA isolates are present at the time of hospital admission, suggesting that MRSA is found in both the community and the hospital. In addition, DNA typing studies have documented the heterogeneity of MRSA isolates in both hospital and community isolates. Because of these changes in the epidemiology of MRSA, infection control programs using MRSA cases for surveillance must determine whether cases are nosocomial and must use a marker of strain identity, such as DNA typing, to determine whether cross-transmission actually is occurring. Emerging reports of vancomycin intermediate *S. aureus* (glycopeptide intermediate *S. aureus*; GISA) are of particular concern. Such isolates reported to date have also been methicillin-resistant, raising therapeutic dilemmas and justifying stringent control measures if these organisms are identified.

The prevalence of *C. albicans* in the hospital continues to increase, particularly in ICUs and among immunocompromised patients. Studies also have shown a worrisome increase in other species of *Candida*, some of which are intrinsically resistant to azoles or amphotericin B. Among *Enterobacter* species, resistance to third-generation cephalosporins has increased during the past decade, and many reports exist of the emergence of resistance on therapy with these agents. Extended-spectrum β-lactamases

TABLE 338.1. PATHOGEN DISTRIBUTION (PERCENTAGE) FOR MAJOR SITES OF NOSOCOMIAL INFECTIONS 1986–1989 NATIONAL NOSOCOMIAL INFECTIONS SURVEILLANCE SYSTEM

Pathogen	Urinary Tract Infection	Wound	Pneumonia	Bloodstream	Total
Escherichia coli	26[a]	10	6	6	16
Enterococci	16	13	2	8	12
Pseudomonas aeruginosa	12	8	17	4	11
Staphylococcus aureus	2	17	16	16	10
Coagulase-negative staphylococci	4	12	2	27	9
Enterobacter species	6	8	11	5	7
Klebsiella pneumoniae	6	3	7	4	5
Candida albicans	7	2	4	5	5
Proteus mirabilis	5	4	3	1	4
Streptococcal species	0	3	1	4	2
Citrobacter species	2	2	1	1	2
Candida species	2	0	1	3	2
Serratia marcescens	1	1	4	1	2

have emerged in *Klebsiella pneumoniae* and other Enterobacteriaciae, conferring resistance to broad-spectrum cephalosporins and other agents. Many of these evolving patterns of antimicrobial resistance in nosocomial pathogens represent a response to patterns of antimicrobial drug use in the hospital. The hospital epidemiology program is an important link to the hospital antibiotic use program.

NOSOCOMIAL PNEUMONIA

Nosocomial pneumonia is a substantial cause of morbidity and mortality and is the second most common nosocomial infection in US hospitals. It accounts for 15% to 24% of nosocomial infections overall with higher rates in the ICU, but it may be responsible for up to 60% of those that are fatal. Major patient risk factors include endotracheal intubation or mechanical ventilation, severe underlying disease, decreased mental status, cardiac or pulmonary disease, immunosuppression, thoracoabdominal surgery, and age over 70 years. Other risk factors are ventilator circuit changes every 24 hours, fall or winter season, stress ulcer prophylaxis with a histamine-2 (H_2) antagonist with or without an antacid, use of a nasogastric tube, and recent bronchoscopy. After stratifying the incidence density of ventilator-associated pneumonias by ventilator days, the NNIS reported that the median rate of ventilator-associated pneumonia ranged from 4.2 per 1,000 ventilator days in pediatric ICUs to 21.1 per 1,000 ventilator days in burn ICUs. Reported mortality rates include crude rates of 20% to 50% and attributable rates of 30%.

The diagnosis of nosocomial pneumonia is difficult, and the criteria used for surveillance have been based on clinical findings of fever, cough, and the development of purulent sputum in combination with a new or progressive infiltrate. Sputum cultures are nonspecific, especially in ventilated patients, but often are monitored in conjunction with clinical criteria to detect potentially cross-transmitted organisms. Blood or pleural fluid cultures are more specific, but are not sensitive methods of detection. Consensus recommendations for standardizing more specific methods of diagnosing pneumonia for clinical research studies include the use of bronchoscopic techniques, such as quantitative cultures of protected specimen brushings, bronchoalveolar lavage, and protected bronchoalveolar lavage. The reported sensitivity and specificity of these methods are 70% to 100% and 60% to 100%, respectively. These techniques are invasive and are not used routinely in all institutions; many institutions still rely on clinical criteria for the surveillance of nosocomial pneumonia.

The microbial causes of nosocomial pneumonia vary somewhat, depending on the diagnostic method used. Most documented organisms are aerobic bacteria, but anaerobic and viral cultures are not done routinely. Using clinical criteria, enteric gram-negative bacilli (e.g., *Enterobacter* species, *Klebsiella pneumoniae*, *E. coli*) account for most cases. *S. aureus*, particularly MRSA, and *P. aeruginosa* also are important causes. In addition, *Streptococcus pneumoniae* and *Haemophilus influenzae* are recognized as significant isolates. In studies using bronchoscopic criteria for diagnosis, enteric gram-negative bacilli are less common,

and *S. aureus, S. pneumoniae,* and *H. influenzae* are more common.

Control measures are difficult to assess because many risk factors are related to the severity of the patient's illness. Gastric bacterial overgrowth resulting from antacids or H_2 antagonists given as prophylaxis against stress gastritis has been implicated as a preventable risk factor. Sucralfate has been studied as a substitute because it has a cytoprotective effect on the gastric mucosa without affecting gastric pH. However, clinical trials comparing the two regimens have produced variable results. In most studies, mechanically ventilated patients in the ICU who are given antacids with or without H_2 blockers have increased gastric pH, high gastric bacterial counts, and an increased risk of pneumonia compared with patients who are given sucralfate. Meta-analyses of several studies and a study comparing ranitidine with sucralfate have not shown a significant difference.

Selective decontamination of the digestive tract also has been studied as a way of decreasing oropharyngeal and gastric bacterial colonization, and the incidence of lower respiratory tract infections in the ICU. A combination of a nonabsorbable antimicrobial agent (i.e., polymyxin, an aminoglycoside, quinolone) and nystatin or amphotericin B is administered locally to the oropharynx and orally or by nasogastric tube. In many studies, a systemic antibiotic such as cefotaxime or trimethoprim also is administered intravenously. Although most studies have demonstrated reduced rates of nosocomial pneumonia, study designs and patient populations have varied and follow-up periods have been short.

The diagnosis of pneumonia is based on clinical criteria in most studies. In addition, two large trials have demonstrated no benefit with selective decontamination of the digestive tract. An extensive meta-analysis shows this technique to be expensive and to have only an equivocal effect on patient mortality. Further, there are significant concerns regarding the development of antibiotic-resistant bacteria with these regimens. Selective decontamination of the digestive tract is not recommended for routine use in all patients in the ICU, but may be beneficial in certain high-risk subsets such as patients with severe immunosuppression.

Routine measures such as elevating the head of the bed and withholding enteral feedings when there is gastric residue are recommended to minimize aspiration. Devices used in the respiratory tract, particularly in mechanically ventilated patients, may be a reservoir for nosocomial pathogens. Proper cleaning and disinfection or sterilization of reusable respiratory equipment is important. The use of an aseptic technique during suctioning and proper maintenance of the ventilator circuit also are recommended. In many hospitals, ventilator circuit condensate is emptied periodically. Another option is to use a heat–moisture exchanger within the ventilator circuit that eliminates condensate formation. Earlier studies showed that ventilator circuit changes every 48 hours were advantageous compared with changes every 24 hours. More recent studies have shown no increase in the rate of ventilator-associated pneumonia when the interval for circuit changes is longer than 48 hours. CDC recommendations call for ventilator circuit changes every 48 hours or more. The maximum time a circuit may be left unchanged is unknown.

NOSOCOMIAL LEGIONNAIRES' DISEASE

Because the environment is the reservoir for infections caused by *Legionella* species, a nosocomial case of legionellosis warrants further investigation to prevent such infections in other patients. The mortality rate of patients with nosocomial *Legionella* pneumonia is twice that of patients with community-acquired disease, probably because of the increased severity of illness in hospitalized patients. To determine whether a case is nosocomial, the incubation period of 2 to 10 days for legionnaires' disease must be considered. By CDC guidelines, a case of laboratory-confirmed legionellosis occurring in a patient who has been hospitalized at least 10 days before the onset of illness is a definite nosocomial case of legionnaires' disease. A case of laboratory-confirmed infection occurring 2 to 10 days after hospitalization is a possible nosocomial case. The inhalation or aspiration of water contaminated with *Legionella* species is thought to be the major mode of entry of these organisms into the respiratory tract. In early hospital outbreaks, suspected environmental sources were cooling towers, showers, room air humidifiers, and respiratory therapy equipment. More recent investigations identify contaminated potable water supplies as significant reservoirs.

The diagnosis of *Legionella* pneumonia requires laboratory confirmation by one of the following methods: culture isolation from a respiratory specimen, visualization by immunofluorescent microscopy from a respiratory specimen, detection of *Legionella* urinary antigen on radioimmunoassay, or a fourfold rise in antibody titer to 1:128 or higher on an indirect immunofluorescent antibody test.

Prevention and control strategies vary by institution and depend on the identification of nosocomial cases, the immunologic status of the patients, the design and construction of the facility, and the available resources. One approach is routine, periodic culturing of the hospital's potable water supply for *Legionella* species. When a threshold level of 30% of samples are positive, decontamination of the water supply is undertaken, and active laboratory surveillance of cases begins. Advantages of this approach are that active surveillance of patient cases is driven by environmental surveillance, and infrequent periodic environmental sampling may be less expensive than routine laboratory testing for *Legionella*. Uncertainties of this approach include the unclear relation between water culture results and the risk of legionellosis in an institution without detected cases. *Legionella* occurs commonly in water systems, including those of hospitals, without causing disease.

A second approach is to maintain a high index of suspicion in patients at risk for the disease, particularly if a nosocomial pneumonia is unresponsive to routine empiric antibiotic therapy. Epidemiologic investigation is initiated for one laboratory-confirmed definite nosocomial case or for two laboratory-confirmed possible cases. The advantage of this approach is that environmental and epidemiologic investigation is problem-focused. The disadvantage is that cases may be missed if an index of suspicion is not maintained and laboratory diagnoses are not made.

Decontamination of the hospital's potable water supply is a formidable task. Options include superheating, pulse thermal disinfection (flushing the system for several minutes with water at 65° C or higher), and hyperchlorination (flushing the system with water containing at least 10 mg per liter of free residual chlorine). All these methods are difficult and expensive and should be considered in collaboration with the engineering department. Physical cleaning of water storage tanks, water heaters, faucets, and showerheads also may be required. For patients with severe immunosuppression, such as bone marrow transplant recipients, a combination of sterile water for ingestion or systemic decontamination and point-of-use decontamination (i.e., filtration or ultraviolet treatment) may be considered.

NOSOCOMIAL ASPERGILLOSIS

Nosocomial aspergillosis also is associated with environmental reservoirs and is a particular problem for immunocompromised patients. Those at highest risk include patients with bone marrow transplants or hematologic malignancies. However, *Aspergillus* infection also occurs in patients with solid organ transplants, corticosteroid regimens, AIDS, and no apparent immunodeficiency. Pulmonary infection results from the inhalation of *Aspergillus* fungal spores.

Outbreaks have been associated with hospital renovation, contaminated ventilation systems, and high airborne fungal spore counts. The diagnosis of *Aspergillus* pneumonia is difficult without an invasive procedure and often is presumptive. Although bronchoalveolar lavage is useful, transbronchial biopsy is the most reliable means of diagnosis. The isolation of *Aspergillus* species may represent colonization or contamination in many samples from patients with intact immune systems, but positive cultures for *Aspergillus* in immunocompromised (particularly granulocytopenic) patients must be considered significant.

Preventive measures are directed toward those at highest risk, including bone marrow transplant recipients and other severely immunocompromised patients. Patient care areas designed for these patients should include high-efficiency particulate filtration systems that are 99.97% efficient for the filtration of particles measuring 0.3 μm or larger, directed air flow, positive-pressure rooms, and high rates of room air exchange (at least 15 air changes per hour).

VIRAL PNEUMONIAS

Nosocomial outbreaks of viral respiratory diseases usually are associated with respiratory diseases in the community. Respiratory syncytial virus is a problem in the hospital during its peak season, because it spreads readily among patients and health care workers. Although infants and young children are affected most commonly, the disease can occur in adults. The diagnosis is based on laboratory evaluation by culture or antigen detection. Respiratory droplets are the mode of spread, with contaminated hands of health care workers or fomites serving as vectors of transmission. A combination of cohorting, contact isolation, emphasis on compliance with control measures, limitation of visitors, and the temporary exclusion of health care workers with respiratory diseases has contributed to successful control in hospital outbreaks of respiratory syncytial virus.

Influenza viruses also are seasonal and pose a significant threat to hospitalized immunocompromised patients. Cohorting and contact isolation can be used to control outbreaks. Antiviral therapy or prophylaxis with amantadine hydrochloride or rimantadine can be used for influenza A, but not influenza B. Routine seasonal vaccination should be emphasized each year for high-risk patients and the health care workers who care for them.

CATHETER-RELATED BLOODSTREAM INFECTIONS

Catheter-related (or primary) bloodstream infections are a major cause of high costs and long stays in the hospital and of morbidity and mortality. According to CDC NNIS data, they account for 8% of all nosocomial infections. Significant increases in these infections were observed during the past decade in every type of hospital monitored by the NNIS (small nonteaching, small teaching, large nonteaching, and large teaching). The increases resulted largely from the following pathogens: coagulase-negative staphylococci, *S. aureus,* enterococci, and *Candida* species. The rate of bloodstream infections caused by gram-negative bacilli was the same in all types of hospitals. Although the rate of nosocomial secondary bacteremia (caused by urinary tract infection, surgical site infection, and pneumonia) has remained the same over the past decade, the rate of nosocomial primary bacteremia (primarily caused by intravascular devices) has doubled.

Short-term, noncuffed central venous catheters (CVCs) are associated with the highest rates of bacteremia, ranging from 1% to 10%. Peripheral intravenous catheters, arterial catheters, and long-term catheters are associated with substantially lower rates of infection (Table 338.2). The highest rates of CVC septicemia are associated with hemodialysis catheters, and the lowest with subcutaneous central venous ports.

Definitions of catheter-related infections vary, complicating surveillance for these nosocomial infections and making comparison of various clinical studies difficult. Local catheter infections include exit or insertion site infections, tunnel infections, and significant catheter colonizations. Using a semiquantitative roll-plate culture technique, Maki and colleagues showed a correlation between the recovery of 15 or more colony-forming units from a catheter tip and inflammation of the catheter site. For routine nosocomial infection surveillance of primary catheter-related bacteremias, many institutions use the definitions provided in the CDC guidelines. Most infections detected by this method have positive blood cultures or signs of infection at the catheter site, evidence of clinical sepsis, and 15 or more colony-forming units recovered from an intravascular catheter tip using the semiquantitative method. The CDC Guidelines for Nosocomial Infections should be consulted for specific criteria.

Definitions of systemic catheter-related bacteremias are more rigorous in some research studies. Many hospitals report rates of catheter-related bacteremias in terms of device days (number of infections per 1,000 central catheter days), as suggested by the CDC. According to NNIS data, these rates range from 5 to 10 per 1,000 central-line days, depending on the type of ICU monitored.

Quantitative catheter culture techniques have proved useful in differentiating colonization from infection. In addition, quantitative blood cultures have been used to identify sepsis associated with a central line. In this technique, quantitative blood cultures are drawn simultaneously through the central catheter and a peripheral vein. Sepsis associated with a CVC is suggested by a differential colony count of 10:1 when the central catheter specimen is compared with the peripheral vein specimen.

TABLE 338.2.	APPROXIMATE RISKS OF SEPTICEMIA ASSOCIATED WITH INTRAVASCULAR ACCESS DEVICES		
Type of Device	**Representative Rate**	**Range**	
Short-Term Temporary Access (Number of Septicemias Per 100 Devices)			
Peripheral IV cannulas			
Winged steel needles	<0.2	0–1	
Peripheral IV catheters			
Percutaneously inserted	0.2	0–1	
Cutdown	6	—	
Arterial catheters	1	0–1	
Central venous catheters			
All-purpose, multilumen	3	1–7	
Swan–Ganz	1	0–5	
Hemodialysis	10	3–18	
Long-Term Indefinite Access (Number of Septicemias Per 100 Devices-Days)			
Peripherally inserted central venous catheters	0.20	—	
Cuffed central catheters (e.g., Hickman, Broviac)	0.20	0.10–0.53	
Subcutaneous central venous ports (e.g., Infuse-A-Port, Port-A-Cath)	0.04	0.00–.10	

Adapted from Maki DG. Infections due to infusion therapy. In Bennett JV, Brachman PS (eds): Hospital infections. Third ed. Boston: Little, Brown, 1992.

The pathogenesis of catheter-related infections is important in the selection and implementation of preventive measures. The skin insertion site and the catheter hub are thought to be the most important initial sources of infecting pathogens. It is hypothesized that skin flora, such as coagulase-negative staphylococci and *S. aureus,* migrate from the skin insertion site to the catheter tip, resulting in catheter colonization and infection. In addition, pathogens introduced into the catheter hub by health care workers can migrate internally along the catheter, resulting in bloodstream infection. Decreasing the colonization of pathogens at the skin insertion site and interrupting the migration of microorganisms along the catheter are important preventive measures. Hematogenous seeding of the central catheter from a secondary site, such as the urinary tract, has been suggested but appears to be uncommon. Episodes of bacteremia related to contaminated infusate may appear as local or regional epidemics. In addition, these bacteremias usually are caused by gram-negative bacilli (*Serratia, Enterobacter, Citrobacter,* and *Pseudomonas* species other than *P. aeruginosa*).

Proposed risk factors for catheter-related infections include catheter location, use of aseptic technique during insertion or maintenance of the line, number of catheter lumina, number of catheter manipulations, type of catheter dressing, and contamination or lack of effectiveness of antiseptic solutions. Short-term CVCs present a greater risk for infection than do peripheral or tunneled CVCs. In addition, some studies suggest that internal jugular CVCs have higher rates of infection than do subclavian CVCs, although other studies have produced contradictory evidence. Several investigations have documented higher rates of infection with triple-lumen compared with single-lumen CVCs, whereas others have found no significant differences. Certain types of impermeable transparent dressings have proved to be risk factors compared with gauze dressings. However, newer transparent dressings with greater permeability and less moisture retention are under evaluation and appear promising. The number of catheter manipulations appears to be important, particularly with Swan–Ganz catheters. Prolonged catheterization also is a well-documented risk factor for certain types of CVCs. The risk of infection increases at 72 hours with peripheral venous catheters and at 96 hours with Swan–Ganz and peripheral arterial catheters. Many institutions have policies limiting the amount of time these catheters can be used, but few agree on the optimal duration of use for short-term CVCs because infection rates related to length of placement have varied among studies based on institution-specific factors. Most investigators believe that signs of infection warrant the removal of short-term CVCs. Exchanging CVCs over guide wires is a controversial practice because some investigators have documented colonization of the new CVCs with pathogens from the previous CVCs.

Several protective factors have been documented to help prevent catheter-related infections. Placement and maintenance of peripheral and central catheters by infusion therapy teams have been associated with significantly lower rates of infection in many studies. An aseptic technique incorporating maximal sterile barriers for the insertion of CVCs has been documented by Raad and associates to decrease infection rates. Maki and colleagues also have demonstrated the superiority of chlorhexidine gluconate for antisepsis at the skin insertion site compared

with 70% alcohol and 10% povidone-iodine. The rate of catheter-related bacteremia is about four times lower with chlorhexidine gluconate antisepsis than with the other two agents. An attachable silver-impregnated cuff that prevents the migration of pathogens on the surface of the catheter has been shown to reduce short-term CVC bacteremia but has not been as helpful for long-term tunneled catheters.

■ SURGICAL SITE INFECTIONS

Surgical wound surveillance is a routine part of nosocomial infection surveillance at many hospitals, and several large studies have shown that sharing such data with surgeons helps reduce infection rates. National infection control organizations such as SHEA and APIC recommend surgical wound infection surveillance, and the Joint Commission for Accreditation of Healthcare Organizations has proposed that it be made a mandatory practice. Definitions for surgical site infections vary, but most institutions use those established by the CDC. The CDC definitions were modified in 1992, and the term was changed from *surgical wound infection* to *surgical site infection.* The changes were made so that the anatomical site of a deep infection could be specified and because the word "wound" connoted only the incision from the skin to the deep soft tissues, whereas a postoperative infection may involve an organ or space other than the incision that is opened or manipulated during the operative procedure. Surgical site infections are divided into superficial incisional surgical site infections, deep incisional surgical site infections, and organ/space surgical site infections. To be classified as a surgical site infection, the infection must occur within 30 days of the operative procedure if no implant is in place or within 1 year if an implant is in place. Postdischarge surveillance (a method of detecting surgical site infections after hospital discharge) is an important component of surgical site infection surveillance programs now that hospital stays are becoming shorter. The confidential and timely reporting of specialty-specific wound rates and surgeon-specific wound rates is endorsed by the Surgical Infection Society and recommended by a consensus panel with representatives from the Surgical Infection Society, SHEA, APIC, and CDC.

Surgeons and nurses have been classifying surgical wounds in the operating room for 30 years, ever since the National Research Council study on surgical wounds that introduced the use of four wound classes. The National Research Council classification is based on the risk level and type of contamination that are expected or observed at the time of operation. A surgical wound classified as clean (class I) is one in which only exogenous, airborne contamination is expected; the predicted wound infection rate is 2% or less; and anticipated pathogens are primarily gram-positive organisms such as *S. aureus.* Clean-contaminated wounds (class II) are those in which endogenous and exogenous contamination is anticipated or observed. These infections usually are caused by polymicrobial endogenous (aerobic and anaerobic) flora and occur at a predicted rate of 5% to 15%. Wounds are classified as contaminated (class III) when early endogenous leakage or delayed exogenous contamination occurs without a clinical infection at the time of surgery. These wounds are associated with a 15% or higher infection rate. Dirty (class IV) wounds are those in which active infection is present in the operating field at the time of surgery, and postoperative infection rates are high (30% or higher).

In the 1980s, problems were identified with this wound classification system because of differences in the risk of infection and the severity of illness among patients in each wound class. There are recognized host and operative risk factors for surgical wound infection. Host risk factors include obesity, infection at other sites, diabetes mellitus, malnutrition, immunosuppressant therapy, American Society of Anesthesiology class higher than 3, and severity of illness. Operative risk factors include prolonged duration of surgery, surgical wound class, emergency surgery, lack of surgical experience or skill, low procedure volume, tissue trauma, prolonged hospital stay, timing of preoperative shaving, intraoperative microbial contamination, surgical wound class, lack of prophylactic antibiotics, and number of persons in the operating room. A composite risk index for predicting surgical site infections more accurately than the National Research Council classification has been sought. The SENIC proposed that patients be stratified according to the number of discharge diagnoses, presence of abdominal surgery, duration of surgery, and wound class. However, the use of discharge diagnoses as criteria made the SENIC index difficult to use for timely analysis. A CDC NNIS risk index that stratifies patients by the American Society of Anesthesiology score, surgical wound class, and duration of surgery (specific to type of surgery) is easier to use and is being assessed in the NNIS program.

URINARY TRACT INFECTIONS

Catheter-associated urinary tract infections are the most common nosocomial infections, accounting for about 40% of all cases. The pathogenesis of these infections is the migration of pathogens into the catheterized urinary tract by the periurethral route in women and the intraluminal route in men. *E. coli* is the most common pathogen, followed by enterococci, *P. aeruginosa,* and enteric gram-negative bacilli. Studies consistently reveal four independently significant risk factors for catheter-associated urinary tract infections: female gender, absence of systemic antibiotics, duration of catheterization, and violations in catheter care and drainage. Systemic antimicrobial agents have been shown to decrease the risk of urinary tract infection during the first 4 to 5 days of catheterization. However, their routine use is precluded by concern over antimicrobial resistance, superinfection with pathogens such as enterococci and *Candida,* cost, and potential adverse drug reactions. These antibiotics may be helpful in high-risk patients who require short-term catheterization. Catheters coated with silver ions have not been consistently effective in reducing bacteriuria. Likewise, catheter bag decontamination can be accomplished with various agents (e.g., hydrogen peroxide, iodophors, chlorhexidine) but does not decrease urinary tract infection rates, suggesting that the bag rarely is the source of infection. Disconnection of catheter junctions and other errors in catheter care are common and have been identified as risk factors, necessitating ongoing staff education regard-

ing catheter care. Sealed junctions have been proposed as an alternative approach.

GASTROINTESTINAL INFECTIONS

Routine microbiologic surveillance of enteric pathogens is worthwhile to facilitate the early detection of potential outbreaks of enteric pathogens. Nosocomial outbreaks of *Salmonella* species have been well documented and are common in health care institutions. These outbreaks usually derive from index cases that are acquired in the community, then cross-transmitted in the hospital, particularly on the pediatric ward. Cross-transmission usually results from transient hand carriage by health care personnel. Occasionally, however, personnel become colonized in the gastrointestinal tract. In some cases, health care workers have acquired infection in the community and become chronic carriers of *Salmonella* species. Many states have public health laws that prohibit health care workers who carry *Salmonella* from having direct patient contact. In addition, food-borne outbreaks are relatively uncommon in health care institutions, but food workers who carry *Salmonella* usually are restricted from food preparation. Hospital employees who have stool cultures that are positive for *Salmonella* should undergo serial cultures every 1 to 2 months or until they are established as chronic carriers (i.e., cultures are positive for more than 1 year). State law may forbid certain personnel such as food workers from returning to work until their culture results are negative. If epidemiologic evidence implicates a chronic carrier as the source of an outbreak, the worker should be removed from the site until carriage is eliminated or should be reassigned to a low-risk area. Personnel with acute disease should be restricted from patient care and personnel contact until they are asymptomatic. *Shigella* infections also can be transmitted in the institutional setting, but are less common than *Salmonella* infections. Outbreaks of *E. coli* O157:H7 have been reported in extended-care facilities and should be suspected and ruled out in investigations of diarrhea in this setting. Nosocomial transmission of diarrhea caused by rotavirus has been reported on numerous occasions, primarily on pediatric, maternity, and geriatric wards. Transmission is difficult to prevent because viral shedding can occur and persist for long periods in asymptomatic personnel and immunocompromised patients. Cohorting of patients and personnel is useful in controlling such outbreaks.

For all patients with enteric pathogens, barrier precautions should be used for contact with feces and other body fluids and secretions. Because such precautions are now standard for all patients in most institutions, the previously used CDC isolation category of "Enteric Precautions" is superfluous, but standard precautions should be reviewed and emphasized with hospital staff when an enteric pathogen is identified on a unit. If patient compliance or hygiene is poor, a private room may be required for management.

The nosocomial transmission of *Clostridium difficile* has been well documented and presents a difficult problem. Although the use of systemic antibiotics may select for *C. difficile* colitis, cross-transmission related to environmental reservoirs and transient hand carriage has been documented with molecular typing techniques. High-level disinfection with 2% glutaraldehyde for appropriate intervals is performed routinely for semicritical equipment, such as endoscopes, and reduces the possibility of transmission by this route. However, this spore-forming organism survives readily on environmental surfaces in affected patients' rooms and serves as a persistent reservoir for hand carriage by transient personnel. Surveillance for *C. difficile* toxin titers may be helpful in determining whether a cluster of patients with *C. difficile* colitis occurs on a specific ward or unit, suggesting potential cross-transmission of this pathogen. In these instances, contact precautions, with particular regard to environmental cleaning or special organism isolation, may be helpful in controlling transmission. Daily environmental cleaning of horizontal surfaces in proximity to affected patients using hospital-grade disinfectants may limit the endemicity of this organism. In addition, barrier precautions and hand-washing measures must be reemphasized to personnel.

OUTBREAK INVESTIGATION

Effective surveillance methods should lead to the early identification of increased rates or outbreaks of problem nosocomial infections or organisms. The primary objective of outbreak investigation is to identify ways of preventing further transmission of or exposure to the disease-causing agent. In the investigation of any outbreak or cluster, the principles of epidemic investigation apply. The first question to be answered is whether an epidemic is occurring. An *epidemic* is an increase in the number of cases compared with past experience for a given population, time, and place. To answer this question, the previous endemic, baseline rate of the problem must be known. This can be determined easily for infections or microorganisms that are surveyed routinely. For other identified problems, computerized laboratory records or discharge diagnoses may be required to establish previous rates. A timeline of cases and statistical determination of whether the perceived increase is significant is warranted at this stage. For specific pathogens, laboratory typing methods are critical. If DNA typing techniques are available in a timely fashion, these should be used early. For instance, if DNA typing techniques suggest that the isolates in question are distinct strains, further epidemiologic investigation may not be warranted. Likewise, if a common strain is documented, epidemiologic investigation should proceed.

When a problem is documented, several steps should be taken immediately (Table 338.3). During the first 24 hours, the extent of the outbreak should be determined, the cause should be identified if possible, persons at risk should be recognized, and the key clinical and epidemiologic features of the cases should be described. For pathogens that are identified and the mode of spread known, appropriate isolation precautions should be used and hospital staff should be educated regarding the situation and intervention measures. The laboratory should be notified and asked to save any relevant isolates or clinical specimens. Data on environmental samples should be obtained if pertinent. The investigative team should be organized, including the hospital epidemiologist, the infection control staff, clinicians, the lab-

TABLE 338.3.	INITIAL STEPS IN OUTBREAK INVESTIGATION

Is It An Outbreak?

Assess previous rate of problem
Use laboratory typing to determine strain identity

Initial Steps

Make a timeline
Define cases
Identify key clinical and epidemiologic features
Institute isolation precautions if appropriate
Notify laboratory and ask them to save isolates
Organize investigative team
Depending on extent and seriousness:
    Arrange for public relations
    Notify local and state health departments, and the Centers for Disease Control and Prevention

oratory, and, possibly, an environmentalist. Depending on the extent and seriousness of the outbreak, public relations must be arranged. Additional help should be requested if needed from local and state health departments and the CDC.

Existing data should be assessed and a case definition developed. The potential mode of transmission, incubation period, and common denominators or unusual exceptions among the cases must be determined. The outbreak should be characterized by time, place, and patient. Case-control study methods commonly are used at this point in hospital outbreak investigations to identify specific risk factors that can be modified or prevented. A hypothesis should be formulated regarding the source of infection and method of spread, and control measures such as vaccines or prophylaxis should be instituted, if relevant. The hypothesis should be tested using the case-control study and relevant laboratory investigations such as DNA typing of further isolates or serologic tests. Finally, a report documenting the investigation, interventions, outcome, and plans for future surveillance and prevention should be written and documented with the institution's infection control committee or quality improvement committee. Such feedback also should be given directly to the wards or units involved in the outbreak.

ISOLATION PRECAUTIONS

The CDC first published isolation guidelines in 1970, and substantial changes were made in the 1983 CDC Guidelines for Isolation Precautions in Hospitals. Category-specific isolation was simplified to include contact isolation, tuberculosis isolation, drainage/secretion precautions, and blood/body fluid precautions. Disease-specific isolation also was offered as an alternative for hospitals that wanted to direct precautions at specific, identified diseases. Recognition of the AIDS epidemic drastically affected precautions in all United States health care institutions. The 1987 CDC document, "Recommendations for Prevention of HIV Transmission in Health Care Settings," outlined blood and body fluid precautions for all patients. Barrier precautions were recommended for blood, certain body fluids, and body fluids containing blood.

The application of blood and body fluid precautions to all patients was referred to as *universal blood and body fluid precautions* or *universal precautions*. In 1988, the CDC published an update, "Universal Precautions for Prevention of Transmission of Human Immunodeficiency Virus, Hepatitis B Virus, and Other Bloodborne Pathogens in Health Care Settings." This document clarified that the potential transmission of blood-borne pathogens other than the human immunodeficiency virus, such as hepatitis B, also should be prevented. Category- or disease-specific guidelines were recommended for dealing with non–blood-borne pathogens. The Occupational Safety and Health Administration became involved in the regulation and enforcement of these guidelines. Many infection control programs recognized the need to reduce the transmission of non–blood-borne pathogens because CDC-defined universal precautions were directed primarily at blood-borne pathogens. A system of "Body Substance Isolation" previously had been introduced by Jackson and Lynch to control the transmission of non–blood-borne pathogens. This system designated all body fluids and tissue as potentially infectious and provided an alternative to the category- and disease-specific system. Confusion ensued in many institutions because the term "universal precautions" was used to apply to barrier precautions for all body fluids, not just blood and certain body fluid, as originally defined.

STANDARD PRECAUTIONS

CDC isolation guidelines underwent revision by the CDC's Hospital Infection Control Practices Advisory Committee and were published in 1996. The guidelines contain two levels of precautions. The first is termed *standard precautions* and combines the major features of universal precautions and body substance isolation. These precautions apply to all patients, regardless of disease or known infection status. Standard precautions apply to blood; all body fluids, secretions, and excretions, regardless of whether they contain visible blood; nonintact skin; and mucous membranes. This first level of precautions decreases the risk of transmission from recognized or unrecognized infection.

TRANSMISSION-BASED PRECAUTIONS

The second level of precautions apply to patients with documented or suspected transmissible or epidemiologically significant pathogens that require more than standard precautions to prevent cross-transmission. Transmission-based precautions are of three types: airborne precautions, droplet precautions, and contact precautions. These can be combined for diseases that have several routes of transmission. Each type is used in addition to standard precautions. The previous category-specific types of isolation (strict isolation, contact isolation, respiratory isolation, tuberculosis isolation, enteric precautions, and drainage/secretion precautions) and disease-specific isolation precautions have been combined into the three types of transmission-based precautions. As with previous guidelines, the CDC acknowledges that no guidelines address every hospital's needs. Hospitals are encouraged to review the guidelines and to modify them as necessary.

AIRBORNE PRECAUTIONS

Airborne precautions are designed to decrease the risk of transmitting infection by the airborne route, through airborne droplet nuclei (measuring 5 μm or less) or dust particles containing the infectious agent. Organisms that are transmissible by this route can be dispersed widely by air currents. Diseases in this category include varicella, measles, and tuberculosis. Patients should be kept in private rooms with monitored negative airflow, a minimum of six air changes per hour, and exhaust that is directed outside or to a high-efficiency particulate air filtration system. Doors should be kept closed. Patients should leave their rooms wearing masks and for necessary purposes only. Respiratory protection should be worn for patients with known or suspected tuberculosis according to current guidelines. The type of mask or respirator that should be worn for tuberculosis protection is controversial. Persons who are susceptible to measles or varicella (chickenpox or disseminated varicella) should not enter the rooms of patients who have these infections.

DROPLET PRECAUTIONS

Droplet transmission occurs when the mucous membranes of the nose, mouth, or conjunctivae of susceptible persons come in contact with large particle droplets (measuring more than 5 μm) from individuals colonized or infected with the infectious agent. Transmission through large-droplet nuclei differs from airborne transmission in that it requires close contact between sources and recipients, because droplet nuclei do not remain suspended in the air and usually travel only short distances. Some diseases that require droplet precautions are meningococcal meningitis, multiply drug-resistant pneumococcal meningitis or pneumonia, pertussis, streptococcal pharyngitis or pneumonia, influenza, and parvovirus B19 (with aplastic crisis or chronic infection). Patients should be placed in private rooms. If this is not possible, cohorting may be done with patients who have active infections with the same microorganisms but no other infections. If private rooms or cohorting are not available, spatial separation of at least 3 feet between infected patients and other patients is suggested. Patients should leave their rooms only when necessary and should wear masks.

CONTACT PRECAUTIONS

Contact precautions are used for patients who are known or suspected to harbor epidemiologically significant microorganisms that are transmitted by direct patient contact (by hand or skin contact that occurs during routine patient care or indirect contact [touching] of environmental surfaces). Patients should be placed in private rooms when possible. If this is not feasible, cohorting is recommended. If neither private rooms nor cohorting is possible, the epidemiology of the organism must be considered and infection control professionals consulted. Gloves should be used as a barrier against contact with blood and body substances, as in standard precautions. In addition, gloves should be changed after contact with infective material carrying high concentrations of microorganisms (i.e., feces, wound drainage), as in contact precautions. Gloves should be removed before leaving patients' rooms and hands should be washed using antiseptic solution. Clean, nonsterile gowns should be worn if substantial patient contact is anticipated.

Diseases for which contact precautions are recommended include infection or colonization with multiply drug-resistant bacteria; *C. difficile* colitis; respiratory syncytial virus in children; skin infections caused by scabies, impetigo, or herpes zoster (disseminated); and viral hemorrhagic fevers (Lassa fever or Marburg virus). Disseminated varicella is an example of an infection that requires two transmission-based precautions—airborne and contact.

Vancomycin-resistant enterococci have emerged and are prevalent in many areas. Patients colonized or infected with these organisms are cared for according to contact precautions in some institutions. Guidelines for preventing the transmission of vancomycin-resistant enterococci have been published by the CDC and emphasize the use of contact precautions and designated patient equipment or careful disinfection between patients. In addition, a multidisciplinary approach to controlling this organism is recommended, including appropriate vancomycin use. Because the guidelines are in transition, some have found it helpful to use a category of *special organism isolation*. This may be used for multiply resistant organisms, including some vancomycin-resistant *Enterococcus faecium, Acinetobacter anitratus,* and epidemiologically significant organisms such as *C. difficile.* The policy includes barrier precautions for all contact with the patient, the bedside equipment, and the patient's immediate environment. Special emphasis is placed on environmental control measures, such as designating individual rather than shared equipment and carefully cleaning the environment, because these are important with organisms such as vancomycin-resistant enterococci and *C. difficile.*

THE NEW HOSPITAL EPIDEMIOLOGY: EXPANSION TO OTHER INTERESTS

Infection control and classic hospital epidemiology techniques have served as an early model for the quality improvement process in hospitals. The field of hospital epidemiology has expanded to health care epidemiology. Epidemiologic methods and hospital epidemiologists now evaluate noninfectious quality of care issues using the same principles: surveillance, prevention, and control. This time-tested methodology, enhanced in the computer age and exercised by personnel with experience in the field, will lead to continued improvement in all areas of health care delivery and efficiency.

BIBLIOGRAPHY

Bennett JV, Brachman PS, eds. *Hospital infections,* third ed. Boston: Little, Brown, 1992.
Centers for Disease Control and Prevention. National Nosocomial Infections Surveillance (NNIS) report, data summary from October 1986–April 1998. Issued June 1998. http://www.cdc.gov/ncidod/hip/NNIS/sar98net.PDF
Garner JS, Hospital Infection Control Practices Advisory Committee (HICPAC). Guideline for isolation precautions in hospitals. *Infect Control Hosp Epidemiol* 1996;17:53–80; and *Am J Infect Control* 1996;24:24–52.
Garner JS, Jarvis WR, Emorl TG, et al. CDC definitions for nosocomial infections. *Am J Infect Control* 1988;16:128–140.
HICPAC. Guideline for prevention of nosocomial pneumonia. *Respir Care* 1994;39:1191–1236.
HICPAC. Recommendations for preventing the spread of vancomycin resistance. *Am J Infect Control* 1995;23:87–94.
Kelsey JL, Thompson WD, Evans AS, eds. *Epidemic investigation: methods in observational epidemiology.* New York: Oxford University Press, 1986.
Maki DG. Infections due to infusion therapy. In: Bennett JV, Brachman PS, eds. *Hospital infections,* third ed. Boston: Little, Brown, 1992.
National Nosocomial Infections Surveillance (NNIS) System. Nosocomial infection rates for interhospital comparison: limitations and possible solutions. *Infect Control Hosp Epidemiol* 1991;12:609–621.
Pearson ML, HICPAC. Guideline for the prevention of intravascular device-related infections. *Am J Infect Control* 1996;24:262–293.
Proceedings of the Third Decennial International Conference on Nosocomial Infections. *Am J Med* 1991;91:1S–333S.
Raad II, Hohn DC, Gilbreath BJ, et al. Prevention of central venous catheter-related infections by using maximal sterile barrier precautions during insertion. *Infect Control Hosp Epidemiol* 1994;15:231–238.
Wenzel RP, ed. *Prevention and control of nosocomial infections,* second ed. Baltimore: Williams & Wilkins, 1993.

APPROACH TO THE PATIENT
WITH HIV INFECTION

C H A P T E R
339

APPROACH TO THE PATIENT
WITH HIV EXPOSURE

ELISE M. JOCHIMSEN
DENISE M. CARDO

■ PRESENTATION

The most reliable estimates for the risk of human immunodeficiency virus (HIV) transmission after a single exposure are from occupational exposures involving health care workers (HCWs) studied prospectively after exposure. Such studies have estimated that the risk of HIV infection after a single occupational percutaneous exposure to HIV-infected blood is approximately 0.3% and after a mucous membrane exposure 0.09%. The risk of transmission after skin exposures, while not precisely quantified, is believed to be even smaller. The risk of transmission after a nonoccupational exposure has been more difficult to estimate, due in part to difficulties in determining the time, source, nature, and frequency of exposures. However, available data suggest that the per-episode risk is within the same order of magnitude as that associated with percutaneous exposure.

It must be emphasized that these estimates are averages and may be affected by a variety of factors. For example, a retrospective case–control study found that HCWs who sustained a percutaneous exposure to HIV-infected blood were more likely to become infected if they were exposed to a larger quantity of blood (deep injury, device visibly contaminated with blood, or device previously placed in the patient's vein or artery). In addition, transmission of HIV also was associated with injuries in which the source patient was terminally ill with AIDS. Several risk factors for sexual transmission have been identified, including genital ulcer disease and other coexisting sexually transmitted diseases.

■ PATHOPHYSIOLOGIC FACTORS

Within hours to days after exposure, cutaneous or submucosal dendritic cells are believed to transport HIV to CD4$^+$ T cells in regional lymph nodes, where productive infection is established. The premise underlying postexposure prophylaxis (PEP) is that in the presence of antiretroviral drugs, productive infection may be prevented or inhibited, allowing the host immune system to destroy infectious virions and infected cells while they are localized and relatively small in number. This premise is consistent with knowledge that HIV virions are rapidly cleared by the human immune system while the immune system is still intact. The demonstration of HIV-specific cytotoxic T-lymphocyte activity in a small number of HIV-exposed but non-seroconverting HCWs (and in other groups of HIV-exposed but uninfected persons) is consistent with the possibility that host immune responses may sometimes be able to prevent or eradicate HIV infection after an exposure.

Information from a variety of sources suggests the possibility that PEP may be efficacious in preventing infection after HIV exposure. PEP has prevented or ameliorated retroviral infection in some studies in animals, particularly when administered soon after exposure. However, the application of animal studies using nonhuman retroviruses is uncertain since these viruses have pathogenic mechanisms different from those of HIV. There are some indirect data with which to assess the efficacy of PEP in humans. In a multicenter, double-blind, placebo-controlled clinical trial of zidovudine (ZDV) to prevent maternal–infant HIV transmission, ZDV therapy was associated with a 67% reduction in the risk of mother-to-infant HIV transmission. The protective effect of ZDV was only partly explained by a reduction of HIV titer in maternal blood; ZDV also may have a direct protective effect on the fetus and/or act as postexposure prophylaxis for the infant. Additional studies have shown reductions in the rates of perinatal transmission of HIV even with the use of abbreviated regimens that are begun intrapartum or in the first 48 hours of life. Also, a retrospective case–control study found that PEP with ZDV was associated with a decrease of approximately 81% in the risk for HIV seroconversion among HCWs who had a percutaneous exposure to HIV-infected blood. However, any

STEP 1: DETERMINE THE EXPOSURE CODE (EC)

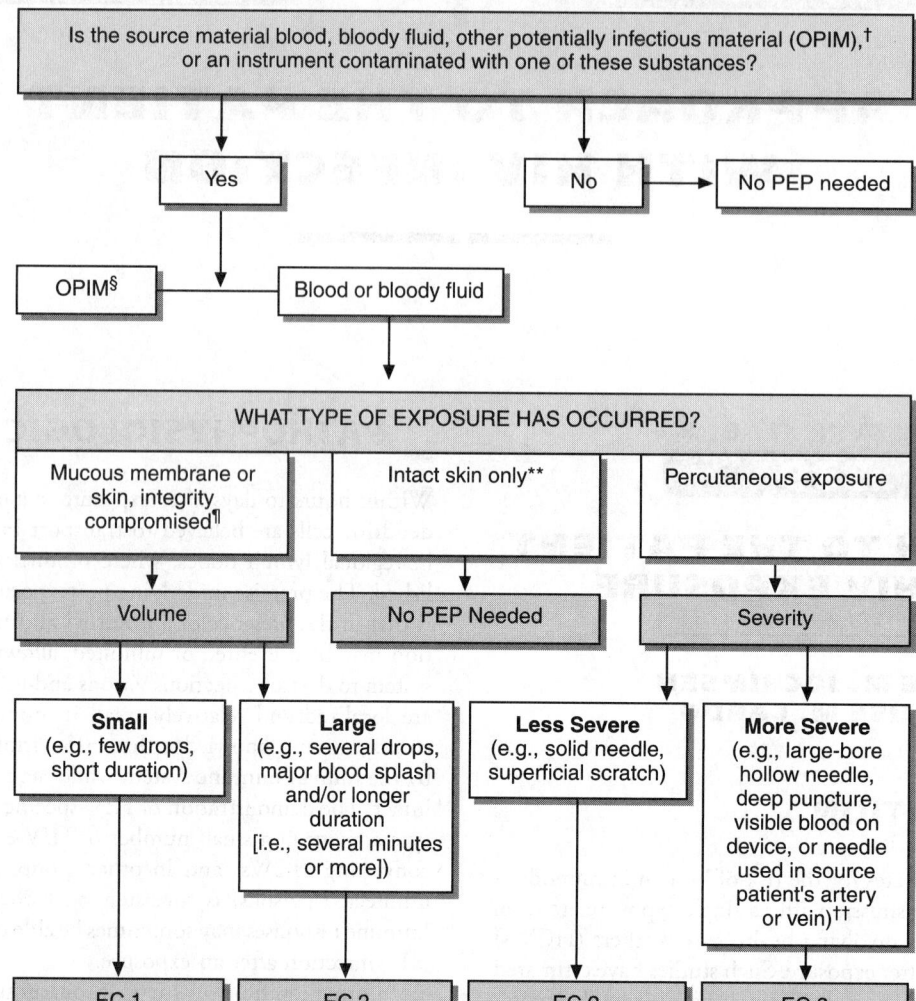

† Semen or vaginal secretions; cerebrospinal, synovial, pleural, peritoneal, pericardial, or amniotic fluids; or tissue.

§ Exposures to OPIM must be evaluated on a case-by-case basis. In general, these body substances are considered a low risk for transmission in health-care settings. Any unprotected contact to concentrated HIV in a research laboratory or production facility is considered an occupational exposure that requires clinical evaluation to determine the need for PEP.

¶ Skin Intergrity is considered compromised if there is evidence of chapped skin, dermatitis, abrasion, or open wound.

** Contact with intact skin is not normally considered a risk for HIV transmission. However, if the exposure was to blood, and the circumstances suggest a higher volume exposure (e.g., an extensive area of skin was exposed or there was prolonged contact with blood), the risk for HIV transmission should be considered.

†† The combination of these severity factors (e.g., large-bore hollow needle **and** deep puncture) contribute to an elevated risk for transmission if the source person is HIV-positive.

FIGURE 339.1. This algorithm is intended to guide initial decisions about PEP and should be used in conjunction with other guidance provided in this report.
EVIDENCE LEVEL: C. Expert Opinion.

STEP 2: DETERMINE THE HIV STATUS CODE (HIV SC)

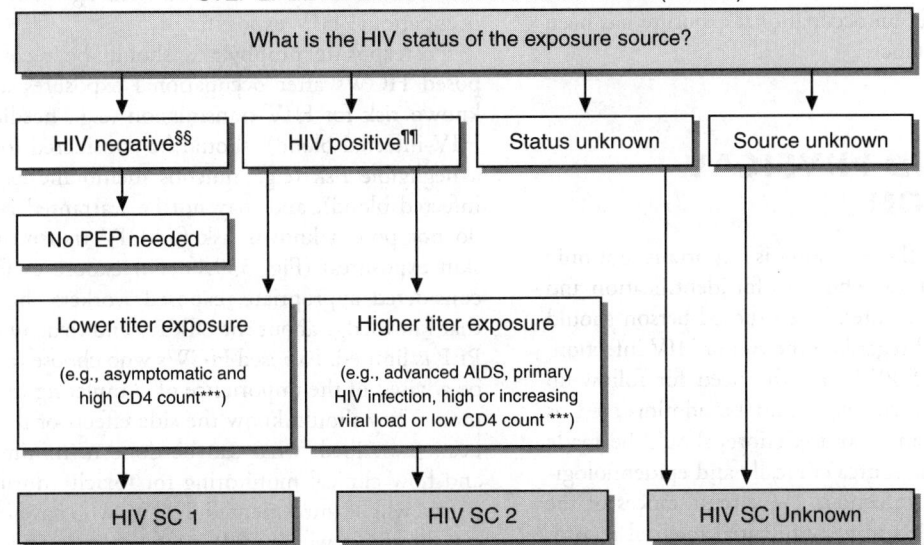

§§ A source is considered negative for HIV infection if there is laboratory documentation of a negative HIV antibody, HIV polymerase chain reaction (PCR), or HIV p24 antigen test result from a specimen collected at or near the time of exposure and there is no clinical evidence of recent retroviral-like illness.

¶¶ A source is considered infected with HIV (HIV positive) if there has been a positive laboratory result for HIV antibody, HIV PCR, or HIV p24 antigen or physician-diagnosed AIDS.

*** Examples are used as surrogates to estimate the HIV titer in an exposure source for purposes of considering PEP regimens and do not reflect all clinical situations that may be observed. Although a high HIV titer (HIV SC 2) in an exposure source has been associated with an increased risk for transmission, the possibility of transmission from a source with low HIV titer also must be considered.

STEP 3: DETERMINE THE PEP RECOMMENDATION

EC	HIV SC	PEP recommendation
1	1	**PEP may not be warranted.** Exposure type does not pose a known risk for HIV transmission. Whether the risk for drug toxicity outweighs the benefit of PEP should be decided by the exposed HCW and treating clinician.
1	2	**Consider basic regimen.** ††† Exposure type poses a negligible risk for HIV transmission. A high HIV titer in the source may justify consideration of PEP. Whether the risk for drug toxicity outweighs the benefit of PEP should be decided by the exposed HCW and treating clinician.
2	1	**Recommend basic regimen.** Most HIV exposures are in this category; no increased risk for HIV transmission has been observed but use of PEP is appropriate.
2	2	**Recommend expanded regimen.** §§§ Exposure types represents an increased HIV transmission risk.
3	1 or 2	**Recommend expanded regimen.** Exposure types represents an increased HIV transmission risk.
Unknown		If the source or, in the case of an unknown source, the setting where the exposure occurred suggests a possible risk for HIV exposure and the EC is 2 or 3, consider PEP basic regimen.

††† Basic regimen is four weeks of zidovudine, 600 mg per day in two or three divided doses, **and** lamivudine, 150 mg twice daily.

§§§ Expanded regimen is the basic regimen plus **either** indinavir, 800 mg every 8 hours, **or** nelfinavir, 750 mg three times a day.

EVIDENCE LEVEL: C. Expert Opinion.

protection afforded is not absolute. Failure of ZDV PEP to prevent HIV infection after an occupational exposure has been reported in at least 18 instances.

HISTORY AND PHYSICAL EXAMINATION

The prompt reporting of HIV exposures is important, not only for management of the exposure but also for identification and evaluation of preventive measures. The exposed person should be evaluated and counseled regarding the risk of HIV infection, the potential usefulness of PEP, and the need for follow-up evaluation. First aid, if necessary, should be administered as quickly as possible. After an exposure, efforts should be made to identify and evaluate the source clinically and epidemiologically for evidence of HIV infection. The circumstances of the exposure should be recorded in a confidential medical record. Data collection should include details about the exposure, information about the source, and details about postexposure management, counseling, and follow-up.

LABORATORY STUDIES AND DIAGNOSTIC TESTS

In persons with known exposure dates, the estimated median time from initial infection to the development of detectable antibody is 2.4 months; 95% of individuals develop antibody within 6 months of infection. The two antibody tests commonly used to detect HIV are the enzyme immunoassay (EIA) for screening and the Western blot for confirmation. Assays for detection of HIV RNA in plasma (e.g., polymerase chain reaction) are sensitive methods for the detection of HIV infection. However, problems with laboratory contamination, false-positive rates, and increased costs limit their routine use. At present, the false-positive and false-negative rates of HIV RNA detection methods are too high to warrant a broader role for them in either routine screening or in the confirmation of diagnosis of HIV infection.

All persons with exposure to HIV should receive postexposure testing. HIV antibody testing should be performed at baseline and for at least 6 months following exposure (e.g., at 6 weeks, 12 weeks, and 6 months). HIV testing using EIA should be performed on any exposed person who has an illness that is consistent with an acute retroviral syndrome.

STRATEGIES FOR OPTIMAL CARE MANAGEMENT

MANAGEMENT

All persons exposed to HIV should receive follow-up counseling and medical evaluation, regardless of whether they receive PEP. The U.S. Public Health Service (PHS) recommends PEP for certain occupational HIV exposures but cannot definitively rec-

ommend for or against antiretroviral agents in preventing non-occupational HIV exposures.

Postexposure prophylaxis should be recommended to exposed HCWs after occupational exposures associated with a known risk for HIV transmission (e.g., needlestick injuries to HIV-infected blood), should be considered for exposures with a negligible risk (e.g., mucous membrane exposures to HIV-infected blood), and may not be warranted for exposures that do not pose a known risk for HIV transmission (e.g., intact skin exposures) (Fig. 339.1). For exposures for which PEP is considered appropriate, exposed workers should be informed that knowledge about the efficacy and toxicity of drugs used for PEP is limited. Exposed HCWs who choose to take PEP should be advised of the importance of completing the prescribed regimen. They should know the side effects of the drugs that have been prescribed, what can be done to minimize these effects, and how clinical monitoring for toxicity during the follow-up period will be implemented. HCWs who have HIV occupational exposures for which PEP is not recommended should be informed that the potential side effects and toxicity of PEP outweigh the negligible risk of transmission posed by the type of exposure.

Most occupational HIV exposures will warrant only a two-drug regimen, using two nucleoside analog reverse transcriptase inhibitors, usually ZDV and lamivudine. The addition of a third drug, usually a protease inhibitor (e.g., indinavir or nelfinavir), should be considered for exposures that pose an increased risk for transmission or when resistance to the other drugs used for PEP is known or suspected. Over time, new antiretroviral agents will be available for the treatment of HIV infection and may offer increased potency for PEP. The inclusion of new drugs in a PEP regimen should be carried out in consultation with a clinical expert in the treatment of HIV infection.

In general, PEP should be initiated as soon as possible (within hours of the exposure). The interval within which PEP should be started for optimal efficacy is not known. The optimal duration of PEP also is unknown. Because 4 weeks of ZDV appears protective in HCWs, PEP probably should be administered for 4 weeks, if tolerated. When PEP is used, drug toxicity monitoring should include a complete blood count and renal and hepatic chemical function tests at baseline and 2 weeks after starting PEP.

The psychological impact of HIV exposure may be considerable and should be addressed during counseling and follow-up. Experts have found that supportive counseling is an important part of management. To prevent the possibility of further transmission to others, the exposed person should be advised to refrain from donating blood, semen, or organs during the follow-up period and to refrain from breast-feeding when safe and effective alternatives are available. To prevent HIV transmission to sexual contacts, all exposed persons should abstain from, or use latex condoms during, sexual intercourse throughout the follow-up period, especially during the first 6 to 12 weeks after the exposure when most HIV-infected persons are expected to sero-convert.

Many of the principles for management of occupational exposures also apply to management of sexual and other nonoccupational HIV exposures, although these instances require the consideration of additional factors. The first step in managing a reported nonoccupational event that may have led to HIV exposure is the determination of the infection status of the reported source. Unlike occupational exposures, the putative source in these cases may not be available to clinicians to provide documentation of HIV status or clinical information on antiretroviral use or viral load. Even in cases where partner notification or timely arrest of assailants (e.g., rape or child abuse) would potentially allow HIV testing of an identified source, delays in seeking care and obtaining test results may necessitate decisions based on estimating the likelihood of infection in the source. If it is determined that the source is, or is likely to be, HIV-infected, the next step is to determine the risk of transmission given the details of the reported exposure. Factors that would either increase (e.g., bleeding and visible mucosal tears in a rape patient) or reduce (e.g., condom used without leak or tear detected) the risk of transmission should be ascertained. If the source is HIV-infected and the exposure event presents an appreciable risk of transmission, it will be important to determine how frequently such exposures occur for a given patient. PEP is not appropriate for persons who frequently put themselves at risk; these patients should be provided or referred urgently for intensive risk reduction intervention.

The use of PEP for nonoccupational exposures should be judicious and only in the context of a comprehensive program of HIV prevention. Results from a program for PEP after nonoccupational exposures in San Francisco, where participants are provided risk reduction counseling in addition to an option to take a 28-day PEP course, have shown that it is possible to provide PEP within 72 hours after exposure and that 80% of persons taking a 4-week PEP regimen completed it.

COMPLICATIONS AND PITFALLS

HIV antiretroviral drug resistance is increasing. Unfortunately, it is difficult to predict the likelihood of drug resistance in the source and the implications for transmission. There are still relatively few data on the prevalence of resistance, and the data are difficult to translate into PEP recommendations. Laboratory evidence of drug resistance does not necessarily imply clinical drug failure. However, a high or rising viral load in the absence of other causes (e.g., treatment discontinuation, intercurrent illness, or vaccination) strongly suggests that drug-resistant virus may be present. Many experts believe that the PEP regimen should include at least two drugs to which the source HIV strain(s) are likely to be susceptible. While probably optimal based on virologic considerations, this recommendation must be tempered by two particularly critical considerations in prescribing PEP: drug toxicity and the complexity of the regimen. Since the great majority of exposed persons will not become infected, even if they receive no PEP, drugs used for PEP should have a very low incidence of moderate or serious toxicity. They also should be well tolerated; incomplete adherence due to unpleasant side effects could render a seemingly highly potent regimen less effective than a less potent regimen. Some side effects that limit adherence (e.g., nausea or diarrhea) can be managed with symptomatic therapy.

When a pregnant woman is exposed to HIV, the evaluation of risk and need for PEP should be approached as with any other person who has had an HIV exposure. The decision to use any antiretroviral drug during pregnancy should be made following discussion between the woman and her health care provider regarding the benefits and potential risks to her and her fetus. Since indinavir may cause indirect hyperbilirubinemia, this drug should not be used in newborns or for PEP in pregnant women if delivery is expected shortly. Efavirenz should not be used during pregnancy.

When the HIV status of the source is unknown or the source cannot be identified, decisions regarding appropriate follow-up and PEP should be individualized, based on factors such as whether potential sources are likely to include an individual at increased risk of HIV infection and the severity of the exposure. If additional information becomes available, these decisions can be modified.

BIBLIOGRAPHY

Busch MP, Satten GA. Time course of viremia and antibody seroconversion following human immunodeficiency virus exposure. *Am J Med 1997;* 102(Suppl 5B):117–124.

Cardo DM, Culver DH, Ciesielski CA, et al. A case–control study of HIV seroconversion in health care workers after percutaneous exposure. *N Engl J Med* 1997;337:1485–1490.

Ippolito G, Puro V, DeCarli G, the Italian Study Group on Occupational Risk of HIV Infection. The risk of occupational human immunodeficiency virus infection in health care workers. *Arch Intern Med* 1993; 153:1451–1458.

Katz MH, Gerberding JL. Postexposure treatment of people exposed to the human immunodeficiency virus through sexual contact or injection-drug use. *N Engl J Med* 1997;336:1097–1100.

Mastro TD, de Vincenzi I. Probabilities of sexual HIV-1 transmission. *AIDS* 1996;10(Suppl A):S75–S82.

Perelson AS, Neumann AU, Markowitz M, et al. HIV-1 dynamics in vivo: virion clearance rate, infected cell life-span, and viral generation time. *Science* 1996;271:1582–-1586.

Tokars JI, Marcus RA, Culver DH, et al. Surveillance of human immunodeficiency virus (HIV) infection and zidovudine use among health care workers with occupational exposure to HIV-infected blood. *Ann Intern Med* 1993;118:913–919.

U.S. Centers for Disease Control and Prevention. Decision aid: determining the need for HIV postexposure prophylaxis (PEP) after an occupational exposure. Public Health Service guidelines for the management of health-care worker exposures to HIV and recommendations for postexposure prophylaxis. *MMWR* 1998;47(RR-7):14–15.

U.S. Centers for Disease Control and Prevention. Management of possible sexual, injecting-drug-use, or other nonoccupational exposure to HIV, including considerations related to antiretroviral therapy. *MMWR* 1998; 47(RR-17):1–14.

U.S. Centers for Disease Control and Prevention. Public Health Service guidelines for the management of health-care worker exposures to HIV and recommendations for postexposure prophylaxis. *MMWR* 1998; 47(RR-7):1–34.

Wade NA, Birkhead GS, Warren BL, et al. Abbreviated regimens of zidovudine prophylaxis and perinatal transmission of the human immunodeficiency virus. *N Engl J Med* 1998;339:1409–1414.

Kelley's Textbook of Internal Medicine, fourth edition. Edited by H. David Humes. Lippincott Williams & Wilkins, Philadelphia © 2000.

CHAPTER 340

APPROACH TO THE PATIENT WITH ASYMPTOMATIC HIV INFECTION (AND COUNSELING)

ABRAHAM VERGHESE

HIV infection is a disease of young people, many of whom have had little or no prior contact with health care providers. The first visit is critical in establishing a therapeutic patient–physician relationship. Most asymptomatic patients with recently diagnosed HIV infection experience anger, anxiety, guilt, and denial for weeks, months, or even years. Suicidal ideation peaks shortly after diagnosis and may persist over the next year. Identifying the social support available to these patients, such as parents, spouses, lovers, and children, is a critical aspect of patient care. Many patients are unaware of the dramatic new advances in the therapy of HIV that have occurred in the last few years. The laboratory tests that document HIV infection should be scrutinized and repeated if necessary. There have been reports of patients with factitious HIV infections.

PATHOPHYSIOLOGIC FACTORS

Even when patients are clinically asymptomatic, tremendous immunologic activity is occurring within the lymphatic system. Although there may be a period of clinical latency, there is no viral latency. The term *acquired immunodeficiency syndrome,* or "AIDS," is in a sense outmoded and now has only epidemiologic utility, even though it is ingrained in medical parlance. Nonspecific predictors of progression from a clinically latent stage to symptomatic infection or AIDS are listed in Table 340.1. With the availability of tests to measure the viral load in the blood, it has become apparent that the viral load is the best predictor of prognosis. The Multicenter AIDS Cohort Study showed that patients with more than 36,000 viral copies per milliliter had a 62% risk of progressing to AIDS in 5 years compared to those with viral loads less than 4,530 copies per milliliter whose risk was 8%. The CD4$^+$ cell count is also an important clinical predictor of progression, particularly when combined with the viral load. For example, in the Multicenter AIDS Cohort Study, 73% of patients with a CD4 count of less than 350 cells per cubic millimeter who had over 30,000 viral copies per milliliter (measured by B-DNA assays) developed an AIDS-defining event in 3 years, compared to 32% of patients with the same viral load but with more than 500 CD4 cells per cubic millimeter progressed to AIDS in the same time period.

TABLE 340.1.	**CLINICAL AND LABORATORY FEATURES OF HUMAN IMMUNODEFICIENCY VIRUS INFECTION THAT INDICATE DISEASE PROGRESSION**

Clinical

Thrush
Oral hairy leukoplakia
Herpes zoster (?)
Fever, fatigue, weight loss
Peripheral general lymphadenopathy that develops rapidly (?)

Laboratory Studies

High viral load
Decreased CD4 leukocyte count
Anemia
Elevated β$_2$-microglobulin, neopterin
Elevated erythrocyte sedimentation rate
Anergy
Detection of p24 antigenemia
Elevated immunoglobulin levels (IgG and IgA)

HISTORY AND PHYSICAL EXAMINATION

An important element in the history is information regarding risk behaviors, which may continue unless counseling and intervention is provided. Tuberculosis appears to be more common in intravenous drug users, and these patients also may be less compliant with therapy. Kaposi's sarcoma is seen in homosexual and bisexual men. Perianal problems ranging from reactivation of herpes simplex to the development of cloacal cancer are more common in homosexual men.

Patients should be questioned carefully about symptoms that suggest disease progression (Table 340.1). Prior exposure to syphilis, tuberculosis, hepatitis B or C, cytomegalovirus, or *Toxoplasma* should be determined. A detailed history of sexually transmitted disease often is useful in predicting future flare-ups of herpes proctitis, venereal warts, or syphilis. A history of prior immunizations, drug allergies, and medication use must be obtained. Many medications, including methadone, can interact with protease inhibitors.

The goal of the initial physical examination is to establish the patient's baseline status and identify important areas to be followed up at future visits. The weight should be measured carefully on a reliable scale with the patient undressed. A flow chart placed on the front of the patient's chart detailing weight, viral load, CD4$^+$ cell count, vaccination status, medications, and problems makes it easier for different health care providers in the same clinic to track the patient's progress. Careful attention should be given to the eye examination. Cytomegalovirus retinitis is uncommon until the CD4$^+$ count has dropped below 200 cells per microliter. The oral cavity should be examined thoroughly. The tongue is pulled out with a gloved hand and gauze, and the sides are inspected for oral hairy leukoplakia. The oral mucosa is examined for Kaposi's sarcoma, which may be present only in this location. The state of dentition and the health of the gingival tissue should be observed because gingivitis and periodontitis tend to progress in later stages of HIV. Referral for preventive dentistry is helpful. Generalized lymphadenopathy is common in symptomatic patients and does not always indicate disease progression. However, enlargement of one lymph node alone should raise suspicion of lymphoma, tuberculosis, Kaposi's sarcoma, or another process. Enlargement of the liver and spleen are looked for carefully and serve as an important baseline when future abnormalities are detected. Perianal, rectal, and pelvic examinations are performed. Problems such as fistula in ano and perianal abscess should be treated promptly because healing is more difficult at later stages of HIV infection. The presence of ankle and knee reflexes, and intact vibratory sense in the lower extremities, should be established. This provides a baseline for comparison in the event the patient later complains of tingling or numbness in the feet—symptoms that are common side effects of therapy with didanosine and dideoxycytidine, and that can also be caused by HIV and cytomegalovirus. The skin examination is particularly important. Common skin problems include seborrheic dermatitis, molluscum contagiosum, folliculitis, allergic rash, warts, and Kaposi's sarcoma. During the course of the examination, the physician should establish rapport with the patient and try to assess the patient's mental status and coping mechanisms. HIV infection necessitates intense patient–physician interaction, and extra time spent at the initial visit helps gain the patient's confidence. This is also an occasion to educate the spouse, partner, or family members and to help them understand the nature of the illness.

LABORATORY STUDIES AND DIAGNOSTIC TESTS

The laboratory workup of the asymptomatic patient with HIV infection is most extensive at the initial visit. Both routine and less common tests are listed in Table 340.2. The complete blood count is useful to detect unsuspected thrombocytopenia or anemia. The serum lactate dehydrogenase level is a helpful baseline measurement and should be normal; this marker tends to increase during *Pneumocystis carinii* infection.

Most serologic tests are ordered primarily to detect dormant pathogens. Many infections in patients with AIDS result from the reactivation of pathogens already residing in the body, such as *Toxoplasma,* cytomegalovirus, *P. carinii,* herpes simplex, herpes zoster, and *Mycobacterium tuberculosis* (although the last organism is recently acquired in many patients). For example, *Toxoplasma* infection is less probable in a patient who later has encephalopathy or a central nervous system mass lesion if *Toxoplasma* antibodies were not present initially, although newly acquired infection may occur. A purified protein derivative skin test should be done on the first visit. The sensitivity of this test correlates inversely with the degree of immune suppression. Induration of 5 mm is interpreted as indicative of tuberculosis infection and the patient is treated with isoniazid (INH) for 12 months.

Viral load testing is becoming a routine part of HIV care and follow-up. HIV RNA determination can be done by polymerase

TABLE 340.2.	INITIAL EVALUATION OF ASYMPTOMATIC HIV-SEROPOSITIVE PATIENTS

History and physical examination
Complete blood cell count with differential and platelet counts
Erythrocyte sedimentation rate
Serum chemistry profile
Urinalysis
Serologic tests
  Hepatitis B and C
  VDRL
  Toxoplasma gondii[a] antibodies
  Cytomegalovirus antibodies[a]
Stool studies for ova and parasites, if indicated
Chest radiograph
Tuberculin skin test
Glucose-6-phosphate dehydrogenase measurement[a]
Measurement of prognostic serologic markers
  Viral load by branched DNA or polymerase chain reaction
  $CD4^+$ lymphocyte count and percentage of total lymphocytes
  β_2-Microglobulin concentration[a]

[a] = Optional study.
VDRL, Venereal Disease Research Laboratory.

chain reaction (PCR) or branched-chain DNA methods. PCR-based values are up to 2.5 times higher than B-DNA values. The two tests correlate well with each other, but the physician must pick one of the two methodologies and have it performed at the same laboratory in order to make meaningful interpretations of changes over time. Testing for resistance is not routinely done but is increasingly being performed in patients who have failed therapy.

The $CD4^+$ cell count should be done at the same time of day to account for circadian variations. The presence of intercurrent illness affects the results and should delay test performance for 2 to 3 weeks. Patients and physicians often focus excessively on the $CD4^+$ cell count. Trends in the count over time are more useful than are absolute numbers as diurnal variations in CD4 numbers by as much as 100 cells per cubic millimeter have been reported. Some studies have suggested that the CD8 cell count may be useful. Other markers of HIV progression, such as β_2-microglobulin, p24 antigen, and neopterin, are no longer obtained routinely. The Venereal Disease Research Laboratory (VDRL) test is particularly important because patients with HIV are more likely to have a history of syphilis and because early syphilis in these patients is more likely to present as secondary syphilis. If there is a history of incomplete treatment or if the VDRL is reactive, aggressive treatment is indicated.

The second visit takes place a week after the first and allows the patient to obtain test results and meet other members of the HIV health care team (nurses, nurse–practitioners, physician's assistants, social workers, and clinic volunteers). The second visit provides an opportunity to reinforce preventive health care recommendations, such as stopping smoking and joining a support group. At least one study has suggested that belonging to a support group and maintaining an active interest in the treatment program correlates with longevity in patients with HIV infection. The influenza vaccine should be offered at the appropriate time of year and the pneumococcal polysaccharide vaccine should be used. It is not clear as to whether the *Haemophilus influenzae* type B vaccine should be given routinely because most adults are protected. The hepatitis B vaccine should be given if serologic tests show lack of protection. The patient should be advised that children living in the household should receive inactivated polio vaccine rather than live oral vaccine. If the patient has not previously received standard "childhood" immunizations (measles, mumps, and rubella; diphtheria; tetanus; inactivated polio), these should be given.

COUNSELING

GENERAL COUNSELING

It is useful to ask patients what they understand about the disease. Pamphlets and informational brochures can be helpful in patient education. Guidelines for preventing virus transmission and explicit instructions about safe-sex practices should be provided. Sex with other HIV-infected patients often is considered harmless, and patients should be informed that, on the contrary, unprotected intercourse may result in the acquisition of another strain of HIV, another sexually transmitted disease, or an increased viral load. Identifying others who are at risk and arranging for their testing and follow-up also is important. Knowledge of state and local laws concerning confidentiality and disease reporting is essential; social workers can assist with these issues and with housing, funding for medication, and qualifying for state and federal assistance. Women of childbearing age should be counseled about the risk of transmitting HIV to the fetus and encouraged to prevent pregnancy. Patients should be advised to refrain from donating blood, plasma, or other body tissues or organs. Patients should be instructed not to share razors or toothbrushes, and both patients and their family members should be told how to clean up accidental spills of blood or body fluids using household bleach diluted in water at a ratio of 1:10. Patients can be reassured that casual contact with family members and co-workers will not result in HIV transmission. Patients should be questioned about pet ownership, especially cats and birds, and should be advised to exercise care in cleaning cat litter (if serologic tests for *Toxoplasma* are negative) and to seek prompt attention for cat scratches or bites. The consumption of raw fish or meat and of uncooked eggs is discouraged.

PSYCHIATRIC COUNSELING

Patients often manifest signs of emotional distress such as cognitive dysfunction and social withdrawal. Episodic anxiety and depression are common; depression often responds well to antidepressant therapy. Suicidal ideation always must be sought. Many of these problems can be improved remarkably through participation in support groups and use of medications pre-

scribed by the primary physician, but psychotherapy and formal psychiatric consultation occasionally is required.

STRATEGIES FOR OPTIMAL CARE MANAGEMENT

Patients should be encouraged to continue working as long as they are physically able. Physicians should expect patients to approach them aggressively with demands for information about new treatments receiving coverage in the news media. Physicians should not resent these questions, but should attempt to convey what they know while also pointing out the delay between a laboratory observation or a lay press report and a clinically applicable therapy. Patients can obtain additional information from multiple sources; useful newsletters are published by Project Inform and the Gay Men's Health Crisis (GMHC) Department of Medical Information. In addition, the National Directory of AIDS Care and the National Institutes of Health AIDS Clinical Trials Group have toll-free numbers that provide information on resources, services, and clinical trials. A number of web sites (Johns Hopkins, University of San Francisco, and many others) provide current information for both patients and physicians. It is important that physicians adopt nonjudgmental attitudes toward alternative therapies, particularly if such therapies appear to cause no harm to patients and if patients believe in them. Clear evidence of fraud or quackery requires intervention. Practices such as meditation, acupuncture, prayer, and the use of vitamins can be encouraged; the effect of Chinese herbs and other treatments, though probably harmless, may interfere with concomitant antiviral therapy.

SPECIFIC TREATMENT ISSUES

Pneumocystis carinii Pneumonia Prophylaxis

The earliest success in the treatment of HIV disease came with the realization that one could prevent *P. carinii* pneumonia by the administration of antibiotics to patients at risk. The initial popularity of monthly aerosolized pentamidine has given way to some concern about its inability to prevent extrapulmonary *Pneumocystis* infection. Oral trimethoprim–sulfamethoxazole is easier to use and more effective for both primary and secondary prophylaxis. It may also diminish the incidence of *Toxoplasma* infection and *Nocardia* infection, and may prevent some infections with common bacterial pathogens. Dapsone is a useful alternative agent, but patients must be screened for glucose-6-phosphate dehydrogenase deficiency. Prophylaxis of *Mycobacterium avium* complex is discussed in a later section; patients who require such prophylaxis usually have symptoms and CD4$^+$ cell counts of less than 100 cells per microliter.

Antiretroviral Therapy

The discovery of potent new antivirals and the realization that by combining drugs one could suppress viral production heralded a new era in antiviral therapy. The question of when to begin antiretroviral therapy in asymptomatic patients with HIV infection is controversial. Clearly early treatment will control viral replication, prevent immune destruction, and perhaps decrease the risk of viral transmission. On the other hand, early treatment in an asymptomatic patient can cause drug resistance to occur earlier, exposes patients to long-term toxicity of medications, and affects their quality of life. Prior to the advent of routine viral load testing and potent antiviral therapy, a CD4 count of less than 500 cells per cubic millimeter was considered the threshold for beginning treatment. Although there is no clear consensus, most experts agree that patients with more than 500 CD4 cells per cubic millimeter and a viral load less than 10,000 (B-DNA) can be observed. Patients with higher viral loads or a CD4 count below 500 cells per cubic millimeter should probably be offered treatment.

Patients must have a very clear idea of what is involved in treatment. They must understand that they must be committed to the regimen once it begins; noncompliance clearly can result in resistant strains and worsen the prognosis. Patients must realize that they will be taking up to 15 pills a day and will have some side effects, some of which (such as the syndrome of lipodystrophy and insulin resistance) are only beginning to be catalogued. Therapy is expensive, and few patients can afford it without some form of assistance such as the AIDS Drug Assistance Program or Medicaid. Patients who seem unreliable or have ongoing problems with addiction are generally not good candidates, although they may be counseled and could become good candidates for therapy. The final choice about initiating therapy therefore has to be made by the patient.

It seems axiomatic that in beginning therapy three drugs must be used, and it has been typical to use a protease inhibitor (PI) combined with two nucleoside analogs (NRTIs), such as indinavir with zidovudine and lamivudine. New studies, however, suggest that it may be possible to substitute a non-nucleoside reverse transcriptase inhibitor (NNRTI) for the PI and thereby save the PI for later use if there is resistance and disease progression. Newer agents and older agents that can be taken less often will probably continue to simplify therapy and result in fewer pills for the patient to swallow. A major challenge to patients and physicians is to stay abreast of rapid developments in this area. The specific details of therapy are discussed later in this text.

BIBLIOGRAPHY

Merigan TC, Bartlett JG, Bolognesi D. *Textbook of AIDS medicine,* second ed. Baltimore: Williams & Wilkins, 1994.

Mellors J, Munoz A, Giorgi J, et al. Plasma viral load and CD4+ lymphocytes as prognostic markers of HIV-1 infection. *Ann Intern Med* 1997; 126:946–954.

Report of the NIH Panel to Define Principles of Therapy of HIV Infection. *MMWR* April 25, 1998/47(RR-S):1–41.

Sande MA, Volberding PA. *The medical management of AIDS,* fifth ed. Philadelphia: WB Saunders, 1997.

Sexton DJ, Band J, Berman S, et al. Primary care of patients infected with human immunodeficiency virus. *Clin Infect Dis* 1998;26:275–276.

CHAPTER 341

APPROACH TO THE SYMPTOMATIC PATIENT WITH HIV DISEASE

HENRY MASUR

Patients with HIV infection develop a wide range of clinical manifestations due to opportunistic pathogens, immunologic processes, direct effects of HIV, and due to therapies which these patients are administered. These manifestations vary considerably depending on the degree of the patient's immunologic decline, age, sex, pathogen exposure as well as the management strategy that has been pursued. When these patients develop new symptoms, signs, or laboratory abnormalities, it is important to approach them expeditiously and methodically so that complications can be diagnosed and treated early, before disability is severe, which is the time when therapeutic intervention is most likely to be successful. Patients need to be educated about the natural history of their disease, how to recognize complications, and how to participate in management so that they can contribute productively to their health care.

Patients with HIV infection are clearly susceptible to almost all of the infectious and noninfectious disease processes that non–HIV- infected individuals develop. Thus, common infectious causes of pulmonary disease such as influenza, mycoplasmosis, or legionellosis must be considered in patients even though these entities are generally not more severe or more common in HIV-infected patients than in HIV-uninfected patients. Similarly, in patients with central nervous system mass lesions, glioblastoma multiforme must enter into the differential diagnosis regardless of CD4+ T-lymphocyte count, although at low CD4+ T-lymphocyte counts such a diagnosis would be far less likely than other entities.

The best indicator of patient susceptibility to opportunistic infection is still the circulating CD+ T-lymphocyte count (Fig. 341.1). The likelihood of developing an opportunistic infection can be assessed by clinical parameters (e.g., a history of oral

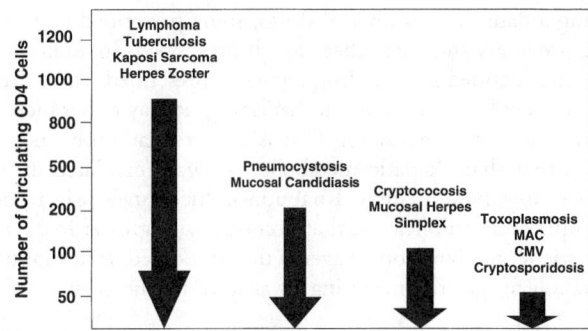

FIGURE 341.1. Typical relationship of clinical manifestations to CD4 count in HIV-infected patients.

EVIDENCE LEVEL: A. Reference: Farizo KM, Buegler JW, Chamberland ME, et al. Spectrum of disease in persons with human immunodeficiency virus infection in the US. *JAMA* 1992;267: 1798–1805.

candidiasis, persistent and unexplained fever, wasting, prior episode of pneumonia, or any prior AIDS-defining disease), by virologic parameters (e.g., HIV RNA viral load as measured by polymerase chain reaction or B-DNA technique is the most commonly employed) or by immunologic parameters. Among the latter, there is considerable interest in lymphocyte proliferation assays, in cytotoxic T-cell assays, and in T-lymphocyte phenotypic assays (e.g., measurements of CD45 RO$^+$ and CD45 RO$^-$ cells), but there is no evidence that these research tools provide clinically relevant information beyond what CD4$^+$ T-cell enumeration provides. The absolute number of circulating CD4$^+$ T-lymphocyte cells is the parameter that most clinicians follow, even though the CD4$^+$ T-lymphocyte percentage (a number that is a direct measurement rather than a number derived from this measurement and the absolute lymphocyte count) is a more reproducible and reliable parameter.

In an era when many patients have responded to highly active antiretroviral therapy in terms of both decreasing their HIV RNA viral load and increasing their CD4$^+$ T-lymphocyte counts, concern has been raised that such counts might no longer be reliable indicators of patient susceptibility. In fact, CD4$^+$ T-lymphocyte counts still appear to be excellent predictors of host susceptibility to infection either in patients receiving antiretroviral therapy or in patients receiving interleukin-2. Patients appear to derive substantial protection from their CD4 cells that is comparable to the protection that same number of cells would have provided a patient with the same count who had never received antiretroviral therapy. If the nadir CD4$^+$ T-lymphocyte count has any influence on host susceptibility to infection, for patients whose counts have risen to a given level, that influence is small. These observations imply that patients who respond to highly active antiretroviral therapy by elevating their CD4$^+$ T lymphocytes well above the CD4$^+$ T-lymphocyte "threshold" for a given infection may be able to discontinue some opportunistic infection primary prophylaxis (e.g., for *Pneumocystis* pneumonia), or even some chronic maintenance regimens (e.g., for cytomegalovirus retinitis), if specific criteria, detailed in Chapters 83 to 87, are met.

As clinicians focus on common diseases, on direct effects of HIV, on immunologically mediated syndromes, and on opportunistic infections, they must have a strong appreciation of the potential for drug toxicities and drug interactions to cause clinically important syndromes. Patients with HIV infection may be taking a daunting number of drugs, some prescribed by health care providers and some that are self-prescribed. In addition to toxicities defined for the drug regimens prescribed, these drugs can interact by a variety of mechanisms that may either increase or decrease drug exposure. This is a particular problem with drugs that share hepatic metabolic pathways mediated by the cytochrome P450 system. Rifabutin-induced uveitis is a good example of a complication that occurred with greater frequency in patients receiving other agents that interfered with rifabutin metabolism, greatly increasing its area under the curve.

■ FEVER AND OTHER CONSTITUTIONAL MANIFESTATIONS

A persistent or intermittent rise in temperature is often one of the first symptomatic manifestations of HIV infection. Virtually

TABLE 341.1.	RADIOLOGIC AND LABORATORY EVALUATION OF FEVER IN PATIENTS WITH HIV INFECTION AND CD4$^+$ LYMPHOCYTE COUNTS OF LESS THAN 200 CELLS/mm³

Initial evaluation
  Chest radiograph
  Blood culture for routine bacteria
  Blood culture for fungus
  Blood culture for mycobacteria
  Serum cryptococcal antigen
  Liver function tests
  Urine analysis
  PPD test
Follow-up evaluation (if initial workup is nonrevealing)
  Abdominal CT scan or MRI
  Chest CT scan or MRI
  Arterial blood gas measurement
  Sinus film (plain film, CT scan, or MRI)
  Lipase and amylase determinations
  Urine for *Histoplasma* antigen
  Stool for culture, ova and parasites, *Clostridium* difficile
  Lumbar puncture
  RPR test
  Lymph node biopsy
  Bone marrow biopsy
  Liver biopsy
  Blood culture or PCR for *Bartonella*
  Dental films

PPD, purified protein derivative; CT, computed tomography; MRI, magnetic resonance imaging; RPR, rapid plasma reagin; PCR, polymerase chain reaction.

every patient experiences episodes of fever at some juncture during his or her disease. A systematic approach including history and physical examination with routine laboratory studies and chest radiograph often reveals a site of infection (Table 341.1). It is important to recognize that the infection may be an ordinary, community-acquired process due to a common virus or bacteria that could respond to conservative management (without antimicrobial therapy) or to a short course of an appropriate narrow spectrum antimicrobial agent. It is also important to be cognizant that drugs such as trimethoprim–sulfamethoxazole, abacavir, or isoniazid may be the cause of fever. Patients may thus warrant a trial off all medications to determine if one of their drugs is the cause of the fever, while obtaining appropriate cultures, stains, and serologic and radiologic tests. However, special caution is necessary before reintroducing abacavir if there is a possibility that the febrile episode represented an "abacavir hypersensitivity syndrome" since rechallenge in that situation has resulted in fatalities.

If a cause is not apparent from this initial evaluation, a more extensive and invasive evaluation is appropriate. The urgency of the evaluation depends on the patient's clinical status (how acutely ill the patient is and if there are concomitant processes, such as substantial inability to perform daily activities, considerable weight loss, or localizing signs). The patient's CD4 count and history of exposure (geographic exposure as well as lifestyle exposure) should also influence the extent and direction of the evaluation. A rapidly rising HIV titer in the circulating blood, as determined by a quantitative method, may also indicate that a patient needs special attention since the CD4 count may be in the process of declining precipitously. Special attention should focus on the pulmonary system because this is often the site of infectious complications; any persistent symptoms should be pursued, even in the absence of radiographic manifestations, as detailed in Chapter 83, especially if the CD4 count is below 200 per cubic millimeter. Subtle neurologic abnormalities, such as persistent headache, aberrant behavior, or cognitive dysfunction, need to be carefully followed (see Chapter 85) with appropriate imaging techniques and cerebrospinal fluid analysis. Gastrointestinal diseases, especially esophagitis, hepatitis, and biliary disease, need to be sought and enteric infections of the small and large bowel considered (see Chapter 84). Evidence for cutaneous disease, such as herpes simplex virus (HSV), varicella-zoster virus (VZV), or *Bartonella,* must also be carefully assessed. Screening laboratory tests are indicated in Table 341.1.

Cultures of the blood, as well as serum cryptococcal antigen determination, are an important part of the evaluation. Routine blood cultures may reveal an enteric pathogen such as *Salmonella,* a complication of intravenous drug abuse such as *Staphylococcus aureus,* a complication of an indwelling line such as *Staphylococcus epidermidis,* or an unsuspected fungus such as *Cryptococcus neoformans* or *Histoplasma capsulatum.* Special blood culture media for mycobacteria may be useful for identifying *Mycobacterium avium* complex (MAC), as well as *M. tuberculosis* or various other atypical mycobacteria. Whether blood should be cultured or assessed by nucleic acid amplification for cytomegalovirus (CMV) is less certain: the presence or absence of CMV does not definitely determine whether fever is due to CMV or whether therapy for CMV is warranted.

Cultures of other sites should be done if there are suggestive symptoms, signs, or laboratory tests. If no source of the fever is apparent, routine histologic studies and culture of a bone marrow aspirate, and perhaps biopsy, is probably worth pursuing with particular attention to fungi, mycobacteria, or lymphoma. Liver biopsies in the absence of suggestive signs or impressive laboratory abnormalities are rarely productive as part of a fever evaluation.

A comprehensive evaluation of a persistent fever also includes a methodical radiologic evaluation, including at least abdominal computed tomography (CT) or magnetic resonance imaging (MRI) with contrast. Some centers would include a CT scan or MRI of the brain and sinuses, and perhaps a chest CT scan as well. However, in the absence of any other suspicious evidence, these are expensive, time consuming, and less likely to be helpful. Nuclear scans such as bone scans, liver scans, gallium scans, or tagged white blood cell studies can be considered, but many clinicians do not find these to be useful or cost-effective.

If fever persists and no cause is discovered, empirical therapy might be considered, focusing on MAC or CMV if the patient's CD4 count is below 75 to 100 per cubic millimeter. Given the broad range of possible causes for fever, however, it is probably preferable to follow the patient carefully and reassess periodically unless the patient is extremely symptomatic, or has substantial concomitant weight loss or "wasting."

Some patients may note fatigue, anorexia, chills, sweats, or weight loss in the absence of fever. These manifestations should probably be approached in a way similar to that for fever, with additional attention given to endocrinologic abnormalities such as thyroid and adrenal dysfunction. The evaluation of wasting is considered in Chapter 84. With regard to patients who describe fatigue or weight loss, the influence of psychological factors such as depression must be considered as one aspect of a methodical and comprehensive evaluation.

LYMPHADENOPATHY

Generalized lymphadenopathy was one of the manifestations of HIV infection recognized early in the history of the AIDS epidemic. Lymphadenopathy may reflect a wide array of infectious agents, including fungi, mycobacteria, and viruses. Lymphadenopathy may also be a manifestation of lymphoma or of an immunologic reaction to HIV itself. Nodes may be apparent by exam in multiple superficial chains, including cervical, axillary, and inguinal. Radiologic evaluation may reveal mediastinal and abdominal nodes as well, although large hilar nodes are not characteristics of the "generalized lymphadenopathy syndrome" caused by HIV. When nodes are less than 1 cm in diameter and symmetrical and stable, it may be reasonable to follow the patient closely without needle aspiration or biopsy if he or she is truly asymptomatic. If the nodes are asymmetrical or tender, or if the patient has fever or fatigue or weight loss, needle aspiration or biopsy for culture and histologic examination (focusing on mycobacterium, fungi, viruses, and lymphoma) is appropriate (Table 341.2). The evaluation often does not reveal a specific pathogen or tumor. Biopsy most often shows a nonspecific follicular hyperplasia. There is no evidence that generalized lymphadenopathy due to HIV correlates with an unfavorable progress.

TABLE 341.2.	RADIOLOGIC AND LABORATORY EVALUATION OF LYMPHADENOPATHY

Asymptomatic patient (symmetrical and homogeneous nodes)
  VDRL test
  PPD test
  Chest radiograph
Symptomatic patient (fever, constitutional manifestations, or nodes that are symptomatic or nonhomogeneous)
  VDRL test
  PPD test
  Chest radiograph
  Chest CT or MRI scan
  Abdominal CT or MRI scan
  Liver function tests
  Blood culture for bacteria
  Blood culture for fungi
  Blood culture for mycobacteria
  Serum cryptococcal antigen test
  Needle aspirate of node
  Bone marrow biopsy
  Urine *Histoplasma* antigen

VDRL, Venereal Disease Research Laboratory; PPD, purified protein derivative; CT, computed tomography; MRI, magnetic resonance imaging.

ORAL AND ESOPHAGEAL DISEASE

Patients commonly complain of white plaques in their oral cavity, altered sensation of taste, pain, foul breath, dental problems such as caries or loosening of teeth, or dysphagia. Careful examination of the oropharynx may reveal white plaques, mucosal ulcers, atrophic mucosa, caries, pyorrhea, or masses arising from mucosal or lymphoid tissue. Mucosal abnormalities should be swabbed; a direct smear should be examined for *Candida;* culture for fungi is not helpful diagnostically regarding *Candida* since many otherwise healthy individuals may grow small quantities of candida from their oropharynx. *Candida* can cause three major types of mucosal abnormalities: the typical white plaques, atrophic mucositis, and angular cheilitis. The oral lesions can usually be distinguished by clinical examination from hairy leukoplakia, a lesion characteristically seen on the lateral aspect of the tongue that is caused by Epstein–Barr virus (EBV). It is important to diagnose these lesions accurately because they have prognostic implications and because candidiasis can be treated specifically. Hairy leukoplakia is a clinical diagnosis; while it is etiologically related to EBV, cultures for EBV and serologies are not helpful. Biopsy is not clinically warranted for hairy leukoplakia, nor is specific therapy. Lesions may regress if patients are given effective antiretroviral therapy, ganciclovir, foscarnet, or high-dose acyclovir for some other indication.

Examination of the oropharynx may also reveal ulcerative lesions. These may be due to herpes simplex, which can be recognized with reasonable accuracy on a clinical basis and can be diagnosed specifically by Tsank prep, by biopsy, or, most commonly and conveniently, by culture. When ulcerative herpetic lesions do not respond to acyclovir therapy, they may be caused by acyclovir-resistant virus, but other causes of the lesions should also be considered, including *Treponema pallidum* and endemic fungi. Ulcers that are large, deep, painful, and few in number (one to three) may be aphthous; biopsies with histologic and microbiologic examination are not specific for identifying aphthous ulcers but are useful to exclude neoplastic processes (lymphoma or Kaposi's sarcoma) or specific infections (fungi, herpesviruses, mycobacteria, and others).

Dental complaints are common. Patients with HIV are clearly predisposed to pyorrhea and gingivitis, which can be quite severe, and which may be associated with fetid breath, tooth decay, dental abscesses, and loss of teeth. These processes can be ameliorated with local therapies and surgical management, and thus their recognition is important.

Dysphagia, a common complaint for patients with HIV, becomes an increasingly frequent occurrence as the CD4 count declines. *Candida* esophagitis is responsible for a large fraction of these cases and may be present even if there is no evidence for oral involvement. Many clinicians treat patients empirically for candidiasis, with an azole such as fluconazole. If there is not prompt symptomatic improvement, usually within 1 to 2 weeks, endoscopy with cultures and biopsies is appropriate since many infectious and neoplastic processes are clinically indistinguishable from *Candida* esophagitis. The differential diagnosis includes CMV, aphthous ulcers of the posterior pharynx and esophagus, herpes simplex virus, mycobacteria, endemic fungi, lymphoma,

and Kaposi's sarcoma, as well as ulcers due to drugs (e.g., zalcitabine, zidovudine, and dapsone) or radiation. There is an increasing incidence of azole-resistant disease due to *Candida albicans* or other *Candida* species. Thus, endoscopy may reveal smears or biopsies consistent with candidal disease despite azole therapy. Susceptibility testing of the candidal isolates can be useful to confirm the need for an alternative therapy such as amphotericin B.

OCULAR MANIFESTATIONS

Patients often complain of "floaters," decreased visual acuity, or reduced field of vision. Dilated fundoscopic examination is indicated. Patients almost never develop retinochoroiditis due to an opportunistic infection until their CD4$^+$ T-lymphocyte count is below 50 to 75 per cubic millimeter. CMV retinitis is responsible for the vast majority of cases of retinochoroiditis and is so characteristic on funduscopic examination that a clinical diagnosis is usually established without further testing. These patients almost all have positive IgG titers for CMV. Retinal lesions due to other pathogens such as *Toxoplasma, Pneumocystis, M. tuberculosis,* VZV, HSV, and endemic fungi do occur. Lymphoma and Kaposi's sarcoma will occasionally present in the globe.

For patients who have been treated for CMV retinitis and who are receiving chronic maintenance therapy when started on highly active antiretroviral therapy, an ocular syndrome, designated as immune restitution vitritis, has been recognized. This syndrome needs to be distinguished from active CMV retinitis since the management of these two disorders is substantially different. Thus, ophthalmologic consultation to confirm the diagnosis of any retinal abnormality is usually appropriate. In difficult cases, microbiologic evaluations may be helpful. If a patient has negative titers against CMV or *Toxoplasma,* for instance, these etiologic factors would be extremely unlikely. Rarely is a vitreal tap or retinal biopsy indicated. Clinicians need to recognize that some drugs such as rifabutin and ethambutal have ocular toxicities that must be considered, either as a predictable result of the administration of a drug or as a result of drug interaction.

HEMATOLOGIC ABNORMALITIES

A wide variety of hematologic abnormalities have been described in patients with HIV infection. Thrombocytopenia often is brought to clinical attention because of a routine screening test and, less commonly, because of petechial bruising or gross bleeding. Thrombocytopenia can be caused by peripheral destruction of platelets (e.g., associated with immune complexes or platelet-associated antibodies) or by decreased production from the bone marrow (e.g., due to infection, tumor, or drugs). Thus, evalua-

TABLE 341.3.	LABORATORY EVALUATION OF CYTOPENIA

Pancytopenia
   Review peripheral smear
   Bone marrow biopsy
   Blood culture for fungi, mycobacteria
Neutropenia
   Review peripheral smear
   Folate level
   Vitamin B_{12} level
   Bone marrow biopsy
Anemia
   Review peripheral smear
   Coombs' test
   Haptoglobin
   Stool guiaic test
   Erythropoietin level
   Bone marrow biopsy
   Blood culture for fungi, mycobacteria
   Antinuclear antibody test
Thrombocytopenia
   Review peripheral smear
   Bone marrow biopsy

tion (Table 341.3) generally includes examination of a peripheral smear for assessment of red cell and platelet morphology and bone marrow examination for megakaryocytes, as well as for infectious and neoplastic processes. Measurement of antiplatelet antibodies is not usually helpful diagnostically. A wide variety of processes can cause thrombocytopenia including opportunistic infections and tumors (e.g., endemic mycoses, tuberculosis, lymphoma), HIV itself, drugs (including prescribed drugs as well as self-administered drugs or alcohol or heroin); thrombotic thrombocytopenic purpura; hypersplenism; disseminated intravascular coagulation; and various other viral infections. The presence of fever or weight loss should suggest an infectious cause, or perhaps lymphoma, especially if there is pancytopenia. Medications may have to be discontinued, depending on the severity of the thrombocytopenia, to assess their role. If patients have a measurable HIV viremia, improved antiretroviral therapy may have a beneficial effect on the platelet count if the thrombocytopenia is related to HIV itself.

Anemia is a common manifestation of HIV disease, especially in advanced stages of AIDS; it can have a substantial impact on quality of life. It is useful to examine a peripheral smear to determine whether the anemia is normocytic, microcytic, or macrocytic, and to search for evidence of hemolysis. Diagnostic evaluation should include assessment for blood loss, nutritional deficiencies, autoimmune processes, hemolysis, and deficient bone marrow production. The influence of concurrent infections, drugs, and splenomegaly must be assessed. A serum erythropoietin level is often useful as part of the diagnostic evaluation and for assessing the likelihood that therapeutic erythropoietin will be useful. A bone marrow aspirate or biopsy is probably most appropriate when the anemia is moderate or severe. A search for the cause of anemia, as well as for other cytopenias, is appropriate before hematopoietic growth factors are utilized.

Neutropenia is associated with an increased incidence of bac-terial infections and is recognized most often in patients with advanced disease. While marrow infiltrative processes due to tumor or infection may occur, most cases are due either to drugs (e.g., zidovudine, ganciclovir, or trimethoprim–sulfamethoxazole) or advanced HIV disease. A trial stopping likely offending agents may be in order, especially if the neutrophil count is below 1,000 per cubic millimeter. Nutritional assessment (e.g., regarding folate and vitamin B_{12}) may also be appropriate. Granulocyte colony-stimulating factor or granulocyte–macrophage colony-stimulating factor can reverse neutropenia and may conceivably have a beneficial effect in terms of reducing the incidence of bacterial infections and prolonging survival.

RENAL ABNORMALITIES

Renal abnormalities often come to medical attention because of abnormal screening tests of blood or urine. Glomerular, tubular, and interstitial processes occur. Proteinuria is particularly common among the observed laboratory abnormalities. Patients with HIV infection need to be approached with the perspective that their renal disease may be due to a process unrelated to HIV, such as hypertension, heroin abuse, or hepatitis B. However, renal dysfunction may be related to opportunistic infection, neoplastic processes, drug toxicity, or HIV itself. Drugs of particular note regarding various forms of nephrotoxicity include trimethoprim-sulfamethoxazole (for *Pneumocystis*), foscarnet (for CMV), pentamidine (for *Pneumocystis*), amphotericin B (for fungi), and intravenous dye (used in radiologic procedures). It may be prudent if patients have renal dysfunction and are receiving drugs capable of causing compatible renal lesions to consider discontinuing drug therapy if feasible alternatives are available. For patients with severe proteinuria and mild to moderate elevation in serum creatinine levels, renal biopsy most often shows focal and segmented glomerulosclerosis. Biopsies are rarely performed, however, because rarely do they influence therapy. Renal calculi have become a well-recognized complication of indinavir therapy: indinavir crystals may develop into calculi, especially in patients who are not optimally hydrated.

SKIN DISORDERS

Dermatologic disorders are common among patients with HIV infection and increase in frequency with greater degrees of immunosuppression. Dermatologic disorders are most often diagnosed by clinical appearance, supplemented in some situations by skin biopsy, culture of fluid or tissue, and/or direct examination of tissue scrapings. Seborrheic dermatitis, psoriasis, and eosinophilic folliculitis require considerable expertise to be diagnosed appropriately. Tinea infections of the skin and nails should be scraped to determine the causative organism, which will guide therapy. Bacterial folliculitis should be cultured to aid in selection of the optimal antibacterial agent. Viral processes such as HSV or VZV infection, or molluscum contagiosum, cause lesions that are highly characteristic. Cultures can be useful to distinguish HSV from VZV lesions or enemic mycoses in atypical cases, or even in a case that appears classic, since therapy will differ depending on which virus is causative. The appearance of molluscum contagiosum lesions is markedly different from that of HSV or VZV lesions; a clinical diagnosis is usually adequate without biopsy or culture. For many patients, clinicians need to have a high index of suspicion for unusual manifestations of syphilis and must perform appropriate serologic and histologic studies as part of their diagnostic evaluation.

Kaposi's sarcoma can usually be diagnosed on a clinical basis by an experienced health care provider. A biopsy can be useful in atypical cases. A few cases of bacillary angiomatosis have been confused with Kaposi's sarcoma. Biopsy of these lesions caused by *Bartonella* infection will show perivascular accumulation of bacilli. Specimens are stained by the Warthin–Starry technique to demonstrate the organism. The diagnosis can be established or confirmed by culture of blood or lesions, or by serum polymerase chain reaction.

GENITAL TRACT DISORDERS

Genital ulcers, genital warts, pelvic inflammatory disease, and other genital lesions, including vaginal candidiasis, need to be

TABLE 341.4.	APPROACH TO THE SYMPTOMATIC PATIENT WITH HIV INFECTION
Finding	**Evaluation/Treatment**
Fever	History, physical examination, and laboratory evaluation to look for infection
Lymphadenopathy	Evaluate for infection: mycobacteria and other bacteria, fungi, viruses (including HIV)
Oral disease	Treat thrush, biopsy lesions of uncertain cause, dental consultation
Esophageal disease	For dysphagia, treat for candida/esophagitis; reserve endoscopy for refractory cases
Ocular disease	Funduscopic examination, serologic testing (cytomegalovirus, *Toxoplasma*), ophthalmologic consultation
Hematologic disease	Review peripheral smear, other laboratory tests (see Table 341.3)
Renal disease	Determine whether caused by hypertension, heroin abuse, hepatitis B, HIV infection, or drugs (trimethoprim/sulfamethoxazole, foscarnet, pentamidine, amphotericin B, intravenous dye)
Skin disease	If not apparent, may need skin biopsy, culture of fluid or tissue, or direct examination of tissue scrapings
Genital disease	The approach should be as in HIV-negative patients; the presentation may vary; cervical examination and Pap smear is advised every 6 months
Musculoskeletal disease	Severe cases require laboratory studies, biopsy, or joint aspiration

approached in HIV-infected patients in a manner similar to that used for other populations. However, clinicians must recognize that syndromes may be more prolonged and more varied in their presentations, thus requiring a methodical diagnostic approach to correctly identify the causative pathogen.

Cervical disease is very common in women with HIV infection. Human papillomavirus has been associated with cervical atypia and squamous intraepithelial lesions. While the evaluation of cervical disease in this population is controversial, it is reasonable to perform a cervical examination and Pap smear every 6 months. Colposcopy should be performed if squamous intraepithelial lesions are found.

MUSCULOSKELETAL DISORDERS

Myalgias, weakness, muscle tenderness, and muscle wasting are commonly reported by patients with HIV infection. Muscle enzymes may be elevated in some asymptomatic patients, particularly after vigorous exercise. Electrophysiologic studies and muscle biopsy are appropriate if the manifestations are severe; these tests often do not lead to a definitive identification of etiologic factors, although they are useful for distinguishing between neuropathy and myopathy (Table 341.4).

Arthralgias and arthropathies are also common manifestations. Evaluation should include serologic testing for rheumatologic disorders, such as aspiration of joint fluid (if any is present). Synovial biopsy is rarely indicated.

REFERENCES

Furrer H, Egger M, Opravil M, et al. Stopping primary antipneumocystis prophylaxis in HIV-1 infected adults treated with combination antiretroviral therapy. *N Engl J Med* 1999 *(in press)*.

Glassock RJ, Cohen AH, Danovitch G, et al. Human immunodeficiency virus and the kidney. *Ann Intern Med* 1990;112:35–49

Hambleton J. Hematologic complications of HIV infection. *Oncology* 1996; 10:671–680.

Jabs D. Ocular manifestations of HIV infection. *Trans Am Ophthalmol Soc* 1995;93:623–683.

Ledergerber B, Effer M, Opravil M, et al. Clinical progression and virologic failure on highly active antiretroviral therapy in HIV-1 patients: a prospective cohort study. *Lancet* 1999;353:868–868.

Miller V, Mocroft A, Reiss P, et al. Relations among CD4 lymphocyte count nadir, antiretroviral therapy, and HIV-1 disease progression: results from the Eurosida study. *Ann Intern Med* 1999;130:570–577.

Murray HW, Godbold JH, Jurica KB, et al. Progression to AIDS in patients with lymphadenopathy or AIDS-related complex: reappraisal of risk and predictive factors. *Am J Med* 1989;86:533–538.

Palella FJ, Delaney KM, Moorman AC, et al. Declining morbidity and mortality among patients with advanced human immunodeficiency virus infection. *N Engl J Med* 1998;338:853–860.

Sepkowitz KA, Telzac EE, Carrow M, et al. Fever among outpatients with advanced human immunodeficiency virus infection. *Arch Intern Med* 1989;153:1909.

U.S. Public Health Service/Infectious Disease Society of America. Guidelines for prevention of opportunistic infections in patients with HIV infection. *MMWR* 1999:xxx–xxx.

Wilcox CM, Straub RF, Clark WS. Prospective evaluation of oropharyngeal finding in human immunodeficiency virus–infected patients with esophageal ulcers. *Am J Gastroenterol* 1995;90:1938.

Kelley's Textbook of Internal Medicine, fourth edition. Edited by H. David Humes. Lippincott Williams & Wilkins, Philadelphia © 2000.

HIV/AIDS: APPROACH TO THE PATIENT WITH PULMONARY DISEASE

PHILIP C. HOPEWELL

PRESENTATION

Pulmonary disorders in patients with HIV infection present with cough, shortness of breath, and, occasionally, chest pain. In addition, infectious disorders usually are marked by fever. Data from a large multicenter study, the Pulmonary Complications of HIV Infection Study (PCHIS), have indicated that screening for lung diseases among patients with HIV infection who do not have respiratory symptoms is not useful. The yield from chest radiographs, examinations of induced sputum for *Pneumocystis carinii* and acid-fast bacilli, pulmonary function tests, and frequent interviews to elicit symptoms was extremely low, and the value of the few instances in which diagnoses were established was offset by false-positive results.

In the PCHIS cohort, an analysis of symptoms showed that cough and shortness of breath were present in a high proportion of patients subsequently shown to have lung disease, whereas constitutional symptoms such as fever and weight loss in the absence of respiratory symptoms were highly unlikely to be associated with lung disease.

In addition to HIV-associated lung diseases, patients with HIV infection may have lung diseases such as asthma or chronic obstructive airway disease, which cause cough, shortness of breath, and wheezing that are not associated with HIV infection. Symptoms and findings caused by these disorders do not entail the same diagnostic approach as symptoms and findings that are suggestive of an HIV-associated disease.

PATHOPHYSIOLOGIC FACTORS

The pulmonary disorders that occur in patients with HIV infection all relate in some fashion to the immune compromise that is produced by the virus. In general, the frequency and types of lung diseases increase with decreasing immune responsiveness, which is reflected most directly by the CD4$^+$ lymphocyte count. Both cell-mediated and humoral immune responsiveness decrease as the CD4 count decreases, making patients with HIV infection progressively more vulnerable to a wide variety of pathogens. Similarly, the degree of immunocompromise increases as the amount of circulating HIV increases.

HISTORY AND PHYSICAL EXAMINATION

The salient points in the history related to presumed HIV-associated lung diseases are listed in Table 342.1. Respiratory disorders

TABLE 342.1.	SALIENT POINTS IN THE HISTORY OF HIV-INFECTED PATIENTS WITH PULMONARY DISEASE

Presence or absence of cough
Production of sputum (purulent or clear?)
Presence or absence of shortness of breath
Presence or absence of fever or chills
Duration, tempo, and severity of symptoms
Previous respiratory diseases
CD4 lymphocyte count (if known)
Presence of weight loss, diarrhea, sore mouth or throat
Use of anti-*Pneumocystis* prophylaxis
Exposure to individuals with tuberculosis
Places of residence currently and in recent past
Previous tuberculin skin tests and results
Use of antituberculous prophylaxis
Previous or current residence in areas endemic for histoplasmosis or coccidioidomycosis

are heralded by the presence of cough and shortness of breath. The rate of symptom progression tends to be more rapid with bacterial pneumonia and slower with *P. carinii* pneumonia. Other infections also tend to be more indolent than bacterial pneumonia. In a patient with acute bronchitis or bacterial pneumonia, the cough usually is productive of purulent sputum. The cough in a patient with *P. carinii* pneumonia typically is nonproductive. This is an important distinction because the diagnostic approach may vary depending on whether a patient produces purulent sputum.

The main risk factor for *P. carinii* pneumonia is a CD4 count of less than 200 cells per microliter. Presumably a high circulating viral burden is also indicative of increased risk, but this presumption is not well quantified. Most patients with diagnosed HIV infection are aware of their most recent CD4 count, indicating whether they are at risk for *P. carinii* infection. *P. carinii* pneumonia developed in a few patients in the PCHIS cohort who had CD4 counts higher than 200 cells per microliter. All but one of these patients had symptoms or findings relating to HIV infection (significant weight loss, unexplained diarrhea, or oral thrush), in addition to respiratory symptoms. It also is important to inquire about the use of prophylactic therapy for *P. carinii*. Although anti-*Pneumocystis* prophylaxis does not entirely prevent *P. carinii* pneumonia, the disease does not occur in patients receiving preventive therapy until there is more advanced immunodeficiency compared with patients who are not receiving prophylaxis.

The history is of particular relevance in the identification of risk factors for tuberculosis. These include exposure to individuals with tuberculosis, a history of a positive tuberculin skin test, residence in an area of high tuberculosis incidence, and previous use of isoniazid preventive therapy. It also is important to determine whether the patient has lived in areas that are endemic for the fungal diseases histoplasmosis and coccidioidomycosis.

Because Kaposi's sarcoma involving the lungs is uncommon in patients who have not had cutaneous lesions, it is important to ask about prior diagnosis of Kaposi's sarcoma and, if present, whether any therapy has been given.

The physical examination of the lungs by itself is not espe-

TABLE 342.2.	RELEVANT FINDINGS ON PHYSICAL EXAMINATION IN PATIENTS WITH HIV INFECTION AND PULMONARY SYMPTOMS

Fever
Evidence of weight loss
Presence or absence of oral candidiasis
Lymphadenopathy
Hepatic and/or splenic enlargement
Cutaneous or mucous membrane Kaposi's sarcoma
Findings related to the lungs (e.g., wheezing, rales, evidence of consolidation or pleural fluid)

cially helpful in elucidating the cause of respiratory symptoms in a patient with HIV infection. However, wheezing suggests airways obstruction as the cause for the symptoms. Other findings add little that is not provided by the chest radiograph.

In contrast, nonpulmonary findings may assist in the formulation of a differential diagnosis. For example, evidence of weight loss or oral thrush is indicative of an increased risk for *P. carinii* pneumonia, even if the CD4 count is higher than 200 cells per microliter. Lymphadenopathy or hepatosplenomegaly suggests that the pulmonary disease may be part of a disseminated infection or neoplastic process. Cutaneous or mucous membrane Kaposi's sarcoma is present in many patients who have pulmonary involvement with the neoplasm. As the listing summarized in Table 342.2 suggests, findings that do not emanate from the lungs themselves often are more helpful than pulmonary findings.

DIFFERENTIAL DIAGNOSIS

The differential diagnosis of respiratory symptoms varies depending on the severity of HIV-induced immune compromise (Table 342.3). Data from the PCHIS cohort indicate that acute bronchitis is the most common cause of pulmonary symptoms

TABLE 342.3.	MOST COMMON CAUSES OF RESPIRATORY SYMPTOMS IN PATIENTS WITH HIV INFECTION

Early (CD4 lymphocyte count ≥500 cells/mm³)
  Acute bronchitis
  Bacterial pneumonia
Midcourse (CD4 lymphocyte count 200–499 cells/mm³)
  Acute bronchitis
  Bacterial pneumonia
  Tuberculosis
Late (CD4 lymphocyte count <200 cells/mm³)
  Pneumocystis carinii pneumonia
  Bacterial pneumonia
  Acute bronchitis
  Tuberculosis
  Fungal infections
  Kaposi's sarcoma

in early (CD4 count 500 cells per microliter or higher) and middle (CD4 count 200 to 499 cells per microliter) HIV disease, and bacterial pneumonia is increasingly common during these stages. When the CD4 count falls below 200 cells per microliter, *P. carinii* pneumonia becomes the most common lung disease and bacterial pneumonia continues to increase in frequency. Acute bronchitis is common, but less common than *P. carinii* pneumonia or bacterial pneumonia. The incidence of tuberculosis also increases as the CD4 cell count declines. In the PCHIS cohort, the median CD4 cell count for the 31 patients in whom tuberculosis developed during the study was 230 cells per microliter. Because of the location of the clinical centers for the PCHIS, neither histoplasmosis nor coccidioidomycosis was seen, but these diseases are common in their endemic areas.

Kaposi's sarcoma involving the lungs is uncommon and occurs when there is advanced immunosuppression. Among 168 patients with pulmonary Kaposi's sarcoma diagnosed during a 7-year period at San Francisco General Hospital, the median CD4 cell count was 19 cells per microliter. Other neoplastic processes involving the lungs are even less common, with non-Hodgkin's lymphoma seen most often.

APPROACH TO THE DIAGNOSTIC EVALUATION

Once it is determined that the history and physical examination suggest an HIV-associated lung disease, the next step usually is to obtain a chest radiograph. If a CD4 cell count has not been performed recently, one should be obtained. The major categories of radiographic findings are a normal film, peribronchial thickening, focal infiltration/consolidation, and diffuse infiltration. Additional findings of interest include intrathoracic lymphadenopathy, pleural effusion, parenchymal cysts or cavities, nodules, and pneumothorax.

The finding of a normal film or peribronchial thickening in a patient who has a productive cough is sufficient to establish a diagnosis of acute bronchitis. The patient should be followed up with or without antimicrobial therapy to ensure that the symptoms resolve.

Focal infiltration in a patient with a productive cough and purulent sputum is most consistent with a diagnosis of bacterial pneumonia. In this setting, sputum should be obtained for Gram stain and culture, and in general a blood specimen should be obtained for culture. A variety of organisms, as shown in Table 342.4, were isolated from patients in the PCHIS cohort who had bacterial pneumonia.

The most likely diagnosis in a patient with a CD4 count of less than 200 cells per microliter who has a pattern of diffuse infiltration is *P. carinii* pneumonia. However, there are many other disorders in the differential diagnosis of this set of circumstances. At this point, essentially three approaches could be used. The most simple is to begin empirical treatment with acute anti-*Pneumocystis* agents, observe the patient closely, and undertake a diagnostic evaluation only if the patient's response is suboptimal. Although this appears to be the least expensive option, the costs of delayed diagnosis must be taken into account. Moreover, the relative frequency of *P. carinii* as a cause of this constellation of findings varies between areas and populations.

TABLE 342.4.	PATHOGENS THAT CAUSE BACTERIAL PNEUMONIA IN PATIENTS WITH HIV INFECTION	
	Number	**Percentage**
Streptococcus pneumoniae	28	42
Haemophilus influenzae	10	15
Staphylococcus aureus	8	12
Gram-negative aerobic bacilli	8	12
Other	12	18

(Hirshtick RE, Glassroth J, Jordan MC, et al. Bacterial pneumonia in persons infected with the human immunodeficiency virus. *N Engl J Med* 1995;333:845, with permission.)

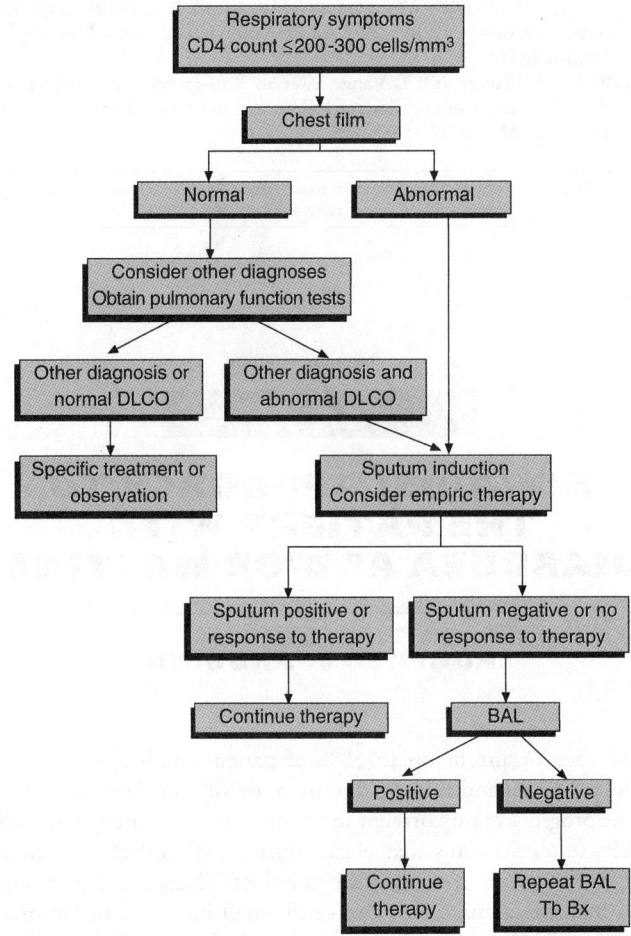

FIGURE 342.1. Algorithm describing the approach to establishing the cause of respiratory symptoms in patients with HIV infection. DLCO, diffusing capacity for carbon monoxide; BAL, bronchoalveolar lavage; Tb Bx, transbronchial lung biopsy. (From Hopewell PC, Masur H. *Pneumocystis carinii* pneumonia: current concepts. In: Sande MA, Volberding PA, eds. *The medical management of AIDS*, fourth ed. Philadelphia: WB Saunders, 1995:367, with permission.)

EVIDENCE LEVEL: B. Reference: Hopewell PC, Masur H. *Pneumocystis carinii* pneumonia: current concepts. In Sande MA, Volberding PA. *The medical management of Aids, fourth edition*. Philadelphia: WB Saunders, 1995:367.

The second approach is to seek a specific diagnosis beginning with an examination of sputum induced by the inhalation of a mist of hypertonic saline generated by an ultrasonic nebulizer. The use of this approach is shown in Fig. 342.1. Sputum obtained in this manner is examined for *P. carinii* and acid-fast bacilli, and is cultured for mycobacteria. If *P. carinii* or acid-fast organisms are not seen and another diagnosis has not been established, fiberoptic bronchoscopy and bronchoalveolar lavage are performed. The lavage specimen is examined for *P. carinii* and acid-fast organisms, and is cultured for mycobacteria and fungi. Transbronchial lung biopsy is not performed unless the radiograph is in some way unusual or no diagnosis is established with the bronchoalveolar lavage.

The third approach to diagnosis is to go directly to fiberoptic bronchoscopy and bronchoalveolar lavage with or without transbronchial lung biopsy. Overall, this method probably is the most costly, but also the most rapid, way to establish a specific diagnosis.

Several approaches have been used to determine whether patients who have convincing respiratory symptoms but normal chest films should undergo further expensive and perhaps invasive diagnostic studies. Data from the PCHIS cohort show that measurement of the diffusing capacity for carbon monoxide is a sensitive means of identifying patients who are likely to have *P. carinii* pneumonia. Gallium citrate lung scanning also has been used to indicate the presence of lung inflammation and the need for further diagnostic studies. However, this test is costly and has a built-in delay of 48 to 72 hours. More recently, high-resolution computed tomographic scanning has been used to identify areas of disease not evident on plain chest radiographs. In an analysis of a small number of patients, this approach provided accurate identification of patients with *P. carinii* pneumonia. Computed tomographic scanning has the advantage of being fast; however, the cost implications of this method have not been fully analyzed.

As long as a system for performing outpatient bronchoscopy is readily available, hospitalization is not required for the evaluation itself. The indications for hospitalization relate to the tempo and severity of the illness, not to the need for evaluation.

The cost-effectiveness of various diagnostic approaches has been subjected to analysis in several reports. However, these analyses are based on assumptions that vary between locales and institutions. What may be more important than cost-effectiveness analyses is for each institution to examine the accuracy of the diagnostic studies it uses and to develop an approach that is accurate and expeditious. Such an approach probably will be the most cost-effective.

BIBLIOGRAPHY

Davis L, Beck JM, Shellito J. Update: HIV infection and pulmonary host defenses. *Semin Respir Infect* 1993;8:75–85.

Hirshtick RE, Glassroth J, Jordan MC, et al. Bacterial pneumonia in persons infected with the human immunodeficiency virus. *N Engl J Med* 1995;333:845–851.

Hopewell PC, Masur H. *Pneumocystis carinii* pneumonia: current concepts. In: Sande MA, Volberding PA, eds. *The medical management of AIDS*, fourth ed. Philadelphia: WB Saunders, 1995:367–380.

Huang L, Hecht FM, Stansell JD, et al. Suspected *Pneumocystis carinii* pneumonia with a negative induced sputum examination: is early bronchoscopy useful? *Am J Respir Crit Care Med* 1995;151:1866–1871.

Ng V, Yajko D, Hadley WK. Update on laboratory tests for the diagnosis of pulmonary disease in HIV-1 infected individuals. *Semin Respir Infect* 1993;8:86–95.

Wallace JM, Hansen NI, LaVange L, et al. Respiratory disease trends in the pulmonary complications of HIV infection study cohort. *Am J Respir Crit Care Med* 1997;155:72–80.

Kelley's Textbook of Internal Medicine, fourth edition. Edited by H. David Humes. Lippincott Williams & Wilkins, Philadelphia © 2000.

C H A P T E R

343

HIV/AIDS: APPROACH TO THE PATIENT WITH DIARRHEA AND/OR WASTING

ROBERTO C. ARDUINO

Diarrhea occurs in up to 50% of patients with AIDS in the United States and Europe, and in up to 90% of those in Africa. The progressive impairment in the mucosal immune system and defense mechanisms that occurs during HIV infection predisposes the host to mucosal histopathologic changes and gastrointestinal infections. Some degree of small intestinal malabsorption, which may contribute to malnutrition and severe wasting, is common in advanced AIDS. HIV wasting syndrome is defined as an involuntary weight loss greater than 10% of baseline body weight plus chronic diarrhea (at least two loose stools per day for more than 30 days) or chronic weakness and documented fever for more than 30 days in the absence of other conditions that could explain these findings. Diarrhea with wasting characterizes 17% of new AIDS cases in the United States and is the most common clinical manifestation of HIV infection in Africa.

Two major mechanisms of enteric disease are seen in patients with HIV infection. The first is intestinal infection by one or more enteric pathogens, including common and opportunistic agents. The second is gut pathophysiologic alteration produced by HIV infection and the resultant immunosuppression, which may lead to atrophic villous changes, crypt hyperplasia, intestinal malabsorption, and diarrhea in the absence of identifiable pathogens.

■ DIFFERENTIAL DIAGNOSIS

In evaluating an HIV-positive patient with diarrhea, the physician should obtain a thorough exposure history and perform a physical examination. Important clues are recent and remote travel; drugs that can cause diarrhea (didanosine, HIV-1 protease inhibitors) or pancreatitis leading to subsequent steatorrhea (didanosine, pentamidine); the simultaneous occurrence of diarrhea

in household or other confined groups; and dietary factors (lactose intolerance, intake of unpasteurized dairy products or raw or uncooked meat or fish). Further diagnostic clues are the duration of the diarrhea, the degree of weight loss, the patient's absolute CD4 count (opportunistic pathogens became more common when CD4 counts are 200 cells per microliter or less), and the distinction between small- and large-bowel diarrhea. Large volume and relatively infrequent or nocturnal diarrhea suggests a small-bowel disorder (enteritis). This often is associated with bloating, gas, and cramping periumbilical pain. Many HIV-infected patients with chronic small bowel diarrhea also have malabsorption, as demonstrated by a decline in the rate of D-xylose or vitamin B_{12} absorption. The chronic diarrhea and wasting syndrome that can result from this process is called "slim disease" in African patients. In contrast, frequent, small-volume stools with abdominal pain often localized to the left or right lower quadrant and rebound tenderness suggests the diagnosis of large-bowel diarrhea (colitis). Fever is common and indicates an inflammatory process. Fecal leukocytes and blood in the stool (dysentery) suggests a diffuse colonic mucosal inflammation rather than a noninflammatory (small-bowel) diarrhea. Patients with colitis can have severe weight loss, often as a complication of the pathogens causing diarrhea rather than as a result of malabsorption. The potential small- and large-bowel pathogens that cause diarrheal disease in relation to the absolute CD4 count are shown in Table 343.1.

In the diagnostic evaluation of diarrhea in a patient with early HIV infection, examination of a stool specimen for pathogenic bacteria (*Salmonella, Shigella, Yersinia,* and *Campylobacter jejuni*), *Clostridium difficile* toxin, and standard ova and parasites (*Giardia lamblia* and *Entamoeba histolytica*) may be sufficient. Modified acid-fast and trichrome staining of the specimen should be performed, particularly in a patient with an absolute CD4 count of 100 cells per microliter or less, to rule out infection with *Cryptosporidium parvum, Isospora belli, Cyclospora cayetanensis,* and microsporidia (*Enterocytozoon bieneusi* and *Encephalitozoon intestinalis*). Routine blood cultures are appropriate in a febrile patient because bacterial pathogens such as *Salmonella* and *Shigella* sometimes can be isolated only from blood. Blood cultures for mycobacteria or fungi are recommended in a febrile patient with an absolute CD4 count of 100 cells per microliter or less. If no pathogen is identified in the stool or blood, the next step is to perform gastroduodenoscopy in a patient with small-bowel diarrhea, colonoscopy in a patient with symptoms suggesting colitis, or both in a patient in whom it is not possible to differentiate between small- and large-bowel diarrhea. Because cytomegalovirus (CMV) disease can be limited to the right colon, full colonoscopy is preferred to flexible sigmoidoscopy. Evaluation of small-bowel biopsy specimens includes culture for CMV and mycobacteria, and histopathologic examination for viral inclusions and, using special stains, acid-fast bacteria, fungi, and parasites. Electron microscopy for microsporidia is reserved for those specimens with negative results up to this point. Duodenal aspirates should be examined for parasites (cryptosporidia and microsporidia) using modified trichrome and acid-fast staining. Evaluation of colon biopsy specimens includes culture for mycobacteria and viruses (CMV, adenovirus, herpes simplex virus); histopathologic examination for viral inclusions, acid-

TABLE 343.1.	COMMON PATHOGENS THAT CAUSE SMALL- OR LARGE-BOWEL DIARRHEAL DISEASE IN RELATION TO THE ABSOLUTE CD4 LEUKOCYTE COUNT		
Absolute CD4 Leukocyte Count (cells/mm³)	**Type of Pathogen**	**Small-Bowel Pathogens**	**Large-Bowel Pathogens**
≥200	Protozoa	*Giardia lamblia*	*Entamoeba histolytica*
	Viruses	Rotavirus, HIV	Herpes simplex virus, adenovirus
	Bacteria	*Salmonella,* EAEC, EPEC, *Mycobacterium tuberculosis*	*Shigella, Campylobacter, Yersinia, Clostridium difficile, Aeromonas, Vibrio parahaemolyticus*
	Fungi		*Histoplasma capsulatum*
≤100	Protozoa	*Cryptosporidium parvum, Isospora belli, Cyclospora, Enterocytozoon bieneusi, Encephalitozoon intestinalis*	
	Viruses		Cytomegalovirus
	Bacteria	*Mycobacterium avium* complex, EAEC, EPEC	
	Fungi	*Cryptococcus neoformans*	

EAEC, enteroadherent *Escherichia coli;* EPEC, enteropathogenic *E. coli.*
(Adapted from Mayer HB, Wanke CA. Diagnostic strategies in HIV-infected patients with diarrhea. *AIDS* 1994;8:1640.)

fast bacteria, and fungi; and electron microscopy for adenovirus when the results of all other studies are negative.

STRATEGIES FOR OPTIMAL CARE

The mainstay of therapy for diarrhea is replacement of fluid and electrolytes. Milk and other dairy products should be avoided because of the intraluminal osmotic load that results from disaccharidase depletion caused by intestinal mucosal damage. The use of antidiarrheal agents, such as loperamide hydrochloride, diphenoxylate, paregoric, or opium, provides symptomatic control of the diarrhea in most patients. Octreotide, a long-acting somatostatin analog given subcutaneously at a dosage of 50 to 500 μg every 8 hours, has a beneficial effect in some patients with AIDS who have diarrhea that is refractory to conventional therapy. Parenteral nutrition may result in temporary weight gain when diarrhea is severe and prolonged, but its role remains controversial because of a lack of controlled data showing that it improves quality of life, its high cost, and difficulties in its administration. Wasting may not respond to enteral feeding because of malabsorption. Treatment with megestrol acetate, a synthetic oral progesterone, has resulted in increased appetite and weight gain in patients with AIDS. Dronabinol, the major psychoactive component of marijuana, also has been reported to increase appetite and promote weight gain in HIV-infected patients with wasting. Anabolic agents (testosterone cypionate or enanthate, nandrolone decanoate or oxandrolone) with or without planned exercise are recommended in patients with adequate caloric intake.

Identifying the cause of diarrhea and treating it with appropriate antimicrobial agents are the goals of therapy in HIV-infected patients. Because a wide array of pathogens can cause diarrhea, and because drug interactions and toxicity are a prob-

lem in patients with AIDS, specific therapy is preferable to empirical treatment. The lack of antimicrobial agents that are active against some pathogens, the development of antimicrobial resistance, and the simultaneous presence of multiple pathogens are problems in these patients. Because of the frequent recurrence of infections in patients with AIDS, lifelong suppressive therapy is necessary for almost all pathogens.

Ganciclovir therapy for CMV colitis in patients with AIDS is associated with weight gain and improved quality of life. The major toxicity associated with ganciclovir is bone marrow suppression with neutropenia and thrombocytopenia, particularly when the agent is used in conjunction with zidovudine. Foscarnet inhibits the DNA polymerase of all herpesviruses, including CMV, and is active against ganciclovir-resistant CMV. Herpes simplex virus infection usually is controlled by oral acyclovir. Foscarnet is indicated for patients who are infected with acyclovir-resistant strains.

No effective antimicrobial agent is available for the treatment of *Cryptosporidium,* although paromomycin and azithromycin have been associated with some clinical improvement. The immune reconstitution associated with the use of highly active antiretroviral therapy can result in a complete clinical and microbiologic resolution of HIV-associated cryptosporidiosis and microsporidiosis. Isosporiasis responds to treatment with trimethoprim–sulfamethoxazole or pyrimethamine, but up to 50% of patients have relapses after the cessation of therapy. Trimethoprim–sulfamethoxazole also has been effective in treating primary *Cyclospora* infection and preventing relapses. The common use of trimethoprim–sulfamethoxazole for the prevention of other opportunistic infections in HIV-infected patients may explain the rarity of isosporiasis and *Cyclospora* infection among these patients in the United States. Albendazole (400 mg twice a day for 1 month) has resulted in resolution of the diarrhea and elimination of the organism in AIDS patients with diarrhea caused by *Encephalitozoon intestinalis.* Studies on *Enterocytozoon bieneusi* infection have not been as successful. Despite the uncertain pathogenic role of *Blastocystis hominis,* metronidazole or iodoquinol may be indicated when high concentrations of *B. hominis* are the only organism found in the stool. Metronidazole is effective to treat giardiasis.

The treatment of *Salmonella, Shigella, Campylobacter,* and *Yersinia* infection in HIV-infected patients follows the standard guidelines. The use of one of the new macrolides (clarithromycin or azithromycin) is an essential component in the treatment of *Mycobacterium avium* complex. Because of the emergence of resistance, a macrolide should be given with at least one or two other drugs that have microbiologic activity against *M. avium* complex, such as ethambutol, rifabutin, rifampin, quinolones (ciprofloxacin and ofloxacin), or amikacin.

BIBLIOGRAPHY

Coodley GO, Loveless MO, Merrill TM. The HIV wasting syndrome: a review. *J AIDS* 1994;7:681–694.

Flanigan TC, Whalen J, Turner R, et al. *Cryptosporidium* infection and CD4 counts. *Ann Intern Med* 1992;116:840–842.

Janoff EN, Orenstein JM, Manischewitz JF, et al. Adenovirus colitis in the acquired immunodeficiency syndrome. *Gastroenterology* 1991;100:976–979.

Kotler DP, Orenstein JM. Chronic diarrhea and malabsorption associated with enteropathogenic bacterial infection in a patient with AIDS. *Ann Intern Med* 1993;119:127–128.

Pape JW, Verdier R, Boncy J, et al. *Cyclospora* infection in adults infected with HIV. Clinical manifestations, treatment, and prophylaxis. *Ann Intern Med* 1994;121:654–657.

Smith PD. Infectious diarrhea in patients with AIDS. *Gastroenterol Clin North Am* 1993;22:535–548.

Smith PD, Lane HC, Gill VJ, et al. Intestinal infections in patients with the acquired immunodeficiency syndrome (AIDS). *Ann Intern Med* 1988;108:328–333.

Kelley's Textbook of Internal Medicine, fourth edition. Edited by H. David Humes. Lippincott Williams & Wilkins, Philadelphia © 2000.

CHAPTER 344

HIV/AIDS: APPROACH TO THE PATIENT WITH NEUROLOGIC SYMPTOMS

RICHARD W. PRICE

Both the central nervous system (CNS) and the peripheral nervous system (PNS) may be injured in the course of HIV-1 (referred to hereinafter simply as HIV) infection as a result of several types of disease processes, including particularly opportunistic infections but also autoimmunity, disturbed systemic organ function, and, more fundamentally, effects of the AIDS retrovirus itself. Despite these several pathways leading to neurologic injury and the potential for perturbed function at all levels of

the neuraxis, a logical and sequential clinical approach usually leads to correct diagnosis. Although it is fortunate that the widespread use of combination antiretroviral therapy has considerably reduced the neurologic burden of HIV infection, this group of diseases remains important, and accurate diagnosis is critical in reducing mortality, preventing important morbidity, and predicting prognosis.

Table 344.1 outlines a classification of the neurologic compli-

TABLE 344.1. CLASSIFICATION OF THE NEUROLOGIC COMPLICATIONS OF HIV INFECTION

Common	Less Common
Central Nervous System	
Meninges and other structures surrounding the CNS	
Early and late-middle course	
Asymptomatic HIV infection	"Aseptic" meningitis
Late	
Cryptococcal meningitis	*Liysteria monocytogenes* meningitis
HIV headache	
Brain	
Focal–middle course	Multiple sclerosis–like disease
Focal–late course	
Cerebral toxoplasmosis	*Mycobacterium tuberculosis*
PCNSL	*Aspergillus*
PML	VZV vasculitis
"Diffuse"—early course	Postinfectious encephalomyelitis
"Diffuse"—late course	
AIDS dementia complex	
CMV encephalitis	
Metabolic/toxic encephalopathies	
Spinal cord	
Late	
Vacuolar myelopathy (part of AIDS dementia complex)	VZV myelitis
Peripheral Nervous System and Muscle	
Nerve and Root	
Early	Brachial plexitis, mono- and polyneuropathies
Middle	
Subacute and chronic inflammatory demyelinating polyneuropathy	Mononeuritis multiplex, "benign" type
Late	
Distal, predominantly sensory polyneuropathy	CMV polyradiculopathy
Nucleoside polyneuropathy	Mononeuritis multiplex (CMV)
Autonomic neuropathy	
Muscle	
Late	
Zidovudine myopathy	Inflammatory myopathy Noninflammatory myopathies

CNS, central nervous system; PCNSL, primary CNS lymphoma; PML, progressive multifocal lymphoma; VZV, varicella-zoster virus; CMV, cytomegalovirus.

cations of HIV infection that combines two of the most useful diagnostic variables: background *stage of systemic HIV infection* and *neuroanatomical localization*. The stage of systemic infection, and particularly the degree of immunosuppression, strongly determines the spectrum of disease vulnerabilities, whereas anatomical localization predicts the range of differential diagnosis because of the predilection of individual disease processes to involve particular parts of the nervous system or in characteristic spacial and temporal patterns.

NEUROLOGIC DISEASE IN "EARLY" HIV INFECTION

A variety of CNS and PNS disorders have been described in the setting of primary HIV infection and seroconversion. Some of these (headache and aseptic meningitis) may relate to direct HIV infection of the meninges and brain as a component of the initial viremia, whereas others (encephalopathy, polyneuropathy, brachial plexitis) likely relate to autoimmune responses triggered by HIV infection and thus resemble other postinfectious encephalitides or neuropathies. Serious or lasting morbidity from these is uncommon and indeed most are insufficiently severe to trigger special medical evaluation.

Despite the direct exposure of the CNS to HIV that begins during primary infection and continues throughout the course of infection, patients usually remain neurologically asymptomatic during the period of "clinical latency." However, examination of cerebrospinal fluid (CSF) often shows evidence of ongoing infection. Viral RNA is detectable in the CSF, although in lower amount than in the plasma, and host responses may be present including mononuclear pleocytosis and protein elevation. While this meningeal infection appears to be clinically benign, these background CSF abnormalities must be taken into account when interpreting results of diagnostic lumbar puncture in this setting.

There are at least two notable exceptions to this freedom from neurologic disease during this phase of systemic infection. One of these is a very rare, multiple sclerosis–like CNS disease in which patients develop demyelinating lesions with remissions and exacerbations and may be responsive to corticosteroid medication. The second exception involves demyelinating polyneuropathies that can evolve either subacutely (Guillain–Barré syndrome) or chronically (chronic idiopathic demyelinating polyneuropathy). These polyneuropathies are sufficiently common as a complication of HIV infection that patients presenting with these conditions should be queried regarding risk of infection and, as appropriate, undergo serologic testing. These neuropathies have an autoimmune pathogenesis and respond to plasma exchange or intravenous immunoglobulin in a fashion similar to that of their non-HIV counterparts.

NEUROLOGIC COMPLICATIONS OF LATE HIV INFECTION

While the incidence of neurologic disease has been reduced by combination antiretroviral therapy, it is still high in those who suffer progressive immunosuppression either because such treatment is unavailable or because this therapy fails. In those who reach the late stage of HIV infection, as measured by reduced $CD4^+$ T-lymphocyte counts, diagnosis begins with anatomical localization of symptoms and signs. The first step involves separating CNS from PNS disease based on the type and distribution of complaints and the findings on examination. Further anatomical subdivision then separates CNS disorders according to presenting manifestations of headache without brain dysfunction, predominantly focal brain dysfunction, predominantly nonfocal brain dysfunction, and myelopathy (which also may be segmentally focal or more diffuse). Likewise, PNS disorders are usefully divided into focal neuropathies and radiculopathies, polyneuropathies, and myopathies.

MAJOR CNS DISEASES COMPLICATING LATE HIV INFECTION

HEADACHE AND MENINGITIS

Headache is common in HIV infection and can be of diverse origin, including both benign and severe conditions. New-onset headache should always be taken seriously and evaluated carefully. If accompanied by focal or nonfocal neurologic dysfunction, it should be approached along a path similar to that used for patients presenting with these abnormalities without headache, although often more rapidly. The clinician must also consider that focal diseases may not present with obvious neurologic dysfunction when they involve "noneloquent" brain regions (e.g., anterior frontal lobes), or are small and multiple; hence, neuroimaging may be needed to rule them out.

In the absence of neurologic dysfunction or focal parenchymal disease, there are a limited number of major considerations. These include meningitis, most notably that due to *Cryptococcus neoformans,* but also an aseptic meningitis seemingly caused by HIV. Cryptococcal meningitis is the most common meningitis afflicting AIDS patients and may present with remarkably mild symptoms; recognition is critical since treatment is usually effective. "Aseptic" meningitis may be acute or chronic in onset and is accompanied by mononuclear pleocytosis and meningeal irritation. So-called "HIV headache" may be clinically similar but is not accompanied by CSF pleocytosis. It can nonetheless be quite severe and difficult to treat.

FOCAL CNS DISORDERS

Nearly all of the common focal CNS disorders complicating AIDS evolve subacutely. In contrast, acute CNS disease is uncommon in AIDS, although it can be caused by ischemic stroke, hemorrhage, or migraine-like disease. While transient ischemic attacks and strokes can complicate AIDS, their pathogenesis is usually unclear; protein-S disturbance or other coagulopathies may be involved in some patients, and varicella-zoster virus (VZV) may cause CNS vasculitis in some. Hemorrhage uncommonly complicates some of the focal lesions discussed below.

The subacute course of the common focal CNS disorders

relates to similar pathogenetic process, particularly the time course of DNA replication of either invading pathogens or host cells. The three most common focal diseases, comprising perhaps three-fourths or more of such cases, are cerebral toxoplasmosis, primary CNS lymphoma (PCNSL) and progressive multifocal leukoencephalopathy (PML). All of these present subacutely, though they tend to differ somewhat in their temporal profiles. Typically, cerebral toxoplasmosis is the most rapidly evolving, usually presenting within days of onset. PCNSL is intermediary, presenting within several days to two weeks after onset. PML is the most indolent, evolving over several weeks. There are some other differences as well. For example, cerebral toxoplasmosis often has an encephalitic component that produces confusion or lethargy, which in some patients can overshadow focality, as well as fever. The deep location and slow growth of PCNSL may lead to patients being mentally slow along with their focal manifestations (e.g., hemiparesis). In contrast, PML patients usually are alert despite very clear focal abnormalities.

Brain neuroimaging is essential in diagnosis of these focal brain diseases. In general, magnetic resonance imaging (MRI) is superior to computed tomography since it better detects small lesions and white matter abnormalities, and also provides superior definition of the character of lesions. Among the common focal brain diseases, usually the most important issue is to distinguish between toxoplasmosis and PCNSL. Both show focal mass lesions, although the lesions of toxoplasmosis tend to be more numerous, involve cortex and basal ganglia, and exhibit ringlike contrast enhancement at times with an eccentric target sign (a nodule of contrast enhancement at or near the surrounding ring). PCNSL lesions have a predilection for the periventricular white matter and tend to extend along the ventricular ependyma.

However, since these appearances may overlap and may not be distinguished with certainty, most patients require additional diagnostic evaluation. Earlier in the epidemic, it was recommended that all such patients first undergo a trial of anti-*Toxoplasma* therapy before other testing. This has changed with advances in both diagnostic interpretation and methodology along with a relative decrease in the incidence of toxoplasmosis related to antibiotic prophylaxis against *Pneumocystis carinii*, which also effectively reduces the incidence of toxoplasmosis. In brief, we take the current approach. If subjects are *Toxoplasma* antibody–seropositive, not taking prophylaxis, and MRI shows lesions characteristic of *Toxoplasma* abscesses, we begin management with a trial of therapy; if patients respond within a week or two, we consider this diagnostic. However, if the subjects are *Toxoplasma*-seronegative or the MRI lesions are not typical, then PCNSL is considered to be the most likely diagnosis. Polymerase chain reaction (PCR) detection of Epstein–Barr virus (EBV) sequences in CSF has been shown to be highly sensitive and specific for PCNSL, at least in the investigative setting; if this is available, then it can be used to establish this diagnosis. Thallium single photon emission computed tomography (SPECT) scanning has been advocated as helpful as well, though it is not as specific as EBV PCR and in many patients adds little to the information available from MRI. Our current approach in the absence of EBV PCR is to advocate early brain biopsy in those suspected of PCNSL. This avoids needless delay and attendant worsening neurologic status. While the overall prognosis of PCNSL is poor, radiation therapy and concomitant antiretroviral therapy in those not optimally treated can lead to a very gratifying outcome in some.

Progressive multifocal leukoencephalopathy can usually be diagnosed on the basis of the clinical history and examination with gradually evolving distinct focal abnormalities and MRI images showing corresponding focal white matter lesions. PCR detection of nucleic acid of JC virus, the etiologic agent, confirms the diagnosis in 70% to 80% of cases. Where uncertainty continues, brain biopsy may be needed. The remaining, less common causes of focal CNS disease usually are diagnosed by the presence of disease in other organs, characteristic neuroimaging, or direct brain biopsy.

NONFOCAL CNS DISORDERS

It is helpful to subdivide the nonfocal disorders into two subgroups: those in which patients remain fully awake and those in which there is reduced alertness. The most important disorder in the first category is the AIDS dementia complex (ADC, also called HIV-associated cognitive–motor complex), a subacutely or indolently progressive CNS disorder affecting cognition, motor performance, and behavior. The salient aspects of the cognitive dysfunction in these patients include difficulty with speed of thought, attention, and concentration. When mildly affected, patients complain of difficulty remembering appointments or attending to tasks such as reading, as well as needing to remind themselves with notes or by repeating the same task. When more severe, most aspects of mentation are compromised, so that daily activities and self-care no longer are possible. While motor symptoms usually occur later, the concomitant involvement of motor systems can usually be detected earlier on examination by looking for slowing of rapid finger opposition, toe tapping, or ocular saccades. Later, particularly in those with the vacuolar myelopathy variant (see below), gait may be compromised with spasticity and ataxia, and may progress to an end stage of paraparesis. Deep tendon reflexes are increased and abnormal "release" reflexes including a snout response appear. Behavioral manifestations include apathy, blunting of personality and drive, and, in those most severely affected, mutism.

Several pathogenetic questions remain, but the most widely prevalent theory is that the AIDS dementia complex is caused by HIV itself rather than another opportunistic pathogen. This may involve "indirect" mechanisms of brain injury whereby infection of brain macrophages and microglia leads to activation of cytokine and other endogenous neurotoxic pathways in the brain. Antiretroviral therapy has been reported to reverse, arrest, and prevent ADC and likely accounts for its declining incidence.

Among the nonfocal disorders that concomitantly suppress alertness and cognition, metabolic and toxic encephalopathies related to systemic organ compromise and neuroactive drugs are most important. As noted, in some patients with cerebral toxoplasmosis, diffuse encephalopathy may characterize presentation, usually due to widespread small lesions. Cryptococcal meningitis may also present in this way. Cytomegalovirus (CMV) encephalitis is another important cause of nonfocal brain dysfunction. Its presentation can range from impaired cognition with little focality or impairment of consciousness to impaired consciousness with nystagmus and other minor focal abnormalities. Diagnosis may be difficult but is essential to implement specific treatment. Some patients may have a characteristic MRI image showing altered signal adjacent to the ventricles related to subependymal infection, and some will exhibit CSF pleocytosis, including the presence of neutrophils. With or without these findings, detection of CMV nucleic acid using PCR or other amplification techniques has greatly aided diagnosis.

MYELOPATHIES

Myelopathies are also divided into focal and diffuse types. The most common cause of focal (or segmental) myelopathy is VZV in which the level of spinal cord dysfunction is usually centered at or near the level corresponding to a preceding dermatomal rash. Onset is usually delayed for days to a week or two after the rash. The pathogenesis involves a varying combination of direct spinal cord infection and local vasculitis, which may account for the explosive onset or progression in some. Other rare focal myelopathies may relate to spinal or meningeal lymphoma or to the infections described above that characteristically cause focal brain lesions. Tuberculosis of the spine also can cause cord compression. In active intravenous drug abusers, spinal epidural abscess may enter into differential diagnosis but its incidence is independent of the CD4$^+$ T-cell count.

Vacuolar myelopathy was defined as part of the AIDS dementia complex, although it can be clinically segregated in some because of the prominence of gait impairment in relation to that of cognition. It is a nonfocal myelopathy in that it is usually symmetrical and without clear definition of a segmental level of spinal cord involvement. Motor abnormalities predominate with spasticity and hyperreflexia, whereas sensation is relatively preserved unless there is concomitant neuropathy. Bladder and bowel dysfunction are usually late manifestations. Diagnosis depends largely on clinical findings since MRI of the spinal cord is usually unremarkable. Human T-lymphotrophic virus types I and II can cause a similar nonfocal myelopathy, although this is independent of the stage of HIV infection and develops in the same population because of overlapping transmission risk; serology is helpful in this diagnosis.

MAJOR PERIPHERAL NERVOUS SYSTEM AND MUSCLE DISEASES

FOCAL NEUROPATHIES

The focal neuropathies are of several types, and most are uncommon. They include facial palsy, at times associated with aseptic meningitis. Peripheral root or nerve involvement may also complicate metastatic systemic lymphoma. Of greater importance is more widespread nerve involvement with mononeuritis multiplex, which can be of two types, differing in cause, prognosis, and treatment. The first occurs earlier in HIV infection, when blood CD4$^+$ T-lymphocyte counts are in the 150 to 400 cells per cubic millimeter range. It is more benign and self-limited, may relate to a vasculitis involving immune complex formation, and may respond to immunosuppression. The second is more

severe, occurs at very low CD4$^+$ cell counts, and is caused by CMV infection. If recognized and treated early, it may respond to anti-CMV therapy.

A second type of severe CMV infection of nerve is also important. This is a severe, subacute ascending radiculopathy or radiculomyelopathy. It usually begins with sacral involvement and spreads rostrally. It is painful and induces a nearly pathognomonic neutrophil-predominant CSF pleocytosis. Its progression can be arrested and partially reversed by aggressive anti-CMV treatment.

POLYNEUROPATHIES

The most common and important polyneuropathy—indeed the most common neuropathy overall in HIV infection—is a distal sensory polyneuropathy. This disorder affects axons and their sensory ganglion cell bodies rather than myelin and presents with paresthesias and pain in the feet. Indeed, the discomfort ("positive symptom") of the sensory nerve involvement exceeds the extent of functional impairment related to sensory loss or weakness ("negative symptoms"). In mild form this neuropathy is very common. In its less common severe form it can be a source of great morbidity related to intractable, disabling neuropathic pain. Its etiologic process and pathogenesis are uncertain, although speculation now centers on a triggering role of HIV and the effects of dysregulated local production of cytokines. Autonomic neuropathy also occurs and may involve similar processes.

A second type of sensory neuropathy relates to the toxicity of some of the antiretroviral nucleosides, including zalcitabine, didanosine, and stavudine. This axonal neuropathy is dose-related, largely reversible if the medication is stopped early, and may be mediated by an effect of these drugs on the DNA polymerase of nerve mitochondria. It may also be difficult to distinguish clinically from the spontaneous HIV-related distal sensory polyneuropathy and may require drug interruption for diagnosis.

These and other neuropathies can usually be diagnosed clinically but may require help from the electrophysiology laboratory evaluating electromyograms and nerve conduction. Other than those related to CMV infection or drug effects, treatment is often symptomatic.

MYOPATHIES

While uncommon, several types of myopathy have been identified in AIDS patients. These include an inflammatory polymyositis and non-inflammatory myopathy, at times with nemaline rods noted pathologically. There is controversy as to whether these both respond favorably to corticosteroid medication. Zidovudine also can cause a myopathy after prolonged use, perhaps related to a toxic effect on muscle mitochondrion DNA polymerase; this seems far less common than earlier in the epidemic when higher doses of this drug were used. Many patients with this condition, but perhaps not all, will show ragged red fibers on muscle biopsy and abnormal mitochondria ultrastructurally. Diagnosis of myopathy often involves assessment of blood creatine kinase and electromyographic examination to confirm its presence and biopsy to establish more definitive diagnosis.

BIBLIOGRAPHY

Antinori A, De Rossi G, Ammassari A, et al. Value of combined approach with thallium-201 single-photon emission computed tomography and Epstein–Barr virus DNA polymerase chain reaction in CSF for the diagnosis of AIDS-related primary CNS lymphoma. *J Clin Oncol* 1999; 17(2):554–560.

Berger JR, Levy RM. *AIDS and the nervous system.* Philadelphia: Lippincott-Raven, 1997.

Gendelman HE, Lipton SA, Epstein L, et al. *The neurology of AIDS.* New York: Chapman & Hall, 1998.

Hall CD, Dafni U, Simpson D, et al. Failure of cytarabine in progressive multifocal leukoencephalopathy associated with human immunodeficiency virus infection. *N Engl J Med* 1998;338:1345–1351.

Harrison MJG, McArthur JC. *AIDS and neurology.* (Clinical neurology and neurosurgery monographs.) New York: Churchill Livingstone, 1995.

Price RW. Neurologic disease. In: Dolin R, Masur H, Saag MS, eds. *AIDS therapy.* New York: Churchill Livingstone, 1999:620–638.

Simpson DM, Tagliati M. Nucleoside analogue–associated peripheral neuropathy in human immunodeficiency virus infection [Review]. *J AIDS Hum Retrovirol* 1995;9(2):153–161.

Staprans S, Inkina N, Glidden D, et al. Time course of cerebrospinal fluid (CSF) responses to antiretroviral therapy: evidence for variable compartmentalization of infection. *AIDS* 1999;13:1051–1061.

Kelley's Textbook of Internal Medicine, fourth edition. Edited by H. David Humes. Lippincott Williams & Wilkins, Philadelphia © 2000.

CHAPTER 345

PATHOGENESIS OF HIV INFECTION

SHARON LEWIN
MARTIN MARKOWITZ

HIV ENTRY

Human immunodeficiency virus 1 (hereinafter referred to simply as HIV) enters its target cells by interaction of the virion glycoproteins (gp120/41) with the CD4 molecule and an additional receptor now known to be a chemokine receptor. Chemokines are small proteins that serve as chemoattractants in inflammation. The two most important chemoreceptors for HIV are CXCR4 (also called fusin or LESTR) and CCR5. Macrophage tropic (M-tropic) strains of HIV replicate in macrophages and CD4$^+$ T cells and use the chemokine receptor CCR5. T tropic viruses replicate in primary CD4$^+$ T cells, established CD4$^+$ T-cell lines but not macrophages. T-tropic viruses use the chemokine receptor CXCR4 but can also use CCR5. Fusion of infected and uninfected cells leads to the formation of multinucleated giant cells, or syncytia. Most commonly, isolates derived early in the course of infection are non-syncytium-inducing (NSI), while isolates from approximately 50% of late stage patients have a syncytium-inducing (SI) phenotype. HIV viruses are now classified on the basis of their coreceptor usage (Fig. 345.1). The classification includes R5 (CCR5-tropic viruses or previously M-tropic, NSI viruses); X4 (CXCR4-tropic viruses or previously T-tropic, SI viruses); and R5X4 (using both receptors with comparable efficiency and those previously called dual tropic).

TRANSMISSION

HIV is transmitted by contact with infected body fluids, including blood or blood products; semen; vaginal and cervical secretions; amniotic fluid and breast milk. The precise mechanism of transmission of HIV is not completely understood. The R5 viruses are the strains most commonly transmitted and are present early in the disease. The most likely cellular target in the mucosa for initial viral infection is antigen-presenting cells, particularly macrophage-related cells of the dendritic cell lineage. Dendritic cells residing in skin are called Langerhans' cells (LCs), whereas those in the circulation are known as blood dendritic cells. Even though LCs are not highly permissive to HIV infection, both blood dendritic cells and Langerhans' cells are able to transmit HIV to T cells very efficiently (Fig. 345.2).

CLINICAL COURSE OF INFECTION

PRIMARY INFECTION

Primary HIV infection is associated with a rapid rise in plasma viremia, often to levels in excess of 1 million RNA molecules per milliliter. This is followed by a marked reduction in plasma viremia to a "steady-state" level of viral replication. The peak in viral load is associated with a fall in the level of CD4$^+$ T cells in the first 2 to 8 weeks following infection. The levels of CD4$^+$ T cells usually rebound toward normal but rarely return to preinfection levels (Fig. 345.3).

The decrease in viral load following acute infection is largely due to virus-specific immune responses that limit viral replication. These include cellular and humoral immunity, the secretion of virus-suppressing cytokines, and the possible exhaustion of suitable CD4$^+$ target cells. There is a strong temporal relationship between the appearance of HIV-specific cytotoxic T lymphocytes (CTL) responses and the striking fall in plasma viremia. Although HIV envelope–binding antibodies can be detected in the sera of HIV-infected individuals by 2 to 3 weeks following infection, most of these antibodies lack the ability to inhibit virus infection (Fig. 345.3).

CLINICAL LATENCY

Following primary infection, there is usually a relatively long period that is characterized by few, if any, clinical manifestations. In adults, the average time between infection and development of AIDS is 7 to 10 years. However, a small number of individuals progress rapidly to AIDS within 5 years. At the other extreme,

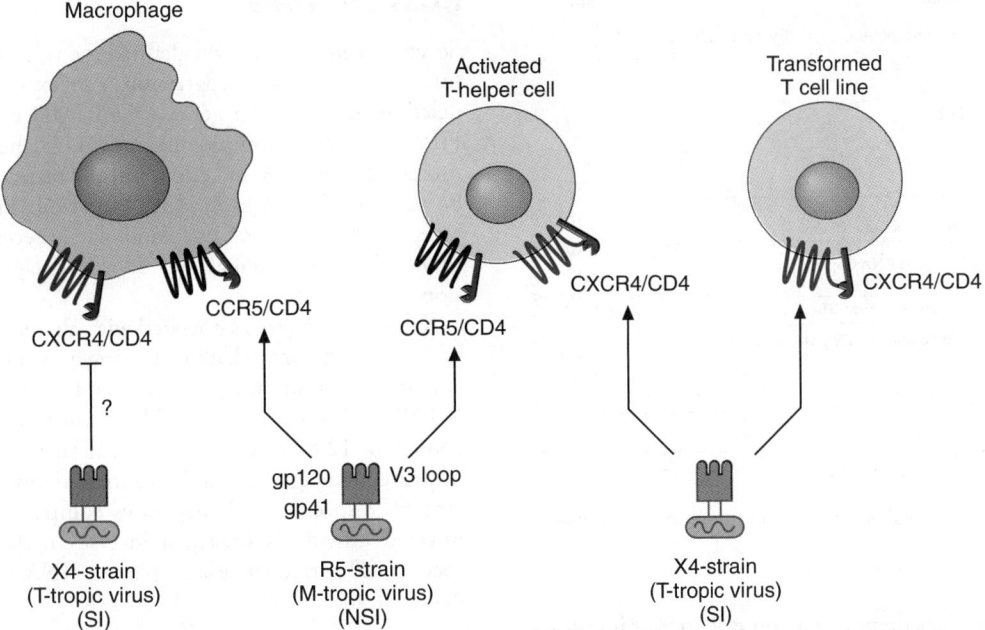

FIGURE 345.1. Basis of HIV cellular tropism. Previous nomenclature for viral tropism is noted at the bottom. R5 strains were previously named macrophage-tropic or NSI (non-syncytium-inducing in T-cell lines), whereas X4 isolates were known as T–cell line–tropic or SI (syncytium inducing). (Adapted from Littman D. Chemokine receptors: keys to AIDS pathogenesis? *Cell* 1998;93:677–680.)

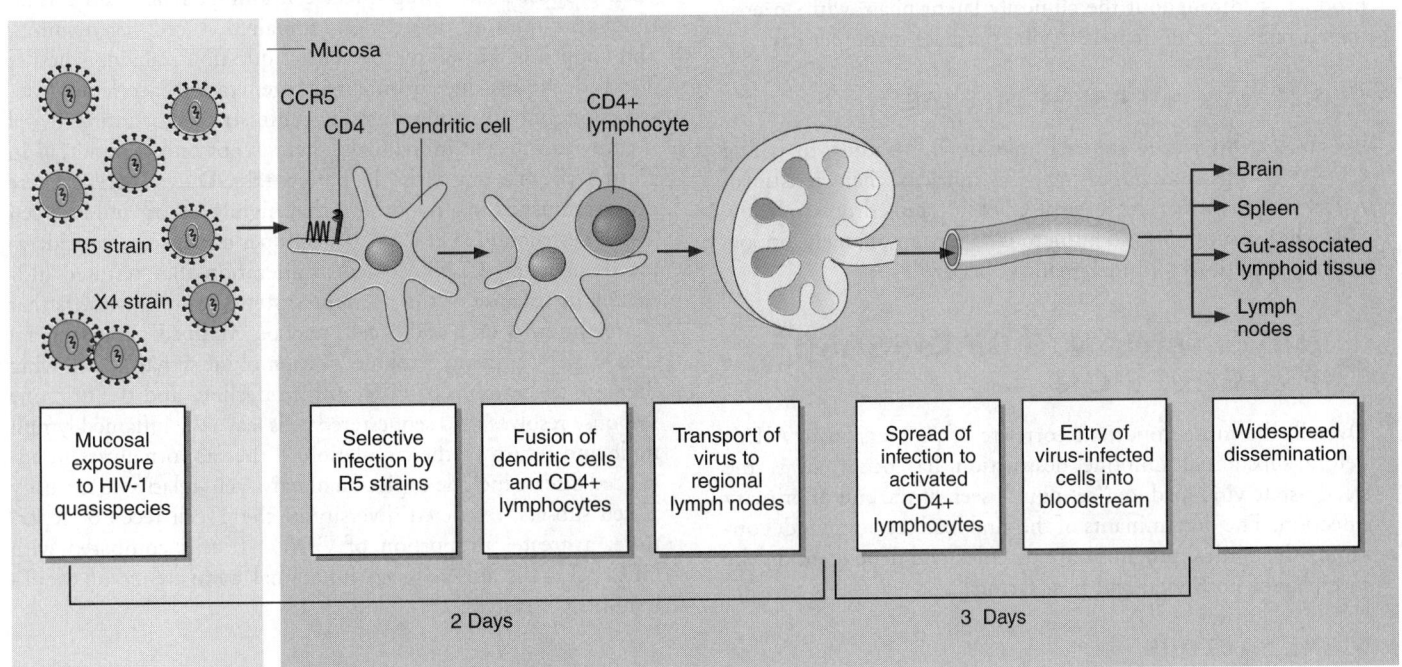

FIGURE 345.2. Early events following transmission of HIV. The arrows indicate the path of the virus. Dendritic cells, which express the viral coreceptors CD4 and CCR5, are selectively infected by R5 strains. Within 2 days after mucosal exposure, virus can be detected in the lymph nodes. Within another 3 days, it can be cultured from the plasma (based on experiments with SIV). (From Kahn J, Walker B. Current concepts: acute human immunodeficiency virus type 1 infection. *N Engl J Med* 1998;339:33–40, with permission.)

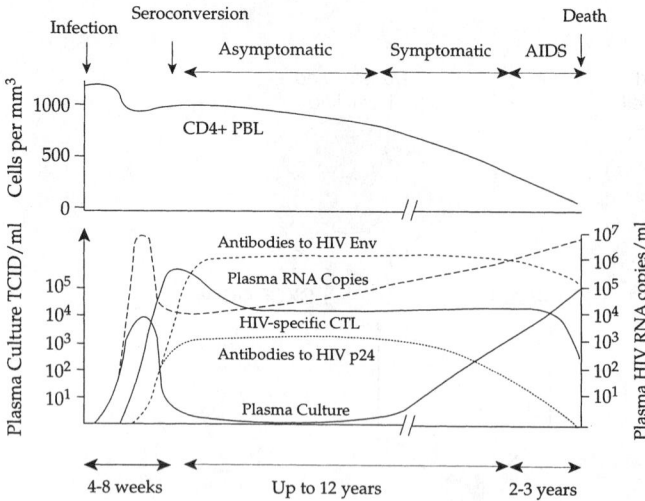

FIGURE 345.3. Typical clinical, virologic, and immunologic course of HIV infection.

some infected individuals demonstrate no evidence of immunopathologic processes for more than 16 years.

Although there is an asymptomatic phase in nearly all infected individuals, there is undisputed evidence that throughout this period there is continuous ongoing viral replication. The level of plasma HIV RNA is reasonably stable reflecting a "quasi-steady state" in which virus production was predicted to equal viral clearance. In fact, there is an extremely high rate of viral production throughout the clinically latent phase with an estimated rate of more than 10^{10} viral particles made per day.

CLINICALLY APPARENT DISEASE

Eventually this steady state "breaks down" leading to falling CD4$^+$ T cells and increasing viral burdens characteristic of AIDS (Fig. 345.3). The level of CD4$^+$ T cells drops to below 200 cells per milliliter and numerous conditions, namely, opportunistic infections and malignancies occur.

DETERMINANTS OF DISEASE PROGRESSION

Overall, the most important correlate of progression to AIDS, before substantial immune destruction has occurred, is the steady-state viral load, or "set point" seen at the end of primary infection. The determinants of the viral load set point and, consequently, clinical prognosis are complex and dependent on the interplay of both viral and host factors.

VIRAL FACTORS

HIV isolates from the infected individual change over time. Isolates from patients early in the course of HIV infection are generally M-tropic, NSI, R5 viruses. The emergence of T-tropic, SI isolates correlates with increasing viral burden and increasing rate of CD4$^+$ T-cell decline. There are also rare examples of genetic defects in the infecting virus playing a role in nonprogression.

HOST FACTORS

Several recent reports have defined the role of chemokine receptors in HIV disease progression. For example, a 32-base-pair deletion in the *CCR5* gene (*CCR5 D32*) confers resistance to HIV infection in homozygotes. *CCR5 D32* heterozygotes are not protected from HIV infection, but the onset of AIDS appears to be postponed by 2 to 4 years. Mutations in other chemokine receptors (e.g., *CCR2 64I*) and chemoreceptor ligands (e.g., *SDF-1*) have also been associated with delays in disease progression.

Other host factors associated with altered disease progression have included human leukocyte antigen types, as well as humoral and cellular immunity. Studies in long-term nonprogressors (LTNPs; HIV-infected individuals with normal CD4$^+$ T-cell counts for 12 to 15 years) show neutralizing antibody responses improved in magnitude and breadth and more robust and persistent HIV-specific CTL responses compared with other HIV-infected individuals. In fact, an inverse correlation between HIV-specific CTL frequency and plasma RNA viral load has been demonstrated.

T-CELL DYNAMICS

The central immunopathogenic hallmark of HIV disease is the progressive loss of CD4$^+$ T cells. The exact mechanism of this is still incompletely understood. Numerous mechanisms have been proposed, including direct cell killing, syncytium formation, autoimmune destruction, impaired T-cell regeneration, and apoptosis. However, the central question remains whether T-cell decline is due to impaired regeneration, accelerated destruction, or both. Following the administration of antiretroviral therapy to infected individuals, there is not only a rapid fall in plasma viremia but a rise in peripheral CD4$^+$ T cells. These observations led to a hypothesis that high levels of viral induced T-cell destruction (1 to 2 $\times$ 10^9 cells per day) placed considerable demand on CD4$^+$ T-cell proliferation that resulted ultimately in collapse of the immune system. Another view is that a large number of T and B cells may be "trapped" in peripheral sites (e.g., by antigen, cytokine, or chemokine signals). Following therapy, the amount of HIV antigen declines and the immune response resolves, and sequestered cells leave the inflamed lymph node and return to the circulation. Other abnormalities in advanced disease include depletion of naive cells relative to memory T-cell subsets; restricted diversity of the T-cell receptor repertoire; a greater proportion of CD8$^+$ T cells compared with CD4$^+$ T cells and reduced functional competence of the T-lymphocyte system.

RESPONSE TO ANTIVIRAL THERAPY

Following effective antiviral therapy, there is an initial rapid fall in plasma viremia with a reduction in plasma virus of approximately 100-fold in the first 2 weeks of therapy. This reflects two processes: the clearance of free virions and the loss of the infected cells that produce most of the plasma virus. Plasma virus then declines at a slower rate, reflecting the turnover of a longer lived viral reservoir, such as macrophages and dendritic cells. Despite the fact that virus is often no longer detectable in the periphery after this phase, recent studies have demonstrated that infectious HIV persists in resting $CD4^+$ memory T cells despite 1 to 2 years of combination therapy. This so-called "latent reservoir" is small (estimated to be no larger than 10^7 cells) but is the main obstacle to eradication of HIV infection as it remains uncertain as to how quickly this reservoir decays in patients on effective antiviral therapy. Despite the persistence of HIV, there is clear evidence of immune reconstitution following antiviral therapy as demonstrated by an early rise in memory $CD4^+$ T cells, a reduction in T-cell activation with an improved $CD4^+$ T-cell reactivity to recall antigens, and, finally, a late rise in naive cells. However, more significantly, effective antiviral therapy has been shown to have a beneficial effect on patient prognosis as demonstrated by a decrease in morbidity and mortality.

BIBLIOGRAPHY

Cao Y, Qin L, Zhang L, Safrit J, et al. Virologic and immunologic characterization of long-term survivors of human immunodeficiency virus type 1 infection. *N Engl J Med* 1995;332:201–208.

Ho D, Neumann A, Perelson A, et al. Rapid turnover of plasma virions and CD4 lymphocytes in HIV-1 infection. *Nature* 1995;373:123–126.

Kahn J, Walker B. Current concepts: acute human immunodeficiency virus type 1 infection. *N Engl J Med* 1998;339:33–40.

Koup R, Safrit J, Cao Y, et al. Temporal association of cellular immune responses with the initial control of viremia in primary human immunodeficiency virus type 1 syndrome. *J Virol* 1994;68:4650–4655.

Littman D. Chemokine receptors: keys to AIDS pathogenesis? *Cell* 1998; 93:677–680.

Mellors J, Rinaldo C, Gupta P, et al. Prognosis in HIV-1 infection predicted by the quantity of virus in plasma. *Science* 1996;272:1167–1170.

Ogg G, Bonhoeffer S, Dunbar P, et al. Quantification of HIV-specific cytotoxic T lymphocytes and plasma load of viral RNA. *Science* 1998; 279:2103–2106.

Palella FJ Jr, Delaney KM, Moorman AC, et al. Declining morbidity and mortality among patients with advanced human immunodeficiency virus infection. HIV Outpatient Study Investigators. *N Engl J Med* 1998;338:853–860.

Perelson A, Neumann A, Markowitz M, et al. HIV-1 dynamics in vivo: virion clearance rate, infected cell life-span, and viral generation time. *Science* 1996;271:1582–1586.

Wei X, Ghosh S, Taylor M, et al. Viral dynamics in human immunodeficiency virus type 1 infection. *Nature* 1995;373:117–122.

Kelley's Textbook of Internal Medicine, fourth edition. Edited by H. David Humes.
Lippincott Williams & Wilkins, Philadelphia © 2000.

DISORDERS OF HIV INFECTION

HIV/AIDS: CLINICAL CONSIDERATIONS

STEPHEN B. GREENBERG
CHRISTOPHER J. LAHART

The AIDS pandemic has altered the world's medical system and precipitated a national and international crisis. This pandemic has changed our concepts of immunology and microbiology, and has called into question the responsiveness of our health care system. In the past 20 years, the quantity of information concerning the causative virus, the clinical manifestations of the syndrome, and our therapeutic options have increased greatly. In the coming years, physicians will be challenged to appropriately manage AIDS patients with their myriad complications and provide humane care in this ultimately fatal illness.

ETIOLOGIC AND PATHOPHYSIOLOGIC FACTORS

Since the first reports in 1981, AIDS has been identified as a primarily sexually transmitted disease that also can be transmitted through blood exposure. By 1986, a lentivirus linked to the syndrome was named the human immunodeficiency virus (HIV). HIV is similar to other retroviruses in that it is composed of single-stranded, positively sensed RNA surrounded by a protein envelope. This virus primarily infects cells with a $CD4^+$ cell membrane glycoprotein but may infect other cells that do not express $CD4^+$. Two recently described coreceptors, CCR5 and CXCR4, appear to be necessary for HIV-1 entry into macrophage-tropic, non–syncytium-inducing strains and lymphocyte-tropic, syncytium-inducing strains, respectively. Once the virus enters the cells, uncoating occurs. A reverse transcriptase enzyme transcribes viral RNA into double-stranded DNA, which is inserted into the host cell chromosome. With activation of the cell by antigenic or viral stimulation, DNA transcription occurs and new viral particles are assembled at the cell surface. The infected cell then dies by mechanisms that are not clearly understood. Potential mechanisms for $CD4^+$ cell destruction may include direct lysis, killing of progenitor cells in the thymus and bone marrow, syncytium formation between uninfected and infected cells, apoptosis (programmed cell death), and/or immune-mediated lysis.

Following the initial infection of monocytes, macrophages, and dendritic cells, virus disseminates through the bloodstream and lymphatics to the germinal center of lymph nodes. Most of the virus in the lymph nodes is extracellular and in the form of virus–antibody immune complexes. In lymphoid tissues, the frequency of HIV-infected $CD4^+$ cells is approximately tenfold higher than in peripheral blood. Thus, the germinal centers of lymph nodes serve as a large reservoir of replicating virus. With the use of quantitative RNA polymerase chain reaction it has been demonstrated that a relatively constant level of virus can be detected in plasma at all stages of clinical disease.

It is currently believed that quantitative measurement of HIV RNA in plasma is a marker for total body HIV replication and a measure of viral load. Using these quantitative viral load measurements, the half-life of HIV-infected cells in blood has been calculated as 1.1 days. The number of HIV virions produced each day has been estimated at 1×10^{10}. Clearance of the virus and virus-infected cells is quite efficient and effective until late in the disease. Where viral loads have been reduced with effective antiretroviral therapies, $CD4^+$ cell counts have increased and life expectancy has been prolonged.

EPIDEMIOLOGIC FACTORS

An estimated 40 million persons have been infected worldwide. In the United States, over 600,000 persons with AIDS have been reported and more than half have died. The mean time from HIV infection to clinical AIDS has been calculated to be 8 to 10 years. High-risk individuals continue to be reported primarily in homosexual and bisexual men, injection drug users, hemophiliacs, blood-product recipients, and sexual partners of these groups. In the United States, new cases of AIDS per 100,000 population were highest in cities with population greater than 500,000, in men (70%), and in black, non-Hispanic individuals (56%). In 1996, there was a 15% decline in mortality due to AIDS compared with 1995 rates, reflecting the impact of new therapies.

Outside the United States, the major route of HIV transmission has been during heterosexual vaginal intercourse. Although transmission efficiency is low, increased transmission has been associated with the presence of genital ulcers or other sexually transmitted diseases and infrequent use of condoms. Male-to-female transmission is more efficient than female-to-male transmission. Sexual intercourse between men accounts for approximately 40% of current AIDS cases in the United States. Orogenital sex is an uncommon route for HIV infection. However, there have been rare cases of HIV transmission by oral secretions. The probability of transmission from an infected pregnant woman to her infant is about 25%. Neonates have been infected through breast-feeding. Approximately 25% of United States AIDS cases have been related to injection drug use. The majority of cases in heterosexual men has been related to drug use. The risk of receiving an HIV-contaminated unit of blood in the United States is 1 in 500,000. In developing countries with fewer screening resources, the risk of transmission through blood products continues to be high. No credible evidence has been presented to support the transmission of HIV by close or causal contact or by fomites.

HIV-1 transmission in health care workers has been documented by the U.S. Centers for Disease Control and Prevention (CDC) in over 100 cases. Needle-stick injuries among laboratory technicians and nurses have accounted for most of the infections. The risk following percutaneous exposure from a known HIV-infected individual is approximately 2.5 in 1,000 exposures. Mucocutaneous exposures have a lower risk of transmission (1 in 1,000 exposures). Viable HIV-1 has been detected in human tissue up to 16 days post mortem.

CLINICAL DEFINITION OF HIV INFECTION

Depending on the stage of HIV infection, individuals may be asymptomatic or have severe opportunistic infections or cancers. A revised CDC classification system for HIV infection emphasized the CD4$^+$ cell count as a marker of disease progression. Three CD4$^+$ cell ranges and three clinical groups are arranged into nine categories (Table 346.1). The CD4$^+$ cell categories are (500 per cubic millimeter, 200 to 499 per cubic millimeter, and less than 200 per cubic millimeter. Clinical category A includes (a) asymptomatic HIV infection, (b) persistent generalized lymphadenopathy (PGL), and/or (c) primary HIV illness. Clinical category C includes infections and malignancies that meet the criteria for AIDS. Clinical category B includes symptomatic patients who do not have conditions outlined in categories A or C. Examples of clinical category B conditions include bacillary angiomatosis, poorly responsive vulvovaginal candidiasis, orophayngeal candidiasis, cervical dysplasia, carcinoma in situ, or unexplained fever or diarrhea for more than a month. Categories A3, B3 and C are reported as AIDS. With this revised classification revision, new AIDS-defining conditions included invasive cervical cancer, pulmonary *Mycobacterium* tuberculosis,

and recurrent pneumonias (≥ 2 episodes in one year). No CDC definitions currently utilize viral load calculations.

CLINICAL PRESENTATIONS OF PATIENTS WITH SYMPTOMATIC HIV DISEASE

ACUTE HIV INFECTION SYNDROME

Although many individuals are asymptomatically infected, approximately 20% will report an acute seroconversion syndrome (Table 346.2). Typically, there is a mononucleosis-like illness of sudden onset. Fever, lethargy, headaches, lymphadenopathy, sore throat, and macular rash are the most common signs and symptoms. Symptoms usually last for 5 to 10 days, but lethargy and malaise are commonly experienced for up to several months. The sore throat is usually not associated with exudates or enlargement of the tonsils. A macular rash may involve the palms and soles. Odynophagia and mucosal ulcers are found in about 50% of patients. A meningitis syndrome has been associated with the acute HIV syndrome and HIV has been recovered from cerebrospinal fluid (CSF) during acute illness. Uncommon clinical manifestations during acute symptomatic HIV infections have included esophageal candidiasis, hepatitis, vasculitis, rhabdomyolysis, myositis, splenomegaly, and red cell aplasia.

Laboratory abnormalities during the acute HIV infection syndrome include lymphopenia (40%), thrombocytopenia (45%), and elevated hepatic enzymes (20%). Atypical lymphocytes are uncommonly detected. CD4$^+$ cell counts usually are in the normal range until several weeks later when the CD4$^+$ cell count will decrease and the CD8$^+$ cell count will increase.

FEVER

The most common complaint in HIV-infected persons is fever. The causes of fever in AIDS include *Pneumocystis carinii* pneumonia, *Mycobacterium avium* complex (MAC), bacterial pneumonia, sinusitis, lymphoma, catheter infection, drug allergy, and, occasionally, cytomegalovirus (CMV) infection. Unexplained fever usually lasting for 1 to 2 weeks has been reported in 15% to 30% of AIDS patients. In Spain, the most frequently identified causes of fever were *Mycobacterium* tuberculosis, leishmaniasis, and MAC infection. *Bartonella henselae* and *Bartonella quintana* have been recovered from blood cultures of AIDS patients in certain regions of the United States.

Blood cultures are positive for pathogens in less than 20% of hospitalized febrile AIDS patients. Blood cultures are more likely to be positive if pneumonia, abscess, urinary tract infection, central line leukopenia, or neutropenia is present. Fungi are uncommonly recovered from blood cultures in these patients. When the fever remains unexplained, the most common identifiable causes appear to be MAC, lymphoma, bartonella, *P. carinii* pneumonia, or fungus. When fever is accompanied by hypotension, hyponatremia, and hyperkalemia, adrenal insufficiency should be suspected. When this occurs, HIV, CMV, or MAC adrenalitis may be the cause.

TABLE 346.1. **1993 REVISED CDC HIV CLASSIFICATION SYSTEM AND EXPANDED AIDS SURVEILLANCE DEFINITION FOR ADOLESCENTS AND ADULTS**[a]

Classification System

CD4 Cell Category[b]	Clinical Category			Clinical Category A	Clinical Category B	Clinical Category C
	A	B	C			
(1) ≥500/mm³	A1	B1	C1	Asymptomatic HIV infection	Symptomatic, not A or C conditions	Candidiasis: esophageal, tracheal, bronchial
(2) 200–499/mm³	A2	B2	C2	Persistent generalized lymphadenopathy	Examples include but not limited to:	Coccidioidomycosis, extrapulmonary
(3) <200/mm³	A3	B3	C3	Acute (primary) HIV illness	Bacillary angiomatosis	Cryptococcosis, extrapulmonary
					Candidiasis, vulvovaginal: persistent >1 mo., poorly responsive to rx	Cervical cancer, invasive[c]
					Candidiasis, oropharyngeal	Cryptosporidosis, chronic intestinal (>1 month)
					Cervical dysplasia, severe, or carcinoma in situ	CMV retinitis, or CMV in other than liver, spleen, nodes
					Constitutional sx, eg, fever (38.5°C) or diarrhea >1 month	HIV encephalopathy
						Herpes simplex with mucocutaneous ulcer >1 mo, bronchitis, pneumonia
						Histoplasmosis: disseminated, extrapulmonary
						Isosporiasis, chronic, >1 mo
						Kaposi's sarcoma
						Lymphoma: Burkitt's, immunoblastic, primary in brain
						M. avium or *M. kansasli* extrapulmonary
						M. tuberculosis, [c]pulmonary or extrapulmonary
						P. carinii pneumonia
						Pneumonia, recurrent (≥2 episodes in 1 yr)[c]
						Progressive multifocal leukoencephalopathy
						Salmonella bacteremia, recurrent
						Toxoplasmosis, cerebral
						Wasting syndrome due to HIV

[a] See table for clinical definitions.
The above must be attributed to HIV infection or have a clinical course or management complicated by HIV.
[b] There is a diurnal variation in CD4 counts averaging 60/mm³ higher in the afternoon in HIV-positive individuals and 500/mm³ in HIV-negative persons. Blood for sequential CD4 counts should be drawn at about the same time of day each time. The equivalence between CD4 counts and CD4 % of total lymphocytes is ≥500 = ≥29%, 200–499 = 14–28%, <200 = <14%.

LYMPHADENOPATHY

Lymph node enlargement is common in HIV-infected persons. Diffuse lymphadenopathy involving the axillary, inguinal, and cervical areas is common. Generalized lymphadenopathy can be seen in acute HIV infection, with mycobacterial or fungal infections, as well as lymphoma, Kaposi's sarcoma, syphilis, toxoplasmosis, Epstein–Barr virus, and CMV infections. If lymph nodes are fluctuant, aspiration should be performed and material stained and cultured. In patients receiving highly active antiretroviral therapy (HAART), fever and generalized lymphadenopathy have been found secondary to coinfection with MAC. In asymptomatic patients, persistent generalized lymphadenopathy is usually not an indication for lymph node biopsy. If patients have adenopathy detected on chest radiography or abdominal computed tomography, then enlarged peripheral lymph nodes should be biopsied to evaluate for possible lymphoma or oppor-tunistic infection. Lymph nodes tend to decrease in size as HIV infection progresses.

CUTANEOUS MANIFESTATIONS

Both infectious and noninfectious dermatologic complications are common in HIV-infected patients. A wide variety of bacteria, viruses, and fungi have been implicated in several cutaneous infections. The most commonly reported maculopapular rashes include molluscum contagiosum, secondary syphilis, cryptococcosis, histoplasmosis, candidiasis, atypical mycobacteria, and warts. Less common infectious agents include *Penicillium marneffei* and cutaneous *P. carinii*. *P. carinii* has been found in patients who lived or traveled in Southeast Asia. Cutaneous *P. carinii*, though reported rarely, is usually seen with pulmonary symptoms. The most common causes of nodular lesions include bacillary angiomatosis, MAC infection, and Kaposi's sarcoma.

TABLE 346.2.	SYMPTOMS AND FINDINGS ASSOCIATED WITH ACUTE HIV-1 INFECTION IN SYMPTOMATIC PATIENTS

Symptom or Finding	Percentage of Patients
Fever	>80–90
Fatigue	>70–90
Rash	>40–80
Headache	32–70
Lymphadenopathy	40–70
Pharyngitis	50–70
Myalgia or arthralgia	50–70
Nausea, vomiting, or diarrhea	30–60
Night sweats	50
Aseptic meningitis	24
Oral ulcers	10–20
Genital ulcers	5–15
Thrombocytopenia	45
Leukopenia	40
Elevated hepatic enzyme levels	21

Kahn JO, Walker BD. Acute human immunodeficiency virus type 1 infection. *N Engl J Med* 1998;339(1):33–39, with permission.)

Vesiculopustular lesions are typical of herpes simplex and varicella-zoster virus infections. These infectious agents can present at any stage of the HIV infection.

Noninfectious skin disorders include minor conditions, such as dry skin or telangiectasia, or major problems, such as severe psoriasis or extensive seborrheic dermatitis. The prevalence of seborrheic dermatitis, the most common noninfectious skin disorder in HIV, ranges from 7% to 50% in HIV-infected patients. Seborrheic dermatitis is generally more difficult to treat and less responsive to therapy in HIV-infected patients than non–HIV-infected patients. Psoriasis is not more prevalent in HIV-infected patients, but it has different features in these patients. Psoriasis may be the first clinical manifestation of HIV infection. With declining CD4$^+$ cell counts, psoriasis appears to become more severe with atypical skin lesions being common. Streptococcal pharyngitis has been reported to precede guttate psoriasis. Acquired ichthyosis involving the lower extremities is common in HIV-infected patients. Other uncommon but associated skin disorders in HIV-infected individuals include porphyria cutanea tarda, eosinophilic pustular folliculitis, and pityriasis rubra pilaris.

Changes in the nails and hair of patients with progressive HIV infection are common. Onychomycosis is often present. A yellow discoloration of the nails has been reported with *P. carinii* pneumonia. Thinning of the hair has been observed in addition to alopecia, sudden premature graying, and elongation of eyelashes.

NERVOUS SYSTEM SIGNS AND SYMPTOMS

Dementia

Brain dysfunction has been reported in HIV-1-infected patients throughout all stages of the disease. An AIDS dementia complex

has been diagnosed in one-third of adults and half of children with AIDS. Early cognitive changes include inattention and forgetfulness. With declining mental activity, a global dementia may ensue. In 30% of asymptomatic HIV-positive patients, CSF abnormalities have been documented. The severity of AIDS–dementia complex may correlate with the cerebrospinal fluid HIV RNA. Although normal early, magnetic resonance images can show variable cerebral atrophy later in the infection. Other causes of declining mental activity but without decreases in consciousness include depression or progressive multifocal leukoencephalopathy during its early stages.

Causes of cognitive impairment with alterations in consciousness include advanced AIDS–dementia complex; bacterial, viral, or fungal meningitis; lymphoma; and toxic–metabolic systemic disorder. The most common infectious causes include cryptococcal meningitis, *Toxoplasma* encephalitis, CMV encephalitis, tuberculous meningitis, and herpes simplex encephalitis. Less commonly reported infectious causes include *B. henselae* encephalitis, central involvement with *P. carinii*, and neurosyphilis. Primary central nervous system (CNS) lymphoma usually has focal neurologic findings, but clinical presentation and radiographic abnormalities are similar to those of *Toxoplasma* encephalitis.

HIV-infected patients can manifest depressed consciousness because of drugs, hypoxemia, or metabolic abnormalities. Therefore, it is important to look for noninfectious factors in HIV-positive patients with altered levels of consciousness.

Focal Neurologic Signs and Symptoms

The sudden onset of focal neurologic signs, such as hemiparesis and blindness, has been reported in HIV-infected patients. Transient ischemic attacks are usually without long-term neurologic sequelae and are postulated to be secondary to a hypercoagulable state. Illicit drugs such as cocaine are associated with ischemic events. Cerebrovascular accidents have also been reported. Focal neurologic signs developing over several days can be the presentation for *Toxoplasma* encephalitis, primary CNS lymphoma, tuberculosis, and/or cryptococcoma. In *Toxoplasma* encephalitis, altered mental status, hemiparesis and other focal signs, headache, and seizures are commonly reported. The higher the serum IgG antibody to *Toxoplasma* organisms ratio, the greater the incidence of *Toxoplasma* encephalitis. Common radiographic findings include multiple ring-enhancing lesions in the cortex and basal ganglia. Magnetic resonance imaging (MRI) is more sensitive than computed tomography (CT) in detecting cerebral lesions in *Toxoplasma* encephalitis. As the incidence of *Toxoplasma* encephalitis declines secondary to trimethoprim–sulfamethoxazole prophylaxis, primary CNS lymphoma is becoming an increasing cause of focal neurologic disease in AIDS patients. CMV and herpes simplex encephalitis are two viruses that can present with focal neurologic signs and seizures.

Progressive multifocal leukoencephalopathy is caused by a papovavirus, the JC virus. It presents slowly in AIDS patients with CD4$^+$ counts ≤100 per cubic millimeter. The patient develops altered mentation late in the course. Limb weakness and visual defects are found in less than half of patients. Seizures have been reported in approximately 20%. The findings on MRI or CT scan often appear worse than the clinical condition. Multiple diffuse hypodense non–contrast-enhancing lesions in subcortical white matter without mass effect are the typical findings.

Seizures are usually secondary to mass lesions, encephalopathy, meningitis, or electrolyte disorders, such as hyponatremia. The majority of cerebral mass lesions are due to *Toxoplasma* infection or lymphoma.

Headaches are a commonly reported symptom in AIDS patients. A focal brain pathology can be associated with headaches. In early HIV infection, headaches can be a presenting symptom. A common side effect of antiretroviral drugs is headache. Bacterial and fungal meningitis are frequently associated with headaches as a chief complaint.

Peripheral nerve syndromes are found in early HIV infections. Mononeuritis multiplex, a demyelinating polyneuropathy, and a rare multiple sclerosis–like syndrome have been described. Later in HIV infection, peripheral weakness and spasticity have been observed secondary to either a vacuolar myopathy or CMV polyradiculopathy. An axonal neuropathy has been reported with nucleoside antiretroviral drugs. Non–drug-related, distal sensory symmetrical polyneuropathy with burning feet, distal numbness, and depressed DTRs has also been seen late in symptomatic HIV infections.

Visual Loss

Acute loss of vision in HIV-infected individuals is most commonly due to CMV papillitis, varicella-zoster virus retinitis, secondary syphilis, cryptococcal meningitis, and bacterial/fungal endophthalmitis (Table 346.3). With CMV papillitis, there is rapid loss of visual activity that may respond to ganciclovir or foscarnet and steroids, if administered early in the course. Peripheral retinitis due to CMV has a more gradual loss of vision

heralded by "floaters" across the visual field of one eye. The acute retinal necrosis syndrome secondary to herpes zoster can lead to loss of vision in one or both eyes. Secondary syphilis can be associated with necrotizing retinitis with hemorrhage that is similar clinically to CMV retinitis. Several cases of rapid visual loss with optic nerve involvement have been reported with cryptococcal meningitis. In addition to antifungal therapy for these patients, repeated CSF drainage has been found to be effective in reducing high intracranial pressure, which often accompanies the visual changes. Uveitis secondary to rifabutin has been seen with increased frequency in those patients receiving concomitant protease inhibitors. Bacterial retinitis secondary to MAC and *Rhodococcus equi* infection has been reported in a few patients.

GASTROINTESTINAL SIGNS AND SYMPTOMS

Oral Lesions

Oral lesions may involve the lips, buccal mucosa, gums, tongue, and/or pharynx. Both infectious and noninfectious conditions are more common and/or more clinically severe in HIV-infected individuals. The most common infectious cause of oral and pharyngeal lesions is candidiasis. This fungal infection can be asymptomatic or associated with soreness, burning, and dysphagia. Periodontitis may be severe and involve necrosis of the gingiva or may be mild presenting as linear gingival erythema. Good oral hygiene is usually effective in mild cases, but necrotizing periodontitis will require dental surgery, irrigation, and antibiotics.

Oral ulcers may be due to herpes simplex virus or CMV. Aphthous ulcers are seen with increased frequency in HIV infection and usually respond clinically to topical steroids. On rare occasions, non-Hodgkin's lymphoma may present with an oral swelling or nonhealing ulcer. Kaposi's sarcoma may be seen on the gingiva or palate. Oral hairy leukoplakia involves the tongue epithelium and involves Epstein–Barr virus infections of these cells. Although it is not painful and can be treated with acyclovir, recurrences are common.

Dysphagia and Odynophagia

Difficulty and/or pain on swallowing are common symptoms in AIDS patients which should prompt further evaluation by x-ray and/or endoscopy. The most common cause of dysphagia, candidiasis, is often found with oral thrush. Large plaques are usually detected in the esophagus by endoscopy. CMV esophagitis usually presents with odynophagia and little dysphagia. Large, superficial ulcers in the distal esophagus show the typical intranuclear inclusions on histology. Herpes simplex virus can also cause erosive ulcers. Idiopathic esophageal ulcerations are a common cause of odynophagia and respond to 4 weeks of steroids. A few cases have responded to thalidomide. Other rarer causes of esophageal ulcerations include drugs (zalcitabine), lymphoma, Kaposi's sarcoma, and squamous cell carcinoma.

Acute Abdominal Pain

Diffuse abdominal pain without other associated symptoms may be due to pancreatitis or peritonitis. The drugs associated with

TABLE 346.3.	CD4+ T-LYMPHOCYTE COUNTS IN PATIENTS PRESENTING WITH COMMON HIV-ASSOCIATED DISORDERS INVOLVING THE EYES
CD4+ Count	**Disorder**
<500 cells/mm³	Kaposi's sarcoma
	Lymphoma
	Tuberculosis
<250 cells/mm³	Pneumocystosis
	Toxoplasmosis
<100 cells/mm³	Retinal or conjunctival microvasculopathy
	Cytomegalovirus retinitis
	Keratoconjunctivitis sicca
	Varicella-zoster virus retinitis
	Mycobacterium avium complex infection
	Cryptococcosis
	Microsporidiosis
	HIV encephalopathy
	Progressive multifocal leukoencephalopathy

Cunningham ET Jr, Margolis TP. Ocular manifestations of HIV infection. *N Engl J Med* 1998;339(4):236–244, with permission.)

pancreatitis include didanosine, pentamidine, and lamivudine. Intestinal perforations can be seen with lymphoma, typhilitis, Kaposi's sarcoma, tuberculosis, or salmonellosis. In advanced AIDS, CMV may be a cause of bowel perforations and peritonitis.

Diarrhea and Weight Loss

Both acute and chronic diarrhea are commonly seen during the clinical course of AIDS. The evaluation for the cause of diarrhea depends on persistence of symptoms. Microscopic examination of the stool should include wet mount, modified acid-fast stain, and modified trichrome stain. Stool cultures for routine pathogens and *Clostridium difficile* should also be ordered. Endoscopy of the colon and small bowel is necessary if the cultures and stains are negative. Watery diarrhea with fever and fecal leukocytes has been found with *Campylobacter, C. difficile, Salmonella, Shigella,* and CMV. Chronic watery diarrhea and enteritis are more commonly seen with cryptosporidia, *Cyclospora, Giardia, Isospora belli,* microsporidia, and MAC. Malabsorption and wasting syndromes can be seen in association with chronic diarrhea. Other, less common causes include bacterial overgrowth, enteric viral infection, Crohn's disease, and HIV disease.

Weight loss is commonly seen in AIDS patients. Once treatable causes of the wasting syndrome are ruled out, then HIV itself may be the cause.

RESPIRATORY TRACT SIGNS AND SYMPTOMS

Sinusitis

Symptoms of nasal congestion, postnasal drip, facial pain, and fever are found in many patients. The diagnosis of sinusitis can be made clinically, but radiographic changes are usually found. The maxillary and ethmoid sinuses are most commonly involved. Although isolates of *Streptococcus pneumoniae* and *Haemophilus influenzae* are often recovered, *Pseudomonas aeruginosa* and *Staphylococcus aureus* are also reported with increased frequency. Chronic sinusitis in HIV-infected patients often have *Moraxella catarrhalis,* gram-negative bacilli, and/or anaerobes recovered in sinus cultures. The severity of sinusitis is greater in patients with low CD4$^+$ counts. Treatment with antibiotics may be necessary for periods longer than the usual 10 to 14 days.

Cough and Fever

The HIV-infected patient with cough and fever requires a careful history, physical examination, and chest radiography. If the patient's CD4$^+$ count is greater than 200 per cubic millimeter and the chest radiograph is clear, then the patient should be treated for acute bronchitis or sinusitis. If the patient's CD4$^+$ count is under 200 per cubic millimeter and the chest radiograph is clear, then bronchitis, sinusitis, as well as *P. carinii* pneumonia, tuberculosis, cryptococcosis, and MAC infection should be ruled out. If infiltrates are found by chest radiograph, then the bacteria associated with community-acquired pneumonia should be con-

sidered. Active tuberculosis is increased significantly in HIV-infected patients compared to the general population.

Bacteria pneumonia, the most common cause of death in AIDS patients, is caused by *S. pneumoniae, H. influenzae, P. aeruginosa,* and, uncommonly, *S. aureus. S. pneumoniae* has a 150-fold increased incidence over that of healthy controls. Clinically, HIV-infected patients with pneumonia are similar to other patients without HIV. Antibiotic treatment usually leads to good responses if there are no resistant organisms.

Dyspnea

The most common underlying cause of dyspnea in HIV-infected patients is *P. carinii* pneumonia. Dyspnea is usually present with other symptoms such as cough and fatigue. Fever and weight loss are reported frequently. Although examination of the chest is usually normal, chest radiographs often reveal diffuse interstitial infiltrates. Less common findings are lobar infiltrates, nodular densities, and pulmonary edema. Respiratory alkalosis with a widened alveolar–arterial gradient is the usual arterial blood gas finding. Induced sputum is positive for *P. carinii* in approximately 70% of cases, with the other 30% requiring bronchoalveolar lavage or biopsy for diagnosis.

Dyspnea is also a common symptom in other lung infections, such as community-acquired pneumonia due to *S. pneumoniae* and *H. influenzae.* In patients with AIDS, bacterial pneumonia will present with other typical signs and symptoms and respond to appropriate antimicrobial treatment. Other respiratory pathogens, such as fungi and mycobacteria, can also present with dyspnea as a major symptom.

Noninfectious causes of dyspnea include pulmonary lymphoma, Kaposi's sarcoma in the lung, primary pulmonary hypertension, and cardiomyopathy. Pulmonary Kaposi's sarcoma is usually observed when skin lesions are present, but in 10% to 15% of cases there may be lung involvement without cutaneous lesions. Both diffuse interstitial infiltrates and pleural effusions are frequently identified. Examining for lesions on bronchoscopy is the most common diagnostic method. Primary pulmonary hypertension has been reported with increased frequency in AIDS patients, with resultant right-sided heart failure being reported. No good treatment is available for this unusual complication.

MUSCULOSKELETAL SIGNS AND SYMPTOMS

Arthralgia may be the initial symptom in patients with septic arthritis. Although of low incidence in HIV-infected patients, septic arthritis is the most common infection of the musculoskeletal system in these patients. *S. aureus* is the most commonly isolated organism. Reiter's syndrome is more prevalent in HIV-infected individuals than in the general population. Arthritis is one of the three classic findings in Reiter's syndrome, with the other two being urethritis and conjunctivitis. Symptoms of arthritis may precede other clinical manifestations of HIV infection by several months. The joints of the lower extremities or the sacroiliac joint are most commonly affected. Skin manifestations commonly seen in Reiter's syndrome include keratoderma blennorrhagicum and circinate balanitis. Etretinate and topical steroids are effective treatments in Reiter's syndrome in HIV-infected individuals.

Other musculoskeletal infections include osteomyelitis, pyomyositis, and septic bursitis. *S. aureus* is the most commonly identified pathogen in these infections. As with septic arthritis, clinical presentation, prevalence and treatment outcome do not appear to be different in HIV-infected patients compared with uninfected individuals.

COMMON LABORATORY ABNORMALITIES

Routine laboratory tests often are abnormal in HIV-infected patients (Table 346.4). The most common electrolyte abnormality is hyponatremia. Extrarenal loss of sodium due to diarrhea and vomiting is common in hospitalized patients. Pulmonary and CNS diseases are also associated with hyponatremia due to the syndrome of inappropriate secretion of antidiuretic hormone.

With severe diarrhea, volume depletion, hypokalemia, and metabolic acidosis are common. Replacement of the fluid losses and potassium supplements are necessary for clinical improvement, but treatment of the cause of diarrhea is most important. Drugs that affect renal tubular function can also lead to hypokalemia.

Renal insufficiency, whether acute or chronic, can lead to hyperkalemia. Type IV renal tubular acidosis, adrenal insufficiency, and isolated mineralocorticoid deficiency are causes of hyperkalemia. Drugs such as trimethoprim and pentamidine can lead to severe hyperkalemia.

Other electrolyte abnormalities have included hypocalcemia secondary to drugs, hypercalcemia secondary to infection or malignancy, and hyperphosphatemia secondary to drug (foscarnet) therapy. Increased uric acid concentration has been reported with the use of antituberculosis drugs and didanosine.

The most common causes of acute renal failure with elevated blood urea nitrogen and serum creatinine in HIV-infected patients are drug toxicity, volume depletion, and shock. The underlying cause of the acute renal failure usually is more important to the outcome than the HIV status of the individual. HIV-associated nephropathy (HIVAN) is thought to be a result of HIV in the kidney. HIVAN is common in African Americans, in men more than in women, and in individuals with a history of intravenous drug use. There is rapid progression to renal failure without treatment. Newer antiretroviral therapies appear to help maintain renal function if begun early. Immune-mediated renal diseases are also reported in HIV-infected individuals. Whether the renal disease is related to HIV immune responses is unclear. The most common pathologic factor found on kidney biopsy has been IgA nephropathy, focal proliferative or membranoproliferative glomerulonephritis. Coinfection with

---

TABLE 346.4.	COMMON ABNORMALITIES FOUND IN ROUTINE LABORATORY TESTS FROM AIDS PATIENTS	
Laboratory Tests	**Abnormality**	**Differential Diagnosis**
Electrolytes	Hyponatremia	Volume depletion, SIADH, Adrenal insufficiency, hyporeninemic hypoaldosteronism, nephrogenic diabetes insipidus, nephrotoxic drugs
	Hyperkalemia	Drugs: TMP, ketoconazole, adrenal insufficiency, hypoaldosteronism
	Hypercalcemia	Lymphoma
	Hypocalcemia	Drugs: foscarnet, ketoconazole, amphotericin B, aminoglycosides
Hematologic	Anemia of chronic disease	HIV opportunistic infection, malignancy
	Iron deficiency anemia	GI bleeding secondary to Kaposi's sarcoma, lymphoma, or carcinoma
	Bone marrow infiltration	*Mycobacterium avium* complex
	Red cell aplasia	Parvovirus B19
	Drug-induced G-6-PD-deficient hemolysis	Dapsone, primaquine, sulfonamides, TMP-SMX
	Megalobastic anemia	Zidovudine
	Myelosuppression	Ganciclovir, foscarnet, flucytosine, sulfonamides, TMP, pyrimethamine, pentamidine, interferon-α, neoplastic drugs
	Granulocytopenia	Ineffective granulopoiesis, antiretrovirals
	Thrombocytopenia	ITP drugs, TTP and hemolytic-uremic syndrome
	Eosinophilia	HIV drug reactions, parasitic infections, Hodgkin's disease, coccidioidomycosis
	Coagulation abnormality	Prolonged PTT, lupus anticoagulant/antiphospholipid absent
Liver function tests	Elevated transaminases	Cholecystitis, cholangiopathy, viral hepatitis, hepatomegaly with severe steatosis, peliosis hepatitis, drug-associated
	Elevated alkaline phosphatase	Histoplasmosis, lymphoma
Urinalysis	Proteinuria	HIV-associated glomerulosclerosis, HIV-associated IgA nephropathy, amyloidosis, heroin nephropathy, drugs

HCV may lead to cryoglobulinemia and membranoproliferative glomerulonephritis.

COMPLICATIONS RELATED TO ANTIRETROVIRAL THERAPY

The advent of more effective antiretroviral therapy has dramatically altered the course of disease in HIV-infected individuals. The potential for extended survival is now very real for the majority of patients treated with HAART. Along with extended survival, however, comes extended exposure to the therapeutic agents, many of which were approved and released for use after relatively short-term clinical trials. Several common and fairly predictable adverse reactions have been described for several of the antiretroviral drugs. Other new reactions are only now becoming apparent. Active investigations are under way to determine prevalence, incidence, etiologic mechanisms, and treatment of these reactions. With multiple therapeutic options available, the choice of which regimen to prescribe in an individual patient will often be based on presumed tolerance of the regimen and its anticipated toxicity.

NEUROPATHY

Several nucleoside analogue reverse transcriptase inhibitors (NRTIs) cause a distal symmetrical polyneuropathy that is indistinguishable from that caused by HIV itself. This is most commonly seen with the dideoxynucleoside analogues didanosine, zalcitabine, and stavudine. The primary symptoms are numbness, tingling, or burning in the feet. Paresthesias and hyperesthesia of the lower extremities can also occur. In more advanced cases, the upper extremities may be affected, although it is very unusual for there to be upper extremity involvement without lower extremity symptoms. On physical exam, there may be decreased or absent ankle reflexes and decreased sensation in a stocking distribution in response to vibration, pin prick, and temperature. Objective weakness is rare. The diagnosis can be confirmed by nerve conduction studies.

It is important to consider other causes of neuropathic symptoms in this setting, and evaluation for diabetes, vitamin deficiency, and alcohol use should take place. Other neurotoxic drugs (e.g., isoniazid) should also be considered as potential etiologic factors.

Initial treatment is withdrawal or dose reduction of the known neurotoxic drugs. Symptomatic improvement may be reported by the patient within 2 to 3 weeks following dose alteration, but resolution may take 2 to 3 months. Complete resolution does not happen in all cases, but is more likely in those whose drug was not continued for a prolonged period despite increasing neuropathic symptoms. Management of the painful neuropathies should be individualized. Nonsteroidal agents should be the initial symptomatic treatment. Tricyclic antidepressants, such as amitriptyline, can be added for those patients with incomplete relief, although efficacy has not been fully demonstrated in HIV-related disease. The anticonvulsants phenytoin and carbamazepine also have a role in advanced cases, and a newer agent, gabapentin, with demonstrated effect in diabetic neuropathy, has shown early promise.

PANCREATITIS

Didanosine and zalcitabine have also been associated with episodes of clinical and subclinical pancreatitis. The cause of this reaction is unclear, but it is more common in those patients with advanced HIV infection and those with prior pancreatic injury or chronic alcohol use. The symptoms are identical to pancreatitis from any other cause. In some cases, asymptomatic hyperamylasemia may be detected. Permanent drug discontinuation, with no rechallenge in the future, should be done immediately. Treatment of this drug-induced pancreatitis is general clinical support as with pancreatitis from other causes.

RASH

Although rash is possible with any medication, it is somewhat common with the use of the non-NRTIs, occurring in 10% to 20% of those treated. It is most common and most important during the use of nevirapine. Both nevirapine and delavirdine are associated with the development of rash in approximately one of five persons taking either medication. With delavirdine the rash is usually mild and many patients can be treated for it. During nevirapine therapy the rash may progress to a severe reaction including widespread dissemination, constitutional symptoms, and mucosal involvement. This occurs in approximately 6% to 7% of treated patients. Stevens–Johnson syndrome can be seen, but it develops in less than 1% of patients. If severe rash develops, discontinuation of nevirapine is necessary and rechallenge should not be attempted.

HYPERGLYCEMIA

The use of protease inhibitors has been associated with the development of hyperglycemia in up to 6% of patients. There may be symptoms related to the hyperglycemia, including ketoacidosis. The onset of hyperglycemia is usually within 6 months of initiation of protease inhibitor therapy, and has been seen within the first week. Laboratory studies indicate a possible insulin resistance in these patients. The use of oral hypoglycemic drugs is generally successful in managing this disorder, and the use of protease inhibitors can usually be continued. Some patients may respond to exercise and diet modification without specific drug therapy.

HYPERTRIGLYCERIDEMIA

Elevated levels of triglycerides are seen in untreated HIV infection; however, the use of protease inhibitors has exacerbated this metabolic complication. Levels of 1,000 mg per deciliter or greater are not uncommon. This abnormality has been seen with all of the protease inhibitors, although it appears to be more common in those patients on ritonavir. Despite remarkably high levels of triglycerides, little in the way of clinical complications has been reported, with no clearly related cases of cardiovascular events or pancreatitis. The long-term significance of hypertriglyceridemia in the setting of HIV infection is unknown. Current guidelines for the management of hypertriglyceridemia in the cardiovascular patient can be applied to HIV-infected patients. Due to the concern of drug interactions with either fibric acid derivatives or 3-hydroxy-3-methylglutaryl reductase coenzyme A inhibitors and protease inhibitors, the use of these agents should be reserved for those patients at higher risk for pancreatitis or those with multiple cardiac risk factors.

MALDISTRIBUTION OF FAT

Several seemingly unrelated disorders of fat distribution have been increasingly described in the era of HAART. Although more common in patients taking regimens including protease inhibitors, these disorders have been seen in HIV-infected patients on all combinations of therapy or none at all. The most common alteration in fat distribution is a wasting, or thinning, of the arms and legs with or without thinning of the face. Also commonly seen is accumulation of abdominal fat. Many women experience breast enlargement of a bra cup size or more. This can be uncomfortable in general or actually locally tender. Less common is an accumulation of fat just at and below the posterior neck, the so-called buffalo hump. No common cause or therapy is apparent for these disorders. Some patients have experienced a regression of these changes upon the withdrawal of protease inhibitor therapy.

BIBLIOGRAPHY

Cunningham ET Jr, Margolis TP. Ocular manifestations of HIV infection. *N Engl J Med* 1998;339(4):236–244.

Farber BF, Lesser M, Kaplan MH, et al. Clinical significance of neutropenia in patients with human immunodeficiency virus infection. *Infect Control Hosp Epidemiol* 1991;12(7):429–434.

Havlir DV, Barnes PF. Tuberculosis in patients with human immunodeficiency virus infection. *N Engl J Med* 1999;340(5):367–373.

Jacobson MA, French M. Altered natural history of AIDS-related opportunistic infections in the era of potent combination antiretroviral therapy. *AIDS* 1998;12 Suppl A:S157–S163.

Kahn JO, Walker BD. Acute human immunodeficiency virus type 1 infection. *N Engl J Med* 1998;339(1):33–39.

Kroll MH, Shandera WX. AIDS-associated Kaposi's sarcoma. *Hosp Pract* (Off Ed) 1998;33(4):85–88, 95–96, 99–102.

Tumbarello M, Tacconelli E, de Gaetano K, et al. Bacterial pneumonia in HIV-infected patients: analysis of risk factors and prognostic indicators. *J AIDS Hum Retrovirol* 1998;18(1):39–45.

U.S. Centers for Disease Control and Prevention. 1993 Revised classification system for HIV infection and expanded surveillance case definition for AIDS among adolescents and adults. *MMWR* 1992 Dec 18;41(RR-17):1–19.

Vassilopoulos D, Chalasani P, Jurado RL, et al. Musculoskeletal infections in patients with human immunodeficiency virus infection. *Medicine* (Baltimore) 1997;76(4):284–294.

Yunis NA, Stone VE. Cardiac manifestations of HIV/AIDS: a review of disease spectrum and clinical management. *J AIDS Hum Retrovirol* 1998; 18(2):145–154.

Kelley's Textbook of Internal Medicine, fourth edition. Edited by H. David Humes. Lippincott Williams & Wilkins, Philadelphia © 2000.

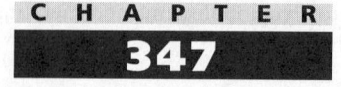

CHAPTER 347

NEOPLASMS IN AIDS

DAVID M. ABOULAFIA
RONALD T. MITSUYASU

Kaposi's sarcoma (KS), intermediate- and high-grade peripheral non-Hodgkin's lymphoma (NHL), primary central nervous system (CNS) lymphoma, and invasive squamous cell carcinoma of the cervix are included in the U.S. Centers for Disease Control and Prevention case definition of AIDS. A variety of other non–AIDS-defining neoplasms are occasionally seen in the setting of HIV infection.

▬ KAPOSI'S SARCOMA

DEFINITION

The lesions of KS are multifocal, vascular proliferative neoplasms of mesenchymal origin that are characterized by abnormal angiogenesis, leukocytic infiltration, and proliferation of spindle cells, fibroblasts, and endothelial cells.

INCIDENCE AND EPIDEMIOLOGIC FACTORS

Unique aspects of the epidemiology of KS include its association with sexually transmitted HIV infection, its male-to-female ratio of roughly 20:1, its rare appearance in individuals at risk for HIV infection but without detectable HIV, and its declining incidence among male homosexuals. It is now presumed that a new herpes virus, termed Kaposi's sarcoma–associated herpesvirus (KSHV), or human herpesvirus 8 (HHV-8), is involved in the pathogenesis of KS. HHV-8 sequences are present in peripheral blood mononuclear cells, spermatozoa, and seminal fluid of AIDS–KS patients but is found infrequently in sputum and stool samples.

Assuming that HHV-8 is acquired through the mucosa during anal intercourse, the declining incidence of KS among male homosexuals may be related to the gradual adoption of safer sex practices that minimize transmission. Partial restoration of the immune system that occurs following the implementation of highly active antiretroviral therapy (HAART) may also contribute to the declining incidence of AIDS-associated KS.

ETIOLOGIC FACTORS AND PATHOGENESIS

Although HIV infection is not required for the development of KS, it clearly increases the risk and greatly influences the clinical pattern of the disease. There may be several mechanisms behind this, including decreased immune surveillance and enhanced production of KS-inducing cytokines and growth factors. The KS spindle cells secrete paracrine factors that appear to mediate angiogenesis and the mononuclear cell infiltrate. The mononuclear cells, in turn, may secrete cytokines that stimulate growth of KS cells, setting up an autocrine–paracrine loop.

CLINICAL FINDINGS

The initial evaluation of the patient with KS includes a complete history with a focus on the rate of progression of new KS lesions, HIV-related opportunistic infections, overall immune status, and treatment history. The clinical features of epidemic KS differ markedly from those of classic, iatrogenic, and endemic forms of the disease. In patients with AIDS, KS tends to be multicentric. It may appear as a single, seemingly innocuous skin blemish that is easily overlooked. Alternatively, larger confluent skin lesions, manifested as red, purple, or brown patches, plaques, or nodules, may spread randomly over the body surface. In some patients, only a few lesions are apparent, and they remain unchanged for years; in others, lesions proliferate rapidly. In most patients, new lesions develop gradually over several weeks to months.

Kaposi's sarcoma lesions of the head, the neck, and the tip of the nose are often disfiguring. Lymphatic involvement may produce debilitating and cosmetically unacceptable edema, particularly when the periorbital area, genitalia, and lower extremities are involved. About 30% of patients with cutaneous KS have gastrointestinal involvement. Examination of the oropharynx may uncover asymptomatic lesions on the palate, pharynx, or tongue; if allowed to grow, these lesions can interfere with eating or breathing. Fortunately, KS rarely causes gastrointestinal hemorrhage or obstruction. KS involvement of the tracheobronchial tree, pulmonary parenchyma and pleura may cause dyspnea, chest pain, pleural effusions, and fevers.

LABORATORY EVALUATION

Essential laboratory tests include a baseline $CD4^+$ count and HIV viral load. The diagnosis of KS is relatively straightforward in HIV-infected individuals presenting with numerous erythematous or violaceous cutaneous or mucosal lesions. However, bacillary angiomatosis caused by *Rochalimaea* species and other conditions may mimic the appearance of KS. This latter condition is treatable with antibiotics and should be excluded by Warthin–Starry stain of biopsied material. A chest radiograph is useful when screening for asymptomatic pulmonary disease. Suspicious pulmonary lesions should be further evaluated by bronchoscopy. Symptomatic gastrointestinal involvement is best evaluated by endoscopy with biopsy of mucosal lesions.

OPTIMAL MANAGEMENT

Immediate therapeutic intervention is rarely necessary at the time of KS diagnosis, although many patients require some form of palliative treatment during the course of their disease. Small, localized lesions of limited number may be observed or treated with regional therapy, including intralesional vinblastine, topical liquid nitrogen, and 9-*cis*-retinoic acid gel. Radiation therapy is especially useful in treating tumors that are complicated by edema involving the extremities and periorbital areas. Painful lesions on the soles of the feet and those on the conjunctivae, nose, and ears can also be palliated with this modality. However, HIV-infected patients have heightened susceptibility to radiation-induced mucositis. Oral and genitorectal lesions probably are managed best by other modalities.

Extensive or rapidly progressive KS, particularly involving visceral organs, requires a more aggressive systemic approach. Single and combination chemotherapy consisting of *Vinca* alkaloids, etoposide, anthracyclines, and bleomycin are active against KS and produce response rates varying from 25% to 80%. Interferon-α in conjunction with HAART produces objective response rates of 30% to 60% when used in patients with $CD4^+$ counts greater than 100 per cubic millimeter. Because liposomal anthracyclines are rarely associated with mucositis or alopecia, they have become a first-line treatment for patients who have progressive or symptomatic disease. Paclitaxel is another active agent that is often used when tumors progress following initial therapies. Important in all approaches to the treatment of patients with AIDS-associated KS is an effective antiretroviral regimen that limits HIV replication. When HIV viral loads are reduced, lesions will occasionally regress, and KS therapy can sometimes be scaled back without recrudescence of tumors.

NON-HODGKIN'S LYMPHOMA

DEFINITION

About 90% of AIDS-related NHLs are of B-cell origin. The histologic patterns are representative of aggressive lymphomas and fall into two groups: large-cell lymphomas, which include intermediate-grade large-cell and high-grade immunoblastic lymphomas, and high-grade, small, noncleaved lymphomas (often classified as Burkitt's or Burkitt-like lymphomas). Low-grade NHL and T-cell phenotypes rarely are seen in patients with HIV disease and are not considered to be AIDS-defining illnesses.

INCIDENCE AND EPIDEMIOLOGIC FACTORS

The risk for development of NHL appears to be constant over time and is not confined primarily to a single group, as is the case with KS. NHL may occur at any level of immune function. The median $CD4^+$ count is approximately 100 per cubic millimeter. In contrast, primary CNS lymphoma occurs almost exclusively in severely immunocompromised individuals. The median $CD4^+$ cell count is 30 per cubic millimeter.

ETIOLOGIC FACTORS AND PATHOGENESIS

The reason for the high incidence of NHL in patients with AIDS remains poorly understood. In one model, severe immunodeficiency leads to the reactivation of latent Epstein–Barr virus (EBV) infection. Chronic antigenic stimulation of B lymphocytes and macrophages by EBV and other pathogens elicits the release of various growth factors and cytokines, promoting B-cell growth and activation and facilitating malignant transformation of these cells. The usual T-cell suppressive factors called into play to limit B-cell proliferation are ineffective and, by a multistep process, in 25% to 50% of cases, proto-oncogenes such as c-*myc* are activated following specific chromosomal translocations.

CLINICAL FINDINGS

Sixty percent to 95% of AIDS-related NHL patients present with extranodal involvement. Common extranodal sites include the bone marrow in 33% of patients, the leptomeninges in 20%, the gastrointestinal tract in 17%, and the oral and anorectal mucosa in 7%. Patients with primary CNS involvement may appear confused, lethargic, or complain of headache. Such tumors almost always are composed of immunoblastic or large-cell lymphocytes and invariably are associated with EBV.

More than 80% of patients with AIDS-related NHL have significant fever, weight loss, and night sweats. Yet the diagnosis of NHL is often obscured by the presence of constitutional symptoms related to other non-neoplastic causes.

LABORATORY FINDINGS

HIV viral load and $CD4^+$ T-cell count are routinely obtained in conjunction with a complete blood count, sedimentation rate, chemistry panel (including lactate dehydrogenase), and bilateral bone marrow aspirate and biopsy. Various cultures, stains, and additional radiographic studies may be required to evaluate the extent of disease and complicating infections. Unusual or suspicious growths mandate additional evaluation, often culminating in tissue biopsy. In the absence of a space-occupying CNS lesion, a spinal puncture is performed and fluid is collected for cytologic analysis. Patients with primary CNS lymphomas may have single or multiple contrast-enhancing and hypodense lesions on computed tomography and magnetic resonance imaging. For patients with focal neurologic defects and normal computed tomographic scans, magnetic resonance imaging may be more sensitive in the detection of occult disease. Although solitary lesions are more likely to be lymphoma, imaging alone cannot reliably distinguish between tumor and cerebral toxoplasmosis. The presence of polymerase chain reaction–amplified EBV DNA in spinal fluid appears to be a sensitive and specific test for primary CNS lymphoma.

OPTIMAL MANAGEMENT

Despite intensive chemotherapy, the median survival for HIV-infected patients with NHL and low $CD4^+$ counts is only 4 to 6 months. However, patients with $CD4^+$ counts greater than 100 cells per cubic millimeter may achieve response rates as high as 72% and disease-free intervals exceeding 15 months. Treatment strategies usually incorporate several paradigms: the use of systemic chemotherapy, even in patients with apparently localized disease on staging evaluation; the use of low-dose chemotherapy with or without hematopoietic growth factors in patients with lymphomatous bone marrow involvement, $CD4^+$ T-cell counts less than 100 cells per cubic millimeter, or constitu-

tional symptoms; the early use of prophylactic intrathecal methotrexate or cytarabine to prevent CNS relapse; the use of prophylactic antibiotics and antifungal agents to reduce the occurrence of opportunistic infections; and the use of non-myelosuppressive antiretroviral drugs to reduce HIV viral burden during periods of heightened immunosuppression.

Because toxoplasmosis is the cause of 90% of focal cerebral lesions, patients with focal neurologic defects or abnormal brain scans often are treated empirically with antitoxoplasmosis regimens while undergoing close observation. Failure to improve radiographically or clinically within 7 to 10 days mandates reconsideration of the diagnosis. Patients diagnosed with primary CNS lymphoma are most often treated with whole-brain radiation. Patients may achieve short-term palliation, but survival rarely exceeds 4 months.

■ MISCELLANEOUS CANCERS

In the setting of HIV infection, Hodgkin's disease is more commonly associated with advanced stage at diagnosis, lymphocyte depleted or mixed cellularity, and a propensity to involve extranodal locations. Patients respond to conventional chemotherapy, but tumors often recur. Consequently, patients have a median survival of only 12 to 16 months.

Anal cancer and cervical cancer, neoplasms associated with human papillomavirus infection, may occur with higher incidence in HIV-infected patients. This is due to the high prevalence of human papillomavirus infection in groups at risk for HIV and the high frequency of the premalignant condition, intraepithelial neoplasia in HIV-infected women. While the incidence of an abnormal Pap smear of the cervix is only 5% in otherwise healthy women, the incidence of abnormal cervical smears in women with HIV infection is 60%. Ongoing studies of infected individuals using Pap smears on cells obtained from the transitional zone of the anus and cervix should provide more data regarding the increasing incidence and optimum surveillance programs for these cancers in this population.

Although anecdotal reports of other malignancies reported in HIV-infected individuals abound, it is unclear as to whether these occur above the background prevalence in the general population. These malignancies include tumors of the skin, lung, brain, testes, and, in children, the mesenchyma.

Acknowledgment

Supported in part by a grant from the Universitywide AIDS Research Program to the UCLA CARE Center (CC96-LA-175) and by USPHS, NIH grants AI-27660, AI-28697, CA-70080, and RR-00865.

BIBLIOGRAPHY

Aboulafia DM. Epidemiology and pathogenesis of AIDS-related lymphomas. *Oncology* 1998;12:1068–1081.

Brodt HR, Kamps BS, Helm EB, et al. Kaposi's sarcoma in HIV infection: impact on opportunistic infections and survival. *AIDS* 1998;12: 1475–1481.

Cottrill CP, Bottomley DM, Phillips RH. Cancer and HIV infection. *Clin Oncol* 1997;9:365–380.

Fruchter RG, Maiman M, Sedlis A, et al. Recurrent cervical intraepithelial neoplasia in women with the human immunodeficiency virus infection. *Obstet Gynecol* 1996;87:338–344.

Kaplan LD, Strauss DJ, Testa MA, et al. Low dose compared with standard-dose m-BACOD chemotherapy for non-Hodgkin's lymphoma associated with human immunodeficiency virus infection. *N Engl J Med* 1997; 336:1641–1648.

Palefsky JM. Anal human papilloma virus infection and anal cancer in HIV-positive individuals: an emerging problem. *AIDS* 1994;8:283–295.

Siranni M, Vincenzi L, Fiorelli V, et al. Gamma-interferon production in peripheral blood mononuclear cells and tumor infiltrating lymphocytes from Kaposi's sarcoma patients: correlation with the presence of human herpesvirus-8 in peripheral blood mononuclear cells and lesional macrophages. *Blood* 1998;91:968–976.

Von roenn J, Krown SE, Benson CA et al. Management of AIDS-associated Kaposi's sarcoma: a multidisciplinary perspective. *Oncology* 1998; 12(Suppl 3):1–24.

Kelley's Textbook of Internal Medicine, fourth edition. Edited by H. David Humes.
Lippincott Williams & Wilkins, Philadelphia © 2000.

MANAGEMENT, PREVENTION, AND CONTROL

PRINCIPLES OF ANTIRETROVIRAL TREATMENT AND VACCINES

CHRISTOPHER J. LAHART

During the late 1990s, HIV-infected patients have benefited from a propitious confluence of events. Based on years of research into the pathogenesis of HIV infection, therapeutic and diagnostic approaches representing dramatic improvements over previous methods have come into general use. Development of the non-nucleoside reverse transcriptase inhibitors and the protease inhibitors heralded a new era in the treatment of HIV infection. Broad use of plasma HIV RNA levels allowed further fine tuning of therapeutic interventions prior to clinical progression or loss of $CD4^+$ lymphocytes. As a result, in the United States the mortality attributed to HIV infection and AIDS decreased by over 60% during 1996–1998. Despite these tremendous changes in our approach to antiretroviral therapy, the optimal timing of therapy initiation and the preferred agents with which to start therapy are still unknown. Additionally, even in the setting of perfect adherence to the therapeutic regimen, the ultimate durability of these new therapies is unknown at this time. There are also multiple barriers to perfect adherence with the need for multiple medications, difficult dosing schedules, varying dietary restrictions for some medications, and, for many persons living with HIV, lack of ready access to medications and physicians with the expertise necessary to properly prescribe the medications. The decrease in mortality seen in the most recent years may represent merely a delay in progression of disease rather than true disease containment.

GENERAL PRINCIPLES IN THE THERAPEUTIC APPROACH

As outlined in Table 348.1, the harm to an individual with HIV infection stems from the continual replication of HIV and the resultant immune system dysfunction. Many pharmaceutical agents have been developed for use in antiretroviral therapy based on their ability to impair viral replication (Table 348.2). Unfortunately, no single agent with the ability to completely suppress viral replication has been found. Thus, the use of a single agent, or even most combinations of two agents, is associated with impaired, but still active, viral replication. In this setting there is transient benefit reflected in laboratory measures or actual clinical outcomes; however, this benefit is not durable. The transient nature of this benefit is due to the development and selection of resistant HIV viral mutants that then return viral replication to its previous level despite continued therapy. The end result is continued high-level viral replication and further immunologic decline.

The recent development and use of combinations of three or more effective antiretroviral medications has accomplished what was not possible before: the suppression of HIV viral replication as evidenced by plasma HIV RNA levels falling below the level of detection using highly sensitive assays. This approach has come to be known as "highly active antiretroviral therapy (HAART). However, this is not to say that viral replication has been halted in all body compartments, particularly the lymphatic tissues. Indeed, there is evidence that a residual amount of replication does take place, although the clinical repercussions are not yet known. Even in the most successful trials, 20% to 40% of patients do not attain the goal of undetectable viral load. The reasons for such a high failure rate are not clear but should give pause to a practitioner recommending therapy in a more reluctant patient. Success is far from certain with these therapies, and failure implies resistant virus and limited future options. However, the rational use of these multidrug combinations has been demonstrated to suppress the plasma HIV RNA levels to below attainable levels of detection for over 3 years in over half of patients. These patients appear to continue to accumulate clinical and immunologic benefit. Even in those patients experiencing a treatment failure from the virologic standpoint, clear clinical benefit is seen in most. Studies designed to examine the approach of more intensive induction therapy with less intensive maintenance therapy have recently been presented. In the case of using three- or four-drug combination therapy as induction and then dropping medications to move into a maintenance mode, the maintenance therapy did not continue viral suppression for a large minority of the study participants. For the time being, it would appear that treatment must be continued

TABLE 348.1.	**PRINCIPLES OF THERAPY OF HIV INFECTION (NIH PANEL)**

Principle 1:
HIV replication leads to immune system damage and development of AIDS. HIV infection is always harmful. Long-term survival free of immune system dysfunction is rare.

Principle 2:
Plasma HIV RNA levels reflect the magnitude of HIV replication and its associated rate of CD4+-lymphocyte count decline. CD4+-lymphocyte counts indicate the current level of immune system damage. Periodic measurement of plasma HIV RNA level and CD4+-lymphocyte count is needed to assess risk for disease progression and to determine the need to initiate or alter antiretroviral therapy.

Principle 3:
Rates of disease progression vary among HIV-infected persons. Treatment decisions should be individualized based on risk of progression as indicated by plasma HIV RNA levels and CD4+-lymphocyte counts.

Principle 4:
Maximum achievable suppression of HIV replication should be the goal of therapy. The use of combinations of antiretroviral agents to suppress HIV replication to below the level of detection of plasma HIV RNA assays decreases the potential for selection of drug-resistant HIV variants.

Principle 5:
Durable suppression of HIV replication is most likely with the simultaneous initiation of combinations of antiretroviral agents with which the patient has not been previously treated and that are not cross-resistant with agents previously used.

Principle 6:
Each of the antiretroviral agents used in combination should be used according to the optimum dosages and frequencies.

Principle 7:
Any change in antiretroviral therapy decreases future therapeutic options due to the limited number of agents and significant cross-resistance between specific agents.

Principle 8:
Women should receive optimum antiretroviral therapy regardless of pregnancy.

Principle 9:
These same principles apply to children, adolescents, and adults.

Principle 10:
Acute primary HIV infection should be treated with combination antiretroviral therapy to suppress viral replication to below the level of detection of plasma HIV RNA assays.

Principle 11:
All HIV-infected persons should be considered infectious, even if the plasma HIV RNA level is below the level of detection. Counseling against activities associated with HIV transmission should continue.

EVIDENCE LEVEL: A. Reference: Report of the NIH panel to define the principles of therapy for HIV infection. *MMWR Recommendations and Reports* **1998;47:1–41.**

USE OF PLASMA HIV RNA LEVELS: VIRAL LOAD TESTING

The level of plasma HIV RNA detected by specific assays directly correlates with the total viral burden in the infected individual. The pretreatment, or baseline, measurement of this level is the single best prognostic indicator in HIV infection. Higher levels are associated with more rapid disease progression, more rapid CD4+ lymphocyte decline, and the development of AIDS or death. Following an acute elevation during initial HIV infection, the plasma HIV RNA level usually decreases to a plateau, or set point, within 6 months. This level remains fairly constant over months to years and is the prognostically significant value. Although the range of values for the commercially available viral load tests generally extends up to 750,000 or 1 million copies of viral RNA per milliliter, prognostic studies in large cohorts of patients have shown that the highest risk quintile contains those individuals with values greater than 30,000 to 55,000, depending on the type of assay used. Thus, the groups with the best prognoses are concentrated in the lower end of the viral load spectrum. With the initiation of effective antiretroviral therapy, this viral load measurement shows a rapid decline. This initial decline is used to assess the efficacy of the newly administered therapy. When repeated 3 to 6 weeks after the initiation of therapy, a three- to tenfold (0.5 to 1.0 log) decrease in the viral load should be seen. The plasma HIV RNA assay is then repeated on a regular basis to confirm continued efficacy of the therapeutic regimen. The durability of the response to treatment is directly related to the viral load nadir that is achieved. The most durable responses are in those individuals in whom the viral load has declined to below the limit of detection, which has been under 400 to 500 copies per milliliter in standard testing and under 50 copies per milliliter in highly sensitive assays.

INITIATION OF ANTIRETROVIRAL THERAPY

Since the approval of the first antiretroviral agent (zidovudine in 1987) there has been continual debate over the optimal time to initiate antiretroviral therapy. At this time there is general consensus that any patient with an AIDS diagnosis has endured too much immune system damage and is at too high a risk for progression to more advanced disease, hospitalization, or death for any further delay in therapy. There is also consensus, with minimal dissension, that any symptomatic HIV infection should be treated, regardless of CD4+ lymphocyte count and plasma HIV RNA level. Where substantial debate continues is in the patient who is free of any symptoms of HIV infection. Two sets of recommendations have recently been put forward; one by the International AIDS Society–USA and the other by the U.S. Department of Health and Human Services (DHHS). Although these recommendations do not totally agree on a level of plasma HIV RNA at which therapy should be started, the difference is inconsequential. A plasma HIV RNA level of greater than 5,000 to 20,000 copies per milliliter is deemed to be associated with a high enough risk of progression to AIDS (6% to 9% within

on a life-long basis at the more intensive level. Studies of the utility of viral resistance testing to assess the baseline resistance profile of a particular patient's virus prior to the initiation of any therapy are under way. Perhaps this possibility of baseline resistance will help explain the relatively high rate of virologic failure.

TABLE 348.2.	APPROVED ANTIRETROVIRAL AGENTS AND INVESTIGATIONAL AGENTS IN ADVANCED PHASES OF DEVELOPMENT				
Generic Name	**Brand Name**	**Also Known As:**		**FDA Approval Date**	**Comments**
Nucleoside analogue reverse transcriptase inhibitors					
zidovudine	Retrovir	ZDV, AZT		March 1987	
didanosine	Videx	ddI		October 1991	
zalcitabine	Hivid	ddC		June 1992	
stavudine	Zerit	d4T		June 1994	
lamivudine	Epivir	3TC		November 1995	
abacavir	Ziagen	ABC, 1592		December 1998	
	Combivir	AZT/3TC			Fixed dose
Nucleoside analogue reverse transcriptase inhibitors					
adefovir dipivoxil	Preveon	ADV, bis-POM PMEA			In development
PMPA					In development
Non-nucleoside reverse transcriptase inhibitors					
nevirapine	Viramune	NVP		June 1996	
delavirdine	Rescriptor	DLV		April 1997	
efavirenz	Sustiva	EFV, DMP-266		September 1998	
Protease inhibitors					
saquinavir	Invirase	SQV-HGC		October 1995	Hard-gel caps
ritonavir	Norvir	RTV		March 1996	
indinavir	Crixivan	IDV		March 1996	
nelfinavir	Viracept	NFV		March 1997	
saquinavir	Fortovase	SQV-SGC		November 1997	Soft-gel capsules
amprenavir	Agenerase	VX-478, 141W94			In FDA review
ABT-378					In development

3 years) to warrant therapy, regardless of $CD4^+$ lymphocyte count. For those individuals with a plasma HIV RNA level below this range, treatment is advised if the $CD4^+$ lymphocyte count is less than 500 cells per cubic millimeter. Thus, a practitioner may consider delaying or withholding therapy in those individuals with both a $CD4^+$ lymphocyte count above 500 cells per cubic millimeter *and* a plasma HIV RNA level below 5,000 copies per milliliter. In most clinical practices this is a small minority of patients.

In individuals with symptomatic HIV infection, an examination of the risk/benefit ratio clearly favors the use of antiretroviral therapy due to the advanced state of infection indicated by the presence of symptoms and the likelihood that the symptoms will be addressed by enhanced viral control and immunologic improvement. In the asymptomatic patient, the risk/benefit analysis can be more difficult to perform, particularly if there is a higher $CD4^+$ lymphocyte count or a lower viral load. Potential benefits include the control of viral replication and thus decreased viral mutation and less selection of resistant virus, immune system maintenance or improvement, delayed disease progression, prolonged survival, lower risk of drug toxicity when used in less advanced infection, and possibly a decreased risk of viral transmission to contacts. Potential risks to the asymptomatic patient considering therapy include adverse drug reactions, decline in quality of life due to pill taking and scheduling, development of resistant virus, transmission of resistant virus, decreased options for future therapy and the unknown durability of current therapy, as well as the development of currently unknown long-term toxicity.

Due to the rather complicated nature of the combination therapies and the potential for side effects in someone previously asymptomatic, both physician and patient need to consider the difficulties of long-term adherence to the treatment regimen prior to the initiation of such a regimen. Incomplete adherence is associated with incomplete viral suppression and the development of resistance. Significant cross-resistance in both the non-nucleoside agents and the protease inhibitors can then develop, creating a severe limitation in any future therapies. This point cannot be emphasized enough. Clinical studies performed thus far indicate a need for 90% to 95% adherence to the dosing schedule to maintain viral suppression. This implies the need for an ongoing clinical relationship and a mechanism to ensure continued access to medication—two difficult propositions in today's health care environment (Table 348.3).

THERAPEUTIC AGENTS

Currently available antiretroviral therapies can be divided into two broad categories: inhibitors of HIV reverse transcriptase and inhibitors of HIV protease. Although other aspects of the viral life cycle are amenable to therapeutic attack, these two areas are the sole targets exploited thus far. Within the category of reverse transcriptase inhibitors (RTIs) there are two subcategories: the nucleoside analogue reverse transcriptase inhibitors (nRTIs), and the non-nucleoside reverse transcriptase inhibitors (NNRTIs). Clinical experience with nRTIs dates back to 1987, whereas with NNRTIs there is only 3 years' experience, and less than 4 years'

| TABLE 348.3. | DOSING RECOMMENDATIONS AND TOXICITIES | | | |

Class	Drug	Dosing	Toxicity	Comments
Nucleoside analogues	Zidovudine	300 mg b.i.d.	GI upset, headache, anemia, leukopenia	Marrow suppression more common in advanced disease
	Didanosine	200 mg b.i.d., avoiding food	Peripheral neuropathy, pancreatitis, diarrhea	Interaction of buffer with other drugs; early data on qd dosing
	Zalcitabine	0.75 mg t.i.d.	Peripheral neuropathy, stomatitis	Most neurotoxic
	Stavudine	40 mg b.i.d.	Peripheral neuropathy	
	Lamivudine	150 mg b.i.d.	Minimal GI upset	May help maintain viral sensitivity to other nucleosides
	Abacavir	300 mg b.i.d.	Hypersensitivity, GI upset	Never rechallenge after hypersensitivity
Non-nucleoside analogues	Nevirapine	200 mg b.i.d.	Rash, hepatitis, Stevens–Johnson	200 mg qd × 14 days, then b.i.d. to decrease rash; class-wide resistance; inducer of cytochrome P450
	Delavirdine	400 mg t.i.d.	Rash, headache	Class-wide resistance; inhibitor of cytochrome P450
	Efavirenz	600 mg qhs	Dizziness, somnolence, confusion	Class-wide resistance; mixed effect on cytochrome P450
Protease inhibitors	Saquinavir	1,200 mg t.i.d. (400 mg q12h with ritonavir), with meal	GI upset, headache	
	Ritonavir	600 mg q12h (400 mg q12h with saquinavir)	GI upset, emesis, parestheias, hepatitis, elevated triglycerides	Strong cytochrome P450 inhibitor, many drug interactions
	Indinavir	800 mg q8h, on empty stomach or a low-fat snack	GI upset, nephrolithiasis, elevated bilirubin	q8h, not t.i.d., dosing; hydration to prevent stones
	Nelfinavir	750 mg t.i.d. with food	Diarrhea	Early data on 1,250 mg b.i.d.
	Amprenavir	1,200 mg b.i.d.	GI upset	FDA approval pending

with protease inhibitors (PIs). There remains much to be learned about the use of each category of antiretroviral agents as well as how to best combine them in effective therapy. Since the release of ritonavir and indinavir in early 1996, most antiretroviral treatment recommendations have utilized a combination of two nucleoside analogue reverse transcriptase inhibitors and one protease inhibitor as the starting point from which all therapy goes forward. The recent recognition of several adverse reactions that if not actually caused by protease inhibitors are at least more prevalent in patients on protease inhibitors has caused some rethinking about these treatment recommendations.

NUCLEOSIDE ANALOGUE REVERSE TRANSCRIPTASE INHIBITORS

The six agents in this class of antiretrovirals are all nucleoside derivatives that act on HIV reverse transcriptase through competitive binding to reverse transcriptase in place of endogenous nucleosides and by inducing the termination of the elongating viral DNA. They all require phosphorylation to attain the active triphosphate form and are thus dependent on intracellular metabolic pathways. In planning therapy with nRTIs, it is important

to consider combining a thymidine analogue (zidovudine or stavudine) with a non-thymidine analogue (didanosine, zalcitabine, lamivudine, or abacavir). Thymidine analogues are most active in virally activated cells, whereas nonthymidine analogues are active in resting cells.

Zidovudine

Zidovudine, a thymidine analogue, was the first antiretroviral agent approved for use against HIV. It was quickly demonstrated to have dramatic effects when compared to placebo in persons with advanced stage disease. Clinical and survival benefits were shown in multiple clinical trials. It remains a mainstay in combination therapy. Zidovudine is rapidly absorbed from the gastrointestinal tract and crosses the blood–brain barrier. No dietary restrictions complicate zidovudine use. The most common side effects are headache, fatigue, malaise, nausea, anemia, and leukopenia. The constitutional symptoms are greatest during the initial 2 to 4 weeks of therapy and generally improve afterward, although they may not resolve completely. Symptomatic therapy can be directed at these side effects. Side effects are also more common in those patients whose disease is more advanced at the time of drug initiation.

When initially approved for use, zidovudine was prescribed at a dose of 200 mg every 4 hours around the clock. The current recommended dose is 300 mg twice daily. The older dose was associated with much greater toxicity, particularly since it was being prescribed for prolonged periods of time in advanced infection. Since it was the only antiretroviral available for approximately 4 years, many patients took no other antiretroviral and progressed through their illness to death, despite zidovudine use. This issue is still raised by many patients presenting for initial care in this era. It should be addressed directly to facilitate patient adherence to an important component of many regimens.

Zidovudine used in the perinatal period has shown a significant decrease in the perinatal, or vertical, transmission of HIV infection. In the major controlled trial, transmission in the zidovudine-treated group was 8.3%, whereas the placebo group had a transmission rate of 25.5%. In this trial zidovudine was prescribed after the first trimester, given intravenously intrapartum, and then administered to the newborn for the first 6 weeks of life. Shorter course studies have confirmed benefit with decreased transmission.

Didanosine

Didanosine, an adenosine analogue, was initially made available for compassionate use in those patients failing zidovudine therapy. So the initial experiences with the drug were in advanced, treatment-exposed patients. Clinically, it was shown to be more effective than continuing zidovudine in those patients who had already received more than 16 weeks of zidovudine. The drug is acid-labile and is packaged with buffers to prevent degradation in the stomach. For the best effect of these buffers, didanosine should be taken at least 30 minutes before a meal or 2 hours after a meal. Since didanosine is a twice-daily medication, this can often be handled by taking the medication prior to the first meal of the day and after the last. This dietary restriction offers a hurdle to be addressed when planning combination therapy. It would not be advisable to combine didanosine with a drug whose absorption is increased with food or a drug that requires the normally acidic stomach, thereby increasing the number of drug-taking episodes per day. For many patients the poor palatability of the buffered tablets is reason enough to stop the medication. This can often be avoided by dissolving the tablets in water and drinking the suspension. The main side effects of didanosine are a distal symmetrical polyneuropathy, pancreatitis, and diarrhea. Neuropathic symptoms generally improve over a period of weeks following discontinuation of the drug. Pancreatitis necessitates drug withdrawal, although asymptomatic elevations of amylase, lipase, and triglycerides are seen and can be followed. Once amylase levels surpass two times the upper limit of normal, the drug should be stopped. The diarrhea is thought to be related to the buffers and can be treated symptomatically.

Zalcitabine

Zalcitabine, a cytidine analogue, was initially approved as the first combination therapy. Clinical benefit was seen for patients in whom zalcitabine was added to ongoing zidovudine therapy. It was later demonstrated that this benefit was due to zalcitabine and not to the continued zidovudine, so that zalcitabine was given an indication outside of this combination therapy. Zalcitabine is administered every 8 hours and has no dietary restrictions, although when taken with food the maximum plasma concentration is reduced by a third. A dose-related distal symmetrical polyneuropathy is the most common side effect seen with zalcitabine use. This makes therapy combining didanosine and zalcitabine inadvisable from a tolerance standpoint. As with didanosine, the neuropathic symptoms are addressed by drug withdrawal and symptomatic medications. Stomatitis with ulcerations of the buccal mucosa, soft palate, pharynx, and tongue can occur. These are usually self-limited and treatment need not be interrupted. Pancreatitis is also listed as a side effect of zalcitabine, but this is unusual.

Stavudine

Stavudine, another thymidine analogue, was quickly adopted for general use due to its relatively easy dosing schedule and light toxicity profile. Although peripheral neuropathy is its main adverse effect, stavudine is less neurotoxic than zalcitabine and didanosine. Stavudine and zidovudine should not be administered together because of possible antagonism. This may be due to competition for activation by thymidine kinase since these are the two thymidine analogues. Zidovudine-resistant mutants are susceptible to stavudine. Extensive studies have demonstrated the effectiveness of stavudine in combination with didanosine or lamivudine. Stavudine resistance is seen clinically, but the exact mechanism of this resistance has not been fully elucidated. It appears that an insertion mutation rather than substitution may be responsible.

Lamivudine

Lamivudine is the second cytidine analogue approved for use against HIV. Lamivudine is very well tolerated and has no major toxicity. Resistance to lamivudine develops rapidly, although the development of this resistance seems to delay the development of resistance to zidovudine. Also, in zidovudine-resistant virus, the administration of lamivudine seems to resensitize the virus to zidovudine. Lamivudine is also available as a fixed-dose combination tablet with zidovudine, allowing combination nucleoside therapy with the convenience of a single tablet twice daily.

Abacavir

Abacavir is the first guanosine analogue and received FDA approval in late 1998. At this time there is limited information on its use in the general HIV-infected population. Abacavir has the highest anti-viral potency of any of the nucleoside analogues when examined as monotherapy for short durations. Studies examining its use in highly treatment-experienced patients are under way to determine its efficacy in various resistance situations. This drug is generally well tolerated, with gastrointestinal upset and headache being the most common side effects. A clinically important adverse reaction despite its occurrence in less than 5% of patients studied thus far is a hypersensitivity reaction. Characterized by fever, nausea, malaise, and with or without a rash, the severity of this symptom complex increases with continued dosing. Drug discontinuation is necessary. There should be no effort at rechallenge with this drug since a fatal reaction has been reported in that setting.

NON-NUCLEOSIDE REVERSE TRANSCRIPTASE INHIBITORS

This group of medications is related by their antiretroviral activity and not by chemical structure. These drugs bind to reverse transcriptase near the enzyme's catalytic site, leading to a conformational change that inactivates the enzyme. The NNRTIs are not dependent on intracellular mechanisms for any phosphorylation. Resistance to this class of antiretrovirals develops quickly and easily when they are used in suboptimal treatment regimens. The resistance that develops is usually class-wide, causing the loss of this whole class of drugs if virologic failure occurs while taking one. For this reason, extra care must be taken when incorporating NNRTIs into the treatment plan. At least one, if not two, new agents should be used in addition to the NNRTI. Rash is also a class-wide phenomenon as the most common adverse event.

The non-nucleoside reverse transcriptase inhibitors were overshadowed by the release of the protease inhibitors and the accompanying revolution in treatment. At the time of the release of nevirapine and delavirdine, these drugs were not properly appreciated for what they could offer in terms of therapeutic options. It is only now, in the face of possible long-term toxicity due to protease inhibitors and the recent approval of efavirenz, that they are being reevaluated as a group.

Nevirapine

Nevirapine is currently recommended in a twice-daily dosing schedule but has a pharmacokinetic profile that lends it to once-daily dosing. Such clinical trials are under way. Nevirapine is generally well tolerated, with rash being the primary treatment-limiting reaction. Nevirapine induces its own metabolism and is begun at a half-dose initially in an attempt to minimize the occurrence of rash. Some clinicians have prescribed a short course of steroids to further minimize the chance of rash. If treatment is continued despite the onset of rash, the reaction may progress to Stevens–Johnson syndrome. However, the majority of rashes remain mild to moderate and do not necessitate drug withdrawal. Resolution of the rash is rapid after drug discontinuation. In many clinics, nevirapine has been a part of the so-called salvage treatment of patients failing prior therapy. In combination with ritonavir and saquinavir, nevirapine can help achieve strong antiretroviral effect.

Delavirdine

Like nevirapine, delavirdine is generally well tolerated with rash as the primary adverse event. The rash seen with delavirdine

seems to be milder than that sometimes observed with nevirapine. Unlike nevirapine, which is an inducer of the cytochrome P450 system, delavirdine is an inhibitor of this metabolic pathway. Delavirdine should not be taken shortly after antacids or didanosine since this will impair its absorption. Dosing of delavirdine is three times daily and each dose is four tablets. For persons having difficulty swallowing four tablets, they are readily dissolved in 3 or more ounces of water. Like the other NNRTIs, the place of delavirdine in treatment plans is undergoing reevaluation. Combined with nucleoside analogues, it offers potent antiretroviral activity. Head-to-head trials comparing the antiviral effect with that of protease inhibitors have not been completed; thus, neither delavirdine nor nevirapine is listed as a preferred initial regimen in the DHHS recommendations (Table 348.4).

Efavirenz

Efavirenz is the newest member of the NNRTI class, receiving FDA approval in late 1998. Efavirenz offers the attraction of once-per-day dosing. In addition to rash, patients taking efavirenz can experience a variety of central nervous system effects: dizziness, somnolence, confusion, impaired concentration. To help avoid these symptoms, most patients are advised to take efavirenz at bedtime. These symptoms will wane over the course of the first 2 weeks of therapy. Clinical data have shown that efavirenz compares favorably with protease inhibitor therapy when combined with nucleoside analogues. Additionally, a trial of efavirez with indinavir alone demonstrated strong and durable anti-HIV effect without the use of nucleoside analogues.

PROTEASE INHIBITORS

The protease inhibitors burst onto the scene of HIV therapy in late 1995 and early 1996 with impressive clinical data, including dramatic clinical outcomes and large decreases in mortality in advanced patients when a single protease inhibitor was added to ongoing therapy. This occurred just as combination therapy with nucleoside analogues was gaining general acceptance. Protease inhibitors also represented the first opportunity to attack the productive aspect of the HIV viral life cycle. By initiating triple therapy instead of monotherapy or dual therapy, patients experienced remarkable turnarounds. Some of the luster has come off the protease inhibitors as metabolic complications have developed during their use. Initially seen in early clinical trials as many patients experiencing an elevation of serum triglycerides and/or cholesterol, the spectrum of alterations has grown. Following the release of the protease inhibitors, the FDA began to receive reports of glucose intolerance and frank diabetes mellitus related to protease inhibitor use. Subsequently, there has been much debate about the relationship of protease inhibitors to body habitus changes, including facial and extremity wasting, abdominal fat accumulation or truncal obesity, breast enlargement, and the development of fat pads over the lower neck/upper shoulders ("buffalo hump"). These developments have moderated the early enthusiasm for protease inhibitor use and, as noted above, have brought about a reexamination of the place for non-nucleoside combination therapy or other "protease-sparing" regimens.

TABLE 348.4.	DHHS[a] RECOMMENDATIONS FOR INITIAL TREATMENT OF HIV INFECTION	
	One Choice Each from Column A and Column B	
Preferred Regimens	**Column A**	**Column B**
	Indinavir	ZDV + ddI
	Nelfinavir	D4T + ddI
	Ritonavir	ZDV + ddC
	Saquinavir–SGC	ZDV + 3TC
	Ritonavir + saquinavir–SGC or HGC	D4T + 3TC
	Efavirenz	
Alternative regimens	Less likely to provide sustained viral suppression, or data inadequate	
	Nevirapine or delavirdine + one choice from column B	

[a] Department of Health and Human Services.

Saquinavir

Saquinavir was first released in a hard-gel formulation that suffered from very poor bioavailability. This formulation is known as Invirase and has generally been replaced by a soft-gel formulation known as Fortovase. Both are well tolerated with gastrointestinal upset as the primary side effect. Due to its poor bioavailability, Invirase was not listed as a preferred agent in the DHHS recommendations (Table 348.4). Subsequent studies of the ritonavir/saquinavir combination have elevated Invirase to this list as part of the combination. There is little reason, however, to continue to use Invirase since the release of Fortovase. Fortovase is a preferred agent, although it does require three-times-a-day dosing with six capsules each time.

Ritonavir

Ritonavir is probably the most potent antiretroviral agent yet released, but it is also the least well tolerated. Many individuals can tolerate ritonavir with no problem at all, and for them it is an extremely effective part of their regimen. However, a large minority are unable to continue therapy due to gastrointestinal upset and circumoral paresthesias. Some of this intolerance can be addressed by a dose escalation strategy during the first 2 weeks of therapy as the cytochrome P450 system compensates for ritonavir's strong inhibition of this metabolic pathway. This inhibition can also be utilized in combination therapy, as has been done with the ritonavir/saquinavir combination. Taking advantage of this pharmacologic interaction allows for twice-daily dosing of saquinavir at a much lower total-milligram dose. During 1998 and 1999, the capsule formulation of ritonavir has been unavailable. Ritonavir has been distributed in a solution that has been unpalatable for many patients. This difficulty is being addressed with the development of a new capsule.

Indinavir

The release of indinavir marked a turning point in the presentation and reception of antiretroviral data. Since then discussion has focused on what percentage of persons on a particular regimen have obtained plasma HIV RNA levels below the level of detection. The data show a potent and very durable suppression of viral replication. Indinavir use is limited by a dosing schedule required to be every 8 hours with attention to avoiding meals. Attempts to modify the dose and the frequency to accommodate twice-daily administration have been unsuccessful. The tolerance of indinavir is quite good with some gastrointestinal upset. Nephrolithiasis and renal colic are the main adverse events of real clinical significance. This can be minimized through adequate hydration but does require about a half liter with each dose.

Nelfinavir

Nelfinavir use has progressively increased due to both its own characteristics and those of the other protease inhibitors. It has a more flexible three-times-a-day dosing recommendation and can be taken with food. Studies of twice-a-day dosing are very advanced and promising. It is well tolerated, with the main side effect being diarrhea. For most persons this is a dose initiation phenomenon with improvement following the first 2 weeks of treatment. Symptomatic treatment is usually effective.

CHOICE OF ANTIRETROVIRAL REGIMEN

Current published guidelines (Table 348.4) suggest only two approaches to antiretroviral therapy for initial consideration: two nucleosides with a protease inhibitor (or the ritonavir/saquinavir protease inhibitor combination), or two nucleosides with efavirenz (preferred list) or nevirapine or delavirdine (alternative list). Several recent studies may make a practitioner also consider the options of triple-nucleoside combination therapy using abacavir, or a non-nucleoside (efavirenz) with a protease inhibitor (indinavir or nelfinavir). Ultimately, the prescribing practitioner must take into account the very real possibility that the patient will need to alter therapy in the future due to toxicity or treatment failure. Because successful trials still show 20% to 40% of participants not obtaining an undetectable viral load, possible cross-resistance must be taken into consideration when planning the initial regimen. Beyond the purely pharmacologic considerations, care must be taken to consider the real-life scenario in which the medications will be taken. The patient's lifestyle must be part of the equation up front. Is there a rigid or flexible work schedule? Is food available at medication dosing intervals? How about refrigeration? What about hydration and the resultant urination? Is there a problem with pill swallowing, or is a solution or slurry preferred? Because adherence to the regimen is a most important factor, all of these issues need assessment.

CHANGING THERAPY

Once therapy has been initiated there may be a need to change it later in the course of care. A Change in therapy due to toxicity related to a particular drug can be accomplished by switching out the toxic drug for an alternate. There is no need to change the other components of the regimen. In the face of treatment failure, however, a single drug should never be switched or added. Much like the lessons learned over years of antituberculosis treatments, the entire failing regimen must be addressed. In HIV care it is not clear how helpful some of the available resistance testing may be. Results of such tests may help the practitioner know which drugs are more likely to *not* work but cannot assure the practitioner that any particular drug will be effective. To change a failing regimen, the entire past treatment history should be investigated. An effort must be made to avoid new drugs with significant potential for cross-resistance. Information about optimal combinations and the sequence of a particular regimen is changing rapidly and would be out of date prior to the publication of this text. Patients failing their initial regimen should be cared for by practitioners highly experienced in the delivery of HIV care.

VACCINES

It appears that the development of a preventive vaccine for HIV is still little more than a hope. There are multiple obstacles to overcome, although some progress has been made. The virus itself offers many challenges with its multiple subtypes and high mutability. Examination of the host response to infection has not yielded clear indications to the immune responses that correlate to control of infection. Animal models of HIV infection are few and complicated by cost or scarcity of the animals themselves. Despite these problems, several vaccine candidates have made it into clinical trials. In general, the subunit vaccines have demonstrated the ability to generate neutralizing antibodies to the vaccine strain of the virus. Primary isolates of HIV, however, have not been neutralized.

Immune-based therapy of established HIV infection using so-called therapeutic vaccines is also in development. The idea here is to stimulate better immunologic control of the virus in an infected individual rather than attempting to prevent infec-

tion in the first place. This approach has gotten increased attention with the development of drug therapies able to bring the plasma HIV RNA levels to the undetectable range. In trials performed thus far, it has been difficult to demonstrate any clinical benefit to the use of this type of agent.

BIBLIOGRAPHY

Carpenter CCJ, Fischl MA, Hammer SM, et al. Antiretroviral therapy for HIV infection in 1998: updated recommendations of the International AIDS Society–USA Panel. *JAMA* 1998;280:78–86.

Cohen PT, Sande MA, Volberding PA. *The AIDS knowledge base.* Philadelphia: Lippincott Williams & Wilkins, 1999.

Hirsch MS, Conway B, D'Aquilla RT, et al. Antiretroviral drug resistance testing in adults with HIV infection: implications for clinical management. *JAMA* 1998;279:1984–1991.

Mellors JW, Munoz A, Giorgi JV, et al. Plasma viral load and CD4+ lymphocytes as prognostic markers of HIV-1 infection. *Ann Intern Med* 1997;126:946–954.

Sande MA, Volberding PA. *The medical management of AIDS.* Philadelphia: WB Saunders, 1999.

U.S. Department of Health and Human Services and the Henry J. Kaiser Family Foundation. Guidelines for the use of antiretroviral agents in HIV-infected adults and adolescents. *Ann Intern Med* 1998;128: 1079–1100.

Kelley's Textbook of Internal Medicine, fourth edition. Edited by H. David Humes. Lippincott Williams & Wilkins, Philadelphia © 2000.

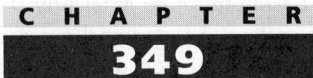

C H A P T E R

349

HIV/AIDS: EPIDEMIOLOGY, PREVENTION, AND CONTROL

SUBHASH K. HIRA

EPIDEMIOLOGY

AIDS was recognized as a clinical entity in 1981, and within the next few years important advances were made in the understanding of its epidemiology, cause, and natural history. HIV-1 is responsible for most of the AIDS cases reported throughout the world; HIV-2 is prevalent in western Africa and parts of Asia, including India, and is reported to be less pathogenic. HIV-1 is broken down to ten subtypes: A–J and O. The latter (the "O" stands for "outlier" and is considered to be the primitive form of HIV-1) is reported to be responsible for nine cases of AIDS that occurred in Cameroon in 1993 (P. Zekeng, personal communication, 1994). These subtypes are unevenly distributed throughout the world. For instance, subtype B is mostly found in the Americas, Japan, Australia, the Caribbean, and Europe; subtypes A and D predominate in sub-Saharan Africa; subtype C in South Africa and India; and subtype E in Central African Republic, Thailand, and other countries of Southeast Asia (Fig.

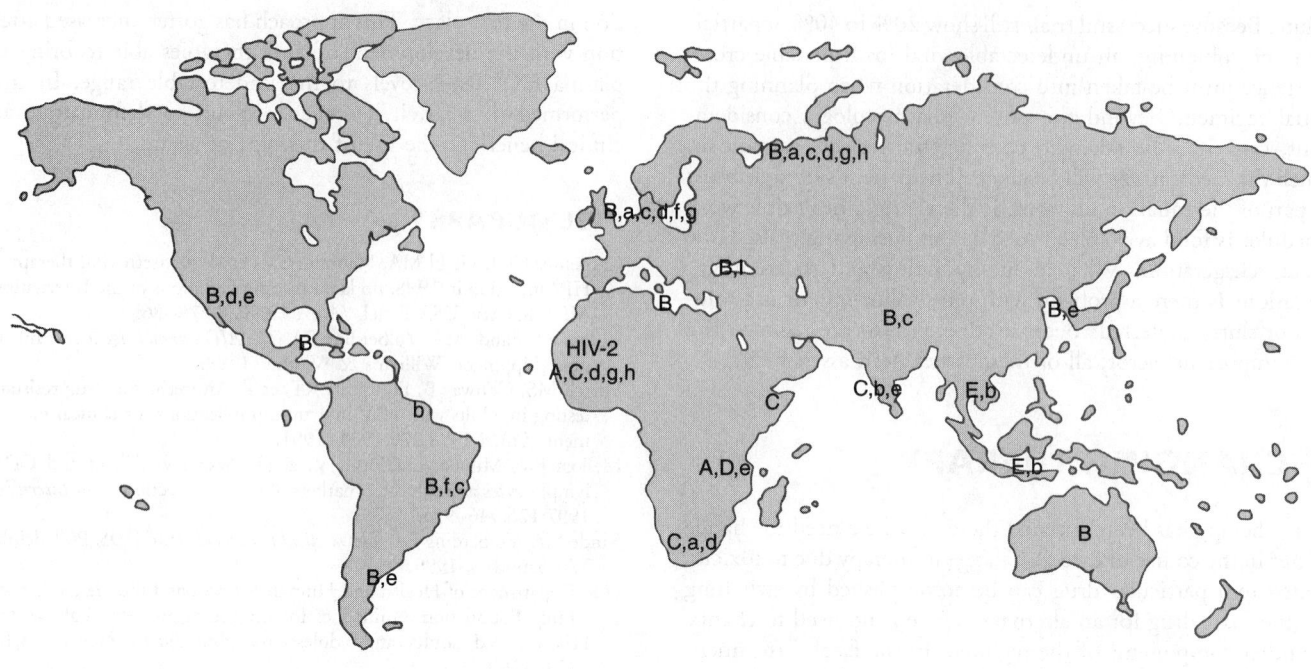

Source: UN AIDS

FIGURE 349.1. Global distribution of HIV-1 subtypes. A–I, HIV genetic subtypes of high prevalence in a region; a–i, HIV genetic subtypes of low prevalence in a region.

349.1). Laboratory studies have demonstrated that subtypes C and E infect and replicate more efficiently than subtype B in Langerhans' cells present in the vaginal mucosa, cervix, and the foreskin of the penis but not on the wall of the rectum. It is likely that HIV subtypes C and E have a higher potential for heterosexual transmission than subtype B. However, other variables that affect the risk of transmission, such as the stage of HIV disease, the frequency of exposure, condom use, and the presence of other sexually transmitted diseases (STDs), are equally important.

HIV is transmitted in three ways: sexually, by anal or vaginal intercourse; parenterally, by transfusion with contaminated blood or injection with contaminated needles; and perinatally, by passage of infection from mothers to their infants (Fig. 349.2). However, these modes of transmission are not equally

efficient. Transfusion with contaminated blood is a highly efficient means of transmission; about 95% of those who receive infected blood become infected. A study conducted by the U.S. Centers for Disease Control and Prevention showed that seroconversion occurred in 4 of every 1,000 health care workers who were inadvertently inoculated by contaminated hollow needles used on patients with HIV infection. No health care workers who were pricked by solid (suture) needles used in HIV-infected patients became infected. Male homosexual (anal) intercourse is an efficient means of virus transmission, as shown by the epidemiologic pattern observed in the United States and Western Europe. The efficiency of transmission in heterosexual (vaginal) intercourse is reported to range from 0.1% to 1%. However, this rate may be augmented four to eight times by the presence of a cofactor, such as genital ulcer disease, to 0.4% to 8%. This

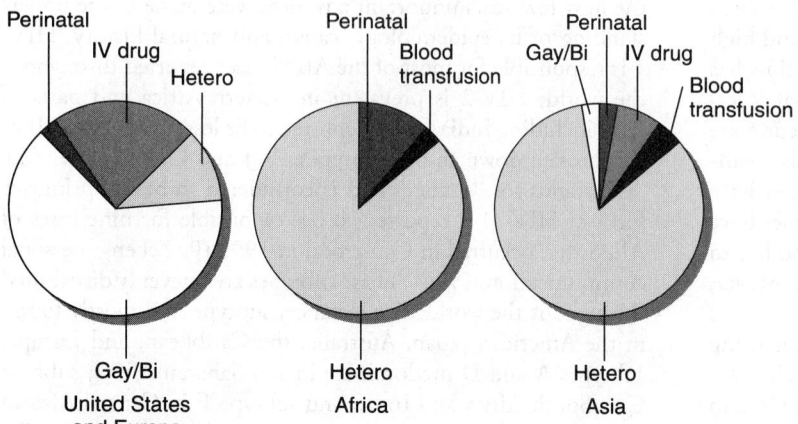

FIGURE 349.2. Modes of HIV transmission. Hetero, heterosexual; gay/bi, homosexual/bisexual; IV drug, intravenous drug use; blood trans, blood transfusion.

mechanism of heterosexual transmission accounts for the 1:1 ratio of AIDS cases among men and women in Africa and Asia, in contrast to the predominance of the disease in men in industrialized Western countries. Perinatal transmission is the third mechanism of virus spread. About 25% to 45% of children born to infected mothers are actively infected with HIV, and AIDS develops in most of them within the first 2 years of life. The virus transmission through infected breast milk has been attributed in 10% to 33% of mother–baby transmission.

HIV transmission has not been documented to occur with any other type of exposure. Intensive studies of household contacts of HIV-infected patients have demonstrated virus transmission only to sexual partners. There is no public health concern regarding possible HIV transmission in the usual school, community, or employment settings.

As of December 1998, the Joint United Nations Program on HIV/AIDS estimated that, since the start of the epidemic two decades ago, at least 47 million individuals were infected with HIV worldwide. Of these, 13.9 million have died of AIDS, including 4.7 million women and 3.2 million children. Presently, there are 33.4 million individuals living with HIV/AIDS across the world; more than 95% of them live in developing countries (Table 349.1). Each day, about 7,000 young adults aged 15 to 24 get infected with HIV, mostly in developing countries of Africa and Asia.

At least 1 million individuals are infected in the United States, and AIDS has developed in half of them. African Americans bear a disproportionate burden of this epidemic. They are eight times more likely than whites to have HIV. Among black men, the national HIV prevalence is estimated to have reached 2%, and AIDS has become the leading killer in the 25–44 age group. For black women in the same age group, AIDS takes second place as cause of death. Since the widespread introduction of new combinations of antiretroviral drugs 2 years ago, the death rate for persons with AIDS continues to decrease to almost two-thirds below rates recorded in 1996. India has an estimated 4 million HIV-infected individuals. The seroprevalence of HIV in major Indian cities is rising steadily. In Mumbai, which has a population of 12 million, the seroprevalence among antenatal clinic attendants increased from 0.8% in 1992 and 2.4% in 1994 to 4.2% in 1998. It is estimated that by the year 2000 at least 46 million individuals will be living with HIV/AIDS worldwide and that more than 95% of these individuals will be living in developing countries.

Tuberculosis, the second biggest infectious killer, is on the increase, partially driven by the HIV epidemic. Individuals with dual HIV/tuberculosis infections are at greater risk of activation of tuberculosis and consequent death. About 30% of all AIDS deaths are attributable to tuberculosis.

The HIV epidemic has visible and less visible consequences.

TABLE 349.1. REGIONAL HIV/AIDS STATISTICS AND FEATURES, DECEMBER 1998

Region	Epidemic Started	Adults and Children Living with HIV/AIDS	Adults and Children Newly Infected with HIV	% Prevalence Rate[a]	% HIV-Positive Adults Who Are Women	Main Mode(s) of Transmission for Adults Living with HIV/AIDS
Sub-Saharan Africa	Late '70–early '80s	22.5 million	4.0 million	8.0	50	Hetero
North Africa and Middle East	Late '80s	210,000	19,000	0.1	20	IDU, Hetero
South and Southeast Asia	Late '80s	6.7 million	1.2 million	0.7	25	Hetero
East Asia and Pacific	Late '80s	560,000	200,000	0.07	15	IDU, Hetero, MSM
Latin America	Late '70s–early '80s	1.4 million	160,000	0.6	20	MSM, IDU, Hetero
Caribbean	Late '70s–early '80s	330,000	45,000	2	35	Hetero, MSM
Eastern Europe and Central Asia	Early '90s	270,000	80,000	0.1	20	IDU, MSM
Western Europe	Late '70s–early '80s	500,000	30,000	0.3	20	MSM, IDU
North America	Late '70s–early '80s	890,000	44,000	0.6	20	MSM, IDU, Hetero
Australia and New Zealand	Late '70s–early '80s	12,000	600	0.1	5	MSM, IDU
Total		33.4 million	5.8 million	1.1	43	

[a] The proportion of adults (15–49 years of age) living with HIV/AIDS in 1998.
MSM, men having sex with men.
IDU, Intravenous drug users.

In several countries of sub-Saharan Africa, AIDS is causing highly visible damage. For example, the Rakai district of Uganda has lost a significant number of adults to AIDS. This has led to scores of AIDS orphans being cared for by aging grandparents while loss of productive work force has deepened poverty. Families struggle to find money to pay for funerals, and employers struggle to train new staff to replace the sick. The less visible consequences show that AIDS has reduced average life expectancy by 17 years and wiped out gains in child survival rates.

PREVENTION AND CONTROL

Because there is no known cure or vaccine for HIV infection, prevention and control strategies are extremely important. The early dramatic rise in HIV in the United States was reversed by the late 1980s due to prevention campaigns that increased condom use among gay men. However, during the last decade the rate of new infections has remained stable instead of continuing to decrease. In 1998, an estimated 75,000 persons became infected in the United States. Hence, prevention challenges are greater than before. The main approaches are as follows:

1. *Promotion of safer sexual behaviors.* Since the onset of the pandemic, information, education, and communication campaigns have been vital in reducing behaviors that put individuals at high risk for infection. These campaigns are of two types: broad mass communication for the general public, and targeted, more intensive behavioral change communication strategies aimed at vulnerable groups. Person-to-person education programs are important for certain vulnerable groups because such programs increase the level of knowledge about AIDS and high-risk behaviors.
2. *Promotion of condom use.* The promotion of safer sexual behaviors, including the use of condoms, is an integral part of prevention and control strategies. Condom use is encouraged through programs that involve market research, product importation, brand name packaging, advertising, media promotion, distribution, and management.
3. *Prevention and treatment of STDs.* Conventional STDs facilitate the transmission of HIV. Because of its adverse effect on the immune system, HIV infection can alter the incidence, natural history, and response to treatment of other STDs. In addition, these diseases rank among the top ten most important health problems in nonindustrialized countries in terms of years of healthy life lost (Over and Piot, personal communication, 1990). The early diagnosis and treatment of sexually transmitted diseases combined with behavioral intervention is recommended.
4. *Prevention of unsafe drug use behavior.* Prevention strategies for injected drug users in drug abuse treatment programs are successful but expensive. Community-based outreach programs that include education regarding the need to eliminate needle sharing, instruction in the disinfection of contaminated injection equipment, bleach distribution, and needle exchange are less expensive and equally successful. Each interaction with a client provides an opportunity for risk reduction education.
5. *Provision of a safe blood supply.* Transfusion-induced HIV infection can be prevented by safe blood initiatives, including rational use of blood. Yet as many as 3% to 5% of HIV-infected individuals in sub-Saharan Africa and parts of Asia become infected by contaminated blood. This is attributed to the low effectiveness of safe-blood programs in these countries.
6. *Targeted interventions.* For individuals at high risk of HIV infection, an epidemiologically sound set of preventive activities (interventions) are put together as a package. These interventions not only are easy to implement but they are cost-efficient and their impact is measurable.

BIBLIOGRAPHY

Confronting AIDS. Public priorities in a global epidemic. A World Bank policy research report. New York: Oxford University Press, 1997.

Hira SK, Dholakia YN, Lanjewar DN, et al. Severe weight loss: the predominant clinical presentation of tuberculosis in patients with HIV infection in India. *Natl Med J India* 1998;11:256–258.

Hira SK, Kamanga J, Macuacua R, et al. Genital ulcers and male circumcision as risk factors for acquiring HIV-1 in Zambia. *J Infect Dis* 1990; 161:584–585.

Hira SK, Mangrola U, Kamanga J, et al. Apparent vertical transmission of human immunodeficiency virus type 1 by breast feeding in Zambia. *J Pediatrics* 1990;117:421–424.

Hunter DJ. AIDS in sub-Saharan Africa: the epidemiology of heterosexual transmission and the prospects for prevention. *Epidemiology* 1993;4: 63–72.

Jamkhedkar PP, Hira SK, Shroff HJ, et al. Clinico-epidemiologic features of granuloma inguinale in the era of acquired immune deficiency syndrome. *Sex Transm Dis* 1998;25:196–200.

Mann J, Tarantola D, eds. *AIDS in the world II.* New York: Oxford University Press, 1996.

Salunke SR, Shaukat M, Hira SK, et al. HIV/AIDS: a country responds to a challenge. *AIDS* 1998;12(S):S27–S31.

United Nations. *Report on the global HIV/AIDS epidemic,* Geneva, December 1998.

PULMONARY AND CRITICAL CARE MEDICINE

Talmadge E. King, Jr., Editor

APPROACH TO THE PATIENT WITH RESPIRATORY DISEASE OR CRITICAL ILLNESS

APPROACH TO THE PATIENT WITH HYPOXEMIA

DAVID H. INGBAR

Hypoxemia is a common sign of pulmonary or cardiac disease. It may be suspected from clinical symptoms or physical examination, but laboratory testing is required to confirm its presence. The identification and differential diagnosis of hypoxemia are considered in this chapter.

Hypoxemia is defined as decreased arterial partial pressure of oxygen (PaO2) that decreases the oxygen saturation of hemoglobin; consequently, hypoxemia is defined as a PaO_2 of less than 60 mm Hg. When the PaO_2 is less than 50 to 55 mm Hg, hypoxemia is life threatening because the oxygen content of hemoglobin drops rapidly with even small decreases in oxygen partial pressure. Some experts use the term "relative hypoxemia" to indicate that the PaO_2 is lower than normal but not low enough to decrease the hemoglobin oxygen saturation.

Oxygenation normally decreases somewhat with increasing age. The efficacy of oxygen transfer from the alveolus to the pulmonary capillaries can be expressed as the gradient or difference between the alveolar and arterial oxygen partial pressures ($PAO_2 - PaO_2$). The normal gradient is less than 10 mm Hg but rises slightly with age.

The normal levels of PAO_2 and PaO_2 are determined in part by the amount of alveolar ventilation. Changes in the alveolar ventilation alter the alveolar PO_2 and PCO_2, thereby changing the end-pulmonary capillary gas pressures. The alveolar CO_2 partial pressure ($PACO_2$) directly relates to the rate of CO_2 production ($\dot{V}CO_2$) and the alveolar ventilation per minute ($\dot{V}A$), as determined by the formula $PACO_2 = (\dot{V}CO_2/\dot{V}A)/(P_b - 47)$, where P_b is the barometric pressure and 47 is the water vapor pressure. The extent of change in the alveolar PO_2, and consequently the arterial PO_2, is predicted by the alveolar gas equation: $PAO_2 = FIO_2 (P_{atm} - P_b) - (PaCO_2/0.8)$, where P_{atm} is the atmospheric pressure. The first term—$FIO_2 (P_{atm} - P_b)$—represents the inspired oxygen partial pressure (PIO_2). For patients breathing room air at sea level, the $PIO_2 = 150$ mm Hg and the alveolar gas equation simplifies to $PAO_2 = 150 - (PaCO_2/0.8)$. The inspired PO_2 falls with altitude: in Denver, it is about 120 mm Hg; in high mountain villages in the Andes and Himalayas, it is about 100 mm Hg; and on the summit of Mount Everest, it is about 38 mm Hg.

Alveolar hypoventilation, as evidenced by hypercapnia, decreases the PaO_2 even when lung function is completely normal. For example, a patient who overdoses on narcotics with normal lungs might hypoventilate with a $PaCO_2$ level rising to 80 mm Hg. The predicted PAO_2 then would be 50 mm Hg. With an alveolar–arterial O_2 gradient of 8, the PaO_2 would be 42 mm Hg. Similarly, hyperventilation increases the PaO_2 in normal persons. Hyperventilation to a $PaCO_2$ of 24 mm Hg would lead to a PAO_2 of 120 mm Hg and a PaO_2 of 112 mm Hg.

CLINICAL SIGNS AND CONSEQUENCES

Hypoxemia sometimes is obvious, as in the patient who is cyanotic, tachypneic, and tachycardic, is audibly wheezing, and is using accessory muscles of respiration. The physiologic consequences and the associated signs and symptoms of different degrees of hypoxemia are outlined in Table 350.1. However, some patients who seem comfortable and not in distress may still have life-threatening hypoxemia.

Respiratory distress often is indicated by tachypnea, cyanosis, or use of the intercostal, sternocleidomastoid, and scaleni muscles. However, not all patients with these findings are hypoxemic. Some patients may be able to compensate for their lung problems and maintain a PaO_2 of more than 60 mm Hg due to their rapid ventilation. For example, many patients with interstitial disease or restrictive lung disease adopt a rapid, shallow breathing pattern, expending high energy in their work of breathing. Their arterial blood gases often show relative hypoxemia with a PaO_2 of 60 to 75 mm Hg and hypocapnia (e.g., $PaCO_2$ 30 to 36 mm Hg).

Cyanosis may be detectable when there is more than 5 g % of deoxygenated hemoglobin in the blood. Central cyanosis is

TABLE 350.1.	PHYSIOLOGIC EFFECTS OF HYPOXEMIA	
Pao$_2$ (mm Hg)	**Abnormality in Function**	**Sign or Symptom**
<60	Heart rate	Increased tachycardia
	Respiratory rate	Increased tachypnea
	Na$^+$ and H$_2$O excretion	Decreased edema
<55	Cardiac output	Increased bounding pulses
	Dysrhythmias	Tachyarrhythmias
		Bradyarrhythmias
	Mentation	Increased somnolence
		Confusion
		Pinpoint pupils
	Red blood cell mass	Increased plethora
		Erythrocythemia
		Thromboemboli
	Pulmonary arterial pressure	Increased jugular venous pressure
		Edema
		Right ventricular S$_4$
		Hepatomegaly
		Abnormal ECG indicating cor pulmonale[a]
<30	Cardiac output	Shock
		Decreased pulse pressure
	Metabolism	Increased lactic acidosis

[a] Right atrial enlargement, right ventricular enlargement, rightward shift in ventricular or atrial vectors.

detected in the perioral area and is most common in patients with cyanotic congenital heart disease. Peripheral cyanosis is detected in the nail beds. It is a much more subjective physical finding, and there often is interobserver disagreement. In addition, many seriously ill hypoxemic patients do not have cyanosis because they have anemia.

Tachycardia may be the sole manifestation of hypoxemia. The increased catecholamines released in response to tissue hypoxia increase cardiac output and systemic oxygen delivery through increased heart rate and stroke volume. In addition, peripheral tissues vasodilate, increasing the number of open capillaries in response to local tissue hypoxia. Although this does not increase the oxygen content of blood, it decreases the diffusion distance for oxygen and increases tissue P$_{O_2}$. The decreased systemic vascular resistance also promotes tachycardia.

Tachypnea commonly occurs with hypoxemia. Patients may increase both their respiratory rate and their tidal volume. However, even experienced physicians cannot reliably estimate minute ventilation at the bedside.

The brain is very sensitive to decreased oxygen delivery. Consequently, agitation, seizures, or changes in mental status should raise the question of hypoxemia.

Cardiac consequences of hypoxemia are a major concern because they include myocardial ischemia, dysrhythmias, and decreased cardiac output.

Hypoxemia per se may indicate patients at risk for increased mortality. One study of inpatients at a tertiary care center who underwent continuous oximetry monitoring demonstrated increased postdischarge mortality in patients with episodic hypoxemia.

In summary the signs and symptoms of hypoxemia are very non-specific and easily attributed to other causes. Some patients may have essentially none of the above manifestations, and thus hypoxemia must be suspected and sought in patients at risk.

DIAGNOSIS

Hypoxemia may be diagnosed directly through arterial blood gas measurement of Pao$_2$ or oximetry measurement of percentage of hemoglobin saturated with oxygen. Arterial blood samples must be rapidly placed on ice or analyzed immediately; otherwise, cells in the sample may metabolize oxygen, yielding falsely low Pao$_2$ measurements. For example, patients with leukemia and circulating white blood cell counts above 60,000 cells per microliter may have falsely low measurements if they are not analyzed immediately or if cell metabolism is not abolished. Samples are placed in heparinized syringes, but the amount of residual heparin should be minimized because its volume dilutes the gas partial pressure and it is acidic. The patient's temperature and, if used, supplemental oxygen always should be noted on the laboratory request. The former is important in calculating the percentage of hemoglobin saturated with oxygen since it shifts the position of the hemoglobin–oxygen dissociation curve. Some laboratories calculate the percentage of hemoglobin that is saturated with oxygen based on a normal hemoglobin–oxygen dissociation curve, whereas others measure this directly with a cooximeter. Hyperlipidemia also may interfere with accurate measurement.

There is significant variability in arterial blood gas (ABG) results in clinically stable intensive care unit patients. In multiple studies, PaO_2 had a mean coefficient of variation of 5% to 6% over 1 hour. Therefore, clinical decision making should be based on trends and on large changes in arterial blood gas values.

Technology for continuous measurement of arterial PO_2, PCO_2, and pH has been developed, but the clinical value of these continuous measurements is not well established. They may be useful for earlier detection of desaturation, but they may alert caregivers too frequently, leading to time and dollars spent investigating brief desaturations without clinical significance.

Oximetry, a noninvasive method for assessing hypoxemia, uses the spectrophotometric changes in hemoglobin absorption of ultraviolet light upon oxygenation and deoxygenation. This measurement can be performed on arterialized blood in the heated ear lobe or through pulse oximetry. In pulse oximetry, the background absorption present during the nonfilling phase of blood flow is subtracted from the absorption during arterial pulsations to determine the absorption from arterial blood. It may be performed on the finger, toe, ear lobe, or bridge of the nose. Oximetry directly measures the percentage of hemoglobin saturated with oxygen. Above 85% saturation, most oximeters are accurate within 3%, but for oxygen saturations below 85% they are less accurate. Consequently, for oxygen saturations above 90% where the hemoglobin–oxygen dissociation curve flattens, a given oximetry measurement may correspond with a relatively wide range of PaO_2 values. Thus, oximetry is not a sensitive method to detect changes in PaO_2 for patients with a PaO_2 of more than 65 to 70 mm Hg.

Oximetry also may be inaccurate when there are high levels of bilirubin or other ultraviolet light–absorbing compounds in the bloodstream. Different oximeters measure absorption with different numbers of simultaneous wavelengths of light. Therefore, measurements by some, but not all, oximeters are inaccurate in the presence of methemoglobin or carboxyhemoglobin. Poor perfusion of the tissue measurement site also promotes inaccuracy and may require use of well-perfused sites such as the bridge of the nose.

Most oximeters average the percentage of oxygen saturation over multiple cardiac cycles. This gives more accurate and stable measurements; however, in patients with rapid or transient oxygen desaturation, this may delay or blunt the machine's readout indication that the patient has become hypoxemic. Many oximeters permit adjustment of the window of time averaging for the values reported, and it may be important to adjust this based on the patient's instability. This also is important to accurately assess hypoxemia in patients with apneic episodes.

PATHOPHYSIOLOGIC FACTORS

Hypoxemia can arise from multiple pathophysiologic mechanisms, but the four standard mechanisms are hypoventilation, shunt, ventilation–perfusion mismatch, and diffusion block or limitation. An additional rare mechanism is a low FIO_2, but this is relevant only in unusual environments, such as at very high altitude. Finally, a low mixed venous PO_2 can contribute to arterial hypoxemia when other significant abnormalities, such as shunt, are present. This is discussed further after consideration of shunt physiology.

HYPOVENTILATION

Alveolar hypoventilation lowers PAO_2 and raises $PaCO_2$ due to decreased minute ventilation. Because with pure hypoventilation the lung parenchyma is normal, the alveolar–arterial oxygen gradient remains normal. Hypoventilation commonly occurs when ventilatory drive is decreased by drugs, endocrine abnormalities, central nervous system disorders, or diseases of the neuromuscular system or chest wall. Narcotics, benzodiazepines, and other sedatives are common drug-related causes. Severe hypothyroidism or hypopituitarism can decrease ventilatory drive and cause hypoventilation. Diaphragm paralysis, muscular dystrophy, Guillain–Barré syndrome, fibrothorax, and kyphoscoliosis are examples of restrictive abnormalities that may result in hypoventilation. Essentially, the normal closely coupled relation between $PaCO_2$ and minute ventilation is disrupted in either the sensing or effector limbs. Supplemental oxygen improves the hypoxemia of alveolar hypoventilation but does not decrease the hypercapnia.

SHUNT

Peripheral vascular shunts have little effect on oxygenation, but may increase venous PO_2. Intracardiac shunts can cause severe hypoxemia if there is right-to-left shunting, as may occur when pulmonary hypertension with the Eisenmenger complex is combined with an atrial or ventricular septal defect. Intrapulmonary shunts may be macroscopic (vascular) or microscopic (parenchymal). Arteriovenous malformations within the pulmonary arterial circulation are an example of the former that can cause hypoxemia. Finally, microscopic parenchymal shunts occur when blood flows through the capillaries of nonventilated alveoli; examples are flooded or atelectatic alveoli. When shunt is discussed as the physiologic cause of hypoxemia, microscopic parenchymal shunts usually are assumed to be the cause.

Hypoxemia due to shunt does not respond significantly to high-level supplemental oxygen because the alveolar PO_2 does not affect the oxygenation of blood flowing through the shunted alveolar capillary units. Shunt pathophysiologic processes commonly occur in pulmonary edema, acute lung injury (acute respiratory distress syndrome), pneumonia, or atelectasis. It also can occur in patients with sepsis or in association with hepatic cirrhosis. Therapy for the hypoxemia must be directed at the underlying cause of the shunt. When shunts are more than 30%, even 100% oxygen usually has relatively little benefit on oxygenation. In patients with hypoxemia from shunt physiologic factors, increasing cardiac output may worsen hypoxemia.

Normal persons have 1% to 3% of blood flow shunted past the lungs through the thesbian and bronchial circulations. Many clinicians calculate shunt at the bedside in the intensive care unit from ABG results obtained on supplemental oxygen. These calculations attribute all the hypoxemia to shunt physiologic factors and then yield a percentage shunt that would cause the observed hypoxemia. Strictly speaking, this is a calculation of venous admixture rather than a true measurement of shunt. To measure shunt, the patient should be breathing 100% oxygen so that all contributions of hypoventilation, diffusion block, and ventilation–perfusion mismatch are eliminated.

Hypercapnia is uncommon with shunt physiology, provided that minute ventilation increases in compensation for the hypoxemia. Hypercapnia sometimes occurs clinically in shunt from acute lung injury or severe pneumonia, but often it is multifactorial and CO_2 production is also increased.

VENTILATION–PERFUSION MISMATCHING

Ventilation–perfusion (V/Q) mismatch, the most common cause of hypoxemia, often confuses physicians and students. The normal lung has alveolar–capillary units with a broad range of V/Q ratios. The bases of the lungs receive more ventilation and more perfusion than the apices. The perfusion gradient results from gravity and is pronounced, whereas the ventilation gradient is less significant. Consequently, basal alveoli tend to have low V/Q ratios, whereas apical alveoli usually have relatively high V/Q ratios. The dispersion of V/Q ratios in the normal lung increases with age, leading to the slight increases in PaO_2 − PaO_2.

Patients with hypoxemia from V/Q mismatching usually have more of both low- and high-V/Q units than normal. Alveolar capillary units with low V/Q ratios are well perfused but relatively underventilated; consequently, the venous blood leaving them still is partially deoxygenated. Low-V/Q units usually result from underventilation, as occurs in both obstructive and restrictive lung disease. Less commonly, these units result from overperfusion, as occurs when massive pulmonary emboli shunt high blood flow through small amounts of remaining normal pulmonary vascular bed. The extreme form of low-V/Q unit is shunt alveoli that are perfused but not ventilated. In contrast, units with high V/Q are relatively overventilated and their venous effluent is fully saturated. High-V/Q units may result from overventilation or underperfusion. These units waste alveolar ventilation and work of breathing but do not make patients hypoxemic. High-V/Q units are common in patients with emphysema and in those receiving positive-pressure mechanical ventilation. The extreme form of high-V/Q unit is dead-space alveoli that are ventilated but not perfused. The systemic arterial PO_2 is determined by the relative numbers and distribution of high- and low-V/Q units and by the absolute blood flows to them.

V/Q mismatch often causes hypoxemia and less often causes hypercapnia. Hypoxemia results from increasing numbers of low-V/Q units. This form of hypoxemia corrects easily with small amounts of supplemental oxygen because a small increase in FIO_2 significantly increases the inspired PO_2 and hence the PaO_2 in the low-V/Q units. In turn, this increases the venous PO_2 in the blood exiting these units. There is no significant effect on the high-V/Q units.

V/Q mismatch also interferes with CO_2 excretion. Low-V/Q units have relatively high alveolar PCO_2, but high-V/Q units have low $PaCO_2$. Thus, once again, the low-V/Q units lead to blood gas abnormalities, in this case hypercapnia. However, two factors combine to make hypercapnia less common than hypoxemia. First, even a small increase in $PaCO_2$ often triggers increased minute ventilation, which diminishes the tendency toward hypercapnia. Second, the carboxyhemoglobin dissociation curve is relatively linear and does not plateau in a fashion similar to the oxyhemoglobin dissociation curve. This allows red blood cells to load large amounts of CO_2. The red blood cells that perfuse the high-V/Q units can transfer large amounts of CO_2 to the alveolus but can pick up only a limited quantity of oxygen. Thus, V/Q mismatch causes hypoxemia more readily than hypercapnia.

A clinical measure of the impact of low-V/Q units is the physiologic dead space or the ratio of dead space to tidal volume (VDS or VDS/VT). Normal persons have about 150 mL of anatomic dead space obligated by the conducting airways. By measuring the end-expiratory PCO_2 ($PECO_2$) and assuming that the arterial PCO_2 accurately reflects the end-capillary PCO_2 in the perfused alveoli, one can calculate the VDS/VT ratio by the Bohr equation:

$$VDS/VT = (PaCO_2 − PECO_2)/PaCO_2$$

This equation attributes all the hypercapnia to dead space but in reality includes the contribution of low-V/Q alveolar–capillary units.

Patients with asthma and chronic obstructive pulmonary disease (COPD) typically have hypoxemia due to V/Q mismatch. When these patients have a high $PaCO_2$, usually there is a combination of severe V/Q mismatch and a diminished increase in minute ventilation to compensate for the respiratory acidemia. Supplemental oxygen readily corrects hypoxemia in patients with COPD, but some COPD patients given supplemental oxygen have significant increases in $PaCO_2$. The mechanism of the rise in CO_2 is controversial; two alternatives are suppression of hypoxic ventilatory drive in patients with blunted hypercapnic ventilatory drive; or alveolar oxygen increasing perfusion to poorly ventilated alveoli with high $PaCO_2$.

From a practical standpoint, patients with acute exacerbations of COPD need to be given enough oxygen to get their PaO_2 above 50 mm Hg, even if they are at risk for CO_2 retention. This should be done by starting with low levels of supplemental oxygen and increasing it in small increments to avoid preventable hypercapnia and acidosis. Even so, some patients require intubation and mechanical ventilation.

DIFFUSION BLOCK

Oxygen and carbon dioxide move passively between the alveolus and the capillary blood. The amount of diffusive gas transfer is determined by Fick's law: gas transfer = D (PA − Pc), where Pc is the capillary gas partial pressure and the diffusing capacity, D, is a combined coefficient determined by the thickness and properties of the intermediate structures (endothelial and epithelial cells and their basement membranes) and the gas exchange surface area. It is difficult to measure D for O_2 or CO_2. As a clinical approximation, the diffusing capacity for carbon monoxide (CO) is measured; the oxygen diffusing capacity normally is 20% to 25% greater than for CO.

Gas diffusion usually does not limit gas exchange and hence diffusion block is an unusual sole cause of hypoxemia. The red blood cell normally spends 0.75 second traversing the pulmonary capillary and alveolar gas pressures are completely equilibrated after 0.25 second. Thus, there is a large reserve that can accommodate increased blood flow or greater barriers to diffusion. For example, even a threefold increase in cardiac output does not lead to desaturation from diffusion abnormality. Pulmonary fibrosis previously was believed to cause diffusion block. Most authorities now believe that there is a loss of alveolar capillary gas exchange surface but that diffusion block does not contribute significantly to hypoxemia at rest.

Occasionally gas transfer becomes limiting, usually when there is a combination of decreased transit time, abnormal thickening of the alveolar wall, and decreased PaO_2 as a driving force. Clinically this most commonly occurs when patients with interstitial lung disease exercise; it also may occur at high altitude. Hypoxemia from diffusion abnormality is corrected relatively easily with supplemental oxygen.

MIXED VENOUS HYPOXIA

In patients with underlying shunt pathophysiologic states, much of the blood flowing out of the lungs still is at mixed venous PO_2. When this blood combines with better oxygenated blood from other units, the oxyhemoglobin dissociation curve requires that the oxygen content of the arterial blood be significantly decreased. Thus, when shunt physiology is present, the mixed venous PO_2 significantly affects the arterial PO_2. Similar effects occur in low-V/Q units of the lung, but to a lesser degree. One clinical situation where this is relevant is exercise in patients with cardiac or lung disease. Some cardiac patients may be at risk because of low mixed venous PO_2 from poor tissue perfusion, combined with a tendency to develop pulmonary edema.

The mixed venous PO_2 is a function of tissue oxygen delivery, the distribution between organ beds, and the peripheral oxygen utilization. Because oxygen delivery is determined by the cardiac output and the oxygen content of the arterial blood, the arterial and mixed venous PO_2 measurements are closely linked.

There are several therapeutic implications of these relations. First, changes in PaO_2 may due not to altered lung function but to changes in cardiac output or tissue oxygen use. For example, decreased cardiac output might lower PaO_2 by lowering mixed venous PO_2. Second, increasing the mixed venous PO_2 may increase the PaO_2 in some clinical situations, such as severe acute lung injury. For example, transfusing acute respiratory distress syndrome patients to increase the oxygen-carrying capacity of the blood may increase the mixed venous, and hence the arterial, PO_2.

■ APPROACH TO THE PATIENT

The two most important steps are to suspect that a patient may be hypoxemic and to assess oxygenation, preferably with an ABG measurement. Oximetry is rapid and inexpensive but can be misleading. First, as long as the patient's PaO_2 is above 60 mm Hg, the oxygen saturation will be adequate and may be falsely reassuring. For example, if the patient is hyperventilating to a $PaCO_2$ of 25 to 30 mm Hg, a PaO_2 of even 65 may indicate severe difficulty with oxygenation. Also, supplemental oxygenation often already has been started as symptomatic treatment for respiratory distress, making oximetry more misleading. Second, hypercapnia and acid–base disorders will be missed if oximetry alone is performed.

TABLE 350.2. RAPID DIFFERENTIAL DIAGNOSTIC APPROACH TO THE HYPOXEMIC PATIENT

Normal Chest Radiograph	Abnormal Chest Radiograph
Increased $PaCO_2$	
Severe asthma	Severe COPD
Neuromuscular disease	Diaphragm impairment
Ventilatory drive problem	Thorax abnormality
Normal or Low $PaCO_2$	
Pulmonary embolus	Heart failure
Sepsis	Pneumonia
Moderate COPD	ARDS
Moderate asthma	Interstitial fibrosis

COPD, chronic obstructive pulmonary disease; ARDS, acute respiratory distress syndrome.

Once hypoxemia is determined to be present, then the clinical cause must be ascertained. A rapid approach to the differential diagnosis of common clinical entities is presented in Table 350.2; the specific entities are discussed elsewhere.

Finally, when the PaO_2 is less than 60 mm Hg and the patient is in respiratory distress, or if myocardial ischemia may be present, then supplemental oxygen should be initiated. Oximetry may be useful to assess the response while the amount of supplemental oxygen is increased. Care must be taken when treating COPD patients to avoid worsening hypercapnia and respiratory acidemia. In this particular setting, it is essential to obtain repeat arterial blood gas measurements.

BIBLIOGRAPHY

Bowton DL, Scuderi PE, Haponik EF. The incidence and effect on outcome of hypoxemia in hospitalized medical patients. *Am J Med* 1994;97: 38–46.

Bowton DL, Scuderi PE, Harris L, et al. Pulse oximetry monitoring outside the intensive care unit: progress or problem? *Ann Intern Med* 1991;115: 450–454.

Mahutte CK, Holody M, Maxwell TP, et al. Development of a patient-dedicated, on-demand blood gas monitor. *Am J Respir Crit Care Med* 1994;149:852–859.

Raffin TA. Indications for blood gas analysis. *Ann Intern Med* 1986;105: 390–398.

Sassoon CSH, Hassell KT, Mahutte CK. Hyperoxic-induced hypercapnia in stable chronic obstructive pulmonary disease. *Am Rev Respir Dis* 1987; 135:907–911.

Severinghaus JW, Naifeh KH. Accuracy of response of six pulse oximeters to profound hypoxia. *Anesthesiology* 1987;67:551–558.

Sherter CB, Jabbour SM, Kovnat DM, et al. Prolonged rate of decay of arterial PO_2 following oxygen breathing in chronic airway obstruction. *Chest* 1975;67:259–261.

Thorson SH, Marini JJ, Pierson DH, et al. Variability of arterial blood gas values in stable patients in the ICU. *Chest* 1983;84:14–18.

Kelley's Textbook of Internal Medicine, fourth edition. Edited by H. David Humes. Lippincott Williams & Wilkins, Philadelphia © 2000.

C H A P T E R
351

APPROACH TO THE PATIENT WITH DYSPNEA

KATHY E. SIETSEMA

The term *dyspnea* is used to describe perceptions of difficulty or distress related to breathing. Some degree of dyspnea is considered normal in the appropriate context of activities or environment, such as during vigorous exercise or on ascent to higher altitude. However, dyspnea is recognized as symptomatic of disease when it occurs under inappropriate circumstances. Dyspnea is a presenting complaint of patients with a wide variety of medical diseases and undoubtedly arises by multiple mechanisms.

■ PATHOPHYSIOLOGIC FACTORS

Experimental models of dyspnea have demonstrated that the intensity of this symptom correlates with the ratio of *ventilatory requirement* at a given time to the *ventilatory capacity* of the individual. Ventilatory requirement is closely tied to the rate of CO_2 production and so is dictated by metabolic rate and activity level. The ventilation required for a given rate of CO_2 production is determined by the efficiency of ventilation, which reflects how well regional ventilation and perfusion are matched in the lung, and by the level of arterial CO_2. Ventilatory capacity is a function of the mechanical and neuromuscular properties of the thorax as well as the lungs, and may be therefore be reduced by extrapulmonary processes as well as by intrinsic lung disease. Even when ventilatory requirements are within an individual's capacity, the sense of *ventilatory effort* needed to meet those requirements may be increased by such factors as abnormal lung mechanics or respiratory muscle fatigue. For any condition to cause dyspnea there must be *sensory perceptions* related to breathing and ventilatory stimuli. To appreciate the range of conditions that can cause dyspnea, it is valuable to review the physiologic stimuli that give rise to respiratory sensations.

■ SENSORY PERCEPTIONS RELATED TO VENTILATION

Sensory perception involves a series of processes: activation of sensory receptors, transmission of information to the central nervous system (CNS), integration and processing of these inputs, and, finally, perception at higher brain levels. No discrete area of the cortex appears responsible for dyspnea perception, however, nor are there unique sensory receptors producing dyspnea when stimulated. Thus, although considerable insight has been gained into the stimuli that cause respiratory sensations and the conditions that modulate these sensations, the mechanisms

responsible for dyspnea in many disease states remain incompletely understood.

RESPIRATORY CHEMORECEPTORS

Chemoreceptors provide feedback to brain stem respiratory centers for the control of ventilation. The carotid bodies, the principal peripheral chemoreceptors in humans, respond primarily to reductions in arterial PO_2, whereas central chemoreceptors are sensitive to PCO_2 and pH. There is controversy as to whether dyspnea can result solely from stimulation of chemoreceptors, or whether it depends instead on the resulting reflex increases in CNS ventilatory effort or ventilatory motor activity. Despite intersubject variability in chemoreceptor responsiveness, increases in chemoreceptor stimulation increase the level of dyspnea experienced at a given level of ventilation.

LUNG AND THORACIC CAGE SENSORY RECEPTORS

Afferent inputs from the airways and lung parenchyma are carried by the vagus nerve and include signals from irritant receptors, pulmonary stretch receptors, and J receptors. These pathways may be activated by lung inflammation, edema, or changes in lung volume. The diaphragm and intercostals are skeletal muscles and are the source of a rich array of sensory information. Muscle spindles respond to changes in muscle length or displacement, and tendon organs respond to tension developed within the muscle. These respiratory muscle mechanoreceptors appear to be important in the perception of dyspnea related to respiratory pattern or mechanics. Reflex increases in ventilation occur in response to pressure or stretch stimulation in the heart or pulmonary arteries. These observations provide circumstantial evidence to support a role for vascular mechanoreceptors in the pathogenesis of dyspnea, particularly in pulmonary hypertension and other cardiovascular disorders.

CENTRAL MOTOR COMMAND

Efferent output from the CNS to the respiratory apparatus has been termed "motor command." There is evidence that the magnitude of motor command can be sensed. This has led to the concept that brain stem respiratory centers send a copy of their efferent traffic to the cortex as well as to the respiratory apparatus.

INTEGRATION OF SENSORY INPUT

The sensory signals described above are part of a complex, redundant system that provides feedback for perceiving and controlling ventilation. Like many sensations, the severity of dyspnea is quantitatively related to the stimulus inducing it. In addition, the multiplicity of potential combinations of input from differential stimulation of each sensory receptor provides a mechanism for producing qualitative as well as quantitative differences in respiratory sensation.

It is likely that lung volume is sensed principally through

muscle spindle and joint proprioceptors, and respiratory muscle tension through tendon organs. Many abnormalities of lung mechanics (e.g., lung compliance, impedance, or volume) resulting from cardiorespiratory disease can thus be derived from the relations between factors, or their time integrals, to which these receptors are sensitive. The sensation of ventilatory effort is proposed to be related to motor command, i.e., the efferent output of the respiratory center. A major postulate arising from research of dyspnea is that dyspnea results from consciousness of discrepancies between sensory input from the lungs and chest wall related to respiratory activity, and the expected perceptions based on motor command.

SPECTRUM OF CLINICAL CONDITIONS PRESENTING WITH DYSPNEA

Acute dyspnea, developing over minutes to days, most often reflects an acute cardiac or pulmonary process requiring urgent evaluation and treatment. Pulmonary processes in this context include diffuse airflow obstruction, pneumonia, upper airway obstruction, compression of the lung by chest trauma or pleural processes, rapidly progressive inflammatory disease, or diffuse lung injury with noncardiogenic pulmonary edema. Cardiovascular diseases causing acute dyspnea include pulmonary edema due to myocardial or valve dysfunction, thromboembolism, or pericardial disease. Chronic dyspnea, which is more likely to present diagnostic difficulty than acute dyspnea, is the focus of most of the following discussion. Disease categories to be considered in patients with chronic dyspnea, along with disease examples, are summarized in Table 351.1.

OBSTRUCTIVE AIRFLOW DISEASES

Obstructive airflow diseases are characterized by a reduction in expiratory flow rates for a given lung volume. A common consequence is end-expiratory hyperinflation, resulting in alteration of the position of the respiratory muscles (principally foreshortening of the diaphragm, which decreases muscle efficiency, increases respiratory work, and can lead to muscle fatigue). Regional mismatching of pulmonary ventilation to perfusion due to heterogeneity of airflow obstruction increases ventilatory requirements and may result in arterial hypoxemia. Total ventilatory capacity is usually reduced. Thus, decreased capacity and increased requirements and effort may all contribute to dyspnea in patients with airflow obstruction.

Episodic worsening of dyspnea results from worsened airflow obstruction due to airway inflammation or bronchoconstriction. Temporal variability of airflow obstruction is particularly characteristic of asthmatics, whose lung mechanics may be entirely normal between exacerbations. Diurnal variation of airway tone is exaggerated in asthmatics and may be manifest as nocturnal dyspnea or cough. Dyspnea due to bronchospasm may follow exercise or exposure to irritants or allergens. Chest tightness is

a common complaint in asthma and has been attributed to stimulation of irritant receptors in the lung.

Although much less common than diffuse airway disease, focal lesions such as tumor, stricture, or aspirated foreign body may cause obstruction of large airways. In the larynx or trachea, obstructing lesions may present with inspiratory stridor. An increasingly recognized cause of variable airflow obstruction is vocal cord dysfunction consisting of inappropriate adduction of the vocal cords during inspiration. This condition is often mistaken for asthma due to the intermittent nature of the symptoms.

INTERSTITIAL LUNG DISEASES

Progressive dyspnea on exertion is the most common presentation of interstitial lung diseases of any cause, and may sometimes begin before abnormalities are detectable on chest radiograph and before lung volumes are measurably reduced. Alterations in lung mechanics, sensed through either vagal or respiratory muscle afferents, are probably responsible for dyspnea early in the course of disease. Inflammation or fibrosis due to interstitial disease affecting the pulmonary capillaries can reduce the total alveolar–capillary interface and result in hypoxemia and, ultimately, pulmonary hypertension. As is true for obstructive diseases, with increasing severity of disease total ventilatory capacity decreases, while ventilatory requirements increase due to progressive ventilation to perfusion mismatching.

CARDIOVASCULAR DISEASES

Left ventricular dysfunction results in increased pulmonary venous pressure and vascular congestion, with attendant reduction in lung and pulmonary vascular compliance. With overt pulmonary edema, there is compromised gas exchange and arterial hypoxemia. In addition, reduction of maximal cardiac output reduces O_2 delivery and results in an earlier onset of lactic acidosis during exercise. This increases ventilatory requirements due to the need to compensate for metabolic acidosis and can cause dyspnea even in the absence of pulmonary congestion. Bronchial hyperreactivity or "cardiac asthma" may further contribute to dyspnea in heart failure. The mechanisms of dyspnea in pericardial disease and pulmonary vascular disease are not clear: dyspnea can occur even in the absence of hypoxemia or altered lung mechanics, thus suggesting a role for mechanical receptors (stretch receptors and/or baroreceptors) in the central circulation.

Many cardiovascular diseases, including cardiomyopathy, valvular disease, and pulmonary hypertension, present first with exertional dyspnea. Although coronary ischemia is typically manifest as angina, exertional breathlessness may be predominant, presumably due to ischemic ventricular dysfunction. Orthopnea and paroxysmal nocturnal dyspnea are additional manifestations of elevated pulmonary venous pressure. Pulmonary vascular diseases may be particularly difficult to diagnose. With acute pulmonary embolism, the onset of dyspnea is usually acute and unrelated to exertion; there is frequently associated anxiety,

TABLE 351.1.	SOME DISORDERS PRESENTING WITH CHRONIC DYSPNEA

Category	Examples
Impaired Pulmonary Function	
Airflow obstruction	
Diffuse	Asthma
	Chronic obstructive pulmonary disease
Focal	Vocal cord paralysis or dysfunction
	Tracheal stenosis
	Endobronchial tumor
Restriction of lung mechanics	
Interstitial lung disease	Idiopathic pulmonary fibrosis
	Pneumoconioses
	Lymphangitic carcinomatosis
Extrapulmonary thoracic restriction	Kyphoscoliosis
	Pleural effusion or fibrothorax
Neuromuscular weakness	Amyotrophic lateral sclerosis
	Phrenic nerve paralysis
Gas exchange abnormalities with normal lung	
mechanics	
Right-to-left shunt	Pulmonary arteriovenous malformation
Impaired Cardiovascular Function	
Myocardial disease	Dilated cardiomyopathy
Valvular disease	Aortic or mitral stenosis
	Aortic or mitral regurgitation
Pericardial disease	Restrictive pericarditis
Pulmonary vascular disease	Thromboembolism
	Idiopathic pulmonary hypertension
	Central venous obstruction
Congenital anomolies	Intracardiac right-to-left shunt
	Pulmonary vascular abnormalities
Altered Central Ventilatory Drive or Perception	
	Idiopathic hyperventilation
Systemic or Metabolic Disorders	
Increased metabolic requirements	Hyperthyroidism
	Obesity
Anemia	Chronic blood loss
Metabolic acidosis	Renal failure
	Mitochondrial myopathy
Physiologic Processes Causing Dyspnea	
Deconditioning	
Hypoxic air breathing at altitude	
Vigorous exercise	
Pregnancy	

sometimes described as a sense of impending doom. Chronic forms of pulmonary hypertension are first manifest by exertional dyspnea and often are not diagnosed until secondary right ventricular hypertrophy or failure has developed. Exertional lightheadedness or syncope, due to limited cardiac output, are ominous signs in this setting.

NEUROMUSCULAR WEAKNESS

Neurologic or myopathic diseases affecting the muscles of respiration can lead to respiratory insufficiency. The occurrence of dyspnea in these conditions depends primarily on the relation between ventilatory requirement and capacity, although there may be a heightened sense of respiratory effort, even when breathing capacity is adequate. Because the underlying neuromuscular disease may restrict the patient's activity, dyspnea is often not noted until ventilatory capacity is severely reduced. Phrenic nerve paralysis, either unilateral or bilateral, is a focal neurologic defect that can cause distressing dyspnea, typically worsened with recumbency as the weight of the abdominal contents displaces the diaphragm cephalad.

HYPERVENTILATION SYNDROMES

Hyperventilation, with no apparent cause, is a relatively common condition. It is frequently attributed to, but is not invariably associated with, anxiety or other psychological symptom. When idiopathic hyperventilation is the cause of dyspnea, it may be described as "air hunger" or inability to take a deep breath. The dyspnea is usually episodic; it often occurs at rest and may not worsen with exercise. As the basis for this condition is unclear, the diagnosis of psychogenic hyperventilation as the cause of unexplained dyspnea should be made with caution, and only after other potential causes have been considered.

METABOLIC AND OTHER CONDITIONS

Anemia reduces the blood's O_2-carrying capacity, so that a greater proportion of the cardiac reserve is needed for a given metabolic rate. Lactic acidosis is incurred at a lower level of exertion, thereby increasing ventilatory requirements. Other, poorly understood mechanisms may also contribute to dyspnea caused by anemia. Metabolic acidosis from renal insufficiency, myopathy, or other causes can similarly lead to dyspnea due to increased ventilatory requirements. Progesterone, a ventilatory stimulant, is responsible for chronic respiratory alkalosis and exertional dyspnea associated with pregnancy. Obesity causes increased ventilatory requirements because of the added metabolic work of supporting excess weight during ambulatory activity; it can lead to exertional dyspnea on this basis. Dyspnea may be a symptom of hypo- or hyperthyroidism, which in either case may be due to respiratory muscle weakness or cardiovascular impairment, and in the latter also to increased metabolic rate or respiratory drive.

PREVALENCE OF CONDITIONS CAUSING DYSPNEA IN MEDICAL PRACTICE

The prevalence of the above diagnoses in patients presenting with chronic dyspnea depends on the patient population and practice setting. Two published reports tabulated diagnoses for a total of 162 patients referred to pulmonary specialists for evaluation of dyspnea. Combining results of these two studies, 48% of patients were found to have diseases of the lungs or airways, including (in order of frequency) asthma, chronic obstructive airway diseases, interstitial diseases, upper-airway obstruction, and lung cancer. Cardiovascular diseases accounted for 15%, including cardiomyopathy, coronary artery disease, pulmonary vascular disease, dysrhythmia, valvular and pericardial diseases. In 11% of patients, hyperventilation syndrome or psychogenic dyspnea was diagnosed. In 8%, dyspnea improved after treatment of gastroesophageal reflux or postnasal drip. Neuromuscular or extrapulmonary restriction of lung mechanics was identified in 4%, deconditioning in 4%, and metabolic diseases in 2%. Nine percent remained undiagnosed despite extensive evaluation. Despite the selection biases and the limited number of patients represented by these studies, this is probably a reasonable estimate of the distribution of causes of chronic dyspnea for which a diagnosis is not immediately apparent.

■ CLINICAL EVALUATION

HISTORY AND PHYSICAL EXAMINATION

Because a careful history and physical examination often identifies the cause of dyspnea, this is the essential starting point for clinical evaluations.

It is important to establish the acuity of symptoms, as this bears on the differential diagnosis and dictates how rapidly a diagnosis must be established and therapy instituted. Normally, the ventilatory system has a large functional reserve, and resting ventilation requires only a small percentage of the maximum capacity. Increases in ventilatory requirements and effort may not be noticed by the patient at rest. Therefore, in addition to the onset, character, and severity of dyspnea, information regarding current and past activity levels are needed to establish the context of the symptoms. Questioning should be specific, as patients may have difficulty quantifying their activity levels or may have unconsciously reduced activity levels over time to avoid symptoms of breathlessness. Because the magnitude of dyspnea associated with a particular physiologic stimulus is reproducible for a given person, a recent change in dyspnea during a particular activity is meaningful and an important part of the history.

Most patients do not complain of "dyspnea", but use a variety of descriptors for discomfort or difficulty with breathing. Different descriptors are used with varying frequency among patients with different underlying diseases, supporting the concept that the perception of dyspnea results from a variety of sensations arising from multiple mechanisms. Although distinct clusterings of respiratory symptoms characterize different diseases, most descriptors are not unique to a particular condition. Personal, cultural, and linguistic factors can also affect how symptoms are described, limiting the utility of these distinctions in the evaluation of individual patients.

The differential diagnosis for chronic dyspnea is broad, and the physical examination needs to be similarly comprehensive. Careful attention should be directed to cardiorespiratory findings. Observation of the patient's appearance and respiratory rate while walking or moving about the room is of particular value. Signs of systemic conditions, such as collagen vascular disorders, thyroid disease, or neurologic deficits, can also provide important direction to subsequent testing and should be sought systematically.

LABORATORY STUDIES AND DIAGNOSTIC TESTS

Acute Dyspnea

For acutely ill patients, a chest radiograph to evaluate for lung infiltrates or edema and arterial blood gas analysis to assess the adequacy of gas exchange are almost always indicated (Table 351.2). Peak expiratory flow rates are readily measured and provide an objective measure of the severity of obstruction in airway disease. An electrocardiogram (ECG) is indicated whenever cardiac disease is known or suspected. Additional studies that might be indicated on the basis of the initial evaluation include perfu-

TABLE 351.2.	COMMON DIAGNOSTIC STUDIES USED IN EVALUATION OF DYSPNEA

Acute Dyspnea

Indicated Initially in Nearly All Patients
  Chest radiograph
  Arterial blood gas analysis
  ECG
Commonly Indicated
  Measurement of peak flow or spirometry
Indicated for Selected Patients (Based on Clinical Suspicion and Initial Findings)
  Perfusion lung scanning
  Echocardiogram
  Respiratory secretion analysis

Chronic Dyspnea

Indicated Initially in Most Patients
  Pulmonary function tests (spirometry, with or without additional measures of lung volumes, diffusing capacity, and arterial blood gases)
  Chest radiograph
  Blood hemoglobin concentration and chemistries
Consider If Initial Evaluation Is Nondiagnostic
  Bronchoprovocation testing
  Exercise testing
Indicated for Selected Patients (Based on Clinical Suspicion and Initial Findings)
  Chest CT scanning
  Echocardiogram
  Other cardiac imaging procedures
  Laryngoscopy or bronchoscopy
  Esophageal pH monitoring
  Thyroid function tests
  Biopsy of lung tissue

sion lung scanning to evaluate for thromboembolism, echocardiography to assess valvular or ventricular dysfunction, and analysis of respiratory secretions or lung tissue to identify infectious agents or noninfectious inflammatory processes.

Chronic Dyspnea

The cause of chronic dyspnea is often evident from the history, examination, and basic screening studies, such as hematocrit and blood chemistries. Additional tests should be selected with specific goals: to confirm the clinical impression, follow up abnormal findings, investigate cases of uncertain cause, or quantify impairment.

No set sequence of diagnostic studies can be recommended in all cases, as the selection of tests is guided by the clinical presentation and diagnostic probabilities. However, given the high prevalence of pulmonary conditions among dyspneic patients, the most useful tests for initial evaluation are usually measures of pulmonary function. Simple spirometry can demonstrate airflow obstruction, which characterizes the most common diseases presenting with dyspnea. The flow volume loop may further distinguish extrathoracic from intrathoracic obstruction. Restrictive processes can be suspected from spirometry and con-

firmed with measurement of lung volumes. The diffusing capacity is often reduced in interstitial or pulmonary vascular diseases. Chest radiographs are usually indicated to identify focal or diffuse disease of lung parenchyma and to assess cardiac size. The ECG may reflect chamber enlargement or evidence of prior infarction. Evaluation of serum thyroid-stimulating hormone is helpful to screen for thyroid disorders.

If the initial evaluation does not point definitively to a diagnosis, exercise testing often helps direct the workup further. The rationale is straightforward: Most dyspnea is worsened by exercise because of the increased requirements for cardiac and ventilatory outputs to support an increased metabolic rate. Therefore, exercise may uncover impairment in an organ system that had been adequately compensated at rest. Measurements of respiratory gas exchange, ventilation, heart rate, blood pressure, ECG, and, where appropriate, arterial blood gases during a graded exercise stress allow identification of limitations in the O_2 transport system and its components. At the same time, functional capacity or impairment can be quantified.

Other specific tests may be indicated by the initial evaluation. Bronchoprovocation testing is highly sensitive for reactive airway disease and should be performed if asthma is suspected despite normal pulmonary function tests. While pulse oximetry may detect overt arterial desaturation, blood gas analysis provides more precise assessment of oxygenation and is essential for characterization of acid–base disturbances. Echocardiography is a valuable starting point for suspected cardiac causes of dyspnea and is particularly sensitive for identifying valvular lesions. The presence of resting or exercise ventricular dysfunction can also be assessed in most subjects by echocardiography. Esophageal pH monitoring to identify gastroesophageal reflux, or radiography to identify sinus disease, may be obtained when occult upper-airway causes of dyspnea are suspected. Laryngoscopy is the diagnostic procedure of choice when vocal cord dysfunction is suspected. High-resolution computed tomography may be useful to establish the presence of interstitial diseases, especially if findings are equivocal on plain radiograph. Histologic examination of lung tissue is sometimes ultimately required for diagnosis of specific interstitial diseases.

■ STRATEGIES FOR OPTIMAL CARE

Treatment of dyspnea is directed at the underlying condition and is detailed in the relevant chapters of this text. For many conditions, however, treatment may be unable to reverse the disease or fully relieve dyspnea. This is particularly true in cases of lung involvement by malignancy, but it also applies to some patients with chronic obstructive pulmonary disease, interstitial lung disease, and pulmonary hypertension. thus, palliative relief of dyspnea may be needed.

PHARMACOLOGIC APPROACHES

Increasing arterial P_{O_2} specifically suppresses carotid body output. Because the carotid bodies sense P_{O_2} over a wide range, extending well above the normal level of around 100 mm Hg, supplemental O_2 may reduce dyspnea for some patients, even if the arterial P_{O_2} is normal. Narcotic analgesics and anxiolytics can also suppress ventilatory drive, by altering the sensitivity of the chemoreceptors or through central mechanisms. Anecdotal success has been reported with the use of these agents in conjunction with appropriate O_2 therapy for treatment of patients with intolerable dyspnea due to chronic lung disease, but chronic use of these is usually limited by the undesirable side effects. Fear of narcotic side effects should not dissuade clinicians from their use for palliating dyspnea in patients with end-stage untreatable malignant or nonmalignant disease.

PULMONARY REHABILITATION

An integrated approach to coping with chronic lung disease, particularly obstructive disease, is found in pulmonary rehabilitation programs that combine education, optimal medication and oxygen therapy, exercise conditioning, and psychological support. Such programs cannot reverse abnormalities of lung mechanics but are successful in reducing dyspnea. These effects are achieved in part by behavior modification, such as learning to pace activities so as to work within the range of ventilatory capacity, or altering breathing patterns to minimize dead-space ventilation. Physiologic effects of exercise conditioning allow some patients to do ambulatory activities with less lactic acidosis, thereby reducing ventilatory requirements. Educational and psychological aspects of rehabilitation also appear beneficial. Understanding the disease and its treatment offers patients more personal control over its impact on their lives. Becoming familiar with the bounds of exertional dyspnea and reassurance that dyspnea is predictable and not intrinsically dangerous may help patients desensitize themselves to this symptom when other treatments are exhausted.

BIBLIOGRAPHY

Dyspnea: mechanisms, assessment, and management—a consensus statement. *Am J Respir Crit Care Med* 1999;159:321–340.

Bass C, Gardner W. Emotional influences on breathing and breathlessness. *J Psychosom Res* 1985;29:599–609.

DePaso WJ, Winterbauer RH, Lusk JA, et al. Chronic dyspnea unexplained by history, physical examination, chest roentgenogram, and spirometry. *Chest* 1991;100:1293–1299.

Elliott MW, Adams L, Cockcroft A, et al. The language of breathlessness. Use of verbal descriptors by patients with cardiopulmonary disease. *Am Rev Respir Dis* 1991;144:826–832.

Manning HL, Schwartzstein RM. Pathophysiology of dyspnea. *N Engl J Med* 1995;333:1547–1553.

Pratter MR, Curley FJ, Dubois J, et al. Cause and evaluation of chronic dyspnea in a pulmonary disease clinic. *Arch Intern Med* 1989;149: 2277–2282.

Tobin MJ. Dyspnea. Pathophysiologic basis, clinical presentation, and management. *Arch Intern Med* 1990;150:1604–1613.

Wasserman K, Hansen JE, Sue DY, et al. *Principles of exercise testing and interpretation*, second ed. Philadelphia: Lea & Febiger, 1994.

C H A P T E R

352

APPROACH TO THE PATIENT WITH COUGH

K. F. CHUNG

THE CLINICAL PROBLEM OF COUGH

Cough is an important natural defensive mechanism and protective reflex for clearing the upper and lower airways of excessive secretions such as mucus and inhaled particles or foreign materials. Healthy people do not cough frequently, but cough is a common symptom of most respiratory disorders and is a very common reason for patients of all ages to consult their doctor, particularly when the cough is chronic and persistent. The prevalence of chronic cough in the community is estimated to be 14% to 23% of nonsmoking adults and of children. In the United States, cough is the fifth most common symptom in patients presenting at outpatient clinics.

Cough has both beneficial and detrimental effects. Clearing of secretions or of foreign particles or material is an important

TABLE 352.1.	POTENTIAL COMPLICATIONS RESULTING FROM EXCESSIVE COUGH

Respiratory
  Pneumothorax
  Subcutaneous emphysema
  Pneumomediastinum
  Pneumoperitoneum
  Laryngeal damage
Cardiovascular
  Cardiac dysrhythmias
  Loss of consciousness
  Subconjunctival hemorrhage
Central nervous system
  Syncope
  Headaches
  Cerebral air embolism
Musculoskeletal
  Intercostal muscle pain
  Rupture of rectus abdominis muscle
  Increase in serum creatine phosphokinase
  Cervical disc prolapse
Gastrointestinal
  Esophageal perforation
Other
  Social embarassment
  Depression
  Urinary incontinence
  Disruption of surgical wounds
  Petechiae
  Purpura

| **TABLE 352.2.** | **COMMON CAUSES OF COUGH** |

Acute infections
  Tracheobronchitis
  Bronchopneumonia
  Viral pneumonia
  Acute-on-chronic bronchitis
  Pertussis
Chronic infections
  Bronchiectasis
  Tuberculosis
  Cystic fibrosis
Airway disease
  Asthma
  Chronic bronchitis
  Chronic postnasal drip
Parenchymal disease
  Chronic interstitial lung fibrosis
  Emphysema
  Sarcoidosis
Tumors
  Bronchogenic carcinoma
  Alveolar cell carcinoma
  Benign airway tumors
  Mediastinal tumors
Foreign body
Cardiovascular
  Left ventricular failure
  Pulmonary infarction
  Aortic aneurysm
Other disease
  Reflux esophagitis
  Recurrent aspiration
  Endobronchial sutures
Drugs
  Angiotensin-converting enzyme inhibitor

benefit. However, excessive coughing may be associated with injury to the patient since the sudden repetitive excessive muscular activities can generate large intrathoracic pressures and expiratory flows to induce musculoskeletal, pulmonary, cardiovascular, and neurologic complications (Table 352.1). Persistent cough commonly interferes with quality of life to cause social embarrassment and deranged sleep.

Cough may be indicative of trivial to very serious airway or lung pathology. The differential diagnosis of chronic cough is extensive and includes infections, inflammatory and neoplastic conditions, and many pulmonary conditions (Table 352.2). The protocol for investigating cough, particularly for a cough that has persisted for more than a month, takes into account several factors pertaining to the pathophysiology of cough and the most common causes of cough. Persistent cough may be due to the presence of excessive secretions or to the establishment of a sensitive cough reflex, or both.

■ PHYSIOLOGY OF COUGH

AFFERENT LIMB

The cough reflex is subserved by vagal afferent pathways arising from the trachea and intrapulmonary airways, and also by the larynx whose afferent nerves pass into the superior laryngeal nerves. Cough receptors have also been described in the tympanic membrane and the external auditory meatus, which are subserved by the auricular branch of the vagus nerve. Cough-sensitive nerves in the lower airways extend to the division of segmental bronchi and possibly beyond, although it is difficult to induce coughing from the smaller airways. The most important tussigenic zones are at the level of the larynx and trachea, especially in the region around the carina and other distal branching points. Rapidly adapting irritant nerve receptors (RARs) in the larynx can be activated by both mechanical and chemical stimuli, such as mucus, dust, probing with a catheter, cigarette smoke, ammonia, acid, hypo- or hypertonic saline, and inflammatory mediators. Irritant RARs are also found in the trachea and proximal bronchi. Sensory nerve fibers presumed to mediate cough are present close to the airway epithelium, and are also activated by a similar range of mechanical and chemical stimuli as for laryngeal receptors. Pulmonary congestion, lung collapse, and bronchoconstriction can also stimulate RARs. Other afferent nerve endings of the tracheobronchial tree, such as slow-adapting pulmonary stretch receptors and pulmonary and bronchial C fibers, may also participate in cough. The slow-adapting stretch receptors responsible for the Hering–Breuer reflex enhance cough, but there is controversy as to whether C fibers receptors, found in the bronchial and alveolar wall, can induce cough. Chemical agents, such as citric acid, capsaicin, and low-chloride solutions, may activate C fibers, but they are not selective.

CENTRAL NERVOUS CONTROL

The afferent pathways for cough are carried to the medulla oblongata in the brain stem, where the signals are integrated. These fibers relay into the nucleus tractus solitarius, and the motor outputs are in the ventral respiratory group. Motoneurons to the respiratory muscles are sent from the nucleus retroambigualis, and those to the larynx and bronchial tree from the nucleus ambiguus. There is little information concerning the neurotransmitters involved in the cough center. Neurotransmitters, such as 5-hydroxytryptamine (5-HT) and (γ-aminobutyric acid (GABA), have been implicated, and the antitussive effects of opiates may be mediated through an effect on these neurotransmitters. Specific GABA agonists, including baclofen, have antitussive effects in experimentally induced cough in animals.

EFFERENT LIMB

Cough usually starts with a deep inspiration, followed by a forced expiration against a closed glottis. Following this compressive phase, the glottis opens allowing an expulsive phase (Fig. 352.1). Cough initiated in the tracheobronchial tree is accompanied by a large inflation, while initiation in the larynx may not be accompanied by any inflation. During the compressive phase, the expiratory muscles contract against a closed glottis, allowing intrapleural and intra-alveolar pressures to rise to levels as high as 40 kPa for about 200 milliseconds. The expiratory phase occurs as the glottis opens and this expulsive phase may be long-lasting, with a large expiratory tidal volume or by a series of short expiratory efforts. Dynamic compression of the airways

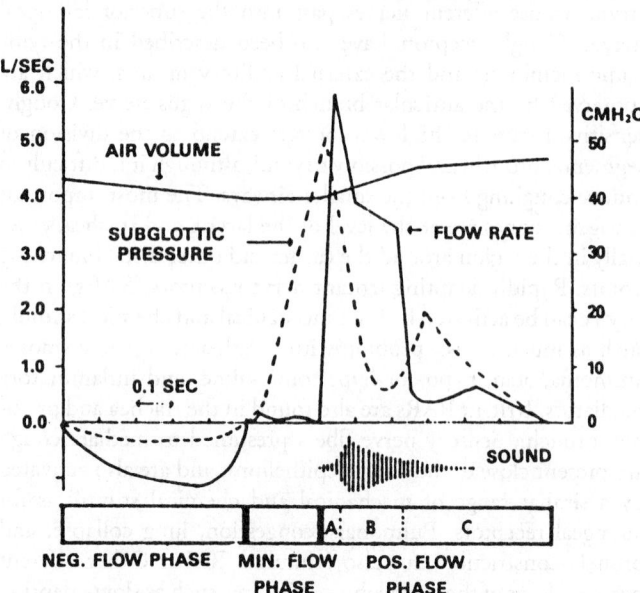

FIGURE 352.1. Changes in flow rate, volume, subglottic pressure, and sound level during a representative cough. During inspiration, the flow rate is negative; at the glottic closure, the flow rate is zero; and during the expiration phase, the flow rate is positive. (From Yanagihara N, von Leden H, Werner-Kukuk E. The physical parameters of cough: the larynx in a normal single cough. *Acta Oto-laryngol* 1996;61:495–502, with permission.)

occurs downstream of the "equal pressure point" where intraluminal and extraluminal pressures across the bronchial wall are equal. Starting at high lung volumes, the equal pressure point is near the trachea, but it moves toward the smaller airways as the lung empties and the elastic lung recoil is diminished. As this occurs, the airflow velocity and kinetic energy of the air passing through the proximal airways increase, thereby improving the clearance of the airways. This may be further improved by a series of short expiratory efforts. Coughing at large lung volumes causes dynamic compression of larger airways, while coughing at low lung volumes induces dynamic compression of the lower airways. This may allow secretions to be moved from the smaller airways into the larger airways, and finally cleared from the tracheobronchial tree.

Coughing may be accompanied by bronchoconstriction since the stimuli that cause cough, such as chemical irritants and inflammatory mediators, can also induce reflex bronchoconstriction. Afferent receptors for cough also cause reflex secretion of mucus from airway submucosal glands. Both bronchoconstriction and intraluminal mucus would narrow the luminal diameter and increase the linear velocity of airflow, resulting in more turbulence and central impaction of inhaled particles. Mucus also may trap inhaled particles and irritant chemicals.

INEFFECTIVE COUGH

Because cough is important in preventing foreign inhaled materials to enter the lower respiratory tract and in clearing lower

respiratory tract secretions, an ineffective cough may lead to lower respiratory tract infections with pneumonia or bronchiectasis and lung collapse. This usually results from any condition associated with diminished expiratory flow rates or reduced ability to compress airways. These pathologic conditions may interfere with either the inspiratory or expiratory phases of cough or both, and include extrapulmonary causes such as rib fractures, disorders of respiratory muscles such as myasthenia gravis, depression of the cough reflex such as during postoperative anesthesia, and a variety of pulmonary causes such as asthma and bronchiectasis. Closure of the glottis is not essential for the production of an effective cough, but the muscles of expiration are the most important determinant of the production of elevated intrathoracic pressures.

MEASURING COUGH SEVERITY

Assessment of cough severity traditionally rests on asking the patient for his or her perception of the symptom. Measurement of the cough reflex can be done by counting the cough responses to inhalation of tussive agents such as capsaicin, the hot extract of peppers, and low-chloride solutions. Although cough can be induced directly by airway secretions and irritants, persistent cough may also result from an increase in the sensitivity of the cough receptor. Most patients with a nonproductive persistent cough due to a range of causes have an enhanced cough reflex to capsaicin when compared to healthy non-coughing subjects. Successful treatment of the primary condition underlying the chronic cough often leads to a normalization of the cough reflex. In contrast, patients with a productive cough, such as that associated with bronchiectasis and chronic bronchitis, do not usually demonstrate an enhanced cough reflex. The degree of the cough responsiveness to inhaled capsaicin may be a reflection of the severity of the cough, but this has yet to be examined. Of relevance to the evaluation and treatment strategies for persistent dry cough is the fact that the cough response can be augmented by various mediators of inflammation such as the prostaglandins PGE_2 and $PGF_{2\alpha}$, and bradykinin through a process of sensitization.

Direct measurement of the number of coughs as a measure of severity has not been extensively assessed. A significant correlation between daytime cough numbers and daytime cough symptom scores has been shown for a group of chronic dry coughers. In both patients with cough of unknown cause or associated with asthma, the number of coughs counted were highest during the daytime, and very few coughs were observed at night during sleep. Both ambulatory monitoring of cough and measurement of the cough reflex are not routinely used in the clinical setting.

CAUSES OF COUGH: ACUTE AND CHRONIC

A useful clinical classification is to consider whether the cough is acute or chronic. Acute cough is usually due to a viral or bacterial upper respiratory tract infection. The cough of the common cold is usually self-limiting and accompanies the cold in 83% of sufferers within the first 48 hours. Other symptoms of postnasal drip—throat clearing, nasal obstruction, and nasal discharge—also accompany the cough, which usually resolves within 2 weeks, sometimes longer. Bronchial epithelial inflammation and damage is present in children with chronic cough following lower respiratory tract illness. Irritants may penetrate more readily through the damaged epithelium.

Acute onset of cough can also be the presenting symptom of more life-threatening respiratory conditions, such as acute bacterial pneumonia, congestive cardiac failure, pulmonary embolism or aspiration. These conditions are usually accompanied by other symptoms, such as shortness of breath and fever, but cough may be the predominant or, rarely, the only symptom.

Chronic cough (cough that persists for more than a month) can be caused by many diseases, but it is most commonly due to asthma, gastroesophageal reflux, postnasal drip, chronic bronchitis, and bronchiectasis. Smoking is a common independent determinant of cough with or without mucus hypersecretion. A smoker may also develop a chronic cough due to other causes that may or may not directly relate to cigarette smoke, such as an endobronchial tumor or the development of asthma. The definitive diagnosis of cough can be established if the specific treatment aimed at the condition is successful.

■ CONDITIONS ASSOCIATED WITH CHRONIC COUGH

POSTNASAL DRIP (RHINOSINUSITIS)

The strong association between postnasal drip (rhinosinusitis) and chronic persistent cough is based on epidemiologic evidence and on a prospective study in adults. Postnasal drip ("nasal catarrh") is characterized by a sensation of nasal secretions or of a "drip" at the back of the throat, often accompanied by frequent throat clearing. There may be a nasal quality to the voice due to concomitant nasal blockage and congestion. Physical examination of the pharynx is often unremarkable, although infrequently a "cobblestoning" appearance of the mucosa and draining secretions are observed. Computed tomography (CT) of the sinuses may reveal mucosal thickening or sinus opacification and air–fluid levels. There may be an extrathoracic variable upper-airway obstruction presumably arising from upper-airway inflammation.

Topical administration of corticosteroid drops in the head-down position is the best treatment, sometimes with the concomitant use of antihistamines. Topical decongestant vasoconstrictor sprays may be useful adjunct therapy for a few days, but rebound nasal obstruction may occur after prolonged use. Antibiotic therapy is advisable when mucopurulent secretions are present. Postnasal drip is a very common cause of cough, and empirical therapy is justified in the presence of suggestive symptoms.

ASTHMA

Chronic dry cough may occur in asthma under different clinical settings. Asthma may present predominantly with cough, often nocturnal, and the diagnosis is supported by reversible airflow limitation and bronchial hyper-responsiveness. This condition of "cough-variant" asthma is a common type of asthma in children. Elderly asthmatics may give a history of clinic cough prior to a diagnosis of asthma made on the basis of episodic wheeze. Cough may also occur as a sign of worsening of asthma, usually presenting first at night, associated with other symptoms such as wheeze and shortness of breath with falls in early morning peak flows. On the other hand, some patients with asthma develop a persistent dry cough despite good control of their asthma with antiasthma therapy.

Patients with asthma usually do not have an enhanced cough reflex, although a subgroup with persistent cough may. In these patients, cough receptors may be sensitized by inflammatory mediators such as bradykinin, tachykinins, and prostaglandins. Induction of sputum by inhalation of hypertonic saline often reveals a predominance of eosinophils, and bronchial hyper-responsiveness is invariably present.

Cough associated with asthma should be treated with antiasthma medication, including inhaled corticosteroid therapy and bronchodilators such as β_2-adrenergic agonists. Often a trial of oral corticosteroids (e.g., prednisolone 40 mg per day for 2 weeks) is recommended. Treatment with nedocromil sodium can be a useful addition.

CHRONIC BRONCHITIS

Most patients with cough due to chronic bronchitis from cigarette smoking do not usually seek medical attention. Chronic bronchitis should be considered in a patient who produces phlegm on most days over at least three consecutive months, particularly during the winter months over at least 2 consecutive years. Often, the productive cough is exacerbated by upper respiratory infections with common viruses or by exposure to irritating dusts. Other causes of productive cough should be excluded, such as bronchiectasis or postnasal drip. Cessation of cigarette smoking is usually successful in reducing the cough. Treatment of any associated chronic obstructive pulmonary disease with β_2-adrenergic agonists and anticholinergic agents may be indicated.

BRONCHIECTASIS

The cough of bronchiectasis is associated with excessive secretions from overproduction together with reduced clearance of airway secretions. Usually, the patient produces 30 mL or more of purulent sputum per day, sometimes accompanied by fever, hemoptysis, and weight loss. In early bronchiectasis, the condition may only present with a persistent productive cough. The chest roentgenogram may show increased bronchial wall thickening, particularly in the lower lobes in advanced cases, but thin-section CT of the chest can reveal early changes of intrapulmonary airway wall thickening, dilatation, and distortion.

The cough due to bronchiectasis may be successfully controlled with inhaled β_2-agonist, which improves mucociliary clearance and reverses any associated bronchoconstriction, postural drainage of airway secretions, and use of intermittent antibiotic therapy.

GASTROESOPHAGEAL REFLUX

Patients with symptoms of gastroesophageal reflux, such as heartburn, chest pain, a sour taste, or regurgitation, may also complain of a chronic persistent cough. Not infrequently, there may be no symptoms of gastroesophageal reflux or impaired clearance of esophageal acid. An esophageal–tracheobronchial cough reflex mechanism has been proposed on the basis of studies in which distal esophageal acid perfusion induced coughing episodes in such patients. Local distal esophageal perfusion of lidocaine suppressed the acid-induced cough in patients with chronic cough, and the inhaled anticholinergic agent ipratropium bromide was also effective. Over 90% of the cough episodes are temporally related to reflux episodes. Significant reflux occurs in both supine and upright positions. A high proportion of patients with gastroesophageal reflux also appear to have gastrohypopharyngeal reflux, and there may be a direct effect of acid reflux on cough receptors in the larynx and trachea. Continuous monitoring of tracheal and esophageal pH in patients with symptomatic gastroesophageal reflux has demonstrated significant increases in tracheal acidity, with pH values falling to 4.10 during episodes of reflux. Other components of the refluxate apart from acid may also contribute to stimulating cough.

Evidence for gastroesophageal reflux can be obtained by upper gastrointestinal contrast series that show reflux of barium into the esophagus, or by esophageal pH monitoring revealing pH values in the lower esophagus outside normal values. Sometimes cough may coincide with the presence of reflux episodes. Treatment of gastroesophageal reflux consists of using either H_2-histamine blockers or proton pump inhibitors, together with advice about elevation of the head of bed.

ANGIOTENSIN-CONVERTING ENZYME INHIBITOR COUGH

Angiotensin-converting enzyme (ACE) inhibitors are often prescribed for the treatment of hypertension and heart failure, and cough has been observed in 2% to 33% of patients. The cough is typically described as dry, associated with a tickling, irritating sensation in the throat. It may appear within a few hours of taking the drug but may also only become apparent after weeks or even months. The cough disappears within days or weeks following withdrawal of drug. Patients with ACE inhibitor cough demonstrate an enhanced response to capsaicin inhalation challenge. The mechanisms underlying ACE inhibitor cough are not clear, but accumulation of bradykinin and prostaglandins, which sensitize cough receptors directly, has been implicated. The best treatment for ACE inhibitor cough is to discontinue the treatment and to replace it with alternative therapies (such as an angiotensin II receptor antagonist, which does not cause cough).

CHRONIC PERSISTENT COUGH OF UNKNOWN CAUSE

Identification of a potential cause of cough has been reported in 78% to 99% of patients presenting at a specialized cough clinic. Treatment of identifiable causes may also not be successful. These patients present in a way similar to that of others in whom a cause has been identified. An enhanced cough reflex is found. Patients often complain of a persistent tickling sensation in the throat that often leads to paroxysms of coughing. This sensation can be triggered by factors such as a change in ambient temperature, the taking of a deep breath, and the presence of cigarette smoke or other irritants such as aerosol sprays or perfumes. These symptoms are typical of a sensitized cough reflex. Mucosal biopsies taken from a group of nonasthmatic patients with chronic dry cough showed evidence of epithelial desquamation and inflammatory cells, particularly mononuclear cells. These changes could represent the sequelae of chronic trauma to the airway wall following intractable cough and lead to sensitization of the cough reflex. Because no clear effective and safe antitussives are available, the control of persistent cough without associated cause remains difficult. Antitussive therapy may be instituted.

OTHER CONDITIONS

Other conditions causing cough include bronchogenic carcinoma, metastatic carcinoma, sarcoidosis, chronic aspiration, or left ventricular failure. These conditions can be excluded by chest roentgenogram. Psychogenic or habit cough is not uncommon, particularly in children, and is usually a diagnosis arrived at after exclusion of other causes. Habit cough is a throat-clearing noise made by a person who is nervous and self-conscious. Cough may be associated with a depressive illness.

■ PRACTICAL APPROACH TO CHRONIC PERSISTENT COUGH

The clinical approach to cough is first to identify and then to treat the cause(s) (Tables 251.3 and 251.4). The history and examination will often indicate likely associated diagnosis or diagnoses, and the timing of various investigations may vary according to presentation. Initial investigation may be limited to a chest roentgenogram, particularly if there is a high suspicion of a tumor, particularly in a smoker. A period of observation of 3 to 4 weeks in a patient who provides a good history of an upper respiratory tract infection prior to further investigation or therapeutic trial is adequate, although institution of an anti-inflammatory therapy such as inhaled corticosteroids can be useful in controlling this type of cough.

Postnasal drip, asthma, and gastroesophageal reflux are the three most common conditions associated with a chronic dry cough. It would be sensible in the diagnostic approach to exclude these conditions first. Direct inspection of the nasal passages and throat together with a CT scan of the sinuses may be indicated, and ambulatory pH monitoring, with possible fiberoptic esophageal–gastroscopic examination. The diagnosis of asthma is sup-

TABLE 352.3.	DIAGNOSTIC EVALUATION OF CHRONIC COUGH

1. History and physical examination
2. Chest roentgenogram for all patients
3. Initial evaluation leads to diagnosis of chronic bronchitis in cigarette smokers and of ACE inhibitor cough. Discontinue cigarette smoking and offending drug.
4. Further diagnostic evaluation on basis of initial evaluation:
   (i) If suggestive of postsatal drip, order a CT scan of sinuses, and allergy tests.
   (ii) If suggestive of asthma, request a record of peak expiratory flow measurements at home for 2 weeks and a bronchoprovocation test with histamine/methacholine, and/ or a trial of antiasthma treatment.
   (iii) If suggestive of gastroesophageal reflux disease, request 24-hour pH monitoring, and if necessary, an endoscopic examination of the esophagus, or a barium swallow series.
   (iv) If the chest roentgenogram is abnormal, consider examination of sputum and a fiberoptic bronchoscopy. In some cases, a CT scan of the thorax and further lung function evaluation may be necessary.
5. Treat specifically for associated conditions. The cause(s) of cough is(are) determined when specific therapies eliminate or improve the cough.

ACE, angiotensin-converting enzyme; CT, computed tomographny.

TABLE 352.4.	TREATMENTS FOR COUGH

1. Treatment of specific underlying cause(s)

Asthma	Bronchodilators and inhaled corticosteroids
Allergic rhinitis and postnasal drip	Topical nasal steroids and antihistamines (with antibiotics, if indicated)
Esophageal reflux	H_2-histamine antagonist or proton pump inhibitor
Angiotensin-converting enzyme inhibitor	Alternative drug such as angiotensin II receptor antagonist
Chronic bronchitis	Smoking cessation
Bronchiectasis	Postural drainage. Treat infective exacerbation and airway obstruction
Infective tracheobronchitis	Appropriate antibiotic therapy

2. Symptomatic treatment (only after consideration of cause of cough)

Acute cough likely to be transient, e.g., upper respiratory viral infection	Simple linctus
Persistent cough particular nocturnal	Opiates (codeine or pholcodeine)
Persistent intractable cough due to terminal incurable disease	Opiates (morphine or diamorphine). Local anesthetic aerosol
Cough in children	Simple linctus (pediatric)

ported by the presence of diurnal variation in peak flow measurements, bronchial hyper-responsiveness to histamine or methacholine challenge, and the presence of eosinophils in sputum. However, a therapeutic trial may be the best initial approach, particularly when the history and examination provide supportive clues. It is important that effective doses of medication over a sufficient period of time be given. Sometimes a longer-than-usual period of treatment is necessary to control the cough. Postnasal drip is an often overlooked condition, and aggressive treatment should consist of corticosteroid nasal drops with an antihistamine, with the possibility of adding antibiotic therapy and a short period of treatment with a nasal decongestant. Often more than one of these conditions may coexist, and cough may only respond with concomitant treatment of these. For example, inhaled steroid therapy and acid suppression with H_2-histamine blockers or a proton pump inhibitor would be indicated for the coexistence of asthma and gastroesophageal reflux.

Bearing in mind that there are a myriad of other, less common causes of a chronic cough, investigations must proceed further if the above causes are excluded. Full lung function tests to include lung volumes and gas transfer factor, along with a CT scan of the lungs, should be considered in case of bronchiolar or parenchymal disease or unsuspected bronchiectasis. Fiberoptic bronchoscopy should be considered and apart from excluding small central tumors provides mucosal biopsies for histologic examination.

THERAPIES AIMED SPECIFICALLY TOWARDS COUGH SUPPRESSION

When the treatment of the cause of cough is unavailable or ineffective, therapies specifically directed at eliminating the symptom of cough should be tried. Drugs that affect the complex mechanism of the cough reflex may act in several ways (Fig. 352.2). They may act by inhibition of central mechanisms within the cough center or by reducing the response of cough receptors in the airways. Opiates, demulcents, expectorants, local anesthetics, and antiasthma drugs have been used as antitussive agents with varying degrees of success.

NARCOTIC AND NON-NARCOTIC ANTITUSSIVES

Opiates, including morphine, diamorphine, and codeine, are the most effective antitussive agents. At their effective doses they cause physical dependence, respiratory depression, and gastrointestinal colic. Morphine and diamorphine are reserved for the control of cough and pain of terminal bronchial cancer patients, but codeine, dihydrocodeine, and pholcodeine can be tried in other cases of chronic cough. These drugs may cause some physical dependence and drowsiness; nausea, vomiting, and constipation may be important side effects.

Non-narcotic antitussives include dextromethorphan, which is a synthetic derivative of morphine with no analgesic or sedative properties and which is usually included as a constituent of many

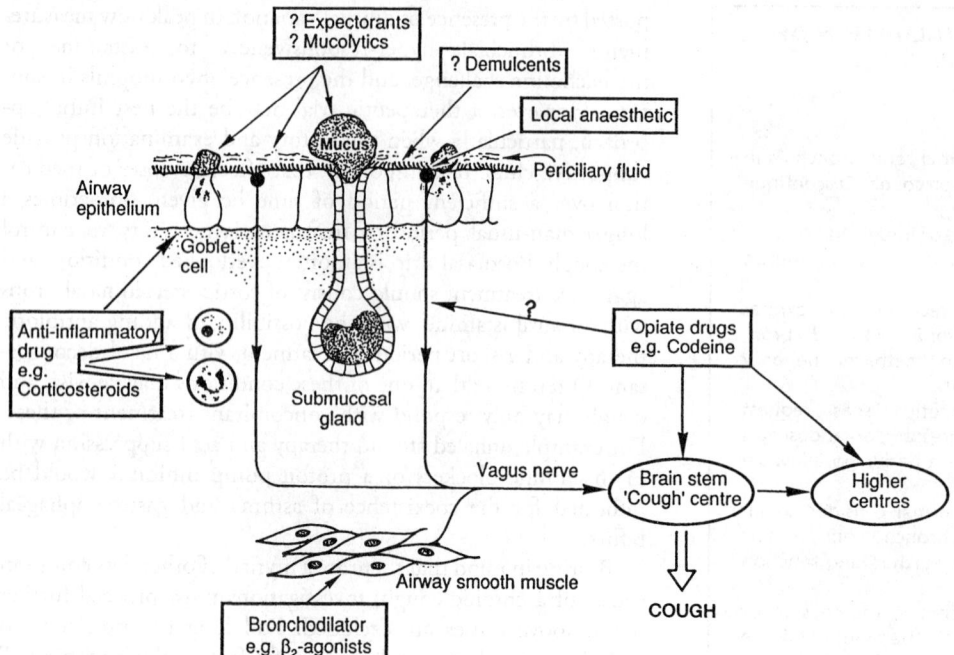

FIGURE 352.2. Afferent pathways of the cough reflex and some potential sites of action of antitussive drugs.

compound cough preparations sold over the counter. Other non-narcotic preparations include noscapine and levopropoxyphene, although their antitussive efficacy has not been proven.

EXPECTORANTS AND MUCOLYTICS

The basis for using these agents as antitussives lies in the belief that altering the volume of secretions or their composition leads to suppression of the cough reflex. Despite the lack of proof, mucolytic agents, such as acetylcysteine, carbocysteine, bromhexine, and methylcysteine, are often used to facilitate expectoration by reducing sputum viscosity in patients with chronic bronchitis. Aromatic agents, such as eucalyptus and menthol, have decongestant effects in the nose and can be useful in short-term relief of cough. Demulcents also form an important component of many proprietary cough preparations and may be useful because the thick sugary preparation may act as a protective layer on the mucosal surface.

LOCAL ANESTHETICS

Lidocaine aerosol has been administered to patients with intractable cough with variable results and should be reserved for such patients. They work by inhibiting sensory neural activity but also remove reflexes that protect the lung from noxious substances. Their effects are transient, and they should be avoided in patients with asthma or a past history of asthma because they can induce severe bronchoconstriction.

ANTIASTHMA THERAPY

Often antiasthma therapy (β_2-agonist and anticholinergic therapy or corticosteroid therapy) may be tried even in the absence

of symptoms or tests supporting asthma. Cough may be accompanied by bronchoconstriction, which in turn can worsen cough—an effect that can be prevented by an inhaled β_2-agonist. In addition, airway inflammation may be present in the airways as a contributory factor and could be controlled by an inhaled corticosteroid. Such treatment should be instituted as a trial after diagnostic evaluation has excluded most causes associated with the cough.

BIBLIOGRAPHY

Carrao WM, Braman SS, Irwin RS. Chronic cough as the sole presenting manifestation of bronchial asthma. *N Engl J Med* 1979;300:633–637.
Chung KF. Cough. In: Crystal RG, et al. *The lung: scientific foundations,* second ed. Philadelphia: Lippincott–Raven Publishers, 1997: 2309–2323.
Hsu J-Y, Stone RA, Logan-Sinclair R, et al. Coughing frequency in patients with persistent cough using a 24-hour ambulatory recorder. *Eur Respir J* 1994;7:1246–1253.
Ing AJ, Ngu MC, Breslin AB. Pathogenesis of chronic persistent cough associated with gastroesophageal reflux. *Am J Respir Crit Care Med* 1994; 149:160–167.
Irwin RS, Curley FJ, French CL. Chronic cough: the spectrum and frequency of causes, key components of the diagnostic evaluation, and outcome of specific therapy. *Am Rev Respir Dis* 1990;141:640–647.
Ninan TK, MacDonald I, Russell G. Persistent nocturnal cough in childhood: a population-based study. *Arch Dis Child* 1995;73:403–407.
O'Connell F, Thomas VE, Pride NB, et al. Capsaicin cough sensitivity decreases with successful treatment of chronic cough. *Am J Respir Crit Care Med* 1994;150:374–380.
Pratter MR, Bartter T, Akers S, et al. An algorithmic approach to chronic cough. *Ann Intern Med* 1993;119:977–983.
Wynder EL, Lemon FR, Mantel N. Epidemiology of persistent cough. *Am Rev Respir Dis* 1965;91:679–700.

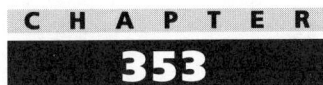

APPROACH TO THE PATIENT WITH HEMOPTYSIS

EDWARD F. HAPONIK

Hemoptysis is a common sign and symptom of respiratory and systemic disease, although its precise incidence is unknown. Expectoration of blood usually signals a condition that requires recognition and treatment, but the bleeding itself is self-limited. At the other extreme, severe pulmonary hemorrhage is a medical and surgical emergency. Thus, clinical challenges range from the reassurance of an ambulatory patient with an alarming but innocuous problem to the resuscitation of a drowning person. Judgments about the extent, pace, and priorities of the evaluation are highly individualized (Table 353.1); the pattern and degree of bleeding and its physiologic impact influence the clinical presentation and determine the approach to diagnosis and therapy.

PATHOPHYSIOLOGIC FACTORS, CAUSES, AND CLASSIFICATIONS

Although there are more than 100 causes of hemoptysis, the most commonly encountered problems and their presentations are summarized in Fig. 353.1. Causes of bronchoscopically confirmed bleeding have changed during the past three decades; the likelihood of tuberculosis has decreased and that of lung cancer has increased. This shift reflects changes in the prevalence of these conditions and refinements of fiberoptic bronchoscopy, radiologic imaging, and other diagnostic tools.

The dual blood supply to the lung from the pulmonary and bronchial arterial systems, the proximity of all airways to vessels, and the diversity of conditions affecting the respiratory tract can lead to hemoptysis in various ways. Bleeding can originate from vascular disruption at any anatomical level, but the bronchial arterial system is the predominant source in most patients. Acute inflammatory disease (e.g., bronchitis) commonly causes mucosal hyperemia associated with superficial bleeding; blood-streaked sputum may worsen after coughing paroxysms. Chronic inflammation (e.g., bronchiectasis) and neoplasms may result in extensive, friable neovascular networks, often with systemic collateral communications. Bleeding occurs in the lower pressure pulmonary circulation less often (e.g., Rasmussen's aneurysm with tuberculosis, mycotic aneurysm with lung abscess, or endocarditis) and may worsen with pulmonary arterial hypertension. Acute and chronic destructive processes may erode large central vessels (e.g., bronchogenic carcinoma, cavitary tuberculosis, lung abscess, necrotizing pneumonia). Less often, congenital and acquired arteriovenous communications are the cause. Vessels may be lacerated by chest trauma and complicate increasingly performed invasive diagnostic procedures such as lung biopsy or Swan–Ganz catheterization.

Because the lung is, in effect, a sheet of blood, numerous injuries to either side of the alveolar–capillary membrane can cause varying degrees of hemoptysis. Capillary hemorrhage associated with pulmonary venous hypertension commonly results in bloody pulmonary edema fluid in patients with congestive heart failure. Alternatively, microvascular oozing might reflect

TABLE 353.1.	SOME MAJOR CLINICAL DISTINCTIONS BETWEEN MILD AND MASSIVE HEMOPTYSIS	
	Mild Hemoptysis	**Massive Hemoptysis**
Relative frequency	Common (precise frequency unknown)	Uncommon
Major causes	Chronic bronchitis, unexplained (cryptogenic); cancer more common; tuberculosis less common	Lung cancer, necrotizing pneumonia, tuberculosis, mycetonia common; bronchitis, idiopathic uncommon
Pathogenesis of bleeding	Superficial mucosal inflammation, erosion	Major vascular disruption, extensive neovascularization
Clinical setting	Gradual onset of bleeding in ambulatory outpatients	Abrupt onset, often superimposed on chronic illness
Typical course	Usually mild, self-limited, rapid spontaneous resolution expected	Unpredictable, often fatal, medical and surgical emergency
Roentgenographic findings	Chest radiograph usually nonlocalizing; focal abnormalities, often nondiagnostic	Chest radiograph more often reveals definitive abnormalities
Arterial blood gases	Usually normal or mildly abnormal	Combined hypoxemic and hypoventilatory respiratory failure common
Timing of diagnostic tests, pace of evaluation	Elective; sequential diagnostic tests precede therapeutic planning	Urgent: resuscitation, definitive diagnosis, and therapy, usually simultaneous
Usual focus of workup	Exclude lung cancer	Prevent drowning
Levels of clinical uncertainty, risks	Relatively low	Extremely high

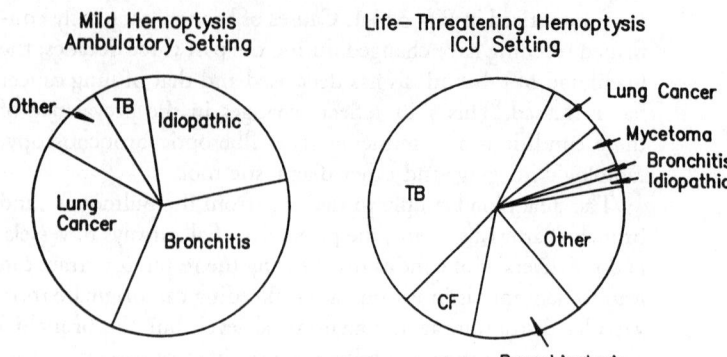

FIGURE 353.1. Relative frequencies of conditions associated with hemoptysis vary with the clinical settings in which bleeding occurs. Life-threatening hemorrhage more often complicates diseases, producing major lung parenchymal destruction or vascular disruption.

diffuse immunologically mediated injury (e.g., vasculitis, pulmonary–renal syndromes), inhalation or aspiration of irritants (e.g., trimellitic anhydride), drugs (e.g., D-penicillamine), or infectious agents, or may represent diffuse alveolar damage following organ transplantation (e.g., cardiac or bone marrow transplants). Pulmonary capillaritis (Table 353.2) has been caused by various potentially treatable systemic diseases, and its incidence may be increasing. In immunocompromised patients, alveolar hemorrhage has been associated with thrombocytopenia, other coagulation abnormalities, and renal insufficiency, and is usually associated with infectious pneumonias. Cigarette smoking appears to predispose to alveolar hemorrhage.

Bleeding rates in the range of 400 to 600 mL expectorated during a 16- to 24-hour period have arbitrarily defined "massive" hemoptysis, but considerably less hemorrhage presents a major threat to the patient whose ability to clear the airway effectively is compromised. Patients with altered mental status, severe preexisting lung disease, or ineffective cough are especially vulnerable, and the term "life-threatening" rather than "massive" applies. Severe hemorrhage has profound physiologic sequelae: alveolar filling or atelectasis due to aspirated blood causes hypoxemia due to ventilation–perfusion mismatch (and, with severe bleeding, physiologic shunt). Proximal airway obstruction by clot causes alveolar hypoventilation; with massive bleeding,

TABLE 353.2.	CAUSES OF PULMONARY CAPILLARITIS

Common
  Wegener's granulomatosis
  Microscopic polyangitis
  Systemic lupus erythematosus
Uncommon
  Primary capillaritis without systemic disease
  Capillaritis associated with idiopathic pulmonary fibrosis
  Rheumatoid arthritis
  Scleroderma
  Mixed connective tissue disease
  Primary antiphospholipid syndrome
  Henoch–Schönlein purpura
  Mixed cryoglobulinemia
  Behçet's syndrome
  Pauci-immune glomerulonephritis
  Autologous bone marrow transplantation

death is usually caused by asphyxiation rather than by exsanguination, although the latter can occur in patients who survive the immediate respiratory collapse or after great vessel injuries.

DIAGNOSTIC APPROACH

Knowledge of the setting and patient population in which bleeding occurs (i.e., the pretest probabilities of disease) influences the differential diagnostic considerations (see Table 353.1 and Fig. 353.1). The signs and symptoms of diverse pulmonary diseases are detailed elsewhere. Despite the nonspecificity of many of these manifestations, they help to assess the likelihood of particular pulmonary or systemic causes of hemoptysis and the patient's overall physiologic reserve. Generally, clinical manifestations of the primary disease causing hemoptysis dominate the clinical presentation. Coagulopathies further predispose to bleeding, and coexisting nonpulmonary illnesses compromise the patient's ability to tolerate it. In most patients, a carefully performed history, physical examination, chest roentgenogram, selectively used laboratory tests, and diagnostic bronchoscopy prove sufficient to guide management.

Evaluation begins with the detailed medical history and physical examination. The subglottic origin of expectorated blood is usually obvious, but bleeding from the upper airway (e.g., sinusitis, nasal polyps, nasopharyngeal and laryngeal neoplasms) or aspirated from the gastrointestinal tract must be considered. The latter might be suggested by associated nausea and vomiting or by the dark color and acidic character of blood. Less often, "pseudohemoptysis" due to foods, pigment-producing microbes (e.g., *Serratia marcescens*), or medications (oxidized Bronkosol) mimic bloody sputum. Historical and bedside clues might strongly suggest the cause of bleeding, but usually further objective information is necessary to localize the source of bleeding and to identify its specific cause, or at least to exclude serious treatable disease.

RADIOLOGIC STUDIES

The chest roentgenogram is a basic component of evaluation and often directs the highest-yield diagnostic approach. Characteristic apical cavitary disease might strongly suggest tuberculosis or central mass lesions bronchogenic carcinoma; focal consolidation might suggest bacterial pneumonia; diffuse radiographic infiltration should suggest widespread aspiration of blood or microvascular bleeding. Readily appreciated findings include broncholiths; "middle-lobe" syndrome; extensive cystic bronchiectasis; "crescent" signs of intracavitary mycetomas, clot, or necrosing lung or tumor; and vascular malformations. Abnormal roentgenograms are more often found in patients with severe, protracted bleeding. Especially when previous films are available for comparison, the extent of radiographic abnormalities also helps assess chronic anatomical abnormalities that might predict limited physiologic reserve. Serial chest films help to monitor the course or identify new hazards; for example, the abrupt opacification of a preexisting cavity is an ominous radiographic sign.

For carefully selected patients with unexplained hemoptysis or particular predispositions to disease, other imaging procedures have complementary applications. Their optimal, integrated roles continue to evolve. Historically, bronchography has helped document bronchiectasis, which when localized might benefit from surgical resection. Fewer than 10% of patients carefully evaluated in this manner have bronchiectasis, perhaps reflecting increased use of empirical antimicrobials in patients with bacterial infection and the decreased prevalence of tuberculosis.

Chest computed tomography (CT), which has supplanted bronchography at most centers, may also reveal occult masses or cavities, mycetomas, arteriovenous malformations, or parenchymal bleeding sites. Because of the high prevalence of self-limited, benign causes of bleeding, chest CT is not routinely indicated in all patients with hemoptysis. CT is most useful in patients at risk for lung cancer, in whom it may identify the neoplasm and assist in its staging.

Magnetic resonance imaging has documented bronchogenic cysts or vascular causes of bleeding (e.g., pulmonary arterial aneurysms) but is used less often than CT or chest x-rays. Defining the precise vascular source of bleeding by bronchial or pulmonary arteriographic examination may have major therapeutic implications in selected patients with chronic, recurrent, or life-threatening hemoptysis. Infrequently, use of radionuclides or radiolabeled autologous erythrocytes helps in the localization of occult chronic bleeding.

LABORATORY TESTS

Several laboratory studies may contribute to patient evaluation and are used selectively, according to clinical suspicions. Examination of expectorated sputum may identify infectious causes of hemoptysis (e.g., Gram stain, smears for mycobacteria and fungi) but usually is nondefinitive. Sputum cytopathologic evaluation is valuable in patients at risk for cancer, especially in the presence of suggestive central radiographic abnormalities. Hemosiderin-laden alveolar macrophages have been associated with chronic or occult pulmonary hemorrhage (e.g., in immunocompromised hosts with coagulopathies or fungal infections) but are not routinely useful. Serologic studies (e.g., collagen vascular disease profiles, anti–glomerular basement membrane or antineutrophil cytoplasmic antibodies) may help clarify systemic diseases and direct subsequent diagnostic and therapeutic procedures. Coagulation tests are often obtained in search of correctable abnormalities but usually have a low yield in the absence of a clinically

obvious propensity for bleeding. Spirometry and arterial blood measurements provide useful estimates of pulmonary reserve and the physiologic impact of bleeding. An elevated carbon monoxide diffusion capacity may suggest pulmonary hemorrhage but does not define the cause of bleeding, and the procedure has limited value in the acute setting. Other tests (e.g., pulmonary ventilation–perfusion scanning to assess pulmonary embolism with infarction, hemodynamic measurements, echocardiography to exclude mitral stenosis) are useful when clinical findings suggest particular conditions. Routine otolaryngologic evaluations of all patients with hemoptysis has been advocated, but the yield is low in the absence of other signs or symptoms of upper-airway disease.

BRONCHOSCOPY

Careful upper- and lower-airway examination by fiberoptic bronchoscopy is indicated when hemoptysis is clinically significant, the simple database is nondiagnostic, and the test results will influence management. This relatively noninvasive outpatient procedure helps to localize bleeding and can identify a spectrum of conditions with specific (e.g., bronchial adenoma, bronchogenic carcinoma) and nonspecific (e.g., bronchitis) manifestations. Often, only focal or diffuse blood or even a normal tracheobronchial tree is seen; the precise cause of bleeding is unknown and is often considered to be occult bronchitis or bronchiectasis. Such patients are more properly regarded as having hemoptysis of unknown cause (e.g., essential or cryptogenic bleeding). Even such nondiagnostic bronchoscopy is clinically useful, however: few such patients subsequently are found to have lung cancer. Hemoptysis spontaneously abates by 1 month in about 75% of patients with nonlocalizing x-rays and nondiagnostic bronchoscopy and in over 90% of patients over the following year.

Repeat bronchoscopy is generally well tolerated and is indicated if the initial endobronchial examination was incomplete, if bleeding persists, or when follow-up radiographic studies or clinical risk factors suggest treatable disease (e.g., lung cancer, granulomatous infection).

Patient selection for fiberoptic bronchoscopy varies among institutions, but retrospective investigations suggest several useful criteria: bleeding that exceeds 1 to 2 weeks' duration, expectoration of more than 30 mL of blood daily, older age (more than 40 years), abnormal chest roentgenograms (especially with central abnormalities), smoking history, chronic cough, and anemia all suggest lung cancer. Lung cancer occurs in about 5% to 8% of patients with normal or nonlocalizing chest x-rays and unexplained, significant hemoptysis. The high clinical benefit of detecting resectable lung cancer and the low risk of fiberoptic bronchoscopy generally favor the procedure in patients at risk. In contrast, young persons (under 35 years) with brief (less than 1 week), mild (less than 30 mL) bleeding are less likely to have lung cancer. Combinations of these negative findings have a high negative predictive value. Bronchoscopy is also deferred when the patient's clinical status is prohibitively fragile, when bleeding originates from extrapulmonary sites or obvious non-neoplastic disease (e.g., pneumonia, pulmonary infarction), or with systemic etiologies.

The optimum timing of bronchoscopy for nonmassive hemoptysis is unclear. A bleeding site is identified bronchoscopically more often during the first 24 hours of presentation, but it has not been shown that outcomes are compromised when bronchoscopy is delayed for several days as bleeding abates.

Some patients with extensive airspace filling by blood (e.g., due to thrombocytopenia, diffuse alveolar damage, lung contusion) have had minimal hemoptysis; in these instances, bronchoalveolar lavage has helped clarify the nature of bleeding. In general, the diagnostic yield is lower and the risk higher in patients with diffuse disease. Although transbronchial forceps biopsy has been diagnostic in this setting (e.g., with Wegener's granulomatosis, Goodpasture's syndrome), open or thoracoscopic lung biopsy or sampling of an extrapulmonary site of systemic involvement is more often helpful when definitive histologic diagnosis is essential to management.

■ LIFE-THREATENING HEMOPTYSIS

In fewer than 5% of patients with hemoptysis, pulmonary hemorrhage is life threatening and requires the diagnostic approach to be merged with therapy (Fig. 353.2). The clinician must simultaneously recognize the conditions associated with massive bleeding, protect the airway to maintain alveolar ventilation and preserve function of the nonhemorrhaging lung, and determine whether the patient is a candidate for urgent definitive treatment. Tuberculosis, lung cancer, bronchiectasis (including cystic fibrosis), and mycetomas are the leading causes of life-threatening bleeding (Fig. 353.1).

While oxygenation and general support are provided, airway maintenance is a focus of acute management. In most instances, insertion of a large, single-lumen tube is the initial approach. Placement of a double-lumen endotracheal tube permits selective lung ventilation and suctioning but requires considerable technical expertise. The patient is positioned with the bleeding side dependent in efforts to minimize aspiration into the more functional, nonhemorrhaging lung. Because accurate localization of the bleeding site determines subsequent therapy, bronchoscopy is usually performed urgently but carries increased risk. Rigid

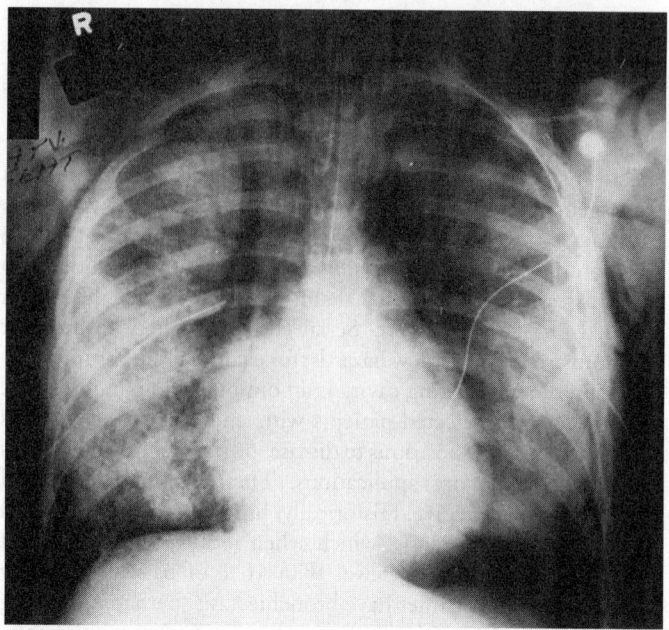

FIGURE 353.3. Diffuse air space filling due to Goodpasture's syndrome in a patient with hemoptysis. (Note the coexisting bilateral pneumothoraxes and extensive subcutaneous emphysema due to barotrauma.)

bronchoscopy is preferred because the open-tube instrument ensures an airway and permits several temporizing interventions: the insertion of large suction catheters; tamponade of bleeding or occlusion of the bronchus of the hemorrhaging lung by balloon catheters or blockers; and endobronchial instillation of iced saline, topical vasoconstrictors (e.g., vasopressin, epinephrine), or clot-promoting agents (e.g., thrombin).

Prospective comparisons of the outcomes of surgically and nonsurgically managed patients are unavailable. Controversies about the prognoses of patients with massive bleeding relate to institutional selection factors and the heterogeneity of patients reported in retrospective studies. Conditions associated with extensive lung necrosis and erosion of major vessels (e.g., lung cancer, lung abscess, cavitary tuberculosis, mycotic aneurysms) consistently have exceedingly high mortality (30% to 80%); patients with self-limited, superficial mucosal disease, such as bronchitis, have a good outcome with conservative management (Fig. 353.3). The overall mortality of life-threatening hemoptysis is about 10% in large, surgically treated populations; 30% in operable, medically supported patients; and 50% in inoperable patients treated medically.

Recurrent bleeding of unpredictable onset is the natural history of massive hemoptysis complicating destructive parenchymal disease. Accordingly, surgical resection of the bleeding site remains the established, definitive approach for operable patients. Estimates of the patient's functional status before the onset of bleeding and, when available, objective pulmonary function measurements are key components of the acute assessment. Once the decision for operative treatment has been made, it is advisable to proceed directly to surgery rather than to risk massive rebleeding.

Surgery is contraindicated when the patient's pulmonary re-

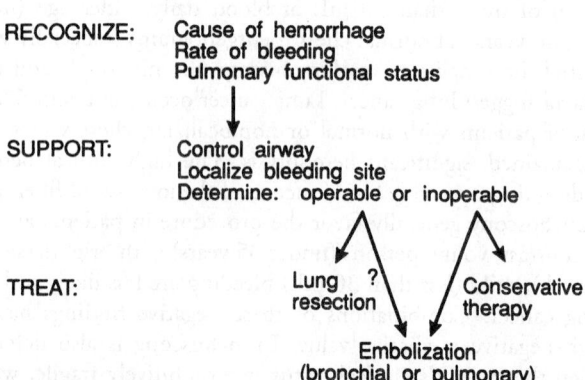

RECOGNIZE: Cause of hemorrhage
                    Rate of bleeding
                    Pulmonary functional status

SUPPORT: Control airway
              Localize bleeding site
              Determine: operable or inoperable

TREAT: Lung resection ?   Conservative therapy
              Embolization (bronchial or pulmonary)

FIGURE 353.2. Effective management of patients with life-threatening hemoptysis requires the timely integration of diagnostic and therapeutic approaches.

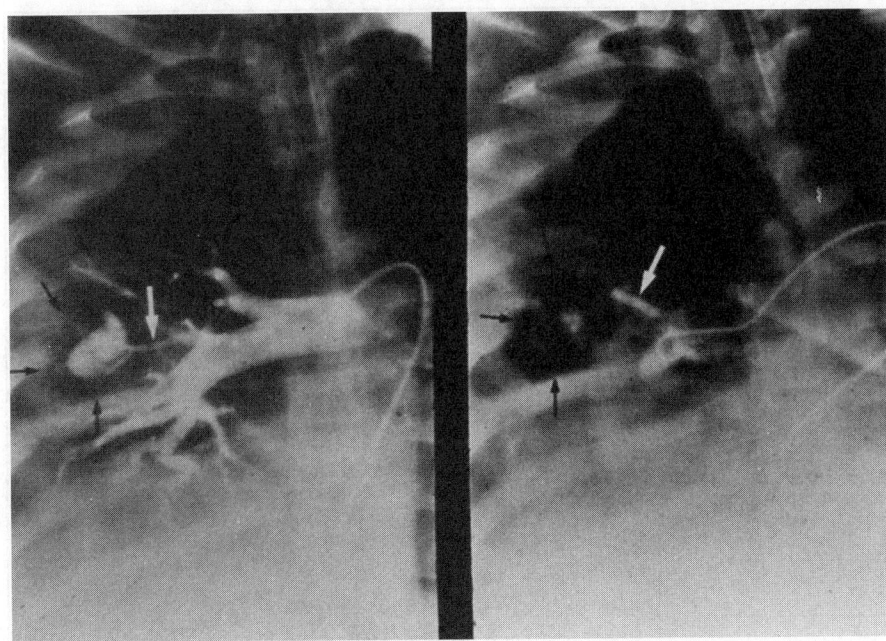

FIGURE 353.4. The pulmonary arteriogram in a patient with life-threatening hemoptysis due to lung abscess demonstrated a mycotic aneurysm *(left)*. Bleeding abated after occlusion of the feeding vessel with a silicone balloon *(right)*.

serve is marginal, when coexisting illness makes operative risks prohibitively high, when the bleeding site is diffuse or unidentified, in the presence of uncontrollable coagulopathy, or when bleeding is caused by unresectable cancer or systemic disease.

Angiographic identification of the vascular source of bleeding provides more active intervention for inoperable patients and is a temporizing option for surgical candidates (Fig. 353.4). Bleeding vessels may be occluded therapeutically by autologous clot, balloons, or synthetic agents. Cessation of bleeding is often immediate and in up to 75% of patients is definitive. The long-term efficacy of this procedure suggests that interventional angiography has a role as first-line therapy even in operable patients, but more data are needed.

Massive bleeding due to systemic or diffuse microvascular disease (Table 353.1) is approached by treating the primary disorder, rather than by surgery or embolization. Corticosteroids for systemic lupus erythematosus, cyclophosphamide and corticosteroids for Wegener's granulomatosis, and plasmapheresis for Goodpasture's syndrome have successfully controlled bleeding. Emergency mitral valve replacement in patients with mitral stenosis is a classic disease-specific therapy. Pulmonary embolism with infarction or parenchymal hemorrhage may cause hemoptysis but seldom precludes anticoagulation. For severe bleeding in this setting, temporary discontinuation of anticoagulation and insertion of a caval interruption device may be necessary. Development of hemoptysis, pleurisy, and pulmonary infiltrates in leukopenic leukemia patients represents invasive aspergillosis until proven otherwise; the outcome depends on effective antifungal therapy and, even more importantly, on restoration of host defenses by treatment of the primary neoplasm. When hemoptysis complicates penetrating or blunt chest trauma, diagnostic procedures such as percutaneous needle or transbronchial lung biopsies, Swan–Ganz catheterization, or intraoperative accidents, the cause and high risk of bleeding are usually obvious

and the management approach is directed by the primary clinical condition.

Several adjunctive measures have been used in patients with hemoptysis, but their efficacy has not been documented. Antitussives and sedatives may diminish cough, but they also compromise airway clearance and must be used cautiously. Empirical antimicrobials are often prescribed for tracheobronchial inflammation, but their benefits are unknown. Radiation therapy has palliated hemorrhage due to unresectable lung cancer and occasionally in patients with mycetomas. Less often, laser photocoagulation has been used to control bleeding from endobronchial tumors.

BIBLIOGRAPHY

Adelman M, Haponik EF, Bleecker ER, et al. Cryptogenic hemoptysis. Clinical features, bronchoscopic findings, and natural history in 67 patients. *Ann Intern Med* 1985;102:829–834.

Arney KL, Judson MA, Sahn SA. Airway obstruction arising from blood clot: three reports and a review of the literature. *Chest* 1999;115: 293–300.

Conlan AA. Massive hemoptysis—diagnostic and therapeutic implications. *Surg Ann* 1985;17:337–354.

De Lassence A, Fleury-Feith J, Escudier E, et al. Alveolar hemorrhage. Diagnostic criteria and results in 194 immunocompromised hosts. *Am J Respir Crit Care Med* 1995;151:157–163.

Dweik RA, Stoller JK. Role of bronchoscopy in massive hemoptysis. *Clin Chest Med* 1999;20:89–105.

Green RJ, Ruoss SJ, Kraft SA. Pulmonary capillaritis and alveolar hemorrhage. Update on diagnosis and management. *Chest* 1996;110: 1305–1316.

Haponik EF, Chin R. Hemoptysis: clinicians' perspectives. *Chest* 1990;97: 469–475.

Hirshberg B, Biran I, Glazer M, et al. Hemoptysis: etiology, evaluation, and outcome in a tertiary referral hospital. *Chest* 1997;112:440–444.

Jones DK, Cavanagh P, Shneerson JM, et al. Does bronchography have a role in the assessment of patients with hemoptysis? *Thorax* 1985;40: 668–670.

Knott-Craig C, Oostuizen G, Rossouw G, et al. Management and prognosis of massive hemoptysis. Recent experience with 120 patients. *J Thorac Cardiovasc Surg* 1993;105:394–397.

Marshall TJ, Jackson JE. Vascular intervention in the thorax: bronchial artery embolization for haemoptysis. *Eur Radiol* 1997: 7:1221–1227.

Marshall TJ, Flower CD, Jackson JE. The role of radiology in the investigation and management of patients with haemoptysis. *Clin Radiol* 1996; 51:391–400.

McGuinness G, Bech JR, Harkin TJ, et al. Hemoptysis: prospective high-resolution CT/bronchoscopic correlation. *Chest* 1994;105:1155–1162.

Poe RH, Israel RH, Marin MG, et al. Utility of fiberoptic bronchoscopy in patients with hemoptysis and a nonlocalizing chest roentgenogram. *Chest* 1988;98:70–75.

Primack SL, Miller RR, Müller NL. Diffuse pulmonary hemorrhage: clinical, pathologic, and imaging features. *AJR* 1995;164:295–300.

Rabkin JE, Astafjer VI, Gothman LN, et al. Transcatheter embolization in the management of pulmonary hemorrhage. *Radiology* 1987;163: 361–365.

Weaver LJ, Solliday N, Cugell D. Selection of patients with hemoptysis for fiberoptic bronchoscopy. *Chest* 1979;76:7–10.

Winter SM, Ingbar DH. Massive hemoptysis: pathogenesis and management. *J Intens Care Med* 1988;3:171.

Kelley's Textbook of Internal Medicine, fourth edition. Edited by H. David Humes. Lippincott Williams & Wilkins, Philadelphia © 2000.

C H A P T E R

354

APPROACH TO THE CRITICALLY ILL PATIENT

LEONARD D. HUDSON
KENNETH P. STEINBERG

TABLE 354.1.   APPROACH TO THE CRITICALLY ILL PATIENT

Initial Assessment

Rapid assessment of the life-threatening problems requiring immediate attention and institution of therapy
Rapid directed history from patient and family and friends
Rapid directed physical examination
Full history and physical examination repeated after immediate danger to life is addressed

Therapeutic Decisions and Plan

Definite and clear therapeutic decisions (maybe to not treat) and plan necessary
Dynamic database (initial database usually incomplete)
Flexible plan, based on dynamic database
Plan includes specific endpoints
  Desired goals to each therapy
  Possible adverse effects
  Limits for each end point that would lead to change in therapy
  Means of monitoring and assessing end points and frequency of assessments

Dynamic Management Process

Each treatment decision regarded as a therapeutic trial
Frequent reassessment of decisions included in the plan

Appreciation of Multiple Problems

Recognition that multiple problems (e.g., multiple organ failure, multiple diseases) are common
Appreciation of interaction of multiple problems or diseases
Assessment of, and adjustments to, plan made accordingly

Prevention of Complications

Prevent complications of the disease process
Minimize complications of the therapy
Avoid iatrogenic procedural complications
Minimize drug interactions
Recognize balance of benefits and harms of invasive monitoring techniques and potential therapies

Critical care medicine is a relatively new discipline of medicine. The name is self-explanatory: a field of medicine and surgery devoted to care of the critically ill patient—that is, the patient with any illness or injury the nature and severity of which either (a) pose a direct threat to life or (b) place the patient at high risk for complications that are life threatening. This life-threatening nature implies either the high risk or actual presence of single or multiple organ failure. Whether critical care medicine is a distinct discipline has been debated, but the debate is largely a semantic one. Critical care medicine actually involves multiple disciplines, not only in medicine and many of its various subspecialties, surgery, anesthesiology, and pediatrics, but also in nursing and other health care disciplines such as respiratory care, social work, and nutrition. In addition, a body of knowledge in critical care medicine has developed that includes management approaches to the critically ill patient, increased knowledge of particular disease processes that either cause a threat to life or are common complications in the critically ill patient, and specific therapies frequently applied to the critically ill patient (particularly life support measures such as mechanical ventilation and pharmacologic hemodynamic support).

The philosophy of the approach to management of the critically ill patient is similar to that applied to other patients with less severe illnesses, but the circumstances of the critically ill patient dictate certain changes in the way this philosophy is carried out and particularly affect the time frame of diagnosis and therapy. Several implications are discussed here and summarized in Table 354.1.

One concept that has developed from the field of critical care medicine is that of multiple organ dysfunction syndrome (MODS), also known as multiple organ system failure. MODS is often a result of a systemic inflammatory process. The severity of the threat to life posed by MODS appears to be greater than the sum of any of its parts; that is, even though each individual organ failure may be potentially reversible, there appears to be a threshold of total number of failing organs (at least in certain clinical settings) beyond which survival is unprecedented. The approach to the critically ill patient with MODS is discussed in detail in Chapter 355.

HISTORY OF CRITICAL CARE MEDICINE

The practice of medicine has always included care of the critically ill patient. However, a body of knowledge dealing specifically with care of critically ill patients evolved since the mid-1960s as critical care units or intensive care units (ICUs) developed across North America. Development of these units paralleled or lagged slightly behind the proliferation of coronary care units, which were devoted to a single-organ problem and especially treatment of a single disease manifestation (acute myocardial infarction). Significant development of early ICUs occurred in the 1960s, and ICUs became commonplace in the 1970s. Currently, 90% of hospitals have an ICU and almost all hospitals with more than 200 beds have at least one ICU. (Whether this high prevalence of ICUs in hospitals of all sizes is justified in this era of managed care and medical cost containment is debatable. Certainly, a case can be made on the basis of cost-effectiveness that fully equipped and staffed ICUs may be warranted only in tertiary referral centers; smaller hospitals may require only the ability and facilities to stabilize and support a patient who is expected to be unstable for a short and finite period or to support a critically ill patient until transfer to a tertiary center can be arranged.)

Growth in the field of critical care medicine paralleled the development of both practical life support systems and procedures and systems for monitoring the function of critical organs. Experience during wartime in the management of military casualties and experience in the management of critically ill civilians were both important factors in the growth of critical care medicine. Experience in caring for critically injured patients in the Vietnam War provided information on managing patients with severe trauma.

Training in critical care medicine developed in several specialties, especially medicine, surgery, anesthesiology, and pediatrics. Means of certifying for special clinical competence in critical care medicine were developed during the 1980s. An attempt was made to form a joint board or certifying test committee, with representatives from the primary boards of those specialties plus representatives from the Society of Critical Care Medicine. The goal of this joint committee was to develop a common procedure and test to certify, for expertise in critical care medicine, all critical care specialists regardless of their primary discipline. Members of this committee could not agree on training eligibility criteria, however, and the committee was disbanded. Subsequently, critical care medicine subspecialty boards or test committees were formed within the American boards of internal medicine, surgery, anesthesiology, and pediatrics. Eligibility criteria have been established for each primary discipline, and each of these primary boards awards certificates for special competence in critical care.

The American Board of Internal Medicine has established two training pathways, following general internal medicine training, that enable the trainee to sit for the examination for critical care medicine: (a) 3 years of combined training in an established subspecialty (usually pulmonary diseases) plus critical care medicine; or (b) 2 years in a critical care medicine training program within a department of medicine. Experience from the early examinations indicates that the most frequently chosen pathway is a combination of pulmonary and critical care medicine training. Two years of critical care medicine fellowship training is the next most common pathway, followed by a relatively small number of applicants with combined training in

critical care medicine and a subspecialty other than pulmonary (e.g., cardiology or nephrology).

APPROACH TO THE CRITICALLY ILL PATIENT

Acuity and severity of illness and the potential threat to life markedly affect the approach to management of the critically ill patient compared with the approach to patients with less severe illness. The major effects are on the time frame within which steps in management must occur and the dynamic nature of the management process. Other characteristics exist, including the likelihood of multiple disease or organ problems, but time sequence and the need for frequent reassessment are the major distinguishing characteristics of critical care medicine (Table 354.1.) The common need to institute nearly immediate therapy after rapid assessment of life-threatening problems means that the database on which actions are taken is incomplete. That database is also dynamic; not only is additional information becoming available, but changes are occurring in previously acquired data. After institution of therapy for acute life-threatening problems, the next assessment step, a directed history and physical examination, should be carried out rapidly. This step requires the physician to remember to repeat a full history and physical examination when the immediate dangers to life have been treated.

The approach to the critically ill patient requires that definite therapeutic decisions and plans be made. The therapeutic decision may be to do nothing (other than to carry out certain common supportive measures), but even this decision should be a firm one with a plan for evaluation. The patient's situation and the resulting database are dynamic; therefore, the plan must be flexible. The plan must include elucidation of end points (the desired beneficial effects of therapy as well as possible adverse effects). Limits for these end points, which would lead to a change in therapy, must be determined, as must means of monitoring the end points. In this way, the monitoring or assessment of the patient is individualized to the patient's specific situation. The dynamic process also requires that reassessment be performed frequently. Again, the frequency of reassessment or monitoring should be tailored to the patient's specific situation. Management of the critically ill patient requires that each treatment decision be thought of as a true therapeutic trial, with frequent reassessment to determine whether the goals of therapy are being achieved or whether adverse effects have occurred. In some cases, lack of change in the patient should be considered an adverse outcome. A critically ill patient who fails to improve over time may be at increasing risk for development of complications and, thus, for higher morbidity and mortality. Even such standard decisions as fluid therapy must be individually tailored and frequently reassessed. For example, fluid orders should not written for the standard 24-hour period but rather for 4 or 8 hours initially, with reassessment and new orders at the end of those time periods.

Although current practice of critical care medicine involves an understanding of cellular biology (particularly with regard to the systemic inflammation involved in MODS) and molecular biology (especially with certain proposed therapies), evaluation of the patient and of the effects of therapy continues to be based primarily on an understanding of normal physiologic and pathophysiologic processes. The process of monitoring organ function in the critically ill patient is essentially an exercise in practical clinical application of the principles of physiology and pathophysiology. Although many monitoring elements are performed in nearly every case, none of these should be considered routine but rather should be designed to provide information relevant to understanding the physiologic factors specific to the individual patient.

Finally, it must be recognized that the critically ill patient frequently has multiple problems that interact. This interaction may take the form of multiple organ failure, such as acute respiratory distress syndrome coupled with acute renal failure, with the resulting changes in intravascular fluid volume status related to the renal failure having significant effects on the pulmonary condition. Interaction may take the form of more than one disease. For example, many medical ICU patients have a chronic illness with a superimposed acute illness, which leads to worsening organ failure in organs affected by the chronic disease. The more aggressive treatments required may have more profound systemic effects or effects on multiple organs compared with most treatments for less severely ill patients. Finally, drug interactions, both known and unsuspected, are more likely to occur by abnormal drug metabolism related to organ dysfunctions (which also contributes to increased risk).

ELEMENTS OF CRITICAL CARE MEDICINE

Not only does the management of the critically ill patient necessitate a different approach; it also requires that several elements be in place. These elements are listed in Table 354.2. The multi-

---

TABLE 354.2.   ELEMENTS OF CRITICAL CARE MEDICINE

- Physician specialists in critical care and appropriate consultants available
- Nurse specialists in critical care
- Health care professionals with expertise in critical care, including respiratory care practitioners, social workers, physical therapists, nutritionists, and spiritual and emotional support staff
- Physical plant

Monitoring Systems: necessary knowledge, equipment, and experience to obtain and interpret monitoring data on hemodynamic, respiratory, central nervous, and other systems

Life Support Systems: ventilatory and oxygenation support; dialysis and hemofiltration; cardiovascular support, including pacemaking, cardiopulmonary resuscitation, and pharmacologic and mechanical hemodynamic support; and nutritional support

Systems for Effective Communication: Communication among all health care providers, especially between physicians and nurses, and between critical care team and patient and patient surrogates

- Means of resolving conflicts: medical issues and medical/ethical dilemmas

---

disciplinary nature of the team of caregivers and a functioning system for good communication between the caregivers are perhaps the most essential of these elements. The multidisciplinary approach, with specific roles for each type of health care provider but with a collegial working relationship and interchange between caregivers, must be emphasized. A recent study compares several critical care units and shows that improved patient outcome is related to the relationship between the physicians and nurses. The physician has the responsibility of determining the initial therapy and plan, and synthesizing the dynamic database, as well as the ultimate responsibility for ordering therapy and its evaluation. However, the wise physician includes the nurse's assessment of the patient's condition as one of the most important, perhaps the dominant, element in reassessment and listens carefully to any suggestions from the nurse. The nurse has the professional responsibility of converting many of the therapeutic goals to specific action plans and then implementing those plans. Optimal nursing care includes understanding the physiologic principles of the therapy, as well as the pathophysiology of the disease process, and appropriately questioning the therapeutic plan when the rationale is not clear or understood. Fostering clear communication between the various health care givers as well as between the health care team and the patient or patient's family and friends is extremely important. This includes creating an appropriate environment to encourage free communication, as well as establishing certain times and settings at which communication affecting management decisions is expected. The physical plant is secondary to the knowledge and skill of the critical care health providers but is still important to optimal management.

Bioethical dilemmas or problems appear to be more common, or at least more dramatic, in the management of the critically ill patient, probably because of the life-or-death nature of many of the decisions involved. It is important that the entire critical care team be alert to these issues and that a consistent approach to identification of problems and to possible resolution be maintained. If there is a willingness to understand various viewpoints, clear communication, and sufficient time, most problems can be managed to the satisfaction of all parties involved. Occasionally, however, ethical dilemmas arise involving conflicts of values that cannot be resolved in this manner. When conflicts arise, either between health care providers or between the critical care team and the patient or—more often—the patient's surrogate, a means of resolution (or frequently several alternative means) should be available. An approach to medical ethical issues is discussed further in Chapter 2.

BIBLIOGRAPHY

American Thoracic Society. Withholding and withdrawal of life-sustaining therapy. *Am Rev Respir Dis* 1991;144:726–731.

Ayres SM, Grenvik A, Holbrook PR, et al., eds. *Textbook of critical care*, third ed. Philadelphia: WB Saunders, 1995.

Chernow B, ed. *The pharmacologic approach to the critically ill patient*, third ed. Baltimore: Williams & Wilkins, 1994.

Curtis JR, Park DR, Krone MR, et al. Use of the medical futility rationale in do-not-attempt-resuscitation orders. *JAMA* 1995;273:124–128.

Groeger JS, Guntupalli KK, Strosberg M, et al. Descriptive analysis of critical care units in the United States: patient characteristics and intensive care unit utilization. *Crit Care Med* 1993;21:279–291.

Hall JB, Schmidt GA, Wood LDH, eds. *Principles of critical care.* New York: McGraw-Hill, 1992.

Lanken PN. Critical care medicine at a new crossroads: the intersection of economics and ethics in the intensive care unit. *Am J Respir Crit Care Med* 1994;149:3–5.

Luce JM. The changing physician–patient relationship in critical care medicine under health care reform. *Am J Respir Crit Care Med* 1994;150: 266–270.

Zimmerman JE, Shortell SM, Knaus WA, et al. Value and cost of teaching hospitals: a prospective, multicenter, inception cohort study. *Crit Care Med* 1993;21:1432–1442.

Zimmerman JE, Shortell SM, Rousseau DM, et al. Improving intensive care: observations based on organizational case studies in nine intensive care units—a prospective, multicenter study. *Crit Care Med* 1993;21: 1443–1451.

Kelley's Textbook of Internal Medicine, fourth edition. Edited by H. David Humes. Lippincott Williams & Wilkins, Philadelphia © 2000.

C H A P T E R

355

MANAGEMENT OF THE CRITICALLY ILL PATIENT WITH MULTIPLE ORGAN DYSFUNCTION

PAUL M. DORINSKY
MICHAEL A. MATTHAY

One of the earliest descriptions of multiple organ failure, now referred to as the multiple organ dysfunction syndrome (MODS), has been credited to Baue in an editorial that he wrote in 1975:

> The sequence of events often begins with a period of shock or circulatory failure at some point during the initial injury, accompanied sooner or later by failure of ventilation and the need for ventilatory support. This may be followed by renal failure, hepatic failure (jaundice and decreasing albumin levels), gastrointestinal (GI) failure (stress ulcers and GI bleeding), and metabolic failure (decrease in lean body mass and weakness due to progressive catabolism). Our ability to support a single system that has failed, transiently at least, is reasonably good. The support of two or more failed units, however, stresses our knowledge and capability. Survivors of multiple systems failure are infrequent.

Since this description was published, a number of medical and surgical studies have reported a high mortality rate associated with MODS in critically ill patients. Sepsis syndrome is clearly the most frequently encountered clinical problem associated with the development of MODS. Some patients, however, develop MODS and do not seem to have a clear-cut infectious cause. The best support for this possibility comes from data in studies of patients treated with interleukin-2 for malignant disorders. These patients frequently develop renal failure, GI

failure, neurologic disturbances, and sometimes even acute respiratory failure. These observations suggest that release of potent endogenous humoral factors during noninfectious disorders (e.g., severe hypovolemic shock) may produce the clinical manifestations of the sepsis syndrome without necessarily being related to infection. Finally, primary lung injury itself can lead to the development of MODS. In any case, sepsis often complicates MODS even if sepsis is not the initial clinical disorder.

In the first part of this chapter, the definition and epidemiology of MODS are discussed with an emphasis on specific guidelines for defining the failure or dysfunction of the respiratory, cardiovascular, renal, hepatic, central nervous, and hematologic systems. In the second part, the pathogenesis of MODS is considered. In the third part, guidelines are provided for the management of patients with MODS, with an emphasis on practical issues related to therapy with fluids, colloid, blood, and vasoactive agents as well as anti-inflammatory agents. In the final section, the prevention and early recognition of MODS and sepsis syndrome are discussed.

■ DEFINITION AND EPIDEMIOLOGY

Multiple organ dysfunction syndrome refers to the pattern of altered organ function that occurs in acutely ill patients, especially patients with shock from sepsis, major trauma, severe pancreatitis, drug overdose, or thermal injury. The extent to which an individual organ is likely to be damaged in these clinical settings depends on numerous factors, including age, preexisting medical illnesses, severity of illness on admission to the intensive care unit (ICU), and the specific precipitating event. However, it is clear that organ dysfunction affects overall mortality, especially when the organ dysfunction is present before the patient is admitted to the intensive care unit. In fact, one recent study demonstrated that the presence of systemic organ dysfunction before ICU admission was one of the most significant predictors of nonsurvival for acute lung injury (ALI) patients.

The clinical manifestations of organ dysfunction in this patient group are also variable and have been defined by different criteria. Specifically, organ dysfunction in acutely ill patients ranges from minor biochemical abnormalities to irreversible organ failure. Nonetheless, the incidence of cardiac, renal, GI, hepatic, central nervous, and hematologic system failure has been studied especially in patients with acute respiratory failure. The definition and incidence of acute respiratory failure are discussed later in this chapter, after the criteria for failure of the nonpulmonary organ systems have been considered.

CARDIOVASCULAR DYSFUNCTION

The incidence of cardiovascular failure among critically ill patients varies from approximately 10% to 23%. Although a uniform definition in critically ill patients has not been established, most clinicians agree that cardiovascular failure exists when one or more of the following factors are present: (a) mean arterial pressure of 60 mm Hg or less; (b) cardiac index of 2.0 L per minute per square meter or less; or (c) reversible ventricular fibrillation or asystole. This definition could include a patient with an acute myocardial infarction and severe pump failure. However, it could also include a patient with septic shock who has high cardiac output, low systemic vascular resistance, and low mean arterial blood pressure. Cardiovascular failure therefore includes those disturbances that cause a major decrease in myocardial function as well as those clinical disorders associated primarily with abnormalities in the peripheral circulation.

Among the various critical illnesses that may present clinically with cardiovascular failure, the myocardial dysfunction that occurs with sepsis has been the most thoroughly investigated. Although human septic shock is usually characterized by elevated cardiac output and reduced systemic vascular resistance, it is also associated with a decrease in the left ventricular ejection fraction. In addition, recent studies have shown that septic patients have increased left ventricular end-systolic and end-diastolic volumes, normal or decreased stroke work, and decreased right ventricular ejection fraction. Among patients who survive, these cardiovascular parameters normalize.

The mechanism of myocardial dysfunction during sepsis is not entirely known. Nonetheless, serum obtained from patients with septic shock has been shown to depress myocardial cell contractility in vitro. Moreover, evidence suggests that tumor necrosis factor (TNF), an important humoral mediator of sepsis, is capable of depressing myocardial cell contractility. It is likely that one or more of these myocardial depressant substances is responsible for the reduction in ejection fraction and the ventricular volume changes that occur during sepsis.

Given the complexities associated with the diagnosis and management of cardiovascular dysfunction in acutely ill patients, the use of right heart catheterization has become routine for many physicians caring for ICU patients. However, a recent prospective study suggested that the use of right heart catheters was associated with both an increase in 30-day mortality (odds ratio = 1.24; 95% confidence interval = 1.03 to 1.49) and resource utilization. Although this study has been widely criticized on the basis of its design and conclusions, it has stimulated an intense dialogue on the role of these catheters in acutely ill patients. In addition, it has served as a catalyst for an upcoming, prospective, National Institutes of Health (NIH)–sponsored study on the role of right heart catheterization in the management of critically ill patients.

RENAL DYSFUNCTION

Renal dysfunction is a common complication in critically ill patients (40% to 55% incidence) and is manifested by reductions in urine output or a rise in the serum blood urea nitrogen and creatinine. Specifically, renal failure may be defined in this patient group as a serum creatinine in excess of 2 mg per deciliter, a urine output below 600 mL per 24 hours, or both.

The three most important risk factors for the development of renal failure in critically ill patients are hypotension, sepsis, and nephrotoxic drugs. Acute nonoliguric renal failure associated primarily with nephrotoxic drugs has a better prognosis than acute oliguric renal failure that occurs with septic shock or following major cardiovascular surgery.

GASTROINTESTINAL DYSFUNCTION

Alterations in GI tract function are estimated to occur in 7% to 30% of critically ill patients. The pathologic basis for GI dysfunction appears to be both an alteration in microvascular permeability and mucosal ischemia. For example, TNF causes necrosis of intestinal villi when infused into experimental animals. These morphologic observations suggest a pathologic basis for the functional abnormalities of the GI tract that occur in critically ill patients.

The clinical manifestations of GI tract dysfunction are variable and include hemorrhage, ileus, malabsorption (e.g., inability to tolerate enteral feedings), and, occasionally, acalculous cholecystitis or pancreatitis. Among these complications, GI blood loss in excess of 1 g per deciliter of hemoglobin per 24 hours is generally accepted as clinically significant.

An intact GI tract mucosa provides an essential barrier to the entry of bacteria into the systemic circulation. Because GI mucosal integrity is frequently impaired in critically ill patients, bacterial growth may be increased in areas of bowel that are normally sterile. In addition, bacteria may translocate or migrate from the bowel lumen into the peritoneal cavity, regional lymph nodes, and the portosystemic circulation. To the extent that this migration occurs, the process of bacterial translocation may propagate septic shock and result in further lung and systemic organ injury.

Clinical data in support of a central role for the GI tract in the pathogenesis of MODS in acutely ill patients is increasing. In this regard, marked alterations in GI permeability were demonstrated to occur in a prospectively studied group of ICU patients using monosaccharide and disaccharide probes. Perhaps even more significant, however, was the observation that the patients who developed MODS had significantly greater alterations in intestinal permeability upon ICU admission than those who did not ultimately develop MODS. Taken together, these observations suggest that altered GI tract function plays an important if not a central role in the pathogenesis of MODS in critically ill patients.

HEPATIC DYSFUNCTION

Fulminant hepatic failure is uncommon in critically ill patients and occurs in less than 10% of these patients. By contrast, reversible elevations in serum transaminases or elevations in serum bilirubin or clotting parameters are common and may be found in as many as 95% of critically ill patients. Criteria for hepatic dysfunction in critically patients are in a state of evolution. Nonetheless, elevation in serum bilirubin that exceeds 4 to 5 mg per deciliter, a prothrombin time that is greater than 1.5 times control, or a serum albumin that is below 2.0 g per deciliter is indicative of significant hepatic dysfunction.

As a complication of septic shock or other critical illnesses, hepatic dysfunction is of more than academic interest. The liver is an important reticuloendothelial organ, the function of which is also altered when the liver is damaged. In this context, there is compelling clinical evidence in support of the notion that liver dysfunction is a major determinant of survival in patients with ALI. For example, it has been shown that mortality from septic shock approaches 100% in patients with severe hepatic damage. Likewise, when hepatic failure occurs in the setting of acute respiratory failure, the prognosis for recovery from the ALI is exceedingly poor. Thus, evidence is accumulating to suggest the various systemic organs are not merely targets of damage during critical illnesses. Rather, once these organs are damaged, they have a substantial impact on host defense, the propagation of injury to other organs, and survival.

CENTRAL NERVOUS SYSTEM DYSFUNCTION

Abnormalities of central nervous system (CNS) function are frequently described in critically ill patients. For example, CNS dysfunction, including disorientation, confusion, agitation, obtundation, and seizures, occurs commonly in septic patients. One study reports a 9% incidence of CNS dysfunction, defined as an inability to follow simple commands, in 106 patients with intra-abdominal sepsis. By contrast, another recent study, using an altered sensorium as the criteria for CNS dysfunction, reports a 33% incidence of CNS abnormalities in sepsis.

Use of the Glasgow Coma Scale helps to provide a more uniform, standard approach to defining CNS function. The scale provides a measurement of visual, motor, and verbal (e.g., orientation) responsiveness (Table 355.1). The Glasgow Coma Scale can be used in intubated patients; the CNS function is considered abnormal in critically ill patients with a score of less than 6 to 8 (maximal score = 15). Using these criteria, abnormalities of CNS function have been found to occur in 7% to 30% of critically ill patients. The factors that underlie CNS dysfunction in this patient population are unclear but may include the production of false neurotransmitters, direct microvascular injury, or brain ischemia from global or regional reductions in cerebral blood flow.

TABLE 355.1.	**GLASGOW COMA SCALE**

Parameter	Score
Eye Opening	
Spontaneous	4
To speech	3
To pain	2
None	1
Motor Response	
Obeys verbal commands	6
Responds appropriately to painful stimuli (localizes pain)	5
Withdraws to pain (e.g., flexion withdrawal)	4
Decorticate posturing	3
Decerebrate posturing	2
No response	1
Verbal Responses	
Oriented and conversant	5
Disoriented but conversant	4
Inappropriate response	3
Incomprehensible sounds	2
No response	1

HEMATOLOGIC DYSFUNCTION

The frequency of hematologic abnormalities among critically ill patients ranges from approximately 0% to 26%. There is little clinical consensus, however, regarding the definition of hematologic failure in this patient group. A number of parameters, including platelet count, white blood cell count, fibrinogen levels, and coagulation parameters, have been used to assess the adequacy of the hematologic system in these patients. Despite some differences, most clinical studies employ criteria that include a platelet count of 50,000 per cubic millimeter or fewer, a white blood cell count of 1,000 per cubic millimeter or fewer, or a fibrinogen level below 100 mg per deciliter to define hematologic failure. Obviously, the presence of severe neutropenia decreases host resistance to infection, whereas thrombocytopenia increases the risk of bleeding and the need for transfusion of blood products.

ACUTE RESPIRATORY FAILURE

The incidence of acute respiratory failure in critically ill patients varies considerably depending on the criteria used to define failure of the respiratory system. Although the term *acute respiratory disease syndrome* (ARDS) has been very useful for designating the clinical syndrome, a more quantitative definition has been needed. A recent North American–European consensus conference proposed a simplified, uniform definition of ALI and ARDS. Acute lung injury is defined as that existing in a patient with a PaO_2/FIO_2 less than 300 with chest radiographic evidence of bilateral pulmonary infiltrates. Exclusion criteria include the presence of interstitial lung disease or left ventricular failure assessed by history, physical examination, or laboratory criteria. As previously noted, the role of right heart catheterization in the management of patients with ARDS is controversial and will be the subject of an upcoming, NIH-sponsored clinical trial. However, at the present time it appears prudent to recommend that a pulmonary arterial catheter be inserted only when it is clinically necessary to determine if the patient has a pulmonary arterial wedge pressure less than 18 mm Hg.

ARDS is defined with the same criteria as ALI except the PaO_2/FIO_2 ratio is less than 200. As such, the distinction between ALI and ARDS is based entirely on the severity of the gas exchange alterations. The clinical relevance of this distinction remains to be proven. Nonetheless, the notion that the distinction between ALI and ARDS may not be relevant was underscored by a recent study in which the overall mortality in medical patients with ALI was 58% and was identical to the mortality in the subset of these patients who had ARDS.

A quantitative scoring system for assessing ALI has also been used to evaluate the severity of lung injury (Table 355.2). This system is based on the severity of hypoxemia and the extent of infiltrates on the chest radiograph. If the patient is mechanically ventilated, abnormalities in the compliance of the lungs and the level of positive end-expiratory pressure are also scored. Using these criteria, patients can be classified as having mild, moderate, or severe lung injury.

SPECIAL CONSIDERATIONS

Although not unique to any particular organ system, a number of serious problems exist with respect to MODS. Because there

TABLE 355.2.	COMPONENTS OF THE ACUTE LUNG INJURY SCORE[a]	
Score Components		**Value**
Chest Radiograph		
No alveolar consolidation		0
Alveolar consolidation in 1 quadrant		1
Alveolar consolidation in 2 quadrants		2
Alveolar consolidation in 3 quadrants		3
Alveolar consolidation in all 4 quadrants		4
Hypoxemia		
$Pao_2/Fio_2 \geq 300$		0
Pao_2/Fio_2 225–299		1
Pao_2/Fio_2 175–224		2
Pao_2/Fio_2 100–174		3
$Pao_2/Fio_2 < 100$		4
Respiratory System Compliance (When Ventilated)		
Compliance ≥ 80 mL/cm H_2O		0
Compliance 60–79 mL/cm H_2O		1
Compliance 40–59 mL/cm H_2O		2
Compliance 20–39 mL/cm H_2O		3
Compliance ≤ 19 mL/cm H_2O		4
Positive End-expiratory Pressure (PEEP) (When Ventilated)		
PEEP ≤ 5 cm H_2O		0
PEEP 6–8 cm H_2O		1
PEEP 9–11 cm H_2O		2
PEEP 12–14 cm H_2O		3
PEEP ≥ 15 cm H_2O		4
		Score
No lung injury		0
Mild to moderate lung injury		0.1–2.5
Severe lung injury (acute respiratory distress syndrome)		>2.5

[a] The final value is obtained by dividing the aggregate sum by the number of components used.
(From Murray JF, Matthay MA, Luce J, Flick MR. An expanded definition of the adult respiratory distress syndrome. *Am Rev Respir Dis* 1988;138:720, with permission.)

is a general lack of consensus regarding the criteria for individual organ system failure, the incidence of organ failure is variable among different study centers and contributes to the general confusion in this area. Until more uniform criteria are established, the true incidence and natural history of MODS remains unclear. The new criteria for ALI and ARDS, discussed previously, are a good example of progress in this area. Prospective studies of these criteria and definitions of liver, renal, gastric, hematologic, cardiac, and CNS dysfunction are needed.

Despite the current uncertainties, a number of important issues regarding MODS in critically ill patients have been resolved. First, the number of involved organ systems impacts significantly on patient mortality. Mortality for a single-organ failure ranges from 15% to 30% and for two-organ failure from 45% to 55%. By contrast, mortality exceeds 80% when three or more organ systems fail and reaches 100% if the MODS persists beyond four hospital days. Second, certain organ systems (e.g., heart, kidney, lung, and liver) are involved more frequently

than other organ systems. Third, the presence of organ dysfunction before a patient is admitted to the ICU is a major predictive factor for nonsurvival in patients with ALI. Finally, early detection and treatment of the underlying cause of the MODS may offer the best hope for treatment of this potentially fatal disorder.

PATHOGENESIS

Multiple organ dysfunction syndrome occurs in a variety of clinical settings, including infection, severe hypotension, and multiple trauma. Prototypic among the risk factors for MODS is septic shock. Moreover, evidence is accumulating to suggest that MODS during sepsis and other critical illnesses is caused by widespread organ injury that in turn is caused by activated inflammatory cells and a variety of humoral mediators. However, any theory regarding the pathogenesis of MODS during sepsis or other acute, catastrophic illnesses must take into account the abnormalities in systemic gas exchange that occur in these disorders and manifest as an abnormal relation between oxygen uptake (Vo_2) and oxygen delivery (Do_2).

As illustrated in Fig. 355.1, whole-body oxygen uptake is normally maintained at a constant level over wide ranges of oxygen delivery. This is accomplished by means of local compensatory mechanisms, which include increases in oxygen extraction and increases in recruitable capillary reserves (the cross-sectional area of perfused capillaries within an individual organ). Once these mechanisms for the preservation of oxygen uptake are exhausted, Vo_2 falls in a manner that is directly related to the reductions in oxygen delivery. The level of oxygen delivery below

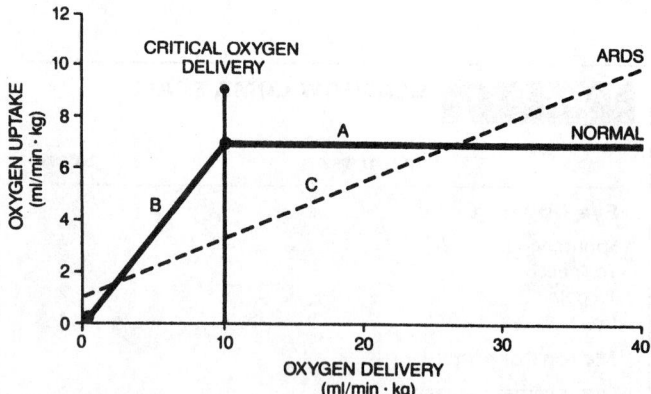

FIGURE 355.1. Oxygen uptake–oxygen delivery (Vo_2–Qo_2) relation in normal subjects and in patients with ARDS. Vo_2 is regulated by whole-body metabolic demand and is normally constant over a wide range of Qo_2 values (line A). Constancy is accomplished by local compensatory mechanisms, including increases in oxygen extraction and increases in the cross-sectional density of perfused capillaries. Once these compensatory mechanisms are exhausted, further reductions in Qo_2 are accompanied by reductions in Vo_2 (line B). The Qo_2 below which Vo_2 begins to decrease is termed the critical threshold for Qo_2 (Qo_{2c}). In contrast to the normal situation, Vo_2 is dependent on Qo_2 at nearly all levels of Qo_2 in ARDS. This finding indicates that an oxygen supply–demand imbalance exists at all levels of Qo_2 in ARDS patients. ARDS, acute respiratory distress syndrome. (From Dorinsky PM, Gadek JE. Mechanisms of multiple nonpulmonary organ failure in ARDS. *Chest* 1989;96:885–892, with permission.)

which oxygen uptake begins to fall is termed Do_{2c} (critical threshold for oxygen delivery), and it signifies the level of Do_2 below which oxygen supply–demand imbalances exist.

In contrast to the situation described for the normal Vo_2–Do_2 relationship, the relation between Vo_2 and Do_2 in critically ill patients is often markedly altered. For example, in many critically ill patients, Vo_2 is dependent on Do_2 at nearly all levels of oxygen delivery, including levels that would normally be more than adequate to meet tissue metabolic demands. These abnormalities indicate that oxygen supply–demand imbalances may exist at all levels of Do_2 in these patients.

In recent years, the concept that the Vo_2–Do_2 relationship is altered in the critically ill patient has been challenged. In particular, whether Vo_2 is calculated using the Fick equation [Vo_2 = cardiac output $\times$ (A − Vo_2 content difference)] or measured using a metabolic cart may affect whether or not an abnormal Vo_2–Do_2 relationship is observed in these patients. The explanation for differences in measured versus calculated Vo_2–Do_2 is not intuitively obvious. However, when both Vo_2 and Do_2 are calculated, it is believed that an artifactual mathematical coupling occurs because both Vo_2 and Do_2 share the variables of cardiac output and arterial oxygen content. This problem may be avoided by measuring Vo_2 directly, using a metabolic cart. However, in some studies, an abnormal relationship between Vo_2 and Do_2 was observed whether or not Vo_2 was measured using a metabolic cart or calculated using the Fick equation. As such, criticisms of the method by which Vo_2 was determined do not negate the concept that Vo_2–Do_2 relationships can be altered in the setting of sepsis or ALI—a fact that has been well established experimentally. Rather, these observations underscore the notion that whole-body Vo_2–Do_2 relations in humans may be unreliable and that a better method for assessing oxygenation in individual tissues needs to be established.

Despite remaining uncertainties, a number of mechanisms exist that may explain both the nonpulmonary organ failure and the Vo_2–Do_2 abnormalities that occur in this patient population. These mechanisms may be divided into two broad categories: (a) altered blood flow distribution and (b) endothelial or parenchymal injury.

ALTERED BLOOD FLOW DISTRIBUTION

Oxygenated blood that bypasses nutrient capillary beds could alter Vo_2–Do_2 relationships and cause organ damage. This sequence of events may result from (a) a redistribution of cardiac output to organs with inherently low O_2 extraction fractions (e.g., skeletal muscle), (b) an increase in the fraction of cardiac output that bypasses nutrient capillaries through anatomical, precapillary arteriovenous channels (e.g., shunt flow), (c) local blood flow heterogeneities such that tissue oxygen supply and demand are unbalanced, or (d) a reduction in recruitable capillary reserves that would prevent effective compensation for reductions in oxygen supply.

ENDOTHELIAL OR PARENCHYMAL INJURY

Endothelial injury may be accompanied by local edema formation, with subsequent increases in diffusion distances for oxygen or reductions in capillary surface area (e.g., reduced recruitable capillary reserves), or both. Alternatively, direct parenchymal cell injury may impair O_2 use at any level of oxygen delivery by impairing cellular oxidative metabolism.

POSSIBLE MECHANISMS OF INJURY

Little direct experimental evidence supports the hypothesis that either MODS or the systemic Vo_2–Do_2 abnormalities in ARDS, septic shock, and other critical illnesses are caused by primary alterations in the distribution of cardiac output (e.g., increased anatomical shunt flow or increased blood flow to organs with low O_2 extraction). By contrast, evidence indicates that nonpulmonary organs sustain significant structural and functional damage in these disorders, including alterations in individual organ Vo_2–Do_2 matching.

The best studied experimental model for MODS has been septic shock, produced either by live bacterial organisms or by endotoxin. Bacteria or bacterial products have a variety of direct effects on endothelial cells. For example, structural studies of endothelial monolayers exposed to endotoxin show that these cells undergo contraction, become pyknotic, and finally die.

Endotoxin or live bacteria can also induce the release of a variety of mediators that can cause cell injury. Considerable experimental evidence indicates that both cyclooxygenase and lipoxygenase products of arachidonic acid metabolism participate in the hemodynamic, pathologic, and metabolic derangements that occur during sepsis. Also, complement is activated in sepsis. In one study, the elevated levels of a C5a derivative correlated with the severity of hypotension and metabolic acidosis. There has also been considerable recent interest in the possible role of cytokines (e.g., TNF) in mediating systemic organ injury. In one recent study, anti-TNF antibodies prevented in rabbits the development of endotoxin-mediated hypotension, fibrin deposition, and death. In addition, anti-TNF antibody prevented shock and death in baboons given live *Escherichia coli* organisms, but only when given 2 hours before the bacteremia.

Many studies (but not all) report a central role for neutrophils in mediating both the systemic and pulmonary injury from bacteria or endotoxin. In recent animal studies, a monoclonal antibody to the adherence-promoting leukocyte glycoprotein CD18 prevented systemic organ injury after acid-induced ALI and reduced systemic organ injury from hemorrhagic shock and improved survival. Although many schemes have been proposed to explain the mechanism by which neutrophils cause tissue injury, recent work suggests that there may be important interactions between elastases and toxic oxygen radicals elaborated by neutrophils.

Finally, evidence from several sources suggest that there is a link between the organ injury that occurs during sepsis and other critical illnesses and the Vo_2–Do_2 alterations that occur in these settings. It has generally been presumed that the mechanism for the altered Vo_2–Do_2 relationships in these disorders is insufficient delivery of oxygen to metabolically active tissues. However, altered oxygen metabolism, especially during sepsis, cannot be totally accounted for by this proposed mechanism. This may explain the fact that several clinical trials have shown that augmentation of oxygen delivery in the setting of established sepsis or ALI failed to reduce mortality and in some studies actually increased mortality. This apparent clinical paradox may be reconciled by a hypothesis that proposes that both organ injury and Vo_2–Do_2 alterations during sepsis and other critical illnesses are the result of mitochondrial injury. Experimental data in support of this notion is increasing. However, future studies are needed to more definitively address the validity of this compelling hypothesis.

MANAGEMENT OF THE PATIENT WITH MULTIPLE ORGAN FAILURE

Critically ill patients at risk for developing MODS generally present with one or more of the following clinical signs: shock (hypovolemic, cardiac, or septic), acute respiratory failure, or a major alteration in mental status. These clinical problems initially require a prompt therapeutic response to stabilize the patient. In general, initial management is directed to maintaining an adequate blood pressure and supporting gas exchange. For example, patients who present with hypovolemic shock, either from trauma or from GI bleeding, require rapid intravascular volume expansion with blood and crystalloid or colloid. Likewise, patients who have severe alterations in mental status with failure to protect the airway or progressive respiratory failure require prompt endotracheal intubation and mechanical ventilation. It is very important that the physician caring for critically ill patients recognize that the initial priority must be to stabilize the patient's circulatory and respiratory status. For example, the decision to insert a pulmonary arterial catheter should not take precedence over initial management of hypotension and respiratory failure. Once the patient is stabilized and appropriate support given to the circulatory and respiratory systems, careful assessment of the likely cause of the patient's condition should then be undertaken.

A logical starting point in evaluating critically ill patients is a search for the usual causes of shock, which include sepsis, cardiac failure (especially acute myocardial infarction), GI bleeding, acute pancreatitis, drug overdose, and occult bleeding from recent trauma. The physician, however, must always maintain a high index of suspicion for the presence of septicemia and should have a low threshold for obtaining blood cultures and appropriate cultures of other possible sources of infection. In addition, patients with even presumptive evidence for infection should be promptly placed on broad-spectrum antibiotics. General supportive measures have been discussed; the remainder of this section addresses specific issues related to support of the circulatory system and the respiratory system, as well as longer term measures, including appropriate support of the patient's nutritional status. The primary emphasis is on patients with sepsis and acute respiratory failure. Management of shock associated with acute myocardial infarction is covered in Chapter 73.

GUIDELINES FOR FLUID THERAPY

Except for patients with acute blood loss, who need blood transfusion to maintain the hematocrit between 25% and 35%, most patients need crystalloid or colloid therapy. At the present time, most medical and surgical centers favor the use of crystalloid over colloid for volume expansion. This preference is based in part on the ability of crystalloid (unlike colloid) to restore both the intravascular and the interstitial component of the extracellular fluid space. Some physicians do administer colloid in an attempt to maintain circulating plasma protein osmotic pressure; however, large volumes of colloid are often needed to achieve this objective, and the clearance of infused protein from the intravascular space is usually quite rapid. Despite the advantages of crystalloid versus colloid, red blood cells remain the ideal volume expander because they both increase oxygen transport to the tissues and maintain intravascular volume.

The timing of fluid resuscitation in hypotensive patients with acute blood loss has been examined recently. One study concluded that a delay of aggressive fluid resuscitation until surgical intervention improves outcome in patients with shock from penetrating injuries to the torso. These results, however, need to be confirmed in other medical centers before they can be accepted as optimal guidelines for the timing of fluid resuscitation.

In general, the appropriate fluid therapy depends on the cause of the patient's shock. For the patient with an acute myocardial infarction, fluid replacement should be titrated to maintain the pulmonary arterial wedge pressure between 15 and 20 mm Hg. By contrast, for patients with hypovolemic shock, traumatic shock, or septic shock, an increase in the central venous pressure or pulmonary arterial wedge pressure to 15 to 20 mm Hg may not be optimal. For example, in one study that examined volume resuscitation in patients with septic shock, the investigators found that increases in pulmonary arterial wedge pressure beyond 11 to 12 mm Hg did not result in a higher cardiac output.

Ideally, optimal fluid resuscitation in any form of shock should include the restoration of euvolemia; however, euvolemia is often difficult to define in critically ill patients. In addition, the adjustment of fluid therapy depends on the use of vasoactive agents, a topic discussed in the next section. Finally, although invasive hemodynamic monitoring with a pulmonary arterial catheter is frequently used to assist in the management of patients with septic shock, there is no evidence that this kind of monitoring changes outcome. Given these uncertainties, the best indexes for evaluating fluid replacement therapy are the patient's acid–base status, mental status, skin perfusion, and, perhaps most importantly, urine flow and renal function.

VASOACTIVE AGENTS

The most useful vasopressor for treating patients with septic shock is dopamine. Dopamine improves cardiac output via a positive chronotropic effect, an increase in preload to the heart, and an increase in contractility. This agent is particularly efficacious in septic shock because it both increases cardiac output and improves blood flow to the kidneys when given at doses below 10 μg per kilogram per minute. Moreover, dopamine, in contrast to fluid replacement therapy, has the additional advantage of increasing the cardiac output without increasing the pulmonary arterial wedge pressure. Finally, dopamine, unlike dobutamine, does not cause vasodilatation, thus making it preferable in shock caused by factors other than primary cardiac failure.

In some patients, septic shock will be unresponsive to even high doses of dopamine. In these patients, norepinephrine can be added to provide an increase in systemic arterial pressure. Epinephrine is another catecholamine that can be used for blood pressure support in severe septic shock. In doses greater than 10 μg per minute, epinephrine causes primarily α stimulation. High doses of any of these potent vasopressors cause vasoconstriction that may maintain systemic blood pressure, but blood flow to the kidneys, the splanchnic bed, muscles, and skin may be markedly reduced.

It is often difficult to determine the level of mean arterial pressure or cardiac output that is optimal in septic shock. In general, our recommendation is to try to adjust the mean arterial pressure and cardiac output to a level that stabilizes the metabolic acidosis associated with sepsis and improves tissue perfusion, particularly as indicated by urine flow. However, some patients with severe septic shock will require very high doses of dopamine, norepinephrine, or epinephrine to maintain even a barely adequate blood pressure.

In most patients, vasodilator therapy is not appropriate in the setting of septic shock. In a minority of cases, patients with primary cardiac disease may present with hypotension and an elevation of systemic vascular resistance associated with septicemia. These patients may benefit from dobutamine and, occasionally, from low doses of afterload reduction with a vasodilator, such as nitroprusside or nitroglycerin. With the exception of these patients, the use of vasodilators in the setting of multiple organ dysfunction and septic shock remains experimental.

ANTI-INFLAMMATORY AGENTS

A large number of animal model studies have demonstrated the potential value of various anti-inflammatory agents for the treatment of septic shock. In many of these studies, however, the pharmacologic agents were effective only for prevention, not as treatment. A recent multicenter trial of the prostaglandin inhibitor ibuprofen showed no benefit on reducing mortality in patients with sepsis. Also, ibuprofen treatment had no effect on the incidence of ARDS from sepsis. Thus, there are no clinically proven anti-inflammatory agents that decrease morbidity or improve mortality in patients with ARDS, septicemia, or MODS.

Corticosteroids had been used for a number of years in the management of patients with septicemia and ARDS, based largely on the unproven clinical impression that they might be beneficial. In the last few years, however, a number of prospective, well-controlled studies have demonstrated that corticosteroids are of no therapeutic value in patients with either septic shock or ARDS. Specifically, these clinical studies demonstrate that corticosteroids do not prevent the development of ARDS in patients with sepsis, nor do they prevent MODS, and they have no favorable effect on mortality.

IMMUNOTHERAPY

The most promising new therapeutic approach for the treatment of sepsis derives from recent studies using immunotherapy plus antibiotics. In two clinical trials, administration of hyperimmune sera to *E. coli* was given to patients with gram-negative bacteremia or to patients at risk for gram-negative bacteremia. In both studies there was a substantial decrease in morbidity and mortality. These two studies marked the beginning of an era of immunotherapy for ARDS, sepsis, and MODS. Since that time, numerous immunotherapeutic agents have been developed, synthesized, and tested in large, multicenter clinical trials (Table 355.3). The results of most studies that involve these agents have been reviewed. Unfortunately, none of these agents have been shown to prevent MODS or to improve outcome in patients with ARDS or sepsis. Perhaps as our ability to identify patients with ARDS or sepsis earlier in their clinical course improves, so too will the efficacy of these innovative immunotherapeutic agents.

TABLE 355.3.   IMMUNOLOGIC THERAPY FOR MODS

Immunotherapeutic Agent	Site of Action	Outcome in Animals	Status and Outcome of Clinical Trials
HA-IA	LPS	Efficacious in most	Completed No benefit
E5	LPS	Efficacious	Completed No benefit
TNF mAb	TNF	Efficacious	Completed No benefit
IL-1 RA	IL-1 receptor	Efficacious	Completed, No benefit
IL-6 mAb	IL-6	Efficacious	
IL-8 mAb	IL-8	Efficacious	Pending
mAb 60.3	CD11/CD18	Efficacious	Planned
BPI	LPS	Efficacious	Pending
TF mAb	TF	Efficacious	Planned

LPS, lipopolysaccharide; TNF, tumor necrosis factor; mAb, monoclonal antibody; IL-1, RA, interleukin-1 receptor antagonist; IL-1, interleukin-1; IL-6, interleukin-6; IL-8, interleukin-8; BPI, bactericidal permeability increasing factor; TF, tissue factor.

ANTIBIOTICS

Selection of appropriate antibiotics for patients with septic shock and MODS is very important. In general, a careful search for the likely source of sepsis should be undertaken and then appropriate broad-spectrum antibiotics instituted. Although antibiotic therapy is an important part of the treatment of patients with confirmed or suspected septic shock, the guidelines for specific selection of antibiotics are covered in Chapter 335.

NUTRITIONAL SUPPORT

Nutritional and metabolic support is an essential part of the management of patients with MODS. Hypermetabolism develops early in the syndrome, and severe malnutrition can become a prominent feature within days after the onset of illness. The characteristics of the hypermetabolic state include (a) increased resting energy expenditure and oxygen consumption, (b) increased use of carbohydrate, fat, and amino acids as energy substrates, and (c) increased loss of nitrogen in the urine. The hypermetabolic state results in profound protein catabolism, which is associated with a decrease in total body protein synthesis. The mechanism for the alteration of metabolism observed in patients with multiple organ failure appears to be related to the inflammatory mediators and the hormonal response to injury. Unfortunately, these fundamental alterations in metabolism do not appear to be readily altered by therapy. If adequate nutritional support is not provided, however, it is likely that organ dysfunction will be accelerated.

The goal of nutritional support in patients with, or at risk for, MODS is to prevent substrate-limited metabolism and to support, rather than attempt to alter, the hypermetabolism (see Chapter 130 for a detailed discussion of nutritional support).

In general, nutrition should be provided by the enteral route whenever possible. Enteral feedings eliminate cholestasis and reduce the risk of acalculous cholecystitis. Enteral alimentation may also offer some protection against GI hemorrhage in mechanically ventilated patients.

For patients who cannot tolerate enteral feeding, parenteral nutrition is a viable therapeutic alternative. The standard regimens of hyperalimentation, however, may not meet metabolic needs and can actually be harmful. Improved support can usually be achieved by decreasing the caloric and glucose load and by increasing the load of protein. For example, a regimen of 35 to 40 nonprotein calories per kilogram per day with 2 to 3 g per kilograms per day of amino acids has been described as an initial starting point. The regimen is then adjusted by determination of resting energy expenditures or the respiratory quotient. Intravenous fat emulsions can also be included to reduce the problems of excess glucose administration and to prevent essential fatty acid deficiency. Fatty emulsions can be used to provide 30% to 40% of the nonprotein calories.

In some patients, the amino acid load associated with hyperalimentation may worsen renal failure and accelerate the need for dialysis. Clinical judgment must be exercised to determine the potential benefits of initiating early hyperalimentation versus delaying dialysis in patients with MODS and renal failure. In general, we recommend providing adequate alimentation and dialysis, as needed.

ETHICAL SUPPORT

It is very important for physicians to assess carefully the likelihood of meaningful recovery in each critically ill patient with MODS. This assessment will depend on the natural history of the patient's underlying disease, as well as the extent and severity of organ failure. There is a growing awareness among the medical community that reasonable limits should be exercised by physicians and patients' families in supporting patients with critical illnesses and MODS. Recent studies demonstrate that some patient groups have a particularly poor prognosis for recovery. For example, bone marrow transplantation patients and those with ARDS have a less than 5% chance for recovery, whereas patients with a combination of hepatic failure and ALI have nearly 100% mortality. In addition, one study in two ICUs at the University of California Medical Center showed that withdrawal of life support was the mechanism for death in approximately 80% of patients in the ICU setting. As more information becomes available regarding prognostic indexes for specific disease processes, it may help guide decisions to discontinue life support in patients who do not have a reasonable chance for meaningful recovery.

■ EARLY RECOGNITION AND PREVENTION OF MULTIPLE ORGAN FAILURE

EARLY RECOGNITION

A number of studies have been published that identify patients who are at the highest risk for developing MODS. Patients with multiple trauma and hypotension who require emergency surgery and multiple transfusions are one common group of patients at high risk. Other patients considered to be at high risk for the development of MODS include patients with septic shock, patients with advanced chronic diseases (e.g., chronic liver disease or chronic renal failure) who are hospitalized for cardiac failure or a primary infection, and patients with AIDS. Finally, patients who are immunosuppressed because of an underlying malignancy or its treatment may be at particularly high risk for MODS, from both the toxic effects of the chemotherapy and the increased susceptibility to septicemia.

Some investigators have evaluated clinical factors as well as easily measurable plasma factors that might predict which patients with nonpulmonary sepsis syndrome would progress to develop ALI. One study focused on the possible value of a product of endothelial cells for predicting ALI. This study was based on the premise that endothelial cell injury is a ubiquitous, early event in the pathogenesis of sepsis. A variety of in vitro and in vivo studies have shown that both pulmonary and systemic endothelial cell injury occur during endotoxemia and septicemia. The investigators measured plasma levels of von Willebrand's factor–antigen (vWf-Ag) because vWf-Ag has been shown to be released from endothelial cells in vitro when they are injured and because two prior clinical studies demonstrated that plasma vWF-Ag levels are markedly elevated in patients with established acute respiratory failure. Plasma vWF-Ag levels were increased twofold in patients with nonpulmonary sepsis who subsequently developed ALI, compared with those in patients with nonpulmonary sepsis who did not progress to ALI. Moreover, of the 15 patients who developed ALI from sepsis, 14 patients died (93% mortality). An elevated vWF-Ag level above 450 (% of control) was predictive of the development of ALI (87% sensitivity, 77% specificity) and had a positive predictive value of 80% for identifying septic patients who were not likely to survive. In a subsequent study, plasma vWf-Ag was elevated in most patients at risk for ALI from both sepsis and nonseptic causes but did not have a significant predictive value for identifying which patients would develop ARDS. This study differed from the previous study cited in the heterogeneity of patient risks included. Thus, plasma vWf-Ag has some predictive value for identifying risk of developing ARDS and MODS in the more homogeneous risk group of patients with sepsis. Other studies have indicated that elevation of plasma ICAM-1, an endothelial and epithelial adhesion molecule, also has predictive value for identifying sepsis patients who will have the highest mortality.

More studies are needed to combine clinical factors and readily measurable plasma factors to identify those patients with sepsis syndrome at the greatest risk of developing ALI. These patients would be reasonable candidates for early treatment with immunotherapy, anti-inflammatory agents, and other new treatments that may become available in the near future.

PREVENTION OF MULTIPLE ORGAN DYSFUNCTION

Interest has grown in various approaches to reducing the risk of MODS, particularly because outcome is so poor once a patient develops MODS. Although specific treatment approaches have yet to be established, a number of general supportive measures are available. Perhaps the most important supportive measure is prevention of infection. Nosocomial infection can be reduced by good hand washing, removal of unnecessary intravascular and urinary catheters, and prevention of skin ulcers. Moreover, it is important to change central venous catheters in a timely manner (e.g., every 3 to 4 days) and to remain diligent to the possibility of surgically treatable infections.

Some studies suggest that an additional approach to preventing nosocomial infections in critically ill patients may be the use of selective decontamination. This approach involves the use of nonabsorbable antibiotics (orally or topically) to the oral pharynx as well as the administration of intravenous antibiotics. Although mortality has not been significantly reduced in the studies published to date, the incidence of late nosocomial infections was decreased in the patients who receive selective decontamination..

Finally, it may be important that some patients receive prophylaxis for upper GI bleeding (see Chapter 107). Prophylaxis can be provided with enteral feedings, antacids, sucralfate, or histamine blockers. Sucralfate may have an additional advantage over antacids in its being associated with a lower incidence of nosocomial pneumonia. One study indicated that respiratory failure and coagulopathy were the two most important independent risk factors for GI bleeding in critically ill patients.

BIBLIOGRAPHY

Artigas A, Bernard GR, Carlet J, et al., and the Consensus Committee. The American-Europen Consensus Conference on ARDS, Part 2. *Am J Respir Crit Care Med* 1998;157:1332–1347.

ATS Board of Directors. Round table conference on acute lung injury. *Am J Respir Crit Care Med* 1998;158:675–679.

Connors AF, Speroff T, Dawson NV, et al. The effectiveness of right heart catheterization in the initial care of critcally ill patients. *JAMA* 1996;276:889–897.

Cook DJ, Fuller HD, Gordon MB, et al. Risk factors for gastrointestinal bleeding in critically ill patients. *N Engl J Med* 1994;330:377–381.

Doyle RL, Szaflarski N, Modin GW, et al. Identification of patients with acute lung injury—predictors of mortality. *Am J Respir Crit Care Med* 1995;152:1818–1824.

Hayes MA, Timmins AC, Yau E, et al. Elevation of systemic oxygen delivery in the treatment of critically ill patients. *N Engl J Med* 1994;330:1717–1722.

Knaus WA, Wagner DP. Multiple systems organ failure: epidemiology and prognosis. *Crit Care Clin* 1989;5:221–232.

Macho JR, Luce JM. Rational approach to the management of multiple systems organ failure. *Crit Care Clin* 1989;5:379–392.

Moss M, Ackerman L, Gillespie MK, et al. von Willebrand factor antigen levels are not predictive for the development of adult respiratory distress syndrome. *Am J Respir Crit Care Med* 1995;151:15–20.

Parsons PE, Moss M. Early detection and markers of sepsis. In: Dorinsky PM, ed. *Clinics in chest medicine*, vol. 17. Philadelphia: WB Saunders, 1996:199–212.

Pittet JF, Mackersie RC, Martin TR, et al. Biologic markers of acute lung injury: prognostic and pathogenetic significance. *Am J Respir Crit Care Med* 1997;155:1187–1205.

Ralston DR, St. John RC. Immunotherapy for sepsis. In: Dorinsky PM, ed. *Clinics in chest medicine*, vol. 17. Philadelphia: WB Saunders, 1996:307–317.

Ronco JJ, Fenwick JC, Tweeddale MG, et al. Identification of the critical oxygen delivery for anaerobic metabolism in critically ill septic and nonseptic humans. *JAMA* 1993;270:1724–1730.

Rubin DB, Wiener-Kronish JP, Murray JF, et al. Elevated von Willebrand factor antigen is an early plasma predictor of impending acute lung injury and death in non-pulmonary sepsis syndrome. *J Clin Invest* 1990;86:474–480.

Smedira N, Evans B, Grais L, et al. Withholding and withdrawing of life support from the critically ill. *N Engl J Med* 1990;322:309–315.

St. John RC, Dorinsky PM. An overview of the multiple organ dysfunction syndrome. *J Lab Clin Med* 1994;124:478–483.

Wheeler AP, Bernard GR. Treating patients with severe sepsis. *N Engl J Med* 1999;340:207–214.

Zilberberg MD, Epstein SK. Acute lung injury in the medical ICU—comorbid conditions, age, etiology, and hospital outcome. *Am J Respir Crit Care Med* 1998;157:1159–1164.

Kelley's Textbook of Internal Medicine, fourth edition. Edited by H. David Humes. Lippincott Williams & Wilkins, Philadelphia © 2000.

C H A P T E R
356

APPROACH TO THE PATIENT WITH ACUTE RESPIRATORY FAILURE

THOMAS CORBRIDGE

Acute respiratory failure (ARF) is defined as a sudden deterioration in the ability of the respiratory system to maintain adequate gas exchange. It may occur in the previously healthy (e.g., pneumonia), or in the setting of chronic respiratory failure (e.g., acute exacerbation of chronic obstructive pulmonary disease)—a state commonly referred to as acute-on-chronic respiratory failure. A primary disturbance of oxygenation is called acute hypoxemic respiratory failure; a sudden rise in carbon dioxide tension defines acute hypercapnic respiratory failure. Implicit in all of these terms is the fact that there has been an acute decline in the patient's usual condition.

PRESENTATION

Respiratory distress is the hallmark of ARF. However, hypoxemia may present solely as an alteration in mental status or tachycardia; and in some cases hypercapnia may present only as a change in mental status, tachycardia, hypertension, or papilledema.

There are no clear cutoff values for PaO_2 or $PaCO_2$ that define ARF. Commonly accepted values are PaO_2 below 60 mm Hg and $PaCO_2$ above 50 mm Hg while breathing room air. However, these values are influenced by age, altitude, preexisting lung disease, and other nonrespiratory factors. For example, consider that an 80-year-old person living in Denver, Colorado normally has a PaO_2 of 60 mm Hg, and that a 60-year-old with chronic obstructive pulmonary disease (COPD) at sea level may have a baseline PaO_2 of 60 mm Hg and a $PaCO_2$ of 50 mm Hg. Conversely, a PaO_2 of 70 mm Hg in a 20-year-old hypocapnic patient is distinctly abnormal (see below). Therefore, to be consistent with ARF, hypoxemia or hypercapnia must be significant and acutely different from baseline.

Acute respiratory insufficiency (ARI) is distinguished from ARF by the lack of significant blood gas deterioration. These terms are descriptors of common pathophysiologic processes, with ARI referring to illness of lesser severity or better physiologic compensation. Serial blood gas measurements help discern the transition from ARI to ARF.

PATHOPHYSIOLOGIC FACTORS

Although oxygenation and ventilation are unavoidably linked, it is helpful to consider the determinates of each separately and to establish whether the problem is primarily one of oxygenation or ventilation.

DETERMINATES OF OXYGENATION

An understanding of the alveolar gas equation is mandatory for understanding hypoxemic states. A simplified and commonly used version of this equation is as follows:

$$PAO_2 = (P_b - PAH_2O)FIO_2 - PACO_2/RQ$$

where PAO_2 is alveolar oxygen tension; P_b, barometric pressure; PAH_2O, alveolar water vapor pressure; FIO_2, fraction of inspired oxygen; RQ, respiratory quotient (ratio of CO_2 production to O_2 consumption); and $PACO_2$ is alveolar CO_2 (assumed

to equal $PaCO_2$). In a normal subject breathing room air at sea level, P_b is 760 mm Hg, PAH_2O is 47 mm Hg, FIO_2 is 0.21, $PaCO_2$ is 40 mm Hg, and RQ is assumed to be 0.8 (although it can be measured by inspiratory and expiratory gas analysis). Under these conditions, the predicted PAO_2 is 100 mm Hg.

In health, PaO_2 approaches PAO_2, so that the difference between the two, $P(A-a)O_2$, is small (less than 10 mm Hg in a young adult). Calculation of $P(A-a)O_2$ helps prevent misinterpretations of PaO_2. For example, a room air, sea level PaO_2 of 90 mm Hg is too low in a 20-year-old with a $PaCO_2$ of 20 mm Hg because $P(A-a)O_2$ is 25 mm Hg.

$P(A-a)O_2$ increases normally with age according to the formula: $P(A-a)O_2 = 2.5 + 0.25(age)$. $P(A-a)O_2$ also increases as FIO_2 increases, complicating its use in patients on supplemental oxygen. In such cases, an estimate of gas exchange may be obtained by relating the arterial to the alveolar oxygen tension (PaO_2/PAO_2). A ratio of 0.8 or greater indicates adequate gas exchange. An even simpler estimate can be obtained by dividing PaO_2 by FIO_2. This ratio is normally greater than 400.

The alveolar gas equation predicts four causes for a low PAO_2 (and thereby a low PaO_2) that do not elevate $P(A-a)O_2$: low barometric pressure, low FIO_2, high $PaCO_2$, and low RQ (Table 356.1). Only high altitude and hypercapnia are important in common clinical practice. Consider, for example, the effects of a $PaCO_2$ of 60 mm Hg in a patient with heroin overdose and a room air PaO_2 of 60 mm Hg. In this case, hypoxemia occurs because alveolar CO_2 displaces oxygen and the rate of oxygen removal from alveoli may exceed its resupply. The $P(A-a)O_2$ is normal so hypoxemia is entirely explained by the elevated $PaCO_2$.

States that elevate $P(A-a)O_2$ include disorders that lower ventilation (V) to perfusion (Q) ratios, or impair diffusion. Under normal conditions, ventilation and perfusion are closely matched (i.e., V/Q approaches 1). A V/Q of zero defines shunt. In the lung, alveolar filling processes (such as pneumonia, pulmonary edema, and alveolar hemorrhage), and acute lobar atelectasis cause shunt (Fig. 356.1). Right-to-left intracardiac shunt similarly isolates venous blood from inspired oxygen. Indeed oxygen

TABLE 356.1.	COMMON CAUSES OF HYPOXEMIA	
Conditions with Normal $P(A-a)O_2$	**Conditions Elevating $P(A-a)O_2$**	**Conditions Associated with Low $Pv O_2$**
High altitude	Intrapulmonary shunt (pneumonia, pulmonary edema, alveolar hemorrhage, lobar atelectasis)	Low cardiac output
Hypercapnia	Low-V/Q states (asthma, COPD, PE)	High oxygen consumption
Low respiratory quotient	Diffusion limitation	Anemia
Low F_iO_2		Low P_aO_2

COPD, chronic obstructive pulmonary disease; PE, pulmonary embolism.

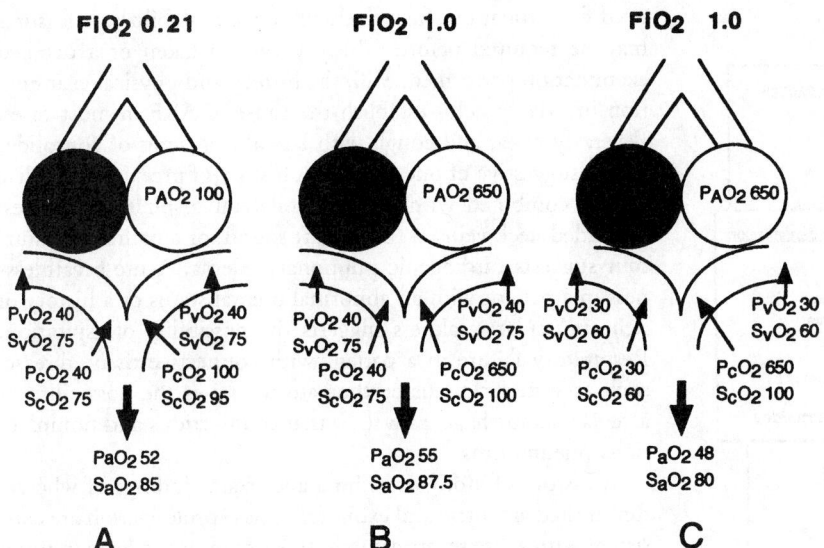

FIGURE 356.1. Effects of 50% intrapulmonary shunt on PaO$_2$ in a two-lung-unit model, each receiving 50% of the cardiac output, during three experimental conditions: on room air with a normal PvO$_2$ **(A)**, on 100% oxygen with a normal PvO$_2$ **(B)**, and on 100% oxygen with a low PvO$_2$ **(C)**. Three points along the transit of blood are noted: the mixed venous entry point, the end-capillary point and the arterial blood. For simplicity, effects of dissolved oxygen have been ignored. SaO$_2$ is determined by averaging S$_c$O$_2$, not P$_c$O$_2$, from each lung unit. Note how little PaO$_2$ increases despite 100% oxygen. Note also how lowering PvO$_2$ affects PaO$_2$. PvO$_2$, partial pressure of oxygen, mixed venous blood; SvO$_2$, oxygen saturation, mixed venous blood; P$_c$O$_2$, partial pressure of oxygen, end-capillary blood; S$_c$O$_2$, oxygen saturation, end-capillary; PaO$_2$, partial pressure, arterial blood; SaO$_2$, oxygen saturation, arterial blood.

supplementation may have minimal effects in a patient with significant shunt physiology.

Disorders lowering V/Q (but not to zero) include asthma and COPD, diseases of the airways that lower ventilation to perfused lung units. Low V/Q is also important in the hypoxemia of pulmonary embolism (PE), in part because nonobstructed vessels receive more blood flow. PE occasionally causes shunt when a foramen ovale opens in the setting of acute right heart strain. Unlike shunt, low V/Q states respond well to supplemental oxygen because poorly ventilated lung units still supply oxygen to passing blood.

Diffusion limitation refers to pathologic processes that increase the distance between a functional alveolus and the pulmonary capillary bed (as in pulmonary fibrosis), or to processes that decrease the oxygen diffusion gradient (as in carbon monoxide intoxication, hemoglobinopathy, and anemia). The importance of diffusion limitation in routine clinical practice is debated.

Perfusing low-V/Q units with a low PvO$_2$ (the PO$_2$ of venous blood in the precapillary bed) also causes hypoxemia (Fig. 356.1). Causes of low PvO$_2$ are listed in Table 356.1. Low PvO$_2$ does not affect PaO$_2$ in the normal lung, which can adequately oxygenate even severely desaturated venous blood.

DETERMINATES OF HYPERCAPNIA

PaCO$_2$ is set by the ratio of carbon dioxide production (VCO$_2$) to carbon dioxide elimination, modified by a constant (K). CO$_2$ elimination is determined by alveolar ventilation (VA), where VA is the portion of minute ventilation (Ve = respiratory rate × tidal volume) that participates in gas exchange. In other words, VA equals Ve times a fraction that accounts for deadspace ventilation (1 − Vd/Vt), where Vd is the volume of dead space and Vt is tidal volume. Dead space (defined as V/Q of infinity) does not participate in gas exchange and consists mainly of large airways. Normally, Vd/Vt is less than 0.25. If Vd/Vt is 0.25, then 1 − Vd/Vt is 0.75 and 75% of Ve eliminates CO$_2$. The constant K (0.863) is necessary to convert CO$_2$ elimination

in the gas phase, measured in BTPS, to STPD, and to convert fractional concentration to partial pressure. Thus:

$$PaCO_2 = VCO_2 \; (0.863)/[Ve(1 - Vd/Vt)]$$

PaCO$_2$ is about 40 mm Hg under normal conditions of VCO$_2$, 220 mL per minute; Ve, 7 L per minute; Vd, 125 mL; and Vt, 500 mL.

This formula predicts three causes for hypercapnia: low Ve, high VCO$_2$, and high Vd/Vt. Disorders that lower Ve may be understood by considering the relationship between respiratory muscle strength and respiratory system load (Fig. 356.2). The neuromuscular apparatus must generate enough negative intrathoracic pressure to overcome two major obstacles: the resistance to airflow in the conducting airways, and the elastance of the lungs and chest wall (which includes the abdomen). As long as the pressure generated is able to overcome these two mechanical loads, adequate alveolar ventilation will be sustained. If not, CO$_2$ accumulates.

Patients with normal neuromuscular function may develop hypercapnic respiratory failure in the face of markedly altered lung mechanics (e.g., a young patient with acute asthma). Alternatively, hypercapnia may develop in a patient with normal lung mechanics when neuromuscular strength is markedly decreased (e.g., drug overdose or amyotrophic lateral sclerosis). Often both strength and load are affected. In an exacerbation of COPD, resistive load is increased by secretions and bronchospasm and elastic load is increased by auto-PEEP and lung hyperinflation. Auto-PEEP (auto–positive end-expiratory pressure) occurs when expiratory airflow limitation prevents complete emptying of alveolar gas. Auto-PEEP represents a threshold pressure that must be overcome before inspiratory airflow can occur. Auto-PEEP thus increases inspiratory work of breathing. The hyperinflated lung is also harder to inflate if it is operating at a flatter portion of its pressure–volume relationship (i.e., it has a lower compliance). At the same time, diaphragm force generation is decreased by hyperinflaton (which places the diaphragm in a mechanically disadvantageous position), acute respiratory acido-

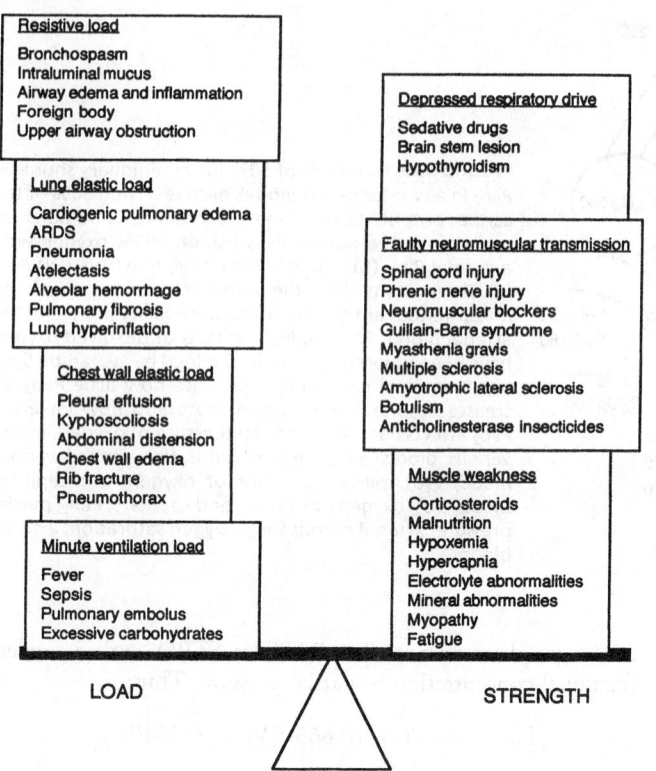

FIGURE 356.2. Conditions associated with hypercapnic respiratory failure may be divided into conditions affecting neuromuscular strength and conditions affecting respiratory system load. In order to maintain minute ventilation, adequate strength must be present to handle the given load. (Adapted from Schmidt GA, Hall JB. Acute-on-chronic-respiratory-failure. In: Hall JB, Schmidt GA, Wood LDH, eds. Principles of critical care, second ed. New York: McGraw-Hill, 1998: 565–594.)

sis, and a lack of substrate delivery to the diaphragm due to hypoxemia, abnormalities of electrolytes and minerals, or shock. Malnutrition and corticosteroid therapy may also decrease diaphragm function.

As Vd/Vt increases, so will $PaCO_2$ for a given Ve and VCO_2. In some conditions, such as emphysema or PE, dead space is high because of obliteration or obstruction of blood vessels continuing to receive ventilation. In other cases, dead space increases because high alveolar pressure decreases adjacent blood flow, a state aggravated by low intravascular hydrostatic pressure. Examples include a severely hyperinflated asthmatic and a patient with the acute respiratory distress syndrome (ARDS) requiring high levels of PEEP.

Carbon dioxide production is increased in patients who are working excessively to breathe and in patients who are febrile, septic, or receiving carbohydrate-rich diets. High CO_2 production contributes to hypercapnia when a compensatory increase in Ve does not occur (as in a mechanically ventilated patient receiving a fixed Ve or in a patient with severe COPD).

HISTORY AND PHYSICAL EXAMINATION

The general appearance of the patient (posture, speech, diaphoresis, alertness) provides a quick guide to disease severity and

need for intubation. In severely ill patients, stabilizing measures may be required before a history can be taken or a detailed examination performed. Still, the history and physical examination invariably helps establish the cause of ARF in most cases. Fever, dyspnea, and cough with lateralizing signs of consolidation is suggestive of pneumonia. A history of preexisting cardiac disease combined with dyspnea, bilateral inspiratory crackles, distended neck veins, a third heart sound, or a pathologic murmur suggests cardiogenic pulmonary edema. Acute breathlessness in a patient with an abnormal mental status or a history of neuromuscular weakness suggests the possibility of aspiration. Respiratory failure in a patient with connective tissue disease, such as systemic lupus erythematosus, raises the possibility of alveolar hemorrhage, as well as that of infectious and noninfectious pneumonitis.

A history of atopy or asthma and exam findings of wheeze, diminished air entry, and expiratory phase prolongation are consistent with acute severe asthma. It is important to keep in mind that severely obstructed patients have a silent chest. That is, they may not wheeze at all because there is insufficient flow for wheeze to occur. Accessory muscle use and pulsus paradoxus indicate severe airflow obstruction, but the absence of these findings does not exclude a severe attack. A "mediastinal crunch" or subcutaneous emphysema (crepitus) suggests pneumomediastinum or pneumothorax and a potentially worse clinical course.

It is important to keep in mind that "all that wheezes is not asthma." An extensive smoking history suggests COPD, which may be associated with variable degrees of fixed and reversible airflow obstruction, pulmonary hypertension, and chronic respiratory acidosis. Cardiac asthma refers to airway hyperreactivity stemming from congestive heart failure. Heart failure is usually discernible on examination, but the distinction between heart failure and primary airway disease can be difficult, particularly in the elderly. The presence of a foreign body must be considered in children and in adults with poor swallowing, altered mental status, or recent dental work. Foreign body obstruction may cause atelectasis with or without ipsilateral tracheal deviation. Tracheal deviation is also caused by contralateral volume expanding lesions such as pneumothorax or pleural effusion. Upper airway obstruction from granulation tissue, tumor, infection, laryngeal edema, or vocal cord dysfunction may also be mistaken for acute asthma. Stridor is not always distinguishable from wheeze, and wheezes may be heard best over the trachea. Inspiratory phase prolongation is a useful sign of upper airway obstruction.

Pulmonary embolism should be considered in all breathless patients, unless there is another convincing cause of ARF. Historical features worrisome for PE include recent surgery, malignancy, prior thromboembolic disease, a family history of thromboembolic disease, pregnancy, the use of oral contraceptives in a smoker, right heart failure, and prolonged immobility (including recent long travel). Dyspnea is invariably present. Hemoptysis, pleuritic chest pain, syncope, and shock also occur. Examination classically reveals tachypnea and tachycardia. The lungs may be clear or there may be basilar crackles. Wheezes are rare. Significant pulmonary hypertension is signaled by accentuation of the pulmonic component of the second heart sound or a third heart sound. The finding of a swollen or erythematous extremity is suspicious but not diagnostic of thromboembolic disease. Likewise, normal extremities do not exclude clot.

Assessment of neuromuscular function is important in patients with ARF, keeping in mind that it is the imbalance between strength and load that leads to hypercapnic respiratory failure. The examiner should seek evidence for an underlying neuromuscular disease and for other factors associated with weakness, such as fatigue, malnutrition, electrolyte disorders, and chronic use of corticosteroids.

LABORATORY STUDIES AND DIAGNOSTIC TESTS

If circumstances permit, the initial blood gas should be obtained on room air to allow for determination of $P(A\text{-}a)O_2$. If the patient is receiving supplemental oxygen by nasal cannula or face mask, $P(A\text{-}a)O_2$ cannot be measured accurately because FIO_2 is not precisely known. A rough calculation, however, still suggests whether $P(A\text{-}a)O_2$ is normal or not. In intubated patients, the FIO_2 is known and $P(A\text{-}a)O_2$ can be measured, but because $P(A\text{-}a)O_2$ varies with FIO_2, it is less useful than PaO_2/PAO_2 or PaO_2/FIO_2. Whenever possible, comparison with a baseline blood gas is helpful. It is also important to measure hemoglobin (which is important for oxygen delivery) and white cell count (which helps assess the possibility of infection).

Pulse oximetry allows for continuous, noninvasive readings of arterial saturation. However, it has several limitations. First, the 95% confidence interval for measurements is $\pm 4\%$ for SaO_2 greater than 70%. Pulse oximetry is even less accurate in severe hypoxemia. Thus, a value of 92% could correspond to a SaO_2 by blood gas between 88% and 96% (roughly corresponding to a PaO_2 between 55 mm Hg and 95 mm Hg). Second, accuracy is affected by a number of factors that overestimate (carboxyhemoglobinemia, methemoglobinemia), underestimate (methylene blue, jaundice, dark nail polish), and have variable effects (patient temperature, hypoperfusion, skin pigmentation) on measured values. Third, $PaCO_2$ and pH are not measured by pulse oximetry.

The relationship between serum pH and $PaCO_2$ is crucial in the evaluation of patients with hypercapnic respiratory failure. For every 10 mm Hg rise in $PaCO_2$ acutely, pH falls by 0.08 unit. Thus, an acute increase in $PaCO_2$ from 40 to 60 mm Hg should drop the arterial pH from 7.40 to 7.24. If this is not the case, additional factors should be considered including compensation and other primary acid–base disturbances. Accurate interpretation of the acid–base status requires simultaneous measurement of electrolytes and calculation of the anion gap.

A chest radiograph should be obtained and compared (if possible) with previous films for the detection of infiltrates, pneumothorax, hyperinflation, atelectasis, pleural effusion, and change in heart size. Radiographic patterns associated with ARF are listed in Table 356.2. Measurement of expiratory airflow by a peak flowmeter or spirometer helps assess the severity of obstruction in patients with acute asthma; and a normal peak flow helps direct the clinician away from an obstructive process. Echocardiography helps to delineate right- and left-sided ventricular function, valvular integrity, and the presence of pericar-

TABLE 356.2.	SELECTED DISORDERS AND RADIOGRAPHIC PATTERNS ASSOCIATED WITH HYPOXEMIA	
Lucent	**Diffuse**	**Focal**
Intracardiac shunt	Diffuse pneumonia	Pulmonary infarction
Arteriovenous malformation	Bronchopulmonary dysplasia	Lung mass
Cirrhosis	Alveolar hemorrhage	Pneumonia
Asthma	Acute respiratory distress syndrome	Aspiration
Pulmonary embolism	Cardiogenic pulmonary edema	Mucus plug
Pneumothorax	Aspiration pneumonitis	Contusion
	Lymphangietic spread of cancer	Reexpansion or dependent pulmonary edema
Microatelectasis	Drug reaction Interstitial lung disease	Atelectasis

dial disease. Noninvasive tests for deep venous thrombosis, such as duplex ultrasonography, are useful in evaluating patients with suspected thromboembolic disease. These studies are helpful when positive, but 30% to 40% of patients with acute PE have negative studies. Ventilation–perfusion scans are useful in some cases, but the majority of studies are indeterminate. In selected patients, spiral CT scanning with a PE protocol or pulmonary angiography is required to establish a diagnosis of PE.

STRATEGIES FOR OPTIMAL CARE MANAGEMENT

The primary responsibility of the treating clinician is to identify and treat life-threatening conditions, beginning with sequential assessment of the ABCs (airway, breathing, and circulation). The foremost goal is immediate correction of arterial hypoxemia. In nonintubated patients, the fraction of inspired oxygen should be increased until an oxygen saturation of 90% to 92% is achieved. A pulse oximeter allows for initial rapid titration of oxygen, but the adequacy of oxygenation should be confirmed by blood gas. Supplemental oxygen can be delivered by nasal cannula or face mask with the highest FIO_2 achieved by delivering 100% oxygen through a tight-fitting, non-rebreathing face mask. Refractory hypoxemia identifies patients with shunt physiology. When this is caused by cardiogenic pulmonary edema, continuous positive airway pressure (CPAP) by nasal or full-face mask is particularly effective because it reduces venous return to the right-sided heart, decreases left ventricular afterload, and redistributes alveolar fluid. CPAP is less reliable in patients with ARDS and pneumonia, but it still works in selected patients.

If adequate oxygenation cannot be achieved quickly by noninvasive means, intubation and mechanical ventilation are indicated. During the peri-intubation period, FiO_2 should be 1.0, though it should be decreased as soon as possible to no greater than 0.6 to avoid oxygen toxicity. Strategies that allow for a nontoxic FiO_2 in most cases include (a) the use of PEEP, (b) therapies that increase PvO_2, and (c) positional changes. Other strategies (most often considered in ARDS) include the use of nitric oxide, partial-liquid ventilation, and surfactant. Discussion of these therapies is beyond the scope of this chapter.

PEEP is synonymous with CPAP in a mechanically ventilated patient. In diffuse lung disorders (such as cardiogenic pulmonary edema and ARDS), PEEP lowers shunt by the mechanisms specified above. By maintaining a higher end-exhalation lung volume, PEEP may also prevent the closing and opening of lung units with each tidal breath, a situation that generates significant shear forces and may contribute to ventilator-induced lung injury. When using PEEP, care must be taken to limit Vt excursions above the set PEEP to avoid lung over-distention. In focal lung disease (such as pneumonia), PEEP may preferentially distend normal lung units, thereby diverting blood flow from them to diseased areas and worsening V/Q inequality. PEEP is also detrimental to gas exchange when it decreases cardiac output and PvO_2 by decreasing venous return or when it increases dead-space ventilation.

Strategies that elevate PvO_2 may improve PaO_2. These include (a) the use of sedatives and/or paralytics to decrease oxygen consumption, (b) fluid resuscitation and/or use of inotropes and vasodilators to increase cardiac output, and (c) blood transfusion.

The purpose of positional maneuvers is to improve V/Q inequality by increasing blood flow to healthier lung units. In lobar pneumonia, this goal may be achieved by placing the "good lung down." In ARDS, prone positioning improves oxygenation two-thirds of the time, but it has not yet been shown to affect outcome.

Concurrent with supportive measures, it is necessary to treat the underlying disorder responsible for ARF. Examples include the use of antibiotics for pneumonia, diuretics and afterload reducers for congestive heart failure, and immunosuppressants for some cases of alveolar hemorrhage. It is beyond the scope of this chapter to discuss all of these therapies in detail.

Successful treatment of acute hypercapnic respiratory failure requires restoration of the balance between the neuromuscular strength and respiratory system load. When the problem is strictly one of decreased neuromuscular function (e.g., drug overdose), restoring neuromuscular competence is all that is required (e.g., naloxone infusion). When hypercapnia results primarily from abnormal lung mechanics (e.g., acute severe asthma in an otherwise healthy person), the primary strategy should be to decrease respiratory system load (see bibliography for suggested readings on the management of acute severe asthma). Often both strength and load must be addressed, as in the case of acute exacerbations of COPD. An expanded discussion of the care of patients with COPD exacerbation is included because this condition is a common cause of respiratory failure.

In COPD, hypercapnic respiratory failure results when the precarious balance between decreased patient strength and increased load on the respiratory system is tipped in the wrong direction, often by a relatively trivial insult. To restore this bal-ance, the treating clinician should first achieve 90% saturation of arterial blood. Adequate oxygen saturation is important for respiratory muscle function and to further decrease the risk of myocardial ischemia, arrhythmia, cerebral injury, and respiratory arrest. Clinicians are often hesitant to supply oxygen, fearing that patients will stop breathing. It is now known, however, that supplemental oxygen does not stop patients from breathing; rather, oxygen elevates $PaCO_2$ by increasing Vd/Vt and the haldane effect. Oxygen causes a small and insignificant fall in Ve, and respiratory drive remains supranormal despite oxygen. Substrates other than oxygen are important for adequate muscle function. Electrolytes and minerals should be corrected and nutritional supplementation provided early in the course of acute illness. CPAP decreases the inspiratory work of breathing in patients with air trapping by decreasing the pressure gradient required for inspiratory gas flow. Additional support can be achieved by adding pressure support to CPAP (commonly referred to as noninvasive positive pressure ventilation, or NPPV). Considerable data support the use of NPPV in acute COPD exacerbations.

Several pharmacologic agents are available to lower respiratory system load. Bronchodilators are used to decrease airway resistance. While much of the airflow obstruction of COPD is fixed, many patients have a reversible component that responds to bronchodilators. Available data demonstrate that the combination of a β-agonist and ipratropium bromide is better than either drug used alone. Bronchodilators may also decrease lung inflation by improving expiratory airflow. This places the diaphragm in a better position and may improve lung compliance. The available data do not support the use of theophylline in the initial management of exacerbations of COPD. Systemic corticosteroids are beneficial, and antibiotics should be used whenever there is an increase in sputum amount or purulence.

Patients failing pharmacotherapy and NPPV should be intubated and mechanically ventilated. During mechanical ventilation, it is important to avoid excessive lung hyperinflation and high levels of auto-PEEP. Setting a short inspiratory time and low Ve extends exhalation time and achieves this goal. It is also important to ensure patient–ventilator synchrony and adequate rest of fatigued respiratory muscles. The goal of ventilatory support is to return the arterial pH to normal, not to return the $PaCO_2$ to normal. In a patient with compensated respiratory acidosis, returning $PaCO_2$ to normal levels could result in deleterious lung hyperinflation and significant metabolic alkalosis.

PROGNOSIS AND OUTCOME

The outcome of ARF is frequently good, but it depends on multiple host and disease factors, including age, presence of comorbid conditions, and severity and nature of the acute insult. For instance, asthmatics who develop ARF and arrest out of hospital have a poor prognosis for meaningful recovery if they arrive with anoxic brain injury. On the other hand, asthmatics who are intubated in hospital rarely die if a ventilator strategy is used that limits lung hyperinflation. Patients with acute exacerbations of COPD similarly do well, although intubated patients do have a 20% to 30% mortality rate. In ARDS, mortality is approximately 40%. Preliminary data suggest that mortality in ARDS is less if a small tidal volume is used during mechanical ventilation. If ARDS is associated with other organ dysfunction, mortality increases, so that by the time three major organs have failed for three consecutive days, mortality exceeds 90%.

Because the prognosis of ARF is generally good, an initial plan to deliver critical care, including intubation, is appropriate unless the patient had previously decided to forego life-sustaining therapies. It is important to monitor patient progress (or lack thereof) and maintain open communication with the patient and/or surrogate so that good decisions can be made regarding the utility of critical care. Finally, for patients who recover, it is important to consider whether measures can be taken to prevent a recurrent episode of ARF.

BIBLIOGRAPHY

Corbridge T, Hall JB. Assessment and management of adults with status asthmaticus: state-of-the-art. *Am J Respir Crit Care Med* 1995;151:1296–1316.

Goldner M, Shapiro R. Acute respiratory failure: today's approach. *J Respir Dis* 1998;19:825–833.

Goldner M, Shapiro R. Acute respiratory failure: update on management. *J Respir Dis* 1998;19:1058–1068.

Goldner M, Shapiro R. Acute respiratory failure: ventilatory support strategies. *J Respir Dis* 1999;20:158–167.

Marini JJ, Wright LA. Acute respiratory failure. In: Baum GL, Crapo JD, Celli BR, et al., eds. *Textbook of pulmonary diseases*, sixth ed. Philadelphia: Lippincott–Raven Publishers, 1998:919–939.

O'Connor MF, Hall JB, Schmidt GA, et al. Acute hypoxemic respiratory failure. In: Hall JB, Schmidt GA, Wood LDH, eds. *Principles of critical care*, second ed. New York: McGraw-Hill, 1998:537–564.

Schmidt GA, Hall JB. Acute-on-chronic-respiratory-failure. In: Hall JB, Schmidt GA, Wood LDH, eds. *Principles of critical care*, second ed. New York: McGraw-Hill, 1998:565–594.

Kelley's Textbook of Internal Medicine, fourth edition. Edited by H. David Humes. Lippincott Williams & Wilkins, Philadelphia © 2000.

C H A P T E R
357

APPROACH TO THE PATIENT WITH ACUTE RESPIRATORY DISTRESS SYNDROME

KENNETH P. STEINBERG
LEONARD D. HUDSON

Acute respiratory distress syndrome (ARDS) (previously called adult respiratory distress syndrome) represents the abrupt onset of diffuse lung injury characterized by severe hypoxemia and generalized pulmonary infiltrates in the absence of cardiac failure. Although the syndrome may be initiated by a wide variety of illnesses or injuries, the clinical picture and histopathologic factors are remarkably uniform. The incidence of ARDS has been variably estimated at 15,000 to 150,000 cases per year in the United States. Despite the sophisticated monitoring and support systems available in intensive care units, progress has been slow. However, the survival rates do appear to have improved from about 40% in the 1970s and 1980s to about 60% in the 1990s. Most recently, a large clinical trial of mechanical ventilation demonstrated further improvement in survival from 60% to 70% with the use of small tidal volumes. Nevertheless, even with this improvement the death rate remains regrettably high and, because a large proportion of ARDS victims are relatively young previously healthy adults, the effect in terms of productive life lost is immense.

ETIOLOGIC FACTORS

Acute respiratory distress syndrome has been associated with a diversity of precipitating clinical events, the most common of which are listed in Table 357.1. Infectious causes appear to be the most common, with sepsis syndrome and bacterial or viral pneumonia leading the list. Approximately 40% of patients with sepsis syndrome or severe sepsis will develop ARDS. Major traumatic injury, often involving extensive soft-tissue damage, is also a common cause with approximately 25% of victims developing ARDS. Aspiration of gastric contents is an etiologic picture frequently seen in patients with an altered level of consciousness. Other risk factors include massive transfusion, inhalation injury, pancreatitis, near-drowning, and drug overdose. Many other causes of ARDS have been described in case reports and small series.

CLINICAL PRESENTATION AND DIAGNOSIS

Acute respiratory distress syndrome usually develops rapidly, occurring most often within 12 to 72 hours of the predisposing

TABLE 357.1. CLINICAL DISORDERS ASSOCIATED WITH ARDS[a]

Disorder	Estimated Incidence (%)
Direct or primary causes:	
Aspiration of gastric contents	22–36
Diffuse pneumonia	a
Pulmonary contusion	17–22
Inhalation injury	a
Near-drowning	a
Indirect or secondary causes:	
Sepsis	
Bacteremia without sepsis	4
Severe sepsis/sepsis syndrome	35–45
Major trauma	25
Hypertransfusion	5–36
Drug overdose	5–8
Pancreatitis	a

[a] Incident not known.

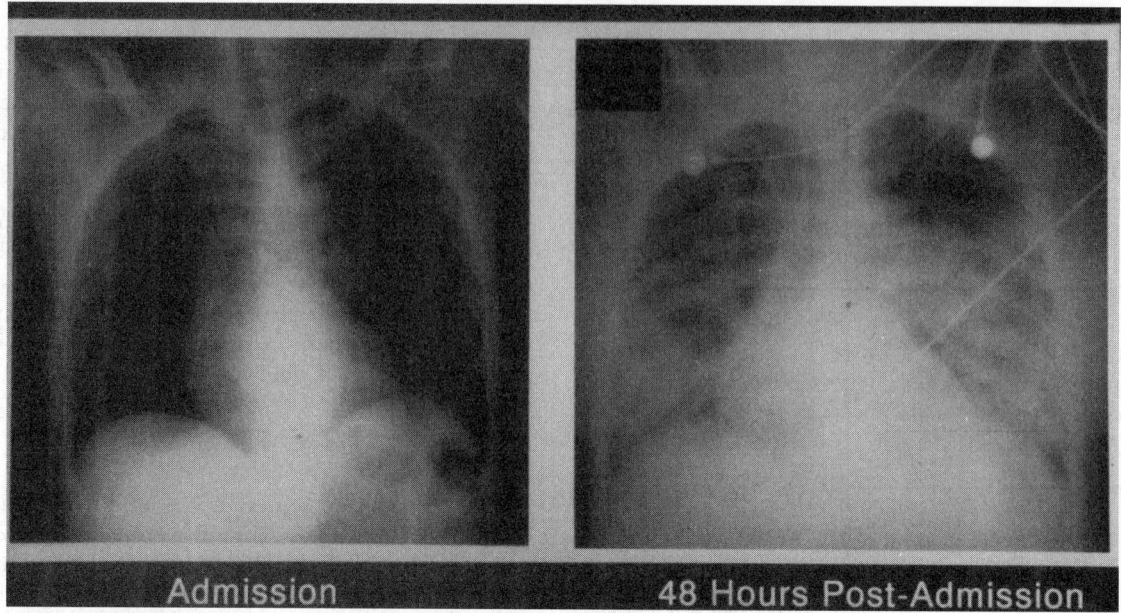

FIGURE 357.1. The presence of bilateral pulmonary infiltrates in a patient with sepsis is consistent with the development of acute respiratory distress syndrome within 48 hours of admission to the intensive care unit (*right*).

event. Respiratory distress, severe hypoxemia, and generalized pulmonary infiltrates are all necessary for the diagnosis of ARDS (Fig. 357.1). Because the arterial partial pressure of oxygen (Pa_{O_2}) is influenced by the fraction of inspired oxygen (FI_{O_2}), most ARDS definitions have defined hypoxemia in terms of a Pa_{O_2}/FI_{O_2} ratio or ratio between arterial and alveolar oxygen tensions (Pa_{O_2}/PA_{O_2} ratio). The specific definition of ARDS varies depending on the author and the attempt to describe the severity of the disease. The most widely accepted definition was developed by a joint American–European consensus committee in 1994. The concept of acute lung injury (ALI) as a spectrum of severity, with ARDS as the most severe end of the spectrum, was formulated by this group (Table 357.2). Bilateral pulmonary infiltrates must be present on chest radiographs, although correlation between the roentgenographic abnormalities and the de-

gree of hypoxemia varies widely. Hypoxemia with a Pa_{O_2}/FI_{O_2} ratio less than 300 defines ALI; a ratio of less than 200 describes ARDS. Congestive heart failure as a possible explanation of the pulmonary findings should be excluded either by a pulmonary artery occlusion pressure measurement of less than 18 mm Hg or clinically. Total respiratory compliance is usually reduced, but this is generally not required for the diagnosis.

To date, no specific laboratory findings of ARDS have been described other than those necessary to meet the criteria of the syndrome. Although certain blood and bronchoalveolar lavage (BAL) fluid abnormalities are common or universal in ARDS, such as evidence of activation of inflammatory pathways with elevation of multiple cytokines or reduction in plasma fibronectin levels, these findings are not specific to ARDS. Patients with similar underlying illnesses or injuries who do not develop

TABLE 357.2.	CRITERIA FOR ACUTE LUNG INJURY AND ACUTE RESPIRATORY DISTRESS SYNDROME			
	Onset	**Oxygenation**[a]	**Chest Radiograph**	**PAOP**[b]
ALI criteria	Acute	$Pa_{O_2}/FI_{O_2} \leq 300$ mm Hg	Bilateral interstitial or alveolar infiltrates	≤18 mm Hg if measured or no clinical evidence of left atrial hypertension
ARDS criteria	Acute	$Pa_{O_2}/FI_{O_2} \leq 200$ mm Hg	Bilateral interstitial or alveolar infiltrates	≤18 mm Hg if measured or no clinical evidence of left atrial hypertension

Adapted from Bernard GR, Artigas A, Brigham KL, et al. The American–European Concensus Conference on ARDS: definitions, mechanisms, relevant outcomes, and clinical trial coordination. *Am J Respir Crit Care Med* 1994;149:818.
[a] Regardless of level of positive end-expiratory pressure.
[b] Pulmonary artery occlusion pressure.
[c] ALI, acute lung injury; ARDS, acute respiratory distress syndrome.

ARDS may also have the same findings. Although they may be pathogenetically important, these findings are not yet helpful clinically in predicting the course or outcome of ARDS.

ARDS may develop as a part of the fat embolism syndrome after long-bone fractures. Fat embolism syndrome is characterized by mental status changes, conjunctival and axillary petechiae, anemia, thrombocytopenia, and diffuse lung injury with hypoxemia occurring 24 to 72 hours after injury. The pathogenesis has not been clearly elucidated but is believed to involve the release of toxic free fatty acids from bone marrow fat after trauma. ALI follows long-bone fractures in 5% to 10% of patients. The incidence of full-blown fat embolism syndrome has declined dramatically in recent years, however, presumably because of earlier stabilization of fractures.

Occasionally, a patient develops ARDS without recognition of any of the processes known to be associated with the syndrome. This occurs in 5% to 10% of the ARDS patients we see. If other processes in the differential diagnosis have been excluded, the patient still should be considered to have ARDS. In such patients, a careful search for precipitating causes of the syndrome should be undertaken. This especially includes ruling out occult sources of sepsis such as intra-abdominal abscess. BAL may be helpful as well to rule out unusual pathogens, acute eosinophilic pneumonia, and other intrinsic pulmonary processes such as severe hypersensitivity pneumonitis, bronchiolitis obliterans–organizing pneumonia, and diffuse pulmonary hemorrhage syndromes.

The term ARDS is used because it denotes a common syndrome despite multiple etiologic factors or associated illnesses. It implies similar if not identical pathophysiologic processes. Whether or not this is true is unclear. The etiologies of ARDS can be grouped into direct (primary) and indirect (secondary) causes of lung injury (Table 357.1). Indirect lung injury is believed to develop after an extrapulmonary process leads to systemic inflammation and blood-borne inflammatory mediators that secondarily cause injury to pulmonary capillary endothelial cells. This vascular injury then leads to interstitial and alveolar epithelial injury. Primary or direct lung injury develops in the opposite sequence, with alveolar inflammation and injury progressing to capillary injury. There is some evidence that primary and secondary lung injury respond differently to clinical interventions such as administration of positive end-expiratory pressure (PEEP) and prone positioning. More work needs to be done, however, before different strategies of care for ARDS of different causes can be recommended. Moreover, it may be difficult to distinguish between diffuse lung inflammation due to diffuse pneumonia with generalized involvement of the lung by microorganisms (direct injury) and a localized pneumonia that leads to sepsis with resultant widespread intravascular (indirect) injury.

Hantavirus pulmonary syndrome (HPS), a viral disease first described in 1993, is a unique cause of severe acute respiratory failure. The virus is thought to be transmitted by aerosols of the infected feces and urine of the deer mouse. This syndrome is discussed in Chapter 308. Signs and symptoms of HPS include fever, hypotension secondary to profound volume depletion from increased vascular permeability and third-spacing of fluids,

thrombocytopenia, neutrophilia, and increased hematocrit (secondary to volume depletion). As the illness progresses, dyspnea, pleuritic chest pain, hemoptysis, and diffuse rales develop rapidly. Respiratory failure results from the accumulation of highly proteinaceous noncardiogenic edema in the lungs. The chest radiograph reveals diffuse alveolar infiltrates. The reported case fatality rate is approximately 60%. Autopsy studies have revealed diffuse alveolar damage with edema, hyaline membranes, and a marked, mononuclear, interstitial inflammatory infiltrate. Unlike ARDS, polymorphonuclear leukocytes are generally not seen.

Because of the unique clinical syndrome, viral cause and pathologic picture (lack of polymorphonuclear leukocytes), it is not clear as to whether HPS should be considered to be ARDS. However, HPS is a cause of ALI with noncardiogenic pulmonary edema secondary to epithelial and endothelial lung injury and is associated with a high mortality. Treatment consists of aggressive supportive care. For these reasons, as with diffuse infection, HPS is similar to ARDS, hence its inclusion in this chapter.

High-altitude pulmonary edema (HAPE) has been established as an increased permeability form of pulmonary edema, but the constituents of alveolar fluid obtained by BAL and the pathologic factors differ from those of other forms of ARDS. The time course after therapy also varies. Therefore, HAPE is not considered a classic form of ARDS. One possible difference is that HAPE is associated with less surfactant abnormality and thus with less extensive diffuse microatelectasis.

PATHOPHYSIOLOGIC FACTORS

PHYSIOLOGIC CHANGES

The physiologic abnormalities associated with ARDS include impaired gas exchange, altered lung mechanics, and pulmonary vascular changes. Hypoxemia is seen early in the course and is believed to be caused by intrapulmonary venoarterial shunting due to alveolar flooding and collapse. These phenomena, along with septal edema and fibrosis, lead to a reduction in lung compliance, low functional residual capacity, and increased work of breathing. The loss of microvasculature in the later stages of ARDS leads to pulmonary hypertension and increased dead space with impaired carbon dioxide elimination, even while oxygenation may be improving.

STRUCTURAL CHANGES

The histologic changes in the lung that characterize ARDS represent a relatively nonspecific response to injury and have been termed *diffuse alveolar damage* by pathologists. These changes are found in other disease processes, such as fibrosing alveolitis or drug-induced pulmonary disease, and the pattern shows little variability, even among cases of ARDS associated with widely divergent causes. Inflammatory cells, especially neutrophils, accumulate within the alveolar space and are believed to contribute to the lung injury by releasing of granular enzymes and oxidants. Type I alveolar epithelial cells appear to be the most susceptible to injury, undergoing cytopathic changes extremely early, with resultant damage to the alveolar basement membrane. Pulmonary vascular endothelial cells are also affected, although the histologic changes are less striking and occur more slowly. Endothelial and epithelial cells undergo changes in permeability, allowing interstitial and alveolar edema to develop. Hyaline membranes, identical to those seen in premature infants with respiratory distress syndrome, are caused by the aggregation of fibrin and other proteins in the alveolar space. Alveolar flooding occurs, accompanied by distortion of the alveoli by septal edema and impairment of surfactant function with the loss of functional lung units through microatelectasis. These phenomena lead to hypoxemia as well as to abnormalities in lung mechanics (low lung compliance and reduced functional residual capacity).

As the process continues, there is loss of pulmonary microvasculature, intravascular thrombosis, and distortion of septal architecture due to fibrosis. Vascular damage is believed to be responsible for pulmonary hypertension, increased dead-space ventilation, and a reduction in carbon monoxide diffusing capacity.

Lung scarring is well documented in patients with ARDS and appears to be associated with both fibroblast proliferation and increased collagen synthesis. Increased amounts of lung collagen have been documented as early as a few days after the onset of ARDS. The regulation of collagen deposition appears to be a dynamic process, as evidenced by a shift from predominantly type III collagen in the earlier stages to type I collagen in the later stages of ARDS. The recovery of normal lung function in many survivors of ARDS has been taken as evidence that pulmonary fibrosis complicating ARDS is not necessarily permanent. Studies have correlated the degree of the fibrotic response in the lung with mortality.

PATHOGENESIS OF LUNG INJURY

Pulmonary inflammation is a prominent feature of ARDS, and inflammatory cells and biochemical markers have been implicated in the lung injury process, much as they have in arthritis and other diseases. Neutrophils are found in the lungs of ARDS patients, and investigators have also found evidence that toxic neutrophil products have been released into the alveolar space. Although prior depletion of neutrophils in experimental animals has led to amelioration of the lung injury induced by certain stimuli, there are many clinical reports of patients with profound neutropenia who have developed ARDS. Neutrophils may not be required for the development of lung injury, but they appear to represent at least one major mechanism by which tissue damage is initiated or amplified during ARDS.

Although attention has been focused on neutrophil-derived oxygen radicals and proteolytic enzymes, other inflammatory pathways and other cell types may also be involved. Proteins in the complement cascade, kinin system, and coagulation system are susceptible to the action of proteases, generating products with proinflammatory activity. Phospholipase products, including platelet-activating factor, prostaglandins, and lipoxygenase products of arachidonic acid, have also been studied as potential mediators of lung inflammation. The potential role of free fatty acids in the pathogenesis of lung injury after long-bone fractures

has been mentioned previously. Tumor necrosis factor and other cytokines (e.g., interleukins 1 and 8) may be important intermediates, particularly in cases of ARDS associated with sepsis. In addition, the lipopolysaccharide molecule itself appears to have direct cytotoxic effects, along with a multitude of actions mediated indirectly through the activation or priming of inflammatory cells.

◼ THERAPY

GOALS

The therapy for ARDS is primarily supportive. However, there is strong evidence that traditional approaches to mechanical ventilation may contribute to and propagate both pulmonary and systemic inflammation. Therefore, therapy is directed at the correction of physiologic abnormalities presenting a threat to life or organ function while simultaneously minimizing the risk of ventilator-associated lung injury (VALI). Although some patients respond to oxygen therapy alone, mechanical ventilation is usually required, along with PEEP. Newer modes of mechanical ventilation offer an alternative when conventional therapy is inadequate or associated with complications. Fluid management must balance the need for adequate cardiac output and prevention of renal failure against the potential for exacerbation of pulmonary edema.

Therapeutic controversies include the following:

- The level of FIO_2 that is nontoxic to the lung
- The risk/benefit ratio of higher PEEP and lower FIO_2 versus lower PEEP and higher FIO_2
- The risk/benefit ratio of high PEEP with maintenance of cardiac output by volume administration or vasoactive agents
- The preferred mode of mechanical ventilation
- The philosophy of fluid management (whether to "dry out" the patient and run the risk of increased lung water)
- The use of colloid versus crystalloid solutions in fluid management

VENTILATORY MANAGEMENT
Oxygen Therapy and Mechanical Ventilation

The major physiologic abnormality in ARDS is hypoxemia due to intrapulmonary shunt. The work of breathing is increased by reduced lung compliance and by the increased minute ventilation requirement imposed by the associated hypermetabolic state and increase in physiologic dead space. These factors contribute to patient discomfort and may further impair oxygenation by increasing oxygen consumption. The majority of patients with ARDS require tracheal intubation and mechanical ventilation either to overcome hypoxemia or to alleviate ventilatory failure due to excessive work of breathing. Although supplemental oxygen therapy alone is rarely adequate, the application of continuous positive airway pressure (CPAP) through a tight-fitting mask is sometimes sufficient to improve both oxygenation and comfort.

High concentrations of oxygen can be injurious to the lung,

potentially intensifying ARDS. Although an FIO_2 of 0.8 or higher has been demonstrated to cause direct injury to lung tissue, there is no clear agreement as to what level of FIO_2 is nontoxic. In general, the lowest FIO_2 achieving adequate oxygenation (generally, an arterial oxygen saturation less than or equal to 88% to 90%), should be used. Administration of PEEP can improve arterial oxygenation and allow a reduction in FIO_2. PEEP may also play a role in protecting against VALI, as discussed below.

Until recently it was conventional to use tidal volumes of 10 to 15 mL per kilogram in persons with ARDS. A body of evidence now strongly suggests that conventional ventilatory techniques can worsen lung injury in previously injured lungs. Two mechanisms have been identified as the cause of VALI: (a) overdistention of alveoli from the use of high VT; and 2) cyclical opening and closure of alveoli with each breath that creates shear forces on alveolar epithelium. This theory arose from animal model studies in the 1970s and 1980s but the evidence was largely ignored as irrelevant by clinicians. Recent human studies now suggest that VALI is a clinically relevant process that can contribute to lung and systemic inflammation and patient mortality.

The clinical evidence began with uncontrolled reports of small VT ventilation (5 to 6 mL per kilogram) with permissive hypercapnia. These case series reported remarkable survival rates and were followed by a relatively small randomized controlled trial in which reducing VT as part of a "lung-protective" mechanical ventilation strategy decreased 28-day mortality but not hospital discharge mortality. Other studies in which the VT was limited were disappointingly negative.

The recently completed large randomized controlled trial conducted by the NIH/NHLBI ARDS Clinical Trials Network now provides strong evidence that VALI is likely to occur in humans. That study compared 6 mL per kilogram tidal volume to 12 mL per kilogram and was stopped early for efficacy with a significant survival benefit in the low tidal volume group. Patients enrolled in the study were placed on volume-controlled ventilation in the assist/control (A/C) mode (Table 357.3). Their ideal body weights (IBWs) were calculated and their tidal volumes were set at either 12 mL per kilogram IBW or 8 mL per kilogram IBW. The VT was then reduced in the small-VT group by 1 mL per kilogram increments over 4 hours to 6 mL per kilogram IBW. If the plateau pressure (inspiratory hold pressure) exceeded 30 cm H_2O in the 6 mL per kilogram group, the VT could be reduced further to a minimum of 4 mL per kilogram IBW. Hypercapnia and respiratory acidosis were tolerated, but if the pH dropped to less than 7.15 despite sodium bicarbonate infusion, the VT could be increased. The mortality in the 12 mL per kilogram group was 40%, and this was reduced to 30% in the 6 mL per kilogram group—a difference that is both clinically and statistically significant.

In addition to VT, another major clinical decision includes the mode of ventilation to be used. The conventional approach has been to use volume-controlled ventilation in either the A/C mode, as in the NIH trial, or the intermittent mandatory ventilation (IMV) mode. One advantage of the A/C mode is that if minute ventilation requirements increase (e.g., due to fever, sepsis, or changes in dead-space ventilation), the patient

TABLE 357.3.	INITIAL VENTILATOR SETUP AND ADJUSTMENT

Calculate ideal body weight (IBW)
- Male IBW = 50 + 2.3 [height (in.) − 60]
- Female IBW = 45.5 + 2.3 [height (in.) − 60]

Select assist–control mode

Set initial V_T to 8 mL/kg IBW

Reduce V_T by 1 mL/kg at intervals ≤2 hours until V_T = 6 mL/kg IBW

Set initial respiratory rate to approximate baseline minute ventilation (maximum rate ≤35 beats/min)

Set inspiratory flow rate above patient demand (usually >80 L/min)

Adjust respiratory rate and V_T to achieve pH and plateau pressure (P_{PLAT}) goals
- If P_{PLAT} >30 cm H_2O: decrease V_T by 1 mL/kg (minimum = 4 mL/kg)
- pH goal: 7.30–7.45
- If pH 7.15–7.30, increase RR
- If pH <7.15, consider $NaHCO_3$ or increase V_T in 1 mL/kg increments until pH >7.15

(Adapted from the NIH/NHLB1 ARDS Clinical Trials Network Respiratory Management of ARDS Study protocol.)

will be able to meet them by triggering the machine at a higher rate. The A/C mode is theoretically associated with a lower work of breathing, although some patients continue to perform inspiratory work even during ventilator-assisted breathing. The A/C mode, though, can lead to air trapping and auto-PEEP, and on some ventilators the inspiratory flow rate can be slow at low respiratory rates. In these instances, other modes of ventilation, such as IMV, may be advantageous. Some authors and clinicians recommend the use of pressure-controlled ventilation (PC) in ARDS patients, but no mode of mechanical ventilation when used properly has been proven to decrease mortality in ARDS. Given the data provided by the NIH trial, we recommend A/C as the mode of choice and only use another mode if there are strong specific indications in an individual case. Because of potential adverse effects, other modes, such as inverse ratio ventilation (IRV) or airway pressure release ventilation (APRV), should be applied only with careful monitoring by experienced personnel.

Positive End-Expiratory Pressure

PEEP remains a mainstay of ventilatory management in patients with ARDS. The beneficial effect of PEEP on arterial ozygenation in ARDS, allowing a reduction in the FIO_2 thus potentially reducing the risk of oxygen toxicity, was reported when the syndrome was first described clearly in 1967. The improvement in arterial PaO_2 with PEEP is associated with an increase in lung volume, measured as functional residual capacity, which results from either opening of previously collapsed lung units or increasing the size of some acini such that the volume of edema fluid present no longer totally fills the acinus, thus making some portion available for gas exchange. PEEP does not decrease extravascular lung water, in fact, total lung water may increase with PEEP.

Achieving the "optimal level of PEEP"—the level that best balances potential benefits with potential risks—has been an elusive goal. The major risk of PEEP is a reduction in cardiac output mediated primarily through a decrease in venous return related to the increase in intrathoracic pressure. It has not been clearly demonstrated that PEEP is associated with an increased risk of pneumothorax. Although improvement in oxygenation and reduction in the F_{IO_2} appears to be a desirable goal, choosing the best PEEP is limited by our incomplete knowledge on the risk of oxygen toxicity in patients with lung injury. Animal model studies suggest that prior lung injury may produce tolerance to the toxic tissue effects of high levels of inspired oxygen; whether this is true in humans with ARDS is unknown. Of course, the ultimate desired benefit is a reduction in mortality in these patients, a goal that has not yet been clearly demonstrated in a large controlled trial with any particular PEEP strategy.

Animal model studies have demonstrated that PEEP has a protective effect against VALI. The lungs of animals ventilated with high tidal volumes but with PEEP show considerably less injury than the lungs of animals given the same high tidal volumes but without PEEP. It is hypothesized that PEEP prevents the cyclical opening and closing of alveoli, which can lead to a stress injury of the alveolar wall and thus diffuse lung injury. A strategy for choosing a level of PEEP to prevent this cyclical opening and closing has been suggested—that of measuring a pressure–volume curve of the respiratory system in a patient with ARDS. As the lung volume is increased, a deflection is seen from a relatively flat slope where an increase in pressure results in very little change in volume to a much steeper slope where pressure and volume increase proportionally. One relatively small two-center study found that utilizing a PEEP level 2 cm H_2O above this so-called lower inflection point combined with limiting tidal volume (6 mL per kilogram) compared to much lower PEEP values and more traditional tidal volumes resulted in improved 28-day mortality. Although we find the theoretical basis for this strategy compelling, confirmation of a beneficial outcome in a large multicenter trial is needed before the results can be generalized to a wide variety of patients with ARDS and before we can recommend its routine use. In the meantime, we continue to favor selection of a PEEP level from data obtained in a PEEP trial. In such a trial, PEEP is increased in increments at relatively short (15 to 30 minutes) intervals with measurement of arterial blood gases and hemodynamics. A PEEP level is then selected that incorporates the bias of the clinician regarding available data, the severity of the ARDS, the F_{IO_2} required, and the hemodynamic status. The detrimental effect of PEEP on cardiac output is sensitive to the intravascular volume status. If blood pressure falls (or if cardiac output drops when a pulmonary artery catheter is in place) before a PEEP level is reached that achieves the oxygenation goals or would be likely to prevent considerable areas of lung from cyclical collapse and reopening, then intravascular volume can be increased and the PEEP trial repeated.

PHARMACOLOGIC THERAPY

Corticosteroid therapy has been widely used in the treatment of respiratory failure, but well-controlled clinical trials have failed to demonstrate any clear benefit either in the early treatment or in the prevention of ARDS. Randomized controlled trials have also failed to confirm a previous report suggesting a beneficial effect of large-dose corticosteroids in sepsis. Four small uncontrolled series and one small randomized trial of methylprednisolone therapy in nonresolving, late-phase (more than 7 days' duration) ARDS suggested possible benefit. This treatment carries with it potential harm with an increased risk of infection, hyperglycemia, and prolonged neuromuscular weakness. A large-scale, well-controlled clinical trial is now under way. Currently, the routine use of corticosteroids is not recommended in patients with ARDS. Recent randomized controlled trials of stress dose hydrocortisone (e.g., 100 mg t.i.d., a considerably lower dose than used in most previous sepsis trials) in patients with sepsis and hypotension requiring vasopressors have suggested a mortality benefit compared to placebo. These trials have been relatively small and require confirmation in a large multicenter trial.

Prostaglandin E_1 is a vasodilator with anti-inflammatory properties that lowers pulmonary artery pressures and increases cardiac output in ARDS. Because the drug is 95% metabolized during a single pass through the lung, vasodilatation of the systemic vasculature is usually minimal. Despite an earlier report of improved survival in ARDS patients treated with prostaglandin E_1, a subsequent multicenter controlled trial showed no reduction in ARDS severity, duration, or mortality. Other modulators of the inflammatory response, including ketoconazole, lisophylline, pentoxifylline, ibuprofen, antioxidants, and antibodies directed against endotoxin, complement fragments, and tumor necrosis factor, have been studied without evidence of benefit. Surfactant replacement, so successful in infant respiratory distress syndrome, is also being evaluated in ARDS. Nitric oxide, an inhaled selective pulmonary vasodilator, is being studied as a means to improve gas exchange. It has been shown to improve oxygenation and reduce pulmonary artery pressures in ARDS, but no survival benefit has yet been demonstrated in a controlled clinical trial. So far, none of these therapies can be recommended for the routine treatment of ARDS.

COURSE, OUTCOME, AND COMPLICATIONS

Once a patient develops ARDS, the course is variable, lasting from a few days to several months. The average duration of mechanical ventilation is approximately 10 to 12 days, and about 10% to 20% of patients remain ventilator-dependent for longer than 3 weeks. Even in patients who resolve their underlying illness or injury and respond readily to supportive therapy, the course usually lasts several days, in contrast to patients with cardiogenic pulmonary edema, who typically respond to therapy much more rapidly, improving in a few hours or at most in 1 to 2 days. The primary determinants of outcome appear to be age, underlying disease process, degree of the fibrotic response, prevention of VALI by an appropriate ventilation strategy, and development of complications, especially infection and multiple organ dysfunction.

One-third of the deaths in ARDS patients are related to the underlying disease or injury; that is, death is caused by events occurring before the onset of ARDS. The remaining two-thirds of ARDS deaths are due to complications that have their onset either coincident with or after ARDS onset. Only about 15% of nonsurvivors die a respiratory death (i.e., due to hypoxemia or respiratory acidosis that is refractory to treatment).

Three-fourths of those who die of complications have clinical evidence of sepsis syndrome (septic shock) and associated multiple organ system failure. The specific cause of death may vary, but sepsis syndrome and extrapulmonary organ system failure seem to be the common link. Although these patients do not die a respiratory death, most of them still meet the criteria for respiratory failure at the time of death. The exact process leading to death in these patients is unknown.

Sepsis syndrome is much more common in patients with ARDS than in critically ill patients who do not have respiratory failure, even when differences in duration of endotracheal intubation and mechanical ventilation are considered. This may reflect a higher incidence of nosocomial lung infection due to disturbances in local defense mechanisms, or significant defects in systemic cellular and humoral immune function associated with the syndrome. Sepsis syndrome does not always have an infectious cause; the systemic manifestations of pulmonary inflammation can produce the sepsis syndrome. This may explain why, in one series, outcome in patients with ARDS with infectious complications was not influenced by whether appropriate antibiotic therapy had been administered. Nevertheless, a careful search for infectious foci is always warranted.

Another significant complication in patients with ARDS is pulmonary barotrauma with resultant pneumothorax. Although the term *barotrauma* implies that this complication is caused by high pressures in the lung, other factors are probably operative as well. The incidence of barotrauma has been correlated with the level of peak airway pressure and to the use of large V_T values in mechanically ventilated patients. The pathogenesis probably involves overdistention of lung regions that have already been structurally weakened by alveolar inflammation. Subsequent alveolar rupture leads to the tracking of gas along bronchial and vascular bundles into the mediastinum. The continued air leakage may result in further soft-tissue dissection into retroperitoneal and subcutaneous tissues, or the accumulated mediastinal emphysema may rupture across the thin mediastinal pleura, causing pneumothorax. In patients on positive-pressure ventilation, immediate placement of a chest tube is essential to avoid the life-threatening complications of a tension pneumothorax.

Patients can and do survive prolonged courses of ARDS, even when complicated by sepsis, barotrauma, and pulmonary fibrosis. The recently described decline in mortality speaks to the importance of supportive care, including the use of lung-protective mechanical ventilation strategies, and prevention and treatment of complications. Advances in specific therapies may lead to a further decline in mortality.

BIBLIOGRAPHY

Amato MB, Barbas CSV, Medeiros DN, et al. Effect of a lung-protection approach on mortality in the acute respiratory distress syndrome. *N Engl J Med* 1998;338:347–354.

Bernard GR, Artigas A, Brigham KL, et al. The American–European Consensus Conference on ARDS: definitions, mechanisms, relevant outcomes, and clinical trial coordination. *Am J Respir Crit Care Med* 1994; 149:818–824.

Hudson LD. New therapies for ARDS. *Chest* 1995;108(Suppl):79S–91S.

Hudson LD, Milberg JA, Anardi D, et al. Clinical risks for development of ARDS. *Am J Respir Crit Care Med* 1995;151:293–301.

Hudson LD, Steinberg KP. Epidemiology of acute lung injury and ARDS. *Chest* 1999;116:74S–82S.

Kollef MH, Schuster DP. The acute respiratory distress syndrome. *N Engl J Med* 1995;332:27–37.

Milberg JA, Davis DR, Steinberg KP, et al. Improved survival of patients with ARDS, 1983–1993. *JAMA* 1995;273:306–309.

Meduri GU, Headley AS, Golden E, et al. Effect of prolonged methylprednisolone therapy in unresolving acute respiratory distress syndrome: a randomized controlled trial. *JAMA* 1998;280:159–165.

National Institutes of Health. National Heart, Lung and Blood Institute ARDS Clinical Trials Network: www.hedwig.mgh.harvard.edu.

Ranieri VM, Suter PM, Tortorella C. Effect of mechanical ventilation on inflammatory mediators in patients with acute respiratory distress syndrome: a randomized controlled trial. *JAMA* 1999;282:54–61.

Kelley's Textbook of Internal Medicine, fourth edition. Edited by H. David Humes. Lippincott Williams & Wilkins, Philadelphia © 2000.

CHAPTER
358

APPROACH TO THE PATIENT WITH PLEURAL DISEASE

STEVEN A. SAHN
JOHN E. HEFFNER

▮ PLEURISY

Pleurisy denotes inflammation of the pleura with or without pleural effusion. Pleurisy can result from direct trauma to the chest wall, but it most commonly occurs from extension of localized disease of the lung (pneumonia), mediastinum (esophageal rupture), pericardium (pericarditis), or abdomen (subphrenic abscess), or from systemic disease (lupus erythematosus). Patients who present with pleurisy usually have an associated pleural effusion; the presence or absence of pleural fluid may be a helpful differential finding. For example, viral pleurisy, rheumatoid pleurisy, and sarcoid involvement of the pleura often lack pleural effusions, whereas bacterial pneumonia, lupus pleuritis, and postcardiac injury syndrome usually have associated pleural fluid.

PATHOPHYSIOLOGY

A scant nerve supply exists in the lung distal to the bronchi, primarily composed of efferent twigs of sympathetic and vagal origin. Therefore, stimulation of the visceral pleura and lung usually does not produce pain. The parietal pleura, in contrast, is a highly sensitive surface, supplied extensively with sensory afferents from intercostal, sympathetic, phrenic, and vagus nerves.

Injury to the costal parietal pleura produces sharp, localized pain at the site of irritation. Inflammation of the peripheral diaphragmatic pleura also results in localized pain but tends to extend over a greater area of the chest wall, back, or abdomen. The area of perceived pain expands in relation to the intensity of the injury. Irritation of the central portion of the diaphragmatic pleura does not elicit pain in the immediate area but results in referred pain to the ipsilateral posterior neck, shoulder, and trapezius muscle. Stimulation of the mediastinal parietal pleura over the pericardium also may result in pain referred to the neck. This referred pain results because most of the sensory fibers of the phrenic nerve enter at the C4 level of the spinal cord, the usual entry point of sensation from the shoulder.

CLINICAL FEATURES

The patient with pleurisy complains of pain on breathing that may be minimal or severe, depending on the degree of inflammation. The patient may describe the chest pain as stabbing or shooting, or as a stitch in the side. It is exacerbated by deep breathing, coughing, sneezing, or even talking. Pleuritic pain may be relieved by manual pressure against the chest wall that causes splinting. However, this maneuver does not differentiate pleural inflammation from other causes of pleuritic-like pain caused by rib fractures, myositis, or neuritis, which also can respond to a diminution in chest wall motion.

The pain of costal pleural inflammation is located directly over the site of irritation, with associated tenderness to deep palpation. Cutaneous hypersensitivity and abdominal pain are notably absent. In contrast, irritation of the lateral anterior and portions of the posterior diaphragmatic pleura results in a more diffuse area of pain over the lower thorax, back, and abdomen, accompanied by cutaneous hyperesthesia, exacerbation by pressure, and muscle rigidity. The neck and shoulder pain from irritation of the central diaphragmatic pleura is associated with tenderness, hyperesthesia, hyperalgesia, and muscle spasm.

Dyspnea, a common complaint, results partially from the voluntary and involuntary restriction in respiration imposed by the pain. An accompanying large pleural effusion, pneumonia, or other underlying lung disease may aggravate shortness of breath. Other presenting symptoms depend on the cause of the pleurisy. For example, a shaking chill, fever, and purulent sputum suggest bacterial pneumonia as the cause of the pleurisy, whereas isolated acute pleuritic pain and dyspnea may indicate spontaneous pneumothorax.

The patient generally has shallow and rapid breathing and ipsilateral restriction of chest wall motion, and often lies on the affected side to limit chest expansion. Palpation verifies the limited ipsilateral movement of the hemithorax and rarely demonstrates a friction rub. The percussion note may be flat owing to underlying consolidation or pleural effusion; fremitus may be increased or diminished, depending on the presence or absence of consolidation.

A pleural friction rub confirms the diagnosis of pleurisy. The succinct description by Hippocrates that in pneumonia "the lung . . . squeaks like a leather strap" is difficult to improve on.

A pleural friction rub, which is often evanescent, can vary in intensity from a faint scratchy sound to a loud creak that is appreciated close to the ear. The presence of pleural fluid may modify or abolish the pleural rub. A pleural friction rub usually is audible during both phases of respiration but is best heard at or near the end of inspiration; the rub disappears with breath holding, in contrast to a pericardial rub. The pleural friction rub may be localized or heard over a wide area, and is most frequently appreciated over the lateral and posterior regions of the inferior thorax. It is rarely heard over the upper thorax and apex because of limited movement of the lung in the apexes relative to the bases. In the patient with acute pleurisy, splinting diminishes the friction rub; only when the patient is encouraged to take a deep breath is the rub "discovered" by the clinician.

The clinician may hear a false friction rub if the stethoscope is allowed to slide over the skin; firm pressure eliminates this problem and increases the intensity of the rub. It is sometimes difficult to differentiate crackles from a friction rub; cough may diminish or ablate crackles but has no effect on the rub.

DIFFERENTIAL DIAGNOSIS

The symptoms associated with pleurisy are nonspecific, and the documentation of a pleural friction rub simply confirms pleural inflammation. The remaining history, physical findings, and pertinent laboratory tests enable the clinician to narrow the differential diagnosis of pleurisy (Table 358.1). The history may suggest empyema (alcoholism, loss of consciousness 10 days previously, fever), pulmonary embolism (recent leg fracture with cast, acute onset of dyspnea), postcardiac injury syndrome (myocardial infarction 2 weeks previously, fever, dyspnea), or asbestos pleurisy (shipyard worker for the past 15 years). A history of vomiting, retching, and chest or upper abdominal pain should raise the possibility of esophageal rupture. A known diagnosis of systemic lupus erythematosus or a history of taking drugs (procainamide, hydralazine, quinidine, phenytoin) associated with the lupus syndrome, sarcoidosis, rheumatoid disease, or uremia should alert the clinician to a potential cause of pleurisy. Drugs such as nitrofurantoin, methysergide, methotrexate, and procarbazine have been associated with pleurisy.

An elevated leukocyte count with a shift to the left suggests a bacterial infection such as pneumonia, subphrenic abscess, esophageal rupture (mediastinitis and empyema), hepatic or splenic abscess, or severe inflammation (pancreatitis). Leukopenia may be seen with viral pleurisy or systemic lupus erythematosus.

The chest radiograph may establish the diagnosis of pneumothorax or suggest bacterial pneumonia (lobar consolidation with effusion), esophageal rupture (left hydropneumothorax with mediastinal and subcutaneous emphysema), or pathologic process originating below the diaphragm (subphrenic abscess: elevated hemidiaphragm, small effusion, air-fluid level below the diaphragm).

Pleural fluid analysis is the most helpful diagnostic test in establishing the presumptive or definitive diagnosis in most cases of pleurisy (Table 358.2). Thoracentesis should be performed as soon as the presence of a pleural effusion is documented by

| **TABLE 358.1.** | **CLINICAL FEATURES OF COMMON DISEASES THAT CAUSE PLEURISY** | | | |

Diagnosis	Clinical Findings	Chest Radiograph	Pleural Fluid Characteristics	Course
Infection				
Viral pleurisy	Abrupt pleuritic pain, constitutional symptoms; WBC <10,000/μL	Small pleural effusion (10%–20%); infiltrate (20%)	Serous exudate, low nucleated cells, PMNs, or mononuclears	Effusions transient; pleuritic pain may persist for several days
Bacterial pneumonia	Acute pleuritic pain (60%), fever, chills, purulent sputum; WBC >15,000/μL	Alveolar opacities; small to large free-flowing or loculated effusion	PMN-predominant exudate, nucleated cells >10,000/μL; may evolve into empyema ($\downarrow$ pH, $\downarrow$ glucose, $\uparrow$ LDH)	Effusion resolves in 2–8 wk with antibiotics; empyema requires drainage, pleuritic pain may be transient but tends to persist longer in empyema
Tuberculous pleurisy	Abrupt or insidious onset; cough, pleuritic pain (75%), fever; pleuritic pain precedes cough; friction rub unusual	Small to moderate unilateral pleural effusion; coexisting parenchymal disease (33%)	Serous exudate (protein >5 g/dL); nucleated cells <5,000/μL; 80%–90% lymphocytes; acute—may be PMN-predominant; >5% mesothelial cells or eosinophilia makes TB unlikely; low glucose and pH (20%)	Pleuritic pain resolves in days; effusion resolves in 2–4 mo with or without treatment
Esophageal rupture	Vomiting, severe chest pain, fever, hematemesis, dyspnea, subcutaneous emphysema	Left pleural effusion; widened mediastinum; mediastinal and subcutaneous air, pneumothorax	Turbid to purulent exudate; $\uparrow$ amylase; pH 6.00; squamous epithelial cells	Anaerobic empyema; contrast study of esophagus confirms diagnosis; early drainage and primary closure has excellent prognosis
Immunologic				
Lupus pleuritis	Known SLE; pleuritic pain (>85%), dyspnea, cough, pleural rub, fever	Unilateral or bilateral small to moderate effusions; alveolar infiltrates; atelectasis	Serous to serosanguineous exudate, nucleated cells 5,000/gmL; PMN-predominant early; pH and glucose low (20%); +LE cells; PF/S ANA > 1	Rapid response (within 2 wk) to corticosteroids
Rheumatoid pleurisy	Males, 6th decade: within 5 y of onset of articular disease; subcutaneous nodules; moderate to severe arthritis, pleuritis pain, dyspnea; asymptomatic chest radiograph finding	Small to moderate unilateral pleural effusion: up to 33% have other manifestations of rheumatoid lung disease	Straw-colored, turbid, "debris": glucose 10 mg/dL, pH 7.00, LDH >1000 IU/L; $\downarrow$ complement; RF $\geq$1:320	Variable; spontaneous resolution over months; recurrences common; dry pleurisy; some develop marked pleural fibrosis
Postcardiac injury syndrome	Pleuritic pain (>90%), fever; pleural and pericardial rub, dyspnea; 3 wk (days to months) after cardiac surgery or myocardial infarction; $\uparrow$ ESR	Small to moderate left or bilateral pleural effusion (85%); alveolar opacities on left	Bloody (70%) exudate; PMN-predominant; normal pH and glucose	Resolves 1–5 wk, spontaneously, or with NSAIDs or corticosteroids
Sarcoidosis	Pleuritic or nonpleuritic chest pain, dyspnea; stage II or III disease	Unilateral, small to moderate pleural effusion; hilar and medastinal adenopathy and interstitial opacities	Straw-colored exudate; low nucleated cells; >90% lymphocytes	Spontaneous resolution or with corticosteroids (1–3 mo); "dry" pleurisy

(continued)

TABLE 358.1. *Continued*

Diagnosis	Clinical Findings	Chest Radiograph	Pleural Fluid Characteristics	Course
Diseases that Originate Below the Diaphragm				
Pancreatitis	Abdominal symptoms, pleuritic pain and dyspnea in alcoholic or biliary tract disease	Small to moderate left pleural effusion; elevated diaphragm and basilar opacities	Serous to bloody exudate; ↑ nucleated cells; PMN-predominant; ↑ amylase, pH 7.30–7.40	Effusion and pleuritic pain resolve as pancreatitis subsides; no resolution in 2 wk, consider abscess or pseudocyst
Subphrenic abscess	After abdominal surgery; chest or abdominal symptoms, pleuritic pain, fever	Unilateral, small to moderate pleural effusion; basilar opacities; elevated diaphragm	Turbid exudate; ↑ nucleated cells, PMN-predominant; pH >7.20; glucose >50 mg/dL	Diagnosis suggested by routine chest or abdominal films; abdominal CT most sensitive; drainage and antibiotics
Other				
Pneumothorax	Young, thin, tall male; COPD, interstitial lung disease; acute chest pain (>90%), may be pleuritic, dyspnea	Detection of visceral pleural line; small effusion (10%)	Sanguineous because of ruptured vessels	Chest pain may be transient but may progress if air leak continues
Pulmonary embolism	Predisposing factor; acute dyspnea, pleuritic pain (>80%), hemoptysis	Small, unilateral effusion present on admission (90%); reaches maximum size by 3 days	Bloody (65%), exudate (75%), bloody, PMN exudate (25%)	Effusion regresses over several days if consolidation not present; resolves slower with consolidation
Benign asbestos pleural effusion	Males, 5th decade; within 20 y of first asbestos exposure; asymptomatic, pleuritic pain (20%), dyspnea	Small to moderate unilateral pleural effusion; other manifestations of asbestos exposure uncommon	Serous to bloody exudate; PMN or mononuclear-predominant; eosinophilia (25% of cases)	Pleural effusion resolves over several months; recurrence ipsilateral or contralateral
Uremic pleural effusion	Fever, chest pain (30%), transient pleural and pericardial friction rub in patient with uremia for months to years	Small to large unilateral pleural effusion; cardiomegaly; minimal pulmonary congestion	Serous to bloody exudate; low nucleated cells, predominantly lymphocytes	Resolves in 4–6 wk with continued dialysis; 20% develop progressive pleural fibrosis

ANA, antinuclear antibody; COPD, chronic obstructive pulmonary disease; CT, computer tomography; ESR, electron spin resonance; LDH, lactate dehydrogenase; LE, lupus erythematosus; NSAID, nonsteroidal anti-inflammatory drug; PF/S, pleural fluid/serum; PMN, polymorphonuclear cell; RF, rheumatoid factor; R/O TB, rules out tuberculosis; SLE, systemic lupus erythematosus. TB, tuberculosis; WBC, white blood cell count.

chest radiograph. Cell counts, protein/lactate dehydrogenase (LDH)/glucose/amylase concentrations, pH, and appropriate cultures should be obtained on most patients who present with pleuritic chest pain. Essentially all patients with pleurisy have exudative effusions. Bloody effusions are suggestive of pulmonary embolism, postcardiac injury syndrome, neoplasm involving the pleura, uremic pleural effusion, pleural endometriosis, or asbestos pleural effusion. Pus aspirated from the pleural space confirms the diagnosis of empyema, either related to pneumonia or from esophageal rupture (anaerobic empyema). An increased pleural fluid amylase (greater than serum amylase) level in the setting of pleurisy is found with acute pancreatitis and esophageal rupture; pleural fluid associated with esophageal rupture has a low pH (often 6.00 or less), whereas that associated with pancreatitis has a pH between 7.30 and 7.40. The pleural fluid nucleated cell count is increased (more than 10,000 per microliter) with a polymorphonuclear predominance in bacterial pneumonia, esophageal rupture, pancreatitis, and subphrenic abscess. A low (less than 5,000 per microliter) nucleated cell count with a lymphocyte predominance usually is observed in tuberculous pleurisy. Causes of pleurisy with pleural effusions of low pH (less than 7.30) and a glucose level below 60 mg per deciliter include empyema, esophageal rupture, rheumatoid pleurisy, lupus pleuritis, and tuberculous pleurisy.

If the cause of the pleurisy remains unclear after pleural fluid analysis, then other appropriate studies should be done. These include a ventilation–perfusion lung scan and possibly angiography if pulmonary embolism is a consideration, a pleural biopsy to diagnose suggested tuberculous pleurisy, a contrast study of the esophagus to confirm a suspected diagnosis of esophageal

TABLE 358.2.	DIAGNOSES THAT CAN BE ESTABLISHED DEFINITIVELY BY PLEURAL FLUID ANALYSIS
Disease	**Diagnostic Pleural Fluid Tests**
Empyema	Observation (pus, putrid odor); culture
Malignancy	Positive cytology
Lupus pleuritis	LE cells present; ANA (pleural fluid/serum ratio >1.0)
Tuberculous pleurisy	Positive AFB stain, culture
Esophageal rupture	High amylase, pleural fluid acidosis (often as low as 6.00)
Fungal pleurisy	Positive KOH stain, culture
Chylothorax	Triglycerides (>110 mg/dL); lipoprotein electrophoresis (chylomicrons)
Hemothorax	Hematocrit (pleural fluid/blood ratio >0.5)
Urinothorax	Creatinine (pleural fluid/serum ratio >1.0)
Peritoneal dialysis	Protein (<1 g/dL), glucose (300–400 mg/dL)
Extravascular migration of a central venous catheter	Observation (milky if lipid is infused); glucose PF/serum >1.0 if glucose is infused
Rheumatoid pleurisy	Characteristic cytologic findings (pH 7.00, glucose 10 mg/dL, LDH 1000 IU/L)

AFB, acid-fast bacillus; ANA, anti-nuclear antibody; LE, lupus erythematosus; PF, pleural fluid.

rupture, or an abdominal computed tomography (CT) scan if subphrenic abscess is a likely possibility.

The treatment and course of pleurisy vary with the underlying disease. Drainage of the pleural space is necessary in postpneumonic empyema and esophageal rupture, and in some patients with pneumothorax. Patients with lupus pleuritis and postcardiac injury syndrome respond rapidly to corticosteroids, whereas many patients with pleuritic pain obtain relief from the nonsteroidal anti-inflammatory drugs. With appropriate and prompt treatment, most patients with pleurisy have successful outcomes, as it is unusual for patients with malignant pleural effusions or mesothelioma to manifest pleuritic chest pain.

■ PLEURAL EFFUSIONS

The clinical recognition of a pleural effusion signifies that an abnormal physiologic state exists whereby there is a dysequilibrium in the formation and removal of pleural fluid. The pleural fluid commonly is the sequela of primary pulmonary disease, but it can also result from disease in an extrapulmonic focus, such as the heart (congestive heart failure), the kidneys (nephrotic syndrome), the liver (cirrhosis), and the pancreas (acute pancreatitis). Pleural effusions also can occur with systemic diseases (systemic lupus erythematosus, yellow-nail syndrome), meta-

static malignancy, and iatrogenic causes such as drug therapy (nitrofurantoin) and extravascular migration of central venous catheters. Therefore, patients with pleural effusions may present not only to the pulmonologist but to the general internist, medical subspecialist, family physician, dermatologist, and surgeon.

VALUE OF PLEURAL FLUID ANALYSIS

The discovery of pleural fluid provides the opportunity to verify the disease, procedure, or drug that has caused the pleural effusion. With thoracentesis at the bedside, the fluid can be rapidly sampled and observed, its constituents examined microscopically, and its cells and biochemistry quantified. A comprehensive and systematic approach to analysis of the fluid in conjunction with the clinical presentation should allow the clinician to diagnose the cause of the pleural effusion in 75% of patients at the initial thoracentesis. A definitive diagnosis, such as finding malignant cells or specific organisms in pleural fluid, can be established only in about 25% of patients, but a presumptive diagnosis, based on the prethoracentesis clinical impression, can be substantiated by pleural fluid analysis in an additional 50% of patients. However, even with a nondiagnostic thoracentesis, pleural fluid analysis is useful in excluding other causes of the pleural effusion, such as infection. Therefore, in 75% of patients, the cause of the effusion can be "diagnosed," and in over 90% of patients clinical decision making–related information can be gained by pleural fluid analysis.

DIAGNOSTIC THORACENTESIS: INDICATIONS, CONTRAINDICATIONS, AND COMPLICATIONS

When a pleural effusion is suspected on physical examination and confirmed radiographically, a diagnostic thoracentesis should be performed in an attempt to establish the cause of the effusion. Instances where observation is warranted, in lieu of thoracentesis, include uncomplicated congestive heart failure and viral pleurisy. In the former the clinical diagnosis is usually secure, and in the latter there is typically only a small amount of fluid. However, if the clinical situation is atypical or does not progress as anticipated, thoracentesis should be performed without delay. When the sampling of pleural fluid is indicated clinically but the volume of the pleural effusion is small on a standard chest radiograph, thoracentesis should be performed under ultrasonographic guidance.

There are no absolute contraindications to diagnostic thoracentesis. Relative contraindications include a bleeding diathesis, anticoagulation, small volume of pleural fluid, mechanical ventilation, and active skin infection. The patient on mechanical ventilation is not at increased risk of pneumothorax from thoracentesis but is more likely to develop tension pneumothorax if the lung is punctured.

Complications of diagnostic thoracentesis include pain at the needle insertion site, bleeding, pneumothorax, empyema, and spleen or liver puncture.

DIAGNOSES THAT CAN BE ESTABLISHED DEFINITIVELY BY PLEURAL FLUID ANALYSIS

The select number of diagnoses that can be established definitively by thoracentesis are shown in Table 358.2. Confirming the diagnosis of chylothorax does not establish its cause but provides evidence that the thoracic duct has been violated; lymphoma is the cause of more than 50% of chylothoraxes. Esophageal rupture is one of two diagnoses (the other is malignancy) that causes a pleural effusion with a high amylase (salivary) concentration and pleural fluid acidosis (pH less than 7.30); the pleural fluid pH usually approaches 6.00 by 48 to 72 hours after rupture as a result of anaerobic empyema. Empyema, tuberculous pleurisy, rheumatoid disease, and lupus pleuritis all can be associated with a low pleural fluid pH (less than 7.30), but the pleural fluid amylase concentration is less than the concomitant serum amylase. In 10% to 14% of patients with malignant effusions, the fluid may be salivary amylase-rich; however, the pleural fluid pH is usually not below 7.05. With extravascular migration of a central venous catheter, the resultant pleural effusion can have characteristics similar to those of the infusate (milky if lipid is being given) and may be hemorrhagic and neutrophil-predominant due to trauma and inflammation. The ratio of pleural fluid to serum glucose exceeds 1.0 if glucose is being infused; however, the pleural fluid glucose level is usually lower than the infusate, as glucose is transported rapidly from the pleural space.

OBSERVATION OF PLEURAL FLUID ASPIRATE

Initial diagnostic clues can be obtained by gross inspection of pleural fluid as it is being aspirated from the patient's chest (Table 358.3). A straw-colored fluid is typical of all transudates and minimally inflammatory effusions that are borderline exudates, as occur with early malignancy, tuberculous pleurisy, and yellow-nail syndrome. A bloody fluid in the absence of trauma suggests malignancy, benign asbestos pleural effusion, postcardiac injury syndrome, or pulmonary infarction. A milky effusion suggests a chylothorax but could be caused by a chyliform effusion (with or without a high cholesterol level) or an empyema. A chylothorax signifies leakage of chyle from the thoracic duct. A pleural fluid triglyceride concentration of more than 110 mg per deciliter signifies a high likelihood of chylothorax, whereas a triglyceride concentration below 50 mg per deciliter makes chylothorax highly unlikely. A nonchylous or chyliform effusion occurs with chronic (an average of 5 years) pleural disease, usually associated with a trapped lung from rheumatoid pleurisy, tuberculous pleurisy, empyema, or the result of pneumothorax therapy for tuberculosis. The diagnosis of a chyliform (cholesterol) effusion can be established by identifying cholesterol crystals on smears of sediment; these rhomboid crystals impart a lustrous sheen to the pleural fluid. To differentiate a chylothorax from a lipid effusion that does not demonstrate cholesterol crystals, or when the triglyceride concentration is between 50 and 110 mg per deciliter, a lipoprotein electrophoresis should be performed to evaluate for the presence of chylomicrons, which is diagnostic of a chylothorax.

When an amebic liver abscess has ruptured into the pleural space, it will produce an anchovy paste–like pleural aspirate that represents a mixture of lysed hepatic tissue cells, small pieces of liver parenchyma, and blood. However, the color may vary from pink to red and pale yellow to dark brown, and it may be mistaken for frank blood. Amebas can be demonstrated in pleural

TABLE 358.3.	OBSERVATIONS OF PLEURAL FLUID HELPFUL IN DIAGNOSIS
Observation	**Suggested Diagnosis**
Color of Fluid	
Pale yellow (straw)	Transudate, some exudates
Red (bloody)	Malignancy, BAPE, PCIS, or pulmonary infarction in absence of trauma
White (milky)	Chylothorax or cholesterol effusion
Brown	Long-standing bloody effusion; amebic liver abscess
Black	*Aspergillus*
Yellow–green	Rheumatoid pleurisy
Color of enteral tube feeding or central venous line infusate	Feeding tube has entered pleural space; extravascular catheter migration
Character of Fluid	
Pus	Empyema
Viscous	Mesothelioma
Debris	Rheumatoid pleurisy
Turbid	Inflammatory exudate or lipid effusion
Anchovy paste	Amebic liver abscess rupture
Odor of Fluid	
Putrid	Anaerobic empyema
Ammonia	Urinothorax

BAPE; benign asbestos pleural effusion; PCIS, postcardiac injury syndrome.

fluid in less than 10% of patients with these right-sided effusions. Patients with rheumatoid pleurisy may have a yellowish green tint to the effusion, or the fluid may appear to contain debris that results from exfoliation of necrotic visceral pleural rheumatoid nodules.

When fluid with the color of the enteral feeding is aspirated from the pleural space, it confirms that the narrow-bore enteral feeding tube has passed through the tracheobronchial tree and into the pleural space. When the pleural fluid is similar to the infusate in the central venous line, extravascular catheter migration, most commonly associated with left-sided catheter placement through the jugular veins, has occurred. A viscous effusion suggests malignant mesothelioma due to the high levels of hyaluronic acid. A putrid odor is diagnostic of an anaerobic empyema; an ammonia smell suggests ipsilateral obstructive uropathy producing a urinothorax.

TRANSUDATES VERSUS EXUDATES

The characterization of pleural fluid as a transudate or an exudate is the next deductive step in pleural fluid analysis after observation of the aspirate. Transudates, due to imbalances in hydrostatic and oncotic pressures in the chest, can also result from movement of fluid from the peritoneal (cirrhosis) or retroperitoneal (urinothorax) spaces or iatrogenic causes, such as crystalloid

TABLE 358.4.	CAUSES OF TRANSUDATIVE PLEURAL EFFUSIONS
Cause	**Comment**
Effusion Virtually Always Transudative	
Congestive heart failure	Acute diuresis can result in pseudoexudate
Cirrhosis	Rare without clinical ascites
Nephrotic syndrome	Usually subpulmonic and bilateral
Peritoneal dialysis	Develops within 48 h of initiating dialysis
Hypoalbuminemia	Edema fluid never isolated to pleural space
Urinothorax	Caused by ipsilateral obstructive uropathy
Atelectasis	Caused by increased intrapleural negative pressure
Constrictive pericarditis	Bilateral effusions, distended neck veins
Trapped lung	Result of remote or chronic inflammation
Superior vena caval obstruction	May be due to acute systemic venous hypertension or acute blockage of thoracic lymph flow
"Classic" Exudates That Can Be Transudates	
Malignancy	Due to early lymphatic obstruction, obstructive atelectasis, or concomitant disease (CHF)
Pulmonary embolism	23% incidence; due to atelectasis
Sarcoidosis	Stage II and III disease
Hypothyroid pleural effusion	Transudates secondary to hypothyroid heart disease

CHF, congestive heart failure.

infusion into an extravascular central line. Nevertheless, transudates have a limited number of diagnostic possibilities that can usually be easily discerned from the clinical presentation (Table 358.4).

In contrast, exudative effusions can be caused by various diseases and present more of a diagnostic dilemma. Exudates result primarily from pleural and lung inflammation (pneumonia) or impaired lymphatic drainage of the pleural space (malignancy) that results in either a capillary protein leak or decreased protein removal from the pleural space, respectively. Exudates can also occur from movement of fluid from the peritoneal space, as seen with acute or chronic pancreatitis, chylous ascites, and peritoneal carcinomatosis. Disease in virtually any organ can cause exudative pleural effusions through various mechanisms, including infection, malignancy, immunologic responses, lymphatic abnormalities, noninfectious inflammation, iatrogenic causes, and movement from below the diaphragm (Table 358.5).

The most practical method of separating transudates and exudates is to measure serum and pleural fluid protein, LDH, and cholesterol concentrations. If at least one of the following criteria is present, the fluid has a high likelihood of being an exudate; if none is present, the fluid has a high likelihood of being a transudate.

Ratio of pleural fluid protein to serum protein more than 0.5

Pleural fluid protein greater than 2.9 g per deciliter

Ratio of pleural fluid LDH to serum LDH more than 0.6

Pleural fluid LDH more than 0.45 of the upper limits of normal of serum LDH

Ratio of pleural fluid cholesterol to serum cholesterol more than 0.3

Pleural fluid cholesterol greater than 45 mg per deciliter

Transudates have characteristic but nondiagnostic cellular and biochemical characteristics that support their noninflammatory pathogenesis. These effusions are usually straw-colored, nonviscous, and odorless. In about 80% of cases, the nucleated cell count is less than 1,000 per microliter; it is rare to find a transudative effusion with a nucleated cell count of above 10,000 per microliter. Eighty-five percent of transudative effusions have red blood cell counts up to 10,000 per microliter, so the clinician cannot exclude a serosanguineous effusion as a transudate.

Transudative effusions are composed primarily of lymphocytes, mesothelial cells, and macrophages. It is unusual for transudates to be neutrophil-predominant; if found, this should suggest a dual diagnosis. A low pleural fluid glucose level (less than 60 mg per deciliter) is not found in transudative effusions (with the exception of urinothorax), and the pleural fluid pH is alkaline and exceeds the simultaneously obtained arterial blood pH, usually in the range of 7.45 to 7.55.

PLEURAL FLUID PROTEINS

Although most transudates have absolute total protein concentrations below 2.9 g per deciliter, acute diuresis in congestive heart failure can elevate protein levels into the exudative range. Tuberculous pleural effusions virtually always have total protein concentrations above 4.0 g per deciliter, although protein concentrations vary widely in parapneumonic effusions and malignant effusions. However, the clinician should consider lymphoproliferative disorders such as Waldenström's macroglobulinemia and multiple myeloma when pleural fluid protein concentrations of 7.0 to 8.0 g per deciliter are discovered. When exudative criteria are met by LDH but not protein measurements, malignancy and parapneumonic effusions should be considered. Very high concentrations of pleural fluid LDH (more than 1,000 IU per liter) are characteristically found with empyema, rheumatoid pleurisy, and paragonimiasis; they are sometimes observed with malignancy and rarely with tuberculosis. Pleural effusions secondary to *Pneumocystis carinii* pneumonia often have a pleural fluid/serum LDH ratio of more than 1.0 and a pleural fluid/serum protein ratio of less than 0.5.

NUCLEATED CELLS

The total pleural fluid nucleated cell count is virtually never diagnostic; however, counts above 50,000 per microliter are usually found only in complicated parapneumonic effusions, which are loculated effusions with positive bacteriology and a low pleural fluid pH (less than 7.30). When the pleural fluid is grossly purulent, the nucleated cell count may be less than antici-

| TABLE 358.5. | CAUSES OF EXUDATIVE PLEURAL EFFUSIONS |

Infectious
Bacterial pneumonia
Tuberculous pleurisy
Parasites
Fungal disease
Atypical pneumonias
Nocardia, Actinomyces
Subphrenic abscess
Hepatic abscess
Splenic abscess
Hepatitis
Spontaneous esophageal rupture

Malignancy
Carcinoma
Lymphoma
Mesothelioma
Leukemia
Chylothorax

Other Inflammatory
Pancreatitis
Benign asbestos pleural effusion
Pulmonary embolism
Radiation therapy
Uremic pleurisy
Sarcoidosis
Postcardiac injury syndrome
Hemothorax
Acute respiratory distress syndrome

Connective Tissue Disease
Lupus pleuritis
Rheumatoid pleurisy
Mixed connective tissue disease
Churg–Strauss syndrome
Wegener's granulomatosis
Familial Mediterranean fever

Iatrogenic
Drug-induced
Esophageal perforation
Esophageal sclerotherapy
Central venous catheter
   misplacement/migration
Enteral feeding tube in pleural space

Lymphatic Abnormalities
Malignancy
Yellow-nail syndrome
Lymphangiomyomatosis

Endocrine Dysfunction
Hypothyroidism
Ovarian hyperstimulation syndrome

Increased Negative Intrapleural Pressure
Atelectasis
Trapped lung
Cholesterol effusion

Movement of Fluid from Abdomen to Pleural Space
Pancreatitis
Pancreatic pseudocyst
Meigs' syndrome
Carcinoma
Chylous ascites
Urinothorax

pated because the neutrophils have undergone lysis; cellular debris, fibrin, and coagulated pleural fluid account for the purulence of the fluid. Exudative pleural effusions from bacterial pneumonia, acute pancreatitis, and lupus pleuritis usually have total nucleated cell counts of more than 10,000 per microliter. Chronic exudates, typified by tuberculous pleurisy and malignancy, usually have nucleated cell counts of below 5,000 per microliter.

The timing of thoracentesis in relation to the acute pleural injury determines the cellular predominance. The early cellular response to pleural injury is neutrophilic. As the time from the acute insult lengthens, the effusion evolves to a mononuclear predominance if pleural injury does not persist or recur. Therefore, in diseases in which the patient presents shortly after the onset of symptoms, such as bacterial pneumonia, pulmonary embolism with infarction, and acute pancreatitis, effusions are usually neutrophil-predominant. Diseases with an insidious onset, such as malignancy and tuberculous pleurisy, usually have lymphocyte-predominant effusions.

Pleural fluid lymphocytosis, particularly with lymphocyte counts of 85% to 95% of the total nucleated cells, suggests tuberculous pleurisy, lymphoma, sarcoidosis, chronic rheumatoid pleurisy, yellow-nail syndrome, chylothorax, or acute lung rejection. Carcinomatous pleural effusions are lymphocyte-pre-dominant in over half of cases, usually in the range of 50% to 70%. As some lymphocytic effusions can be diagnosed by pleural biopsy, an undiagnosed lymphocytic exudate is the most appropriate indication for this procedure. However, the finding of a lymphocyte-predominant transudate is not such an indication.

Pleural fluid eosinophilia (ratio of pleural fluid eosinophils to total nucleated cells greater than 10%) is commonly associated with air or blood in the pleural space (Table 358.6). Pleural fluid eosinophilia is rare with tuberculous pleurisy. The prevalence of malignancy is similar in eosinophilic and noneosinophilic pleural effusions. About a third of patients with eosinophilic pleural effusions are considered "idiopathic"—many of these effusions are probably due to occult pulmonary embolism or benign asbestos pleural effusion. The mechanism for pleural fluid eosinophilia is unknown; however, a common finding in patients with spontaneous pneumothorax is reactive eosinophilic pleuritis. Patients with eosinophilic parapneumonic effusions usually do not become infected, do not develop complicated effusions, and do not require pleural space drainage for resolution. Pleural fluid basophilia (ratio of pleural fluid basophils to total nucleated cells greater than 10%) has been found only with leukemic involvement of the pleura.

Mesothelial cells are found in small numbers in normal pleural fluid. They are prominent in transudative pleural effu-

TABLE 358.6.	PLEURAL FLUID EOSINOPHILIA

Disease	Comment
Pneumothorax	Most common cause of PFE
Hemothorax	May take 1–2 wk for PFE to develop
Benign asbestos pleural effusion	Up to 50%; probably a common cause of idiopathic PFE
Pulmonary embolism	Associated with radiographic infarction and hemorrhagic effusion
Previous thoracentesis	Usually due to pneumothorax or bleeding
Parasitic disease	Paragonimiasis, hydatid disease, amebiasis, ascariasis
Fungal disease	Histoplasmosis, coccidioidomycosis
Drug-induced	Dantrolene, bromocriptine, nitrofurantoin
Lymphoma	Hodgkin's disease
Carcinoma	Not excluded by PFE
Tuberculous pleurisy	Rare

PF, eosinophils/total nucleated PF cells > 10%.
PFE, pleural fluid eosinophilia.

TABLE 358.7.	DIAGNOSES ASSOCIATED WITH PLEURAL FLUID ACIDOSIS (pH < 7.30) AND LOW GLUCOSE CONCENTRATION (PF/S < 0.5)

Diagnosis	Usual pH (Incidence)	Usual Glucose Concentration (mg/dL)
Empyema	5.50–7.29 (~100%)	<40
Esophageal rupture	6.00 (~100% by 48 h)	<60
Rheumatoid pleurisy	7.00 (80%)	0–30
Malignancy	6.95–7.29 (33%)	30–59
Tuberculous pleurisy	7.00–7.29 (20%)	30–59
Lupus pleuritis	7.00–7.29 (20%)	30–59

sions and are variable in exudative effusions. The major clinical significance of mesothelial cells in exudates is that a finding of more than 5% mesothelial cells makes tuberculous pleurisy unlikely. Mesothelial cells may be confused with malignant cells. A paucity of mesothelial cells in pleural fluid is noted with diffuse pleural injury or fibrosis that inhibits exfoliation into the pleural space. In addition to tuberculous pleurisy, this finding is common with empyema, rheumatoid pleurisy, and chronic malignant pleural effusions, and after the use of sclerosing agents.

The pleural fluid macrophage has its origin in the circulating blood monocyte. Its importance in the pleural space may be as a modulator of pleural injury, being called to the pleural space by neutrophil-released chemotaxins. The presence of macrophages is not of diagnostic value, but differentiation from mesothelial cells is important, as the presence of macrophages does not exclude tuberculous pleurisy.

The presence of numerous plasma cells in pleural fluid is suggestive of multiple myeloma with pleural involvement. The presence of few plasma cells in serous fluid is nondiagnostic and has been observed in several nonmalignant diseases.

PLEURAL FLUID GLUCOSE AND PH

A low pleural fluid glucose concentration, defined as a glucose concentration below 60 mg per deciliter or a pleural fluid/serum glucose ratio of below 0.5, narrows the differential diagnosis of the exudate to rheumatoid pleurisy, complicated parapneumonic effusion or empyema, malignant effusion, tuberculous pleurisy, lupus pleuritis, and esophageal rupture (Table 358.7). All transudates and most exudates have pleural fluid glucose concentrations similar to that of blood glucose. The mechanism responsi-

ble for a low pleural fluid glucose level depends on the underlying disease and includes decreased transport of glucose from blood to pleural fluid (rheumatoid pleurisy, malignancy) and increased use by constituents of pleural fluid, namely, neutrophils, bacteria (empyema), and malignant cells. The lowest glucose concentrations are found in rheumatoid pleurisy and empyema, with glucose being undetectable in some cases. When the glucose concentration is low in tuberculous pleurisy, lupus pleuritis, and malignancy, it usually falls in the range of 30 to 50 mg per deciliter.

Pleural fluid for glucose measurement should be placed immediately in a tube containing sodium fluoride to stop glycolysis; failing to do so may falsely decrease the glucose concentration, especially in fluids containing a large number of metabolically active granulocytes. A falsely low glucose effusion can lead the clinician down a confusing diagnostic pathway.

A pleural fluid pH below 7.30 with a normal blood pH is found with the same diagnoses associated with a low pleural fluid glucose concentration (Table 358.7). A pH below 7.30 represents a substantial accumulation of hydrogen ions, as pH in normal pleural fluid is about 7.60 due to a bicarbonate gradient between pleural fluid and blood. Transudates generally have a pleural fluid pH in the range of 7.40 to 7.55; most exudates range from 7.30 to 7.45. Pleural fluid acidosis (pH less than 7.30) has been found with esophageal rupture, empyema, rheumatoid pleurisy, malignancy, tuberculous pleurisy, and lupus pleuritis.

The mechanisms responsible for pleural fluid acidosis include increased acid production by pleural fluid cells and bacteria (empyema, esophageal rupture) and decreased hydrogen ion efflux from the pleural space due to pleuritis, tumor, or pleural fibrosis (malignancy, rheumatoid pleurisy, and tuberculous pleurisy). A low pleural fluid pH has diagnostic, prognostic, and therapeutic implications in parapneumonic and malignant effusions. In parapneumonic effusions, a pH below 7.20, usually in association with a glucose level below 40 mg per deciliter and an LDH level above 1,000 IU per liter, indicates with a high likelihood that pleural space drainage will be necessary to resolve pleural sepsis and prevent pleural fibrosis. When the pleural fluid pH is 7.30 or higher, a parapneumonic effusion usually can be treated with antibiotics alone, directed at the pneumonia. With a malignant pleural effusion, a pH below 7.30 is associated with a poorer survival, a high yield on pleural biopsy and cytology, and less successful chemical pleurodesis. However, the pleural fluid pH should not be the sole criterion for a decision concerning pleurodesis. The general health, functional status, and extent of metastases should be considered. Furthermore, a high percentage of patients with a low pleural fluid pH will have successful pleurodesis.

PLEURAL FLUID AMYLASE

The finding of an amylase-rich pleural effusion, defined as a pleural fluid amylase level greater than the upper limits of normal for serum amylase or a pleural fluid/serum amylase ratio greater than 1.0, narrows the differential diagnosis of the exudative effusion to acute pancreatitis, chronic pancreatic pleural effusion (usually with pseudocyst formation), esophageal rupture, and malignancy. Mechanisms that may be operational in the pathogenesis of a pancreatic pleural effusion include direct contact of pancreatic enzymes with the diaphragm, transfer of ascitic fluid via transdiaphragmatic lymphatics or diaphragmatic defects, communication of a fistulous tract between a pseudocyst and the pleural space, and retroperitoneal movement of fluid into the mediastinum with mediastinitis or rupture into the pleural space. Of the possible factors involved in the increased pleural fluid amylase concentration, movement of the enzyme from the peritoneal to the pleural cavity by lymphatics appears to be of considerable importance. Furthermore, impaired lymphatic drainage from the pleural space, in combination with amylase clearance by the kidney, explains why the pleural fluid/serum amylase ratio is greater than unity.

The pleural fluid amylase concentration may be normal in early acute pancreatitis but it increases over time. In contrast to acute pancreatitis, the amylase concentration in chronic pancreatic effusions is always elevated and may reach levels above 100,000 IU per liter; the serum amylase level may be elevated due to back-effusion or may be normal.

Ten percent to 14 percent of patients with malignant pleural effusion have increased pleural fluid amylase concentrations. The most common malignancy causing amylase-rich effusions is adenocarcinoma of the lung, followed by adenocarcinoma of the ovary. However, other cell types of lung cancer as well as lymphoma and leukemia have been associated with amylase-rich effusions. Patients with malignant amylase-rich effusions have predominantly salivary-type isoamylase; thus, the finding of a salivary isoamylase-rich effusion is virtually diagnostic of malignancy in the absence of esophageal perforation. Furthermore, it is highly suggestive of adenocarcinoma of the pleura, as mesothelioma has not been reported to produce salivary amylase.

PLEURAL FLUID CYTOLOGIC EXAMINATION

Pleural fluid cytologic examination has a positive diagnostic yield in 40% to 90% of patients with malignancy. The most important reason for the variability in diagnostic yield is that the effusion is paramalignant. Paramalignant effusions are effusions associated with a known malignancy but are not due to pleural involvement with the tumor. These effusions are due to local

effects of the tumor (obstructive atelectasis, obstructive pneumonia with parapneumonic effusion, and impaired lymphatic drainage of the pleural space), systemic effects (pulmonary embolism), and results of therapy (radiation). Additional reasons for the variability in cytologic diagnosis are the tumor type (high positivity with adenocarcinoma, low with Hodgkin's disease), the number of specimens submitted (yields tend to increase with additional specimens due to exfoliation of fresher cells), and the interest and expertise of the cytopathologist.

OTHER TESTS

Immunologic markers in pleural fluid are helpful in the diagnosis of rheumatoid pleurisy and lupus pleuritis but, except for the finding of lupus erythematosus (LE) cells, are nondiagnostic. A rheumatoid factor in pleural fluid of 1:320 or higher, or a measurement greater than the serum rheumatoid factor, is suggestive of rheumatoid pleurisy. A pleural fluid antinuclear antibody (ANA) level of 1:320 or higher, or a measurement greater than serum ANA with a homogenous staining pattern, is suggestive but not diagnostic of lupus pleuritis. The finding of LE cells in pleural fluid is specific for the diagnosis of lupus pleuritis, but the sensitivity of the test is unknown. The likelihood of finding pleural fluid LE cells appears to increase if the fluid is allowed to stand at room temperature for several hours before examination by Wright's stain. Pleural fluid complement levels are low in most patients with lupus pleuritis and rheumatoid pleurisy; this is true whether total hemolytic complement or complement components are measured. Some overlap exists in pleural fluid complement levels between lupus pleuritis and rheumatoid pleurisy and other exudative effusions; however, very low complement levels are found only in the two connective tissue diseases.

UNDIAGNOSED PLEURAL EFFUSION

An understanding of the pathogenesis of pleural fluid formation and knowledge of pleural fluid analysis in conjunction with the clinical presentation should allow the cause of the pleural effusion to be determined in most cases. Sometimes, however, the clinical presentation and stage of disease do not allow a diagnosis to be established. Observation of the patient and repeat pleural fluid analysis are often diagnostic. The decision to pursue more invasive procedures to establish the cause of the pleural effusion depends on the clinical course and the patient's urgency to have a diagnosis established. If symptoms are minimal or improving, a less aggressive approach is indicated, but if the patient has anxiety concerning the undiagnosed effusion, a more aggressive approach may be pursued.

Percutaneous needle biopsy of the pleura is of diagnostic value in tuberculous pleurisy and malignant involvement of the pleura. Suspicion of these diagnoses is the main indication for its use. Culture and histologic examination of the pleural tissue is positive in 50% to 80% of patients with tuberculous pleurisy; the yield in malignant pleural effusions is 40% to 50%. It may be helpful in the diagnosis of fungal pleurisy, particularly coccidioidomycosis, but it is rarely positive in rheumatoid pleurisy. In the patient with suspected malignancy, pleural fluid cytologic examination should be the initial diagnostic approach, as its sensitivity is greater than that of pleural biopsy. However, if the initial cytologic examination is negative, a repeat cytologic examination several days later in conjunction with percutaneous pleural biopsy provides an increased diagnostic yield.

The yield of fiberoptic bronchoscopy in the patient who has a pleural effusion as the only abnormality on chest radiograph and who does not have clinical symptoms of tracheobronchial disease (hemoptysis, cough) is exceedingly low. However, when there are clinical signs (hemoptysis) or radiographic evidence (mass lesion, atelectasis, mediastinal and hilar adenopathy) that suggest tracheobronchial or parenchymal abnormalities, the yield of bronchoscopy is considerably higher.

Thoracoscopy establishes the diagnosis in virtually all patients with malignant pleural effusions. It is of minimal value in the diagnosis of nonmalignant pleural effusions and is unnecessary for the diagnosis of tuberculous pleurisy, as percutaneous pleural biopsy has a high diagnostic yield. Pleural biopsy culture and histologic examination in conjunction with pleural fluid culture and sputum analysis will diagnose about 90% of patients with tuberculous pleural effusions. However, if the tuberculin skin test is positive in the patient with a lymphocyte-predominant exudative pleural effusion who has a negative histologic and bacteriologic evaluation, the patient still needs to be treated for tuberculous pleurisy. All tuberculous effusions resolve in 2 to 4 months with or without chemotherapy; however, there is a high risk (about 70%) that the patient will develop pulmonary or extrapulmonary tuberculosis within the next 5 years.

The value of chest CT is limited in establishing the cause of an undiagnosed pleural effusion. However, a CT scan may demonstrate abnormalities suggestive of asbestos-related pleural disease, empyema, mesothelioma, metastatic adenocarcinoma, or fibrothorax. Furthermore, finding mediastinal or hilar adenopathy and parenchymal lesions that are not clearly delineated by the standard chest radiograph can guide further diagnostic procedures.

With improved instrumentation, thoracoscopy has virtually replaced open pleural biopsy for the diagnosis of unknown pleural disease. One possible exception is mesothelioma, where a large amount of tissue may be necessary for diagnosis. However, many thoracoscopists have demonstrated a high yield in the diagnosis of mesothelioma.

BIBLIOGRAPHY

Good JT Jr, Antony VB, King TE Jr, et al. Lupus pleuritis. Clinical features and pleural fluid characteristics with special reference to antinuclear antibody titers. *Chest* 1983;84:714–718.

Heffner JE, Brown LK, Barbieri CA. Diagnostic value of tests that discriminate between exudative and transudative pleural effusions. Primary Study Investigators. *Chest* 1997;111:970–980.

Heffner JE, Nietert PG, Barbieri C. Pleural fluid pH as a predictor of pleurodesis failure. *Chest* 2000;117:87–95.

Heffner JE, Nietert PG, Barbieri C. Pleural fluid pH as a predictor of survival for patients with malignant pleural effusions. *Chest* 2000;117:79–86.

Joseph J, Sahn SA. Connective tissue diseases and the pleura. *Chest* 1993;104:262–270.

Light RW. *Pleural diseases,* third ed. Philadelphia: Lea & Febiger, 1995.

Sahn SA. Pleural fluid pH in the normal state and in diseases affecting the pleural space, and pathogenesis and clinical features of diseases associated with a low pleural fluid glucose. In: Chretien J, Bignon J, Hirsch A,

eds. *The pleura in health and disease.* New York: Marcel Dekker, 1985:253–266.

Sahn SA. State of the art. The pleura. *Am Rev Respir Dis* 1988;138:184–234.

Sahn SA. Management of complicated parapneumonic effusions. *Am Rev Respir Dis* 1993;148:813–817.

Sahn SA. The diagnostic value of pleural fluid analysis. *Semin Respir Med* 1995;16:269–278.

Sahn SA. Malignancy metastatic to the pleura. *Clin Chest Med* 1998;119:351–361.

Stelzner TJ, King TE, Antony VB, et al. The pleuropulmonary manifestations of the postcardiac injury syndrome. *Chest* 1983;84:383–387.

Kelley's Textbook of Internal Medicine, fourth edition. Edited by H. David Humes. Lippincott Williams & Wilkins, Philadelphia © 2000.

CHAPTER

359

APPROACH TO THE PATIENT WITH A SOLITARY PULMONARY NODULE

JOSEPH P. LYNCH III
ELLA A. KAZEROONI

A solitary pulmonary nodule (SPN) is a single, circumscribed nodular opacity within the lung parenchyma that should be sufficiently discrete to allow measurement of the diameter in two planes. Because nodules larger than 3 cm almost invariably are malignant, they are excluded from this discussion. SPNs with specific patterns of calcification on plain chest radiographs virtually always are benign and do not require additional evaluation. An aggressive evaluation is warranted for all noncalcified SPNs, however, because an asymptomatic SPN may be the presenting feature of bronchogenic carcinoma, for which prompt surgical excision may be curative. Many of the same differential diagnostic considerations and tests used for SPN evaluation also may be applied to the evaluation of several pulmonary nodules, but there are significant differences in management. A thorough discussion of the approach to several nodules is beyond the scope of this chapter and is addressed only briefly.

Infectious granulomas and primary bronchogenic carcinomas each account for between 30% and 60% of SPNs in most series. Hamartomas constitute about 6% of SPNs; bronchial adenomas, 2%; metastatic malignancies, 3% to 5%; and miscellaneous causes, such as intrapulmonary lymph nodes, pulmonary infarction, and arteriovenous malformations, less than 5%. When bronchogenic carcinomas take the form of asymptomatic SPNs, complete surgical resection of the lesion can be achieved in up to 90% of cases, with the 5-year survival rate approaching 50%. Because a delay in resection of bronchogenic carcinoma may lessen or eliminate the chance for cure, an aggressive diagnostic approach—to include possible thoracotomy and SPN resection—is warranted unless specific contraindications to surgery exist. Nearly half of SPNs are benign, however, and would not require resection if a benign diagnosis could be established with less invasive or noninvasive techniques. In an attempt to limit the number of unnecessary thoracotomies, several criteria have been used to differentiate benign from malignant lesions more reliably. At least one center has reported an increase in the percentage of resected SPNs that are malignant, from 55% to 60% in the early 1980s to 90% to 100% in the early to mid-1990s. This is likely due to the advancement of imaging technologies, such as computed tomography (CT) and positron emission tomography (PET), that allow more benign nodules to be diagnosed without surgical intervention.

FACTORS THAT PREDICT A BENIGN (VERSUS MALIGNANT) SOURCE

CLINICAL FEATURES

The probability that a lesion is malignant increases progressively with advancing age. SPNs in patients less than 35 years old are malignant in fewer than 1% to 2% of cases. In contrast, SPNs are malignant in 15% to 30% of patients 35 to 45 years old and in more than 50% of patients over age 50. The presence or absence of symptoms cannot distinguish benign from malignant lesions. The history, physical examination, serologic tests, and skin tests for purified protein derivative and fungi are often appropriate in the evaluation of an SPN, but they do not reliably exclude malignancy. Smoking history has some predictive value, since the risk of carcinoma rises considerably with increasing number of pack-years. The risk of carcinoma in nonsmokers over age 35, however, is sufficiently high to justify an aggressive evaluation even in this group.

CHEST RADIOGRAPHY

Various radiographic criteria have been applied to differentiate benign and malignant SPNs. They include the size and growth rate of the lesion, the presence or absence of calcification within the lesion, satellite lesions, and the smoothness of the margin. Once an SPN is detected on plain chest radiographs, obtaining any previous chest radiographs is important, since the review of previous chest radiography reports alone may be misleading. The growth rate on serial radiographs may suggest the nature of the lesion. Lesions that are stable in size for 2 or more years are so rarely malignant that they may be followed with repeated radiographs at 6 and 12 months. New SPNs, lesions that have increased in size, or lesions in which stability can be documented for less than 2 years should be examined promptly by biopsy or resected to establish a specific diagnosis. Because doubling times for carcinomas vary widely (30 to 400 days), obtaining serial radiographs prospectively to assess the rate of growth before confirming the nature of the lesion is not recommended.

The likelihood of malignancy grows with increasing size of the lesion. SPNs smaller than 1 cm in diameter are benign in more than 90% of cases. Seventy percent of SPNs exceeding 2 cm in diameter and more than 90% of lesions larger than 3 cm are malignant. Overlap exists, however, and 5% to 10% of

TABLE 359.1.	**SOLITARY PULMONARY NODULE: CHEST RADIOGRAPHY OF PROGNOSTIC IMPORTANCE**

Almost Certainly Benign

Distinctive pattern of calcification (dense, central, popcorn or laminated)
Radiographic stability for at least 2 y

Very Likely Malignant

>2.5 cm in size
Grossly irregular or spiculated margin

Indeterminate

Eccentric, smudgy or punctate calcification
Smooth margins or sharp edge
Cavitation
Satellite lesions
<2.5 cm in size

bronchogenic carcinomas are smaller than 1 cm when they first are identified.

Calcification within an SPN markedly lessens but does not exclude the chance of malignancy. The specific pattern of calcification is of critical importance. There are four benign patterns of calcification: dense and solid, central, popcorn or lobulated, and laminated. A clump of lobulated calcification within a nodule (a popcorn pattern) is essentially pathognomonic of hamartoma. Patterns of calcification that should be considered indeterminate of benignity or malignancy include eccentric, smudgy and stippled, or punctate. Eccentric calcification is sometimes seen with carcinomas, for instance, a carcinoma that surrounds a nearby calcified granuloma, and cannot be used to differentiate benign from malignant lesions. Satellite lesions, or several smaller radiopacities surrounding a central nodule, are more often associated with a benign origin, but because exceptions exist, this feature has marginal discriminatory value.

The smoothness or regularity of the SPN margins may provide a clue to the nature of the lesion. The margins of most carcinomas are irregular or spiculated, while most benign lesions have smooth or sharp, rounded margins. A smooth margin may be seen in more than 40% of carcinomas, however, so this is an unreliable single sign of benignity. Although assessment of size, growth rate, pattern of calcification, and margin characteristics may be useful in estimating the probability that a lesion is benign or malignant, these features can be misleading. The only chest radiographic criteria that are reliable in certifying that a lesion is benign are the four described patterns of calcification (dense and solid, central, popcorn or lobulated, and laminated) and lack of growth for at least 2 years (Table 359.1).

COMPUTED TOMOGRAPHY

CT of the chest is far more sensitive than plain chest radiographs or standard tomography for detecting calcification and may provide additional information as to the benign or malignant nature of an SPN. When the specific benign features are not seen on chest radiographs, thin-section CT through the lesion is carried out. Thin-section CT scanning using 1- to 3-mm sections is

TABLE 359.2.	SOLITARY PULMONARY NODULE: CT FEATURES OF PROGNOSTIC OR DIAGNOSTIC IMPORTANCE

Almost Certainly Benign

Distinctive pattern of calcification (dense, central, popcorn or laminated)

Fat

Likely Benign if *All* the Following are Present:

Diffuse calcification (attenuation >164 HU), calcification occupying ≥10%

Smooth margin

Diameter <2.5 cm

Likely a Hamartoma if *All* the Following are Present:

Diameter <2.5 cm

Smooth edge

Focal collections of fat, or fat alternating with areas of calcification

---

HU, Hounsfield units.

superior to conventional CT scans, with sections at 8 to 10 mm thickness, for evaluating the attenuation (density) of nodules, since the partial volume-averaging effect that may be evident with larger sections is eliminated. The CT features of nodules are categorized in Table 359.2. If one of the four benign patterns of calcification can be identified on thin-section CT, the nodule is considered benign, and the CT examination can be terminated without requiring intravenous contrast and the risk of contrast-related complications. Localized or eccentric foci of calcification have no discriminatory value, because localized calcification in an otherwise low-density lesion is evident on CT in 10% to 15% of carcinomas. An additional benign feature that can be seen on thin section is fat attenuation within a nodule, indicating a hamartoma. More than 50% of hamartomas can be diagnosed on CT by using the following criteria: diameter less than 2.5 cm, a smooth margin, and focal collections of fat or fat and calcification.

If a nodule does not meet the specific criteria for benign features on CT, it must be considered possibly malignant. Although the precise role of chest CT in the evaluation of SPN remains the subject of controversy, the next logical step is complete chest CT of the thorax and upper abdomen, including the adrenal glands, to search for suspected bronchogenic carcinoma. CT may detect additional nodules, enlarged lymph nodes, or liver, adrenal, or bone lesions suggestive of metastases, which subsequently can be sampled as part of lung cancer staging.

The characteristics used to evaluate nodules on chest radiographs, such as lesion size and margin, also are used for CT scans. Individually, these features lack sufficient sensitivity to exclude malignancy. The size of the lesion has predictive value, however. In one series, 35 of 36 lesions larger than 3 cm were malignant, whereas only 20% of benign SPNs were larger than 2 cm. In a separate study, only 16 of 279 benign SPNs (6%) exceeded 2.5 cm in diameter. The smoothness and sharpness of the edge of the margin of the lesion are also important prognostically. In a multicenter study of 384 SPNs, 97% of the 188 benign nodules had smooth or relatively smooth borders on CT

scan, whereas 80 of 91 SPNs with an irregular or spiculated border were malignant. Accordingly, any SPN exhibiting an irregular margin on chest CT scan should not be characterized as benign, regardless of other CT characteristics. A smooth, sharp margin has no discriminatory value, since 60% of SPNs in one series with smooth margins were carcinomas.

Other techniques have been used to classify nodules on CT as benign or malignant, including CT nodule densitometry and CT nodule enhancement. With respect to the former method, tissue attenuation values on CT range from $-1,024$ Hounsfield units (HU) to $+1,024$ HU, with 0 HU representing water, $-1,024$ HU representing air, and $+1,024$ HU representing dense mineral. CT scanners must be calibrated regularly to ensure that these values do not drift. The higher the CT number of a nodule, the more likely that it contains calcification. CT nodule densitometry was first reported for the evaluation of SPNs by Siegelman et al. in 1980. CT numbers were measured for 91 noncalcified nodules seen on chest radiographs. The mean CT number of the 58 malignant lesions was 92 HU; none exceeded 147 HU. In contrast, the mean CT number exceeded 164 HU in 20 of 33, or 61%, of benign lesions. Calcified nodules seen on chest radiographs typically have CT numbers ranging from 600 to 1,200 HU. The authors suggested that SPNs with CT numbers exceeding 164 HU can be presumed to be benign, whereas lesions with CT numbers less than 164 HU should be classified as indeterminate. High attenuation values (calcification) distributed diffusely throughout a lesion and occupying at least 10% of the cross-sectional area strongly suggest a benign origin. In two large series encompassing more than 500 malignant lesions, no malignancy exhibited diffuse calcification or had representative CT numbers above 164. Among 166 SPNs categorized as benign by CT criteria, none proved to be malignant at operation or after prolonged follow-up. Lesions assessed by CT as indeterminate were malignant in 355 of 458 (78%) and 176 of 229 (77%) cases, respectively.

Several technical factors, including kilovoltage, slice thickness, size of the nodule, position of the nodule within the thorax, type of scanner, and the algorithm used to construct images, may influence quantitative CT densitometry measurements. Since quantitative CT data obtained from different centers may vary considerably, an absolute CT number (such as 164 HU) cannot be used to distinguish benign from malignant lesions reliably across different centers. In the mid-1980s, a technique was developed in which reference nodules of known density were inserted into a chest phantom to determine more accurately the density of nodules on CT. Lesions denser than the reference phantom were likely to be benign, and the remaining lesions were indeterminate. The use of the phantom was transient, and because of the technical factors previously discussed, most centers no longer use the reference phantom.

Lung nodule contrast enhancement on CT after intravenous contrast administration has been investigated in the evaluation of SPNs. In a series of 107 indeterminate SPNs measuring 7 to 30 mm in diameter (52 malignant, 55 benign), Swensen et al. (1996) found that a 20-HU increase in attenuation (or higher) from baseline was an indicator of malignancy; this technique was 98% sensitive and 73% specific for malignancy. Pathologic correlation showed that the degree of nodule enhancement was related to the amount of central vascular staining. More widespread application of this technique is necessary before conclusions can be drawn regarding the role of this technique in SPN evaluation.

POSITRON EMISSION TOMOGRAPHY

PET using fluorodeoxyglucose or [^{11}C]methionine has been investigated in the evaluation of SPNs. Increased tracer uptake is characteristic, but not pathognomonic, of malignant lesions, because some infectious and inflammatory lesions also evidence uptake. Absent tracer uptake is more useful and is a strong negative predictor of malignancy. A lesion without uptake is almost certainly benign, with one caveat. One limitation of PET scanning is the inability to evaluate consistently lesions less than 2 cm in size. While a lesion less than 2 cm with positive uptake may be malignant, lesions of this size without uptake are not consistently benign. Therefore, PET cannot be recommended for the evaluation of nodules less than 2 cm. In one series of 50 patients with nodules 3 cm or smaller in size, PET was 90% sensitive and 83% specific for malignancy; 10% of malignant lesions were incorrectly classified as benign, and 17% of benign lesions were erroneously categorized as malignant. In the same series, CT was 100% sensitive and 52% specific for malignancy. How PET fits into the algorithm for SPN evaluation is unclear, and PET scanners are not as widely available as the other technologies described here.

OTHER RADIOLOGIC IMAGING

Magnetic resonance imaging, digital or planar tomographic imaging, and single photon emission tomography have no advantage over CT scanning and are not recommended. Radioimmunoscintigraphy using technetium Tc 99m–or indium In 111–labeled monoclonal antibodies is an exciting area of research investigation, but this method is of unproven clinical value.

■ OTHER DIAGNOSTIC STUDIES

FIBEROPTIC BRONCHOSCOPY

Sputum smears and cultures for specific pathogens or sputum cytologic evaluations are diagnostic in only 1% to 3% of asymptomatic SPNs and have no role in routine management because of their expense. They may be indicated, however, for patients with serious underlying disease who are not candidates for thoracotomy and are marginal candidates for invasive diagnostic procedures. Flexible fiberoptic bronchoscopy (FFB) or percutaneous needle aspiration sometimes can be helpful in the evaluation of SPNs, because thoracotomy may be avoided if a specific benign source can be established by either of these techniques. A thoracotomy still is required, however, if the biopsy result is nonspecific or negative. FFB establishes the diagnosis in 40% to 80% of malignant SPNs but in only 5% to 20% of benign SPNs. Size and nodule location strongly influences the yield. Diagnostic accuracy is less than 30% for lesions smaller than 2 cm but exceeds 60% in lesions larger than 3 cm in diameter. Central lesions are diagnosed

more accurately with FFB (more than 60%) than lesions within 2 cm of the peripheral pleural surface (20% to 30%). The diagnostic yield from bronchoscopy is greater when a positive bronchus sign is noted on CT, that is, when a bronchus can be identified extending into the lesion to be sampled.

PERCUTANEOUS NEEDLE ASPIRATION

Percutaneous needle aspiration performed under fluoroscopic or CT guidance has a higher yield but a greater complication rate than FFB. Pneumothoraxes complicate needle aspiration in 10% to 20% of cases (compared with a 1% to 2% complication rate with FFB). Nodules clearly visible in two planes are usually approached with fluoroscopy, whereas CT is used for nodules not visible in two planes (usually smaller nodules) and for nodules in difficult locations (abutting the great vessels or aorta). The diagnostic accuracy of needle aspiration is especially high for malignant lesions, ranging from 85% to 97%. The diagnostic yield can be increased by the use of immediate cytologic study to determine the adequacy of the specimen, so that additional needle passes can be taken during the same procedure if further sampling is required.

As with FFB, the rate of positive diagnoses correlates with the size of the lesion, with a yield of 50% to 70% for lesions smaller than 1 cm but more than 90% for lesions exceeding 4 cm in diameter. There is no need to perform needle aspiration simply to corroborate the diagnosis of carcinoma in patients who are acceptable candidates for thoracotomy. Needle aspiration may be advantageous if a specific benign diagnosis is suspected, such as infection, but it is in this context that needle aspiration has shown the least impressive results. In most medical centers, fine-needle aspiration has had a high diagnostic accuracy in terms of malignant lesions, but it less frequently establishes a specific diagnosis in the context of benign lesions. Using a cutting needle to obtain a core of tissue may increase the yield for benign diagnoses. With percutaneous core-needle biopsies, specific diagnostic yields of 60% to 97% have been reported, even for benign lesions.

VIDEO-ASSISTED THORACOSCOPIC BIOPSY AND MINITHORACOTOMY

An SPN usually can be resected with video-assisted thoracoscopic (VATS) techniques or minithoracotomy. These techniques have lower rates of morbidity than standard posterolateral thoracotomy and are ideally suited to the identification and resection of SPNs suspected of being benign. For small nodules deep to the pleural surface, CT-guided methylene blue injection or hook-wire placement can be used during VATS to guide the surgeon to the lesion, because surgeons lose the tactile sensation of palpation of the lungs that accompanies thoracotomy. If the lesion proves to be malignant at the time of surgery, many surgeons extend the incision and perform standard thoracotomy with curative intent. Studies suggest that high rates of curative resections can be achieved with VATS. In one large series of 388 patients undergoing VATS, 217 nodules were diagnosed as malignant and 171 as benign. Methylene blue or hook-wire localization was used in 76 patients (20%) for guidance. In 67 patients (17%) the procedure was converted into a thoracotomy, primarily owing to an inability to resect the lesion completely (n = 33) or to carry out a lobectomy (n = 30). In this same series, 21 lobectomies were successfully carried out without requiring conversion to open thoracotomy.

MANAGEMENT

The decision to proceed with surgery (VATS or thoracotomy) for the diagnosis of SPNs depends on several factors, including the likelihood that a lesion is malignant, the patient's overall physical condition and ability to withstand surgery, and the patient's desires. Although the axiom When in Doubt, Take It Out generally applies, the physician should avoid being overly dogmatic and should assess the factors cited earlier before arriving at a treatment strategy. For example, for a patient with asymptomatic SPN but such severe pulmonary disease that thoracic resection would be impossible, one could justify following the lesion with serial chest radiographs as the initial step. In contrast, watching a noncalcified SPN of indeterminate cause in a healthy 50-year-old patient cannot be justified. In some cases, the appropriate management strategy may not be obvious. For a 30-year-old nonsmoker who has a 1-cm SPN with a smooth margin, in whom the risk of malignancy is less than 1%, the decision to repeat a chest roentgenogram at 3 months would be reasonable. This approach would be ill advised, however, if the same person had a strong smoking history, a larger nodule, or a lesion with irregular borders.

Lillington and colleagues pointed out that by applying Bayes theorem and analyzing multiple (presumably independent) variables, such as age, smoking history, and size of the lesion, one could arrive at a better estimate of likelihood of malignancy than by using any single variable. This approach is intriguing but still establishes only probabilities and not actual risk. Hence, in the final analysis, thoracotomy (or VATS) may be required to substantiate the diagnosis. Owing to the low risk of surgery for benign lesions and the potentially fatal outcome if malignant lesions should fail to be promptly resected, the prudent approach is to resect any SPNs that are not clearly calcified on chest radiographs (or CT) and when ancillary tests (e.g., FFB or needle aspiration) have failed to achieve a specific benign diagnosis.

SEVERAL PULMONARY NODULES

Several small parenchymal nodules (often less than 5 mm) may be evident on chest CT scan performed as part of the evaluation of an SPN. At least 30% to 50% of incidental nodules noted on CT are benign, even when the SPN is carcinoma. In patients who are otherwise able to undergo resection, we usually proceed with thoracotomy but look for and take biopsy specimens of any additional nodules noted at the time of operation. In patients who are marginal candidates for operation, needle aspiration biopsy of one or more of the nodules may be considered as an alternative to immediate thoracotomy. Additional nodules

detected on CT scan should not be considered definitely malignant unless specific histologic confirmation has been obtained.

BIBLIOGRAPHY

Bernard A. Resection of pulmonary nodules using video-assisted thoracic surgery. The Thorax Group. *Ann Thorac Surg* 1996;61:202–205.

Khan A, Herman PG, Vorwerk P, et al. Solitary pulmonary nodules: comparison of classification with standard, thin-section, and reference phantom CT. *Radiology* 1991;179:477–481.

Lillington GA, Caskey CI. Evaluation and management of solitary and multiple pulmonary nodules. *Clin Chest Med* 1993;14(1):111–119.

Midthun DE, Swensen SJ, Jett JR. Clinical strategies for solitary pulmonary nodule. *Ann Rev Med* 1992;41:195–208.

Prauer HW, Weber WA, Romer W, et al. Controlled prospective study of positron emission tomography using the glucose analogue 18f-fluorodeoxyglucose in the evaluation of pulmonary nodules. *Br J Surg* 1998; 85:1506–1511.

Rubins JB, Rubins HB. Temporal trends in the prevalence of malignancy in resected solitary pulmonary lesions. *Chest* 1996;109:100–103.

Salazar AM, Westcott JL. The role of transthoracic needle biopsy for the diagnosis and staging of lung cancer. *Clin Chest Med* 1993;14(1): 99–110.

Siegelman SS, Zerhouni EA, Leo FP, et al. CT of the solitary pulmonary nodule. *AJR* 1980;135:1–13.

Siegelman SS, Khouri NF, Leo FP, et al. Solitary pulmonary nodules: CT assessment. *Radiology* 1986;160:307–312.

Swensen SJ, Brown LR, Colby TV, et al. Lung nodule enhancement at CT: prospective findings. *Radiology* 1996;201:447–455.

Zerhouni EA, Stitik FP, Siegelman SS, et al. CT of the pulmonary nodule: a cooperative study. *Radiology* 1986;160:319–327.

Kelley's Textbook of Internal Medicine, fourth edition. Edited by H. David Humes. Lippincott Williams & Wilkins, Philadelphia © 2000.

C H A P T E R

360

APPROACH TO THE PATIENT WITH INTERSTITIAL LUNG DISEASE

KEVIN K. BROWN

The clinician evaluating the patient with known or suspected interstitial lung disease (ILD) faces a diagnostic challenge, with a long and heterogeneous list of potential causes to consider (Table 360.1). To complicate the evaluation, the majority of these disorders have nonspecific initial pulmonary symptoms, noncharacteristic parenchymal shadowing on chest radiography, and a similar restrictive pulmonary physiologic picture. Moreover, the majority of the ILDs are of unknown origin, the most common causes being sarcoidosis, the idiopathic interstitial pneumonias (such as idiopathic pulmonary fibrosis, or IPF), and connective tissue disease–related ILD. Of the ILDs of known cause, those related to occupational and environmental expo-

TABLE 360.1. ETIOLOGIC CLASSIFICATION OF INTERSTITIAL LUNG DISEASE

Idiopathic interstitial pneumonias
  Idiopathic pulmonary fibrosis
  Desquamative interstitial pneumonia
  Acute interstitial pneumonia (Hamman-Rich syndrome)
  Respiratory bronchiolitis–interstitial lung disease
  Cryptogenic organizing pneumonia (idiopathic bronchiolitis obliterans with organizing pneumonia)
Occupational and environmental exposures
  Inorganic
    Silica
    Silicates (asbestos, talc, mica, vermiculite, kaolin, or "china clay")
    Hard metal dusts (cobalt)
    Beryllium, aluminum, titanium
    Coal dust, mixed inert dust
  Organic (hypersensitivity pneumonitis or extrinsic allergic alveolitis)
    Microbial agents
      Bacteria (farmer's lung, humidifier lung)
        Thermophilic bacteria (species, *Micropolyspora* species, *Thermactinomyces* species)
        Other bacteria (*Bacillus* species, *Pseudomonas fluorescens*)
      Fungi (farmer's lung, hot-tub lung: e.g., *Aspergillus, Alternaria, Faeni, Cryptostroma, Cladosporium, Aureobasidium,* and, *Penicillin* species)
      Amoebae (humidifier lung: *Naegleria* and *Acanthamoeba* species)
    Animal/insect proteins
      Avian droppings, feathers, serum (bird breeder's disease)
      Pelts, urine, serum (animal handler's lung)
      Sitophilus species (miller's lung)
    Chemicals
      Isocyanates (chemical worker's lung)
      Trimellitic anhydride (chemical worker's lung)
      Copper sulfate (vineyard sprayer's lung)
Drugs, poisons, radiation
  Chemotherapeutic agents (busulfan, bleomycin, methotrexate)
  Antibiotics (nitrofurantoin, sulfasalazine)
  Cardiovascular drugs (amiodarone, tocainide, angiotensin-converting enzyme inhibitors)
  Anti-inflammatories (gold salts, penicillamine)
  Neurotropics/psychotropics

Miscellaneous
  Paraquat, cocaine
  Radiation, oxygen
Rheumatologic and autoimmune diseases
  Systemic lupus erythematosus
  Rheumatoid arthritis
  Progressive systemic sclerosis
  Sjögren's syndrome
  Polymyositis and dermatomyositis
  Mixed connective tissue disease
  Ankylosing spondylitis
  Behçet's syndrome
  Wegener's granulomatosis
  Churg–Strauss syndrome
  Goodpasture's syndrome
Unclassified disease
  Sarcoidosis
  Pulmonary histiocytosis X (eosinophilic granuloma of the lung)
  Chronic gastric aspiration
  Lymphangioleiomyomatosis, tuberous sclerosis
  Alveolar proteinosis
  Eosinophilic pneumonia
  Lipoid pneumonia
  Diffuse alveolar hemorrhage
  Amyloidosis
Lymphoproliferative and neoplastic diseases
  Lymphocytic interstitial pneumonia
  Angiocentric immunoproliferative lesion (lymphomatoid granulomatosis)
  Pseudolymphoma
  Pulmonary lymphoma
  Lymphangitic carcinomatosis
  Bronchoalveolar cell carcinoma
Infections (active or remote)
  Mycobacterial, fungal, viral, bacterial
Cardiovascular
  Chronic left ventricular failure
  Mitral stenosis
  Pulmonary veno-occlusive disease

sures predominate. Despite these obstacles, almost every case of ILD can be confidently diagnosed with the appropriate combination of clinical, radiologic, physiologic, and histologic data.

PATHOPHYSIOLOGY

The underlying source for most of these disorders is unknown, and the mechanisms of action responsible for the transition from normal lung to fibrosis remain a focus of active ongoing investigation. In those diseases characterized by progressive fibrosis, however, a common pathogenetic sequence is proposed. Injury to the alveolar and/or endothelial cells may occur through inhalation or via the vasculature, with resultant recruitment of local and circulating inflammatory cells. T lymphocytes and macrophages appear to have a central role in the transition from acute injury to chronic inflammation; depending upon the type or stage of disease, excess numbers of neutrophils, plasma cells, or even eosinophils can be found. Why this inflammation persists is not known, though continued exposure to an inciting agent or antigen or failure of the lung's intrinsic anti-inflammatory mechanisms have both been hypothesized.

This chronic inflammation progresses to a fibrotic response characterized by fibroblast proliferation and excess production of collagen and extracellular matrix. This process leads to architectural distortion and disruption of gas-exchange units, with ensuing physiologic disturbance. While they are characterized as "interstitial," these disorders also can involve the alveolar space, the vasculature, the small membranous airways, and even the pleura. Sometimes this process can be checked and even reversed (such as in cryptogenic organizing pneumonia) but in the majority of patients the process proceeds uninhibited. Ultimately, it results in the development of "honeycomb lung" or end-stage fibrosis, with large cystic spaces separated by thick bands of fibrous tissue.

For those ILDs that are not characterized by progressive irreversible fibrosis, different pathophysiologic events take place. An alveolar filling process with lipoproteinaceous material (alveolar proteinosis), blood (diffuse alveolar hemorrhage, or DAH), malignant cells (e.g., alveolar cell carcinoma or lymphoma), or eosinophils (eosinophilic pneumonia) develops in some of these disorders. The unexplained proliferation of local smooth-muscle cells is seen in lymphangioleiomyomatosis (LAM) and the genetically related tuberous sclerosis. As with other organs, amyloid protein can be deposited in many compartments, including the alveolus, the vessels, and the alveolar capillary membrane.

HISTORY AND PHYSICAL EXAMINATION

The importance of a detailed history in the evaluation of ILD cannot be overemphasized. The most common initial symptoms are slowly progressive (often over several months) exertional breathlessness and a chronic nonproductive cough. Often, the indolent development of exertional breathlessness is overlooked and is incorrectly attributed to the general aging process or lack of physical conditioning. Many patients will note that they have just "slowed down." The cough is often attributed to recurrent upper respiratory tract infections, postnasal drip, or asthma. The breathlessness and cough sometimes develop so insidiously that the patient fails to notice until a spouse or friend points out the symptoms. The cough can be particularly troublesome in those ILDs that also affect the airways, including respiratory bronchiolitis (RB), cryptogenic organizing pneumonia, sarcoidosis, hypersensitivity pneumonitis (HP), eosinophilic granuloma (EG or pulmonary histiocytosis X), bronchiolitis, and lymphangitic carcinomatosis.

Wheezing is uncommon, but when it is present it can be an important clue to associated airways involvement, with such conditions as RB, HP, eosinophilic pneumonia, or the Churg–Strauss syndrome. Sputum production is unusual, though hemoptysis can be noted and may be an early feature of LAM, EG, vasculitis, or one of the DAH syndromes. Hemoptysis seen in the context of a known ILD can be due to a superimposed infection, pulmonary embolus, or malignancy. Chest pain is atypical, though pleurisy can accompany almost any of the connective tissue diseases, some drug-induced disorders, and the pneumothoraxes that complicate LAM or EG. Atypical, nonpleuritic, midsternal chest pain occasionally is seen in sarcoidosis.

The symptoms in the majority of ILDs are chronic and progressive over months to years. Some take the form of acute illness that arises in just days (acute interstitial pneumonia, acute eosinophilic pneumonia); others progress as subacute illness over the course of weeks (cryptogenic organizing pneumonia, DAH, and some drug-induced ILDs). These acute forms of ILD must be differentiated from atypical respiratory infections, cardiac decompensation, and pulmonary emboli. Gender and age can be helpful in making a diagnosis. Most patients with IPF are older than 60, whereas patients with connective tissue diseases and sarcoidosis tend to be younger than 50. LAM develops only in premenopausal women, and the ILD that complicates connective tissue disease is more common in women—except for RA, which more commonly afflicts men.

A review of systems must be performed, with a particular focus on the systemic complaints seen in such autoimmune diseases as arthralgias or joint swelling, Raynaud's phenomena, dry eyes and dry mouth, myalgias, or exanthems. Even in the context of a previously diagnosed ILD, examination for these symptoms is useful, since lung disease can precede the development of a definable connective tissue disease by years. The medical history often gives clues to other pulmonary (such as lung cancer) or systemic illnesses (such as rheumatoid arthritis) or to therapies (such as chemotherapy or radiation) that could have resulted in lung injury. Information concerning current medications, including over-the-counter and nontraditional oral or inhaled therapies, vitamins, food supplements, and recreational drugs, should be solicited.

Previous medications (of any sort) taken for an appreciable length of time also should be reviewed, because the signs or symptoms of drug-induced lung disease may not appear for months or years after the exposure. The use of tobacco products should be explored, since some ILDs are seen primarily in smokers (desquamative interstitial pneumonia, RB, EG, pulmonary hemorrhage in Goodpasture's syndrome). Occasionally, a family history of similar chest or systemic illnesses will be found, because some ILDs have shown evidence of familial association either through genetic mechanisms of action (IPF, tuberous sclerosis, and perhaps sarcoidosis) or common exposures (HP).

Among the most common causes of ILD are occupational and environmental exposures. Diagnosis requires an exhaustive review of current and previous occupations, an understanding of the actual job performed, the likely exposures encountered, and whether or not protective equipment was used. The same is true of the environmental history in terms of exposures in the home as well as potential exposures preceding the initial symptoms or radiographic abnormalities. The presence of hot tubs, swimming pools, humidifiers, water damage, or pets in the home should be examined. Exposures during the pursuit of hobbies or avocations, such as bird breeding, are of special importance for the diagnosis of HP. The development of symptoms in relation to particular exposures, such as the workplace or a home workshop, or the improvement in symptoms over the weekend or on vacation away from the home suggests a potential environmental exposure as the cause.

Physical findings of a skin rash, eye changes, adenopathy, salivary or lacrimal gland enlargement, hepatosplenomegaly, synovitis, or muscle tenderness can be useful hints to an underlying connective tissue disease, malignancy, vasculitis, or sarcoidosis (Table 360.2). Clubbing most often occurs in IPF. The chest auscultatory examination often shows fine, mid-to-end inspiratory crackles (dry rales) in IPF, asbestosis, CTD-related ILD, and the chronic form of HP, whereas fewer abnormal sounds are heard in other granulomatous and eosinophilic lung disease.

TABLE 360.2.	EXTRATHORACIC PHYSICAL FINDINGS IN THE INTERSTITIAL LUNG DISEASES

Abnormality	Associated ILD
Systemic arterial hypertension	Connective tissue disease, some diffuse alveolar hemorrhage syndromes
Skin changes	
Erythema nodosum	Sarcoidosis, connective tissue disease, Behçet's syndrome
Maculopapular rash	Drug-induced, amyloidosis, lipoidosis, connective tissue disease, Gaucher's disease
Heliotrope rash	Dermatomyositis
Telangiectasia	Scleroderma
Palpable purpura (cutaneous vasculitis)	Systemic vasculitides, connective tissue disease
Subcutaneous nodules	Rheumatoid arthritis
Calcinosis	Dermatomyositis, scleroderma
Eye changes	
Uveitis	Sarcoidosis, Behçet's syndrome, ankylosing spondylitis
Scleritis	Systemic vasculitis, systemic lupus erythematosus, scleroderma, sarcoidosis
Keratoconjunctivitis sicca	Connective tissue disease, lymphocytic interstitial pneumonia
Other findings	
Salivary gland enlargement	Sarcoidosis, lymphocytic interstitial pneumonia
Peripheral lymphadenopathy	Sarcoidosis, lymphangitic carcinomatosis, lymphocytic interstitial pneumonia, lymphoma
Hepatosplenomegaly	Sarcoidosis, eosinophilic granuloma, connective tissue disease, amyloidosis, lymphocytic interstitial pneumonia
Pericarditis	Radiation pneumonitis, connective tissue disease
Myositis	Connective tissue disease, drugs (tryptophan)
Synovitis	Connective tissue disease

ILD, interstitial lung disease.

LABORATORY STUDIES AND DIAGNOSTIC TESTS

IMAGING STUDIES

Chest Radiography

Abnormal results on a chest radiograph (CXR) discovered during a routine physical exam, in preoperative evaluation, or in response to respiratory symptoms are the common initial finding that precipitates evaluation for ILD. The usefulness of the CXR is limited, however, because up to 10% of patients with symptomatic and histologically proven ILD are said to have normal results on CXR. While the CXR is only occasionally useful in making a specific diagnosis, recognition of a radiographic pattern narrows the differential diagnosis (Table 360.3). For example,

TABLE 360.3.	USEFUL CHEST RADIOGRAPHIC PATTERNS

Pattern	Common Diagnoses
Decreased lung volumes	IPF, CTD related, chronic hypersensitivity pneumonitis, asbestosis
Increased lung volumes	LAM, tuberous sclerosis, EG, bronchiolitis
Mid-upper zone predominance	Sarcoidosis, silicosis, coal workers' pneumoconiosis, hypersensitivity pneumonitis, EG
Lower zone predominance	IPF, CTD-related, asbestosis
Peripheral zone	Cryptogenic organizing pneumonia, eosinophilic pneumonia
Micronodules	Infection, sarcoidosis, hypersensitivity pneumonitis
Septal thickening	Malignancy, chronic congestive heart failure, infection, pulmonary veno-occlusive disease
Honeycombing	IPF, asbestosis, CTD related, sarcoidosis, chronic hypersensitivity pneumonitis
Migratory or remitting infiltrates	Cryptogenic organizing pneumonia, hypersensitivity pneumonitis, allergic bronchopulmonary aspergillosis, Löffler's syndrome
Pleural disease	CTD related, asbestosis, malignancy
Pneumothorax	LAM, EG, tuberous sclerosis
Adenopathy	Sarcoidosis, malignancy, silicosis, infection, chronic beryllium disease
Normal	Hypersensitivity pneumonitis, IPF, CTD related, bronchiolitis

IPF, idiopathic pulmonary fibrosis; CTD, ▪▪▪; LAM, lymphangioleiomyomatosis; EG, eosinophilic granuloma.

Mid-inspiratory musical crackles are often noted in HP and other diseases that affect the small airways (bronchioles). Wheezing suggests an associated airway abnormality, such as eosinophilic pneumonia or RB-ILD. Pleural or pericardial rubs are occasionally noted in CTD-related disease. In the late stage of any ILD, there may be findings of right ventricular failure with increased intensity of the pulmonic component of the second heart sound, elevated jugulovenous pressure, and peripheral edema. Examination of the joints may show deformities or synovitis characteristic of a particular autoimmune disease.

the presence of bilateral basilar reticular markings and pleural plaque suggests asbestosis. Radiographic patterns in ILD traditionally have been divided into alveolar-filling and interstitial infiltrates. This approach is limited, since many ILDs have a pattern that combines both features. While the general availability of high-resolution computed tomography (HRCT) has diminished the importance of the CXR in defining ILD, the CXR is still a good starting point.

High-resolution Computed Tomography

HRCT should be considered a standard method for the initial evaluation of most patients with ILD. It is more sensitive than plain radiography in identifying ILD (particularly in those symptomatic patients with a normal or near-normal CXR), with a sensitivity greater than 90% in diffuse lung disease compared with 80% for the CXR. The radiographic pattern on HRCT often suggests a particular set of diagnostic possibilities (Table 360.4). HRCT also more easily identifies mixed patterns of disease (such as ILD plus emphysema) or additional pleural, hilar,

TABLE 360.4. USEFUL HRCT PATTERNS IN THE DIAGNOSIS OF ILD

By Type of Radiographic Abnormality

Finding	Common Diagnoses
Reticular lines, honeycombing	CTD related, IPF, asbestosis, sarcoidosis, chronic hypersensitivity pneumonitis
Airspace opacity, "ground glass" appearance	BOOP, CEP, pulmonary alveolar proteinosis, consolidation lymphoma, sarcoidosis
Nodules	Granulomatous diseases, pneumoconioses, malignancy
Septal thickening	Infection, edema, malignancy, drug reaction, pulmonary veno-occlusive disease
Cystic changes	Eosinophilic granuloma, LAM

By anatomic distribution of abnormality

Location	Common Diagnoses
Mid-upper lung zone	Hypersensitivity pneumonitis, sarcoidosis, EG, chronic beryllium disease
Lower lung zone	CTD related, IPF, asbestosis
Peripheral	BOOP, IPF, eosinophilic pneumonia
Perihilar	Sarcoidosis, malignancy
Along bronchovascular sheath	Sarcoidosis

HRCT, high-resolution computed tomography; ILD, interstitial lung disease; CTD, ■■■; IPF, idiopathic pulmonary fibrosis; BOOP, ■■■; CEP, ■■■; LAM, lymphangioleiomyomatosis; EG, eosinophilic granuloma.
(From Lynch D, Gamsu G. Imaging of diffuse parenchymal lung diseases. In: Schwarz MI, King TE Jr, eds. *Interstitial lung disease,* third ed. Hamilton: BC Decker, 1998.)

or mediastinal abnormalities. It has a better correlation with physiologic impairment and can be used more easily as a road map for either transbronchial or open biopsy.

Gallium Scanning

In general, gallium scanning is not useful in the diagnosis or management of ILD. From a diagnostic perspective, the abnormal lung accumulation of gallium citrate Ga 67 24 and 48 hours after intravenous injection will occur in a variety of ILDs. This finding is therefore nonspecific, since it is seen in infections, drug-induced lung disease, IPF, sarcoidosis, CTD-related ILD, and others. Whole-body scanning may be of use in the evaluation of some patients with suspected sarcoidosis, to confirm extrathoracic organ involvement.

PHYSIOLOGY

Pulmonary Function Testing

Pulmonary function testing is necessary for the evaluation of ILD. While ILD can be accompanied by a variety of physiologic abnormalities, including normal function, the classic separation of restrictive and obstructive disease helps categorize the patient's illness and narrows the differential diagnostic possibilities. The majority of ILDs have a restrictive ventilatory defect, though occasionally an obstructive (such as in LAM or EG) or a mixed restrictive–obstructive defect (as in HP, RB, or mixed IPF/emphysema) may be present.

Lung Volumes

Patients usually show symptoms of generally symmetric reduction in the total lung capacity, functional residual volume, and residual volume, which defines the restrictive ventilatory defect. Patients with LAM, EG, or bronchiolitis may have normal or even increased lung volumes, particularly the residual volume.

Spirometry

Airway function in ILD is typically well preserved. Both the forced expiratory volume in 1 second (FEV_1) and the forced vital capacity (FVC) are reduced in a restrictive defect, with the FEV_1/FVC ratio and the expiratory flow rates normal and often supranormal except in the context of concomitant small airway disease. Airflow limitation can be detected if diseases that affect the small airways, such as HP, bronchiolitis, LAM or EG, are present.

Diffusing Capacity of the Lung for Carbon Monoxide

The diffusing capacity of the lung for carbon monoxide (D_{LCO}) is usually decreased, sometimes to very low values. This decrease is related primarily to ventilation-perfusion ratio mismatch, with a poorly ventilated fibrotic lung still being adequately perfused. Marked declines in oxygenation can occur even with a normal

DLCO, and, for this reason, DLCO cannot substitute for an actual measure of arterial blood gases, particularly with exercise. Marked reduction of DLCO with relative maintenance of lung volumes suggests concomitant pulmonary vascular disease such as that seen in progressive systemic sclerosis, emphysema, or a cystic lung disease (LAM, EG). In DAH the DLCO may be normal or even elevated, since intra-alveolar hemoglobin absorbs the inhaled carbon monoxide.

Pressure-volume Curve

A reduction in lung compliance or an increase in the elastic recoil or stiffness of the lung is a common finding in those ILD patients with a restrictive ventilatory defect. The measurement of the lung's pressure-volume curve can be useful when radiographic or other physiologic information is difficult to interpret or shows conflicting evidence. Such testing is technically demanding, making it generally less practical except in specialized centers.

Gas Exchange

Gas exchange in an identified ILD is almost always abnormal, particularly with exercise. Pulse oximetry to identify the presence of oxygen desaturation either at rest or with exertion is a good screening method, but it is not as reliable or sensitive as direct measures of gas exchange. Hypoxemia with an elevated alveolar–arterial oxygen tension gradient is the rule. There is sometimes accompanying respiratory alkalosis, and in the late stages of any ILD increased carbon dioxide can be found. Measurements of gas exchange during walking or stationary bicycling are practical and helpful in assessing the severity of disease as well as defining the adequacy of supplemental oxygen replacement. Direct measures of gas exchange (arterial blood gases) are more sensitive, reliable, and reproducible than those relying on ear- or finger-probe oximetry, though the latter measures are less invasive and less expensive.

LABORATORY EVALUATION

Laboratory studies are generally nonspecific, though there are exceptions (Table 360.5). Serologic studies to detect autoimmune disease are often helpful, in particular, antinuclear antibody, rheumatoid factor, and, in the appropriate clinical context, antinuclear cytoplasmic antibody. While subtle elevations in both the antinuclear antibody and rheumatoid factor are seen in several ILDs, significant elevations, even in the absence of systemic disease, may suggest an evolving connective tissue disease. A complete blood count and biochemical evaluation of liver and renal function should be carried out to look for evidence of systemic disease. Elevated erythrocyte sedimentation rates, C-reactive protein titers, and hypergammaglobulinemia are relatively common nonspecific findings. Elevated lactic dehydrogenase can be present in a variety of ILDs (IPF, alveolar proteinosis, acute interstitial pneumonia).

An elevated angiotensin-converting enzyme level suggests sarcoidosis but is nonspecific, since it also is found in HP, silicosis,

TABLE 360.5.	LABORATORY FINDINGS IN THE INTERSTITIAL LUNG DISEASES
Abnormality	**Associated ILD**
Leukopenia	Sarcoidosis, connective tissue disease, lymphoma, drug induced
Eosinophilia	Eosinophilic pneumonia, sarcoidosis, systemic vasculitis, drug induced (sulfa, methotrexate)
Thrombocytopenia	Sarcoidosis, connective tissue disease, drug induced, Gaucher's disease
Hemolytic anemia	Connective tissue disease, sarcoidosis, lymphoma, drug induced
Normocytic anemia	Diffuse alveolar hemorrhage syndromes, connective tissue disease, lymphangitic carcinomatosis
Urinary sediment abnormalities	Connective tissue disease, systemic vasculitis, drug induced
Hypogammaglobulinemia	Lymphocytic interstitial pneumonitis
Hypergammaglobulinemia	Connective tissue disease, sarcoidosis, systemic vasculitis, lymphocytic interstitial pneumonia, lymphoma
Serum immune complexes	Idiopathic pulmonary fibrosis, lymphocytic interstitial pneumonitis, systemic vasculitis, connective tissue disease, eosinophilic granuloma
Serum angiotensin-converting enzyme	Sarcoidosis, hypersensitivity pneumonitis, silicosis, Gaucher's disease
Anti–basement membrane antibody	Goodpasture's syndrome
Antineutrophil cytoplasmic antibody	Wegener's granulomatosis, Churg–Strauss syndrome, microscopic polyangiitis
Serum precipitating antibodies	Hypersensitivity pneumonitis
Lymphocyte transformation test to specific antigens	Chronic beryllium disease, aluminum, potroom worker's disease, gold-induced pneumonitis

ILD, interstitial lung disease.

lymphocytic interstitial pneumonia, and the adult respiratory distress syndrome, among other disorders. Serum precipitin testing to antigens known to cause HP is useful but not diagnostic, and rarely does a random hypersensitivity panel provide insight in the absence of an identified antigen exposure. Identification of circulating serum precipitins to a known organic exposure in a patient with pathologically proven HP helps cement the relationship between the exposure and the disease. The identification of antibodies to organic antigens can merely mean exposure to the antigen, however, without indicating disease; the absence of antibodies does not exclude HP. The blood beryllium lymphocyte proliferation test has high specificity and sensitivity for chronic beryllium disease and can be used to distinguish this disorder from other granulomatous ILDs.

BRONCHOALVEOLAR LAVAGE

Bronchoalveolar lavage (BAL), used previously primarily for investigational purposes, appears to have a limited role in the initial evaluation and diagnosis of ILD. The ability to use the available data regarding BAL in ILD is limited by the lack of standardized techniques in both the performance of the procedure and the laboratory analysis of the lavagate. The primary clinical usefulness of BAL is to narrow the differential diagnosis, though it can provide a definitive diagnosis in rare cases. Particular patterns of the cellular differential allow one to focus on a small group of potential diagnoses, while different lavage abnormalities may point to others (Table 360.6). Lavage is also helpful in excluding infectious diseases.

A standard fiberoptic bronchoscope is passed through successive airways until its tip is wedged, usually in a third- or fourth-generation bronchus. In ILD the right-middle lobe or lingula typically is used. Once the bronchoscope is wedged, aliquots of saline (usually 20 to 60 ml) are infused and withdrawn individually, and the collected specimen is sent for evaluation. In normal subjects, about 60% of the infused saline will be retrieved

and 10 to 15 $\times$ 106 overall cells obtained, with a differential of 85% macrophages, 10% lymphocytes, 2% polymorphonuclear cells, and less than 1% eosinophils or basophils. Eosinophilia or lymphocytosis in lavage fluid can significantly narrow the differential diagnosis. Eosinophilia of more than 35% or lymphocytosis of more than 35% is generally helpful. In the idiopathic interstitial pneumonias the lavage findings are nondiagnostic, with generally greater overall numbers of cells and often a near normal differential.

LUNG BIOPSY

Given the number of potential diagnoses and the generally nonspecific nature of clinical, physiologic, radiographic, and laboratory findings, a lung biopsy is often necessary for definitive diagnosis. Histopathologic evaluation of lung tissue remains the most sensitive and specific test to determine accurately the diagnosis and prognosis of the underlying disease.

A transbronchial lung biopsy specimen often is obtained at the time BAL is performed. It is possible to make a histologic diagnosis with transbronchial biopsy, but it is not usual. The technique is helpful for the diagnosis of granulomatous diseases, in patients with peribronchovascular disease (such as lymphangitic spread of carcinoma), and in some airspace-filling diseases, such as eosinophilic pneumonia, bronchoalveolar carcinoma, or alveolar proteinosis. It is very unusual to establish a diagnosis of any of the idiopathic interstitial pneumonias (usual interstitial pneumonia, desquamative interstitial pneumonia, cryptogenic organizing pneumonia, acute interstitial pneumonia, nonspecific interstitial pneumonia) from a transbronchial biopsy specimen. If findings from a transbronchial biopsy specimen are nonspecific, an open or video-assisted thoracoscopic lung biopsy is indicated. This approach should be considered if diagnostic uncertainty persists after noninvasive evaluation and the patient is not at high risk for a surgical procedure or if therapeutic decisions would change given a particular histologic finding. While some ILDs have unique histologic findings (desquamative interstitial pneumonia or EG), others (rheumatoid arthritis) can produce a variety of abnormal pulmonary histologic patterns (UIP, honeycombing, BOOP, NSIP, bronchiolitis, vasculitis). Some histologic patterns (UIP) are seen in several ILDs (IPF, chronic HP, asbestosis, connective tissue disease–related ILD).

The appropriate management of ILD requires a specific diagnosis, which generally necessitates histologic information. While many of these disorders have poor prospects for long-term survival, there are important differences in prognosis and therapy. A firm diagnosis gives both the physician and the patient a sense of confidence when evaluating the available options based on the untreated natural history of the disease, the likelihood of response to therapy, and the risk of disease and therapy-related complications.

TABLE 360.6.	USEFUL BRONCHOALVEOLAR LAVAGE FINDINGS	
Findings	**Potential or Real Diagnoses**	
Cellular differential		
Eosinophilia (>35%)	Eosinophilic pneumonias	
Lymphocytosis (>35%)	Sarcoidosis, hypersensitivity pneumonitis, LIP, lymphoma, malignancy, drug-induced lung disease	
Bloody lavage with hemosiderin-laden macrophages	Diffuse alveolar hemorrhage	
Organisms on stain or culture	Infection	
Positive cytologic results	Malignancy	
Lipid-laden macrophages	Lipoid pneumonia	
PAS-positive lipoproteinaceous material	Alveolar proteinosis	
Ferruginous bodies (asbestosis), dust particles	Pneumoconioses	
Lymphocyte transformation test	Berylliosis	
Birbeck granules on electron microscopy of mononuclear cells	Eosinophilic granuloma	

LIP, lymphocytic interstitial pneumonia; PAS, periodic acid–Schiff.

STRATEGIES FOR OPTIMAL CARE

MANAGEMENT

Since the natural history of most untreated ILDs is progression of fibrosis with its attendant physiologic and lifestyle impairment, most clinicians feel that at least a time-limited trial of therapy is warranted even in the absence of well-designed controlled trials. End-stage lung disease or honeycomb lung can occur in the vast majority of the ILDs and is irreversible. The goal of therapy should be to prevent its development or progression. Lesser degrees of pathologic change usually include a combination of mature fibrosis, granulation tissue (organizing pneumonia), and chronic inflammation. It is the granulation tissue and chronic inflammation that are potentially reversible. A major goal of therapy is to suppress this chronic inflammatory response and reverse the deposition of granulation tissue. The earliest possible diagnosis and institution of therapy is likely to offer the best chance of a response.

The initial intervention should include a vigorous search to identify an etiologic agent and, if found, to avoid it. A patient with HP may need no more than removal from the pertinent exposure to recover completely, while failure to avoid the exposure will lead to recurrent or chronic progressive disease. The patient with RB-ILD may stabilize or improve with cessation of tobacco smoking, whereas one with drug-induced lung disease may respond to cessation of the medication and a short course of corticosteroids. In most of the ILDs, such as IPF, CTD-related ILD, and sarcoidosis, however, the source is unknown, and therapy is directed at the chronic inflammatory response presumed to be responsible for the progressive fibrosis.

Almost all ILD patients need treatment. Control of inflammation requires immunosuppressive medications. Corticosteroid therapy is still considered the standard approach. The response can vary widely, from near complete response (eosinophilic pneumonia) to limited or no response (asbestosis). Unfortunately, corticosteroids have significant side effects, particularly at the doses used in ILD. Even in responsive patients, side effects of therapy may warrant a decrease in dose or even cessation of therapy. Cytotoxic agents—cyclophosphamide and azathioprine—are common treatments for ILD. The beneficial effect noted in Wegener's granulomatosis is one example of how they can consolidate and amplify the benefits of corticosteroids. Many clinicians now add a cytotoxic drug after initial high-dose corticosteroid therapy as a steroid-sparing agent, to allow for maintenance of a response at a much lower steroid dose. Others may initiate therapy with lower doses (10 to 20 mg per day of prednisone) of corticosteroids and a cytotoxic agent simultaneously, taking advantage of their differing mechanisms of antiinflammatory action. When immunosuppressive therapy is used, particularly combination therapy, *Pneumocystis carinii* prophylaxis should be considered. Colchicine also has been proposed to offer modest therapeutic benefit in IPF.

Both the dose and length of therapy depend upon the specific ILD. While some may respond within days (eosinophilic pneumonia) and others within weeks (sarcoidosis and cryptogenic organizing pneumonia), disorders such as IPF require months (often 3 to 6 months) of therapy before a response can be detected. Response to therapy usually is defined by improvement of symptoms and stabilization or improvement in functional, gas exchange, and radiographic abnormalities. Objective evaluations should be carried out on a scheduled basis and as clinically indicated.

A major contributor to death in ILD is hypoxemia, which also can lead to secondary complications, such as pulmonary hyper-

---

TABLE 360.7. CLINICAL DETERIORATION IN PATIENTS WITH ILD

Progression of ILD

Clinical manifestations
Symptoms
Increased dyspnea or cough, reduced exercise capacity
Physical examination
Progression of crackles from basilar regions throughout the lung fields
Worsening right-sided ventricular failure
Pulmonary function
Progressive restrictive ventilatory defect
Decreasing D$_{LCO}$
Worsening hypoxemia
Increased supplemental oxygen requirement
Increased alveolar–arterial oxygen gradient at rest or with exercise
Chest radiography
Progressive volume loss
Progression of interstitial opacities
Honeycombing
Pulmonary arterial hypertension
Progressive cardiomegaly

Complications of ILD

Cardiovascular disease
Right ventricular hypertrophy and cor pulmonale due to progressive pulmonary hypertension or chronic hypoxemia
Left ventricular failure also common, generally due to concurrent ischemic heart disease
Pulmonary infections
Slight increased incidence in many of the interstitial lung disorders
Risk heightened by immunosuppressive therapy
Pulmonary embolism
Sudden worsening of dyspnea with unexplained deterioration in gas exchange and without evidence of superimposed infection should prompt the clinician to consider lung ventilation–perfusion scan or pulmonary angiography.
Malignancy
Idiopathic pulmonary fibrosis and scleroderma carry slight increased risk of lung cancer (all cell types, but particularly adenocarcinoma).
Pneumothorax
Often very difficult to manage

Complications of therapy

Prolonged high-dose corticosteroids
Myopathy with proximal muscle weakness, cataracts, osteoporosis, peptic ulcer, fluid/electrolyte abnormalities, hyperglycemia, weight gain, increased susceptibility to infection
Cytotoxic agents
Increased susceptibility to infection, bone marrow suppression, hepatitis, hemorrhagic cystitis

ILD, interstitial lung disease.

tension and right ventricular failure. Supplemental oxygen to help maintain normoxia at rest, exercise, and sleep can improve significantly a patient's sense of well-being and help prevent hypoxia-related complications. The use of supplemental oxygen also may be necessary to allow a patient to engage in exercise or a pulmonary rehabilitation program. A routine exercise program is important in maintaining aerobic cardiovascular fitness, weight control, bone mass on corticosteroid therapy, and an overall sense of well-being. Any patient with chronic lung disease should receive a pneumococcal vaccine and a yearly influenzae vaccine.

COMPLICATIONS AND PITFALLS

Clinical deterioration in patients with ILD is common and can be life-threatening. Deterioration generally is caused by progression of the primary disease, a disease-related complication, or a complication associated with therapy (Table 360.7). Disease progression usually takes the form of progressive respiratory symptoms with increased dyspnea and cough. Radiologic and physiologic deterioration and worsening gas exchange accompany the symptoms. Worsening of symptoms does not in itself define progression of disease, however, since disease-related complications can be heralded in the same fashion. Right and/or left ventricular dysfunction, pulmonary embolism, respiratory infection, pulmonary malignancy, and pneumothorax all can mimic the progression of an underlying ILD. Complications of treatment include infection, respiratory and peripheral muscle weakness, and osteoporosis.

The most common pitfall in the management of ILD is the failure to establish a diagnosis. At the first sign of disease, patients with IPF may have had abnormal CXR results for more than 5 years. It is not unusual to find that by the time the diagnosis is established, end-stage fibrosis is present. With the currently available therapies, initiation of treatment before development of end-stage fibrosis offers the only hope for response. In some patients a generic diagnosis of ILD is made on the basis of symptoms and a CXR. Corticosteroid therapy is instituted, and the patient responds—but the abnormalities recur after cessation of therapy, or significant complications arise. Without a fully characterized diagnosis, the appropriate dose and length of therapy, alternative medications, and risk of recurrence or complications cannot be intelligently considered.

Indications for REFERRAL

The initial evaluation of a patient with known or suspected ILD should include an exhaustive history and complete physical examination. A plain CXR, an HRCT scan, and pulmonary function testing with lung volumes, spirometry, and a DLCO should be obtained. Gas exchange should be assessed with a resting arterial blood gas analysis and exercise oximetry. A complete blood count, blood chemistry panel, urinalysis, and serologies are undertaken as dictated by the history (anti-

nuclear antibody, rheumatoid factor, antineutrophil cytoplasmic antibodies, anti–basement membrane antibody, and so forth). It is important to review all available old CXRs and pulmonary function studies. The type and pace of change over time often provide insight into the diagnosis and activity of the disease. Common chest diseases (chronic obstructive pulmonary disease, heart failure, atypical pneumonia, asthma, mycobacterial or fungal disease) can mimic ILD, and it is important to consider them as the evaluation evolves. It is likely that most patients ultimately will require lung biopsy to characterize their disease fully, though this decision might be left for the consultant.

Almost all patients with a suspected or known diagnosis of ILD would benefit from referral to a pulmonologist, since pulmonologists are in the best position to combine the clinical, radiographic, physiologic, and pathologic findings of a particular case into a coherent diagnosis. This is particularly true if there are questions regarding the relationship of a lung disease to an occupational or environmental exposure or if a therapeutic immunosuppressive or cytotoxic drug trial is contemplated. Patients with a deteriorating clinical status after initiation of therapy also would benefit from referral, since progression of the underlying disease, complications of the primary disease, and complications of therapy can all manifest in a similar fashion.

A pulmonologist can perform and/or interpret specialized tests, such as open, thorascopic, or transbronchial lung biopsy; BAL; a pressure-volume curve; and cardiopulmonary testing (exercise testing with arterial blood gas analysis to determine if physiologic limitation exists, whether its cause is cardiac or pulmonary, and the degree of hypoxemia with exertion). They also can determine whether additional testing, such as radionuclide scans, right-sided heart catheterization, pulmonary angiography, or studies of respiratory drive would be useful.

BIBLIOGRAPHY

BAL Cooperative Group. Bronchoalveolar lavage constituents in healthy individuals, idiopathic pulmonary fibrosis, and selected comparison groups. *Am Rev Respir Dis* 1990;141:S169–S202.

Bjoraker JA, Ryu JH, Edwin MK, et al. Prognostic significance of histopathologic subsets in idiopathic pulmonary fibrosis. *Am J Respir Crit Care Med* 1998;157(1):199–203.

Coultas DB, Zumwalt RE, Black WC, et al. The epidemiology of interstitial lung disease. *Am Rev Respir Crit Care Med* 1994;150:967–972.

Hogg JC. Chronic interstitial lung disease of unknown cause: a new classification based on pathogenesis. *AJR* 1991;156:225–233.

Katzenstein AL, Myers JL. Idiopathic pulmonary fibrosis: clinical relevance of pathologic classification. *Am J Respir Crit Care Med* 1998;157(4 Pt 1):1301–1315.

King TE Jr. Connective tissue disease. In: Schwarz MI, King TE Jr, eds. *Interstitial lung disease*, third ed. Hamilton: BC Decker, 1998.

Panos RJ, Mortenson R, Niccoli SA, et al. Clinical deterioration in patients with idiopathic pulmonary fibrosis: causes and assessment. *Am J Med* 1990;88:396–404.

Ryu JH, Colby TV, Hartman TE. Idiopathic pulmonary fibrosis: current concepts. *Mayo Clin Proc* 1998;73:1085–1101.

Schwarz MI, King TE Jr, eds. *Interstitial lung disease*, third ed. Hamilton: BC Decker, 1998.

Kelley's Textbook of Internal Medicine, fourth edition. Edited by H. David Humes. Lippincott Williams & Wilkins, Philadelphia © 2000.

C H A P T E R

361

APPROACH TO THE PATIENT WITH SUSPECTED PNEUMONIA

GALEN B. TOEWS

PRESENTATION

Pneumonia is defined as an acute inflammatory process of the lung parenchyma. The inflammatory process is associated with symptoms of acute infection, auscultatory findings consistent with airspace filling and/or lobar consolidation, and an acute infiltrate visible on a chest radiograph. The goals of treating a patient with suspected pneumonia are to establish the presence of an intrapulmonary process, to determine that infection is present, to identify the causative agent, to assess the severity of illness, and to initiate appropriate therapy. Determining the exact causative agent of acute pneumonia is difficult. Therefore, the clinician must collect and correctly interpret various clinical, epidemiologic, and laboratory clues to make a presumptive initial diagnosis. The initial treatment usually is based on the clinical signs and symptoms, an estimate of the severity of illness, the need for hospitalization, evidence of coexisting disease, the patient's age, and the relative frequency of specific pathogens in the at-risk population. The clinical picture of pneumonia classically has been categorized into four syndromes: bacterial or typical, atypical, anaerobic/cavitary, and opportunistic. Nonetheless, some studies have found no convincing associations between symptoms, physical findings, or laboratory test results and specific etiologic factors.

Lower respiratory tract infections are the leading cause of death from infectious diseases in the United States. Community-acquired pneumonia affects three million patients and results in approximately ten million physician visits, 5,000 hospitalizations, and 45,000 deaths in the United States annually. Pneumonia is the sixth most common cause of death in the United States. Death rates associated with pneumonia and influenza increased by 59% between 1979 and 1994. The growing proportion of persons who are at least 65 years of age accounts for much of this increase. Age-adjusted rates also rose by 22%, suggesting the importance of comorbid conditions in a greater percentage of the population. Financial costs associated with pneumonia are estimated at $14 million in direct costs and $9 million

in lost wages annually. Mortality rates are estimated to be less than 1% for patients who are not hospitalized, but they are approximately 14% for hospitalized patients. Thus, a sense of clinical urgency often exists in the early management of acute pneumonia because of the potential for a fatal outcome.

PATHOPHYSIOLOGY

The lungs are inoculated repeatedly with microorganisms from the upper airways and from inhaled aerosols. Inoculum size, bacterial virulence, and the state of host defenses determine the pathogenetic potential of a microbial challenge. The development of a clinical infectious disease of the lungs is determined largely by the success or failure of pulmonary defense mechanisms.

Several factors combine to protect the lower respiratory tract against infection that might result from inhalation or aspiration of infective organisms. The configuration of the upper airway passages ensures that a thin, laminar flow of air passes close to hairs and sticky surfaces that can trap potentially infectious particles. Secretory immunoglobulin A, which constitutes 10% of protein in nasal secretions, binds to and neutralizes certain viruses and may even protect against bacterial colonization by blocking the adherence of bacteria to mucosal surfaces. The epiglottis is the major organ that prevents particles from entering the trachea; its closure during swallowing ensures that mouth contents pass down the esophagus. Similarly, the larynx prevents the passage of secretions down into the trachea and allows the generation of the intrapulmonic pressure needed for an effective cough. If particles succeed in entering the trachea, ciliary action and coughing work together to clear them from the bronchi, the former by steadily moving particles toward the larynx and the latter by propelling them rapidly, bypassing ciliary action.

When bacteria bypass these mechanisms, noncellular and cellular host factors at the level of the alveolus provide further protection. Bacterial cell wall components, such as peptidoglycan in gram-positive bacteria, can activate the complement cascade and generate C3b on the bacterial surface. Three sets of reactions result. First, C3b is recognized by polymorphonuclear leukocytes (PMNs) and macrophages, thus serving as an opsonizing factor; second, C5a is generated, providing a potent chemotactic force for attracting PMNs into the area; and third, membrane attack complexes may be generated on the bacterial surfaces. In the absence of antibody that reacts with the bacterial surface, the alternative complement pathway, a relatively slow and inefficient process, is responsible. These reactions proceed far more vigorously through the classic complement pathway in the presence of immunoglobulin that reacts specifically with antigenic sites on the bacterial surfaces. Cellular defenses depend on alveolar macrophages and recruited PMNs, which can ingest infectious organisms. Inflammatory cell recruitment is dependent on chemokines, a supergene family of small, inducible, protein mediators. Immune and nonimmune cells (epithelial cells, fibroblasts, endothelial cells) generate chemokines in response to microbial products (lipopolysaccharides) or host-derived mediators, such as tumor necrosis factor α or interleukin-1. Virulent bacteria resist attempts at phagocytosis in the absence of relevant antibodies, usually because of the presence of an exopolysaccharide capsule or slime layer. Other microorganisms, such as mycobacteria and fungi, are eradicated only by activated macrophages and, therefore, require intact cell-mediated immunity.

HISTORY AND PHYSICAL EXAMINATION

COMMUNITY-ACQUIRED PNEUMONIA

Symptoms of acute lower respiratory tract infection include cough, with or without sputum production; change in the color of respiratory secretions; dyspnea; chest discomfort; fever or hypothermia; shaking chills; sweats; and pleuritic chest pain. Nonspecific symptoms of abdominal pain, anorexia, fatigue, myalgias, and headache also may be present.

Physical examination may document fever, tachycardia, and tachypnea. In advanced cases, confusion, cyanosis, splinting, and labored breathing may be noted. Localized, fine crepitant rales are noted initially over the involved portion of lung, and signs of lobar consolidation (bronchial breath sounds, whispered pectoriloquy, vocal fremitus, and dullness to percussion) may be found as the disease progresses. Extension of pneumonia to pleural surfaces is associated with pleuritic pain and signs suggestive of a pleural effusion. Lower-lobe pneumonias may cause referral of pain to the abdomen; the clinical symptoms of these patients can mimic those of an acute intra-abdominal process. The white blood cell count is elevated in most patients with bacterial pneumonia. Leukopenia, if present, is a poor prognostic sign.

A chest radiograph is critical to making the diagnosis of pneumonia; however, it is almost never diagnostic of the specific infectious agent causing pneumonia. A localized bronchopneumonia pattern is the most typical radiographic finding. Nevertheless, dense lobar or multilobar consolidation, cavitation, or large pleural effusions also are found in patients with bacterial pneumonia. Certain radiographic features may aid diagnosis. Several bilateral, cavitary infiltrates suggest infection caused by *Staphylococcus aureus*. Ill-defined, thin-walled cavities (pneumatoceles); bronchopleural fistulas; and empyema also develop in the context of *S. aureus* infections. Cavitation also indicates gram-negative infection, *Streptococcus pneumoniae* type 3, or anaerobic infection.

ANAEROBIC/CAVITARY PNEUMONIA SYNDROME

Anaerobic infections usually take the form of subacute or chronic constitutional and pulmonary symptoms. Symptoms often are present for 3 to 5 weeks. Chronic cough, usually productive or containing purulent sputum, is reported by virtually all patients. A putrid odor of the sputum is present in 33% to 60% of patients and is virtually diagnostic of anaerobic infection. Fever (about 102°F) and chest pain occur in half of patients. The chest pain may be pleuritic or a dull, aching pain. About one-third of patients experience hemoptysis and weight loss (about 20 pounds).

About 75% of patients have a predisposition to aspiration of oropharyngeal secretions. Alcoholism is the most common predisposition; others include seizure disorders, dysphagia, cerebrovascular accidents, and general anesthesia. Poor dental hygiene and periodontal disease are often present. Patients who experience anaerobic infections stemming from aspiration almost always have some teeth. Physical examination of the chest usually is not helpful. Laboratory findings are nonspecific; leukocytosis and anemia are noted in most patients.

Lung abscesses are associated with bronchogenic carcinoma in 10% to 30% of cases. Certain signs and symptoms may be useful in differentiating patients who have carcinoma from those who have abscess alone. The presence of systemic symptoms (chills, sweats, general malaise), predisposition to aspiration, an initial oral temperature above normal, and a white blood cell count greater than 10,900 per milliliter are associated with a high probability of no underlying malignancy.

Numerous organisms other than anaerobes can result in these symptoms. The possibility of involvement of extrapulmonary organs always should be explored, because it suggests a cause other than anaerobes and may even indicate a specific origin of infection. Several verrucous or ulcerative skin lesions frequently are seen in blastomycosis and coccidioidomycosis and may be the first complaint. Skin lesions also are seen with cryptococcosis and nocardiosis, but much less frequently. Oral ulcers (painful or painless) are a characteristic manifestation of histoplasmosis and also are noted in cases of blastomycosis, coccidioidomycosis, and tuberculosis. Headache or the presence of abnormal spinal fluid points to coccidioidomycosis, tuberculosis, or cryptococcosis. Focal neurologic symptoms or signs in a patient with a cavitary lung lesion suggest the possibility of brain abscess associated with anaerobic disease or nocardiosis. Bone involvement indicates tuberculosis, blastomycosis, or coccidioidomycosis; the spine is affected most often. Blastomycosis and tuberculosis can involve both the upper and the lower genitourinary tracts.

The chest radiograph provides important clues. Anaerobes typically cause cavitary lesions (lung abscess), necrotizing pneumonia, or empyema. Lesions usually are found in dependent segments, and the right lung is involved in 75% of cases. The posterior segment of the right-upper lobe often is affected. About two-thirds of lesions are found in the posterior segments of the upper lobes or the superior segments of the lower lobes. A prominent infiltrate frequently surrounds the cavity, and the wall of the cavity is thick (more than 4 mm) and ragged. An air-fluid level strongly suggests anaerobic disease. Although gram-negative bacilli and *S. aureus* produce similar radiographic manifestations, anaerobic infections can be pinpointed by their indolent clinical course and association with aspiration. Anaerobes also can cause acute pneumonitis that is clinically and radiographically indistinguishable from pneumococcal pneumonia.

Typical and atypical tuberculosis, histoplasmosis, coccidioidomycosis, sporotrichosis, and melioidosis all characteristically produce unilateral upper-lobe fibrocavitary disease that looks like tuberculosis. Prominent infiltrates often surround cavities in tuberculosis and melioidosis. A thin-walled cavity is suggestive of coccidioidomycosis or sporotrichosis. Cryptococcosis and actinomycosis take the initial form of masslike nodular infiltrates, whereas nocardiosis has manifestations that resemble consolidative segmental pneumonia. Lesions of nocardiosis and actinomycosis tend to cavitate eventually. Pleural effusions, chest wall abscesses, and osteomyelitis of an adjacent rib also suggest infection with *Nocardia* or *Actinomyces* organisms. Calcification commonly occurs in tuberculosis, histoplasmosis, and coccidioidomycosis, but it is rare in actinomycosis, blastomycosis, cryptococcosis, nocardiosis, or sporotrichosis.

OPPORTUNISTIC PNEUMONIA SYNDROME

For a discussion of opportunistic pneumonia syndrome, see Chapter 362.

LABORATORY STUDIES AND DIAGNOSTIC TESTS

GRAM'S STAIN OF SPUTUM

A Gram's stain of expectorated sputum is the only diagnostic tool available to all physicians at the outset of therapy. The value of examining expectorated sputum is the subject of debate, since no studies have correlated data from Gram's stains to cultures of alveolar secretions in large numbers of patients with community-acquired pneumonia.

If a Gram's stain is part of the clinical evaluation, the patient must be instructed properly regarding sample collection, and the sample collection should be supervised directly by a physician. If sputum is collected without supervision, there is a 75% chance that the specimen will be of poor quality. Gram-stained sputum should first be examined under low-power magnification $(100 \times)$ and the number of epithelial cells and neutrophils determined. Large numbers of epithelial cells (more than 25 per low-power field) reflect contamination of the specimen with oral contents; in this case, another specimen should be collected, regardless of the number of visible neutrophils. Even if these criteria are applied, the usefulness of Gram's stain data is uncertain. No studies have demonstrated clearly the cost-effectiveness or other advantages of attempts to identify the etiologic pathogen.

In the appropriate clinical context, a predominance of gram-positive, lancet-shaped diplococci reflects *S. pneumoniae* infection. The presence of more than 10 diplococci per oil-immersion field $(1,000 \times)$ reportedly predicts the isolation of pneumococci in sputum with a specificity of 85% and a sensitivity of 62%. Similarly, the presence of small, gram-negative coccobacillary organisms suggests *Haemophilus influenzae* infection, whereas the presence of gram-positive cocci in tetrads and grapelike clusters denotes *S. aureus* infection. The presence of more than 12 organisms resembling *H. influenzae* distinguishes patients with acute bacterial exacerbations from those who have recovered from pneumonia or are well.

Special stains or preparations of sputum frequently are required in the evaluation of cavitary pneumonias. An acid-fast smear should be carried out in all cases of subacute, chronic, or cavitary pneumonia, because it provides the first evidence of infection in about half of patients who show culture-positive results for *Mycobacterium tuberculosis*. A modified acid-fast stain

(sulfuric rather than hydrochloric acid in the decolorizer) should be used if the partially acid-fast *Nocardia* species is sought. Examination of a potassium hydroxide wet-mount preparation may allow rapid diagnosis of blastomycosis, coccidioidomycosis, and cryptococcosis. A Gomori's methenamine-silver or periodic acid–Schiff stain may be useful for identifying fungal elements.

SPUTUM CULTURES

Culture of expectorated sputum is neither specific nor sensitive. If isolation of penicillin-resistant pneumococci is anticipated in light of local epidemiologic and sensitivity data, sputum culture and sensitivity data are useful. Half of patients with bacteremic pneumococcal pneumonia have negative results on sputum cultures, even when large numbers of organisms are present on Gram's stain. Furthermore, expectorated sputum is contaminated with oropharyngeal flora. Because organisms that produce pneumonia often colonize the oropharynx of the uninfected patient, sputum cultures may erroneously suggest pneumonia infection.

Sputum cultures are valuable in the diagnosis of certain subacute/cavitary pneumonias. Mycobacteria grow well on culture media, and it has been estimated that sputum cultures can detect as few as 10 acid-fast bacilli per milliliter of concentrated, digested sputum. A period of 4 to 8 weeks is required for growth. Interpretation of positive sputum cultures for *Mycobacterium avium* complex is difficult, because this organism can colonize patients without causing disease.

The yield of fungal cultures varies with the organism and the stage of disease. Chronic forms of coccidioidomycosis and blastomycosis yield positive culture results in 70% to 100% of cases if several specimens are collected. In histoplasmosis, the yield depends on the stage of illness. In the early stages, characterized by a clinical picture of nonbacterial pneumonia and an interstitial infiltrate, the yield is only 30%; in the chronic cavitary stage, the yield approaches 70%. In cryptococcosis, less than 50% of patients have positive results on sputum culture. Transtracheal aspirates or percutaneous aspirates are required as culture sources for *Actinomyces*, because this organism is part of the normal oral flora. Anaerobic culture conditions must be requested for this organism. Isolation of *Nocardia* organisms also requires special considerations. Although this organism can grow aerobically, it rarely is recovered from routine sputum cultures, because the cultures are discarded before the 3 to 5 days required for this organism's growth. The laboratory should be requested to hold cultures longer than usual if *Nocardia* is the suspected culprit. *Nocardia* organisms also may be isolated in fungal or tuberculosis cultures, because it grows well on the media used in these cultures.

BLOOD AND SEROLOGIC STUDIES

Blood cultures (two sets) should be obtained from all patients who require hospitalization for suspected bacterial pneumonia. A positive blood culture finding offers definitive proof of the cause of pneumonia. Blood culture results are positive in 20% to 30% of patients with pneumococcal pneumonia and gram-negative bacillary pneumonia.

DNA PROBES AND AMPLIFICATION

Rapid diagnostic tests that use nucleic acid amplification for detecting microbes that cause pneumonia are under development. The greatest potential usefulness for these tests will be in detection of *Mycoplasma pneumoniae*, *Legionella* species, and selected pathogens that infrequently colonize the upper airways in the absence of disease. Polymerase chain reaction for detection of *M. tuberculosis* is the only such assay for a respiratory pathogen approved by the Food and Drug Administration.

DIFFERENTIAL DIAGNOSIS

The clinical signs and symptoms, including history, physical examination, and routine laboratory tests and roentgenographic examination, do not allow the clinician to pinpoint a specific diagnosis and source of infection in patients with community-acquired pneumonia. *H. influenzae*, *S. aureus*, and *S. pneumoniae* produce indistinguishable clinical syndromes. Bacterial and viral agents bring about subacute illness indistinguishable from that caused by *M. pneumoniae*. *Legionella* species and influenza can provoke subacute pneumonia or even life-threatening pneumonia.

Certain pathogens cause pneumonia more often in patients with specific risk factors. Pneumococcal pneumonia develops more frequently in the elderly and in patients with a variety of comorbid conditions, including chronic obstructive pulmonary disease, cardiovascular disease, HIV infection, immunoglobulin deficiency, asplenia, and hematologic malignancy. *S. pneumoniae* is the second most common cause of acute pneumonia in patients with AIDS. *Legionella* is an opportunistic pathogen; it is an important cause of pneumonia in patients with chronic obstructive pulmonary disease who smoke, patients with renal failure, and organ transplant recipients.

Parenteral drug abusers often suffer pneumonia as a result of hematogenous dissemination of organisms from an infected injection site or from right-sided endocarditis. The onset of this form of pneumonia can mimic acute pulmonary embolism with pleuritic chest pain, dyspnea, and fever. Insufficiency murmurs of the tricuspid, aortic, and mitral valves may be present. *S. aureus* is the most common cause of pneumonia in these patients, but disease may stem from infection with *S. pneumoniae* and gram-negative bacilli, such as *Pseudomonas*, *Serratia*, and *Proteus*.

Bacterial pneumonia that arises in the convalescent phase of influenza deserves special attention. Symptoms of typical pneumonia (shaking, chills, pleuritic chest pain, cough productive of purulent sputum) appear in these patients 2 to 14 days after the onset of signs and symptoms of influenza. In many instances, the symptoms of the viral illness have nearly resolved, and the patient complains of a relapse. This type of pneumonia, which is sometimes life-threatening, most often is caused by *S. pneumoniae*, but *S. aureus* also is seen more commonly than in patients without influenza.

Seasonal differences exist in the incidence of community-acquired pneumonia. *S. pneumoniae* and *H. influenzae* infections and influenza occur predominantly in the winter. *Chlamydia pneumoniae* organisms cause pneumonia year round. The incidence of *Legionella* infections is highest in the summer. An increase in the incidence of *Mycoplasma* infection occurs every 3 to 6 years. Viral agents associated with pneumonia in adults include influenza A and B and adenovirus types 3, 4, and 7. Adenoviral infections are found primarily in military recruits, and outbreaks are most common between January and April. Influenza triggers disease in an epidemic pattern, though sporadic cases also occur. Respiratory syncytial virus, rhinovirus, enterovirus, and parainfluenza are unusual pathogens in adult patients.

Although it is ideal to make a specific diagnosis and pinpoint the source of disease in the management of community-acquired pneumonia, limitations in diagnostic testing usually make this goal impossible. The responsible microbe is not identified in about 50% of patients, even when extensive diagnostic tests are undertaken. Accordingly, an empiric approach to initial antibiotic therapy is often required.

Upper respiratory tract infections should be distinguished from lower respiratory tract infections; most upper respiratory tract infections are of viral origin and do not require antimicrobial therapy. Chest radiographs are particularly valuable for documenting the presence of lower respiratory tract infection, detecting alternative diagnoses or associated conditions, and assessing the severity of pneumonia; radiographs are occasionally useful in determining the origin of pneumonia. Pulmonary infections also must be differentiated from other pulmonary diseases. Pulmonary pathologic conditions have a limited number of signs and symptoms; accordingly, the majority are nonspecific (Table 361.1). This is a particularly important consideration in

TABLE 361.1.	DIFFERENTIAL DIAGNOSIS OF CLINICAL MANIFESTATIONS OF PNEUMONIA
Cough	Asthma
	Chronic bronchitis
	Upper respiratory tract infection
	Bronchogenic carcinoma
	Interstitial lung disease
	Drugs (captoprin)
Dyspnea	Asthma
	Chronic bronchitis
	Emphysema
	Congestive heart failure
	Interstitial lung disease
	Pulmonary vascular disease
Sputum production	Chronic bronchitis
	Asthma
	Bronchiectasis
Fever	Upper respiratory tract infection
	Non-respiratory tract infection
	Rheumatic diseases
Pulmonary infiltrates	Congestive heart failure
	Bronchiolitis obliterans–organizing pneumonia
	Pulmonary carcinoma
	Pulmonary hemorrhage
	Pulmonary vasculitis
	Atelectasis

the evaluation of outpatients, for whom laboratory and radiographic investigations are limited.

STRATEGIES FOR OPTIMAL CARE

Indications for HOSPITALIZATION

The initial task in the treatment of patients with community-acquired pneumonia is to determine whether the patient can be treated as an outpatient or whether hospitalization is re-

quired. This decision has a significant impact on the cost and outcome of therapy. There are no firm guidelines concerning the time at which a patient should be admitted, but factors that raise the risk of death or the risk of a complicated course have been identified (Table 361.2). A prediction rule has been developed to predict the risk of dying within 30 days of presentation in patients with community-acquired pneumonia. This scoring system employs 19 variables that stratify patients into groups I to V according to risk of death (Table 361.2). While these groups were validated as predictors of death, they serve as a rational foundation for decision making regarding hospitalization. Prognosis is sufficiently good in categories I or II to consider outpatient care. Category III patients might be hospitalized briefly or treated as outpatients. Patients in categories IV or V require hospitalization. The availability and quality of home support and the proba-

TABLE 361.2.   A STORING SYSTEM FOR PREDICTION OF MORTALITY

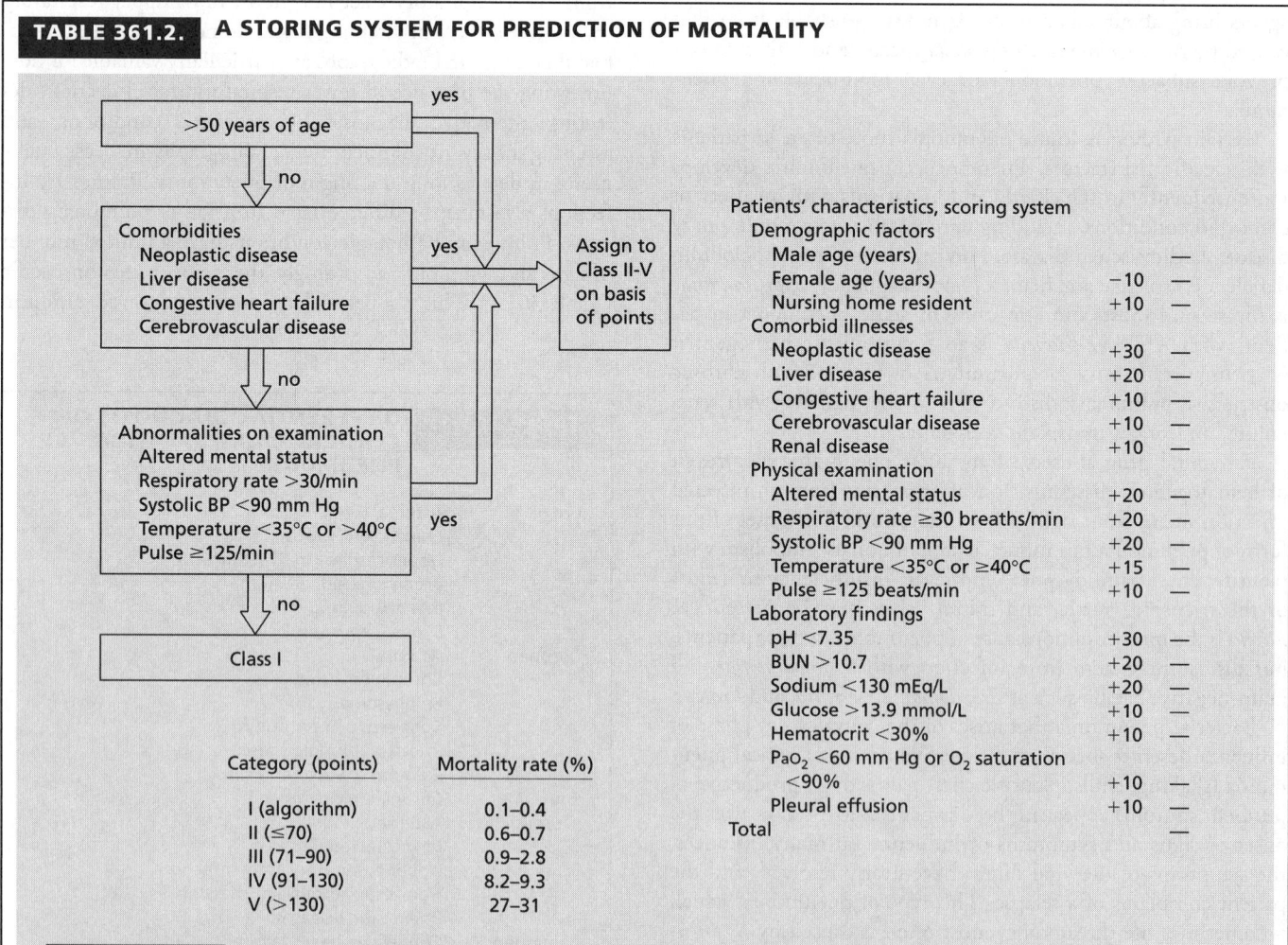

Category (points)	Mortality rate (%)
I (algorithm)	0.1–0.4
II (≤70)	0.6–0.7
III (71–90)	0.9–2.8
IV (91–130)	8.2–9.3
V (>130)	27–31

BP, blood pressure; BUN, blood urea nitrogen.
(From Fine MJ, Auble TE, Yealy DM, et al. A prediction rule to identify low-risk patients with community acquired pneumonia. *N Engl J Med* 1997;336:243–250, with permission.)
EVIDENCE LEVEL: A. Reference: Fine MJ, Auble TE, Yealy DM, et al. A prediction rule to identify low-risk patients with community acquired pneumonia. *N Engl J Med* 1997;336:243–250.

TABLE 361.3.	FINDINGS SUGGESTING SEVERE COMMUNITY-ACQUIRED PNEUMONIA

Respiratory rate >30 breaths/min
Systolic BP <90 mm Hg or diastolic BP <60 mm Hg
Bilateral or multilobe involvement
Severe respiratory failure—Pao$_2$/Fio$_2$ ratio <250 mm Hg
Requirement for mechanical ventilation
Requirement of vasopressors for >4 hr
Urine output <20 mL/hr, acute renal failure requiring dialysis

BP, blood pressure.

TABLE 361.4.	ORGANISMS THAT CAUSE PNEUMONIA

Common	Uncommon
Outpatient pneumonia	
Streptococcus pneumoniae	*Legionella* species
Mycoplasma pneumoniae	*Staphylococcus aureus*
Respiratory viruses	*Mycobacterium*
Chlamydia pneumoniae	*tuberculosis*
Haemophilus influenzae	*Fungi*
	Klebsiella pneumoniae
Community-acquired pneumonia requiring hospitalization	
Streptococcus pneumoniae	*Mycoplasma pneumoniae*
Haemophilus influenzae	*Moraxella catarrhalis*
Polymicrobial	*Mycobacterium*
Anaerobic bacteria	*tuberculosis*
Aerobic gram-negative bacilli	*Fungi*
Legionella species	
Staphylococcus aureus	
Chlamydia pneumoniae	
Respiratory viruses	
Severe community-acquired pneumonia requiring hospitalization	
Streptococcus pneumoniae	*Haemophilus influenzae*
Legionella species	*Mycobacterium*
Aerobic gram-negative bacilli	*tuberculosis*
	Fungi
Mycoplasma pneumoniae	
Respiratory viruses	

bility of compliance are crucial variables. Prognostic scores are complex and should not supercede clinical judgment.

Patients with severe community-acquired pneumonia should be separated from those with pneumonia that is less severe but still requires hospitalization. Although no universally accepted definition of severe community-acquired pneumonia exists, the presence of one of the conditions shown in Table 361.3 defines pneumonia as severe. These patients have a mortality rate of about 50% and must be identified immediately for intensive care. The most common pathogens associated with community-acquired pneumonia treated on an outpatient basis, community-acquired pneumonia treated on an inpatient basis, and severe community-acquired pneumonia are shown in Table 361.4. An unusual cause of community-acquired pneumonia should be considered if the history provides epidemiologic clues (exposure, occupation, geography, travel) (Table 361.5).

MANAGEMENT

Selection of antibiotics is straightforward if a causative agent has been pinpointed. Initial therapy for community-acquired pneumonia is necessarily empiric, however, because clinical and radiographic findings are nonspecific and diagnostic tests cannot identify the responsible microbe in most instances. Initial empiric therapy must be broad, so that several different possible microbes are inhibited. Antimicrobial treatment should be initiated promptly after the diagnosis of pneumonia is established; a delay from the time of admission to initiation of antibiotic therapy exceeding 8 hours is associated with rising death rates. Antimicrobial therapy can be adjusted to specific narrow-spectrum agents if an etiologic agent is identified and antimicrobial susceptibility tests are available.

COMMUNITY-ACQUIRED PNEUMONIA TREATED ON AN OUTPATIENT BASIS

A macrolide antibiotic is reasonable empiric therapy for outpatients. Erythromycin (250 mg taken orally every 6 hours for 14 days) provides excellent coverage for *S. pneumoniae*, *M. pneumoniae*, *C. pneumoniae*, and *Legionella pneumophila* but is relatively inactive against *H. influenzae*. Clarithromycin (500 mg taken orally every 12 hours for 14 days) or azithromycin (500 mg administered orally on day 1 and then 250 mg taken orally

each day for 4 days) is an alternative for patients who experience unacceptable gastrointestinal symptoms with erythromycin. Clarithromycin and azithromycin have in vitro activity against *H. influenzae* as well as *S. pneumoniae*, *M. pneumoniae*, *C. pneumoniae*, and *L. pneumophila*; the latter agents could be considered for patients likely to be harboring *H. influenzae* (those with a history of smoking). Clarithromycin should not be given to pregnant women.

Doxycycline (100 mg taken orally twice daily for 14 days) is also acceptable therapy for these patients, because it is inexpensive, produces few side effects, and can be administered once or twice a day. Reluctance to use doxycycline is based on the concern that a substantial percentage of *S. pneumoniae* organisms are resistant; contemporary studies show that 5% to 8% of these organisms are resistant to doxycycline. Fluoroquinolones (which have enhanced activity against *S. pneumoniae*), such as levofloxacin (500 mg administered orally every 24 hours for 7 to 14 days), trovafloxacin (200 mg taken orally every 24 hours for 7 to 14 days), sparfloxacin (400 mg ingested orally as a loading dose followed by 200 mg every 24 hours for 7 to 14 days), or grepafloxacin (600 mg administered every 24 hours for 7 to 14 days), are also appropriate therapy. These drugs are active against most aerobic gram-positive cocci, gram-negative bacilli, *H. influenzae*, *Moraxella catarrhalis*, *Legionella* species, *M. pneumoniae*, and *C. pneumoniae*. Morbidity and mortality rates and the need for subsequent hospitalization are no higher among outpatients treated with less expensive agents.

TABLE 361.5.	HISTORICAL CLUES TO UNUSUAL PNEUMONIAS	
Type of Pneumonia	**Exposure History**	**Occupational or Risk Population**
Anthrax	Cattle, horses, swine, wools, hides	Butchers, tanners, wool carders, agricultural workers
Brucellosis	Cattle, swine, goats, raw milk products	Abattoir workers, recent Mexican immigrants from Mexico, veterinarians, agricultural workers
Coccidioidomycosis	Travel to San Joaquin Valley, southern California, southwest Texas, New Mexico, Arizona	Agricultural workers, construction workers
Cryptococcosis	Pigeon droppings, HIV	AIDS
Hantavirus pulmonary syndrome	Deer mouse (*Peromyscus maniculatus*)	Residents/traveler in Four Corners Region (New Mexico, Arizona, Utah, Colorado)
Histoplasmosis	Chicken or bat droppings, travel to Ohio or Mississippi River valley	Agricultural workers, construction workers
Legionnaires' disease	Contaminated air coolers or hospital water supply	Office workers, maintenance workers, hospitalized patients
Melioidosis	Travel to Southeast Asia, Australia, South and Central America, Guam	Military personnel
Plague	Ground squirrels, prairie dogs, rabbits, rats in endemic areas (western United States)	Hunters, campers, agricultural workers
Psittacosis	Budgerigars, cockatoos, parrots, parakeets, pigeons, turkeys	Bird fanciers, agricultural workers
Q fever	Cattle, sheep, or goat milk, placentas, or feces	Agricultural workers
Sporotrichosis	Rose thorns	Gardeners, florists
Tularemia	Tissue of rabbits or squirrels, bite of infected ticks or flies	Hunters, campers

COMMUNITY-ACQUIRED PNEUMONIA TREATED ON AN INPATIENT BASIS

Patients with community-acquired pneumonia who require hospitalization are usually treated with parenteral antibiotics. Intravenous β-lactam agents with activity against *S. pneumoniae*, such as cefuroxime (750 to 1,500 mg administered intravenously every 8 hours), ceftriaxone (1 g taken intravenously every 12 hours), or cefotaxime (1 g taken intravenously every 8 hours) plus erythromycin (1 g administered intravenously every 6 hours), are appropriate therapy for hospitalized patients. This regimen is effective antimicrobial treatment against *S. pneumoniae*, *H. influenzae*, anaerobes, gram-negative bacilli (*Klebsiella pneumoniae*, non-pseudomonads), and *L. pneumophila*. Intravenous treatment with levofloxacin (500 mg daily) or trovafloxacin (200 mg daily) alone also is appropriate.

SEVERE COMMUNITY-ACQUIRED PNEUMONIA

Certain pathogens have a strong relationship to severe community-acquired pneumonia (Table 361.4), so antibiotic therapy must be tailored to inhibit these microbes. *S. pneumoniae* and *L. pneumophila* are the most common organisms responsible for these types of pneumonia. Gram-negative bacilli cause severe pneumonia almost exclusively in patients with chronic obstructive pulmonary disease, alcoholism, and diabetes mellitus. Ceftiaxone (1 g taken intravenously every 12 hours), cefotaxime (1 g delivered intravenously every 8 hours), or piperacillin tazobactam (3.375 g dispensed intravenously every 6 hours) plus erythromycin (1 g taken intravenously every 6 hours) or azithromycin (500 mg administered intravenously daily) is appropriate therapy. Treatment with levofloxacin (500 mg administered intravenously daily) or trovafloxacin (200 mg dispensed intravenously daily) is also effective therapy.

P. aeruginosa is rare except in patients with bronchiectasis, patients who have received broad-spectrum antibiotics for 1 week or patients who have undergone phagocyte-suppressive therapy. Patients with risk factors for *P. aeruginosa* infection should be given piperacillin/tazobactam (3.375 g taken intravenously every 6 hours), imipenem (500 mg taken intravenously every 6 hours), meropenem (1.0 g dispensed intravenously every 6 hours), or cefepime (1.0 to 2.0 g administered intravenously every 6 hours) plus erythromycin (1 g delivered intravenously every 6 hours), azithromycin (500 mg given intravenously daily), levofloxacin (500 mg taken intravenously daily), or trovafloxacin (200 mg administered intravenously daily) plus gentamycin or tobramycin (1.7 mg per kilogram delivered intravenously every 8 hours).

The therapy for anaerobic/cavitary pneumonia depends on the pace of the illness and the degree of clinical toxicity. Clindamycin is effective for most patients with anaerobic pulmonary disease and is the drug of choice. If tuberculosis is a strong possibility in light of clinical symptoms, antituberculosis therapy should be initiated while waiting for culture results. Treatment of other causes of chronic cavitary pneumonia is postponed until a diagnosis is established.

COMPLICATIONS

Pleural fluid can be detected on radiography in 40% of patients hospitalized for pneumonia. In most cases, the amount is so small that needle aspiration is unsuccessful. When fluid can be obtained, in about 90% of cases, it is not purulent, microorganisms cannot be seen on Gram's stain, and the pH is above 7.2. In these patients, fluid removal (if enough is present) and implementation of appropriate antibiotics seem to be associated with uneventful recovery. This state is called uncomplicated parapneumonic effusion.

When radiography shows loculated fluid, or if the fluid is frankly purulent, gives a positive result on Gram's stain, or has a pH less than 7.1, the diagnosis of empyema or complicated parapneumonic effusion is made. This condition is associated with a substantially greater risk of serious morbidity. Pneumococcal and anaerobic pneumonias appear to cause most empyemas, though pneumonia due to *Streptococcus pyogenes* is associated with a disproportionately high incidence of empyema. The essence of therapy for complicated empyema is to remove the infected material from the pleural space by whatever means is required—needle aspiration, thoracentesis tube, or thoracotomy. Delay of this essential treatment is likely to lead to a prolonged hospital course and the eventual need for thoracotomy. See Chapter 358 for further discussion of pleural effusions. Aside from empyema, other complications of bacterial pneumonia are rare. Metastatic infection may affect the meninges, heart valves, pericardium, bones, and joints. Cases of purulent pericarditis and vertebral osteomyelitis are seen infrequently.

COST-EFFECTIVENESS

The initial decision to hospitalize patients with pneumonia or to treat them as outpatients in the ambulatory care setting is the major determinant of cost of treatment. Judicious use of antibiotics can clearly lower costs, but these costs are trivial when compared with hospital costs. Average costs of treating community-acquired pneumonia in the hospital are 17 to 51 times higher than in the ambulatory setting. Thus, limiting the need for hospitalization or the length of stay offers the greatest opportunity to reduce health care costs.

No controlled trials have addressed specifically the question of length of therapy for pneumonia. It is reasonable to treat *S. pneumoniae* infections until a patient is afebrile for 72 hours. Pneumonia caused by *M. pneumoniae*, *C. pneumoniae*, and *Legionella* species should be treated for at least 2 weeks. Shorter courses of therapy should be used if azithromycin is given. Changing from intravenous to oral therapy is associated with economic and social benefits. This adjustment can be made if the patient's clinical symptoms are improving and if he or she is hemodynamically stable, able to swallow drugs, and has a functioning gastrointestinal tract. These conditions are usually met within 2 to 4 days. Broad-spectrum cephalosporins, newer macrolides, and fluoroquinolones have been used successfully as oral therapy. Patients failing to improve within this time frame should be evaluated for reasons for failure. Possible reasons include an incorrect diagnosis (Table 361.1), a resistant pathogen, host defense abnormalities, medication error, poor compliance, or an unusual pathogen (Table 361.5). Complications or extension of disease (empyema) should be considered. Radiographic signs of improvement may be delayed; follow-up radiographs should be obtained 7 to 12 weeks after initiation of treatment.

PREVENTION OF PNEUMONIA

Influenza vaccine should be given annually to persons at risk for complications and to health care workers. The currently available 23-valent pneumococcal vaccine should be administered, as suggested by the Centers for Disease Control Guidelines.

BIBLIOGRAPHY

Bartlett JG, Breiman RF, Mandell LA, et al. Community acquired pneumonia in adults: guidelines for management. *Clin Infect Dis* 1998;26: 811–838.

Bartlett JG, Mundy LM. Community-acquired pneumonia. *N Engl J Med* 1995;333:1618–1623.

Fine MJ, Auble TE, Yealy DM, et al. A prediction rule to identify low-risk patients with community acquired pneumonia. *N Engl J Med* 1997; 336:243–250.

Gilbert K, Gleason PP, Singer DE, et al. Variations in antimicrobial use and cost in more than 2,000 patients with community acquired pneumonia. *Am J Med* 1998;104:17–27.

Huchon G, Woodhead M, ESOCAP Committee. Guidelines for the management of adult community-acquired lower respiratory tract infections: European Study of Community Acquired Pneumonia (ESOCAP) Committee. *Eur Respir J* 1998;11:986–991.

Marrie TJ, Durant H, Yates L. Community-acquired pneumonia requiring hospitalization: a 5 year prospective study. *Rev Infect Dis* 1989;11: 586–599.

Marrie TJ, Peeling RW, Fine MJ, et al. Ambulatory patients with community-acquired pneumonia: the frequency of atypical agents and clinical course. *Am J Med* 1996;101:508–515.

Niederman MS, Bass JB, Campbell GD, et al. Guidelines for the initial management of community-acquired pneumonia: diagnosis, assessment of severity, and initial antimicrobial therapy. *Am Rev Respir Dis* 1993; 148:1418–1426.

Torres A, Serra-Batlles J, Ferrer A, et al. Severe community-acquired pneumonia: epidemiologic and prognostic factors. *Am Rev Respir Dis* 1991; 144:312–318.

Weingarten SR, Riedinger MS, Hobson P, et al. Evaluation of a pneumonia practice guideline in an interventional trial. *Am J Respir Crit Care Med* 1996;153:1110–1115.

Kelley's Textbook of Internal Medicine, fourth edition. Edited by H. David Humes. Lippincott Williams & Wilkins, Philadelphia © 2000.

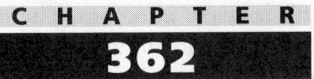

CHAPTER
362

EVALUATION OF PULMONARY DISEASE IN THE IMMUNOCOMPROMISED HOST

PHILIP C. HOPEWELL

This chapter defines the diagnostic strategies applicable to patients with disorders that result in a reduction in the functional capabilities of the immune system in the broad sense. These disorders include abnormalities in polymorphonuclear leukocyte (PMN) number or function, dysfunction of the humoral immune system, and alterations in cell-mediated immunity. In many instances, defects may exist in more than one component of lung defenses, and nonimmunologic factors may compound these abnormalities further.

FACTORS AFFECTING LUNG DEFENSES

QUANTITATIVE OR QUALITATIVE NEUTROPHIL DEFECTS

A decline in the number of circulating PMNs is particularly common in patients undergoing chemotherapy for malignancies, in patients with acute leukemia, and in patients who have undergone bone marrow transplantation. If the cells function normally, serious infections generally are not seen until the absolute PMN count falls below 500 per microliter. The incidence of infection also seems to be directly related to the rate of reduction in PMN counts.

Qualitative defects in PMN function can occur as a result of abnormalities in any of the steps involved in the ingesting and killing of infecting organisms. Most of the primary disorders in which PMN function is impaired are congenital, recognized in childhood, and uncommon. They include chronic granulomatous disease, Chédiak-Higashi syndrome, and Job syndrome. Myeloperoxidase deficiency, though common, is not usually associated with an increased rate of infection unless another abnormality is present as well.

Of greater relevance to this discussion are the acquired disorders of neutrophil function. Corticosteroids, antineoplastic drugs, irradiation, and alcohol all can impair the effectiveness of PMNs by decreasing chemotaxis or adherence. In addition, alterations in neutrophil chemotaxis caused by a circulating inhibitor have been described in the context of cirrhosis, renal failure, and Hodgkin's disease. Various complement-deficiency states also are associated with reduction in chemotaxis.

Abnormalities in the number or function of PMNs are associated with pyogenic bacterial infections. The specific organisms encountered relate to the circumstances of the patient and his or her environment. Because granulocytopenia more commonly develops in hospitalized patients, who may have been receiving antimicrobial therapy and who may have cofactors predisposing to pulmonary infections, organisms such as *Staphylococcus aureus* and aerobic gram-negative bacteria tend to predominate. Much less often, neutropenic patients may experience respiratory tract infection caused by *Candida*, *Mucor*, and *Aspergillus* species.

HUMORAL IMMUNODEFICIENCY

Antibody production is a function of B lymphocytes; thus, decreased antibody production results when the number of B cells is critically reduced or when their ability to respond to specific antigens is impaired. The prototypic example is X-linked agam-

maglobulinemia, in which there is complete absence of B lymphocytes. Common variable immunodeficiency is not necessarily associated with an overall decline in B cells. In both of these situations, IgG is most affected, and sinopulmonary infections with both gram-positive and gram-negative encapsulated bacteria are commonplace.

Patients infected with the human immunodeficiency virus (HIV) are in many ways similar to patients with common variable immunodeficiency. Although B cells are present, they do not respond effectively to specific antigens. This presumably is the basis for the increased incidence of severe bacterial infections (particularly those caused by *Streptococcus pneumoniae* and *Haemophilus influenzae*) in these patients. Other conditions associated with defective antibody production include multiple myeloma, chronic lymphocytic leukemia, and the splenectomized state. In each of these conditions, pneumococcal pneumonia, often with bacteremia, frequently develops, and infections with other encapsulated organisms have been reported.

CELLULAR IMMUNODEFICIENCY

Cell-mediated immunity is mainly responsible for fending off intracellular pathogens. Killing of these organisms within the lung is accomplished primarily by alveolar macrophages and secondarily by cytotoxic lymphocytes. Primary abnormalities of cell-mediated immunity are uncommon and become evident early in life. They include severe combined immunodeficiency, DiGeorge syndrome, ataxia telangiectasia, and Wiskott-Aldrich syndrome. Far more common are defects produced by various diseases and therapeutic interventions. Acquired immunodeficiency syndrome (AIDS) is characterized by a progressive and ultimately profound reduction in cell-mediated immunity produced by HIV infection. Untreated Hodgkin's disease also uniformly impairs cell-mediated responses. A large number of other disorders cause reductions in cell-mediated immunity but do not predictably predispose to infection. In addition to diseases, therapeutic agents, such as corticosteroids, azathioprine, cytotoxic drugs, and radiography, have a dose-related effect on cell-mediated immunity.

Because many of the infectious diseases that develop as a consequence of alterations in cell-mediated immunity are reactivations of latent infections, their incidence is determined by the prevalence of the underlying infection. This is especially true for tuberculosis, nontuberculous mycobacterial diseases, and fungal processes. In addition, infections with other bacteria, particularly *Listeria monocytogenes*, *Salmonella* species, and *Legionella* species, and with parasites, especially *Strongyloides stercoralis*, may develop in persons with deficient cell-mediated immunity.

RECOGNITION AND QUANTIFICATION OF IMMUNOCOMPROMISE

Initial recognition that a patient is immunocompromised generally results from a knowledge of the clinical conditions and therapies that interfere with host responsiveness. Neutropenia is identified easily and quantified simply by an accurate total white blood cell and differential count. As observed previously, the risk of infection is increased with counts of less than 500 per microliter when there has been a rapid decline in PMNs and when there are factors that interfere with PMN function. Although there are tests that measure different aspects of PMN function, they are of limited clinical relevance under usual circumstances. It can be assumed, however, that alcoholism, cirrhosis, diabetes, and treatment with corticosteroids, antineoplastic drugs, and radiography cause impairment of PMN function.

A reduction of immunoglobulin concentration should be suspected in patients who have recurrent sinopulmonary infections. The abnormality can be identified and quantified by measurement of serum immunoglobulins and immunoglobulin subsets using immunoelectrophoresis. Total B-cell counts also may quantify the defect. Cellular immunodeficiency can be assumed in patients who have conditions that are known to suppress cell-mediated immunity, as discussed previously. In patients with HIV infection, the best means of quantifying the degree of immunosuppression is the total CD4 lymphocyte count. The rate of opportunistic infections relates inversely to the total CD4 lymphocyte count, with a striking increase associated with CD4 lymphocyte counts less than 200 per microliter.

DIFFERENTIAL DIAGNOSIS OF RESPIRATORY DISEASE IN IMMUNOCOMPROMISED PATIENTS

As shown in Table 362.1, several other categories of conditions, in addition to infections, should enter the differential diagnosis. Within the differential diagnosis, opportunistic infections are the most important disorders of which to be aware, because they often are treatable and, without treatment, may progress rapidly. As mentioned previously and as indicated in Table 362.2, the pathogens can be predicted to a certain extent from a knowledge of the underlying disease and the abnormalities in host defenses that the disease or its treatment can produce. Knowledge of the likely organisms also allows for selection of appropriate diagnostic studies and rational empiric therapy. Respiratory disorders, either preexisting or new, that are unrelated to the underlying disorder or its treatment figure into the differential diagnosis. A variety of chronic lung diseases may worsen during the course of another illness. Asthma, which is common in the general population, is likely to develop in a population of immunocompromised patients. Because immunocompromised patients are often on bed rest and because some have neoplastic conditions, they may be predisposed to pulmonary embolism. Left ventricular failure with cardiogenic pulmonary edema also may occur and is related to intrinsic heart disease and, occasionally, fluid overload or cardiotoxic drugs.

Many of the primary disorders can involve the lungs or intrathoracic lymph nodes directly, for example, leukemia, Hodgkin's disease, non-Hodgkin's lymphoma, and metastatic solid tumors. In addition to direct involvement by tumors, there may be secondary hematologic effects. In patients who have major coagulation defects, there may be spontaneous bleeding into the lung. Intrapulmonary leukostasis is believed to account for dyspnea and hypoxemia in patients with both acute and chronic non-lymphocytic leukemia. This condition usually has developed in patients with white blood cell counts of more than 200,000 per microliter. A syndrome suggestive of diffuse lung damage has been reported after administration of chemotherapy. This so-called leukemic cell lysis pneumonopathy is believed to result from destruction of white blood cells within the lungs, with subsequent liberation of white cell enzymes causing lung damage.

Lung disease caused by agents used to treat neoplastic processes can mimic many of the other conditions listed in the differential diagnosis. Confounding the problem is the fact that there is no test that can provide a positive diagnosis of drug-induced lung disease, though the histopathologic features may be highly suggestive in some instances. Bleomycin most often is associated with lung disease, probably followed in frequency by methotrexate.

Several idiopathic processes can affect the lungs in immunosuppressed patients. These disorders presumably are caused by immunosuppression itself or by the primary condition underlying immunosuppression. Kaposi's sarcoma is common in patients with AIDS, but it also may develop with other forms of immunosuppression. Nonspecific interstitial pneumonitis is seen in patients with HIV infection but is found in other immunocompromised patients as well. The condition is characterized by interstitial inflammatory changes without a specific histologic pattern. Lymphoid interstitial pneumonitis is a typical finding in children with HIV infection but also develops in both immunosuppressed and nonimmunosuppressed patients without HIV infection. The histopathologic picture shows interstitial infiltration with lymphocytes, peripheral lymphoid aggregates, and

---

TABLE 362.1.   DIFFERENTIAL DIAGNOSIS OF PULMONARY PROCESSES IN IMMUNOCOMPROMISED PATIENTS

Opportunistic infections: all categories of pathogens

Preexisting or new lung disease unrelated to immunosuppression: asthma, chronic obstructive pulmonary disease, pulmonary embolism, cardiogenic pulmonary edema

Lung involvement by the primary disease process: leukemic infiltration, Hodgkin's disease with lymph node or parenchymal involvement, plasmacytoma, lymphangitic metastases

Hematologic processes related to primary disease or its treatment: intrapulmonary hemorrhage, intrapulmonary leukostasis, leukemic cell lysis pneumonopathy

Pulmonary reactions to agents used to treat the primary process: bleomycin, methotrexate, radiation

Idiopathic processes presumably related to immunosuppression or to the immunosuppressive process: Kaposi's sarcoma, lymphoid interstitial pneumonia, nonspecific interstitial pneumonia

Graft-versus-host disease

TABLE 362.2.	DEFECTS IN HOST DEFENSES, UNDERLYING ASSOCIATED DISEASES, AND LIKELY PULMONARY INFECTIONS	
Defect	**Disease**	**Pulmonary Infection**
Neutropenia	Primary chronic or cyclic neutropenia	Community-acquired bacterial pneumonia, sinusitis, otitis
	Acute-leukemia and myelosuppressive chemotherapy, bone marrow transplant	Aerobic gram-negative bacteria, especially *Pseudomonas aeruginosa*, *Staphylococcus aureus*, *Staphylococcus epidermidis*, *Candida* species, *Aspergillus* species, *Mucor*
Complement abnormalities	Primary C3 or C5 deficiency	*Staphylococcus aureus*, *Streptococcus pneumoniae*, aerobic gram-negative bacteria
	Sickle cell disease (defect in alternate pathway)	*Streptococcus pneumoniae*
Antibody deficiencies	Primary immunoglobulin deficiencies	Aerobic gram-negative bacteria, *Staphylococcus aureus*, *Streptococcus pneumoniae*
	Human immunodeficiency virus infection	*Streptococcus pneumoniae*, *Haemophilus influenzae*, *Staphylococcus aureus*
Cellular immunodeficiency	Human immunodeficiency virus infection, Hodgkin's disease, immunosuppressive therapy, bone marrow transplantation	*Pneumocystis carinii*; *Mycobacterium tuberculosis*; nontuberculous mycobacteria, *Legionella* species; *Listeria monocytogenes*; cytomegalovirus; fungi, especially *Cryptococcus neoformans*, *Coccidioides immitis*, *Histoplasma capsulatum*, *Aspergillus* species

small amounts of fibrosis. Both nonspecific pneumonitis and lymphoid interstitial pneumonitis are diagnoses of exclusion, even when the histopathologic characteristics are consistent. Only after the other diseases, particularly opportunistic infections, have been ruled out can these idiopathic disorders be diagnosed. Graft-versus-host disease occurs only in patients who have had bone marrow transplantation. Pulmonary involvement is seen in the chronic form of the disease, which begins about 3 months after transplantation. The disease usually manifests as a nonproductive cough, dyspnea, and bronchospasm.

DIAGNOSTIC APPROACH

HISTORY, PHYSICAL EXAMINATION, AND INITIAL LABORATORY EVALUATION

The diagnostic evaluation for pulmonary disease in an immunosuppressed patient may be initiated by respiratory symptoms, fever, or the discovery of an abnormality on chest radiography. In patients who are capable of providing a history, this information can yield important clues with regard to the severity of the pulmonary process and the nature of the immunosuppression. Pertinent historical information includes a description of the kind of respiratory symptoms, usually cough and shortness of breath; their duration; and their functional effects. Whether or not the cough is productive of sputum, its amount, and its color should be determined. It is important to gauge the severity of shortness of breath. Obviously, shortness of breath that progresses rapidly and produces marked limitation in activity indicates that the evaluation must be pursued with some urgency, whereas a condition with a more indolent course can be evaluated at a more leisurely pace. Other important symptomatic manifestations of pulmonary conditions are chest pain and fever. In assessing any fever, one should determine its duration, magni-

tude (if known), and association with chills. The severity and nature of chest pain, especially whether it is pleuritic, should be ascertained.

In many instances, it is not known that the patient is immunosuppressed at the time of initial evaluation. Thus, pertinent historical information would include previously diagnosed diseases associated with immunosuppression; drug therapy that could impair immune responsiveness, especially glucocorticoids or cytotoxic agents; and membership in a recognized HIV transmission category. In addition, it is important to determine whether the patient was taking antimicrobial drug therapy before the evaluation.

The physical examination, like the history, can provide useful data concerning the presence and severity of lung disease as well as inferential evidence of an immunosuppressive disorder. In addition to the routine examination, particular attention should be paid to detecting oral lesions, such as thrush (oral candidiasis) or hairy leukoplakia; cutaneous findings, such as Kaposi's sarcoma or herpetic lesions; lymphadenopathy, as might be indicative of HIV infection or a hematologic or reticuloendothelial malignancy; and liver or splenic enlargement, which is also suggestive of a malignant process.

Routine laboratory studies, particularly a complete blood cell count and differential, can be extremely useful in suggesting the presence of an underlying immunosuppressive process and perhaps its cause, such as leukemia. Leukocytosis can reflect a standard bacterial infection. Tests of liver and kidney function are of value in identifying disorders that in themselves are associated with weakening of host defenses or can compound other immunosuppressive disorders.

As a general rule, serologic studies have not been found to be of much assistance in identifying infecting organisms. An exception to this rule, however, is the detection of circulating cryptococcal antigen, which provides strong evidence of cryptococcal infection. Likewise, detection of precipitating antibodies (IgM) to *Coccidioides immitis* or a high titer (more than 1:16) of complement-fixing antibody (IgG) is highly suggestive of infection with this organism.

ROENTGENOGRAPHIC STUDIES

Roentgenography of the chest should be carried out for all patients who are being evaluated for respiratory symptoms or physical findings. Although radiographic abnormalities can never establish etiologic sources, they can be extremely helpful in narrowing the differential diagnosis and providing guidance for subsequent diagnostic studies. A wide variety of radiographic patterns can be encountered in immunocompromised patients. Diffuse interstitial infiltration is the most common pattern produced by opportunistic lung infections. (The term *interstitial* is used to describe the roentgenographic pattern, not to indicate the anatomic location of the process within the lungs.) This pattern is particularly common in *Pneumocystis carinii* pneumonia and also is seen with cytomegalovirus, *Mycobacterium tuberculosis*, and infection with nontuberculosis mycobacteria and with fungi, especially *Histoplasma capsulatum* and *C. immitis*. As any of these conditions becomes more severe, there may be diffuse airspace consolidation, occasionally with air bronchograms.

Diffuse infiltration is the rule in drug-related lung disease, leukemic infiltration, lymphangitic metastases, intrapulmonary hemorrhage, leukostasis, leukemic cell lysis pneumonopathy, lymphocytic interstitial pneumonia, and nonspecific interstitial pneumonia. Pulmonary edema, both cardiogenic and noncardiogenic, also must be included in the differential diagnosis. Localized infiltration is more consistent with pyogenic bacterial pneumonia, legionellosis, fungal infection (especially with *Cryptococcus neoformans* and *Aspergillus* species), lymphoma, and lung infarction. Virtually all of the conditions that cause diffuse infiltration can produce localized abnormalities, but they are less likely to do so.

Single or several nodular lesions most likely are caused by primary or metastatic neoplasms, including lymphoma, fungal infections (especially *C. neoformans*), and mycobacterial infections. Cavitation may occur in these lesions as well as in staphylococcal pneumonia and in pneumonia provoked by *Klebsiella*, anaerobic bacteria, and *Aspergillus*. *P. carinii* has been reported to produce cavitary lesions and pneumatocele formation. Although *M. tuberculosis* frequently causes cavitary lesions in immunocompetent patients, it rarely does so in patients with advanced HIV infection.

Pleural effusion is not typically associated with opportunistic infections or drug-induced lung diseases. It may develop in the context of metastatic neoplasia, Kaposi's sarcoma, pyogenic bacterial pneumonias, and tuberculosis as well as heart failure and pulmonary infarction. Intrathoracic adenopathy usually is caused by lymphomas and by infectious processes, in particular, mycobacterial and fungal infections. Metastatic malignancies also can cause lymph node enlargement. The presence of adenopathy is strong evidence arguing against *P. carinii* infection as the only pulmonary disease. In patients with respiratory symptoms and normal chest film results, high-resolution computed tomography scans may show evidence of lung disease. This is especially true for *P. carinii* pneumonia.

PULMONARY FUNCTION STUDIES AND GALLIUM LUNG SCANS

Because the evaluation of respiratory symptoms in immunocompromised patients often requires invasive and expensive studies, there must be some objective indication that lung disease is present. In most patients, the chest film shows abnormal results and thus provides the objective evidence. In some patients who have subsequently been found to have lung disease, however, the chest film has shown normal findings. In these patients, measurements of pulmonary function, including arterial blood gas determination and calculation of the alveolar to arterial Po_2 difference ($P[A - a]o_2$), have been of value. Of the routine pulmonary function tests, the diffusing capacity of the lung for carbon monoxide (D_{LCO}) is the most sensitive to the presence of opportunistic pulmonary disease. Many unrelated disorders can cause a reduced D_{LCO} value (less than 80% of the predicted value), including emphysema, pulmonary vascular disease, pulmonary fibrosis, and intravenous drug abuse. Nevertheless, a decline in the D_{LCO} in an immunocompromised patient with respiratory symptoms should be accepted as an objective indicator of lung disease, prompting further evaluation. Similar sensitivity has been noted for measurements of gas exchange with exercise. These measurements assess arterial blood gases at rest and with a standard level of exercise and then determine the difference in the $P(A - a)o_2$. Failure of the $P(A - a)o_2$ to decrease by at least 5 mm Hg with exercise is regarded as a positive test result, indicating the presence of lung disease.

Radionuclide imaging of the lungs by gallium citrate Ga 67 is also a sensitive means of detecting pulmonary inflammation. Lung scanning is performed 48 to 72 hours after injection of 5 to 7 mCi of gallium, and any pulmonary uptake is regarded as abnormal. Conditions such as *P. carinii* pneumonia are generally associated with diffuse uptake. In addition to uptake in the pulmonary parenchyma, uptake may be noted in intrathoracic lymph nodes.

SPUTUM EXAMINATION

Examination of sputum, either spontaneously produced or induced by inhalation of hypertonic (3% to 5%) saline, is extremely valuable in identifying organisms in patients with opportunistic pulmonary infections. Most patients with pyogenic bacterial pneumonia have sputum production, as do some patients with other infectious diseases. Sputum specimens produced spontaneously should be smeared promptly and stained with Gram and acid-fast stains. A portion should be submitted for culture for pyogenic bacteria and mycobacteria. Definitive identification of the organisms present is not possible from examination of the smear, but there may be strong presumptive evidence of the organism.

In addition to bacteria, the presence and number of PMNs,

alveolar macrophages, and squamous epithelial cells should be noted. Alveolar macrophages are indicative of a lower respiratory tract origin, and PMNs are associated with acute inflammation. Squamous epithelial cells indicate contamination with oropharyngeal contents. An obvious limitation is in the diagnosis of pyogenic bacterial infections in which contamination with oropharyngeal flora precludes interpretation of an organism as originating from the lungs. Even with regard to the potential for contamination, however, isolation of a bacterial pathogen in the sputum from a patient who has a pulmonary condition that could be caused by the organism is often sufficient information on which to base therapy. Sputum examination is of greater value when an organism that is not normally present in the oropharynx is seen or isolated in culture. Finding an acid-fast organism on smear is adequate evidence to prompt initiation of antimycobacterial therapy. In patients with AIDS, examination of induced sputum has a sensitivity for *P. carinii* of about 70%. By using Giemsa stain or other rapid-staining techniques, a result can be obtained promptly, thus avoiding the need for more invasive procedures.

Culture of sputum often provides definitive identification of organisms seen on smear, though these organisms may still represent oropharyngeal flora. A routine culture can identify most pyogenic bacterial organisms within 48 hours. Mycobacterial cultures take considerably longer, but with the use of radiolabeled substrates, growth can be detected in 5 to 14 days. Standard culture media require 2 to 6 weeks for growth. Identification of species often requires another 2 weeks, but the use of specific DNA probes may shorten the process to a few hours. Identification and speciation of *M. tuberculosis* is now possible using rapid amplification techniques. At present, however, the approved use of such methods is limited to specimens in which acid-fast organisms have been seen on microscopic examination.

ROLE OF EMPIRIC TREATMENT

The evaluation described thus far is only minimally invasive; however, the next steps that can be undertaken to identify a specific condition require more invasive studies. An option that can be considered at this point is the use of an empiric treatment trial. This option is based on the assumption that the process is most likely an infection and that the infection is the most serious and most treatable of all of the possible diagnoses. Based on the nature of the defect in host defenses, the pathogens likely to cause infection in a particular context can be predicted and an antimicrobial regimen selected. If the patient is neutropenic, agents to cover aerobic gram-negative organisms, including *Pseudomonas aeruginosa* and also *S. aureus*, should be used. Patients with altered cell-mediated immunity are likely to be infected with *P. carinii* as well as mycobacteria, fungi, and *Legionella* species.

Because of the long-term nature of antimycobacterial treatment and the toxicity of amphotericin B, empiric therapy for mycobacteria and fungi should not be started except while awaiting results of cultures. Empiric treatment of this group of patients with trimethoprim-sulfamethoxazole and perhaps erythromycin is a rational approach. If empiric therapy is undertaken,

it is important to monitor the patient carefully for indications of improvement or deterioration. If there is no improvement or if the patient's condition worsens, more definitive studies should be done. How long the empiric trial should go on before moving ahead to more definitive procedures depends on a number of factors, including the severity of the condition, the rapidity of its progression, and the patient's wishes.

BRONCHOSCOPIC PROCEDURES

The flexible fiberoptic bronchoscope provides ready access to the lower respiratory tract for making visible the endobronchial anatomy and sampling material for histologic and microbiologic evaluations. The procedure itself is minimally invasive and can be performed in awake patients using conscious sedation and topical anesthesia. Any bronchoscopic procedure should begin with a careful examination of the airway. A variety of endobronchial lesions can be seen, including granulomas from mycobacterial or fungal diseases and tumors. In patients with AIDS, findings of typical hemorrhagic-appearing submucosal lesions of Kaposi's sarcoma is sufficiently definitive to establish a diagnosis.

The samples that should be obtained with the bronchoscope vary somewhat, depending on the underlying disorder and the pulmonary diseases that are believed to be present. In patients who likely have pyogenic bacterial pneumonia, the specimens should include a sampling of material from the involved area with the use of a protected brush. The protected brush is contained within two catheters, the outer one sealed at its distal end by a small wax plug. The system enables uncontaminated specimens to be collected from lower airways. The diagnostic specificity of protected brush catheter specimens is increased by quantitative cultures of the material obtained. Colony counts of more than 105 more likely indicate that the infection is caused by the isolated organism.

In patients thought to have HIV-related opportunistic infections, bronchoalveolar lavage is highly sensitive. This procedure samples material from a large number of alveoli; thus, it is likely to detect intra-alveolar infections. The lavage specimen should be centrifuged, smeared, and stained for *P. carinii* and acid-fast organisms. Immunofluorescent staining for *Legionella* species also can be carried out. The specimen should be cultured for mycobacteria and fungi and perhaps for viruses, *Legionella* species, and *Mycoplasma* organisms. In patients with HIV infection, the sensitivity of bronchoalveolar lavage for the common infecting organisms, especially *P. carinii*, approaches 100%. The sensitivity in other immunocompromised patients is not so high, but it is still good for the organisms described previously.

In patients in whom disorders other than infections rank high in the differential diagnosis, bronchoalveolar lavage should be supplemented by transbronchial biopsy. The biopsy adds considerably to the risk of the bronchoscopic procedure and cannot be performed in the context of an uncorrectable coagulation disorder. This limits the usefulness of the procedure in some immunosuppressed patients. Bleeding is also a risk for patients with pulmonary hypertension, and patients receiving mechanical ventilation have a risk of tension pneumothorax.

Tissue obtained by transbronchial biopsy should be subjected to histologic and microbiologic examinations. Touch imprints of fresh, moist tissue should be stained and examined for *P. carinii*. An unfixed portion of the tissue should be cultured for mycobacteria, fungi, and perhaps viruses. Fixed tissue sections should have standard hematoxylin-eosin staining as well as acid-fast and methenamine silver stains. Immunofluorescent stains and cultures for *Legionella* also should be undertaken if the epidemiologic and chemical features are consistent with legionellosis. Special stains may be necessary, depending on the findings on hematoxylin-eosin–stained sections.

When there is enlargement of the mediastinal or hilar lymph nodes with or without pulmonary parenchymal involvement, transtracheal needle aspiration may be used to sample material from the nodes. This is most easily accomplished when the subcarinal nodes are affected, but right-sided paratracheal and hilar nodes also can be aspirated. This technique can be used to aspirate mass lesions in the lungs. Specimens obtained by transbronchial aspiration should be examined as cytologic preparations. In addition, stains and cultures for mycobacteria and fungi should be carried out.

NEEDLE ASPIRATION LUNG BIOPSY

Needle aspiration of the lung has been used for many years, especially in children, to provide material for diagnosing infections. The technique also can be used in evaluating localized mass lesions that may be either infectious or neoplastic. The sensitivity of the procedure is fairly high for both infections and tumors. Unfortunately, the rate of complications is also high. Both pneumothorax and bleeding may occur, at an overall rate of about 40%.

OPEN LUNG BIOPSY

Open lung biopsy can be accomplished either via the traditional limited thoracotomy incision or using a thoracoscope. Because of its lesser degree of invasiveness, the thoracoscopic approach is favored in many centers. If it can be performed promptly, the major advantage offered by open lung biopsy is that it is the most expeditious means of arriving at a diagnosis without concern that a condition is being overlooked. A nondiagnostic open lung biopsy is accepted as being nondiagnostic, whereas failure to obtain a diagnosis using less invasive studies often leaves the physician with doubts about the validity of the negative result. Additional advantages of open lung biopsy are that the area to be sampled can be selected while it is directly visible and effective hemostasis can be achieved even in the presence of coagulopathy. The procedure can be undertaken in severely ill patients who require mechanical ventilation.

The disadvantages of open lung biopsy are several. It requires an operating room and, usually, general anesthesia; the potential exists for infection and for chronic air leak; and the patient is left with postoperative pain and a thoracostomy tube, which, in immunocompromised patients, can serve as a nidus for infection. For all of these reasons, the decision to perform an open lung biopsy should not be made lightly but only after the benefits and risks have been thoroughly assessed. These complications

are substantially less likely with a thoracoscopy procedure. Tissue specimens obtained by open lung biopsy should be examined as described for tissue from transbronchial biopsy, including making touch imprints and culturing the tissue. For this reason, the tissue specimen should not be immersed immediately in fixative; instead, a portion should be placed on moistened sterile gauze in an airtight container for transport to the laboratory.

AN INTEGRATED DIAGNOSTIC STRATEGY

The first step in formulating an integrated diagnostic strategy for the immunocompromised patient with lung disease is to assess the immune defect and determine the differential diagnosis based on the underlying disease and the nature of the abnormality in host defenses. Routine diagnostic evaluation, including chest radiography, can assist in narrowing the differential diagnosis. The rapidity or urgency with which the evaluation proceeds should be determined by the overall assessment of the severity of the illness and the pace at which it is progressing. If infection is possible, a sputum specimen should be obtained using inhalation of hypertonic saline if necessary. In patients who have respiratory symptoms but normal results on chest radiograms, pulmonary function tests, especially measurement of the D_{LCO} and gas exchange with exercise, may provide the necessary objective indication of lung disease. A high-resolution computed tomography scan can be useful in this situation. If these test results are normal, a gallium lung scan may be helpful.

At this point, if no specific diagnosis is established, the decision can be made to embark on an empiric course of antimicrobial treatment with close observation of the response. Alternatively, a specific diagnosis may be sought using a bronchoscopic technique. This course should be taken in patients who have failed to respond to empiric therapy as well. The particular bronchoscopic procedure should be determined by the differential diagnosis based on the underlying disorder and the immune defect. If a pyogenic bacterial infection is possible, a specimen should be obtained from the involved area by the protected brush technique. In the context of a defect in cell-mediated immunity, bronchoalveolar lavage should be conducted and transbronchial biopsy considered. If the lavage result is negative or if the differential diagnosis includes noninfectious disorders, a transbronchial biopsy should be carried out, unless there is a contraindication. When all studies are inconclusive or when transbronchial biopsy is contraindicated, a decision concerning open lung biopsy must be made. At this point, if the lung disease is not progressing rapidly, a second bronchoscopic procedure can be undertaken. The value of open lung biopsy in this context is not well established, and the risk may outweigh the gain.

BIBLIOGRAPHY

Ettinger NA. Invasive diagnostic approaches to pulmonary infiltrates. *Semin Respir Infect* 1993;8:168–176.

Fishman JA, Rubin RH. Infection in organ-transplant recipients. *N Engl J Med* 1998;338:1741–1751.

Ginsberg SJ, Comis RL. The pulmonary toxicity of antineoplastic agents. *Semin Oncol* 1982;9:34–51.

Melero MJ, Brodsky AL. Pulmonary infiltrates in acute leukemia. *Clin Pulm Med* 1998;5:165.

Ng VL, Gartner I, Weymouth LA, et al. The use of mucolysed induced sputum for the identification of pulmonary pathogens associated with human immunodeficiency virus infection. *Arch Pathol Lab Med* 1989; 113:488–493.

Potter D, Pasa HI, Brower S. Prospective randomized study of open lung biopsy versus empirical antibiotic therapy for acute pneumonitis in non-neutropenic cancer patients. *Ann Thorac Surg* 1985;40:422–428.

Rosenow EC III, Wilson WR, Cockerill FR III. Pulmonary disease in the immunocompromised host. 1. *Mayo Clin Proc* 1985;60:473–487.

Superdock KR, Helderman JH. Immunosuppressive drugs and their effects. *Semin Respir Infect* 1993;8:152–159.

Toews GB. Pulmonary defense mechanisms. *Semin Respir Infect* 1993;8: 160–167.

Wilson WR, Cockerill FR III, Rosenow EC III. Pulmonary disease in the immunocompromised host. 2. *Mayo Clin Proc* 1985;60:610–631.

Kelley's Textbook of Internal Medicine, fourth edition. Edited by H. David Humes.
Lippincott Williams & Wilkins, Philadelphia © 2000.

CHAPTER

363

ASTHMA

SALLY E. WENZEL

DEFINITION

Asthma is defined as intermittent, reversible airway obstruction in association with increased nonspecific bronchial reactivity. These physiologic changes are now known to exist in the context of airway inflammation. The addition of inflammation to the definition has shifted the understanding of asthma from a disease of airway nerves and smooth muscle to one that identifies inflammation as the driving force for the symptoms associated with the disease. This realization has led to a dramatic shift in the treatment of the disease in the past 10 years.

NATURAL HISTORY AND EPIDEMIOLOGY

Asthma is one of the most common and expensive chronic illnesses in the United States, affecting between 5% and 10% of the population. Annual health care costs were about six to seven billion dollars in 1990, and costs have risen since then. Development of asthma follows a bimodal distribution, with an early peak in the pediatric years (4 to 10 years of age) and a second peak after 40 years of age. A male predominance in childhood disappears by adolescence and reverses after age 40. A large percentage (80% to 85%) of early childhood wheezers (less than 2 years of age) will not progress to definitive asthma later in childhood. Many of these children with asthma may even "outgrow" their illness later in life, but a large percentage of children continue to experience asthma into adulthood. In adulthood, mean pulmonary function appears to decline at a greater than normal rate.

The incidence and severity of asthma have been increasing, but there is some evidence that we have reached a plateau in the past two to three years. The reasons for these increases in incidence and severity are not clear but likely include growing awareness of the disease, socioeconomic factors, and increases in indoor and outdoor air pollution. Outdoor air pollution (ozone, sulfur dioxide, particulates) does not appear to be causative but may exacerbate asthma and lead to increases in the subsequent reporting of it. African-American and Hispanic populations have higher incidence rates of asthma compared with other racial/ethnic groups, but perhaps more important, the African-American and Puerto Rican populations, specifically these populations in inner city areas, have considerably higher morbidity and mortality rates than other ethnic and socioeconomic groups. The factors that play a part in this higher incidence and severity are likely both environmental and genetic in nature.

The understanding of the genetics of asthma is at a very preliminary stage. Unlike such diseases as cystic fibrosis, which has been identified as the result of a single abnormal gene, the heterogeneity of asthma suggests that the genetic factors will prove to be multifactorial and strongly influenced by environment. Atopy appears to raise the risk of asthma. Since a majority of atopic/allergic individuals do not have asthma, however, other genetic and environmental factors likely play a part. Several chromosomes, including chromosomes 11 and 5, have been highlighted as containing potential genes (generally related to atopy) that could modify hereditary aspects of asthma. There is emerging information that certain genes may be more important in some racial/ethnic groups than in others.

ENVIRONMENTAL RISK FACTORS FOR THE DEVELOPMENT OF ASTHMA

In a child with atopic characteristics, exposure to indoor allergens, such as the house dust mite, cockroaches, and cats appears to increase the risk of asthma. In regions of lower humidity, cats and molds, such as *Alternaria*, may play a more important role. Outdoor allergens have not been linked to the development of chronic asthma. Removing susceptible individuals from their allergic environment may have a positive impact on the disease. Exposure to viruses, such as respiratory syncytial virus, during infancy/early childhood, also can influence the development of asthma in susceptible individuals. The most preventable risk factor is cigarette smoking by the mother, which likely poses the greatest risk prenatally through age 5 years. Occupational asthma can develop after exposure to either low- or high-molecular-weight compounds in the workplace. The disease is especially prevalent in the lumber, plastics, and paint industries and can develop de novo in patients with no history of it. Asthma has become more prevalent among hospital workers because of the prevalence of latex use and the attendant subsequent development of allergies and asthma. Although the disease usually improves after departure from the workplace, certain occupational stimuli (western red cedar) have been shown to induce a disease that does not fully resolve once the patient is separated from the initiating stimulus.

PHYSIOLOGY

Airflow limitation in asthma is based on a reduction in the ratio of forced expiratory volume in 1 second (FEV_1) to forced vital capacity (FVC). This ratio is normally over 75% in adults and 85% in children. Reversibility is defined as an improvement in FEV_1 of more than 12% to 15% after inhalation of a β-agonist, but this response may not always be seen. There may be naturally occurring changes in airflow throughout the day as well. Even though individuals with normal lungs will have some circadian variation in airflow, asthmatics often have exaggerated changes in peak flows over a 24-hour period (10% to 30%).

In addition to a decline in airflow, other physiologic changes include hyperinflation (increased thoracic gas volume, residual volume) and increased airway resistance. Routine measurement of these parameters is not indicated for most patients with asthma. Airway hyperresponsiveness is determined through methacholine, histamine, and/or exercise testing. A positive methacholine challenge demonstrates a fall in FEV_1 of 20% or more [provocation concentration (PC) 20] with 8 mg per milliliter or less of methacholine, but by itself this result is not adequate for diagnosis. Other diseases can cause increases in nonspecific airway responsiveness, including chronic obstructive pulmonary disease, congestive heart failure, bronchiectasis, and seasonal allergic rhinitis. Therefore, the methacholine test should be used as a confirmatory test in the appropriate clinical situation.

PATHOLOGY

It is now recognized that inflammation is a salient feature of asthma, present in mild and even newly diagnosed cases. Although many cell types may be involved in asthma, the predominant ones include lymphocytes, eosinophils, and mast cells. It is believed that for asthma to develop, a complex immunologic reaction must be initiated and maintained. Early on, naive T lymphocytes in the airways must be sensitized to specific allergens/antigens by antigen-presenting cells (perhaps monocytes, macrophages, or dendritic cells). The naive lymphocyte then alters its phenotype to that of a helper T cell type of lymphocyte (TH2), which produces cytokines (autocrine- and paracrine-acting proteins) that drive an IgE-associated, eosinophilic process. These cytokines include interleukin (IL)-4, IL-5, and IL-13. Functionally, these cytokines are involved in IgE production, mast cell and eosinophil migration, and survival and further generation of TH2 cells.

In contrast to TH2 cells, TH1 cells are active in other disease states (i.e., granulomatous diseases) and produce larger numbers of cytokines, such as IL-2 and interferon-γ. The IgE produced binds to mast cells (and perhaps other cells), which then can be activated by allergen cross-linking. Allergen exposure prompts mast cells to release preformed mediators, such as histamine, several proteases, and stored cytokines, and to generate lipid mediators, such as the cysteinyl leukotrienes (LTs) C_4, D_4, and E_4 and prostaglandin (PG) D_2. In addition to mast cell activation, asthmatic airways show broad up-regulation of activated lymphocytes and other cells, leading to increased amounts of tumor necrosis factor α, granulocyte–macrophage colony-stimulating factor (GM-CSF) and more typical TH2 cytokines, such as IL-4, IL-5, and IL-13. This up-regulation, which likely perpetuates the inflammatory process even after exposure to the allergen has ceased, increases the migration and the survival of eosinophils, neutrophils, and monocytes in the airways. This migration is thought to be under the control of chemotactic signals released by resident and nonresident airway cells and up-regulation of adhesion molecules on the surface of inflammatory cells and the endothelium/epithelium.

Potential chemotactic agents include the cytokines and chemokines (GM-CSF, RANTES, eotaxin, IL-5, and IL-8) and the LTs (both the cysteinyl LTs and LT B_4). Adhesion molecules, which appear to be specific for eosinophil migration (such as very late cellular adhesion molecule-1, expressed on endothelium, and its ligand, very late antigen-4, expressed on eosinophils), also are modulated by the TH2 cytokines. Once in the tissue, these cells can release tissue-inflaming substances, such as eosinophilic cationic protein, major basic protein, the cysteinyl LTs, platelet-activating factor, proteases, and superoxides. This release of eosinophil and other inflammatory cell products leads to tissue damage and destruction involving the epithelium and the submucosal space. This continuous, active wounding of the airways likely provokes poorly defined structural responses in the airways that have been termed *remodeling*.

The sub-basement membrane, a band of collagen lying just beneath the basement membrane, is generally thickened in asthma, which is thought to be indicative of the remodeling process. An additional structural change is smooth-muscle hypertrophy/hyperplasia throughout the airways. How much these structural changes contribute to the inability to completely restore normal pulmonary function in more severe cases of asthma is not fully understood, but correlations (even when significant) between sub-basement membrane thickening and measures of airway physiology and clinical severity have generally been poor. At present, there are no reliable clinical markers for the activity of the inflammation in asthma.

ASTHMA DIAGNOSIS

The symptoms of asthma include cough, wheezing, chest tightness, and shortness of breath, but symptoms alone are not adequate for diagnosis (Fig. 363.1). The diagnosis of asthma should be made by documenting reversible airway obstruction, with FEV_1 as the gold standard for physiologic measurement of reversibility in the context of symptoms suggestive of asthma. Because of the intermittent nature of the disease, however, an occasional patient may have normal spirometry results and, therefore,

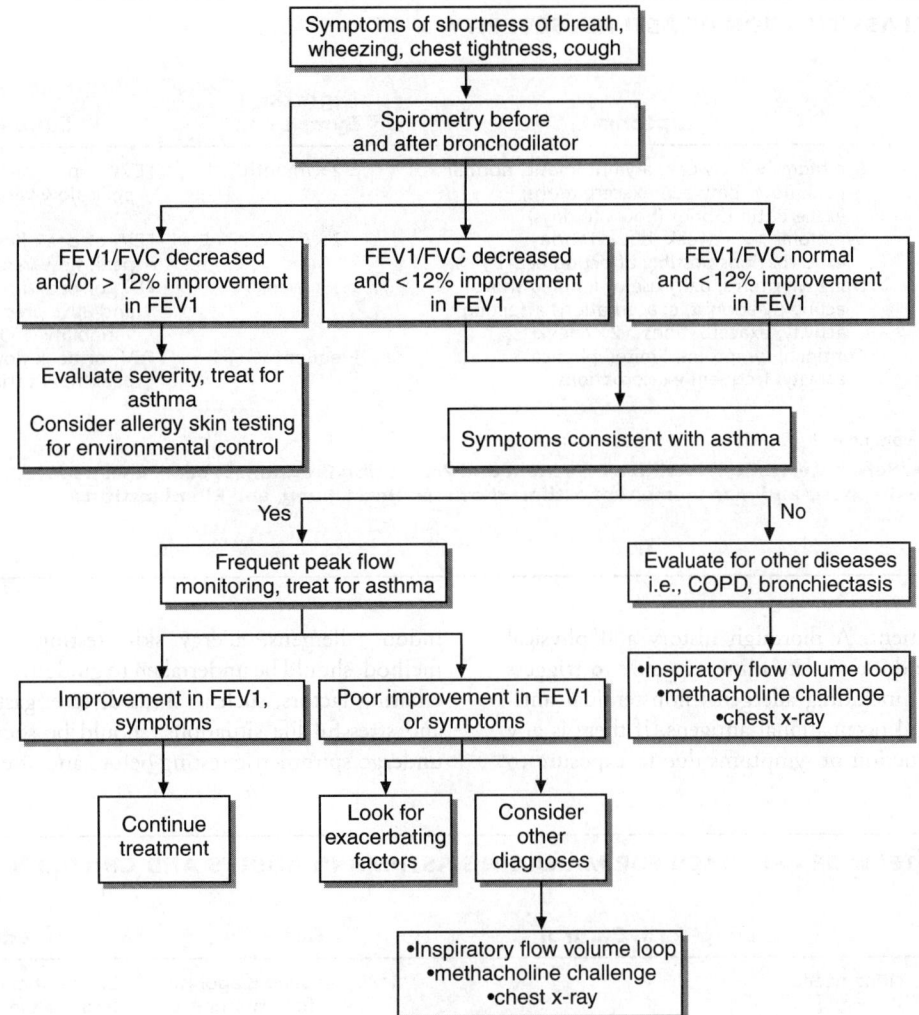

FIGURE 363.1. Strategy for the diagnosis and initial management of asthma.
EVIDENCE LEVEL: C. Expert Opinion.

no reversibility. If the history suggests asthma, the patient's peak flow can be monitored at home. Generally, a more than 10% variation in peak flows is considered diagnostic of asthma. If this variation is not present and the patient is still symptomatic, the next step in diagnosis is a methacholine challenge. A fall in FEV$_1$ of more than 20% at a methacholine concentration of less than 8 mg per milliliter supports the diagnosis. However, false-positive results may be seen if other diseases are present, including chronic bronchitis, cystic fibrosis, bronchiectasis, and vocal cord dysfunction. The methacholine challenge may be particularly helpful in patients with so-called cough-variant asthma. These patients often show initial signs of cough alone and normal results on spirometry.

Certain diseases are difficult to differentiate from asthma. One of the most common situations arises when there is a history of smoking or when the patient currently smokes (typically more than 10 pack-years). When the spirometry and methacholine results mimic asthma, the possible confounding conditions often can be distinguished on the basis of a decreased diffusing capacity [seen in chronic obstructive pulmonary disease (COPD), but not asthma]. A second confounding condition is vocal cord dys-

function (VCD). VCD involves involuntary closure of the vocal cords, classically during inspiration but occasionally on expiration as well. VCD is often misdiagnosed as asthma for years. The diagnosis is made through laryngoscopic confirmation of inappropriate closure of the vocal cords during inspiration or flattening of the inspiratory limb of a flow-volume loop. Upper airway obstruction due to tumors or strictures also can induce symptoms similar to asthma. Flow-volume loops in fixed upper airway obstruction, however, show flattening on both inspiration and expiration. Cardiac failure can lead to a form of wheezing known as *cardiac asthma*. This condition normally is relatively easy to detect on the basis of exam and chest radiography.

■ APPROACH TO THE MANAGEMENT OF ASTHMA

The appropriate management of asthma requires a broad-based approach with contributions from physicians, nurses, and other health care workers as well as active involvement and acceptance

TABLE 363.1.	CLASSIFICATION OF ASTHMA SEVERITY		

	Symptoms	Nighttime Symptoms	Lung Function
Step 1: mild, intermittent	Symptoms ≤2×/week; asymptomatic, normal peak flows between exacerbations; exacerbations brief (hours to days)	≤2×/month	FEV$_1$ or peak flow >80% predicted, peak flow variability <20%
Step 2: mild, persistent	Symptoms >2×/week, but <1×/day; exacerbations possibly affecting activity	>2×/month	FEV$_1$ or peak flow ≥80% predicted, peak flow variability 20–30%
Step 3: moderate, persistent	Daily symptoms, daily use of inhaled short-acting β$_2$-agonist, exacerbations affecting activity, exacerbations >2×/week	>1×/week	FEV$_1$ or peak flow between 60% and 80% predicted, peak flow variability >30%
Step 4: severe, persistent	Continual symptoms, limited physical activity, frequent exacerbations	Frequent	FEV$_1$ or peak flow <60% predicted, peak flow variability >30%

FEV$_1$, forced expiratory volume in 1 second.

EVIDENCE LEVEL: A. Reference: National Asthma Education and Prevention Program. Expert Panel Report II: Guidelines for the diagnosis and management of asthma. National Heart, Lung, and Blood Institute 1997;146.

on the part of the patient. A thorough history and physical examination should be done to determine exposure to triggers or inducers of asthma, including allergens, nonsteroidal anti-inflammatory drugs, and occupational antigens. If there is any question regarding induction of symptoms due to exposure to indoor allergens, allergy skin testing, using the skin-prick method, should be undertaken to guide avoidance therapy. Exacerbating factors, such as sinus disease, gastroesophageal reflux, and stressful life situations, should be sought. Patients should undergo spirometric testing before and after using a bronchodi-

TABLE 363.2.	STEPWISE APPROACH FOR MANAGING ASTHMA IN ADULTS AND CHILDREN >5 YEARS OLD		

	Long-Term Control	Quick Relief	Education
Step 1: mild, intermittent	None needed	Inhaled β-agonist for symptom relief	Basic asthma facts Basic inhaler/spacer techniques Discuss roles of medications Develop self-management plan Develop asthma action plan Discuss environmental control

Step 2: mild, persistent	One daily medication
	  Anti-inflammatory: inhaled corticosteroid (low doses)
	  Cromolyn/nedocromil
	Alternatively
	  Theophylline
	  Leukotriene modulator
		Inhaled β-agonist for symptom relief	Step 1 actions plus
			  Teach self-monitoring
			  Refer to group education
			  Review/update self-management plan

Step 3: moderate, persistent	Daily medications
	  Anti-inflammatory: medium dose inhaled corticosteroid
	or
	  Inhaled corticosteroid (low- to medium dose) with long-acting bronchodilator (long-acting β$_2$-agonist or theophylline)
	If needed
	  Medium to high dose of inhaled corticosteroids and long-acting bronchodilator (as above)
		Inhaled β-agonist for symptom relief	As for step 2

Step 4: severe, persistent	Daily medications
	  Anti-inflammatory
	  Inhaled corticosteroids (high dose) and long-acting bronchodilator (long-acting β-agonist or theophylline) and oral corticosteroids
		Inhaled β-agonist for symptom relief	As for steps 1–3
			Refer to individual education/counseling

EVIDENCE LEVEL: A. Reference: National Asthma Education and Prevention Program. Expert Panel Report II: Guidelines for the diagnosis and management of asthma. National Heart, Lung, and Blood Institute 1997;146.

TABLE 363.3.	ASTHMA MEDICATIONS

Long-term Controllers	Quick-relief Medications
Inhaled corticosteriods	β-agonists
Beclomethasone	Anticholinergics (atropine,
Triamcinolone	ipratroprium)
Flunisolide	Systemic corticosteroids
Fluticasone	(oral, intravenous,
Budeseonide	intramuscular)
Theophylline	
Cromones (cromolyn, nedocromil)	
Long-acting β-agonists	
(salmeterol, formoterol)	
Leukotriene-modulating drugs	
Zafirlukast	
Montelukast	
Zileuton	

lator, to make an objective determination of baseline pulmonary function and reversibility as an important guide to therapy. In addition, peak flow monitoring can be used to guide therapy, especially in moderate and severe cases of asthma.

Several studies have suggested that the patient's perception of airflow limitation does not correlate well with the actual degree of physiologic obstruction. A more than 20% fall in peak flow is an indication for increased attention and treatment, whereas a 50% fall from the patient's baseline always requires an aggressive approach. For further recommendations, the reader is encouraged to refer to the National Institutes of Health's Expert Panel 2 report *Guidelines for the Diagnosis and Management of Asthma*. Patients should be categorized by severity based on their initial symptoms and treated appropriately for that clinical picture, based on a step-therapy paradigm. The characteristics of the different severity levels of asthma are described in Table 363.1, with the appropriate treatments for each given in Table 363.2. Pharmacologic agents have been divided into two groups, known as long-term control medications and quick-relief medications (Table 363.3). This approach to the management of asthma is based on the latest Expert 2 Panel report.

LONG-TERM CONTROL MEDICATIONS

Inhaled Corticosteroids

This class of drugs forms the cornerstone of the management of all but the most mild asthma. Inhaled corticosteroids (ICs) are effective and, in general, safe treatments for asthma. They are potent anti-inflammatory agents, decreasing both eosinophil and lymphocyte numbers in the airways after treatment. Corticosteroids also can affect the production of such cytokines as IL-4 and 5 and the up-regulation of adhesion molecules. ICs directly improve FEV_1 and airway hyperreactivity at doses ranging from about 200 μg per day to 2,000 μg per day. Higher doses (more than 1,000 μg per day) have been studied only rarely, but systemic side effects begin to increase at about that dose. Although ICs improve airway obstruction, reactivity, and

inflammation, discontinuation of therapy often leads to relapse; complete cures do not occur. Nonetheless, ICs remain the most clinically useful and cost-effective anti-inflammatory treatment available for asthma.

Although they are highly effective in children, inhaled corticosteroids remain a controversial treatment owing to issues of bone growth and the unknown potential for long-term residual effects. In adults, low to moderate doses of ICs have proved safe in clinical practice. The 5% incidence of oral thrush can be minimized by use of a spacer device, which diminishes oral deposition, as well as by rinsing the mouth after use. IC-induced dysphonia affects a small portion of the treated population. It is a trivial problem to most patients, but it can be a considerable annoyance to patients whose voice is an important aspect of their careers. Only about 10% of the inhaled dose of IC actually reaches the lung, but systemic effects can result from this inhaled portion or through absorption of the 90% that enters the gastrointestinal tract. The effect of ICs on the adrenal axis is related to dose and potency, as is the effect on osteoporosis. Older women treated with ICs are at greater risk of increased skin thinning and bruisability. Cataract formation and glaucoma have been associated with IC use in retrospective studies. The biggest limiting factor to ICs remains compliance with therapy on the part of patients.

It is likely that differences in potency (with subsequent differences in both efficacy and safety) exist among the five available corticosteroids. Although few direct comparisons exist, fluticasone, budesonide, and beclomethasone are likely more potent than flunisolide or triamcinolone. It is recommended that the patient start at a higher dose (more than 1,000 μg per day) to relieve symptoms and then taper the dose as symptoms resolve (step-up/step-down therapy). The evidence to support this approach is minimal, however.

Cromones (Nedocromil Sodium, Cromolyn Sodium)

Despite the use of these compounds for more than 20 years, little is known regarding their mechanism of action. Although they are potent mast cell stabilizers in vitro, the clinical importance of this effect is less clear. Cromones are moderately efficacious drugs for controlling asthma symptoms. They protect against physiologic bronchoconstriction after challenges with allergens, ozone, sulfur dioxide, and exercise. Comparative studies have shown ICs to be more efficacious, but this class of drugs has proved remarkably safe. For this reason, cromolyn sodium has been the first-line controller for asthmatic children with mild to moderate disease, while it is second-line therapy for adults. There likely is very little difference between cromolyn and nedocromil. There may be a mild steroid-sparing effect with nedocromil. The anti-inflammatory or disease-modifying effects of this class of drugs remain doubtful.

Theophyllines

Theophyllines are nonspecific phosphodiesterase inhibitors with weak bronchodilating effects and some anti-inflammatory properties. They are effective for the treatment of asthma and are classified as second-line controller drugs for mild and moderate, persistent asthma. Inhaled corticosteroids, however, are more effective anti-inflammatory drugs. Seizures and arrythmias can develop when recommended therapeutic concentrations are exceeded. Theophylline dosage is based on body weight and serum concentrations. Since many drugs interfere with the metabolism of theophylline by the P-450 enzyme system (erythromycin, cimetidine, zileuton, etc.), appropriate dosage adjustments should be made and drug levels monitored with any changes.

Long-acting Inhaled β-agonists (Salmeterol, Formoterol)

These compounds are classified as controllers on the basis of their long duration of action, but there is minimal evidence to suggest that they have anti-inflammatory properties. Salmeterol is an effective bronchodilator for up to 12 hours (and beyond in some asthmatics). It has shown efficacy in preventing nocturnal symptoms and diurnal peak flow changes. Although these drugs were once recommended for long-term protection against exercise-induced bronchospasm, recent studies suggest that protection against bronchospasm associated with exercise that occurs several hours after dosing decreases within 1 to 2 weeks of initiating therapy. Long-acting β-agonists should always be prescribed with a short-acting β-agonist and with an anti-inflammatory agent (ICs). In several studies, the addition of a long-acting β-agonist to ICs was more effective therapy than increasing the dose of ICs. For these reasons, long-acting β-agonists are recommended for use primarily with ICs in moderate, persistent asthma.

Leukotriene Modulators (Zafirlukast, Montelukast, Zileuton)

LT modulators fall into two categories: LT D_4 receptor antagonists (zafirlukast, montelukast) and a 5-lipoxygenase (5-LO) inhibitor (zileuton). The LT D_4 receptor antagonists antagonize the cysteinyl LTs (LT C_4, D_4, and E_4), while the 5-LO inhibitors block production of both cysteinyl leukotrienes and LT B_4, giving them a potentially broader spectrum of activity. LT modulators have shown efficacy in allergen-, exercise-, and aspirin-induced asthma. There may be some anti-inflammatory effect, with reduction in inflammatory cells in lung fluids and tissue. There is a small (10% to 15%), immediate effect on FEV_1. Long-term improvement in FEV_1 continues for the first 1 to 3 weeks and then plateaus. Studies comparing LT drugs, such as montelukast and zafirlukast, to low-dose ICs show a greater effect on FEV_1 with ICs, but the improvement in symptom scores, β-agonist use, and exacerbations are more comparable. They may be particularly helpful for patients with aspirin-sensitive asthma—long-term studies have shown additional improvement in both upper and lower airway disease when these drugs are added to inhaled and even oral corticosteroids.

Few side effects have been reported with the receptor antagonists. However, Churg-Strauss syndrome, a type of eosinophilic vasculitis that presents with eosinophilia, pulmonary infiltrates, and/or cardiac, neurologic, and dermatologic changes, has been reported in patients treated with the receptor antagonists. Cause and effect is unclear, but practitioners should be aware of the association. The 5-LO inhibitor zileuton may cause abnormal liver function elevations in 3% of patients, and monitoring (at least in the first year) is suggested. The most recent National Institutes of Health guidelines suggest that these drugs be used in patients with mild, persistent asthma as alternatives to ICs, theophylline, and cromones. Recent studies in more severely affected patients suggest that these drugs may have a wider applicability as "add-on" therapy than was described originally.

QUICK-RELIEF MEDICATIONS

Short-acting β-agonists

Short-acting β_2-agonists increase levels of intracellular cyclic AMP, causing smooth-muscle relaxation and bronchodilation. They also may stabilize mast cells but do not reduce airway inflammation. Short-acting β-agonists remain the acute bronchodilator of choice and the most effective pretreatment for exercise-induced asthma. There does not appear to be any added benefit to regular dosing, and there are some data to suggest that regular dosing may be detrimental.

Anticholinergics (Ipratroprium, Atropine)

Anticholinergic agents inhibit increased vagal tone in the airways of patients with asthma through antagonism of muscarinic receptors (specifically the M3 receptor). About 50% of asthmatics experience bronchodilation with the use of anticholinergic agents, but, in general, the bronchodilating response is weaker than that seen with β-agonists. Anticholinergics have shown small additive effects to β-agonists in the treatment of status asthmaticus and are effective for therapy of β-blocker-induced bronchospasm.

Systemic Corticosteroids

Systemic corticosteroids are the most effective anti-inflammatory treatment for asthma. The onset of action is within 4 to 6 hours, and there does not appear to be a difference between intravenous and oral therapy. Although systemic corticosteroids are the most effective treatment for asthma, they are also probably the most toxic; every effort should be made to limit their long-term use.

SPECIAL SITUATIONS

Pregnancy

Symptoms improve in approximately one-third of asthmatic patients during pregnancy, worsen in one-third, and do not change at all in one-third. Treatment of pregnant women requires good medical control of asthma. It is likely that poor asthma control during pregnancy is more detrimental to the fetus than treatment with available drugs. Most drugs are poorly classified regarding risk in pregnancy, since very little reliable data exist in humans. The β-agonists have strong tocolytic effects, which may result in delayed or prolonged labor.

Status Asthmaticus

Asthma exacerbations can be initiated by a variety of factors, including noncompliance with medication; exposure to allergens, aspirin, and β-blockers; sinus and viral infections; and stress. Viral infections may account for up to 40% to 50% of exacerbations; rhinovirus is likely the most common factor. Although the best management of asthma exacerbations is prevention, the acute situation demands objective diagnosis and rapid treatment. All patients seen regularly by a physician for their asthma should have an action plan to begin treatment at home, including increased use of β-agonists and oral corticosteroid therapy if there is no initial response to β-agonists. Objective measures of lung function should always be obtained before treatment. Patients should continue to receive inhaled or nebulized β-agonist therapy at home and/or in the emergency room until they experience a favorable response.

The usefulness of other bronchodilating medications for the treatment of status asthmaticus in the emergency room is the subject of controversy. Anticholinergic (ipratropium bromide) solution has shown varying effects in improving FEV_1 beyond that of β-agonists alone, but an effect on hospitalization has not been established. Unless a patient is already on theophylline (in which case it should be continued), there is no indication for theophylline in the emergency management of asthma. Systemic corticosteroids have become a mainstay of therapy for those patients who fail initial treatment with β-agonists. The effects will not be seen until 6 to 8 hours after dosing, however. Dosing should be started at 60 to 120 mg of prednisone or the equivalent. A distinct dose response does not exist for steroid use in the emergency room, and there is no difference in oral or intravenous delivery. Patients who receive steroids in the emergency department should be given corticosteroids (likely both oral and inhaled) on discharge to limit a second exacerbation. These patients also need good long-term follow-up, since they are likely to be at higher risk for exacerbations in the future.

Exercise-induced Asthma

The mechanisms of exercise-induced asthma (EIA) remain incompletely defined, but they likely involve bronchoconstrictive effects stemming from abnormal heat and water fluxes in the bronchial tree. EIA normally develops 10 to 20 minutes after discontinuation of exercise. It is usually self-limited, resolving within 1 hour. It is exacerbated by exercise in cold, dry air. An initial warm-up period can induce a state of refractoriness, which limits bronchospasm during the planned exercise. In mild or intermittent cases, EIA is best treated with an inhaled β-agonist 15 to 30 minutes before exercise. Refractory or chronic cases require long-term therapy with ICs. Cromolyn and LT modulator drugs also are efficacious in this syndrome.

BIBLIOGRAPHY

Corbridge TC, Hall JB. The assessment and management of adults with status asthmaticus. *Am J Respir Crit Care Med* 1995;151:1296–1316.
Djukonovic R, Wilson TW, Britten KM, et al. Effect of an inhaled corticosteroid on airway inflammation and symptoms of asthma. *Am Rev Respir Dis* 1992;145:669–674.
Expert Panel Report 2. *Guidelines for the diagnosis and management of asthma.* Bethesda, Md.: National Institutes of Health, 1997. NIH publication no. 97–4051.
Haahtela T, Jarvinen M, Kava T, et al. Effects of reducing or discontinuing inhaled budesonide in patients with mild asthma. *N Engl J Med* 1994; 331:700–705.
Lange P, Parner J, Vestbo J, et al. A 15-year follow-up study of ventilatory function in adults with asthma. *N Engl J Med* 1998;339:1194–1200.
Martinez FD, Wright AL, Taussig LM, et al. Asthma and wheezing in the first six years of life. *N Engl J Med* 1995;332:133–138.
Sly RM, O'Donnell R. Stabilization of asthma mortality. *Ann Allergy Asthma Immunol* 1997;78:347–354.
Wenzel S. Antileukotriene drugs in the management of asthma. *JAMA* 1998;280:2068–2069.
Woolcock A, Lundback B, Ringdal N, et al. Comparison of addition of salmeterol to inhaled steroids with doubling of the dose of inhaled steroid. *Am J Respir Crit Care Med* 1996;153:1481–1488.
Ying S, Humbert M, Barkans J, et al. Expression of IL-4 and IL-5 mRNA and protein product by CD4 + and CD8 + T-cells, eosinophils and mast cells in bronchial biopsies obtained from atopic and nonatopic (intrinsic) asthmatics. *J Immunol* 1997;158:3539–3544.

Kelley's Textbook of Internal Medicine, fourth edition. Edited by H. David Humes. Lippincott Williams & Wilkins, Philadelphia © 2000.

CHAPTER 364

CHRONIC OBSTRUCTIVE PULMONARY DISEASE

ANDREW L. RIES

Chronic obstructive pulmonary disease (COPD) refers to a group of disorders that have in common the presence of persistent airflow obstruction. Specific conditions may be defined on the basis of clinical, anatomic, or physiologic criteria—such as chronic bronchitis, emphysema, and asthma—that may or may not be associated with chronic airflow obstruction. Chronic bronchitis typically is defined clinically by chronic cough and sputum production for at least 3 months for 2 successive years without other known causes. Emphysema is an anatomic, pathologic condition with abnormal permanent enlargement of airspaces distal to the terminal bronchioles, accompanied by destruction of walls but without fibrosis. Asthma is characterized by reversible airway narrowing and increased responsiveness to various stimuli. The overlapping diagnostic categories are illustrated in Fig. 364.1.

From a clinical perspective, the term *COPD* has gained widespread use for several reasons. Many patients exhibit features of more than one disease (e.g., emphysema and chronic bronchitis or asthmatic bronchitis); it is often difficult to establish clearly one predominant source. Precise diagnosis is difficult, particularly in early-stage disease. Moreover, the clinical approaches to management are similar. Other terms may be encountered, such as chronic obstructive airways disease, chronic obstructive lung

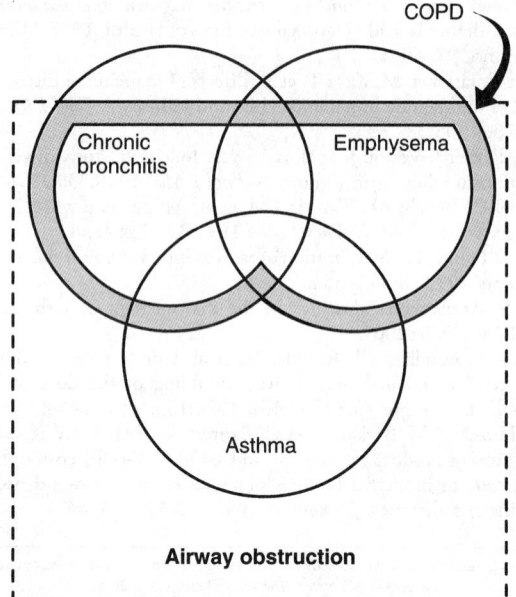

FIGURE 364.1. Nonproportional Venn diagram of the spectrum of overlapping conditions that make up chronic obstructive pulmonary disease (COPD). COPD includes airway obstruction and chronic bronchitis, emphysema, or irreversible asthma. Some persons with clinical or radiographic features of chronic bronchitis or emphysema may not have evidence of airway obstruction. (From Snider GL, Faling LJ, Rennard SI. Chronic bronchitis and emphysema. In: Murray JR, Nadel JA, eds. *Textbook of respiratory medicine*, second ed. Philadelphia: WB Saunders, 1994:1331–1397, with permission.)

disease, chronic airflow obstruction or chronic airways obstruction, and chronic airflow limitation, but in this discussion they are considered identical to COPD. Specifically excluded are localized airways diseases, cystic fibrosis, bronchiectasis, and asthma without chronic airway obstruction.

INCIDENCE AND EPIDEMIOLOGY

COPD is a major cause of death and disability. Because COPD is insidious, with a long latency period before clinical recognition, official statistics underestimate morbidity and mortality rates. As of 1990, COPD had become the fourth leading cause of death in the United States. COPD was listed as the underlying cause of more than 106,000 deaths in 1996, accounting for about 4% of all deaths and contributing to an additional 5%. This represents an age-adjusted death rate of 21 per 100,000 in the population. In persons age 55 to 74, COPD as cause of death ranks third among men and fourth among women. More than 95% of deaths from COPD occur after the age of 55 years. In contrast to other major diseases, death rates from COPD have increased considerably in recent years—the rate was 47% between 1979 and 1993.

In the United States, the overall disease prevalence is about 4% to 6% in men and 1% to 3% in women; in adults older than 55, COPD is recognized in about 10% to 15%. The 1994 National Health Interview Survey estimated that 14 million

adults had chronic bronchitis and two million had emphysema. In that year, the prevalence rates for COPD in older adults (65 years or older) were 119 per 1,000 men and 97 per 1,000 women. Recent trends indicate that prevalence rates are stable or declining among men but increasing among women. The impact of COPD on morbidity is even greater than on mortality. In the National Health Interview Survey in 1985, COPD accounted for 5% of doctors' office visits and more than 13% of all hospitalizations. COPD is an enormous cause of disability and reduced function among affected persons.

Epidemiologic studies have identified two main syndromes, with different risk factors and natural histories. The "usual" emphysematous form is associated closely with cigarette smoking. Airflow obstruction develops insidiously over many years with minimal symptoms, followed by clinical disease in later years with progressive symptoms and high morbidity and mortality rates. The second form of COPD, chronic asthmatic bronchitis, is associated with risk factors of atopy, high serum IgE levels, and bronchial hyperreactivity. Patients experience chronic airflow obstruction independent of smoking, though smoking may add to the risk. Asthmatic bronchitis is more amenable to medical therapy and has a better prognosis and survival rate than the emphysematous type.

Morbidity and mortality rates from COPD continue to rise despite declining smoking rates; this discrepancy is due to the long latency period between smoking exposure and clinical disease. Lower smoking rates ultimately will reduce the burden of COPD, but not for many years. With higher overall life expectancy and lower death rates from other major diseases, the impact of COPD will be magnified in our aging population.

ETIOLOGY

Cigarette smoking is the major risk factor and accounts for nearly 90% of COPD cases. Compared with nonsmokers, current smokers have about ten times the relative risk of COPD. The risk is equal for men and women. Previously, COPD was more common in men owing to their higher smoking rates, but in recent years the disease has manifested more gender equality, reflecting similar smoking rates for men and women. There is marked individual variation in susceptibility, and host factors play an important role. Only about 10% to 15% of smokers experience significant obstructive lung disease. In susceptible persons, smoking is associated with an accelerated decline in lung function over many years that is related to the amount of smoking (Fig. 364.2). Because of the large reserve in healthy lungs, disease typically is not recognized until later in life. From then on, progressive symptoms, disability, and death predominate. Figure 364.2 also indicates the benefit of smoking cessation. Although lung function does not improve, the subsequent rate of decline slows to that in nonsmokers, which can significantly delay the onset of death and disability and justifies the emphasis on smoking cessation, even in persons with recognized disease.

Exposure of nonsmokers to the smoke of others in an indoor environment (second-hand smoke) is associated with an increase in respiratory infections and lung disease in children and with

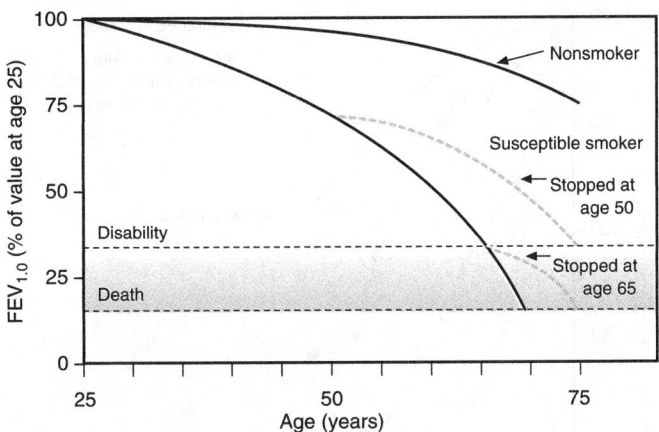

FIGURE 364.2. Age-related rate of decline in lung function ($FEV_{1.0}$) in a nonsmoker (*top*) and susceptible smoker (*bottom*). The dashed lines indicate the beneficial effects of smoking cessation with moderate and severe disease. The accelerated decline in lung function approaches the normal rate, significantly delaying the onset of disability and death. $FEV_{1.0}$, forced expiratory volume in 1 second. (From Fletcher CM, Peto R. The natural history of chronic airflow obstruction. *Br Med J* 1977;1: 1645, with permission.)

modest changes in lung function in adults. It has not been established clearly, however, that passive smoke exposure leads to clinically significant obstructive lung disease. There is some evidence that environmental exposures, such as air pollution and occupational dusts and fumes, are harmful for persons with underlying lung disease and may increase the risk of COPD, but it is unclear whether the effects are independent of smoking. There is also growing evidence that a history of childhood respiratory infections amplifies the risk of COPD in later life.

PATHOGENESIS

It is well established that cigarette smoking is the major risk factor for COPD, but the manner in which smoke produces airway disease is not entirely understood. In susceptible persons, smoking is associated with pathologic evidence of emphysema as well as inflammatory changes in the large and small airways. There is wide variability between persons, and there are poor correlations between the amount of cigarette smoking and the degree of emphysema, bronchiolar inflammation, and airway obstruction.

One credible theory about the pathogenesis of emphysema is that disease results from an imbalance between lung proteases and antiproteases, enzymes that promote injury and protect the lung against injury, respectively. An inherited deficiency of $\alpha_1$protease inhibitor (Pi) is associated with premature emphysema. α_1-Pi is found in serum and alveolar fluid and is an acute-phase reactant in inflammatory states. Diagnosis of α_1-Pi deficiency can be made by measuring the serum level and by phenotyping. The gene is inherited in an autosomal recessive pattern—Pi MM is the normal phenotype and Pi ZZ the most common phenotype of homozygous deficiency. Although heterozygous persons have reduced levels of α_1-Pi, they do not have

a clearly increased risk of disease. In congenital emphysema, anatomic changes predominate at the lung bases rather than in the upper lung fields. Additional evidence about the role of proteolytic enzymes in emphysema comes from animal studies in which human neutrophil elastase instilled into the lungs caused emphysema. The exact role of cigarette smoke in promoting enzymatic proteases or inhibiting the action of antiproteases is unknown.

In chronic bronchitis, pathologic changes in the airways include an inflammatory cell response, squamous metaplasia of ciliated epithelial cells, goblet cell proliferation, enlargement in submucosal glands with dilatation of ducts, and an increase in smooth muscle. These processes result in clinical symptoms of cough and sputum and sometimes airflow obstruction. There is controversy about whether asthma itself is part of the spectrum of COPD. Nonspecific airway hyperresponsiveness has been proposed as a risk factor that predisposes smokers to developing COPD (the "Dutch hypothesis"). Asthmatic bronchitis is one of the recognized epidemiologic patterns of COPD. Asthma can result in chronic airflow obstruction and should probably be included within the clinical spectrum of COPD (Fig. 364.1).

CLINICAL FINDINGS

COPD typically develops later in life. Dyspnea is the hallmark symptom that brings the patient to medical attention and leads to diagnosis. A careful history of the insidious onset of breathlessness on exertion, with or without a history of cough, sputum, or frequent lung infections, often provides the clue to diagnosis. Because of the slowly progressive course of disease and the large reserve in lung function, there is a long preclinical period in which the person who has smoked for years "without a problem" begins to note breathlessness with physical activities previously accomplished without difficulty. This breathlessness may be attributed to getting older or being out of shape. Reduced expiratory flow rates may be detected at this stage. Later, the patient often comes to medical attention after a critical event, such as a winter cold from which he or she never quite recovers. The person attributes the onset of illness to this time, but in truth this event simply pushed the already diseased lungs over the clinical edge, so to speak, much like a rope weakened by progressive fraying breaks when only a small weight is attached.

Cough (often called *smoker's cough*) is a common symptom early in the course of disease. It is usually productive; sputum is described as mucoid. There may be a history of frequent respiratory infections associated with increased cough, purulent sputum, and breathlessness. The patient may note that it takes longer than usual to recover. Some patients with COPD experience abnormal gas exchange with hypoxemia or hypercapnia. Hypoxemia may be associated with cognitive or personality changes, polycythemia, and cyanosis. Chronic hypercapnia may cause headache, particularly on arising, and increased somnolence. During exercise, the PaO_2 may change significantly and unpredictably from the resting level. In many patients, the PaO_2 declines with physical activity; in others, it does not change or actually may increase.

On physical examination, it is important to assess maximum expiratory flow in high-risk persons (i.e., smokers). In early-stage disease, the examination may show normal results, but prolonged expiration or wheezing can be detected on forced exhalation at later stages. This symptom can be assessed easily with the forced expiratory time, a useful screening test for expiratory obstruction. In this maneuver, the patient exhales with maximal effort through an open mouth after a full inspiration. The examiner listens with the bell of the stethoscope over the trachea in the suprasternal notch and records the time in seconds until airflow ceases. Normal persons can exhale completely within 4 seconds. A forced expiratory time longer than 6 seconds signifies significant expiratory obstruction.

Other physical signs of COPD often are not present until the disease becomes moderate to severe. Overinflation of the lungs may result in an increased anteroposterior diameter of the thorax and a low, flat diaphragm with limited respiratory excursion. The flattened diaphragm contributes less to inspiration, placing more burden on the accessory breathing muscles (neck and intercostals) and producing greater respiratory movement in the upper chest. With severe hyperinflation, the diaphragm may even become inverted and move paradoxically—up on inspiration, down on expiration. This can be detected best with the patient supine, noting the inward movement of the lower rib cage and abdomen during inspiration. With advanced emphysema, the breath sounds are diminished owing to reduced flow and increased lung inflation. Signs of pulmonary hypertension and right-sided heart failure, such as peripheral edema and hepatic congestion, usually are not detected until an advanced stage of disease.

LABORATORY FINDINGS

The central diagnostic feature of COPD is reduced expiratory airflow resulting from increased airway resistance due to airway narrowing. Spirometry is the standard test for measuring maximal airflow and is relatively simple, reliable, and reproducible. It is useful for detecting airflow obstruction, staging severity, and following the disease course. A reduction in the forced expiratory volume in 1 second (FEV_1) in relation to the forced vital capacity (FVC)—the FEV_1/FVC ratio—is a standard bench mark of obstruction. The FEV_1 is the best measure of disease severity; it correlates with exercise tolerance and survival (Fig. 364.3). Other assessments of expiratory airflow also may be helpful (see Chapter 387). Peak expiratory flow can be calculated with relatively inexpensive peak flow meters that patients can be taught to use. It is most helpful for following changes over time, particularly in patients with reactive (i.e., asthmatic) disease.

Measures of lung volumes show an increase in residual volume, functional residual capacity, and, sometimes, total lung capacity in COPD. These tests can help confirm the diagnosis suspected on the basis of spirometry results. Emphysema produces a greater increase in total lung capacity than other obstructive diseases as well as a reduced carbon monoxide diffusing capacity of the lung (D_{LCO}), primarily as the result of the loss of alveolar-capillary surface area. Nevertheless, D_{LCO} is neither specific nor sensitive for emphysema.

Chest radiographs have limited usefulness in diagnosing or staging COPD. Early in the course of disease, they may show

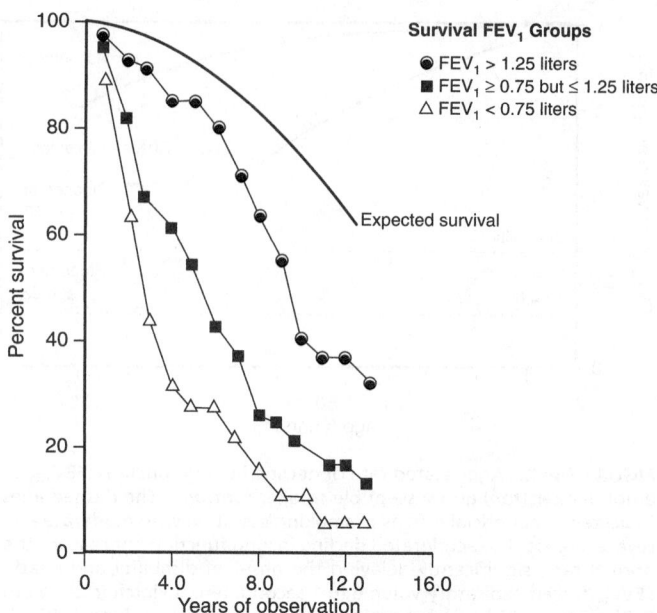

FIGURE 364.3. Long-term survival of 200 patients with chronic obstructive pulmonary disease grouped by initial FEV_1. (From Diener CF, Burrows B. Further observations on the course and prognosis of chronic obstructive lung disease. *Am Rev Respir Dis* 1975;111:719–724, with permission.)

normal results. Their main use is in detecting other parenchymal lung or cardiovascular diseases that may have similar symptoms. In the context of advanced emphysema, the chest radiograph may evidence overinflation of the lungs, with a low, flat diaphragm and an increase in the retrosternal airspace (anterior to the heart) on the lateral film. The emphysematous lungs also can appear radiolucent, owing to bullous changes and a paucity of vascular shadows. High-resolution computed tomography may be useful in documenting pathologic evidence of emphysema, but the clinical usefulness of this test is unproved.

Arterial blood gas analysis may document hypoxemia and hypercapnia, particularly in advanced disease. The relationship between gas exchange abnormalities and other measures of lung function is poor. Hypoxemia can worsen with exercise, sleep, or changes in body position. Two characteristic clinical patterns of disease can be defined by blood gas findings. Patients with severe dyspnea, mild hypoxemia, and normal to low $PaCO_2$ have been termed *pink puffers* (type A COPD), reflecting their color and increased breathing effort. Patients with severe hypoxemia, carbon dioxide retention, right-sided heart failure, and little dyspnea are called *blue bloaters* (type B COPD), indicating their bloated, cyanotic appearance and low ventilation. These differences may reflect variations in ventilation–perfusion ($\dot{V}/\dot{Q}$) mismatching and central respiratory drive. In clinical practice, most patients with COPD fall between these two extremes. The ECG usually shows normal results early in the course of disease; later, there may be signs of right-sided heart strain, including right axis shift, increased R waves over the right precordial leads (V_1 and V_2), and peaked P waves (so-called P pulmonale). These changes do not correlate well with the level of pulmonary hypertension.

OPTIMAL MANAGEMENT

COPD is by and large a chronic, progressive, and irreversible disease, so the primary goals of management should be directed toward preventive health strategies to slow progression and minimize complications. Secondary goals are to improve symptoms and function and treat reversible components of the disease. Optimal treatment depends on the stage of disease. For patients with mild to moderate disease, early detection and diagnosis and counseling regarding appropriate preventive health strategies are important. For patients with moderate to severe disease, symptomatic treatment also is indicated.

PREVENTION

There are several effective prevention strategies for patients with COPD throughout the natural history of disease (Table 364.1). Primary prevention strategies focus on suppressing the development of disease. Secondary prevention emphasizes early detection and halting of the course of clinical disease. Tertiary prevention methods involve minimizing complications for patients with symptomatic disease.

Cigarette Smoking

Controlling smoking behavior is the most important preventive strategy at all phases of disease. Physicians can play an important role by setting a smoke-free example in their personal lives, offices, and health care settings and by supporting social and political antismoking efforts (see Chapter 33). Public policies that encourage youths, who are the prime target of tobacco marketing, not to smoke can eliminate the epidemic of COPD, just as public health measures can control certain infectious diseases.

Smoking cessation should be a high priority for all patients with COPD. Although much of the disease is irreversible, there are clear, important benefits to quitting. Lung function may not improve after smoking cessation, but the accelerated loss of function due to smoking will slow and approach the normal,

TABLE 364.1. PREVENTION STRATEGIES IN COPD

Primary: preventing development of disease
  Prevent cigarette smoking—support public policy, encourage nonsmokers
  Smoking cessation
Secondary: early detection and prevention of clinical disease
  Smoking cessation
  Expiratory flow rate measurement in high-risk persons (smokers)
  α_1-protease inhibitor replacement for persons with proven genetic deficiency
Tertiary: minimizing complications in symptomatic disease
  Smoking cessation
  Influenza and pneumococcal vaccination
  Pulmonary rehabilitation
  Oxygen therapy for persons with hypoxemia

age-related rate of decline (Fig. 364.2). The Lung Health Study, a multicenter randomized clinical trial of 5,887 middle-aged smokers with spirometric evidence of early COPD, established that an aggressive smoking intervention program significantly lessened the age-related decline in FEV_1 over 5 years of follow-up.

The advice of physicians is important and effective in inducing smokers to quit. Several studies have found that only a few minutes of a physician's time inquiring about smoking status and providing advice to quit can achieve abstinence rates of up to 10% to 20% at 1 year. Physician counseling for high-risk smokers is even more effective. Even in patients with symptomatic and advanced disease, smoking cessation is important in delaying progression and limiting the consequences of the disease.

Preventing Influenza and Pneumonia

Patients with COPD are particularly vulnerable to lung infections. Influenza can be prevented or minimized in severity by immunization or chemoprophylaxis. Moreover, some bacterial pneumonias caused by pneumococci can be prevented by immunization. An annual influenza vaccine is produced from the strains of influenza A and B viruses expected to be most prevalent during the next flu season. Made from inactivated virus, it cannot cause infection. Persons at high risk should be vaccinated annually because of changes in the viral strains each year.

Amantadine is an antibiotic that is effective for prophylaxis of influenza A infection. It can be used during epidemics or with exposure, but it is effective only for the duration of administration. The usual dose is 100 mg taken orally twice daily for persons older than 10 years. It is particularly useful when vaccination is contraindicated and can be used with the vaccine during epidemics in the several weeks necessary to mount an antibody response. Side effects develop in about 10% of patients, including insomnia, nervousness, or difficulty concentrating. Rimantadine, a newer derivative, may have fewer side effects. Amantadine also may shorten the duration of influenza A infection, if started within 48 hours of symptom onset.

Pneumococcal vaccine should be given once to the same high-risk groups as for the influenza vaccine. In addition, patients over age 2 years with sickle cell disease or other causes of splenic dysfunction should be vaccinated. The current vaccine contains capsular polysaccharide antigens of the 23 serotypes of pneumococci responsible for more than 80% of serious, bacteremic pneumococcal infections. Although antibody levels decline over time, routine revaccination is not recommended because of the risk of allergic reactions.

Pulmonary Rehabilitation

Pulmonary rehabilitation is an established preventive health strategy that enhances standard therapy for persons with chronic lung disease to control and alleviate symptoms, optimize function, and limit the medical and economic burdens of disease. Multidisciplinary programs include education, respiratory and chest physiotherapy instruction, psychosocial support, and exercise training. As with other rehabilitation programs, the primary goal is to restore the patient to the highest possible level of independent function. This can be accomplished by helping patients become more knowledgeable about their disease, more actively involved in their own health care, more independent in daily care activities, and less dependent on family, friends, and health professionals and other expensive medical resources.

Benefits of pulmonary rehabilitation include improved exercise tolerance and symptoms and reduced hospitalizations and use of expensive medical resources. Patients report improved quality of life with a decline in respiratory symptoms, an increase in exercise tolerance and ability to perform physical activities of daily living, and improved psychological functioning, with less anxiety and depression and elevated feelings of hope, control, and self-esteem.

OXYGEN THERAPY

Long-term, continuous oxygen therapy has been shown to improve survival and lower morbidity in hypoxemic patients with COPD; in fact, this is the only treatment proven to prolong survival. Possible benefits of supplemental oxygen for nonhypoxemic patients or for patients who experience hypoxemia only under certain conditions (e.g., exercise, sleep) are less clearly defined. The results of two multicenter randomized clinical trials (one in Great Britain and the other in the United States) justify long-term oxygen therapy for patients with significant resting hypoxemia (PaO_2 55 of mm Hg or less or oxygen saturation of 88% or less). For patients with a PaO_2 between 56 and 59 mm Hg, oxygen is indicated if there is erythrocytosis (hematocrit of 55 or more) or cor pulmonale. The decision for long-term therapy should be made only in stable patients on optimal treatment for at least 30 days. Patients recovering from an acute illness should be reevaluated after a period of stability before committing to this expensive treatment. There are several options for long-term oxygen therapy. Home-care providers, respiratory therapy personnel, and pulmonary rehabilitation professionals are excellent sources of information about available options, including gas sources (liquid, compressed gas, concentrators) and delivery devices (nasal, transtracheal, or conserving catheters and inspiratory demand regulators).

α₁-PROTEASE INHIBITOR REPLACEMENT

For patients with verified deficiency of α_1-Pi, replacement therapy with the purified human protein is available. This treatment has presumed but not proven efficacy in slowing the progression of emphysematous lung destruction. The current treatment regimen is expensive: the drug alone can cost more than $25,000 per year. According to American Thoracic Society guidelines, treatment should be reserved for patients with proven α_1-Pi deficiency and abnormal lung function.

SYMPTOMATIC TREATMENT

Bronchodilators

For patients with recognized COPD, medical treatment is directed toward the reversible component of airway obstruction and control of secretions. Bronchodilators used to improve symptoms and increase airway caliber include sympathomimetic

β-agonists, anticholinergics, and methylxanthines (theophylline). The decision to treat a patient with a bronchodilator should not depend on evidence of an acute response, because many patients respond later to regular therapy. Furthermore, these medications may have effects beyond just bronchodilation.

Sympathomimetic bronchodilators are used routinely. Newer β_2 agents are more selective and longer acting and have fewer side effects than older, nonselective drugs. The preferred method of administration is by inhalation with a metered-dose inhaler (MDI). This produces more bronchodilation with fewer side effects than administration via oral or other systemic routes. Used properly, an MDI is just as effective as and less expensive than a liquid nebulizer and can be used in acute-care and emergency department settings. Extensions or spacers can help persons who have difficulty coordinating the MDI, particularly children and older adults. The key to MDI use is proper technique (Table 364.2). In addition to bronchodilation, β-agonists also can minimize airway hyperresponsiveness and enhance mucociliary clearance. The most common side effects are tachycardia and skeletal muscle tremor.

Anticholinergics have gained prominence in the treatment of COPD. Although their bronchodilating effects have been known for many years, the selectivity and few side effects of newer agents, such as ipratropium bromide, have enhanced their usefulness. Bronchodilation is thought to be due to inhibition of cholinergic-mediated bronchomotor tone. The drugs are reported to be more effective in larger airways, making them particularly useful for patients with COPD.

Theophylline preparations have been used in treating patients with COPD for many years, but their usage has declined because of frequent problems with toxicity, the need for regular monitoring of blood levels, and the advent of newer, more selective bronchodilating agents. The mechanism of bronchodilation from theophylline is not clearly defined. Theophylline has other potentially beneficial effects, such as improved diaphragmatic function, decreased dyspnea, increased mucociliary clearance, and stimulation of respiratory drive. Because of individual variability in metabolism and the many factors that can alter metabolism, monitoring blood levels is necessary with long-term therapy. The target therapeutic level is typically 10 to 20 μg per milliliter. Minor side effects, such as tremor, insomnia, irritability, and gastrointestinal upset, can develop with levels well below 20 μg per milliliter. More serious side effects, including vomiting, dysrhythmias, hypotension, and seizures, generally develop at higher blood levels. Older patients are particularly susceptible to toxicity.

TABLE 364.2.	PROPER USE OF A METERED-DOSE INHALER

Shake inhaler, remove cap, and hold upright.
Place inhaler 2–4 cm in front of open mouth.
Exhale to functional residual capacity or below.
Activate inhaler once just after the start of a slow, deep inhalation.
Hold breath for 5–10 seconds.
Exhale slowly.
Wait at least 1 minute before next puff.

Corticosteroids

Corticosteroids can be beneficial for some patients with COPD. A meta-analysis of 16 clinical trials of oral steroid therapy for stable patients found that a 20% improvement in FEV_1 occurred in about 10% more patients on steroids than on placebo. Many patients on corticosteroids report subjective symptom improvement, but long-term steroid use is associated with numerous serious adverse effects. A limited trial of corticosteroids probably is justified for patients who cannot be treated with standard bronchodilators alone. A single morning dose of 20 to 40 mg of prednisone for 5 to 7 days is a typical starting point. Treatment beyond a few weeks should be continued only if there is significant improvement in pulmonary function and symptoms. For long-term therapy, the dose should be kept as low as possible, to minimize side effects. Inhaled steroids, best taken in through a spacer device to minimize oral deposition, are safer, but their effectiveness in COPD has not been established.

Control of Secretions

For patients with chronic cough and sputum, techniques to control secretions are important. Patients should be encouraged to drink several glasses of fluid per day, but excessive hydration is not warranted. They also should be taught the technique of controlled coughing, which involves a deep inspiration, breath-holding for a few seconds, and then coughing two or three times. Postural drainage is effective in patients with heavy sputum production. The use of mucolytic agents to thin secretions and promote clearance is the subject of controversy. Theoretically, therapy with such drugs as oral iodinated glycerol, nebulized acetylcysteine, or, more recently, recombinant human DNase, works best in thinning secretions that are thick, mucoid, and heavy. Whether this produces physiologic or symptomatic improvement is unclear. Cough-suppressant therapy is generally not recommended, since cough is an essential protective mechanism.

Because of impaired mucociliary clearance and less effective cough, secretions may pool in dependent portions of the lung and be difficult to clear. For acute exacerbations, when sputum changes color and increases in volume, treatment with antibiotics is indicated. In many cases, a specific bacterial pathogen cannot be identified from purulent sputum. For such episodes of acute bronchitis, it is appropriate to institute a 7- to 10-day course of antibiotics empirically, without a sputum culture. Oral antibiotics, such as trimethoprim-sulfamethoxazole, ampicillin, amoxicillin-clavulanate, tetracycline, or erythromycin, often are chosen to cover pathogens colonizing the respiratory tract, including *Haemophilus influenzae*, *Streptococcus pneumoniae*, and *Moraxella catarrhalis*.

BIBLIOGRAPHY

American College of Chest Physicians (ACCP)/American Association of Cardiovascular and Pulmonary Rehabilitation (AACVPR) Pulmonary Rehabilitation Guidelines Panel. Pulmonary rehabilitation: joint ACCP/AACVPR evidence-based guidelines. *Chest* 1997;112:1363–1396; *J Cardiopulmonary Rehabil* 1997;17:371–405.
Adams PF, Marano MA. Current estimates from the National Health Interview Survey, 1994. National Center for Health Statistics. *Vital Health Stat* 1995;10(193):83–84.
American Thoracic Society. Guidelines for the approach to the patient with severe hereditary α_1-antitrypsin deficiency. *Am Rev Respir Dis* 1989;140:1494–1497.
American Thoracic Society. Standards for the diagnosis and care of patients with chronic obstructive pulmonary disease. *Am J Respir Crit Care Med* 1995;152:S77–S120.
Anthonisen NR, Connett JE, Kiley JP, et al. Effects of smoking intervention and the use of an inhaled anticholinergic bronchodilator on the rate of decline of FEV_1. *JAMA* 1994;272:1497–1505.
Burrows B. Epidemiologic evidence for different types of chronic airflow obstruction. *Am Rev Respir Dis* 1991;143:1452–1455.
Diener CF, Burrows B. Further observations on the course and prognosis of chronic obstructive lung disease. *Am Rev Respir Dis* 1975;111:719–724.
Feinleib M, Rosenberg HM, Collins JG, et al. Trends in COPD morbidity and mortality in the United States. *Am Rev Respir Dis* 1989;140:S9–S18.
Fletcher CM, Peto R. The natural history of chronic airflow obstruction. *Br Med J* 1977;1:1645–1648.
Murphy TF, Sethi S. Bacterial infection in COPD. *Am Rev Respir Dis* 1992;146:1067–1083.
Ries AL. Preventing COPD: you can make a difference. *J Respir Dis* 1993;14:739–749.
Snider GL, Faling LJ, Rennard SI. Chronic bronchitis and emphysema. In: Murray JF, Nadel JA, eds. *Textbook of respiratory medicine*, second ed. Philadelphia: WB Saunders, 1994:1331–1397.
Tiep BL. Long-term home oxygen therapy. *Clin Chest Med* 1990;11:505–521.

Kelley's Textbook of Internal Medicine, fourth edition. Edited by H. David Humes. Lippincott Williams & Wilkins, Philadelphia © 2000.

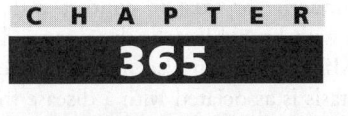

BRONCHIECTASIS

JOHN M. LUCE
ROBERT M. JASMER

The term *bronchiectasis* derives from the Greek words *bronkos*, meaning windpipe, and *ektasis*, signifying stretching or extension. It refers to an abnormal dilatation of the proximal medium-size bronchi greater than 2 mm in diameter due to destruction of the muscular and elastic components of their walls. This dilatation typically is associated with chronic bacterial infection and the production of large quantities of foul-smelling sputum. Bronchiectasis need not always be associated with purulent expectoration, especially when it involves areas of the lung with dependent drainage, such as the upper lobes, which frequently are involved in patients with pulmonary tuberculosis. In this circumstance, the bronchiectasis is called "dry" to distinguish it from the more common "wet," or productive, variety.

CLASSIFICATION

Several systems have been used to classify bronchiectasis, most of them based on anatomic abnormalities of the bronchi seen on bronchography or at autopsy. One common classification system developed by Reid consists of cylindrical bronchiectasis, in which sections of the bronchi are consistently widened; varicose bronchiectasis, in which local constrictions in cylindrical bronchiectatic sections cause an irregularity resembling that of varicose veins; and saccular or cystic bronchiectasis, in which dilatation increases toward the lung periphery so that the bronchi terminate in balloon-like structures. Note that few clinical, epidemiologic, or pathophysiologic differences have been found between cylindrical, varicose, and saccular bronchiectasis.

EPIDEMIOLOGY

Infectious bronchiectasis once was a common disease in the United States. However, it has become rare since the introduction of antibiotics and now is seen in very few Americans. Most affected persons have bronchiectasis in association with systemic disorders. Despite its decline in the United States and in other developed nations, infectious bronchiectasis persists in less developed parts of the world.

PULMONARY FUNCTION ABNORMALITIES

The pulmonary function abnormalities attributable to bronchiectasis are difficult to differentiate from those caused by the diseases that underlie or exist in concert with this condition. Most patients with bronchiectasis show some degree of airflow obstruction. Mild restriction also may be present, especially if the bronchiectasis is associated with a disease that reduces lung volumes. The diffusing capacity for carbon monoxide also may be diminished. Most patients have mild hypoxemia owing to ventilation–perfusion mismatching and intrapulmonary shunt. Normocapnia or hypocapnia is observed in all but the most advanced cases. Cor pulmonale occurs in only a minority of patients with bronchiectasis, because their hypoxemia is often not severe.

SYMPTOMS

Patients with bronchiectasis may have symptoms referable to the bronchiectatic process alone or to underlying disorders. Symptoms caused by bronchiectasis itself include chronic cough, purulent expectoration, fever, weakness, and weight loss. Sputum production often increases during acute respiratory infections. Dyspnea is reported by some patients with bronchiectasis but is not a universal finding. As might be expected, breathlessness is especially common among patients with extensive bronchiectasis seen on chest radiographs. Hemoptysis is also a typical finding among patients with bronchiectasis. It is generally mild, most often consisting of the expectoration of purulent sputum flecked with blood. Because the bleeding usually originates from bronchial arteries or bronchial-pulmonary anastamoses under systemic pressures, however, it may become massive, that is, in excess of 250 mL per day.

PHYSICAL FINDINGS

The physical signs of patients with bronchiectasis are neither sensitive nor specific for that process. The breath is fetid in some but not all patients. Digital clubbing also is an inconsistent finding, as are cyanosis and plethora reflective of polycythemia. Nasal polyps and signs of chronic sinusitis may be present. Rales are often found at the lung bases; rhonchi may be encountered, especially if active infection is present; and scattered wheezes may be heard.

DIAGNOSIS AND PATIENT EVALUATION

Bronchiectasis may be suspected on the basis of clinical signs and symptoms, especially if the process involves purulent expectoration and if such disorders as pneumonia, emphysema, and lung abscess have been ruled out. The onset of bronchiectasis may be traced to a clear-cut aspiration or febrile illness, especially in patients with postobstructive or infectious bronchiectasis. Sputum analysis should reinforce the clinical impression of bronchiectasis. Such analysis often includes visual inspection of expectorated sputum that has been allowed to settle into the characteristic three layers: an upper frothy and watery layer, a middle layer that is turbid and mucopurulent, and a bottom layer that is purulent and opaque. Bacteriologic studies of bronchiectatic sputum may confirm the presence of such microorganisms as *Streptococcus pneumoniae*, *Haemophilus influenzae*, and *Staphylococcus aureus*, but these pathogens also can be present in the sputum of patients with chronic bronchitis. The finding of *Aspergillus* species is suggestive, but not diagnostic, of allergic bronchopulmonary aspergillosis.

Radiographic studies have long been the means by which the diagnosis of bronchiectasis is firmly established. Results of plain chest radiography may be normal in some patients with bronchiectasis, but most often radiography shows characteristic patterns. When cylindrical bronchiectasis is present, these patterns involve linear radiolucencies and thin parallel markings that radiate from the hili and are called tram tracks or tram lines (Fig. 365.1). The dilated bronchi may appear as thick parallel markings or so-called toothpaste lines.

Computed tomography (CT) of the chest, which involves little discomfort and few adverse complications, has virtually replaced bronchography in diagnosing bronchiectasis, especially among patients with generalized disease (Fig. 365.2). Thin-section high-resolution chest CT (HRCT) has a sensitivity and a specificity each in excess of 90% in detecting bronchiectasis at a segmental level. Bronchiectasis results in six characteristic HRCT findings, as originally described by Naidich et al.: bronchial dilatation, bronchial wall thickening, lack of normal bronchial tapering, gross irregularities in airway contact, and air-fluid levels in distended bronchi.

Bronchoscopy is less helpful than bronchography or HRCT in making visible entire bronchiectatic segments. Bronchoscopy may, however, be useful in detecting aspirated foreign bodies and other obstructing lesions and is indicated when such lesions are suspected. Bronchoscopy also may be indicated for patients

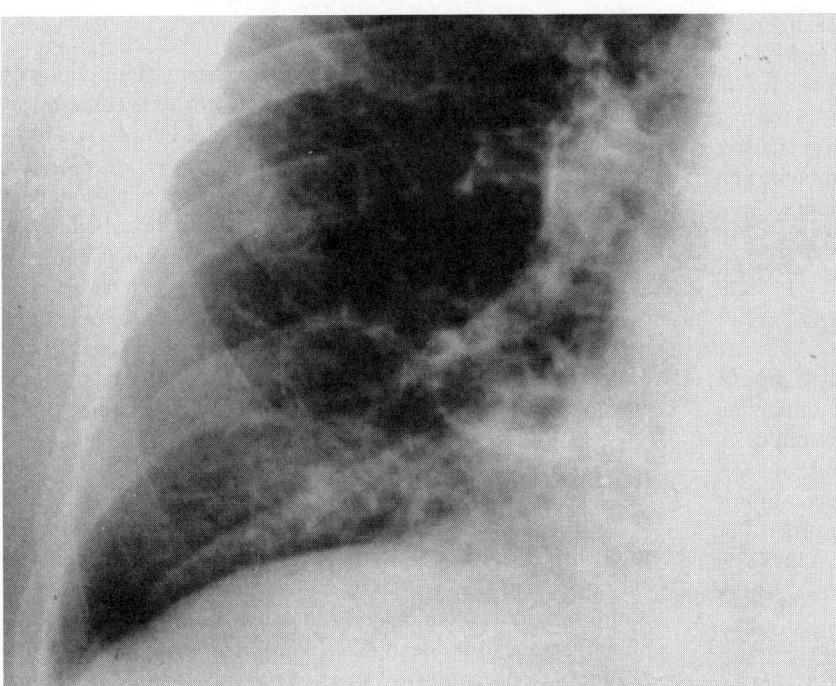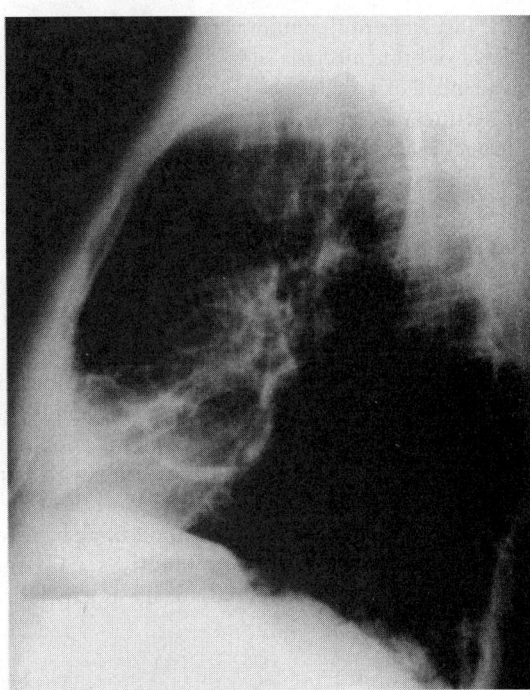

FIGURE 365.1. Tram tracks or tram lines. When cylindrical bronchiectasis is present, radiography shows patterns involving linear radiolucencies and thin parallel markings radiating from the hili.

with hemoptysis, to localize the bleeding site or to determine from which lung blood is coming. In the United States and other developed countries, however, the detection of de novo bronchiectasis should prompt a search for its underlying cause. Depending on the type of patient, this search might include some or all of the following possibilities: serum protein electro-

phoresis for α_1-antitrypsin deficiency; immunoglobulin levels, including IgG subclasses, for hypogammaglobulinemia; pilocarpine iontophoresis (sweat test) for cystic fibrosis; determination of immunoglobulins and *Aspergillus* precipitins for allergic bronchopulmonary aspergillosis; and electron microscopic examination of sperm or respiratory epithelium for primary ciliary dyskinesia.

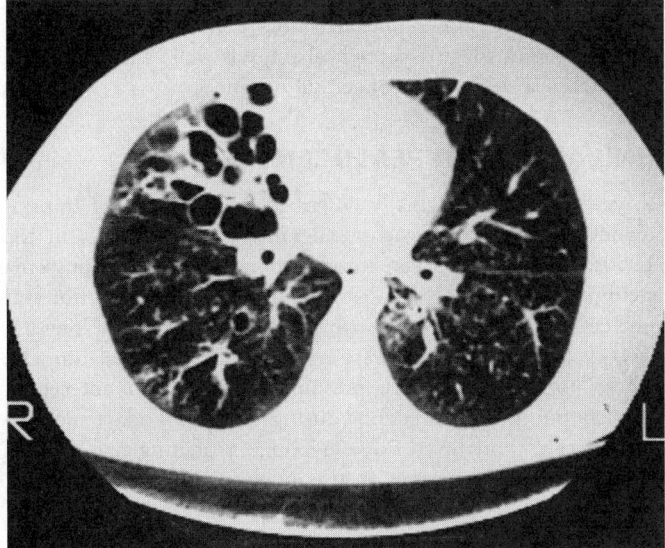

FIGURE 365.2. Computed tomography (CT) of the chest showing extensive cystic bronchiectasis of the right middle lobe and mucoid impaction of the left lower lobe.

PRINCIPLES OF MANAGEMENT

Antimicrobials have been the mainstay of treatment of bronchiectasis since their introduction more than 40 years ago. The choice of specific agents should be dictated by sputum or bronchoalveolar lavage fluid culture for aerobes, anaerobes, and mycobacteria whenever possible. If mixed flora are present, as is often the case, treatment consists of a broad-spectrum antibiotic such as amoxycillin, tetracycline, or trimethoprim-sulfamethoxazole. Most clinicians prefer to give antimicrobial agents during acute exacerbations of bronchiectasis, but some physicians prescribe them on a regular basis or during a given number of weeks each month, as is done for chronic bronchitis. Chest physical therapy with postural drainage, chest clapping, humidification, the use of mucolytics, and other measures to promote clearance of secretions also has been recommended.

In addition to these general measures, specific therapies may be appropriate when the underlying cause of bronchiectasis has been identified. For example, the regular administration of immunoglobulin in patients with immunodeficiency may lessen the incidence of sinopulmonary infection. The medical management of bronchiectasis should prove effective in the majority of patients. Nevertheless, consideration should be given to surgical resection in certain instances. Surgery is rarely indicated for bronchiectasis and should be limited to patients with massive hemoptysis who do not respond to bronchial artery embolization or patients with local disease unresponsive to antibiotics.

ASSOCIATED CONDITIONS

In countries such as the United States, the pathologic process called bronchiectasis usually develops in patients with underlying systemic disorders upon which airway infection is superimposed. Bronchiectasis often occurs in association with systemic diseases and other conditions (Table 365.1). Several of these conditions are reviewed in the following section in alphabetical order. For further information on cystic fibrosis, see Chapter 370; for a review of allergic bronchopulmonary aspergillosis, see Chapter 369.

BRONCHIAL OBSTRUCTION

Investigators once assumed that a common pathogenetic factor was proximal airway obstruction with distal infection of the bronchial walls and, in many cases, the surrounding lung parenchyma. Although this assumption has proved to be incorrect, focal postobstructive bronchiectasis may indeed occur in patients with endobronchial tumors, broncholithiasis, bronchial stenosis from inflammatory disorders such as tuberculosis, and aspirated foreign bodies such as coins, nuts, and timothy grass heads. It also may develop as part of the middle lobe syndrome. This syndrome presumably results from the angulation of the lobar bronchus at its origin, impingement on the right middle lobe bronchus by enlarged lymph nodes, and a lack of collateral ventilation to that lobe. Although some patients with the middle lobe syndrome are symptomatic, the condition is frequently detected on a plain chest roentgenogram taken for other purposes.

TABLE 365.1.	CONDITIONS ASSOCIATED WITH BRONCHIECTASIS

Allergic bronchopulmonary aspergillosis
α_1-antitrypsin deficiency
Bronchial obstruction (including middle lobe syndrome)
Bronchopulmonary sequestration
Congenital cartilage deficiency (Williams-Campbell syndrome)
Cystic fibrosis
Human immunodeficiency virus infection
Immunodeficiency
Infection
Inflammation
Primary ciliary dyskinesia
Rheumatoid arthritis
Tracheobronchomegaly (Mounier-Kuhn syndrome)
Unilateral hyperlucent lung (Swyer-James-MacLeod syndrome)
Yellow nail syndrome

IMMUNODEFICIENCY

Bronchiectasis and other chronic or recurrent sinopulmonary infections are common among patients with congenital or acquired immunodeficiency. Abnormalities of B-lymphocyte function most frequently are associated with bronchiectasis. Congenital or acquired hypogammaglobulinemia characterized by a decline or absence of circulating IgG has been described in several patients with bronchiectasis. Immunodeficiency states involving one or more of the four IgG subclasses in the context of normal total IgG levels are associated perhaps even more often with bronchiectasis. IgG subclass deficiencies are a typical cause of bronchiectasis, and serum subclass levels should be obtained whenever other causes of bronchiectasis have been ruled out.

INFECTION

In third world countries (and historically in developed countries), bronchiectasis typically results from necrotizing pulmonary infections that are poorly treated, if at all. Rosenzweig and Stead first drew attention to bronchiectasis following bronchopulmonary necrosis due to *Klebsiella*, *Staphylococcus aureus*, other aerobic bacteria, and *Mycobacterium tuberculosis*. Since that time, bronchiectasis has been reported in patients with pulmonary disease caused by nontuberculous mycobacteria and aerobic bacteria, such as *Mycoplasma pneumoniae*.

TRACHEOBRONCHOMEGALY

Tracheobronchomegaly, also known as Mounier-Kuhn syndrome, is characterized by a striking dilatation of the intrathoracic trachea and major bronchi. Enlargement of the airways and the deep corrugations produced by redundant musculomembranous tissues between the cartilaginous rings gives a roentgenographic appearance of multiple diverticulae. The diagnosis is often made on CT scan. The cause of tracheobronchomegaly is unknown; although it has been attributed to severe, chronic bronchopulmonary suppuration, the latter condition may be a result of tracheobronchomegaly rather than its cause. Enlargement of the cartilaginous tracheal rings as well as the membranous trachea supports a congenital origin.

UNILATERAL HYPERLUCENT LUNG

Swyer and James originally described "unilateral lung transradiancy" on the chest roentgenograms of ten patients in the 1950s. These patients were initially thought to have emphysema stemming from bronchial obstruction, but such obstruction was not confirmed by bronchoscopy or bronchography. Nonetheless, cystic abnormalities were noted in the proximal bronchi. These abnormalities were presumably related to antecedent bronchopulmonary infections during infancy. Today, such infections are thought to cause hypoplasia of lung parenchyma and the pulmonary artery on the involved side.

YELLOW NAIL SYNDROME

The term *yellow nail syndrome* was coined in 1964 to describe the association of yellow discoloration of the fingernails and lymphedema. Since then, some, but not all, patients with these findings have been reported to have pleural effusions and bronchiectasis as well. In these cases, bronchiectasis has been attributed either to hypoplasia of the lymphatic system with altered lung drainage or to immunologic deficiencies that have been found in certain patients.

BIBLIOGRAPHY

Barker AF, Bardana EJ. Bronchiectasis: update of an orphan disease. *Am Rev Respir Dis* 1988;137:969–978.

De Gracia J, Rodrigo MJ, Morell F, et al. IgG subclass deficiencies associated with bronchiectasis. *Am J Respir Crit Care Med* 1996;153:650–655.

Heard BE, Khatchatourov V, Otto H, et al. The morphology of emphysema, chronic bronchitis, and bronchiectasis: definition, nomenclature, and classification. *J Clin Pathol* 1979;32:882–892.

Lucidarme O, Grenier P, Coche E, et al. Bronchiectasis: comparative assessment with thin-section CT and helical CT. *Radiology* 1996;200:673–679.

Lynch DA, Newell J, Hale V, et al. Correlation of CT findings with clinical evaluations in 261 patients with symptomatic bronchiectasis. *AJR* 1999;173:53–58.

Naidich DP, McCauley DI, Khouri NF, et al. Computed tomography of bronchiectasis. *J Comput Assist Tomogr* 1982;6:437–444.

Roditi GH, Weir J. The association of tracheomegaly and bronchiectasis. *Clin Radiol* 1994;49:608–611.

Rosenzweig DY, Stead WW. The role of tuberculosis and other forms of broncho-pulmonary necrosis in the pathogenesis of bronchiectasis. *Am Rev Respir Dis* 1966;93:769–785.

Swyer PR, James GCW. A case of unilateral pulmonary emphysema. *Thorax* 1953;8:133–136.

Webb WR. Radiology of obstructive pulmonary disease. *AJR* 1997;169:637–647.

Kelley's Textbook of Internal Medicine, fourth edition. Edited by H. David Humes. Lippincott Williams & Wilkins, Philadelphia © 2000.

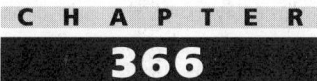

CHAPTER 366

DISEASES OF THE UPPER AIRWAY

MICHAEL G. GLENN
ERNEST A. WEYMULLER, JR.

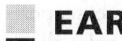 EAR

EXTERNAL OTITIS

Infection of the external auditory canal is characterized by progressive pain, itching, and discharge. There is often an antecedent history of local trauma or water in the ear canal. Characteristically, pressure on the tragus or auricular cartilage produces exquisite pain. The ear canal is erythematous and swollen, often to the point of obscuring the eardrum. In severe infections, peri-

auricular cellulitis and even regional lymphadenopathy develop. Conductive hearing loss may result from severe edema of the external ear canal.

Pseudomonas aeruginosa and *Staphylococcus aureus* are most frequently responsible for the infection. Culture of the discharge is not necessary for routine cases. The key to successful treatment is removal of wax and desquamated debris from the ear canal by suction or irrigation. Any foreign body should be removed as well. If the ear canal is not occluded by edema, treatment with antibiotic eardrops for 7 to 10 days should resolve the infection. If the ear canal is narrowed, a wick can be inserted to ensure adequate distribution of antibiotic drops to the medial portion of the ear canal. Systemic antibiotics are not recommended unless the patient has periauricular cellulitis or regional lymphadenopathy. Patients should be cautioned to refrain from instrumentation of the external ear canal and to protect the ear canal during showering or hair washing by means of a cotton ball saturated with petrolatum ointment.

External otitis may be a much more severe problem in elderly diabetic patients, in whom the infection may extend into the surrounding soft tissues and bone. If standard therapy fails to control external ear canal drainage and pain after 1 or 2 weeks, so-called malignant external otitis should be considered. Careful examination shows granulation tissue at the junction of the bony and cartilaginous portions of the external ear canal. In addition, patients may evidence progressive cranial nerve deficits. Besides aggressive local care of the ear canal, treatment with intravenous antipseudomonal antibiotics is indicated. Several weeks of antibiotic therapy is necessary, and occasionally surgical debridement is required to remove sequestered bone.

OTITIS MEDIA

Although it is most prevalent in children, otitis media can occur at any age. It usually follows an upper respiratory tract infection. It is characterized by pain and conductive hearing loss. On physical examination, the landmarks of the eardrum are distorted by erythema, thickening, and bulging of the tympanic membrane. In advanced cases, a perforation of the eardrum with purulent discharge may be noted. Blockage or dysfunction of the eustachian tube is believed to be the pathophysiologic basis for otitis media. *Streptococcus pneumoniae* and *Haemophilus influenzae* are the bacteria most frequently isolated from middle ear effusions in acute otitis media. Gram-negative enteric bacilli often are isolated from the effusions in neonates and infants up to 6 weeks of age; they are rarely present in the effusions of older children. Myringocentesis with aspiration of middle ear effusion is useful when treating infection in severely immunocompromised patients or nonresolving infections; otherwise empiric treatment with oral antibiotics effective against *H. influenzae* is appropriate for children and adolescents. The duration of treatment should be between 10 and 14 days.

Serous Otitis Media

Failure of fluid to clear from the middle ear cleft after acute otitis media may result in serous otitis media. In serous otitis media, the eardrum may vary in color from gray to blue to yellow. It may be retracted, and air bubbles may be visible behind it. A mild to moderate conductive hearing loss (10 to 30 dB) is also noted. Most serous effusions clear spontaneously or with the use of nonoperative therapy, including antihistamines and decongestants, antibiotics, or autoinflation (modified Valsalva maneuver). Pressure equalization tubes may be inserted in patients with effusions that persist more than 12 weeks or that fail to respond to medical therapy. These tubes are also useful in preventing recurrent infections in young children. Adults with persistent unilateral serous otitis media should be referred to a head and neck surgeon to exclude the possibility that nasopharyngeal carcinoma is the cause of eustachian tube blockage.

Chronic Otitis Media

Persistent eustachian tube dysfunction and recurrent acute infection may result in chronic perforation of the tympanic membrane with a recurring foul-smelling discharge. Occasionally, the eardrum is intact between periods of drainage, and the only evidence of disease is squamous debris or cholesteatoma in the pars flaccida of the eardrum. Patients should be referred for possible surgical management. Many small tympanic perforations and watery otorrhea should raise the suspicion of tuberculous otitis media.

Complications of Acute and Chronic Otitis Media

Acute mastoiditis classically occurs 1 to 2 weeks after an episode of acute otitis media. In a patient with chronic perforation, chronic drainage, or cholesteatoma, mastoiditis can develop at any time. The most common symptom is persistent discharge from the affected ear. Ordinarily, pain is not significant; when there is pain, abscess formation should be suspected. The patient may have a slight fever but frequently does not seem extremely ill. Severe pain and tenderness or systemic toxemia suggests a complication of mastoiditis. These complications result from extension of infection to involve structures adjacent to the temporal bone. Subperiosteal abscess, an extension of infection within the mastoid bone to the mastoid tip (Bezold's abscess) or to the root of the zygomatic bone, produces localized pain and swelling. Surgical drainage is typically required. Extension of infection through dehiscent bone or by destruction of bone overlying the facial nerve can result in facial nerve paralysis. Labyrinthitis and even fistulization of the semicircular canals can evolve through a similar process. Petrositis or Gradenigo syndrome is a result of an abscess or osteomyelitis at the apex of the petrous portion of the temporal bone and consists of a persistently draining ear with ipsilateral sixth cranial nerve palsy and pain behind the ipsilateral orbit.

Intracranial complications of otitis media include extradural abscess, subdural abscess, brain abscess, lateral sinus thrombophlebitis, and meningitis. In meningitis after acute otitis media, the usual infecting organism is either a gram-positive coccus or *H. influenzae*. Meningitis is a rare complication of chronic otitis media; the agent is usually a gram-negative organism. Initial management should be directed at identifying the organism and treating the meningitis. Once meningitis is under control, the otologic disease can be addressed. An extradural abscess in either the middle or the posterior cranial fossa produces symptoms of localized headache, fever, and meningismus. Signs of increased intracranial pressure also may be noted. Surgical intervention usually is required. Lateral sinus thrombophlebitis arises as a consequence of erosion by chronic infection through the lateral venous sinus plate, causing a focus of phlebitis. Usual organisms are group A streptococci and *S. pneumoniae*. The primary symptom is a persistent spiking fever. Between bouts of fever the patient is often well.

HEARING LOSS

Hearing loss is typically divided into two categories: sensorineural and conductive. Abnormalities of the cochlea, eighth cranial nerve, or central nervous system are responsible for sensorineural hearing loss. Processes affecting the external ear canal, tympanic membrane, and middle ear are responsible for conductive hearing loss.

Conductive Hearing Loss

The most common cause of conductive hearing loss is obstruction of the ear canal by cerumen or foreign body, typically associated with external otitis. Removal of the obstruction and treatment of external otitis readily reverse the hearing loss. Middle ear effusion associated with acute or serous otitis media results in a mild to moderate conductive hearing loss. Chronic otitis media leads to hearing loss either by destruction of the tympanic membrane or by erosion of the ossicular chain.

Otosclerosis is a bony disorder of the otic capsule that causes conductive hearing loss owing to fixation of the stapes within the oval window. It is similar in histopathologic features to Paget's disease, except that involvement is limited to the temporal bone and involves all three layers of the otic capsule (endosteum, endochondral bone, and periosteum). Stapes fixation is also noted in patients with osteogenesis imperfecta tarda. Van der Hoeve syndrome is the constellation of conductive hearing loss, blue sclerae, and history of multiple fractures. Surgical replacement of the stapes can be successful in restoring normal hearing, though a hearing aid is also effective.

Sensorineural Hearing Loss

Sudden sensorineural hearing loss is a well-recognized entity. It is most commonly idiopathic, but patients must be evaluated thoroughly to exclude such conditions as Ménière's disease, perilymphatic fistula, or acoustic neuroma. As a general rule, about one-third of patients recover completely, one-third improve somewhat, and the remaining one-third fail to recover any hearing in the affected ear. High doses of glucocorticoids are frequently prescribed, but there are no conclusive studies that establish their benefit (except in patients with certain audiometric patterns).

Association of acute hearing loss with sudden exertion or

head trauma should raise the suspicion of a rupture of the oval or round window membrane. In addition to hearing loss, these patients experience disequilibrium and occasionally nystagmus. When this condition is suspected, patients should immediately be referred for consideration of middle ear exploration.

Presbycusis is hearing loss resulting from degenerative changes associated with aging, which can be due to atrophy of the organ of Corti, loss of neural elements of the eighth cranial nerve, degeneration of the stria vascularis, or defects in the basilar membrane. Characteristically, higher frequencies are lost first. Patients typically complain of difficulty in understanding speech, especially in noisy situations, but the speech may seem loud enough. Any elderly patient complaining of hearing difficulties should be referred for audiometric examination. Sensorineural losses are not reversible, but hearing aid amplification provides invaluable benefit.

Noise-related hearing loss may stem from immediate or long-term effects. The first effect of exposure to excessive noise is a temporary loss of hearing accompanied by tinnitus. This is known as a temporary threshold shift and is maximal at about 4 kHz. If the exposure to a noise is repeated and prolonged, permanent hearing loss may result. Permanent loss is caused by damage of the hair cells in the organ of Corti and is not reversible.

Hearing loss due to syphilis is more likely to be a complication of congenital syphilis than of late-acquired syphilis. The deafness is bilateral, progressive, and usually associated with vestibular dysfunction. Diagnosis is important, because treatment with corticosteroids and antibiotics may be effective in controlling disequilibrium and in preserving or even improving hearing. Serologic tests for syphilis should be performed on all patients who have fluctuating or progressive hearing loss.

Ménière's disease is a syndrome characterized by fluctuating sensorineural hearing loss, intermittent tinnitus, and an episodic sensation of fullness in the affected ear. As these symptoms intensify, they may be followed by an attack of severe vertigo that lasts for several hours. The disease has a varying course and may remit spontaneously or progress to recurrent disabling vertigo and profound hearing loss. Bilateral involvement occurs 17% of the time. The hearing loss is typically most pronounced in the low frequencies. The characteristic histopathologic finding is hydrops (edema) of the endolymphatic space. Medical therapy involves diuretics and dietary salt restriction as well as the use of vestibular suppressants, such as antihistamines, benzodiazepine, or scopolamine. Surgical therapy is reserved for cases in which vertigo is unresponsive to aggressive medical management.

Tumors of the cerebellopontine angle can cause sensory hearing loss through direct pressure on the eighth cranial nerve. A diagnostic imaging scan of the temporal bone and brain stem is usually indicated in patients who show signs of asymmetric sensorineural hearing loss. The most common toxins associated with a hearing loss are aminoglycoside antibiotics and diuretics. Aspirin and other salicylates, quinine, nitrogen mustards, and cisplatin are also well-described ototoxic agents. Timely withdrawal of the offending agent can result in reversal of the hearing loss.

SINUSES AND THE FACE

Sinusitis is one of the most common causes of facial pain. Dental problems are another typical source. Acute unilateral facial pain in the absence of either of these disorders suggests a pathologic process of the fifth cranial nerve. Neurologic diseases, such as trigeminal neuralgia (tic douloureux) or herpes zoster, must be considered. If anesthesia is present in the area of pain, a comprehensive evaluation is indicated, to exclude an occult neoplasm of the affected branch of the trigeminal nerve.

SINUSITIS

Sinusitis is most often a complication of acute upper respiratory tract infection or allergic rhinitis. Pain is frequently described as a steady pressure and may be severe. It may be experienced in the anterior portion of the face or behind the eye; typically, the pain is exacerbated by hanging the head down. Fever is not a consistent finding. Intranasal examination may show purulent mucus draining from the sinus ostia, but the absence of discharge does not exclude sinusitis. The examiner should search for nasal polyps, foreign body, or tumor as possible causes of sinusitis, particularly in cases of disease limited to one side. Because infection in the upper teeth can produce symptoms similar to those of maxillary sinusitis, the mouth should be examined carefully. Transillumination of the sinuses may find a unilateral opacification, further aiding diagnosis. Sinus radiographs are not indicated for uncomplicated cases.

S. pneumoniae and *H. influenzae* are the usual infecting organisms. Antibiotics should be prescribed for a minimum of 14 days. Phenylephrine or oxymetazoline nasal spray administered for 3 to 5 days is also useful in minimizing edema of the nasal mucosa, allowing drainage and aeration of the involved sinuses. For severely immunocompromised patients or for patients in whom infection fails to respond to empiric antibiotic therapy, puncture of the anterior wall of the maxillary sinus is helpful in obtaining material for culture to identify the infecting organism and to wash out residual purulent debris.

Periorbital cellulitis or orbital abscess may result from extension of infection from the ethmoid sinuses, particularly in young children. The diagnosis is suggested by worsening pain in and behind the eye, erythema and swelling of the upper and lower eyelids, proptosis, chemosis, and diminishing ocular motility. Aggressive intravenous antibiotic treatment and appropriate surgical intervention aided by localization by computed tomography scanning is required. Osteomyelitis of the skull base, meningitis, epidural abscess, brain abscess, and cavernous sinus thrombosis can develop as well.

Aspergillus infection can develop in the maxillary sinus, particularly in diabetic patients with chronic sinusitis. The fungus is rarely invasive and usually responds well to local surgical debridement and drainage. In contrast, rhinocerebral mucormycosis is a severe acute fungal infection of the paranasal sinuses occurring in debilitated immunocompromised patients. It spreads rapidly to involve the eye and central nervous system. Therapy includes aggressive surgical debridement and amphotericin B. Even with optimal therapy there is a high mortality rate.

FACIAL PARALYSIS

Any lesion of the facial nerve from its nucleus in the brain stem to the motor end plate is considered peripheral. A peripheral lesion usually causes total unilateral facial paralysis, except when the lesion is distal to the branching of the nerve within the parotid gland. A lesion proximal to the facial nerve nucleus in the brain stem is considered central and provokes ipsilateral weakness in the lower two-thirds of the face. The forehead typically is unaffected because of its bilateral crossed motor innervation.

Bell's palsy is a diagnosis of exclusion, which can be made only after other treatable causes of facial weakness have been excluded. The origin is believed to be viral. Typically, the unilateral facial weakness progresses over 1 to 3 days and occasionally is associated with facial numbness or pain at the mastoid tip. Varying degrees of facial paralysis ensue, ranging from partial to complete. When the patient is asked to close the eye on the affected side, it closes incompletely, and the globe rotates upward (Bell's phenomenon). Further evaluation should include stapedius reflex testing, a Schirmer test, testing for taste sensation, and, for cases of complete paralysis, transcutaneous electrical stimulation of the main trunk of the facial nerve to determine stimulation threshold, which may help indicate the prognosis.

A short course of oral corticosteroids is believed to be helpful, but their use is the subject of controversy. A key aspect of management is protection of the affected eye from the drying effects of constant corneal exposure. Methylcellulose drops in the eye every 2 to 4 hours during the day and taping the eyelid shut during sleep should prevent corneal ulceration. In Bell's palsy, the facial paralysis invariably improves to a greater or lesser degree over the ensuing 3 months. Patients who fail to improve by 3 months or patients with recurrent episodes of facial paralysis should be evaluated further, to exclude the possibility of intracranial or temporal bone tumors or even multiple sclerosis.

Patients with a variant of Bell's palsy, herpes zoster oticus (Ramsay Hunt syndrome), have painful herpetic eruptions of the ear canal and pinna associated with facial paralysis. Occasionally, there is sensorineural hearing loss. The cause is herpetic involvement of the ganglia of the seventh and eighth cranial nerves. There is no specific therapy for this problem, though acyclovir may help. Ramsay Hunt syndrome generally is considered to have a poor prognosis for eventual complete recovery of facial nerve function.

Partial or complete facial paralysis may develop during the course of acute otitis media. A patient with this complication should undergo myringotomy to decompress the middle ear space. Facial paralysis should lessen as the ear infection resolves with antibiotic therapy. Facial paralysis in a patient with chronic otitis media and cholesteatoma usually progresses slowly over several days. The patient should be evaluated for surgical decompression of the involved portion of the facial nerve.

Malignant parotid tumors may cause gradual paralysis of any of several peripheral branches of the facial nerve. The tumor frequently can be palpated on physical examination. Gradual paralysis of the nerve over several weeks suggests the possibility of a facial nerve neuroma. Acoustic neuroma, a benign tumor of the vestibular nerve, also can take the initial form of facial paralysis, but the patient's primary complaints are usually vertigo and hearing loss. Glomus jugulare tumor may be suspected in patients with facial paralysis associated with pulsatile tinnitus and conductive hearing loss. On examination, a pulsatile reddish mass may be evident behind the eardrum, and the ninth, tenth, or twelfth cranial nerve may be involved. Other rare tumors of the temporal bone causing facial paralysis include eosinophilic granuloma and metastatic tumors (most commonly from the breast, kidney, or lung). In these instances, lytic or blastic lesions of the temporal bone may be identified on computed tomography. Disorders of the central nervous system, such as multiple sclerosis, stroke, or arachnoiditis, can manifest as facial paralysis, though other signs and symptoms usually make these diagnoses apparent.

■ SALIVARY GLANDS AND ORAL CAVITY

Sialolithiasis with local ductal obstruction can lead to recurrent sialadenitis, the most common cause of sudden salivary gland swelling. Conversely, recurrent inflammation may lead to stone formation. Stones composed of inorganic calcium and sodium phosphate salts are believed to develop around the nidus of a small mucus plug. Salivary stones prompt recurrent episodes of acute pain with associated swelling of the involved gland.

Acute suppurative sialadenitis is uncommon. It can involve either the parotid or the submaxillary gland and typically develops in patients with general debility because of uncontrolled diabetes, dehydration, or cardiovascular disease. Progressive pain and swelling of the affected gland occurs over 1 to 3 days. There is often associated fever and leukocytosis. The salivary gland is firm, indurated, and tender; palpation may express pus from the ductal orifice. Any available discharge from the duct should be evaluated by Gram stain and culture. The most common causative organism is coagulase-positive *Staphylococcus*. Treatment involves vigorous rehydration and control of any systemic conditions, such as diabetes. An appropriate cephalosporin or antistaphylococcal penicillin antibiotic should be prescribed. Local application of warm, moist heat; massage of the affected gland, and sialagogues (such as lemon drops) are useful adjunctive measures. Open surgical drainage should be considered if response is not rapid.

Both benign and malignant tumors of the salivary gland can manifest as gland swelling. A discrete mass is usually palpable. Facial paralysis in association with a parotid neoplasm suggests a malignant process. Salivary gland swelling also is seen in the context of tuberculosis, sarcoidosis, and Sjögren's syndrome. Other causative factors include toxic inflammation from ingestion of heavy metals, such as lead, copper, or mercury, or halogens, such as bromide or iodide, in which case the glandular swelling is frequently diffuse and bilateral.

Ludwig angina is a painful swelling in the anterior floor of the mouth that causes dysphagia and eventually respiratory obstruction. It often follows a dental infection or dental extraction. Lymphadenopathy typically is minimal, but the patient may show signs of sepsis. The airway obstruction that can result from edema and displacement of the tongue caused by progression of the infection makes Ludwig angina a life-threatening disease. A mixture of mouth organisms often is responsible for the infection. Treatment is high-dose corticosteroids and broad-spectrum intravenous antibiotics with careful monitoring of the airway. Intervention with intubation or tracheotomy may be needed for airway control. Incision and drainage are indicated if antibiotic treatment fails to bring about rapid resolution. Fluctuance is rarely evident, but surgical exploration and drainage of the sublingual space may effect control of the progressive soft-tissue infection.

The most common malignancy of the upper digestive tract is squamous cell carcinoma. Minor salivary gland tumors, melanomas, and sarcomas are found from time to time. Squamous cell carcinoma of the oral cavity is related to excessive use of alcohol and tobacco, particularly chewing tobacco. It also is associated with the use of betel nut. The outcome of treatment of oral cavity carcinomas is related directly to the size and extent of the lesion, highlighting the need for careful evaluation of any suspicious lesions and early referral for treatment. Leukoplakia (white patch) or erythroplasia (red patch) on the oral mucosa may indicate a malignant lesion. Full-thickness biopsy is necessary to determine whether dysplasia, carcinoma in situ, or invasive carcinoma is present; it is best done by the specialist who is treating the cancer. Therapeutic options range from local excision to irradiation or a combination of surgery and irradiation for advanced lesions.

NOSE

EPISTAXIS

Local irritation and excessive dryness of the blood vessels of the anterior portion of the nasal septum is the most common cause for epistaxis. Other important sources to consider include hypertension, coagulopathy, foreign body, and acute upper respiratory tract infection or exacerbation of allergic rhinitis. Benign nasal tumors infrequently bleed, but malignant tumors may cause unilateral bleeding. Nasopharyngeal angiofibroma, a tumor most often found in adolescent males, may manifest in the form of epistaxis and nasal obstruction. It should be considered in the differential diagnosis of epistaxis in these patients. Hereditary hemorrhagic telangiectasia (Rendu-Osler-Weber syndrome) is an autosomal dominant trait causing dilated thin-walled capillaries and veins throughout the body. The syndrome is characterized by recurrent nasal bleeding and telangiectasia of the lip and oral mucosa.

Localization of the specific bleeding point is of utmost importance in the management of epistaxis. If the identified bleeding point is anterior, it can be cauterized with silver nitrate or electrocautery. Posterior bleeding is typically more severe and more difficult to control. Before placing a nasal pack, the examiner should attempt to determine whether bleeding is from the upper or lower half of the nose, because specific arterial ligation may be necessary later if packing fails to control the bleeding. In patients with coagulopathy or immunosuppression, all attempts short of placing a pack should be made to control the bleeding.

Nasal packing is usually left in place for 3 to 5 days. If bleed-ing is severe enough to require placement of a pack in the posterior nasopharynx, the patient should be hospitalized and undergo monitoring of oxygenation status. Placement of a posterior pack is known to cause hypoventilation and hypoxia. Prophylactic antibiotics should be administered while the nasal packing is in place, with the specific aim of preventing the possibility of sinusitis and toxic shock syndrome. Should these conservative attempts at hemostasis be unsuccessful, direct ligation of branches of the internal maxillary artery can be carried out. The anterior ethmoid artery may be ligated through an external approach for superior bleeding sites. An alternative in patients with coagulopathy or severe anesthetic risk is selective embolization of the bleeding vessel.

NASAL OBSTRUCTION

The most common cause of acute nasal obstruction is the common cold. A patient in the first stages of a cold usually has nasal discharge and possibly a low-grade fever with minimal clinical findings. As viral infection spreads from the portal of entry to adjacent mucous membranes, the nose becomes progressively more obstructed with associated sneezing and watery rhinorrhea. A sore throat may develop, which typically persists for 3 to 5 days. A mild infection begins to resolve at this time, but with bacterial superinfection, increased mucopurulent nasal discharge and signs of systemic illness may progress. Bacterial superinfection causes a rise in temperature, sinus tenderness, mucopurulent nasal discharge, erythema of the throat, and possibly regional adenopathy. The symptoms of allergic rhinitis, vasomotor rhinitis, and rhinitis medicamentosa may all be confused with those of the initial stages of a cold.

There is no specific therapy for a cold; symptomatic treatment should be adjusted to the age and general medical condition of the patient. Antihistamines, decongestants, and topical vasoconstrictive agents aid in the relief of symptoms and may prevent the complications of sinusitis and otitis media. Nasal drops containing phenylephrine or oxymetazoline may be administered, but the patient should be warned not to use them for more than 1 week. Antibiotics should not be prescribed in the initial stages of a cold.

Allergic rhinitis (hay fever) classically manifests as nasal irritation, itching, nasal obstruction with frequent sneezing, and copious clear rhinorrhea (see also Chapter 174). The patient also may have a history of other allergic traits, such as asthma or eczema. Episodes are usually seasonal, and there may be a strong family history of allergic disease. On examination, the patient has a watery nasal discharge and pale, swollen nasal mucosa. The turbinates may have a bluish appearance because of venous engorgement. Often the conjunctivae are red, which is associated with increased lacrimation. Similar, usually milder symptoms may be caused by perennial allergens, typically foods in children and inhalants, such as dust and molds, in adults. Drugs that may produce allergic reactions include salicylates, iodides, quinidine, sulfa compounds, and penicillins. A test to identify the specific allergens, followed by desensitization, is the most specific form of therapy. For most patients whose symptoms are not severe enough to warrant this evaluation, symptomatic treatment with oral antihistamines, corticosteroid nasal sprays, or nasal inhalation of cromolyn is usually sufficient.

At times, it may be difficult to differentiate allergic rhinitis and vasomotor rhinitis. A patient with vasomotor rhinitis lacks a history of other allergic tendencies, and there is no family history of allergic rhinitis. Typically, the patient complains of exacerbation of nasal obstruction and discharge on exposure to heat, cold, or nonspecific irritants, such as smoke or dust. A nasal smear for eosinophils may help distinguish allergic from vasomotor rhinitis. Oral decongestants may be helpful in providing relief, as are corticosteroid nasal sprays or aerosolized atropine.

Use of decongestant nasal sprays, such as oxymetazoline or phenylephrine, for an extended period can result in a condition known as rhinitis medicamentosa. With repeated use, tachyphylaxis (decreased sensitivity to the medication) develops, as does a rebound phenomenon in which the nasal obstruction and discharge become progressively more severe on loss of the vasoconstrictor effect. On examination, severe congestion of the nasal mucosa, with a profuse watery discharge, is evident. Treatment centers on gradual withdrawal of the offending agent, often aided by interim use of a corticosteroid nasal spray. Occasionally, a short course of oral corticosteroids may be helpful in providing relief during the period of withdrawal from topical decongestant sprays.

Persistent unilateral nasal obstruction is most often due to an anatomic abnormality of the nasal septum. This can be readily documented by examination after application of a topical vasoconstrictor. In small children with unilateral obstruction and nasal discharge, a foreign body in the nose should be suspected. If the object is not visible and cannot be removed in the outpatient clinic, examination under anesthesia may be required. Similarly, in adults with persistent unilateral symptoms, a careful examination must be carried out, to rule out the possibility of a tumor of the nose or paranasal sinuses.

ANOSMIA

The most common sources of absent or diminished sensation of smell are nasal obstruction by polyps, damage to the sensory epithelium after an upper respiratory tract infection, and damage from blunt head trauma to first cranial nerve fibers at the point where they pass through the cribriform plate. A less typical cause is a tumor of the frontal lobe or optic chiasm. Shrinkage of nasal polyps with topical or systemic corticosteroids or treatment by surgical removal often restores the sensation of smell. Oral corticosteroids may be useful for patients with anosmia after an upper respiratory tract infection.

◼ THROAT

ACUTE UPPER AIRWAY OBSTRUCTION

In most cases of acute upper airway obstruction, there is a clear-cut history suggesting foreign body, infection, or trauma. It is important to determine whether the patient has experienced stridor or hoarseness for an extended time, because this symptom implies a chronic infection, tumor, or other long-standing laryngeal problem that tends to be less rapidly progressive in terms of acute airway obstruction. In general, a patient with upper airway obstruction has stridor on inspiration. As obstruction progresses, suprasternal retraction, tachycardia, and biphasic (inspiratory and expiratory) stridor develop. Particularly in patients with previously compromised cardiopulmonary function, complete airway obstruction may evolve rapidly as respiratory muscle fatigue and airway edema progress.

In treating a patient with acute upper airway obstruction, every effort short of tracheotomy should be made to secure an airway. A true emergency tracheotomy or cricothyrotomy is a difficult and dangerous procedure; endotracheal intubation is preferred if at all feasible. A fiberoptic endoscope specifically designed for use with intubation may be helpful for transoral or transnasal intubation of patients with an abnormal upper airway. Like any technical procedure, however, intubation requires practice to be effective in the emergency situation. If it is recognized that a tracheotomy will be required for long-term airway management, it is still preferable to undertake the procedure after endotracheal intubation rather than on a patient with an uncontrolled airway. Tracheotomy under local anesthesia is an acceptable alternative in the hands of an experienced surgeon.

In the event that endotracheal intubation is not possible, the most expeditious way to secure an airway is by emergency cricothyrotomy. Common indications for this procedure are foreign-body obstruction, facial or laryngotracheal trauma, inhalation thermal injury or caustic injury of the upper airway, angioneurotic edema, upper airway hemorrhage, epiglottitis, or croup. The patient is placed in a supine position with support under the shoulders and hyperextension of the neck. The spaces between the thyroid and cricoid cartilages are identified by palpation. A skin incision is made over the cricothyroid membrane, and the subcutaneous tissues are bluntly dissected. A 1-cm horizontal incision is made between the cricoid and thyroid cartilages. Any flat instrument, such as a scalpel handle, is inserted in the incision and rotated 90° to hold the incision open. The incision can be kept open by introduction of a small endotracheal tube.

As soon as the patient's condition permits, this temporary airway should be replaced by a standard tracheotomy placed between the second and third tracheal rings. Although cricothyrotomy is an excellent method for securing an airway rapidly with minimal blood loss, it risks significant damage to the cricoid cartilage, the thyroid cartilage, and the vocal cords. This damage can result in chronic laryngeal stenosis with airway obstruction and hoarseness. Standard tracheotomy involves dissection through considerably more subcutaneous tissue as well as the need to divide and ligate the isthmus of the thyroid gland. It is advisable to take a postoperative chest radiograph, because pneumothorax can complicate an emergency cricothyrotomy or tracheotomy, especially in children, in whom the apical pleura lies close to the trachea proximal to the clavicle.

A poorly secured tracheotomy tube may become dislodged.

If this happens in the first 48 to 72 hours, urgent re-intubation or a second tracheotomy may be required. After 3 or 4 days, the tracheotomy track is established, and the tube can be reinserted easily. The tube can become occluded. To prevent accumulation of a dry mucous crust, the inner cannula is removed and cleaned every 6 to 8 hours. Inspired air should be well humidified, because this also minimizes obstruction of the tube.

HOARSENESS

Acute inflammation of the larynx from bacterial or viral infection may develop in isolation or in conjunction with other signs of upper respiratory tract infection. It also can result from inhaled irritants. It may even be due to simple overuse of the voice, especially in singers, other performers, and children. Treatment consists of voice rest and avoidance of irritants, such as tobacco smoke. Cough suppressants are useful in preventing recurrent irritation of the vocal cords with harsh coughing. Hoarseness persisting for more than 2 weeks should be evaluated by indirect or fiberoptic laryngoscopy.

The differential diagnosis of chronic hoarseness is extensive. Long-term vocal abuse with formation of nodules on the vocal cords, prolonged inhalation of irritants (including smoking), chronic sinus and throat infection with postnasal discharge, recurrent acute laryngitis, laryngeal papillomas, chronic reflux of gastric acid into the posterior pharynx, tuberculosis, syphilis, and laryngeal cancer all can manifest with the chief complaint of hoarseness. The most common tumor of the larynx is squamous cell carcinoma. Lesions on the vocal cords first appear in the form of hoarseness and are thus more likely to be diagnosed at an early stage. Tumors in the region of the tongue base, epiglottis, and supraglottic larynx may become symptomatic only when they are large, owing to their lack of effect on the voice or airway at earlier stages. These tumors are more likely to be associated with pain (including referred otalgia), dysphagia, or odynophagia early in the course of disease. Pharyngeal carcinomas also are more likely to show signs of regional lymphatic metastases at the time of diagnosis.

◼ NECK

DEEP INFECTIONS

A deep neck infection usually stems from infection of one of three areas: a tooth, the pharynx, or the parotid gland. Often the patient has been taking antibiotics for tonsillitis or an infected dental extraction site. Signs of progression include fever, swelling and tenderness of the neck or submaxillary area, trismus, pain on motion of the neck or tongue, and stridor. The physician should search for an obvious primary site of infection, such as tonsillitis, peritonsillar abscess, infected tooth, dental extraction site, or parotitis. Antibiotics can mask obvious signs of sepsis. Infection of the pharyngomaxillary space as an extension of tonsillitis or mastoid infection is common in children. Signs include trismus and swelling of the parotid region, the lateral pharyngeal

wall, or both. The anterior part of the neck usually is infected after esophageal or hypopharyngeal trauma. Symptoms include tenderness along the sulcus between the sternocleidomastoid muscle and larynx, hoarseness, stridor, and dysphagia. Anteroposterior and lateral radiographs of the neck may aid in evaluation of the airway. Fluid replacement and broad-spectrum antibiotics should be given, and the patient should be hospitalized for intensive therapy and possible operative drainage. Early surgical consultation should be obtained. If airway compromise is present, intubation may be required.

Retropharyngeal abscess is a deep space infection that develops most often in infants. Infection occurs in the fascial space between the posterior pharyngeal wall and the prevertebral fascia, usually after an upper respiratory tract or tonsil infection. Airway management and supportive care, along with possible surgical drainage, are appropriate.

Peritonsillar abscess is a complication of acute tonsillitis resulting from spread of infection into the peritonsillar space (between the tonsil capsule and the pharyngeal constrictor muscle). Dysphagia, trismus, and severe pain are present. The swelling may extend to the soft palate and displace the uvula to the contralateral side. Needle aspiration can determine if an abscess is indeed present and provide material for culture and sensitivity testing. Repeated aspirations and intravenous antibiotics may be adequate therapy. Alternatively, drainage through a small incision in the soft palate just above the tonsil or even a tonsillectomy may be required to drain the abscess adequately. Hospitalization is indicated for administration of intravenous antibiotics as well as monitoring of the status of the airway. Intravenous antibiotics are given until there is significant reduction in trismus.

NECK MASS

Any patient with a new neck mass of more than 2 weeks' duration needs evaluation, depending on the size and location of the mass as well as the relative risk factors for cancer in the patient's history. The physician must be more vigilant in the case of older patients with a history of tobacco and alcohol abuse than for young, otherwise healthy persons. Masses that have progressed in size, masses larger than 2 cm, hard or fixed lesions, and lesions in the anteroinferior triangle of the neck deserve more aggressive evaluation. The most common midline lesion is a thyroglossal duct cyst; another possibility is a dermoid cyst. In the anterosuperior triangle of the neck, the most common cause is inflammation of lymph nodes from tuberculosis or atypical microbacterial infection. Metastatic carcinoma from the upper aerodigestive tract as well as a primary tumor of the parotid or submaxillary gland are also possibilities.

Rarer lesions include Zenker's diverticulum, laryngocele, chemodectoma, and carotid artery aneurysm. Adenopathy due to lymphoma can be found in any part of the neck. The primary considerations for posterior triangle neck masses include nasopharyngeal tumor metastases, lymphoma, local skin infections, metastatic thyroid disease, and neurofibroma. Lesions in the supraclavicular or anteroinferior triangle suggest metastatic carcinoma from the lung, breast, or gastrointestinal tract. Thyroid tumors and aneurysm of the great vessels may take the form of a mass in this region. Branchial cleft cysts characteristically are located along the anterior border of the sternocleidomastoid muscle.

In the patient with a neck mass, careful measurement and documentation of the precise size and location of the lesion is important. Particular attention should be paid to whether the lesion is fixed to the deep tissues and whether it is tender or mobile or fluctuant. A complete examination of the upper aerodigestive tract, including the nasopharynx, hypopharynx, and larynx, is mandatory. Inspection of the gingiva after removal of any dentures or partial plates as well as close scrutiny of the ventral surface of the tongue are important in identifying early-stage oral cavity lesions. Even small oropharyngeal carcinomas may have extensive neck metastases. Needle aspiration should be undertaken in the case of any nonpulsatile lesion that enlarges or fails to resolve or is suggestive of malignancy. If fluid is aspirated, it should be sent not only for cytologic study but also for culture and sensitivity testing. Skin tests for tuberculosis should also be done. Incisional or excisional biopsy of neck masses should be carried out only by a surgeon familiar with treating head and neck cancer.

BIBLIOGRAPHY

Bailey BJ, Calhoun KH. *Head and neck surgery: otolaryngology*, second ed. Philadelphia: Lippincott Williams & Wilkins, 1998.

Biel MA, Brown CA, Levinson RM, et al. Evaluation of the microbiology of chronic maxillary sinusitis. *Ann Otol Rhinol Laryngol* 1998;107: 942–945.

Blomquist IK, Bayer AS. Life-threatening deep fascial space infections of the head and neck. *Infect Dis Clin North Am* 1988;2:237–264.

Cummings CW, Frederickson AE, Harker LA, et al. *Otolaryngology: head and neck surgery*, second ed. St Louis: CV Mosby, 1993.

Gwaltney JM Jr. Acute community acquired bacterial sinusitis: to treat or not to treat. *Can Respir J* 1999;6(suppl A):46A–50A.

Hughes GB. Practical management of Bell's palsy. *Otolaryngol Head Neck Surg* 1990;102:658–663.

Osguthorpe JD, Hadley JA. Rhinosinusitis: current concepts in evaluation and management. *Med Clin North Am* 1999;83:27–41.

Paradise JL, Bluestone CD, Bachman RZ, et al. Efficacy of tonsillectomy for recurrent throat infection in severely affected children: results of parallel randomized and unrandomized clinical trials. *N Engl J Med* 1984;310:674–683.

Poole MD. A focus on acute sinusitis in adults: changes in disease management. *Am J Med* 1999;106:38S–47S.

Rachelefsky GS. National guidelines needed to manage rhinitis and prevent complications. *Ann Allergy Asthma Immunol* 1999;82:296–305.

Ramsey PG, Weymuller EA. Complications of bacterial infection of the ears, paranasal sinuses and oral pharynx in adults. *Emerg Med Clin North Am* 1985;3:143–160.

Stammberger H. Surgical treatment of nasal polyps: past, present, and future. *Allergy* 1999;54(suppl 53):7–11.

Stewart MH, Siff JE, Cydulka RK. Evaluation of the patient with sore throat, earache, and sinusitis: an evidence based approach. *Emerg Med Clin North Am* 1999;17:153–187.

Tan LK, Calhoun KH. Epistaxis. *Med Clin North Am* 1999;83:43–56.

Vaughan CW. Diagnosis and treatment of organic voice disorders. *N Engl J Med* 1982;307:863–866.

Kelley's Textbook of Internal Medicine, fourth edition. Edited by H. David Humes. Lippincott Williams & Wilkins, Philadelphia © 2000.

CHAPTER 367

LUNG ABSCESS

HUGH A. CASSIERE
MICHAEL S. NIEDERMAN

A lung abscess is a localized (usually more than 2 cm in diameter), suppurative necrotizing process within the pulmonary parenchyma. Several processes, either respiratory or systemic, can lead to abscess formation. Most abscesses are primary and result from necrosis in an existing parenchymal process (usually an infectious pneumonia). Among the causes of necrotizing pneumonitis, infections and neoplasms are the most commonly identified. When an abscess complicates septic vascular emboli (e.g., right-sided endocarditis), bronchial emboli (e.g., aspirated foreign bodies), or rupture of an extrapulmonary abscess into the lung (e.g., empyema), it is termed secondary.

Numerous infectious agents can be responsible for abscess formation, but classically anaerobes are the most common, although aerobic bacilli, fungi, parasites, and mycobacteria may also be responsible. Primary squamous carcinoma of the lung is the most common malignancy associated with abscess formation. Between 8% and 18% of lung abscesses are associated with neoplasms in all age groups, but as many as 30% of patients over age 45 have an associated cancer.

In the postantibiotic era, the incidence of lung abscess has declined, presumably as a result of improved treatment regimens for pneumonia. In fact, over the past 40 years, the incidence has declined tenfold, while the mortality rate has fallen to 5% to 10%. Diagnosis and treatment have changed little over the years and are largely dictated by past clinical practices, as lung abscesses are uncommon and it is difficult to obtain enough patients to perform controlled clinical trials. Nonetheless, the mainstay of therapy is antibiotics, and surgery is rarely needed. The role of newer antimicrobials is still controversial, but they may represent an advance over traditional therapeutic agents (penicillin), especially as drug-resistant bacteria become more prevalent.

PATHOGENESIS

Most lung abscesses are caused by infectious agents, including bacteria, fungi, parasites, and mycobacteria. However, most cases involve a mixed bacterial flora that includes anaerobes up to 90% of the time. Aerobic bacilli may be present in up to 50% of patients, but in most cases they coexist with anaerobes. The proposed pathogenesis is a combination of infective orogingival material in a host who has a predisposition to aspirate this material into a lung that cannot adequately clear the infectious challenge. The first pathogenetic factor, aspiration, is more likely to occur in patients who have altered consciousness or oropharyngeal/esophageal dysfunction. This includes patients with alcoholism, seizure disorders, drug overdose, general anesthesia, protracted vomiting, or neurologic disorders such as cerebrovascular accident, myasthenia gravis, amyotrophic lateral sclerosis, and other bulbar processes. As the second required factor, the material aspirated must contain a large concentration of potentially pathogenic bacteria. Aspiration of gastric contents may not always lead to infection, especially if the aspirate is only acid, in which case a chemical pneumonitis will result. On the other hand, orogingival material often contains a large bacterial inoculum and can lead to lung abscess, especially if the inoculum size is enhanced by the presence of poor dentition or gingival disease.

Bartlett and Finegold found that about 73% of patients with lung abscess had at least one predisposing factor for aspiration, and many had gingival disease found after careful dental evaluation. Obviously, not all patients with risk factors develop abscesses, and other factors, particularly underlying comorbidities and impaired host defenses, also play a key role in the development of lung abscess. In patients with HIV infection, the risk factors for lung abscess include advanced illness (CD4 cell count less than 50 per cubic millimeter), prior pulmonary infection, and other opportunistic infections, but gingivitis is not common in this population and therefore anaerobic abscess is uncommon in this group.

According to animal and some human data, the development of a lung abscess occurs 7 to 14 days after aspiration of infectious orogingival material into the terminal bronchioles. When aspirated in large amounts, a single species of anaerobic bacteria, or a combination of multiple organisms, can cause a necrotizing pneumonitis that, if progressive, can become a lung abscess. The location of the abscess is determined by gravity and body position at the time of aspiration. As most patients aspirate while upright or supine, a lung abscess is typically located in the basal segments of the lower lobes, the superior segment of the lower lobe, or the posterior segments of the upper lobes. With these pathogenetic principles in mind, it is clear that an abscess arising in an edentulous patient (without oral anaerobes) or in a location other than the ones mentioned should raise suspicion of another pathogenic process, involving either a nonanaerobic infection or an endobronchial obstructive lesion.

MICROBIOLOGY AND CLASSIFICATION

About 90% of lung abscesses are associated with anaerobic bacteria, either as the primary pathogens or in combination with aerobic bacterial agents. This observation may be explained by the fact that anaerobic bacteria commonly cause necrosing infection, but other bacteria that can cause lung abscess include *Staphylococcus aureus, Escherichia coli, Klebsiella pneumoniae, Pseudomonas aeruginosa,* other gram-negative bacilli, *Streptococcus pyogenes, Pseudomonas pseudomallei* (melioidosis), *Haemophilus influenzae* (especially type b), *Legionella pneumophila, Nocardia asteroides, Actinomyces* species, and, rarely, *Pneumococcus.* Parasites *(Paragonimus westermani, Entamoeba histolytica),* fungi, and mycobacteria may also cause lung abscess.

In infections caused only by anaerobes, the average number

of different organisms isolated is three; thus, most lung abscesses are polymicrobial infections, involving either strictly anaerobes or a combination of aerobic and anaerobic bacteria. In only 10% of lung abscesses are anaerobes not involved; these are caused by aerobes only. Although the bacteria involved this process have not changed much in recent years, the taxonomy of the bacteria has changed, and the current names of the most clinically relevant organisms are *Peptostreptococcus* species (anaerobic gram-negative cocci), *Fusobacterium nucleatum, Fusobacterium necrophorum, Porphyromonia* species (formerly classified in the genus *Bacteroides*), and *Prevotella melanogenicus* (also formerly classified in the genus *Bacteroides*).

The bacteria involved in lung abscess may differ in the HIV-infected patient. In this population, anaerobes do not play an important role, and the infection often involves a mix of aerobic bacteria. However, 25% of this population can have a lung abscess involving fungi and protozoa. In one series of lung abscess patients with HIV infection, the most commonly identified pathogen was *P. aeruginosa,* but other pathogens included other gram-negatives, *Pneumocystis carinii,* and fungi such as *Aspergillus* species and *Cryptococcus neoformans.*

Lung abscesses have been categorized using several methods, but the separation between acute and chronic has the most clinical utility. This distinction is not absolute but can aid the clinician by helping in the planning of treatment regimens and by identifying patients who may need further diagnostic evaluation, such as bronchoscopy. A patient with an acute lung abscess presents with symptoms of less than 2 weeks' duration; he or she is less likely to have an underlying neoplastic process and is more likely to have infection caused by a virulent aerobic bacterial agent such as *S. aureus* or *K. pneumoniae.* A patient with a chronic lung abscess (symptoms lasting more than 4 to 6 weeks) has an underlying cancer or an infection with a less virulent anaerobic agent. There may be some overlap in this classification scheme, as it does not take into account host defense factors or serious comorbidities. However, this scheme can be useful during the initial patient evaluation to help plan a diagnostic and therapeutic approach.

CLINICAL FEATURES

SIGNS AND SYMPTOMS

Most patients with lung abscess have an insidious presentation, with symptoms lasting at least 2 weeks before evaluation. Signs and symptoms include cough, foul-smelling sputum that forms layers on standing, hemoptysis (in 25% of patients), fever, chills, night sweats, anorexia, pleuritic chest pain (in 60% of patients), weight loss, and clubbing. Patients with HIV infection have the same constellation of symptoms with lung abscess as other populations. Although most of these signs and symptoms are sensitive, their specificity is extremely low. However, foul-smelling or putrid sputum is a highly specific sign that is pathognomonic for anaerobic infection, although it is found in only 50% to 60% of patients. A history of weight loss is also common, occurring in 60% of patients, with an average loss of between 15 and 20 pounds. As described earlier, historical data may also include risk factors for aspiration such as alcoholism, drug overdose, seizures, head injury, or stroke, and the absence of such risk factors should prompt a search for a diagnosis other than primary lung abscess.

PHYSICAL EXAMINATION

Physical examination may reveal fever, altered sensorium, poor dental hygiene, and clubbing. Fever is found in about 60% to 90% of patients with lung abscess, with an average maximal temperature of 39.1°C. Clubbing is present in about 20% of patients but, like other findings, it lacks sensitivity and specificity.

LABORATORY DATA

Laboratory data are also nonspecific, showing an elevated erythrocyte sedimentation rate, anemia of chronic inflammation, and leukocytosis. Culture and microbiologic information are generally not helpful unless the abscess is caused by nonanaerobic agents such as mycobacteria, fungi, or aerobic bacteria. Sputum examination is useful only in helping to diagnose nonanaerobic pulmonary infections because sputum can pick up anaerobes as it is expectorated through the oral cavity; thus, the finding of these organisms is not specific. More invasive methods are available for microbiologic diagnosis (transtracheal aspiration and bronchoscopy) but are rarely used because most patients are treated empirically and invasive diagnostic procedures are usually not justified. If the patient presents in an atypical way or is not responding to therapy, then invasive techniques are justified to look for an endobronchial obstructive lesion. If the abscess is associated with an empyema, as is the case 30% of the time, then culture of the empyema fluid may yield reliable bacteriologic data.

RADIOLOGIC DATA

Although certain historical information may suggest the presence of a lung abscess, a radiograph is needed to define the presence of a cavitary lung lesion (Table 367.1). The typical chest radiograph reveals a solitary cavitary lesion measuring about 4 cm in diameter with an air-fluid level. Some studies reported that the size of the cavity is helpful in distinguishing neoplastic versus nonneoplastic lung abscesses, but others have not found such a correlation. Instead, the amount of inflammation, seen radiographically surrounding the abscess, can help to identify patients more likely to have an underlying nonmalignant abscess. In contrast to an infectious abscess, neoplasms tend to have less surrounding radiographic infiltrate.

Radiographically, empyema and lung abscess are sometimes difficult to distinguish from one another. An empyema is a purulent infection usually confined to the pleural space, although it can develop as a complication of or serve as a cause of a lung abscess. Both entities can have air-fluid levels, but one is intraparenchymal (lung abscess) and the other is extraparenchymal (empyema). If an empyema contains an air-fluid level, then a bronchopleural fistula is usually present.

TABLE 367.1.	DIFFERENTIAL DIAGNOSIS OF CAVITARY LESION ON CHEST RADIOGRAPH
Infectious	**Neoplastic**
Anaerobic abscess	Bronchogenic carcinoma
Aerobic abscess	Squamous cell
Infected bulla	Metastatic carcinoma
Infected pulmonary infarct	Colorectal
Empyema	Renal
Tuberculosis	Lymphoma
Actinomycosis	Hodgkin's disease
Fungi	
Coccidioidomycosis	**Inflammatory**
Histoplasmosis	Wegener's granulomatosis
Blastomycosis	Sarcoidosis
Aspergillosis	
Cryptococcus	
Parasitic	
Echinococcus	
Amebiasis	

When the chest radiograph cannot distinguish these entities, a computed tomography scan should be performed. On the computed tomography scan, a lung abscess usually appears as a thick, irregular-walled cavity with no associated lung compression; an empyema has a thin, smooth wall with compression of the uninvolved lung. The real difficulty arises when one tries to differentiate a lung abscess from an empyema with a bronchopleural fistula, as both may be radiographically similar. The radiographic characteristics that help identify an empyema with a bronchopleural fistula are listed in Table 367.2.

If a lung abscess fails to communicate with a bronchus, the characteristic cavity with an air-fluid level will not be seen radiographically. This often leads to initial misdiagnosis because no clear abscess can be visualized. If no air-fluid level is seen, then the radiographic appearance is one of a focal, ground-glass infiltrate with indistinct borders. Given the history of illness and this radiographic picture, the differential diagnosis includes other chronic pulmonary infections such as postobstructive bacterial pneumonia, nocardiosis, fungal pneumonia, tuberculosis, and actinomycosis. Various noninfectious pulmonary processes can also be confused with a noncavitary lung abscess. These include bronchiolitis obliterans organizing pneumonia, radiation pneumonitis, chronic eosinophilic pneumonia, and allergic bronchopulmonary aspergillosis. When a lung abscess presents in this

TABLE 367.2.	RADIOGRAPHIC CHARACTERISTICS OF AN EMPYEMA WITH A BRONCHOPLEURAL FISTULA
Prior pleural fluid on chest radiograph	
Extension of the air-fluid level toward the chest wall	
Extension of the air-fluid level across a fissure	
Tapering of the air-fluid collection	

manner, it is usually necessary to do further diagnostic workup, such as bronchoscopy or lung biopsy.

When the radiograph reveals multiple cavitary lesions, it usually indicates that a necrotizing pneumonitis is present. This type of presentation is usually acute and fulminant, and secondary to virulent aerobic bacteria such as *S. aureus* or *K. pneumoniae*. The presence of multiple bilateral cavities should raise suspicion of a hematogenously disseminated process such as a right-sided endocarditis. Multiple cavities are rarely secondary to an anaerobic process unless the patient is severely immunocompromised or recurrently aspirating, or the anaerobe is virulent, causing a necrotizing pneumonitis, instead of the typical lung abscess.

■ TREATMENT

In the preantibiotic era, three treatment modalities were available for lung abscesses: supportive care, postural drainage with or without bronchoscopy, and surgery. All three led to the same mortality rate, 30% to 35%. Currently, the mainstay of therapy for lung abscess is antimicrobial therapy that targets orogingival anaerobes, the organisms present in 90% of lung abscesses. The initial antibiotic is usually intravenous penicillin or clindamycin, although in the past oral antibiotics have been used (usually 3 g per day of penicillin V). Penicillin has historically been the first choice of therapy since it was first used in the 1950s, with a cure rate of 95%. With the growing concern over penicillin-resistant anaerobes, two trials compared clindamycin to penicillin in a prospective study design. Both found that clindamycin therapy was associated with fewer treatment failures and a shorter time to symptom resolution. Metronidazole, when evaluated as a single treatment modality, was found to have a 43% rate of treatment failure and hence is not recommended for single-agent therapy. Metronidazole in combination with penicillin is considered an appropriate treatment regimen for lung abscess because the penicillin is active against the aerobic and micro-aerophilic streptococci that are often resistant to metronidazole.

Many other antibiotics have in vitro activity against orogingival anaerobes but have never been evaluated in clinical trials to gain U.S. Food and Drug Administration approval for use in these infections. These antibiotics include chloramphenicol, imipenem, meropenem, erythromycin, azithromycin, clarithromycin, the new fluoroquinolone trovafloxacin, and β-lactams with a β-lactamase inhibitor (e.g., ampicillin with sulbactam, piperacillin with tazobactam).

After selecting the appropriate antimicrobial agent, the next issue is determining the length of therapy. Although there is controversy in the literature, the approach taken by Bartlett seems the most conservative and appropriate. He recommends treating most patients until the pulmonary infiltrates have resolved or until the residual lesion is small and stable. In the initial stage of treatment, intravenous antibiotics are given until the patient is afebrile and shows clinical improvement (4 to 8 days). This is followed by the use of oral medications, usually for a prolonged time, although the length of time needed varies from patient to patient. Many patients require a total of 6 to 8 weeks of antimicrobial therapy.

In the past, bronchoscopy was part of the standard of care of patients with lung abscess. Its uses included helping to promote drainage and ruling out underlying malignancy. Currently, bronchoscopy is reserved for patients with atypical presentations who are suspected of having an underlying malignancy or an aspirated or obstructing foreign body. Bronchoscopy is no longer routinely used for abscess drainage because most abscesses communicate spontaneously with the airways and drain. There is also a possibility of rupturing an abscess during bronchoscopy and causing contamination of previously uninvolved lung segments. In regard to bronchoscopy's use to rule out underlying malignancy, Sosenko and Glassroth have identified several patient characteristics that correlate with underlying carcinoma. The criteria for bronchoscopy in patients with lung cavities included mean oral temperature below 100°F, absence of systemic symptoms, absence of predisposing factors for aspiration, and a mean leukocyte count below 11,000 per cubic millimeter. If a patient with a lung abscess had more than three of these factors, then an underlying carcinoma was a strong possibility. Other factors that should prompt bronchoscopic evaluation include atypical clinical presentation (noncavitary lesion, fulminant time course), atypical abscess location (especially those located in the anterior half of the lung), abscess formation in an edentulous patient, failure to respond to antibiotics, and lung abscess associated with mediastinal adenopathy, which is not commonly found in anaerobic lung infection.

Complications of lung abscess include empyema formation resulting from a bronchopleural fistula, massive hemoptysis, spontaneous rupture into uninvolved lung segments, and nonresolution of the abscess cavity. Although uncommon, these complications often require prolonged medical therapy as well as surgical intervention, either with tube thoracostomy (in the case of empyema) or lung resection (in the case of massive hemoptysis).

Surgical treatment for lung abscess is usually reserved for complications such as massive hemoptysis, bronchopleural fistula, and empyema. It is also used in the setting of fulminant infection and in patients who fail medical therapy. About 10% of lung abscesses require surgical intervention. Prognostic factors associated with medical treatment failures include recurrent aspiration, large cavity size (more than 6 cm), prolonged symptom complex before presentation, abscess associated with an obstructing lesion, abscesses with thick-walled cavities, and serious comorbidities such as advanced age, neoplasm, and other chronic medical conditions. Patients with HIV infection have a greater than 50% rate of recurrence or death due to lung abscess. Certain organisms are also associated with a high mortality, probably as a reflection of underlying comorbid illness. These include *P. aeruginosa*, *S. aureus*, and *K. pneumoniae*. An alternative to surgical drainage is percutaneous catheter placement into the abscess cavity, which should be reserved for patients who are unresponsive to medical therapy and have lung abscesses located peripherally. This is not a standard therapy, but some investigators have successfully treated patients in this manner, without patients developing a bronchopleural fistula. These patients should also continue to receive intravenous antibiotics during and after percutaneous drainage.

BIBLIOGRAPHY

Bartlett JG. Antibiotics in lung abscess. *Semin Respir Infect* 1991;6(2):103–111.

Bartlett JG. Anaerobic bacterial infections of the lung and pleural space. *Clin Infect Dis* 1993;16S:S248–S255.

Bartlett JG, Gorbach SL. The triple threat of aspiration pneumonia. *Chest* 1975;68:560–566.

Furman A, Jacobs J, Sepkowitz K. Lung abscess in patients with AIDS. *Clin Infect Dis* 1996;22:81–85.

Geppert EF. Lung abscess and other subacute pulmonary infections. In: Niederman MS, ed. *Respiratory infections.* Philadelphia: WB Saunders, 1994:291–304.

Ha HK, Kang MW, Park JM, et al. Lung abscess. Percutaneous catheter therapy. *Acta Radiol* 1993;34:362–365.

Hirshberg B, Sklair-Levi M, Nir-Paz R, et al. Factors predicting mortality of patients with lung abscess. *Chest* 1999;115:746–750.

Levison ME, Mangura CT, Lorber B, et al. Clindamycin compared with penicillin for the treatment of anaerobic lung abscess. *Ann Intern Med* 1983;98:466–471.

Sosenko A, Glassroth J. Fiberoptic bronchoscopy in the evaluation of lung abscesses. *Chest* 1985;87:489–494.

Kelley's Textbook of Internal Medicine, fourth edition. Edited by H. David Humes. Lippincott Williams & Wilkins, Philadelphia © 2000.

CHAPTER

368

PULMONARY TUBERCULOSIS

CHARLES L. DALEY

Tuberculosis (TB) is caused by bacteria of the *Mycobacterium tuberculosis* complex, which includes *M. tuberculosis* (MTB), *M. africanum,* and *M. bovis.* Infection with these organisms occurs primarily through inhalation of infected aerosols that are generated when persons with infectious TB cough. TB may occur shortly after infection or decades later. Clinical manifestations are protean, and although the lungs are most commonly affected, TB may occur at extrapulmonary sites. Persons coinfected with HIV are at increased risk of developing TB, and coinfection is known to alter the clinical and radiographic presentation of TB. This chapter reviews the epidemiology, pathogenesis, clinical presentation, and treatment of pulmonary TB and latent tuberculous infection.

INCIDENCE AND EPIDEMIOLOGIC FACTORS

An estimated 30% of adults are infected with organisms in the *M. tuberculosis* complex. Worldwide, there are about 9 million cases of TB annually, with over 3 million deaths attributable to the disease. In fact, TB is the leading cause of death from an infectious or parasitic disease worldwide, and it is the number one killer of HIV-infected individuals. High population growth

TABLE 368.1.	HIGH-PREVALENCE AND HIGH-RISK GROUPS
High-Prevalence Groups	**High-Risk Groups**
Persons born in countries with high prevalence of tuberculosis	Persons with HIV coinfection
Low-income populations	Close contacts of persons with infectious tuberculosis
Injection drug users	Persons whose tuberculin skin test results converted to positive within the past 2 years
Persons who live or spend time in some facilities (nursing homes, correctional institutions, homeless shelters, drug treatment centers)	Children <4 years of age
	Persons who have chest radiographs suggestive of old tuberculosis
	Injection drug users
	Persons with certain medical conditions[a]
	Recent immigrants (≤5 years)

[a] Diabetes mellitus, silicosis, prolonged therapy with corticosteroids, immunosuppressive therapy, leukemia, Hodgkin's disease, head and neck cancers, end-stage renal disease, certain intestinal conditions, malnutrition.
(From U.S. Centers for Disease Control and Prevention Core Curriculum on Tuberculosis. *What the clinician should know,* third edition, 1994.)

rates and coinfection with HIV are expected to worsen the global morbidity and mortality caused by TB.

In the United States, the TB case rate declined 3% to 5% per year from 1953 to 1984. Between 1986 and 1992, the numbers of TB cases increased by approximately 20%. This increase in the number of cases was the result of at least four major factors: (a) inadequate public-health measures; (b) immigration from countries where TB is prevalent; (c) coinfection with HIV; and (d) the emergence of multidrug-resistant strains of MTB. Fortunately, since 1992 cases are again on the decline.

Certain individuals are at higher risk of developing TB simply because they are more likely to be exposed and thus infected with MTB (Table 368.1). For example, approximately 40% of reported TB cases in the United States and 70% of cases in California occur in foreign-born individuals who come from areas where the disease is endemic. Other populations with an increased prevalence of tuberculous infection include low-income populations, the homeless, and injection drug users.

Anyone infected with MTB can develop TB disease, but certain groups have a higher than normal risk for progressing to active disease (Table 368.1). HIV coinfection is the strongest known risk factor for the development of TB, but there are also other medical conditions associated with an increased risk of developing disease. Persons who were recently infected with MTB are at greater risk of progressing to active disease within the next 1 to 2 years than persons infected in the distant past.

PATHOGENESIS

TB is spread from person to person through the air by droplet nuclei; particles 1 to 5 μm in diameter that contain viable MTB.

Droplet nuclei are expelled into the air when patients with infectious TB create an aerosol by talking, coughing, or singing. Three factors determine the likelihood of transmitting TB: the number of bacilli being expelled into the air, the concentration of organisms in the air, and the length of time the contact breathes the infected air. Whether or not an inhaled tubercle bacillus establishes an infection in the contact's lung depends on both the bacterial virulence and the inherent microbicidal ability of the alveolar macrophage that ingests it. If the bacillus survives the initial defenses, it can multiply in the alveolar macrophage.

The tubercle bacillus grows slowly, dividing approximately every 18 to 24 hours. The organisms grow essentially unimpeded until a cellular immune reaction develops after 2 to 8 weeks. However, before the development of cellular immunity, an inflammatory response appears and is associated with the spread of tubercle bacilli through the lymphatics to the hilar lymph nodes or through the bloodstream. Small numbers of MTB organisms are deposited in other organs that act as potential sites for disease.

Once cell-mediated immunity develops, collections of activated T cells and macrophages form granulomas that wall off the MTB organisms. Antibodies against MTB are formed but do not appear to be protective. For most persons with normal immune function, infection with MTB appears to be arrested once cell-mediated immunity develops, even though small numbers of viable bacilli remain in the granuloma. Although a primary complex can sometimes be seen on chest radiograph, most tuberculous infections are inapparent. A positive tuberculin skin test (TST) is the only way to detect latent infection with MTB. Persons with tuberculous infection who do not have active disease are not infectious and thus cannot spread the disease to others.

If cell-mediated immunity cannot contain MTB, the infected person progresses to active disease. Untreated, about 10% of persons with normal immunity develop active TB, 5% within the first 1 to 2 years of infection. In contrast, persons who are coinfected with HIV have a 5% to 10% annual risk of developing active disease. When active TB develops soon after infection with MTB, the disease is referred to as primary tuberculosis. In contrast, when TB develops years or even decades after the initial tuberculous infection, the disease is referred to as postprimary or reactivation disease. Exogenous reinfection, due to acquisition of a second strain of MTB, appears to be relatively uncommon in immunocompetent individuals but may be more common in HIV-infected persons.

CLINICAL PRESENTATION

The clinical manifestations of TB may vary depending on whether the disease is primary or reactivation in nature. However, it is important to note that the clinical manifestations of active TB are the result of a balance between host defenses and bacterial virulence; therefore, there may be a continuum of disease and the clinical presentation of disease may be altered in severely immunocompromised patients.

PRIMARY TUBERCULOSIS

The initial infection in the lung, referred to as primary infection, may cause an inflammatory infiltrate that may be seen on a chest radiograph: the middle or lower lung zones are often affected. The draining lymph nodes may enlarge and compress adjacent bronchi, particularly in infants and children. Parenchymal disease usually clears as cell-mediated immunity develops, and it tends to clear more rapidly than nodal involvement. If the parenchymal disease persists beyond the development of cell-mediated immunity, cavitation may occur, although this is uncommon.

Pleural effusions are a common manifestation of primary TB. Presumably this results when a peripheral, caseous focus ruptures into the pleural space. Initially, the pleural fluid has characteristics of acute inflammation, with a predominance of polymorphonuclear cells. Later, the pleural fluid has a predominance of mononuclear cells, including large numbers of TB-specific CD4$^+$ T lymphocytes. Pleuritis due to tuberculosis may present as an acute illness characterized by cough, fever, and pleuritic chest pain. Without treatment, the pleuritis resolves, but about half of all patients develop active TB later.

REACTIVATION TUBERCULOSIS

During most initial infections with MTB, small numbers of organisms are disseminated hematogenously and some become seeded in the apexes of the lung. The organisms appear to grow preferentially in this well-oxygenated environment and can progress to active disease months or years after the initial infection. This accounts for the characteristic radiographic location of reactivation disease, which in most cases occurs in the apical or posterior segments of the upper lobes. In areas of chronic infection or areas of caseation, fibrosis may occur. Fibrocaseous lesions may contain live mycobacteria for many years, and these are the lesions that may reactivate years later.

EXTRAPULMONARY TUBERCULOSIS

As tubercle bacilli spread throughout the body during the initial infection, they can lodge in any organ and produce a focus of disease: 17% of patients with TB have an extrapulmonary form of disease only. HIV-infected patients are more likely to develop an extrapulmonary site of infection than HIV-seronegative persons, and the risk increases as the CD4 lymphocyte count decreases. The two most commonly involved extrapulmonary sites are peripheral lymph nodes and the pleura. Other common sites for extrapulmonary TB are those in well-vascularized areas, such as the kidney, the meninges, the spine, and the growing ends of long bones.

MILIARY TUBERCULOSIS

Miliary or disseminated TB occurs when tubercle bacilli spread throughout the body, via the bloodstream, resulting in small (about 2 to 5 mm) granulomatous lesions. Miliary TB is seen more commonly in infants, children under 4 years old, and immunocompromised individuals. Disseminated TB usually develops insidiously with systemic symptoms such as fever, weakness, weight loss, fatigue, and anorexia. Cough and dyspnea may also be prominent symptoms. The mean duration of symptoms approaches 16 weeks, but some patients may go undiagnosed for over 2 years.

■ DIAGNOSTIC METHODS AND LABORATORY FINDINGS

In order to diagnose TB, the disease must first be suspected. TB should be suspected in certain high-risk groups (Table 368.1) and when the clinical and/or radiographic presentation is consistent with TB.

MEDICAL HISTORY

The medical history should elicit whether or not the person suspected of having TB has been exposed to MTB or has a previous history of tuberculous infection or disease. Symptoms that are compatible with active TB include fever, chills, night sweats, fatigue, cough, and weight loss occurring over several weeks to a year. Of note, up to 20% of patients with pulmonary disease are asymptomatic. Because patients coinfected with HIV are at increased risk of developing TB, and the signs and symptoms of active disease may be atypical in this group, TB should be considered when any respiratory infection occurs in these patients or when there is a fever of unknown origin.

TUBERCULIN SKIN TEST

The tuberculin skin test (TST), utilizing purified protein derivative (PPD), is the only way to identify persons with latent tuberculous infection. The intracutaneous Mantoux method is performed by injecting 0.1 mL of PPD containing 5 tuberculin units (TU) into the volar surface of the forearm. The TST is read by noting the transverse diameter of induration (not erythema) at the site of injection at 48 to 72 hours. The sensitivity of tuberculin testing in patients with proven pulmonary tuberculosis is 80% to 95%. Multiple puncture (Tine) PPD skin tests are unreliable and not recommended.

The TST should not be used to screen the general population. Instead, the test should be used to screen populations that have

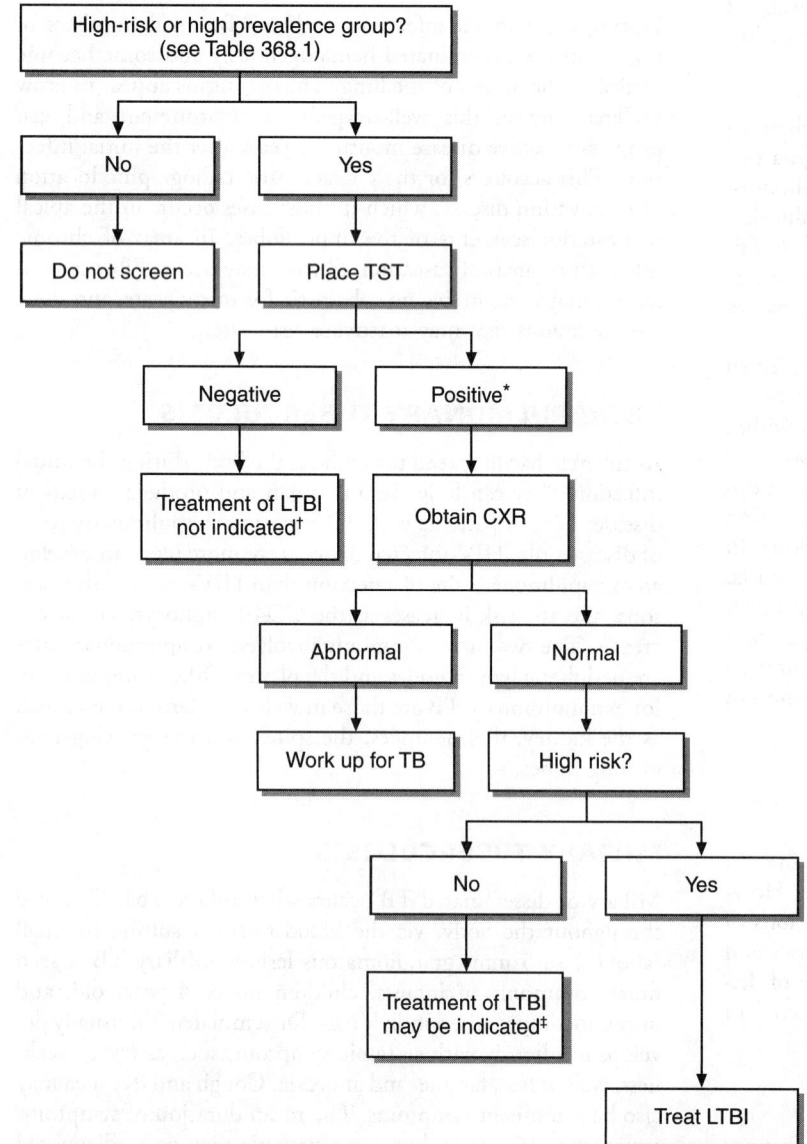

FIGURE 368.1. Management of latent tuberculous infection. TST, tuberculin skin test; CXR, chest radiograph; TB, tuberculosis; LTBI, latent tuberculous infection.

*TST more than or equal to 5 mm is considered positive for persons with HIV infection, close contacts to infectious cases, and persons with an abnormal CXR consistent with old TB. TST more than or equal to 10 mm is considered positive for other high-risk and high prevalence groups. TST more than or equal to 15 mm is considered positive for low-risk reactors (who should not be screened).

†Treatment of LTBI may be indicated for close contacts to infectious persons, even if the initial tuberculin skin test is negative. In persons with symptoms consistent with TB, a CXR should be obtained even if the skin test is negative.

‡Depending on local epidemiologic circumstances, treatment may be indicated.

an increased prevalence of tuberculous infection or an increased risk of progressing to TB once infected. Examples of these two categories are listed in Table 368.1.

The TST must be interpreted in the context of a person's risk factors and the prevalence of TB in the community (Fig. 368.1). False-positive results occur more often in persons living in areas with a high prevalence of nontuberculous mycobacterial infections and in persons recently vaccinated with BCG. False-negative reactions may be due to anergy and often occur in children less than 6 months old and in persons with HIV infection. Up to 20% of patients with active tuberculosis have a negative TST skin test that may convert to positive shortly after initiation of therapy. Thus, the diagnosis of TB should never be excluded because of a negative TST.

CHEST RADIOGRAPH

The chest radiograph is useful for determining if there are radiographic findings consistent with TB. However, a chest radiograph alone cannot confirm or exclude the diagnosis of TB. The radiographic manifestations may vary, depending on when the initial infection occurred and whether or not the patient is coinfected with HIV. Patients coinfected with HIV may sometimes have a normal chest radiograph but still be coughing up large numbers of tubercle bacilli.

BACTERIOLOGIC EXAMINATION

Sputum specimens, material from fiberoptic bronchoscopy, gastric washings, or other body fluids can be stained for the presence of acid-fast bacillus (AFB) and cultured for MTB. Direct acid-fast smears are generally positive when there are at least 10^5 organisms per milliliter, but fluorescent staining for mycobacteria can detect fewer organisms. Three early-morning sputum specimens are preferred. Because other nontuberculous mycobacteria are also acid-fast, staining with nucleic acid probes specific for MTB complex can be helpful. Nucleic acid amplification tests are more sensitive in detecting small numbers of MTB and offer promise for a more rapid diagnosis of TB. The tests available currently perform best with AFB smear–positive specimens. However, depending on the clinical suspicion of active disease, direct nucleic amplification tests may be useful, even in AFB smear–negative cases.

Culture of MTB remains the only means for confirming the diagnosis of TB. Because of the growth characteristics of MTB, traditional culture methods take 2 to 8 weeks. Radiometric methods using liquid media take less time, but mixed cultures of MTB and nontuberculous mycobacteria are possible. MTB can be identified from cultures and distinguished from other nontuberculous mycobacteria by chemical means or with nucleic acid probes.

DRUG SUSCEPTIBILITY TESTING

Drug susceptibility studies should be performed on all initial isolates and only by laboratories that have experience in culturing mycobacteria and a sufficient volume of such tests. Traditional susceptibility studies involve the proportions method, and careful control is required for meaningful results. Automated radiometric procedures for drug susceptibility testing offer more rapid results. In the near future, nucleic amplification or other molecular techniques may allow for the rapid identification of drug resistance.

OPTIMAL MANAGEMENT

TREATMENT OF TUBERCULOSIS DISEASE

Identifying and treating patients with TB is the most effective way of preventing transmission in the community. TB must be treated with at least two drugs to which the organism is susceptible to prevent the emergence of drug resistance. Dosages of commonly used drugs are shown in Table 368.2. A regimen containing isoniazid (INH) and rifampin for 6 months, plus pyrazinamide for the initial 2 months, is considered standard short-course therapy. Ethambutol or streptomycin should be added to the initial regimen if drug resistance is suspected or the patient comes from an area or population in which the prevalence of INH resistance is 4% or higher. In most urban areas of the country, levels of INH resistance are above 4%.

Other treatment regimens require at least 9 to 24 months of therapy, depending on the drugs used. In addition to the first-line agents noted in Table 368.2, there are other drugs available for the treatment of TB that are needed to treat patients with multidrug-resistant disease. These medications include the quinolones, *para*-aminosalicylic acid, ethionamide, cycloserine, clofazamine, and injectables such as kanamycin, capreomycin, and amikacin. A review of the treatment of multidrug-resistant disease is beyond the scope of this chapter. However, if any drug is stopped due to underlying drug resistance or drug toxicity, expert consultation should be obtained to determine the appropriate duration of therapy.

In order to prevent acquired drug resistance, clinicians must prescribe an adequate regimen and ensure that patients adhere to therapy. Directly observed therapy (DOT) should be used whenever possible. If DOT is not available, combined preparations that include INH and rifampin (Rifamate), or INH, rifampin, and pyrazinamide (Rifater), should be considered.

Persons with active untreated pulmonary TB are infectious, particularly those who have AFB identified in a sputum specimen. Treatment of TB rapidly renders these patients noninfectious. According to the U.S. Centers for Disease Control and Prevention (CDC), patients are not considered infectious if they have been receiving adequate therapy for 2 weeks or longer, have a favorable clinical response to therapy, and have three consecutive negative sputum smear results from sputum collected on different days.

Special Circumstances

HIV Coinfection

Despite being immunocompromised, HIV-infected individuals with TB respond well to regimens containing INH and rifampin (see Chapter 294). Thus, the current recommendations are to

TABLE 368.2.	**DOSAGE RECOMMENDATIONS FOR THE TREATMENT OF TUBERCULOSIS IN ADULTS**				
Drug	**Dose in mg/kg (Maximum Dose)**			**Adverse Reactions**	**Comments**
	Daily	**2/Week**[a]	**3/Week**[a]		
Isoniazid	5 (300 mg)	15 (900 mg)	15 (900 mg)	Hepatic enzyme elevation Hepatitis Peripheral neuropathy CNS (mild) Drug interactions	Hepatitis risk increases with age and alcohol consumption Pyridoxine can prevent peripheral neuropathy
Rifampin	10 (600 mg)	10 (600 mg)	10 (600 mg)	GI upset Drug interactions Hepatitis Bleeding problems Flulike symptoms Rash	Significant interactions with many drugs Colors body fluids orange May discolor soft contact lenses
Rifabutin	5 (300 mg)	NA	NA	Rash Hepatitis Fever Thrombocytopenia	Significant interactions with many drugs Colors body fluids orange May discolor soft contact lenses With increased levels, severe arthralgias, uveitis, leukopenia
Pyrazinamide	15–30 (2 g)	50–70 (4 g)	50–70 (3 g)	Hepatitis Rash GI upset Joint aches Hyperuricemia Gout (rare)	Treat hyperuricemia only if patient has symptoms
Ethambutol	15–25	50	25–30	Optic neuritis	Not recommended for children too young to be monitored for changes in vision unless tuberculosis is drug-resistant
Streptomycin	15 (1 g)	25–30 (1.5 g)	25–30 (1.5 g)	Ototoxicity Renal toxicity	Avoid or reduce dose in adults >60 years old

[a] All regimens administered 2 or 3 times a week must be used with directly observed therapy.
(From U.S. Centers for Disease Control and Prevention Core Curriculum on Tuberculosis. *What the clinician should know,* third edition, 1994.)

begin the same antituberculosis regimens as used in HIV-seronegative cases. Therapy should be initiated as soon as TB is suspected because delays in treatment have been associated with a high mortality rate.

Recently, the treatment of TB in HIV-infected individuals has become more complicated because of the availability of highly effective antiretroviral agents, such as the protease inhibitors (PIs) and non-nucleoside reverse transcriptase inhibitors (NNRTIs). These drug have bidirectional pharmacokinetic interactions with rifamycin derivatives, such as rifampin, rifapentine, and rifabutin. Some combinations of these drugs are contraindicated, and for other combinations dosages must be adjusted. Therefore, consultation with an expert in the field is necessary to determine the best treatment regimens for HIV-infected patients with TB.

Children

Children should be treated with the same regimens as those recommended for adults, but doses should be adjusted appropri-

ately. Some experts do not recommend the use of ethambutol until the child can be monitored accurately for optic neuritis (the primary drug toxicity associated with this drug). Additionally, some experts recommend increasing the duration of therapy to 12 months in children with disseminated, meningeal, or bone and joint disease.

Pregnancy

Pregnant women with active TB must be treated because the risk of transmitting TB to the fetus is always greater than any small risks of therapy. However, streptomycin and the quinolones should be avoided if possible because of potential fetal toxicity. Pyrazinamide is not recommended currently by the U.S. Food and Drug Administration in the setting of pregnancy because of a lack of data regarding teratogenicity.

Monitoring For Adverse Reactions

All patients receiving antituberculosis therapy must be educated about possible drug-related adverse reactions. The patients should be warned about insignificant side effects, such as the orange discoloration of urine from rifampin, as well as the symptoms of potentially serious side effects (Table 368.2). Patients must be instructed to seek medical attention immediately if they have symptoms of a serious side effect. Baseline measurements of hepatic enzymes, bilirubin, serum creatinine, and blood urea nitrogen, as well as a complete blood cell count including platelets, are obtained before drug therapy is begun. A serum uric acid level is obtained if pyrazinamide is included in the drug regimen. Visual acuity and red/green color discrimination are monitored in patients receiving ethambutol. Although routine laboratory monitoring for drug toxicity may not be necessary, many centers repeat liver function tests after a month of therapy and thereafter if symptoms develop or the liver function tests are elevated significantly.

Evaluating Response to Therapy

Sputum examinations at monthly intervals are important to monitor response to therapy. Smears and cultures should be negative after 3 months of therapy. If the sputum remains positive after 3 months, the patient must be reevaluated; special attention is given to monitoring adherence and ruling out acquired drug resistance. Drug susceptibility tests are repeated, and the appropriateness of the drug regimen is reassessed. Most patients with HIV coinfection respond well to treatment. However, the duration of therapy is extended if response is delayed or incomplete. These patients must be carefully monitored after completing therapy for possible recurrence of disease.

TREATMENT OF LATENT TUBERCULOUS INFECTION (PREVENTIVE THERAPY)

Persons who are infected with MTB but do not have active disease should be considered for treatment of their latent infection. However, treatment is not recommended for all persons with a positive TST. Instead, therapy should be provided to those persons at higher risk for tuberculous infection and/or TB (Fig. 368.1). For persons who are at increased risk of progressing to disease, treatment of latent infection is indicated, regardless of age. However, for persons who have a positive TST but who are not at increased risk of developing TB, therapy is generally reserved for younger individuals. Everyone being considered for therapy should receive a clinical and radiographic evaluation to exclude the possibility of active disease

Historically, the primary treatment regimen for latent tuberculous infection has been INH 300 mg given daily (or 900 mg per day given twice a week) for 6 to 12 months. Recently, other options have become available as well (Table 368.3). The CDC currently recommends 9 months of INH, 2 months of rifampin and pyrazinamide, or 4 months of rifampin for all persons with evidence of tuberculous infection, regardless of HIV status. Patients with parenchymal abnormalities on the chest radiograph due to prior inadequately treated TB should be given 9 to 12 months of INH, 4 months of rifampin (with or without INH), or 2 months of rifampin and pyrazinamide, once active disease has been ruled out. For persons exposed to an INH-resistant

TABLE 368.3.	RECOMMENDED REGIMENS FOR TREATMENT OF LATENT TUBERCULOUS INFECTION IN ADULTS

Drug	Frequency and Duration	Comments
Isoniazid	Daily or twice weekly[a] for 6–9 mo	Nine months is the preferred duration
Rifampin plus pyrazinamide	Daily or twice weekly[a] for 2 mo	Rifabutin may be substituted in patients receiving PIs or NNRTIs[b]
Rifampin	Daily for 4 mo	For persons who cannot tolerate pyrazinamide

[a] DOT must be used for twice-weekly regimens
[b] Rifabutin may be used with certain PIs or NNRTIs, dose adjustment of rifabutin and/or the PIs may be necessary. DOT, directly observed therapy; PI, protease inhibitor; NNRTI, non-nucleoside reverse transcriptase inhibitor.
EVIDENCE LEVEL: A. Reference: American Thoracic Society. Targeted tuberculin testing and treatment of latent tuberculosis infection. *Am J Respir Crit Care Med* 2000; 161:S221–S247.

patient, rifampin alone for 4 months or rifampin and pyrazinamide for 2 months may be used.

Monitoring for Adverse Effects

Patients should be informed of the possible drug-related toxicities and told to return to the clinic as soon as any of these symptoms develop. Most persons taking INH do not require routine laboratory monitoring of liver function tests. Persons who have other risk factors of hepatoxicity (e.g., HIV infection, pregnant or post-partum, taking concurrent hepatotoxic medications, significant alcohol use, chronic or acute liver disease) should have baseline liver function tests measured. These tests should be repeated periodically in particularly high-risk individuals or if the baseline liver function tests are abnormal. Whether or not regimens containing rifampin and pyrazinamide require more intensive monitoring is not yet known. Routine chest radiographs are not recommended as follow-up for persons with a positive TST; rather, periodic review of symptoms is indicated.

ROLE OF PUBLIC HEALTH IN TUBERCULOSIS CONTROL

Control of TB transmission is possible only with the coordinated efforts of the private medical community and public health departments. All patients with suspected TB must be reported to the local department of public health as soon as possible (exact reporting requirements vary from jurisdiction to jurisdiction).

Outpatient management of TB and the timely identification and treatment of contacts of patients with TB need to be coordinated with appropriate public health personnel. The local health department often has resources that are not available to the private medical community, such as the ability to provide DOT. In some jurisdictions, incentives and enablers such as housing, food, and transportation may be provided to help ensure completion of therapy. In addition, most jurisdictions have laws that can assist with the management of cases involving nonadherent infectious persons.

BIBLIOGRAPHY

American Thoracic Society. Treatment of tuberculosis and tuberculosis infection in adults and children. *Am J Respir Crit Care Med* 1994;149: 1359–1374.

American Thoracic Society. Diagnostic standards and classification of tuberculosis. *Am Rev Respir Dis* 1990;142:725–735.

American Thoracic Society. Rapid diagnostic tests for tuberculosis. *Am J Respir Crit Care Med* 1997;155:1804–1814.

Bloom BR. *TB: pathogenesis, protection, and control.* Washington, DC: American Society of Microbiology Press, 1994.

Huebner R, Schein MF, Bass JB Jr. The tuberculin skin test. *Clin Infect Dis* 1993;17:968–975.

U.S. Centers for Disease Control and Prevention. The tuberculin skin test, 1981. *Am Rev Respir Dis* 1981;124:1–8.

U.S. Centers for Disease Control and Prevention. Core curriculum on tuberculosis. *What the clinician should know,* third edition, 1994.

U.S. Centers for Disease Control and Prevention. Prevention and treatment of tuberculosis among patients infected with human immunodeficiency virus: principles of therapy and revised recommendations. *MMWR* 1998;47:1–58.

American Thoracic Society. Targeted tuberculin testing and treatment of latent tuberculosis infection. *Am J Respir Crit Care Med* 2000; 161: S221–S247.

Kelley's Textbook of Internal Medicine, fourth edition. Edited by H. David Humes. Lippincott Williams & Wilkins, Philadelphia © 2000.

C H A P T E R
369

BRONCHOPULMONARY ASPERGILLOSIS

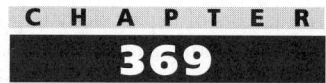

ALAN F. BARKER

DEFINITIONS AND INCIDENCE

Bronchopulmonary aspergillosis (BPA) occurs in persons with damaged airways, as found in those with asthma and cystic fibrosis. In North America, an estimated 5% to 10% of steroid-dependent asthmatic patients have BPA, whereas in Great Britain the percentage approaches 20% or higher. Because wheezing, cough with phlegm, and dyspnea are typical features of patients with asthma, a heightened awareness or different diagnostic cri-

TABLE 369.1.	DIAGNOSTIC FEATURES OF BRONCHOPULMONARY ASPERGILLOSIS

History of asthma or cystic fibrosis
Migratory pulmonary infiltrates on chest radiographs
Type I wheal-and-flare reaction to *Aspergillus* antigen
Serum precipitins against *Aspergillus* antigen
Blood eosinophilia
Very high serum concentrations of total IgE[a]
Central bronchiectasis[a]

[a] Most specific laboratory features.

teria may partly explain differences in prevalence. Debate is ongoing regarding whether the entity is strictly a hypersensitivity reaction to fungal *(Aspergillus)* spores or is an actual infection due to *Aspergillus*.

Immune features include the setting of usually atopic asthma, peripheral and airway eosinophilia, very high IgE levels, type I skin test positivity to *Aspergillus* protein, and minimal airway mucosal damage in the early stages. Features favoring an infectious component include viscid airway secretions containing fungal hyphae and spores, airway mycotoxins and lysozomal enzymes such as elastase, and cytokines such as interleukins 4 and 5. In addition, in later stages neutrophilic airway damage occurs and is sometimes accompanied by invasion of the organism into the mucosa leading to the entity of semi-invasive or limited invasive aspergillosis. The major hallmarks of BPA are listed in the Table 369.1 and include an appropriate clinical setting, chest imaging, blood laboratory testing, and a single skin-prick test.

PATHOGENESIS

Bronchopulmonary aspergillosis is most commonly caused by a reaction to the fungus *Aspergillus fumigatus* (but other species of *Aspergillus* have been noted), although rarely other fungi such as *Candida* and *Penicillium* have been implicated. *Aspergillus* is a ubiquitous aeroallergen. When inhaled in persons with normal airways, it is cleared rapidly from the upper and lower airways by mechanical defense mechanisms. In those individuals with damaged airways or excessive mucus such as with asthma, spores are retained, resulting in prolonged exposure to phagocytic cells and bronchus associated lymphoid tissue. In atopic individuals an intense IgE and a lesser IgG antibody response are elicited, triggering mast cell degranulation in migration of eosinophils with subsequent discharge of inflammatory mediators and cytotoxic proteins. Recent experimental work suggests incremental involvement of the T-helper type 2 lymphocyte capable of releasing interleukins 4 and 5 into airway secretions. Finally the fungi themselves release mycotoxins and proteolytic enzymes. The combination of these potent inflammatory mediators causes sustained mucous gland hypersecretion and mucosal epithelial damage releasing debris that becomes inspissated. This causes blocking of small and sometimes large airways and contributes to the mucous plugs and parenchymal infiltrates seen on chest imaging.

Although *Aspergillus* may be cultured from sputum in patients with BPA, it is not a required because airway secretions are not uniform and the intense inflammatory reaction is not related to the quantity of fungal organisms.

CLINICAL FINDINGS

Specific clinical clues include expectoration of viscid brown phlegm, sometimes with hardened mucous plugs. Patients may report frequent episodes of decompensation simulating a respiratory tract infection. These may be accompanied by reduced peak flow recordings, increased use of stabilizing aerosol corticosteroids or bronchodilators, increased use of rescue medication such as albuterol, or increased need for systemic prednisone. No single or combination of physical findings, including chest auscultation, indicates BPA in an asthmatic patient. Gross examination of phlegm for mucous plugs should raise suspicion that laboratory analysis can be performed for infectious pathogens (*Aspergillus*) and eosinophils and their breakdown products such as Curschmann's spirals or Charcot–Leyden crystals.

LABORATORY FINDINGS

Judicious use of laboratory testing as outlined in Table 369.1 establishes or refines the diagnosis. Although the leukocyte count is normal or slightly elevated, eosinophils are almost always high. In asthmatic patients without BPA the eosinophil percentage is often 4% to 9%, and the absolute number is 400 to 900 per cubic millimeter. In patients with BPA the eosinophil percentage is often 10% to 20%, with an absolute number of 1,000 to 2,000 per cubic millimeter. A unique feature of BPA is an extremely high total IgE. The normal range for IgE is 0 to 100 ng per milliliter. In asthmatic patients values of 100 to 400 ng per milliliter may be seen. Almost all patients with BPA have values greater than 1,000 ng per milliliter, with values of 3,000 to 5,000 ng per milliliter often noted. Serum immunoglobulins IgG, IgM, and IgA are normal. Specific IgE and IgG antibodies against *Aspergillus* are elevated in those with BPA, but assays are not routinely available. Serum precipitins to *Aspergillus* are present in about 10% of asthmatic patients and in most patients with BPA. The immediate cutaneous reactivity to *Aspergillus* antigen is positive in up to 4% of the general population, 10% to 40% of an asthmatic population, and almost 100% of patients with BPA. The eosinophilia, high IgE, and precipitins reaction all are reduced in the presence of corticosteroids at the time of suspected diagnosis or during therapy with corticosteroids. Other tests of immune function, such as antinuclear antibody (ANA), rheumatoid factor, and antinuclear cytoplasmic antibody (ANCA) have not been studied in proven cases of BPA.

IMAGING

Chest imaging plays a key role in confirming the diagnosis of BPA. The chest radiograph is usually normal without infiltrates in asthma. The presence of patchy infiltrates, atelectasis, thickened airway (tram lines or ring shadows) are certainly nonspecific but should raise suspicion of BPA or bronchiectasis. Infiltrates, focal consolidations, and subsegmental atelectasis raise the suspicion of proximal airways obstruction by mucous plugging. Broad or tubular (2 to 7 mm wide) infiltrates may be seen representing actual mucous plugs that appear and disappear with coughing and expectoration. High-resolution computed tomography (HRCT) without contrast has become the standard imaging test for bronchiectasis. The characteristic distribution of bronchiectasis in BPA is usually central or proximal airway, but review of large numbers of patients with bronchiectasis has shown the central distribution to be neither sensitive nor specific. On HRCT, bronchial wall thickening can be seen in asthmatic patients, reflecting mucosal edema and inflammation. In BPA patients, other changes are seen on HRCT, such as airway dilatation detected by the finding of parallel (tram) lines or end-on ring shadows. Cysts off the bronchial wall are a more destructive feature of bronchiectasis. Mucous plugs may be observed as on chest radiographs with proximal tapering from the periphery like an arrow.

CULTURES AND PULMONARY FUNCTION TESTS

Positive fungal cultures for *A. fumigatus* are not a cardinal feature of the diagnosis. The usefulness of cultures is in looking for bacterial and nontuberculous mycobacterial pathogens that may be seen in a similar clinical setting. A patient with asthma and an infiltrate may have bacterial pneumonia. In patients with bronchiectasis, *Mycobacterium avium* complex may be a colonizing or even infecting organism.

Pulmonary function tests are normal or show obstructive impairment persons with asthma. Decrements in spirometry should raise an alarm that complications such as BPA are present. Spirometry can be a useful adjunct as therapy is administered.

In summary, the most characteristic confirmatory laboratory features are very high serum IgE, positive skin-prick tests to *Aspergillus,* and HRCT evidence of central bronchiectasis.

DIFFERENTIAL DIAGNOSIS

The differential diagnosis of a patient with asthma and deteriorating function is often triggered when a complete blood cell count shows eosinophilia, or there is an abnormal chest radiograph. Other confounding diseases include eosinophilic pneumonia, extrinsic allergic alveolitis (e.g. bird fancier's lung or farmer's lung), Churg–Strauss vasculitis, particularly in the setting of leukotriene modifier use or corticosteroid tapering, other drug-induced pulmonary eosinophilia (methotrexate, nitrofurantoin), mucoid impaction, bronchocentric granulomatosis, and parasitic infection. Testing for specific bird antigens or thermophilic fungi assists the diagnosis of extrinsic allergic alveolitis. Churg–Strauss vasculitis is often accompanied by neuropathy, skin lesions, or cardiomyopathy, and patients have a positive perinuclear ANCA. Mucoid impaction and bronchocentric granulomatosis have many features of BPA but lack high IgE. Airway or lung biopsy may be needed to confirm bronchocentric granulomatosis. Confirming parasite infection of the lung requires sputum or bronchoscopic lavage with wet mount preparation.

BPA occurs in patients with cystic fibrosis. BPA should be suspected when a patient fails to respond to seemingly appropriate antibacterial therapy (for *Pseudomonas*), develops a new chest radiographic infiltrate, or has *Aspergillus* in the sputum. Tests for BPA should be considered to include *Aspergillus precipitins* and IgE levels with the same diagnostic criteria as for asthmatics. Making the diagnosis of BPA is important because corticosteroids will be helpful in treatment.

OPTIMAL MANAGEMENT AND PROGNOSIS

Treatment for BPA requires reducing the intense inflammatory airway response and the mucous viscidity of the secretions and plugs. With the multifaceted inflammatory response in BPA, broad and systemic anti-inflammatory therapy is the mainstay. Although there has always been a hypothetical concern that aerosol corticosteroids might promote lower airway fungal colonization and predispose to BPA, this has never been proved. Nevertheless, prednisone at 0.75 to 1.0 mg per kilogram per day is the beginning recommended treatment of choice to be continued for 2 to 6 weeks. If the patient is already taking prednisone, higher doses many be needed initially. Dosage reductions are guided by improved symptoms and peak flows, reductions in IgE levels, and decreasing chest radiograph opacities. Tapering over 3 to 6 months is recommended. Although some clinicians recommend early switch to every-other-day dosing to reduce side effects, the off-steroid day is often accompanied by increased symptoms such that slow daily reductions are more effective. There are no large studies of the use of nonsteroid immune-altering agents such as azathioprine and cyclophosphamide. Because *Aspergillus* may be an infectious pathogen as well as an intense immune modifier, itraconazole has been reported as an adjunctive agent to reduce the colonizing load of *Aspergillus*.

Mechanical measures as used in bronchiectasis to loosen viscid secretions may be helpful. Examples are maintaining systemic and airway hydration with bland aerosols, chest physical therapy with postural drainage, and positive expiratory pressure or flutter valve maneuvers.

The prognosis of patients with BPA varies widely. Some patients worsen in spite of high-dose prednisone or as corticosteroids are lowered. Other *Aspergillus*-complicating diseases may develop, such as mycetoma or even the semi-invasive aspergillosis. A rising IgE level is probably the best index to deterioration and may precede clinical or radiographic worsening.

BIBLIOGRAPHY

Angus RM, Davies ML, Cowan MD, et al. Computed tomographic scanning of the lung in patients with allergic bronchopulmonary aspergillosis and in asthmatic patients with a positive skin test to *Aspergillus fumigatus*. *Thorax* 1994;49:586–589.

Becker JW, Burke W, McDonald G, et al. Prevalence of allergic bronchopul-
monary aspergillosis and atopy in adult patients with cystic fibrosis. *Chest* 1996;109;1536–1540.

Chauhan B, Knutsen AP, Hutcheson PS, et al. T cell subsets. Epitope mapping and HLA-restriction in patients with allergic bronchopulmonary aspergillosis. *J Clin Invest* 1996;97:2324–2331.

Greenberger PA. Immunologic aspects of lung diseases and cystic fibrosis. *JAMA* 1997;278:1924–1930.

Kauffman HF, Tomee JF, van der Werf TS, et al. Review of fungus-induced asthmatic reactions. *Am J Respir Crit Care Med* 1995;151:2109–2116.

Knutsen A, Slavin R. Allergic bronchopulmonary mycosis complicating cystic fibrosis. *Semin Respir Infect* 1992;7:179–192.

Lynch DA. Imaging of asthma and allergic bronchopulmonary mycosis. *Radiol Clin North Am* 1998;36:129–142.

Reiff DB, Wells AU, Carr PJ, et al. CT findings in bronchiectasis: limited value in distinguishing between idiopathic and specific types. *AJR Am J Roentgenol* 1995;165:261–267.

Schwartz HJ, Greenberger PA. The prevalence of allergic bronchopulmonary aspergillosis in patients with asthma, determined by serologic and radiologic criteria in patients at risk. *J Lab Clin Med* 1991;117:138–142.

Stevens DA, Schwartz HJ, Lee JV, et al. A randomized trial of itraconazole in allergic bronchopulmonary aspergillosis. *N Engl J Med* 2000;342:756–762.

Kelley's Textbook of Internal Medicine, fourth edition. Edited by H. David Humes. Lippincott Williams & Wilkins, Philadelphia © 2000.

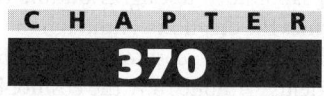

CHAPTER 370

CYSTIC FIBROSIS

MOIRA L. AITKEN

DEFINITION

DIAGNOSIS

The diagnosis of cystic fibrosis (CF) is based on a positive sweat test (greater than 60 mEq per liter) or genetic testing demonstrating two CF alleles and symptoms compatible with CF. When performed correctly, the sweat test is highly sensitive (96% of adults) and specific for CF. False-positive sweat tests can be seen in hypoadrenalism, hypothyroidism, or renal diabetes insipidus.

GENETICS

The *CF* gene is located on the long arm of chromosome 7. The deletion of three base pairs (ΔF508) accounts for approximately 70% of all the *CF* alleles. There are over 700 other alleles, none of which is found on more than 5% of CF chromosomes. Clinical laboratories can screen for up to 70 alleles, accounting for 87% of abnormal genes; thus, a negative screening test does not exclude carrier status. The high prevalence of CF suggests a survival advantage of carrying one copy of this gene, which may be protection against chloride-secreting diarrheas, such as cholera.

INCIDENCE AND EPIDEMIOLOGIC FACTORS

Cystic fibrosis is an autosomal recessive disorder and approximately 1 in 30 persons of European descent are carriers. It affects 1 in 3,000 whites, 1 in 15,000 blacks, and 1 in 90,000 Asians.

ETIOLOGIC FACTORS

The *CF* gene product is expressed in cells of epithelial origin with disease manifest in the lungs, sinuses, pancreas, gastrointestinal (GI) tract, hepatobiliary system, sweat glands, and reproductive tract. The term cystic fibrosis refers to the original description of the pathologic appearance of disease in the pancreas.

PATHOGENESIS

The *CF* gene encodes for the cystic fibrosis transmembrane conductance regulator (CFTR), a membrane glycoprotein that is a chloride ion channel. In CF, one of the chloride ion channels present on the apical membrane of the epithelial cells either is absent or does not open under appropriate stimuli. The apical membrane of the airway epithelial cells also shows increased sodium ion absorption. The pathophysiologic mechanism by which these ion channel defects lead to organ disease is incompletely understood. In the lung, increased sodium absorption and decreased chloride secretion reduce the water content of the periciliary fluid. The osmolality of the periciliary fluid in CF has not been measured, but hyperosmolar periciliary fluid would lead to unhydrated mucin and increased mucus viscosity. This in turn may slow mucociliary transport, but slowed mucociliary transport per se is probably not the only abnormal process involved in the disease process. Another mechanism postulated is that CFTR may also be expressed in the intracellular organelles by the production of many abnormal proteins, such as epithelial cell receptors that have a predilection for *Pseudomonas* attachment. This phenomenon may be the explanation for the increased sulfation of CF mucin, leading to increased viscosity of the mucus, and for increased bacterial adherence to the altered mucin. More recently, a third mechanism has been postulated. Airway epithelial cells secrete antimicrobial peptides (defensins) that are capable of killing bacteria at low salt concentrations. Human β-defensin-1 is salt-sensitive and may be inactivated in CF. Human β-defensin-2 is also expressed in the airway and may contribute to the pathogenesis of CF disease.

CLINICAL FINDINGS AND MANAGEMENT

SWEAT DEFECT

The sweat duct ion-channel dysfunction is different from that of respiratory epithelia. Like the respiratory epithelia, the sweat duct has a reduced chloride ion permeability, but sodium ion transport across the CF sweat duct is not raised. In the secretary coil of the sweat gland, sweat is isotonic or slightly hypertonic. As it moves through the duct, sodium is conserved by being pumped out of the fluid, and chloride passively follows sodium. In CF, impermeability to the chloride ion prevents chloride from leaving the duct and results in an elevated concentration of chloride in the sweat. Electro-neutrality causes a greater amount of sodium concentration in the sweat.

PULMONARY DISEASE

Over 95% of CF patients die from respiratory failure. Histologically the lung is normal at birth. The earliest pathologic change is plugging of submucosal gland ducts in the large airways. Recent evidence from bronchoalveolar lavage fluid in infants suggests that infection is preceded by an inflammatory response with neutrophil influx to the airways. Once infection is present, the chronic presence of potent neutrophil chemoattractants leads to a self-perpetuating destructive inflammatory reaction in the CF lung. Neutrophils release chemoattractants and elastase, which cause tissue destruction directly; interfere with phagocytosis as well as complement and immunoglobulin function; and perpetuate airway infection. Disease can progress rapidly, causing bronchiolitis and bronchitis, with some degree of bronchiectasis usually demonstrated by 6 to 24 months. Although the severity of pathologic changes often varies greatly within each lobe or segment, the upper lobes (and particularly the right upper lobe) tend to be the earliest and most severely affected.

PULMONARY COMPLICATIONS

Acute Exacerbation

A diagnosis of acute exacerbation is made on the basis of subjective symptoms: increased cough, sputum production, and shortness of breath, sometimes associated with anorexia and weight loss. Fever or leukocytosis may be seen (but not invariably) in the adult population. An objective way to assess an exacerbation is by improvement in spirometric values with treatment for the exacerbation. Sputum quantitative cultures and DNA concentration are not precise in the individual patient.

Infection

Global T-cell and B-cell function, complement function, and phagocytosis is normal in CF. Infection is predominantly caused by *Staphylococcus aureus*, *Haemophilus influenzae*, and *Pseudomonas aeruginosa*. *S. aureus* and *H. influenzae* are often recovered from respiratory secretions of children with CF. *P. aeruginosa* eventually becomes the dominant organism in at least 90% of CF patients. Colonization of the respiratory tract with *P. aeruginosa* almost always begins with the morphologically classic (nonmucoid) strain. Onset of *P. aeruginosa* colonization often begins while *S. aureus* is still present. A variety of morphologic variants can occasionally be detected thereafter; however, eventually a smooth mucoid strain appears, and it is this strain that ultimately dominates or totally replaces the other *P. aeruginosa* variants and, often, all other pathogens as well. *B. cepacia* is not an inevitable colonizer, but in some patients it can become the dominant pathogen, replacing all others, including *P. aeruginosa*. Infection with *B. cepacia* can be associated with a rapid decline in pulmonary status. There is also strong epidemiologic evidence of person-to-person transmission of *B. cepacia*; clinical isolation between those infected with *B. cepacia* and those not infected is advocated.

Colonization with nontuberculous mycobacteria has been reported in up to 20% of patients with CF. Rarely does nontuberculous mycobacteria cause disease that requires chemotherapy. *Aspergillus*, usually *Aspergillus fumigatus*, is frequently recovered from CF respiratory secretions. Allergic bronchopulmonary aspergillosis occurs in 2% of patients with CF. Invasive aspergillosis has been reported in CF but is quite rare.

Common respiratory viruses, including respiratory syncytial virus and influenza, and measles can be associated with pulmonary exacerbations.

Hemoptysis

Blood streaking of the sputum is very common in CF patients over 10 years of age, and massive hemoptysis occurs in up to 10% of adults, leading to death in 1% of that population. Mild streaking hemoptysis is caused by mucosal irritation in the airway and is often associated with an acute pulmonary exacerbation. Streaking hemoptysis should prompt a check of coagulation. Massive hemoptysis is due to bleeding from the bronchial circulation, which becomes tortuous and enlarged with the chronic infection of CF. Patients should be warned of the potential of massive hemoptysis and urged to seek emergency treatment if it occurs. (See Chapter 353 for a discussion of the management of massive hemoptysis.)

Pneumothorax

Pneumothorax occurs in 8% to 23% of older CF patients who have more severe pulmonary disease. The incidence in men and women is equal, and appearance is as common on the right as the left. Because of a 50% to 70% chance of recurrence in pneumothorax, obliteration of the pleural space is the treatment of choice but may depend on whether the patient is a candidate for lung transplantation. If the patient is a lung transplantation candidate, intercostal drainage, chemical pleurodesis, ligation of bullae, or limited surgical pleurodesis should be performed in preference to pleurectomy. The majority of CF patients develop pleural adhesions spontaneously, presumably because of air or bacterial leakage into the pleural space.

Clubbing and Hypertrophic Osteoarthropathy

Clubbing of the fingers and toes is eventually a universal finding in CF patients with pulmonary disease, but the severity is variable. Hypertrophic osteoarthropathy is occasionally seen in older patients.

Respiratory Failure and Cor Pulmonale

Secondary pulmonary hypertension leading to cor pulmonale occurs late in the course of disease, with a mean survival of 8 months once right heart failure develops. The indications for oxygen therapy are primarily extrapolated from the Nocturnal Oxygen Therapy Trial group in the chronic obstructive pulmonary disease population, which suggested that oxygen reduced mortality, preserved exercise capacity, and improved neuropsychologic function. In small studies, no improvement in these parameters has been shown in CF patients, but improved quality of life has been demonstrated.

Patients can very rarely be weaned from mechanical ventilation instituted for end-stage disease. A handful of CF patients have successfully undergone lung transplantation from mechanical ventilation, but only a minority of transplantation centers perform transplantation on patients receiving mechanical ventilation. BiPAP has been shown to improve ventilation and oxygenation, and can be a bridge for patients awaiting transplantation.

TREATMENT OF PULMONARY DISEASE

Antibiotics

The mainstay of treatment for pulmonary disease in CF has been chest physical therapy and antibiotics, although the bacterial pathogen is rarely eradicated from the airway. Antibiotics are usually given for 2 weeks for exacerbation of disease, but no trials have been conducted to ascertain the optimum duration of treatment. Several studies have shown that intravenous antibiotic therapy in the home may be as effective as hospitalization. The advantages of cost savings and reduced psychosocial disruption are weighed against more intensive chest physical therapy and more rest in the hospital.

There is no consensus as to whether prophylactic antibiotics should be used in CF. A 5-year multicenter study of prophylactic continuous antistaphylococcal therapy showed no benefit. Prophylactic aerosolized antibiotics (penicillin, carbenicillin, aminoglycosides, colistin, neomycin, and ceftazidime) have also been used in studies. Collectively, these studies showed an initial improvement in spirometry lasting up to 6 months and a decreased number of acute exacerbations over several months. The disadvantage of prophylactic treatment is the emergence of drug-resistant organisms.

Chest Physical Therapy

The results of pulmonary function tests (PFTs) improve following treatment of an exacerbation with chest physical therapy alone. Postural drainage usually accompanied by percussion, deep breathing exercises, directed cough, forced-expiration technique, positive expiratory pressure, flutter and vest devices, as well as exercise have all been used in clinical practice. The optimal chest physical therapy is somewhat controversial and should be the one with which the patient is most compliant.

Bronchodilators

Airway hyperreactivity with a positive methacholine challenge test is present in 50% to 60% of CF patients. β-Agonists may be indicated for those who are clinically wheezy or demonstrate a significant bronchodilator response; it must be recognized that reversible airway obstruction caused by secretions and edema in the airway wall is a universal finding in CF patients with pulmonary disease. Ipratropium bromide may be equally efficacious to β-agonists in this population. There are variable reports on the benefit of theophylline on pulmonary function in CF patients. Theophylline improves diaphragmatic contractility and may assist patients with air trapping and hyperexpansion.

Cromolyn

Small studies suggest that cromolyn sodium is not an effective treatment in cystic fibrosis, which appears counterintuitive as there is a high prevalence of atopy and airway hyperresponsiveness.

Airway Clearance Agents

N-Acetylcysteine, taken by inhalation, may cause bronchospasm, and iodinated therapy and glyceryl guaiacolate are unproven in CF. Recombinant human DNase alters the rheologic properties of sputum by cutting the size of DNA molecules in sputum. Clinical trials have shown a sustained 5% improvement in pulmonary function with this drug.

Anti-inflammatory Drugs

Anti-inflammatory agents, including corticosteroids, ibuprofen, and antiprotease, have been examined in CF. High-dose corticosteroids (1 to 2 mg per kilogram 4 times a day) have been shown to ameliorate the decline in PFTs over a 4-year period, but not without significant side effects. Whether a lower dose would be beneficial has not been studied. Large randomized trials of inhaled steroids in CF have not been completed, but inhaling steroids seems reasonable in patients with an asthmatic component to their disease. The administration of high doses of ibuprofen has shown a more modest decline in PFTs compared to placebo over a 4-year period in a small clinical trial.

Therapeutic options being developed for CF are those meant to correct the basic defect of CF by increasing gene expression or by activating abnormal CFTR.

Lung Transplantation

A final therapeutic option for a few CF patients may be lung transplantation. As of 1998, more than 700 CF patients in the United States had received a heart–lung or double-lung transplant. The 3-year survival is 60%. There is no CF pulmonary disease recurrence as demonstrated by a normal transepithelial potential difference in the transplanted lung. In a very small number of cases, transplantation of unilateral lower lobes has been performed for CF, necessitating two living donors (see Chapter 391 for further discussion of this procedure).

SINUS COMPLICATIONS

The pathophysiologic factors involved in sinus disease are similar to those involved in pulmonary disease. Alteration in mucus,

impaired mucociliary transport, and mechanical obstruction of the sinus ostia occur. Obstruction is followed by bacterial infection. Pan-opacification of the paranasal sinuses is present on the sinus radiographs in 90% to 100% of patients. The frontal sinuses rarely develop in CF patients. It is believed that the early onset of sinusitis prevents pneumatization. Nasal polyposis is found in up to 30% of patients, more commonly seen in the pediatric group. Surgical removal of polyps is associated with a 50% to 90% recurrence rate. Acute symptoms of sinusitis are far less common than the radiologic appearance. Treatment is with antibiotics, nasal irrigation, and nasal steroids, and, if necessary, surgical drainage. Whether the organisms giving rise to sinusitis are the same as those in the sputum is controversial but may not correlate.

PANCREATIC DISEASE
Exocrine Pancreatic Insufficiency

Up to 90% of CF patients have exocrine pancreatic insufficiency, and failure to thrive is a common presenting symptom of the disease. The pancreatic lesion appears to be the result of obstruction of the pancreatic ducts with eosinophilic inspissated secretions. Intraluminal calcifications may develop but are rarely large enough to be seen on plain abdominal films. The diagnosis of pancreatic dysfunction is made by clinical symptoms of malabsorption and measurements of the serum levels of fat-soluble vitamins and sometimes of fecal fat. The quantity of enzymes used with each meal varies from patient to patient and is based on the number of calories consumed; the number, volume, and quality of the stools; and the presence of cramping abdominal pain.

Pancreatitis

Acute pancreatitis occurs in up to 10% of patients. Cholelithiasis should be sought as a precipitating factor. The clinical course of pancreatitis in CF patients appears more benign than in the general population, possibly because the pancreas is scarred and replaced with fatty tissue and because development of a pseudocyst is rare.

Diabetes Mellitus

Diabetes mellitus occurs in up to 15% of CF patients and glucose intolerance in up to 75% of CF patients, contributing to malnutrition in this population. The clinical course and metabolic patterns seen in diabetes associated with CF is distinct from those associated with type I or type II diabetes. This diabetes differs from type I in that it is of slow onset and nonketotic, some insulin secretion persists, intermittent episodes of hyperglycemia occur between prolonged episodes of euglycemia, and markers for islet cell autoimmunity are absent. It differs from type II in that patients are underweight and hypoinsulinemic, and its onset is early in life. It differs from both type I and type II in that glucagon secretion varies, ranging from hypoglucagonemia to hyperglucagonemia. Although the complications of diabetes have not frequently been reported in CF diabetes, typical com-

PART 8: PULMONARY AND CRITICAL CARE MEDICINE

plications of diabetes are expected to occur over time in a group of patients whose median survival is rising. Treatment is with diet and insulin. The only controversy over treatment is about the use of oral hypoglycemic agents and whether they have any role in CF-associated diabetes control.

GASTROINTESTINAL DISEASE

Meconium Ileus and Meconium Ileus Equivalent

Meconium ileus, present in up to 10% of CF neonates at birth, is diagnostic of CF. Meconium ileus is caused by meconium plugging the lumen of the small intestine, usually near the ileocecal valve. Meconium ileus equivalent and distal intestinal obstruction syndrome are the terms used to describe partial or complete intestinal obstruction beyond the neonatal period. It occurs in 10% to 20% of adult CF patients. The cause of meconium ileus is multifactorial. Intestinal mucoproteins may be more viscous; the increased acid in the small intestine may precipitate proteins; undigested fat stimulates enteroglucagon release, which may further slow intestinal transit. Meconium ileus equivalent can present as an acute intestinal obstruction. Often there are recurrent episodes of colicky abdominal pain, with some distention and relative constipation. A soft, mobile, non-tender mass in the right iliac fossa is sometimes present. Patients with chronic symptoms often recognize the precipitating events and alter their behavior to avoid them. Precipitating causes include abrupt cessation of pancreatic enzymes, pulmonary exacerbation, dehydration, or change in diet. Acute episodes are treated with rehydration and hyperosmolar enemas, e.g., diatrizoate meglumine (Gastrografin) and nasogastric suction. If partial obstruction is present, oral hyperosmolar solutions (GoLytely), 5% N-acetylcysteine, and pancreatic supplement may be given orally. Surgery is rarely required.

Gastroesophageal Reflux

Clinically apparent reflux is present in up to 14% of patients. The predominant reflux mechanism is a transient inappropriate lower esophageal sphincter relaxation. Gastroesophageal reflux may contribute to poor pulmonary function because of recurrent aspiration. Patients respond well to cisapride and antireflux therapy.

Peptic Ulceration

Peptic ulcers are found in up to 13% of CF patients. The increased incidence of peptic ulcer disease is related to the decreased pH of the luminal contents secondary to decreased pancreatic bicarbonate secretion. Endoscopic evaluation is the procedure of choice in CF patients with peptic ulcer disease. Contrast radiography is inaccurate because the duodenal mucosa typically appears nodular and distorted with poor definition of the mucosal folds. The ulcers heal well (90%) with H_2 receptor antagonists.

Crohn's Disease and Bowel Strictures

The incidence of Crohn's disease is higher in this population than in the general population. Large quantities of high-strength enteric-coated pancreatic enzymes appear to be associated with nongranulomatous bowel strictures. Currently, no pathophysiologic explanations exist for either of these clinical observations. Concomitant use of H_2 blockers to increase gastric pH allows release of enteric-coated enzyme preparations and thus decreases the total amount of enzymes used.

Intussusception and Rectal Prolapse

Intussusception occurs in 1% of pediatric CF patients, and rectal prolapse is seen in up to 20% of pediatric patients 6 to 36 months of age.

HEPATOBILIARY DISEASE

Hepatomegaly, splenomegaly, or both are found in 1% to 5% of CF patients. The pathogenesis of multilobular cirrhosis is thought to be a response to the accumulation of thickened secretions in the bile ductules, leading to plugging, ductular proliferation, inflammation, and, finally, fibrosis. Patients with overt liver disease often have stricture of the distal common bile duct. Abnormal liver function tests (transaminases two to three times normal values) are frequently found in CF patients with no clinically apparent disease. There is no specific regimen to prevent progression of the hepatic lesions, although treatment with ursodeoxycholic acid has shown improvement in liver function tests and weight gain. Cholelithiasis is found in up to 12% of CF patients; symptomatic presentation is rare before adolescence.

OSTEOPOROSIS

Patients with CF are susceptible to osteopenia and osteoporosis because of malabsorption of vitamin D, calcium, and other nutrients, possible hypogonadism, corticosteroid use, physical inactivity, and circulating cytokines from chronic pulmonary infection. Management includes giving adequate nutritional support, implementing vitamin D and calcium replacement, ensuring appropriate gonadal hormonal levels, encouraging exercise, and using corticosteroids only when necessary. It remains unclear as to when to initiate screening with a DEXA scan. Certainly CF patients being assessed for lung transplantation and those who fall below ideal body weight should have a DEXA scan.

MALIGNANCY

The rate of GI cancer is increased in CF. The increased incidence of tumors is found throughout the GI tract. Routine screening for GI malignancy is not recommended because malignancy is rare. There is only speculation as to the pathophysiologic factors involved in the development of these tumors.

REPRODUCTIVE ISSUES

Of men with CF, 98% to 99% have obstructive azospermia. The abnormalities are confined to the derivatives of the embryonic wolffian duct: the vas deferens, seminal vesicles, and body and tail of the epididymis, with absence or atresia of some or all of these structures. Testicular histologic examination is normal and active spermatogenesis occurs, albeit with production of an increased number of abnormal and immature forms. Microscopic epididymal sperm aspiration may offer men with CF the opportunity to father their own genetic children.

Women with CF have anatomically normal reproductive tracts. Fertility rates among CF women have never been documented, but there is no evidence that fertility is decreased in female CF patients. Cervical mucus viscosity is increased but has not been shown to be less permeable for sperm penetration. Oral contraceptives possess a number of potential side effects that could exacerbate preexisting CF-associated conditions, such as diabetes, malabsorption, cholelithiasis, and hepatic dysfunction, but clinical experience with oral contraceptives has been favorable. Women considering pregnancy should undergo formal evaluation. Those women with mild airflow obstruction and good nutritional status usually tolerate pregnancy well. For women with more severe but stable disease, pregnancy may be endorsed, but with the understanding that close medical observation is essential. Pregnancy does not appear to adversely affect long-term prognosis.

Genetic counseling should be offered to all CF patients who are contemplating starting a family. All offspring will be carriers; the risk of having a CF-affected child is 2% if the spouse is of European decent. A final issue to be considered before conception is the shortened life expectancy of the CF parent; patients should make plans as to who will raise the child in the event of their premature death.

ARTHROPATHY

Immune-mediated episodic arthritis most commonly involving the lower limbs and fingers may start in adolescence. This episodic arthritis is usually a nondestructive arthritis, but erosive changes have been reported. A high fever and erythema nodosum may accompany the arthropathy. Attacks last for several days and respond to nonsteroidal anti-inflammatory drugs, although systemic corticosteroids are sometimes necessary. Hypertrophic pulmonary osteoarthropathy is occasionally seen in CF.

PHARMACOKINETICS

Cystic fibrosis patients have altered pharmacokinetics due to a variety of mechanisms. CFTR may alter renal and hepatic cells directly by altering ion channels and by affecting intracellular pH. Loss of bile salts increases hepatic cytochrome P450. The drugs affected range widely from those that are extensively metabolized, such as sulfamethoxazole and theophylline, to those that are excreted unchanged in the urine, such as the penicillins. The increased clearance of sulfamethoxazole is attributable to increased hepatic N-acetylation. The increased clearance of trimethoprim is primarily increased tubular secretion. Aminoglycoside requirement is increased secondary to increased volume of distribution, increased total body clearance, and aminoglycosides binding to DNA in the purulent secretions.

PROGNOSIS

In the United States in 1997, the median survival was 30.6 years (Fig. 370.1). Prognosis has some correlation to genotype. Patients homozygous for the ΔF508 mutation are diagnosed at an earlier age and die, on average, 3 years earlier than those with other genotypes; however, clinical outcome does not entirely depend on genotype. Other important factors include nutritional status and the number of respiratory viral infections. Prognostic clinical scoring systems that include evaluation of pulmonary function, chest radiograph, and nutritional status have been developed and the forced expiratory volume in 1 second (FEV_1) is the single most sensitive predictor of mortality, with an FEV_1 of less than 30% predicted having a 45% 2-year risk of mortality.

NUTRITIONAL MANAGEMENT

Cystic fibrosis patients often have poor weight gain, growth retardation, delayed puberty; muscle wasting; and vitamin, mineral, essential fatty acid, and taurine deficiencies. Nutrition deficiencies occur because of malabsorption, decreased food intake, and increased metabolic requirements secondary to the disease. Improved nutrition should enhance respiratory muscle strength and immunity, and evidence suggests that it may have important long-term effects on lung function and prognosis.

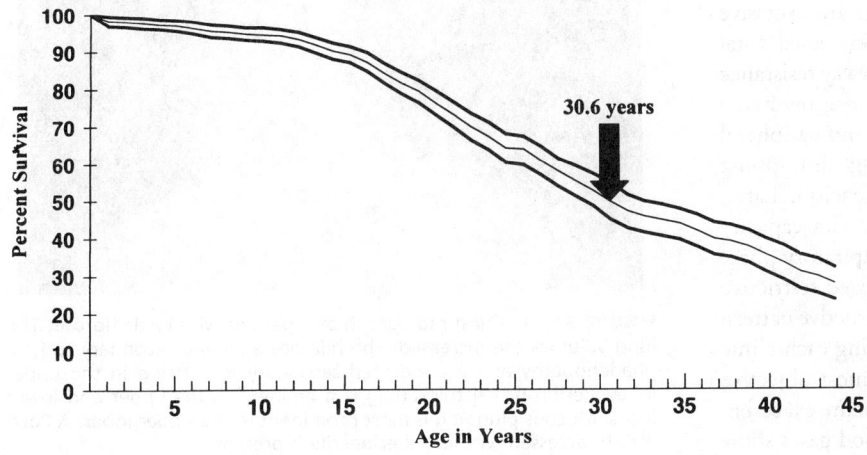

FIGURE 370.2. Median survival of patients with cystic fibrosis in the United States in 1997. Thirty-six percent of patients are 18 years of age or older. (Data from National Cystic Fibrosis Patient Registry, Cystic Fibrosis Foundation, Baltimore, MD, 1998.)

Management includes a dietary intake history and assessment of malabsorption. A 3-day fecal fat collection may be necessary. Pancreatic enzyme replacement therapy should be given to patients with pancreatic insufficiency before each meal and snack. Most patients require vitamin A and E supplement. Enteral feeding should be offered to patients who lose weight despite aggressive dietary measures. Nasogastric tubes, gastrostomy tubes, and jejunostomy tubes have all been used successfully in patients who have been unable to maintain an adequate calorie intake. Gastrostomy tubes carry the risk of increasing gastroesophageal reflux in this susceptible population.

GENE THERAPY

As of 1999, there have been numerous trials using CFTR vectors trials to the nose, lungs, or sinuses. Vectors used in these clinical trials include adenoviruses, adeno-associated viruses, and liposomes. Outcomes have shown CFTR RNA expression and, rarely, CFTR protein expression by alteration in electrophysiologic measurement across the airway. It is anticipated that it will be many years before any of these vectors are clinically useful.

GENETIC COUNSELING

The American Society of Genetics recommends that patients and their relatives be offered nondirective genetic counseling concerning carrier testing and the risk of having a CF-affected child. A major question is whether population-based screening for CF carriers could or should be implemented at present. The current test detects only approximately 85% to 90% of carriers; therefore, only half of the couples in the general population can be identified. Concern has been expressed about false-negative results that occur in any population screening program. For relatives of CF-affected individuals, accuracy of testing is increased because carrier testing can be performed with linkage analysis in addition to mutation analysis when there is a DNA sample available from an affected person in a family.

◼ LABORATORY FINDINGS

PULMONARY FUNCTION

The newborn with CF probably will have normal pulmonary function until peripheral airways are obstructed by excessive mucus. Infant CF patients often demonstrate increased total respiratory resistance, but as the child grows the airway resistance may again have normal values because with lung growth the relative distribution of resistance between central and peripheral airways changes. As lung disease progresses, initially air trapping is seen (increased residual volume/total lung capacity). Later, airflow obstruction predominates [decreased forced vital capacity (FVC), FEV_1, force expiratory flow (FEF), midexpiratory phase (FEF 25% to 75%), and peak flow]. Finally, a mixed restrictive pattern (decreased total lung capacity) and an obstructive pattern are seen. Spirometric testing should be done during each clinic visit. Changes in spirometric values may be the most objective way to determine whether a patient is having an acute exacerbation of his or her pulmonary disease. Arterial blood gases show

progressive widening of the alveolar to arterial oxygen difference with disease progression, and the presence of CO_2 retention is an ominous sign. A PcO_2 greater than 50 torr has a 2-year survival rate of approximately 50%.

MICROBIOLOGIC EXAMINATION

Sputum should be checked during each clinic visit or following a course of antibiotics. The microbiology laboratory should be aware that the sample comes from a CF patient and should have special procedures in the laboratory to deal with the increased viscosity and the organisms found in CF sputum.

RADIOLOGIC EXAMINATION

Overinflation, peribronchial cuffing, and small infiltrates (mucous plugging) are early findings on the chest radiograph. With disease progression, there is bronchiectasis and diffuse fibrosis, most marked in the upper lobes, with scarring and upward retraction of the hila (Fig. 370.2). During an acute exacerbation there may be no obvious changes on chest radiograph. Mucus plugging and increased peribronchial thickening may inconsistently be found. Pneumothorax, pneumomediastinum, lobar and segmental atelectasis, pleural fluid, and large cysts or blebs (particularly in the apexes) may be present. Hilar and mediastinal adenopathy secondary to chronic infection and enlargement of the pulmonary arteries is present later in the disease course. Bronchiectasis is observed at a much earlier stage with computer tomography scanning; airway structure is demonstrated to the level of the subsegmental bronchi. It is also sensitive for small cysts (3 mm), bullae, peribronchial thickening, fibrosis, and early infiltrates.

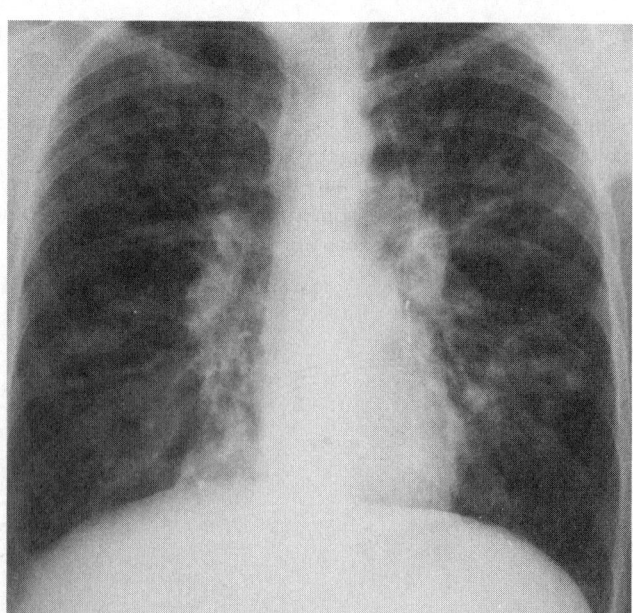

FIGURE 370.1. Chest radiograph of a patient with cystic fibrosis. The lung volumes are increased. The hila are enlarged secondary to lymphadenopathy and are elevated secondary to scarring in the upper lobes. Peribronchial thickening is prominent in the upper and lower lobes. Mucous plugging is most prominent in the upper lobes. A Port-A-Cath accessed with a Huber needle is present.

NUTRITIONAL ASSESSMENT

The Cystic Fibrosis Foundation Clinical Practice Guidelines recommend that complete blood count and liver function testing be performed at least annually. It is not uncommon for adult patients with CF to have anemia of chronic disease. It is also common for them to have a hepatic enzyme rise of two to three times normal values. Vitamin A and vitamin E levels should be monitored at least annually. This may monitor both adequate pancreatic enzyme and vitamin supplementation.

DIABETES SCREENING

The Cystic Fibrosis Foundation consensus statement recommends that a random blood sugar be done annually and, if it is above 126 mg per liter, that a fasting blood sugar follow. A confirmed fasting blood sugar above 126 mg per liter indicates that diabetes treatment should be started.

BIBLIOGRAPHY

Aitken ML, Beall RJ, Bergman D, et al. *Clinical practice guidelines for cystic fibrosis.* Bethesda, MD: Cystic Fibrosis Foundation, 1997.

Barasch J, Kiss B, Prince A, et al. Defective acidification of intracellular organelles in cystic fibrosis. *Nature* 1991;325:70–73.

Bourke S, Rooney M, Fitzgerald M, et al. Episodic arthropathy in adult cystic fibrosis. *Q J Med* 1987;64;651–659.

Burke W, Aitken ML, Chen S-H, et al. Variable severity of pulmonary disease in adults with identical cystic fibrosis mutations. *Chest* 1992; 102;506–509.

Gabriel S, Brigman K, Koller B, et al. Cystic fibrosis heterozygote resistance to cholera toxin in the cystic fibrosis mouse model. *Science* 1994;266: 107–109.

Gaskin KJ, Waters DL, Howman GR, et al. Liver disease and common-bile-duct stenosis in cystic fibrosis. *N Engl J Med* 1988;318:340–346.

Goldman M, Anderson G, Stolzenberg E, et al. Human β-defensin-1 is a salt-sensitive antibiotic in lung that is inactivated in cystic fibrosis. *Cell* 1997:88: 553–560.

Greene K, Takasugi J, Godwin J, et al. Radiographic changes seen in acute exacerbations of cystic fibrosis in adults: a pilot study. *Am J Radiol* 1994; 163:557–562.

Hilman BC, Aitken ML, Constantinesu M. Pregnancy in patients with cystic fibrosis. *Clin Obstet Gynecol* 1996;39:70–86.

Kerem E, Reisman J, Corey M, et al. Prediction of mortality in patients with cystic fibrosis. *N Engl J Med* 1992;326:1187–1191.

Knowles MR, Hohneker KW, Zhou Z, et al. A controlled study of adenoviral-vector-mediated gene transfer in the nasal epithelium of patients with cystic fibrosis. *N Engl J Med* 1995:333:823–831.

Lanng S, Thorsteinsson B, Erichsen G, et al. Glucose tolerance in cystic fibrosis. *Arch Dis Child* 1991:66:612–616.

Nakagawa M, Colombo C, Setchell K. Comprehensive study of the biliary bile acid composition of patients with cystic fibrosis and associated liver disease before and after UDCA administration. *Hepatology* 1990;12: 322–334.

Ott SM, Aitken ML. Osteoporosis in patients with cystic fibrosis. *Clin Chest Med* 1998;Sept:555–567.

Ramsey BW, Pepe MS, Otto KL, et al., and the Cystic Fibrosis Inhaled Tobramycin Writing Committee (ML Aitken, member). Intermittent administration of inhaled tobramycin in patients with cystic fibrosis. *N Engl J Med* 1999:340:23–30.

Redding G, Restuccia R, Cotton E, et al. Serial changes in pulmonary functions in children hospitalized with cystic fibrosis. *Am Rev Respir Dis* 1982;126:31–36.

Rommens J, Iannuzzi M, Kerem B-S, et al. Identification of the cystic fibrosis gene: chromosome walking and jumping. *Science* 1989;245: 1059–1065.

U.S. National Institutes of Health. Workshop on population screening for the cystic fibrosis gene. *N Engl J Med* 1990;323:70–71.

Yankaskas JR, Knowles MR, eds. *Cystic fibrosis in adults.* Philadelphia: Lippincott-Raven Publishers, 1999.

Yankaskas J, Mallory G, and the Consensus Committee. Lung transplantation in cystic fibrosis. *Chest* 1998:113:217–226.

Kelley's Textbook of Internal Medicine, fourth edition. Edited by H. David Humes. Lippincott Williams & Wilkins, Philadelphia © 2000.

CHAPTER 371

IDIOPATHIC INTERSTITIAL PNEUMONIAS

TALMADGE E. KING, JR.

The idiopathic interstitial pneumonias represent a common and important group of interstitial lung diseases. Liebow proposed a pathologic classification for interstitial pneumonia that included usual interstitial pneumonia (UIP), desquamative interstitial pneumonia (DIP), bronchiolitis obliterans interstitial pneumonia (BIP), lymphocytic interstitial pneumonia (LIP), and giant cell interstitial pneumonia (GIP). It was recognized that these entities had no identifiable cause, so the term "idiopathic" was added. Subsequent additional studies showed that LIP represented a group of lymphoproliferative disorders and most cases of GIP were associated with hard-metal (cobalt) pneumoconiosis. Consequently, over the last decade these entities were excluded from the group of idiopathic interstitial pneumonias (IIPs). In addition, other histologic subtypes have been better recognized and are now included in this group: idiopathic bronchiolitis obliterans–organizing pneumonia (BOOP), acute interstitial pneumonia (AIP), and nonspecific interstitial pneumonia (NSIP). Recently, Katzenstein proposed revisions of the classification of idiopathic interstitial pneumonias to include the following entities: UIP, DIP, respiratory bronchiolitis-interstitial lung disease (RB-ILD), AIP, and NSIP. Most experts combine RB-ILD and DIP because it is believed that they represent different stages of the same process. It remains unsettled as to whether or not to include idiopathic BOOP among the IIPs because most of the connective tissue proliferation characteristic of this process is within airspaces rather than the interstitium.

The histologic patterns seen in UIP, DIP, and AIP are distinctive; unfortunately, they are not specific and can be seen in a variety of conditions. Consequently, the diagnosis of the specific entities requires careful clinical, radiologic, and pathologic correlation (Table 371.1). This chapter presents an approach to the diagnosis and management of these disorders. Further discussion can be found in Chapters 360 and 376.

| TABLE 371.1. | IDIOPATHIC INTERSTITIAL PNEUMONIAS: DIFFERENTIAL DIAGNSIS |

Histologic Pattern	Prodrome	Chest X-Ray	HRCT	Pathology	Treatment	Prognosis
UIP	Chronic (>12 mo)	• Bilateral reticular opacities • Lower zone predominance • Honeycombing	• Intralobular interstitial opacities • Irregular interlobular septal thickening • Traction bronchiectasis and honeycombing • Lower zone predominance	• Variegated, patchy, subpleural interstitial fibrosis • Fibroblastic foci, • Mild to moderate interstitial inflammation • Honeycombing	Poor response	50–70% mortality in 5 yr
DIP/RB-ILD	Subacute (weeks to months)	• Ground-glass opacities in lower lung zones	• Diffuse ground-glass opacity in middle and lower lung zones	• Diffuse • Prominent accumulation of alveolar macrophages in alveolar spaces • Mild interstitial inflammation	Corticosteroid responsiveness	5% mortality in 5 yr
AIP	Abrupt (1 to 2 wk)	• Diffuse, bilateral, airspace opacification	• Bilateral, symmetrical ground-glass opacities • Bilateral airspace consolidation	• Diffuse, temporally uniform • Alveolar septal thickening due to organizing fibrosis, usually diffuse • Airspace organization • Hyaline membranes (focal or diffuse)	• Mechanical ventilation • Corticosteroid responsiveness	60% mortality in ≤6 mo
NSIP	Subacute (weeks to months)	• Bilateral patchy opacities • Lower zone predominance	• Patchy ground-glass opacity • Cystic changes	• Diffuse, temporally uniform, • Mild to moderate interstitial chronic inflammation • Type II pneumocyte hyperplasia in areas of inflammation	Corticosteroid responsiveness	15–20% mortality in 5 yr

HRCT, high-resolution computed tomography scan.
UIP, usual interstitial pneumonia; AIP, acute interstitial pneumonia; DIP, desquamative interstitial pneumonia; RB-ILD, respiratory bronchiolitis–interstitial lung disease; NSIP, nonspecific interstitial pneumonia.

IDIOPATHIC PULMONARY FIBROSIS/USUAL INTERSTITIAL PNEUMONIA

DEFINITION

Idiopathic pulmonary fibrosis (IPF) is the prototypical interstitial lung disease (ILD), and it is characterized by progressive pulmonary parenchymal inflammation and fibrosis. These changes result in exertional dyspnea, bibasilar interstitial opacities on chest radiograph, and restrictive physiologic impairment, and can eventually cause respiratory failure and cor pulmonale. IPF is the preferred term for this disease in North America, but there are many descriptive synonyms, including cryptogenic fibrosing alveolitis, Hamman–Rich syndrome, diffuse interstitial fibrosis, "honeycomb lung," Osler–Charcot disease, diffuse pulmonary alveolar fibrosis, and idiopathic interstitial pneumonitis.

Until recently, reports of IPF included cases with the histologic patterns of UIP, DIP, idiopathic BOOP, AIP, and NSIP because most investigators tended to "lump" these under this diagnosis. In the last decade there has been a move to narrow the definition of IPF to include only cases of UIP. This paradigm shift has been largely influenced by the identification of different clinical and radiologic (especially high-resolution CT, or HRCT, scanning) features among the other histologic subtypes and, most importantly, a strikingly different response to treatment and thus to survival. For example, it was shown that median survival of patients with the UIP pattern was significantly worse than that for patients with the other chronic interstitial pneumonias.

INCIDENCE AND EPIDEMIOLOGIC FACTORS

The incidence of IPF is unknown. It is thought to occur in 3 to 5 persons per 100,000, but recent data suggest that the incidence may be much higher. Most patients are diagnosed in the fifth to seventh decades of life. No racial, seasonal, or geographic associations have been noted. Males appear to have a slightly greater likelihood of developing IPF in some studies.

ETIOLOGIC FACTORS AND PATHOGENESIS

The cause of IPF is unknown. Its pathogenesis is highly complex and probably multifactorial; genetic, viral, environmental, and autoimmune factors have been implicated. Cigarette smoking has been proposed as a contributory/confounding factor in IPF, but no controlled studies have confirmed this association. A variety of cell, cytokine, and matrix interactions appear to contribute to the parenchymal inflammation and fibrosis seen in IPF; the exact mechanisms of this complex interaction are unclear. Regardless of the inciting cause, much evidence suggests a role for the immune response in the pathogenesis of IPF. A genetic predisposition is strongly supported by the recognition of familial forms of many ILDs, including familial IPF, which appears to have an autosomal dominant inheritance pattern with variable penetrance. A search for "fibrosis susceptibility genes" in the major histocompatibility complex has produced contradictory results. More promising is the association of IPF with the Z and S α_1-antitrypsin inhibitor alleles and immunoglobulin allotypes on chromosome 14. Efforts to confirm a respiratory viral cause for IPF have been unsuccessful. Other viruses, such as hepatitis C virus, may be implicated in some cases. Airborne environmental factors (other than the known fibrogenic agents inhaled in the occupational environment such as asbestos or silica) may be linked to the development of IPF.

CLINICAL FINDINGS

The symptoms of IPF are nonspecific. Most patients note the insidious development of exertional dyspnea. A nonproductive cough may be present. Constitutional symptoms, such as fatigue, malaise, or weight loss, are less common. As the disease progresses, patients may become dyspneic at rest and develop sputum production. Exertional chest discomfort and peripheral edema are associated with the development of pulmonary hypertension and cor pulmonale. Most patients present for care more than 6 months after the onset of symptoms.

Physical examination of the IPF patient is similarly nonspecific or it may be entirely normal in early stages of the disease. Chest auscultation usually reveals basilar inspiratory crackles. As the disease progresses, crackles become coarser and more widespread; digital clubbing and cyanosis may become apparent. A prominent pulmonic closure sound, palpable pulmonary arterial impulse, or right ventricular heave suggests pulmonary arterial hypertension; jugular venous distention, hepatomegaly, and peripheral edema signal the development of cor pulmonale.

LABORATORY FINDINGS

Routine Laboratory Studies

Laboratory studies may reveal the nonspecific presence of rheumatoid factor, antinuclear antibody, or cryoglobulins, usually in low titers. Complete blood counts are usually normal.

Chest Imaging Studies

Radiographic findings in IPF are not specific. Typically there are bibasilar reticular opacities with reduced lung volumes. As the disease progresses, the upper lung fields become involved, coarse polygonal markings become apparent (honeycombed lung), and pulmonary arterial enlargement and cardiomegaly may be seen. Hilar and mediastinal adenopathy and pleural effusions are not evident in routine cases of IPF and should suggest an alternative diagnosis.

HRCT scans are more sensitive at detecting parenchymal abnormalities. Typical HRCT findings in IPF include peripheral, subpleural, basal distribution; reticular opacities; honeycombing; traction bronchiectasis and bronchiolectasis; focal areas of ground-glass opacities; and architectural distortion (Fig. 371.1). Unrelated coexistent lung diseases such as smoking-related emphysema are often present in IPF.

The gallium lung scan is insensitive and nonspecific, and it correlates poorly with lung biopsy tissue cellularity or response to therapy in IPF. Technetium Tc 99m diethylenetriamine pentaacetate (^{99m}Tc-DTPA) scanning is an index of lung epithelial

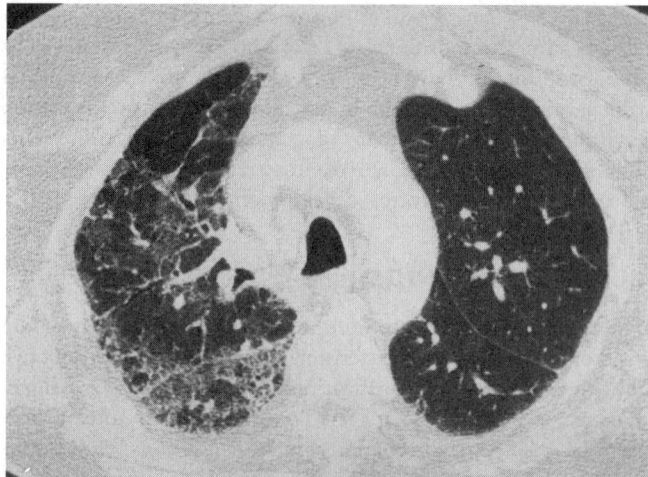

FIGURE 371.1. High-resolution chest computed tomography scan from a patient with idiopathic pulmonary fibrosis. The opacities are patchy and asymmetrical but worse in the dorsal segments of the right lung (lower left), where early honeycombing is present. Fine hazy opacities (ground-glass appearance) are interspersed with relatively normal-appearing areas in the remainder of the right lung and left lung.

permeability. Increased permeability results from inflammation. A normal ^{99m}Tc-DTPA clearance at initial measurement in IPF predicted stable disease and rapid clearance identified patients at risk for deterioration. Insufficient data exist to support the routine use of either method in the routine assessment of ILD.

Lung Function Studies

Static pulmonary function testing in IPF typically reveals a reduced forced expiratory volume in 1 second (FEV$_1$), vital capacity (VC), and total lung capacity; the FEV$_1$/VC ratio is usually normal or increased (consistent with a restrictive ventilatory impairment due to decreased lung compliance). The single-breath diffusing capacity for carbon monoxide (corrected for hemoglobin) is reduced, reflecting a loss of functional alveolar capillary gas exchange area. Arterial blood gas measurements may be normal at rest but typically reveal varying degrees of hypoxemia and respiratory alkalosis. Carbon dioxide retention causing respiratory acidosis is a late finding. Patients with IPF and coexisting chronic pulmonary obstructive disease may have normal airflow measurements and lung volumes due to the offsetting effects of these two diseases on lung mechanics yet may have severe functional impairment. The diffusing capacity in these patients is usually markedly diminished.

Cardiopulmonary exercise testing in IPF reveals diminished maximal oxygen consumption and exercise capacity. Increased ventilatory equivalents for oxygen and carbon dioxide, elevated physiologic dead space with progressive exertion, widening of the alveolar–arterial oxygen difference, and oxygen desaturation are typical physiologic characteristics in patients subjected to an exercise test. Most patients stop due to dyspnea and fatigue, and demonstrate oxygen desaturation. Occasionally, patients with exertional dyspnea have normal radiographic studies, pulmonary function tests, and arterial blood gas measurements at rest. In these cases, physiologic abnormalities may surface during pro-

gressive cardiopulmonary exercise testing and prompt further diagnostic evaluation and lung biopsy.

Bronchoalveolar Lavage

Bronchoalveolar lavage (BAL) findings in IPF are highly variable and are nondiagnostic. Lymphocytes, macrophages, neutrophils, and eosinophils may be increased in varying proportions. Certain soluble factors, such as surfactant phospholipids, may be reduced; others, such as procollagen III peptides, may be increased. The clinical utility of these findings is undetermined.

Lung Biopsy and Histopathologic Examination

There is a tendency to be overconfident of one's ability to make a correct clinical diagnosis of IPF-UIP. Lung biopsy improves the accuracy of the diagnosis and appears most important when an HRCT pattern consistent with UIP is uncertain or unlikely. Fiberoptic bronchoscopy with BAL and transbronchial lung biopsy cause little morbidity and can provide useful information if definitive diagnostic findings are recovered (i.e., infection, granulomatous inflammation, or malignancy). However, findings of nonspecific interstitial fibrosis must not be considered

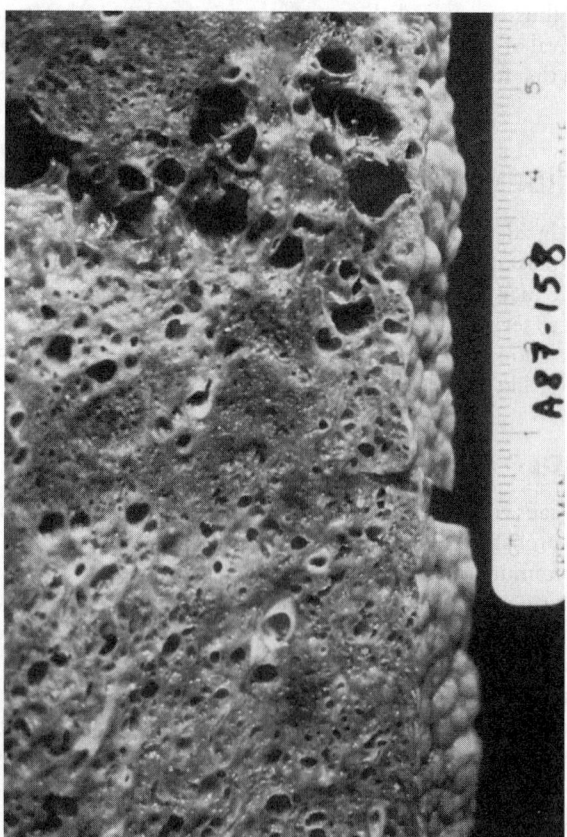

FIGURE 371.2. Gross view of honeycombed lung. The cut surface reveals distortion by irregular dense bands of fibrosis separating numerous cystic spaces of varying size. The pleural surface (adjacent to the label) has an irregular cobbled appearance, reflecting the underlying parenchymal changes.

conclusive for identification of IPF because of the sampling error inherent in the technique.

Some controversy exists as to the need for surgical lung biopsy in the diagnosis of ILD. However, examination of representative lung tissue confirms a specific diagnosis, justifies long-term therapy with drugs having significant adverse effects, and may predict the response to therapy and prognosis. Lung biopsy via thoracotomy is the gold standard diagnostic procedure in ILD, and recent experience with video-assisted thoracoscopic lung biopsy suggests that it is equally effective, less morbid, and better tolerated by patients. Biopsies should be obtained from multiple sites, including areas of involved lung and relatively normal lung because of the patchy distribution of the disease and the nondiagnostic histopathologic findings in areas of advanced honeycombed lung. HRCT may help to select locations for surgical lung biopsy and to identify other findings appropriate for biopsy (especially adenopathy and pleural abnormalities). Careful handling and review of the biopsy specimens by an experienced lung pathologist who is aware of the clinical features enhances diagnostic yields.

Gross structural changes occur as the alveolar walls become progressively thickened by fibrosis. Alveolar spaces and vascular beds become obliterated, and the parenchymal architecture becomes distorted into multiple cystic structures surrounded by dense bands of fibrotic tissue known as "honeycombed lung" (Fig. 371.2). The histopathologic changes of UIP are patchy. Usually the abnormalities are more advanced in the periphery of the basilar lung segments. UIP is characterized by increased fibroblasts, excessive deposition of collagen, and expansion of lymphocyte and plasma cell populations within the alveolar wall. Fibroblasts, alveolar type II epithelial cells, fibrin, and collagen deposition also are present in alveolar spaces (intra-alveolar fibrosis) (Fig. 371.3). Distortion of airway walls by retracting fibrotic parenchymal tissue can result in "traction bronchiectasis," and the vascular changes of secondary pulmonary hypertension are a late finding in IPF.

There are no pathognomonic histologic features that distin-guish IPF from most other forms of ILD. Scattered foci of proliferating fibroblasts (so-called fibroblastic foci) are a consistent finding in UIP. The extent of fibroblastic proliferation is predictive of disease progression. Granulomatous and vasculitic changes are incompatible with a diagnosis of IPF, and some other forms of IIP can be excluded by histopathologic study. Honeycombed lung is the final common pathway for all advanced ILD and may be devoid of specific diagnostic features, regardless of the underlying cause.

OPTIMAL MANAGEMENT

The nonspecific clinical, laboratory, and radiographic features described above should suggest the diagnosis of an ILD but do not confirm the diagnosis of IPF. A detailed medical history, meticulous physical examination, and directed laboratory evaluation are essential steps in the diagnosis of IPF, primarily by excluding other forms of ILD (see Chapter 360). Evaluation of IPF disease progression and therapeutic responses should be based on objective criteria. Static pulmonary function tests and radiographic changes prove insensitive to significant functional changes in the IPF patient. Serial cardiopulmonary exercise tests may be a more sensitive measure of global function. The best measure of disease status in an individual patient is probably a combined clinical, radiographic (HRCT), physiologic, and pathologic index. BAL has contributed enormously to our understanding of the pathogenesis of IPF, but its routine clinical use in the management of IPF patients is controversial. BAL lymphocytosis has been associated with a favorable prognosis, and elevated neutrophil or eosinophil counts or procollagen peptide levels appear to predict a worse prognosis in some patients with IPF; however, the reliability of these observations in individual patients is uncertain.

In most series (combining treated and untreated patients), the median survival after the onset of symptoms is less than 5 years. However, with the narrowing of the diagnosis to cases involving the UIP lesion, the median survival has declined to approximately 3 years following diagnosis. There is no evidence for spontaneous remission in biopsy-proven IPF, and most patients experience a steadily progressive deterioration. In a few patients, treatment appears to lead to stabilization or retardation of disease progression. Rapid clinical deterioration over weeks or months, historically called the Hamman–Rich syndrome, is uncommon and may represent a different process (see section "Acute Interstitial Pneumonia"). Factors that appear to increase survival include younger age, female gender, lesser degrees of radiographic abnormality, more cellular or inflammatory changes on the lung biopsy, and an early response to treatment.

The goal of therapy for IPF is to prevent disease progression and improve survival. No curative therapy exists, but efforts to suppress the inflammatory response appear justified based on the immunopathogenesis of the disease. There are no controlled studies to guide the dosage and duration of therapy. Because only a few IPF patients improve significantly on corticosteroids alone, combined therapy with an immunosuppressive agent (azathioprine or cyclophosphamide) has been recommended as initial treatment. Treatment with prednisone is usually initiated at 40 to 60 mg per day and continued for 4 to 6 months. If the

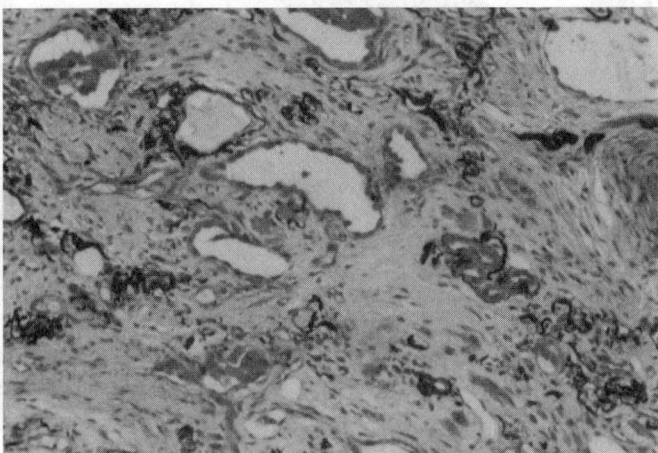

FIGURE 371.3. Photomicrograph of histologic features of usual interstitial pneumonitis. The lung architecture is markedly distorted by fibrosis, involving the replacement of normal alveolar structures by bands of collagen and fibroblasts and scattered cystic spaces.

patient stabilizes or shows objective improvement, the dose is gradually tapered to the minimum effective level (usually 0.25 mg per kilogram per day). Azathioprine or cyclophosphamide at 2 to 3 mg per kilogram per day lean body weight (LBW) to a maximum dose of 150 mg per day orally is recommended as part of the initial regimen. Dosing should begin at 25 to 50 mg per day and increase gradually, by 25-mg increments every 7 to 14 days until the maximum dose is reached. Clear response to therapy may not be evident until the patient has received 3 months or more of therapy. Consequently, in the absence of complications or adverse effects of the medications, combined therapy should be continued for at least 6 months. At that time, repeat studies should be performed to determine the response to therapy. Therapy with alternative agents such as colchicine, interferon gamma, pirfenidone, methotrexate, D-penicillamine, antioxidants, and cyclosporine may be helpful, but there is little data available to justify their routine use.

Treatment for IPF is generally lifelong for patients who respond, and complications of therapy must be considered at the outset. A tuberculin skin test should be performed and preventive antituberculous therapy offered to positive reactors before corticosteroid therapy. The routine use of trimethoprim–sulfamethoxazole (one single-strength tablet thrice weekly) as prophylaxis against *Pneumocystis carinii* has been recommended for patients receiving immunosuppressive therapy. In addition to cushingoid features, the possibility of developing cataracts, hypertension, hyperglycemia, hyperlipidemia, myopathy, osteoporosis, osteonecrosis, opportunistic infection, psychosis, and other adverse effects should be considered. Patients receiving cytotoxic therapy should be closely monitored for evidence of hematologic or hepatic toxicity.

Basic medical management can help alleviate many of the clinical manifestations of IPF. Smoking cessation is vital. Oxygen should be prescribed when the resting PaO_2 falls below 60 mm Hg or when exercise oxygen desaturation below 90% occurs. Judicious diuretic therapy can help manage cor pulmonale, and opiates may be palliative measures for the relief of terminal dyspnea or intractable cough. Pneumococcal and influenza vaccinations should be administered. New symptoms and focal radiographic abnormalities should be evaluated for infectious and malignant causes. IPF patients have an extraordinarily high incidence of lung cancer (10% to 15%). Lung transplantation is a realistic option for many patients with IPF who do not respond to medical therapy. Referral to a transplant center should be timed to avoid a long and fruitless course of corticosteroids in patients with advanced fibrosis, or premature demise during the pretransplantation evaluation and inevitable wait for organ availability.

DESQUAMATIVE INTERSTITIAL PNEUMONIA AND RESPIRATORY BRONCHIOLITIS–ASSOCIATED INTERSTITIAL LUNG DISEASE

DEFINITION

Like UIP, the term desquamative interstitial pneumonia (DIP) is used to describe both an idiopathic clinicopathologic entity

and a histologic pattern. Previously, under the clinical concept of IPF, the cellular DIP and fibrotic UIP were considered part of the spectrum of the same disease. Currently, each is viewed as a separate clinicopathologic entity with the radiographic and histologic pattern of UIP being required for the diagnosis of IPF. The term respiratory bronchiolitis–associated interstitial lung disease (RB-ILD) is more anatomically accurate as is it conveys important pathogenetic implications, which the older term, DIP, does not.

The histologic criteria for diagnosis of DIP has been narrowed following the description of the histologic pattern of RB-ILD and refinement of the criteria for UIP. Consequently, the clinicopathologic entity of DIP is very rare, whereas RB-ILD and UIP are more common. The cause is unknown. However, DIP/RB-ILD is seen almost exclusively in cigarette smokers or persons exposed to passive cigarette smoke.

CLINICAL FINDINGS AND LABORATORY FINDINGS

Most patients are in the fourth to fifth decade of life. It is more common in men than women (2:1). Most patients present with a subacute (weeks to months) illness characterized by dyspnea and cough. The chest radiograph may be normal in up to 20% of cases. The chest radiograph and HRCT scan pattern shows diffuse ground-glass opacity in the middle and lower lung zones (Fig. 371.4). Lung function testing shows a restrictive pattern with reduced single-breath diffusing capacity of carbon monoxide and hypoxemia on blood gas analysis.

The histologic hallmark of DIP is diffuse marked intra-alveolar macrophage accumulation—smoker's macrophages with a golden brown pigment with numerous tiny black particles (Fig.

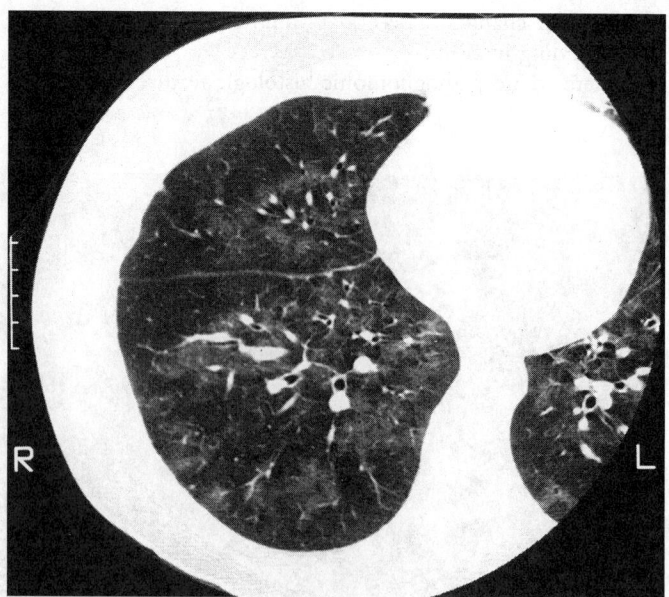

FIGURE 371.4. A high-resolution computed tomography (HRCT) scan of the chest from a patient with respiratory bronchiolitis–associated interstitial lung disease showing extensive ground-glass opacities. The diagnosis was confirmed by thoracoscopic lung biopsy. The symptoms and HRCT scan improved following cessation of smoking.

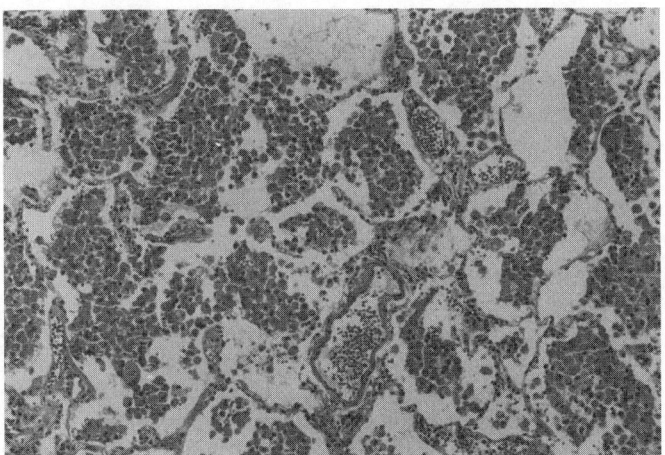

FIGURE 371.5. Photomicrograph of histologic features of desquamative interstitial pneumonitis. The lung architecture is relatively preserved, with minimal thickening or inflammation of the alveolar walls, but the alveolar spaces are filled with alveolar macrophages.

371.5). Lung biopsy reveals a uniform, diffuse, intra-alveolar macrophage accumulation. The macrophage accumulation is accentuated around respiratory bronchioles and extends diffusely throughout the lung parenchyma. There is little fibrosis, with only mild or moderate thickening of alveolar walls. Unlike UIP, there is no scarring fibrosis causing remodeling of the lung architecture. Fibroblastic foci are absent or inconspicuous, and the fibrous connective tissue that is present appears about the same age. Interstitial inflammation is usually mild in extent and severity, consisting of lymphocytes and a few plasma cells.

A DIP-like reaction can occur as a nonspecific reaction adjacent to a variety of pathologic lesions: pulmonary Langerhans' cell histiocytosis, IPF, drug reactions (e.g., amiodarone), chronic alveolar hemorrhage, eosinophilic pneumonia, pneumoconioses (e.g., talcosis, hard-metal disease, asbestosis), obstructive pneumonias, exogenous lipoid pneumonia, histiocyte-rich infections (e.g., *Mycobacterium avium* complex, HIV infection). Chronic eosinophilic pneumonia without eosinophils may resemble DIP.

OPTIMAL MANAGEMENT

Clinical recognition of DIP/RB-ILD is important because the process is associated with a better prognosis than IPF, with an overall survival of about 70% after 10 years. Smoking cessation should be required treatment. Corticosteroid administration, which is occasionally required, usually results in improved function and resolution of DIP/RB-ILD.

ACUTE INTERSTITIAL PNEUMONIA

DEFINITION

AIP is a rare fulminant form of lung injury causing rapidly progressive parenchymal fibrosis. AIP likely represents the subset of cases of idiopathic adult respiratory distress syndrome (ARDS). The cases of pulmonary fibrosis originally reported by Hamman

and Rich had clinical and histopathologic features of AIP rather than IPF. AIP is rare. The pathogenesis is unknown and appears to involve a complex array of cellular events involving a wide variety of cells such as epithelial cells, endothelial cells, neutrophils, histiocytes, fibroblasts, and smooth muscle cells as well as the extracellular matrix.

CLINICAL FINDINGS AND LABORATORY FINDINGS

AIP presents acutely (days to weeks from onset of symptoms) in a previously healthy person usually over the age of 40 years. There is no sexual predilection. A prodromal illness, lasting usually 7 to 14 days before presentation, is common. The clinical signs and symptoms include fever, cough and shortness of breath.

Routine laboratory studies are nonspecific and generally not helpful. Most patients have moderate to severe hypoxemia and develop respiratory failure. Mechanical ventilation is often required. A rigorous search for infectious and inflammatory conditions causing acute lung injury is essential. The radiographic findings are similar to those seen in ARDS. Diffuse, bilateral, air-space opacification is seen on chest radiograph. CT scans show bilateral, patchy, symmetric areas of ground-glass attenuation. Bilateral areas of air space consolidation may also be present. A predominantly subpleural distribution may be seen. Mild honeycombing, usually involving <10% of the lung may be seen on CT examination. A surgical lung biopsy is required to confirm the diagnosis. The histopathologic features are typical of diffuse alveolar damage, with extensive hyaline membranes and varying degrees of interstitial and alveolar organization with fibrosis.

OPTIMAL MANAGEMENT

The mortality from AIP is high (>60%) with the majority of patients dying within 3 months of presentation. It is not clear that corticosteroid therapy is effective in AIP. The main treatment is supportive care because unlike other chronic forms of IIP, AIP may regress or resolve with supportive therapy. In fact, those who recover usually do not have recurrence of the disease and most have substantial or complete recovery of lung function.

NONSPECIFIC INTERSTITIAL PNEUMONIA

DEFINITION

Nonspecific interstitial pneumonia does not appear to be a discrete entity, and the risk is that it will become a "wastebasket" designation for any interstitial inflammatory and fibrotic processes that does not have the classical clinical or histopathologic features of other IIPs. The importance in recognizing NSIP is to separate these cases from UIP since the overall survival is substantially better in NSIP than in UIP. The incidence and pathogenesis are unknown.

CLINICAL FINDINGS AND LABORATORY FINDINGS

Most patients are middle-aged adults with a subacute onset of symptoms of approximately 8 months prior to diagnosis. There appears to be a slight female predominance (1.4:1). Dyspnea and cough are the most common presenting complaints. Fever and systemic flulike symptoms are common.

The chest radiograph usually shows bilateral reticular or hazy opacities. HRCT scan findings in NSIP include bilateral patchy ground-glass attenuation, bilateral areas of consolidation, irregular lines, and bronchial dilatation.

Surgical lung biopsy is required to confirm the diagnosis. NSIP is characterized by the presence of varying degrees of inflammation and fibrosis within alveolar walls. The changes are temporally uniform, but the process may be patchy with intervening areas of unaffected lung. The process is frequently accentuated in the peribronchiolar interstitium and the density of the inflammatory infiltrate is considerably greater than that occurring other IIPs. The fibrotic cases of NSIP involve dense interstitial fibrosis with a diffuse or patchy pattern. Type II cell hyperplasia often accompanies the interstitial inflammation and may be prominent. Fibroblastic foci are far less common than that seen in UIP. However, foci of honeycomb fibrosis may be present.

OPTIMAL MANAGEMENT

Patients with this lesion appear to have different clinical outcomes compared to patients with AIP, UIP, DIP, or BOOP. Importantly, unlike patients with IPF/UIP, the majority of patients with NSIP have a good prognosis, with most showing improvement after treatment with corticosteroids. The prognosis appears to depend on the extent of fibrosis.

■ LYMPHOCYTIC INTERSTITIAL PNEUMONITIS

DEFINITION

Lymphocytic interstitial pneumonia is an uncommon pathologic process characterized by the presence of widespread, monotonous sheets of lymphocytic infiltration in the interstitium of the lung. LIP is no longer included among the IIPs, but it is included in the chapter because it can have similar modes of presentation. In addition to being differentiated from IPF, it must be distinguished from lymphocytic infiltrations associated with pseudolymphoma, primary lymphomas, lymphomatoid granulomatosis, benign lymphocytic angiitis and granulomatosis, plasma cell interstitial pneumonia, and angioimmunoblastic lymphadenopathy. LIP is associated with autoimmune conditions such as Sjögren's syndrome and has been found with hypogammaglobulinemia and HIV infection and after allogeneic bone marrow or solid organ transplantation.

CLINICAL FINDINGS

Lymphocytic interstitial pneumonia occurs more commonly in women, usually in the fourth to sixth decade of life. It is also seen in children, particularly those with hypogammaglobulinemia or AIDS. The clinical manifestations of LIP are dominated by those related to the underlying disease, such as Sjögren's syndrome. Progressive dyspnea and cough are the most common presenting symptoms, while weight loss, pleuritic pain, arthralgias, and fever also occur. Bibasilar rales on chest examination, cyanosis, and finger clubbing are common physical findings.

LABORATORY FINDINGS

The chest roentgenogram is nonspecific, with reticular opacities being the most common abnormality. A mixed alveolar–interstitial pattern appears as the disease progresses, as a result of the coalescence of the opacities. Cysts, honeycombing, and pulmonary hypertension are also late manifestations. Pleural effusions are uncommon and are suggestive of a complicating lymphoma. A restrictive defect is commonly seen, often associated with a reduction in the carbon monoxide diffusing capacity and arterial hypoxemia. A striking T-cell lymphocytosis is seen on bronchoalveolar lavage.

Surgical lung biopsy is required for the diagnosis in almost all cases. The lymphocytic infiltration involves the alveolar septa and peribronchiolar and perivascular interstitium, and is usually extensive and severe. The lymphocytes are polytypic (both B and T cells may be found), distinguishing them from the monotypic lymphocytic infiltrates characteristic of pulmonary lymphoma. The number of plasma cells and macrophages is also increased in these infiltrates. Other prominent histopathologic features include the accumulation of large interstitial reticuloendothelial cells, mononuclear cells, and giant cells forming noncaseating granulomas, as well as the presence of perivascular and paraseptal amyloid deposition and well-formed lymphoid germinal centers.

OPTIMAL MANAGEMENT

The clinical course of idiopathic LIP is unknown. In cases where LIP is associated with another disease, the underlying disease largely determines the outcome. Progression to end-stage fibrosis can occur, and the development of lymphoma is a recognized complication of LIP. Marked improvement or complete resolution followed corticosteroid therapy in many cases. Progressive pulmonary fibrosis, cor pulmonale, and death can occur despite therapy. Infection is a common complication in such patients, especially those with an associated dysproteinemia.

BIBLIOGRAPHY

American Thoracic Society. Idiopathic pulmonary fibrosis: diagnosis and treatment. International consensus statement. *Am J Respir Crit Care Med* 2000;161:646–664.

Bjoraker JA, Ryu JH, Edwin MK, et al. Prognostic significance of histopathologic subsets in idiopathic pulmonary fibrosis. *Am J Respir Crit Care Med* 1998;157:199–203.

British Thoracic Society. The diagnosis, assessment and treatment of diffuse parenchymal lung disease in adults. *Thorax* 1999;54(Suppl 1):S1–S28.

Daniil ZD, Gilchrist FC, Nicholson AG, et al. A histologic pattern of nonspecific interstitial pneumonia is associated with a better prognosis than usual interstitial pneumonia in patients with cryptogenic fibrosing alveolitis. *Am J Respir Crit Care Med* 1999;160:899–905.

Johnston IDA, Prescott RJ, Chalmers JC, et al., for the Fibrosing Alveolitis

Subcommittee of the Research Committee of the British Thoracic Society. British Thoracic Society study of cryptogenic fibrosing alveolitis: current presentation and initial management. *Thorax* 1997;52:38–44.

Katzenstein ALA, Myers JL. Idiopathic pulmonary fibrosis. Clinical relevance of pathologic classification. *Am J Respir Crit Care Med* 1998;157:1301–1315.

Katoh T, Andoh T, Mikawa K, et al. Computed tomographic findings in non-specific interstitial pneumonia/fibrosis. *Respirology* 1998;3:69–75.

Mapel DW, Samet JM, Coultas DB. Corticosteroids and the treatment of idiopathic pulmonary fibrosis. Past, present, and future. *Chest* 1996;110:1058–1067.

Muller NL, Colby TV. Idiopathic interstitial pneumonias: high-resolution CT and histologic findings. *Radiographics* 1997;17:1016–1022.

Nagai S, Kitaichi M, Itoh H, et al. Idiopathic nonspecific interstitial pneumonia/fibrosis: comparison with idiopathic pulmonary fibrosis and BOOP. *Eur Respir J* 1998;12:1010–1019.

Primack SL, Hartman TE, Ikezoe J, et al. Acute interstitial pneumonia: radiographic and CT findings in nine patients. *Radiology* 1993;188:817–820.

Schwarz MI, King TE Jr. *Interstitial lung diseases*, third ed. Hamilton: BC Decker, 1998.

Kelley's Textbook of Internal Medicine, fourth edition. Edited by H. David Humes. Lippincott Williams & Wilkins, Philadelphia © 2000.

CHAPTER 372

HYPERSENSITIVITY PNEUMONITIS

WILLIAM W. MERRILL

The air that we breathe usually appears to be a clear, homogeneous gas mixture. The gas, however, contains small amounts of foreign materials of various sizes. Some of this complex mixture can be inhaled to the lower respiratory tract. Although the amount of foreign material per volume per day of air is small, the total volume of air inhaled is large—about 10,000 per day on average—and therefore significant amounts of this debris can reach the lower airways. The lung has a variety of mechanisms to deal with these substances, and usually these are effective.

Some people, however, when confronted by a large amount of inhaled foreign antigen substance are unable to cope and contract a lung disease caused by immune reaction to the inhaled antigen. Although much is known about the immune reaction and the relevant antigens, the diagnosis of hypersensitivity pneumonitis still rests on an astute clinician's recognizing the pattern of a clinical syndrome. Therefore, making a correct diagnosis is intellectually challenging. Furthermore, because treatment is usually effective, the clinician's diagnostic acumen may be rewarded by a beneficial outcome.

■ ETIOLOGIC FACTORS AND PATHOGENESIS

This group of diseases represents an inflammatory host response subsequent to inhalation of a foreign substance. As indicated in Table 372.1, the potential clinical causes of such reactions are diverse. The occupational exposure to mold dusts during farming operations was the first of these syndromes to be reported and still represents a common cause of illness. Almost any situation that generates high concentrations of respirable foreign material can cause illness. In fact, this is an important common feature of these illnesses—all are associated with the delivery of large amounts of antigen to the lung. Farmers with disease were found to be exposed to 2.6×10^9 mold spore per cubic meter of air during farm work.

Sometimes the reaction occurs as the result of exposure to a substance that the patient knows to be present in his or her environment. The reactions of some workers who manufacture laundry detergent to *Bacillus subtilis* enzymes and of others to hapten fumes from vaporizing plastics are appropriate examples. Frequently, however, the illness is caused by contamination of the environment with molds or, less commonly, bacteria, and subsequent inhalation of contaminated dusts or aerosols generated by work, hobbies, recreation, heaters, air conditioners, or humidifiers. Although everyone in the environment is exposed during the generation of antigenic dusts, illness develops in only a fraction of exposed subjects. This allows an epidemiologic separation of the exposed population into two groups: exposed-diseased (ED) and exposed-nondiseased (END).

Careful study of these two groups has aided our understanding of the immunopathogenesis of the chronic phase of this illness. When human beings are exposed to respirable antigen, some clearance of antigen occurs by nonimmune mechanisms. When the amount of antigen inhaled is large, some type of reaction ensues. For example, Semenzato and co-workers assessed peripheral blood, lung lavage, and lung biopsy lymphocytes in ED and END farmers. These data, shown in Table 372.2, demonstrate that the most impressive difference is an expansion of lung cytotoxic lymphocytes (HNK-1) in the ED group. This expansion was mirrored by the presence of cytotoxic functional activity in ED but not END subjects. Possibly these cells can mediate part of the illness.

Humoral immune responses are also stimulated by inhaled antigen. Precipitating antibodies to the relevant antigen are almost always detected in the serum of diseased subjects who have experienced recent exposure (within a few months). As with indexes of cellular immunity, there is overlap between ED and END patients. About half of END patients have detectable antibodies.

The precise mechanism by which the immune response injures the lung is uncertain. Acute exposure of ED patients to antigen results in a neutrophilic granulocyte response in the lung, suggesting that antibody–antigen complex interactions might be important in the genesis of the acute syndrome. By contrast, the presence of parenchymal granulomas and increased numbers of cytotoxic lymphocytes in lavage cell populations of ED patients in the subacute period of illness suggests that mononuclear cells have a role in this phase. Likewise, the factors that predispose to disease have not been revealed by study of ED and END subject groups. Preliminary studies do not support a critical difference in immune response gene phenotype. Other nonimmune host defense characteristics (e.g., breathing pattern, ciliary clearance, cough) may play a role.

TABLE 372.1.	AGENTS OF HYPERSENSITIVITY PNEUMONITIS	
Agent	**Exposure**	**Disease**
Thermophilic Actinomycetes		
Saccharopolyspora rectivirgula	Moldy compost	Farmer's lung
Thermoactinomyces sacchari	Moldy sugar cane	Bagassosis
Thermoactinomyces vulgaris		
Thermoactinomyces viridis	Moldy compost	Mushroom worker's lung
Thermoactinomyces candidus	Contaminated forced-air systems	Ventilation pneumonitis
Fungi		
Alternaria sp.	Moldy wood chips	Woodworker's lung
Pullularia pullulans	Moldy redwood dust	Sequoiosis
Aspergillus clavatus	Moldy malt	Malt worker's lung
Penicillium frequentans	Moldy work dust	Suberosis
Penicillium caseii		
Penicillium roqueforti	Cheese mold	Cheese worker's lung
Phoma sp.	Moldy shower curtain	Shower curtain lung
Mucor stolonifer	Paprika dust	Paprika splitter's lung
Cryptostoma corticale	Moldy maple bark	Maple bark stripper's lung
Animal Proteins		
Avian proteins	Avian droppings	Bird breeder's lung
Bovine and porcine	Heterologous proteins	Pituitary snuff user's lung
Rodent urinary proteins	Rodent urine	Laboratory animal worker's lung
Sea snail shells	Shell dust	Mollusk shell hypersensitivity
Arthropods		
Sitophilus grainarius	Infested wheat	Wheat weevil
Chemicals		
Phthalic anhydride	Epoxy resin	Epoxy resin worker's lung
Toluene diisocyanate	Paint catalyst	Porcelain refinisher's lung
Trimellitic anhydride	Trimellitic anhydride	Plastic worker's lung
Other Agents		
Ameba, various fungi	Contaminated systems	Ventilation pneumonitis
Bacillus subtilis	Detergent enzymes	Enzyme worker's lung
Hair dust	Animal proteins	Furrier's lung
Coffee dust	?	Coffee worker's lung
Thatched-roof dust	?	New Guinea lung
Shitake mushroom spores	Mushroom cultivation	Mushroom worker's lung

Finally, one host factor has clearly been isolated: cigarette smoking. Curiously, the smoking habit seems to be protective because attack rates among smokers are dramatically lower than rates among nonsmokers. A recent study shows that smoking reduces serum IgG antibody titers to inhaled antigen. Mucosal IgA responses were unaffected as were responses to parenteral injection of antigens.

PATHOLOGIC FACTORS

Clinical hypersensitivity pneumonitis is often a benign illness in which the history is of paramount importance in making the diagnosis. Pathologic specimens are obtained in general only from unusual examples of the syndrome (when the diagnosis is in doubt or when the lesion is unusually severe). Pathologic series of cases from the literature are plagued with this problem; there is no prospective series. In one large series reported from an area endemic for farmer's lung, a useful, lucid description of

the incidence of specific lesions detected in 60 biopsy specimens is provided.

The most common finding (100% of specimens) was an interstitial infiltrate composed predominantly of lymphocytes but containing variable numbers of neutrophils and eosinophils. Granulomas were detected in 70% of specimens. Some evidence of foreign-body accumulation was present in 60% of specimens, and there was a component of bronchiolitis in half of the cases. In this series vasculitis was not noted, and it is rare in other descriptions as well. These histologic findings are not specific, but the constellation of a pleomorphic interstitial infiltrate, predominantly of lymphocytes, with some granuloma formation and a component of bronchiolitis should be suggestive of the diagnosis. Some overlapping may be seen with sarcoidosis and with the more recently described entity of bronchiolitis obliterans with organizing pneumonia. Granulomas are not a feature of bronchiolitis obliterans with organizing pneumonia, however, and lymphocyte subset analysis of lavage or biopsy specimens would allow some discrimination between hypersensitivity pneumonitis and sarcoidosis (T8 cells are increased in hypersen-

Cell Type[a]	ED	END	Control Subjects
% Lymphocytes	78	36	7.5
% CD4	25	28	43
% CD8	61	38	22
CD4:CD8	0.47	0.88	2.0
% HNK1	30	21	10
NK function	+ +	−	−

TABLE 372.2. LUNG CELL CHANGES ASSOCIATED WITH HYPERSENSITIVITY PNEUMONITIS AND WITH CHRONIC EXPOSURE TO ANTIGEN

[a] Cell type refers to percentages of lymphocytes and lymphocytes staining positively for CD4 (helper subtype), CD8 (supressor/cytotoxic), and HNK1 (cytotoxic cells) recovered from the lower respiratory tract of patients with hypersensitivity pneumonitis (ED), control subjects chronically exposed to similar antigens (END), and nonexposed control subjects. NK function refers to killing of cell targets by lung lymphocytes.
ED, exposed-disased subjects; END, exposed-nondiseased subjects; NK, natural killer cell.
(Data abstracted from Semenzato G, et al. Lung T cells in hypersensitivity pneumonitis: phenotypic and functional analyses. *J Immunol* 1986;137:1164.)

sitivity pneumonitis and T4 cells are expanded in sarcoidosis). The pathologic process also mirrors the common physiologic finding of restriction (interstitial infiltrate) with varying amounts of obstruction (bronchiolitis), described later.

CLINICAL FINDINGS

Patients with exposure to relevant antigens may develop a variety of symptoms. Although these presentations can be divided into three groups, these groups constitute a spectrum of clinical cases, and considerable overlap is seen for individual patients. Important in the clinical presentation is the tendency for the illness to attack nonsmokers. Epidemiologic studies indicate that the disease is two- fold to ten-fold more common in nonsmokers. Although a similar "protective" effect of smoking is seen in sarcoidosis, the mechanism of this effect is unknown.

ACUTE PNEUMONITIS

Heavy acute exposure may result in sudden onset of clinical illness. Symptoms include fever, chills, malaise, headache, and dyspnea. Cough is variable. Although the chief lung insult is to the alveolar zone and small airways, occasionally patients with prior history of allergies (e.g., rhinitis or asthma) may present with a component of wheezing indicative of large-airway involvement. This syndrome usually peaks in intensity 3 to 6 hours after initial exposure. The degree of disability at the peak of symptoms may range from moderate illness reminiscent of influenza to noncardiogenic pulmonary edema requiring mechanical ventilatory support. Death has been reported.

This illness should be distinguished from another, similar clinical syndrome: organic dust toxic syndrome. This illness is characterized by fever beginning a few hours after exposure to dust contaminated by endotoxins. Immunity to organic antigens is absent. The patient may experience flulike symptoms. However, dyspnea is absent. Workers in several occupations that involve exposure to dust have reported these symptoms. Some of these occupations also are associated with hypersensitivity pneumonitis.

SUBACUTE ILLNESS

Some patients may have minimal symptoms at the time of acute exposures. These subjects may note only vague malaise and chilliness after exposure—symptoms similar to those of a mild viral syndrome. With recurrent exposure these symptoms continue, and weight loss, anorexia, night sweats, and headache may develop. Respiratory symptoms of chest tightness and cough gradually dominate the illness. Some hemoptysis has been noted in up to one-fourth of patients. As in the acute syndrome, the constitutional symptoms and chest tightness tend to peak about 6 hours after each exposure. Furthermore, the patient may feel remarkably better after avoiding exposure for several days. For example, subjects with occupational exposure may note gradual progressive improvement during vacation periods. Eliciting a history of such symptom fluctuation is of paramount importance in establishing a firm diagnosis.

CHRONIC FIBROSIS

Some exposed individuals may have chronic lung scarring after prolonged exposure to the relevant stimulus. Dyspnea becomes chronic, and the symptom fluctuation with exposure may be lost. However, all of these patients have clear histories of chronic exposure to large amounts of antigen and of previous acute or subacute bouts of illness. At this point, the disease is otherwise indistinguishable from other chronic inflammatory lung diseases. The outcome from the chronic phase of the illness is similar to that described for idiopathic pulmonary fibrosis.

LABORATORY FINDINGS

Although a welter of tests is available, none of these tests is specific for this illness. This nonspecificity results from both the intrinsic nonspecificity of the tests (e.g., chest radiograph, leukocyte count) and from the tendency for most END subjects to have some reaction to the antigen (e.g., serum precipitins). Because no test is diagnostic per se, the diagnosis rests on construction of the elements of a clinical syndrome. The foundation for this syndrome is a careful clinical history of exacerbation of symptoms that occurs 3 to 6 hours after acute exposure and a remission in symptoms that follows avoidance of contact with the antigen. A history of potential sources of antigen in the workplace (e.g., antigenic dust, hapten fumes, or farming) or at home (e.g., pigeon cooups, humidifiers) is necessary. It is important to remember that certain sources of antigens (humidifiers, heaters, and air conditioners) are not obvious. Although symptoms develop in only about 10% to 20% of those exposed, a history of others in the same environment with similar symptoms may be helpful in these cases. A history of antigen exposure, coupled with the constitutional and respiratory tract symptoms listed earlier, is mandatory for the diagnosis.

STANDARD LABORATORY TESTS

Standard laboratory tests are nonspecific. Leukocytosis is usually found after acute exposure to antigen. Polymorphonuclear leukocytes (PMNs) are most prominent, but an increase in circulating eosinophils is occasionally reported. The erythrocyte sedimentation rate is elevated, and polyclonal hypergammaglobulinemia is noted. Chest radiographs disclose a variety of findings. These include a normal examination, patchy alveolar shadows, diffuse alveolar opacities, and miliary nodules. Significant adenopathy and pleural reaction are rare. Some reports suggest that computed tomography imaging provides useful information. Computed tomography scans show widespread groundglass changes and poorly defined small nodular densities. These findings should suggest the diagnosis. They are not definitive but are seen in most patients.

SEROLOGIC TESTING

Serologic testing is an important adjunct to the diagnosis. Although all exposed persons may react to the offending antigen, antibody reactions are highest in patients with active disease. Virtually all acutely or subacutely ill patients have circulating precipitating antibodies when screened with the appropriate antigen. Unfortunately, the antigen panels for hypersensitivity screening contain only the more common antigens (e.g., pigeon serum, *Saccharopolyspora rectivergula,* and thermophilic *Actinomycetes*). Other antigens that have been described are not commercially available, and there is no uniform method to test for hapten antigens. Finally, about half of the group of subjects with chronic disease test negative for antibody. Many of these subjects have not had recent exposure, and it is believed that the intensity of the antibody response wanes during this interval.

PULMONARY PHYSIOLOGY

Pulmonary physiology is usually that of a restrictive ventilatory defect. This is most dramatic after acute exposure to antigen. Lung volumes and diffusing capacity are reduced in most patients. The signs of restriction may be accompanied by varying amounts of small-airway obstruction, as suggested by the pathologic distribution of the lesions. Some patients may have evidence of significant amounts of airway obstruction because of asthma, predominant bronchiolitis with minimal alveolitis, or even emphysema. These abnormalities in lung function are usually associated with significant arterial oxygen desaturation.

BRONCHOALVEOLAR LAVAGE

Bronchoalveolar lavage is indicated for most patients suspected of having this syndrome. These patients often have complex

histories and laboratory findings that are nonspecific. In many patients, the diagnosis is not obvious, and the physician is forced to consider the differential diagnosis of diffuse parenchymal lung lesions. Furthermore, treatment options may be associated with some morbidity and with significant alterations in lifestyle, and therefore should not be recommended without an attempt to elucidate the diagnosis fully. A reasonable approach in these patients is to perform a bronchoscopy with wedged lavage and transbronchoscopic biopsy. The recovered material is processed to exclude infectious causes of the syndrome. Specifically, mycobacterial, parasitic, and fungal pathogens should be sought in recovered fluids and biopsy specimens. Cytologic examination of recovered cells is most useful. Pathogens are absent (e.g., mycobacteria and *P. carinii*). Differential counts of recovered cells obtained from the lungs of subacutely ill patients reveal the classic finding of lymphocytosis, which may be striking (often more than 60% of recovered cells are lymphocytes; Table 372.3). Small numbers of PMNs, including neutrophils and eosinophils, may be seen as well. Patients who have had acute exposure (within 24 hours) have higher numbers of PMNs. If access to assessment of lymphocyte surface markers is available, lymphocytes in recently exposed patients are of the suppressor–cytotoxic subset, and cytotoxic cells predominate. Transbronchoscopic biopsy specimens tend to show a pleomorphic alveolitis. Infectious pathogens must be absent. Although these bronchoscopic findings of hypersensitivity pneumonitis are never diagnostic, they may significantly increase the physician's confidence in the diagnosis and reduce the diagnostic possibility of infection.

Some confusion may result, with the lavage finding of at least two other relatively common diagnoses: sarcoidosis and AIDS. Sarcoid lavage fluid contains an increased number of lymphocytes, although usually fewer lymphocytes than in hypersensitivity pneumonitis. These cells are predominantly of the helper phenotype. Many patients with AIDS have some degree of lymphocytosis of the lower respiratory tract during their illness and,

| TABLE 372.3. | LOWER RESPIRATORY TRACT CELLS FROM PATIENTS WITH LYMPHOCYTIC ALVEOLAR INFLAMMATION |

Patient Group	% PMN[a]	% Lys	CD4/CD8
Hypersensitivity pneumonitis			
Acute	41	38	NA
Subacute	2	78	0.41
Sarcoidosis	2[b]	40	>2
HIV infection	2[c]	53	0.02
Tuberculosis	4[d]	11	3.6

[a] %PMN and %Lys are the percentages of polymorphonuclear leukocytes and lymphocytes, respectively, among lower respiratory tract cells. CD4/CD8 is the ratio of lower respiratory tract cells staining positive for CD4 and CD8.
[b] May be increased in stage III sarcoidosis.
[c] May be increased in infected patients.
[d] Quite variable in this disease and in fungal infection.
NA, not available.

similar to findings in the peripheral blood, the suppressor–cytotoxic subset predominates. Symptomatic lung disease in these patients is most commonly associated with infection, and such infections are readily sampled by lavage.

OPEN-LUNG BIOPSY

Some patients may need to undergo open-lung biopsy. This procedure should be used in patients whose diagnosis is still uncertain owing to atypical history or confusing lavage findings. Again, the tissue findings are not diagnostic by themselves. They exclude other diagnoses and refocus attention on the possibility of hypersensitivity pneumonitis. Renewed attempts at eliciting a compatible history may now meet with success.

RESPIRATORY TRACT ALLERGEN CHALLENGE TESTING

Challenge testing has been used in some cases. The subject is exposed to the suspected antigen, and a clear response of reduction in lung function and the evolution of constitutional symptoms usually occurs 4 to 8 hours after inhalation. Unfortunately, antigens are not commercially available for these tests, and the tests themselves are not standardized. Furthermore, the clinical reactions to laboratory challenge can be severe. These factors argue against routine use of this potentially useful diagnostic modality.

▮ OPTIMAL MANAGEMENT

Hypersensitivity pneumonitis is initiated and perpetuated by exposure to organic antigens or hapten. Because of its dependence on antigen exposure, the disease may be controlled by antigen avoidance. For example, once the offending agent has been identified, the environment may be purged, as in the case of contaminated humidifiers or car heaters. In some cases, the environment cannot be controlled easily. Farmers who deal with stored hay are unable to prevent fungal contamination. In such instances, a change in work habits could be considered. Because total avoidance of antigen is the best approach, a change in occupation may be necessary. For some patients this is unrealistic. For patients who must continue their exposure, commercial respirators may reduce the amount of inhaled antigen to a sufficient degree as to prevent recurrence of the illness. Electrostatic particle removal devices have successfully cleaned home air.

A period of corticosteroid therapy has been advocated for patients with constitutional symptoms and reduction in lung function. Treated patients usually show a dramatic improvement in symptomatology and lung function. Furthermore, corticosteroid therapy prevents the late symptoms and drops in lung function attendant to antigen challenge testing. Although patients may indeed feel better, corticosteroid treatment is not an ideal therapy. In one randomized trial, treated patients improved more rapidly. However, 5 years later both groups had similar lung function. Treated patients were found to have an excess number of relapses in comparison with untreated subjects. Thus,

therapy should probably be reserved for patients with severe acute symptoms or significant lung dysfunction. The optimum dose and duration of treatment are also uncertain. Initial doses of 30 to 60 mg of prednisone daily and a 2-month treatment course (including a period of taper) have been most frequently advocated. Corticosteroid therapy does not absolve the patient and physician from attempting to control exposure. Corticosteroids are merely an adjunct to the primary therapy—avoidance of the antigens responsible for the illness.

BIBLIOGRAPHY

Anonymous. Respiratory health hazards in agriculture. *Am J Respir Crit Care Med* 1998;158(5 Part 2):S31–41.

Baldwin CI, Todd A, et al. Pigeon fanciers lung: effects of smoking on serum and salivary antibody responses to pigeon antigens. *Clin Exp Immunol* 1998;113:166–172.

Dickey HA, Rankin JA. Farmer's lung: an acute granulomatous interstitial pneumonitis occurring in agricultural workers. *JAMA* 1958;167:1069–1076.

Erkinjuntti-Pekkanen R, Rytkonen H, Kokkarinen JI, et al. Long-term risk of emphysema in patients with farmer's lung and matched control farmers. *Am J Respir Crit Care Med* 1998;158:662–665.

Jacobs RC, Andrews CP, Jacobs FO. Hypersensitivity pneumonitis treated with an electrostatic dust filter. *Ann Intern Med* 1989;110:115–118.

Kokkarinen JI, Tukiainen HO, Terho EO. Effect of corticosteroid treatment on the recovery of pulmonary function in farmer's lung. *Am Rev Respir Dis* 1992;145:3–5.

Kokkarinen JI, Tukiainen HO, Terho EO. Mortality due to farmer's lung in Finland. *Chest* 1994;106:509–512.

Lynch DA, Newell JD, Logan PM, et al. Can CT distinguish hypersensitivity pneumonitis from idiopathic pulmonary fibrosis? *AJR Am J Roentgenol* 1995;165:807–811.

Rameriz-Venegas AR, Sansores RH, et al. Utility of a provocation test for diagnosis of pigeon breeders disease. *Am J Respir Crit Care Med* 1998;158:862–869.

Reyes CN, Wenzel FJ, Lawton BR, et al. The pulmonary pathology of farmer's lung. *Chest* 1982;81:142–146.

Kelley's Textbook of Internal Medicine, fourth edition. Edited by H. David Humes. Lippincott Williams & Wilkins, Philadelphia © 2000.

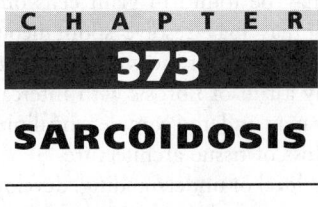

CHAPTER

373

SARCOIDOSIS

LEE S. NEWMAN
CECILE S. ROSE

▮ DEFINITION

Sarcoidosis is a systemic granulomatous disorder of unknown cause that most commonly affects adults. Its manifestations are diverse, affecting virtually any organ, especially the lungs, lymphatics, eyes, and skin.

INCIDENCE

Sarcoidosis occurs worldwide, affecting persons of all ages, races, and gender. It may be more common in Scandinavian countries, the United Kingdom, Ireland, the United States, and Japan. Estimated prevalence rates range from 1 to 40 per 100,000 population, with age-adjusted annual incidence rate of 10.9 per 100,000 for whites and 35.5 per 100,000 for blacks in the United States. Because the disease is often misdiagnosed or goes unrecognized, these rates likely underestimate the frequency of this disorder.

ETIOLOGIC FACTORS

The cause or causes of sarcoidosis remain unknown. Reports of work-related risk for health care workers, community outbreaks, and studies tracing case contacts to previously diagnosed cases suggest either shared environmental exposures or spread by person-to-person transmission. Careful environmental investigation of new cases can uncover clusters of disease cases and sometimes point to sources of antigen exposure. No infective agent or single antigen has been consistently linked to sarcoidosis. The disease most likely represents a hypersensitivity response to one or many agents (bacteria, fungi, virus, chemicals) by a person with either an inherited or acquired predisposition. It is likely that multiple genetic factors play a part in the pathogenesis. Associations with human leukocyte antigen genes have been reported, but specifics vary with the population studied. Excess rates among twins and in African-American families suggest genetic risk.

PATHOGENESIS

The basic pathologic lesion in sarcoidosis is the noncaseating granuloma made up of radially arranged epithelioid cells with pale nuclei, a few multinucleated giant cells, and lymphocytic infiltration. Caseation is absent; occasionally, a small area of fibrinoid necrosis may be present. Schaumann and asteroid inclusion bodies may be found in giant cells of the granuloma. Sarcoidal granulomas may resolve spontaneously, leaving no scar; may persist for a long time with little or no fibrosis; may be surrounded by a rim of fibrosis with intercalated fibroblasts and mast cells; or may undergo complete hyalinization and fibrosis, resulting in loss of tissue architecture.

At our present level of understanding, development of sarcoidal granulomas requires at least three events to occur: (a) antigen exposure; (b) a cellular immune response directed against the antigen; and (c) a more nonspecific inflammatory response that amplifies the antigen-specific immunologic reaction. An overexuberant reaction by antigen-specific T cells and other accessory cells, including macrophages, dendritic cells, mast cells, and fibroblasts, results in eventual tissue injury and physiologic dysfunction if the cellular immune hypersensitivity response fails to abate spontaneously or with immunosuppressive medications. For example, in the lung, a T-cell alveolitis occurs, followed by granuloma formation. $CD4^+$ T cells usually predominate,

associated with excessive production of interleukin-2, interferon-γ, and tumor necrosis factor–α, among other proinflammatory cytokines. Further inflammation is propagated by changes in vascular/alveolar permeability and the influx or local proliferation and activation of inflammatory macrophages and other cells.

CLINICAL FINDINGS

Sarcoidosis may involve one organ system or several. Routine chest radiography may identify asymptomatic cases of sarcoidosis. However, the majority of patients present with nonspecific systemic symptoms, such as fatigue, weight loss, fever, anorexia, and, occasionally, chills and night sweats.

ORGAN INVOLVEMENT

RESPIRATORY TRACT

The respiratory tract is involved in over 90% of patients. Chest symptoms typically include dyspnea, retrosternal chest discomfort, and nonproductive cough. Hemoptysis is rare but may occur with endobronchial disease or when mycetomas complicate stage IV disease. Interstitial involvement results in clinical findings of inspiratory crackles in fewer than 20% of patients, with restricted lung volumes and abnormalities of gas exchange on pulmonary function testing. Bronchial involvement often results in airflow limitation and bronchial hyperreactivity. Sarcoidosis of the upper respiratory tract occurs in 2% to 18% of patients, producing nasal obstruction, recurrent or persistent sinusitis, hoarseness, and, rarely, palatal destruction. Uncommon lung manifestations include pleural effusion, pneumothorax, chylothorax, pleural thickening and calcification, lymph node calcification, and cavity formation.

The modified Scadding classification of lung involvement based on chest radiograph findings, which is widely accepted, is as follows:

Stage 0, no abnormality
Stage I, bilateral hilar adenopathy without parenchymal opacities
Stage II, hilar adenopathy with parenchymal opacities
Stage III, parenchymal infiltrates without hilar adenopathy, and
Stage IV, fibrosis with honeycombing, hilar retraction, bullae, cysts, or emphysema

The Scadding system scores radiographic appearance only; it does not score the extent of disease. Radiographic evidence of disease does not necessarily progress through all stages or in a linear manner. The differential diagnosis of the chest radiograph, by stage, is summarized in Table 373.1.

LYMPHATIC AND HEMATOLOGIC SYSTEMS

Palpable peripheral lymphadenopathy occurs in 5% to 30%, and glands are discrete, mobile, and nontender. Cervical, epitrochlear, axillary, and inguinal lymph nodes are the most fre-

TABLE 373.1.	RADIOGRAPHIC MANIFESTATIONS OF SARCOIDOSIS	
Chest Radiograph Stage	**Differential Diagnosis**	
I. Bilateral hilar lymphadenopathy	Lymphoma, tuberculosis, coccidioidomycosis, histoplasmosis, brucellosis, metastatic carcinoma	
II. Bilateral hilar lymphadenopathy and parenchymal opacities	Same as stage I, chronic beryllium disease	
III. Pulmonary opacities without hilar lymphadenopathy	Extrinsic allergic alveolitis, fibrosing alveolitis, histiocytosis, systemic lupus erythematosus, rheumatoid lung, scleroderma, tuberculosis, chronic beryllium disease	
IV. Advanced fibrosis, bullae, cysts	Advanced tuberculosis, bullous emphysema, melioidosis, bronchiectasis	

quently affected. Splenomegaly occurs in about 10% of patients, often resulting in mild leukopenia or thrombocytopenia due to splenic sequestration. Peripheral lymphopenia is the most common hematologic manifestation. Mild anemia occurs due either to granulomatous bone marrow involvement or to the chronic disease state. Thrombocytopenia can be observed in association with splenomegaly or bone marrow involvement.

HEART

Serious cardiac involvement is detected in 5% to 10% of patients, although the autopsy incidence appears to be much higher. Symptoms may include chest pain and palpitations, and previously asymptomatic sudden death occurs occasionally. Half of patients with cardiac sarcoidosis have electrocardiographic abnormalities of rhythm, conduction, and repolarization, more easily detected with 24-hour cardiac event or Holter monitoring than with routine electrocardiography. Other manifestations include infiltrative cardiomyopathy with congestive heart failure, pericarditis, and papillary muscle dysfunction. Echocardiography can identify valvular abnormalities, left ventricular dysfunction, pericardial effusion, and ventricular aneurysms. Thallium 201 myocardial scintigraphy may reveal segmental defects from granulomatous or fibrous infiltrates, although findings are nonspecific. The diagnostic yield of endomyocardial biopsies is low. Early suspicion and diagnosis of myocardial sarcoidosis is essential, since treatment improves the prognosis. Management includes systemic corticosteroids, pacemakers, implantable defibrillators, and antiarrhythmic agents.

EYES

Ocular lesions occur in approximately 25% of patients, with granulomatous uveitis being the most common finding. Symp-toms of acute uveitis include blurred vision, photophobia, and excessive lacrimation. Anterior uveitis may respond to local corticosteroid drops and ointments, but posterior disease requires systemic corticosteroids. Chronic uveitis may lead to cataracts, glaucoma, and blindness. Other ocular lesions include conjunctival follicles, lacrimal gland enlargement, keratoconjunctivitis sicca, retinal vasculitis, dacryocystitis, and optic nerve involvement.

SKIN

Approximately 25% of patients will have dermal manifestations of sarcoidosis. Definite cutaneous findings include (a) erythema nodosum, a vasculitic lesion manifesting as painful, 1- to 2-cm, red bumps over the shins, often accompanied by arthralgias and occasionally fever; (b) lupus pernio, a characteristic violaceous nodular or plaque-like lesion over the nose, cheeks, and ears; (c) purple–red, indurated, annular skin lesions; and (d) any skin lesion showing granulomas on biopsy. In the setting of biopsy-confirmed sarcoidosis, new areas of hyper- or hypopigmentation, macules, papules, nodules, and keloids, especially if changed in appearance, indicate probable dermal sarcoidosis.

CENTRAL NERVOUS SYSTEM

Neurologic manifestations of sarcoidosis, affecting less than 10% of patients, may involve cranial nerves, brain, leptomeninges, or peripheral nerves. Though any cranial nerve can be affected, unilateral facial nerve palsy from seventh-nerve involvement is the most common. Syndromes related to hypothalamic disease include hypopituitarism, diabetes insipidus, and hyperprolactin secretion. Headache, confusion, and malaise, usually accompanied by cerebrospinal fluid lymphocytosis and elevated protein level and magnetic resonance imaging abnormalities, reflect leptomeningeal sarcoidosis. Unexplained peripheral neuropathy, myopathy, and abnormal electromyographic test results suggest possible neuromuscular sarcoidosis.

RENAL

Kidney disease is usually related to nephrolithiasis associated with overproduction of calcitriol, leading to hypercalciuria with or without hypercalcemia. Severe granulomatous kidney disease causing renal dysfunction is rare.

LIVER

Although liver biopsy reveals granulomatous involvement in two-thirds of patients, clinically significant hepatic dysfunction is uncommon. Up to one-third of patients have hepatomegaly or a cholestatic pattern of biochemical abnormalities, with elevations in serum alkaline phosphatase, total bilirubin, and aminotransferase levels.

OTHER ORGAN SYSTEMS

Salivary and parotid gland involvement may cause dry mouth, and probably occurs in about 10% of patients. Symmetrical parotid swelling associated with uveitis, with or without facial nerve palsy, is termed Heerfordt's syndrome. Arthritis most commonly occurs as symmetrical swelling and tenderness of ankles, knees, and fingers. Löfgren's syndrome is distinguished by fever, arthralgias, erythema nodosum, and bihilar lymphadenopathy, and portends a generally good prognosis. Muscle involvement is rare and may include nodules, acute polymyositis, or chronic myopathy.

LABORATORY FINDINGS

Since there is no single or specific diagnostic test for sarcoidosis, diagnosis depends on a compatible clinical picture, histologic findings of noncaseating granulomas in affected organs, and the exclusion of other granulomatous diseases. The evaluation of patients with sarcoidosis must (a) provide histologic confirmation of disease; (b) assess extent and severity of organ system involvement; (c) map which organs are clinically involved; (d) determine whether disease is stable or likely to progress; and (e) assess the need for treatment. Table 373.3 summarizes the baseline tests recommended for any patient with newly diagnosed sarcoidosis. Asymptomatic organ system involvement may be missed without sophisticated and expensive testing. Such involvement is usually mild and of little clinical significance except for uveitis. A slit-lamp examination is recommended for all patients with sarcoidosis. Subclinical hypercalciuria is associated with risk for kidney stones, and baseline 24-hour urine calcium measurement is useful.

BIOPSY CONFIRMATION

Transbronchial lung biopsy is the usual procedure of choice, with a diagnostic yield of up to 90%. Examination of the patient may disclose other possible biopsy sites such as conjunctiva, skin, lip, or peripheral lymph node. When transbronchial biopsies are nondiagnostic and no other biopsy site has been identified, biopsy of enlarged mediastinal lymph nodes and surgical lung biopsy have high diagnostic yields. Biopsies should be carefully examined and cultured for infectious organisms capable of causing granulomatous diseases.

BLOOD TESTS

Baseline complete blood count is recommended to evaluate the presence of anemia, leukopenia, and thrombocytopenia. Assessment of serum calcium and liver function may show abnormalities reflecting organ system involvement that affect treatment decisions. Serum angiotensin converting enzyme level is elevated in more than half of patients with sarcoidosis but can be found in many other diseases as well. Thus, the test has limited diagnostic value but may be useful in monitoring the course of disease.

PULMONARY FUNCTION TESTS

Pulmonary function tests (PFTs) are required to assess lung function impairment and to monitor disease progression or remis-

sion. PFT abnormalities are found in approximately 20% of those with stage I disease compared with 40% to 70% of patients with stage II, III, or IV disease. Exercise physiology testing is a sensitive means for evaluating dyspnea on exertion and for determining the presence of hypoxia. In the lung, the granulomatous infiltration and fibrosis occurring in some patients with sarcoidosis results in low lung compliance, impaired diffusing capacity, and reduced lung volume. Many patients have a low forced expiratory volume in 1 second/forced vital capacity ratio and increased airway resistance. Ventilation–perfusion imbalance and widening of the alveolar–arterial oxygen difference are common. In the early stages, PaO_2 may be within normal limits at rest but decreases with exercise.

CHEST RADIOGRAPHY

Chest roentgenography is necessary and usually sufficient to determine extent of radiographic disease. High-resolution lung computed tomography scanning may be indicated to detect complications of more advanced disease such as bronchiectasis, mycetoma or pulmonary fibrosis, or to evaluate an atypical chest radiograph or superimposed infection or malignancy.

OTHER DIAGNOSTIC TESTS

Kveim–Stilzbach skin testing, in which spleen or lymph node homogenate from a patient with sarcoidosis is injected intradermally and later biopsied, is not widely available, not well standardized, and not approved for general use by the U.S. Food and Drug Administration. Gallium 67 scanning adds little of diagnostic value due to poor specificity. Analyses of bronchoalveolar lavage fluid and cells has provided insight into disease pathogenesis, but none of the findings are specific to sarcoidosis,

TABLE 373.2.	COMPARISON OF SARCOIDOSIS AND CHRONIC BERYLLIUM DISEASE	
Feature	**Sarcoidosis**	**Berylliosis**
Hilar adenopathy	Common	Common but less pronounced
Erythema nodosum	Common in acute stage	Absent
Parotid involvement	May be present	Absent
Bone changes	May be present in chronic stage	Absent
Beryllium lymphocyte proliferation test (blood or bronchoalveolar lavage)	Negative	Positive
Clinical course	Remission common	Remission rare
Response to therapy	Good	Good

including the ratio of CD4 to CD8 lymphocytes. Lavage may be helpful in excluding infection or chronic beryllium disease. A comparison of sarcoidosis and chronic beryllium disease is presented in Table 373.2.

DIFFERENTIAL DIAGNOSIS

The major categories of disease which may mimic sarcoidosis are (a) infections, including those caused by mycobacteria, fungi, bacteria, and parasites capable of inducing a granulomatous disease; (b) occupational or environmental lung diseases, including hypersensitivity pneumonitis, chronic beryllium disease, and other metal-induced lung diseases; (c) drug-induced granulomatous pneumonitides; and (d) autoimmune disorders associated with granulomatous lesions such as Wegener's granulomatosis, primary biliary cirrhosis, and Churg–Strauss syndrome. A complete occupational, environmental, and pharmacologic history is necessary for all patients who may have sarcoidosis to exclude exposure to known antigens. Other specific diagnostic tests should be used where appropriate, such as the blood or bronchoalveolar lavage beryllium lymphocyte proliferation test for chronic beryllium disease, antineutrophil cytoplasmic antibody tests for Wegener's granulomatosis and related vasculitides, antimitochondrial antibody tests for primary biliary cirrhosis, and serologic or culture technique tests for fungal or mycobacterial infections. Some neoplasias are associated with sarcoid-like granulomatous reactions in regional lymph nodes, spleen, or liver. The term *granulomatous lesions of unknown significance* describes patients in whom isolated granulomatous involvement of liver or lymph node is found. Therefore, isolated lymph node granulomas are not definitive for diagnosing sarcoidosis.

NATURAL HISTORY OF UNTREATED PULMONARY SARCOIDOSIS

It is not known why some sarcoidosis patients recover spontaneously while others progress. Even after apparent recovery, recrudescence of disease can occur months to years later, although more commonly sarcoidosis is thought to resolve without relapse. Stage I disease remits in 60% to 80% of cases; stage II in 50% to 60%; and stage III in less than 30%, without treatment. Factors associated with poorer prognosis include older age at onset, black race, symptoms lasting more than 6 months, splenomegaly, lupus pernio, and multiorgan and extrathoracic involvement. In a Swedish study, patients with acute disease who expressed human leukocyte antigens DR3 and DQ2 had a particularly favorable prognosis, whether or not they had erythema nodosum. Pulmonary infiltration, if it persists for more than 2 years, is unlikely to remit without therapy.

OPTIMAL MANAGEMENT

Important considerations and tests to be performed as part of the baseline evaluation of any newly suspected sarcoidosis patient

TABLE 373.3.	RECOMMENDED BASELINE CLINICAL EVALUATION

Occupational/environmental history
Medication history
Exam emphasizing lung, lymphatics, skin, eye, liver, heart
Biopsy of an affected organ, with special stains, cultures
Chest radiography
Pulmonary function tests, including gas exchange
Electrocardiogram
Slit-lamp exam
Liver function tests, renal function tests
Serum calcium
Other tests, depending on clinical/organ system presentation

are summarized in Table 373.3. Corticosteroids are the mainstay of therapy for sarcoidosis and its complications. In most cases, a 3-month period of observation prior to treatment allows for assessment of disease activity. If there is interval deterioration in lung function or gas exchange, oral corticosteroids can be started. Usual dosage starts at prednisone 40 mg per day for 6 weeks to 3 months with gradual taper to a lower dose (5 to 10 mg daily or alternate-day) for 6 to 12 months. There is no single well-established regimen for corticosteroid dosing. Factors that

TABLE 373.4.	GUIDELINES AND INDICATIONS FOR THERAPY

Disease Status	Recommendation
Asymptomatic, no organ dysfunction	No treatment, observe
Mild to moderate pulmonary dysfunction, symptoms	Observe ×3 months and reassess
Airflow limitation and/or cough	Consider trial of high-dose inhaled steroids
Erythema nodosum (generally good prognosis)	Observe
Symptomatic pulmonary disease, with moderate to severe pulmonary dysfunction	Treatment with corticosteroids
Extrapulmonary disease affecting vital organs, including but not limited to heart, CNS, eyes, liver	Treatment with corticosteroids
Deterioration during observation period	Treatment with corticosteroids
Moderate to severe disease that fails to respond to corticosteroids	Add another immunosuppressive to corticosteroid regimen (e.g., methotrexate)
End-stage pulmonary disease	Lung allograft
Cardiac sarcoidosis with arrhythmia	Consider pacemaker or implanted cardioverter defibrillator in addition to corticosteroids
Dermatologic sarcoidosis	Hydroxychlorquine and/or corticosteroids, especially for disfiguring lesions

warrant more immediate or more prolonged therapy are presented in Table 373.4. Alternative forms of treatment may be required if corticosteroids fail to control the disease or if significant side effects occur. Of the alternative immunosuppressives, methotrexate (7.5 to 15 mg per week orally) has been best studied as a corticosteroid-sparing agent, often in combination with lower dose prednisone. Hydroxychloroquine has efficacy for cutaneous sarcoidosis and for hypercalcemia (200 mg twice daily orally). Other agents have yielded varying results or have been studied less thoroughly, including azathioprine, cyclosporine, chlorambucil, and cyclophosphamide.

Before implementing therapy, it is important to establish objective measures that can be followed serially to assess therapeutic response. Where possible, it is more valuable to monitor physiologic alterations in vital organs. For example, gas exchange alterations are more sensitive than chest radiographic changes for monitoring pulmonary involvement and response to therapy.

SPECIAL SITUATIONS

PREGNANCY

Many patients improve and are able to discontinue or curtail corticosteroid therapy during pregnancy. The disease does not have any damaging effect on gestation or on the fetus. In some patients the disease worsens after parturition. Certain immunosuppressive agents used to treat sarcoidosis, including methotrexate and azathioprine, can cause miscarriage or damage to the fetus.

INFECTION

The frequency of bacterial and viral infections in patients with sarcoidosis is not greater than in the general population. Aspergilloma is the common fungal colonizer in chronic fibrotic sarcoidosis.

SARCOIDOSIS, MALIGNANCY, AND LYMPHOMA

Sarcoid-like granulomatous lesions may be found in regional lymph nodes draining a carcinoma or even among the tumor cells at the site of the primary neoplasm. It is important that the local "sarcoid reaction" be differentiated from multisystem sarcoidosis. Large population–based studies suggest increased risk of lymphoproliferative malignancy in patients with chronic sarcoidosis.

LUNG TRANSPLANTATION

Transplantation can improve quality of life for some patients, although sarcoidosis patients may have a higher than normal rate of rejection. Sarcoidosis granulomas can develop in the pulmonary allograft.

BIBLIOGRAPHY

Johns CJ, Michele TM. The clinical management of sarcoidosis. A 50-year experience at the Johns Hopkins Hospital. *Medicine* 1999;78:65–111.

Judson MA. An approach to the treatment of pulmonary sarcoidosis with corticosteroids: the six phases of treatment. *Chest* 1999;115:1158–1165.
Newman LS, Rose CS, Maier LA. Medical progress: sarcoidosis. *N Engl J Med* 1997;336:1224–1234.
Stirling RB, Gullinan P, du Bois RM. Sarcoidosis. In: Schwartz MI, King TE Jr, eds. *Interstitial lung disease*, third edition. Hamilton, Ontario, Canada: BC Decker, 1998:279–323.
Vourlekis JS, Sawyer RT, Newman LS. Sarcoidosis: developments in etiology, immunology, and therapeutics. In: Schrier RW, ed. *Advances in internal medicine*, Vol. 45. Chicago: Mosby, 2000:209–257.

Kelley's Textbook of Internal Medicine, fourth edition. Edited by H. David Humes. Lippincott Williams & Wilkins, Philadelphia © 2000.

CHAPTER
374

THE GRANULOMATOUS VASCULITIDES

ULRICH SPECKS

The term *granulomatous vasculitis* refers to a very heterogeneous group of disorders consisting of Wegener's granulomatosis (WG), Churg–Strauss syndrome (allergic angiitis and granulomatosis), bronchocentric granulomatosis, necrotizing sarcoid granulomatosis, and lymphomatoid granulomatosis. This grouping is merely of historic interest and does not reflect our current understanding of the nosoly of these diseases. The term *pulmonary angiitis and granulomatosis* applied to this group of disorders was coined by Liebow because they share the infiltration of blood vessels by inflammatory cells (angiitis) and necrotizing inflammation of the pulmonary parenchyma, resulting in nodules or masses with variable degrees of cavitation (granulomatosis). The clinical presentations—particularly the pulmonary manifestations of these disorders—may occasionally resemble one another. However, in most instances the clinical and histopathologic differentiation is no longer a problem. New serologic markers, such as antineutrophil cytoplasmic antibody (ANCA) and the application of immunohistochemical techniques, have facilitated the clinicopathologic differentiation of these disorders and contributed to a more appropriate classification that reflects an enhanced understanding of their pathogenesis.

Wegener's granulomatosis and Churg–Strauss syndrome are granulomatous inflammatory processes that usually originate in the respiratory tract and evolve into systemic vasculitis, affecting predominantly small vessels and capillaries. Therefore, they are classified together with microscopic polyangiitis in the group of primary necrotizing small-vessel vasculitides, which are usually associated with ANCA (Table 374.1). Bronchocentric granulomatosis and necrotizing sarcoid granulomatosis are extremely rare granulomatous inflammatory processes that are limited to the lung. They need to be differentiated primarily from infec-

TABLE 374.1.	SYSTEMIC VASCULITIDES DEFINED BY THE 1992 CHAPEL HILL INTERNATIONAL CONSENSUS CONFERENCE ON THE NOMENCLATURE OF SYSTEMIC VASCULITIS[a]

Large-vessel vasculitis
    Giant cell (temporal) arteritis
    Takayasu's arteritis
Medium-size vessel vasculitis
    Classic polyarteritis nodosa
    Kawasaki's disease
Small-vessel vasculitis
    Wegener's granulomatosis[b]
    Churg–Strauss syndrome[b]
    Microscopic polyangiitis[b]
    Henoch–Schönlein purpura
    Essential cryoglobulinemic vasculitis
    Cutaneous leukocytoclastic angiitis

[a] *Arthritis Rheum* 1994;37:180–182.
[b] Antineutrophil cytoplasmic autoantibody–associated.

TABLE 374.2.	ACR 1990 CRITERIA FOR WEGENER'S GRANULOMATOSIS[a]	
Criterion	**Definition**	
(1) Nasal or oral inflammation	Development of painful nasal or oral ulcers or purulent or bloody nasal discharge	
(2) Abnormal chest radiograph	Nodules, fixed infiltrates, or cavities	
(3) Urinary sediment	Microhematuria (>5 red cells per high-power field) or red cell casts	
(4) Granulomatous inflammation on biopsy	Histologic changes showing granulomatous inflammation within the wall of an artery or in the perivascular or extravascular area	

[a] *Arthritis Rheum* 1990;33:1121–1127.
Note: A patient with vasculitis is said to have Wegener's granulomatosis if two or more of the four criteria have been satisfied.

tious granulomatous diseases. Vascular inflammation in these two disorders is secondary. It occurs as the result of extension of the inflammatory process from adjacent areas (bronchocentric granulomatosis) or in the form of non-necrotizing granulomas infiltrating or replacing portions of the vessel walls (necrotizing sarcoid granulomatosis). Both processes respond favorably to corticosteroids and may occasionally even resolve spontaneously. Some authors have argued that bronchocentric granulomatosis and necrotizing sarcoid granulomatosis represent atypical tissue reactions, rather than separate disease entities, and are part of the spectrum of allergic bronchopulmonary aspergillosis and of sarcoidosis, respectively. The term *lymphomatoid granulomatosis* was originally introduced to reflect the clinical and radiographic similarities of this disorder with WG in association with histopathologic features of lymphomas. The prolonged misclassification of lymphomatoid granulomatosis among the vasculitides is the result of the prominent vascular infiltration by lymphoid cells. Advanced immunohistochemical staining techniques now allow most cases of lymphomatoid granulomatosis to be appropriately classified as true lymphomas.

WEGENER'S GRANULOMATOSIS

DEFINITION

Wegener's granulomatosis is a multisystem disorder that is characterized histopathologically by the presence of necrotizing granulomatous inflammation and vasculitis affecting predominantly the small and medium-size vessels. The upper and/or lower respiratory tracts are most frequently involved, followed by the kidneys. However, any organ system may be involved. WG is unique among the systemic vasculitides because its clinical and histologic findings cannot be explained solely on the basis of the inflammation of the vessels, and a primary necrotizing granu-

lomatosis of the tissues (particularly of the respiratory tract) is an integral part of the lesion, frequently overshadowing the vasculitis. Correspondingly, the clinical course of WG is highly variable. It may range from a protracted illness limited to the respiratory tract with predominantly necrotizing granulomatous pathology to a rapidly progressive illness in which capillaritis is the predominant histopathologic feature, resulting in acute renal or respiratory failure.

The American College of Rheumatology put forth diagnostic criteria that allow the differentiation of WG from other forms of vasculitis (Table 374.2). The Chapel Hill Consensus Conference (Table 374.1) proposed the following definition of Wegener's granulomatosis: "granulomatous inflammation involving the respiratory tract, and necrotizing vasculitis affecting small to medium-sized vessels (i.e., capillaries, venules, arterioles, and arteries)." WG is closely associated with the presence of ANCA (particularly cytoplasmic-staining ANCA, C-ANCA, with specificity for proteinase 3, PR3). The diagnosis of WG depends on a correlation of clinical, pathologic, and serologic features.

INCIDENCE AND EPIDEMIOLOGIC FACTORS

The exact incidence and prevalence of WG are unknown. The available limited epidemiologic studies suggest that the incidence is increasing. However, this may be the result of heightened awareness about the disease, changes in diagnostic criteria, and the availability of ANCA testing. The annual incidence is estimated to be 2.8 to 5 per million. Women and men are affected equally. WG can affect patients of any age, with a median onset at age 45 to 55. In contrast to microscopic polyangiitis, WG is more common in patients of Northern European descent, compared to those with Mediterranean background. The disease is rare in African Americans. Whether this reflects a genetic predisposition or environmental factors remains unclear.

ETIOLOGIC FACTORS AND PATHOGENESIS

The cause of WG remains unknown. The pathogenesis of the symptoms and clinical manifestations is linked to the nature and evolution of the histopathologic lesions. The characteristic histopathologic features of WG are (a) vasculitis, (b) necrosis, and (c) inflammatory background. The vasculitis typically involves medium-size and small vessels, including arteries, arterioles, capillaries, venules, and veins. The large vessels are rarely affected. There may be simply a mural cellular infiltrate or fibrinoid necrosis. More frequently, an intramural eccentric necrotizing granulomatous lesion is found. The capillaritis may be neutrophilic or, rarely, granulomatous. The necrosis is granulomatous in nature. Microabscesses appear to be the initial lesion. They enlarge and coalesce until the typical geographic and basophilic appearance of the necrosis has developed. The necrotic center is surrounded by palisading histiocytes and scattered giant cells. Occasionally, the necrosis may be bronchocentric. The inflammatory background of the granulomatous necrosis and vasculitis can cause extensive parenchymal consolidation mimicking organizing pneumonia. The cellular infiltrates are mixed, consisting of lymphocytes, plasma cells, scattered giant cells, and eosinophils. Sarcoid-like non-necrotizing granulomas are absent. Several atypical histopathologic patterns have also been described.

There is increasing evidence that the interaction of monocytes and T cells is significant in the pathogenesis of WG. T cells from patients with active disease overproduce interferon-γ and tumor necrosis factor-α, apparently due to dysregulated interleukin-12 production by monocytes. In addition, the ANCA target antigen, PR3, was shown to enhance T-lymphocyte proliferation in WG patients compared to controls.

Clinical, in vitro, and even some animal model observations support a pathogenic role for ANCA in the development of small-vessel vasculitis. ANCA is present in most patients with active generalized WG; however, they cannot be detected in about a third of patients with biopsy-proven active WG limited to the respiratory tract. ANCA titers change in relation to disease activity in most patients. Finally, patients in complete remission do not appear to relapse in the absence of ANCA, even though the converse is not always the case. Many in vitro studies have shown proinflammatory effects of ANCA on neutrophils, monocytes, and endothelial cells such as oxygen radical release, degranulation, cytokine release, and expression of cell adhesion molecules, all of which, directly or indirectly, alone and in combination, may contribute to cell injury and tissue destruction. While ANCA may not be essential for the initiation of WG, its presence seems to play a crucial role in the modulation of the inflammatory cascade leading to small-vessel vasculitis.

Upper respiratory tract infections have been implicated in the pathogenesis of WG, but the exact mechanisms by which they may trigger the initial onset of disease or subsequent relapses remain unclear.

CLINICAL FINDINGS

Wegener's granulomatosis usually affects the respiratory tract first. Symptoms caused by predominantly necrotizing granulo-

matous inflammation of the upper airways and/or the lung may predominate and persist for variable amounts of time (limited phase of the disease) before progressing to the generalized phase of the disease, during which the organ injury caused by small-vessel vasculitis determines the clinical picture and outcome. The limited phase of the disease may be associated with minimal morbidity. Usually it is associated with few constitutional symptoms, and nonspecific markers of inflammatory activity such as the erythrocyte sedimentation rate and the C-reactive protein are only minimally elevated. The generalized vasculitic phase of the disease is usually associated with prominent constitutional symptoms such as malaise, fevers, night sweats, and weight loss. The presence of migratory arthralgias affecting the large joints is also a sign of generalized disease. The erythrocyte sedimentation rate and the C-reactive protein are markedly elevated, as are other markers of acute-phase reaction. While most patients, if untreated, will progress from limited disease to generalized disease with kidney involvement, this progression does not occur in every patient. The presence of C-ANCA appears to be a prognostic indicator in this context.

The clinical manifestations of WG may be highly heterogeneous (Table 374.3), and any organ system can be affected. At first, when all of these symptoms may occur in isolation, a positive PR3–ANCA test may be the only indicator of an impending systemic disease.

Eye involvement occurs in about 40% to 70% of patients over the course of their disease, and the frequency and type of eye involvement do not differ between patients with limited and generalized disease. The "red eye" may be the initial manifestation of the disease. Conjunctivitis, scleritis, episcleritis, corneal ulcerations, and uveitis may all persist as the only organ manifestation of the disease for protracted periods of time. Inflammatory pseudotumor of the orbit associated with proptosis, lid swelling, chemosis, and limitations of ocular movement can affect one or both eyes and should be differentiated from metastatic malignancies, lymphoma, and sarcoidosis of the orbit. Retinal vasculitis and optic neuropathy are more commonly encountered in patients with generalized disease. Involvement of the nasolacrimal system can be the cause of epiphora, dacryocystitis, and draining fistulas.

Most frequently, chronic rhinitis with or without epistaxis and nasal crusting, chronic sinusitis, and recurrent or chronic serous otitis are the first symptoms of the disease. Destruction of the nasal cartilage may be the cause of the typical nasal septal perforation or saddle-nose deformity. Ulcerations of the oropharynx, gingival hyperplasia with clefting and petechiae, and salivary gland involvement are other potential manifestations of otorhinogologic inflammation and may represent a convenient site for a diagnostic tissue biopsy. Tracheobronchial involvement can cause symptoms that may initially be mistaken for asthma. The inspiratory and expiratory flow–volume loop allows a preliminary determination of the location of the airway obstruction. The acute inflammation of the airways may present as tracheobronchial ulceration, intraluminal inflammatory pseudotumor, or, if the cartilage is involved, bronchomalacia. The most common location of tracheobronchial involvement is the immediate subglottic area. The healing of tracheobronchial lesions may result in significant scarring and be the cause of persistent morbid-

TABLE 374.3.	ORGAN-SPECIFIC SYMPTOMS AND FINDINGS OF WEGENER'S GRANULOMATOSIS

Organ	Predominantly Caused by Necrotizing Granulomatous Inflammation	Predominantly Caused by Small-Vessel Vasculitis[a]
Eye	Orbital pseudotumor, lacrimal duct stenosis	Conjunctivitis, episcleritis–scleritis, corneoscleral ulceration, uveitis, retinal vasculitis, optic neuritis, central artery occlusion
Ear	Serous otitis, chronic/subacute otitis or mastoiditis (conductive hearing loss)	Sensorineural hearing loss
Nose	Epistaxis, narcotizing inflammation with crusting, chondritis, septum perforation, saddle-nose deformity	
Sinuses	Mucosal thickening, pansinusitis, bony destruction	
Oral cavity	Hyperplastic gingivitis, ulcerations, jaw pain	
Salivary glands	Salivary gland swelling	
Trachea, bronchi	Subglottic stenosis, inflammatory pseudotumor, ulceration, bronchomalacia	
Lung	Solitary or multiple nodules, thick- or thin-walled cavities, localized or diffuse opacities, atelectasis, lobar collapse	Alveolar hemorrhage, respiratory failure
Pleura	Effusion, inflammatory pseudotumor	
Heart	Granulomatous valvulitis of aortic or mitral valves*	Coronariitis, myocardial infarct, pericarditis, pancarditis
Kidney	Periglomerular granulomatosis	Focal, segmental necrotizing glomerulonephritis, rapidly progressive glomerulonephritis (with crescent formation), renal insufficiency
Genital tract	Orchitis, epididymitis, prostatitis	
Spleen	Splenomegaly	Splenic infarcts
Gastrointestinal tract		Bowel perforation
Skin	Pyoderma gangrenosum	Urticaria, papules, vesicles, erythema, petechiae, ulcerations, palpable purpura
Joints	Arthralgias (frequently migratory)	Oligo- or monoarthritis (usually migratory, rarely destructive), polyarthritis of small and large joints
Central nervous system		Multiple mononeuropathy, cranial nerve palsies, symmetric peripheral neuropathies, cerebral infarcts, seizures, transverse myelitis, aseptic meningitis

[a] Clinical manifestations resulting predominantly from small-vessel vasculitis usually require therapeutic regimens that include cyclophosphamide. If the clinical manifestations are limited to symptoms caused predominantly by necrotizing granulomatous inflammation, less aggressive treatment regimens may be preferable, unless the location of the inflammation mandates the most aggressive approach (*).

ity, such as airway obstruction, bronchomalacia, and recurrent postobstructive pneumonia. The airway lesions observed in WG may be identical to those observed more rarely in microscopic polyangiitis and difficult to differentiate from those associated with relapsing polychondritis.

Necrotizing granulomatous lesions of the lung may present as solitary pulmonary nodules or masses. More frequently these lesions are multiple, and characteristically they cavitate. While these granulomatous lesions of the lung can be the cause of mild hemoptysis, they are usually somewhat asymptomatic. The differential diagnosis of the lung nodules or masses of WG include primary or metastatic malignancies of the lung, including lymphomatoid granulomatosis, infectious processes such as fungal or nocardia infections, and other idiopathic pulmonary processes such as necrotizing sarcoid granulomatosis.

Alveolar hemorrhage resulting from capillaritis of the lung is a less frequent pulmonary manifestation of WG. It may rapidly lead to respiratory failure and is associated with a mortality of about 50%. While alveolar hemorrhage may occur as an isolated disease manifestation, it is usually associated with renal involvement. In the absence of other granulomatous features of WG, such a presentation is clinically indistinguishable from microscopic polyangiitis or Goodpasture's syndrome, and only the serologic detection of ANCA reacting with PR3 may allow a nosologic distinction from these other syndromes. Pleural effusions (small, exudative), pleural inflammatory pseudotumors (rare), and hilar adenopathy (usually only detectable by computed tomography scan) occur in less than 10% of patients.

Skin involvement may develop in up to 50% of patients over the course of their disease. In 10% it is part of the initial presentation. Leukocytoclastic vasculitis presenting as palpable purpura with or without petechial lesions is the most common manifestation and usually an indicator of the generalized phase of the disease. The presence of PR3–ANCA in patients with isolated leukocytoclastic vasculitis can predict the later development of other characteristic lesions of WG. Necrotizing granulomatous lesions of the skin or pyoderma gangrenosum–like lesions are encountered more rarely.

Nervous system involvement is rarely an initial presentation of WG, but during the course of the disease it affects up to one-third of patients. Peripheral neuropathy, frequently in the form of multiple mononeuropathy, is the most common abnormality, followed by cranial neuropathies. The neuropathy of WG is thought to be caused by vasculitis of the vasa nervorum and consequently to be an indicator of generalized disease. Contiguous spread of the granulomatous inflammation from the respiratory tract can also lead to neurologic symptoms, particularly cranial nerve palsies. Granulomatous infiltration of the pituitary gland can cause diabetes insipidus. Cerebrovascular events, seizures, and meningeal involvement are other rare complications of nervous system involvement.

The glomerulonephritis of WG affects up to 70% of patients and is the result of capillaritis. It requires prompt immunosuppressive therapy to prevent irreversible loss of renal function. The characteristic renal lesion is focal, segmental necrotizing glomerulonephritis with or without crescent formation. This lesion is not specific for WG and is also found in microscopic polyangiitis, Goodpasture's syndrome, or systemic lupus erythematosus (SLE). Immunofluorescence microscopy shows no or only scant immune deposits in WG and microscopic polyangiitis ("pauci-immune"), in contrast to the linear distribution of immune deposits along the basement membranes in Goodpasture's syndrome or the granular immune complex deposits in SLE and other forms of glomerulonephritis. Granulomatous lesions that would allow a distinction between WG and microscopic polyangiitis are rarely detected on renal biopsy specimens. On rare occasions, renal involvement precedes other specific organ manifestations of WG.

The clinical course of WG is unpredictable and the degree and extent of organ involvement determine the outcome. Renal involvement and alveolar hemorrhage carry the worst prognosis.

LABORATORY FINDINGS

Laboratory tests that should be obtained on all patients with suspected WG include an erythrocyte sedimentation rate (ESR), C-reactive protein, a complete blood count, a serum chemistry group, urinalysis, and urine microscopy. If renal involvement becomes apparent on urine testing or if impaired renal function is suspected based on serum chemistry abnormalities, the renal function should be assessed quantitatively. In patients with limited-phase WG most of these parameters are within normal limits, with the exception of a mildly elevated ESR or C-reactive protein. Patients with active small-vessel vasculitis, i.e., generalized-phase WG, usually display a high ESR (more than 70 mm per hour), as well as mild anemia and elevated white blood cell and platelet counts. Active renal involvement is indicated by microhematuria (more than 10 red blood cells per high-power field), red blood cell casts, or serum creatinine rise (more than 25%). Proteinuria is the result of renal injury that may persist after the active inflammation has subsided.

The greatest advance in laboratory testing for WG has come about with the discovery of ANCA. C-ANCA directed against PR3 as target antigen are highly specific for WG. The sensitivity of C-ANCA for WG is affected by the extent of the disease, its activity at the time of sampling, and the methodology used for detection.

OPTIMAL MANAGEMENT

Optimal management of patients with WG requires a close collaboration between the patient's primary care provider and subspecialists who have experience with the clinical heterogeneity of this disease. Early diagnosis and implementation of appropriate therapy are crucial determinants of outcome. Treatment regimens should be individualized depending on organ systems involved, severity of disease, and rate of progression at the time of diagnosis. Complete remissions can be induced in the majority of patients within 6 months of therapy.

Immunosuppression remains the principal mode of therapy for WG. Combined use of oral prednisone and cyclophosphamide is still the most effective therapy and is required for all patients who have rapidly progressive disease and organ involvement associated with the risk of irreversible damage, particularly renal involvement. Patients with alveolar hemorrhage or rapidly progressive glomerulonephritis should receive intravenous methylprednisolone (1 g per day for 3 days) as initial therapy, followed by standard oral therapy. The combination of oral prednisone with low-dose weekly methotrexate (orally or subcutaneously) appears to be equally effective for patients with more limited disease that is sparing the kidneys. Patients with necrotizing granulomatous pathology limited to the respiratory tract lacking evidence of rapid disease progression, and particularly those who are ANCA-negative, may be treated with co-trimoxazole (800/160 mg twice daily), with or without oral prednisone, under careful clinical observation. Other treatment modalities, including plasmapheresis, intravenous gammaglobulin, newer drugs such as mycophenolate mofetil, etanercept, interleukin-10, or luflinomide, remain under investigation and should only be applied on a protocol basis or under specific circumstances by an experienced subspecialist.

Once complete remission has been achieved, prevention of relapse and avoidance of complications of long-term prednisone and cyclophosphamide use become the major goals of therapy. Following successful prednisone dose reduction, cyclophosphamide can be switched to a less toxic agent, such as methotrexate or azathioprine, after about 6 to 9 months of therapy. Long-term co-trimoxazole therapy has also been shown to significantly reduce the rate of relapses.

As most patients with WG require prolonged and repeated courses of immunosuppressive therapy, the prevention and treatment of therapy-related complications becomes a significant aspect of disease management. Infectious complications can be minimized if the white blood count is monitored frequently (no less then every 2 weeks) during cytotoxic therapy and dose adjustments are implemented promptly. White blood counts should not drop below 3.5×10^9 per liter. *Pneumocystis carinii* pneumonia prevention is mandatory during the entire period of immunosuppressive therapy, even if methotrexate is the only agent used. Symptoms of infection should be evaluated immediately and treated accordingly. Diabetes and hypertension should be managed aggressively, particularly in patients who have had renal involvement. Appropriate osteoporosis prevention measures need to be implemented at the onset of corticosteroid therapy. Patients who have received cyclophosphamide require lifelong surveillance for their significant risk of developing cancers of the urinary tract. To preserve future fertility in young patients, consideration should be given to the use of pulse intravenous instead of oral cyclophosphamide application, as well as to sperm banking and ovarian protection measures for male and female patients, respectively.

CHURG–STRAUSS SYNDROME

DEFINITION

Churg–Strauss syndrome was originally called allergic granulomatosis and angiitis and was thought to be related to, yet clearly distinct from, classic polyarteritis nodosa. It is characterized by severe asthma, fever, and hypereosinophilia in association with a systemic vasculitis. The histopathologic features comprise necrosis in association with an eosinophilic exudate, severe "fibrinoid" collagen alteration, and granuloma formation with accumulation of epithelioid and giant cells that Churg and Strauss termed "allergic" granuloma. These granulomatous changes could be found in the connective tissue of any organ, as well as in vessel walls. The most common histopathologic features include prominent eosinophilia of vessels and perivascular tissues with accompanying lymphocytes, plasma cells, and some histiocytes, as well as necrotizing vasculitis of the small arteries and veins, necrotizing extravascular granulomatosis, and, occasionally, fibrinoid necrosis of vessel walls.

The diagnosis of Churg–Strauss syndrome cannot be established based on histopathologic findings alone. The "allergic" Churg–Strauss granuloma may occur as a nonspecific cutaneous reaction in association with a wide range of systemic diseases. At times, Churg–Strauss syndrome may be associated with eosinophilic pulmonary infiltrates indistinguishable from Löffler's eosinophilic pneumonia, and indeed, Churg and Strauss themselves have considered Löffler's eosinophilic pneumonia a limited form of Churg–Strauss syndrome. In addition, cases involving eosinophilic vasculitis and/or extravascular granuloma in isolated organs, particularly the gastrointestinal tract, without evidence of systemic disease have been reported. The term "limited forms of Churg–Strauss syndrome" has been proposed for such cases. Finally, the necrotizing vasculitis of Churg–Strauss syndrome may be indistinguishable from that of microscopic polyangiitis or WG, and prominent tissue eosinophilia has been described in some cases of WG. Consequently, Churg–Strauss syndrome is a clinicopathologic diagnosis, and other forms of systemic vasculitis or eosinophilic syndromes need to be excluded. A study of the American College of Rheumatology (ACR) found that criteria proposed by Lanham and co-workers were more than 95% sensitive and specific for the distinction of Churg–Strauss syndrome from other forms of vasculitis. To be diagnosed with Churg–Strauss syndrome, a patient must have at least four of the six ACR criteria listed in Table 374.4.

At the Chapel Hill Consensus Conference (Table 374.1), Churg–Strauss syndrome was defined as "an eosinophil-rich and

TABLE 374.4	ACR 1990 CRITERIA FOR CHURG–STRAUSS SYNDROME[a]

(1) Asthma
(2) Eosinophilia (>10% on differential white blood cell count)
(3) Mono- or polyneuropathy attributable to a systemic vasculitis
(4) Migratory or transient pulmonary infiltrates
(5) Paranasal sinus abnormalities
(6) Extravascular eosinophils on a biopsy including artery, arteriole, or venule

---

[a] *Arthritis Rheum* 1990;33:1094–1100.
Note: A patient with vasculitis is said to have Churg–Strauss syndrome rather than another form of vasculitis if four or more of the six criteria have been met.

granulomatous inflammation involving the respiratory tract, and necrotizing vasculitis affecting small to medium-sized vessels, and associated with asthma and eosinophilia."

INCIDENCE AND EPIDEMIOLOGIC FACTORS

Churg–Strauss syndrome is distinctly rare. Between 1950 and 1992, 77 patients have been diagnosed with Churg–Strauss syndrome at the Mayo Clinic. Only 20 of the 807 patients with vasculitic syndromes submitted to the ACR classification study had Churg–Strauss syndrome. For the adult population of 414,000 of the Norwich Health Authority, an annual incidence of 2.4 per million has been reported for Churg–Strauss syndrome. Both sexes are affected equally.

ETIOLOGIC FACTORS AND PATHOGENESIS

The cause and pathogenesis of Churg–Strauss syndrome remain unknown. It appears that the allergic background and associated eosinophilia play a significant role in the modulation of the clinical disease manifestations. Serum markers of T-cell activation (soluble interleukin-2 receptor), eosinophil activation (eosinophil cationic protein), and endothelial damage (soluble thrombomodulin) are markedly elevated during active disease, suggesting a close relationship between T-cell and eosinophil activation and vascular damage. It is unclear as to what extent ANCA also contributes to the pathogenesis of the vasculitic complications of this syndrome. Recent reports of Churg–Strauss syndrome in asthmatic patients who used the leukotriene receptor antagonist zafirlukast are intriguing. They raise the question of whether this association is a consequence of steroid dose reduction or of a unique effect of this drug not shared with other steroid-sparing agents used for the treatment of asthma.

CLINICAL FEATURES

Lanham and co-workers gave a detailed description of the clinical features and course of the disease. They identified three phases of the disease: a prodromal phase that may persist for years, consisting of allergic disease (allergic rhinitis, nasal polyposis, frequently followed by asthma). The second phase of the disease is characterized by the onset of peripheral blood and tissue eosinophilia, frequently causing a picture resembling Löffler's syndrome, chronic eosinophilic pneumonia, or eosinophilic gastroenteritis associated with abdominal pain, diarrhea, or gastrointestinal bleeding. Nonspecific constitutional symptoms including fever, malaise, and weight loss are common at this stage of the disease. The eosinophilic infiltrative disease may remit and recur over years before the third phase is reached, which consists of a life-threatening systemic vasculitis. However, these three phases do not necessarily follow one another in that order. In 20% of cases asthma, eosinophilia and vasculitis develop simultaneously.

Most deaths from Churg–Strauss syndrome are caused by cardiac involvement. This may present as pericarditis, eosinophilic infiltrative myocarditis giving rise to congestive heart failure or mural thrombus formation, or coronaritis causing ischemia. Skin lesions, such as granulomas or palpable purpura typical for leukocytoclastic vasculitis, are common. Neurologic manifestations occur in two-thirds of patients with Churg–Strauss syndrome. Peripheral neuropathy is the most common finding, usually in the form of multiple mononeuropathy. Cerebral infarction is a rare feature of Churg–Strauss syndrome (less than 10%) and is usually a consequence of thromboembolism.

Churg–Strauss syndrome must be differentiated from other granulomatous processes and vasculitis conditions, as well as from other hypereosinophilic syndromes. Peripheral blood eosinophilia, a defining feature of Churg–Strauss syndrome, is only an occasional and minimal finding in WG, and an allergic background is no more common in WG than in the general population. Whereas the upper respiratory tract frequently manifests allergic rhinitis in Churg–Strauss syndrome, necrotizing lesions as seen characteristically in WG are rare. Renal involvement in Churg–Strauss syndrome is much less prominent than in WG or microscopic polyangiitis.

LABORATORY FINDINGS

Peripheral blood eosinophilia (more than 10% of total white blood cell count) is a defining feature of the Churg–Strauss syndrome. The degree of eosinophilia appears to correlate well with systemic disease activity, with the exception of the asthmatic component. Churg–Strauss syndrome is classified as part of the ANCA-associated vasculitides, yet data on ANCA testing in Churg–Strauss syndrome and its clinical value for the differential diagnosis are limited. However, most Churg–Strauss syndrome patients have perinuclear ANCA (P-ANCA) with specificity for myeloperoxidase (MPO). Only few patients have been reported to have C-ANCA. However, many patients with Churg–Strauss syndrome do not have detectable ANCA. If present, MPO–ANCA levels seem to correlate with disease activity in Churg–Strauss syndrome patients. Other laboratory abnormalities, including elevation of erythrocyte sedimentation rate and C-reactive protein, leukocytosis, hypergammaglobulinemia, and elevated IgE levels, nonspecifically reflect the degree of inflammatory activity.

Pulmonary function testing usually shows reversible airways obstruction consistent with asthma. Serial peak flow measurements are useful for monitoring the asthma activity and treatment response. Chest roentgenographic abnormalities are also nonspecific. Transient alveolar infiltrates of various intensity, location, and distribution are the most common abnormality, but interstitial infiltrates and multiple nodules (usually without cavitation) can also be encountered. Eosinophilic pleural effusions (usually small) occur in up to 30% of patients. Electromyography is helpful in assessing the degree and course of neuropathies associated with Churg–Strauss syndrome.

OPTIMAL MANAGEMENT

The systemic vasculitis of Churg–Strauss syndrome responds generally well to corticosteroids. The challenge in the management of patients with Churg–Strauss syndrome is to minimize the cumulative prednisone dose and its associated morbidity. The asthma symptoms should be managed according to asthma treatment principles. Zafirlukast should be avoided as steroid-sparing agent because of its reported association with Churg–Strauss syndrome. The role of cytotoxic agents, such as cyclophosphamide, is not as clearly defined as in WG. Azathioprine is the steroid-sparing immunosuppressive agent of choice for Churg–Strauss syndrome, and cyclophosphamide should be reserved for patients with refractory vasculitis symptoms.

■ BRONCHOCENTRIC GRANULOMATOSIS

DEFINITION

Bronchocentric granulomatosis is a necrotizing granulomatous inflammation that is limited to the lung. Characteristically, the inflammatory process originates in the wall of the bronchiole and remains mostly confined to the peribronchiolar tissue. There is minimal extension of inflammation to the surrounding lung parenchyma. Occasionally, the inflammation extends to adjacent vessel walls; however, this does not represent a form of vasculitis. Consistent with the clinical history, histopathologic changes of asthma, such as mucoid impaction, increased numbers of goblet cells, thickened basement membrane, and dense eosinophilic infiltrates, are typically seen.

ETIOLOGIC FACTORS AND PATHOGENESIS

The cause of bronchocentric granulomatosis is unknown. However, it is suspected that this type of inflammatory response represents a hypersensitivity reaction to fungal antigens, particularly from *Aspergillus,* but also *Candida* and *Mucor* species.

CLINICAL FINDINGS

The clinical symptoms are somewhat nonspecific. Younger patients usually present with cough, hemoptysis, pleuritic chest pains, and dyspnea in association with asthma and peripheral blood eosinophilia. In elderly patients, asthma and eosinophilia may be less prominent. Constitutional symptoms, such as fever and night sweats, are common. Most patients satisfy the diagnostic criteria for allergic bronchopulmonary aspergillosis. Chest roentgenograms usually show well-circumscribed, solitary segmental or lobar consolidations or atelectasis.

OPTIMAL MANAGEMENT

As the illness is closely related to allergic bronchopulmonary aspergillosis and usually occurs in asthmatics, the diagnosis should be questioned in the absence of asthma. Bronchocentric granulomatosis needs to be carefully differentiated from a variety of granulomatous infections (fungal, mycobacterial, and parasitic), particularly since similar tissue reactions have been reported in association with such infections. Occasionally, bronchocentric granulomatous inflammation has also been reported in association with rheumatoid arthritis and WG.

Bronchocentric granulomatosis responds promptly to short-term, high-dose oral corticosteroid therapy. Relapses requiring repeated courses of therapy are frequent. Consequently, long-term follow-up is indicated. If the inflammatory reaction is localized and always recurs in the same location, resection of the involved segment or lobe should be considered. Nonasthmatic patients and those without other underlying condition may recover without therapy.

■ NECROTIZING SARCOID GRANULOMATOSIS

DEFINITION

Necrotizing sarcoid granulomatosis was originally described as a separate disease entity by Liebow in 1973. This extremely rare disorder is characterized by multiple large confluent necrotizing granulomas and nonnecrotizing vasculitis, usually limited to the lung. Whether necrotizing sarcoid granulomatosis is a unique disorder has been the subject of debate. Some authors have argued that cases of necrotizing sarcoid granulomatosis represent variants of nodular sarcoidosis. Other cases may represent granulomatous infection in which the organisms are no longer detectable. Necrotizing sarcoid granulomatosis remains a diagnosis of exclusion, particularly of granulomatous infections but also of WG and lymphomatoid granulomatosis limited to the lung.

ETIOLOGIC FACTORS AND PATHOGENESIS

The cause and pathogenesis are completely unknown. Histopathologically, necrotizing sarcoid granulomatosis is characterized by aggregate-forming necrotizing epithelioid cell granulomas and prominent vasculitis. The granulomas are surrounded by lymphocytes and plasma cells. Langerhans-type multinucleated giant cells are always found; granulocytic necrosis and eosinophilia are rare. In distinction to the necrotizing granulomatous inflammation of WG, the inflammatory areas of necrotizing sarcoid granulomatosis are well circumscribed and clearly demarcated from normal lung tissue. The inflammatory infiltrate can contiguously affect bronchial walls and may cause bronchial obstruction. Three types of vasculitis are distinguishable: an epithelioid–granulomatous form; a giant cell reaction resembling giant cell arteritis; and a lymphocytic form lacking granuloma formation and giant cells. Small foci of fibrinoid necrosis may be encountered in vessel walls, but, in contrast to WG, the vasculitis is not necrotizing. Both arteries and veins may be affected. Even though vascular involvement is often seen in sarcoidosis, the degree of vasculitis and necrosis characteristic of necrotizing sarcoid granulomatosis would be unusual for sarcoidosis.

CLINICAL FINDINGS

The characteristic pulmonary nodules, which are usually bilateral, may be an incidental finding in asymptomatic patients. Alternatively, patients may complain of cough, phlegm production, dyspnea, or pleuritic chest pains. Generalized constitutional symptoms occur rarely. Patients of any age may be affected, and a female predominance of 4 : 1 has been suggested.

Chest roentgenographic findings consist of usually bilateral, potentially cavitating, and rarely solitary nodules. Hilar adenopathy is usually not prominent. Pleural effusions are uncommon. Pulmonary nodules or masses, and pleural involvement, are unusual for sarcoidosis. Extrapulmonary involvement has only rarely been documented in necrotizing sarcoid granulomatosis.

OPTIMAL MANAGEMENT

The differential diagnosis includes primarily infectious processes. Special sputum and tissue stains and cultures should always be obtained to exclude mycobacterial or fungal disease. The therapy of necrotizing sarcoid granulomatosis can be approached in the same fashion as that of chronic pulmonary sarcoidosis. Decisions about the use of oral corticosteroid therapy should be individualized based on symptoms, pulmonary function data, and their evolution over time. The prognosis is good and spontaneous remissions may occur.

■ LYMPHOMATOID GRANULOMATOSIS

DEFINITION

Lymphomatoid granulomatosis was first described as a distinct entity by Liebow in 1972. It is defined as an angiocentric lymphoproliferative process with predominant involvement of the lungs, skin, and central nervous system. Many cases previously described as *lethal midline granuloma* and those with the destructive lymphomatoid upper respiratory tract process referred to as *polymorphic reticulosis* represent the same disease process. The nomenclature of lymphomatoid granulomatosis continues to be the subject of debate. The application of the term *granulomatosis* by Liebow to describe the focal necrosis that is part of the lymphocytic inflammatory nodules is misleading, should not be confused with granulomas in the classical sense, and does not reflect the lymphomatous nature of the lesion. However, Katzenstein proposed to preserve the term *lymphomatoid granulomatosis* as it implies that the patient has lung involvement associated with certain characteristic clinical features. The term *angiocentric immunoproliferative lesion,* graded from 1 to 3 depending on the degree of cellular atypia, has been proposed for the same disease process, irrespective of pulmonary involvement. Myers and co-workers suggested doing away with both terms and using terms according to the National Cancer Institute's working formulation instead (*angiocentric mixed small- and large-cell lymphoma* and *angiocentric large-cell lymphoma*). Despite their merits, the different terminologies complicate the interpretation of the literature for clinical practice. The most important message is that lymphomatoid granulomatosis is neither a granulomatous disease nor a vasculitis; rather, it must be understood as a malignant lymphoproliferative process with a wide spectrum of clinical manifestations and a variable course.

INCIDENCE AND EPIDEMIOLOGIC FACTORS

Lymphomatoid granulomatosis is extremely rare. Population-based studies that would allow an estimation of incidence and prevalence are not available. Between 1979 and 1989 only 28 cases were diagnosed as lymphomatoid granulomatosis at the Mayo Clinic. The largest reported series includes 152 cases. Patients of all ages ranging from 20 to 80 years may be affected, and men are affected 1.7 to 3 times more often than women.

ETIOLOGIC FACTORS AND PATHOGENESIS

Lymphomatoid granulomatosis is characterized by lymphocytic infiltrates consisting of predominantly small lymphocytes and plasma cells and variable amounts of atypical mononuclear cells. These infiltrates can form centrally necrotizing nodules. The term *angiitis* was used for the transmural lymphocytic infiltration of vessel walls affecting arteries and veins. Subsequent immunophenotyping studies indicated that the predominant cell type consisted of mature T cells. Because of these pathologic and clinical similarities to angiocentric T-cell/natural killer cell lymphoma, lymphomatoid granulomatosis was thought to be part of the same disease spectrum until recently. Most recent studies have identified the large lymphoid cells in the infiltrate as B cells, leading to the classification of most cases as T-cell-rich B-cell lymphoma. However, in a few cases the large lymphoid cells have been identified as T cells, indicating that some cases of lymphomatoid granulomatosis represent T-cell lymphomas and that different types of lymphoma may present as the clinical syndrome of lymphomatoid granulomatosis. A relationship between lymphomatoid granulomatosis and Epstein–Barr virus infection could be confirmed for most cases of apparent B-cell origin but not for those of T-cell origin. The chemokines interferon-inducible protein-10(IP-10) and monokine induced by interferon-γ (Mig) appear to mediate the Epstein–Barr virus–associated necrosis and vascular damage observed in lymphomatoid granulomatosis.

CLINICAL FINDINGS

Constitutional symptoms, such as fever, malaise, and weight loss, are common. Dyspnea, productive or nonproductive cough, and, occasionally, pleuritic-type chest pains are symptoms of pulmonary involvement encountered in most patients with lymphomatoid granulomatosis. Hemoptysis may occur transiently and is rarely fatal. Chest roentgenograms reveal multiple peripheral, usually bilateral, but occasionally unilateral (20%) nodules predominantly in the lower lungs. Cavitation occurs in about one-third of cases. Massive diffuse infiltrates leading to acute respiratory insufficiency are observed rarely. Small pleural effusion may occur in one-third of patients. Hilar adenopathy is rare.

Involvement of the upper respiratory tract may precede systemic involvement and rarely occurs in isolation. A prodrome of nonspecific nasal and sinus congestion is followed by erythematous swelling of the facial skin and infiltration of the oropharyngeal mucosa. This sequentially leads to ulcerations of the skin and mucosa, with subsequent destruction of the facial cartilaginous and bony structures.

Skin involvement occurs in 43% of patients, typically in the form of erythematous macular lesions or subcutaneous nodules. Skin lesions usually occur simultaneously with lung lesions, but may precede them by days to years, and rarely occur later. The presence of skin lesions does not affect the overall prognosis.

Confusion, ataxia, hemiparesis, seizures, amaurosis fugax, sensorineural hearing loss, or vertigo are suggestive of central nervous system involvement affecting about one-third of patients. These symptoms are caused by infiltration of the meninges, blood vessels, and brain parenchyma associated with occasional tumor formation. Cranial nerve palsies and paresthesias may result from infiltration of cranial nerves or peripheral neuropathies. The prognosis associated with central nervous system involvement is poor, and most patients die despite immunosuppressive therapy.

Any organ system may be involved in lymphomatoid granulomatosis. Hepato- and splenomegaly, bone marrow, cardiac, adrenal, pancreatic, and gastrointestinal involvement have been found at autopsy in 7% to 9% of cases. Renal parenchymal infiltration is detectable histopathologically in 40% of patients but, in contrast to WG, clinically relevant loss of renal function is extremely rare. Glomerulonephritis does not occur.

The differential diagnosis includes chronic infectious granulomatous process, WG, other lymphomatous process, or solid malignancy. If the destructive process is isolated to facial structures, chronic cocaine abuse also needs to be excluded, as it can cause significant nonspecific necrotizing inflammation, with destruction of facial structures on rare occasions. Chest roentgenographic abnormalities are similar to those encountered in WG. Skin lesions that occur on the lower extremities should be differentiated from erythema nodosum.

LABORATORY FINDINGS

Laboratory abnormalities are nonspecific, such as elevation of erythrocyte sedimentation rate, hypochromic anemia, polyclonal hypergammaglobulinemia, or relative monocytosis. ANCA testing may help in the differentiation from WG. The few cases of lymphomatoid granulomatosis tested have all been negative for C-ANCA with PR3 specificity. The diagnosis of lymphomatoid granulomatosis is based on the histopathologic and immunohistochemical findings. Gene rearrangement studies to identify monoclonal proliferation of lymphocytes on bronchoalveolar lavage specimens may facilitate the diagnosis.

OPTIMAL MANAGEMENT

When a diagnosis of lymphomatoid granulomatosis or pulmonary lymphoma is suspected clinically, an open-lung biopsy procedure, such as video-assisted thoracoscopic biopsy, promises the highest yield. In one study, the histopathologic diagnosis of lymphomatoid granulomatosis was established in all of 20 open-lung, but only in 3 of 11 transbronchial lung, biopsy specimens. Significant histopathologic heterogeneity and different degrees of cellular atypia may be detected within the same biopsy specimen as well as at different sites sampled at the same time. Consequently, biopsy specimens should be obtained from all apparent sites of disease before therapy is initiated.

The prognosis of lymphomatoid granulomatosis is generally poor. The median survival of the disease is estimated to be about 2 years; however, the clinical course is highly variable. Patients with limited disease or those who are asymptomatic at the time of diagnosis appear to have a better prognosis. The degree of atypia of inflammatory cells detected on the biopsy specimen appears to determine the outcome. Most patients die of respiratory failure resulting from extensive parenchymal necrosis, hemorrhage, or infectious complications. The combined use of prednisone and cyclophosphamide is not nearly as effective as in WG. This fact and the more appropriate classification and staging according to lymphoma classification systems has lead to the application of aggressive combination chemotherapy regimens early in the course of the disease. However, patients presenting with few symptoms and displaying low levels of cellular atypia may be treated with prednisone alone for prolonged periods. Surgical debridement and radiation therapy may control disease activity localized to the upper respiratory tract and facial structures. Interferon alfa-2b has been used because of its antiviral, antiproliferative, and immunomodulatory effects. Success with cyclosporin A in otherwise refractory patients has also been reported.

BIBLIOGRAPHY

Churg A. Pulmonary angiitis and granulomatosis revisited. *Hum Pathol* 1983;14:868–883.

Cordier J-F, Valeyre D, Guillevin L, et al. Pulmonary Wegener's granulomatosis: a clinical and imaging study of 77 cases. *Chest* 1990;77:906–912.

Hoffman GS, Kerr GS, Leavitt RY, et al. Wegener granulomatosis: an analysis of 158 patients. *Ann Intern Med* 1992;116:488–498.

Hoffman GS, Specks U. Anti-neutrophil cytoplasmic antibodies. *Arthritis Rheum* 1998;41:1521–1537.

Jaffe ES, Wilson WH. Lymphomatoid granulomatosis: pathogenesis, pathology, and clinical implications. *Cancer Surveys* 1997;30:233–248.

Langford CA. Chronic immunosuppressive therapy for systemic vasculitis. *Curr Opinion Rheumatol* 1997;9:41–47.

Lanham JG, Elkon KB, Pusey CD, et al. Systemic vasculitis with asthma an eosinophilia: a clinical approach to the Churg–Strauss syndrome. *Medicine* 1984;63:65–81.

Liebow AA. The J. Burns Amberson Lecture. Pulmonary angiitis and granulomatosis. *Amer Rev Respir Dis* 1973;108:178–182.

Myers JL, Kurtin PJ, Katzenstein AL, et al. Lymphomatoid granulomatosis. Evidence of immunophenotypic diversity and relationship to Epstein–Barr virus infection. *Am J Surg Path* 1995;19:1300–1312.

Stegeman CA, Tervaert JWC, de Jong PE, et al. Trimethoprim–sulfamethoxazole (cotrimoxazole) for the prevention of relapses of Wegener's granulomatosis. *N Engl J Med* 1996;335:16–20.

Kelley's Textbook of Internal Medicine, fourth edition. Edited by H. David Humes. Lippincott Williams & Wilkins, Philadelphia © 2000.

C H A P T E R

375

OCCUPATIONAL LUNG DISEASE

PATRICK G. HARTLEY
DAVID A. SCHWARTZ

There are several reasons for clinicians and clinical investigators to be interested in occupational lung disease. First, the identification of an etiologic agent can result in the resolution of a disease process. This is perhaps best illustrated for occupational asthma, where diminishing the exposure to the inciting agent can improve and even cure the underlying disease process. In contrast, persistent exposure to the causative agent may exacerbate the need for medications and accelerate the progression of airway disease. Second, detection of occupational or environmental causes of lung disease provides the opportunity to minimize or even prevent disease in a similarly exposed larger group of individuals. Further evaluation of a patient's home or workplace may lead to identification of the causative agent, recognition of other affected and at-risk individuals, and recommendations for specific interventions in the local environment that would reduce future exposures. Third, occupational lung diseases provide ideal models for the study of pathophysiologic processes for which the cause is less well known (Table 375.1). Models of occupational asthma have been used to advance our understanding of the physiologic and biologic mechanisms that cause airflow obstruction, and these findings have proven relevant to other forms of asthma. Similarly, the pneumoconioses have provided substantial clinical, physiologic, and pathogenic findings that appear to be applicable to nonoccupational forms of pulmonary fibrosis. Thus, understanding the occupational and environmental contribution to lung disease will potentially have a substantial impact on the burden of lung disease in our society. Finally, this discipline is intellectually stimulating, focusing on the etiologic factors and biologic responses that account for the development of lung disease. It is very likely that this interface between the host and the environment is largely responsible for the development of most forms of lung disease. This point is even illustrated in genetic diseases, such as cystic fibrosis, which have a diverse clinical expression despite a well-defined genetic abnormality. Moreover, investigating the interaction between host and environment will allow us to understand the individual development and expression of lung disease.

TABLE 375.1.	POTENTIAL CAUSES OF SPECIFIC TYPES OF LUNG DISEASE

Lung Disease	Occupational and Environment Factors
Asthma	Aeroallergens, organic dusts, chemicals (isocyanates), metals, and irritants
Chronic obstructive lung disease	Cigarette smoke and cadmium
Bronchitis	Chronic dust inhalation
Granulomatous lung disease	Beryllium
Hypersensitivity pneumonitis	Organic dusts
Pulmonary alveolar proteinosis	Silica
Acute respiratory distress syndrome	Noxious gases
Pulmonary fibrosis	Asbestos, silica, tungsten carbide, and paraquot
Bronchogenic carcinoma	Asbestos, bischloromethyl ether, and radon

The lung is a common site of occupationally induced disease, primarily because of its direct contact with the external environment. Thousands of environmental toxins and commercial chemicals are in use today, the particles of which may become aerosolized or airborne in the form of fibers, fumes, mists, or dust. Individuals living in major metropolitan areas may inhale more than 2 mg of dust every day, and workers in occupations involving exposure to dust may inhale up to 100 times that amount. Despite these circumstances, pulmonary function in most individuals is rarely affected because the lung is equipped with a complex system to reduce the effect of potentially harmful inhaled toxins and to preserve the sensitive gas-exchange mechanism of the alveolar surface.

The development of occupational lung disease in an individual worker is dependent on the toxicity of the inhaled substance, the intensity and duration of exposure, and the physiologic and biologic susceptibility of the host. The physical state of the inhaled substance (e.g., solid, fume, or mixture) and its solubility and aerodynamic dimensions principally determine the initial location of disease activity. Smaller particles (0.1 to 1.0 μm) are more likely to reach the alveoli, but airborne toxins, up to 5 μm, have been demonstrated in the alveolus. In general, larger particles (10 μm or greater) are trapped and removed by the mucous and ciliated epithelia of the upper respiratory tract. Although the respiratory tract is resilient in its response to the plethora of agents contacted in the environment, disruption of the alveolar clearance mechanism may occur if the individual is exposed to highly concentrated particles under certain working conditions, or if exposure occurs during strenuous labor when minute ventilation is increased and mouth breathing is more likely. Depending on the solubility and reactivity of the inhaled substance, acute or chronic reactions occur as particles are deposited on the alveolar surface. Acute reactions with associated edema or inflammation, or more chronic reactions, characterized

by fibrosis or granuloma formation, have been demonstrated following inhalation of many environmental agents.

Several factors may increase an individual's susceptibility to inhaled toxins in the workplace. These include genetic factors related to inflammation and fibrosis, an individual's ability to clear substances from the lower respiratory tract, the presence of coexisting pulmonary diseases, and the effects of coexisting exposures such as cigarette smoking. Occupational lung disease can be challenging to diagnose and even more difficult to study epidemiologically because of the extended time from exposure to clinical expression of disease, often ranging from years to decades. In addition, most individuals are exposed to a variety of substances at one time and may participate in a number of occupations in their lifetime. Thus, many factors may be involved in the development of occupational lung disease. In this chapter, we first address the importance of an organized approach to the patient with suspected inhalation exposure in the workplace and then discuss several specific forms of occupational pulmonary disease.

CLINICAL EVALUATION AND MANAGEMENT

The diagnosis of a work- or occupation-related form of lung disease requires three distinct pieces of information: a relevant exposure history, definitive diagnosis of a specific type of lung disease, and literature supporting an association between the exposure and the disease process. The physician involved in the diagnosis of an occupational lung disease needs to approach these three domains objectively, fully and critically assessing the available data.

Assessment of exposure is unique to the diagnosis of occupational lung disease. Since the clinical presentations of occupational forms of lung disease are not pathognomonic, the exposure history has become an essential component of the medical evaluation for occupational lung disease and should be included in any examination of a patient with lung disease. In cases where the inhaled agent is acutely toxic, little additional information may be needed. However, even under these circumstances, details of the exposure, such as the chemical agent, the extent of the exposure, and its inherent toxicity, contribute substantially to the clinical evaluation. Because of the highly variable period of time between exposure and onset of lung disease, a detailed exposure history should be administered to all individuals with lung disease. The essential features of an occupational history include the following:

- Characterizing the job process
- Listing known toxic exposures
- Assessing the degree of exposure
- Ascertaining temporal relationships between exposures and symptoms, and
- Identifying the use of respiratory protective equipment

Many workers have part-time or summer employment, have been enlisted in the military, or have hobbies that may account for additional exposure risks. Other nonoccupational risk factors, such as cigarette smoking, should be fully characterized.

The goal of this history is to establish a list of agents that potentially cause or exacerbate the lung disease.

With few exceptions, the diagnosis of occupational pulmonary disease is based on standard diagnostic procedures in pulmonary medicine. Measurement of lung function, although nonspecific in regard to diagnosis, is essential for characterizing the functional correlates of occupational lung disease. However, care must be exercised in the use of standard nomograms to interpret lung function. Factors that select workers for a specific job and the healthy-worker effect, which allows them to maintain their job, may contribute to higher baseline measures of lung function in the individual who is being evaluated for occupational lung disease when compared to standard reference populations. Clearly, the most useful approach to the assessment of lung function is to have more than one measure over time and to define whether the rate of change is within the expected or acceptable range. Although the chest radiograph is currently the cornerstone of our diagnostic armamentarium for the pneumoconioses, the chest radiograph is neither a sensitive nor a specific method for identifying the parenchymal or pleural manifestations of these diseases. For example, 15% to 20% of individuals with pathologic evidence of asbestosis will have normal-appearing parenchyma on the chest radiograph. In addition, autopsy studies and studies using computed tomography (CT) scans indicate that the chest radiograph can identify 50% to 80% of pleural plaques. Moreover, the chest radiograph is not particularly effective in distinguishing asbestos-induced pleural fibrosis from subpleural fat (specificity = 71% in comparison to conventional CT scans). In this context, CT scanning of the chest represents a potentially important advance that may substantially improve our ability to noninvasively identify and quantify early and more advanced parenchymal and pleural lesions caused by inhalation of fibrogenic agents (Fig. 375.1). While the high-resolution CT (HRCT) scan can identify parenchymal abnormalities that are not evident on the plain chest film, visual interpretation of the HRCT scan is prone to the same problems observed with the chest film. A reliable and valid system has not been developed to evaluate the type and extent of interstitial or pleural lung disease identified on the HRCT scan. Although attempts have been made to apply the International Labor Organization (ILO) criteria to the interpretation of CT scans, these criteria have inherent problems with reliability and validity. Moreover, the ILO criteria may not be applicable to the CT scan.

The medical literature establishing a clear relationship between occupational exposures and specific forms of lung disease is readily accessible through the standard sources (medical texts and primary literature referenced by Medline). The clinician can obtain additional information from the Material Safety Data Sheet (MSDS), which contains information about the potential health effects of toxic agents and is now required by federal law to be available in the workplace. Occasionally, other less commonly used databases, such as Toxline or Chemline, are needed to access the relevant medical literature. The literature linking exposures with diseases is readily available and should be accessed when one is considering the diagnosis of occupational lung disease. In cases where the temporal sequence of events or the histopathologic picture strongly supports an occupational cause but convincing literature does not exist, the clini-

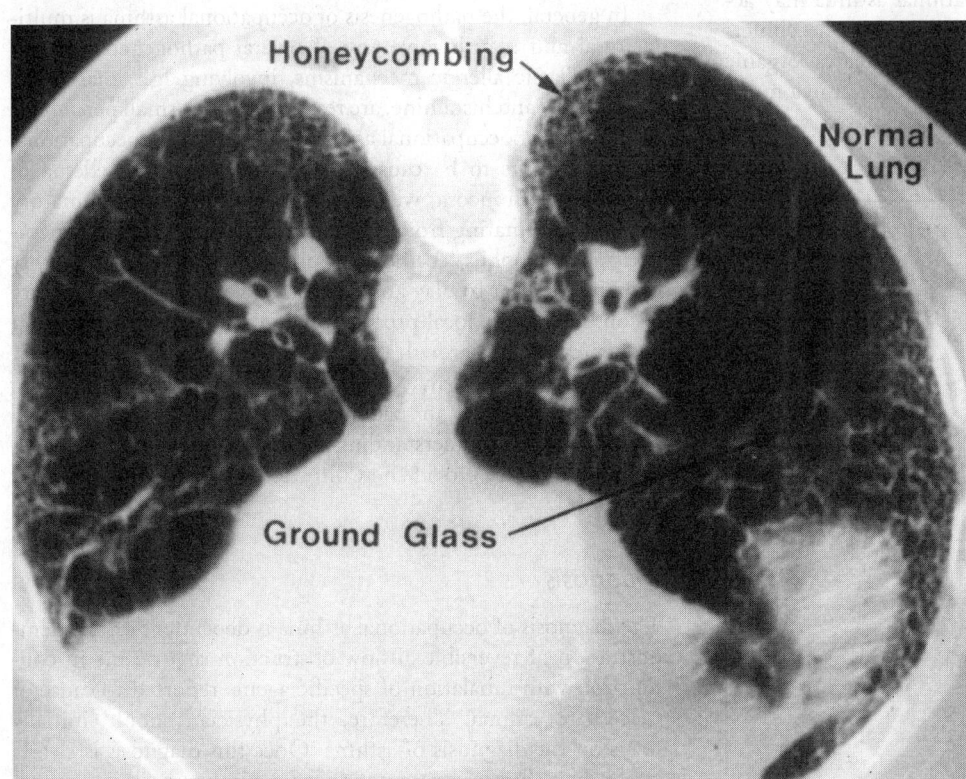

FIGURE 375.1. High-resolution computed tomography scan (HRCT). HRCT is becoming increasingly useful as a more sensitive test than chest x-ray for evaluating workers with occupational exposures. This HRCT from a patient with severe asbestosis demonstrates both honeycombing and an area of ground-glass infiltrate. Importantly, this HRCT scan also demonstrates that asbestosis is a heterogeneous disease with radiologically abnormal lung adjacent to normal-appearing lung parenchyma.

cian should consider referral to an academic center for further evaluation and consideration.

SPECIFIC OCCUPATIONAL PULMONARY DISORDERS

Occupational lung disease can arise from a vast array of occupational exposures, representing every major industrial sector. As mentioned previously, the spectrum of occupational pulmonary disease may be a continuum of several pathologic processes, with severity and onset of symptoms dependent on length and types of exposures and associated individual risk factors. Disease classification is divided into occupational airways disease, parenchymal lung disease, mixed airway and parenchymal disease, and occupational neoplastic diseases (Table 375.2).

OCCUPATIONAL AIRWAYS DISEASE

Occupational Asthma

Definition and Epidemiologic Factors

Occupational asthma may be defined as reversible airflow obstruction associated with hyperreactivity of the airways either caused or exacerbated by exposure to excessive concentrations of irritants or contact with sensitizing agents in the workplace. Increased mucus production, cough, and bronchospasm are hallmarks of this disorder, with symptoms initially evident after exposure to inhaled dusts, gases, fumes, or vapors. Although the incidence of occupational asthma is not known, the prevalence has been estimated to be approximately 5% of all cases of asthma; however, one study suggests that occupational asthma may account for as many as one-fourth of cases seen in the clinical setting. Importantly, some agents, such as isocyanates, organic dusts, and high concentrations of irritant gases, result in a much higher proportion of airway disease among exposed workers.

TABLE 375.2.	OCCUPATIONAL PULMONARY DISORDERS

Airways Disease
  Occupational asthma
  Industrial bronchitis
  Byssinosis
  Reactive airways dysfunction syndrome
Parenchymal Lung Disease
  Asbestosis
  Silicosis
  Coal worker's pneumoconiosis
  Silicate pneumoconioses
  Miscellaneous pneumoconioses and other conditions
Mixed Airway and Parenchymal Diseases
  Hypersensitivity pneumonitis
  Bronchiolitis
  Berylliosis
Neoplastic Diseases
  Bronchogenic carcinoma
  Mesothelioma

Recognition of the occupational factors that contribute to the development or exacerbation of asthma assists in the treatment and control of the disease process.

Pathogenesis

It has been reported that more than 200 chemicals or agents are known to cause or precipitate occupational asthma. These compounds have been divided into three groups: (a) high molecular weight compounds, (b) low molecular weight compounds, and (c) high-concentrate gaseous or particulate toxic irritants. High molecular weight compounds, consisting mainly of biologic proteins, are often the inciting agents responsible for airway hyperreactivity associated with allergic mechanisms. Specific examples include exposure to animal dander, *Bacillis subtilis* enzymes, organic dusts, castor beans, or vegetable gums. Patients are usually atopic and have a positive skin-prick test in reaction to dust extracts. Specific IgE antibodies to dust antigens may be identified using radioallergosorbent tests. Importantly, nonallergic mechanisms may contribute to the development of airflow obstruction in individuals exposed to high molecular weight compounds. Conversely, low molecular weight substances (less than 2,000 d) are usually inorganic compounds and are not commonly mediated by acute inflammatory mechanisms. Examples of low molecular weight agents that cause occupational asthma include platinum compounds, concentrated fumes of epoxy resins, nickel sulfate, isocyanates, and other chemicals (e.g., formaldehyde). Several exceptions to this have been noted with IgE or IgG antibodies identified in workers exposed to phthalic anhydrides, trimetallic anhydrides, and plicatic acid (the agent responsible for asthma in workers exposed to Western red cedar dust).

In general, the pathogenesis of occupational asthma is multifactorial and may involve any of several pathogenetic mechanisms. Classic allergic mechanisms, involving IgE, mast cells, eosinophils, and histamine, are responsible for a small percentage of the cases of occupational asthma. In most cases, occupational asthma appears to be caused by inflammation and edema of the bronchial mucosa, with the stimulus for the inflammatory response originating from airway macrophages and airway epithelia. Neutrophils, eosinophils, and specific proinflammatory cytokines appear to play an important role in the inflammatory lesion. Moreover, local production and release of inflammatory agents (cytokines, growth factors, arachidonic acid metabolites, and oxygen radicals) may contribute to the chronic remodeling of airway observed in patients with persistent occupational asthma. Further understanding of the acute inflammatory response is likely to provide new directions for treatment and early diagnosis.

Diagnosis

The diagnosis of occupational asthma is dependent on the demonstration of reversible airflow obstruction that occurs in conjunction with inhalation of specific agents reported to cause or exacerbate asthma. Therefore, the physician should initially focus on the diagnosis of asthma. Once this diagnosis is clearly established, further examination of environmental or occupational causes should be considered. Pulmonary function testing is an essential component in the evaluation of patients suspected of having occupational asthma. Spirometric patterns of airflow obstruction (see Chapter 388) and the physiologic changes typical of asthma (see Chapter 363) are identical to those of occupational asthma. However, unlike nonoccupational forms of asthma, obstructive airways disease induced or exacerbated by workplace exposures is temporally related to specific occupational exposures. Physiologic testing, either by spirometry, peak flow measurements, or periodic nonspecific bronchoprovocative challenge, can and should be used to evaluate the temporal relation between occupational exposures or environmental agents and the development of airflow obstruction. For instance, demonstration of consistent decreases in peak flows of at least 20% following exposure to a specific agent in the workplace not only helps to establish the diagnosis of occupational asthma but also may assist in identifying the agent. Although specific airway challenges are the most definitive method of making the diagnosis, this test is not entirely accurate, and very few centers are equipped to perform these potentially hazardous exposure–response studies.

Several laboratory tests have been proposed to evaluate patients with suspected or proven occupational asthma; however, their ultimate clinical usefulness is questionable. Serologic or immunologic testing can assist in determining atopic status with respect to environmental allergens. Reactions to specific allergens are limited to the relatively few that have been completely purified, such as extracts of flour and grain dusts, animal products, and certain chemicals. Serum IgG or IgE antibodies may also be measured by radioimmunoassay or enzyme-linked immunosorbent assay methods. Unfortunately, these tests lack the sensitivity and specificity required for making a definitive diagnosis; however, when used in conjunction with other testing methods and a careful patient history, these tests may help document a specific cause.

Optimal Management

Once standard medical treatments have been initiated, including inhaled β-sympathomimetics, anticholinergics, inhaled or oral corticosteroids, cromolyn sodium, or leukotreine antagonists, emphasis should be placed on avoiding or minimizing further exposure. Isocyanates and other sensitizers must be completely eliminated from the environment of those with occupational asthma caused by these agents. However, individuals with irritant-induced asthma may continue to be exposed as long as the concentration of the exposure is reduced to tolerable levels. A majority of individuals have persistent symptoms despite their completely avoiding the offending agent. It has been observed that patients with the most severe symptoms have the longest exposure histories and the most abnormal pulmonary function tests. When complete avoidance of the offending agent is impractical or if the exposure is occasional, the use of respirators or, preferably, improved local ventilation may alleviate symptoms. However, it is uncertain as to whether these measures halt airway injury; therefore, these patients must be monitored very closely.

Industrial Bronchitis

Industrial bronchitis, a disorder characterized by dyspnea and cough productive of sputum at least 3 months each year, is associated with occupational exposure to high concentrations of airborne dusts or where mixed exposures occur. Industries where there are significant mixed-dust exposures include construction and demolition, mining and smelting, food processing, and animal confinement. Workers in industries that manufacture complex materials, such as ceramics, furniture, or rubber, are exposed to a variety of agents that may contribute to increased airway symptoms. Firefighters and emergency response workers are frequently exposed to complex mixtures of potentially harmful agents by inhalation. Confounding the occupational exposures may be a history of cigarette smoking, which further contributes to morbidity. Impaired pulmonary function may result in hypersecretion of mucus in the more proximal airways. Although not all workers are affected by industrial bronchitis and those who are affected often become less symptomatic once removed from the source of irritation, treatment should be directed to minimizing airway irritants, including smoking cessation, and using antibiotics with postural drainage to decrease any infected airway secretions.

Byssinosis

Workers exposed to dust from cotton, flax, hemp, or jute used in the textile industry may experience chest discomfort, cough, or dyspnea. Characteristically, patients complain of Monday-morning fever, referring to the onset of symptoms immediately upon exposure after some time away from the work environment. A majority of patients with these symptoms experience a decreased forced expiratory volume in the first second (FEV_1) over the course of a work shift and, at least initially, develop symptoms to exposures only after having been away from the inciting agent. As the disease progresses, the symptoms of dyspnea, wheezing, and cough persist and are exacerbated throughout the work week.

These organic dusts contain live microorganisms, endotoxins, mycotoxins, and tannins, all of which are capable of initiating an inflammatory response. Direct epithelial cell injury may occur, and inflammatory cells such as macrophages may actively participate in the inflammatory response by releasing proinflammatory cytokine. Although most workers do not develop chronic byssinosis for 10 years or more after inhaling cotton dust, presenting symptoms may vary from mild cough and occasional chest discomfort to marked respiratory failure with dyspnea at rest. Byssinosis, like most inflammations caused by inhaled irritants, is managed by minimization of future exposures and treatment of airway inflammation.

Reactive Airways Dysfunction Syndrome

Definition and Clinical Presentation

The persistence of airway reactivity following acute exposure to respiratory irritants has been termed *reactive airways dysfunction syndrome* (RADS). A variety of inhaled irritants have been associated with this syndrome, including sulfuric acid, chlorine, am-

TABLE 375.3.	PHYSICAL PROPERTIES AND MECHANISMS OF LUNG INJURY OF GASEOUS RESPIRATORY IRRITANTS	
Irritant Gas	**Water Solubility**	**Mechanism of Injury**
Ammonia	High	Alkali burns
Chlorine	Intermediate	Acid burns, reactive oxygen species
Hydrogen chloride	High	Acid burns
Oxides of nitrogen	Low	Acid burns, reactive oxygen species
Ozone	Low	Reactive oxygen species
Phosgene	Low	Acid burns
Sulfur dioxide	High	Acid burns

monia, household cleaners, and smoke. Most often, the initial inhalation injury is due to a single, acute, high-intensity exposure. Symptoms of airflow obstruction, including cough, dyspnea, and wheezing, are reported immediately or several hours after the end of the exposure, and may persist for months to years. Previous exposure or sensitization to the toxic agent does not appear to be necessary. By definition, individuals who develop RADS have no history of respiratory illness. Pulmonary function tests may be normal or they may demonstrate airflow obstruction. Individuals with RADS have persistent, positive responses to methacholine challenge testing, even in the presence of normal pulmonary function tests. Nonspecific bronchial reactivity may persist for months to years following the initial inhalation injury.

Pathogenesis

Inhaled toxins exist in many forms and may be categorized by taking into account their physical properties. General categories include gases, vapors, fumes, aerosols, and smoke. Tables 375.3 and 375.4 summarize the physical properties and clinical manifestations of these inhalants. The initial pathologic responses to a harmful inhaled agent depend on a number of factors, including the concentration of the substance in the ambient air, the pH of the inhaled substance, the presence and size of particles, the relative water solubility of the inhaled agent, the duration of exposure, and whether the exposure occurs in an enclosed space versus an area with adequate ventilation and free circulation of fresh air. In addition, an undetermined number of host factors, including age, smoking status, presence of preexisting pulmonary or extrapulmonary disease, and the use of respirators or other protective breathing apparatus, all impact on an individual's response to the inhalation of a toxic substance.

Inhaled gases with potential irritant effects manifest their actions at different anatomical locations in the respiratory system. In general, substances that are highly water-soluble, such as ammonia, sulfur dioxide, and hydrogen chloride, can cause immediate irritant injury to the upper airway. The acute effects of highly water-soluble irritants on the upper airway, exposed skin, and other mucous membranes often produce such unpleasant symptoms that exposed persons quickly leave the area of exposure, thus avoiding continued inhalation of the harmful toxins. In contrast, inhaled toxins that have low water solubility, such as phosgene, ozone, and oxides of nitrogen, often have little or no acute effect on the upper airway and instead produce irritant effects at the level of the terminal bronchiole and alveolus. Because agents of low water solubility do not produce immediately

TABLE 375.4.	PULMONARY MANIFESTATIONS OF TOXIN INHALATION					
	Acute Clinical Manifestations			**Chronic Clinical Manifestations**		
Substance	**Onset**	**Upper-Airway Irritation**	**Pneumonitis, ARDS**	**Bronchiolitis Obliterans, BOOP**	**Obstructive Lung Disease**	**RADS**
Irritant gases						
Ammonia	Minutes	Severe	+	+	+	+
Chlorine	Minutes to hours	Moderate	+	+	+	+
Hydrogen chloride	Minutes	Severe	+	−	−	−
Oxides of nitrogen	Hours	Mild	+	+	+	+
Ozone	Minutes to hours	Mild	+	+	−	−
Phosgene	Hours	Mild	+	+	+	−
Sulfur dioxide	Minutes	Severe	+	+	+	+
Metals						
Cadmium	Hours	Mild	+	−	+	−
Mercury	Hours	Mild	+	+	−	−
Zinc chloride	Minutes	Mild	+	−	−	−
Zinc oxide	Hours	Mild	+	+	−	−

+, Exposure reported to be associated with clinical entity; −, exposure as yet not reported to be associated with clinical entity.
ARDS, acute respiratory distress syndrome; BOOP, broncholitis obliterans–organizing pneumonia; RADS, reactive airways dysfunction syndrome.

noticeable upper-airway irritation (except in episodes of massive acute exposure), exposed persons may inadvertently remain in the area of exposure and thus increase their duration of exposure to harmful inhalants. Agents that exhibit intermediate water solubility, such as chlorine, can have pathologic effects throughout the respiratory system. However, extreme exposure to any one of these irritants may result in upper and lower respiratory tract involvement. Furthermore, absorption of any one of these irritants on particulate matter may also alter the area of involvement.

Bronchial biopsies of patients with RADS demonstrate an inflammatory response characterized by epithelial desquamation and mucus cell hyperplasia. The exact mechanisms of the pathophysiologic processes involved in RADS are unclear, but implicated mechanisms include altered neural tone and vagal reflexes, modified β-adrenergic sympathetic tone, and influences of a number of proinflammatory mediators. The direct irritant injury may expose and damage subepithelial irritant receptors. Subsequently, repair mechanisms that are not fully understood may result in alteration of the irritant receptor threshold and lead to airway hyperreactivity. Changes in epithelial permeability may also contribute to the resultant hyperreactivity. None of these proposed mechanisms is completely understood at this time.

Optimal Management

Treatment of RADS includes the use of corticosteroids to help minimize inflammatory mechanisms and bronchodilators to reverse bronchospasm. There is limited, mostly anecdotal, evidence for the efficacy of corticosteroids. Bronchodilators may only partially reverse airflow obstruction, especially in later, chronic stages of the syndrome. Despite treatment with corticosteroids and bronchodilators, many exposed individuals are left with persistent asthma-like symptoms, airflow obstruction, and nonspecific bronchial hyperreactivity.

OCCUPATIONAL PARENCHYMAL DISEASE

Parenchymal lung disease may arise from a vast array of occupational exposures that represents every major industrial sector. The most important class of occupational lung diseases is the pneumoconioses, which result from the inhalation of and tissue reactions to various naturally occurring or synthetic mineral dusts. Pneumoconiosis is still relatively common among older men who have been employed in jobs with exposure to mineral dust. In fact, interstitial lung disease (ILD) is much more common than previously thought, and the pneumoconioses account for approximately 14% of the incident cases of ILD. Prior to 1970, when the federal government began regulating the amount of concentrated particulate material to which workers could be legally exposed, dust levels were often extremely high; those exposures that occurred 20 to 30 years ago are reflected in the manifestation of various pneumoconioses today.

Asbestosis and Asbestos-Induced Pleural Fibrosis

Definition and Epidemiologic Factors

Exposure to asbestos (occupational and nonoccupational) constitutes the most pervasive of the mineral dust exposures and

has had the greatest impact on morbidity and mortality in these exposed workers. The National Institute for Occupational Safety and Health (NIOSH) estimated that in 1990 alone more than 40,000 workers were directly exposed to asbestos while working with insulation and that between 3 million and 5 million individuals were indirectly exposed. As many as 25 million more Americans have had occupational exposure to asbestos in the past 40 years and remain at increased risk for asbestos-related diseases. Many millions more have environmental exposures to asbestos from insulation, building products in homes and public buildings, brake and clutch facings, and demolition of asbestos-containing buildings in urban areas. Asbestos has been federally regulated by the Occupational Safety and Health Administration (OSHA) of the Department of Labor since its inception in 1972.

Asbestos refers to a group of six separate fibrous mineral silicates that can be woven and contain properties that allow for resistance to heat and acids. The vast majority of asbestos produced in North America, called *chrysotile* or *white asbestos,* consists of hydrated magnesium silicate. Other forms of asbestos include crocidolite, amosite, anthophyllite, tremolite, and actinolite. Despite decreased demand for asbestos in Europe and North America, its production has remained stable secondary to continued use of this material in developing nations. Most exposures to asbestos occur during the milling and manufacture of asbestos, while installing and replacing insulated packing around heating pipes and furnaces, or while using asbestos-containing cement. All of these applications cause the fibrous asbestos particles to become airborne.

Pathogenesis

The pathogenesis of asbestos-induced fibrosis of the lung parenchyma is unknown. Despite the absence of definitive knowledge regarding the biologic mechanisms that result in pulmonary fibrosis, it is very clear that the chronic inflammatory response is progressive, the inflammation and fibrosis are distributed heterogeneously throughout the lung, and the chronic inflammatory process is associated with extensive remodeling and fibrosis of the lower respiratory tract. Retention of fibers in the lung parenchyma appears to be associated with the severity of disease. Cigarette smoking, which may reduce the clearance of fibers, has been shown to enhance the risk of developing asbestosis. In the lung parenchyma, this chronic inflammatory process eventually leads to proliferation of mesenchymal cells, intra-alveolar fibrosis, and loss of alveolar capillary units. The mechanisms for asbestos-induced lung fibrosis are complex and likely to involve several lung cells and cell mediators (Fig. 375.2). Inflammatory cells (neutrophils and macrophages) and lung epithelial cells are affected by asbestos.

Clinical Presentation

Asbestosis and asbestos-induced pleural fibrosis, unlike silicosis or coal worker's pneumoconiosis, often present clinically as progressive dyspnea. Among patients with asbestosis, dyspnea is often a more prominent complaint than tests of lung function would suggest. These patients complain of a dry cough and pleuritic chest pain. Physical findings include rales, which may

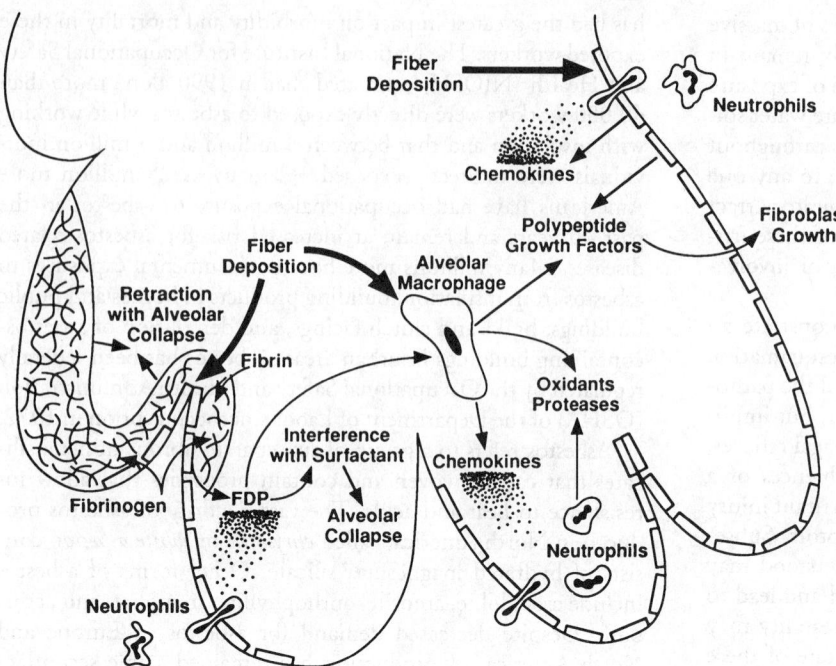

FIGURE 375.2. The predominant biologic processes involved in the development of fiber-induced pulmonary fibrosis. Fiber deposition stimulates alveolar macrophages and terminal airway and type I alveolar epithelial cells to release chemotactic factors that attract neutrophils to the alveolar duct. Oxidants, myeloperoxidase, and proteolytic enzymes directly injure the alveolar wall, growth factors enhance mesenchymal proliferation and collagen production, and alveolar injury increases permeability to fibrinogen and other plasma proteins which ultimately result in induration and collapse of the bronchoalveolar unit.

be absent in early asbestosis and are best heard laterally over the lower thoracic wall. In advanced cases of asbestosis, clubbing and cyanosis may be observed.

Radiographic Abnormalities

Pleural fibrosis with circumscribed pleural plaques and diffuse pleural thickening is the most common radiographic abnormality among persons who have been exposed to asbestos, and these chest wall lesions have recently been found to be independently associated with progressive restrictive function. Asbestosis tends to radiographically progress slowly over several years, even in the absence of additional exposure. The chest radiograph may reveal only pleural plaques and no clear evidence of the small linear opacities in the lower lung zones that are classically seen in asbestosis. Using the chest HRCT scan, several groups of investigators have shown that clinically significant interstitial abnormalities are missed by the standard chest radiograph. With more advanced disease, diffuse linear opacities, often in association with pleural plaques, are observed in middle and lower lung zones. A pleural effusion may be caused by asbestos exposure and is believed to contribute to the formation of diffuse pleural thickening. In those patients who develop diffuse pleural thickening, the lower lung zones have a ground-glass appearance, making interpretation of small linear opacities difficult without the use of the HRCT scan.

Physiologic Abnormalities

Because asbestosis initially involves the respiratory bronchiole, early stages of the disease may involve airflow obstruction. Alternatively, no detectable abnormalities may be demonstrated on routine pulmonary function testing. As the disease progresses, both asbestosis and asbestos-induced pleural fibrosis may result in the development of restrictive lung function. Asbestosis may also involve abnormalities in gas exchange (decreases in the diffusing capacity or increases in the alveolar–arterial oxygen difference).

Diagnosis

The diagnosis of asbestosis is based on objective evidence of both exposure (history, fibers in bronchoalveolar lavage fluid, fibers in lung parenchyma, or bilateral pleural fibrosis) and disease (characteristic radiographic findings on chest radiograph or HRCT, restrictive lung function, or reduced diffusing capacity), without other explanations for the radiographic or physiologic abnormalities. In most cases, the diagnosis is based on a clear exposure history occurring at least 15 years before the onset of disease and on typical radiographic features on the standard chest radiograph. Because the risk of lung cancer is known to decrease with cessation of smoking, it is critical that the physician provide strong incentives for asbestos-exposed workers to stop smoking.

Optimal Management and Prevention

Although there appears to be no effective treatment for asbestosis other than providing supportive therapy for patients who develop respiratory compromise, physicians should consider treating for progressive asbestosis in patients just as they treat for other forms of interstitial lung disease (see Chapter 360). Despite the fact that all new mining and application of asbestos have been restricted by federal regulating agencies, existing structures containing asbestos remain a potential source of exposure in the United States. In addition, use of asbestos continues in developing countries because it remains a very inexpensive form of insulation.

Silicosis

Definition and Epidemiologic Factors

The diagnosis of silicosis dates back to the times of Hippocrates and the ancient Egyptians. Despite being recognized for centuries as a preventable disease, both classic nodular silicosis and the rapidly fatal acute form, silicoproteinosis, continue to be diagnosed around the world. In the United States, a diverse working population numbering more than 2 million is at risk of developing silicosis from exposure to "free" or crystalline silica. Those at risk include persons working with silica abrasives, refractories, or ceramics and those involved in coal mining and milling, metal and nonmetal mining and milling, foundry work, filler manufacture and handling, quarrying, tunneling, and many other occupations.

Pathogenesis

Silicosis typically progresses slowly over many years, even in the absence of further exposure. Recent reports indicate, however, that workers without clinical or physiologic abnormalities and with lesions less than 5 mm have long-term survival similar to that of the general population. Once silica is inhaled and penetrates into the alveoli, a series of inflammatory events is postulated to involve the alveolar macrophage. Macrophages ingest the foreign antigens and package the material into phagosomes that in turn release lytic enzymes, rupturing the phagosome and allowing the irritant to interact with the cytoplasm. The cell is autolyzed when inflammatory mediators are released and the silica is reingested by additional macrophages, which perpetuate the inflammatory cycle. Tumor necrosis factor, released primarily by alveolar macrophages, may be an essential component of the inflammatory response to inhaled silica. In fact, one provocative animal study has shown that antibodies to tumor necrosis factor prevent the development of silica-induced pulmonary fibrosis. Chronic inflammatory responses lead to fibrosis. Over time, collagenous fibers are deposited in concentric layers and undergo hyalinization, becoming a whorled nodule encapsulated by a mostly acellular, discrete layer of collagen (Fig. 375.3). Silicotic particles may be seen pathologically as birefringent material under polarized light. Although the exact mechanisms of pathogenesis are unclear, recent reports have suggested that the electrostatic charge on the surface of the silica particle is an important component of the inflammatory response.

Clinical Presentation

Clinically, silicosis may appear in many different forms. *Chronic or pure nodular silicosis* typically occurs after 20 to 40 years of low or moderate exposure to silica-containing dust with less than 35% quartz. Chronic silicosis is often first detected by a routine chest radiograph and in the early stages may have no respiratory symptoms apart from possibly a cough. With more advanced silicosis, the patient is more often dyspneic and frequently complains of chronic cough and phlegm production. Lung sounds are usually normal or reflect concurrent airway disease. Radiographically, chronic silicosis is characterized by symmetrical, rounded opacities in the upper and middle lung zones. Hilar

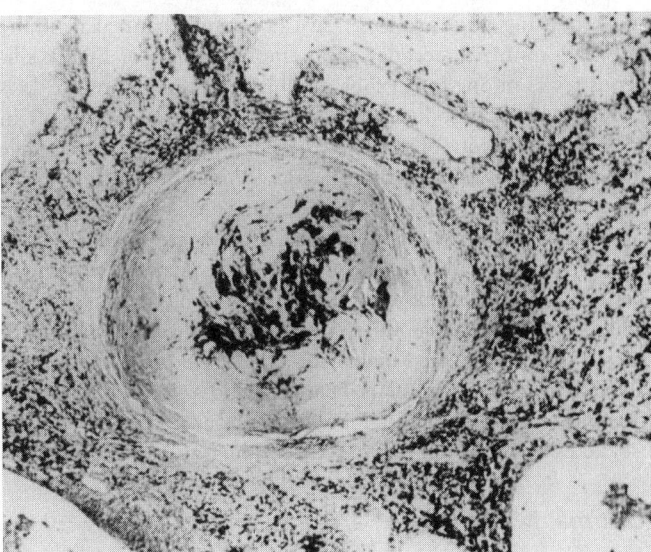

FIGURE 375.3. Light microscopic view of a typical silicotic nodule demonstrating a whorled fibrous center (original magnification ×70).

lymph nodes rimmed with calcium may also be seen on chest radiograph; these opacities are termed *eggshell calcifications.* It is well recognized, however, that a patient with somewhat dramatic radiographic evidence of silicosis may remain free of symptoms and functional impairment. Physiologically, patients with silicosis typically present with a restrictive pulmonary impairment but may have a mixed obstructive–restrictive pattern or a purely obstructive pattern. In fact, epidemiologic studies have shown that workers exposed to silica may develop mild airflow obstruction, independent of the effect of cigarette smoking.

Progressive massive fibrosis (also known as complicated or conglomerate silicosis) may develop in a small percentage (less than 5%) of patients with silicosis. These lesions result from coalescence of the initial fibrotic nodules, which engulf obliterated blood vessels and bronchi. The conglomerate masses typically appear symmetrically in the upper lung zones, may assume a *butterfly* distribution, and may develop cavitates; they are typically associated with scar emphysema. Patients with progressive massive fibrosis are severely impaired by end-stage dyspnea, which is the predominant symptom. The disease is usually progressive despite removal from the inciting agent. Pulmonary function evaluation usually reveals both marked obstructive and restrictive pulmonary impairment. Patients with this disease are at increased risk for tuberculosis and other respiratory infections (influenza virus and *Pneumococcus*). In fact, it has been suggested that tuberculosis may contribute to the development of progressive massive fibrosis.

Accelerated silicosis is seen in workers, such as sandblasters, who receive more concentrated exposures of dust containing greater than 50% quartz. Lesions may develop after only 5 years of exposure, with nodules appearing on radiographs somewhat smaller than those of classic silicosis and concentrated in the middle zones of the lung.

Very high concentrations of silica may result in *acute silicosis,* also known as silicoproteinosis. This rapidly progressive and often fatal disease has been reported in the United States among workers using sand as an abrasive (a practice banned in many Western countries decades ago), among drillers of highly siliceous rock, among tombstone sandblasters, and among workers milling silica to produce silica flour. These processes result in high concentrations of respirable particles with a high percentage of *free* silica—two important factors influencing silica toxicity. Within months of exposure, patients may present with profound dyspnea, weight loss, and fatigue that may progress to death from respiratory failure. Lipids and proteinaceous material reactive to periodic Schiff reagent are found histologically in the alveoli. Milky-appearing lavage fluid containing high concentrations of surfactant is considered diagnostic of silica-induced pulmonary alveolar proteinosis. Similar to patients who have idiopathic alveolar proteinosis, whole-lung lavage has been successfully used in isolated cases to reverse the excess production of surfactant.

Optimal Management and Prevention

Removal from the exposure site and elimination of exacerbating factors, such as cigarette smoking, are the mainstays of therapy. In individuals with progressive disease, tuberculosis should be considered and, if present, treated aggressively.

Coal Worker's Pneumoconiosis

Definition and Epidemiologic Factors

For many years, coal miners were believed to be suffering from silicosis. Surveys of coal tipplers and graphite workers exposed to either coal dust or graphite, but not silica, revealed a form of pneumoconiosis that is radiographically indistinguishable from chronic silicosis but pathologically quite different. Although many miners are also exposed to silica and may therefore have both silicosis and coal worker's pneumoconiosis (CWP), the latter is recognized as a distinct form of pneumoconiosis with its own natural history and pathology.

About 300,000 miners in the United States are exposed to coal dust each year. However, an increasing proportion of these workers are involved in strip mining, in which exposures are considerably lower than in underground mining. The exposure to coal dust for underground miners was greatly reduced as a result of the Federal Coal Mine Health and Safety Act of 1969, which provided benefits for miners with documented exposures and mandated that employers prevent workers from receiving exposures of coal dust greater than 2 mg per cubic meter. The act was subsequently revised to include workers suffering disabilities not only from pneumoconiosis but also from chronic obstructive pulmonary disease arising from coal dust exposures. Today more than 90% of mine sections are in compliance with federal standards. NIOSH provides an ongoing medical surveillance program for underground coal miners and reports that less than 5% of working miners have radiographic evidence of CWP. Those with advanced simple CWP or progressive massive fibrosis (PMF) typically have had mine exposures of 20 years or more.

Clinical Presentation

As with silicosis, the risk of CWP depends on the cumulative dose of exposure (the amount of dust concentration multiplied by the duration of exposure). Simple CWP, in the absence of other respiratory disease, usually is detected radiographically and most often is not accompanied by respiratory symptoms. Industrial bronchitis is common among coal miners (20% to 50%) and is clearly related to the cumulative dose of coal dust. Similarly, airflow obstruction and progressive loss in lung function have been observed to be dose-related in cohorts of miners with high exposure to coal dust. Smoking does not appear to increase the incidence of simple CWP or PMF, but it does act in an additive fashion to increase the risk of developing airflow obstruction and bronchitis among coal miners. As in silicosis, CWP may present as a restrictive impairment, although obstructive and mixed patterns are more often observed. Simple CWP typically presents without dyspnea, but the patient often complains of chronic cough and phlegm production.

The chest examination is usually not helpful but may reveal breath sounds arising from airway obstruction. The combination of peribronchiolar deposition of coal dust, macrophages, and fibrosis, together with adjacent focal emphysema, makes up the classic coal macule, the earliest pathologic lesion of CWP (Fig. 375.4). Particle deposits continue to accumulate and typically form rounded micronodules (less than 7 mm in diameter) and later macronodules (more than 7 mm in diameter). Nodular pneumoconiosis arising from coal dust exposures typically occurs symmetrically and predominantly in the upper lobes of the lung. Rapidly developing nodules in the presence of CWP with rheumatoid arthritis is recognized as *Caplan's syndrome*.

Unlike silicosis, simple CWP tends not to progress with removal from dust exposure. A small proportion (less than 5%) of those with simple CWP may progress to PMF. The risk of developing PMF depends on the extent of simple CWP and previous exposure to silica. Although those with early PMF (one or more large radiographic opacities greater than 1 cm in diameter) may not be impaired, those with more advanced PMF are typically severely impaired with progressive dyspnea and mixed

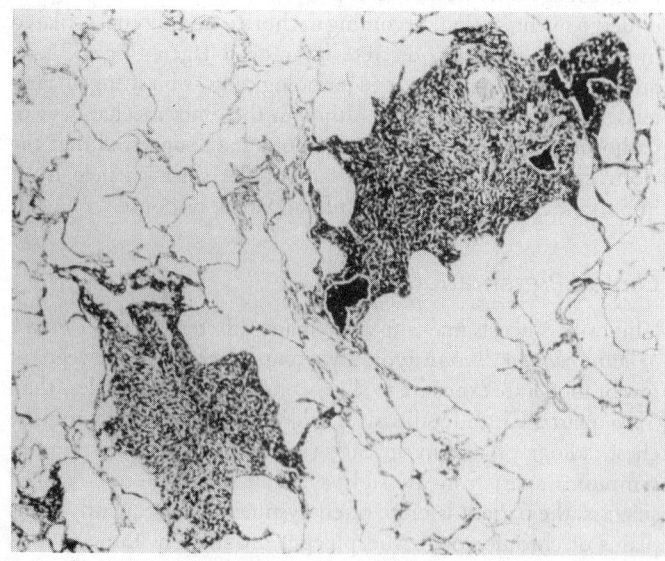

FIGURE 375.4. Histologic section demonstrates a coal macule (heavily pigmented lesion comprised of dust-laden macrophages) surrounded by emphysema (light microscopic magnification, ×70.)

obstructive–restrictive physiology. The lesions of PMF appear histologically as encapsulated dense fibrotic tissue surrounding coalesced coal macules, destroyed vascular tissue, collagen-containing scars, and proteinaceous acellular material saturated with coal dust (see Fig. 375.4). Investigators have recently suggested that alveolar macrophages contribute to pulmonary injury in CWP through generation of a superoxide anion, although the precise mechanisms involved in the disease pathogenesis remain unclear.

Optimal Management and Prevention

Therapy for symptomatic CWP is limited to treatment of complications; clinical intervention should focus on removal from the exposure site, discontinuation of additional exacerbating factors such as cigarette smoking, and treatment of the bronchitic phase of this disease. In addition, the presence of tuberculosis should be carefully considered among those with progressive disease.

Silicate Pneumoconioses

In addition to asbestos, other silicates may cause pneumoconiosis, given sufficient dust concentration and duration of exposure. The occupational populations at risk for these exposures are diverse because of the wide distribution of these products in consumer goods. For most of these exposures, limited environmental and epidemiologic data are available. The pneumoconioses arising from mining, milling, or subsequent processing of minerals are often more closely related to the more toxic "contaminants" of the host rock, such as crystalline silica or fibrous amphibole asbestos. As a result, silicate pneumoconiosis may closely resemble silicosis or asbestosis. Of particular importance is talc, a widely used consumer product and industrial material. NIOSH estimated the population occupationally exposed to talc in 1980 to be 1.8 million. Cosmetic talcs, now regulated by the Food and Drug Administration to prevent fiber contamination, consist of platy talcs, which may produce a reticulonodular form of pneumoconiosis known as talcosis. Exposure to this type of talc has not been associated with lung cancer. Fibrous talcs, commonly contaminated with significant amounts of asbestiform fibers, produce lung lesions that are typical of the asbestos-related lung diseases and include interstitial fibrosis, pleural plaques, diffuse pleural thickening, lung cancer, and mesothelioma.

Other silicates are being more widely used as asbestos substitutes in the absence of adequate data on health effects. A fibrous calcium silicate, wollastonite, appears to be relatively nontoxic, causing at most mild pneumoconiosis in the small work forces mining and milling it in the United States and Finland. Some vermiculite sources have been found to be contaminated with asbestiform fibers, resulting in lung fibrosis, lung cancer, and mesothelioma.

Miscellaneous Pneumoconiosis and Other Conditions

Occupational exposure to aluminum, barium, iron, and tin dusts may result in pneumoconiosis. These exposures result in nodular pneumoconiosis, often with striking chest radiographs due to the deposition of metal in the lung. In most cases, in the absence of other respiratory risk factors, the radiographic findings are not associated with symptoms, physical findings, or impairment.

Exposure to cemented tungsten carbide (hard metal), commonly used as an abrasive or metal cutting tool, may result in hard-metal lung disease. Patients with hard-metal lung disease can present with either airflow obstruction or diffuse interstitial fibrosis. The asthma-like syndrome is characterized by cough and chest tightness, which usually develop toward the end of the work shift or in the evening. This pneumoconiosis may develop rapidly within a year of employment, with the onset of cough, sputum, and dyspnea on exertion. Physical examination reveals basilar rales. The chest radiograph is characterized by irregular opacities with some hilar prominence.

Manufactured mineral fibers include slag wools, rock wools, glass wools and filaments, and ceramic fibers. These materials have numerous industrial applications and are frequently used as asbestos substitutes. Because the morphology of these fibers is similar to that of asbestos, there has been a good deal of concern about their potential for causing interstitial fibrosis, lung cancer, and mesothelioma. Epidemiologic studies reveal some linear opacities, similar to those of mild asbestosis, in a low prevalence among fiberglass manufacturing workers. However, exposure to manufactured mineral fibers does not appear to be associated with an excess risk of either lung cancer or mesothelioma.

MIXED OBSTRUCTIVE–PARENCHYMAL DISEASE

Hypersensitivity Pneumonitis

Definition

Hypersensitivity pneumonitis, also referred to as extrinsic allergic alveolitis, is a syndrome characterized by a granulomatous inflammatory reaction of the interstitium and terminal bronchioles. A complete description of hypersensitivity pneumonitis, including a discussion of its pathogenesis, diagnostic evaluation, and treatment, is found in Chapter 372. The lung disease in hypersensitivity pneumonitis is often accompanied by systemic symptoms and is caused by exposure to airborne organic dusts and other agents. This disorder differs from allergic asthma in that the immunologically mediated inflammatory response is in the terminal bronchioles and interstitium rather than in the more proximal airways; however, the two disorders are caused by many of the same organic dusts. A wide variety of offending agents has been identified, but most agents are rare and the majority of reported cases comprise a few well-substantiated syndromes. Diagnosis of hypersensitivity pneumonitis is based on recognition of a pattern of clinical, radiographic, and pathophysiologic criteria. Farmer's lung and pigeon breeder's disease are the prototypic syndromes in hypersensitivity pneumonitis (see Chapter 372 for further discussion).

Depending on the frequency and intensity of exposure to the causative agent, the clinical presentation differs from worker to worker. Acute, subacute, and chronic forms of hypersensitivity pneumonitis have been used to describe the variety of presentations. Acute disease is associated with such symptoms as cough, fever, chills, malaise, and dyspnea, which may begin 6 to 8 hours after the initial exposure to the antigen and spontaneously resolve once further exposure has ceased. This latent period makes it difficult for the patient to directly relate the exposure to the symptoms. Pulmonary examination often reveals tachypnea and bibasilar crackles, but wheezes are usually absent. The subacute pattern is characterized by progressively worsening cough and dyspnea that occurs over weeks and may progress to severe dyspnea and cyanosis, requiring hospitalization if the worker has been exposed repeatedly to the antigen. Typically, these patients have fleeting infiltrates and a history of being treated for recurrent episodes of suspected pneumonia. Fewer numbers of individuals develop the chronic pattern of disease, which involves progressive dyspnea with clinical features of interstitial fibrosis occurring after multiple symptomatic exposures. Fever is uncommon in the chronic form of hypersensitivity pneumonitis; however, evidence of cor pulmonale has been reported in advanced cases of pulmonary fibrosis associated with hypersensitivity pneumonitis.

Laboratory and Physiologic Findings

A leukocytosis with neutrophil predominance is often seen in acute cases, with white blood cell counts approaching 30,000 per milliliter. Most patients have acquired specific IgG antibodies to the antigen responsible for their symptoms, measurable as precipitins using radioimmunoassay or enzyme-linked immunosorbent assay. Establishing the quantity of a specific precipitin, although providing valuable clues to the clinician in making a diagnosis, is not alone diagnostic of the syndrome and simply indicates that an individual has been exposed to a potentially hazardous organic dust. Pulmonary function testing often reveals a decrease in the forced vital capacity (FVC) and a corresponding elevation of the FEV_1/FVC ratio. Total lung capacity is usually decreased. Impairment of the carbon monoxide diffusion in the lung may also be observed with associated low arterial PO_2 levels measured at rest. Importantly, in the acute phase of the disease all of the physiologic changes are reversible. Radiographically, there are no findings specific for hypersensitivity pneumonitis, although many cases reveal bilateral alveolar infiltrates with involvement of both upper and lower lung fields. Occasionally, these infiltrates present in different locations when imaged over time, but long-term exposures frequently show interstitial infiltrates appearing much like other forms of interstitial lung disease.

Optimal Management and Prevention

Absolute avoidance of the inciting antigen is the mainstay of therapy. If the work environment cannot be significantly altered to eliminate exposure to the antigen, respiratory protection is of little value because small amounts of inhaled antigen may cause acute symptoms in a sensitized individual. Although corticosteroids and supplemental oxygen may be administered for acute attacks, chronic treatment should focus on the prevention of antigenic exposures.

Bronchiolitis

Definition

Bronchiolitis represents an inflammatory injury to the bronchiolar epithelium that results in fibrosis and obliteration of the airway. Post injury, the subsequent healing leads to excessive proliferation of granulation tissue within the airway walls, lumen, or both. The nomenclature for bronchiolitis is quite large; other diagnostic entities that are used to describe this condition include bronchiolitis obliterans, bronchiolitis fibrosa obliterans, bronchiolitis obliterans–organizing pneumonia (BOOP), cryptogenic-organizing pneumonia, and follicular bronchiolitis. While a more complete description of this disease is outlined elsewhere (see Chapter 376), we have included it in this chapter because bronchiolitis is associated with occupation-related exposure to toxic fumes.

Pathogenesis

There are two classification systems used to characterize bronchiolitis—a clinical system based on cause [inhalation (Table 375.4), infection, drug reaction, and idiopathic] and a system based on histopathologic signs. The histopathologic signs can be separated into those associated with proliferative bronchiolitis and those associated with constrictive bronchiolitis. Proliferative bronchiolitis is more common and is characterized by organizing intraluminal exudate with intraluminal fibrotic buds (Masson bodies) in respiratory bronchioles, alveolar ducts, and alveoli. This is primarily an inflammatory condition associated with collagen vascular diseases, acute infections, hypersensitivity pneumonitis, organ transplantation, or a reaction to drugs. Constrictive bronchiolitis is characterized by damage to the membranous and respiratory bronchioles, with concentric narrowing or complete obliteration of the airway lumen; the alveolar ducts may be spared. Step sections are often required to make the diagnosis. In addition to the causes listed for proliferative bronchiolitis, constrictive bronchiolitis may be caused by inhalation of toxic fumes (Table 375.4) (nitrogen dioxide, sulfur dioxide, ammonia, chlorine, phosgene, ozone, chloropicrin, trichlorethylene, cadmium oxide, methyl sulfate, hydrogen sulfide, and hydrogen fluoride), mineral dust–induced airway disease (asbestos, silica, iron oxide, aluminum oxide, talc, mica, and coal), or cigarette smoke.

Although the pathogenesis of bronchiolitis is unknown, it has been hypothesized that whereas constrictive bronchiolitis is initiated by injury to the airway epithelia, proliferative bronchiolitis primarily involves an alveolitis. In constrictive bronchiolitis, it is thought that the initial airway injury is followed by neutrophilic inflammation and that the repair process results in intramural and intraluminal fibrosis. In proliferative bronchiolitis, the primary alveolitis results in an inflammatory exudate in the distal airspace. Fibroblast proliferation forms Masson bodies and extracellular matrix that further occlude the lumen of the respiratory bronchioles and alveolar ducts.

Diagnosis

Although a lung biopsy is essential for the diagnosis of bronchiolitis (see above), several clinical features are suggestive of this disorder. The history is essential to establish the specific exposures or inflammatory conditions that are associated with either constrictive or proliferative bronchiolitis. In constrictive bronchiolitis, the chest radiograph is often normal, whereas the HRCT scan may show marked heterogeneity in lung density (e.g., ground-glass infiltrates). In contrast, the radiographs in proliferative bronchiolitis demonstrate interstitial opacities that may be migratory. While the lung physiology in constrictive bronchiolitis is obstructive, the typical lung physiology in proliferative bronchiolitis is restrictive or mixed. However, there is no clear separation between the diagnostic categories of bronchiolitis, and overlap clearly exists between constrictive and proliferative bronchiolitis.

Optimal Management

Corticosteroids are the mainstay of treatment for bronchiolitis. Proliferative bronchiolitis is steroid-responsive and can be cured with an extensive course of treatment (usually requiring a year of therapy). Although corticosteroids should be used in constrictive bronchiolitis, this condition is relatively unresponsive and progressive, despite aggressive treatment.

Berylliosis

Definition

Metallic beryllium, simple salts of beryllium, and complex beryllium silicates, commonly referred to as beryllium compounds, cause both acute and chronic lung disease. Beryllium is widely used in the production of copper and nickel alloys, dental alloys, computers, x-ray tubes, electronic and nuclear reactors, and foundry products; in tool and die manufacturing; and in the aerospace industry. NIOSH estimated in 1990 that as many as 1 million U.S. workers are potentially exposed to beryllium oxides.

Beryllium lung disease may be divided into acute and chronic forms. The acute disease comprises those beryllium-related conditions that last for less than 1 year and that occur during beryllium exposure. Acute manifestation appear to be dose-related and include dermatitis (which may ulcerate), conjunctivitis, nasopharyngitis, tracheobronchitis, and acute chemical pneumonia. Chemical pneumonitis is rare but can be fulminant and fatal. Patients present with dyspnea, cough, fatigue, blood-tinged sputum, and substernal pain. Rales, tachypnea, and cyanosis are seen in advanced cases. Radiographic findings include diffuse or patchy infiltrates. Lung volumes are reduced, and hypoxemia is common. Of the 892 cases of beryllium-induced lung disease in the Beryllium Case Registry, 212 were acute, and of these only 17% progressed to chronic beryllium disease.

Chronic beryllium disease (berylliosis) is both a pulmonary and a systemic granulomatous disease. Clinically, berylliosis is very similar to sarcoidosis. However, berylliosis can be distinguished from sarcoidosis by exposure history and the absence of either central nervous system disease or altered calcium metabolism. The duration of exposures may vary from months to years, with a latent period from initial exposure to disease manifestations of 10 to 15 years. As with uncomplicated pneumoconiosis,

chronic beryllium disease may present as a radiographic finding without respiratory symptoms. Chronic berylliosis, however, may result in severe dyspnea and end-stage pulmonary fibrosis. Physical findings include bibasilar rales, peripheral lymphadenopathy, hepatosplenomegaly, clubbing, and skin lesions. Lung function abnormalities may include airflow obstruction, reduced lung volume, and isolated diffusion defects. Bronchoalveolar lavage with measurement of the proliferative response of the lung lymphocytes to beryllium salts has been shown to be a sensitive marker for determination of chronic beryllium disease. The disease course is highly variable: with cessation of exposure some patients progress, some remain stable, and some improve. It is thought that corticosteroid treatment promotes resolution of chronic beryllium disease, but no controlled trial data are currently available.

Pathogenesis

Chronic beryllium disease is an immune-mediated systemic disorder. This position is strongly supported by the variable susceptibility to this metal, the presence of noncaseating granulomas with mononuclear cell infiltrates on histologic examination of the lung, an antigen-specific immune response, and the accumulation of major histocompatibility complex (MHC) class II–restricted beryllium-specific CD4$^+$ T lymphocytes in the lungs of patients with chronic beryllium disease. Furthermore, peripheral mononuclear cells and lung T cells proliferate and release lymphokines (tumor necrosis factor–α, interleukin-2, interleukin-6) when exposed to beryllium salts *ex vivo*. However, CD4$^+$ T lymphocytes from the lung exhibit enhanced beryllium-induced proliferation when compared to peripheral T cells, and the magnitude of the antigen-specific cellular response in the lung is strongly associated with the degree of the local inflammatory process. These findings suggest that the pulmonary immune response in chronic beryllium disease is compartmentalized, and this inflammatory response is antigen-specific and mediated by activated CD4$^+$ T lymphocytes. However, the immunogenicity of this innocuous-appearing metal is not understood. It has been hypothesized that macrophages ingest aggregates of this metal, slowly releasing it and thus causing a chronic granulomatous response. Alternatively, beryllium has been hypothesized to complex with proteins and act as a hapten. However, there are no data to support either hypothesis.

Understanding these beryllium-specific immunologic responses has provided a reliable method to distinguish chronic beryllium disease from sarcoidosis. This is particularly important because the presence or absence of beryllium in lung tissue does not prove or refute the diagnosis of berylliosis. The beryllium lymphocyte proliferation test (BeLPT) has been standardized, is an essential component of the diagnostic criteria for berylliosis, and results in negative findings in patients with sarcoidosis. The BeLPT quantifies the cellular proliferative immune response to beryllium and is positive in peripheral blood specimens in over 90% of patients with berylliosis. The remaining individuals with chronic beryllium disease will have abnormal BeLPT responses in lymphocytes obtained by bronchoalveolar lavage. The BeLPT also appears to function as a screening test, since exposed workers with a positive BeLPT may have subclinical granulomatous lung disease and are at excess risk of developing beryllium disease. In fact, a longitudinal study has shown that approximately 50% of those with a positive BeLPT go on to develop chronic beryllium disease.

A recent study suggests that allelic substitution of the *HLA-DP* gene may place individuals at higher risk of developing beryllium disease. Specifically, chronic beryllium disease was found to be strongly associated with a base-pair substitution that resulted in glutamic acid (rather than lysine) at position 69 of the *HLA-DP* gene. It was further postulated that residue 69 of the *HLA-DP* gene, which is a negatively charged site when glutamic acid is present, may directly interact with beryllium and be involved in the immunopathogenesis of this disease. The finding that allelic alteration of the *HLA-DP* gene is associated with enhanced susceptibility to an immune-mediated lung disease is consistent with the finding that alterations in MHC class II genes (*HLA-DR, HLA-DQ,* and *HLA-DP*) are associated with susceptibility to autoimmune diseases. These findings in the HLA-DP *gene* may be relevant to other forms of granulomatous lung disease. Moreover, these observations provide further evidence that host susceptibility may be an important determinant of occupational lung disease and indicate that minor alterations in the human genome may substantially modify the biological response to environmental stimuli. Given the tools available in human molecular genetics, gene–environment interactions represent a feasible and very important area for further investigation in chronic beryllium disease, as well as other forms of occupational lung disease.

OCCUPATIONAL NEOPLASTIC DISEASES OF THE LUNG

Lung cancer is the leading cause of cancer deaths in the United States and in many other industrialized countries. Importantly, occupational exposures can play an important role in the development of bronchogenic carcinoma. Although the clinical aspects of lung cancer will be discussed elsewhere in this text (see Chapter 377), we focus on the etiologic considerations of bronchogenic carcinoma. Mesothelioma, a malignancy originating from the cells that line the pulmonary surface (mesothelium), is exclusively associated with previous exposure to asbestos and is discussed in detail later.

Bronchogenic Carcinoma

In 1987, approximately 100,000 men and 50,000 women in the United States developed lung cancer. The disease accounts for nearly one-fourth of all cancer deaths. The four major malignant cell types of bronchogenic carcinoma are large-cell, small-cell, squamous cell, and adenocarcinoma. Occupational exposures may involve any one of these cell types, and all forms of neoplasia are increased with cigarette smoking. Signs and symptoms, laboratory findings, and diagnosis of lung tumors are discussed elsewhere in this text (see Chap. 377). Therapy for occupation-related lung tumors is dependent on the cell type and is no different from treatment of lung cancer due to other exposures.

Cigarette smoking is the most important risk factor for developing pulmonary malignancies in the general population. In more recent studies, passive exposure to cigarette smoke was also found to contribute to development of lung cancer deaths. This trend is expected to decline gradually, however, as smoking decreases and as cigarette manufacturers develop products containing less nicotine and tar. Occupational exposures to cigarette smoke are important to consider because the carcinogenic potential of several substances encountered in the workplace can be greatly enhanced by concomitant exposure to cigarette smoke.

Asbestos inhalation is generally considered to have the highest carcinogenic risk in the workplace. Many studies have documented an increase in all forms of bronchogenic carcinoma in workers exposed to asbestos, and all fiber types have been implicated in carcinogenesis. Most asbestos-related pulmonary tumors have a long latency period (20 to 30 years) and a dose–response relationship has been observed between the exposure and development of the tumor. Investigators estimate a 6- to 8-fold increase in lung cancer risk in nonsmoking workers exposed to asbestos and 50- to 100-fold excess risk in asbestos workers who are heavy smokers. Lung cancer accounts for up to 25% of all deaths in asbestos-exposed workers.

Excess mortality rates from lung carcinoma have also been reported in workers exposed to other compounds and chemicals. Uranium miners were discovered to develop lung disease by inhaling the breakdown products of uranium ore, one of which is radon, an inert gas found to increase the risk of lung cancer in a dose-dependent fashion. The risk related to domestic radon exposures, however, remains controversial.

Chloromethyl ethers are one example of chemical carcinogens in the workplace. These substances, which are used in the process of manufacturing a number of organic substances such as water repellents, fireproofing agents, and pesticides, have been implicated in increasing small-cell lung cancer rates. Chloromethyl ether causes small-cell lung carcinoma even among individuals who have never smoked.

Workers exposed to chromium, beryllium, nickel, and cadmium have higher lung cancer rates, and these metals are considered to be carcinogenic in humans by the International Agency for Research on Cancer (IARC).

Mesothelioma

Mesothelioma, a rare tumor of the cells lining the lung surface, was first reported in the 1940s. The annual incidence, although small, continues to increase with rates of approximately 2.5 cases per million for men and 0.7 case per million for women in North America. Asbestos exposure has been directly linked as a causative agent in almost all cases of this disease; isolated exposures to erionite (a mineral in the silicate zeolite family) and radiation may possibly contribute to the development of mesothelioma. Unlike bronchogenic carcinoma, no specific association between mesothelioma development and cigarette smoking has been established. The latency period for this disease often is greater than 30 years.

Pathogenesis

Although all fiber types have been found to cause mesothelioma, crocidolite has been noted to be the most carcinogenic. Since chrysotile was the primary asbestos fiber to which U.S. workers were exposed, chrysotile asbestos accounts for a disproportionate number of cases of mesothelioma in the United States. Formation of mesothelioma appears to be dependent on the size of the fiber and its dimensions, but the exact mechanism of tumor development is not known.

Pathologic Factors

Mesotheliomas often may appear grossly as multiple gray or white nodules or granules on the visceral or parietal pleura. As the tumor load multiplies, the affected pleura becomes progressively thicker and in its later stages may eventually encase the entire hemithorax. The tumor may advance and spread to the diaphragm, liver, the parietal pleura of the opposite side, or even the pericardium. Hematologic spread has been identified in approximately half of affected patients.

The tumor is classified into three discrete types: epithelial (50% of all cases), mesenchymal (16%), or mixed (34%). Epithelial tumors may appear in cordlike or sheetlike patterns, but may also show papillary or tubular arrangements. Mesenchymal tumors have been described as having cells that are spindle-like and contain elongated nuclei. The mixed form has both spindle-shaped cells and features of the epithelial tumor.

Clinical Presentation

Malignant mesothelioma most commonly presents in the sixth decade of life. Patients often present with nonpleuritic chest pain and dyspnea, although complaints of shoulder or upper abdominal pain referred from areas of diaphragmatic involvement may be observed. Pleural effusions are common at presentation and patients may also have fever and weight loss.

Diagnostic Testing

On radiographs, pleural effusions are commonly seen and pleural plaques are often present in the opposite hemithorax. Mediasti-

nal widening, soft-tissue masses, and enlargement of the cardiac silhouette is seen on chest radiograph with progression of the disease. Chest CT scans are valuable in the evaluation of mesothelioma because large pleural effusions may make evaluation of pleural lesions quite difficult. The chest CT shows thickened pleura with a somewhat nodular margin. The major fissure may also be abnormal secondary to fibrosis or tumor invasion. Evaluation of pleural fluid reveals a cellular serosanguinous exudate that contains not only benign and malignant mesothelial cells but also varying numbers of lymphocytes and polymorphonuclear leukocytes. Pleural fluid pH and glucose levels may be significantly diminished in patients with mesothelioma. Occasionally, patients may present with skin deposits, which, after biopsy, can be used to establish a diagnosis.

Diagnostic tissue for malignant mesothelioma is obtained in nearly all patients by thoracoscopy or open thoracotomy. Because of the varying microscopic features in isolated lesions, multiple biopsies should be obtained. Histochemical staining using the periodic acid–Schiff method, immunohistochemical testing with monoclonal antibodies, and electron microscopy have all been used to differentiate malignant mesothelioma from metastatic adenocarcinoma. Definite pathologic diagnosis of a mesothelioma, however, relies on electron microscopic findings. Long microvilli, identified by electron microscopy (Fig. 375.5), are characteristic of a mesothelioma and distinguish it from an adenocarcinoma, which characteristically has very short microvilli.

Optimal Management

Although chemotherapy, gene therapy, and surgical interventions have been attempted, no effective life-prolonging therapy is currently known for malignant mesothelioma. Mesotheliomas are not responsive to radiation. The median survival of patients with malignant mesothelioma has been reported at about 18 months.

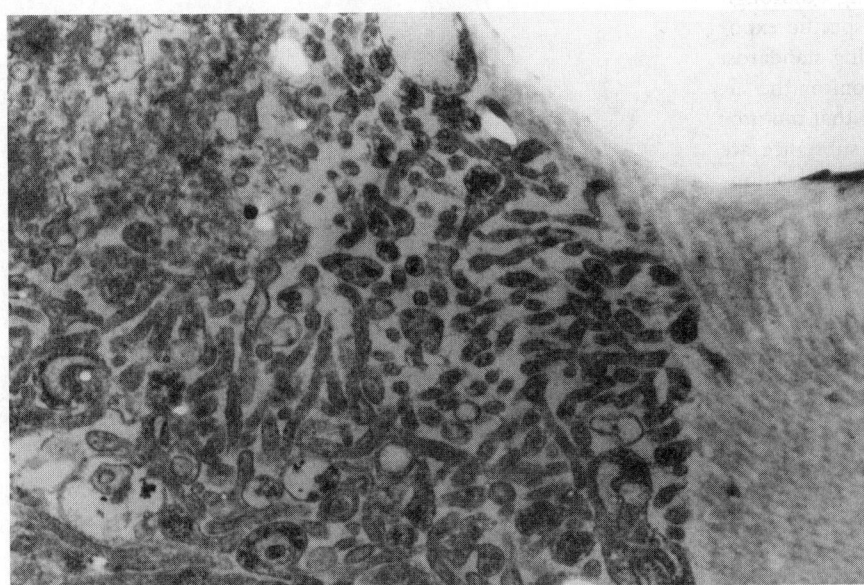

FIGURE 375.5. Electron microscopy reveals long microvilli, characteristic of malignant mesothelioma (magnification ×15,300.)

IMPAIRMENT/DISABILITY EVALUATION

Physicians involved in the evaluation of patients with occupational lung disease are frequently asked to provide an impairment rating and to make determinations regarding causation. Impairment is defined as a measurable decrement in a physiologic function and is based on objective clinical tests. Disability, on the other hand, considers not only the physical and mental impairment but also the social, psychological, or vocational factors associated with a person's ability to work. The latter is an administrative assessment and is generally not performed by a physician. Using guidelines established by the American Medical Association (AMA) and American Thoracic Society (ATS), percentage impairment can be calculated based on the results of a clinical evaluation, spirometric testing, and diffusion capacity assessment. In circumstances where spirometry and diffusion capacity are thought to underestimate the degree of impairment, an exercise test with measurement of maximal exercise capacity (Vo_2) can be performed. The standard AMA impairment guidelines generally address patients with stable, irreversible pulmonary disorders and are not suitable for rating patients with reversible airflow obstruction. Consequently, the ATS has developed guidelines for impairment rating in patients with asthma, which takes into account factors such as post-bronchodilator FEV_1, reversibility of airflow obstruction, degree of airway hyperresponsiveness, and medication usage. It is recommended that physicians performing impairment ratings familiarize themselves with relevant AMA or ATS guidelines on this topic.

PREVENTION: CONTROLLING OCCUPATIONAL HEALTH HAZARDS

Industrial hygiene involves recognizing and testing for hazards and modifying the work environment where occupational health hazards exist. Once a complete survey of the manufacturing or production process involved is completed (including a thorough understanding of the workplace environment), specific exposures can be measured and compared with existing standards. Exposures may be measured by devices that monitor the air immediately surrounding an individual worker or that monitor an entire work area. If unacceptable levels of a substance are identified, all possibilities of replacing that substance with a nontoxic product should be explored. Recommendations should be made for encouraging employers to minimize exposures among all employees through engineering controls and improved ventilation.

For potentially damaging occupational pulmonary disease, personal respiratory protection may be required, but this is less desirable than other methods (substitution and ventilation) because it is difficult to ensure that the equipment is properly used by each worker. Respirators provide a method of temporary protection from airborne hazards, from benign odoriferous fumes to toxic materials, that are potentially life threatening. Employers are responsible for instituting the use of respiratory protection, providing appropriate equipment, and ensuring that

the equipment meets established standards. Programs for proper maintenance and inspection of the respirator must also be implemented. Three general classifications of respirators are as follows: (a) air-purifying respirators, (b) atmosphere-supplying respirators, and (c) a combination of the two. Air-purifying respirators contain a mechanical filter that removes particulate matter from the air, using a fibrous padded mesh. Inhaled air is drawn in through filters before entering the face piece, and exhaled air is guided out through a different pathway, using a system of valves in the mask itself or through air-tight tubing. Cartridges and canisters are occasionally used for removal of specific gases or vapors. Atmosphere-supplying respirators provide a portable external source of oxygen and virtually eliminate exposure to work site air.

In summary, a well-supervised control program emphasizes replacement of the inciting agent as a first line of therapy. If substitution is unrealistic or infeasible, then isolating the substance from the majority of workers through administrative controls, local exhaust ventilation, or personal protection may be required.

BIBLIOGRAPHY

American College of Chest Physicians. Consensus statement: Assessment of asthma in the workplace. *Chest* 1995;1084–1117.

American Medical Association. *Guides to the evaluation of permanent impairment,* fourth ed. Chicago, 1993.

American Thoracic Society. Guidelines for the evaluation of impairment/disability in patients with asthma. *Am Rev Respir Dis* 1993;1056–1061.

Harber P, Schenker MB, Balmes JR. *Occupational and environmental respiratory disease.* St. Louis: Mosby, 1996.

Rom WN, ed. Environmental and occupational medicine, third ed. Philadelphia: Lippincott–Raven Publishers, 1992.

Rosenstock L, Cullen M, eds. *Textbook of clinical occupational and environmental medicine.* Philadelphia: WB Saunders, 1994.

Kelley's Textbook of Internal Medicine, fourth edition. Edited by H. David Humes.
Lippincott Williams & Wilkins, Philadelphia © 2000.

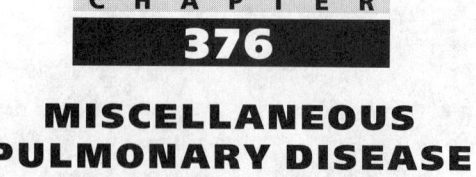

MISCELLANEOUS PULMONARY DISEASE

LESLIE ZIMMERMAN

AMYLOIDOSIS

DEFINITION

Amyloidosis is a term applied to disorders associated with extracellular tissue deposition of amyloid, an insoluble homogeneous proteinaceous material that typically has apple-green birefringence with polarized light after staining with Congo red. Amyloidosis can be classified into subtypes according to the composition of the protein component. Examples are immunoglobulin light chains, amyloid A protein, and transthyretin related protein. Many different fibril proteins have been associated with both systemic and localized amyloidosis; however, all protein subtypes share a β-pleated sheet configuration.

ETIOLOGY AND PATHOGENESIS

Amyloidosis may be a primary systemic disorder in which amyloid (in this case, monoclonal light chains) is produced by a clone of bone marrow–derived plasma cells, or it may be secondarily associated with inflammatory, infectious, or other neoplastic diseases. Familial amyloidosis is the rarest form of systemic amyloidosis. The most common of these autosomal dominant diseases is associated with a mutant transthyretin, a liver transport protein. Generally in systemic amyloidosis, many organs, including the lung, have amyloid protein deposition. Diffuse infiltration interferes with organ function. Much more rarely, fibril deposition is limited to a single organ, such as the bladder, eye, tongue, or respiratory tract.

CLINICAL FINDINGS AND STRATEGIES FOR OPTIMAL CARE

In primary and secondary systemic amyloidosis, as many as 30% of patients have dyspnea, a cough, or both. Although the lung parenchyma may be infiltrated with amyloid, clinical symptoms usually are dominated by cardiac involvement. Congestive heart failure from cardiac infiltration can cause dyspnea, pulmonary infiltrates, and pleural effusion. The prognosis of systemic amyloidosis once was poor—a median survival period of 1 year, but therapeutic options have improved in the past few years. Therapy is tailored to the specific underlying disease mechanism, and survival rates have increased. Unlike systemic amyloidosis, localized pulmonary amyloidosis typically has a good prognosis. The most common respiratory tract manifestation is hoarseness from laryngeal deposition. In the lower respiratory tract, tracheobronchial involvement includes submucosal plaques and pseudotumors; parenchymal involvement includes nodules and diffuse septal deposition. Plaques and pseudotumors may be asymptomatic, incidental findings at bronchoscopy or cause hemoptysis, wheezing, or obstruction with atelectasis. Patients with symptomatic lesions have been successfully treated with endoscopic laser resection, although recurrence is common.

Alveolar deposition may cause single or multiple pulmonary nodules that can cavitate or calcify. Although benign and generally asymptomatic lesions, these nodules are difficult to differentiate radiographically from malignant or tubercular lesions and so are frequently resected. The rarest form of localized disease is diffuse alveolar septal deposition. Patients typically have progressive dyspnea and a cough that often progress to respiratory failure. Pulmonary function tests show a restrictive pattern. Like advances in the management of some types of systemic amyloidosis, therapeutic options for localized disease are emerging. If diffuse alveolar septal deposition of amyloid is found, a search

for a subtle form of a primary systemic amyloidosis and a subspecialty consultation may be warranted.

■ BRONCHIOLITIS OBLITERANS–ORGANIZING PNEUMONIA

DEFINITION

Bronchiolitis obliterans–organizing pneumonia (BOOP) is a clinical pathologic entity characterized by a subacute respiratory illness with plugs of loose granulation tissue in distal airways and associated organizing pneumonitis. Although the term *bronchiolitis obliterans–organizing pneumonia* was proposed in the 1980s, the disease is not new, having been recognized pathologically since the beginning of the twentieth century. Unfortunately, the term *bronchiolitis obliterans* sometimes is used to imply BOOP or a different airway disease, obliterative bronchiolitis. The distinction is important. BOOP is a relatively benign disease that resolves completely in most patients. Obliterative bronchiolitis typically is a progressive disease that irreversibly scars the airways. Adding to the confusion, in Europe the idiopathic form of BOOP is called *cryptogenic organizing pneumonia* (COP).

INCIDENCE AND EPIDEMIOLOGY

The overall incidence of BOOP is unknown. Most reported cases of BOOP are idiopathic. Idiopathic BOOP occurs among men and women equally, the incidence peaking in the fourth through sixth decades of life. In the idiopathic form, there is no common pattern of occupational exposure, and smoking does not appear to be a risk factor. Secondary BOOP has been associated with viral infection, *Legionella* and *Mycoplasma* infections, exposure to toxic fumes, HIV infection, inflammatory bowel disease, connective tissue disease (especially rheumatoid arthritis and dermatomyositis-polymyositis), radiation therapy, myelodysplasia syndrome, bone marrow transplantation, and use of various drugs. Although some rare cases of secondary BOOP have been associated with pulmonary infection, in most cases culture results from biopsy specimens are negative, and results of viral serologic testing do not suggest recent infection.

ETIOLOGY AND PATHOGENESIS

BOOP may represent a reparative process to a variety of insults to the distal airways. In the most distal airways, the respiratory bronchioles and alveolar ducts, extensive loose granulation tissue protrudes from the airway wall into the lumen to form tufts or plugs. These intraluminal polypoid masses extend into alveolar ducts and alveoli, and organizing pneumonitis develops (Fig 376.1). Alveoli contain a fibrinous exudate, and alveolar macrophages appear foamy from endogenous lipid ingestion characteristic of airway obstruction. The adjacent alveolar walls have mild chronic inflammatory infiltration, but generally there is an absence of extensive interstitial fibrosis. The process is patchy and

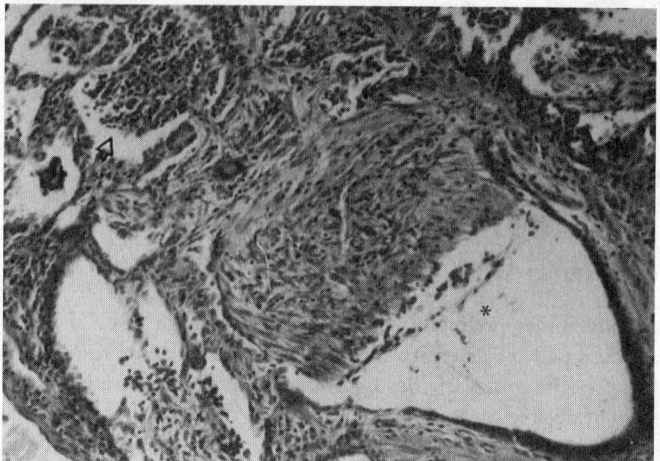

FIGURE 376.1. Bronchiolitis obliterans organizing pneumonia. Thoracoscopic lung biopsy specimen contains a bronchiole with intraluminal granulation tissue (*asterisk*). An adjacent alveolus (*arrow*) is filled with inflammatory cells. (Pathology slide courtesy of Martha L. Warnock, MD.)

of uniform, generally recent age; mature collagen deposition is unusual.

CLINICAL PRESENTATION

In idiopathic BOOP, patients have a subacute, flulike illness with mild dyspnea, a nonproductive to mildly productive cough, fatigue, and fever. They may have mild weight loss. Hemoptysis is rare, but it does occur. Duration of symptoms typically is 2 to 3 months before diagnosis. Physical examination reveals inspiratory rales in two-thirds of patients and wheezing or normal auscultatory findings in the others. Cyanosis is unusual; clubbing is not associated with this disease.

LABORATORY AND RADIOGRAPHIC FINDINGS

Laboratory abnormalities in BOOP may include mild to moderate hypoxemia, an elevated erythrocyte sedimentation rate, and an elevated peripheral white blood cell count. BOOP is a restrictive not an obstructive physiologic process in that only the most peripheral airways are affected. Pulmonary function testing reveals reduced lung volume and reduced diffusion capacity for carbon monoxide. Airflow obstruction does not occur, except among current or former smokers. Chest radiographs reveal bilateral, patchy, often peripheral, alveolar infiltrates. Infiltrates may be dense or partially opaque with a ground glass appearance. Nodules or linear opacities are present in one-third of cases but are rarely the sole radiographic manifestation. Infiltrates may resolve spontaneously and reappear in different lung segments, so-called *fleeting infiltrates.* Computed tomography (CT) and high-resolution CT also reveal the patchy dense and ground glass alveolar infiltrates that have a predilection for subpleural and perivascular areas. Although it does not provide enough information to confirm a diagnosis, CT may help differentiate BOOP from interstitial pulmonary fibrosis and can help direct

the pulmonologist or surgeon to optimal sites for biopsy. Pleural effusions, cavities, and lymphadenopathy are rare.

STRATEGIES FOR OPTIMAL CARE

BOOP may be suspected when an adult has a prolonged viral-like respiratory illness that does not respond to antibiotics. Lung biopsy is recommended because of the wide differential diagnosis and the prolonged corticosteroid therapy required in most cases. Results of transbronchial biopsy confirm the diagnosis if a piece of tissue of sufficient size is obtained that contains all the elements of the lesion. However, most patients need either thoracoscopic or open lung biopsy. Diagnosis is made when the defining pathologic characteristics are found in the appropriate clinical setting.

Although spontaneous improvement can occur, most patients need a prolonged course of corticosteroids. Prednisone, 1 mg per kilogram per day for 1 to 3 months then a very gradual taper, is recommended. The duration of therapy is empiric, but because relapses are common in courses of less than 3 months, most authors recommend a total course of 6 months to 1 year. Relapse after steroid dosage is reduced or stopped is not uncommon, but BOOP responds favorably to a second course of treatment. With corticosteroids, symptomatic relief is rapid, over days to weeks, and can be dramatic; physiologic and radiographic improvements take longer. More than 80% of treated patients respond to therapy, and approximately 65% have complete resolution. Death of respiratory failure occurs among less than 5% of patients and is caused by a progressive illness that results in end-stage fibrosis. Clear benefit of cytotoxic agents has not been established. BOOP occasionally can be localized or focal, and surgical resection appears to be curative. BOOP also can be a reactive process that forms around a tumor, abscess, or infarct. Pathologic specimens from bronchoscopic transbronchial biopsy of or near solitary lesions should be interpreted within the context of the clinical scenario.

◼ OBLITERATIVE BRONCHIOLITIS

DEFINITION

Obliterative bronchiolitis is an inflammatory disease with concentrically scarred or stenotic small airways from extrinsic bronchiolar and peribronchiolar narrowing. This process is a lesion confined to the bronchioles and usually lacks an associated organizing pneumonitis. A more precise term is *constrictive bronchiolitis.*

EPIDEMIOLOGY AND PATHOGENESIS

Obliterative bronchiolitis is a rare disease, less common than BOOP. Most instances are idiopathic and occur mostly among women in their fifth through seventh decades. Secondary causes include viral infection, exposure to toxins and fumes, drug reaction, and connective tissue disease, especially rheumatoid arthritis. Why a toxin, infection, or other secondary cause triggers the relatively benign reaction of BOOP in some or obliterative bronchiolitis in others is unknown. Obliterative bronchiolitis also occurs after bone marrow, heart-lung, and lung transplantation. With obliterative bronchiolitis after bone marrow transplantation, most patients have clinical evidence of graft versus host disease. The incidence of obliterative bronchiolitis among patients with chronic graft versus host disease is approximately 10%. There is a high case fatality rate despite aggressive therapy with steroids, immunosuppressive agents, and bronchodilators. Obliterative bronchiolitis develops among 30% to 50% of long-term survivors of heart-lung or lung transplantation and is the leading cause of death. There may be many cofactors, but the primary event appears to be chronic transplant rejection.

CLINICAL, LABORATORY, AND RADIOGRAPHIC PRESENTATION

Patients have progressive dyspnea and a nonproductive cough that can develop over months to years in idiopathic cases or within months after transplantation. Fever is rare. Findings at physical examination may be unremarkable or reveal diffuse expiratory wheezing. Chest radiographs may be normal or have evidence of hyperinflation with or without interstitial infiltrates. Pulmonary function usually reveals an obstructive pattern. Because small airways are irreversibly scarred and occluded, little improvement occurs with use of bronchodilators.

STRATEGIES FOR OPTIMAL CARE

The diagnosis of obliterative bronchiolitis usually is made when lung biopsy reveals concentrically scarred small airways in the appropriate clinical setting. Presumptive diagnosis without biopsy may be appropriate in the care of patients with graft versus host disease after bone marrow transplantation who have new onset of obstructive airway disease. Bronchoalveolar lavage is recommended to exclude opportunistic infection.

The clinical course of obliterative bronchiolitis is variable, but the disease tends to be progressive, often ending in respiratory failure, especially among patients with underlying rheumatoid arthritis. Most patients have little response to steroids, although a therapeutic trial is warranted for most. Although many airways may be irreversibly scarred, some may be in earlier stages of the inflammatory process. For patients who have undergone bone marrow, lung, or heart-lung transplantation, augmentation in immunosuppression and vigilance for opportunistic infection may slow or stabilize the lung disease.

■ IDIOPATHIC EOSINOPHILIC PNEUMONIA: SIMPLE, ACUTE, AND CHRONIC

DEFINITION

Eosinophilic pneumonia is pneumonia with infiltration of the lung parenchyma by eosinophils that may or may not be accompanied by excess eosinophils in the peripheral blood. This type of pneumonia is associated with helminthic, bacterial, and fungal infection, drug reactions, connective tissue disease, vasculitis,

Hodgkin's disease, sarcoidosis, systemic hypereosinophilic syndrome, Churg–Strauss syndrome, allergic bronchopulmonary aspergillosis, and other forms of bronchocentric granulomatosis. When underlying diseases or specific causes are excluded, there remain the idiopathic eosinophilic types of pneumonia, which have no discernible cause but do have distinctive clinical and radiographic presentations. The classification of eosinophilic pneumonia has changed over the past several decades to include such terms as *Loffler's syndrome* for simple pulmonary eosinophilia and pulmonary infiltrates with eosinophilia (PIE) syndrome to describe a broad range of eosinophilic types of pneumonia. Because these terms denote mixed idiopathic and secondary eosinophilic types of pneumonia, the terms *acute* and *chronic eosinophilic pneumonia* are now used to mean the idiopathic forms of these types of pneumonia. The distinction between these idiopathic forms is based on differences in clinical observation and may be arbitrary or valid. Most patients with simple eosinophilic pneumonia have a parasitic infection or drug reaction; however, no cause is found in as many as one-third of these patients.

INCIDENCE AND EPIDEMIOLOGY

All eosinophilic types of pneumonia are rare disorders. Although these diseases can occur at any age and affect either sex, case series suggest a male predominance that peaks in the third decade of life for the acute form and a female predominance that peaks in the fifth decade for the chronic form. There does not appear to be any regional or geographic clustering.

ETIOLOGY AND PATHOGENESIS

Idiopathic eosinophilic pneumonia is a diagnosis made after drugs, infection, and associated diseases are excluded as etiologic factors. Patients with the acute form typically have been healthy before the onset of disease. A high percentage of patients with the simple idiopathic form have atopy or allergic diathesis found with skin testing to common antigens. Most patients with chronic eosinophilic pneumonia have established or new-onset asthma, allergic rhinitis, or another form of atopy.

In eosinophilic pneumonia, eosinophils mixed with alveolar macrophages, lymphocytes, and neutrophils accumulate in the airway, interstitium, and alveoli for unknown reasons. The eosinophils may be nonspecific markers of inflammation or the direct perpetrators of lung injury. In the acute form, inflammatory cells and edema occur within the alveolar and bronchial walls. In the chronic variant, alveolar walls may be thickened; interstitial fibrosis occurs in one-half of cases.

CLINICAL FINDINGS

Acute Eosinophilic Pneumonia

Patients with acute eosinophilic pneumonia have rapidly progressive pulmonary disease with dyspnea, a nonproductive cough, fever, and myalgia. The time from onset of symptoms to respiratory failure that necessitates mechanical ventilation may

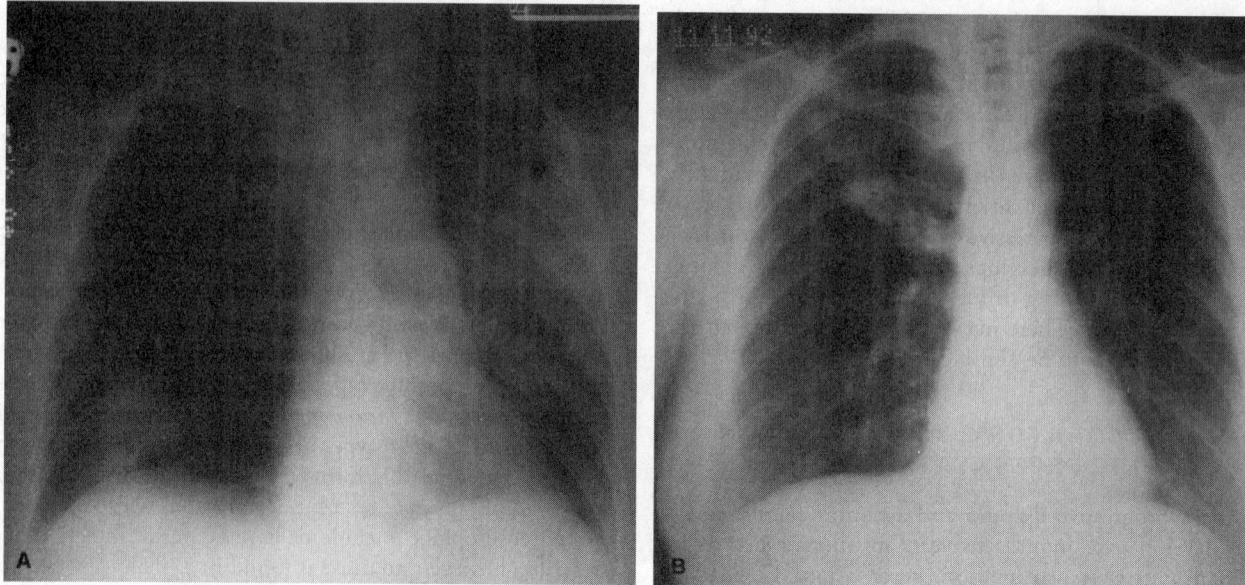

FIGURE 376.2. Chronic eosinophilic pneumonia. A 42-year-old woman had dyspnea, a nonproductive cough, and a low-grade fever. Eosinophilia was present in the serum and bronchoalveolar lavage fluid. Chest radiograph **(A)** shows peripheral infiltrates in the left upper and right lower lobes. Symptoms and infiltrates resolved with glucocorticoid therapy. Several months later, during steroid taper, the patient had a flare of symptoms, elevation of serum eosinophil count, and a new right upper lobe infiltrate **(B)**. Symptoms and infiltrate resolved with resumption of steroid therapy. (Radiographs courtesy of Marcia McCowin, MD).

be as rapid as a few days. Physical examination typically reveals rales and rarely wheezes on chest auscultation.

Simple Eosinophilic Pneumonia

Patients with simple eosinophilic pneumonia can have an asymptomatic presentation with an unexpected elevated eosinophil count, an abnormal chest radiograph, mild dyspnea, or a cough typically of less than 1 month's duration. Fever may be present. Findings at physical examination may be normal or reveal rare rales or wheezes on chest auscultation.

Chronic Eosinophilic Pneumonia

Patients with chronic eosinophilic pneumonia have an insidious onset, usually lasting more than 2 months, of dyspnea, cough occasionally productive of mucoid sputum, low-grade fevers, and malaise (Fig 376.2). Wheezing and weight loss may be present. Physical examination may reveal rales, wheezes, and occasionally hepatomegaly from eosinophil infiltration of the liver.

LABORATORY AND RADIOGRAPHIC FINDINGS

Acute Eosinophilic Pneumonia

The number of eosinophils in peripheral blood typically is normal or is minimally elevated when the patient comes to medical attention, although most patients have some elevation during the clinical course. Total peripheral blood white blood cell count, erythrocyte sedimentation rate, and IgE level may be elevated.

In the acute form as opposed to the simple and chronic forms, hypoxemia may be marked. Chest radiographs may reveal unilateral or bilateral, diffuse or patchy, interstitial or alveolar infiltrates. Small pleural effusions are common.

Simple Eosinophilic Pneumonia

Simple eosinophilic pneumonia is much less well-described than the acute and chronic forms. Many patients with simple eosinophilic pneumonia have peripheral blood eosinophilia. Chest radiographs characteristically show transient, migratory, peripheral infiltrates.

Chronic Eosinophilic Pneumonia

Mild to moderate elevation of eosinophil count in the peripheral blood is typical; the count usually is higher than in the acute variety. Total peripheral blood white blood cell count, erythrocyte sedimentation rate, and IgE level may be elevated. Hypoxemia or an elevated alveolar-arterial gradient may be present. On radiographs the classic pattern of chronic eosinophilic pneumonia—migratory, dense, bilateral, peripheral infiltrates—occurs among only 25% of patients; however, the infiltrates are peripheral (outer two-thirds of the lung field) in 65% of patients. CT findings confirm the typically peripheral nature of the infiltrates. Some patients also have hilar or mediastinal adenopathy. In both forms, reduced lung volume and a decreased diffusion capacity for carbon monoxide occur. Although more frequent among patients with asthma, an obstructive pattern may occur among patients without such a history. In all forms, even though peripheral blood eosinophilia may be absent or minimal, lung eosinophil count is invariably elevated. The number of eosinophils recovered at bronchoalveolar lavage by means of bronchoscopy correlates well with the presence of lung eosinophils.

STRATEGIES FOR OPTIMAL CARE

Secondary causes should be considered when a patient has any type of eosinophilic pneumonia, especially that caused by a drug reaction or parasitic infection. Patients with simple eosinophilic pneumonia may have spontaneous resolution of symptoms, eosinophilia, and radiographic abnormalities within several weeks even without glucocorticoid treatment. Relapse is unusual. Among patients with fulminant acute eosinophilic pneumonia, the rapid progression mimics that of acute respiratory distress syndrome ARDS or rapidly progressive community-acquired pneumonia. Bronchoalveolar lavage, which reveals eosinophilia and allows exclusion of infectious causes for the infiltrates, may be the most opportune way to make a rapid diagnosis. High-dose steroid therapy causes rapid reversal of the disease. Steroids are tapered over several weeks, and recurrence is not a feature of this form of eosinophilic pneumonia.

Patients with chronic eosinophilic pneumonia need glucocorticoid therapy because spontaneous resolution occurs among less than 10% of patients. Patients with classic bilateral peripheral infiltrates on radiographs, an elevated peripheral eosinophil count, and typical symptoms do not need lung biopsy. Marked eosinophilia (more than 25% of recovered cells; normal is less than 1%) at bronchoalveolar lavage supports the diagnosis of eosinophilic pneumonia. Therapy for chronic eosinophilic pneumonia with prednisone 1 mg per kilogram per day brings about rapid improvement of symptoms within several days and radiographic improvement over 1 to 2 weeks. The dramatic clinical response to steroids supports a presumptive diagnosis. Steroid therapy for chronic eosinophilic pneumonia should continue for approximately 6 months. Relapse after withdrawal of steroids is common, but not predictable. Many patients need long-term daily or alternate-day therapy. The long-term prognosis is good. Relapses typically respond to re-initiation of steroid therapy.

■ GOODPASTURE'S SYNDROME

DEFINITION

Goodpasture's syndrome is alveolar hemorrhage and glomerulonephritis associated with the presence of anti–glomerular basement membrane (GBM) antibody in serum or evident on immunofluorescent stains of renal or lung tissue. *Anti–glomerular basement membrane antibody disease* is the preferred term because it clearly differentiates Goodpasture's syndrome from other pulmonary–renal syndromes and includes patients with isolated anti-GBM antibody renal disease.

INCIDENCE AND EPIDEMIOLOGY

Anti-GBM antibody disease is a rare disorder. The true incidence is unknown, but this disease has been estimated to account for 1% to 5% of all cases of glomerulonephritis. Case reports suggest the disease is more prevalent among whites and men, although the male to female ratio varies from 2:1 to 9:1 in different reports. Although the disease occurs among persons of all ages, the peak incidence is in the twenties through fifties.

ETIOLOGY AND PATHOGENESIS

Anti-GBM antibody disease is a true autoimmune disorder in which antibodies form against basement membrane for unknown reasons. Possible triggers include viral upper respiratory tract infection (20% to 60% of patients) and exposure to hydrocarbon solvent (less than 5% of patients). This disease is strongly associated with smoking (75% to 80% of patients), especially among patients with pulmonary hemorrhage. It has been postulated that a noxious event, such as infection or exposure to a toxin, among genetically predisposed persons damages basement membrane and exposes an antigen that triggers IgG autoantibody production.

Basement membrane is heterogeneous in the body; anti-GBM antibody appears to have specificity for an α3 domain on type IV collagen present in high concentrations in alveolar and GBM. This binding specificity may account for the organ specificity of this disease. Once formed, the circulating autoantibody has direct access to GBM. In contrast, alveolar capillaries lack the large fenestrations of glomeruli. An increase in capillary permeability appears to be necessary for antibodies to gain access to alveolar basement membrane. This hypothesis is supported by the clinical observations that alveolar hemorrhage is more common among smokers and that episodes of hemoptysis often occur after infection and fluid overload. Once the anti-GBM antibody is bound to basement membrane, complement binding occurs, and there is an influx of neutrophils and other inflammatory cells. Light microscopic examination of the kidney tissue reveals focal segmental necrotizing glomerulonephritis with epithelial crescents. Lung findings include alveolar red blood cells, hemosiderin-laden macrophages, and type II cell hyperplasia. In both the kidney and lung, immunofluorescent microscopic examination reveals linear deposits of IgG along the basement membrane.

CLINICAL FINDINGS

The most common presenting symptom is hemoptysis (80% to 90% of patients), which can be mild to life threatening. Most patients also have dyspnea, a cough, and fatigue. Patients may report fever and chills, chest pain, weight loss, and for 10% to 40% of patients, gross hematuria. Unlike the situation with systemic vasculitis, joint pain and skin rashes are uncommon. At physical examination, pallor from anemia is common (50% to 90% of patients). Lung examination may have normal findings or reveal rales, rhonchi, or decreased breath sounds. Patients with advanced renal disease may have peripheral edema. Unlike the situation with many other forms of active glomerulonephritis, systemic hypertension is uncommon. Hemoptysis can precede clinically apparent renal disease by months to years, although renal involvement usually is evident on immunofluorescent staining of renal biopsy specimens. Ten percent to 20%

of patients with anti-GBM disease have renal manifestations only.

LABORATORY AND RADIOGRAPHIC FINDINGS

Circulating anti-GBM antibodies found with enzyme-linked immunosorbent assay can be detected among more than 90% of patients. The finding of these antibodies appears to have a specificity of more than 95%. Anemia occurs among 90% of patients and is caused primarily by pulmonary blood loss. Serum iron levels may be decreased, though microcytic anemia is not common. The white blood cell count may be elevated. One-half of patients have some degree of azotemia. Urinalysis reveals hematuria or proteinuria (not in the nephrotic range) among 80% to 100% of patients. Radiographs of patients with alveolar hemorrhage show nonspecific patchy or diffuse alveolar infiltrates that typically, though not invariably, spare the apexes and bases. Several days after a bout of alveolar hemorrhage, a reticulonodular pattern may emerge that is thought to reflect clearance of hemoglobin by macrophages into lymphatic vessels and the interstitium. After repeated bouts of hemorrhage, interstitial fibrosis may occur. CT does not appear to add any clinically relevant information. Pulmonary function testing may reveal an elevated diffusion capacity for carbon monoxide consistent with recent alveolar hemorrhage. Many patients are too dyspneic for the breath holding required for this maneuver. Serious pulmonary hemorrhage sometimes occurs without apparent hemoptysis. Bronchoscopy performed to investigate an undiagnosed infiltrate suggests alveolar hemorrhage if the recovered lavage material is or becomes increasingly bloody during lavage. Lavage typically reveals hemosiderin-laden macrophages; this is a nonspecific finding that occurs with any type of bleeding in the lung.

STRATEGIES FOR OPTIMAL CARE

Because the disease can have a rapidly progressive and fulminant course, prompt diagnosis and initiation of therapy for anti-GBM antibody disease are extremely important. An elevated anti-GBM antibody level in the appropriate clinical setting establishes the diagnosis. When uncertainty exists, or if there is delay in obtaining antibody levels, tissue may be obtained for immunofluorescent staining. The kidney is the preferred biopsy site because use of lung tissue is associated with higher reported false-positive and false-negative rates of immunofluorescent staining. Therapy, a combination of immunosuppression and plasma exchange, is directed at removal of the pathogenic anti-GBM antibodies and suppression of future production. Compared with results for historical controls, who had 75% to 90% mortality, the survival rate for combination therapy is 50% to 85%. Prednisone 1 to 2 mg per kilogram per day and cyclophosphamide 2 mg per kilogram per day are recommended. Some authors recommend 1 to 3 days of higher doses of glucocorticoids initially and for additional bouts of alveolar hemorrhage.

Plasmapheresis should be repeated every 1 to 3 days until circulating anti-GBM antibodies disappear (approximately 2 weeks). The addition of plasmapheresis to immunosuppression is associated with a faster decline in circulating antibody levels

and better recovery of renal function. Renal failure with poor chance of recovery occurs among patients who come to medical attention with anuria, a creatinine level greater than 7 mg per deciliter, or more than 50% glomeruli with crescent formation at renal biopsy. Early relapse is not uncommon and has been associated with concurrent infection, fluid overload, resumption of cigarette smoking, and taper of immunosuppression. Late recurrence is very rare.

■ PULMONARY ALVEOLAR PROTEINOSIS

DEFINITION

Pulmonary alveolar proteinosis (PAP) is a disorder of unknown causation characterized by alveolar accumulation of an acellular amorphous insoluble lipoproteinaceous material that resembles surfactant. Although complicated in rare instances by secondary right heart failure, the disease is otherwise limited to the lungs.

INCIDENCE AND EPIDEMIOLOGY

PAP appears to be a rare disease. Although the disease has distinct pathologic findings, PAP was not reported in the medical literature until the late 1950s. The disease appears to be twice as common among men as among women. The typical age at onset is in the third to sixth decades. Primary or idiopathic PAP occurs among previously healthy persons. Secondary PAP has been associated with hematologic malignant disease, especially myeloid leukemia; immunosuppression, including HIV disease; and acute exposure to dust and fumes, especially silica in sandblasting.

ETIOLOGY AND PATHOGENESIS

The cause of PAP is unknown. The association between some exposures and secondary PAP suggests a nonspecific alveolar injury response from known and as yet unknown factors. At light microscopic examination, alveoli and small airways are filled with large amounts of an acellular eosinophilic material that stains with periodic acid–Schiff (PAS) reagent. The main components of this material are phospholipids and proteins that appear to be mainly derived from lung surfactant. Alveolar macrophages are vacuolated (filled with ingested lipoproteinaceous material), giant, and poorly mobile. Inflammation and fibrosis have been detected in some cases but are not prominent features. Electron microscopic examination reveals numerous lamellar bodies composed of layers of phospholipids in the alveolar material and in the vacuoles of alveolar macrophages. Overaccumulation of surfactant or surfactant-like material in alveoli may be caused by overproduction, oversecretion, or abnormal reabsorption by type II pneumocytes, poor clearance by alveolar macrophages, or a combination of several dysfunctions.

Pneumocystis carinii infection is characterized by the presence of foamy eosinophilic alveolar material containing cysts, trophozoites, and macrophages. Although *P. carinii* pneumonia is typically pathologically distinct from PAP, in some cases extracellular material has PAP-like lamellar structures evident at electron microscopic examination.

CLINICAL PRESENTATION

Patients most commonly notice a gradual onset of exertional dyspnea and coughing, usually nonproductive but occasionally productive of gummy or chunky sputum. Patients may also have low-grade fevers, pleuritic chest pain, scant hemoptysis, and weight loss. Physical examination may reveal rales or lack of breath sounds in densely consolidated lung segments. Cyanosis and clubbing have been reported among about one-fourth of patients. Some patients have no symptoms and have radiographic abnormalities only. Some patients may have a sudden onset of fever, coughing, and dyspnea from PAP or a superimposed infection. Patients with PAP appear to be prone to pulmonary infection with *Nocardia* organisms, mycobacterial species, fungi, and viruses. Alveolar macrophages in PAP exhibit poor phagocytic function. This acquired defect may be caused by overingestion of the surfactant material. Filling of alveoli with this insoluble material may impede other infectious clearance mechanisms.

LABORATORY AND RADIOGRAPHIC PRESENTATION

Most patients with PAP have a mildly elevated lactate dehydrogenase level. Serum levels of lung surfactant proteins A and D can be markedly elevated, but these levels may be elevated with idiopathic pulmonary fibrosis and interstitial lung disease associated with connective tissue disease. Hypoxemia may be present and worsens with exercise. Pulmonary function testing typically reveals an increased shunt fraction, a mildly restrictive defect with a disproportionate decrease in diffusion capacity for carbon monoxide. Chest radiographs typically show bilateral, symmetrical alveolar infiltrates with air bronchograms that are worse in the bases but spare costophrenic angles. Unilateral infiltrates also are present. Pleural effusions and lymphadenopathy are unusual and suggest another pathologic or infectious process. In long-standing cases of PAP, fibrosis may occur, and an interstitial or reticulonodular pattern may be seen. High-resolution CT (Fig 376.3) may reveal a characteristic, though not pathognomonic crazy paving pattern of polygonal areas of ground-glass opacification next to radiographically uninvolved tissue.

STRATEGIES FOR OPTIMAL CARE

The diagnosis of PAP is made most conveniently by means of bronchoalveolar lavage. The lavage material is turbid, opaque, and opalescent and has a tan, dense sediment after gravity centrifugation. Under a light microscope, the sediment stains pink with PAS reagent. Results of transbronchial or open lung biopsy confirm the diagnosis when characteristically acellular, eosinophilic, PAS-positive material fills the alveoli (Fig 376.4). Electron microscopic demonstration of lamellar bodies also confirms the diagnosis. Because PAP can histologically mimic and perhaps be triggered by *P. carinii* infection, lavage material should be examined for this organism. Lavage material also should be cultured for fungi, *Nocardia* organisms, and mycobacterial species, because PAP may be a predisposing factor for these infections. The incidence, however, of these coexistent infections is lower in more recent case series.

PAP occasionally resolves spontaneously; therefore observation for several months may be appropriate, especially when a patient has no symptoms or mild symptoms. Therapy is indi-

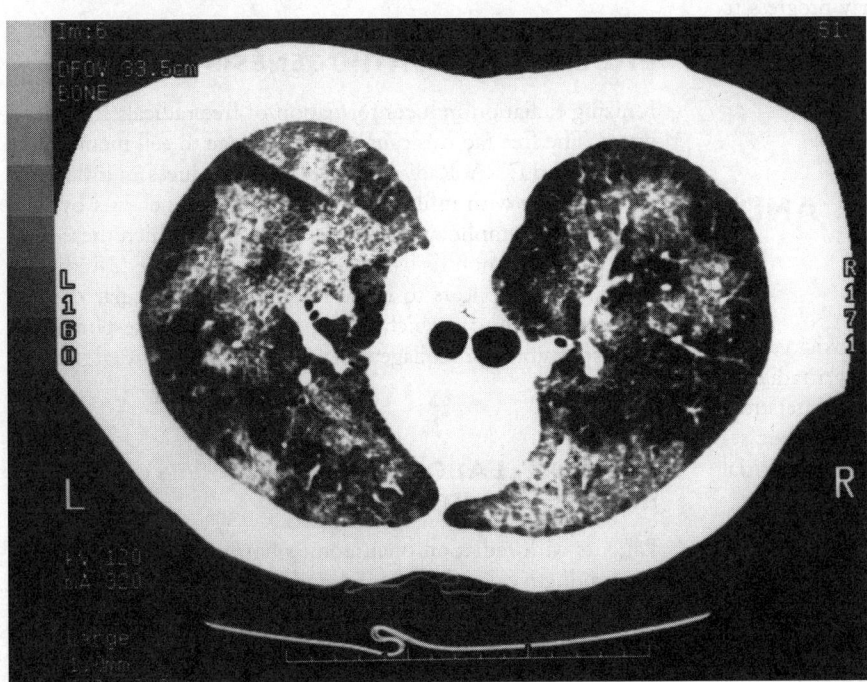

FIGURE 376.3. Pulmonary alveolar proteinosis. A 39-year-old man had gradual onset of dyspnea and a nonproductive cough. High-resolution CT scan shows the characteristic crazy paving pattern that corresponds to polygonal areas of ground-glass opacification next to areas that are closer to normal. The diagnosis was confirmed through examination of bronchoalveolar lavage fluid. The patient's condition improved after whole-lung lavage therapy. (Image courtesy of Marcia McCowin, MD).

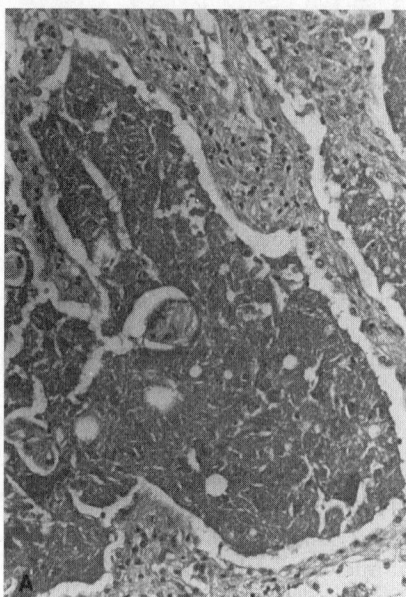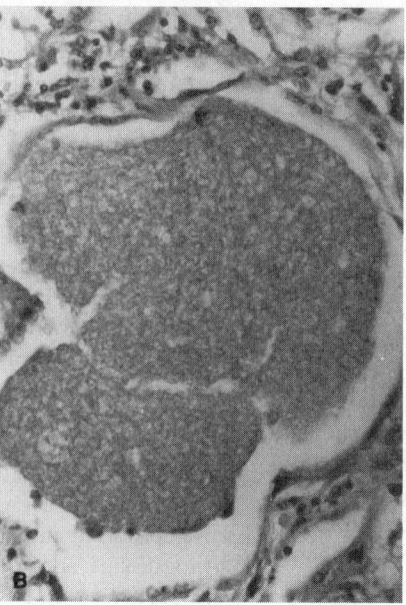

FIGURE 376.4. Pulmonary alveolar proteinosis. Lung biopsy specimens from a patient with pulmonary alveolar proteinosis **(A)** and a patient with *Pneumocystis carinii* pneumonia **(B)**. Both specimens reveal alveolar filling of an amorphous, acellular material that stains pink with routine hematoxylin and eosin stain. The distinction is important. The exudate in **B** appears foamy. Silver stain of this specimen demonstrated characteristic cysts of *P. carinii* organisms. (Pathology slides courtesy of Martha L. Warnock, MD).

cated for moderate to severe symptoms, failure of resolution, progression of symptoms, or physiologic abnormalities such as resting or exertional hypoxemia. Therapy is unique and consists of endotracheal intubation with a double-lumen tube and single whole-lung lavage with sterile saline solution with the aid of general anesthesia. The therapeutic efficacy of lavage is largely due to the mechanical removal of intra-alveolar phospholipids. Substantial symptomatic and physiologic improvement is typical, and lavage of the contralateral lung can be performed at a later time. One-third to one-half of patients who need whole-lung lavage need additional lavage because of recurrences until the disease dissipates, usually within a few years. As many as 20% of patients do not respond to lavage and may progress to pulmonary fibrosis and respiratory failure or die of pulmonary infection. Glucocorticoids are not effective therapy for this disease.

RADIATION PNEUMONITIS AND RADIATION FIBROSIS

DEFINITION

Radiation pneumonitis is a syndrome of radiation toxicity, generally in lung tissue unintentionally or unavoidably irradiated. It is characterized by localized interstitial edema and interstitial and alveolar inflammation. Radiation fibrosis is a late toxic sequela of this inflammatory process characterized by interstitial fibrosis.

INCIDENCE AND EPIDEMIOLOGY

Radiation therapy for malignant disease in the thorax is associated with early acute pneumonitis in 5% to 15% of patients

and with late fibrosis in as many as 75% of patients. Pneumonitis typically develops 6 to 12 weeks after completion of therapy of 4,000 cGy or more, although cases have been reported as early as 2 weeks and as late as 6 months after therapy. Earlier onset usually is associated with higher radiation doses. Pneumonitis is unusual at doses less than 3,000 cGy. Risk factors for the development of pneumonitis include daily radiation dosage, rate of delivery, total radiation dose, volume of lung irradiated, prior radiation, older age, presence of collagen vascular disease, recent withdrawal from steroid therapy, and previous sensitizing or concurrently administered chemotherapeutic agents, especially bleomycin, doxorubicin, cyclophosphamide, and mitomycin.

ETIOLOGY AND PATHOGENESIS

Ionizing radiation induces formation of free radicals from lung water. The free radicals cause direct damage to cell membranes, protein, and DNA. Radiation therapy also induces an inflammatory response with infiltration of the lung parenchyma by neutrophils and lymphocytes. The mechanism by which these injuries cause pneumonitis has not been fully elucidated. Radiation exposure also appears to cause microcapillary vascular damage and ischemic injury, which with the inflammatory response may be responsible for collagen deposition and eventual fibrotic healing.

CLINICAL, LABORATORY, AND RADIOGRAPHIC FINDINGS

Patients with radiation pneumonitis have a subacute onset of a nonproductive cough, dyspnea, and fever. Physical examination may reveal rales or consolidation on the affected side. Hyperpigmentation of the skin within the radiation port is common but does not correlate with the presence or severity of pneumonitis.

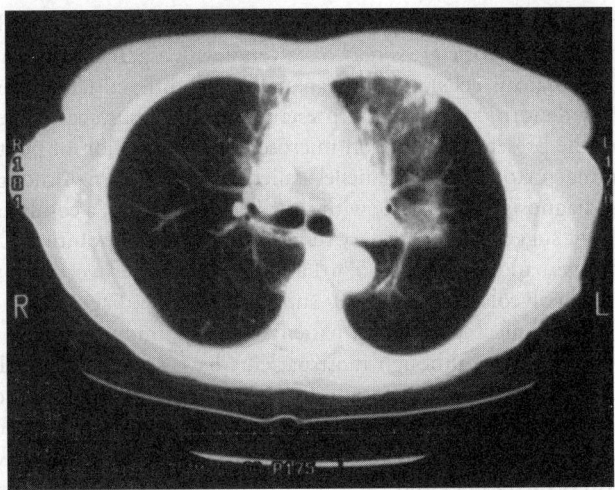

FIGURE 376.5. Radiation pneumonitis. A 77-year-old woman underwent radiation therapy to the left upper hemithorax and mediastinum for lung cancer. Two months after therapy, she reported dyspnea and a dry cough. CT scan shows an area of increased opacity in left upper lobe with a straight edge, which corresponded to the radiation port. (Image courtesy of Marcia McCowin, MD).

Laboratory studies may reveal hypoxemia, an elevated white blood cell count, and elevated erythrocyte sedimentation rate. Chest radiographs and CT scans show homogeneous or patchy alveolar infiltrates, which classically coalesce to have sharp borders that corresponding to radiation ports and not to anatomical lung segments (Fig 376.5). Radiographic changes may occur in patients who do not have symptoms.

STRATEGIES FOR OPTIMAL CARE

The differential diagnosis of radiation pneumonitis includes infection, local tumor reoccurrence, or lymphangitic spread of tumor. The condition of most patients gradually improves over the course of several weeks. With time the involved area contracts, and fibrosis, scarring, and volume loss occur. Therapy consists of symptomatic relief with cough suppressants, analgesics, and antipyretics. Although there are no controlled trials of steroid use by humans, most clinicians agree that in severe cases, prednisone 1 mg per kilogram per day should be instituted. Guidelines for tapering steroids are not well defined, but because radiation pneumonitis has been reported during steroid withdrawal, slow tapering over weeks is advisable. Steroid prophylaxis has not been shown to be beneficial. Pneumonitis may occasionally involve areas outside the radiation port, even the contralateral lung. Several theories, such as radiation scatter, unsuspected infection, including viral infection, and obstruction of lymphatic flow have been proposed to explain cases of bilateral pneumonitis after unilateral radiation. Bronchoalveolar lavage studies have found activated T lymphocytes in segments of lung within and outside the radiation port. This finding suggests that ionizing radiation may stimulate a generalized lymphocyte-mediated reaction.

Some degree of lung fibrosis and scarring within the radiation field occurs in most patients undergoing thoracic irradiation, even in patients without clinically apparent radiation pneumonitis. Nearly all patients with radiation pneumonitis eventually have fibrosis in the region of the radiographic abnormality. Fibrotic radiographic changes usually are present within 1 year of completion of therapy and consist of linear interstitial thickening. Volume loss may cause tracheal deviation and mediastinal shift toward the affected area. Most patients have no symptoms, and stable fibrosis is evident only on radiographs. A few patients, especially those with previous severe pneumonitis, have widespread scarring with physiologic abnormalities. Patients with severe underlying lung disease may have symptomatic pneumonitis with otherwise tolerable amounts of radiation fibrosis. Patients have an insidious onset of dyspnea, which may progress to marked hypoxemia and respiratory failure. Glucocorticoids do not appear to be effective in the management of radiation fibrosis.

HISTIOCYTOSIS X OR LANGERHANS CELL HISTIOCYTOSIS

DEFINITION

Histiocytosis X or Langerhans cell histiocytosis (LCH) is a group of disorders characterized by excessive proliferation of Langerhans cells. Clinical presentations are varied and include Letterer–Siwe disease, a fulminant visceral form that occurs mainly among infants; Hand–Schüller–Christian disease, a multifocal form with lytic bone lesions, exophthalmus, and diabetes insipidus; isolated bony lesions; and pulmonary LCH, sometimes called *eosinophilic granuloma of the lung.*

INCIDENCE AND EPIDEMIOLOGY

Pulmonary LCH is a rare disorder, thought to represent approximately 1% to 5% of all cases of interstitial lung disease. Although LCH can occur at any age, pulmonary LCH typically occurs in the third to fifth decade. Most case series but not all suggest a male predominance. The disease appears to be less common among African Americans and very rare among Asians.

ETIOLOGY AND PATHOGENESIS

The cause of pulmonary LCH is unknown. More than 90% of patients are smokers and frequently heavy smokers. There is no known association with any other environmental or infectious agent. All forms of LCH are thought to represent clonal proliferation of Langerhans cells. Langerhans cells are histiocytes derived from bone marrow precursors and are related to dendritic cells. They occur normally in the skin and sparsely in oral, esophageal, and colonic mucosa and the peribronchiolar interstitium. The function of these cells includes presentation of antigen to lymphocytes. LCH is thought to represent an uncontrolled immune response or hypersensitivity reaction initiated by Langerhans cells to some unknown antigen. Despite the monoclonal nature of the proliferation, the disease appears to be more consistent with a reactive rather than a neoplastic process. The primary lesion in the lung is an accumulation of Langerhans cells at terminal and respiratory bronchioles surrounded by lymphocytes, neutrophils, and eosinophils. This granulomatous lesion destroys nearby bronchiolar walls and causes bronchiolitis, which may cavitate. As the lesions progress, stellate scarring occurs with surrounding traction emphysema or cyst formation. Often in advanced fibrotic lesions, only rare Langerhans cells remain.

CLINICAL FINDINGS

The clinical presentation of pulmonary LCH among adults is variable. Although most patients have a cough and exertional dyspnea with or without constitutional symptoms such as fatigue, fever, and weight loss, approximately 25% have no symptoms, and the condition is found when a chest radiograph is abnormal. Ten percent to 20% of patients have chest pain, most commonly from a spontaneous pneumothorax and occasionally from a lytic rib lesion. Fifteen percent to 20% of patients have focal lytic bony lesions in long bones, the spine, the jaw, and most commonly the skull. As many as 5% of patients initially or eventually have diabetes insipidus from posterior pituitary involvement. The findings at physical examination may be normal, or the patient may have rales and rarely wheezes at chest auscultation. In rare instances clubbing may be present. With advanced fibrotic lung disease, right-sided heart failure and cor pulmonale may develop.

LABORATORY AND RADIOGRAPHIC FINDINGS

Laboratory findings of mild anemia, elevated white blood cell count, low positive titers of rheumatoid factor and antinuclear antibodies may be present but are nonspecific. Blood eosinophilia is not a feature of this disease. A bone scan may be useful to identify bony lesions. Chest radiographs typically reveal a diffuse, bilateral micronodular and cystic process, especially in mid and upper lung zones, that spare costophrenic angles and preserve lung volume. In advanced disease, honeycombing may be present. Enlarged hilar lymph nodes are not present. Pleural abnormalities are unusual unless there is current or previous pneumothorax. High-resolution CT can depict the characteristic combination of cysts and nodular lesions even if a chest radiograph appears normal or reveals only a reticular–nodular pattern. Pulmonary function tests reveal a combination of restriction and obstruction, the latter becoming worse if the disease progresses. Bronchoalveolar lavage can recover increased numbers of Langerhans cells among nonaffected smokers and those with pulmonary LCH. Lavage cell counts with more than 5% Langerhans cells support the diagnosis of pulmonary LCH. Because of sampling error, a low cell count of Langerhans cells does not rule out the diagnosis.

STRATEGIES FOR OPTIMAL CARE

Definitive diagnosis requires tissue biopsy. Transbronchial biopsy typically is inadequate; pathologic diagnosis usually requires open lung or thoracoscopic biopsy. Biopsy specimens reveal

bronchiolar-centric granulomatous lesions with Langerhans cells (end-stage fibrotic areas may have very few Langerhans or other inflammatory cells). Langerhans cells are differentiated from other dendritic cells by the presence of CD1a surface antigen and the presence at electron microscopic examination of penti-laminar cytoplasmic organelles called *Birbeck bodies*. Although the diagnosis can be made with confidence at biopsy, a combination of suggestive pulmonary function tests, high-resolution CT findings, and more than 5% Langerhans cells recovered from bronchoalveolar lavage is very supportive of the diagnosis.

The clinical course for patients with pulmonary LCH is highly variable, although most patients have a good prognosis. Many of those without symptoms and only radiographic or pathologic abnormalities have a self-limited course with radiographic resolution. Patients with symptomatic disease may have periods of stability and even remission. A minority of patients progress to end-stage pulmonary fibrosis and right heart failure; the overall mortality is 2% to 6%. Therapy has included smoking cessation, steroids, and cytotoxic therapy. Though smoking cessation has many beneficial health effects and theoretical support (a strong epidemiologic association and the peribronchiolar location of the lesions suggest an inhaled antigen as the trigger for inflammation), the effect of smoking cessation on the course of pulmonary LCH is unclear.

BIBLIOGRAPHY

Alasaly K, Muller N, Ostrow DN, et al. Cryptogenic organizing pneumonia: a report of 25 cases and a review of the literature. *Medicine (Baltimore)* 1995;74:201–211.

Ambruse JL, Sridhar NR. Immunologic aspects of renal disease. *JAMA* 1997;278:1938–1945.

Epler GR. Bronchiolitis obliterans organizing pneumonia: definition and clinical features. *Chest* 1992;102:2S–6S.

Falk RH, Comenzo RL, Skinner M. The systemic amyloidoses. *N Engl J Med* 1997;337:898–909.

Goldstein LS, Kavuru MS, Curtis-McCarthy P, et al. Pulmonary alveolar proteinosis: clinical features and outcomes. *Chest* 1998;114:1357–1362.

Howarth DM, Gilchrist GS, Mullan BP, et al. Langerhans cell histiocytosis: diagnosis, natural history, management, and outcome. *Cancer* 1999;85: 2278–2290.

Lohr RH, Boland BJ, Douglas WW, et al. Organizing pneumonia: features and prognosis of cryptogenic, secondary, and focal variants. *Arch Intern Med* 1997:157:1323–1329.

Marchand E, Reynaud-Gaubert M, Lauque D, et al. Idiopathic chronic eosinophilic pneumonia: a clinical follow-up study of 62 cases. *Medicine (Baltimore)* 1998;77:299–312.

Movas B, Raffin TA, Epstein AH, et al. Pulmonary radiation injury. *Chest* 1997;111:1061–1076.

Pope-Harman AL, Davis WB, Allen ED, et al. Acute eosinophilic pneumonia: a summary of 15 cases and review of the literature. *Medicine (Baltimore)* 1996;75:334–342.

Roberts CM, Foulcher E, Zaunders JJ, et al. Radiation pneumonitis: a possible lymphocyte mediated hypersensitivity reaction. *Ann Intern Med* 1993;118:696–700.

Utz JP, Swenson SJ, Gertz MA. Pulmonary amyloidosis: the Mayo Clinic experience from 1980 to 1993. *Ann Intern Med* 1996;124:407–413.

Wang BM, Stern EJ, Schmidt RA, et al. Diagnosing pulmonary alveolar proteinosis: a review and update. *Chest* 1997;111:460–466.

Kelley's Textbook of Internal Medicine, fourth edition. Edited by H. David Humes. Lippincott Williams & Wilkins, Philadelphia © 2000.

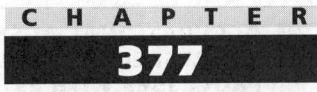

LUNG CANCER

ERIC J. OLSON
JAMES R. JETT

DEFINITION

The term *lung cancer* usually applies to neoplasms arising from the respiratory epithelium called *bronchogenic carcinoma*. Bronchogenic carcinoma accounts for more than 90% of pulmonary tumors (Table 377.1). To account for differences in clinical and pathologic characteristics, bronchogenic carcinoma is divided into two main types—small-cell lung carcinoma (SCLC) and non–small cell lung carcinoma (NSCLC). SCLC is part of the spectrum of neuroendocrine tumors and has a notable propensity for early metastases. The mainstays of treatment are chemotherapy and radiation therapy. NSCLC includes adenocarcinoma, squamous cell carcinoma, large-cell carcinoma, and their subtypes. Surgery is the therapy of choice for early-stage disease. Smoking is the preeminent risk factor for lung cancer. Outcome depends on the cell type of the tumor, the stage of disease, and the performance status of the patient.

INCIDENCE AND EPIDEMIOLOGY

During the twentieth century, lung cancer became one of the most common and lethal forms of cancer worldwide. Lung cancer is now the second most common malignant disease diagnosed among both men and women in the United States. At present, 170,000 to 180,000 new cases are diagnosed each year, an incidence of approximately 60 per 100,000 of the U.S. population. Lung cancer remains more common among men, but the sex difference is narrowing. The incidence among men has declined since peaking in 1984, whereas the incidence among women continues to climb. The result is that 47% of all new cases of lung cancer occur among women. Fortunately, the annual rate of increase in incidence among women is slowing. The age-adjusted incidence of lung cancer is consistently higher among

TABLE 377.1.	WORLD HEALTH ORGANIZATION HISTOLOGIC CLASSIFICATION OF LUNG CANCER
Squamous cell carcinoma	Carcinoid tumor
Small-cell carcinoma	Bronchial gland carcinoma
Adenocarcinoma	Adenoid cystic carcinoma
Large-cell carcinoma	Mucoepidermoid carcinoma
Adenosquamous carcinoma	Other

black men than among white men. The disparity may be caused by differences in smoking behavior, socioeconomic factors, and susceptibility to tobacco smoke. Lung cancer is most commonly diagnosed among persons 55 to 74 years of age. Diagnoses before the age of 35 years are rare. NCSLC is the histologic type in 75% of cases. Adenocarcinoma has increased in incidence in recent years faster than any other cell type.

No other cancer currently claims more lives each year than lung cancer. One-third of all cancer deaths are attributable to lung cancer. The overall 5-year survival rate is a disappointing 14%. The worldwide incidence and mortality rate of lung cancer will continue to increase as a result of ongoing use of tobacco products.

ETIOLOGY

TOBACCO SMOKING

Tobacco smoking is undeniably the leading risk factor for lung cancer. It is estimated that smoking is responsible for 80% to 90% of cases of lung cancer. The evidence establishing a causal relation between tobacco smoking and lung cancer among men was initially summarized in the landmark 1964 report of the U.S. Surgeon General. The association among women was delineated in a 1980 report of the U.S. Surgeon General. The risk of lung cancer is related to the number of cigarettes smoked, age at starting to smoke, and the duration of smoking. The relative risk for death of lung cancer is 9 to 15 times greater among current smokers than among never smokers, and may be as high as 25 times greater among persons who smoke more than 25 cigarettes per day. Greater cigarette consumption or longer, more frequent puffs may negate the use of lower-tar or filtered cigarettes.

Women appear to be more susceptible to the carcinogenic effects of cigarette smoking. Odds ratios for lung cancer are 1.2 to 1.7 times higher among women smokers than among men. This disparity is not simply due to differences in smoking habits or anthropomorphic factors. Pipe and cigar smoking increase the risk of lung cancer, but the risk ratios are generally lower than for cigarette smoking. Approximately 25% of the U.S. population smoke cigarettes, almost all having started before 21 years of age. Use of cigarettes be teenagers has risen in recent years.

The relative risk of lung cancer actually increases for 1 to 4 years after smoking cessation, presumably because some cessation is motivated by symptoms of occult lung cancer. Relative risk then declines substantially. Whether the risk of lung cancer among former smokers ever equals that of nonsmokers remains unclear. In a 40-year study of smoking among British physicians it was concluded that the degree of risk reduction was greater among those who smoked fewer cigarettes for a shorter period of time and who stopped at a younger age. For example, smokers who stopped before the age of 35 years had a survival rate similar to that of nonsmokers.

ENVIRONMENTAL TOBACCO SMOKE

Environmental tobacco smoke is composed of sidestream smoke that emanates from the burning end of cigarettes and of mainstream smoke exhaled by smokers. Some components of tobacco smoke may be more concentrated in sidestream smoke than in mainstream smoke. The cumulative data on environmental tobacco smoke indicate that nonsmokers living with smokers have a 20% to 30% higher risk of lung cancer than do persons in smoke-free homes. In 1992 the U.S. Environmental Protection Agency estimated that environmental tobacco smoke accounts for 3,000 new cases of lung cancer each year in the United States.

RADON

The link between radon, a breakdown product of uranium, and lung cancer was initially established among underground miners of uranium, tin, and iron ore in areas of high radioactivity. Exposures now occur in residences as radon and its decay progeny pervade basements. Extrapolating from the mining experience is difficult, but in a meta-analysis of eight case-control studies it was concluded that indoor radon exposure caused a 1.14 increased relative risk of lung cancer. It has been estimated by the Committee on Biologic Effects of Ionizing Radiation that radon is responsible for 10% of cases of lung cancer in the United States.

OCCUPATIONAL EXPOSURE

The International Agency for Research on Cancer of the World Health Organization classifies chemicals and industrial processes with respect to their association with lung cancer (Table 377.2). Industrial carcinogens usually are not exclusively associated with a specific lung cancer cell type. Typically there are synergistic effects between exposure to occupational agents and smoking, and there are prolonged latency periods (years) between occupational exposure and the clinical emergence of lung cancer.

Asbestos includes a group of naturally occurring serpentine or straight, needlelike silicates, the unique properties of which have broad commercial application. Inhalation of asbestos fibers increases risk of pulmonary parenchymal fibrosis (asbestosis), pleural abnormalities (pleural plaques, pleural thickening, effusions, rounded atelectasis) and malignant tumors (lung cancer, mesothelioma). It is estimated that nonsmokers exposed to asbestos are at fivefold greater risk of lung cancer than are nonsmokers not exposed to asbestos. The combination of tobacco smoking and asbestos exposure may increase lung cancer risk 50-fold. Risk of lung cancer usually increases 20 to 30 years after the initial exposure. Amphibole (straight) fibers are considered more carcinogenic than chrysotile (serpentine) fibers. Whether a threshold asbestos exposure level exists for lung cancer remains unclear.

OTHERS

Chronic obstructive pulmonary disease (COPD) is an independent risk factor for lung cancer. The relative risk of lung cancer is 4 to 6 times greater in the setting of airway obstruction. This risk increases in proportion to the magnitude of airway obstruction. A genetic predisposition is suggested by numerous investigators who have demonstrated increased risk of lung cancer

TABLE 377.2.	OCCUPATIONAL AGENTS AND THE RESPECTIVE INDUSTRIAL PROCESSES WITH ESTABLISHED LINKS TO LUNG CANCER[a]
Agent	**Industrial Process**
Arsenic	Ore (copper, lead, zinc) smelting; pesticide use
Asbestos	Mining, milling, manufacturing, installation, or removal of asbestos-containing products (pipe fitters, boilermakers, ship builders, textile workers, cement workers, automotive brake workers)
bis (chloromethyl) ether	Manufacturing of ion exchange resins, plastics
Chromium	Alloy production; dye and paint manufacturing; welding; electroplating
Nickel	Electroplating; steel and alloy production; manufacture of ceramics or storage batteries; petroleum refining; manufacture of electric circuits
Polycyclic aromatic hydrocarbons	Smelting of nickel-containing ores; iron and steel founding; coke oven emissions; organic material combustion
Radon	Mining
Vinyl chloride	Manufacture of plastics or packaging materials

[a] Classification of the International Agency for Research on Cancer.

among close relatives of patients with lung cancer. This familial clustering may be caused by shared tobacco smoke, common environmental factors, or heritable elements. Genes proposed to increase susceptibility for lung cancer include those coding for enzymes that metabolize procarcinogens, such as the cytochrome P450 constituents *CYP1A1* and *CYP2D6*. Air pollution, principally with polycyclic hydrocarbons generated from fossil fuel combustion, may be associated with an increased risk of lung cancer, but establishing a causal link has been methodologically challenging. An inverse relation has been found between fresh fruit and vegetable consumption and risk of lung cancer. Major attention has focused on the vitamin A–related compounds, especially beta carotene, in light of their abilities to neutralize reactive oxygen species and regulate gene expression. However, several randomized chemoprevention trials of use of beta carotene alone or with other antioxidants by subjects at increased risk of lung cancer have shown a higher incidence of lung cancer among the actively treated groups. The preventive agent or agents in fruits and vegetables remains elusive.

PATHOGENESIS

Lung cancer is thought to arise from pluripotent respiratory epithelial stem cells that undergo neoplastic transformation as a result of the accumulation of numerous carcinogen-induced genetic mutations. The exact sequence of events remains to be elucidated, but the putative stages are initiation, promotion, and progression. Genetic alterations caused by radicals produced by the various compounds of the tar and gas phases of cigarette smoke are major initiators and promoters of lung cancer. Pertinent genes affected are believed to be those that regulate cell growth, namely tumor suppressor genes, such as p53 and *RB,* and oncogenes, such as c-*myc,* K-*ras,* and *her2/neu.* The frequently observed chromosomal deletions of 3p, 5q, 9p, and 17p in both SCLC and NSCLC occur at locations of known or suspected tumor suppressor genes. Loss or inactivation of tumor suppressor genes may be integral to development of lung cancer, but the causal relation of these mutations remains unproved. Oncogene activation may be associated with abnormal expression of growth factors, which may have mitogenic effects on the parent cell (autocrine stimulation) and neighboring cells (paracrine stimulation).

The multistep model of lung carcinogenesis is consistent with the myriad cytogenetic abnormalities demonstrated in resected lung cancer, the increase in incidence of lung cancer with age, and the progressive histologic changes of metaplasia, dysplasia, and carcinoma in situ that occur during malignant transformation (at least in the case of squamous cell carcinoma). The proposed pluripotent respiratory epithelial stem cell that gives rise to lung cancer has yet to be identified, but the concept is supported by the histologic variability in tumor specimens. Major heterogeneity (features of more than one histologic type) can be identified in as many as 45% of cases of lung cancer.

CLINICAL FINDINGS

Most cases of lung cancer are symptomatic at diagnosis. Locoregional effects of lung cancer, metastasis, or paraneoplastic phenomena may cause symptoms and physical signs (Tables 377.3 and 377.4).

LOCOREGIONAL EFFECTS

A cough, the most common symptom of lung cancer, occurs among as many as 75% of patients and may be caused by invasion of the bronchial mucosa by tumor, postobstructive pneumonitis or atelectasis, tumor cavitation, or pleural effusion. A cough is a universal symptom among smokers, but a change in character of the cough may signal a cause other than smoking-related bronchitis. Fifty percent of patients with lung cancer have dyspnea, which may arise from large airway obstruction with or without pneumonitis or atelectasis. Patients also may have pleural effusion, lymphangitic metastasis, pericardial effusion, thromboembolism, or concurrent COPD. Hemoptysis also occurs among 50% of patients and usually consists of blood-streaked sputum. Causes include tumor necrosis, mucosal ulceration, erosion into thoracic blood vessels, postobstructive pneumonia, and thromboembolism. Lung cancer occurs among only 2% to 9% of patients who have hemoptysis and a normal chest

TABLE 377.3.	PRESENTATION OF LUNG CANCER: LOCOREGIONAL AND METASTATIC CONSIDERATIONS

Locoregional
  Cough
  Dyspnea
  Hemoptysis
  Chest pain
  Hemidiaphragm paralysis
  Hoarseness
  Pericardium effusions, tamponade
  Dysrhythmias
  Intrathoracic metastases
    Nodules
    Lymphangitic carcinomatosis
  Pleural effusion
  Superior vena cava syndrome
  Pancoast's syndrome
Sites of metastasis
  Adrenal glands
  Liver
  Central nervous system
  Bone

radiograph. Forty percent of patients have chest pain. Tumor involvement of the parietal pleura, chest wall, and mediastinum may cause aching chest pain. Pleuritic pain may be caused by infection, extension of tumor into the chest wall, or thromboembolic disease. Extension of the lung cancer to the mediastinum also may cause ipsilateral diaphragmatic paralysis due to phrenic nerve involvement or hoarseness due to entrapment of the left recurrent laryngeal nerve along its intrathoracic course. Extension to the pericardium may produce effusion, tamponade, or dysrhythmia. Jugular venous hypertension, paradoxical pulse, and an enlarged cardiac silhouette on a chest radiograph that suggests pericardial involvement. Patterns of spread of lung cancer within the lung include lymphangitic spread and nodular or mass lesions.

Pleural effusion occurs among 10% of patients with lung cancer because of impaired lymphatic drainage, pleural metastasis, postobstructive pneumonitis or atelectasis, thromboembolism, hypoalbuminemia, or illnesses unrelated to lung cancer, such as congestive heart failure. Pleural effusion is suggested at examination by the combination of percussed dullness, diminished breath sounds, and reduced fremitus. These findings, however, also occur with hemidiaphragmatic dysfunction from phrenic nerve involvement or postobstructive pneumonitis or atelectasis. Malignant effusions usually are exudative, lymphocytic predominant, ipsilateral to the main tumor, and moderate to large in size, and they reaccumulate quickly after thoracentesis. The cytologic yield from initial thoracentesis of a malignant effusion is 50% and increases to 65% and 70% on the second and third cytologic evaluations. Closed pleural biopsy adds slightly to the diagnostic yield when combined with cytologic examination (7% in one retrospective series). A second thoracentesis is advised in the evaluation of a potentially malignant effusion. Consideration should be given to closed pleural biopsy. For NSCLC, positive results of pleural fluid cytologic examination

TABLE 377.4.	LUNG CANCER: PARANEOPLASTIC SYNDROMES

Endocrine or metabolic
  Hypercalcemia
  Syndrome of inappropriate secretion of antidiuretic hormone
  Cushing's syndrome
  Anorexia, weight loss
  Carcinoid syndrome
  Hyperglycemia or hypoglycemia
  Hypophosphatemia
  Hypouricemia
  Acromegaly
  Galactorrhea
  Hyperthyroidism
Neurologic
  Eaton–Lambert myasthenic syndrome
  Peripheral neuropathy
  Cerebellar degeneration
  Limbic encephalitis
  Polyradiculopathy
  Myelopathy
  Opsoclonus, myoclonus
  Gastrointestinal dysmotility
  Retinopathy
Dermatologic
  Clubbing
  Hypertrophic pulmonary osteoarthropathy
  Bazex's syndrome (acrokeratosis)
  Acquired icthyosis (dry skin)
  Dermatomyositis
  Tylosis (thickened skin of palms)
  Erythema annulare centrifugum
  Acanthosis nigricans
  Erythema gyratum repens
  Erythroderma
  Urticaria
  Vasculitis
  Pruritis
  Leser–Trélat sign (abrupt onset of multiple seborrheic keratoses)
Musculoskeletal
  Polymyositis
  Myopathy
Hematologic
  Anemia
  Polycythemia
  Hypercoagulable state
    Migratory thrombophlebitis
    Disseminated intravascular coagulation
    Nonbacterial thrombotic endocarditis
  Dysproteinemia
  Eosinophilia
Renal
  Glomerulonephritis
  Nephrotic syndrome
  Tubulointerstitial disorders

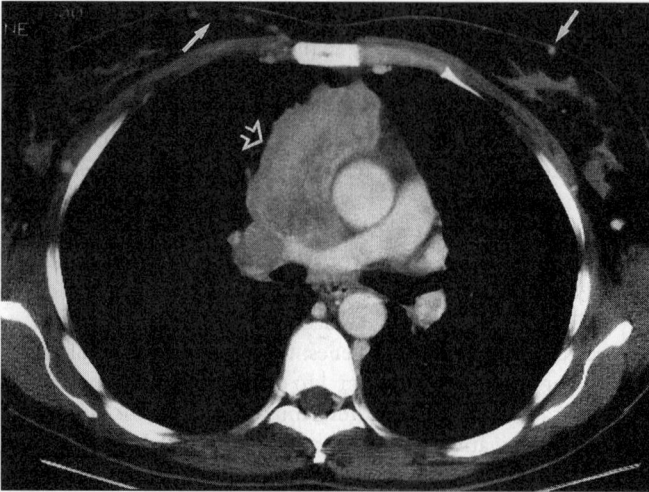

FIGURE 377.1. Superior vena cava syndrome. CT scan shows small-cell carcinoma (*open arrow*) engulfing the superior vena cava and causing dilatation of collateral veins of the chest wall (*solid arrows*). (Image courtesy of Thomas E. Hartman, MD, Mayo Clinic.)

channels over the upper chest. Superior vena cava syndrome is no longer considered a medical emergency. A tissue diagnosis should be obtained before therapy is initiated. Radiation or chemotherapy relieves symptoms in most cases. Pain in the ipsilateral shoulder and scapula, pain with or without muscle atrophy in the ulnar nerve distribution, and Horner's syndrome (ptosis, miosis, and ipsilateral facial anhidrosis) resulting from invasion of the chest wall, brachial plexus, and sympathetic ganglion by tumors in the superior sulcus characterize Pancoast's syndrome. NSCLC is the most common histologic type of superior sulcus tumor. Magnetic resonance imaging (MRI) more accurately defines the local magnitude of the superior sulcus tumor than does computed tomography (CT).

METASTATIC EFFECTS

Common sites of metastatic spread are the adrenal glands, liver, central nervous system (CNS), and bone. Adrenal metastasis usually is asymptomatic and is detected as unilateral adrenal enlargement during staging chest CT extended to the upper abdomen. This scenario occurs in approximately 8% of lung cancer evaluations, and 2% of lesions found to be metastatic. The differential diagnosis is adrenal adenoma, which usually appears as a well-circumscribed, homogenous, low-attenuation lesion less than 3 cm in diameter at CT. An indeterminate adrenal lesion in a patient with NSCLC should be sampled by means of CT-guided biopsy before an attempt is made at curative thoracic surgery. Liver metastasis is more common with SCLC. It is present in 25% of patients when they come to medical attention as opposed to 5% of patients with NSCLC.

Metastases to the CNS may involve the cerebral hemispheres, spinal cord, or meninges. The most common cause of cerebral metastasis is lung cancer. SCLC and adenocarcinoma are most likely to metastasize to the brain; squamous cell carcinoma is least likely. Cerebral metastatic lesions cause focal (seizures) or

eliminate surgical resection as an option. It therefore is imperative that the clinician thoroughly evaluate pleural effusion for patients with NSCLC that is otherwise resectable.

Superior vena cava syndrome is caused by lung cancer in 65% to 80% of cases (Fig 377.1). Manifestations include headache, facial fullness, swelling of the face, neck, and upper extremities, jugular venous congestion, and prominent collateral venous

nonfocal (headache) symptoms. Intraspinal lesions usually cause persistent back pain aggravated by movement, straining, and supine positioning. Spinal cord compression, heralded by a sensorimotor deficit at or below the level of the lesion and bowel or bladder incontinence, is an emergency for which steroids should be administered pending definitive diagnosis and treatment. Skeletal metastatic lesions typically take the form of osteolytic lesions of the vertebral bodies, ribs, and long bones of the extremities. SCLC has the highest propensity for bony metastasis; 20% to 30% of patients are found to have skeletal involvement at initial staging.

PARANEOPLASTIC EFFECTS

Ten percent to 20% of patients with lung cancer have a paraneoplastic syndrome, a diverse set of conditions most commonly associated with SCLC that is caused by effects of lung cancer apart from the physical presence of the primary or metastatic lesions (Table 377.5). Paraneoplastic symptoms may be the initial feature of lung carcinoma, a tumor that sometimes is small and otherwise difficult to detect. Hypercalcemia is the most frequent paraneoplastic effect, and squamous cell carcinoma usually is responsible. Hypercalcemia is caused primarily by tumor production of parathyroid hormone–related peptide (PTHrP), which mimics the action of endogenous parathyroid hormone (PTH). It causes hypercalcemia by increasing osteoclastic bone breakdown, decreasing bone formation, and decreasing renal excretion of calcium. The diagnosis is suggested by the combination of increased serum levels of ionized calcium (or a disproportionate increase in total serum calcium level relative to serum albumin level), normal or low PTH level at immunoassay, and exclusion of other causes of hypercalcemia (such as bone metastasis). PTH can be differentiated from PTHrP by carboxy and amino terminal PTH assays. Patients with hypercalcemia caused by ectopic PTHrP usually have extensive disease with liver involvement. Treatment includes volume repletion with normal saline solution, loop diuretics to increase calcium excretion, bi-

phosphonates or calcitonin to decrease bony resorption, and therapy for the malignant disease.

In the setting of cancer, the syndrome of inappropriate secretion of antidiuretic hormone (SIADH) is nearly always caused by SCLC. Antidiuretic hormone promotes free water retention in the distal renal tubule. The diagnostic criteria for SIADH are hyponatremia, serum hypo-osmolality (<275 mOsm per kilogram), inappropriately increased urine osmolality (>200 mosm per kilogram), inappropriately increased urine sodium concentration (>20 mEq per liter), clinical euvolemia without edema, and normal thyroid, adrenal, and renal function. Fluid restriction (less than 1 L per day) is the initial treatment of patients with no or mild symptoms. Demeclocycline, which blocks the renal effects of antidiuretic hormone, may be added if necessary. More serious symptoms, such as changes in mental status and seizures or more profound hyponatremia (serum sodium concentration <120 mEq per liter) necessitate administration of normal saline solution with a loop diuretic. Serum sodium level should be increased at a maximum rate of 2 mEq per liter per hour (maximum 20 mEq per liter per day) to a target of 120 to 125 mEq per liter. More aggressive sodium correction can cause central pontine myelinolysis, a neurologic insult characterized by flaccid quadriplegia and usually death. SIADH occurs among approximately 10% of patients with SCLC. Serum sodium level normalizes for 80% to 90% of patients within 6 weeks after initiation of chemotherapy.

SCLC and carcinoids can cause Cushing's syndrome through ectopic production of corticotropin (ACTH) or corticotropin-releasing hormone. The 5% of patients with SCLC who have Cushing's syndrome have a poor prognosis. The presence of Cushing's syndrome is confirmed by elevation of 24-hour urinary free cortisol level and failure to suppress cortisol production during low-dose dexamethasone challenge. Ectopic production of ACTH as a cause of Cushing's syndrome is suggested by lack of cortisol suppression with high-dose dexamethasone and plasma ACTH levels greater than 200 pg per milliliter. Treatment options include management of the underlying tumor (surgery for carcinoid and chemoradiation therapy for SCLC), bilateral adrenalectomy, or pharmacologic adrenal suppression. All patients with Cushing's syndrome should undergo CT of the chest and entire abdomen to find occult carcinoid tumor in the lung, thymus, or pancreas.

The paraneoplastic neurologic manifestations of lung cancer include a group of conditions thought to be autoimmune phenomena. Ectopic expression by tumor cells of antigens homologous to those normally present in the nervous system triggers an immune response. Neural tissue expressing the same antigen is attacked. The result is clinical deficits ranging from focal deficits to more widespread dysfunction. An example is Eaton–Lambert myasthenic syndrome, a condition that occurs among 1% to 3% of patients with SCLC and is characterized by proximal muscle weakness, hyporeflexia, and autonomic dysfunction. SCLC cells express P/Q type voltage-gated calcium channels similar to those normally found at presynaptic cholinergic synapses. These channels mediate the release of acetylcholine by allowing influx of calcium on arrival of an action potential. Anti–calcium channel antibodies are generated and are demonstrated in the serum.

TABLE 377.5.	CAUSES OF SOLITARY PULMONARY NODULES
Benign	**Malignant**
Infectious granulomas	Bronchogenic carcinoma
Histoplasmosis	Metastatic lesion
Coccidiomycosis	Carcinoid
Tuberculosis	
Hamartoma	
Pneumonia	
Wegener's granulomatosis	
Rheumatoid arthritis	
Arteriovenous malformation	
Pulmonary infarct	
Amyloidoma	
Dirofiliariasis	
Abscess	
Scar	

The clinical manifestations of Eaton–Lambert myasthenic syndrome are caused by the interference of acetylcholine release by the antibody–calcium channel interaction. Approximately one-third to one-half of patients with Eaton–Lambert myasthenic syndrome improve with therapy for SCLC. Other examples include the diverse set of neurologic manifestations associated with antineuronal nuclear autoantibodies (ANNA-1). These polyclonal IgG antibodies, also known as anti-Hu, recognize a family of nuclear mRNA-binding proteins expressed in SCLC cells and throughout the nervous system. The pathogenetic role of ANNA-1 remains undefined.

The neurologic manifestations associated with ANNA-1 precede the cancer diagnosis more than 90% of the time and usually progress subacutely. These manifestations include neuropathy (sensory, mixed somatic, autonomic, cranial nerve, motor), cerebellar ataxia, limbic encephalitis (neurocognitive and neurobehavioral deficits with or without seizures), polyradiculopathy, Eaton–Lambert myasthenic syndrome, myopathy, myelopathy, opsoclonus or myoclonus, motor neuronopathy, abnormality of the brachial plexus, aphasia, and gastrointestinal dysmotility. Antiretinal antibodies have been found in some patients with cancer-associated retinopathy, a condition of reduced visual acuity caused by the strikingly focal loss of retinal cells among patients with SCLC. The autoimmune response also may be directed at the tumor itself. This may explain why the underlying SCLC can be localized and difficult to detect with noninvasive imaging. There are no standard, effective therapies for these syndromes.

Cachexia is a common paraneoplastic syndrome and is of multifactorial causation. Clubbing of the fingers and toes is characterized by flattening of the angle between the base of the nail bed and cuticle, curved nails, and bulbous enlargement of the digit tips. Clubbing may be accompanied hypertrophic osteoarthropathy, which is painful periosteal inflammation of the long bones of the arms and legs. The affected bones have periosteal elevations on plain radiographs and symmetrically increased uptake on radionuclide studies. Hypertrophic osteoarthropathy is managed with aspirin or nonsteroidal anti-inflammatory drugs and therapy for the underlying lung cancer. Lung cancer may increase thrombotic potential, which manifests as nonbacterial thrombotic (marantic) endocarditis or recurrent thrombophlebitis (Trousseau's syndrome). An extensive search for a malignant tumor is unjustified when venous thromboembolism develops without conventional risk factors. However, patients with idiopathic venous thromboembolism have a 10% to 15% likelihood of having cancer, so additional investigations for cancer are warranted when the findings of the history, examination, and routine laboratory studies suggest the diagnosis.

SCREENING

To the extent that symptomatic lung cancer has a worse prognosis than cancer detected among persons without symptoms and that the outcome of lung cancer depends heavily on the extent of disease at diagnosis, there has been considerable interest in lung cancer screening. The American Cancer Society does not currently recommend routine screening for lung cancer because multiple studies, including three large prospective, randomized U.S. studies sponsored by the National Cancer Institute in the 1970s did not demonstrate decreased lung cancer mortality in populations screened with sputum cytologic examination and chest radiography. Lung cancer screening is being reassessed as groups at high risk of lung cancer become more clearly defined, understanding of lung carcinogenesis increases, and newer technologies become available (such as monoclonal antibodies to detect malignancy-associated antigens in sputum, spiral CT to obtain rapid and detailed images of the lung, and autofluorescence bronchoscopy to detect early malignant tumors through the differential mucosal uptake of photosensitizing agents).

DIAGNOSIS

The essential aspects of the lung cancer evaluation are histologic distinction of SCLC from NSCLC, accurate appraisal of the extent of disease, and determination of the patient's performance status. This information is obtained through a combination of clinical findings, imaging modalities, and procedures to procure specimens for cytologic or histologic analysis. Difficulties with histologic differentiation of SCLC from NSCLC are infrequent (<5% cases), but SCLC may be mistaken for carcinoid tumor, lymphoma, or NSCLC in the presence of crush artifact or improper specimen processing. Differentiation of primary lung cancer from pulmonary metastasis from an extrapulmonary neoplasm may require special immunohistochemical tests of the tissue, but even then differentiation may not be possible. Obtaining correct information is crucial given the profound effects on treatment and prognosis.

IMAGING STUDIES

Conventional chest radiography usually is the first study to suggest lung cancer. Chest radiography is 70% to 80% accurate in the detection of lung cancer. Certain radiographic appearances may suggest histologic types of lung cancer, although these generalizations are not absolute. Squamous cell carcinoma often manifests as a large perihilar mass that may cavitate, adenocarcinoma as a peripheral solitary nodule or mass, large cell carcinoma as a large peripheral mass, and bronchioloalveolar carcinoma as either a slow-growing nodule or an alveolar infiltrate that may be diffuse. SCLC classically appears as a rapidly enlarging central mass with early hilar and mediastinal spread. Specificity limitations (that is, determining the relevance of abnormalities on chest radiographs) can be partially overcome by comparing current chest radiographs with previous chest radiographs. The sensitivity of chest radiography is low for detection of lymph node metastasis or invasion of the chest wall or mediastinum.

CT provides further definition of the appearance of the primary lesion, may depict concurrent parenchymal or pleural disease, and guides diagnostic maneuvers. CT is limited in its ability to define the extent of lung cancer. For example, the reported sensitivity and specificity of CT in the detection of hilar and mediastinal lymph node metastasis are 60% to 70% because of the inherent constraints of relying on lymph node size as the main measure of normality. The consensus is that intrathoracic lymph nodes larger than 1 cm in diameter on CT scans are abnormal, yet microscopic metastases occur. Benign etiologic factors such as reactive hyperplasia and granulomatous inflammation can cause lymph node enlargement. CT also is less than ideal in the accurate diagnosis of invasion of the chest wall or mediastinal structures, detection of endobronchial lesions, and differentiation of tumor from adjacent atelectasis or pneumonia. CT is not a substitute for pathologic information. Patients must not be denied surgery for NSCLC simply on the basis of CT findings without tissue confirmation.

A common clinicoradiologic problem is a solitary pulmonary nodule (SPN), defined as a singular rounded lesion less than 3 cm in diameter entirely surrounded by normal lung parenchyma and without associated lymphadenopathy. SPNs may be benign or malignant (Table 377.5). Most are benign. Most malignant SPNs are early stage lung cancer. Accurate differentiation is crucial so that malignant lesions are promptly resected and benign nodules are not unnecessarily removed. Clinical factors predictive of high risk of malignancy include smoking, advanced age, prior malignant tumors, and larger nodule size (SPNs larger than 3 cm in diameter are malignant more than 90% of the time). The evaluation proceeds, if possible, with a review of previous chest radiographs. An SPN that has been stable for at least 2 years is considered benign, and no further testing is necessary. An enlarging nodule is considered malignant, and immediate resection is indicated.

When comparison studies are insufficient, the next step is CT with thin sections through the nodule to assess the SPN for calcification, contour, and fat. Central, concentric, and popcorn calcification are reliable indicators that the lesion is benign. Eccentric calcification does not rule out malignancy. The more irregular the edge of the SPN, the greater is the likelihood of malignancy. Spiculation increases the likelihood of malignancy. Fat density within an SPN suggests hamartoma, a benign neoplasm, and nothing further need be done.

Additional radiographic modalities may help clarify the nature of an SPN. Positron emission tomography (PET) with [^{18}F]fluorodeoxyglucose may help detect malignant lesions with 90% to 100% sensitivity and 80% to 89% specificity. The expense and availability of PET are serious limitations. The presence of granulomatous disease may cause false-positive results of PET scans. Lesions less than 1 cm in diameter and slowly growing cancer such as bronchioloalveolar cell carcinoma may be false-negative findings. CT contrast enhancement studies, which entail thin-section evaluation of SPN density before and after administration of iodinated contrast material, help identify malignant SPNs through accentuated enhancement (>15 Hounsfield units) with a sensitivity of 98% and a specificity of 58%.

If the clinical features and radiographic studies are inconclusive, the options are resection, biopsy, or observation of the SPN. The patient's wishes must be considered in decision making. Proceeding directly to resection is reasonable when concern about malignancy is high because surgery would be anticipated regardless of the biopsy results. Observation typically involves serial CT every 3 months for the first year and every 6 months during the second year. If the nodule enlarges, resection is indicated.

SPUTUM CYTOLOGY

The yield of sputum cytologic examination depends on the tumor type, size, and relation to major airways. Sensitivity is highest for central squamous cell carcinoma but less than 20% for peripheral nodules. Collection of one to three consecutive, early morning samples or a 3-day pooled sputum specimen is generally recommended, but the appropriate number of specimens to collect is unclear. Malignant cells may be from unsuspected head and neck cancer, so bronchoscopy is needed for a positive cytologic result if chest radiographs do not localize the tumor. If the bronchoscopic findings are normal, an otorhinolaryngologist should perform a careful examination of the upper airway. False-positive cytologic findings can be caused by pulmonary infection and inflammation.

FLEXIBLE FIBEROPTIC BRONCHOSCOPY

Flexible fiberoptic bronchoscopy is used for diagnostic and staging purposes. Diagnostic techniques include forceps biopsy, brushing, and washing. The diagnostic yield depends on tumor location and size. For central NSCLC or SCLC lesions, the overall yield is 70%. The yield climbs to approximately 90% if the tumor is visible at endoscopy. For peripheral lesions, the diagnostic yield of fluoroscopic bronchoscopy is 10% to 20% for nodules less than 2 cm in diameter, 50% to 60% for lesions 2 to 4 cm, and 80% for lesions larger than 4 cm. The chief complications of forceps biopsy are life-threatening bleeding and pneumothorax, which occur in less than 1% of procedures. Diagnostic and staging information may be obtained by means of transbronchial needle aspiration biopsy of paratracheal, subcarinal, and hilar lymph nodes. The outcome of transbronchial needle aspiration biopsy depends heavily on technique. Chest CT to direct location of the biopsy specimen can improve results. The overall sensitivity is 50%. Thus normal findings at transbronchial needle aspiration biopsy do not rule out lymph node metastasis. Bronchoscopy also provides local staging information through assessment of the proximal extent of tumor and occasionally through detection of synchronous neoplasms (1% to 3%).

TRANSTHORACIC NEEDLE ASPIRATION BIOPSY

Peripheral lesions or those with extension to the mediastinum, pleura, or chest wall may be sampled by means of fluoroscopically or CT-guided transthoracic needle aspiration biopsy (TTNA). TTNA usually is performed on patients who need a tissue diagnosis but cannot or should not undergo surgery, will not consent to an operation until a tissue diagnosis is made, have undergone bronchoscopy that did not provide enough information for a diagnosis, or are not able to undergo bronchoscopy. The yield of TTNA for peripheral lesions is 80% to 95%. There is a substantial false-negative rate (10% to 20% of patients with normal findings on TTNA may have a malignant lesion), so a normal TTNA result cannot be interpreted as a diagnostic end point unless a specific benign diagnosis is made from the aspirate. Pneumothorax occurs among 15% to 30% of patients, and approximately one-half of those patients need a chest tube. Massive bleeding or death is rare. Percutaneous radiographically guided needle aspiration is used in the diagnosis of extrapulmonary metastasis.

THORACIC SURGICAL PROCEDURES

Pathologic evaluation of mediastinal lymph nodes larger than 1 cm in diameter should be performed for any NSCLC patient who is considered a candidate for thoracotomy and surgical resection. Right paratracheal and subcarinal lymph nodes traditionally have been approached with cervical mediastinoscopy. Biopsy of left paratracheal, supraaortic, and aortopulmonary window nodes has been through anterior mediastinotomy

(Chamberlain procedure). Indeterminate peripheral nodules and pleural abnormalities can be explored by means of video-assisted thoracoscopic surgery (VATS). Pleurodesis of malignant effusions can be accomplished at the time of VATS. Complication rates for mediastinoscopy, mediastinotomy, and VATS are low.

▉ STAGING

NON–SMALL CELL LUNG CANCER

Staging for NSCLC is based on the TNM classification (Table 377.6). The T component refers to the size, location, and extent of locoregional invasion of the primary tumor. The N element describes locoregional lymph node involvement. The M constituent identifies whether distant metastatic lesions are present. The TNM stage is the most important prognostic factor in NSCLC. The various TNM components can be grouped to identify subsets of patients who have similar prognoses and treat-

---

TABLE 377.6.	**TNM INTERNATIONAL STAGING SYSTEM**

T: Primary Tumor

TX	Primary tumor cannot be assessed or tumor proved by the presence of malignant cells in sputum or bronchial washings but not visualized by imaging or bronchoscopy
T0	No evidence of primary tumor
Tis	Carcinoma in situ
T1	Tumor ≤3 cm in greatest dimension, surrounded by lung or visceral pleura, without bronchoscopic evidence of invasion more proximal than the lobar bronchus[a] (i.e., not in the main bronchus)
T2	Tumor with any of the following features of size or extent: • More than 3 cm in greatest dimension • Involves main bronchus, 2 cm or more distal to the carina • Invades the visceral pleura • Associated with atelectasis or obstructive pneumonitis that extends to the hilar region but does not involve the entire lung
T3	Tumor of any size that directly invades any of the following: chest wall (including superior sulcus tumors), diaphragm, mediastinal pleura, parietal pericardium; or tumor in the main bronchus less than 2 cm distal to the carina, but without involvement of the carina; or associated atelectasis or obstructive pneumonitis of the entire lung
T4	Tumor of any size that invades any of the following: mediastinum, heart, great vessels, trachea, esophagus, vertebral body, carina; or tumor with a malignant pleural or pericardial effusion,[b] or with satellite tumor nodule(s) within the ipsilateral primary-tumor lobe of the lung, and is not an exudate. When these elements and clinical judgment dictate that the effusion is not related to the tumor, the effusion should be excluded as a staging element and the patient should be staged T1, T2, or T3. Pericardial effusion is classified according to the same rules.

N: Regional Lymph Nodes

NX	Regional lymph nodes cannot be assessed
N0	No regional lymph node metastasis
N1	Metastasis to ipsilateral peribronchial and/or ipsilateral hilar lymph nodes, and intrapulmonary nodes involved by direct extension of the primary tumor
N2	Metastasis to ipsilateral mediastinal and/or subcarinal lymph node(s)
N3	Metastasis to contralateral mediastinal, contralateral hilar, ipsilateral or contralateral scalene, or supraclavicular lymph node(s)

M: Distant Metastasis

MX	Presence of distant metastasis cannot be assessed
M0	No distant metastasis
M1	Distant metastasis present[c]

---

[a] The uncommon superficial tumor of any size with its invasive component limited to the bronchial wall, which may extend proximal to the main bronchus, is also classified T1.
[b] Most pleural effusions associated with lung cancer are caused by tumor. However, there are a few patients in whom multiple cytopathologic examinations of pleural fluid are negative for tumor. In these cases, the fluid is non-bloody.
[c] Separate metastatic tumor nodule(s) in the ipsilateral nonprimary-tumor lobe(s) of the lung also are classified M1. From Mountain CF. Revisions in the international system for staging lung cancer. *Chest* 1997;111:1710–1717, with permission.

TABLE 377.7.	STAGE GROUPING AND FIVE-YEAR SURVIVAL OF TNM SUBSETS	
Stage	**TNM Subset**	**5-Year Survival Rate (%)**
0	Carcinoma in situ	
IA	T1 N0 M0	67
IB	T2 N0 M0	57
IIA	T1 N1 M0	55
IIB	T2 N1 M0	39
	T3 N0 M0	38
IIIA	T3 N1 M0	25
	T1-3 N2 M0	23
IIIB	T4 N1-2 M0	7
	Any T N3 M0	3
IV	Any T Any N M1	1

Adapted from Mountain CF. Revisions in the international system for staging lung cancer. *Chest* 1997;111:1710–1717, with permission.

ment options (Table 377.7). In general, the more advanced the stage, the worse is the prognosis. The observation that patients with lesions at identical stages can have widely varying outcomes emphasizes that the TNM system has limitations. The intrinsic sensitivity problems of all staging tests leaves open the chance for understaging. The TNM system does not take into account various clinical factors, such as weight loss or comorbid conditions, nor does it factor in biologic properties, such as tumor genetic markers or histologic subtypes.

Given the superiority of surgery for NSLC, the pretreatment evaluation must discern whether the extent of disease prevents resection. Two meta-analyses have revealed that the likelihood of metastatic disease is sufficiently low if a carefully conducted clinical evaluation has normal findings. The American Thoracic Society recommends that all patients with NSCLC undergo a thorough history interview and physical examination, complete blood cell count, serum chemistry profile (electrolytes, alkaline phosphatase, albumin, aspartate aminotransferase, alanine aminotransferase, total bilirubin, and creatinine), chest radiography, and chest CT through the adrenal glands. If results of these evaluations are normal, no further tests are necessary. Further testing should proceed surgery if the evaluation findings are abnormal. Clues to the presence of metastasis include weight loss and anemia. CT of the liver with contrast enhancement or hepatic ultrasonography is indicated if hepatomegaly is detected or results of liver function tests are abnormal. New neurologic symptoms or focal deficits justify performing head CT with contrast enhancement or head MRI. Radionuclide bone scanning is warranted in the presence of hypercalcemia, focal abnormalities of bone, or elevated alkaline phosphatase level (bone fraction).

If NSCLC is believed to be resectable, the patient must be assessed for medical contraindications to surgical treatment. It must be determined whether there is adequate pulmonary reserve for curative lung resection. Tobacco smoking is a risk factor for cardiovascular and cerebrovascular disease. Eighty to ninety percent of patients with lung cancer have COPD; 20% to 30% of these have severe disease. Preoperative spirometry and measurement of the diffusing capacity of the lung for carbon monoxide are strongly recommended. Patients with forced expiratory volume in one second (FEV_1) less than 1.5 to 2 L or more than 60% of predicted normal value, maximal voluntary ventilation more than 50% of predicted normal value, and diffusing capacity greater than 60% of predicted value can proceed directly to thoracotomy. Patients with lower values need quantitative ventilation-perfusion lung scanning (postoperative FEV_1 is estimated by multiplying the preoperative FEV_1 by the percentage of tracer in the area to be resected), measurement of arterial blood gases, or exercise testing. Although no value categorically precludes surgery, predicted postoperative FEV_1 less than 0.8 L or less than 40% of predicted value, hypercapnia ($P_{CO_2} > 45$), or maximal exercise oxygen consumption less than 10 mL per kilogram per minute indicate high risk of postoperative problems. Consultation with a pulmonologist, thoracic surgeon, radiation oncologist, and medical oncologist, especially in a multimodality clinic, is ideal in borderline cases.

SMALL-CELL LUNG CANCER

The TNM staging system of NSCLC usually is not applied to SCLC because of the limited role of surgery and because more than 90% of patients have locally advanced (stage III) or metastatic (stage IV) disease when they come to medical attention. SCLC is classified with the Veterans Affairs staging system of *limited* and *extensive* disease. *Limited disease* refers to tumor confined to one radiation port (disease within one hemithorax and its regional lymph nodes). *Extensive disease* encompasses everything else. Pretreatment evaluation should include a careful history and physical examination, complete blood cell count, serum chemistry profile (electrolytes, alkaline phosphatase, albumin, aspartate aminotransferase, alanine aminotransferase, total bilirubin, and creatinine), chest radiography, and chest CT. Testing for extensive disease should be directed by the understanding that two-thirds of patients with SCLC have extensive disease when they come to medical attention and that the most common sites of metastatic lesions from SCLC are the liver (25% at initial diagnosis), bone (20–30%), and brain (10%). It is generally recommended that patients with SCLC undergo head CT or MRI of the brain and isotope bone scanning before initiation of treatment.

STRATEGIES FOR OPTIMAL CARE

NON–SMALL CELL LUNG CANCER STAGES 0 THROUGH II

Stage 0 (carcinoma in situ) is uncommon, and the recommended treatments range from surgery to photodynamic therapy, external beam radiation therapy, or brachytherapy (intraluminal radiation therapy). Surgical resection with curative intent is the therapy of choice for stage I and II cancer. Stage 0 to II categorization can only be applied to 20% to 25% of patients with NSCLC when they come to medical attention. The standard operation is thoracotomy with mediastinal lymph node sampling combined with lobectomy, bilobectomy, or pneumonectomy. Less extensive resections are associated with higher rates of local recurrence and should be reserved for patients whose lung status will not allow lobectomy. Operative mortality is 2% to 3% for lobectomy and 5% to 6% for pneumonectomy.

In the latest TNM classification scheme, T3 N0 M0 lesions are downgraded from stage IIIA to IIB because of the reasonable response to en bloc resection of the tumor and adjacent structures. Expected 5-year survivals are shown in Table 377.7. Adjuvant chemotherapy has not been shown to improve survival. Postoperative radiation therapy for resected stage I and II disease has a detrimental effect on survival. Patients who have undergone resection have a 3% to 4% risk per year of development of a second primary lung cancer, so follow-up chest radiographs every 3 to 4 months for the first 2 years and every 6 to 12 months thereafter are recommended. There are no proven chemopreventive agents, although several agents are currently in clinical trials (*cis*-retinoic acid and selenium).

NON–SMALL CELL LUNG CANCER STAGE III

Optimal management of potentially resectable disease remains controversial. Results of phase II studies have suggested but not definitively shown that neoadjuvant (preoperative) chemotherapy with or without radiation therapy followed by surgery improves survival among patients with stage IIIA disease and carefully selected patients with stage IIIB disease. Neoadjuvant therapy may be associated with greater perioperative morbidity and mortality. Thoracic radiation therapy combined with platinum-based chemotherapy is recommended for inoperable stage IIIA and IIIB disease and has been shown to be superior to radiation therapy alone. Palliative radiation therapy alone is an option for patients with limited medical reserve. Expected 5-year survival rates are shown in Table 377.7. Pancoast tumors usually are stage IIB, IIIA, or IIIB. The typical regimen is preoperative radiation therapy with or without chemotherapy followed if possible by surgical resection. The 5-year survival rate is approximately 35%.

NON–SMALL CELL LUNG CANCER STAGE IV

Approximately 50% of patients with NSCLC have M1 disease at presentation. There are no curative options; the goal is to control the disease and palliate symptoms. The median survival period is 5 to 7 months. Radiation therapy may be used to control brain or bone metastasis or to relieve bronchial or superior vena caval obstruction. Airway obstruction can be palliated with bronchoscopic neodymium:yttrium-aluminum-garnet (Nd:YAG) laser tumor resection, stent placement, or brachytherapy. Chemotherapy provides a modest survival benefit (median

increase of 1.5 months) over supportive care. Patients who respond to therapy generally have improvement in cancer-related symptoms and quality of life. Persons with poor performance scores or multiple comorbid conditions may not be candidates for systemic therapy.

SMALL-CELL LUNG CANCER

SCLC is highly responsive to systemic therapy. The response rate is 80% to 90%. Therapy for limited disease consists of 4 cycles of chemotherapy with etoposide and cisplatin or carboplatin with concurrent thoracic radiation therapy given in at least 2 of the cycles. Concurrent therapy is thought to be superior to sequential chemoradiation therapy. Complete responses can be obtained by 50% of patients with a median survival time of 18 to 20 months, 2-year survival rate of 40%, and 5-year survival (cure) rate of 15% to 20%. There are no data to show that chemotherapy beyond 4 to 6 cycles is of benefit, but it does increase toxicity.

Extensive disease responds to the same chemotherapeutic agents as limited disease. Complete responses are obtained by 25% of patients, for a median survival time of 9 months and a 2-year survival rate of 10% or less. Almost no one survives 5 years. Thoracic radiation therapy is not recommended for extensive disease.

Prophylactic cranial irradiation (PCI) is controversial and should not be considered unless the disease is in complete remission. It is well established that the chance of CNS relapse is 50% if the patient survives 2 years. PCI decreases the rate of CNS metastasis but it may not prolong survival. PCI may be associated with the late sequelae of cognitive dysfunction and ataxia.

BIBLIOGRAPHY

American Thoracic Society and European Respiratory Society. Pretreatment evaluation of non-small-cell lung cancer. *Am J Respir Crit Care Med* 1997;156:320–332.

Arcasoy SM, Jett JR. Superior sulcus tumors and Pancoast's syndrome. *N Engl J Med* 1997;337:1370–1376.

Doll R, Peto R, Wheatley K, et al. Mortality in relation to smoking: 40 years observation on male British doctors. *BMJ* 1994;309:901–911.

Lucchinetti, CF, Kimmel DW, Lennon VA. Paraneoplastic and oncologic profiles of patients seropositive for antineuronal nuclear autoantibodies. *Neurology* 1998;50:652–657.

Lubin JH, Boice JD Jr. Lung cancer risk from residential radon: meta-analysis of eight epidemiologic studies. *J Natl Cancer Inst* 1996;88:49–57.

Midthun DE, Swenson SJ, Jett JR. Approach to the solitary pulmonary nodule. *Mayo Clin Proc* 1993;68:378–385.

Mountain CF. Revisions in the international system for staging lung cancer. *Chest* 1997;111:1710–1717.

Mountain CF, Dressler CM. Regional lymph node classification for lung cancer staging. *Chest* 1997;111:1718–1723.

Patel AM, Davila DG, Peters SG. Paraneoplastic syndromes associated with lung cancer. *Mayo Clin Proc* 1993;68:278–287.

Patel AM, Peters SG. Clinical manifestations of lung cancer. *Mayo Clin Proc* 1993;68:273–277.

Pritchard RS, Anthony SP. Chemotherapy plus radiotherapy compared with radiotherapy alone in the treatment of locally advanced, unresectable, non-small-cell lung cancer: a meta-analysis. *Ann Intern Med* 1996;125: 723–729.

Silvestri JA, Littenberg B, Colice GL. The clinical evaluation for detecting metastatic lung cancer: a meta-analysis. *Am J Respir Crit Care Med* 1995; 152:225–230.

Swenson SJ, Brown LR, Colby TV, et al. Lung nodule enhancement at CT: prospective findings. *Radiology* 1996;201:447–455.

Kelley's Textbook of Internal Medicine, fourth edition. Edited by H. David Humes.
Lippincott Williams & Wilkins, Philadelphia © 2000.

CHAPTER 378

PULMONARY THROMBOEMBOLISM

THOMAS M. HYERS

Venous thromboembolism has two major clinical manifestations: deep venous thrombosis (DVT), most often found in the deep veins of the leg, and pulmonary embolism (PE), which develops as a complication in approximately 50% of persons with DVT. DVT typically originates in a venous valve cusp in a deep calf vein. Approximately one-third of persons with calf vein thrombi have propagation in the direction of venous return into the deep veins of the thigh and pelvis. When the thrombus involves the deep veins of the knee and above, the condition is called *proximal DVT*. Proximal deep venous thrombi are larger and are more likely to dislodge and traverse the venous system to embolize the pulmonary arteries. Larger pulmonary emboli can be life threatening. The patient is most likely to die when the acute embolic burden obstructs more than 50% of the cross-sectional area of the pulmonary arteries.

Venous thromboembolism occurs in approximately one person per 1,000 yearly in North America and Europe. The disease can occur at any age, but its frequency is strongly linked to advanced age. Other acquired risk factors are immobility and any form of trauma, including surgery and childbirth. With the exception of pregnancy, there is no sex predilection. Both inherited and acquired risk factors predispose a person to venous thromboembolism. The leading risk factors are shown in Table 378.1. Risk factors are cumulative. A common scenario is the occurrence of venous thromboembolism in a patient with an unidentified genetic risk factor and a recent surgical procedure (Table 378.1).

Of the genetic risk factors, the condition known as factor V Leiden is particularly prevalent. The point mutation at position 506 on blood coagulation factor V causes substitution of glutamine for arginine. The substituted glutamine occurs at one of three cleavage sites for activated protein C and renders factor V relatively resistant to degradation. This mutation also is known as *activated protein C resistance,* and the heterozygous state is present in approximately 5% of whites. The mutation is quite

TABLE 378.1.	RISK FACTORS FOR VENOUS THROMBOEMBOLISM	
Inherited	**Acquired**
Factor V Leiden	Trauma (surgery, childbirth)
Prothrombin variant	Immobilization (bedrest, paralysis)
Hyperhomocysteinemia	Cancer
Protein C deficiency	Lupus anticoagulant
Protein S deficiency	(antiphospholipid antibody
Antithrombin	syndrome)
deficiency	Pregnancy
	Estrogen use

rare among native Asians and Africans but is present in 1% to 2% of African Americans. Factor V Leiden increases risk of venous thromboembolism approximately fivefold. It should be suspected when a patient has idiopathic venous thromboembolism, venous thromboembolism that occurs early in life, or recurrent venous thromboembolism. Genetic abnormalities such as deficiency of antithrombin, protein C, or protein S are quite rare. Through an entire career, an individual clinician might encounter only one or two affected persons.

PREVENTION

Acute PE is estimated to cause 50,000 deaths in the United States each year. Because most deaths of PE happen suddenly before therapy can be given, ascertaining who is at high risk and instituting effective prevention is extremely important. Preventive therapy includes anticoagulant drugs and mechanical compressive methods that stimulate venous return and fibrinolysis in the lower extremities. Some preventive therapies are more effective than others. Table 378.2 shows recommended preventive measures according to risk of venous thromboembolism. In some studies, combinations of pharmacologic and mechanical methods have proved more effective than either approach alone (Table 378.2).

No single preventive measure or combination is completely effective. Results of studies with patients at high risk indicate that preventive therapy provides tenfold risk reduction for both clinical events and death. Unfortunately, practice audits show that for many patients at high risk, either preventive therapy is not prescribed or ineffective methods are used. Innovative approaches to prevention are needed.

Vena caval filters are mechanical devices that allow venous return but obstruct the passage of large emboli. The filter usually is placed in the inferior vena cava below the renal veins. These devices prevent fatal PE but do not prevent DVT. Vena caval filters are used when DVT is present and anticoagulation cannot be given or when treatment has failed after an adequate trial.

DIAGNOSIS

Symptoms and signs of DVT and PE are maddeningly nonspecific, so clinical diagnosis is unreliable. Patients with DVT can have nonspecific symptoms of leg pain, swelling, or skin discoloration, but approximately 50% have no symptoms, and the

TABLE 378.2	PREVENTION OF VENOUS THROMBOEMBOLISM				
	Without Prophylaxis		**Recommended Prophylactic Methods**	**With Prophylaxis**	
Risk Group	**Proximal DVT (%)**	**Fatal PE (%)**		**Proximal DVT (%)**	**Fatal PE (%)**
Hip replacement	20–30	2–4	War, LMWH	5	0.1–0.2
Knee replacement	20–30	2–4	War, LMWH, IPC	5	0.1–0.2
Hip fracture	25–35	2–4	War, LMWH	10	0.2–0.4
Major trauma	20	0.5–1.0	LMWH, IPC	10	<0.1
Abdominal or pelvic cancer surgery	20	0.5–1.0	LMWH, IPC, WAR	10	<0.1
Abdominal surgery, coronary artery bypass graft	5–7	0.5	UH, LMWH, IPC, War, ES	<1	<0.1
Medical patients 40 yr or older with immobilization	5	<0.5	UH, ES, LMWH	<1	<0.1

War, Warfarin; LMWH, low-molecular–weight heparin; IPC, intermittent pneumatic compression; UH, unfractionated heparin; ES, graded elastic stockings.
From Hyers TM. Venous thromboembolism state of the art. *Am J Respir Crit Care Med* 1999;159:1–14.

leg appears normal at physical examination. Measurement of circumference at midthigh and midcalf is helpful. A difference in circumference of 1 cm or more is abnormal and mandates further testing. All of these symptoms and findings can be associated with other conditions such as cellulitis, ruptured Baker's cyst, heart failure with edema, and chronic venous insufficiency.

DEEP VENOUS THROMBOSIS

Although findings of a carefully taken history and physical examination cannot confirm the diagnosis of DVT, the information allows the clinician to estimate the probability of disease. The clinician should consider the presence of risk factors, symptoms, and physical findings. Before objective testing, the clinician should assign a probability to the likelihood of disease: low (1% to 19% probability) or high (80% to 100% probability). Indeterminate status (20% to 79% probability) is assigned to instances that fit into neither the low nor the high category. This pretest probability is useful in assessment of the results of objective testing.

The most commonly used diagnostic test for DVT is duplex ultrasonography with manual compression. The study incorporates Doppler flow measurement and B-mode imaging of the vein in question. Although venous thrombi often cannot be imaged directly, the noncompressibility of a venous segment on the B-mode image is good indirect evidence of the presence of a thrombus. This test is most reliable in the knee and thigh, where the veins course near the surface. The test is less reliable in the calf with its multiple overlapping veins and in the pelvis, where the veins cannot be easily compressed.

In contrast venography, radiographic contrast material is injected into a foot vein and plain-film images are obtained as the contrast material ascends through the deep veins of the leg. This test is used when findings at duplex ultrasonography are equivocal and when pretest probability is high and the results of duplex ultrasonography are normal. Figure 378.1 shows a common approach to the diagnosis of DVT with clinical inference and objective testing. Magnetic resonance imaging has shown promise in the diagnosis of DVT, but this technique has been insufficiently tested to be substituted for duplex ultrasonography in the algorithm shown in Figure 378.1.

PULMONARY EMBOLISM

Patients with PE most often report dyspnea, pleuritic chest pain, or hemoptysis. Physical examination most commonly reveals tachypnea or tachycardia. Each of these symptoms and findings can be associated with other diseases. Although the history and physical findings cannot be used to confirm the diagnosis, patients with PE nearly always have at least dyspnea, pleuritic chest pain, or a respiratory rate faster than 20 breaths per minute. This triad is a sensitive screening tool to help rule out the possibility of PE. That is, patients who have none of these findings are unlikely to have PE. As with the clinical diagnosis of DVT, the clinician should assign a pretest probability for PE before proceeding to more objective testing. The pretest probability should incorporate the history, including risk factors, physical findings, and the presence of other heart or lung diseases that might explain any abnormal findings. A high, low, or indeterminate probability is assigned before objective testing.

Results of routine laboratory tests often are abnormal but cannot be used to confirm the diagnosis of PE. A chest radiograph may show nonspecific findings of hemidiaphragmatic elevation, small pleural effusions, or ill-defined parenchymal infiltrates. Arterial blood gas analysis may show widening of the alveolar to arterial oxygen gradient, often with a low Po_2. The electrocardiogram most often shows tachycardia with nonspecific ST-segment and T-wave changes.

The most commonly used diagnostic test for PE is ventilation and perfusion lung scanning ($\dot{V}/\dot{Q}$ scans). The perfusion scan shows the distribution of microvascular blood flow in the lungs after intravenous injection of a radionuclide, and the ventilation scan shows distribution of ventilation in the small airways after inhalation of a radioactive gas or aerosol. Normal scans show uniform distribution of the radionuclides throughout both

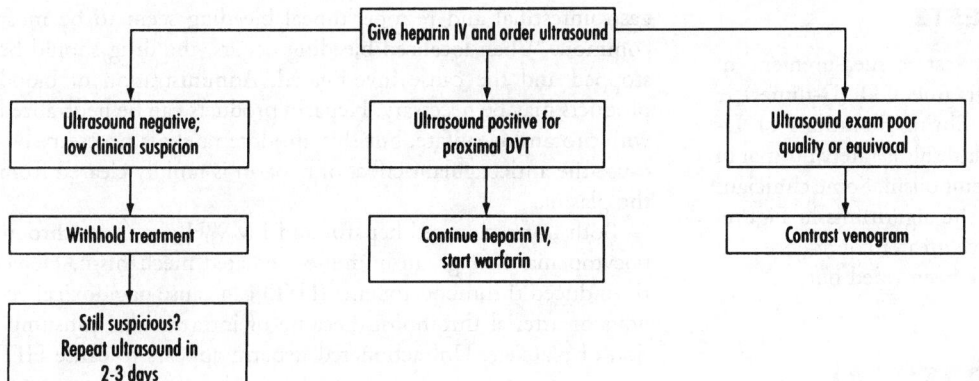

FIGURE 378.1. Clinical pathway for evaluation of deep venous thrombosis (DVT).

lungs. If the V̇/Q̇ scan findings are normal, PE is highly unlikely. The diagnostic hallmark of PE on a V̇/Q̇ scan is a normal ventilation pattern with two or more large perfusion defects (>25% of an anatomic lung segment). This pattern is commonly called a *V̇/Q̇ mismatch* and is highly diagnostic of PE, particularly if the patient has a high pretest probability of PE. Unfortunately, fewer than 50% of patients with PE have this classic V̇/Q̇ mismatch because they also have preexisting lung or heart disease, which can cause ventilation abnormalities or small perfusion defects. Most patients with PE have abnormal V̇/Q̇ scans, but this is not enough information for a diagnosis, and further testing often is necessary.

Pulmonary angiography involves the injection of radiographic contrast material into the main pulmonary artery with subsequent radiographic imaging of the material as it traverses the pulmonary arterial tree. In a patient with a high or indeterminate pretest probability, demonstration of a consistent pulmonary arterial filling defect or vascular cutoff confirms the diagnosis of PE. The test is expensive, invasive, and occasionally difficult to perform and interpret. Many smaller hospitals are

not equipped to perform pulmonary angiography. Pulmonary angiography is most often performed when results of V̇/Q̇ scans are indeterminate or when there is disagreement with the pretest probability. Spiral computed tomography with radiographic contrast material has shown promise for the diagnosis of PE, particularly emboli that lodge in segmental or larger pulmonary vessels. Further evaluation of this diagnostic modality is needed before it can be widely recommended.

THE COMBINED APPROACH

Because PE is nearly always preceded by DVT in the leg, clinicians often use a combined approach of both leg and lung diagnostic studies. This approach is particularly useful when results of V̇/Q̇ scans are indeterminate. If duplex ultrasonography shows DVT, the diagnosis of venous thromboembolism is assured, and treatment can be given with confidence. If the findings of the leg study are normal, pulmonary angiography likely is necessary. Figure 378.2 shows a stepwise approach to the diagnosis of venous thromboembolism using both leg and lung studies.

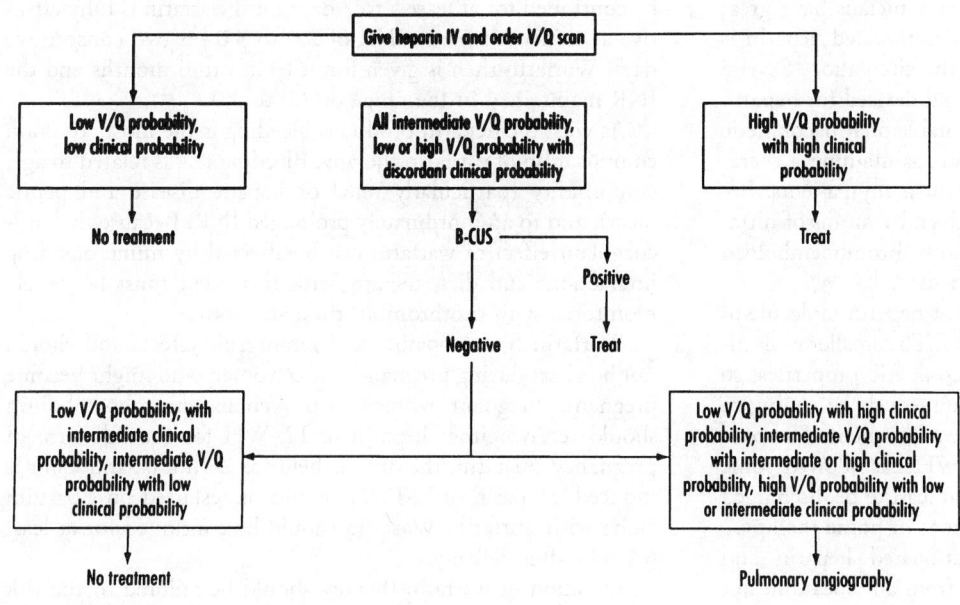

FIGURE 378.2. Clinical pathway for evaluation of pulmonary embolism. *B-CUS,* compressive B-mode ultrasonography.

ANCILLARY DIAGNOSTIC TESTS

The most commonly used ancillary test is measurement of plasma levels of dimerized plasmin fragment D (D-dimer), a degradation product of cross-linked fibrin. Elevations of D-dimer level are nonspecific, but the test result is rarely normal in the presence of acute venous thromboembolism. Some clinicians thus incorporate D-dimer levels into the algorithms in Figures 378.1 and 378.2 in an effort to achieve greater confidence that venous thromboembolism has actually been ruled out.

■ STRATEGIES FOR OPTIMAL CARE

Unfractionated heparin and low-molecular-weight heparin (LMWH) are rapidly acting anticoagulants that provide effective management of acute venous thromboembolism. The drugs enhance the effect of a circulating coagulation inhibitor, antithrombin, so that the inhibitor combines with and inactivates thrombin, factor IX, and factor X. Both drugs must be given parenterally. When venous thromboembolism is suspected, anticoagulation with heparin or LMWH should be administered until the diagnostic evaluation is complete. If the presence of PE or proximal DVT is confirmed, one or the other drug should be given in a therapeutic dose for 5 to 7 days or until an oral anticoagulant such as warfarin is shown to be fully effective. Patients with symptomatic DVT in the calf should be treated in the same way.

HEPARIN

Unfractionated heparin usually is administered by means of intravenous infusion. The effect is monitored with activated partial thromboplastin time (aPTT). The goal is to maintain the heparin infusion at a rate that keeps aPTT in the therapeutic range. This range is commonly quoted to be a time in seconds that corresponds to a plasma heparin level of about 0.3 to 0.6 IU per milliliter. Even the most experienced clinicians have great difficulty achieving this goal because unfractionated heparin is cleared rapidly and unpredictably from the circulation. Several nomograms and dosing schemes have been devised for heparin administration, but because of the unfavorable pharmacokinetic characteristics of the drug, achieving and maintaining a therapeutic effect continues to be a problem for many patients. Because unfractionated heparin usually is given by means of intravenous infusion, most patients with venous thromboembolism have to stay in the hospital for at least 5 days.

LMWH is fractionated from the parent heparin molecule to have a mean molecular weight of 4 to 5 kd. The smaller molecular size confers more favorable pharmacokinetic properties, so that LMWH can be administered subcutaneously according to body weight without monitoring or dose adjustment. The convenience and portability of use of LMWH has allowed some patients to receive treatment at home or at least to be discharged from the hospital earlier with a component of home therapy.

The worst complication of unfractionated heparin and LMWH is bleeding. Patients can bleed from any location, but gastrointestinal and retroperitoneal bleeding seem to be most common. When localized bleeding occurs, the drug should be stopped and the cause investigated. Administration of blood products may be necessary. Heparin products can be neutralized with protamine sulfate, but this antidote rarely is necessary because the anticoagulant effect of heparin is rapidly cleared from the plasma.

Both unfractionated heparin and LMWH can cause thrombocytopenia through an immune-mediated mechanism. Heparin-induced thrombocytopenia (HIT) can cause paradoxical venous or arterial thrombosis because of intravascular consumption of platelets. Unfractionated heparin appears to cause HIT among 2% to 3% of patients who receive the drug for more than 5 days. LMWH is less likely to cause this complication but should not be substituted for unfractionated heparin if HIT develops. A precipitous decrease in platelet count, usually occurring 5 to 10 days after the start of therapy, signals the onset of HIT. When HIT is suspected, heparin or LMWH should be stopped immediately. The first direct thrombin inhibitor, recombinant hirudin, has become available for anticoagulation of patients with HIT and acute thrombosis.

Long-term administration of unfractionated heparin in high doses can cause severe osteoporosis. This complication is particularly worrisome for pregnant women with venous thromboembolism, who cannot take warfarin. LMWH appears to cause less osteoporosis than unfractionated heparin and should be considered in the care of pregnant patients with venous thromboembolism who need anticoagulation throughout pregnancy.

WARFARIN

Warfarin is an oral agent that interferes with effective synthesis of vitamin K–dependent coagulation factors II, VII, IX, and X. Warfarin also inhibits synthesis of the anticoagulant proteins C and S. The drug is given daily and monitored with prothrombin time as standardized with the international normalized ratio (INR). Daily platelet counts should be monitored during administration of unfractionated heparin. Heparin or LMWH should be continued for at least 5 to 7 days until warfarin is fully effective as evidenced by an INR of 2.0 to 3.0 on two consecutive days. Warfarin then is given for at least 3 to 6 months and the INR maintained in the range of 2.0 to 3.0.

As with the heparin products, bleeding is the most common complication of warfarin therapy. Bleeding risk is related to age, comorbidity (particularly renal or hepatic disease and peptic ulcer), and to an inordinately prolonged INR. Because the anticoagulant effect of warfarin can be affected by numerous drug interactions and diet, therapy with this agent must be closely monitored with prothrombin time and INR.

Warfarin has fetopathic and teratogenic effects and should not be given during pregnancy or to women who might become pregnant. Pregnant women with venous thromboembolism should receive either heparin or LMWH for the full term of pregnancy. At term, the drug is held for 24 hours, and labor is induced. Heparin or LMWH should be restarted post partum along with warfarin. Warfarin should be continued for at least 6 weeks after delivery.

Duration of warfarin therapy should be tailored to the risk

of recurrence of venous thromboembolism. Patients who experience venous thromboembolism after a time-limited risk factor such as surgery or transient immobilization probably need no more than 3 months of therapy. Patients who have venous thromboembolism without a risk factor should be treated for at least 6 months. Patients with ongoing risk factors such as cancer, lupus anticoagulant, or one of the genetic causes listed in Table 378.1 should be treated indefinitely because the risk of recurrence is high. Patients with recurrent venous thromboembolism, no matter what the putative risk factor, should receive indefinite therapy. Many times the prescription for therapy of indefinite duration commits a patient to a lifetime of anticoagulation. Therefore the diagnosis of recurrent venous thromboembolism should be firmly established before the recommendation is made.

THROMBOLYTIC AGENTS

Thrombolytic agents dissolve fibrin thrombi by activating the plasma proenzyme, plasminogen, to the active enzyme, plasmin. Plasmin then degrades fibrin, fibrinogen, and several other coagulation proteins. Several thrombolytic agents are available for management of venous thromboembolism. These include streptokinase, a bacterial product, and the human-derived products urokinase and tissue plasminogen activator. Each of these agents causes more thrombolysis than heparin or LMWH, although there is no clear evidence that one thrombolytic agent is preferred over another for treatment of venous thromboembolism. There also is no clear evidence that treatment of patients with venous thromboembolism with thrombolytic agents improves survival. Thrombolytic agents are more likely to cause bleeding than are heparin products. Thrombolytic agents consequently are usually reserved for patients with life-threatening PE or massive iliofemoral thrombosis in which compromise of the adjacent arterial circulation seems imminent. When a thrombolytic agent is infused, heparin or LMWH is held until the fibrinolytic effect has cleared. The heparin product is restarted and given with warfarin as described earlier.

CHRONIC THROMBOEMBOLIC PULMONARY HYPERTENSION

In some patients PE does not resolve even with proper treatment. Other patients seem to have episodes of PE and never come to medical attention. These persons are at risk of chronic thromboembolic pulmonary hypertension (CTPH), a syndrome characterized by progressive dyspnea with normal chest radiographs and results of pulmonary function tests. CTPH develops in less than 1% of patients with PE. Half of patients with CTPH have never received medical care for PE but when questioned give a history of an event that is compatible with the diagnosis. The presence of lupus anticoagulant appears to confer the highest risk, but in one series this abnormality was present in only 10% of patients with CTPH. The hallmark of the syndrome is dyspnea, which progresses from dyspnea with exertion to continuous dyspnea present even at rest. The diagnosis is strongly suggested when a V̇/Q̇ scan shows large perfusion defects with relatively normal ventilation. Medical therapy is ineffective, but

pulmonary endarterectomy can be lifesaving when performed by an experienced surgeon with a skilled support team.

CURRENT PROBLEMS AND NEW DIRECTIONS

Two unsolved problems with venous thromboembolism are failure to use preventive therapy in the care of patients at high risk and failure to diagnose the condition in the face of suggestive symptoms and findings. Many patients undergoing high-risk surgical procedure still do not receive adequate preventive therapy despite widespread promulgation of preventive guidelines. When venous thromboembolism occurs in such a patient, medical-legal action is likely, particularly if the patient dies. Innovative methods are needed to ensure that adequate preventive therapy is provided when indicated.

The problem of failure of diagnosis relates to clinician error and to inherent deficiencies of the major diagnostic tests, particularly V̇/Q̇ lung scanning. Venous thromboembolism can be an insidious disease, and even the most experienced clinician can overlook this diagnosis, especially in the care of younger persons without clear risk factors. Unexplained dyspnea is the most common initial manifestation of PE, and clinicians should always be alert to the possibility of this disease unless there is another plausible explanation for shortness of breath. When a patient dies of undiagnosed venous thromboembolism after seeking medical attention with suggestive symptoms and findings, a lawsuit is likely. If venous thromboembolism is suspected, objective testing must be performed and the results assessed in a timely manner by the responsible physician. If results of first-line diagnostic tests are indeterminate and clinical suspicion is high or indeterminate, further invasive testing with venography and pulmonary angiography should be pursued. In this regard, additional evaluation of spiral computed tomography for the diagnosis of PE is urgently needed, because this modality is available in most hospitals, and pulmonary angiography is not.

Patients with cancer or lupus anticoagulant who have venous thromboembolism are especially difficult to treat because of high risk of both recurrence and bleeding. New methods are needed to prevent venous thromboembolism among cancer patients at high risk. The potential benefits of LMWH in the management of venous thromboembolism among cancer patients should be investigated. Patients with lupus anticoagulant seem to need more intensive warfarin therapy than the usual patient with venous thromboembolism. Many authorities recommend that the INR be maintained above 3.0 for such patients.

Approval of the LMWH enoxaparin for the treatment of patients with venous thromboembolism in the United States has opened the door to outpatient therapy. Physicians should develop and implement algorithms and pathways for outpatient treatment, specifically identifying patients who need hospitalization. Not all patients are good candidates for home therapy, although cost-containment efforts put great pressure on physicians to treat everyone as an outpatient.

Although LMWH offers greater convenience than unfractionated heparin, LMWH still must be given by means of parenteral injection. New derivatives of heparin and LMWH that can be given orally are being developed and when available should offer added convenience and ease of dosing. As these and other new therapeutic agents enter clinical use, the opportunity for enhanced efficacy and greater cost savings should be realized.

BIBLIOGRAPHY

Hyers TM. Venous thromboembolism-state of the art. *Am J Respir Crit Care Med* 1999;159:1–14.

Kearon C, Ginsberg JS, Hirsh J. The role of venous ultrasonography in the diagnosis of suspected deep venous thrombosis and pulmonary embolism. *Ann Intern Med* 1998;129:1044–1049.

Poort R Rosendaal FR, Reitsma PH, et al. A common genetic variation in the 3′-untranslated region of the prothrombin gene is associated with elevated plasma prothrombin levels and an increase in venous thrombosis. *Blood* 1996;88:3698–3703.

Price DT, Ridker PM. Factor V Leiden mutation and the risks for thromboembolic disease: a clinical perspective. *Ann Intern Med* 1997;127: 985–903.

Weitz JI. Low-molecular-weight heparins. *N Engl J Med* 1997;337: 688–698.

Wells PS, Ginsberg JS, Anderson DR, et al. Use of a clinical model for safe management of patients with suspected pulmonary embolism. *Ann Intern Med* 1998;129:997–1005.

Kelley's Textbook of Internal Medicine, fourth edition. Edited by H. David Humes. Lippincott Williams & Wilkins, Philadelphia © 2000.

C H A P T E R

379

DISEASES OF THE MEDIASTINUM AND CHEST WALL

CAMERON D. WRIGHT

■ DISORDERS OF THE MEDIASTINUM

The mediastinum is the potential space between the pleural cavities. It is bounded by the sternum anteriorly, the vertebral bodies and costal arches posteriorly, the thoracic inlet superiorly, and the diaphragm inferiorly. The major structures contained are the heart and great vessels, trachea and main bronchi, esophagus, and thymus along with fat, connective tissue, and lymph nodes. Fascial planes connect the mediastinum with the neck and retroperitoneum and allow movement of air, infection, or a mass from one location to another.

The mediastinum is commonly divided into anterior, middle, and posterior compartments (Fig 379.1). These boundaries are not strictly anatomic but do allow simple classification of masses, which facilitates a proper differential diagnosis. The anterior compartment is bounded by the pericardium and great vessels posteriorly and the sternum anteriorly. It normally contains the thymus, fat, and some lymph nodes. The middle compartment is shaped like a triangle with the diaphragm base. The anterior

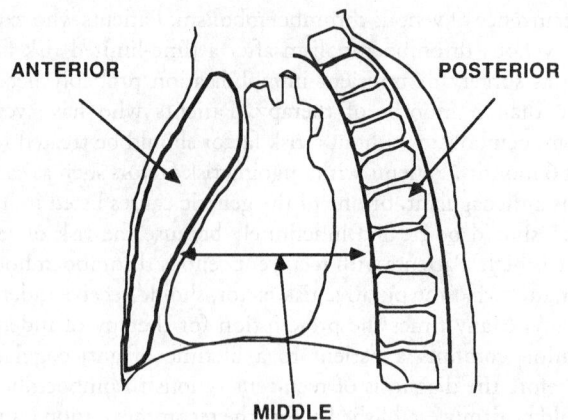

FIGURE 379.1. Anatomic location of mediastinal compartments on an idealized lateral radiograph.

margin is the heart and great vessels running from the diaphragm to the thoracic inlet. The posterior margin is the anterior vertebral border. It normally contains the pericardium, heart and great vessels, trachea and pulmonary hila, numerous lymph nodes, and the vagus and phrenic nerves. The posterior compartment is bordered by the projection of the vertebral body as seen on a lateral chest radiograph and contains the descending thoracic aorta, esophagus, azygous vein, thoracic duct, autonomic ganglia, and fat.

PRESENTATION

Pneumomediastinum

The presence of air in the mediastinum is most commonly caused by barotrauma from mechanical ventilation. Other causes include spontaneous, trauma, esophageal rupture, Valsalva maneuvers, or severe asthma. Substernal pain, often aggravated by breathing, is the most common symptom. Dyspnea, dysphagia, dysphonia, and subcutaneous crepitus are other symptoms. Patients undergoing mechanical ventilation need close observation with radiographs to search for occult pneumothoraxes. Prophylactic intercostal drainage should be considered for patients with high inspiratory pressures or those in tenuous clinical condition.

Mediastinitis

Acute mediastinitis is usually caused by esophageal rupture from instrumentation, vomiting (Boerhaave's syndrome), an impacted foreign body, trauma, or surrounding necrotizing infection. Descending necrotizing mediastinitis originates from the head or neck, usually either the teeth or hypopharynx, and dissects down contiguous fascial planes into the chest. Most patients with mediastinitis appear acutely ill with fever, chills, dyspnea, pleuritic chest pain, and systemic toxicity. Hamman's sign (crunching sound of the auscultated heart tones) occasionally may be heard. Cervical subcutaneous emphysema may be palpated from extension of the associated pneumomediastinum. Most patients have abnormal chest radiographs. Radiographic findings include pneumomediastinum, mediastinal widening, pneumothorax, and pleural effusion. Computed tomography (CT) of the chest is more sensitive in picking up all of these radiographic findings. If esophageal rupture is suspected, a radiographic study with a swallow of water-soluble contrast medium is required, and the findings usually confirm the diagnosis. Most patients with esophageal rupture need urgent surgical repair. Descending necrotizing mediastinitis necessitates urgent drainage of the causative neck infection and of the affected areas of the mediastinum. Mediastinitis after sternotomy, usually in cardiac surgery, usually presents within the first week after the operation with fever, wound pain, redness, and drainage. Prompt surgical re-exploration with drainage and debridement usually is curative.

Chronic mediastinitis usually is caused by granulomatous disease from histoplasmosis, although tuberculosis may cause a smoldering infection. Most commonly this condition is asymptomatic and found as mediastinal widening on a chest radiograph. Chest CT usually shows mediastinal adenopathy, most commonly concentrated in the right paratracheal area. Scattered calcified lymph nodes or lung granuloma may be present. The lymph node mass sometimes enlarges enough to compress the airway or superior vena cava to cause symptoms. Mediastinoscopy with biopsy and culture are needed to confirm the diagnosis. Some patients have an excessive host reaction, and acellular fibrosis develops. Mediastinal fibrosis may then compress and obstruct important hollow mediastinal structures and cause clinical syndromes, such as dyspnea, wheezing or stridor, superior vena cava (SVC) syndrome, and dysphagia.

CLINICAL EFFECTS

Most mediastinal masses are asymptomatic and are diagnosed when chest radiography is performed for another reason. About 80% of malignant masses are symptomatic, and only 40% of benign masses are symptomatic. Compression of adjacent structures may cause symptoms that lead to identification of the problem. Symptoms include chest pain, cough, dysphagia, SVC syndrome, hoarseness (from pressure on the recurrent laryngeal nerve), and dyspnea (from mass effect, pleural effusion, or phrenic nerve paralysis). Fever, night sweats, and weight loss may be associated with lymphoma. Myasthenia gravis often is associated with thymoma.

DIAGNOSIS

The presence of a mediastinal mass requires a diagnosis. Old chest radiographs may be helpful, especially if the mass is seen in retrospect. The presence of a characteristic air-fluid level on a lateral radiograph of a hiatal hernia usually indicates a mass. Contrast chest CT is useful to refine the differential diagnosis of most masses. Size, shape, calcification, vascular structures, soft-tissue density (fluid, blood, fat), enhancement, homogeneity, edge characteristics, and effects on surrounding structures can be assessed to generate a probable diagnosis. Magnetic resonance imaging (MRI) is of no additional benefit except to assess spinal cord impingement of neurogenic tumors, evaluate high-density foregut cysts that contain blood or mucus, and assess chest wall invasion.

The location of a mediastinal mass is helpful in making a

diagnosis, although a mass may abut or transgress another compartment (Table 379.1). Once a vascular lesion (a true or false aneurysm or a congenital vascular lesion) is excluded with CT and a short list of possible causes is generated on the basis of location and symptoms, an approach to biopsy can be chosen. CT-guided needle aspiration is helpful in diagnosing metastatic carcinoma but is often unreliable in differentiating lymphoma from thymoma. Anterior mediastinotomy (Chamberlain procedure) provides access to anterior mediastinal masses through a small parasternal transverse incision. Cervical mediastinoscopy provides access to the paratracheal and subcarinal nodal areas in the middle mediastinum and can reliably provide the diagnosis of granulomatous, cancerous, or lymphomatous involvement of these areas. A common misconception is that mediastinoscopy provides ready access to anterior lymphoma or thymoma, but it does not. Both mediastinoscopy and anterior mediastinotomy can be performed as outpatient procedures. Small, encapsulated typical mediastinal tumors (thymoma, neurogenic tumors) should be excised for both diagnosis and treatment.

■ DISORDERS OF THE CHEST WALL

CONGENITAL ABNORMALITIES

Congenital abnormalities of the chest wall include pectus excavatum (funnel chest), pectus carinatum (pigeon breast), and Poland's syndrome (unilateral absence of the pectoral muscles and breast). These are corrected in childhood if severe. Patients with pectus excavatum often report exercise intolerance. It has been reported that this condition can be improved with repair, but most studies do not show measurable improvement with cardiopulmonary function after repair. Severe kyphoscoliosis causes restrictive pulmonary impairment that can lead to respiratory failure later in life. Costochondritis (Tietze's syndrome) is a relatively common cause of localized anterior chest wall pain that can be confused with more serious chest pain syndromes. The pseudojoint between the bony rib and costal cartilage is peculiarly susceptible to painful inflammation. There is usually point tenderness of the affected cartilage with no overlying redness or swelling. The diagnosis is one of exclusion. Treatment usually is successful with nonsteroidal anti-inflammatory agents.

INFECTION

Infectious processes may affect the chest wall. Herpes zoster commonly involves the chest wall and can cause exquisite pain before the characteristic skin lesions appear. The distribution of the clinical findings over the dermatome of an intercostal nerve facilitates diagnosis. Empyema necessitans usually is the result of neglected chronic empyema that burrows through the chest wall and manifests as a fluctuant subcutaneous abscess. Actinomycosis is characteristic for traversing the chest wall if extensive parenchymal or pleural disease is present. Tuberculosis manifests as a cold (no redness or warmth) chest wall abscess when it involves the chest wall. Infection of the sternoclavicular joint appearing as overlying soft-tissue inflammation is a common

PART 8: PULMONARY AND CRITICAL CARE MEDICINE

TABLE 379.1.	CLINICAL FEATURES OF MEDIASTINAL MASSES	
Location	Clinical Features	Treatment
Anterior Mediastinum		
Thymoma	Most common tumor; incidence same for men and women, average age at onset 50 yr; 33% of patients have myasthenia gravis.	Encapsulated tumor should be resected without preoperative biopsy.
Thymic cyst	Rare, usually multiloculated; may be neoplastic	Excision
Lymphoma	Common, often symptomatic; nodular sclerosing Hodgkin's disease most common type; biopsy of tumor arising from thymus or prevascular nodes usually performed by means of limited anterior mediastinotomy (Chamberlain procedure).	Radiotherapy and/or chemotherapy
Thyroid	Common; patients usually older women; often asymptomatic; most are benign multinodular goiters	All symptomatic tumors and those with marked tracheal narrowing should be removed (usually through a cervical approach).
Germ Cell Tumors		
Teratoma	Uncommon; usually asymptomatic; teeth, hair, bone often present	Resection
Seminoma	Uncommon; 90% of patients men; often symptomatic; tumor markers negative	Small tumors treated by resection and radiation; large tumors with cisplatin-based chemotherapy.
Nonseminomatous tumor	Rare; 90% of patients men; usually symptomatic; 90% of patients have elevated tumor markers (β-human chorionic gonadotropin or α-fetoprotein)	All treated with cisplatin-based chemotherapy; resection reserved for residual marker-negative masses after chemotherapy.
Middle Mediastinum		
Lymphoma	See above. Mediastinoscopy (for paratracheal and subcarinal masses) usually is the biopsy route of choice.	Radiotherapy and/or chemotherapy
Lymph node mass	Common; metastatic cancer; sarcoidosis, granulomatous infection usual cause; mediastinoscopy usually provides diagnosis	Medical treatment of underlying condition
Pericardial cyst	Uncommon; never symptomatic; reliably diagnosed with CT	Excision rarely warranted
Foregut cyst	Uncommon; usually asymptomatic; usually centered on the carina; infection or hemmorhage into cyst possible	Most should be excised.
Paraganglioma	Rare; often asymptomatic; locally invasive with high local recurrence rate	Resection, possibly with cardiopulmonary bypass
Posterior Mediastinum		
Neurogenic tumor	Common; usually asymptomatic; most adult tumors benign; may arise from peripheral nerve, sympathetic ganglia, parasympathetic ganglia; may grow into spinal canal (dumbbell tumor)	Resection
Lateral thoracic meningocele	Rare; usually asymptomatic; 75% of patients have neurofibromatosis; filled with cerebrospinal fluid; diagnosed with magnetic resonance imaging	No treatment required

complication of intravenous drug abuse. Debridement of the joint usually is needed in addition to antibiotics.

CHEST WALL TUMORS

Chest wall neoplasms may be benign or malignant, primary or metastatic. Malignant tumors usually cause pain or a mass, and most benign tumors are asymptomatic. Plain radiography, CT, MRI, and bone scans are helpful in making a diagnosis and assessing the extent of tumor. If rib metastasis is suspected and tissue diagnosis is important for decision making, results of CT-guided needle biopsy often confirm the diagnosis. Most soft-tissue tumors of the chest wall are sarcoma. An incisional biopsy (with an incision designed to be resected later) usually should be performed to establish a diagnosis. Treatment often involves

chemotherapy, radiation therapy, and wide resection with soft-tissue reconstruction. Desmoid tumors are rare benign soft-tissue tumors that nonetheless locally involve surrounding structures. They must be managed with aggressive wide local resection. Small, clinically benign solitary rib tumors usually are excised for diagnosis and treatment. Benign rib tumors include fibrous dysplasia of the rib and chondroma. Two malignant chest wall tumors are treated nonsurgically—Ewing's sarcoma and solitary plasmacytoma. Ewing's sarcoma is diagnosed by means of incisional biopsy and is managed with chemotherapy. Solitary plasmacytoma is managed with incisional biopsy and radiation therapy. Survival is limited by the eventual development of multiple myeloma. Chondrosarcoma and osteosarcoma of the chest wall are managed by means of wide local resection with selective adjuvant therapy.

BIBLIOGRAPHY

Brown K, Aberle DR, Batra P, et al. Current use of imaging in the evaluation of primary mediastinal masses. *Chest* 1990;98:466–473.
Burt M. Primary malignant tumors of the chest wall. The Memorial Sloan-Kettering Cancer Center experience. *Chest Surg Clin N Am* 1994;4:137–154.
Cioffi U, Bonavina L, De Simone M, et al. Presentation and surgical management of bronchogenic and esophageal duplication cysts in adults. *Chest* 1998;113:1492–1496.
Strollo DC, Rosado de Christenson ML, Jett JR. Primary mediastinal tumors, I: tumors of the anterior mediastinum. *Chest* 1997;112:511–522.
Strollo DC, Rosado de Christenson ML, Jett JR. Primary mediastinal tumors, II: tumors of the middle and posterior mediastinum. *Chest* 1997;112:1344–1357.
Wright CD. Nonneoplastic disorders of the mediastinum. In: Fishman AP, ed. *Pulmonary diseases and disorders,* 3d ed. New York, McGraw-Hill, 1998:1485–1498.

Kelley's Textbook of Internal Medicine, fourth edition. Edited by H. David Humes. Lippincott Williams & Wilkins, Philadelphia © 2000.

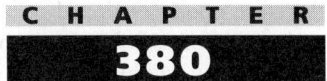

DISEASES OF RESPIRATORY MUSCLES

THOMAS K. ALDRICH

Disease can affect both inspiratory and expiratory muscles. Most respiratory work, however, is performed by the inspiratory muscles, and most of the energy required for expiratory airflow is stored as potential energy during the inspiratory phase and released as elastic recoil of lungs and chest wall during the largely passive expiratory phase. Even in the presence of acute asthma or chronic airway obstruction, the inspiratory muscles do most of the work. Expiratory muscle strength is vital, however, for effective coughing. Comfortable breathing requires enough respiratory muscle endurance to manage the respiratory workload. Any disease or condition that weakens respiratory muscles or that increases their workload can contribute to the symptoms and complications of respiratory insufficiency.

■ CAUSES OF RESPIRATORY MUSCLE INSUFFICIENCY

CHRONIC LUNG DISEASE

In chronic lung disease, the respiratory muscles must contend with major increases in workload. In chronic obstructive pulmonary disease or asthma, and especially in upper airway obstruction, the excessive airway resistance directly increases the work of breathing. When expiratory airway resistance is markedly impaired, as by dynamic airway compression in emphysema, and when dyspnea provokes premature onset of the inspiratory

phase, dynamic hyperinflation and intrinsic positive end-expiratory pressure are produced. The result is an inspiratory threshold load, often the most important contributor to the inspiratory work of breathing. Elastic workloads contribute to respiratory muscle overload in congestive heart failure, pneumonia, pleural effusion, and especially in chest wall-restrictive disorders such as kyphoscoliosis. In obesity-hypoventilation syndrome, inertial respiratory loads are prominent.

Although excessive respiratory load is the main contributor to respiratory symptoms and exercise intolerance in chronic lung disease, several factors may impair respiratory muscle endurance. As with all skeletal muscles, respiratory muscle strength increases as the precontraction length of the muscle fibers increases. The pulmonary hyperinflation common in airway obstruction shortens the inspiratory muscles and decreases their strength. It has been suggested that chronic hyperinflation may prompt adaptive drop-out of diaphragmatic sarcomeres and cause a right shift of the length-tension curve of the diaphragm to maintain good diaphragmatic strength despite hyperinflation. However, acute hyperinflation always weakens the diaphragm and perhaps other inspiratory muscles. When hyperinflation is severe, as in advanced emphysema, the diaphragm becomes almost flat, completely losing its effectiveness as a generator of intrathoracic vacuum. Patients with chronic lung disease often are sedentary, and the lack of activity leads to detraining of respiratory and other muscles. To make matters worse, malnutrition, hypoxemia, electrolyte disorders, and several commonly used drugs can impair respiratory muscle function in chronic lung disease.

NEUROMUSCULAR DISEASE

Weakness, the hallmark of generalized neuromuscular disease, usually affects the respiratory muscles as well as other muscles. These diseases also are frequently associated with increased workload. The typical rapid, shallow pattern of breathing in neuromuscular disease can lead to microatelectasis, which decreases lung compliance and increases the work of breathing. When the laryngeal muscles are paretic, vigorous inspiratory efforts may cause paradoxical inspiratory adduction of the vocal cords and functional upper airway obstruction, especially during sleep. Kyphoscoliosis is a complication of many neuromuscular diseases. When severe, this condition dramatically restricts expansion of the chest wall and increases the inspiratory load on the muscles. Impaired cough effectiveness, recurrent aspiration of gastric contents, and the resulting pulmonary infection among patients with generalized neuromuscular diseases can cause inflammatory or fibrotic changes in the bronchi and lungs. These changes increase both the resistive and the elastic work of breathing.

■ SPECIFIC CONDITIONS THAT AFFECT RESPIRATORY MUSCLES

SPINAL CORD INJURIES

The diaphragm can support breathing in spinal cord injuries below C5 because the phrenic nerves originate from the C3 to C5 roots. Such patients often have recurrent pulmonary infections, however, because of the almost complete absence of expiratory muscle activity and the resulting ineffective cough. Higher levels of cervical injuries affect almost all the respiratory muscles, in many cases causing intractable respiratory failure.

DISEASES OF THE ANTERIOR HORN CELLS

Diseases of anterior horn cells commonly cause respiratory failure because the respiratory muscles are effectively denervated and in many cases because bulbar involvement causes recurrent aspiration pneumonia. Amyotrophic lateral sclerosis usually causes particularly severe and relentless respiratory insufficiency, and death occurs in 1 to 3 years. Bilateral diaphragmatic paralysis, with its characteristic severe orthopnea, sometimes is the presenting manifestation of amyotrophic lateral sclerosis.

NEUROPATHY

Guillain-Barré syndrome often follows a viral infection, especially influenza. Most cases start with leg weakness and progress over 1 to 4 weeks, until, in 20% to 50% of cases, mechanical ventilation is required. Although there is no specific treatment, the prognosis for at least partial respiratory muscle recovery is good. Unilateral diaphragmatic paralysis may be the result of traumatic or neoplastic phrenic nerve injury, but in many cases, no cause can be established. In the absence of pulmonary disease, the paralysis usually is well tolerated, often asymptomatic, and detected only when the characteristic elevated hemidiaphragm is an incidental finding on a chest radiograph. Bilateral diaphragmatic paralysis usually causes severe orthopnea.

DISORDERS OF NEUROMUSCULAR TRANSMISSION

Myasthenia gravis involves the respiratory muscles in most instances but usually not until months or years after the onset of the disease. Myasthenia gravis is characterized by marked muscle weakness after repeated contraction and improvement with rest, but such pathologic fatigability is not clearly demonstrated for the diaphragm. Although they may be less severely affected by myasthenic weakening than are other muscles, respiratory muscles often are more sensitive to the cholinergic toxicity of anticholinesterase inhibitors. This sensitivity can lead to the insidious onset of respiratory insufficiency when other symptoms are responding to treatment.

MYOPATHY

The respiratory muscles are involved in almost all forms of generalized myopathy. Respiratory failure is particularly common with Duchenne's muscular dystrophy, especially when it is complicated by scoliosis and cardiac failure. Dystrophic weakening of the respiratory muscles is the main factor contributing to respiratory insufficiency in myotonic dystrophy. Another possible but as yet speculative factor may be myotonia (delayed relaxation) of the respiratory muscles, which may promote hyperinflation and further weakening of inspiratory muscles. Although no specific therapy is available for any of the dystrophies, dystrophic muscles are capable of improved strength with training and are susceptible to atrophy with disuse.

The inflammatory forms of myopathy, polymyositis and dermatomyositis, affect the respiratory muscles in a high percentage of cases. In 5% to 10% of cases, interstitial lung disease occurs and may contribute to respiratory insufficiency. Acid maltase deficiency is the most important form of glycogen storage myopathy. In the childhood form, respiratory failure causes death by 20 years of age. In the adult form, respiratory muscle involvement usually parallels slowly progressive weakening of peripheral muscles.

RESPIRATORY MUSCLE WEAKNESS DUE TO NONNEUROLOGIC CONDITIONS

Respiratory muscle weakness occurs in many conditions, including thyroid disease (both thyrotoxicosis and myxedema), malnutrition, cancer, alcoholism, and disorders of potassium, phosphate, calcium, and magnesium homeostasis. A number of drugs, including adrenocorticosteroids, aminoglycoside antibiotics, and possibly calcium channel blockers, can impair respiratory muscle function. Some of these agents are commonly used to treat seriously ill patients who have compromised respiratory reserve and are therefore poorly equipped to handle a decrease in respiratory muscle endurance. Polyneuropathy and polymyopathy, probably mediated by cytokines, are common in serious acute and chronic illnesses. The respiratory muscles, especially the diaphragm, frequently appear to be weakened by such effects. The respiratory muscles are subject to fatigue when the work of breathing is too much for respiratory muscle endurance and is sustained for long periods. Such fatigue may play an important role in the chronic symptoms of patients who have little or no respiratory reserve and may be particularly important in preventing successful weaning from mechanical ventilation.

METHODS FOR MEASURING RESPIRATORY MUSCLE FUNCTION

Tachypnea is a sensitive but nonspecific sign of respiratory insufficiency. An important physical finding that suggests respiratory muscle overload is visible or palpable contraction of accessory muscles. Such contractions can be detected through observation of sternocleidomastoid or intercostal retraction or palpation of scalene muscle activity deep in the posterior aspect of the neck. Active expiratory muscle (abdominal) contractions generally indicate respiratory muscle overload, often with hyperinflation.

Qualitative information about the strength of diaphragmatic contraction can be obtained by means of abdominal palpation if excessive expiratory muscle activity is not present. Paradoxical inward inspiratory motion of the abdomen can be observed in most cases of bilateral diaphragmatic paralysis. Reversible or intermittent abdominal paradoxical breathing is a sign of diaphragmatic fatigue or overload.

Quantitative assessment of respiratory muscle function can be made with a few simple pulmonary function tests, either at the bedside or in the laboratory. Inspiratory muscle strength can be measured as maximal static inspiratory pressure, and expiratory muscle strength can be measured as maximum static expiratory pressure. Both tests are highly effort dependent and unreliable in seriously ill patients. Measurement of transdiaphragmatic twitch pressure, painlessly elicited by means of magnetic stimulation of the phrenic nerves, offers a possible objective test of diaphragmatic strength.

Fluoroscopy of the diaphragm can help confirm suspected diaphragmatic paralysis by revealing paradoxical cephalic motion during the inspiratory phase of respiration. When the results are equivocal, measurement of transdiaphragmatic pressure with gastric and esophageal balloon catheters or measurement of phrenic nerve latency and conduction times may help in the evaluation of diaphragmatic paresis.

STRATEGIES FOR OPTIMAL CARE

Specific therapy for respiratory muscle weakness is available for only a few conditions. In myasthenia gravis, cholinesterase inhibitors prolong the time that acetylcholine is in neuromuscular junctions, improving neuromuscular transmission. For patients with thymoma in association with myasthenia gravis, thymectomy often causes dramatic improvement. For polymyositis, adrenocorticosteroid therapy is often helpful. For myopathy associated with hyperthyroidism and hypothyroidism, malnutrition, electrolyte disorders, and the presence of drugs, management of the underlying condition, if successful, causes improved respiratory muscle function. For most patients with respiratory muscle weakness, however, there is no specific therapy.

For all patients with respiratory muscle weakness, it is important to ensure adequate arterial oxygenation, cardiac output, nutritional intake, acid–base balance, and electrolyte status. Efforts should be made to prevent aspiration of gastric contents. For patients at bed rest, prophylactic low-dose heparin should be given to prevent pulmonary emboli. Coexisting or complicating conditions that increase respiratory workload, such as asthma, atelectasis, or pneumonia, should be actively sought, identified, and corrected.

Three types of treatment—drugs, training, and rest—have been recommended for improving respiratory muscle strength and endurance in a variety of clinical conditions. Methylxanthine drugs such as caffeine and theophylline can immediately improve the diaphragmatic tension elicited by low-freqeuncy phrenic nerve stimulation and possibly improve the strength of submaximal inspiratory efforts. The clinical implications of such effects are uncertain. More chronic improvements in respiratory muscle strength and endurance have been suggested by preliminary studies of treatment with anabolic steroids or human growth hormone. However, results of detailed studies with objective measurements of strength by means of phrenic nerve stimulation have not yet been reported. There has been little experience with methylxanthines, anabolic steroids, or growth hormone in the management of neuropathic or myopathic disease. Thus the role of drugs as respiratory muscle tonics remains uncertain.

Respiratory muscle training has been used to augment respiratory muscle endurance. Therapy entails repeated 15- to 30-minute sessions of isocapnic hyperventilation or inspiratory resistive loading. Although promising results have been obtained in several studies of patients with chronic lung diseases and in a few studies of patients with neuromuscular disease, especially spinal cord injuries and muscular dystrophy, the weight of the evidence suggests that most patients gain little or nothing from respiratory muscle training, at least in part because of poor compliance. It is not clear whether respiratory muscle training is more effective than less specific exercise training. There also is reason to believe that respiratory muscle overuse resulting from training might be harmful to some patients with neuromuscular disease.

Regular nocturnal mechanical ventilation by means of intermittent positive-pressure ventilation delivered through tracheostomy or a nasal mask may help some patients with respiratory muscle insufficiency. Assisted ventilation can allow these patients to sleep without nocturnal dyspnea or sleep apnea. It also provides them with adequate oxygenation for at least part of the day, potentially preventing cor pulmonale. It has been suggested, without definitive proof that nocturnal mechanical ventilation may relieve chronic respiratory muscle fatigue and allow patients to breathe more comfortably off the respirator during the day.

BIBLIOGRAPHY

Aldrich TK, Rochester DF. The lungs and neuromuscular disease. In: Murray JF, Nadel JA, eds. *Textbook of respiratory medicine,* 3d ed. Philadelphia: WB Saunders, 2000 (*in press*).
Begin P, Grassino A. Inspiratory muscle dysfunction and chronic hypercapnia in chronic obstructive pulmonary disease. *Am Rev Respir Dis* 1991; 143:905–912.
Belman MJ, ed. Respiratory muscles: function in health and disease. *Clin Chest Med* 1988;9(2):1–361.
Elliott M, Moxham J. Noninvasive mechanical ventilation by nasal or face mask. In: Tobin MJ, ed. Principles and practice of mechanical ventilation. New York: McGraw-Hill, 1994:427–453.
Roussos C, ed. *The thorax 2nd ed. (Lung biology in health and disease,* vol 85). New York: Marcel Dekker, 1995.
Smith K, Cook D, Guyatt GH, et al. Respiratory muscle training in chronic airflow limitation: a meta-analysis. *Am Rev Respir Dis* 1992;145: 533–539.

Kelley's Textbook of Internal Medicine, fourth edition. Edited by H. David Humes. Lippincott Williams & Wilkins, Philadelphia © 2000.

CHAPTER 381

DISEASES OF VENTILATORY CONTROL

CLIFFORD W. ZWILLICH
SOGOL NOWBAR

Advances have been made in understanding the control of breathing. This chapter reviews modern physiologic concepts that explain pathophysiologic events and clinical characteristics

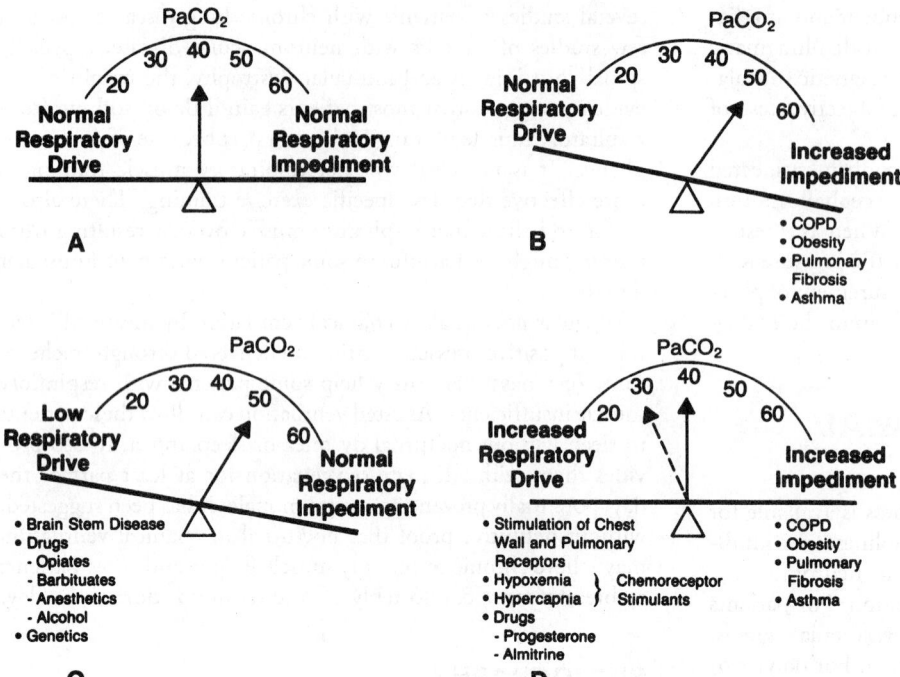

FIGURE 381.1. Interaction between respiratory drive and the impediment to breathing and the effect on arterial carbon dioxide tension ($Paco_2$). **A:** Normal $Paco_2$ as the result of a balance between normal respiratory drive and normal respiratory impediment. **B:** High $Paco_2$ (hypoventilation) is caused by increased respiratory impediment if respiratory drive remains at baseline (normal) value. **C:** High $Paco_2$ is the result of abnormally low ventilatory drive even though the respiratory impediment is normal. **D:** Common clinical situation in which alveolar ventilation ($Paco_2$) remains normal or even slightly increased (low $Paco_2$) in response to frequently encountered respiratory impediments. Alveolar ventilation is maintained because respiratory drive increases as a result of the reflex mechanism shown or in response to drug administration.

of disorders in which abnormalities of ventilatory control appear to play an important role. Fundamental to this discussion is the concept that the adequacy of alveolar ventilation depends on the balance between the impediment to breathing (obstructive and restrictive respiratory disorders) and respiratory drive. Both impediment and drive may rapidly change in response to normal physiologic adaptations or disease or as a result of therapy. Alveolar hypoventilation occurs when ventilatory drive is insufficient to counterbalance the influence of respiratory impediment (Fig 381.1).

When abnormal blood gas values (hypoxemia and hypercapnia) seem out of proportion to the degree of respiratory impediment, an abnormality in ventilatory drive should be considered. This discussion begins with a description of unusual disorders in which hypoventilation occurs among patients with normal respiratory function and markedly deficient drives. Next more common disorders are described, such as hypothyroidism and obesity, in which respiratory impediment is greater than normal but insufficient by itself to cause hypoventilation. When respiratory impediment is combined with attenuation of drive, however, hypoventilation occurs. Asthma and chronic obstructive pulmonary disease (COPD) are discussed last. These are high respiratory impediment states in which alveolar ventilation usually is maintained because of reflex stimulation of ventilatory drive mechanisms. Some patients have a low drive, and hypoventilation occurs.

IDIOPATHIC ALVEOLAR HYPOVENTILATION

A rare disorder in which attenuated ventilatory drive appears to be fundamental in causing alveolar hypoventilation is called

idiopathic alveolar hypoventilation. This disorder may become clinically apparent in infancy or in adulthood. The most common manifestation is caused by hypercapnia and hypoxemia. Accordingly, these patients have cor pulmonale, polycythemia, or alteration in consciousness. The last is explained in part by the central nervous system dysfunction caused by blood gas derangements and abnormal breathing during sleep. No identifiable central nervous system disease is present to explain the dysfunction in respiratory control. It is interesting that patients with chronic hypercapnia and hypoxemia can normalize the blood gas derangements with a few minutes of voluntary hyperventilation. Careful measurement of respiratory function typically discloses no abnormality of the lung parenchyma, respiratory muscles, or chest-wall mechanics, which suggests that abnormal impediment does not have a role in the pathogenesis of hypoventilation in this disorder.

When challenged in the laboratory with additional carbon dioxide or hypoxia, these patients do not have reflex hyperventilation. Great care must be used to ensure patient safety because unheralded unconsciousness may occur with this form of testing. It is not clear why these patients have this degree of attenuation in ventilatory responses to chemical stimuli. Postmortem brain and spinal cord examination usually is not revealing. Healthy family members of a few of these patients have had attenuated chemosensitivity, which suggests a genetic cause.

CENTRAL ALVEOLAR HYPOVENTILATION

Central alveolar hypoventilation is similar to the idiopathic disorder in that neither respiratory disease nor neuromuscular weakness is present to explain inadequate breathing. As in the idiopathic disorder, abnormalities in respiratory rhythm during wakefulness may be present, but these are typically amplified during sleep, when cortical influences no longer have a strong role in modulating respiratory rhythm. Hypoventilation, apnea, or another form of dysrhythmic breathing therefore is severe during sleep. Unlike patients with idiopathic disease, those with central alveolar hypoventilation have primary central nervous system abnormalities, which are thought to be causative. Intrinsic medullary disorders such as infarction, hemorrhage, encephalitis, polio, tumors, and multiple sclerosis have been implicated in this disorder. Brain stem herniation, cerebellar mass lesions, and bacterial meningitis have been causal. Traumatic injuries to the cervical spine or ventrolateral cordotomy may cause this breathing disorder. Numerous other central nervous system and peripheral neuropathic and myopathic syndromes cause hypoventilation. The cause of hypoventilation among patients with intrinsic brain stem disease is multifactorial. Some patients have anatomic abnormalities in medullary regions in which respiratory motor neuron cells are present. Others have disease in brain stem zones in which both vagal and carotid body chemoreceptor afferents are known to converge. In many such cases, abnormalities in the chemical control of breathing (ventilatory responses to hypoxia and hypercapnia) have been found.

Dyspnea is not prominent among patients with hypoventilation and no lung dysfunction, a contrast to the dyspnea present among patients with hypoventilation caused by severe lung disease. Patients with central hypoventilation have attenuated ventilatory drive and little or no reflex respiratory muscular effort in response to the blood gas derangement. High work of breathing and dyspnea are absent.

Successful treatment of patients with central alveolar hypoventilation is difficult. Many patients need assisted mechanical ventilation, particularly during sleep, when respiration worsens. For some patients, low-flow oxygen improves arterial hypoxemia without worsening hypercapnia. Partial or complete reversal of polycythemia, cor pulmonale, and cognitive dysfunction may result. Great care must be used in the initial administration of oxygen because when alveolar ventilation is low, a further small decrement induced by supplemental oxygen may cause life-threatening hypercapnia. Phrenic nerve pacing may be useful. In summary, idiopathic and central alveolar hypoventilation represent disorders in which underbreathing is present because of markedly attenuated drive but normal respiratory impediment (Fig 381.1C).

OBESITY HYPOVENTILATION SYNDROME

Most obese people compensate for the increased chest-wall elastic load by augmenting inspiratory drive and maintaining normal alveolar ventilation (Fig 381.1D). A minority hypoventilate in response to obesity and come to medical attention with the typical clinical abnormalities caused by hypoxemia and hypercapnia. In addition to polycythemia, cor pulmonale, and cognitive disability, these patients frequently have daytime hypersomnolence, probably caused by coexistent obstructive sleep apnea.

They characteristically have a long history of sonorous snoring and morning fatigue.

A disorder of ventilatory control is thought to be present in obesity hypoventilation syndrome (OHS) for numerous reasons. As a group, these patients can typically normalize hypercapnic and hypoxemic blood gas values during voluntary hyperventilation. Although the impediment to breathing is high because of obesity, it usually is not severe enough to explain the blood gas derangement. In OHS, neural respiratory drive to the ventilatory muscles may be greater than that of healthy controls, but it usually is much less than that of equally obese persons who maintain adequate alveolar ventilation. Several studies have demonstrated low ventilatory and attenuated neuromuscular responses to additional (laboratory-induced) hypercapnic and hypoxemic stimuli among persons with OHS. The occasional obese person with hypoventilation appears to have an imbalance between impediment (obesity) and the amount of ventilatory drive necessary to maintain adequate breathing (Fig. 381.1D). Considerable weight reduction, as with gastric surgery, results in less restriction, improvement in arterial blood gas abnormalities, and reduction of pulmonary hypertension.

The causes of attenuated ventilatory drive among persons with OHS are unknown. Some patients have low drive after weight reduction when blood gas values are normal. This suggests a premorbid attenuation in drive. Among other patients with OHS, continuous positive airway pressure (CPAP) therapy for the accompanying obstructive sleep apnea improves respiratory drive and blood gas values measured during wakefulness even though no loss in body weight or improvement in lung function was found. For some patients CPAP does not affect respiratory drive until the patient has been treated with a period of nasal intermittent positive pressure ventilation (bilevel). Among these patients effective nasal ventilation ameliorates apnea and hypoventilation during all sleep states, which leads to improved respiratory drive. This result suggests that the attenuation in ventilatory drive that causes hypoventilation may have been the result of severe blood gas derangements during sleep or other apnea-related abnormalities such as sleep fragmentation.

Normalization of alveolar ventilation with reversal of polycythemia and cor pulmonale occurs in OHS when the ventilatory drive stimulant progesterone (medroxyprogesterone acetate) is administered. This drug significantly increases the ventilatory response to hypoxemia. Progesterone is believed to be the cause of the alveolar hyperventilation present among normal women during the luteal phase of the menstrual cycle and during pregnancy.

THYROID HORMONE INSUFFICIENCY

Hypercapnic respiratory failure and coma have been documented among some patients with myxedema, although lung disease and chest-wall mechanics (obesity) are not severe enough to explain its occurrence. Patients with thyroid insufficiency have concomitant hypometabolism, which is believed to decrease respiratory drive. Specifically, patients with hypothyroidism have low ventilatory responses to chemical stimuli. Thyroxine replacement raises metabolic rate and improves ventilatory chemosensitivity, suggesting that a cause of hypercapnic respiratory failure complicating myxedema may be related in part to attenuated chemosensitivity. Patients with hypothyroidism do not have adequate inspiratory muscular responses to experimentally increased respiratory resistance loading. Accordingly, several abnormalities in the ventilatory control system are present during wakefulness among persons with inadequate thyroid function.

Derangements in ventilatory control and blood gas abnormalities recorded during wakefulness may be mild compared with those found during sleep. Such appears to be the case for persons with hypothyroidism, among whom severe obstructive sleep apnea is common. These persons have hundreds of nightly occurrences of apnea with associated hypercapnia, oxyhemoglobin desaturation, and bradycardia. An obese patient with hypothyroidism is particularly prone to sleep apnea. Thyroid hormone replacement greatly diminishes the frequency of sleep apnea even if weight reduction is not achieved.

CONTROL OF BREATHING AMONG PERSONS WITH ASTHMA

The diffuse bronchoconstriction of asthma increases resistive respiratory impediment, hyperinflation, and stimulation of intrapulmonary vagal afferent reflexes. These derangements predictably increase ventilatory drive and the sensation of breathlessness. Patients are dyspneic and display alveolar hyperventilation (hypocapnia). Ventilatory control testing among persons with moderately severe but stable asthma has demonstrated greatly increased diaphragmatic neural drive. Most persons with asthma have hypoxemia during severe exacerbations, suggesting that it may cause their high drive to breathe, dyspnea, and hyperventilation. This appears not be the case, however, because reversing the hypoxemia with supplemental oxygen usually has only a minor effect on dyspnea and hyperventilation. Intrapulmonary vagal afferent stimulation and hyperinflation during asthma may be responsible for both the high drive and dyspnea. Some persons with asthma who have severe bronchoconstriction also have hypercapnic respiratory failure, but most do not. Therefore the severity of the impediment to breathing (bronchoconstriction) does not completely explain this complication.

Persons with asthma who have had an episode of hypercapnic respiratory failure have low ventilatory chemosensitivity and attenuated perception of dyspnea. Studies with persons fully recovered from asthma have shown that those who had had hypercapnic respiratory failure during an asthma attack had much lower ventilatory and neuromuscular response to experimental hypoxemia than did healthy persons or persons with asthma who did not have respiratory failure during an attack. Persons with asthma who are prone to respiratory failure have little dyspnea during externally applied resistive breathing loads designed to simulate bronchoconstriction. These observations may explain why some persons with severe asthma have respiratory failure without the apparent warning suggested by progressive dyspnea. These new findings place additional emphasis on the need for home self-monitoring of lung function by persons with asthma when decrements in peak expiratory flow signal the need for accelerated antiasthma therapy.

VENTILATORY CONTROL IN CHRONIC OBSTRUCTIVE LUNG DISEASE

During the course of progressive COPD, airflow obstruction typically worsens, so that on average, the forced expiratory volume in 1 second (FEV_1) decreases about 80 mL per year. This eventually causes a large mechanical load against which the patient must breathe. Arterial hypoxemia is a frequent finding among persons with progressive airflow obstruction. These features of severe COPD explain the high respiratory drive and dyspnea that occur among most such patients.

Some patients with chronic airflow obstruction are less likely to detect and respond to additional respiratory resistive loads when compared to healthy persons or to persons with asthma. This loss of load compensation appears to be caused by increased endogenous endorphin activity because naloxone transiently reestablishes respiratory load compensation. Numerous factors may influence the control of breathing among persons with COPD.

The fundamental cause of hypoventilation among this population is of great interest because its presence is associated with severe hypoxemia and a worse prognosis. There is wide variability between the impediment to breathing, measured with FEV_1, and the occurrence of hypoventilation, measured with $Paco_2$. Although some patients with COPD and carbon dioxide retention fit the profile for having chronic bronchitis and patients with normocapnia often have emphysema, this correlation is weak. Patients with carbon dioxide retention generally have a breathing pattern of rapid and shallow respiration that enhances dead-space rebreathing and may help explain carbon dioxide retention. Respiratory muscle fatigue and the inappropriate use of sedatives and analgesics cause hypoventilation among some patients.

Persons with hypercapnia generally have a lower ventilatory response to laboratory-induced hypercapnia than do patients with the same amount of obstruction but normocapnia. In addition, measures of neural respiratory drive are different for the two groups. All patients with COPD typically have high resting electromyographic diaphragm signals (drive). Patients with normocapnic COPD, however, usually have a greater enhancement of drive to the respiratory muscles in response to added hypercapnia than do patients with COPD and chronic hypercapnia. Similar experimental results are found for laboratory-induced hypoxemia. In general, patients with hypercapnia have lower but clearly measurable responses to laboratory-induced hypoxemia than do normocapnic patients with COPD.

Factors that may explain attenuated ventilatory drive among some patients with COPD include acquired and genetic influences. The hypercapnic patients with COPD may have attenuated drives because of chronic hypoxic depression of ventilatory autonomic function. Although acute hypoxemia is a ventilatory stimulant, it is known that chronic hypoxemia may act as a ventilatory depressant if severe and prolonged. This influence appears to explain the low hypoxic drive to breathe among patients with cyanotic congenital heart disease and among people living at high altitudes for prolonged periods.

Genetic differences also may have a role in explaining attenuated drive and hypoventilation in COPD. Healthy offspring of hypercapnic persons with COPD have lower ventilatory responses to hypoxia than do healthy offspring of patients with COPD who have maintained normal ventilation. Neither of these two mechanistic possibilities (chronic hypoxic depression or genetic factors) has been proved unequivocally to be the cause of altered drive and hypercapnia among patients with COPD.

Hypercapnia induced by oxygen therapy is a problem in the management of severe COPD. Patients most likely to retain carbon dioxide are those with an acute exacerbation associated with severe hypoxemia or the presence of hypercapnia before oxygen is administered. Of concern is that use of high-flow oxygen unnecessarily elevates arterial oxygen tension. New-onset hypercapnia or worsening hypercapnia may occur within minutes to hours of oxygen initiation. The main clinical manifestation of this complication is alteration in consciousness caused by hypercapnia.

The causes of carbon dioxide retention during administration of oxygen are incompletely understood. It was initially believed that such patients had absent hypercapnic ventilatory sensitivity and breathed solely because of hypoxic drive. Eliminating hypoxic drive with oxygen administration would therefore cause hypoventilation and carbon dioxide retention. This explanation appears to be too simplistic in that only a small decrement in ventilation occurs during hypercapnia induced by oxygen administration and does not explain the degree of hypercapnia. High-flow oxygen administration reverses alveolar hypoxia and its local pulmonary vasoconstriction. This reversal may initiate or enhance pulmonary capillary perfusion of poorly ventilated, and therefore hypercapnic, lung units. The presence of hypercapnic blood draining these units may increase $PaCO_2$. Low-flow oxygen that raises PaO_2 only to the 55 to 65 mm Hg (SaO_2 90%) is sufficient to reverse many hypoxemic abnormalities but reduces the risk of severe hypercapnia. Serial clinical and blood gas evaluations during administration of oxygen to patients with clinical exacerbations of COPD seem to be the most effective means of avoiding hypercapnic coma and death.

Therapeutic options for the management of acute severe hypoventilation in the presence of exacerbations of COPD vary from assisted mechanical ventilation to pharmacologic intervention. Endotracheal intubation often is not necessary when mechanical assistance is needed. Nasal mask or full face mask bilevel ventilation has been used successfully in the care of cooperative patients. Use of bilevel mask ventilation as a substitute for endotracheal intubation improves in-hospital mortality and shortens time spent in an intensive care unit. The notion that decreasing the respiratory impediment associated with COPD improves ventilation, particularly if respiratory muscle fatigue is present, is fundamental. Bronchodilators, glucocorticoids, chest physical therapy, and antibiotics should be started early.

BIBLIOGRAPHY

Bott J, Carroll MP, Conway JH, et al. Randomized controlled trial of nasal ventilation in acute ventilatory failure due to chronic obstructive airways disease. *Lancet* 1993;341:1555–1557.

Kikuchi Y, Okabe S, Tamura G, et al. Chemosensitivity and perception of dyspnea in patients with a history of near-fatal asthma. *N Engl J Med* 1994;330:1329–1334.

Lourenco RV, Miranda JM. Drive and performance of the ventilatory apparatus in chronic obstructive lung disease. *N Engl J Med* 1968;279:53–59.

Moore GC, Zwillich CW, Battagia JD, et al. Respiratory failure associated with familial depression of ventilatory response to hypoxia and hypercapnia. *N Engl J Med* 1976;295:861–865.

Piper AJ, Sullivan CE. Effects of short-term NIPPV in the treatment of patients with severe obstructive sleep apnea and hypercapnia. *Chest* 1994;105:434–440.

Robinson R, Zwillich CW. Hypoventilation, central apnea, and disordered breathing patterns. In: Bone R, et al, eds. *Pulmonary and critical care medicine*, part Q. St Louis: Mosby, 1993:1.

Sampson M, Grassino A. Neuromechanical properties in obese patients during carbon dioxide rebreathing. *Am J Med* 1983;75:81–90.

Santiago TV, Remolina C, Scoles V III, et al. Endorphins and the control of breathing. *N Engl J Med* 1981;304:1190–1195.

Sugerman HJ, Fairman RP, Rakesh KS, et al. Long-term effects of gastric surgery for treating respiratory insufficiency of obesity. *Am J Clin Nutr* 1992;55:597S–601S.

Zwillich CW, Sutton FD, Pierson DJ, et al. Decreased hypoxic ventilatory drive in the obesity-hypoventilation syndrome. *Am J Med* 1975;59:343–348.

Kelley's Textbook of Internal Medicine, fourth edition. Edited by H. David Humes. Lippincott Williams & Wilkins, Philadelphia © 2000.

CHAPTER 382

SLEEP APNEA SYNDROME, HYPERSOMNOLENCE, AND OTHER SLEEP DISORDERS

DAVID P. WHITE

It has been only in the last 20 to 30 years that physicians have recognized sleep disorders with any frequency and only in the last 10 to 15 years that sleep laboratory evaluations have been common. Over this time period, substantial knowledge has emerged regarding normal sleep and the disorders that affect it. Specific diagnoses and effective treatment plans can be implemented for most patients. To accomplish this physicians must ask patients specifically about sleep as they would any other physiologic system and then approach identified problems in a systematic way. If this is done, the quality of life of many persons can be substantially improved.

Most sleep disorders can be grouped into one of three general categories (Table 382.1) and then further defined on the basis of historical findings, findings on physical examination, and possibly a formal sleep study (polysomnography). The general categories are excessive daytime sleepiness (hypersomnolence), inability to initiate or maintain sleep (insomnia), or unusual events or movements during sleep (parasomnia). Once the general category has been identified, the various causes of the problem can

TABLE 382.1.	GENERAL CATEGORIES OF SLEEP DISORDERS	
Excessive Daytime Sleepiness (Hypersomnolence)	**Inability to Sleep (Insomnia)**	**Unusual Events at Night (Parasomnia)**
Sleep apnea	Acute	Sleep terrors
Narcolepsy	Psychological stress	Sleep walking or talking
Primary CNS hypersomnolence	Physical illness	REM behavior disorder
Inadequate sleep time	Time zone travel	Nocturnal seizures
Periodic limb movement disorder	Chronic	
Severe depression	Psychiatric disorder	
Drugs	Conditioned insomnia	
	Poor sleep hygiene	
	Circadian rhythm disorders	
	Pain or medical disorder	
	Restless leg syndrome	

REM, rapid eye movement.
EVIDENCE LEVEL: C. Expert Opinion.

be systematically ruled out until a correct diagnosis has been reached.

EXCESSIVE DAYTIME SLEEPINESS (HYPERSOMNOLENCE)

Defining when daytime sleepiness becomes excessive may be difficult because everyone has periods of sleepiness after a poor night's sleep or a particularly strenuous period of work with inadequate sleep time. However, frequently falling asleep when not actively stimulated or in passive situations (watching television, reading, attending the theater, driving) is likely excessive and should be pursued. Sleepiness generally develops slowly over time and the person may not recognize a change or believes everyone feels the same way. In this case, the spouse may provide useful information about the severity of the problem. Many patients use the generic term *fatigue* to describe sleepiness. In this case, the physician must differentiate sleepiness, which is manifested by a desire or drive to fall asleep, from fatigue, which may be caused by a physical condition such as heart failure, anemia, or lung disease. Fatigue produces not a desire to sleep but a lack of energy or a reduced wish to be active. It is the tendency to fall asleep that differentiates hypersomnolence from fatigue.

Once excessive sleepiness has been identified, the various disorders listed in Table 382.1 should be considered. The first to be ruled out should be inadequate sleep time, which can be determined from the history. Most persons need at least 7 hours of sleep per night and often closer to 8 hours. Patients sleeping less than this should increase their total sleep time before other diagnoses are considered or while other possibilities are being explored. Severe depression and use of drugs that cause sleepiness should be excluded in a careful history. The other causes of daytime sleepiness generally require a sleep study for formal documentation of the diagnosis.

SLEEP APNEA SYNDROME

Although there are several types of apnea (primarily obstructive or central), most patients with this syndrome have obstructive sleep apnea (OSA). This disorder is characterized by recurrent collapse of the pharyngeal airway during sleep. Arousal is needed to reestablish airway patency and resume breathing (Fig. 382.1). Thus the patient experiences both sleep fragmentation (recurrent arousal) and the consequences of recurrent hypoxia and hypercapnia caused by the respiratory pause. Results of epidemiologic studies suggest that this is a common disorder. Approximately 4% of men and 2% of women have more than five events (apneas plus hypopneas, defined later) per hour of sleep in association with daytime sleepiness. If these numbers are correct, most cases of OSA remain undiagnosed, and most patients remain untreated.

Pathophysiology

The principal event in the development of OSA is collapse of the pharyngeal airway during sleep, either at the onset of sleep or during rapid eye movement (REM) sleep (Fig. 382.2). Patency of the pharyngeal airway (from the end of the nasal septum to the epiglottis) is modulated by both structural anatomic features and activation of dilator muscles. This portion of the airway has little bony or rigid support and therefore depends on these dilator muscles to maintain patency. If the pharyngeal airway is large, little muscle activity may be needed to keep it open. A small airway needs substantial muscle activation to maintain patency. Thus there is a direct interaction between anatomic features and muscle function.

There is convincing evidence that most patients with OSA have a small pharyngeal airway, usually because of obesity. Other causes are anatomic features such as small size of the mandible, posterior position of the mandible, or tonsillar hypertrophy. This deficiency of the airways of persons with apnea has been demonstrated with numerous techniques, including computed

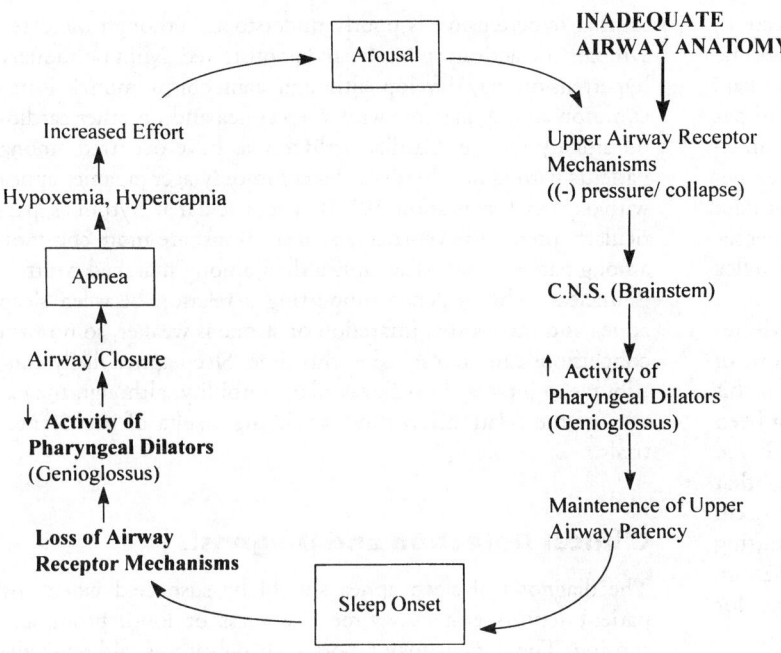

FIGURE 382.1. Pathophysiologic series of events that characterize the obstructive sleep apnea cycle. (From Fogel RB, White DP. Obstructive sleep apnea. In: Schrier RW, Baxter JD, Dzau VJ, et al., eds. *Advances in internal medicine.* St. Louis, MO: Mosby, 2000;45:351–389, with permission.

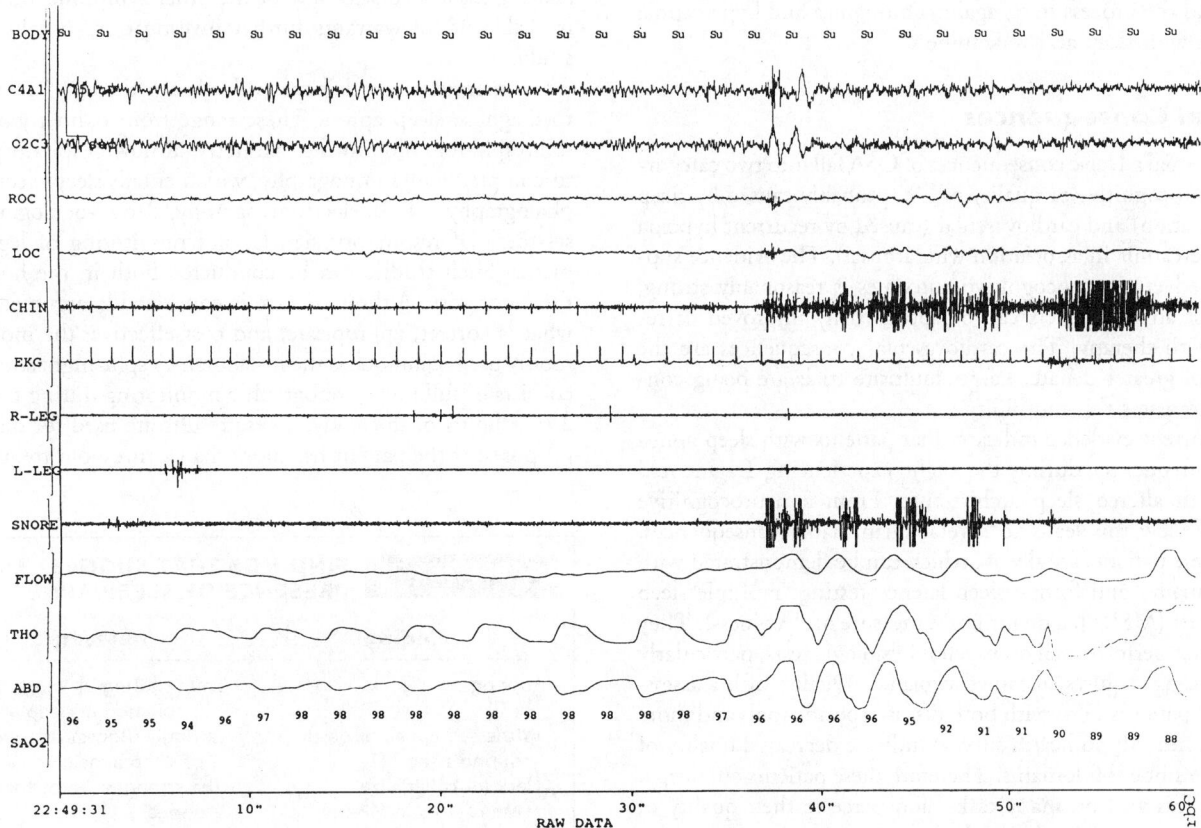

FIGURE 382.2. Thirty-second page from a polysomnogram shows apnea with arousal and apnea termination. Tracing shows absence of flow with paradoxical chest–abdominal wall motion and a decrease in oxygen saturation during apnea. With arousal there is snoring and resumption of ventilation. (From Fogel RB, White DP. Obstructive sleep apnea. In: Schrier RW, Baxter JD, Dzau VJ, et al., eds. *Advances in internal medicine.* St. Louis, MO: Mosby, 2000;45:351–389, with permission.)

tomography, magnetic resonance imaging, acoustic reflection, and endoscopy. Most data suggest that this deficient anatomic configuration activates reflexes in the upper airway that stimulate pharyngeal dilator muscles. Thus the pharyngeal muscles of patients with apnea are more active during wakefulness (neuromuscular compensation) than those of persons without apnea because they must overcome anatomic limitations to maintain airway patency. The stimulus to this neuromuscular compensation remains unclear but likely is activation of a pharyngeal reflex sensitive to negative pressure.

During sleep patients with apnea have a substantial decrement in dilator muscle activation in association with collapse of the pharyngeal airway. Although the precise explanation for this loss of muscle activity among patients with apnea has not been defined, evidence suggests the problem is a loss of reflex-driven neuromuscular compensation present during wakefulness that is a product of a sleep-induced decrement in the reflex itself. The negative pressure reflex clearly is diminished or lost during sleep. To the extent that it drives neuromuscular compensation, the loss minimizes the ability of the muscles to compensate for the deficient anatomic features. Thus the airway collapses.

Over the course of the apnea, hypoxia and hypercapnia progress and stimulate increasing respiratory effort. This rising effort awakens the patient; pharyngeal muscle activity returns and opens the airway with a resumption of ventilation. Hypoxia and hypercapnia are quickly corrected, the patient returns to sleep, and the process starts again. Thus apnea and hypercapnia alternate with sleep and wakefulness.

Clinical Consequences

The potential adverse consequences of OSA fall into two categories—neurocognitive or quality of life (probably caused by sleep fragmentation) and cardiovascular (caused by recurrent hypoxia and hypercapnia in association with arousal). The evidence supporting adverse neurocognitive outcomes is reasonably strong, and most adverse effects can be substantially improved or reversed with therapy. The cardiovascular consequences are the subject of greater debate. Large, multisite trials are being conducted to assess this morbidity.

All current evidence indicates that patients with sleep apnea awaken frequently during the night experiencing fragmented sleep with altered sleep architecture. From a neurocognitive point of view this leads to several quantifiable consequences. First, these patients are sleepy, which can be demonstrated with questionnaires and formal sleep latency testing (multiple sleep latency test [MSLT], a quantitative measure of sleepiness). They also do not perform well on psychophysiologic tests, particularly when testing requires sustained vigilance. Quality of life assessments of patients OSA with both disease-specific tools and more general ones (SF-36 health survey) indicate decreased quality of life in a number of domains. Therefore these patients are sleepy, perform less well on many tasks, and perceive their quality of life to be substantially diminished.

Evolving data also support adverse cardiovascular outcomes among patients with OSA. It seems clear that sleep apnea can contribute to the development of hypertension, although the effect size probably is relatively small. The mechanism driving diurnal hypertension is poorly understood, although increased sympathetic activation has been demonstrated. Mild pulmonary hypertension may develop, although frank cor pulmonale is uncommon among patients with sleep apnea and no other cardiopulmonary disease. Cardiac arrhythmias have occurred among patients with apnea; bradycardia commonly accompanies apnea with oxygen desaturation. Whether ventricular arrhythmias, particularly premature ventricular contractions, are more common among patients with sleep apnea than among matched controls is unclear. The evidence supporting a relation between sleep apnea and myocardial infarction or stroke is weaker, so no firm conclusions can be reached at this time. Sleep apnea likely contributes to increased cardiovascular morbidity, although the extent of the relationship must await the results of multicenter trials.

Clinical Detection and Diagnosis

The diagnosis of sleep apnea should be suspected when any patient reports either daytime sleepiness or loud, prominent snoring. The patient may report such symptoms, although the spouse or bed partner also may point them out. Once suspicion of apnea arises, certain components drive the decision to pursue this diagnosis (Table 382.2). Snoring alone unless it is a social nuisance rarely requires further testing or treatment. However, snoring associated with any of the other symptoms or findings in Table 382.2 warrants further investigation, usually a sleep study.

Numerous methods have evolved over the last 5 to 10 years to diagnose sleep apnea. These range from oximetry alone to full respiratory monitoring (oximetry, airflow, respiratory effort) to complete polysomnography, which entails sleep electroencephalography (EEG), electromyography, electro-oculography, assessment of respiratory signals, and monitoring of leg movements. Such studies can be conducted both in the home and the laboratory. Although there is considerable argument about what is correct, appropriate, and cost-effective; the most commonly used technique is the in-laboratory split-night study. This consists of full polysomnographic monitoring during the initial 2 to 3 hours of the study. These results are used for diagnostic purposes. If the patient has more than a threshold frequency of

TABLE 382.2.	FINDINGS THAT SUGGEST THE PRESENCE OF SLEEP APNEA
Finding	**Relevance**
Snoring	Loud snoring on most nights is common in sleep apnea
Witnessed apnea or gasping during sleep	Strongly suggests diagnosis of sleep apnea
Neck (or collar) size Men >16.5 in (42 cm) Women >15.5 in (39 cm)	The strongest predictor of apnea
Occasional dozing or falling asleep during the day when not busy or active	A weak but clear indicator of apnea

apneas plus hypopneas per hour of sleep (generally 20 to 30), continuous positive airway pressure (CPAP) is begun and titrated to the appropriate pressure to abolish disordered breathing. Thus diagnosis and the initiation of one form of therapy can be accomplished in one night. There are other valid approaches as well.

A sleep study can provide substantial information. The measurement on which most therapeutic decisions are based is the number of apneas (complete cessation of ventilation for longer than 10 seconds) plus hypopneas (decrements in ventilation, generally more than 50%, associated with desaturation (>3% to 4%) or arousal) per hour of sleep (apnea-hypopnea index [AHI] or respiratory disturbance index [RDI]). There is no absolute threshold to define normal and abnormal. Generally more than 5 events per hour is considered abnormal, although therapy has not commonly been instituted until 15 to 20 events per hour are encountered. Results of several studies suggest that treatment of patients with mild sleep apnea (5 to 15 events per hour) leads to improved outcome and quality of life. Patients with symptoms and more than 5 events per hour probably need therapy. Some patients have high upper airway resistance during sleep and recurrent arousal yet do not demonstrate quantifiable apneas or hypopneas according to the aforementioned criteria. They are considered to have *upper airway resistance syndrome.* Improved methods of quantifying airflow are revealing most such events to be subtle hypopneas; thus this syndrome likely represents one end of the spectrum of OSA.

Strategies for Optimal Care

The treatment of patients with sleep apnea should be tailored to the severity of the disorder and the tolerance of the patient. For patients with mild disease, behavioral or simple approaches can be considered. These include weight loss if appropriate, maximizing of nasal patency, avoidance of alcohol or sedatives near bedtime, and avoidance of sleeping supine. These remedies also may be appropriate for patients with more frequent apnea generally in conjunction with the other approaches described later. For more severe disease, the three main therapeutic options are nasal CPAP, dental appliances, and upper airway surgery.

Nasal CPAP applies positive pressure through the nose to the pharyngeal airway to pneumatically splint the airway open. It is highly effective for most patients, but compliance is difficult. Only 50% to 60% of patients use CPAP for more than 5 hours per night. Compliance can likely be enhanced by means of maximizing mask comfort, addressing nasal problems (humidification of inhaled air, nasal steroids or anticholinergics), and possibly by reducing expiratory pressure (bilevel pressure device). Newer CPAP devices can automatically adjust pressure breath by breath as needed to maintain airway patency. Whether this will lead to improved compliance or more effective treatment is unclear.

Should CPAP prove ineffective or intolerable, dental appliances can be considered. Most such devices are fabricated by a dentist. They advance the mandible thereby pulling the tongue apparatus off the posterior pharyngeal wall. Although commonly better tolerated than CPAP, such oral appliances are not always effective, particularly among patients with severe apnea.

Upper airway surgery is aimed at enlarging the pharyngeal airway so that sleep-induced decrements in muscle activity do not lead to airway collapse. Most procedures include removal of the uvula and portions of the soft palate with or without advancing the genioglossus muscle (the tongue) or mandible. Success rates (reduction of apnea-hypopnea index to less than 10 to 20) vary from 30% with laser-assisted uvuloplasty to 42% with uvulopalatopharyngoplasty (UPPP) to 60% when UPPP is combined with genioglossal advancement to 90% when UPPP is combined with mandibular–maxillary advancement. The newly evolved radio frequency reduction of the soft palate or tongue base has been minimally tested on patients with apnea, so no conclusions are possible. There are no particularly effective methods of determining who will or will not respond to these various surgical procedures.

Central Sleep Apnea

Central sleep apnea is a much less common disorder than OSA. It is characterized by recurrent cessation of ventilation during sleep with no associated ventilatory effort. This disorder occurs under a variety of seemingly unrelated circumstances. Therapy is directed at the specific pathophysiologic condition that produced the respiratory instability. The characteristics of these disorders, the sequelae, and treatment are outlined in Table 382.3.

NARCOLEPSY AND PRIMARY CENTRAL NERVOUS SYSTEM HYPERSOMNOLENCE

If a patient is spending adequate time in bed and sleep is not disrupted (sleep apnea, periodic limb movement disorder) yet substantial somnolence is present during wakefulness, a diagnosis of narcolepsy or primary central nervous system (CNS) hypersomnolence is entertained.

Narcolepsy

Narcolepsy is a neurologic condition characterized primarily by extreme sleepiness during the day. This disorder is strongly associated with the major histocompatibility antigen DQB1 0602 and has an onset of symptoms generally in the teens or twenties. This hypersomnolence may or may not be accompanied by one or all of the following symptoms: cataplexy, the sudden onset and transient loss of muscle strength generally in association with strong emotion (laughter or anger); sleep paralysis, transient inability to move on awakening; and hypnogogic hallucinations, visual or auditory hallucinations during drowsiness. The diagnosis requires full night polysomnography to exclude disruptors of sleep and an MSLT the following day. A patient with narcolepsy has characteristic, somewhat fragmented sleep with no clear cause, a short MSLT (generally less than 5 or 6 minutes) and the onset of REM sleep during two or more of the five naps. If all these results are encountered, one can generally be quite comfortable with the diagnosis of narcolepsy.

Treatment of patients with narcolepsy is aimed at the symptoms. Hypersomnolence is managed with stimulants (pemoline, methylphenidate, dextroamphetamine sulfate) or modafinil.

TABLE 382.3.	CENTRAL SLEEP APNEA		
	Idiopathic		
	Waking Hypercapnia	**Waking Hypocapnia**	**Cheyne–Stokes Ventilation**
Nocturnal ventilatory pattern	Central apnea plus sustained hypoventilation	Central apnea in wake-sleep transition	Crescendo-decrescendo ventilation with apnea or hypopnea at nadir
Hypercapnic ventilatory response	Reduced	Increased	Increased
Associated disorders	Obesity–hypoventilation syndrome Central alveolar hypoventilation Neuromuscular disease	None	Congestive heart failure (most patients) Possibly cerebrovascular disease
Sequelae	Disrupted sleep Consequences of chronic hypoxia	Disrupted sleep Insomnia	Disrupted sleep Possibly decreased survival
Treatment	Nocturnal noninvasive ventilation	Oxygen Hypnotics Acetazolamide	Continuous positive airway pressure Maximize cardiac function Oxygen Theophylline

Cataplexy is managed with REM-suppressing antidepressants such as tricyclic compounds or selective serotonin reuptake inhibitors (SSRI). Short naps frequently are refreshing for a patient with narcolepsy, although the effect is of fairly short duration.

Primary Central Nervous System Hypersomnolence

Primary CNS hypersomnolence is characterized by extreme daytime sleepiness, although the other symptoms commonly encountered with narcolepsy (cataplexy, sleep paralysis) do not occur in this disorder. There are several other distinguishing characteristics. Primary CNS hypersomnolence generally begins later in life and is not improved by napping. Naps that lead to transiently reduced sleepiness for persons with narcolepsy often leave a patient with primary CNS hypersomnolence quite lethargic. This diagnosis requires sleep laboratory documentation with full-night polysomnography and MSLT. Polysomnography most often shows sustained high-quality sleep without frequent disruption, whereas the MSLT demonstrates a shortened sleep-onset latency (certainly less than 10 minutes and commonly less than 6 minutes) with no onset of REM. Thus the findings are different from those encountered with narcolepsy. As with narcolepsy, treatment is symptomatic with the use of stimulants to reduce or eliminate sleepiness over the course of the day.

RESTLESS LEG SYNDROME AND PERIODIC LIMB MOVEMENT DISORDER

Restless leg syndrome (RLS) is a disorder generally characterized by leg paresthesias that is improved by moving the legs. The formal diagnosis requires the patient to have the set of symptoms listed in Table 382.4. Because the symptoms of RLS generally occur in the evening or night, they can affect the ability to fall asleep and lead to sleep onset insomnia.

Periodic limb movement disorder (PLMD) is characterized by repetitive periodic contraction of the anterior tibialis muscle during sleep that leads to dorsal flexion of the foot and great

toe. Other muscles sometimes are involved. Current definitions require the contractions to be more than 0.5 second in duration with an interval of 5 to 90 seconds (generally 20 to 40 seconds) and that least four contractions occur sequentially before these events are scored on a sleep study. Occasional contractions or periods of contractions are common among healthy persons. As a result, the number of such events required to define a pathologic condition is controversial. In addition, the periodic limb movements lead to symptoms (insomnia or hypersomnolence) only if they disrupt sleep. Therefore, in assessing the importance of periodic limb movements, one is interested in both the frequency and how often they lead to arousal from sleep.

The cause of RLS and PLMD is unknown, although a number of clear associations with other diseases have been observed. Both disorders occur more commonly among patients with renal failure, myelopathy, peripheral neuropathy, and iron deficiency anemia. Medications such as tricyclic antidepressants and selective serotonin reuptake inhibitors have been found to cause PLMD. Efforts should be made to control iron deficiency anemia if present and to eliminate the medications if possible.

If a patient has symptoms of RLS (Table 382.4), treatment is indicated. PLMD, on the other hand, is a sleep laboratory diagnosis. Although there are no absolute standards to define a normal and abnormal frequency of periodic limb movements, more than 10 movements per hour of sleep generally are considered abnormal. This is particularly the case if arousals are commonly associated with the periodic limb movements. If the pa-

TABLE 382.4.	DIAGNOSTIC CRITERIA FOR RESTLESS LEG SYNDROME

Need to move the extremities, commonly associated with paresthesias
Motor restlessness (leg rubbing, pacing)
Symptoms worse at rest and relieved with activity
Symptoms worse in the evening and during the night

tient reports insomnia or hypersomnolence and the sleep study reveals more than 10 periodic limb movements per hour of sleep with no other clear disruptors, a trial of therapy seems indicated.

Therapy for both RLS and PLMD usually is pharmacologic, although behavioral approaches such as avoiding caffeine may be mildly helpful. The most commonly used medications are dopaminergic agonists (levodopa, bromocriptine, pergolide, and primapexole), which reduce symptoms of RLS and decrease the frequency of periodic limb movements. Narcotics may also prove useful, although they are often less effective than the dopamine agonists. If PLMD is the principal problem, several benzodiazepines (clonazepam, temazepam) have proved useful in either allowing the patient to sleep through the movements without arousal or actually reducing the frequency of movements. Efficacy of therapy is based on relief of symptoms, although in some instances a sleep study may be indicated to assess periodic limb movements.

INABILITY TO SLEEP (INSOMNIA)

ACUTE INSOMNIA

Most persons at some time in life have difficulty sleeping. The difficulty usually is caused by psychological stress, physical illness, or travel over a number of time zones. Most such patients never seek help, and the problem resolves spontaneously. If the person visits a physician, the transient insomnia often can be managed with a hypnotic agent. However, duration of use of hypnotic agents should be limited to avoid habituation or dependence. In the case of insomnia due to crossing multiple time zones, sleep quality often can be maximized with a number of maneuvers. First, the traveler should rapidly adopt the clock time of the destination site and get as much light exposure as possible (preferably evening light for westerly travel and morning light for easterly travel). Short-acting hypnotics can be used to facilitate sleep at the new bedtime. Some data suggest that taking melatonin before bedtime at the new location may speed circadian phase shifts and facilitate adaptation to the new clock time.

CHRONIC INSOMNIA

There are many causes of chronic insomnia (Table 382.1). Only with careful questioning can the specific one be identified. Rarely is a sleep study needed to diagnose the cause of insomnia. About one-half of patients with chronic insomnia have a psychiatric disorder such as depression, anxiety, post-traumatic stress, or panic disorder. In most instances, if the psychiatric problem is identified and managed appropriately, the insomnia generally improves or resolves completely. This concept also applies to insomnia caused by medical problems or pain. If the primary problem can be addressed, the sleep disorder should improve.

Conditioned Insomnia

After psychiatric disorders, conditioned or psychophysiologic insomnia is probably the most common cause of difficulty sleep-

TABLE 382.5.	BEHAVIORAL THERAPY FOR INSOMNIA

Maintain regular bedtimes and waketimes.
Do not nap during the day.
If sleep does not come, read or watch television in another room until drowsy.
Do not keep clocks visible in the bedroom.
Exercise regularly, but not within 3 to 4 hours of bedtime.
Do not drink alcohol within 5 hours of bedtime or caffeine after about 2:00 P.M.
Engage in relaxing activities for the 2 hours before bedtime.

ing. Conditioned insomnia is an adaptive response to acute insomnia of any cause. The person becomes so focused on or concerned about the sleep problem that sleep is inhibited. These patients, in an attempt to address the inability to sleep, also commonly develop poor sleep habits that exacerbate the problem.

Treatment of most patients with chronic insomnia is behavioral, although hypnotic agents have been used. Behavioral therapy is aimed at improving sleep hygiene and reducing concern over sleep issues. This approach is outlined in Table 382.5. The use of hypnotic agents on a long-term basis for this and other causes of insomnia has been minimally studied and is generally not recommended. However, short-term (3 to 4 weeks) use of hypnotic agents by patients with chronic insomnia has been shown to be effective. Some clinicians advocate use of these agents, at least intermittently, in the management of conditioned insomnia.

The hypnotic agents commonly prescribed are benzodiazepines, an imidiazopyridine (zolpidem), and sedating antidepressants such as trazodone. For benzodiazepines, half-life is the principal consideration. Agents with a rapid onset and short half-life are preferable for patients with sleep onset insomnia (difficulty falling asleep). Longer-acting agents are more appropriate for patients who awaken and have difficulty returning to sleep (sleep maintenance insomnia). The agents and half-lives are listed in Table 382.6. Longer-acting agents have the disadvantage of potential daytime sedation. Shorter-acting agents may not sustain sleep throughout the night. Trazodone is a sedating antidepressant that has become popular as a hypnotic agent because it is believed to cause less habituation. There are limited data on the hypnotic efficacy of antidepressants. Zolpidem is a short-acting agent with potentially reduced tolerance and rebound insomnia.

TABLE 382.6.	HALF-LIVES OF BENZODIAZEPINE HYPNOTICS AND ZOLPIDEM

Short (1.5–5 hr)	Medium (10–20 hr)	Long (20–100 hr)
Zolpidem	Temazepam	Flurazepam
Triazolam	Estazolam	Clonazepam
	Lorazepam	

The use of melatonin as a hypnotic in the treatment of patients with insomnia is controversial. Because melatonin has both modest sleep-promoting actions and can influence circadian phase, it probably is effective in the management of circadian rhythm disorders (delayed phase syndrome, jet lag). However, there is little consistent evidence that melatonin is effective in noncircadian insomnia. Use of this agent cannot be advocated for persons with conditioned insomnia.

Circadian Rhythm Disorders

The most common chronic circadian rhythm disorders are the advanced and delayed sleep phase syndromes. In the former, patients tend to fall asleep early (8:00 or 9:00 P.M.) and waken early (3:00 to 4:00 A.M.). In the delayed sleep phase syndrome the opposite is true—falling asleep late (1:00 to 3:00 A.M.) and awakening late (9:00 to 11:00 A.M.). Whether these disorders are acquired genetically or evolve from behavioral preference is unclear. It does appear that adolescents tend to adopt a delayed circadian sleep schedule and the elderly acquire an advanced one.

These disorders are identified from the history. Patients have little difficulty sleeping within their circadian sleep phases (advanced or delayed) but great difficulty sleeping during conventional sleep hours. Once the problem is identified, there are several potential therapeutic options. One is based on the use of light, which has been demonstrated to be the strongest circadian modulator. Morning light tends to advance the circadian system and allow a patient with a delayed-phase syndrome to fall asleep and awaken earlier. Late evening light delays the circadian system so that a patient with an advanced-phase syndrome can go to sleep earlier and waken later. Although these general principles regarding light exposure have been unambiguously demonstrated, exactly how much light (lux) and for what duration (hours) it is needed remain poorly delineated. Precise recommendations are difficult.

The other plausible approach to the treatment of patients with chronic circadian rhythm disorders is use of melatonin. Melatonin has weak hypnotic effects and can influence circadian phase. It can be taken early in the evening by patients with the delayed-phase syndrome and may help advance the circadian system. However, only a few clinical trials have assessed the efficacy of this approach in the care of patients. The data that do exist indicate this to be a reasonable approach, although the strength of the circadian effect of melatonin is modest.

■ PARASOMNIA (UNUSUAL EVENTS AT NIGHT)

Parasomnias are unusual events or movements during the night that would generally not be associated with the sleeping state. Although there are numerous such disorders, only a few are addressed herein.

Sleep terrors, sleep walking, and sleep talking are grouped as disorders of arousal. They occur out of deep non-REM sleep (stages 3 and 4) and thus take place in the first third of the night, when these sleep stages are most common. The patient is believed to be in a state between sleep and waking with some behavioral and EEG characteristics of each. The events occurring during sleep walking and sleep talking are reflected in the names. Sleep terrors are characterized by sudden arousal from sleep often with screaming and intense fear manifested by heightened sympathetic activation (tachycardia, hyperpnea). Once fully alert, the patient generally has amnesia of the sleep event. Therapy for any of the disorders of arousal, if needed, is aimed at avoiding sleep deprivation and eliminating disrupting events during sleep, such as apnea and PLMD. Sleep deprivation or fragmentation seems to worsen these disorders. Whether a sleep study is needed for diagnosis and institution of therapy depends on the severity of the problem, the ability to reach a clear diagnosis from the history, and the level of concern regarding sleep-disrupting events.

REM behavior disorder, unlike the disorders of arousal, evolves out of REM sleep and thus tends to occur in the later third of the night, when REM sleep is most common. One of the principal characteristics of REM sleep is skeletal muscle paralysis (atonia), the neurophysiologic process of which has been reasonably well characterized. Among patients with REM behavior disorder, the atonia of REM sleep is absent, and the patient can move about, presumably in response to events occurring in a dream. Such movements can be violent. This disorder often requires polysomnography for formal diagnosis, but once the diagnosis is established, it responds well, for unclear reasons, to benzodiazepine hypnotics, usually clonazepam.

In many cases a seizure disorder may manifest itself more commonly during sleep than during wakefulness, although such events are most often observed during both behavioral states. A sleep evaluation is not needed to define the cause or characteristics of the event because this can be accomplished by recording the events during the day. In some cases, however, the seizures occur only during sleep and necessitate polysomnography with extensive EEG monitoring for formal diagnosis. Nocturnal seizures may take many forms and are commonly confused with other forms of parasomnia. However, the events tend to be consistent and stereotypical. Because therapy for nocturnal seizures is quite different from that of other forms of parasomnia, definitive EEG diagnosis is required.

BIBLIOGRAPHY

Brzezinski A. Melatonin in humans. *N Engl J Med* 1997;336:184–195.
Choo KL, Guilleminault C. Narcolepsy and idiopathic hypersomnolence. *Clin Chest Med* 1998;19:169–181.
Engelman HM, Kingshott RN, Wraith PK, et al. Randomized placebo-controlled crossover trial of continuous positive airway pressure for mild sleep apnea/hypopnea syndrome. *Am J Respir Crit Care Med* 1999;159:461–467.
Mahowald MW, Schenck CH. Parasomnias including the restless leg syndrome. *Clin Chest Med* 1998;19:183–202.
Nowell PD, Mazumdar S, Buysse DJ, et al. Benzodiazepines and zolpidem for chronic insomnia: a meta-analysis of treatment efficacy. *JAMA* 1997;278:2170–2177.
Redline S, Strohl KP. Recognition and consequences of obstructive sleep apnea hypopnea syndrome. *Clin Chest Med* 1998;19:1–20.
Trenkwalder C, Walters AS, Hening W. Periodic limb movements and restless leg syndrome. *Neurol Clin* 1996;14:629–650.

White DP. The pathophysiology of obstructive sleep apnea. *Thorax* 1995;
50:797–804.

Kelley's Textbook of Internal Medicine, fourth edition. Edited by H. David Humes.
Lippincott Williams & Wilkins, Philadelphia © 2000.

CHAPTER 383

INHALATION AND ASPIRATION SYNDROMES

NORMAN E. ADAIR
EDWARD F. HAPONIK

When respiratory defenses are overwhelmed by inhaled or aspirated materials, a spectrum of potentially life threatening but treatable injuries may occur. Clinical uncertainty is high because of the diversity of injurious agents, variations in exposure scenarios and in patients' functional reserve, and the delayed onset of many clinically important sequelae. The clinician may be confronted by problems such as triage of multiple workers after an industrial accident or of victims of smoke inhalation after a residential or hotel fire, resuscitation of someone who has almost drowned, or treatment of a chronically ill, hospitalized patient with unwitnessed aspiration. Effective management requires familiarity with common clinical presentations and advanced preparation to deal with multiple levels of respiratory injury.

■ PATHOGENESIS AND CLINICAL FINDINGS

The anatomic level, severity of damage, and timing of onset are key determinants of the symptoms, signs, and therapeutic priorities (Fig 383.1). Thus rapid characterization of the extent of injury to the upper and lower airways, distal lung parenchyma, or their combinations is essential. Possible systemic effects of absorbed toxins, secondary multiple organ failure, or exacerbation of preexisting medical illnesses all have additional practical implications. The upper airway may be obstructed mechanically by impacted foreign bodies such as vomitus or food, by severe inflammation such as supraglottitis or laryngitis due to water-soluble irritant gases or heat, or by reflex laryngospasm, such as dry drowning. Acute tracheitis, bronchitis, and bronchiolitis with associated bronchorrhea and true bronchospasm may mimic status asthmaticus and cause hypoventilatory respiratory failure. More focal tracheobronchial obstruction such as aspirated food or inspissated secretions may cause atelectasis or postobstructive pneumonia. Aspiration of acidic gastric contents, near drowning, or inhalation of irritant gases with low water solubility often cause diffuse alveolar capillary membrane injury with development of permeability (noncardiogenic) pulmonary edema (acute respiratory distress syndrome [ARDS]). In the latter instances, massive physiologic shunt causes hypoxemic respiratory failure.

Direct cellular damage is caused by exposure to highly reactive chemicals such as acids and bases that lead to oxidation or denaturation of cellular constituents. Lipid peroxidation is an important common pathway of many of these injuries. The ciliated epithelium of the respiratory tract and type I pneumocytes are particularly vulnerable. In addition to their primary effects, inhaled or aspirated chemicals precipitate an inflammatory response. Recruitment of polymorphonuclear neutrophils into pulmonary capillaries may lead to neutrophilic alveolitis with further alveolar capillary injury caused by proteases and elastases and perpetuated by activation of interacting cytokines. Such cellular events prime the lung, further predisposing to catastrophic permeability edema (ARDS) in the presence of another, superimposed stimulus, such as burn injury, aspiration, nosocomial pneumonia, or sepsis.

Acute
- Rhinitis
- Supraglottic edema
- Laryngospasm
- Obstruction

Chronic
- Stenosis

Acute
- Bronchitis
- Bronchospasm
- Obstruction
- Atelectasis

Chronic
- Reactive airways
- Obliterative Bronchiolitis
- Bronchiectasis

Acute
- Chemical pneumonitis
- Atelectasis
- Acute Respiratory Distress Syndrome

Chronic
- Pulmonary fibrosis

Acute and Chronic
- Central nervous system and cardiovascular dysfunction
- Renal injury
- Hepatic injury
- Tissue asphyxia

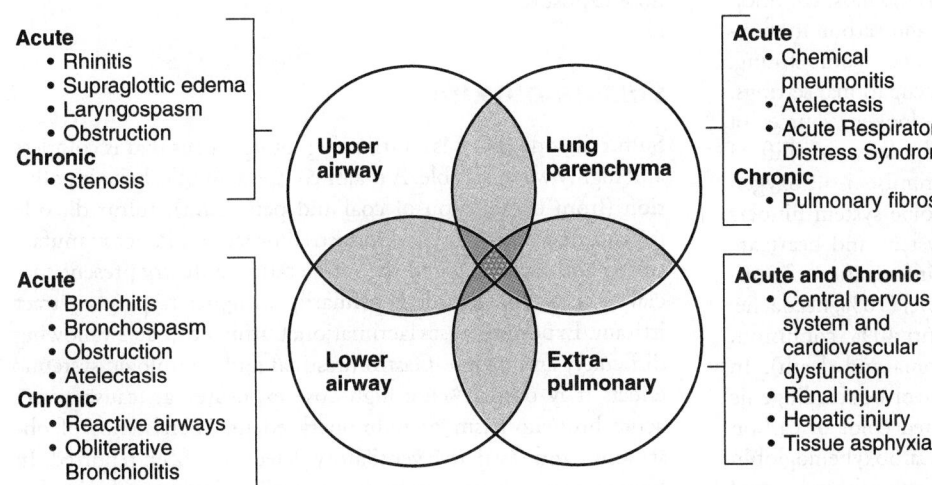

FIGURE 383.1. Clinical spectrum of inhalation injury.

ACUTE INHALATION INJURY

Despite the diversity of potentially toxic inhalants, the tissue responses are stereotypical, and management principles are supportive and usually nonspecific. Although the setting of exposure, such as residential fire or industrial accident, may aid in determining that an inhalation injury is probable, the injurious agent may not be identifiable. Inhalation injury may involve the upper airway (stridor, choking, laryngospasm, rhinorrhea), conducting airways (cough, bronchospasm, bronchorrhea, luminal impaction), alveoli (hypoxemia, noncardiogenic pulmonary edema), and systemic toxicity (tissue asphyxia, central nervous system or cardiovascular toxicity). When exposures are especially severe or the injurious agent extremely noxious, global respiratory damage may occur. The site and extent of respiratory injury depend on the chemical reactivity, pH, water solubility, and concentration of the agent, and the duration of exposure. Chemical reactivity and water solubility are particularly important: Inhalant gases with high water solubility, such as ammonia and sulfur dioxide, tend to irritate the conjunctiva, nasal passages, and upper airway; those with lower water solubility, such as phosgene and oxides of nitrogen, tend to penetrate farther into the respiratory tract to injure distal airways and alveoli. Low water solubility also minimizes upper airway mucosal irritation, thus recognition of and escape from the hazardous exposure are delayed until severe injury has developed.

Asphyxiation implies impairment of tissue oxygen delivery or utilization and may be multifactorial. Inhaled methane and natural gas displace alveolar oxygen, causing direct asphyxia. Cyanide, carbon monoxide, and hydrogen sulfide interfere with mitochondrial oxygen utilization and are tissue asphyxiants. Systemic toxicity, especially of the central nervous system, may occur after inhalation of certain hydrocarbons or heavy metals, such as mercury. Immunologically mediated injuries also are possible after inhalation of platinum salts, isocyanates, and anhydrides.

CARBON MONOXIDE

Carbon monoxide (CO) intoxication may occur in any setting in which incomplete combustion occurs. It is the most common cause of death after acute smoke inhalation, and carbon monoxide may be the most common inhaled toxin. Petroleum refining, mining, and foundry work are important occupational settings. Home heaters are frequent, potentially overlooked, sources of exposure. Avid binding to hemoglobin and a leftward shift of the oxyhemoglobin dissociation curve compromise tissue oxygen delivery, and interference with the cytochrome system hinders cellular respiration. The central nervous system and heart are especially vulnerable to carbon monoxide intoxication. Symptoms relate broadly to carboxyhemoglobin level (10%, headache; 30%, severe headache and visual impairment; 40%, confusion, lethargy, and collapse; more than 60%, coma and death). In addition to systemic effects, both cardiogenic or noncardiogenic pulmonary edema may occur. The cherry-red color of carbon monoxide intoxication is seldom present. Carboxyhemoglobin measurements should be obtained for all patients with suspected smoke inhalation or other exposures. Levels are influenced by the time elapsed after exposure (half-time is about 6 hours) and oxygen therapy. The risk of acute and long-term neurologic effects heightens the importance of prompt treatment with high concentrations of supplemental oxygen.

CYANIDE

Cyanide (CN) toxicity is an important hazard in the electroplating and steel industries. Acrylonitrile and propionitrile are used in plastics manufacturing and are metabolized to cyanide. Cyanide intoxication also occurs after smoke inhalation, and cyanide may have synergistic morbidity with carbon monoxide. The presence of neurologic dysfunction, unexplained metabolic (lactic) acidosis, and, occasionally, the odor of bitter almonds on the patient's breath suggest cyanide intoxication (more than 0.5 mg is toxic and 1 to 3 mg per liter is the lethal range). Because rapid measurement of cyanide levels may not be possible, empiric treatment often is necessary.

AMMONIA

Ammonia (NH_4) is a highly water soluble, colorless gas that because of its caustic properties is extremely irritating. When ammonia combines with water on the respiratory mucosa, the resulting alkaline solution can produce tissue liquefaction. Mild exposures such as encountered with household cleaners often produce irritant effects, including rhinorrhea, cough, headache, occasional bronchospasm, and nausea. Severe inhalation sufficient to damage tissues usually occurs when pressurized ammonia is leaked during transportation or in fertilizer, refrigerator, explosive, and chemical industry accidents. Immediate asphyxia is possible at high concentrations. Upper airway obstruction from edema or laryngospasm, severe desquamative chemical bronchitis, and noncardiogenic pulmonary edema all may occur. Corneal damage can lead to blindness and may delay escape from the exposure scene, resulting in more serious respiratory damage. Long-term pulmonary effects, including bronchiectasis, bronchiolitis, and reactive airways disease, have followed high-dose exposures.

SULFUR DIOXIDE

Sulfur dioxide (SO_2) is an irritating, pungent gas that is colorless and highly water soluble. A major component of urban air pollution (from combustion of coal and petroleum), sulfur dioxide is generated during myriad industrial processes. Paper manufacturing and bleaching and the refrigeration industry present special risks. Sulfur dioxide is primarily an upper respiratory tract irritant. Exposure causes lacrimation, burning throat, swallowing difficulty, and cough. Gastrointestinal and neurologic systemic effects may occur. Acute high-dose exposure can cause severe acute bronchospasm or pulmonary edema. Persistence of obstructive and restrictive ventilatory defects has been reported. In lower doses, sulfur dioxide may contribute to exacerbations of chronic obstructive lung disorders.

HYDROGEN FLUORIDE

Hydrogen fluoride (HF) is used widely in etching of glass and ceramics and in the semiconductor industry. It is highly water soluble. Upper and lower airway obstruction and pulmonary edema may occur after inhalation. Hydrogen fluoride also may cause severe cutaneous burns. Skin necrosis may appear deceptively minor at first. Hydrogen fluoride may bind calcium and magnesium in tissues, resulting in hypocalcemia and hypomagnesemia that necessitate therapy.

CHLORINE

Chlorine (Cl_2) is a yellowish-green reactive gas that is intermediate in water solubility and denser than air. Used as a chemical warfare agent in World War I, it is now used widely in water and sewer purification, bleaching processes, and chemical manufacturing. Accidental home exposures often are caused by swimming pool care and mixture of cleaning agents. Chlorine interacts with water in the respiratory tract to produce hydrochloric acid and other highly reactive compounds that can denature and coagulate tissues. Necrosis and sloughing of the respiratory epithelium, upper airway obstruction, and pulmonary edema may develop after acute exposure. Severe respiratory symptoms may be delayed several hours after exposure. Most acute exposures, however, are not fatal, and pulmonary function usually normalizes within several months.

PHOSGENE

Phosgene ($COCl_2$) is a dense gas that was used as a warfare agent in World War I but is now encountered during isocyanate production, synthesis of dyes, insecticides, and drugs, and as a byproduct in arc welding or burning of polyvinyl chloride. Phosgene is more toxic than chlorine and has lower water solubility and thus has an increased propensity to damage the pulmonary parenchyma. A latent period from one-half to several hours may pass after exposure before pulmonary symptoms develop. Phosgene produces chemical pneumonitis and pulmonary edema.

OXIDES OF NITROGEN

Nitrogen dioxide (NO_2) and related oxides of nitrogen are potent oxidants that in aqueous solution form nitrous and nitric acids. Inhalation of nitrogen dioxide may occur during the storage of silage (silo-filler's disease), chemical manufacturing, arc welding, and fire fighting. Nitrogen dioxide is heavier than air, yellow to reddish-brown, and has low water solubility. The odor is similar to that of chlorine bleach but is not especially irritating. Low water solubility and minimal warning signs may prolong exposure sufficiently to cause a severe, delayed lung injury, including pulmonary edema. The permissible exposure limit is 5 parts per million. Concentrations 10 times that level may not be immediately irritating yet may lead to serious lung injury within 2 to 24 hours. Multiphasic clinical illnesses may occur. Bronchiolitis obliterans has been reported as a late sequela, developing within weeks of acute exposure. Symptoms include recurrent fever, cough, dyspnea, and diffuse nodular or reticulonodular opacities on chest radiographs. Corticosteroids have been used to manage the acute event and to prevent bronchiolar fibrotic changes, although the efficacy remains unproved.

HYDROGEN SULFIDE

Hydrogen sulfide (H_2S) may be encountered in waste disposal and in oil and natural gas drilling and refining. Not only an irritant but also an asphyxiant, hydrogen sulfide can cause cyanosis and metabolic acidosis, often with severe neurologic dysfunction.

METALLIC COMPOUNDS

Exposure to high concentrations of fumes from metals, often in the form of metal oxides, can cause acute pulmonary and systemic injury. Cadmium oxide may be volatilized during welding or smelting and produces delayed-onset noncardiogenic pulmonary edema that occasionally is associated with renal failure. Less severe chemical pneumonitis or bronchitis also follows inhalation of cadmium, cobalt, manganese, nickel carbonyl, vanadium, and mercury. Platinum halide complexes may cause occupational asthma.

Exposures to metal hydrides, such as arsine, phosphine, and diborine, occur increasingly as a result of their use in the semiconductor industry. Arsine, an arsenical, is associated with intravascular hemolysis, renal failure, bilirubinemia, abdominal pain, and hematuria. Hemodialysis often is necessary for renal failure, and exchange transfusion often is required to clear arsenic–hemoglobin complex. Phosphine and diborine can cause pulmonary edema and central nervous system dysfunction.

Metal fume fever is a relatively benign systemic response to inhalation of certain metallic fumes, especially zinc oxide. Exposure typically occurs during welding in closed spaces or smelting of metals. Symptoms include fever, chills, myalgia, and malaise, which occur 4 to 6 hours after exposure. Leukocytosis accompanies these symptoms and may suggest infection. There usually are no respiratory symptoms or radiographic abnormalities. Tolerance of exposure is characteristic. Symptoms decrease as the work week progresses, only to recur after a weekend without exposure. The pathogenesis of metal fume fever is unknown, but long-term sequelae are not recognized.

ISOCYANATES AND ANHYDRIDES

Isocyanates and anhydrides are very reactive compounds. Despite chemical differences, they elicit similar respiratory responses. Toluene disodium is the prototype of its class, encountered in the manufacture of polyurethane foams, fibers, and coatings. Trimellitic anhydride is used as an anticorrosive on metals and in the manufacture of epoxy resins. High-dose exposures produce upper airway irritation and a cough, which is chemically mediated. A second syndrome of occupational asthma and rhinitis develops after a latent period, appears to be immunologically mediated, and can be provoked at extremely low concentrations. A third syndrome is similar to hypersensitivity pneumonitis; systemic and respiratory symptoms developing after a lag period of 4 to 12 hours. An uncommon but severe syndrome characterized by pulmonary hemorrhage and anemia may develop after a latent period. Symptoms include dyspnea, a cough, and hemoptysis. This syndrome is believed to be immunologically mediated and may respond to corticosteroid therapy. Avoidance is important because recurrences are possible.

SMOKE INHALATION

Smoke inhalation epitomizes the clinical challenges of inhalation injury. The spectrum of clinical features ranges from inconsequential, self-limited coughing or mild exacerbations of intrinsic airways disease to life-threatening respiratory failure. Smoke is a heterogenous product of thermal demutation that evolves through pyrolysis (smoldering in a low-oxygen environment) or combustion (burning with visible flame). True thermal lung injury is unusual, but inhalation of steam, with its higher heat-carrying capacity, and the burning ether vehicle from the crack form of cocaine are noteworthy exceptions. Most damage is caused by a mixture of toxic products of incomplete combustion that varies with the fuels burned and other aspects of each fire scenario. Acrolein is an aldehyde particularly important in residential fires, but combinations of irritant gases are generated during most fires, probably with synergistic toxicity. The association of smoke inhalation with cutaneous burns considerably increases morbidity and mortality. With progress in burn resuscitation, inhalation injury and related infections have become the leading causes of death.

Respiratory problems vary with time after smoke exposure. Early complications (initial 24 hours) include carbon monoxide and cyanide intoxication and upper airway and tracheobronchial obstruction. Delayed complications (2 to 5 days) include pulmonary edema and, less often, pneumonia. Late complications (more than 5 days after exposure) include nosocomial pneumonia, ARDS (often due to sepsis), and, less often, pulmonary embolism. The clinical diagnosis of smoke inhalation is suggested by a closed-space setting of exposure, unconsciousness at the fire scene (often with alcohol or other drug intoxication), and facial burns, especially involving the respiratory area—the area around the face and mouth—or circumferential burns of the neck. Carbonaceous sputum is a nonspecific marker of exposure and has no prognostic importance. The presence of respiratory signs or symptoms, such as obvious hoarseness or stridor, or the finding of pharyngeal edema at physical examination is a more reliable predictor of serious smoke inhalation.

▮ ASPIRATION SYNDROMES

Aspiration syndromes are caused by introduction of liquid or solid material into the respiratory tract and may be acute or chronic. Common scenarios include oropharyngeal aspiration (disorders of deglutition), regurgitation (aspiration of gastric contents), and immersion accidents (near drowning; see Chapter 59). The extent of respiratory injury and the nature and anatomic distribution of the tissue response depend on the volume of the aspirate, its physical properties, the duration of aspiration,

and the patient's posture at the time of the event. Dependent lung zones are typically involved most severely; posterior segmental and lower lobe disease is especially common. Secondary complications such as atelectasis or infection are frequent; predisposing factors are aspiration-related damage, decreased airway clearance, and the condition that led originally to the aspiration.

OROPHARYNGEAL ASPIRATION

Small volumes of saliva often are aspirated during sleep or anesthesia with no adverse impact. Clinically important aspiration of food or saliva usually is associated with anatomic oropharyngeal lesions such as neoplasms or hypopharyngeal diverticulum, esophageal obstruction such as achalasia or carcinoma, esophageal dysfunction such as reflux, or neuromuscular disorders. Impaction of food or other solid materials within the glottis may cause acute upper airway obstruction with asphyxia (cafe coronary). Lesser amounts of aspirated solid material may lodge in lower airways and produce a syndrome of obstructive pneumonia (often recurrent) or chronic wheeze mimicking asthma.

Lipoid pneumonia is a syndrome associated with oropharyngeal aspiration of oils from mineral or vegetable sources. Oily nose drops or castor oil taken at bedtime may cause this syndrome, especially among elderly patients. Use of these agents may not be reported in the medical history because they are not regarded as medications. Oil mists used in industrial processes also may produce this condition. Typically there are few signs or symptoms, but radiographs show opacities that suggest infection or neoplasia. The diagnosis is made after biopsy, usually performed to exclude cancer. The low density of lipoidal infiltrates seen on computed tomographic scans of the chest may suggest the diagnosis.

Aspiration of oropharyngeal contents is particularly common when consciousness is reduced and upper airway protective reflexes become impaired, such as after seizures, intoxication, or therapeutic use of sedative-hypnotic agents. The inoculum of aspirated oropharyngeal bacteria may be sufficient to cause pneumonia, which often is characterized by tissue necrosis, lung abscess formation, or extension to the pleural space (empyema). Such infections often are polymicrobial with a high proportion of anaerobic pathogens. Among debilitated hospitalized patients the oropharynx is readily colonized with gram-negative enteric organisms and staphylococci; aspiration leads to potentially lethal nosocomial pneumonia (see Chapter 361).

REGURGITATION (ASPIRATION OF GASTRIC CONTENTS)

Gastric contents may be acutely and massively aspirated whenever consciousness is impaired, especially during anesthetic procedures and cardiopulmonary resuscitation. The severity of this syndrome varies with the volume of aspirate, its pH, and its particulate content. Milder episodes are manifested predominantly by wheezing and cough. The most serious presentation is acid aspiration syndrome (aspiration pneumonitis or Mendelson's syndrome), characterized by severe hypoxemia, reduced lung compliance, and the presence of bilateral alveolar infiltrates caused by noncardiogenic pulmonary edema (ARDS). This syndrome is most likely when pH is less than 2.0 and aspirate volume exceeds 50 mL. Dependent distribution, asymmetry of infiltrates, and associated volume loss are among the radiographic signs of massive aspiration.

Recurrent episodes of gastroesophageal reflux have been implicated as a cause of upper and lower airway inflammation, extending the spectrum of acid-mediated airway injury. Tracheal microaspiration or esophageal irritant reflexes may be involved in some instances of chronic cough or asthma. Control of the respiratory symptom is facilitated by antireflux measures and modification of esophageal acidity. The role of gastroesophageal reflux in producing respiratory symptoms may be evaluated with intraesophageal pH probe studies and nasopharyngoscopic examination of the upper airway.

GENERAL DIAGNOSTIC CONSIDERATIONS

The severity, and sometimes the cause, of inhalation- and aspiration-mediated injury usually is apparent after acute massive exposures, when the classic clinical history, often coupled with the patient's predisposition to injury, establishes the diagnosis. More difficult, however, is determining the ultimate extent of injury, prediction of the clinical course, and how these will be modified by the patient's previous health status. The severity of injury often is underestimated at first, or a lag before the onset of life-threatening sequelae complicates triage decisions. Chronic low-dose or subacute inhalation or aspiration may produce enigmatic illnesses. Assessment of chronic cough, dyspnea, and unexplained radiographic abnormalities requires consideration of such exposures.

Patient and rescue personnel often provide essential information regarding exposures. The anatomic and physiologic effects may be assessed by means of physical examination. Arterial blood gas measurements and chest radiographs are essential, but results may be normal soon after the injury. Nevertheless, they provide baseline information needed for follow-up care. The extent of laboratory testing and monitoring is individualized. In the pertinent clinical setting, assays relevant to certain asphyxiants (carboxyhemoglobin, cyanide, methemoglobin, and sulfhemoglobin) should be performed. End-organ dysfunction, such as abnormal results of neuropsychologic tests in association with carbon monoxide intoxication, rather than a single blood measurement, is a more sensitive indicator of intoxication. Administration of antidotes to cyanide toxicity should be undertaken presumptively if clinical suspicions warrant.

After smoke inhalation, simple spirometry and flow-volume curves have shown patterns of extrathoracic or intrathoracic airway obstruction or restrictive defects and have a high negative predictive value. Peak flow measurements may be useful in the emergency department. Radionuclide scans demonstrating maldistribution or delayed clearance of inhaled tracer have documented acute inhalation injury, but the technology is not available in many facilities. The lethal potential and treatable nature of acute upper airway obstruction demand careful supraglottic examination by an experienced person. Upper airway injury may be evaluated by means of fiberoptic laryngoscopy if obstruction

is not immediately life threatening. Bronchoscopy reveals nonspecific tracheobronchial inflammation, carbonaceous material, or food particles after, respectively, irritant gas exposure, smoke inhalation, or aspiration, but these findings seldom define management or are predictive of the clinical course. Preliminary studies of bronchoalveolar lavage after smoke inhalation suggest that the presence and persistence of alveolitis may have prognostic value.

STRATEGIES FOR OPTIMAL CARE

Diagnostic evaluation is merged with immediate supportive care. Initial priorities include removal from further harm, establishing an airway, supplying supplemental oxygen, and arranging immediate transportation to a health care facility. Decontamination of skin and clothes may be performed in the field or the emergency department. The decision to admit the patient to the hospital should be based on symptoms and clinical findings. The presence of signs or symptoms indicating toxicity warrants hospitalization. The potential for delayed onset of injury, as with exposure to low-solubility inhalants, necessitates a cautious approach to discharging persons who do not have symptoms. The presence of comorbid illnesses, limited access to medical care, and extremes of patient age also favor hospitalization. The clinician must seek associated traumatic injuries sustained at the scene.

Because inhalation and aspiration injuries share common tissue responses and clinical features, management priorities are similar. Specific antidotes rarely are available. Carbon monoxide intoxication requires high-flow oxygen inhalation with a tight-fitting mask with a reservoir bag. The role of hyperbaric oxygen therapy is controversial, but this treatment may benefit patients with neurologic impairment, prolonged exposure, lactic acidosis, cardiac dysfunction, or carboxyhemoglobin levels greater than 25%. Whether hyperbaric therapy prevents delayed neurologic sequelae remains unclear. Patients with cyanide intoxication are treated by means of sequential administration of drugs. Inhaled amyl nitrite and intravenous sodium nitrite are administered to generate cyanomethemoglobin; sodium thiosulfate is then given to produce thiocyanate, which will be excreted. Patients with methemoglobinemia after oxidant exposure, as with oxides of nitrogen, may be treated with methylene blue.

Abdominal compression may help dislodge a mechanical upper airway obstruction but is not otherwise advocated. For persons who have almost drowned or those with gastric distention, this maneuver might accentuate aspiration. Clinically significant upper airway obstruction, signaled by stridor and labored accessory respiratory muscle recruitment, usually is managed by means of translaryngeal intubation. Intubation should be performed early and electively for patients at risk, such as those with facial burns of the respiratory area. Fiberoptic nasopharyngoscopy may facilitate difficult intubation. Tracheotomy may be necessary when pharyngeal edema is severe.

For symptomatic cases, supplemental oxygen is continued and upper airway patency and oxygenation are monitored. Use of an aerosolized bronchodilator may be of value. Respiratory failure from pulmonary edema and desquamative bronchitis necessitates supportive care with positive-pressure ventilation, including positive end-expiratory pressure. The administration of positive end-expiratory pressure may be essential in the management of severe shunt-related hypoxemia in established ARDS, but it is of no prophylactic benefits to patients at risk. The management of acute respiratory failure is detailed in Chapter 356. In essence, the patient is supported until the primary injury heals. Avoidance of superimposed iatrogenic problems, especially nosocomial pneumonia, assumes special importance. If the patient survives the respiratory failure, recovery may be complete, although there is potential for residual respiratory dysfunction. Overall outcome usually depends on the severity of the exposure, the extent of preexisting illness, and timeliness of initial therapy.

Mechanical airway obstruction by mucus, cellular debris, or particulates is managed by means of maintaining hydration, effective coughing, postural drainage, and airway suction. Respiratory therapy maneuvers such as chest percussion and use of the upright posture are advisable. Mucolytic agents and expectorants have an unknown role. Intratracheal instillation of buffers or diluents to neutralize inhaled gases or aspirated acid is not effective. Only rarely is therapeutic bronchoscopy of additional value in mechanically clearing the airways; it is reserved for patients for whom conservative approaches have failed. For severe atelectasis, bronchoscopy may be necessary to identify and remove a foreign body or central mucous plug.

Corticosteroids usually are not indicated to modify the acute injury or to reduce the risk of sequelae. Clinical observation of patients with smoke inhalation in the presence of cutaneous burns, acid aspiration, and near drowning has indicated that steroids do not improve outcome and may increase the risk of infection. Steroids have been used to treat patients with intractable bronchospasm and may reduce inflammation and the likelihood of bronchiolitis obliterans after inhalation of nitrogen dioxide. Antioxidants, free radical scavengers, surfactants, and antiproteases are theoretically attractive but of unproven clinical value. Inhalation and aspiration injuries are predispositions for infection, but prophylactic antibiotics do not appear to prevent pneumonia. Unnecessary use of antibiotics can promote infection by resistant organisms. Close monitoring of clinical signs, respiratory secretions, and radiographic features helps determine whether antimicrobial agents are indicated, but definitive diagnosis of superimposed infection remains difficult.

■ PREVENTION

Because of the severity of inhalation and aspiration syndromes and the limited therapeutic options (Table 383.1), emphasis is on prevention. Job safety programs and industrial hygiene surveillance should decrease the likelihood of industrial accidents. Clinicians should be familiar with the potential industrial risks within their communities and participate actively in public education, disaster planning, and triage. Public education regarding the hazards of smoke inhalation injury, carbon monoxide exposure, and the management of acute mechanical upper airway obstruction (Heimlich maneuver) should be emphasized. Use of home smoke detectors and safety policies at public swim-

TABLE 383.1.	PREVENTION OF INHALATION- AND ASPIRATION-INDUCED RESPIRATORY INJURY

Smoke detectors in home, office, and other work sites
Heating system inspection (wood, coal, gas)
Adequate engine exhaust systems
Adequate ventilation for smoke and volatiles
Respiratory protective equipment around high-risk exposure sites
Air monitoring at industrial sites

ming pools have been shown to reduce fatalities from fires and near drowning, respectively. Basic fire safety practices and familiarity with escape routes are other important general preventive measures.

Enhanced physician awareness of risk of aspiration of gastric contents has led to routine practices regarding food abstinence before general anesthesia, caution in the use of sedative-hypnotic agents, and increased use of antacids and histamine-2 antagonists to alter gastric acidity. Simple nonpharmacologic measures, such as maintenance of an upright posture in bed, the use of bed blocks during sleep, and for hospitalized patients, early mobilization, should minimize the likelihood of aspiration. For patients receiving enteral nutrition, the use of continuous low-volume feedings, rather than large-bolus administration, and avoidance of large gastric residuals may be effective prophylactic measures.

Oropharyngeal aspiration can be a recurrent problem, depending on the cause. When substantial aspiration has occurred and the patient has recovered from the acute episode, a search for correctable predispositions is important to minimize the likelihood of another event. A multidisciplinary approach has been helpful that includes combined neurologic, otolaryngologic, and speech assessments and radiologic swallowing studies.

BIBLIOGRAPHY

Bartlett JG, Gorbach SL. The triple threat of aspiration pneumonia. *Chest* 1975;68:560–566.

Bynum LJ, Pierce AK. Pulmonary aspiration of gastric contents. *Am Rev Respir Dis* 1976;114:1129–1136.

Collier BD. Detection of aspiration: scintigraphic techniques. *Am J Med* 1997;103:135S–137S.

Finland M, Davidson CS, Levenson SM. Clinical therapeutic aspects of conflagration injuries to respiratory tract sustained by victims of Coconut Grove disaster. *Medicine (Baltimore)* 1946;25:215.

Fitzpatrick JC, Cioffi WG Jr. Ventilatory support following burns and smoke inhalation injury. *Respir Care Clin N Am* 1997;3:21–49.

Haponik EF. Acute inhalation injury. In: Sivak ED, Higgins TL, Seiver A, eds. *The high risk patient: management of the critically ill.* Malvern, PA: Lea & Febiger, 1995:315.

Kimmel EC, Still KR. Acute lung injury, acute respiratory distress syndrome and inhalation injury: an overview. *Drug Chem Toxicol* 1999;22:91–128.

King TE Jr. Bronchiolitis. In: Schwarz MI, King TE Jr, eds. *Interstitial lung diseases.* Hamilton: BC Decker, 1998:645–684.

Lentz CW, Peterson HD. Smoke inhalation is a multilevel insult to the pulmonary system. *Curr Opin Pulm Med* 1997;3:221–226.

Mendelson CL. The aspiration of stomach contents into the lungs during obstetric anesthesia. *Am J Obstet Gynecol* 1946;52:191.

Pruitt BA Jr, Cioffi WG. Diagnosis and treatment of smoke inhalation. *J Intensive Care Med* 1995;10:117–127.

Seaton A, Morgan WKC. Toxic gases and fumes. In: Morgan WKC, Seaton A, eds. *Occupational lung diseases,* 3d ed. Philadelphia: WB Saunders, 1995.

Shifrin RY, Choplin RH. Aspiration in patients in critical care units. *Radiol Clin North Am* 1996;34:83–96.

Tietgen PA, Kaner RJ, Quinn CE. Aspiration emergencies. *Clin Chest Med* 1994;15:117.

Wald PH, Balmes JR. Respiratory effects of short-term, high-intensity toxic inhalations: smoke, gases, and fumes. *J Intensive Care Med* 1987;2:260.

Weiss SM, Lakshminarayan S. Acute inhalation injury. *Clin Chest Med* 1994;15:103–116.

Wynne JW, Modell JH. Respiratory aspiration of stomach contents. *Ann Intern Med* 1977;87:466–474.

Kelley's Textbook of Internal Medicine, fourth edition. Edited by H. David Humes.
Lippincott Williams & Wilkins, Philadelphia © 2000.

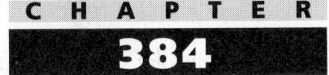

DISEASES OF HIGH ALTITUDE

ROBERT B. SCHOENE

Aided by the speed of modern travel, sojourners to high altitudes have unrivaled access to mountains for recreation and work. Awareness of high-altitude illnesses is even more important for medical practitioners today than it was as recently as 30 to 40 years ago. This chapter discusses adaptation and maladaptation to high altitude, the clinical signs and symptoms of altitude-related illness, and the treatment of healthy sojourners, the high-altitude dwellers, and persons with medical problems at low altitude who go to high altitude.

ADAPTATION

Understanding the acute and chronic adaptations to high altitude provides a sound basis for comprehending the complex series of physiologic events that occur in patients at lower altitudes who have hypoxemia from heart, lung, or blood disease. At high altitude, the problem begins with the lower inspired partial pressure of oxygen, a result of the lower barometric pressure. For example, despite a fixed fraction of oxygen in the earth's atmosphere (0.2093), the oxygen available in the inspired air (PIO_2) at 14,000 feet (4,200 m) (barometric pressure at 450 mm Hg) is approximately 94 mm Hg, whereas at sea level (barometric pressure at 760 mm Hg), the PIO_2 is about 150 mm Hg. The PIO_2 is the beginning of the oxygen cascade, in which oxygen from the atmosphere goes to the lungs to the blood to the cells. A number of mechanisms are invoked along this cascade that compensate in part for the lower PIO_2.

The first immediate response is an increase in ventilation, which is caused by stimulation of the carotid body by hypo-xemia. At any attained altitude, this process continues to augment ventilation for several weeks after arrival, effects a higher alveolar and arterial oxygen content, and is called *ventilatory acclimatization.*

The next step is transfer of oxygen by means of diffusion across the alveolar–capillary membrane. This process is limited at high altitude because of the decreased driving pressure of oxygen from air to blood and is particularly impaired during exercise, when a decreased transit time of blood across the blood–gas interphase allows less time for diffusion. Oxygen then becomes bound to hemoglobin, the carrier that takes oxygen to the tissues. Two further adaptive mechanisms take place. First, the number of red blood cells increases over 2 to 3 weeks owing to the erythropoietic stimulus from hypoxia. Second, the oxygen–hemoglobin dissociation curve shifts to the left because of progressive respiratory alkalosis, which facilitates loading of oxygen at the lung, where there is a lower pressure gradient from the air to the blood. This leftward shift is presumed not to impair unloading to the cells. Tissue adaptation is not fully understood. It is known to involve an increase in capillary and mitochondrial density and a decrease in muscle cell size, especially at very high altitudes. The result is a decrease in diffusion distance from the capillary to the mitochondria. Failure to undergo this complex series of events or individual variations in making these changes may lead to maladaptation and altitude illness.

CLINICAL SYNDROMES

THE SOJOURNER

If not enough time is allowed for adaptations, altitude illness can occur. For example, sudden ascent to 26,000 feet can cause death. However, a climber who takes weeks or months to arrive at that altitude on foot can work and function remarkably well. To minimize the risk of altitude illness, one should allow time to acclimatize. All altitude illnesses, from mild to severe, are probably a continuum. A unifying hypothesis is that hypoxia causes fluid to extravasate from the vascular to extravascular space. This process leads to tissue edema and accounts for neurologic and pulmonary symptoms. The initial leak may be in the brain and may cause increased intracerebral pressure and the symptoms of acute mountain sickness.

ACUTE MOUNTAIN SICKNESS

Presentation

Acute mountain sickness usually occurs within the first 12 to 72 hours of ascent above 2,500 m and may affect 25% to 40% of sojourners from low altitude who ascend rapidly. It is a mild form of altitude illness. Headache is the primary symptom. The headache may be mild or severe, constant or pounding, and may be accompanied by fatigue, lethargy, anorexia, nausea, and vomiting. Resting tachycardia, a sign of lack of acclimatization, decreased urine output, and fluid retention, signified by puffiness of hands and face, also may be present. Mild arterial oxygen desaturation greater than expected for the altitude and a widened alveolar to arterial oxygen difference are common. Periodic breathing at night and insomnia go hand in hand with acute mountain sickness. If one remains at that altitude, the symptoms usually abate in 24 to 48 hours and allow one to ascend. If symptoms do not subside, or if they worsen, one should descend before severe altitude illness ensues.

Treatment

A high index of suspicion and knowledge of the symptoms of acute mountain sickness allow one to avoid severe altitude illness and enjoy a sojourn to the mountains. Once acute mountain sickness is diagnosed, one should rest and not ascend higher until symptoms have improved. If symptoms do not abate or if they worsen, the patient must descend as far as necessary (more than 300 to 500 m) while he or she can still walk. Failure to do so can lead to severe altitude illness, inability to help oneself, and danger to colleagues.

Mild analgesics (aspirin, acetaminophen, and codeine) usually are effective in managing the symptoms of acute mountain sickness. If these measures do not work, other diagnoses or severe altitude illness should be considered. Acetazolamide is effective in preventing and controlling acute mountain sickness if taken during ascent (125 to 250 mg twice a day). The drug also may be taken when symptoms begin or before sleep. It prevents periodic breathing and decreases in arterial oxygen saturation during the night. The mechanism of action is not known but may be secondary to its role as a respiratory stimulant, mild diuretic, and carbonic anhydrase inhibitor—all of which may facilitate some of the normal mechanisms of acclimatization. A sojourner who has recurrent AMS should take acetazolamide prophylactically on ascent; otherwise, the drug should be carried as a treatment. Persons allergic to sulfa drugs should not take acetazolamide.

Dexamethasone, 4 mg by mouth every 6 hours, also is effective in controlling or preventing symptoms of mild to severe acute mountain sickness but does not aid acclimatization. It may convert a severely ill, nonambulatory patient into one who can descend and improve on his or her own. One should not, however, be lulled into false security, because relapses occur if the drug is stopped and descent is not undertaken. The drug is most appropriately used as a rescue drug if symptoms are worsening, especially in a remote environment. The mechanism of action of dexamethasone may be related to its effect on stabilization of the endothelium and prevention of tissue edema. Use of portable, inflatable hyperbaric bags also is effective if descent is not possible.

HIGH-ALTITUDE CEREBRAL EDEMA

High-altitude cerebral edema occurs in the presence of acute mountain sickness and usually includes a severe headache not relieved with analgesic, confusion, and truncal and gait ataxia; it can proceed to coma and death. Autopsy examinations demonstrate diffuse brain edema with microhemorrhages. Because all altitude illnesses have some neurogenic components, there is reason to believe that high-altitude cerebral edema is merely a worsening of acute mountain sickness. It is therefore important to be vigilant in all cases of acute mountain sickness. If definite neurologic signs appear, one must descend. Oxygen administra-

tion is helpful, and dexamethasone is effective in ameliorating symptoms so that the victim can descend. There should never be a delay in descent when high-altitude cerebral edema occurs unless severe weather or orthopedic trauma prevents descent.

HIGH-ALTITUDE PULMONARY EDEMA

High-altitude pulmonary edema is a severe and potentially fatal form of altitude illness. About 1% to 2% of sojourners above 10,000 feet (3,000 m) experience high-altitude pulmonary edema. High-altitude pulmonary edema was thought to be pneumonia or cardiac edema, but in the 1960s, subjects were studied and found to have normal pulmonary artery wedge pressures, which suggested that high-altitude pulmonary edema is a noncardiogenic form of pulmonary edema. Associated characteristics may include a blunted ventilatory response to high altitude, paradoxical fluid retention, and an accentuated pulmonary vascular response to hypoxia—all of which may lead to an increased pressure and stress on the pulmonary microvasculature and leakage into the interstitial and alveolar space. Examination of bronchoalveolar lavage fluid of persons with high-altitude pulmonary edema at 4,400 m on Mount McKinley showed very high concentrations of protein and cells similar to other forms of permeability pulmonary edema except that the cells were primarily alveolar macrophages rather than neutrophils. Because high pulmonary artery pressures appear to play a role in the development of high-altitude pulmonary edema, therapy that attenuates hypoxic pulmonary vasoconstriction, as with nifedipine, helps to prevent high-altitude pulmonary edema among susceptible subjects. Complete understanding of the underlying mechanism has not been achieved.

Dyspnea at rest and a dry cough accompanied by symptoms of acute mountain sickness begin 1 to 4 days after arrival at high altitude and evolve into severe dyspnea, confusion, worsening cough productive of pink frothy sputum, and death. These symptoms are accompanied by low-grade fever, tachypnea, tachycardia, and cyanosis. Varying degrees of neurologic dysfunction also may be present, underscoring the relation between high-altitude pulmonary edema and high-altitude cerebral edema. A chest radiograph shows diffuse bilateral infiltrates and a normal cardiac silhouette.

Slow ascent prevents high-altitude pulmonary edema, and early recognition of symptoms and descent are the best treatment. Patients with severe hypoxemia and illness usually recover within a couple of days of descent without apparent residual pulmonary dysfunction and can reascend after adequate acclimatization. Use of sedatives and hypnotic agents should be avoided, because respiratory depression worsens hypoxemia. Where medical care is available at moderate altitude, oxygen therapy for several days is adequate when arterial oxygen saturation can be raised to more than 90%. Patients can return home or to hotels with family or friends for observation and be seen daily by a physician until recovered. This approach is safe and economical for all but those with the most severe high-altitude pulmonary edema, who should be evacuated if possible. Nifedipine-XL (20 mg once or twice a day) should be used to prevent high-altitude pulmonary edema among susceptible persons who anticipate rapid ascent without time for adequate acclimatization. Diuretics, morphine, and nitroglycerin may have theoretic efficacy. All these drugs may have some beneficial effect on right-sided pressure but should not be used in the field. Unless severe weather or concomitant illness or trauma prevents descent, no one should die of high-altitude pulmonary edema.

OPHTHALMOLOGIC ABNORMALITIES

A number of visual symptoms have been reported, including transient blindness and blurring of vision, that may be caused by vascular spasm and clear without residual impairment. Retinal hemorrhage is common above 15,000 feet (4,500 m) but is usually asymptomatic unless it occurs over the macula. The hemorrhage resolves within 10 to 14 days. The underlying mechanism is not understood but may reflect microvascular leakage that occurs elsewhere, especially in the brain.

HIGH-ALTITUDE NATIVES

CHRONIC MOUNTAIN SICKNESS

The incidence of chronic mountain sickness is unknown. The illness is more prevalent in some high-altitude populations than in others. For example, it is more prevalent in the Andes and the North American Rocky Mountains and almost unheard of in Tibet. Chronic mountain sickness affects both highland natives and lowlanders who move to high altitude.

The clinical manifestations of chronic mountain sickness are similar to those that occur among lowlanders with chronic hypoxemia. The primary finding is excessive erythrocytosis in which hematocrit may reach 70% to 90%. Pulmonary hypertension, cor pulmonale, mental slowing, hypersomnolence, cyanosis, and plethora also are present. Patients have blunted ventilation, which may be a contributing factor to their accentuated hypoxemia. It is not clear whether this relative hypoventilation is a result of chronic high-altitude exposure or a contributing factor to the disease. Not all high-altitude natives with blunted ventilation have chronic mountain sickness.

Therapy for chronic mountain sickness requires reversal of the hypoxemia. Relocating to low altitude is ideal but often not practical. Most natives with chronic mountain sickness languish the remainder of their days, unrecognized as being ill. Oxygen therapy, especially at night, is helpful in reversing the syndrome but is often impractical and unavailable in remote mountain regions. Respiratory stimulants, such as acetazolamide, 125 mg twice a day, or medroxyprogesterone acetate, 20 mg three times a day, improve oxygen saturation when the patient is awake and reverse nocturnal periodic breathing and profound arterial oxygen desaturation. Phlebotomy is helpful as a temporary measure, especially to reverse the mental lassitude and decrease pulmonary vascular resistance.

REENTRY PULMONARY EDEMA

In North and South America, pulmonary edema occurs, especially among children and young adults, when high-altitude natives descend to low altitudes and then return to their high-altitude homes. The cause of this syndrome is not known but may be related to chronic hypertrophy of the pulmonary arteries, which become hyper-reactive on re-exposure to the hypoxic stress.

CLINICAL DISEASES AT HIGH ALTITUDE

Physicians should be aware of the detrimental effects that patients may undergo at high altitude. Although few data are available to document these effects, it is important to advise patients who live or who are going to high altitude, especially if they have pulmonary, cardiovascular, hematologic (e.g., sickle cell), or hypertensive disease or are pregnant. Patients with stable diseases cope with ascents and activities to moderate altitudes quite well. A better understanding of the adaptations and maladaptations to the hypoxic environment should allow the practitioners to help their patients make more judicious decisions.

LUNG DISEASE

Asthma

Although the cold, dry air of high altitude often is associated with greater airway reactivity, the scant literature that is available suggests that persons with asthma who live at high altitude or travel to high altitude do quite well. This may be because there are fewer allergens and less pollution in the high-altitude environment. Patients with asthma who ascend to high altitude should be advised about the potential risks and be armed with a spectrum of drugs, including bronchodilators and inhaled and oral steroids. Most studies of asthma among adults and children suggest that these agents are rarely necessary.

Chronic Obstructive Pulmonary Disease

Patients with chronic obstructive pulmonary disease (COPD) who live at high altitude have greater morbidity, and many of these patients migrate to lower altitudes as symptoms worsen. Patients with COPD who live at low altitude encounter environmental hypoxia with both air travel and more extended stays for recreation or family visits. With respect to air travel, patients who are hypoxemic and need oxygen therapy at low altitude and are not hypercapnic at low altitude should make arrangements for supplemental oxygen during the flight. Several studies have suggested ways to calculate the dose of oxygen, but these techniques usually are impractical and inaccurate; a reasonable estimate of an increase in usual oxygen dose is adequate. These patient should follow similar recommendations during a stay at high altitude because it is conceivable that several days of exaggerated hypoxemia can be potentially dangerous. Treatment of patients with chronic carbon dioxide retention, hypoxemia, and pulmonary hypertension is particularly problematic because too much oxygen may blunt their ventilation further and accentuate the manifestations of disease. Patients with COPD but without cardiac disease and not using oxygen therapy at low altitude should tolerate a flight of several hours or less.

Sleep Disorders

Little information is available regarding the effect of ascent to high altitude on patients with sleep disorders at low altitude. Anecdotal evidence suggests that the stimulus of hypoxia actually improves periodic breathing during sleep, but it is reasonable to have patients, particularly those with obstructive sleep apnea, continue their usual regimen.

CARDIOVASCULAR DISEASE

Systemic Hypertension

Upon acute exposure to high altitude, catecholamines increase proportionally and increase systemic blood pressure. Within a few days both catecholamines and blood pressure decrease toward sea level values. Among patients with pre-existing hypertension, the response is variable. For those with recalcitrant blood pressure going to higher altitude (3,000 ms) the increase in blood pressure can become quite accentuated and potentially dangerous. Although data are scant and clinical guidelines in the literature are lacking, patients should be advised to continue their blood pressure medications and check their blood pressure every couple of days during their sojourn to high altitude. It may be necessary for them to increase their regimen to maintain acceptable blood pressures during more prolonged stays at high altitude.

Coronary Artery Disease

Evidence suggests that there may be a lower incidence of coronary artery disease among persons with long-time residence at high altitude. The reasons for such an association are not clear. The myocardium can withstand very low levels of oxygen, but theoretically the ambient hypoxia may unmask previously unknown coronary artery disease, turn angina to unstable disease, accentuate risk of myocardial infarction or sudden death, and provoke dysrhythmia. Studies to substantiate these possibilities do not exist. The threshold for angina among patients with coronary artery disease may be a lower level of exercise on acute ascent to high altitude, around 2,500 to 3,000 meters, but this finding does not preclude patients with stable angina from going to high altitude for recreation if moderate exercise is undertaken. Several studies with large cohorts of patients in the age range susceptible to myocardial infarction who were visitors to high-altitude resort areas or were trekkers to high altitude in Nepal did not show an increased prevalence of cardiac events. Clinicians must use clinical judgment in advising patients who want to go to high altitude. Except for those with unstable angina or difficult-to-manage dysrhythmias, there seems little additional risk to persons with pre-existing coronary artery disease or in those who have undergone coronary artery bypass surgery.

Pulmonary Vascular Disorders

Many times the symptoms of primary pulmonary hypertension are first realized during trips to moderate altitudes. Symptoms of dyspnea are sometimes quite striking. These patients should be counseled not to go to high altitude. Patients with pulmonary hypertension caused by chronic hypoxemic lung disease may be more susceptible to high-altitude pulmonary edema. The use of pulmonary vasodilators, such as nifedipine, might be indicated. Few studies have been performed to substantiate these conjectures.

Miscellaneous Disorders

Blood disorders such as sickle cell disease may be easily unmasked at even modest altitudes. It therefore is prudent to counsel patients with sickle cell disease or trait not to ascend even as high as 1,000 m. Little information is available on patients with cerebrovascular disease, epilepsy, or diabetes.

What clearly emerges from these cursory surveys is the need for good clinical studies to describe what happens to common medical problems among patients who live for many years at high altitude and among low-altitude residents who ascend to high altitude for recreation. This dearth of data is frustrating and begs for simple descriptive and epidemiologic studies of a number of diseases and long-term prospective studies to understand the underlying pathophysiologic processes so that clinicians can be better equipped to advise patients.

BIBLIOGRAPHY

Bartsch P, Maggionni M, Ritter M, et al. Prevention of high altitude pulmonary edema by nifedipine. *N Engl J Med* 1991;325:1284–1289.

Brammell HL, Morgan BJ, Niccoli SA, et al. Exercise tolerances reduced with altitude in patients with coronary artery disease. *Circulation* 1982; 66:366–371.

Dillard T, Moores L, Bilello K, et al. The preflight evaluation: a comparison of the hypoxia inhalation test with hypobaric exposure. *Chest* 1995;107: 352–357.

Hackett PH, Roach RC, Wood RA, et al. Dexamethasone for prevention and treatment of acute mountain sickness. *Aviat Space Environ Med* 1988;59:950–954.

Halhuber M, Humpeler E, Inama K, et al. Does altitude cause exhaustion of the heart and circulatory system? *Med Sport Sci* 1985;19:192–202.

Larson EB, Roach RC, Schoene RB, et al. Acute moutain sickness and acetazolamide: clinical efficacy and effect on ventilation. *JAMA* 1982; 248:328–332.

Moore L, Rohra, Maisenbach J, et al. Emphysema mortality is increased in Colorado residents at high altitude. *Am Rev Respir Dis* 1982;126: 225–228.

Schoene RB, Hackett PH, Hornbein TF. High altitude. In: Murray JF, Nadel JA, eds. *Textbook of respiratory medicine,* 3d ed. Philadelphia: WB Saunders (*in press*).

Schoene RB, Swenson ER, Pizzo CJ, et al. The lung at high altitude: bronchoalveolar lavage in acute mountain sickness and pulmonary edema. *J Appl Physiol* 1988;64:2605–2613.

Sly R, O'Donnell R. Lack of effect of geographic elevation on mortality from asthma. *Ann Allergy* 1989;63:495–497.

Winslow RM Monge C. *Hypoxia, polycythemia, and chronic mountain sickness.* Baltimore: Johns Hopkins University Press, 1987.

Kelley's Textbook of Internal Medicine, fourth edition. Edited by H. David Humes. Lippincott Williams & Wilkins, Philadelphia © 2000.

DIAGNOSTIC AND THERAPEUTIC MODALITIES

ESSENTIAL POINTS OF THE HISTORY AND PHYSICAL EXAMINATION

MICHAEL E. HANLEY

▌ MEDICAL HISTORY

Most patients with respiratory disorders initially seek medical evaluation because they have signs or symptoms of respiratory illness or have an abnormality that is identified during routine health screening, evaluation of an unrelated medical problem, or epidemiologic surveys. A thorough and complete medical history is critical to the evaluation of all such disorders. Evaluation of abnormal but asymptomatic physical, laboratory, or radiographic findings requires a history of risk factors for pulmonary disease, including a thorough occupational, environmental, social including use of recreational and therapeutic drugs, and family history.

Patients with symptoms usually have one or more of the four cardinal respiratory symptoms of chest pain, cough with or without sputum production or hemoptysis, dyspnea, and wheezing. When evaluating symptoms, the clinician must ask the patient specific questions to elicit the character, chronology, severity, and, most important, pattern of the symptoms. Although the medical interview should be specific and detailed, the physician must avoid asking leading questions or questions that are too direct. Whenever possible, patients should be allowed to describe symptoms in their own words.

CHEST PAIN

Chest pain is one of the most common symptoms that prompt patients to seek medical assistance. Although the evaluation often focuses on whether the pain is caused by myocardial ischemia, pain localized to the thorax may originate from disease of any thoracic structure. It is crucial to have patients describe

the pain in their own words. Diagnosis of the cause of pain, however, depends on identifying specific characteristics of the pain, including quality, location, radiation, severity, duration, frequency, and factors that precipitate, worsen, or relieve it. The differential diagnosis of chest pain is summarized in Table 385.1.

The quality and location of chest pain are related to the sensory innervation of the anatomic origin of the pain. In general, chest pain can be functionally classified into two main diagnostic categories: visceral cardiac and somatic pleuritic pain. The heart, pericardium, and mediastinal structures are innervated through autonomic pathways that travel through the vagus nerve. Patients with cardiac and mediastinal abnormalities perceive pain in a visceral rather than a somatic pattern. The pain usually is described as dull, heavy, constricting, or squeezing, a pressure sensation, or, if severe, crushing.

The intensity of cardiac pain ranges from mild to severe and has no value in identifying the underlying cause. Cardiac pain is central in location, usually substernal or epigastric, and radiates to either arm and the neck. Although chest pain that is lateral or precordial does not exclude myocardial ischemia, pain in this location usually indicates cardiac anxiety or a left anterior pleural or chest wall process. Classic angina pectoris from myocardial ischemia is caused by an imbalance between myocardial oxygen supply and demand. Angina pectoris is precipitated by any activity that increases cardiac demand or induces coronary arterial spasm, such as exertion, exposure to cold air, heavy meals, or emotional upset, and is relieved by rest and vasodilating medications. Persistent, intense pain of a cardiac quality that is not relieved by rest or vasodilating medications suggests a diagnosis of myocardial infarction. In myocardial infarction, the pain frequently is associated with sweating, palpitations, syncope, nausea, vomiting, and hypotension.

Pericardial pain has both cardiac and pleuritic quality because the adjacent visceral mediastinal and parietal chest wall pleura often are involved. Chest pain from pericarditis is a steady substernal pain worsened by breathing. The pain also typically increases with swallowing, hiccuping, or lying in a recumbent position, especially on the left side. It is improved by sitting or leaning forward and lying on the right side. When the diaphragmatic pleural pericardial surfaces are involved, the pain is referred to the shoulder blades or neck through the phrenic nerves. If pericarditis is suspected, it is important to evaluate for signs of abnormal cardiac hemodynamics due to cardiac tamponade. These include tachycardia, jugular venous distention, Kuss-

TABLE 385.1.	DIFFERENTIAL DIAGNOSIS OF CHEST PAIN
Source	**Common Characteristics**
Ischemic heart disease	Precipitated by activity or ↑ cardiac demand
	Relieved by rest or vasodilators
Pericardial disease	Steady, substernal
	↑ with swallowing or recumbency
	Relieved by sitting forward
Diseases of chest wall	Localized; ↑ with movement
Diseases of pleura	Pleuritic; often acute or crescendo pattern
Esophageal, upper GI, or subdiaphragmatic disease	Burning or achy; ↑ or ↓ with meals; relieved by antacids or H$_2$-antagonists.

maul's sign (persistent or paradoxical increase of jugular venous distention during inspiration), paradoxical pulse, and hypotension. The presence of these signs warrants emergency evaluation and intervention, including echocardiography, right-sided heart catheterization, or pericardiocentesis.

The sensory innervation of the chest wall and diaphragmatic parietal pleural is through afferent fibers in the intercostal nerves. Disease that involves these structures typically manifests as an achy or sharp pain well localized to the involved area, usually is unilateral, and is worsened by torso or chest movement, such as coughing, sneezing, and deep breathing. The pain is ameliorated by shallow breathing or breath holding. Patients with pleuritic pain may report dyspnea because of a pain-induced increased awareness of breathing and may have evidence of chest wall splinting at physical examination. Pleuritic pain from inflammation or irritation of the diaphragmatic parietal pleura commonly radiates to the ipsilateral shoulder or side of the neck. Important additional clues in the evaluation of pleuritic chest pain are recent thoracic trauma or paroxysmal coughing, acuity of the pain, presence of systemic symptoms, and presence of localizing signs at physical examination. The speed of onset of pleurisy depends on the speed of development of the underlying disease.

Pain from pneumothorax, fractured ribs, or pulmonary embolism with lung ischemia or infarction develops suddenly. The intensity of the pain has a crescendo pattern in pulmonary embolism. Chest pain from acute infectious causes of pleurisy, such as viral epidemic pleurodynia, coxsackievirus B infection, or bacterial pneumonia, is slower but still rapid in onset and is characteristically associated with systemic inflammatory signs and symptoms, including fever, sweats, chills, myalgia, arthralgia, and malaise. Pain from chronic conditions, such as tuberculous pleuritis, asbestos-induced pleural disease, metastatic cancer, and occasionally anaerobic pleuropulmonary infection, has a more insidious onset.

Examination of the involved chest wall area and adjacent structures, including the lung and upper abdomen, may lead to a specific diagnosis. Point tenderness over a rib after trauma or a coughing paroxysm suggests a rib fracture. Point tenderness

over one or more costochondral junctions, especially associated with localized warmth and erythema, may indicate costochondritis or infectious costal arthritis. The approach to pleuritic pain is discussed in Chapter 358.

Esophageal, upper gastrointestinal, and subdiaphragmatic diseases often produce chest pain that can be mistaken for cardiac or lung disease. A primary abdominal process such as pancreatitis or cholecystitis should be considered in the differential diagnosis of lower chest pain or pleurisy, including pleural effusions of obscure causation. Esophagitis and esophageal spasm usually are associated with a history of heartburn, reflux, dysphagia, and odynophagia. If symptoms suggest an esophageal origin, a trial antacid-antireflux regimen should be undertaken before a more expensive and invasive evaluation is initiated.

Diseases involving only lung parenchyma or visceral pleura, such as a solitary pulmonary nodule, usually are not painful because these structures lack pain fibers. The development of pain with such a condition suggests that the disease has spread outside the lung or that a second process exists.

COUGH

Coughing protects the lungs from injury and infection by clearing large bronchial airways of accumulated secretions and foreign material. The normal cough reflex is caused by afferent stimuli from cough receptors transmitted through sensory nerves to the central nervous system cough center and is mediated through motor nerves. Cough receptors are located throughout the respiratory tract and in extrapulmonary sites, including the pleura and pericardium, ear canals, paranasal sinuses, stomach, and diaphragm. Activation of the reflex occurs through receptor stimulation by inflammatory, mechanical, chemical, and thermal stimuli.

The most common causes of coughing are acute viral respiratory tract infections and smoking. Most patients with acute viral respiratory tract infections do not seek medical evaluation because their symptoms are self-limited and easily explained. A chronic cough is defined as a troublesome cough that lasts more than 3 weeks. The most common causes of chronic cough are tobacco-related chronic bronchitis, postnasal drip, occult asthma, and gastroesophageal reflux. Less common causes are pneumoconiosis, idiopathic interstitial lung disease such as sarcoidosis or idiopathic pulmonary fibrosis, bronchiectasis, bronchogenic carcinoma, drugs, chronic infection, and nonpulmonary disorders such as left ventricular failure, esophageal diverticula, and recurrent aspiration. The medical history suggests a specific diagnosis for 70% of patients with a chronic cough. Historical factors to be considered in the evaluation of a cough are shown in Table 385.2.

The evaluation of a cough among tobacco users is a challenge. Although all smokers with a cough should not be presumed to have only smoker's bronchitis, evaluating a cough for this population may lead to multiple unnecessary and expensive diagnostic tests. Full evaluation of chronic coughing among smokers should be considered when the cough is persistent and severe or if it is accompanied by a change in or development of sputum production, an increase in the frequency of coughing, hemoptysis, or constitutional symptoms such as weight loss and fatigue. The evaluation in this setting should focus on the diagnosis of chronic bronchitis, emphysema, or bronchogenic carcinoma.

TABLE 385.2.	MEDICAL HISTORY FACTORS IN THE DIAGNOSIS OF CHRONIC COUGH

Tobacco use
Recent change in pattern or character of cough
Presence and quantity of sputum production
Hemoptysis
Environmental and occupational exposure through inhalation
History of allergy or atopy
Nocturnal cough
Sinus symptoms
New drug exposure, especially to angiotensin-converting enzyme inhibitors and β-blocking agents
Substance abuse, especially of crack cocaine

A history of sputum production narrows the differential diagnosis of chronic cough to primary pulmonary conditions. Expectoration of sputum is caused by a combination of increased production of sputum by irritant stimulation of mucous glands and decreased mucociliary clearance. When patients have sputum production, the amount and quality of sputum should be characterized. This is best accomplished by giving the patient a specimen cup and collecting all sputum produced over 24 hours.

Sputum can be microscopically classified into five categories: clear and mucoid; purulent; putrid with three layers; rusty or blood-stained; and miscellaneous. Clear or mucoid sputum usually is caused by an irritative inhalant source, is not infected, and rarely requires antibiotic treatment. Purulent sputum suggests bacterial bronchitis or pneumonia and clinically mandates antibiotic therapy. Copious putrid sputum strongly indicates an anaerobic process such as a lung abscess or necrotizing pneumonia. Severe bronchiectasis commonly is associated with production of copious amounts of purulent sputum that classically settles into three layers: a mucous layer above, a watery layer in the middle, and purulent sediment below. Rusty or uniformly blood-stained sputum indicates the presence of red blood cells or hemoglobin. Cardiac causes and primary pulmonary inflammatory conditions should be considered. Two rare but characteristic types of sputum that suggest specific diagnoses are the clear, golden-yellow sputum that accompanies biliary tract–bronchial fistula and the copious, watery sputum that suggests alveolar cell carcinoma.

Cough accompanied by hemoptysis is a potential medical emergency and warrants immediate evaluation. Hemoptysis is expectoration of blood from the lower respiratory tract. When hemoptysis occurs, symptoms and signs of upper airway and gastrointestinal disease should be sought to exclude pseudohemoptysis (expectoration of blood from a source other than the lower respiratory tract, such as aspirated blood from epistaxis or upper gastrointestinal hemorrhage). Direct oral examination should be carefully performed, because a minor oral or gingival lesion may be overlooked. A simple maneuver to diagnose pseudohemoptysis in this situation is to collect an expectorated specimen of clear water that the patient has orally swished and gargled. Persistent fresh blood in the immediately expectorated specimen is highly confirmatory of pseudohemoptysis.

The differential diagnosis of hemoptysis depends on several factors, including the amount and duration of bleeding, the patient's age and smoking history, and accompanying symptoms such as weight loss, chest pain, and fever. It is important to measure the amount of blood in true hemoptysis. Massive hemoptysis is expectoration of more than 600 mL of blood in a 24-hour period. Expectoration of less than 600 mL, but more than blood streaking, is referred to as *frank* or *gross hemoptysis*. Scant hemoptysis is characterized by blood streaking of sputum.

Acute bronchitis is the most common cause of hemoptysis in the United States. Hemoptysis due to acute bronchitis resolves with antibiotic therapy and does not necessitate invasive evaluation other than chest radiography unless the hemoptysis persists despite use of antibiotics or if the radiographic findings are abnormal. Bronchogenic carcinoma is uncommon among nonsmokers and patients younger than 35 years. Patients with bronchogenic carcinoma usually also have a history of recent change in the severity and character of the cough and constitutional symptoms such as weight loss, fever, and anorexia.

Chronic coughing sometimes is caused by nonpulmonary disorders. If symptoms do not suggest a pulmonary source, additional questions should be asked to find a nonpulmonary or systemic chronic disease. The patient should be evaluated for evidence of heart disease that leads to pulmonary venous hypertension, such as cryptic mitral stenosis or left ventricular failure. Ear, nose, and throat disorders, including chronic sinusitis with postnasal drip, should not be overlooked. Symptoms of neurologic or gastrointestinal disease that leads to silent reflux and cryptic aspiration should be pursued. A useful test to detect aspiration is to watch the patient swallow a glass of water. Immediate coughing suggests aspiration. The rapidity and severity of the cough are directly related to the size and severity of aspiration. Evaluation of coughing is discussed in Chapter 352.

DYSPNEA

Dyspnea is an awareness or perception of labored breathing. Most patients describe it as shortness of breath or breathlessness, but some describe a sensation of choking, tightness, or suffocation. If symptoms are sudden or severe, the patient may notice dyspnea at rest, but when dyspnea is mild or insidious, it is initially noticed only with considerable exertion.

The evaluation of patients with dyspnea should focus on quantifying the severity of shortness of breath, identifying the pattern of symptoms by determining the circumstances in which they occur, and searching for associated symptoms. Although quantifying the degree of dyspnea rarely leads to a specific diagnosis, it may yield clues to the cause and is valuable in monitoring the response to therapy and performing disability evaluations. Several issues should be considered when grading the degree of dyspnea. Does the severity of symptoms correlate with objective evidence of pulmonary disease, such as results of pulmonary function tests or chest radiographic findings? If it does not, there may be a second contributing process or an altogether new diagnosis. What is the tempo of illness? Are symptoms stable or slowly progressive? Dyspnea is graded according to the amount of exertion needed to produce symptoms. A simple scale recommended by the American College of Chest Physicians is shown in Table 385.3.

One of the most important clues in determining a specific cause of dyspnea is determining the pattern of symptoms and

TABLE 385.3.	DYSPNEA SCALE
Grade	**Description**
I	No dyspnea with keeping pace with healthy persons of the same age and body build on level ground but shortness of breath on climbing hills or stairs
II	Can walk a mile at own pace without dyspnea but cannot keep pace with a healthy person on level ground
III	Shortness of breath on walking about 100 yards (90 m) or for a few minutes, even on level ground
IV	Shortness of breath on slight exertion, such as when dressing or talking

American College of Chest Physicians modification of British Medical Research Council Scale

the circumstances in which it occurs. The diagnosis frequently focuses on differentiating left-sided heart disease with left ventricular dysfunction and elevated pulmonary venous pressure from a primary lung disease. Specific types of dyspnea such as paroxysmal nocturnal dyspnea (PND; dyspnea that awakens a patient from sleep) and orthopnea (dyspnea on assuming a supine position) strongly suggest a cardiac cause. However, PND-like symptoms also occur with nocturnal asthma, esophageal reflux with aspiration, and sudden "choking" from accumulated bronchopulmonary secretions obstructing large airways. Orthopnea also occasionally occurs among patients with chronic obstructive pulmonary disease, asthma, and neuromuscular disease. Additional history may help differentiate heart disease from primary pulmonary disease in these situations, and physical signs of left ventricular failure should be aggressively pursued. For example, although patients with cardiac PND may have a cough, the cough usually is dry and nonproductive. Patients with pulmonary-induced PND, however, have a productive cough and improvement in dyspnea with expectoration. Most patients with reflux and nocturnal aspiration also give a history of considerable heartburn. Nocturnal bronchial asthma causing PND may be accompanied by allergic or atopic clues and blood or sputum eosinophilia.

Other patterns of dyspnea suggest other diseases. Platypnea is the development or worsening of dyspnea after assuming an upright position. Although nonspecific, it often occurs among patients with pulmonary manifestations of chronic liver disease and patients with poor abdominal muscle tone. Sudden onset of dyspnea at rest may be associated with pulmonary emboli, gastric aspiration, or pneumothorax. A history of more severe dyspnea developing toward the end of the workday or work week with improvement during periods away from work suggests an occupational exposure. Seasonal variation or worsening after exercise or exposure to cold dry air or nonspecific irritants may indicate reactive airway disease. Because the cause of dyspnea is often a nonpulmonary condition, the physician must search for signs and symptoms of extrapulmonary disease, such as neuromuscular disease or hyperthyroidism.

The cause of dyspnea due to pulmonary disease usually can be accurately diagnosed with a careful history and physical examination, chest radiography, spirometry, and analysis of carbon monoxide–diffusing capacity or arterial blood gas measurements. If the results of this evaluation are normal or do not provide enough information for diagnosis and the symptoms are not considered psychogenic, a cardiopulmonary exercise test is warranted.

AUDIBLE RESPIRATORY SOUNDS

Some patients seek treatment with wheezing, stridor, or snoring. These abnormal respiratory sounds indicate abnormal turbulent airflow and increased airway resistance. Wheezes are high-pitched musical sounds generated by rapid passage of air through airways that are narrowed to the point of closure. Wheezes are generated by narrowing of either large or small airways. The quality of the wheeze does not differentiate the site of obstruction. Wheezes may occur in either phase of the respiratory cycle but tend to occur more commonly and are more prominent during expiration, when the airway caliber is smaller. Although wheezes are most commonly noticed by patients with acute asthma, wheezing may be produced by any cause of bronchial narrowing, including bronchospasm, mucosal edema and congestion, intraluminal accumulation of mucus, external airway compression, or dynamic airway narrowing or collapse. When the wheeze is localized to a specific site in the chest, focal obstruction of a larger bronchus by a neoplasm or foreign body should be considered.

Stridor is an especially harsh, loud musical sound of constant pitch. Although it may be heard throughout the respiratory cycle, it is most common during inspiration, when extrathoracic airways are typically narrowed. This sound is generated by critical obstruction of large airways, usually at the larynx but occasionally involving the trachea or a main stem bronchus. Stridor should be considered a medical emergency with the potential for complete airway obstruction and asphyxiation. Emergency airway evaluation with direct laryngoscopy and bronchoscopy and preparation for emergency establishment of an airway must be performed. All patients with stridor should be under constant direct observation and monitoring in an intensive care unit until the situation is resolved.

Snoring is a coarse sound generated in the nasopharynx, oropharynx, or hypopharynx during sleep. Snoring of oropharyngeal or hypopharyngeal origin is more likely to be pathologic than is snoring that is nasally produced. Snoring is more common among men than among women and should not be considered pathologic or in need of further medical evaluation unless the patient has additional clinical features of sleep-disordered breathing. These include otherwise unexplained pulmonary hypertension, cor pulmonale, polycythemia, severe morning headaches, excessive daytime somnolence or frank narcolepsy, intellectual deterioration, poor job performance, and personality changes (see Chapter 382).

OTHER MEDICAL HISTORY

Although most of the medical interview should focus on specific evaluation of the chief problem and present illness, important additional clues to the cause of the patient's pulmonary illness can be gathered from other aspects of the medical history. The most valuable of these include the history of previous illnesses and the social, family, occupational, and environmental histories. These parts of the medical history frequently are considered discrete components when the complete history is organized. However, when pertinent, these portions of the medical history are obtained during the characterization of the chief problem.

History of Previous Illnesses

Many chronic diseases follow cycles of remission and exacerbation. Symptoms often are caused by pulmonary complications of extrapulmonary disease. A thorough review of previous hospitalizations, medical evaluations, and other illnesses should be performed for all patients with pulmonary symptoms. This should include an inquiry about the existence of previous chest radiographs.

Social and Family History

A confidential inquiry regarding lifestyle and habits should be pursued, including sexual behavior, substance abuse, pet exposure, and hobbies. When necessary, the data obtained may require confirmation through interviews with family and friends. Clues to the diagnosis of atypical infection include travel to an area endemic for the infection, such as coccidioidomycosis, or a hobby that involves exposure to sites or animals that are vectors for the infectious agent. If the patient is immunosuppressed, the physician should ask about remote residence in endemic areas, because the infection may manifest as dissemination of a previously acquired but dormant infection.

Although genetically transmitted pulmonary diseases are uncommon, a family history of diseases such as cystic fibrosis or α_1-antiprotease deficiency should be pursued when appropriate. The immediate family history is more helpful in identifying illness due to common exposures, especially infection. This should include a history of recent exposure to adults, children, or animals with known or suspected transmittable infections such as measles, chickenpox, influenza, tuberculosis, tularemia, Q fever, and psittacosis.

Occupational and Environmental History

Information about potential exposures through occupation or the environment is especially important in the evaluation of diffuse interstitial lung disease and asthma. General questions regarding changes in the severity of symptoms when exposed to or removed from various environments may provide a clue that the illness is environmentally mediated. Identification of specific agents that may contribute to illness requires specialized knowledge of workplace environments and may necessitate referral to an occupational medicine specialist. The occupational and environmental interview requires a detailed, systematic approach, because many exposure histories may be subtle or forgotten. Questionnaires that require patients to review systematically their employment record, hobbies and recreational activities, home environment, and other potential exposures are helpful.

PHYSICAL EXAMINATION OF PATIENTS WITH RESPIRATORY DISEASE

The ready availability and utility of chest radiography and the limitations of physical examination of the thorax have deemphasized physical examination of the chest. Many patients, however, such as those with asthma, have normal chest radiographs but significant findings at physical examination. Overdependence on chest radiographs, especially in monitoring, is wasteful and not cost-effective. Chest radiographs and physical examination supplement each other in the evaluation of chest abnormalities. The chest examination is not complete without review of a current, high-quality chest radiograph. Clinicians also need well-developed physical examination skills to diagnose pulmonary disease and to monitor the response to therapy.

DIRECT CHEST EXAMINATION

Because of the common association between pulmonary and cardiac disease, every evaluation for a chest disorder includes a thorough evaluation of the cardiovascular system. Details of this examination are described in Chapter 63. The chest examination is based on the four basic skills of inspection, palpation, percussion, and auscultation. In general, palpation and percussion are the most helpful in confirming and clarifying the pathophysiologic mechanism associated with abnormal breath sounds detected at auscultation. Palpation also is useful in evaluating chest wall pain, swelling, or trauma. Palpation of subcutaneous crepitus is pathognomonic of subcutaneous emphysema and is always pathologic. Crepitus is most commonly found over the neck and upper chest or over sites of chest wall trauma. Subcutaneous emphysema is commonly associated with pneumothorax, pneumomediastinum, or laceration of the pharynx, esophagus, or large airway. The presence of crepitus should trigger a search for signs of these conditions.

Inspection can produce useful information about pulmonary symptoms. It includes assessment of respiratory distress, the presence of clubbing, and skin color and direct chest examination. The use of accessory muscles of respiration should be assessed, and the presence of plethora or cyanosis documented. Cyanosis is a bluish discoloration of the skin and mucous membranes associated with an increased percentage of reduced hemoglobin in the capillaries of those tissues. Central cyanosis, cyanosis occurring in both the skin and mucous membranes, suggests generalized arterial oxygen desaturation. Peripheral cyanosis, cyanosis localized to the skin, usually indicates marked tissue hypoperfusion. Clinical differentiation of one form from another often is difficult, and considerable arterial oxygen desaturation can occur in the absence of clinically detectable cyanosis. Measurement of arterial oxygen saturation by means of pulse oximetry or analysis of arterial blood gases should be considered for all patients with respiratory distress.

Although direct chest inspection should include assessment of the general shape, symmetry, and movement of the thorax, it is most valuable in evaluating the dynamics of breathing, especially for patients with respiratory distress. Of particular importance are the depth of tidal volume breaths and respiratory rate and pattern. Rapid, shallow breathing, especially with respiratory rates greater than 40 breaths per minute for adults, and paradoxical thoracic–upper abdominal movement (inward abdominal retraction during inspiration) often are associated with impending or frank respiratory collapse.

AUSCULTATION

The most useful physical examination technique applied to the chest is auscultation. Auscultation should be performed over the anterior, posterior, and midaxillary chest regions with careful comparison of the left and right hemithoraxes. The examiner must determine whether breath sounds are normal or abnormal and whether adventitial sounds are present. Normal breath sounds include tracheal, bronchial, bronchovesicular, and vesicular sounds. Determining whether breath sounds are abnormal requires assessment of the relative duration of each phase of the respiratory cycle and the intensity, pitch, and quality of the sounds. Evidence of increased transmission of breath sounds, such as detection of bronchial breath sounds at a site where vesicular sounds are expected, should alert the examiner to the existence of lung consolidation. Consolidation can be confirmed by means of detecting egophony in the involved area. Egophony is the increased transmission of voice-generated sounds through the chest. When spoken words are transmitted clearly and distinctly, egophony is characterized as either bronchophony (if the words were spoken) or whispered pectoriloquy (if the words were whispered).

Adventitial lung sounds are sounds that are not naturally associated with the breathing process. Adventitial sounds include rales, wheezes, rhonchi, and pleural rubs. Laennec originally referred to all adventitial lung sounds as *rales,* further categorizing them as sibilant, sonorous, or crepitant. In modern parlance, however, adventitial lung sounds are categorized as continuous or discontinuous on the basis of sound wave analysis. The term *rales* is restricted to discontinuous sounds characterized as crackly, short, explosive, and nonmusical, typically superimposed on the underlying breath sounds. Synonyms are *crackles* and *crepitation.* Rales, which may be further categorized as fine or coarse, are commonly heard in infiltrative lung disease and in conditions associated with increased airway secretions.

Continuous sounds include wheezes (sometimes called as *sibilant rhonchi*) and rhonchi. Wheezes have a high-pitched, sibilant quality; rhonchi are low in pitch and are sonorous. Wheezes and rhonchi typically are detected in diseases characterized by airway narrowing. Wheezes and rhonchi associated with mild degrees of airway narrowing may not be readily detectable during tidal volume breathing but can be accentuated by having the patient perform a cough or forced expiratory maneuver. The degree of airflow limitation can be accurately estimated at the bedside by means of grading the intensity of breath sounds. The examiner listens to the intensity of the breath sounds over six lung zones (upper anterior, midaxillary, and posterior bases) during repeated maximal inspiratory efforts by the patient. The intensity of the breath sounds is graded on a simple 5-point scale, 0 being absent sounds, 3+ normal, and 4+ louder than usual, normal. The total score (16 to 20 is normal, 6 to 10 severely abnormal) has an excellent correlation with forced expiratory volume in 1

second (FEV_1) measured during concomitant spirometry. An alternative is to use a simple peak flowmeter to estimate the degree of airflow limitation. Expiratory peak flow rates of 100, 200, 300, and 400 L per minute are roughly equal to FEV_1 of 1, 2, 3, and 4 L and breath sound intensities of 1, 2, 3, and 4+.

Pleural rubs are loud, coarse, evanescent sounds that typically have a rough or leathery quality. They usually are heard throughout the respiratory cycle but may be limited to one component of it. A pleural rub typically indicates a thickened pleura, usually caused by an inflammatory or neoplastic process.

EXTRATHORACIC EXAMINATION

Many respiratory diseases actually are multisystemic or generalized systemic processes and therefore often have extrathoracic features. Often the most critical part of the lung physical examination is careful attention to the evaluation of extrathoracic sites. On the first encounter with a patient with undiagnosed respiratory symptoms or disease, a complete physical examination is often performed by rote, not surprisingly with minimal return. As specific differential diagnoses are entertained and more diagnostic information is collected, experienced physicians have learned the value of returning to reexamine the patient for subtle new or previously missed signs and symptoms. The physician should be compulsive, comprehensive, and complete on the first encounter but should return to recheck the patient with a high index of suspicion for new disease or previously missed subtle abnormalities.

ACKNOWLEDGMENT

This chapter is an adaptation of the one written by Thomas A. Neff, M.D., for the second edition of this textbook. Dr. Neff was a professor of medicine in the pulmonary and critical care section of the University of Colorado School of Medicine for many years and was highly regarded for his skills as a clinician and his many contributions to the understanding of respiratory illness. He passed away in December 1994 and will be missed.

BIBLIOGRAPHY

American Thoracic Society. Dyspnea. Mechanisms, assessment, and management: a consensus statement. *Am J Respir Crit Care Med* 1999;159: 321–340.

Hirschberg B, Biran I, Glazer M, et al. Hemoptysis: etiology, evaluation, and outcome in a tertiary referral hospital. *Chest* 1997;112:440–444.

Irwin RS, Boulet LP, Cloutier MM, et al. Managing cough as a defense mechanism and as a symptom: a consensus panel report of the American College of Chest Physicians. *Chest* 1998;114:133S–181S.

Jouriles NJ. Atypical chest pain. *Emerg Med Clin North Am* 1998;16: 717–740.

Loudon RG. The lung exam. *Clin Chest Med* 1987;8:265–272.

Michelson E, Hollrah S. Evaluation of the patient with shortness of breath: an evidence-based approach. *Emerg Med Clin North Am* 1999;17: 221–237.

Pardee NE, Martin CJ, Morgan EH. A test of the practical value of estimating breath sound intensity. *Chest* 1976;70:341–344.

Warley ARH, Finnegan OC, Nicholson EM, et al. Grading of dyspnoea and walking speed in cardiac disease and in chronic airflow obstruction. *Br J Dis Chest* 1987;81:349–355.

Kelley's Textbook of Internal Medicine, fourth edition. Edited by H. David Humes. Lippincott Williams & Wilkins, Philadelphia © 2000.

C H A P T E R
386

APPROACH TO IMAGING OF THE CHEST

DAVID A. LYNCH

The purposes of this chapter are to outline the techniques available for imaging the chest, to review normal imaging anatomy, to illustrate the common radiographic signs of lung disease, and to describe the imaging approach to common clinical problems.

CHEST RADIOGRAPH

The chest radiograph is the first and often the only technique used in the patient with known or suspected lung disease. Radiographs must be obtained using a reproducible high-quality technique. Abnormalities are often simulated by an underexposed radiograph or by a radiograph with an inadequate inspiration. A reproducible inspiration close to total lung capacity can be ensured by having the patient breathe in, then breathe out as far as possible, and then breathe in as far as possible. Photo-timed exposure, with appropriate positioning of photocells, provides consistent radiographic density. Meticulous quality control of the film processor is also important.

If possible, the chest radiograph is obtained in the erect position with the patient's chest against the film cassette, so that the beam passes from back to front (posteroanterior, or PA). Because the heart is close to the front of the chest, it is less magnified on a PA radiograph than on an anteroposterior (AP) radiograph. AP radiographs are obtained in patients who are too sick to stand and in those who require portable radiographs. Lateral radiographs are obtained with the left side against the film cassette, which minimizes cardiac magnification.

NORMAL ANATOMY

FRONTAL CHEST RADIOGRAPH (FIG. 386.1)

The trachea is visible in the midline, inclining to the right at the level of the aortic arch. The right lung is immediately in contact with the right wall of the trachea, forming the right paratracheal line or stripe, which is usually less than 5 mm in thickness. The azygos vein is seen at the lower end of the right

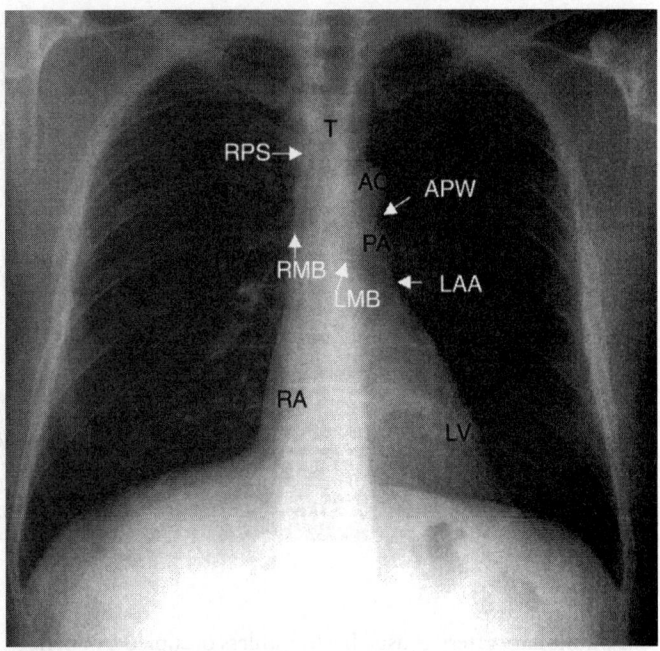

FIGURE 386.1. Normal anatomy on the frontal chest radiograph. T, trachea; RPS, right paratracheal stripe; Ao, aorta; APW, aortopulmonary window; PA, main pulmonary artery; LAA, left atrial appendage; RA, right atrium; LV, left ventricle.

paratracheal line, as it arches over the right main bronchus. The left wall of trachea is separated from the left lung by the aortic arch and its branches.

Because the left pulmonary artery arches over the left main bronchus, the left hilum is usually higher than the right, and the left main bronchus is twice as long as the right. Both hila have concave lateral margins. The horizontal minor fissure is visible in the right lung, at the level of the hilum. The left hemidiaphragm is usually lower than the right.

The convex right heart border is formed by the right atrium. The left heart border begins at the convex aortic arch. The next convexity is due to the main pulmonary artery, and the concavity between the aortic arch and main pulmonary artery is called the aortopulmonary window. A concavity below the main pulmonary artery is occupied by the left atrial appendage. The remainder of the left heart border is formed by the left ventricle.

LATERAL CHEST RADIOGRAPH (FIG. 386.2)

On the lateral radiograph, the useful landmarks are the trachea, the aortic arch, the heart, the sternum, and the spine. The upper two-thirds of the retrosternal space is usually clear, but it may be occupied by fat in obese patients, and it may be obscured by the patient's arms if they are insufficiently elevated. The major and minor fissures are usually visible.

As on the frontal view, the hilar opacity on the lateral view is composed primarily of the pulmonary arteries. The arch of the left pulmonary artery passes over the left main bronchus just below and parallel to the aortic arch. The right interlobar pulmonary artery is seen end-on, as it passes in front of the bronchus intermedius. The area immediately below the interlo-

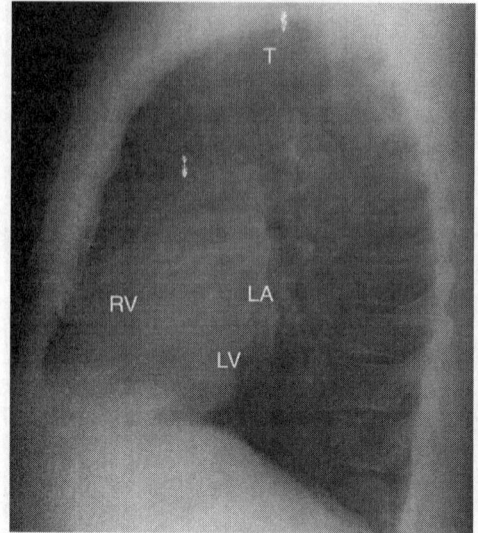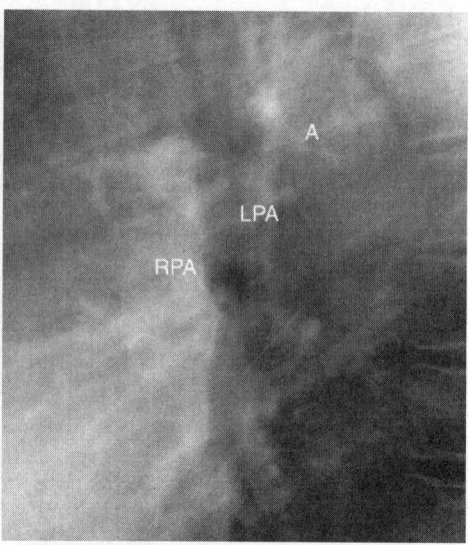

A,B

FIGURE 386.2. A, B: Normal anatomy on lateral chest radiograph, with detailed view of hila. T, trachea; RV, right ventricle; LV, left ventricle; LA, left atrium; RPA, oval composite shadow of right interlobar pulmonary artery and right superior pulmonary vein; LPA, left pulmonary artery, arching over the left main bronchus, parallel to aorta (A).

bar pulmonary artery is usually clear unless occupied by adenopathy.

The anterior border of the heart is formed by the right ventricle. The posterior border of the heart is formed by the left atrium and left ventricle.

APPROACH TO THE CHEST RADIOGRAPH

An ordered approach to the chest radiograph includes assessment of its technical adequacy (Fig. 386.3), a systematic search for

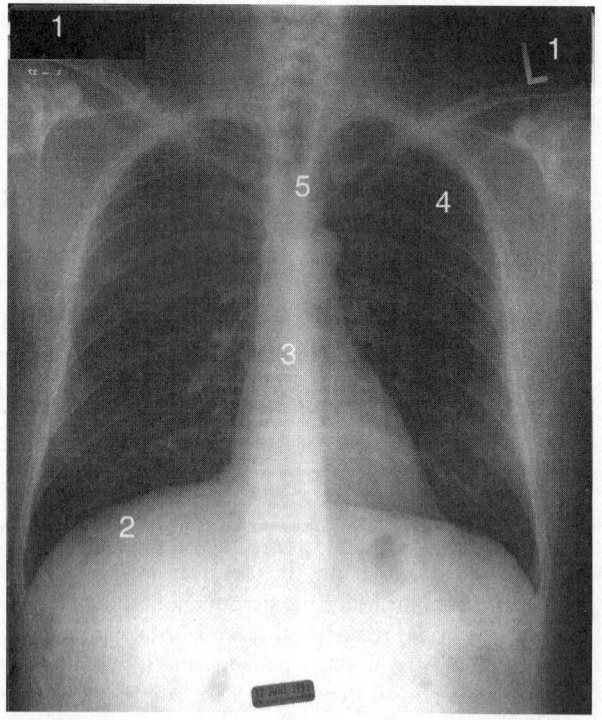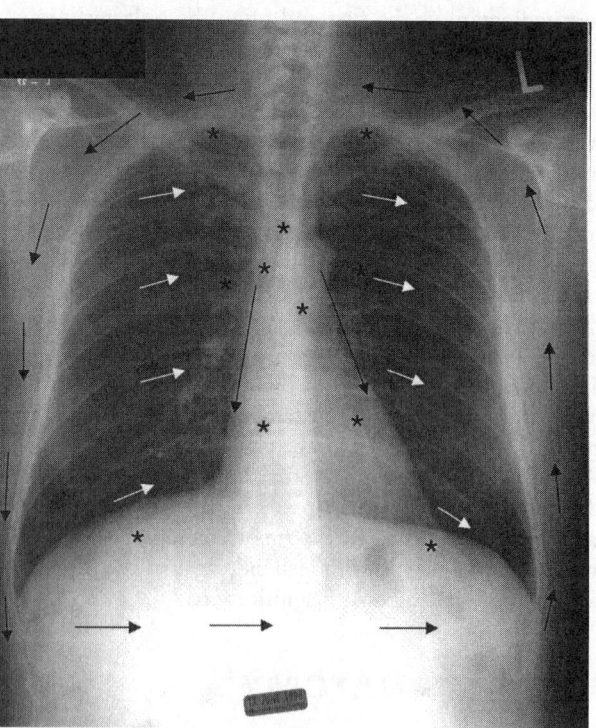

A   B

FIGURE 386.3. A: The review of a chest radiograph begins with analysis of technical adequacy. A technically adequate chest radiograph should be labeled with the patient's name, the date, and a side marker (1). The midportion of the right hemidiaphragm should be below the right tenth rib (2). The exposure should allow visualization of the vertebral bodies through the spine (3), and the pulmonary vessels should be visible to the outer third of the lung (4). The thoracic spinous processes should be midway between the heads of the clavicles (5). **B:** The systematic search of the chest radiograph, beginning at the periphery of the image (1), then systematically scanning the lungs (2), evaluating the mediastinal borders (3), and reviewing the six miss areas (*) (see text).

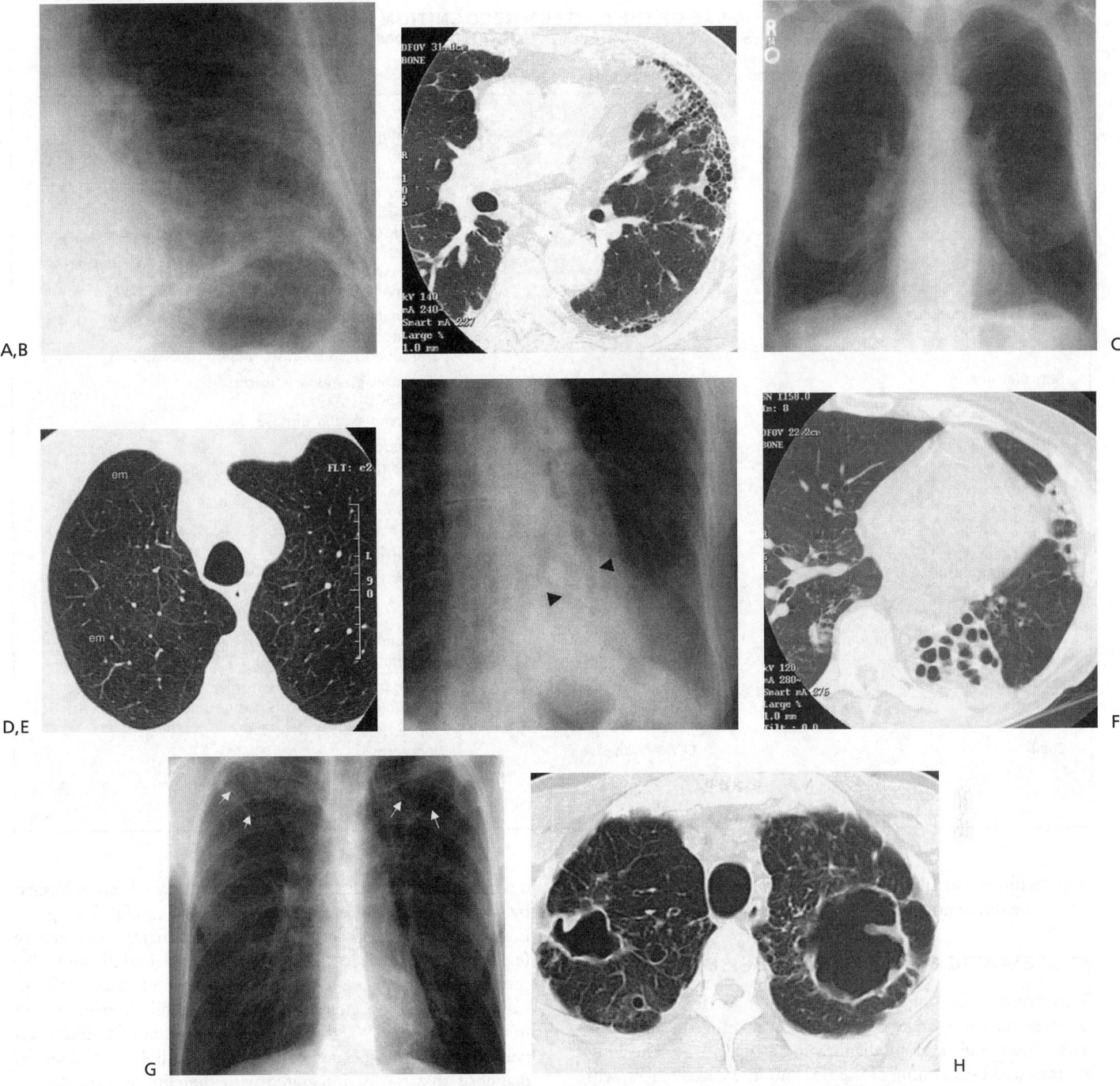

FIGURE 386.4. Radiologic signs of lung disease on chest radiograph and high-resolution CT (HRCT). **A, B:** Detailed chest radiograph in a 64-year-old man with idiopathic pulmonary fibrosis shows fine honeycomb cysts, best seen at the periphery of the lung *(arrows)*, and confirmed on HRCT. **C, D:** Chest radiograph in a 78-year-old man shows hyperinflation with diaphragmatic flattening. Upper lobe hyperlucency and decreased vascularity is strongly suggestive of emphysema. HRCT shows numerous poorly defined black holes due to emphysema (em). The vessels are splayed around the emphysematous areas. **E, F:** Chest radiograph in a 75-year-old woman shows multiple dilated tubular structures evident as "train tracks" *(arrows)*. HRCT shows multiple dilated bronchi within a collapsed left lower lobe. **G, H:** Chest radiograph in a 50-year-old man with tuberculosis shows multiple thin-walled cavities in the upper lobes *(arrows)*, associated with upper lobe volume loss. CT confirms thin-walled cavities.

TABLE 386.1.	EXAMPLES OF THE USE OF THE PATTERN RECOGNITION APPROACH TO DIAGNOSE LUNG DISEASE BY CHEST RADIOGRAPH AND COMPUTED TOMOGRAPHY	
Radiographic and CT Observations	**Category (Inference)**	**Common Causes**
Poorly defined opacities Coalescence Air bronchograms	Airspace (alveolar) disease	*Acute:* Pneumonia Edema Aspiration Hemorrhage *Chronic:* Chronic infection (mycobacterial, fungal) Infiltrative disease (chronic obstructive pulmonary disease eosinophilic pneumonia, sarcoidosis) Malignancy (bronchioloalveolar carcinoma, lymphoma)
Well-defined nodules	Interstitial nodules	Malignancy Pneumoconiosis Granulomas (sarcoidosis, miliary tuberculosis)
Reticular lines Honeycombing	Interstitial fibrosis	Idiopathic pulmonary fibrosis Asbestosis Collagen vascular disease
Kerley A, B, C lines	Septal thickening	Lung edema Lymphangitic spread
Ring shadows Train tracks Hyperinflation	Airway disease	Asthma Bronchitis Cystic fibrosis
Hyperlucency Decreased number and branching of vessels Vascular "stretching"	Emphysema	Cigarette smoking α_1-Antitrypsin deficiency
Amorphous increased lung density Vascular indistinctness	Ground-glass opacity	Early airspace or interstitial disease (e.g., edema, *Pneumocystis* infection)
Poorly defined nodules	Fuzzy nodules	*Malignancy* (bronchioloalveolar, metastases) *Granulomas* (sarcoidosis, Langerhans' histiocytosis) Mycobacterial, fungal, or viral infection
Cavity	Cavitary disease	Neoplasm Vasculitis or thromboembolism Infection

abnormalities, careful description of the radiographic abnormalities, and a differential diagnosis based on radiologic appearance.

SYSTEMATIC SEARCH (FIG. 386.3B)

After noting gross abnormalities and asymmetries, it is best to begin at the outer edges of the film, evaluating the shoulders, neck, chest wall, and subdiaphragmatic structures. The lungs are reviewed by scanning of the ribs and intercostal spaces, with comparison of right and left. The eye sweeps down along the right and left mediastinal borders. Finally, one reviews the six areas where abnormalities are most likely to be missed because of low contrast or because of overlapping structures: the lung apexes, the hila and suprahilar regions, the trachea and main bronchi, the right and left retrocardiac region, and the retrodiaphragmatic lung.

DESCRIPTION, CATEGORIZATION, AND DIFFERENTIAL DIAGNOSIS

Radiologists are trained to describe abnormalities in standard terms. Glossaries of recommended descriptors for the chest ra-

diograph and computed tomography (CT) have been published by the Fleischner Society. The advantage of careful description is that it often allows allocation of the abnormality to a category (e.g., airspace disease, cavitary disease, extrapleural disease). The process of description is distinct from that of categorization. Categorization is an inference based on careful observation and must not be forced when the observations do not fit. Each category of disease is associated with a specific radiologic differential diagnosis that can be integrated with the clinical information. Table 386.1 illustrates how the pattern recognition approach progresses from observation to inference to differential diagnosis. This table is not intended to be comprehensive. Common patterns of lung disease are illustrated in Fig. 386.4.

ADDITIONAL RADIOGRAPHIC TECHNIQUES

Expiration radiographs have traditionally been performed to detect pneumothorax but in fact are rarely indicated because inspiration views are equally sensitive for pneumothorax. They may sometimes be helpful in detecting air trapping due to large-

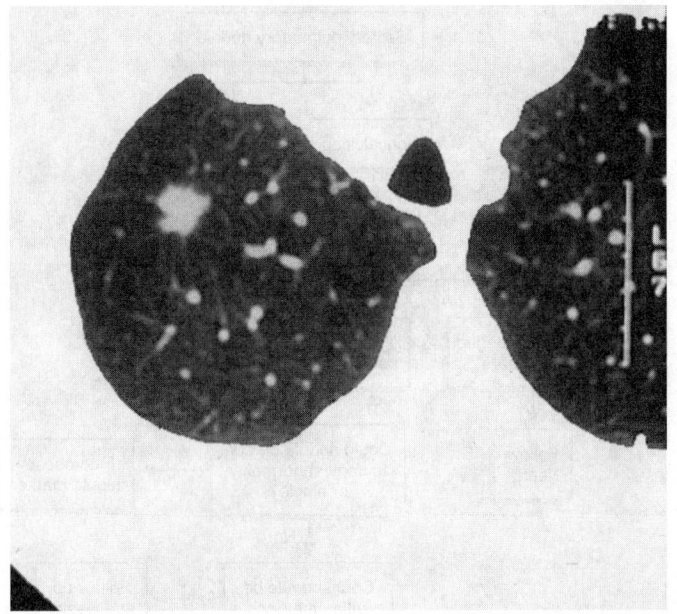

A

FIGURE 386.5. Solitary pulmonary nodule due to adenocarcinoma in a 62-year-old woman. **A:** Computed tomography shows solitary irregular pulmonary nodule, which was noncalcified. **B:** The nodule enhances by more than 15 Hounsfield units, indicating that it is not benign. Some inflammatory lesions may have a similar enhancement pattern.

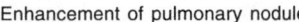

Enhancement of pulmonary nodule

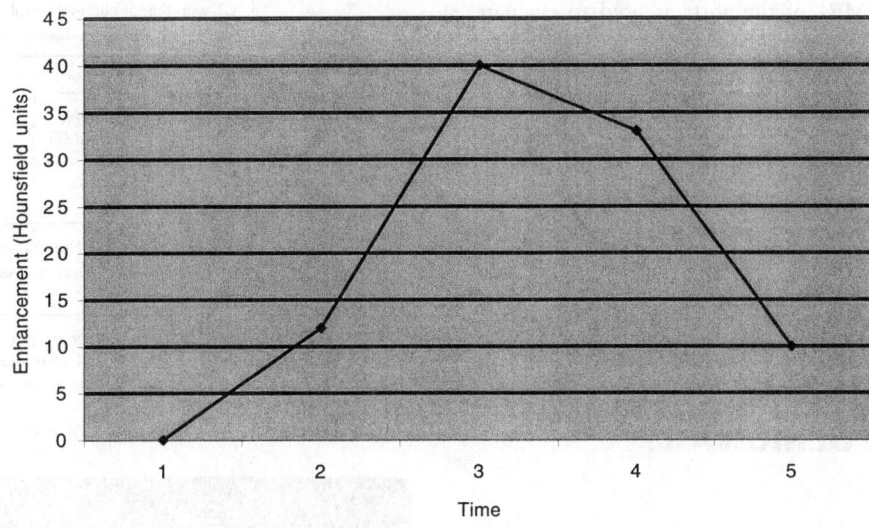

B

airway obstruction. Decubitus views are helpful in showing mobile pleural effusions and in showing pneumothorax in supine patients. Lordotic views were commonly used to identify tuberculous lesions at the lung apexes, but their value is declining with the decrease in prevalence of tuberculosis.

Fluoroscopy remains a useful technique for distinguishing between pulmonary nodules and extrapulmonary lesions, such as rib fractures, and for evaluating the movement of the diaphragm using a "sniff" test.

▌ CT OF THE CHEST

The changing terminology of computed tomography requires some clarification. *Helical or spiral CT* is a technique by which

the entire lung can be imaged as a three-dimensional dataset during one or two breath holds. It is the technique of choice for surveying the chest for nodules and other focal abnormalities. It is also useful for constructing images of airways or vessels in sagittal, coronal, or other planes. Contrast-enhanced helical CT is increasingly being used for direct visualization of emboli in the main, lobar, and segmental pulmonary arteries. Low-dose helical CT is being studied as a method for screening for lung cancer in high-risk individuals.

High-resolution CT (HRCT) is optimized to visualize fine detail within the lung, using thin sections (1 mm rather than 7 or 10 mm) and an edge-enhancing reconstruction algorithm. This technique is the primary method for diagnosis of bronchiectasis, and for diagnosis and characterization of infiltrative lung diseases and small-airway disease. Because the thin sections of

HRCT are usually separated by 1 to 4 cm, this technique is not suitable for detecting lung nodules. However, a set of HRCT images obtained through a focal lung abnormality or nodule may help to characterize the abnormality.

Expiratory HRCT may be useful to detect air trapping in patients with emphysema, asthma, or small-airway disease.

Indications for administration of intravenous contrast during chest CT include visualization of the heart, aorta, hila, or pulmonary vessels, and characterization of lung nodules. Contrast is not usually indicated for evaluation of diffuse lung disease or for screening for metastases.

In general, the physician requesting a chest CT scan should not be too concerned about the details of chest CT technique. If the clinical question is clear from the requisition, the radiologist can usually determine the protocol and assess the need for intravenous contrast.

OTHER IMAGING MODALITIES

The clinical usefulness of magnetic resonance imaging (MRI) of the chest is limited. MRI of the aorta is used to evaluate dissection or aneurysm. MRI can help evaluate cardiac or paracardiac masses. MRI is more sensitive than CT for detection of chest wall invasion by tumor (particularly Pancoast tumor). Although magnetic resonance angiography of the pulmonary arteries may diagnose pulmonary emboli, it has been difficult to develop a robust technique for this purpose.

Nuclear imaging of the lung is primarily used to diagnose pulmonary embolism. Gallium imaging is occasionally used to help diagnose sarcoidosis. The use of ultrasonography of the chest is discussed below.

SOLITARY PULMONARY NODULE

Lung cancer is often first detected as an asymptomatic nodule on the chest radiograph. For this reason, solitary pulmonary nodules must never be ignored. Algorithm 1 (Fig. 386.6) shows that the most useful single test in the evaluation of a solitary pulmonary nodule is that of obtaining old films. Although nodules that have been stable for more than 2 years are likely to be benign, slow-growing lung cancers may take up to 5 years to develop. Other causes of noncalcified pulmonary nodules include noncalcified granulomas (due to tuberculosis or histoplasmosis), hamartomas, arteriovenous malformations, round pneumonia, and solitary metastasis. Hamartomas can often be recognized on CT by the presence of fat in the nodule. Arteriovenous malformations are identified by the presence of feeding or draining vessels. The technique of dynamic nodule CT is an important recent advance in the evaluation of the indeterminate solitary pulmonary nodule (Fig. 386.5). Nodules that fail to enhance by more than 15 Hounsfield CT units following a bolus of intravenous contrast are likely to be benign.

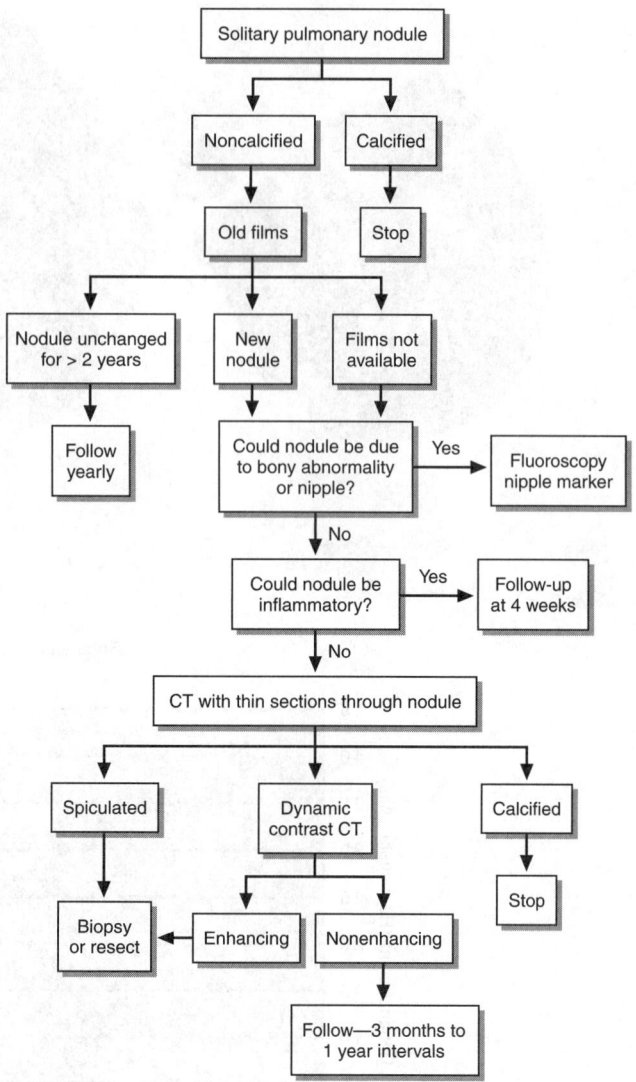

FIGURE 386.6. The evaluation of a solitary pulmonary nodule.

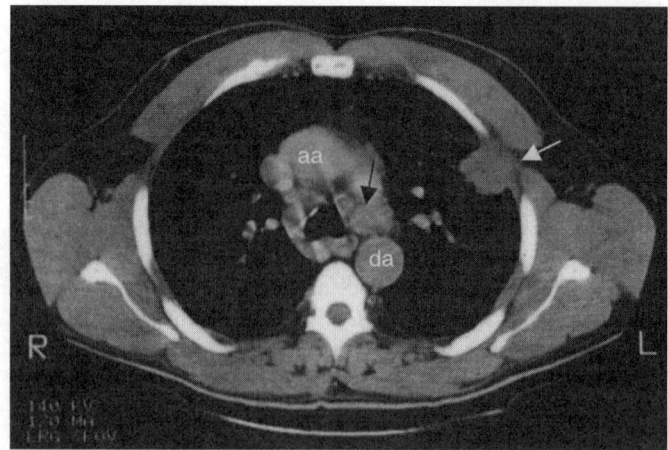

FIGURE 386.7. Computed tomography staging of lung cancer. Unenhanced chest computed tomogram in a 70-year-old man shows a 2.5-cm left upper lobe nodule with invasion of the chest wall *(white arrow).* There is a 2-cm lymph node *(black arrow)* in the aortopulmonary window lateral to the trachea. aa, ascending aorta; da, descending aorta. The radiologic staging of T3 N2 (stage IIIA) was confirmed histologically.

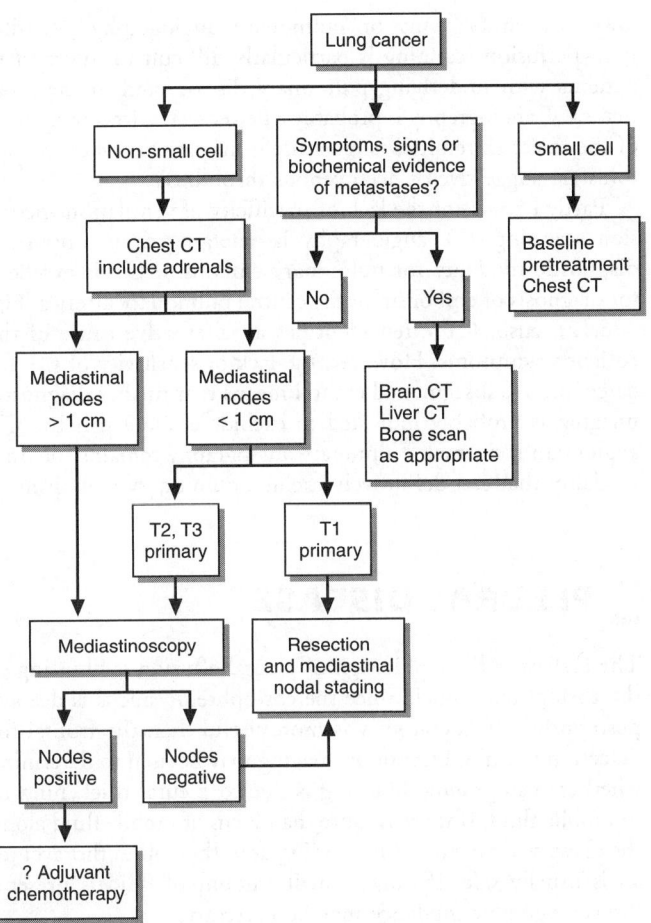

FIGURE 386.8. Approach to the patient with suspected or confirmed lung cancer.

STAGING OF LUNG CANCER

In a patient with suspected or confirmed lung cancer, algorithm 2 (Fig. 386.8) shows that CT scanning is currently the pivotal investigation (Fig. 386.7). Positron emission tomography scanning using ^{17}F-deoxyglucose to detect metabolically active tumor is emerging as a valuable test for detection of occult mediastinal and distal metastasis, thereby distinguishing resectable from unresectable tumor with greater accuracy than CT. However, further clinical trials of this modality are required before can be introduced into clinical practice.

DIFFUSE LUNG DISEASE

Asthma, probably the commonest diffuse lung disease, may be associated with radiologic evidence of airway wall thickening or hyperinflation, but the chest radiograph is otherwise normal. Acute exacerbations of asthma can be associated with pneumomediastinum, pneumothorax or atelectasis. Allergic bronchopulmonary aspergillosis, an uncommon complication of asthma, is associated with central bronchiectasis, best seen on CT.

Moderate or severe emphysema is diagnosed on the chest

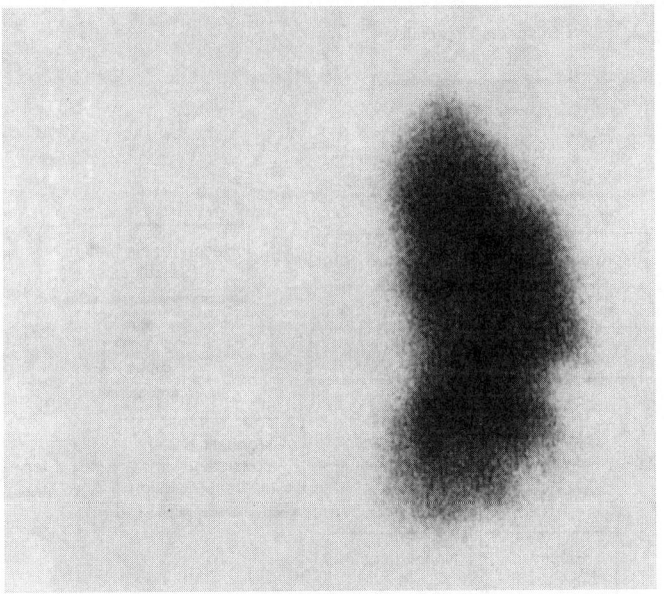

A

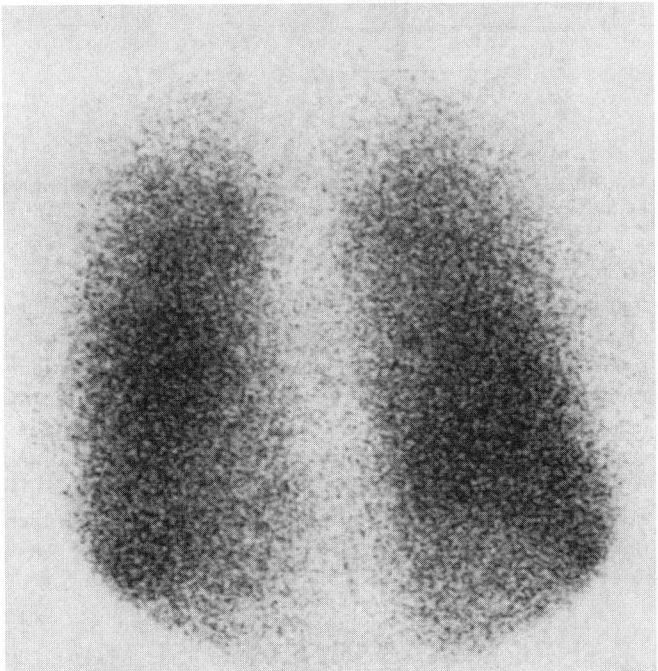

B

FIGURE 386.9. High probability lung scan in patient with suspected pulmonary embolism. **A:** Perfusion image (posterior view) obtained following intravenous administration of ^{99m}Tc-labeled macroalbumin particles shows absent perfusion in the left lung and multiple large defects in the right lung. **B:** Ventilation image obtained following inhalation of xenon 133 is near-normal.

radiograph by the presence of hyperlucency and vascular obliteration. Smoking-related emphysema is most marked in the upper lobes, while emphysema related to α_1-antitrypsin deficiency is more marked in the lower lobes. CT is more sensitive for detection of emphysema and can be used to classify emphysema into centrilobular, panlobular, and paraseptal patterns.

Table 386.1 and Algorithm 3 (Fig. 386.10) indicates how the chest radiograph and CT can be used to characterize infiltra-

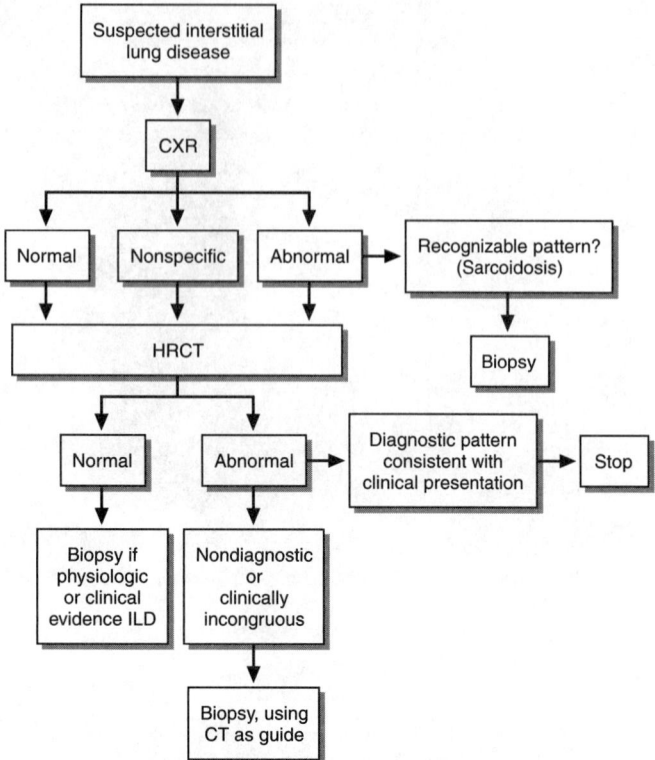

FIGURE 386.10. Imaging approach to characterization of infiltrative lung disease.

tive lung diseases. HRCT is significantly more accurate than chest radiography for disease characterization. HRCT can be used to identify certain diffuse diseases, such as idiopathic pulmonary fibrosis, lymphangiomyomatosis, pulmonary histiocytosis X, and sarcoidosis, with a high degree of accuracy. However, the HRCT appearance of individual patients should always be considered in association with the clinical features. If the radiologic pattern or the clinical presentation is atypical, then biopsy should always be performed.

THROMBOEMBOLIC DISEASE (ALGORITHM 4, FIG. 386.11)

The chest radiograph is usually abnormal, though nonspecific, in patients with pulmonary thromboembolism. The commonest abnormality is a decrease in lung volumes, often associated with linear atelectasis. Wedge-shaped peripheral consolidation due to pulmonary infarction is substantially less common.

Ventilation–perfusion lung scanning is the traditional next step in the diagnostic pathway. A normal perfusion scan is associated with a very low likelihood of pulmonary embolism. A high-probability scan (Fig. 386.9) in patients with a high clinical suspicion for pulmonary embolism is associated with a 96% prevalence of pulmonary embolism. However, only 40% of patients with pulmonary embolism have high-probability scans. Most of the remaining patients have inconclusive scans and will require further investigation, such as ultrasonography of the

lower extremity veins or pulmonary angiography. Ventilation–perfusion scanning is particularly difficult to interpret in patients with underlying pulmonary disease, and in these patients CT angiography is probably a better test. Ultrasonography of the lower extremities is most useful in patients whose symptoms are suggestive of deep venous thrombosis.

Partly because of the lack of specificity of ventilation–perfusion scanning, CT angiography is emerging as an important diagnostic modality for pulmonary embolism. CT is excellent for diagnosis of embolism in the central pulmonary arteries (Fig. 386.12). Also, CT often identifies an alternative cause of the patient's symptoms. However, the lack of sensitivity of CT for detection of subsegmental emboli means that further diagnostic imaging is probably indicated to exclude embolism if the CT angiogram is normal. Pulmonary angiography remains the only modality that can definitively exclude pulmonary embolism.

PLEURAL DISEASE

The earliest radiographic sign of pleural effusion is blunting of the costophrenic sulci. Since the costophrenic sulcus is deepest posteriorly, the lateral view is more useful than the frontal for detection of fluid. Decubitus imaging may be used to determine whether costophrenic blunting is due to pleural thickening or to mobile fluid. If there is more than 2 cm of mobile fluid along the chest wall on a decubitus radiograph, then blind thoracentesis is usually safe. If only a small amount of fluid is present, ultrasonographic guidance may be necessary.

A thin white line conforming to the expected shape of the pleura is the only specific radiologic sign of pneumothorax (Fig. 386.13). This line corresponds to the visceral pleura. Lung vessels are usually not visible outside the pleural line.

CHEST RADIOLOGY IN THE INTENSIVE CARE UNIT

The major roles of the chest radiograph in critically ill patients are to identify the positions of tubes and lines and to detect and follow pulmonary complications such as pneumonia, pulmonary edema, pneumothorax, and acute respiratory distress syndrome. Chest radiographs are indicated in these patients when a new tube or line is placed, or when there are clinical signs of deterioration, such as an increasing oxygen requirement. Routine daily chest radiographs are indicated only in the sickest patients.

Interpretation of radiographs in critical care patients is compromised by the fact that these are usually portable AP radiographs obtained in the supine position, often with an inadequate inspiration. Comparison of serial radiographs must take account of technical factors influencing radiographic appearances, including radiographic exposure, erect or supine positioning, depth of inspiration, and positive-pressure ventilation.

Pneumothorax and pleural effusions are more difficult to detect in the supine than in the erect position. In the supine patient, pneumothorax is usually anterobasal, while pleural effu-

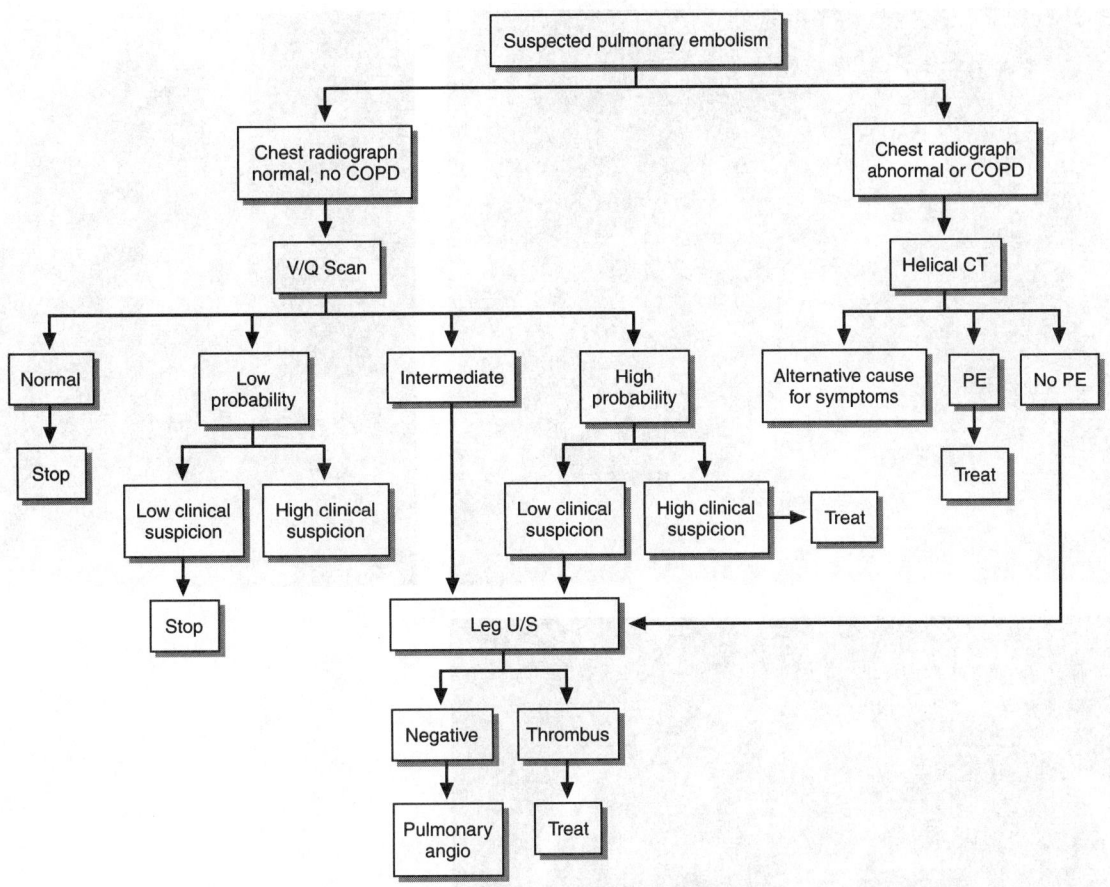

FIGURE 386.11. Imaging approach to thromboembolic disease.

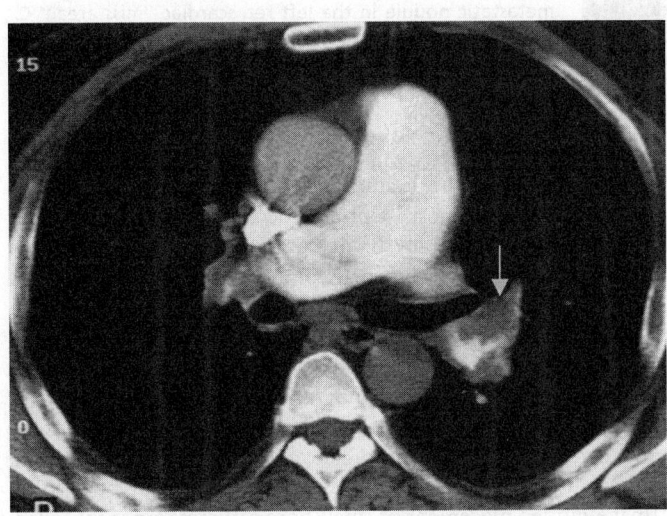

FIGURE 386.12. Acute pulmonary embolism on computed tomography (CT). Contrast-enhanced helical CT scan shows an irregular large thrombus in the dilated descending left pulmonary artery, extending into a segmental branch *(arrow)*. The main pulmonary artery is mildly enlarged.

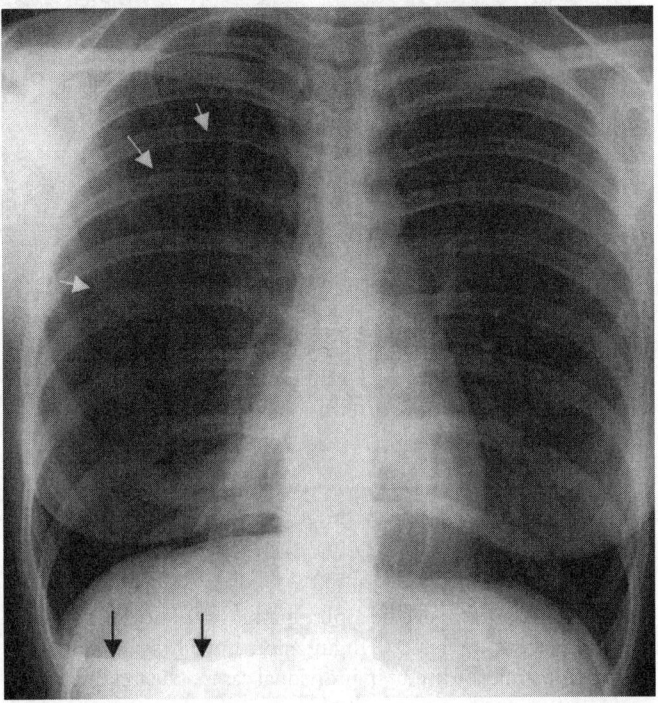

FIGURE 386.13. Spontaneous right hydropneumothorax in 25-year-old man. The pleural line is clearly visible *(white arrows)*. An air–fluid level behind the diaphragm *(black arrows)* indicates that there is fluid as well as air in the right pleural space.

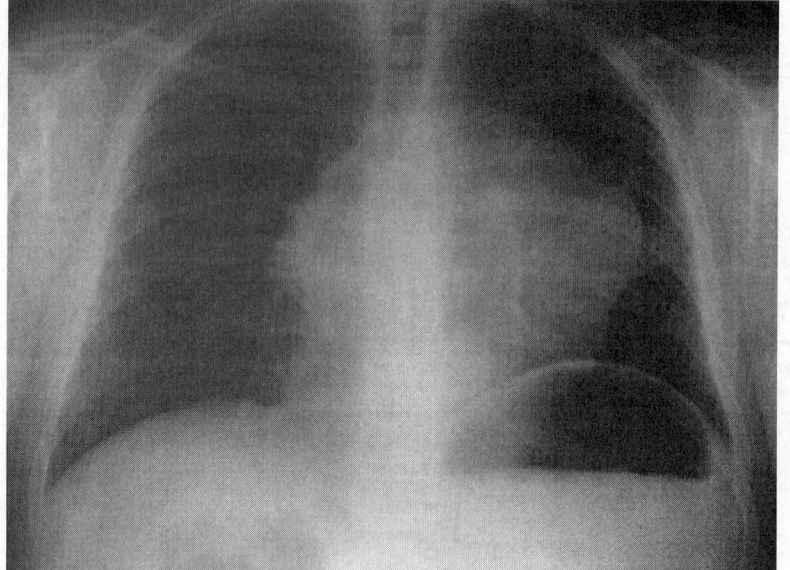
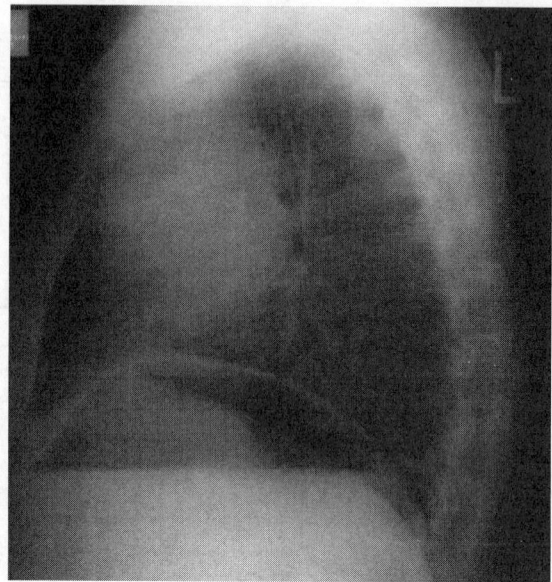
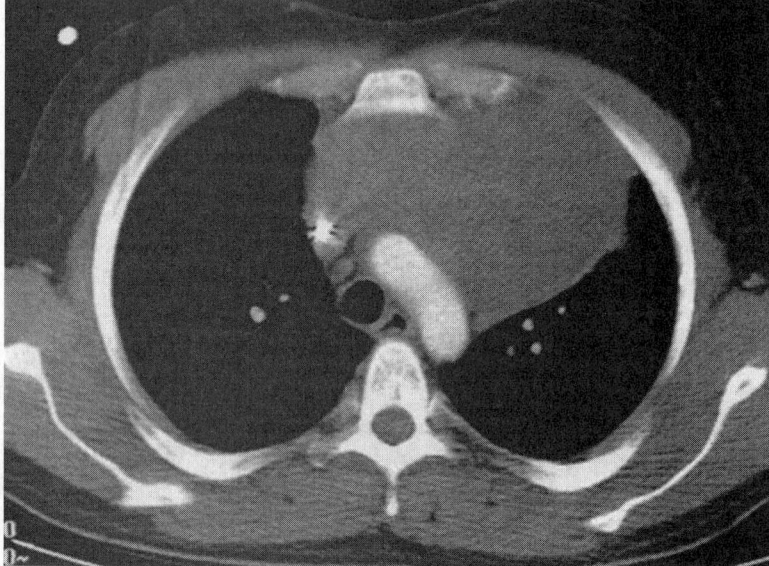

FIGURE 386.14. Anterior mediastinal mass in 25-year-old man. **A, B:** Posteroanterior and lateral chest radiographs show a mass in the anterior mediastinum. There is also a metastatic nodule in the left retrocardiac "miss area." **C:** Computed tomography shows that the mass is composed of water density material. Biopsy confirmed germ cell tumor.

sions layering posteriorly are evident as an increase in density superimposed on the lung. Decubitus imaging may be useful in detecting pneumothorax or effusion.

INTERVENTIONAL CHEST RADIOLOGY

Most pulmonary and mediastinal masses are amenable to image-guided transthoracic needle aspiration biopsy. These biopsies are usually performed using CT guidance, but ultrasonography or fluoroscopy may be useful in individual cases. The major complication of percutaneous needle biopsy is pneumothorax, which occurs in about 20% of cases but is usually self-limited, with chest tube drainage being required in only 5%. The risk of pneumothorax increases with the presence of emphysema, with in-

creasing depth of the lesion, and with decreasing size of the lesion. CT can be most helpful in deciding whether to biopsy a mass bronchoscopically or percutaneously. If CT shows the mass to have an endobronchial component, or to have a bronchus leading directly to it (bronchus sign), then bronchoscopic biopsy is preferable, using the CT as a road map.

Imaging is increasingly used to guide diagnostic and therapeutic interventions. Ultrasonography is the ideal modality for guiding aspiration of pleural effusions. Ultrasonography excels at showing loculations and organization in a pleural collection. When ultrasonographic access is difficult, CT may be helpful. Image-guided placement of small-bore catheters is a viable alternative to surgical chest tubes for drainage of most pneumothoraxes and fluid collections. Drainage of empyemas or complicated, loculated fluid collections can be enhanced by intrapleural administration of thrombolytics (streptokinase or urokinase).

Pleurodesis may also be effectively accomplished using small-bore catheters.

BIBLIOGRAPHY

Austin J, Muller N, Friedman P, et al. Glossary of terms for CT of the lungs: recommendations of the nomenclature committee of the Fleischner Society. *Radiology* 1996;200:327–331.

Klein JS, Schultz S, Heffner JE. Interventional radiology of the chest: image-guided percutaneous drainage of pleural effusions, lung abscess, and pneumothorax. *AJR Am J Roentgenol* 1995;164:581–588.

Muller N, Miller R. Computed tomography of chronic diffuse infiltrative lung disease. 1. *Am Rev Respir Dis* 1990;142:1206–1215.

Muller N, Miller R. Computed tomography of chronic diffuse infiltrative lung disease. 2. *Am Rev Respir Dis* 1990;142:1440–1448.

Steinert HC, Hauser M, Allemann F, et al. Non–small cell lung cancer: nodal staging with FDG PET versus CT with correlative lymph node mapping and sampling. *Radiology* 1997;202:441–446.

Swensen S, Aughenbaugh G, Myers J. Diffuse lung disease: diagnostic accuracy of CT in patients undergoing surgical biopsy of the lung. *Radiology* 1997;205:229–234.

Swensen S, Brown L, Colby T, et al. Lung nodule enhancement on CT: prospective findings. *Radiology* 1996;201:447–455.

Tuddenham WJ. Glossary of terms for thoracic radiology: recommendations of the Nomenclature Committee of the Fleischner Society. *AJR Am J Roentgenol* 1984;143:509–517.

Kelley's Textbook of Internal Medicine, fourth edition. Edited by H. David Humes. Lippincott Williams & Wilkins, Philadelphia © 2000.

C H A P T E R

387

PULMONARY FUNCTION TESTING

JACK L. CLAUSEN

In addition to testing lung function, pulmonary function tests assess other determinants of effective ventilation (e.g., upper airway patency, respiratory muscles, chemoreceptors). Our focus in this chapter is on those tests commonly used to assess pulmonary function with emphasis on what is required to maximize clinical usefulness.

■ P_{O_2}, P_{CO_2}, $\%S_{O_2}$ OF ARTERIAL BLOOD

Measurements of the P_{O_2} of arterial blood (Pa_{O_2}) are often useful for the detection of mild lung disease, especially when measured during exercise. Predicted values for Pa_{O_2} decline with the normal changes of adult aging and must be adjusted for altitudes above sea level. The Pa_{O_2} is also useful for following *changes* in lung function. However, relatively small changes in shunts (e.g., from localized atelectasis or an airway obstructed from secretions) can result in substantial changes in the Pa_{O_2}, which might be misinterpreted as changes in overall lung function.

The alveolar–arterial oxygen gradient, $P(A-a)_{O_2}$, is less dependent on variations in ventilation than the Pa_{O_2} and often is more useful for the detection of mild disease. The PA_{O_2} can be derived from the equation:

$$PA_{O_2} = PI_{O_2} - \frac{PA_{CO_2}}{R}$$

By assuming that alveolar equals arterial P_{CO_2}; that the respiratory exchange ratio is 0.8, as in normal dietary conditions; and that water vapor pressure is 47 mm Hg, at sea level (760 mm Hg barometric pressure), $PA_{O_2} = (760 - 47) (0.21) - Pa_{CO_2}/0.8 = 150 - 1.2 (Pa_{CO_2})$.

Measurements of Pa_{CO_2} are important for assessing the acid–base status and as indicators of the effectiveness of alveolar ventilation. Elevations of Pa_{CO_2} above the upper limit of normal (46 mm Hg) indicate that alveolar clearance of CO_2 is reduced and may be a valuable indicator of severe lung dysfunction. However, Pa_{CO_2} can also be elevated secondary to reduced central drive, including adaptive responses to excessive work of breathing and/or inspiratory muscle fatigue. Consequently, there is growing recognition that elevation of Pa_{CO_2}, either at rest or during exercise, may not always be the bad prognostic sign it was once considered. Because of the large functional reserve of the lungs and the normal increase in ventilation in response to hypoxemia, elevation of Pa_{CO_2} is not a sensitive sign of mild lung disease.

Terminology regarding oxyhemoglobin saturation is frequently misused. Percent oxyhemoglobin ($\%Hb_{O_2}$) is defined as oxyhemoglobin expressed as a percentage of total hemoglobin. In contrast, percentage oxygen saturation ($\%S_{O_2}$) is oxyhemoglobin expressed as a percentage of hemoglobin available for oxygenation (the sum of deoxyhemoglobin and oxyhemoglobin). If a patient has an HbCO of 20%, a deoxyhemoglobin of 10%, and an Hb_{O_2} of 70%, the $\%S_{O_2}$ would be 87.5% (70/80).

Pulse oximeters are devices with miniaturized sensors that attach to an ear or digit and estimate $\%Sa_{O_2}$ from measurements of changes in light absorption associated with systolic pulsations of blood flow. Because such devices respond within 60 seconds to changes in $\%Sa_{O_2}$, they are valuable noninvasive monitors of oxygenation during surgery and other procedures, in unstable patients in intensive care units, and for studies of sleep disorders. It is important to appreciate the limitations of this new technology. Because the 95% confidence interval for the accuracy of $\%Sa_{O_2}$ from most pulse oximeters is $\pm 4\%$, and because of the shape of the oxyhemoglobin saturation curve, cutaneous oximeters have limited use for the detection of mild disease when compared with direct measurements of Pa_{O_2}. Inherent inaccuracies in pulse oximeters also limit their use for other applications based on Pa_{O_2}, such as prescription of home oxygen therapy. Their measurements are somewhat less accurate in the presence of carboxyhemoglobin and significantly less accurate with high levels of methemoglobin.

■ SPIROMETRY, FLOW–VOLUME CURVES

Figure 387.1 illustrates relevant terminology and time and flow–volume curves from a normal subject. Although the devel-

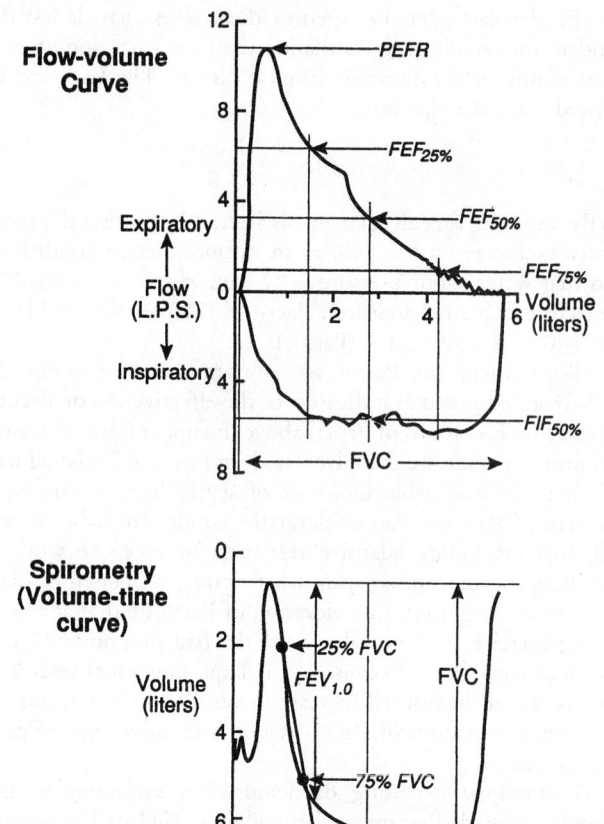

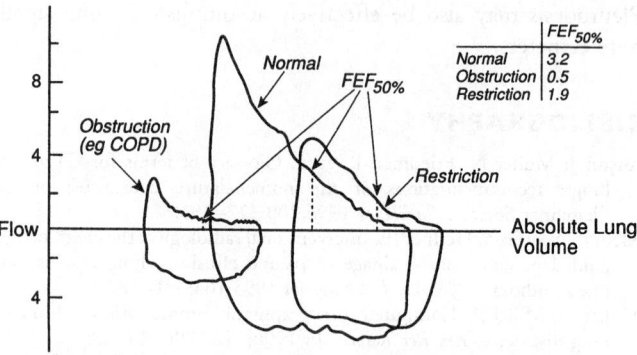

FIGURE 387.2. Examples of flow–volume curves in a patient with obstructive disease and a patient with restriction (diffuse interstitial fibrosis), as compared with a normal person. Volumes on the axis are absolute volumes to better demonstrate the relation of flows (e.g., FEF$_{50\%}$) to hyperinflation and restriction. COPD, chronic obstructive pulmonary disease; FEF$_{50\%}$, forced expiratory flow rate of 50%.

FIGURE 387.1. Flow–volume curve and spirometry tracing (volume–time curve) from a normal subject, with both curves from the same expiratory effort. FVC, forced vital capacity; FEV$_1$, forced expiratory volume in the first second of expiration; PEFR, peak expiratory flow rate. FEF$_{25\%}$, forced expiratory flow rate at 25% VC. For this and other flows, the subscript indicates that the flow is measured at the volume expired, usually expressed as a percentage of the vital capacity.

opment of equipment standards has improved the availability of spirometers with acceptable accuracy, attention to calibrations and other quality control steps are still important for acquiring clinically useful results.

With time tracings, the duration of the expiratory effort can be assessed. Flow–volume tracings offer easier visual assessments of changes of flow rates with repeat testing, appreciation of the relation between flow rates and expired volumes (Figs 387.1 and Figure 387.2), and recognition of patterns characteristic of localized and upper airway obstruction (Fig. 387.3).

The forced expiratory volume in 1 second (FEV$_1$) and the ratio of FEV$_1$ to the forced vital capacity (FVC) are the best parameters for the identification of patients with obstructive lung disease. Declines in FEV$_1$ with time is commonly used for assessing the rate of progression of obstructive lung disease; a normal decline in FEV$_1$ with aging of adults is 25 to 30 mL per year.

The FEV$_1$-to-FVC ratio is useful when evaluating patients who have reductions of both the FVC and FEV$_1$. A normal or

high value for the ratio suggests that the FVC and FEV$_1$ are reduced because of a restrictive process rather than obstruction, whereas a low value indicates obstructive disease. For evaluating the progression of disease or responses to therapy, FEV$_1$ is more useful than the FEV$_1$-to-FVC ratio. For example, bronchodilators may cause a greater increase in FVC than FEV$_1$, causing a paradoxical decrease in the FEV$_1$-to-FVC ratio.

Studies from the 1970s suggest that flow rates later in expiration (e.g., FEF$_{25\%-75\%}$, FEF$_{50\%}$) might be more useful than the

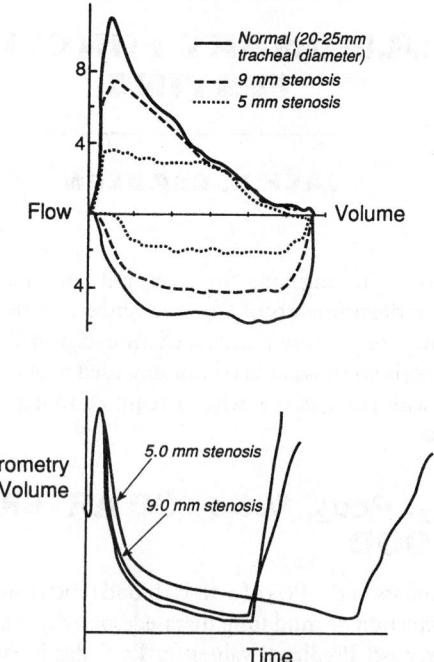

FIGURE 387.3. Effects of fixed obstruction of central airways (e.g., tracheal stenosis) on flow–volume curves. The 5-mm stenosis curve represents the characteristic flattened loop. The 9-mm-diameter stenosis (a 75% reduction in tracheal cross-sectional area) shows only a mild reduction in peak flows. Also notable for both examples of stenosis is the difficulty in recognizing the abnormalities from inspection of the volume vs time tracings.

FEV_1 for the identification of patients with early obstructive lung disease. However, several disadvantages of these flow rates limit their clinical usefulness, including larger variability on repeat testing, wider ranges of predicted values, and lack of evidence that isolated reductions in these flow rates (reductions when the FEV_1 is within normal limits) predict who develops clinically significant chronic obstructive pulmonary disease (COPD) in the future.

Reductions in expiratory flow rates must be interpreted with caution in patients with reduction of total lung capacity (TLC) because of the relation between lung volume and airway size. In Figure 387.2, the volume axis of the flow–volume curves is expressed in terms of absolute lung volumes; although the loops from the patients with obstruction and restriction both have reduced values for $FEF_{50\%}$, if one compares flows at the same lung volumes, the restricted patient's $FEF_{50\%}$ is slightly *above* the value predicted from a normal patient.

Figure 387.3 illustrates the changes in flow–volume loops from a fixed localized obstruction of the trachea. The classic configuration is a loop flattened in both inspiration and expiration, as observed in the curve representing a severe stenosis of 5-mm tracheal diameter. Less severe obstruction may cause a mild blunting of the peak expiratory flow rates, a pattern difficult to distinguish from normal. Although a flattened flow–volume curve is a specific sign of localized central airway obstruction, it is not sensitive and its absence does not rule out significant localized obstruction of central airways. Variable intrathoracic obstruction, as seen with tracheomalacia where luminal diameters increase with inspiration and decrease during expiration, produce curves that may be difficult to distinguish from loops that are suggestive of COPD. Variable extrathoracic airway obstruction (e.g., paralyzed vocal cords) results in reductions in maximal inspiratory flows with normal maximal expiratory flows. (This picture is, however, most commonly artifactual and the result of an inadequate inspiratory effort or, occasionally, inspiratory muscle weakness).

RESPONSE TO BRONCHODILATORS

Testing the response to bronchodilators seldom requires more than repeat measurements of spirometry 15 to 30 minutes after inhalation of a bronchodilator. An increase in FEV_1 of at least 12% and 200 mL is a standard criterion of response. The absence of an acute response, however, does not obviate the need for a clinical trial of bronchodilator therapy. Testing bronchodilator response is frequently not indicated; clinicians should carefully consider when it is necessary.

BRONCHIAL CHALLENGE

A decrease in FEV_1 of 20% or more after low doses of inhaled methacholine or histamine is common in patients with asthma and is a useful test of bronchial hyperresponsiveness (see Chapter 363). Responses to higher doses can also occur in patients with allergic rhinitis, chronic bronchitis, and congestive heart failure.

Inhalation challenges using specific antigens can be useful in confirming that a suspected inhalant is the cause of lung dysfunction.

LUNG VOLUMES

Lung volume measurements can be useful for evaluating patients with restrictive or obstructive lung diseases. Restrictive lung disease is defined physiologically as a reduction in TLC. Obstructive disease is a disorder with reduced maximal inspiratory or expiratory flow rates, which is frequently accompanied by hyperinflation of residual volume (RV), functional residual capacity (FRC), and sometimes TLC. Figure 387.3 illustrates that both obstructive and restrictive diseases can cause reductions of vital capacity (VC) of similar magnitude; the measurements of TLC distinguish the two processes. If spirometry shows a reduced FVC, but no reduction in the FEV_1-to-FVC ratio or other flows (e.g., $FEF_{25-75\%}$), it is reasonable to assume that the FVC is reduced because of restrictive disease even in the absence of measurements of TLC. However, if the FEV_1-to-FVC ratio is reduced without measurements of TLC, one cannot determine whether the VC is reduced as a result of the obstructive disease or restrictive disease superimposed on obstruction.

In clinical practice, absolute lung volumes (TLC, FRC, and RV) can be measured by one of three techniques: gas dilution or washout, body plethysmography, or surface measurements of thoracic borders on conventional posteroanterior and lateral chest radiographs. All three techniques give comparable results in normal subjects, but the results can differ in patients with disease.

Helium dilution or nitrogen washout techniques are the lung volume techniques most commonly available, but they may un-

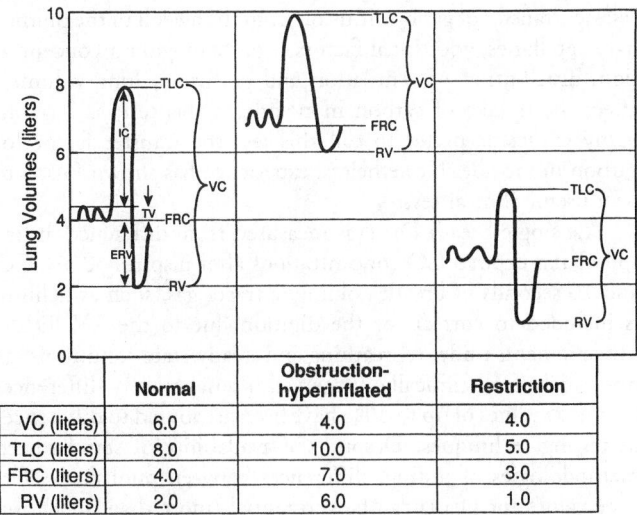

	Normal	Obstruction-hyperinflated	Restriction
VC (liters)	6.0	4.0	4.0
TLC (liters)	8.0	10.0	5.0
FRC (liters)	4.0	7.0	3.0
RV (liters)	2.0	6.0	1.0

FIGURE 387.4. Absolute lung volumes in a normal person, a patient with hyperinflation secondary to obstructive airways disease, and a patient with restrictive lung disease. VC, vital capacity (the volume expired from a maximal inspiration); TLC, total lung capacity (to full expiration); RV, residual volume; FRC, functional residual capacity (volume at end of a normal tidal breath); IC, inspiratory capacity; TV, tidal volume; ERV, expiratory reserve volume.

derestimate volumes in patients with obstructive airway or bullous diseases because of impaired communication between proximal airways and distal airspaces. Body plethysmography can measure lung volumes accurately in such patients but requires equipment and levels of technical expertise that are not available in many hospitals. The accuracy of radiographic TLC measurements (15% or greater) limits their clinical usefulness in individual patients, except when determining changes in volumes from serial radiographs.

Accurate measurements of RV, FRC, and TLC give a better appreciation of the impressive hyperinflation of lung volumes that can occur in severe obstructive lung disease (Fig. 387.4). Measurements of TLC facilitate recognition of restrictive processes superimposed on obstructive disease and increase the detection of mild obstructive disease in some patients.

MAXIMAL INSPIRATORY PRESSURES

Maximal inspiratory pressures (MIP) is more specific for neuromuscular disease than reductions in VC and is useful for identifying patients weanable from mechanical ventilation. MIP may also be decreased by severe hyperinflation, electrolyte derangements, or nutrition deficiencies. The wide range of predictive values limits the sensitivity of these tests. Tests for the early recognition of respiratory muscle fatigue, a significant determinant of dyspnea, are complex and available only in specialized laboratories.

DIFFUSING CAPACITY OF CARBON MONOXIDE

Although the diffusing capacity of carbon monoxide (D_{LCO}) assesses transfer of gas by diffusion from the alveoli to the pulmonary capillaries, additional factors (e.g., hemoglobin concentration, distribution of ventilation and perfusion, lung volumes) affect the uptake of carbon monoxide in this test; as a result, many clinicians prefer to call this test the transfer factor for carbon monoxide. Nonetheless, experience has shown D_{LCO} to be a useful clinical test.

The single-breath D_{LCO} is measured from differences in inspired and expired CO concentrations after inspiring 0.3% CO and 10 seconds of breath holding; a tracer gas, such as helium, is included to correct for the dilution due to the RV. D_{LCO} measurements under rebreathing and steady-state conditions are not widely used clinically. Observed interlaboratory differences for D_{LCO} values of up to 40% have been attributed to differences in testing techniques. Despite the availability of standardized methodologies of testing, differences between published reference values for D_{LCO} can be substantial (more than 30%) and necessitate confirmation that the predicted values used are appropriate for specific testing systems.

The D_{LCO} is increased in pulmonary hemorrhage, polycythemia, and some cases of asthma or early congestive heart failure. The D_{LCO} is frequently decreased in severe anemia, interstitial diseases, emphysema, congestive heart failure, and pulmonary

vascular diseases (e.g., emboli). Although the D_{LCO} is often the most sensitive standard pulmonary function test for detecting early interstitial or pulmonary vascular disease, a normal test does not rule out these disorders. Although nonspecific, the D_{LCO} is a reasonable early test for the evaluation of a patient complaining of dyspnea.

EXERCISE TESTING

Spirometry before and after exercise identifies exercise-induced asthma. Observing simple tests of exercise capacity (e.g., the distance walked in 12 minutes) often clarifies the specific symptoms that limit exercise and the severity of exercise limitation and dyspnea.

Measurement of exercise PaO_2 and $PaCO_2$ detects dysfunction not present at rest and identifies the need for ambulatory oxygen supplementation. Increased physiologic dead space (V_{DS}) as measured by the V_{DS}-to-V_T ratio can be a sensitive but nonspecific indicator of lung dysfunction during exercise. Increases in $PaCO_2$ during exercise may reflect limited lung reserve but can also reflect alterations in ventilatory drive. Oxygen uptake during maximal exercise (VO_2max), a measure of maximal work, may be useful in assessing patients being considered for disability compensation, cardiac surgery, resectional lung surgery, or heart or lung transplantation. Assessments of changes in FRC and flow limitation of tidal volumes during exercise can identify causes of dyspnea not detected during conventional testing but are currently available in relatively few centers.

OTHER TESTS

Tests for small-airway disease (e.g., closing volume, flow–volume curves before and after inhalation of helium–oxygen mixtures, and frequency dependence of compliance) now play a limited role in clinical practice because they do not identify those patients whose airway disease will progress to disabling disease. Tests of distribution of ventilation (e.g., from multiple-breath nitrogen washout measurements of lung volumes) may be helpful in identifying patients with mild obstructive airway disease. Other specialized tests (e.g., physiologic dead space, airway resistance, lung compliance, tests of control of ventilation) have clinical applications but are often available only in specialized tertiary laboratories, such as at centers involved with lung volume reduction surgery.

SCREENING TESTS

The use of pulmonary function tests to screen for early airway disease is not recommended because there is no evidence that earlier therapy has an effect on long-range outcome. However, when appropriately utilized, screening can be useful for persons facing future occupational exposure to noxious inhalants, for the preoperative evaluation of selected patients, and for patients undergoing therapy that could cause pulmonary dysfunction (e.g., therapy with bleomycin).

INTERPRETATION OF RESULTS

Few medical tests are as dependent on patient cooperation as many tests of pulmonary function. Reductions of VC, TLC, or FEV_1 can readily be caused by inadequate patient effort or a patient's poor understanding of the ventilatory maneuvers required. Test reports should always be reviewed for comments regarding such factors that might influence their validity. Additional clues may be the reproducibility of duplicate maneuvers and whether the actual tracings are consistent with adequate effort.

After confirming that the tests were performed adequately and that the predicted values are appropriate for the specific patient being studied, the interpretation should address the following four basic questions:

- Is the test normal?
- Does the pattern of abnormalities suggest a specific category of disease?
- What is the severity of disease?
- What changes have been observed since previous tests?

Is the Test Normal?

Normal values for most pulmonary function tests should be adjusted for relevant determinants (age, height, race, and sex). If predicted values of FVC, FEV_1, and TLC from studies of white subjects are used for black or Asian patients, they should be reduced by 12%, or prediction equations specific for Asian and blacks can be used. For spirometry and most pulmonary function tests, predicted values from commonly used published studies are reasonably comparable. For other tests (e.g., D_{LCO}, MIP), predicted values may differ substantially, most likely because of differences in testing methodologies and possibly also from differences in the subjects tested. Until standardization of testing methodologies is sufficiently widespread to allow standardized prediction equations appropriate for all laboratories, the adequacy of prediction equations (and testing methodologies) is best confirmed by testing disease-free subjects representative of a hospital's patient population.

For most pulmonary function tests, results from normal subjects fall in a gaussian distribution that allows prediction of limits of normal from the predicted value and the standard deviation of the predicted values for that specific patient. For nongaussian distributions, limits of normal can be defined by analysis of percentiles of the study population. The 95% confidence limits for the range of normal values are determined by a 2-tailed t test; 2.5% of a normal population fall below the lower limit of normal. In most cases, however, disease only causes changes in one direction (e.g., reduced FEV_1 in COPD). In such situations, it is more appropriate to define only the lower limit of normal by a 1-tailed t test; 5% of a normal population is expected to have values below this limit.

Caution must be used in interpreting results that are near

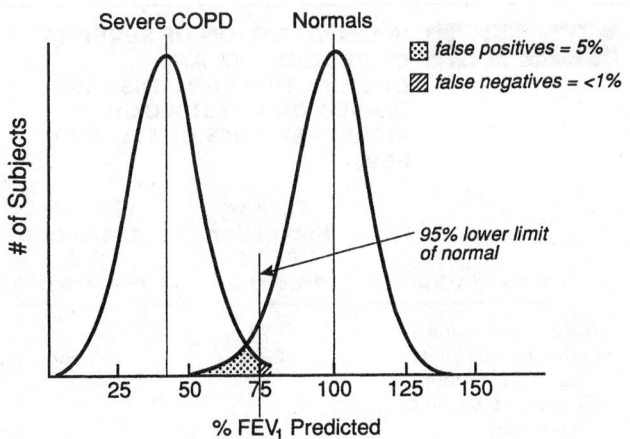

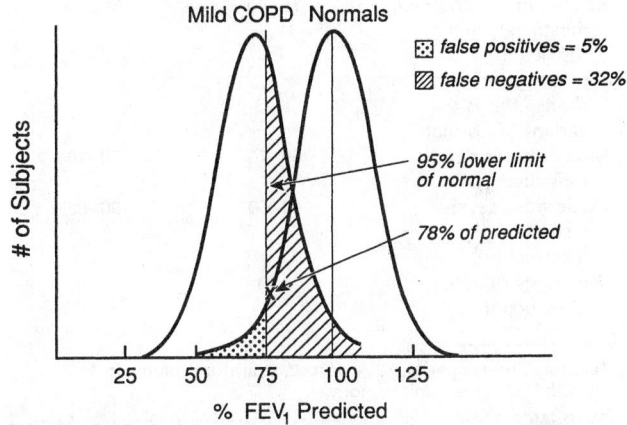

FIGURE 387.5. Comparison of distribution of FEV_1 values in a sample of normal adults and a sample of patients with severe COPD. In contrast to the top graph, in the bottom graph the sample of patients with mild COPD (mean FEV_1 = 68% of predicted) shows considerable overlap with a normal population. More than 30% of patients with mild disease are falsely labeled as normal, using the conventional lower limit of normal (p = .05). FEV_1, forced expiratory volume in the first second of expiration; COPD, chronic obstructive pulmonary disease.

the limits of normal. As illustrated in Fig. 387.5, the 95% lower limit of normal for FEV_1 would be a relatively good criterion for identifying patients with severe COPD because there is relatively little overlap with normal subjects. In contrast, because of the overlap in FEV_1 between patients with mild COPD and normal subjects, over 30% of a population of patients with mild COPD may have FEV_1 greater than the lower limit of normal. If a patient's result is just above the lower limits of normal (e.g., 78% of predicted), it would be misleading to conclude that the patient is normal—the result could represent a low normal and could also represent mild COPD. Table 387.1 illustrates how interpretations can be worded to reflect this overlap of mild dysfunction and limits of normalcy.

A second important consideration regarding limits of normal is that they do not predict the probability of disease but rather the probability that the value would occur in a sample of normal subjects. To predict the probability of disease, one would need to know both the distribution of values in a sample of patients with disease and the prevalence of disease in the patients being

TABLE 387.1.	INTERPRETATION OF SEVERITY OF RESTRICTIVE AND OBSTRUCTIVE LUNG DISEASE (BASED ON PHYSIOLOGIC MEASUREMENTS OF TLC AND FEV$_1$)

Interpretation	TLC for Restriction (% of Predicted)	FEV$_1$ for Obstruction (% of Predicted)
Within normal limits	≥90	≥90
Within normal limits but is a low-normal: could also be mild restriction (obstruction)	80–90	LLN–90
Below limits of normal; most likely mild restriction (obstruction); small chance this is a variant of normal	70–80	70–LLN
Moderate restriction (obstruction)	60–70	60–70
Moderately severe restriction (obstruction)	50–60	50–60
Severe restriction (obstruction)	<50	<50

TLC, total lung capacity; FEV$_1$, forced expiratory volume in 1 second; LLN, lower limit of normal.

EVIDENCE LEVEL: B. Reference: American Thoracic Society Official Statement: Lung function testing: selection of reference values and interpretative strategies. *Am Rev Respir Dis* 1991;144:1202–1218.

tested—information that is seldom available. If an FEV$_1$ of 78% of predicted (Fig. 387.5) was from an asymptomatic student in a screening survey, the probability is higher that the subject is normal than it would be if the result was from a clinic patient with complaints of wheezing.

Does the Dysfunction Suggest a Specific Category of Disease?

The symptom that usually leads to an assessment of lung function is dyspnea, a ubiquitous symptom with a complex differential diagnosis. Although it is rare that pulmonary function testing indicates a specific diagnosis, the results frequently suggest a category of diseases that substantially narrows the differential diagnosis.

Lung dysfunction leading to dyspnea can be divided into three basic physiologic categories: obstructive, restrictive, and vascular. Patients with obstructive lung disease are identified from reductions of flow rates during maximal inspiration and expiration. Then, based on additional clinical information, the disease can be subdivided into the following subcategories: localized obstruction (e.g., tracheal stenosis), asthma, chronic bronchitis, emphysema, and other diseases causing obstruction of small airways such as bronchiolitis.

Restrictive lung diseases are characterized physiologically by a reduction in TLC. This broad category can then be subdivided into pleural diseases; alveolar filling processes; interstitial diseases; neuromuscular involvement of respiratory muscles; and thoracic cage abnormalities, which include intra-abdominal processes such as pregnancy or tense ascites as well as chest wall problems such as scoliosis.

Diseases involving the pulmonary vascular bed (e.g., emboli, vasculitis) do not result in patterns of gas exchange or ventilatory dysfunction specific for these disorders. Instead, they are suggested from pulmonary function tests by their typical abnormalities (reduced PaO$_2$ at rest or during exercise, reduced DLCO, increased VDS-to-VT ratio) in the absence of evidence of other lung diseases.

How Severe Is the Disease?

Table 387.1 provides a guideline for interpreting the severity of dysfunction for both restrictive and obstructive lung disease based on measurements of TLC and FEV$_1$, respectively. Such guidelines are, however, somewhat arbitrary and may not meaningfully reflect the severity of the disease process in individual patients. For example, if a patient had a high-normal TLC of 115% of that predicted before developing pulmonary fibrosis, a decrease in the TLC to 72% of that predicted could represent much more severe disease than if the healthy baseline value was 84% of that predicted.

Assigning a patient's disease to somewhat simplistic categories of severity may be much less useful clinically than using physiologic data to answer more meaningful questions. Such questions include the following: What is the estimated 5-year survival rate if the patient is not treated? Is the severity of airway obstruction consistent with the patient's PaCO$_2$ of 55 mm Hg? What is the risk of lung resection in this patient?

Are There Significant Changes Since Previous Testing?

When interpreting serial studies, consideration must be given to possible interlaboratory differences, normal variability on repeat testing, and the effects of growth or aging (which, ideally, should be based on cross-sectional rather than longitudinal studies).

BIBLIOGRAPHY

American Thoracic Society. Lung function testing: selection of reference values and interpretative strategies. *Am Rev Respir Dis* 1991;144:1202–1218.

American Thoracic Society. Standardization of spirometry, 1994 Update. *Am J Respir Crit Care Med* 1995;152:1107–1136.

American Thoracic Society. Single-breath carbon monoxide diffusing capacity (transfer factor): recommendations for a standard technique—1995 update. *Am J Respir Crit Care Med* 1995;152:2185–2198.

Babb TG, Rodarte JR. Exercise capacity and breathing mechanics in patients with airflow limitation. *Med Sci Sports Exerc* 1992;24:967–974.

Carlin BW, Clausen JL, Ries AL. The use of cutaneous oximetry in the prescription of long-term oxygen therapy. *Chest* 1988;94:239–241.

Cotes JE. *Lung function: assessment and application in medicine*, fifth edition. Oxford: Blackwell Scientific Publications, 1993.

Crapo RO. Pulmonary function testing. *N Engl J Med* 1994;331:25–30.

O'Brien GM, Furukawa S, Kuzma AM, et al. Improvements in lung function, exercise, and quality of life in hypercapnic COPD patients after lung volume reduction surgery. *Chest* 1999;115:75–84.

Rochester DF. Respiratory muscles and ventilatory failure: 1993 perspective. *Am J Med Sci* 1993;305:394–402.

Simard AA, Maltais F, LeBlanc P. Functional outcome of patients with chronic obstructive pulmonary disease and exercise hypercapnia. *Eur Respir J* 1995;8:1339–1344.

Kelley's Textbook of Internal Medicine, fourth edition. Edited by H. David Humes.
Lippincott Williams & Wilkins, Philadelphia © 2000.

C H A P T E R

388

HEMODYNAMIC AND RESPIRATORY MONITORING IN CRITICAL CARE

BARBARA A. COCKRILL

Critically ill patients often suffer from derangements in the cardiovascular and respiratory systems. The field of critical care has developed in large part because of the relatively recent ability of the clinician to monitor and intervene in these derangements. This chapter will discuss monitoring techniques frequently used in critical care medicine. The first section discusses hemodynamic pressure measurements, the second covers ventilation and carbon dioxide exchange, and the third discusses monitoring parameters of oxygenation.

▌ MONITORING HEMODYNAMIC PRESSURES

ARTERIAL PRESSURE

All patients in the intensive care unit (ICU) should have frequent assessment of peripheral blood pressure. For many, an automated blood pressure cuff, which automatically inflates at regular intervals, is sufficient. The cuff is placed on the upper arm, and pressure is recorded digitally on a screen.

Placement of an intra-arterial catheter for invasive monitoring of peripheral blood pressure is indicated for patients with the potential for rapid changes in hemodynamic status, those in whom vasoactive drugs are being used, or in patients with respiratory failure who need frequent blood gas analysis. The most common site for an arterial line is the radial artery. This site is easily accessible, relatively comfortable for the patient, and carries a low risk of ischemic injury. Before cannulating a radial artery, an Allen test should be performed to confirm adequate collateral flow via the ulnar artery. The examiner manually compresses both arteries until the patient's hand becomes pale. Pressure on the ulnar artery is released: the hand should flush pink

within 5 to 7 seconds, indicating adequate perfusion from the ulnar artery. If not, another site should be used for the arterial access. If the Allen test has been properly performed, the risk of ischemic damage to the hand is low. Other potential sites include the ulnar, brachial, femoral, and dorsalis pedis arteries. The contour of the arterial waveform changes depending on the site of measurement (Fig. 388.1). At sites more distal to the aorta the systolic pressure will be higher and the diastolic pressure lower; however, the *mean* arterial blood pressure (MAP) is essentially constant. Systolic pressure in the dorsal pedis artery may be as much as 25 mm Hg higher than that recorded from the radial artery.

Inaccurate transmission of pressures due to "overdamping" is a frequent pitfall in pressure monitoring. Overdamping results in a waveform that is blunted: systolic pressure appears lower than the actual pressure, and diastolic appears higher. The presence of air bubbles in the pressure tubing is the most common cause. Because the air is compressible, the bubble will "cushion" the transmission of pressure. The mean pressure is still accurate, but systolic hypertension and/or diastolic hypotension will be missed. The latter becomes critically important for patients with myocardial hypoperfusion. The left ventricle is primarily perfused during diastole; isolated diastolic hypotension may result in cardiac ischemia.

Local hemorrhage, infection, and thrombosis are all potentially serious complications of arterial catheters. Hemorrhage is best controlled with local compression as most sites are superficial. The risk of bacteremia with arterial catheters is roughly 4% in large series, although local colonization rates are higher. Risk factors for infection include (a) placement by surgical cut-down

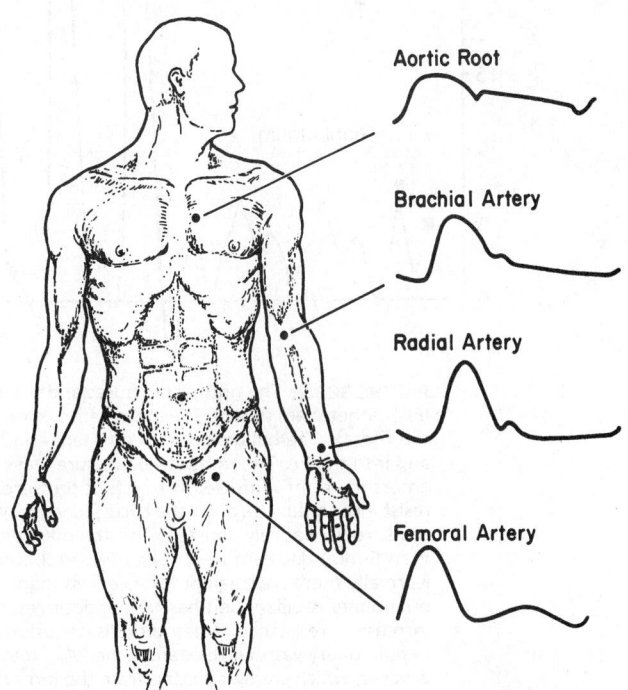

FIGURE 388.1. The arterial waveform recorded from different parts of the arterial tree. (From Marino PL. *The ICU book*. Philadelphia: Lea & Febiger 1991:91, with permission.)

(ninefold increase); (b) local inflammation; and (c) a longer duration of cannulation. A catheter should not be placed through inflamed skin and should be removed as soon as it is no longer needed. In most studies, the infection rate is similar for femoral lines as compared with radial lines.

The incidence of clinically significant arterial occlusion is low (less than 1% in large series), although radiographic occlusion is present in 25%. Risk factors for ischemia include (a) a large-bore cannula; (b) systemic hypotension; (c) severe peripheral vascular disease; and (d) the use of systemic vasopressor agents. An 18-gauge catheter is associated with a fourfold increase in radial artery occlusion, as compared with a 20-gauge catheter. It is recommended that a 20-gauge line be used, especially in a smaller individual. Patients with vasospastic disease, such as severe Raynaud's phenomenon, may also be at increased risk and must be monitored closely.

PULMONARY ARTERY CATHETERS

Pulmonary artery (PA) or Swan–Ganz catheters are long, flow-directed, balloon-tipped catheters that are inserted via the central venous circulation through the right heart and into the PA. Most catheters also have a thermistor at the distal end to allow the measurement of thermodilution cardiac output. Pulmonary vascular resistance (PVR) and systemic vascular resistance (SVR) are derived from the measured pressure and cardiac output values. Mixed venous blood from the pulmonary artery may also be obtained.

Clinical Indications

In complicated critically ill patients, the hemodynamic profile is difficult to assess by clinical examination alone. In one study, clinicians accurately predicted the hemodynamic profile less than 50% of the time in patients who subsequently had PA catheters inserted. Furthermore, the information gained from PA monitoring frequently resulted in a change in therapy. The situations in which a PA catheter may be useful include (a) hypotension despite adequate fluid resuscitation; (b) pulmonary edema unresponsive to empirical diuresis; (c) pulmonary edema associated with hypotension and/or pulmonary hypertension; and (d) respiratory failure in which high levels of positive end-expiratory pressure (PEEP) are required. The information gained from a

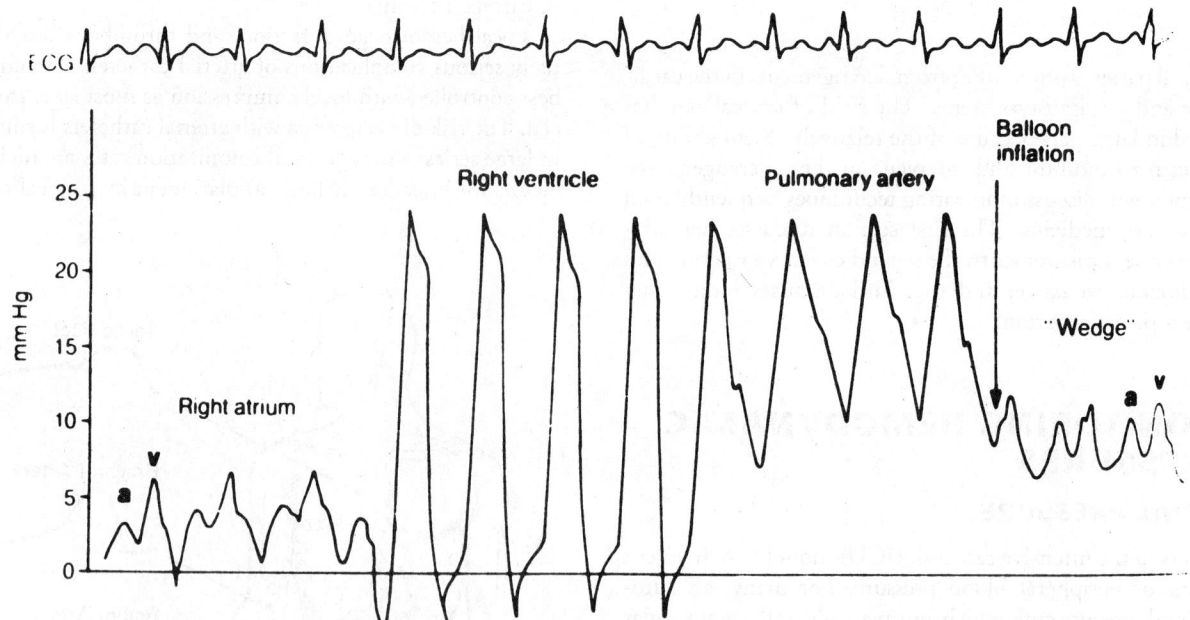

FIGURE 388.2. The normal pressures and waveforms demonstrated on insertion of a pulmonary artery (PA) catheter are shown. The appearance of respiratory variation indicates that the catheter has entered the thorax. The balloon is then inflated, and blood flow directs the catheter through the right heart and into the PA. The right atrial pressure waveform shows characteristic a and v waves. As the catheter enters the right ventricle (RV), systolic pressure rises and diastolic pressure is unchanged due to the low resistance to flow through the tricuspid valve. When the catheter traverses the pulmonary valve, systolic pressure is relatively constant and the diastolic pressure rises. It is not unusual to observe a small (less than 5 mm) decrease in systolic pressure between the RV and PA (PA), especially in high-flow states. Normally there is a small difference (less than 5 mm Hg) between PA_{dia} and left atrial pressure (LA). The pulmonary capillary bed has tremendous reserve, so that increases in flow are not associated with an increase in resistance. When there is occlusion or loss of the pulmonary capillary bed and an elevation in pulmonary vascular resistance, the PA_{dia} may exceed LA significantly. The wedge tracing shows a and v waves, which are transmitted from the left atrium. The v wave occurs after the T wave on a simultaneously recorded electrocardiogram (see text). Pulmonary and systemic vascular resistance (PVR and SVR) are calculated using the cardiac output (CO): PVR = (PA_{mean} − PAOP)/CO; SVR = (MAP − RA)/CO. (From Mathay MA. Invasive hemodynamic monitoring in critically ill patients. *Clin Chest Med* 1983;4:233, with permission.)

PA catheter is probably most helpful in balancing two often opposing goals: (a) minimizing pulmonary venous pressure and edema; and (b) optimizing left-heart filling pressures.

The subclavian and internal jugular veins are the most common insertion sites. The subclavian is more comfortable for the patient but carries an increased risk of pneumothorax (1% to 2%) and bleeding (because the subclavian artery is not compressible). The internal jugular route is preferred in patients with hyperinflation or on mechanical ventilation due to the lower incidence of pneumothorax.

The pressure tracing should be continuously displayed and recorded during insertion to allow complete analysis (Fig. 388.2). The catheter is advanced though the right heart into the PA until the balloon lodges in a smaller branch and the typical "wedge" tracing appears. Once the balloon is wedged, a static column of blood develops between the catheter tip and the next junction between flowing and nonflowing blood: the junction or "J" point (Fig. 388.3). Because of the static column of blood, the pressure measured at the catheter tip (pulmonary artery occlusion pressure, PAOP) is equal to the pressure at the J point. The J point is usually at the level of the pulmonary veins. Under normal circumstances, the PAOP accurately reflects left ventricular end-diastolic pressure (LVEDP) because there is no obstruction between the pulmonary veins and the left ventricle at end diastole when the pulmonary veins and mitral valve are normal. Thus, the PAOP is equal to the J-point pressure, which is equal to the LVEDP.

In a number of conditions, the PAOP does not accurately reflect the LVEDP (Fig. 388.3). The easiest circumstance to

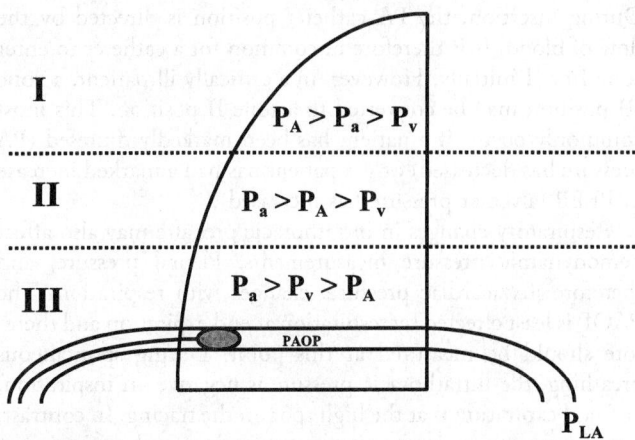

FIGURE 388.4. The lung is partitioned into three zones based on the relationship between the alveolar pressure (P_A), the mean pulmonary arterial pressure (P_a), and the pulmonary venous pressure (P_v). The pulmonary artery occlusion pressure (PAOP) is an accurate measurement of the downstream left atrial pressure (P_{LA}) *only* when P_v exceeds P_A (zone III). (Adapted from Marino PL. *The ICU book.* Philadelphia: Lea & Febiger, 1991:125, with permission.)

understand is that of mitral stenosis. In the presence of mitral stenosis, the pressure at the J point is higher than LVEDP due to obstruction to blood flow at the mitral valve. The pressure in the left atrium (LA) is accurately measured in mitral stenosis. Pulmonary edema may be present in mitral stenosis due to elevated pulmonary capillary pressures up-stream from the site of obstruction. If the obstruction to flow is distal to the J point but proximal to the LA (such as with an obstructing left atrial myxoma), the PAOP will be higher than both the LA pressure and the LVEDP.

The term pulmonary capillary wedge pressure (PCWP) is often used interchangeably with PAOP and is so much part of medical jargon that it is likely to prevail. Note that pulmonary *capillary* wedge pressure is not correct in that the occlusion pressure reflects pulmonary capillary pressure only when the catheter is wedged. Once the balloon is deflated and flow continues through the pulmonary capillaries, the actual capillary pressure (and tendency for edema formation) may be higher. This is why patients with pulmonary veno-occlusive disease (a rare disorder characterized by obstruction at the site of the pulmonary venules) will have pulmonary edema with a normal PAOP (Fig. 388.3).

The use of positive-pressure mechanical ventilation may also affect the accuracy of PAOP measurement. The lung can be divided into three zones based on the relative pressures of the pulmonary arteries, pulmonary veins, and the alveoli. Note that the PAOP reflects the J-point pressure only if the catheter is in zone III (Fig. 388.4). If the catheter enters zone I or II (alveolar pressure less than pulmonary venous pressure), when the balloon is up and the catheter is wedged, the pulmonary capillary pressure is equal to the pulmonary venous pressure, and the capillaries will therefore be compressed by alveolar pressure. Thus, alveolar pressure will be measured, not the downstream J-point pressure. Most of the lung is under zone III conditions in the supine patient, and most of the blood flows through zone III.

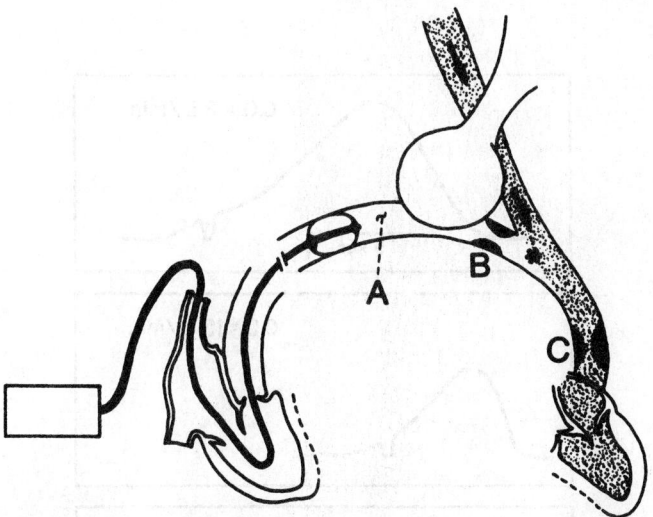

FIGURE 388.3. Definition of the pulmonary artery occlusion pressure (PAOP). The PAOP measured at point A is nearly identical to the pressure at the junction of static and flowing venous blood (J point, *). This site is generally in a pulmonary vein of equal size to the artery that has been occluded. The PAOP will not be influenced by partial occlusions of the static column (B), as would be seen in the rare disorder pulmonary veno-occlusive disease. However, obstructions (C) downstream of the junction point dissipate pressure, causing PAOP to significantly exceed the mean left atrial pressure, as is seen in an obstructing left atrial myxoma or mitral stenosis. (From Marini JJ, Wheeler AP. *Critical care medicine: the essentials.* Baltimore: Williams & Wilkins, 1989:17, with permission.)

During insertion, the PA catheter position is directed by the flow of blood. It is therefore uncommon for a catheter to enter zone I or II initially. However, in a critically ill patient, a zone III position may be converted to a zone II position. This most commonly occurs if a patient has been markedly diuresed (PA pressure has decreased) or if a patient has had a marked increase in PEEP (alveolar pressure has increased).

Respiratory changes in intrathoracic pressure may also affect hemodynamic pressure measurements. Pleural pressure, and therefore juxtacardiac pressure, changes with respiration. The PAOP is least effected by respiration at end expiration and therefore should be measured at this point. During spontaneous breathing, the intrathoracic pressure is negative on inspiration, and end expiration is at the high spot on the tracing. In contrast, for patients on positive pressure ventilation, end expiration is represented at the low spot on the tracing.

By definition, PEEP applies positive pressure at end expiration. In compliant lungs this pressure will be transmitted and raise pleural and juxtacardiac pressure at end expiration, and therefore could be reflected in the measured PAOP. However, in clinical practice it is unusual for transmitted PEEP to account a large part of the measured PAOP. With less than 10 cm PEEP transmission is not clinically significant. In general, only patients with low pulmonary compliance require high levels of PEEP, and in this case typically 25% or less of PEEP is transmitted. Furthermore, it must be remembered that PEEP is measured in centimeters of H_2O and PAOP in millimeters of Hg. Fourteen cm H_2O approximately equals 10 mm Hg. This means that on 14 cm of PEEP the typical pressure that may be reflected in the PAOP would be 0.25 × 10 mm Hg = 2.5 mm Hg. A PEEP trial is helpful when high levels (more than 12 cm) are used.

Complications

The complications of PA catheters can be divided into complications of insertion and those associated with an indwelling line. Pneumothorax and infection are complications common to any central line. Because the PA catheter traverses the right heart, arrhythmias may develop but usually are transient. All patients must have a continuous ECG monitor during insertion and while the PA catheter is in place. Premature atrial and ventricular complexes are generally well tolerated, but ventricular tachycardia requiring countershock does occur. Right bundle-branch block develops in a small percentage of patients, and anyone with a preexisting left bundle-branch block should have an external or temporary internal pacemaker in place prior to insertion.

Pulmonary infarction is a serious complication of PA catheters. The risk is increased in patients with poor cardiac output. The risk is reduced by minimizing the time in the wedge position and keeping the catheter from migrating too distally. Daily chest roentgenograms are necessary to check catheter position. The tip of the catheter should be within the shadow of the pulmonary artery. The full 1.5 cm³ of air should be required for balloon inflation to obtain the wedge, and inflation should always be done slowly.

The most devastating complication is pulmonary artery rup-

ture, which has a 75% mortality in some series. Pulmonary hypertension and anticoagulation are the major risk factors, but above-noted factors associated with infarction are also associated with rupture. A contained perforation must be considered in any patient who develops hemoptysis with a pulmonary artery line in place. A contrast chest computed tomography scan will demonstrate a pseudoaneurysm in patients with a contained rupture, which requires radiographically directed embolization or surgery.

THERMODILUTION CARDIAC OUTPUT

Another important function of a PA catheter is to provide thermodilution cardiac output measurements. Cool saline (iced or room temperature) is injected via the catheter into the right atrium where it mixes with and cools the blood. As the cooler blood (and saline) is pumped through the heart and enters the PA, the change in temperature caused by injection of saline will be detected by the thermistor at the distal tip of the catheter. A high cardiac output will cause a rapid change in temperature, as the injectate is rapidly pumped past the thermistor; a low cardiac output will cause a slower change in temperature. The cardiac output is inversely proportional to the area under the curve of the plotted temperature change (Fig. 388.5).

Does the PA catheter help us to treat patients more effectively? Despite the widespread use of the PA catheter and its substantial cost, data to confirm that the procedure is beneficial to patients are lacking. In fact, some recent studies (all observational in design) have suggested that the use of the PA catheter is associated with increased mortality. A large prospective cohort study that examined the association between right heart catheter-

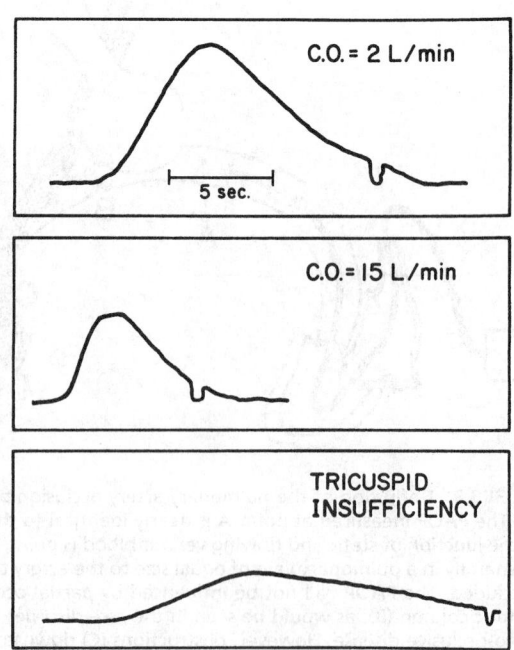

FIGURE 388.5. Thermodilution curves for low cardiac output *(upper)*, high cardiac output *(middle)*, and tricuspid valve insufficiency *(lower)*. (From Marino PL. *The ICU book*. Philadelphia: Lea & Febiger, 1991:125, with permission.)

ization in the first 24 hours of care in the ICU and subsequent survival found a significantly increased 30-day mortality in patients who underwent right heart catheterization. The differences could not be explained by any measure of severity of illness (propensity score, APACHE III score). The following explanations have been suggested for the following sobering results:

■ PA catheterization may be a marker for an aggressive or invasive style of care that may be associated with a higher mortality rate.
■ The information gained from PA catheterization may have been misunderstood or misused.
■ The therapy selected on the basis of the information provided by PA catheterization may lead to a higher mortality.
■ The study may not have adjusted for a confounding variable.

This study reinitiated a long-standing debate about the risk: benefit ratio of PA catheters. The American Thoracic Society, the Society of Critical Care Medicine, the American Association of Critical Care Nurses, the American College of Chest Physicians, and the European Society of Intensive Care Medicine have issued a consensus statement with the following recommendations:

There is currently no indication for a moratorium on the use of PA catheters. Prospective randomized trials of PA catheters are indicated, ethical, and appropriate. The decision to insert a PA catheter should continue to be based on the specific clinical circumstances of a given patient.

■ MONITORING VENTILATION

MECHANICS OF VENTILATION

During normal spontaneous respiration, negative pressure is generated by contraction of the diaphragm, while the intercostals stabilize the rib cage. Exhalation is passive, relying on the intrinsic elastic recoil of the lungs. During respiratory distress, both inspiratory and expiratory accessory muscles are recruited, and exhalation becomes active. In the mechanically ventilated patient, positive inspiratory pressure is generated by the ventilator, and exhalation is either passive or active depending on the patient. Negative-pressure mechanical ventilators, such as the iron lung, are rare in current clinical use.

The most basic form of respiratory monitoring is simple observation. Patients in respiratory distress usually assume a breathing pattern of a rapid rate and small tidal volume (VT). In the setting of diaphragmatic weakness or fatigue, the patient may also develop *abdominal paradox*. This refers to the inward motion of the abdomen on inspiration, and occurs because the diaphragm is not moving normally on inspiration. The term *respiratory alternans* describes the patient who is alternating between a normal pattern (abdomen moves down and out on inspiration) and abdominal paradox. Both of these patterns may be a sign of fatigue and impending hypercapneic respiratory failure.

A maximal inspiratory pressure (MIP) measurement is direct assessment inspiratory muscle strength. This is measured having the patient maximally inspire against an occluded airway. For intubated patients who are unable to cooperate, the endotracheal tube is occluded for 20 seconds or 10 inspiratory efforts, and the maximum force generated is recorded. The MIP is useful for following patients with neuromuscular disease, such as myasthenia gravis, to assess the need for mechanical ventilation, and for patients weaning from the ventilator to assess readiness for discontinuation of mechanical ventilation. The patient who cannot generate an inspiratory force of -20 cm H_2O or less is unlikely to be able to breathe without mechanical support. A single value which is more negative than -20 cm H_2O is not a definite indicator of successful weaning. The MIP measures strength, not endurance; the patient with a very high respiratory load may be unable to sustain adequate ventilation over a long period.

COMPLIANCE

The compliance of the respiratory system (Crs) is a measure of the pressure needed to inflate the lungs and chest wall with a given volume of gas. Intuitively, compliance can be considered as the relative "stiffness" of the respiratory system. Compliance is calculated as change in volume divided by the change in pressure:

$$Crs = \Delta V / \Delta P$$

Static compliance (Cstat) is a measure of the airway pressure required to hold the lungs and chest wall inflated at a given VT. It is determined by stopping flow at end inspiration, allowing a short period for equilibration, and measuring the pressure at the airway (plateau pressure). Because it is measured during a no-flow state, airway resistance does not influence Cstat. When using Cstat clinically, it is assumed that the contribution from the chest wall is fairly constant. In ICU patients, however, chest wall compliance may be variable due to level of sedation, surgery, pain, abdominal distention, respiratory muscle contraction, chest wall edema, and the use of paralytic drugs. Therefore, while determination of the Cstat is a useful parameter, changes do not necessarily indicate a change in the status of the pulmonary parenchyma, and the rest of the clinical picture must be considered.

AIRWAY PRESSURE AND LUNG VOLUMES

The airway pressure parameters that are most important to monitor depend on the mode of ventilation being used. A few points deserve emphasis. There are two basic modes in clinical use: pressure-limited and volume-limited.

During pressure-limited ventilation, the ventilator delivers a set inspiratory pressure. In this case, the tidal volume is the dependent variable. Therefore, changes in respiratory status will be reflected in the tidal volume. The inspiratory pressure will be unchanged because it is set by the ventilator. There are many determinants of the tidal volume, including set pressure level, Crs, inspiratory time, and inspiratory flow rate. Monitoring the tidal volume for a patient on pressure-limited ventilation will provide immediate clues to changes in the respiratory status.

During volume-limited ventilation, the ventilator delivers a set tidal volume. The inspiratory pressure is determined by the airways resistance, Crs, V_T, and the inspiratory flow rate. Peak inspiratory pressure (PIP) is a key parameter to follow in patients on volume-limited ventilation because nonaltered ventilator settings are an indicator of airways resistance and lung compliance. High PIP is associated with barotrauma (including pneumothorax and pneumomediastinum) and overdistention (which causes ongoing pulmonary parenchymal injury). A sudden increase in PIP must be investigated. Comparison of the peak and plateau pressures can provide a clue to the etiology. If plateau pressure is unchanged from baseline (or significantly less than peak), then an increase in airways resistance from bronchospasm, retained secretions, or a kink in ventilator tubing is the major culprit. If plateau pressure is also increased, then atelectasis, pneumothorax, or a right main-stem intubation are possible, as are causes of acute decreases in lung compliance such as congestive heart failure.

DEAD SPACE

The partial pressure of carbon dioxide (CO_2) in the arterial blood (Pa_{CO_2}) is determined by the balance between CO_2 production ($\dot{V}_{CO_2}$) and CO_2 elimination by the lungs. The amount of CO_2 excreted by the lungs is dependent on the alveolar ventilation ($\dot{V}_A$). Thus:

$$Pa_{CO_2} - \dot{V}_{CO_2}/\dot{V}_A$$

Not all of the gas that enters the lungs is active in the exchange of carbon dioxide and oxygen. The tidal volume can be divided into two components: that which participates in gas exchange ($\dot{V}_A$) and that which does not (dead space ventilation, $\dot{V}_{DS}$). That is:

$$V_T = \dot{V}_{DS} + \dot{V}_A$$

The alveolar ventilation is the volume of gas that is in contact with pulmonary capillary blood and is active in gas exchange. Dead space ventilation includes the volume that is in the conducting airways (anatomical dead space) and in alveoli that are not perfused by capillary blood (alveolar dead space). If the fraction of ventilation that goes to dead space ($\dot{V}_{DS}/V_T$) increases, then the total minute ventilation ($\dot{V}_E$) must increase in order to maintain the same $\dot{V}_A$ (and Pa_{CO_2}). This ratio increases in patients on positive-pressure mechanical ventilation but is overcome by increasing total ventilation. The fraction of ventilation that goes to dead space can be approximated as follows:

$$\dot{V}_{DS}/V_T = (Pa_{CO_2} - P_{ECO_2})/Pa_{CO_2}$$

where P_{ECO_2} is the partial pressure of CO_2 in mixed expired gas. This determination requires collection of expired gas and measurement of CO_2, which is time consuming, expensive, and technically difficult. For patients on mechanical ventilation, $\dot{V}_{DS}/V_T$ can be approximated. The condensate in the expiratory circuit trap is constantly exposed to expired gas; therefore the partial pressure of CO_2 of the fluid is the same as that of the expired gas. Thus determination of the P_{CO_2} in the fluid will give an estimate of the P_{ECO_2}. This is done by simply obtaining a "blood gas" analysis on the fluid. Care should be taken to use fresh water, allow equilibration for 5 minutes, and collect the fluid anaerobically. If water that has been sitting in the tap is used, bacterial contamination may cause an artificially high P_{CO_2}, and thus dead space will be underestimated. If exposed to room air, the fluid P_{CO_2} will be artificially low. Dead space is a useful parameter to evaluate in mechanically ventilated patients with respiratory failure. A patient with a dead space ratio of more than 0.6 will generally not be able to sustain the high $\dot{V}_E$ required to wean successfully from mechanical ventilation. (For a more complete discussion of ventilation, see Chapter 10.)

■ MONITORING OXYGEN EXCHANGE

OXIMETRY

The pulse oximeter is an electronic monitoring device that allows noninvasive assessment of hemoglobin saturation. The oximeter transmits two wavelengths of light through pulsating tissue via a probe that usually is applied to the finger or ear lobe. By comparing the light absorption at the two wavelengths, the degree to which hemoglobin is saturated (Sa_{O_2}) can be determined. The four common hemoglobin species are oxyhemoglobin, reduced hemoglobin, carboxyhemoglobin, and methemoglobin. The pulse oximeter, which emits only two wavelengths of light, does not detect carboxyhemoglobin or methemoglobin. This is especially important to consider in the emergency room setting and for patients with smoke inhalation injury. Hemoglobin molecules with CO at the binding sites may register as "saturated" hemoglobin and thus will give a falsely elevated Sa_{O_2}. Methemoglobin may also cause inaccuracies. Some drugs, especially nitrates and inhaled nitric oxide, may elevate methemoglobin. The hallmark of methemoglobinemia is cyanosis despite apparently adequate arterial oxygen levels. If carboxyhemoglobinemia or methemoglobinemia is suspected, blood should be analyzed on a co-oximeter. This device can accurately measure hemoglobin, oxyhemoglobin, carboxyhemoglobin, and methemoglobin.

Pulse oximetry is very useful for monitoring trends in individual patients. It has pitfalls and does not replace arterial blood gas determinations. The reading is accurate at ± 4 percentage points if the saturation is above 75%, but the accuracy decreases at saturations below 75%. The oximeter uses the difference between systolic and diastolic values to factor out the absorption due to tissues; in low perfusion states, a lack of pulse differential may lead to incorrect values. If a good pulse tracing is not obtained, the reading should not be considered accurate. Darkly pigmented skin may also cause inaccuracies: one study found that when titrating oxygen therapy a higher pulse oximetry saturation target is needed (more than 95%) in black individuals. Other factors that may cause an incorrect saturation determination include the use of intravascular dyes such as methylene blue and indocyanine green, high levels of ambient light, and dark-colored nail polish. The oximeter may be inaccurate by four percentage points or more under the best circumstances. In addition, the pulse oximeter gives no information regarding $PaCO_2$. Hypoventilation and hypercarbia are often present without coexisting falls in SaO_2.

BLOOD GAS ANALYSIS

A blood gas refers to the measurement of the partial pressures of oxygen (PaO_2), carbon dioxide ($PaCO_2$), and pH. Blood gases may be monitored either by a single sample drawn via needle puncture, or by drawing from an indwelling arterial catheter. Specimens drawn from a catheter more accurately reflect the steady-state blood gas because the patient is less likely to experience an acute change in breathing patterns as with an arterial puncture.

To ensure a steady state, arterial blood gases should be drawn after at least 10 minutes on a stable inspired oxygen (FiO_2), and more time may be required in patients with severe lung disease. Specimens are placed on ice and analyzed within 30 minutes. Leaving a blood sample at room temperature or a delay in analysis may lead to falsely low values of PaO_2 and/or falsely high values of $PaCO_2$, because leukocytes in the blood continue to be metabolically active, consuming oxygen and producing carbon dioxide. In the presence of very high leukocyte (more than 100,000 K) counts, falsely low PaO_2 is common because of the rapid oxygen consumption by the leukocytes ("leukocyte larceny"). In this case, samples must be run immediately in order to obtain an accurate PaO_2. In cases of marginal oxygenation, recognition of the patient's positional effects on oxygenation may help with management.

ALVEOLAR/ARTERIAL OXYGEN GRADIENT

The alveolar/arterial gradient [$P(A-a)O_2$] refers to the difference between alveolar and arterial oxygen, and quantifies the efficiency of transfer of oxygen from alveoli to blood. In order to determine the gradient, the partial pressure of oxygen in the alveoli (PAO_2) is calculated from the modified alveolar gas equation. On room air at sea level, this equation simplifies to

$$PAO_2 = 150 - 1.25(PaCO_2)$$

The $P(A-a)O_2$ gradient is calculated by subtracting the measured PaO_2 obtained by blood gas from the *derived* value for PAO_2. The $P(A-a)O_2$ calculation takes alveolar CO_2 partial pressure into account and therefore is most useful in distinguishing hypoxia due to hypercarbia from hypoxia due to other causes. Patients with hypoxia due to hypercarbia will still have a normal $P(A-a)O_2$. On room air the normal value is less than 10 mm Hg. Because the normal $P(A-a)O_2$ is effected by increasing FiO_2 and changes in mixed venous oxygen saturation, it is much less helpful in patients on supplemental oxygen. The PaO_2/FiO_2 ratio is also a commonly used index in critical care, but it is influenced by changes in FiO_2 and is therefore imprecise.

SHUNT FRACTION

The shunt fraction ($\dot{Q}s/\dot{Q}t$) is the fraction of the systemic cardiac output ($\dot{Q}t$) that reaches the arterial circulation without exposure

to alveolar oxygen. The oxygen content of shunted blood is therefore equal to that of mixed venous blood. In normals, $\dot{Q}s/\dot{Q}t$ is less than 5% and comprises venous return to the left atrium from bronchial, pleural, and thebesian veins. Determination of shunt fraction is a useful exercise in the hypoxic ICU patient. Hypoxia due to large shunt fractions (more than 25%) is unresponsive to increases in FiO_2; therefore, the presence of a large shunt should encourage the clinician to decrease FiO_2 to levels below the toxic range. Elevated levels should also alert the clinician to search for intracardiac shunts and/or pulmonary arteriovenous malformations. Right to left shunting may develop through the patent foramen in the setting of severe pulmonary hypertension and elevated right-sided pressures. Efforts to decrease the elevated right-sided pressures or, occasionally, to increase the left heart pressures may be useful in decreasing the degree of shunt. Approximately 30% of adults have a probe patent foramen ovale.

Most patients in the ICU are hypoxic due to a combination of ventilation–perfusion ($\dot{V}/\dot{Q}$) mismatching and shunt, and occasionally a low mixed venous oxygen. In order to determine the "true" shunt, blood gases must be drawn while the patient is breathing 100% oxygen, or areas of $\dot{V}/\dot{Q}$ mismatching will also contribute to the hypoxia. Fifteen minutes of 100% FiO_2 must be allowed prior to drawing arterial and mixed venous blood gases. If inhalation of 100% O_2 is prolonged, absorption atelectasis will develop, further contributing to the shunt fraction. The shunt fraction is calculated as follows:

$$\dot{Q}s/\dot{Q}t = (Cc'O_2 - CaO_2)/(Cc'O_2 - CvO2)$$

where CaO_2 is the oxygen content of arterial blood, CvO_2 is the oxygen content of mixed venous blood, and $Cc'O_2$ is the oxygen content of end-capillary blood in the lungs. End-capillary blood is assumed to have a PO_2 equal to that of PAO_2 (calculated with the alveolar gas equation), and the saturation is determined by the oxygen dissociation curve.

OXYGEN CONTENT

The oxygen content of blood refers to the total amount of oxygen in the blood and is composed of oxygen that is dissolved in the plasma and oxygen that is bound to hemoglobin. The partial pressure of oxygen (PaO_2) reflects the amount dissolved in plasma. The amount of oxygen bound to hemoglobin is typically quantified as the percentage of hemoglobin that is saturated with oxygen (SaO_2). The formula for arterial oxygen content is as follows (amount dissolved + amount bound to hemoglobin):

$$CaO_2 \text{ (mL/dL)} = (0.003 \times PaO_2) + (1.39 + [Hb] + SaO_2)$$

Factors that lead to fewer binding sites on hemoglobin molecules include anemia and binding by substances that have a higher affinity for hemoglobin than oxygen, such as carbon monoxide. The affinity of hemoglobin for oxygen is decreased with abnormal hemoglobins and by the factors associated with shifting the oxyhemoglobin dissociation curve to the left (Fig. 388.6). Note that when the number of binding sites on hemoglobin is

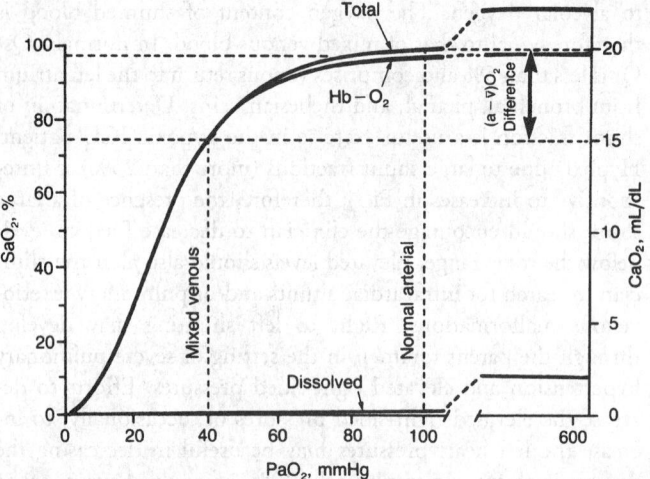

FIGURE 388.6. The oxyhemoglobin dissociation curve, relating the partial pressure of oxygen (O_2) in systemic arterial blood (Pa_{O_2}), in millimeters of mercury, to systemic arterial saturation (Sa_{O_2}), in percent, and to the O_2 content of systemic arterial blood (Ca_{O_2}), in milliliters per deciliter of blood. A normal hemoglobin (Hb) concentration of 15 g per deciliter is assumed, as is an unshifted dissociation curve. The curve descends steeply below Pa_{O_2} values of 50 to 60 mm Hg, indicating severely reduced O_2-carrying capacity by Hb below this Pa_{O_2}. The lower line represents O_2 bound to Hb plus O_2 dissolved. Dissolved O_2 contributes little to Ca_{O_2} at a Pa_{O_2} in the normal range. (From Luce JM, Tyler ML, Pierson DJ. *Intensive respiratory care.* Philadelphia: WB Saunders, 1984:26, with permission.)

decreased, it follows that the oxygen content will be decreased even if the hemoglobin saturation is normal!

OXYGEN DELIVERY

Two components are involved in providing delivery of oxygen to the tissues: arterial oxygen content and cardiac output ($\dot{Q}$). The oxygen delivery (D_{O_2}) is equal to the arterial oxygen content multiplied by the cardiac output:

$$D_{O_2} = Ca_{O_2} \times \dot{Q}$$

When oxygen demand is increased, the normal response is an increase in cardiac output. With further stress, the tissues increase oxygen extraction such that the oxygen content of mixed venous blood decreases. The normal arterial content is approximately 20 mL O_2 per 100 mL of blood, and the resting difference between arterial and venous oxygen content is approximately 5 mL per 100 mL (Fig. 388.6). Therefore, the extraction ratio is 25%; only one-fourth of the total oxygen that is delivered is actually taken up by the tissue. This ratio rises when more oxygen is extracted peripherally, and consequently the oxygen content of mixed venous blood (Cv_{O_2}) falls. In most clinical situations, low-oxygen mixed venous content is a reliable indicator that the extraction ratio is increased and oxygen delivery is inadequate. This can be confirmed by measuring lactic acid: an increase in lactic acid provides clear evidence that cells are not receiving enough oxygen to maintain aerobic metabolism. In this setting, clinical interventions to increase oxygen delivery, either through increases in oxygen content or cardiac output, are reasonable.

In sepsis, however, there may be a peripheral defect in cellular oxygen utilization such that lactic acid will be produced even if sufficient oxygen is being delivered. In this setting the Cv_{O_2} will not be low; adequate oxygen is being delivered but the tissues are unable to use it.

MIXED VENOUS OXYGEN

The normal value for mixed venous oxygen saturation (Sv_{O_2}) is about 75%. Values below this level indicate that O_2 delivery is not keeping up with O_2 demand. Continuous monitoring of Sv_{O_2} may allow the early detection of changes in this balance—especially when associated with an increased lactic acid level. Sv_{O_2} influences Sa_{O_2} when there is a high degree of shunt or $\dot{V}/\dot{Q}$ mismatch. Thus a fall in Sa_{O_2} should not be immediately attributed to changes in pulmonary function, as the determinants of Sv_{O_2} may also be contributing.

Some PA lines are equipped with an oximeter for continuous monitoring; otherwise a sample drawn from the PA is needed for measurement of Sv_{O_2}. The sample is drawn slowly with the balloon down from the distal port of the catheter after an initial 3 cm^3 has been discarded. If blood is drawn too rapidly or if the catheter is too distal, the sample will be contaminated by pulmonary capillary blood and therefore overestimate the mixed venous oxygenation.

Decreased Sv_{O_2} has been associated with increased mortality in acute myocardial infarction and shock. In sepsis and acute respiratory distress syndrome, however, the Sv_{O_2} may remain increased despite serious tissue hypoxemia due to a cellular defect in oxygen uptake. There is controversy regarding the value of continuous monitoring of mixed venous blood. Currently, the best use of continuous Sv_{O_2} monitoring is as an early warning to prompt investigation of changes (i.e., cardiac output, oxygen demand).

BIBLIOGRAPHY

Connors AF, Speroff T, Dawson NV, et al. The effectivenss of right heart catheterization in the intial care of critically ill patients. *JAMA* 1996; 276:889–897.

Eisenberg PR, Jaffe AS, Schuster DP. Clinical evaluation compared to pulmonary artery catheterization in the hemodynamic assessment of critically ill patients. *Crit Care Med* 1984;12:549–553.

Jubran A, Tobin M. Reliability of pulse oximetry in titrating supplemental oxygen therapy in ventilator-dependent patients. *Chest* 1990;97: 1420–1425.

Kacmarek RM. Assessment of gas exchange and acid–base balance. In: Pierson DJ, Kacmarek RM, eds. *Foundations of respiratory care.* New York: Churchill-Livingstone, 1992:477.

Marini JJ. Monitoring during mechanical ventilation. *Clin Chest Med* 1988; 9:73–100.

Mermel LA, Maki DG. Infectious complication of Swan–Ganz pulmonary artery catheters. Pathogenesis, epidemiology, prevention, and management. *Am J Respir Crit Care Med* 1994;149:1020–1036.

O'Quin R, Marini JJ. Pulmonary artery occlusion pressure: clinical physiology, measurement and interpretation. *Am Rev Respir Dis* 1983;128: 319–326.

Pulmonary Artery Catheter Consensus Conference Participants. Pulmonary artery catheter consensus conference: consensus statement. *Crit Care Med* 1997;25:910–925.

von Pohle WR, Anholm JD, McMillan J. Carbon dioxide and oxygen partial pressure in expiratory water condensate are equivalent to mixed expired carbon dioxide and oxygen. *Chest* 1992;101:1601–1604.

Wiesel RD, Berger RL, Hechtman HB. Current concepts: measurement of cardiac output by thermodilution. *N Engl J Med* 1975;292:682–684.

C H A P T E R

389

DIAGNOSTIC PROCEDURES IN PULMONARY AND CRITICAL CARE MEDICINE

SUZETTE GAROFANO
DIANE E. STOVER

DIAGNOSTIC PROCEDURES IN PULMONARY AND CRITICAL CARE MEDICINE

A wide variety of noninvasive and invasive procedures are useful in the diagnosis of diseases affecting the respiratory tract. A knowledge of these procedures, their indications, complications, and limitations is essential for formulating a rational approach to the evaluation of patients with pulmonary disease. Chest imaging, pulmonary function testing, and hemodynamic and respiratory monitoring in the critically ill patient are covered in other chapters (see Chapters 386 to 388). The remaining most common diagnostic procedures are discussed in this chapter.

EVALUATION OF THE LUNG PARENCHYMA AND AIRWAYS

SPUTUM EXAMINATION

Examination and culture of expectorated sputum is usually the first step in evaluating patients with pulmonary symptoms or chest roentgenographic abnormalities. The proper collection and handling of the specimen is essential to maximize diagnostic yield, especially if a bacterial pneumonia is suspected. Because sputum specimens are contaminated by upper airway–colonizing organisms, examination of expectorated sputum may not accurately reflect lower respiratory pathogens, especially in patients with bacterial pneumonia. This is less of a problem in the diagnosis of malignancies or infections caused by organisms that do not normally colonize the oropharynx, such as *Mycobacterium tuberculosis* and *Pneumocystis carinii*. To minimize oropharyngeal contamination, patients should be instructed to first rinse their mouths or brush their teeth. They should cough deeply and expectorate directly into a sterile, leak-proof container. The spec-

imen should be transported immediately to the microbiology laboratory. In cases of suspected tuberculosis, three fresh morning specimens should be collected for the best diagnostic yield.

The gross characteristics of the sputum specimen may suggest specific diagnoses. Copious purulent sputum is generally suggestive of pyogenic bacterial infection. However, a purulent appearance may be caused by any inflammatory process, including asthma caused by the presence of numerous eosinophils. Pneumococcal infection has classically been described to produce rusty sputum. Dark red currant jelly sputum has been associated with *Klebsiella pneumoniae*. Foul-smelling sputum suggests the presence of an anaerobic or mixed anaerobic and aerobic bacterial infection. Hemoptysis is a nonspecific finding that is often associated with bronchitis or pneumonia; however, it should raise the suspicion of an underlying malignancy, especially if signs and symptoms of an infection are lacking.

Gram's stain of the sputum can be used to assess the quality of the specimen and should be performed on all specimens obtained from patients with a suspected bacterial pneumonia. A specimen is considered satisfactory if fewer than 10 squamous epithelial cells per low-power field are seen. In patients with a suspected bacterial pneumonia, more than 25 polymorphonuclear cells per low-power field and the presence of elastin fibers on KOH wet mount of the specimen are supportive evidence that the specimen originated from the lower respiratory tract. However, one should not exclude the possibility of oropharyngeal contamination. An unsatisfactory specimen should not be submitted for bacterial culture.

Because of difficulties in performing and interpreting the sputum Gram stain and problems with oropharyngeal contamination, the value of the Gram stain in the initial evaluation of a patient with pneumonia has recently been questioned. Yet most authorities agree that, when examined by someone with experience, a properly performed Gram stain on a good-quality specimen with a predominant intracellular organism is useful in suggesting the likely diagnosis and guiding initial antibiotic choice while awaiting culture results. Likewise, in a febrile patient with a pulmonary infiltrate, Gram's stain of a satisfactory specimen without a predominant organism may indicate an atypical bacterial infection, such as *Mycoplasma*, *Legionella*, or *Chlamydia*, or a viral process.

The diagnostic usefulness of a sputum specimen may be maximized by a variety of special staining and immunologic techniques. Direct staining of sputum can be diagnostic for several infectious processes (Table 389.1). Acid-fast stains of expectorated sputum are frequently positive for tuberculosis. In early, noncavitary disease, sputum smears reveal acid-fast bacilli in 20% to 40% of cases, with up to 95% yield in cases of advanced cavitary disease. The direct fluorescent antibody stain is a rapid method of identifying *Legionella* species in sputum. The sensitivity of the direct fluorescent antibody stain has been reported to range from 30% to 70%, with a specificity of approximately 95%. The polymerase chain reaction and DNA probes are newer techniques currently being developed for the rapid, sensitive, and specific diagnosis of infections, especially those caused by organisms that may not be detected by direct microscopic examination or are slow-growing in culture. Early studies using polymerase chain reaction probe for the diagnosis of *M. tuberculosis*

TABLE 389.1. **RESPIRATORY PATHOGENS THAT MAY BE DETECTED BY DIRECT STAINING OF EXPECTORATED SPUTUM**

Pathogen	Stain
Fungi	Grocott–Gomori methenamine-silver
Legionella	Direct fluorescent antibody
Mycobacterium tuberculosis	Acid-fast stain
Nocardia	Modified acid-fast stain
Pneumocystis carinii	Toluidine blue O
	Grocott–Gomori methenamine-silver
	Weigert–Gram
	Giemsa
	Fluorescent monoclonal antibody
Viruses:	
Respiratory syncytial virus	Fluorescent monoclonal antibody
Influenza	
Parainfluenza	
Adenovirus	

infection report sensitivities equal to or greater than culture, ranging from 39% to 100% and specificities of more than 90%.

If a spontaneously expectorated sputum cannot be obtained, sputum induction using nebulized hypertonic (3%) saline may be useful. Sputum induction has been of value in diagnosing *P. carinii* pneumonia in patients with AIDS. The sensitivity of stained induced specimens in this population ranges from 55% to 92%, the highest yields obtained with the use of immunofluorescent monoclonal antibodies. The diagnostic use of sputum induction for other infectious processes or malignancies is not known, but it probably should be performed in those circumstances if patients cannot provide a satisfactory specimen spontaneously.

Cytologic examination of sputum should be performed when malignancy is suspected. The diagnostic yield of cytologic examination ranges from 50% to 90%. Recovery rates can be improved by sending multiple early-morning specimens. Yield improves sequentially when sending up to five specimens. Recent studies suggest that overexpression by sputum cells of the protein heterogeneous nuclear ribonucleoprotein A2/B2 may be a marker of lung carcinoma. Examination of expectorated sputum samples for this protein by monoclonal antibody staining may be a potentially useful means for detecting preclinical lung cancer. These studies are preliminary, and the sensitivity and specificity of this technique for the early detection of lung cancer are not known.

TRANSTRACHEAL ASPIRATE

Transtracheal aspirate is a technique used to obtain specimens from the lower respiratory tract for microbiologic examination without contamination by oropharyngeal flora. In this technique, a plastic catheter is passed through the cricothyroid membrane into the trachea. As the patient coughs, a specimen is aspirated into an attached syringe.

False-negative results of bacterial cultures are rare using this technique unless the patient is receiving concurrent antibiotic therapy. However, a significant false-positive rate may occur in patients with chronic respiratory diseases such as chronic bronchitis, bronchiectasis, bronchogenic carcinoma, and symptomatic asthma who may have bacterial colonization of the lower respiratory tract without true infection. The risk of serious complications, including hemorrhage, worsening hypoxemia, and, rarely, death, has also limited the usefulness of this technique.

BRONCHOSCOPY

Since its introduction in the late 1960s, flexible fiberoptic bronchoscopy (FOB) has become one of the most commonly used diagnostic tools in pulmonary medicine. FOB allows direct visualization of the tracheobronchial tree and sampling of the lower respiratory tract and lung parenchyma for microbiologic, cytologic, and pathologic evaluation.

Flexible fiberoptic bronchoscopy can be performed on inpatients, outpatients, and mechanically ventilated patients. Although bronchoscopy may be performed comfortably without premedication in some patients, most commonly some combination of parenteral atropine and an analgesic or benzodiazepine is administered. After the application of topical anesthesia to the upper airway mucosa, the bronchoscope is passed through the nose or mouth and then through the vocal cords into the trachea. After inspection of the tracheobronchial tree, a variety of attendant procedures may be performed. Bronchial washings are obtained by instilling small amounts of saline into the airway and suctioning back the saline. Bronchial and transbronchial brushings are obtained by inserting a small brush through the bronchoscope and moving it back and forth over an endobronchial lesion or by advancing the brush into the lung parenchyma, entrapping fragments of tissue between the bristles. The specimens are then transferred onto a glass slide for cytologic and microbiologic evaluation. Bronchoalveolar lavage (BAL) is performed by wedging the bronchoscope into a subsegmental bronchus, usually in the lingula or right middle lobe. Aliquots of saline (30 to 60 mL) are instilled through the bronchoscope and then gently aspirated back into a syringe or suction trap. Approximately 40% to 60% of the infused fluid is recovered. Bronchial biopsies can be performed under direct vision of lesions that are endoscopically visible. Transbronchial biopsies (TBBs) of the lung parenchyma are usually performed under fluoroscopic guidance. Transbronchial needle aspiration (TBNA) allows tissue sampling from the lung parenchyma as well as paratracheal, hilar, and subcarinal lymph nodes.

The protected specimen brush and protected BAL are two techniques developed in an attempt to improve the diagnosis of bacterial pneumonia, especially nosocomial or ventilator-associated pneumonia. Specimens are obtained from the lower respiratory tract, without upper airway contamination, through protected, sealed catheters advanced through the bronchoscope into the distal bronchial tree. These techniques have been found to be useful in diagnosing bacterial infections in the absence of concurrent antibiotic therapy when quantitative bacterial culture thresholds of more than 103 colony-forming units per milliliter

TABLE 389.2.	INDICATIONS FOR BRONCHOSCOPY

Diagnostic

Abnormal chest radiograph
  Atelectasis
  Interstitial lung disease
  Cavitary lesion
  Diffuse infiltrates in the immunocompromised host
Suspected bronchogenic carcinoma
Staging of bronchogenic carcinoma
Cough
Hemoptysis
Suspected tracheobronchial foreign body
Wheeze and stridor
Assessment of endotracheal tube position

Therapeutic

Removal of tracheobronchial foreign body, retained secretions, or mucous plugs
Control of massive hemoptysis
Treatment of endobronchial neoplasms
  Laser therapy
  Brachytherapy
  Photodynamic therapy
  Tracheobroncial stent placement
  Therapeutic lavage in pulmonary alveolar proteinosis
  Insertion of endobronchial tubes

TABLE 389.3.	PATHOGENS IN WHICH ISOLATION FROM BRONCHOALVEOLAR LAVAGE IS DIAGNOSTIC FOR INFECTION

Pneumocystis carini	*Histoplasma*
Mycobacterium tuberculosis	*Toxoplasma*
Nocardia	*Strongyloides*
Mycoplasma	*Influenza*
Legionella	*Respiratory syncytial virus*

for protected specimen brush and more than 104 colony-forming units per milliliter for protected BAL are used.

Flexible FOB has a wide variety of diagnostic and therapeutic applications. Some of the most common uses are listed in Table 389.2. FOB is very useful in the diagnosis of bronchogenic carcinoma. A diagnostic yield of 95% has been reported with biopsy and brushings of endobronchial lesions. The diagnosis of lung carcinoma can be made in approximately 80% of cases that present as parenchymal masses larger than 2 cm. BAL has recently been reported to be valuable in diagnosing peripheral primary lung carcinomas, revealing malignant cells in up to 64% of cases. The diagnostic yield was higher with larger lesions and with bronchoalveolar carcinoma cell type.

The major clinical application for TBNA is to obtain mediastinal or hilar lymph node tissue for the diagnosis and staging of lung cancer. The sensitivity of TBNA for this indication has been reported to range for 50% to 80% with the specificity approaching 100%. TBNA may also be useful for the diagnosis of granulomatous diseases associated with intrathoracic adenopathy. TBNA has been found to have a yield of up to 90% for the diagnosis of sarcoidosis. A recent study found TBNA to be particularly useful for the diagnosis of mycobacterial infection in HIV-positive patients. TBNA established the diagnosis of mycobacterial disease in 87% of patients and was the only positive bronchoscopic specimen in 48% of cases.

Fluorescent bronchoscopy using a device termed the lung-imaging fluorescent endoscopy (LIFE) bronchoscope is a recently introduced technique to detect small, superficial endobronchial precancerous and carcinoma-in-situ lesions that are not readily visible with conventional bronchoscopy. This technique is based on differences in autofluorescence patterns be-

tween premalignant and malignant tissue and normal bronchial tissue. In one study, the use of LIFE bronchoscopy improved the detection of carcinoma in situ from 40% with conventional bronchoscopy to 91%. The ultimate role for this technique in the surveillance, diagnosis, and treatment of early carcinoma remains to be determined.

BAL can be diagnostic in several infectious processes (Table 389.3). The isolation of other organisms, such as cytomegalovirus and *Aspergillus*, in susceptible hosts with compatible clinical presentations can be considered diagnostic for invasive pulmonary infection. BAL can also be diagnostic for a few noninfectious processes, whereas several others can be presumptively diagnosed in the proper clinical setting (Table 389.4).

The diagnostic accuracy of FOB with or without TBB for diffuse lung disease of noninfectious etiologic process varies with the underlying disease process. Sarcoidosis can be diagnosed in a majority of cases, but the sensitivity of FOB for other disorders, such as eosinophilic granuloma, pulmonary alveolar proteinosis, and bronchiolitis obliterans with organizing pneumonia, may be low. FOB should be the initial invasive diagnostic procedure

TABLE 389.4.	BRONCHOALVEOLAR LAVAGE ANALYSIS OF NONINFECTIOUS PROCESSES

Diagnosis	BAL Findings
Malignancy	Neoplastic cells
Pulmonary alveolar proteinosis	Opaque, milky BAL fluid
	Periodic acid–Schiff staining
	Lamellar structures on electron microscopy
Eosinophilic granuloma	Langerhans cells
	Birbeck's granules on electron microscopy
	OKT6 monoclonal antibody staining
Asbestos exposure	Asbestos bodies
Pulmonary hemorrhage[a]	Hemosiderin-laden macrophages
Sarcoidosis[a]	Noncaseating granuloma
Lipid pneumonia[a]	Fat globules in macrophages
Eosinophilic pneumonia[a]	Increased percentage of eosinophils
Amiodarone exposure or toxicity[a]	Large macrophages with lamellar inclusion bodies

[a] Suggested diagnosis in the proper clinical setting.
BAL, bronchoalveolar lavage.

performed in most cases of diffuse lung diseases to exclude an infectious process or sarcoid, but a surgical procedure may be required for a definitive diagnosis.

Fiberoptic bronchoscopy has become an invaluable tool in the evaluation of diffuse pulmonary infiltrates in the immunocompromised host. Bronchoscopy with BAL and TBB has been reported to have about 90% sensitivity for the diagnosis of an infectious process in this setting, with an overall diagnostic yield of 70%. Bronchoscopy has a particularly high yield for *P. carinii* pneumonia; 94% in non–AIDS-immunocompromised patients with bilateral BAL and close to 100% in patients with AIDS if both BAL and TBB are performed. BAL is also an excellent technique for the diagnosis of cytomegalovirus pneumonia in bone marrow transplant recipients with a sensitivity of more than 90% when stained with immunofluorescent cytomegalovirus monoclonal antibodies.

Rigid bronchoscopy that uses a large-diameter, straight metal tube is less frequently performed. In comparison with flexible FOB, rigid bronchoscopy usually requires general anesthesia and allows good visualization of only the lobar bronchi. It remains the procedure of choice in several clinical settings, however, including foreign-body retrieval, massive hemoptysis, and dilatation of tracheobronchial stenosis.

Fiberoptic bronchoscopy is a safe and well-tolerated procedure. Major complication rates range from 0.08% to 5% and mortality rates from 0.01% to 0.5%. The most serious complications are respiratory depression and hypotension caused by excessive sedation, laryngospasm, bronchospasm (especially in patients with a history of bronchospasm), hypoxemia, and pneumothorax and bleeding following biopsy procedures. Postbronchoscopy fever may occur in approximately 25% of patients and usually follows BAL. It is generally self-limited and not associated with infection. Flexible FOB carries an extremely low risk of bacteremia, and prophylaxis with antibiotics is not routinely recommended, even in the immunocompromised host. In contrast, bacteremia has been documented following rigid bronchoscopy, and prophylactic antibiotics are recommended in patients at risk for bacterial endocarditis. Transient radiographic abnormalities may occur in the area where BAL was performed.

In general, an oxygen tension of at least 75 mm Hg on 50% or less supplemental oxygen should be present before proceeding with FOB. The PO_2 may decrease by up to 25 mm Hg during the procedure. All patients should be continuously monitored by pulse oximetry and receive supplemental oxygen. The procedure should be terminated if a PO_2 of at least 60 mm Hg and an oxygen saturation of 90% cannot be maintained. Any further decrease in the PO_2 may lead to severe hypoxemia because of the location of this value near the steep portion of the oxyhemoglobin dissociation curve.

Fiberoptic bronchoscopy is absolutely contraindicated without intubation in the presence of bilateral vocal cord paralysis because of the potential for complete occlusion of the airway. Other contraindications to FOB include inability of the patient to cooperate with the procedure, hemodynamic instability, recent myocardial infarction or unstable angina, and severe uncorrectable coagulopathy. Biopsy procedures should not be performed with a platelet count below 50,000 per millimeter.

Bleeding complications during FOB with BAL are rare even, with platelet counts of fewer than 50,000 per millimeter.

TRANSTHORACIC NEEDLE ASPIRATION

Transthoracic needle aspiration (TTNA) is an important means of diagnosing thoracic and mediastinal disease. The procedure may be performed on an outpatient basis. Sedation is usually not required. The lesion for biopsy is localized using either fluoroscopy or computed tomography (CT) scan. The patient is appropriately positioned; local anesthesia is administered to the skin, subcutaneous tissue, and parietal pleura. The needle is advanced into the lesion under fluoroscopic or CT guidance. The specimen is aspirated into a syringe attached to the needle. It is often useful to have a cytologist present during the procedure to assess whether diagnostic material has been obtained or a second needle pass is required. Stains and culture of the aspirated material should be obtained if clinically indicated. Newer types of needles allow procurement of core specimens of tissue for histologic examination as well. A chest radiograph is usually performed immediately after the procedure and 2 to 4 hours later to detect the presence of a pneumothorax.

TTNA is indicated in the diagnosis of pulmonary nodules, especially if peripheral and smaller than 2 cm. In this setting, the diagnostic yield for TTNA is higher than for FOB. Other indications for TTNA include the diagnosis of central (hilar and mediastinal) masses and pleural-based masses and the diagnosis of suspected infectious processes, especially if bronchoscopy has failed to reveal a definitive diagnosis and the lesion is localized or nodular. TTNA is generally not useful in the diagnosis of diffuse or interstitial lung diseases; such processes tend to involve the lung parenchyma in a patchy manner in varying stages of evolution and require pathologic examination of larger tissue specimens for diagnosis.

The sensitivity of TTNA for the diagnosis of malignancy is high, ranging from 64% to 97%. False-positive results for malignancy are extremely low. The diagnostic yield for infections ranges from 40% to 90%, with the higher yields reported for nonbacterial processes. A negative result or specific nonmalignant diagnosis, such as hamartoma, amyloid, granulomatous disease, or infection, is made in approximately 5% to 25% of patients undergoing this procedure. However, such findings do not necessarily exclude the possibility of malignancy. If the clinical suspicion for malignancy is great, the decision must be made as to whether to repeat the TTNA, which yields a diagnosis in 35% to 40% of cases, or proceed to a surgical procedure. Some physicians recommend surgery as the initial procedure of choice if the clinical presentation is highly suggestive of malignancy and the patient is an acceptable surgical candidate. If the clinical picture is consistent with a benign process, the patient may be followed closely with serial chest radiographs.

The most common complication of TTNA is pneumothorax, which occurs in 10% to 37% of procedures. Chest tube placement is required in less than 50% of such cases. The risk of pneumothorax appears to increase with an increasing number of needle passes, increased depth of the lesion, presence of cavitation, advanced patient age, and underlying chronic obstructive pulmonary disease or bullous disease. Other, less common complications include hemoptysis, which is usually self-limited; intraparenchymal hemorrhage; venous air embolism; subcutaneous emphysema; and hemopericardium with tamponade when lesions are located near the pulmonary artery. Reports of tumor seeding of the needle tract exist but are exceedingly rare. Reported mortality rates of this procedure are less than 0.2%.

Contraindications to performing TTNA include an uncooperative patient or excessive coughing, uncorrectable coagulopathy, thrombocytopenia with platelet counts less than 50,000 per millimeter, and hydatid cyst. Relative contraindications include severe emphysema, previous pneumonectomy, pulmonary artery hypertension, mechanical ventilation, and suspected vascular lesion. However, TTNA has been performed safely in patients with these conditions.

THORACOSCOPY

The technique of thoracoscopy (pleuroscopy) was introduced in the early 1900s and used primarily for the lysis of pleural adhesions to create a pneumothorax for the treatment of tuberculosis. With the advent of antituberculosis therapy, thoracoscopy became rarely used, except for the diagnosis of pleural diseases and pleurodesis of malignant effusions. With recent technical advances in video imaging and endoscopic instrumentation, video-assisted thoracoscopic surgery (VATS) has rapidly emerged as a technique with many potential diagnostic and therapeutic applications.

VATS requires general anesthesia and endotracheal intubation. In contrast to simple thoracoscopy, VATS requires single-lung ventilation with collapse of the lung to be examined. The patient is placed in the lateral decubitus position and a video thoracoscope is introduced through a 1-inch incision. Images are projected on a video monitor. Various instruments for dissection, resection, and stapling of the lung parenchyma, as well as for talc insufflation for pleurodesis, are introduced through two or three additional small incision sites. At the end of the procedure, a chest tube is inserted in one of the sites and the other sites are closed.

Using this technique, the surgeon can visualize the entire pleural space and parenchymal surface. A large number of potential indications for VATS has been advanced, but the currently accepted applications in the management of pleuropulmonary diseases are listed in Table 389.5. Thoracoscopy (simple or VATS) remains a very effective means of diagnosing and managing pleural diseases. The vast majority of undiagnosed exudative pleural effusions can be diagnosed using thoracoscopy. Pleurodesis of malignant effusions with talc insufflation is effective in 85% to 90% of cases using thoracoscopic techniques. Pleurodesis is less successful when using other sclerosing agents such as tetracycline or bleomycin.

At what point thoracoscopy should be considered in the evaluation of patients with pulmonary nodules or diffuse lung disease is a more controversial issue. Many physicians either proceed directly to thoracoscopy or follow a nondiagnostic TTNA with thoracoscopy when evaluating an indeterminate pulmonary nodule, especially if the index of suspicion is high for malignancy. If a malignancy is detected at the time of thoracoscopy, the patient should undergo proper staging and thoracotomy with

TABLE 389.5.	INDICATIONS FOR VIDEO-ASSISTED THORACOSCOPIC SURGERY

Diagnostic
Evaluation of undiagnosed exudative pleural effusions
Diagnosis of indeterminate pulmonary nodules
Lung biopsy in diffuse lung disease
Biopsy of pleural-based or peripheral lung masses
Biopsy of mediastinal nodes or masses

Therapeutic
Pleurodesis of malignant pleural effusion
Treatment of spontaneous pneumothorax
Resection of pulmonary metastases
Thoracic sympathectomy

definitive resection (lobectomy or pneumonectomy), unless he or she is unable to tolerate an extensive resection because of underlying pulmonary compromise or is inoperable for another reason.

VATS may supplant open-lung biopsy (OLB) as the method of choice for the definitive diagnosis of diffuse lung disease when less invasive techniques have failed to determine a cause. Few studies directly comparing VATS and OLB exist, but VATS appears to be of equal diagnostic accuracy (more than 90%). VATS is less invasive than standard thoracotomy and results in less postoperative morbidity. Respiratory compromise, pain, length of time for which chest tube drainage is required, and length of hospital stay are all reduced following VATS, compared with thoracotomy.

Preliminary studies indicate that VATS can be performed safely in thrombocytopenic immunocompromised patients to establish the diagnosis of a variety of infectious and noninfectious diseases. VATS has been reported to have a diagnostic yield of up to 100% in the immunocompromised patient population, with postoperative morbidity comparable to that of conventional OLB.

Lesions located deep within the lung parenchyma or in the hilum, upper mediastinum, or posterior paravertebral area are frequently not amenable to biopsy or resection by VATS. VATS cannot be performed in the presence of dense pleural scarring or severe coagulopathy. Patients who require mechanical ventilation or have severe pulmonary compromise are usually not candidates for VATS because they often cannot tolerate single-lung ventilation.

OPEN-LUNG BIOPSY

Open-lung biopsy has been considered the most reliable procedure for obtaining lung tissue for examination, with an overall diagnostic accuracy of more than 90%. It is performed under general anesthesia. Usually biopsies are taken through a small, anterior intercostal incision. In diffuse lung processes, lung specimens are typically obtained from the anteriorly located right middle lobe or lingula. It is important that both normal-appearing and abnormal-appearing lungs are biopsied because severely affected, fibrotic regions may be of little diagnostic use. For lesions localized laterally or posteriorly, a full posterolateral thoracotomy incision may be required.

Complications from OLB occur infrequently (7%) and include bleeding, infection, and problems related to general anesthesia. Mortality rates range from 0.5% to 1.8%. There are relatively few absolute contraindications to performing an OLB, but they do include hemodynamic instability and severe coagulopathy that cannot be corrected by blood product support.

OLB has historically been performed after less invasive procedures have been exhausted or when a rapidly deteriorating clinical picture mandates that a definitive diagnosis be expediently obtained. More studies are required that directly compare the diagnostic accuracy of OLB with that of VATS, particularly in the patient who is immunocompromised. The less invasive VATS may ultimately replace OLB as the diagnostic procedure of choice when surgical intervention is necessary for the diagnosis of parenchymal lung disease.

EVALUATION OF PLEURAL EFFUSIONS

THORACENTESIS

Thoracentesis is the most commonly performed procedure to diagnose and manage pleural effusions. A thoracentesis should be performed in most cases of an undiagnosed pleural effusion. In certain circumstances, such as obvious congestive heart failure, following thoracic or abdominal surgery, or following the postpartum period, pleural effusions are common and thoracentesis generally is not necessary if the clinical picture is typical. A thoracentesis may be performed therapeutically for relief of dyspnea in patients with large effusions.

Before a thoracentesis can be performed, lateral decubitus chest radiographs should be obtained. If the pleural effusion is freely layering and the distance between the inner chest wall and the outer lung on the decubitus film is more than 10 mm, ample fluid is present to support the safe performance of a thoracentesis. If there is a small amount of fluid or the fluid does not freely layer, ultrasonography of the chest should be performed prior to thoracentesis for fluid localization or guidance during the procedure.

The patient should be sitting upright with arms resting on a bedside table and his or her back relatively straight to maximize layering of the pleural effusion posteriorly. The site of needle insertion is identified by locating the point at which dullness to percussion or decreased tactile fremitus occurs because this indicates the superior border of the effusion. The thoracentesis should be performed posterolaterally, one interspace below this point. The area is cleansed with an antiseptic solution and a sterile field created. The skin is anesthetized using a small (25-gauge) needle. A larger 22-gauge needle is then used to anesthetize the periosteum of the underlying rib and moved over its superior aspect to avoid the neurovascular bundle running along the inferior rib border. The needle is slowly advanced toward the pleural space with aspiration followed by injection of small

amounts of anesthesia every few millimeters. Once pleural fluid is aspirated, the needle is withdrawn. Then another needle, attached to a 60-mL syringe, is advanced over the same path as the anesthetic needle and a sample of the pleural fluid is aspirated into the syringe. For a therapeutic thoracentesis, a plastic catheter that threads over or through the needle may be advanced into the pleural space. The needle is then withdrawn and the catheter attached to a drainage bag or vacuum bottle. Following the procedure, an expiratory chest radiograph should be obtained to check for the presence of a pneumothorax.

The gross features of the pleural fluid should be noted. A putrid odor is suggestive of an anaerobic infection. Frank pus indicates the presence of an empyema. A grossly bloody effusion with a hematocrit of more than 50% of the peripheral value is consistent with a hemothorax. Milky-appearing fluid may be caused by a chylous or pseudochylous effusion.

Analysis of pleural fluid of unknown cause should consist of a protein and lactate dehydrogenase (LDH) determination, glucose level, pH, cell count, cytologic examination, and Gram's stain with culture. Determining whether the pleural fluid is a transudate or an exudate is useful in formulating a differential diagnosis. An exudative pleural effusion meets one of following criteria set forth by Light and colleagues: pleural fluid protein/serum protein more than 0.5, pleural fluid LDH/serum LDH more than 0.6, pleural fluid LDH more than two-thirds of the upper limit of normal for the serum LDH. The pleural effusion is transudative if none of the above criteria is met. Several recent studies have proposed other laboratory values to identify exudative pleural effusions. The parameters include cholesterol more than 55 mg per deciliter, pleural fluid bilirubin/serum bilirubin 0.6 or more, and serum and pleural fluid albumin gradient less than 1.2 g per deciliter. However, none of these values has been found to be more accurate than the LDH and protein criteria.

A transudative pleural effusion may be caused by a limited number of disorders. The most common cause is congestive heart failure. Pleural effusions caused by congestive heart failure are usually right-sided or bilateral. About 25% of pleural effusions secondary to pulmonary emboli are transudative. The differential diagnosis of an exudative pleural effusion is much more extensive. Some of the more common causes are listed in Table 389.6. Other pleural fluid values that may aid in narrowing the diagnostic possibilities of an exudative effusion are listed in Table 389.7. (See Chapter 358 for a more detailed discussion of laboratory evaluation of pleural effusion fluid.)

Three of the most common causes of an exudative pleural effusion are a parapneumonic effusion, malignancy, and tuberculosis. Parapneumonic effusions should be analyzed to determine the need for chest tube placement. An empyema (frank pus in the pleural space) or the presence of organisms on Gram's stain of the fluid requires immediate drainage. A complicated pleural effusion has been defined as one that does not resolve with antibiotic therapy alone and requires chest tube drainage either for control of infection or to prevent the development of a fibrothorax. The criteria used to determine whether a parapneumonic effusion requires chest tube drainage include presence of loculation, pH less than 7.10, glucose less than 40, or LDH more than 1,000, or any combination of the latter three

TABLE 389.6.	DIFFERENTIAL DIAGNOSIS OF PLEURAL EFFUSIONS

Transudates

Congestive heart failure
Pericardial disease
Cirrhosis
Nephrotic syndrome
Myxedema
Atelectasis
Pulmonary embolism

Exudates

Malignancy
Infection
Pulmonary embolism
Pancreatitis and other pancreatic diseases
Esophageal perforation
Postabdominal surgery
Intra-abdominal abscess
Splenic infarct/hematoma
Collagen vascular disease
   Rheumatoid arthritis
   Systemic lupus erythematosus
Drug- or radiation-induced
Asbestos exposure (benign effusion)
Sarcoid

TABLE 389.7.	DIFFERENTIAL DIAGNOSIS OF EXUDATIVE PLEURAL EFFUSIONS

Pleural Fluid Parameter	Differential Diagnosis
Total WBC >10,000/μL	Empyema Pulmonary embolism Pancreatitis Malignancy Collagen vascular disease Tuberculosis
Lymphocytes >50% of WBC	Lymphoma and other malignancies Tuberculosis Fungal infections Sarcoidosis Postpericardiotomy syndrome
Eosinophils >10% of WBC	Blood or air in pleural space Fungal infections Parasitic disease Drug reaction (nitrofurantoin, bromocriptine, dantrolene) Benign asbestos effusion Churg–Strauss syndrome
RBC HCT >50% of peripheral blood	Hemothorax
HCT >100,000/mm³	Malignancy Pulmonary embolism Trauma
pH <7.20	Empyema Complicated parapneumonic effusion Systemic acidosis Esophageal rupture Rheumatoid pleuritis Tuberculosis Malignancy Hemothorax Paragonimiasis Churg–Strauss syndrome
Glucose <60 mg/dL	Parapneumonic effusion Malignancy Tuberculosis Rheumatoid pleuritis Hemothorax Churg–Strauss syndrome Paragonimiasis
Amylase > upper limit of normal in serum	Pancreatic disease Malignancy (adenocarcinoma of lung most common) Esophageal rupture Ruptured ectopic pregnancy
Antinuclear antibody Titer ≥ 1:160 or serum titer	Lupus pleuritis
Rheumatoid factor Titer ≥ 1:320 or serum titer	Rheumatoid pleuritis
Chylothorax (>110 mg/dL triglycerides or presence of chylomicrons)	Malignancy (especially lymphoma) Traumatic rupture of thoracic, duct Idiopathic lymphangioleiomyomatosis

WBC, white blood cell count; RBC, red blood cell count; HCT, hematocrit.

factors. If the initial pH is between 7.10 and 7.20, the thoracentesis should be repeated in 12 to 24 hours.

Pleural fluid cytologic examination can provide a diagnosis of malignancy in 54% to 63% of cases. Obtaining a second and third sample for cytologic examination increases the yield to 72% and 77%, respectively.

Acid-fast smears of the pleural fluid yield a diagnosis of tuberculosis in less than 10% of cases. Pleural fluid cultures identify tuberculosis in 13% to 75% of patients. An elevated adenosine deaminase level of more than 70 units per liter has been reported to be diagnostic of tuberculous pleuritis. The presence of more than 5% mesothelial cells in the pleural fluid virtually excludes the possibility of tuberculosis; their absence, however, is not specific for tuberculosis.

The most common complication of thoracentesis is pneumothorax, which occurs in approximately 10% of procedures. Most pneumothoraxes do not require chest tube insertion. Vasovagal reactions may occur, and some physicians routinely administer atropine before the procedure to reduce vagal tone. Reexpansion pulmonary edema has been described after removal of large amounts of fluid. It is recommended that no more than 1.0 to 1.5 L of fluid be removed at one sitting. Data regarding the mechanism by which reexpansion pulmonary edema develops are inconclusive. Some have speculated that its development is related to increasing negative pleural pressures generated during the procedure and that draining large volumes of fluid can be accomplished safely if the pleural pressure can be monitored and maintained at more than −20 cm H_2O. Reexpansion pulmonary edema usually develops in the ipsilateral lung but may involve the contralateral lung as well. Other more serious but rarely occurring complications include laceration of the intercostal artery, splenic rupture, and air embolism.

There are few contraindications to performing a thoracentesis, and the decision to proceed must be guided by the clinical circumstances. Relative contraindications include severe coagulopathy, small volume of fluid, mechanical ventilation, and cutaneous infection at the site of needle entry.

PLEURAL BIOPSY

A percutaneous pleural biopsy is indicated for further evaluation of an undiagnosed exudative pleural effusion. A pleural biopsy is performed in a manner similar to that of a thoracentesis. Special larger bore needles (Abrams and Cope) designed with a hook and cutting edge are used to ensnare the parietal pleura. Contraindications and complications of the procedure are essentially the same as those for a thoracentesis.

Pleural biopsy is most useful in establishing the diagnosis of tuberculosis and malignancy. Histologic examination and culture of pleural biopsy specimens provide the diagnosis of tuberculosis in more than 75% of patients. The addition of pleural biopsy histology and culture to pleural fluid studies increases the diagnostic yield for tuberculous pleuritis to approximately 90%. If tuberculosis is highly suspected, pleural biopsy should be performed at the time of initial thoracentesis.

Pleural biopsy is less useful than pleural fluid cytology in the diagnosis of malignancy. Biopsy reveals malignancy in 40% to 50% of cases but is rarely the sole positive result. Adding pleural biopsy to pleural fluid cytology increases the diagnostic yield by only 7%. Although opinions vary, if a malignant pleural effusion is suspected, pleural biopsy may be performed either at the time of the initial thoracentesis or on repeat thoracentesis if the results of the first are nondiagnostic.

An exudative pleural effusion that remains undiagnosed after two to three thoracenteses and a pleural biopsy presents a clinical dilemma. In patients with underlying lung parenchymal abnormalities on chest radiograph or CT scan, a bronchoscopy should be the next diagnostic procedure attempted. It has been suggested that a conservative approach be considered in patients in whom a low index of suspicion for tuberculosis or malignancy exists if the following criteria are met: clinical stability, no weight loss, negative purified protein derivative, afebrile, less than 95% lymphocytes in the pleural fluid, and an effusion size less than 50% of the hemithorax. If a patient does not meet these criteria, a more aggressive evaluation is warranted. Thoracoscopy, as described previously, is usually selected as the next diagnostic procedure; it reveals the cause of the effusion in approximately 90% of cases. Lymphoma and malignant mesothelioma are the most common causes of pleural effusions that remain undiagnosed even after surgical evaluation.

■ CERVICAL MEDIASTINOSCOPY AND ANTERIOR MEDIASTINOTOMY

Cervical mediastinoscopy and anterior mediastinotomy are complementary procedures that allow evaluation of mediastinal structures. These procedures are most commonly performed for staging of mediastinal lymph nodes in patients with non–small cell lung carcinoma prior to thoracotomy. Other indications include biopsy of enlarged mediastinal lymph nodes in patients suspected of having lymphoma, granulomatous disorders, infections, or mediastinal malignancies; drainage of mediastinal cysts; and staging of patients with esophageal carcinoma.

Both procedures require general anesthesia. Cervical mediastinoscopy is performed through a small incision in the suprasternal notch. The pretracheal fascia is opened and blunt dissection continued anteriorly and laterally to the trachea, extending distally to the carina. A lighted mediastinoscope is advanced through the created space. Paratracheal, superior tracheobronchial, azygous, and anterior subcarinal lymph nodes are accessible through this approach. An anterior mediastinotomy (Chamberlain's procedure) is usually performed through a 3- to 5-cm incision in the second intercostal space just lateral to the sternum. This procedure is preferred by some surgeons in patients with lung carcinomas located in left upper lobe because it allows access to anterior mediastinal and aortopulmonary lymph nodes, which are common sites of metastases from such lesions.

Whether these procedures should be performed in all patients with non–small cell carcinoma before thoracotomy is controversial. CT evaluation of the mediastinum has about an 80% sensitivity and specificity for detecting nodal metastases using a node size threshold of more than 1 cm. Most surgeons reserve mediastinoscopy and mediastinotomy for those patients with radiographic evidence of lymph node enlargement, as well as for those with centrally located tumors and large locally advanced tumors.

Major complications occur in less than 1% of procedures. The principal risk is of hemorrhage caused by injury or inadvertent biopsy of one of the intrathoracic vessels. Less common complications include vocal cord paralysis from recurrent laryngeal nerve injury and chylothorax following injury to the thoracic duct.

Severe bleeding diathesis and inability to tolerate general anesthesia are the major contraindications to the performance of these procedures. Relative contraindications include the superior vena cava syndrome, because vessel engorgement may increase the risk of significant bleeding, and previous mediastinal procedures including tracheostomy and mediastinal irradiation, which cause scarring and obliteration of mediastinal fascial planes.

BIBLIOGRAPHY

Bartter T, Santarelli R, Akers SM, et al. The evaluation of pleural effusion. *Chest* 1994;106:1209–1214.

Bensard DD, McIntyre RC, Waring BJ, et al. Comparison of video thoracoscopic lung biopsy to open lung biopsy in the diagnosis of interstitial lung disease. *Chest* 1993;103:765–770.

Cazzadori A, DiPerri G, Todeschini G, et al. Transbronchial biopsy in the diagnosis of pulmonary infiltrates in immunocompromised patients. *Chest* 1995;107:101–106.

Daniel TM, Kern JA, Tribble CG, et al. Thoracoscopic surgery for diseases of the lung and pleura. Effectiveness, changing indications and limitations. *Ann Surg* 1993;217:566–575.

Goldstein RA, Rohtagi PK, Bergofsky EH, et al. Clinical role of bronchoalveolar lavage in adults with pulmonary disease. *Am Rev Respir Dis* 1990; 142:481–486.

Harkin TJ, Ciotoli C, Addrizzo-Harris DJ, et al. Transbronchial needle aspiration (TBNA) in patients infected with HIV. *Am J Respir Crit Care Med* 1998;157:1913–1918.

Harrow EM, Wang KP. The staging of lung cancer by bronchoscopic transbronchial needle aspiration. *Chest Surg Clin North Am* 1996;6(2): 223–135.

Light RW, Macgregor I, Luchsinger PC, et al. Pleural effusion: the diagnostic separation of transudates and exudates. *Ann Intern Med* 1992;77: 507–513.

Tockman MS, Mulshine JL, Piantadosi S, et al. Prospective detection of preclinical lung cancer: results from two studies of heterogeneous nuclear ribonucleoprotein A2/B1 overexpression. *Clin Cancer Res* 1997;3: 2237–2246.

Weisbrod GL. Transthoracic percutaneous lung biopsy. *Radiol Clin North Am* 1990;28:647–655.

Kelley's Textbook of Internal Medicine, fourth edition. Edited by H. David Humes. Lippincott Williams & Wilkins, Philadelphia © 2000.

CHAPTER 390

RESPIRATORY THERAPY TECHNIQUES

CAROLYN H. WELSH

Respiratory therapy is a specialty in which trained practitioners operate under medical guidance to provide evaluation and treatment of persons with cardiopulmonary disease. Most respiratory therapy techniques and devices are designed and used to achieve one or more of the following goals: to improve oxygenation, to increase ventilation, to expand lung volume, or to clear secretions. Other techniques involve delivery of medications via the airway for treatment of respiratory and systemic diseases. Respiratory therapy techniques are used not only in intensive care units but also on hospital wards, clinics, and at home. Recently, practice guidelines have been developed by the National Board for Respiratory Care to enhance standard high-quality respiratory care practice throughout the United States. Some techniques are supported by good-outcome data, whereas others, such as humidification, are often used based on tradition rather than proof of benefit. Where outcome data are available, they are provided in this chapter. If information on relative cost is available, it is also provided.

■ SUPPLEMENTAL OXYGEN THERAPY

Oxygen therapy has been used extensively during the past 20 years, on the basis of information provided by the Nocturnal Oxygen Therapy Trial and the British Medical Research Council studies. Both these trials demonstrated that for hypoxemic patients, longer use of oxygen each day significantly prolongs survival. Current criteria for supplemental oxygen use in hypoxemic patients include a low PaO_2 (less than 50 to 55 mm Hg), or an oxygen saturation less than or equal to 85%. When PaO_2 is in the 55 to 60 mm Hg range, long-term oxygen therapy is also warranted if there is clinical evidence of right-heart failure, as demonstrated by jugular venous distention, a right-sided S_3 gallop, pedal edema, erythrocytosis, or electrocardiographic manifestations such as P pulmonale, right axis deviation, and right ventricular hypertrophy. Methods for oxygen delivery are listed in Table 390.1. The choice of oxygen delivery technique and device is based on both the severity of hypoxemia and patient comfort.

For either the hospitalized or home patient, oxygen orders should specify a delivery method, flow rate or FiO_2, and duration of therapy during a 24-hour cycle. Oxygen may be prescribed, as needed, for nocturnal use only, for use with exercise, or for 24 hours per day. Monitoring to assess safety and efficacy can be performed using a finger oximeter, and flow rate can be appropriately titrated. For the acutely ill patient, the lack of a carbon dioxide tension ($PaCO_2$) measurement from an oximeter limits its usefulness. The acutely ill patient generally requires the full arterial blood gas (ABG) analysis, which measures pH, $PaCO_2$, PaO_2, calculated bicarbonate, base excess and oxygen saturation. The additional acid–base information from the ABG aids in the assessment of respiratory fatigue and a potential decision to intubate. An arterial blood gas specimen should also be taken after starting oxygen therapy in a CO_2-retaining patient to check for worsening hypercarbia and 20 to 30 minutes after starting mechanical ventilation to assess the impact of treatment on oxygenation and acid–base status.

Gas enriched in oxygen can be supplied in one of three ways for home use: by concentrator, tank, or compressed liquid. Concentrators purify oxygen from the atmosphere and require a functioning electrical power source. Cylindrical tanks of compressed gas can be delivered to the home for stationary or portable use. These are heavy and have the potential to explode with decompression. A third source, liquid oxygen, can be supplied in a large reservoir with light-weight portable tanks filled from this stationary source. In general, the liquid is lighter to carry and thus often preferred, but it is also considerably more expensive.

To conserve oxygen supply from either a tank or a liquid system, a trigger or demand valve can be inserted in-line, which limits release of oxygen to the inspiratory phase of the breathing cycle. Duration of portable supplies can be doubled or tripled with use of this valve. To increase the FiO_2 for a patient chronically requiring high flow rates, a small reservoir can be attached in-line with the oxygen tubing so that less room air is entrained with a breath and the actual FiO_2 reaching the pharynx is higher. On rare occasions, transtracheal oxygen delivery may be useful to increase the PaO_2 to an acceptable level, or to improve acceptability of oxygen therapy to a patient by improving cosmetic appeal or lessening nasal irritation or sinus symptoms. Good outcome data are lacking to support the superiority of transtracheal oxygen over other methods of delivery.

Oxygen is not only expensive; it is also potentially hazardous. Severe hypoxemia in a patient must be addressed immediately. However, for the chronic obstructive lung disease (COPD) patient, overly vigorous treatment with oxygen may lead to progressive hypoventilation from suppression of the hypoxic respiratory drive and induce respiratory acidosis. Therefore, it is important to start therapy with the lowest flow of oxygen needed

TABLE 390.1.	CHARACTERISTICS OF OXYGEN ADMINISTRATION DEVICES				
	Oxygen Administration Device				
Characteristic	**Nasal Cannula**	**Venturi Mask**	**Simple Face Mask**	**Non-Rebreathing Mask**	**Endotracheal or Tracheostomy Tube**
How ordered	0.5–6 L/min	24%, 28%, 35% O_2, etc.	1–10 L/min[a]	50–100% O_2	21–100% O_2
Effective delivery range	0.5–6 L/min[b]	Variable, up to ordered FIO_2[c]	Variable, up to 50–60% O_2[c]	Highly variable, up to 70–80% O_2[a,c]	21–100% O_2[a,d]
Actual (tracheal) FIO_2 known?	No	No	No	No	Yes[d]
Humidification and heating required?	No[e]	No	No[e]	No[e]	Yes
Constancy of FIO_2 to patient?	++	+	+	+	+++[d]
Inconvenience or discomfort to patient	+	++	++	+++	+++

[a] May be as high as 100 L/min when high-flow generator is used.
[b] FIO_2 not known but usually constant.
[c] Varies, depending on amount of room air is entrained, which is increased by high minute ventilation, poor mask fit, agitation, and so on.
[d] Assumes correct circuit assembly, including downstream extension tube to prevent inspiratory entrainment of room air.
[e] In low-humidity environments some patients are more comfortable with added humidity when flows exceed 4 L/min.
FIO_2, fraction inspired oxygen.

and proceed cautiously. Such patients cannot be given oxygen and then left in an unmonitored situation but must be observed for overt or insidious onset of respiratory acidosis. Supplemental oxygen is said to lead to parenchymal oxygen toxicity, but actual clinical relevance of oxygen toxicity is unclear and its incidence is probably overestimated.

ARTIFICIAL AIRWAYS

An endotracheal tube is inserted in the nose or mouth to facilitate mechanical ventilation in the treatment of acute respiratory failure. Other indications for intubation are to relieve upper airway obstruction, to allow removal of excessive secretions by suction catheter, and to protect the airways from aspiration of gastric contents. Unfortunately, intubation fails to completely protect a patient from aspiration. To minimize the risk of aspiration, patients should be kept in a semi-upright position while intubated. Use of a large tube will decrease the work of breathing during ventilator weaning. An additional choice is that of tube insertion site. Orotracheal tubes move around more in the mouth and are less well tolerated by the patient. Nasotracheal tubes are both more comfortable and smaller, but they are associated with a higher incidence of sinusitis. Because of the perceived risk of sinusitis, nasotracheal tubes are now being used less often.

Tracheostomy has been advocated at an early time point after endotracheal intubation for the patient needing long-term ventilation, with the premise that tracheostomy leads to fewer complications than the endotracheal tube and shortens the duration of ventilation. The lower number of complications is not well documented, although patient comfort is said to be improved

with tracheostomy placement. The timing of tracheostomy is thus a clinical decision. Clinical practice varies, with tracheostomy performed 2 to 6 weeks after the initial intubation.

Complications of endotracheal intubation and tracheostomy include aspiration, lower respiratory tract infection, bleeding from erosions induced by the tube or a suction catheter, sinusitis, intraluminal scar formation that narrows the trachea, or tracheal collapse. It is important to remove these tubes as soon as they are no longer needed in order to minimize such side effects.

Similar to its use for obstruction in the vascular bed, stent placement in an airway or balloon dilatation of the airway can be tried to relieve significant airway obstruction or collapse in the trachea or large bronchi. Conditions that may merit this treatment include post-transplantation or postirradiation bronchial stenosis, bronchomalacia, malignant obstruction of large airways, respiratory–esophageal fistula, or congenital tracheobronchomegaly.

MECHANICAL VENTILATION

Mechanical ventilation is initiated most often for patients who fail to ventilate adequately due to conditions such as drug overdose, operative anesthetics, neuromuscular disease, or asthma and COPD exacerbations. In this setting, $PaCO_2$ is acutely elevated such that the pH falls to less than 7.20 to 7.25. The second major category of patients who merit mechanical ventilation comprises primarily hypoxemic patients who may have a condition such as pneumonia, aspiration, cardiogenic pulmonary edema, or acute respiratory distress syndrome (ARDS) and need ventilation mainly to support oxygenation. Often, mechanical ventilation is required when $P(A-a)O_2$ is more than 350 mm Hg while the patient is receiving 100% oxygen. Some persons may also require ventilation if they are experiencing excessive work of breathing.

Mechanical ventilation through an endotracheal tube delivers positive pressure during inspiration and expiration, in contrast to normal breathing whereby inspiration is accompanied by negative intrathoracic pressure. Standard ventilation is most often volume-limited where a preset volume of air is delivered to the patient (volume-controlled, pressure- or time-cycled), but it can also be pressure-limited, whereby the tidal volume is determined by a preset pressure and the volume varies with chest wall and lung compliance (pressure-controlled, volume- or time-cycled). Several different means of delivering ventilation to a patient are available; these are called *modes* (Table 390.2). Frequently used

TABLE 390.2	TYPES AND MODES OF MECHANICAL VENTILATION	
Type	**Mode**	**Description**
Conventional positive-pressure ventilation: tidal volume preset (volume or time cycled)	Assisted mechanical ventilation (AMV) or assist control (AC)	All breaths machine delivered at preset tidal volume; patient can increase rate (and thus minute ventilation) by triggering additional machine breaths if desired
	Controlled mechanical ventilation (CMV)	All breaths machine delivered at preset tidal volume; fixed rate (and minute ventilation) cannot be increased by patient effort
	Intermittent mandatory ventilation (IMV)	Fixed rate of machine-delivered, set-tidal-volume breaths; patient can also breathe spontaneously between machine-delivered breaths if desired
	Synchronized intermittent mandatory ventilation (SIMV)	As in IMV, except that machine-delivered breaths are initiated only after patient exhales, preventing "stacking" on spontaneous breaths
Conventional positive-pressure ventilation; peak pressure preset (flow or time cycled)	Pressure support (PS)	Patient breathes spontaneously and determines rate; tidal volume is determined by inflation pressure used and patient's lung–thorax compliance; minute ventilation varies, depending on inflation pressure used
	Pressure control ventilation (PCV)	Inflation pressure, inspiratory time, and rate are fixed, with tidal volume (and thus minute ventilation) determined by patient's lung–thorax compliance
	Pressure control with inverse-ratio ventilation (PCIRV)	As with PCV, but with inspiratory time exceeding expiratory time, thus increasing proportion of ventilatory cycle spent at peak inflation volume
	Airway pressure release ventilation (APRV)	Patient breathes spontaneously at high level of continuous positive airway pressure (CPAP), which is released intermittently to allow brief passive exhalation to lower lung volume; minute ventilation determined by patient's spontaneous rate and inspiratory effort plus CPAP level and frequency of pressure release
High-frequency ventilation	High-frequency positive-pressure ventilation (HFPPV)	Preset (usually small) tidal volume, as with AMV, CMV, or IMV, at cycling frequencies of 60–110 breaths/min
	High-frequency jet ventilation (HFJV)	Bursts of high-pressure (jet) gas flow directly into patient's trachea at rates of 60–150 bursts/min: delivered tidal volume augmented by entrainment from a second, humidified gas source; tidal volume and minute ventilation are unknown
	High-frequency oscillation (HFO)	Oscillation of gas in the respiratory tract at 600–1,200 cycles/min (10–20 Hz) with both inspiration and expiration active
	High-frequency body surface oscillation (HFBSO); also called external chest wall oscillation (ECWO)	Oscillation applied to the chest wall at frequencies of 60–300 cycles/min (1–5 Hz), with both inspiration and expiration active
Negative-pressure ventilation		Intermittently applied subatmospheric pressure to the chest and abdomen, either by a rigid tank into which the patient is placed with head protruding (tank ventilator; "iron lung"), a less extensive shell covering only the thorax (chest cuirass), or a rigid chest piece covered by a "pneumo-wrap" or "poncho" sealed at neck, arms, and feet
Ventilation by displacement of abdominal contents	Rocking bed	Patient is rocked back and forth through an arc of approximately 45 degrees, using the force of gravity to produce diaphragmatic motion
	Pneumo-belt	Periodic inflation and deflation of a rubber bladder contained in a wide abdominal corset, causing upward diaphragmatic motion

modes of volume-limited ventilation include assist control (AC) and synchronized intermittent mandatory ventilation (SIMV). Most ventilation is accomplished using one of these two modes. AC may result in higher ventilation because each initiated breath is a full tidal volume but usually induces a lower work of breathing. SIMV generates less alkalosis but induces a higher work of breathing. Frequently used pressure-limited modes are pressure support ventilation (PSV), where pressure support is given only during the inspiratory phase with spontaneous breathing, and pressure control where pressure truly limits ventilation. PSV heightens patient–ventilator synchrony but relies on an intact drive; therefore, it should not be used for patients who require high-level sedation. It is, however, a well-tolerated and commonly used mode of weaning. Pressure control is most often implemented for the severely hypoxemic patient. The concept that barotrauma is induced by high volumes or large swings in intra-alveolar pressure, and the fact that this is deleterious favors use of this mode for the complicated ARDS, trauma, or sepsis patient.

Initial ventilator settings are chosen to minimize peak and mean airway pressures while delivering adequate oxygen. This may often be accomplished with volume-cycled ventilation using a tidal volume of 6 to 8 mL per kilogram (400 to 600 cm^3 for the average adult), a respiratory rate of 10 to 20, and an FIO_2 of 100%, with either an AC or an SIMV mode. Initial settings, including flow rate, are adjusted to keep peak airway pressure below 35 to 40 cm H_2O. The aim is also to improve patient synchrony with the ventilator and to decrease the work of breathing (the energy expended to breathe). Increased availability of microprocessor technology on ventilators has been helpful in achieving these goals.

Complications from mechanical ventilation and endotracheal intubation are common. This realization led to recent attempts to switch to noninvasive ventilation whenever possible. Positive-pressure ventilation may adversely affect every organ system. The most important complications are barotrauma, hemodynamic compromise, and nosocomial infection. Barotrauma results from overdistention of alveoli under positive pressure, with pneumothorax being one common manifestation. The alveoli can rupture, forcing gas into adjacent interstitium, with subsequent tracking into the pleural space, mediastinum, or peritoneum as well as into vessels, which may cause air emboli. Keeping peak pressures as low as possible, below 35 to 40 cm H_2O, minimizes this complication. In general, application of positive-pressure ventilation decreases venous return to the heart and thus lowers cardiac output, which may lead to hypotension and impaired oxygen delivery. Persistent hypotension can worsen renal and other organ function, thus escalating multiorgan failure. The third major complication, nosocomial infection (especially ventilator-associated pneumonia), remains a common problem for as many as 10% to 15% of ventilated patients.

Since there is a potential for oxygen toxicity on FIO_2 of 60% or greater, the lowest necessary FIO_2 should be selected. To lower the FIO_2, positive end-expiratory pressure (PEEP) can be used. PEEP works by increasing the lung volume, thereby opening collapsed alveoli and improving ventilation/perfusion matching. Potential problems with PEEP are an increased likelihood of barotrauma and hypotension, similar to that of positive-pressure ventilation itself.

Auto-PEEP, or intrinsic PEEP, is the development of hyperinflation within the alveolus during mechanical ventilation. It should be routinely monitored in ventilated patients. It is caused by the ventilator delivery of positive-pressure breaths before complete exhalation of the previous breath has occurred. It is most common in conditions with a high minute ventilation

---

TABLE 390.3. WEANING FROM MECHANICAL VENTILATION

1. Determine that the patient's clinical condition is appropriate for a weaning attempt:
   a. Disorder or situation precipitating need for mechanical ventilation has resolved or improved
   b. FIO_2 requirement for acceptable PaO_2 is ≤0.40–0.50
   c. Ventilation requirement for normal or desired $PaCO_2$ is <10–12 L/min
   d. Patient's ventilatory mechanics and drive are adequate for spontaneous ventilation:
      Spontaneous vital capacity >10 mL/kg
      Maximum inspiratory force >20–25 cm H_2O
      Rapid shallow breathing index (f/V_T) <100[a]
      If feasible, patient can double resting ventilation requirement during brief (10–12 s) maximum voluntary ventilation maneuver
2. Choose an appropriate time for the weaning attempt:
   a. Adequate support personnel (respiratory care practitioner; nurse) available at bedside
   b. No other procedures or manipulations of the patient expected during the period of the weaning attempt
3. Reduce or discontinue respiratory depressant drugs (e.g., narcotics, benzodiazepines, hypnotics)
4. Clear airway using endotracheal suction as needed
5. Position patient upright or semiupright if feasible
6. Switch patient from mechanical to spontaneous ventilation, using same FIO_2 or increasing it by 0.10[b]
7. Monitor patient appropriately during weaning trial:
   a. Bedside observation and reassurance
   b. Arterial blood gas measurement after 20–30 min[c]
   c. Continue spontaneous ventilation if PaO_2 is >80% of pre-weaning value with adequate arterial hemoglobin saturation, and arterial pH is acceptable (e.g., 7.30 or higher)
8. Extubate patient after 20–30 min of spontaneous breathing, provided:
   a. Oxygenation and ventilation are adequate, as above
   b. Patient is awake and responsive, with gag reflex present
   c. Patient can cough
   d. Airway secretions are manageable in amount and consistency
   e. Signs of upper airway obstruction are absent (e.g., patient can exhale around deflated endotracheal tube cuff)

---

[a] Example: While breathing spontaneously at 20 breaths/min with V_T 0.4 L/breath, the value for this index would be 20/0.4 = 50.
[b] Leaving patient attached to ventilator and turning rate to 0 breaths/min is adequate in many settings, although breathing through ventilator circuit may impose excessive work of breathing in patients with marginal reserve, especially with some ventilator models in such patients, a separate T-piece circuit should be used.
[c] Pulse oximetry is insufficient in most instances because it does not detect changes in $PaCO_2$ and pH on which the success or failure of a weaning attempt usually rest.
FIO_2, fraction of inspired oxygen; f/V_T, breath frequency divided by tidal volume.

(amount of air breathed per minute), such as in ARDS and in diseases of airflow limitation (asthma and COPD). Since the ventilator manometer will not register auto-PEEP, detection involves occlusion of the expiratory port at end exhalation, allowing equilibration of the airway and circuit pressure. The complications of auto-PEEP are similar to those of applied PEEP: diminished cardiac output and actual hypotension, increased intracranial pressure, increased risk of barotrauma, and inaccurate pulmonary artery catheter measurements, including false elevation of the wedge pressure which may lead to inappropriate fluid and vasopressor management. Strategies to reduce auto-PEEP include use of a large-bore endotracheal tube, slowing of respiratory rate, lowering of minute ventilation, increasing of inspiratory flow rates and thereby allowing for more exhalation time, use of bronchodilators if appropriate, sedation, paralysis, and addition of PEEP equivalent to the original auto-PEEP.

There are many ways to wean a patient from the ventilator. The first task for the clinician is to assess the patient's readiness to wean with spontaneous ventilatory parameters or the even more useful rapid shallow breathing index (Table 390.3). The rapid shallow breathing index can distinguish persons with a high likelihood of weaning failure. It is the ratio of breaths per minute to tidal volume for a spontaneously breathing patient. If a patient breathing spontaneously has an index greater than 100 breaths per minute per liter, the chance of weaning success is negligible. The observation of excessive accessory muscle use and paradoxical breathing during weaning is a useful physical examination adjunct to assessment of high likelihood of weaning failure.

There are several choices of weaning technique. A routine healthy postoperative patient may need little or no weaning from mechanical ventilation. For the patient in whom success is less certain, initial weaning choice may be either with a T piece, whereby a patient's endotracheal tube is connected to oxygen but separate from ventilator circuit; with sequentially diminishing levels of pressure support and assessment of tidal volume adequacy; or with lowering of SIMV breaths from 10 to 12 L per minute to less than 1 L per minute. Favored type of wean varies. Randomized trials indicated that both pressure support ventilation (PSV) and daily T-piece trials are good options for weaning. In general, patients will wean from mechanical ventilation as the underlying medical conditions that precipitated the need for starting ventilation resolve.

NONINVASIVE POSITIVE-PRESSURE VENTILATION

Noninvasive positive-pressure ventilation (NIPPV) consists of mask delivery of air or oxygen under positive pressure, but it is otherwise similar to standard mechanical ventilation by an endotracheal tube. This technique is advocated in acute respiratory failure to avoid the complications of endotracheal intubation and mechanical ventilation, particularly those of nosocomial infections. During the past few years, NIPPV use has risen in hospitalized patients in three settings: (a) treatment of acute respiratory failure, especially respiratory failure due to chronic obstructive lung disease exacerbations; (b) weaning; and (c) post-

operative support of ventilation. There is some evidence that NIPPV shortens the length of ICU stay, and a recent meta-analysis of seven randomized controlled trials showed that use of NIPPV decreased the need for endotracheal intubation and improved survival in persons with respiratory failure due to acute exacerbations of COPD. In addition, the use of early extubation with subsequent noninvasive ventilation weans in acute respiratory failure/COPD decreased weaning times, diminished nosocomial pneumonia, and improved 60-day survival. For chronic home use, patients may receive nocturnal positive-pressure ventilation either for chronic respiratory failure due to neuromuscular disease or for obstructive sleep apnea therapy where treatment increases upper airway pressure, keeps the airway patent, and prevents apneas.

NIPPV can be delivered as either continuous positive airway pressure (CPAP) or bilevel positive airway pressure (Bi-PAP). CPAP is the application of positive pressure at one level throughout the respiratory cycle. Bi-PAP consists of separately set inspiratory and expiratory pressures, with the difference between these two set pressures being a driving pressure for ventilation. Bi-PAP can be administered with or without time-cycled breaths, similar to standard mechanical ventilation. Use of either of these methods of NIPPV may be achieved via nasal mask or full-face mask, and oxygen can be administered simultaneously. The importance of coaching and talking patients through the setup and implementation of NIPPV cannot be overemphasized. If a patient cannot cooperate, the success rate of this therapy drops dramatically. Mask fit is especially important to the success of this therapy. Initiation of this technique is time consuming for therapists, nurses, and doctors, which has limited its use in some settings (e.g., emergency room).

OTHER RESPIRATORY THERAPY TECHNIQUES

Two goals of treatment underlie many of the standard respiratory therapy techniques: removal of secretions and expansion of lung volume to diminish atelectasis. Both of these goals may lead to improved oxygenation and reduced infection rates. Therapies that address these two objectives are interrelated. Sputum removal may be a particularly important strategy for the patient with bronchiectasis or chronic bronchitis. Chest physiotherapy, renamed postural drainage therapy (PDT) in the recently published National Board for Respiratory Care practice guidelines, includes techniques of postural drainage, chest wall percussion and vibration, coughing, suctioning, breathing exercises, and patient mobilization. These sputum removal techniques are listed in Table 390.4. Although postural drainage is thought to be an important component of PDT, measurement of efficacy of PDT is difficult as there is little standardization of protocols and published studies include only small numbers of patients. Cook and colleagues undertook comparison of several PDT techniques with a meta-analysis to address efficacy and cost containment. Despite use of percussion and vibration techniques for many years, there is little evidence to support their use. Additionally, they are labor-intensive, requiring a trained therapist to assist the patient. Ultrasonic therapy is similarly labor-intensive

TABLE 390.4.	RESPIRATORY THERAPY TECHNIQUES
Technique	**Description**
Techniques to Enhance Removal of Secretions: Airway Clearance Techniques	
• Postural drainage	Positioning to increase secretion and drainage
• Cough	
• Chest wall percussion and vibration	Chest wall pounding by a skilled assistant
• Ultrasonic vibration	Delivery of high-frequency vibration the thorax
• Flutter valve	Hand-held device that, upon exhalation, induces oscillations in pressure and flow, thus vibrating the airway walls and loosening mucus. Decreased need for assistance
• ThAirapy vest	Bronchial drainage system that allows for self-administered high-frequency chest compressions
• Mucolytics	Medications such as rhDNAase and n-acetylcysteine, which decrease viscosity of secretions
• Suctioning	Useful when upper airway bypassed
• Humidification	Moisture delivery by mask or tube
• Aerosol therapy	Medication delivery by airway
Maneuvers to Increase Lung Expansion, Which May Also Improve Secretion Removal	
• Cough	
• Voluntary deep breathing exercises	Used in spontaneously breathing patients
• Forced expiratory technique	Huff cough
• Autogenic drainage	Breathing maneuvers with cough suppression
• Diaphragmatic breathing	
• Positive expiratory pressure valve	Increases expiratory expansion
• Incentive spirometry	Increases inspiratory volume
• Intermittent positive-pressure breathing	Delivery of positive-pressure breaths by mask or mouthpiece, often for medication delivery
• Continuous positive airway pressure	Improves oxygenation, treats atelectasis
• Bilevel positive airway pressure	Useful for preventing atelectasis in postoperative obese patients
• Patient mobilization	Exercise (such as walking) to increase likelihood of deep breathing

without proven efficacy beyond other PDT techniques. Use of a flutter valve during exhalation induces oscillations in pressure and flow, which vibrate the airway walls and loosen mucus. This has received much recent attention, as has the ThAirapy vest, a new device that allows a patient to self-administer high-frequency chest compressions. The advantages of the flutter valve

and the vest are the capacity for self-administration and the resulting lower associated personnel cost. Mucolytic drugs, such as acetylcysteine or rhDNAase delivered into the airway, may also enhance secretion removal, although survival efficacy is unproven.

Techniques to increase lung expansion are also listed in Table 390.4. These, in addition to postural drainage itself, are thought to be the major useful components of chest physiotherapy. The huff or forced expiratory technique (FET) is controlled diaphragmatic breathing interspersed with forced expirations from mid- to low-lung volume. It is more effective than either manual techniques or intermittent positive-pressure breathing (IPPB) to increase sputum production in cystic fibrosis patients. Since after initial instruction it involves using the efforts of the patient only, rather than the services of an additional therapist, it is time- and cost-effective for many patients. Positive expiratory pressure (PEP) therapy uses exhalation through a fixed-orifice resistor at an expiratory pressure of 10 to 20 cm H_2O. PEP splints airways open so that the patient can expectorate secretions using the huff technique. It is simple to use, and is an inexpensive way to remove secretions and expand lungs. In cystic fibrosis patients, PEP mask breathing with FET was compared both to postural drainage and FET and to exercise bicycle and FET. All were effective in sputum removal.

Patient mobilization and exercise are important not only for sputum removal in the chronically infected patient but also for avoidance of postoperative atelectasis. Intermittent positive-pressure breathing, incentive spirometry, and CPAP have all been shown to reduce postoperative atelectasis. Supplemental oxygen therapy should not be interrupted to deliver these treatments.

Undesirable effects of PDT and related procedures include hypoxemia, pain, dehiscence of wounds, arrhythmias, or displacement of lines, endotracheal tubes, and chest tubes. Pain can be assessed and pretreated with analgesia. When chest physiotherapy is poorly tolerated or accompanied by pain, patient compliance diminishes to about 40%.

AIRWAY SUCTIONING

Suctioning with a catheter through the nose, mouth, or endotracheal or tracheostomy tube is another therapy implemented to remove secretions from the airways. Its use should be limited to situations where the patient is mechanically ventilated or where other physiotherapy modes to remove secretions have been ineffective. Secondary goals of suctioning include improving oxygenation and lowering the work of breathing. All patients on ventilators whose upper airways are bypassed with an endotracheal tube undergo routine suctioning. Patients may also need suctioning if they are producing copious secretions due to bronchiectasis or pneumonia, where the secretions cannot be mobilized with less invasive techniques, such as a cough or a forced breathing maneuver. If a patient is bleeding or vomiting, or has lost the cough reflex due to underlying neurologic disease, sedatives, overdose, or stroke, intermittent suctioning is often indicated.

A rigid suction catheter is used for removal of oral secretions and a flexible catheter is used for airway suctioning to avoid airway trauma and abrasions. The airway catheter is inserted using sterile technique to minimize the risk of nosocomial pneumonia. Normal saline instillation before suctioning is practiced routinely for ventilated patients, without much data to suggest its benefit. Some hospitals have recently implemented suctioning without normal saline unless secretions are too viscid. Complications of suctioning include hypoxemia, arrhythmias, and hemodynamic instability. A closed-system, in-line suction catheter is frequently placed into mechanical ventilator circuits to minimize these complications and to reduce the aerosol spread of infectious particles into the atmosphere.

HUMIDITY AND AEROSOL THERAPY

Humidity is delivered to the airways for several theoretical reasons, mostly to avoid excessive drying when the glottis and upper airway are bypassed, as happens with endotracheal or tracheostomy tube placement. Humidity may also improve mucus transport or provide passive heating for a hypothermic patient. Humidification therapy is most commonly used for mechanically ventilated patients, but whether there is benefit from humidity alone in any other situation is unclear. Two categories of humidification devices are available for the ventilated patient; a heat moisture exchanger, which allows passive heat production and high flow, and a heated humidifier, such as a cascade or the bubble-through-wick apparatus. Potential complications and relative cost in part decide the choice of device. Heat moisture exchangers have the potential for high airway resistance, which may hamper weaning for a patient with underlying respiratory disease. In contrast, heated humidifiers are easily colonized with bacteria, may also develop high resistance from the pooled condensate in the circuit, and can burn airway mucosa if the heater malfunctions.

MEDICATION VIA AEROSOL THERAPY

The medications that can be administered by aerosol therapy are numerous and the list is growing. These include bronchodilators, anti-inflammatory medications, corticosteroids, morphine, topical anesthetics, mucolytic agents, insulin, other hormones, epinephrine, antibiotics, and antiviral therapy. Many of these can also be given by mouth or vein. Reasons to choose an inhaled method of delivery include better penetration of a drug delivered by the aerosol route to the site of action, often the lungs or airways. In addition, some medications may be given by aerosol on an emergency basis, even in the absence of intravenous access.

Three types of devices are used for aerosolized medication delivery: a small-volume nebulizer, a metered-dose inhaler, or a dry-powder inhaler. The small-volume nebulizer requires a higher dose of drug than the metered-dose inhaler and is correspondingly more costly. Its major benefit is that less mastery of technique is required for successful delivery of medications. Years of emergency room visits and home use for persons with asthma and COPD exacerbations have convinced patients that nebulizers are superior to metered-dose inhalers. Despite this bias, data

of Mandelberg et al. suggest that metered-dose inhalers are subjectively and objectively comparable, if not superior, for emergency room therapy and perhaps even ventilator use when used correctly.

Most anticholinergic agents, β-agonists, and anti-inflammatory therapy for asthma can be delivered with a metered-dose inhaler. The importance of good technique cannot be overestimated. Components of delivery include the following steps: inversion and shaking of the canister, normal exhalation, an activation push starting halfway through inhalation, and sustaining of a breath-hold for 4 to 10 seconds. Problems with technique happen at each step. Patients routinely misuse metered-dose inhalers and thus limit the efficacy of medication. At most, 10% of the solution is delivered to the lungs; however, doses are usually tenfold lower than for the nebulizer devices, since less drug is deposited in the large airways. For the elderly and the young infant, hand–mouth coordination is more difficult and the inhaler is often activated improperly, resulting in inadequate medication delivery. Use of a spacer attached to the inhaler, either 6 inches of ventilator tubing or a specially designed chamber device, improves drug delivery to the lungs. For arthritic adults, special adapters improve the ability to initiate dispensation. Dry-powder inhaler delivery systems are under development to meet the federal mandate to minimize fluorocarbon release into the atmosphere and avoid ozone depletion. In contrast to the metered-dose inhaler, these devices are easy to use; however, they are not available for ventilator attachment.

BIBLIOGRAPHY

Brochard L, Rauss A, Benito S, et al. Comparison of three methods of gradual withdrawal from ventilatory support during weaning from mechanical ventilation. *Am J Respir Crit Care Med* 1994;150:896–903.

Celli BR, Rodriguez KS, Snider GL. A controlled trial of intermittent positive pressure breathing, incentive spirometry, and deep breathing exercises in preventing pulmonary complications after abdominal surgery. *Am Rev Respir Dis* 1984;130:12–15.

Esteban A, Frutos F, Tobin MJ, et al. A comparison of four methods of weaning patients from mechanical ventilation. Spanish Lung Failure Collaborative Group. *N Engl J Med* 1995;332:345–350.

Keenan SP, Kernerman PD, Cook DJ, et al. Effect of noninvasive positive pressure ventilation on mortality in patients admitted with acute respiratory failure: a meta-analysis. *Crit Care Med* 1997;25:1685–1692.

Lannefors L, Wollmer P. Mucus clearance with three chest physiotherapy regimes in cystic fibrosis: comparison between postural drainage, PEP and physical exercise. *Eur Respir J* 1992;5:748–753.

Mandelberg A, Chen E, Novishi N, et al. Nebulized wet aerosol treatment in emergency department—is it essential? Comparison with large space device for metered-dose inhaler. *Chest* 1997;112:1501–1505.

Maziak DE, Meade MO, Todd TR. The timing of tracheotomy: a systematic review. *Chest* 1998;114:605–609.

Nava S, Ambrosino N, Clini E, et al. Noninvasive mechanical ventilation in weaning patients with respiratory failure due to chronic obstructive pulmonary disease. A randomized controlled trial. *Ann Intern Med* 1998; 128:721–728.

Nocturnal Oxygen Therapy Trial Group. Continuous or nocturnal oxygen therapy in hypoxemic chronic obstructive lung disease: a clinical trial. *Ann Intern Med* 1980;93:391–398.

Thomas J, Cook DJ, Brooks D. Chest physical therapy. Management of patients with cystic fibrosis: a meta-analysis. *Am J Respir Crit Care Med* 1995;151:846–850.

Kelley's Textbook of Internal Medicine, fourth edition. Edited by H. David Humes. Lippincott Williams & Wilkins, Philadelphia © 2000.

C H A P T E R
391

LUNG TRANSPLANTATION

ROBERT M. KOTLOFF

Human lung transplantation was first attempted in 1963, but it was not until two decades later that extended survival was achieved. Further refinements in patient selection, surgical technique, and postoperative care have since facilitated the successful application of lung transplantation to a wide variety of advanced disorders of the airways, lung parenchyma, and pulmonary vasculature. There has been a marked proliferation of lung transplant centers worldwide, and as of 1999 more than 9,000 procedures had been performed.

Although lung transplantation has assumed an important role in the therapeutic approach to select patients with advanced lung disease, several serious problems remain that limit its efficacy. There is a severe shortage of suitable donor organs at a level that is increasingly insufficient to meet current demands. Immunosuppressive therapy is associated with a number of troubling side effects, most notably a significant risk of infection and malignancy. Rejection occurs frequently and continually threatens organ function. Though lung transplantation offers the prospect of improved quality of life, long-term survival remains an elusive goal, with less than half of recipients living beyond 5 years. To optimize outcomes in the face of these shortcomings, it is essential that candidates be selected judiciously and that care of recipients be rendered in a meticulous and vigilant fashion.

CURRENT TRENDS IN TRANSPLANT ACTIVITY

Following the initial technical successes of the 1980s, the field of lung transplantation realized tremendous growth in both the number of procedures performed and the number of candidates listed (Fig. 391.1). Over the past several years, however, lung transplant activity in the United States has leveled off at an approximate rate of 800 to 900 procedures annually, representing one-third the volume of heart transplants and one-fourth the volume of liver transplants performed. This limitation reflects a fixed cadaveric organ donor pool, accentuated by the fact that only 15% of cadaveric donors have lungs suitable for harvest. As a result of the current donor constraints, the number of registered candidates now exceeds the annual number of procedures by threefold (Fig. 391.1), the median waiting time has escalated to 18 months, and an increasing number of candidates are dying on the waiting list.

INDICATIONS

The range of diseases amenable to transplantation is broad. Chronic obstructive pulmonary disease (including α_1-antityp-

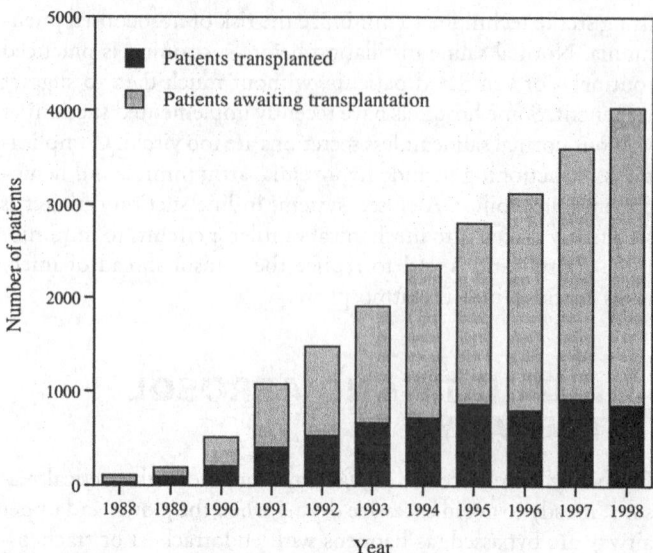

FIGURE 391.1. Lung transplantation–related activity in the United States between 1988 and 1998. There is a widening discrepancy between the number of patients awaiting transplantation and the number of procedures performed annually. (Data from the United Network for Organ Sharing U.S. Scientific Registry.)

sin deficiency) represents the most common indication, accounting for approximately 40% of all procedures. Other established indications are idiopathic pulmonary fibrosis, primary pulmonary hypertension, Eisenmenger's syndrome, and cystic fibrosis. Less common disorders for which transplantation has been successfully applied include lymphangioleiomyomatosis, eosinophilic granuloma, bronchiectasis unrelated to cystic fibrosis, and pulmonary fibrosis due to radiation or drugs. Transplantation of patients with lung disease due to a systemic process remains controversial. In this regard, reports of frequent disease recurrence in patients with sarcoidosis and of extrapulmonary complications in patients with collagen vascular disease have raised concern about the suitability of such patients for transplantation. Nonetheless, short-term functional outcomes and survival following transplantation are comparable to those of other patient populations, and most centers are willing to offer transplantation to carefully selected patients without significant extrapulmonary organ dysfunction.

TIMING OF REFERRAL

Several considerations impact on the timing of referral for lung transplantation. The inherent risks of transplantation, including a 50% mortality rate by 5 years, dictate that this option be reserved for patients with advanced, life-threatening disease for which alternative therapies are unavailable or unsuccessful. On the other hand, patients who have progressed to a stage of profound debility are poor candidates at high risk for perioperative morbidity and mortality and for inferior functional recovery. Thus, patients should be referred during the "transplant window" when they are sufficiently ill to warrant the risks of transplantation but not so ill as to compromise the likelihood of a

TABLE 391.1.	DISEASE-SPECIFIC GUIDELINES FOR LISTING FOR LUNG TRANSPLANTATION

Chronic Obstructive Pulmonary Disease

- Postbronchodilator forced expiratory volume in 1 second (FEV_1) <25% of predicted and/or presence of cor pulmonale and/or P_{CO_2} > 55 mm Hg

Idiopathic Pulmonary Fibrosis

- Symptomatic, progressive disease unresponsive to medical therapy
- Vital capacity below 60–70% of predicted
- Resting or exercise oxygen desaturation

Cystic fibrosis

- FEV_1 <30% of predicted, or rapidly declining lung function if FEV_1 >30%
- Females and patients <18 years of age have a poorer prognosis; consider earlier referral

Primary Pulmonary Hypertension

- New York Heart Association functional class III or IV despite optimal medical therapy (including intravenous prostacyclin)
- Parameters portending a high risk of death include mean pulmonary arterial pressure >55 mm Hg, mean right atrial pressure >15 mm Hg, and cardiac index <2 L/min/m²

Eisenmenger's Syndrome

- New York Heart Association functional class III or IV despite optimal medical therapy

(Modified from Maurer JR, Frost AE, Estenne M, et al. International guidelines for the selection of lung transplant candidates. *J Heart Lung Transplant* 1998;17:703.)

PATIENT SELECTION

Selection criteria are necessarily stringent in order to maximize the likelihood of successful outcomes. Indiscriminate transplantation of poor candidates willing to accept any degree of risk cannot be justified in the face of current severe organ shortages. Recommended selection criteria are listed in Table 391.2. The scarcity of organs and the somewhat inferior outcomes achieved with increasing age have prompted the establishment of recom-

TABLE 391.2.	GENERAL GUIDELINES FOR TRANSPLANT RECIPIENT SELECTION

Indications

- Advanced obstructive, fibrotic, or pulmonary vascular disease with a high risk of death within 2–3 years
- Alternative therapies unsuccessful or unavailable
- Ambulatory but with severe functional limitation (New York Heart Association class III or IV)
- Age ≤55 years for heart lung; ≤60 years for bilateral lung; ≤65 years for single lung

Absolute Contraindications

- Severe extrapulmonary organ dysfunction including:
  - Renal insufficiency with creatinine clearance <50 mL/min
  - Hepatic dysfunction with coagulopathy or portal hypertension
  - Left ventricular dysfunction or severe coronary artery disease (consider heart–lung transplantation)
- Acute, critical illness
- Active malignancy, or recent history of malignancy with significant likelihood of recurrence (except for basal and squamous cell carcinoma of the skin)
- Hepatitis B antigen positivity
- Hepatitis C with histologic evidence of liver disease
- Infection with HIV
- Severe psychiatric illness; drug or alcohol abuse
- Active or recent (past 6 months) cigarette smoking
- Nonambulatory with poor rehabilitation potential
- Extremes of weight (<70% or >130% of ideal body weight)

Relative Contraindications (considered on an individual basis)

- Chronic medical conditions that are poorly controlled or associated with target organ damage
- History of noncompliance with medical care
- Daily corticosteroid requirements in excess of 20 mg of prednisone (or equivalent)
- Mechanical ventilation (excluding noninvasive ventilation)
- Prior thoracic surgery
- Aspergillomas, especially when associated with significant pleural reaction
- Active collagen vascular disease, particulary with extrapulmonary manifestations
- Preoperative colonization of the airways with pan-resistant bacteria (presence of *Burkholderia cepacia* considered an absolute contraindication by some centers)[a]

(Modified from Maurer JR, Frost AE, Estenne M, et al. International guidelines for the selection of lung transplant candidates. *J Heart Lung Transplant* 1998;17:703.)
[a] Applies to patients with cystic fibrosis.

successful outcome. An additional factor that must be considered is an anticipated waiting time of 12 to 24 months at most centers, during which the patient must remain functionally suitable for transplantation.

Disease-specific guidelines for timely referral and listing of patients, based on available prognostic indexes, are listed in Table 391.1. The patient's perception of an unacceptably poor quality of life is an important additional factor to consider but should not serve as the sole justification for referral of a patient whose disease is not deemed to be at a life-threatening stage. The imprecise nature of predictive indexes must be acknowledged, particularly with respect to chronic obstructive pulmonary disease and Eisenmenger's syndrome, which tend to follow highly variable and often protracted courses even in the advanced stages. In contrast, idiopathic pulmonary fibrosis is usually a rapidly progressive and highly lethal disease without effective medical treatment; early referral of such patients for transplantation is prudent. The availability of continuous intravenous prostacyclin for treatment of primary pulmonary hypertension has influenced the timing of transplantation for this group of patients. The use of prostacylin has been associated with improvement in hemodynamics, exercise tolerance, and survival. While previously viewed as a "bridge" to transplantation, this therapeutic modality can actually obviate the need for transplantation for those patients who demonstrate a dramatic and sustained response.

mended age cutoffs: 55 years for heart–lung, 60 years for bilateral lung, and 65 years for single-lung transplantation. Candidates should be functionally disabled (New York Heart Association class III or IV) but still ambulatory and able to participate in preoperative pulmonary rehabilitation. They should be free of significant extrapulmonary end-organ dysfunction. In particular, renal function must be normal or only mildly impaired since the chronic use of cyclosporine or tacrolimus following transplantation invariably causes significant renal insufficiency. Adequate hepatic function is necessary to minimize the risk of postoperative bleeding, liver failure, and drug toxicity. This issue has been most closely examined in patients with pulmonary hypertension and passive hepatic congestion, for whom a preoperative bilirubin level exceeding 2.1 mg per deciliter is associated with an early post-transplantation mortality rate approaching 60%, as compared to 16% for those with normal bilirubin levels. Severe left ventricular dysfunction or extensive coronary artery disease contraindicates isolated lung transplantation but warrants consideration of heart–lung transplantation for younger candidates. Other absolute contraindications include active infection with HIV or hepatitis B virus infection with hepatitis C virus with evidence of significant liver damage; active or recent cigarette smoking, drug abuse, or alcohol abuse; and extremes of weight. Current or recent history of malignancy (other than skin cancer) is also considered an absolute contraindication, though there have been several recent attempts to utilize lung transplantation with curative intent for patients with bronchoalveolar cell carcinoma restricted to the lungs. The risk posed by other chronic medical conditions, such as diabetes mellitus, hypertension, osteoporosis, and limited coronary artery disease, must be assessed individually based on severity of disease, presence of end-organ damage, and ease of control with standard therapies.

Selection criteria have been liberalized in several important areas. Preoperative corticosteroid therapy was once considered an absolute contraindication as it was believed to impair healing of the bronchial anastomosis. Refinement in the surgical handling of this precarious anastomosis now permits transplantation to be safely performed in patients maintained on moderate doses of steroids. Prior thoracic surgery or pleurodesis renders the native lung more difficult to explant and increases the risk of perioperative bleeding, particularly when cardiopulmonary bypass is required, but does not contraindicate transplantation in most instances. As discussed previously, transplantation of carefully selected patients with active collagen vascular disease is now considered appropriate by many centers as long as there are no major extrathoracic manifestations that could compromise outcomes. Perhaps most controversial is the transplantation of mechanically ventilated patients. In the absence of an allocation system that preferentially diverts lungs to patients with respiratory failure, expeditious transplantation is feasible only for those patients whose accrued time places them at the top of the waiting list. In these circumstances, some centers are willing to offer transplantation until the time that progressive debility or superimposed complications necessitate deactivation of the ventilator-dependent patient. Although successful outcomes have been reported, preoperative mechanical ventilation is associated with an increased likelihood of death in the first post-transplantation year.

The presence of chronic infection of the airways and sinuses poses unique risks for patients with cystic fibrosis. In general, however, the incidence of post-transplantation infection in the cystic fibrosis population is similar to that of other groups. Some centers exclude patients harboring pan-resistant *Pseudomonas aeruginosa*, but recent evidence demonstrating similar infection rates and survival compared to patients colonized with sensitive strains has challenged this policy. The experience with *Burkholderia cepacia* has been much more ominous. This organism is intrinsically resistant to available classes of antibiotics and has a propensity to reemerge in the post-transplantation period as a cause of life-threatening infections. Because of its association with inferior survival rates, an increasing number of centers consider preoperative colonization with *B. cepacia* to be an absolute contraindication to transplantation. Colonization of the respiratory tract with *Aspergillus* organisms, while common among cystic fibrosis patients, does not appear to portend an increased risk of post-transplantation infection. Exclusion of patients on the basis of positive preoperative cultures is therefore not justified. Furthermore, the merits of attempting to eradicate the organism prior to transplantation, a strategy advocated by some programs, remain uncertain.

■ DONOR SELECTION AND ORGAN ALLOCATION

In addition to meeting strict criteria for declaration of brain death, cadaveric lung donors are selected on the basis of established guidelines (Table 391.3). Unfortunately, the lungs are a particularly fragile organ in the brain-dead patient and are frequently compromised by volume overload, contusion, aspiration of gastric contents, or pneumonia. The extreme scarcity of organs has prompted some programs to liberalize selection criteria to include older donors, more extensive smoking histories

TABLE 391.3.	**STANDARD DONOR CRITERIA FOR LUNG TRANSPLANTATION**

Age <55 years
Negative for HIV antibody and hepatitis B surface antigen
No active or recent history of malignancy (excluding localized squamous or basal cell skin cancer, localized cervical cancer, and primary brain tumors with low metastatic potential)
Cigarette smoking history of ≤20 pack-years
No history of significant chronic lung disease
No prior thoracic surgery on side of harvest
Absence of significant chest trauma
No evidence for aspiration or sepsis
Clear chest radiograph
Pao_2 ≥300 mm Hg on Fio_2 1.0, PEEP 5 cm H_2O
Absence of purulent secretions or gastric contents at bronchoscopy

---

Pao_2, partial pressure of oxygen; arterial; Fio_2, fraction of inspired oxygen; PEEP, positive end-expiratory pressure.

(in the absence of significant smoking-related lung disease), and contralateral organ harvest in the setting of a unilateral pneumonia or contusion.

Allocation of lungs to candidates awaiting transplantation is governed by time accrued rather than medical urgency. The only variance to this principle is a 90-day "credit" granted to patients with idiopathic pulmonary fibrosis at the time of listing, in deference to the rapidly deteriorating course associated with this disease. Specific donor–recipient matching is based on size and ABO blood group compatibility. Some centers also consider cytomegalovirus (CMV) serologic status, avoiding the use of a CMV-positive organ in a CMV-negative recipient. The relatively brief ischemic time tolerated by the lung allograft (typically less than 6 hours) precludes prospective human leukocyte antigen (HLA) matching. However, candidates identified through standard screening to have preformed circulating antibodies to foreign HLA antigens—arising from prior pregnancy, blood transfusions, or transplantation—require prospective donor–recipient lymphocytotoxic cross-matching to ensure compatibility.

AVAILABLE SURGICAL TECHNIQUES

Four techniques are currently utilized: heart–lung, single-lung, bilateral lung, and living donor bilobar transplantation. The choice of procedure is dictated by such factors as the underlying disease, age of the patient, and center-specific preferences.

Heart–lung transplantation was the first procedure to be successfully performed, but it has largely been supplanted by techniques to replace the lungs alone. Current indications are principally restricted to Eisenmenger's syndrome with surgically irreparable cardiac lesions, and advanced lung disease with concurrent left ventricular dysfunction or severe coronary artery disease. Previously, the presence of severe right ventricular dysfunction was deemed to be an indication for heart–lung transplantation. However, subsequent experience with isolated lung transplantation has demonstrated the remarkable ability of the right ventricle to recover once pulmonary artery pressures are normalized. Patients requiring heart–lung transplantation in the United States face a median waiting time of approximately 2.5 years, due to the preferential allocation of heart allografts to "status 1" cardiac transplantation candidates.

Single-lung transplantation is the most commonly performed procedure. A standard posterolateral thoracotomy incision is employed and three anastomoses are accomplished—main-stem bronchus, pulmonary artery, and left atrium (incorporating the two pulmonary veins). Major advantages of the procedure are its technical ease and its efficient use of the limited donor pool, permitting two recipients to benefit from a single donor. It is the procedure of choice for pulmonary fibrosis and for most patients with chronic obstructive pulmonary disease but is contraindicated in patients with suppurative lung disorders, such as cystic fibrosis. Debate persists on the role of single-lung transplantation for pulmonary hypertension. In this setting, nearly the entire cardiac output is diverted through the allograft due to the high vascular resistance in the remaining native lung. In the immediate postoperative period, this may predispose to

exaggerated reperfusion pulmonary edema in the allograft. Moreover, the extreme maldistribution of blood flow creates ventilation–perfusion mismatching that magnifies the degree of hypoxemia associated with episodes of graft dysfunction due to edema, pneumonia, or rejection. Although these potential pitfalls have led many to advocate against single-lung transplantation for these patients, some centers have reported excellent results, with the strong caveat that only organs deemed flawless at the time of harvest should be utilized.

Bilateral sequential lung transplantation involves the performance of two single-lung transplant procedures in succession during a single operative session. A bilateral thoracosternotomy ("clam-shell") incision, spanning the entire anterior thorax, is employed. In the absence of severe pulmonary hypertension, cardiopulmonary bypass can often be avoided by sustaining the patient on the contralateral lung during implantation of each allograft. The primary indications for this procedure are cystic fibrosis, other forms of bronchiectasis, and pulmonary vascular disorders. Additionally, some programs have advocated its use for younger patients with emphysema, arguing that it offers functional and survival advantages over single-lung transplantation.

Living donor bilateral lobar transplantation is a recently developed but still uncommonly performed procedure involving the implantation of lower lobes derived from each of two living, blood group–compatible donors. The procedure is most appropriately utilized for candidates whose deteriorating status does not permit them to wait for a cadaveric donor. In order to assure that the lobes will accommodate the size of the hemithoraxes, it is preferable that the donors be taller than the recipient. Patients with cystic fibrosis are particularly well suited as a target population since even as adults they tend to be of small stature. Intermediate-term functional outcomes and survival among recipients are similar to those achieved with cadaveric transplantation. Concerns about excessive risk to the donor have thus far proven unfounded. In the largest experience reported to date, there were no deaths among 120 donors and only four complications of sufficient magnitude to warrant surgical re-exploration. Donation of a lobe results in an average decrement in vital capacity of 15%, a degree of loss that is clinically inconsequential in an otherwise normal individual.

ROUTINE POST-TRANSPLANTATION MANAGEMENT

Care of the lung transplant recipient involves close surveillance to ensure that the allograft is functioning properly, that immunosuppressive medications are properly administered and adequately tolerated, and that complications are detected early and treated expeditiously. Most centers require patients to return frequently for office visits, blood tests, and chest radiographs during the initial 2 to 3 months following transplantation. Analogous to home glucose monitoring of the diabetic patient, lung transplant recipients chart their pulmonary function on a daily basis with a hand-held microspirometer and are instructed to contact the transplant center if a sustained fall of greater than

TABLE 391.4.	COMMONLY USED IMMUNOSUPPRESSIVE MEDICATIONS		
Medication	**Dosing[a]**	**Common Adverse Effects**	**Comments**
Cyclosporine/ tacrolimus	Cyclosporine: dosed to achieve a whole-blood trough level of 250–350 ng/mL (1st year), then 200–300 ng/mL Tacrolimus: dosed to achieve a whole-blood trough level of 10–20 ng/mL	Nephrotoxicity Hypertension Neurotoxicity (tremor, seizures, white-matter disease, headache) Hyperlipidemia Hyperkalemia, hypomagnesemia, hyperuricemia Hemolytic-uremic syndrome Hirsutism, gingival hyperplasia (cyclosporine) Osteoporosis (cyclosporine) Gastroparesis (cyclosporine) Hyperglycemia (tacrolimus)	*Blood levels are increased by:* Macrolide antibiotics Azole antifungals Calcium channel blockers (except nifedipine) *Blood levels are decreased by:* Anticonvulsants Rifampin
Azathioprine	2–2.5 mg/kg/d Adjust dose if WBC < 4,000/mm³	Leukopenia, anemia, thrombocytopenia Hepatotoxicity Pancreatitis Hair loss	Enhanced bone marrow suppression with allopurinol
Mycophenolate mofetil	1,000–1,500 mg b.i.d.	Diarrhea, nausea, vomiting Leukopenia	Used as an alternative to azathioprine
Prednisone	0.5 mg/kg/d for 3–6 mo, then tapered to a dose of 0.15 mg/kg/d	Hyperglycemia Hypertension Hyperlipidemia Weight gain Osteoporosis Myopathy Mood changes, insomnia Cataracts	
Equine polyclonal antilymphocyte globulin (Atgam)	10–15 mg/kg/d, adjusted to an absolute CD3 count of 50–100 cells/ mm³	Fever and chills Thrombocytopenia, leukopenia Serum sickness Anaphylaxis	May increase risk of cytomegalovirus reactivation and posttransplantation lymphopoliferative disorder

[a] Dosing is based on the protocol used at the University of Pennsylvania Medical Center; dosing may vary among transplantation centers.
[b] Measured by high-performance liquid chromatography assay.

10% in the forced expiratory volume in 1 second (FEV_1) or forced vital capacity is documented.

Many transplantation programs employ frequent surveillance bronchoscopies and transbronchial lung biopsies within the first post-transplantation year as a means of monitoring the allograft. Such an approach has been demonstrated to detect low-grade rejection in up to 39% and subclinical CMV pneumonia in 16% of asymptomatic, clinically stable patients. However, it has yet to be determined as to whether treatment of clinically silent disease has a beneficial impact on long-term graft functioning.

Immunosuppressive therapy is initiated immediately following transplantation and is maintained throughout the patient's lifetime. The most common regimen consists of cyclosporine, azathioprine or mycophenolate, and prednisone. Tacrolimus, a more potent inhibitor of lymphocyte proliferation than cyclosporine, is often substituted for cyclosporine in the setting of refractory or recurrent acute rejection and as salvage therapy for patients who develop chronic rejection (bronchiolitis obliterans). Antilymphocyte antibody preparations are used by some centers as part of the induction phase of immunosuppression and as definitive therapy for acute and chronic rejection refractory to pulse steroids.

Individuals providing care to transplant recipients must be familiar with the administration, side effects, and drug interactions of these immunosuppressive agents (Table 391.4). While serving as the cornerstone of therapy, the use of cyclosporine and tacrolimus is particularly problematic. When administered orally, the bioavailability of these agents is poor and unpredictable, necessitating that dosing be based on trough blood levels. Both drugs are metabolized via the hepatic cytochrome P450 system, and blood levels are influenced by the concurrent administration of other drugs that affect this enzymatic pathway. Adverse effects of these two agents, as well as of the other drugs that are commonly utilized, are legion and contribute significantly to the morbidity associated with transplantation.

OUTCOMES

SURVIVAL

The Registry of the International Society for Heart and Lung Transplantation contains data on more than 8,000 patients from 150 centers worldwide who have undergone lung transplantation since 1985. Actuarial survival rates for this large cohort are 71% at 1 year, 55% at 3 years, 43% at 5 years, and 32% at 7 years, with a median survival of 3.8 years. Collective survival rates have not improved substantially since 1991 and remain inferior to those achieved with liver and heart transplantation, for which 5-year actuarial survival approximates 70%. Long-term survival following bilateral lung transplantation is moderately superior to that following single lung transplantation. Older recipients (55 years and older) have inferior long-term survival rates compared to their younger counterparts.

Mortality is highest during the first year, with primary graft failure and infection representing the most common causes of deaths. Factors portending an increased risk of early death include ventilator dependence prior to transplantation, an underlying diagnosis other than emphysema, and advanced recipient or donor age. Beyond the first year, attrition slows to an annual rate of approximately 5% to 10%. Most late deaths are attributable to the development of bronchiolitis obliterans, the lethal effects of which are due to both progressive respiratory failure and to an increased susceptibility to infection.

PULMONARY FUNCTION

The peak effect of lung transplantation on pulmonary function parameters is usually not realized until 3 to 6 months following the procedure, at which time the adverse impact of such factors as postoperative pain, weakness, altered chest wall mechanics, and reimplantation lung injury has dissipated. Complete normalization of pulmonary function is the anticipated result of bilateral lung transplantation. Following single-lung transplantation for chronic obstructive pulmonary disease, the FEV_1 increases several fold to a level of approximately 50% to 60% of the predicted normal value. Similarly, single-lung transplantation for pulmonary fibrosis results in marked but incomplete improvement in lung volumes, with persistence of a mild restrictive pattern.

Transplantation also leads to correction of gas exchange abnormalities. Oxygenation improves rapidly, permitting the majority of patients to be weaned from supplemental oxygen within the first week. Hypercapnia may take longer to resolve due to lingering abnormalities in the ventilatory response to CO_2.

EXERCISE CAPACITY

Exercise tolerance improves sufficiently to permit the majority of transplant recipients to resume an active lifestyle. Although free of limitations to usual activity, transplant recipients demonstrate a characteristic reduction in peak exercise performance as assessed by cardiopulmonary exercise testing. Specifically, patients typically achieve a maximum oxygen consumption at peak exercise of only 40% to 60% of that predicted, despite a normal ventilatory response, maintenance of normal oxygenation, and essentially normal cardiac response. Suboptimal exercise performance persists in subjects tested as late as 1 to 2 years following transplantation. Despite the greater magnitude of improvement in pulmonary function associated with the bilateral procedure, there is no significant difference in peak exercise performance between single and bilateral lung transplant recipients. Emerging

evidence suggests that the limitation to exercise may be due to skeletal muscle dysfunction caused by cyclosporine-induced impairment in mitochondrial respiration.

HEMODYNAMICS

When performed in patients with pulmonary hypertension, both single and bilateral lung transplantation lead to immediate and sustained normalization of pulmonary arterial pressure and enhanced cardiac output. In response to a decrease in afterload, right ventricular performance gradually normalizes in the majority of patients. A threshold of right ventricular dysfunction, below which recovery will not occur, has yet to be defined.

COMPLICATIONS

PRIMARY GRAFT FAILURE

Primary graft failure describes a severe form of acute allograft dysfunction that appears within the first hours to days following transplantation and is presumed to represent a manifestation of ischemia–reperfusion injury. Histologically, a pattern of diffuse alveolar damage is seen, identical to that associated with acute respiratory distress syndrome. The incidence of this complication varies from 15% to 35% in contemporary clinical series. The diagnosis rests on the presence within 72 hours of transplantation of widespread radiographic infiltrates and impaired oxygenation, and the exclusion of other causes of early graft dysfunction such as volume overload, pneumonia, rejection, and pulmonary venous outflow obstruction. Treatment is supportive, relying on conventional mechanical ventilatory techniques as well as on the use of such adjunct measures as nitric oxide, independent lung ventilation, and extracorporeal life support for those who cannot be otherwise stabilized. With mortality rates of up to 60%, primary graft failure ranks second only to infection as a leading cause of early deaths among transplant recipients. Recovery in survivors is often protracted and incomplete, though attainment of normal lung function and exercise tolerance is possible. Results of emergent retransplantation in this setting have been poor.

AIRWAY COMPLICATIONS

With implantation of the allograft, no attempt is routinely made to reestablish the bronchial arterial circulation. As a result, the donor bronchus is precariously dependent on retrograde blood flow through low-pressure pulmonary venous to bronchial vascular collaterals, placing it at risk for ischemic injury. Because dehiscense of the airway was initially a common sequela, techniques have evolved to buttress the bronchial anastomosis and provide a nurturing blood supply. A telescoping technique is currently employed that intussuscepts donor and recipient bronchi, overlapping by one to two cartilaginous rings. Life-threatening dehiscence is now rare; partial dehiscence is still occasionally encountered but typically heals with expectant management only. The most common form of airway complication that remains is anastomotic stenosis, which may result from stricture, excessive granulation tissue, or bronchomalacia. Stenosis typically becomes manifest several weeks following transplantation. Clues to its presence include focal wheezing on the involved side, recurrent bouts of pneumonia or purulent bronchitis, abnormally low spirometric values, and a flow–volume loop demonstrating flattening of the midexpiratory limb. Airway stenosis is now readily correctable in most cases with bronchoscopically placed stents.

INFECTION

Infection rates among lung transplant recipients are several fold higher than among recipients of other solid organs. The greater risk is likely related to the unique exposure of the lung allograft to microorganisms via inhalation and aspiration. Bacterial pathogens account for the majority of infections. Bacterial pneumonia, often due to gram-negative organisms, is most commonly encountered in the immediate postoperative period. Predisposing factors include immunosuppression, blunted cough due to pain and lung denervation, disruption of lymphatic drainage, impaired mucociliary clearance from widespread mucosal ischemic injury, narrowing of the bronchial anastomosis, and passive transfer of organisms with the donor lung. Bacterial infections reemerge as a later complication among recipients who develop chronic rejection. Notably, despite persistent carriage of pathogenic bacteria in the sinuses and proximal airways, recipients with cystic fibrosis are not at greater risk for lower respiratory tract infections than other recipient populations.

CMV is the most common viral pathogen encountered in the post-transplantation period. Active infection can occur by transfer of virus with the lung allograft or blood products, or by reactivation of latent virus remotely acquired by the recipient. Seronegative recipients who acquire primary infection from a seropositive donor are at greatest risk for serious CMV disease, particularly pneumonitis.

CMV infection typically emerges within the first 3 months. Infection can be subclinical, manifested as asymptomatic viremia or shedding of virus in the respiratory tract or urine. Clinical disease can assume a number of forms, including a mononucleosis-like syndrome with fever and malaise, and organ-specific involvement of the lungs, gastrointestinal tract, liver, and central nervous system. Treatment of clinically significant disease with ganciclovir is usually effective, although relapses may occur.

Although rarely lethal, CMV infections contribute substantially to post-transplantation morbidity and have been linked with an increased risk of chronic rejection. In an attempt to minimize the adverse impact of this infection, many centers have adopted prophylactic strategies. For seronegative recipients, the most effective strategy is matching with seronegative donors and use of screened blood products. However, this strategy is associated with prolonged waiting times since the majority of the donor pool is serologically positive. Antiviral prophylaxis of seronegative recipients of seropositive organs, as well as of seropositive recipients, is an alternative strategy in widespread use. Current data suggest that such an approach delays the onset and may attenuate the severity of infection.

Aspergillus species commonly colonize the airways of lung transplant recipients, but only a minority of patients develop invasive disease. Due to the presence of devitalized cartilage and suture material, the bronchial anastomosis is particularly vulnerable to localized invasion. *Aspergillus* may also cause more diffuse airways infection, characterized by mucosal ulceration and formation of pseudomembranes. Infection restricted to the airway is usually responsive to itraconazole or to inhaled or parenteral amphotericin B, but fatal erosion into the pulmonary artery and widespread fungal dissemination have been reported. In contrast to airway infection, invasive disease of the lung parenchyma and extrapulmonary aspergillosis are associated with high mortality.

REJECTION

Despite the use of potent immunosuppressive agents, allograft rejection remains a pervasive problem. Features of acute and chronic forms of rejection are summarized in Table 391.5 and elaborated on below.

Frequent surveillance of the allograft by transbronchial biopsies has demonstrated that most transplant recipients experience at least one episode of acute rejection in the first several months. Beyond this initial period, the risk of acute rejection declines steadily, reaching a low but not negligible rate by the end of the first year. Episodes of acute rejection may be clinically silent; biopsies from asymptomatic and functionally stable recipients have demonstrated evidence of acute rejection in up to one-third of cases. When present, clinical manifestations are nonspecific and include malaise, low-grade fever, dyspnea, cough, and leukocytosis. Radiographic infiltrates, a decline in arterial oxygenation at rest or with exercise, and an abrupt fall of greater than 10% in spirometric values are important clues to the possible presence of rejection; however, similar findings accompany bouts of infection.

Reliance on clinical criteria alone runs the risk of misdiagnosis and unnecessary augmentation of immunosuppression. In one study, acute rejection was confirmed histologically in only two-thirds of patients in whom it was suspected on clinical grounds. Transbronchial lung biopsy has emerged as the gold standard for diagnosis of acute rejection. The procedure is safe, can be performed in serial fashion over time, and has a sensitivity and specificity in excess of 90% for the diagnosis of acute rejection. To achieve this degree of diagnostic accuracy, at least five pieces of alveolated lung parenchyma, each containing bronchioles and more than 100 alveoli, must be obtained. The hallmark of acute rejection is the presence of perivascular lymphocytic infiltrates, which in more severe cases spill over into the adjacent interstitium and alveolar airspaces. A lymphocytic bronchitis or bronchiolitis may accompany the parenchymal involvement.

Treatment of acute rejection consists of a 3-day pulse of intravenous solumedrol at a daily dose of 15 mg per kilogram and, in some centers, by a transient increase and subsequent taper of maintenance prednisone. In most cases, this results in rapid improvement in symptoms, pulmonary function, and radiographic abnormalities, but follow-up biopsies show persistent histologic evidence of rejection in 30% of mild rejection episodes and 48% of moderate episodes. A variety of modalities have been employed for refractory or recurrent acute rejection, including

TABLE 391.5.   FEATURES OF ACUTE AND CHRONIC ALLOGRAFT REJECTION

Feature	Acute Rejection	Chronic Rejection
Onset	Initial 3 months	Beyond first year
Risk factors	HLA mismatching	Recurrent or severe acute rejection, cytomegalovirus infection, airway ischemia, HLA mismatching
Histology	Perivascular lymphocytic infiltrates	Bronchiolar submucosal inflammation and fibrosis; luminal obliteration
Signs and symptoms	Malaise, low-grade fever, dyspnea, cough, impaired oxygenation, leukocytosis	Dyspnea, chronic cough, recurrent bouts of purulent bronchitis
Chest radiograph	Alveolar or interstitial opacities, pleural effusions	Clear lung fields (may show hyperinflation)
High-resolution computed tomography	Ground-glass or alveolar opacities	Attenuation of peripheral vascular markings, bronchiectasis, air trapping (on expiratory images)
Pulmonary function testing	Proportional decline in both FEV_1 and FVC	Disproportionate decline in FEV_1 with worsening obstructive pattern
Yield of transbronchial biopsy	High	Low
Response to treatment	Rapid improvement	Refractory; treatment may slow rate of decline

HLA, human leukocyte antigen; FEV_1, forced expiratory volume in 1 second; FVC, forced vital capacity.

antilymphocyte antibody preparations, tacrolimus, methotrexate, and photopheresis.

Chronic rejection represents the major impediment to long-term graft function and patient survival following lung transplantation. It is manifested histologically as bronchiolitis obliterans, a fibroproliferative process characterized by submucosal inflammation and fibrosis of the bronchiolar walls ultimately progressing to complete obliteration of the airway lumen. Although presumed to represent an immunologically mediated process, the pathogenesis of bronchiolitis obliterans remains poorly understood. Acute rejection, particularly when recurrent or severe, has been consistently identified as the major risk factor for development of bronchiolitis obliterans. Other proposed risk factors include CMV infection, airway ischemia, and HLA mismatching.

Unlike acute rejection, bronchiolitis obliterans is difficult to diagnose by transbronchial biopsy, with reported sensitivity as low as 17%. For this reason, diagnosis now rests on demonstration of physiologic rather than histologic criteria. The term *bronchiolitis obliterans syndrome* has thus evolved, defined as an otherwise unexplained and sustained decline in FEV_1 of at least 20% below the peak post-transplantation baseline.

Bronchiolitis obliterans syndrome is rarely encountered in the initial year but its prevalence increases steadily beyond that point, involving approximately two-thirds of recipients by the fifth year. Onset of disease is typically insidious and heralded by dyspnea and cough. Recurrent bouts of purulent tracheobronchitis, with recovery of *P. aeruginosa* from sputum cultures, are highly characteristic. Spirometry demonstrates evidence of airflow obstruction, with a disproportionate fall in the FEV_1 and consequent fall in the ratio of FEV_1 to forced vital capacity. The plain chest radiograph is unrevealing, but high-resolution computed tomography of the chest often demonstrates decreased peripheral vascular markings, bronchiectasis, and evidence of air trapping on expiratory images.

Progressive decline in lung function is the rule, although the pace of decline is highly variable and the course may be inter-rupted by periods of functional stability. A wide range of therapies have been employed, all of which center on augmentation of immunosuppression. Options include high-dose corticosteroids, antilymphocyte antibodies, tacrolimus, inhaled cyclosporine, methotrexate, and total lymphoid irradiation. Current data are insufficient to support the conclusion that treatment impacts favorably on the natural history of bronchiolitis obliterans, and consensus on the optimal therapeutic strategy is lacking. At best, treatment appears to slow the rate of decline rather than to fully arrest or reverse the process. The prognosis is generally poor, with a 40% mortality rate within 2 years of onset. The only definitive treatment is retransplantation, but this strategy remains highly controversial in the context of a scarce donor organ pool.

POST-TRANSPLANTATION LYMPHOPROLIFERATIVE DISORDER

Post-transplantation lymphoproliferative disorder (PTLD) encompasses a group of abnormal B-cell proliferative responses ranging from benign polyclonal hyperplasia to malignant lymphomas. The reported incidence of PTLD in the lung transplant recipient population ranges from 6% to 9%, and most cases occur within the first post-transplantation year. The pathogenesis of PTLD involves Epstein–Barr virus–mediated B-cell proliferation that is permitted to proceed in an uncontained fashion in a host lacking the necessary cellular immune response. Previously unexposed recipients who acquire primary infection are at greatest risk for this complication. In this regard, the incidence of PTLD is 33% to 50% among Epstein–Barr virus–seronegative recipients compared to less than 2% among seropositive recipients. Intrathoracic involvement is most commonly encountered, typically assuming the form of single or multiple pulmonary nodules and/or mediastinal lymphadenopathy. Extrapulmonary sites of involvement include tonsils, intra-abdominal lymph nodes, and gastrointestinal tract as well as widely disseminated disease.

Initial treatment centers on reduction in the magnitude of immunosuppression to permit partial restoration of host cellular immunity. PTLD presenting within the first year is most likely to respond to this strategy. Treatment modalities reserved for refractory cases include chemotherapy, radiation, surgical resection, interferon-α, and anti–B-cell monoclonal antibodies. Antiviral therapy is often concurrently employed but is of unproven efficacy. Mortality related to PTLD or complications of treatment is on the order of 30% for those who develop disease within the first year but rises to 70% for those with later onset of disease.

REFERENCES

Bando K, Paradis IL, Similo S, et al. Obliterative bronchiolitis after lung and heart–lung transplantation: an analysis of risk factors and management. *J Thorac Cardiovasc Surg* 1995;110:4–14.

Barr ML, Schenkel FA, Cohen RG, et al. Recipient and donor outcomes in living related and unrelated lobar transplantation. *Transplant Proc* 1998;30:2261–2263.

Boehler A, Kesten S, Weder W, et al. Bronchiolitis obliterans after lung transplantation. *Chest* 1998;114:1411–1426.

Christie JD, Bavaria JE, Palevsky HI, et al. Primary graft failure following lung transplantation. *Chest* 1998;114:51–60.

Edelman J, Kotloff RM. Lung transplantation: a disease-specific approach. *Clin Chest Med* 1997;18:627–644.

Hosenpud JD, Bennett LE, Keck BM, et al. The registry of the International Society for Heart and Lung Transplantation: sixteenth official report—1999. *J Heart Lung Transplant* 1999;18:611–626.

Kshettry VR, Kroshus TJ, Hertz MI, et al. Early and late airway complications after lung transplantation: incidence and management. *Ann Thorac Surg* 1997;63:1576–1583.

Maurer JR, Frost AE, Estenne M, et al. International guidelines for the selection of lung transplant candidates. *J Heart Lung Transplant* 1998; 17:703–709.

Sibley RK, Berry GJ, Tazelaar HD, et al. The role of transbronchial biopsies in the management of lung transplant recipients. *J Heart Lung Transplant* 1993;12:308–324.

Trulock EP. Lung transplantation. *Am J Respir Crit Care* 1997;155: 789–818.

Kelley's Textbook of Internal Medicine, fourth edition. Edited by H. David Humes. Lippincott Williams & Wilkins, Philadelphia © 2000.

9

ENDOCRINOLOGY, METABOLISM, AND GENETICS

D. Lynn Loriaux, Editor

APPROACH TO THE PATIENT WITH ENDOCRINOLOGIC, METABOLIC, AND GENETIC DISORDERS

APPROACH TO THE PATIENT WITH A THYROID NODULE

JAMES A. FAGIN

Thyroid nodules are discrete swellings in the thyroid gland. They are considered as solitary if they are found within an otherwise normal palpable thyroid. Thyroid nodules are present in about 5% of the adult population. Prevalence increases with age, and nodules are more common in women. When prevalence is ascertained by high-resolution ultrasonography, unsuspected thyroid nodules are found in up to 44% of women and 20% of men. Frequency of nodularity is even higher in autopsy studies. By contrast, annual age-adjusted incidence of thyroid cancer in the United States is 2.2 and 5.8 per 100,000 males and females, respectively. The diagnostic challenge is to identify correctly those rare patients with thyroid nodules that are caused by thyroid cancer.

ETIOLOGIC FACTORS

Adenomatous colloid nodules are the most common cause of discrete thyroid enlargement. These hyperplastic lesions are histologic features of multinodular goiters, which can occasionally present with a large dominant nodule that gives the false appearance of being the sole abnormality by palpation. Follicular adenomas are benign neoplasms that are somewhat less prevalent than hyperplastic nodules. Primary thyroid cancers represent fewer than 10% of all clinically apparent nodules. Most of these are papillary thyroid carcinomas. Follicular carcinomas are comparatively uncommon, although their prevalence is higher in iodine-deficient populations. Anaplastic carcinomas are the most malignant form of thyroid cancer and very rare. Medullary thyroid carcinomas are also infrequent and derive from calcitonin-secreting C cells. Occasionally, lymphocytic or subacute thyroiditis can present with regional or nodular thyroid enlargement. Additional causes include thyroid lymphomas, cancers metastasizing to the thyroid, abscesses, and infiltrative/granulomatous diseases.

PRESENTATION

Thyroid nodules are usually asymptomatic and discovered as a visible or palpable neck mass by the physician or patient. Few patients complain of dysphagia, hoarseness, or rapid tumor growth, symptoms that increase the likelihood of cancer. Pain, which is uncommon, is suggestive of subacute thyroiditis or spontaneous bleeding into a preexisting nodule. Risk of cancer is higher in children, male individuals, and older patients. The most significant risk factor for thyroid cancer is a history of radiation exposure, particularly during childhood. Patients receiving external radiation to the head or neck for benign conditions such as thymic or tonsillar enlargement, acne, or tinea capitis are at greater risk for benign nodules as well as thyroid cancer. Although the practice of administering radiation for benign conditions has ceased, the risk persists for several decades after exposure. Also at risk are patients treated with high doses of radiation for Hodgkin's disease, children exposed to internal radiation by radioiodines, such as those living in areas contaminated by fallout from the Chernobyl nuclear accident, and atomic bomb survivors. Radiation exposure is associated specifically with papillary thyroid carcinomas. A family history of medullary thyroid carcinoma, or of multiple endocrine neoplasia type 2 (medullary thyroid carcinomas, pheochromocytomas, and parathyroid adenomas, with or without mucosal neuromas) places patients at a 50% risk of this disease, conferred by inheritance of germ line mutations of the *ret* oncogene. Risk of papillary carcinoma is higher in patients with a family history of adenomatous polyposis coli, Gardner's syndrome, Cowden's disease, or papillary thyroid cancer. The great majority of patients with thyroid nodules, however, have no specific risk factors.

Nodules greater than 1.5 cm can usually be palpated if they are located close to the surface of the gland. Most are of soft or firm consistency. Physical characteristics of the nodule are not usually helpful in differential diagnosis, as most cancers are found within lesions that are clinically indistinguishable from benign tumors. However, presence of a hard nodule, fixation to adjacent structures, vocal cord paralysis, and palpable enlargement of regional lymph nodes are highly indicative of malignancy. Dominant nodules from multinodular goiters can be malignant and should be evaluated in the same manner as solitary nodules. Increasingly, thyroid nodules are discovered incidentally during carotid ultrasonography, neck computed tomography, or magnetic resonance imaging studies. Solitary nodules that are greater than 1 cm in diameter should be evaluated.

LABORATORY EVALUATION

Thyroid function should be routinely assessed in patients with thyroid nodules. If such nodules are thought to be euthyroid based on their clinical presentation, as is most often the case, measurement of thyroid-stimulating hormone (TSH) levels is sufficient. Patients with clinical suspicion of hyperthyroidism or hypothyroidism should also have measurements of serum free T_4 and T_3. Patients with lymphocytic (Hashimoto's) thyroiditis may present occasionally with regional thyroid enlargement giving the appearance of a discrete thyroid nodule. Determination of antithyroid antibodies is helpful in these cases. Patients confirmed to be thyrotoxic should have a radionuclide scan with iodine 131, technetium Tc 99m pertechnetate, or iodine 123 to determine whether the nodule is "hot" (i.e., incorporates higher levels of the isotope than the surrounding gland). This is caused by autonomously functioning thyroid nodules, which are usually benign. Alternatively, hyperthyroidism may be associated with diffusely increased thyroid uptake, with the nodule appearing as a hypofunctioning ("cold") lesion; this unlikely eventuality is of concern, as thyroid cancers may run an aggressive course in patients with Graves' disease. Because of this, cold nodules in this setting should be evaluated carefully by fine-needle aspiration (FNA) biopsy (see below).

Most patients with thyroid nodules have no abnormalities in thyroid function. Here an FNA biopsy is the initial procedure of choice. This is also the case for thyroid nodules discovered incidentally as a consequence of imaging studies of the neck. Solitary nodules greater than 1 cm should be biopsied, under ultrasonographic guidance if necessary. Cytologic evaluation of the aspirate indicates whether the nodule is benign (i.e., features consistent with colloid nodules, thyroiditis, or benign cysts), suspicious (hypercellular follicular lesions, Hürthle cell changes without lymphocytic infiltration), or malignant. When the smear does not contain at least five or six groups of well-preserved cells, the aspirate is considered unsatisfactory or nondiagnostic. In this event, a repeat aspirate may be diagnostic in about 50% of cases. The false-negative rate of a benign cytologic diagnosis is about 5%, whereas false-positive tests are seen in about

1% of aspirates classified as malignant. Classification of aspirates as indeterminate or suspicious stems from the inability to distinguish benign follicular or Hürthle cell adenomas from their malignant counterparts (i.e., follicular or Hürthle cell carcinomas) based on their cytologic appearance. About 25% of all aspirates fall into this category, and 10% to 15% ultimately prove to be malignant. As mentioned above, likelihood of cancer is considerably diminished in autonomously functioning nodules, which are also follicular neoplasms, and thus give rise to suspicious aspirates. It is therefore prudent to perform radionuclide scans and exclude hyperthyroidism in patients with suspicious or indeterminate cytology. Aspirates from patients with medullary thyroid carcinomas are often not diagnostic, particularly if not followed by immunostaining for calcitonin. The diagnostic accuracy and cost-effectiveness of screening all patients with thyroid nodules for medullary thyroid carcinoma by determining plasma basal calcitonin levels has not been established conclusively, and this test is therefore not performed on a routine basis.

High-resolution ultrasonography is not recommended in the initial evaluation of a thyroid nodule, as it does not help to distinguish benign from malignant tumors. Furthermore, as this technique allows imaging of lesions of 1 to 2 mm, its use in screening could result in inappropriate evaluation of subclinical conditions. Occasionally, ultrasonography-guided FNA biopsy is indicated to assess nodules that are difficult to palpate or embedded deeply within the gland. It is also useful when conventional FNA has failed to provide a diagnostic specimen and to help direct the biopsy needle to the solid component of cystic nodules. In patients with cystic lesions, aspiration decreases the size of nodules and cures many of them. There is a place for ultrasonography in the management of patients with presumed benign nodular disease when palpation is not sufficient to track lesion size during prolonged follow-up, as discussed below.

OPTIMAL MANAGEMENT

About 60% to 70% of patients will prove to have a benign thyroid aspirate, in many cases corresponding to colloid adenomas. These patients are best managed expectantly, i.e., by monitoring changes in nodule size over time. Nodules showing significant growth during the observation period should be rebiopsied. As cells from colloid adenomas are thought to retain responsiveness to TSH, some physicians treat these patients with *l*-thyroxine to suppress TSH levels below the normal range, and hence reduce the size of the nodule. (*Note:* a *suppressive* dose of thyroid hormone is one that reduces TSH to levels below the normal range, as opposed to a *replacement* dose in which TSH levels are maintained within the normal range). The use of suppressive doses of thyroid hormone for benign nodules is controversial. Short-term treatment (about 6 months) with *l*-thyroxine was formerly advocated to help identify those nodules most likely to be malignant based on their failure to decrease in size when TSH levels were low. However, the good predictive power of FNA cytology and the fact that many benign nodules do not shrink with *l*-thyroxine suppressive therapy have largely rendered this practice outmoded. Long-term TSH-suppressive therapy to prevent growth of benign nodules is also of uncertain efficacy. It is unknown as to whether this practice decreases the likelihood that benign tumors will become malignant over time, a rare occurrence in these nodules. Furthermore, supraphysiologic doses of thyroid hormone are associated with osteopenia and cardiac arrhythmias, and should therefore be avoided in post-menopausal women and older patients. In summary, suppressive therapy with thyroid hormone is usually not indicated for benign nodules, which are best followed by clinical observation (with or without ultrasonography) over time. Suppressive therapy should be restricted to selected patients with large nodules, particularly if they cause symptoms (dysphagia, stridor) or are cosmetically disfiguring, and possibly to prevent recurrence of nodules in irradiated patients previously treated with partial thyroidectomy.

Patients with suspicious or indeterminate aspirates should be referred for surgery, as the possibility of malignancy cannot be excluded. Intraoperative histologic evaluation of frozen sections of the nodule may help determine the extent of operation but is often still not sufficient to distinguish benign from malignant follicular neoplasms. In this event, a lobectomy and isthmectomy are appropriate. A completion thyroidectomy is performed at a later date if malignancy is diagnosed on the permanent sections (see Chapter). Another circumstance in which surgery is advisable is for clinically significant nodules in which FNA biopsy has been repeatedly non-diagnostic. Cysts that are greater than 4 cm in size or that recur after drainage may also require surgery.

Nodules from patients with a history of radiation exposure have a higher likelihood of being malignant (about 30%), and therefore merit closer surveillance and a lower threshold for surgical referral. In solitary nodules from irradiated patients, FNA biopsy with multiple sampling of the lesion is appropriate. If the patient has multiple nodules, particularly if many of them are larger than 1 cm, FNA sampling becomes more cumbersome, and these patients should be treated with a near-total thyroidectomy. Treatment with suppressive doses of TSH may prevent recurrence of nodules after partial thyroid removal in these patients.

Patients with malignant aspirates are treated surgically. Although most require a total or near-total thyroidectomy, the type of surgery is dependent on the size of the nodule and the histologic diagnosis. In those in whom medullary thyroid carcinoma is suspected based on FNA, family history, or calcitonin levels, it is important to redouble efforts to make this diagnosis preoperatively, as this cancer requires more extensive surgery.

BIBLIOGRAPHY

Burch HB. Evaluation and management of the solid thyroid nodule. *Endocrinol Metab Clin North Am (Thyroid Cancer 1)* 1995;24:663–710.

Cooper DS. Clinical Review 66: Thyroxine suppression therapy for benign nodular disease. *J Clin Endocrinol Metab* 1985;80:331.

Daniels GH. Thyroid nodules and nodular thyroids: a clinical overview. *Compr Ther* 1996;22(4):239–250.

Gharib H, Mazzaferri EL. Thyroxine suppressive therapy in patients with nodular thyroid disease. *Ann Intern Med* 1998;128:386–394.

Mazzaferri EL. Management of a solitary thyroid nodule. *N Engl J Med* 1993;328(8):553–559.

Kelley's Textbook of Internal Medicine, fourth edition. Edited by H. David Humes. Lippincott Williams & Wilkins, Philadelphia © 2000.

CHAPTER

393

APPROACH TO MENSTRUAL DISORDERS AND GALACTORRHEA

ROBERT L. BARBIERI

The menstrual cycle is controlled by the interaction of the hypothalamus [pulsatile secretion of gonadotropin-releasing hormone (GnRH)], pituitary [secretion of luteinizing hormone and follicle-stimulating hormone (FSH)], ovary (follicular growth, ovulation, and corpus luteum formation), and uterus (cyclic growth and shedding of the endometrium). Abnormalities in any of these systems can result in menstrual abnormalities, including primary amenorrhea, secondary amenorrhea, and oligomenorrhea.

PRIMARY AMENORRHEA

Primary amenorrhea is present when a girl's first menses has not occurred by 16 years of age. Girls who reach 14 years of age and have not had breast development should undergo an evaluation similar to that for primary amenorrhea. Primary amenorrhea usually is caused by a genetic or congenital defect and often is associated with disorders of puberty.

In large case series, the most common causes of primary amenorrhea are gonadal dysgenesis resulting from chromosomal abnormalities such as 45,X, 45,X/46,XX, and 46,XY (45%); physiologic delay of puberty (20%); müllerian agenesis (15%); transverse vaginal septum or imperforate hymen (5%); absence of hypothalamic GnRH production, such as in Kallmann's syndrome (5%); anorexia nervosa (2%); and hypopituitarism (2%). Less common causes of primary amenorrhea are found in Fig. 393.1.

Primary amenorrhea is evaluated most efficiently by focusing on the presence or absence of breast development, the presence or absence of the uterus and cervix, and the FSH level. If there is no breast development and the FSH level is elevated, the probable diagnosis is gonadal dysgenesis (Fig. 393.1). If the uterus is absent, the probable diagnosis is müllerian agenesis. If the FSH level is elevated, a karyotype must be obtained. An elevated FSH level with a 46,XY karyotype indicates a high risk for the development of gonadoblastoma and dysgerminoma, and

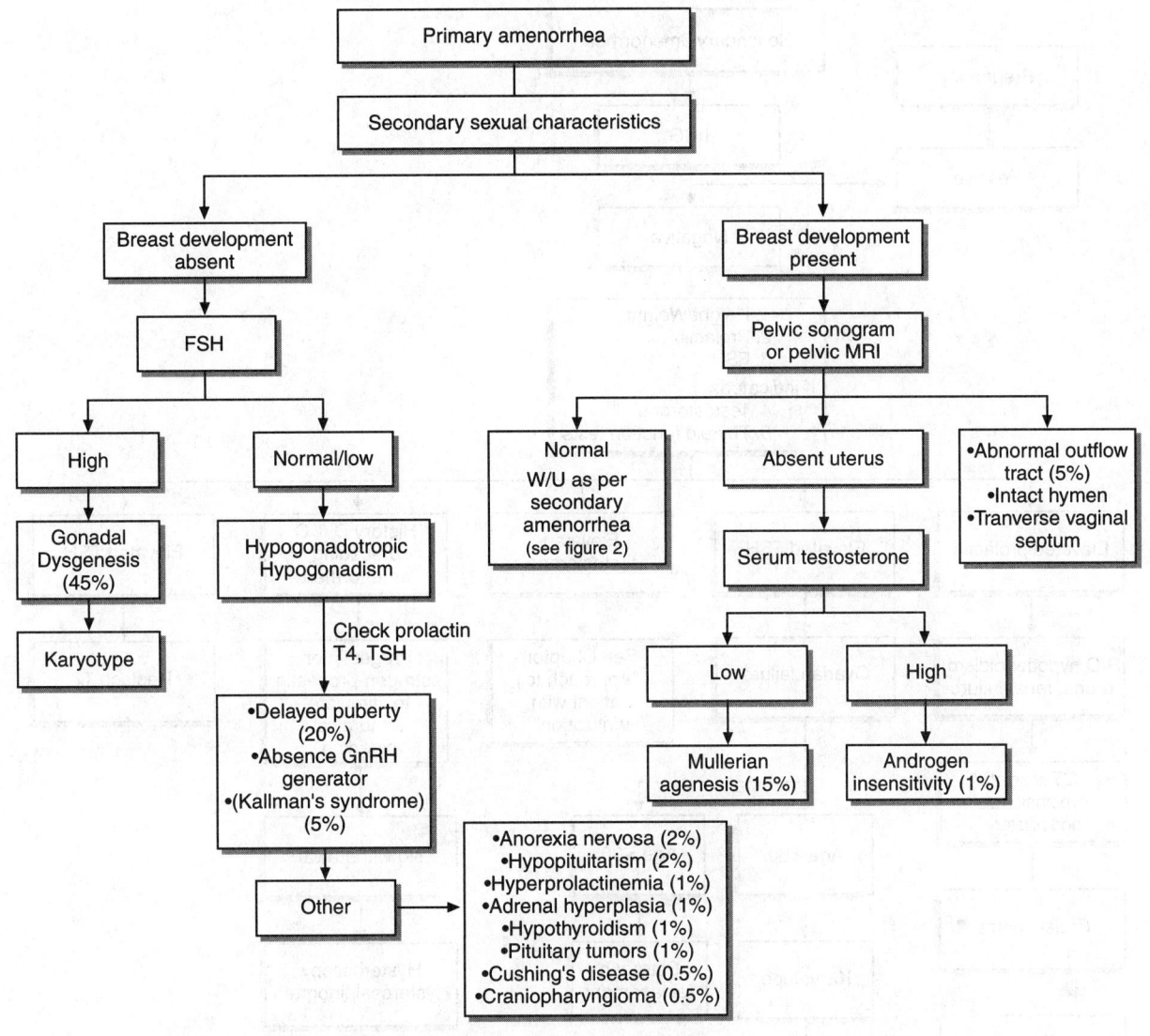

FIGURE 393.1. Causes of primary amenorrhea. FSH, follicle-stimulating hormone; GnRH, gonadotropin-releasing hormone; T$_4$, thyroxine; TSH, thyroid-stimulating hormone.
EVIDENCE LEVEL: C. Expert Opinion.

surgical removal of the gonads is necessary. In many cases of primary amenorrhea, long-term therapy with estrogen and progesterone is required to stimulate the development of secondary sex characteristics and to protect bone mass. Women with gonadal dysgenesis due to 45,X are at high risk for developing thyroid disease and diabetes mellitus.

SECONDARY AMENORRHEA

Secondary amenorrhea is present when a women who has been menstruating experiences the absence of periods for a time greater than three of her previous cycle intervals, or 6 months.

A common cause of secondary amenorrhea is pregnancy, and this possibility can be eliminated by measuring the serum human chorionic gonadotropin level (Fig. 393.2). Once pregnancy is excluded, the major causes of secondary amenorrhea are as follows:

Hypothalamic dysfunction (35%). This category includes problems associated with decreased GnRH pulse frequency and amplitude, such as abnormalities of weight and nutrition (including anorexia nervosa), stress, strenuous exercise, and infiltrative diseases of the hypothalamus (lymphoma, histiocytosis). Hypothyroidism occasionally presents as secondary amenorrhea, probably because of changes in hypothalamic GnRH production. Elite athletes and ballet dancers commonly have anovulation and amenorrhea.

Pituitary disease (17%). The single most common cause of secondary amenorrhea is hyperprolactinemia (13%). Hyperprolactinemia causes amenorrhea by decreasing GnRH production.

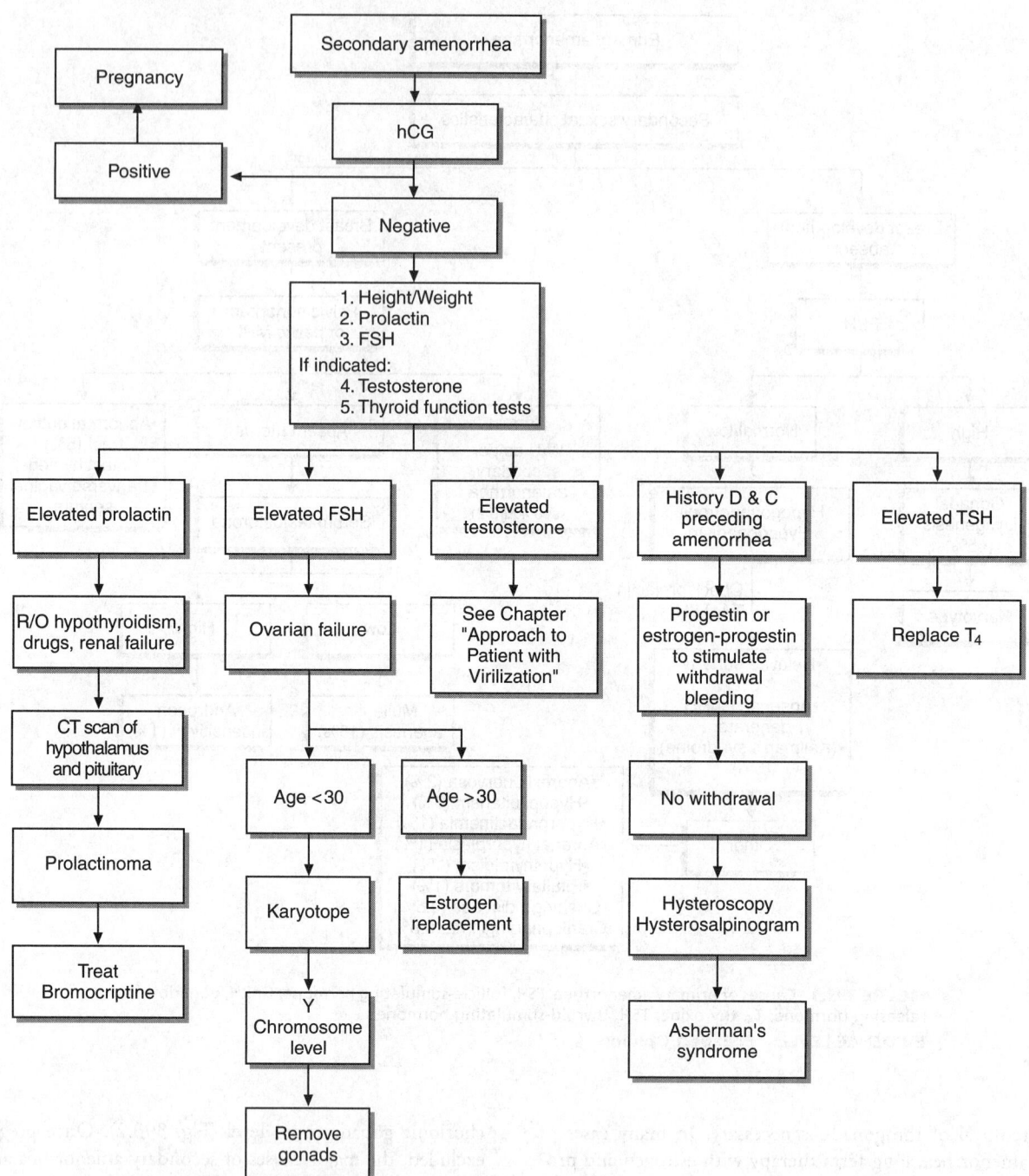

FIGURE 393.2. Major causes of secondary amenorrhea. CT, computed tomography; D&C, dilation and curettage; FSH, follicle-stimulating hormone; hCG, human chorionic gonadotropin; R/O, rule out; T₄, thyroxine.

EVIDENCE LEVEL: C. Expert Opinion.

Empty-sella syndrome, (1.5%), Sheehan's syndrome (1.5%), and Cushing's disease (1%) also can cause amenorrhea.

Ovarian disease (40%). Both ovarian failure (10%) and the polycystic ovary syndrome (PCOS) (30%) can cause amenorrhea. Ovarian failure occurs with the loss of all follicles, which are the source of 95% of the estradiol produced in women. Hypoestrogenic women often have hot flashes. Women with

ovarian PCOS often have insulin resistance and hirsutism and/or acne.

Uterine disease (7%). Asherman's syndrome (intrauterine synechiae), which typically occurs after curettage of the uterus, often presents as amenorrhea.

Other causes. Adrenal hyperplasia, hypothyroidism, and ovarian and adrenal tumors also can cause secondary amenorrhea.

On physical examination, height and weight should be measured and recorded. Women who are more than 10% below their ideal body weight need to be evaluated for anorexia nervosa. The laboratory evaluation of secondary amenorrhea includes measurement of prolactin and FSH levels, and a progestin withdrawal test. The progestin withdrawal test is performed by administering progesterone in oil (100 mg intramuscularly) or medroxyprogesterone acetate (10 mg per day orally for 5 days) and monitoring any uterine bleeding. The absence of uterine bleeding after a progestin challenge suggests that endogenous estrogen levels are particularly low or that Asherman's syndrome is present. The presence of uterine bleeding after an estrogen–progestin withdrawal test indicates that Asherman's syndrome is not present. Some women with amenorrhea and low endogenous estrogen (negative progestin challenge) have a hypothalamic or pituitary tumor.

In women with secondary amenorrhea and hyperprolactinemia caused by a pituitary tumor, the therapeutic goals are to reduce the hyperprolactinemia, preserve pituitary function, and prevent tumor growth. This often can be achieved with bromocriptine therapy. Bromocriptine is an ergot alkaloid that is a dopamine agonist. Administered at a dosage of 2.5 mg orally twice a day, it reduces prolactin levels and decreases tumor size in most patients with prolactinoma. Nausea, vomiting, and orthostatic hypotension are common initial side effects, so that bromocriptine therapy should be started at a low dosage (0.625 mg orally once a day) and titrated upward.

Women with secondary amenorrhea are at risk for developing osteoporosis. Some authorities recommend that all women with secondary amenorrhea be treated with estrogen–progestin hormone replacement. Others suggest that bone density be measured and only those women who have a low bone density measurement receive therapy.

GALACTORRHEA

Galactorrhea is the secretion of breast milk not associated with nursing. Galactorrhea can be caused by a distant pregnancy, oral contraceptive use, hyperprolactinemia, or hypothyroidism. Measurement of the prolactin level and thyroid function is useful. Of all women with galactorrhea, 20% have hyperprolactinemia and a few have hypothyroidism. Women with galactorrhea and regular, ovulatory menses seldom have hyperprolactinemia or hypothyroidism. In these women, a distant pregnancy or oral contraceptive use has sensitized the breast to be stimulated by normal levels of circulating prolactin. In contrast, 80% of women with galactorrhea and secondary amenorrhea have hyperprolactinemia. Irrespective of its cause, galactorrhea usually can be managed with bromocriptine.

BIBLIOGRAPHY

Frisch RE, Snow RC, Johnson LA, et al. Magnetic resonance imaging of overall and regional body fat, estrogen metabolism and ovulation of athletes compared to controls. *J Clin Endocrinol Metab* 1993;77:471–477.

Hull MGR, Knuth VA, Murray MAF, et al. The practical value of the progesterone challenge test in the assessment of the estrogen state and response to clomiphene in amenorrhea. *Br J Obstet Gynaecol* 1979;86:799–805.

Laughlin GA, Dominguez CE, Yen SS. Nutritional and endocrine–metabolic aberrations in women with functional hypothalamic amenorrhea. *J Clin Endocrinol Metab* 1998;83:25–32.

Mashchak CA, Kletzky OA, Davajan V. Clinical and laboratory evaluation of patients with primary amenorrhea. *Obstet Gynecol* 1981;57:715–721.

Miller KK, Parulekar MS, Schoenfeld E, et al. Decreased leptin levels in normal weight women with hypothalamic amenorrhea: the effects of body composition and nutritional intake.

Putukian M. The female triad. Eating disorders, amenorrhea and osteoporosis. *Med Clin North Am* 1994;78:345–356.

Reindollar RH, Byrd JR, McDonough PG. Delayed sexual development: a study of 252 patients. *Am J Obstet Gynecol* 1981;140:371–380.

Reindollar RH, Novak M, Tho SPT, et al. Adult onset amenorrhea: a study of 262 patients. *Am J Obstet Gynecol* 1986;155:531–543.

Reinhold C, Hricak H, Forstner R, et al. Primary amenorrhea: evaluation with MR imaging. *Radiology* 1997;203:383–390.

Young N, Formica C, Szmukler G, et al. Bone density at weight bearing and nonweight bearing sites in ballet dancers: the effects of exercise, hypogonadism and body weight. *J Clin Endocrinol Metab* 1994;78:449–454.

Kelley's Textbook of Internal Medicine, fourth edition. Edited by H. David Humes. Lippincott Williams & Wilkins, Philadelphia © 2000.

CHAPTER 394

APPROACH TO THE PATIENT WITH VIRILIZATION

RICHARD S. LEGRO

PRESENTATION

Virilization in an adult women is a rare disorder and must be separated from more common and less severe causes of androgen excess in women, such as polycystic ovary syndrome (PCOS). This chapter focuses primarily on virilization in an adult woman, acknowledging that the differential diagnosis is broader for a newborn infant or young child. Virilization includes the common signs of acne and hirsutism but is also accompanied by other peripheral effects such as temporal balding, clitoromegaly, deepening of the voice, breast atrophy, and changes in body contour. Amenorrhea may occur in a premenopausal woman. A rapid presentation of the virilization often leads to a speedy evaluation and diagnosis, whereas the more lingering forms may be overlooked until there is marked masculinization. Virilization is never "idiopathic," and all cases must be investigated until a cause is discovered (Table 394.1). Virilization rarely occurs with the common forms of androgen excess that present in postmenarchal women, such as PCOS or nonclassical congenital adrenal hyperplasia (NC-CAH). These disorders rarely produce androgen excess to the degree of virilization.

Virilization presents with a variety of peripheral effects. Acne and hirsutism are invariably present. A deepening of the voice has been reported in women with androgen-secreting tumors or

TABLE 394.1.	CAUSES OF VIRILIZATION IN AN ADULT WOMAN	
Cause	**Onset**	**Diagnosis**
Ovarian tumor	Rapid, but gradual possible	Pelvic exam, transvaginal ultrasonography, elevated testosterone level
Adrenal tumor	Rapid, but gradual possible	CT or MRI, elevated cortisol or DHEA-S
Hyperthecosis	Gradual, but rapid possible	Ultrasonography, elevated testosterone, insulin, and lipid levels
Hyperprolactinemia	Gradual or rapid	Elevated prolactin levels, CT or MRI of pituitary
Polycystic ovary syndrome	Gradual, perimenarchal onset	Elevated testosterone and/or DHEA-S levels, menstrual irregularity, exclusion of the other causes above

CT, computed tomography; MRI, magnetic resonance imaging; DHEA-S, dehydroepiandrosterone sulfate.

undergoing exogenous androgen treatment. Increase in the size of the larynx is one factor in the voice change. Clitoromegaly is defined as a clitoral index greater than 35 mm² (the clitoral index is the product of the sagittal and transverse diameters of the glans of the clitoris). In a normal woman these diameters are in the range of 5 mm each. The degree of clitoral enlargement correlates with the degree of androgen excess. Androgens can lead to body composition changes, especially in the upper body, with increased muscle mass and decreased fat mass. This is accompanied by breast atrophy.

PATHOPHYSIOLOGIC FACTORS

The degree of androgen excess that can result in virilization almost always has its source in increased production (or intake) of androgens. However, other factors, such as the potency of the androgen produced [dihydrotestosterone (DHT) > testosterone > androstenedione > dehydroepiandrosterone (DHEA)], the amount of androgen that is free or weakly bound in serum and thus bioavailable [sex hormone–binding globulin (SHBG) preferentially binds more potent androgens], and the peripheral metabolism of androgens (primarily the intracellular production of DHT from prehormones), all figure in the phenotype of virilization.

Both the adrenal glands and ovaries contribute to the circulating androgen pool in women. The adrenal preferentially secretes weak androgens such as DHEA and DHEA-S (the latter referring to the sulfate preparation) (up to 90% of adrenal origin). These hormones, in addition to androstenedione, may serve as prohormones for more potent androgens, such as testosterone or DHT. The ovary is the preferential source of testosterone, and it is estimated that 75% of circulating testosterone originates from the ovary (mainly through peripheral conversion of prohormones by liver, fat, and skin; but also through direct secretion). Androstenedione, largely of ovarian origin, is the only circulating androgen that is higher in premenopausal women than men, yet its androgenic potency is only 10% of that of testosterone. DHT is the most potent androgen, though it circulates in negligible quantities and results primarily from the intracellular 5α reduction of testosterone.

Androgen excess is most commonly evident in its effects on the pilosebaceous unit. Hirsutism occurs when androgens stimulate the transformation of fine, unpigmented vellus hair to coarse, pigmented, thickened terminal hair. This is thought to be mediated by the intracellular actions of enzymes 17-ketosteroid reductase, which converts androstenedione to testosterone, and 5α-reductase, which converts testosterone to DHT. Androgen-dependent hair is midline hair: that on the upper lip, chin, and cheeks, intermammary hair; and hair in the escutcheon, inner thighs, and lower back attributable to the intergluteal area. Paradoxically, androgens can exert opposite effects in hair follicles on the scalp, causing conversion of terminal follicles to velus-like follicles and leading to male pattern baldness characterized by frontal and temporal balding. Androgens can also cause increased sebum production and abnormal keratinization in the pilosebaceous unit, contributing to the development of acne.

It is important to note that factors other than androgens may contribute to the development of signs and symptoms of virilization. Hyperinsulinemia, which accompanies many benign forms of virilization, can also stimulate the pilosebaceous unit both directly and indirectly (the latter by acting as a cogonadotropin in the ovary to stimulate thecal and stromal androgen production). Both hyperinsulinemia and androgen excess suppress SHBG, leading to a greater pool of bioavailable androgens.

LABORATORY STUDIES AND DIAGNOSTIC TESTS

The purposes of the physical and laboratory evaluations are to rule out adrenal and ovarian tumors, assess the severity of the androgen excess, and evaluate the source of the hyperandrogenism (adrenal vs. ovarian). The history and physical examination are essential to arriving at a diagnosis of virilization. The history should focus on the onset and duration of the various symptoms of virilization, menstrual background, and concomitant medications. During physical examination, the physician should carefully check the patient for balding and body hair distribution. The presence and severity of acne should be noted. Acanthosis nigricans (a velvety, verrucous, brownish skin lesion frequently noted on the nape of the neck, axilla, and under the breasts) is a peripheral skin manifestation of circulating hyperinsulinemia. Coexisting signs of Cushing's syndrome, including moon facies, buffalo hump, abdominal striae, centripetal fat distribution, and hypertension, should be documented. A pelvic examination should be performed on all women with virilization, as 90% of ovarian tumors present with unilateral enlargement. A transvaginal ultrasonographic exam, increasingly office-based, should be sufficient to identify ovarian masses less than 1 cm in diameter, although physiologic follicular and cystic developments throughout the normal menstrual cycle, especially a corpus luteal cyst, can masquerade as more serious pathologic lesions.

Androgen-secreting tumors, primarily of ovarian and secondarily of adrenal origin, are invariably accompanied by elevated circulating androgen levels. However, there is no absolute level that is pathognomonic for a tumor, just as there is no minimum androgen level that excludes a tumor. In the past, testosterone levels greater than 2 ng per milliliter and DHEA-S levels greater than 700 mg per deciliter were regarded as indicative of a tumor of ovarian and adrenal origin, respectively, but these cutoffs display poor sensitivity and specificity. Nonetheless, they are useful to quantify the amount of circulating androgen excess and potential source. Diagnostic tests that involve suppression or stimulation of the ovary or adrenal to identify the source of androgen production are not generally useful. Both functional states of androgen excess and tumors can variably respond or not respond to these dynamic challenges. However, a prolonged course of dexamethasone (1 mg t.i.d. for 5 days because androgens are suppressed less readily than cortisol) that fails to suppress androgens may potentially identify an adrenal tumor. A fasting insulin level may be useful in suspected cases of stromal hyperthecosis, and a prolactin level can identify prolactinomas that secrete massive amounts of prolactin, which can stimulate ovarian androgen production.

The preferred screening tool for an ovarian tumor is transvaginal ultrasonography. For an adrenal tumor, transabdominal ultrasonography is less sensitive. Computed tomography scan or magnetic resonance imaging can detect adrenal nodules less than 5 mm in diameter, providing a greater resolution than ultrasonography. However, about 2% of the population harbors a clinically insignificant adrenal adenoma (i.e., incidentaloma) such that their localization is not diagnostic for an androgen-secreting adrenal tumor. Functional radiologic techniques, such as selective venous catheterization or scintigraphy with [131]iodomethyl norcholesterol, are rarely used for the initial screening for such tumors.

DIFFERENTIAL DIAGNOSIS

The differential diagnosis of androgen excess leading to virilization, especially combined with a sudden onset and rapid progression, will always begin and end with tumors or dysfunctional states, usually of the ovary and less commonly of the adrenal gland. The most common androgen-producing tumor in a pre-

menopausal woman is a Sertoli–Leydig cell tumor. Other common tumors are thecomas and hilus cell tumors. Hilus cell tumors are often small (even less than 1 cm) and theoretically below the range of imaging visualization. Tumors may also present with a more indolent history, such as granulosa cell tumors, 10% of which primarily secrete androgens instead of estrogens. Any large ovarian tumor can produce androgens indirectly by causing hyperplasia of the surrounding normal stroma (benign cystic teratomas, dysgerminomas, epithelial tumors). The vast majority of ovarian androgen-secreting tumors are benign. Adrenal tumors are rare, with an estimated incidence of two cases per one million persons per year, which are equally divided among adenomas and carcinomas. The age of onset in adults peaks in the fifth decade. Virilization can accompany both tumors that primarily produce androgens and tumors that primarily produce cortisol (Cushing's syndrome). A long history of symptoms, as in the case of an ovarian tumor, does not preclude the presence of an adrenocortical neoplasm.

Dysfunctional states of the ovary, primarily hyperthecosis, may also result in virilization. In stromal hyperthecosis, most of the ovarian androgen overproduction results from hyperplasia of the ovarian stroma and not from the accumulation of small follicles, as is the case with PCOS. Most women with stromal hyperthecosis have severe hyperinsulinemia, which may be the stimulus for stromal androgen overproduction. It has been reported in both premenopausal and postmenopausal women, often with coexisting sequelae of the insulin resistance syndrome such as dyslipidemia and glucose intolerance.

The differential diagnosis of virilization in a woman must also consider the use of exogenous androgens, such as anabolic steroids in a body builder or an overdose of androgens in a postmenopausal woman. Virilization that occurs during pregnancy has its own unique differential diagnosis, including benign ovarian sources such as hyperreactio luteinalis (gestational ovarian theca–lutein cysts) or luteomas, and extremely rare fetoplacental sources such as aromatase deficiency, resulting in androgen excess due to the placental inability to convert precursor androgens to estrogens.

OPTIMAL MANAGEMENT

Congenital causes of virilization rarely present in an adult woman, and most causes of virilization in the adult are acquired. Thus, the ideal treatment involves removal of the acquired insult. This may mean stopping or revising exogenous medications. For the vast majority of women, treatment of virilization involves surgical removal of the tumor or gland(s), depending on the cause of the androgen production and the menopausal status of the woman. Almost all ovarian androgen-secreting tumors or hyperfunctioning states can be treated initially with surgery. In patients with inoperable adrenal tumors, chemotherapy may be the primary therapy. Choice of medical or surgical treatment of a prolactinoma with virilization is not clear. Many of the peripheral effects of virilization may require additional treatment, such as electrolysis for the hirsutism or a clitoral reduction for massive clitoromegaly. Changes in the voice are also thought to be permanent.

For those rare cases of virilization associated with common causes of androgen excess such as PCOS or NC-CAH, treatment involves suppression of the hyperfunctioning gland (ovary with the oral contraceptive pill and/or a gonadotropin hormone–releasing hormone agonist, or the adrenal with a glucocorticoid) combined with peripheral antagonism of androgen action through an androgen receptor antagonist such as spironolactone. This treatment may also be utilized in a premenopausal woman with hyperthecosis who desires to preserve ovarian function, though response must be closely monitored. There is no current evidence to suggest that the use of insulin-sensitizing agents can improve signs of virilization in women with marked androgen excess, although they are theoretically appealing.

BIBLIOGRAPHY

Barbieri RL, Ryan KJ. Hyperandrogenism, insulin resistance and acanthosis nigricans: a common endocrinopathy with unique pathophysiologic features. *Am J Obstet Gynecol* 1983;147:90–101.

Barth JH, Jenkins M, Belchetz PE. Ovarian hyperthecosis, diabetes, and hirsuties in post-menopausal women. *Clin Endocrinol* 1997;46:123–128.

Derksen J, Nagesser SK, Meinders AE, et al. Identification of virilizing adrenal tumors in hirsute women. *N Engl J Med* 1994;331:968–973.

Dunaif A, Hoffman AR, Scully RE, et al. Clinical, biochemical, and ovarian morphologic features in women with acanthosis nigricans and masculinization. *Obstet Gynecol* 1985;66:545–552.

Freeman, DA. Steroid hormone–producing tumors in man. *Endocr Rev* 1986;7:204–220.

Legro RS. Polycystic ovary syndrome treatment paradigms. *Am J Obstet Gynecol* 1998;179:S101–S108.

Lobo RA. Ovarian hyperandrogenism and androgen-producing tumors. *Endcrinol Metab Clin North Am* 1991;20:773–805.

McKenna TJ, Cunningham SK, Loughlin T. The adrenal cortex and virilization. *Clin Endocrinol Metab* 1985;14:997–1020.

Pittaway DE. Neoplastic causes of hyperandrogenism. *Infertil Reprod Med Clin North Am* 1991;2:295.

Ross NS, Aron DC. Hormonal evaluation of the patient with an incidentally discovered adrenal mass. *N Engl J Med* 1990;323:1401–1405.

Verkauf BS, Von Thron J, O'Brien WF. Clitoral size in normal women. *Obstet Gynecol* 1992;80:41–44.

Kelley's Textbook of Internal Medicine, fourth edition. Edited by H. David Humes. Lippincott Williams & Wilkins, Philadelphia © 2000.

C H A P T E R
395

APPROACH TO THE PATIENT WITH GYNECOMASTIA

GLENN D. BRAUNSTEIN

Gynecomastia represents the benign proliferation of breast glandular tissue that begins beneath the nipple–areolar complex and spreads laterally. It is a common condition that is found in approximately two-thirds of pubertal boys and at least one-third of adults.

PATHOPHYSIOLOGIC FACTORS

Estrogen stimulates breast glandular epithelium growth, an effect that is antagonized by androgens. Therefore, gynecomastia results when there is an imbalance between estrogen and androgen action at the breast tissue level. This can occur through increased serum free estrogen concentrations resulting from exogenous estrogen exposure, increased endogenous production through secretion or conversion of androgens to estrogens by the widely distributed aromatase enzyme complex, displacement of estrogens from sex hormone–binding globulin (SHBG), decreased androgen secretion, or abnormalities of the androgen receptor (Table 395.1). In many instances the gynecomastia is multifactorial, as, for example, with aging. Aging is associated with an enhanced activity of the aromatase enzyme in fat cells, as well as an increase in the proportion of fat to lean body mass. In addition, many men have a slight decrease in their testosterone production rate, which reduces their free testosterone level. Fi-

TABLE 395.1.	MECHANISMS AND CAUSES OF GYNECOMASTIA	
Mechanism	**Specific Causes**
Increased Serum Estrogens	
Exogenous	Topical estrogen creams and lotions
	Ingestion of estrogens
	Use of aromatizable androgens
	Environmental exposure
Increased aromatization in testes, adrenals, or peripheral tissues	Testicular tumors
	Adrenal tumors
	Obesity
	Liver disease
	Hyperthyroidism
	Aging
	Familial or sporadic excessive aromatase activity
Displacement of estrogens from SHBG	Spironolactone
	Ketoconazole
hCG-secreting tumors	Choriocarcinoma
	Lung, liver, renal, gastric carcinoma
Decreased testosterone synthesis	Primary hypogonadism
	Secondary hypogonadism
	Drug-induced: Spironolactone Ketoconazole
Androgen receptor defects	Congenital mutations
	Drug interference: Cimetidine Cyproterone Flutamide Spironolactone

SHBG, sex hormone–binding globulin; hCG, human chorionic gonadotropin.

nally, older men may be ingesting medications that can alter androgen production or action.

HISTORY AND PHYSICAL EXAMINATION

Inquiries into medication and recreational drug (e.g., ethanol, marijuana) use, the circumstances surrounding the onset of gynecomastia, and the presence of breast tenderness, which indicates recent onset of the condition, should be made. Symptoms suggestive of renal or hepatic insufficiency, hyperthyroidism, pituitary dysfunction, and hypogonadism should be sought. Examination for these conditions as well as a careful breast examination to confirm the presence of gynecomastia, along with testicular palpation for masses or atrophy should be carried out.

LABORATORY STUDIES AND DIAGNOSTIC TESTS

If the cause of gynecomastia is not readily apparent from the history and physical examination, measurement of serum concentrations of human chorionic gonadotropin (hCG), luteinizing hormone (LH), testosterone, and estradiol can help differentiate among the various causes (Fig. 395.1).

An elevated hCG concentration is found with gonadal or extragonadal germ cell tumors or with nontrophoblastic neoplasms, such as lung, liver, or kidney tumors. A suppressed testosterone with elevated LH indicates primary hypogonadism, whereas low levels of both is indicative of a hypothalamic or pituitary disorder. Elevations of both LH and testosterone are found in patients with hyperthyroidism as well as those with androgen resistance, which can be distinguished through measurements of thyroid function tests. Elevations of estradiol may be found with Leydig or Sertoli cell tumors of the testes, feminizing adrenocortical neoplasms, or in situations in which the extraglandular aromatization of androgens is increased (Table 395.1). If all tests are normal, then the patient is considered to have idiopathic gynecomastia.

DIFFERENTIAL DIAGNOSIS

It is important to differentiate gynecomastia from pseudogynecomastia, which reflects an enlargement of the breast subcutaneous fat. This can be accomplished by having the patient lie on his back with hands behind the head. The examiner places his or her thumb and forefinger on either side of the breast and gradually brings the fingers together. If gynecomastia is present, a ridge of rubbery tissue will be felt spreading radially from the nipple, whereas in pseudogynecomastia, the fingers will not meet any resistance until they touch the nipple. The most important condition to differentiate is breast carcinoma. Breast carcinoma often presents as a unilateral, painless, hard, eccentric mass, which may be associated with dimpling of the skin and axillary adenopathy, rather than the concentric subareolar rubbery tissue that may be tender and is often bilateral in patients with gyneco-

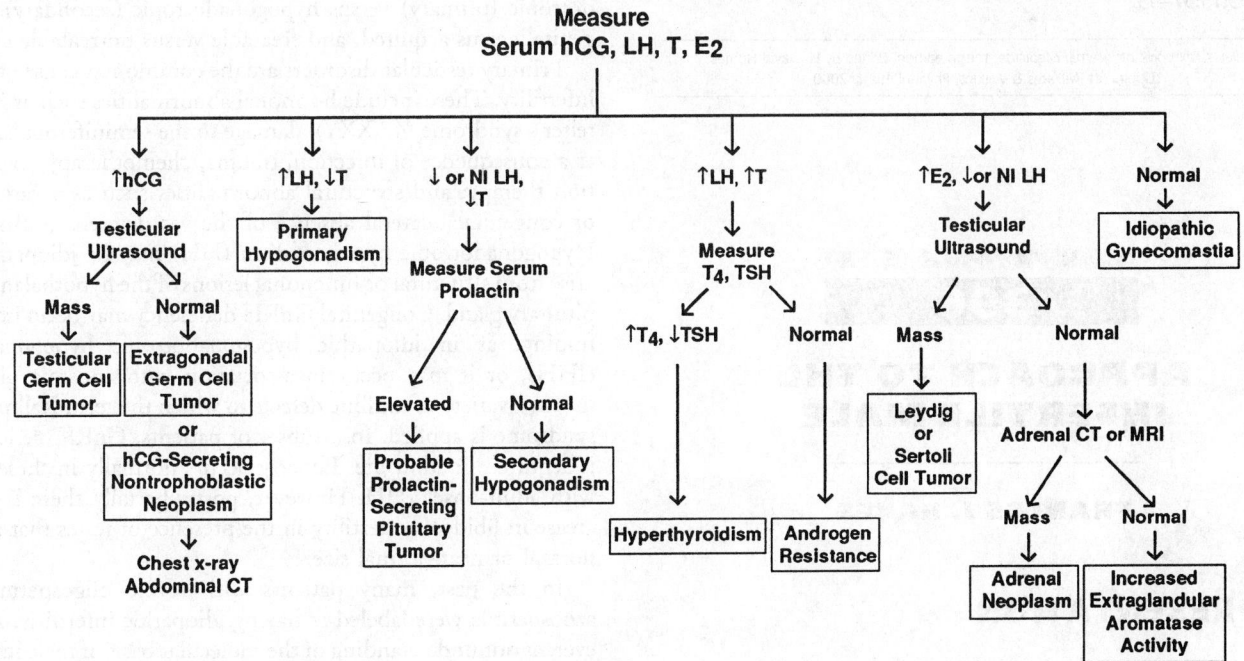

FIGURE 395.1. Evaluation of gynecomastia. hCG, human chorionic gonadotropin; LH, luteinizing hormone; T, testosterone; E₂, estradiol; T₄, thyroxine; TSH, thyroid-stimulating hormone; ↑, increased; ↓, decreased; Nl, normal. (From Braunstein GD. Gynecomastia. *N Engl J Med* 1993;328:490–495, with permission.)

EVIDENCE LEVEL: C. Expert Opinion.

mastia. If uncertainty exists after the examination, mammography or fine-needle aspiration biopsy may be performed.

OPTIMAL MANAGEMENT

Correction of the identified inciting cause of the gynecomastia will lead to a resolution of the breast enlargement if the gynecomastia is of recent onset. However, if the gynecomastia has been present for over a year, much of the hyperplastic glandular component can be replaced by fibrous tissue that will not regress. The indications for specific medical or surgical treatment of the gynecomastia include persistent pain as well as intense emotional discomfort and/or embarrassment. Medical therapies are generally useful only during the early proliferative phase of the condition (when pain and tenderness are prominent). The antiestrogen tamoxifen citrate or aromatase inhibitors, such as testolactone or anastrozole, may be tried for up to 3 months. If they fail to reduce the breast size sufficiently or if the gynecomastia is in the fibrotic stage, the only curative therapy is reduction mammoplasty, which can be accomplished by excision of the glandular tissue through a periareolar incision accompanied by liposuction to remove the subcutaneous fat and contour the breast.

BIBLIOGRAPHY

Mathur R, Braunstein GD: Gynecomastia: pathomechanisms and treatment strategies. *Horm Res* 1997;48:95.
Thompson DF, Carter JR: Drug-induced gynecomastia. *Pharmacotherapy* 1993;13:37–45.

Kelley's Textbook of Internal Medicine, fourth edition. Edited by H. David Humes.
Lippincott Williams & Wilkins, Philadelphia © 2000.

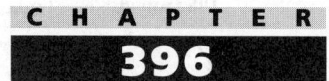

396

APPROACH TO THE INFERTILE MALE

FRANCES J. HAYES

PRESENTATION

Using the definition of failure to conceive after a year of regular unprotected intercourse, 10% to 15% of couples in the United States are infertile. Of these, a male factor is the sole abnormality in 30% of cases and a contributory factor in an additional 20%.

Given this high prevalence of male factor infertility, obtaining a semen analysis is an essential component of the workup of every infertile couple. While male infertility is typically diagnosed in the setting of a couple who fail to conceive, the diagnosis may be made earlier in the subset of infertile men presenting with concomitant symptoms of hypogonadism.

PATHOPHYSIOLOGIC FACTORS

NORMAL SPERMATOGENESIS

Reproductive competence in the male requires the integration of a normal hypothalamic–pituitary–testicular (HPT) axis. Pulsatile secretion of gonadotropin-releasing hormone (GnRH) from the hypothalamus stimulates release of luteinizing hormone (LH) and follicle-stimulating hormone (FSH) from the pituitary. LH stimulates the testicular Leydig cells to produce testosterone, which is important for virilization and normal sexual function. In addition, high intratesticular levels of testosterone are necessary for spermatogenesis. FSH plays a critical role in the initiation and, to a lesser extent, maintenance of spermatogenesis. The process of spermatogenesis, which occurs in the seminiferous tubules, takes approximately 75 days. Once spermatogenesis is complete, sperm are transported through the epididymis to the ejaculatory duct. During this period of 12 to 21 days, sperm acquire the capacity for sustained motility.

DISORDERS OF SPERMATOGENESIS

The differential diagnosis of male infertility includes hypergonadotropic (primary) versus hypogonadotropic (secondary), congenital versus acquired, and treatable versus untreatable causes.

Primary testicular disorders are the commonest cause of male infertility. These include hormonal abnormalities such as Klinefelter's syndrome (47,XXY); damage to the seminiferous tubules as a consequence of infection, trauma, chemotherapy, or radiation therapy; and structural abnormalities such as a varicocele or congenital bilateral absence of the vas deferens (CBAVD). Hypogonadotropic hypogonadism (HH) may be idiopathic or arise from structural or functional lesions of the hypothalamus or pituitary gland. Congenital GnRH deficiency may be an isolated finding, as in idiopathic hypogonadotropic hypogonadism (IHH), or it may occur in association with anosmia plus or minus a variety of midline defects to which the term Kallmann's syndrome is applied. In a subset of patients, GnRH deficiency is acquired in adult life. Puberty occurs normally in these men with adult-onset IHH. However, postpubertally there is a decrease in libido and fertility in the presence of testes that are of normal or near-normal size.

In the past, many patients with severe oligospermia or azoospermia were labeled as having idiopathic infertility. However, as our understanding of the molecular basis of male infertility increases, the percentage of patients in the idiopathic category has decreased. In fact, careful genetic screening of men with "idiopathic" azoospermia indicates that approximately 15% of these men have microdeletions in the Y chromosome.

HISTORY AND PHYSICAL EXAMINATION

A careful history and physical examination are essential to the workup of the infertile male patient. In the history one should ask specifically about problems with libido, potency, or ejaculation. It is important to determine if there is a history of congenital defects, such as cryptorchidism and micropenis, or of delayed puberty, anosmia, or orchitis. The physician should also inquire about ingestion of drugs or exposure to toxins known to interfere with testosterone production or spermatogenesis. On physical examination, it is important to look for features of hypogonadism (eunuchoid body habitus, i.e., upper/lower body ratio less than 1 with an arm span 6 cm greater than standing height, absence of virilization, gynecomastia). Testicular volume should be estimated with a Prader orchidometer (normal ≥ 15 mL) and the presence of a varicocele excluded.

LABORATORY STUDIES AND DIAGNOSTIC TESTS

A semen analysis is the single most important diagnostic test and may be all that is required if the history and physical examination are normal (Fig. 396.1). A normal semen analysis (volume greater than 2 mL, count greater than 20 million per milliliter, motility greater than 50%, morphology greater than 30% normal, *WHO Criteria, 1992*) excludes male factor infertility provided that libido and potency are normal. If an abnormal semen analysis is obtained, an additional sample should be examined after 2 to 3 months. If no sperm are present in the ejaculate (azoospermia), an obstructive cause, such as CBAVD, must be distinguished from a seminiferous tubular defect. If an obstruction is causing azoospermia, seminal fructose, which is produced by seminal vesicles, is low. In azoospermic men in whom the diagnosis of CBAVD has been made, screening for the cystic fibrosis gene should be performed as mutations in the *CFTR* gene have been reported in up to 70% of such patients.

In men with oligo- or azoospermia in whom obstruction has been excluded, an endocrine evaluation, comprising measurement of testosterone, LH, FSH, and prolactin, should be undertaken. If the hormonal pattern is consistent with HH (low testosterone with low or inappropriately normal gonadotropin levels) or if serum prolactin is elevated, magnetic resonance imaging of the hypothalamic–pituitary region is indicated. The commonest hormonal abnormality seen in infertile men is an elevated FSH level in association with normal LH and testosterone levels, reflecting selective seminiferous tubular damage. Serum inhibin B is inversely related to FSH in infertile men, suggesting that it may serve as a useful marker of Sertoli cell function. However, the clinical utility of serum inhibin B measurements in the routine assessment of the infertile male has yet to be definitively established. The role of genetic analysis of the Y chromosome is controversial and presently limited to specialist centers. Genetic testing is particularly important in couples contemplating assisted reproductive technology so that appropriate genetic counseling can be provided. In men with gynecomastia, small testes, and an elevated FSH level, a karyotype should be obtained to screen for Klinefelter's syndrome.

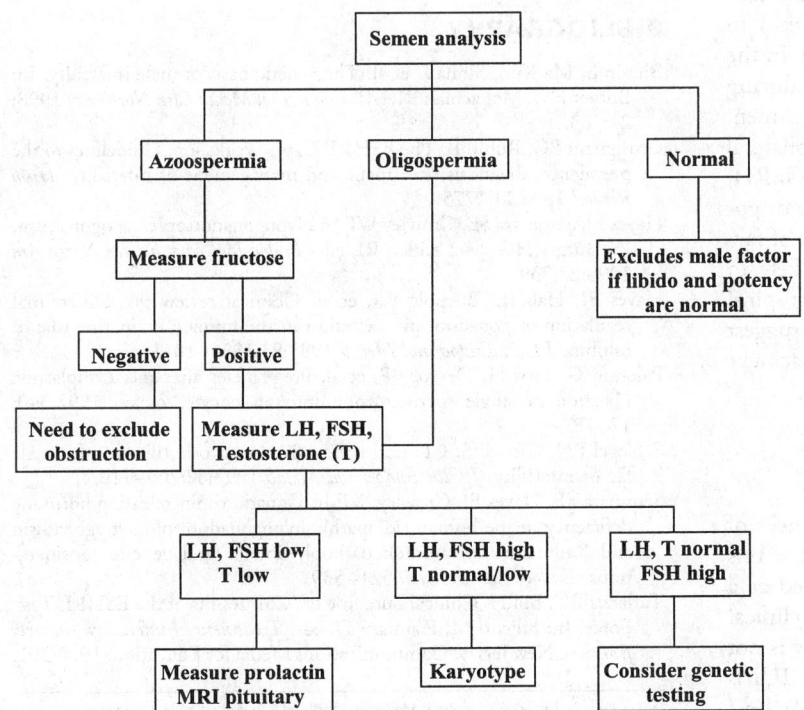

FIGURE 396.1. Approach to the evaluation of an infertile man.

EVIDENCE LEVEL: C. Expert Opinion.

■ OPTIMAL MANAGEMENT

Treatment of male infertility is guided by the underlying diagnosis. While HH is a relatively uncommon cause of infertility in men, it is an important diagnosis to make as exogenous gonadotropins or pulsatile GnRH can be used to stimulate spermatogenesis. In contrast, men with normal testosterone levels and severe oligo- or azoospermia require assisted reproductive technology to achieve fertility. For men with primary testicular failure, therapeutic options are limited to donor insemination or adoption.

INDUCTION OF SPERMATOGENESIS

Gonadotropin therapy consists of administration of human chorionic gonadotropin (hCG) in combination with human menopausal urinary gonadotropin (hMG) or recombinant FSH formulations. Therapy with hCG is usually initiated with a dose of 500 to 1,000 IU subcutaneously on alternate days and titrated based on testicular growth and trough testosterone levels. Most patients also require FSH to stimulate spermatogenesis. Because hMG contains both LH and FSH, when administered in combination with hCG, estradiol concentrations may become disproportionately elevated, thus leading to gynecomastia. Gynecomastia can be avoided by reducing the hCG dose prior to the addition of hMG so that serum testosterone levels are maintained at the lower end of the normal range. Alternatively, recombinant FSH may confer an advantage in this clinical setting.

Although not approved by the U.S. Food and Drug Administration for use in hypogonadotropic men, pulsatile GnRH is a highly effective therapy for inducing spermatogenesis. GnRH is administered subcutaneously by a portable mini-infusion pump at a frequency of every 2 hour. Most patients require treatment for 1 to 2 years (depending on pretherapy testicular size) to maximize testicular growth and achieve spermatogenesis. In the authors' experience, pulsatile GnRH is successful in inducing spermatogenesis in the vast majority of hypogonadotropic men, with the exceptions tending to be those with a history of bilateral cryptorchidism, rare patients who develop antibodies to GnRH, or patients with GnRH receptor mutations. The choice of gonadotropin versus GnRH therapy depends on a number of factors. Patients with extensive pituitary damage are unlikely to respond to GnRH and should be treated with gonadotropins. While both are very effective therapeutic modalities, data suggest that testicular growth is greater and the time taken to achieve spermatogenesis shorter in patients treated with GnRH.

ASSISTED REPRODUCTIVE TECHNOLOGY

It is intuited that when sperm counts are low, the chances of sperm–egg interaction in vivo are reduced. To overcome this difficulty, intrauterine insemination (IUI) was developed as a means of bringing sperm closer to the egg. However, the clinical effectiveness of IUI in couples with male factor infertility is not significantly different from that of no treatment, unless IUI is coupled to ovulation induction in the female partner. At least 1 million to 2 million motile sperm are required for IUI to be successful. If pregnancy does not ensue within the first three cycles, more invasive forms of assisted reproduction should be considered.

As a result of exciting advances in the treatment of male infertility in recent years, couples who would previously have been offered donor insemination or adoption are now achieving pregnancy. While male factor infertility was initially considered a contraindication to in vitro fertilization (IVF), IVF is now viewed as an acceptable treatment option for infertile men. However, for men with severe male factor infertility, the main drawback of IVF is that at least 100,000 sperm must be inseminated per oocyte for fertilization to occur. This has led to the development of a number of micromanipulation techniques to assist fertilization, including intracytoplasmic sperm injection (ICSI).

The first pregnancy to result from the direct injection of a single sperm into the cytoplasm of an oocyte using the technique of ICSI occurred in 1992. ICSI is now recommend in the following circumstances: (a) fertilization failure with standard IVF; (b) severe male factor infertility (i.e., sperm count greater than 2 million per milliliter, normal morphology less than 4%, sperm motility less than 5%; and (c) the use of surgically retrieved spermatozoa. Sperm for ICSI can be retrieved from the ejaculate, from epididymal aspiration, or from testicular aspiration/biopsy. The clinical outcome of ICSI to date has been very encouraging, with fertilization rates of 50% to 60% and pregnancy rates of 30% per cycle. The incidence of congenital malformations does not appear to be increased. However, a slight increase in chromosomal aberrations, especially of the sex chromosomes, has been observed. The increase in chromosomal abnormalities underscores the importance of proper genetic counseling of couples contemplating ICSI.

BIBLIOGRAPHY

Bhasin S, Ma Kun, Sinha I, et al. The genetic basis of male infertility. In: Burger HG, McLachlan RI, eds. *Endocrinol Metab Clin North Am* 1998; 27:783.

Crosignani PG, Rubin B. The ESHRE Capri Workshop. Guidelines to the prevalence, diagnosis, treatment and management of infertility. *Hum Reprod* 1996;11:1775.

Hayes FJ, Seminara SB, Crowley WF Jr. Hypogonadotropic hypogonadism. In: Burger HG, McLachlan RI, eds. *Endocrinol Metab Clin North Am* 1998;27:739.

Hayes FJ, Hall JE, Boepple PA, et al. CLinical review 96: Differential regulation of gonadotropin secretion in the human: endocrine role of inhibin. *J Clin Endocrinol Metab* 1998;83:1835–1841.

Palermo G, Joris H, Devroey P, et al. Pregnancies after intracytoplasmic injection of single spermatozoon into an oocyte. *Lancet* 1992;340: 17–18.

Schlegel PN, Girardi S. CLinical review 87: In vitro fertilization for male factor infertility. *J Clin Endocrinol Metab* 1997;82:709–716.

Seminara SB, Hayes FJ, Crowley WF Jr. Gonadotropin-releasing hormone deficiency in the human (idiopathic hypogonadotropic hypogonadism and Kallmann's syndrome): pathophysiologic and genetic considerations. *Endocr Rev* 1998;19:521–539.

Tarlatzis BC, Bili H. Clinical outcome of ICSI: results of the ESHRE Task Force. In: Filicori M, Flamigni D, eds. *Treatment of infertility: the new frontiers.* New Jersey: Communications Media for Education, 1998;301.

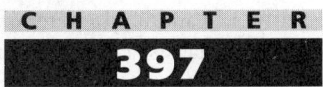

APPROACH TO SEXUAL DYSFUNCTION IN THE FEMALE

ROBERT L. BARBIERI

Sexual function allows individuals to come together to bond, enjoy each other, and reproduce; it is influenced by physical, emotional, and social factors. Fewer than half of all women discuss issues of sexuality with their physicians. Although a comprehensive examination is not complete unless the patient is given the opportunity to discuss this topic, many physicians are too busy and most patients too anxious to initiate such a discussion. By creating a supportive and nonjudgmental atmosphere and by initiating a discussion of sexuality, physicians can determine quickly whether sexual problems requiring further attention are present.

SEXUAL RESPONSE CYCLE

Masters and Johnson first characterized the female sexual response as consisting of four successive phases: excitement, plateau, orgasm, and resolution. Kaplan proposed sexual desire, or libido, as the first phase in the female sexual response cycle. The excitement phase is initiated by psychological (fantasy) and physiologic (kissing) stimuli. During this phase, the woman experiences nipple erection, hyperemia of the clitoris and labia minor, swelling of the labia, an increase in vaginal fluid, expansion of the vaginal cavity, and elevation of the uterus. In the plateau phase, the shaft of the clitoris retracts, vaginal transudation occurs, and the outer third of the vagina contracts. Orgasm typically lasts 5 to 30 seconds and is associated with rhythmic contractions of the vagina, uterus, and pelvic musculature. In the resolution phase, the hyperemia of the genitalia slowly resolves.

SEXUAL HISTORY

For the premenopausal woman, a discussion of sexuality can be approached as part of a discussion of contraceptive practices using the following types of questions: Are you sexually active? Do you need birth control? Are sexual relations enjoyable and comfortable? Are you having pain with sexual relations? Is there any aspect of your sexual life that is not satisfactory? For the menopausal woman, a discussion of sexuality can be initiated as part of the interview pertaining to the effects of hypoestrogenism. This line of questioning leads naturally to questions pertaining to libido (sexual desire), sensation, vaginal dryness, and pain with sexual relations.

SEXUAL PAIN DISORDERS

In premenopausal women, vaginismus, the involuntary contraction of the perineal muscles in the outer third of the vagina, may cause pain with sexual relations. If genital anatomy is normal, vaginismus is best treated by desensitization training; allowing the woman to self-insert vaginal dilators of increasing length and diameter. In postmenopausal women, vaginal dryness resulting from low estrogen concentration can contribute to pain with sexual relations. Estrogen replacement therapy can improve vaginal lubrication and sexual function. In postmenopausal women, estrogen replacement enhances clitoral and vaginal vibration and pressure thresholds, and increases blood flow to the pelvic tissues. For menopausal women with contraindications to systemic estrogen treatment, vaginal rings that release estradiol can often improve vaginal function. Insufficient foreplay and performance anxiety can also result in insufficient vaginal secretions, contributing to pain with sexual relations.

DECREASED SEXUAL DESIRE

During the perimenopause and menopause, some women report a decrease in sexual desire. Low estrogen and testosterone levels may contribute to decreased sexual desire. In one study of sexual desire and function after surgical oophorectomy, androgen plus estrogen treatment was reported to be more effective in enhancing sexual desire than estrogen alone. Oral combinations of conjugated estrogen (estrone sulfate) and androgen (methyl testosterone; Estratest) may be effective in enhancing libido in some menopausal women. Health status, past level of sexual activity, partner availability, and social status are also important determinants of libido in menopausal women.

In both pre- and postmenopausal women, psychoactive agents such as selective serotonin reuptake inhibitors, tranquilizers, and excess quantities of alcohol can impair sexual desire. Conditions such as severe rheumatoid arthritis, diabetes, and HIV disease can have a major impact on sexual functioning in a couple.

ADVANCES IN PHARMACOLOGIC TREATMENT

Sildenafil (Viagra) is a selective type 5 (cGMP-specific) phosphodiesterase inhibitor that increases cGMP levels, resulting in relaxation of clitoral and vaginal smooth muscle, enhancing blood flow into these tissues. Sildenafil is approved for the treatment of erectile dysfunction in men but is not currently approved for use in women. Recent data indicate that central nervous system dopamine may mediate libido and sexual excitement. Apomorphine may prove useful in the treatment of disorders of libido.

SEXUAL ABUSE

Approximately 25% of adult women report a previous history of sexual abuse, including undesired vaginal penetration and other undesired direct contact with the genitals. In some cases, a result of sexual abuse can be sexual dysfunction and chronic pelvic pain syndromes. Childhood sexual abuse is especially likely to result in sexual dysfunction, depression, and chronic pelvic pain.

BIBLIOGRAPHY

Ayton RA, Darling GM, Murkies AL, et al. A comparative study of safety and efficacy of continuous low dose oestradiol released from a vaginal ring compared with conjugated equine oestrogen vaginal cream in the treatment of postmenopausal urogenital atrophy. *Br J Obstet Gynecol* 1996;103:351–358.

Bachmann GA, Moeller TP, Bennett J. Childhood sexual abuse and the consequences in adult women. *Obstet Gynecol* 1988;71:631–642.

Kaplan HS. *The new sex therapy.* London: Bailliere Tindall, 1974.

Lief HI. Sexology. *JAMA* 1989;261:2889–2890.

Masters EH, Johnson VE. *Human sexual response.* Boston: Little, Brown and Company, 1966.

Semmens JP, Wagner G. Estrogen deprivation and vaginal function in postmenopausal women. *JAMA* 1982;248:445–448.

Sherwin BB, Gelfand MM. Differential symptom response to parenteral estrogen and androgen in the surgical menopause. *Am J Obstet Gynecol* 1985;151:153–160.

Tutten A, Laan E, Panhuysen G, et al. Discrepancies between genital responses and subjective sexual function during testosterone substitution in women with hypothalamic amenorrhea. *Psychosom Med* 1996;58:234–241.

Walling MK, Reiter RC, O'Hara MW, et al. Abuse history and chronic pelvic pain in women: I. Prevalence of sexual abuse and physical abuse. *Obstet Gynecol* 1994;84:193–199.

Kelley's Textbook of Internal Medicine, fourth edition. Edited by H. David Humes. Lippincott Williams & Wilkins, Philadelphia © 2000.

C H A P T E R

398

APPROACH TO SEXUAL DYSFUNCTION IN THE MALE

MAX HIRSHKOWITZ
GLENN R. CUNNINGHAM

Four fundamental processes are involved in male human sexuality: desire, arousal (both attaining and maintaining erections), ejaculation/orgasm, and fertilization. In men, problems with arousal [(erectile dysfunction (ED)] and desire (loss of libido) are common. Among 1,290 noninstitutionalized men between the ages of 40 and 70 years, an estimated 5% to 15% reported severe ED and 17% to 34% reported moderate ED. The age-adjusted probabilities calculated for *complete ED* were 39% in men treated for heart disease, 28% in treated diabetes, and 15% in treated hypertension. Smoking and lower HDL cholesterol also correlated with increased ED.

Until fairly recently, ED and libido were infrequently evaluated or treated by nonspecialists. Evaluation and treatment of sexual dysfunction has become common practice because of increasing emphasis on maximizing quality of life, more precise diagnostics, and improved therapeutics. After the U.S. Food and Drug Administration's approval of sildenafil (Viagra), an orally administered agent for treating ED, widespread media attention produced a flood of patients seeking treatment. Physicians administered the drug as an empirical challenge with little regard for etiology or diagnosis. When it proved effective and well tolerated, it was continued. Thus, we have witnessed a revolutionary change in who seeks treatment, who administers treatment, and the approach to treatment.

■ EVALUATION OF ERECTILE DYSFUNCTION

Ideally, etiology should direct therapeutic selection. However, ED diagnostic techniques are not readily available to many physicians, are not fully refined, and are expensive. Thus, available noninvasive therapies make it more practical to administer a therapeutic challenge than to perform extensive diagnostic procedures. Nonetheless, evaluation should begin with a careful history and physical examination (Fig. 398.1). Sexual functioning inventories and psychometric tests can be extremely valuable for delineating ED type, severity, and complication by relationship or psychiatric problems. Appropriate referrals for counseling, behavioral therapy, and/or psychiatric treatment should be made. The patient's medication regimen should be reviewed because iatrogenic ED must be considered. Furthermore, ED as a medication side effect tends to foster noncompliance with needed medications. Drugs adversely affecting erectile function include antiandrogens (cimetidine, cyproterone acetate, estrogens, finasteride, ketoconazole, progestins, spironolactone), anticholinergics (atropine, butyrophenones, disopyramide, ganglionic blocking agents), antidepressants (monoamine oxidase inhibitors, tricyclic antidepressants, selective serotonin reuptake inhibitors), antihypertensives (α-methyldopa, reserpine, clonidine, propranolol, thiazides, prazosin, phenoxybenzamine, phentolamine), antipsychotics (phenothiazines, thioridazine), central nervous system depressants (barbiturates, benzodiazepines, carbamazepine, methadone, morphine, phenytoin, primidone), and substances of abuse (amphetamines, cocaine, heroin, ethanol, tobacco).

Laboratory tests should be ordered to exclude a systemic disease or testosterone deficiency. Placebo-controlled trials repeatedly demonstrate that testosterone replacement therapy improves libido and erectile function in men with hypogonadism. However, comorbid diseases may limit testosterone's effectiveness in improving ED, particularly in men over 50. Normalizing hyperprolactinemia with dopamine agonists or surgically removing a prolactinoma may increase serum testosterone level and restore potency. Dopaminergic erectogenic properties likely derive from D_2 receptors and oxytocin neuronal action. Apomorphine has been shown to produce erections in a small sample

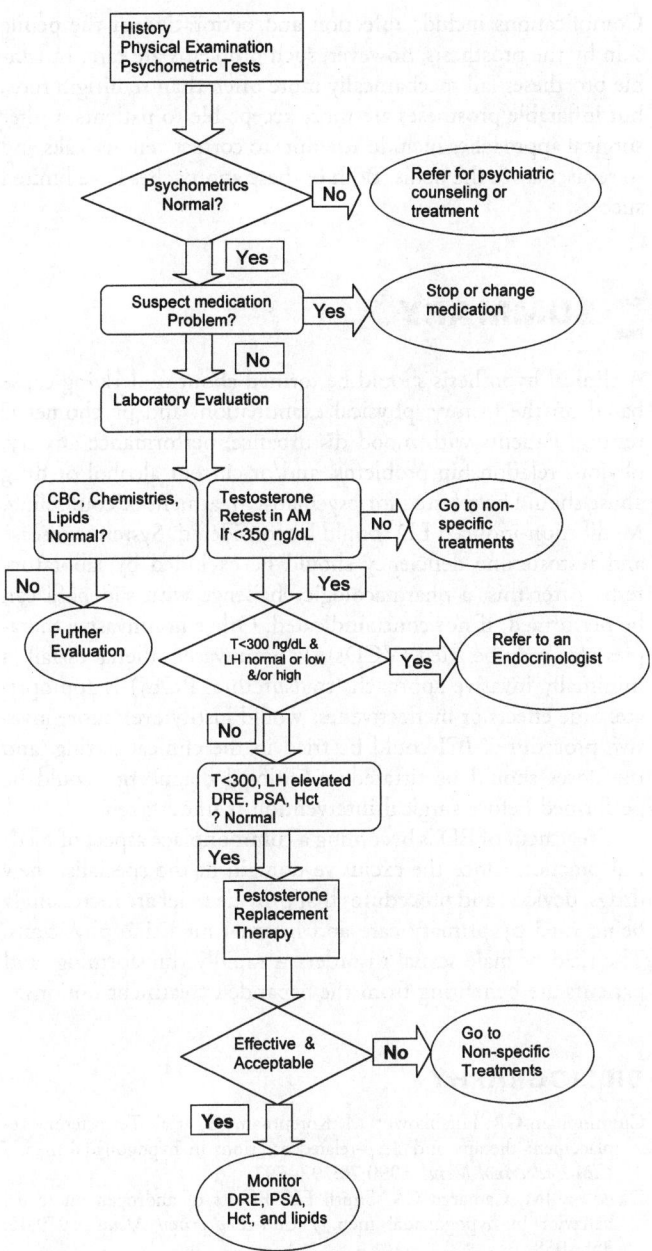

FIGURE 398.1. Evaluation and treatment of erectile dysfunction.

Other approaches to nonspecific treatment are outlined in Fig. 398.2. A general purpose, orally administered agent to treat ED has long been sought, and in 1998 sildenafil was approved for use. Smooth-muscle relaxation in cavernosal bodies is triggered by sexual stimuli. This leads to nitric oxide (NO) release from nonadrenergic, noncholinergic nerves; NO innervates the cavernosal smooth muscle. Sildenafil is a selective inhibitor of cGMP-specific phosphodiesterase type 5. It appears to potentiate erections induced by physiologic mechanisms as opposed to directly stimulating corporal smooth-muscle relaxation.

Sildenafil reportedly improved erectile function in men with presumed organic, psychogenic, or mixed causes. Outcome data were self-reported assessments. The study did not measure erections physiologically. Dose escalation increased the chance of

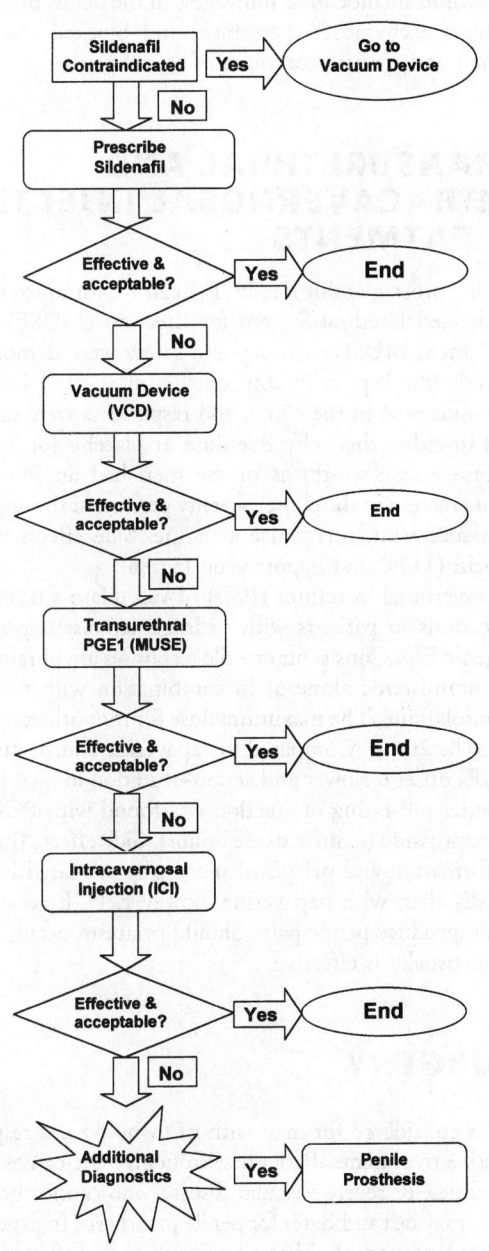

FIGURE 398.2. Nonspecific treatments for erectile dysfunction.

of men with ED. Larger clinical trials are under way; however, at present its therapeutic role is not defined.

■ NONSPECIFIC TREATMENT WITH NONINVASIVE THERAPIES

Topically applied preparations represent another approach and formulations of nitroglycerin, prostaglandins E_2 and E_1, papaverine, stearyl vasoactive intestinal peptide, and minoxidil are being evaluated. They show promise; however, these agents tend to have systemic effects when applied in quantities sufficient to affect erections.

headaches, flushing, dyspepsia, rhinitis, and visual disturbances; however, priapism was not a problem. The Food and Drug Administration issued an advisory warning against using both sildenafil and nitrates after several deaths were attributed to sildenafil. Additionally, sildenafil should be used very cautiously in men with significant cardiac disease.

If sildenafil is either ineffective or contraindicated, an external vacuum constriction device (VCD) can be tried. This device is a cylinder-like chamber in which a vacuum is created around the penis with a suction pump. The negative pressure induces blood flow into the corpora cavernosa, thereby producing an erection. Erection is maintained by placing a constricting band at the penile base to restrict outflow. VCDs have been used with success by many patients with ED, especially men with venous leaks and neurologic disorders (traumatic and nontraumatic). Complications include mild numbness in the penis, mild cyanosis, painless ecchymoses, petechiae, and blocked ejaculation. Some men and spouses complain of a cool penis.

TRANSURETHRAL AND INTRACAVERNOSAL INJECTION TREATMENTS

Aprostadil (prostaglandin E1, PGE$_1$) can be administered with the Medicated Urethral System for Erection (MUSE). Tested in 1,511 men, MUSE's efficacy and safety were demonstrated in a double-blind, placebo-controlled clinical trial. Trial doses were administered in the clinic, and responders were randomly assigned to either their effective dose or placebo for 3 months of in-home use. Two-thirds of the men had an intercourse-sufficient erection in the clinic. Seventy percent of the responders reported successful intercourse at home. Side effects included penile pain (11%) and hypotension (3.3%).

Intracavernosal injections (ICIs) of vasodilators usually produce erections in patients with neurogenic, vasculogenic, and psychogenic ED. Consistent erectile responses are obtained with PGE$_1$, administered alone or in combination with papaverine and phentolamine. The maximum dose for monotherapy is considered to be 20 µg. Compared to papaverine and/or nitroprusside, PGE$_1$ onset is slower and action–duration longer. Furthermore, better self-rating of erection was found with PGE1 than with nitroprusside (a nitric oxide donor). Side effects (including plaque formation and priapism) reportedly appeared less often with PGE$_1$ than with papaverine; however, PGE$_1$ costs more. PGE$_1$ can produce penile pain. Should priapism occur, medical treatment usually is effective.

SURGERY

Surgery is considered for men with ED who do not respond to less invasive treatments. Patients with neurologic causes, genital abnormalities, or severe vascular disease who cannot be treated medically may be candidates for penile prosthesis. In experienced hands, implantation of either a semirigid or an inflatable penile prosthesis achieves satisfactory results in 74% to 95% of patients.

Complications include infection and perforation of the penile skin by the prosthesis; however, such problems are rare. Inflatable prostheses fail mechanically more often than semirigid rods, but inflatable prostheses are more acceptable to patients. Other surgical approaches include attempts to correct venous leaks and to revascularize the penis. Both of these approaches have limited success.

SUMMARY

A clinical hypothesis should be formed about underlying cause based on the history, physical examination, and psychometric testing. Patients with mood disturbance, performance anxiety, obvious relationship problems, and/or current alcohol or drug abuse should be referred for psychiatric treatment or counseling. Medication-induced ED should be considered. Systemic disease and testosterone deficiency should be excluded by laboratory tests. After this, a pharmacologic challenge with sildenafil can be performed, if not contraindicated. Other noninvasive therapies also may be tried (VCDs). If noninvasive therapies fail, a minimally invasive approach (transurethral PGE$_1$) is appropriate. Side effects or ineffectiveness would justify even more invasive procedures. ICI could be tried in the clinical setting, and the doses should be titrated. Additional diagnostics could be performed before surgical intervention is undertaken.

Treatment of ED is becoming a commonplace aspect of medical practice. Once the exclusive domain of the specialist, new drugs, devices, and procedures that provide relief are increasingly being used by primary care and internal medicine physicians. The field of male sexual disorders is rapidly transforming, and patients are benefiting from the expanded treatment options.

BIBLIOGRAPHY

Cunningham GR, Hirshkowitz M, Korenman SG, et al. Testosterone replacement therapy and sleep-related erections in hypogonadal men. *J Clin Endocrinol Metab* 1990;70:792–797.

Davidson JM, Camargo CA, Smith ER. Effects of androgen on sexual behavior in hypogonadal men. *J Clin Endocrinol Metab* 1979;45:955–958.

Feldman HA, Goldstein I, Hatzichristou DG, et al. Impotence and its medical and psychosocial correlates: results of the Massachusetts Male Aging Study. *J Urol* 1994;151:54–61.

Goldstein I, Lue TF, Padma-Nathan H, et al. Oral sildenafil in the treatment of erectile dysfunction. *N Engl J Med* 1998;338:1397–1404.

Heaton JP, Morales A, Adams MA, et al. Recovery of erectile function by the oral administration of apomorphine. *Urology* 1995;45:200–206.

Kulmala R. Treatment of priapism: primary results and complications in 207 patients. *Ann Chir Gynaecol* 1994;83:309–314.

Padma-Nathan H, Hellstrom WF, Kaiser FE, et al. Treatment of men with erectile dysfunction with transurethral alprostadil. Medicated Urethral System for Erection (MUSE) Study Group. *N Engl J Med* 1997;336:1–7.

U.S. Food and Drug Administration (FDA) Web page: http://www.fda.gov/.

Witherington R. Vacuum constriction device for management of erectile impotence. *J Urol* 1989;141:320–322.

C H A P T E R

399

APPROACH TO HYPERGLYCEMIA IN THE PATIENT WITH DIABETES MELLITUS

JAY S. SKYLER

This chapter addresses the therapeutic approach to hyperglycemia in patients with diabetes. The discussion is divided into three sections: therapy of hyperglycemia in type I diabetes, therapy of hyperglycemia in type II diabetes, and therapy of acute decompensated diabetes (diabetic ketoacidosis and hyperosmolar hyperglycemic nonketotic coma). The pathophysiologic characteristics of these conditions are discussed in Chapter 411, as is the treatment of chronic diabetic complications.

■ THERAPY OF TYPE I DIABETES

Patients with type I diabetes do not produce insulin and thus depend on exogenous insulin for survival. The diabetic state is recognized and characterized by virtue of the hyperglycemia that ensues as a consequence of insulin deficiency. Physiologic insulin secretion includes both continuous basal insulin secretion and substrate-related incremental insulin secretion after meal consumption (see Fig. 411.2 in Chapter 411). Basal insulin secretion modulates hepatic glucose production and metabolic homeostasis in the postabsorptive period. Thus, basal insulinemia restrains hepatic glucose production and keeps it in equilibrium with basal glucose utilization by the brain and other tissues that are obligate glucose consumers. After meals, substrate-related incremental insulin secretion stimulates glucose utilization and storage, while inhibiting hepatic glucose output.

Insulin is essential for the physiologic use of all substrates and therefore is the primary regulator of energy metabolism. Thus, underlying the management of type I diabetes is the necessity to balance energy availability (food intake) with energy expenditure (activity) and insulin dosage. From this framework, three components of therapy emerge: the nutritional plan, exercise, and insulin dosage. Successful treatment of diabetes, by definition, involves balancing these three components and carefully monitoring that balance (self-monitoring of blood glucose by the patient). The attainment of an equilibrium of food intake, activity, and insulin assumes that neither physical nor emotional stress alters this balance by stress-induced secretion of glucose counterregulatory hormones (catecholamines, glucagon, cortisol, growth hormone). Because the patient must be engaged in maintaining this equilibrium on a daily basis, two additional critical principles emerge: education of patients is essential to successful therapy, and the treatment program must be suffi-

ciently flexible and dynamic to allow for highly varied and changing lifestyles without sacrificing careful metabolic control.

THERAPEUTIC OBJECTIVES IN TYPE I DIABETES

Table 399.1 lists three levels of treatment for type I diabetes, as developed by the American Diabetes Association (ADA), along with the characteristics of metabolic control in each of these categories. Given the demonstration by the Diabetes Control and Complications Trial that intensive therapy markedly lessens the risks of the chronic complications of diabetes, the goal for most patients should be the achievement of the intensive level of control. Specific glycemic targets for this level are listed in Table 399.2. Blood glucose targets must be individualized for each patient, however, and must be explicitly defined to be achieved. For otherwise healthy, young patients who readily recognize hypoglycemic symptoms and who spontaneously recover from hypoglycemia, targets may be similar to those listed in Table 399.2. Targets need to be lowered during pregnancy and raised in patients who have difficulty perceiving hypoglycemic symptoms, who do not spontaneously recover from hypoglycemia, or in whom hypoglycemia might be particularly dangerous (e.g., patients with angina pectoris or transient ischemic attacks). In motivated patients, realistic targets are achievable 70% to 80% of the time.

TREATMENTS FOR TYPE I DIABETES

As noted, the management of type I diabetes entails balancing the three components of therapy: the nutritional plan, exercise, and insulin dosage.

TABLE 399.1.	**LEVELS OF TREATMENT FOR TYPE I DIABETIC PATIENTS: BIOCHEMICAL AND CLINICAL CHARACTERISTICS**

Minimal (unacceptable under all normal circumstances)
  HbA$_{1c}$ 11–13% or GHb 13–15%
  Many SMBG values >300 mg/dL (>16.7 mmol/L)
  Intermittent ketonuria
  Mean blood glucose level >300 mg/dL (>16.7 mmol/L)
Average (improvement should be attempted if the patient's clinical and personal situations permit)
  HB$_{Alc}$ 8–9% or GHb 10–11%
  Premeal SMBG 160–200 mg/dL (8.9–11.1 mmol/L)
  Rare ketonuria
  Mean blood glucose level 160–240 mg/dL (8.9–13.3 mmol/L)
Intensive (desired, if possible to achieve without significant serious side effects)
  HbA$_{1c}$ 6–7% or GHb 7–9%
  Before SMBG 80–120 mg/dL (4.4–6.7 mmol/L)
  Bedtime SMBG 100–140 mg/dL (5.6–7.8 mmol/L)
  Essentially no ketonuria
  Mean blood glucose level 120–160 mg/dL (6.7–8.9 mmol/L)

Hb A$_{1c}$, the major fraction of glycosylated hemoglobin; SMBG, Self-monitored blood glucose.
(From Skyler JS, ed. Medical management of type 1 diabetes, third ed. Alexandria, Va: American Diabetes Association, 1998, with permission.)

TABLE 399.2.	REPRESENTATIVE TARGET LEVELS FOR SELF-MONITORING OF BLOOD GLUCOSE LEVELS SUITABLE FOR A YOUNG, OTHERWISE HEALTHY PATIENT WITH TYPE I DIABETES IN A PROGRAM OF INTENSIVE THERAPY

Time	Ideal[a]	Acceptable[a]
Fasting/preprandial	70–105 mg/dL (3.9–5.8 mmol/L)	70–130 mg/dL (3.9–7.2 mmol/L)
Postprandial (1 hr)	100–160 mg/dL (5.6–8.9 mmol/L)	100–180 mg/dL (5.6–10.0 mmol/L)
Postprandial (2 hr)	80–120 mg/dL (4.4–6.7 mmol/L)	80–150 mg/dL (4.4–8.3 mmol/L)
Bedtime	100–140 mg/dL (5.6–7.8 mmol/L)	100–160 mg/dL (5.6–8.9 mmol/L)
2:00–4:00 a.m.	70–105 mg/dL (3.9–5.8 mmol/L)	70–130 mg/dL (3.9–7.2 mmol/L)

[a] Ideal values approximate those seen in nondiabetic individuals; they are included for illustrative purposes. Acceptable values are attainable in a reasonable number of patients without provoking undue hypoglycemia; they are provided to appropriate patients.

EVIDENCE LEVEL: C. Expert Opinion.

Nutritional Plan

There should be careful balance of food intake, activity, and insulin dosage. A meal plan based on the person's usual food intake should be determined and used as a basis for integrating insulin therapy into the usual eating and exercise patterns. To accomplish this, patients (and their families) need to learn a system that incorporates the calorie and nutrient content of foods (carbohydrate content or exchanges). They also should learn general principles of the influence of various foods and of activity on glycemia and the balancing of these factors to achieve glycemic control.

In the past, it was common to recommend an insulin program and dosage, a particular pattern of food intake, and perhaps an exercise or activity prescription. The pattern of food intake almost invariably included three meals (breakfast, lunch, and supper) and one or more (often three) snacks. The dietary prescription usually included a specific calorie intake, proportions of nutrients (carbohydrate, fat, and protein distribution), and specified distribution of calories into meals. It was recommended that patients eat at consistent times synchronized with the time-action profile of the insulin preparation used. Unfortunately, such dietary prescriptions often were at odds with the previous habits of patients or families. Many patients prefer to eat at different hours some days, to skip meals either routinely or occasionally, or to vary portion sizes or meal composition. This created conflict between dietary prescriptions and a patient's desires, frequently leading to frustration or abandonment of the dietary prescription.

Contemporary dietary practices are considerably more flexible. Intensified insulin therapy allows flexibility in when and what patients eat. With intensified therapy, insulin regimens are integrated with lifestyle and doses calculated for the amount of food usually eaten. Patients monitor blood glucose levels and adjust insulin for variations in blood glucose and for deviations from usual eating and exercise habits.

Diabetic patients should follow sound general nutritional practices. In particular, this means avoiding excess intake of saturated fats and cholesterol, which influence serum lipids, which, in turn, also may be elevated if there is suboptimal diabetic control. It also means limiting salt consumption, which can aggravate the risk of blood pressure elevation and alter vascular reactivity.

Dietary protein should contribute approximately 10% to 20% of the total caloric content of the diet, leaving 80% to 90% of the calories to be distributed between dietary fat and carbohydrate. For people who have normal lipid levels and maintain a reasonable weight—and for normal growth and development in children and adolescents—the appropriate recommendations are those of the Dietary Guidelines for Americans (that 30% or less of the calories come from total fat). Less than 10% of calories should be derived from saturated fats and up to 10% calories from polyunsaturated fats, leaving 60% to 70% of total calories from monounsaturated fats and carbohydrates. The distribution of calories from fat and carbohydrate can vary and is individualized based on the nutrition assessment and treatment goals. Dietary cholesterol should be limited to 300 mg or less daily. Sucrose and sucrose-containing foods, when used, must be substituted for other carbohydrates and not simply added to the meal plan.

In making such substitutions, the nutrient content of concentrated sweets and sucrose-containing foods, as well as the presence of other nutrients frequently ingested with sucrose, such as fat, must be considered. Saccharin, aspartame, sucralose, and acesulfame-K may be used as non-nutritive sweeteners. There should be a tendency to avoid foods that have a high glycemic index (those that cause rapid rises in plasma glucose), while also favoring foods relatively high in fiber. There is no need to limit disproportionately the intake of complex carbohydrates or foods that have a low glycemic index. If the patient is not overweight (most patients with type I diabetes are not), there is no need to limit calorie consumption arbitrarily.

Exercise

Many variables, including fitness, duration and intensity of exercise, and time of exercise in relationship to insulin administration and meals, affect the metabolic response to exercise. The energy expended in the patient's usual daily routine determines the calorie content of the diet and influences the insulin dose and regimen. Regular physical activity is factored into this balance. On the other hand, for sporadic physical activity that is a departure from the daily routine, patients must take action to avert hypoglycemia. Patients might want to take in extra food to provide energy for increased activity, initially perhaps 10 to 15 g of carbohydrates every 30 to 45 minutes during the activity. Blood glucose is monitored before, during, and after exercise to determine the effectiveness of the extra carbohydrate. Insulin dose reductions may be used in addition to or instead of extra carbohydrate. All patients should have quick-acting, rapidly absorbed carbohydrate available during activity in case of hypoglycemia. Patients should realize that moderately intensive exercise may deplete glycogen stores, resulting in a sustained food requirement to replace the glycogen. As a consequence, hypoglycemia may develop well after exercise (e.g., 12 hours after jogging). For this reason, patients should be cautious when planning vigorous physical activity in the evening hours; nocturnal hypoglycemia may ensue.

INSULIN IN TYPE I DIABETES

Patients with type I diabetes lack both basal and prandial insulin secretion. Contemporary flexible insulin programs have multiple components that attempt to mimic these two types of endogenous physiologic insulin secretion by providing components that give prandial insulin coinciding with each meal and separate components that provide basal insulinemia overnight and between meals. All insulin treatment programs at best approximate normal physiology, because they are contingent on the time-action profiles of available insulin preparations (Table 399.3).

Prandial Insulin Therapy

Prandial incremental insulin secretion is best duplicated by giving preprandial rapid-onset insulin before each meal, by syringe, pen, or infusion pump. Each preprandial insulin dose is adjusted individually to provide insulinemia appropriate to the size of the meal. The use of preprandial insulin doses permits total flexibility in meal timing. The timing of meals need not be fixed, and meals may be omitted along with the accompanying preprandial insulin dose.

Regular human insulin administered subcutaneously is relatively rapid in its onset of action, but not immediate. Thus, if preprandial regular insulin is used, it is best to administer it at least 20 to 30 minutes before eating a given meal, in an attempt to have prandial insulinemia parallel meal-related glycemic excursions. With the very rapid-onset human insulin analogs, insulin lispro and insulin aspart, this waiting period is not needed. As a consequence, insulin lispro and insulin aspart are becoming the standard prandial insulins.

Basal Insulin Therapy

Basal insulinemia is given either as intermediate-acting human insulin (NPH or lente) at bedtime and in a small morning dose (Fig. 399.1A) or, occasionally, just as a bedtime dose (Fig. 399.1B); one (Fig. 399.2A) or two (Fig. 399.2B) daily injections of long-acting ultralente human insulin can also be administered, which in most patients is relatively peakless after steady state has been attained.

The intermediate-acting human insulins NPH (neutral protamine Hagedorn—also known as isophane insulin suspension) and lente have an onset of action about 2 hours after injection and produce peak insulin levels after 8 to 10 hours. Bedtime intermediate-acting insulin provides overnight basal insulinemia with peak serum insulin levels before breakfast, a time of relative insulin resistance known as the "dawn phenomenon." Bedtime administration of intermediate-acting insulin also eliminates nocturnal peaks of insulin action, thus lessening the risk of noc-

| TABLE 399.3. | TIME COURSE OF ACTION OF INSULIN PREPARATIONS |

Insulin Preparation	Onset of Action (hours)	Peak Action (hours)	Duration of Action (hours)
Rapid onset			
Lipro	¼–½	1–2	3–5
Aspart	¼–½	1–2	3–5
Short acting			
Regular	½–1	2–4	4–6
Intermediate acting			
NPH	1–4	8–10	12–20
Lente	2–4	8–12	12–20
Long acting			
Ultralente	3–5	10–16	18–24
Glargine	2–4	None obvious	20–26
Combinations			
70/30—70% NPH, 30% regular	½–1	Dual	12–20
50/50—50% NPH, 50% regular	½–1	Dual	12–20

This table summarizes the typical time course of action of various insulin preparations. It is based on doses of 0.1–0.2 u/kg, in the abdomen, for human insulin. These values vary among individuals, depending on the site and depth of injection, skin temperature, and level of exercise.

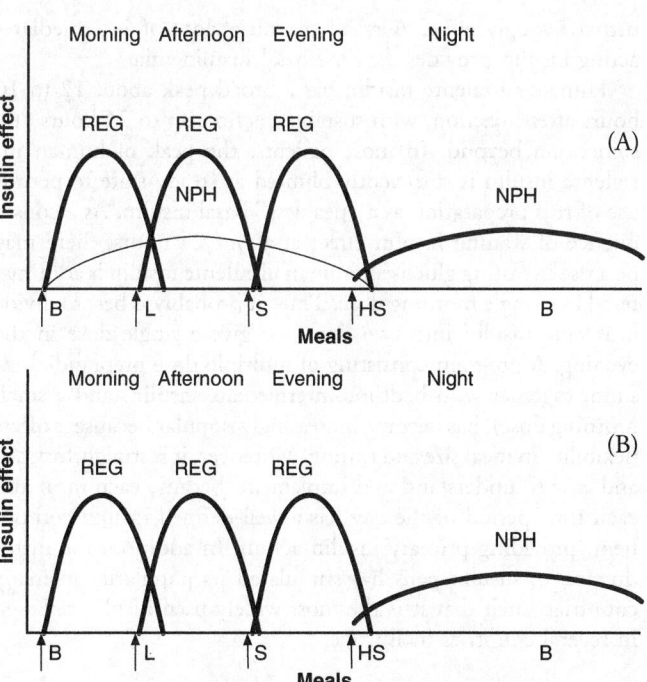

FIGURE 399.1. Schematic representation of the idealized insulin effect provided by a multiple-dose regimen of preprandial injections of regular (REG) insulin before meals and a basal regimen consisting of two daily injections of intermediate-acting insulin (NPH) **(A)** or basal intermediate-acting insulin (NPH) just at bedtime **(B)**. B, breakfast; L, lunch; S, supper; HS, bedtime snack. Arrows indicate time of insulin injection, 30 minutes before meals.

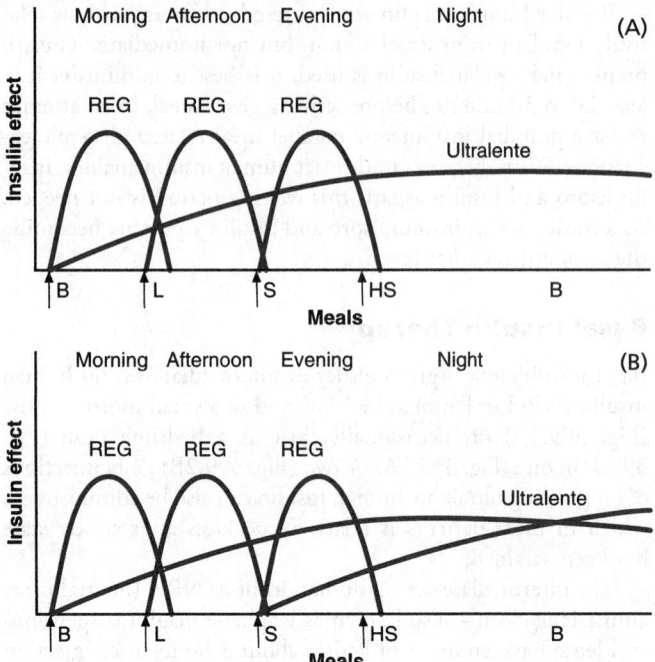

FIGURE 399.2. Schematic representation of the idealized insulin effect provided by a multiple-dose regimen of preprandial injections of regular (REG) insulin before meals and basal long-acting ultralente insulin either once daily (**A**) or twice daily (**B**). B, breakfast; L, lunch; S, supper; HS, bedtime snack. Arrows indicate time of insulin injection, 30 minutes before meals.

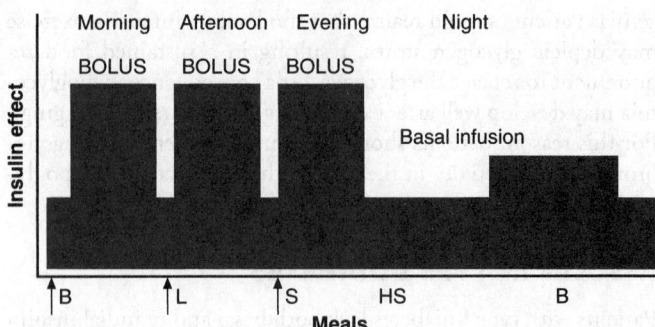

FIGURE 399.3. Schematic representation of idealized insulin effect provided by continuous subcutaneous insulin infusion. B, breakfast; L, lunch; S, supper; HS, bedtime snack.

turnal hypoglycemia. A small morning dose of intermediate-acting insulin provides daytime basal insulinemia.

Human ultralente insulin has a broad peak about 12 to 16 hours after injection, with sustained action up to 24 hours and sometimes beyond. In most patients, the peak of human ultralente insulin is sufficiently blunted at steady state to permit use of this preparation as a "peakless" basal insulin. As a consequence of waning insulin effect at about 24 hours, there may be a rise in fasting glucose if human ultralente insulin is administered in a single morning dose. Thus, it probably is best to divide ultralente insulin into two doses, or give a single dose in the evening. A program consisting of multiple-dose preprandial insulin, together with bedtime intermediate insulin (and a small morning dose), has become increasingly popular because it offers flexibility in meal size and timing. Moreover, it is straightforward and easy to understand and implement, because each meal and each time period of the day has a well-defined insulin component, providing primary insulin action. In addition, the introduction of insulin pens has stimulated its popularity in many countries, such that it is the most widely used insulin regimen in several countries in Europe.

Continuous Subcutaneous Insulin Infusion

The most precise way to mimic normal insulin secretion in clinical practice is to use an insulin pump in a program of continuous subcutaneous insulin infusion (Fig. 399.3). The pump delivers microliter amounts of insulin on a continual basis, thus replicat-

ing basal insulin secretion. With many pumps, the basal rate can be programmed to vary at times of diurnal variation in insulin sensitivity, if these variations result in disruption of glycemic control. Thus, the basal infusion rate may be decreased overnight to avert nocturnal hypoglycemia or increased to counteract the dawn phenomenon that often results in hyperglycemia on awakening. The pump is activated before meals to provide increments of insulin as meal boluses or "boosts," allowing total flexibility in meal timing. If a meal is skipped, the insulin bolus is omitted. If a meal is larger or smaller than usual, a larger or smaller insulin bolus is selected. With increased physical activity, patients may either suspend insulin delivery or use the quick-release option of disconnecting the pump from its indwelling catheter, thus lowering the risk of exercise-related hypoglycemia.

Other Insulin Programs

Separately considering prandial and basal insulin needs permits flexibility in eating and activity. Such an approach requires motivated, educated patients who carefully monitor blood glucose several (four or more) times daily. In the absence of motivation, education, or frequent blood glucose monitoring, an alternative (and clearly not optimal) approach is to maintain day-to-day consistency both of activity and of timing and quantity of food intake and thus permit prescription of a relatively constant insulin dose. This approach allows the patient to use either twice-daily administration of mixtures of regular insulin and intermediate-acting insulin (NPH or lente)—the so-called split-and-mixed insulin regimen (Fig. 399.4A), or morning administration of a mixture of regular insulin and intermediate-acting insulin with regular insulin before supper and intermediate-acting insulin at bedtime (Fig. 399.4B), a method used to minimize nocturnal hypoglycemia and to counteract the dawn phenomenon. In general, it is not possible to control glycemia in type I diabetes adequately using one or two injections of intermediate-acting insulin alone. The exception may be early in the course of the disease, when some endogenous insulin secretion remains.

Initial Insulin Doses and Distribution

The insulin dosage required for meticulous glycemic control in typical patients with type I diabetes who are within 20% of their

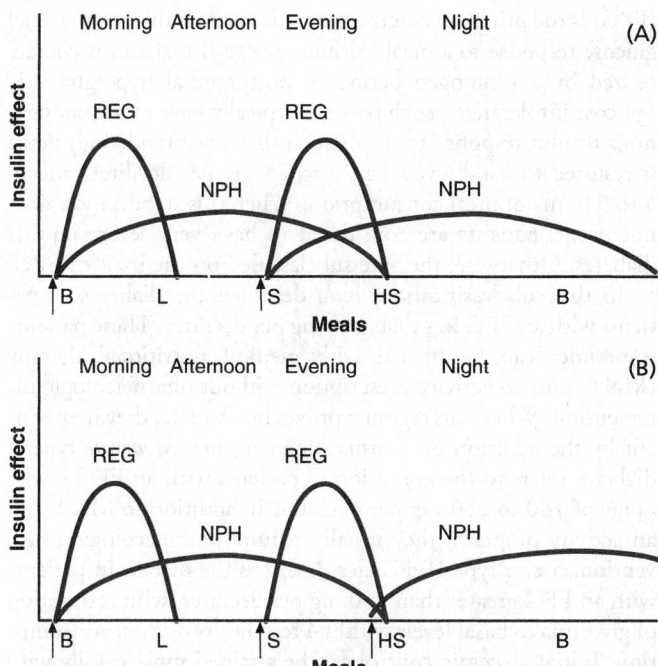

FIGURE 399.4. **(A)** Schematic representation of the idealized insulin effect provided by an insulin regimen consisting of two daily injections of regular (REG) insulin and intermediate-acting insulin (NPH). **(B)** A similar program, with the evening insulin dose divided into an injection of regular insulin before supper and a bedtime injection of intermediate-acting insulin. B, breakfast; L, lunch; S, supper; HS, bedtime snack. Arrows indicate time of insulin injection, 30 minutes before meals.

ideal body weight, in the absence of intercurrent infections or other periods of instability, approximates 0.5 to 1.0 U per kilogram per day. During the "honeymoon" period of relative remission early in the course of disease, insulin requirements are lower. In the context of intercurrent illness, the dosage may increase markedly. Dosage needs rise during the adolescent growth spurt, and some adolescents have a sustained increased dose requirement. About 40% to 50% of the total daily insulin dose is used to provide basal insulinemia. The remainder is divided among the meals empirically, proportionate to the relative carbohydrate content of the meals, or by initially giving (adults) approximately 1.0 to 1.2 U of insulin for every 10 g of carbohydrate consumed.

Alteration of Insulin Doses

Patients are provided with an action plan to alter therapy to achieve individually defined blood glucose targets. Actions are guided by self-monitored blood glucose determinations and daily records. Specific action depends on answers to several questions the patients ask at the time of insulin administration before meals: What is my blood glucose level now? What do I plan to eat now (usual meal, large meal, or small meal and the amount of carbohydrate)? What do I plan to do after eating (usual activity, increased level of activity, decreased level of activity)? What has happened under these circumstances previously? The answers dictate the treatment response. The actions include changes in food intake (altering the size or content of food), activity, insulin dosage, and timing of injections in relation to meals. The plan

also should call for separate measures in response to a *pattern* of glycemia occurring over several days, assuming the patient has a relatively stable pattern of meals and activities, has no intercurrent illness, and is free from unusual stress.

ASSESSMENT AND MONITORING OF TYPE I DIABETES

Glycosylated hemoglobin determination (Hb A_{Ic} or Hb A_1) is carried out quarterly to monitor long-term glycemic control. The value obtained from a random plasma glucose test is used to compare with that obtained simultaneously by the patient using his or her own monitoring system. A lipid profile should be determined for patients older than 2 years, after diagnosis of diabetes and when glucose control has been stabilized. If values fall within accepted risk levels, the assessment should be repeated every 2 years for adults or every 5 years for children. Treatment should be instituted if there are abnormalities, and patients should be followed appropriately.

Patient self-monitoring of blood glucose levels must be done on a daily basis, four times per day most days (before meals and at bedtime), with additional samples obtained in the middle of the night (2:00 to 4:00 a.m.) once every 1 to 2 weeks and any time that overnight insulin dosage is to be altered. Additional samples are obtained any time hypoglycemia is suspected. Periodically, postprandial samples should be taken as well, particularly if there is a disparity between preprandial results and Hb A_{Ic} determinations. The patient should keep a careful diary of daily blood glucose measurements, insulin doses, hypoglycemic episodes, and departures from daily routine (unusually large meals, increased physical activity, intercurrent illness). The patient's record is the focus of discussion at follow-up visits. Patient-determined blood glucose values are part of treatment, not assessment (but should be compared with the glycosylated hemoglobin value). In addition, the patient's compliance and responsibility for diabetes management should be assessed on a regular basis.

EDUCATION AND SUPPORT

To implement the management plan, considerable education of the patient is necessary. Moreover, the patient needs continued access to and interaction with a specialized diabetes management team, if successful control is to be achieved. Thus, the control of type I diabetes with a contemporary flexible insulin program mandates management by an expert multidisciplinary diabetes team. Successful participation in a demanding treatment program requires a committed, motivated patient. The team must take extra effort to help maintain motivation. This is often the most difficult component of treatment. Patients and families with new-onset type I diabetes need psychological support to adjust to having diabetes. Additional support is required to aid in the management program. To this end, ongoing psychological support, such as regular diabetes support group meetings, may be desirable for all patients with type I diabetes.

SPECIAL CONSIDERATIONS CONCERNING PREGNANCY

To lower the risk of fetal malformations and maternal and fetal complications, pregnant women and women planning preg-

TABLE 399.4.	REPRESENTATIVE TARGET LEVELS FOR SELF-MONITORING OF BLOOD GLUCOSE LEVELS SUITABLE FOR A PREGNANT WOMAN WITH TYPE I DIABETES

Time	Glucose
Fasting	60–90 mg/dL (3.3–5.0 mmol/L)
Preprandial	60–105 mg/dL (3.3–5.8 mmol/L)
Postprandial (1 hr)	70–140 mg/dL (3.9–7.8 mmol/L)
Postprandial (2 hr)	60–120 mg/dL (3.3–6.7 mmol/L)
Bedtime	60–120 mg/dL (3.3–6.7 mmol/L)
2:00–4:00 a.m.	60–100 mg/dL (3.3–5.5 mmol/L)

nancy need to have excellent control of blood glucose levels. Because of the need for prepregnancy planning and excellent glucose control, pregnancy in women with diabetes should be planned in advance. Therefore, women not attempting to conceive should use effective methods of contraception.

Glycemic targets during pregnancy are more stringent than otherwise because of the profound potential adverse impact of even modest hyperglycemia on the fetus (Table 399.4). Treatment should include more frequent self-monitoring of blood glucose values, extra snacks to avert hypoglycemia, and the expectation of a progressive increase in insulin requirement during the course of gestation, as a consequence of insulin resistance induced by placental hormones.

THERAPY OF TYPE II DIABETES

For clinical purposes, the severity of type II diabetes can be related to the degree of hyperglycemia on a stable diet and activity program. This clinical subclassification has four categories: mild, moderate, severe, and very severe (Table 399.5). Because basal (fasting) glycemia is relatively constant from day to day on a stable diet and activity program, the fasting plasma glucose

TABLE 399.5.	SUBCLASSIFICATION OF TYPE II DIABETES

Category	Fasting (Basal) Plasma Glucose[a]	Postprandial Glucose Response to Meals[b]
Mild	<140 mg/dL (<7.8 mmol/L)	Restored to basal
Moderate	140–250 mg/dL (7.8–13.9 mmol/L)	Restored to basal
Severe	>250 mg/dL (>13.9 mmol/L)	Restored to basal
Very severe	>250–300 mg/dL (>13.9–16.7 mmol/L)	NOT restored to basal

[a] On a stable diet and activity program.
[b] Within 4–5 hours, within 20–25 mg/dL.

(FPG) is the principal determinant. Also used is the postprandial glucose response to a meal. Although type II diabetes is characterized by a prolonged period of postprandial hyperglycemia (glucose intolerance), such patients typically have intact endogenous insulin response to meals such that postprandial glycemia is restored to basal levels (±20 to 25 mg per deciliter) within 4 to 5 hours of meal consumption. When this stabilization does not occur, patients are considered to have very severe type II diabetes. Otherwise, they are subclassified on the basis of FPG.

In this subclassification, *mild* describes the diabetes of patients with an FPG less than 140 mg per deciliter. These patients sometimes can be treated with medical nutritional therapy (MNT) and an activity prescription without pharmacologic intervention. When this regimen proves inadequate, they may benefit by the addition of pharmacologic agents. *Moderate* type II diabetes refers to the condition of patients with an FPG in the range of 140 to 250 mg per deciliter. In addition to MNT and an activity program, they usually require pharmacologic intervention. *Severe* type II diabetes describes the disease in patients with an FPG greater than 250 mg per deciliter, with restoration of glycemia to basal levels within 4 to 5 hours of meal consumption. Initial glycemic control can be attained most readily with insulin therapy that provides around-the-clock insulinization. Long-term glycemic control then can be maintained either with oral pharmacologic agents or with insulin.

Patients with a nonintact endogenous insulin response to meals, such that postprandial glycemia is not restored to basal levels within 5 hours of meal consumption have *very severe* type II diabetes. The FPG usually is quite elevated as well (above the 250 to 300 mg per deciliter range), but it may not be. There is such profound insulin deficiency that these patients initially may be difficult to distinguish from patients with type I diabetes, though in general they do not manifest ketosis. Initially they are best treated like type I patients. In all four subcategories of type II diabetes, it should be recognized that with adequate treatment there can be improvement both in islet B-cell function and in peripheral insulin action at target cells. As a consequence, there may be sufficient improvement in glucose homeostasis for a patient to be reclassified to a less severe subcategory, with glycemic control maintained by a treatment program typical for that category.

THERAPEUTIC OBJECTIVES IN TYPE II DIABETES

The Diabetes Control and Complications Trial (DCCT) and the United Kingdom Prospective Diabetes Study (UKPDS) have shown that meticulous glycemic control is important in both type I and type II diabetes. Results from the DCCT and UKPDS serve as the basis for recommendations of glycemic targets in diabetes management. Table 399.6 lists the biochemical indexes of glycemic control for type II diabetes suggested by the ADA. The recommended treatment goals are fasting and preprandial glucose levels below 120 mg per deciliter, with a glycosylated hemoglobin (Hb A_{Ic} or Hb A_1) level normal or near normal. Furthermore, it is desirable to minimize excessive postprandial hyperglycemia and obviate glycosuria. Ideally, patients should strive for normal fasting and preprandial levels (less than 110

TABLE 399.6.	INDEXES OF GLYCEMIC CONTROL IN TYPE II DIABETES		
Index	Ideal	Goal	Not Acceptable
Fasting/preprandial plasma glucose	<110 mg/dL (<6.1 mmol/L)	<120 mg/dL (<7.8 mmol/L)	<80 or >140 mg/dL (≥7.8 mmol/L)
Postprandial (2 hr) plasma glucose	<140 mg/dL (<7.8 mmol/L)	<180 mg/dL (<10.0 mmol/L)	>200 mg/dL (>11.1 mmol/L)
Bedtime plasma glucose	<140 mg/dL (<7.8 mmol/L)	100–140 mg/dL (5.6–8.9 mmol/L)	<100 or >160 mg/dL (<5.6 or >8.9 mmol/L)
Hb A$_{Ic}$ (%)[a]	<6.0%	<7.0%	>8.0%
GHb (%)[b]	<7.0%	<8.0%	>9.5%

Hb A$_{Ic}$, the major fraction of glycosylated hemoglobin.
[a] Referenced to a nondiabetic range of 4–6%.
[b] Referenced to a nondiabetic range of 4.5–7%.
EVIDENCE LEVEL: C. Expert Opinion.

mg per deciliter) and normal glycosylated hemoglobin (Hb A$_{Ic}$ or Hb A$_1$). Various therapies should be used progressively until the glycemic treatment goals are attained. Such goal-based therapy is the basis for contemporary management of type II diabetes.

In addition to glycemic goals, attention must be paid to other variables, particularly those related to atherosclerotic risk, which is substantial (Table 399.7). Thus, lipids and blood pressure need careful control, and smoking cessation should be promoted. A final objective is to attain and maintain weight as close as possible to ideal body weight. Normalizing weight in obese patients with type II diabetes is as crucial as controlling glycemia, because success with the former often leads to success with the latter.

TREATMENTS FOR TYPE II DIABETES

MNT and the promotion of physical activity are the cornerstones of management of type II diabetes. Pharmacologic therapy is required for most patients.

Medical Nutritional Therapy

MNT is integral to total diabetes care and management. Although adherence to nutrition and meal-planning principles is

TABLE 399.7.	OTHER THERAPEUTIC GOALS IN TYPE II DIABETES

Aglycosuria
Freedom from symptoms
Normalize plasma total cholesterol
Normalize plasma LDL cholesterol
Normalize plasma triglycerides
Normalize blood pressure
Smoking cessation
Body weight stable and as close to normal as possible

LDL, low-density lipoprotein.

one of the most challenging aspects of diabetes care, MNT is an essential component of successful diabetes management. The emphasis of MNT in type II diabetes should be placed on achieving glucose, lipid, and blood pressure goals. In obese patients with type II diabetes, a major nutritional principle is promotion of weight reduction by restriction of total calorie intake. Unfortunately, most patients are unable to adhere to a calorie-restricted diet to attain an ideal body weight. Even mild to moderate weight loss (10 to 20 pounds [5 to 10 kg]) has been shown to improve short-term glycemic control, even if desirable body weight is not achieved. It also has the potential to increase long-term metabolic control.

Weight loss is best attempted through a moderate decrease in caloric intake and an increase in caloric expenditure. Moderate caloric restriction (250 to 500 calories less than the average daily intake) usually is recommended, though very-low-calorie diets may be needed to achieve weight loss. If so, this diet should be monitored carefully. Although weight loss is desirable, and some people are able to lose weight and maintain the loss, several additional MNT strategies can be implemented to improve metabolic control.

In type II diabetes patients who are not obese and in those who have either completed weight reduction or who are unable to lose additional weight, different MNT principles apply. There are five such principles: a balanced nutrient intake; emphasis on appropriate alterations for achieving lipid and blood pressure goals; adequate spacing between meals (4 to 5 hours apart); consideration for additional consumption of dietary fiber; and avoidance of excessive intake of rapidly absorbed, simple sugars (sucrose, glucose, maltose), confining their use to substitution for other carbohydrates and not simply as additions to the meal plan. Although these principles are seemingly straightforward, each is the subject of controversy.

The nutrient proportions recommended by the ADA and American Dietetic Association emphasize the need to correct lipid abnormalities and lessen the risk of accelerated atherosclerosis, which remains the major cause of death in type II diabetes. These recommended proportions are listed in Table 399.8. The current ADA recommendations do not curtail the use of rapidly absorbed sugars, provided these are substituted for other carbo-

TABLE 399.8.	RECOMMENDED NUTRIENT INTAKE FOR AMERICANS
Nutrient	**Content**
Proteins	10–20% of calories
Total fats	≤30% of calories
Saturated fats	≤10% of calories
	<7% with elevated LDL
Polyunsaturated fats	≤10% of calories
Carbohydrates and menounsaturated fats	60–70% of calories
Cholesterol	<300 mg/day
Fiber	20–35 g/day
Sodium	<3,000 mg/day
Alcohol	<2 alcoholic beverages daily

LDL, low-density lipoprotein.
EVIDENCE LEVEL: C. Expert Opinion.

hydrates. Many experts disagree with such liberalization, unless there is careful measurement of glycemic excursions by the patient, to ensure that there is no deterioration of glucose control. The basis for the concern is that in type II diabetes endogenous insulin secretion is delayed, and consumption of rapidly absorbed simple sugars may result in rapid incremental increases in plasma glucose. The need for adequate spacing between meals is perhaps the most neglected nutritional principle in the management of type II diabetes. Because the period of postprandial hyperglycemia is prolonged in patients with type II diabetes, necessitating 4 to 5 hours before glucose levels are restored to preprandial (basal) levels, it is important to space meals at a like interval. Initial meal planning should thus include a 5-hour interval between food consumption, unless there is documentation that glycemia is restored to basal levels in a shorter interval for any given patient.

Coexisting conditions may require alteration in nutrient content. Particular attention needs to be paid to dyslipidemia, which may mandate even greater restriction of saturated fats (to less than 7% of calories) and cholesterol (to less than 200 mg per day) or use of monounsaturated fats. The presence of renal disease may require reduction of protein intake to less than 0.8 g per kilogram ideal body weight per day, approximately 10% of total calories. The presence of hypertension may result in the reduction of sodium intake.

Exercise

Exercise in patients with type II diabetes has several potential benefits. Moderate exercise has been shown to improve insulin sensitivity and facilitate insulin action, thus improving glucose tolerance even in the absence of weight loss. Moreover, increased physical activity has the benefit of intensifying energy expenditure in a relatively sedentary population, thus augmenting the effects of calorie restriction to promote weight loss when used in combination with a proper diet program. In addition, exercise may lower the risk of macrovascular disease by improving cardiovascular conditioning, facilitating control of hypertension, and

improving dyslipidemia. In the latter regard, exercise may increase levels of high-density lipoprotein (HDL) cholesterol and also lower levels of triglycerides and low-density lipoprotein (LDL) cholesterol. The greatest beneficial effects are seen with regular (at least three times per week), moderate, sustained exercise. Regular exercise also can improve psychological well-being.

It must be recognized, however, that most patients with type II diabetes are older, usually are obese, and often have significant coexisting medical conditions, all of which makes initiation of an exercise program more complicated. Nevertheless, all patients with type II diabetes should be encouraged to increase physical activity to a level that is tolerable to them. For some patients, it may be acceptable only to expand familiar daily activities, such as walking or climbing stairs. Any program of increased physical activity taken up by these patients should start slowly and build up gradually. If a serious exercise program is contemplated, it should be preceded by an evaluation specifically designed to uncover previously undiagnosed hypertension, neuropathy, retinopathy, and nephropathy. If neuropathy or peripheral vascular disease is present, the activity program should be designed to avoid lower extremity injury and the feet should be carefully inspected after conclusion of each activity period. Evaluation should include an exercise-stress electrocardiogram in all individuals older than 35 years of age to detect silent ischemic heart disease. Patients should self-monitor their glycemic response to exercise.

Pharmacologic Agents

There are now five classes of oral antidiabetic drugs. Those available in the United States are listed in Table 399.9.

Insulin Secretagogues

Insulin secretagogues act to stimulate insulin secretion and improve B-cell function, thus correcting one of the two fundamental defects that characterize type II diabetes. There are two classes of insulin secretagogues available at present—the sulfonylureas and the meglitinides. The sulfonylureas include older, first-generation drugs (tolbutamide, chlorpropamide, acetohexamide, and tolazamide) and newer, second-generation drugs (glyburide, glipizide, and glimepiride). There are two drugs in the meglitinide class, though they are structurally different both from meglitinide and from each other: repaglinide is a benzoic acid derivative, while nateglinide is a phenylalanine derivative.

The primary mechanism of action of insulin secretagogues is binding to the SUR subunit of an adenosine triphosphate (ATP)–dependent potassium (K) ion channel (K-ATP channel) on the membrane of the pancreatic islet B cell. This results in closure of the K-ATP channel, causing membrane depolarization and influx of calcium. Calcium entry leads to migration of insulin secretory granules down microtubules to the B cell, thus improving B-cell function and facilitating insulin secretion. Insulin secretion occurs primarily in response to plasma glucose, though with longer-acting sulfonylureas there may be spontaneous insulin secretion. Although insulin is secreted in response to glycemic excursions with meals, there is modulation of hepatic glucose production as well, since insulin is secreted into the hepatic portal circulation. Secretagogues are ineffective in the

TABLE 399.9.	CHARACTERISTICS OF ORAL ANTIDIABETIC AGENTS AVAILABLE IN THE UNITED STATES				
Generic Name	Brand Name	Dosage Range (mg/day)	Duration of Action (hr)	Dosing Frequency (per day)	Excretion
Sulfonylureas					
Tolbutamide	Orinase	500–3,000	6–12	2–3 times	Urine
Chlorpropamide	Diabinese	100–500	60	Once	Urine
Tolazamide	Tolinase	100–1,000	12–24	Twice	Urine
Acetohexamide	Dymelor	250–1,500	12–18	Twice	Urine
Glipizide	Glucotrol	2.5–40	12–24	Twice	Urine (Bile 20%)
Glipizide-GITS	Glucotrol XL	5–20	24	Once	Urine (bile 20%)
Glyburide	Diabeta micronase	1.25–20	16–24	Twice	Urine 50%, bile 50%
Glyburide (micronized)	Glynase	0.75–12	12–24	Twice	Urine 50%, bile 50%
Glimiperide	Amaryl	1–8	24	Once	Urine (bile 20%)
Miglitinides					
Repaglinide	Prandin	1.5–16	4–6	2–4 times ac	Bile
Nateglinide	Starlix	60–240	2–4	2–4 times ac	Urine
Biguanide					
Metformin	Glucophage	1,000–2,550	5–12	2–4 times	Urine
Thiazolidinediones					
Troglitazone	Rezulin	200–600	24	Once	Bile
Rosiglitazone	Avandia	4–8	15–25	1–2 times	Urine 70%, bile 30%
Pioglitazone	Actos	15–45	24–48	Once	Bile
α-Glucosidase inhibitor					
Acarbose	Precose	150–300	6	2–4 times ac	—
Miglitol	Glyset	75–600	6	2–4 times ac	—

absence of concomitant adherence to diet, and their effects are enhanced by promotion of physical activity. Secretagogues are efficacious only in patients with some retention of endogenous insulin secretion and thus have no role in the management of type I diabetes.

Sulfonylureas

Sulfonylureas were first introduced in the 1950s and have long played an important role in the management of type II diabetes. In fact, as of the early 1990s, sulfonylureas were the only class of oral antidiabetic medication available in the United States. As a consequence of their long usage, convenient dosing, rapidity of response, and low price, they still command a large share of the market of antidiabetic medications. Sulfonylureas are indicated for patients with mild or moderate type II diabetes who have not experienced correction of fasting hyperglycemia with MNT and physical activity; they are used in combination with any other class of antidiabetic medication when adequate glycemic control has not been attained with one medication.

When initiating sulfonylurea therapy, it is desirable to use the second-generation drugs. In contrast to the first-generation drugs, which are prescribed only rarely, the second-generation drugs have fewer overall side effects and less potential for interaction with other drugs. The newest sulfonylurea formulations—glipizide-GITS and glimepiride—have resulted in long-acting sulfonylureas that can be taken once daily to achieve both effective control of fasting glycemia and improvement of meal-related insulin secretion. The traditional formulations of second-

generation drugs—glyburide and glipizide—must be taken two to four times daily; less adequately control fasting glycemia; and increase the risk for hypoglycemia due to large, sustained postprandial peaks of drug. In fact, satisfactory glycemic control can be achieved with glipizide-GITS using a lower total daily dose than with the traditional formulation. The sulfonylureas available in the United States are listed in Table 399.9, along with other oral antidiabetic drugs.

After an initial response, effectiveness of therapy may not be sustained. Most of the time this decline stems from progression of the disease process rather than loss of pharmacologic effect. As a consequence, the sulfonylurea should not be discontinued when another drug is added. Other potential explanations for loss of glycemic control are lack of dietary adherence and deterioration in control due to intercurrent illness. In view of the possibility of secondary failure, plasma glucose should be monitored frequently to regulate dosage and to verify that any beneficial effects are sustained.

Advantages of sulfonylureas include improvement in a primary pathophysiologic impairment, that of insulin secretion; a physiologic route of insulin delivery (from the pancreas into the hepatic portal circulation); a high initial response rate (80% to 90% of subjects showing a response of at least a 30 mg per deciliter decrement in plasma glucose); a rapid response time (improvement in glycemia within 24 to 48 hours); and no intolerance to initiation. The effect on glycemia is quite good, with an Hb A_{Ic} decrease of about 1.5% to 2% when used in monotherapy. Disadvantages of sulfonylureas include the risk of hypoglycemia (which in some instances may be prolonged or severe), weight gain, drug interactions (especially with first-generation compounds), and hyponatremia with chlorpropamide. The major side effects are weight gain and hypoglycemia.

Meglitinides

This relatively new class of drugs, the non-sulfonylurea insulin secretagogues, were first introduced in the late 1990s. They also bind to the SUR subunit of the K-ATP channel, though apparently at different sites than the sulfonylureas. Meglitinide was the first such agent studied in the laboratory, and the class has been given that designation. As noted, however, the two drugs in the class have different chemical structures from meglitinide and also differ from each other. Repaglinide is a benzoic acid derivative, and nateglinide is a phenylalanine derivative. Both are ultrashort in duration of action, stimulating insulin to coincide with meals. Therefore, these agents need to be taken together with any meal consumed. This regimen offers flexibility in dosing and allows meals to be skipped easily (omitting the medication as well), which some patients may find advantageous. The effect is primarily on postprandial glucose, though repaglinide (but not nateglinide) also lowers the fasting glucose.

Advantages of meglitinides include improvement in a primary pathophysiologic impairment, that of insulin secretion; a physiologic route of insulin delivery (from the pancreas into the hepatic portal circulation); a high initial response rate; a rapid response time; flexible dosing in relationship to meals; no intolerance to initiation; and the fact that they can be used in the context of renal insufficiency. Disadvantages of meglitinides include the risk of hypoglycemia, weight gain, and unknown long-term side effects of these new agents.

Insulin Sensitizers

Insulin sensitizers improve insulin action at target cells, thus correcting one of the two fundamental defects that characterize type II diabetes. There are two classes of insulin sensitizers available at present—the biguanides and the thiazolidinediones. The only biguanide available in the United States is metformin. There are three available drugs in the thiazolidinediones class, though many others are in development. The available thiazolidinediones are troglitazone, rosiglitazone, and pioglitazone.

Biguanides

Biguanides have had a long history; they were shown to lower glucose in the nineteenth century and were introduced clinically in the 1950s. One biguanide, phenformin, was sold in the United States until 1977, when it was withdrawn by the Food and Drug Administration because of its propensity to lead to lactic acidosis. Another biguanide, metformin, which had been available throughout the world, except in the United States, for nearly four decades, was finally released in the United States in 1995. The molecular mechanism of action of metformin is complex and poorly understood. The drug appears to affect glucose metabolism directly. Thus, it lowers blood glucose levels by decreasing hepatic glucose output, increasing glucose uptake, and enhancing peripheral glucose utilization. Metformin is an "antihyperglycemic" agent that does not cause hypoglycemia.

Metformin often is used as initial monotherapy in type II diabetes, particularly in obese patients, because, unlike secretagogues, it is not associated with weight gain upon improvement in glycemia; in fact, modest weight loss may ensue. It is particularly effective in combination with secretagogues, since biguanides and secretagogues have complementary mechanisms of action. Indeed, most patients require this combination to achieve glycemic targets. On the other hand, in the context of inadequate glycemic regulation, switching from a secretagogue to metformin, or vice versa, does not result in improvement of glycemic control. For this reason, several formulations combining metformin with a secretagogue are under development. The earliest available data suggest that these combination drugs are highly effective in lowering glucose levels.

In treating patients, it should be appreciated that because of the need for slow-dose titration (to minimize the gastrointestinal side effects of nausea, abdominal discomfort, and, less frequently, diarrhea that arise with initiation of therapy), the full effectiveness of metformin may not be seen for 4 to 6 weeks. It also is important to ensure that patients receive adequate doses of metformin. One dose-response study showed that maximum glucose lowering was achieved with a dose of 1,000 mg twice daily, which is substantially higher than that prescribed by most physicians.

Advantages of metformin include improvement in a primary pathophysiologic impairment, that of insulin resistance; a high initial response rate (80% to 90% of subjects show a response); a long record (40 years) of relative safety; absence of weight gain (even modest weight loss); and beneficial effects on plasma lipids. Disadvantages of metformin include gastrointestinal side effects on initiation of metformin, which forces administration of gradually rising dose increments, and the risk of lactic acidosis in patients with elevated serum creatinine, hepatic disease, congestive heart failure, or cardiovascular compromise. After radiographic procedures that use contrast dyes, metformin should be withheld until it is ensured that acute renal insufficiency has not been induced by the contrast media. Unlike phenformin, metformin rarely is associated with lactic acidosis if attention is paid to proper selection of patients.

Thiazolidinediones

Thiazolidinediones (TZDs), also known as glitazones, are a relatively new class of oral agents for the treatment of diabetes, first introduced in the late 1990s. In the United States, troglitazone became available in 1997 and rosiglitazone and pioglitazone in 1999, with several other TZDs in various stages of development. These agents act by binding to nuclear receptors called peroxisome proliferator–activated receptors (PPARs), specifically to the PPARγ subtype (PPARγ). This results in the expression of a number of gene-encoding proteins that enhance cellular insulin action on glucose and lipid metabolism. As a consequence, there is improvement in insulin sensitivity, particularly resulting in increased peripheral (muscle and adipose) glucose uptake and utilization, with a modest effect on the liver to inhibit glucose production. The TZDs have been shown to improve insulin action in type II diabetes, in impaired glucose tolerance, and in obese people with normal glucose tolerance.

TZDs are most effective in combination with insulin in type II diabetes. This combination can achieve both lowering of insulin dose and improvement in glycemic control. In fact, some patients previously refractory to glucose lowering in spite of large doses of insulin may experience control of their diabetes on this regimen. TZDs are also effective in combination with secretagogues, metformin, or both (so-called triple therapy). Unfortunately, in monotherapy the response rate varies, and there is no easy way to anticipate who will be a responder. Rosiglitazone and pioglitazone appear to have a higher response rate than troglitazone, but troglitazone is no longer labeled as approved for monotherapy.

Advantages of TZDs include improvement in a primary pathophysiologic impairment, that of insulin resistance; a unique mechanism of action that allows it to be combined with any other class of glucose-lowering agent; once-daily dosing; lowering of serum triglycerides and increase in HDL cholesterol; and the fact that some agents may be used in the context of renal insufficiency. The biggest disadvantage is that troglitazone has been associated with idiosyncratic liver disease, which in some cases has led to acute hepatic necrosis, resulting either in death or the need for liver transplantation. As a consequence, the product label notes the recommendation that liver enzyme levels be measured at the start of therapy and monthly thereafter. Nonetheless, in spite of monitoring, some cases of severe liver dysfunction have been missed. Although this is a rare problem, it is unpredictable. Fortunately, however, the clinical trial experience with rosiglitazone and pioglitazone suggests that these agents may not carry this risk of liver disease. It is hoped that this finding will be confirmed in the clinical arena. Other disadvantages of TZDs include the fact that there is a delayed onset of action (up to 3 weeks) and a prolonged time before the full effect becomes evident (up to 8 to 12 weeks); weight gain; a relatively high lack-of-response rate in monotherapy; increased levels of LDL cholesterol; and unknown long-term side effects (stemming from the fact that this is a relatively new class of drugs).

α-Glucosidase Inhibitors

The α-glucosidase inhibitors compete with carbohydrates for binding to the α-glucosidase enzymes (sucrase, maltase, isomaltase, amylase, glucoamylase) in the intestinal brush border. This results in slowing of digestion of complex carbohydrates, oligosaccharides, and disaccharides, with consequent retardation of gastrointestinal glucose absorption and reduction in postprandial glycemic excursions. There is a consequent modest improvement in Hb A_{Ic}, which, on average, is about 0.5% to 1%. Although these inhibitors occasionally are used alone, their primary role is in combination with other agents when glycemic targets are not met. There are several α-glucosidase inhibitors. In the United States, acarbose became available in 1996 and miglitol in 1999; volglibose is in clinical trials. Carbohydrates are retained in the gastrointestinal tract. As a consequence, there frequently are gastrointestinal side effects, including a high rate of flatulence, which often is severe; nausea; abdominal discomfort; borb-

orygmi; and diarrhea. These effects can be minimized, to some extent, by slow-dose titration to therapeutic levels.

Advantages of α-glucosidase inhibitors include a good safety profile, lack of weight gain with improved glycemic control, and a unique mechanism of action that allows these drugs to be combined with any other class of glucose-lowering agent. Disadvantages of α-glucosidase inhibitors include the need for a high-carbohydrate diet for efficacy, since these are competitive enzyme inhibitors; flatulence and other gastrointestinal side effects; a limited impact on FPG; and the necessity for caution in the treatment of hypoglycemia. Because the enzymes are inhibited, hypoglycemia cannot be treated with sucrose, maltose, or starch, since glucose is not readily available for absorption. Lactose (milk) may be used to treat hypoglycemia, however, because lactase is a α-glucosidase. Monosaccharides (glucose or fructose) may be used to correct hypoglycemia.

Weight Loss Agents

Effective control of weight leads to improved glucose control as well. Therefore, agents that expedite weight loss may be helpful in facilitating glycemic control. There are two weight-loss agents available in the United States—sibutramine, an inhibitor of serotonin and norepinephrine reuptake that limits food intake, and orlistat, an inhibitor of gastrointestinal lipases that blocks systemic absorption of dietary fat. Both have been used in patients with type II diabetes with modest success. One disadvantage is that sibutramine is associated with blood pressure elevation. Another is that because of retained fat in the gastrointestinal tract, orlistat often causes fat loss in stools, with resulting greasy bowel movements.

Other Pharmacologic Approaches

A number of therapeutic agents are under development. These agents include compounds that overcome insulin resistance, enhance insulin secretion, retard glucose absorption, increase thermogenesis (facilitating weight loss), inhibit gluconeogenesis, and suppress fatty acid oxidation. All have potential glucose-lowering effects.

INSULIN IN TYPE II DIABETES

The primary pathophysiologic defects in type II diabetes are impairment in B-cell function and resistance to insulin action. Although it has been argued that insulin is not an effective therapy in type II diabetes because insulin deficiency per se is not the primary defect, it is possible with insulin therapy to overcome insulin resistance and to ensure insulin availability in the face of islet B-cell dysfunction. Moreover, given the aggravation of the pathophysiologic defects with glucose toxicity, insulin therapy can be used effectively to overcome glucose toxicity and restore the potential effectiveness of other therapies, making maintenance of the improved metabolic state easier. Such a "feed-forward" system would explain the clinical aphorism that it is *much easier to maintain glucose control than it is to attain glucose control.*

Temporary Insulin Therapy

One important use of insulin is as temporary initial therapy to attain glycemic control in patients with severe type II diabetes, to overcome glucose toxicity, and to re-regulate decompensated patients. Indeed, type II diabetes may be considered a disease of periodic decompensation with the need for re-regulation, usually with insulin therapy. For this reason, all patients with type II diabetes should learn insulin administration techniques and be prepared to initiate insulin therapy in the face of expected periodic decompensation, which occurs spontaneously and particularly with intercurrent illness or stress.

Combination Insulin Therapy

Over the past several decades, the use of combinations of insulin and oral antidiabetic agents has grown in popularity. One popular program has combined oral medication with the use of bedtime intermediate-acting insulin to control fasting hyperglycemia. All of the classes of oral medication have been used successfully with insulin. In particular, the combination of metformin with bedtime intermediate-acting insulin is effective in improving glycemic control and does so without hypoglycemia or weight gain. By restoring responsiveness to insulin, the TZDs are quite successful in improving glycemic control in patients on large doses of insulin.

Ongoing Insulin Therapy

If insulin therapy is used for patients with moderate type II diabetes (FPG 140 to 250 mg per deciliter), it is often sufficient to use basal insulin therapy to correct fasting hyperglycemia, with endogenous insulin secretion being adequate to control meal-related, postprandial glucose excursions. Basal insulin therapy may be provided as a bedtime dose of intermediate-acting insulin (NPH or lente), as long-acting ultralente insulin to supplement basal insulin secretion, or as a continuous insulin infusion. Doses required usually are in the range of 0.3 to 0.6 U per kilogram per day. When intermediate-acting insulin is administered at bedtime, its peak effect 8 to 10 hours later coincides with the period before breakfast, thus controlling basal (fasting) glycemia.

For patients with severe type II diabetes (FPG more than 250 mg per deciliter), clinical experience has shown that around-the-clock administration of insulin is necessary. Thus, in contrast to patients with moderate type II diabetes, bedtime intermediate-acting insulin cannot be used (though twice-daily intermediate-acting insulin may be used). Most patients with severe type II diabetes require a more intensive insulin program (with addition of regular insulin) to attain glucose control. Necessary doses are usually in the range of 0.5 to 1.2 U per kilogram per day. Large doses, even in excess of 1.5 U per kilogram per day, may be needed, at least initially, to overcome prevailing insulin resistance. Such high-dose therapy may be necessary only to attain control, with subsequent control maintained on lower doses—on a basal insulin program or with oral hypoglycemic agents. Often, insulin therapy is continued at doses in the range of 0.3 to 1.0 U per kilogram per day. The use of premixed insulin preparations (70/30, which contains 70% NPH and 30% regular insulin) may facilitate implementation of such programs. Another option is to attain glycemic control through the use of continuous insulin infusion, with subsequent maintenance of control as outlined previously. Patients with very severe type II diabetes are severely insulin deficient and need to be treated like patients with type I diabetes.

In all categories of patients with type II diabetes, there is improvement of the pathophysiologic defects as glycemic control is attained and maintained. This facilitates ease of control and may permit patients initially treated with insulin to be maintained on oral hypoglycemic therapy or even a diet and activity program alone. The insulin dose can be adjusted to lower and lower amounts; when the dosage reaches less than 0.3 to 0.4 U per day, maintenance on oral antidiabetic agents can be considered. For most patients, type II diabetes can be controlled with insulin, if adequate doses are given and if the patient follows an appropriate MNT and exercise program. The latter factors facilitate the action of insulin. Failure to follow a proper diet may counter the effects of insulin and lead to a vicious cycle of progressively increasing insulin doses, yet failure to control glycemia. In patients already on insulin therapy who are experiencing inadequate glycemic control, it is often desirable to add an insulin sensitizer—either metformin or a TZD—in an effort to improve insulin action and gain better glycemic control.

ASSESSMENT AND MONITORING OF TYPE II DIABETES

Office measurement of glycosylated hemoglobin (Hb A_{Ic} or Hb A_1) and FPG should be carried out quarterly to judge glycemic control in patients with type II diabetes. The level obtained from a laboratory plasma glucose measurement may be useful for comparison with the value obtained simultaneously by the patient using his or her own monitoring system. A lipid profile (total cholesterol, fasting triglycerides, high-density lipoprotein cholesterol, and low-density lipoprotein cholesterol) should be assessed annually. If treatment is instituted for dyslipidemia, the appropriate laboratory measurement should be repeated as needed to monitor therapy. If all values are within acceptable limits, the clinician may consider obtaining this lipid profile less frequently. The patient should monitor fasting blood glucose levels on a daily basis. In addition, insulin-treated patients should take at least one additional daily reading—either before meals or at bedtime. Once every 1 to 2 weeks, patients should take a profile, including fasting, preprandial, and bedtime measurements.

THERAPY OF ACUTE DECOMPENSATED DIABETES

THERAPY OF DIABETIC KETOACIDOSIS

The first priority of treatment of diabetic ketoacidosis (DKA) is to restore intravascular volume to normalize tissue perfusion and aid in the delivery of insulin to target organs. Treatment is aimed at restoration of body water and electrolytes. There must be provision of adequate insulin to correct the defects in carbohydrate, fat, and protein metabolism. Other priorities are the treatment of infection and circulatory collapse, if present. Treatment must be energetic yet not so vigorous as to result in hypoglycemia, hypokalemia, or cerebral edema, all of which are potentially disastrous complications of therapy.

Patients with DKA and mild degrees of acidemia who are able to tolerate increased oral fluids can be treated at home, with supplemental regular insulin before meals in addition to their usual daily regimen. With moderate to severe ketoacidosis, volume depletion, or vomiting, the patient requires hospitalization. Fluid and electrolyte replacement is critical and should be vigorously pursued. Average fluid losses are 10% of body weight. Electrolyte losses, notably of sodium and chloride but also of potassium and phosphate, need to be corrected as well. Close, careful clinical and biochemical monitoring of the patient is a mandatory component of therapy. A prospective flow sheet should be used.

Isotonic solutions are the fluids of choice; hypotonic solutions run the risk of rapid reduction of plasma osmolality, with large fluid shifts precipitating cerebral edema and hypovolemia. Appropriate solutions are either 0.9% saline or, alternatively, one ampule (50 mEq) of sodium bicarbonate (plus appropriate potassium supplements) added to each liter of 0.45% saline. The latter solution has several advantages. First, its osmolality is close to physiologic but hypotonic relative to plasma, thus minimizing fluid shifts. Second, it provides sodium at a higher rate than chloride, thus minimizing the likelihood of the development of hyperchloremic acidosis with treatment. Last, when given slowly over an hour or more, bicarbonate therapy does not cause any of the adverse consequences sometimes associated with a bolus dose. In adult patients with DKA, fluid is given at a rate of 1 to 2 L over the first hour and 1 L per hour for the next 3 to 4 hours, then decreased and maintained according to intake and output measurements and clinical assessment of the patient's state of hydration, supplemented by central venous pressure readings (if available). When the plasma glucose level falls to 250 to 300 mg per deciliter, glucose is included in the intravenous fluids to prevent hypoglycemia and to permit intravenous insulin infusion to be continued until acidosis is resolved. The goal is to restore the normal metabolic state gradually, without creating complications due to treatment.

Serum potassium levels do not reflect total body levels accurately. Potassium deficiency puts patients at risk for cardiac arrhythmias or arrest, particularly if potassium levels decline further with correction of acidosis and hyperglycemia. Therefore, unless the patient has anuria, potassium supplementation is initiated immediately in the course of treatment, at a rate of 10 to 40 mEq per hour in adult patients, depending on initial and subsequent repeated potassium determinations, the degree of acidosis, and the development of electrocardiographic changes. The goal is to aim for a serum potassium of 4 to 5 mEq per liter, as follows:

- If the serum K^+ is less than 3 mEq per liter, potassium is infused at 40 mEq per hour.

- If the serum K^+ is 3 to 4 mEq per liter, potassium is infused at 30 mEq per hour.
- If the serum K^+ is 4 to 5 mEq per liter, potassium is infused at 20 mEq per hour.
- If the serum K^+ is 5 to 6 mEq per liter, potassium is infused at 10 mEq per hour.
- If the serum K^+ is greater than 6 mEq per liter or there are hyperkalemic T-wave changes on the electrocardiogram, potassium infusion is withheld.

Although deficient total body levels of phosphate invariably exist in DKA, serum phosphate levels do not accurately reflect them. Phosphate deficiency is associated with low 2,3-diphosphoglycerate levels, rhabdomyolysis, and respiratory muscle weakness, particularly if phosphate levels decline further with treatment of acidosis and correction of fluid depletion and hyperglycemia. Nevertheless, the issue of phosphate supplementation is the subject of controversy. The major concern is the potential of inducing hyperphosphatemia and resultant hypocalcemia. Therefore, phosphate should be withheld during the initial few hours of treatment of DKA, to avoid aggravation of preexisting hypocalcemia. Afterward, phosphate supplementation can be initiated using half potassium phosphate and half potassium chloride.

The use of bicarbonate in the treatment of DKA also is debated. There are good arguments on both sides of the issue. On the one hand, there are severe potential adverse effects of acidosis, including depressed cardiac and respiratory function, arrhythmias, and hypotension. On the other hand, overzealous bolus bicarbonate use aggravates hypokalemia, may lead to metabolic alkalosis, can result in paradoxical induction of cerebral spinal fluid acidosis (due to disparities in the rates by which HCO_3^- and carbon dioxide cross the blood–brain barrier), and may contribute to the development of cerebral edema. Early bolus administration of bicarbonate also can prolong ketonemia. Therefore, universally accepted guidelines for bolus bicarbonate administration are difficult to formulate. Its use probably should be restricted to cases of very severe acidemia (pH less than 7.0) or less severe acidemia (pH 7.0 to 7.1) with severe underlying medical problems (myocardial infarction, cardiac arrhythmias, sepsis).

Insulin administration is vital to treatment and is initiated immediately, unless there is evidence of severe hypovolemia or hypokalemia. Low doses of insulin are as effective as high doses for treating hyperglycemia and ketoacidosis; they help avoid the development of hypoglycemia and hypokalemia, which may occur with high doses. An initial priming dose of 0.1 U of regular insulin per kilogram body weight as an intravenous bolus is followed by a continuous infusion of regular insulin at a rate of 0.1 U per kilogram per hour. This infusion may be adjusted approximately every 2 hours according to glycemic levels, which should fall at a rate of 50 to 100 mg per deciliter per hour. The infusion is continued until the plasma glucose level falls to 200 to 300 mg per deciliter, after which it may be cut back to 0.05 U per kilogram per hour, with the infusion maintained for at least 6 hours after acidosis has resolved.

THERAPY OF HYPEROSMOLAR HYPERGLYCEMIC NONKETOTIC COMA

The first priority of therapy is to restore intravascular volume. Fluid replacement also lowers plasma glucose levels by hemodilution and by improvement in renal blood flow and glucose excretion. Fluid replacement considerations are similar to those in the management of DKA, but fluid typically is replaced at slower rates because of the fragility of these usually elderly patients, who often have compromised cardiovascular or renal systems. The actual rate of fluid replacement is individualized, based on clinical assessment of the patient's status. The initial rate of fluid replacement generally is restricted to 1 L per hour until peripheral perfusion is normalized. Hypotonic fluids then are given at a rate approximately equal to twice urine output. The goal is gradual restoration of a normal metabolic state. In patients with hyperosmolar hyperglycemic nonketotic coma, who are profoundly volume depleted and often hypotensive, insulin therapy is withheld until the volume status is normalized, because the movement of glucose and water from the extracellular to the intracellular fluid compartment may precipitate shock. Low doses of insulin are used.

BIBLIOGRAPHY

American Diabetes Association. Nutrition recommendations and principles for people with diabetes mellitus. *Diabetes Care* 1999;22(suppl 1): S42.

American Diabetes Association. Standards of medical care for patients with diabetes mellitus. *Diabetes Care* 1999;22(suppl 1):S32.

Bailey CJ. New pharmacological approaches to glycemic control. *Diabetes Rev* 1999;7:94.

Balfour JA, Plosker GL. Rosiglitazone. *Drugs* 1999;57:921–932.

Cryer PE. Banting Lecture. Hypoglycemia: the limiting factor in the management of IDDM. *Diabetes* 1994;43:1378–1389.

Cusi K, DeFronzo RA. Metformin: a review of its metabolic effects. *Diabetes Rev* 1998;6:89.

Farkas-Hirsch RM, ed. *Intensive diabetes management*, second ed. Alexandria, Va.: American Diabetes Association, 1998.

Franz MJ, Bantle JP, eds. *American Diabetes Association guide to medical nutrition therapy for diabetes.* Alexandria, Va.: American Diabetes Association, 1999.

Jovanovic L, ed. *Medical management of pregnancy complicated by diabetes*, second ed. Alexandria, Va.: American Diabetes Association, 1998.

Lebovitz HE. α-Glucosidase inhibitors as agents in the treatment of diabetes. *Diabetes Rev* 1998;6:132.

Lebovitz HE. Insulin secretagogues: old and new. *Diabetes Rev* 1999;7: xxx–xxx.

Saleh YM, Mudaliar SR, Henry RR. Metabolic and vascular effects of the thiazolidinedione troglitazone. *Diabetes Rev* 1999;7:55.

Scheen AJ, Lefebvre PJ. Management of the obese diabetic patient. *Diabetes Rev* 1999;7:77–93.

Skyler J, ed. *Medical management of type 1 diabetes mellitus*, third ed. Alexandria, Va.: American Diabetes Association, 1998.

Yki-Järvinen H, Ryysy L, Nikkilä K, et al. Comparison of bedtime insulin regimens in patients with type 2 diabetes mellitus: a randomized, controlled trial. *Ann Intern Med* 1999;130:389–396.

Zimmerman B, ed. *Medical management of type 2 diabetes mellitus*, fifth ed. Alexandria, Va.: American Diabetes Association, 1998.

Kelley's Textbook of Internal Medicine, fourth edition. Edited by H. David Humes. Lippincott Williams & Wilkins, Philadelphia © 2000.

CHAPTER 400

APPROACH TO THE PATIENT WITH HYPOGLYCEMIA

F. JOHN SERVICE

DEFINITION

Hypoglycemia is a clinical syndrome arising from diverse causes, in which low levels of plasma glucose eventually lead to neuroglycopenia.

SYMPTOMS

Symptoms of hypoglycemia may begin at plasma glucose levels of approximately 60 mg per deciliter and impairment of brain function at approximately 50 mg per deciliter. The rate of plasma glucose decline does not influence the occurrence of symptoms. Hypoglycemic symptoms have been classified into two major groups: autonomic and neuroglycopenic. Symptoms of hypoglycemia differ among patients but are usually consistent from episode to episode for each patient. Autonomic symptoms (sweating, trembling, anxiety, nausea, palpitation, hunger, tingling) do not always precede neuroglycopenic symptoms (confusion, abnormal behavior, visual disturbance, seizure). In many patients, neuroglycopenic symptoms are the only ones experienced. None of the previously listed symptoms is specific to hypoglycemia; the presence of one or several may be due to other causes.

CLASSIFICATION

The long-established classification of hypoglycemia as fasting is no longer useful because segregation by timing does not result in different nosologic entities. A more useful approach is a classification based on clinical characteristics (Table 400.1). Persons who appear healthy are likely to have different hypoglycemic disorders from those experienced by persons who are ill. Hospitalized patients are at additional risk for hypoglycemia, often from iatrogenic factors. Hypoglycemia may stem from accidental drug ingestion in healthy persons, the mistaken dispensing of a sulfonylurea, or the idiosyncratic actions of some of the drugs used in the treatment of seriously ill patients. The occurrence of symptoms in a patient with an illness known to be associated with hypoglycemia requires little, if any, investigation, only recognition of the association of the disease with the risk for hypoglycemia. Asymptomatic patients may have artifactual hypoglycemia due to leukemia or severe hemolysis or may have adapted to lifelong hypoglycemia caused by glycogen storage disease.

TABLE 400.1.	CLINICAL CLASSIFICATION OF HYPOGLYCEMIC DISORDERS

Healthy-appearing patient
  No coexisting disease
    Cause or predisposing condition
      Drugs
        Ethanol
        Salicylates
        Quinine
        Haloperidol
      Insulinoma
      Islet hyperplasia/nesidioblastosis
        Persistent hyperinsulinemic hypoglycemia of infancy
        Noninsulinoma pancreatogenous hypoglycemia syndrome
      Factitious hypoglycemia induced by insulin or sulfonylurea
      Intense exercise
      Ketotic hypoglycemia
  Coexisting disease under treatment
    Cause or predisposing condition
      Drugs
        Dispensing error
        Disopyramide
        β-adrenergic-blocking agents
        Drugs containing sulfhydryl or thiol and insulin autoimmune hypoglycemia
        Ackee-fruit poisoning and undernutrition
Ill-appearing patient
  Cause or predisposing condition
    Drugs
      Pentamidine for *Pneumocystis* pneumonia
      Trimethoprim-sulfamethoxazole and renal failure
      Propoxyphene and renal failure
      Quinine for cerebral malaria
      Quinidine for malaria
      Topical salicylates and renal failure
    Illness or condition
      Small size for gestational age in infants
      Beckwith–Wiedermmann syndrome
      Erythroblastosis fetalis
      Hyperinsulinemia in infants due to maternal diabetes
      Glycogen storage disease
      Defects in amino acid and fatty acid metabolism
      Reye syndrome
      Cyanotic congenital heart disease
      Hypopituitarism
      Isolated growth hormone deficiency
      Isolated corticotropin deficiency
      Addison disease
      Galactosemia
      Hereditary fructose intolerance
      Carnitine deficiency
      Defective type 1 glucose transporter in the brain
      Acquired severe liver disease
      Large non-β-cell tumor
      Sepsis
      Renal failure
      Congestive heart failure
      Lactic acidosis
      Starvation
      Anorexia nervosa
      Surgical removal of pheochromocytoma
      Insulin-antibody hypoglycemia
Hospitalized patient
  Cause or predisposing condition
    Hospitalization for a predisposing illness
    Total parenteral nutrition and insulin therapy
    Interference of cholestyramine with glucocorticoid absorption
    Shock

EVALUATION

A healthy-appearing patient with no coexisting disease who has a history of neuroglycopenic spells requires an approach quite different from that taken for a hospitalized patient with acute hypoglycemia.

THE HEALTHY-APPEARING PATIENT

Plasma Glucose Levels

Because symptoms of hypoglycemia are nonspecific, it is necessary to verify a low plasma glucose level at the time that spontaneous symptoms arise and to establish that symptoms are relieved through correction of the low glucose level ("Whipple's triad"). A normal plasma glucose level, reliably obtained when spontaneous symptoms are present, eliminates the possibility of a hypoglycemic disorder; no further evaluation is required. Glucose measurements made by the patient with a reflectance meter while experiencing spontaneous symptoms are likely to provide false information. Often, the measurement of the plasma glucose level is not feasible when spontaneous symptoms occur during the activities of ordinary life. Under such circumstances, a judgment by the physician about whether to proceed with further evaluation depends on a detailed history. A history of neuroglycopenic symptoms or a confirmed low (less than 50 mg per deciliter) plasma glucose level warrants further testing.

The Prolonged (72 Hour) Fast

The prolonged (72 hour) fast is the classic diagnostic test for hypoglycemia. It should be conducted following standardized procedures. A suggested protocol is shown in Table 400.2. For patients who have neither symptoms nor signs of hypoglycemia

TABLE 400.2.	PROTOCOL FOR PROLONGED SUPERVISED FASTS

1. Date the onset of the fast as of the last ingestion of calories. Discontinue all nonessential medications.
2. Allow the patient to drink calorie-free and caffeine-free beverages.
3. Ensure that the patient is active during waking hours.
4. Measure plasma glucose, insulin, and C-peptide levels and, if an assay is available, proinsulin in the same specimen; repeat measurements every 6 hours until the plasma glucose is <60 mg/dL, when the interval should be reduced to every 1–2 hours.
5. End the fast when the plasma glucose is <45 mg/dL and the patient has symptoms and/or signs of hypoglycemia or <55 mg/dL when Whipple's triad is not the goal.
6. At the end of the fast, measure plasma glucose, insulin, C-peptide, proinsulin, β-hydroxybutyrate, and sulfonylurea levels in the same specimen; then inject 1 mg of glucagon IV and measure plasma glucose after 10, 20, and 30 minutes. Then feed the patient.
7. When a deficiency is suspected, measure plasma cortisol, growth hormone, or glucagon at the beginning and end of the fast.

and who do not show signs of severely depressed plasma glucose concentrations (less than 40 mg per deciliter), the fast should be terminated at 72 hours. Fasting, however, should be terminated before 72 hours should a patient have both symptoms of hypoglycemia and a plasma glucose level in the hypoglycemic range or, in the case of a patient previously shown to satisfy Whipple's triad, a plasma glucose level less than 55 mg per deciliter. The decision to end the fast may not be easy for the house officer to make. Because of possible delays in the availability of the results of plasma glucose testing, the bedside reflectance meter may have to serve as a guide to glucose levels. Careful examination and testing for subtle signs or symptoms of hypoglycemia should be carried out repeatedly when the patient's plasma glucose level is near or in the hypoglycemic range.

Criteria for hyperinsulinemic hypoglycemia are the following: a plasma insulin level $\geq 6 \mu U$ per milliliter (radioimmunoassay) or $\geq 3 \mu U$ per milliliter (ICMA), a C-peptide value ≥ 200 pmol per milliliter (ICMA), a proinsulin level ≥ 5 pmol per milliliter (ICMA), a β-hydroxybutyrate level ≤ 2.7 mmol per liter, an increment of plasma glucose in response to 1 mg glucagon i.v. ≥ 25 mg per deciliter, and absence from the plasma of first- and second-generation sulfonylureas. These criteria apply whether hypoglycemia develops in the fasting state or after meals, that is, 2 to 4 hours pc.

Ratios of glucose to insulin are useless for identification of relative hyperinsulinemia. Not infrequently, it becomes apparent that a patient undergoing a history and physical examination after fasting overnight is frankly hypoglycemic at that time or has a plasma glucose close to the hypoglycemic range. In the former instance, all the measurements recommended for the end of the prolonged supervised fast should be made at that time in the outpatient setting. In the latter instance, the fast protocol should be initiated in the outpatient setting. Often, Whipple's triad can be verified (i.e., completion of the fast) before the end of the business day; if not, the patient is admitted to the hospital to complete the fast.

C-Peptide Suppression Test

The C-peptide suppression test may be used as a screening test. Interpretation of the C-peptide suppression test requires normative data appropriately adjusted for the patient's body mass index and age.

Insulin Antibodies

The presence of insulin antibodies, once considered to be firm evidence of factitious hypoglycemia due to self-administered insulin, (when animal insulin was the only type commercially available), at present (in the era of human insulin use) is diagnostic of insulin autoimmune hypoglycemia, especially if titers are high.

Localization Studies

Once a diagnosis of endogenous hyperinsulinemic hypoglycemia has been made, an attempt should be made to localize the tumor. Success with various procedures—transabdominal ultrasonogra-phy, endoscopic ultrasonography, triple-phase computed tomography, angiography, octreoscan—varies with local skill and experience. Transhepatic portal venous sampling has been abandoned in most tertiary centers. The selective arterial calcium stimulation test not only regionalizes the lesion but also is a useful dynamic test to identify hyperfunctioning islet cell tissue.

Clinical Features

Insulinoma may develop at any age; it is more common in women and has an estimated incidence of one case per 250,000 patient-years. Multiple endocrine neoplasia type 1 syndrome (MEN1), multiplicity, and malignancy occur in less than 10% of cases. The tumor recurrence rate is less than 10% without MEN1 and 20% with MEN1. Long-term survival in the context of benign insulinoma is normal. Treatment is surgical removal.

Factitial hypoglycemia, whether from sulfonylurea or insulin use, is probably more common than reported. It may result from self-injury or may play a part in suicide, homicide, or child abuse. Perpetrators are more frequently women in a health-related occupation or those who have diabetes. Treatment is discontinuation of the drug. Insulin autoimmune hypoglycemia is extraordinarily rare, reported mostly but not exclusively in Asians of all ages without gender preference. Often, there is a history of antecedent autoimmune disease or use of drugs containing sulfhydril. Insulin antibody titers are high. Often spontaneous remission occurs. There is no known effective treatment. Noninsulin pancreatogenous hypoglycemia syndrome is a newly described entity of neuroglycopenia occurring postprandially primarily in men who have negative results on 72-hour fast, negative results on radiologic localization studies, positive outcomes on calcium stimulation tests, amelioration of symptoms by gradient-guided partial pancreatectomy, and presence of islet hyperplasia and nesidioblastosis in resected pancreata.

THE ILL-APPEARING PATIENT

In persons with coexisting disease, it may be sufficient to recognize the underlying disease and its association with hypoglycemia and to take action to minimize recurrences of hypoglycemia. Confirmation of the suspected source of hypoglycemia may be sought, for example, low insulin and C-peptide levels in ethanol hypoglycemia, elevated insulin-like growth factor II levels in non-B-cell tumor hypoglycemia, low levels of cortisol in adrenal insufficiency, and blunted plasma glucose responses to intravenous glucagon in hypoglycemias due to abnormal liver function (glycogen storage disease, sepsis, and congestive heart failure).

Hospitalized patients are often severely ill with multisystem disease. They are at risk for iatrogenic forms of hypoglycemia (insulin added to total parenteral nutrition) as well as for any type of hypoglycemia that may be produced by the underlying disease. In determining the cause of hypoglycemia in a hospitalized seriously ill patient, diligent examination of the record may be more profitable than examination of the patient.

CONCLUSION

The diagnosis of a hypoglycemic disorder requires a high level of suspicion, careful assessment of the patient for the presence of mediating drugs or a predisposing illness, and, where indicated, methodical evaluation of the basis of well-defined diagnostic criteria. The diagnostic burden is heaviest for healthy-appearing persons with episodes of confirmed neuroglycopenia. The insulin mediation of hypoglycemia are a plasma insulin level ≥ 6 μU per milliliter (radioimmunoassay), a C-peptide value ≥ 200 pmol per liter (ICMA), a proinsulin level ≥ 5 pmol per liter (ICMA), a β-hydroxybutyrate value ≤ 2.7 mmol per liter, and generous (≥ 25 mg per deciliter) response of plasma glucose to i.v. glucagon administered when the patient is hypoglycemic. Sulfonylurea should be sought in the plasma of any hypoglycemic patient, especially by an assay that can detect the second-generation of these drugs.

BIBLIOGRAPHY

Archambeaud-Mouveroux F, Huc MC, Nadalon S, et al. Autoimmune insulin syndrome. *Biomed Pharmacother* 1989;43:581–586.

Doppman JL, Chang R, Fraker DL, et al. Localization of insulinomas to regions of the pancreas by intra-arterial stimulation with calcium. *Ann Intern Med* 1995;123:269–273.

O'Brien T, O'Brien PC, Service FJ. Insulin surrogates in insulinoma. *J Clin Endocrinol Metab* 1993;77:448–451.

Palardy J, Havrankova J, Lepage R, et al. Blood glucose measurements during symptomatic episodes in patients with suspected postprandial hypoglycemia. *N Engl J Med* 1989;321:1421–1425.

Service FJ. Hypoglycemic disorders. *N Engl J Med* 1995;332:1144–1152.

Service FJ, McMahon MM, O'Brien PC, Ballard DJ. Functioning insulinoma—incidence, recurrence, and long-term survival of patients: a 60-year study. *Mayo Clin Proc* 1991;66:711–719.

Service FJ, Natt N, Thompson GB, et al. Noninsulinoma pancreatogenous hypoglycemia: a novel syndrome of hyperinsulinemic hypoglycemia in adults independent of mutations in *Kir6.2* and *SUR1* genes. *J Clin Endocrinol Metab* 1999;84:1582–1589.

Kelley's Textbook of Internal Medicine, fourth edition. Edited by H. David Humes.
Lippincott Williams & Wilkins, Philadelphia © 2000.

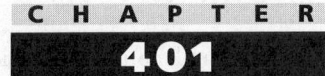

CHAPTER 401

APPROACH TO THE PATIENT WITH FLUSHING

JEROME M. FELDMAN

Flushing, or blushing, is a transient reddening of the skin resulting from vasodilation. Although it occurs most commonly in the face and neck, the chest, abdomen, arms, and legs can be affected. Facial flushing often is accompanied by increased facial perspiration and a subjective feeling of facial warmth. The flushing can last for minutes, hours, or even days. The cause of flushing in most patients is not serious. In a few patients, however, it is the first sign of a neoplasm. Not all patients with a red face have flushing; patients with lupus erythematosus, seborrhea, or drug-induced photosensitivity reactions may have red faces without flushing.

PATHOPHYSIOLOGY

In some individuals, vasodilation of the superficial capillary loops of the skin is caused by altered sympathetic tone from the central nervous system. In others, it results from a circulating neurohumor released by a normal or pathologic condition. The neurohumors that have been suggested to play a role in flushing include histamine, serotonin, bradykinin, substance P, prostaglandins, and endorphins.

PHYSIOLOGIC FLUSHING

In response to embarrassment or nervousness, healthy individuals may flush. In an attempt to dissipate heat, they also may flush after drinking a hot beverage or during a febrile illness. Individuals who flush can be divided into three types: psychologically sensitive, physiologically sensitive, and anatomically predisposed. At the time of spontaneous menopause, 40% to 50% of women experience flushing. This type of flushing also is common after surgical removal of the ovaries and after damage to or surgical removal of the testes. Although the mechanism of the vasomotor instability that develops after the loss of gonadal function is not completely understood, flushing usually responds dramatically to the replacement of estrogen in women and testosterone in men.

ETHANOL INGESTION

The ingestion of ethanol can provoke flushing in normal individuals, particularly those of Asian ancestry. Medications such as nicotinic acid, β-adrenergic antagonists, calcium channel antagonists, and nitroglycerin can produce spontaneous flushing. Other groups of medications sensitize patients to ethanol-induced flushing. These include antimicrobial agents, such as cephalosporins, chloramphenicol, griseofulvin, quinacrine, furazolidone, and metronidazole; drugs used to treat chronic alcohol abuse, such as disulfiram and calcium carbamide; the calcium channel blockers, such as verapamil and nifedipine; and sildenafil, a medication for erectile dysfunction. Medications that interfere with gonadal function, such as leuprolide, flutamide, danazol, tamoxifen, and clomiphene citrate, also provoke flushing.

NEOPLASTIC DISEASES

Patients with islet cell tumors that secrete vasoactive intestinal polypeptide, gastrin, or insulin occasionally have attacks of facial flushing. Although most patients with pheochromocytoma have facial pallor, a few patients with these catecholamine-secreting tumors experience flushing. Patients with medullary carcinoma or even lymphoma sometimes have facial flushing after ethanol ingestion. Some patients with systemic mastocytosis have attacks of facial flushing. The neoplastic condition most often associated with episodes of flushing is carcinoid tumor and the carcinoid syndrome. Carcinoid tumors have been reported to originate in virtually every organ in the body. The two most common sites are the ileum and the bronchus. In some patients who ultimately prove to have carcinoid syndrome, episodes of facial flushing precede the diagnosis by 15 years. If a patient describes flushing attacks within 10 minutes of ingesting ethanol, the rapidity of onset is suggestive of carcinoid syndrome.

The character of flushing attacks in carcinoid syndrome varies. One type lasts a few minutes and leaves no residual redness. Another type lasts only a few minutes but results in residual telangiectasia. A third type lasts for hours to days and causes lacrimation and furrowing and edema of the brow, and a fourth type produces a bright red, but patchy flush. The first two types of flushing can be caused by a carcinoid tumor arising from any anatomic site, the third type can originate in the bronchus, and the fourth type can originate in the stomach.

DIAGNOSTIC TESTS

The most serious diseases to be ruled out in a patient with flushing are systemic mastocytosis and carcinoid syndrome. Systemic mastocytosis can be excluded by measuring histamine in plasma and urine or by measuring methylhistamine or imidazole acetic acid in urine. Punch biopsy of the skin with stains for mast cells also is helpful. Carcinoid syndrome can be dismissed by measuring serotonin in platelets, serum, or urine or by measuring 5-hydroxyindoleacetic acid, the principal metabolite of serotonin, in urine.

BIBLIOGRAPHY

Kulke MH, Mayer RJ. Carcinoid tumors. *N Engl J Med* 1999;340: 858–868.
Mohyi D, Tabassi K, Simon J. Differential diagnosis of hot flashes. *Maturitas* 1997;27:203–214.

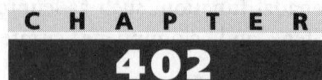

C H A P T E R
402

APPROACH TO HYPERCALCEMIA AND HYPOCALCEMIA

BRUCE LOBAUGH
MARC K. DREZNER

Skeletal and mineral homeostasis depends on precise regulation of the small, but crucial circulating pool of calcium and the considerably larger skeletal reserve. The dynamics of both pools are affected by the entry of calcium into and excretion from the system, processes that are modified by nonhormonally mediated exchanges of calcium between the bone fluid, which is rich in calcium, and the extracellular fluid and by the actions of parathyroid hormone (PTH), calcitonin, and calcitriol. Hypercalcemia can result from primary disturbances of these calcitropic hormones or from abnormal processes directly affecting bone resorption, intestinal absorption, or mineral excretion that overcome homeostatic compensatory mechanisms. In contrast, defects in bioactive PTH secretion or resistance to the action of this hormone are the primary causes of permanent hypocalcemia. In the complete absence of PTH, serum calcium is maintained at a basal level of about 5.5 mg per deciliter by fluxes of calcium between the bone fluid/bone surface and extracellular fluid, whereas bioactive PTH is required to increase the total serum calcium level to the normal range (about 8.9 to 10.1 mg per deciliter).

In general, about 47% of the circulating calcium is ionized or "free" calcium, an equivalent amount is protein bound, and the remainder is complexed to phosphate, citrate, bicarbonate, and other ions. Whereas both free and complexed calcium are ultrafilterable, only the former is metabolically active (i.e., available for uptake by cells). The bound calcium is associated with albumin (75%) and a variety of globulins.

Sometimes a careful history and physical examination reveal an apparent cause for an abnormal serum calcium concentration. Often, however, confirmation of the diagnosis requires the use of appropriate laboratory tests. Because numerous diseases, therapeutic agents, and physiologic states can affect calcium homeostasis, every effort should be made to determine the mechanism of action underlying any change in the serum calcium concentration, to allow a rational choice of appropriate therapy.

HYPERCALCEMIA

Many parathyroid-related and non–parathyroid-related disorders can result in hypercalcemia. Most commonly, elevated serum calcium levels develop in association with primary hyperparathyroidism or malignant disorders. The other potential causes of hypercalcemia (Table 402.1) usually are not considered seriously unless primary hyperparathyroidism and malignancy have been excluded or the preliminary evaluation clearly suggests an alternative pathogenesis.

PARATHYROID-RELATED HYPERCALCEMIA

Primary Hyperparathyroidism

Primary hyperparathyroidism is a disorder of bone and mineral metabolism resulting from excessive, abnormally regulated secretion of PTH from the parathyroid glands. In most cases (80%), a hyperfunctioning adenoma of a single parathyroid gland underlies the disease. Less frequently (15% to 20%), diffuse hyperplasia of all four parathyroid glands produces the disorder. Such four-gland hyperplasia may occur sporadically or, more often, in association with multiple endocrine neoplasia, type 1 or 2A.

TABLE 402.1.   CAUSES OF HYPERCALCEMIA

Parathyroid-related
  Primary hyperparathyroidism
    Adenoma
    Hyperplasia
    Spontaneous
    Familial
    Multiple endocrine neoplasia type 1 or 2
    Carcinoma
  Familial hypocalciuric hypercalcemia
  Lithium therapy
  Severe secondary hyperparathyroidism (chronic renal failure)
Non–parathyroid-related
  Malignancy-associated hypercalcemia
    Local osteolytic (tumor/hematologic malignancy with bone metastases)
    Humoral hypercalcemia
    PTHrP
    Calcitriol mediated
    Other factors (growth factors, cytokines, or HTLV-1)
  Vitamin D related
    Vitamin D intoxication
    Granulomatous diseases (excessive calcitriol production)
    Idiopathic hypercalcemia of infancy (Williams syndrome)
  Increased bone turnover
    Hyperthyroidism
    Immobilization
    Vitamin A intoxication
    Benzothiadiazide therapy
  Decreased bone mineralization
    Aluminum intoxication
  Endocrinopathy
    Pheochromocytoma
    Addisonian crisis
    Pancreatic VIPoma syndrome
  Milk-alkali syndrome
  Parenteral nutrition

PTHrP, parathyroid hormone–related protein; HTLV-1, human T-cell leukemia/lymphoma virus 1; VIP, vasoactive intestinal polypeptide.

Rarely, patients with primary hyperparathyroidism harbor several adenomas and, less often (less than 0.5%), parathyroid carcinoma. Furthermore, several unique familial diseases infrequently underlie hyperparathyroidism, including the hyperparathyroidism-jaw tumor syndrome, localized to chromosome 1q21-q31, and isolated familial hyperparathyroidism.

Etiology

Although an alteration of the calcium-dependent regulatory control of parathyroid secretion is the mechanism of action underlying all forms of primary hyperparathyroidism, the cellular basis for this abnormality is multifactorial. In fact, studies indicating that parathyroid adenomas are monoclonal neoplasms suggest that there is a fundamental biologic difference between single-gland disease and multiple-gland hyperplasia. In single-gland disease, caused by adenoma, an altered set point for calcium regulation of parathyroid secretion and an increased number of cells appear to be operative factors. Conversely, in disease caused

by hyperplasia, the set point seems to be closer to normal, and abnormal hormone secretion results from an increase in cell number alone. Although the pathophysiologic basis for the proliferative defect and altered calcium set point that underlie these variants of the disorder remains incompletely defined, an understanding of the molecular genetics of parathyroid gland neoplasia is evolving. Indeed, the clonal origin of most parathyroid adenomas suggests a defect at the level of the gene controlling growth of the parathyroid cell or the expression of PTH.

In this regard, the *MEN1* gene for multiple endocrine neoplasia type 1 has been linked to chromosome 11q13, and a high percentage of the monoclonal parathyroid gland tumors in this disease show loss of alleles at this site. This suggests that the *MEN1* gene may be a "tumor suppressor," the loss of which leads to tumorigenesis. A significant percentage of sporadic parathyroid tumors also manifest allele loss at this locus, suggesting a similar pathogenesis. In contrast, parathyroid hyperplasia in multiple endocrine neoplasia type 2A is associated with mutations of the *RET* proto-oncogene on chromosome 10q11, the expression of which confers unregulated cell growth on the parathyroid tissue. Finally, studies have shown the relatively rare occurrence of genetic rearrangements between the *PTH* gene and the *PRAD1* oncogene in patients with parathyroid adenomas. Juxtaposing the *PTH* gene with the *PRAD1* oncogene, such that this growth promoter may fall under the influence of the *PTH* gene regulatory apparatus, likely results in enhanced expression of *PRAD1* in parathyroid glands and excessive cellular proliferation without conferring the phenotypes of invasiveness or metastasis on the tumor cell.

Incidence and Epidemiology

Before serum calcium determinations were carried out routinely, primary hyperparathyroidism was an infrequently diagnosed disease. This disorder now is discovered in one in 500 to 1,000 of the general population, and the number of recognized cases closely approximates the prevalence of the disease. Although the disorder occurs at all ages, it is distinctly unusual in children and has a peak incidence in the sixth to seventh decades of life, with a female-to-male ratio variably reported as 2:1 or 3:2. When the disease develops in children, it is likely a component of one of several endocrinopathies with a genetic basis, such as multiple endocrine neoplasia type 1 or 2. Even though there are no clearly defined risk factors for primary hyperparathyroidism, 15% to 25% of patients have a remote history of external irradiation to the head and neck region.

Clinical Features and Prognosis

The widespread use of multiphasic screening has had a significant effect on the modern clinical features of primary hyperparathyroidism. Whereas patients with this disorder traditionally had symptoms of kidney (nephrolithiasis) or bone disease or protean symptoms referable to prolonged hypercalcemia, today they often have no symptoms whatsoever. Eighty percent of patients with primary hyperparathyroidism have no complaints at the time of diagnosis, and it is common for mild, asymptomatic hypercalcemia to persist for years with little progression. In some patients, however, symptoms attributable to the disease develop insidiously.

Nephrolithiasis causes renal colic, hematuria, and passage of stones or gravel. Although the incidence of this complication has declined over the years, it still occurs in 15% to 20% of the population at risk. The incidence of hypercalciuria has remained constant (35% to 40%), however, and urinary calcium excretion is no higher in patients with primary hyperparathyroidism who have renal stones than in those who do not. Rarely, affected patients also have nephrocalcinosis, radiographic features of diffuse renal calcification, and a diminished glomerular filtration rate.

Bone symptoms, when present, include pain and tenderness, usually over areas of increased bone turnover, such as the tibial periosteum; recurrent back pain stemming from vertebral compression fractures or progressive kyphosis; and abnormal fractures at the sites of bone cysts. This complication is rare (less than 2%), however, and subperiosteal resorption, salt-and-pepper changes in the skull, bone cysts, and brown tumors are so unusual that skeletal radiographs no longer are taken routinely in the diagnostic evaluation of patients with primary hyperparathyroidism.

Nonspecific symptoms or those related to hypercalcemia can include muscle weakness, depression, memory impairment, personality changes, pruritus, anorexia, constipation, polyuria, and polydipsia. Occasionally, intercurrent illness, dehydration, or immobilization triggers an episode of acute hypercalcemia. Serum calcium in these cases can climb rapidly to levels of 15 to 20 mg per deciliter. In addition, an inordinate concurrence has been found between primary hyperparathyroidism and other disease states, such as peptic ulcer, chondrocalcinosis, pancreatitis, and hypertension. It remains difficult to associate these complications directly with the hyperparathyroid state itself. With severe or prolonged hypercalcemia, corneal calcification (band keratopathy), anemia, weight loss, mental obtuseness, or coma and death can occur.

Although many biochemical tests have been advocated for the identification of parathyroid-related disorders, none are as discriminating as PTH immunoassays. More than 90% of patients with primary hyperparathyroidism found at surgery have elevated intact PTH levels. Assays for intact PTH involve the immunoradiometric technique, which uses two different antibodies against two different regions of the 84-amino-acid peptide. Immunoradiometric assays have substantial sensitivity and can detect levels of intact PTH within the normal range. These assays are helpful in distinguishing primary hyperparathyroidism from virtually all other causes of hypercalcemia. The only exceptions are hypercalcemia resulting from thiazide diuretic and lithium use and familial hypocalciuric hypercalcemia. Hypercalcemic patients taking lithium or thiazides should be retested when drugs are discontinued, if possible, since both drugs can alter serum calcium and PTH secretion. In young, asymptomatic individuals who have mild hypercalcemia, a marginally elevated PTH determination may be due to familial hypocalciuric hypercalcemia rather than hyperparathyroidism (see later discussion).

The medical treatment of hyperparathyroidism is largely dependent on the serum calcium concentration. If hypercalcemia is severe and symptomatic, the calcium level must be lowered rapidly (see Medical Management of Hypercalcemia). In the absence of marked hypercalcemia, primary hyperparathyroidism presents a dilemma in management because most patients have no symptoms. Surgical resection of parathyroid tissue is the treatment of choice, but it is unclear whether it should be used for asymptomatic patients. Indications for parathyroidectomy are a history of renal stones, progressive bone disease, symptoms attributable to hypercalcemia, or a serum calcium level greater than 11.5 mg per deciliter. In less severe cases, the potential for increased bone loss, mental impairment, or hypercalcemic crisis with advancing age must be weighed against the risk of surgery. Evidence suggests that many asymptomatic patients with primary hyperparathyroidism do not experience progressive increases in serum calcium levels or reductions in bone mass. Nevertheless, serum calcium levels greater than 12 mg per deciliter; hypercalciuria; bone mineral density at cortical sites more than two standard deviations below age- and sex-matched control values; or specific complications, such as nephrolithiasis or bone disease, develop in at least 50% of asymptomatic patients and are clear indications for surgery. Because many asymptomatic patients eventually become surgical candidates, early surgical intervention may be most appropriate.

Unfortunately, we still lack an effective and safe therapeutic agent for the medical treatment of primary hyperparathyroidism. While oral phosphate will lower the serum calcium concentration in affected patients, the development of ectopic calcification in soft tissues, stemming from an increased calcium-phosphate product, and further elevation of the serum PTH levels have limited extensive use of this therapy. Estrogen has been advocated for postmenopausal women, but the known antagonism of this agent on PTH-mediated bone resorption has limited effects on the serum calcium concentration. More recently, bisphosphonates have been considered as a therapeutic intervention. Unexpectedly, studies of etidronate have proved this drug ineffective in the treatment of hypercalcemia, whereas investigations of dichloromethylene bisphosphonate show that this agent does not have sustained effects on the serum calcium concentration. Whether alendronate will prove efficacious in the management of primary hyperparathyroidism remains unknown. Finally, a new class of drugs, termed calcimimetics, is under study to determine whether altering the function of the extracellular calcium-sensing receptor might reduce PTH levels in primary hyperparathyroidism. Pilot studies have given credence to this approach, and larger clinical studies are under way to determine the usefulness of this management strategy.

Between 5% and 10% of patients who undergo cervical exploration for primary hyperparathyroidism have persistent or recurrent hyperparathyroidism requiring re-operation. Recent studies indicate, however, that the incidence of surgical failure may be lessened markedly through the use of intraoperative PTH immunoassay as a determinant of satisfactory resolution of the disease state. This procedure is cost-effective and accurate and may minimize the morbidity of surgical intervention in revision procedures. Indeed, given the increased risk of morbidity in re-operative parathyroid exploration and the higher probability of ectopic gland location after failed parathyroid exploration, preoperative localization of parathyroid tissue usually is warranted when an initial attempt at parathyroidectomy has been unsuccessful. Technetium-sestamibi localization studies are the most efficacious way to pinpoint cervical and mediastinal ectopic glands.

After successful surgery, transient mild hypocalcemia occasionally occurs but rarely requires treatment. In patients with extensive bone disease, however, severe and persistent hypocalcemia can arise as the result of "bone hunger." Acute treatment with calcium infusions and long-term management with oral calcium and vitamin D may be necessary. If normal parathyroid tissue remains, patients generally tolerate cessation of therapy.

Familial Hypocalciuric Hypercalcemia

Familial hypocalciuric hypercalcemia is a benign disorder with an autosomal dominant pattern of inheritance. It has a high rate of penetrance and is characterized by hypercalcemia and relative hypocalciuria. In the vast majority of patients the disease is caused by mutations in a gene on the long arm of chromosome 3 encoding a calcium-sensing receptor. Hypercalcemia often manifests during childhood, but patients usually remain asymptomatic throughout life. The PTH concentration usually is elevated slightly, though normal levels have been reported. Not surprisingly, subtotal parathyroidectomy does not resolve hypercalcemia.

The mildly elevated serum calcium level of familial hypocalciuric hypercalcemia results from enhanced renal tubular reabsorption of calcium. The defect in the calcium-sensing receptor, located in the parathyroid glands and kidneys, leads to exaggerated renal reabsorption of filtered calcium (and magnesium) and failure of the resultant hypercalcemia to suppress PTH secretion fully. As a consequence, the parathyroid glands invariably display pathologic changes suggestive of chief cell hyperplasia.

The finding of hypercalcemia in relatively young patients, with only a slight elevation of the serum PTH level and a family history of unsuccessful neck exploration for presumed parathyroid disease, should raise suspicion regarding the presence of this disorder. Hypermagnesemia and urinary calcium/creatinine ratios of less than 0.01:1 strongly support the diagnosis, as does documentation of hypercalcemia in first-degree relatives. In affected families, specific genetic diagnosis is possible by screening for mutations in the calcium-sensing receptor gene. Because nephrolithiasis, bone disease, and other complications of primary hyperparathyroidism or hypercalcemia do not occur often, conservative treatment is indicated. In general, these patients should not undergo neck exploration because subtotal parathyroidectomy fails to resolve hypercalcemia. Instead, once the diagnosis is made, continued observation for unexpected complications and avoidance of aggressive intervention are appropriate therapeutic strategies. In the rare situation where an adult has a complication, such as relapsing pancreatitis or a serum calcium level consistently greater than 14 mg per deciliter, total parathyroidectomy is recommended.

NON–PARATHYROID-RELATED HYPERCALCEMIA

Malignancy-associated Hypercalcemia

Many malignant diseases are complicated by the development of hypercalcemia. This complication results from osteolytic metastases (local osteolytic hypercalcemia), most often associated with solid tumors, such as carcinoma of the breast, kidney, lung, or thyroid; from hematologic malignant disorders with skeletal infiltration, such as multiple myeloma; or from humoral hypercalcemia, in which a humoral agent that causes hypercalcemia is produced and secreted by tumors not of parathyroid origin, such as squamous cell carcinomas (head and neck, esophagus, lung, cervix, vulva, skin), renal or bladder carcinomas, and ovarian malignancies.

Etiology

The mechanisms of action responsible for hypercalcemia associated with malignancy are heterogeneous, but the final common pathway leading to hypercalcemia in most cases is osteoclastic bone resorption. The agency underlying osteoclast-mediated acceleration of bone turnover in local osteolytic hypercalcemia remains uncertain. Most investigators agree that the osteolytic metastases probably produce paracrine or local cell-to-cell chemical messengers that activate or increase the production of osteoclasts. Several lymphokines, including tumor necrosis factor α (cachectin), tumor necrosis factor β (lymphotoxin), and interleukin-1, have been identified as potential osteoclast-activating factors involved in hypercalcemia associated with lymphoma and multiple myeloma. The production of these factors appears to be mediated by the local production of prostaglandin E_2. Less commonly, hypercalcemia caused by osteolytic metastases can result, in part, from direct bone resorption by tumor cells.

In humoral hypercalcemia of malignancy, extensive evidence supports the role of a tumor-derived humoral agent in osteoclast activation, bone resorption, and consequent hypercalcemia. Most notably, affected patients have little or no evidence of skeletal tumor involvement, and resection of the primary tumor, when possible, leads to resolution of the hypercalcemia. Identification of the presumptive humoral factor has been impaired by the apparent heterogeneity of the syndrome. Nevertheless, several substances have been identified as mediators of humoral hypercalcemia. Although these substances include ectopically produced PTH, which was once considered to be the primary mediator of the syndrome, investigators have documented the production of authentic PTH by a source other than parathyroid tumor in a few patients. Instead, observations suggest that two classes of proteins mediate hypercalcemia in most patients with this paraneoplastic syndrome: PTH-related protein (PTHrP) and tumor-derived growth factors.

PTHrP has been identified in tumors of patients who have the humoral hypercalcemia of malignancy syndrome and displays biologic activity remarkably similar to that of PTH. This protein is larger than PTH, however. Even though it manifests partial homology, it does not react with antibodies directed at PTH and is derived from a gene distinct from that which encodes PTH. Moreover, antisera to PTHrP reverse many of the biochemical manifestations of the syndrome in vitro and in vivo, whereas those to PTH usually do not. Nevertheless, PTHrP and PTH bind with equivalent affinities to a common receptor, accounting for the very similar ranges of biologic activities of these hormones. Studies indicate that PTHrP is almost ubiquitous in normal tissues. It appears that PTHrP may play roles different from those initially identified, including differentiation of the skin and skin appendages, lactation, placental calcium transport, fetal calcium regulation, smooth-muscle function, and bone and chondrocyte development. PTHrP probably is a multi-purpose autocrine–paracrine factor that is produced in excess amounts by the malignant transformation of normal squamous epithelial cells.

Tumor-derived growth factors (α and β classes) also have been identified in tumors of patients with humoral hypercalcemia of malignancy. These agents cause hypercalcemia when injected in vivo and are powerful stimulants of osteoclastic bone resorption. Moreover, they impair osteoblast function and probably decrease the bone formation rate, a common complication observed in the humoral hypercalcemia of malignancy syndrome. These agents can be extracted from virtually all tumors, however, including those that produce PTHrP, and their role in the paraneoplastic syndrome is uncertain. Nevertheless, it is probable that the tumor-derived growth factors and the PTHrPs act synergistically to produce the full spectrum of the malignancy-associated hypercalcemic syndrome.

Less often, the humoral hypercalcemia syndrome results from the elaboration of lymphotoxin, a multifunctional cytokine that is produced under normal circumstances by activated T lymphocytes. Convincing evidence suggests that this factor plays an important role in the bone destruction and hypercalcemia that occur in multiple myeloma. Established cultures of human myeloma cells produce this factor, and a major portion of bone-resorbing activity generated by these cells in vitro is accounted for by lymphotoxin. Lymphotoxin is not the only cytokine that has been implicated in myeloma, however. Several studies suggest that interleukin-1 and interleukin-6 have roles in bone destruction. Further investigations are necessary to indict these factors. Even though essentially all patients with myeloma experience extensive bone destruction, less than 40% become hypercalcemic. The explanation for this disparity rests with the observation that increased bone resorption likely leads to hypercalcemia only in the context of impaired glomerular filtration, a common abnormality in multiple myeloma.

In a small subset of patients with humoral hypercalcemia of malignancy, the elevated serum calcium concentration does not result from increased bone resorption but from enhanced production of calcitriol and consequent intestinal hyperabsorption of calcium. This mechanism has been described in some patients with T-cell lymphoma, B-cell lymphoma, Hodgkin's disease, and other types of lymphoproliferative disorders in which the neoplastic cells are the source of the active vitamin D metabolite. In most patients with lymphoma and hypercalcemia, increased calcitriol production is not a factor.

Incidence and Epidemiology

Studies indicate that hypercalcemia complicates various malignant disorders in 5% to 10% of hospitalized patients, and the incidence of humoral hypercalcemia of malignancy is equal to or greater than that of local osteolytic hypercalcemia, depending on the series of patients examined. Regardless of syndrome type, an elevated serum calcium concentration is a marker of advanced cancer in affected patients. Consequently, uncontrolled hyper-

calcemia contributes directly to death in only 25% of cases. Most patients die of progressive cancer or its complications, with only slightly elevated serum calcium values before death.

Clinical Features and Prognosis

Hypercalcemia of malignancy in general has clinical features similar to those of hyperparathyroidism per se but modified by symptoms referable to the underlying cancer. The complications of long-term primary hyperparathyroidism (nephrolithiasis and subperiosteal resorption of bone) rarely are encountered in these patients. This probably relates to the relatively short course of the malignant disease. Polyuria, polydipsia, dehydration, renal compromise, constipation, and varying degrees of neurologic dysfunction ranging from lethargy to coma are common symptoms, and patients with skeletal metastases often have significant bone pain or abnormal fractures. Although the relationship between tumor size and the presence of hypercalcemia is unclear, small occult tumors rarely cause malignancy-associated hypercalcemia. In contrast, osteolytic lesions can be the initial signs of malignancy in multiple myeloma or lymphoma.

In some patients with cancer, the onset of hypercalcemia seems to be unrelated to the malignancy. In these cases, the elevated serum calcium level may be provoked by recent immobilization, the use of thiazide drugs, prerenal or renal azotemia leading to inadequate renal calcium clearance, coincident hypophosphatemia, gastrointestinal fluid loss, or the administration of calcium as part of a hyperalimentation regimen. Such patients do not have the hypercalcemia of malignancy syndrome, and the serum calcium concentration normalizes with correction of the ancillary event. In less than 5% of patients, coincident primary hyperparathyroidism is the cause of hypercalcemia.

Abnormal or suppressed levels of immunoactive PTH in conjunction with elevated urinary cyclic adenosine monophosphate (cAMP) excretion favors the presence of malignancy-associated hypercalcemia. The level of PTH observed is largely dependent upon the assay employed. Using a two-site immunoradiometric assay for PTH (1-84), several groups have found virtually universal suppression of PTH levels to values below normal. In contrast, levels that approach (within 25%) only the lower limits of the reference range are obtained with midregion-specific immunoassays. Conversely, immunoreactive PTHrP values are elevated in the majority of patients with malignancy-associated hypercalcemia. In this regard, immunoradiometric assays measuring large N-terminal species of PTHrP discriminate affected patients most effectively. Nonetheless, not all patients with hypercalcemia caused by malignancy will have elevated levels of PTHrP. Approximately 20% of patients, generally those with decreased urinary cAMP excretion (and likely osteolytic hypercalcemia), will have normal or suppressed values. Discrimination of malignancy-associated hypercalcemia is also limited by increased levels of C-terminal PTHrP in renal insufficiency, elevated N-terminal levels associated with nonmalignant pheochromocytomas, and increased PTHrP in a few patients with mammary hypertrophy or lymphedema.

Despite the suppressed PTH concentration, the hypercalcemia of malignancy syndrome bears a strong clinical resemblance to the hyperparathyroid state. In this regard, patients with both clinical disorders manifest reduced renal tubular reabsorption of phosphorus and consequent phosphaturia, a lower serum phosphorus concentration, elevated urinary cAMP levels, and increased markers of bone resorption. Several clinical features distinguish hypercalcemia of malignancy from primary hyperparathyroidism. While osteoblastic bone formation is amplified and coupled to the increased bone resorption rate in patients with hyperparathyroidism, in patients with malignancy and hypercalcemia, osteoblastic bone formation is diminished. In addition, patients with hypercalcemia of malignancy often have low-normal to frankly low calcitriol levels, in contrast to patients with primary hyperparathyroidism, who have high-normal or elevated calcitriol levels. However, this discrepancy is not invariable. Studies suggest that in the absence of bone metastases, patients with malignancy-associated hypercalcemia may show an elevated serum calcitriol level. A significant correlation between serum PTHrP and calcitriol concentrations in patients without bone metastases supports this possibility. These findings suggest that in metastatic disease, locally produced factors can override the effects of PTHrP on vitamin D metabolism.

In general, hypercalcemia in patients with cancer has grave prognostic significance. Many studies indicate that the median survival term of such patients varies from 1 to 6 months. In most cases, the shortened life span is not related to uncontrolled hypercalcemia. The elevated serum calcium level is a marker of advanced cancer, and death results from the progress of this disease or its complications. Treatment of hypercalcemia has little effect on the patient's survival,, but it does ameliorate polyuria, polydipsia, central nervous system abnormalities, nausea, vomiting, and constipation and often allows patients to be cared for at home during the terminal phases of their illnesses. Standard therapies for hypercalcemia are applicable in these cases, but patients with malignancy-associated hypercalcemia who have high circulating levels of PTHrP respond less well to treatment with such agents as bisphosphonates than do those who have normal levels of PTHrP. Concomitant elevation of calcitriol concentrations further compromises therapy.

MEDICAL MANAGEMENT OF HYPERCALCEMIA

Short-term Treatment

The short-term treatment of life-threatening hypercalcemia often is successful, resulting in a 2 to 7.5 mg per deciliter decline of the serum calcium value within 24 to 48 hours. The necessity for such therapy is signaled by the occurrence of anorexia, nausea, mental status changes, hypertension, or deterioration of renal function in association with a serum calcium level greater than 13.5 mg per deciliter. An understanding of the pathogenesis of such profound hypercalcemia can guide appropriate intervention. For example, the high serum calcium concentration observed in vitamin D intoxication results in part from excessive gastrointestinal calcium absorption. In such cases, dietary restriction of calcium intake may be beneficial. Alternatively, when hypercalcemia results from excessive osteolytic destruction stemming from metastatic tumor or prolonged immobilization, drug-induced blockade of bone resorption may be preferable.

Regardless of its pathogenesis, the clinical picture of a hypercalcemic crisis often includes superimposed dehydration, which reduces renal calcium excretion. The initial therapy for this disorder should be restoration of hydration. This normalizes the glomerular filtration rate and increases renal tubular sodium and calcium clearance, resulting in a 100- to 300-mg increment per day of urinary calcium excretion. After the volume deficit has been restored, calciuresis can be enhanced further with a saline diuresis induced by the administration of large volumes of isotonic saline (up to 6 L per day) plus intravenous furosemide (in doses up to 100 mg every 2 hours). Urine volume and sodium and potassium concentrations must be monitored throughout this aggressive treatment and maintained to preserve euvolemia and prevent hyponatremia and hypokalemia. Pulmonary edema can be precipitated, and appropriate measures must be taken to prevent this effect.

Alternative or adjunctive forms of therapy have emerged for the life-threatening hypercalcemic state. Bisphosphonates have become some of the principal agents used in the treatment of severe hypercalcemia. These drugs are osteoclast inhibitors and effectively block the mobilization of calcium from bone, influencing an important pathophysiologic mechanism of action underlying hypercalcemia. Four bisphosphonates are available: etidronate, pamidronate, alendronate, and clodronate. Of these four, pamidronate is the preferred agent for the urgent treatment of acute hypercalcemia, because of its potency, efficacy, and formal Food and Drug Administration approval as a single intravenous therapy. The effective dose of pamidronate is between 30 and 90 mg administered as a single intravenous infusion over 24 hours. The 90-mg dose is recommended only for the most severe hypercalcemic states. For most patients, 30 to 60 mg is adequate and minimizes the hypocalcemia that can arise when the highest dose is used. Treatment with this drug leads to normalization of the serum calcium level in 70% to 100% of patients. Adverse effects, which develop in up to one-third of treated patients, include transient fever, a small decline in the serum phosphorus level, and myalgia. Administering the drug over a prolonged period (no less than 2 hours) prevents potential nephrotoxicity.

Other pharmacologic interventions for hypercalcemia include glucocorticoids, calcitonin, and indomethacin. These agents are of particular value in the treatment of acutely elevated serum calcium levels resulting from specific causes. Glucocorticoids enhance urinary calcium excretion, decrease gastrointestinal calcium absorption, and diminish renal $25(OH)D$-1α-hydroxylase activity. Consequently, they are effective in combating hypercalcemia resulting from vitamin D intoxication (by blocking end-organ effects) and granulomatous diseases (by impairing extrarenal calcitriol production). In general, the hypercalcemic action of glucocorticoids manifests over several days, and the usual dosage is 40 to 100 mg of prednisone (or its equivalent) given in four divided doses per day. In contrast, calcitonin diminishes the skeletal resorption of calcium and phosphorus within minutes of administration and is particularly suited for the treatment of hypercalcemia caused by rapid bone turnover.

The most impressive results are seen in patients with vitamin D intoxication, thyrotoxicosis, or immobilization hypercalcemia, disease states that are characterized by a high rate of bone mobilization. Nevertheless, many patients with malignancy-associated hypercalcemia resulting from osteolysis do not respond to treatment. Calcitonin is administered parenterally at doses of 25 to 50 U every 6 to 8 hours. In patients who receive continuous therapy for 1 to 5 days, escape from drug action often occurs via an unknown mechanism of action. Because the humoral factor that causes hypercalcemia in some patients with malignancy is a prostaglandin, indomethacin can be useful in combating hypercalcemia in selected cases. Responsive patients manifest a decline in the serum calcium concentration in response to the administration of 25 mg orally every 6 hours.

Plicamycin (mithramycin) at one time was a first-line drug for the treatment of hypercalcemia, particularly the form caused by bone dissolution and refractory to adequate hydration. A dose of 2.5 g per kilogram is administered intravenously and often results in the restoration of normocalcemia. One or two doses per week usually are sufficient, with treatment withheld until hypercalcemia recurs. If there is no response during the first 24 to 48 hours after initial treatment, the 2.5 g per kilogram dose can be given daily until the serum calcium level begins to fall. Because toxicity to plicamycin can be striking, careful monitoring is necessary when repeated doses are administered. Major side effects include thrombocytopenia, hepatocellular necrosis, and decreased clotting factors. Hypocalcemia, hypophosphatemia, and hypokalemia also can develop, as can nausea, vomiting, and stomatitis. Other concerns include nephrotoxicity. Because of these adverse effects and the emergence of other effective therapies, this drug is reserved for particularly difficult and unusual situations.

In life-threatening emergencies, when other medicines have failed, oral (2,000 mg per day) or intravenous (1,500 mg over 6 to 8 hours) phosphorus may be advantageous. This treatment can be dramatically effective, causing a decrement in the serum calcium level ranging from 4 to 7 mg per deciliter. Phosphorus should be used only in extreme emergencies, however, because overdose can result in fatal hypocalcemia. The serum calcium concentration must be monitored frequently during treatment. Phosphate does not remove calcium from the body. Instead, colloidal calcium-phosphate precipitation results in a redistribution of the total body calcium and inevitable soft-tissue calcification. Alternatively, treatment of life-threatening hypercalcemic emergencies can include peritoneal or hemodialysis. This therapy generally is reserved for the severely hypercalcemic patient who has not responded adequately to various drug-related interventions. Use of a low- or zero calcium dialysate frequently will lower the serum calcium level rapidly in those patients who are refractory to other measures (or who have renal insufficiency).

Long-term Treatment

In general, long-term outpatient therapy for hypercalcemia is ineffective. Mild hypercalcemia can be treated with modest success using hydration with or without furosemide or ethacrynic acid, moderate-dose oral phosphate (maintaining normophosphatemia), estrogens, or indomethacin. More potent remedies (mithramycin, glucocorticoids, and high-dose phosphate) have significant long-term toxicity or side effects. Long-term treatment is directed more appropriately at management of the un-

derlying disease. This approach is best when hyperparathyroidism, thyrotoxicosis, or other disorders that respond to surgical or pharmacologic intervention are the cause of hypercalcemia.

Elevated serum calcium concentrations resulting from intractable diseases (e.g., malignancy) often do not respond to such treatment. In these cases, long-term combination therapy with calcitonin and low-dose glucocorticoids may be beneficial. Calcitonin (salmon or human) is administered by subcutaneous injection at a dose of 25 to 50 U every 6 to 8 hours on an alternate-week schedule. Prednisone is given concurrently, without interruption, at a dosage of 10 mg per day. This program permits long-term delivery of calcitonin without the rapid development of refractoriness to the drug. Although the serum calcium value may remain elevated after the initiation of therapy, an adequate therapeutic response usually occurs, precluding recurrent episodes of life-threatening hypercalcemia. Bisphosphonates are another option in the long-term treatment of hypercalcemia. The availability of these drugs in oral formulations and experience in their use will define the future role of this therapeutic approach.

■ HYPOCALCEMIA

Although numerous mechanisms of action are involved in the genesis of hypercalcemia and homeostatic compensatory responses are easily overwhelmed, adequate parathyroid function and end-organ responsiveness to PTH normally ensure the maintenance of ionized calcium concentrations within normal limits when hypocalcemic challenges are encountered. A defect in bioactive PTH secretion or a primary or acquired (e.g., vitamin D deficiency, hypomagnesemia) resistance to the action of the hormone, however, can result in chronic hypocalcemia.

The most common hypocalcemic disorders seen in clinical practice are hypoparathyroidism and vitamin D–related diseases, including chronic renal failure. Other causes of hypocalcemia include pseudohypoparathyroidism (PHP), magnesium deficiency, drug-induced hypocalcemia, malignancy, neonatal hypocalcemia, and acute pancreatitis (Tables 402.2 and 402.3). False hypocalcemia (normal levels of ionized calcium with low levels of albumin-bound and total serum calcium) is common among chronically ill, hospitalized patients. True hypocalcemia (decreased levels of ionized calcium, which may produce symptoms of neuromuscular excitability) is less common but more important. Because the evaluation of a patient with hypocalcemia always involves determination of the specific causative disease entity, this section focuses on the major diseases in which hypocalcemia plays an important role, including idiopathic and surgical hypoparathyroidism and PHP. Other disorders associated with hypocalcemia are reviewed in the chapters devoted to malignant disease of the prostate (Chapters 207 and 223) and breast (Chapters 205 and 220), acute pancreatitis (Chapter 117), and vitamin D abnormalities (Chapter 412).

HYPOPARATHYROIDISM

Idiopathic hypoparathyroidism is a disorder of mineral metabolism caused by the diminished secretion of PTH from the parathyroid glands or impaired parathyroid gland function due to

TABLE 402.2.	CAUSES OF HYPOPARATHYROIDISM

Hypoparathyroidism
  Idiopathic
    Sporadic
    Autoimmune
      Late onset
      Polyglandular syndrome
      Familial
    Failure of parathyroid gland development
      Autosomal recessive
      DiGeorge syndrome
      Kenny–Caffey syndrome
      Kearns–Sayre syndrome
      Barakat syndrome
      Hypoparathyroidism with short stature, mental retardation, and siezures
    Reduced parathyroid gland function stemming from altered regulation
      Primary
        Calcium sensor mutation
        PTH mutation
      Secondary
        Maternal hyperparathyroidism
        Hypomagnesemia
  Acquired
    Postsurgical
    Infiltration
      Hemochromatosis
      Thalassemia
      Wilson's disease
      Metastatic carcinoma
    Postirradiation
    Reversible
      Alcohol
      Transient neonatal
Pseudohypoparathyroidism
  Abnormal Gsα protein
    Pseudohypoparathyroidism type Ia
    Pseudo-pseudohypoparathyroidism
  Abnormal Gs protein
    Pseudohypoparathyroidism type Ib
  Etiology unknown
    Pseudohypoparathyroidism type Ic
  Abnormal cyclic AMP–dependent protein kinase A
    Pseudohypoparathyroidism type II

PTH, parathyroid hormone; AMP, adenosine monophosphate.

TABLE 402.3.	NONPARATHYROID CAUSES OF HYPOCALCEMIA

Deficiency of vitamin D and abnormalities of vitamin D metabolism
  Decreased precursors
    Dietary deficiency
    Malabsorption
    Liver disease
    Abnormal enterohepatic circulation
    Drugs
      Phenytoin, phenobarbital
    Nephrotic syndrome
  Decreased production of active metabolite
    Vitamin D–dependent rickets type I
Resistance to vitamin D
  Vitamin D–dependent rickets type II
Medications
  Plicamycin, calcitonin, bisphosphonates, phosphate
  Fluoride
  Foscarnet, pentamidine
  Citrated blood, radiographic contrast dye
Malignancy
  Osteoblastic metastases
Phosphate excess
  Exogenous
    Dietary
    Intravenous
    Enemas
    White phosphorus burns
  Endogenous
    Rhabdomyolysis
    Tumor lysis
    Malignant hyperthermia
Altered bone remodeling
  "Hungry bone" syndrome (postparathyroidectomy)
Renal failure

Etiology

Autoimmune destruction of the parathyroid glands is the most common cause of idiopathic hypoparathyroidism; it is a sporadic (late-onset hypoparathyroidism) or familial (autoimmune polyglandular failure) disorder. In the sporadic form, dysfunction of the parathyroid glands is an isolated abnormality mediated by organ-specific autoantibodies. Autosomal recessive inheritance, hypofunction of several endocrine glands (parathyroids, ovaries, and adrenals), and recurrent mucocutaneous candidal infections usually mark the familial version. Less frequently, idiopathic hypoparathyroidism results from primary hypoplasia of the parathyroid glands, which is associated with congenital absence of the thymus in DiGeorge syndrome and with a variable inheritance pattern in affected kindred in familial hypoparathyroidism.

In addition, autosomal dominant inheritance of hypoparathyroidism (familial benign hypocalcemia) has been recognized in families with distinct activating mutations of the calcium receptor gene. A mutation in the sensor, resulting in constitutive activation, chronically suppresses PTH secretion and induces hypercalciuria. No doubt other molecular genetic abnormalities are operative in other families with autosomal dominant and recessive isolated hypoparathyroidism.

Acquired hypoparathyroidism (permanent or transient) oc-

altered regulation of hormone secretion or the congenital absence of the parathyroid glands. In general, this term refers to all cases of PTH deficiency that do not result from surgical damage or another well-defined cause. Within this group, several distinct syndromes have been defined: congenital absence of the parathyroid glands, late-onset hypoparathyroidism, branchial dysembryogenesis (DiGeorge syndrome), Kenny–Caffey syndrome, autoimmune polyglandular failure type I, and familial hypoparathyroidism (persistent neonatal). The acquired form of hypoparathyroidism occurs most often as a result of surgical extirpation of the parathyroid glands, but damage caused by irradiation and infiltrative diseases (metastatic carcinoma, Wilson's disease, hemochromatosis, and thalassemia) also provokes diminished parathyroid function.

curs in up to 3.5% of patients undergoing neck surgery for hyperparathyroidism, goiter, or cancer or extensive parathyroidectomy. Incidental or purposeful removal of the parathyroid glands results in hypocalcemia within 24 hours and leaves patients with hypoparathyroidism for the remainder of their lives. In contrast, ischemic vascular damage or trauma can cause transient hypocalcemia lasting from 2 weeks to 6 months. Such patients may have impaired parathyroid reserve and experience periodic hypocalcemia during stress. In patients with severe hyperparathyroidism and osteitis fibrosa cystica, surgical removal of one or more of the parathyroid glands can prompt hypocalcemia as a result of "hungry bone" syndrome. In this case, the deposition of available calcium into healing bone lesions leads to a transient relative hypoparathyroidism.

Much less often, infiltrative disease or sclerosis stemming from radiation compromises gland function. Hypoparathyroidism can develop after external radiation to the neck or, rarely, low-dose radioactive iodine therapy for Graves' disease. Magnesium deficiency also can result in impaired PTH secretion and resistance to the action of PTH on the target organs (bone and kidney). This usually occurs in poorly nourished alcoholic patients who have been binge drinking.

Hypocalcemia in hypoparathyroidism results from a drop in the level of the blood–bone equilibrium of calcium and from reduced renal reabsorption of calcium, both of which are direct consequences of PTH deficiency. In addition, resultant impairment of renal 25(OH)D-1α-hydroxylase activity limits the serum calcitriol concentration, diminishing gastrointestinal calcium absorption and further compromising mobilization of calcium from bone and tubular reabsorption of calcium. The absence of PTH also increases the renal threshold for phosphorus, resulting in hyperphosphatemia.

Incidence and Epidemiology

Idiopathic hypoparathyroidism is a rare disorder, but its prevalence has never been determined accurately. In the most extensive study, Hsien-Yi and colleagues detected 12 cases among 25,311 admissions to Tientsin Medical College Hospital, an overall incidence of one in 2,100. In contrast, systematic screening of serum calcium values in the outpatient setting confirmed idiopathic hypoparathyroidism in one of every 8,666 patients. The average interval between the onset of symptoms and the diagnosis of idiopathic hypoparathyroidism is 6.3 years. The gender distribution appears to be equal, except in the case of autoimmune polyglandular failure type I, in which there is a slight female preponderance. At major medical centers, the incidence of surgical hypoparathyroidism has declined dramatically as iodine 131 treatment of hyperthyroidism has increased and thyroid operations have diminished. In contrast, the incidence of the disorder in the general community has remained unchanged.

Clinical Features and Prognosis

The onset of symptoms in idiopathic hypoparathyroidism typically is insidious, with a slow increase in the number of episodes related to the neuromuscular and neurologic systems. Patients experience paresthesia (particularly in the oral area), muscle spasm, carpopedal spasm, facial grimacing, and, in extreme cases, laryngeal spasm and convulsion. Common central nervous system manifestations include irritability, depression, impaired memory, and psychosis. Often, the symptoms are precipitated or intensified by physical or emotional stress-induced hyperventilation and consequent alkalosis. With long-standing hypocalcemia, patients variably manifest increased intracranial pressure, often in association with papilledema, subcapsular cataracts, and calcification of the basal ganglia. In addition, the skin and hair become dry, and the teeth may be hypoplastic or have ridges stemming from enamel hypoplasia.

Hypocalcemia also can lead to the exacerbation of psoriasis. Cardiovascular manifestations of a decreased serum calcium level include arrhythmias, bradycardia, hypotension, and impaired cardiac contractility. Hypotension is unresponsive to the use of fluids and pressors until calcium is administered. Similarly, impaired cardiac contractility responds poorly to inotropic agents unless hypocalcemia is corrected. On physical examination, Chvostek's or Trousseau's signs can be used to confirm latent tetany. A false-positive Chvostek's sign is present in about 10% of the normal population.

Serum calcium concentrations in affected individuals vary from about 5.5 mg per deciliter to low-normal levels, depending on the degree of PTH deficiency. Serum phosphorus concentrations usually rise to values as high as 7.5 mg per deciliter. Two-site immunoradiometric and immunochemiluminometric assays for intact PTH are now sensitive enough that low or undetectable values are obtained routinely. In contrast, older PTH radioimmunoassays that measure midregion or C-terminal peptides of PTH sometimes yield inappropriately low results for the prevailing serum calcium concentration but often falsely elevated levels that do not distinguish between idiopathic hypoparathyroidism and nonparathyroid causes of hypocalcemia. Serum calcitriol levels are low, and bone remodeling is markedly impaired. When the diagnosis is suspected but unproved, PTH provocation of urinary cAMP excretion (an increase of four to ten times) can be used to confirm normal end-organ responsiveness.

Treatment with vitamin D (50,000 to 100,000 U per day) or calcitriol (0.5 to 1.5 μg per day) with calcium supplements (1 to 2 g per day) effectively restores serum calcium levels to normal in most patients and lowers serum phosphorus levels. Although vitamin D is the least expensive form of therapy, it has the longest duration of action and can result in prolonged toxicity. Thus, calcitriol is the contemporary treatment of choice. Therapy in the absence of PTH effects on the renal tubule often results in hypercalciuria, however, and the potential for renal toxicity exists when serum calcium levels are maintained within the normal range. Therefore, a therapeutic balance must be found between minimizing episodes of hypocalcemia with their attendant symptoms and stimulating hypercalciuria with the consequent risks of nephrolithiasis and nephrocalcinosis. Chlorthalidone often is added to the treatment regimen and is effective in lowering urinary calcium concentrations. Careful monitoring of renal function is essential. Occasionally, the disease is refractory to treatment, and serum calcium levels remain well below the normal range. In some cases, a coincident magnesium deficiency underlies such refractoriness. Treatment with intravenous magnesium sulfate or oral magnesium citrate may restore responsiveness. Close monitoring of the urine and serum calcium is essential in the treated patient until stable laboratory values are reached, generally in 1 to 3 months. Thereafter, follow-up at 3- to 6-month intervals usually is adequate.

PSEUDOHYPOPARATHYROIDISM

PHP refers to a heterogeneous group of disorders characterized by end-organ unresponsiveness to PTH. In its prototypic form, the disease is a hereditary syndrome of short stature, mental retardation, distinctive skeletal abnormalities, hypocalcemia, and hyperphosphatemia, which are present despite excessive secretion of PTH. These manifestations are found in different combinations in various forms of the disorder, reflecting both biochemical and genetic heterogeneity.

PHP can be subdivided into several syndromes according to a classification scheme based on signs of ineffective PTH action (low calcium, high phosphorus levels), blunted urinary cAMP and phosphate response to exogenous PTH, the presence or absence of Albright's hereditary osteodystrophy, and assays of the Gs subunits and enzyme activity of the adenylate cyclase moiety (Table 402.4). Using these criteria, there are five well-characterized forms of the disease: PHP type I, subdivided into a, b and c categories; PHP type II; and pseudo-PHP. Patients with PHP type I have a diminished nephrogenous cAMP response to PTH. In the Ia variant of the disease, this defect stems from a decreased amount of the stimulatory G proteins (Gsα) and occurs in association with the constellation of somatic abnormalities referred to as Albright's hereditary osteodystrophy. These patients also exhibit resistance to a variety of other hormones, such as thyroid-stimulating hormone and gonadotropins, the effects of which are mediated through the G proteins. Unexpectedly, a subgroup of these patients, with the phenotype of Albright's hereditary osteodystrophy and a deficiency of Gsα, have no evidence of hormone resistance and a normal nephrogenous cAMP response to PTH. This disease subtype, referred to as pseudo-PHP, exists in the same kindreds as does PHP Ia, and mutations in the gene encoding Gsα have been described in affected patients. Studies indicate that genomic imprinting may explain the alternative phenotypes that result from identical Gsα mutations. Male transmission of the gene results in pseudo-PHP, whereas female transmission results in PHP type Ia.

Patients with PHP type Ib lack Albright's hereditary osteodystrophy and manifest hormone resistance that is limited to the PTH target organs. Normal Gsα activity in some tissues has been documented in patients with this disease variant. Hence, speculation has focused on the possibility that the defect underlying this disorder may involve abnormal regulation of PTH receptor messenger RNA expression. Nonetheless, a genome-wide search in four PHP type Ib kindreds has established linkage to a small telomeric region on chromosome 20q, which contains the stimulatory G protein gene. Moreover, the genetic defect is imprinted paternally, as is the genetic defect underlying PHP type Ia and pseudo-PHP.

Thus, it appears possible that the PTH-resistant hypocalcemia found in patients with PHP type Ib is caused by a tissue- or cell-specific defect in Gs gene expression. Since Gs transcripts are derived from only one parental allele—at least in some tissues or cells—mutations in a promoter or enhancer of the Gs gene could explain the kidney-specific resistance toward PTH and the resulting hypocalcemia in patients with PHP type Ib. In PHP type Ic, there is resistance to several hormones in the absence of a defect in Gsα, for reasons that are unclear. Patients with PHP type II have a normal nephrogenous cAMP response to PTH and normal Gsα activity, but a subnormal phosphaturic response to PTH. There is no clear genetic basis for this disorder. Several investigators postulate that a defect exists between the generation of cAMP in the renal tubular cell and the effect of this increase in cAMP on phosphate reabsorption.

Clinical Features and Prognosis

Most of the symptoms of PHP reflect enhanced neuromuscular excitability, a consequence of a reduced serum calcium concentration. Symptoms appear, on average, at about 8 years of age but usually persist for 9 to 12 years before the correct diagnosis is made. Many patients remain essentially asymptomatic for many years, and the diagnosis is not established until late in life. In patients with PHP types Ia and Ic, signs and symptoms of associ-

| TABLE 402.4. | CLASSIFICATION OF PSEUDOHYPOPARATHYROIDISM |

	Serum			PTH-Responsive Cyclic AMP		PTH-Responsive Urine Phosphate	GS Deficiency	Generalized Hormone Resistance	AHO
	Ca	P	PTH	Urine	Fibroblasts				
PHP Ia	⇓	⇑	⇑	⇓	⇓	⇓	Yes	Yes	Yes
PHP Ib	⇓	⇑	⇑	⇓	⇑/N	⇓	No	No	No
PHP Ic	⇓	⇑	⇑	⇓	⇓	⇓	No	Yes	Yes
PHP II	⇓	⇑	⇑	⇓	?	⇓	No	No	No
PPHP	N	N	⇑	⇓	N	⇓	Yes	No	Yes

AHO, Albright's hereditary osteodystrophy; AMP, adenosine monophosphate; Ca, calcium; P, phosphorus; PHP, pseudohypoparathyroidism; PPHP, pseudo-pseudohypoparathyroidism; PTH, parathyroid hormone.

ated endocrine abnormalities can be initial features of the disease. The spectrum of these abnormalities is wide, but it can include mild hypothyroidism and primary amenorrhea or oligomenorrhea.

On physical examination, patients have evidence of tetany or developmental defects referable to Albright's hereditary osteodystrophy. Most notably, the physiognomic changes, primarily in patients with type Ia disease, include short stature, obesity, and brachydactyly (unilateral or bilateral, involving the hands or feet). Posterior subcapsular cataracts can develop in patients with long-standing hypocalcemia, resulting in poor vision. Basal ganglion calcification occurs in nearly half of all patients and occasionally is associated with extrapyramidal movement disorders. Although hypocalcemia is characteristic, normocalcemia can be present, particularly in children. Hypocalcemia can lead to emotional derangements varying from depression to schizophrenia. Cognitive defects often are observed.

Laboratory test abnormalities in most patients include hypocalcemia, hyperphosphatemia, an elevated PTH concentration, and a defective urinary cAMP response to PTH. Urinary hydroxyproline excretion is universally high, consistent with PTH-mediated bone resorption. Although bone cells are presumed to be unresponsive to PTH, evidence has been inferential. Studies of bone density in the radius show that patients with PHP have reduced bone mass. Moreover, bone biopsy evidence of increased resorption or decreased mineralization is common, and a few patients have severe osteitis fibrosis cystica. The hypocalcemia in PHP may not result solely from intrinsic resistance but from a deficiency of calcitriol as well, which can compromise the bone homeostatic mechanisms.

The treatment of PHP is similar to that of hypoparathyroidism, except that the dosages of vitamin D and calcium required usually are lower. Lesser amounts of medication are needed because vitamin D or its metabolites restores bone responsiveness to PTH in part in many patients. The decreased serum calcitriol concentrations in patients with PHP and the role of this metabolite in maintaining bone homeostasis indicate that improved therapy might be achieved by using physiologic replacement doses of this active metabolite.

MEDICAL MANAGEMENT OF HYPOCALCEMIA

Short-term Treatment

The objectives of emergency therapy for hypocalcemia with tetany are to relieve symptoms and prevent laryngeal obstruction. These complications are unlikely if the serum calcium concentration is maintained at more than 7 mg per deciliter. In adults, 10 to 20 mL of 10% calcium gluconate is given by intravenous push at a rate of at least 10 mL per minute. In patients receiving digitalis, caution is essential and electrocardiographic control advisable. If a patient can take oral medications, 100 mg of calcium should be given every 2 hours, increasing the dose to

500 mg if necessary. Repeated intravenous administration of calcium, if it is essential, should be accomplished by the continuous infusion of 10 mL of a 10% solution added to 500 mL of intravenous fluids over 6 hours. After acute hypocalcemia has been controlled, persistent decrements of the serum calcium concentration are managed appropriately through long-term therapy for the underlying disease.

Long-term Treatment

The long-term treatment of hypocalcemia depends largely on the specific cause of the disorder. In diseases marked by a deficiency of vitamin D, treatment requires provision of this substance in amounts sufficient to overcome the inadequate vitamin stores. When the underlying disease involves abnormal metabolism of the parent vitamin or resistance to the active metabolite, the use of vitamin D metabolites in physiologic or pharmacologic amounts often is required. In states of parathyroid deficiency or resistance, maintenance of a normal serum calcium level can be achieved by the administration of vitamin D (or its metabolites) and calcium supplements.

BIBLIOGRAPHY

Berger AC, Libutti SK, Bartlett DL, et al. Heterogeneous gland size in sporadic multiple gland parathyroid hyperplasia. *J Am Coll Surg* 1999; 188:382–389.

Blind E, Schmidt-Gayk H, Scharla S, et al. Two-site assay of intact parathyroid hormone in the investigation of primary hyperparathyroidism and other disorders of calcium metabolism compared with a midregion assay. *J Clin Endocrinol Metab* 1988;67:353–360.

Duan Y, DeLuca V, Seeman E. Parathyroid hormone deficiency and excess: similar effects on trabecular bone but differing effects on cortical bone. *J Clin Endocrinol Metab* 1999;84:718–722.

Guise TA, Mundy GR. Evaluation of hypocalcemia in children and adults. *J Clin Endocrinol Metab* 1995;80:1473–1478.

Heath III H. Primary hyperparathyroidism: recent advances in pathogenesis, diagnosis and management. *Adv Intern Med* 1991;37:275.

Hindie E, Melliere D, Simon D, et al. Primary hyperparathyroidism: is technetium 99m-sestamibi/iodine-123 subtraction scanning the best procedure to locate enlarged glands before surgery? *J Clin Endocrinol Metab* 1995;80:302–307.

Horwitz MJ, Bilezikian JP. Primary hyperparathyroidism and parathyroid hormone–related protein. *Curr Opin Rheumatol* 1994;6:321–328.

Juppner H, Schipani E, Bastepe M, et al. The gene responsible for pseudohypoparathyroidism type Ib is paternally imprinted and maps in four unrelated kindreds to chromosome 20q13.3. *Proc Natl Acad Sci USA* 1998; 95:11798–11803.

Levine MA, Jap T, Mauseth RS, et al. Activity of the stimulatory guanine nucleotide-binding protein is reduced in erythrocytes from patients with pseudohypoparathyroidism and pseudopseudohypoparathyroidism: biochemical, endocrine and genetic analysis of Albright's hereditary osteodystrophy in six kindreds. *J Clin Endocrinol Metab* 1986;62: 497–502.

Wilson LC, Oude Luttiukhuis EM, Clayton PT, et al. Parental origin of Gs alpha gene mutations in Albright's hereditary osteodystrophy. *J Med Genet* 1994;31:835–839.

Kelley's Textbook of Internal Medicine, fourth edition. Edited by H. David Humes. Lippincott Williams & Wilkins, Philadelphia © 2000.

DISORDERS OF ENDOCRINOLOGY, METABOLISM, AND GENETICS

CHAPTER

403

DISORDERS OF THE HYPOTHALAMUS AND ANTERIOR PITUITARY

JOHN C. MARSHALL
ARIEL L. BARKAN

HYPOTHALAMIC–PITUITARY–END-ORGAN INTERACTIONS

Pituitary hormone secretion is controlled by the central nervous system (CNS). The neurons involved in the final regulatory pathways are located in the ventral hypothalamus (Fig. 403.1). Hypothalamic regulation of pituitary function occurs by two distinct pathways. The first is a neuroendocrine system. Amine-secreting and peptide-secreting neurons release their products from axon terminals in the median eminence into capillaries of the hypothalamic-hypophyseal-portal system. The peptides travel to the anterior lobe of the pituitary and stimulate or inhibit pituitary hormone secretion by interacting with specific receptors on pituitary cells. Most hypothalamic peptides stimulate pituitary hormone synthesis and secretion, but somatostatin and dopamine exert inhibitory actions. Thus, medications that interfere with the synthesis of monoamines or peptides and lesions that destroy the median eminence or pituitary stalk result in reduced secretion of luteinizing hormone (LH), follicle-stimulating hormone (FSH), thyroid-stimulating hormone (thyrotropin, TSH), adrenocorticotropic hormone (corticotropin, ACTH), and growth hormone (GH), but secretion of prolactin, which is inhibited by dopamine, is increased.

The second pathway, a neurosecretory system, is involved in osmoregulation and control of the onset of labor and subsequent nursing. Large neurons of the magnocellular system are located in the supraoptic nuclei of the anterior hypothalamus and in the paraventricular nuclei (adjacent to the third ventricle). Some axons from these neurons terminate in the median eminence, but others pass down the pituitary stalk and terminate on modi-

fied neural (glial) cells in the posterior pituitary. These cells store arginine vasopressin and oxytocin. Because their function is storage only, removal of the posterior pituitary does not cause diabetes insipidus as long as the neuronal perikarya and the median eminence remain intact. Regulation of arginine vasopressin secretion is discussed elsewhere in this text (see Chapter 404).

ANATOMY

HYPOTHALAMUS AND PITUITARY STALK

The hypothalamus extends from the optic chiasm anteriorly to the mammillary bodies posteriorly. The hypothalamic sulcus of the third ventricle separates the thalamus above. Inferiorly, the hypothalamus forms a tubular structure, the tuber cinereum, which contains the infundibular recess of the third ventricle. The median eminence (infundibulum) continues down to form the pituitary stalk. The portal capillaries form from a capillary plexus in the median eminence, become the veins of the pituitary stalk (six to eight in all), and form a second capillary plexus interspersed among the cells of the anterior pituitary. Thus, most of the blood supply to the anterior pituitary (about 1 mL per gram per minute) originates from the superior hypophyseal arteries and has passed through the median eminence before reaching the pituitary. The blood–brain barrier is relatively permeable in the median eminence, allowing circulating hormones to gain access to the axon terminals, which respond by modifying release of hypothalamic regulatory hormones.

The cell bodies of hypothalamic secretory neurons are not in discrete nuclei but are distributed throughout the hypophysiotropic area of the hypothalamus. Gonadotropin-releasing hormone (GnRH) neurons are located in the arcuate nucleus and in the anterior hypothalamus, corticotropin-releasing hormone (CRH) neurons in the paraventricular area, somatostatin neurons in the anterior hypothalamus, growth hormone–releasing hormone (GH-RH) neurons in the ventromedial arcuate nuclei, and thyrotropin-releasing hormones (TRH) neurons in the anterior hypothalamus. The hypothalamic secretory neurons are influenced by neural input from other areas of the brain, but function often is maintained after hypothalamic deafferentation, indicating that the neurons are relatively autonomous.

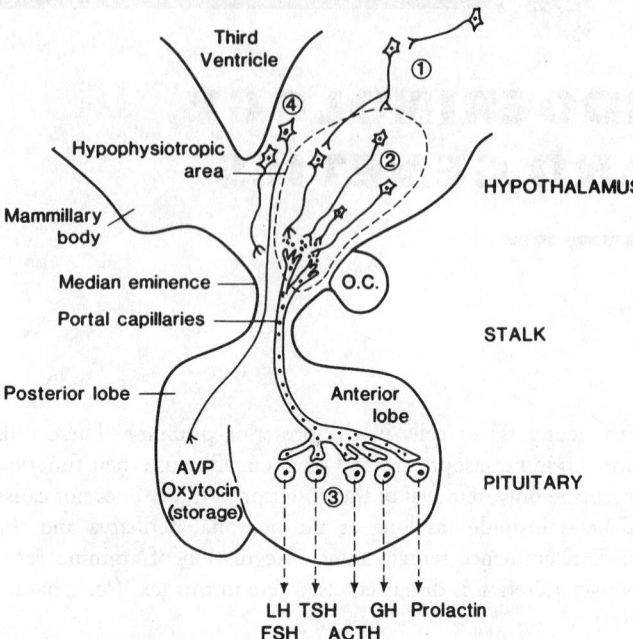

FIGURE 403.1. Hypothalamic-pituitary connections: (1) Intermediary neurons secrete neurotransmitters. (2) Hypophysiotropic neurons located in the hypophysiotropic area secrete releasing and inhibiting hormones. (3) Anterior pituitary cells. (4) neurons in the paraventricular and supraoptic nuclei secrete AVP and oxytocin. *ACTH*, adrenocorticotropic hormone; *AVP*, arginine vasopressin; *GH*, growth hormone; *FSH*, follicle-stimulating hormone; *LH*, luteinizing hormone; *O.C.*, optic chiasm; *TSH*, thyroid-stimulating hormone.

PITUITARY GLAND

The human pituitary consists of three parts: an anterior lobe (adenohypophysis), an intermediate lobe (poorly developed in humans except during fetal life), and a posterior lobe (the neurohypophysis). The gland weighs 0.5 to 1 g; measures 15 mm across, 6 mm deep, and 10 mm long; and lies within the sella turcica ("Turkish saddle"), a depression in the sphenoid bone. The roof of the sella turcica is formed by dura mater, the diaphragma sellae, through which the pituitary stalk passes. The posterior wall of the sella is formed by the bony dorsum sellae, but the lateral walls are fibrous and include the medial wall of the cavernous sinus. The proximity of the optic chiasm above and the presence of cranial nerves III, IV, V, and VI in the cavernous sinus are important. Pituitary tumors may impinge on these nerves and manifest clinically as visual field defects or cranial nerve palsies.

The anterior and posterior lobes of the pituitary are functionally independent and have distinct embryologic origins. The anterior lobe is formed from an upward extension of ectoderm from the primitive oral cavity (Rathke's pouch). The posterior lobe arises as a downgrowth of the diencephalon and fuses with Rathke's pouch. The cystic center of Rathke's pouch usually is obliterated, but small cystic structures may persist, typically in the superior part of the pituitary. Tumors arising from these cystic remnants form craniopharyngiomas, which may be intrasellar or suprasellar in position. Remnants of Rathke's pouch often are present in or below the sphenoid bone, forming a pharyngeal pituitary that can be the site of tumor formation in rare instances.

Pituitary cells were originally classified as acidophils, basophils, or chromophobes based on the staining properties of the cytoplasmic granules; this system is now outmoded. Five distinct pituitary cell types have been identified in the anterior pituitary by electron microscopy and immunocytochemistry. The various cell types are scattered throughout the anterior pituitary, though some areas of the gland contain a predominance of one cell type. The characteristics and location of the pituitary cell types, together with their secretory products, are shown in Table 403.1.

HYPOTHALAMIC HORMONES

Regulation of Hypophysiotropic Hormone Secretion

Secretion of hormones by the hypophysiotropic neurons is regulated by neurotransmitters from intermediary neurons and by the negative or positive feedback effects of target gland hormones (Figs. 403.1 and 403.2). The feedback actions of target gland hormones are usually negative and may be exerted directly on the hypophysiotropic neurons or through modification of the secretion of neurotransmitters, including catecholamines, indoleamines, and other neuropeptides. In humans, the exact pathways are uncertain, and, in particular, the role of other neuropeptides is unclear. Many peptides have been shown to be distributed widely in the hypothalamus and throughout the CNS, and some have been shown to function as neurotransmitters. Neuropeptides that have been identified in the CNS include TRH, somatostatin, enkephalins, endorphins and dynorphin, neuropeptide PYY, substance P, calcitonin, and angiotensin. Peptides originally identified in the gastrointestinal tract are also present in the CNS, including insulin, glucagon, pancreatic polypeptide, gastrin, cholecystokinin, vasoactive intestinal peptide, secretin, and motilin. The function of these peptides and their role as neurotransmitters are unclear, but their presence in the CNS has led to the hypothesis of a *brain–gut axis* that may be involved in regulation of nutritional and metabolic function.

Catecholamines (dopamine, norepinephrine, epinephrine) are all derived from tyrosine. Tyrosine hydroxylase converts tyrosine to L-dihydroxyphenylalanine (L-dopa), which is decarboxylated to dopamine. Dopamine is stored in the secretory granules of dopaminergic neurons but is converted to norepinephrine by dopamine-fl-hydroxylase in noradrenergic neurons. Adrenergic neurons contain phenylethanolamine *N*-methyltransferase, which converts norepinephrine to epinephrine. Catecholamines are released into the synaptic cleft and act on postsynaptic receptors. After dissociation from postsynaptic receptors, catecholamines can be taken up by the presynaptic neuron (reuptake) or can be degraded by the enzymes monoamine oxidase and catechol-*O*-methyltransferase. The actions of catecholamines are enhanced by drugs that inhibit the reuptake process (tricyclic antidepressants, cocaine) or by monoamine oxidase inhibitors (pargyline).

Indoleamines (serotonin, melatonin) are formed by hydroxylation and decarboxylation of tryptophan, and the rate of serotonin synthesis depends on the serum levels of tryptophan. Seroto-

TABLE 403.1.	CHARACTERISTICS OF CELL TYPES IN THE ANTERIOR PITUITARY				
Cell Type	Original Classification	Percentage of Cells	Secretion Granules	Secreted Hormone	Location and Other Features
Thyrotrope	Basophil	5–7	Heterogeneous (150–250 nm)	TSH	Anteromedial areas; increased in primary thyroid failure
Gonadotrope	Chromophobe or basophil	5–7	Varying size	LH FSH	Dispersed throughout the gland and often adjacent to lactotropes. Some cells may secrete only LH or FSH. Increased in gonadal failure and reduced in pregnancy
Corticotrope	Chromophobe or basophil	18–20	Large (300–400 nm) in intermediate lobe cells Smaller (200–300 nm) in anterior lobe cells	ACTH β-Lipotropin β-Endorphin Other POMC-derived hormones	One group is in the intermediate lobe. Other cells are in the anteromedial part of the pituitary. These cells increase in adrenal failure and degranulate (Crooke's changes) with cortisol excess, suggesting that they are the site of ACTH secretion.
Somatotrope	Acidophil or chromophobe	45–50	Dense, 250–500 nm	Growth hormone	Lateral areas of gland
Lactotrope	Acidophil or chromophobe	10–20	Large, varying in size (600–1,000 nm)	Prolactin	Dispersed through the gland, most in lateral areas; increased in pregnancy to 60–70% of cells and to a lesser degree with estrogen therapy
Other		10–15	Often granulated	?	Not identified as hormone secreting by present techniques. May represent undifferentiated cells or may secrete unidentified hormones

ACTH, adrenocorticotropic hormone; FSH, follicle-stimulating hormone; LH, luteinizing hormone; POMC; prooplomelanocortin; TSH, thyroid-stimulating hormone.

nin is a precursor for melatonin synthesis in the pineal and also functions as a neurotransmitter; its storage, release, and reuptake processes are similar to those of catecholamines. Cyproheptadine and methysergide are serotonin antagonists, and lysergic acid diethylamide acts as an agonist; serotonin effects are potentiated by monoamine oxidase inhibitors and some tricyclic drugs. Endogenous opioid peptides (endorphins, enkephalins, and dynorphin) are present in the hypothalamus and exert predominantly inhibitory effects, mainly on GnRH secretion. Endorphins appear to be the principle product of proopiomelanocortin metabolism in the brain, and dynorphin is secreted by the magnocellular neurons that secrete arginine vasopressin.

There are other neurotransmitters. Histamine acts through two types of receptors: H_1, blocked by such antihistamines as diphenhydramine, and H_2, blocked by cimetidine and ranitidine. Acetylcholine also acts through two receptor types, muscarinic and nicotinic, with muscarinic effects being blocked by atropine. Gamma-aminobutyric acid (GABA) is formed from L-glutamate and appears to function as an inhibitory neurotransmitter, though it may have a stimulatory role in GH regulation.

Hypophysiotropic Hormones

TRH was the first hypothalamic hormone to be isolated and characterized and has subsequently been shown to be widely distributed throughout the CNS and the gut. TRH release is stimulated by norepinephrine and dopamine and is inhibited by serotonin. TRH causes release of TSH and prolactin, though the physiologic importance of its action on prolactin secretion is uncertain. TRH-stimulated secretion of TSH is inhibited by somatostatin, by thyroxine and triiodothyronine, and by dopamine and high levels of glucocorticoids. TRH is used in the clinical assessment of pituitary function and in the evaluation of thyrotoxicosis. In acromegalic patients, TRH induces secretion of GH.

GnRH stimulates the synthesis and release of LH and FSH (Fig. 403.3). GnRH is secreted in a series of pulses, and regulation of secretion is discussed in detail later. GnRH is available for clinical assessment of pituitary gonadotrope responsiveness, but its value is limited. Because GnRH is required to stimulate LH synthesis, the absence of LH release with GnRH stimulation may result from deficient endogenous GnRH secretion or from absence of functional gonadotropes.

CRH is the major regulator of ACTH release and is secreted in pulses that occur more frequently during sleep and produce the nocturnal increase in ACTH and cortisol secretion. Secretion of CRH is influenced by numerous neurotransmitters. Acetylcholine stimulates CRH release and is involved in the so-called stress-induced increase in CRH secretion. Serotonin also stimu-

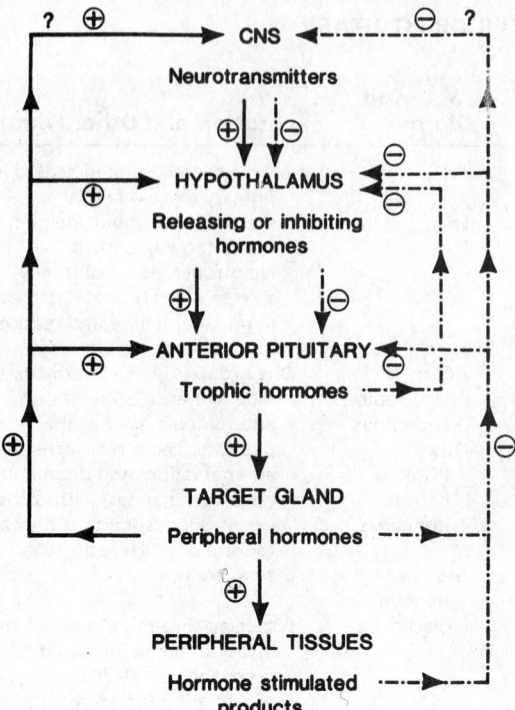

FIGURE 403.2. Feedback regulation of hypothalamic and anterior pituitary function. Stimulatory (+) feedback pathways are shown as solid lines; inhibitory (−) pathways, as dashed lines. Question marks indicate presumed pathways.

lates CRH secretion, but GABA, norepinephrine, enkephalin, and melatonin are inhibitory, and melatonin may be involved in reducing CRH secretion during periods of daylight. CRH stimulation of ACTH secretion is enhanced by vasopressin and is blocked by somatostatin and elevated levels of glucocorticoids. CRH can be used in the assessment of excess cortisol secretion. ACTH responses to CRH are enhanced in Cushing's disease despite the elevated levels of plasma cortisol, but they are reduced

or absent in Cushing's syndrome stemming from adrenal tumors or ectopic ACTH secretion.

GH-RH was originally isolated from a GH-RH-secreting pancreatic tumor in a patient with acromegaly. Somatotrope hyperplasia was present in the pituitary gland, which was the clue to the presence of an ectopic GH-RH-secreting tumor. Subsequently, GH-RH has been identified in the hypothalamus and is also present in the pancreas. GH-RH shows structural homology to a family of hormones that includes glucagon, secretin, vasoactive intestinal peptide, and gastric inhibitory peptide. Hypothalamic GH-RH secretion is stimulated by dopamine, norepinephrine, epinephrine, GABA, acetylcholine, and serotonin. GH-RH stimulates GH secretion, and this action is blocked by somatostatin. The regulation of GH release involves a complex interplay between GH-RH and somatostatin; however, GH-RH appears to play the predominant role, because GH levels fall after pituitary stalk section. GH-RH has been used in clinical testing of pituitary function and has been shown to be effective in stimulating growth in GH-RH-deficient children.

Somatostatin originally was isolated from the hypothalamus, but it is now known to be widely distributed throughout the CNS and to function as a neurotransmitter in the cerebral cortex and spinal cord. Somatostatin also is present in the gut and in the D cells of the pancreatic islets; it regulates secretion of insulin and glucagon. Stimulation of hypothalamic somatostatin release is complex and not well understood. Norepinephrine, epinephrine, dopamine, GABA, and acetylcholine all have been found to increase somatostatin secretion. Hypothalamic somatostatin blocks the actions of GH-RH and blunts TRH-induced TSH release. The latter effect may be responsible for the TSH deficiency that can develop during GH therapy of GH-deficient children (GH stimulates somatostatin release). Somatostatin, and particularly long-acting analogues of somatostatin (octreotide), have been used successfully in the treatment of acromegaly and TSH-secreting pituitary tumors.

A family of small peptides and of their non-peptidyl analogues, collectively called GH secretagogues (GHS), have been

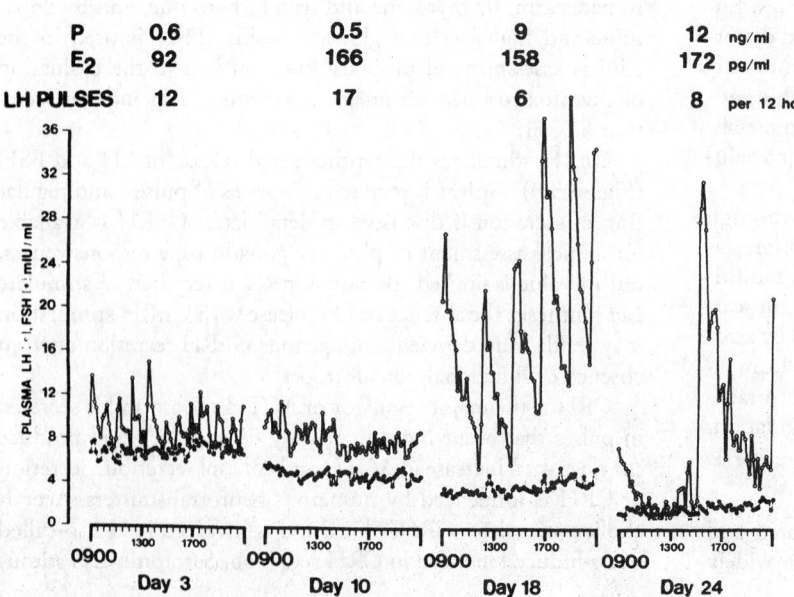

FIGURE 403.3. Patterns of pulsatile luteinizing hormone (LH; ○) and follicle stimulating hormone (FSH; ●)secretion and ovarian steroid concentrations during the early and late follicular (days 3 and 10) and luteal phases (days 18 and 24) of an ovulatory menstrual cycle. The first day of menstrual bleeding is designated day 1 of the cycle, and ovulation occurred on day 14. LH and FSH were measured in samples drawn every 10 minutes. P, progesterone, E_2, estradiol. (Marshall JC, Kelch RP, Saunder SE, et al. Pulsatile GnRH—studies of puberty and the menstrual cycle. In: Labrie F, ed. *Endocrinology. International Congress Series 655.* Amsterdam:Elsevier BV, 1984:25.)

TABLE 403.2.	ANTERIOR PITUITARY HORMONES AND THEIR ACTIONS		
Hormone	**Molecular Weight (d)**	**Structure**	**Stimulatory Action**
Glycoproteins			
TSH	29,000	All consist of two glycosylated subunit, α and β.	Thyroid hormone secretion
LH[a]	29,000	The α subunit is identical, and the β subunit	Gonadal steroid secretion
FSH	29,000	confers biologic specificity.	Ovarian follicle development and testicular spermatogenesis
POMC-derived hormones			
POMC	29,000	Precursor hormone	
ACTH	4500	Midportion of POMC	Adrenocortical hormone secretion
α-MSH	1800	N-terminal amino acids of ACTH	Uncertain
CLIP	2400	C-terminal amino acids of ACTH	Uncertain
β-Lipotropin	11,200	C-terminal portion of POMC	Uncertain
β-Endorphin	4000	C-terminal amino acids of β-lipotropin	Uncertain
Somatomammotropins			
GHT[b]	22,000	Single-chain proteins with disulfide bridges	Somatomedin-C production and direct metabolic effects
Prolactin	23,000		Lactation

[a] Chorionic gonadotropin has actions similar to those of LH and also consists of α and β subunits.
[b] Placental lactogen (chorionic somatomammotrophin) has a structure (80% homology) similar to that of GH.
ACTH, adrenocorticropic hormone; CLIP, corticotropin-like intermediate lobe peptide; FSH, follicle-stimulating hormone; GH, growth hormone; LH, luteinizing hormone; α-MSH, α-melanocyte stimulating hormone; POMC, proopiomelanocortin, TSH, thyroid-stimulating hormone.

shown to stimulate GH secretion. A specific receptor for GHS has been found in the hypothalamus and the pituitary. The GHS receptor and its intracellular second messenger system leading to GH release are distinct from GH-RH, which strongly supports the existence of a still unidentified endogenous hypothalamic peptide that serves as a "third regulator" of GH secretion. Dopamine is the predominant regulator of prolactin secretion, but evidence suggests that a prolactin-releasing hormone, not yet identified, is present in the hypothalamus. The role of these compounds in regulating prolactin secretion is discussed later.

The actions of hypophysiotropic hormones are modified by circulating levels of the respective target gland hormones, cortisol, somatomedin C, thyroxine, androgens, and estrogens. These hormones can modify hypophysiotropic hormone modulation of the number of hypophysiotropic hormone receptors on specific pituitary cells. They also exert effects at postreceptor sites, including regulation of transcription, though the exact mechanisms of action remain to be identified.

ANTERIOR PITUITARY HORMONES

The hormones produced by the anterior pituitary can be grouped into three types: glycoproteins (TSH, LH, FSH), proopiomelanocortin-derived peptides, and somatomammotropins (GH and prolactin). The structural characteristics of the hormones and their main actions are shown in Table 403.2.

DISORDERS OF THE HYPOTHALAMUS AND ANTERIOR PITUITARY

Disorders of the hypothalamus and pituitary may take the form of endocrine or neurologic dysfunction. Hyposecretion or hyper-

secretion of one or more pituitary hormones can occur, and neurologic manifestations are caused by pressure effects from tumors or reflect abnormal autonomic function. The clinical endocrine manifestations of hypothalamic and pituitary disorders are similar, and it may be difficult to differentiate hypothalamic and pituitary causes of abnormal hormone secretion.

HYPOTHALAMIC DISORDERS

The hypothalamus regulates both endocrine and autonomic function. Small lesions may cause symptoms if they affect a specific hypothalamic nucleus, but lesions are often large and bilateral before clinical evidence becomes apparent. Hypothalamic tumors are commonly slow growing and usually cause endocrine abnormalities, eating disturbances, or cognitive dysfunction. Patients with rapidly expanding lesions often experience autonomic dysfunction or coma. Diseases that may show initial symptoms of hypothalamic disorders are shown in Table 403.3.

Clinical Findings

Hypothalamic disorders may be neurologic, endocrine, or a mixture of the two. In some instances, endocrine failure may result in symptoms similar to neurologic dysfunction. If temperature regulation is abnormal, hypothyroidism and cortisol deficiency should be excluded before attributing the symptoms to neurologic causes.

Neurologic Findings

Eating Behavior

Lesions of the ventromedial nuclei lead to loss of satiety, hyperphagia, and progressive obesity. Hypothalamic lesions are a rare

TABLE 403.3.   DISEASES THAT MAY HAVE INITIAL SIGNS OF ABNORMAL HYPOTHALAMIC FUNCTION

Idiopathic
  Isolated or multiple hypophysiotropic hormone deficiency[a]
Tumors
  Craniopharyngiomas and ependymomas
  Gliomas (particularly of the optic nerve)
  Pituitary tumors (with suprasellar extension)
  Meningiomas
  Germinomas (includes pinealomas)
  Hamartomas and gangliocytomas
  Lymphomas and leukemia
  Metastases
Granulomatous diseases
  Sarcoidosis
  Tuberculosis
  Histiocytosis X (children)
Vascular abnormalities
  Aneurysms
  Infarction
  Subarachnoid hemorrhage (late complication)
Infections
  Bacterial meningitis (especially tuberculosis)
  Viral encephalitis
Others
  Hydrocephalus
  Colloid cysts of the third ventricle
  Postradiation therapy (to nasopharynx or pituitary)
  Demyelinating diseases
  Trauma
  Wernicke's disease
  Laurence-Moon-Biedl syndrome
  Prader-Willi syndrome
  Anorexia nervosa

[a] These disorders appear as deficiencies of pituitary hormone secretion and are discussed in the section on hypopituitarism.

cause of obesity, but unidentified abnormalities of satiety regulation may be present in some obese patients. The lateral hypothalamus monitors hunger, and bilateral lesions result in anorexia. In men with apparent anorexia nervosa, a hypothalamic lesion should be sought actively.

Temperature Regulation

The hypothalamus monitors and increases core temperature. Prostaglandin E is involved in raising the set point, which results in increased heat production (shivering) and reduced heat loss (vasoconstriction). Hypothalamic diseases also may alter temperature regulation in cycles lasting days to weeks. Hyperthermia with paroxysms of fever, shaking, chills, and sweating may be interspersed with periods of normal temperature regulation. Hypothermia occasionally is reported and may be associated with sweating and flushing. More often, sustained hypothermia reflects hypothyroidism, which may also be of hypothalamic origin.

Thirst

Hypothalamic osmoreceptors monitor serum osmolality and regulate water excretion through secretion of antidiuretic hormone (ADH). The syndrome of inappropriate ADH secretion may develop in association with hypothalamic lesions, meningitis, or subarachnoid hemorrhage. Hypothalamic lesions also may inhibit ADH release, and if perception of thirst is lost, it may lead to hypernatremia and dehydration. Now and then, primary polydipsia may occur, which is difficult to distinguish from diabetes insipidus.

Memory, Behavior, and Sleep

In Wernicke's encephalopathy, hemorrhage into the mammillary bodies and hypothalamus may occur and is associated with short-term memory loss. Ventromedial lesions can lead to expressions of rage, whereas lateral lesions typically result in apathy. Dementia may be a symptom of bilateral lesions. Sleep patterns also can be disturbed; agitation and insomnia are features of anterior hypothalamic lesions, and marked somnolence or coma occur with posterior lesions.

Autonomic Nervous System Functions

Diencephalic epilepsy is a rare condition characterized by episodes of increased autonomic activity. Anterior hypothalamic lesions usually affect parasympathetic outflow, whereas posterior lesions result in sympathetic manifestations.

Endocrine Findings

Endocrine manifestations of hypothalamic disease reflect altered secretion of hypothalamic hormones. Usually, secretion is reduced. Because most hypothalamic hormones stimulate pituitary secretion, the typical clinical picture is hypopituitarism. A hypothalamic origin of deficiencies of TSH, GH, ACTH, and gonadotropin can be differentiated from pituitary causes by the injection of hypophysiotropic hormones. Normal increases in plasma TSH after injection of TRH, in GH after injection of GH-RH, in ACTH after injection of CRH, and in LH and FSH after repeated injections of GnRH indicate a hypothalamic origin.

Pituitary Hypofunction

Deficiency of hypophysiotropic hormones usually is reported in children as *idiopathic hypopituitarism* and commonly involves several hypothalamic hormones. Hypothalamic lesions can produce single or several hormone deficiencies. Isolated deficiencies of TRH, CRH, and, most often, GnRH or GH-RH also may be seen in the absence of demonstrable hypothalamic disease.

On occasion, hypophysiotropic hormone deficiency may be functional and reversible. In emotional deprivation syndromes (psychosocial dwarfism), spontaneous GH secretion may be impaired, and GH responses to provocative stimuli are subnormal. After several days in a better home environment, GH secretion is restored, and linear growth resumes. This finding probably reflects restoration of normal neurotransmitter regulation of GH-RH secretion. Similarly, GnRH deficiency may develop after severe weight loss (to less than 70% of ideal body weight) from any cause and is reversible after weight gain. Amenorrhea seen in female athletes results from reduced GnRH secretion, which may be provoked by excess hypothalamic opioid activity and consequent suppression of GnRH pulse frequency. Reduced GnRH pulse frequency is the cause of amenorrhea in the context of hyperprolactinemia. GnRH secretion returns to normal after suppression of prolactin by bromocriptine or removal of a prolactinoma.

Pituitary Hyperfunction

Less commonly, hypothalamic diseases may appear in the form of pituitary hypersecretion. Idiopathic hyperprolactinemia is a disorder in which serum prolactin is elevated (usually to more than 100 ng per milliliter) in the absence of established pituitary or hypothalamic disease. Irregular ovulation and amenorrhea are noted, and the disorder is rare in women older than 40 years of age. The abnormality presumably reflects reduced dopamine secretion, and in many cases the disorder appears to be self-limiting. Serum prolactin levels do not rise, and in half the patients they tend to fall over 5 to 10 years of follow-up.

Precocious puberty may be the initial feature of hypothalamic disease in children. In girls, anatomic lesions usually are not found, but in boys a tumor should always be sought. The presence of hypothalamic tumors may initiate the early onset of normal mechanisms of pubertal maturation. Other tumors have been shown to contain GnRH or human chorionic gonadotropin (hCG). GnRH stimulates pituitary LH and FSH secretion, whereas hCG acts on the gonad to increase steroid synthesis.

Acromegaly or gigantism also may result from hypothalamic tumors; some tumors have been shown to secrete GH-RH, with consequent GH release. Cerebral gigantism is a syndrome in children characterized by rapid growth, accelerated bone age, clumsiness, and sometimes mental retardation. Enlarged cerebral ventricles may be seen on computed tomographic (CT) scan, but hypothalamic tumors are not found. Hormone data are limited, but GH secretion appears to be normal and the mechanisms of rapid growth are unknown.

Polycystic ovarian disease may result from increased GnRH pulse frequency, leading to enhanced LH secretion with consequent development of ovarian cysts and excess ovarian androgen secretion. This would explain the hirsutism, amenorrhea, and elevated serum LH levels usually found in this syndrome, but definite evidence of abnormal GnRH regulation is lacking.

Hypothalamic Tumors

Hypothalamic tumors usually are located in the midline beneath the third ventricle. The most common tumors are craniopharyngiomas and their variants (epidermoid cysts and ependymomas), followed by gliomas and germinomas. The tumors may lead to any of the neurologic or endocrine manifestations described previously, but the common symptoms are visual abnormalities, raised intracranial pressure, diabetes insipidus, hypogonadism, or delayed puberty and growth retardation.

Craniopharyngiomas

Craniopharyngiomas arise from remnants of Rathke's pouch and hence are of ectodermal origin. Most tumors are suprasellar and have features of a hypothalamic disorder, though others are partly intrasellar and partly suprasellar. Craniopharyngiomas may appear in childhood, but more than half the patients are older than 20 years of age at diagnosis. The tumors are benign and usually cystic. They contain a thick, cholesterol-rich fluid, and half are calcified.

In children, the usual manifestations are headache, vomiting, and papilledema due to increased intracranial pressure or hydrocephalus. Visual field defects are often present; less common findings are short stature, delayed puberty, and diabetes insipidus. In adults, visual abnormalities and field defects are present in 80% to 90% of cases. Papilledema is less typical, but headaches, hypogonadism, and mental or behavioral changes occur in 20% to 40% of patients. The serum prolactin level is elevated (less than 150 ng per milliliter) in about half the patients; diabetes insipidus, weight gain, and panhypopituitarism occur less frequently (10% to 20%). The presence of curvilinear suprasellar calcification on skull roentgenography or CT scan suggests a craniopharyngioma, but other hypothalamic tumors may calcify. Treatment of craniopharyngiomas is difficult. If feasible, total removal of the lesion is preferred and is often associated with long remissions. Complete removal usually is not possible, however; in that case, drainage of the cyst fluid or partial removal is carried out, followed by postoperative radiation therapy to reduce the rate of tumor regrowth. For predominantly cystic craniopharyngiomas, stereotactic intracavitary instillation of phosphorus-32 appears to be effective.

Germinomas

Germinomas (atypical teratomas, pinealomas, ectopic pinealomas) are often adjacent to the lower part of the third ventricle and usually infiltrate the hypothalamus. The tumors may metastasize through the cerebrospinal fluid (CSF) to the meninges and form distal deposits. Diabetes insipidus is a common initial feature, as is precocious puberty in boys. The mechanisms of sexual precocity are unclear. Some tumors infiltrate the hypothalamus and remove the normal prepubertal inhibition of GnRH secretion. Human chorionic gonadotropin has been found in other tumors, and plasma levels of hCG may be elevated. The management of these tumors is difficult—surgical removal usually is not possible. Tumors containing mainly germinal elements are radiosensitive, but those with a predominantly teratomatous component may be resistant.

Hamartomas and Gangliocytomas

Hamartomas typically are located in the posterior hypothalamus, are capsulated, and contain disorganized neuronal and glial tissue. The neurons may incorporate neurosecretory granules. GnRH often is secreted by the tumor, and increased LH and FSH release may cause precocious puberty. Treatment is directed toward inhibiting pubertal maturation, preventing premature epiphyseal fusion, and restoring growth potential. Long-acting GnRH agonists, which desensitize gonadotrope responses to GnRH, have been shown to be effective in arresting pubertal maturation and slowing accelerated bone maturation. Some hypothalamic hamartomas have been shown to contain GH-RH and to result in GH hypersecretion and acromegaly. A similar tumor, the gangliocytoma, has been found within the pituitary and may contain GH-RH or CRH. These tumors are rare causes of acromegaly or Cushing's disease.

Granulomatous Diseases

Histiocytosis X

Histiocytosis X is a histiocytic/eosinophilic granulomatous disorder that manifests as different clinical types. Hand-Schüller-Christian disease is the type commonly associated with hypothalamic deposits and usually is accompanied by diabetes insipidus (50%), defects in bone, and exophthalmos. GH deficiency, hypogonadism, and panhypopituitarism also may develop; they are usually permanent and require replacement hormonal therapy. Diagnosis rests on biopsy findings, and treatment consists of glucocorticoids or chemotherapy.

Sarcoidosis

Hypothalamic or suprasellar deposits are uncommon in sarcoidosis. When they arise, they typically manifest as a thickening of the stalk, which enhances on the MRI after gadolinium contrast administration. CNS involvement is suggested by the presence of diabetes insipidus, an elevated serum prolactin level (less than 150 ng per milliliter), or galactorrhea or by varying degrees of hypopituitarism. Endocrine dysfunction rarely improves with glucocorticoid therapy for sarcoidosis.

Radiation Therapy

Hypothalamic and pituitary abnormalities may appear several years after radiation therapy for nasopharyngeal or intracranial tumors. The effects of radiation are rarely evident until 1 to 3 years after treatment and may arise 10 or more years later. Hypopituitarism often develops after radiation therapy in children; GH and LH-FSH deficiencies are the most common side effects. Radiation may involve both the hypothalamus and the pituitary, but studies using releasing hormones suggest that the major lesion is one of hypothalamic dysfunction.

Trauma

Head injuries that result in coma may be associated with hypothalamic-pituitary failure. Gonadotropin and TSH deficiencies have been described, presumably as a result of defective releasing hormone secretion; these effects may improve with time. If the pituitary stalk has been severed, anterior pituitary hormone deficiency is usually permanent, and diabetes insipidus is also present. Stalk damage often is seen in the context of basal skull fractures.

Syndromes Associated with Hypothalamic Dysfunction

Laurence-Moon-Biedl and Prader–Willi Syndromes

Laurence-Moon-Biedl and Prader–Willi syndromes are familial disorders associated with characteristic facies, mental retardation, and hypotonia. The Laurence-Moon-Biedl syndrome is characterized by retinitis pigmentosa, polydactyly, and congenital heart defects. Abnormalities of hypothalamic function include hyperphagia, resulting in severe obesity, disordered diurnal rhythms, temperature dysregulation, and hypogonadism. The latter is caused by reduced GnRH secretion, but other hypophysiotropic hormones are usually intact.

Anorexia Nervosa

Anorexia nervosa is a disorder of unknown origin that typically takes the form of anorexia, severe weight loss, and amenorrhea (see Chapter 37). Several aspects of hypothalamic-pituitary function are abnormal. Amenorrhea results from reduced GnRH secretion, which reverts to the low-amplitude, slow-frequency pattern seen in prepubertal girls. If weight is regained, GnRH secretion returns to the adult pattern by rising first during sleep and later during the day, a progression identical to that seen in normal pubertal maturation.

Approach to the Patient with Suspected Hypothalamic Dysfunction

The initial features of hypothalamic dysfunction vary widely (for example, with the age of the patient) and may be endocrine or neurologic in nature. In adults, the presence of diabetes insipidus, alone or in association with hypopituitarism, is suggestive of hypothalamic disease. Pituitary hormone secretion should be assessed; a head CT or magnetic resonance imaging (MRI) test is needed to exclude a pituitary or hypothalamic mass lesion. If individual hormone deficiencies are found, the diagnosis of hypothalamic failure can be confirmed by normal pituitary responses to releasing hormones. Treatment is directed to replacing deficient hormones, particularly cortisol and thyroxine and, if appropriate, by surgical removal of a tumor.

PITUITARY TUMORS

Pituitary tumors represent 10% to 15% of intracranial tumors diagnosed during life. They may be more common, however, because small adenomas have been reported in up to 30% of autopsy series. In most cases, the cause is unknown, though some hormone-secreting tumors may stem from enhanced stimulation by hypophysiotropic hormones. Studies have indicated that most, if not all, pituitary tumors are monoclonal (they appear to arise from a single cell). A single-cell somatic mutation, rather than diffuse hypothalamic stimulation, is likely to be the initiating event in pituitary tumorigenesis. Pituitary tumors are almost always benign in histologic manifestations and usually expand slowly over a period of years. On occasion, tumors may be aggressive and invade surrounding structures, but true pituitary carcinomas are rare.

Tumors are classified based on immunocytochemical staining for pituitary hormones, which characterizes the cell type, identifies the tumor product, and allows correlation with serum hormone levels. With this system, 15% to 20% of pituitary adenomas are apparently nonfunctioning. Classification by size is based on radiologic findings. Stage I tumors are microadenomas (less than 1 cm) without sella expansion, stage II tumors are macroadenomas (more than 1 cm) and may extend above the sella, stage III tumors are macroadenomas with enlargement and invasion of the sella floor or with suprasellar extension, and stage IV tumors are macroadenomas with extensive invasion or destruction of the sella turcica.

Clinical Findings

Patients with pituitary adenomas may have initial endocrine symptoms or neurologic features due to pressure effects; alternatively, the lesion may be found incidentally on skull roentgenography or CT scan. In the past, tumors were large at diagnosis, and patients usually first experienced neurologic symptoms. Improvements in hormone assays have led to earlier diagnosis, and fewer than 20% of patients now have visual field defects as a first symptom.

Endocrine Findings

Endocrine features may be those of hypopituitarism, hypersecretion of one or more hormones, or a mixture of hypofunction and hyperfunction. Patients with nonfunctioning tumors usually have initial symptoms of hypopituitarism. Hypogonadism may reflect destruction of pituitary gonadotropes but more often results from suppression of GnRH secretion by an elevated prolactin level. The most common functioning pituitary tumors are prolactinomas, followed by GH- and ACTH-secreting tumors. TSH- and gonadotropin-secreting tumors are rare. Tumors may secrete more than one hormone; immunocytochemical studies have shown that 10% to 20% of tumors fall into this category. GH and prolactin commonly are co-secreted, and GH-TSH and ACTH-prolactin secretion also has been described.

Functioning tumors produce symptoms early. ACTH-secreting tumors in both sexes and prolactinomas in women typically are diagnosed as microadenomas. In men, the early symptoms of hypogonadism are impotence and loss of libido. These symptoms often are not investigated; as a consequence, prolactinomas and nonfunctioning tumors often are large at the time of diagnosis. Symptoms of acromegaly also are not recognized early in men, and GH-secreting tumors are frequently large at diagnosis. Pituitary tumors may develop as part of the multiple endocrine neoplasia type 1 syndrome (see Chapter 415). Generally, GH-secreting or prolactin-secreting tumors are found, but nonfunctioning tumors also may be associated with parathyroid and pancreatic tumors.

Neurologic Findings

Headache is the most common symptom of pituitary tumor and is usually present in patients with large tumors. The headache is often generalized, tends to be of a dull character, and frequently is not relieved by analgesics. It is believed to result from pressure on the diaphragma sellae, and sudden cessation of headache may signal rupture of the diaphragma.

Visual field defects develop in patients with large tumors with suprasellar extensions—they are the initial symptom in 20% of cases. The classic defect is a bitemporal hemianopsia, but field defects vary and often are asymmetric. In 80% of patients, the optic chiasm lies 0.5 to 1 cm above the diaphragma sellae, but it may be prefixed (anterior to the tuberculum sellae) or postfixed (overlying the dorsum sellae) in the other 20%. Visual field defects depend on the relative positions of the optic chiasm and the tumor, and they range in character from small, uniocular scotomata to varying degrees of field loss in both eyes. Consequently, clinical testing of peripheral fields is not adequate, and formal assessment by Goldman perimetry should be undertaken.

Oculomotor nerve palsies occur if the tumor extends laterally into the cavernous sinus. Palsies typically are unilateral, and diplopia due to third cranial nerve involvement is most common. Fourth and fifth cranial nerve palsies may be seen alone or together. Diminished sensation or pain in the face indicates involvement of the fifth cranial nerve. Pituitary adenomas rarely cause papilledema, which, when present, suggests a craniopharyngioma. Suprasellar extension of pituitary tumors may be large (3 to 5 cm), and patients have initial symptoms of hypothalamic dysfunction. Rarely, tumors extend over or through the dorsum sella, compress the brain stem, and manifest as long tract signs. Occasionally, compression of the temporal lobe produces seizures, and erosion down into the sphenoid sinus may appear in the form of CSF rhinorrhea or nasopharyngeal bleeding.

Pituitary Apoplexy

Infarction may occur after hemorrhage into a tumor and is more common in large tumors and after radiation therapy. The clinical manifestations vary, ranging from the acute onset of severe headache that resolves spontaneously over a few days to progression to coma and circulatory collapse. Mild forms of the syndrome are probably more common than is recognized. Patients with large tumors often have a history of acute headache, fever, and mild meningismus. Frequently, the history shows that the patient visited an emergency department and that spinal tap confirmed the presence of a few white or red blood cells or xanthochromia. In these circumstances, a diagnosis of viral encephalitis often is made, and symptoms resolve spontaneously over the next few days.

Severe forms of pituitary apoplexy are life-threatening situations. Onset is dramatic, with severe headache, vomiting, and progressive loss of consciousness. Meningismus is marked, and there may be third, fourth, and sixth cranial nerve paresis with periorbital hemorrhage, suggesting cavernous sinus thrombosis. CSF examination shows several hundred white and red blood cells, which may suggest subarachnoid hemorrhage. Angiography may be required to exclude a leaking aneurysm, but the presence of an enlarged sella on roentgenography strongly suggests the diagnosis. Acute hypopituitarism with hypotension requires immediate replacement of fluids and hydrocortisone. Deficiency of thyroid and gonadal function may develop over days to weeks.

Acute surgical decompression by the transsphenoidal route is indicated in the context of acute neurologic pressure symptoms. Studies have suggested, however, that this treatment may not be necessary in all cases, and recovery has been reported after supportive therapy with intravenous fluids and hydrocortisone. If visual symptoms are pronounced, however, decompression reduces pressure on the optic or oculomotor nerves.

After recovery of pituitary apoplexy, pituitary function may be normal or partially or completely deficient. Formal assessment of pituitary function should be carried out. Infarction of a functioning pituitary tumor may result in diminution of pituitary hypersecretion, but true normalization of secretion or "spontaneous cure" of pituitary tumors is exceedingly rare.

Diagnosis

Evaluation of pituitary tumors consists of assessment of pituitary function, assessment of tumor anatomy by radiologic procedures, and differentiation of pituitary tumors from extrasellar or parasellar lesions or the empty sella syndrome. Endocrine tests should be conducted before therapy, because the results influence subsequent treatment. In hormone-secreting tumors (particularly prolactinomas), medical therapy may be the optimal approach. Basal hormone studies always should be obtained before treatment, and appropriate replacement therapy should be given before surgery. If progressive visual loss or other neurologic symptoms necessitate immediate surgery, preoperative hydrocortisone in stress doses should be administered.

Radiologic Assessment of the Pituitary

Plain roentgenograms of the skull identify an enlarged sella and show bony erosions due to a large tumor (Fig. 403.4). Irregulari-

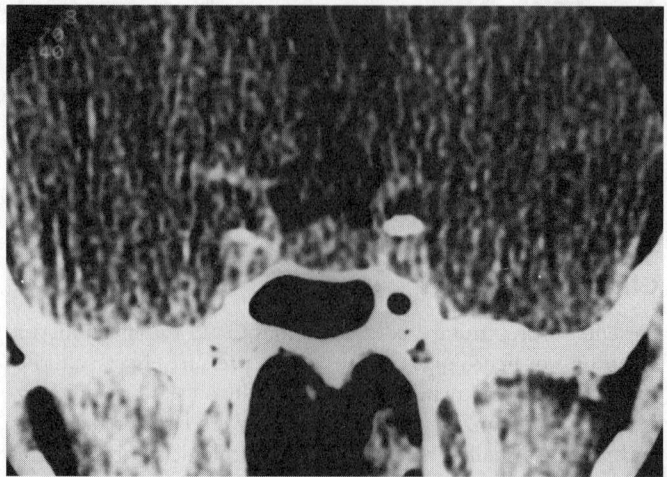

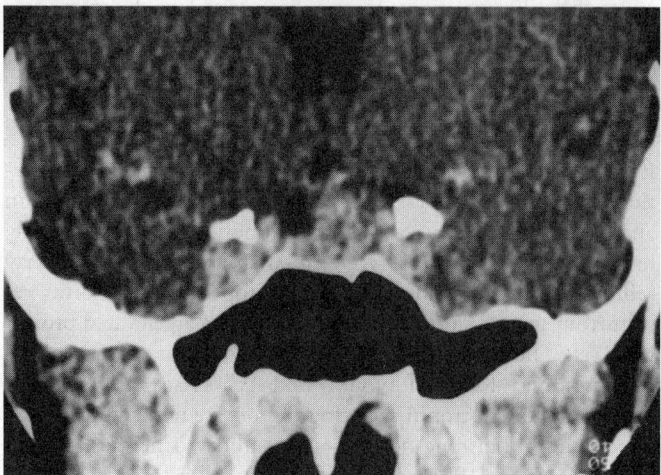

FIGURE 403.5. Computed tomography scans showing pituitary tumors. Both scans were taken in the coronal plane after contrast injection in patients with acromegaly. In the upper panel, the tumor was small and intrasellar and is seen as an upward bulging on the upper surface of the center of the pituitary. The lower panel shows a large tumor with a suprasellar extension on the right side and in the midline. The nonenhancing area on the left side of the fossa is cerebrospinal fluid in a partially empty sella.

ties of the sella floor, particularly the presence of a double floor, may suggest the presence of an intrasellar tumor. CT scanning or MRI is needed to verify intrasellar lesions and to define the extent of any suprasellar extension. CT scans with contrast enhancement usually show homogeneous enhancement of the pituitary, but areas of low density are seen in 20% of normal subjects, which can cause problems in the diagnosis of microadenomas. In coronal views, microadenomas typically appear as hypodense areas within the pituitary, though small lesions (less than 3 mm) are difficult to detect (Fig. 403.5). Macroadenomas generally manifest as an enhancing intrasellar mass, though the center may be hypodense or the sella partially empty, suggesting previous infarction. MRI offers better delineation of the tumor and the surrounding soft tissues, such as the optic chiasm and the cavernous sinus content (internal carotid artery and cranial nerves) (Fig. 403.6). This is facilitated by gadolinium enhancement. MRI does not provide direct information about surround-

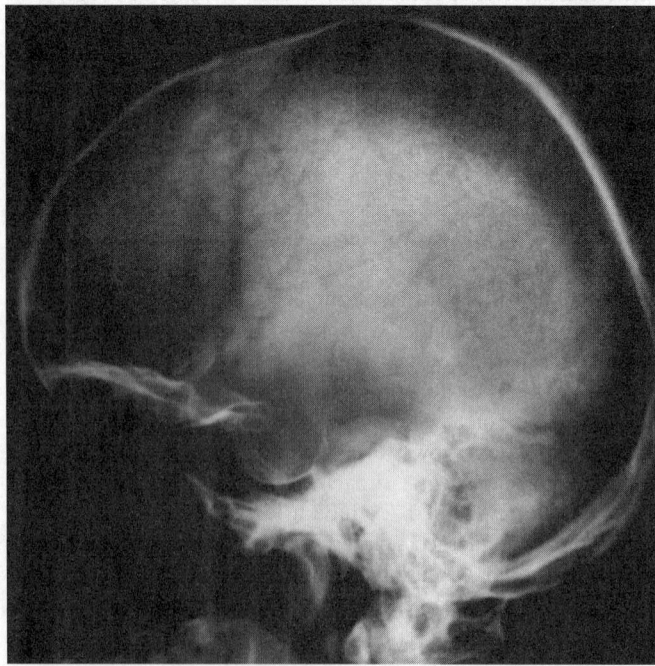

FIGURE 403.4. Lateral skull roentgenogram in a 57-year-old man who presented with bitemporal hemianopia and hypogonadism due to a nonfunctioning pituitary tumor. The sella is enlarged, a double floor is present, and the dorsum sella has been eroded by the tumor. (Courtesy of T.O. Gabrielsen, M.D.)

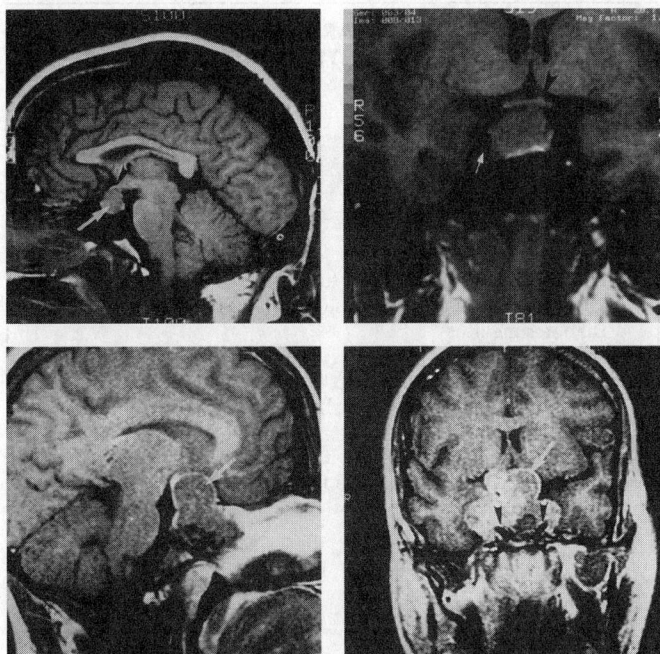

FIGURE 403.6. Magnetic resonance imaging scans in two patients with acromegaly. The upper panel shows coronal and sagittal images of a generous macroadenoma (*thick white arrow*) that reaches the optic chiasm (*black arrow*) and borders on the right internal carotid artery (*thin white arrow*). The lower panel shows coronal and sagittal images of a giant tumor. Optic chiasm is not discernible, and both cavernous sinus are invaded. Integral carotid arteries (*black arrows*) are firmly embedded within the tumor.

ing bone structures, however. In some instances, homogeneous enhancement of suprasellar or parasellar areas may be difficult to differentiate from aneurysms, and angiography is required to establish the diagnosis.

Secondary Pituitary Enlargement

Failure of a target gland (thyroid, adrenals, gonads) results in loss of negative feedback and resultant hyperplasia of the corresponding pituitary cells. Occasionally, this leads to significant pituitary enlargement, which may compromise other pituitary function in rare cases. The finding of an enlarged sella, together with evidence of target gland hypofunction, may lead to erroneous diagnosis of a true pituitary tumor. This is especially pertinent in the context of primary hypothyroidism, in which the serum prolactin level may be elevated. The finding of an elevated trophic hormone level provides the clue to the true nature of the process; appropriate replacement therapy is followed by the shrinkage of the hyperplastic pituitary and restoration of pituitary function.

Empty Sella Syndrome

The usual clinical picture in empty sella syndrome is the finding of an enlarged sella turcica on roentgenography. It is important to consider this syndrome in the differential diagnosis of pituitary tumors. In the primary empty sella syndrome, the sella is symmetrically enlarged and partially filled with CSF. The pituitary gland is flattened to a crescent of tissue in the lower posterior part of the sella. The origin of the syndrome is unknown; it may be associated with previous raised intracranial pressure. In most instances, the abnormality is believed to result from a defect in the diaphragma sellae, which allows CSF pressure to herniate the arachnoid down into the sella turcica, resulting in ballooning of the bony sella. The primary empty sella syndrome should be distinguished from a partially empty sella resulting from infarction of the pituitary tumor. The latter condition is suggested by an irregularly enlarged sella and by a double floor or erosions of the surrounding bone.

The primary empty sella syndrome usually develops in women, and headaches may be the initial feature. Most patients are obese and multiparous, and one-third have hypertension. CSF rhinorrhea occurs from time to time, and a minority of patients have a history of pseudotumor cerebri. Pituitary function is typically normal, but sometimes mild hyperprolactinemia may be present, perhaps because of stretching of the pituitary stalk. Dynamic testing may show impairment of TSH and GH reserve, which may reflect concomitant obesity. The diagnosis is established by CT scan or MRI and the presence of normal endocrine function. No therapy is required in most cases, though CSF rhinorrhea needs surgical correction.

Optimal Management

Treatment of pituitary tumors is aimed at limiting hormonal oversecretion, preventing progressive loss of pituitary function, and halting progression of tumor size. Medical therapy is often successful in hyperprolactinemia and in some patients with acromegaly. In other hormone-secreting tumors and in nonfunctioning tumors, medical therapy is ineffective, and treatment consists of pituitary surgery or radiation therapy. The optimal mode of therapy is the subject of controversy and often depends on experience in different centers. In considering treatment, the benefits and risks of therapy should be weighed against the present and future risks of the pituitary tumor. In Cushing's disease and acromegaly, it is important to prevent the progression of the metabolic effects of hormonal hypersecretion, and more aggressive approaches are appropriate. In nonfunctioning tumors without neurologic manifestations, expansion of the tumor takes place slowly. In an elderly patient, replacement of the hormone deficiency may be the most efficacious approach. In general, good results are obtained with microadenomas, but it is rarely possible to cure large tumors by surgery.

Surgery

Except for patients with large suprasellar extensions, pituitary surgery is carried out by the transsphenoidal route. This approach is safe, with a mortality rate of less than 0.5%; morbidity due to such complications as CSF rhinorrhea is also low (less than 2%). The transsphenoidal approach allows visualization of the sella contents, and microadenomas often can be removed selectively without impairment of other pituitary function. Glucocorticoids always should be administered during the perioperative period, even if preoperative testing does not show ACTH deficiency. Hydrocortisone, 100 mg, should be administered intravenously immediately before surgery, followed by 50 mg intramuscularly every 6 hours during the subsequent 2 or 3 days. A replacement hydrocortisone dose (usually 25 mg per day) typically is administered on discharge and continued before formal assessment of pituitary function 2 to 3 months later. Polyuria due to diabetes insipidus commonly is seen during the first 2 to 3 postoperative days and may require treatment with oral or intranasal desmopressin. Diabetes insipidus usually is transient and results from mild trauma to the pituitary stalk. If polyuria persists beyond 7 to 10 days after surgery, it suggests the presence of permanent stalk damage.

The results of surgery for microadenomas that secrete prolactin, GH, and ACTH are good; normalization of hypersecretion has been reported in 70% to 80% of cases. Results are not as good for macroadenomas. Excess secretion is abolished in less than 50% of patients, and a high proportion (10% to 20%) experience postoperative hypopituitarism. The efficacy of pituitary surgery is highly operator-dependent. Several studies have shown that in the hands of an experienced pituitary neurosurgeon (more than 200 to 500 previous operations), elimination of hormone hypersecretion is three to four times more common, and the complication rate is three to four times lower, than after intervention by a general neurosurgeon with only limited pituitary experience. Surgery is rarely successful in curing the mass effects of large tumors, and symptoms recur in 70% to 80% of patients. This rate can be lowered to 10% to 20% if postoperative radiation therapy is given.

Radiation Therapy

Radiation therapy often is used as an adjunct to surgical therapy of macroadenomas, but it also can be used as primary treatment. A major disadvantage is that the effects of radiation are delayed and suppression of pituitary hypersecretion may not be evident until 3 to 5 years after treatment. In addition, a growing body of evidence suggests that hypopituitarism, in part as a result of effects on the hypothalamus, is common after radiation therapy; as many as 50% of patients may experience it. Conventional radiation is given using a rotational technique, and 20 to 25 treatments over 4 to 6 weeks are required to deliver the total dose of 45 to 50 Gy. Heavy-particle therapy with proton beams or ?? -particles also can be used; this treatment has the advantage of delivering a higher radiation dose (up to 140 Gy) to the pituitary. This treatment allows somewhat improved results in limiting hypersecretion, but the full effects are still not manifest until several years after treatment, and the incidence of hypopituitarism may be higher than after conventional radiation therapy. This type of radiation therapy is contraindicated if significant suprasellar expansion is present, because it may lead to optic nerve damage. Stereotactic radiosurgery utilizing ?? -knife is rapidly becoming more widespread owing to the commercial availability of the equipment. Nevertheless, direct comparison of its efficacy versus conventional radiotherapy is still largely unavailable.

HYPOPITUITARISM

Hypopituitarism results from impaired secretion of one or more pituitary hormones. It may be caused by primary pituitary dis-

TABLE 403.4.	PITUITARY LESIONS CAUSING HYPOPITUITARISM

Tumors
 Pituitary adenoma
 Craniopharyngioma
 Metastatic carcinoma
 Primary pituitary carcinoma
 Meningioma
Pituitary infarction
 Pituitary apoplexy (pituitary tumor)
 Postpartum pituitary necrosis (Sheehan's syndrome)
 Diabetes mellitus
 Shock
 Sickle cell anemia (crisis)
 Infections (malaria, epidemic hemorrhagic fever)
 Cavernous sinus thrombosis
 Vasculitis (temporal arteritis, Takayasu's arteritis)
 Trauma (stalk section or sella fracture)
Infiltrative diseases
 Sarcoidosis
 Tuberculosis
 Leukemia
 Lymphoma
 Hemochromatosis
 Autoimmune hypophysitis
Miscellaneous
 Hypophysectomy
 Radiation necrosis
 Carotid artery aneurysm
 Pituitary abscess
 Congenital anomalies (hypoplasia, aplasia)

ease or abnormal hypothalamic hormone secretion. Patients with pituitary and hypothalamic diseases have clinical features similar to endocrine manifestations. Radiologic investigation and pituitary responses to hypothalamic hormones are useful in localizing the site of the lesion, but it is not always possible to distinguish between hypothalamic and pituitary disorders. Hypothalamic and pituitary causes of hypopituitarism are listed in Tables 403.3 and 403.4, respectively.

In patients with functioning pituitary tumors, hypersecretion of one hormone may coexist with reduced function of other pituitary cells. Hypopituitarism may be permanent (pituitary necrosis or hypophysectomy) or reversible (function may be restored after removal of a pituitary tumor). As a rule, GH and gonadotropin secretion is lost early, followed by failure of TSH, ACTH, and prolactin later in the course of the disease. In practice, however, any permutation of hormonal deficiencies may be seen, and the effects of individual hormone failure should be considered separately.

Clinical Findings

Patients with hypopituitarism typically are well nourished, and the skin is often pale and waxy with increased wrinkling around the eyes and mouth. General apathy and mental slowing often occur and may not be recognized because of the insidious nature of their onset. Mild anemia is common and usually is normochromic and normocytic, probably reflecting deficiency of thyroid and gonadal hormones. Hypoglycemia is rare in adults, but it may develop in diabetic patients who require insulin, because GH and ACTH deficiency leads to increased sensitivity to insulin.

Growth Hormone Deficiency

In adults, GH deficiency is the most frequently encountered component of hypopituitarism stemming from pituitary tumors, surgery, and irradiation. In the past, GH deficiency in the adult patient was believed to be devoid of any appreciable clinical significance. Studies using recombinant GH preparations, however, have suggested that daily administration of GH to hypopituitary patients increases lean body mass, decreases body fat content, and strengthens bone density. Many additional studies have to be done to validate GH use in various clinical situations. Until that time, there is no justification for using GH for the treatment of obesity, for the purpose of bodybuilding, or for other unproven indications.

In children, isolated GH deficiency likely is caused by isolated GH-RH deficiency. This is often a familial disease, and autosomal recessive (type I), autosomal dominant (type II), and X-linked recessive (type III) modes of transmission have been documented. No abnormalities in GH or GH-RH genes have been detected. A special form of GH deficiency (type IA) has been reported in Switzerland; these children appear to lack a gene for GH. Administration of exogenous human GH in these patients leads to a rapid rise in the titer of GH-blocking antibodies and attenuation or cessation of clinical responses to exogenous GH, because GH is regarded by the immune system as a completely foreign substance.

Other causes of congenital GH deficiency include defective GH-RH receptor and mutations in the transcription factors pit-1 and prop-1. In the latter cases, GH deficiency may coexist with partial or complete prolactin and TSH deficiencies. GH deficiency also may be seen in patients with several hormonal deficits stemming from hypothalamic or pituitary tumors, pituitary hypoplasia (or aplasia), or the so-called midline brain syndrome. In this congenital condition, hormonal abnormalities are associated with hypoplasia of the optic nerves, absent septum pellucidum, cleft palate, and a single central incisor. Increasingly, cranial irradiation for malignant diseases is being seen as a cause of clinically apparent GH deficiency because of the longer survival of affected children.

The hallmark of GH deficiency in childhood is short stature with progressive downward deviation from the predicted growth curve. Classically, these children are short and appear to be somewhat fat. The genitalia may be small, and the presence of micropenis at birth always should alert the clinician to the possibility of combined GH and gonadotropin deficiency. Bone age typically is delayed. Severe hypoglycemia may be a feature of GH deficiency in children, especially when ACTH also is missing.

Gonadotropin Deficiency

The clinical picture of gonadotropin deficiency depends on the age at onset of the disease. Failure of LH and FSH secretion before puberty results in absent or incomplete sexual maturation. In men, the testes are small (less than 2 cm), as is the penis, and scrotal rugosity, facial and pubic hair, and the laryngeal notch are absent. Women have primary amenorrhea, and the breasts and uterus are underdeveloped. Body proportions are eunuchoid, with long extremities (arm span exceeds height by more than 5 cm) due to failure of epiphyseal closure. Isolated gonadotropin deficiency of prepubertal onset may be associated with anosmia (Kallmann's syndrome, olfactory-genital dysplasia). The disorder is more common in boys and is caused by GnRH deficiency, which may be complete or partial. Other congenital abnormalities, such as color blindness and midline facial defects, also may be present. GnRH deficiency also is seen in the absence of other defects. In individual members of an affected family, GnRH deficiency and anosmia may be present together or as isolated abnormalities. The disease apparently results from the embryologic failure of GnRH cells to migrate from the olfactory placode into the brain during fetal life. Mutations in the *KAL* gene, normally coding for a neural cell adhesion molecule, which normally "guides" the embryologic migration of GnRH and olfactory neurons, have been documented in these patients.

Postpubertal gonadotropin deficiency in men takes the form of impotence, infrequent need to shave, infertility, and general weakness. Examination shows a normal penis, testicular atrophy initially manifest as soft testes, sparse pubic hair, atrophic skin, and poor muscle development. Fine radial wrinkling of the skin around the mouth is evident, and gynecomastia may be present. Women have amenorrhea and decreased vaginal lubrication and may have atrophic breasts and uterine involution. Osteoporosis is common in both sexes.

Thyroid-Stimulating Hormone Deficiency

Cold intolerance, fatigue, somnolence, dry skin, constipation, bradycardia, and mental impairment are common in both primary and secondary hypothyroidism. The symptoms are usually less severe in TSH deficiency, and a goiter does not develop.

Adrenocorticotropic Hormone Deficiency

Isolated ACTH deficiency leads to diminished cortisol secretion. Aldosterone secretion typically is intact, because the renin–angiotensin system continues to function normally. Patients with ACTH deficiency do not experience severe volume depletion, hyperkalemia, and hyponatremia. In contrast to Addison's disease, the skin is pale and does not tan, because melanocyte-stimulating hormone also is deficient. ACTH deficiency usually appears as weakness, fatigue, and orthostatic hypotension. Patients often describe the clinical course of minor illnesses, such as a common cold, as unusually severe and exhausting. Surgery or intercurrent illness increase cortisol demand and may precipitate nausea, vomiting, abdominal pain, and vascular collapse.

Prolactin Deficiency

Failure to lactate is the only known consequence of prolactin deficiency in women and is the usual clinical feature of postpartum pituitary necrosis (Sheehan's syndrome). In men, prolactin deficiency is of no known physiologic or clinical consequence. Isolated prolactin deficiency has been reported rarely, but it may be more common, owing to the lack of clinical manifestations.

Disease Syndromes

Pituitary tumors are the most common cause of hypopituitarism. Postpartum pituitary necrosis (Sheehan's syndrome) has become a rare cause of hypopituitarism because of improved obstetric care. In nonindustrialized countries, however, it remains a common cause of pituitary failure when delivery is associated with severe hemorrhage and shock. Pituitary hypertrophy during pregnancy makes the gland especially vulnerable to reduced blood flow, and spasm of the superior hypophyseal artery results in anterior pituitary necrosis. Occasionally, necrosis is complete, and if ACTH deficiency is not treated immediately, the postpartum mortality rate is high. More often, necrosis is partial and takes the form of failure of lactation and amenorrhea. Pituitary fibrosis leads to progressive loss of pituitary function during subsequent months, and a partial or completely empty sella becomes evident on CT scan. Endocrine testing usually shows panhypopituitarism, though partial or selective loss of anterior pituitary secretion may occur. Clinical ADH deficiency is rare. Pituitary necrosis can develop in any patient with profound shock, but it is most common in diabetics, because of microangiopathy and macroangiopathy. Pregnancy and ketoacidosis are important predisposing factors. Rarely, necrosis can develop in patients with infectious diseases, sickle cell anemia, or arteritis or after trauma to the pituitary stalk.

Infiltrative Diseases

The pituitary may be affected by the same diseases that produce infiltrative lesions in the hypothalamus (Table 403.3). Autoimmune hypophysitis typically occurs during the third trimester of pregnancy or in the first few months postpartum. The cause is unknown, but it is believed to result from the autoimmune destruction of pituitary cells. Histologic examination shows diffuse lymphocytic infiltration of the anterior pituitary. Another form of autoimmune hypophysitis is associated with other autoimmune endocrine diseases, such as Addison's disease, Hashimoto's thyroiditis, pernicious anemia, hypoparathyroidism, or gonadal failure. In some cases, circulating antibodies directed against prolactin-secreting cells have been found.

Miscellaneous Causes

Radiation therapy of the head is often followed by hypopituitarism that may not become evident for months to years after treatment. Deficiencies of GH in children and gonadotropins in adults are the most common manifestations. Carotid artery aneurysms may simulate a pituitary tumor on CT scan but seldom cause pituitary compression. Congenital pituitary anomalies are rare and usually are recognized in childhood during the workup to assess growth retardation.

Diagnosis

The clinical suggestion of hypopituitarism should be substantiated by endocrine testing. The presence of low pituitary and corresponding target gland hormone levels establishes the diagnosis. Differentiation of pituitary from hypothalamic failure and assessment of the degree of the pituitary impairment require appropriate stimulation tests (see Chapter 417).

Approach to the Patient With Suggested Hypopituitarism

The clinical history in a patient believed to have hypopituitarism is of paramount importance. A history of pituitary surgery, head radiation or trauma, a traumatic delivery, or existing systemic diseases may provide valuable clues. Several questions should be addressed:

Is the patient truly hypopituitary? Growth failure in a child may result from causes other than GH deficiency, and short stature is most often constitutional. Similarly, delayed sexual maturation may be provoked by gonadotropin deficiency or primary gonadal failure, but more often it is of constitutional origin or the result of systemic illness. In adults, organic causes of hypopituitarism are more likely, and symptoms and signs of hormonal failure should not be attributed to functional causes. Basal assessment of thyroid, gonadal, and adrenal function always should be performed, and low or borderline values must be followed by assessment of pituitary hormone secretion.

What is the origin of hypopituitarism? History and examination may provide important clues to the source of pituitary failure. Concomitant diseases, such as blood dyscrasias, hemochromatosis, or granulomatous diseases, in a patient with hypopituitarism suggest a common origin. Absent sexual maturation indicates a prepubertal onset of hypogonadism, and the presence of anosmia strongly suggests Kallmann's syndrome. Visual field defects or ophthalmoplegia indicate a mass lesion. CT scans or MRI always should be performed in the context of hypopituitarism, to exclude mass lesions.

Should dynamic tests of pituitary function be performed? If hypopituitarism is caused by a lesion that requires surgery, preoperative dynamic tests of pituitary function are unnecessary, because they may not reflect the postoperative situation. Before surgery, all patients should be viewed as having ACTH deficiency and treated with stress doses of glucocorticoids during the perioperative period. Dynamic assessment of pituitary function should be performed 2 to 3 months after surgery, and appropriate hormonal replacement must be given. If surgery is not indicated, assessment of pituitary reserve should be carried out via a combined pituitary function test (see Chapter 417). Diminished ACTH or TSH reserve is an indication for replacement therapy with glucocorticoids or thyroxine, even when the basal plasma cortisol or thyroxine levels are apparently normal. In patients with potentially progressive diseases (radiation damage, infiltrative diseases, vasculitis), residual pituitary function should be assessed on a semiannual basis with basal tests. Dynamic tests should be undertaken if a decline in basal function is observed.

Optimal Management

Treatment of hypopituitarism should be directed toward the underlying cause and to replacement of hormonal deficiencies.

The first objective is usually possible only with mass lesions, such as pituitary tumors. Pituitary function may improve after surgery, but more often it remains deficient or deteriorates further. Replacement therapy should take into account the patient's age, sex, and desire for fertility.

Adrenocorticotropic Hormone Deficiency

Maintenance therapy consists of hydrocortisone, 25 mg per day, generally administered in split doses: 10 to 15 mg in the morning, 10 mg with lunch, and 5 mg with dinner. If the patient experiences insomnia and restlessness in the late evening, the evening dose may be omitted or given earlier. Prednisone, 7.5 mg per day, can be used as an alternative; mineralocorticoid replacement usually is not required. If an intercurrent disease develops, especially one associated with fever, the daily dose of hydrocortisone should be doubled until recovery is complete. Nausea, vomiting, or diarrhea may require parenteral therapy. Acute surgery or severe illness should be covered by stress doses of parenteral hydrocortisone, 200 mg per day. As the patient's condition improves, the dose should be tapered to replacement levels over 3 to 7 days. All patients with ACTH deficiency should wear an identification necklace or bracelet.

Thyroid-Stimulating Hormone Deficiency

Thyroid hormone replacement consists of 0.1 to 0.2 mg per day of L-thyroxine; the individual dosage is determined on the basis of serum thyroxine levels, since TSH is not a reliable marker in hypothalamic or pituitary disease. Desiccated thyroid or triiodothyronine should not be used. In elderly individuals (older than 70 years) or in patients with coronary artery disease or dysrhythmias, the initial dose should be lower, 0.025 mg per day, and gradually increased by 0.025 mg each week to full replacement dosage. In otherwise healthy individuals and in those with recent-onset hypothyroidism (postpituitary surgery), full replacement doses can be started immediately. Thyroid replacement increases cortisol degradation and basal metabolism and may precipitate adrenal insufficiency in patients with diminished ACTH reserve. If the ACTH or cortisol reserve is impaired, hydrocortisone must be administered before thyroxine replacement.

Gonadotropin Deficiency

If fertility is not desired, gonadal steroid replacement therapy is given. Women should be treated with 17α-estradiol in the form of skin patches (Estraderm) or taken orally (Estrace), 1 to 2 mg per day, which allows monitoring of plasma estradiol (80 to 100 pg per milliliter). Estrogens are administered on a cyclical basis for the first 3 weeks of each month; medroxyprogesterone acetate (Provera), 5 to 10 mg per day, is added during the third week. This regimen induces regular withdrawal bleeding during the week off therapy and avoids the risk of endometrial cancer. Cyclical therapy is not required in women who have had a hysterectomy. Men should be treated with long-acting testosterone preparations (testosterone enanthate or cypionate), 200 to 300 mg administered intramuscularly every 2 to 3 weeks. Transdermal testosterone delivery systems are available, but the theoretical advantage of constant plasma hormone levels often is outweighed by lower efficacy (due to only low-normal hormone levels), high cost, and skin irritation. Oral testosterone preparations are weak androgens and are rarely effective. At adequate dosage they may cause cholestatic jaundice or hepatitis. In men older than 50 years, testosterone may produce prostatic hyperplasia, and the prostate should be examined at regular intervals.

In pituitary failure, fertility can be achieved only by using exogenous gonadotropins. Human chorionic gonadotropin exerts LH-like actions, whereas human menopausal gonadotropin is a mixture of LH and FSH. In men, hCG, 2,000 IU, should be administered intramuscularly three times a week for at least 4 months, followed by the addition of human menopausal gonadotropin, 75 IU administered intramuscularly three times a week. Therapy generally is required for more than a year to induce adequate spermatogenesis, and the best results occur when gonadotropin deficiency develops after puberty. In prepubertal women, sexual maturation and uterine growth should be induced by estrogen treatment for 4 to 6 months. Cyclical estrogen and progesterone therapy is then given for 3 to 4 months, to induce menses before gonadotropin therapy. Human menopausal gonadotropin, 75 to 150 IU per day, is administered for up to 2 weeks, and follicular maturation is monitored by estradiol assays and ovarian ultrasonography. Ovulation then is induced by intramuscular injection of hCG (2,000 IU). Recombinant FSH is replacing hCG as a drug of choice. Care should be taken to avoid ovarian hyperstimulation. This therapy should be reserved for use in medical centers where rapid estradiol assays and ovarian ultrasonography are available.

In GnRH deficiency, sexual maturation and fertility can be induced in both sexes by pulsatile GnRH therapy. Pituitary responsiveness to exogenous GnRH should be determined before long-term treatment. GnRH pulses are given every 60 to 120 minutes by portable pump, either intravenously at a dose of 25 to 50 ng per kilogram or subcutaneously at a dose of 50 to 100 ng per kilogram. Ovulatory cycles can be induced rapidly in women, but restoration of spermatogenesis in men requires a year or more of therapy.

Growth Hormone

No area of clinical endocrinology is as controversial as diagnosis and treatment of GH deficiency. First, the definition of a "short" child should take into account racial and familial backgrounds. Stature correction for parental height may be helpful when appropriate tables are consulted. Because idiopathic GH deficiency is often a genetic disease, however, cursory consideration of parental height may be misleading. Growth velocity (centimeters per year) may be influenced by gonadal status, and delayed puberty often is associated with slow statural growth.

Second, it may be difficult to define "abnormal" GH secretion, because of the pulsatile nature of hormone secretion. Several samples should be taken, and stimulation tests should be used. A normal GH rise to hypoglycemia or any other pharmacologic test, however, does not necessarily mean that a child can have endogenous GH pulses of normal frequency and amplitude.

A diagnosis of so-called GH neurosecretory dysfunction is suggested for short children with normal provocative GH test results but an abnormal spontaneous secretory pattern. Plasma insulin-like growth factor I (IGF-I) appears to be lower in short children than tall children, but the within-group variability is significant, and overlaps are common. Even when the biochemical diagnosis was based on the most sophisticated tests with seemingly unquestionable results, 30% to 70% of these children exhibited perfectly normal GH secretion when retested several years later. In this group, GH deficiency might have been functional and transient, akin to gonadotropin deficiency in delayed puberty.

Third, introduction of high-resolution CT scans and MRI showed that more than 90% of children with "idiopathic" GH deficiency have some radiologic evidence of abnormality, most often pituitary hypoplasia. The meaning of these findings is uncertain. Fourth, the question of who should be treated with exogenous GH is still subject to debate. Although it is agreed that an otherwise healthy short child with low growth velocity, delayed bone age, absent GH rises to provocative stimuli, and low IGF-I should be given GH injections, there is no consensus on the use of GH in a much larger group of children with equivocal clinical and biochemical findings. Moreover, in these children the response to GH substitution is less dramatic. In children whose GH deficiency is caused by surgery or radiation for intracranial neoplasm, the benefits of GH replacement should be weighed carefully against the theoretical possibility of induction of tumor-promoting growth factors. The cost of GH replacement is in excess of $10,000 per year, and the long-term consequences of unnecessary GH therapy are still unknown. A decision to start GH replacement in a child should never be taken lightly and is best accomplished in a pediatric endocrine center specializing in this problem.

GH replacement has been approved for use in GH-deficient adults. Whereas it improves body composition (decrease in fat mass and increase in lean body mass) and bone density, there is still no evidence of tangible benefits, such as a decline in the incidence of cardiovascular events or bone fractures. The purported improvement in the quality of life must be viewed with caution, since many studies were done in an unblinded fashion, the psychometric evaluations were imprecise, and the quality of life in some studies of GH-deficient adults either was normal or, when impaired, was attributed not to GH deficiency itself but rather to previous interventions, such as surgery and, more often, cranial irradiation.

The differential diagnosis of isolated GH deficiency should include chronic diseases, especially those associated with poor nutritional status (cardiopulmonary diseases, celiac disease, inflammatory bowel disease), hypothyroidism, poorly controlled diabetes, Cushing's syndrome, delayed puberty, psychosocial deprivation, and Laron's dwarfism. In the latter condition, GH receptors are missing or defective, and the resultant peripheral GH insensitivity manifests as high GH and low IGF-I levels. High-resolution CT scan or MRI should be carried out, to exclude cranial neoplasm. Assessment of GH secretion should include lists of the dynamic responses of GH to provocative stimuli. Only recombinant human GH is available in the United States for therapeutic purposes, and it is likely to supplant the pituitary-derived preparations worldwide. Optimally, GH should be administered intramuscularly once a day, at a dose between 0.02 and 0.04 mg per kilogram. Treatment should start as early as possible, to capitalize on the maximal growth potential, and continue until epiphyseal fusion is documented. Maximal growth velocity happens during the first year of therapy (*catch-up growth*). Development of GH-RH and its analogues opens a new avenue for treatment of children with GH-RH deficiency.

PITUITARY HYPERFUNCTION

Hyperprolactinemia

Hyperprolactinemia, the elevation of the serum prolactin level to more than 20 ng per milliliter in men or nonpregnant women who are not nursing, is the most common form of pituitary hyperfunction. Disorders causing hyperprolactinemia are shown in Table 403.5. Prolactin secretion normally is inhibited by dopamine. Therefore, any disorder or medication that interferes with the synthesis or secretion of dopamine, reduces the amount of dopamine reaching the pituitary, or blocks dopamine binding to its receptor results in hyperprolactinemia. Occasionally, elevated prolactin levels are evident in severe primary hypothyroidism and are believed to result from increased TRH secretion.

TABLE 403.5.   CAUSES OF HYPERPROLACTINEMIA

Physiologic
  Pregnancy
  Breast-feeding (first 6 wks)
  Sleep
  Nipple stimulation
  Stress
Medications
  Dopamine receptor antagonists
    Phenothiazines
    Butyrophenones
    Metoclopramide
    Thioxanthines
  Inhibitors of dopamine synthesis or storage
    α-Methyldopa
    Reserpine
    Tricyclic antidepressants
  Estrogens
Pituitary tumors
  Prolactinomas
  Growth hormone–secreting tumors (30%)
  Nonfunctioning tumors with suprasellar extension and stalk compression
Hypothalamic/pituitary stalk abnormalities
  Granulomas (sarcoidosis, histiocytosis X)
  Craniopharyngiomas and other suprasellar tumors
  Stalk section
  Empty sella syndrome
  Postradiation therapy
Idiopathic hyperprolactinemia
Other causes
  Primary hypothyroidism
  Chronic renal failure
  Chest wall lesions (postsurgery or herpes zoster)

Hypothalamic or stalk disorders produce modest elevations of prolactin (less than 150 ng per milliliter). Similar elevations of prolactin occur in renal failure, because of reduced prolactin metabolism and diminished pituitary sensitivity to dopamine. Now and then, the combination of renal failure and such medications as phenothiazines or methyldopa increases prolactin levels to higher than 150 ng per milliliter. Elevation of serum prolactin above 200 ng per milliliter almost always is caused by a prolactinoma. The differentiation of idiopathic hyperprolactinemia from a prolactinoma, however, rests on the ability to find evidence of a pituitary tumor on CT scanning or MRI.

Hyperprolactinemia is more common in women and is the underlying abnormality in 20% to 25% of women with amenorrhea. Prolactin is elevated in 25% of women with amenorrhea after discontinuing oral contraceptives, but there is no evidence that the estrogen component of the pill is a causative factor. In men, the incidence of hyperprolactinemia is not well documented, though in some series prolactin levels have been elevated in up to 10% of impotent men and 60% to 70% of those harboring prolactinomas. In both sexes, an elevated prolactin level results in reduced GnRH secretion, and the initial symptoms are those of hypogonadism. In most cases, hypogonadism associated with hyperprolactinemia is reversible after suppression of prolactin secretion.

Clinical Findings

In women, hyperprolactinemia causes oligomenorrhea or amenorrhea, infertility, and galactorrhea. Amenorrhea usually is present if serum prolactin levels exceed 100 ng per milliliter. Galactorrhea, the production of milk in nonpostpartum women, is evident in only 30% to 40% of hyperprolactinemic women, because both an elevated prolactin level and normal or near-normal ovarian steroid levels are needed for sustained milk production. Hyperprolactinemia should be suspected in all amenorrheic women. If amenorrhea and galactorrhea are both present, an elevated prolactin level is found in 80% of patients and a prolactinoma can be confirmed in half these women. Galactorrhea in the presence of normal menses often is not associated with an elevated prolactin value. The mechanisms of action are unclear, but they may relate to the fact that prolactin levels are not elevated after the first 6 weeks of breast-feeding, yet milk production is maintained. A transient elevation of prolactin may initiate milk secretion, which continues, perhaps maintained by nipple stimulation, even though the prolactin level has returned to normal. Diminished gonadotropin secretion leads to anovulation and estrogen deficiency, which takes the form of reduced vaginal lubrication and dyspareunia—or osteoporosis, if it is of prolonged duration. Hirsutism is sometimes present and may reflect a combination of estrogen deficiency and, possibly, increased androgen production.

In men, prolactin excess results in impotence, diminished libido, infertility, and hypogonadism. Hyperprolactinemia should be considered in all impotent men, especially if the serum testosterone is low or low-normal. Impotence in men often is not investigated early. Consequently, hyperprolactinemia may be missed, and prolactinomas are commonly large at the time of diagnosis. The serum testosterone value is typically low, but impotence and reduced libido sometimes have been reported in men with hyperprolactinemia and normal testosterone levels.

Differential Diagnosis

Investigation of hyperprolactinemia should identify the underlying cause if possible and establish whether a prolactinoma is present. An outline of the investigation of an elevated prolactin level is given in Chapter 417. Minor elevations of prolactin (less than 30 ng per milliliter) may be related to stress or to samples being drawn in the early morning, before the sleep-associated rise in prolactin has declined. A careful drug history should be taken, hypothyroidism and renal failure should be excluded, and a pregnancy test should be carried out in amenorrheic women. Serum prolactin values of less than 150 ng per milliliter may be caused by medications, by nonfunctioning pituitary tumors, or by a small prolactinoma, and careful attention should be paid to the possible presence of hypothalamic disease. Prolactin values more than 200 ng per milliliter are virtually diagnostic of a prolactinoma. The degree of hyperprolactinemia reflects the size of the tumor, and levels may reach 20,000 ng per milliliter in patients with large macroadenomas.

Tests using TRH or metoclopramide to stimulate prolactin or dopamine agonists to suppress prolactin are not helpful in distinguishing prolactinomas from other causes of hyperprolactinemia. The presence of a prolactinoma is confirmed by a CT scan or MRI, and in most women the tumor is a microadenoma (less than 1 cm in size). If the scan result is negative and no other cause for the elevated prolactin value is found, the patient is said to have idiopathic hyperprolactinemia. Small tumors cannot be excluded by MRI, however, and follow-up, with measurement of prolactin at 6-month intervals, and an annual scan are recommended. Microadenomas do not compromise other aspects of pituitary function, and formal testing of pituitary reserve is not needed. Macroadenomas may cause hypopituitarism, and pituitary function should be assessed by a combined pituitary function test. If a macroadenoma is present on scanning and the serum prolactin value is less than 150 ng per milliliter, the tumor is unlikely to be a prolactinoma, and a nonfunctioning pituitary tumor with suprasellar extension should be suspected.

Optimal Management

Considerable change has occurred in the management of hyperprolactinemia, which reflects the availability of dopamine agonists and recognition of the fact that most microadenomas do not progress to form macroadenomas. In addition, though surgery results in an initial remission in 80% to 90% of microadenomas, follow-up has shown that up to 50% of patients have a recurrence of hyperprolactinemia within 5 to 6 years. Surgery may be required for large tumors—to reduce tumor mass and relieve pressure symptoms—but rarely results in normalization of serum prolactin levels. The management of hyperprolactinemia may involve observation only; drug therapy; or a combination of dopamine agonist, surgery, and radiation therapy. The approach used should reflect the patient's age and sex, their desire for fertility, and the need to preserve pituitary function and avoid the consequences of tumor growth.

If a woman with idiopathic hyperprolactinemia or a microadenoma experiences regular menses and fertility is not desired, a case can be made for observation. Series have suggested that many microadenomas do not enlarge over 5 to 8 years. With idiopathic elevation of prolactin to the range of 30 to 60 ng per milliliter, prolactin levels have been shown to decline in 50% of women over 3 to 5 years and occasionally fall to normal. If fertility is desired and the CT scan result is negative or shows a microadenoma, then dopamine agonist therapy should be given. Bromocriptine suppresses serum prolactin values to normal in 95% of women, menses resume within 6 to 8 weeks in 90%, and galactorrhea is reduced or abolished in 80%. The usual dose required is 2.5 mg three times daily, but a total dose of 5 mg per day or less is effective in some women.

Side effects include nausea, anorexia, fatigue, nasal congestion, and postural hypotension. These side effects usually can be prevented by starting therapy at a low dose of 1.25 mg administered at bedtime and increasing by 1.25-mg increments every 2 or 3 days, to a total dose of 2.5 mg three times daily taken with meals. Occasionally, the side effects of bromocriptine persist and prevent the use of doses needed to suppress prolactin to normal levels. In such patients, an alternative is to use pergolide mesylate, 25 to 50 g per day. Pergolide is a dopamine agonist that has been shown to be effective in clinical research studies. A newer dopamine agonist, cabergoline, is effective as a once- or twice-weekly dose (0.25 to 1 mg each) and has a lower incidence of reported side effects.

The patient should avoid pregnancy until at least one spontaneous menstrual period has occurred, to allow more accurate dating of conception. Bromocriptine or cabergoline have not been shown to have adverse effects on the fetus. The drug is usually stopped when menses are overdue, however, and not restarted if the patient is pregnant. Microadenomas may enlarge during pregnancy but rarely cause symptoms. In 15% to 20% of women with larger tumors, however, headaches and visual field defects occur, and visual fields should be carefully checked during the first trimester. Minor field defects generally do not progress, and specific therapy often is not required. Progression of visual field defects is found occasionally and usually responds to reinitiation of dopamine agonist during the remainder of the pregnancy.

In amenorrheic women who do not desire fertility, treatment of microadenomas is more controversial. Suppression of prolactin secretion is needed to restore ovarian function and to prevent the possible development of osteoporosis. Dopamine agonists restore gonadal function and prevent tumor growth for as long as the medication is taken, but prolactin levels typically rebound to previous values when the drug is discontinued. These drugs are effective in suppressing prolactin, but they are expensive and rarely curative. For these reasons, some centers prefer to remove the microadenoma, even though the disorder may recur after an apparently successful operation. Surgery also may be indicated for patients who are intolerant of drugs. Treatment is required for all patients with macroadenomas and may consist of dopamine agonists, surgery, radiation therapy, or a combination of all three. Bromocriptine is effective in suppressing prolactin in 95% of macroadenomas, and tumor size usually decreases by up to 50%.

Suprasellar extensions are reduced in size and visual fields usually become normal within a few days to weeks, though doses up to 20 mg per day may be needed to produce these effects. In moderate-sized macroadenomas, dopamine agonists are a reasonable choice for initial therapy. In women, menses typically resume. In men, testosterone levels increase within 3 months as a rule but may not rise to normal until after 9 months of treatment. Dopamine agonists are not curative, however, and tumors expand rapidly with recurrence of field defects if the drug is discontinued. Surgery may be needed for patients who do not respond or who are intolerant of dopamine agonists. Radiation is reserved for patients with unusually aggressive lesions or for those whose tumors continue to grow despite surgery and/or dopamine agonists.

Acromegaly

Acromegaly is a chronic debilitating disorder caused by hypersecretion of GH and secondary overproduction of IGF-I, which was formerly called somatomedin C. The clinical manifestations are overgrowth of bone and soft tissues, metabolic abnormalities, and mass effects of the GH-secreting pituitary tumor. The annual incidence of acromegaly is three new cases per million, and the overall prevalence is 40 cases per million. Acromegaly occurs with equal frequency in both sexes, and most patients are diagnosed in the third or fourth decade of life. A careful history usually shows a 5- to 10-year lag between the onset of symptoms and diagnosis. During this interval, pituitary tumors enlarge, and at diagnosis 70% to 80% are macroadenomas. The pathologic processes causing acromegaly are listed in Table 403.6.

Pituitary GH-secreting tumors account for virtually all cases of acromegaly. Most are benign adenomas, though they often exhibit rather aggressive behavior, with infiltration of peripituitary tissues. GH-producing adenomas account for 25% to 30% of pituitary tumors and exhibit substantial clinicopathologic heterogeneity, with 20% to 25% producing prolactin, ACTH, or TSH in addition to GH. GH-producing pituitary adenomas may develop in a remnant of Rathke's pouch, but ectopic GH secretion by bronchial or pancreatic islet cell carcinomas is rare. Ectopic GH-RH secretion resulting in somatotrope hyperplasia

TABLE 403.6.	PATHOLOGIC PROCESSES CAUSING ACROMEGALY	
Process		**Percentage**
Pituitary GH-producing adenoma		>99
Pituitary GH-producing carcinoma		
Adenoma of the ectopic pharyngeal pituitary		
Ectopic GH-producing tumor		
Hypothalamic or pituitary GHRH-producing gangliocytoma		<1
Ectopic GHRH-producing tumor		
Autonomous production of insulin-like growth factor I (not yet described)		

GH; growth hormone, GHRH; growth-hormone–releasing hormone.

has been described in pancreatic islet cell carcinomas, carcinoid tumors, and pheochromocytomas. Plasma GH-RH levels are higher than 300 pg per milliliter (normal, less than 50) and usually exceed 1 ng per milliliter. Hypothalamic or pituitary gangliocytomas also may produce GH-RH. In these patients, pituitary adenoma rather than hyperplasia is usually present, which may reflect the longer duration of GH-RH stimulation. GH-independent overproduction of IGF-I has not yet been clearly documented. The pathogenesis of GH-producing pituitary tumors is uncertain. In theory, they may arise de novo as an autonomous pituitary tumor or result from chronic hypothalamic overstimulation of pituitary somatotropes by increased GH-RH or deficient somatostatin secretion. Evidence supports both possibilities, and a clear consensus is not available.

Clinical Findings

The clinical picture of GH excess depends on the age at onset. Before puberty, GH excess results in accelerated linear growth and pituitary gigantism. Because patients often become hypogonadal as a result of tumor-induced hypopituitarism, the epiphyses remain open, and somatic growth may persist after the expected age of puberty. After puberty, GH excess results in acromegaly (large extremities). The somatic changes result from increased production of IGF-I, but some metabolic changes may be caused by a direct action of GH. The clinical features of GH excess are shown in Fig. 403.7.

A history of changes in shoe, glove, or ring sizes and coarsening of facial features is characteristic of acromegaly. A large nose, thick lips, accentuated nasolabial and frontal furrows, and frontal bossing are usually obvious. Comparison of earlier photographs is of great help in establishing the approximate age at onset of the disease. Most patients notice oily skin and malodorous perspiration, and the degree of sweating is an index of disease activity. Skin tags, hypertrichosis, and increased pigmentation with acanthosis nigricans are common. Prognathism and malocclusion lead to difficulties in chewing and frequent changes of dentures. Voice changes result from hypertrophy of the larynx, edema of the vocal cords, and enlarged sinuses. Almost all patients experience severe snoring, and sleep apnea is very common. Arthralgias are typical, and arthropathy is caused by overgrowth of the cartilage plates and joint deformities. There is often visceral hypertrophy, and the salivary glands and thyroid are enlarged. Cardiac hypertrophy is common, in part because of hypertension, and frequently is associated with dysrhythmias and congestive heart failure. Acroparesthesias frequently are caused by nerve entrapment, and the carpal tunnel syndrome is present in most patients.

About 80% of patients with acromegaly are insulin resistant, and overt diabetes mellitus is present in 15%, usually those with a family history of diabetes. Hyperphosphatemia, hyperphosphaturia, and hypercalciuria are frequently present, but hypercalcemia suggests the coexistence of hyperparathyroidism. Hyperlipidemia results from inhibition of plasma lipoprotein lipase

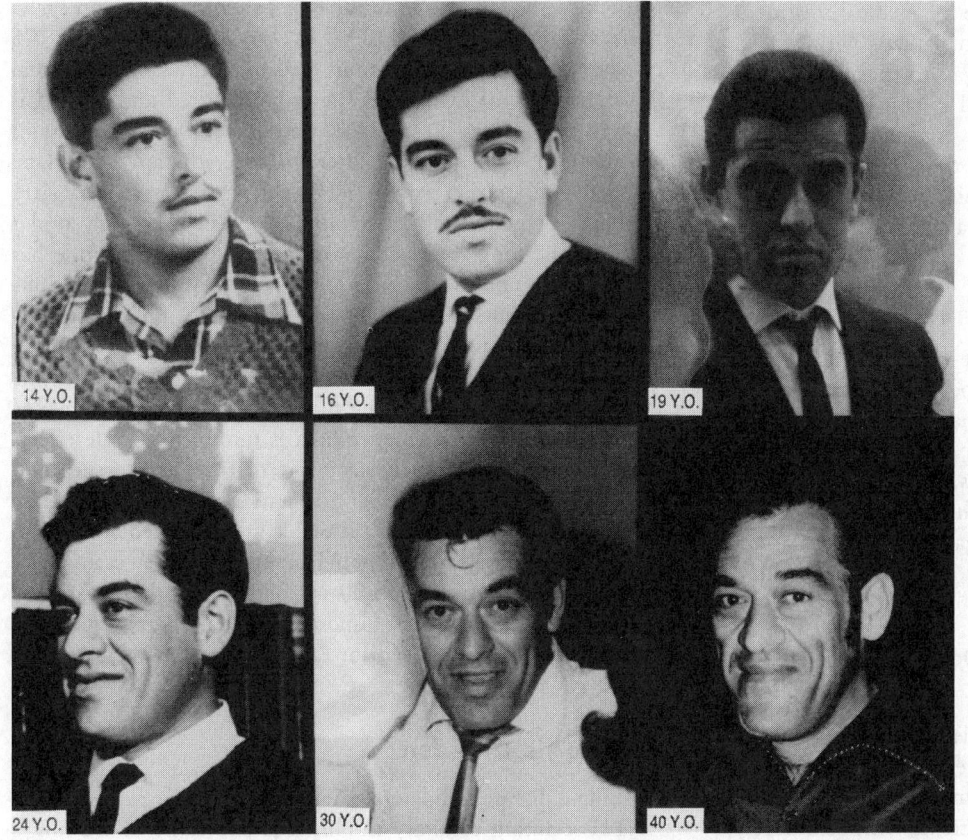

FIGURE 403.7. Appearance and progression of acromegalic features in a young man. Mild coarsening of facial features is noticeable at age 16 years, but at that time it could have easily been attributed to pubertal changes. The patient became unmistakably acromegalic at age 19 years, and the disease progressed relentlessly until 40 years of age, when the diagnosis was made by a *blind* physician who shook the patient's hand. At that time, plasma growth hormone was in excess of 200 ng/mL, and invasive pituitary macroadenoma was found. Coarse facial features, frontal bossing, overdevelopment of lower jaw, and prominent frontal and nasolabial furrows are apparent.

and hepatic triglyceride lipase. Hypopituitarism is typical with large tumors. A low serum testosterone level in men may reflect the inhibitory action of GH on synthesis of testosterone-binding globulin rather than hypogonadism; they can be differentiated by measurement of the binding protein or bioavailable testosterone. Hyperprolactinemia may be caused by stalk compression or by concomitant secretion of prolactin from a mixed pituitary tumor. Acromegaly is associated with an increased frequency of colonic polyps. The disease may be part of the multiple endocrine neoplasia type 1 syndrome, but familial acromegaly, not associated with other neoplasia, has been described.

Laboratory Findings

The diagnostic criteria of acromegaly have been redefined as a result of the introduction of sensitive GH assays. In normal individuals, most plasma GH values are within the 0.05 to 0.5 ng per milliliter range; they are always above 1 ng per milliliter in untreated patients, however, and most often are frankly elevated, reaching values as high as 500 ng per milliliter. Owing to the normally occurring GH pulsatility, random GH values up to 20 to 30 ng per milliliter are nondiagnostic. The presence of an elevated IGF-I level confirms GH hypersecretion. The hallmark of acromegaly is the nonsuppression of plasma GH below 1 ng per milliliter in a sensitive GH assay after an oral glucose load. TRH stimulates GH secretion in 60% to 80% of patients with acromegaly, and this test is helpful when plasma GH is relatively low. GnRH has a similar effect in 20% to 30% of patients. In contrast to healthy subjects, L-dopa or bromocriptine suppress plasma GH in half the patients, and both are helpful in assessing whether bromocriptine may be of value for medical treatment. Plasma GH-RH should be measured in patients with lung or abdominal tumors. This is the only way to diagnose ectopic GH-RH secretion, because dynamic GH responses are indistinguishable from those in pituitary tumors. A pituitary CT scan or MRI is required to assess tumor size, and the degree of extrasellar expansion. Chest radiography or abdominal CT scan should be considered if lung or gastrointestinal malignancy is suspected.

Differential Diagnosis

The clinical features of acromegaly are characteristic and are rarely confused with other diseases. On occasion, pachydermoperiostosis (skin hypertrophy and large hands) can mimic some features of acromegaly, but GH secretion is normal. Plasma GH levels may be elevated in other diseases, such as renal failure, cirrhosis, uncontrolled diabetes, and malnutrition. In these conditions, the clinical features of acromegaly are not present and the IGF-I value is either normal or low.

Natural History, Prognosis, and Optimal Management

Acromegaly is a slowly progressive disease, and appreciable changes in the patient's status occur over years. Therefore, aggressive therapy may not be required in elderly patients with mild disease. The mortality rate for patients with acromegaly, however, is two to three times that of the general population and is mainly the result of cardiovascular and respiratory diseases. Lowering GH secretion below 2.5 ng per milliliter has been associated statistically with the normalization of mortality rates. Pituitary apoplexy occurs in 30% of untreated patients, but this rarely results in complete tumor necrosis, and the GH level remains elevated. Treatment always should be considered in young patients with acromegaly.

Normalization of GH secretion results in reduced somatic growth and reversal of metabolic abnormalities. Shrinkage of soft tissues takes place rapidly (even within 24 to 48 hours after surgery), and skin changes and hyperhydrosis improve markedly over time. Transsphenoidal surgery is the treatment of choice in most patients. The results depend on tumor size, and intrasellar lesions can be removed successfully in 60% to 80% of patients. Long-term follow-up (up to 8 years) has shown that recurrence is unusual when normal basal GH and IGF-I levels and normal GH responses to provocative stimuli are present after surgery. Pituitary irradiation is reserved for patients with elevated GH and IGF-I levels after surgery or for those in whom surgery is contraindicated. In patients who respond to therapy, GH declines by 50% over the first 1 to 2 years and by 10% to 20% per year for the next 5 to 7 years. Patients with GH levels in excess of 50 ng per milliliter are unlikely to respond to radiation therapy. Despite plasma GH suppression below 0.5 to 1 ng per milliliter, many patients retain high IGF-I levels. Normalization of IGF-I is seen in less than 5% of patients after a 5- to 10-year interval after external radiation. Whether stereotactic radiosurgery is more effective in this regard remains unknown.

Bromocriptine is effective in suppressing the plasma GH level to the near-normal range in 20% of patients with acromegaly; however, normalization of IGF-I levels occurs in less than 10% of patients. The drug is administered four times a day. A total dose of up to 40 mg per day may be required and is used if surgery is unsuccessful or while waiting for the full effects of radiation to occur. In the latter instance, therapy should be stopped temporarily every 1 to 2 years to assess residual GH secretion. Pergolide and cabergoline have been used with similar success. The long-acting somatostatin analogue octreotide has been shown to be effective in normalizing GH secretion in 50% to 70% of patients with acromegaly. Shrinkage of pituitary GH-producing tumors has been noted regularly using 50 to 250 g by subcutaneous injection two to four times a day. Octreotide is also effective in suppressing plasma GH in ectopic GH-RH secretion, and pituitary hyperplasia is diminished. Side effects include nausea, abdominal discomfort, diarrhea, steatorrhea, and formation of gallstones. Newer preparations include slow-release octreotide (Sandostatin LAR, available in the United States) and lanreotide (available in Europe). The former is given as an intramuscular injection of 10 to 30 mg once a month. Since these preparations also shrink the tumors and/or halt their progression, they often obviate the need for radiotherapy.

Cushing's Disease

Cushing's disease is bilateral adrenal hyperplasia caused by an ACTH-secreting pituitary tumor; it is one cause of Cushing's syndrome. The presentation, diagnosis, and management of Cushing's disease are discussed in Chapter 407.

Thyroid-stimulating Hormone Hypersecretion

Rarely, hyperthyroidism results from pituitary TSH hypersecretion due to a TSH-secreting tumor or to selective pituitary resistance to thyroid hormone. In both disorders, the patient has hyperthyroidism and a goiter. Plasma thyroid hormone levels are elevated, and thyroid scan shows diffusely increased radioiodine uptake. Many patients initially are diagnosed as having Graves' disease and treated accordingly. Hyperthyroidism and goiter may recur, however, because of continuing stimulation by the elevated TSH. The absence of ophthalmopathy in a hyperthyroid patient with a diffuse goiter suggests TSH hypersecretion, and the serum TSH should be measured.

TSH-secreting pituitary tumors are usually large and do not respond to TRH with an increase in TSH. Pituitary surgery with subsequent radiation is not always effective. The somatostatin analogue octreotide has been shown to be effective in suppressing TSH and restoring euthyroidism. Selective pituitary resistance to thyroid hormone is often familial. A pituitary tumor is not found on CT scan, and TRH elicits normal or augmented TSH release in the context of hyperthyroidism. Several therapies have been tried, including triiodothyronine, inactive triiodothyronine analogues, bromocriptine, and propylthiouracil, but they are only partially effective.

GONADOTROPIN HYPERSECRETION

Gonadotropin-secreting pituitary tumors are being recognized with increasing frequency. Most tumors are large and take the form of field defects in middle-aged men. Most tumors secrete free α subunit or FSH; LH secretion is either normal or low and is reflected by a normal or low plasma testosterone level. Rarely, hypersecretion of intact LH is accompanied by high testosterone concentrations. Surgery is required to salvage vision, usually followed by irradiation. Bromocriptine may suppress hormonal secretion and slightly reduce tumor size.

BIBLIOGRAPHY

Antoni FA. Hypothalamic control of adrenocorticotropin secretion: advances since the discovery of 41 residue corticotropin-releasing hormone. *Endocr Rev* 1986;7:351–378.

Barkan AL. Acromegaly. Diagnosis and treatment. *Endocrinol Metab Clin North Am* 1989;18:277–310.

Barkan AL, Halasz I, Dornfeld KJ, et al. Pituitary irradiation is ineffective in normalizing plasma insulin-like growth factor I in patients with acromegaly. *J Clin Endocrinol Metab* 1997;82:3187–3191.

Ben-Jonathan N. Dopamine: a prolactin-inhibiting hormone. *Endocr Rev* 1985;6:564–589.

Carbezudo JM, Vaquero J, Arietio E, et al. Craniopharyngiomas: a critical approach to treatment. *J Neurosurg* 1981;55:371–375.

Carroll PV, Christ ER, Bengtsson BA, et al. Growth hormone deficiency in adulthood and the effects of growth hormone replacement: a review. Growth Hormone Research Society Scientific Committee. *J Clin Endocrinol Metab* 1998;83:382–394.

Conn PM, ed. Gonadotropin-releasing hormone. *Endocr Rev* 1986;7.

Dalkin AC, Marshall JC. Medical therapy of hyperprolactinemia. *Endocrinol Metab Clin North Am* 1989;18:259–276.

Davies PH, Stewart SE, Lancranjan I, et al. Long-term therapy with long-acting octreotide (Sandostatin-LAR) for the management of acromegaly. *Clin Endocrinol* 1998;48:311–316.

Frohman LA, Jansson JO. Growth hormone-releasing hormone. *Endocr Rev* 1986;7:223–253.

Giustina A, Veldhuis JD. Pathophysiology of the neuroregulation of growth hormone secretion in experimental animals and the human. *Endocr Rev* 1998;19:717–797.

Haisenleder DJ, Dalkin AC, Marshall JC. Regulation of gonadotropin gene expression. In: Knobil E, Neill JD, eds. *The physiology of reproduction*, second ed. New York: Raven Press, 1994:1793.

Lamberts SW, de Herder WW, van der Lely AJ. Pituitary insufficiency. *Lancet* 1998;352:127–134.

Lam KSL, Tse VKC, Wang C, et al. Early effects of cranial irradiation on hypothalamic-pituitary function. *J Clin Endocrinol Metab* 1987;64: 418–424.

Littley MD, Shalet SM, Beardwell CG, et al. Radiation-induced hypopituitarism is dose-dependent. *Clin Endocrinol* 1989;31:363–373.

Marshall JC, Dalkin AC, Haisenleder DJ, et al. GnRH pulses: regulators of gonadotropin synthesis and ovulatory cycles. *Recent Prog Horm Res* 1991;47:155.

Martini L, ed. *Frontiers in neuroendocrinology*, ninth ed. New York: Raven Press, 1986:31.

Melmed S, ed. *The pituitary*. Blackwell Scientific, 1995.

Melmed S, Braunstein GD, Horvath E, et al. Pathophysiology of acromegaly. *Endocr Rev* 1983;4:271.

Molitch ME. Pregnancy and the hyperprolactinemia woman. *N Engl J Med* 1985;321:1364–1370.

Morley JE. Neuroendocrine control of thyrotropin secretion. *Endocr Rev* 1981;2:396–436.

Newman CB, Melmed S, Snyder PJ, et al. Safety and efficacy of long-term octreotide therapy of acromegaly: results of a multicenter trial in 103 patients. *J Clin Endocrinol Metab* 1996;80:2768–2775.

Oppenheim DS, Klibanski A. Medical therapy of glycoprotein hormone–secreting tumors. *Endocrinol Metab Clin North Am* 1989;18: 339–358.

Prager O, Braunstein GD. X-chromosome-linked Kallmann's syndrome: pathology at the molecular level. *J Clin Endocrinol Metab* 1993;76: 824–826.

Sano T, Asa SL, Kovacs K. Growth hormone-producing tumors: clinical, biochemical and morphological manifestations. *Endocr Rev* 1988;9: 357–373.

Schlechte JA. Clinical impact of hyperprolactinemia. *Baillieres Clin Endocrinol Metab* 1995;9:359–366.

Seminara SB, Hayes FJ, Crowley WF. Gonadotropin-releasing hormone deficiency in the human (idiopathic hypogonadotropic hypogonadism and Kallmann's syndrome): pathophysiological and genetic considerations. *Endocr Rev* 1998;5:521–539.

Serri O, Rasio E, Beauregard H, et al. Recurrence of hyperprolactinemia after selective transsphenoidal adenomectomy in women with prolactinomas. *N Engl J Med* 1983;309:280–283.

Snyder PJ. Gonadotroph cell adenomas of the pituitary. *Endocr Rev* 1985; 6:552–563.

Veldhuis JD, Hammond JM. Endocrine function after spontaneous infarction of the human pituitary: report, review and reappraisal. *Endocr Rev* 1980;1:100–107.

Webster J, Piscitelli G, Polli A, et al. A comparison of cabergoline and bromocriptine in the treatment of hyperprolactinemic amenorrhea. *N Engl J Med* 1994;331:904–909.

Ying SY. Inhibins, activins and follistatins: gonadal proteins modulating the secretion of follicle-stimulating hormone. *Endocr Rev* 1988;9:267–293.

C H A P T E R

404

DISORDERS OF POSTERIOR PITUITARY FUNCTION

ALAN G. ROBINSON

SYNTHESIS AND ANATOMY

The hormones of the posterior pituitary, oxytocin and vasopressin, are synthesized in individual oxytocin cells and vasopressin cells of the paired supraoptic nuclei and paraventricular nuclei in the hypothalamus. The paraventricular nuclei are located in a middle position just lateral to the walls of the third ventricle. The supraoptic nuclei are located bilaterally above the lateral extremes of the optic chiasm. In these nuclei are large neurons (magnocellular) in which the hormones are synthesized. Axons extend from the paraventricular nuclei anterolaterally and inferiorly, passing around and through the supraoptic nucleus. Then, with the axons of the magnocellular neurons of the supraoptic nuclei, they pass medially to the midline, where they join the tracks from the opposite side and extend together as the supraopticohypophyseal track down the pituitary stalk to axon storage terminals in the posterior pituitary. Hormones are stored in the axon terminals until stimulated exocytosis releases the hormones into the systemic circulation.

For vasopressin, in addition to the pathways to the posterior pituitary, there are additional axons that extend from the paraventricular nuclei to the median eminence to terminate on the initial capillary plexus of the hypothalamic pituitary portal system. Vasopressin is secreted into the capillaries, which drain via the long portal veins to the second capillary system in the anterior pituitary. Vasopressin secreted by this pathway acts on pituitary coricotrophs to stimulate release of adrenocorticotropic hormone (ACTH). For both hormones there are ill-defined pathways that terminate in the wall of the third ventricle and secrete into the cerebrospinal fluid. There is no known function for the hormones in cerebrospinal fluid.

In the magnocellular neurons, the hormone vasopressin or oxytocin (1,100 dalton) is synthesized as part of a precursor molecule including a 10,000-dalton neurophysin that is specific for oxytocin or vasopressin. For vasopressin, but not oxytocin, there is a third component of the precursor molecule, a 12,000-dalton glycopeptide. After synthesis, the precursor is packaged into neurosecretory granules, and in the granules the precursor is enzymatically cleaved into the hormone, the neurophysin, and (for vasopressin) the glycopeptide. In the granules, the neurophysins form complexes with the hormone, which stabilizes the hormone during axon transport and storage.

At the time of release, the entire contents of the neurosecretory granule are liberated by exocytosis into the perivascular space, and each component of the neurosecretory granule can be detected in the bloodstream. Although the neurophysins (or glycopeptide) might serve in the plasma as surrogate markers for the hormone, they have not been found to have any physiologic function after release from the neuron. The gross anatomy of this system is localized entirely in the pituitary fossa and the basal hypothalamus. The osmoreceptor that is described later herein is located just anterior to the third ventricle in this same anatomic region. The discrete location of the osmoreceptor and the sites of synthesis and secretion of vasopressin have important implications for pathophysiology, as explained later.

VASOPRESSIN

OSMOTIC REGULATION

Sensation of thirst and secretion of vasopressin are the main mechanisms whereby the body controls water balance and osmolality. Although the range of serum osmolality, 275 to 295 mOsm per kilogram, is relatively broad for the normal human population, for each individual, osmolality is tightly regulated around that individual's normal value. When water is lost in excess of solute, there is an increase in plasma osmolality. As little as a 1% increase in osmolality will cause secretion of vasopressin, which stimulates renal conservation of water. Increased osmolality also induces thirst, to replace the water deficit. Thirst is less well studied in humans and is generally thought to have a somewhat higher threshold for stimulation of water intake. In fact, because of social custom, most people drink adequate fluid during the day without experiencing severe thirst. Some studies in animals indicate that thirst is regulated tightly, similarly to secretion of vasopressin. It may be that thirst in humans is more tightly regulated physiologically but is overridden by social custom. Nonetheless, water intake is an important and necessary component to replete loss of water. The action of vasopressin on the kidney only conserves that water which is present in the body, while repletion of water loss requires water intake.

The role of vasopressin in the relationship between plasma osmolality and urine output is illustrated in Fig. 404.1. There is a direct linear and sensitive relationship between plasma osmolality and levels of plasma vasopressin, and there is a similar linear and sensitive relationship between plasma vasopressin and urine osmolality. These relationships (Fig. 404.1) illustrate why there is a sensitive and linear relationship between plasma osmolality and urine osmolality. Thus, measure of urine osmolality often can serve as an internal "bioassay" for the level of plasma vasopressin. In pathologic situations, there may be wider than normal excursions of plasma osmolality—as in abnormal states of water retention at the low end of the osmolality scale or abnormal states of dehydration at the high end of the osmolality scale.

At plasma osmolality below the threshold for release of vasopressin, vasopressin is absent, and there is maximum dilution of the urine and excretion of the abnormal water content. Alternatively, markedly elevated levels of osmolality will produce superphysiologic levels of vasopressin in plasma. These abnormally high levels of vasopressin will not, however, produce a urine osmolality above the normal physiologic ceiling. This is because the maximum concentration of the urine is determined by the

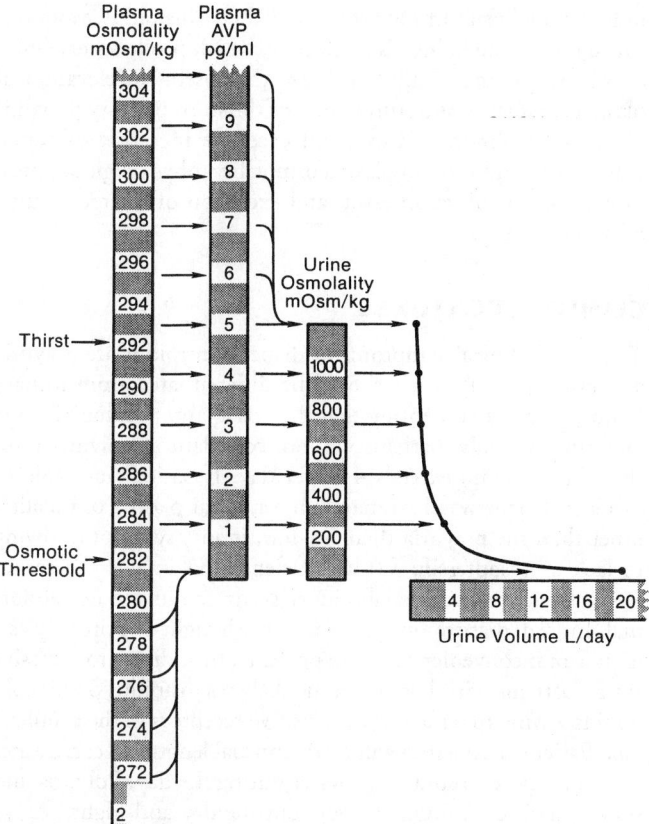

FIGURE 404.1. Idealized schematic of normal physiologic relationships, showing the direct relationship between plasma osmolality and plasma vasopressin. At low levels of osmolality, however, there may be no subsequent lowering of vasopressin because it is completely suppressed. There is also a direct relationship between plasma vasopressin and urine osmolality, except that once maximum concentration of the urine is obtained, further elevations of plasma vasopressin will not produce a higher urine osmolality. Urine volume is plotted as a horizontal scale to emphasize the geometric relationship of urine volume to urine osmolality. Urine volume is relatively well maintained until urine osmolality is compromised severely by an extremely low level of vasopressin in plasma. At the far left the osmotic threshold is illustrated as a floor for plasma osmolality below which the plasma osmolality will not normally fall because of excretion of a high volume of dilute urine. Thirst is illustrated as a physiologic ceiling for plasma osmolality, because above this level thirst will be sensed and water imbibed to avoid further elevation of plasma osmolality. (From Robinson AG. Disorders of antidiuretic hormone secretion. *Clin Endocr Metab* 1985;14:55.)

osmolality of the inner medulla of the kidney (see later description of vasopressin action on renal tubules). The relationship of urine volume to urine osmolality and, hence, the relationship of urine volume to plasma vasopressin and plasma osmolality are distinctly different. Urine volume is illustrated as a horizontal bar in Fig. 404.1.

Urine volume is related to urine osmolality logarithmically. Thus, urine volume will change very little as plasma vasopressin levels decline from a level producing maximum urine concentration until very low levels of plasma vasopressin are reached. For example, in the idealized schema a reduction of plasma vasopressin from 5 pg per milliliter to 2 pg per milliliter results in a marked decrease in urine osmolality but only a modest increase in urine volume. Nevertheless, when plasma vasopressin is com-

pletely suppressed and urine osmolality becomes maximally dilute, there is a dramatic exponential increase in urine volume to approximately 18 L per day (which represents the quantity of fluid delivered to the collecting duct). In summary, normally osmolality is regulated within a small range, and this is accomplished by a small range of levels of plasma vasopressin. Urine osmolality has a wider range, but there is not a dramatic change in urine volume until plasma vasopressin levels are extremely low.

RENAL RESPONSE TO VASOPRESSIN

See Chapter 9 for a description of the normal physiology of glomerular filtration of fluid and regulation of fluid and electrolyte absorption in the renal tubules. At the end of the physiologic processes of filtration and reabsorption in the descending and ascending loops of Henley, approximately 18 L of dilute fluid enters the collecting duct, which passes back through the inner medulla of the kidney. Acting on specific vasopressin receptors in the collecting duct, V_2 receptors, vasopressin causes water to move from the lumina of the duct across the ductal epithelium and into the concentrated inner medulla. This reabsorption conserves water and concentrates the urine. The vasopressin-stimulated movement of water is facilitated by aquaporin 2 water channels. When V_2 receptors are activated by the binding of vasopressin, cyclic AMP levels inside the cell rise; cAMP activates protein kinase A and, subsequently, phosphorylation of aquaporin 2. Aquaporin 2 water channels then move from the cytoplasm to the apical membrane of the collecting duct. This allows transport of water from the collecting duct into the cytoplasm. The water then exits from the basolateral surface through aquaporin 3 and aquaporin 4 water channels. Aquaporin 3 and 4 are constitutively synthesized, whereas the synthesis of aquaporin 2 is controlled by vasopressin (as is the shuttle movement in and out of the membrane). When the action of vasopressin dissipates, the aquaporin 2 channels move out of the membrane back to the cytoplasm.

VOLUME REGULATION

While the body regulates volume primarily through retention and excretion of sodium, there is also regulation of secretion of vasopressin in response to volume. The volume receptors are located in the chest, with low-pressure volume receptors in the atrium and pulmonary vessels and pressure receptors in the aorta. Signals from these receptors are carried via the ninth and tenth cranial nerves to the brain stem, through the medulla, and through synapses to terminate on the perikarya of the magnocellular neurons in the hypothalamus. The primary action of volume receptors is to inhibit secretion of vasopressin. When pressure falls or volume declines, the amount of inhibition is decreased, and vasopressin is released. The released vasopressin acts to restore pressure and/or volume. The effector mechanism for volume-regulated release of vasopressin is the V_1 receptors in blood vessels. Acting on V_1 receptors, vasopressin produces increased intracellular calcium and contraction of vascular smooth-muscle cells to raise pressure. Increased pressure will close the loop by raising pressure in the chest and restoring the inhibition of release of vasopressin. The vasopressin that is released in response to hypovolemia also will stimulate V_2 receptors in the kidney to provoke water retention, as described earlier. The water retention will help restore volume. Not described here is the retention of sodium to maintain and restore extracellular fluid volume through mechanisms of action that are discussed in Chapter 9.

INTERACTION OF REGULATION OF OSMOLALITY AND REGULATION OF VOLUME

In most physiologic situations there is concurrence between increased osmolality and decreased volume (or pressure), which produces additive effects to enhance release of vasopressin. Similarly, expanded volume and hypo-osmolality would lessen the secretion of vasopressin and cause water excretion. These mechanisms of action are usually complimentary, but in some conditions either system can augment pathologic conditions. For example, in excessive loss of salt by the kidney or gut or through sweat, there may be hyponatremia, yet vasopressin levels will be high because of the diminished volume. With excess secretion of vasopressin, water retention causes dilutional hyponatremia. Hyponatremia may be worsened, however, by sodium excretion in response to the volume expansion produced by water retention.

ANTERIOR PITUITARY FUNCTION

As mentioned previously, in addition to the secretion of vasopressin from the posterior pituitary, there are axons predominantly of the paraventricular nuclei that terminate on the portal capillary vessels in the hypothalamus. Vasopressin released at this site traverses the long portal capillaries to the anterior pituitary, where V_{1a} receptors are present on pituitary corticotrope cells. Acting on the V_{1a} receptor, vasopressin stimulates release of ACTH. The importance of vasopressin in regulating ACTH varies among animal species. While response of the V_{1a} receptors can be verified in humans using experimental manipulations, the physiologic function of this action of vasopressin in humans has not been determined.

■ DIABETES INSIPIDUS—HYPOSECRETION OF VASOPRESSIN

Diabetes insipidus is the excretion of an excess volume of dilute insipid (tasteless) urine. Hypotonic polyuria can be induced by the absence of vasopressin (hypothalamic diabetes insipidus), lack of renal response to vasopressin (nephrogenic diabetes insipidus), or physiologic suppression of vasopressin in response to excessive ingestion of water (primary polydipsia). The pathophysiologic condition that produces polyuria and polydipsia in each of the three is easily distinguished. In the case of hypothalamic diabetes insipidus, there is a lack of vasopressin, which causes excretion of dilute urine, subsequent concentration of plasma with increased osmolality, and stimulation of thirst to induce polydipsia. In nephrogenic diabetes insipidus, vasopressin action on the kidney is ineffective, which produces excretion of a large volume of dilute urine with subsequent elevation of plasma osmolality and stimulation of thirst. In primary polydipsia, there is abnormal thirst and excessive ingestion of water, which causes dilution of plasma osmolality, physiologic suppression of release of vasopressin, and excretion of a large volume of dilute urine.

CLINICAL FEATURES

The initial clinical symptoms of diabetes insipidus are polyuria and polydipsia. Polyuria should be differentiated from urinary frequency by documenting that there is a large volume of urine excretion. Usually, patients will not complain of polyuria until the urine volume exceeds 4 L per day. If patients are able to drink sufficient water to maintain a normal plasma osmolality, other than the polyuria there are few, if any, symptoms, owing to lack of vasopressin. With sufficient fluid intake, the serum electrolytes and routine laboratory study results are not abnormal. Indeed, diabetes insipidus may be thought of primarily as a disease of inconvenience due to polyuria. In addition to excessive thirst, patients with hypothalamic diabetes insipidus prefer cold liquids, owing to temperature-sensitive receptors in the oropharynx. Patients frequently will go to unusual lengths to carry water and to be close to sources of water during the day. Polyuria and polydipsia is continuous throughout the day and night.

In patients who have primary polydipsia with a psychological or psychiatric basis, thirst and secondary polyuria may decline during times of diminished stress or at night. The increased urine volume caused by absent vasopressin does not exceed 18 to 20 L per day, which is the maximum urine volume delivered to the distal diluting segment. Patients with diabetes insipidus often are chronically mildly dehydrated, with a subsequent modest decrease in urine volume (to 6 to 12 L per day) by vasopressin-independent mechanisms of action. When urine volumes exceed 18 L per day, the possibility of a primary disorder of thirst should be considered. In cases of partial diabetes insipidus, formal testing with dehydration may verify the patient's ability to produce isotonic or hypertonic urine osmolality, even though the patient drinks sufficient water so that the urine osmolality never reaches this maximum and there is a corresponding large urine volume.

In these cases, there is no normal relationship of plasma osmolality to plasma vasopressin, as shown in Fig. 404.1. Instead, there is a shift upward in the level of plasma osmolality required to stimulate a given level of vasopressin release. For example, a plasma osmolality level above 295 may be required to stimulate maximum AVP release. If there is no shift in the threshold for thirst, the patient will sense thirst at a plasma osmolality that is not sufficient to stimulate release of vasopressin and will drink sufficient fluid to assuage thirst. Thus, thirst will maintain a plasma osmolality that is below that necessary to stimulate release of vasopressin. There will then be an excessive volume of dilute urine, similar to the situation with patients who have more complete diabetes insipidus.

As a group, patients with complete diabetes insipidus may have a slightly greater than normal serum sodium level; there may be a slightly lower serum sodium level in patients with primary polydipsia. For an individual patient, however, the concentration of sodium is frequently within the normal range. Loss of posterior pituitary function may be associated with loss of anterior pituitary function, and, therefore, endocrine deficits related to the anterior pituitary should be sought, and anterior pituitary testing should be undertaken as indicated. In patients with a large pituitary tumor and a history of diabetes insipidus, it should be noted that both adrenal insufficiency and severe myxedema can impair the ability to excrete free water and mask manifestations of diabetes insipidus. Replacement with thyroid hormone, but especially adrenal steroids, can result in sudden massive excretion of dilute urine and abrupt manifestation of diabetes insipidus in a patient who previously had no polyuria. In patients with diabetes insipidus and an associated disruption of the hypothalamic portal vascular system leading to the anterior pituitary, there may be increased levels of prolactin because of diminished hypothalamic inhibition of prolactin. Symptoms related to a tumor or other disease in the hypothalamus or symptoms related to systemic disease that also involves the hypothalamus may appear as manifestations of the pathologic process. With adequate water intake, the course may be benign, but in any situation in which a patient with diabetes insipidus is unable to take in sufficient fluid, marked and severe dehydration can develop, leading to vascular collapse, coma, and death.

DIAGNOSIS

The diagnosis of diabetes insipidus is established when it is determined that a patient is unable to concentrate the urine in response to normal physiologic input. As mentioned earlier, physiologic input is from osmoreceptors and baroreceptors (volume receptors). If the patient is dehydrated when he or she is first seen, with an elevated plasma osmolality and dilute urine unexplained by osmotic diuresis, the diagnosis of diabetes insipidus is made. Measuring the plasma vasopressin and determining the response to an administered vasopressin agonist (desmopressin) will distinguish nephrogenic from hypothalamic diabetes insipidus. In hypothalamic diabetes insipidus, the plasma vasopressin level is absent or low, and there is a prompt response to administered vasopressin, whereas in nephrogenic diabetes insipidus, the plasma vasopressin level is elevated, and there is little or no response to administered vasopressin.

Most patients are conscious when first seen, and on ad lib fluids with an intact thirst mechanism these patients will drink a sufficient amount to maintain a normal plasma osmolality and dilute urine. In this case, it is necessary to carry out a test to stimulate secretion of vasopressin. The best described and easiest test to administer is the dehydration test outlined in Chapter 137. The test is done under controlled conditions with no fluid intake while observing urine osmolality. Patients are dehydrated to a weight loss of 2% of body weight and a constant urine osmolality. At this state of dehydration the plasma vasopressin level is obtained, and the patient is given 2 μg of desmopressin intravenously. Normal patients concentrate urine with dehydration and have less than a 5% increase in urine osmolality in response to the administered desmopressin.

Patients with complete hypothalamic diabetes insipidus have little increase in urine osmolality with dehydration and then experience a greater than 50% increase in urine osmolality in response to administered desmopressin. Patients with nephrogenic diabetes insipidus show little concentration of the urine with dehydration but may have some response to the pharmacologic dose of desmopressin. Nephrogenic diabetes insipidus is distinguished by the elevated level of plasma vasopressin. There has been some debate as to whether the standard dehydration test distinguishes partial hypothalamic diabetes insipidus from primary polydipsia. If patients with partial diabetes insipidus are severely dehydrated, they may secrete sufficient vasopressin to reach their own maximum urine concentration and not respond to desmopressin. On the other hand, patients with primary polydipsia may reach a plateau in urine osmolality before there is maximum secretion of vasopressin and, hence, may respond to administered desmopressin. These conditions can be distinguished by a reliable and sensitive assay of vasopressin in plasma but may not be adequately differentiated by the vasopressin levels available from commercial laboratories. Any patient started on desmopressin therapy who experiences hyponatremia should be assessed for an abnormality of thirst; attention should be given to the potential diagnosis of primary polydipsia rather than partial diabetes insipidus.

ETIOLOGY

In rare cases, hypothalamic diabetes insipidus is a congenital disorder that develops in children with a family history of the disease. In other situations a specific cause is first sought by an evaluation of hypothalamic anatomy. Because of the discrete location of synthesis described earlier, hypothalamic diabetes insipidus always involves the area of the hypothalamus above the sella and around the base of the third ventricle. Pathologic lesions in the hypothalamus are not usually subtle. As noted, V_2 receptors in the kidney are extremely sensitive to plasma levels of vasopressin, and even low levels of vasopressin maintain urine volume in a normal range. Thus, more than 90% of the vasopressin cells must be lost before symptomatic diabetes insipidus occurs. Lesions in the hypothalamus must be sufficiently large to destroy the paired paraventricular and supraoptic nuclei on both sides of the hypothalamus or must be located in a discrete position just above the diaphragma sella, where there is convergence of the axons from the paired right and left nuclei into the supraopticohypophyseal track, which courses through the infundibular stalk to the posterior pituitary.

Magnetic resonance imaging of the hypothalamus is the best initial test of anatomy. Primary tumors in this area include dysgerminoma (ectopic pinealoma), craniopharyngioma, and pituitary tumors (but only with suprasellar extension). Infiltrative lesions of the hypothalamus, such as sarcoidosis, hysticytosis X, or tuberculosis, may be found, usually with accompanying peripheral manifestations of the disease. Metastatic lesions to the hypothalamic area stemming from carcinoma elsewhere, especially of the lung and breast, may cause diabetes insipidus. On T1-weighted magnetic resonance images, the normal posterior pituitary shows a high-intensity (white) signal. This high-intensity signal is due to stored hormone content and is present in most (but not all) normal subjects and absent in most (but not all) patients with diabetes insipidus. Widening of the posterior

TABLE 404.1.	DRUGS THAT AFFECT VASOPRESSIN RELEASE OR ACTION	
Level of Action	**Enhance Vasopressin**	**Inhibit Vasopressin**
Hypothalamus (secretion)	Nicotine Vincristine Chlorpropamide Phenothiazine Clofibrate Morphine Carbamazepine Amitriptyline	Ethanol Vinblastin Narcotic antagonists Phenytoin
Kidney (action)	Oxytocin dDAVP Chlorpropamide Prostaglandin inhibitors Cyclophosphamide	Lithium Demeclocycline Tolazamide Darvon Acetohexamide Cisplatinum Hypokalemia Hypercalcemia

pituitary stalk has been reported in inflammatory diseases of the neurohypophysis and may be seen in the context of recent-onset diabetes insipidus for which no other source is found (idiopathic). A thickened stalk with absence of the posterior pituitary bright spot should prompt a thorough body search for the infiltrative systemic diseases described previously. Most often, diabetes insipidus is provoked by pituitary surgery or a readily identified tumor, or else it is idiopathic diabetes insipidus. If no suprasellar mass is identified and no systemic disease is found in the course of 4 years of follow-up, the patient probably has idiopathic diabetes insipidus.

Nephrogenic diabetes insipidus is most often due to pharmacologic agents (Table 404.1), such as lithium, demeclocycline, or cisplatinum, or electrolyte disturbances, such as hypercalcemia or hypokalemia. With the exception of lithium, which may produce permanent defects, diabetes insipidus usually abates when the offending agent is withdrawn. Inability to concentrate the urine maximally also may be caused by a variety of structural lesions in the kidney, including sickle cell disease and inflammatory disorders, as described in Chapter 152. Hereditary nephrogenic diabetes insipidus due to abnormalities of the V_2 receptor or abnormalities of the aquaporin gene also have been described. Patients with inherited nephrogenic diabetes insipidus usually show signs of profound dehydration, fever, and vomiting in childhood. Severe hypernatremia with hypotonic polyuria and absent response to desmopressin confirm the diagnosis.

SPECIAL CONSIDERATIONS
Triphasic Diabetes Insipidus

In trauma-induced diabetes insipidus or diabetes insipidus developing after surgery of the hypothalamic area, there is the possibility of a "triphasic" pattern. In the first phase, the patient experiences diabetes insipidus due to axon shock and lack of function of the damaged neurohypophyseal neurons. This lasts a few

hours to several days and is followed by the second antidiuretic phase, which stems from uncontrolled release of vasopressin from the disconnected posterior pituitary or from the remaining severed neurons. Excess fluid intake during the second phase does not suppress the vasopressin and leads to hyponatremia. Antidiuresis lasts 2 to 14 days and is followed by the third phase, when the store of hormone is depleted and there is return of diabetes insipidus.

Essential Hypernatremia

Some patients with diabetes insipidus have normal synthesis of vasopressin but inadequate secretion, because they lack the osmoreceptor input to the neurohypophysis. Volume receptors are intact. These cases are described as "essential hypernatremia." In response to increased osmolality (serum sodium), the patient does not secrete vasopressin to concentrate the urine and similarly does not develop thirst to stimulate drinking. Therefore, dehydration with hypernatremia ensues. When dehydration becomes sufficient to stimulate volume receptors, vasopressin is secreted, and the urine is concentrated. The patients may not have a large urine volume at first, but only a high serum sodium with modest dehydration. Administration of fluids to replace the volume deficit turns off the release of vasopressin stimulated by the volume receptor and causes excretion of dilute urine owing to absence of the vasopressin response to osmolality. These patients require replacement with desmopressin and often a prescribed intake of fluid, which is taken regardless of the absence of thirst.

Diabetes Insipidus in Pregnancy

The normal serum sodium level in pregnancy is as low as 136 mEq per liter; thus, pregnant patients with symptoms of diabetes insipidus and a serum sodium level in the normal range may, in fact, have severe dehydration. The diagnosis of diabetes insipidus in pregnancy is complicated by a cystine aminopeptidase in the plasma of pregnant women. This enzyme, oxytocinase, also destroys vasopressin in plasma, which speeds the clearance of vasopressin but also may produce artifactually elevated measures of vasopressin by radioimmunoassay. The shortened half-life of vasopressin during pregnancy may cause partial hypothalamic diabetes insipidus or mild, asymptomatic nephrogenic diabetes insipidus to become overtly symptomatic, with excessive polyuria and polydipsia.

TREATMENT

Water diuresis is the primary manifestation of diabetes insipidus, and drinking water in sufficient quantity will correct the metabolic abnormalities. Pharmacologic therapies are designed to limit the amount of necessary water intake to a tolerable level and to decrease polyuria to an acceptably low volume and frequency. Desmopressin is the treatment of choice for diabetes insipidus. This analogue acts predominantly on the antidiuretic V_2 receptors of the kidney, with little action on the V_1 pressor receptors. Desmopressin is available in tablets of 0.1 and 0.2 mg for oral administration, a metered spray bottle that delivers 10 μg per spray, or a dropper bottle with a rhinal catheter that can deliver doses of 5 to 20 μg. Most new patients will want to try the tablets first.

When beginning therapy it is desirable to determine the duration of action of the chosen dose in each patient, because there is considerable individual variation. This can be done by having the patient record the time and volume of each voided urine after an administered dose. A decline in urine volume is usually noted 30 to 60 minutes after the dose and reaches a maximum in 1 to 2 hours. The return of polyuria is rapid and is readily determined by the increased excretion of a large volume of urine. Therapy is initiated with a low dose, 0.05 mg (half a tablet) orally, one spray intranasally, or 50 μL (5 μg) intranasally via rhinal catheter. The dose is increased to achieve a convenient schedule of two (most common with intranasally administered medication) or three (most common with orally administered medication) doses per day. Raising the dose above 0.2 mg for an oral dose or 20 μg for an intranasal dose usually does not result in significant prolongation of the effect.

If the patient never becomes polyuric on a fixed dose, it may be advantageous, at least once a week, for the patient to delay an administered dose of desmopressin to ensure that he or she does not become water intoxicated. Recurrent episodes of hyponatremia may indicate abnormal thirst and should prompt re-evaluation of the patient. Desmopressin is also available as a solution of 4 μg/mL to be given parenterally. The usual dose is 0.5 to 2 μg and may be given during surgical procedures or if a patient develops an allergy to other routes of administration. Desmopressin is the preferred agent in pregnancy because dDAVP is not destroyed by the cystine aminopeptidase.

Orally administered pharmacologic agents (Table 404.1) are effective in some patients with diabetes insipidus, especially those with partial hypothalamic diabetes insipidus. Chlorpropamide in a dose of 100 to 500 mg per day enhances the renal action of vasopressin and often reduces urine volume to an acceptable level. Carbamazepine and chlofibrate cause release of vasopressin from the pituitary. Thiazide diuretics and amiloride lessen urine volume as the result of volume contraction. Prostaglandin inhibitors enhance the action of vasopressin by suppressing the normal action of prostaglandin E to suppress the action of vasopressin on the kidney. The diuretics (especially potassium-sparing amiloride) and prostaglandin inhibitors are useful in nephrogenic diabetes insipidus. For each of these pharmacologic agents, the "antidiuretic" action is not the primary therapeutic action of the drug and potential side effects and toxicity should be noted. Complicated cases of diabetes insipidus, for example, with anterior pituitary deficits, in children, with associated electrolyte imbalance, or during pregnancy should be evaluated in consultation with an endocrinologist or other physician familiar with the disorder.

PROGNOSIS

The prognosis of diabetes insipidus per se is excellent. If the disease is not treated, patients may experience problems with bladder enlargement and dilatation of the ureters and renal pelvis; when treatment is adequate, however, the disorder does not predispose to other disease or influence longevity. The ultimate prognosis may depend more on the pathologic condition that caused the diabetes insipidus. The long-term prognosis of diabetes insipidus due to trauma or surgery varies. Some patients eventually regain sufficient function (usually within 1 year) and are able to come off replacement therapy. For this reason, such patients should be periodically withdrawn from vasopressin replacement to determine whether there has been return of function.

■ SYNDROME OF INAPPROPRIATE SECRETION OF ANTIDIURETIC HORMONE—HYPERSECRETION OF VASOPRESSIN

The diagnosis of inappropriate secretion of antidiuretic hormone, vasopressin (SIADH), is considered in the differential diagnosis of hyponatremia. The differential diagnosis of hyponatremia is discussed in detail in Chapter 144. With the exceedingly rare exception of someone drinking more than 20 L of water per day, causes of hyponatremia are associated with impaired renal diluting ability and a urine osmolality that is greater than the maximum urine dilution, that is, greater than 100 mOsm per kilogram. Thus, urine osmolality is uniformly elevated and is not useful in the differential diagnosis. Instead, the first consideration in the differential diagnosis of hyponatremia is the extracellular fluid volume, and the second is urinary sodium.

If the extracellular fluid volume is diminished and the urinary sodium level is low, less than 10 mEq per liter, the patient has had extra renal loss of sodium, for example, from sweat or gastrointestinal losses, and is showing a normal physiologic accommodation by retaining sodium via the kidney. If the patient has decreased extracellular fluid volume but inappropriately high urinary sodium values, more than 20 mEq per liter, the problem is renal loss of sodium due to an intrinsic renal defect caused by diuretics, osmotic diuresis, or renal disease or due to an inappropriate signal to the kidney caused by decreased aldosterone (as in Addison's disease). If the extracellular fluid volume is high but the urinary sodium is low, the cause is usually an edematous disorder such as occurs in congestive heart failure, cirrhosis, or nephrotic syndrome. If the extracellular volume is normal but the urine sodium is inappropriately high, the diagnosis is SIADH. In SIADH the pathophysiologic condition is related to expanded extracellular fluid volume, but the extracellular fluid volume may be normal at the time the patient is seen. Similarly, urinary sodium loss is a part of the pathophysiologic picture, but urinary sodium may be in balance with intake at the time the patient is examined. Nonetheless, the urinary sodium level is inappropriately elevated for the degree of hyponatremia. In SIADH, in addition to the low levels of serum sodium, decreased blood urea nitrogen and low uric acid levels may be noted as a consequence of volume expansion and natriuresis.

PATHOPHYSIOLOGY

The pathophysiologic picture of hyponatremia in SIADH is initially that of water retention, volume expansion, and dilution of serum sodium. In response to volume expansion, the body undergoes physiologic reactions in an attempt to bring the extracellular fluid volume back to normal. These physiologic responses to provoke excretion of sodium include an increased glomerular filtration rate, suppression of aldosterone, and initiation of natriuretic factors, most notably, atrial natriuretic peptide. When the excretion of sodium and water by the kidney brings the extracellular fluid volume back to normal, the stimulus to natriuresis ceases, and the patient may be in sodium balance at this new lower level of serum sodium. Ingestion of salt (and water) reproduces the cycle of extracellular fluid volume expansion and natriuresis, to maintain the serum sodium at the new low level. Further ingestion of water reproduces the expansion and dilution of sodium and prompts sodium loss, to further diminish serum sodium. Note, however, that the excretion of sodium produces correction only in the extracellular fluid volume.

All cellular spaces participate in volume expansion produced by water retention, and intracellular fluid volume remains expanded after sodium excretion. Subsequently, the body attempts to return the intracellular fluid volume to normal by excreting potassium, the major intracellular electrolyte, and other intracellular osmoles, such as creatinine, glutamate, glutamine, taurine, myoinositol, and glycerophosphorycholine. While the correction of extracellular fluid volume in response to volume expansion is immediate, it takes about 48 hours to see a correction of the intracellular fluid volume expansion. It should be noted that when the intracellular organic osmoles are lost, there is a decline in the ability of the intracellular fluid compartments to buffer volume in response to a rise in extracellular fluid osmolality. This has important therapeutic implications, as discussed later.

ETIOLOGY

The three major causes of excess secretion of vasopressin to produce SIADH are ectopic secretion by a tumor, a pharmacologic agent that affects vasopressin release or action, and secretion from the normal store of vasopressin in the neurohypophysis. A variety of tumors can cause ectopic production of vasopressin and should be considered in the case of any patient with hyponatremia and malignancy. Among the most common tumors are carcinoma of the lung, thymus, duodenum, and pancreas. Drugs that affect the release or action of vasopressin are illustrated in Table 404.1.

Secretion of vasopressin by the neurohypophysis may be caused by pressure or irritation of the magnocellular neurons. Essentially any pathogenetic mechanism in the hypothalamic area that, in some cases, causes diabetes insipidus may provoke excess secretion of vasopressin, in other situations, if the neurons are "irritated" rather than destroyed. Similarly, head trauma, subarachnoid hemorrhage, stroke, encephalitis, meningitis, and other central nervous system disorders can produce excess secretion of vasopressin in this manner. A more common cause of excess secretion of vasopressin by the neurohypophysis is, however, interruption of the normal inhibitory input of the volume receptor system. As noted previously, both low-pressure volume receptors and high-pressure receptors are located in the chest. These receptors usually inhibit the release of vasopressin, and

when their input to the central nervous system is interrupted, there is excess secretion of vasopressin. Thus, numerous pulmonary diseases, including granulomatus diseases, acute and chronic infections, infiltrative diseases and positive pressure ventilation (by decreasing venous return), can cause SIADH.

The so-called syndrome of inappropriate secretion of antidiuretic hormone develops only if sufficient fluid is ingested to initiate volume expansion and the pathogenetic sequence described previously that leads to clinical hyponatremia. All of the clinical features of the disorder are related to hyponatremia and range from no symptoms in mild long-standing cases to weakness, lethargy, anorexia, vomiting, convulsions, and coma in more severe cases. Usually the symptoms are more severe if there is a rapid decline in the serum sodium level. One form of SIADH that is frequently asymptomatic is the reset osmostat. Patients with this condition have chronic hyponatremia and often some history of excess water ingestion. With dehydration they concentrate urine, and with a water load they dilute urine—but both occur at a lower than normal level of serum sodium. These patients do not require specific therapy. The cause of hyponatremia in myxedema and glucocorticoid insufficiency may be confused with SIADH, and these conditions must be excluded in the differential diagnosis.

TREATMENT

Just as administration of water is the primary form of therapy for diabetes insipidus, so water restriction is the primary therapy for SIADH. This treatment must be accompanied by some repletion of the depleted body sodium. Typically, sodium repletion is accomplished by dietary salt intake, but occasionally supplementation is necessary. The amount of fluid to be restricted varies from patient to patient and depends on the level of vasopressin. This is all that is required in most cases of chronic and asymptomatic hyponatremia. Treatment of extremely low serum sodium levels, that is, less than 120 mEq per liter, especially when accompanied by neurologic symptoms and signs, may require more aggressive therapy. The rapidity of therapeutic correction depends upon the chronic nature of hyponatremia.

Where it is known that hyponatremia has occurred over several hours, for example, during fluid administration for a surgical procedure, cerebral edema may be present, and it may be lifesaving to bring the sodium level rapidly back to the low 120s, with careful monitoring of central nervous system signs and symptoms. In the context of chronic profound hyponatremia, studies have indicated that abrupt correction may produce an osmotic demyelination syndrome that is characterized by gradual neurologic deterioration several days after alleviation of hyponatremia. There is fluctuating consciousness, convulsions, hypoventilation, and hypotension. Eventually, pseudobulbar palsy with swallowing dysfunction, inability to speak, and quadraparesis may develop. Recovery varies. Osmotic demyelination probably occurs only in situations in which hyponatremia has been present for longer than 48 hours and the neurons have accommodated chronic hyponatremia by extruding potassium and intracellular organic osmoles.

Extrusion of intracellular osmoles allows the neurons that were expanded by extracellular osmolality to shrink back to normal size but also removes any buffering capacity for the neurons to respond to increased extracellular fluid osmolality that may be caused by aggressively treating the low serum sodium. Overly rapid correction (increase) of extracellular osmolality causes osmotic loss of intracellular fluid and shrinkage of central nervous system cells and, by unknown mechanisms, may produce osmotic myelinolysis. The recommendation for patients with chronic hyponatremia is to correct at a rate no more than 0.5 mEq per hour, not to exceed 12 mEq over 24 hours. One might start with an initial correction of 5% to 10% of the measured sodium, to remedy residual cerebral edema. Because of the rigidity of the skull, the brain can enlarge a maximum of 10%—this is the maximum brain expansion. A slower rate of correction is continued after this minimal rapid increase in serum sodium.

Although fluid restriction is the most physiologic treatment, chronic cases may require additional therapy. One might consider demeclocycline at doses of 600 to 1,200 mg per day. This treatment provokes nephrogenic diabetes insipidus by inhibiting the action of vasopressin at the kidney. A maximum clinical response is not noted until approximately 4 days after adjusting the dosage. The serum sodium level should be followed, to determine that patients do not become hypernatremic. It should be noted that the drug may worsen liver disease.

BIBLIOGRAPHY

Martin PY, Schrier RW. Role of aquaporin-2 water channels in urinary concentration and dilution defects. *Kidney Int* 1998;53(suppl)65: S57–S62.

Reeves WB, Bichet DG, Andreoli TE. The posterior pituitary and water metabolism. In: Wilson JD, Foster DW, Kronenberg HM, et al., eds. *Williams textbook of endocrinology*, ninth ed. Philadelphia: WB Saunders, 1998:341–387.

Robinson AG. Disorders of antidiuretic hormone secretion. *Clin Endocrinol Metab* 1985;14(1):55–88.

Robinson AG, Verbalis JG. Diabetes insipidus. In: Bardin CW, ed. *Current therapy in endocrinology and metabolism*, sixth ed. St. Louis: CV Mosby, 1997:1–7.

Robertson GL. Diabetes insipidus. *Endocrinol Metab Clin North Am* 1995; 24(3):549–572.

Kelley's Textbook of Internal Medicine, fourth edition. Edited by H. David Humes. Lippincott Williams & Wilkins, Philadelphia © 2000.

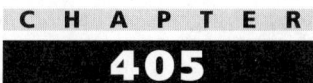

CHAPTER 405

DISORDERS OF THE PINEAL GLAND

WARNER BURCH

ANATOMY

The pineal gland, a pine cone–shaped structure that measures 4 × 8 mm and weighs 100 to 180 mg in adults, is attached to the posterior roof of the third ventricle. It rests in a groove between the superior colliculi and lies very close to the opening of the cerebral aqueduct connecting the third and fourth ventricles. Thus, any pineal enlargement may paralyze upward conjugate gaze by pressure on the superior colliculi (Parinaud's syndrome) or impair the flow of cerebrospinal fluid (CSF), leading to obstructive hydrocephalus.

The pineal consists of lobules of parenchymal cells (pinealocytes) that are separated by nonparenchymal connective tissue septa (mostly astrocytes). The pineal gland has no direct neural attachment to the brain. Its innervation comes from sympathetic postganglionic fibers of the superior cervical ganglia. Historically, the pineal was thought to be a vestigial third eye because in anamniotic animals (fish, amphibia) it contains cells similar to the neuroepithelial cells of the retina that respond directly to light. In mammals, the direct photic response is lost and a complex neural pathway is established through the autonomic nervous system.

PHYSIOLOGY

The major secretory product of the pinealocytes is melatonin (*N*-acetyl-5-methoxytryptamine). Other pineal hormones include the biogenic amines (norepinephrine, serotonin, histamine, and other indoleamines) and peptides (thyrotropin-releasing hormone, luteinizing hormone–releasing hormone, somatostatin, and vasotocin). Serotonin is converted to melatonin by two rate-limiting enzymes that are unique to the pineal.

Lighting conditions regulate melatonin synthesis. Darkness leads to increased sympathetic outflow, causing adrenergic discharge to the pineal, which stimulates melatonin synthesis. Maximal pineal melatonin production occurs during the dark phase of the photoperiod regardless of whether the animal is nocturnally or diurnally active. Light is inhibitory to melatonin secretion. Ablating the superior cervical ganglion or ingesting propranolol causes decreased melatonin levels. Melatonin is secreted primarily into the blood in adult humans, with the highest levels at night reaching 500 to 700 pg per milliliter, compared with daylight values of 50 to 300 pg per milliliter. Much lower levels of melatonin are found in the CSF. Melatonin is metabolized by the liver to 6-hydroxylmelatonin, which is excreted in the urine. Unfortunately, plasma or urine melatonin levels have not proved helpful in diagnosing or treating pineal tumors. Although pineal physiology has been extensively studied in vertebrates (particularly rat and hamster), the pineal's role in human physiology remains largely unknown.

CLINICAL SIGNIFICANCE

The clinical relevance of the pineal relates to tumor formation and to calcification of the pineal gland. No symptoms or signs can be attributed to changes in melatonin secretion.

PINEAL TUMORS

Pineal tumors represent less than 1% of intracranial tumors. Tumors of the pineal region fall into three categories: 20% are parenchymal tumors of the pinealocyte (pineocytoma or pineoblastoma, depending on degree of differentiation); 25% are nonparenchymal tumors of glial origin (astrocytoma, glioblastoma, or ependymoma); and 55% are germ cell tumors (germinoma or teratoma). These latter tumors develop from primordial or embryonic rests of germ cells, similar to germinomas of the testes (seminoma), ovary, or anterior mediastinum. Often, germinomas arise from the floor of the third ventricle and appear histologically similar to germinomas derived from the pineal; hence the term "ectopic pinealoma." Intracranial germinomas frequently spread locally, infiltrate the hypothalamus, and metastasize to the spinal cord. Teratomas contain evidence of two or more germ lines and often include chorionic tissue that secretes human chorionic gonadotropin (hCG). Pineal tumors may present at any age, but most are found in the second decade of life and more often in males than females (3 : 1).

Patients with pineal tumors present with neurologic or endocrine manifestations; neurologic symptoms and signs are more common. Increased intracranial pressure causing headache, nausea, vomiting, and altered mental status occurs in nearly 85% of patients with tumors in the pineal region. About half of pineal tumors press against the quadrigeminal plate, leading to Parinaud's syndrome, which consists of paresis of upward gaze, pupillary areflexia to light, paralysis of convergence, and wide-based gait. Endocrine manifestations due to hypothalamic involvement (pressure or invasion) lead to precocious or delayed puberty or anterior pituitary insufficiency. Some pineal tumors are teratomas that secrete abundant quantities of hCG; hCG stimulates testosterone production in males but not estrogen secretion in females, leading to precocious puberty in boys. Precocious puberty is not a common finding in pineal disease (one series of 65 pineal tumors reported no precocious puberty, and another reported that only 10% of 177 patients had precocious puberty). Hypogonadism due to infiltration of tumor in the hypothalamus leads to delayed pubescence, but it has been postulated that pineal tumors secrete an antigonadotropic hormone that may also cause hypogonadism. Diabetes insipidus, visual impairment, and anterior pituitary insufficiency associated with polyphagia and obesity are common in the ectopic pinealoma.

For years, the treatment of tumors in the pineal region consisted of ventricular shunting to relieve the hydrocephalus and radiation therapy without a tissue diagnosis. Germinomas, the most common pineal tumor, are very radiosensitive (in contrast to most tumors of the third ventricle), so that pineal tumors carried a better prognosis than most forms of brain cancer, with 5-year survivals ranging from 60% to 80% and with 10-year survivals of 60%. Surgery was generally avoided because this area was relatively inaccessible. With the advent of better preoperative localization techniques [computed tomography (CT) and magnetic resonance imaging (MRI)] and intraoperative use of the microscope, many neurosurgeons recommend surgical exploration, which may permit total resection of benign encapsulated tumors, provide histologic identification of nonresectable tumors, and identify whether the tumor has spread locally or seeded throughout the CSF. This information permits optimization of the adjunctive therapy (radiation or chemotherapy). Germinomas frequently seed the meninges; thus, whole-brain and

spinal irradiation must be considered. Seeding of germinoma cells to the peritoneum from ventriculoperitoneal shunts is not uncommon. Chemotherapy with bleomycin, vinblastine, and cisplatin has been advocated for metastatic germinoma. Ectopic pinealomas in the chiasmal region usually are explored because these procedures are relatively safe, provide tissue diagnosis, and offer the possibility of removing or debulking tumors that are not as radiosensitive as germinomas.

PINEAL CALCIFICATION

Calcium deposits increase with age such that calcification of the pineal gland is evident often in the second decade of life. Pineal calcification serves as a midline marker on routine skull radiographs. Deposition of calcium within the pineal does not interfere with pineal function.

EVALUATION FOR PINEAL DISEASE

The workup of the patient begins with a high index of suspicion for an intracranial process. Signs and symptoms of increased intracranial pressure (headache, vomiting, somnolence, gait disturbance, papilledema), visual impairment, diabetes insipidus, precocious puberty in boys, and delayed puberty point to possible tumors of the third ventricle. Parinaud's syndrome localizes the process to the pineal region. Routine skull radiographs are seldom helpful, although suprasellar calcification is often seen in craniopharyngiomas. Enhanced CT or MRI scans yield important clues as to presence and localization of tumor. Radiographic criteria to differentiate between benign and malignant tumors have not been substantiated. The differential diagnosis of third ventricular tumors is diverse. A significant number are benign, encapsulated, and potentially resectable; these include simple non-neoplastic cysts, ependymal cysts, colloid cysts, dermoids, teratomas, craniopharyngiomas, meningiomas, and certain ependymomas. A large group of gliomas found in this area usually are not resectable. Levels of β-hCG should be determined in serum and in CSF obtained at ventricular shunting. Plasma levels of β-hCG correlate with tumor growth and regression. Unfortunately, most germ cell tumors do not secrete β-hCG.

BIBLIOGRAPHY

Erlich SS, Apuzzo MLJ. The pineal gland: anatomy, physiology, and clinical significance. *J Neurosurg* 1985;63:321–341.

Preslock JP. The pineal gland: basic implications and clinical correlations. *Endocr Rev* 1984;5:282–308.

Reichlin S. Neuroendocrinology. In: Wilson JD, Foster DW, eds. *Textbook of endocrinology*, seventh ed. Philadelphia: WB Saunders, 1985:492.

Schild SE, Scheithauer BW, Schomberg PJ, et al. Pineal parenchymal tumors: clinical, pathologic, and therapeutic aspects. *Cancer* 1993;72:870–880.

DISORDERS OF THE THYROID GLAND

LEONARD WARTOFSKY

THYROID HORMONE PRODUCTION, TRANSPORT, AND ACTION

ANATOMY

The thyroid gland consists of two lobes and a connecting isthmus, and lies just anterior to and below the larynx. The glandular tissue is arranged in acini, or follicles, composed of cuboidal epithelium surrounded by a capillary network. Within the lumen of the follicles is a proteinaceous substance—colloid—in which the protein, thyroglobulin, is stored. Other parafollicular or C cells are also present and are the source of calcitonin; their malignant transformation may give rise to medullary thyroid cancer. Thyroglobulin is a 660,000-d glycoprotein that constitutes approximately 75% of the protein content of the thyroid.

THYROID HORMONE BIOSYNTHESIS AND SECRETION

The normal function of the thyroid gland is directed to the secretion of thyroxine (T_4) and triiodothyronine (T_3), the active thyroid hormones that influence diverse metabolic processes. Synthesis of T_4 and T_3 depends on entry into the thyroid of adequate quantities of iodine, on iodine metabolism within the gland, and on thyroglobulin synthesis in which iodination and synthesis of T_4 and T_3 occurs. Iodine enters the thyroid as inorganic iodide, usually derived from dietary sources (Fig. 406.1). Dietary iodide is rapidly absorbed and distributed into extracellular fluid from which it is trapped by the thyroid or excreted by the kidneys as a function of glomerular filtration rate. In the United States, a dietary iodine intake of 200 to 300 μg per day is generally sufficient to sustain a plasma iodide concentration of approximately 40 nmol per liter (0.5 per deciliter). The thyroid also concentrates other monovalent anions, such as pertechnetate, which is available as the radioactive isotope sodium technetium Tc 99m pertechnetate. Unlike iodide, little pertechnetate is organically bound; hence, its duration of stay in the thyroid is short. This property, together with its short physical half-life, makes pertechnetate a valuable radionuclide for imaging the thyroid by scintillation scanning.

Synthesis and secretion of T_4 and T_3 can be divided into four phases, each under the control of thyroid-stimulating hormone (TSH). The first involves active transport of iodide into the thyroid cell, a process mediated by the Na^+/I^- symporter, a protein in the plasma membrane of thyroid cells. Iodide is actively transported such that the thyroid maintains an iodide con-

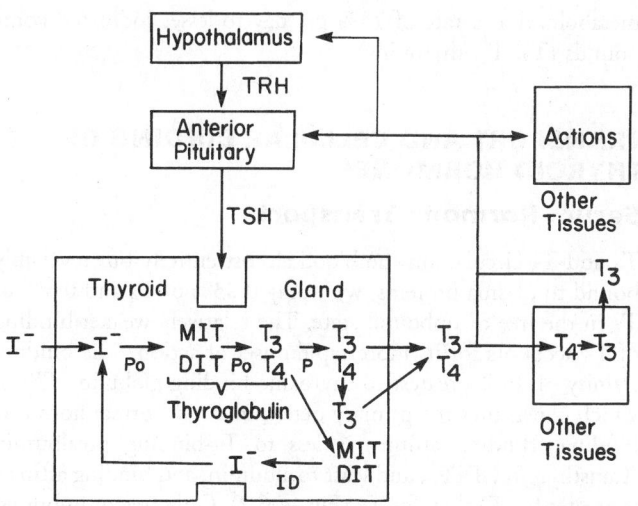

Figure 406.1. Iodine enters the thyroid as inorganic iodide, usually derived from dietary sources. Dietary iodide is rapidly absorbed and distributed into extracellular fluid from which it is trapped by the thyroid or excreted by the kidneys as a function of glomerular filtration rate.

centration gradient (thyroid/plasma) of 25 or greater. The second phase of hormone biosynthesis involves the oxidation of iodide mediated by thyroidal peroxidase, with the oxidized iodide serving to iodinate tyrosine residues within thyroglobulin to form the hormone precursors monoiodotyrosine (MIT) and diiodotyrosine (DIT). MIT and DIT undergo oxidative condensation or coupling as the third phase of hormone synthesis, again via mediation by peroxidase, to yield the iodothyronines T_4 and T_3. Phase 4 consists of hormonal secretion of T_4 and T_3 into the blood and involves pinocytosis of follicular colloid at the apical end of the cells into colloid droplets that merge with cellular lysosomes to form phagolysosomes, within which thyroglobulin is hydrolyzed by proteases. Thyroidal secretion is the sole source of circulating T_4 whereas only about 20% of circulating T_3 is produced in the thyroid, with the remainder being generated in extraglandular tissues by deiodination of the 5′-iodine.

The foregoing steps in hormone synthesis may be inhibited by a variety of agents, which may be called goitrogens, and which may include inorganic anions such as perchlorate and thiocyanate, or the thiourea antithyroid agents propylthiouracil or mercaptoimidazole, which are commonly employed in the treatment of hyperthyroidism. Iodine itself, when given in large doses, blocks the organic binding and coupling reactions, a phenomenon known as the Wolff–Chaikoff effect that is normally transient. Iodide in large doses is capable of inhibiting proteolysis of thyroglobulin and hormone release, an effect responsible for the ameliorative action of iodides in hyperthyroidism. Excess iodide also may induce either hypothyroidism or thyrotoxicosis in susceptible individuals, as discussed below.

Approximately 80 to 100 μg of T_4 is produced daily. T_4 is metabolized via deiodination to either T_3 or reverse T_3 (see below). The total extrathyroidal pool of T_4 (in serum and tissues) approximates 600 to 800 μg and is metabolized at a rate of 10% daily. The total extrathyroidal pool of T_3 is 50 to 60 μg and is metabolized at a rate of 75% per day to lesser iodinated compounds (T_2, T_1, thyronine).

TRANSPORT AND CELLULAR BINDING OF THYROID HORMONES

Serum Hormone Transport

T_4 and T_3 circulate in the blood almost entirely but reversibly bound to plasma proteins, with only 0.03% of T_4 and 0.3% of T_3 in the free or unbound state. The relatively weaker binding of T_3 accounts for its more rapid onset of action. The binding affinity of T_4 is greatest to thyroxine-binding globulin (TBG), which constitutes the primary determinant of normal hormone binding. Binding affinity is less to T_4-binding prealbumin (transthyretin, TTR), and least to albumin, and binding affinity is greater for T_4 than for T_3 (Fig. 406.2). Only free or unbound T_4 or T_3 is available to tissues, and as a consequence, metolic state correlates more closely with the concentration of plasma free hormone than with total hormone. Homeostatic regulation of thyroid function by the hypothalamic–pituitary axis, and in part by peripheral rates of hormonal deiodination in peripheral tissues, is directed to maintenance of a normal concentration of free hormone. Eighty percent of circulating T_4 is bound to TBG, 15% to TTR, and 5% to albumin. In the case of T_3, 90% is bound to TBG, 5% to TTR, and 5% to albumin.

Because nearly all T_4 and T_3 is protein-bound, any change in the capacity or affinity of TBG or TTR will result in changes in measured total T_4 or T_3. Alterations in the interaction between T_4/T_3 and the binding proteins are of two general types. In one case, there is an intrinsically normal pituitary–thyroid axis with intact thyroid-stimulating hormone (THS) regulation of thyroid hormone production and secretion. When an increase in the TBG concentration occurs, there is a shift of free hormone

TABLE 406.1.	CONDITIONS INVOLVING INCREASED OR DECREASED SERUM THYROXINE DUE TO ALTERATIONS IN THYROID HORMONE BINDING
Decreased TBG	**Increased TBG**
On genetic basis	Newborn
High-dose glucocorticoids	Estrogens
Androgens	Pregnancy
Nephrotic syndrome	Tamoxifen
Acromegaly	Perphenazine
Cirrhosis	Acute hepatitis
Severe systemic illness	Chronic active hepatitis
Asparaginase	Biliary cirrhosis
	Acute intermittent porphyria
	On genetic basis

TBG, thyroxine-binding globulin.

to the increased binding sites, thereby lowering the concentration of free hormone and reducing the quantity of hormone available to tissues. Ultimately, a new equilibrium is established, with an increased total hormone concentration but a smaller proportion of hormone that is free, resulting in restoration of the absolute concentration of free hormone (product of total hormone and free fraction) to normal, as well as the metabolic state. With a reduction in TBG concentration, the opposite occurs. Various conditions associated with increases or decreases in the concentration of TBG are listed in Table 406.1. The serum TBG concentration is approximately 20 mg per liter and can bind approximately 200 µg of T_4. Serum TTR concentration is some tenfold higher, averaging 250 mg per liter and binding up to 2,000 µg of T_4.

A second type of altered binding interaction occurs when there is a primary increase or decrease in the concentration of thyroid hormones in the blood, as in thyrotoxicosis or hypothyroidism. In such cases, there are only minor changes in the concentration of TBG, but there can be major alterations in the concentrations of both total and free hormones. The abnormal secretion of thyroid hormone precludes homeostatic restoration of free-hormone levels or the metabolic state back to normal.

Thyroid Hormone Metabolism

T_4 and T_3 bound to TBG or TTR dissociate readily and the free hormone diffuses into cells where sequential removal of a single iodine atom (5′-monodeiodination) yields T_3. There are two 5′-deiodinases. Most T_4-to-T_3 conversion is effected by the type I isoenzyme in liver and kidney and the thyroid itself. The type II enzyme is localized in the pituitary, central nervous system, placenta, and brown fat. The type I enzyme is inactive during systemic illness and during normal fetal life, leading to low levels of serum T_3. Generation of T_3 from T_4 in brain and pituitary is continued in hypothyroidism due to an increase in activity of type II enzyme activity. Approximately 30% of all T_4 is converted to T_3 and the T_3 generated accounts for approxi-

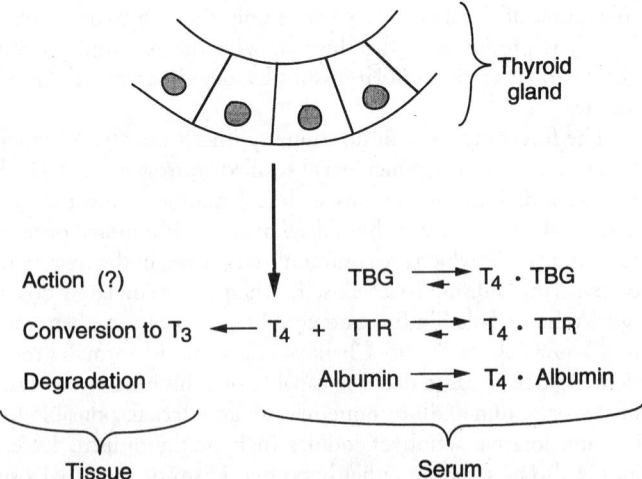

Figure 406.2. T_4 and T_3 circulate in the blood almost entirely but reversibly bound to plasma proteins. Relatively weaker binding of T_3 accounts for its more rapid onset of action. Binding affinity of T_4 is greatest to thyroxine-binding globulin (TBG), which constitutes the primary determinant of normal hormone binding. Binding affinity is less to T_4-binding prealbumin, and least to albumin, and binding affinity is greater for T_4 than for T_3.

mately 80% of total T_3 production. The remaining 20% is secreted directly from the thyroid gland. Since T_3 has approximately three times the metabolic potency of T_4, virtually all the metabolic action of T_4 can be attributed to T_3.

An additional 40% of T_4 is disposed of by monodeiodination at the 5-position of its inner ring to yield reverse T_3 (rT_3). There is very little rT_3 produced by the thyroid, and rT_3 has neglible metabolic potency. As a consequence, 5'-deiodination has been termed the activating pathway of T_4 metabolism, and 5-deiodination at the inner ring as the inactivating pathway, and the relative rates of 5- and 5'-monodeiodination of T_4 determine the metabolic state by governing the availability of active hormone.

REGULATION OF THYROID FUNCTION

TSH and the TSH Receptor

Thyroid function is regulated by TSH, a 28-kd glycoprotein secreted by basophilic (thyrotropic) cells in the anterior pituitary. TSH consists of an α subunit common to other glycoprotein hormones and a unique β subunit. TSH controls thyroid function by binding to TSH receptors on the basolateral membrane of thyroid follicular cells. The TSH receptor is an 85-kd glycoprotein member of the guanyl nucleotide (G) protein–coupled receptor family and is organized into an extracellular and intracellular domains. TSH-R binding leads to activation of adenylate cyclase and phospholipase C pathways of intracellular signaling that regulate thyroid function and growth. Effects of TSH stimulation include thyroid hypertrophy, hyperplasia, and goitrogenesis mediated by protein synthesis; acceleration of most aspects of intermediary metabolism (glucose and fatty acid utilization) in the thyroid; enhanced synthesis of nucleic acids and proteins, including synthesis and proteolysis of thyroglobulin; enhanced activity of 5'-deiodinase; increased oxygen consumption by follicular cells; and stimulation of the biosynthesis and secretion of thyroid hormones. Somatic mutations and clonal expansion of the gene for the TSH receptor have been shown to account for development of some types of toxic follicular adenomas presumably due to chronic stimulation of the cyclic adenosine monophosphate (cAMP) cascade.

TSH and TRH

TSH secretion is regulated by two opposing influences at the level of the thyrotropic cell. TSH stimulation is mediated by thyrotropin-releasing hormone (TRH), a tripeptide (pyroglutamyl-histidyl-prolineamide) that is produced from the hypothalamus in the median eminence and paraventricular and arcuate nuclei. TRH reaches the pituitary via the hypophyseal portal blood system and binds to specific high-affinity receptors on the plasma membrane of the thyrotropic cell and via activation of the adenylate cyclase system; in addition, increased calcium flux stimulates the secretion and synthesis of TSH. Along with stimulating release of stored TSH, TRH enhances the synthesis of TSH via transcription and translation of the β-subunit gene. Negative regulation of TSH is mediated by the thyroid hormones, which both antagonize TRH action and directly inhibit the TSH secretory mechanism. Thyroid hormone homeostatic

control of TSH secretion is exerted by negative feedback at the level of the thyrotropic cell, with the threshold for feedback inhibition set by TRH. Thyroid hormone inhibition is unopposed and more effective in the absence of TRH due to hypothalamic disease. Experimentally, thyroid hormones both inhibit production of TRH messenger RNA (mRNA) and TRH prohormone and reduce the number of TRH receptors on the thyrotropic cell, thus impairing the cell's responsiveness to TRH. The major negative-feedback action of the thyroid hormones is at the pituitary level, mediated by binding of the hormones to thyroxine in the nucleus of the thyrotropic cell, resulting in reduced expression of the genes for the α and β subunits of TSH. The principal arbiter of thyroid hormone action in the pituitary is T_3, both that generated in the pituitary from T_4 and that derived from plasma.

Thyroid Hormone Action

Thyroid hormone bound to its transport proteins dissociates very readily, and the free fractions of T_4 and T_3 enter the cell primarily by diffusion and, to a lesser extent, by active transport. Some T_3 that is derived from intracellular T_4 via type II T_4-5'-deiodinase activity will diffuse back into the circulation, but most will bind to the nuclear receptors mediating hormone action. Thyroid hormone influences growth and maturation of tissues, cell respiration and total energy expenditure, and the turnover of essentially all substrates, vitamins, and hormones, including the thyroid hormones themselves. Some actions of these hormones on cell metabolism may be mediated at the level of the mitochondrion to influence oxidative metabolism or at the level of the plasma membrane and endoplasmic reticulum to influence the synthesis and activity of Ca^{2+} ATPase and NA^+,K^+ adenosine triphosphatase, as well as several lipogenic and mitochondrial enzymes. Increased activity of these enzymes leads to increased cellular sodium transport, mitochondrial oxidative metabolism, and glucose utilization, accounting for the thermogenic action of T_3.

THYROID HORMONE RESISTANCE

Generalized thyroid hormone resistance (GTHR) is a rare autosomal recessive syndrome characterized by reduced responsiveness to elevated levels of thyroid hormone. The resistance to thyroid hormone action is due to mutations of the T_3 nuclear receptor with varied phenotypes due to a heterogeneous series of mutations of the $Tr\beta$. The mutation results in a reduced affinity of the receptor for T_3 and consequently to reduced hormone action. Reduced T_3 effectiveness is compensated for by increases in thyroidal hormone production, and the syndrome is marked by elevated circulating levels of free T_4 and free T_3, appropriately normal or elevated (nonsuppressed) serum TSH, and intact TSH responsiveness to TRH. Kindreds have been described whose members express variable patterns of resistance, and the responsiveness of target tissues may vary within an individual. The clinical features suggestive of hypothyroidism include short stature, attention deficits with mental deficiency or learning disability, deafness, and goiter. Other features suggestive of hyperthyroidism include hyperactivity, weakness, and tachycardia. While GTHR patients are either euthyroid or hypothyroid, the differential diagnosis includes isolated pituitary resistance to thyroid hormone and a TSH-secreting pituitary tumor, disorders usually associated with hyperthyroidism. The presence of increased serum TSH suggests the need for treatment with supplemental thyroid hormone, and the dosage requirement may be titrated against several parameters of tissue responses to thyroid hormone.

DISEASES OF THE THYROID

HYPOTHYROIDISM

Thyroid hormone deficiency from any cause results in hypothyroidism. The thyroid deficiency may either be due to a primary defect in the thyroid gland or be secondary to TSH deficiency resulting from pituitary or hypothalamic disease. Cretinism refers to hypothyroidism dating from birth, which is usually accompanied by intellectual impairment and developmental abnormalities. Although the term *myxedema* is often used synonymously with hypothyroidism, it originally connoted a more severe hypothyroidism in which patients had a tendency to generalized edema with characteristically puffy facies and a doughy, almost peau d'orange induration of the skin due to infiltration of the skin with hydrophilic mucopolysaccharides.

Causes of Hypothyroidism

Of all cases of hypothyroidism, 95% are due to primary disease of the thyroid gland leading to inadequate production of the thyroid hormones, with the remainder being due to hypothalamic–pituitary disease. The various specific causes of hypothyroidism are listed in Table 406.2. In the United States, the most

TABLE 406.2.	CAUSES OF HYPOTHYROIDISM

Primary (thyroidal) hypothyroidism
  Chronic autoimmune thyroiditis[a]
  ^{131}I or external-beam radiation therapy
  Postoperative hypothyroidism
  Transient hypothyroidism
  Infiltrative, diseases[a]
  Thyroid dysgenesis
  Defective thyroid hormone biosynthesis:
    Congenital defects[a]
    Iodide deficiency[a]
    Antithyroid agents[a]
    Iodine excess[a]
Secondary (central, hypothyrotropic) hypothyroidism
  Thyroid-stimulating hormone deficiency
  Thyrotropin-releasing hormone deficiency
  Generalized resistance to thyroid hormone[a]

---

[a] Goiter often present.
EVIDENCE LEVEL: C. Expert Opinion.

common cause of primary thyroid deficiencies is autoimmunity due to lymphocytic (Hashimoto's) thyroiditis in which cytotoxic antibodies are directed against thyroid follicular cells, leading to thyroid atrophy and fibrosis. Another variant of autoimmune hypothyroidism is due to TSH receptor antibodies which are of a blocking type. Probably next in frequency are those patients with Graves' disease who have undergone ablative therapy by either radioiodine or thyroidectomy. Both Hashimoto's disease and Graves' disease are primary autoimmune disorders of the thyroid that often coexist with diabetes mellitus and other diseases in which circulating autoantibodies are found, such as Sjögren's syndrome, pernicious anemia, systemic lupus erythematosus, rheumatoid arthritis, primary biliary cirrhosis, and chronic hepatitis. Rarely, hypothyroidism may also be a manifestation of a polyglandular endocrine deficiency state in which various autoantibodies cause impaired function of the thyroid, adrenal, parathyroid, and gonads.

A number of hereditary defects in the various steps of thyroid hormone biosynthesis can occur at birth and constitute the entity of sporadic goitrous cretinism, and incomplete forms of the same disorders may account for cases of milder hypothyroidism presenting later in adult life. Certain drugs may also induce defects in hormone biosynthesis, such as aminosalicylic acid and lithium. Lithium may cause both goiter and hypothyroidism, and patients with underlying Hashimoto's disease may be particularly susceptible. Endemic iodine deficiency as a cause of goiter, hypothyroidism, or cretinism is discussed elsewhere (see section "Goiter"). As described below (see section "Thyroiditis"), there typically is a self-limited or transient interval of hypothyroidism that occurs as part of the natural course of de Quervain's (subacute) thyroiditis as well as in lymphocytic "painless" thyroiditis and lymphocytic "postpartum" thyroiditis. Patients who have taken long-term thyroxine therapy in doses sufficient to fully suppress TSH (e.g., for goiter suppression) but who have underlying functional thyroid glands will pass through a period of transient hypothyroidism when the exogenous thyroxine might be discontinued. This interval may last for weeks to as long as a month and represents the time required for recovery first of the pituitary (TSH synthesis and release) and then of the thyroid to trap iodide and synthesize thyroid hormone.

Other than in cases of thyroidal atrophy and fibrosis or congenital athyreosis, the failure to synthesize adequate amounts of thyroid hormone for physiologic needs will lead to goiter mediated by increased secretion of TSH. If thyroid hormone production is sufficient, euthyroidism may ensue, but at the cost of chronic mild TSH elevation maintaining the goiter (see section "Goiter"). However, both goiter and hypothyroidism will occur when the thyroid gland cannot provide an adequate response. In the United States, the most common cause of goitrous hypothyroidism is Hashimoto's thyroiditis, early in its course prior to its evolution into an atrophic gland. Some of the goiter is actually due to lymphocytic infiltrates rather than thyroid follicular tissue, and the disorder is usually diagnosed on the basis of serologic tests for thyroid autoantibodies. Euthyroid patients with Hashimoto's disease may be uniquely sensitive to exposure to exogenous iodine excess and develop iodine-induced hypothyroidism. Other patients may also develop iodine-induced hypothyroidism, presumably on the basis of incomplete defects in the ability of their thyroid to organically bind iodide and to escape from the Wolff–Chaikoff effect (see section "Physiology," above). Another category of euthyroid patients who are susceptible to iodine-induced hypothyroidism comprises patients with Graves' disease who have been treated by partial thyroidectomy or radioiodine, as well as normal fetuses in utero. The latter may be unusually susceptible to large doses of iodine that may be given during pregnancy and can develop both hypothyroidism and goiter, sometimes large enough to result in neonatal asphyxiation.

Hypothyroidism may be on a secondary (pituitary) or tertiary (hypothalamic) basis, in which case circulating levels of total and free T_4 will be reduced but TSH concentrations will not be increased. In these patients, the thyroid gland is intrinsically normal, as can be demonstrated by increases in serum T_4 or radioiodine uptake that follow injection of recombinant human TSH. A pituitary basis for hypothyroidism may be due to pituitary tumor, postpartum pituitary necrosis (Sheehan's syndrome), or autoimmune hypophysitis. More rarely, hypothyroidism is due to hypothalamic TRH deficiency such as may be caused by a craniopharyngioma, or granulomatous infiltration seen with sarcoidosis or tuberculosis.

Clinical Presentation

Signs and symptoms of hypothyroidism will vary greatly depending on the severity and duration of the thyroid deficiency, the age of the patient, and the possible coincidence of other systemic illness. Neonatal screening programs have disclosed that hypothyroidism is present in approximately 1 of every 5,000 neonates; it may be manifested as persistent physiologic jaundice, a hoarse cry, constipation, somnolence, and feeding problems. Early diagnosis and treatment is mandatory to achieve normal intellectual development, and consequently all neonates are routinely screened for hypothyroidism with measurements of serum T_4 and/or TSH. The manifestations of hypothyroidism in older children depend on the age at which the deficiency began, and the presence of any residual problems may depend on the promptness with which replacement thyroxine therapy was instituted. Cretinism may be detected at birth but usually becomes manifest several months after birth, depending on the extent of thyroid failure. As the child gets older, a delay in reaching the normal milestones of development becomes evident, and more of the classic physical characteristics of the cretin appear. These include short stature; coarse features with a protruding tongue; a broad, flat nose and widely set eyes; sparse hair and dry skin; delayed dentition; a protuberant abdomen often with an umbilical hernia; and impaired mental development. Sexual precocity has been described, whereas retardation of linear growth and delayed puberty may be seen in the older child. Intellectual deficiency and poor performance at school may first call attention to the potential diagnosis. X-ray examinations may reveal retarded bone age, epiphyseal dysgenesis, and delayed union of the epiphyses.

In adults, early symptoms of hypothyroidism (Table 406.3) are often nonspecific and insidious in onset, and may include

TABLE 406.3.	SYMPTOMS AND SIGNS OF HYPOTHYROIDISM

Symptoms

Weakness and fatigue
Lethargy
Decreased mental activity
Decreased physical activity
Dry skin
Decrease perspiration
Cold intolerance
Weight gain
Constipation
Paresthesia
Myalgia
Muscle and joint stiffness

Signs

Slow movements
Hoarse voice
Dry, cool skin
Periorbital edema
Edema of hands and feet
Goiter
Bradycardia
Slow relaxation of tendon reflexes
EVIDENCE LEVEL: C. Expert Opinion.

fatigue, lethargy, constipation, cold intolerance, muscle stiffness and cramping, carpal tunnel syndrome, and menorrhagia. In the very elderly, the symptoms may be erroneously attributed to the aging process or to other common disorders of the elderly, such as Parkinson's disease, depression, or Alzheimer's disease. Along with apathy, there is slowing in mental agility and motor activity, reduced memory, and weight gain in spite of a reduced appetite. The skin and hair become dry, and the hair becomes thinner as it falls out. Hearing becomes impaired, and edema of the vocal cords may account for deepening of the voice. Somnolence is common, and enlargement of the tongue contributes to a tendency to obstructive sleep apnea. With little functional thyroid reserve, the severity of hypothyroidism progresses to a clinical picture of florid myxedema. At this stage, patients appear pallid, depressed, and hypokinetic, with a hoarse voice, a dull and expressionless facies, sparse hair, and a large tongue. The skin is both cool to touch and dry, rough, or scaly; there is facial and periorbital puffiness, often accompanied by generalized edema. Fluid may collect in various body compartments, and pleural effusion, pericardial effusion, or ascites is not uncommon. Goiter may or may not be present depending on the cause of the hypothyroidism. With so-called primary myxedema due to burned-out Hashimoto's disease, the gland is atrophic and usually not palpable. On physical examination or chest x-ray, the cardiac silhouette will appear enlarged, which may be due to either chamber dilatation or pericardial effusion. A small cardiac silhouette should bring adrenal insufficiency to mind, either on a pituitary basis or due to coincident primary adrenal insufficiency (Schmidt's syndrome). Constipation is common due to slowed gastrointestinal motility, and adynamic ileus may cause megacolon or intestinal obstruction. A psychiatric syndrome ("myxedema madness") has been described, and neurologic findings include a delayed or "hung-up" relaxation phase of deep tendon reflexes, muscle weakness, and ataxia.

Laboratory Diagnosis

The single most important diagnostic test is measurement of the serum TSH, which is increased in patients with primary thyroid disease of any kind, and is in the low-normal to undetectable range in patients with pituitary or hypothalamic disease. Serum total and free T_4 will be decreased in all forms of hypothyroidism. Measurement of serum total T_3 is less useful and will be within the normal range in the majority of patients with hypothyroidism. This may be due to a relatively augmented rate of conversion of available circulating T_4 to T_3 in peripheral tissues, or to a relative preponderance of T_3 over T_4 secretion from the thyroid as a response to elevated serum levels of TSH. Free T_3 concentration may be low. Thyroid autoantibodies will be detectable in the majority of patients with underlying Hashimoto's disease as the basis for their hypothyroidism. Although the radioiodine uptake may be normal to elevated in the latter patients, it is usually decreased when there is another cause of thyroprivic hypothyroidism and may be of limited diagnostic utility because of the low value for the lower limit of the normal range.

Other nonthyroid laboratory tests may provide further clues to the presence of hypothyroidism. Serum triglycerides, along with total and low-density lipoprotein (LDL) cholesterol level, are usually elevated in hypothyroidism, although not necessarily in hypothyroidism of pituitary origin. Serum levels of carotene may be elevated, thus contributing to the yellow complexion of these patients. Serum levels of creatine phosphokinase (CPK), aspartate transaminase, and lactate dehydrogenase (LDH) will be increased. Anemia may be present on the basis of impaired iron utilization, which can be corrected by thyroxine administration. In patients with Hashimoto's disease, there may be coincident pernicious anemia in about 10% of patients. Electrocardiographic changes include bradycardia, low-amplitude QRS complexes, and flattened or inverted T waves—findings that may be most pronounced in the presence of a pericardial effusion. Cardiac contractility is reduced, as can be assessed by systolic time intervals demonstrating a prolonged pre-ejection period and an increased ratio of the pre-ejection period to the left ventricular ejection time.

"Subclinical" (Mild) Hypothyroidism

As with many disorders, patients with hypothyroidism may present earlier or later in the course of their disease. In its earliest, mild form, hypothyroidism has been called "subclinical" because the symptoms may be so mild as to be overlooked. Moreover, routine thyroid function tests, such as total and free T_4 or T_3, will still be within the normal range, albeit probably lower than when the patients were truly euthyroid. The diagnosis of subclinical disease rests on the finding of a slight elevation in TSH concentration, and the TSH response to TRH may be augmented. With a normal range for TSH of 0.3 to 4.0 milliunits

per liter, patients may have TSH levels between 4 and 10 milliunits per liter with adequate remaining thyroid reserve to maintain T_4 measurably normal. Often, the mild TSH elevation is ignored because of the normal T_4 and T_3 levels, and follow-up of such patients indicates that approximately half will progress to overt hypothyroidism within 5 to 7 years. Subclinical hypothyroidism is most often seen in patients with Hashimoto's disease or those with Graves' disease who have been treated with iodine 131 or surgery, and can be viewed as a stage in the evolution to overt hypothyroidism. Because many studies have shown mild abnormalities in lipoproteins with elevations in total and LDL cholesterol and other atherogenic moieties, such as apolipoproteins (a) and (b), early initiation of thyroxine replacement in low dosage has been recommended. Therapy may eliminate the progression from mild to overt disease, ameliorate symptoms, and possibly reduce cardiovascular risks of ongoing atherogenesis.

Treatment

The overwhelming majority of patients with hypothyroidism are treated with a single daily dose of synthetic levothyroxine. Only once-daily therapy is required because of the long (6 to 7 days) half-life of thyroxine. Other thyroid hormone preparations are available, including desiccated thyroid extract, USP, a T_3 preparation, and a mixture of thyroxine and T_3 (liotrix). While once in popular use, the thyroid extract preparation is no longer recommended because of its content of T_3, which is so rapidly absorbed that the resultant high serum T_3 can cause worrisome tachycardias or arrhythmias in elderly patients or those with underlying cardiac disease. The levothyroxine products also are more stable, with a longer and more predictable shelf life. Since T_4 is converted to T_3, ultimately near-normal concentrations of serum T_3 can be restored by the administration of thyroxine alone. In order to more closely mimic thyroidal T_3 secretion and normal blood levels, oral supplements of T_3 would need to be given in frequent divided dosage, a regimen that makes good compliance problematic. Moreover, convincing arguments or data demonstrating benefit of concomitant T_3 administration are lacking. When initially diagnosed, most patients with hypothyroidism have had the condition for some time, and there is usually (with the exception of myxedema coma) no reason to rapidly correct the thyroid deficiency with aggressive therapy. Rather, the dosage generally is gradually incremented with an initial daily dose of 25 to 50 μg thyroxine increased by 25 to 50 μg at 4- to 6-week intervals until a normal metabolic state is attained. This is especially true in elderly patients and in patients with heart disease, since a sudden increase in metabolic rate may tax cardiac or coronary reserve. The best indication that a normal metabolic state has been attained is normalization of the TSH level down to the range of 0.5 to 1.5 milliunits per liter. On average, this will equate to an ultimate full replacement dose of approximately 1.7 μg per kilogram per day.

In some circumstances a previously stable dosage of levothyroxine may need to be increased or decreased. Increases of 25 to 50 μg per day may be required during pregnancy, as evidenced by increases in serum TSH. Progressive increases in dose may be required as further atrophy of the gland occurs in patients

TABLE 406.4.	FACTORS ALTERING THYROXINE DOSAGE NEEDED FOR ADEQUATE REPLACEMENT THERAPY IN HYPOTHYROID PATIENTS

Decreased dosage requirement
  T_4 production normally decreased
    Androgen therapy
  Decreased T_4 clearance
    Older age
  Remaining autonomous thyroid tissue
    Graves' disease
    Multinodular goiter
Increased dosage requirement
  T_4 production normally increased
    Pregnancy and estrogen therapy
    Obesity
  Decreased gastrointestinal absorption of T_4
    Malabsorption and short-bowel syndromes
    Therapy with agents that bind T_4 in the intestinal tract
      Sucralfate, ferrous sulfate, aluminum hydroxide, cholestyramine, colestipol
  Increased T_4 clearance
    Young age
    Therapy with phenytoin, carbamazepine, rifampin
  Decreased extrathyroidal T_4 conversion to T_3
    Therapy amiodarone
Apparent increase in dosage requirement (pseudomalabsorption)
  Poor adherence

T_4, thyroxine; T_3, triiodothyronine.

with Hashimoto's disease or in patients with Graves' disease who have been treated with surgery or radioiodine. On the other hand, spontaneous disappearance of TSH receptor–blocking antibodies in Hashimoto's disease or increases in stimulating TSH receptor antibodies leading to evolution of autonomy in a previously treated Graves' gland can necessitate a reduction in dosage. Thyroxine absorption may be minimally reduced when taken with food or certain other pharmacologic agents that interfere with gastrointestinal absorption or enhance the metabolic clearance of levothyroxine (Table 406.4). Similarly, decreases in dosage may be required with the emergence of autonomous hyperfunction in a uninodular or multinodular goiter.

In known or suspected cases of pituitary or hypothalamic hypothyroidism, it is traditional not to begin thyroid hormone replacement without concomitant corticosteroid administration. This practice is based on the theoretical risk of precipitating acute adrenocortical insufficiency by augmenting the metabolism of plasma cortisol in a patient with sluggish adrenal output as a result of long-standing hypothyroidism. The exogenous steroid would be continued for perhaps 10 to 14 days or until euthyroidism was reestablished. More rapid treatment of hypothyroidism may be indicated in certain patients, such as those in whom myxedema coma is suspected (see below), and perhaps in hypothyroid patients who are being prepared for emergency surgery, out of concern for their sensitivity to anesthesia and central nervous system depressants. In these patients, intravenous administration of levothyroxine, in conjunction with the use of hydrocortisone, may be employed. Patients discovered to be hypothyroid prior to scheduled or urgent coronary artery bypass grafting or angioplasty need not be started on their thyroxine replacement urgently. There is some risk of infarction or arrhythmia with rapid hormone replacement in the setting of coronary ischemia. Outcomes are generally more satisfactory when the coronary revascularization is done first to ensure vessel patency and thyroid hormone therapy is initiated postoperatively. In such patients, special intraoperative and postoperative attention to airway and ventilation is necessary to prevent carbon dioxide retention and coma, as is attention to fluid and electrolyte balance to avoid hyponatremia. In the neonate or small child, thyroxine replacement dosage will be disproportionately greater than the 1.7 μg per kilogram per day described above, and should be begun as soon as possible to avoid impairment of normal intellectual development and growth.

Myxedema Coma

Myxedema coma represents the extreme clinical expression of hypothyroidism and constitutes a life-threatening emergency. The presentation is typically an elderly woman with a history of radioiodine therapy or surgery who had discontinued or never started thyroxine replacement. Presentation is often in winter, and the patient appears profoundly myxedematous, with hypothermia, hypotension, bradycardia, and altered mental status ranging from disorientation and confusion to somnolence and frank coma. Any patient with profound long-standing hypothyroidism is at risk for evolution into a stuporous precomatose to comatose state if left untreated, and ultimately to a fatal outcome. Even with aggressive management, mortality may average 30% to 60%, and patients should be admitted to and treated in an intensive care unit. Factors that predispose to myxedema coma include cold exposure, trauma, infection, respiratory disease, and administration of central nervous system depressants such as hypnotics, narcotics, and sedatives. With narcosis, respiratory depression occurs and CO_2 retention is an important component of the pathophysiology of the coma. Patients may present with hypothermia, hypotension, hypoglycemia, hyponatremia, hypoventilation with hypercapnia, respiratory acidosis, progressive stupor, coma, and seizures. When myxedema coma is suspected, blood should be drawn for measurements of TSH, free T_4, and cortisol, but therapy should be initiated immediately without waiting for the results if a disastrous outcome is to be avoided. Hydrocortisone is given intravenously because of the frequency of concomitant adrenal insufficiency. The latter may be due to pituitary disease (secondary hypothyroidism and adrenocorticotropic hormone deficiency) or to primary autoimmune adrenal insufficiency associated with Hashimoto's disease and hypothyroidism (Schmidt's syndrome). Often the patients have some underlying infection or systemic illness that may have precipitated the coma, but which also causes a reduced conversion rate of T_4 to T_3, as in the sick euthyroid syndrome. For this reason, in addition to vigorous thyroxine therapy, supplementary small doses of T_3 may be warranted. Treatment with T_3 alone is not recommended in view of the potential for cardiovascular risk. In the comatose patient unable to take oral medications, parenteral forms of both levothyroxine and liothyronine are available. One regimen could be to immediately administer 3 to 4 μg of thyroxine per kilogram intravenously followed by 100 μg per day thereafter, along with 10 μg of liothyronine every 8 hours. Both parenteral preparations are discontinued when the patient becomes able to take oral medications. Supportive therapy is essential with special attention to ventilation. Warming should be done gently with blankets to avoid sudden peripheral vasodilatation and secondary shock. Water restriction with judicious saline administration will be required to reverse hyponatremia, which is usually related to impaired water excretion and disordered regulation of vasopressin secretion. Mental status, blood pressure, temperature, and pulse rate should improve within the first 24 hours. Treatment of any precipitating or coincident illness will be indicated as in the management of any other elderly patient with multisystemic problems. This may include treatment of any underlying infectious processes, congestive heart failure, diabetes, hypertension, and so forth. It should be kept in mind that the dosage of specific medications (e.g., digoxin for congestive heart failure) may have to be modified based on their altered distribution and slowed metabolism in profound hypothyroidism.

THYROTOXICOSIS AND HYPERTHYROIDISM

Thyrotoxicosis is the term applied to the clinical, physiologic, and biochemical findings that result when the tissues are exposed to, and respond to, excess thyroid hormone. Rather than being a specific disease, thyrotoxicosis can occur in a variety of ways (Table 406.5), and it may be temporary or permanent until treated. Of the various causes, the most important are those that lead to sustained overproduction of hormone by the thyroid gland itself ("hyperthyroidism"). Rarely, this hyperfunction results from excessive secretion to TSH by a pituitary tumor or as a result of resistance to thyroid hormone in the pituitary but not in peripheral tissues. Other than the normal thyroid stimulator (TSH), stimulators of extrapituitary origin occur as

TABLE 406.5.	CAUSES OF HYPERTHYROIDISM

Graves' disease
Multinodular goiter
Hyperfunctioning thyroid adenoma (toxic adenoma)
Thyroiditis
    Subacute thyroiditis
    Painless (silent, postpartum) thyroiditis
Exogenous hyperthyroidism
    Thyroid hormone–induced hyperthyroidism
    Iodide-induced hyperthyroidism
Rare causes of hyperthyroidism
    TSH-secreting pituitary adenomas
    Trophoblastic tumors
    Struma ovarii
    Thyroid carcinoma
    Familial nonautoimmune hyperthyroidism

TSH, thyroid-stimulating hormone.
EVIDENCE LEVEL: C. Expert Opinion.

in Graves' disease, Hashimoto's disease, and trophoblastic tumors. The thyroid gland may also develop hyperfunctioning areas (or nodules) within the gland itself that are autonomous and not dependent on TSH. Thyrotoxicosis not associated with hyperthyroidism per se occurs in subacute thyroiditis and the syndrome called chronic thyroiditis with transient thyrotoxicosis. In these disorders, an inflammatory (or an autoimmune) process leads to leakage of an excess of preformed hormone from the gland. New hormone formation is decreased because of the suppression of TSH secretion by the circulating hormone excess as well as because of the inflammatory process the thyroid. Thyrotoxicosis due to thyroiditis is only a transient phenomenon because the stores of preformed hormone are eventually depleted. Recovery of hormone synthesis and secretion after the thyrotoxicosis may take weeks to months; as a consequence, the thyrotoxic state is often followed by a transient period of thyroid hormone deficiency. Thyrotoxicosis without true hyperthyroidism can also occur with exogenous sources of excess hormone, as in thyrotoxicosis factitia or the ingestion of meat contaminated with animal thyroids ("hamburger toxicosis"), or from thyroid hormone derived from follicular cells outside of the thyroid gland, such as functioning metastatic thyroid carcinoma and struma ovarii.

The distinction between *thyrotoxicosis* and *hyperthyroidism* has implications for both diagnosis and treatment. Because hyperthyroidism denotes sustained hyperfunction of the thyroid gland, there is usually an increased radioiodine uptake (RAIU), whereas in the nonhyperthyroid thyrotoxic states, thyroid function (as reflected in the RAIU) is subnormal. Furthermore, treatment of thyrotoxicosis by means intended to decrease hormone synthesis (antithyroid agents, surgery, or radioiodine) is appropriate in hyperthyroidism but is inappropriate and ineffective in other forms of thyrotoxicosis. Overt hyperthyroidism will be marked by clinical signs and symptoms, elevated serum T_4 and T_3, and suppressed serum TSH. "Subclinical" hyperthyroidism reflects a term utilized to describe early or mild thyrotoxicosis and is defined as having few signs or symptoms, normal serum total and free T_4 or T_3, but a suppressed serum TSH. Subclinical hyperthyroidism is common and is often due to degrees of excessive thyroid hormone replacement taken by hypothyroid patients. The prevalence of all types of thyrotoxicosis may range from 5 to 20 per 1000 population, being highest in the elderly. The most common variety of true thyroid hyperfunction is Graves' disease.

GRAVES' DISEASE

Graves' disease or diffuse toxic goiter, also known as Parry's or Basedow's disease, is a disorder that in its full-blown state has three major manifestations: hyperthyroidism, diffuse goiter, and ophthalmopathy. A peculiar localized myxedema or infiltrative dermopathy may also occur. These manifestations need not appear together. Indeed, one or two need never appear, and the three may run largely independent courses. The expression "euthyroid Graves' disease" has been applied to patients who present with clear evidence of thyroid autoimmunity, such as proptosis due to infiltrative ophthalmopathy or dermopathy, but do not have thyrotoxicosis as indicated by normal serum levels of T_4 or T_3. They may, however, have low serum TSH and minimal goiter.

Prevalence

Graves' disease occurs most commonly in women (6–8:1) in their third or fourth decade but can occur in men and children, and at virtually any age. Genetic factors play an important role; there is an increased incidence of haplotypes HLA-B8 and DRw3 in Caucasian, HLA-Bw36 in Japanese, and HLA-Bw46 in Chinese patients with the disease. Not surprisingly, there is a familial predisposition. In addition, among family members, a clinical and immunologic overlap exists with respect to Hashimoto's disease, primary thyroprivic hypothyroidism, and pernicious anemia, and probably with respect to other autoimmune disorders as well. Concordance rates in monozygotic twins are high, and both Graves' disease and Hashimoto's thyroiditis occur frequently in other family members. In occasional patients the picture may change from Graves' disease to Hashimoto's disease or vice versa; rarely, patients with primary myxedema later become hyperthyroid. Thus, in view of the concordance of the two disorders in families, and their serologic and pathologic similarities, Graves' disease, Hashimoto's disease, and primary myxedema can be considered as closely related autoimmune thyroid diseases. Other than genetic predisposition, other risk factors may include smoking, female sex, and psychological or physical stress.

Pathogenesis and Pathology

The precise initiating cause of Graves' disease remains unknown, and no one factor may be responsible for the entire syndrome. With respect to the goiter and hyperthyroidism, the central cause is the production by lymphocytes of TSH receptor–stimulating autoantibodies (TSH-R-Ab; TSAb), also known as thyroid-stimulating immunoglobulins (TSIs) of the IgG class. It is speculated that exogenous initiating factors such as bacteria or retroviruses may activate an immunologic cascade leading to activation of lymphocytes in susceptible individuals with an inherited abnormality in immune surveillance. The defect allows thyroid-specific T lymphocytes to stimulate quiescent B lymphocytes to proliferate and secrete the immunoglobulins that are stimulatory to the TSH receptor. By binding to the TSH receptor and continuously stimulating thyroid hormone synthesis and release, these antibodies disrupt homeostatic mechanisms that normally control hormone secretion (Fig. 406.3) Some thyroid-directed antibodies may be of a TSH-blocking type rather than of the stimulating type and can be identified in the serum of some patients with euthyroid ophthalmic Graves' disease, occasional patients with Hashimoto's disease, and some euthyroid relatives of patients with Graves' disease. Pathologically, the thyroid is diffusely enlarged, demonstrating both hypertrophy and hyperplasia, characterized by increased epithelial height and redundant follicular walls causing papillary infoldings. The gland is soft, vascular, and infiltrated with lymphocytes. Occasional patients will show generalized lymphoid hyperplasia with enlargement of the spleen or thymus as well.

The pathogenesis of Graves' ophthalmopathy is even more

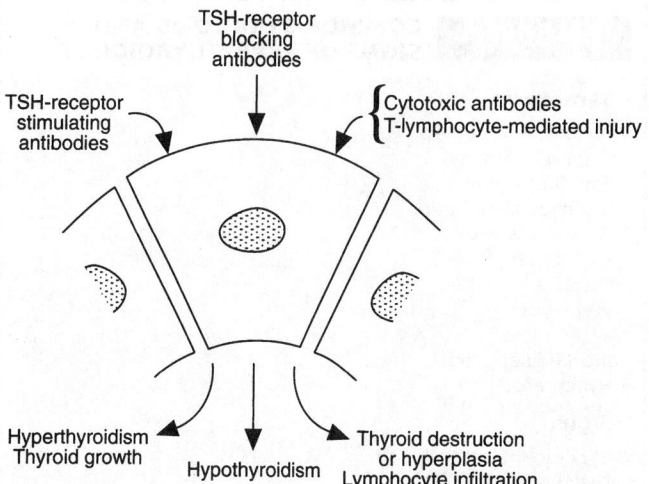

Figure 406.3. While the precise initiating cause of Graves' disease is unknown, the central cause of the goiter and hyperthyroidism is the production by lymphocytes of TSH receptor–stimulating autoantibodies, also known as thyroid-stimulating immunoglobulins (TSIs) of the IgG class. Bacteria or retroviruses may activate an immunologic cascade leading to activation of lymphocytes in susceptible individuals with an inherited abnormality in immune surveillance.

enigmatic, but both cellular and humoral immunity may have a role. It has been suggested that an antigen in orbital tissues cross-reacts with the thyroid, and intraorbital fibroblasts produce a protein that reacts with antibodies to the TSH receptor. The T cells release cytokines or growth factors that provoke an inflammatory reaction with proliferation of more fibroblasts and production of glycosaminoglycans. On pathologic examination, there is an inflammatory infiltrate of the orbital contents, with lymphocytes, mast cells, and plasma cells. Early on, the orbital musculature is enlarged owing to infiltration with lymphocytes, mucopolysaccharides, and edema, whereas with time the muscles show degeneration and loss of striations and become more fibrotic and bound down, leading to restrictive eye movement. The increased retrobulbar fat and infiltration of the eye muscles with lymphocytes and inflammatory edema cause an increased soft-tissue volume of the orbit; with the confinement imposed by the four bony walls of the orbit, the orbital contents protrude through the orbital fissure, leading to proptosis. Even less is known about the pathogenesis of the pretibial myxedema or infiltrative dermopathy that is characterized both by thickening of the dermis and by infiltration with lymphocytes and hydrophilic mucopolysaccharides.

Clinical Findings

Graves' disease is a multisystem disease reflecting the ubiquity of thyroid hormone receptors, and the clinical manifestations may involve virtually every tissue in the body (Table 406.6). On presentation, often the most prominent manifestations are nervousness, tremors, frequent bowel movements, excessive sweating, emotional lability, inability to sleep, and heat intolerance. Weight loss is usual despite a well-maintained or increased appetite, but actual weight gain may occur due to the dramatically stimulated appetite. Difficulty in arising from a sitting or

TABLE 406.6.	COMMON SYMPTOMS AND SIGNS OF HYPERTHYROIDISM

Symptoms

Anxiety, nervousness
Emotional lability
Easy fatigability
Increased perspiration
Heat intolerance
Palpitation
Dyspnea
Weakness
Weight loss
Increased appetite
Hyperdefecation

Signs

Hyperactivity
Eyelid retraction
Thyroid enlargement
Tachycardia (>90 beats/min)
Atrial fibrillation
Tremor
Muscle weakness
Hyperreflexia
EVIDENCE LEVEL: C. Expert Opinion.

squatting position or in climbing stairs is a manifestation of proximal muscle weakness. In premenopausal women, infertility, loss of libido, oligomenorrhea, and amenorrhea are common. The cardiac manifestations of chronic excesses of thyroid hormone include tachycardia, palpitations, dyspnea with exertion, and, in older patients, a lowered threshold for ischemic chest pain or congestive heart failure. Symptom complexes may be age-dependent, with weight loss, atrial fibrillation, or cardiac failure more common in the elderly, and irritability, heat intolerance, and increased appetite more common in younger individuals. The nervousness, anxiety, and emotional lability will often lead to poor school or job performance, impaired decision making, volatile interpersonal relations, and rarely even to sociopathic behaviors. Paradoxically, in some older patients, the clinical picture is one of apathy rather than hyperactivity ("apathetic thyrotoxicosis"), and myopathic features may be prominent. In elderly patients, the cardiovascular manifestations predominate, and it is generally wise to evaluate any patient with atrial arrhythmias or unexplained cardiac failure thyrotoxicosis.

On physical examination, patients appear anxious, restless, and fidgety. The hair is fine and may be thinned due to hair loss, and there may be premature graying as is also seen in Hashimoto's thyroiditis. A fine tremor of the fingers and tongue, together with hyperreflexia, is characteristic. The skin is warm and moist with a velvety texture, and patchy vitiligo and palmar erythema may be present. Separation of the fingernail from the nailbed (onycholysis, Plummer's nail) may be seen. There may be lid retraction with a characteristic stare with widened palpebral fissures, infrequent blinking, lid lag, and failure to wrinkle the brow on upward gaze. These signs result from sympathetic overstimulation; they often subside with correction of the thyrotoxicosis and should be distinguished from infiltrative ophthalmopathy. The latter, which is characteristic of Graves' disease,

is marked by impaired eye muscle movement and periorbital edema, with or without proptosis. The exophthalmos may be unilateral early on but usually becomes bilateral with time. With moderate to advancing severity, the proptosis will be accompanied by varying degrees of ophthalmoplegia and congestive oculopathy characterized by chemosis, conjunctivitis, and periorbital swelling. The most dreaded potential complications are corneal ulceration, optic neuritis, and optic atrophy. When exophthalmos becomes more severe and progresses rapidly to this point, it has been termed *malignant exophthalmos.* The term *exophthalmic ophthalmoplegia* refers to the ocular muscle weakness that results in impaired upward gaze and convergence and strabismus with varying degrees of diplopia. The thyroid is usually enlarged, sometimes asymmetrically; it is beefy in texture and may have an enlarged pyramidal lobe, audible bruit, and a palpable thrill. Effects on the cardiovascular system may be manifest as sinus tachycardia, atrial arrhythmias (especially atrial fibrillation), systolic flow murmurs, increased intensity of the apical first sound, cardiac enlargement, and, at times, overt heart failure. Blood pressure is usually normal but with a widened pulse pressure due to peripheral vasodilatation with reduced peripheral resistance. A to-and-fro, high-pitched sound simulating a pericardial friction rub (Means–Lerman scratch) has been described as heard best in the pulmonic area. Infiltrative dermopathy, when present, usually occurs over the dorsum of the legs or feet and has been called "pretibial myxedema." The affected area is usually raised, plaquelike, nodular, or polypoid, and hyperpigmented with a peau d'orange appearance. Thyroid acropachy, manifest as clubbing of the fingers and toes with bony changes, may be associated with the dermopathy. Deep tendon reflexes are brisk and unsustained clonus may be seen. Choreoathetoid movements have been described. Thyrotoxic periodic paralysis appears to occur rarely, primarily in men of Asian or Latin American extraction.

Diagnosis and Laboratory Findings

In its full-blown clinical presentation as described above, Graves' disease presents little difficulty in diagnosis. Distinction of Graves' disease from other causes of thyrotoxicosis is rendered relatively easy in the presence of typical diffuse thyroid enlargement and ophthalmopathy. Absence of thyroid enlargement makes the diagnosis of Graves' disease less likely but does not exclude it. The laboratory evaluation of patients suspected of having thyrotoxicosis is described in Chapter 418. Laboratory tests will confirm the diagnosis by documenting that TSH levels are undetectable by a sensitive technique and that the measured values for RAIU and serum total and free T_4 and T_3 are increased. Patients may rarely have a TSH-producing tumor with TSH-induced hyperthyroidism manifest as a measurable low-normal to normal TSH level, or so-called T_3 toxicosis in which the levels of serum T_4 and free T_4 are within normal limits but the values for total and free T_3 are elevated. Serum thyroglobulin should be elevated in endogenous hyperthyroidism of all causes, and its measurement, when found to be low, may be useful to detect exogenous or factitial thyrotoxicosis. Other aberrated laboratory parameters in thyrotoxicosis may relate to the effects of excess thyroid hormone on bone and include increases in serum calcium, urine calcium, osteocalcin, and alkaline phosphatase, with osteopenia or osteoporosis on bone densitometry. Liver function tests may be abnormal, with elevated aminotransferases, LDH, angiotensin-converting enzyme activity, and sex hormone–binding globulin. In contrast, CPK is decreased.

Differential Diagnosis

While the constellation of symptoms of tachycardia, tremulousness, irritability, weakness, and fatigue is typical of thyrotoxicosis, an anxiety state or pheochromocytoma may have to be ruled out. Pheochromocytoma and thyrotoxicosis may share symptoms of heat intolerance, sweating, tachycardia with palpitations, and a hypermetabolic state. In anxiety, the skin is usually cold and clammy rather than warm and moist. Weight loss in anxiety disorders is usually accompanied by anorexia rather than the increased appetite of thyrotoxicosis. Proptosis accompanying signs and symptoms of thyrotoxicosis invariably represents Graves' disease, particularly when the eye disease is bilateral. But apparent euthyroid Graves' ophthalmopathy must be distinguished from intraorbital or intracranial disease, such as retrobulbar tumors, cavernous sinus thrombosis, sphenoidal ridge meningioma, or pseudotumor oculi. Proptosis also may be seen in systemic disorders such as uremia, accelerated hypertension, chronic alcoholism, chronic obstructive pulmonary disease, superior mediastinal obstruction, and Cushing's syndrome. Ophthalmoplegia in the absence of infiltrative manifestations can be confused with that in diabetes mellitus or myasthenia gravis. When doubt exists about the cause of ophthalmopathy, the demonstration of significant titers of TSH receptor antibody or an immeasurably low TSH suggests that the cause is Graves' disease. Changes in the extraocular muscles characteristic of Graves' disease may be seen by ultrasonography, magnetic resonance imaging, or computed tomography of the orbit.

When the laboratory results and signs and symptoms indicate thyrotoxicosis but there are no signs of Graves' disease, such as ophthalmopathy or infiltrative dermopathy, other causes of thyrotoxicosis must be considered. Palpation of the thyroid, ultrasonography, or radionuclide scanning will disclose whether the problem is a hyperfunctioning autonomous nodule or a toxic multinodular goiter. The absence of radioactive iodine uptake by the thyroid suggests factitial thyrotoxicosis, subacute thyroiditis, or the extremely rare struma ovarii. Tenderness of the thyroid is suggestive of subacute thyroiditis, and an immeasurably low thyroglobulin is suggestive of an exogenous factitial source of thyroid hormone. In struma ovarii, the RAIU measured over the thyroid is low, since TSH secretion is suppressed, and the struma as the source of the circulating high levels of thyroid hormone can be identified by scintillation scanning over the pelvis. The unusual presentation of thyrotoxicosis due to inappropriate TSH production (associated with a pituitary tumor or resistance to feedback suppression of TSH secretion) or an abnormal stimulator of trophoblastic origin (hydatidiform mole, choriocarcinoma) may be ruled out by measurements of TSH or human chorionic gonadotropin (hCG). Demonstration of elevated titers of thyroid-stimulating immunoglobulins in the blood also provides strong evidence that Graves' disease is the cause of thyrotoxicosis.

Course and Treatment of Thyrotoxicosis

There is no cure for Graves' disease. The thyrotoxicosis may spontaneously remit, but neither the likelihood nor the duration of remission can be predicted. The principal therapy of hyperthyroidism is directed to reducing the production of thyroid hormone from the gland. For this purpose, antithyroid agents that chemically block hormone synthesis may be employed. An alternative therapy for thyrotoxicosis could be to functionally destroy the ability of the thyroid gland to manufacture hormone via the ablation of thyroid tissue by either surgical thyroidectomy or the use of radioactive iodine. With the latter therapy, advantage is taken of the fact that the thyroid normally actively traps iodine, and the uptake of iodine (or radioiodine) is further accelerated in hyperthyroidism. Based on the size of the goiter and the measured radioiodine uptake, doses of radioactive iodine can be standardized sufficiently to ensure attainment of at least euthyroidism, and more often transformation into hypothyroidism. The transition with time into hypothyroidism after thyroidectomy or radioiodine ablation is generally deemed to be a more acceptable trade-off than the alternative of the possibility of less than permanent remissions with antithyroid drugs with subsequent exacerbation or recurrence of thyrotoxicosis. The choice of which of the three available therapies (Tables 406.7 and 406.8) might be most appropriate in a given patient varies depending on a number of factors; it represents a decision that should be individualized after adequate discussion and education of the patient on the pros and cons of each approach. The patient should be made aware that the thyrotoxicosis of Graves' disease is often characterized by cyclic phases of exacerbation and remission, which are of unpredictable onset and duration.

Antithyroid Drug Therapy

The primary advantage of antithyroid drug therapy is that patients have an opportunity to remain euthyroid after therapy is discontinued, providing that they enter a sustained remission. Since the thyrotoxicosis may recur at any time after remission, patients must be followed indefinitely or made aware of the possibility of recurrence so that they will recognize the signs and symptoms. Choices for long-term antithyroid drug therapy include either methimazole (Tapazole) or propylthiouracil (PTU) in the United States and carbimazole in Europe and elsewhere. Initial daily dosage often averages 300 to 450 μg of

TABLE 406.7.	THERAPY FOR HYPERTHYROIDISM

Antithyroid therapy
  Drugs
    Methimazole (carbimazole)
    Propylthiouracil
    Iodide
  Radioactive iodine (^{131}I)
  Subtotal thyroidectomy
Amelioration of thyroid hormone action
  β-Adrenergic antagonist drugs

TABLE 406.8.	FEATURES OF ANTITHYROID DRUG AND IODINE 131 THERAPY FOR HYPERTHYROIDISM CAUSED BY GRAVES' DISEASE	
	Drug Therapy	**Iodine 131**
Dosage	Daily	Single dose[a]
Initial response	2–6 wk	8–12 wk
Side effects[b]	Uncommon	Rare
Hypothyroidism	Uncommon	Common
Therapy inadequate	Uncommon	Rare
Need for continuous or repeated courses of therapy	Common	Rare
Long-term outcome	Euthyroidism or hyperthyroidism	Hypothyroidism
Outcome dependent on continued TSAb production	Yes	No
Use during pregnancy	Indicated	Never

[a] If dose is small, one or more additional doses may be required.
[b] Toxic drug effects (rash, fever, arthralgia; arthritis, hepatitis, agranulocytosis) and radiation thyroiditis or radiation–induced exacerbation of hyperthyroidism.
TSAb, thyroid-stimulating hormone receptor–stimulating autoantibodies.

PTU or 30 to 45 μg of methimazole, in divided doses every 8 hours or t.i.d., but relatively mild disease can be treated with as little as 50 to 100 μg of PTU or 5 to 10 μg of methimazole daily. Some clinical improvement may be seen as early as 2 weeks, although such improvement may be due largely to the use of concomitant β-adrenergic blocking agents. Usually, it takes as long as 4 to 8 weeks to achieve clinical and laboratory evidence of euthyroidism, at which time the daily dosage can be titrated downward by as much as 50% to a lower "maintenance" dose. Adequate satisfactory control of symptoms with restoration of normal levels of T_4 and T_3 can virtually always be attained, given sufficient drug dosage and a compliant patient. Monitoring of TSH levels may be useful as well, but this should not be relied on because TSH levels can remain suppressed for months after attainment of a euthyroid state. Overdosage with serum total or free T_4 below the normal range (with or without elevated TSH) should be avoided in view of some observations of worsening ophthalmopathy when this occurs. In some patients with more severe thyrotoxicosis, doses of PTU greater than 150 mg every 6 or 8 hours may be required for initial control.

Approximately 4% to 8% of patients will have adverse side effects with either methimazole or PTU. Side effects, which tend to occur within the first month or two of therapy, are frequently dose-dependent and usually promptly reversible with discontinuation. The most serious and fortunately rare adverse reactions include agranulocytosis, aplastic anemia, hepatitis, and a lupus-like syndrome with vasculitis, arthralgias, and fever. These occur in no more than 0.1% to 0.2% of patients. Nevertheless, it may be useful to monitor blood counts during therapy with routine blood counts, including white blood cell count, differential, and

platelet count obtained before commencement of thiourea drug therapy in order to distinguish between patients whose leukopenia is due to Graves' disease and those whose leukopenia is a side effect of antithyroid drug therapy. Given availability of alternative therapies, antithyroid drug therapy can be discontinued as soon as leukopenia is detected in follow-up evaluations, although a mild transient leukopenia may occur with antithyroid drugs in perhaps 10% of patients. Discontinuing a drug is often simpler than attempting to document that a leukopenia is transient by serial testing, which might allow continuation of drug therapy. Clearly, however, antithyroid medication should be discontinued when the absolute number of polymorphonuclear leukocytes reaches ≤1,500 per microliter. Other more minor adverse reactions to the antithyroid drugs, such as pruritus, urticaria, or other skin rashes, often disappear with concomitant antihistamine therapy. Nevertheless, it is probably wiser to at least change to the alternative thiourea agent in the event of a sensitivity reaction. Antithyroid drug therapy should be terminated when severe sensitivity reactions occur, and radioactive iodine therapy may be the next best option.

In addition to the thiourea antithyroid drugs, there are a number of other pharmacologic agents that may be used to ameliorate the thyrotoxic state. Several different β-*adrenergic blocking agents* have been used routinely in thyrotoxicosis in view of the dramatic salutary response obtained on the adrenergic component of the thyrotoxicosis, which may include amelioration of hyperkinesis, tremor, tachycardia, insomnia, nervousness, and lid retraction. The first agent available for this purpose, propranolol, is still widely used, but usually is required to be given in divided dosage of 10 to 30 μg every 6 hours. Other, longer acting adrenergic antagonists, such as atenolol, may be equally effective in doses of 50 to 100 μg once daily, and both agents are relatively free of adverse side effects. While some studies have demonstrated reduction of T_4 to T_3 conversion by propranolol, this is only a modest effect with probably minimal clinical importance. Thus, the β-adrenergic blocking agents are very useful as adjunctive therapy while awaiting responses to antithyroid drugs or radioiodine, and may provide dramatic clinical improvement while not affecting the underlying thyrotoxicosis per se. Cautious use of these agents is recommended in patients with congestive heart failure other than rate-related failure, in whom further reduction in myocardial contractility will further compromise cardiac function. Several studies have demonstrated the utility of propranolol as the sole agent in preparation of patients for thyroidectomy. While this may rarely be necessary in patients who manifest significant allergy to all antithyroid agents, or in thyrotoxic patients with a nonthyroid surgical emergency, more routine use of propranolol alone is not recommended since its use will not eliminate the risk of thyroid storm in the perioperative period. β-Adrenergic blocking agents are particularly useful for symptomatic control during the transient thyrotoxic phase of thyroiditis.

Administration of *iodide* (100 to 200 μg per day) in the form of saturated solution of potassium iodide (50 μg per drop) or Lugol's solution will acutely inhibit proteolysis of colloid within the gland, thereby reducing release of hormone. Because the effect is virtually immediate, improvement in serum T_4 or T_3 is seen more rapidly than occurs with the antithyroid drugs that act by inhibiting hormone synthesis. An important application for the use of iodides is in life-threatening severe thyrotoxicosis (*thyrotoxic crisis*) and in patients who cannot tolerate prolonged thyrotoxicosis, such as those with underlying severe cardiac disease. Sole therapy with iodide without concomitant antithyroid drug may be hazardous because inhibition of hormone release without blockade of new-hormone synthesis allows continuing new-hormone synthesis (with the iodide substrate provided), thereby expanding intrathyroidal stores of hormone. In cases of severe thyrotoxicosis in which iodide administration may be required, *antithyroid drug therapy should be initiated first* in relatively large doses to block hormone synthesis prior to administration of iodide. Another drawback of sole therapy with iodine is that the patients will escape from the inhibitory effect on hormone secretion in 2 to 4 weeks, which can be followed by secretion of the iodine-augmented hormone stores and worsening thyrotoxicosis. Iodide therapy also complicates subsequent management by two potential mechanisms. First, planned treatment with radioactive iodine (iodine 131, or ^{131}I) may have to be postponed pending clearance of the increased thyroidal and blood pool of stable iodine, which serves to dilute the radioactive iodine and reduce thyroid uptake; second, the increased intrathyroidal iodine resulting from iodide treatment may prolong the period of initial response to the thiourea drugs, which act in part by depleting intrathyroidal iodine. On the other hand, iodide may be administered *after* radioiodine therapy has been given in order to achieve a more rapid clinical response while awaiting the longer term destructive effect of ^{131}I. The iodide-induced inhibition of hormone release serves to retain the ^{131}I within the thyroid gland and provides a greater degree of ablation. In patients allergic to iodides, lithium carbonate is an alternative agent with much the same effect. Other agents that may be employed in cases of severe thyrotoxicosis believed to represent actual or impending thyrotoxic crisis are glucocorticoids in relatively large doses. Dexamethasone (2 mg every 6 hours) reduces the serum T_3 concentration by inhibition of T_4 to T_3 conversion, as will the iodinated x-ray contrast agent sodium ipodate. Ipodate has been given as an initial loading dose of 2 to 3 g followed by a single daily dose of 0.5 to 1.0 g. The rich iodine content of this agent also has the adjunctive effect of inhibiting thyroidal secretion of both T_4 and T_3.

Radioactive iodine (^{131}I) Therapy

Radioiodine is generally considered to be the most efficient and cost-effective treatment for thyrotoxicosis. The usual therapeutic dose of ^{131}I for Graves' disease is approximately 5.9 MBq (160 μCi) per gram of estimated gland weight. This generally delivers 50 to 150 Gy (5,000 to 15,000 rad) to the thyroid. Significantly larger doses than those employed for thyrotoxicosis have been given for thyroid cancer, and the doses given for hyperthyroidism in adults have not been shown to lead to an increased incidence of leukemia or other malignancy later in life. However, the thyroid in children may be more susceptible to radiation-induced carcinogenesis, as was clearly shown by the marked increase in thyroid neoplasms in children exposed to radioactive fallout following the 1986 Chernobyl disaster. As a result, many physicians reserve radioiodine therapy for patients over 25 years of age.

Women of childbearing age are generally advised to avoid pregnancy for at least a year following treatment. Some physicians prefer to not treat patients still desiring children even though no adverse or mutagenic effects have been shown.

The outcome after a dose of ^{131}I therapy may be post-radioiodine hypothyroidism, euthyroidism, or persistent hyperthyroidism requiring a second dose. Eventually and increasingly with time, hypothyroidism will supervene in the overwhelming majority of patients necessitating lifelong thyroxine replacement therapy. Smaller doses of approximately 3.0 to 4.5 mBq per gram (80 to 120 μCi per gram) have been given in an attempt to avoid hypothyroidism; but these lower doses merely delay the onset of hypothyroidism without reducing its frequency. Within 10 to 15 years after treatment, approximately 50% to 75% of patients will be hypothyroid. Because the insidious evolution into hypothyroidism over years may evade detection, and in view of the morbidity of untreated hypothyroidism, many expert clinicians have suggested that all patients be treated with a relatively large doses of ^{131}I to predictably achieve hypothyroidism earlier so that replacement therapy can be initiated immediately thereafter. This approach to management is particularly applicable to the elderly. Surgical thyroidectomy would be the choice for therapy in younger patients in whom it may be desirable to avoid long-term effects of radioiodine. However, younger patients can be considered candidates for radioiodine therapy in the event of recurrent thyrotoxicosis following an initial surgery, or in patients who refuse surgery or have a complicating illness that renders surgery a greater risk.

Controversy remains at present regarding whether or not patients with Graves' disease may experience an exacerbation of ophthalmopathy following radioiodine therapy. Patients who may be at greater risk include smokers, those with preexisting ophthalmopathy, and those with severe thyrotoxicosis. The theoretical basis for this phenomenon may be radiation thyroiditis with release of antigen, provoking increases in TSH receptor antibody which binds to orbital fibroblasts and muscle, thereby eliciting an inflammatory response. Studies have demonstrated less propensity to post-radioiodine worsening of ophthalmopathy when glucocorticoids are administered for approximately 2 weeks before and 6 weeks after the ^{131}I dose.

On average, the peak effect of radioiodine in regard to restoration of iodothyronine levels to normal may not be reached before 6 to 12 weeks. Most patients will be too symptomatic to wait this long for improvement, nor would it be necessarily safe to do so. As a consequence, given the latent period for radioiodine effect, the majority of patients benefit from a course of antithyroid drug therapy to render them euthyroid prior to radioiodine therapy. This serves to accelerate the attainment of a eumetabolic state and to preclude the possibility of a posttreatment radiation thyroiditis causing thyrotoxic crisis. Simultaneously, propranolol can be given to relieve the hyperadrenergic symptoms. Since the thiourea drugs will impede organic binding of the radioiodine within the thyroid and diminish its therapeutic effect, it is necessary that the drugs be discontinued approximately 2 to 3 days prior to treatment with radioiodine. In patients with a large thyroid gland and a history of moderate to severe thyrotoxicosis, resumption of antithyroid drugs after the radioiodine therapy will be necessary but should not be initiated until at least 3 days after therapy to permit adequate accumulation and retention of administered ^{131}I. It is mandatory to perform a radioiodine uptake test prior to administration of the treatment dose to ensure that the uptake is adequate for therapy, as well as to use the observed value to calculate the treatment dose. Hypothyroidism due to radiation necrosis of the gland is a virtually inevitable consequence of radioactive iodine therapy and may occur in months to years depending on the dose. Given the above doses, approximately 50% of patients will be hypothyroid within the first 6 to 9 months, and additional patients will become so at a rate of 1.5% to 2.5% per year thereafter. An alternative outcome to post-radioiodine hypothyroidism is persistent hyperthyroidism, particularly if a relatively low dose of radioiodine was administered. In such cases, a second and rarely a third therapeutic dose is required.

A post-radioiodine radiation thyroiditis may follow ^{131}I therapy (usually within a week if it occurs) that may be associated with accelerated release of hormone into the blood. Optimally, given the risk of radiation-related release of hormone into the circulation and exacerbation of thyrotoxicosis, values for serum T_4 and/or T_3 should be relatively normal prior to administration of the treatment dose. While radiation thyroiditis–related thyrotoxic crisis is rare, it appears to occur more frequently in elderly thyrotoxic patients with other systemic illness. For these reasons, patients with severe hyperthyroidism or underlying cardiorespiratory disease first should be rendered eumetabolic with antithyroid agents before therapy with ^{131}I. Large doses of ^{131}I should be used with caution in patients with large retrosternal goiters because of the potential for radiation-related tissue edema with swelling that may cause tracheoesophageal compression.

Surgery

Subtotal thyroidectomy in the hands of a skilled surgeon who is experienced in this procedure remains an effective and relatively safe choice of therapy albeit infrequently employed today for Graves' disease. Prior to the advent of radioiodine, thyroidectomy was often employed and surgeons were able to develop sufficient expertise with the procedure to avoid anticipated risks and complications. Given the few procedures performed during surgical training today, experienced surgeons tend to be confined to major medical centers, and it is these surgeons to whom patients should be referred. Complications seen following procedures done by less experienced surgeons include hemorrhage leading to respiratory obstruction, hoarseness or voice loss due to recurrent laryngeal nerve injury and vocal cord paralysis, and hypoparathyroidism necessitating lifelong calcium and vitamin D supplementation. Sufficient tissue may be left behind to cause persistent or recurrent thyrotoxicosis. Just as with radioiodine therapy, hypothyroidism is likely to occur when sufficient thyroid tissue is removed to avoid a postoperative recurrence of thyrotoxicosis, and it is simply treated with thyroxine replacement. Prior to surgery, patients should first be rendered euthyroid by means of antithyroid agents. Some surgeons prefer that iodides be administered along with the antithyroid drugs for an additional week (e.g., five drops of Lugol's solution per day), which is said to reduce the vascularity and subsequent blood loss during the procedure. Candidates for surgical therapy may include those patients who have had major allergic reactions to antithyroid drugs or who are habitually noncompliant but decline radioiodine therapy, pregnant patients who cannot tolerate antithyroid therapy or who require very large doses, and patients with unusually large goiters.

TOXIC MULTINODULAR GOITER

After Graves' disease, toxic multinodular goiter represents the next most common cause of hyperthyroidism. Thyroid hyperfunction is believed to develop as a gradual transition over years from a benign, nontoxic, or simple goiter into one with scattered foci characterized by functional autonomy (i.e., independence from control by TSH stimulation). These foci can be demonstrated by radioisotopic scan as "hot" in two general types of patterns. Usually tracer is concentrated in patchy foci diffusely throughout the gland, or less frequently the isotope will be concentrated in several discrete nodules with the remainder of the gland being essentially "cold" or nonfunctional. Studies on thyroid slices following radioiodine administration permit autoradiographic mapping of functional activity and demonstrate marked irregularity and heterogeneity of both structure and function in these glands. However, there do not appear to be specific pathologic features that distinguish nontoxic from toxic multinodular goiter. Not uncommonly, toxic multinodular goiter arises in patients residing in areas of endemic iodine deficiency. Typically, the native thyroglobulin in these glands is characterized by a relatively low iodination, due to either long-standing iodine deficiency or an intrinsically impaired ability to normally incorporate iodine. Functional hyperactivity leading to thyrotoxicosis may develop slowly over years or relatively acutely after exposure to excess iodine. The latter phenomenon (jod-Basedow) occurs typically in patients with this type of endemic multinodular goiter, as well as those with sporadic nontoxic goiter.

The functional autonomy of this disorder does not appear to be governed by stimulation by TSH receptor antibodies as in Graves' disease. And there are several other clinical differences from Graves' disease as well. On average, Graves' patients tend to be in their third or fourth decade, whereas those with toxic multinodular goiter tend to be elderly, largely due to the years of evolution inherent to the natural history of toxic multinodular goiter. Because the latter patients are more elderly, they are more likely to manifest clinically more apparent muscle wasting, weakness, and cardiac decompensation with arrhythmias and/or congestive heart failure. The hyperadrenergic features of Graves' disease are often lacking in these patients, and their thyrotoxicosis in not infrequently incidentally discovered by a T_4 or TSH measurement performed as part of a screen for weight loss. This has led to use of the designation "apathetic thyrotoxicosis." Importantly, the features of Graves' disease generally associated with autoimmunity and the TSH receptor antibodies are lacking in toxic multinodular goiter, such as ophthalmopathy and infiltrative dermopathy.

A definitive diagnosis of toxic multinodular goiter should not be difficult to establish in the majority of patients. If the multinodular goiter cannot be appreciated on physical examination due to the anatomy of the patient's neck or a substernal location of the gland, a radioiodine uptake and scintiscan should demonstrate both hyperfunction and the typical scan appearance. As in thyrotoxicosis of any cause, the key to the diagnosis is an immeasurably low TSH value by a sensitive assay. Serum total and free T_4 or T_3 levels may be only mildly increased, but these slight increases may be more significant in an elderly patient in view of the usually observed trend toward physiologically lower levels with aging. Serum thyroglobulin levels may be increased as well.

In regard to treatment, the age of these patients may preclude thyroidectomy as an option, particularly since the ease of administration of radioactive iodine and the absence of any contraindications in the elderly tends to make it almost invariably the treatment of choice. In contrast to Graves' disease, there is little indication for antithyroid drugs in toxic multinodular goiter other than as perhaps a therapeutic trial when the diagnosis may be uncertain, or to render the patient euthyroid prior to radioiodine treatment. Long-term use of antithyroid drugs will effectively maintain euthyroidism, but the spontaneous remission typical of Graves' disease will not occur, and lifelong use of antithyroid agents is generally not acceptable therapy. As in the thyrotoxicosis of Graves' disease, adrenergic blockers such as propranolol are useful unless contraindicated, for control of the manifestations of thyrotoxicosis both before and after radioiodine therapy, while awaiting its therapeutic effect. For therapeutic ablation with radioiodine, typically larger doses than are employed for Graves' disease are required to satisfactorily return the patient to euthyroidism. The administered dose is often as high as 600 to 1,200 MBq (16 to 32 mCi) because of the relatively lower radioiodine uptake in these glands. In contrast to the post-radioiodine hypothyroidism that is ultimately so common in Graves' patients, the thyroid gland of patients with toxic multinodular goiter is more resistant. This may be because of the heterogeneous function in differing segments of the gland, which allows those segments that were previously less functional to augment their function after the hot areas are destroyed by ^{131}I.

UNUSUAL CAUSES AND PRESENTATIONS OF THYROTOXICOSIS

Thyrotoxicosis Factitia

Many of the clinical manifestations of thyrotoxicosis are the same whether the excess circulating concentrations of T_4 or T_3 responsible for the syndrome are derived from an exogenous source, such as thyroid medications, or from endogenous hyperthyroidism. The former results from either the intentional or the inadvertent ingestion of large amounts of thyroid hormone. Commonly, the syndrome is seen in women with the mistaken belief that the excess thyroid hormone will allow them to lose weight safely. In other patients, thyroid hormone ingestion may constitute a form of Munchausen syndrome or malingering, which implies an underlying psychiatric disorder. When excessive exogenous thyroid hormone is ingested, the resultant elevation in hormone levels suppresses pituitary TSH production, thereby secondarily suppressing endogenous thyroid function. This results in low values for radioiodine uptake and serum

thyroglobulin concentration. When the subject takes a preparation containing T_3 only, serum T_3 will be elevated but serum T_4 will be reduced. Since T_4 is converted to T_3 physiologically, ingestion of supraphysiologic amounts of any preparation containing T_4 will result in elevated levels of both T_4 and T_3, and of course a suppressed TSH.

TSH-Mediated Hyperthyroidism

In animal models, continuous administration of TRH or TSH results in hyperthyroidism. In man, continuous hypersecretion of TSH from a TSH-secreting pituitary adenoma can result in thyrotoxicosis. Another form of TSH-driven hyperthyroidism results from selective resistance of the pituitary to feedback inhibition by thyroid hormone (discussed above). The distinction between resistance syndromes and a pituitary tumor may be based on evidence of a pituitary adenoma on CT scan or MRI, and presence of a higher than normal ratio of free α subunit of TSH to total assayable TSH. TRH testing may also be useful in that the TSH response to TRH will be blunted or absent with tumors.

Trophoblastic Thyrotoxicosis

Human chorionic gonadotrophin (hCG) is a thyroid stimulator, albeit a weak one, but sufficient to induce thyrotoxicosis when continuously present in relatively high serum levels. Such levels can be achieved in patients with trophoblastic tumor such as choriocarcinoma or hydatidiform mole, and patients with these tumors may demonstrate increased levels of total and free T_4 and T_3 and suppressed, immeasurable levels of TSH. These patients manifest all of the typical hyperadrenergic signs and symptoms of thyrotoxicosis as might be seen in Graves' disease, but dermopathy or ophthalmopathy is absent. The cause of the thyroid hyperfunction may be confirmed by measurement of serum hCG, whereas titers of TSH receptor antibody, if measured, will be negative. Removal of the source of origin of the hCG (the tumor) restores thyroid function tests to normal limits.

Thyrotoxicosis Ectopia

Rarely, thyrotoxicosis may result from excess circulating levels of thyroid hormone that are derived not from the thyroid gland but from an ectopic focus of thyroid tissue. One such lesion is struma ovarii, which is the presence of autonomously hyperfunctioning thyroid tissue within a benign cystic teratoma of one or both ovaries. TSH levels and, as a consequence, the thyroid gland in the neck are suppressed by the high T_4 or T_3 levels derived from the ovary, and the thyroid gland demonstrates a low radioiodine uptake and fails to be visualized on thyroid scintiscan. However, scanning over the pelvis will disclose uptake in the struma, and its surgical removal will be followed by recovery of function in the cervical thyroid. Even more rare is the occurrence of thyroid malignancy in a struma, or the coincidence of goiter or Graves' disease along with a pelvic struma. Another cause of thyrotoxicosis due to ectopic thyroid hormone production is that due to widespread functioning metastases of thyroid carcinoma. The tumor type is usually of the follicular variety, which by virtue of the sheer mass of metastases present can produce enough T_4 to cause thyrotoxicosis.

Iodine-Induced Thyrotoxicosis

As described above, the jod-Basedow phenomenon refers to the induction of thyrotoxicosis in a previously euthyroid patient as a result of exposure to excess iodine. The thyrotoxicosis is triggered by avid uptake and hormone synthesis by thyroid tissue that either has been chronically exposed to endemic iodine deficiency or has underlying functionally autonomous tissue as in multinodular goiter or Graves' disease, or both. In addition to sanctioned dietary supplements, such as iodized salt, iodine is so ubiquitously available as to constitute an omnipresent risk of excess ingestion, at least in the United States. Iodide or other salts of iodine are in common use as a preservative in baked goods, as an antiseptic in public water supplies, in food dyes, and of course, in organic contrast agents commonly employed for radiographic procedures such as CT scans, cholecystography, myelography, pyelography, and, most commonly today, coronary angiography. Patients undergoing the latter procedures tend to be elderly and at greater risk of serious cardiovascular manifestations should they become thyrotoxic. Consequently, these sources of iodine should be avoided in patients known to have underlying autonomous function, multinodular goiter, or autoimmune thyroid disease. When pharmaceuticals containing iodine or x-ray contrast media must be employed, patients should be carefully monitored for evolution into hypo- or hyperthyroidism and promptly treated accordingly. Indeed, where risk of thyrotoxicosis is high, therapy with an antithyroid agent such as PTU (450 mg per day in divided dosage) should be considered both for a week prior to and for 1 to 2 weeks after the procedure.

Amiodarone is an antiarrhythmic drug that has effects at multiple sites in thyroid economy, in part due to its high (37%) iodine content but also due to specific effects of the drug and its metabolites on cellular receptors. Effects of the drug include inhibition of the conversion of T_4 to T_3 and displacement of T_4 from its binding sites leading to high serum T_4 levels whether or not thyrotoxicosis is also present. Due to an intrapituitary block on T_4 to T_3 conversion, TSH levels will ordinarily be normal to high-normal in euthyroid individuals. Serum total and free T_3 will be low. Thyrotoxicosis is indicated by elevated (or even merely high normal) levels of T_3 and by a suppressed TSH. The high iodine content will induce hyperthyroidism in susceptible individuals, such as those with underlying autonomously functioning glands (e.g., patients with multinodular goiters or Graves' disease). This type of amiodarone-induced thyrotoxicosis is consistent with the jod-Basedow phenomenon and is characterized by goiter with low to low-normal values for radioiodine uptake, normal levels of interleukin-6 (IL-6), and a normal erythrocyte sedimentation rate (ESR). A second type of amiodarone-induced thyrotoxicosis represents a thyroiditic syndrome consequent to a drug-related acute inflammatory response and aspiration cytologic examination will demonstrate necrosis with polymorphonuclear cell and histiocytes. This disorder is not associated with goiter, radioiodine uptake is negligible, and IL-6 levels and ESR are elevated. Therapy should consist of discontinuation of the amiodarone, if possible, along with measures to deplete intrathyroidal iodine stores, such as the thiourea antithyroid drugs, often in conjunction with perchlorate. Short-term, moderate to high-dose corticosteroids have proven useful for the acute inflammatory type of amiodarone-related thyrotoxicosis. The high iodine content of the drug may also induce hypothyroidism in susceptible individuals, such as those with underlying Hashimoto's disease. Clinical manifestations may rarely oscillate between hypothyroidism and hyperthyroidism constituting a therapeutic dilemma. Assuming that the amiodarone cannot be discontinued because of the underlying problem with arrhythmias, management may sometimes be resolved by thyroidectomy followed by stable-dose thyroxine replacement.

T_3 Toxicosis

In euthyroid individuals under certain conditions, such as with iodine deficiency, the thyroid gland preferentially produces more T_3 relative to T_4. In general, hyperthyroidism results in overproduction and oversecretion of both thyroid hormones T_4 and T_3. However, in almost all types of hyperthyroidism, the thyroidal T_3 production rate is relatively greater than it is in the euthyroid state. This disproportionate T_3 production can be exaggerated in some thyrotoxic states, again perhaps related to relative iodine deficiency. Excluding a binding defect such as TBG deficiency, which would cause a low serum T_4, the presence of a low serum T_4 and a relatively high T_3 in a thyrotoxic patient has been called "T_3 toxicosis." This diagnosis applies to patients with clinical manifestations of thyrotoxicosis in whom the serum T_4 and free T_4 are normal or low and the RAIU is high-normal to increased. The distinction between endogenous T_3 toxicosis due to Graves' disease or toxic nodular goiter and T_3 thyrotoxicosis factitia can be based on findings of low radioiodine uptake and low serum thyroglobulin in the latter case. Often T_3 toxicosis represents the earliest manifestation of Graves' thyrotoxicosis, either during its initial presentation or in relapse following discontinuation of antithyroid drug therapy.

T_4 Toxicosis

As described above, most patients with hyperthyroidism have elevations in both serum T_4 and serum T_3 although the ratio of T_3 to T_4 may be slightly higher than in euthyroid individuals. The higher T_3 results from increased generation both from the thyroid gland and from peripheral conversion of the relatively high serum T_4 levels in thyrotoxicosis. On rare occasions, a higher serum T_4 level relative to that of T_3 may be seen in thyrotoxicosis, or the serum T_3 may be frankly normal. This presentation of laboratory parameters has been called T_4 toxicosis. Just as T_3 toxicosis tends to occur in the setting of iodine deficiency, T_4 toxicosis is seen most commonly in a milieu of prior excess iodine exposure (which favors T_4 biosynthesis) and may be more prevalent in elderly patients.

Thyrotoxic Storm

Thyrotoxic storm or crisis is a syndrome of exaggerated signs and symptoms of thyrotoxicosis with systemic decompensation that is likely to be fatal unless vigorously treated. The diagnosis is a clinical one based on the identification of the typical cardinal manifestations, which include fever (temperature usually more than 38.5°C); tachycardia out of proportion to the fever; central nervous system signs, varying from extreme irritability, delirium, or confusion to apathy and even coma; and gastrointestinal dysfunction, which can include nausea, vomiting, diarrhea, and, in severe cases, jaundice. The earliest possible diagnosis and subsequent implementation of therapy are required to avoid a fatal outcome. Even with early diagnosis death can occur, and reported mortality rates have ranged from 10% to 75% in hospitalized patients. The syndrome may be less common today than in the past, perhaps because of earlier diagnosis and treatment of thyrotoxicosis, thereby precluding its progression to the stage of crisis. Nevertheless, it is likely that the syndrome still occurs in 1% to 2% of hospital admissions for thyrotoxicosis. It is not possible to distinguish those with thyrotoxic storm from those with uncomplicated thyrotoxicosis simply on the basis of routine function tests. Often there is a history of previously partially treated thyrotoxicosis, but the initiation of the decompensation into thyrotoxic crisis usually follows some specific precipitating event, as listed in Table 406.9. The overwhelming majority of patients will have rather obvious signs and symptoms of thyrotoxicosis, including goiter and Graves' ophthalmopathy. Older patients, particularly those who may have an underlying toxic multinodular goiter rather than Graves' disease, may present as so-called masked or "apathetic" thyrotoxicosis.

Treatment must be swift and aggressive to avoid a disastrous outcome and includes both supportive measures and specific therapy of the thyrotoxicosis. Supportive therapy includes treatment of dehydration and the intravenous administration of glucose and saline, vitamin B complex, and glucocorticoids. Patients should be treated in an intensive care unit and placed in a cooled, humidified oxygen tent, with a cooling blanket if hyperpyrexia is present. Digitalis or other appropriate cardiac medications are employed to control ventricular rate in those with atrial fibrillation. In addition to vigorous fluid replacement, intravenous pressor agents may be needed for hypotension. Treatment of hyperthyroidism consists of blockade of hormone synthesis by the immediate and continued administration of large doses of anti-

thyroid agent (e.g., 100 mg PTU every 2 hours). In comatose patients unable to swallow the medication, tablets can be crushed and given by nasogastric tube or per rectum, since parenteral preparations are unavailable. Shortly after antithyroid drugs are started, stable iodine as Lugol's solution or saturated solution of potassium iodide is given to block further hormone release from the gland. Sodium ipodate can be administered (1 g per day) instead of iodine; it has the added advantage of inhibiting peripheral conversion of T_4 to T_3. In severe cases, attempts may be made to remove thyroid hormone from the peripheral circulation by peritoneal dialysis, plasmapheresis, or hemoperfusion through a resin or charcoal bed, and cholestyramine resin may be used to bind T_4 and T_3 within the gastrointestinal tract. β-Adrenergic antagonists are a critical part of the therapeutic regimen and must be used with caution in the presence of cardiac failure. Propranolol can be administered in doses of 40 to 80 mg every 6 hours. If medications cannot be taken orally, propranolol may be given intravenously. A plasma propranolol level in excess of 50 ng per milliliter may have to be maintained to establish clinical response. When used intravenously, an initial dose of 0.5 to 1 mg should be given cautiously while the patient's cardiac rhythm is continuously monitored. Subsequent doses of 2 to 3 mg may be given intravenously over 10 to 15 minutes every several hours, while one awaits the effect of the orally administered drug. Use of a Swan–Ganz catheter to monitor central hemodynamics is recommended in patients receiving high-dose propranolol, pressors, digoxin, diuretics, and fluids. A very short-acting β-adrenergic blocker, esmolol, has also been used in thyrotoxic storm with success. An initial loading dose of 0.25 to 0.5 mg per kilogram is followed by continuous infusion of 0.05 to 0.1 mg per kilogram per minute. Large doses of dexamethasone (e.g., 2 mg every 6 hours) should be administered based on the belief that there are increased glucocorticoid requirements in thyrotoxicosis and because adrenal reserve may be reduced. Steroids will also impair the peripheral generation of T_3 from T_4. With the combined use of PTU, iodine, and dexamethasone, the serum T_3 concentration generally returns to normal within 36 to 48 hours. Dexamethasone may be tapered thereafter, while antithyroid therapy and iodine must be continued until a normal metabolic state is achieved, at which time iodine is progressively withdrawn and plans are made for definitive treatment.

EUTHYROID SICK SYNDROME

The euthyroid sick syndrome is really not a syndrome at all, but the designation has become firmly entrenched in the literature and represents observed abnormalities in tests of thyroid function in patients with systemic illness. The abnormalities tend to assume a typical pattern that is seen in virtually any severe illness, or after physical trauma or physiologic stress, and is due to alterations in the peripheral transport and metabolism of the thyroid hormones, in regulation of TSH secretion, and, occasionally, in thyroid function itself. Acting alone or together, these alterations lead to changes in the concentrations of both total and free T_4 and T_3. Because the most dramatic effect is a reduction in serum T_3 concentration, the entity is also known as the low-T_3 syndrome. Given the frequency and variety of nonthyroid disease

---

TABLE 406.9.	EVENTS ASSOCIATED WITH PRECIPITATION OF THYROTOXIC STORM

Withdrawal of antithyroid drug therapy
Iodine 131 (^{131}I) therapy
Sepsis: infection
Surgery; trauma
Iodinated contrast dyes
Hypoglycemia
Parturition
Vigorous palpation of thyroid
Emotional stress
Burn injury
Diabetic ketoacidosis
Pulmonary thromboembolism
Cerebrovascular accident; seizure disorder

associated with changes of the euthyroid sick syndrome, it likely is a more common cause of abnormalities in thyroid function tests than is intrinsic thyroid disease.

Under normal circumstances, circulating T_4 undergoes 5'-monodeiodination (see section "Thyroid Hormone Metabolism," above) which generates 80% of circulating T_3. With illness or any perturbation from normal physiology, activity of 5'-deiodinase is inhibited, resulting in dramatic reductions in T_3 production rates and in serum T_3, the degree of which varies with the severity of the underlying illness. The same 5'-deiodinase is responsible for the clearance of reverse rT_3, and rT_3 levels are increased as a result of the decreased activity of the enzyme. In mild to moderate illness, serum T_3 falls but T_4 remains within the normal range. Another aspect of the euthyroid sick syndrome is the presence of circulating inhibitors to hormone binding to both serum transport proteins and cellular receptors. As a result of the inhibition of binding to its transport proteins, values for the resin T_3 uptake test will be increased and unbound or free T_4 will be increased, at least initially. Thus, the low serum T_3 should not be taken to indicate hypothyroidism, particularly because serum T_3 tends to be within normal limits in most hypothyroid patients and is not a useful measurement in those patients. The designation "euthyroid sick" is based on the belief that the patients are indeed euthyroid in spite of often dramatic abnormalities in serum T_4 and T_3, and this belief is strongly supported by measured values for TSH that are normal. A euthyroid state is also implied by the serum rT_3 levels, which are increased due to slowing of rT_3 degradation but would be decreased in most (albeit not all) cases of primary or pituitary hypothyroidism. Moreover, patients with primary hypothyroidism and systemic illness tend to still have elevated serum TSH levels, although generally somewhat lower than prior to becoming ill. TSH responses to TRH administration are usually blunted, rather than being exaggerated as is seen in hypothyroidism. With more prolonged and severe systemic illness, TSH levels are more suppressed; serum T_4 levels fall as well, probably as a result of both inhibition of binding and reduced thyroidal production secondary to the low TSH levels, and to circulating cytokines such as IL-1 and tumor necrosis factor. It is controversial as to whether this stage of illness reflects some degree of hypothyroidism with inappropriately low TSH response. There is a correlation between the severity of the aberrated thyroid function tests and survival from the underlying illness. With recovery from the illness, TSH levels rise, often transiently into an elevated range of 10 to 20 milliunits per liter, and thyroid hormone production resumes. Intervention with thyroid hormone therapy is generally neither necessary nor recommended and does not improve survival, with the possible exception of patients with an extremely prolonged course of illness, such as coma.

Rarely, a variant of the euthyroid sick syndrome is seen in which the serum total T_4 is elevated, as least initially. This may be seen in critically ill patients on admission to an intensive care unit, in patients with psychiatric disorders on admission to hospital, and in patients who have received exogenous iodine. The latter may represent a transiently augmented production of T_4 relative to T_3 and must be distinguished from so-called T_4 toxicosis (see above). The high T_4 generally resolves within days to a week with treatment of the underlying critical or psychiatric illness and with no specific thyroid therapy. A thyrotoxic patient with superimposed illness may have lower than baseline values for T_4 and T_3, but in general the values for total and free T_3 will be elevated or at least be high-normal (in contrast to the low or immeasurable levels in uncomplicated illness), and TSH will be immeasurably low.

Patients with AIDS may have a pattern of thyroid function test abnormalities that do not differ significantly from other causes of the euthyroid sick syndrome except that rT_3 may not be increased. Most patients, with the exception of those who may be severely cachectic, will have normal total and free T_4 and low-normal total T_3. As the disease progresses and CD4 counts fall and other infections supervene, serum T_4 as well as T_3 will fall, but serum TSH may remain normal. Observed increases in TBG may account for maintenance of normal serum T_4 at least early in the course of the disease. Rarely, AIDS patients develop hypothyroidism due to opportunistic infections of the gland itself, such as *Pneumocystis carinii* thyroiditis, or due to involvement of the thyroid by Kaposi's sarcoma.

SIMPLE (NONTOXIC) GOITER

The thyroid gland normally weighs 14 to 18 g in adults, and enlargement due to any cause may be called goiter. Although the cause of goiter may be a diffuse or generalized process, it may not result in symmetrical enlargement for the right lobe tends to be larger than the left. Goiter may be associated with increased, normal, or decreased hormone secretion, depending on the underlying process. The overwhelming majority of patients with simple or sporadic goiter are euthyroid. A focal enlargement manifested as a nodule usually implies a neoplasm, which may be benign or malignant. Any cause of goiter may lead to compression of adjacent structures in the neck or mediastinum and cause difficulty with swallowing or with breathing. Goiter may be classified as "endemic" when it is present in more than 10% of a given population, whereas the designation of "sporadic" refers to thyroid enlargement that occurs in nonendemic areas and is due to other factors. The commonly used designation of simple or nontoxic goiter is employed for any enlargement of the thyroid that is not attributable to an inflammatory or neoplastic process and is not initially associated with hypothyroidism or thyrotoxicosis, and may occur in either an endemic or a nonendemic area. On pathologic examination, there is either diffuse thyroid follicular cell hyperplasia or hyperplastic follicles and larger, quiescent ones. The goiters may change little during follow-up periods of years but may become more multinodular with time.

Pathogenesis

For most patients presenting with simple goiter, the underlying cause is never known. Occasionally, it can be documented that the goiter is being driven by an elevated TSH secondary to impaired thyroid hormone synthesis such as might be seen with iodine deficiency, ingestion of a goitrogen, or a defect in hormone biosynthesis. On the other hand, TSH levels are often perfectly within normal limits, and another goitrogenic influence will be operative. The cause is likely heterogeneous, but whatever it is, the underlying pathogenesis usually relates to factors that impair the capacity of the thyroid to secrete insufficient hormones to meet the needs of peripheral tissues.

Clinical Presentation

In simple goiter without associated hypothyroidism, the clinical manifestations are due only to the thyroid enlargement of the thyroid. In goitrous hypothyroidism, symptoms of thyroid hormone deficiency accompany those caused by thyromegaly. Early compressive symptoms may include a sensation of pressure discomfort that may be positional. As the goiter enlarges, displacement of the trachea or esophagus occurs and may cause obstructive symptoms such as dysphagia or odynophagia. Respiratory compromise can result from tracheal compression and hoarseness can result from compression of one or both recurrent laryngeal nerves. A low-lying goiter may enlarge inferiorly to below the jugular notch and sternum (substernal or retrosternal goiter) and lead to superior mediastinal obstruction and a superior vena caval syndrome. A diagnostic clinical sign of thoracic outlet obstruction by a large retrosternal goiter can be demonstrated by having the patient raise his or her arms above the head, which causes a plethoric suffusion of the face, light-headedness, and, rarely, syncope (Pemberton's sign). The sudden appearance of painful swelling in the neck with compressive symptoms is often due to hemorrhage within the goiter or within a dominant nodule in the goiter. Hyperthyroidism may supervene in long-standing multinodular goiter (see section "Toxic Multinodular Goiter") as autonomous foci of hyperfunctioning tissue may develop with time, especially after exposure to excess iodide (jod-Basedow phenomenon).

Goitrous hypothyroidism may be present in areas of severe endemic iodine deficiency, and the children of goitrous parents in these regions are at greater risk of having cretinism. Other goitrogenic factors appear to play a role in the etiologic process of endemic goiter, since the frequency and severity of goiter will vary among persons with equally severe iodine deficiency. Nutritional or water-borne goitrogens can represent important conditioning factors, or these goitrogens may cause goiter in the absence of iodine deficiency. In parts of Africa, for example, the cassava root, which is highly goitrogenic, is a dietary staple, and a history of chronic cassava ingestion is often obtained from patients who have emigrated from Africa.

Diagnosis and Treatment

The extent of a substernal goiter may be assessed by performance of CT scan or MRI imaging, and the degree of possible upper airway obstruction should be evaluated by respiratory flow-loop studies. A diagnosis of simple goiter per se implies the presence of a euthyroid state with normal levels of serum TSH, T_4, and T_3. Not uncommonly, a multinodular goiter may be associated with normal serum T_4 and T_3 but with an undetectable TSH (see section "Subclinical Hyperthyroidism"). This is particularly the case in elderly patients in whom clinical manifestations of thyrotoxicosis may be quite subtle (see section "Toxic Multinodular Goiter"). A number of these patients have underlying Ha-

shimoto's thyroiditis, which can be confirmed by measurement of antithyroglobulin and/or antithyroperoxidase antibodies. The radioiodine uptake test is usually within normal limits but may be increased with Hashimoto's disease or in the context of iodine insufficiency. A dominant nodule may be apparent in a multinodular goiter and should be managed no differently than a single nodule in a nongoitrous gland (see section "The Thyroid Nodule"). Such a nodule may harbor a carcinoma, and diagnosis is facilitated by fine-needle aspiration cytology. Hemorrhage within either a benign or a malignant nodule may be the cause of a sudden increase in size and, if infarction is extensive, will result in loss of radiotracer concentrating ability and the appearance of a cold nodule on scintiscan.

Treatment of goiter with thyroxine replacement is intended to diminish the size of the goiter by both inhibiting supraphysiologic TSH production and by supplying sufficient product of the thyroid gland to put the thyroid gland to rest. Exposure to known goitrogens should be eliminated and iodine deficiency addressed as applicable. While a daily dose of iodide may prove efficacious for iodine deficiency goiter, often thyroxine replacement is equally or more practical. In young patients, treatment can be initiated with a dose of 0.1 mg of levothyroxine daily, with the dose increased at four to six weekly intervals based on measurements of TSH. In older patients, a starting dose of 0.050 mg will suffice. Ultimately, no more than 0.125 to 0.15 mg per day is required (average dose 1.7 µg per kilogram per day) to achieve a TSH level between 0.3 and 1.5 mU per liter. There is little need to administer higher doses of thyroxine to achieve complete TSH suppression (less than 0.1 milliunit per liter), which would imply risk for loss of bone mineral and possible atrial fibrillation. While measurement of TSH alone should suffice, adequacy of thyroxine dosage has been assessed as well by measurement of the 24-hour radioiodine uptake, with the desired level being less than 5%.

In many multinodular goiters of long standing, areas of functional autonomy arise that are by definition nonsuppressible. Hence, the radioiodine uptake will not decrease to less than 5%, and often these patients will have subclinical hyperthyroidism with undetectable or very low TSH levels. This constitutes the rationale for TSH measurement prior to initiation of thyroxine therapy, for if autonomy or low TSH is present, there is no point in attempting further TSH suppression. In fact, supplemental thyroxine is contraindicated because it would create overt thyrotoxicosis. In such patients, optimal management would consist of radioiodine ablation. Efficacy of thyroxine therapy in terms of goiter shrinkage varies widely. Diffuse, hyperplastic goiters in younger adults may regress in size by 50% to 70% in 3 to 6 months, whereas the multinodular goiter of the elderly rarely responds very well, with some reduction in goiter achieved in perhaps 25% of patients. Thyroidectomy may be indicated when a goiter fails to shrink with therapy, for unrelieved compressive symptoms, or when a cytology report indicates findings indicating of malignancy. While radioactive iodine has traditionally been employed for toxic multinodular goiter (or Graves' disease), several studies have shown that therapeutic doses of 60 to 100 mCi may be employed safely for large nontoxic goiters, especially when substernal and causing partial upper airway obstruction.

THYROIDITIS

The clinically most important types of thyroiditis are subacute and chronic lymphocytic thyroiditis (Hashimoto's disease) and subacute granulomatous thyroiditis. All of these disorders may be associated at some time in their course with either euthyroidism, thyrotoxicosis, or hypothyroidism. Discussion here will necessarily be brief for both acute infectious pyogenic thyroiditis and chronic fibrosing (Riedel's) thyroiditis because of their rarity. *Acute pyogenic thyroiditis* is generally the result of an acute bacterial infection in the pharynx or hypopharynx that is believed to spread via the pyriform sinuses or connecting soft-tissue planes to the thyroid gland by direct extension. The presentation is one of acute bacterial infection with fever, high white blood cell count, and erythema and warmth overlying the thyroid gland, which is enlarged and tender. The ESR may be increased, thyroid function tests in serum will be normal, but a radioiodine uptake or scan will demonstrate patchy distribution of radionuclide. A scintiscan cold area may represent an abscess, which can be imaged by ultrasonography or MRI. Therapy should be symptomatic for the pain and fever with appropriate antibiotics, usually with gram-positive and anaerobic coverage pending culture results. Cultures of the throat and of fine-needle aspirates of the thyroid may guide antibiotic choice, and incisional drainage is indicated for any abscesses or fluctuant areas within the thyroid or perithyroid tissues. Unusual organisms may cause acute thyroiditis in immunosuppressed patients, such as those on high-dose corticosteroids, or those with AIDS or cachexia due to widespread malignancy. Organisms such as *Mycobacterium tuberculosis, P. carinii,* cytomegalic inclusion virus, and various fungal infections have been seen. *Riedel's struma* or thyroiditis is even more uncommon, and some pathologists even doubt its existence as a distinct disorder, suggesting instead that it may be part of the spectrum of retroperitoneal and mediastinal fibrosis. The thyroid gland is entirely replaced by dense, fibrotic tissue that extends through the gland capsule into the surrounding structures of the neck. The neck is indurated and may be tender to palpation, and there may be associated mediastinal fibrosis. Biopsy is indicated to rule out primary or metastatic malignancy of the thyroid, and surgery may be required to relieve tracheal or esophageal compressive symptoms.

Subacute Granulomatous Thyroiditis

This form of thyroiditis is relatively common and is believed to usually represent a viral or postviral disorder. It is also known as de Quervain's or granulomatous giant cell thyroiditis, and the typical presentation is of a pain or pressure sensation in the thyroid gland that may involve first one lobe and then the other. The discomfort frequently radiates to the chin, jaw, ears, or mastoid area and may be associated with dysphagia or odynophagia. The painful thyroid often follows a nonspecific mild febrile illness, such as an upper respiratory infection, and constitutional symptoms may include low-grade fever, fatigue, malaise, and anorexia. Not infrequently, these symptoms are mild enough to be tolerated without medical attention, until symptoms of thyrotoxicosis such as nervousness, palpitations, and insomnia develop. On physical examination, the patient demonstrates

findings of thyrotoxicosis, such as warm and moist skin, tachycardia, tremor, and so forth, but without the stigmata of Graves' disease such as ophthalmopathy or dermopathy. Depending on when in the course of the illness the patient is seen, the thyroid gland may or may not be tender. Classically, the gland will be moderately to exquisitely tender and its palpation is often not tolerated by the patient. Palpation may disclose a diffuse or multinodular goiter.

The illness is said to pass through four phases: thyrotoxicosis, transition, hypothyroidism, and, finally, recovery with euthyroidism. The thyrotoxic phase may last for 2 to 6 weeks, and patients seen after this time may have normal to low values for T_4 and T_3 depending on the stage of the illness. The hypothyroid phase of the illness is due to the latency of thyroid gland recovery based on several mechanisms. First, TSH has been suppressed by the thyrotoxicosis and may take weeks to recover. Second, the iodide-trapping mechanism of the gland was inhibited (as reflected by the low radioiodine uptake) by the inflammation and recovers slowly under stimulation by a rising TSH level. This may take several weeks, and sufficient hormone biosynthesis to generate adequate T_3 and T_4 secretion into the blood pool is the final step in the recovery process. As a consequence, the hypothyroid phase may last for 6 weeks to 6 months.

The white blood cell count may be normal or slightly increased with a lymphocytic predominance, although leukopenia typical of viral infection is common. The distinction between the thyrotoxicosis of thyroiditis and that due to diffuse or multinodular toxic goiter can best be made by performance of a radioiodine uptake measurement and an erythrocyte sedimentation rate. The radioiodine uptake will be virtually zero, and any uptake greater than 10% should raise doubt as to the diagnosis. The antiarrhythmic agent amiodarone may cause thyrotoxicosis with low radioiodine uptake as well. The mechanism may be of two types, either a jod-Basedow phenomenon (see section "Iodine-Induced Thyrotoxicosis") or an acute, necrotic thyroiditis related to drug toxicity itself.

In most cases, aspirin or a nonsteroidal analgesic is all that is required for alleviation of the symptoms of pain and pressure in the neck. Generally all that is needed to combat the thyrotoxic symptoms is β-adrenergic blocker therapy for the duration of the thyrotoxic phase of the illness. Occasionally, patients are seen in whom the thyroid pain is not relieved by analgesics alone, and a short (7- to 10-day) course of prednisone (20 to 40 mg per day) may be required. Thyroxine therapy is indicated once the patient enters the hypothyroid phase of the illness. Although the gland ultimately spontaneously recovers, patients clearly benefit symptomatically from a short, self-limited course of thyroid hormone replacement. After 6 to 9 months, the thyroxine is gradually tapered during monitoring of serum TSH levels. Once free T_4 and TSH levels remain normal ???or minimal (50 μg or less) doses of thyroxine, it should be possible to discontinue the replacement therapy.

Subacute Lymphocytic Thyroiditis

In contrast to granulocytic thyroiditis, lymphocytic thyroiditis is likely to progress to a chronic variant (Hashimoto's disease), often culminating in hypothyroidism. Early presentations of lymphocytic thyroiditis may be associated with thyrotoxicosis, of either a transient variety much like that seen in viral subacute granulomatous thyroiditis or a longer lasting variant, similar to Graves' disease, which has been called "hashitoxicosis." The short, self-limited variant differs from subacute thyroiditis in that it is painless and not associated with systemic signs of viral infection; it has been called "silent thyroiditis." Histologically, there is lymphocytic infiltration of the thyroid gland as in Hashimoto's disease, but the areas of patchy fibrosis and atrophy are lacking. Like subacute thyroiditis, there is no thyroid hyperfunction per se, and the thyrotoxicosis is due to discharge or leak of T_4 and T_3 into the circulation. There may or may not be goiter and, if so, the thyroid tends to be firm and without nodules. The radioiodine uptake is typically low, but may be normal to high in the hashitoxicosis variant, making distinction from Graves' disease difficult. Indeed, describing a distinction may be artificial, for the two disorders may represent different presentations along a spectrum of autoimmune thyroid disease. As in subacute painful thyroiditis with thyrotoxicosis, the sedimentation rate is increased, and serum total and free T_4 and T_3, along with thyroglobulin, are elevated. Antithyroglobulin or antithyroperoxidase antibodies will be positive in modest to high titers, in contrast to subacute postviral thyroiditis in which antibodies are rarely detectable. Silent thyroiditis may occur at any age but is, like all autoimmune thyroid disease, more common in women. The pathogenesis of silent lymphocytic thyroiditis is unknown, but a postviral etiologic process has not been documented as in granulomatous thyroiditis. The reduced radioiodine uptake may be due in part to TSH suppression by high T_4/T_3, and perhaps less so to any inflammatory process as is the case for subacute thyroiditis. Unlike Graves' disease, there is no TSH receptor antibody present to provide ongoing stimulation of the radioiodine uptake. The duration of the thyrotoxic state in lymphomatous thyroiditis varies from 6 weeks to 6 months, and, like subacute postviral thyroiditis, the thyrotoxicosis may be followed by a hypothyroid phase of the illness. Also, as in subacute thyroiditis, there is recovery and return to normal thyroid function, although it is more likely that these patients will ultimately progress to burned-out Hashimoto's disease later in life.

Postpartum Thyroiditis

Postpartum thyroiditis is a variant of lymphocytic painless thyroiditis that presents after pregnancy, usually within 2 to 6 months of delivery in 5% to 6% of otherwise normal women. It is particularly common in women with type 1 diabetes mellitus, 25% of whom will develop postpartum hypothyroidism or thyrotoxicosis, and may present with postpartum depression. There is usually a small, diffuse goiter and a family history of thyroid disease. Approximately 6% of normal pregnant women have positive antithyroid antibodies at their first prenatal visit, and about 20% of them go to symptomatic postpartum thyroiditis, which may occur as late as 6 to 8 months after delivery. Typically, the first phase of the illness is thyrotoxicosis during which patients will have the usual symptoms of fatigue, palpitations, emotional lability, and heat intolerance, and then usually transition into a subsequent hypothyroid phase, as in granuloma-

tous thyroiditis. However, postpartum thyroiditis may present with only hypothyroidism, or with hyperthyroidism that evolves back to euthyroidism without ever going through a hypothyroid phase. Laboratory findings may include an elevated serum level of T_4 and T_3, suppressed TSH, elevated titers of antithyroid antibodies, and low radioiodine uptake. During the hypothyroid phase (from 4 to 8 months post partum), patients usually manifest a low serum T_4 level, elevated TSH, and high titers of autoantibodies. These patients usually require no treatment other than (a) symptomatic management or (b) β-adrenergic blockers while thyrotoxic and levothyroxine while hypothyroid until the thyroid recovers.

Chronic Lymphocytic (Hashimoto's) Thyroiditis

Chronic autoimmune thyroiditis or lymphadenoid goiter, is the most common form of thyroiditis, the most common basis for hypothyroidism, and arguably the most common of all thyroid disorders. It is a chronic inflammatory disease of the thyroid in which cytotoxic T lymphocytes and antithyroid antibodies play a prominent role. While seen in men as well, it occurs most frequently in women of middle age and is the most common cause of sporadic goiter in children, especially adolescents. The risk factors are female sex, family history or inherited susceptibility, and advancing age. There are said to be two forms of the disease, a goitrous and a nongoitrous, atrophic form, but the latter is likely only the end stage of the earlier, goitrous form. Both are characterized by lymphocytic infiltration and varying degrees of fibrosis, with the atrophic form having the most fibrosis. In the goitrous form, there is thyroid follicular cell hyperplasia, and greater degrees of lymphocytic infiltration with actual lymphoid germinal centers. The progressive atrophy is presumed to be due to both antibody- and cell-mediated injury to the follicular cells. The hallmark of the disease is the antibodies, which are now routinely measured in serum as two types: antithyroglobulin antibody, detected by the tanned red cell agglutination test, and antithyroid peroxidase (anti-TPO or antimicrosomal) antibody, detected by immunofluorescence, complement fixation, or enzyme-linked immunosorbent assay (ELISA). Cytotoxic T lymphocytes and these autoantibodies reflect and also may cause the thyroid follicular cell destruction. In addition, there may be antibodies present to the TSH receptor that inhibit the binding of TSH, thereby blocking its action. In this way, the hypothyroidism may be the result of either (or both) follicular cell destruction and impaired TSH action. Qualitative and quantitative differences in antibody production and activation of the cytotoxic T lymphocytes likely account for the extent of thyroid cellular destruction and resulting hypofunction.

In younger patients presenting with goiter, generalized thyroid enlargement is seen, which typically also involves the pyramidal lobe, and the patients are usually euthyroid. The consistency is that of rubber, but as the disease progresses, there is progressive replacement of thyroid parenchyma by lymphocytes or fibrous tissue, and hypothyroidism supervenes. At this stage, the goiter is usually smaller and finely nodular or so atrophic as to be barely palpable. Between first presentation and development of overt hypothyroidism, there may be years or even decades of falling thyroid reserve and a state described as "subclinical hypothyroidism," which represents simply early or mild thyroid failure. The hallmark of this state of the disease is the presence of an increased TSH level but normal values for circulating total and free T_4 and T_3. Perhaps 5% to 10% progress to hypothyroidism per year of follow-up. What may appear to be paradoxical is the finding of an elevated radioiodine uptake in Hashimoto patients with mild to moderate thyroid failure. This phenomenon reflects the continued integrity of the iodide trap, particularly when under more intense TSH stimulation, while thyroid hormonogenesis is failing.

Chronic Hashimoto's thyroiditis may account for as many as 90% of cases of hypothyroidism. Clinicians may argue about whether to start levothyroxine therapy when the TSH is only mildly elevated (e.g., between 4 to 10 microunits per liter), but controlled studies indicate statistically significant improvement in profile or well-being and in objective parameters such as lipid profiles. Since the presence of positive antibodies predicts inexorable thyroid failure in patients with mild TSH elevations, our practice is to initiate treatment. A small reduction in goiter size may be seen with treatment, but the lymphocytic components to the goiter would not be expected to shrink with therapy. Presentation during pregnancy of mild hypothyroidism due to chronic thyroiditis is common, probably precipitated by the increased demands for thyroid hormone during gestation. High antibody titers are associated with a greater frequency of postpartum thyroiditis and with miscarriage. Euthyroid patients with Hashimoto's disease are sensitive to iodine exposure, which can induce a reversible form of hypothyroidism. Rarely, Hashimoto's disease may present as thyrotoxicosis, likely representing patients with an overlap autoimmune syndrome reflecting the presence of both Graves' disease and its TSH receptor antibodies and Hashimoto's disease with cytotoxic autoantibodies. This presentation has been called hashitoxicosis, and the clinical picture includes a more firm or even nodular goiter than that seen in Graves' disease, but with the same profile of laboratory tests, including elevated serum T_4 and T_3, high radioiodine uptake, and high titers of circulating antithyroid antibodies. Equally rare is the transition of a euthyroid or even a hypothyroid patient with Hashimoto's disease to Graves' disease with thyrotoxicosis. This latter phenomenon suggests the emergence of clones of lymphocytes that produce stimulatory anti-TSH receptor antibodies. Both of these forms of autoimmune thyrotoxicosis tend to progress more readily to spontaneous remission than is seen in the usual patient with Graves' disease, probably because of the presence of intrathyroidal cytotoxic T lymphocytes. As a consequence, short-term therapy of the hyperthyroidism with antithyroid drugs is preferable to ablative therapy by either radioiodine or surgery.

THYROID NODULES AND NEOPLASMS

Epidemiology and Pathogenesis

Solitary nodules of the thyroid gland are present in about 6.4% of women and 1.5% of men. The incidence is low in children (about 1.5%), and increases with age. Many single palpable nodules thought to be solitary are actually in a multinodular thyroid gland. Autopsy studies indicate thyroid nodules in as many as 50% of consecutive necropsies, although many may be small and clinically inapparent. High-resolution ultrasonography has identified nodules in 13% to 40% of patients under evaluation for nonthyroid problems. The prevalence of nonpalpable nodules incidentally detected by ultrasonography ("incidentalomas") is 30% to 60% in autopsy studies and 19% to 67% in clinical studies, with an average risk for malignancy of 4%.

Although the cause of thyroid nodules is not known, some association with iodine deficiency and states of TSH stimulation has been noted. Radiation exposure can cause thyroid neoplasia, with a linear relationship between radiation doses up to 1,800 cGy and the incidence of thyroid nodules and cancer. Radiation exposure as a child is more likely to produce thyroid neoplasia than similar exposure at a later age, possibly related to greater cellular mitotic activity at the earlier age of insult. Among individuals in the United States receiving head and neck irradiation in childhood, palpable nodules are found in 16% to 29% and carcinoma in one-third of these nodules. Most nodules tend to occur within 10 to 20 years of exposure, but the risk may exist for more than 40 years. The increase in thyroid nodules and thyroid cancer occurring in Belarus after the 1986 Chernobyl nuclear disaster has been dramatic. Higher doses of irradiation, such as those used for Hodgkin's disease (more than 2,000 rads), and ^{131}I therapy do not appear related to subsequent thyroid carcinoma.

Diagnosis and Differential Diagnosis

The differential diagnosis of apparent thyroid nodules is indicated in Table 406.10. Most (27% to 60%) true intrathyroidal nodules will represent colloid adenomas or simple follicular ade-

TABLE 406.10.	**DIFFERENTIAL DIAGNOSIS OF APPARENT THYROID NODULES**
Benign Thyroid Neoplasms	Nonthyroidal Lesions
Follicular adenoma	Thyroglossal duct cyst
Colloid	Lymphadenopathy
Simple	Aneurysm
Fetal	Parathyroid adenoma
Embryonal	Parathyroid cyst
Hürthle cell	Cystic hygroma
Lipoma	Laryngocele
Papillary adenoma	
C-cell adenoma	
Teratoma	
Dermoid cyst	
Malignant Thyroid Neoplasms	
Papillary carcinoma	
Follicular carcinoma	
Metastatic carcinoma	
Medullary thyroid carcinoma	
Anaplastic carcinoma	
Lymphoma	
Sarcoma	
Other Thyroid Abnormalities	
Thyroiditis	
Thyroid cyst	
Hemiagenetic thyroid	
Infectious	
Granulomatous disease (e.g., sarcoidosis)	

nomas (26% to 40%). About 5% of thyroid nodules are classified as hot on the basis of a relative increased ability to trap iodide (see below). Hot nodules rarely represent malignancy; warm nodules carry an intermediate risk of around 5%; and cold nodules, while having the highest risk of malignancy, still represent benign pathology in more than 80% of cases. Since the morbidity of thyroid nodules is related to those lesions representing carcinoma, the diagnostic evaluation is focused on identification of those nodules that may be malignant. The single most important historical risk factor for cancer is exposure to radiation. It is important to determine the age at time of exposure, exact region of the body irradiated, and, if possible, the type and dose of radiation to the thyroid. Although women are more prone to thyroid nodules and cancer than men, the probability of cancer is higher among men with nodules. The incidence of thyroid cancer increases with age, but a higher percentage of nodules in patients younger than 20 years are malignant. Thyroid lymphoma should be considered in patients with rapid thyroid enlargement and a previous diagnosis of Hashimoto's thyroiditis, especially in women over age 50 with coincident diabetes mellitus. A family history of pheochromocytoma, hypercalcemia, mucosal abnormalities, or medullary thyroid carcinoma raises suspicion of the latter diagnosis as part of a MEN syndrome. While a family history of benign goiter may be reassuring, the rare Pendred's syndrome of familial goiter and deaf mutism is associated with a higher cancer risk. Most thyroid nodules are discovered incidentally in asymptomatic patients. As noted in Table 406.11, a number of symptoms or physical findings are felt to be more common in malignant than benign nodules, although as few as 5% to 10% of patients with malignancy present with symptoms. Patients with advanced disease may present with lymphadenopathy, growth of hard nodules, thyroid pain and tenderness, and vocal cord paralysis, all of which point to the likelihood of malignancy.

Routine thyroid function tests are of little value in the evaluation of thyroid nodules. The best preoperative method to identify a malignancy is to obtain cells from the nodule for cytopathologic examination by a fine-needle aspiration (FNA) technique. The results of FNA of a thyroid nodule will be generally categorized as "benign," "suspicious," "malignant," or "inadequate for diagnosis." Use of ultrasonographically guided

| TABLE 406.11. | PHYSICAL AND HISTORICAL FEATURES SUGGESTING INCREASING RISK OF CARCINOMA IN A THYROID NODULE |

History	Physical Exam
Dysphagia	Documented growth
Rapid growth	Vocal cord paralysis
Hoarseness	Cervical lymphadenopathy
Pain	Firm-to-hard consistency
Family history of multiple endocrine neoplasia	Tenderness
	Fixation
History of irradiation	Horner's syndrome
Growth on levothyroxine therapy	
Respiratory obstructive symptoms	

| TABLE 406.12. | POTENTIAL UTILITY OF ULTRASONOGRAPHY OF THYROID NODULES |

Differentiation of solid vs. cystic consistency
Detection of multinodularity
Guidance for needle biopsy in difficult selected cases
Monitoring nodule size, including response to suppressive therapy
Determination of solid vs. hemorrhagic expansion in thyroid lesions showing rapid increase in size
Monitoring irradiated thyroids
Monitoring for local recurrence of thyroid carcinoma
Detection of occult thyroid malignancy in cases of metastatic cervical lymphadenopathy from unknown primary

FNA has been shown to be effective for the detection of malignancy in nonpalpable lesions (Table 406.12). Some studies have sought to use cytometric DNA analysis to improve the predictive value of FNA. While it has not been found to be entirely successful in separating benign from malignant disease, it does correlate with outcome and survival in patients with proven malignancy. Polymerase chain reaction amplification of TSH receptor or thyroglobulin transcripts on material obtained by FNA of cervical lymph nodes has facilitated earlier diagnosis of metastatic malignancy. FNA carries no significant risk, and no cases of tumor seeding have been reported.

Thyroid Adenomas

True adenomas, as opposed to localized adenomatous areas, are typically monoclonal, encapsulated cellular tumors that compress contiguous tissue and are composed of thyroid follicular cells. Adenomas vary in size and are classified into three histologic types: papillary, follicular, and Hürthle cell. The follicular adenomas can be subdivided, according to the size of the follicles, into colloid or macrofollicular, fetal or microfollicular, and embryonal varieties. Adenomas very in physiologic differentiation, as judged by their ability to concentrate radioiodine. The more highly differentiated adenomas (follicular) are most likely to mimic the function of normal thyroid tissue and be responsive to TSH stimulation except when autonomous and/or hyperfunctioning. On scintiscan, an adenoma may be seen to accumulate radiotracer sufficient to constitute an area of increased density within the still functioning extranodular tissue (a warm nodule). With time, the nodule may grow larger and ultimately increase function to the point of suppressing TSH secretion. Consequently, the remainder of the gland undergoes relative atrophy and loss of function, and the scintiscan reveals radioiodine accumulation only in the region of the nodule (See section The Hyperfunctioning ("Hot") Thyroid Nodule below).

Management

Thyroid hormone therapy has been used for many years to reduce the size of thyroid lesions thought to be dependent on TSH stimulation. Typically, patients are given a 3- to 6-month trial of *l*-thyroxine at a dose titrated to result in TSH suppression to below the lower limit of normal of a sensitive TSH assay.

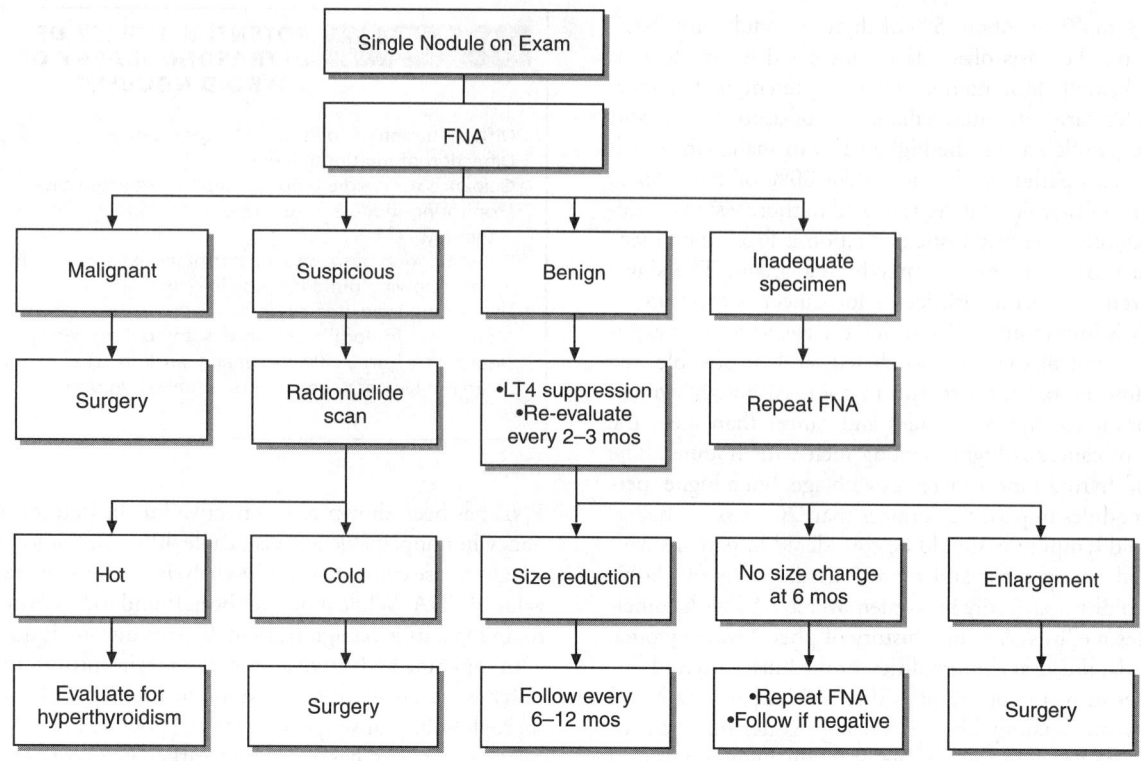

Figure 406.4. Approach to fine-needle aspiration (FNA).
EVIDENCE LEVEL: A. Reference: Singer PA, Cooper DA, Daniels GH, et al. Treatment guidelines for patients with thyroid nodules and well-differentiated thyroid cancer. *Arch Int Med* **1996; 156:2165–2172.**

Growth of a nodule or lack of reduction in size during therapy raises suspicion of malignancy. Complete responses probably occur in less than 10% of cases, whereas 50% reduction in size has been reported in an average of 30% of cases. The benefit of thyroxine therapy remains controversial, with some studies failing to show significant shrinkage and others reporting both a reduction in size and possible prevention of the appearance of new nodules. Possible risk of osteopenia after long-term suppressive doses of thyroid hormone is a concern, especially in postmenopausal women, but either replacement dosage or mild suppressive doses of thyroxine has not been shown to cause osteopenia. An elevated serum TSH indicates that dosage is insufficient and an elevated serum T_3 that it is excessive. Levothyroxine treatment is contraindicated for autonomous hyperfunctioning adenomata. FNA biopsy should be repeated immediately when a nodule is found to be enlarging on suppressive therapy, and surgical exploration should be deemed inevitable unless cystic fluid or hemorrhage with benign cytology is obtained. FNA should also be repeated when there is failure to obtain significant reduction in nodule size after 6 to 12 months of suppressive therapy. Figure 406.4 suggests an algorithm that may be useful in a practice where FNA is frequently utilized with experienced cytopathologic support.

The Hyperfunctioning ("hot") Thyroid Nodule

Hyperfunctioning thyroid adenomas result from genetic alterations in either the $G_s\alpha$ protein or the TSH receptor. Most of these hot nodules are autonomously functioning, and more than half in patients over age 60 will cause hyperthyroidism. Twenty percent of nodules greater than 3 cm in diameter are associated with hyperthyroidism, compared with 2% of smaller lesions. Although most toxic autonomous nodules secrete both T_4 and T_3, elevations of T_3 or T_4 alone occasionally may be seen. Moreover, even when T_3 and T_4 levels are "normal," low serum TSH by a highly sensitive assay indicates supraphysiologic iodothyronine production ("subclinical" hyperthyroidism).

Although hyperfunctioning nodules are rarely the seat of carcinoma, one advantage of surgical excision (usually lobectomy) is the acquisition of definitive histopathologic diagnosis, which is lacking with radioiodine therapy or ethanol injection. Nevertheless, surgery is infrequently recommended for hyperfunctioning nodules because of its own associated risks, the low incidence of cancer, and the efficacy of radioiodine. One exception may be those very large (greater than 4 cm diameter) nodules for which the required dose of radioiodine is so great as to itself provide the contralateral lobe with a risk of radiation-induced neoplasia.

■ MALIGNANT TUMORS OF THE THYROID

Cancers are found in 10% to 14% of patients presenting with palpable thyroid nodules. In the United States, papillary carcinomas account for about 70% of all thyroid cancer, with follicular being the next most common (20% to 25%), and anaplastic and medullary thyroid carcinomas each composing 3% to 5%. The frequency of diagnosis of new thyroid cancer cases appears to be increasing with about 11,300 cases and 1,000 thyroid cancer–related deaths occurring in the United States in 1989, whereas the American Cancer Society projected 18,800 new cases in 1999 with perhaps 1,500 deaths. Autopsy studies have revealed occult thyroid cancer in 6% of autopsies in North American series. There is general agreement that these small, occult, and mostly papillary cancers are of little or no clinical significance, and their increased prevalence does not correlate with an increase in the death rate from thyroid carcinoma.

Owing to its rich vascular supply, the thyroid is a common site of secondary or metastatic cancers from primary tumors elsewhere. Some common sources include malignant melanoma and carcinomas of the lung, breast, kidney, and esophagus. The thyroid also may be the site of lymphoproliferative disease, namely, thyroid lymphoma (see below). Primary thyroid carcinomas may be classified into two varieties depending on whether the lesion arises in thyroid follicular epithelium or from the parafollicular or C cells. The latter disorder, medullary thyroid carcinoma, is described below.

CARCINOMAS OF FOLLICULAR EPITHELIUM

Of the three general histologic types, papillary and follicular carcinomas, which tend to be slow growing, account for 75% and 15% of all thyroid cancers, respectively, while anaplastic carcinoma is the least common. Some tumors will have both papillary and follicular features. Follicular carcinoma, because of its tendency to metastasize to distant sites, is considered to have a less favorable prognosis. But the management, prognosis, and outcome are similar for papillary or follicular cancer providing that patients are of similar age, sex, and stage of disease (Table 406.13).

TABLE 406.13.	**CHARACTERISTICS OF DIFFERENT TYPES OF DIFFERENTIATED THYROID CARCINOMA**	
	Papillary	**Follicular**
Peak ages (y)	30–50	40–60
Women/men	W > M	W > M
Risk factors	Head–neck irradiation	—
Primary tumor	Solitary nodule	Solitary nodule
Usual size of primary tumor (cm)	1–3	2–5
Multicentricity	25%	50%
Recurrence		
Cervical lymph nodes	20–40%	5–10%
Distant metastases	2–5%	15–20%
Pattern of spread	Through lymphatics	Through bloodstream
Sites of metastasis	Cervical lymph nodes, lungs, bone	Lungs, bone, brain

Follicular carcinoma tends to occur in older individuals, resembles normal thyroid epithelium histologically, is encapsulated, and differs from benign follicular adenoma only by the presence of capsular and/or vascular invasion. These tumors can be classified as minimally, moderately, or highly invasive, and prognosis varies accordingly. One subtype of follicular carcinoma, the Hürthle cell tumor, tends to be more invasive, to metastasize frequently to bone, and to have a less favorable clinical course. Follicular carcinoma undergoes early hematogenous spread, and the patient may present with a distant metastasis, usually in lung, bone, or the central nervous system. Lesions in bone are osteolytic. Large primary lesions are associated with worse prognosis, but even small lesions may metastasize widely. Rarely, the functioning mass of metastatic follicular carcinoma may produce sufficient thyroid hormone as to cause increased serum levels of T_4 and/or T_3 and clinical thyrotoxicosis.

Papillary carcinoma is the most common type of thyroid cancer. It tends to have a good prognosis, with a 5% mortality at 20 years for patients with no local invasion or distant metastases at diagnosis. There is a bimodal frequency of occurrence, with peaks in the second and third decades and again in later life. This lesion is slow growing and usually unencapsulated, and it may spread through the thyroid capsule to structures in the surrounding neck, especially to regional lymph nodes, where it may remain indolent for many years. The prognosis depends on the size of the original lesion, with tumors less than 2 cm in diameter having a potentially excellent outcome. The presence of involved lymph nodes may be associated with a greater risk of recurrence but not necessarily with increased mortality. Acceleration of the disease may take place at any time. Follicular elements are usually present in both the primary lesion and its metastases. Papillary carcinoma is the most common thyroid malignancy to develop after exposure of the head and neck to radiation in childhood. Tumors in this setting are usually multicentric, thereby meriting more extensive thyroidectomy, but are associated with a good prognosis.

The diagnosis of thyroid cancer usually begins with the palpation of an asymptomatic thyroid nodule, and the evaluation is described above (see section "Thyroid Nodule"). Fine-needle aspiration for cytology is the initial procedure of choice in the evaluation of most patients and provides a reliable means of differentiating between benign and malignant nodules in all but highly cellular lesions or follicular lesions, where evidence of vascular invasion (as may only be seen on tissue sections) may be required to differentiate benign from malignant forms. Typically, aspirates of papillary carcinoma appear as very cellular smears, with psammoma bodies, and large pink follicular cells with large pale nuclei and nuclear inclusions ("Orphan Annie cells") with numerous nucleoli. Ultrasonography and nuclear scintiscanning may be also useful, with the former indicating a solid tumor and the latter a nonfunctioning, or cold, lesion.

When the cytologic results are equivocal, suppressive doses of thyroid hormone may be tried in an attempt to shrink the suspect nodule, or one can proceed to thyroidectomy. Candidates for surgery include those with a history of radiation to the thyroid and one or more clearly palpable nodules, as well as young men and women with solitary cold nodules, particularly nodules that are hard, nontender, and changing rapidly in size. In the remainder, thyroid hormone therapy with repeat aspiration cytology in 3 to 6 months is recommended. Opinions vary as to the preferable procedure when carcinoma is found. In skilled hands the preferred procedure may be near-total thyroidectomy, especially for lesions larger than 2 cm in view of the high incidence of multicentric tumor and the evidence that both recurrence rates and subsequent mortality are lower following this more extensive operation. Regional lymph nodes should be explored and removed if there is evidence of involvement, but radical neck dissection is not justified. When the initial surgical procedure was not a near-total thyroidectomy and the permanent sections reveal carcinoma when frozen sections failed to do so, a second surgery for a completion thyroidectomy should be undertaken. A total thyroidectomy is warranted for follicular carcinoma in view of its tendency for distant metastasis. This is so because the metastases do not concentrate adequate ^{131}I in the presence of residual normal thyroid tissue, which both competes for the ^{131}I and prevents the increase in serum TSH required to stimulate uptake by tumor cells.

The need for postoperative ablation of the thyroid remnant with radioiodine and for subsequent periodic radioisotopic scanning for residual or current disease varies with the histologic type of cancer, size of lesion, presence of metastases, and other indications of invasiveness or aggressiveness.

Total body scintiscanning with ^{131}I is the method employed to evaluate for residual normal or malignant thyroid tissue in the neck and for distant metastases, and is only done when the TSH is sufficiently elevated to stimulate good uptake and imaging. One concern is that high doses of ^{131}I (a β-particle emitter) used for diagnostic scanning may have an adverse effect on the subsequent uptake of the therapeutic dose, a phenomenon that has been called "stunning." As a precaution against stunning, ^{123}I (a pure τ-ray emitter) or ^{99m}Tc may be used instead for initial scans, reserving ^{131}I for actual therapy, or for scanning when the ^{123}I scan is negative but residual disease is suspected on the basis of elevated serum thyroglobulin levels. Postoperatively, the patient is not started on *l*-thyroxine replacement and is allowed to become hypothyroid with the resultant increase in serum TSH. With the recent availability of recombinant TSH for parenteral injection, it is no longer necessary to discontinue thyroid hormone therapy for follow-up scanning. Some patients may be monitored for recurrence by measuring serum thyroglobulin only.

Patients are reexamined approximately 6 months after the initial operation and at least every 6 months for several years thereafter. At these examinations, the neck is palpated for evidence of recurrence, which often can be surgically removed. Serum thyroglobulin is measured, and elevated values in patients receiving suppressive therapy signal the presence of metastatic disease. At the initial 6-month examination, patients in whom metastases had previously been found are prepared for wholebody scan as described above. Patients with relatively small initial ("low risk") lesions, in whom no metastases have been demonstrated by earlier scan, may not require rescanning unless the serum thyroglobulin is shown to increase (either basally or after recombinant TSH administration). Patients in whom wholebody scans are positive are reentered into the therapeutic algorithm, as described above. Those in whom scans are negative continue to be reexamined and have measurements of serum thyroglobulin concentrations at regular intervals. If both serum thyroglobulin concentrations and scans fail to disclose residual tumor, patients are scanned for possibly the last time after approximately 3 to 5 years, unless serum thyroglobulin concentrations subsequently rise. In some patients, serum thyroglobulin may be elevated despite the absence of demonstrable functioning metastases, and empirical therapy has been given. Reduction in serum thyroglobulin in such patients is presumed to represent therapeutic benefit. In scan-negative patients, alternative imaging to identify tumor may be feasible by CT or MRI or other radionuclides such as fluorodeoxyglucose–polyethylene terephthalate, thallium 201 or technetium-99m MIBI to determine whether the site of the thyroglobulin-secreting metastases may be amenable to surgery or external radiation. This management program with near-total thyroidectomy, long-term suppressive therapy, and treatment of functioning metastases with radioiodine reduces the recurrence rate and prolongs survival in patients with papillary carcinoma of the thyroid. Follicular carcinoma should be treated with even greater vigor, since the outcome with this tumor is generally less favorable. Because follicular carcinoma metastasizes to lung and bone, appropriate followup radiography and measurements of serum thyroglobulin should be performed. Mixed differentiated tumors with both follicular and papillary elements tend to behave biologically as papillary tumors and should be so managed.

CARCINOMAS OF PARAFOLLICULAR EPITHELIUM

Medullary thyroid carcinoma (MTC) arises from the thyroid parafollicular C cells, clustered in the upper two-thirds of the thyroid lobes, and is traditionally classified as sporadic versus hereditary. There are four presentations, with the sporadic form accounting for 80% of cases, and three autosomal dominant hereditary forms, which account for the remaining 20%.

Hereditary Medullary Thyroid Carcinoma

Hereditary medullary thyroid carcinomas are thought to begin as C-cell hyperplasia and are usually multifocal. Two of the familial forms of MTC occur as MEN 2A and 2B. MEN 2A is the most common form, representing perhaps 95% of affected individuals, 50% of whom will have associated pheochromocytoma and 15% to 25% of whom will also have hyperparathyroidism. MEN 2A is rarely associated with Hirschsprung's disease or with cutaneous lichen amyloidosis. Patients with MEN 2B, the second most common syndrome, do not have hyperparathyroidism. MEN 2B includes MTC, pheochromocytoma, and ganglioneuromas of the oral mucosa and gastrointestinal tract. Familial MTC is the least common hereditary form and has no extrathyroidal (MEN) manifestations. Each of the hereditary syndromes is associated with a germ line mutation of the *ret* gene on chromosome 10. In familial forms, the disease may be diagnosed early in family members by means of screening DNA analysis of the *ret* gene, precluding the necessity for periodic tests of calcitonin secretion in family members at risk. Thyroidectomy is recommended for gene carriers starting at age 5 years.

Sporadic Medullary Thyroid Carcinoma

There is a peak incidence of the sporadic form in the sixth and seventh decades of life. At presentation, patients may already have cervical lymph node metastases, which often demonstrate calcification on routine radiographic examination of the neck. Local symptoms of dysphagia or hoarseness may be due to tissue compression or invasion of the recurrent laryngeal nerves. Paraneoplastic manifestations of flushing, secretory diarrhea, or hypercortisolism occur rarely. FNA biopsy is the diagnostic procedure of choice, and correct preoperative diagnosis is essential to screen for pheochromocytoma and plan an appropriate staging evaluation. Staging may include scintigraphic imaging of the neck and mediastinum, and CT or MRI of the neck and chest. The preoperative evaluation should also include a basal calcitonin and carcinogenic embryonic antigen level, serum calcium, and 24-hour urine catecholamines or metanephrines to rule out pheochromocytoma. The preoperative diagnosis of MTC prepares the surgeon to search for regional metastases and perform extensive lymph node dissection. Postoperatively, serum calcitonin serves as a tumor marker for residual disease, and the serum levels correlate with tumor burden.

Anaplastic Carcinoma

Anaplastic carcinoma, aggressive tumor, constitutes approximately 5% of thyroid cancers and usually occurs in the sixth or seventh decade of life. The tumor is histologically undifferentiated, composed largely of spindle and giant cells, and is fast growing and highly malignant. Despite radical surgery, the prognosis is dismal, with survival in months rather than years, although survival is slightly better in younger patients with early disease. The rapidly fatal character of the lesion is due to extensive local invasion that is refractory to both external-beam radiation therapy and radioiodine therapy (because the tumor does not concentrate iodine). The fact that many patients have coexisting differentiated carcinoma suggests that anaplastic tumors arise from the former, and metastases of papillary or follicular carcinoma have been known to undergo late malignant dedifferentiation.

Lymphoma

Primary thyroidal lymphoma constitutes about 5% of all thyroid malignancies. Of the various cell types, large-cell histiocytic (or immunoblastic) lymphoma is the most common and typically occurs in women between the ages of 55 and 75, who often have underlying chronic lymphocytic thyroiditis with positive serum antithyroglobulin or anti-TPO antibodies. Patients with Hashimoto's disease have an approximate 60-fold relative risk for developing non-Hodgkin's lymphoma of the thyroid, a risk so high that any enlarging thyroid mass in an elderly patient with Hashimoto's thyroiditis should be considered to be thyroid lymphoma until ruled out. While occasional T-cell lymphomas have been reported, primary thyroidal lymphoma is almost always of B-cell lineage. Because of histologic and prognostic similarities, some workers have grouped B-cell thyroid lymphomas with mucosa-associated lymphoid tissue (MALT) lymphomas. Molecular abnormalities reportedly associated with both thyroid and MALT lymphomas include loss of expression of bcl-2 and increased p53 inactivation.

Symptoms of thyroid lymphoma typically include dysphagia, odynophagia, and hoarseness (those of a rapidly enlarging goiter, with compression of surrounding structures, and substernal extension is common). Many patients also have cervical or supraclavicular lymphadenopathy. Hypothyroidism, when present, is due to both the underlying Hashimoto's thyroiditis and possible replacement of functioning follicular tissue with the lymphoma. The tumor may completely encircle the trachea giving rise to a "donut sign" on CT. The mass will be cold on radioiodine scanning but frequently may be made visible with either gallium 67, thallium 201, or technetium 99m MIBI. The diagnosis is usually confirmed by fine needle aspiration cytology but rarely a surgical biopsy may be required. Because of the tendency of this tumor to grow rapidly, airway management is usually a principal focus of management. Prognosis depends on the cell type and the extent of disease beyond the neck. Variable success rates have been reported with combinations of surgery, radiation, and chemotherapy. External-beam radiation therapy with approximately 4,000 cGy usually provides a 5-year survival of 10% to 70%, and whether or not aggressive surgery may further benefit survival is controversial. More advanced disease may benefit from chemotherapy or combined-modality therapy.

BIBLIOGRAPHY

Browne-Martin K, Emerson CH. Postpartum thyroid dysfunction. *Clin Obstet Gynecol* 1997;40:90–101.

Burch HB. Evaluation and management of the solid thyroid nodule. *Endocrinol Metab Clin North Am* 1995;24:663–710.

Dayan CM, Daniels GH. Chronic autoimmune thyroiditis. *N Engl J Med* 1996;335:99–107.

Franklyn JA. The management of hyperthyroidism. *N Engl J Med* 1994; 330:1731–1738.

Hermus AR, Huysmans DA. Treatment of benign nodular thyroid disease. *N Engl J Med* 1998;338:1438–1447.

Heshmati HM, Gharib H, van Heerden JA, et al. Advances and controversies in the diagnosis and management of medullary thyroid carcinoma. *Am J Med* 1997;103:60–69.

McIver B, Gorman CA. Euthyroid sick syndrome: an overview. *Thyroid* 1997;7:125–132.

Schlumberger MJ. Papillary and follicular thyroid carcinoma. *N Engl J Med* 1998;338:297–306.

Singer PA, Cooper DS, Daniels GH, et al. Treatment guidelines for patients with thyroid nodules and well-differentiated thyroid cancer. American Thyroid Association. *Arch Intern Med* 1996;156:2165–2172.

Singer PA, Cooper DS, Levy EG, et al. Treatment guidelines for patients with hyperthyroidism and hypothyroidism. Standards of Care Committee, American Thyroid Association. *JAMA* 1995;273:808–812.

Woeber KA. Subclinical thyroid dysfunction. *Arch Intern Med* 1997;157: 1065–1068.

Kelley's Textbook of Internal Medicine, fourth edition. Edited by H. David Humes. Lippincott Williams & Wilkins, Philadelphia © 2000.

407

DISORDERS OF THE ADRENAL GLAND

DAVID E. SCHTEINGART

▮ NORMAL ADRENAL FUNCTION

The adrenal cortex is the source of three types of steroid hormones: cortisol, aldosterone, and sex steroids. Cortisol is synthesized in the zona fasciculata and its secretion is regulated by adrenocorticotropic hormone (ACTH; also called adrenocorticotropin, or corticotropin). ACTH binds to specific receptors in the adrenocortical cell membrane where it activates adenyl cyclase. In turn, cyclic AMP activates a protein kinase that increases the activity of cholesterol esterase and the hydrolysis of cholesteryl esters, making cholesterol available to the mitochondria for initiation of steroidogenesis. The rate-limiting step in the activation of steroidogenesis by ACTH is the transport of cholesterol from the outer to the inner mitochondrial membrane, a process that is regulated by a steroidogenic acute regulatory protein (StAR). ACTH also activates the conversion of cholesterol to pregnenolone, a step catalyzed by the cholesterol side-chain cleavage enzyme. A series of four enzyme-catalyzed steps then converts pregnenolone to cortisol. The four key enzymes that regulate this process belong to the cytochrome P450 family. They are 3βol dehydrogenase-δ5-4 isomerase, which catalyzes the conversion of pregnenolone to progesterone; and 17α, 21, and 11β-hydroxylases, which sequentially act on the various carbons to introduce hydroxyl groups and convert progesterone to 17a-hydroxyprogesterone, 11-deoxycortisol, and cortisol, respectively. Cortisol is secreted into the blood where 94% of it is transported in association with two plasma proteins: corticosteroid-binding globulin (CBG) and albumin. The remaining 6% is a biologically active free fraction of small molecular size that is capable of moving freely across cell membranes. CBG is primarily of hepatic origin, but it may also be produced in smaller quantities in other organs, including lung, kidney, and testis. The major source of physiologic variation of CBG is pregnancy. CBG levels start to increase from 10 weeks on and a marked two- to threefold increase is observed during the last trimester. The concentration of CBG can also vary in families in which there is an inherited deficiency of CBG leading to a decrease in total cortisol level. Cortisol is metabolized in the liver by reduction and converted to dihydro and tetrahydro derivatives. Small amounts of cortisol are metabolized by hydroxylation. Cortisol metabolites are cleared through glomerular filtration. Conditions that diminish filtration, such as renal insufficiency, can alter cortisol clearance. The following situations also affect cortisol metabolism: estrogen therapy, which increases the binding capacity of CBG; thyroxine therapy, which accelerates the rate of reduction of cortisol by the liver; and liver disease, which decreases the rate of cortisol turnover.

Aldosterone synthesis takes place in the zona glomerulosa and its secretion is regulated by the renin–angiotensin system, potassium, and ACTH in the short term. The pathway of aldosterone synthesis involves the synthesis of progesterone and the subsequent hydroxylation on carbons 21 and 11 to produce 11-deoxycorticosterone and corticosterone. Aldosterone synthase catalyzes the final steps in aldosterone synthesis.

Adrenal androgen synthesis takes place in the zona reticularis under ACTH control. The main adrenal androgens produced are dehydroepiandrosterone (DHEA) and Δ^4-androstenedione. Small amounts of testosterone are synthesized and secreted by the adrenal cortex.

Cortisol secretion is regulated by ACTH. In turn, ACTH secretion depends on the integrated function of the limbic system, the anteromedial hypothalamus, and the anterior pituitary gland. Activation of the hypothalamic neurons is mediated by release of serotonergic, dopaminergic, and cholinergic neurotransmitters. The various physiologic characteristics of ACTH release (basal secretion, circadian rhythm, and feedback regulation), as well as the activation or suppression of ACTH release under conditions of stress, depend on specific neuronal pathways located in the limbic system. Hypothalamic corticotropin-releasing hormone (CRH)–secreting neurons are the final common pathway for these various inputs. CRH, a 41-amino-acid peptide, is released into the hypothalamic–hypophysial portal system, through which it reaches pituitary corticotropes in the anterior pituitary gland causing the release of pro-opiomelanocortin (POMC)-derived peptides [ACTH, β-lipotropic pituitary hormone (β-LPH), β-endorphin, melanocyte-stimulating hormone (MSH)]. This release involves CRH binding to specific receptors in the corticotrope cell membrane and activation through adenyl cyclase and G proteins of a protein kinase, which regulates gene expression for the synthesis of POMC. POMC is processed in the pituitary corticotropes through a series of steps regulated by endopeptidases that cleave POMC into β-LPH (a 91-amino-acid peptide) and ACTH (a 39-amino-acid peptide). Two important functions of the neurohypothalamus determine the normal physiology of ACTH secretion. They are a circadian rhythm whereby ACTH reaches a peak between 6 and 8 a.m. and a nadir at midnight. In addition, the secretion of ACTH is subject to negative feedback whereby a decrease in cortisol increases ACTH secretion and a rise in cortisol suppresses ACTH release.

Renin is synthesized in the afferent arteriole of the renal glomerulus. Stretch receptors in the wall of the afferent arteriole respond to changes in arterial pressure and stimulate the release of renin. Renin, acting on renin substrate produced in the liver, generates angiotensin I, a decapeptide that is further processed in the lung under the effect of converting enzyme to the octapeptide angiotensin II. Angiotensin II has both direct pressor effects on the peripheral vasculature and endocrine effects through which it stimulates glomerulosa cells to secrete aldosterone. Factors that stimulate the secretion of renin, angiotensin, and aldosterone are volume depletion (hemorrhage, low sodium intake, dehydration, and diuretics) and assuming the upright posture. Factors that inhibit renin, angiotensin, and aldosterone secretion include those associated with volume expansion. In addition, aldosterone secretion can be directly stimulated by the concentration of potassium and ACTH reaching the adrenal cortex.

MECHANISM OF ACTION OF ADRENOCORTICAL STEROIDS

Most steroid effects involve penetration of the cell membrane by the steroid molecule and its binding to specific intracellular protein receptors. These receptors are found in the cytosol and/or nucleus of steroid-responsive cells. This initial interaction is necessary for a subsequent hormonal response. The steroid–receptor complex then binds reversibly to specific sites in the cell nucleus, resulting in transcriptional activation.

The tissue response to cortisol is catabolic in most tissues (muscle, skin, lymphoid, adipose, or connective) but anabolic in the liver where it stimulates gluconeogenesis. The general response is due to specific stimulation or inhibition of a number of individual enzymes, each of which contributes to the total catabolic or anabolic pattern. The resulting effect is protein catabolism, stimulation of gluconeogenesis and hepatic glucose production, and redistribution of fat with development of truncal obesity.

Glucocorticoids have a major anti-inflammatory and immunosuppressive role, although it is not clear if this role occurs within a physiologic range of secretion. They inhibit the initial inflammatory reaction by suppressing hyperemia, extravasation, cellular migration, and cellular permeability; they also inhibit the release of vasoactive kinins from plasma proteins and suppress the phagocytic mechanism. They decrease histamine synthesis by mast cells, which in turn inhibits the acute anaphylactic reaction based on antibody-mediated hypersensitivity. They have a suppressive effect on wound healing and scar formation.

Mineralocorticoids stimulate sodium pump activity, causing sodium retention, potassium excretion, metabolic alkalosis, and increased blood pressure. Androgens induce protein anabolism and development of male secondary sexual characteristics.

CUSHING'S SYNDROME

DEFINITION

Cushing's syndrome is the clinical expression of the metabolic effects of persistent, inappropriate hypercortisolism. The diagnosis can be precisely established by biochemical means, by noninvasive imaging of pituitary and adrenal lesions, and by selective identification of the source of ACTH in the ACTH-dependent types.

ETIOLOGIC FACTORS

The cause of Cushing's syndrome can be exogenous, resulting from the administration of glucocorticoids or ACTH, or endogenous, resulting from a primary increased secretion of cortisol or ACTH (Fig. 407.1).

Pituitary ACTH hypersecretion occurs in 60% of patients with Cushing's syndrome. This condition is also called Cushing's disease. About 85% of patients with Cushing's disease have pituitary microadenomas. In most cases, the microadenomas are located in the periphery of the gland and can be identified by imaging techniques or transsphenoidal pituitary exploration. Occasionally, they are located deep in the central wedge of the pituitary and can be missed on imaging or at surgery. It has been suggested that excessive ACTH secretion may develop from corticotrope hyperplasia caused by neurohypothalamic stimulation and CRH hypersecretion. Clonal analyses of the pituitary tissue obtained from patients with Cushing's syndrome show that ACTH-secreting microadenomas have a monoclonal pattern consistent with a monoclonal proliferation of a genetically altered cell. In contrast, corticotrope hyperplasia such as that seen in patients with CRH-secreting bronchial carcinoids is polyclonal. Thus, a spontaneous somatic mutation in pituitary corticotropes is the primary pathogenetic mechanism in this disorder. In the few patients in whom CRH levels have been measured in the spinal fluid, low levels have been found, suggesting suppressed CRH secretion.

The association of Cushing's syndrome with nonadrenal neoplasms is called ectopic ACTH or paraneoplastic ACTH syn-

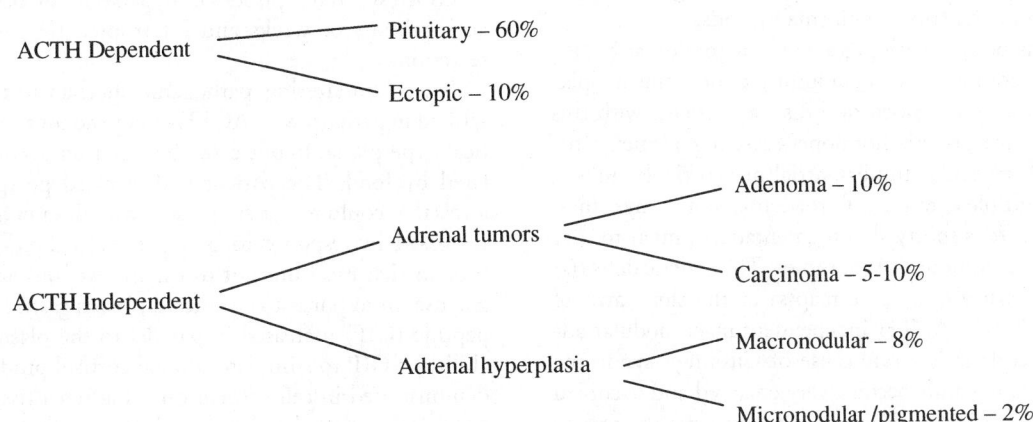

FIGURE 407.1. Etiologic classification of Cushing's syndrome.

drome. Typically, a rapidly developing malignancy causes the autonomous secretion of high levels of ACTH and cortisol, with clinical manifestations of Cushing's syndrome and pigmentation. Approximately 50% of these ectopic ACTH-secreting tumors are in the lung, and the remainder occur in a variety of tissues. In addition to ACTH, these tumors may contain other hormones, such as insulin, gastrin, and glucagon, which are not produced in sufficient amounts to cause a metabolic syndrome. Less frequent causes of ectopic ACTH syndrome include thymic carcinoids; gastric and appendicular carcinomas; pheochromocytomas; adrenal medullary paragangliomas; cyst adenomas of the pancreas; epithelial carcinomas of the thymus; medullary thyroid carcinomas; prostatic carcinomas; carcinomas of the esophagus, ileum, and colon; ovarian tumors; squamous cell carcinoma of the lung, larynx, and cervix; and melanomas. Although the relationship between the more commonly occurring tumors and ectopic ACTH production has been well established, the production of ACTH by the less commonly occurring tumors has not been absolutely proven. An unusual cause of ectopic ACTH production is an ectopic pituitary adenoma. In some cases, normal pituitary tissue occurs in an ectopic location and not in continuity with intrasellar pituitary tissue. Occasionally, adenomas may develop in this ectopic pituitary tissue, causing excessive ACTH production.

Ectopic CRH production can cause Cushing's syndrome. Tumors associated with ectopic CRH secretion include bronchial carcinoids, medullary thyroid carcinoma, and metastatic prostatic carcinoma.

Primary nodular hyperplasia, adrenocortical adenomas, and carcinomas, and rare cases of ectopic cortisol production by tumor, are found in 30% of patients presenting with Cushing's syndrome. Primary bilateral micronodular hyperplasia is characterized by the presence in the adrenal cortex of one of more yellow nodules visible to the naked eye and 2 to 3 cm in diameter. Its pathogenesis is unknown. Histologically, the nodules consist of clear cells arranged in acini and cords, and are occasionally encapsulated and surrounded by simple or micronodular cortical hyperplasia. The incidence of mitotic figures is low. A form of ACTH-independent micronodular adrenal disease is characterized by darkly pigmented micronodules in the presence of atrophy of the perinodular adrenal tissue, disorganization of normal zonation of the cortex, and small glands.

A condition associated with pigmented micronodular hyperplasia is Carney's complex, a form of multiple endocrine neoplasia. In addition to the adrenocortical disease, patients with this condition may have growth hormone–secreting pituitary tumors, Sertoli cell testicular tumors, atrial or ventricular myxomas, single or multiple cutaneous fibroadenomas and myxomas. A prominent feature is spotty skin pigmentation similar to that observed in several lentiginosis syndromes. The genetic defect(s) responsible for Carney's complex map(s) to the short arm of chromosome 2 (2PIG). ACTH-independent macronodular adrenocortical hyperplasia is a rare cause of Cushing's syndrome in which the adrenal glands become very enlarged and occupied by multiple large cortical nodules. In some patients the masses can be extremely large and weigh close to 100 g each. Histologically the nodules are mostly composed of clear cells, and no

cortical architecture has been observed in the internodular regions.

Adrenal adenomas are unilateral, well-circumscribed, brown-to-yellow tumors with a homogeneous appearance, weighing less than 30 g. Histologically, they have the characteristics of normal adrenal cortex, with compact and clear cells arranged in cords. Adrenal carcinomas are large neoplasms with irregularly shaped nodules, exhibiting areas of necrosis or hemorrhage. Histologically, the cells are small, with nuclear pleomorphism and mitotic figures, and there is evidence of capsular and angioinvasion by tumor. Adrenocortical carcinomas can develop in patients with hereditary cancer syndromes. The Li–Fraumeni syndrome is characterized by cancers involving all three types of germinal cells and includes sarcomas, brain tumors, leukemia, lymphoma, and adrenocortical carcinoma, in addition to early-onset breast cancer. Mutations in the P53 tumor suppressor gene have been identified in patients with cancer associated with the Li–Fraumeni syndrome.

PATHOGENESIS

In the ACTH-dependent types of Cushing's syndrome, ACTH is secreted by the pituitary gland or by an extrapituitary neoplasm capable of producing peptide hormones, including ACTH and CRH (see Fig. 407.2). In pituitary-dependent Cushing's disease, the feedback relationship between the pituitary and the adrenal glands is maintained but is abnormal. In the ectopic ACTH syndrome, pituitary ACTH release is suppressed by excessive production of cortisol, which is stimulated by an unsuppressible overproduction of ACTH by the ectopic source. In ectopic CRH syndrome, tumor CRH stimulates ACTH secretion by the pituitary corticotropes; this causes an excessive production of cortisol that is not sufficient to suppress ACTH secretion. In patients with ACTH-independent Cushing's syndrome, pituitary ACTH secretion is suppressed by excessive cortisol production that originates in adrenocortical tumors (adenomas or carcinomas) or in autonomous nodular hyperplastic glands.

The manifestations of abnormal ACTH secretion in Cushing's disease are a loss of normal negative feedback and a blunted circadian rhythm of ACTH and cortisol secretion. Unusual abnormal patterns of release of ACTH and cortisol have been described whereby episodes of hypersecretion occur periodically, lasting hours or weeks and interrupted by periods of normal secretion.

Several interesting pathogenic mechanisms have been described in patients with ACTH-independent nodular adrenocortical hyperplasia. In one case, the secretion of cortisol was stimulated by food. The patient had elevated postprandial cortisol levels that could not be suppressed with dexamethasone. Cortisol increased in response to oral glucose, a lipid-rich meal, or a protein-rich meal but not to the intravenous administration of glucose. In response to test meals, plasma gastric inhibitory polypeptide (GIP) increased in parallel to the plasma cortisol. The ability of GIP to stimulate adrenal cortisol production could be demonstrated in cell suspensions of adrenal tissue from the patient. It was postulated that nodular adrenocortical hyperplasia and Cushing's syndrome was food-dependent and resulted from abnormal responsiveness of adrenal cells to the physiologic secre-

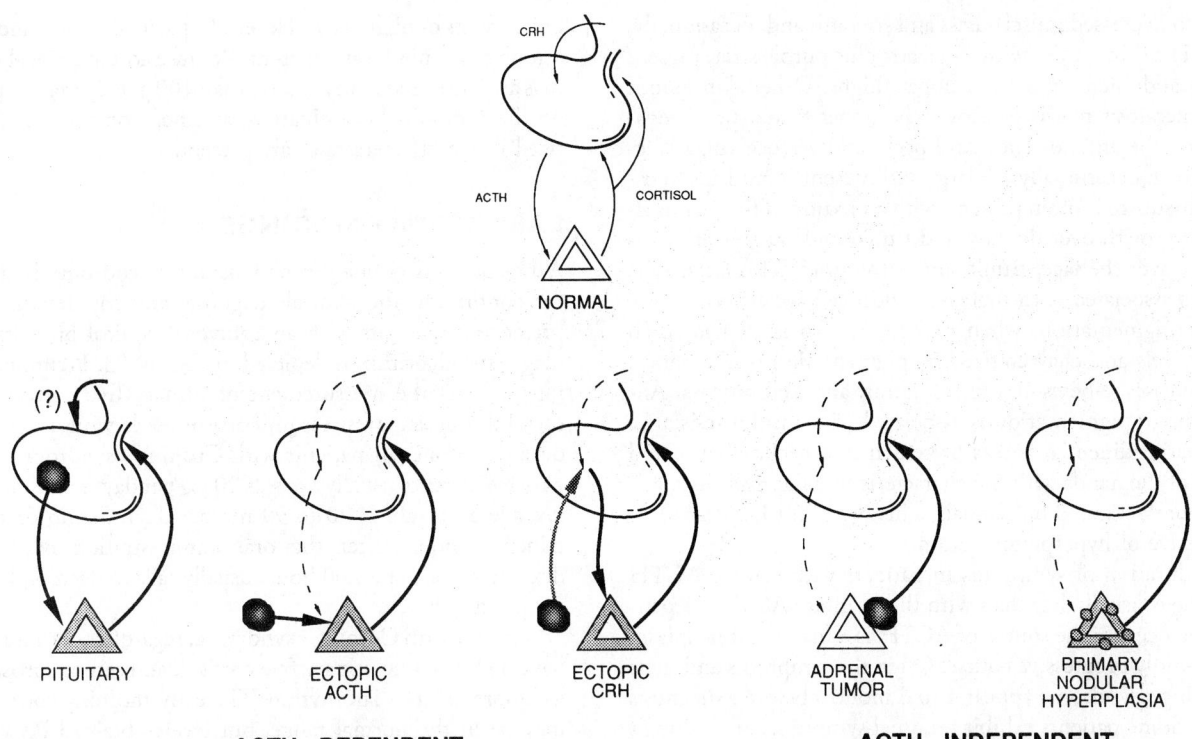

FIGURE 407.2. Changes in ACTH and cortisol secretion observed in patients with ACTH-dependent and ACTH-independent Cushing's syndrome.

tion of GIP. Ectopic expression of GIP receptors in the adrenal cells was felt to mediate this disorder. A case of Cushing's syndrome secondary to ACTH-independent bilateral adrenal hyperplasia was also described that responded to catecholamines acting through ectopic adrenal β-receptors. This increased cortisol secretion was responsive to changes in posture and inhibited by β-blockade with propranolol.

CLINICAL FINDINGS

The clinical manifestations of Cushing's syndrome involve many organ systems and metabolic processes. Hypertension, obesity, diabetes, androgen-type hirsutism, and acne are commonly seen in these patients. When present, the following findings increase the suspicion of Cushing's syndrome: symptoms and signs of protein catabolism (e.g., ecchymoses, myopathy, osteopenia); truncal obesity; lanugal hirsutism; cutaneous lesions (wide, purple striae; tinea versicolor; verrucus vulgaris); hyperpigmentation; and psychiatric manifestations (impairment of affect, cognition, and vegetative functions). In some instances, the diagnosis of Cushing's syndrome can be strongly suspected on clinical grounds alone, but confirmation of the diagnosis requires specific laboratory studies. The clinical manifestations of Cushing's syndrome are determined by the increased abnormal secretion of cortisol, ACTH, and other adrenocortical steroids under ACTH control. However, the clinical presentation varies among the different types.

Patients with pituitary ACTH–dependent disease have a history of 2- to 3-year duration. In milder cases, symptoms may

be present for 5 to 10 years. Earliest symptoms include weight gain, progressive changes in physical appearance, hypertension, and glucose intolerance. Patients may have been treated for these conditions with weight reduction diets, antihypertensive drugs, and oral hypoglycemic agents. The response to diet is frequently unsuccessful. Those who do not experience actual weight gain notice redistribution of adipose tissue resulting in changes in appearance, with facial rounding, increased central adiposity, and thinning of upper and lower extremities. After 2 to 3 years of mild symptoms, additional symptoms or increased severity of the initial symptoms draw patients to the attention of the physician. Patients relate the appearance of striae, easy bruising, and increased body hair growth; women may complain of irregular menses or amenorrhea and men of gynecomastia. Proximal muscle weakness and atrophy are common, and some patients exhibit manifestations of a steroid myopathy. A history of increased skin pigmentation is uncommon in patients with pituitary ACTH–dependent Cushing's disease because ACTH levels are not sufficiently elevated to induce hyperpigmentation. Other manifestations include peripheral edema, back pain, and loss of height if patients have developed severe osteoporosis and compression fractures of their vertebrae.

The physical examination reveals plethora, a round face with pre-auricular fullness, a prominent upper lip (cupid's bow), supraclavicular fossa fullness, and a cervicodorsal fat pad (buffalo hump) disproportionate to the degree of obesity. Patients exhibit truncal obesity, with large breasts or gynecomastia and a protuberant abdomen. This protuberance is the result of an increased omental fat and relaxed abdominal muscles. The extremities are thin, with decreased muscle mass and strength and, occasionally, edema. The skin is thin, with wide, atrophic purple striae present over the abdomen, chest, and upper thighs. Other skin lesions include keratosis pilaris seen over the upper trunk, tinea versicolor over the anterior chest and back, and verruca vulgaris lesions, which occasionally are large and present in multiple locations. Hirsutism is often present, with a mixture of fine, lanugal-type hair growth over the face and trunk, and coarse, terminal-type hair over the face, trunk, and extremities. This latter type of hair is associated with increased androgen secretion.

Hyperpigmentation, when present, is associated with high ACTH levels and characterized by pigmentation of the hands, palmar creases, elbows and knees, gums, and oral mucosa. Another type of pigmentation is associated with insulin resistance and hyperinsulinemia, and is present in the neck, elbows, and dorsum of the hands with the characteristics of acanthosis nigricans. In dark-skinned individuals, a history of further darkening is suggestive of hyperpigmentation.

The duration of symptoms in patients with ectopic ACTH syndrome is usually less than with the pituitary ACTH–dependent type because the source of ACTH is a malignant neoplasm with a rapidly progressive course. Often the symptoms and signs of Cushing's syndrome appear 4 to 6 months before a diagnosis is made. Some patients exhibit minimal symptoms of Cushing's syndrome because of the short duration of hypercortisolemia. In these patients, very high cortisol levels are often associated with manifestations of mineralocorticoid excess, including hypernatremia, hypokalemia, and metabolic alkalosis. Because the levels of ACTH in these patients are 5 to 10 times higher than those with pituitary ACTH–dependent disease, hyperpigmentation of the skin and oral mucosa may be an early manifestation. Severe hypokalemia may also lead to significant muscle weakness. The manifestations of the underlying malignant neoplasm, including anorexia, weight loss, and focal symptoms of organ involvement, may occur together with manifestations of cortisol excess. Some patients with ectopic ACTH syndrome have a more protracted course. These are patients with bronchial or mediastinal carcinoids whose clinical course may last for several years before detection and whose clinical and biochemical features are similar to those with pituitary ACTH–dependent disease.

Patients with benign adrenocortical adenomas usually have a long history of manifestations of cortisol excess before a definitive diagnosis is made. Because adrenocortical adenomas are often purely cortisol-secreting tumors, the predominant clinical manifestations are those related to the protein catabolic effects of cortisol unopposed by androgen excess. These include skin and muscle atrophy, easy bruising, and osteopenia. Patients have the typical fat distribution associated with hypercortisolism, but acne and coarse, terminal-type hair growth are unusual. Patients with primary nodular adrenocortical hyperplasia are clinically indistinguishable from patients with benign adrenocortical adenomas or pituitary ACTH–dependent disease.

Patients with adrenocortical carcinoma have a history of shorter duration, typically 4 to 6 months. The severity of the clinical manifestations depends on the degree of hypercortisolemia. These patients also exhibit manifestations of androgen excess, including hirsutism, acne, scalp hair loss, and clitoromegaly. The androgen excess can moderate the severity of the cata-

bolic effects of high cortisol levels. In particular, skin and muscle atrophy may not be as apparent. Because adrenocortical carcinomas are large, frequently greater than 100 g, they may be palpable on the abdominal examination, and hepatomegaly may be noticed if hepatic metastases are present.

LABORATORY FINDINGS

A biochemical evaluation of Cushing's syndrome is necessary for confirming the clinical diagnosis and for determining its presence in patients with an equivocal clinical presentation. A diagnostic algorithm is depicted in Fig. 407.3. Preliminary testing includes the measurement of urinary free cortisol and of the ability to suppress serum cortisol levels with a low dose of dexamethasone. In patients with Cushing's syndrome, the urinary free cortisol usually exceeds 90 μg per day (radioimmunoassay reference values: 20 to 90 mg per day). Serum cortisol obtained 9 hours after the oral administration of 1 mg of dexamethasone at 23:00 hours usually fails to decrease below 10 μg per deciliter.

Patients with Cushing's syndrome, regardless of cause or type, have high baseline urinary free cortisol, and serum cortisol levels lack normal circadian rhythm. The early-morning cortisol levels may be in the normal range, but levels obtained between 22:00 hours and midnight are higher than in normal persons. A convenient procedure to test the circadian rhythm is the measurement of salivary cortisol at 08:00 and 22:00 hours or midnight. Salivary cortisol correlates well with plasma free-cortisol levels. Patients with Cushing's syndrome have high evening salivary cortisol levels.

The pituitary response to dexamethasone is measured to detect abnormal feedback regulation of ACTH and cortisol secretion. Dexamethasone is given in doses of 0.5 mg every 6 hours for eight doses, followed by 2 mg every 6 hours for eight doses. A lack of normal suppression of cortisol with low doses of dexamethasone is found in all types of Cushing's syndrome, but most patients with pituitary ACTH–dependent Cushing's syndrome (Cushing's disease) suppress with high doses of dexamethasone to values below 50% of the baseline levels. Fewer than 10% of patients with ectopic ACTH syndrome respond in this manner. In patients with ACTH-dependent Cushing's syndrome, high ACTH levels and lack of response to dexamethasone should strongly raise the possibility of ectopic ACTH syndrome.

Benign and malignant adrenocortical tumors can be differentiated biochemically. Malignant neoplasms often have partial enzymatic deficiencies in the steroid biosynthetic pathway. When this occurs, steroid biosynthetic intermediates or other metabolites are found in increased quantity in serum or urine. Impaired activities of 3-β-hydroxysteroid dehydrogenase and 11β-hydroxylase are the most common. These deficiencies lead to increased serum levels of pregnenolone, DHEA, and 11-deoxycortisol.

After the diagnosis of Cushing's disease is established on clinical and biochemical grounds, the presence of pituitary lesions should be further determined by magnetic resonance imaging (MRI) of the pituitary and hypothalamus. Pituitary adenomas can be found by MRI in about 70% of patients with Cushing's disease using gadolinium contrast with coronal cuts. Petrosal

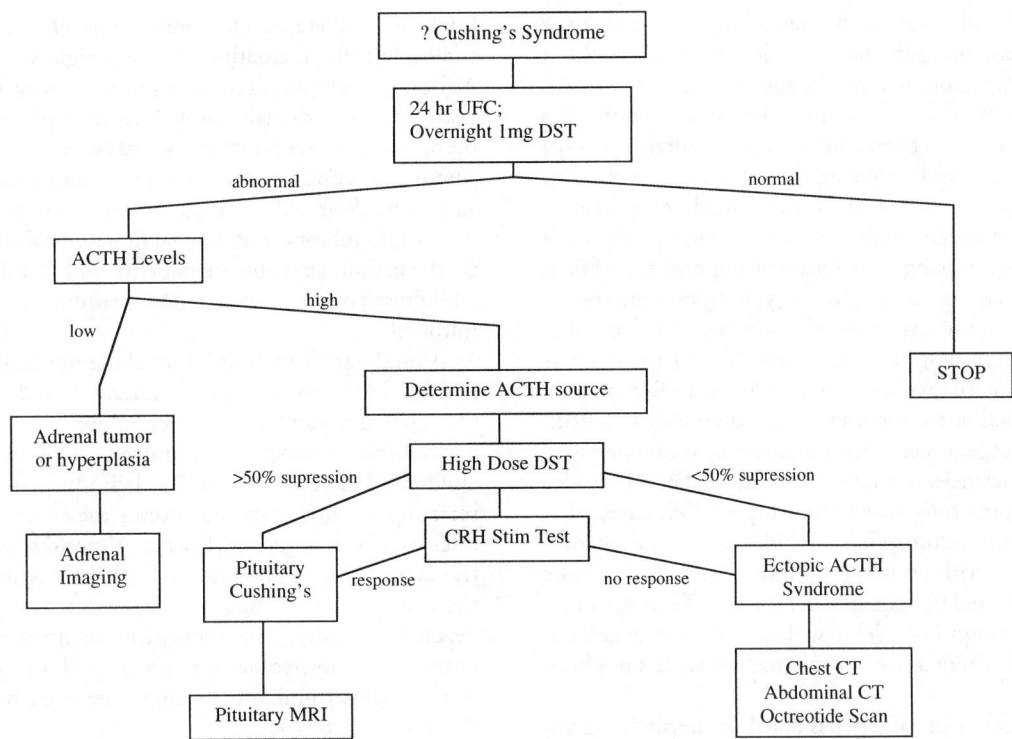

FIGURE 407.3. Algorithm for diagnosis of Cushing's syndrome.
EVIDENCE LEVEL: C. Expert Opinion.

sinus sampling with CRH stimulation can be used to localize pituitary tumors. Through a percutaneous unilateral or bilateral femoral approach, catheters are placed in the left and right inferior petrosal sinuses, and blood for ACTH is withdrawn simultaneously from both catheters and a peripheral vein. To account for fluctuations in levels caused by the pulsatile nature of ACTH secretion, sequential samples are drawn at 2- to 5-minute intervals. A plasma ACTH concentration gradient (petrosal sinus/peripheral vein ACTH $\geq$ 3.0) verifies the pituitary source of ACTH. A right-to-left discrepancy may also help to lateralize ACTH secretion and aids in the preoperative localization of the lesion. A lateralization of the source of ACTH by this procedure can help in cases in which a tumor is not found at the time of surgery. Partial resection of the side of the pituitary where the highest ACTH levels are recorded can result in remission of the disease.

Techniques for the anatomical localization of adrenal lesions include abdominal computed tomography (CT) scans and MRI, ultrasonography, and adrenal scintigraphy with iodine I 131 6β-iodomethyl-19-norcholesterol. These techniques are noninvasive and provide good definition of the pathology of the adrenal glands.

Scintigraphy with iodocholesterol provides information about the structure of the adrenal gland and its function. Patients with bilateral adrenocortical hyperplasia demonstrate bilateral increased adrenal uptake of iodocholesterol. Patients with cortisol-secreting adrenocortical adenomas, which suppress pituitary ACTH secretion and the function of the contralateral gland, demonstrate unilateral concentration of the tracer. Patients with

Cushing's syndrome secondary to an adrenocortical carcinoma fail to show tracer uptake on either side.

The localization of ectopic sources of ACTH involves a variety of procedures, including CT of the chest, CT or MRI of the abdomen, thyroid scan, octreotide scan, and selective venous catheterization and sampling in search of concentration gradients of ACTH. Approximately 50% of these tumors are within the thorax (e.g., small-cell carcinomas, bronchial carcinoids, thymomas), and thoracic CT scanning usually can localize the lesion. Other ACTH-secreting tumors are found in the pancreas (islet cell tumors), the thyroid (medullary carcinoma), and the adrenal medulla (pheochromocytoma). Small carcinoid tumors may escape detection by any of the available imaging procedures.

OPTIMAL MANAGEMENT

Optimal treatment of Cushing's disease depends on an accurate diagnosis of the underlying pathologic process. Four approaches are used in the management of pituitary ACTH–dependent Cushing's disease: pituitary surgery, pituitary irradiation, adrenal surgery, and drug therapy.

The treatment of choice is surgical removal of the pituitary tumor in Cushing's disease. The transsphenoidal selective resection of ACTH-secreting pituitary microadenomas is the most common treatment of Cushing's disease and comes closest to the ideal form of treatment for this condition. It is a reasonably safe procedure with a mortality rate of less than 1% and a high cure rate. The main complications are anterior pituitary insufficiency in 19% and diabetes insipidus in 18%. If a microadenoma can be identified and resected, the remaining pituitary tissue remains functional, and patients can enjoy remission without loss of endocrine function. If a specific adenoma cannot be identified during surgery, the decision must be made to perform a partial or total hypophysectomy. If preoperative inferior petrosal sinus sampling is clearly lateralizing, hemiresection of the side with the highest concentration of ACTH should be performed. If the endocrine studies strongly indicate a pituitary origin but the petrosal sinus sampling is not lateralizing and the patient does not wish to have children, a total hypophysectomy should be considered, but only after a lengthy preoperative discussion with the patient regarding this possibility. If the patient wants to have children, alternative forms of therapy including medical treatment or a total adrenalectomy must be considered. With transsphenoidal surgery, permanent anterior or posterior pituitary hormone deficiencies are rare. Transient diabetes insipidus may occur during the early weeks after surgery. Permanent diabetes insipidus and cerebrospinal fluid rhinorrhea are uncommon complications with an initial procedure but may be more common with repeated transsphenoidal surgery. Treatment failures are most common in patients with pituitary macroadenomas or in those in whom a distinct microadenoma has not been found.

When transsphenoidal surgery has failed or alternative forms of treatment are desired, pituitary irradiation is an option. The most widely used type is high-voltage fractionated irradiation provided by cobalt 60 in a total dose of 40 to 50 Gy. Remission is achieved in about 50% of patients. The best responses are observed in patients with the juvenile form of the disease or in adults younger than 40 years.

When successful, ^{60}Co irradiation has several advantages. Remission occurs with preservation of pituitary and adrenal function; panhypopituitarism develops infrequently; normal reproductive function is usually restored when the patient is in remission; corticosteroid replacement therapy is not needed; recurrence is rare; and normal cortisol secretion may be restored (circadian rhythm, normal suppressibility on dexamethasone). The major disadvantage is the slow therapeutic response; 6 to 18 months may elapse before a clinical and biochemical remission is achieved. ^{60}Co irradiation alone is not adequate in patients who have severe Cushing's syndrome. Symptoms may progress while the patient waits for remission, and severe complications may result. Heavy particle beam irradiation and Bragg peak proton irradiation therapy, which can deliver a higher radiation dose, is more effective than ^{60}Co irradiation, with a rate of improvement or remission as high as 80%. There is a higher incidence of postirradiation side effects, including radiation necrosis of the brain, with a higher dosage. Another method of focally targeted radiation therapy is stereotactic radiosurgery or gamma knife therapy. These techniques have been applied to patients with residual tumor who experience recurrence of Cushing's disease after transsphenoidal resection of pituitary adenomas.

In patients with advanced Cushing's disease in whom transsphenoidal surgery or pituitary irradiation have failed, bilateral total adrenalectomy is the preferred treatment. The major disadvantage of adrenalectomy is that it fails to remove the ACTH-secreting pituitary tumor, which may continue to grow and become locally invasive and difficult to control either by surgery or by radiation therapy. The combination of an enlarging pituitary tumor, hyperpigmentation, and very high ACTH levels is called Nelson's syndrome. This complication may occur months or years after the adrenalectomy. Laparoscopic adrenalectomy has become a common procedure for resecting benign adrenocortical tumors. In contrast, resection of an adrenocortical carcinoma should be done only through an open procedure.

Various inhibitors of adrenal function have been used to suppress cortisol secretion in patients with Cushing's syndrome. The most common are aminoglutethimide, ketoconazole, and mitotane.

Aminoglutethimide inhibits cholesterol side-chain cleavage and blocks the conversion of cholesterol to Δ^5-pregnenolone in the adrenal cortex. This causes inhibition of the synthesis of cortisol, aldosterone, and androgens. It is used in adults and children in doses of 0.5 to 2 g daily. In persons with cortisol-secreting adrenocortical carcinoma, the effect of aminoglutethimide can be maintained for many months, with regression of the clinical manifestations of Cushing's syndrome. However, the drug is only transiently effective in patients with ACTH-dependent Cushing's syndrome, in whom the inhibitory effect of the drug is overcome by the high levels of ACTH. The effect of aminoglutethimide is promptly reversed by interruption of therapy.

Ketoconazole is an imidazole derivative that inhibits mitochondrial cytochrome P450-dependent enzymes, such as 11β-hydroxylase and the enzymes needed for cholesterol side-chain cleavage. Ketoconazole inhibits abnormal cortisol production in patients with adrenal adenoma and Cushing's syndrome. These patients respond promptly, with disappearance of the clinical and metabolic manifestations of the disease within 4 to 6 weeks of treatment. When patients are treated with ketoconazole, adrenal insufficiency is avoided by decreasing the dose sufficiently to maintain normal cortisol levels.

Mitotane inhibits biosynthesis of corticosteroids and destroys adrenocortical cells that secrete cortisol, producing a long-lasting effect. Mitotane acts on adrenocortical cell mitochondria, where it inhibits 11β-hydroxylase and cholesterol side-chain cleavage enzymes. As a result of this inhibition, the production of cortisol, aldosterone, and DHEA is suppressed. Mitotane appears to require metabolism for its action. Under the effect of mitochondrial P450 monooxygenases, the drug is probably transformed into an acyl chloride that covalently binds to important macromolecules in the cell mitochondria. The result is destruction of the mitochondria with necrosis of the adrenal cortex. The zona reticularis of the adrenal cortex appears to be most sensitive to the action of mitotane, and the glomerulosa is the least sensitive.

A combination of ^{60}Co irradiation of the pituitary gland and selective suppression of cortisol secretion with low doses of mitotane has resulted in clinical and biochemical remission in 80% of patients with Cushing's disease.

Treatment of ectopic ACTH syndrome involves the surgical resection of the primary tumor, followed by radiation therapy or chemotherapy, depending on the type of neoplasm producing the illness. In patients whose neoplasms cannot be resected, the use of adrenal inhibitors, such as aminoglutethimide and ketoconazole, may ameliorate the clinical manifestations of Cushing's syndrome. However, the very high ACTH levels may overcome the suppressive effect of these drugs. Bilateral surgical adrenalectomy is an alternative approach but is not a practical form of treatment for patients who have rapidly progressive metastatic disease. Because the underlying tumors (bronchial carcinoids) may be slow growing, an adrenalectomy followed by replacement therapy with normal amounts of hydrocortisone can lead to remission of Cushing's syndrome.

Adrenocortical adenomas should be surgically removed. Because of suppression of the hypothalamic–pituitary–adrenal axis in these patients, adrenal insufficiency occurs postoperatively and patients require replacement therapy with physiologic doses of cortisol until recovery of the hypothalamic–pituitary–adrenal axis takes place.

Adrenal carcinomas causing Cushing's syndrome are highly malignant neoplasms resulting in a shortened life expectancy. Their treatment has not been well standardized, and the prognosis has been poor regardless of therapy.

Several approaches to therapy have been used. One method is surgical excision of the primary tumor and of large neoplastic abdominal masses. Although temporary remission of the disease frequently occurs with this approach, recurrence and eventual death from metastatic disease is the rule. Another approach is nonspecific chemotherapy, but the neoplasm is generally resistant to therapy.

PRIMARY ALDOSTERONISM

DEFINITION

Primary aldosteronism or Conn's syndrome results from a renin-independent, inappropriate hypersecretion of aldosterone. Patients with secondary aldosteronism have an increase in aldosterone production in response to volume depletion or decrease in effective renal perfusion pressure. In contrast, patients with primary aldosteronism secrete aldosterone in the presence of volume expansion and hypertension.

INCIDENCE AND EPIDEMIOLOGIC FACTORS

Hypokalemic primary aldosteronism is present in 1% to 3% of patients with hypertension. Other reports based on observations in patients with minimal hypokalemia or normal serum potassium levels suggest an incidence of up to 10% of patients with hypertension.

ETIOLOGIC FACTORS

Approximately 60% of patients with primary aldosteronism have a single, benign adrenocortical adenoma as the cause of excessive aldosterone production; 40% exhibit bilateral adrenocortical hyperplasia. Aldosterone-secreting adrenocortical carcinomas are very rare.

PATHOGENESIS

The excessive production of aldosterone by an adrenocortical tumor or hyperplasia leads to increase sodium retention and volume expansion. This causes suppression of plasma renin and decreased generation of angiotensin II. The aldosterone secretion continues in the absence of renin. The high levels of aldosterone act on the distal nephron to promote sodium reabsorption in exchange for potassium and hydrogen ions. Acting on sodium-transporting epithelial cells, aldosterone binds to the mineralocorticoid receptor and causes transcriptional activation of an aldosterone-induced protein thought to increase the apical to basal sodium flux. Aldosterone also activates Na^+,K^+-ATPase, promoting the exchange of sodium for potassium. The consequence of these events is the development of hypertension accompanied by hypokalemia and metabolic alkalosis.

CLINICAL FINDINGS

The principal clinical findings in primary aldosteronism are hypertension and hypokalemia. Hypertension is moderate to severe and may be complicated by stroke and proteinuria. Symptoms of hypokalemia include muscular weakness and tetany; renal loss of concentrating ability due to kaliopenic nephropathy and subsequent polyuria; and changes in β-cell function which result in abnormal glucose tolerance.

LABORATORY FINDINGS

Measurement of serum electrolytes reveals hypernatremia (serum sodium 142 to 150 mEq per liter), hypokalemia (serum potassium 1.6 to 3.2 mEq per liter), and metabolic alkalosis (serum bicarbonate 28 to 38 mEq per liter). Hypokalemia is present in 90% of patients with adenoma and in 70% of patients with hyperplasia. A high aldosterone/renin ratio is diagnostic of primary aldosteronism. Figure 407.4 depicts a diagnostic algorithm for patients suspected of primary aldosteronism. The aldosterone/renin ratio is greater than 50 in patients with primary aldosteronism and less than 50 in patients with essential hypertension.

Once the diagnosis has been established, tests are available for localization of an adrenocortical adenoma. CT or MRI of the adrenal glands usually demonstrates a small adrenocortical tumor. Adrenal scintigraphy with ^{131}I-6β-iodomethyl-19-norcholesterol allows for detection of an aldosterone-secreting tumor. The scintigraphy is enhanced by the administration of dexamethasone that suppresses uptake by the normal adrenal cortex but not by the tumor. Occasionally, localization by these procedures is equivocal and more definitive localization requires selective adrenal venous catheterization and sampling. For this procedure, catheters are placed in the right and left adrenal veins through a transfemoral approach. Blood samples are obtained for aldosterone and cortisol. The side with an aldosterone-producing tumor will show much higher aldosterone levels than the contralateral side. This difference will not be noted in patients with primary aldosteronism secondary to bilateral adrenocortical hyperplasia.

OPTIMAL MANAGEMENT

The treatment of choice for patients with a single aldosterone-secreting adrenocortical adenoma is laparoscopic unilateral adre-

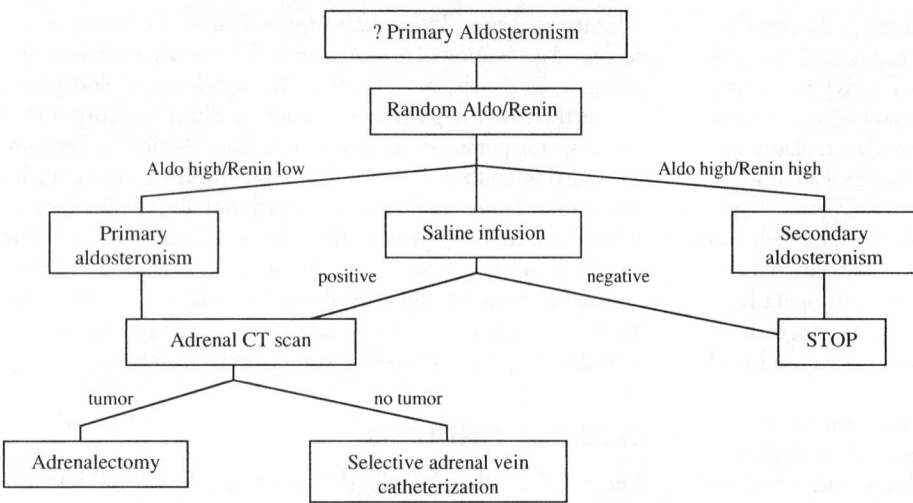

FIGURE 407.4. Diagnostic algorithm for patients suspected of having primary aldosteronism.
EVIDENCE LEVEL: C. Expert Opinion.

nalectomy. Since these tumors are usually less than 2 cm, laparoscopic surgery is ideal because of its relatively low morbidity. Removal of an aldosterone-producing adrenocortical adenoma results in cure of the hypertension in 50% to 70% of cases and the electrolyte abnormality in every case. In contrast, patients with bilateral adrenocortical hyperplasia do not benefit from a bilateral adrenalectomy. Although hypertension improves, most patients continue to be hypertensive. Treatment with high doses of spironolactone, an aldosterone antagonist, is effective. Side effects in men are gynecomastia and impotence.

ADRENAL INSUFFICIENCY

DEFINITION

Adrenal insufficiency occurs when the cessation of normal secretion of the two major adrenocortical hormones, cortisol and aldosterone, is deficient. It can develop as a consequence of destruction or suppression of the adrenal cortex (primary adrenocortical insufficiency) or as a result of failure of pituitary ACTH secretion (secondary adrenal insufficiency).

INCIDENCE AND EPIDEMIOLOGIC FACTORS

Primary adrenocortical insufficiency is uncommon; it has been reported with a prevalence rate of 4 to 6 per 100,000 population.

Adrenal insufficiency is usually sporadic, but certain forms, especially those with an autoimmune cause, occur in families in which siblings can be affected. An infectious cause is found in some patients, including tuberculosis, coccidioidomycosis, histoplasmosis, blastomycosis, and HIV-2 infection.

ETIOLOGIC FACTORS

Autoimmune primary adrenocortical insufficiency is the most common form of adrenal insufficiency in the United States. Patients with autoimmune Addison's disease show familial prevalence of this condition and other associated autoimmune endo-

crinopathies, including Hashimoto's thyroiditis with primary hypothyroidism (Schmidt's syndrome), Graves' disease, type 1 diabetes mellitus, idiopathic hypoparathyroidism, pernicious anemia, primary gonadal failure, and pituitary insufficiency. These patients show a statistical association with human leukocyte antigen (HLA) haplotypes, especially HLA-B8 and Dw3. Other causes of primary adrenocortical insufficiency are infectious (tuberculosis, coccidioidomycosis, histoplasmosis, and blastomycosis). Bilateral adrenal hemorrhage with consequent adrenocortical insufficiency can occur with severe sepsis, pneumonia, recent abdominal surgery, heparin therapy, and coagulopathies. These patients usually present with clinical manifestations of adrenal insufficiency and a CT scan of the abdomen showing bilateral adrenal masses that regress over time. Adrenocortical involvement can occur in patients with HIV infection. The adrenal insufficiency observed with HIV infection appears to be related to superimposed cytomegalovirus infection, which is found in 84% of autopsy cases of patients with AIDS. Infiltrative diseases involving the adrenal glands can lead to adrenocortical insufficiency. These include lymphomas, primary amyloidosis, and metastatic neoplastic disease. In some cases, adrenal insufficiency is the first manifestation of lymphoma. The involvement of the adrenals by infiltrative diseases has to be severe and bilateral to induce clinical manifestations of adrenal insufficiency. Congenital adrenocortical hypoplasia has been described in children who present with adrenocortical insufficiency. Iatrogenic diseases leading to adrenal insufficiency include bilateral adrenalectomy, treatment with adrenalytic drugs (e.g., mitotane), and administration of anticoagulants, which in the presence of severe stress lead to bilateral adrenal hemorrhage. Enzyme deficiencies are also associated with adrenal insufficiency. These may be congenital and involve 21-, 11β-, and 17α-hydroxylases or iatrogenically induced by the administration of adrenal inhibitors. The most common cause of secondary adrenocortical insufficiency is chronic suppression of ACTH secretion by chronic glucocorticoid therapy. Other causes include pituitary tumors (which destroy normal pituitary cells), pituitary infarction resulting from cerebrovascular thrombosis, or postpartum necrosis of the pituitary gland. Surgical hypophysectomy for the treatment of pituitary disease also results in panhypopituitarism and secondary adrenal insufficiency. In these cases, renin and aldosterone secretion is preserved, and patients exhibit only the clinical manifestations of cortisol deficiency. In patients with isolated renin deficiency, aldosteronopenia may be the presenting disorder. Renin deficiency is seen in patients who develop hyporeninemic hypoaldosteronism as a consequence of diabetic nephropathy, chronic renal failure, or the administration of indomethacin or angiotensin- converting enzyme (ACE) inhibitor. The main clinical expression of this deficiency is hyperkalemia. A rare familial variety of primary adrenal insufficiency is adrenoleukodystrophy, a condition in which general adrenocortical failure is present together with destruction of the cerebral white matter. This condition, which has an X-linked transmission, shows large areas of cerebral demyelination and accumulation of specific lipid-like material in the adrenocortical cells.

PATHOGENESIS

Adrenocortical insufficiency results from cessation of normal secretion of adrenocortical hormones. In primary adrenal insufficiency there is a destruction of the adrenal cortex with inability to synthesize and secrete all major adrenocortical steroid hormones. In contrast, secondary adrenal insufficiency develops as a result of either ACTH or renin deficiency, leading to isolated cortisol or aldosterone deficiency. Cortisol insufficiency leads to depletion of gluconeogenic substrates as well as suppressed gluconeogenesis and hepatic glucose production. In addition, there is increased sensitivity of the liver and peripheral tissues to the action of insulin, resulting in increased glucose transport. A clinical consequence of these changes is the development of fasting hypoglycemia with possible neuroglucopenia. Lack of cortisol also leads to decreased renin substrate production, decreased vascular sensitivity to the effect of angiotensin II and norepinephrine, and increased vasodilator prostaglandin E_2 and kallikrein. These changes lead to the development of hypotension. A decrease in the feedback suppression of pro-opiomelanocortin synthesis by cortisol leads to high ACTH and MSH levels and the development of hyperpigmentation. In addition, there are major changes that occur with aldosteronopenia, including natriuresis, iso-osmotic water loss, and increased potassium and hydrogen ion reabsorption. The clinical consequence of these changes is hyponatremia, development of extracellular fluid volume depletion and hypotension, hyperkalemia, metabolic acidosis, and cardiac arrhythmias. Volume depletion also leads to stimulation of renin release. The decrease in cortisol leads to increased arginine vasopressin secretion and a decrease in free-water clearance. While restoring volume, the water retention is likely to further depress sodium levels. Finally, a decrease in androgen production is particularly significant in women in whom there is a decrease in axillary and pubic hair growth.

CLINICAL FINDINGS

The diagnosis of primary adrenal insufficiency is suspected in patients who present with anorexia, weight loss, nausea, vomiting, chronic fatigue, and increased pigmentation of the skin. Secondary adrenal insufficiency should be considered in patients

who have received therapy with glucocorticoids for long periods of time, have pituitary tumors, or have undergone pituitary surgery.

Symptoms associated with primary adrenal insufficiency, such as fatigue, pigmentation, anorexia, weight loss. and hypotension, occur in more than 90% of patients. The fatigue appears to be present constantly and is aggravated by physical activity. Patients describe profound asthenia and difficulty in getting out of bed. The pigmentation is a persistent tan over sun-exposed areas and darkening of areas not normally exposed such as nipples, scars, and genitalia. Dark-skinned individuals relate increased depth of their natural skin pigmentation. Occasionally, patients have vitiligo. Dizziness is most prominent when patients are upright and when they change from the recumbent to the standing position. Generalized muscle and joint pains and abdominal pain are also described. Patients with secondary adrenal insufficiency have similar symptoms, except for the absence of pigmentation and postural dizziness. In fact, patients may notice decrease in skin pigmentation and ability to tan when exposed to sunlight. Associated with symptoms of adrenal insufficiency are symptoms related to the deficiency of other pituitary hormones, including amenorrhea in women, impotence in men, dry skin, cold intolerance, and increased lethargy.

Patients with primary adrenal insufficiency may have associated endocrine deficiencies caused by autoimmune pluriglandular failure. Thus, clinical findings of hypothyroidism and hypogonadism in patients with adrenal insufficiency do not necessarily indicate panhypopituitarism. In contrast to the hypopigmentation observed in patients with panhypopituitarism, those with autoimmune pluriglandular failure are usually hyperpigmented.

LABORATORY FINDINGS

Laboratory findings include manifestations of aldosterone and cortisol deficiency. Prominent manifestations of aldosterone deficiency are hyponatremia, hyperkalemia, metabolic acidosis, and urinary sodium excretion in excess of 20 mEq per liter. Because of intravascular volume contraction, serum urea and creatinine are increased. The most severe electrolyte and renal changes are observed in patients with chronic adrenal failure who have developed acute adrenal insufficiency as a consequence of stress with vomiting and diarrhea. Patients with secondary adrenal insufficiency who have normal aldosterone secretion may also develop hyponatremia as a result of impaired free-water clearance. Cortisol deficiency is associated with hematologic changes, including normochromic normocytic anemia, leukopenia with relative lymphocytosis, and eosinophilia. Fasting hypoglycemia is seen in patients who have been eating poorly.

Radiographic examination reveals a small heart. Adrenal calcifications can be seen on a plain radiograph of the abdomen in patients in whom the cause of the adrenal insufficiency is granulomatous disease. Abdominal computerized CT scanning shows small adrenals in patients with autoimmune disease and enlarged adrenals or adrenal masses in patients with either granulomatous disease or adrenal hemorrhage.

Figure 407.5 depicts a diagnostic algorithm for the evaluation of patients suspected of having adrenal insufficiency. Hormonal

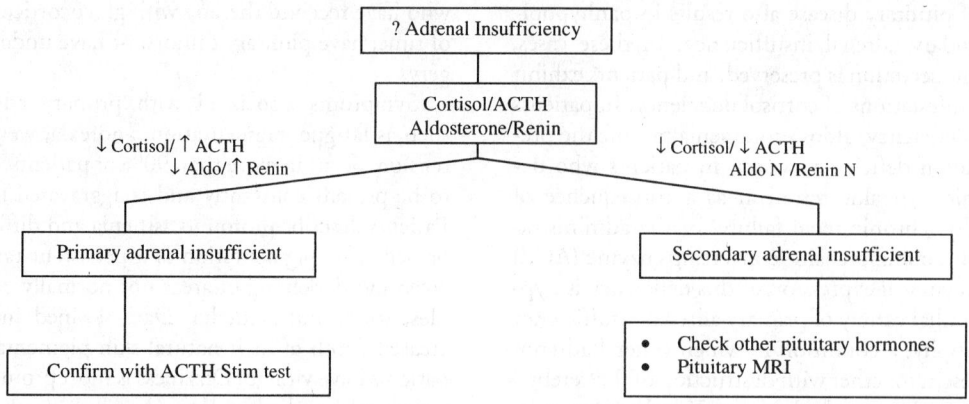

FIGURE 407.5. Diagnostic algorithm for patients suspected of having adrenal insufficiency.
EVIDENCE LEVEL: C. Expert Opinion.

measurements reveal low serum and urine cortisol levels in all patients with adrenocortical insufficiency. Serum aldosterone levels are low in patients with primary adrenal insufficiency and normal or low in patients with secondary adrenal insufficiency. When aldosterone levels are low, plasma renin levels are usually high. In the presence of low cortisol levels, the level of plasma ACTH defines the type of adrenal insufficiency. Patients with primary adrenal insufficiency have high ACTH levels, whereas levels are low in patients with adrenal insufficiency secondary to hypopituitarism.

Patients whose clinical features suggest adrenal insufficiency should have biochemical confirmation and a definitive diagnosis established prior to institution of long-term therapy. Since this biochemical confirmation may take some time before it is completed and severe adrenal insufficiency may develop while the patient is awaiting results, therapy should be initiated immediately and either continued or discontinued once a definitive diagnosis has been made. A diagnosis of primary adrenal insufficiency is based on the finding of low random cortisol and aldosterone levels together with high ACTH and renin levels. This combination of findings is unique for primary adrenocortical insufficiency. Other conditions that increase ACTH, such as stress, also increase cortisol levels, whereas those that increase renin, such as a low-sodium diet, will correspondingly increase aldosterone levels. Conversely, low cortisol levels obtained in the late evening hours are associated with low ACTH levels whereas low aldosterone levels in patients on high sodium intake are associated with correspondingly low renin values. Immediately after obtaining a basal sample, patients should receive 250 μg of synthetic corticotropin intravenously. Blood samples for cortisol are obtained 30 and 60 minutes thereafter. A peak value above 20 μg per milliliter usually rules out adrenal insufficiency.

Patients who have been on chronic glucocorticoid therapy have suppressed ACTH and cortisol levels and may develop secondary adrenal insufficiency when corticosteroid therapy is discontinued. A diagnosis of concomitant primary adrenocortical insufficiency in such patients is difficult and may require the demonstration of failure to respond to prolonged ACTH stimulation. In such cases, a corticotropin stimulation test should be performed by administering 250 μg of synthetic corticotropin over a 12-hour period on 2 to 3 consecutive days.

Patients with suppressed ACTH levels secondary to glucocorticoid therapy exhibit a gradually increasing cortisol response, whereas patients with primary adrenal insufficiency fail to respond.

Additional studies can be performed to evaluate the cause of adrenal insufficiency. This includes imaging of the adrenals by CT scanning, thyroid function tests and a serum calcium and phosphorus to investigate for associated autoimmune endocrinopathies, and a combined pituitary function test to evaluate for panhypopituitarism.

OPTIMAL MANAGEMENT
Chronic Adrenal Insufficiency

Treatment of chronic adrenal adrenal insufficiency requires the administration of cortisol in physiologic replacement amounts. The most commonly used preparation is hydrocortisone given in amounts of 20 to 30 mg daily in unequally divided doses to mimic the normal circadian rhythm of cortisol secretion. The largest dose of 10 to 15 mg is given upon arising and the smallest dose, 5 mg, is given shortly before bedtime. Larger doses given at bedtime may cause insomnia. Alternatively, patients may be treated with two doses daily, with the largest dose being given in the morning and the other dose in the evening. The optimal replacement dose of cortisol may be established by measuring urinary free-cortisol levels, which should be in the mid-normal range. Cortisol replacement is preferable to other synthetic glucocorticoid analogs with low sodium retention activity because it helps maintain a better sodium balance. In addition to cortisol, patients with primary adrenal insufficiency require replacement with fludrocortisol, a preparation similar to aldosterone in its mineralocorticoid activity The usual dose is 0.05 to 0.2 mg daily, adjusted according to serum electrolyte and blood pressure response. The dose given should be sufficient to eliminate orthostatic hypotension or tachycardia, but hypokalemia or hypertension should be avoided. Patients with essential hypertension may have an exaggerated sensitivity to mineralocorticoids and develop sodium retention and hypertension. In those patients, the dose of fludrocortisol should be reduced. Patients with associated endocrinopathies or hypopituitarism may require concomitant replacement with thyroxine and gonadal hormones.

Patients with secondary adrenal insufficiency usually require replacement therapy with cortisol alone. Occasionally, prolonged ACTH deficiency can cause marked adrenocortical atrophy and impaired aldosterone secretion. In those cases, replacement therapy with fludrocortisol is also indicated.

Acute Adrenal Insufficiency

Acute adrenal failure is a medical emergency. It may develop as a result of progression of undiagnosed or untreated chronic adrenocortical insufficiency, or it may occur in patients with chronic adrenal insufficiency who develop acute stress for which appropriate adjustments in cortisol therapy have not been made. Frequently, these patients have suffered intercurrent infection, trauma, or acute surgical stress. Undiagnosed patients present with nausea, vomiting, rapid weight loss, and hypotension. The presence of hyperpigmentation in this setting should raise suspicion of primary adrenal insufficiency. Laboratory studies should be obtained immediately, including serum electrolytes, urea, creatinine, cortisol, aldosterone, ACTH, and renin. An intravenous line is then established through which patients receive an infusion of a 5% dextrose in 0.9% sodium chloride solution at a rate sufficient to deliver 1 liter over the next hour. Simultaneously, a dose of 250 μg of synthetic corticotropin is injected as an intravenous bolus and blood samples for cortisol are obtained 30 and 60 minutes later. Once the samples have been obtained, patients should receive hydrocortisone, 100 mg, followed by a continuous infusion with hydrocortisone to be administered at a rate of 10 mg per hour for the next 5 hours. Patients may require additional intravenous fluids as needed to restore intravascular volume and correct the abnormal electrolyte findings. Restoration of normal blood pressure and heart rate should be the goal of this replacement therapy. Patients with more severe hyperkalemia whose serum potassium levels are greater than 6 mEq per liter may require, in addition to hydrocortisone, glucose and insulin or potassium-binding resins in order to rapidly lower serum potassium. Once patients have recovered from the acute manifestations of adrenocortical insufficiency, the dose of cortisol and fludrocortisol should be gradually reduced to the replacement dosages described above. The maintenance steroid therapy should be altered under conditions of stress. Physical stress, such as fever-producing systemic infections, trauma, or major surgery with general anesthesia, requires an increase in the dose of cortisol. The dose and duration of this increment varies with the type of stress. Systemic infections causing fever require a doubling of the replacement amount of cortisol until the infectious process is brought under control and the patient is no longer febrile. Patients undergoing surgery with general anesthesia should receive larger doses of cortisol as follows: 50 mg is injected intramuscularly in each buttock, on call to the operating room. A solution of 5% dextrose in water with 100 mg of cortisol is started with induction of anesthesia and infused intravenously at a rate of 10 mg per hour. The steroid coverage is completed with intramuscular injections of cortisol, 50 mg every 6 hours for the rest of the first postoperative day. This dose of cortisol is subsequently tapered back to replacement doses within the

next 3 to 4 days if the patient is free of surgical complications. Sustained administration of large doses of cortisol should be avoided since they can induce undesirable metabolic side effects. These include protein catabolism, delayed wound healing, immune suppression, suppression of inflammation, increased susceptibility to infection, sodium and water retention, hypertension, and hyperglycemia. Psychological stress usually does not require increases in the maintenance dose of cortisol. During hot, humid weather, patients with primary adrenal insufficiency may experience increased sweating with consequent increased sodium and water losses. It may be necessary to increase the dose of fludrocortisol to maintain normal electrolytes and intravascular volume.

If left untreated, patients with adrenocortical insufficiency may develop progression of symptoms leading to acute adrenal failure, a condition that is fatal if not treated. Patients who are adequately treated with steroid replacement therapy can live a normal life and have a normal life expectancy. In its early stages, patients may present with loss of adrenocortical reserve such that they are able to maintain normal cortisol levels under unstressed conditions. However, they fail to respond to stress and may become acutely adrenal-insufficient in the face of stressful events. If early stages of adrenal insufficiency are diagnosed, patients should receive full therapy to prevent more severe manifestations of adrenal insufficiency. Patients with autoimmune disease may develop other endocrinopathies as a consequence of autoimmune involvement of other endocrine glands. The physician should check the patient periodically for such occurrences. In most cases, a medical history focused on these other endocrine conditions should determine the extent of laboratory testing. Patients with secondary adrenal insufficiency frequently require replacement with other hormones to treat thyroid or gonadal failure. When panhypopituitarism is caused by a pituitary tumor, the prognosis of the adrenal insufficiency is determined by the clinical course of the pituitary disease.

CONGENITAL ADRENAL HYPERPLASIA

DEFINITION

Congenital adrenal hyperplasia is an inborn error of metabolism due to enzymatic deficiencies in the pathway of adrenocortical steroid biosynthesis. As a consequence of these deficiencies, patients present with various phenotypes, depending on the type of enzyme involved. While any of the enzymes may be affected, the most common type results from 21-hydroxylase deficiency. The more severe forms express themselves in utero and result in the classic form of the disease. Milder forms are recognized postnatally and produce the nonclassic form.

INCIDENCE AND EPIDEMIOLOGIC FACTORS

The incidence by screening has been calculated as 1 in 10,000 to 1 in 18,000, but the incidence is much higher in selected groups, such as Ashkenazi Jews in whom the incidence can be as high as 1:30.

ETIOLOGIC FACTORS

The most common form of CAH, accounting for more than 90% of cases, is due to 21-hydroxylase deficiency. The gene responsible for this syndrome, the *CYP21* gene, is located in chromosome 6 within the HLA complex, and mutations in this gene have been determined in large number of families with CAH. Depending on the type of mutation, various degrees of enzyme deficiency have been identified. In the classic, salt-losing type, no enzyme activity is detected; in the simple virilizing type, 2% enzyme activity is present. In nonclassic 21-hydroxylase deficiency, 10% to 20% enzyme activity is present, leading to a much milder form of the disease.

PATHOGENESIS

The impairment in cortisol biosynthesis leads to a decrease in cortisol secretion, as well as adrenocortical hyperplasia and activation of the androgen pathway through increased secretion of ACTH. Five enzymes are responsible for the transformation of cholesterol to cortisol under ACTH control (Fig. 407.6). Decreased action of any of these enzymes produces accumulation of steroid precursors prior to the enzymatic block. The products accumulated will follow alternative pathways that are not blocked, such as androgen biosynthesis. Deficiency of P450 cholesterol scc and P450 c17 do not lead to accumulation of androgens. In contrast, deficiency of 3β-hydroxysteroid dehydrogenase, 21-hydroxylase, or 11β-hydroxylase results in shunting of precursors to androgen production and produces virilization.

CLINICAL FINDINGS

Clinical findings of patients with CAH depend on which enzyme is defective and the severity of the deficiency. The more severe forms are diagnosed prenatally or at birth, and are associated with severe virilization and electrolyte disturbance. Female newborns with 21-hydroxylase deficiency exhibit pseudohermaphroditism with virilization of the external genitalia, consisting of clitoromegaly and various degrees of genital ambiguity. In the salt-losing variety, dehydration and volume depletion may be a serious complication shortly after birth. The milder forms of 21-hydroxylase deficiency, also known as nonclassic CAH, are diagnosed post puberty and are characterized by hirsutism, menstrual irregularity, and infertility. Nonclassic CAH shares many phenotypical features with polycystic ovary syndrome, including acne, hirsutism, and menstrual disturbance. Both may have onset at puberty and a positive family history. Similarly, polycystic ovaries can be present in nonclassic CAH in response to chronic androgen excess and disturbance of gonadotropic function.

LABORATORY FINDINGS

The biochemical diagnosis of CAH is based on the finding of increased plasma concentration of cortisol precursors and of adrenal androgens, such as DHEA, androstenedione, and testosterone. Baseline levels of immediate precursors of the blocked enzymatic step may be high. It includes 17α-hydroxyprogesterone in cases of 21-hydroxylase deficiency, 17α-hydroxypregnenolone in cases of 3β-hydroxysteroid dehydrogenase deficiency, and 11-deoxycortisol in cases of 11β-hydroxylase deficiency. However, because in nonclassic CAH the defect is mild, baseline levels may be normal or high-normal but show an exaggerated response to stimulation with synthetic ACTH. This test is performed with 250 mg of ACTH injected intravenously as a bolus. A blood sample for cortisol, 17α-hydroxyprogesterone, 17α-hydroxypregnenolone, and 11-deoxycortisol is obtained both before and 30 and 60 minutes after the injection. The cortisol response is usually within normal limits. Patients with 3β-hydroxysteroid dehydrogenase deficiency exhibit a 17α-hydroxypregnenolone and a 17α-hydroxypregnenolone/17α-hydroxy-

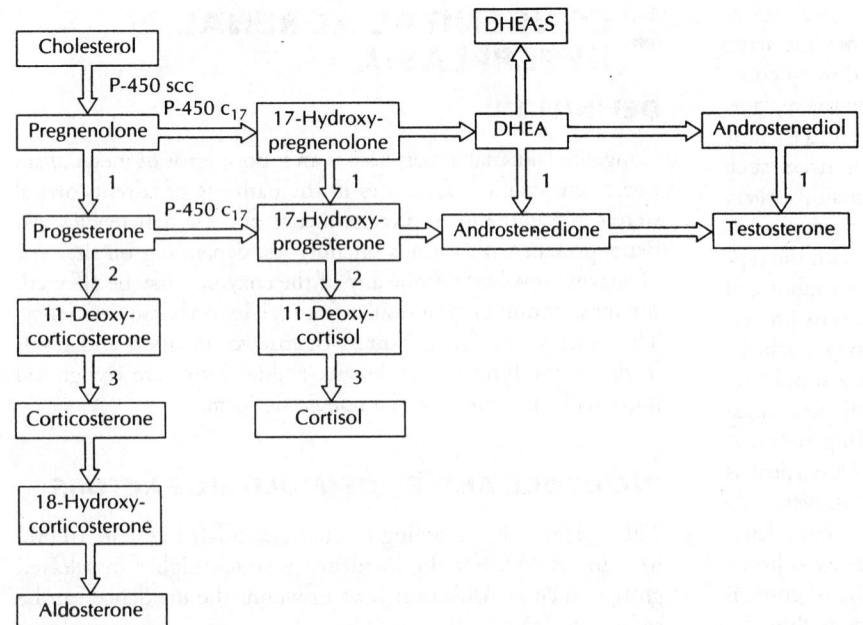

FIGURE 407.6. Adrenal steroid biosynthetic pathways.

progesterone ratio response greater than 2 standard deviations (SD) above the normal mean response. In patients with 21-hydroxylase deficiency, the 17α-hydroxyprogesterone response to ACTH is greater than 2 SD above the normal mean response or 1,200 mg per deciliter. Similarly, in patients with 11β-hydroxylase deficiency, the serum 11-deoxycortisol and the 11-deoxycortisol/cortisol ratio response is greater than 2 SD above the normal mean response.

OPTIMAL MANAGEMENT

Treatment of patients with CAH involves suppression of ACTH and the abnormal cortisol steroidogenic pathway with corticosteroids. Dexamethasone, in doses of 0.5 mg at bedtime, or prednisone, in doses of 5.0 to 7.5 mg daily, suppresses endogenous ACTH and excessive androgen secretion. Caution should be used in selecting doses of glucocorticoids that do not result in Cushing's syndrome. Occasionally, patients develop these side effects while receiving standard physiologic doses. Patients with the salt-losing form of CAH should also be treated with mineralocorticoids. Patients in whom hirsutism is the main concern can be treated with oral contraceptives and spironolactone in a manner similar to that for idiopathic hirsutism. Because of the side effects that may occur with even low doses of glucocorticoids, this type of therapy should be reserved for patients who do not respond optimally to other types of antiandrogen therapy. Androgen receptor antagonists, such as spironolactone, cyproterone acetate, flutamide, and 5α-reductase inhibitors such as finasteride, may be preferable to glucocorticoids as primary treatment of mild 21-hydroxylase deficiency. Ovarian suppression with the GnRH analog luprolide has been effective in patients with nonclassic CAH, but this type of treatment requires injections and is expensive. Patients with pseudohermaphroditism require corrective surgery of their ambiguous genitalia.

▬ INCIDENTALLY FOUND ADRENAL MASSES

DEFINITION

Adrenal masses are discovered radiographically during the evaluation of nonspecific abdominal complaints. These masses are not usually uncovered as a result of investigation for symptoms associated with adrenal hormone production.

INCIDENCE AND EPIDEMIOLOGIC FACTORS

Various reports place the prevalence of such masses at 1% to 3% of abdominal CT scans. This figure is consistent with the finding of nonfunctioning adrenocortical adenomas or nodules in 1.45% to 2.85% of autopsies. Adrenal tumors can be found in 71% of patients with non-classic CAH. Occasionally, these patients reach older age undiagnosed and are found to have incidentally discovered adrenal masses in the course of investigation for other unrelated complaints.

ETIOLOGIC FACTORS

Adrenal masses are (a) benign or malignant adrenocortical tumors, (b) pheochromocytomas, (c) myelolipomas, and (d) cysts and hematomas.

CLINICAL FINDINGS

While the great majority of incidentally discovered masses are clinically silent, 20% to 30% are hormone-secreting and associated with subtle symptoms of hormone excess. Approximately 7% of these hormone-secreting masses secrete cortisol. The clinical manifestations are nonspecific, such as generalized obesity, hypertension, abnormal glucose tolerance, and depression. The daily amount of cortisol produced is within normal limits, but secretion is ACTH-independent, without a normal circadian rhythm, and resistant to suppression with dexamethasone. This combination of clinical and biochemical findings has been called subclinical Cushing's syndrome.

Autonomous aldosterone production by otherwise clinically silent, incidentally found adrenal masses is rare. Some patients have been described who are either normotensive or hypertensive but without hypokalemia. Pheochromocytomas may also present as a silent mass, without a history of hypertension or typical symptoms of catecholamine excess.

LABORATORY FINDINGS

Preliminary studies to determine if the adrenal mass is functioning or silent should include measurement of cortisol and ACTH levels, serum electrolytes, plasma renin and aldosterone, and urinary metanephrines and normetanephrines.

Normal cortisol with suppressed ACTH levels is consistent with subclinical Cushing's syndrome. Characteristically, these patients have normal urinary free cortisol, similar 8 a.m. and midnight cortisol levels, and undetectable or low ACTH levels. Cortisol levels following a 1-mg overnight dexamethasone suppression test exceed 3 mg per deciliter. Patients with aldosterone-secreting tumors have low renin concentrations, but aldosterone levels are not in a diagnostic range and fail to suppress with fludrocortisol. Patients with pheochromocytomas, even if not hypertensive, have elevated urinary metanephrine and normetanephrine levels.

The major concern in the evaluation of an incidentally discovered adrenal mass is to determine if the mass is malignant and requires surgical resection. Primary adrenocortical carcinomas are rare, and many of the lesions that are malignant are metastatic from extra-adrenal neoplasms. Adrenocortical adenomas are 60 times more common than primary adrenocortical carcinomas. Size is a significant factor in determining the probability that a lesion is benign or malignant. There is consensus that most benign lesions are smaller than 3 cm, whereas most malignant lesions are larger than 6 cm. Uncertainty remains for masses measuring 3 to 6 cm. The importance of determining if a small tumor is benign or malignant has to do with the fact that patients with primary adrenocortical carcinomas have the best life expectancy when subject to curative resection in Mac-Farlane stage 1, when the tumor is less than 5 cm. The malignant or benign character of a lesion can be defined by CT, MRI, adrenal scintigraphy with ^{31}I-6β-iodomethyl-19-norcholesterol and CT or ultrasonographically guided fine-needle biopsy (FNB). CT and MRI of the adrenal mass can help determine if the mass is lipid-rich or lipid-poor. Lipid-rich masses have a high probability of being benign, whereas lipid-poor masses have a high probability of being malignant. Occasionally, a benign adrenocortical adenoma is lipid-poor and may be confused with a malignant lesion. With unenhanced CT, an attenuation of less than 10 Hounsfield units is consistent with an adenoma, whereas nonadenomas have unenhanced attenuation of greater than 30 Hounsfield units. With contrast enhancement, a major distinguishing characteristic appears to be a different retention of contrast by benign and malignant lesions. Benign lesions exhibit more than 50 % wash-out of contrast within the first 15 minutes after injection, while malignant lesions tend to retain the contrast with a much slower wash-out phase. Using chemical-shift MRI, lipid-rich adenomas show a decrease in relative signal intensity of 34%, whereas nonadenomas show no significant change in relative signal intensity. Benign tumors appear to be homogeneously enhancing, while malignant tumors are inhomogeneous because of areas of necrosis. Ultrasonographic scanning of an adrenal mass may help distinguish cystic from solid masses. A homogeneous mass with a thin, noncomplex wall is consistent

with a benign adenoma. ^{131}I-6β-iodomethyl-19-norcholesterol scintigraphy can be combined with CT to evaluate euadrenal masses of less than 4 cm. Concordant images (increased uptake on the side of the mass) are 100% benign, whereas discordant images (uptake contralateral to the mass) are frequently associated with malignant lesions. Metaiodobenzylguanidine scintigraphy is highly specific for the detection of pheochromocytomas.

FNBs of adrenal masses may be helpful, particularly in the detection of metastatic disease to the adrenal. Occasionally, the primary tumor is unknown, but the adrenal metastasis is found incidentally and can direct attention to the site of the primary neoplasm. Neoplasms that frequently metastasize to the adrenal are lung cancer, renal cell carcinoma, melanoma, and breast, prostate, and pancreatic carcinoma. Of importance is that the cytologic characteristics of the metastases are similar to those of the primary tumor and help to determine the origin of the primary tumor. FNB can be useful in documenting metastatic disease and determining resectability of the primary lesion. A potential serious complication of FNB in patients with suspected primary adrenocortical carcinoma is tracking and seeding neoplastic cells along the path of the needle, with consequent dissemination of the tumor. If based on size or imaging characteristics a mass is likely to be malignant, the approach should be to have the mass surgically removed. FNB should not be necessary.

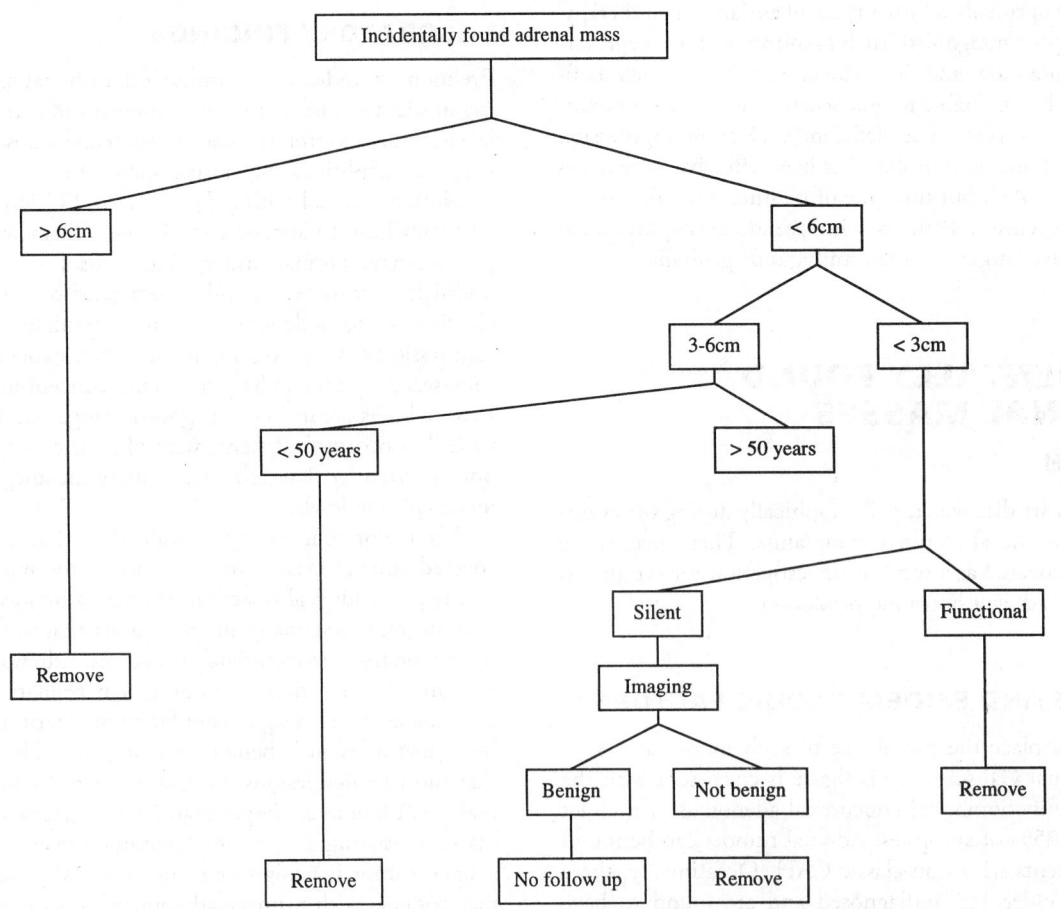

FIGURE 407.7. Algorithm for managing incidentally found adrenal masses.
EVIDENCE LEVEL: C. Expert Opinion.

OPTIMAL MANAGEMENT

The following strategy (Fig. 407.7) can be used in managing incidentally found adrenal masses: (a) remove hormone-secreting or large (more than 6 cm) masses; (b) follow masses smaller than 3 cm if they are silent; (c) follow masses 3 to 6 cm in size if patients are 50 years of age or older; (d) consider surgical resection in younger patients with masses between 3 and 6 cm; (e) masses between 3 and 6 cm can be further evaluated with FNB. However, other radiographic and scintigraphic techniques can be used to determine whether a mass is benign or malignant.

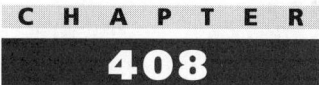

CHAPTER 408

ADRENAL MEDULLARY DISORDERS

BRAHM SHAPIRO
MILTON D. GROSS

UNDERLYING PHYSIOLOGIC PRINCIPLES

EMBRYOLOGY AND ANATOMY

In fetal life, neural crest cells migrate to form sympathetic and other ganglia, and they invade the adrenal cortex to form the adrenal medulla. This sympathochromaffin system, which includes the carotid bodies, aortic arch, paravertebral sympathetic ganglia, aortic bifurcation (Zuckerkandl's organ), and vagus nerve ganglia, is one component of the neuroendocrine system derived from the neural crest that has amine precursor uptake and decarboxylation (APUD) properties.

PHYSIOLOGY OF CATECHOLAMINE SYNTHESIS, STORAGE, RELEASE, AND METABOLISM

Amines with the 3,4-dihydroxyphenyl structure are termed *catecholamines* and include dopamine, norepinephrine, and epinephrine. Within the central nervous system, they act as neurotransmitters; norepinephrine is the neurotransmitter of peripheral adrenergic axons. Both norepinephrine and epinephrine from the adrenal medulla are true hormones.

Catecholamines are synthesized from tyrosine derived from the diet or converted from phenylalanine (Fig. 408.1). Tyrosine hydroxylase converts tyrosine to dihydroxyphenylalanine (dopa) and is rate limiting. The enzyme is stimulated by acetylcholine and inhibited by its own product. Aromatic L-amino acid decarboxylase (ALAAD) converts dopa to dopamine. Dopamine β-hydroxylase acts on dopamine to form norepinephrine, the final product in sympathetic and central noradrenergic neurons. Phenylethanolamine-*N*-methyltransferase (PNMT) promotes methylation of norepinephrine to form epinephrine and is induced by glucocorticoids, which the adrenal medulla receives in high concentrations from the adrenal cortex.

Tyrosine hydroxylase and ALAAD are cytoplasmic enzymes in chromaffin cells and postganglionic neurons. Dopamine formed by their action is transported by a specific uptake mechanism into storage vesicles, where it is converted to norepinephrine by dopamine β-hydroxylase. Where conversion to epinephrine occurs, PNMT is present in the cytoplasm, norepinephrine leaves the vesicle, and epinephrine is then taken up.

Catecholamine release occurs by exocytosis, whereby vesicle contents are discharged into the extracellular space adjacent to a capillary, in the case of the adrenal medulla, or into the synapse in neurotransmission. This requires an influx of calcium mediated by an acetylcholine-induced action potential.

In neurotransmission, after release, a small fraction of the catecholamines binds to the postganglionic receptors and produces the effect appropriate to the specific receptor. Some is metabolized and some enters the circulation (thus, plasma norepinephrine is an index of sympathetic neuronal function), but most is taken into the preganglionic neuron by a specific energy-dependent mechanism (uptake I) and stored in cytoplasmic vesicles.

Catecholamines have a short half-life in plasma (1 to 2 minutes) because of either cellular uptake or enzymatic degradation (Fig. 408.1). The major pathways are catalyzed by catechol *O*-methyltransferase (COMT) and monoamine oxidase (MAO). COMT converts epinephrine to metanephrine, norepinephrine to normetanephrine, and dopamine to 3-methoxytyramine. The former are converted by MAO and aldehyde oxidase to 3-methoxy-4-hydroxymandelic acid [or vanillylmandelic acid (VMA)]. Alternatively, MAO first converts norepinephrine and epinephrine to 3,4-dihydroxymandelaldehyde, and aldehyde oxidase converts this to 3,4-dihydroxymandelic acid, which is converted via COMT methylation to VMA. Another pathway is by COMT and alcohol dehydrogenase on 3,4-dihydroxymandelaldehyde to yield 3-methoxy-4-hydroxyglycol, much of which is metabolized to VMA. In the case of dopamine, the final product is 3-methoxy-4-hydroxyphenylacetic acid (or homovanillic acid). Conjugation, primarily to sulfates, also occurs. The concentrations of conjugated catecholamines excreted in urine are several fold greater than those of free catecholamines.

Catecholamines act through cell surface receptors. These are divided into α_1-, α_2-, β_1-, and β_2-adrenergic and D_1- and D_2-dopaminergic receptors on the basis of responsiveness to agonist and antagonist drugs. Norepinephrine, epinephrine, and dopamine are all mixed agonists. Adrenergic receptors are subject to down- and up-regulation in the presence of high and low catecholamine levels, respectively. Receptors are also classified by location: *prejunctional* (presynaptic) receptors, on the axonal

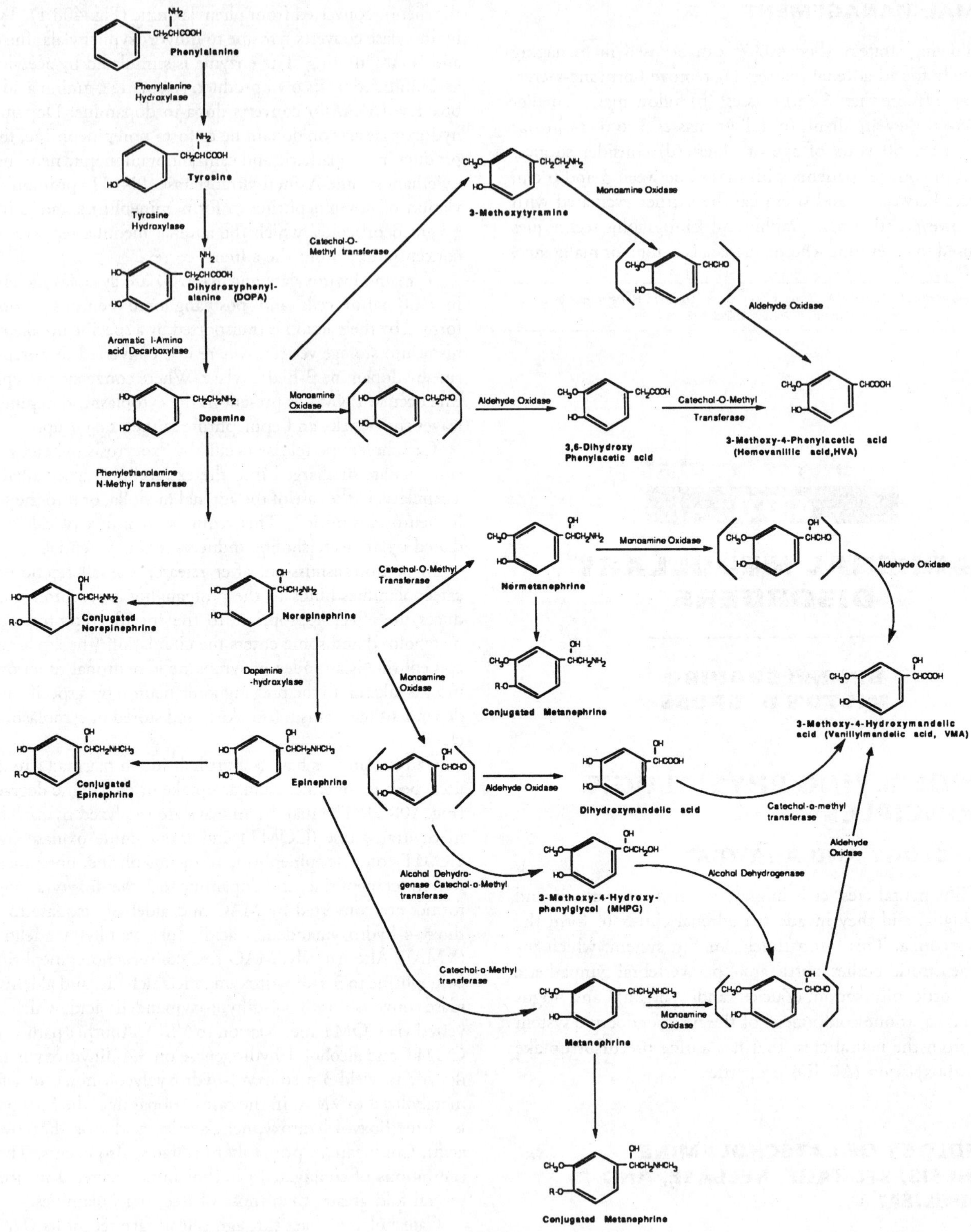

FIGURE 408.1. Biosynthesis of catecholamines and the metabolic pathways for their degradation.

terminal itself, which autoregulate catecholamine release; *post-junctional* (postsynaptic) receptors in the synapse opposite the axonal terminal; and *extrajunctional* receptors on noninnervated cells, where catecholamines act as true hormones.

Agonist binding to receptors does not result in hormonal action directly but induces second messengers. For β_1 and β_2 receptors, there is linkage by a guanine nucleotide–regulatory protein to a cell membrane adenylate cyclase, and a rise in intracellular cyclic adenosine monophosphate induces a series of protein kinase activations resulting in hormone action. D_1 receptors are linked to stimulation of adenylate cyclase, and D_2 receptors are linked to its inhibition. The β_2 receptors are linked to an inhibitory guanine nucleotide regulatory protein and inhibit adenylate cyclase. For α_1 receptors, the coupling to intracellular events is not yet elucidated but results in calcium influx.

Upright posture, pain, anxiety, exercise, hypovolemia, hypotension, sodium depletion, and hypoglycemia all elevate the catecholamine levels, as does acute myocardial infarction, diabetic ketoacidosis, surgical trauma, burns, and chronic processes, including cardiac failure, anemia, respiratory failure, and hypothyroidism. Decreased levels (especially in response to normal stimuli) occur in autonomic neuropathy, after depletion of stores by reserpine, inhibition of synthesis by methylparatyrosine, and reduction of central sympathetic tone by clonidine.

Hemodynamic effects include vasoconstriction (α), vasodilatation (β_2), and positive chronotropic and inotropic effects on the heart (β_1). Norepinephrine causes generalized vasoconstriction, systolic and diastolic hypertension, and reflex bradycardia. Epinephrine, by β_2 effect, causes vasodilatation, systolic hypertension, and diastolic hypotension, and cardiac rate and output are increased. Dopamine increases cardiac output and systolic blood pressure with little effect on diastolic blood pressure, and (at low concentrations) causes renal and mesenteric vasodilatation. Peripheral infusion of norepinephrine must achieve concentrations greater than 1,000 pg per milliliter to cause significant metabolic and hemodynamic effects. With epinephrine, 50 to 200 pg per milliliter is required. Metabolic effects include increased glycogenolysis and gluconeogenesis by liver and muscle; reduced glucose utilization outside the central nervous system; stimulation of lipolysis, hepatic ketogenesis, and amino acid release from muscle; and increased thermogenesis. Hypokalemia and hypophosphatemia result from cellular potassium and phosphate uptake. Smooth-muscle relaxation of bronchi and uterus is mediated by β_2 receptors. Other effects are mydriasis (α) and reduction of gastrointestinal motility (β_1). Catecholamines modulate the secretion of hormones, including insulin (suppressed by α_2 effect and to a lesser degree stimulated by β_2). Stimulation of glucagon (β), growth hormone (α), and renin (β_1) dopamine receptors has been reported. Stimulation of the pituitary reduces prolactin secretion.

SPECIFIC DISORDERS OF THE SYMPATHOADRENAL SYSTEM: PHEOCHROMOCYTOMA

Only the tumorous hypersecretion of catecholamine is considered in this section. A functional increase in sympathetic tone

may play a role in essential hypertension and defective catecholamine release in autonomic neuropathy, which is discussed elsewhere in this text.

DEFINITION

Catecholamine-secreting tumors derived from the adrenal medulla or sympathetic autonomic paraganglia frequently stain brown with chromium salts, leading to the name *pheochromocytoma*. There are two nomenclatures. "Pheochromocytoma" may be used for all catecholamine-secreting tumors, adrenal and extra-adrenal; alternatively, the term "pheochromocytoma" is reserved for adrenal lesions, and extra-adrenal tumors are termed *functional paragangliomas*. The embryologically related, highly malignant neuroblastoma occurs almost exclusively in childhood.

INCIDENCE AND EPIDEMIOLOGY

Pheochromocytomas are not rare tumors. The true incidence is not known, but such tumors may be present in 0.1% to 0.5% of hypertensive patients. Ten percent to 20% of patients have associated neurocristopathies (Table 408.1). No age group is exempt, and 10% of cases occur in childhood.

ETIOLOGIC FACTORS

Most cases are sporadic with unknown cause. The responsible regulatory genes for a number of the autosomal dominant familial syndromes have been identified, e.g., the *RET* oncogene in multiple endocrine neoplasia type 2 (MEN 2) syndromes, which

TABLE 408-1.	NEUROCRISTOPATHIC SYNDROMES ASSOCIATED WITH PHEOCHROMOCYTOMA
Syndrome	**Component Features**
Multiple endocrine neoplasia type 2a	Medullary thyroid carcinoma, hyperparathyroidis, pheochromocytoma (usually bilateral intraadrenal)
Multiple endocrine neoplasia type 2b	Medullary thyroid carcinoma, ganglioneuromatosis pheochromocytoma (usually bilateral intraadrenal)
von Hippel–Lindau disease	Retinal hemangiomatosis, cerebellar hemangioblastoma, visceral tumors and cysts including pheochromocytoma
von Recklinghausen's neurofibromatosis	Café-au-lait spots, neurofibromata, plexiform neuromas and occasional pheochromocytoma
Simple familial pheochromocytoma	Familial pheochromocytoma without other lesions

provides a tool for early diagnosis, family screening, and insights regarding cause of disease.

PATHOGENESIS

Pheochromocytomas may arise from chromaffin tissue anywhere from the base of the skull to the bladder. Most (90%) are intra-adrenal. The most common extra-adrenal site is the organ of Zuckerkandl near the aortic bifurcation. In addition, tumors may arise in the urinary bladder; paravertebral and celiac ganglia; sympathetic jugular chain; paracardiac, aortic, and carotid bodies; and the glomus jugulare. They are typically chromaffin-positive and stain for neuron-specific enolase and chromogranin. Characteristic dense-core granules are observed on electron microscopy. As in other endocrine neoplasms, it is difficult to distinguish benign from malignant lesions in the absence of frank metastasis.

Catecholamine hypersecretion accounts for most symptoms and signs in pheochromocytoma. The relative proportions of epinephrine and norepinephrine affect the clinical presentation. Excessive epinephrine, usually from an intra-adrenal lesion, leads to tachycardia, diastolic hypotension, and cardiac arrhythmia. Metabolic effects, including increased metabolic rate, glucose intolerance due to decreased insulin secretion, and insulin resistance, are common, but frank diabetes is unusual. More commonly, norepinephrine secretion predominates and accounts for most symptoms and signs. A number of manifestations are not explained by catecholamine excess, including hypercalcemia and polycythemia. Many neuropeptides have been described in pheochromocytomas and may contribute to the individual symptom complex. Ectopic adrenocorticotropic hormone production occasionally leads to Cushing's syndrome.

CLINICAL FINDINGS

Hypertension is the cardinal abnormality. In many patients it is sustained, whereas in the remainder baseline hypertension is associated with paroxysms of greater severity. Truly intermittent hypertension is unusual. Rarely, hypotension may alternate with hypertension, usually with epinephrine-secreting neoplasms. Other features of the hypertension include severity, early onset, resistance to conventional therapy, and exacerbation by β blockers. Hypertension may lead to all the complications of elevated blood pressure. In addition, paroxysms occur, characterized by various combinations of throbbing headache, anxiety, drenching sweats, tachycardia, palpitations, chest and abdominal pain, nausea and vomiting, syncope, tremor, and blanching followed by flushing. These episodes may occur spontaneously or after exercise, meals, or other provocative stimuli. Bladder lesions are associated with hematuria in 50% of patients, and paroxysmal headache, hypertension, or other symptoms are related to micturition. Glomus jugulare tumors invade the base of the skull. Extra-adrenal primary tumors have a greater tendency to metastasize than intra-adrenal lesions. Metastases spread to bone, lymph nodes, and liver, where they lead to local symptoms. Diagnostic physical signs in pheochromocytoma are few. The most important sign is hypertension during and between typical episodes. Hypertension may follow abdominal palpation. Intra-

vascular volume constriction may lead to postural hypotension. Hypertensive changes and, in von Hippel–Lindau disease, angiomatosis may be observed in the retina. Other signs include neurofibromas and café au lait spots in neurofibromatosis. Goiter due to medullary carcinoma of the thyroid occurs in all types of MEN. Hypertrophy of corneal nerves and ganglioneuromatosis occur in MEN type 2b.

The clinical features of pheochromocytoma are protean and overlap with those of many other disorders, including essential, secondary, and paroxysmal hypertension (e.g., after withdrawal of medications, clonidine, or adverse reactions to MAO inhibitors). Other manifestations may overlap with thyrotoxicosis, anxiety states (including panic attacks), carcinoid syndrome, mastocytosis, paroxysmal tachycardia, vasodilatory headaches, intracranial lesions, atypical diencephalic seizures, and hypoglycemia. Also included in the differential diagnosis are related tumors, including neuroblastoma, ganglioneuroblastoma, and ganglioneuroma. Pheochromocytoma may go unrecognized for years and is often not diagnosed in life. Left untreated, it may lead to chronic complications of hypertension or, rarely, sudden death. Unanticipated, potentially lethal presentation may occur with anesthesia, pregnancy and delivery, or trauma. Multifocal pheochromocytomas, most commonly bilateral intra-adrenal, may present simultaneously or evolve over decades, warranting lifelong surveillance. Malignancy is uncommon, occurring in about 10% of cases. The natural history of these lesions is highly variable, and if the effects of catecholamine excess are controlled, patients may tolerate large tumor burdens for extended periods. Death may then occur from local invasion of critical organs.

LABORATORY FINDINGS

Plasma catecholamines are labile, and samples must be obtained in the fasting, rested, and supine state via an indwelling needle. Because of a multitude of potential interferences and alterations due to drug use, studies should be performed with subjects in a drug-free state whenever possible. Many drugs may interfere with assays of catecholamines depending on the methodology used. Twenty-four-hour urine collections serve to integrate the overall daily excretion; 12-hour overnight collections have the advantage of excluding the effect of upright posture.

PLASMA AND URINARY MEASUREMENTS

Once clinically suspected, the diagnosis of pheochromocytoma is made by demonstrating excessive catecholamine secretion. The choice of biochemical studies is controversial, with much depending on availability, quality, and costs of assays at a given institution. Urinary catecholamines or metabolites (e.g., metanephrines or VMA) provide a logistically convenient index. Only the free fraction of urinary catecholamines should be determined. Many consider a single, spot, unfractionated urine metanephrine to be an adequate screen for hypertensive persons without typical symptoms. Plasma catecholamine measurements, performed under appropriate conditions, provide a sensitive alternative. About 80% of patients with pheochromocytoma have unequivocal elevations (e.g., more than 2,000 pg per milliliter of norepinephrine), but some, especially those with paroxysmal patterns or asymptomatic patients at risk due to familial syndromes, may have normal or borderline values. In these cases, multiple determinations or provocative or suppressive tests are indicated. In the absence of the characteristic clinical picture, the yield from biochemical investigations is low, and false positives are common.

SUPPRESSION TESTS

Clonidine reduces sympathetic tone and plasma catecholamine levels. The autonomous hypercatecholaminemia of pheochromocytoma is not suppressed by clonidine (oral dose of 300 μg with blood samples both before and 0.5, 1, 1.5, and 2 hours later). The test is superfluous when plasma catecholamines exceed 2,000 pg per milliliter. Tyramine-, glucagon-, and histamine-provocative tests are potentially dangerous, have high false-negative and false-positive rates, and are obsolete.

PREOPERATIVE TUMOR LOCATION

Accurate preoperative identification of all pheochromocytoma deposits is a prerequisite for curative surgery. Localizing procedures are justified only when a clinical and biochemical diagnosis has been made. Plain radiography, intravenous urography, retroperitoneal air insufflation, and ultrasonography are obsolete. Angiography and venography with sampling are invasive, may trigger crisis, and, while effective, have in most cases been replaced by computed tomography (CT), magnetic resonance imaging (MRI), and scintigraphy with metaiodobenzylguanidine (MIBG). CT is highly effective in adrenal pheochromocytomas (greater than 95% sensitivity) but is less so for extra-adrenal lesions (75% sensitivity). Adequate technique requires the use of modern scanners, thin sections, and oral contrast agents. CT may fail in thin patients and in the presence of metallic clips and other postoperative artifacts. With MRI the high T2-weighted signal from pheochromocytoma permits distinction from adrenocortical lesions but not from metastases. MIBG and radiolabeled somatostatin analogs both permit noninvasive scintigraphy of the entire body in a single procedure and are effective in locating pheochromocytomas of all types (sensitivity 88%, specificity 98%). Both radiopharmaceuticals are now available commercially in the United States.

OPTIMAL MANAGEMENT
Preoperative Management

Acute crisis is best managed with 1 mg intravenous phentolamine followed by an infusion, titrated against blood pressure. An alternative is a nitroprusside infusion. The only definitive cure for pheochromocytoma is surgical extirpation. To achieve acceptable morbidity and mortality requires meticulous preoperative preparation. Radiologic procedures requiring contrast media need similar preparation. The time-honored agent is phenoxybenzamine, an oral, noncompetitive α-adrenergic blocker. The full effect occurs 12 hours after administration, and action

accumulates over several days. An initial dose of 10 mg twice daily is increased by 10 mg every other day. The goal is control of hypertension without symptomatic postural hypotension. If paroxysms predominate, the dose should be that which eliminates or significantly blunts attacks without causing symptomatic postural hypotension. Nasal congestion and failure of ejaculation are common side effects of α blockade. Prazosin is an alternative with shorter action that may be titrated more rapidly. An α blockade for about 2 weeks permits reexpansion of the contracted plasma volume; β blockade is only occasionally required for tachycardia or tachyarrhythmia. Either a nonspecific β blocker (propranolol) or a β_1-selective blocker (metoprolol) may be used. Although risks have probably been overemphasized, β blockade should not be induced before α blockade because this can lead to severe, even lethal, hypertensive crisis as a result of unopposed α-adrenergic agonism. Occasionally, adrenergic blockade cannot control symptoms, and inhibition of catecholamine synthesis by α-methylparatyrosine is required. It is seldom completely effective but permits lower doses of α blockers. Calcium channel antagonists may also be effective. Heart failure sometimes encountered with pheochromocytoma responds to α blockade and α-methylparatyrosine, and diuretics and digitalis are seldom indicated.

Presentation in Pregnancy

Pheochromocytoma may present as a crisis during pregnancy or delivery, and it carries a poor prognosis for both infant and mother even when recognized. It must be distinguished from eclampsia. Rapid induction of α blockade and the use of nitroprusside infusion with delivery by cesarean section are required.

Intraoperative Management and Surgery

The purpose of surgery is total extirpation and requires close collaboration between anesthesiologist and surgeon. A rapid, stress-free induction of anesthesia is best achieved with pentobarbital and succinylcholine followed by methoxyflurane or enflurane, oxygen, and nitrous oxide. Endotracheal intubation, muscle relaxation, and mechanical ventilation are essential. Electrocardiographic monitoring and intra-arterial pressure and urinary output measurement are mandatory, and a central venous pressure or Swan–Ganz catheter may be required. Preoperative α blockade is seldom complete, and intraoperative tumor manipulation frequently leads to hypertension, best managed by gentle dissection, phentolamine, or nitroprusside. Tachycardia or supraventricular arrhythmia is controlled by β blockers, and ventricular arrhythmia by lidocaine. When venous drainage from the tumor is interrupted, catecholamines and blood pressure may fall precipitously. This is minimized by preoperative α blockade and liberal administration of intravenous fluids. Pressors are seldom required. Intra-abdominal lesions require an anterior abdominal approach with thorough exploration of the entire retroperitoneum. Laparoscopic surgery is currently gaining popularity and speeds recovery. Bladder lesions require partial cystectomy with ureteric reimplantation. Posterior mediastinal lesions are approached through posterior thoracotomy, whereas paracardiac lesions require median sternotomy and, often, cardiopulmonary bypass.

Postoperative Follow-up

Catecholamine levels fall within minutes of tumor resection. Complete return to normal requires as long as 2 weeks because of large amounts of catecholamines stored in peripheral sympathetic nerve endings. Failure to do so indicates residual, second primary, or metastatic tumor. The histology of the primary tumor may not predict long-term behavior. Even lesions that are not strictly malignant may not be resectable. Up to one-third of patients are left with some sustained hypertension despite normal catecholamine levels, probably because of damage to renal vasculature. All patients require lifelong follow-up because metastases or second primary tumors may manifest after long periods. Control of hypercatecholaminemia effects by long-term adrenergic blockade or methylparatyrosine is the mainstay of management. This controls most disabling and potentially life-threatening effects; tumor growth, though unaltered, is often slow and may be tolerated for years with good quality of life. Painful skeletal metastases may be palliated by radiation therapy. Experimental therapy with large doses of iodine 131–labeled MIBG has been attempted with some success. Large doses of indium 111–or yttrium 90–labeled somatostatin analogs may also be effective. The combination of vincristine, cyclophosphamide, and dacarbazine (a commonly used combination for the embryologically related neuroblastoma) has shown promise.

BIBLIOGRAPHY

Atuk NO, Stolle C, Owen JA Jr, et al. Pheochromocytoma in von Hippel–Lindau disease: clinical presentation and mutational analysis in a large, multigenerational kindred. *J Clin Endocrinol Metab* 1998;83: 117–120.

Bravo EL. Evolving concepts in the pathophysiology, diagnosis, and treatment of pheochromocytoma. *Endocr Rev* 1994;15:356–368.

Heshmati HM, Gharib H, Khosla S, et al. Genetic testing in medullary thyroid carcinoma syndromes: mutation types and clinical significance. *Mayo Clin Proc* 1997;72:430–436.

Hoefnagel CA. MIBG and radiolabeled octreotide in neuroendocrine tumors. *Q J Nucl Med* 1995;39:137–139.

Jalil ND, Pattou FN, Combemale F, et al. Effectiveness and limits of preoperative imaging studies for the localisation of pheochromocytomas and paragangliomas: a review of 282 cases. *Eur J Surg* 1998;164:23–28.

Kebebew E, Duh UY. Benign and malignant pheochromocytoma: diagnosis, treatment and follow up. *Surg Oncol Clin North Am* 1998;7: 765–789.

Lenz T, Ross A, Schumm-Draeger P, et al. Clonidine suppression test revisited. *Blood Pressure* 3998;7:153–159.

Luh KC, Fitzgerald PA, Matthay KK, et al. The treatment of malignant pheochromocytoma with iodine-131 metaiodobenzylguanidine; a comprehensive review of 116 patients. *J Endorinol Invest* 1997;20:648–658.

Mobius E, Nies C, Rothmund M. Surgical treatment of pheochromocytomas; laparoscopic or conventional? *Surg Endosc* 1999;13: 35–39.

Russell WJ, Metcalfe IR, Tonkin AL, et al. The preoperative management of pheochromocytoma. *Anaesth Intensive Care* 1998;26:196–200.

Shapiro B, Fig LM. Management of pheochromocytoma. *Endocrinol Metab Clin North Am* 1989;18:443–481.

Ulchaker JC, Goldfarb DA, Bravo EL, et al. Successful outcomes in pheochromocytoma surgery in the modern era. *J Urol* 1999;161:764–767.

Kelley's Textbook of Internal Medicine, fourth edition. Edited by H. David Humes.
Lippincott Williams & Wilkins, Philadelphia © 2000.

CHAPTER 409

DISORDERS OF THE REPRODUCTIVE CYCLE IN WOMEN

ROBERT L. BARBIERI

The reproductive endocrine environment of the female depends on the complex interaction of hypothalamic, pituitary, ovarian, and uterine events. In contrast to the male, the critical and unique aspect of this system is cyclic ovarian function, which is responsible for the production of gametes and the sex steroids, estradiol and progesterone. An inherent feature of the female reproductive system is that depletion of gametes and cessation of estrogen and progesterone production usually occurs by 55 years of age. The resulting hypoestrogenic state is associated with important changes in lipid and bone metabolism. Common clinical problems requiring intervention to alter the production and action of estradiol and progesterone are discussed in this chapter.

HORMONAL CONTROL OF FEMALE FERTILITY

The major structural components of the female reproductive system and their functions are the hypothalamus, which controls the pulsatile release of gonadotropin-releasing hormone (GnRH); the pituitary, which controls the pulsatile release of luteinizing hormone (LH) and follicle-stimulating hormone (FSH); the ovary, which controls follicular development, with cyclic secretion of estradiol and progesterone, and gamete maturation; and the uterus, which controls cyclic endometrial growth, maturation, and shedding in response to ovarian estradiol and progesterone secretion (Fig. 409.1).

The most widely used reversible birth control method remains the combined estrogen–progestin (E-P) oral contraceptive. The E-P oral contraceptive contains a synthetic estrogen and a synthetic progestin. Ethinyl estradiol is the synthetic estrogen in most E-P contraceptives. Many E-P contraceptives contain a synthetic progestin related to norethindrone or norgestrel. The synthetic progestins norethindrone acetate and ethynodiol diacetate are converted to norethindrone in vivo. Norethindrone and norgestrel are structurally related to progesterone and testosterone and have progestogenic and androgenic properties. More recently, three "nonandrogenic" synthetic progestins have become available: desogestrel, norgestimate, and gestodene. Unlike norgestrel, these nonandrogenic progestins do not suppress hepatic sex hormone–binding globulin or high-density lipoprotein (HDL) cholesterol production.

The most commonly used E-P oral contraceptives are available in packages containing 28 pills. Twenty-one pills contain

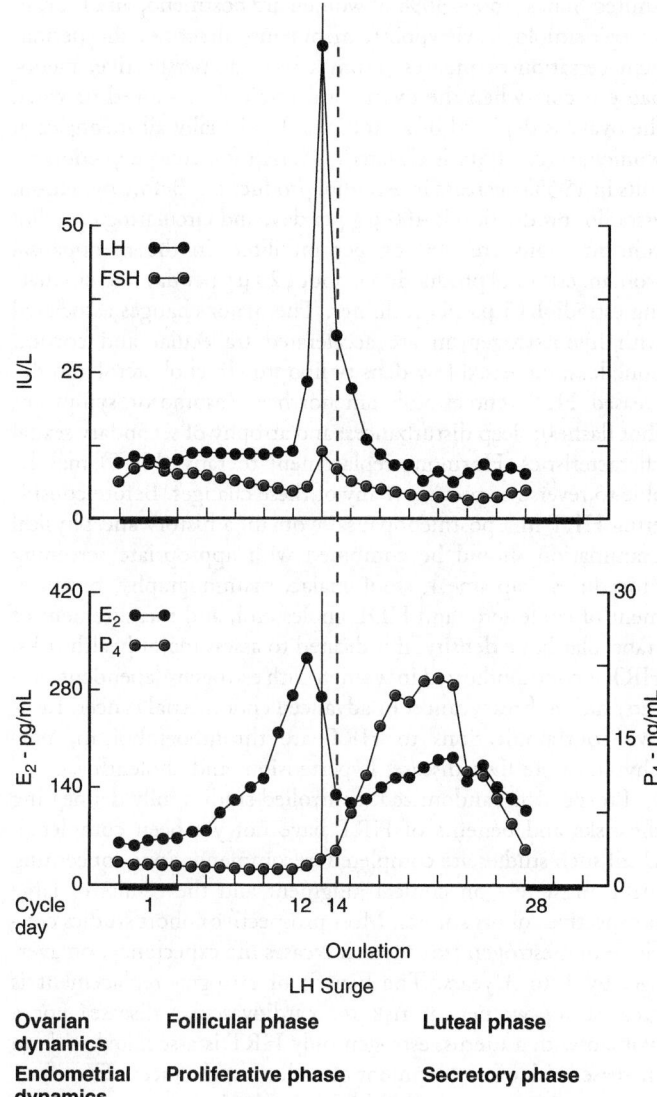

FIGURE 409.1. Circulating luteinizing hormone (LH), follicle-stimulating hormone (FSH), estradiol (E₂), and progesterone (P₄) throughout the normal ovulatory menstrual cycle.

the synthetic E-P hormones and seven pills contain inert ingredients. Menses usually occurs while the user is taking the seven inert pills owing to the withdrawal of E-P hormones. E-P contraceptives prevent conception by inhibiting hypothalamic GnRH secretion, inhibiting pituitary response to GnRH, preventing normal endometrial maturation, and blocking sperm entry to the upper reproductive tract by producing a hostile cervical mucus. Because E-P contraceptives block fertility by redundant and overlapping mechanisms, they are extremely efficacious and have failure rates in the range of one to two pregnancies per 100 woman-years of use.

The major serious side effects of the birth control pill are cerebrovascular accidents (thromboembolic stroke, subarachnoid hemorrhage), myocardial infarction, and venous thrombosis with pulmonary embolism. In women younger than 35 years of age who do not smoke, these life-threatening complications

of oral contraceptives are exceedingly rare. Women younger than 35 years who do not smoke have a fourfold greater risk of dying of a pregnancy than of dying as the result of a complication of oral contraceptive use. Women older than 35 years of age who smoke should not be prescribed oral contraceptives. Activated protein C resistance caused by factor V Leiden mutation is an important risk factor for venous thromboembolism in women using oral contraceptives. Other medical problems that can be associated with oral contraceptive use include hepatic adenoma, gallbladder disease, elevated blood pressure, and increased risk of cervical dysplasia.

Studies suggest that oral contraceptives *decrease* the risk of development of endometrial cancer, ovarian cancer, pelvic inflammatory disease, and breast cysts. Oral contraceptives appear to decrease the risk of development of endometrial cancer by 60%. It is likely that the continuous exposure of the endometrium to the synthetic progestins contained in the pill, which prevent endometrial growth (mitosis), accounts for this effect. Oral contraceptives decrease the risk of ovarian cancer in both low-risk and high-risk women by approximately 50%. For example, in women with the *BRCA1* mutation (high risk for ovarian cancer) oral contraceptive use reduced the risk of ovarian cancer by 50%. Epidemiologic studies suggest that ovarian cancer is related to both elevated gonadotropin levels and incessant ovulation. Oral contraceptives may decrease the risk of development of ovarian cancer by decreasing gonadotropin secretion and preventing ovulation.

POSTCOITAL CONTRACEPTION

Women who are the victims of sexual assault or who have a failure of a barrier contraceptive method (e.g., condom rupture) may be offered postcoital contraception. Pregnancy can often be prevented in women with unprotected intercourse at midcycle by administering 100 μg ethinyl estradiol and 0.5 mg levonorgestrel immediately and repeating the dose in 12 hours. The failure rate is approximately 1%. Human chorionic gonadotropin should be assayed before therapy, and therapy must be instituted within 72 hours of exposure. These high doses of E-P appear to prevent pregnancy by disrupting endometrial maturation and implantation. Many experts recommend that all women at risk for pregnancy (e.g., sexually active, using a barrier contraceptive) should be prescribed a postcoital contraceptive to keep in their home, so that they have easy access to this form of contraception should a failure of a nonhormonal contraceptive occur. Economic modeling suggests that preemptive prescription of postcoital contraceptives to all sexually active women using a barrier contraceptive can save health care resources by preventing undesired pregnancies.

PREVENTION OF MENSES

In many clinical settings, such as severe thrombocytopenia, cyclic uterine bleeding is undesirable. Hormones can be used to stabilize the endometrium and prevent menses. Four hormonal agents are available to prevent or delay menses: E-P contraceptives used in a "pseudopregnancy" regimen, danazol, high-dose progestin, and GnRH agonist analogs. Each cycle of E-P contraceptives contains 21 hormone pills and 7 inert pills. Menses can often be prevented by the continuous administration of one hormone pill daily for 3 to 12 months without using the inert pills (pseudopregnancy regimen). The main complication of this regimen is irregular uterine spotting or bleeding. Danazol at doses of 800 mg per day, medroxyprogesterone acetate at doses of 30 to 100 mg per day, and leuprolide acetate at doses of 3.75 or 7.5 mg by intramuscular injection every 4 weeks can also prevent menses.

For the thrombocytopenic patient who is already bleeding, E-P contraceptives, one to four pills per day, until bleeding is controlled, can be instituted. Before initiating hormone therapy, the possibility of pregnancy or a structural abnormality of the uterus should be assessed.

DYSMENORRHEA

Dysmenorrhea is often divided into two broad categories: primary and secondary. Primary dysmenorrhea is the presence of painful menstruation in the absence of a demonstrable pelvic pathologic process. Secondary dysmenorrhea is the occurrence of painful menstruation due to a pelvic lesion, such as endometriosis, chronic pelvic inflammatory disease, or uterine leiomyomas. In primary dysmenorrhea, the pain characteristically begins with the onset of menstruation and lasts for 12 to 72 hours. The pain is usually confined to the lower abdomen and is most intense in the midline. It is often described as crampy and intermittent in intensity. Evidence suggests that prostaglandin $F_{2\alpha}$ and prostaglandin E_2 released from the endometrium at the time of menstruation cause primary dysmenorrhea. Prostaglandins induce smooth-muscle contraction in many tissues. Prostaglandin-induced uterine contractions can last many minutes and may produce intrauterine pressures greater than 60 mm Hg. When uterine pressure exceeds mean arterial pressure for a prolonged period, uterine ischemia may occur.

In a woman with dysmenorrhea, a history consistent with primary dysmenorrhea, and a negative pelvic examination, a trial of antiprostaglandins or E-P contraceptives is warranted. Initial therapy for dysmenorrhea consists of ibuprofen at doses up to 2,400 mg daily. Therapy is initiated just before menses, for those women who can accurately predict the onset of menses, or at the onset of menses. Therapy usually lasts for 3 or 4 days. If ibuprofen (an arylpropionic acid derivative) is not effective, a trial with a drug in the fenamate class (mefenamic acid) or an E-P contraceptive may be warranted. Nifedipine at doses of 20 to 40 mg daily has also been demonstrated to be effective in the treatment of primary dysmenorrhea. If aggressive therapy for primary dysmenorrhea fails, the patient should be evaluated by a gynecologist to consider if laparoscopy is warranted.

TREATMENT OF HYPOESTROGENIC STATES

The rapid aging of the population is one of the most dramatic demographic changes occurring in developed countries. In the United States, about 30% of women are postmenopausal. From an epidemiologic viewpoint, menopause describes the permanent cessation of menses. From a biologic perspective, menopause occurs when the ovaries are surgically removed or when the ovary is depleted of all follicles. In virtually all menopausal women, serum FSH is elevated. Ovarian follicular depletion results in a 95% decrease in estradiol production. Before ovulation, estradiol production is 400 μg per day, and circulating estradiol concentrations are 300 pg per milliliter. In the menopausal woman, estradiol production is about 20 μg per day and circulating estradiol 15 pg per milliliter. The major changes associated with hypoestrogenism are accelerated trabecular and cortical bone loss; increased low-density lipoprotein cholesterol and decreased HDL cholesterol; amenorrhea; vasomotor symptoms (hot flashes); sleep disturbances; and atrophy of secondary sexual characteristics. Hormone replacement therapy (HRT) may be able to reverse or prevent many of these changes. Before considering HRT in a postmenopausal woman, a history and physical examination should be combined with appropriate screening procedures: Pap smear, stool guaiac, mammography, measurement of cholesterol and HDL cholesterol, and measurement of trabecular bone density, if indicated to assess major health risks. HRT is contraindicated in women with estrogen-dependent cancers, such as breast cancer or advanced endometrial cancer. Relative contraindications to HRT are thromboembolism, porphyria, severe liver disease, hypertension, and cholelithiasis.

Prospective, randomized, controlled studies fully delineating the risks and benefits of HRT have not yet been completed. Until such studies are completed, recommendations concerning HRT must rely on clinical judgment and the results of large prospective cohort studies. Most prospective cohort studies conclude that estrogen treatment increases life expectancy, on average, by 1 to 3 years. The benefit of estrogen replacement is greatest for women at risk for cardiovascular disease. For a woman with a uterus, estrogen-only HRT is associated with an increased risk of development of endometrial cancer. Therefore, women with a uterus should receive both an estrogen and a progestin. A typical cyclic regimen consists of conjugated equine estrogens, 0.625 mg every day of the year, and medroxyprogesterone acetate, 5 mg per day for calendar days 1 to 12 of each month (Fig. 409.2). Most women younger than 70 years can expect to have uterine bleeding each month, typically lasting 3 to 5 days and occurring sometime between day 9 and day 17 of the month. Many menopausal women dislike the resumption of menses produced by cyclic HRT. An alternative continuous regimen is conjugated equine estrogens, 0.625 mg, and medroxyprogesterone 2.5 or 5 mg every day of the year. About half of women become amenorrheic on this regimen. Unfortunately, the others have irregular menses. Endometrial biopsy is warranted in any menopausal woman, on or off HRT, who has irregular or heavy uterine bleeding.

Epidemiologic studies suggest that estrogen plus progestin HRT is associated with a decreased risk of development of coronary heart disease (relative risk of 0.6). HRT also appears to decrease the rate of bone loss that occurs in aging hypoestrogenic women. Long-term HRT may be associated with a small increase in risk of development of breast cancer. These data are controversial and require confirmation.

Cyclic

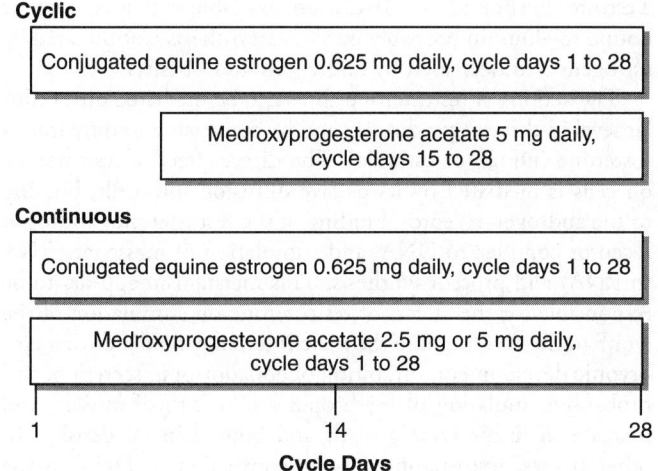

Conjugated equine estrogen 0.625 mg daily, cycle days 1 to 28

Medroxyprogesterone acetate 5 mg daily, cycle days 15 to 28

Continuous

Conjugated equine estrogen 0.625 mg daily, cycle days 1 to 28

Medroxyprogesterone acetate 2.5 mg or 5 mg daily, cycle days 1 to 28

1   14   28
Cycle Days

FIGURE 409.2. Cyclic and continuous hormone replacement therapy.

The discovery of selective estrogen receptor modulators (SERMs) has opened a new era in hormone replacement. SERMs interact with the estrogen receptor but can act as estrogen agonists in some tissues and estrogen antagonists in other tissues.

In hypoestrogenic women, the SERM raloxifene is an estrogen agonist in the liver (decreases LDL cholesterol) and bone (decreases osteoclast activity), but is an estrogen antagonist in the breast. In menopausal women, raloxifene treatment (60 mg daily) decreases the risk of osteoporotic fracture and appears to decrease the risk of breast cancer. Raloxifene treatment does not cause uterine bleeding.

BIBLIOGRAPHY

American College of Physicians. Guidelines for counseling postmenopausal women about preventive hormone therapy. *Ann Intern Med* 1992;117: 1038–1041.

Andersson KE, Ulmsten V. Effects of nifedipine on myometrial activity and lower abdominal pain in women with primary dysmenorrhoea. *Br J Obstet Gynaecol* 1978;85:142–148.

Colditz GA, Egan KM, Stampfer MJ. Hormone replacement therapy and risk of breast cancer: results from epidemiologic studies. *Am J Obstet Gynecol* 1993;168:1473–1480.

Collaborative Group on Hormonal Factors in Breast Cancer. Breast cancer and hormone replacement therapy: collaborative reanalysis of data from 51 epidemiologic studies of 52,705 women with breast cancer and 108,411 women without breast cancer. *Lancet* 1997;350:1047–1059.

Delmas PD, Bjarnason NH, Mitlak BH, et al. Effects of raloxifene on bone mineral density, serum cholesterol concentrations and uterine endometrium in postmenopausal women. *N Engl J Med* 1997;337:1641–1647.

Glasier A, Baird D. The effects of self-administering emergency contraception. *N Engl J Med* 1998;339:1–4.

Glasier A, Thong KJ, Dewar M, et al. Mifepristone compared with high-dose estrogen and progestogen for emergency postcoital contraception. *N Engl J Med* 1992;327:1041–1044.

Grodstein F, Stampfer MJ, Colditz GA, et al. Postmenopausal hormone therapy and mortality. *N Engl J Med* 1997;336:1769–1775.

Hirsch DR, Mikkola KM, Marks PW, et al. Pulmonary embolism and deep venous thrombosis during pregnancy or oral contraceptive use: prevalence of factor V Leiden. *Am Heart J* 1996;131:1145–1148.

Narod SA, Risch H, Moslehi R, et al. Oral contraceptives and the risk of hereditary ovarian cancer. *N Engl J Med* 1998;339:424–428.

Stampfer MJ, Colditz GA, Willett WC, et al. Postmenopausal estrogen therapy and cardiovascular disease: ten year follow up from the Nurses' Health Study. *N Engl J Med* 1991;325:756–762.

Kelley's Textbook of Internal Medicine, fourth edition. Edited by H. David Humes. Lippincott Williams & Wilkins, Philadelphia © 2000.

C H A P T E R
410

DISORDERS OF GONADAL FUNCTION IN MEN

PETER J. SNYDER

NORMAL MALE REPRODUCTIVE ENDOCRINOLOGY

The male gonads are the testes, whose two major functions are production of testosterone by the Leydig cells and production of sperm in the seminiferous tubules. Testosterone secreted into the systemic circulation affects many tissues, mostly by binding to the androgen receptor, and the cumulative effect is to produce a phenotypic male. Testosterone within the testes is the principal hormonal stimulus to sperm production. Both functions of the testes are controlled by the gonadotropins, luteinizing hormone (LH), and follicle-stimulating hormone (FSH), which are secreted by the gonadotroph cells of the pituitary gland. LH stimulates the Leydig cells to secrete testosterone, and FSH stimulates the Sertoli cells of the seminiferous tubules. LH and FSH, in turn, are both stimulated by gonadotropin-releasing hormone (GnRH), which is secreted by the hypothalamus into the hypothalamic–pituitary portal circulation. Testosterone inhibits the gonadotroph cell from secreting both LH and FSH. Inhibin, secreted by the Sertoli cells, also inhibits FSH secretion (Fig. 410.1).

SYNTHESIS AND SECRETION OF GONADOTROPINS AND THEIR CONTROL

FSH and LH are both synthesized in the gonadotroph cells of the pituitary. Both are heterodimeric glycopeptides, consisting of a common α subunit and a unique β subunit. The α subunit has two aspartic acid (Asp)–linked oligosaccharide chains, and both β subunits have one.

Both LH and FSH are stimulated by GnRH, a decapeptide that is cleaved from a larger precursor peptide, which is synthesized in the arcuate nucleus of the hypothalamus. GnRH is released into the hypothalamic–pituitary portal circulation and binds to specific cell-surface G-protein-coupled receptors, which triggers a cascade of intracellular signaling pathways and stimulates LH and FSH release. GnRH cannot be measured readily in the portal or peripheral circulation of humans, but its secretion is

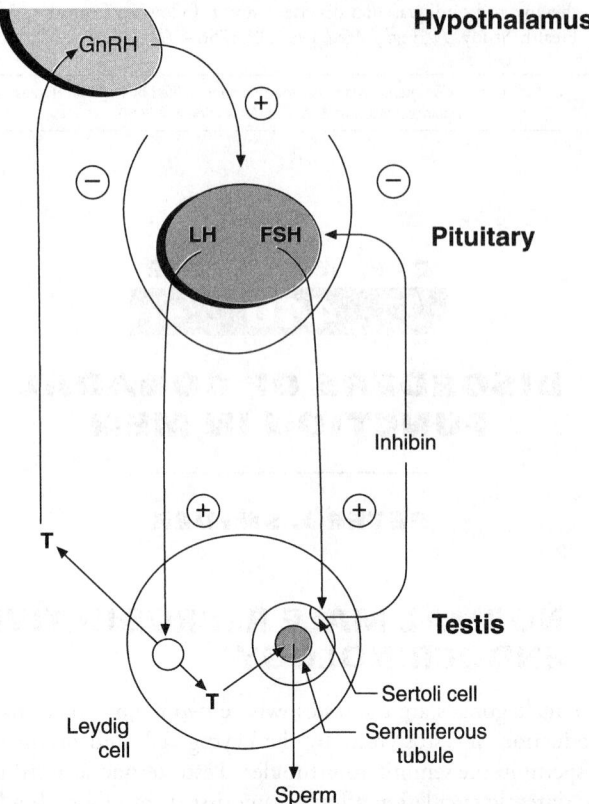

FIGURE 410.1. The hypothalamic–pituitary–testicular axis. The hypothalamus secretes gonadotropin-releasing hormone (GnRH) into the portal circulation, and GnRH stimulates the gonadotroph cells of the pituitary to secrete luteinizing hormone (LH) and follicle-stimulating hormone (FSH). LH stimulates the Leydig cells of the testes to secrete testosterone into the systemic circulation, and testosterone within the testes is also the principal hormonal stimulus to spermatogenesis. FSH stimulates the Sertoli cells of the seminiferous tubules to secrete inhibin and other peptides, which also stimulate spermatogenesis. Testosterone inhibits GnRH secretion and thereby LH and FSH secretion, and inhibin inhibits FSH directly.

thought to be pulsatile because secretion of LH is pulsatile. In addition, administration of GnRH to men who are unable to secrete it by themselves increases LH secretion to normal if the GnRH is administered in pulses, but not if it is administered continuously, and continuous administration of GnRH to men whose own secretion is normal decreases LH secretion to subnormal.

TESTOSTERONE SYNTHESIS, SECRETION, TRANSPORT, AND ACTION

LH stimulates testosterone synthesis by binding to a cell-surface receptor on the Leydig cells and activating a cyclic adenosine monophosphate (cAMP)–mediated mechanism that increases cholesterol side-chain cleavage and conversion to pregnenolone and, eventually, to testosterone. Daily synthesis of testosterone is 5 to 7 mg.

Testosterone secreted into the systemic circulation is 98% to 99% bound, about half to sex hormone–binding globulin (SHBG) with high affinity and half to albumin with low affinity.

Testosterone bound to SHBG is not available to tissues, but that bound to albumin probably is. SHBG synthesis is stimulated by estrogens and decreased by androgens and obesity.

The actions of testosterone appear to be mediated on a cellular level in three ways: directly and by conversion to dihydrotestosterone (DHT) or estradiol. The direct effect of testosterone on cells is mediated by its passive diffusion into cells, binding to the androgen receptor, binding of the testosterone–androgen receptor complex to DNA, and stimulation of messenger RNA (mRNA) and protein synthesis. This mechanism appears to be responsible for the effects of testosterone on stimulation of the wolffian ducts to become the male internal genitalia during embryonic development, inhibition of gonadotropin secretion, and probably stimulation of erythropoiesis, growth of muscle, and increase in linear bone growth and bone mineral density. In other tissues, testosterone acts by conversion to DHT in the target cell cytoplasm by the enzyme 5α-reductase. DHT is then bound to the androgen receptor, and the DHT–receptor complex binds to DNA, stimulating mRNA and protein synthesis. DHT binds to the androgen receptor with greater affinity than does testosterone and so has a greater effect. This mechanism appears to be responsible for the effects of testosterone in male sexual differentiation of the external genitalia in utero, enlargement of the external genitalia during puberty, and the development of sexual hair during puberty. Testosterone may also act in some tissues through conversion to estradiol by the enzyme aromatase, which is found in greatest concentrations in some hypothalamic nuclei, adipose tissue, and liver. This mechanism appears to mediate the effect of testosterone on epiphysial closure, since the epiphyses of males who have mutations either of the gene coding for the estrogen receptor or the aromatase enzyme do not close. This mechanism appears to partially mediate the inhibition of LH secretion, since administration of an aromatase inhibitor to men increases their serum LH concentrations.

SPERMATOGENESIS

Spermatogenesis occurs in the seminiferous tubules of the testes. The principal hormonal stimulus of spermatogenesis is testosterone, whose concentration in the testes is 100 times that in the peripheral circulation. This relatively high testosterone concentration, which is essential for spermatogenesis, is likely the consequence of both the LH-stimulated production of testosterone nearby in the Leydig cells and the binding of testosterone by androgen-binding protein, produced by the Sertoli cells of the seminiferous tubules. FSH stimulates the Sertoli cells to secrete androgen-binding protein and also inhibin, which inhibits FSH secretion by the pituitary, and activin, which stimulates spermatogenesis. Maturation of a spermatogonium to a mature spermatozoon takes approximately 75 days, and passage through the epididymis, where motility is acquired, takes another 14 days—a total of approximately 3 months.

THE AGES OF MAN: IN UTERO, PUBERTY, SENESCENCE

The preceding description of male reproductive function is that found in the young adult. The development of adult function occurs primarily in utero and during puberty, and that function declines in the male senescence.

In Utero

During the first trimester in utero, sexual differentiation occurs. In the presence of the sex-determining region of the Y chromosome, SRY, the indifferent gonads become testes. The Sertoli cells of the testes secrete anti-müllerian hormone, which suppresses the müllerian ducts so that they do not become female internal genitalia. The Leydig cells of the testes, stimulated by human chorionic gonadotropin from the placenta, secrete testosterone, which stimulates the nearby wolffian ducts to become the male internal genitalia (vas deferens and seminal vesicles). In addition, testosterone is converted to DHT by the anlage of the external genitalia, and DHT influences them to become the penis, scrotum, and prostate. During the third trimester in utero, LH from the fetal pituitary stimulates the fetal Leydig cells to secrete testosterone, which results in penile growth. During the first few months post partum there is a third testosterone elevation, but the consequences of this elevation are not known. Thereafter, the serum testosterone concentration falls to relatively low values until puberty.

Puberty

Puberty in boys begins at a mean age of 11.4 ± 1.1 years with an increase in the secretion of LH and FSH by the gonadotroph cells of the pituitary, presumably stimulated by an increase in GnRH secretion by the hypothalamus. The initial consequence is an increase in testicular length, from 2 cm to, eventually, 4 to 7 cm. The increase in LH stimulates an increase in testosterone secretion; causes an increase in the size of the phallus; growth of pubic, axillary, and, eventually, body and facial hair; and regression of temporal scalp hair. Testosterone also causes an increase in long-bone growth and height, thickening of the vocal cords and lowering of the voice, and increase in hemoglobin concentration. Most of these changes are completed within 4 to 5 years, but full development of body hair and beard may take several more years, and temporal scalp hair regression continues for decades.

Senescence

As men age, their serum total testosterone concentration decreases and their estradiol increases, increasing their SHBG. The consequence is that their free-testosterone concentration decreases to a greater degree than the total, so that by age 80 years the free testosterone is one-half to one-third of that at age 20 years (Fig. 410.2). The cause appears to be both decreased LH secretion and decreased responsiveness of the Leydig cells. These changes, unlike the female menopause, occur very slowly. What is uncertain is whether the decrease in testosterone causes any deleterious effects. Because some of the changes that occur in the male senescence are similar to those that occur in male hypogonadism, such as decreases in libido, energy, muscle mass and strength, and bone mineral density, testosterone deficiency could be a cause of these changes during the male senescence.

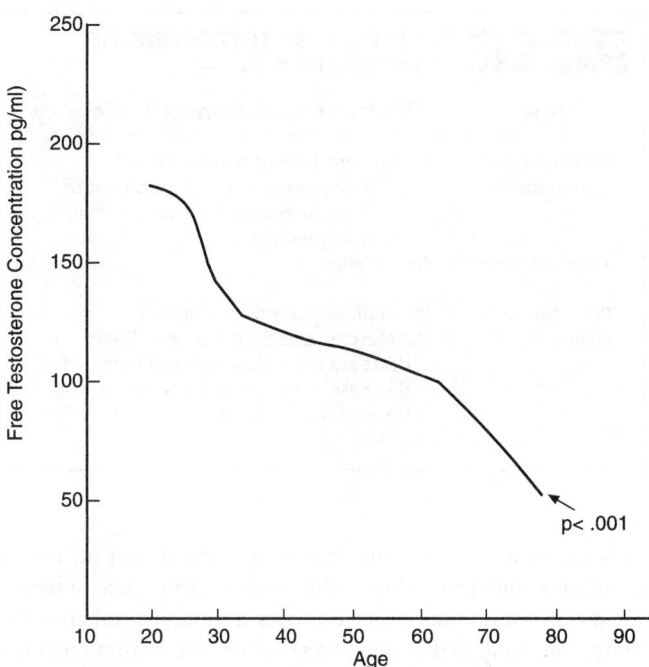

FIGURE 410.2. Serum free testosterone concentrations throughout adult life. (Adapted from Purifoy FE, Koopmans LH, Mayes DM. Age differences in serum androgen levels in normal adult males. *Hum Biol* 1981;53:499–511.)

MALE HYPOGONADISM

DEFINITION

Abnormalities of reproductive function in a genetic male can occur as a consequence of diseases of the testes, called primary hypogonadism, or of the pituitary or hypothalamus, called secondary hypogonadism. The physician suspects the diagnosis of hypogonadism on the basis of certain symptoms and signs and confirms it by laboratory tests. Treatment of testosterone deficiency is usually satisfactory whether the hypogonadism is primary or secondary, but treatment of spermatogenesis is satisfactory only if the hypogonadism is secondary.

CLINICAL FINDINGS

The clinical features of hypogonadism depend on whether spermatogenesis alone is impaired or testosterone secretion is also impaired. The one clinical feature of decreased spermatogenesis is infertility. In contrast, the clinical features of testosterone deficiency vary widely, depending on when the deficiency is manifested (Table 410.1). When testosterone deficiency is manifested in the first trimester in utero, male sexual differentiation is incomplete. Complete lack of testosterone during this period results in female external genitalia (clitoris and labia). Incomplete testosterone deficiency causes partial virilization, from posterior labial fusion when testosterone deficiency is severe to hypospadias when testosterone deficiency is mild. When testosterone deficiency is not manifested until the third trimester in utero, the result is normal male sexual differentiation but microphallus

2746 PART 9: ENDOCRINOLOGY, METABOLISM, AND GENETICS

TABLE 410.1.	EFFECTS OF TESTOSTERONE DEFICIENCY BY AGE
Age	**Effects of Testosterone Deficiency**
First trimester in utero	Incomplete virilization of external genitalia; incomplete development of wölffian ducts and therefore of male internal genitalia
Third trimester in utero	Micropenis
Prepubertal	Incomplete pubertal maturation
Postpubertal	Decrease in energy, mood, and libido; decrease in hemoglobin and hematocrit; decrease in muscle mass, strength, and bone mineral density

at birth. When testosterone deficiency is manifested before the anticipated onset of puberty, the result is incomplete puberty.

When testosterone deficiency does not occur until after puberty, some pubertal changes regress, but even of those that do, most do so slowly. Although decreases in energy and libido can be recognized within days to weeks of the decrease in testosterone and a decrease in hemoglobin and hematocrit within a few months, decreases in sexual hair, muscle mass, and bone mineral density are usually not recognized for several years.

PHYSICAL EXAMINATION

Physical examination focuses primarily on whether sexual development is consistent with the patient's age. If the patient is an adult, the testes should be 4 to 7 cm in length (20 to 25 mL in volume), musculature should be normal for a man, pubic hair should be dense and in a diamond pattern, chest and other body hair should be present, and temporal scalp hair should be receding appropriately for the patient's age and family pattern. If the patient is an adolescent, development should be appropriate for his age. If a child, the testes should be descended and no hypospadias present.

Physical examination should also include evaluation of the possibility of eunuchoid proportions and gynecomastia. An adult male usually has an upper body segment approximately equal to his lower segment and an arm span equal to his height. The absence of testosterone and the continued presence of growth hormone during puberty causes a delay in epiphysial closure and increased length of the long bones, so that the lower body segment is longer than the upper and the arms are longer than the legs, a relationship known as eunuchoid proportions. This relationship persists even after testosterone treatment, so when an adult of any age has a heel-to-pubis measurement more than 2 cm longer than his pubis-to-crown measurement and when his arm span is more than 2 cm longer than his height, he was probably hypogonadal during adolescence. Gynecomastia, the presence of glandular breast tissue in a man, may occur as a consequence of many abnormalities (see Chapter 395), one of which is hypogonadism, especially primary hypogonadism.

LABORATORY FINDINGS

Although hypogonadism can be suspected on the basis of symptoms, and strongly suspected on the basis of signs, the diagnosis can be confirmed only by documenting decreased production of sperm or testosterone. If hypogonadism is confirmed, supranormal serum concentrations of LH or FSH indicate primary hypogonadism, and "inappropriately normal" or subnormal values indicate secondary hypogonadism.

Spermatogenesis

Sperm production can be assessed most readily by counting how many sperm are present in an ejaculated semen specimen. Normal men produce at least 20×10^6 sperm per milliliter of ejaculate and at least 40×10^6 sperm per ejaculation. More than 60% of the sperm in a fertile man are motile. A severely subnormal sperm count (e.g., less than 5×10^6 sperm per specimen) can occur as a consequence of either primary or secondary hypogonadism. A normal or mildly subnormal sperm count (e.g., 35×10^6 sperm per specimen) associated with a markedly abnormal sperm motility is most likely the result of a primary spermatogenic abnormality and almost certainly not a result of secondary hypogonadism.

Testicular biopsy can also provide information about the status of the seminiferous tubules, but usually no more than number and motility of ejaculated sperm because the variety of histologic responses of the testes to injury is limited. The one situation in which testicular biopsy may be helpful is when there are no sperm in the ejaculated semen but testicular size and the serum concentrations of testosterone, LH, and FSH are normal. This situation could occur as a consequence of obstruction of the ejaculatory outflow or of damage to the seminiferous tubules sufficient to impair spermatogenesis but not sufficient to elevate the serum FSH concentration. A testicular biopsy showing normal seminiferous tubules would favor the former diagnosis and suggest that the next step in diagnosis be evaluation of the patency of the ejaculatory outflow.

Testosterone Concentration

Testosterone secretion is most readily evaluated by measuring the serum concentration of total testosterone because the total testosterone usually reflects accurately the free testosterone and because current assay techniques for free testosterone are usually not as accurate as those for total testosterone. Measurement of free testosterone and SHBG may be helpful in situations where the total testosterone does not accurately reflect the free testosterone, such as obesity.

Gonadotropins

If the testosterone concentration is subnormal, the finding that the serum LH and FSH concentrations are supranormal indicates that the patient has primary hypogonadism, and the finding that they are not supranormal indicates that he has secondary hypogonadism. If the sperm count is distinctly subnormal but the serum testosterone is normal, a supranormal FSH and normal LH indicates that there has been damage to the seminiferous tubules but that the Leydig cells have not been affected. If the hypogonadism is secondary, magnetic resonance imaging of the sellar region will show if the cause is a mass lesion and, if so, whether it is in the pituitary or hypothalamus, or is a parasellar lesion. Measuring the LH responses to a single dose of exogenous GnRH, however, does not distinguish between a pituitary and a hypothalamic lesion. The reason for this is that a normal LH response to GnRH depends on normal up-regulation of GnRH receptors on the gonadotroph cells, which in turn requires the episodic exposure of the cells to GnRH. Severe hypothalamic disease leads to diminished GnRH secretion and therefore to down-regulation of GnRH receptors, so that there is a poor LH response to a single-bolus dose of exogenous GnRH, just as occurs in severe pituitary disease. Repeated administration of exogenous GnRH for many days leads to a normal LH response to a single-bolus dose of GnRH in patients who have hypothalamic disease, but not in patients who have pituitary disease.

DISEASES THAT CAUSE HYPOGONADISM

Once a patient's hypogonadism has been identified as primary or secondary, the specific cause can be sought.

Primary Hypogonadism

Taken together, the causes of primary hypogonadism (Table 410.2) are more common than those of secondary hypogonadism (Table 410.3). Of the congenital abnormalities that cause primary hypogonadism, the most common is Klinefelter's syndrome, which occurs in approximately 0.2% of newborns. It is the phenotypic presentation of a male with an extra X chromosome. The most common genotype is 47,XXY, but additional X chromosomes (e.g., 48,XXXY) and mosaics (e.g., 46,XY/

TABLE 410.2.	CAUSES OF PRIMARY HYPOGONADISM

Congenital

Chromosomal abnormalities
   Klinefelter's syndrome
   46,XX male
   Noonan's and male Turner's syndrome
Cryptorchidism
Disorders of androgen biosynthesis
Myotonic dystrophy

Acquired

Orchitis (e.g., mumps)
X irradiation
Drugs
   Alkylating agents
   Ketoconazole
   Cyclophosphamide
   Alcohol
Trauma
Torsion
Autoimmune damage
AIDS

TABLE 410.3.	CAUSES OF SECONDARY HYPOGONADISM

Congenital

Isolated gonadotropin-releasing hormone deficiency
   With anosmia (Kallmann's syndrome)
   With other abnormalities (Prader–Willi, Lawrence–Moon–Biedl syndromes)
   Without other abnormalities
Mutations of *LHβ* and *DAX-1* genes
Multiple hypothalamic and pituitary hormone deficiencies

Acquired

Benign tumors and cysts:
   Pituitary adenomas
   Craniopharyngiomas, dysgerminomas, Rathke's pouch cysts
Malignant tumors:
   Metastases from lung, breast, and other malignancies
   Meningiomas, gliomas
   Lymphomas
Infiltrative diseases (e.g., sarcoidosis, Langerhans' cell histiocytosis, hemochromatosis)
Infectious diseases (e.g., tuberculosis, histoplasmosis)
Infarction of the pituitary (e.g., Sheehan's syndrome)
Lymphocytic hypophysitis
Trauma
Surgery
Radiation
Aneurysm of the internal carotid artery
Systemic illness (starvation, anorexia, acute and chronic illness)
Medications (glucocorticoids megestrol acetate, suramin)
Drugs (opiates)
Hyperprolactinemia
Isolated acquired gonadotropin-releasing hormone deficiency
Delayed puberty (physiologic)

47,XXY) have also been reported. The 47,XXY genotype occurs from the nondisjunction of the sex chromosomes of either parent during meiotic division. Mosaicism probably results from nondisjunctive mitotic division after conception. The phenotypic consequences usually are more severe the greater the number of extra X chromosomes. The gonadal consequence is usually severe damage to the seminiferous tubules and variable damage, from minimal to severe, to the Leydig cells. Individuals who have this syndrome therefore usually have very small testes, no sperm in the ejaculate, infertility, and markedly high serum FSH concentrations. Their serum testosterone concentrations vary from normal to subnormal, so that their virilization varies from normal to subnormal and their serum LH from normal to supranormal. Persons with this condition also usually exhibit behavioral and long-bone abnormalities not directly related to the gonadal abnormalities. The behavioral abnormality causes difficulty in social interactions that are recognized in childhood and leads to problems in school and eventually in work. The long-bone abnormality is increased length of the legs, but not the arms, and occurs independently of increased length of both the arms and legs due to testosterone deficiency. The diagnosis can usually be made by determining the karyotype of the peripheral leukocytes. Testosterone deficiency, if present, can be treated as described later. The behavioral abnormality cannot be treated satisfactorily, but a support group can be helpful to the person's family, and school counselors should be advised of the diagnosis.

Cryptorchidism, or undescended testes, is also associated with damage to the testes, as well as with greater damage to the seminiferous tubules than to the Leydig cells. More than one mechanism may cause the damage; damage or testosterone deficiency in utero may cause the lack of descent, and the heat of the abdomen may cause further damage to the testis that has not descended. Some clinical consequences depend on whether one or both testes are undescended. If only one, the chances are 25% to 33% that the sperm count will be subnormal and the serum FSH slightly high. If both, the sperm count is likely to be severely subnormal and the patient infertile, and he may have a subnormal serum testosterone and be undervirilized as well. A neoplasm is also 50 times more likely to develop in cryptorchid testes. The diagnosis is made by failing to palpate a testis that is within the scrotum or that can be manipulated manually from the inguinal canal into the scrotum by 1 year of age. The initial treatment is administration of small doses of human chorionic gonadotropin or a GnRH agonist, based on the rationale that descent depends on testosterone. If this treatment is unsuccessful, the next step is orchiopexy (surgically bringing the testis into the scrotum and attaching it there). This procedure is performed before the age of 2 years in an attempt to minimize testicular damage, although there is little evidence that early surgery reduces the amount of testicular damage or the risk of testicular neoplasm. Securing the testis within the scrotum allows it to be palpated more readily.

The possibility that a varicocele, which is a varicosity of the venous plexus within the scrotum, can cause damage to the seminiferous tubules has been considered for decades, and varicoceles of infertile men are often ligated in an attempt to improve their fertility. The proposed mechanism by which a varicocele causes infertility is increased blood flow, which in turn causes a higher than normal temperature in the scrotum, and the higher than normal temperature impairs spermatogenesis. However, since infertile men who do not have varicoceles have scrotal temperatures similar to those with varicoceles, and infertile men are not much more likely to have a varicocele than fertile men, it is not certain that varicocele is a cause of infertility. More important, when men who are infertile and have a varicocele are randomized to ligation and no-treatment groups, eventual fertility in the ligated group is no better than in the no-treatment group. Therefore, varicocele ligation cannot be recommended to improve fertility.

Congenital deficiency of testosterone production can also result from mutations of genes that encode enzymes necessary for androgen biosynthesis. These disorders are rare. Two of them, deficiencies of the cholesterol side-chain cleavage enzymes β-hydroxysteroid dehydrogenase and 17α-hydroxylase, occur in the adrenal as well as in the testes, and so lead to deficient cortisol secretion as well. Deficiency of 17β-hydroxysteroid oxidoreductase occurs only in the testes. All three disorders result in deficient testosterone secretion beginning in the first trimester in utero, resulting in incomplete virilization. The degree of incompleteness, especially of phallic development, influences the sex of rearing. The testosterone deficiency itself can be treated as testosterone deficiency of any other cause.

Many acquired illnesses also cause primary hypogonadism. One is various infections, including mumps orchitis. Mumps usually does not cause orchitis, but when it does the testes initially become markedly swollen and severely painful, followed by gradual atrophy. Diminished sperm production is common; decreased testosterone secretion is less common. Diagnosis is made by eliciting a history of painful swelling of the testes during systemic mumps infection.

Treatment of neoplasms by chemotherapeutic drugs, especially by alkylating agents or by radiation therapy to the inguinal lymph nodes, often damages the seminiferous tubules and, less often, the Leydig cells. Radiation causes damage in spite of shielding of the testes because of radiation scatter. The degree of damage is usually proportional to the extent of treatment and, in cases of less extensive treatment, the damage may be reversible. However, no specific treatment is available. Other drugs that damage the testes include alcohol, the antifungal agent ketoconazole, and the nematocide dibromochloropropane.

HIV infection and AIDS wasting are commonly associated with hypogonadism, and more than one mechanism appears to be involved. Some men who have AIDS and subnormal serum testosterone concentrations have inappropriately low serum concentrations of LH, which may be the result of concomitant illnesses and drugs, such as malnutrition, opiate use, and megestrol acetate administration, which are known to cause secondary hypogonadism. Other men with AIDS who do not have those associated illnesses have elevated serum concentrations of LH, indicating primary hypogonadism.

Trauma to the testes can sometimes be sufficiently severe as to damage them. Bilateral castration is a treatment for bilateral testicular cancer, and, unlike castration for prostatic cancer, there is no reason not to withhold testosterone treatment.

More men who have primary hypogonadism have no identifiable cause than do all of those who have one of the known causes given here. Presumably, many causes are yet unknown.

Secondary Hypogonadism

When a man has secondary hypogonadism, it is especially important to identify the cause because the cause of secondary hypogonadism, unlike that of most primary hypogonadism, often can be treated specifically (Table 410.3). Pituitary adenomas, other benign tumors and cysts of the sellar area, and malignancies that metastasize to the hypothalamus or parasellar area can usually be detected by magnetic resonance imaging. Infiltrative diseases can usually be detected by their simultaneous presence elsewhere. Tumors, cysts, and infiltrative lesions are often accompanied by deficiencies of other hypothalamic or pituitary hormones.

Secondary hypogonadism that is not associated with any other hormonal abnormalities (isolated) is probably caused by deficiency of GnRH secretion by the hypothalamus and can be either congenital or acquired. When congenital, it may or may not be an aspect of Kallmann's syndrome. Kallmann's syndrome is the association of deficient GnRH secretion with, variably, anosmia, cryptorchidism, red–green color blindness, and long-bone and urogenital tract abnormalities. It may occur sporadically or in families, and when familial can be inherited in an autosomal dominant pattern with expression mostly limited to males, or in an X-linked recessive pattern. The genetic defect responsible both for the deficiency in GnRH secretion and for anosmia in some patients who have the X-linked recessive form of Kallmann's syndrome is a mutation in the *KAL-1* gene, which encodes the neural cell adhesion protein anosmin. Without this protein during embryogenesis, GnRH-secreting neurons do not migrate from the olfactory placode to the olfactory bulb and then to the hypothalamus, resulting in both anosmia and hypogonadotropic hypogonadism. Other causes of a congenital inability to secrete LH include a mutation of the *LHβ* gene and a mutation of the *DAX-1* gene.

Any systemic illness or hyperprolactinemia inhibits gonadotropin secretion, but reversibly. The effect of medications and drugs, such as glucocorticoids, suramin, and opiates, is also reversible. Damage to the pituitary from surgery or radiation, in contrast, is usually permanent.

Delayed puberty differs from all other causes of secondary hypogonadism in that it is always transient. The difficulty in making the diagnosis is in knowing when an adolescent male whose pubertal development is delayed more than 2 standard deviations from the mean has one of the previously mentioned diseases or merely a delay in the onset of puberty that will eventually correct itself spontaneously. The degree of hypogonadism is usually not helpful in making this distinction, nor is any biochemical test. A family history of delayed puberty or constitutional short stature increases the chance of delayed puberty. The finding of anosmia, symptoms of a chiasmal lesion, or other indications of a specific hypothalamic or pituitary disease increases the chance of an organic lesion.

Subnormal serum testosterone concentration due to no recognizable cause other than aging can be considered another form of secondary hypogonadism, and administration of testosterone to elderly men who have subnormal serum testosterone concentrations may increase their bone mineral density and lean body mass. Whether or not this treatment will increase their risk of prostate disease, however, has not yet been determined.

OPTIMAL MANAGEMENT

Testosterone Replacement

Testosterone can be replaced whether the hypogonadism is primary or secondary. Testosterone itself cannot be readily replaced orally because after it is absorbed into the portal circulation it is rapidly catabolized during its first pass through the liver. Several derivatives of testosterone that are alkylated in the 17α position were introduced several decades ago to obviate such rapid hepatic catabolism, and they do, but they appear to lack the full virilizing effect of testosterone. In addition, they may cause hepatic toxicity, including cholestatic jaundice, a cystic condition of the liver called peliosis, and, possibly, hepatocellular carcinoma. For all of these reasons, and because the other preparations described below are preferable, the 17α alkylated androgens rarely should be used to treat testosterone deficiency.

Long-acting esters of testosterone, enanthate, or cypionate, produced by esterifying the hydroxyl group in the 17β position with a fatty acid, have also been available for decades. These produce full virilization. They are usually administered in 150- to 200-mg doses by deep intramuscular injection every 2 weeks. This regimen results in peak serum testosterone values within a

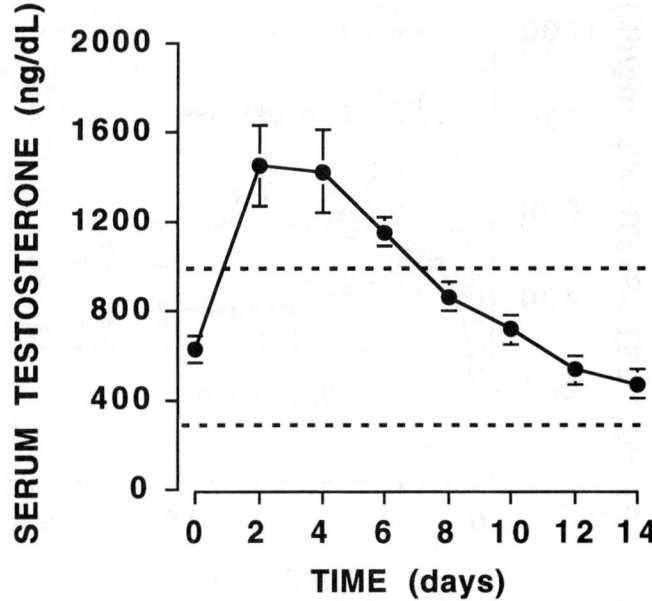

FIGURE 410.3. Serum testosterone concentrations during the 14 days following an injection of a 200-mg dose of testosterone enanthate to hypogonadal men. The serum testosterone concentration was highest just after the injection and lowest just before the next injection. The dashed lines represent the range of normal. (Adapted from Snyder PJ, Lawrence DA. Treatment of male hypogonadism with testosterone enanthate. *J Clin Endocrinol Metab* 1980;51:1335–1339.)

day or two after the injection and fall to a nadir just before the next injection (Fig. 410.3). These fluctuations are noted by some patients as fluctuations in energy, mood, and libido.

A new way of replacing testosterone is by transdermal means, using patches, gels, or creams that contain testosterone. These preparations usually produce serum testosterone concentrations that are within the normal range in most hypogonadal men and that fluctuate no more than is physiologically normal (Fig. 410.4). These relatively stable serum testosterone concentrations result in relative stability of energy, mood, and libido.

Men who are being treated with testosterone should be monitored for efficacy and side effects. Efficacy should be monitored by measurement of the serum testosterone concentration, which should be midnormal midway between injections of testosterone esters or at any time after application of a transdermal preparation. Men who are older than 40 years should be monitored for testosterone-dependent diseases, such as prostate cancer, benign prostatic hyperplasia, and erythrocytosis. No evidence yet presented, however, shows that testosterone administered exogenously is more likely to exacerbate any of these conditions than is testosterone produced endogenously.

Stimulation of Spermatogenesis

When sperm production is impaired by damage to the seminiferous tubules, no treatment can improve it, although any mature sperm produced may be used for in vitro fertilization. When sperm production is subnormal due to diseases of the pituitary or hypothalamus, it can be stimulated by administration of exogenous gonadotropins if the cause is pituitary or hypothalamic

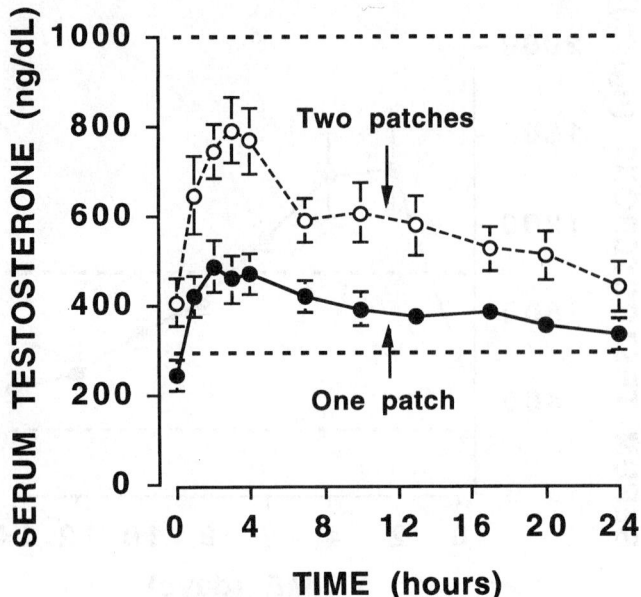

FIGURE 410.4. Serum testosterone concentrations during a 24-hour period in hypogonadal men treated with testosterone transdermally. One or two testosterone patches increased the mean serum testosterone concentration to within the normal range, which is indicated by the dashed lines. (Adapted from Yu Z, Gupta SK, Hwang SS, et al. Testosterone pharmacokinetics after application of an investigational transdermal system in hypogonadal men. *J Clin Pharmacol* 1997;37: 1139–1145.)

disease, or by administration of gonadotropin-releasing hormone if the cause is hypothalamic disease.

ANDROGEN RESISTANCE

Not surprisingly, generalized tissue resistance to the action of androgens results in abnormalities similar to those of testosterone deficiency. Two kinds of biochemical abnormalities can prevent testosterone from having its usual effects: an abnormal androgen receptor and an abnormal 5α-reductase type 2 enzyme, so that testosterone cannot be converted to DHT. Both conditions result from genetic mutations, both are rare, and both result in incomplete virilization of the external genitalia.

Many different mutations of the androgen receptor gene have been described, and most are limited to a single family. These mutations lead to several kinds of abnormalities in the androgen receptor. Some of the receptor abnormalities result in absent or subnormal binding of androgen to the receptor and others in lack of binding of the androgen–receptor complex to DNA. The clinical presentations of the different receptor abnormalities also vary but do not correlate with the receptor abnormality. In the most severe clinical presentation, called complete testicular feminization, the affected person is born with testes in the inguinal canals, no internal genitalia, and female external genitalia. At puberty the serum testosterone concentration increases to high-normal or slightly higher than normal, but sexual hair does not develop because of the absence of functional androgen receptors. Breasts develop because testosterone can still be converted

to estradiol. In the next most severe form of the disorder—incomplete testicular feminization—there is partial fusion of the posterior labial folds, but the genitalia are still more female than male; in Reifenstein's syndrome, a greater degree of labial fusion occurs, so that the genitalia are more appropriately called incompletely male. The least severe form of androgen resistance is manifested only by infertility and, perhaps, gynecomastia. Serum testosterone and LH concentrations are high-normal to slightly high in all of these forms of androgen resistance.

Many different mutations of the 5α-reductase type 2 gene also lead to incomplete virilization of the external genitalia because virilization requires conversion of testosterone to DHT. At birth, the external genitalia are usually predominantly female, so that the sex of rearing is usually female. At puberty, the serum testosterone concentration increases and overcomes to some degree the lack of DHT by binding to the androgen receptor to cause phallic enlargement and development of sexual hair in an adult male pattern. If the sex of rearing is female, the testes should be removed before the anticipated age of puberty to prevent these events. Subsequently, estradiol should be administered.

BIBLIOGRAPHY

Findlay JC, Place V, Snyder PJ. Treatment of primary hypogonadism in men by the transdermal administration of testosterone. *J Clin Endocrinol Metab* 1989;68:369–373.

Finkel DM, Phillips JL, Snyder PJ. Stimulation of spermatogenesis by gonadotropins in men with hypogonadotropic hypogonadism. *N Engl J Med* 1985;313:651–655.

Griffin JE. Androgen resistance: the clinical and molecular spectrum. *N Engl J Med* 1992;326:611–618.

Katznelson L, Finkelstein JS, Schoenfeld DA, et al. Increase in bone density and lean body mass during testosterone administration in men with acquired hypogonadism. *J Clin Endocrinol Metab* 1996;81:4358–4365.

Lee MM, Donahoe PK. Müllerian inhibiting substance: a gonadal hormone with multiple functions. *Endocr Rev* 1993;14:152–164.

Lipshultz LI, Caminos-Torres R, Greenspan CS, et al. Testicular function after orchiopexy for unilaterally undescended testis. *N Engl J Med* 1976; 295:15–18.

Sellmeyer DE, Grunfeld C. Endocrine and metabolic disturbances in human immunodeficiency virus infection and the acquired immune deficiency syndrome. *Endocr Rev* 1996;17:518–532.

Seminara SB, Hayes FJ, Crowley WF Jr. Gonadotropin-releasing hormone deficiency in the human (idiopathic hypogonadotropic hypogonadism and Kallmann's syndrome): pathophysiological and genetic considerations. *Endocr Rev* 1998;19:521–539.

Smith EP, Boyd J, Frank GR, et al. Estrogen resistance caused by a mutation in the estrogen-receptor gene in a man. *N Engl J Med* 1994;331: 1056–1061.

Snyder PJ, Lawrence DA. Treatment of male hypogonadism with testosterone enanthate. *J Clin Endocrinol Metab* 1980;51:1335–1339.

Stanik S, Dornfeld LP, Maxwell MH, et al. The effect of weight loss on reproductive hormones in obese men. *J Clin Endocrinol Metab* 1981: 53:828–832.

Vermeulen A. Androgens in the aging male. *J Clin Endocrinol Metab* 1991; 73:221–224.

Wilson JD, Griffin JE, Russell DW. Steroid 5α-reductase 2 deficiency. *Endocr Rev* 1993;14:577–593.

411

DIABETES MELLITUS, TYPES I AND II

JAY S. SKYLER

Diabetes mellitus is a chronic metabolic syndrome. The metabolic dysregulation is a consequence of relative or absolute deficiency of insulin. Diabetes mellitus is recognized when there are elevated levels of plasma glucose (hyperglycemia) and is monitored by means of measurement of variations in glycemia. The metabolic dysregulation is pervasive, involving deranged metabolism of carbohydrates, fats, and proteins. As a function of time and the metabolic disruption, many patients with diabetes have chronic complications of the disease, including accelerated vascular disease, neurologic deficits, and other organ-specific, particularly retinal and renal, degenerative disorders.

Diabetes mellitus is an important public health problem. Worldwide, more than 120 million persons have diabetes. One in every 20 Americans has diabetes—an estimated 15.7 million persons. Five million of these cases of diabetes are undiagnosed. Approximately 10% of the population has either an impaired fasting glucose or an impaired glucose tolerance state, in which glucose homeostasis is disrupted. These conditions often are harbingers of the overt clinical syndrome of diabetes. Diabetes, with its complications, is the seventh leading cause of death of disease in the United States. Persons with diabetes are two to four times more likely to have coronary and cerebral vascular disease than the general population. In the United States, the economic burden of diabetes in 1995 was estimated at $92 billion in direct health care costs and $138 billion in combined direct and indirect costs.

■ CLASSIFICATION AND DIAGNOSIS

CLASSIFICATION

Diabetes mellitus is a heterogeneous syndrome. The primary manifestation, hyperglycemia, can have from various causes. The currently used classification of diabetes was revised by an expert committee of the American Diabetes Association (ADA) and a World Health Organization (WHO) consultation group (Table 411.1). It divides primary diabetes mellitus into two major categories. These are type I diabetes mellitus, which accounts for 5% to 10% of cases of diabetes in the United States, and type II diabetes mellitus, which accounts for 90% to 95% of cases of diabetes in the United States. These two main clinical patterns of the diabetic syndrome are distinct in terms of etiology, pathogenesis, clinical presentation, and treatment.

Type I diabetes is characterized by immune-mediated pancreatic islet β-cell destruction, absolute insulin deficiency, and dependence on insulin therapy for the preservation of life. The previous term *insulin-dependent diabetes* denoted the dependence on daily insulin administration for survival. Because of absolute insulinopenia, patients with type I diabetes are prone to ketosis and possibly ketoacidosis even under basal conditions. In the past the disease had been called *ketosis-prone diabetes.* In most cases of type I diabetes the β-cell destruction is caused by an immune attack and thus is called *immune-mediated type I diabetes.* This form of type I diabetes is most common among Europids. However, a minority of patients with type I diabetes, particularly those of other than Europid ancestry, have no evidence of autoimmunity, and the disease is classified as *idiopathic type I diabetes.* This includes a variant that occurs most often among young blacks, labeled *atypical diabetes,* in which there are some features of both type I and type II diabetes and fluctuation in β-cell function.

The onset of type I diabetes usually is in the first two decades of life. The peak incidence is between 10 and 13 years of age (hence the previous name *juvenile-onset diabetes*) but may occur at any age. A slowly evolving variant of type I diabetes is called *latent autoimmune diabetes among adults.*

Type II diabetes is the common form of diabetes caused by defects in insulin secretion, almost always with a major contribution from insulin resistance. One subclassification divides this entity into obese and nonobese subtypes. Most patients (80% to 90% in the United States) are obese. The characteristics of type II diabetes are altered insulin secretory dynamics but retention of endogenous pancreatic insulin secretion; absence of ketosis (the disease therefore in the past has been called *ketosis-resistant diabetes*); and insulin resistance caused by diminished target cell action of insulin. Patients with type II diabetes usually are not dependent on insulin for prevention of ketosis or maintenance of life (hence the previous term *non–insulin-dependent diabetes*), but insulin may be necessary to control symptoms or correct disordered metabolism. Temporary insulin therapy can be used to re-regulate glycemic control. Type II diabetes usually begins after the age of 40 years (hence the previous name *maturity-onset diabetes*), and the frequency increases with aging, although the disease is increasingly making its appearance in adolescence and early adulthood, especially among obese sedentary persons at high genetic risk.

A number of other specific types of diabetes are caused by genetic defects in insulin secretion or insulin action. The best characterized of these are a group of mutations in which diabetes is caused by monogenetic defects in β-cell function. These familial autosomal dominant forms of diabetes frequently are characterized by onset of mild hyperglycemia at an early age (generally before 25 years) and were previously called *maturity-onset diabetes of the young.* These forms of diabetes are characterized by impaired insulin secretion with minimal or no defects in insulin action. Abnormalities at several genetic loci on different chromosomes have been identified, including mutations on chromosome 12 in a hepatic transcription factor (HNF-1α) gene region, mutations on chromosome 7p in the glucokinase gene, and mutations on chromosome 20q in a hepatic transcription factor (HNF-4α) gene region.

Gestational diabetes mellitus (GDM) begins or is first recognized during pregnancy, although it is possible that glucose intolerance may antedate the pregnancy but have been previously

TABLE 411.1.	ETIOLOGIC CLASSIFICATION OF DIABETES MELLITUS

I. Type I (β-cell destruction usually leading to absolute insulin deficiency)
  A. Immune-mediated
  B. Idiopathic
II. Type II (may range from predominant insulin resistance with relative insulin deficiency to a predominantly secretory defect with or without insulin resistance)
III. Other specific types of diabetes
  A. Genetic defects of β-cell function
    1. Chromosome 20, HNF4α (*MODY1*)
    2. Chromosome 7, glucokinase (*MODY2*)
    3. Chromosome 12, HNF1α (*MODY3*)
    4. Chromosome 13, IPF 1 (*MODY4*)
    5. Mitochondrial DNA 3243 mutation
    6. Others
  B. Genetic defects in insulin action
    1. Type A insulin resistance
    2. Leprechaunism
    3. Rabson–Mendenhall syndrome
    4. Lipoatrophic diabetes
    5. Others
  C. Diseases of the exocrine pancreas
    1. Pancreatitis
    2. Trauma, pancreatectomy
    3. Neoplasia
    4. Cystic fibrosis
    5. Hemochromatosis
    6. Fibrocalculous pancreatopathy
    7. Others
  D. Endocrinopathy
    1. Acromegaly
    2. Cushing's syndrome
    3. Glucagonoma
    4. Pheochromocytoma
    5. Hyperthyroidism
    6. Somatostatinoma
    7. Aldosteronoma
    8. Others

  E. Drug or chemical-induced diabetes
    1. Vacor (*N*-3-pyridylmethyl-*N-p*-nitrophenyl urea)
    2. Pentamidine
    3. Nicotinic acid
    4. Glucocorticoids
    5. Thyroid hormone
    6. Diazoxide
    7. β-Adrenergic agonists
    8. Thiazides
    9. Phenytoin (Dilantin)
    10. Interferon-α therapy
    11. Others
  F. Infections
    1. Congenital rubella
    2. Cytomegalovirus
    3. Others
  G. Uncommon forms of immune-mediated diabetes
    1. "Stiff man" syndrome
    2. Anti–insulin receptor antibodies
    3. Insulin autoimmune syndrome (antibodies to insulin)
    4. Others
  H. Other genetic syndromes sometimes associated with diabetes
    1. Down syndrome
    2. Klinefelter's syndrome
    3. Turner's syndrome
    4. Wolfram's syndrome
    5. Friedreich's ataxia
    6. Huntington's chorea
    7. Lawrence–Moon–Biedel syndrome
    8. Myotonic dystrophy
    9. Porphyria
    10. Prader–Willi syndrome
    11. Others
IV. Gestational diabetes mellitus (GDM)

unrecognized. Almost all women with GDM have normal glucose tolerance after parturition but are at markedly increased risk of future diabetes. Women with known diabetes who become pregnant do not have GDM.

Secondary diabetes mellitus refers to hyperglycemia caused by another condition, such as pancreatic surgery, chronic pancreatitis, chronic liver disease, or various forms of endocrinopathy, such as Cushing's syndrome, acromegaly, pheochromocytoma, or aldosteronism, or by medication use, such as chronic glucocorticoid therapy. Diabetes mellitus also is associated with a number of relatively uncommon genetic conditions.

Impaired fasting glucose (IFG) and *impaired glucose tolerance* (IGT) refer to abnormalities in glucose homeostasis with glucose values intermediate between normal and overt diabetes. Persons with these conditions are at increased risk of overt diabetes and of coronary artery disease. Results of serial testing may show worsening to diabetes, improvement toward normal, or no change.

Metabolic syndrome (insulin resistance syndrome, deadly quartet) is a precursor of diabetes that confers increased risk of coronary disease and atherosclerosis. The components are as follows: impaired glucose regulation or diabetes; insulin resistance (under hyperinsulinemic euglycemic conditions, glucose uptake below lowest quartile for background population under investigation); high arterial pressure (more than 140/90 mm Hg); dyslipidemia (plasma triglyceride level more than 150 mg per deciliter or high-density lipoprotein cholesterol level less than 35 mg per deciliter for men, less than 39 mg per deciliter for women); central obesity (more than 120% ideal body weight, body mass index [mass in kilograms divided by square of height in meters] greater than 30, or waist to hip ratio more than 0.90 for men or more than 0.85 for women); and microalbuminuria (urinary albumin excretion rate more than 20 μg per minute). Although there is no international standard for the definition of *metabolic syndrome*, WHO suggests as a working definition, which does not imply causal relations, the following: glucose intolerance (IGT, IFG, or diabetes mellitus) or insulin resistance, or both, with two or more of the other components.

DIAGNOSTIC CRITERIA

Diabetes mellitus is recognized on the basis of elevated plasma glucose levels. The criteria for diagnosis of diabetes are as follows:

- Unequivocal symptoms (polyuria, polydipsia, polyphagia, unexplained weight loss) *and* casual (any time of day without regard to time since last meal) plasma glucose levels of 200 mg per deciliter or more; *or*
- Fasting (no caloric intake for at least 8 hours) plasma glucose (FPG) level 126 mg per deciliter or more; *or*
- Two-hour plasma glucose level 200 mg per deciliter or more during an oral glucose tolerance test (OGTT; ingestion of 75 g glucose)

In the absence of unequivocal hyperglycemia with acute metabolic decompensation, such as ketoacidosis, these criteria should be confirmed through repetition of the test on a different day. The preparation and procedure for an OGTT are summarized in Table 411.2.

Persons with IFG and IGT are recognized as intermediate groups in whom glucose levels, although not meeting criteria for diabetes, are too high to be considered normal. IFG is defined as FPG levels more than 110 mg per deciliter but less than 126 mg per deciliter. IGT is defined as 2-hour OGTT values greater than 140 mg per deciliter but less than 200 mg per deciliter during an OGTT involving ingestion of 75 g glucose.

Because 35% to 40% of cases of type II diabetes are undiag-

TABLE 411.2. ORAL GLUCOSE TOLERANCE TEST

Preparation

If the patient has not consumed sufficient dietary carbohydrate before the test, the insulin secretory response to the oral glucose stimulus may not be as great as it should be, and the test results may be unreliable. Therefore the patient must consume a high-carbohydrate diet for a minimum of 3 full days before testing. The requirements are as follows:

- High carbohydrate (>150 g) diet for at least 3 days before the test
- 10–16 hour fast
- 10 hour abstinence from coffee, tea, caffeine-containing drinks, cigarettes, alcohol, vigorous exercise
- Water consumption

The patient should remain seated during the test. The test is started the morning after a night's sleep (6:00–10:00 A.M.) Patients may not work the night before the test.
The test should be postponed at least 1 week after any intercurrent infectious illness or other stress.

Procedure

Oral glucose is administered to adults in a dose of 1.75 g/kg body weight to a maximum of 75 g and to children as a solution in a concentration no greater than 35 g/dL of flavored water consumed within 5 min. A fasting baseline blood sample is obtained before glucose is consumed (0 min). Blood samples are obtained 30, 60, 90, and 120 minutes after glucose consumption for measurement of plasma glucose.

TABLE 411.3. DIAGNOSTIC CRITERIA: GESTATIONAL DIABETES MELLITUS

Procedure

Oral glucose is administered in a dose of 100 g (adults). A fasting baseline blood sample is obtained before glucose is consumed (0 min). Blood samples are obtained 60, 120, and 180 min after glucose consumption for measurement of plasma glucose.

Interpretation

Gestational diabetes mellitus is diagnosed if two or more values equal or exceed the following:

Time	Glucose
Fasting	105 mg/dL (5.8 mmol/L)
1 h	190 mg/dL (10.6 mmol/L)
2 h	165 mg/dL (9.2 mmol/L)
3 h	145 mg/dL (8.1 mmol/L)

---

nosed, screening is an important public health measure. Testing for diabetes among persons without symptoms is recommended by the ADA for everyone older than 45 years. If FPG level is normal, the test should be repeated within 3 years. FPG testing at a younger age and more frequently and follow-up OGTT testing should be considered by persons who have any risk factors of diabetes. These factors are IFG or IGT; parents or siblings with diabetes; obesity (more than 120% ideal body weight or body mass index of 27); high-risk ethnicity (African American, Hispanic, Native American); hypertension (blood pressure 140/90 mm Hg or more); dyslipidemia (plasma triglyceride level more than 150 mg per deciliter or high-density lipoprotein cholesterol level less than 35 mg per deciliter for men, less than 39 mg per deciliter for women); and for women, a history of GDM or giving birth to an infant weighing more than 9 pounds (4 kg).

Because GDM endangers the fetus, it is recommended that all or most pregnant women undergo screening for abnormal glucose levels at approximately 26 to 28 weeks' gestation. The ADA recommends starting with a screening test to measure plasma glucose 1 hour after consumption of 50 g glucose. Values of at least 140 mg per deciliter on the screening test warrant a full OGTT. The ADA still advises use of the 100-g OGTT during pregnancy and interprets the results according to the O'Sullivan criteria (pregnancy protocol and interpretation; Table 411.3). The WHO criteria are the same as those for nonpregnant adults.

PATHOPHYSIOLOGY OF HYPERGLYCEMIA

Insulin is a protein hormone of approximately 5,800 kd synthesized in the β-cells of the pancreatic islets. The insulin molecule consists of two peptide chains, a 21-amino-acid A chain connected by two disulfide bridges to a 30-amino-acid B chain. There also is a third disulfide bond within the A chain. Insulin is produced from proinsulin, a high-molecular-weight, single-

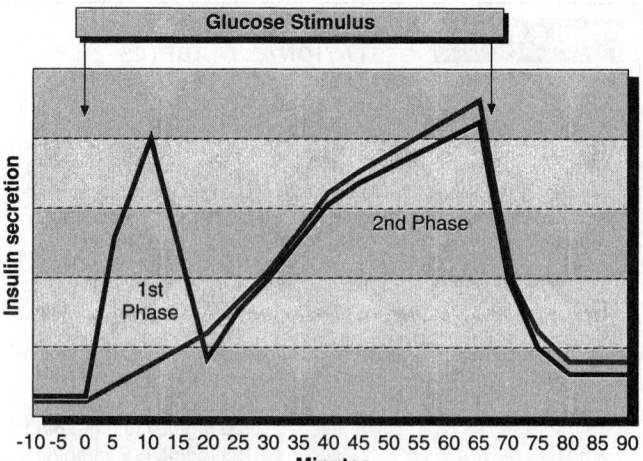

FIGURE 411.1. Insulin secretory response to intravenous glucose. *Dark line,* normal biphasic response. *Light line,* response typical of both type II diabetes and evolving type I diabetes during the prediabetic phase.

chain precursor molecule, in which the A and B chains are linked by an additional 31-amino acid sequence, C-peptide. Proinsulin is packaged into secretory granules, where specific peptidases cleave it into insulin and C-peptide. These are released into the circulation concomitantly when the secretory granules liberate their contents, a process known as *exocytosis.*

Glucose is the primary physiologic stimulus for insulin secretion. Asynchronous biphasic secretion of insulin occurs after a glycemic challenge (Fig. 411.1). The first phase of insulin secretion is from a pool that can be rapidly mobilized. Second-phase release is from a larger compartment that is replenished by newly synthesized insulin if the stimulus is prolonged. Other factors that influence insulin secretion include gastrointestinal hormones, protein ingestion, and neural control mechanisms. The important physiologic event is that in response to nutrient ingestion there is substrate-mediated (particularly glucose-mediated) insulin secretion. Insulin secretion is timely, occurring in concert with glycemic challenge, and decreases abruptly as glycemia diminishes and the signal abates (Fig. 411.2). Nevertheless, in the absence of substrate stimulation, insulin secretion is not absent but continues at a low basal rate (basal insulin secretion) that is crucial in modulating intermediary metabolism, particularly in maintaining hepatic glucose production equivalent to

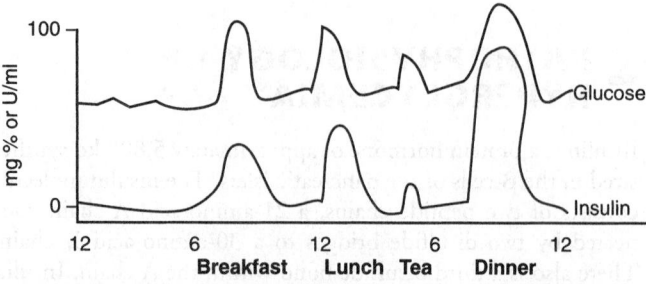

FIGURE 411.2. Schematic representation of 24-hour plasma glucose and insulin profiles of a hypothetical person without diabetes.

non–insulin-mediated basal glucose utilization, principally in the brain and nervous system.

Circulating insulin concentration is the primary regulator of fuel metabolism. It coordinates the mobilization of fuel into and out of the various fuel storage depots to meet the needs of the organism depending on the availability or lack of fuel in the environment. The net effect of insulin action is facilitation of utilization and storage of substrates. Decrements in insulin secretion allow mobilization of depot substrate at precisely the rate needed by the body. Such precision is modulated in part by continued basal insulin secretion, which dampens the rate of substrate mobilization. In addition, several hormones have biologic effects directly or indirectly antagonistic to the effects of insulin. These are the so-called glucose counterregulatory hormones, including glucagon, catecholamines (epinephrine and norepinephrine), growth hormone, and cortisol. Collectively these hormones counteract the effects of insulin, prevent hypoglycemia, and maintain adequate substrate availability in the fasted state.

In the diabetic state, the normal adaptations to fasting are amplified. Relative or absolute insulin deficiency leads to aberrations in fuel metabolism during periods of eating and of fasting. With milder degrees of insulin deficiency, the abnormalities may be manifest only during the fed state, when plasma insulin levels are normally high. With more severe degrees of insulin deficiency, the normal effects of insulin in the fasted state (modulation of hepatic glucose production and inhibition of catabolism) are impaired and the metabolic derangement is more severe.

■ TYPE I DIABETES

PATHOGENESIS

The pathogenesis of type I diabetes involves, first, a genetic predisposition, conferred principally by "diabetogenic" genes in the major histocompatibility complex (MHC) on the short arm of chromosome 6, although multiple other genetic loci modulate disease risk; second, nongenetic (environmental) factors that appear to act as triggers in genetically susceptible persons; and third, activation of immune mechanisms targeted against pancreatic islet β-cells. The initial immune response appears to engender secondary and tertiary immune responses, which collectively cause progressive destruction of pancreatic islet β-cells and consequent development of type I diabetes. The insidious process of immune-mediated destruction of the pancreatic islet insulin-secreting β-cells may precede the overt expression of clinical symptoms by many years, because these effects become apparent only when most of the β-cells have been destroyed (Fig. 411.3).

Genetics

The familial predisposition to type I diabetes has long been known. A specific mode of genetic transmission has not been established. There is a higher concordance rate for type I diabetes between monozygotic twins (35% to 50%) than between dizygotic twins (5% to 10%). The empirical risk of type I diabetes is higher among first-degree relatives of probands with the disease.

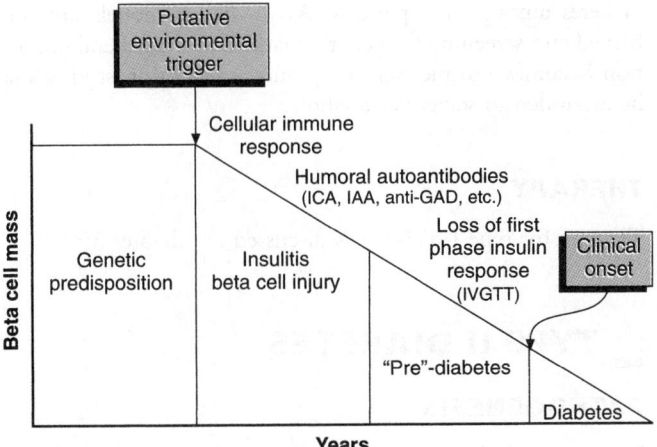

FIGURE 411.3. Schematic representation of the slow, progressive loss of β-cell mass during the development of type I diabetes. The process is divided into four phases: genetic predisposition, β-cell injury (insulitis), prediabetes, and overt diabetes. Accompanying features include an anti–β-cell cellular immune response, the appearance of humoral markers (antibodies), and loss of first-phase insulin response. *GAD,* glutamic acid decarboxylase; *IAA,* insulin autoantibodies; *ICA,* islet cell antibodies; *IVGTT,* intravenous glucose tolerance test.

Among whites in the United States, the overall risk is 0.2% to 0.4%. However, among siblings of probands with type I diabetes, the risk is about 5%. Offspring of diabetic parents have a 3% risk if the mother has the disease and 6% risk if the father has the disease.

About 40% to 50% of the genetic predisposition to type I diabetes is conferred by genes on the short arm of chromosome 6, either within or close to the class II human leukocyte antigen (HLA) region of the MHC. It has been suggested that at least a dozen other loci are involved, the largest contribution (about 10% of the genetic predisposition) accounted for by the flanking region of the insulin gene on chromosome 11.

The relation between type I diabetes and specific HLA region alleles is complex. There is a strong positive relation with HLA-DR3 and HLA-DR4 and a strong negative relation with HLA-DR2. More than 90% of whites with type I diabetes are HLA-DR3 or HLA-DR4. There is an even stronger relation with type I diabetes when DQ loci (DQα and DQβ) are considered with DR loci. That is, the predisposition to type I diabetes among whites is associated with HLA-DR3,DQB1*0201 and with HLA-DR4,DQB1*0302, the strongest association being the DQαDQβ combination DQA1*0501–DQB1*0302. Other DQ alleles appear to confer protection from type I diabetes; for example, DQA1*0201–DQB1*0602 provides protection even in the presence of DQ susceptibility alleles. This suggests that protection is dominant over susceptibility. Because class II MHC genes regulate the immune response, the susceptibility and protective alleles could be involved differentially in antigen presentation of peptides that establish and maintain tolerance or influence the immune response.

Environmental Factors

The role of environmental factors in type I diabetes among humans is uncertain. It has been argued that the substantial dis-

cordance between identical twins mandates that environmental factors play a role. However, the potential genetic diversity between such "identical" twins eliminates the need to include environmental events in the disease sequence. Yet the prevailing view is that environmental factors at least influence the probability of development of type I diabetes in a given person. One potential environmental influence is nutrition in the neonatal period and early infancy. There is a reciprocal relation between breast-feeding and frequency of type I diabetes. A Finnish study suggests that exclusive breast-feeding may reduce the likelihood of development of disease. It has been proposed that consumption of cow's milk proteins, particularly early in life, may lead to initiation of the immunologic attack against pancreatic islet β-cells and increase susceptibility to type I diabetes. Another theory is that consumption of breast milk may lead to disease protection.

Several chemical toxins can destroy β-cells, including nitrosourea compounds such as streptozotocin and the rodenticide Vacor (*N*-3-pyridilmethyl-*N*-*p*-nitrophenyl urea). Results of one study suggested that maternal consumption of nitrates and nitrites around the time of conception may influence eventual development of type I diabetes. A developing embryo exposed to toxins may suffer an initial β-cell insult, enhancing the risk of diabetes, which appears years later.

Exposure to a variety of viruses may influence development of type I diabetes. A number of viral infections contracted by humans can damage β-cells in vitro. The role of viruses in disease pathogenesis is unclear. However, type I diabetes develops in 10% to 15% of children with congenital rubella. As with maternal periconceptual nitrate and nitrite consumption, exposure is remote in time from the clinical onset of diabetes. It is not clear whether this is a direct effect of the virus, whether the virus initiates an immune mechanism, or whether involvement is magnified because exposure occurs during embryonic and fetal development. Whether or not viruses initiate the disease sequence, viral infection may bring type I diabetes to clinical recognition without playing a specific role in β-cell destruction.

Environmental factors may influence the immune response through molecular mimicry. There is homology between glutamic acid decarboxylase and coxsackievirus protein P2-C; insulin and a retrovirus sequence; a 52-kd islet protein and a rubella protein; β-cell protein IA-2 and a rotavirus sequence; and the β-cell surface protein ICA-69 and a 17-amino-acid sequence of bovine serum albumin.

Immunologic Factors

Specific cell-mediated T-lymphocyte immune processes appear responsible for the destruction of β-cells, although the exact mechanisms have not yet been clearly defined. Immune activation seems to involve presentation of a diabetogenic peptide to the immune system and activation of a helper subset ($T_H 1$) of $CD_4 +$ T lymphocytes. The cytokines produced by $T_H 1$ cell activation, interleukin-$_2$ and interferon-γ, activate cytotoxic T lymphocytes and macrophages to kill β-cells. The killing mechanism involves oxygen free radicals, nitric oxide, destructive cytokines (interleukin-$_1$, tumor necrosis factors α and β, and interferon-γ), and $CD_8 +$ cytotoxic T lymphocytes that interact with a β-cell autoantigen–MHC class I complex. Once initial immune destruction begins, secondary and tertiary immune responses are activated, compounding interpretation of the sequence of events.

The cell-mediated immune reaction is seen as a mononuclear cell infiltration of islets (insulitis) and is a pathognomonic lesion in pancreases examined near time of onset of type I diabetes. However, at the time of diagnosis of type I diabetes, only a few islets show the insulitis lesion. Some normal islets and rarely a hyperplastic islet can be seen. Most islets are pseudoatrophic small islets, devoid of β-cells and without mononuclear infiltration but with intact glucagon-secreting α-cells and somatostatin-secreting δ cells. It is presumed that these islets already have had their β-cells destroyed and that the immunologic attack has abated. Type I diabetes appears when enough β-cells are destroyed that glucose tolerance can no longer be maintained.

Because β-cell destruction is immunologically mediated, attempts have been made to interdict the disease by means of immune intervention in new-onset type I diabetes in an effort to preserve any residual β-cell function that may be present. Although immune intervention does alter the course of the disease, providing compelling support that immune mechanisms are important in disease pathogenesis, studies of new-onset diabetes have failed to show convincing long-term benefit. It may be that at this stage in the disease it is already too late to preserve sufficient β-cell function to be clinically important.

A number of circulating autoantibodies to islet cell markers are detected at diagnosis of type I diabetes, including cytoplasmic islet cell antibodies, antibodies directed against insulin, glutamic acid decarboxylase, β-cell protein IA-2, and a variety of others. These antibodies usually are not thought to mediate β-cell destruction through humoral mechanisms. Rather it is likely that as β-cells are destroyed, multiple antigens are exposed to the immune system and antibodies directed against these components are generated. Thus these antibodies serve as markers of immune activity or of β-cell damage and are useful in heralding the disease through the appearance of various antibodies several years before the onset of overt clinical hyperglycemia and type I diabetes. Because β-cell function is lost and total diabetes evolves, antibodies tend to decrease in titer or disappear.

Persons destined to have type I diabetes have a progressive metabolic defect measured as a decline in β-cell function detected by a decrease in early first-phase insulin release during an intravenous glucose tolerance test. Thus it is possible to predict development of type I diabetes through identification of genetic, immunologic, and metabolic markers in persons without symptoms. Screening programs are in place for identifying such individuals among relatives of persons with type I diabetes, because empiric risk of type I diabetes (about 3% to 6% among first-degree relatives) is 10- to 20-fold that in the general population (prevalence about 0.3%). This has led to a strategy aimed at prevention or delay of disease among susceptible persons by means of alteration of the pathogenetic sequence early in its course, before clinical manifestation of type I diabetes. Such intervention is contingent on effective case finding. This involves screening of persons at high risk, such as relatives of persons with type I diabetes. In the United States and Canada, the Diabetes Prevention Trial–Type 1 is designed to test whether antigen-based therapies can prevent or delay the development of clinical

diabetes among such persons. As predictive models are confirmed and screening for genetic markers in the general population becomes feasible, screening and intervention studies may be expanded to society as a whole.

THERAPY

Therapy for type I diabetes is discussed in Chapter 399.

TYPE II DIABETES

PATHOGENESIS

Two major pathogenetic mechanisms are operative in type II diabetes: impaired islet β-cell function (impaired insulin secretion) and impaired insulin action (insulin resistance or decreased insulin sensitivity). Although type II diabetes is a heterogeneous disorder, there is invariable impairment in insulin secretion, almost always with a major contribution from impairment in insulin action. However, different patients manifest variable degrees of insulin resistance and impairment in β-cell function. Current thinking is that separate genetic defects are responsible for each of these. In addition, environmental factors cause further insulin resistance. There is progressive decrease in insulin sensitivity with age, and insulin resistance is induced by adiposity and a sedentary lifestyle. It is not surprising that the incidence of type II diabetes increases after 40 years of age and that there is a higher prevalence among older patients, particularly those who are overweight or sedentary. Yet there are growing numbers of younger persons, even adolescents, with type II diabetes, a manifestation of the modern lifestyle characterized by low levels of physical activity and high levels of adiposity. In addition, hyperglycemia per se can further impair both β-cell function and the action of insulin, creating a vicious circle that aggravates hyperglycemia.

Impaired Islet β-Cell Function

Impairment in β-cell function is manifest in at least three ways. First, there is blunted or absent first-phase insulin response to glucose (see Fig. 411.1), so that insulin secretion is delayed and fails to restore prandial glycemic excursions in a timely manner. The first phase of the normally biphasic insulin response is the critical determinant of the magnitude of hyperglycemia after carbohydrate intake. The decrease in first-phase insulin secretion results in an overall delayed insulin secretory response to glucose. Although variable, in most circumstances the second-phase insulin response is sufficient to restore postprandial plasma glucose excursions to basal (preprandial) levels before the next meal, albeit after a prolonged interval. Second, the sensitivity of the insulin response to glucose decreases such that hyperglycemia may not trigger an appropriate insulin response. The insulin response to glucose is attenuated so that the β-cells have a relative blindness to hyperglycemia and do not generate an adequate insulin response. The blindness is selective for glucose in that the β-cells respond to nonglucose stimuli, such as amino acids (e.g., arginine), glucagon, secretin, sulfonylureas, theophylline,

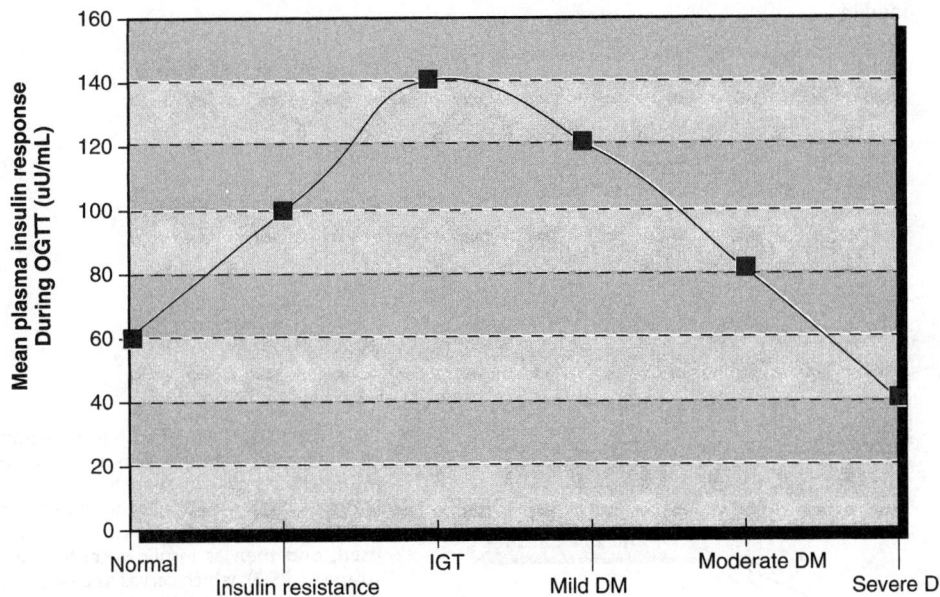

FIGURE 411.4. Mean plasma insulin response during oral glucose tolerance test (*OGTT*) for six groups of subjects: nondiabetic insulin-sensitive (normal), nondiabetic insulin resistant, impaired glucose tolerance (IGT), mild type II diabetes, moderate type II diabetes, and severe type II diabetes. *DM,* diabetes mellitus.

and isoproterenol. Third, there is a progressive decline in overall insulin secretory capacity, particularly in severe type II diabetes. This declining insulin response is illustrated by Starling's law of the pancreas (Fig. 411.4). There is compensatory insulin release in response to increasing hyperglycemia among persons without diabetes and among patients with IGT but a decreased insulin response to increasing hyperglycemia once type II diabetes is present.

The impairment in insulin secretory response is not static. It is dynamic such that chronic hyperglycemia may itself aggravate the impairment in insulin secretion, so-called glucose toxicity. Thus with progressive hyperglycemia in type II diabetes, there is concomitant deterioration in insulin secretory response. Moreover, and most important, when hyperglycemia is corrected, there is some reversal of the impairment in endogenous insulin response to a meal challenge, that is, there is demonstrable improvement in insulin secretion. Attainment of glucose control therefore facilitates maintenance of glucose control.

At the cellular level, mutations in the glucokinase gene on chromosome 7 have been found in about 60% of families with maturity-onset diabetes of the young. Because the mutant enzyme has a low affinity for glucose, glucose-stimulated insulin secretion is impaired. Glucokinase mutations do not appear to be involved in typical type II diabetes. Likewise, normal coding sequences for the insulin gene on chromosome 11 and the predominant glucose transporter in islets, GLUT2, have been found in typical type II diabetes. Thus the genetic basis of altered β-cell function in typical type II diabetes remains to be defined.

Impaired Insulin Action

Patients with type II diabetes have impaired insulin action (insulin resistance) at target cells. Insulin resistance may be defined as being present whenever normal concentrations of insulin elicit a less-than-normal biologic response. Among persons without diabetes, insulin resistance is recognized through the presence

of hyperinsulinemia in the absence of hypoglycemia. In anyone insulin resistance can be demonstrated through a subnormal response to exogenous insulin. Most insulin resistance is a consequence of impaired insulin action at the level of target cells (hepatocytes, adipocytes, myocytes). This is the case for the most common causes of insulin resistance, obesity and type II diabetes.

Insulin action may be quantified in vivo with measurement of the biologic response to exogenous insulin under controlled conditions. A number of protocols have been devised to standardize the conditions for insulin administration (the challenge) and to provide uniformity of measurement of the response variables. One of the most commonly used methods to assess insulin action is the insulin clamp technique, in which insulin is infused at a fixed rate designed to achieve a steady-state plasma insulin concentration. Plasma glucose level is kept constant (clamped) at a predetermined level (usually either euglycemia or the basal plasma glucose level, depending on the protocol) by means of continuous infusion of a variable amount of glucose, the amount determined by measurement of plasma glucose every 5 minutes. Once steady-state glucose infusion rates are achieved, these are considered a measure of insulin action, because the glucose infusion rate equals the rate of glucose metabolism (less any urinary glucose losses). If clamping is performed at basal glucose concentration, glucose clearance (glucose infusion rate divided by plasma glucose level) reflects insulin action. With the insulin clamp technique, decreased insulin action (insulin resistance) has been demonstrated among persons with type II diabetes, among those with IGT, and among many first-degree relatives of persons with type II diabetes although they have normal glucose tolerance. Chronic hyperglycemia may of itself aggravate the impairment in insulin action (glucose toxicity). With decompensation of glycemic control, there is a concomitant decrease in the action of insulin. When hyperglycemia is corrected, there is some reversal of the impairment in insulin action.

Quantitatively, impairment of insulin-stimulated glucose uptake principally affects skeletal muscle, specifically the nonoxida-

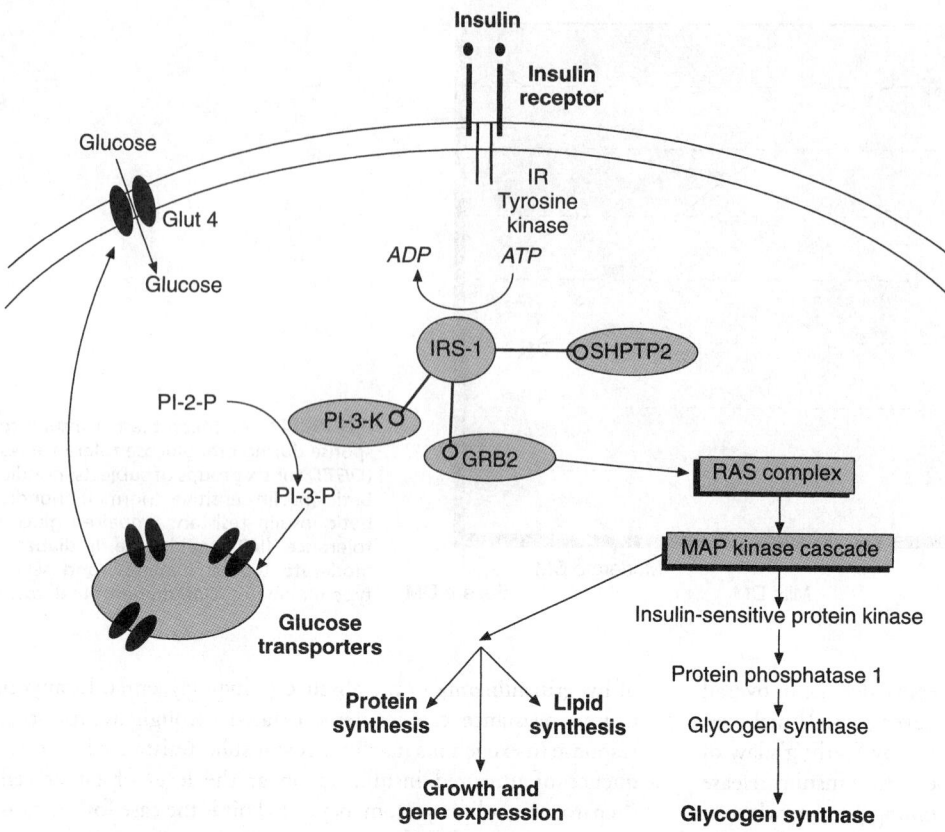

FIGURE 411.5. Cellular scheme of action of insulin. Circulating insulin binds to the insulin receptor (*IR*), which spans the plasma membrane. The IR then functions as a tyrosine kinase, first phosphorylating itself, and then as insulin receptor substrate-1 (*IRS-1*), which serves as a docking protein for several molecules important in the action of insulin. These include SH protein tyrosine phosphatase 2 (*SHPTP2*), growth factor receptor-binding protein 2 (*GRB2*), and phosphatidylinositol-3-kinase (*PI-3-K*), which further propagate insulin signaling. *ADP*, adenosine diphosphate; *ATP*, adenosine triphosphate; *GLUT4*, glucose transporter 4; *MAP*, mitogen-activated protein.

tive pathway of glucose metabolism. The result is diminished glucose storage (glycogen synthesis). To a lesser degree, glucose oxidation is reduced, the liver resists the action of insulin, and enhanced hepatic glucose production is not inhibited by insulin.

The sequential steps in the action of insulin at the cellular level are depicted in Fig. 411.5. The first step in the action of insulin at target cells is binding of insulin to its cellular receptor. The receptor spans the plasma membrane of the cell and is a tetrameric protein composed of two α subunits responsible for insulin binding and serving a regulatory function and two β subunits with inherent kinase activity responsible for transmembrane signaling. The receptor itself undergoes autophosphorylation and causes phosphorylation of insulin receptor substrates (IRS-1 and IRS-2). IRS-1 and IRS-2 serve as docking proteins, intracellular ligands that bind noncovalently to other specific proteins, including phosphatidylinositol-3-kinase, which phosphorylates phosphatidylinositol-2-P to phosphatidylinositol-3-P, which appear to be involved in translocation of the glucose transporter GLUT4 (stored in cytoplasmic vesicles) to the cell surface in skeletal muscle and adipose cells; SHPTP2, a phosphotyrosine phosphatase potentially capable of dephosphorylating the insulin receptor IRS-1 or IRS-2 to modulate the insulin signal; and growth factor receptor-binding protein 2 (GRB2), which links IRS-1 and IRS-2 to the Ras signaling pathway, activating a cascade that includes the mitogen-activated protein kinases, which initiate a sequence resulting in glycogen and lipid synthesis and transcriptional expression of enzymes stimulated by insulin.

Among patients with type II diabetes, defects have been identified in insulin receptor binding of insulin, in receptor tyrosine kinase activity for both autophosphorylation and for phosphorylation of substrates, in translocation of GLUT4 glucose transporters from their intracellular pool to the plasma membrane and their activation therein, and in the total number of glucose transporters per cell. However, most of these defects are at least partly reversible with one or another intervention. In addition to these, some patients have been found to have increased levels of either a member of the Ras superfamily named *Rad* or a membrane glycoprotein inhibitor of insulin tyrosine kinase action named *PC-1*. Whether the increased levels of these factors have a role in the pathogenesis of type II diabetes is not yet known. Thus the primary cellular mechanisms responsible for insulin resistance in type II diabetes and other conditions are still being clarified.

THERAPY

Therapy for type II diabetes is discussed in Chapter 399.

◼ ACUTE COMPLICATIONS

DIABETIC KETOACIDOSIS

Diabetic ketoacidosis (DKA) is acute, life-threatening metabolic acidosis, the most extreme result of uncontrolled diabetes mellitus. DKA is most commonly a complication of type I diabetes and occasionally occurs as the initial manifestation of undiagnosed diabetes. DKA occurs infrequently in type II diabetes, particularly when the patient is decompensated by severe intercurrent illness.

Pathophysiology

Diabetic ketoacidosis develops as a consequence of severe insulin deficiency and an excess of the glucose counterregulatory hormones (glucagon, the catecholamines, cortisol, and growth hormone). The result is a disturbance of glucose and fatty acid metabolism. Insulin deficiency decreases glucose uptake and utilization. Insulin deficiency combined with glucagon excess increases glucose production because glucagon promotes glycogenolysis and gluconeogenesis in the liver. Insulin deficiency enhances proteolysis and causes muscle breakdown and release of amino acids, which are used by the liver for gluconeogenesis. Glucose overproduction is perpetuated, and concomitant urinary nitrogen loss occurs. Hyperglycemia and hyperosmolality develop, and water shifts from the intracellular to the extracellular compartment. Glycosuria occurs, as does osmotic diuresis accompanied by large urinary losses of potassium and phosphorus and hypovolemia. This process can have several consequences, including tissue hypoxia, which produces both lactic acidosis and loss of cellular potassium; hypotension and decreased blood flow; hyperviscosity; and in rare instances, thrombosis. Decreased renal blood flow leads to acidosis and without intervention, anuria. Decreased cerebral blood flow leads to stupor and contributes to coma.

Insulin deficiency also leads to lack of inhibition of lipolysis and mobilization of free fatty acids and glycerol. In the presence of severe insulin deficiency and availability of free fatty acids, glucagon stimulates gluconeogenesis and ketogenesis. In the liver, free fatty acids are activated to their fatty-acyl-coenzyme A derivatives, transported by carnitine into the mitochondria, and oxidized to acetyl-coenzyme A, with coupling to form acetoacetate. Acetoacetate can diffuse into the circulation or be reduced to β-hydroxybutyrate or spontaneously to decarboxylate to form acetone. With the rapid oxidation of free fatty acids, dihydronicotinamide adenine dinucleotide (NADH) accumulates, so that most of the acetoacetate is converted to β-hydroxybutyrate. Although acetoacetate, β-hydroxybutyrate, and acetone are used for energy by many tissues, in severe insulin deficiency the rate of production exceeds the capacity of extrahepatic tissues to use them. The consequence is ketonemia and severe acidosis. Hyperpnea ensues in a compensatory attempt to eliminate both carbon dioxide and acetone. Ketonuria develops and aggravates osmotic diuresis and the consequences described earlier.

Diagnostic Criteria

The cardinal diagnostic features of DKA are hyperglycemia (250 mg per deciliter or greater), ketosis (ketonemia or ketonuria), and acidosis (arterial pH less than 7.3 and serum bicarbonate concentration less than 15 mEq per liter). DKA is metabolic acidosis with an elevated anion gap. Volume depletion frequently is present. A quick diagnosis can be made at the bedside by means of demonstrating hyperglycemia and ketonemia in a patient with evidence of volume depletion and Kussmaul's respirations, from which acidosis can be inferred. It is not always appreciated that the degree of hyperglycemia need not be great—a large proportion of patients with DKA have glucose concentrations less than 350 mg per deciliter.

Therapy

Therapy for DKA is discussed in Chapter 399.

HYPEROSMOLAR HYPERGLYCEMIC NONKETOTIC COMA

Hyperosmolar hyperglycemic nonketotic coma (HHNC) is an acute syndrome that may occur with uncontrolled type II diabetes. The hyperglycemia, hyperosmolality, and dehydration of HHNC usually are more severe than those of diabetic ketoacidosis, and there is no ketosis.

Pathophysiology

The increased severity of hyperglycemia, hyperosmolality, and dehydration is probably related to a more prolonged period of osmotic diuresis. Perhaps because there are no symptoms of ketosis and acidosis, the syndrome is not readily recognized. Insulin levels usually are somewhat higher than those of persons with ketoacidosis, and they may be sufficient to suppress lipolysis and ketogenesis. Some researchers have postulated that the dehydration and hyperosmolality per se may have antilipolytic effects. The elevations of growth hormone and cortisol usually are less than those that occur with ketoacidosis. Changes in mental status associated with lesser degrees of hyperosmolarity also occur and comprise a range of hyperosmolar hyperglycemic nonketotic states that can be called *hyperosmolar hyperglycemic syndrome*. HHNC develops most often among older patients with or without a known history of type II diabetes. Patients at risk often are elderly and often have other underlying medical problems, including cardiac and renal disease. HHNC frequently is precipitated by infection, which augments fluid losses. Patients become severely hyperglycemic and profoundly dehydrated because of osmotic diuresis and inadequate fluid replacement. Extreme hyperosmolality leads to brain dehydration. This may account for focal neurologic deficits and hallucinations, which are frequent. Marked dehydration and postural hypotension occur, and the mortality is high.

Diagnostic Criteria

The diagnosis of HHNC is made when a patient with abnormal mental status has severe hyperglycemia (usually 600 to 1200 mg per deciliter), elevated serum osmolality (more than 350 mOsm per kilogram), and minimal or absent ketonemia or ketonuria.

Therapy

Therapy for HHNC is discussed in Chapter 399.

CHRONIC COMPLICATIONS

The chronic complications of diabetes include accelerated vascular disease, neurologic deficits (diabetic neuropathy), and other organ-specific degenerative processes. The vascular disease is of two types. *Microangiopathy* is a disease of the capillaries specifically associated with diabetes, characterized by thickening of capillary basement membranes, and clinically manifested principally in the retina and kidney. *Macroangiopathy* is the accelerated frequency and severity of atherosclerotic disease of the arteries clinically manifested principally in the coronary arteries, cerebral arteries, and peripheral vessels of the lower extremities.

EFFECTS OF GLYCEMIC CONTROL

Over the years, extensive evidence has mounted suggesting that careful control of glycemia can reduce the risk of diabetic complications, particularly retinopathy, nephropathy, and neuropathy. The beneficial effects and effect of effective glycemic control on chronic complications of type I diabetes were firmly established with the results of the Diabetes Control and Complications Trial (DCCT) and the Stockholm Diabetes Intervention Study (SDIS). The overall results of the DCCT dramatically exceeded all expectations. Clinically important progression of diabetic retinopathy was reduced by more than 70%. The incidence of clinical renal disease (proteinuria) was reduced 54%, of early renal damage (microalbuminuria) 39%, and of clinically significant neuropathy 64%.

The United Kingdom Prospective Diabetes Study (UKPDS) also demonstrated the effect of effective glycemic control on chronic complications among patients with type II diabetes. In the UKPDS, intensive treatment decreased the risk of any diabetes-related end point 12%, of microvascular end points 25%, and of myocardial infarction 16%. The small Kumomoto Study in Japan showed similar results.

Epidemiologic studies, such as the Wisconsin Study, point to a relation between glycemia and diabetic complications for both type I and type II diabetes. The results of all of these studies have resolved the long-standing debate on whether glycemia is important. Now the debate focuses on the best means of attaining effective glycemic control and on the therapeutic targets that should be sought. It is ironic that the goal articulated by the DCCT investigators of maintaining glycemic status as close to normal as safely as possible is identical to that recommended in 1923, soon after the discovery of insulin.

MECHANISMS LEADING TO COMPLICATIONS

A variety of pathways contribute to the pathogenesis of one or more of the major complications.

Protein Glycation

Nonenzymatic glycation of proteins occurs at both N-terminal amino groups and at ε-amino groups of intrachain amino acids, such as lysine, with the slow, continuous addition of glucose to protein by means of a reaction that is a function of the duration

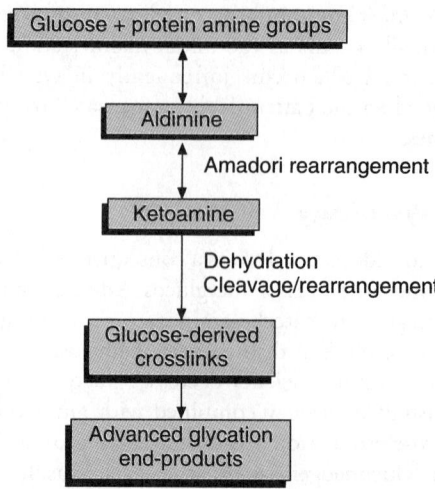

FIGURE 411.6. Steps in pathway of nonenzymatic glycation, with subsequent cross-linking to form advanced glycation end products.

of contact between the reactants and the integrated glucose concentration during the time of contact (Fig. 411.6). The first product is an aldimine, or Schiff base, which undergoes internal rearrangement of the double bond, an Amadori rearrangement, to form a ketoamine, a relatively irreversible reaction. The nonenzymatic glycation reaction occurs in essentially all tissues, leading to the genesis of many functional abnormalities. There may be further essentially irreversible transformation by cross-linking of glycated proteins to form advanced glycation end products (AGEs). This results in profound alteration of protein function and structure and leads to diabetic complications. Glycation reaction inhibitors (GRIs), such as aminoguanidine and its derivatives, have been shown to block the cross-linking that results in AGEs. Clinical trials with GRIs are underway.

Dicarbonyl Pathway

Another potential mechanism of complications is generation of dicarbonyl compounds to form methylglyoxal and 3-deoxyglucosone. Methylglyoxal is produced by means of fragmentation of triose phosphates, and 3-deoxyglucosone is formed from 3-phosphofructose or frucotose–lysine. These reactive α-dicarbonyls are extremely reactive as glycating agents for collagen, enzymes, and other important cellular components and have been shown to be toxic to cultured cells. They are thought to contribute to diabetic complications either as direct toxins or as precursors for AGEs, because their effects include inhibition of cell growth, inhibition of cell DNA synthesis, mutagenic effects on DNA, inhibition of cell enzymatic activity, protein fragmentation, protein cross-linking, and precursors of AGE formation. Methylglyoxal and 3-deoxyglucosone are elevated in the plasma of persons with diabetes and are found in increased levels in patients who have evidence of early diabetic nephropathy and retinopathy.

Polyol Pathway Activity

Glucose is converted to its sugar alcohol, sorbitol, by the enzyme aldose reductase (Fig. 411.7). In cells where insulin-mediated

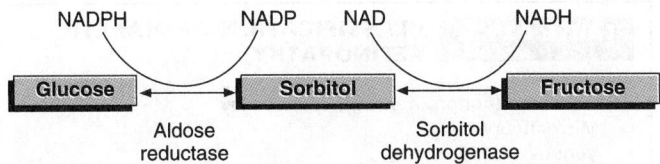

FIGURE 411.7. Polyol pathway by which glucose is converted to sorbitol and then slowly to fructose. Thicknesses of *arrows* and *lines* are proportional to reaction rates.

glucose transport is not rate limiting, and glucose is freely permeable, the presence of the polyol pathway enzymes aldose reductase and sorbitol dehydrogenase leads to intracellular accumulation of sorbitol and fructose in direct proportion to the degree of hyperglycemia. The result is a high intracellular glucose concentration. The reaction also consumes dihydronicotinamide-adenine dinucleotide phosphate (NADPH), resulting in a change in intracellular redox potential. Sorbitol accumulation has osmotic effects in the lens and is associated with changes in nerve function, mediated through alteration of Na^+-K^+-adenosine triphosphatase (Na^+-K^+-ATPase) activity, depletion of intracellular myoinositol, impairment of nerve conduction, and nerve fiber loss. In addition, hyperglycemia causes competitive inhibition of sodium-dependent myoinositol uptake, reduces the intracellular level of myoinositol, decreases membrane content of phosphatidylinositol, and further reduces Na^+-K^+-ATPase activity. The altered redox potential in vaso nervorum (from NADPH depletion) decreases local vasodilatation and reduces blood flow to the nerves and other tissues. All these abnormalities may be reversible with the use of aldose reductase inhibitors, which are in clinical trials.

Endothelial Cell Proliferation

The activation of protein kinase C (PKC) and increase in diacylglycerol (DAG) levels initiated by hyperglycemia are associated with many vascular abnormalities in retinal, renal, and cardiovascular tissue. The glucose-induced activation of PKC has been shown to increase production of extracellular matrix and cytokines; to enhance contractility, permeability, and vascular cell proliferation; to induce activation of cytosolic phospholipase A_2; and to inhibit Na^+-K^+-ATPase. PKC activation may also regulate vascular permeability and neovascularization through expression of growth factors, such as vascular endothelial cell growth factor (VEGF), which interacts with endothelial cell membrane receptors to initiate a series of events, including activation of intracellular PKC, that result in endothelial cell mitosis and proliferation. The level of VEGF–vascular permeability factor (VPF) is increased in the ocular fluid of patients with diabetes. This substance has been implicated in the neovascularization of proliferative retinopathy. Production of VEGF by hypoxic retinal tissue leads to neovascularization.

In the kidney, expression of transforming growth factor β (TGF-β) has been shown to be increased in the glomeruli of patients with diabetes and those of experimental animals. The secondary metabolic products of glucose, such as glycation products and oxidants, also can increase DAG-PKC, suggesting that the activation of DAG-PKC may be a common downstream mechanism by which multiple by-products of glucose exert their adverse effects. In experiments, inhibitors of PKC block endothelial tube formation in vitro and block intraocular neovascularization caused by retinal ischemia. Clinical trials are being conducted to test the effects of an orally effective β-isoform-selective inhibitor of PKC.

Enzymatic Glycosylation of Basement Membranes

The hallmark of diabetic microangiopathy is thickening of capillary basement membranes. Hyperglycemia enhances the rate of biosynthesis of capillary basement membranes. Renal glomerular capillary basement membranes contain increased carbohydrate in two types: complex heteropolysaccharide and disaccharide (galactose and glucose) bound to hydroxylysine. There is an increased proportion of disaccharide units in diabetic tissue.

Platelet and Endothelial Function

Alterations in platelet or endothelial function, including increased platelet aggregation, increased platelet metabolism of arachidonic acid, decreased platelet survival, decreased prostacyclin production by endothelial cells, diminished fibrinolytic activity, increased levels of plasminogen activator inhibitor-1 (PAI-1), and increased levels of von Willebrand's factor, may contribute to the vascular complications of diabetes. Hyperglycemia may influence arachidonic acid metabolism through inhibition of myoinositol uptake and reduction of membrane phosphatidylinositol and other membrane phospholipids, of which arachidonic acid is a component. The availability of arachidonic acid for prostaglandin or prostacyclin synthesis is decreased, resulting in an imbalance between these substances. Antiplatelet agents, such as salicylates, dipyridamole, and similar agents, decrease platelet aggregation and may reduce vascular risk.

Hemorheologic Abnormalities

Vasodilatation is limited. The viscosity or fluidity of blood is a limiting factor in perfusion and oxygen delivery to tissues. Factors contributing to fluidity include erythrocyte aggregation and deformability, whole blood viscosity, and plasma viscosity, which is determined from levels of high-molecular-weight plasma proteins, such as fibrinogen, levels of which are increased among persons with diabetes. When fluidity is lost, erythrocyte deformability is decreased. Pentoxifylline and its congeners may influence the rheologic characteristics of blood and improve flow.

Hemodynamic Alterations

Hemodynamic alterations in the microcirculation (hyperfiltration) are important in initiating and perpetuating diabetic nephropathy. Moderate hyperglycemia increases blood volume, glomerular plasma flow rate, and perfusion, causes hyperfiltration, and increases glomerular transcapillary hydraulic pressure.

The high capillary pressures and flows, if sustained, cause direct cellular injury, increase mesangial matrix, and cause proteinuria and glomerulosclerosis. Progressive renal injury causes selective changes in the glomerular barrier and aggravate proteinuria. Factors that lessen the effect of hyperfiltration include careful control of hyperglycemia; aggressive control of systemic blood pressure; selective efferent arteriolar dilation with angiotensin-converting enzyme (ACE) inhibitors, which decrease trans-glomerular capillary pressure; and restriction of dietary protein, because high protein intake increases renal perfusion rate.

Growth Factors

Decreases in nerve growth factor may have a role in diabetic neuropathy. Studies with animals show improvement in nerve function with administration of nerve growth factor. Retinal neovascularization develops as a consequence of retinal hypoxia, which liberates a local vasoproliferative or angiogenesis factor. There may be an imbalance between retinal vasoproliferative factors and their inhibitors.

MANIFESTATIONS AND MANAGEMENT OF COMPLICATIONS

Diabetic Retinopathy

Diabetic retinopathy is the leading cause of blindness in the United States among working-age adults (20 to 65 years of age). An estimated 24,000 persons lose vision each year as a consequence. The National Eye Institute estimates that 90% of such blindness is preventable.

The earliest clinically apparent manifestations of diabetic retinopathy are classified as nonproliferative or background diabetic retinopathy (Table 411.4). At this stage, there may be microaneurysms, dot and blot hemorrhages, hard and soft exudates, venous dilatation and beading, and intraretinal microvascular abnormalities. These changes do not impair vision. Background diabetic retinopathy affects 80% of patients with type I diabetes 10 years after onset and almost 100% of patients with type I diabetes 15 to 20 years after onset. Background diabetic retinopathy affects 50% to 80% of patients with type II diabetes 15 to 20 years after onset. The more severe form of diabetic retinopathy is classified as proliferative diabetic retinopathy (PDR) because of the presence of neovascularization as the hallmark of this type of retinopathy. There also may be fibrous proliferation and preretinal and vitreous hemorrhages. After 20 to 25 years of diabetes, 50% to 60% of patients with type I diabetes and 15% to 20% of patients with type II diabetes have PDR. PDR is relentlessly progressive and impairs vision, causing blindness if not treated. The mainstay of treatment is panretinal laser photocoagulation. Vitrectomy has become an important therapeutic modality for advanced diabetic eye disease, in which there is severe vitreous hemorrhage or fibrosis, often with retinal detachment. The eye disease eventually becomes quiescent, a stage called *involutional retinopathy.*

A separate subtype of retinopathy is diabetic maculopathy, in which severe macular edema impairs central vision and for which focal laser photocoagulation may be effective.

TABLE 411.4.	CLASSIFICATION OF DIABETIC RETINOPATHY

Background (nonproliferative) retinopathy
  Microaneurysms
  Venous dilatation
  Hemorrhages
  Exudates
  No effect on vision
Background with maculopathy
  Macular edema
  May impair central vision
  Focal laser photocoagulation effective
Proliferative retinopathy
  Neovascularization (cardinal feature)
  Fibrous proliferation
  Preretinal hemorrhage
  Vitreous hemorrhage
  Panretinal laser photocoagulation effective
Advanced diabetic eye disease
  Vitreous opacities (hemorrhage and fibrous tissues)
  Retinal detachment
  Vitrectomy effective
  Retinal reattachment possible
Involutional retinopathy
  Residual scarring from previously active proliferative retinopathy
  No treatment indicated

Glycemic control has been shown to be important in slowing the course of diabetic retinopathy. The DCCT and the UKPDS showed that intensive therapy has major beneficial effects on type I and type II diabetes. In the DCCT, the rate of clinically important progression of diabetic retinopathy (a sustained three-step change on the quantitative grading scale) was significantly reduced 70.3% overall, 78.5% among patients with no retinopathy at enrollment, and 64.5% among those with some retinopathy at enrollment. In the cohort with some retinopathy at entry, the rate of progression of retinopathy to proliferative or severe nonproliferative retinopathy (necessitating referral to an ophthalmologist for evaluation and treatment) was significantly reduced 60.8% overall. The rate of need for laser photocoagulation, an index of progression to vision-threatening retinopathy, was significantly reduced 56% overall. The rate of initial appearance of any retinopathy in the cohort with no retinopathy at enrollment was significantly reduced 27%. In the UKPDS, the rate of retinal photocoagulation was reduced 29%, of cataract extraction 24%, and of deterioration in retinopathy 21% after 12 years of follow-up study.

A number of pharmacologic therapies have been assessed, but none has been shown beneficial in controlled clinical trials. Both aspirin and the aldose reductase inhibitor sorbinil were found to be without benefit.

The Diabetic Retinopathy Study (DRS) demonstrated the dramatic effects (more than 50% reduction in visual loss) of laser photocoagulation on preventing vision loss due to diabetic retinopathy. The DRS results defined criteria for high risk in which generalized panretinal laser photocoagulation is indicated. These high-risk criteria are PDR with new vessels on disc greater than 25% of the disc diameter; new vessels on disc with preretinal hemorrhage; or new vessels elsewhere with preretinal hemorrhage. Because panretinal photocoagulation is associated with side effects, such as decreased peripheral vision and decreased night vision, it should not be used routinely unless criteria of high risk are present.

The Early Treatment Diabetic Retinopathy Study (ETDRS) showed that focal laser photocoagulation, in which only the vessels responsible for leakage are destroyed, was effective (more than 50% reduction in visual loss) therapy for diabetic maculopathy with clinically significant macular edema. For advanced diabetic eye disease not amenable to photocoagulation, the Diabetic Retinopathy Vitrectomy Study (DRVS) established guidelines for the timing of pars plana vitrectomy by showing that early vitrectomy reduces approximately 50% the 1-year rate of blindness from vitreous hemorrhage or retinal detachment.

The effect of diabetic retinopathy may be minimized and blindness prevented with a strategy that includes careful glycemic control; aggressive control of coexisting hypertension; and annual, comprehensive, dilated eye and vision examinations by an ophthalmologist for all patients 12 years and older who have had diabetes for 5 years, all patients older than 30 years, and any patient with visual symptoms or abnormalities. It is recommended that such examinations be performed by ophthalmologists because of the difficulty in assessing diabetic retinopathy. In one study the rate of serious errors in assessment was 52% for general internists, 50% for medical residents, and 33% for diabetologists but only 9% for general ophthalmologists and 0% for retinal specialists. Underlying this strategy is the aggressive use of argon laser photocoagulation when criteria of high risk are detected.

Diabetic Nephropathy

Diabetic nephropathy is the leading known cause of end-stage renal disease (ESRD) in the United States. It accounts for an estimated 28,000 new cases of ESRD per year. However, most if not all future ESRD from diabetic nephropathy is preventable. Diabetic nephropathy affects 20% to 40% of patients with type I diabetes 20 years after onset. Although a lower percentage (less than 20%) of patients with type II diabetes have nephropathy, still about one-half of patients with ESRD and diabetes have type II diabetes. Although diabetes accounts for more than 40% of cases of ESRD in the United States, patients with diabetes consume 75% of ESRD costs, principally because the renal disease is associated with other complications. Data from Denmark suggest that the increased mortality risk for type I diabetes may be confined to patients with nephropathy. The risk of nephropathy increases with duration of diabetes to 25 to 30 years' duration (after which this complication rarely begins) and with family history of essential hypertension. Some authorities contend the appearance of diabetic nephropathy is the result of the combination of diabetes and genetic predisposition to hypertension.

The course of diabetic nephropathy is slow. It once was thought that there was a long silent period in which no changes were demonstrated. Now, through demonstration of an increased albumin excretion rate, so-called *microalbuminuria* (urine albumin levels of 30 to 300 mg per 24 hours), it is possible to identify diabetic nephropathy during this period, a stage

TABLE 411.5.	CLASSIFICATION OF DIABETIC NEPHROPATHY

Incipient diabetic nephropathy
  Increased albumin excretion rate (microalbuminuria)
  Hyperfiltration possible
  Blood pressure elevation
Early (overt) diabetic nephropathy
  Clinical-grade proteinuria
  Hypertension
Advanced diabetic nephropathy
  Progressive proteinuria
  Hypertension
  Declining glomerular filtration rate (decreased creatinine clearance, increased blood urea nitrogen and creatinine levels)
End-stage renal disease
  Uremia
  Nephrotic syndrome
  Need for renal replacement therapy (transplantation or dialysis)

known as *incipient diabetic nephropathy* (Table 411.5). During this stage, there may be hyperfiltration or blood pressure elevation as well. This is followed by the development of clinical-grade proteinuria (urine albumin levels more than 300 mg per 24 hours, also detectable with standard reagent dipstick tests for protein), which defines the presence of overt diabetic nephropathy and is usually accompanied by the appearance of hypertension. Advanced diabetic nephropathy is defined by a progressive decline in renal function (declining glomerular filtration rate [GFR] measured according to decreases in creatinine clearance and increases in serum levels of blood urea nitrogen and creatinine), progressive proteinuria, and hypertension. Progression to ESRD is recognized with the appearance of uremia, the nephrotic syndrome, and the need for renal replacement therapy (transplantation or dialysis).

Glycemic control has been shown to be important in slowing the evolution of diabetic nephropathy. The DCCT showed that intensive therapy yields a 39% reduction in development of microalbuminuria and a 54% reduction in development of clinical-grade proteinuria. The UKPDS showed that glycemic control resulted in a 33% reduction in microalbuminuria after 12 years of follow-up study. Pancreatic transplantation accompanied by normoglycemia has been shown to prevent the recurrence of diabetic nephropathy in kidney grafts. Other interventions also may slow the appearance or progression of nephropathy, particularly aggressive, effective control of coexisting hypertension, which slows the rate of decline in GFR in early (overt) or advanced nephropathy. Dramatic slowing has been achieved with ACE inhibitors. For patients with microalbuminuria, the European Microalbuminuria Captopril Study showed a 66% reduction in rate of progression to clinical-grade proteinuria with an ACE inhibitor. Among patients with proteinuria, the U.S. Collaborative Study Group found that with an ACE inhibitor there was a 48% reduction in the rate of doubling of serum creatinine level and a 50% reduction in the rate of death, dialysis, or transplantation. Angiotensin receptor blockers probably share these effects. Use of calcium channel blockers also has reduced the rate of microalbuminuria. Restriction of dietary protein may delay the decline in GFR that occurs with diabetic nephropathy. Aldose reductase inhibitors may decrease or prevent an increase in albumin excretion rate. Cross-link blockers, such as aminoguanidine, have been effective in slowing renal disease in animal models of diabetes and are in clinical trials as therapy for diabetes among humans. In a provocative but uncontrolled study, pentoxifylline was found to decrease albumin excretion rate.

It may be possible to prevent diabetic nephropathy with a strategy that includes careful glycemic control and aggressive control of coexisting hypertension. Routine urinalysis should be performed yearly for adults. Postpubertal patients who have had diabetes for 5 years should undergo annual measurement of either albumin excretion rate in a timed urine collection specimen (24 hours or overnight) or albumin-to-creatinine ratio. If abnormal albumin or protein excretion is detected, serum creatinine or urea nitrogen concentrations should be measured and GFR assessed. There should be appropriate use of dietary protein restriction, early use of ACE inhibitors, and potential use of other emerging strategies.

As renal disease progresses, careful attention should be paid to all aspects of the medical renal plan, particularly that aimed at prevention of renal osteodystrophy. Protein intake for patients with evidence of nephropathy should be no more than 0.8 g per kilogram per day, or approximately 10% of daily calories. The presence of diabetes is not a contraindication to dialysis, as once was asserted. Chronic ambulatory peritoneal dialysis has been advocated by some authorities, but experience is limited. The most effective therapy for ESRD due to diabetes is renal transplantation, which often is performed at an earlier stage than with other forms of renal disease because of the accelerated catabolism that occurs when diabetes and uremia coexist. These patients ideally should undergo simultaneous renal and pancreatic transplantation, which reduces the risk of recurrent nephropathy in the transplanted kidney and takes advantage of the need for immunosuppression to prevent renal allograft rejection to allow reversal of the hyperglycemic state by the pancreatic graft.

Diabetic Neuropathy

Diabetic neuropathy may be manifested both by peripheral neurologic deficits and by autonomic dysfunction, which may involve a variety of organ systems, including the cardiovascular, gastrointestinal, and genitourinary systems. A variety of clinical syndromes occur (Table 411.6). The nature of the clinical syndrome dictates treatment.

Glycemic control has been shown to be important in slowing the evolution of diabetic neuropathy. The DCCT showed that intensive therapy yields a 64% overall reduction in the 5-year incidence of clinically significant neuropathy, defined as concordance between clinical diagnosis by a certified neurologist plus either peripheral nerve conduction abnormalities or autonomic nerve testing abnormalities. Aldose reductase inhibitors slow the progression of neuropathy. Other strategies aimed at interdicting the pathways leading to neuropathy also seem to show promise.

TABLE 411.6.	**CLASSIFICATION OF DIABETIC NEUROPATHY**

Peripheral Neuropathy

Distal symmetrical neuropathy
  Sensory loss with numbness
  Dysesthesia
  Paresthesia
  Muscle pain
  Neuropathic foot ulceration
  Neuroarthropathy (Charcot's joint)
Mononeuropathy
  Mononeuropathy
    Cranial neuropathy
    Compression or entrapment neuropathy
  Mononeuropathy multiplex
  Plexopathy
  Diabetic truncal neuropathy or radiculopathy

Autonomic Neuropathy

Cardiovascular autonomic neuropathy
  Cardiac denervation syndrome
  Postural hypotension
Gastrointestinal neuropathy
  Gastroparesis diabeticorum
  Diabetic diarrhea
  Fecal incontinence
  Constipation
Genitourinary neuropathy
  Diabetic cystopathy
  Erectile dysfunction
  Female sexual dysfunction
Sudomotor dysfunction
Pupillary abnormalities

Peripheral Neuropathy

Distal Symmetrical Neuropathy

The most common of the diabetic neuropathies is diabetic peripheral sensorimotor polyneuropathy. This is usually distal symmetrical neuropathy. Although it involves all nerves, this condition manifests in a glove-and-stocking distribution. Motor or sensory loss may occur. Distal symmetrical neuropathy can be divided clinically into three stages—early, symptomatic, and severe or disabling. Early neuropathy usually is asymptomatic, although a careful neurologic examination may elicit sensory loss. Neurologic electrophysiologic abnormalities can be demonstrated to establish the diagnosis.

The hallmark of the clinical presentation of the symptomatic stage of peripheral neuropathy is clinically detectable sensory loss with numbness. Other possible symptoms include dysesthesia, paresthesia, and muscle pain. Tendon reflexes may be diminished. Sensory loss is detectable at clinical examination, usually in a stocking-and-glove distribution. Intervention at this stage is designed to relieve symptoms, such as to manage pain, and to halt disease progression. Therapies aimed at the pathophysiologic alterations may transiently worsen symptoms because of nerve cross-talk during regeneration.

In the severe stage of peripheral neuropathy, symptoms can be disabling. Neuropathic foot ulceration and neuroarthropathy (Charcot's joint) may occur, both of which are caused by injury from sensory impairment. Progressive ulceration may lead to potential loss of limb. In this stage, the diagnosis is obvious. Therapy is directed at relieving symptoms, preventing loss of limb, and providing appropriate rehabilitation to overcome disability.

Diabetic neuropathy may lead to amputation, often in collaboration with coexisting peripheral vascular disease. Diabetes is the leading cause of nontraumatic amputations in the United States. An estimated 67,000 limbs are lost each year as a consequence of diabetes. The ADA, however, estimates that 75% to 85% of such limb loss is preventable through use of a primary care strategy that includes patient education in foot care, regular inspection of the feet by patients and health care providers, use of appropriate shoes and footwear, careful glycemic control, podiatric and pedorthic referral, aggressive early management of foot ulcers, and use of vascular surgical intervention if needed.

Current management of neuropathy is aimed at improving symptoms. Prevention and education constitute the first line of treatment. The patient should be educated about methods for and the importance of preventing foot injury. Improving glycemic control often provides some relief. Management of painful neuropathy depends on the type of pain present—dysesthesia, paresthesia, or muscular pain. Dysesthetic pain, induced by contact with objects that do not usually cause pain, such as bed sheets or clothing, can be managed with gabapentin or tricyclic antidepressant drugs, such as amitriptyline, often in high doses. Dysesthesia also can be relieved with capsaicin cream, a topical treatment that depletes the pain-modulating neurotransmitter substance P from type C nociceptive fibers.

Paresthetic pain, manifested as a burning sensation or pins and needles, also can be relieved with gabapentin or tricyclic antidepressants, such as amitriptyline or imipramine, or with mexiletine. If these approaches fail, carbamazepine should be tried. Muscular pain, manifested as shooting pain, aching night cramps, or a band-like feeling, can be relieved with physical therapy (stretching exercises) perhaps accompanied by a nonsteroidal anti-inflammatory drug or skeletal muscle relaxant. For severe pain, analgesics may be needed, but narcotics should be avoided at all costs because of the high risk of addiction in this setting and a predictable loss of effectiveness due to tachyphylaxis.

Mononeuropathy

Other types of peripheral diabetic neuropathy are focal and multifocal neuropathy. These types are characterized by neurologic deficits confined to the distribution of single or multiple nerves (mononeuropathy or mononeuropathy multiplex), brachial or lumbosacral nerve plexuses (plexopathy), or nerve roots (radiculopathy).

Isolated cranial neuropathy is not rare among elderly patients with diabetes. Cranial nerves, particularly III, IV, and VI, often are affected by mononeuropathy (cranial neuropathy). Characteristic third cranial nerve palsy occurs with diabetic ophthalmoplegia (unilateral pain, diplopia, and ptosis with pupillary sparing). Management of cranial neuropathy is palliative because of its self-limited nature.

Diabetic truncal neuropathy or radiculopathy manifests as

bandlike thoracic or abdominal pain often misdiagnosed as an acute intrathoracic or intra-abdominal emergency. Diabetic femoral neuropathy results in both motor and sensory deficits at the sacral plexus and femoral nerve. Some types of mononeuropathy mimic compression or entrapment neuropathy, such as carpal tunnel syndrome. Compression and entrapment palsy responds to standard conservative management or a surgical release procedure. Diabetic plexopathy is a diagnosis of exclusion. Other causes must be carefully excluded in consultation with a specialist.

All of these focal neuropathic syndromes mimic similar neurologic conditions of nondiabetic origin. Mononeuropathy tends to occur among older patients with diabetes, is relatively uncommon, and usually has an acute clinical onset. Management of mononeuropathy is essentially supportive. Recovery (complete or partial) usually occurs, so these syndromes usually but not always are self-limited. The acute onset and complete or partial recovery suggest a vascular or traumatic basis.

Autonomic Neuropathy

A multitude of clinical syndromes compose diabetic autonomic neuropathy. Management of autonomic neuropathy depends on the manifestations.

Cardiovascular Autonomic Neuropathy

Cardiovascular autonomic neuropathy manifests as increased heart rate, altered heart rate control (a fixed heart rate of 80 to 90 beats per minute that does not respond to stress, mild exercise, sleep, or postural changes), and the possibility of exercise intolerance, postural hypotension, or cardiac denervation syndrome.

Cardiac Denervation Syndrome
Cardiac denervation syndrome manifests as silent myocardial ischemia and painless myocardial infarction, increased incidence of sudden death, increased incidence of cardiac arrhythmia, poor exercise tolerance, a higher incidence of cardiovascular lability during anesthesia, denervation hypersensitivity to autonomic drugs or medicines that contain autonomic drugs (e.g., procaine hydrochloride with epinephrine), poor survival after myocardial infarction, increased morbidity during pregnancy, and poor prognosis for 5-year survival. There is no therapy for cardiac denervation syndrome. However, it is important to ascertain whether a patient has this problem, particularly before surgical anesthesia or before commencement of an exercise program. Measurement of R-R variation and evaluation of heart rate responses to the Valsalva maneuver (during which the patient blows against a standardized pressure) are simple, reliable, and noninvasive tests with which to screen patients for cardiovascular autonomic neuropathy. An exercise stress test should be performed before patients with autonomic neuropathy begin an exercise program. Patients may fatigue easily or have painless ischemia. Painless ischemia precludes participation in strenuous exercise.

Postural Hypotension
A severe manifestation of cardiovascular sympathetic neuropathy is postural hypotension. Overt postural hypotension is uncom-

mon and usually appears as a late complication. Postural hypotension is defined as a decrease in systolic blood pressure greater than 30 mm Hg or any fall in diastolic blood pressure on standing. The clinical definition is any decrease in arterial blood pressure soon after standing that produces symptoms such as blurry vision, pain in the neck, light-headedness, or transient loss of consciousness. Two additional factors may precipitate hypotension among patients with autonomic failure. First, meals lower blood pressure dramatically among patients with autonomic failure and may provoke symptomatic postprandial postural hypotension. Second, insulin lowers blood pressure among patients with diabetes and autonomic neuropathy. The presence of postural tachycardia usually indicates that the postural hypotension may be caused by potentially reversible factors, such as hypovolemia or pharmacologic agents.

Postural hypotension from cardiovascular neuropathy can be managed with mechanical maneuvers (head-up tilting of the bed during the night, use of waist-high custom-fitted elastic support stockings during the day), increased salt intake, fludrocortisone, and in rare instances, short-acting pressor agents. It may be necessary to give vasodilators, such as hydralazine, minoxidil, or transdermal nitrates, at bedtime. Patients who take these agents should be advised against getting up during the night without assistance.

Gastrointestinal Neuropathy

Diabetic neuropathic involvement of the gastrointestinal tract, mostly causing motility disturbances, extends from the esophagus to the anorectum. In addition, acute hyperglycemia, especially with ketoacidosis, may inhibit gastrointestinal motility with resulting anorexia, nausea, vomiting, and abdominal pain, all of which resolve as the metabolic derangements are controlled.

Esophageal motor disorders are rare. For most patients, esophageal dysfunction is mild and nonspecific and does not produce symptoms. Some patients may have dysphagia, chest pain, and gastroesophageal reflux.

Gastroparesis can be detected among as many as one-fourth of persons with diabetes. In most patients it is clinically silent. However, severe diabetic gastroparesis can be quite debilitating. Typical symptoms include anorexia, early satiety, nausea, vomiting, abdominal bloating, and epigastric discomfort. A classic symptom is postprandial vomiting of undigested food, although morning nausea or dry heaves also may occur. Disruption of nutrient delivery to the small intestine upsets the relation between glucose absorption and insulin administration, with resulting wide swings of glucose levels and unexpected episodes of postprandial hypoglycemia. Diagnosis is made with upper gastrointestinal endoscopy when retained food is found in the stomach after an 8- to 12-hour fast in the absence of obstruction or with a nuclear solid-phase gastric emptying study. Treatment is careful attention to blood glucose control, a low-fat diet, and several small meals throughout the day. Pharmacologic therapy involves prokinetic agents, such as metoclopramide, bethanechol, and cisapride.

Intestinal autonomic neuropathy may cause diarrhea through effects on motility or on enterocyte absorption. Diarrhea among patients with diabetes typically is frequent and watery and may be persistent, intermittent, or alternating with constipation. Fecal incontinence among these patients also is caused by neuropathic damage with loss of internal sphincter control and anorectal sensation. Constipation is the most common gastrointestinal symptom and is assumed to be caused by generalized autonomic neuropathy.

Management of diabetic diarrhea depends on the specific cause, but the common bacterial overgrowth syndrome often responds to rotating antibiotics, which should be used if bacterial overgrowth is found or cannot be ruled out. A hydrophilic fiber supplement (psyllium) may be useful if diarrhea alternates with constipation. Synthetic, nonaddicting antidiarrheal opiates, such as diphenoxylate or loperamide, can be tried. The long-acting somatostatin analog octreotide may be effective in the care of patients with severe refractory symptoms. Management of fecal incontinence should include sphincter-strengthening exercises. Clonidine, an α_2 agonist, may reverse adrenergic nerve dysfunction and improve diarrhea and particularly fecal incontinence. Constipation can be managed with adequate hydration and a high-fiber diet supplemented with a hydrophilic colloid such as psyllium or perhaps with a promotility drug. Patients with more severe symptoms may need intermittent use of saline or osmotic laxatives.

Genitourinary Neuropathy

Diabetic Cystopathy
Diabetic neuropathy affects the genitourinary system, particularly the urinary bladder (diabetic cystopathy), and involves a spectrum of voiding dysfunction. Initial symptoms usually are related to impaired bladder sensation, which causes a gradual change in voiding pattern—increased intervoiding interval, voiding only once or twice a day, the need to strain abdominally with resulting slow urinary stream and terminal dribbling, and increased difficulty in initiating or maintaining micturition with possible urinary incontinence. As decreased bladder sensation progresses, there are incomplete emptying, impaired bladder contractility with increased bladder capacity, an increased amount of postvoid residual urine, impaired urinary flow rate, and proneness to infection. Management of diabetic cystopathy entails scheduled voiding (voiding every 3 to 4 hours), double or triple voiding to reduce large postvoid residual volumes, abdominal straining (Credé's maneuver), intermittent self-catheterization, and use of cholinergic agents, such as bethanechol, to stimulate bladder contractility.

Erectile Dysfunction
Erectile dysfunction is one of the most common problems among men with diabetes. Erectile dysfunction may be psychogenic or organic in origin, the latter usually caused by both neurologic and vascular impairment. Autonomic neuropathy decreases penile smooth-muscle relaxation. Arterial stenosis, particularly of the internal pudendal artery, venous leaks, and microvascular abnormalities may be present. Psychological factors may contribute to erectile dysfunction among men with diabetes as they do in the general population. In addition, fear of diabetic

erectile dysfunction may induce erectile dysfunction. In rare instances, testosterone deficiency may cause erectile dysfunction.

The onset of organic erectile dysfunction is gradual and progressive, beginning with decreased rigidity and reduced frequency of erection and followed by incomplete tumescence and eventually by complete erectile dysfunction. Libido usually remains unchanged. In contrast, the most obvious symptom of psychogenic erectile dysfunction is sudden onset or problems related to isolated situations or persons. Monitoring of nocturnal penile tumescence may be useful in determining whether a man is capable of having an erection.

Theoretical treatment depends on the cause of erectile dysfunction. However, many clinicians start treatment with a therapeutic trial of sildenafil, which is straightforward, provided the patient does not have coronary artery disease and is not using nitrates. Improved glycemic control may improve erectile function among patients with very poor control. Psychogenic erectile dysfunction often can be successfully treated by a therapist with expertise in sexual dysfunction. Vascular surgery may improve blood supply or repair venous leaks, when present. Injection directly into the corpora cavernosa of vasodilators (phentolamine, prostaglandins) produces an erection. A variety of mechanical vacuum devices can produce an erection, and there are several types of penile prostheses.

Female Sexual Dysfunction

Sexual problems among women with diabetes include inadequate vaginal lubrication; alteration in desire, arousal, or orgasm; and pain during sexual intercourse. Poor lubrication most closely parallels erectile dysfunction among men in that both depend on genital vasocongestion during sexual arousal. Along with vaginal dryness and lack of expansion, inadequate genital vasocongestive responses can cause poor vaginal lubrication with vaginal irritation or painful intercourse. Older women with type II diabetes have more problems than do healthy women in terms of low sexual desire, poor vaginal lubrication, dyspareunia, and difficulty reaching orgasm.

It often is easy to manage the arousal-phase problem of poor vaginal lubrication. For women with low estrogen levels, estrogen replacement should be prescribed as a pill, patch, or vaginal cream. Estrogen replacement can improve vaginal elasticity and lubrication, but additional supplementation with androgens is more likely directly to increase sexual desire. Clinical trials of sildenafil are in progress. For premenopausal women and postmenopausal women who have risk factors that prevent estrogen replacement, vaginal lubricants are useful. For sexual activity, a water-based gel lubricant may be used. For severe dryness, a vaginal suppository inserted before foreplay can be helpful.

Probably the most common causes of sexual problems among women with diabetes are psychological, such as depression, anxiety about attractiveness, poor sexual communication, relational conflict, or a history of a traumatic sexual experience. Loss of desire for sex often is related to depression. Antidepressant drugs and brief symptom-focused psychotherapy are effective. Many women can be successfully treated by a therapist with expertise in sexual dysfunction.

Sudomotor Dysfunction

Sudomotor dysfunction occurs because the sweat glands are innervated by autonomic nerves, and function may be compromised by diabetic neuropathy. Longer nerves tend to be impaired before shorter nerves are, resulting in anhidrosis in the lower extremities, with compensatory hyperhidrosis in the upper body. The main symptom of sudomotor dysfunction is excessive perspiration on the torso and face. There also may be gustatory sweating during eating. Anhidrosis in the lower extremities may contribute to the development of foot and leg ulcers. Loss of the ability to regulate core temperature may cause heat exhaustion and heat stroke. The most important aspect of treatment is education about the causes of the increased upper-body sweating and awareness of the risk of heat exhaustion and heat stroke.

Pupillary Abnormalities

Sympathetic nerves dilate the pupil, and parasympathetic nerves constrict the pupil; thus pupil adapts to the level of illumination. Autonomic neuropathy reduces pupil size and inhibits the ability of the pupil to adapt to changes in illumination. Symptoms include night blindness and poor adaptation to darkness. Decreased pupil diameter also is associated with reduced anterior chamber depth and is a predisposition to glaucoma.

■ OTHER COMPLICATIONS

SKIN LESIONS
Diabetic Dermopathy

Diabetic dermopathy, also known as *shin spots* or *pigmented pretibial patches,* usually occurs on the extensor surfaces of the distal lower extremities. It is characterized by multiple, asymptomatic, hyperpigmented, oval or circular macules, which may be atrophic or scaly. No treatment is needed.

Necrobiosis Lipoidica Diabeticorum

Necrobiosis lipoidica diabeticorum is a relatively rare form of atrophic degeneration of dermal and epidermal tissue. It occurs most commonly on the shin. This condition is characterized by shiny, transparent skin with reddish-brown to violet plaques that frequently become yellow in the center; dermal vessels can be seen under the plaques. The lesions may ulcerate. Treatment is difficult, but has been attempted with intralesional glucocorticoids, pentoxifylline, dipyridamole, and salicylates.

INFECTIONS UNIQUE TO DIABETES
Malignant Otitis Externa

Malignant otitis externa is a chronic, potentially fatal erosive infection of the soft tissue and cartilage around the external auditory canal; it is caused by *Pseudomonas aeruginosa*. The infection is characterized by pain, purulent drainage, and progressive destruction of the temporal, petrous, and mastoid bones that ultimately reaches the cranial nerves (V, VII, or VIII), meninges, or sigmoid sinus. Treatment involves vigorous debridement of necrotic tissue and a prolonged course (at least 4 weeks) of antibiotics.

Mucormycosis

Rhinocerebral mucormycosis is a phenomenally rapid necrotizing invasive process caused by the mycelia of the genera *Mucor, Absidia, Rhizopus,* and *Cunninghamella.* The organisms are essentially nonpathogenic in a healthy host because they are unable to regenerate if ingested by normal macrophages. In the presence of high concentrations of glucose and in an acid environment, however, these fungi grow remarkably rapidly. The process may extend from a small eschar on the nasal septum to the paranasal sinuses, orbit, and brain. The infection erodes into the nerves and blood vessels. It often is lethal. Diagnosis requires aggressive surgical biopsy. Treatment includes vigorous repeated debridement and aggressive antifungal therapy with amphotericin B.

PERSPECTIVE

A patient with diabetes mellitus lives with a number of impositions. Not the least of these is simply having to contend with daily administration of treatment and monitoring therapy while walking the tightrope of metabolic balance. A well-educated patient with type I diabetes who responds appropriately to early cues of impending metabolic decompensation can avert diabetic ketoacidosis. Likewise, the increased susceptibility to infection and the retardation of growth and maturation characteristic of uncontrolled diabetes can be obviated with careful metabolic control. Although the chronic complications of diabetes are related wholly or partly to metabolic control, they remain an immutable threat to persons with diabetes. The leading cause of death among patients with diabetes with onset of disease before age 20 years is diabetic nephropathy. An analysis of mortality factors for patients with diabetes applying for life insurance between 1951 and 1970 revealed an actuarial projection of 33 years' life expectancy from onset of disease if younger than 30 years at onset of disease. It is doubtful that such a bleak projection now applies. Therapy has improved, and there is clearer recognition of the effect of glycemic control on risk of complications and on mortality, which was 2½ times greater in among patients with poorly controlled diabetes than among those with well-controlled disease. With further therapeutic advances likely, one can be optimistic that risk will be lessened further.

Patients with diabetes, particularly those with type I diabetes, still are targets of discrimination in employment. Although there is a rational basis for excluding persons who may have unexpected hypoglycemic episodes from occupations such as commercial pilot or truck driver, patients with diabetes can engage in most occupations successfully and need not be excluded from employment solely because they have diabetes. Educational opportunities for patients with diabetes are unlimited. Patients with diabetes can successfully pursue athletics. Diabetes per se should not be a reason for exclusion from many activities, and a person with diabetes can do almost anything a person without diabetes can with very little restraint, provided attention is paid to not sabotaging diabetes therapy.

Although the threats inherent in diabetes persist, there is reason for optimism that progress in medical research will continue to improve approaches to therapy for diabetes, lessen the impact of the disease, and ultimately eradicate it.

Treatment of patients with diabetes and their families requires that physicians muster all of their skills and resources and that they recruit nurse educators, dietitians, psychologists, and physician assistants to become part of the comprehensive management team. The expenditure of time and effort can be enormous, but the results of such expenditure make it worthwhile.

BIBLIOGRAPHY

Alberti KG, Zimmet PZ. Definition, diagnosis and classification of diabetes mellitus and its complications, I: diagnosis and classification of diabetes mellitus provisional report of a WHO consultation. *Diabet Med* 1998; 15:539–553.

American Diabetes Association. Report of The Expert Committee on the Diagnosis and Classification of Diabetes Mellitus. *Diabetes Care* 1997; 20:1183–1197.

Atkinson MA, Maclaren NK. The pathogenesis of insulin dependent diabetes mellitus. *N Engl J Med* 1994;331:1428–1436.

Bach JF. Insulin-dependent diabetes mellitus as an autoimmune disease. *Endocr Rev* 1994;15:516–542.

Beck-Nielsen H, Groop LC. Metabolic and genetic characterization of prediabetic states: sequence of events leading to non-insulin-dependent diabetes mellitus. *J Clin Invest* 1994;94:1714–1721.

Brownlee M. Lilly Lecture 1993. Glycation and diabetic complications. *Diabetes* 1994;43:836–841.

Clark CM Jr, Lee DA. Prevention and treatment of the complications of diabetes mellitus. *N Engl J Med* 1995;332:1210–1217.

Davis MD. Diabetic retinopathy. A clinical overview. *Diabetes Care* 1992; 15:1844–1874.

DeFronzo RA, Bonadonna RC, Ferrannini E. Pathogenesis of NIDDM: a balanced overview. *Diabetes Care* 1992;15:318–368.

Diabetes Control and Complications Trial Research Group. The effect of intensive treatment of diabetes on the development and progression of long-term complications in insulin-dependent diabetes mellitus. *N Engl J Med* 1993;329:977–986.

Gerich JE. The genetic basis of type II diabetes mellitus: impaired insulin secretion versus impaired insulin sensitivity. *Endocr Rev* 1998;19: 491–503.

Greene DA, Sima AAF, Stevens MJ, et al. Aldose reductase inhibitors: an approach to the treatment of diabetic nerve damage. *Diabetes Metab Rev* 1993;9:189–217.

Hostetter TH. Diabetic nephropathy: metabolic versus hemodynamic considerations. *Diabetes Care* 1992;15:1205–1215.

Kahn CR. Banting Lecture. Insulin action, diabetogenes, and the cause of type II diabetes. *Diabetes* 1994;43:1066–1084.

Klein R. Hyperglycemia and microvascular and macrovascular disease in diabetes. *Diabetes Care* 1995;18:258–268.

Lebovitz H, ed. *Therapy for diabetes mellitus and related disorders,* 3rd ed. Alexandria, VA: American Diabetes Association, 1998.

Nathan DM. Long-term complications of diabetes mellitus. *N Engl J Med* 1993;328:1676–1685.

Ohkubo Y, Kishikawa H, Araki E, et al. The Kumomoto Study: intensive insulin therapy prevents the progression of diabetic microvascular complications in Japanese patients with non-insulin-dependent diabetes mellitus—a randomized prospective 6-year study. *Diabetes Res Clin Pract* 1995;28:103–117.

Permutt MA, Chiu K, Ferrer J, et al. Genetics of type II diabetes. *Recent Prog Horm Res* 1998;53:201–216.

Pugliese A. Unraveling the genetics of insulin-dependent type 1A diabetes: the search must go on. *Diabetes Rev* 1999;7:39.

Rabinovitch A. An update on cytokines in the pathogenesis of insulin-dependent diabetes mellitus. *Diabetes Metab Rev* 1998;14:129–151.

Reichard P, Nilsson BY, Rosenqvist U. The effect of long-term intensified insulin treatment on the development of microvascular complications of diabetes mellitus. *N Engl J Med* 1993;329:304–309.

Rosenbloom AL, Joe JR, Young RS, et al. Emerging epidemic of type II diabetes in youth. *Diabetes Care* 1999;22:345–354.

Skyler JS. Prevention & treatment of diabetes and its complications. *Med Clin North Am* 1998;82:665.

Skyler JS, Marks JB. Immune intervention in type I diabetes mellitus. *Diabetes Rev* 1993;1:15.

Tattersall RB. The quest for normoglycaemia: a historical perspective. *Diabet Med* 1994;11:618–635.

UK Prospective Diabetes Study (UKPDS) Group. Effect of intensive blood glucose control with metformin on complications in overweight patients with type II diabetes (UKPDS 34). *Lancet* 1998;352:854–865.

Vinik AI, Holland MT, LeBeau JM, et al. Diabetic neuropathies. *Diabetes Care* 1992;15:1926–1975.

Yki-Jarvinen H. Glucose toxicity. *Endocr Rev* 1992;13:415–431.

Kelley's Textbook of Internal Medicine, fourth edition. Edited by H. David Humes. Lippincott Williams & Wilkins, Philadelphia © 2000.

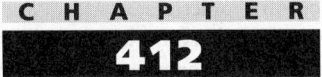

METABOLIC BONE DISEASE

DOLORES SHOBACK
COLEMAN GROSS

NORMAL SKELETON

STRUCTURE

The skeleton is composed of several tissues, including bone, cartilage, and bone marrow. Bone itself is a highly organized and complex connective tissue made up of many cell types and a noncellular matrix (osteoid) rich in collagenous and noncollagenous proteins. Bone is unique among the connective tissues in that it undergoes a regulated and organized process of mineralization. Two principal types of bone are present in the skeleton—cortical and trabecular (also called *cancellous*). Although cortical bone and trabecular bone are composed of the same cellular and noncellular components, there are many differences between the two bone types. Cortical bone is compact mineralized tissue, whereas trabecular bone is composed of a rich latticework of bone struts. The axial skeleton is mainly trabecular bone, and the long bones of the peripheral skeleton are predominantly cortical bone.

FUNCTION

Trabecular bone and cortical bone are made up of the same cellular and noncellular components. The functional differences between these two types of bone are largely related to differences in structure. Cortical bone is highly compact; approximately 90% of its volume is calcified. Only 15% to 25% of the trabecular bone volume is calcified. The mechanical function of the skeleton is to provide sites for ligamentous attachment of muscles and to protect the viscera. The skeleton also serves an important metabolic function. It is the main reservoir for exchangeable calcium, phosphorus, and buffering molecules. The rich latticework of trabecular bone increases the surface area in contact with the marrow space and available for remodeling. As a result trabecular bone is highly metabolically active. Because of its compact structure, cortical bone is less metabolically active than trabecular bone, but it plays a critical mechanical role. Because it constitutes 80% of the skeletal mass, cortical bone makes a substantial contribution to the metabolic activity of the skeleton.

BONE MODELING AND REMODELING

Skeletal growth begins during fetal life and continues through the second decade. The skeleton is modeled by a variety of processes that include endocrine, paracrine, and mechanical factors. Bone formation occurs by means of endochondral ossification at the epiphyseal growth plates in the long bones or by means of intramembranous ossification from mesenchyme in the flat bones such as the skull, ribs, and pelvis.

Even though skeletal growth ceases in adults, bone remodeling continues in a regulated and organized way. The process of remodeling includes cyclic phases of bone resorption and formation. The temporal and spatial coordination of these two phases of the remodeling cycle has been called *coupling*. Under normal physiologic conditions, resorptive activity is essentially equally balanced by formative activity through this coupling mechanism. The relative constancy of bone mass during life under normal steady-state physiologic conditions attests to this fact. The processes that regulate resorptive and formative activities and their coupling are not clearly understood. A growing body of data implicates a large variety of factors, including steroid hormones, peptide hormones, prostaglandins, growth factors, and cytokines.

Osteoblasts are responsible for the production of osteoid and its subsequent mineralization to form new bone. Osteoblasts synthesize and secrete the various substances that compose osteoid, such as collagen. The osteoblast then directs the initial process of mineralization several days after initial deposition of osteoid matrix. During this time, several changes occur in the matrix, such as cross-linking of collagen fibrils, which facilitate the mineralization process. Under normal circumstances, the process of mineralization of newly formed osteoid takes several days. The mineralization lag time can be greatly increased in certain metabolic derangements, such as vitamin D deficiency (see later). The fate of the osteoblast is "sealed"; a large proportion of these cells encase themselves in newly formed mineralized bone and become osteocytes. These cells have numerous processes that penetrate bone within canaliculi. It is thought that these tubules may participate in cell–cell communication, may constitute a nutrient network, and may sense mechanical strain in bone. Another portion of osteoblasts appears to undergo apoptosis, which is a highly regulated process of programmed cell death.

The primary bone-resorbing cell of the skeleton is the osteoclast, a multinucleated giant cell derived from the monocyte-macrophage lineage. Its ability to resorb mineralized bone is the result of several highly specialized characteristics. Activated osteoclasts are polarized such that a portion of their membrane forms a ruffled border, which consists of deep folds of the plasma membrane. This membrane is anchored to the bone surface through specific interactions between integrin receptors in the osteoclast plasma membrane and collagen in bone matrix. Bone is resorbed through the action of hydrogen ions and proteolytic enzymes secreted by the osteoblast into the secondary lysosome formed by the osteoblast membrane on one side and the surface of bone on the other.

Metabolic bone disorders often occur when remodeling activity is altered from underlying pathophysiologic conditions. In healthy persons, the proportion of skeleton undergoing remodeling at any one time is regulated and on the order of 2% to 4%. Removal of old bone is a normal process necessary to maintain the structural integrity of bone. The resorption pit, or Howship's lacuna, is produced by the osteoclast and reaches a depth of approximately 50 μm after 7 to 10 days. After the resorption phase, osteoblasts begin the process of bone formation with the production of matrix, which starts mineralization 10 days later. The process of formation takes 3 to 4 months. The signals responsible for recruitment of osteoblasts to areas of resorption are poorly understood, yet it is clear that this is a tightly regulated process. A variety of signaling molecules have been suggested as potential coupling factors, including the newly described osteoprotegerin and its ligand.

METABOLIC BONE DISEASE

Metabolic bone disease consists of a diverse group of disorders. These conditions arise as a result of disordered bone formation, resorption, or mineralization. Often multiple defects occur as part of the pathophysiologic mechanism of a particular disease. The pattern of defects in any given disease is the result of the initial derangement and the metabolic and hormonal response to it.

The concept of bone turnover is helpful in understanding and categorizing metabolic bone diseases. *Turnover* refers to the balance of rates of formation and resorption. In metabolic disorders of bone, turnover may be increased or decreased often with relative uncoupling of the rates of formation and resorption which leads to increments or decrements in bone mass. Defective mineralization may be the predominant derangement, as in vitamin D deficiency osteomalacia, or it may be a minor histologic feature.

Osteoporosis is the most common metabolic bone disease. It is a multifactorial disease in which bone resorption exceeds formation (see Chapter 465). The focus of this chapter is on the other common forms of metabolic bone disease: osteomalacia, rickets, renal osteodystrophy, Paget's disease, and osteosclerosis.

RICKETS AND OSTEOMALACIA
Definition

Rickets and osteomalacia describe a clinical, radiographic, and histologic phenotype caused by a variety of disorders the patho-

physiologic mechanisms of which decrease mineralization of cartilage and osteoid. Rickets affects children and is caused by abnormal calcification of epiphyseal cartilage and osteoid. Osteomalacia, the counterpart of rickets among adults because of the absence of longitudinal growth, is caused by a defect in mineralization of osteoid.

Incidence and Epidemiology

In the early part of this century, vitamin D deficiency was by far the most common cause of rickets and osteomalacia. Over the last 80 years, rickets and osteomalacia have greatly decreased in incidence in industrialized western countries. This decreased incidence is largely the result of understanding of the role of vitamin D in the prevention of this disease and the fortification of foodstuffs. In the developing world, however, rickets continues to be a serious public health problem. The incidence may be as high as 20%. This high incidence is caused primarily by inadequate access to fortified foods, limited exposure to sunlight because of cultural practices, and dark racial pigmentation that limits cutaneous production of vitamin D. Recent immigrants to western countries may have a high incidence of rickets because of adherence to cultural practices.

In recent years, it has become increasingly appreciated that subclinical vitamin D deficiency is common in western countries, particularly among the elderly. Dietary restrictions (avoidance of dairy products), limited access to nutritious meals, limited mobility, and an age-related decline in cutaneous vitamin D production are contributing factors. Subclinical vitamin D deficiency may have a role in as many as 50% of hip fractures.

With the decrease in incidence of rickets in western nations, attention to other, heretofore less common types of osteomalacia has increased (Table 412.1). These disorders have diverse pathophysiologic mechanisms and include acquired and genetic disorders. Many of these diseases have similar clinical signs and symptoms. The challenge for the clinician is to dissect out the pertinent findings that lead to the precise diagnoses and ultimately to tailored therapy.

Etiology and Pathogenesis

Rickets and osteomalacia are caused by inadequate mineralization of epiphyseal cartilage or bone matrix. The diseases that lead to osteomalacia and rickets are extensive and are listed in Table 412.1. Although the process of mineralization is complex and still poorly understood, it is clear that adequate local concentrations of calcium and phosphorus are an absolute requirement for formation of hydroxyapatite crystals, the predominant form of calcium phosphate in bone. Increasing evidence suggests an important role for osteoblasts in mineralization. Alkaline phosphatase produced locally by osteoblasts cleaves inorganic phosphate from phosphoproteins and pyrophosphate, a natural inhibitor of mineralization. In the process, inorganic phosphate levels are increased locally, and the increase contributes to a milieu conducive to the formation of hydroxyapatite crystals $[Ca_{10}(PO_4)_6(OH)_2]$. Other requirements include a neutral pH and type I collagen that has been properly matured by means of formation of cross-links and other modifications.

TABLE 412.1.	**CAUSES OF RICKETS AND OSTEOMALACIA**

Vitamin D deficiency
  Dietary deficiency
  Ineffective endogenous production
  Loss of vitamin D and metabolites
    Nephrotic syndrome
    Peritoneal dialysis
Calcium deficiency
  Nutritional calcium deficiency
  Dietary calcium binders
    Phytate, chapatti
Vitamin D malabsorption
  Gastrointestinal disorders
    Gastrectomy, partial or total
    Ileojejunal bypass
    Celiac disease
    Inflammatory bowel disease
  Pancreatic insufficiency
  Hepatobiliary disease
    Biliary atresia
    Cholestatic liver disease
    Alcoholic liver disease
    Cirrhosis
  Drugs
    Bile acid sequesterants
Disordered vitamin D metabolism
  Increased catabolism of vitamin D
    metabolites

Phenytoin
Phenobarbital
Impaired 1α-hydroxylation
  Pseudo–vitamin D resistant rickets
  Chronic renal failure
Impaired 25-hydroxylation
  End-stage liver disease
Target tissue resistance to vitamin D
  Hereditary vitamin D–resistant rickets
Phosphate depletion
  Dietary
    Low phosphate intake
    Phosphate binding agents
  Genetic
    X-linked hypophosphatemic rickets or
      osteomalacia
    Hereditary hypophosphatemic rickets
      with hypercalciuria
    Autosomal dominant
      hypophosphatemic rickets
  Acquired
    Tumor-induced osteomalacia
    Sporadic hypophosphatemic
      osteomalacia
Renal disease
  Renal tubular disorders (Fanconi's
    syndrome)

Genetic
  Wilson's disease
  Cystinosis
  Tyrosinemia
Acquired
  Multiple myeloma
  Amyloidosis
  Nephrotic syndrome
Drugs and toxic agents
  Heavy metals
  Ifosfamide
  Mercaptopurine
  Outdated tetracycline
  Aminoglycosides
Osteomalacia of chronic renal disease
Primary mineralization defects
  Hypophosphatasia
  Drugs
    Fluoride
    Etidronate, first-generation
      biphosphonates
Defective bone matrix synthesis
  Fibrogenesis imperfecta ossium
Miscellaneous
  Aluminum bone disease
  Total parenteral nutrition

Other noncollagenous proteins also may play an important role in the regulation of mineralization. The elongated hydroxyapatite crystals are deposited linearly along collagen fibrils. Diminished supply of either calcium or phosphorus limits normal mineralization. Under such conditions, osteoid is no longer mineralized at the normal rate, and the amount of osteoid that accumulates and covers the surface of bone increases. The histomorphometric appearance indicates prolongation of mineralization lag time—the time required for mineralization of newly formed osteoid (Fig. 412.1).

Although increased amounts of osteoid may be present in states of high bone turnover, such as hyperthyroidism and hyperparathyroidism, because of accelerated bone formation, the presence of defective mineralization occurs only in osteomalacia. In addition to the presence of increased osteoid, the diagnosis of osteomalacia also requires abnormal mineralization. A presumptive diagnosis of osteomalacia can be based on clinical and laboratory findings (see later). Establishing the presence of this condition often necessitates histologic examination of a bone biopsy specimen.

Vitamin D has long been thought to play a central role in mineralization of bone and thus prevention of osteomalacia and rickets. More specifically, the active hormonal form of vitamin D, 1,25-dihydroxyvitamin D ($1,25(OH)_2D_3$ or calcitriol), has been thought to have a central role in mineralization. Recent evidence from a variety of sources suggests that vitamin D may play a more permissive role in mineralization and may act predominantly by increasing intestinal absorption of calcium and phosphorus and enhancing mineralization. Children with a genetic form of rickets due to mutations in the nuclear receptor for vitamin D may have their bony abnormalities cured with intravenous infusions of calcium. The bony abnormalities associated in the vitamin D receptor gene disruption mouse model likewise may be rescued by a high calcium diet. Calcium treatment of children with nutritional rickets has been shown to be as effective as vitamin D and calcium. These data do not diminish the importance of vitamin D in bone homeostasis but indicate a complex and somewhat redundant system reminiscent of other hormonal axes.

Clinical Findings

Rickets generally becomes apparent by the age of 2 years. The children have short stature, delayed motor development, and skeletal abnormalities. Hypotonia and proximal muscle weakness may be present, and children often are listless and irritable. Tetany may be caused by profound hypocalcemia.

Because rachitic bones are soft, they bow under mechanical loads. This causes the typical deformities of the long bones—bowed legs (genu varum) and knock-knees (genu valgum). A characteristic prominence of the costochondral junction, the rachitic rosary, may be caused by widening of the growth plate of the anterior ribs. Because of chest wall deformities and muscle weakness, respiratory compromise and pneumonia can occur in severe cases of rickets. Calvarial deformities also can occur; they include softening of the skull (craniotabes), frontal bossing, and basilar invagination.

The clinical findings of osteomalacia are more subtle than

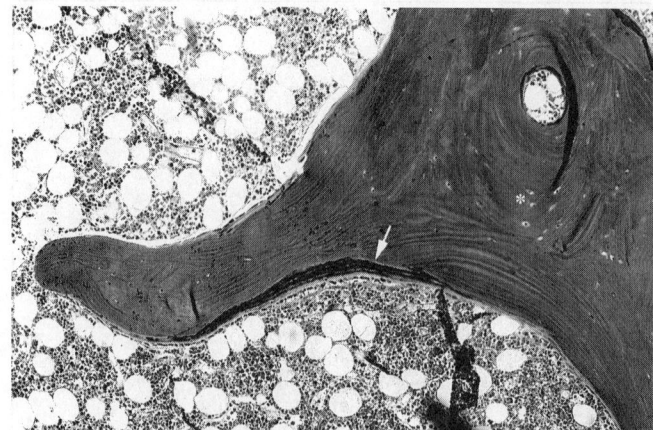

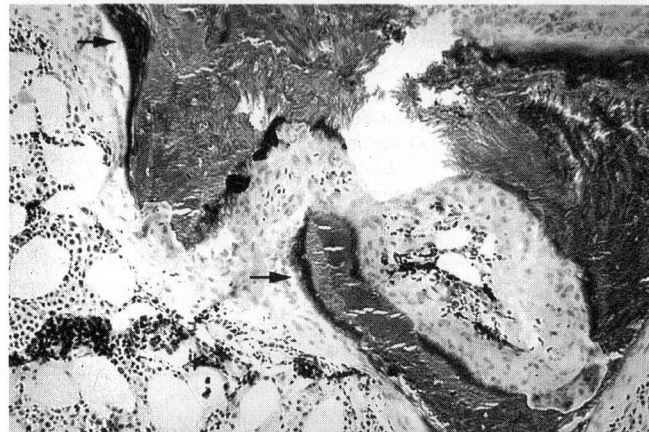

FIGURE 412.1. Specimen of trabecular bone, Goldner stain. *Top,* Normal bone. *Arrowhead* indicates osteoid, which appears darker than mineralized bone in black and white photograph. Goldner staining makes mineralized bone appear green, and unmineralized bone, orange. *Asterisk* indicates a collection of osteocytes. Cuboidal osteoblasts are visible along the mineralizing surface. Lamellar organization of bone is apparent. *Bottom,* biopsy specimen shows findings of osteomalacia with widened osteoid seams (*arrowhead*) that cover a larger amount of bone surfaces than normal.

those of rickets. Bone pain and proximal muscle weakness may predominate. Pressure on bony areas may elicit tenderness. Lower back pain is a common symptom of osteomalacia, and spinal abnormalities such as absence of normal lordosis may occur. A waddling gait may be caused by weakness and bony abnormalities, which can include the pelvis. In severe cases, hypocalcemia can occur and cause paresthesia and tetany.

Radiographic Findings

The characteristic radiologic findings of rickets are caused by disordered mineralization in the hypertrophic zone of epiphyseal cartilage. The expansion of cells in this zone widens the growth plate. Inadequate mineralization produces irregular margins at the metaphysis and causes a frayed appearance on radiographs. Cupping of the metaphysis can be caused by continued expansion of the cartilaginous growth plate into the soft metaphysis,

and metaphyseal widening occurs (Fig. 412.2). The epiphyseal bone also may have a similar appearance with irregular edges. These abnormalities are most common in areas of greatest growth, such as the knees, wrist, anterior ribs, proximal femur, and distal tibia. The bones usually are osteopenic. Because of weakness, bowing deformities may occur and predominate in the weight-bearing bones. Scoliosis may be present, as may slipped epiphyses, protrusio acetabuli, and a triradiate pelvis. Other radiographic changes include characteristic osteomalacic changes in mature bone (see later).

The radiographic findings of osteomalacia are caused by excessive amounts of poorly mineralized osteoid. Lucent areas that appear as linear areas of rarefaction perpendicular to the cortical surface of the bone may be present and are known as *Looser's zones* or *pseudofractures* (Fig. 412.2). These areas are caused by accumulation of osteoid, often are symmetric, and occur at the medial aspect of long bones such as the femur near the femoral head or neck. Trabecular bone may appear to be coarsened and fuzzy. Vertebral collapse can occur and produce a biconcave appearance (codfish deformity) caused by pressure exerted by the intervertebral disks. Softening of the bone may cause basilar invagination, protrusio acetabuli, and a triradiate pelvis. In general, the bones are osteopenic and susceptible to fracture. Skeletal changes of secondary hyperparathyroidism such as brown tumors of osteitis fibrosa cystica may be seen.

Laboratory Findings

The laboratory findings of rickets and osteomalacia reflect the underlying pathophysiologic condition. A useful framework is to consider the abnormalities associated with the calciopenic and phosphopenic disorders. The calciopenic disorders are largely caused by nutritional deficiencies of calcium, vitamin D, or both or by inborn errors of vitamin D metabolism. Characteristic of these conditions are frankly low or low normal serum calcium and phosphate concentrations. In the presence of vitamin D deficiency, 25-hydroxyvitamin D (25-OHD) levels are low. Although 25-OHD levels of 4 ng per milliliter or less can cause osteomalacia, levels in the lower range of normal can be associated with histologic evidence of osteomalacia. Because of an increase in renal 1α-hydroxylase activity due to low serum levels of phosphorus or compensatory increases in parathyroid hormone (PTH) levels, serum levels of calcitriol are typically normal. In severe vitamin D deficiency, in which 25-OHD is very limited, calcitriol levels may be low. The compensatory normalization of calcitriol levels and elevated PTH level may result in normal serum calcium and low serum phosphate levels, which may contribute to osteomalacia (see later). The bone-specific isoform of alkaline phosphatase is elevated in both rickets and osteomalacia.

Phosphopenic disorders usually are caused by primary or secondary renal defects that cause abnormal transport of phosphate in the nephron and thus cause phosphate wasting. These disorders include X-linked hypophosphatemic rickets, Fanconi's syndrome, and tumor-induced osteomalacia. Renal phosphate wasting leads to hypophosphatemia. Serum levels of calcium, PTH, and 25-OHD are characteristically normal. Levels of calcitriol

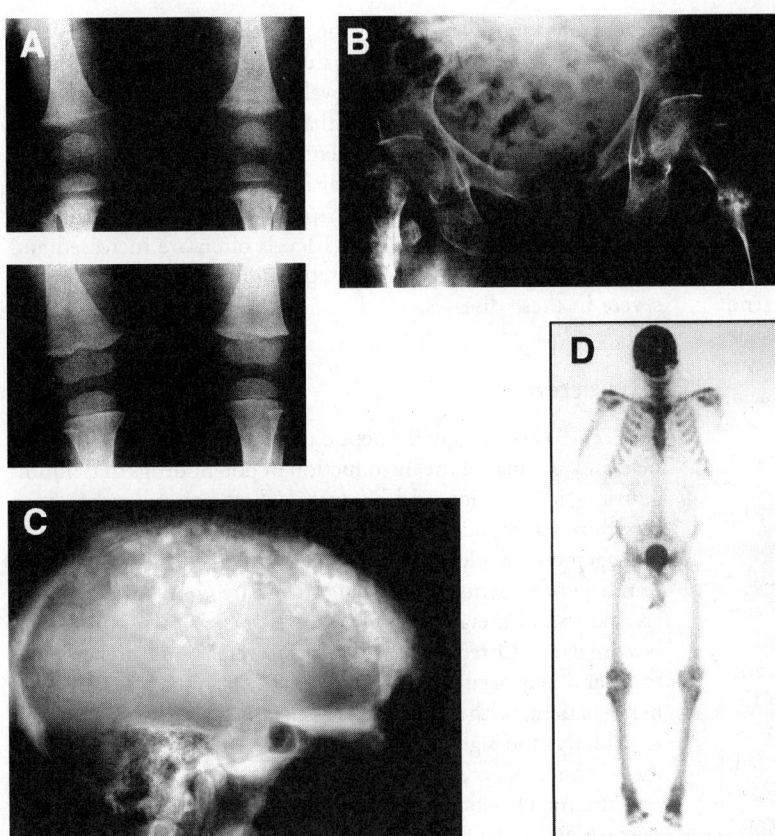

FIGURE 412.2. Radiographic findings in metabolic bone disorders. **A:** Epiphyseal fraying, cupping, and widening in rickets. **B:** Pseudofracture (Looser's zone) of the femur in osteomalacia. **C:** Cotton wool appearance and osteoporosis circumscripta in the skull in Paget's disease. **D:** Bone scintigraphy in Paget's disease showing increased uptake in the skull and spine.

also are within the normal range. They are said to be inappropriately normal because of the attendant hypophosphatemia, which normally increases renal 1α-hydroxylase activity and raises calcitriol levels (see later).

Strategies for Optimal Care

Therapy for rickets and osteomalacia depends on an accurate diagnosis of the particular disease or syndrome that causes the skeletal abnormalities. When possible, efforts should be to remove or ameliorate precipitating causes of the disease. This is not always possible, because the etiologic factor can be elusive, genetic, or structural. Several syndromes may necessitate adjunctive surgical procedures to restore function. Many of the diseases that cause rickets or osteomalacia necessitate treatment with high doses of vitamin D, calcium, or phosphorus, and toxicities may occur in the course of therapy. To limit toxicity, pharmacologic intervention should be initiated at low doses and titrated upward guided by biochemical measurements, such as serum levels of vitamin D metabolites and PTH. The length of treatment can vary from a few months to a lifetime and must be based on the underlying pathophysiologic mechanism and clinical response.

RACHITIC AND OSTEOMALACIC DISORDERS
Vitamin D Deficiency

Natural sources of vitamin D are mainly limited to fish liver products and egg yolks. Fortified dairy products, however, are

the main sources of dietary vitamin D. The best measure of nutritional vitamin D status is serum level of 25-OHD, the main circulating vitamin D metabolite. In general, rickets or osteomalacia is associated with a decrease in 25-OHD level to less than 5 ng per milliliter. At this level, other associated metabolic derangements are present, including secondary hyperparathyroidism and decreased serum calcium levels. Levels of 25-OHD toward the lower end of the normal range (10 to 20 ng per milliliter) also may be associated with the histologic changes of osteomalacia. Numerous commercial clinical laboratories provide reliable assays for measuring this vitamin D metabolite, thus making a diagnosis of vitamin D deficiency straightforward.

Several therapeutic regimens for rickets and osteomalacia have been evaluated and found to be effective. Vitamin D (ergocalciferol or cholecalciferol) is the agent of choice. Therapy usually consists of 5,000 to 15,000 international units (IU) of vitamin D daily for 3 or 4 weeks. Normalization of calcium, phosphorus, and PTH levels occurs within a few weeks, as does evidence of healing of rickets. Other changes, such as elevations in alkaline phosphatase level, may lag. Oral doses of vitamin D at higher doses once a month or periodic intramuscular injections are used less frequently, and only in specific cases. Once vitamin D stores have been normalized, adequate maintenance therapy should be supplied (400 IU daily or greater). Adults with osteomalacia likewise should have vitamin D stores normalized to effect a cure. Adequate vitamin D supplementation (400 to 800 IU per day) can be effective in preventing bone loss and fracture among elderly persons at risk of vitamin D deficiency. Calcium supplementation also should be provided.

Nutritional Calcium Deficiency

It has become increasingly clear that dietary calcium deficiency may cause rickets and osteomalacia. Both environmental and dietary practices, such as vegetarianism, contribute to low calcium intake and absorption, particularly among some African and Asian populations. The diets of these cultural groups tend to be low in calcium but may be rich in substances that interfere with the absorption of calcium, such as phytate. Unlike persons with the vitamin D deficiency form of rickets and osteomalacia, those with calcium-deficiency rickets often have normal or near normal levels of 25-OHD. Serum calcium level is frankly low among these patients, and there is a compensatory increase in PTH level. Serum phosphorus level is variable and may not be decreased as it is in vitamin D deficiency rickets. Urinary excretion of calcium is low. It has been suggested that the muscular weakness associated with vitamin D deficiency is absent in calcium-deficiency rickets. Patients with this condition have radiographic evidence of osteopenia and hyperparathyroidism and have the typical metaphyseal changes of children, although the latter finding is variable. Management of this form of rickets or osteomalacia is centered on restoring calcium balance to normal. Vitamin D replacement is advisable (400 to 800 IU daily) to enhance calcium absorption, although recent evidence indicates healing of rickets with calcium supplementation alone.

Vitamin D Malabsorption

Severe gastrointestinal and hepatobiliary diseases may cause malabsorption of vitamin D. As a result of impaired mucosal integrity or biliary function, the lipid-soluble vitamin is poorly absorbed from the proximal small intestine, and osteomalacia may develop. Because substantial amounts of vitamin D are derived from cutaneous synthesis, malabsorption of vitamin D plays a lesser role in vitamin D economy. Other factors associated with these diseases may limit a person's exposure to sunlight, and dietary sources of vitamin D become more important. In such a scenario, malabsorption of limited dietary vitamin D plays a greater role in leading to metabolic bone disease.

It had been thought that impairment of enterohepatic circulation of vitamin D was the putative factor leading to vitamin D deficiency and osteomalacia in these disorders. Now, however, the etiologic importance of such a circulatory route is being questioned. Although metabolites of vitamin D can be recirculated, they are largely inactive. It is more likely that biliary secretion of vitamin D is the main excretory pathway for this molecule and limits toxicity from high doses of vitamin D. Another alternative mechanism is that increased production of calcitriol increases turnover of 25-OHD and eventually exhausts this substrate for the production of active hormone. In this scenario, vitamin D malabsorption decreases 25-OHD and calcitriol levels, decreases intestinal calcium absorption, and causes secondary hyperparathyroidism. The increase in PTH level accelerates calcitriol synthesis from the limited substrate 25-OHD and stimulates catabolism of 25-OHD. Although calcium absorption improves temporarily, ultimately the active hormone, calcitriol, becomes insufficient for adequate calcium and phosphorus absorption, and osteomalacia develops. Potential problems with this construct include the fact that calcitriol levels circulate at 1/100th to 1/1,000th the concentration of 25-OHD and that calcitriol levels often are normal in persons with osteomalacia caused by gastrointestinal and hepatobiliary diseases. Whatever the proximate mechanism, PTH levels often are increased and the effects of secondary hyperparathyroidism on the skeleton are severe in these diseases.

Gastrectomy

In recent years therapy for peptic ulcer disease has changed dramatically because of the introduction of potent drugs that inhibit gastric acid secretion and because *Helicobacter pylori* has been recognized as an etiologic agent. As a result, the role of surgical management of ulcer disease is decreasing. Nonetheless, large numbers of patients have undergone gastrectomy and are at increased risk of metabolic bone disease, such as osteoporosis and osteomalacia. Osteomalacia develops several years after gastrectomy and may occur among as many as 20% of patients. Because many patients with bone disease associated with gastric resection are elderly, the signs and symptoms often are complicated by the presence of osteoporosis.

Vitamin D deficiency, secondary hyperparathyroidism, and calcium malabsorption have pathophysiologic roles in the development of osteomalacia after gastrectomy. Therapy should be directed at normalizing the biochemical abnormalities. Vitamin D may have to be supplemented at high oral doses (1,000 to 5,000 IU daily) to overcome limited absorption. An alternative is parenteral administration of vitamin D. Levels of 25-OHD should be maintained in the normal range with such therapy. Calcium should be supplemented at 1 to 2 g daily. Adequate vitamin D and calcium nutrition can be gauged by following the decline of elevated PTH levels to normal. When osteoporosis coexists, antiresorptive therapy with a second-generation bisphosphonate can be considered. Intravenous dosing may be needed because of the inherently poor absorption of these agents.

Ileojejunal Bypass

Ileojejunal bypass surgery has been used to manage morbid obesity. This procedure is associated with several morbidities, including osteomalacia, which may develop after several years. Absorption of calcium and vitamin D, which occurs in the proximal small intestine, is disturbed, and the disturbance contributes to the development of osteomalacia. Management is similar to that of postgastrectomy osteomalacia, but parenteral administration of therapeutic agents is necessary more often because of the absence of functional proximal small intestine.

Celiac Disease

It is now appreciated that celiac disease is commonly associated with decreased bone mass and osteoporosis. As many as 26% to 36% of persons with celiac sprue may have osteoporosis, and many patients with osteoporosis have asymptomatic sprue. Because of the involvement of the duodenum and jejunum, vitamin D malabsorption can cause osteomalacia. Defective calcium absorption also is caused by vitamin D deficiency and villous atrophy. Levels of 25-OHD are low among persons with osteomalacia, but not all persons with sprue and low bone mass have frank vitamin D deficiency. Secondary hyperparathyroidism usually is present. Management of the underlying condition with a gluten-free diet should resolve the metabolic abnormalities of vitamin D absorption. Some patients may remain in a state of secondary hyperparathyroidism, indicating a defect in calcium absorption. If metabolic derangements persist after gluten restriction, vitamin D and calcium supplementation may be necessary. PTH may be a guide to monitoring of therapy.

Inflammatory Bowel Disease

Metabolic bone disease is associated more commonly with Crohn's disease than it is with ulcerative colitis because of the relative sparing of the small intestine in the latter disease. Nonetheless, glucocorticoids used in the management of both conditions may cause osteoporosis. Even in the absence of glucocorticoid therapy, osteoporosis is common in Crohn's disease. It may occur among as many as 30% of persons with this disease. Because the proximal small bowel commonly is affected, malabsorption of vitamin D and calcium occur in Crohn's disease and may cause osteomalacia. Levels of 25-OHD are low in approximately 65% of patients with Crohn's disease and can be in the osteomalacic range (≤ 10 ng per milliliter) in as many as 25% of patients. Persons who undergo small-bowel resection may have additional derangements in vitamin D and calcium absorption that complicate their care. Patients with osteomalacia from inflammatory bowel disease should be treated in the same way as those with other skeletal disorders due to gastrointestinal diseases.

Hepatic Osteodystrophy

Metabolic bone disease is common among patients with hepatic diseases such as cholestatic liver disease, especially primary biliary cirrhosis, alcoholic liver disease, and chronic active hepatitis. The most common abnormality is osteoporosis. However, osteomalacia can occur with primary biliary cirrhosis and alcoholic liver disease. Biliary atresia has been reported to cause rickets among children. Bile facilitates absorption of vitamin D, and disruption of the enterohepatic circulation of vitamin D has been suggested to be the cause of the low 25-OHD levels that sometimes are encountered (see earlier). The 25-hydroxylation of vitamin D, which occurs in hepatocytes, is maintained until very late in the stage of hepatic disease and likely does not have a central role in the pathophysiologic mechanism of hepatic osteodystrophy. The use of cholestyramine decreases the availability of vitamin D by binding the vitamin in the intestine. Decreased cutaneous synthesis of vitamin D, because of jaundice and avoidance of sunlight, also may contribute to vitamin D deficiency. Persons with alcoholism may have poor overall nutrition and vitamin D deficiency. Management of osteomalacia should be directed at correcting the vitamin D deficiency by means of supplementa-

tion with vitamin D or one of its hydroxylated metabolites. 25-OHD is more polar that vitamin D and is more readily absorbed. It may be useful in some cases. Serum 25-OHD levels should be maintained in the normal range (20 to 45 ng per milliliter) with either form of vitamin D therapy. Adequate calcium nutrition should be supplied with supplements if necessary.

Disorders of Vitamin D Metabolism

Drugs

Commonly used medications may interfere with the absorption and metabolism of vitamin D and contribute to vitamin D deficiency and metabolic bone disease. Bile acid sequestrants such as cholestyramine impede vitamin D absorption. Use of these agents to treat persons otherwise not at risk of vitamin D deficiency and osteomalacia is not be expected to cause clinically significant deficiency. Other agents may interfere with vitamin D metabolism primarily by increasing its catabolism. The anticonvulsants phenytoin and phenobarbital induce hepatic cytochrome P450 enzymes, which catabolize 25-OHD. Osteomalacia and rickets have been reported to occur among patients living in institutions who take these drugs and have been associated with increased fracture risk during seizures. On the other hand, osteomalacia rarely is a complication of outpatient anticonvulsant therapy. Nonetheless, monitoring 25-OHD levels for patients taking phenytoin or phenobarbital is prudent, and vitamin D supplementation should be considered.

Pseudo–Vitamin D Deficiency Rickets

Also called *vitamin D–dependent rickets type I,* pseudo–vitamin D deficiency rickets is caused by an inborn error of metabolism in which 25-OHD is not converted to the active hormonal form of vitamin D, calcitriol. The gene encoding 25-hydroxyvitamin D 1α-hydroxylase, the enzyme responsible for this conversion, has been cloned. Mutations have been identified in this gene in families with this disease, confirming the molecular pathogenesis of this disorder long predicted with clinical observation. The genetic defect is transmitted as an autosomal recessive trait, and affected children are homozygous for mutations in the 1α-hydroxylase gene. At an early age these children come to medical attention with hypocalcemia, secondary hyperparathyroidism, and rickets. Growth retardation, hypotonia, tetany, and respiratory compromise may complicate the clinical course. Serum 25-OHD levels are normal in untreated patients, and calcitriol levels are very low. PTH level is elevated to compensate for hypocalcemia and the low calcitriol level, which has an inhibitory effect on PTH secretion. Normal replacement doses of calcitriol (0.25 to 1.0 μg daily) are sufficient to manage the bone disease.

Hereditary Vitamin D–Resistant Rickets

Hereditary vitamin D–resistant rickets, also called *vitamin D–dependent rickets type II,* manifests in a manner similar to that of pseudo–vitamin D deficiency rickets. In contrast to children with pseudo–vitamin D deficiency rickets. The patient is resistant to calcitriol because of mutations in the gene that codes for the nuclear vitamin D receptor. As a result, these persons have cellular resistance to vitamin D at the target tissue level (e.g., intestine, kidney) and cannot respond to even supraphysiologic doses of calcitriol. Affected persons are homozygous for the autosomal trait and often are the products of consanguineous parents. Children come to medical attention at an early age with hypocalcemia and rickets. Tetany, muscular weakness, and dental abnormalities occur as they do in pseudo–vitamin D deficiency rickets. Alopecia totalis often occurs, but the pathogenesis is not understood. Unlike in pseudo–vitamin D deficiency rickets, in hereditary vitamin D–resistant rickets, calcitriol levels are elevated if the person is not treated. This finding reflects the increase in 25-hydroxyvitamin D 1α-hydroxylase activity in response to hyperparathyroidism and hypophosphatemia. Some patients with this disorder have responded to treatment with very high doses of vitamin D (40,000 IU vitamin D, 20 μg calcitriol daily) indicating a milder defect in the vitamin D receptor than is present in patients who do not respond to any amount of the vitamin. High-dose oral calcium (3 to 4 g daily) or long-term intravenous infusion of calcium has been shown to improve clinical status.

Phosphate Depletion

Chronic phosphate depletion may cause rickets and osteomalacia. Although hypophosphatemia can be caused by decreases in intake or absorption or by increases in urinary losses, metabolic bone disease caused by disordered phosphate economy usually is caused by defects in renal proximal tubular function. These diseases may be caused by a congenital or an acquired defect, which causes renal phosphate wasting and hypophosphatemia. Unlike the calciopenic causes of rickets and osteomalacia, the hypophosphatemic disorders are characterized by the absence of secondary hyperparathyroidism among untreated persons. Patients also may have quantitatively normal bone mass, but because of the mineralization defect, the skeleton is susceptible to deformity and fracture. Table 412.1 lists disorders of phosphate depletion that cause metabolic bone disease.

X-linked Hypophosphatemic Rickets

X-linked hypophosphatemic rickets, also called *hypophosphatemic vitamin D–resistant rickets* is inherited as an X-linked dominant trait. The disease is most robustly expressed among hemizygous boys who come to medical attention with impaired growth, rachitic skeletal deformities, and hypophosphatemia. The patients usually have hypophosphatemia at birth. Skeletal deformities usually develop later, when the child begins weight bearing. The expression of the disease is quite variable. It ranges from isolated hypophosphatemia to severe rickets and osteomalacia. Among untreated persons, serum levels of 25-OHD are normal, and levels of calcitriol are low-normal. Because of hypophosphatemia, which would otherwise induce 1α-hydroxylase, calcitriol concentrations are inappropriately normal among these patients. This suggests abnormal regulation of 1α-hydroxylase, which is an important aspect of this disease. A large body of work with HYP mice, a murine homologue of this disease, has greatly contributed to an improved understanding of the patho-

genesis of X-linked hypophosphatemia and phosphate conservation.

Genetic linkage studies and positional cloning strategies have led to the isolation of a candidate gene called *PEX* or *PHEX.* Mutations in the human gene have been identified among persons with X-linked hypophosphatemia. The gene codes for a membrane-bound endopeptidase. It has been suggested that this enzyme is normally responsible for proteolytic inactivation of a phosphate-lowering factor called *phosphotonin.* Among persons with X-linked hypophosphatemia, the *PHEX* gene product does not function normally and is unable to inactivate phosphotonin, and renal phosphate wasting occurs. This hypothesis is being addressed in several laboratories. Sporadic mutations may cause a nonfamilial form of X-linked hypophosphatemia. Similar disorders, such as hereditary hypophosphatemic rickets with hypercalciuria and autosomal dominant hypophosphatemic rickets, have similar physiologic mechanisms.

Tumor-induced Osteomalacia

Several patients have been described who had hypophosphatemia, hyperphosphaturia, and osteomalacia that reversed after resection of a tumor. These tumors were generally of mesenchymal origin, were benign, and often had vascular features. In rare instances the syndrome has been reported to be part of a paraneoplastic process associated with breast cancer, prostate cancer, small-cell carcinoma, and hematologic malignant disease. As in X-linked hypophosphatemia, the tubular maximum for phosphate reabsorption is abnormally reduced, and the deficiency causes renal phosphate wasting and hypophosphatemia. Patients often have bone pain, muscle weakness, and fractures. Rickets and decreased growth velocities may be present in children. The diagnosis may be delayed for several years because of the lack of awareness of the syndrome, small size and obscure location of the tumor, such as popliteal or nasopharyngeal tumors. Most patients are middle-aged when the condition is diagnosed; however, persons of any age can be affected. The diagnosis of this condition is confirmed when hypophosphatemia and osteomalacia reverse after resection of the tumor. A phosphaturic substance from tumor tissue of patients with this disorder has been isolated and partially characterized as a polypeptide. It is believed that tumor tissue in this disease is responsible for ectopic production of phosphatonin, which increases the phosphate excretion that underlies the pathophysiologic mechanisms of this disorder.

Fanconi's Syndrome

Fanconi's syndrome is generalized tubulopathy that occurs in association with inherited metabolic disorders or is acquired as the result of a toxic insult to the proximal nephron. Offending agents include toxic protein products associated with diseases such as amyloidosis, nephrotic syndrome, and myeloma; heavy metal exposure; and various drugs such as ifosfamide, aminoglycosides, and mercaptopurine. The tubulopathy of this disorder is characterized by phosphate wasting; defective reabsorption of glucose, amino acids, bicarbonate, uric acid; and proteinuria. Calcium also may be excreted in excess. Hyperphosphaturia, which leads to hypophosphatemia, may end in osteomalacia. Attendant acidosis and hypercalciuria also have a detrimental effect on the skeleton. In some forms of the syndrome, levels of calcitriol are low or low-normal, which may signify abnormal 1α-hydroxylase regulation reminiscent of X-linked hypophosphatemia.

Strategies for Optimal Care

Therapy for tumor-induced osteomalacia centers on resection of the tumor. Calcitriol and phosphate supplementation may be a useful adjunct until the tumor is removed. For Fanconi's syndrome, the offending agent is removed if possible. Often the syndrome is not reversible. Therapy should provide oral phosphate supplementation of 1 to 4 g per day in divided doses with a neutral phosphate preparation. If levels of calcitriol are inappropriate, supplementation with calcitriol is advisable. Acidosis should be controlled. These measures often improve the clinical signs and symptoms of metabolic bone disease. Therapy for X-linked hypophosphatemia among children centers on phosphate supplementation. This usually requires 1 to 3 g of phosphorus a day in several divided doses. Vitamin D also is given, primarily as a means to prevent hypocalcemia from the increased phosphate load and to prevent secondary hyperparathyroidism. Calcitriol is the preferred form of vitamin D, and generally is provided at 1 to 3 μg daily. Because of concern about nephrocalcinosis with this regimen, periodic renal ultrasonography and urinary calcium measurements are prudent. Therapy often is associated with improvement in signs and symptoms. Improving growth rates is an important therapeutic end point. Recent data suggest a benefit from recombinant human growth hormone therapy. The importance of continuing therapy through adult life is debatable, but therapy probably provides ongoing skeletal benefit.

RENAL OSTEODYSTROPHY

Definition

Uremic osteodystrophy represents the inevitable skeletal complications of end-stage renal disease. Because patients are surviving for many more years because of improvements in dialysis techniques and medical management, nearly all patients with chronic renal failure encounter some form of skeletal complications. Uremic osteodystrophy comprises the syndromes of secondary hyperparathyroidism, osteomalacia, aluminum overload, adynamic bone disease, and mixed lesions.

Incidence and Epidemiology

Uremic osteodystrophy is a common metabolic complication of uremia. All patients in whom renal functional capacity begins to decline experience the skeletal consequences of the reduced capacity to excrete dietary phosphate and ability to make the active form of vitamin D, calcitriol. The different clinical characteristics of an individual patient influence the type of presentation and the underlying histologic lesions present.

Etiology and Pathogenesis

Broadly defined, uremic osteodystrophy comprises high- and low-turnover forms of bone disease. The pathogenetic mechanisms responsible for the wide spectrum of bone histomorphometric findings and clinical and laboratory alterations in the forms of renal bone disease are complex. These mechanisms include the following physiologic derangements directly or indirectly caused by decreases in renal mass and function.

Phosphate Retention

Declining nephron function causes inability to excrete dietary phosphorus, a predominant component of dietary protein. This is evident as soon as renal function decreases to a glomerular filtration rate less than 50 mL per minute. As serum phosphate level increases, serum calcium level declines, and the serum calcium deficiency stimulates PTH secretion to maintain serum calcium homeostasis. The eventual result of hyperphosphatemia is the development of secondary hyperparathyroidism.

Calcitriol Deficiency

As glomerular filtration rate decreases to less than about 40 mL per minute, the ability of the kidney to produce calcitriol declines. This is further exacerbated by hyperphosphatemia, which suppresses calcitriol formation. The calcitriol deficiency impairs intestinal calcium absorption, which further decreases calcium availability.

Secondary Hyperparathyroidism

Low serum calcium concentrations and the calcitriol deficiency promote PTH secretion and parathyroid gland hyperplasia. Under normal physiologic circumstances, calcitriol exerts a negative effect on the transcription and translation of the PTH gene. Once parathyroid gland mass expands chronically, the calcium-nonsuppressible component of PTH secretion becomes progressively dominant. As the parathyroid glands grow, nodular hyperplasia can occur, as can clonal outgrowths of nodules that express mutations in growth-controlling genes such as cyclins.

Aluminum Accumulation

The aluminum present in dialysate and in phosphate-binding antacids can accumulate in bone along mineralizing surfaces and in parathyroid tissue. Aluminum accumulation in bone suppresses bone formation and produces a low turnover state. In the parathyroid glands, this impairs hormone secretion. The deficiency of PTH, which stimulates bone formation, is considered to be a key etiologic factor in low turnover states.

Acidosis

Progressive renal dysfunction is accompanied by the inability to buffer endogenously generated acid. Bone, because it is a reservoir of ions, is affected by acidosis. Physicochemical dissolution of bone matrix occurs and releases bicarbonate, carbonate, and phosphate anions as well positively charged calcium ions. Bone mineral is progressively lost if acidosis is not addressed through dialysis or dietary supplementation.

Resistance to Parathyroid Hormone

Resistance to parathyroid hormone has been ascribed to the chronically high levels of PTH resulting from the other derangements in mineral metabolism (hypocalcemia and perhaps phosphate retention) that accompany uremia. PTH receptors in bone are thought to be down-regulated by the chronically high hormone levels.

Other Uremic Toxins

In addition to aluminum, iron deposits can be present in the bone of uremic patients and have been implicated in the pathogenesis of low-turnover bone disease. Iron deposits in the parathyroid gland may induce a state of PTH insufficiency. Patients with diabetes mellitus, without stainable aluminum or iron, often have low-turnover bone disease. The pathogenesis of this condition is unknown, although roles for hyperglycemia and PTH suppression have been suggested. Deposition of β-2-amyloid can occur in patients uremia, especially after many years of dialysis, and predisposes these persons to fractures, bone cysts, arthropathy, and carpal tunnel syndrome.

High-turnover bone disease, the classic skeletal lesion of uremia, typically manifests in its early stages with mild secondary hyperparathyroidism. It progresses, if unaddressed, to full-blown osteitis fibrosa cystica. Along with this progression is a steady increase in serum intact PTH levels. The pathogenetic mechanisms cited earlier likely contribute to the development of this disorder along with a decrease in the number of calcitriol receptors in uremic parathyroid tissue.

Low-turnover bone disease in uremia can have several causes, such as aluminum intoxication. Because aluminum has been eliminated from dialysates, and long-term therapy with aluminum-containing antacids is rarely used, this form of low-turnover bone disease is now rare. In the past, before the central role of the kidney in the production of calcitriol was appreciated, patients with low-turnover bone disease had osteomalacia caused by vitamin D deficiency. The last type of low-turnover disease is an adynamic bone lesion of unknown causation. This form of low turnover often is associated with diabetes mellitus and is more common among elderly persons undergoing long-term dialysis than it is among other persons.

Mixed uremic osteodystrophy is a combination of low- and high-turnover bone lesions. The pathogenesis is uncertain. One suggestion has been that dietary deficiencies of calcium and phosphate can alter the composition of the bone formed. In such a situation, even under the influence of secondary hyperparathyroidism, the bone matrix is undermineralized. The appearance of the bone biopsy specimen in such a would include features of high-turnover bone disease along with poorly mineralized osteoid, which is characteristic of low turnover. Some patients with mixed lesions may have partially treated examples of both aluminum toxicity and secondary hyperparathyroidism.

Clinical Findings

Differentiating low- from high-turnover renal bone disease on the basis of clinical findings is challenging. Patients with most forms of renal osteodystrophy may have bone pain, weakness, and fractures. Bone pain occurs especially in the lower extremities and with weight bearing. Especially in cases of osteomalacia and low turnover, the muscle weakness accompanying renal osteodystrophy can be profound. That along with the bone pain can produce a waddling gait and great difficulty with walking. Patients with secondary hyperparathyroidism, especially in its severe forms, may report intractable itching. Depending on the magnitude of the calcium to phosphate product, especially if greater than 70, persons with uremia may have ectopic calcifications. These can occur in any soft-tissue site, including the periarticular areas, lung, and heart and can be painful and even life threatening depending on the location. The most severe form of ectopic calcification is calciphylaxis. This condition usually affects the digits, is caused by severe vascular calcification, and can cause ischemic necrosis of the involved digits. Fractures also can occur in any form of renal osteodystrophy, especially if it is severe. In osteomalacia and low-turnover bone disease, pseudofractures can be present (Fig. 412.2). Any site weakened by high-turnover bone disease or replaced by cystic lesions or fibrous tissue instead of normal bone can fracture with minimal trauma.

Laboratory Findings

The laboratory abnormalities in a given patient with uremic bone disease reflect the duration of chronic renal failure, the therapy used, and the underlying bone histologic lesions present. Patients with uremia may have reduced serum levels of total and ionized calcium, especially after many years of renal failure, when resistance to PTH and decreased production and action of calcitriol are evident. Hypocalcemia often occurs with severe secondary hyperparathyroidism before dialysis and therapy become effective. Because of underlying parathyroid hyperplasia and autonomy, some patients have hypercalcemia after dialysis becomes effective. Patients with low-turnover bone disease often maintain normal calcium levels, are very sensitive to therapy with calcitriol and calcium salts, and can have hypercalcemia.

Serum phosphorus level usually is in the normal or high-normal range early in renal insufficiency and may increase progressively with the decrease in glomerular filtration rate. Phosphorus level can be lowered through dialysis, judicious reduction of dietary protein intake, and the use of calcium salts as phosphate-binding therapy.

The measurement of plasma intact PTH levels is critical in the assessment of all forms of renal osteodystrophy. Early in renal functional decline, PTH levels begin to increase. Unless carefully controlled, these levels increase progressively to concentrations greater than tenfold normal. Several investigators have examined the relation between plasma PTH levels and underlying histomorphometric characteristics of bone in patients with chronic renal failure. In general, the highest PTH levels are related most closely to the presence of osteitis fibrosa and secondary hyperparathyroidism at bone biopsy and to a lesser extent with mixed bone lesion. Patients with low-turnover bone disease have the lowest PTH levels among patients with renal failure. Lowering these levels further with dialysis and calcium and calcitriol therapy has been implicated in the exacerbation of the low turnover–adynamic bone formation state. These general predictions hold for measurements of intact PTH. If only midregion or carboxyterminal PTH assays are available for clinical use, then the degree of elevation in PTH values is much more difficult to relate to the underlying bone lesion. This is because fragments of PTH detected with such assays accumulate progressively with renal functional decline.

Aluminum toxicity can be investigated for persons who have received aluminum-binding antacids. Serum aluminum levels or the response in aluminum 24 or 48 hours after an infusion of deferoxamine can be measured. The aluminum content of bone can be estimated in bone biopsy specimens and is typically elevated in states of aluminum excess.

An elevated level of serum alkaline phosphatase, an osteoblast-derived enzyme, usually indicates the presence at bone biopsy of increased bone turnover, as occurs in secondary hyperparathyroidism. The degree of elevation usually reflects the severity of the hyperparathyroidism. Alkaline phosphatase measurements are neither sensitive nor specific. Marked elevations in alkaline phosphatase are unlikely, however, to be found among patients with adynamic bone disease.

Histomorphometric analysis of bone by means of bone biopsy is the definitive means by which the underlying skeletal lesion and its severity can be best assessed for patients with chronic renal failure. This study is best performed after tetracycline labeling to assess rates of bone formation and mineralization. Proper analysis of bone biopsy specimens can be performed only at centers equipped for histomorphometry. Bone biopsy, although invasive, may be the only way to exclude aluminum osteodystrophy with certainty and to enable definitive therapy.

Radiologic Findings

A variety of radiologic features can be seen on images of patients with uremic osteodystrophy, although few signs are pathognomonic. Osteosclerosis, typified by "rugger jersey" spine, usually is caused by high-turnover bone disease and chronic excessive secretion of PTH. Pseudofractures are typical of osteomalacia and low-turnover bone disease but occur infrequently (Fig. 412.2). Subperiosteal resorption of bone, typically detected in the phalanges and distal clavicles, can occur at a variety of sites and is not confined to secondary hyperparathyroidism. β-2-Amyloid deposition often is accompanied by cystic changes in bones such as the femur, humerus, hands, and tibia. Osteitis fibrosa cystica, a once common skeletal presentation among patients with end-stage renal disease, is now seen in only the most severe cases of secondary hyperparathyroidism. It is manifested by multiple cystic lesions (brown tumors) throughout the skeleton at which pathologic fractures can occur.

Strategies for Optimal Care

Successful management of renal osteodystrophy involves a combination of dietary measurements, drug therapy, and dialysis. The spectrum of renal bone disease has a complex pathogenesis

and can evolve over time, rendering this complication of uremia highly challenging for physicians to control. The goals of treating these patients can be broadly stated as follows: to maintain serum calcium and phosphorus levels as close to normal as possible; to regulate the level of parathyroid activity such that substantial increases in intact PTH and parathyroid hyperplasia are prevented; to maintain adequate vitamin D levels so that mineralization, given the proper complement of calcium and phosphorus, can proceed normally; and to avoid the accumulation of aluminum in bone and parathyroid glands.

Despite our understanding of the pathogenesis of several aspects of uremic osteodystrophy, successful therapy for this condition is difficult. Early in renal failure, dietary efforts should be made to ensure adequate calcium intake (1,500 mg per day) and restrict phosphorus ingestion (1,000 mg per day). Calcium carbonate or calcium acetate taken with meals can be used effectively to reduce serum phosphorus concentrations should the former maneuvers not be successful. Sevelamer hydrochloride (Renagel), a calcium- and aluminum-free phosphorus binding gel can be used to reduce serum phosphorus levels.

Vitamin D metabolites, particularly calcitriol, can be used to boost intestinal calcium absorption if dietary supplements are less than satisfactory. Calcitriol therapy in oral or intravenous bolus dosage forms has been used widely to control extant secondary hyperparathyroidism among patients with uremia. Calcitriol can effectively suppress PTH levels through either route of administration. Extremely judicious follow-up care of these patients is needed to prevent serious elevations in calcium–phosphorus product, extraskeletal calcifications, and frank hypercalcemia. Less calcemic analogs of calcitriol have become available for use in suppressing PTH secretion.

Patients with low-turnover bone disease caused by aluminum and symptoms related to accumulation of aluminum are best treated by means of chelation therapy with deferoxamine infusion. Relief from bone pain and muscle weakness, a decrease in the bone burden of aluminum, and improvement in bone formation rate can be achieved with this therapy. PTH levels also often increase after this therapy.

OSTEOSCLEROSIS

Definition

Osteosclerosis comprises a group of disorders that increase bone mass. Many of these disorders cause diffuse thickening of the bone in trabecular sites. Others cause localized sclerotic lesions or predominantly affect cortical sites (hyperostosis). The types of osteosclerosis are listed in Table 412.2. Paget's disease of bone is relatively common, but many other types of osteosclerosis are quite rare and poorly characterized. The pathophysiologic mechanism of osteosclerosis involves excessive formation of new bone or decreased resorption of previously formed bone. When new bone formation is rapid, the newly deposited bone is woven. The new bone can be so voluminous that it occupies the medullary space and compromises hematopoiesis.

Paget's Disease of Bone

Paget's disease of bone is one of the most common metabolic bone disorders among the the elderly. It is characterized by single

TABLE 412.2.	CAUSES OF OSTEOSCLEROSIS

Congenital

Osteopetrosis
  Infantile
  Adult
  Intermediate
  Carbonic anhydrase deficiency type II
Endosteal hyperostosis (Van Buchem's syndrome)
Pycnodysostosis
Progressive diaphyseal dysplasia (Englemann's disease)

Acquired

Toxic exposure
  Fluoride
  Lead
Malignant disease
  Skeletal metastasis
  Myeloproliferative disorders
    Leukemia
    Multiple myeloma
Hematologic disease
  Sickle cell anemia
Endocrine disease
  Hyperparathyroidism
  Hypoparathyroidism
  Milk–alkalai syndrome
  Hypervitaminosis A, D
Renal disease
  Renal osteodystrophy
Miscellaneous diseases
  Paget's disease
  Hepatitis C
  Mastocytosis
  Sarcoidosis

or multiple bone involvement by a progressive lytic process followed by sclerosis. Paget's disease has a remarkable geographic distribution. The disease is common in some areas of the British Isles, for example, and distinctly rare in places such as sub-Saharan Africa and Asia. The cause of Paget's disease continues to be debated, but the most widely favored theories of causation involve a viral mechanism.

Incidence and Epidemiology

Paget's disease typically manifests among persons older than 50 years with a slight predominance of men over women. It is estimated that the disease may be present among 2% to 3% of the U.S. population older than 50 years. In some areas of the British Isles, the incidence is as high as 7% or 8% of elderly persons. Paget's disease also is common in Australia, New Zealand, and western Europe.

Etiology and Pathogenesis

The etiology and pathogenesis of Paget's disease are unknown, but viral infection of osteoclasts or their precursors is a preferred hypothesis. In many cases, genetics plays a critical role in the development of Paget's disease. A large percentage of patients

have a family history of the disease. In some kindreds, there appears to be an autosomal dominant form of inheritance. It is thought that viral infection of osteoclasts occurs early in life in a person with a genetic susceptibility to the disease. The disease may remain dormant for many years, and then in later life, unknown precipitating factors initiate the process in localized sites within the skeleton.

Bone remodeling is a highly ordered series of events in which the formation of new bone closely follows resorption of a unit of bone. In Paget's disease, bone remodeling is highly abnormal. This is reflected in the pathologic findings in affected bones. First, the rate of bone remodeling in this disease is accelerated and loosely coupled. Osteoclasts in pagetic lesions can be described as abnormally activated. The cytologic hallmarks of overactivity include generalized enlargement of the cells and a marked increase in the number of nuclei per cell. Second, an important pathologic feature of these osteoclasts is the presence of viral nucleocapsids in both the nuclei and the cytoplasm of these cells. The virus thought to be responsible for these inclusion bodies appears to come from the family of paramyxoviruses. Candidates include measles, respiratory syncytial, and canine distemper virus. A feature of infection with these viruses is formation of multinucleated cells.

The activated state of the osteoclast in Paget's disease stimulates bone resorption within pagetic lesions. This causes areas of bone matrix dissolution or lysis in a highly localized manner. Because bone formation and resorption are coupled, this primary stimulation of resorption increases bone formation. Paget's lesions are characterized first by areas of lysis and subsequently by areas of active new bone formation. The lytic lesions that are characteristic of Paget's disease include the blade-of-grass lesion and osteoporosis circumscripta. The former lesion typically occurs in a long bone in which the advancing front of bone resorption, led by osteoclasts, produces what appears to be a lytic edge. This lytic front can advance through the shaft of the long bone and eventually involve it in its entirety. *Osteoporosis circumscripta* is the description given to the classical lytic appearance of the skull of a patient with Paget's disease (Fig. 412.2).

After the initial and sometimes quite rapid phase of bone resorption in a pagetic lesion, new bone matrix is laid down at sites of prior resorption. The new bone formed in the area of these lesions is quite abnormal, consisting of woven bone and not typical adult lamellar bone (Fig. 412.1). The collagen fiber arrangement is abnormal and disordered in this woven bone. At the tissue level, a fibrotic response appears in the areas of bone involved by Paget's disease, such that dense connective tissue expands into these areas and blood vessels develop. The result is dense, hypervascular infiltration with connective tissue. With time, bone turnover ceases in the pagetic lesion, cellularity and vascularity decrease, and the remaining bone at the site becomes dense and sclerotic. This end-stage appearance has been called *burned-out Paget's disease.* Because of the intense new bone formation, long-standing pagetic involvement often enlarges the bone itself.

Clinical Findings

What has never been satisfactorily explained about Paget's disease is the propensity to involve certain bones over others and to be monostotic in one patient and polyostotic in another. In general, when the diagnosis is made, the sites involved are the ones that are affected throughout the course of the disease. It is distinctly uncommon for a new site to emerge even over many years of follow-up care of patients with classic Paget's disease. Most patients with this condition have no symptoms. The disease is detected when an evaluation is performed because of elevated alkaline phosphatase activity or when radiographs are obtained for another reason.

A striking feature of Paget's disease is its localized nature. The condition can affect one or several bones. The most common sites are the pelvis, skull, spine, and long bones, including the femur and tibia. Involvement of the upper extremities and ribs is uncommon, and the hands and feet are essentially spared. The clinical presentation and objective findings reflect the sites of involvement and intensity of disease activity. Symptoms of Paget's disease include bone pain, adjacent joint pain, warmth and dysesthesia over an involved bone, headache, and a variety of neurologic syndromes. Many patients also have concomitant degenerative arthritis. Differentiating arthritic pain from bone pain caused by Paget's disease can be challenging.

Neurologic complications, including hearing loss and cranial nerve compression syndromes, affect patients with skull involvement. Hearing loss can be conductive or sensorineural or both. If there is extreme involvement of the skull, softening of the bone at the base of the skull can occur and cause platybasia and in rare instances basilar impression. Brain stem or cerebellar complications are uncommon but can occur, as can obstruction to the flow of cerebrospinal fluid, which leads to obstructive hydrocephalus. Other neurologic syndromes, such as nerve root compression, can result in radiculopathy. If vertebral involvement is extensive, spinal cord compression can occur but is rare. The neurologic sequelae of Paget's disease can be serious, even life threatening, and often are strong indications for immediate therapy.

Other complications of Paget's disease are fractures, bone deformity, cardiac failure, and malignant degeneration. Fractures can be caused by softening of bone by the excessive resorption and lysis characteristic of Paget's disease. The most common fractures are of long bones, especially the femur. Bone deformity may progress in an insidious manner and may come to medical attention only after serious abnormality, gait disturbance, and limb shortening have developed. Congestive heart failure due to Paget's disease is extremely rare. It occurs when multiple bones are involved and is believed to be the result of an increase in blood flow to hypervascularized bone. Malignant degeneration within a pagetoid lesion can cause osteosarcoma, chondrosarcoma, or fibrosarcoma. This occurs among no more than 1% of patients and is heralded by an increase in alkaline phosphatase activity, an increase in bone pain, and development of a soft-tissue mass. The prognosis when sarcomatous degeneration occurs is poor because of the advanced age of these patients and their uniformly poor response to treatment.

Laboratory Findings

The disordered and localized nature of the bone remodeling defects of Paget's disease is reflected in these typical laboratory features. The laboratory abnormalities of Paget's disease are caused by its effects on bone remodeling. Because of the enhanced rate of bone resorption, biochemical markers of bone resorption become elevated. These markers reflect the increased breakdown of bone collagen matrix. They include urinary hydroxyproline, deoxypyridinoline, pyridinoline, and N-telopeptide. Because of the coupling of bone resorption and formation, markers of bone formation, such as alkaline phosphatase activity and osteocalcin, also are increased in Paget's disease. Osteocalcin is a highly specific protein product of osteoblasts. Measures of bone formation and resorption generally increase and correspond to disease activity and the extent of bone involvement. The values are elevated more typically in polyostotic disease and more variably in a monostotic presentation. Which value to measure has been a subject of debate. It has become clear that follow-up evaluation of disease activity and the effect of treatment can be accomplished with serial measurement of alkaline phosphatase activity in combination with clinical, radiologic, and scintigraphic assessment of disease activity.

Paget's disease does not typically alter serum calcium levels. Immobilization, however, for a patient with active bone remodeling can cause hypercalcemia (and hypercalciuria) and is an indication for therapy. A patient with Paget's disease who is found to have hypercalcemia should be evaluated for the presence of primary hyperparathyroidism. Secondary hyperparathyroidism can occur among patients with active Paget's disease. The elevation in PTH level in this situation presumably is caused by the intense stimulus to calcium accretion at sites of highly active bone formation and the inability of dietary calcium intake and intestinal absorption to meet the needs of the overactive bone remodeling state. Such patients need calcium supplementation to compensate for the increased calcium demand, and specific therapy for Paget's disease also should be provided. Because of the increased frequency of vitamin D deficiency among elderly patients, who are the typical patients with Paget's disease, it is sound practice to assess vitamin D sufficiency by measuring the 25-OHD levels of patients with secondary hyperparathyroidism and Paget's disease. Specific therapy can be directed at achieving vitamin D sufficiency for these persons and potentially better healing of the osseous lesions.

Radiographic Findings

The radiographic findings of Paget's disease often are characteristic and readily suggest the diagnosis. Skull involvement can cause osteoporosis circumscripta or a "cotton wool" appearance of intense blastic involvement with thickening of the bony cortex (Fig. 412.2). Involvement of long bones, for example, can be seen in the tibia and spare the adjacent fibula. Often the entire shaft of a long bone is affected. The radiographic findings are mixed areas of lucency and sclerosis. The entire bone typically is enlarged with thickened cortices and clear-cut bowed deformity. Pagetic involvement of the pelvis includes thickening of the iliopectineal (Brimmer's sign) and ilioischial lines and typical sclerosis, trabecular accentuation and thickening, and expansion of the bones. Paget's disease in the spine can affect several contiguous vertebral bodies but often is isolated to one level. The dense, sclerotic radiographic appearance of these bones has led to use of the term *ivory vertebrae* because of the striking radiodense appearance.

Scintigraphic studies can be quite helpful in assessing the extent of involvement and the level of disease activity and should be performed in the initial evaluation of all patients. Isotopic bone scanning can direct the clinician to the affected bones, which can then be assessed radiographically for features of Paget's disease (Fig. 412.2). The bone expansion and deformity and typical pattern of bone involvement can be readily appreciated on bone scans. A typical disease pattern often is helpful in differentiating other pathologic entities from Paget's disease.

The diagnosis of Paget's disease is made on the basis of a compatible history, physical examination, laboratory tests, radiographs, and bone scan. Radiographic findings often are characteristic of Paget's disease and sometimes are enough to confirm the diagnosis. Elevated alkaline phosphatase activity in the absence of liver disease provides strong support for the diagnosis. The level of alkaline phosphatase activity corresponds roughly with disease activity but is low in the presence of burned-out Paget's disease. The value can be only mildly abnormal or even normal in the presence of monostotic disease. Other differential diagnoses to consider are metastasis to bone, especially from carcinoma of the prostate, and fibrous dysplasia of bone, which does not share the osteoblastic or osteosclerotic appearance of Paget's disease.

Strategies for Optimal Care

Therapy for Paget's disease is becoming increasingly effective as new agents are developed that have enhanced therapeutic efficacy. The agents used include calcitonin, bisphosphonates, and nonsteroidal anti-inflammatory agents.

Calcitonin, an agent that selectively inhibits osteoclastic bone resorption, has been used in therapy for Paget's disease for more than 20 years. At present, the only form of calcitonin available in the United States is salmon calcitonin, which must be administered parenterally. It is given as a subcutaneous injection once a day (100 IU). Improvement in symptoms can occur within the first several weeks of therapy, and treatment usually is continued at this level for 6 months. On average, 60% to 70% of patients have 50% reduction in a measure of disease activity, such as an elevated alkaline phosphatase activity. After evidence of disease amelioration, the dose of calcitonin is reduced to 50 or 100 IU three times a week. Many patients continue with this dose for 1 to 2 years or indefinitely. It can be expected that once the medication is discontinued, relapse will occur that may or may not respond to repeated cycles of calcitonin therapy. It has been widely observed that patients readily become resistant to the effects of calcitonin and that all the abnormal biochemical indexes of active disease recur. In the past, calcitonin has been helpful in preparing patients with active Paget's disease for elective bone or joint surgery. This drug rapidly diminishes bone vascularity and the accelerated remodeling characteristic of the disease. Advantages of calcitonin therapy include a relatively low toxicity and rapid onset of action. The major disadvantages include parenteral administration and risk of resistance to the agent. Side effects include itching, flushing, nausea, and head-

ache. These troublesome effects can occur among 10% to 20% of patients.

Therapy for Paget's disease has been revolutionized by several potent bisphosphonate compounds. These agents inhibit bone resorption and can expeditiously achieve biochemical and clinical remission of disease in a high proportion of patients. The first bisphosphonate used for management of Paget's disease was etidronate. This agent, at a dose of 400 mg per day (5 mg per kilogram) for 6 months, is as efficacious as calcitonin, producing approximately 50% reductions in alkaline phosphatase activity. Therapy with this agent must be cycled every 6 to 12 months because of the risk of inducing a mineralization defect in normal bone due to the deposition of etidronate in bone matrix. Etidronate is well tolerated except for occasional diarrhea.

Many patients with extensive polyostotic disease respond only partially to either etidronate or calcitonin. Such persons need more potent bisphosphonates. These needs have been met to a considerable extent by intravenous administration of pamidronate and oral preparations of alendronate and risedronate. These second- and third-generation bisphosphonates are potent antiresorptive agents and are effective at reducing biochemical measures of disease activity, such as alkaline phosphatase activity, to normal in most cases. Pamidronate is given as an intravenous infusion, typically at doses of 60 mg over 3 to 4 hours. Therapy can be given weekly for 3 or 4 weeks or monthly for 3 to 6 months and must be individualized because several regimens are effective and no single regimen has achieved universal acceptance. Alkaline phosphatase activity usually is carefully monitored because levels may decrease, even after one infusion, into the normal range and remain normal for as long as 1 year. The main adverse effect of pamidronate is precipitation of flulike symptoms within 24 to 48 hours of drug administration. This effect is self-limited and occurs among fewer than 10% of patients. Leukopenia and lymphopenia, which are self-limited, also can occur.

The oral bisphosphonates alendronate and risedronate are much more heavily used than all of the other therapies because of ease of administration by the oral route and greater efficacy. Alendronate, given at a dose of 40 mg per day for 3 months, has been shown to induce biochemical remission, defined as normalization of biochemical markers among 50% of patients, with an average decrease of 72% from baseline in alkaline phosphatase activity. Gastrointestinal side effects are the main adverse events. Risedronate, administered at 30 mg per day for 3 months, lowers alkaline phosphatase activity 65% to 70% with normalization among 50%. It also ameliorates bone pain among patients with moderate to severe Paget's disease. These agents have made it possible to achieve striking control of disease and clinical symptoms for most patients. Nonsteroidal anti-inflammatory agents can be combined with antiresorptive therapy for pain control.

An important clinical issue is which patients should be treated. Most clinicians treat patients with congestive heart failure, hypercalcemia, a neurologic syndrome or symptom due to Paget's disease, deformity of a weight-bearing limb, or bone pain referable to a pagetic lesion. Patients also are treated in preparation for a surgical procedure on an affected bone, if they have polyostotic disease, and if long-term bed rest is anticipated after surgery. Most clinicians treat patients at risk of complications such as compression syndromes or deformity because of the sites of involvement. The availability of potent therapies enables more rapid and durable therapeutic responses than were achievable only 10 years ago.

Osteopetrosis

Osteopetrosis comprises a group of related disorders. An autosomal dominant form of the disease often manifests among adults and has few if any symptoms. It is also called a *benign* form of the disease. The other well-characterized form is the autosomal recessive infantile type of the disease. This form of the disease often is fatal and has been called *malignant.* An intermediate form of osteopetrosis is caused by carbonic anhydrase II deficiency and can be associated with renal tubular acidosis.

Etiology and Pathogenesis

The pathogenesis of osteopetrosis is markedly diminished bone resorption caused by qualitative or quantitative osteoclast defects. Evidence from gene disruption experiments on mice indicates that numerous genes can contribute to the osteopetrotic phenotype. This view is supported by the clinical diversity of osteopetrosis among humans. Osteoblast function also is likely important in the pathogenesis of some forms of this disease, perhaps through both direct and indirect mechanisms. It is becoming increasingly clear that control of osteoclast activity and number depends on paracrine signals from osteoblasts, and specific defects in osteoblast gene expression cause osteopetrosis in some animal models.

At histologic examination the absence of osteoclastic bone resorption is characteristic of osteopetrosis. The number of osteoclasts can be low, high, or normal, and normal ruffled borders are absent. Because of defective bone resorption, woven bone is common. Because bone formation rates are preserved in osteopetrosis, the defect in osteoclast function increases bone mass. This can increase the amount of bone in the marrow space and may cause obliteration and functional compromise of the space. Evidence of unresorbed mineralized cartilage within mature bone often is evidence of lack of bone resorption during modeling. The cortex is thickened with disorganized bone. Although the quantity of bone increases, the bone is structurally abnormal, fragile, and susceptible to fracture. Large amounts of osteoid also may be present in some patients with the infantile form of the disease, suggesting the presence of rickets and or osteomalacia.

Clinical Findings

Children with infantile (malignant) osteopetrosis come to medical attention at birth or during infancy. Initial symptoms include nasal congestion due to enlargement of the bony structures of the nose, cranial nerve palsy, including deafness and ophthalmic problems caused by narrowing of the cranial foramina and failure to thrive. Hydrocephalus also can occur. The encroachment of bone into the marrow space causes extramedullary hematopoiesis

and hypersplenism. As a result, anemia, bleeding disorders, and increased susceptibility to infection are commonly encountered. Fractures are a common occurrence, often from minimal trauma. If the patient is not untreated, infantile (malignant) osteopetrosis generally is fatal after the first year of life.

The adult-onset form of osteopetrosis usually is a mild disease. It often is asymptomatic and is diagnosed when radiographs obtained after a low-trauma fracture show increased bone mass. Some patients have cranial nerve entrapment that causes facial palsy and hearing and vision loss.

Carbonic anhydrase II deficiency is an intermediate form of osteopetrosis. Patients may have short stature, failure to thrive, or fractures in childhood. Cranial nerve palsy occurs as with the other forms of the disease. Renal tubular acidosis complicates the disorder. Fractures are a common complication.

Several patients have been described who had hepatitis C and osteosclerosis. A diffuse osteopetrotic skeleton was characteristic. It is likely that cytokines produced as a result of the hepatic infection were responsible for the increase in bone mass. Other forms of osteopetrosis include a variety of rare disorders with varied presentations.

Radiographic Findings

Generalized increased density of bone is the primary radiographic finding of osteopetrosis. Both trabecular and cortical components of the skeleton appear thickened. Although the bones are diffusely dense, alternating areas of lucency and density can be seen, particularly in the long bones. The diaphyseal and metaphyseal portions of the long bones may be widened, giving rise to an Erlenmeyer flask deformity. Thickening of the cranium is visible and is particularly notable at the skull base. The rugger-jersey spine sign is caused by thickening of the cortical end plates of the vertebrae. Evidence of previous fractures is commonly encountered.

Laboratory Findings

Levels of calcitropic hormones usually are normal in patients with osteopetrosis, but abnormalities have been described and include elevations in PTH level, hypocalcemia, hypophosphatemia, and low calcitriol levels. Patients with carbonic anhydrase deficiency have evidence of metabolic acidosis. Patients with the infantile form of the disease often have the hematologic abnormalities described earlier.

Strategies for Optimal Care

The goal of treatment of patients with osteopetrosis is to increase bone resorption. Glucocorticoids, low-calcium diets, and high doses of calcitriol have been tried but have met with limited benefit and serious side effects. Bone marrow transplantation has been an important advance in the management of infantile osteopetrosis. Because osteoclasts are of the monocyte macrophage lineage, this therapy reverses the underlying defect in the most serious form of this disease. Because engraftment may not occur in patients with advanced disease in which there is substantial bony crowding of the marrow space, early transplantation is more likely to be successful. Correction of acidosis should be attempted in the care of patients with carbonic anhydrase deficiency. The mild adult form of the disease does not necessitate specific care. Fracture prevention should be part of the general care of patients with osteopetrosis.

BIBLIOGRAPHY

Andress DL, Sherrard DJ. The osteodystrophy of chronic renal failure. In: Schrier RW, Gottschalk CW, eds. *Diseases of the kidney,* 6th ed. Boston: Little Brown, 1997:2597.

Ankrom MA, Shapiro JR. Paget's disease of bone (osteitis deformans). *J Am Geriatr Soc* 1998;46:1025–1033.

Bushinsky DA. Bone disease in moderate renal failure: cause, nature, and prevention. *Ann Rev Med* 1997;48:167–176.

Delmas PD, Meunier PJ. The management of Paget's disease of bone. *N Engl J Med* 1997;336:558–566.

Drezner MK. Clinical disorders of phosphate homeostasis. In: Feldman D, Glorieux FH, Pike JW, eds. *Vitamin D.* San Diego: Academic Press, 1997.

Favus MJ, ed. *Primer on the metabolic bone diseases and disorders of mineral metabolism,* 4th ed. Philadelphia: Lippincott Williams & Wilkins, 1999.

Leboff MS, Kohlmeier L, Hurwitz S, et al. Occult vitamin D deficiency in postmenopausal US women with acute hip fracture. *JAMA* 1999; 281:1505–1511.

Monegal A, Navasa M, Guanabens N, et al. Osteoporosis and bone mineral metabolism disorders in cirrhotic patients referred for orthotopic liver transplantation. *Calcif Tiss Int* 1997;60:148–154.

Pettifor JM, Daniels ED. Vitamin D deficiency and nutritional rickets in children. In: Feldman D, Glorieux FH, Pike JW, eds. *Vitamin D.* San Diego: Academic Press, 1997.

Siris ES, Canfield RE. Paget's disease of bone. In: Becker KL, ed. *Principles and practice of endocrinology and metabolism,* 2d ed. Philadelphia: JB Lippincott, 1995.

Kelley's Textbook of Internal Medicine, fourth edition. Edited by H. David Humes. Lippincott Williams & Wilkins, Philadelphia © 2000.

C H A P T E R

413

DISORDERS OF CARBOHYDRATE METABOLISM (EXCLUDING DIABETES)

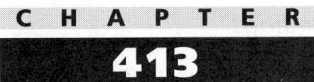

STANTON SEGAL

The disorders of carbohydrate metabolism that are inherited in a mendelian fashion include disorders of galactose metabolism; disorders of fructose metabolism and gluconeogenesis; and glycogen storage disease (GSD). All are rare biochemical genetic diseases with incidences of no more than 1 in 20,000 births. Diabetes mellitus, the most common disorder of metabolism and a result of both environmental and genetic factors, is consid-

ered in Chapter 411. These inborn errors of carbohydrate metabolism are all inherited as autosomal recessive traits, except for the X-linked form of phosphorylase kinase deficiency, a GSD. The GSDs may affect liver, striated muscle, or both tissues. The most common GSDs are glucose-6-phosphatase, debrancher, and phosphorylase kinase deficiencies, which are forms that affect the liver and may result in hypoglycemia. Glucose-6-phosphatase deficiency is not only a hepatic glycogenosis but a disorder of gluconeogenesis. Other examples of the latter include fructose-1,6-bisphosphatase deficiency and, from a functional perspective, hereditary fructose intolerance. The most common inborn error of galactose metabolism is galactose-1-phosphate uridyltransferase deficiency. Diagnosis of most of these disorders requires enzyme analysis in circulating blood elements or affected tissues. In some instances, a molecular diagnostic approach is available. For many of these disorders, prenatal testing can be performed. For any of these testing modalities, consultation with a metabolic specialist is essential.

■ DISORDERS OF GALACTOSE METABOLISM

The galactosemias are toxicity syndromes exhibited by patients with an inherited inability to metabolize the sugar galactose, a constituent of the disaccharide lactose found in milk and milk products. There are three disorders, each resulting from a deficiency of one of the enzymes that catalyze the normal conversion of galactose to glucose. Galactokinase catalyzes the reaction of galactose with adenosine triphosphate (ATP) to form galactose 1-phosphate, which is reacted with uridine diphosphate glucose by galactose 1-phosphate uridyltransferase to form uridine diphosphate galactose and glucose-1-phosphate. The latter is then converted to uridine diphosphoglucose by the enzyme uridine diphosphoglucose. Deficiencies of these enzymes are all autosomal recessive genetic disorders whose genes have been located on chromosomes 17, 9, and 1, respectively. Homozygotes exhibit absent or very little enzyme activity, whereas obligate heterozygotes express about 50% normal activity. The uridyltransferase gene has been cloned and sequenced, revealing a number of mutations responsible for single amino acid substitutions, the most prevalent being the Q188R, occurring in about 70% of alleles in the white population.

Uridyltransferase deficiency occurs in about 1 in 40,000 births and galactokinase in about 1 in 500,000. Epimerase deficiency is extremely rare; a benign form has been found in the African American, Swiss, and Japanese populations, and a symptomatic form, similar to the transferase deficiency described, has been reported in two Pakistani patients.

Cataracts are the principal finding in children with galactokinase deficiency who are otherwise healthy. Opacities have developed in some carriers. People younger than 40 years with cataracts may have lower-than-normal red blood cell galactokinase levels. Uridyltransferase deficiency usually manifests itself shortly after birth or within the first few weeks of birth with growth failure, vomiting, diarrhea, jaundice, hepatomegaly, proteinuria, and renal Fanconi's syndrome. Cataracts, although not easily seen with an ophthalmoscope, may be found by slit-lamp examination. Infants may die in the first few days of life from overwhelming *Escherichia coli* sepsis before other symptoms appear. Severely affected infants die of inanition and liver failure unless galactose is eliminated from the diet.

Galactokinase deficiency should be suspected in an infant or child with cataracts and the diagnosis confirmed by assaying red blood cell galactokinase. The constellation of abnormalities of transferase as well as severe epimerase deficiency also requires enzyme assay of red blood cells or fibroblasts. More than 40 states and some foreign countries screen newborns for galactosemia by analysis of blood spots on filter paper. Non–glucose-reducing substances in urine should make these disorders suspect. A great confusion in differential diagnosis is the distinction between transferase deficiency and primary liver disease because the liver is the major organ for galactose metabolism. Any disruption in hepatocellular function, or diversion of portal blood flow, may result in galactosemia and galactosuria.

A galactose-free diet is the cornerstone of treatment, and early elimination results in resolution of the toxicity syndrome seen in transferase deficiency, with regression of cataracts and jaundice. There is no indication that an ability to metabolize galactose appears with increasing age, so dietary restriction of milk and milk products as well as foods cooked with milk should not be relaxed in older children.

Dietary galactose restriction does not ensure a normal outcome. Despite excellent treatment, many patients with transferase deficiency have below-average mental development with learning defects. More than 60% have speech abnormalities, including verbal dyspraxia, and 80% of girls have hypergonadotropic hypogonadism. An ataxic neurologic syndrome may develop in older patients. Outcome does not differ in patients treated at birth before neonatal symptoms occur and in those recognized to have acute galactose toxicity syndrome within the first several weeks of life. This enigma remains to be unraveled.

■ DISORDERS OF FRUCTOSE METABOLISM, INCLUDING DEFECTS IN GLUCONEOGENESIS

HEREDITARY FRUCTOSE INTOLERANCE

The ingestion of fructose as the disaccharide sucrose is an important dietary habit of industrialized societies. Fructose in large amounts, particularly when administered intravenously, is not necessarily an innocuous dietary constituent, and the metabolic disease known as hereditary fructose intolerance underscores its potential toxicity. The clinical phenotype is variable, and this hereditary disease is thought often to escape detection. The incidence in different countries and in various ethnic groups is unknown, but the incidence in Switzerland was reported to be as high as 1 per 20,000 births.

The deficient enzyme is aldolase B (fructose 1,6-bisphosphate aldolase) located in liver, renal cortical, and small intestinal tissues. The human aldolase B gene has been cloned and is located on chromosome 9. Patients are unable to metabolize fructose beyond fructose 1-phosphate, which accumulates in the previously mentioned tissues. Clinical and laboratory findings depend

on the rate of fructose ingestion. Hypoglycemia is secondary to an inhibition of both glycogenolysis and gluconeogenesis. The toxicity of fructose 1-phosphate accumulation is supported by the fact that patients with the rare entity known as essential fructosuria secondary to fructokinase deficiency manifest increased levels of fructose in blood, urine, and tissues but fail to manufacture fructose 1-phosphate and have no clinical abnormalities.

Hereditary fructose intolerance may be manifest as an acute toxicity syndrome in infants, children, or adults or as a chronic disease. In the latter instance, growth failure may dominate the clinical picture in infancy. However, the full-blown syndrome in infants chronically ingesting fructose consists of poor feeding, recurrent vomiting, jaundice, hepatomegaly, hemorrhage, and renal Fanconi's syndrome. Hypoglycemia usually occurs after acute ingestion of fructose. Acute exposure may result in sweating, tremulousness, dizziness, nausea, vomiting, lethargy, coma, and convulsions. Within 30 minutes, patients given fructose as part of a challenge test experience a depression in blood glucose and serum phosphorus and a rise in serum urate. Subsequently, some patients may display a rise in serum alanine transaminase (ALT), aspartate transaminase (AST), and bilirubin, proteinuria, and a generalized aminoaciduria. These are the chronic albeit intermittent laboratory findings in patients with hereditary fructose intolerance. Liver histologic examination shows steatosis, patchy necrosis of hepatocytes, fibrosis, and, sometimes, frank cirrhosis. Renal findings include dilatation of proximal tubules and possible vacuolization of cells.

The history, particularly as it relates to dietary sucrose or fructose ingestion, and laboratory findings suggest the diagnosis of hereditary fructose intolerance. Occasionally, the clinician may learn that the onset of symptoms occurred after first exposure of an infant to fruits or after administration of a sucrose-containing, soy-based infant formula, or that there is a peculiar aversion to fruits and sweets in the older patients. When the diagnosis is suspected, all exogenous sources of fructose and sucrose should be eliminated. An intravenous fructose tolerance test may reproduce some clinical and laboratory findings. Oral fructose loading should not be performed because of the severe acute reaction referable to gastrointestinal fructose "poisoning." The enzyme may be reliably assayed in liver tissue. Molecular analysis of DNA may establish this diagnosis in most patients. Two point mutations in the aldolase B gene account for 90% of the gene defects in the white population of North America.

The other rare disorders of metabolism that primarily affect gluconeogenesis include fructose-1,6-bisphosphatase, pyruvate carboxylase, and phosphoenolpyruvate carboxykinase deficiencies. Patients with fructose-1,6-bisphosphatase deficiency usually present in infancy with hypoglycemia, lactic acidosis, and ketosis associated with lethargy or coma, seizures, and hyperventilation. Although pyruvate carboxylase is a key enzyme in gluconeogenesis, most patients do not present with hypoglycemia. The most common presentation of this uncommon disease is that of a progressive neurodegenerative disorder with lactic acidosis. Only a few cases of phosphoenolpyruvate carboxykinase deficiency have been reported; some of these patients have displayed liver disease in addition to hypoglycemia and lactic acidosis.

GLYCOGEN STORAGE DISEASE

The liver glycogeneses include type I (glucose-6-phosphatase deficiency or von Gierke's disease), type III (glycogen debrancher enzyme deficiency), type IV (branching enzyme deficiency), and type VI (liver phosphorylase or phosphorylase kinase deficiency) GSDs. The muscle glycogeneses include type II (lysosomal α-1,4-glucosidase deficiency or Pompe's disease), type V (muscle phosphorylase or McArdle's disease), and type VII (phosphofructokinase [PFK] deficiency) GSDs. All of these diseases are rare. Types I, II, III, and VI account for most cases of GSD.

TYPE I GLYCOGEN STORAGE DISEASE

Type I GSD was first described by von Gierke in 1929. Four individual causes of hepatic glycogen storage secondary to defective function of glucose-6-phosphatase have now been reported. The first, termed type Ia, refers to a primary defect in the enzyme. Type Ib refers to defective transport of glucose-6-phosphate into the interior of liver microsomes, where glucose-6-phosphatase resides. Types Ic and Id refer to disorders of microsomal transport of phosphatase and glucose, respectively, which secondarily result in defective glucose-6-phosphatase activity. Defective activity results in glycogen accumulation in liver, kidney, and intestinal mucosa. In the liver, however, neutral lipid accumulation is even more prominent than that of glycogen. Clinical or laboratory findings include poor growth, marked hepatomegaly, hypoglycemia, lactic acidosis, hyperuricemia, and hyperlipidemia. Type Ib is unique in that there is also evidence of recurrent bacterial infections secondary to neutropenia and impaired neutrophil function. Of importance, many patients do not come to clinical attention until after the neonatal period. Hypoglycemia may not be readily detectable, although hypoglycemic seizures after 3 months of age are not uncommon. Physical findings may suggest the disease; the children may manifest doll-like facies with excess adipose tissue in the cheeks, a protuberant abdomen, an accentuated lumbar lordosis, relatively thin extremities, and short stature. Hypoglycemia associated with a rise in blood lactate may occur 4 to 6 hours after a meal. The serum almost always appears lipemic. Liver histologic findings include distention of hepatocytes with glycogen and fat. Long-term complications sometimes develop in the second and third decade of life.

The most important complications include hepatic adenomas and chronic renal disease. The latter is preceded by renal glomerular hyperfiltration, microalbuminuria, and, as in early diabetic nephropathy, histologic evidence of increased glomerular mesangium and focal glomerulosclerosis. Hyperuricemia is also a problem and affects the kidney. Patients may begin to show signs of gout near puberty, which often is delayed. The diagnosis can be suspected based on the clinical presentation and increased levels of blood lactate and serum lipids. A liver biopsy should be performed to demonstrate glycogen accumulation, quantitate its content, and obtain fresh or frozen tissue for glucose-6-phosphatase activity for differentiation of type 1a from the others.

Treatment centers around maintenance of normal blood glucose concentrations. Most of the secondary metabolic abnormalities, such as metabolic acidosis, ketosis, lactic acidosis, hyperuricemia, and severe hypertriglyceridemia, can be eliminated or retarded by maintaining blood glucose levels in the normal range. The use of nocturnal nasogastric infusion of glucose and orally administered, uncooked cornstarch has had a significant impact on metabolic control. These feeding regimens can be used in conjunction with regular formula or meal ingestion.

TYPE III GLYCOGEN STORAGE DISEASE

Most patients with debrancher deficiency have both liver and muscle glycogen accumulation. Clinical findings include hepatomegaly, short stature, variable skeletal myopathy, and cardiomyopathy. However, there is a spectrum of disease involvement. Hypoglycemia, hyperlipidemia, and elevated serum transaminases are usually detected in affected children. Hepatic findings usually abate after puberty. Conversely, skeletal myopathy may become more severe with time. Although hemodynamically significant cardiomyopathy is rare, biventricular hypertrophy with electrocardiographic abnormalities is frequently detected. Serum creatine kinase may be elevated. Liver histologic findings include glycogen accumulation with hepatocytes and fibrosis. Rarely, micronodular cirrhosis is detectable.

The diagnosis is suggested by these findings but, unlike type I GSD, blood lactate elevation is not prominent and there may be evidence of striated muscle dysfunction. In addition, glucagon administration after a meal may result in a rise in blood glucose, whereas in the fasting state the rise is usually absent. In type I disease, it is negative under both conditions. A liver biopsy allows for the demonstration of abnormal glycogen and deficient debrancher enzyme activity. Skin fibroblasts and blood lymphocytes or erythrocytes may also be helpful in measuring enzyme activity, as well as assessing debrancher protein or glycogen content. In particular, with both liver and muscle involvement, the muscle debrancher enzyme activity is also low in muscle biopsy specimens. The human muscle debrancher copy DNA (cDNA) has been cloned and the gene is located on chromosome 1.

As in type I disease, treatment consists of frequent meals with cornstarch supplementation or nocturnal glucose infusions. This regimen usually does not need to be as strict as that in von Gierke's disease.

TYPE IV GLYCOGEN STORAGE DISEASE

Patients with the branching enzyme deficiency accumulate long, unbranched glycogen molecules, which lack the α–1 to 6 side chains in cells or tissues that use glycogen as a storage form of glucose. The features include presentation in early infancy with poor growth and hepatosplenomegaly associated with cirrhosis and portal hypertension, hypotonia, muscle weakness and atrophy, decreased or absent deep tendon reflexes, and cardiomyopathy. Hypoglycemia is not a usual feature. Histologic examination of liver, muscle, heart, skin, intestine, brain, spinal cord, and peripheral nerve reveals the accumulation of abnormal, amylopectin-like material in cells. Presumably, this storage material results in progressive cell or tissue damage, such as diffuse interstitial fibrosis of the liver. Diagnosis requires analysis of a biopsy sample for demonstration of this abnormal glycogen-like species. Enzyme analysis of branching activity can also be performed.

The cDNA for the branching enzyme has been cloned and the gene is on chromosome 3. There is no specific therapy. Although liver transplantation may be effective therapy for the end-stage liver disease, the long-term consequences of extrahepatic tissue involvement remains unknown.

TYPE VI GLYCOGEN STORAGE DISEASE

In this group of disorders, patients have a defect in either the hepatic phosphorylase enzyme itself or one of the four subunits of its regulatory enzyme, phosphorylase kinase. Only a few patients with the former type, which selectively involves the liver and has a relatively mild phenotype, have been reported. The liver phosphorylase gene has been cloned and is on chromosome 14. The most common form is the X-linked liver phosphorylase kinase deficiency. It typically presents in children with hepatomegaly, the characteristic protuberant abdomen of a hepatic glycogenosis, poor growth, and mild elevation of serum lipids and AST and ALT. Although ketosis is prominent during fasting, hypoglycemia is mild or absent. In general, the disease is not very severe and, except for the permanent effect on growth, most of the clinical and laboratory findings abate with age. Liver histologic analysis reveals glycogen accumulation in hepatocytes, but the appearance is somewhat different from that of types I or III GSD. Fibrosis with some inflammatory changes may also be seen. Usually the enzyme deficiency can be detected in erythrocytes, leukocytes, and skin fibroblasts, as well as in liver tissue. A high-carbohydrate diet with frequent feedings is usually sufficient for this type of GSD, which in general has a good prognosis. Other genotypic and phenotypic variants exist. For example, several patients with an autosomal recessive type of phosphorylase kinase deficiency have both liver and skeletal muscle involvement. There are other, rare variants in which the deficiency is restricted to either skeletal muscle or the heart. The basis for these disorders presumably is a specific alteration in one of the four subunits, which perturbs the formation of a tissue-specific phosphorylase kinase isozyme.

TYPE II GLYCOGEN STORAGE DISEASE

A deficiency of lysosomal acid α-glucosidase is the cause of Pompe's disease, which is therefore also a lysosomal storage disease. Disease primarily stems from the involvement of striated muscle tissue. Clinical onset may vary from the first weeks of life to adulthood. In the infantile form, cardiomyopathy and generalized myopathy are evident within the first 6 months of life. The heart, liver, and tongue are enlarged. The electrocardiogram usually shows the characteristic short PR interval and large QRS complexes. Patients usually succumb to cardiopulmonary disease by 2 years of age. In the juvenile and adult forms, skeletal muscle involvement usually dominates the clinical picture. It is a slowly progressive muscular disorder involving the proximal and respiratory muscles. Involvement of the latter is the usual cause of death. The electromyogram shows pseudomyotonic discharges. The serum creatine phosphokinase may be elevated. Histologic studies reveal glycogen accumulation. The α-glucosidase deficiency may be ascertained in skin fibroblasts and in muscle and liver tissue. Several mutations have been de-

scribed in the gene, which has been cloned and localized to chromosome 17. There is no effective treatment for Pompe's disease.

TYPE V GLYCOGEN STORAGE DISEASE

McArdle's disease is caused by a muscle glycogen phosphorylase deficiency. This is primarily a disease of adults, who present with exercise intolerance associated with muscle cramps and, frequently, rhabdomyolysis with myoglobinuria. Muscle fiber injury and secondary complications, such as acute renal failure, appear to correlate with the intensity of exercise. With mild to moderate sustained exercise, the "second-wind" phenomenon is often recognized, presumably the consequence of certain types of muscle fiber being able to sustain or upgrade the aerobic oxidation of fatty acids after increased muscle blood flow. Some patients have been known to complain of weakness and easy fatigability since childhood. Serum creatine phosphokinase is usually normal but increases after exercise. The electromyographic findings may be interpreted as those of a myositis. An ischemic exercise test may lend further support for the diagnosis: blood lactate levels fail to rise in the venous samples that drain an actively contracting muscle bed. Phosphorus (^{31}P) magnetic resonance spectroscopy may also be helpful in establishing the diagnosis. Analysis of a muscle undergoing isometric exercise by this technique fails to show the normal decrease in intracellular pH (acute glycogenolysis should increase lactic acid levels) and reveals an exaggerated decrease in levels of the high-energy compound phosphocreatine. Biochemical analysis of a muscle biopsy sample usually shows extremely low or undetectable phosphorylase activity and glycogen accumulation. As with the phosphorylase kinase enzyme discussed later, phosphorylase also exists in multiple tissue-specific isoforms. The muscle form is the only type found in the muscle of both children and adults. The gene for the muscle type has been cloned and is on chromosome 11. Several mutations have been identified. Approximately half of total enzyme in heart, one-fourth of that in brain, but none in liver is made up of the muscle isoform. There have been rare reports of disease in newborn infants, children, or elderly persons. The most important form of therapy for most patients with McArdle's disease is to avoid moderate to severe exercise. Ingestion of glucose or sucrose may increase exercise capacity in some affected individuals.

TYPE VII GLYCOGEN STORAGE DISEASE

Exercise intolerance in patients with the rare condition known as muscle PFK deficiency, which presents in childhood with muscle pain and easy fatigability, usually is more severe than that in type V GSD. These patients also usually manifest a subclinical hemolytic anemia; the residual enzyme activity in erythrocytes may be reduced, but only to 50% of normal. Carbohydrate intake is of no avail in this glycolytic defect in which muscle glucose cannot be metabolized to lactate and accumulates as glucose-6-phosphate and fructose-6-phosphate. These compounds may be detected in elevated amounts in the exercising muscles of patients using in vivo ^{31}P magnetic resonance spectroscopy. Because of impaired muscle ATP regeneration, serum urate levels may rise markedly during exercise. Histologic analysis of a muscle biopsy sample reveals the presence of an abnormal periodic acid–Schiff–positive, diastase-resistant polysaccharide material, presumably glycogen of long chain length. The mature muscle enzyme exists as a homotetramer of M subunits, the activity of which is decreased in a muscle biopsy specimen. The gene has been cloned and is on chromosome 1. Gene defects have been described, one of which is prevalent in people of Ashkenazic Jewish ancestry. There is also a relatively high prevalence of type VII GSD in the Japanese. A liver isoform of PFK has also been described, with the gene for the L subunit being present on chromosome 21. Erythrocytes express both the M and L subunit with five potential isozyme structures. The PFK activity is therefore not totally absent in erythrocytes because of the presence of the L_4 isoform. Avoidance of strenuous exercise is the only treatment advice that can be provided to these patients.

BIBLIOGRAPHY

Chen YT, Burchell A. Glycogen storage diseases. In: Scriver CR, Beaudet AL, Sly WS, et al., eds. *The metabolic and molecular bases of inherited disease,* seventh ed. New York: McGraw-Hill, 1995:935.

Gitzlemann R, Steinmann B, Van den Berghe G. Disorders of fructose metabolism. In: Scriver CR, Beaudet AL, Sly WS, et al., eds. *The metabolic and molecular bases of inherited disease,* seventh ed. New York: McGraw-Hill, 1995:905.

Hirschhorn R. Glycogen storage disease type II: acid α-glucosidase (acid maltase) deficiency. In: Scriver CR, Beaudet AL, Sly WS, et al., eds. *The metabolic and molecular bases of inherited disease,* seventh ed. New York: McGraw-Hill, 1995:2443.

Segal S. Galactosaemia today: the enigma and the challenge. Komrower Lecture. *J Inher Metab Dis* 1998;21:455–471.

Talente GM, Coleman RA, Alter C, et al. Glycogen storage disease in adults. *Ann Intern Med* 1994;120:218–226.

Kelley's Textbook of Internal Medicine, fourth edition. Edited by H. David Humes. Lippincott Williams & Wilkins, Philadelphia © 2000.

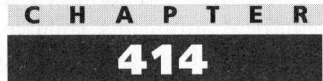

CHAPTER 414

DISORDERS OF AMINO ACID METABOLISM

ROBERT J. SMITH

Amino acids, imino acids (proline and hydroxyproline), and a number of chemically related substances, such as taurine and γ-aminobutyric acid, are a large group of nitrogen-containing compounds that have important structural and metabolic functions in the body. In addition to their roles in protein and peptide structure, amino acids have multiple metabolic functions. To cite a few examples, glutamic acid and glycine are neurotransmitters; glutamine is an important substrate for renal ammoniagenesis pathways that are essential for acid–base balance; alanine

and several other amino acids are endogenous sources of glucose (through gluconeogenesis); tryptophan is a precursor of bioactive amines such as serotonin (5-hydroxytryptamine); methionine is one of the major methyl group donors in the body and thus a precursor for choline, acetylcholine, creatine, and epinephrine; and the nonprotein amino acid ornithine is a key intermediate in the conversion of toxic ammonia to the nontoxic waste product urea.

The provision of adequate quantities of amino acids to serve their diverse metabolic functions is ensured by efficient gastrointestinal absorption (especially important for essential amino acids), resorptive transport of filtered amino acids in the renal tubules, and regulated biosynthetic pathways (in the case of nonessential amino acids). Pools of free amino acids are maintained in the plasma and intracellular compartments. The size of the reserve pools in specific tissues such as skeletal muscle and the transfer of amino acids between pools are determined by regulation of membrane transport and intracellular metabolic processes. The excess accumulation of individual amino acids is prevented by control of flux through the synthetic and catabolic pathways.

Heritable defects in amino acid metabolic and transport pathways account for nearly 100 clinical disorders, most of which occur as rare diseases with autosomal recessive inheritance. Although these disorders occur at increased frequency in consanguineous matings, clinical disease often is a consequence of inheritance from unrelated parents of two alleles with distinct mutations. Table 414.1 is a list of selected disorders and their characteristics. Specific diseases most often have been detected through measurement of elevated amino acid or metabolite levels in the urine or plasma. The former are often referred to with the suffix *-uria* (e.g., iminoglycinuria) and the latter with the suffix *-emia* (e.g., hyperprolinemia). Disorders of amino acid metabolism can be catastrophic. They cause early fetal death; they can cause less severe metabolic disturbances compatible with transient or prolonged survival; or they can be associated with no apparent clinical sequelae. For disorders that cause clinical disease, early diagnosis is often important, because specific dietary therapy or pharmacologic agents may diminish the accumulation of amino acids or their toxic metabolites enough to prevent irreversible tissue injury.

For comprehensive discussions of the many known disorders of amino acid metabolism and transport, a specialized text should be consulted (see Bibliography). This chapter describes representative examples of different types of heritable amino acid disorders.

■ DEFECTS IN AMINO ACID CATABOLISM

EXAMPLE: PHENYLKETONURIA

Hyperphenylalaninemia is a group of heritable disorders characterized by impaired oxidation of the essential amino acid phenylalanine. Although phenylalanine is an essential amino acid and thus is not synthesized endogenously, levels in body pools depend on a balance between dietary intake and rate of conversion

TABLE 414.1.	INHERITED DISORDERS OF AMINO ACID METABOLISM

Amino Acid or Related Substance	Clinical Disorder	Biochemical Defect	Clinical Features	Therapy
Defects in Amino Acid Catabolism				
Arginine	Argininemia	Arginase	Mental retardation, seizures, spastic motor disorder	Protein restriction with essential amino acid supplement, possibly sodium benzoate
Argininosuccinic acid	Argininosuccinic aciduria	Argininosuccinate lyase	Mental retardation, seizures; psychomotor retardation; dry, brittle hair	Protein restriction with arginine supplementation, sodium benzoate
Carbamoyl phosphate	Type I hyperammonemia	Carbamoyl phosphate synthetase	Hyperammonemia, progressive neurologic dysfunction	Protein restriction, essential amino acids, sodium benzoate
Cystathionine	Cystathioninuria	Cystathionase	None proved	Pyridoxine (if responsive)
Citrulline	Citrullinemia	Argininosuccinate synthetase	Mental retardation, seizures, motor weakness, hepatomegaly	Protein restriction, arginine supplementation, sodium benzoate
Glutamic acid	Glutathionemia	γ-Glutamyl-transpeptidase	Possibly mental retardation	None
Glycine	Nonketotic hyperglycinemia	Glycine cleavage system	Mental retardation, seizures	None
Glycine	Hypersarcosinemia	Sarcosine dehydrogenase	None	Not required
Histidine	Histidinemia	Histidase	Mental retardation, speech defect	None
Histidine	Formiminoglutamic aciduria	Cyclodeaminase	Psychomotor dysfunction, possible mental retardation	None
Histidine	Formiminoglutamic aciduria	Formiminotransferase	Same as for cyclodeaminase defect	None
Homocystine	Homocystinuria	Cystathionine β-synthase	Ectopia lentis, osteoporosis, mental retardation, seizures, thromboembolism	Low-methionine, high-cystine diet; pyridoxdine, betaine, choline, dipyridamole, and aspirin
Homocystine	Homocystinuria	Methylene tetrahydrofolate reductase	Psychomotor dysfunction, mental retardation	Occasional response to folate
Hydroxyproline	Hydroxyprolinemia	Hydroxyproline oxidase (probable)	None	Not required
Isoleucine, valine	Methylmalonic acidemia	Methylmalonyl coenzyme mutase	Psychomotor dysfunction, hepatomegaly, hyperammonemia, ketoacidosis	Protein restriction, cobalamin
Isoleucine, valine	α-Methylacetoacetic aciduria	β-Ketothalase	Pyschomotor retardation, ketoacidosis, hyperammonemia	Protein restriction
Isoleucine, valine	Propionic acidemia	Propionyl coenzyme carboxylase	Developmental retardation, ketoacidosis	Protein restriction
Leucine	β-Hydroxy-β-methylglutamic aciduria	β-Hydroxy-β-methylglutaryl coenzyme A lyase	Metabolic acidosis, hypoglycemia	Protein restriction
Leucine	β-Methylcrotonyl glycinuria	β-Methylcrotonyl coenzyme A carboxylase	Metabolic acidosis, developmental retardation	Protein restriction (little benefit)

(continued)

TABLE 414.1. *Continued*

Amino Acid or Related Substance	Clinical Disorder	Biochemical Defect	Clinical Features	Therapy
Leucine	Isovaleric acidemia	Isovaleryl coenzyme dehydrogenase	Ketoacidosis, psychomotor retardation	Protein restriction, glycine, carnitine
Leucine, isoleucine, valine	Branched-chain ketoaciduria (maple syrup urine disease)	Branched-chain ketoacid dehydrogenase	Multiple phenotypes: ketoacidosis, mental retardation, seizures	Low-branched-chain amino acid diet, thiamine, peritoneal dialysis
Lysine	Periodic hyperlysinemia	Lysine dehydrogenase	Episodic hyperammonemia	Protein restriction, fluid therapy for crises
Lysine	Persistent hyperlysinemia	Lysine: α-ketoglutarate reductase (probable)	Possible mental retardation	Protein restriction
Methionine	Hypermethioninemia	Methionine adenosyltransferase	Possible neurologic defects	Not known
Ornithine	Gyrate atrophy	Orithine-δ-aminotransferase	Chorioretinal degeneration with visual loss	Pyridoxine, arginine-restricted diet
Ornithine	Hyperornithinemia–hyperammonemia–homocitrullinuria syndrome	Mitochondrial ornithine transport (?)	Episodic hyperammonemia, psychomotor retardation	Protein restriction, possible ornithine supplementation
Ornithine	Ornithine carbamoyl transferase deficiency	Ornithine carbamoyl transferase	Hyperammonemia with psychomotor consequences, more severe in males	Low-protein diet, essential amino acid supplements, sodium phenylacetate
5-Oxoproline	5-Oxoprolinuria (pyroglutamic aciduria)	Glutathionine synthetase	Mental retardation, hemolysis, acidosis	Sodium bicarbonate, maybe vitamin E
Phenylalanine	Classic phenylketonuria	Phenylalanine hydroxylase	Mental retardation, seizures, hypopigmentation	Phenylalanine-restricted diet
Phenylalanine	Benign hyperphenylalaninemia	Phenylalanine hydroxylase	None	Phenylalanine-restricted diet
Phenylalanine	Transient hyperphenylalaninemia	4α-carbinolamine dehydratase	None	Not required
Phenylalanine	Variant phenylketonuria	Dihydropteridine synthesis	Mental retardation, seizures	Phenylalanine-restriction, possibly levodopa, 5-hydroxytryptophan, carbidopa or folinic acid
Phenylalanine	Variant phenylketonuria	Dihydropteridine reductase	Mental retardation, seizures	Phenylalanine restriction, possibly levodopa, 5-hydroxytryptophan, carbidopa or folinic acid
Proline	Type I hyperprolinemia	Proline oxidase	Uncertain	Not required
Proline	Type II hyperprolinemia	Pyrroline-5-carboxylate dehydrogenase	Uncertain	Not required
Tyrosine	Tyrosinemia II	Tyrosine aminotransferase	Corneal erosions, palm and sole erosions, sometimes mental retardation	Low-tyrosine, low-phenylalanine diet
Tyrosine	Tyrosinosis (tyrosinemia I)	Fumarylacetoacetate hydrolase and maleylacetoacetate hydrolase (probable)	Liver dysfunction, renal tubular dysfunction, vitamin D–resistant rickets	Diet low in tyrosine, phenylalanine, and methionine; liver transplantation
Tyrosine	Tyrosinase-negative albinism	Tyrosinase	No pigmentation, cutaneous neoplasia, blindness	Avoidance of sunlight, sunscreens, protective lenses
Cystine	Cystinosis	Unknown	Cystine accumulation in lysosomes, variable severity, renal dysfunction	Renal transplantation, cysteamine being evaluated

(continued)

TABLE 414.1.	*Continued*

Amino Acid or Related Substance	Clinical Disorder	Biochemical Defect	Clinical Features	Therapy
Storage Diseases				
Glycine	Type I hyperoxaluria	α-Ketoglutarate: glyoxylate carboligase	Calcium oxalate nephrolithiasis, renal failure	Pyridoxine, phosphate, magnesium, high urine volume
Glycine	Type II hyperoxaluria (L-glyceric aciduria)	D-Glyceric dehydrogenase	Calcium oxalate nephrolithiasis	Same as for type I hyperoxaluria
Tyrosine	Alkaptonuria	Homogentisic acid oxidase	Degenerative arthritis (ochronosis), possible increased degenerative cardiovascular disease	Nonspecific management of arthritis
Membrane Transport Defects				
Cystine, lysine, arginine, ornithine	Hypercystinuria	Transport of cystine, arginine, lysine, and ornithine in the renal tubules and intestinal mucosa	Nephrolithiasis	Increased urine volume, alkalinized urine, D-penicillamine
Glutamic acid, aspartic acid	Dicarboxylic aminoaciduria	Transport of dibasic aminoacids in renal tubules and jejunal mucosa	None proved	Not required
Glycine, proline, hydroxyproline	Iminoglycinuria	Renal tubular and jejunal mucosal transport	None	Not required
Histidine	Histidinuria	Renal tubular and jejunal mucosal transport	Mental retardation	None
Lysine	Lysinuria	Renal tubular and jejunal mucosal transport	Mental and growth retardation, seizures	Protein restriction, citrulline supplementation
Lysine, arginine, ornithine	Dibasic amino aciduria, type I	Renal tubular and jejunal mucosal transport	Mental retardation	None
Lysine, arginine, ornithine	Dibasic amino aciduria, type II	Renal tubular and jejunal mucosal transport	Mental retardation, protein imbalance	Protein restriction, citrulline supplementation
Methionine	Methionine malabsorption	Jejunal mucosal transport	Mental retardation hyperpneic attacks, white hair	Methionine-restricted diet
Neutral amino acids	Hartnup disease	Renal tubular and jejunal mucosal transport	Pellagra: red, scaly rash after exposure to sunlight; intermittent cerebellar ataxia	High-protein diet plus nicotinamide

to tyrosine and other products. As shown in Fig. 414.1, phenylalanine is oxidized to tyrosine by the hepatic and renal enzyme phenylalanine hydroxylase (PAH). More than 100 mutations in the PAH gene have been described that result in a deficiency of the enzyme and hyperphenylalaninemia. If the enzyme deficiency is severe and the disease is not controlled, toxic effects of phenylalanine lead to the syndrome of phenylketonuria, which is characterized by progressive central nervous system damage.

PAH activity requires molecular oxygen and a reduction in tetrahydrobiopterin (BH_4) cofactor (Fig. 414.1). This same BH_4 cofactor is required for synthesis of neurotransmitters (dopa-

mine, norepinephrine, and serotonin) from tyrosine and tryptophan. In addition to PAH defects, mutations in the BH_4 recycling enzyme dihydropteridine reductase (DHNR) and the synthetic enzyme 6-pyruvoyl tetrahydropterin synthase (6PTS), as well as presumed mutations in the synthetic enzyme guanosine triphosphate cyclohydrolase (GTP-CH), lead to hyperphenylalaninemia. Central nervous system degeneration with these BH_4 defects tends to be more severe than with PAH mutations, probably because of combined effects of phenylalanine toxicity and neurotransmitter deficiency. Mutations in the 4α-carbinolamine dehydratase (CDH) BH_4 recycling enzyme have been shown to be responsible for occasional cases of hyperphenylalaninemia

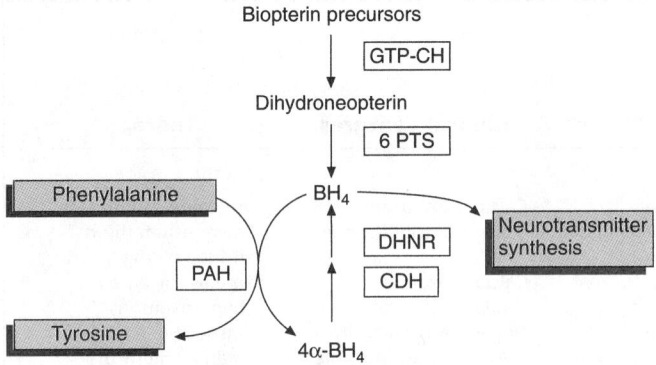

FIGURE 414.1. Pathways of phenylalanine catabolism. Enzymes are *PAH*, phenylalanine hydroxylase; *DHNR*, dihydropteridin reductase; *CDH*, 4α-carbinolamine dehydratase; *6PTS*, 6-pryuvoyl tetrahydropterin synthase; and *GTP-CH*, guanosine triphosphate cyclohydrolase. Mutations in each of these enzymes represent known or putative causes of hyperphenylalaninemia.

that are mild and transient, because this reaction can occur to some extent nonenzymatically.

Most patients with PAH deficiency are homozygotes with two different allelic mutations affecting the enzyme. It is likely that clinical heterogeneity is explained by the effects of different mutations. Some heterozygotes have mild hyperphenylalaninemia, which may be caused by a dominant-negative effect of the mutant allele on the normal gene product. Although homozygous PAH deficiency is uncommon, the incidence of 1 in 10,000 births indicates an unexpectedly high gene frequency of mutations at close to 1%. This suggests the possibility of a heterozygote advantage, which has not been defined.

Although the various forms of phenylketonuria are rare autosomal recessive disorders, most newborns in the United States and Europe are screened for hyperphenylalaninemia because of the severity and lack of reversibility of the central nervous system damage. Early implementation of a phenylalanine-restricted diet can essentially eliminate appreciable central nervous system damage among patients with PAH deficiency. Supplemental therapy with orally administered, recombinant phenylalanine ammonia lyase is being investigated as a means of increasing dietary phenylalanine tolerance. Patients with BH$_4$ deficiency may need not only a restricted diet but also treatment with levodopa, 5-hydroxytryptophan, carbidopa, or folinic acid.

STORAGE DISEASES

EXAMPLE: ALKAPTONURIA

Alkaptonuria is a rare autosomal recessive inherited disorder caused by mutations in the gene that encodes homogentisic acid oxidase. Deficiency of this enzyme, which functions in a pathway of tyrosine metabolism, leads to accumulation and urinary excretion of the metabolic intermediate, homogentisic acid. Fresh urine appears normal initially, but after the urine stands, homogentisic acid becomes oxidized and imparts a characteristic black color to the urine. The presence of homogentisic acid in the urine appears to have no clinical consequences, but gradual dep-

osition of homogentisic acid and its oxidation products in articular cartilage and certain other tissues ultimately causes progressive tissue damage. Pigmented oxidation products impart a bluish-black color to involved tissues that together with the characteristic degenerative arthritis results in the syndrome designated *ochronosis*.

Clinical features include bluish-black discoloration of the sclerae and ears; pigment deposits near the lateral rectus attachment sites in the sclerae; pigmented deposits in the heart valves, larynx, and tympanic membranes; darkening of the skin; and occasional pigmented renal or prostatic calculi. There is a probable increase in degenerative cardiovascular disease among older patients, but the dominant clinical finding is degenerative arthritis that manifests in the fourth and fifth decades with especially marked involvement of the lumbosacral intervertebral disks, dense calcification of disk spaces, fusion of vertebral bodies, and a remarkable absence of osteophyte formation or calcification of intervertebral ligaments. In many patients, the urinary abnormalities are not detected, and the diagnosis is made only during evaluation for arthritis.

Among patients with suspected alkaptonuria, the simplest diagnostic procedure is to alkalinize a urine sample. This accelerates oxidation of the homogentisic acid and generates a bluish-black pigment within several hours. Confirmation of the diagnosis then requires direct assay of homogentisic acid with one of several methods. The only truly effective therapy is nonspecific management of osteoarthritis supplemented with anti-inflammatory agents during episodes of acute arthritis. With the recent proof that mutations in homogentisic acid oxidase cause alkaptonuria, it can be anticipated that efforts will be made to correct this enzymatic deficiency with various approaches to gene therapy.

MEMBRANE TRANSPORT DEFECTS

EXAMPLE: CYSTINURIA

Cystinuria, with a prevalence of about 1 case per 7,000 persons, is the most common of about 10 known disorders of amino acid transport. The renal transporter for resorption of dibasic amino acids in the proximal convoluted tubule is defective. As a result, there is excessive urinary excretion of cystine, lysine, arginine, and ornithine. Cystine is the least soluble of all commonly occurring amino acids. As the urine becomes concentrated, cystine precipitates and forms renal, ureteral, and bladder calculi. More than 30 mutations in the dibasic amino acid transporter gene (r*BAT*) have been related to cystinuria. It is possible that the disease can be caused by mutations in other proteins as well. The inheritance pattern is recessive but complex because of the apparent occurrence of different allelic mutations.

Cystine stones, which account for 1% to 2% of all urinary tract calculi, are responsible for the only known consequences of cystinuria. Clinical features include hematuria, flank pain, obstructive uropathy, urinary tract infection, and for some patients, renal failure. Although there is also a defect in intestinal amino acid transport, adequate amino acid absorption appears to occur through alternative routes. Tissue uptake of dibasic amino acids is mediated by unrelated transporters, so plasma and tissue concentrations of cystine and other amino acids are normal.

The diagnosis of cystinuria should be considered for all patients with urinary tract stones. The diagnosis can be confirmed with the demonstration of typical hexagonal crystals in the urine, cystine excretion in the range of 0.6 to 1.8 g per day, and cystine in urinary stones. In evaluating patients with renal calculi, it should be recognized that stones of mixed composition often occur in cystinuria and that there is an absence of measurable cystine in some stones. The primary treatment is directed at prevention of stone formation by increasing fluid intake and urine volume. Although cystine solubility increases if the urinary pH is greater than 7.5, vigorous measures are needed to achieve this degree of alkalinization with a consequent risk of calcium stone formation or nephrocalcinosis. Dietary restriction has little effect because of endogenous cystine synthesis, but there should be an effort to avoid diets high in the cystine precursor methionine. Penicillamine can be used to treat patients who do not respond to hydration alone. This drug is excreted in the urine, where it forms a mixed disulfide with cystine that has greatly increased solubility. Because the metabolic defect responsible for stone formation is localized to the kidney, patients with renal failure who receive transplants do not have recurrent disease.

CONCLUSION

Although there are many heritable amino acid disorders, acquired diseases of amino acid metabolism or transport rarely occur, presumably reflecting the adaptive capacity of normal pathways. Selected examples of inherited disorders are discussed to illustrate the types of defects and the spectrum of clinical syndromes. As the molecular basis of inherited disorders is better defined, it will undoubtedly become apparent that multiple distinct genetic mutations can cause similar syndromes, perhaps with minor alterations in clinical outcome that may contribute to disease heterogeneity. With better definition of the heritable defects in amino acid pathways, more specific and effective forms of nutritional and pharmacologic therapy have been developed. This has led to improved survival for many patients and a greater need for internists to understand the principles of management of disorders of amino acid metabolism. With the promise of gene therapy, it can be anticipated that the treatment of patients with inherited metabolic defects will become a much more important part of adult medicine.

BIBLIOGRAPHY

Schepartz B. *Regulation of amino acid metabolism in mammals.* Philadelphia: WB Saunders, 1973.

Scriver CR, Beaudet AL, Sly WS, et al., eds. *The metabolic and molecular bases of inherited disease,* 7th ed. New York: McGraw-Hill, 1995.

Scriver CR, Rosenberg LE. *Amino acid metabolism and its disorders.* Philadelphia: WB Saunders, 1973.

C H A P T E R
415

MULTIPLE ENDOCRINE NEOPLASIA

STEPHEN J. MARX

Multiple endocrine neoplasia (MEN) is the occurrence of two or more endocrine tumors in a patient. It has several causes, including chance. Two syndromes stand out, and only these are discussed (Table 415.1). MEN type 1 (MEN1) includes tumors of the parathyroid glands, enteropancreatic neuroendocrine tissue, and anterior pituitary gland. MEN type 2 (MEN2) includes tumors of the calcitonin-secreting thyroid cells (C-cells), the parathyroid glands, and adrenal medulla with three subtypes. The most common subtype of MEN2 is MEN2a with C-cell malignant growth, pheochromocytoma, and hyperparathyroidism. A second syndrome (MEN2b) consists of C-cell malignant growth, pheochromocytoma, ganglioneuromas, and a characteristic body and facial appearance. A third type is familial medullary thyroid cancer only (FMTC).

MEN1 and MEN2 are rare syndromes with disproportionate importance because of their implications for cancer causation and prevention and because of their genes' relevance to some common tumors. Each has a prevalence of about 1 case per 30,000 persons. A substantial fraction of all persons with endocrine tumors has hereditary MEN1: 25% with gastrinoma, 5% with prolactinoma, and 2% with primary hyperparathyroidism.

GENERAL CLINICAL FEATURES

MEN1 or MEN2 can be inherited in an autosomal dominant manner. In general the age of onset is earlier for tumors in MEN1 or MEN2 than for the same tumors in sporadic cases. Another prominent feature in MEN1 or MEN2 is tumor multiplicity. *Multiplicity* means multiple tissues and multiple tumors, which includes bilaterality in a tissue. As in several other multiple neoplasia syndromes, some tumors in MEN1 or MEN2 can become malignant.

PATHOGENESIS

The *MEN1* gene is on chromosome 11; it encodes a nuclear protein that binds to at least one transcription factor (JunD). The *MEN1* gene is a tumor suppressor gene, like the main genes for retinoblastoma, breast cancer, and intestinal polyposis. A tumor suppressor gene contributes to tumors after sequential inactivation of both copies of the gene frees one cell to grow into a clonal tumor.

MEN2 is caused by a gene, *RET*, on chromosome 10 and unrelated to the *MEN1* gene. *RET* encodes a plasma mem-

TABLE 415.1.	COMPARISONS BETWEEN MEN1 AND MEN2	
Feature	Multiple Endocrine Neoplasia Type 1	Multiple Endocrine Neoplasia Type 2 (three subtypes)[a]
Gene and mechanism	*MEN1;* tumor suppressor	*RET;* tumor activator (oncogene)
Tissues affected	Parathyroid glands	1. Parathyroid glands
	Enteropancreatic neuroendocrine (gastrinoma, insulinoma, etc.)	2. Calcitonin-producing parafollicular cells of thyroid (C-cells)
	Anterior pituitary	3. Adrenal medulla
	Carcinoid of foregut	4. Cutaneous lichen amyloidosis
	Lipoma, angiofibroma, collagenoma	5. Ganglioneuroma, marfanoid habitus
Surgery to prevent or cure malignant growth	No good method	Effective at young age for C-cell cancer
Mutation testing	Limited role	Important to prevent malignant growth

[a] Listed tissues are numbered within MEN2 and grouped among the following three MEN2 subtypes: multiple endocrine neoplasia type 2a (MEN2a) (1, 2, 3, 4); multiple endocrine neoplasia type 2b (MEN2b) (2, 3, 5); familial medullary thyroid cancer only (FMTC) (2).

brane–spanning tyrosine kinase. Unlike *MEN1, RET* encodes a direct-acting oncogene that becomes oncogenic by mechanisms of overactivation. Mutation of only highly select *RET* codons can cause *RET* kinase activation and consequently MEN2. There also is a strong relation between the codon of a *RET* mutation and the resulting phenotype. In general, *RET* activation by germ line mutation of codons in a small cysteine-rich extracellular domain causes MEN2a, whereas *RET* germ line mutation at one intracellular codon (methionine to threonine at codon 918) causes MEN2b. A more heterogeneous group of *RET* mutations, overlapping largely with those in MEN2a, occurs in FMTC.

The *RET* gene participates in several other important but only remotely related disorders. *RET* was first discovered because it can be overexpressed from a splicing rearrangement. This is not found in MEN2 but is a frequent contributor to common (nonhereditary) papillary thyroid cancer. *RET* is one of several genes, the inactivation of which can cause aganglionosis of the intestines (Hirschsprung's disease). It is thus paradoxical that MEN2a and Hirschsprung's disease occasionally coexist.

The *MEN1* and *RET* genes each contribute through somatic (nonhereditary) mutation to development of many sporadic tumors of the sorts that occur with the respective hereditary syndrome. For example, somatic inactivation of both copies of *MEN1* is the most frequent mutation in common parathyroid adenoma or in gastrinoma.

MULTIPLE ENDOCRINE NEOPLASIA TYPE 1

PARATHYROID GLANDS

MEN1 or MEN2 tumors are similar to common solitary tumors. This chapter focuses on important differences. Hyperparathyroidism is the most common and usually the first endocrine expression of MEN1. The earliest onset is at approximately 8 years of age with a peak onset at 20 to 25 years (the peak onset of sporadic parathyroid adenoma occurs at 55 years of age). There is approximately 95% expression by 50 years of age. Hy-

perparathyroidism progresses slowly. At early ages, the main surgical indications are degree of elevation of calcium and parathyroid hormone levels and likelihood of urolithiasis. Surgery is more difficult than for sporadic parathyroid adenoma because of tumor multiplicity and likely postoperative recurrence (50% rate of recurrence at 8 to 10 years), quite specific for MEN1. Thus the indications for parathyroid surgery for MEN1 should be somewhat more stringent than those for surgery for sporadic adenoma. The recommended operation is subtotal parathyroidectomy. Some centers cryopreserve fragments of the most normal tumor for possible autograft if hypoparathyroidism develops.

ENTEROPANCREATIC NEUROENDOCRINE TISSUE

Multiple enteropancreatic tumors develop in almost all patients with MEN1 in an age-dependent manner. Almost all MEN1 pancreatic islet tumors stain positively for one or more peptide hormones. The most common are insulin, glucagon, and pancreatic polypeptide. Synthesis of a peptide does not necessarily imply oversecretion of that peptide (for example, clinical glucagonoma is rare in MEN1).

Approximately 40% of patients with MEN1 have Zollinger–Ellison syndrome, the expression of gastrinoma. MEN1 gastrinoma typically develops at 35 years of age, one decade earlier than sporadic gastrinoma. The typical symptoms are those from excess gastric acid: peptic pain, reflux, diarrhea, and altered bowel habits. Hyperparathyroidism, common in MEN1, exacerbates gastrin hypersecretion while euparathyroidism and hypoparathyroidism decrease it. Diagnosis is from a combination of measurement of basal gastrin, secretin-stimulated gastrin, basal acid output, and endoscopy. Achlorhydria is a major differential diagnosis for hypergastrinemia.

Endoscopic examination of patients with MEN1 should include evaluation of the stomach for gastric carcinoids. With gastrinoma, somatostatin receptor imaging is helpful to grade tumor extent and the possibility of hepatic metastasis. Most or all gastrinomas are malignant, though often indolent. The gastrinomas of MEN1 usually are multiple, small, submucosal nodules mainly in the duodenum. Gastrinoma in MEN1 is highly difficult to improve, much less cure, with gastrointestinal surgery. Treatment in most cases should be pharmacologic because drug therapy is highly effective for the humoral component. Pharmacologic treatment is with gastric acid secretion blockers such as omeprazole. Therapy should be monitored with periodic measurements of gastric acid.

Insulinoma with a prevalence of 15% is less common than gastrinoma in MEN1. Insulinoma in MEN1 is usually benign, usually caused by only one tumor, and is imaged poorly with somatostatin receptor scintigraphy. The treatment is surgery. Nonfunctioning tumors are those that do not oversecrete a hormone. They may synthesize but not secrete a hormone, or they may oversecrete a nonhormonal peptide (pancreatic polypeptide or chromogranin A). Nonfunctional tumors are not recognized as often as they occur because they become clinically apparent only when they become large or metastatic. Very uncommon pancreatic endocrine tumors in MEN1 include glucagonoma, vasoactive intestinal peptide–secreting tumor (VIPoma), and growth hormone releasing hormone–secreting tumor (GRH-oma). When recognized, these tumors are generally malignant, large, and metastatic.

ANTERIOR PITUITARY GLAND

Anterior pituitary tumors occur in 30% of cases. Most are prolactinoma, followed by growth hormone or growth hormone–prolactin, then corticotropin, and so-called nonfunctional tumors. The features and management of pituitary tumors in MEN1 are similar to those of sporadic tumors.

OTHER FEATURES

Carcinoid of the foregut (thymus, bronchus, or stomach) occurs in 10% of cases and is frequently malignant. However, it does not cause carcinoid syndrome or ectopic corticotropin syndrome. As a preventive measure, thymectomy is usually done through the neck at initial parathyroid surgery for MEN1. Lipoma occurs in one-third of cases. Subtle skin tumors (angiofibroma and collagenoma) are very common in MEN1. These can contribute to the diagnosis of MEN1 and are best recognized by an experienced dermatologist.

PREVENTION AND MANAGEMENT OF MALIGNANT GROWTH

Approximately half of patients with MEN1 have a malignant MEN1 tumor, but only one-fourth of the tumors grow or metastasize rapidly. Gastrinoma is most frequent, and the rest are other enteropancreatic tumors and foregut carcinoid tumors. About one-third of deaths of MEN1 are caused by these malignant lesions. Unlike the effective malignancy prevention of MEN2, there is no effective prevention or cure of the malignant tumors of MEN1. A common strategy is resection if a pancreatic nodule larger than 2 to 2.5 cm is imaged. Other treatment considerations include debulking surgery, somatostatin analogs to inhibit hormone secretion, interferon-α, and chemotherapy.

DIAGNOSIS OF MEN1 AND FOLLOW-UP CARE

In a sporadic case, the standard criteria for diagnosis are tumor in two of the three major tissues (parathyroid, enteropancreatic, anterior pituitary). Other features, such as multiple parathyroid tumors, render *MEN1* mutation more or less likely. In a family, the clinical criteria for diagnosis are one case with MEN1 plus a first-degree relative with tumor in one of the three major tissues. The principal conditions in differential diagnosis are familial hyperparathyroidism, which can be an expression of MEN1, familial hypocalciuric hypercalcemia, or several less common disorders. Cost-effective biochemical ascertainment can include ionized calcium, parathyroid hormone, and prolactin, measured at 3- to 5-year intervals between the ages of 5 and 50 years. Nonhormonal markers (pancreatic polypeptide and chromogranin A) are not useful. Robust *MEN1* mutation testing could obviate much of this biochemical ascertainment testing.

Follow-up care of an affected patient or carrier is complex. Each tissue must be handled independently. New tumors will arise, and removed ones can recur. A program must be designed to strike a balance of cost and efficacy.

■ MULTIPLE ENDOCRINE NEOPLASIA TYPE 2

CALCITONIN-PRODUCING PARAFOLLICULAR THYROID CELLS (C-CELLS)

C-cell cancer accounts for only 10% of all thyroid cancers; of this minority, 10% to 20% are associated with MEN2. Sporadic tumor is typically recognized around the age of 50 years as a palpable nodule and with metastases. Sporadic MEN2 can have a similarly advanced presentation. Most cases of familial MEN2 are recognized by means of prospective screening, excepting MEN2b, half of which is from new mutation.

The normal C-cells or parafollicular cells are dispersed between the thyroid follicular cells and their basement membranes. The earliest C-cell lesions in MEN2 are benign clumps of C-cells, called *C-cell hyperplasia*. Malignant growth progresses with age. It is expressed subclinically in virtually all cases by 30 years of age but is expressed clinically in only one-third of patients by 70 years of age. C-cell cancer is multifocal and consequently bilateral in MEN2. Calcitonin immunohistologic testing or assay of an aspirated specimen can be specific. The malignant growth spreads to local nodes and occasionally to the liver at a late stage. Although it is a hormone, calcitonin even at high levels in blood causes no symptoms. Thus calcitonin is more correctly considered a useful tumor marker in this context. Almost all C-cell cancers cause hypercalcitoninemia at early stages. Unstimulated calcitonin has limited value for diagnosis because there are many false-positive findings, including some other malignant neoplasms.

Biochemical screening can be conducted by means of measurement of calcitonin after brief infusion of a bolus of pentagastrin, a synthetic secretagogue for calcitonin. However, experience has shown excessive numbers of false-positive results even with careful attention to normal control ranges. The standard of diagnosis is not tumor but *RET* germ line mutation (see later). Tumors are most aggressive in MEN2b and least aggressive in FMTC.

Therapy for C-cell cancer in MEN2 is thyroid surgery. An early operation for prevention is total thyroidectomy with removal of central nodes and with an attempt to preserve parathyroid function. When the likelihood or extent of metastases is higher, the extent of lymph node removal should increase. Calcitonin should be used as a tumor marker for follow-up care. Once C-cell cancer persists or recurs after an extensive operation, gains or even cure from further resection are sometimes still possible.

PHEOCHROMOCYTOMA

Pheochromocytoma, usually benign, occurs in 50% of cases of MEN2a or MEN2b. Pheochromocytoma is functionally similar in MEN2 and in sporadic cases. However, in MEN2 the tumors secrete a higher fraction of epinephrine and are often bilateral. The age at onset is earlier and syndrome dependent: 25 years for MEN2b, 40 years for MEN2a. A danger specific to MEN2 is hypertensive crisis during labor or during thyroidectomy. Pheochromocytoma, because of its unpredictable course and metabolic severity, remains an important cause of mortality due to MEN2. In MEN2, pheochromocytoma can be screened with urine epinephrine and norepinephrine testing. This test should be supplemented with imaging by means of computed tomography or magnetic resonance imaging. Treatment is surgery; experienced teams are divided between unilateral and bilateral adrenalectomy.

PARATHYROID DISORDER

Hyperparathyroidism is a component of MEN2a but not of MEN2b or FMTC. Hyperparathyroidism is uncommon (10–40%) and generally mild and asymptomatic in MEN2a. There may be one or two parathyroid tumors, as opposed to three or four in MEN1. The indications for surgery are the same as for conventional hyperparathyroidism. Prior thyroid surgery for C-cell disease can make this procedure as difficult as a typical parathyroid reoperation. In 20% of cases, asymptomatic parathyroid tumor is encountered during thyroid surgery for MEN2a. Standard treatment is surgical removal of enlarged parathyroid glands. Hyperparathyroidism in MEN2a does not have a high rate of postoperative recurrence in the manner of that in MEN1.

OTHER FEATURES

Patients with MEN2a occasionally have cutaneous lichen amyloidosis. These are intrascapular plaques preceded by pruritus. This condition is limited to occasional MEN2a families, and the associated *RET* mutations are not specific. Patients with MEN2b have a characteristic marfanoid habitus plus hypertelorisim, bumpy lips, and bumpy tongue. They also have characteristic neural lesions—submucosal neuromas, ganglioneuromas, and thickened corneal nerves. Submucosal neuromas cause the bumpy lips and bumpy tongue. Intestinal ganglioneuromas cause bowel motility problems.

PREVENTION AND MANAGEMENT OF MALIGNANT DISEASE

Unlike the malignant growth in MEN1, that in MEN2 often can be prevented or cured with early intervention. *RET* mutation testing is the most effective way to ensure correct diagnosis and early intervention. Although MEN2 is rare, it is a paradigm for early testing and early therapy for malignant neoplasia. This testing once was conducted with mixed results by means of radioimmunoassay for pentagastrin-evoked calcitonin. With the possibility of finding the *RET* mutation in almost all cases, robust DNA diagnostic testing has replaced calcitonin testing for this purpose. For MEN2b and MEN2a the earliest ages at cancer detection are 1 and 5 years. These are the best ages for *RET* mutation testing and preventive thyroid surgery. For these purposes, FMTC is handled as MEN2a.

DIAGNOSIS OF MEN2 AND FOLLOW-UP CARE

Clinical diagnosis in a sporadic case of MEN2 is based on tumor multiplicity or on characteristic histologic features (C-cell hyperplasia and tumor multifocality). Once the diagnosis is suspected, *RET* mutation testing is the critical index. It is possible to identify a *RET* mutation in virtually every case of MEN2. C-cell follow-up testing depends on whether the tumors have been completely extirpated. Carriers and patients with MEN2 should undergo annual tests for pheochromocytoma and tests for hyperparathyroidism every 5 years.

BIBLIOGRAPHY

Eng C. Seminars in medicine of the Beth Israel Hospital, Boston. The *RET* protooncogene in multiple endocrine neoplasia type 2 and Hirschsprung's disease. *N Engl J Med* 1996;335:943–951.

Jensen RT. Management of the Zollinger-Ellison syndrome in patients with multiple endocrine neoplasia type 1. *J Intern Med* 1998;243:477–488.

Lips CJ, Landsvater RM, Hoppener JW, et al. Clinical screening as compared with DNA analysis in families with multiple endocrine neoplasia type 2A. *N Engl J Med* 1994;331:828–835.

Marx SJ, Spiegel AM, Skarulis MC, et al. Multiple endocrine neoplasia type 1: clinical and genetic topics. *Ann Intern Med* 1998;129:484–494.

Skinner MA, Wells SA Jr. Medullary carcinoma of the thyroid gland and the MEN2 syndromes. *Semin Pediatr Surg* 1997;6:134–140.

Kelley's Textbook of Internal Medicine, fourth edition. Edited by H. David Humes. Lippincott Williams & Wilkins, Philadelphia © 2000.

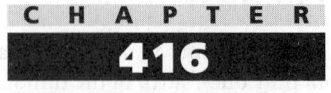

CHAPTER
416

GENETIC DISORDERS

RICHARD W. ERBE

Genetic disorders have traditionally been classified into three major groups—chromosomal disorders, mendelian disorders, and multifactorial disorders. The chromosomal disorders consist of numerical or structural abnormalities in one or more chromosomes that are visible with a light microscope or detected by means of molecular techniques. The phenotypic abnormalities associated with these disorders are caused by the gain or loss of often large numbers of genes produced by structural or numeric chromosomal changes or by inactivation of genes at chromosomal breakpoints. More recently recognized are disorders resulting from imbalance of the paternal and maternal genetic contributions at particular loci, designated parent-of-origin defects. Mendelian disorders are caused by mutations at a single genetic locus. These mutations usually consist of substitutions of a single DNA base or a few bases or the addition or deletion of bases in a region too small to be seen with a light microscope.

In mendelian disorders, one mutant gene or a pair of mutant genes at a single locus is sufficient to produce an abnormal phenotype under the usual environmental conditions. Some mendelian disorders in which the severity of the phenotype characteristically increases in successive generations are known to be caused by expansion in the corresponding locus of a special segment of coding or noncoding DNA known as a trinucleotide repeat. Multifactorial disorders are caused by the collective contributions of mutant genes at several loci acting in concert and with usually unidentified environmental factors. These mutations may be similar to those that produce mendelian disorders, but the loci at which the mutations occur are individually less influential in determining the phenotype. Still other disorders are caused by mutations in the circular 16,569 base pair mitochondrial chromosome or by mutations in somatic cells alone acting in concert with meiotically inherited, or germ line, mutations. Somatic mutations, and combined somatic and germ line mutations, underlie the diverse forms of cancer.

Many references in this chapter, especially in the tables, are to OMIM numbers. These represent the on-line version of the numbering system originated many years ago by Dr. Victor A. McKusick in his book *Mendelian Inheritance in Man.* OMIM and another database of genetic disorders, GeneClinics, are especially useful examples of the wealth of readily accessible, current information about genetic disorders available at the World Wide Web addresses at the end of this chapter.

■ MENDELIAN INHERITANCE AND DISORDERS

Mendelian traits, normal and abnormal, are those that follow the pedigree patterns described in 1865 by Gregor Mendel in research with garden peas and only decades later recognized to apply to humans. Mendelian traits or disorders are determined by genes at a single locus in either the homozygous or heterozygous state. Variant DNA sequences for genes at a given locus are alleles or alternative forms of a gene. A *locus* is a site on a chromosome occupied by a gene or a set of alleles. When the paired genes at a locus on homologous chromosomes are identical, the person is homozygous at that locus and is called a *homozygote.* When the genes differ, the person is heterozygous and called a *heterozygote* or if phenotypically unaffected a *carrier.* The term *compound heterozygote* describes a genotype in which two different mutant, potentially pathogenic alleles are present rather than one mutant allele and one normal allele. The term *hemizygous* applies to the state of men and boys with regard to the X chromosome because the Y chromosome does not provide corresponding paired genes. *Hemizygous* also applies to genes in the region of an autosome for which the corresponding region on the homologous chromosome has been deleted.

The pedigree patterns exhibited by mendelian phenotypes depend on whether the gene responsible is on an autosome or on a sex chromosome and whether the trait is dominant or recessive. They may thus be autosomal dominant, autosomal recessive, or X-linked. Distinctions between dominant and recessive traits apply at the level of the phenotype, the outward expression of the gene, rather than the gene itself. A *dominant trait* is one in which heterozygosity is sufficient to produce a recognizable corresponding phenotype. A *recessive trait* is fully expressed only when the person is homozygous or hemizygous for that allele. According to the formal definition, a recessive gene has no detectable expression in heterozygotes. There are techniques to detect expression at some level of nearly all functional genes. In practice, phenotypes are classified as recessive when they are not evident at clinical examination of a heterozygote. The term *codominant* is used to describe loci at which the products of both alleles are expressed in heterozygotes, generally in regard to serum proteins (e.g., globins), cell-surface markers (e.g., ABO blood groups), and the like.

To illustrate these distinctions, consider the sickling hemoglobin disorders that involve one or more genes for hemoglobin S or its potentially pathogenic alleles, hemoglobin C or β-thalassemia (see Chapters 241 and 244). The homozygous disorder is sickle cell anemia, in which the person's genotype at the β-globin locus is SS. The heterozygote or carrier has sickle cell trait and has the β-globin genotype AS. The compound heterozygote is represented by hemoglobin SC disease, a sickling disorder that is usually less severe than sickle cell anemia, or by Sβ-thalassemia, a variable sickling disorder. The terms *homozygous, heterozygous,* and *compound heterozygote* can be applied either to a person or to a genotype. With regard to whether a trait is considered dominant or recessive, sickle cell anemia is an autosomal recessive disorder, the life-threatening signs and symptoms of which are manifest in the homozygote. In contrast, sickling phenomenon (sickling of erythrocytes in vitro under appropriate test conditions) is dominant, occurring when either one or two genes for hemoglobin S are present.

AUTOSOMAL DOMINANT DISORDERS

Pedigree Patterns

Autosomal dominant disorders typically exhibit generation-to-generation transmission without intervening unaffected offspring, expression among both sexes, a 50% probability that offspring of an affected person will inherit the gene for the disorder, transmission from an affected parent of either sex to offspring of either sex, and absence of the disorder among offspring of persons who have an affected parent but did not themselves inherit the gene. A new mutation often can be inferred to have occurred when a person with clear phenotypic evidence of an autosomal dominant disorder is born to a family in which neither the parents nor other relatives are similarly affected.

Many autosomal dominant disorders, however, exhibit incomplete penetrance and variable expressivity. *Penetrance* is the degree to which a gene is likely to be expressed when it is present. It is an all-or-none phenomenon for any one person but can be expressed as a percentage when large numbers of persons known to have a particular allele are examined. (For example, when one-half of a large number of persons with a mutant allele for a particular disorder express one or more characteristics of that disorder and one-half do not, the penetrance is 50%.) In general, the more thorough the clinical examination, the greater the penetrance proves to be. *Expressivity* is the variability in severity of manifestations of a genetic disorder or trait among different persons with the same genetic disorder as defined with clinical criteria and sometimes additional laboratory, radiographic, and other criteria. In some autosomal disorders the phenotypic severity varies little between affected members of any given family, whereas in others it varies greatly. Factors contributing to greater variability seldom are specifically identified. They may, however, include the effects of other genes, of stochastic factors in one or more steps leading to gene expression, or of environmental factors alone or in combination.

Genetic heterogeneity is the principle that similar phenotypes can be caused by different genotypes. For example, both Charcot–Marie–Tooth disease of hereditary motor and sensory neuropathy and Alport syndrome of hereditary nephritis and sensorineural deafness have both autosomal dominant and X-linked forms. These are examples of locus heterogeneity, because the loci for the two clinically similar forms of these disorders must reside on an autosome and on the X chromosome, respectively. Polycystic kidney disease and osteogenesis imperfecta both have autosomal dominant and recessive forms. *Allelic heterogeneity* is phenotypic differences between affected individuals and families caused by different mutant alleles. For example, 85% of families with cystic fibrosis have pancreatic insufficiency as one of the manifestations; the other 15% do not have pancreatic insufficiency as part of the cystic fibrosis phenotype.

In autosomal dominant disorders, heterozygotes manifest the abnormal features of the disorder. Through various mechanisms, the deficiency or defectiveness of the product of one of two paired alleles produces an abnormal phenotype. In contrast, partial or complete loss of function of one allele in autosomal recessive disorders produces a carrier state and little or no phenotypic change. By definition, a dominant disorder should have its full expression regardless of the presence or absence of a normal allele at the homologous locus. This is rarely the case among humans. When apparent homozygosity for an ordinarily autosomal dominant disorder has been observed, the child is consistently much more severely affected. Examples include familial hypercholesterolemia and achondroplasia. The only known exception to increased severity of expression of an autosomal dominant phenotype in the homozygous state is Huntington's disease. In this disease, there is no observable phenotypic difference between the homozygote and the heterozygote, as it is a truly autosomal dominant disorder.

Examples of Autosomal Dominant Disorders

Table 416.1 presents examples of disorders that illustrate the principles of autosomal dominant inheritance. Achondroplasia is a fully penetrant, dominantly inherited form of dwarfism characterized by short limbs, a large head, and a characteristic habitus. The proportion of persons with achondroplasia caused by new mutation is high, 85% to 90% being born to parents of normal stature. In general, the more severe the phenotypic effect of a disorder, the higher the proportion of new mutations. Achondroplasia poses several major barriers to reproduction. The result is a reduction in *fitness,* the likelihood of reproducing and transmitting one's genes. Achondroplasia due to new mutation, like new mutations in several other autosomal dominant (neurofibromatosis type 1) and X-linked (hemophilia A) disorders, is more likely with increasing age of the father, the paternal age effect.

Charcot–Marie–Tooth disease (CMT) is a group of inherited disorders that together constitute the most common form of hereditary motor and sensory neuropathy. Autosomal dominant, autosomal recessive, and X-linked forms occur. The various forms share clinical features. Diagnostic distinctions are based on findings at physical examination, electromyography, nerve conduction velocity testing, and molecular testing. About one-half of cases of CMT are classified as CMT1, 70% to 80% of which are of the CMT1A type (OMIM 118220), which involve the peripheral myelin protein gene (*PMP22*) on 17p11. These patients exhibit 1.5 million base pair duplications on one copy of chromosome 17. This results in the presence of three, rather than two, copies of this region, which contains *PMP22*. In an unknown manner, the associated gene dosage sensitivity produces the demyelination that underlies this disorder. Within some of these families are persons with a disorder known as *hereditary neuropathy with liability to pressure palsies* (HNPP; OMIM 162500). Affected individuals are predisposed to repeated, reversible, usually mild episodes of pressure neuropathy such as carpal tunnel syndrome and peroneal palsy with foot drop. About 70% to 80% of these persons have a microdeletion of the short arm of chromosome 17p11-p12, which includes the *PMP22* gene. Families segregating both disorders may represent the expected outcomes of misalignment of the paired homologous chromosomes during meiosis with crossing-over in the mispaired region.

Genetic disorders of lipids and lipoproteins are described in Chapters 12 and 31. Of these, familial hypercholesterolemia (FH; OMIM 143890) illustrates the principle that although heterozygotes manifest an autosomal dominant disorders, homozygotes or compound heterozygotes often have even more severe manifestations. FH is inherited in an autosomal dominant pattern and is especially frequent. FH heterozygotes have only half-normal quantities of the cellular receptor for low-density lipoprotein (LDL) cholesterol, resulting in reduced entrance of LDL cholesterol into the cell and therefore reduced degradation and diminished feedback inhibition of endogenous cholesterol biosynthesis. Receptor deficiency increases the circulating level of cholesterol and causes infiltration of lipid into tissues. With a FH heterozygote frequency of 1/500 in the general population, about 1/25,000 matings are between two FH heterozygotes and

TABLE 416.1.   AUTOSOMAL DOMINANT DISORDERS

Disorder	Major Features	Gene and Gene Product	Additional Information	Availability of Molecular Testing
Achondroplasia	Short-limb dwarfism with large head, characteristic facies, exaggerated lumbar lordosis, trident hand, risk of death in infancy from spinal cord or upper-airway obstruction	Fibroblast growth factor receptor 3 gene (*FGFR3*) on 4p16. Most (~98%) involve the same G to A transition at nucleotide 1138 of the cDNA.	OMIM 100800 GeneClinics	Direct DNA, including prenatal
Charcot–Marie–Tooth (CMT) disease	Most common form of hereditary motor and sensory neuropathy; initially weakness, muscle atrophy, loss of deep tendon reflexes, and sensory loss in the lower legs and hands; weakness often leads to progressive foot deformity.	Duplication, frameshift, and other point mutations in the *PMP22* peripheral myelin protein 22 gene in CMT1A. Other genes involved in the other forms of CMT.	OMIM 118220 (CMT1A) GeneClinics	Direct DNA for CMT1A (17p11 duplication), HNPP (17pdeletion) and CMTX (connexin 32)
Familial hypercholesterolemia	Elevated serum low-density lipoprotein (LDL) cholesterol, cholesterol deposits in tissues, premature death of coronary artery disease	Large number and variety of mutations in the LDL receptor gene (*LDLR*) on 19p13, forming five major classes and leading to defective receptor function.	OMIM 143890	Mainly biochemical (see Chapters 12 and 31)
Marfan syndrome	Aortic aneurysm and fatal dissection, ectopia lentis, disproportionately long limbs and digits, other connective tissue abnormalities.	Mutations in the gene for fibrillin (*FBN1*; OMIM 134797), a major component of extracellular microfibrils of both elastic and nonelastic connective tissue, on 15q21.	OMIM 154700	Available but limited
Polycystic kidney disease, autosomal dominant	Renal cysts that increase in number and size with age and cause hypertension and renal failure by middle age; cysts also occur in the liver, pancreas, spleen, and gonads; increased risk of intracranial berry aneurysms and cardiac valve abnormalities	*PKD1* is a large and complex gene close to the α-globin cluster at 16p13.3 and encodes polycystin-1, apparently involved in adhesive protein–protein and protein–carbohydrate interactions in the extracellular compartment. *PKD2* at 4q21-23 encodes polycystin 2.	OMIM 173900 (*PKD1*), OMIM 173910 (*PKD2*)	Linkage

See Online Mendelian Inheritance in Man (OMIM). Center for Medical Genetics, Johns Hopkins University (Baltimore) and National Center for Biotechnology Information, National Library of Medicine (Bethesda, MD), 1999. Available at: http://www.ncbi.nlm.nih.gov/omim/.

about 1 in 1 million persons has two copies of a mutant FH allele. These compound heterozygotes completely lack functional LDL receptors and have extreme elevations in serum cholesterol concentration, extensive tissue deposition, and often fatal coronary artery disease by their teen years. Molecular studies of patients with this disorder have identified more than 350 mutations in the LDL receptor gene, most families having unique mutations that other families do not. Sixty percent of French Canadian patients have a large 5′ deletion, suggesting inheritance of this mutation from an early ancestor of the group, called a *founder effect*.

Marfan syndrome, in its fullest manifestation, produces characteristic changes in the skeletal, ocular, and cardiovascular systems with an autosomal dominant pedigree pattern. Variable expression in Marfan syndrome is the rule both within families and between families. Complete nonpenetrance has not been definitively documented. About one-fourth of affected persons have new mutations; a paternal age effect is present, on average, in sporadic cases. Most Marfan syndrome families carry unique mutations scattered throughout the gene. Although molecular studies have identified mutations in the fibrillin gene on 15q in some patients with Marfan syndrome, the proportion of families with identifiable *FBN1* mutations has ranged from 15% to 80% in large series. Many patients with Marfan syndrome thus do not have a demonstrable mutation in the fibrillin gene. Mutations in *FBN1* have been found in several related connective tissue disorders with different but overlapping phenotypes. Although DNA testing can be used for some families in which a *FBN1* mutant allele has been identified, it is very limited in diagnosing new cases because not all Marfan patients have identifiable *FBN1* mutations; because *FBN1* mutations occur in other disorders; and because identification of a mutant allele may still be a poor predictor of phenotypic severity. As described in Chapter 186, studies of Marfan syndrome, the various autosomal dominant forms of osteogenesis imperfecta, and other inherited connective tissue disorders have shed light on the mechanisms by which heterozygosity for mutant alleles can produce a dominantly inherited disorder and on the often complex genetic heterogeneity of these disorders.

The most frequent forms of polycystic kidney disease are inherited in an autosomal dominant pattern with locus heterogeneity. Autosomal dominant polycystic kidney disease (ADPKD) affects about half a million people and is the reason for renal transplantation for about 10% of the patients undergoing transplantation. With an incidence of approximately 1/800 in all populations, mutations in the *PKD1* gene account for about 85% of cases and those in the *PKD2* gene account for the others. A third possible locus, *PKD3*, remains to be identified. The phenotypes associated with mutations in *PKD1* and *PKD2* are clinically very similar and consist mainly of progressive renal enlargement and cyst formation, which usually leads to end-stage renal disease in later life. Extrarenal manifestations include hepatic and pancreatic cyst and cerebral artery aneurysms. Marked variation in clinical presentation of ADPKD exists between and within families. This may be explained in part by evidence of a genetic two-hit mechanism in renal and hepatic cyst formation. Germ line and somatic inactivating mutations

of the *PKD1* gene have been identified in cyst-lining epithelial cells.

AUTOSOMAL RECESSIVE DISORDERS

Pedigree Patterns

Homozygotes and compound heterozygotes are affected in autosomal recessive disorders. The health and life expectancy of heterozygous carriers of genes for autosomal recessive disorders are normal, although the carrier state may be apparent under special circumstances. Autosomal recessive inheritance is suggested in pedigrees in which siblings with a known or suspected autosomal recessive phenotype are born to unaffected parents, particularly in the case of a rare disorder in a consanguineous mating. In theory, when all of those with the gene are identified and large numbers of families are studied, the sexes are affected in equal numbers, and 25% of the offspring of carrier–carrier couples are affected. In practice, however, large deviations from expected mendelian proportions are common because of chance and the small size of most families.

Autosomal recessive disorders constitute most of the inborn errors of metabolism. The primary biochemical lesions have been identified in about 800 of these disorders, simplifying their identification and sometimes providing a basis for therapy. Many of these defects are demonstrable in skin fibroblasts, peripheral blood lymphocytes, and amniotic fluid cells cultured from those affected. In a growing number of instances, characterization at the DNA level has made it possible to test for these disorders independently of actual gene expression. In other instances, the identification of a large number of alleles, variable expression, and other factors have made biochemical assays the most accurate means of assessing the presence and severity of a disorder.

Autosomal recessive disorders occur in both the homozygous and genetic compound states. Compound heterozygotes may have clinical or laboratory findings that differ from the classic phenotype. Homozygosity is more likely when an allele occurs at high population frequency and in consanguineous matings. Compound heterozygosity is more likely with lower allele frequency and nonconsanguineous matings, as is usually the case.

Examples of Autosomal Recessive Disorders

Various combinations of alleles at a complex locus on chromosome 6 near HLA result in four clinical forms of 21-hydroxylase (CYP21) deficiency, the most frequent cause of congenital adrenal hyperplasia (Table 416.2). Severe CYP21 deficiency causes the salt-losing form of congenital adrenal hyperplasia with marked deficiencies of both mineralocorticoids and glucocorticoids. Lesser CYP21 deficiencies cause the simple virilizing and late-onset forms. Impairment of 21-hydroxylation in the adrenal cortex reduces the conversion of 17-hydroxyprogesterone (17-OHP) to 11-deoxycortisol. The lack of cortisol increases corticotropin, resulting in overproduction and accumulation of cortisol precursors (especially 17-OHP) proximal to the block. This leads to excessive production of androgens, resulting in varying degrees of virilization. Women pregnant with a female fetus found to have inherited the alleles for this autosomal recessive disorder

TABLE 416.2. AUTOSOMAL RECESSIVE DISORDERS

Disorder	Major Features	Gene and Gene Product	Additional Information	Availability of Molecular Testing
Adrenal hyperplasia, congenital, due to 21-hydroxylase deficiency	CYP21 (21-hydroxylase) deficiency accounts for more than 90% of cases of congenital adrenal hyperplasia (CAH) and is manifest in four distinct clinical forms of CAH: salt-wasting, simple virilizing, nonclassic late onset, and cryptic.	The CYP21 gene on 6p21.3 encodes the adrenal microsomal cytochrome P450 responsible for steroid 21-hydroxylation. Nearby is CYP21P, a second 21-hydroxylase gene that is nonfunctional and considered to be a pseudogene. The tandem duplication of this locus is the basis for most of the pathogenic mutations.	OMIM 201910	Direct DNA, prenatal
Albinism, oculocutaneous, tyrosinase related, and tyrosinase-positive	Congenital hypopigmentation of skin, hair and eyes accompanied by reduced retinal pigment with foveal hypoplasia, and misrouting of optic fibers at the chiasm. Symptoms include nystagmus, defective vision, abnormal depth perception, and cutaneous sun sensitivity.	OCA1 results from a variety of mutations in the tyrosinase gene on 11q14-q21; classified into types based on the amount and type of residual tyrosinase activity. OCA2 results from mutations in the gene for the P protein at 15q11-q12.	OMIM 203100 (OCA1), OMIM 203200 (OCA2)	Direct DNA, prenatal (OCA1)
α₁-antitrypsin deficiency	Infantile liver abnormalities in fewer than 20% of cases. Dyspnea, onset 35 years among smokers, 45 years among nonsmokers, associated with small airway and alveolar wall destruction, leading to emphysema especially at bases. Increased risk of hepatocellular carcinoma.	Mutations in PI gene at 14q32.1 resulting in deficiency of serum α_1-antitrypsin. PI Z allele is the most common deficiency allele. ZZ homozygotes are fully affected, MZ heterozygotes are at increased risk of COPD.	OMIM 107400 (protease inhibitor 1, PI)	PI activity assay, PI typing and DNA mutation analysis (direct DNA, linkage, prenatal)
Ataxia–telangiectasia	Progressive cerebellar ataxia beginning in early childhood, choreoathetosis, telangiectasias of the conjunctivae, and increased sensitivity to ionizing radiation followed by immunodeficiency and malignant disease, particularly leukemia and lymphoma.	Large ATM gene on 11q22-q23 appears to function in a signal transduction pathway that controls G1 checkpoint cell cycle arrest following DNA damage. Mutations at the ATM locus have been identified in DNA from many but not all patients having each of the four cell culture complementation groups.	OMIM 208900 GeneClinics	Direct DNA, linkage, prenatal. Also serum AFP, colony survival assay, measures of immunocompetence.
Cystic fibrosis (CF)	Exocrine dysfunction leading to chronic obstructive lung disease, malabsorption and failure to thrive due to pancreatic insufficiency, and aspermia in affected males are characteristic. Many other manifestations occur less frequently, including meconium ileus (about 15%), cirrhosis of the liver, diabetes mellitus, nasal polyposis, and sinusitis.	More than 800 CF-related mutant alleles of the CFTR gene at 7q31.2. Except for the ΔF508 allele, no other single mutation accounts for more than 5% of CF chromosomes in most populations. Among persons of Ashkenazic Jewish ancestry, however, a test for 30 mutations detects 97% of CF carriers.	OMIM 219700	Direct DNA, linkage, prenatal
Gaucher disease types I, II, and III	The most common of the lysosomal storage diseases. Type I (adult, chronic, non-neuronopathic) is characterized by hypersplenism, bone lesions, skin pigmentation, and by the absence of neurologic abnormalities. Types II (infantile, acute) and III (juvenile, subacute) are neuronopathic.	Allelic mutations in the gene for acid β-glucosidase, or glucocerebrosidase, at 1q21 result in 3 clinical types, types 2 and 3 are associated with lower residual enzyme activity. More than 100 mutant alleles have been identified, most single-base changes, but genotype–phenotype correlation is imprecise.	OMIM 230800 (type I), 230900 (type II), and (231000) type III GeneClinics	Direct DNA, prenatal

(continued)

TABLE 416.2. *Continued*

Disorder	Major Features	Gene and Gene Product	Additional Information	Availability of Molecular Testing
Hemochromatosis (HH)	Characterized clinically by the combination of skin pigmentation, hepatic cirrhosis, diabetes mellitus, and cardiac disorders manifest in later life, predominantly in men.	Associated with two missense mutations in the *HFE* gene at 6p21.3. Allele C282Y (G to A at nucleotide 845; Tyr for Cys at amino acid 282) is found in XX% of patients with HH. The role of H63D (C to G at nucleotide 187; Asp for His at amino acid 63) is uncertain.	OMIM 235200	Direct DNA
Phenylketonuria, classic (PKU)	Neonates with PKU have marked hyperphenylalaninemia when they begin to ingest protein, often accompanied by irritability, hypertonicity, seizures, eczema, and a mousy odor. If untreated, they may go on to have severe, irreversible mental retardation and microcephaly.	Classic PKU results from deficiency of phenylalanine hydroxylase (PAH), the locus for which is on 12q24.1. A large number of mutant alleles have been described, three-fourths of which are missense mutations in the *PAH* gene at 12q24.1.	OMIM 261600	Direct DNA, linkage, prenatal
Polycystic kidney disease and hepatic disease (PKDH1)	Severe oligohydramnios and abnormal facies with perinatal presentation; enlarged kidneys, renal failure, and hepatic and biliary abnormalities in infantile and childhood forms.	Prenatal diagnosis with ultrasonography is unreliable but often can be achieved using linkage of DNA markers to the PKDH1 locus at 6p21.1-p12.	OMIM 263200	Linkage
Sickle cell anemia	Septicemia, anemia, episodic painful crises, tissue infarcts, and many other possible abnormalities.	In addition to the missense mutations leading to hemoglobin S, and hemoglobin C and the hemoglobin β locus (OMIM 141900) at 11p15, many other alleles occur, some resulting in clinical abnormalities.	OMIM 603900	Direct DNA, prenatal
Spinal muscular atrophy (SMA)	Muscle weakness and atrophy, hypotonia, and diminished movement of fetus and infant, decreased or absent deep tendon reflexes, respiratory failure. Three types of recessive SMA are based on age at onset, maximum muscular activity achieved, and survival.	Associated in many cases with disruption of the telomeric copy of a duplicated gene called *SMA1* (OMIM 600354) for survival motor neuron at 5q12.2-q13.3. The gene is missing in most patients with SMA, and small intragenic mutations in the gene have been associated with spinal muscular atrophy.	OMIM 253300 (SMA 1, Werdnig–Hoffman disease); OMIM 253550 (SMA II, intermediate form); OMIM 253400 (SMA III, Kugelberg–Welander disease)	Direct DNA, prenatal, linkage
Tay–Sachs disease	Characterized by loss of motor skills beginning at 3–6 months of age with progressive evidence of neurodegeneration, including seizures, blindness, and eventual total incapacitation and death, usually before the age of 4 years. The juvenile, chronic, and adult-onset variants of the GM2 gangliosidoses (HEX A-deficient) have later onsets, slower progression, and more variable neurologic findings.	The infantile form is associated with mutations in the gene for the α-subunit of the enzyme hexosaminidase A (*HEXA*) at 15q23-q24, resulting in severe deficiency. These mutations have been reported worldwide in diverse ethnic groups, but the frequency of the disease and its carrier states is highest in Ashkenazi Jews where three *HEXA* mutations account for 95% to 98% of Jewish heterozygotes.	OMIM 272800	Enzyme assay for HEXA deficiency; direct DNA and prenatal for diagnosis and genetic counseling
Wilson's disease	Manifests as chronic liver or neurologic disease, often with renal disease and a corneal (Kayser–Fleischer) ring, caused by accumulation of toxic levels of copper in tissues, mainly liver, brain, and kidney.	A variety of mutations identified throughout the *ATP7B* locus at 13q14.3. Most affected individuals are compound heterozygotes.	OMIM 277900	Linkage, prenatal

COPD, Chronic obstructive pulmonary disease.
See Online Mendelian Inheritance in Man (OMIM) Center for Medical Genetics, Johns Hopkins University (Baltimore) and National Center for Biotechnology Information, National Library of Medicine (Bethesda, MD), 1999. Available at: http://www.ncbi.nlm.nih.gov/omim/.

can be treated with dexamethasone (because cortisol does not cross the placenta) starting at no later than 5 to 6 weeks of gestation to suppress fetal androgen production and prevent virilization of the external genitalia of affected girls. Reflecting the very high allele frequency, the late-onset form of CYP21 deficiency is a common cause of hirsutism and even infertility among women.

Albinism of the oculocutaneous type manifests as generalized hypopigmentation and nystagmus. More than a dozen forms of oculocutaneous albinism (OCA) have been identified that together occur at an overall frequency of approximately 1 case among 20,000 persons. These are grouped according to several clinical and laboratory findings, especially whether hair bulbs from affected persons can produce melanin when incubated in a tyrosine solution, indicating the presence of the enzyme tyrosinase. Some melanin pigment develops in persons with tyrosinase-positive albinism, as a result of which they have less severe visual defects and sun sensitivity than those with tyrosinase-negative albinism, in whom no pigment develops. In addition to these outward manifestations, persons with OCA have a defect in decussation of the optic pathways, an abnormality that must have originated early in development. OCA1 is caused by a variety of mutations in the tyrosinase gene and is further classified into types based on the amount and type of residual tyrosinase activity and corresponding pigmentation. OCA2 is the most prevalent type of albinism worldwide. It is caused by mutations in the gene for P protein, also called *melanocyte-specific transporter protein*. Disturbances of pigmentation occur in many other single-gene disorders.

Persons with α_1-antitrypsin deficiency lack the major serum protease inhibitor that normally prevents the tissue damage that would otherwise be produced by neutrophil elastase. Many mutant alleles have been characterized, and both homozygotes and compound heterozygotes have been identified. The deficiency is most often associated with the Z allele, the product of which is unable to leave the liver cells in which it is synthesized. Infants and young children with the deficiency may have hepatitis or cirrhosis. For adults, the deficiency is associated with emphysema that develops in the third decade among smokers and the fifth decade among nonsmokers. This disorder is present in about 120,000 persons in the United States.

Ataxia–telangiectasia (Table 416.2) is one of several autosomal recessive disorders that manifest abnormal sensitivity to physical agents, such as light and radiation, or to chemicals, often resulting in somatic chromosomal abnormalities and an increased risk of cancer. Bloom syndrome (OMIM 210900), several forms of xeroderma pigmentosum (OMIM 278700-80), several forms of Fanconi's anemia (OMIM 227650 and others), and hereditary nonpolyposis colon cancer are other examples of severe inherited disorders caused by specific defects in DNA repair.

Cystic fibrosis (CF) affects about 1 in 2,500 white newborns in the United States, and approximately 1 in 25 is a carrier. About 30,000 persons in the United States have CF. Great excitement was generated by the cloning of the CF transmembrane regulator (*CFTR*) gene in 1989 and the observation that a single mutant allele, designated ΔF508, was present on 68% of CF chromosomes (that is, if one were to analyze the mutant CF-related alleles on all of the pairs of number 7 chromosomes in persons affected with CF and the single number 7 chromosome bearing the CF mutation in their carrier parents, the ΔF508 allele would account for 68% of the total). Hopes for the development of a population-based carrier screening and genetic counseling program grew dimmer as an increasing number of low-frequency alleles were found. No other single mutation accounts for more than 5% of CF chromosomes in most populations. At least a dozen alleles must be screened in most situations for the carrier detection rate to approach 90%. Whereas in most autosomal recessive disorders the finding that one parent is not a carrier is enough to reduce the risk of the disorder in that couple's offspring to near zero, a negative result of a CF carrier screen reduces the risk only 90%. In couples in which one parent is a known carrier, a negative CF screen result for the other parent reduces the risk of CF in the fetus to 1/500 ($\frac{1}{2} \times \frac{1}{25} \times \frac{1}{10}$), still five times the a priori risk in the general white population.

Inability to detect all mutant alleles and inability to predict the severity of abnormalities in an affected child have posed obstacles to population screening for CF. Studies of molecular defects resulting from more than 800 mutant *CFTR* alleles have identified a group of mild *CFTR* mutations with residual chloride-channel function in the approximately 15% of patients with a pancreatic-sufficient phenotype rather than pancreatic insufficiency, as is present in the other approximately 85%. The severity of pulmonary involvement is not correlated with the *CFTR* alleles, however, nor is meconium ileus, the severe intestinal obstruction present in approximately 15% of newborns with CF. Studies of the pathogenesis of CF, and of various approaches to conventional and gene therapies are ongoing.

Most men with CF have congenital bilateral absence of the vas deferens (CBAVD) which results in aspermia. CBAVD (OMIM 277180) also occurs, however, among men who are heterozygous for a *CFTR* mutation, especially when associated with a polymorphic sequence of thymidine bases in intron 8, even though they have few if any other evidence of CF. This type of heterozygosity is said to account for about 10% of male infertility in the general population.

Gaucher disease (Table 416.2) is the most common of the lysosomal storage diseases. These are disorders associated with one or more of the approximately 50 lysosomal enzymes needed for catabolism of numerous cellular macromolecules. In Gaucher disease, classified in three types, deficiency of glucocerebrosidase causes lysosomal accumulation of glucosylceramide in mononuclear phagocytes during turnover of cell membranes, resulting in hepatosplenomegaly, skeletal disease, bone-marrow failure, pulmonary infiltration and, in some persons, neurologic disease. Type I (adult, chronic, non-neuronopathic) is characterized by hypersplenism, bone lesions, skin pigmentation, and the absence of neurologic abnormalities. The disorder is particularly frequent among Ashkenazi Jews, among whom the carrier frequency is about 1 in 13. Variable expressivity is prominent, the disease having been diagnosed as early as the first week of life and as late as 86 years. Type II (infantile, acute, neuronopathic) is characterized by infantile onset and severe neurologic involvement. Type III (juvenile, subacute, neuronopathic) is characterized by neuronopathic abnormalities that usually begin later in the first decade and progress more slowly than in the type II disorder. Correlation of genotype with clinical type is imperfect. Affected siblings and even identical twins sometimes manifest different clinical types. Treatment of patients with type I disease by means of enzyme replacement with purified human or recombinant glucocerebrosidase is expensive and widespread despite uncertainties about the variable expression of the various genotypes.

Hereditary hemochromatosis (HH) is among the most common human genetic disorders. The rare classic clinical manifestations of bronzed diabetes caused by widespread iron deposition occur late in life and predominantly among men. The diagnosis of overt HH usually is based on clinical features, elevated serum transferrin saturation, elevated ferritin levels, characteristic findings at liver biopsy, and elevated hepatic iron levels. Measurement of transferrin saturation is the single best screening test. Early molecular studies identified two missense mutations, designated C282Y and H63D, associated with HH in a gene tightly linked to the HLA class I region on chromosome 6. Homozygosity for the C282Y mutation is found among 85% to 90% of persons of northern European origin who have typical HH. Fifteen to 20 percent of the HH patient population is heterozygous for the H63D mutation, which may contribute to increased hepatic iron levels but does not cause iron overload in the absence of the C282Y mutation.

It is not clear whether heterozygosity for C282Y, H63D, or compound heterozygosity increases risk of HH. In HH family studies of relatives of known genotype, as many as one-fourth of those homozygous for the C282Y mutation did not have iron overload. The prevalence of the C282Y allele in the general population approaches 10% among Europeans. The high frequency of the C282Y allele in the target population, the availability of a simple DNA test, and the effectiveness of phlebotomy in preventing or reversing iron overload have led some authorities to urge that a population-based mass screening program be initiated. Uncertainties about genotype–phenotype correlations, reduced penetrance and cost-to-benefit ratios have led others to recommend delaying any such program until more is known.

Phenylketonuria (PKU) is the prototype of treatable inborn errors of metabolism. Occurring in 1 in 13,000 births in the United States, the classic form of PKU is caused by an inherited deficiency of phenylalanine hydroxylase that limits conversion of phenylalanine to tyrosine, resulting in deficient neurotransmitter and melanin synthesis and increasing the concentration of phenylalanine in blood and tissues. Untreated persons with PKU have mental retardation, often severe. Lifelong treatment, however, beginning in early infancy with a phenylalanine-restricted diet, prevents the mental retardation, although other learning and behavioral abnormalities may persist. Adult women with PKU risk damage to the fetal brain and heart if not treated beginning at conception despite the heterozygosity of the fetus. Prenatal diagnosis of classic PKU was not available before the development of DNA methods, because phenylalanine hydroxylase activity is expressed in diagnostically useful amounts only in the liver.

The differential diagnosis of neonatal hyperphenylalaninemia includes other disorders, such as dihydropteridine reductase deficiency (OMIM 261630) and 6-pteroyltetrahydropterin synthase deficiency (OMIM 261640), that elevate blood phenylalanine concentrations by decreasing the amount of cofactor needed by phenylalanine hydroxylase. Unlike classic PKU these disorders cannot be controlled with restriction of phenylalanine intake. Treatment is attempted by means of supplementation with appropriate forms of the missing cofactors. The latter two disorders can be phenotypically severe, and both can be diagnosed for patients and prenatally by means of direct DNA methods.

Forms of polycystic kidney disease with severe manifestations before or soon after birth are inherited in an autosomal recessive pattern (Table 416.2), unlike the ADPKD discussed earlier (Table 416.1), that manifests between 30 and 60 years of age. Designated polycystic kidney and hepatic disease (PKDH1; OMIM 263200), these forms are distinguished by clinical onset before birth, in infancy, or in childhood and by the presence of hepatic fibrosis and involvement of the intrahepatic biliary tree. Prenatal diagnosis by means of ultrasonography is unreliable but often can be achieved with linkage of DNA markers to the PKDH1 locus at 6p21.1-p12. This is an example of the tendency, due to fitness, or likelihood of reproduction, considerations, for phenotypically severe disorders to be inherited in an autosomal recessive pattern. Phenotypically milder disorders with similar types of manifestations are more often inherited in a dominant pattern. Homozygotes or compound heterozygotes for PKDH1, for example, would not reproduce, and thus their mutant genes would be lost to the gene pool. In contrast, the fitness of the much more numerous heterozygous carriers of severe autosomal recessive disorders usually is indistinguishable from that of persons with normal genes. The rarer the autosomal recessive disorder, the greater is the proportion of genes for the disorder that reside in heterozygous carriers rather than homozygous affected persons. Genetic selection against deleterious genes is thus weak in the case of genes for the rarer autosomal recessive disorders.

Sickle cell anemia is present in approximately 1 in 400 to 600 African American newborns and affects about 50,000 persons in the United States. About 1 in 12 African Americans has sickle cell trait. The discovery of hemoglobin S and its mutational basis are landmarks in the history of biochemical genetics. The high gene frequency in an identifiable population, the lack of a cure or fully effective treatment, and the availability of accurate carrier screening and prenatal diagnostic methods have been the bases for the widespread availability of screening and genetic counseling programs for the sickling disorders (hemoglobin disorders SS, SC, and Sβ-thalassemia). The great variability of clinical severity, hopes for effective conventional or gene therapy, and other issues have contributed to the low level of use of such programs in the United States.

Spinal muscular atrophy (SMA) affects 1 in 10,000 live births. The disorder is characterized by degeneration of anterior horn cells of the spinal cord, symmetrical weakness and wasting of the proximal voluntary muscles, and evidence of denervation with normal conduction times. There are three forms of SMA. The acute form of Werdnig–Hoffman disease (SMA 1; OMIM 253300) is characterized by severe, generalized weakness, hypotonia at birth or within the first 3 months, and death of respiratory failure usually before 2 years of age. The intermediate form (SMA 2; OMIM 253550) and the mild form of Kugelberg–Welander disease (SMA 3; OMIM 253400) are characterized by a chronic course with later onset (6 months to teens) and milder muscle weakness ranging from inability to walk to death in the teen years. SMA is caused by disruption of the telomeric copy of a duplicated gene called *SMN1* at 5q12.2-q13.3. Approximately one-half of patients with severe SMA1 also are missing both homologues of a neighboring gene, neuronal apoptosis inhibitory protein (*NAIP*; OMIM 600355). The possible roles of loss of this and possibly other genes in this complex region in the pathogenesis and severity of these disorders is the focus of ongoing studies.

Tay–Sachs disease is a classic inborn error of metabolism due to deficiency of the lysosomal enzyme hexosaminidase A. The disorder is untreatable, and progressive accumulation of the specific glycosphingolipid GM2 ganglioside destroys neural cells in the brain, resulting in death at about 4 years of age. With a carrier frequency of about 1 in 30 among Ashkenazi Jews and 1 in 300 in other groups, the number of children born with Tay–Sachs disease annually in the United States has decreased from about 50 per year to about 6 through the efforts of an extensive program of carrier detection, genetic counseling, and prenatal diagnosis. Juvenile, chronic, and adult-onset variants of GM2 gangliosidosis also occur.

Wilson's disease (Table 416.2), or hepatolenticular degeneration, is an inherited disorder of copper transport that can manifest as hepatic abnormalities from childhood to early adulthood or as neurologic abnormalities after 12 years of age. A related but distinct disorder of copper transport, Menkes' disease (OMIM 309400) manifests in infancy. In Wilson's disease, reduced incorporation of copper into ceruloplasmin and reduced biliary excretion leads to progressive accumulation of copper in the liver with eventual overflow to the brain, cornea (Kayser–Fleischer rings), kidney, heart, and other tissues. If the condition is not diagnosed and the person is not treated with copper chelating agents, potentially fatal hepatic, neurologic, or hematologic complications can occur.

X-LINKED INHERITANCE AND DISORDERS

Pedigree Patterns in the X-Linked Disorders

The key feature of X-linked inheritance is the absence of male-to-male transmission. Because a man transmits his single X chromosome to his daughters and gives his sons his Y chromosome, men do not transmit X-linked disorders to their sons. The presence of male-to-male transmission in a pedigree is evidence that the genetic disorder in this family is not X-linked.

The pedigree patterns of X-linked *recessive* disorders show affected boys and men with affected uncles and nephews when the gene is inherited. Female carriers are not affected, but they may show mild signs and symptoms, and the disorder often can be detected when specific tests exist. X-linked *dominant* disorders are rare but can be recognized because when the disorder occurs among both sexes in successive generations, although without male-to-male transmission, males are more severely affected, sometimes fatally, than females but on the average only one-half as often. Ornithine transcarbamoylase (OTC) deficiency is an example of an X-linked dominant disorder.

In the case of a new X-linked mutation, the pedigree shows one of two possible patterns. In one, a single affected son is born to a woman who is not a carrier. Here the new mutation occurred in a gene on one of the two X chromosomes in the mother's gonadal cells. In the other pattern, one or more affected sons are born to a carrier mother who is the first family member to carry that mutant gene. In this case, the mutation occurred in a gene on the X chromosome in her father's gonad. Recognizing new mutation is thus more complicated for X-linked disorders than for new autosomal mutations.

Examples of X-Linked Disorders

Alport's syndrome manifests as hereditary nephritis and sensorineural deafness associated in some families with ocular abnormalities (Table 416.3). Both renal dysfunction and hearing loss develop earlier and become more severe among affected boys and men than among their affected female relatives. A large number and variety of mutations have been identified in the gene for the α-5 chain of basement membrane collagen. Accordingly, molecular diagnosis entails linkage methods.

Androgen resistance is discussed in Chapter 410. Genetic forms of androgen resistance are now known to include a spectrum of clinical defects associated with mutations in the androgen receptor gene (*AR*) at Xq11-q12. These range from complete androgen insensitivity in the disorder known previously as testicular feminization through Reifenstein's syndrome to various other types of partial androgen resistance. A specific trinucleotide repeat amplification in this gene is responsible for the X-linked neurologic disorder known as *spinal and bulbar muscular atrophy, or Kennedy's syndrome.*

Duchenne type and Becker type muscular dystrophies are caused by different mutant alleles at a single large locus that encodes the essential muscle protein dystrophin at Xp21.2. They differ in severity. Duchenne's muscular dystrophy becomes apparent in childhood and causes death by the early third decade of life. Becker's muscular dystrophy begins later and is compatible with a normal life span. Duchenne's muscular dystrophy exhibits one of the highest mutation rates observed among humans. Studies have shown that Duchenne's and Becker's muscular dystrophies are associated with mutations within the gene for dystrophin on the short arm of the X chromosome. This locus is the largest identified, occupying more than 2,000 kilobases. The gene was one of the first identified by means of positional cloning, an approach in which the approximate location of a particular gene is signaled by cytogenetic abnormalities. Approximately two-thirds of the new mutations at this locus are deletions of various sizes generated through meiotic mispairing and unequal crossing-over events related to the tandem duplication of DNA sequences in this locus. The Duchenne's muscular dystrophy phenotype usually results from deletions that produce frameshifts, changing the protein sequence distal to the mutation, so that a substantial portion of the normal dystrophin sequence is either changed or lost. In contrast, Becker's muscular dystrophy usually is associated with mutations that do not produce frameshifts.

Glucose-6-phosphate dehydrogenase (G6PD) deficiency is the most common inborn error of metabolism, affecting 400 million persons worldwide. More than 400 allelic variants have

TABLE 416.3. X-LINKED DISORDERS

Disorder	Major Features	Gene and Gene Product	Additional Information	Availability of Molecular Testing
Alport's syndrome	Hereditary nephritis and sensorineural deafness; associated in some families with ocular abnormalities.	Many different mutations in gene for type IV α 5 collagen (COL4A5; OMIM 303630) on Xq22.	OMIM 301050	Linkage
Androgen insensitivity syndrome	Abnormalities in males with the various androgen receptor defects range from complete testicular feminization to several recognized clinical variants with partial androgen insensitivity, including Reifenstein syndrome (OMIM 312300).	Caused by mutations in the androgen receptor gene (AR) at Xq11-q12. Mutation in the same gene causes Kennedy spinal and bulbar muscular atrophy.	OMIM 313700	Direct DNA, prenatal
Duchenne's muscular dystrophy (DMD) and Becker's muscular dystrophy (BMD)	Boys affected with DMD have weakness and a tendency to fall as toddlers, cannot climb stairs or arise from the floor by age 4 to 5 y, may have a language and intellectual deficit, need wheelchair assistance by the teens and die by the early third decade. Onset of weakness in BMD occurs later; mental retardation does not occur; ambulation is retained through the teens, and life expectancy is near normal.	Mutation in the dystrophin gene (DMD) at Xp21.2. One-third of DMD cases result from new mutation. Two-thirds of the pathologic alleles are deletions, most frameshift deletions being found in DMD patients and most nonframeshift deletions found in BMD patients.	OMIM 310200	Direct DNA, linkage
Glucose-6-phosphate dehydrogenase deficiency	Neonatal jaundice and acute hemolytic anemia occur with the more severe variants. Others manifest as acute intravascular hemolysis precipitated by certain drugs, infections, or ingestion of fava beans.	About 400 different biochemical variants have been described, reflecting a large number of alleles. Most are missense mutations.	OMIM 305900	Enzyme activity and electrophoretic mobility; direct DNA
Hemophilia A	Affected males have easy bruising, joint and muscle hemorrhage, and prolonged bleeding from wounds resulting from deficiency of active factor VIII in the blood coagulation cascade.	Numerous and varied mutations in the factor VIII gene (F8C) at Xq28.	OMIM 306700	Direct DNA, linkage, prenatal
Ornithine transcarbamylase deficiency	Affected males have acute episodes of hyperammonemic coma with seizures, evidence of cerebral edema, and other neurologic abnormalities, often with incomplete remission. Symptomatic carrier females may present postpartum.	Mutations in the ornithine carbamoyltransferase (OTC) gene at Xp21, most of which are missense mutations. Linkage analysis may be necessary in cases where nonspecific mutation has been identified.	OMIM 311250	Direct DNA, linkage, prenatal

See Online Mendelian Inheritance in Man (OMIM). Center for Medical Genetics, Johns Hopkins University (Baltimore) and National Center for Biotechnology Information, National Library of Medicine (Bethesda, MD), 1999. Available at: http://www.ncbi.nlm.nih.gov/omim/.

been described, making G6PD the most polymorphic human enzyme. Some variants produce no abnormalities, others produce abnormalities under specific conditions, and still others produce abnormalities under all conditions. The A$^-$ deficiency is present in about 12% of male African Americans, and 24% of girls and women are carriers. In this variant, hemolysis occurs in response to agents such as antimalarial drugs. Yet the A$^-$ variant appears to cause little or no mortality among otherwise healthy persons. Most men and boys with other G6PD variants have no symptoms except for hemolytic episodes that may occur with exposures or infection, and many have a normal life expectancy. In rare instances G6PD deficiency causes chronic hemolytic anemia that can be severe. In contrast, the Mediterranean variant is associated with hemolysis without additional stress, and variants such as Canton G6PD produce severe hemolysis that usually is fatal in infancy.

Hemophilia A, or classic hemophilia, occurs among about 1 in 5,000 liveborn male infants (see Chapter 237). New mutations in the *F8C* gene that encodes factor VIII are frequent and varied. Of the 475 mutations presently recorded, 300 are missense or nonsense, 24 affect splicing, 49 are small deletions, 17 are small insertions, 76 are gross deletions, 3 are gross insertions and duplications, and 6 are complex rearrangements. Molecular analysis of this gene was among the first to demonstrate the importance of CpG dinucleotides as a major "hotspot" for point mutations, the spontaneous deamination of a methyl-cytosine causing it to be read as thymine during DNA replication. Remarkably, about 40% to 50% of patients with severe factor VIII deficiency proved to have an inversion of the distal X chromosome that disrupts the factor VIII gene. The inversion is the product of homologous recombination between a small gene, called *gene A,* located within intron 22 of the factor VIII gene and one of the two additional copies of gene A located upstream of factor VIII toward the tip of the X chromosome. This recombination event removes exons 23 through 26 and with them the portion of the factor VIII molecule that they encode, resulting in severe deficiency. This recombination event recurs so often that it constitutes the basis of the severe hemophilia A found in 40% to 50% of unrelated families.

OTC deficiency is one of a group of five hyperammonemic disorders caused by urea cycle enzyme defects. OTC is an X-linked, mitochondrial matrix enzyme expressed almost exclusively in the liver. It catalyzes the second reaction of the urea cycle, the condensation of carbamylphosphate and ornithine to form citrulline. Some cases have an X-linked dominant pattern of inheritance with partial deficiency in heterozygous females and complete deficiency in hemizygous males, for whom it usually is lethal. Male infants with OTC deficiency usually have intractable and lethal neonatal hyperammonemia. Blood ammonia levels always exceed 1,000 μmol per liter. This is accompanied by generalized amino aciduria with particular elevations of glutamine, alanine, and glutamate in the plasma. Citrulline concentration is reduced and may be undetectable. A late-onset form occurs and leads to episodes of hyperammonemia, severe metabolic disturbance, and neurologic abnormalities resulting eventually in developmental delay. Treatment is limitation of the protein content of the diet to the tolerance of the patient and leaching the obligatory excess amino groups with sodium phenylacetate and sodium benzoate as originally described by Brusilow.

Mechanisms of X-Linked Recessive Disorders

Like autosomal recessive disorders, the basic defects are known in many X-linked disorders and frequently consist of amino acid substitutions in enzymes and other proteins. The consequences of these mutations are similar in many respects to those of the autosomal recessive disorders but also differ, primarily because of X-chromosome inactivation. One normal allele and one mutant allele are active in each cell of a male or female carrier of an autosomal recessive disorder. In contrast, carriers of X-linked recessive disorders are always women and girls. Some cells of female carriers have an active normal allele; in other cells, only the mutant allele is active. If the normal gene product cannot be obtained from other cells and used, cells in which the mutant gene is active may become abnormal or even die.

The basic tenets of the single-active-X principle are as follows. In each somatic cell of a girl or woman, one of the two X chromosomes is inactivated for most functions except replication. Some loci on the X chromosome, including the Xg blood group and steroid sulfatase loci, escape inactivation. The inactivated X chromosome condenses as the sex chromatin or Barr body, a darkly staining clump at the periphery of the nucleus. Inactivation occurs early in embryologic development, about 16 days after conception, when the number of stem cells is limited. In normal human female embryos, it is a matter of chance whether the X chromosome inherited from the father or that inherited from the mother is inactivated. Once inactivated during development, that X chromosome remains inactive in that somatic cell and all its progeny. Exceptions to the random inactivation of one of the two X chromosomes in female humans occur in some embryonic tissues and with some cytogenetic abnormalities, especially X-autosome translocations. As a consequence of X inactivation, a normal female human is a mosaic with respect to the X chromosome, some of her cells having the X inherited from the mother as the active X and others having the active X from the father. Male humans are hemizygous with respect to the X chromosome and its genes; their cells contain only one X chromosome, which is inherited from the mother and remains active.

Some female humans with the full complement of manifestations of an X-linked recessive disorder are encountered. This may occur among female progeny of an affected man and a female carrier when the gene frequency is high (e.g., G6PD deficiency), with consanguinity (in which random X inactivation has inactivated most of the X chromosomes bearing the normal allele), or in women with 45,X Turner's syndrome or boys who appear to be girls because of an X-linked androgen receptor defect.

SINGLE-GENE CAUSES OF CANCER

Inherited forms of cancer require special comment (see Chapter 20). The cause of all cancers is fundamentally genetic, but the various forms of cancer differ in regard to whether the genetic contribution is limited to mutations in somatic cells or whether both inherited (germ line) and somatic mutations are involved. Observations regarding retinoblastoma, the most common eye tumor of childhood, led Knudson to postulate the two-hit model, which led to the recognition of tumor suppressor genes. Although initially applied to childhood tumors such as retinoblastoma and Wilms' tumor, far broader relevance has emerged. Many relatively common cancers in some proportion of families follow an autosomal dominant pattern at the level of the pedigree but an autosomal recessive pattern at the level of the cell. A germ line mutation affecting one allele of a tumor suppressor locus is passed from a person in one generation to one or more offspring in an autosomal dominant pattern and is present in all of the cells of the affected offspring. When mutations inactivate the other allele of the tumor suppressor gene in one or more susceptible cells, a tumor may develop from the progeny of those cells in which both copies of the tumor suppressor gene have been inactivated. Indeed, tumor suppressor genes may be first recognized when loci are found that exhibit a high degree of mutation, known as *loss of heterozygosity,* in somatic cells from common cancers.

The proportion of cases caused by combined inherited plus somatic mutations versus somatic mutations alone differs for different forms of cancer. For example, inherited–somatic causation accounts for about two-thirds of cases of retinoblastoma but only a small percentage of cases of colorectal cancer or breast cancer, as currently understood. The mutations underlying most cancers are complex and involve multiple loci as well as environmental factors. Loci that may undergo mutation to contribute to the initiation and progression of cancer include, in addition to tumor suppressors, protooncogenes, mutator genes, and mismatch repair genes.

Single gene disorders associated with a high risk of cancer include familial adenomatous polyposis (FAP; OMIM 175100), hereditary nonpolyposis colon cancer (HNPCC; OMIM 120435), multiple endocrine neoplasia types 1, 2, and 3 [(MEN1; OMIM 131100) (MEN2; OMIM 171400) (MEN3; OMIM 162300)], neurofibromatosis types 1 (NF1; OMIM 162200) and type 2 (NF2; OMIM 101000), retinoblastoma (RB1; OMIM 180200), tuberous sclerosis type 1 (TS1; OMIM 191100) and type 2 (TS2; OMIM 191092), and von Hippel–Lindau syndrome (VHL; OMIM 193300) (see Chapters 19 and 218).

DISORDERS DUE TO TRINUCLEOTIDE REPEAT EXPANSION

The list of disorders associated with trinucleotide repeat expansion has increased in the past few years. Beginning with fragile X syndrome, these disorder now include autosomal dominant, autosomal recessive, and X-linked phenotypes. Some features of the trinucleotide repeat expansion disorders have emerged. A group of autosomal dominantly inherited neurologic disorders appear with the expansion of a CAG trinucleotide located in an exon. In various disorders, the normal allele ranging, for example, from 4 to 16 repeats to 11 to 34 repeats expands to 21 to 27 or 40 to 62 repeats in the fully affected state. Although a normal-sized allele is stable to transmissions through many gen-

erations, an intermediate state of partial expansion known as a *premutation* carries with it a substantial risk of full expansion. This liability to further expansion when the premutation is transmitted between generations gives rise to the phenomenon of anticipation, in which the severity of a particular phenotype worsens in successive generations of an affected family. In some manner, the longer sequence of glutamyl residues in the protein product of this gene produces neurologic abnormalities. This group of disorders includes Huntington disease, spinal and bulbar muscular atrophy, dentatorubral–pallidoluysian atrophy, and more than half a dozen distinguishable forms of spinocerebellar ataxia. In these disorders, the risk of expansion with the resulting abnormality is greater with transmission through the father.

Myotonic dystrophy also is inherited in an autosomal dominant pattern but involves a CTG trinucleotide repeat in the 3′ untranslated portion of the corresponding locus, which is more likely to expand with maternal transmission. Friedreich's ataxia involves expansion of a GAA trinucleotide located in an intron of the corresponding locus. As the only autosomal recessive trinucleotide repeat disorder recognized to date, transmission must be through both parents. Fragile X syndrome (FRAXA) is associated with a dramatic expansion of a CGG trinucleotide in the 5′ untranslated region of the *FMR1* gene from the normal 6 to 52 repeats to 230 to 2,000 repeats, accompanied by methylation and transcriptional silencing of the corresponding region of the X chromosome at Xq27. Although many questions about the pathophysiologic mechanisms of these disorders remain unanswered, DNA testing is available for clinical use.

CHROMOSOMES AND CHROMOSOMAL DISORDERS

THE KARYOTYPE

Diploid human cells normally have 46 nuclear chromosomes occurring in 23 pairs. One pair of chromosomes, the sex chromosomes, consists of the X and the Y. Women and girls have a homologous pair of sex chromosomes (XX), whereas men and boys have a heteromorphic sex chromosome pair (XY). The remaining 22 homologous pairs constitute autosomes. They are numbered 1 through 22 and are grouped according to size and shapes into groups A through G. Although the chromosomes are usually dispersed in the cell nucleus during the cell cycle, during the metaphase stage of mitosis, they are condensed and can be visualized with a light microscope directly or after staining. At this stage each chromosome has already replicated in preparation for the next cell division, but the two separate, replicated strands, called *chromatids,* remain joined at the centromere, the point of attachment of the mitotic spindle.

Chromosome material above the centromere is called the *short arm* (p arm). Material below the centromere is the *long arm* (q arm). The photographed, cut out, and systematic arrangement of pairs 1 to 23 constitutes the *karyotype.* The standard karyotype notation consists of the total number of chromosomes followed by the sex chromosomes followed by a description of any abnormalities. Each term is separated by a comma. According to this convention, the normal male chromosome constitution is 46,XY, and the normal female constitution is 46,XX. In Klinefelter's syndrome, the karyotype is 47,XXY. In Turner's syndrome, it usually is 45,X. The karyotype of a boy with Down syndrome due to trisomy 21 is 47,XY + 21. Cytogenetic analysis can be performed on any cell type that can be induced to undergo mitosis, such as mitogen-stimulated peripheral blood T lymphocytes, or any cell type that spontaneously undergoes mitosis, such as skin fibroblasts, cells from amniotic fluid or chorionic villi, tumor cells, and bone marrow and leukemic cells.

CHROMOSOMAL DISORDERS

Approximately one-third of human conceptuses are chromosomally abnormal, but most are spontaneously eliminated before implantation in the uterus. Whereas chromosomal disorders are present in about 60% of first-trimester abortuses and 6% of perinatal deaths, only 0.6% of live newborns have major chromosomal disorders.

The most common chromosomal disorders are caused by abnormalities of the total chromosome number, or aneuploidy, in which the person has more or fewer than the normal 46 chromosomes. Most chromosomal abnormalities among liveborn infants are detected in childhood because of associated multiple malformations or mental retardation. The features of Down syndrome, the most common autosomal disorder, include microcephaly, small size, hypotonia, flat facial profile, cardiovascular malformations, and an increased incidence of leukemia. In about 95% of cases, Down syndrome is caused by trisomy 21. The other 5% of cases are caused by unbalanced translocation or mosaicism with a trisomy 21 component.

Survival rates from aneuploidy of the sex chromosomes are greater than for autosomal chromosomal aneuploidy. Klinefelter's syndrome (nearly all 47,XXY) is the most prevalent of the sex chromosome anomalies, occurring in 1 in 900 live births of boys but also in about 1 of every 50 stillbirths of boys, and 1 in 10 cases of aspermia. Affected newborns are structurally normal at birth and have normal external genitalia. At the time of expected puberty, however, the testes are functionally deficient in regard to production of androgens and sperm. Fertility is reduced, and affected boys usually have small testes, aspermia, gynecomastia, and elevated levels of plasma and urinary gonadotropins.

Turner's syndrome (most are 45,X) occurs in 1 of 2,500 live births of girls but is many times more frequent in abortions. Girls with Turner's syndrome have primary amenorrhea, short stature, multiple congenital anomalies (small stature, shield-like chest, webbed neck, and coarctation of the aorta), and bilateral streak gonads. About one-half of cases of Turner's syndrome are recognized in childhood because of alterations in morphologic features. The other cases usually come to attention as late as adolescence when a girl is evaluated because of amenorrhea. Other cytogenetic abnormalities, such as isochromosome Xq (two copies of the long arm of an X chromosome joined at the centromere), occur among patients with Turner's syndrome, but all of these have deficiency of a second copy of the X chromosome short arm as a unifying feature. The XYY syndrome is present in 1 in 800 boys. Males with XYY syndrome tend to be tall and to have nodulocystic acne at puberty. XYY males as a group, like XXY males, reportedly are somewhat less intelligent than XY males. This may increase their risk of socialization and academic problems.

Other chromosomal abnormalities relate to abnormalities of chromosomal structure. Translocations are chromosomal abnormalities caused by breakage and rejoining with redistribution of genetic material between chromosomes. Such rearrangements are said to be *unbalanced* translocations when they cause a net gain or loss of genetic material and *balanced* translocations when they produce no net change. About 1 in 500 newborns has a balanced translocation, and about 1 in 1,500 has an unbalanced rearrangement. Even without an apparent gain or loss, translocations occasionally inactivate a critical gene at one of the breakpoints and thereby signal the location of a gene for the resulting mendelian disorder. Balanced chromosome translocations, if detected at all, usually are not recognized until adulthood, when they may cause recurrent abortions or chromosomal imbalances and other abnormalities. Translocation can be detected during pregnancy when, for example, amniocentesis is performed for an indication such as advanced maternal age. A translocation first identified in a fetus usually proves to have been inherited from one of the parents, who is healthy. This unexpected result often causes great anxiety. Specialized knowledge is needed to assess the risk to the fetus in this situation and later to determine which relatives to test for the presence of the translocation.

Mitotic chromosomal abnormalities, which occur after conception, can produce mosaic forms of chromosomal syndromes and somatic chromosomal abnormalities of the types frequently found in leukemia and lymphoma, in which they often involve oncogenes (see Chapters 20, 227, and 251).

MICRODELETIONS, CONTIGUOUS GENE SYNDROMES, AND IMPRINTING

The identification of barely visible small chromosomal deletions in association with some phenotypes, and their subsequent analysis with fluorescence in situ hybridization and other molecular techniques, has led to the recognition of a growing number of microdeletions. Although many of these are smaller than the 5×10^6 base pairs required to be visible with a microscope, they are large enough to remove part or all of several adjacent genes. The complex phenotype thus produced often includes features of more than one mendelian disorder and is known as a *contiguous gene syndrome*. For example, a patient whose X-chromosomal deletion was important in identifying the locus of the Duchenne's muscular dystrophy gene had chronic granulomatous disease, retinitis pigmentosa, and McLeod syndrome, in addition to the muscular dystrophy.

Deletion of portions of autosomal chromosomes causes hemizygosity. The resulting haploinsufficiency of the affected genes often is sufficient to produce a characteristic abnormal phenotype. Microdeletions have been recognized as causing or contributing to several dozen disorders. Examples of disorders due to microdeletions include Williams syndrome (cognitive impairment, unique personality characteristics, distinctive facial features, and cardiovascular disease with or without hypercalcemia; more than 99% of those affected have a contiguous gene deletion of chromosome 7q11, which includes the *ELN* gene), Langer–Gideon syndrome [del(8q24.1)], Miller–Dieker syndrome [del(17p13.3)], and DiGeorge and velocardiofacial syndromes [both associated with del(22q11.2)]. In other instances, however, the associated phenotypic abnormalities differ depending on whether the deletion affects the member of the chromosome pair that was inherited from the person's mother or from the father. For example, deletion of paternal 15q11-13 results in Prader–Willi syndrome (OMIM 176270), whereas deletion of maternal 15q11-13 results in Angelman syndrome (OMIM 234400). Although both syndromes include severe mental retardation and hypopigmentation, Prader–Willi syndrome is differentiated with the presence of severe neonatal hypotonia, distinctive facies with prominent bitemporal depression and almond-shaped eyes, undescended testes or hypoplastic labia, small hands and feet, and massive hyperphagia and obesity that develop in childhood.

Distinctive features of Angelman syndrome include seizures, ataxic gait, bouts of inappropriate laughter, absent language development, and characteristic facies, including prominent jaw, thin upper lip, wide mouth, and protruding tongue. These and other parent-of-origin differences are thought to be caused by a process known as *imprinting* in which methylation and perhaps other processes differentially modify the expression of genes present in some portions of chromosomes 7, 11, 14, 15, and 16. Imprinting is thought to silence the expression of some genes, but the precise mechanism linking imprinting and phenotype is incompletely understood. Both Prader–Willi and Angelman syndromes can be produced by genetic defects other than chromosomal deletions, but the other defects also act through parent-of-origin differences at 15q11-13.

MULTIFACTORIAL INHERITANCE AND DISORDERS

In common medical usage, the term *multifactorial* generally applies to disorders and processes in which several etiologic factors, rather than a single overriding factor, are thought to be involved. The concept in medical genetics is similar but more explicitly defined and based on a quantitative theoretical framework. Multifactorial inheritance generally is divided into continuously varying traits with associated empirical definitions of disease and threshold traits. Threshold traits may be identifiable at birth or may become apparent later. Environmental influences frequently are especially prominent. Multifactorial disorders are thought to be produced by the action of several genes of smaller effect that act in concert in association with an often prominent environmental complement. Multifactorial disorders include congenital malformations (anencephaly, meningomyelocele, and other neural tube defects and most forms of congenital heart disease), metabolic disorders (most forms of diabetes mellitus), and many familial, late-onset disorders (hypertension, most coronary artery disease, most gout, schizophrenia, bipolar depression). Multifactorial inheritance applies to continuously varying traits, such as height, weight, or blood pressure. Measurements within the general population generate a continuous distribution of values that approximates a normal curve. Theoretical formulations of multifactorial inheritance can account for the degree of resemblance of relatives for these traits, depending on the degree of relatedness. Several genetic loci appear to be involved, and environmental factors also contribute to the phenotype.

MITOCHONDRIAL INHERITANCE AND DISORDERS

Unlike the nuclear chromosomes, inheritance of which forms the basis for mendelian inheritance, mitochondrial genes are inherited only from the mother. The mother transmits her mitochondrial DNA (mtDNA) through the cytoplasm of the ovum to all of her offspring. Her daughters transmit their mtDNA to all of their offspring. In contrast, men never transmit their mtDNA. This maternal inheritance pattern produces a distinctive pedigree pattern for mitochondrial disorders in which, if penetrance were complete, all of the sons and daughters of an affected woman would themselves be affected, whereas none of the offspring of an affected man would be affected. Penetrance is, however, rarely complete, and confusing pedigree patterns can result.

Each human cell contains thousands of molecules of mtDNA. Human mtDNA is a closed circular molecule 16,569 base pairs long that contains no introns and in which some genes overlap. The mitochondrial genome encodes 13 of the 80 essential polypeptides that form the five complexes that make up the respiratory chain. It also encodes two ribosomal RNAs and 22 transfer RNAs.

The mutation rate in mitochondrial DNA is 5 to 10 times greater than the mutation rate in nuclear DNA. Cells that contain a mixture of mutant and wild-type mtDNA are said to be *heteroplasmic*. Cells that contain only a single sequence of mtDNA are called *homoplasmic*. During replication of heteroplasmic cells, the mtDNA genotype can shift as the mitochondria and mtDNAs are partitioned randomly into daughter cells. In this way some lineages drift toward becoming homoplasmic for the mutant mtDNA, whereas others become homoplasmic for wild-type mtDNA, and still others remain heteroplasmic. The cell phenotype reflects the relative proportions of constituent mutant and wild-type mtDNA, and the degree to which that cell depends on oxidative phosphorylation. The central nervous system is most dependent on mitochondrial energy, followed by skeletal muscle, heart, kidney, and liver. The mitochondria of cells that contain mutant mtDNA may show distinctive electron micrographic changes.

Molecular studies have identified more than 60 pathogenic mutations of mtDNA associated with multisystemic, maternally inherited syndromes. A database of mtDNA, called MITOMAP, can be found at http://www.gen.emory.edu/mitomap.html. The database contains a wealth of current information about normal and disease-related mtDNA.

BIBLIOGRAPHY

Borgaonkar DS. *Chromosomal variation in man: a catalogue of chromosomal variants and anomalies,* 8th ed. New York: Wiley–Liss, 1997.

Gardner RJM, Sutherland GR. *Chromosome abnormalities and genetic counseling,* 2nd ed. New York: Oxford University Press, 1997.

GeneClinics: Medical Genetics Knowledge Base. University of Washington, Seattle, 1995–. On-line database updated weekly. Available at: http://www.geneclinics.org.

Jones KL. *Smith's recognizable patterns of human malformation,* 4th ed. Philadelphia: WB Saunders, 1988.

MITOMAP: A Human Mitochondrial Genome Database. Center for Molecular Medicine, Emory University, Atlanta, 1999. Available at: http://www.gen.emory.edu/mitomap.html.

Online Mendelian Inheritance in Man, OMIM. Center for Medical Genetics, Johns Hopkins University and National Center for Biotechnology Information, National Library of Medicine, 1999. Available at: http://www.ncbi.nlm.nih.gov/omim/.

Rimoin DL, Connor JM, Pyeritz RE, eds. *Emery and Rimoin's principles and practice of medical genetics,* 3rd ed. Edinburgh: Churchill Livingstone, 1997.

Scriver CR, Beaudet AL, Sly WS, et al, eds. *The metabolic and molecular bases of inherited disease,* 7th ed. New York: McGraw–Hill, 1995.

Kelley's Textbook of Internal Medicine, fourth edition. Edited by H. David Humes. Lippincott Williams & Wilkins, Philadelphia © 2000.

DIAGNOSTIC AND THERAPEUTIC MODALITIES IN ENDOCRINOLOGIC, METABOLIC, AND GENETIC DISORDERS

TESTING AND EVALUATION OF PITUITARY END-ORGAN FUNCTION

ARIEL L. BARKAN
JOHN C. MARSHALL

In the care of every patient with hypothalamic–pituitary disease, the following four questions should be answered:

1. What is the nature of the process?
2. Are there any mass effects?
3. Which hormone is missing?
4. Which hormone is being hypersecreted?

The first two questions usually are answered through a combination of patient history and findings at clinical examination, such as previous trauma, presence of coexistent disease, results of neuroophthalmologic studies and through appropriate radiologic procedures, such as computed tomography (CT) or magnetic resonance imaging (MRI). The latter two questions require performance of basal hormone measurements and dynamic tests.

Pituitary diseases may manifest as pituitary hypofunction or hyperfunction, or a combination of the two. For most patients, the major abnormalities can be identified through clinical assessment and basal measurement of corresponding pituitary (trophic) and peripheral (target gland) hormones. Clinical assessment is most important for planning and interpretation of pituitary function tests. For example, the presence of regular ovulatory cycles in women is evidence of normal hypothalamic-pituitary-ovarian function, and endocrine testing of this system is not indicated. After menopause, low estradiol and high gonadotropin concentrations are normal, but the same findings for a young woman with amenorrhea indicate premature ovarian failure.

When clinical or laboratory features suggest excessive production of pituitary hormone, suppression tests are needed to diagnose autonomy of pituitary function. If hypofunction of the pituitary gland is suspected, appropriate stimulation tests are performed. Blood samples should be drawn from indwelling venous cannulas to minimize the stress of multiple venipunctures. For urinary measurements, the correct procedure for collecting an accurate 24-hour urine sample should be explained to the patient, and creatinine should be measured to assess the completeness of the collection. Important factors for interpreting results of pituitary function tests include age, sex, exposure to acute stress, drug therapy, nutritional status, and timing of the test. Some hormones, such as corticotropin, cortisol, growth hormone (GH), and luteinizing hormone (LH), are secreted in a pulsatile manner, and a single basal estimate may be misleading. In these cases, serial blood sampling or measurement of two or three pooled samples improves diagnostic accuracy.

INVESTIGATION OF PITUITARY HYPOFUNCTION

The presence of low or low-normal levels of tropic and target hormones—such as thyroid-stimulating hormone (TSH) and thyroxine (T_4), corticotropin and cortisol, LH, follicle-stimulating hormone (FSH), and gonadal steroid, or GH and insulin-like growth factor I (IGF-I)—together with appropriate clinical findings suggests pituitary failure. The failure may be caused by deficiency of hypothalamic stimulatory hormones or anterior pituitary cell failure.

The indications for dynamic pituitary function tests include establishment of the diagnosis if basal measurements are borderline low; assessment of the degree of pituitary failure (complete versus partial); localization of the defect (pituitary versus hypothalamic); and assessment of the feasibility of therapy with hypothalamic hormones, such as gonadotropin-releasing hormone (GnRH) or growth hormone-releasing hormone (GH-RH). A combined pituitary function test is used to assess simultaneously secretory reserves of corticotropin, GH, TSH, LH, and FSH. The results of combined stimuli, however, may be confusing in evaluation of some patients with pituitary dysfunction. Administration of several test substances may provoke release of the same hormone by different mechanisms (eg, GH release to insulin, thyrotropin-releasing hormone [TRH], and GnRH in acromegaly; prolactin release to insulin and TRH). When hypopituitarism or nonfunctioning pituitary tumors are suspected, a combined test can be used to assess pituitary reserve. Individual stimulation tests often are more appropriate for assessment of pituitary secretion in the presence of functioning tumors.

SUSPECTED CORTICOTROPIN DEFICIENCY

Whether corticotropin can be secreted in response to stress is important in two clinical situations: when a patient is believed to have hypothalamic-pituitary disease and when a patient has been treated with exogenous glucocorticoids. Assessment of corticotropin secretory reserve is most important and should precede institution of replacement glucocorticoid therapy. During stressful situations, such as pain, fever, or surgery, plasma cortisol level normally rises to more than 20 μg per deciliter, and this can be regarded as the minimal level needed for adaptation to stress. For patients not receiving exogenous glucocorticoids, the finding of a spontaneous basal plasma cortisol greater than 20 μg per deciliter establishes normal function of the hypothalamic–pituitary–adrenal axis, and further testing is unnecessary. Other factors should be considered in interpreting basal measurements of plasma cortisol. The cortisol levels of patients taking hydrocortisone are normal, of patients taking prednisone may be measurable because of cross-reaction in the cortisol assay, and of patients using estrogen therapy are increased because of elevation of cortisol-binding globulin.

Insulin Hypoglycemia Test

Mechanism

The mechanism is a stress-induced increase in hypothalamic corticotropin-releasing hormone (CRH) secretion.

Protocol

If the patient is being treated with dexamethasone or prednisone, replacement therapy should be changed to hydrocortisone, 25 mg per day for 2 to 4 days before testing, with the last dose of hydrocortisone 12 hours before the test. The patient should fast overnight and be recumbent throughout the test. Crystalline (regular) insulin is injected as an intravenous (IV) bolus. The usual insulin dose is 0.15 U per kilogram, but for patients with obesity, cushingoid symptoms, or diabetes, higher doses (0.2 to 0.6 U per kilogram) may be needed to overcome insulin resistance. Patients with suspected hypopituitarism should be given a lower dose (0.1 U per kilogram). Blood glucose is measured with glucose oxidase strips every 15 minutes and as soon as signs of hypoglycemia appear (sense of hunger, perspiration, tachycar-

dia, tremor, confusion). These symptoms are allowed to continue for 5 minutes, and glucose is administered by mouth or IV to correct hypoglycemia. If hypoglycemia (blood glucose level greater than 40 mg per deciliter) does not develop within 45 minutes of insulin injection, a second insulin injection is given at 50% of the initial dose. Cortisol samples are drawn 30, 60, and 90 minutes after the onset of clinical and biochemical hypoglycemia. When the test has been completed, the patient should be given oral carbohydrates and be warned to eat breakfast.

Contraindications

Contraindications to the insulin hypoglycemia test include seizure disorder, history of angina, recent myocardial infarction, arrhythmia, and known or suspected primary adrenal failure.

Interpretation

A plasma cortisol level greater than 20 μg per deciliter in any sample indicates normal function of the hypothalamic–pituitary–adrenal axis. A blunted response is considered abnormal only if adequate hypoglycemia (less than 40 mg per deciliter) was achieved.

Metyrapone Tests

Mechanism

Metyrapone blocks 11-hydroxylation in adrenocortical cells. This leads to a decrease in cortisol production, an increase in corticotropin secretion, and stimulation of synthesis of precursor steroids up to the level of the enzymatic block. The amount of substrate for the 11-hydroxylase enzyme, 11-deoxycortisol (compound S), increases and can be measured directly in plasma or indirectly as urinary 17-hydroxycorticosteroid (17-OHCS).

Standard Test

Protocol
The protocol for the standard metyrapone test is as follows:

Day 1: 8:00 A.M. Collect sample for plasma cortisol; 24-hour urine collection for 17-OHCS and creatinine.

Day 2: Begin metyrapone, 750 mg by mouth every 4 hours (total of six doses); second 24-hour urine collection for 17-OHCS and creatinine.

Day 3: 8:00 A.M. Collect sample for plasma cortisol and 11-deoxycortisol; third 24-hour urine collection for 17-OHCS and creatinine.

Contraindications
Contraindications to the metyrapone test include known corticotropin deficiency or Addison's disease.

Side Effects
Headaches and dizziness may be alleviated with bed rest. Nausea and gastric discomfort are reduced if the drug is taken with

food. Close supervision is needed because patients with partial corticotropin deficiency may have symptoms of cortisol insufficiency. If this occurs, metyrapone should be stopped and hydrocortisone given.

Interpretation

On day 3, the plasma cortisol level should be less than 5 μg per deciliter to confirm suppression of 11-hydroxylation. The level of compound S should increase to more than 7 μg per deciliter, and the urinary level of 17-OHCS should rise at least twofold over baseline on day 2 or 3. Antiepileptic drugs (phenytoin, barbiturates, primidone) increase the metabolism of metyrapone, and responses may be attenuated. Reduced absorption of the drug owing to vomiting or diarrhea also may reduce responses.

Rapid (Overnight) Test

Protocol

Administer a single oral dose of metyrapone (2 g if weight is less than 70 kg; 2.5 g if weight is 70 to 90 kg; 3 g if weight is more than 90 kg) at midnight with a light snack. At 8:00 A.M. the next day, obtain blood for measurement of cortisol and 11-deoxycortisol.

Interpretation

Plasma 11-deoxycortisol level normally increases to more than 7 μg per deciliter. If the increase is blunted, the concomitant plasma cortisol level must be less than 5 μg per deciliter to exclude inadequate suppression of 11-hydroxylation.

Corticotropin Stimulation Tests

Mechanism

Corticotropin stimulates adrenocortical cells.

Short Test

Protocol

Obtain a basal sample for cortisol. Inject synthetic corticotropin 1-24 (cosyntropin [Cortrosyn]), 250 μg IV or intramuscularly. Obtain samples for cortisol measurement 30 and 60 minutes after injection.

Interpretation

A normal response is a plasma cortisol level greater than 20 μg per deciliter in any sample. A blunted response indicates primary or secondary adrenal insufficiency. A normal response excludes primary adrenal failure but does not exclude corticotropin deficiency of recent onset.

Long Test

Mechanism

Repeated stimulation of the adrenal cortex by corticotropin restores cortisol secretion in corticotropin deficiency but not in primary adrenal failure.

Protocol

The protocol for the long test is as follows:

Day 1: 8:00 A.M. Obtain blood specimen for plasma cortisol measurement; obtain a 24-hour urine collection for 17-OHCS and creatinine measurement.

Days 2 through 4: Infuse 250 μg cosyntropin in 500 mL normal saline solution IV over 8 hours. Obtain 24-hour urine collection for measurement of creatinine and 17-OHCS.

Day 4: Measure plasma cortisol at the end of the cosyntropin infusion.

Interpretation

Primary adrenal failure is indicated by an absent or subnormal increase in plasma cortisol and 17-OHCS levels. Corticotropin deficiency is indicated by a plasma cortisol level greater than 20 μg per deciliter and a twofold to threefold increase in urinary 17-OHCS level over baseline on day 4. A normal response to corticotropin infusion does not mean that CRH and corticotropin secretion can respond to stress. This can be assessed only with hypoglycemia or metyrapone tests.

Corticotropin-releasing Hormone Test

CRH stimulates pituitary corticotropic cells. CRH, 1 μg per kilogram, is given IV in the evening, when endogenous cortisol secretion is low. Plasma corticotropin and cortisol levels increase twofold to threefold 30 to 90 minutes after administration of CRH. CRH appears to differentiate endogenous CRH deficiency from pituitary corticotropic failure.

SUSPECTED GROWTH HORMONE DEFICIENCY

Deficiency of GH is a problem in pediatric endocrinologic practice. In the past, GH secretory reserve in adults usually was evaluated to gain information about hypothalamic–pituitary function in general rather than to evaluate GH secretion per se. GH deficiency has come to be associated with increased cardiovascular mortality, abdominal obesity, osteoporosis, and neuropsychiatric abnormalities, even among adults. GH has been approved for treatment of adults with hypopituitarism. Testing of the somatotropic axis became widely used in adult endocrinologic practice.

In children, GH secretion is best assessed with frequent (every 10 to 20 minutes) sampling over 24 hours, especially during sleep. The presence of spontaneous GH pulses (amplitude >10 ng per milliliter) and normal integrated GH concentrations (2 to 4 ng per milliliter) indicates normal GH secretion. This approach is clinically impractical, and stimulation tests of GH secretion are used on an outpatient basis. Screening tests include an exercise test or clonidine hydrochloride 250 μ by mouth. If plasma GH level increases to more than 10 ng per milliliter 15 to 30 minutes after exercise (20 minutes of running or climbing a staircase) or 60 to 90 minutes after clonidine administration, further testing is not needed.

General Considerations

The definition of normalcy of the stimulated GH level is still problematic. It is important to remember that the currently accepted levels of more than 10 ng per milliliter (indicating normalcy) or less than 3 ng per milliliter (indicating severe deficiency) are established by convention rather than from solid physiologic or clinical data.

Ten percent to 20% of healthy persons have impaired responses to any single test, and two different stimuli, preferably including insulin hypoglycemia, should be used to establish the diagnosis of GH deficiency. Obese patients often have blunted responses to all stimuli, and these responses increase after weight loss. Hypothyroidism blunts GH responses, and euthyroidism should be present before GH reserve is tested. GH responses to all stimuli may be blunted by hyperglycemia, high-dose glucocorticoids, and phenoxybenzamine. For boys, GH responses can be augmented by estrogen pretreatment (Premarin 5 mg twice a day for 3 days) or by β-blockers (propranolol 20 to 30 mg per square meter by mouth) given 2 hours before administration of insulin, arginine, or levodopa. Normalization of a blunted GH response is regarded as evidence of normal GH secretory reserve. Some children with short stature and low IGF-I levels may have normal GH responses to provocative stimuli. In this case, the diagnosis of neurosecretory GH dysfunction can be established only with frequent GH sampling (every 10 to 20 minutes) for 24 hours or during sleep.

Levodopa Test

Mechanism

Levodopa probably stimulates hypothalamic secretion of GH-RH.

Protocol

After an overnight fast, the patient is recumbent for 30 minutes. Obtain a basal blood sample for measurement of GH. Administer levodopa (500 mg by mouth for adults, less for children according to body weight). Obtain blood samples for measurement of GH 30, 60, and 90 minutes after administration of levodopa.

Side Effects

Side effects include nausea and vomiting.

Interpretation

A normal response is a GH level of 10 ng per milliliter or more in any sample. Not all healthy subjects respond.

Arginine Tests

Mechanism

The mechanism of the arginine test is unknown, but it requires hypothalamic GH-RH for action.

Protocol

After an overnight fast, the patient remains recumbent for 30 minutes. Obtain a blood sample for basal measurement of GH.

Administer arginine hydrochloride, 0.5 g per kilogram (maximum 30 g) in 200 mL normal saline solution by means of IV infusion over 30 minutes. Obtain blood samples for measurement of GH at the end of infusion and 30 and 60 minutes later.

Contraindications

Contraindications to the arginine test are hepatic or renal failure.

Interpretation

A normal response is a GH level of at least 10 ng per milliliter on any sample. Male subjects, particularly boys, may have lower GH responses.

Insulin Hypoglycemia Test

The insulin hypoglycemia test is the standard for GH stimulation tests. It is especially useful because corticotropin and cortisol reserve can be assessed simultaneously.

Mechanism

The mechanism is complex and requires endogenous hypothalamic GH-RH for its action.

Protocol

After an overnight fast, the patient remains recumbent for 30 to 60 minutes. The insulin dose and glucose sampling are the same as described for testing corticotropin secretory reserve. Measure plasma GH before and 30, 60, and 90 minutes after the onset of hypoglycemic symptoms.

Contraindications

Contraindications include seizure disorder, history of angina, recent myocardial infarction, arrhythmia, and known or suspected primary adrenal failure.

Interpretation

A normal response is a GH level of at least 10 ng per milliliter in any sample. A lower GH response is regarded as abnormal only if adequate hypoglycemia (clinical signs and blood glucose level less than 40 mg per deciliter) is achieved.

Growth Hormone-releasing Factor Test

Growth hormone-releasing factor (GHRF) stimulates somatotroph cells. It is given as an IV bolus, 1 μg per kilogram. Blood samples for measurement of GH are obtained before drug administration and 30, 60, and 90 minutes later. GH responses depend on prevailing somatostatin secretion and may be absent among some healthy persons. Among children with GH deficiency, GH responsiveness to GHRF suggests that GHRF may be used for future therapy.

SUSPECTED DEFICIENCY OF GONADOTROPIN (LUTEINIZING AND FOLLICLE-STIMULATING HORMONES)

Gonadotropin deficiency may be caused by gonadotropic failure or GnRH deficiency. Confirmation of gonadotropic responsiveness to GnRH is necessary when long-term GnRH therapy to induce puberty or restore fertility is contemplated. The test is indicated when amenorrhea for a woman or a low plasma testosterone level for a man is accompanied by low levels of LH and FSH.

Gonadotropin-releasing Hormone Test

Mechanism

The mechanism is direct stimulation of pituitary gonadotropins.

Protocol

Obtain a basal blood sample for measurement of LH and FSH. Administer GnRH 100 μg IV bolus. Obtain samples for measurement of LH and FSH 30, 60, and 90 minutes after injection.

Side Effects

Usually there are no side effects, but transient hot flushing or a metallic taste may occur.

Interpretation

A normal response is an increase in LH level of at least twofold 30 minutes after injection of GnRH. Serum FSH may not respond in adults, but it usually increases at 60 to 90 minutes. LH and FSH responses to GnRH depend on the age (prepubertal, pubertal) and sex of the patient. After a single bolus of GnRH, patients with GnRH deficiency may have absent, subnormal, or normal LH responses, depending on the degree of GnRH deficiency. An absent or subnormal LH response to a single bolus of GnRH does not establish the diagnosis of gonadotropic failure. In GnRH deficiency, LH and FSH increase into the normal range after 3 to 5 days of treatment with GnRH, 25 ng per kilogram IV given in a pulsatile manner every 1 to 2 hours. LH and FSH responses to GnRH may be blunted by exogenous estrogens or androgens and by high levels of glucocorticoids.

Clomiphene Test

Clomiphene binds to hypothalamic receptors and interferes with the negative feedback of estradiol and testosterone. As a result, GnRH secretion and plasma LH and FSH increase. After 5 to 7 days of administration of clomiphene, 50 to 100 mg per day by mouth, LH and gonadal steroid levels increase twofold in adults. No response occurs in among patients with hypopituitarism or GnRH deficiency or among prepubertal children. The clomiphene test is rarely used but is occasionally of value in the diagnosis of suspected GnRH deficiency in adults.

SUSPECTED PROLACTIN DEFICIENCY

Except for lactation, prolactin deficiency has no known clinical significance. Therefore, tests of prolactin secretory reserve are performed not to assess prolactin secretion per se but to gain additional information about pituitary function.

TRH directly stimulates pituitary lactotropic cells, and the test is performed by means of IV infusion of 200 to 500 μg of TRH over 2 to 3 minutes. Serum prolactin level normally increases twofold 30 minutes after administration of TRH, and peak values are greater than 12 ng per milliliter. Metoclopramide (Reglan), 5 to 10 mg IV, blocks dopamine receptors, and serum prolactin level increases twofold 30 to 60 minutes later. Prolactin responses to both stimuli are augmented by estrogen and are higher among women. Serum prolactin level is low in pituitary destruction and does not respond to TRH or metoclopramide. In contrast, patients with a hypothalamic lesion or with a stalk section have elevated prolactin levels that may not respond to metoclopramide but increase after administration of TRH.

Combined Pituitary Function Tests

Concomitant administration of insulin, TRH, and GnRH allows simultaneous testing of corticotropin, GH, TSH, prolactin, LH, and FSH reserve function. Details of normal responses are discussed earlier.

Protocol

After an overnight fast and IV cannulation with the patient recumbent, the protocol is as follows:

30 minutes: Obtain blood samples for measurement of free thyroxine (FT_4), IGF-I, and testosterone (for men).

0 minutes: Sample for glucose, TSH, GH, cortisol, LH, FSH, and prolactin. Inject crystalline (regular) insulin 0.15 U per kilogram (use 0.1 U per kilogram if hypopituitarism is suspected), TRH 200 μg; and GnRH 100 μg IV.

15 minutes: Sample for glucose (glucose oxidase strips)

30 minutes: Sample for glucose, TSH, prolactin, LH, and FSH

60 minutes: Sample for glucose, TSH, prolactin, LH, FSH, cortisol, and GH

90 minutes: Sample for glucose, cortisol, and GH

120 minutes: Sample for glucose, cortisol, and GH. Ensure that adequate hypoglycemia (less than 40 mg per deciliter) is present and allow symptoms to persist for 5 minutes before giving glucose by mouth or IV. If hypoglycemia does not occur within 45 minutes, give additional insulin IV (half the initial dose) and perform cortisol and GH sampling 30, 60, and 90 minutes after the onset of hypoglycemia. If symptoms of cortisol deficiency occur, inject hydrocortisone 100 mg IV and give additional glucose at 120 minutes.

Growth hormone secretion in acromegaly should not be assessed with this test because normal GH responses to hypoglycemia cannot be differentiated from paradoxical responses to TRH or GnRH. A variation of this test involving administration of GHRF and CRH instead of insulin has been described. Although this provides more direct information about the function of GH- and corticotropin-producing pituitary cells, insulin hypoglycemia offers the advantage of testing stress-associated corticotropin secretion and thus is more relevant in clinical practice.

INVESTIGATION OF PITUITARY HYPERFUNCTION

SUSPECTED PROLACTIN HYPERSECRETION

A serum level of prolactin in excess of 200 ng per milliliter almost always indicates the presence of prolactinoma. Serum prolactin elevation to less than 200 ng per milliliter may be caused by prolactinoma or another condition. Dopamine agonists (levodopa, bromocriptine) invariably suppress serum prolactin level and thus have little or no value in the differential diagnosis of hyperprolactinemia. Prolactin responses to stimulation by TRH or dopamine antagonists likewise do not help establish the cause of hyperprolactinemia.

SUSPECTED HYPERSECRETION OF GROWTH HORMONE

Pathologic hypersecretion GH manifests as gigantism or acromegaly, and IGF-I levels are elevated. Patients with malnutrition, chronic renal failure, cirrhosis, uncontrolled diabetes mellitus, and Laron-type dwarfism may have elevated serum GH values, but these are accompanied by low or normal IGF-I levels. A normal GH level is low (less than 0.1 ng per milliliter) during most of the day, but spontaneous GH pulses, postprandial GH pulses (2 to 3 hours after meals), or nocturnal GH pulses (1 to 3 hours after falling asleep) may reach levels of more than 20 ng per milliliter. Stress (physical exercise, anxiety, pain) also cause acute increases in GH level. Testing of GH secretion should be performed after an overnight fast, with a 30-minute rest period after insertion of the IV cannula. Random plasma GH values in excess of 2 ng per milliliter in association with elevated IGF-I concentrations and appropriate clinical findings strongly suggest abnormal GH hypersecretion, but dynamic tests may be needed to confirm the diagnosis.

Glucose Suppression Test

Mechanism

The mechanism of glucose suppression is uncertain but probably is the result of stimulation of hypothalamic somatostatin secretion.

Protocol

Obtain blood samples for basal measurement of GH and glucose. Administer glucose 100 g by mouth. Obtain blood samples for measurement of GH and glucose 30, 60, 90, and 120 minutes later.

Contraindication

Moderate or severe glucose intolerance is a contraindication to the glucose suppression test.

Interpretation

The normal response is a decrease in GH to less than 1 ng per milliliter at any time during the test when sensitive immunoradiometric or immunochemiluminescent assays are used. In acromegaly or gigantism, GH is not suppressed to less than 1 ng per milliliter and may even increase. If basal GH level is not clearly elevated (3 to 5 ng per milliliter), a decrease after glucose administration is difficult to document, and a TRH stimulation test may have to be performed.

Thyrotropin-releasing Hormone Stimulation Test

Mechanism

The mechanism by which TRH stimulates release of GH is unknown.

Protocol

Obtain blood samples for basal measurement of GH and TSH. Inject TRH, 200 μg IV over 15 to 30 seconds. Sample for GH and TSH 15, 30, and 60 minutes later.

Side Effects

Urge to urinate, metallic taste, or flushing may persist for 1 to 2 minutes after injection of TRH.

Interpretation

The normal response is no change in GH concentration. Among 60% to 80% of patients with acromegaly or gigantism, GH increases at least 50% 15 to 30 minutes after administration of TRH. This test may be useful in evaluation of patients with low basal GH concentrations (less than 5 ng per milliliter) when an excess of GH is suspected clinically. The presence of TRH also may increase serum GH level in patients with renal failure, cirrhosis, primary hypothyroidism, uncontrolled diabetes, or malnutrition and in some apparently healthy adolescents with tall stature.

Bromocriptine Suppression Test

Mechanism

The mechanism of the bromocriptine suppression test is uncertain but probably is related to direct pituitary inhibition of GH secretion.

Protocol

Obtain blood samples for basal measurement of GH and prolactin. Administer 2.5 or 5.0 mg bromocriptine, and obtain blood samples for measurement of GH and prolactin at hourly intervals for 6 hours.

Contraindications

Hypotension of any cause is a contraindication to the bromocriptine suppression test.

Side Effects

Orthostatic hypotension, nausea, vomiting, and epigastric discomfort may be caused by administration of bromocriptine.

Interpretation

Bromocriptine suppresses plasma GH level in about one-half of patients with acromegaly or gigantism. This suggests that bromocriptine may be effective for long-term treatment of patients with the disease.

SUSPECTED HYPERSECRETION OF CORTICOTROPIN

Hypersecretion of corticotropin in primary adrenal failure is accompanied by low plasma cortisol values, and further testing is not required. Hypersecretion corticotropin caused by a pituitary tumor leads to bilateral adrenal hyperplasia and elevated cortisol production (Cushing's disease). Cushing's disease is one cause of Cushing's syndrome. *Cushing's syndrome* is the term used to describe the clinical features of glucocorticoid excess. This syndrome may be caused by exogenous glucocorticoid therapy, overproduction of corticotropin (pituitary or ectopic source), or an adrenal tumor. Corticotropin and cortisol levels may be elevated in healthy persons under acute or chronic stress, such as pain, fever, or exercise. Dynamic tests of corticotropin secretion are designed to answer two questions: First, does the patient have endogenous glucocorticoid overproduction? Second, is the glucocorticoid overproduction caused by pituitary or ectopic corticotropin excess or by an autonomous adrenal tumor?

Basal Tests

All basal blood samples should be drawn with minimal stress. Insert an IV cannula and wait 30 minutes before drawing the sample.

Morning and Evening Plasma Corticotropin and Cortisol

Loss of the normal diurnal variation of plasma corticotropin and cortisol levels is the hallmark of endogenous Cushing's syndrome. Obtain samples between 8:00 A.M. and 9:00 A.M. and between 10:00 P.M. and midnight. Normal values for corticotropin and cortisol, respectively, are 20 to 90 pg per milliliter and 10 to 25 µg per deciliter in the morning and less than 20 pg per milliliter and less than 5 µg per deciliter in the evening. When drawn under nonstressful conditions, elevated corticotropin or cortisol levels in the evening suggest Cushing's syndrome.

Plasma corticotropin is undetectable (less than 10 pg per milliliter) in the morning among patients with adrenal tumors or during exogenous glucocorticoid therapy. Evening values are elevated among persons with Cushing's disease. Both morning and evening levels are elevated (100 to 200 pg per milliliter) among persons with the more severe forms of Cushing's disease, but values greater than 200 pg per milliliter suggest an ectopic corticotropin-secreting tumor.

Evening levels of plasma cortisol are greater than 10 to 15 µg per deciliter among 95% of patients with Cushing's syndrome. Both morning and evening cortisol values may be elevated, usually with a preserved diurnal rhythm, in the presence of chronic alcoholism (pseudo-Cushing's syndrome), during estrogen therapy (elevated cortisol-binding globulin levels), and among depressed or malnourished patients. Undetectable levels of cortisol in a patient with Cushing's syndrome indicate exogenous glucocorticoid administration (usually dexamethasone), but cortisol can be measured for patients taking hydrocortisone or prednisone (cross-reaction in cortisol assays).

Urinary Free Cortisol Excretion

The normal range for urinary free cortisol (UFF) excretion in most laboratories is 20 to 100 µg per 24 hours. UFF is elevated (greater than 150 µg per 24 hours) among more than 90% of patients with Cushing's syndrome. Some obese and chronically ill patients may have mildly increased (more than 120 µg per 24 hours) UFF excretion.

Urinary 17-Hydroxycorticosteroid Excretion

The normal range for secretion of 17-OHCS is 5 to 12 mg per 24 hours. In Cushing's syndrome, values exceed 12 mg per 24 hours in 90% of cases, but values also are elevated among 20% of obese patients.

Dynamic Tests

Basal measurements do not always help differentiate patients with true Cushing's syndrome from those with other diseases. Dynamic tests establish the diagnosis and also help differentiate the various forms of the syndrome.

Dexamethasone Suppression Tests

Dexamethasone suppression tests are based on the principle that the negative feedback of glucocorticoids on pituitary corticotropin secretion is intact in healthy persons, defective (high threshold) in Cushing's disease, and already maximally expressed in adrenal tumors or ectopic corticotropin secretion.

Overnight Test

The dexamethasone suppression test can be performed as an outpatient screening procedure by means of administration of 1 mg dexamethasone by mouth at 11:00 P.M. the night before the test. Plasma cortisol is measured at 8:00 A.M. the next morning. For 99% of healthy persons, the plasma cortisol level is less than 5 µg per deciliter. Among persons with Cushing's syndrome, the plasma cortisol value is not suppressed to this level. In addition, 10% to 15% of obese patients and 20% to

25% of sick, hospitalized patients may not have normal suppression in response to dexamethasone. One-half of patients with alcoholism likewise have impaired suppression, but alcohol withdrawal restores normal cortisol suppression within a few days. One-half of the patients with endogenous depression also exhibit impaired suppression, but this condition can be differentiated from Cushing's syndrome with a normal plasma cortisol response to insulin hypoglycemia. This response is absent or blunted in the presence of Cushing's syndrome. Antiepileptic medications (phenytoin, barbiturates, primidone) increase the metabolic degradation of dexamethasone, and cortisol levels may not become normally suppressed among patients taking these drugs.

Low-dose Test

Dexamethasone suppression with a 2-mg dose can confirm the diagnosis of Cushing's syndrome. The protocol for this test is as follows:

Day 1: 8:00 A.M. Measure plasma cortisol. Examine 24-hour urine specimen for 17-OHCS, UFF, and creatinine.

Days 2 and 3: Administer 0.5 mg dexamethasone by mouth every 6 hours (eight doses). Examine 24-hour urine specimen for 17-OHCS, UFF, and creatinine.

Day 4: Measure plasma cortisol at 8:00 A.M. at completion of urine collection.

Normal suppression is present if plasma cortisol is less than 5 μg per deciliter; 17-OHCS less than 4 μg per 24 hours; and UFF less than 20 μg per 24 hours. Fewer than 5% of patients with Cushing's syndrome have normal suppression. Obesity, depression, and use of antiepileptic drugs may cause incomplete suppression (false-positive results).

High-dose Test

To establish the cause of Cushing's syndrome, an 8-mg dose often is administered as a continuation of the low-dose, 2-mg dexamethasone suppression test. The protocol is as follows:

Days 4 and 5: Administer 2 mg dexamethasone by mouth every 6 hours (eight doses). Examine 24-hour urine for 17-OHCS, UFF, and creatinine.

Days 5 and 6: 1:00 A.M. Measure plasma cortisol.

Among 70% to 80% of patients with Cushing's disease (pituitary corticotropin-secreting tumor), plasma cortisol, 17-OHCS, and UFF are suppressed in at least half. The other patients with Cushing's disease show incomplete suppression. Fewer than 10% of adrenal tumors have normal suppression, but results are variable in ectopic corticotropin secretion, and 20% to 30% exhibit normal suppression. The results of this test may be difficult to interpret, and a metyrapone or CRH test may be needed to establish the cause of Cushing's syndrome.

Metyrapone Tests

Mechanism

Blockade of 11-hydroxylation lowers cortisol production. Removal of cortisol-negative feedback augments pituitary corticotropin secretion and 17-OHCS excretion in Cushing's disease but not in adrenal tumors or ectopic corticotropin secretion.

Protocol

See Suspected Corticotropin Deficiency.

Interpretation

Among 98% of patients with Cushing's disease, 17-OHCS excretion increases by more than 10 mg per day. This response may occur among 20% to 50% of patients with other causes of Cushing's syndrome. A negative response almost excludes the presence of a pituitary corticotropin-producing tumor, but a positive response is inconclusive.

Corticotropin-releasing Hormone Test

Plasma corticotropin and cortisol increase twofold to threefold after administration of an IV bolus of CRH (1 μg per kilogram) to patients with Cushing's disease. No increase occurs among most patients with ectopic corticotropin secretion or adrenal tumors.

Suspected Hypersecretion of Thyroid-stimulating Hormone

An elevated serum TSH level most commonly reflects primary hypothyroidism. The diagnosis is made clinically and confirmed by low levels of FT_4. Further testing is not required. Primary TSH hypersecretion is extremely rare and may be caused by TSH-producing pituitary tumors or by pituitary resistance to thyroid hormone. Serum TSH and thyroxine (T_4) levels are elevated, and responses to TRH often differentiate the two conditions. TSH does not respond to TRH in TSH-producing tumors but usually increases more than 30 μU per milliliter in the presence of pituitary resistance to thyroid hormone.

Suspected Hypersecretion of Gonadotropin (Luteinizing and Follicle-stimulating Hormones)

Hypersecretion of LH and FSH occurs most frequently in primary gonadal failure and is accompanied by low concentrations of gonadal steroids. In this situation, dynamic testing is not indicated. In rare instances, gonadotropin-secreting pituitary tumors producing free α subunit, FSH, or LH are encountered. Elevation of plasma α subunit is a helpful sign, but gonadotropin and α subunit responses to GnRH stimulation or gonadal steroid suppression are variable and may not help establish the diagnosis.

■ GUIDELINES FOR THE SELECTION OF PITUITARY FUNCTION TESTS IN CLINICAL SITUATIONS

WITHDRAWAL OF GLUCOCORTICOID THERAPY

Among patients treated with supraphysiologic doses of glucocorticoids (more than 7.5 mg prednisone, more than 0.75 mg dexamethasone) for more than 2 to 3 weeks, the hypothalamic–pituitary–adrenal axis is suppressed. The question often arises whether glucocorticoids can be safely discontinued. The following steps allow safe withdrawal of glucocorticoid therapy:

1. Taper steroid dose to 10 mg prednisone (or equivalent) per day.
2. Change to hydrocortisone 20 mg per day given as a single morning dose, and continue for 3 to 4 days.
3. Measure 8:00 A.M. plasma cortisol before the morning hydrocortisone dose is given. If plasma cortisol level is greater than 10 μg per deciliter, discontinue hydrocortisone. If plasma cortisol level is less than 10 μg per deciliter, continue hydrocortisone replacement and measure cortisol once a month until the 8:00 A.M. cortisol level is greater than 10 μg per deciliter; then discontinue replacement.
4. Perform the short corticotropin test. If plasma cortisol level is greater than 20 μg per deciliter, a normal ability to respond to stress is probable, and steroid coverage is not needed. If cortisol is less than 20 μg per deciliter, steroid cover should be given for any stressful illness or surgery. Repeating the short corticotropin test a few months later may show a normal response, which indicates recovery of the hypothalamic–pituitary–adrenal axis.
5. Perform an insulin hypoglycemia (preferably) or metyrapone test to confirm normal CRH responsiveness to stress. This test often can be omitted if hypothalamic–pituitary disease is not present. If hypothalamic–pituitary disease is suspected, however, the results of the short corticotropin test are not predictive of responsiveness to stress, and an insulin hypoglycemia test should be performed.

SUSPECTED HYPOPITUITARISM

1. Conduct a clinical history interview to elicit information about medications, previous pituitary surgery or irradiation, menstrual history of women, reduced libido and potency among men, and symptoms of hypothyroidism, polyuria, and vision changes.
2. Perform a physical examination to find signs of hypothyroidism or hypogonadism, testicular size and consistency, signs of cortisol or GH excess, and galactorrhea. Examine the visual fields.
3. Obtain basal measurements of prolactin, cortisol (8:00 A.M. to 9:00 A.M.), FT$_4$, TSH, LH, FSH, testosterone, or estradiol. If corticotropin deficiency is strongly suspected on the basis of clinical evidence, administer 10 mg hydrocortisone three times a day by mouth without waiting for the test results.
4. Request CT or MRI of the hypothalamus and pituitary gland.
5. Perform a combined pituitary function test. If a large tumor is present and emergency surgery is needed to reduce pressure symptoms, preoperative dynamic tests are not indicated.
6. If basal measurements suggest deficiency, replace hydrocortisone and T$_4$ before surgery. T$_4$ replacement alone may precipitate cortisol insufficiency among patients with partial corticotropin deficiency.
7. If surgery is not needed, replace hydrocortisone, T$_4$, and gonadal steroids as indicated by the results of the pituitary function tests.

8. Diabetes insipidus may be unmasked by cortisol or T$_4$ replacement.

SUSPECTED PITUITARY HYPERFUNCTION

Elevated Prolactin

1. Assess menses or sexual potency in the history. A drug history is most important. Physical examination should include signs of hypogonadism, galactorrhea, goiter, and chest wall lesions.
2. Conduct biochemical screening to exclude renal failure and hypercalcemia. Measure FT$_4$, TSH, and for men, testosterone.
3. If possible, discontinue any drugs that may elevate prolactin level, and treat the patient as if primary hypothyroidism is present. Reassess prolactin in 1 month.
4. If serum prolactin level remains elevated, request CT or MRI. A serum prolactin level greater than 200 ng per milliliter usually indicates the presence of prolactinoma. Non–prolactin-secreting tumors may elevate prolactin level up to 150 ng per milliliter through compression of the pituitary stalk.

Small prolactinomas (less than 1 cm) rarely compromise other pituitary functions, and dynamic testing is not required. Large tumors may be associated with hypopituitarism, and the approach outlined previously should be followed.

Elevated Levels of Growth Hormone

1. At physical examination, look for changes in the size of the hands and feet, the need for new dentures, an unusual growth pattern, increased perspiration, and characteristic features of elevations in the level of growth hormone.
2. Obtain basal measurements of GH, IGF-I, FT$_4$, 8:00 A.M. cortisol, gonadal steroid (testosterone or estradiol), prolactin, calcium, phosphate, and fasting glucose.
3. Replace cortisol and thyroxine, if required.
4. Request CT or MRI and a visual field examination.
5. If GH and IGF-I are elevated, perform a glucose suppression test (measure GH and glucose). Consider the need for a TRH test (measure GH and TSH), bromocriptine suppression test, and insulin hypoglycemia test to assess corticotropin reserve, if surgery is not planned.
6. If an abdominal or lung tumor is present, suspect ectopic GHRF secretion and measure plasma GHRF.

Cushing's Syndrome

1. Obtain a thorough history and seek characteristic features of Cushing's syndrome at physical examination. Exclude exogenous use of glucocorticoids.
2. Perform a 24-hour urine (10:00 P.M. to 10:00 P.M.) screening test for UFF. At 11:00 P.M., administer 1 mg dexamethasone by mouth. Measure plasma cortisol at 8:00 A.M. the next morning. If UFF is normal (less than 100 μg per 24 hours) and 8:00 A.M. cortisol is less than 5 μg per deciliter, endogenous Cushing's syndrome is excluded.
3. If screening test results are abnormal, schedule the patient

for hospitalization and perform the following tests: morning and evening corticotropin and cortisol; formal dexamethasone suppression tests (2 mg and 8 mg); and maybe a metyrapone or CRH test to define the cause (pituitary, adrenal, ectopic corticotropin). Request appropriate CT or other imaging studies.

BIBLIOGRAPHY

Barkan AL, Reame NE, Kelch RP, et al. Idiopathic hypogonadotropic hypogonadism in man: dependence of the hormone responses on the magnitude of the endogenous GnRH secretory defect. *J Clin Endocrinol Metab* 1985;61:1118.

Bercu BB, Diamond FB. Growth hormone neurosecretory dysfunction. Clin Endocrinol Metab 1986;15:537–590.

Chrousos GP, moderator. Clinical applications of corticotropin-releasing hormone. *Ann Intern Med* 1985;102:344.

Crapo L. Cushing's syndrome: a review of diagnostic tests. *Metabolism* 1979; 28:955.

Fish HR, Chernow B, O'Brien JT. Endocrine and neurophysiologic responses to the pituitary to insulin-induced hypoglycemia: a review. *Metabolism* 1986;35:763.

Harsoulis P, Marshall JC, Kuku SF, et al. A combined test for the assessment of anterior pituitary function. *Br Med J* 1973;4:326.

Sheldon WR, DeBold CR, Evans WS, et al. Rapid sequential intravenous administration of four hypothalamic releasing hormones as a combined anterior pituitary function test in normal subjects. *J Clin Endocrinol Metab* 1985;60:623.

Thorner MD, Vance ML, Evans WS, et al. Clinical studies with GHRH in man. *Horm Res* 1986;24:91.

Utiger RD. Thyrotropin-releasing hormone and thyrotropin secretion. *J Lab Clin Med* 1987;109:327.

Kelley's Textbook of Internal Medicine, fourth edition. Edited by H. David Humes.
Lippincott Williams & Wilkins, Philadelphia © 2000.

C H A P T E R

418

EVALUATION OF THYROID FUNCTION TESTS

RASA KAZLAUSKAITE
BRUCE D. WEINTRAUB
KENNETH D. BURMAN

Secretion of the thyroid hormones thyroxine (T_4) and triiodothyronine (T_3) is regulated by pituitary thyroid-stimulating hormone (thyrotropin; TSH). TSH secretion is controlled through negative feedback by thyroid hormones and both positive and negative hypothalamic factors. This tight interrelation of the hypothalamic–pituitary–thyroid axis allows for convenient and accurate assessment of steady state thyroid function. Laboratory tests of thyroid function have been widely used in clinical practice.

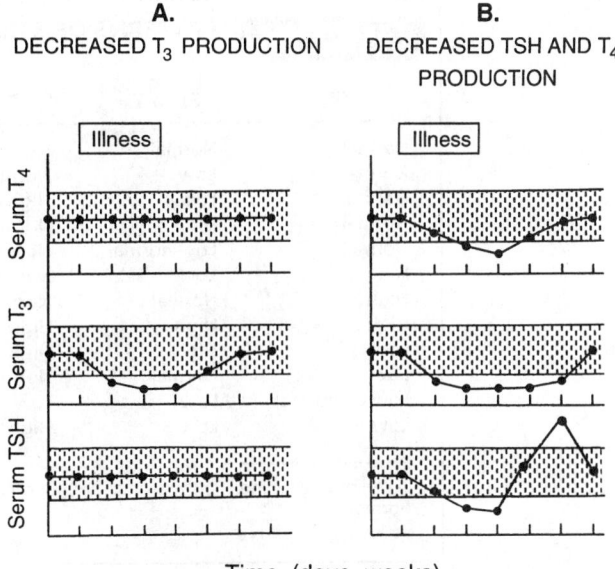

FIGURE 418.1. Thyroid function screening strategies based on results of serum TSH testing. Screening should include a careful history and physical examination. TSH, thyroid-stimulating hormone; T_3, triiodothyronine; T_4, thyroxine; anti-TPO, anti-thyroid peroxidase antibody.

SCREENING FOR THYROID DYSFUNCTION

Screening refers to the testing of thyroid function among persons believed to have thyroid disease but not known to have thyroid disease. The cost-effectiveness of screening of patients without symptoms is a matter of debate. Decision analysis, however, indicates that measurement of serum TSH concentration is as cost-effective as many other preventive medicine measures. The American College of Physicians recommends screening for hypothyroidism among women older than 65 years. Even though in most circumstances a TSH test alone is an appropriate initial screening tool, addition of a free thyroxine (FT_4) test to the screening panel may be indicated (Fig. 418.1). Persons with suspected pituitary or hypothalamic disease cannot be screened with serum TSH measurement alone.

SERUM THYROID-STIMULATING HORMONE CONCENTRATIONS

Measurement of serum TSH is the single best test of thyroid function, in steady state conditions and in the absence of pituitary or hypothalamic disease (Table 418.1). The level of free thyroxine is inversely related to the logarithm of the serum TSH concentration. A small change in FT_4 level may produce a large change in TSH level. Therefore if a single screening test is used to detect primary thyroid dysfunction, third-generation TSH assays are more sensitive and specific than FT_4 measurements for outpatients.

The serum TSH concentration of healthy persons ranges from approximately 0.5 to 5.0 mU per liter. The most common cause of elevated TSH level is primary hypothyroidism caused

TABLE 418.1.	PATTERNS OF STEADY-STATE THYROID FUNCTION TESTS		
TSH	**Free T_4**	**Free T_3**	**Assessment**
Normal	Normal	Normal	Euthyroid
Normal	Low	Normal or low	Central hypothyroidism
Normal	Low	High	T_3 therapy
Normal	High	Normal or high	TSH-mediated hyperthyroidism or RTH
Normal	Low normal	Normal or high	Thyroid extract therapy
High	Low	Normal or low	Primary hypothyroidism
High	Normal	Normal	Subclinical hypothyroidism
High	High	High	TSH-mediated hyperthyroidism or RTH
Low	High	High	Primary hyperthyroidism
Low	Normal	Normal	Subclinical hyperthyroidism
Low or normal	Low	Low	Central hypothyroidism
Low	Low	High	T_3 toxicosis

T_3, triiodothyronine; T_4, thyroxine; TSH, thyroid-stimulating hormone; RTH, resistance to thyroid hormone.

by thyroid gland hypofunction. Patients with overt primary hypothyroidism have TSH values usually greater than 20 mU per liter. Patients with subclinical hypothyroidism, who by definition have few or no symptoms of hypothyroidism and thyroid hormone serum concentrations within the normal range, usually have serum TSH values between 5.0 and 20 mU per liter. The assessment and treatment of patients with subclinical hypothyroidism are controversial.

Inability to detect TSH with a third-generation assay (sensitivity approximately 0.01 mU per liter) is a reliable indicator of the presence of overt primary hyperthyroidism. Subnormal (less than 0.5 mU per liter) serum TSH concentrations with normal serum thyroid hormone concentrations (FT_4 and T_3) in clinically euthyroid patients define subclinical hyperthyroidism (Table 418.1).

If a defect in TSH secretion is present because of hypothalamic or pituitary disease, measurement of TSH levels alone may not be sufficient to define the functional status of the hypothalamic–pituitary–thyroid axis.

SERUM THYROID HORMONE CONCENTRATIONS

Serum FT_4 concentrations should be measured for all patients for diagnosis and follow-up of evaluation of central hypothyroidism, central hyperthyroidism, and thyroid hormone resistance. Measurements of serum TSH and FT_4 levels are the first line tests to investigate thyroid dysfunction for all inpatients, patients with dementia or psychiatric disease, patients with infertility or amenorrhea, patients taking drugs that interfere with thyroid hormone metabolism or function, and patients who need monitoring of thyroid disease.

SERUM FREE THYROXINE CONCENTRATIONS

The serum total thyroxine (TT_4) concentration of healthy adults typically ranges from 4.6 to 11.2 μg per deciliter (64 to 142 nmol per liter). Almost all (99.96%) T_4 in the circulation is bound to carrier proteins, in particular thyroxine-binding globulin (TBG), and to a lesser extent, to transthyretin and albumin. The bound hormone represents a circulating T_4 storage pool; the hormone is not immediately available for uptake into cells. Because drugs and illness (Table 418.2) can alter concentrations of binding proteins or interaction of the binding proteins with T_4 or T_3, the free and total hormone levels may not be concordant.

The FT_4 fraction is responsible for hormonal activity; therefore FT_4 rather than TT_4 concentration is a better estimate of thyroid function in clinical practice. The best laboratory estimate of FT_4 concentration is achieved with an equilibrium dialysis method. In most instances this method is cumbersome and expensive; therefore it is not routinely used in clinical practice. However, some commercial laboratories in the United States (e.g., Nichols) have a good and convenient kit in which FT_4 is measured by means of dialysis.

Because of simplicity of interpretation direct FT_4 measurement by means of radioimmunoassay is used in most clinical laboratories. This method has almost replaced the older methods used to estimate FT_4 concentration. The disadvantage of FT_4 radioimmunoassay is that no currently available kit provides correct FT_4 values for all the binding abnormalities that have been described. However, in most cases this method gives enough information about the hormonal activity of T_4. FT_4 levels are typically 0.7 to 1.9 ng per deciliter, and they vary among the laboratories.

The traditional method was calculation of FT_4 index by use of the thyroid hormone binding ratio or index (THBR or THBI) through measurement of T_3 resin uptake (T_3RU). This method has the advantage that both TT_4 and thyroid hormone binding ratio or index are reported, making it clear when the patient has a potential binding protein abnormality rather than a pathophysiologic condition. It also provides the opportunity to calculate FT_3 index using the thyroid hormone binding ratio or index if total T_3 (TT_3) is measured. Disadvantages of this method are that many clinicians do not understand the calculation and that the FT_4 index, as with direct FT_4 measurement by means of

TABLE 418.2.	DRUGS AFFECTING THYROXINE BINDING IN SERUM	
Increased		**Decreased**

Increased	Decreased
Increased TBG	Decreased TBG
Pregnancy	Inherited complete and partial TBG deficieny
Estrogen excess, including oral	Exogenous androgen and anabolic steroid
contraceptives	hormone excess
Acute and chronic hepatitis, hepatoma	Glucocorticoid excess
HIV infection	Acromegaly
Drugs: 5-fluorouracil, opiates, clofibrate	Drugs: niacin, asparaginase
Familial TBG excess	Nonthyroidal illness
Increased albumin binding	Decreased albumin binding
Familial dysalbuminemic	Nonthyroidal illness
hyperthyroxinemia	Decreased transthyretin binding
Increased transthyretin binding	Nonthyroidal illness
Familial increase	Drug-related inhibition of binding
Islet cell carcinoma	Salicylates
Immunoglobulin binding of thyroxine	Other nonsteroidal anti-inflammatory drugs
Chronic autoimmune thyroiditis	Furosemide

TBG, thyroxine-binding globulin.

radioimmunoassay, does not give correct values for many described binding protein abnormalities. Most important, a small change in the T_3RU result produces a relatively larger change in calculated FT_4 index. These calculated FT_4 values do not consistently correspond to FT_4 values from equilibrium dialysis measurements in many clinical circumstances. We prefer the use of FT_4 measurements over use of a calculated FT_4 index.

The T_3RU was designed to differentiate TBG excess and deficiency from hyperthyroidism and hypothyroidism (Table 418.3). However, the index may not fully correct at the extremes of binding protein abnormalities. In these cases FT_4 may be measured by means of the equilibrium dialysis method, or TBG concentration itself can be measured.

SERUM TRIIODOTHYRONINE CONCENTRATIONS

Total serum T_3 concentration (also called T_3 by radioimmunoassay or stable T_3) in the absence of thyroid binding abnormalities is measured to estimate the severity of hyperthyroidism or to diagnose T_3 toxicosis. T_3 is less tightly bound to TBG but more tightly bound to transthyretin and albumin than is T_4. The normal range typically is 75 to 195 ng per deciliter, and it varies among laboratories.

Serum T_3 concentration changes with alterations in TBG such that, for example, T_3 level increases among euthyroid women taking oral contraceptives. The normal range in this circumstance is different from that among persons not taking estrogen, but the precise normal ranges are not reported on the laboratory slip and must be remembered and recorded by the clinician. It may also be useful to measure T_3 levels for patients who may be having a relapse of Graves' disease after treatment and for patients who are taking exogenous levothyroxine, especially when the dose is sufficiently high to decrease TSH level. A FT_3 index can be calculated with the thyroid hormone binding index. The FT_3 measurements are available commercially and may be used instead of total T_3 if T_3RU is not measured.

ANCILLARY TESTS OF THYROID FUNCTION

The next step after documentation of thyroid function abnormalities is to determine the cause of the abnormality. Valuable information is obtained from the history and physical findings, and any type of thyroid function test must be interpreted in the context of the patient's clinical situation. Ancillary tests may help to isolate the causes of the abnormalities.

ANTI-THYROID ANTIBODY TESTS

The anti-thyroid peroxidase (anti-TPO) antibody test has largely replaced the less sensitive anti-microsomal antibody test. Anti-microsomal antibody was identified as anti-TPO, but the latter is a better test because of the pure recombinant reagents used.

TABLE 418.3.	PATTERNS OF FREE T_4 INDEX ESTIMATE			
Condition	Total T_4	T_3RU or THBI	Free T_4 Index	TSH
Hyperthyroidism	High	High	High	Low
TBG excess	High	Low	Normal	Normal
Hypothyroidism	Low	Low	Low	High
TBG deficiency	Low	High	Normal	Normal

T_3, triiodothyronine; T_4, thyroxine; TSH, thyroid-stimulating hormone; T_3RU, T_3 resin uptake; TBG, thyroxine-binding globulin; THBI, thyroid hormone binding index.

Tests for these antibodies, however, do not contribute direct information about thyroid secretion. Nevertheless, when results of thyroid function tests are ambiguous, evidence of autoimmune thyroid disease may influence the decision regarding therapy versus observation. Low titers of anti-TPO can be found in many thyroid and other autoimmune diseases; however, higher titers suggest Hashimoto's thyroiditis or Graves' disease, or an overlap syndrome called *Hashitoxicosis.* The diagnosis of Hashimoto's thyroiditis among patients with ambiguous thyroid function test results has important clinical implications. The likelihood of the presence or development of hypothyroidism is higher than it is among other patients. The possibility of development of other autoimmune diseases, such as Addison's disease, also increases, as does the possibility of development of thyroid lymphoma.

Thyroid-stimulating immunoglobulin or thyroid binding-inhibiting immunoglobulin assays are an important clinical tool in the care of patients with autoimmune thyroid disease with or without hormone abnormalities. These tests typically are used to determine the likelihood of the presence of transient neonatal thyrotoxicosis or hypothyroidism in the offspring of a mother with autoimmune thyroid disease. Autoimmune thyroid disease may develop in the newborn within the first several weeks of life because of the transplacental passage of IgG antibodies that can stimulate or inhibit the neonatal thyroid gland. Measurement of serum thyroid binding-inhibiting immunoglobulin or thyroid-stimulating immunoglobulin can be used clinically to predict the recurrence of Graves' disease after clinical remission is achieved, to assist in the diagnosis of autoimmune thyroid disease when it is not readily apparent, to help in the diagnosis of Graves' orbitopathy, which can affect any patient with autoimmune thyroid disease, or to differentiate Graves' disease from other causes of orbitopathy.

RADIONUCLIDE TESTS

Many clinicians confuse thyroid scans with uptake tests. These are two different tests that give related but different information. No isotopic test should be performed on a woman who is or may be pregnant.

Thyroid radioiodine uptake among healthy persons in the United States typically ranges from 5% to 15% at 4 hours and 10% to 25% at 24 hours after oral administration of iodine I 131 or iodine I 123. It depends on the iodide intake of a given population. The results usually cannot be interpreted for patients who have substantial exposure to nonradioactive iodide, such as patients who have recently undergone injection of radiographic contrast medium dye for computed tomography scan or angiography. After this kind of exposure, it may take 4 to 6 weeks to clear the iodine load. It seems reasonable to measure 24-hour urine iodine excretion before testing radioiodine uptake. The radioactive iodine test is useful to differentiate hyperthyroidism caused by subacute thyroiditis or exogenous administration of thyroid hormone, in which uptake is low (usually less than 5%), from other causes of hyperthyroidism, such as Graves' disease, multinodular goiter and autonomous nodules, in which it is

TABLE 418.4.	CAUSES OF LOW RADIOIODINE UPTAKE THYROTOXICOSIS

Thyrotoxicosis factitia
Subacute thyroiditis
Silent thyroiditis
Iodine
Ectopic thyroid hormone production (e.g., struma ovarii)
Excess iodine exposure

high (Table 418.4). It is not useful to differentiate hypothyroidism from normal thyroid function.

The radioactive iodine uptake test is not a thyroid function test per se, and it is possible for the uptake to increase even among patients with Hashimoto's thyroiditis, who may be clinically euthyroid or even hypothyroid. This probably occurs because of altered iodine uptake and organification in these patients. For breast-feeding women, a rough estimate of thyroid uptake can be obtained with technetium Tc 99m pertechnetate, which is eliminated faster than iodine I 131. Breast-feeding typically may be resumed 24 hours after the test.

Thyroid radionuclide scanning, which can be performed with technetium Tc 99m pertechnetate, iodine I 123, or iodine I 131, provides information about the function, size, and shape of thyroid nodules but not necessarily about overall thyroid function. Most physicians prefer to use iodine I 123 or technetium for scanning because of the lower radiation dose to the patient.

Thionamide drugs (propylthiouracil, methimazole) and recent administration of iodine or iodide (including amiodarone and iodinated radiocontrast agents) may interfere with the interpretation of results of radionuclide tests.

THYROGLOBULIN

Measurement of serum thyroglobulin in the evaluation of thyroid function is used when factitious ingestion of thyroid hormone preparations is suspected. The thyroglobulin levels of those patients are suppressed, whereas those of patients with thyroiditis are not. Clinicians must be aware not only of prescription thyroid hormone preparations such as levothyroxine (Synthroid, Levoxyl) and liothyronine (Cytomel) but also of thyroid hormone extracts in health foods and food supplements. If a patient has taken a compound that contains thyroglobulin, then serum measurement and interpretation of thyroglobulin levels becomes more problematic.

The most common use of serum thyroglobulin levels is follow-up care of patients with known thyroid cancer to look for recurrence or presence of disease. Most of these patients have undergone complete thyroidectomy and therapy with radioactive iodine. They should have no detectable thyroid tissue, normal or abnormal, and serum thyroglobulin level should be less than 1 ng per milliliter. An increase in serum thyroglobulin level in this circumstance suggests the return of disease. Serum thyroglobulin levels are not useful to detect the presence of thyroid cancer in patients with intact thyroid glands because the normal range is quite wide.

THYROID ULTRASONOGRAPHY

Ultrasonography of the thyroid has minimal value in the evaluation of thyroid function. In some instances it can be helpful in the evaluation of multinodular goiter or autonomous nodules, for example, to help isolate the size and location of nodules and to help ascertain whether nonfunctioning nodules are present that may require aspiration or observation.

PITUITARY AND HYPOTHALAMIC IMAGING STUDIES

Imaging of the pituitary gland and hypothalamus usually is needed after the biochemical diagnosis of central hypothyroidism, which is secondary if caused by pituitary disease or tertiary if caused by hypothalamic disease. In rare instances, hyperthyroidism is caused by a TSH-secreting pituitary tumor, and imaging of the pituitary gland is needed. The optimal imaging study in these circumstances is magnetic resonance imaging of the pituitary and hypothalamic area, although individual circumstances may indicate adjunctive studies, such as high-resolution computed tomography or octreotide scintigraphy.

APPROACH TO THE PATIENT WITH ABNORMAL THYROID FUNCTION TEST RESULTS

Abnormal thyroid function test results for a patient without signs or symptoms of thyroid dysfunction or thyroid function test results discordant with the clinical presentation warrant exclusion of laboratory error, usually through analysis of the clinical context and repetition of the laboratory analysis. Artifacts in

the measurement of TSH may be caused by the presence of heterophilic antibodies against mouse immunoglobulins that interfere with the TSH assay and cause false elevation in many results. Artifactual elevations in T_3 or T_4 may be caused by anti-T_3 or anti-T_4 antibodies (increased titers of anti-thyroglobulin antibody may have some predictive value).

The approach to evaluation of a patient with abnormal thyroid function test results varies with the clinical situation. We recommend evaluation in consultation with an endocrinologist for patients with hyperthyroidism, suspected central causes of thyroid dysfunction, suspected resistance to thyroid hormone or TSH, or abnormal thyroid function test results in the presence or absence of an anatomic abnormality of the thyroid and for pregnant patients with a history of thyroid disease. Consultation should be considered when patients have nonthyroidal illness syndrome, drug-induced thyroid dysfunction or thyroid function test results that are difficult to interpret. When to seek endocrinologic consultation depends on many factors, including the clinical context and laboratory results as well as the background and experience of the referring physician.

PATIENTS WITH SUSPECTED HYPERTHYROIDISM

After a thorough history interview and physical examination, the laboratory evaluation of a patient believed to have hyperthyroidism begins with measurement of serum TSH with or followed by estimation of serum FT_4 and TT_3 or FT_3 (Fig. 418.2). Suppressed undetectable TSH levels with increased FT_4 concentrations help to confirm the diagnosis of primary hyperthyroidism, the most common form of thyrotoxicosis. If serum FT_4 values are normal, serum FT_3 may be elevated, indicating T_3

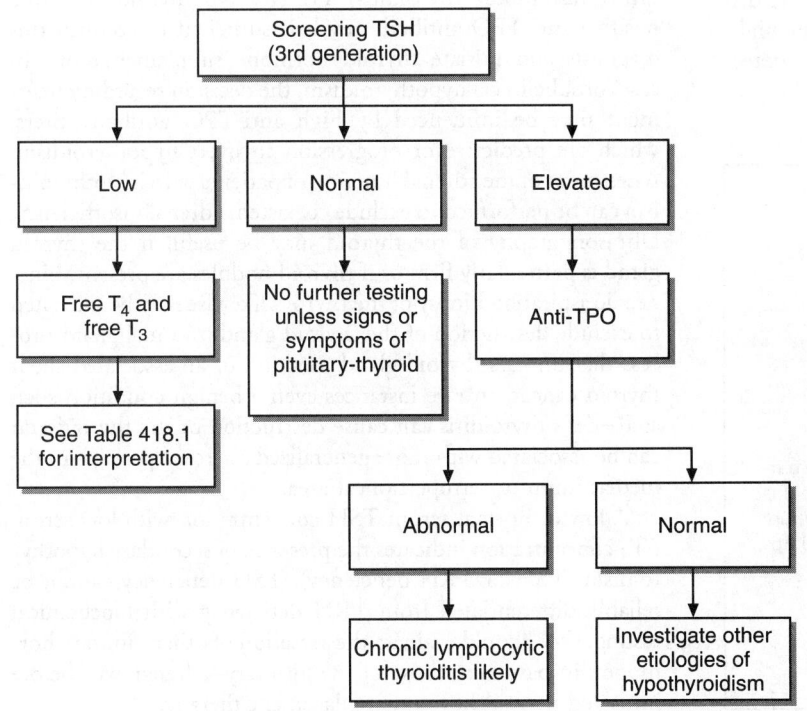

FIGURE 418.2. Strategies for evaluation of thyrotoxicosis. Evaluation should include a careful history and physical examination and should be individualized according to the clinical situation. TSH, thyroid-stimulating hormone; FT_3, free triiodothyronine; FT_4, free thyroxine; RTH, resistance to thyroid hormone; NTIS, nonthyroidal illness syndrome.

EVIDENCE LEVEL: C. Expert Opinion.

toxicosis. A decreased serum TSH level with normal FT_4 and T_3 in the proper clinical context indicates subclinical hyperthyroidism. If TSH level is decreased or undetectable, measurement is best performed with a third-generation TSH assay. Serum TSH levels can vary during the day, and interassay variation can be a factor. As a result, it is important to document a TSH level less than 0.01 mU per liter (undetectable with a third-generation assay), which strongly suggests the presence of hyperthyroidism. If TSH is detectable and slightly below normal range, hyperthyroidism may or may not present.

A normal serum TSH concentration is strong evidence that hyperthyroidism is not present. The exception is the extremely rare instance of TSH-induced hyperthyroidism. Patients with this disorder usually have elevated FT_4 and T_3 levels. Also in rare instances, serum TSH concentration is normal when a patient has secondary hypothyroidism related to a pituitary tumor. The immunoreactive TSH level may be normal, but the pituitary tumor may be producing a form of TSH that is not biologically active but does react with the in vitro antibodies in the TSH assay. As a result, FT_4 and T_3 must be measured when a patient may have secondary hypothyroidism. The two situations just described represent circumstances in which the use of TSH measurement alone as a screening tool can be misleading.

The thyroid gland may be enlarged in primary hyperthyroidism due to Graves' disease or rare cases of secondary hyperthyroidism due to a TSH-producing tumor. The size of the thyroid may decrease in the presence of secondary hypothyroidism or ingestion of thyroid hormone. Subacute thyroiditis may manifest as a painful thyroid gland and hyperthyroidism due to destruction of the thyroid.

After thyrotoxicosis is confirmed, the most cost-effective step may be a referral to an endocrinologist, who chooses the appropriate tests for the differential diagnosis of thyrotoxicosis (Table 418.5) and the mode of treatment. An alternative is to request an anti-TPO antibody titer to test for autoimmune thyroid disease; a thyroid uptake study to differentiate low- from high-uptake thyrotoxicosis; and a thyroid radionuclide scan to detect autonomous (hot) thyroid nodules.

TABLE 418.5.	**CAUSES OF THYROTOXICOSIS**

Toxic diffuse goiter (Graves' disease)
Toxic adenoma
Toxic multinodular goiter
Silent thyroiditis, including lymphocytic and postpartum variations
Subacute painful thyroiditis
Excessive exogenous thyroid hormone ingestion
Drug-induced hyperthyroidism, including iodine-induced
Miscellaneous (TSH hypersecretion, chorionic gonadotropin-induced hyperthyroidism, including pregnancy and trophoblastic disease, struma ovarii, thyroid carcinoma, nonautoimmune autosomal dominant hyperthyroidism, radiation thyroiditis, infarction of thyroid adenoma, congenital thyrotoxicosis, transient neonatal thyrotoxicosis)

TSH, thyroid-stimulating hormone.

TABLE 418.6.	**CAUSES OF HYPOTHYROIDISM**

Chronic autoimmune thyroiditis (atrophic or goitrous)
Radiation therapy (^{131}I therapy–induced, external radiation therapy to the thyroid area, including for head and neck cancer and Hodgkin's lymphoma)
Surgery
Iodine deficiency
Drugs with antithyroid action (including amiodarone and interferon)
Pituitary or hypothalamic hypothyroidism
Silent thyroiditis, including postpartum thyroiditis
Subacute thyroiditis
Riedel's thyroiditis
Withdrawal of thyroid hormone treatment from euthyroid patients
Miscellaneous (congenital, including resistance to TSH, generalized resistance to thyroid hormone, infiltrative disease of the thyroid, including severe granulomatous or cancerous destruction of the thyroid, lymphoma, metastatic disease)

TSH, thyroid-stimulating hormone.

PATIENTS WITH SUSPECTED HYPOTHYROIDISM

After a complete history interview and physical examination, the evaluation of hypothyroidism (Table 418.6) begins with measurement of TSH concentration with or followed by estimation of FT_4 concentration. In most instances serum T_3 levels are not needed in the evaluation of hypothyroidism.

A high serum TSH concentration with low serum FT_4 concentration confirms the diagnosis of primary hypothyroidism, which is most commonly caused by chronic autoimmune thyroiditis (Hashimoto's thyroiditis). Primary hypothyroidism with a positive anti-TPO antibody result is sufficient to confirm this diagnosis and initiate thyroid hormone supplementation. In cases of subclinical hypothyroidism, the decision regarding treatment may be influenced by high anti-TPO antibody titers, which are predictive of progression to overt hypothyroidism. Assessment of the adrenal function of patients with hypothyroidism can be performed to exclude coexistent adrenal insufficiency. Ultrasonography of the thyroid may be useful if the thyroid gland is particularly firm or if thyroid nodules are present. Fine-needle aspiration biopsy of the thyroid likewise may be indicated to exclude destruction of the thyroid gland by a malignant process that impairs thyroid gland function or an associated silent thyroid cancer. In rare instances even a benign condition such as Riedel's thyroiditis can cause destruction of the thyroid and can be associated with more generalized sclerosis, perhaps in the mediastinum or retropertioneal area.

A low or normal serum TSH concentration with low serum FT_4 concentration indicates the presence of secondary hypothyroidism (TSH or TRH deficiency). TSH deficiency cannot be reliably differentiated from TRH deficiency with biochemical testing. One should evaluate the secretion of other pituitary hormones, in particular those of the pituitary–adrenal axis, before initiating thyroid hormone replacement therapy.

TABLE 418.7.	ALTERATIONS IN HYPOTHALAMIC–PITUITARY–THYROID FUNCTION IN NONTHYROIDAL ILLNESS	
Alteration	**Site**	**Cause**
Decreased serum T_3 concentration	Extrathyroidal tissue	Decreased T_4-5'-deiodinase activity
Decreased serum total T_4 concentration	Extrathyroidal tissue	Decreased serum binding of T_4
Decreased serum free T_4 concentration	Thyroid	Decreased TSH secretion
Decreased thyroid responsiveness to TSH	Decreased TSH bioactivity	Altered TSH processing in the pituitary
Pituitary	Decreased TRH secretion	Increased dopamine, somatostatin, or cortisol secretion
Decreased T_3 action	Extrathyroidal tissue	Decreased T_3 receptors or postreceptor actions of T_3
Increased serum T_4 concentrations	Thyroid	Increased TSH secretion Decreased T_4 clearance

T_3, triiodothyronine; T_4, thyroxine; TRH, thyrotropin-releasing hormone; TSH, thyroid-stimulating hormone.

NONTHYROIDAL ILLNESS SYNDROME

Thyroid function should not be routinely assessed for seriously ill patients unless there is a suspicion of abnormal thyroid dysfunction. Screening inpatients is a more difficult problem because of the effects of severe nonthyroidal illness on thyroid hormone, TSH, and TRH homeostasis (Table 418.7). These effects include the following:

- Reduced levels of thyroid hormone binding proteins
- Increased levels of free fatty acids, which displace thyroid hormones from binding proteins
- Acquired central hypothyroidism, a blunted TSH response to low levels of thyroid hormones
- Decreased peripheral conversion of T_4 to T_3, low T_3 levels, and increased reverse T_3
- Alterations in medications that affect hypothalamic–pituitary–thyroid axis and TBG levels (Tables 418.3 and 418.8)
- Increased serum interleukin-6 concentration, which may play a role in alteration of results of thyroid function tests

To assess thyroid function for severely ill inpatients, measurement of both TSH and FT_4 is necessary in conjunction with analysis of the clinical context. Serum T_4 levels usually are normal or low, as is serum FT_4 concentration. TSH level usually is low or normal; however, during recovery from nonthyroidal illness some hospitalized patients have transient elevations in serum TSH concentration (as high as 20 mU per liter). TSH measured with a third-generation assay rarely is undetectable among patients with euthyroid illness syndrome. Administration of a steroid or dopamine may decrease serum TSH level. To further complicate interpretation of thyroid function tests, severe illness may decrease serum TSH levels rapidly. For example, a patient with authentic primary hypothyroidism with a TSH level of perhaps 50 mU per liter may have an apparent TSH value that is lower, 15 mU per liter, for example, measured in the intensive care unit when the patient has other systemic illnesses.

Patients with systemic illnesses who have subnormal but detectable serum TSH concentrations (more than 0.01 but less than 0.3 mU per liter) with a third-generation assay frequently are euthyroid after recovery from the illness. In contrast, approximately 75% of patients with undetectable serum TSH (less than 0.01 mU per liter) are determined to have hyperthyroidism. The TRH stimulation test does not typically give more information than does measurement of basal TSH level with a third-generation assay.

Only about 15% of hospitalized patients with serum TSH values between 5 and 20 mU per liter prove to have hypothyroidism after recovery. Anti-TPO antibody testing may be helpful in evaluating subclinical hypothyroidism for these patients because a positive antibody test result may indicate the presence of autoimmune thyroiditis.

DRUG EFFECTS ON THYROID FUNCTION

Thyroid function itself and results of assays used to measure thyroid hormones can be affected by various drugs (Table 418.8), including those used to manage nonthyroidal illness. Some of those drugs have multiple actions and can cause either hyperthyroidism or hypothyroidism, depending on preexisting thyroid function. Pharmacologic doses of glucocorticoids (equivalent to more than 5 to 10 mg of prednisone daily), dopamine (more than 1 μg per kilogram per minute), and somatostatin analogs (equivalent to more than 100 μg per day) may confound interpretation of TSH results. These drugs usually do not suppress TSH to less than 0.01 mU per liter, although such decreases can occur. Iodine, iodide (including radiocontrast materials), amiodarone, and lithium can cause either hypothyroidism or hyperthyroidism. Both interferon-α and interleukin-2 can initiate or exacerbate autoimmune disease as manifested by hypothyroidism or hyperthyroidism. Patients taking thyroid hormone for replacement may have alterations in thyroid function

TABLE 418.8.	EFFECT OF DRUGS ON CONCENTRATION OF THYROID-STIMULATING HORMONE

Drugs that Increase TSH Concentration	Drug that Decrease TSH Concentration
Well known to affect thyroid function	Well known to affect thyroid hormone
Amiodarone	concentrations and thyroid function
Carbimazole	Amiodarone
Interferon	Interferon
Interleukin-2	Interleukin-2
Iodine and iodide	Iodine and iodide
Lithium	Tetraiodothyrocetic acid (TETRAC)
Methimazole	Thyroxine
Methylthiouracil	Trilodothyroacetic acid (TRIAC)
Propylthiouracil	Triiodothyronine
Drugs that affect absorption of	Other thyroid hormone analogs
thyroid hormone	Drugs with pituitary and hypothalamic action
Cholestyramine	Glucocorticoids
Sucralfate	Somatostatin
Aluminum hydroxide	Dopamine and dopaminergic drugs
Ferrous sulfate	Opiates
Drugs that increase T_4 clearance	Miscellaneous drugs
Carbamazepine	Acetylsalicylic acid
Rifampin	Aminoglutethimide
Possibly phenytoin	Bexarotene
Miscellaneous drugs	Growth hormone
Cimetidine	Heparin
Clomiphene	5-Hydroxytryptophan
Dopamine antagonists and	Neuroleptics
inhibitors	Pyridoxine
Thyrotropin-releasing horone	

TSH, thyroid-stimulating hormone.

tests after taking drugs that interfere with absorption of thyroid hormone.

MONITORING THE ADEQUACY OF LEVOTHYROXINE REPLACEMENT

One of the more common reasons for assessing thyroid function is to monitor levothyroxine (Synthroid, Levothroid, Levoxyl) therapy. Patients with primary hypothyroidism who are taking levothyroxine replacement therapy can be monitored with periodic measurement of serum TSH, usually with T_4 analysis. If the TSH level is high, the dose of levothyroxine has to be increased; if TSH level is low, the dose has to be reduced. The typical goal of treatment in these circumstances is a TSH level of 1 to 3 mU per liter, and monitoring is important. It is preferable that the patient take levothyroxine alone on an empty stomach. Excessive administration of thyroid hormone, as indicated by excessive TSH suppression and concomitant hyperthyroxinemia can increase the risk of both atrial fibrillation and bone disease. For patients with thyroid cancer, whose goal in taking levothyroxine is suppression of thyroid function and of proliferation of thyroid cancer cells, desirable levels of TSH may depend on the risks and benefits of thyroid hormone suppressive therapy in individual clinical circumstances.

After a change in levothyroxine dose, steady state is achieved

in 4 to 6 weeks, because of the 5- to 7-day half-life of T_4 in blood circulation. Therefore, measurement of serum TSH concentration should be performed 4 to 6 weeks after the intervention. Measurement FT_4 alone is insensitive in assessing the appropriateness of the levothyroxine dose in primary hypothyroidism. However, FT_4 concentrations may be helpful to exclude pseudomalabsorption of levothyroxine, which is much more common than true malabsorption, as in severe gastrointestinal disease or with use of some medications (Table 418.8). Patients who are not compliant with thyroid hormone replacement therapy and take thyroid hormone only a few days before a physician appointment may have an elevated TSH and a normal FT_4 concentration. Therefore measurement of both TSH and FT_4 is reasonable in monitoring levothyroxine therapy. The quoted normal range for T_4 or FT_4 does not strictly apply to patients who have primary hypothyroidism and are taking exogenous levothyroxine, presumably because all of T_3 must be converted from T_4 rather than from direct thyroidal secretion. To achieve T_3 levels similar to those of a person with normal thyroid function, a person with hypothyroidism has to have a T_4 level higher than that of a person with a normal thyroid gland and normal physiologic T_4 and T_3 secretion and kinetics.

The one setting in which the FT_4 is used as the primary test to titrate dosage of thyroid hormone is secondary hypothyroidism. These patients do not respond appropriately to hypothyroidism by increasing TSH secretion. In fact, serum T_3 also is measured and used to ensure appropriate levels for the clinical situation.

BIBLIOGRAPHY

Burman KD. Overview of thyroiditis. *UpToDate in Endocrinology*;7(2). Available at: www.uptodate.com.

Burman KD. Hyperthyroidism. In: Baker KL, ed. *Principles and practice of endocrinology and metabolism,* 2d ed. Philadelphia: JB Lippincott–Raven, 1995:367–384.

Garcia M, Baskin HJ, Feld S, et al. *AACE clinical practice guidelines for evaluation and treatment of hyperthyroidism and hypothyroidism.* Available at http://www.aace.com/clinguideindex.htm.

Meier CA, Burger AG. Effects of pharmacologic agents on thyroid hormone homeostasis. In: Braverman L, Utiger RD, eds. *Werner and Ingbar's the thyroid: a fundamental and clinical text,* 7th ed. Philadelphia: Lippincott–Raven, 1996:276–285.

Ross DS. Laboratory assessment of thyroid function. *UpToDate in Endocrinology*;7(2). Available at www.uptodate.com.

Screening for thyroid disease: American College of Physicians clinical guideline parts 1 and 2. *Ann Intern Med* 1998;129:141–158.

Surks MI, Chopra IJ, Mariash CN, et al. American Thyroid Association guidelines for the use of laboratory tests in thyroid disorders. *JAMA* 1990;263:1529–1532.

Weintraub BD, Kazlauskaite R, Grossman M, et al. Thyroid-stimulating hormone and regulation of the thyroid axis. In: De Groot LJ, ed. *Endocrinology,* 4th ed. Philadelphia: WB Saunders.

Kelley's Textbook of Internal Medicine, fourth edition. Edited by H. David Humes. Lippincott Williams & Wilkins, Philadelphia © 2000.

CHAPTER
419

HUMAN GENE THERAPY

JAMES M. WILSON

Advances in our understanding of the molecular basis of human diseases have suggested novel approaches to treatment, such as somatic gene therapy. The two general models of gene therapy are based on gene transfer occurring either ex vivo or directly in vivo. Early models in gene therapy were primarily focused on ex vivo manipulations of autologous cells, such as the hematopoietic stem cell, which are transplanted into the individual from which they were derived after genetic modification. The more practical and effective approach to gene therapy is direct administration of the gene in vivo, a strategy that resembles more traditional pharmacologic therapy.

Critical to the success of gene therapy is the development of efficient and safe gene delivery vehicles. An important concept in the early development of the field was the use of recombinant forms of viruses as gene delivery vehicles. The initial application of this concept was the development of recombinant forms of murine retroviruses for ex vivo gene transfer. Retroviruses can be rendered truly replication defective through deletion of the

gag-pol-env genes. The resulting vectors are grown in appropriate packaging cell lines that provide these functions in trans. An advantage of retroviruses as vectors is that they efficiently integrate their genome into target cells. However, they are difficult to purify and isolate in high yields, and the target cell must be actively dividing at the time of exposure to the virus to achieve gene transfer. A more recently developed virus-based delivery system entails recombinant forms of human adenovirus. Important advantages of this system are that the virus can be grown in extremely high quantities and purified to near homogeneity and is capable of efficiently transferring genes into nondividing target cells. Current limitations of recombinant adenoviruses relate to immunologic responses of the recipient to the virus and virus-infected cells. Consequences of these problematic host responses are immune-mediated clearance of the genetically corrected cells and difficulty in obtaining efficient gene transfer on a second administration of virus because of the development of neutralizing antibody.

Gene delivery vehicles based on synthetic constructs are being developed as an alternative to the virus-based systems. Synthetic complexes of lipid and DNA, called *liposomes,* have undergone extensive analysis in preclinical models with selected experience in clinical trials. Another approach is the development of molecular conjugates constructed through the formation of complexes between DNA and polycationic proteins. The molecular conjugate approach to gene transfer will ultimately prove to be more versatile than liposome technology in that selected components of the gene transfer vehicle can be easily manipulated, as in the development of cell-specific ligands. The nonviral approaches to gene therapy have proved to be extremely inefficient, far outweighing the safety advantages inherent to them.

Several years ago it became clear that the vector systems under development for in vivo gene therapy—adenoviruses and synthetic constructs—did not confer stable expression of the recombinant gene. This made it difficult to treat patients with chronic diseases. Progress has been made in overcoming this limitation through the use of vectors based on recombinant forms of adenoassociated virus (AAV) and lentivirus.

AAV vectors are based on disabled forms of a human parvovirus not associated with human disease. These vectors efficiently transfer their genomes into nondividing cells in vivo (e.g., fibers of skeletal and cardiac muscle, hepatocytes, neuro and photoreceptors) where they randomly integrate into chromosomal DNA. AAV accomplishes efficient in vivo gene transfer without inciting destructive cellular immune responses against the transgene product. Lentiviral vectors are based on certain types of retroviruses, such as HIV, which efficiently infect nondividing cells. The vector is rendered completely defective, and its tropism is expanded by incorporation of a heterologous envelope. Lentivirus performs in much the same way as AAV; there is far less experience with this system.

INHERITED DISEASES

Adenosine Deaminase Deficiency

The best-described model of gene therapy is inherited deficiency of adenosine deaminase (ADA), which leads to severe combined immunodeficiency. The only effective long-term therapy for this disease is allogeneic bone marrow transplantation from a matched donor who expresses normal levels of ADA. The success of allogeneic bone marrow transplantation suggests an alternative therapeutic approach in which the patient is reconstituted with autologous bone marrow that has been genetically modified to express ADA. An attractive aspect of this model is that expression of ADA may confer onto hematopoietic stem cells a selective advantage that facilitates lymphoid reconstitution with ADA-expressing cells. Recombinant retroviruses have been used to transfer the human ADA gene into bone marrow cells from a variety of species. Difficulties working with the human hematopoietic stem cell and lack of an appropriate animal model for ADA deficiency redirected the initial human trials away from bone marrow toward a more accessible and easily characterized cell, the T lymphocyte. The first human trial of gene therapy was performed with ADA-deficient patients. They received autologous T lymphocytes that had been genetically corrected with a recombinant retrovirus ex vivo. Subsequent studies were based on stem cell gene therapy.

Familial Hypercholesterolemia

An inherited defect in the low-density lipoprotein (LDL) receptor gene causes the disease familial hypercholesterolemia (FH), which in its homozygous form leads to fulminant coronary artery disease in childhood. The only effective long-term therapy for FH is orthotopic liver transplantation from an allogeneic donor with normal LDL receptor function. These considerations provide a rationale for development of gene therapies for FH that are based on LDL receptor gene transfer into hepatocytes.

The first attempt at gene therapy directed at the liver was based on an ex vivo strategy in the treatment of patients homozygous for FH. Extensive work in a variety of animal models suggested the feasibility and safety of this protocol. The initial pilot experiment has been completed with modest reductions in LDL realized by most of the patients. Current efforts are directed at development of in vivo approaches to gene therapy to the liver. Recombinant forms of human adenoviruses and AAV have proved to be effective vehicles for accomplishing in vivo directed gene transfer to the liver. There have been substantial reductions in LDL in FH animal models treated with LDL receptor—suppressing adenoviruses. Current limitations of this strategy are immune responses to the virus and viral infection of cells.

Cystic Fibrosis

After isolation of the gene responsible for cystic fibrosis (CF) in 1989, research in this field was redirected at development of a cure based on genetic correction of the disease in the lungs. CF is caused by a defect in a gene that encodes an epithelial cell–specific chloride channel. The defect causes obstructive lung disease. The development of gene therapy for CF proceeded quickly after the isolation of the gene. Recombinant forms of retroviruses and vaccinia viruses were used to transfer a normal version of the CF gene into patient-derived cells and demonstrate functional correction of the chloride secretory defect. Efforts then focused on an in vivo approach to gene therapy in

which the gene delivery vehicle was delivered to airway epithelial cells by means of inhalation techniques. Both recombinant adenovirus and liposome technology have been tested in animal models and human pilot experiments with encouraging results. Problems of immune responses to the vehicle and genetically corrected cells that have been encountered in the in vivo therapies to the liver also have surfaced in the early development of in vivo applications to the lung.

Hemophilia

Genetic deficiencies of blood clotting factors IX or VIII cause bleeding diatheses that are often severe and life threatening. Current treatment involves infusion of normal clotting factors at the time of uncontrolled hemorrhage. Recombinant proteins have largely replaced blood replacement products, which were associated with a high incidence of hepatitis and HIV transmission. Gene therapy for hemophilia involves transfer of a normal factor IX or VIII gene into a somatic cell capable of expressing functional protein, such as liver or skeletal muscle. Stable engraftment of the gene with a vector such as AAV has shown amelioration of the coagulation defect in murine and canine models of factor IX deficiency. Pivotal clinical trials in hemophiliac patients are underway.

ACQUIRED DISEASES

As research in somatic gene therapy has expanded, so has its list of potential clinical applications. Many experts now believe that gene therapy will eventually have its greatest effect on the prevention and control of common acquired diseases. Progress in this area is viewed with specific examples from the general areas of cardiovascular disease, AIDS, and cancer.

Application of gene therapy to cardiovascular diseases is a fast growing area. A promising strategy under evolution in multiple clinical trials is expression of angiogenic factors in limbs or organs compromised by atherosclerosis-induced vascular insufficiency. Site-specific expression of these factors leads to formation of new blood vessels that improve vascular perfusion in animal models. Important data should emerge from several later stage clinical trials.

Several interesting forms of gene therapy have been considered in the management of AIDS. The most promising genetic approach is intracellular immunization, which is an attempt to render the hematopoietic system resistant to infection with HIV by introducing genes into stem cells that interfere with HIV replication. Specific strategies for blocking viral replication by means of gene transfer have been demonstrated in cultured cells. In the initial clinical trials of this approach to HIV an antiviral gene was transferred into peripheral blood T cells. Somatic gene transfer also is being considered in the development of an effective vaccine for HIV. It is hoped that more effective cellular immunity will be elicited with genetically modified autologous cells that express antigenic HIV proteins.

The most extensive investment in gene therapy has been in the context of cancer. The initial clinical application of gene therapy for cancer was a modification of adoptive immunotherapy, which involves infusion of large quantities of autologous tumor-infiltrating lymphocytes directed against the tumor. Somatic gene therapy could enhance the antitumor function of tumor-infiltrating lymphocytes through genetic modification of the cells ex vivo.

Another strategy is to introduce into tumor cells in vivo a gene capable of aborting growth or modifying the program of differentiation. A variety of molecular strategies have been entertained that use molecules such as well-characterized oncogenes. The problem with this strategy is difficulty achieving efficient gene transfer in vivo, especially in the setting of metastatic disease. One approach to overcoming the inherent limitations of in vivo gene transfer is to focus on diseases that cause morbidity and mortality due to local disease. The prototype of this strategy is to transfer a gene, such as thymidine kinase from herpes simplex virus, into the tumor site that renders the cells sensitive to a chemotherapeutic agent, such as ganciclovir in the case of thymidine kinase. This strategy has met with success in animal models. It appears that thymidine kinase–mediated tumor cell ablation is associated with a substantial bystander effect in which adjoining cells also are eliminated. Clinical trials using in vivo gene transfer of thymidine kinase have been initiated for the management of malignant tumors of the central nervous system and mesothelioma, with other types of cancer to follow.

The most versatile strategy for managing metastatic malignant tumors is based on the concept of tumor vaccination. A variety of gene transfer approaches have been considered in an attempt to enhance the patient's immune response to the tumor cells. Ex vivo and in vivo approaches have been developed in which the tumor cell is genetically modified to enhance activation of cellular immunity by one of many strategies, including expressing an allogeneic human leukocyte antigen, secretion of immune regulatory cytokines, and expression of lymphocyte costimulatory molecules.

GENE DELIVERY

The Human Genome Project has revolutionized the way in which new therapeutics are developed in the biopharmaceutical industry. Discovery begins with an analysis of human genes and an assessment of their role in health and disease in a process called *functional genomics*. The traditional pathway for development of therapeutics is to design a small-molecule drug that inhibits or activates the target protein, or the protein itself is manufactured for delivery to the patient. Gene therapy can be use to short-circuit these expensive and time-consuming steps by incorporating the target gene into a vector administered to patients. The therapeutic protein is manufactured in the patient's cells and delivered directly to the site of disease. Use of vectors that confer stable expression eliminates the need for repeated parenteral administration of the protein. Most applications of this strategy, such as erythropoietin for anemia, insulin for diabetes, interferon for cancer, require genes that can be regulated. Development of these so-called molecular rheostats is progressing. Clinical trials are expected in the next 5 years.

FUTURE DIRECTIONS

Somatic gene therapy represents a novel approach to the prevention, management, and cure of diseases of humans. In the past, experiments with animal models completely dominated research in the area of gene therapy. The 1990s have ushered in a new area of expanded basic biology to develop more effective therapy with selective human experimentation. True successes in therapy for multiple diseases are expected in the first decade of the new millenium.

BIBLIOGRAPHY

Blaese RM, Culver KW, Miller AD, et al. T lymphocyte–directed gene therapy for ADA-SCID: initial trial results after 4 years. *Science* 1995; 270:475–480.

Grossman M, Raper SE, Kozarsky K, et al. Successful ex vivo gene therapy directed to liver in a patient with familial hypercholesterolemia. *Nature Genetics* 1994;6:335–341.

Herzog RW, Yang EY, Couto LB, et al. Long-term correction of canine hemophilia B by gene transfer of blood coagulation factor IX mediated by adeno-associated viral vector. *Nature Medicine* 1999;5:56–63.

Rosengart TK, Lee LY, Patel SR, et al. Angiogenesis gene therapy: phase I assessment of direct intramyocardial administration of an adenovirus vector expressing VEGF121 cDNA to individuals with clinically significant severe coronary artery disease. *Circulation* 1999;100:468–474.

Soiffer R, Lynch T, Mihm M, et al. Vaccination with irradiated autologous melanoma cells engineered to secrete human granulocyte-macrophage colony-stimulating factor generates potent antitumor immunity in patients with metastatic melanoma. *Proc Natl Acad Sci USA* 1998;95: 13141–13146.

Ye X, Rivera VM, Zoltick P, et al. Regulated delivery of therapeutic proteins after in vivo somatic cell gene transfer. *Science* 1999;283:88–91.

Zabner J, Couture LA, Gregory RJ, et al. Adenovirus-mediated gene transfer transiently corrects the chloride transport defect in nasal epithelia of patients with cystic fibrosis. *Cell* 1993;75:207–216.

Kelley's Textbook of Internal Medicine, fourth edition. Edited by H. David Humes.
Lippincott Williams & Wilkins, Philadelphia © 2000.

10

NEUROLOGY

John W. Griffin, Editor

APPROACH TO THE PATIENT WITH NEUROLOGIC DISEASES

APPROACH TO THE PATIENT WITH NEUROLOGIC COMPLAINTS

VINCENT P. SWEENEY
DONALD W. PATY

Many physicians approach the problem of neurologic diagnosis and management with trepidation and insecurity. This results in part from the complexity of the nervous system, but it is also related to the wide range of conditions and diseases that affect the central and peripheral nervous systems and muscles. Consequently, the presentation of neurologic complaints and findings is more varied than the clinical features of disorders of other body systems. However, there are certain pathophysiologic considerations and patterns of presentation of neurologic problems that, if understood, can lead to a more confident approach to diagnosis and management. This chapter and the chapter on the patient with sensory loss and weakness (Chapter 430) present a method of rational analysis of symptoms and findings that facilitates neurologic diagnosis.

In the approach to the patient with neurologic complaints, it is important to know the scope of diseases and conditions presenting as neurologic complaints. Such conditions may be primarily located in the nervous system or muscles, or may be based in other organ systems and secondarily alter nervous system function. The primary pathologic processes affecting the nervous system include those occurring in other organs, such as vascular disease, infections, and neoplasms, as well as those more common to the brain, such as inborn errors of metabolism, demyelinating disease, certain degenerative processes, and abiotrophies (e.g., senility, Alzheimer's disease). The vulnerability of the central and peripheral nervous systems and muscles to secondary involvement is related to both their large extent and their metabolic requirements. The requirements for a constant supply of oxygen and glucose make the brain more susceptible than

other organs to hypoxia, ischemia, and hypoglycemia. Similarly, the nervous system is vulnerable to some vitamin deficiencies and to metabolic disturbances, alterations of blood gases, and electrolyte imbalance. Hence, neurologic complaints such as confusion, delirium, stupor, and seizures may be the presenting features of systemic problems that originate outside the nervous system, in the absence of any detectable pathologic process in the brain. Similarly, diffuse weakness may not be caused by a specific lesion of nerves or muscle, but rather by remote effects of such conditions as cancer, thyrotoxicosis, or potassium imbalance.

Other important considerations of neurologic symptoms and findings relate to pathophysiologic processes unique to the nervous system. *Seizures* result from electrophysiologic disturbances affecting cerebral neurons, a process not known to occur elsewhere in the body. Seizures are also unique in producing positive symptoms of cerebral excitation such as convulsions, sensory "march," complex automatic behavior, hallucinations, and other bizarre disturbances. Postseizure cortical dysfunction may present with temporary paralysis or neurologic dysfunction (Todd's palsy). *Syncope* is the brain's reaction to hypoperfusion, designed to compensate for the decrease in blood flow by placing the body flat rather than upright. Again, this is a unique pathophysiologic process determined by specific vulnerability to hypoxia and ischemia. The common phenomenon of *migraine* represents an incompletely understood process primarily affecting the cerebral circulation and metabolism. The central and peripheral nervous systems are vulnerable to *trauma* that may result in irreversible dysfunction.

LOCALIZATION

The traditional teaching in neurologic diagnosis has emphasized the primary consideration of locating the lesion and then determining what the lesion is. Although these considerations are paramount in many situations (focal brain disease, spinal cord compression, nerve root or peripheral nerve root lesions), they do not encompass the full range of neurologic presentation of disease. As discussed earlier, many disturbances of cerebral function and other neurologic dysfunction are not caused by a lesion but are secondary phenomena. With this limitation in mind, the classic tenets of neurologic diagnosis can be applied in a manner that simplifies the process of deductive analysis of complaints and findings. The location of a lesion is determined by relating it to a knowledge of neuroanatomy and neurophysiology. *Such knowledge need not be extensive if certain principles are understood.* Most neurologic symptoms relate to altered nervous system function, which in turn alters the normal activities of daily living. Disorders of thought, memory, speech, and vision reflect dysfunction of cortical neuronal tissues. Essential functions of walking, balance, and coordination result from altered motor, sensory, or cerebellar control. Loss of bladder and bowel control and sexual dysfunctions result from autonomic dysfunction. Thus, if the clinician understands that language disorders are usually related to lesions in the dominant (left) hemisphere of the brain, it follows that an associated weakness of the right side of the body is likely related to the same lesion. A complete right hemiplegia with normal language function is less likely to be cortical in origin, and therefore is probably subcortical, involving white matter pathways rather than neurons. A similar right-sided weakness associated with a symptom or sign pointing to the left side of the brain stem (e.g., left facial weakness or sensory loss, left abducens weakness producing diplopia) accurately locates the site of the lesion to the left brain stem. Lesions in the spinal cord often produce "levels" of involvement. Cervical cord lesions may produce lower motor disturbance in the arms and upper motor neuron weakness in the legs. Bilateral weakness of the legs with sparing of the arms characterizes lesions below the cervical cord. If associated with a sensory level below which pain and temperature sensation are altered, then an accurate diagnosis of the site of the lesion is possible. Conditions affecting spinal roots produce symptoms and findings related to dermatomes and recognized motor disturbances different from those affecting peripheral nerves. Diffuse conditions affecting peripheral nerves preferentially affect long nerve processes, which are more vulnerable. It follows, therefore, that in diffuse polyneuropathy, motor or sensory involvement of the feet first, followed by the fingers and hands, is the usual mode of presentation. Such conditions likely present with clumsy and weak hands and feet and a stocking-and-glove type of sensory loss, usually quickly accompanied by loss of reflexes. On the other hand, large muscles situated proximally are most vulnerable to most conditions presenting as muscle disease. Weakness of the pelvic girdle causing difficulty rising from a chair or weakness of the shoulder girdle causing difficulty with hair grooming are likely presentations. Such muscle weakness is bilateral and symmetric. Sensory loss is not present, and the reflexes are usually preserved in muscle disorders.

ETIOLOGIC CONSIDERATIONS

Determination of *what* the lesion is depends on the nature of the underlying pathologic process and the nervous system's reaction to the lesion. Many pathologic and pathophysiologic processes have a recognized temporal profile in their evolution and clinical presentations (Table 420.1). The most sudden onset of symptoms results from ischemia, seizure, or trauma. Thus, the term *stroke* is related to the sudden onset of symptoms due to either cerebrovascular occlusive disease or hemorrhage. Although frank convulsive seizures or epileptic loss of consciousness can

TABLE 420.1.	TEMPORAL PROFILE IN NEUROLOGIC DIAGNOSIS
Type of Onset	**Most Likely Cause**
Abrupt	
Seconds	Seizure, trauma
Seconds to hours	Vascular disorder
Hours to days	Infection
Subacute	
Days to weeks	Metabolic, inflammatory disorder Neoplasia
Chronic	
Weeks to months	Neoplastic nutritional disorder
Years	Degenerative disorder

be preceded by an aura, the aura is the commencement of the seizure and is itself sudden in origin. The effects of trauma are usually immediate but may also be delayed or progressive if associated with delayed to slow intracranial bleeding. Space-occupying processes present in a temporal manner depending on their speed of expansion and the brain's reaction to the underlying disease. Thus, cerebral abscesses due to bacterial agents with associated cerebral edema are likely to present over a matter of days, in contrast to the slower, more gradual clinical expression of slower-growing neoplasms. The process of brain shift and herniation down through the tentorial notch or foramen magnum adds another dimension of rapidity to the clinical features in many expanding pathologic lesions. Most degenerative processes are slow in the development of clearcut symptoms or findings. Examples include the general motor problems associated with Parkinson's disease or the dementia and personality changes of Alzheimer's disease. The occasional rapid onset of symptoms of such diseases is usually explained by some intercurrent environmental change or associated aggravating illness that brings the condition to light. Multiple sclerosis is unique in the scatter "in time and place" of symptoms and findings, which usually manifest over a number of years.

Demographic characteristics are also helpful in determining the likelihood of underlying disease processes. To a large extent, age determines the distribution of many conditions (Table 420.2). The hereditary and congenital diseases usually present

TABLE 420.2.	RELATION BETWEEN AGE AND CAUSE IN NEUROLOGIC DISEASE
Age	**Cause**
Childhood	Congenital, infectious, genetic, some neoplastic disorders
Adolescence	Genetic, traumatic disorders
Young adulthood	Traumatic, metabolic, inflammatory disorders
Middle age	Metabolic, inflammatory, neoplastic, vascular disorders
Old age	Vascular, metabolic, neoplastic, degenerative disorders

in infancy and childhood. However, hereditary conditions such as polyneuropathies may be recognized only in middle life. Presumably, the nervous system has compensated in some fashion, and the clinical expression of neurologic dysfunction has been so gradual that it has escaped notice for many years. The likely etiology of seizures is also related to age. Congenital anomalies, infections, and trauma account for most seizures in childhood and young adulthood. Tumors become more prominent in causation in middle and older years, closely followed in chronologic sequence by vascular diseases. Metabolic and toxic causes are distributed throughout all ages. Multiple sclerosis has its onset maximally in the third and fourth decades, although epidemiologic studies suggest that exposure to the causative agent takes place in childhood.

A few neurologic conditions are sex specific, such as the X-linked forms of muscular dystrophy. Men are more subject to trauma and have an earlier onset of atherothrombotic cerebrovascular disease than women. Younger women are more prone to development of autoimmune diseases such as myasthenia gravis, systemic lupus erythematosus, and multiple sclerosis and are at risk for the neurologic consequences of pregnancy.

The socioeconomic status of patients may reflect particular vulnerability to the neurologic complications of malnutrition and alcoholism, drug abuse, and sexually transmitted diseases.

Background medical problems are most important in the assessment of patients presenting with neurologic complaints, and no neurologic investigation is complete without a thorough review of a patient's past and current health status and a complete physical examination.

Kelley's Textbook of Internal Medicine, fourth edition. Edited by H. David Humes. Lippincott Williams & Wilkins, Philadelphia © 2000.

C H A P T E R

421

APPROACH TO THE PATIENT WITH HEADACHE

JAMES W. LANCE

Headache is one of the most common symptoms encountered in medical practice, and its differential diagnosis depends mainly on the clinical history. Special investigations are required only if the pattern of headache suggests an underlying organic disorder. The successful management of headache depends on the physician's motivation and knowledge. The process may be exasperating at times, but the outcome is often rewarding.

▪ PRESENTATION

The temporal pattern of headache gives some indication of its cause and whether further investigation is advisable.

ACUTE

The sudden onset of headache, instantaneously or developing over minutes or hours, raises the possibility of some life-threatening condition such as subarachnoid hemorrhage or meningitis that requires prompt investigation and treatment. Acute headache may be accompanied by neck rigidity when there is meningeal irritation and by elevated temperature when there is systemic infection or meningitis.

PROGRESSIVE SUBACUTE

Headache increasing in severity over a period of days, weeks, or months also arouses suspicion of serious organic disturbance. When the headache is aggravated by jarring, coughing, sneezing, or bending forward, it suggests an intracranial origin with dilatation or displacement of intracranial vessels, or obstruction of the ventricular system. If such a headache is associated with drowsiness, mental changes, epileptic seizures, or any form of neurologic deficit, the probability of a progressive intracranial lesion becomes greater. In older patients, temporal arteritis must always be considered.

RECURRENT EPISODIC

Possible causes include the following:

- Migraine, occurring from less than once per year to two or more times each week
- Cluster headache, occurring in bouts lasting from weeks to months in 80% of cases
- Ice cream headache
- Ice pick pains (sudden stabs of pain in the head, more common in migrainous and tension headache patients)
- Paroxysmal hypertension (e.g., pheochromocytoma)
- Transient ischemic attacks (headache is usually a minor component compared with neurologic deficit)
- Tolosa–Hunt syndrome
- Recurrent sinusitis
- Postalcoholic hangover
- Benign recurrent syndromes (benign only if an intracranial lesion has been excluded): headaches associated with coughing, exertion, or orgasm.

CHRONIC CONTINUOUS

Possible causes include the following:

- Tension headache
- Posttraumatic headache
- Postherpetic neuralgia
- Atypical facial pain
- Psychogenic headache

▪ HEADACHE SYNDROMES OF UNCERTAIN ORIGIN

Most headaches encountered in practice are of uncertain origin. A clinical diagnosis can usually be made from the history, but the precise mechanism remains elusive.

MIGRAINE

Migraine is an episodic cerebral disturbance (aura), headache, or both, with intervening periods of relative freedom from headache and no evidence of primary structural abnormality. The headache, usually severe, unilateral, and associated with nausea, vomiting, and photophobia, may recur without any aura (common migraine). About one third of patients experience some attacks in which an aura (blurring, scintillations, or zigzag hallucinations of vision), paresthesias, or speech disturbance precedes the characteristic headache by 5 to 60 minutes (classic migraine). When some neurologic symptoms persist for 24 hours or more after the cessation of headache, ischemia (migrainous infarction) has probably damaged the cortex. Recurrence of the aura phase without ensuing headache (migraine equivalents) can be encountered at any age, even in the elderly, and may be distinguished from transient ischemic attacks by typically gradual onset and resolution. Variations on the migrainous theme have been designated as follows: vertebrobasilar migraine (brain stem and cerebellar symptoms and signs, blurred vision, and impaired consciousness, attributed to ischemia of the hindbrain); retinal migraine (visual disturbance limited to one eye); ophthalmoplegic migraine (paresis of extraocular muscles at the height of headache); facial migraine (episodic pain involving the face more than the head); and hemiplegic migraine (unilateral paresis, not solely paresthesias that are a common feature of classic migraine). Periodic syndromes of childhood, such as recurrent abdominal pain or vomiting, are more common in children who subsequently develop migraine.

Migraine is a common disorder. A U.S. survey showed marked differences in the prevalence of migraine in patients from various ethnic backgrounds. The prevalence in those of Caucasian, African and Asian origin was, respectively, 20.4%, 16.2%, and 9.2% for women and 8.6%, 7.2%, and 4.2% for men. Prevalence is roughly equal between the sexes until puberty, after which it more than doubles in females.

There is a strong hereditary factor in migraine. Twin studies have shown that about half the susceptibility to migraine is of genetic origin with environmental influences determining the other half. Russell and Olesen found that the first degree relatives of patients subject to migraine with aura had nearly four times the risk of this disorder. Relatives of patients without aura had 1.9 times the risk of migraine without aura and 1.4 times the risk of migraine with aura.

The gene responsible for familial hemiplegic migraine, an autosomal dominant, has been localized to chromosome 19 in 55% and chromosome 1 in 15% of families, with the remainder being undetermined at present.

Many patients are subject to attacks at regular intervals of days, weeks, or months as though regulated by some internal clock, whereas others can identify specific trigger factors such as excessive afferent stimuli (flickering light, loud noise, strong perfumes), a sharp blow to the head (footballer's migraine), stress or relaxation after stress, certain foods, the ingestion of alcohol or other vasodilator agents, physical exertion, or menstrual periods (menstrual migraine). About one fourth of all patients recognize certain symptoms, such as a feeling of elation, hunger, or a craving for sweet foods, that anticipate headache by up to 24 hours and may help to plan preemptive treatment.

CLUSTER HEADACHE (MIGRAINOUS NEURALGIA)

Cluster headache has a prevalence of about 3% that of migraine and derives its name from its tendency to recur in bouts or clusters lasting weeks or months, separated by months or years of freedom. It is uncommon to find a family history of cluster headache but cases have been reported in twins, and segregation analysis suggests that cluster headache is transmitted by an autosomal dominant gene with a penetrance of 0.30–0.34 in males and 0.17–0.21 in females. During a bout, patients (85% of whom are male) suffer each day or night from one or more attacks of severe pain in and around the eye or adjacent areas of the head or face, lasting for 10 minutes to hours at a time. The eye on the affected side usually becomes red and waters; the ipsilateral nostril blocks or runs. An ocular Horner's syndrome can be observed during attacks in about one third of cases and may become permanent after repeated episodes.

This typical pattern is known as episodic cluster headache. Some 20% of patients have attacks regularly without remission, called chronic cluster headache. A rare variant, affecting women more than men, is characterized by many brief cluster attacks in one day that are controlled promptly by indomethacin. This entity has been named episodic or chronic paroxysmal hemicrania.

A rare variation of cluster headache is the SUNCT syndrome (Shortlasting Unilateral Neuralgiform headaches attacks with Conjunctival injection and Tearing) with pains lasting less than a minute and recurring 5–30 times each hour.

TENSION HEADACHE

The term *tension headache* is applied to the sensation of tightness around or pressure on top of the head that may recur daily in its chronic form. It affects women more commonly than men and may start at any age.

▋ PATHOPHYSIOLOGY

Peripheral receptors responsible for the registration of pain are present in the proximal parts of the cerebral and dural arteries, the large veins and venous sinuses, and the extracranial arteries. Distention or displacement of these vessels by inflammation, aneurysms, hematomas, tumors, or ventricular dilatation from obstruction of the cerebrospinal fluid (CSF) pathways gives rise to headache. Pain from the internal carotid and middle cerebral arteries is felt behind or around the ipsilateral eye. Pain may also result from irritation of the meninges, cranial nerves, or occipital nerves. Pain originating in the anterior or middle fossa is referred to the distribution of the first division of the trigeminal nerve, in front of a line drawn vertically above the ear. Pain from the posterior fossa is felt behind that line.

Referral of pain from occipital to frontal region and vice versa is common because fibers from the second and third cervical roots, serving pain from the posterior fossa, occiput, ear lobe, and upper neck, converge on second-order neurons of the spinal

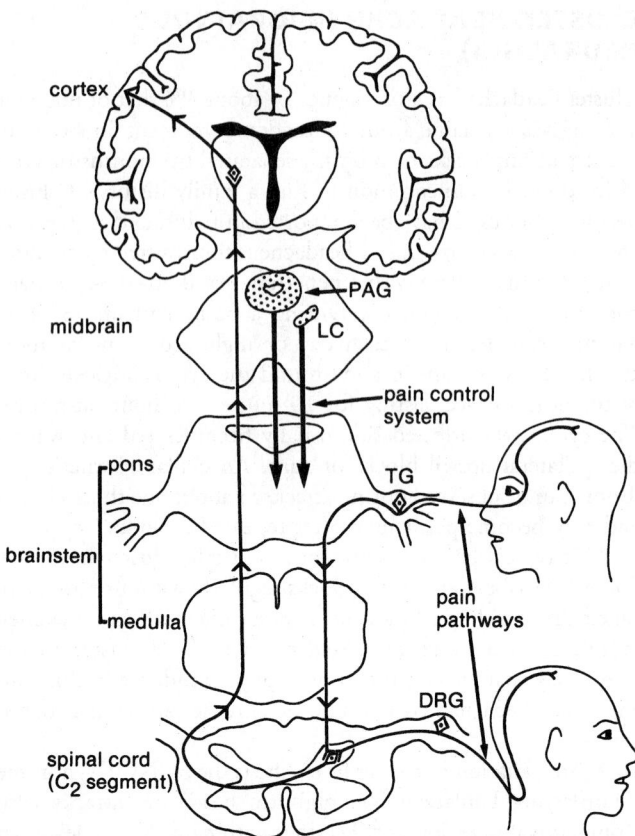

FIGURE 421.1. Pain pathways in the brain. Pain impulses from the front of the head are conveyed to the trigeminal ganglion (TG) and then to the brain stem, where they descend to the upper spinal cord. Here they synapse on the same cells as fibers coming from the back of the head via the dorsal root ganglion (DRG). After this convergence, the combined pathway crosses to the opposite side and travels up to the cerebral cortex. The pain-control system projects down to the brain stem and spinal cord from the periaqueductal gray matter (PAG) and locus ceruleus (LC) to regulate the transmission of pain impulses. (Lance JW. *Migraine and other headaches.* 2d ed. New York: Scribner, 1986: 17.)

trigeminal nucleus in the upper cervical spinal cord (Fig. 421.1). The activity of these neurons is modulated by the endogenous pain-control system, which arises in the periaqueductal gray matter (PAG) and locus ceruleus (see Figure 421.1) and influences transmission at the first-order synapse by inhibitory neurons, using enkephalins and GABA as neurotransmitters as well as projecting upwards to modulate thalamic function. Activity of the pain-control system is thought to play a part in "idiopathic" headaches such as migraine, cluster, and tension headaches.

MIGRAINE AND CLUSTER HEADACHE

PET scanning has shown that the contralateral midbrain surrounding the PAG becomes metabolically active during and after migraine headache, possibly as a "central generator" for migraine, disinhibiting the trigeminothalamic pathway.

Migraine and cluster headaches are accompanied by vascular dilatation that contributes to the headache, which is usually eased by vasoconstrictors such as sumatriptan, related triptans and ergotamine tartrate. Vasodilator substances may induce mi-

graine headache, but more often vasodilatation is secondary to changes in the central nervous system and is thought to be mediated by activation of the parasympathetic pathway via the greater superficial petrosal nerves and sphenopalatine ganglia. The level of the vasodilator agent calcitonin gene-related peptide (CGRP) increases in external jugular venous blood in migraine and cluster headaches with vasoactive intestinal polypeptide (VIP) also being released during cluster pains. Migraine and cluster headache thus appear to involve interaction between the brain and the cerebral, dural and extracranial arteries.

Serotonin (5-hydroxytryptamine, 5-HT) is discharged from blood platelets at the onset of migraine. Free 5-HT could play some part in sensitizing blood vessels to pain, but it is more likely that changes in the peripheral blood mirror changes in central neurotransmission that permit the sustained discharge of central trigeminal pathways to produce headache. The intravenous infusion of 5-HT relieves migraine headache, primarily by inducing vasoconstriction. Serotonin analogs, the triptans, are agonists at the $5-HT_{1B}$ receptor on vessels and the $5-HT_{1D}$ receptor on neurons as well as 1_A and 1_F receptors. Knowledge of the role of these and $5-HT_2$ receptors in the central nervous system and the part that they may play in migraine is incomplete but $5-HT_2$ antagonists such as cyproheptadine and methysergide are useful as prophylactic agents.

In the aura phase of classic migraine, regional cerebral blood flow diminishes, a process that starts in the occipital lobe and spreads anteriorly at 2 to 3 mm/min. This is the same speed as the phenomenon described by Leão as spreading cortical depression in experimental animals as the result of dehydration or other insult to the brain, and could account for the slow march of migrainous symptoms such as fortification spectra and paresthesias that some patients experience.

A similar phenomenon has been found by PET scanning in a patient whose migraine headache was accompanied by blurring of vision but not a classical aura, suggesting that cortical hypoperfusion may underly the impairment of vision and concentration common in migraine attacks. The reason why migraine auras are often followed by headache is unclear since each may occur independently.

Hyperacuity of the special senses (smell, vision and hearing) and hyperesthesia often accompany migraine headache, possibly caused by diminished inhibition of thalamic processing simultaneously with the reduction in efficacy of the endogenous pain control pathway. Nausea and vomiting are probably mediated by dopaminergic receptors in the area postrema.

The nature of the internal clock that begins and ends each bout of cluster headache, and that determines the frequency and timing of episodes in each 24-hour period, remains unknown. The presumption that the hypothalamus is implicated has been strengthened by the demonstration on PET scanning of increased metabolic activity in the ipsilateral hypothalamus during cluster headache but not during migraine. The pain of cluster headache is thought to be caused by a sterile inflammatory response in the wall of the carotid siphon, induced by discharge of vasodilator peptides from fibers of the greater superficial petrosal nerve that end on ganglion cells adjacent to the internal carotid artery. The ocular Horner's syndrome, a common feature of cluster headache, is attributed to edema of the arterial wall that compromises sympathetic fibers in the pericarotid plexus. The autonomic accompaniments (ipsilateral conjunctival injection, lacrimation, and nasal congestion) are abolished by ablation of the greater superficial petrosal nerve or sphenopalatine ganglion.

Tension-type Headache

Some forms of tension headache are associated with overcontraction of frontal and temporal muscles, particularly as a reaction to stress, but some patients may clench their jaws or grind their teeth even during sleep. Certain physical abnormalities, such as temporomandibular joint strain (Costen's syndrome), cervical spondylosis, or eyestrain from ocular muscle imbalance or refractive errors, may aggravate tension headache and warrant specific treatment. Some forms of tension headache are clearly related

to stressful situations, and others are associated with anxiety or depression, but some patients suffer from chronic daily headache following viral infections or without apparent physical or psychological cause. This may represent malfunction of the endogenous pain-control pathway.

▆ HISTORY AND PHYSICAL EXAMINATION

The diagnosis of most headache problems depends on taking a careful history. A suggested sequence is displayed in Table 421.1.

The case history may alert the clinician to look for signs of meningeal irritation, raised intracranial pressure, or other signs

TABLE 421.1.	HEADACHE: TAKING THE CASE HISTORY
Attribute	**Question**
Total duration of headache history	When did the first headache occur? Years, months, days, or hours ago?
Frequency of recurrence	How many attacks have there been in each year or month. Do the headaches recur daily?
Duration of each headache	How long does each headache last? Minutes, hours, or days?
Site	Is the headache unilateral or bilateral, localized or diffuse? Does it radiate to other areas?
Quality	Is the headache constant, or does it throb with each pulse?
	Is the sensation heaviness, tightness, or pressure?
	Is the headache severe (confining the patient in bed), moderate (interfering with work or other daily activities), or mild?
Onset	Does the headache cause awakening from sleep or recur at any particular time of the day?
	Are there premonitory symptoms of elation, hunger, or yawning for hours before the headache?
	Are there any prodromal symptoms (aura) immediately before the headache? If so, describe them. How long do they last?
Associated features	Is the headache accompanied by any of the following?
	Nausea, vomiting, or diarrhea
	Photophobia or hypersensitivity to sounds or smells
	Constriction or dilatation of the ipsilateral pupil
	Neurologic symptoms other than those experienced in the aura
	Vascular features such as redness of one eye, blockage of one nostril, changes in skin color, or prominence of scalp vessels
Precipitating factors	Is the headache triggered by any of the following?
	Stress
	Relaxation after stress
	Ingesting alcohol or vasodilator drugs
	Specific foods
	Menstrual periods
	Cough, sneezing, or straining
	Other factors
Relieving factors	Is the headache eased by any of the following?
	Pressure over affected areas
	Heat or cold
	Ingesting alcohol
	Previous therapy
Previous therapy	Have any of the following treatments been given?
	Pharmamceutical to abort or treat each attack (e.g., analgesics, preparations containing ergotamine)
	Interval (prophylactic) therapy (e.g., amitriptyline; β-blocking drugs; serotonin antagonists such as pizotyline, cyproheptadine, methysergide; nonsteroidal anti inflammatory agents)
	Other treatments (e.g., relaxation therapy, acupuncture, neck mobilization, hypnosis)
Patient history	Are there any illnesses, operations, or head injuries of relevance?
Family history	Is there a familial incidence of the same or other varieties of headache?
Social history	Is there a source of tension at home or work that could be important in causing headaches?
	Is the patient naturally tense—a worrier, frowner, or jaw clencher?
	Does the patient become depressed?
	What is the usual custom of cigarette smoking and intake of alcohol and other drugs?

of organic disease. In such patients, a careful examination of the nervous and other systems is mandatory, looking for localizing neurologic signs and indications of systemic illness. Even when the history is typical of migraine, cluster, or tension headache, a general examination should always be undertaken. It is often completely normal, which is reassuring for patient and clinician.

LABORATORY STUDIES AND DIAGNOSTIC TESTS

Only a few headache patients require investigation other than a careful history and physical examination. Consideration of the differential diagnosis determines which, if any, of these investigations is necessary.

A blood cell count and erythrocyte sedimentation rate is advisable when systemic infection is suggested or when headache is of recent onset in a patient over age 50 years. The erythrocyte sedimentation rate is usually above 40 mm/h in temporal arteritis.

The sudden onset of headache or a progressive course warrants investigation. If a patient with acute headache is febrile and meningitis is suspected, immediate lumbar puncture may be justified, provided there are no signs of raised intracranial pressure. Except for such an emergency, computed tomography (CT) scanning of the brain is usually the first step because it demonstrates blood in the CSF in most cases of subarachnoid hemorrhage and displays or excludes space-occupying lesions, hydrocephalus, and other structural causes of headache. Lumbar puncture is required only rarely; for example, in the investigation of headache for the diagnosis of meningitis or other infections, for confirmation of subarachnoid hemorrhage if the story is typical but the CT scan is negative, or for the measurement of CSF pressure in benign intracranial hypertension. A chest x-ray is always advisable to exclude a carcinoma of the lung or other relevant lesion. Cerebral angiography is reserved for patients with cerebral aneurysm or other cerebrovascular problems. Magnetic resonance imaging (MRI) may help determine the site of obstruction of CSF pathways in patients with hydrocephalus. MR angiography is a noninvasive alternative to contrast-medium angiography in the search for a cerebral aneurysm.

HEADACHE SYNDROMES WITH IDENTIFIABLE CAUSE

PAIN ARISING FROM EXTRACRANIAL STRUCTURES

Temporal Arteritis

See Chapter 182 for a full discussion of vasculitis.

Temporal arteritis occurs in women more than men in the ratio of 3 : 1. It mostly affects persons over age 50. It is probably an immune disorder of the arterial wall, which becomes thickened with cellular infiltration of the media, giant cell formation, deposition of immune complexes, and thrombus formation in the lumen. The scalp arteries are most commonly involved to cause headache and tenderness, but the condition may be more diffuse, with generalized muscle and joint pains (polymyalgia rheumatica). The condition may spread to the ophthalmic arteries, producing sudden blindness, or less commonly to branches of the aorta. Temporal arteritis should be suspected when a constant headache develops in an older patient; the diagnosis is supported by the finding of an erythrocyte sedimentation rate above 40 mm/h. Temporal artery biopsy is advisable to confirm the diagnosis because corticosteroid therapy is specific for the condition and may have to be continued for years. If the index of suspicion is high, corticosteroids should be started immediately while awaiting biopsy results to minimize the risk of blindness, which has been reported in 20% to 50% of cases in different series; this rate is halved by corticosteroid therapy.

OCULAR CAUSES

Acute angle-closure glaucoma may cause severe orbital pain with circumcorneal injection, but it is rare for other ocular conditions to cause headache, although refractive errors and imbalance of the eye muscles may contribute to the muscle-contraction variety of tension headache. Optic (retrobulbar) neuritis is usually associated with a dull ache in the orbit accentuated by eye movement.

SINUSITIS

Frontal and maxillary sinusitis are responsible for pain and tenderness over the appropriate areas, but both sphenoid and ethmoid sinusitis cause midfrontal headache, sometimes in the absence of nasal congestion. Radiography of the sinuses is recommended in any patient with midfrontal pain of recent onset. Recurrent frontal headache of migrainous origin is often misdiagnosed as sinusitis (see Chapters 311 and 368).

DENTAL CAUSES

Apical root infection can cause a constant or jabbing pain in the upper or lower gums. Pain can be referred to the head if the bite is unbalanced so that undue strain is placed on one temporomandibular joint (Costen's syndrome). In this case, pain may radiate from the joint to the temple, face, or neck. A tendency to clench the jaw (bruxism) aggravates the condition, which should be treated as for tension headache as well as by dental management to restore a normal bite.

CERVICAL CAUSES

Any disorder of the upper cervical spine may cause occipital headache in the distribution of the second and third cervical roots and can refer pain to the frontal region and eye by convergence on second-order trigeminal pain neurons. Constant or jabbing pain in one occipital region may be associated with numbness in this area and tenderness over the greater occipital nerve (occipital neuralgia). Provided serious structural changes in the cervical spine, such as fracture, neoplasm, or rheumatoid arthritis, can be excluded, the condition may be managed by the injection of a local anesthetic agent and long-acting corticosteroid preparation around the greater occipital nerve, followed by traction and gentle mobilization of the cervical spine. A light surgical collar may be helpful in some cases. Some patients, usually adolescents, with a tendency to subluxation of the atlantoaxial joints may experience numbness of the tongue on the same side as occipital pain and numbness on sudden head turning (neck-tongue syndrome). The reason is that proprioceptive fibers from the tongue travel with the hypoglossal nerve and transfer to the second cervical root, which is stretched during unilateral subluxation.

PAIN ARISING FROM THE CRANIAL NERVES

Headaches may be caused by excessive stimulation of peripheral branches of the first division of the trigeminal nerve, by exposure to cold, by swallowing cold food or drinks (ice cream headache), or by the pressure of a tight hat or band around the head (swim-goggle headache).

A granuloma in the region of the superior orbital fissure may produce ocular pain and palsies of the third, fourth, or sixth cranial nerves that are responsive to corticosteroids (Tolosa–Hunt syndrome). Any lesion compromising both the trigeminal ganglion and the sympathetic plexus surrounding the internal carotid artery produces pain in one eye and forehead associated with an ipsilateral ocular Horner's syndrome (Raeder's paratrigeminal neuralgia). Involvement of the apex of the petrous temporal bone by inflammation or neoplasm may cause pain in half of the forehead, with an ipsilateral sixth cranial nerve palsy (Gradenigo's syndrome).

Herpes zoster may cause a painful eruption in the distribution of the trigeminal nerve, commonly the first division, and may leave a distressing pain (postherpetic neuralgia) in its wake. Treatment by acyclovir or corticosteroids in the acute phase minimizes the pain. Once established, postherpetic neuralgia can be eased by the administration of amitriptyline as for tension headaches.

TRIGEMINAL AND GLOSSOPHARYNGEAL NEURALGIA

See Chapter 424.

PAIN OF INTRACRANIAL ORIGIN

Headache is a symptom of many intracranial and systemic disorders and may be caused by meningeal irritation or by displacement or dilatation of pain-sensitive blood vessels. Investigation determines whether the patient requires neurosurgical or medical management.

BENIGN INTRACRANIAL HYPERTENSION

Symptoms and signs of raised intracranial pressure (headache, vomiting, transient obscuration of vision, and papilledema) sometimes occur with no obvious systemic or local cause. CT scanning of the brain demonstrates normal or small ventricles and obliteration of the cerebral sulci, and subsequent lumbar puncture confirms the clinical impression of elevated intracranial pressure. This condition is called benign intracranial hypertension (pseudotumor cerebri)—although it is not always benign, as optic atrophy may follow chronic papilledema. It commonly develops in overweight young women with menstrual irregularities for some obscure hormonal reason, but may also be caused by tetracycline and vitamin A (used in the treatment of acne), other drugs such as nalidixic acid, and the withdrawal of corticosteroid therapy.

The probable sequence of events is that a partial thrombosis of the superior sagittal sinus or malfunction of the arachnoid villi leads to reduced CSF absorption, thus increasing intracranial pressure, obstructing venous outflow from the brain, and producing chronic cerebral edema. Management involves repeated lumbar punctures to reduce CSF pressure, diuretics (particularly acetazolamide, which helps reduce CSF formation), and sometimes the administration of corticosteroids. Decompression of the optic nerves or shunting procedures to reduce CSF pressure may be necessary in cases not responding to conservative therapy.

STRATEGIES FOR OPTIMAL CARE MANAGEMENT

The treatment of headache produced by an identifiable organic cause is management of the underlying condition as indicated above, with the use of analgesics or other measures to control pain. Handling migraine, cluster, and tension headaches presents difficulties in the absence of a clearly defined pathophysiology. Despite this, most patients can be helped and many headaches can be relieved completely by using the following measures.

MIGRAINE

The management of migraine relies on psychological counseling, avoidance of trigger factors, relaxation therapy, and pharmacologic agents to treat each attack as it comes (acute therapy) or given daily to reduce the frequency and severity of attacks (interval therapy), as outlined in Figure 421.2.

Mild attacks of migraine may respond to metoclopramide (10 mg intramuscularly (IM) or intravenously (IV), or even orally if given early enough) to promote gastric absorption, followed by effervescent aspirin (600 to 900 mg orally).

The treatment of migraine headache has been transformed by the advent of the triptans, 5-HT$_{1B/D}$ agonists, of which sumatriptan (Imitrex) was the first. Sumatriptan relieves 50–60% of migraine headaches within 2 hours if given as 50–100mg orally or 20mg intranasally and about 75% in one hour by subcutaneous injection of 6mg. Zolmitriptan (Zomig) 2.5–5.0mg has much the same efficacy as sumatriptan and may be effective in some patients who have not responded to sumatriptan. Rizatriptan (Maxalt) 10mg is marginally more effective than both whereas naratriptan (Naramig) 2.5mg is less so although it has a longer action and fewer side-effects. Other triptans such as electriptan are undergoing clinical trials. Because of their vasoconstriction action, they should not be prescribed for patients with suspected coronary disease, Printzmetal's angina, or uncontrolled hypertension; for the same reason they should not be administered for 24 hours after ergotamine tartrate.

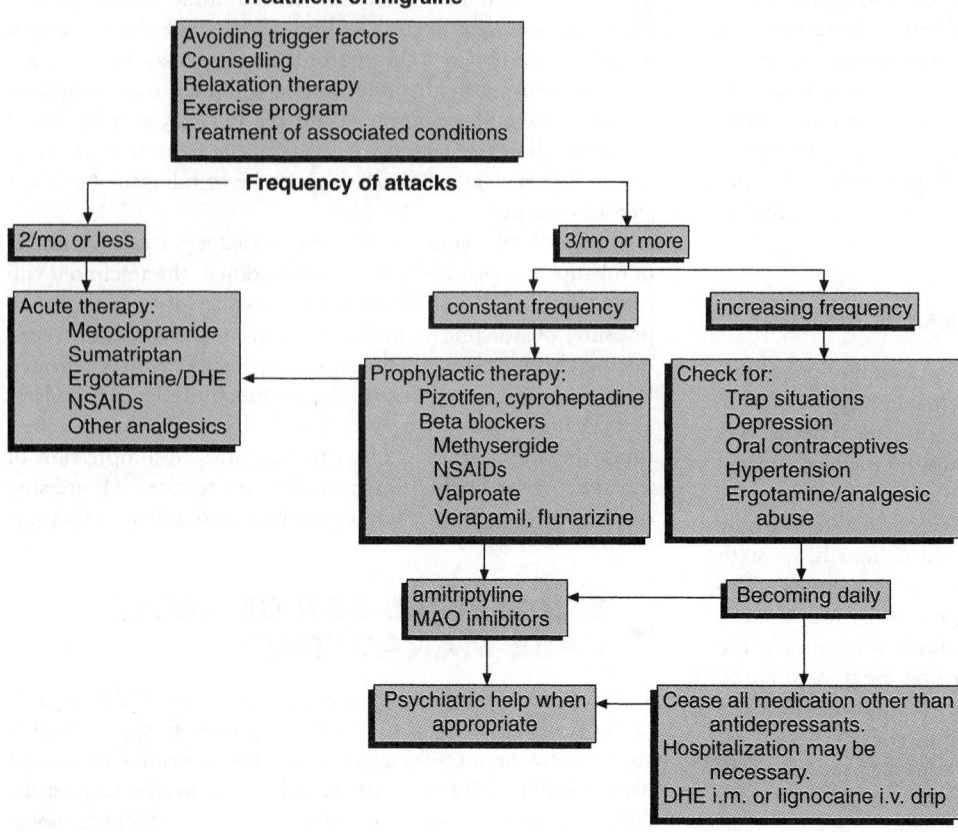

FIGURE 421.2. A logical sequence of therapy in the management of migraine headaches. DHE, dihydroergotamine; NSAIDs, nonsteroidal antiinflammatory drugs; MAO, monoamine oxidase. (Updated from a diagram first published in Current Therapeutics, April 1980. Reproduced by permission of Adis International 1994.)
EVIDENCE LEVEL: B. Reference: Lance JW, Goadsby PJ. *Mechanisms and management of headache,* **sixth edition. Butterworth-Heineman, 1998.**

Ergotamine tartrate (1 to 2 mg) may be given orally at the onset of symptoms, alone or in combination with caffeine (Cafergot) or with antiemetic agents. Ergotamine is more effective if the gastric route of absorption is bypassed by rectal administration (Cafergot suppository) or inhalation. The related drug dihydroergotamine may be given as 1 mg IM or 0.5 mg IV or by inhalation of the powder from a pressure pack at the onset of headache. Patients who do not respond to ergotamine preparations, or become nauseated by them, may find relief from one of the triptans or nonsteroidal antiinflammatory drugs (NSAIDs) such as naproxen (550 mg, repeated in 30 minutes if necessary). Narcotics should be avoided except in the most severe cases because of the risk of habituation.

Patients who are subject to two or more migraine headaches each month that are incompletely relieved by acute therapy may be placed on regular interval therapy (see Fig. 421.2). Provided there is no contraindication, such as asthma, propranolol may be prescribed, increasing from 20 mg twice daily to full β-blocking doses if necessary and if there are no side effects. Nadolol, timolol, atenolol, and metoprolol are also effective in prophylaxis, but not the β-blockers that have partial agonist action (intrinsic sympathomimetic activity). Antiserotonin agents (5-HT$_2$ antagonists) such as pizotifen (pizotyline; Sandomigran) or cyproheptadine, are also useful in prophylaxis and are best given as a single dose at night to avoid daytime drowsiness. The same applies to the administration of amitriptyline (Elavil), which is particularly useful in the prevention of frequent, almost daily, migraine attacks as well as for tension headache. The dos-

age of amitriptyline should be increased slowly from 10 to 75 mg at night, depending on the patient's tolerance, because blood levels vary 10-fold in subjects given the same dose per kilogram of body weight.

If headaches continue despite a conscientious trial of these medications, methysergide (Sansert), 1 to 2 mg, may be given three times daily, starting with a test dose of one half to one tablet to ensure that there are no vasoconstrictive or other side effects. Methysergide therapy should be interrupted for 1 month every 4 to 6 months to minimize the possibility of the rare complication of retroperitoneal fibrosis. Physical examination and blood urea estimation is advisable at 3-month intervals. NSAIDs, the anticonvulsant valproate, and the calcium channel blockers verapamil and flunarizine have also proven useful for the prevention of migraine.

Patients whose headaches prove refractory to all these medications may get relief from the monoamine oxidase inhibitor phenelzine (15 mg two or three times daily), with the usual restriction of the intake of red wine, certain foods, and drugs containing sympathomimetic agents.

Nifedipine is useful in the treatment of migraine equivalents: a few drops from a 10-mg capsule are usually sufficient to abort or shorten the episode.

CLUSTER HEADACHE

As in migraine, there is no cure, but most episodes can be suppressed with ergotamine preparations, timed to anticipate the cluster pains (e.g., ergotamine 2 mg at night to prevent attacks recurring regularly during sleep) or with methysergide (2 mg three times daily). Verapamil 80mg four times daily will often control a bout. The inhalation of 100% oxygen at 7 L/min delivered through a humidifier and a resuscitation mask (without side vents) relieves cluster pains within 10 minutes in two thirds of patients. The subcutaneous injection of sumatriptan (6 mg) stops cluster headache rapidly in about 75% of patients.

Prednisolone (40 to 50 mg/d) interrupts the cluster pattern in most cases. The dose may then be lowered progressively to the minimum necessary to control attacks for the rest of the bout, after which it is slowly tapered off. The slight risk of delayed aseptic hip necrosis after courses of corticosteroid therapy must be weighed against the relief obtained by the suppression of the bout in about 75% of cases.

Chronic cluster headache that does not respond to these measures may be suppressed by lithium carbonate in a dose sufficient to maintain a blood level of 0.7 to 1 mEq/L.

TENSION HEADACHE

The management of tension headache requires psychological counseling, readjustment of physical or emotional stress situations, and muscle relaxation therapy, with or without biofeedback. Amitriptyline or other tricyclics given as a single dose at night as described for frequent migraine headache, is useful in patients who can tolerate an adequate dosage without side effects. Monoamine oxidase inhibitors can be used in patients refractory to other treatment.

COMPLICATIONS AND PITFALLS

Misinterpretation of the acute or progressive subacute onset of headache may have serious consequences. The abrupt onset of pain ("thunderclap headache") may be migrainous in origin, but it is important to exclude subarachnoid hemorrhage, "sentinel headache" (enlargement of a cerebral aneurysm without rupture), meningitis, acute obstruction of the CSF pathways, or a precipitous rise in blood pressure as causes. Intravenous antibiotics should be given immediately if meningitis is suspected because pyogenic meningitis can kill within 24 hours. A CT brain scan detects most cases of subarachnoid hemorrhage; reassurance that there is no shift of midline structures or other contraindications to lumbar puncture enables the CSF to be obtained safely. If the CT scan and CSF are both normal but the suspicion of a sentinel headache remains, MR angiography is a noninvasive way of checking the cerebral circulation.

Temporal arteritis may be overlooked as a cause of headache in the older patient. The erythrocyte sedimentation rate is not always elevated, and a temporal artery biopsy may be warranted if there is localized scalp tenderness. Early diagnosis and the institution of corticosteroid therapy minimizes the possibility of blindness.

There is a tendency to consider headaches or recurrent vomiting attacks in children as psychosomatic because they may develop during excitement or stress. Attention to the symptoms will make it clear that most of these episodes are migrainous and deserve to be treated as such. In adults, migraine headache beginning in the upper neck or occipital region is often misdiagnosed as "cervicogenic," whereas migraine or cluster headache affecting the frontal region or cheek is considered to be caused by sinusitis. Careful consideration of the case history usually leads to the correct diagnosis and appropriate therapy.

Patients found to have a structural abnormality requiring surgical treatment or suspected of having meningitis need hospitalization. Most headaches do not have a sinister cause and can be treated in the office or outpatient department. Patients who suffer chronic daily headaches as the result of excessive consumption of analgesics or ergotamine tartrate may require admission during withdrawal of medication.

Various regimens have been recommended for patients who present to the emergency department with severe continuing migraine headache. These include metoclopramide (10 mg IM or IV), dihydroergotamine (1 mg IM or 0.5 mg IV), the NSAID ketorolac (10 to 30 mg IM; not to be given if renal function is impaired), and chlorpromazine (12.5 mg IV, repeated every 2 hours to a total of 37.5 mg). The use of narcotics is to be avoided whenever possible. Lignocaine (1 mg/kg IV followed by an IV lignocaine drip at 2 mg/min) may be given if the patient is under surveillance in the hospital.

Subarachnoid hemorrhage and meningitis are neurologic emergencies requiring immediate referral for specialist treatment. It is advisable to refer any patient with headaches that are unexplained or not responding to treatment to a neurologist or a physician with a particular interest in headache management.

COST EFFECTIVENESS

The estimates of workdays lost per person each year due to headaches vary from 0.5 to 6.7 in different countries. Effectiveness was reduced for another 10 days each year in the United States. The cost of lost productivity in the United States due to headaches is an estimated $1.4 billion annually. The cost effectiveness of treatment must be assessed by each individual, depending on the rapidity and completeness of response to medication, the cost of medication, and the benefit obtained in working capacity and in enjoyment of life.

BIBLIOGRAPHY

Goadsby PJ, Silverstein SD, eds. *Headache.* Boston: Butterworth-Heinemann, 1997.
Headache Classification Committee of the International Headache Society. Classification and diagnostic criteria for headache disorders, cranial neuralgias and facial pain. *Cephalalgia* 1998;8 (Suppl 7):1–96.
Lance JW, Goadsby PJ. *Mechanism and Management of Headache* 6th ed. Oxford: Butterworth-Heinemann, 1998.
Lipton RB, Stewart WF, eds. The impact of migraine. *Neurology* 1994; 6(Suppl 4).
May A, Bahra A, Buchel C, et al. Hypothalamic activation in cluster headache attacks. *Lancet* 1998;352:275–278.
Russell MB, Andersson PG, Thomsen LL, et al. Cluster headache is an autosomal dominantly inherited disorder in some families: a complex segregation analysis. *J Med Genet* 1995;32:954–956.
Russell MB, Olesen J. Increased familial risk and evidence of genetic factor in migraine. *BMJ* 1995;311:541–544.
Stewart WF, Lipton RB, Liberman J. Variation in migraine prevalence by race. *Neurology* 1996;47:52–59.

Weiller C, May A, Limmroth V, et al. Brainstem activation in spontaneous human migraine attacks. *Nat Med* 1995;1:658–660.

Kelley's Textbook of Internal Medicine, fourth edition. Edited by H. David Humes.
Lippincott Williams & Wilkins, Philadelphia © 2000.

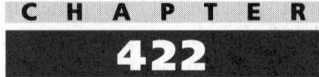

CHAPTER 422

APPROACH TO THE PATIENT WITH DIZZINESS AND VERTIGO

MARK F. WALKER
DAVID S. ZEE

CLINICAL SIGNS AND SYMPTOMS

The complaint of "dizziness" encompasses a variety of symptoms. A feeling of lightheadedness or impending fainting may suggest a cardiovascular cause. *Vertigo* is an illusion of motion of self or of the environment. Patients may describe sensations of spinning or tumbling; perceptions of tilt or linear motion may also occur. Vertigo results from an imbalance in the vestibular inputs from the two labyrinths or in their central connections. Patients with symmetric vestibular lesions (e.g., gentamicin ototoxicity) and those with a slowly developing vestibular imbalance (e.g., vestibular schwannoma), in which adaptation has time to take place, may not have vertigo. *Disequilibrium* is a feeling of imbalance while standing or walking, for example, in the case of bilateral vestibular loss or as the result of cerebellar disease. Patients with nystagmus may have *oscillopsia*, an illusion of back-and-forth movement of the environment produced by movement of visual images across the retina. Symptoms of anxiety, phobias, and panic attacks may be labeled as dizziness. Some patients with otherwise normal vestibular function describe an enhanced sensitivity to visual motion. This perception has been included in the syndrome of psychophysiologic dizziness, often triggered in patients who have or have had recurrent attacks of vertigo. Thus, the first, and sometimes challenging, step in the evaluation of dizziness is to determine which of these symptoms the patient has.

HISTORY AND PHYSICAL EXAMINATION

A careful history is important in the evaluation of vertigo and imbalance. The first questions are whether symptoms are acute or chronic and whether they occurred once or are recurrent. If vertigo is episodic, the duration of each episode is important.

Brief (less than 1 minute) episodes of vertigo, precipitated by a change in the attitude of the head with respect to gravity, are typical of benign paroxysmal positional vertigo (BPPV). Vertigo lasting for several minutes up to an hour suggests transient ischemic attacks (TIAs). Longer episodes may be caused by migraine, Ménière's disease, labyrinthitis, or infarcts. The presence of associated hearing loss and other auditory symptoms (tinnitus, fullness) indicates a peripheral vestibular origin, whereas symptoms of brain stem or cerebellar dysfunction implicate a central cause.

What is the effect of head movement? In general, symptoms provoked by head movements or changes in head position with respect to gravity are the hallmark of a disturbance in the vestibular system. Other factors provoking vertigo, such as loud noises and valsalva maneuvers (coughing, sneezing, straining) should be determined. If oscillopsia is present, does it occur at rest, such as from nystagmus, or only with head movement (e.g., while walking), such as with bilateral vestibular loss? Of course, it is important to be aware of any other medical conditions or medications that may play a contributing role.

A complete neurologic examination must be carried out, with particular attention to eye movements, hearing, other cranial nerves, coordination, gait, and balance. Vestibular function may be tested using rapid, but small-amplitude horizontal head thrusts; a catch-up saccade—a rapid eye movement to "catch up" with the head—indicates an insufficient vestibulo-ocular reflex. Visual acuity during head shaking (dynamic visual acuity) is diminished in patients with an abnormal vestibulo-ocular reflex. The eyes must be observed in the absence of visual fixation, which may suppress spontaneous nystagmus. This may be done either with Frenzel lenses or by looking for movement of the optic disc during direct ophthalmoscopy with the opposite eye occluded. Positioning maneuvers can identify BPPV. Hyperventilation may elicit nystagmus in some patients, such as those with vestibular schwannoma.

DIAGNOSTIC TESTS

Vestibular tests include electronystagmography with caloric or rotatory chair testing and posturography. Every patient with vestibular complaints should have an audiogram. A low-frequency hearing loss is characteristic of Ménière's disease. Unilateral hearing loss raises the possibility of a tumor involving the vestibulocochlear nerve, such as a vestibular schwannoma. Magnetic resonance imaging (always including contrast) of the posterior fossa should be ordered whenever a structural lesion is suspected or if there are symptoms or signs suggesting a brain stem or cerebellar lesion. Patients suspected of having TIAs should undergo magnetic resonance angiography of the head and neck and additional evaluation for stroke, as indicated.

DISORDERS

A summary of the more common and important vestibular disorders follows. For a more comprehensive discussion, the reader is referred to the references listed at the end of the chapter.

BENIGN PAROXYSMAL POSITIONAL VERTIGO

BPPV is the most common cause of recurrent vertigo. It results when calcium carbonate crystals (otoconia) are released from the otolithic membranes and aggregate in a semicircular canal, usually the posterior canal. Many patients can identify a preceding event, such as an episode of labyrinthitis or trauma or a prolonged period of having the head back, such as being at the hairdresser or dentist. Symptoms are produced when a change in position of the head, such as looking up or rolling over in bed, causes the debris to move, creating a shift of endolymph that excites the canal and produces vertigo. Symptoms are usually worse in the morning, perhaps owing to aggregation of debris while the head is relatively still during sleep.

BPPV is diagnosed with the Dix–Hallpike maneuver: with the head turned 45 degrees to one side, the patient is moved rapidly from a seated to a supine position with the head hanging down. This may cause debris to shift within the posterior canal such that a mixed vertical–torsional type of nystagmus is produced: the eyes beat up, and the upper poles of the eyes beat toward the affected (down) ear. There is typically a latency of several seconds to the onset of nystagmus, which then lasts for less than a minute. Fatiguing of nystagmus occurs with repeated maneuvers, presumably owing to dispersion of debris. BPPV occasionally involves the horizontal canals; anterior canal BPPV is rare. BPPV is treated with a particle-repositioning maneuver (e.g., Epley or Semont), which moves the debris out of the canal into the vestibule, where it can be reabsorbed. BPPV must be distinguished from central causes of positional nystagmus, such as craniocervical junction abnormalities, which usually produce a sustained, purely vertical (downbeat) nystagmus.

MIGRAINE

Vestibular migraine is a common cause of recurrent vertigo. Attacks usually last minutes to hours and may or may not be associated with headache. Sometimes there are other associated posterior circulation symptoms or signs (basilar migraine). Other vestibular symptoms of migraine include motion sensitivity and disequilibrium, which may last for hours to days or longer. Benign paroxysmal vertigo of childhood also is probably a form of migraine. Treatment of vestibular migraine consists of the usual migraine prophylactic agents. Antiemetics may be needed for acute treatment of attacks in severe cases.

MÉNIÈRE'S DISEASE

Ménière's disease is attributed to endolymphatic hydrops, which causes increased pressure in the inner ear. Attacks may be difficult to distinguish from vestibular migraine, but characteristic features in addition to vertigo include aural fullness, fluctuating hearing loss in the affected ear, and a low-pitched tinnitus. Occasionally, patients have a sudden loss of balance provoking a fall (otolithic crisis of Tumarkin). Evaluation should include screening for syphilis and autoimmune disorders. Transtympanic electrocochleography may assist in the diagnosis. Treatment is aimed at minimizing hydrops and includes a low sodium diet and diuretics, such as acetazolamide or hydrochlorothiazide. Vestibular

suppressant medications (see later discussion) may be helpful during an attack. Refractory cases may be treated with ablative procedures, such as transtympanic gentamicin or surgical labyrinthectomy. It is important to remember, however, that many patients will go on to experience symptoms in the other ear.

LABYRINTHITIS/VESTIBULAR NEURITIS

Vestibular neuritis often is attributed to a viral infection of the vestibular nerve or labyrinth. Severe vertigo, nausea, and vomiting appear suddenly and improve over several days. Central compensatory mechanisms prompt further improvement over several weeks to months. Important differential diagnoses are labyrinthine and cerebellar infarctions or hemorrhage; patients with risk factors for stroke should have a cerebrovascular evaluation. Cerebellar infarction or hemorrhage is of particular concern, because the resulting mass effect may lead to brain stem compression. Treatment with vestibular suppressants and antiemetics (see later discussion) may be necessary in the initial stages of labyrinthitis, when symptoms are most severe.

TRANSIENT ISCHEMIC ATTACKS

When recurrent vertigo is caused by ischemia, it usually occurs in the context of other posterior circulation symptoms. Rarely, episodes of vertigo may develop in isolation. Recognition of vertebrobasilar TIAs as the source of vertigo is important, because TIAs may herald an impending brain stem or cerebellar infarct. Vertigo caused by TIAs typically lasts minutes but now and then may last longer. Vertigo in older patients and anyone with risk factors should prompt an evaluation for a vascular cause; if vertigo is acute, a computed tomography scan should be undertaken to exclude a hemorrhage or swollen infarct in the cerebellum.

BILATERAL VESTIBULAR LOSS

Patients with bilateral vestibular loss typically have initial symptoms of gait imbalance and oscillopsia during head movement. The most commonly identified cause of bilateral loss is exposure to ototoxic agents, such as aminoglycoside antibiotics and certain chemotherapeutic agents (e.g., cisplatin). Vertigo is uncommon, because vestibular loss is symmetrical. In addition, susceptibilities of the labyrinth and cochlea may differ, such that patients may lose considerable vestibular function with little effect on hearing. Gentamicin ototoxicity has been reported in patients with serum levels and cumulative doses within the accepted ranges. Therefore, patients receiving potentially ototoxic medications should be monitored closely for signs of vestibular toxicity, such as inability to read with the head moving, abnormal head-thrust responses, or a positive Romberg sign. Other causes of bilateral vestibular loss include meningitis, vestibular involvement in hereditary forms of cerebellar degeneration, autoimmune disorders (sarcoid, Cogan's syndrome), hereditary and acquired (vitamin B$_{12}$ deficiency) neuropathies, tumors (bilateral vestibular schwannomas or metastatic disease), bilateral vestibular neuritis, and bilateral Ménière's disease.

TREATMENT

In general, treatment is directed toward the specific diagnosis. Vestibular suppressant and antiemetic medications (diazepam, lorazepam, promethazine, meclizine) may be useful in the initial phase of an acute vestibular syndrome (labyrinthitis) and in the treatment of recurrent attacks of vertigo that last at least several hours, such as in Ménière's disease. Brief episodes of vertigo (BPPV) are not amenable to symptomatic treatment with vestibular suppressants. Long-term prophylactic vestibular suppression may be appropriate when attacks are frequent, but prolonged use following an acute vestibular lesion may impede central adaptation processes and should be avoided.

Vestibular rehabilitation may be beneficial in both acute and chronic vestibular disorders. After an acute vestibular injury, a prompt resumption of normal activity may promote recovery by facilitating central compensation. Specific vestibular exercises may assist in this process. Vestibular therapy also may help patients who have lost vestibular function bilaterally to learn to substitute visual and somatosensory information to maintain balance. When psychiatric factors play a role in patients with complaints of dizziness, either primary (as part of an anxiety disorder or depression) or secondary (as in the case of patients with chronic neurologic diseases) psychiatric intervention, with counseling and medications, is important.

BIBLIOGRAPHY

Baloh RW. Neurotology of migraine. *Headache* 1997;37:615–621.

Baloh RW. *Dizziness, hearing loss, and tinnitus.* Philadelphia: FA Davis, 1998.

Epley JM. Positional vertigo related to semicircular canalithiasis. *Otolaryngol Head Neck Surg* 1995;112:154–161.

Herdman SJ, ed. *Vestibular rehabilitation*, second ed. Philadelphia: FA Davis, 1999.

Hotson JR, Baloh RW. Acute vestibular syndrome. *N Engl J Med* 1998; 339:680–685.

Leigh RJ, Zee DS. *The neurology of eye movements*, third ed. Oxford University Press, 1999.

Minor LB. Gentamicin-induced bilateral vestibular hypofunction. *JAMA* 1998;279:541–544.

Kelley's Textbook of Internal Medicine, fourth edition. Edited by H. David Humes. Lippincott Williams & Wilkins, Philadelphia © 2000.

C H A P T E R
423

APPROACH TO THE PATIENT WITH TUMORS OF THE CENTRAL NERVOUS SYSTEM

LISA M. DEANGELIS
J. GREGORY CAIRNCROSS

The diagnosis and treatment of intracranial and spinal tumors form a major part of neurologic and oncologic practice. Early diagnosis, facilitated by noninvasive imaging techniques, is essential, to minimize neurologic disability. Many central nervous system (CNS) tumors can be controlled or cured with modern treatment.

CLASSIFICATION

Tumors of the CNS are a heterogeneous group of intracranial and intraspinal neoplasms (Table 423.1). Intracranial tumors are divided into two groups, those that grow within the brain (intracerebral) and those that begin outside the brain (extracerebral). Similarly, intraspinal tumors are divided into two groups, those that arise within the cord (intramedullary) and those that originate outside the cord (extramedullary). Extramedullary spinal tumors are subdivided further on the basis of their intradural or extradural location. Primary CNS tumors are then classified by their presumed cell of origin (astrocyte—astrocytoma; arachnoidal cell—meningioma; Schwann cell—acoustic neuroma). Metastatic tumors can be found in either the intracranial or the spinal space and arise from a variety of systemic cancers, the most frequent being lung, breast, and melanoma.

EPIDEMIOLOGY

Most primary intracranial tumors are uncommon or rare illnesses. In North America, primary brain tumors occur in eight to ten people per 100,000 population per year. More than 60% of them are gliomas, and two-thirds of these are clinically aggressive and high-grade tumors. Primary brain tumors have a bimodal incidence distribution, with an early peak in childhood and a second peak after age 50 years. The locations and types of tumors also vary with age. Tumors of the posterior fossa predominate in children (medulloblastoma, ependymoma, cystic cerebellar astrocytoma, brain stem glioma), and those above the tentorium predominate in adults (glioblastoma multiforme, anaplastic glioma, astrocytoma, oligodendroglioma, meningioma, pituitary adenoma). Primary spinal neoplasms are rare at any age, arising in one to two people per 100,000 population per year. Most primary CNS tumors develop more frequently in men, but meningiomas are more common in women. Metastatic brain tumors are fourfold more common than all primary brain tumors combined, and metastatic epidural spinal tumors account for most spinal neoplasms.

ETIOLOGY

The cause of CNS tumors is unknown, though environmental and genetic factors contribute to their development. Cranial and spinal irradiation predispose to meningioma, fibrosarcoma, and glioma but account for less than 1% of these neoplasms. Long-term exposure to chemicals in the petroleum industry may predispose to glioma. Long-term parental exposure to toxic compounds may be a risk factor for CNS tumors in children. Severe head injury may be a risk factor for meningioma and glioma.

TABLE 423.1.	TUMORS OF THE CENTRAL NERVOUS SYSTEM

Intracranial	Extracerebral	Spinal
Intracerebral	Meningeal tumors	Intramedullary
Primitive neuroectodermal tumors	Meningioma	Gliomas
Medulloblastoma	Benign	Astrocytoma
Cerebral neuroblastoma	Papillary	Oligodendroglioma
Neurocytoma	Malignant	Ependymoma
Gliomas	Meningeal sarcoma	Mixed glioma
Glioblastoma multiforme	Fibrosarcoma	Hemangioblastoma
Anaplastic glioma	Hemangiopericytoma	Lymphoma
Astrocytoma	Acoustic neuroma	Metastatic tumor
Oligodendroglioma	Neurofibroma	Extramedullary
Ependymoma	Choroid plexus tumors	Intradural
Astrocytoma	Papilloma	Neurofibroma
Fibrillary	Carcinoma	Meningioma
Hemispheric	Colloid cyst	Ependymoma (conus/filum)
Brain stem	Pituitary tumors	Myxopapillary
Pilocytic	Functioning adenomas	Lipoma
Optic nerve	Growth hormone secreting	Dermoid
Hypothalamic	Prolactin secreting	Metastatic tumor
Cystic cerebellar	Adrenocorticotropic hormone secreting	Leptomeningeal metastasis
Special variants	Thyroid-stimulating hormone secreting	"Drop" metastasis
Xanthoastrocytoma	Follicle-stimulating hormone/luteinizing	(medulloblastoma)
Giant-cell astrocytoma	hormone secreting	Extradural
Oligodendroglioma	Plurihormonal secreting	Metastatic tumor
Ependymoma	Nonfunctioning adenomas	Chordoma
Mixed glioma	Null cell adenoma	Teratoma (sacrococcygeal)
Oligoastrocytoma	Oncocytoma	Vertebral tumors
Ganglioglioma	Carcinoma	(hemangioma, sarcoma)
Pineal tumors	Craniopharyngioma	
Pineocytoma	Dermid/epidermoid	
Pineoblastoma	Chordoma	
Germ cell tumors	Aesthesioneuroblastoma	
Germinoma	Skull tumors	
Nongerminoma	Metastatic tumors	
Teratoma	Dura	
Embryonal carcinoma	Choroid plexus	
Endodermal sinus tumor	Posterior pituitary	
Choriocarcinoma	Leptomeningeal	
Lymphoma		
Hemangioblastoma		
Lipoma		
Metastatic tumor		

Chronic immunosuppression (organ transplantation, AIDS) is associated with primary cerebral lymphoma. RNA viruses (avian sarcoma virus), DNA viruses (simian vacuolating virus), and chemicals (aromatic hydrocarbons, *N*-nitroso compounds) cause gliomas, meningiomas, sarcomas, and other tumors in animals, but no virus or specific chemical has been causally associated with human disease. Most CNS tumors develop sporadically, yet familial aggregations have been noted, and several inherited disorders are associated with CNS neoplasms (Table 423.2).

Brain tumors, like most cancers, arise after mutation or altered expression of several growth-controlling *tumor suppressor genes* and growth-promoting *oncogenes*. The location and nature of these molecular abnormalities are being identified in specific tumor types, especially gliomas and meningiomas. Cytogenetic analyses of high-grade astrocytic gliomas show multiple abnormalities, including extra copies of chromosome 7 and loss of chromosome 10. Genetic losses, identified by Southern blot or polymerase chain reaction–based methods, implicate tumor suppressor gene abnormalities on chromosome 10 in glioblastoma multiforme; chromosomes 9p, 13q, and 19q in glioblastoma and anaplastic astrocytoma; chromosomes 17p (*p53* gene) and 22q in astrocytic gliomas of all malignancy grades; and chromosome 19q in low- and high-grade oligodendrogliomas and mixed gliomas. Studies of gene expression show amplification and rearrangement of several oncogenes in glioblastomas and anaplastic gliomas, notably the epidermal growth factor receptor (*EGFR*) gene, *MYCN, MYC,* and *GLI.* Glioma cells release growth factors (platelet-derived growth factor, transforming growth factor

TABLE 423.2.	DISORDERS ASSOCIATED WITH CENTRAL NERVOUS SYSTEM TUMORS	
Disorder	**Genetic Locus**	**Tumor Types**
Neurofibromatosis type 1	17q11	Neurofibroma
		Glioma
Neurofibromatosis type 2	22q12	Acoustic neuroma (bilateral)
		Meningioma
Tuberous sclerosis	9q34 (50% of families)	Giant-cell astrocytoma (subependymal)
		Glioma
	16p13 (50% of families)	Hamartoma
Von Hippel–Lindau disease	3p25-20	Hemangioblastoma
Multiple endocrine neoplasia type 1	11q13	Pituitary adenoma
Turcot's syndrome	5q21	Glioma
		Medulloblastoma
Basal cell nevus syndrome (Gorlin's syndrome)	9q22-	Medulloblastoma
		Meningioma
Multiple hamartomata syndrome	Unknown	Meningioma
Neurocutaneous melanosis	Unknown	Leptomeningeal melanoma
Li–Fraumeni syndrome	17p13 (p53)	Glioma
		Medulloblastoma

α), angiogenic factors (vascular endothelial growth factor), and proteolytic enzymes, which enhance growth and invasiveness and, like specific genetic abnormalities, are possible targets for novel therapies. Cytogenetic studies and loss-of-heterozygosity analyses in meningiomas point to a critical tumor suppressor gene on chromosome 22, distinct from the bilateral acoustic neurofibromatosis gene.

SYMPTOMS AND SIGNS

Brain tumors produce both generalized and focal neurologic disturbances (see Chapters 427 and 430). Generalized findings stem from raised intracranial pressure and include headache, drowsiness, vomiting, transient visual loss, papilledema, and neck stiffness. Tumor, peritumoral edema, and obstruction of cerebrospinal fluid (CSF) pathways with resulting hydrocephalus are the principal causes of raised intracranial pressure. Intratumoral hemorrhage or cyst formation are less common causes. Focal or lateralizing findings indicate regional abnormalities, such as language dysfunction, hemiparesis, or seizures. Not all focal findings accurately locate the tumor, however; raised intracranial pressure may provoke false localizing signs, such as visual loss, optic atrophy, or sixth nerve palsies. Headache occurs in 50% of patients with brain tumor, particularly younger patients; headache may be lateralizing but does not specifically locate the tumor. Headache is most prominent in the morning upon awakening and usually resolves within 1 to 2 hours. Certain constellations of symptoms and signs pinpoint the tumor and suggest a specific tumor type (Table 423.3). Pituitary and suprasellar tumors also produce non-neurologic symptoms and signs as a result of endocrine dysfunction.

Brain tumors usually cause subacute or chronic symptoms, but they may take the form of acute symptoms of seizures, intra-

tumoral hemorrhage, or ventricular obstruction. Hemorrhage is more common with metastatic than primary tumors (especially melanoma, hypernephroma, choriocarcinoma, and nonseminomatous testicular cancer), but among the primary tumors, glioblastoma multiforme and oligodendroglioma are most likely to bleed. Intratumoral cyst formation is an uncommon cause of acute worsening (gliomas, craniopharyngioma). The tempo at which symptoms and signs evolve may be a clue to the nature of the tumor. Subacute onset over weeks suggests rapid tumor growth and a malignant histologic type (glioblastoma multiforme, medulloblastoma, metastasis), whereas slowly progressive findings over months or years are indicative of benign tumors (meningioma, pituitary adenoma). The rate of growth and typical locations of common CNS tumors are summarized in Table 423.4.

Pain in the neck or back, which may radiate, is the first symptom of spinal tumor in most patients. Within days to years, pain is followed by weakness, sensory loss, and autonomic dysfunction. The interval between pain and other findings is shorter (weeks) with rapidly expanding tumors, such as spinal epidural metastasis, and longer (months or years) with slowly growing tumors, such as astrocytoma, ependymoma, meningioma, and neurofibroma. Cervical, thoracic, and upper lumbar tumors produce a combination of segmental (local) and long tract findings. Segmental symptoms and signs result from damage to local spinal roots and adjacent spinal cord gray matter. Long tract symptoms and signs manifest below the level of the tumor, reflecting damage to motor, sensory, and autonomic fibers descending or ascending the cord. Tumors below L2 compress the cauda equina, not the spinal cord, producing lower back pain, sciatica, muscle wasting, weakness, dermatomal sensory loss, reflex loss in the legs, and autonomic dysfunction by involving single or multiple lumbosacral spinal roots.

Specific spinal tumor syndromes are recognized. Clockwise

| TABLE 423.3. | INTRACRANIAL TUMOR SYNDROMES |

Principal Symptoms	Tumor Location	Tumor Types	Principal Symptoms	Tumor Location	Tumor Types
"Dementia"/ personality change	Frontal lobe	Glioma Metastasis Lymphoma Meningioma	Headache, cranial neuropathy	Subfrontal	Meningioma Aesthesioneuroblastoma
	Temporal lobe (nondominant)	Glioma Metastasis Meningioma		Sellar/suprasellar	Pituitary adenoma Craniopharyngioma Meningioma
	Corpus callosum	Glioma Lymphoma		Brain stem	Glioma Metastasis
	Many sites	Metastasis Lymphoma			Meningioma Dermoid/epidermoid
Headache, vomiting papilledema	Frontal lobe	Glioma Metastasis			Metastasis Optic nerve glioma Chordoma
				Parasellar	Metastasis
	Intraventricular (third, lateral)	Ependymoma Pineal tumor Germ cell tumor Meningioma Choroid plexus papilloma Colloid cyst Craniopharyngioma Neurocytoma		Cerebellopontine angle	Acoustic neuroma Meningioma Ependymoma Choroid plexus papilloma Dermoid/epidermoid Chordoma Paraganglioma Brain stem glioma Metastasis
	Posterior fossa	Medulloblastoma Cerebellar astrocytoma Ependymoma Hemangioblastoma Metastasis		Clivus/base of skull	Chordoma Paraganglioma Meningioma Metastasis Sarcoma (skull)
	Leptomeningeal	Metastasis Lymphoma (primary) Melanoma (primary)		Leptomeningeal	Metastasis Lymphoma (primary) Melanoma (primary)
Lateralizing signs or seizures	Cerebral hemisphere	Glioma Metastasis Lymphoma Meningioma	Headache, endocrinopathy	Sellar/suprasellar	Pituitary adenoma Craniopharyngioma Germ cell tumor Hypothalamic glioma Metastasis
Headache, gait ataxia	Bifrontal/ corpus callosum	Glioma Lymphoma Meningioma	Parinaud's syndrome	Pineal region	Pineal tumor
	Posterior fossa	Medulloblastoma Cerebellar astrocytoma Ependymoma Hemangioblastoma Metastasis			Germ cell tumor Ependymoma Astrocytoma Meningioma Choroid plexus papilloma
	Leptomeningeal	Metastasis Lymphoma (primary) Melanoma (primary)			Metastasis

limb weakness, loss of position and vibration sense in the arms, and atrophy of the hand muscles are characteristic of high cervical and foramen magnum tumors. Dissociated sensory loss (segmental pain and temperature loss with preservation of posterior column function) and sacral sparing are characteristic of cervical and upper thoracic intramedullary tumors. Ipsilateral pyramidal signs and contralateral spinothalamic disturbance (Brown–Séquard syndrome) are features of lateral cervical and thoracic

tumors. Early autonomic dysfunction with relative preservation of leg strength and sensation is characteristic of tumors compressing or invading the conus medullaris. Long-standing lower back and sciatic pain without other neurologic findings is characteristic of slowly growing tumors of the cauda equina. Kyphoscoliosis and deformities of the feet may be the initial features of spinal cord tumors in children. Lumbosacral sinus tract, dimple, tuft of hair, or birthmark may point to an underlying tumor of

TABLE 423.4.	GROWTH CHARACTERISTICS AND LOCATIONS OF COMMON CENTRAL NERVOUS SYSTEM TUMORS	

Tumor Type	Rate of Growth	Location(s)
Glioblastoma multiforme	Fast	Cerebral hemispheres Brain stem (uncommon) Cerebellum (rare)
Medulloblastoma	Fast	Cerebellum
Metastasis[a]	Fast	Cerebral hemispheres (80%) Brain stem Cerebellum Spinal cord (rare)
Lymphoma	Fast-intermediate	Cerebral hemispheres (esp. periventricular) Brain stem Cerebellum Spinal cord (rare)
Germ cell tumors	Fast-intermediate	Pineal region Third ventricle Suprasellar
Anaplastic gliomas	Intermediate	Cerebral hemispheres Brain stem Cerebellum (uncommon) Spinal cord
Astrocytoma, oligodendroglioma	Slow	Cerebral hemispheres Brain stem Cerebellum (children) Spinal cord
Ependymoma	Slow	Intraventricular (esp. fourth) Cerebral hemispheres (uncommon) Spinal cord Filum terminale
Hemangioblastoma	Slow	Cerebellum Spinal cord
Meningioma	Slow	Falx (parasagittal) Hemisphere convexity Subfrontal Tuberculum sellae Tentorium Cerebellopontine angle Clivus Foramen magnum Spinal (esp. thoracic)
Acoustic neuroma	Slow	Cerebellopontine angle
Choroid plexus papilloma	Slow	Intraventricular (esp. third, fourth)
Colloid cyst	Slow	Third ventricle
Pituitary adenoma	Slow	Sella turcica
Craniopharyngioma	Slow	Suprasellar Intrasellar (rare)
Dermoid/epidermoid	Slow	Suprasellar Cerebellopontine angle Spine (lumbosacral)
Chordoma	Slow	Clivus Spine (lumbosacral)

[a] Excluding spinal epidural metastasis.
Fast, growth over weeks; intermediate, growth over months; slow growth over years.

the conus or cauda equina. A combination of cranial and spinal findings, including headache, mental change, cranial neuropathy, polyradiculopathy, and autonomic disturbance, is the hallmark of diffuse leptomeningeal metastasis (leukemia, lymphoma, and solid tumors).

DIAGNOSIS

Advances in neuroimaging have revolutionized the diagnosis of CNS tumors (see Chapter 452). Most tumors of sufficient size to cause symptoms can be seen. Magnetic resonance imaging (MRI), alone and with gadolinium, is the best diagnostic test for brain and spinal tumors. It has largely replaced computed tomography (CT) scanning, though CT is still less expensive than MRI. Radiographic characteristics of brain tumors are comparable on both MRI and CT scans (Table 423.5), except that calcification is better seen on CT. High-grade primary brain tumors and metastases are best seen after the administration of iodinated contrast (CT) or gadolinium (MRI); both CT and MRI locate the tumor precisely, because the blood–brain barrier disruption typical of malignant tumors permits dye extravasation and tumor enhancement. Low-grade tumors (fibrillary astrocytoma) are typically nonenhancing lesions seen as regions of hypodensity on CT or as regions of hypointensity on T1-weighted or hyperintensity on T2-weighted MRI (Fig. 423.1). They are clearly visible on MRI but can be easily missed on CT. Small tumors near the skull base (frontal, intrasellar, suprasellar, clivus,

cerebellopontine angle, foramen magnum) are best imaged by MRI, which eliminates the distortion on CT scan created by adjacent bone. Bone artifact also may obscure small tumors of the brain stem or cerebellum, and MRI may be the only means of identifying tumors in these areas.

Spine MRI is now the optimal test for evaluating patients with suspected spinal tumors (see Chapter 452). Tumors that are extradural (metastases) can be seen on MRI without using gadolinium for enhancement; however, intradural tumors (meningioma, spinal cord glioma) often are more easily made visible after gadolinium administration. Plain films show negative results in most patients with primary spinal neoplasms but positive results in 80% to 90% of patients with spinal epidural metastasis. Vertebral collapse and pedicle erosion are the common findings. Myelography also can identify the level, extent, and nature (extradural, intradural, intramedullary) of most spinal tumors, but it is invasive. Complete myelographic assessment may require lumbar and cervical (lateral C1 to C2) dye injections, to ascertain both the rostral and caudal extent of tumor. Spine CT scans done immediately after myelography help find bone destruction, paraspinal tumor, and the location of an intraspinal tumor. Unlike MRI, myelography permits sampling of the CSF, to assess for leptomeningeal tumor, which may be an important issue for some patients.

Analysis of CSF for malignant cells and tumor markers may be helpful in patients suspected of leptomeningeal metastases, or "drop metastases" from a primary tumor (medulloblastoma, anaplastic ependymoma, germ cell tumor, primary cerebral lym-

| TABLE 423.5. | MAGNETIC RESONANCE IMAGING/COMPUTED TOMOGRAPHY SCAN APPEARANCE OF COMMON BRAIN TUMORS |

Tumor Type	Precontrast	Postcontrast
Astrocytoma	Hypointense (MRI-T1)	No enhancement
Oligodendroglioma	Hypodense (CT)	
Mixed glioma	Hyperintense (MRI-T2)	
Brain stem glioma		
Dermoid/epidermoid		
Pituitary adenoma		
Glioblastoma multiforme	Hypointense (MRI-T1)	Enhancement
Anaplastic glioma	Hypodense (CT)	
Metastasis		
Craniopharyngioma		
Cystic cerebellar astrocytoma		
Metastasis	Isointense or hyperintense (MRI-T1)	Enhancement
Meningioma	Isodense or hyperdense (CT)	
Lymphoma		
Medulloblastoma		
Ependymoma		
Hemangioblastoma (low-density cyst)		
Germinoma		
Choroid plexus papilloma		
Paraganglioma		
Colloid cyst		
Lipoma	Hyperintense (MRI-T1)	No enhancement
Dermoid	Hypodense (CT)	

CT, computed tomography; MR, magnetic resonance.

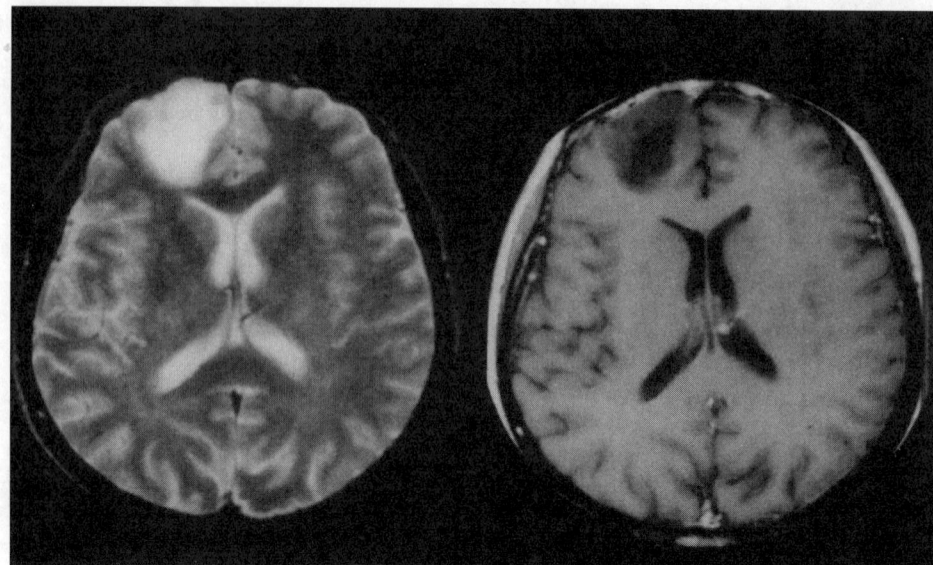

FIGURE 423.1. Magnetic resonance scan of a low-grade right-sided frontal astrocytoma. On the left is a T2-weighted image and, on the right, a T1-weighted image after gadolinium infusion; note the absence of enhancement after gadolinium.

phoma). Lumbar puncture may lead to herniation in patients with brain tumor or cause neurologic deterioration in patients with spinal tumor; it should be undertaken only after cranial imaging and only when necessary. The typical CSF picture in patients with leptomeningeal cancer includes pleocytosis, elevated protein level, low glucose level, and a positive result on cytologic examination. CSF levels of human chorionic gonadotropin and α-fetoprotein may be elevated in the context of intracranial germ cell tumors, and other tumor markers (carcinoembryonic antigen, lactate dehydrogenase isoenzymes) may be high with leptomeningeal metastases from systemic cancers.

TREATMENT—GENERAL CONSIDERATIONS

Treatment for brain and spinal cord tumors can be divided into two broad categories, supportive measures and definitive treatment. Supportive measures are directed at symptom control and include emergency management, corticosteroid administration, and antiseizure medications. Definitive treatments, including surgery, radiation therapy, and chemotherapy, are directed against the neoplasm itself, with the goal of reducing tumor size and controlling subsequent growth.

SUPPORTIVE MEASURES

Threatened cerebral herniation and impending spinal cord compression require emergency treatment (see Chapter 445). Rapid reduction of raised intracranial pressure is the first step in the emergency treatment of patients with brain tumor. Most patients stabilize or improve after intravenous corticosteroids alone, but herniation with coma may require intubation, hyperventilation, intravenous mannitol, and, in some instances, ventricular drainage. Definitive treatment then proceeds under controlled circumstances. Patients with spinal tumors who suddenly have leg weakness, numbness, or urinary retention may improve

with intravenous corticosteroid therapy alone, but usually they require urgent surgical decompression or radiation therapy.

Corticosteroids are highly effective symptomatic treatment for patients with intracranial and spinal neoplasms. Neurologic symptoms and quality of life often improve dramatically within 24 to 48 hours. These agents exert their beneficial effect by controlling peritumoral edema. In addition, corticosteroids control postoperative swelling and lessen the incidence and severity of acute radiation reactions due to perilesional edema incited by radiation therapy. Corticosteroids are administered preoperatively, perioperatively, and often throughout radiation treatment. Subsequently, many patients can be tapered off corticosteroids, though some experience exacerbation of neurologic symptoms at this time and require continued treatment. Corticosteroid dependence is often a poor prognostic sign. Long-term use is associated with many side effects, including mental change (ranging from mild agitation to psychotic delirium), hyperglycemia, opportunistic infection, steroid myopathy (which can be confused with tumor progression), and aseptic necrosis of the femoral head. Acute and chronic corticosteroid toxicities improve with dose reduction and resolve when discontinued, but some side effects, such as steroid myopathy, take weeks to months to disappear.

Anticonvulsants, usually phenytoin, carbamazepine, or phenobarbital, are used for the 20% to 25% of brain tumor patients who have seizures. Prophylactic anticonvulsants are useful in the perioperative period for patients who have not had a seizure. Some physicians continue them indefinitely, but randomized prospective studies show that prophylactic anticonvulsants are ineffective. Pain control; hormone replacement; physical, occupational, and speech therapies; and psychosocial support are other important aspects of treatment.

DEFINITIVE TREATMENT

Surgery and radiation therapy are the principal treatments for most CNS tumors. Surgery, now enhanced by MRI- and CT-guided stereotaxis, is also necessary for diagnosis. Surgery is curative therapy for many, primarily low-grade, tumors (meningioma, pituitary adenoma, acoustic neuroma, cystic cerebellar astrocytoma, choroid plexus papilloma, colloid cyst, neurofibroma). It also plays an important role in the treatment of malignant neoplasms; debulking often improves symptoms, lessens corticosteroid dependence, and prolongs survival. Radiation therapy is standard treatment for most patients with malignant tumors (glioblastoma, anaplastic glioma, primary cerebral lymphoma, malignant meningioma, brain metastasis, germ cell tumor, medulloblastoma, brain stem glioma, epidural spinal metastasis) and may be delivered by external beam, either conventionally or stereotactically (radiosurgery), or by the interstitial technique (brachytherapy). Radiation therapy also may be recommended for some patients with partially resected benign tumors (astrocytoma, oligodendroglioma, ependymoma, meningioma, pituitary adenoma, craniopharyngioma, spinal cord glioma).

Systemic chemotherapy is particularly effective for primary cerebral lymphoma, anaplastic oligodendroglioma, medulloblastoma, and germinoma. Nitrosoureas and procarbazine are the most active drugs for glial tumors, methotrexate for cerebral lymphoma, and the platinum compounds for germ cell tumors and medulloblastoma. Intracarotid chemotherapy is not efficacious and can be neurotoxic. Regional treatment using drug-impregnated, implantable wafers has modest efficacy in the treatment of recurrent malignant gliomas. Antiangiogenesis and gene therapies are investigational approaches under development for glial neoplasms. Intrathecal chemotherapy, through lumbar puncture or Ommaya reservoir, is an effective treatment for leukemic and lymphomatous meningitis. Some patients with carcinomatous meningitis, especially from breast cancer, also improve. Most chemotherapeutic agents are toxic when given intrathecally, but methotrexate, cytarabine, and thiotepa can be used safely.

TREATMENT—SPECIFIC TUMOR TYPES

This section reviews the current management of common CNS tumors and those less common neoplasms for which treatment is either multimodal, changing, or the subject of controversy. Other CNS tumors treated primarily by surgery are summarized in Table 423.6. For all CNS tumors, prognostic factors have a powerful effect upon outcome. The most important factors that are influential in assessing virtually all tumor types are age and performance status; young adults, in good clinical condition at diagnosis, have a significantly better chance of survival than older patients in poor condition. For glial tumors, histologic features and extent of surgical resection also affect outcome. The factors are independent of treatment and, in the case of glial tumors, exert a more profound influence on survival than any therapeutic method.

GLIOBLASTOMA AND ANAPLASTIC ASTROCYTOMA

Glioblastomas and anaplastic astrocytomas are the common primary brain tumors of adults. Optimal treatment includes maximum "safe" surgical resection followed by radiation therapy and systemic chemotherapy. The completeness of surgical removal is dictated largely by tumor location; for example, nondominant frontal lobe tumors can be extensively debulked, whereas tumors in the basal ganglia or thalamus can only be biopsied for diagnosis. Radiation is delivered by external beam using x-rays from a linear accelerator or cobalt unit to a local field that includes tumor and peritumoral tissue only. Tumor control may be enhanced somewhat by a radiosurgical boost, but this is limited to small focal tumors, and efficacy has yet to be established. Several alkylating agents have antiglioma activity, but carmustine given intravenously is the standard chemotherapy drug for the

TABLE 423.6.	**CENTRAL NERVOUS SYSTEM TUMORS PRIMARILY TREATED BY SURGERY**	
Tumor Type	**Treatment**	**Comments**
Cerebellar astrocytoma	Surgery	
Hemangioblastoma	Surgery	
Meningioma	Surgery	
	RT	Focal (atypical/malignant)
Acoustic neuroma	Surgery	
	RT	Radiosurgery (selected patients)
Choroid plexus papilloma	Surgery	
	RT	Focal or neuraxis (malignant)
Pituitary adenoma (macroadenoma)	Surgery	
	RT	Incomplete resection (selected patients)
	Bromocriptine	Prolactin secreting
	Octreotide	Growth hormone secreting
Craniopharyngioma	Surgery	
	RT	Incomplete resection (selected patients)
Dermoid/epidermoid	Surgery	
Chordoma	Surgery	
	RT	Proton beam

RT, radiation therapy.

initial treatment of glioblastoma. PCV, a combination chemotherapy regimen consisting of procarbazine, lomustine (CCNU), and vincristine, may be superior to carmustine for anaplastic astrocytomas but is more toxic. Treatment prolongs life but is seldom curative; the median survival is 10 to 12 months for glioblastoma and 2 to 3 years for anaplastic astrocytoma. Nonrandomized studies of innovative therapies reporting longer-than-expected survivals must be interpreted cautiously; they may have excluded patients with large tumors and unfavorable prognostic factors, such as older age and poor performance status, which can enhance the apparent benefit of the experimental treatment.

ASTROCYTOMA

Several histologic subtypes of astrocytoma, including pilocytic astrocytomas (cystic cerebellar astrocytomas), pleomorphic xanthoastrocytomas, subependymal giant-cell astrocytomas (of tuberous sclerosis), and gangliogliomas, are circumscribed, indolent neoplasms of children and adolescents, curable by surgical resection; radiation is seldom necessary, and malignant degeneration is uncommon. Fibrillary astrocytomas, on the other hand, are diffusely infiltrating tumors of the cerebral hemispheres and spinal cord in adults, rarely curable by surgery alone. Local-field irradiation by conventional external beam enhances tumor control but may be neurotoxic (impaired cognition, myelopathy) in long-term survivors. For hemispheric tumors, the timing of radiation therapy is debated; some advocate early treatment, particularly for symptomatic patients or after partial resection, whereas others prefer to postpone radiation, especially for asymptomatic patients or after gross total removal. Although fibrillary astrocytomas are relatively indolent initially, many progress to anaplastic astrocytomas or glioblastomas. The median duration of survival is 5 to 10 years for patients with fibrillary astrocytomas of the brain.

OLIGODENDROGLIOMA

Oligodendrogliomas may be low grade and exceedingly indolent or high grade (anaplastic) and moderately aggressive; although it is imperfect, this correlation between histologic type and behavior is helpful prognostically and guides treatment. Oligodendrogliomas, most commonly seen in young and middle-aged adults, are frequently amenable to radical surgical resection and re-resection if necessary, because 50% of them are found in the frontal lobe. After surgery, local-field irradiation by conventional external beam has been the standard treatment for anaplastic tumors and often is recommended for symptomatic, partially resected low-grade oligodendrogliomas. The wisdom of early radiation for oligodendrogliomas, a treatment that can be neurotoxic in long-term survivors, is being reconsidered in light of their unusual chemosensitivity; anaplastic oligodendrogliomas and symptomatic, enlarging low-grade tumors respond predictably to PCV. Chemotherapy may soon be the initial nonsurgical treatment for oligodendrogliomas. After surgery and radiation, the median duration of survival is 3 to 5 years for patients with anaplastic tumors and 10 years for those with low-grade oligodendrogliomas.

EPENDYMOMA

Ependymomas occur at all levels of the neuraxis. Intracranial tumors are frequently found in the posterior fossa and are more common in children. Both low-grade and anaplastic intracranial ependymomas seed the leptomeninges occasionally. Treatment includes complete surgical removal, if possible; disease staging by gadolinium-enhanced spinal MRI and CSF cytologic examination; and limited-field irradiation for tumors that are localized or craniospinal irradiation for disseminated disease. Standard initial treatment for older children and adults does not include chemotherapy, but platinum-based regimens have been effective for recurrences. Chemotherapy is used increasingly to postpone radiation in very young children, because they suffer serious developmental side effects after cranial or spinal irradiation. The median duration of survival is 5 years for intracranial ependymomas; very young age, supratentorial location, incomplete resection, anaplastic histologic features, and early dissemination are poor prognostic indicators. Intramedullary spinal ependymomas are often circumscribed and removable by surgery; radiation is recommended after incomplete resection only. Myxopapillary ependymomas of the conus medullaris are difficult to remove completely and may require radiation; those in the filum terminale that can be resected completely require no further treatment.

MEDULLOBLASTOMA

Medulloblastomas are aggressive cerebellar tumors that primarily affect children. Treatment begins with maximum surgical resection. After surgery, the disease is staged by gadolinium-enhanced spinal MRI, CSF for cytologic examination, and bone scan. The extent of surgical resection and tumor stage are helpful prognostic features and guide treatment. Patients with complete resections and no evidence of dissemination have a more favorable prognosis (low or standard risk) compared with those with subtotal resection, brain stem involvement, leptomeningeal spread, or bony metastases (high risk). Subclinical, undetectable leptomeningeal seeding is common with medulloblastoma; for this reason, all patients, except very young children, receive craniospinal irradiation with a boost to the posterior fossa. Overall, the 5-year disease-free survival rate is 65%. High-risk patients are treated with platinum-based adjuvant chemotherapy in addition to radiation, and very young children receive chemotherapy instead of radiation until the musculoskeletal and nervous systems mature more fully. High survival rates (85%) have been reported for aggressively treated, high-risk cases; in light of this, many physicians have added adjuvant chemotherapy for standard-risk patients.

PRIMARY CENTRAL NERVOUS SYSTEM LYMPHOMA

Lymphomas, usually of B-cell origin, once were considered rare tumors of older adults, but they are seen increasingly in younger patients and in the context of iatrogenic or AIDS-associated chronic immunosuppression. Surgery is important for diagnosis but has little therapeutic value for this diffusely infiltrating, multifocal neoplastic process. Many CNS lymphomas are exquisitely corticosteroid sensitive, a property that is advantageous therapeutically but can complicate the diagnostic process; large tumors may regress in the time it takes to organize a stereotactic biopsy procedure. If lymphoma is suspected (clinically or radiologically), corticosteroids should be withheld until the day of surgery. Primary CNS lymphomas are radiosensitive cancers, and for many years whole-brain radiation therapy was the standard treatment. Although some younger patients may have been cured by radiation alone, most died as a result of recurrent tumor 12 to 18 months later.

CNS lymphomas are sensitive to cytotoxic drugs; the addition of systemic chemotherapy to cranial irradiation has doubled median survival (>40 months). Most effective regimens now include high-dose methotrexate and cytarabine; both cross the blood–brain barrier to reach nonenhancing or microscopic tumor. After barrier disruption, chemotherapy with mannitol is an approach used by some, to ensure adequate drug delivery to occult disease. Chemotherapy is given before cranial radiation to assess response and minimize toxicity; however, methotrexate can cause serious neurotoxicity when combined with cranial irradiation. Chemotherapy alone is being investigated in terms of efficacy and reduced CNS toxicity.

GERM CELL TUMORS

Germ cell tumors of the CNS are rare cancers of children and young adults. There are two categories, germinomas and nongerminomatous germ cell tumors; the latter group includes choriocarcinoma, embryonal carcinoma, endodermal sinus tumors, and teratomas. They occur in the pineal and suprasellar regions, where they can be sampled for biopsy but are difficult to remove. They can seed the leptomeninges, necessitating postoperative staging with gadolinium-enhanced spinal MRI, CSF cytologic examination, and CSF biochemistry for the tumor markers α-fetoprotein and β-human chorionic gonadotropin. Germinomas are highly radiosensitive and curable by radiation alone in more than 90% of patients. In an effort to eliminate brain irradiation because of neuropsychological consequences, recent work has focused on the use of combination chemotherapy as initial treatment for germinomas. Platinum-based regimens similar to those for testicular cancer can effect complete responses in many patients; however, these regimens are toxic, and 50% of patients require radiation therapy within 2 years of diagnosis. Therefore, the superiority of this approach has yet to be established. Those with nongerminomatous tumors always require radiation treatment and chemotherapy but are rarely cured.

METASTATIC BRAIN TUMOR

Treatment for metastatic brain tumor depends on the number of lesions and the status of the underlying malignancy. At diagnosis, 50% of patients have single lesions, and an additional 20% have only two. These patients are candidates for focal treatment, whereas those with many brain metastases need whole-brain radiotherapy. Patients with single, surgically accessible tumors and controlled or limited systemic disease should undergo tumor resection. Occasionally, patients with two lesions and limited systemic disease—particularly from radioresistant cancers, such as renal cell carcinoma—are candidates for surgical treatment. Complete resection followed by cranial irradiation prolongs median survival (10 months) compared with radiation alone (4 to 6 months), and some patients are long-term survivors.

The need for radiation therapy after complete resection of a single metastasis from a highly radioresistant primary has been questioned; some physicians postpone radiation therapy and consider reoperation should the tumor recur. Patients with widely disseminated systemic cancer or many brain metastases are treated with whole-brain radiotherapy; although their median survival is short (4 months) and few survive a year, most stabilize or improve neurologically and die as a result of progressive systemic disease. For these palliative cases, radiation therapy usually is delivered over 1 to 2 weeks using large dose fractions. Surgical candidates with the potential for long survival may have fewer late neurologic residual effects if they are irradiated in a more protracted fashion over 3 to 4 weeks using smaller daily fractions. Some patients with few lesions or with recurrent metastases may be candidates for radiosurgery.

METASTATIC EPIDURAL SPINAL CORD COMPRESSION

Epidural spinal metastasis, a common complication of lung, breast, and prostate cancer, is treated with radiation or a combination of surgery and radiation. The indications for surgery include diagnostic uncertainty, tumor in a previously irradiated field, radioresistant primary, and intractable pain. Laminectomy is the most common surgical procedure; it allows for decompression of the cord, but because metastatic tumors typically are located anteriorly in the vertebral body, relatively little tumor is removed. Definitive surgical management requires resection of the vertebral body through an anterolateral approach, followed by spinal reconstruction and stabilization. Occasionally, definitive resection can be accomplished posterolaterally with only partial removal of the vertebral body. Both are major procedures requiring an experienced surgical team and highly selected patients with localized spinal disease and limited systemic tumor.

After surgery, most patients receive radiation if it has not been administered previously. Radiation alone is the treatment of choice for most patients with spinal epidural metastasis. Once the tumor's rostral and caudal extent are known (by MRI), a treatment field is delineated and radiation given by conventional external beam. Radiotherapy is particularly effective for radiosensitive tumors, such as lymphoma and breast cancer, but also for moderately sensitive tumors, such as lung cancer. Radioresistant tumors, such as renal cancer, often are treated surgically—for hypernephroma, typically after an embolization procedure to minimize hemorrhage. Experts debate the intricacies of treatment, but all agree that early diagnosis is essential to good outcome; those patients who are ambulatory at diagnosis usually remain so, but paraplegic patients rarely walk again.

BIBLIOGRAPHY

Abrey LE, DeAngelis LM, Yahalom J. Long-term survival in primary CNS lymphoma. *J Clin Oncol* 1998;16:859–863.

Balmaceda C, Heller G, Rosenblum M, et al. Chemotherapy without irradiation: a novel approach for newly diagnosed CNS germ cell tumors. Results of an international cooperative trial. The First International Central Nervous System Germ Cell Tumor Study. *J Clin Oncol* 1996; 14:2908–2915.

Black PML. Brain tumors (Parts 1 and 2). *N Engl J Med* 1991;324: 1471–1476, 1555–1564.

Byrne TN. Spinal cord compression from epidural metastases. *N Engl J Med* 1992;327:614–619.

Cairncross G, Macdonald D, Ludwin S, et al. Chemotherapy for anaplastic oligodendroglioma. *J Clin Oncol* 1994;12:2013–2021.

DeAngelis LM. Management of brain metastases. *Cancer Invest* 1994;12: 156–165.

Louis DN. The p53 gene and protein in human brain tumors. *J Neuropathol Exp Neurol* 1994;53:11–21.

Packer RJ, Sutton LN, Elterman R, et al. Outcome for children with medulloblastoma treated with radiation and cisplatin, CCNU, and vincristine chemotherapy. *J Neurosurg* 1994;81:690–698.

Patchell RA, Tibbs PA, Walsh JW, et al. A randomized trial of surgery in the treatment of single metastasis to the brain. *N Engl J Med* 1990;322: 494–500.

Plate KH, Breier G, Weich HA, et al. Vascular endothelial growth factor is a potential tumor angiogenesis factor in human gliomas in vivo. *Nature* 1992;359:845–848.

Pollack IF. Brain tumors in children. *N Engl J Med* 1994;331:1500–1507.

Radhakrishnan K, Mokri B, Parisi JE, et al. The trends in incidence of primary brain tumors in the population of Rochester, Minnesota. *Ann Neurol* 1995;37:67–73.

Kelley's Textbook of Internal Medicine, fourth edition. Edited by H. David Humes. Lippincott Williams & Wilkins, Philadelphia © 2000.

CHAPTER

424

APPROACH TO THE PATIENT WITH IMPAIRMENT OF CONSCIOUSNESS

JOHN J. CARONNA

ROLE OF THE BRAIN STEM AND THE HEMISPHERES IN THE REGULATION OF CONSCIOUSNESS

Level of consciousness is defined by both arousal and conscious behavior. Changes in level of consciousness depend on the activities of a brain stem regulatory system called the reticular activating system (RAS). Anatomically, the RAS consists of the paramedian regions of the thalamus, midbrain, and the pons not associated with the cranial nerves or specific ascending or descending pathways. Arousal is a crude function that is simply wakefulness and reflects activation of the RAS by somatosensory stimuli or innate motivational symptoms, such as hunger. In clinical terms, arousal is indicated by eye opening, either spontaneously or in response to stimuli. In some cases, arousal may occur despite complete destruction of the hemispheres. Awareness, that is cognition of self and the environment, implies functioning cerebral hemispheres. Awareness is marked by goal-directed or purposeful motor behavior and the use of language. Mutually sustaining areas of both the RAS and the cerebral hemispheres are required to maintain full consciousness.

DEFINITIONS: COMA, STUPOR, AND THE VEGETATIVE STATE

Coma is a pathologic state in which neither arousal nor awareness is present. The comatose patient maintains a sleeplike unresponsiveness from which he or she cannot be aroused; eye opening does not occur, no comprehensible speech is detected, and the extremities neither move to commands nor respond appropriately to localize or ward off noxious stimuli. Nonpurposive, reflex movements such as flexor (decorticate) or extensor (decerebrate) posturing may be present. Stupor resembles coma, except that the patient remains arousable if strong external stimulation is provided.

Discrete structural lesions in the paramedian areas of the rostral brain stem make arousal impossible by interrupting impulses from the RAS to the hemispheres. Coma induced by depressant drugs, anesthetics, or endogenous metabolic toxins may result from metabolic depression of the RAS alone or depression of both hemispheres. A unilateral lesion in a cerebral hemisphere does not cause coma until brain swelling and herniation impair function either of the opposite hemisphere or, more frequently, of the rostral brain stem and its reticular formation. In some cases, particularly after anoxic–ischemic injury due to cardiac arrest or after head trauma, both hemispheres are severely damaged, but the brain stem RAS is preserved. After a period of coma lasting hours to days, wakefulness returns without evidence of purposive behaviors or cognition. This functionally decorticate state is distinct from coma and is termed the *vegetative state*.

CATEGORIES OF COMA AND DIFFERENTIAL DIAGNOSIS

All types of coma may be divided into three categories: supratentorial lesions, infratentorial lesions, and metabolic encephalopathy. Each has a characteristic clinical evolution. The key to clinical diagnosis when the history is in doubt is to identify the initial anatomic distribution of the lesion and how it evolves (Table 424.1).

SUPRATENTORIAL LESIONS

Mass lesions of the cerebral hemispheres cause coma by herniating beyond the confines of the supratentorial compartment and compressing the brain stem RAS. Two syndromes of herniation associated with supratentorial lesions are recognized.

TABLE 424.1.	PHYSICAL DIAGNOSIS OF COMA: RULES AND EXCEPTIONS

Symmetrical Signs, Brain Stem Functions Intact
  Rule: Cause of coma most likely is metabolic or diffuse. Concentrate on metabolic, toxic, and infectious sources.
  Exception: Early central herniation (see text) due to a supratentorial mass lesion may mimic metabolic encephalopathy.
Asymmetrical Signs, Brain Stem Functions Intact
  Rule: Cause of coma is probably an acute hemisphere mass lesion. Treat urgently to check further herniation.
  Exception: Hypoglycemic and hepatic encephalopathy may produce asymmetrical signs, but usually asymmetries do not persist. Metabolic encephalopathy superimposed on a previous neurological deficit may cause confusion in diagnosis.
Symetrical Signs, Caudal Brain Stem Functions Impaired
  Rule: Cause of coma is most likely intoxication or metabolic encephalopathy.
  Exception: A posterior fossa mass lesion causing rostral to caudal deterioration may mimic metabolic coma.
Asymmetrical Signs of Brain Stem Dysfunction
  Rule: Cause of coma is most likely a structural lesion of the posterior fossa. Consider basilar artery thrombosis, pontine hemorrhage, and cerebellar infarct or hematoma.
  Exception: None
EVIDENCE LEVEL: B. Reference: Stuben JP, Caronna JJ. Coma. In: Parillo JE, ed. *Current therapy in critical care medicine,* third edition. St. Louis: Mosby, 1977:306–310.

Central Downward Transtentorial Herniation

Deep midline tumors, large edematous hemisphere infarcts, and subdural hematomas may compress and shift the supratentorial contents downward through the tentorial opening into the subtentorial compartment. Unless herniation is checked by treatment, there is progressive failure of the rostral brain stem and then the pons and medulla. The initial stages of cerebral herniation are marked by symmetrical signs, which may be mistaken for metabolic encephalopathy. The first clinical signs reflect failure of the hemispheres and subcortical structures and include reduced consciousness, small pupils with preserved reaction to light, bilateral signs of corticospinal and extrapyramidal tract dysfunction, grasp reflexes, decorticate posturing, and periodic (Cheyne–Stokes) respirations. At this stage, downward herniation is potentially reversible by osmotic agents and, if a tumor or hematoma is present, by surgery. When signs of midbrain failure appear (fixed, dilated, or midposition pupils and decerebrate rigidity), it is likely that distortion and compression have led to irreversible infarction of the brain stem.

Herniation of the Temporal Lobe

An expanding mass in one hemisphere or in the lateral middle fossa may displace the uncus of the temporal lobe medially over the edge of the tentorial opening and compress the third cranial nerve, the adjacent midbrain, and the posterior cerebral artery. The earliest sign of uncal herniation is unilateral pupillary dilation with a preserved or sluggish light reaction. As the uncus continues to compress the midbrain, the patient becomes deeply comatose and manifests ipsilateral third nerve palsy and contralateral decerebrate posturing. Bilateral decerebrate rigidity develops when the contralateral cerebral peduncle is compressed

against the tentorial edge opposite the side of herniation. If treatment cannot halt brain displacement at this point, brain stem dysfunction progresses in a manner clinically indistinguishable from that caused by central herniation. In either type of herniation syndrome, destruction of the midbrain RAS results in irreversible coma.

SUBTENTORIAL LESIONS

Two types of posterior fossa lesions produce coma: lesions intrinsic to the brain stem that destroy the RAS (pontine hemorrhage and paramedian infarction of the midbrain or pons) and lesions extrinsic to the brain stem that compress and distort it (cerebral tumor and hematoma). In addition, unconsciousness follows direct blows to the brain stem reticular formation, as occurs in cerebral concussion and rupture of an adjacent cerebral aneurysm.

Hemorrhage into the pontine tegmentum produces coma accompanied by a distinctive clinical pattern. The pupils are pinpoint; horizontal eye movements are impaired, but vertical eye movements may be preserved; and ocular bobbing may occur. Decerebrate rigidity or flaccid quadriplegia, hyperthermia, and progressive slowing of respiration are characteristic. Compressive lesions of the brain stem are often difficult to distinguish from intrinsic lesions, and cerebellar hemorrhage may mimic brain stem stroke in its clinical features. In other cases, the caudal-to-rostral evolution of neurologic signs may resemble the patchy brain stem depression of sedative drug intoxication. Asymmetric motor signs and hypertension due to Cushing's reflex usually serve to identify brain stem compression.

METABOLIC ENCEPHALOPATHY

Metabolic encephalopathy refers to changes in level of consciousness that result from diffuse failure of cerebral metabolism. Metabolic encephalopathy develops acutely or subacutely, commonly produces coma, and is often reversible if the underlying systemic disorder is treated. Examples include anoxia, hypoglycemia, uremia, and drug intoxications. The anatomic locus of metabolic brain disease has not been defined with certainty. The traditional view has been that the neurons of the cerebral cortex are affected first; then, as the metabolic defect becomes more severe, the subcortical structures are affected from the rostral to the caudal end. A second concept is that the neurons of the RAS are affected first and cause the cortical neurons to cease functioning by depriving them of stimulation.

Pathophysiology

In most cases of metabolic encephalopathy, cerebral oxygen uptake is depressed. The degree of brain dysfunction that manifests clinically is proportionate to a decline in cerebral oxygen metabolism. For example, the brain normally consumes about 3.5 mL of oxygen for each 100 g of brain tissue per minute. When this rate declines to 2.5 mL, delirium supervenes; rates of cerebral oxygen metabolism below 2 mL per 100 g per minute are incompatible with an alert state. The mechanisms of action by which systemic illnesses interfere with cerebral metabolism are not known in every case. The relationship between systemic metabolic defects and cerebral dysfunction is clear, however, in two commonly encountered conditions, hypoxia and hypoglycemia.

Hypoxia

Under normal conditions, 90% of the cerebral energy needed to transmit nervous impulses and to maintain ionic gradients across cell membranes is derived from the oxidation of glucose. Because it does not store oxygen, the brain can survive for only a few minutes if oxygen is reduced below critical levels. During acute, total anoxia, consciousness is lost within 15 seconds. In humans, the electroencephalogram shows when there is arterial hypoxemia such that the partial arterial oxygen pressure (PaO_2) falls to 35 mm Hg or when the cerebral blood flow is reduced to 40% of normal. Electrocerebral silence occurs when the cerebral venous partial pressure of oxygen (PO_2) reaches 20 mm Hg or after about 18 seconds of total anoxia. When hypoxia is severe or prolonged, secondary depression of the myocardium supervenes. The clinical importance of hypoxia complicated by hypotension and impaired cerebral perfusion derives from its neurologic consequences; these consequences are more severe than those of uncomplicated hypoxia, perhaps because in the former case the delivery of glucose as well as oxygen is diminished, as is removal of metabolic waste products.

Hypoglycemia

Under physiologic conditions, glucose is the brain's only substrate and crosses the blood–brain barrier by facilitated transport. Each minute, the normal brain uses about 5.5 mg (31 μmol) of glucose per 100 g tissue. The blood glucose level at which cerebral metabolism fails and symptoms develop varies from person to person, but, in general, confusion occurs at levels below 30 mg per deciliter and coma at levels below 10 mg per deciliter. There are about 2 g of glucose and glycogen stores in the brain, so that a hypoglycemic patient in coma may survive for about 90 minutes without suffering irreversible brain damage.

Other Substances Required to Maintain Brain Function

In addition to oxygen and glucose, the brain requires enzymes, vitamins, amino acids, and other substances to function. The functions of the brain include maintaining membrane potentials, transmitting electrical impulses, and synthesizing transmitter substances and structural proteins. Therefore, neuronal excitability may be altered by imbalances in electrolytes and changes in serum osmolality, such as occur in renal disease, diabetic coma, and lithium intoxication. Alterations in the activity of central nervous system biogenic amines, such as happen in cases of psychotropic drug overdose and in hepatic failure, also produce delirium, stupor, and coma.

Clinical Findings

Metabolic encephalopathy is associated with a broad spectrum of disorders of consciousness. Mild metabolic disease can be mistaken for psychiatric disease; severe metabolic brain disease is confused with structural brain damage.

NEUROLOGIC EXAMINATION

The neurologic examination that follows has been derived from the Glasgow Coma Scale developed for head injury by Teasdale and Jennett (Table 424.2) and the techniques for evaluating brain stem function described by Plum and Posner. The neurologic examination consists of an assessment of the level of consciousness, as determined by eye opening, verbal responses, and reflex or purposive movements in response to noxious stimulation of the face, arms, and legs; neuro-ophthalmologic function, as indicated by pupillary size and response to light, spontaneous eye movements, oculocephalic (doll's eyes) and oculovestibular (ice water caloric) responses; and vegetative function, as reflected mainly by the respiratory pattern. Clinical neurologic signs can be correlated with specific anatomic sites, to establish the severity and extent of central nervous system dysfunction (Table 424.3).

LEVEL OF CONSCIOUSNESS

Level of consciousness is best determined by the ease and degree, if any, of behavioral arousal. Attempts should be made to elicit a behavioral motor response by verbal stimulation alone. If no response follows even shouted commands, noxious stimulation can be applied to the face by digital supraorbital pressure and individually to the arms and legs by compression of distal interphalangeal joints with a tongue blade or pen.

TABLE 424.2. **GLASGOW COMA SCALE**[a]	
Parameter	**Score**
Eye opening	
Spontaneous	4
To speech	3
To noxious stimulation	2
None	1
Best Motor Response	
Obeys commands	6
Localizes stimuli	5
Withdraws	4
Abnormal flexion	3
Extensor response	2
None	1
Verbal Response	
Oriented	5
Confused conversation	4
Inappropriate words	3
Incomprehensible sounds	2
None	1

[a] The coma score is the sum of individual scores for eye opening, motor, and verbal response of 3–15.

EVIDENCE LEVEL: A. Reference: Teasdale G, Jennett B. Assessment of coma and impaired consciousness: a practical scale. *Lancet* 1974;2:81.

TABLE 424.3.	CORRELATION BETWEEN LEVELS OF BRAIN FUNCTION AND CLINICAL SIGNS		
Structure	**Function**	**Clinical Sign**	
Cerebral cortex	Conscious behavior	Speech	
		Purposeful movement	
Brain stem sensory pathways	Arousal	Eye opening	
(reticular activating system)		Sleep/wake cycles	
Brain stem motor pathways	Reflex limb postures	Decorticate flexor posturing	
	Muscle tone	Decerebrate extensor posturing	
Midbrain			
CN III	Innervation of ciliary muscle	Pupillary reactivity	
Upper pons			
CN V	Corneal sensation	Corneal reflex—sensory	
CN VII	Facial muscle innervation	Corneal reflex—motor response	
Lower pons			
CN VIII (vestibular portion) connects via	Reflex eye movements	Doll's eyes	
brain stem pathways with CN III, IV, VI		Caloric responses	
Medulla	Regulation of breathing and	Spontaneous breathing	
	blood pressure	Maintained blood pressure	
Spinal cord	Primitive protective responses	Deep tendon reflexes	

CN, cranial nerve.

MOTOR RESPONSE

The absence of motor response, especially if flaccidity and areflexia are also present, indicates severe brain stem depression and is frequently found in terminal coma or in severe sedative intoxication. Decerebrate or extensor responses correlate with destructive lesions of the midbrain and upper pons but also may be present in reversible metabolic states, such as anoxic encephalopathy. Decorticate or flexor responses develop after damage to the hemispheres as well as in metabolic depression of brain function. Withdrawal and localizing responses imply purposeful or voluntary behavior. Obeying commands is the best response and marks the return of consciousness. Generalized or focal repetitive movements, not affected by stimuli, usually represent seizure activity. Focal seizures typically indicate a focal cortical lesion but also may be seen in hypoglycemia, hyperosmolarity, and some drug intoxications (with aminophylline and tricyclic antidepressants).

NEURO-OPHTHALMOLOGIC EXAMINATION

Fundi

The fundus of each eye should be examined for signs of increased intracranial pressure (papilledema and hemorrhage). Subhyaloid hemorrhage indicates the presence of subarachnoid or intracerebral hemorrhage but may follow severe head trauma.

Pupils

In coma due to metabolic brain disease, the pupils as a rule are small but reactive to light. Small, reactive pupils are present in normal people during sleep and are a common finding in elderly people, because of degenerative changes in the iris and ciliary muscles. Small, sluggishly reactive pupils that respond to naloxone administration are characteristic of an overdose of opiates. Pinpoint pupils are seen in pontine hemorrhage.

Bilateral dilated, fixed pupils indicate sympathetic nervous system overactivity because of either an endogenous sympathetic discharge (during anoxia–ischemia) or exogenous catecholamines (dopamine). Similar pupils, dilated or partially dilated, are seen in overdosage with tricyclic antidepressants or other atropine-like agents. In coma due to amphetamine, cocaine, and lysergic acid diethylamide overdosage, the pupils are large but reactive. Midposition, fixed pupils indicate midbrain failure and loss of both sympathetic and parasympathetic pupillary tone, whether caused by structural or metabolic disease. Such fixed and midposition, rather than dilated, pupils are seen in death.

A unilateral dilated, fixed pupil usually means damage to parasympathetic fibers of the third cranial nerve, as described previously in the case of uncal herniation. If the patient has suffered head trauma, an ipsilateral epidural or subdural hematoma is probably present. If there is no evidence of trauma, an intrahemispheric mass lesion (hematoma, tumor, or abscess) is the probable cause of herniation.

Eye Movements

Deeply comatose patients may have no spontaneous eye movements. In such cases, doll's eyes responses and the ice water caloric test can be used to determine the integrity of the eighth, sixth, and third cranial nerves and their interconnecting brain stem pathways. When the cortical influences are depressed but brain stem gaze mechanisms are intact, the eyes deviate conjugately to the opposite side if the head is rotated horizontally to one side. Brisk back-and-forth eye movements, like those of a doll in response to rocking the head to and fro, are characteristic of metabolic coma. Doll's eyes indicate the integrity of proprioceptive fibers from the neck structures, the vestibular nuclei, and the nuclei of the third and sixth cranial nerves. Unilateral lesions of the brain stem eliminate the doll's eyes response to the side of the lesion.

When the doll's eyes responses are absent, it becomes necessary to perform the ice water caloric test. In deep coma, the doll's eyes responses disappear before the ice water caloric responses, because the latter are produced by a stronger stimulus. The caloric response is elicited in comatose patients by irrigating the tympanum with 30 to 50 mL of ice water. When the patient is supine with the head elevated 30 degrees, cold water produces convection currents in the lateral semicircular canal that inhibit the firing of the ipsilateral vestibular nerve. In the absence of cortical influences on the oculovestibular pathways, cold water produces tonic deviation of the eyes to the side of irrigation. Metabolic factors (sedative, hypnotic coma, phenytoin overdose) and structural (brain stem) lesions eliminate the caloric response, as does labyrinthine disease. Dysconjugate ocular deviation implies a unilateral lesion or metabolic depression of brain stem pathways. If one or both eyes fail to adduct, the lesion is in the medial longitudinal fasciculus or third cranial nerve. The distinction between the two can be made by examination of the pupillary size and reaction to light. Failure of abduction indicates a lesion of the sixth cranial nerve.

■ MANAGEMENT OF THE PATIENT IN COMA OF UNKNOWN CAUSE

The initial management of the comatose patient is directed toward stabilization. The first step is to ensure an adequate airway, by intubation if necessary (Table 424.3). The respiratory rate and its pattern should be noted before they are obscured by therapeutic measures, such as intubation and mechanical ventilation.

HYPERVENTILATION

In a comatose patient, hyperventilation represents either compensation for metabolic acidosis or a response to primary respiratory stimulation (respiratory alkalosis). In metabolic acidosis, the arterial blood pH is usually less than 7.3, and the serum bicarbonate concentration is generally below 10 mEq per liter. In respiratory acidosis, lactic acidosis in cerebrospinal fluid stimulates medullary receptors in the absence of any systemic acidosis, so that the arterial pH is high (more than 7.45) and the serum bicarbonate concentration is normal or slightly reduced. In both metabolic acidosis and respiratory alkalosis, the arterial carbon dioxide partial pressure ($PaCO_2$) is often less than 30 mm Hg.

Mixed metabolic acidosis and respiratory alkalosis also can occur, especially in hepatic coma and excessive salicylate ingestion. Metabolic acidosis sufficient to produce coma and increased ventilation is frequently the result of one of the following conditions: uremia, diabetic ketoacidosis, lactic acidosis (anoxic or spontaneous), or ingestion of acidic substances. Diabetes and uremia are diagnosed by appropriate laboratory tests. If acidosis is independent of diabetes and uremia, the patient must have either spontaneous lactic acidosis or poisoning with exogenous toxins, such as methyl alcohol or ethyl glycol. The latter sources of metabolic acidosis can be treated effectively by giving intravenous infusions of sodium bicarbonate to restore the blood pH to normal.

Respiratory alkalosis is found in the context of coma due to salicylate ingestion, hepatic coma, pulmonary disease, and psychogenic hyperventilation. Salicylate poisoning causes combined respiratory alkalosis and metabolic acidosis that lowers the serum bicarbonate level disproportionately to the degree of serum pH elevation. Hepatic coma usually is accompanied by signs of liver dysfunction. Gram-negative sepsis always is associated with hyperventilation, probably because of a direct central effect of the endotoxin. Respiratory alkalosis caused by the pulmonary congestion of pneumonia rarely depresses the serum bicarbonate value. Psychogenic hyperventilation does not lead to coma, but it may be present as a symptom in a patient with psychogenic unresponsiveness.

HYPOVENTILATION

In a comatose patient, hypoventilation means either respiratory compensation for metabolic alkalosis or respiratory depression with consequent acidosis. In metabolic alkalosis, the arterial pH and the serum bicarbonate value are elevated. The $PaCO_2$ is high but is usually less than 50 mm Hg. In untreated respiratory acidosis, the arterial pH is low and the serum bicarbonate level is either normal or high, depending on previous treatment and the rapidity of onset of respiratory failure. The $PaCO_2$ is typically above 55 mm Hg. Metabolic alkalosis results from either excessive ingestion of alkali or excessive loss of acid through gastrointestinal and renal routes. Respiratory acidosis is caused either by severe pulmonary or neuromuscular disease (peripheral respiratory failure) or by damage to or depression of the medullary respiratory center (central respiratory failure). Severe respiratory acidosis of any origin is best treated by artificial respiration.

When adequate ventilation has been established, the following procedures are mandatory: blood should be drawn for a determination of blood glucose, routine chemistries, and toxicologic testing. Immediately afterward, 25 to 50 g of dextrose should be administered intravenously. Bedside glucose determinations are valuable in identifying hypoglycemia and hyperglycemia, but they should never delay the administration of dextrose. Even in cases of hyperosmolar coma, the administration of one ampule of dextrose is not harmful. Naloxone, 0.4 to 0.8 mg, and thiamine, 100 mg, should be administered intravenously to all patients, regardless of whether opiate or alcohol abuse is suggested. At this point, arterial blood gases should be analyzed to confirm that oxygenation is adequate.

Placement of a nasogastric tube may be indicated, to examine the stomach contents. This procedure always puts the patient at risk of aspiration, because the nasogastric tube dilates the gastroesophageal sphincter and permits regurgitation of gastric contents around the tube. Therefore, a cuffed endotracheal tube should be put in place for any patient in a coma or with a depressed gag reflex, before passage of nasogastric tube.

The blood pressure often provides the first clue to the etiologic diagnosis of coma. Hypertension can be a reflex response to the increased intracranial pressure (Cushing's reflex) or brain stem ischemia and commonly accompanies an intracranial hemorrhage. Rarely, hypertension per se may cause coma, as in hypertensive encephalopathy. Hypotension may indicate myocardial infarction, hemorrhagic shock, sepsis, or sedative, hypnotic drug overdose. The pulse rate and rhythm may be additional clues to the cause of coma and should be recorded and monitored. Bradycardia associated with an elevated blood pressure is an ominous sign of brain stem compression, and reversible causes of transtentorial herniation (subdural hematoma) should be considered immediately, before cardiovascular collapse ensues.

Measurement of the patient's temperature should not be neglected in the initial evaluation. Hypothermia can stem from Wernicke's disease, exposure, overdose with sedative drugs, near drowning, and hypothyroidism. This important sign often is not detected, because either the rectal temperature measurement is omitted or an ordinary thermometer is used that cannot detect temperatures below 95°F. Hypothermia below 80°F produces coma by itself; therefore, warming and resuscitative measures are indicated for all hypothermic patients, even if all vital signs are absent. Hypothermic patients have recovered after prolonged cardiorespiratory arrests, presumably because of the protective effects of low body temperature and depressed cerebral metabolism.

The presence of fever in a comatose patient demands an investigation for possible meningitis. If there is no history of trauma, the neck should be flexed to assess the presence of meningismus (stiff neck). When head trauma is a possible cause of coma, cervical spine injury should be assumed until the cervical spine can be examined by radiologic methods. Therefore, the neck should not be flexed but instead should be stabilized immediately by sandbags or headboard, to prevent movement during the physical and radiologic examinations.

A stiff neck may indicate bacterial meningitis or subarachnoid hemorrhage, but in the latter case there is often a delay of up to 12 hours before blood in the subarachnoid cerebrospinal fluid pathways has produced enough chemical irritation of the meninges to be detected by neck flexion. In deep coma, meningismus may be absent, despite the presence of bacterial or chemical meningitis. Other causes of fever include intracranial abscess and subdural empyema.

During this initial stabilization and assessment of the vital signs, the patient should be checked quickly for signs of head trauma (scalp laceration, bleeding from the ears, cerebrospinal fluid rhinorrhea) and spontaneous movements (seizures or posturing). On completion of the initial assessment and treatment, the physician may be able to categorize the cause of coma as either toxic, metabolic central nervous system depression or structural cerebral damage. A systemic physical examination with

special attention to certain key neurologic signs further delineates the cause of coma.

OUTCOME OF COMA AND COST-EFFECTIVENESS OF CARE

The mortality rate for all patients admitted to intensive care units in the United States is 25%; for patients in coma for more than 48 hours, it is 77%. Brain-dead patients who cannot benefit from intensive care must be identified.

CLINICAL CRITERIA OF BRAIN DEATH

Coma of Established Cause

The cerebral lesion must be structural, bearing in mind that an initially metabolic insult, as occurs in prolonged anoxia, can also lead to irreversible structural damage. Any possibility that the patient has drug poisoning or that hypothermia or an electrolyte abnormality is contributing to the depth of coma must be excluded by appropriate laboratory tests. The patient should have no clinical evidence of cerebral function or brain stem reflexes for a period of at least 12 hours, with no demonstrable improvement whatsoever. This period of observation must be extended to 24 or more hours, or until negative toxicology screen results are obtained, if drug overdosage is a possibility. The period of observation may be shortened to as little as 6 hours if, for example, a competent neurosurgeon explores a head wound and finds the brain transected or if one or more supplementary tests (electroencephalography, angiography) confirms the absence of cerebral circulation or electrical activity.

No Cerebral Function

There must be no appropriate response to noxious stimulation, in that the patient must not arouse, groan, grimace, withdraw the head or limbs from an applied stimulus, or attempt to push away the examiner's hand. Reflex responses, such as decerebrate extension or decorticate flexion of the limbs, which are mediated by subcortical but supraspinal cord pathways, cannot be present if a diagnosis of brain death is contemplated. The spinal cord may be intact; therefore, rudimentary reflex responses, such as muscle stretch reflexes, planar flexion, plantar withdrawal (triple flexion), abdominal reflex, and tonic neck reflexes, all of which depend on functions of the spinal cord, may be preserved.

No Brain Stem Reflexes

The pupils must be fixed to light stimulation. The corneal blink reflex must be absent. Both the doll's eyes and ice water caloric responses must be absent. The patient must be apneic and not recover spontaneous ventilatory function after the respirator has been turned off to allow $PaCO_2$ to attain a level high enough maximally to stimulate respiratory drive. Evidence indicates that the threshold for respiratory stimulation may approach a Pa_{CO_2} of 60 mm Hg in patients with brain damage and the rate of rise of Pa_{CO_2} during respiratory arrest is about 3 mm Hg per minute. The duration of respiratory arrest needed to allow Pa_{CO_2} to reach or exceed 60 mm Hg is not constant and varies depending on the level of Pa_{CO_2} before the onset of apnea. Therefore, to confirm absolute apnea, blood gas monitoring is required to verify normocapnia, before beginning apneic oxygenation for 10 minutes, or, if a patient is hypocapnic, Pa_{CO_2} in excess of 60 mm Hg at the end of apnea. No absolute period of apnea sufficient to establish brain death can be recommended in the absence of blood gas determinations. Brain-dead subjects are easily identified and constitute a small population among comatose subjects. A far larger number of comatose patients are those with severe brain damage in whom the prognosis is in doubt. For some patients, intensive care serves only to promote survival in the vegetative state.

PREDICTION OF OUTCOME IN COMA

Studies indicate that despite the best treatment, about 40% of patients unconscious from head trauma and only 15% of those unconscious from nontraumatic causes make a satisfactory neurologic recovery. Critical care physicians have identified certain features that predict a limited response to intensive care of acute illness (advanced age and chronic poor health), but these features do not indicate outcome in individual cases. Several groups of neurologists and neurosurgeons have tried to identify and quantify early indicators that might correlate with prognosis. The results of parallel collaborative studies of 1,500 head-injured and 500 medical coma patients indicate that within a few hours or days after the onset of coma, many patients show neurologic signs that differentiate, with a high degree of probability, the outcome extremes of death or vegetative state from good recovery.

BIBLIOGRAPHY

Jennett B, Bond M. Assessment of outcome after severe brain damage: a practical scale. *Lancet* 1975;1:480–484.

Jennett B, Plum F. Persistent vegetative state after brain damage: a syndrome in search of a name. *Lancet* 1972;1:734–737.

Jennett B, Teasdale G. *Management of head injuries.* Philadelphia: FA Davis, 1981.

Levy DE, Bates D, Caronna JJ, et al. Prognosis in nontraumatic coma. *Ann Intern Med* 1981;94:293–301.

Medical Consultants on the Diagnosis of Death to the President's Commission for the Study of Ethical Problems in Medicine and Biomedical and Behavioral Research. Guidelines for the determination of death. *JAMA* 1981;246:2184–2186.

Plum F, Posner JB. *The diagnosis of stupor and coma,* third ed. Philadelphia: FA Davis, 1982.

Teasdale G, Jennett B. Assessment of coma and impaired consciousness: a practical scale. *Lancet* 1974;2:81–84.

Teres D, Brown RB, Lemeshow S. Predicting mortality of intensive care unit patients. The importance of coma. *Crit Care Med* 1982;10:86–95.

Kelley's Textbook of Internal Medicine, fourth edition. Edited by H. David Humes. Lippincott Williams & Wilkins, Philadelphia © 2000.

APPROACH TO THE PATIENT WITH A SLEEP DISORDER

ROGER J. BROUGHTON

During the 1980s and early 1990s, the clinical importance of sleep became increasingly evident, with the consequent creation of a field of sleep disorders medicine. Epidemiologic studies have shown that at least 10% of people in all decades of life have clinically significant sleep disorders. There are more than 70 discrete sleep disorders. Conditions with symptoms of excessive daytime sleepiness and irresistible sleep attacks unexpectedly have been more common than types of insomnia in patients referred to sleep disorders clinics. In patients with chronic insomnia not caused by sleep hygiene abuse, pulmonary or other medical conditions have been responsible more often than stress-related and other psychogenetic mechanisms.

▉ NORMAL SLEEP

Defining a sleep disorder requires an understanding of normal sleep. Marked changes of sleep occur as a function of age. Neonates sleep in a polyphasic napping fashion around the 24 hours, obtaining an average of close to 8 hours of sleep both at night and in the daytime. They experience lengthy slow-wave sleep (the deepest stages of non–rapid eye movement [NREM] sleep) and rapid eye movement (REM) sleep, and the NREM/REM sleep cycle shows rapid periodicity at 45 to 50 minutes. In childhood, there is rapid consolidation of night sleep, with reduction of daytime napping to three, then two, and finally to a single (almost always afternoon) nap, typically given up at 5 to 6 years of age, when school is attended for the entire day. By adulthood, mean sleep duration is some 6 to 8.5 hours per night, with NREM sleep representing 75% to 80% (deep slow-wave sleep is 5% to 15%) and REM sleep some 20% to 25%; there is little wakefulness after sleep onset. The NREM/REM cycle period slows to 90 to 110 minutes.

In the elderly, sleep fragments, with frequent awakenings, and lightens, with little slow-wave sleep. A return to daytime napping becomes commonplace. The elderly may misperceive this change in night sleep as insomnia and request hypnotics. The normal elderly, however, feel alert in the daytime, and hypnotics only make the quality of night sleep deteriorate and increase daytime sleepiness. Studies under conditions without time cues (*Zeitgebers*) show that the endogenous period of the circadian sleep rhythm is 24.1 to 25.5 hours. Factors (sunlight, alarm clocks, social noise, and so on) that cause awakening at a regular hour entrain sleep to a 24-hour periodicity and keep us from going to sleep later each day. They also confirm the existence of an endogenous twice-daily rhythm, with major and minor sleep periods. In the entrained condition, the latter occurs around midafternoon (the time of the siesta and the last nap given up in ontogeny).

CLASSIFICATION OF SLEEP DISORDERS

Determining the existence of a sleep disorder is not always easy. It is important to recognize the wide variation of normal sleep patterns at all ages. There are morning people (larks) and evening people (owls), light sleepers and deep sleepers, non-nappers and nappers, and short sleepers and long sleepers, all meeting their sleep need per 24 hours. Moreover, events that can constitute a sleep disorder, such as sleep apnea or periodic limb movements, often occur at low frequency in asymptomatic normal people.

A sleep disorder may be said to exist in the context of long-term excessive daytime sleepiness with or without irresistible sleep episodes, significant problems going to sleep or remaining asleep, an undesired change in the circadian timing of sleep/wake states, and episodic behavioral episodes in sleep that disrupt personal or family life or risk injury to self or others. This tetrad of signs and symptoms has formed the basis of a number of classifications of sleep disorders. It has become evident that a single diagnostic entity may take the form of daytime sleepiness, insomnia, or even parasomnia.

The most recent classification of the American Sleep Disorders Association therefore replaces a structure based on symptomatic differential diagnosis by one of final diagnosis. It distinguishes three main groups: *dyssomnias* (subgrouped according to whether the causes are intrinsic or extrinsic to the body or of circadian rhythm origin), *parasomnias* (subgrouped into those involving arousals, sleep/wake transitions, REM sleep, or other), and *sleep disorders associated with medical or psychiatric conditions*. A fourth group lists those proposed sleep disorders that remain incompletely identified. This classification (simplified in Table 425.1) has been accepted by the European and Japanese sleep societies, is compatible with international disease classifications (International Classification of Diseases and World Health Organization), and is recommended.

INVESTIGATION

The value of a careful history for diagnosing sleep disorders cannot be overemphasized. The patient is often unaware of behaviors in sleep, so that information from the sleeping partner is frequently essential. Parents of sleep-disturbed children must be questioned. Sleep-related symptoms must be assessed in terms of intensity and duration. The amount, quality, and temporal stability of nocturnal sleep and of any habitual daytime naps should be documented, as should evidence of daytime sleepiness, brief microsleeps (lapses), amnesic automatic states, and irresistible sleep attacks. Problems getting to sleep both at night and during daytime naps should be sought, to detect sleep-onset forms of insomnia. If awakenings are a problem at night, questions concerning their possible cause (nightmares, full bladder, pain, intense erections, respiratory difficulties) must be posed.

TABLE 425.1.	CLASSIFICATION OF SELECTED SLEEP DISORDERS

Dyssomnias
  Intrinsic sleep disorders
    Psychophysiologic insomnia
    Narcolepsy-cataplexy syndrome[a]
    Idiopathic and symptomatic hypersomnias[a]
    Sleep apnea, syndromes (obstructive, central)[a]
    Periodic limb movement disorders.
  Extrinsic sleep disorders
    Inadequate sleep hygiene
    Environmental sleep disorder
    Sleep-onset insomnia disorder
    Substance-dependent sleep disorders
    Nocturnal eating (drinking) syndrome
  Circadian rhythm sleep disorders
    Time-zone change (jet lag) syndrome
    Shift work sleep disorder
    Irregular sleep/wake pattern
    Delayed sleep phase syndrome
    Advanced sleep phase syndrome
Sleep disorders associated with medical/psychiatric disorders
  Associated with mental disorders (psychoses, anxiety, alcoholism)
  Associated with neurologic disorders (degeneration, epilepsy, headache)[a]
  Associated with other medical disorders (chronic obstructive pulmonary disease, asthma, gastroesophageal reflux)
Parasomnias
  Arousal disorders
    Sleepwalking
    Sleep terrors
  Sleep/wake transition disorders
    Rhythmic movement disorder (jactatio capitis)
    Sleep starts
  Parasomnias usually associated with REM sleep
    Nightmares
    Sleep paralysis (familial, isolated)[a]
    REM sleep behavior disorder
  Other parasomnias
    Sleep bruxism
    Sleep enuresis

[a] These conditions are all of central nervous system origin.
REM, rapid eye movement.
(From Diagnostic Classification Steering Committee *International classification of sleep disorders: diagnostic and coding manual.* Rochester, Minn.: American Sleep Disorders Association, 1990, with permission.)

In patients with daytime sleepiness or sleep attacks, questioning for the presence of cataplexy and sleep paralysis is needed, to arrive at a diagnosis of narcolepsy syndrome. Prolonged 1- to 4-hour daytime sleep episodes, chronic sleepiness, deep night sleep, and marked morning sleep drunkenness all suggest either idiopathic or symptomatic hypersomnia. Breathing problems in sleep are often unrecognized by the patient, who may exhibit loud snoring or visible apneic pauses terminated by inspiratory snorting, which are disturbing to the bed partner. Patients are typically unaware of motor disorders taking place during sleep, such as periodic movements in sleep, or nocturnal paroxysmal dystonia, whereas restless legs or intense hypnagogic jerks (sleep starts) at sleep onset are readily perceived.

Information concerning the circadian timing of sleep may disclose a delayed, advanced, irregular, or about 25-hour sleep/wake periodicity. Occupational questions should quickly determine problems due to rotating shift work or frequent jet lag. There may be episodic behaviors during sleep, which require careful interrogation pertaining to the differentiation of sleep terrors, sleepwalking, confusional arousals, REM nightmares, REM sleep behavior disorder, nocturnal epileptic seizures, sleep talking, bruxism, jactatio capitis (rhythmic movement disorder), and other parasomnias. It is always important to obtain information concerning sleep hygiene, including the regularity of retiring and morning awakening, daily exercise habits, and intake of central nervous system active substances, including caffeine, nicotine, alcohol, and others.

A full physical examination should always be carried out, because a large variety of illnesses may underlie sleep problems. Sleep/wake tests are often indicated for specific diagnosis. Overnight polysomnography combines recording of the electroencephalogram, electrooculogram, and submental electromyogram for sleep/wake state scoring. These variables are combined with leg electromyography to detect movement abnormalities; electrocardiography for cardiac abnormalities; and upper airway airflow, chest and abdominal movement, and transcutaneous oxygen saturation monitoring for (often occult) respiratory problems. Videotaping of behavior is often indicated for analysis of parasomnias and, to permit full movement, preferably is associated with telemetry. Daytime sleepiness and ability to fall asleep can be quantified by the Multiple Sleep Latency Test or Maintenance of Wakefulness Test. Each test has five 20-minute nap periods scheduled every 2 hours across the day. In the former, the subject is requested to fall asleep as rapidly as possible, whereas in the latter, the subject is asked to try to remain awake. Ambulatory monitoring may be indicated for assessment of sleep/wake patterns around the 24 hours. Sleep logs may provide valuable information, especially on sleep timing.

Other laboratory tests are frequently indicated and are tailored to the provisional diagnosis. Daytime pulmonary function tests, though they often show negative results in the context of obstructive and central sleep apnea, may be helpful in chronic obstructive pulmonary disease and other respiratory diseases causing a sleep disorder. Fiberoptic and other examinations of the upper airway for obstruction are often necessary in apneic patients. Radiologic procedures may be needed, including magnetic resonance imaging of the brain stem sleep-regulatory structures. In some patients, metabolic (hepatic, renal) or endocrine (thyroid, hypothalamopituitary) causes may be suggested and assessed by appropriate laboratory tests. Tissue typing of human leukocyte antigen for DR2 and DQW1 haplotypes is helpful to rule out narcolepsy syndrome. Follow-up assessment after some 1 to 2 months of appropriate therapy is important for most sleep disorder patients. Whenever possible, central nervous system active medication should be reduced to the minimal clinically efficacious dose.

BIBLIOGRAPHY

Broughton R. Polygraphic recordings of sleep and sleep disorders. In: Niedermeyer E, Lopes da Silva F, eds. *Electroencephalography*. Baltimore: Urban & Schwartenberg, 1987.

Diagnostic Classification Steering Committee. *International classification of sleep disorders: diagnostic and coding manual.* Rochester, Minn.: American Sleep Disorders Association, 1990.

Guilleminault C. *Sleeping and waking disorders: indications and techniques.* Reading, Mass.: Addison-Wesley, 1982.

Guilleminault C, ed. *Sleep and its disorders in children.* New York: Raven Press, 1987.

Hauri P. *The sleep disorders.* Kalamazoo, Mich.: Upjohn, 1977.

Kryger M, Roth T, Dement WC, eds. *Principles and practice of sleep medicine*, second ed. Philadelphia: WB Saunders, 1994.

Mendelson WB. *Human sleep: research and clinical care.* New York: Plenum, 1987.

Parkes D. *Sleep and its disorders.* Philadelphia: WB Saunders, 1985.

Roffwarg H, Clark RW, Guilleminault C, et al. Diagnostic classification of sleep and arousal disorders. 1979 first edition. Association of Sleep Disorders Centers and the Asociation for the Psychophysiological Study of Sleep. *Sleep* 1979;2:1–154.

Saunders NA, Sullivan CE, eds. *Sleep and breathing*, second ed. New York: Marcel Dekker, 1994.

Kelley's Textbook of Internal Medicine, fourth edition. Edited by H. David Humes. Lippincott Williams & Wilkins, Philadelphia © 2000.

CHAPTER 426

APPROACH TO THE PATIENT WITH SEIZURES

ANTONIO V. DELGADO-ESCUETA

A team approach is vital to the successful treatment of epilepsy. The physician in charge should manage and coordinate the efforts of specialists, including professionals in neurology, pharmacology, psychology, psychiatry, and social services. The physician should foster understanding and support among the patient's family, employer, and school, with the following goals:

1. Verify that seizures are epileptic and differentiate them from syncope, drop attacks, and nonepileptic seizures.
2. Define seizure types and epilepsy syndrome.
3. Determine causes of seizures and block trigger factors.
4. Establish an early treatment plan with choice antiepileptic drugs and understand the clinical context and medical background of the patient.
5. Monitor seizure control and recognize adverse effects on the patient's quality of life; recognize, treat, and hospitalize patients with status epilepticus; advise the patient to seek education and support services from the local chapter of the Epilepsy Foundation.
6. Refer for possible surgical treatment or vagal nerve stimulation when seizures are resistant to antiepileptic drugs.

SIGNS AND SYMPTOMS OF SEIZURES

VERIFY EPILEPSY

When a patient loses consciousness episodically, epilepsy should be distinguished from syncope, pseudoepileptic seizures, drop attacks, and drug-induced or withdrawal seizures. Although closed-circuit television videotaping with biotelemetry of the electroencephalogram (CCTV-EEG) and Holter monitoring of the electrocardiogram have shown important clinical differences among these conditions, the history and context are often the most important determinants of the diagnosis.

Twenty percent of patients believed to have epilepsy actually experience nonepileptic seizures. Four common causes of nonepileptic seizures are hyperventilation, hysteria, alcohol withdrawal, and cocaine use. The provoking factor for hyperventilation is sometimes difficult to discover. Rapid, shallow breathing is present, and the patient feels light-headed, with trembling limbs and often trembling of the whole body. Excessive loss of carbon dioxide produces paresthesias in the hands, face, and feet; carpopedal spasms may develop.

Syncope

Syncope occurs in up to 25% to 30% of young healthy adults. (See Chapter 69 for a more detailed discussion of syncope.) Postural tone and consciousness are suddenly lost, and the patient falls. Most frequently, syncope is due to a temporary decrease in cerebral blood flow, resulting from either a fall in systemic arterial pressure (vasovagal syncope) or a decline in cardiac output (cardiac syncope). The clinical picture of pallor, flaccidity, upward deviation of the eyes, and loss of consciousness in simple syncope is paralleled by the appearance of 2- to 4-Hz high-amplitude slow waves on the EEG. The persistence of cerebral anoxia for more than 15 seconds is reflected by tonic spasms and one or two generalized jerks (convulsive syncope). The EEG becomes slow and low voltage but promptly returns to normal after consciousness is regained. Less often, syncope can be produced by hypoglycemia or hypoxia, characterized by gradual loss and regaining of consciousness. Aortic valvular stenosis, hypersensitive stretch receptors in the carotid sinus, micturition, explosive vigorous coughing, pain, and orthostatic hypotension can all provoke syncope.

Pseudoepileptic Psychogenic Seizures

An audience is usually present during hysterical or psychogenic seizures. Consciousness is preserved, amnesia is absent or patchy, and movements that simulate epileptic convulsions do not have tonic–clonic phases or in-phase clonic movements of the upper extremities. Movements are out of phase, chaotic, and bizarre, without stereotype. Side-to-side head movements are noted in one-third of patients and forward pelvic thrusting in almost half of those experiencing psychogenic seizures. The duration is usually longer than the average 70 seconds of a tonic–clonic convulsion. The attack ends abruptly, with the patient alert and showing no postictal tiredness, sleep, or Todd's paralysis. A psychiatric history is usually present; psychogenic seizures are seldom the sole symptom and sign.

Psychogenic fits and epileptic seizures can exist together in the same patient. The EEG and prolactin levels are especially useful in distinguishing the two. A main indication for CCTV-EEG intensive monitoring is the differentiation of pseudoepileptic from epileptic seizures. During and immediately after epileptic seizures, the EEG almost always shows abnormal results. Between epileptic seizures, the EEG gives abnormal results in 40% to 60% of patients. The EEG is normal between, during, and after hysterical attacks. Serum prolactin levels increase within 20 minutes of a tonic–clonic convulsion or complex partial seizure but do not change with pseudoepileptic hysterical fits.

Drop Attacks

Episodic ischemia of the brain stem, which may occur in elderly patients with insufficient blood flow throughout the vertebrobasilar system, is usually of atherosclerotic origin. Transient ischemic attacks affecting the brain stem can cause episodic loss of tone, with falls. Consciousness usually is preserved, and there are no convulsions. EEGs between episodes show normal results.

Drug-induced or Withdrawal Seizures

A history of psychiatric problems, post-traumatic seizures, and convulsions induced by abstinence is not uncommon in the context of chronic alcoholism. Seizures can be induced by alcohol, but withdrawal seizures are more common. Tonic–clonic seizures appear 24 to 48 hours (up to 7 days) after alcohol withdrawal. Confusion, delusions, and visual, tactile, and auditory hallucinations (alcoholic hallucinosis) accompany agitation and can progress to delirium tremens, lasting up to 5 days. Hypoglycemia can complicate the picture. Subdural or epidural hematoma must be excluded. Smoking of crack or cocaine paste can provoke tonic–clonic convulsions that appear at the height of or immediately after the high. In severe cocaine toxicity, respiratory depression, cardiac dysrhythmias, a hypermetabolic state, and status epilepticus can occur. Alcohol withdrawal convulsions, delirium tremens, and cocaine convulsions are medical emergencies and can be treated effectively with benzodiazepines. Ventricular dysrhythmias in cocaine toxicity can be treated with intravenous propranolol (0.5 to 1 mg).

HISTORY AND PHYSICAL AND LABORATORY EXAMINATION

DEFINE SEIZURE TYPE(S) AND EPILEPSY SYNDROME

A detailed case history and description of the first and subsequent attacks must be obtained from the patient and relatives. Figure 426.1 shows an algorithm for diagnosis and initial management. Are the seizures partial or generalized? Is the epilepsy syndrome idiopathic or symptomatic? In partial epilepsies, the first seizure and its aura can give clues about its site of origin. Changes in character in subsequent attacks may suggest progression of a

A

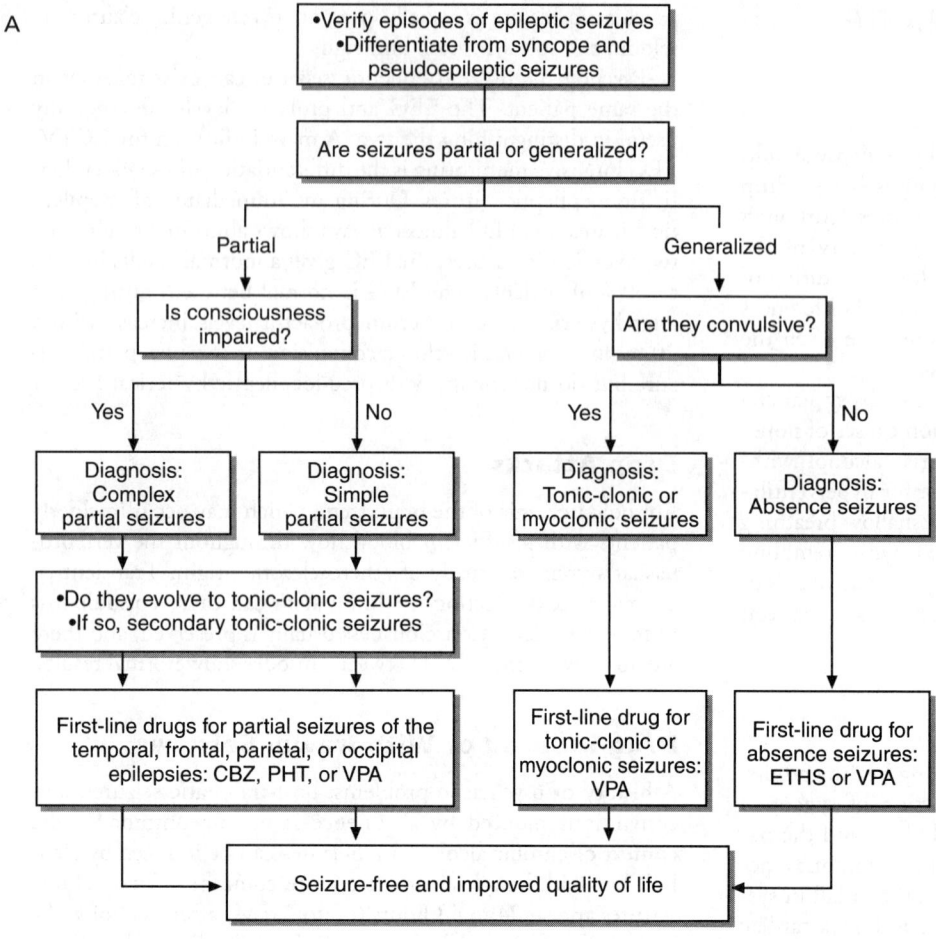

FIGURE 426.1. Diagnosis (**A**) and initial management (**B**) of epileptic seizures. *Continues.*

structural lesion or may reflect the effects of antiepileptic drugs. (See Tables 444.1 to 444.4 in Chapter 444.)

The EEG is indispensable when symptoms point to epilepsy. It should be carried out with the patient awake and asleep and with photic stimulation and hyperventilation. It is typical for sleep to activate epileptogenic paroxysms in both partial and generalized epilepsies. Sleep deprivation is another way to activate EEG abnormalities in the idiopathic generalized epilepsies. Hyperventilation often provokes pyknoleptic absences in the context of childhood absence epilepsy. In complex partial seizures, nasopharyngeal, nasoethmoid, or sphenoid electrodes may be necessary.

IDENTIFY UNDERLYING CAUSES

In most cases of symptomatic epilepsies, the cause(s) of seizures can be identified. Brain magnetic resonance imaging (MRI) or computed tomography (CT) or both are recommended for all adults with symptomatic partial seizures. Positron emission tomography with fluorodeoxyglucose is recommended for surgical candidates. MRI T1- and T2-weighted axial and coronal planes can image neuronal migration disorders, such as cortical dysplasia and hamartomas; clarify the picture of cavernous hemangioma noted earlier on CT as calcifications; and detect low-grade glioma undiagnosed by CT scans. MRI also can show atrophy of the hippocampus by volume measurements of the hippocampus.

Coronal planes can verify hippocampal atrophy and gliosis. Routine MRI is still necessary in benign epilepsy syndromes, such as juvenile myoclonic epilepsy, juvenile or childhood absence epilepsy, or rolandic epilepsy, to rule out symptomatic epilepsies.

Postictal hemiparesis (Todd's paralysis) and postictal dysphasia point to a focal cerebral lesion. Provoking factors, such as sleep deprivation, alcohol, and sleep or awakening states, must be identified. Clusters of seizures before or during menses (catamenial seizures) are often present. When seizures start in childhood, adolescence, and young adulthood, the birth history is of value. Headaches and visual hemisensory or hemimotor complaints suggest a focal lesion. Seizures associated with fever and meningeal signs indicate meningitis or encephalitis and warrant a lumbar puncture.

STRATEGIES FOR OPTIMAL CARE

ESTABLISH AN EARLY TREATMENT PLAN

When to Start Treatment

Antiepileptic therapy is obligatory for generalized or partial epilepsies. The diagnosis of epilepsy implies chronic or recurrent seizures. Uncontrolled convulsions can cause selective cell damage in the cerebral cortex, hippocampus, amygdala, and cerebel-

B

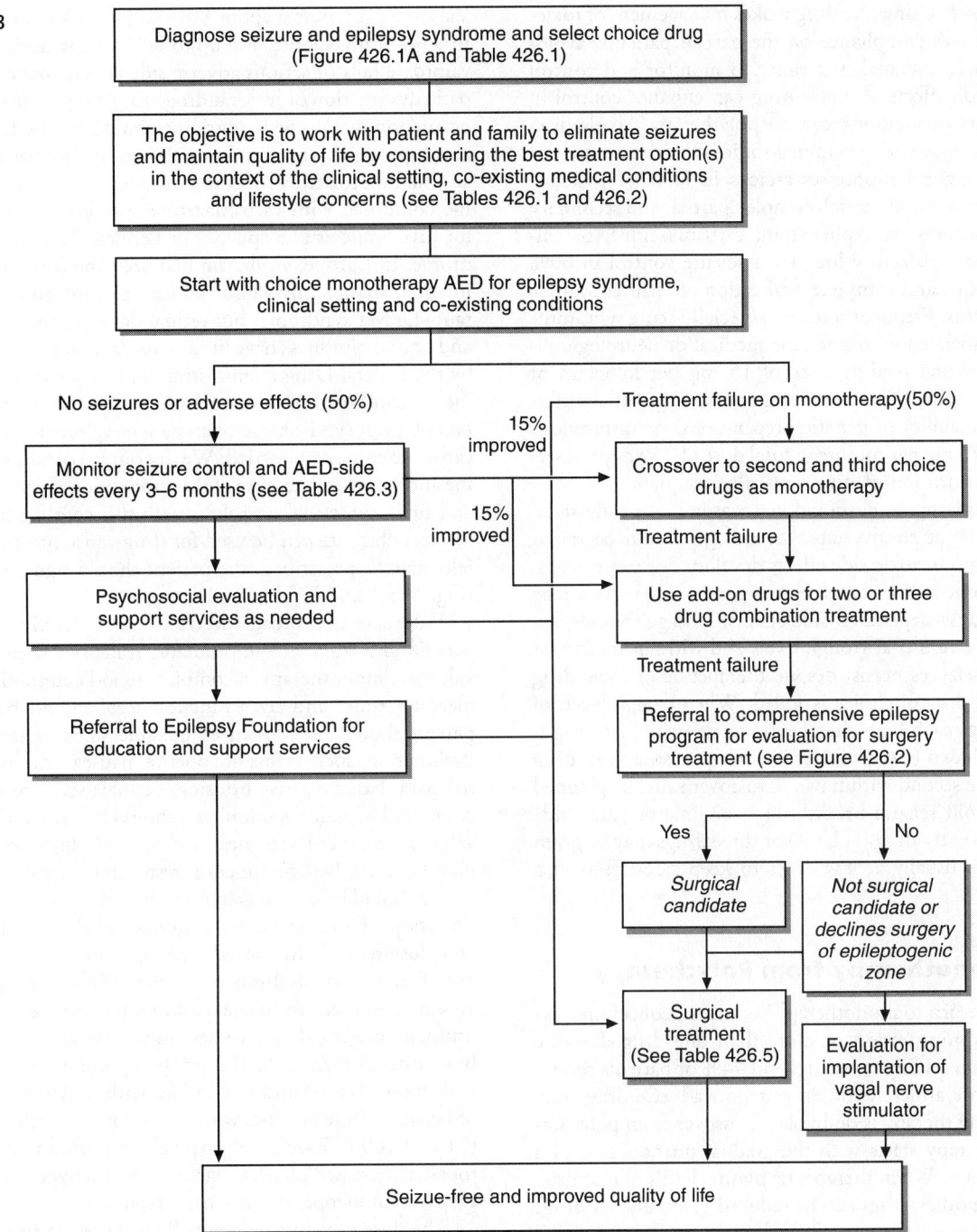

FIGURE 426.1. *Continued.*

lum. Induction of the kindling-mirror focus phenomenon and morphologic evidence of progressive neuronal and dendritic spine degeneration provide even more compelling arguments for the treatment of all forms of epilepsy.

Antiepileptic treatment is seldom indicated, however, after a single tonic–clonic seizure. Most patients who experience such an episode have no risk factors for epilepsy and show normal results on neurologic and EEG examinations, but epilepsy develops in about 25% of them. A strong family history, an aura, absence or complex partial (focal) onset, abnormal neurologic examination findings, and epileptiform EEG patterns require immediate investigation and treatment. Treatment may be postponed if a single tonic–clonic seizure is related to sleep deprivation (more than 36 hours), stress, extreme fatigue, drug or alcohol withdrawal, or use of cocaine.

Start with Monotherapy

The aim of treatment is to control seizures without drug toxicity. Treatment should begin with one antiepileptic drug, preferably the drug of choice. Using one drug makes management of toxicity easier, improves compliance on the part of patients, avoids drug interactions, and makes it easier to monitor and control idiosyncratic side effects. A single drug can enhance control in 40% of patients previously receiving polytherapy. Single-drug treatment of absence with grand mal tonic–clonic seizures and/or myoclonic seizures suppresses attacks in 80% of patients. Single-drug treatment of partial, complex partial, and secondary tonic–clonic seizures with phenytoin, carbamazepine, or valproate results in satisfactory long-term seizure control in 60% to 90% of patients and complete eradication of seizures in 40% to 60% of patients. Frequent seizures, especially acute symptomatic seizures associated with a serious medical or neurologic illness, require an oral loading dose of 15 mg per kilogram of phenytoin (preferably Dilantin, because of the substantial differences in bioavailability of generic preparations) or intravenous fosphenytoin (75 mg per minute to total dose of 750 mg); otherwise, gradual institution of drug is usually adequate.

The trough plasma level should be measured at steady state. If seizures persist at steady state, the dosage should be raised until seizures stop or toxic side effects develop. For some drugs, such as primidone and carbamazepine, peak plasma levels may correlate with dose-dependent side effects. Dosage should produce therapeutic results at trough levels and without toxicity at peak levels. If seizures persist despite therapeutic or toxic drug levels, a second drug of choice is added. When trough levels of the second drug reach high therapeutic ranges, the first drug is gradually withdrawn (crossover). If seizures persist, a third drug is added and the second withdrawn. Crossover must be planned carefully, to avoid seizure breakthrough or unanticipated side effects. If single-entry drugs fail, two or three drugs may be given in combination, usually at low doses to keep side effects at a minimum.

Shift to Monotherapy from Polytherapy

Patients often return to monotherapy because of continuing seizures despite administration of more than one drug. Because 34% of patients receiving two drugs and 44% of patients receiving three or more antiepileptic drugs report adverse drug reactions, single-drug therapy is desirable. Crossover from polytherapy to monotherapy starts with the gradual introduction of a first drug of choice. When therapeutic plasma levels of that drug are reached, the other drugs can be reduced gradually. As drugs are withdrawn, plasma levels of the first drug of choice commonly rise. Nonessential drugs and those with interactions and undesirable side effects are withdrawn first. Withdrawal usually takes place over a 1- to 3-month period, with monitoring of plasma drug levels. An 8-hour outpatient CCTV-EEG monitoring session can be helpful.

CHOOSE FIRST-LINE DRUGS

Primary Generalized Genetic Epilepsies

The first-line drug for primary generalized convulsive epilepsies, such as pure grand mal, juvenile myoclonic, photosensitive, and combined absence/grand mal epilepsies, is sodium valproate.

Valproate suppresses about 80% to 90% of tonic–clonic, 80% to 95% of myoclonic, and up to 90% of absence attacks. When valproate fails or serious adverse side effects (pancreatitis or hepatic dysfunction or hyperandrogenism/polycystic ovary disease) occur, topiramate or lamotrigine should be tried. These drugs also suppress absences and myoclonias. Isolated absence seizures are still best treated with ethosuximide. Topiramate or lamotrigine combined with carbamazepine are now the start-up drugs for myoclonic astatic epilepsy or Lennox–Gastaut–Dravet syndrome. In Europe, vigabatrin had been the first-choice drug for infantile spasms, myoclonic astatic epilepsy, and Lennox–Gastaut–Dravet syndrome, but retinal damage, visual field defects, and partial blindness have limited its use and prevented approval by the Federal Drug Administration. If topiramate or lamotrigine in combination with carbamazepine fails in Lennox–Gastaut–Dravet syndrome, clonazepam or valproate combined with carbamazepine can be tried. We discourage combining lamotrigine and valproate, because of the appearance of generalized rashes and toxic epidermal necrolysis with this combination. As a last resort, felbamate can be used for drug-resistant drop seizures. If felbamate is prescribed, the patient should sign a consent form (Fig. 426.1 and Table 426.1).

Valproate is a broad-spectrum agent effective against both genetic and lesional symptomatic epilepsies. Before initiating valproate monotherapy, a complete blood count, platelet count, bleeding time, and liver function tests should be done. The patient should be warned of possible signs of serious hepatic dysfunction, such as loss of appetite, nausea, vomiting, abdominal pain, lethargy, easy bruising, or malaise. A complete blood count and hepatic function tests should be carried out again and valproate plasma levels measured after 10 days. Serial complete blood counts, hepatic function tests, and careful clinical monitoring should be undertaken every month for the first 6 months. Elevation of the serum transaminase level is usually transient and dose-related. In sporadic cases, it may mean serious and even fatal hepatic dysfunction. Hepatic failure seems to be idiosyncratic and related to age: children less than 2 years old, with unusual congenital syndromes, mental retardation, or organic brain disease, seem to be the group at primary risk (one in 7,000 with monotherapy and one in 500 with polytherapy). The rate of hepatic failure declines with age and is rare with monotherapy (11 in 37,000). Rarely, valproate also has produced thrombocytopenia, increased platelet aggregation, and hypofibrinogenemia. Hyperammonemia also has been reported.

The dose of valproate gradually is increased from 125 mg or 250 mg in capsule form daily, to achieve trough plasma levels of 60 to 80 μg per milliliter (usually 250 mg three times daily). The final dosage may be 500 mg taken three times daily. Valproate is quickly absorbed and eliminated and controls attacks at lower dosages (15 to 18 mg per kilogram) when used alone. Nausea and vomiting appear when the dose is increased too quickly. Gastric irritation can be minimized by taking the capsules after meals. Hair loss and tremors are common side effects. Excessive weight gain, hyperandrogenism, and signs of polycystic ovaries warrant discontinuation.

Ethosuximide controls 60% of cases of childhood absence epilepsy not associated with tonic–clonic seizures. It is absorbed quickly (0.5 to 4 hours), and steady state is reached in 1 week.

	TABLE 426.1.	**COMMON EPILEPSY SYNDROMES WITH CHOICE ANTIEPILEPTIC DRUGS**		
Syndrome		**First-Choice Drug**	**Second-Choice Drug**	**Third-Choice Drug**
Idiopathic				
Absence only		ETHS	VPA or CNZ	LTG
Absence plus grand mal tonic–clonic		VPA	LTG or TPR or ETHS + PHT or ETHS + CBZ	TM + PHT or TM + CBZ
Juvenile myoclonic epilepsy		VPA	LTG or TPR	TM + PHT or TM + CBZ
Benign childhood epilepsy, e.g., rolandic epilepsy		CBZ or PHT	VPA or CNZ	LTG or TPR
Symptomatic				
Lennox-Gastaut-Dravet syndrome		LTG or TPR	GBP + CBZ or LTG + CBZ or VPA + CBZ or TPR + CBZ	FB
Temporal lobe epilepsy		CBZ or PHT	GBP or LTG or TPR	TB
Frontal lobe epilepsy		CBZ or PHT or VPA	GBP or LTG or TPR	TB
Epilepsy in elderly		GBP	PHT or CBZ LTG or TPR	TB

ETHS, ethosuximide (Zarontin); VPA, valproate (Depakote); TPR, topiramate (Topamax); CBZ, carbamazepine (Tegretol); LTG, lamotrigine (Lamictal); PHT, phenytoin (Dilantin); CNZ, clonazepam (Klonopin); TM, trimethadione (Tridione); GBP, gabapentin (Neurontin); FB, felbamate (Felbatol); and TB, tiagabine (Gabitril).

It has an average half-life of 24 to 30 hours in children, with a longer half-life in adults. Dose-dependent side effects include nausea, vomiting, anorexia, dyspepsia, night terrors, motor unrest, agitation, and paranoid psychoses. Rash and thrombocytopenia may suggest uncommon idiosyncratic side effects, such as aplastic anemia and agranulocytosis.

Lamotrigine is also a broad-spectrum agent effective both as monotherapy and as an add-on agent against genetic generalized epilepsies (including JME and absences) and lesional partial, complex partial, and secondary generalized seizures. It is also effective in limiting the atonic drop seizures of Lennox–Gastaut–Dravet syndrome. Sodium valproate inhibits the metabolism of lamotrigine, doubling the elimination half-life from 29 to 60 hours. Cytochrome P450 enzyme-inducing antiepileptic drugs, such as phenytoin, carbamazepine, and phenobarbital, reduce the half-life of lamotrigine by about 50%. Rashes appear in 10% of lamotrigine exposures. Because we are unable to differentiate benign rashes from the rashes of Stevens–Johnson syndrome and toxic epidermal necrolysis, the appearance of generalized maculopapular rashes is a reason for discontinuing lamotrigine. A gradual ascension of dose lowers the incidence of rashes; the dose starts at 25 to 50 mg daily for 2 weeks, rising to 75 to 100 mg daily for 2 weeks until 300 to 500 mg daily is reached.

Topiramate is a novel D-fructose derivative that is useful as monotherapy or as an add-on agent for both genetic and lesional epilepsies, including Lennox–Gastaut syndrome. Topiramate does not change serum carbamazepine or epoxide levels but produces modest to small increases in valproate and phenytoin serum levels. Cytochrome P450 enzyme-inducing antiepileptic drugs accelerate topiramate elimination and decrease its plasma levels. Because it is mostly excreted in the kidneys, renal failure results in higher plasma levels. Adverse effects include nephrolithiasis in 1.5%, depression in 15%, psychoses in 3%, and abnormal cognitive functions in 12% at 200- to 400-mg doses and in 26% at doses over 600 mg. For these reasons, a slow ascension of doses is used, and doses are usually kept between 150 to 300 mg.

Clonazepam can be useful as a third treatment option for atonic drop, myoclonic, and absence seizures. Peak plasma concentrations occur in 1 to 4 hours. The half-life is 20 to 50 hours. Doses start at 0.5 mg daily, increased every 3 to 5 days until seizures are controlled or sedation prohibits further dosage increments. Ataxia and irritability can result. Practitioners should take heed that vigabatrin, gabapentin, and tiagabine, drugs that increase GABA concentrations in the human nervous system, can worsen absences and myoclonias and, in rare cases, produce psychoses.

Symptomatic Partial Epilepsies

Carbamazepine, phenytoin, and valproate are the first-tier monotherapy drugs for partial and secondary generalized epilepsies. The exception is the elderly whose seizures start after 60 years of age; for this group, gabapentin is now recommended. Because of its safety, practitioners favor prescribing gabapentin even in adolescents and young adults, when seizures are mild and infrequent. Gabapentin, lamotrigine, and topiramate are being used earlier in the treatment of symptomatic epilepsy, as monotherapy or as add-on drugs. Thus, they are moving from the group of second-tier drugs to the first tier, depending on the clinical context and coexisting conditions. Because phenobarbital and primidone are less well tolerated and cause ataxia, vertigo, nausea, and drowsiness, these drugs are now prescribed less often.

Drowsiness, dizziness, nystagmus, blurred vision, diplopia, and nausea are pronounced at the onset of carbamazepine, phenobarbital, and primidone therapy and at peak plasma levels (Table 426.2). They can be prevented by starting at lower doses and gradually increasing the dose. Carbamazepine is absorbed slowly, reaching peak plasma levels in 2 to 8 hours (24 hours). Leukopenia occurs in 10% of patients. Idiosyncratic side effects include rash, icterus, anemia, and edema. Bone marrow depression has been reported in rare instances. An incidence of 0.5 cases per 100,000 treatment-years with carbamazepine, or two cases per 75,000 patients, has been reported for aplastic anemia. Hypersensitivity reactions in the form of skin rashes, exfoliative dermatitis, Stevens–Johnson syndrome, and systemic lupus ery-

thematosus occur now and then. It also is important to start lamotrigine and topiramate treatment at low doses and increase them slowly, as indicated earlier.

Ataxia and nystagmus are dose-dependent with phenytoin, but sedation is usually not a problem. Dysmorphic effects, including coarsening of facial features, gum hypertrophy, and hirsutism, appear with long-term use at high doses in children, adolescents, and women. Cerebellar degeneration can develop after long-term high-dose therapy. Stevens–Johnson syndrome occurs in one of 20,000 persons. A lupus-like syndrome, pseudolymphoma, exfoliative dermatitis, and fatal hepatic necrosis also can arise. Exanthema, fever, hepatitis, and lymphadenopathy are indications for withdrawal of the drug. Peak plasma levels appear in 2 to 8 hours; phenytoin has a half-life of 24 hours. Up to 96% is bound to plasma proteins. Phenytoin should not be administered intramuscularly, because it precipitates. Toxic neurologic side effects related to peak plasma levels require reduction of dosage.

Disulfiram (Antabuse), chloramphenicol, sulfamethizole, and phenylbutazone all inhibit the metabolism of phenytoin, increas-

| TABLE 426.2. | ANTIEPILEPTIC DRUGS |

Drug	Usual Total Daily Doses (Divided Doses Given As)[a]	Time Required to Reach Steady State (D)	Therapeutic Range (μg/mL)[b]	Elimination Half-Life (hr)[c]	Protein Binding (%)	Toxicity
Commonly Used Antiepileptic Drugs						
Valproic acid	500–3,000 mg (b.i.d.)	1–2	40–150	6–15	80–95	Nausea, vomiting, somnolence
Ethosuximide	1,000 mg (t.i.d.)	7–10	50–100	20–60	0	Nausea, fatigue, gastrointestinal upset, psychoses
Clonazepam	1–10 mg (o.d. or b.i.d.)	1–2	0.005–0.070	20–40	45	Sedation, ataxia, impaired cognition
Carbamazepine	600–1,600 mg (t.i.d.)	3–6	4–12	18.7 (11–22)	66–89	Dizziness, diplopia, ataxia, blurred vision
Phenytoin	300–400 mg (o.d.)	7–28	10–20	22 (highly variable)	90	Nystagmus, ataxia, somnolence, gastrointestinal discomfort
Primidone	750 mg (b.i.d.)	1–5	4–12	15.6	20–25	Sedation, nausea, dizziness, ataxia
Phenobarbital	120 mg (o.d. or b.i.d.)	10–30	15–40	96	40–60	Sedation, dizziness, hyperactivity in children
New Antiepileptic Drugs[d]						
Gabapentin	900–3,600 mg (t.i.d.)	2–3	2–4	5–7 (100% renal excretion)	0	Somnolence (20%), dizziness (18%), ataxia (13%), fatigue (10%), headaches, diplopia
Lamotrigine	75–500 mg (b.i.d.)	1–3	3–10	29 (14–60) (>50% liver glucorinide)	55	Headaches (30%), nausea (18%), dizziness (38%), diplopia (28%), rash, ataxia (20%)
Topiramate	150–300 mg (b.i.d.)	1–4	3–10	24 (50–60% unchanged in urine)	15	Headaches (30%), nausea (18%), dizziness (38%), diplopia (28%), rash, ataxia (20%)
Tiagabine	30–64 mg per day (b.i.d.)	1–2	??	5–8 (>90% liver metabolism)	96	Dizziness, asthenia, nervousness, tremor, depression, and diarrhea
Felbamate	15–60 mg/kg or 2,400–3,600 (b.i.d.)	7–28	20–80	12–24	25–35	Headaches (25–40%), nausea (35%), decreased appetite (10–20%), insomnia (20%), weight loss, hepatic failure, and bone marrow suppression

[a] This is an eventual dose; a lower dose is necessary when initiating therapy.
[b] Therapeutic levels may change with multiple drugs.
[c] Half-life may change with multiple drugs; half-lives are given for adult dosages. Steady state is reached in four half-lives.
[d] Therapeutic range still being established for newer drugs.

CHAPTER 426: APPROACH TO THE PATIENT WITH SEIZURES

ing the risk of intoxication. Phenytoin accelerates the metabolism of warfarin and dicoumarol. This effect causes a risk of bleeding if phenytoin is withdrawn. Phenytoin lowers serum folate levels, occasionally producing macrocytic anemia. It also interferes with vitamin D metabolism, leading to osteopenia. Antagonism with vitamin K can be important during pregnancy; supplemental vitamin K should be administered to pregnant women and to neonates, to prevent hemorrhagic disease of the newborn. Despite these limitations, 60 years of experience has proved that most adults can use phenytoin safely for effective seizure control.

Gabapentin has an advantage over other antiepileptic agents in that it is not metabolized, is not protein-bound, and does not produce significant pharmacokinetic changes in other antiepileptic agents. For this reason, it has achieved a primary and ideal role in late-onset epilepsy or seizures that start after 60 years of age and in infrequent and mild seizures of young adults. Geriatric patients often are taking various agents for heart disease and hypertension, and thus it is advantageous to prescribe an agent that has little pharmacokinetic effect on other drugs. The sole elimination pathway for gabapentin is renal excretion. As an add-on agent, gabapentin (1,200 to 1,800 mg per day to as much as 3,000 to 4,000 mg per day) lessens the rate of partial, complex partial, and secondary generalized seizures.

Tiagabine is the latest of the new GABAergic antiepileptic drugs developed as add-on drugs. Tiagabine is derived from nipecotic acid, which is a potent anticonvulsant by itself but cannot cross the blood–brain barrier. By inhibiting the reuptake of GABA, tiagabine enhances inhibition and stops seizures. The minimal effective dose is 30 mg daily; higher doses (up to 64 mg) are associated with 50% reduction of seizures in 25% of patients. The most common adverse effects are dizziness, nervousness, tremor, diarrhea, and depression.

Phenobarbital remains useful for nocturnal secondary tonic–clonic convulsions. Because sedation and cognitive impairment can be prominent when the drug is administered in the daytime, it is given as a single dose at the hour of sleep. Sometimes impotence presents a major drawback. Transient sedation is prominent during initiation of treatment, but most patients develop tolerance within a few weeks. Phenobarbital levels of 30 μg per milliliter or higher usually produce drowsiness, but some patients complain of tiredness even at low doses. Hyperactivity, agitation, or sleeplessness can appear as paradoxical reactions, especially in children and the elderly. Systemic toxicity is uncommon.

Primidone may cause listlessness and difficulty in rousing from sleep during the first few months of use. Sixty percent of patients discontinue primidone therapy by the end of the first year. Partial and complex partial seizures are poorly controlled. The initial dose should be low and the dosage increased cautiously. After 1 year, primidone has minimal sedative side effects when used as the sole drug. Patients who remain on the drug successfully for 1 year continue to do so for the next 5 years. It is now considered an acceptable third-tier drug. When primidone is administered in combination with phenytoin, increased biotransformation to phenobarbital can lead to side effects similar to those reported for phenobarbital. Systemic side effects have been rare. Primidone's efficacy may be separate from that of its metabolites. When drugs must be combined, primidone can be used effectively with phenytoin or carbamazepine.

Felbamate should be considered a third-tier agent for symptomatic epilepsy and is recommended as an add-on agent. Felbamate is particularly potent and has a wide clinical spectrum. Felbamate (maximum dose, 45 mg per kilogram per day, or 3,600 mg per day) is particularly effective in limiting atonic seizures, generalized tonic–clonic seizures, and total seizure frequency in the Lennox–Gastaut–Dravet syndrome. Felbamate is also effective as a single-entry drug or as adjunctive therapy in partial seizures. When felbamate is administered with phenytoin, phenytoin concentrations rise. With felbamate administered at 1,800 to 2,400 mg per day, phenytoin should be reduced by 20%; at 3,600 mg per day of felbamate, phenytoin should be reduced by 40%. At 3,600 mg per day of felbamate, mean carbamazepine declines 30%, while carbamazepine epoxide increases 60%. Felbamate given at a dosage of 2,400 mg per day raises steady-state plasma valproic acid concentrations by as much as 50%. Mean felbamate trough concentrations increase with valproate and drop slightly with carbamazepine or phenytoin. Felbamate is limited by hepatic toxicity (one case per 6,000) and bone marrow suppression (one case per 10,000).

■ UNDERSTAND THE CLINICAL SETTINGS UNDER WHICH ANTIEPILEPTIC DRUGS HAVE TO BE USED

Treatment must start with a careful overall assessment of the clinical situation in which epileptic seizures arise. Table 426.3 recommends initial choices for antiepileptic drugs in the context of various clinical pictures and coexisting medical conditions. The age, sex, seizure type, epilepsy syndrome, and medical background of the patient are all important. Is the patient planning pregnancy? Is the patient already pregnant? Is the patient a female adolescent? Is the patient elderly? Does the patient suffer from repeated tonic–clonic seizures or episodes of status epilepticus?

Parenteral administration of antiepileptic drugs is sometimes necessary because of active, repeated tonic–clonic seizures or status epilepticus or when the patient is unable to take drugs by mouth. Intravenous fosphenytoin (75 mg per minute, to reach a total dose of 750 mg) or intravenous valproate (3 mg per kilogram per minute, to reach a total dose of 25 mg per kilogram body weight) is available for rapid loading through the parenteral route when tonic–clonic seizures are frequent. The protocol for treatment of status epilepticus is given in Table 426.4.

EPILEPSY AND PREGNANCY

Carbamazepine, phenytoin, valproate, primidone, phenobarbital, and all the new antiepileptic drugs are potential teratogens when ingested during pregnancy. Major anomalies, such as spina bifida, rarely occur after valproate monotherapy (1.5%) or carbamazepine (0.9%) exposure of the fetus in utero. Urogenital and congenital heart abnormalities are reported with any of the five

TABLE 426.3. **RECOMMENDATIONS FOR INITIAL ANTIEPILEPTIC DRUG, CLINICAL CONTEXTS, AND COEXISTING CONDITIONS**

Clinical Context and/or Coexisting Condition	Valproate	Lamotrigine	Topiramate	Phenytoin	Carbamazepine	Ethosuximide	Gabapentin	Clonazepam
Rapid loading required owing to repetitive tonic–clonic seizures	+ (i.v. infusion 3 mg/kg/min over 1 hr; total dose 25 mg/kg)	No	No	+++ (i.v. fosphenytoin—75 mg per min i.v.; total dose of 750 mg)	No	No	No	No
Unsettled diagnosis of epilepsy syndrome: primary vs. secondary tonic–clonic seizure?	+++ (3–4 weeks to load)	+++ (3–4 weeks to load)	+++ (3–4 weeks to load)	+++ (rapid oral loading possible)	++ (2 weeks to load)	No	++ (1 week to load)	+ (2 weeks to load)
JME and absence plus grand mal in female planning pregnancy	+/+	+ (Use 250–750 mg/d during pregnancy.)	+	+	+/−	+	No	+
JME and absence plus grand mal in prepubertal/ pubertal female	+/−	+++	++	+	+	No	++	++
Absence seizures only in females or males	+++	++	?	No	No	+++	No	++
JME and absence plus grand mal in males	+++	+++	++	+/−	+/−	+	No	+
Lesional or symptomatic epilepsies in females planning pregnancy	+/−	+	+	++	+/−	No	+	+
Lesional or symptomatic epilepsies in males	+++	+++	+++	+++	+++	No	+++	+
Lennox-Gastaut-Dravet syndrome	+	+++	+++	+	++	No	+	++
Infantile spasms	+	+++	+++	No	No	No	No	+
Onset after 60 years	++	++	++	++	++	+/−	+++	++
Liver disease	+	+	+	+	+	+/−	+++	++
Renal disease	++	+	+	+	+	+/−	++	++

older drugs. The incidence of oral palate cleft is increased three- to tenfold after in utero exposure to phenytoin or carbamazepine. Minor craniofacial and limb anomalies, especially epicanthal folds and distal phalangeal hypoplasia, can develop in offspring after use of any of the five drugs during pregnancy. Fortunately, most pregnancies (90% to 95%) in which the fetus is exposed to antiepileptic drugs result in normal offspring. Nevertheless, birth defects are two to three times more common in fetuses exposed to antiepileptic drugs than in those not exposed to anti-epileptic drugs. A family history of birth defects should serve as a warning.

If an antiepileptic drug is necessary, monotherapy with the lowest dose that stops seizures should be used. Genetic epilepsy syndromes are best treated with the lowest effective dose of val-proate during pregnancy. Lesional epilepsies are best treated with the lowest effective dose of phenytoin during pregnancy. Plasma levels of antiepileptic drugs must be monitored monthly. Vitamins, including folic acid (0.8 to 5 mg per day) and vitamin K, are important supplements. Serum and amniotic fluid α-fetoprotein and acetylcholinesterase detect 78% of cases of open spina bifida, but not closed lesions. Ultrasonography detects 96% of cases of open and closed spina bifida. The newborn should receive 1 mg vitamin K (phytonadione) immediately after birth, and clotting factors should be monitored closely.

EPILEPSY IN THE ELDERLY

Epileptic seizures appear for the first time in 52 per 100,000 persons who are 40 to 59 years of age and in 127 per 100,000

TABLE 426.4.	MANAGEMENT OF TONIC–CLONIC AND COMPLEX PARTIAL STATUS EPILEPTICUS	
Step	**Time from Initial Observation and Treatment (min)**	**Procedure**
1	0	Assess cardiorespiratory function. If unsure of diagnosis, observe one tonic–clonic seizure and verify the persistence of unconsciousness after the seizure. Insert oral airway and administer oxygen if necessary. Insert an indwelling intravenous catheter. Draw venous blood for stat levels of anticonvulsants, glucose, electrolytes, and urea. Draw arterial blood for stat pH Po_2, HCO_3. Monitor respiration, blood pressure, and ECG. If possible, monitor EEG.
2	5	Start intravenous infusion through indwelling venous catheter of normal saline containing vitamin B complex. Give a bolus injection of 50 mL 50% glucose.
Three options are available for the first drug regimen		
3	Option 1: i.v. bolus of lorazepam-fosphenytoin combination	
	10–30	Give 0.1 mg/kg lorazepam as intravenous bolus at 4 mg over 2 min. Repeat the same dose in 15 min if control is not achieved. Immediately follow with i.v. fosphenytoin (15–20 mg/kg at rate of 75–150 mg/min)
3	Option 2: diazepam fosphenytoin combination	
	10–30	Infuse diazepam intravenously no faster than 2 mg/min until seizures stop or to total of 20 mg (do not dilute). Also start infusion of fosphenytoin no faster than 75–150 mg/min to a total of 15–20 mg/kg. If hypotension develops, slow infusion rate.
3	Option 3: i.v. phenobarbital	
	10–30	Give intravenous infusion of phenobarbital at 100 mg/min until seizures stop or a total dose of 10 mg/kg is administered. If seizures persist, continue infusing phenobarbital at 50 mg/min until a total dose of 20 mg/kg is reached.
If first-option drugs do not control seizures, EEG monitoring and endotracheal intubation is recommended during the remaining steps.		
4	30–50	If seizures recur or persist and phenobarbital is used as the first option, fosphenytoin can be administered as the second regimen. Fosphenytoin may be increased to 20 mg/kg or to a plasma level above 30 μg/ml. If phenobarbital is used as first option and lorazepam or diazepam is used as second options or vice versa, endotracheal intubation is recommended.
5	60–80	If seizures continue, general anesthesia can be instituted with one of the following regimens. Intravenous pentobarbital loading dose of 15 mg/kg over 1 hr is followed by monitor and infusion of 1–2 mg/kg per hr until seizures stop or EEG burst suppressions. OR Thiopentone may be given at 2 mg/min in normal saline by a microdrip set for 30–60 min. Reduce dose to 0.5 mg/min when controlled. Dose can be increased to anesthetic levels if necessary to achieve control. EEG monitoring to ascertain a burst-suppression pattern and seizure control is required. Alternatively, other anesthetizing barbiturates can be used. OR Halothane and neuromuscular junction blockade can be administered by an anesthesiologist. Once control is achieved, EEG monitoring is recommended continuously or as frequently as is technically possible in the obtunded patient, to ensure that electrographic status has not recurred.

persons age 60 years and older. Epilepsy in persons 65 years and older has twice the prevalence rate of epilepsy in younger adults. The most common identifiable cause of seizures in the elderly is stroke; a silent stroke or an overt completed stroke accounts for one-fourth of all seizures in the elderly. In another one-fourth of patients, no cause can be defined. Less often, a brain tumor, head injury, Alzheimer's disease, or infections are identified. Antiepileptic drug therapy should be initiated at lower doses and at longer intervals in the elderly. Hepatic drug metabolism and the glomerular filtration rate of carbamazepine, phenytoin, valproate, phenobarbital, and primidone decline an average 10% per decade from 40 to 70 years of age, resulting in longer elimination half-lives and diminished clearance. Many elderly have low albumin levels and may require measurements of unbound drug levels. Both therapeutic and adverse effects appear at lower plasma concentrations. Cognitive effects of phenytoin, carbamazepine, valproate, and topiramate appear earlier at lower plasma levels; valproate tremors mimicking parkinsonian tremors occur at relatively low plasma concentrations. Drug interactions are particularly important in the elderly, because these patients often are taking other drugs. Propoxyphene (Darvon) and erythromycin inhibit the metabolism of carbamazepine and phenytoin by the cytochrome P450 system. Carbamazepine and phenytoin can affect cardiac conduction in the elderly.

STATUS EPILEPTICUS

Status epilepticus occurs when seizures persist longer than 30 minutes or when convulsions continue without recovery of consciousness. This medical emergency requires immediate treatment to prevent brain damage or death. There is no single ideal drug for the treatment of convulsive status epilepticus; a step-by-step protocol is given in Table 426.4. Combination treatment with intravenous benzodiazepines (diazepam or lorazepam) and fosphenytoin controls 70% of convulsions and complex partial status. Combination treatment is recommended, because 30%

of status recur after either intravenous diazepam alone or intravenous lorazepam alone. Intravenous fosphenytoin (18 mg per kilogram) or intravenous valproate (25 mg per kilogram) is indicated in tonic status or convulsive status associated with subdural hematoma or subarachnoid hemorrhage. If the patient continues to convulse after 60 minutes, general anesthesia with a barbiturate (usually pentobarbital) should be initiated.

METABOLISM OF ANTIEPILEPTIC DRUGS

To predict the time of drug actions and interactions as well as toxic effects, the physician should be familiar with the absorption, distribution, protein-binding, and elimination characteristics and the half-lives of antiepileptic drugs (Table 426.2). Absorption varies from one drug to another and among patients. Peak plasma concentrations appear most often at 4 to 24 hours. Carbamazepine, primidone, and phenobarbital dosages must be increased slowly, because peak plasma levels may rise quickly. Phenytoin and phenobarbital enhance the metabolism of carbamazepine, reducing its half-life from 20 hours to 10 hours. This may result in early-morning seizures despite drug intoxication in the evening.

Body distribution and full antiepileptic effects depend on plasma protein binding. Only the free, or nonprotein-bound, fraction crosses the blood–brain barrier. Carbamazepine forms an active metabolite (10,11-epoxy-carbamazepine) that may be responsible for some of its clinical action and untoward side effects. Primidone forms two active metabolites, phenylethylmalonamide and phenobarbital. No antiepileptic action of the metabolites of phenytoin has been shown.

The half-life of a drug determines the steady state and the number of doses needed per day (Table 426.1). All antiepileptic drugs are eliminated by first-order kinetics; that is, there is a direct relationship between dosage and plasma levels. The exception is phenytoin, which saturates liver enzyme capacity at high levels. Metabolism depends on plasma levels, so that at the high end of the therapeutic range, dosage should be adjusted by small amounts (25 mg).

Various conditions modify metabolism or protein binding. Adults older than age 65 metabolize drugs more quickly. The dose may be kept unchanged, however, because the unbound protein fraction is larger. Serious kidney failure raises the free fraction of phenytoin, but the absolute plasma concentration is unchanged. Liver dysfunction also can change protein binding and impair metabolism. During serious illnesses and pregnancy, it is wise to track plasma levels carefully. (Dose adjustments in renal failure are discussed in Chapter 143.) The blood levels in newborn infants of treated mothers are similar to the levels in the mothers themselves. Antiepileptic drugs pass into breast milk, but the concentration is significantly lower than in the mother's plasma.

MONITOR TREATMENT AND ASSESS EFFECTS ON QUALITY OF LIFE

Follow-up should be guided by an understanding of the prognosis and psychosocial complications of epilepsy. The prognosis depends to a great extent on the patient's age at onset. An excellent outcome is seen in idiopathic generalized epilepsies of childhood and adolescence. Generalized seizures caused by progressive brain disease have a poor prognosis. Partial epilepsies with psychomotor symptoms can be difficult to treat and may require surgery. Nocturnal tonic–clonic seizures have a good prognosis.

Among patients with absence seizures, 60% to 79% become free of seizures with ethosuximide or valproic acid therapy. Ninety percent of patients with pure grand mal or primary generalized tonic–clonic seizures become free of seizures with valproic acid or lamotrigine therapy. Ninety-five percent of patients with juvenile myoclonic epilepsy are completely free of seizures when receiving valproic acid.

The stigma often associated with epilepsy is still a concern for patients. The burden of epilepsy is not limited to the medical condition. In a study funded by the Epilepsy Foundation, people with epilepsy reported that limits on lifestyle, schooling, driving, and employment were major barriers in their lives. These economic, social, and educational burdens and barriers negatively influence the quality of life and influence the course of epilepsy. For most patients, the single worst thing about epilepsy is the fear of the next seizure. In the past, epilepsy patients were considered to be at high risk for accidents and were thought to have a special tendency toward crime and aggression, but there is no evidence supporting these assumptions. The national Epilepsy Foundation and its affiliates throughout the country can provide a source of support and service to individuals with epilepsy and provide them with opportunities to connect with others who have epilepsy. Physicians are encouraged to refer their patients to the Epilepsy Foundation affiliate in their region.

Persons with epilepsy are often handicapped by depression or cognitive and behavioral problems associated with their condition or with antiepileptic drugs. Emotional immaturity and personality disorders may develop because of defective rearing, overprotection, and rejection. The physician should act as an advocate for the patient and should formulate a support system that includes family, school, and vocational personnel. A multidisciplinary team is needed. The clinician also must be an educator. The patient should have a calendar for recording seizures and a list of drugs and dosages. Follow-up visits should be scheduled at least every 3 months for the first year and every 6 months subsequently. Patients must understand the need for follow-up examinations, complete blood counts, and liver function tests. In a seizure-free condition, patients should experience no mental or psychiatric abnormalities and can have a normal life expectancy. Death can be caused by suicide, status epilepticus, accidents, or brain tumor.

WITHDRAWAL OF ANTIEPILEPTIC DRUG TREATMENT

The prognosis and recurrence of seizures after withdrawal of antiepileptic drugs depend on the specific epilepsy syndrome. The presence of a high rate of seizures, several seizure types, abnormal neurologic signs, abnormally slow EEG background, abnormal mental function during inadequate control of seizures, and repeated tonic–clonic status, as observed in Lennox–Gastaut–Dravet syndrome; severe myoclonic epilepsy of infancy; and the progressive myoclonus encephalopathies all have a poor prognosis. In contrast, 80% of patients whose seizures are completely controlled during the first year of treatment remain free from seizures in the subsequent 3 years. Children older than 5 years who have generalized seizures, such as absence seizures; who have normal neurologic examination results and a normal IQ; and whose seizures have been controlled for 2 to 4 years have a 75% chance of remaining free of seizures after withdrawal of antiepileptic drugs. The exception is the juvenile myoclonic epilepsy of Janz and awakening clonic-tonic-clonic seizures, in which electroclinical traits persist for life. Withdrawal of antiepileptic drugs is not indicated for these patients.

Antiepileptic drugs can be withdrawn gradually after 2 years of complete control in cases of rolandic epilepsy and pure childhood absence and after 4 years of complete control of simple partial epilepsy, complex partial epilepsy, absence associated with tonic–clonic seizures, and grand mal tonic–clonic seizures. A

minimum 5-year follow-up is recommended after withdrawal of therapy. EEGs and clinical visits should be scheduled at 6 months and 1 year. CCTV-EEG monitoring also can be used to confirm the absence of seizures.

REFER TO AN EPILEPSY CENTER FOR SURGICAL TREATMENT IN THE CASE OF DRUG RESISTANCE

Of patients with refractory seizures, about 10% can benefit from tailored resections of epileptogenic zones, anterior temporal lobectomy, amygdalohippocampectomy, or cortectomy. Refractory complex partial seizures can be due to noncompliance, inadequate drug dosage, improper choice of drugs, or the presence of precipitating or aggravating factors (a stressful home or workplace, use of alcohol, sleep deprivation, menses). Structural le-

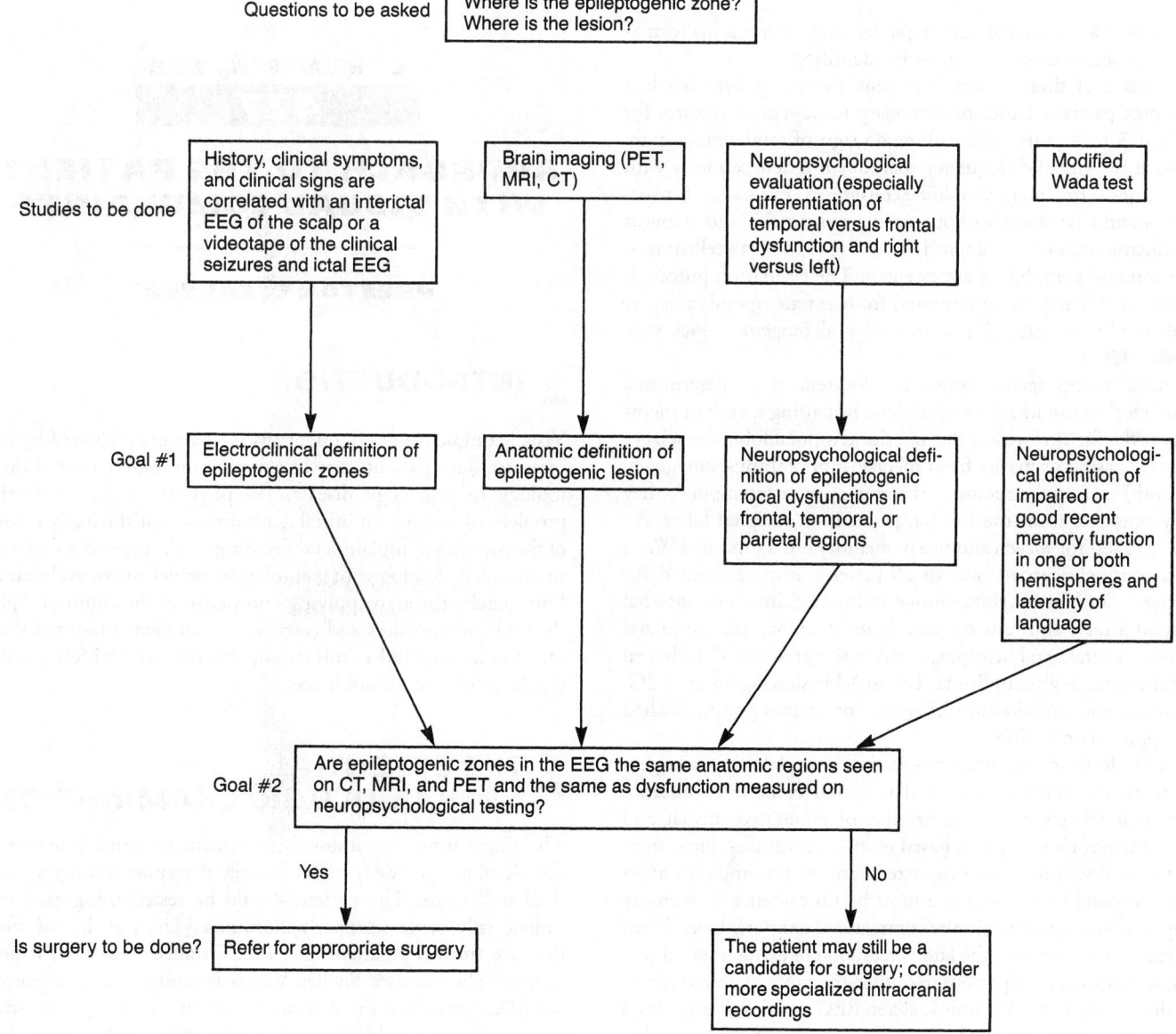

FIGURE 426.2. Presurgical evaluation for medically refractory seizures.

TABLE 426.5.	RESULTS OF TAILORED SURGICAL RESECTION OF EPILEPTOGENIC ZONES

Zone	Complete Elimination or 95% Eradication of Seizures
Temporal lobe epilepsy	
Medial	95%
Lateral	80%
Combined medial–lateral	85%
Combined temporal & frontal	80%
Frontal lobe epilepsy	
Medial	80%
Dorsolateral	
Nondominant hemisphere	70%
Dominant hemisphere	40%
Parietal lobe epilepsy	80%

sions, such as a focal cortical dysplasias, arteriovenous malformation, or occult neoplasm, must be identified.

If none of these factors is present and the patient has had complex partial seizures or secondary tonic–clonic seizures for at least 3 to 4 years, which show no sign of remission and are of such severity and frequency that they interfere seriously with life, surgical treatment should be considered. Evaluation for surgery should be done without undue risk to life and without producing serious neurologic deficits (Fig. 426.2). Excellent motivation and compliance are essential. The evaluation process is aimed at differentiating temporal from extratemporal epilepsy. The results of surgical resection of epileptogenic zones vary (Table 426.5).

After epileptogenic zones are located, it is determined whether they can be removed without impairing speech or memory. If the focus is within the anterior temporal lobe, the seizure may be arising primarily from medial (hippocampus, amygdala, or both) or lateral structures. If seizures are extratemporal, they may originate from the frontal, parietal, or occipital lobes. An essential test for speech and recent memory is the modified Wada test, routinely carried out for all patients being evaluated for surgery. Sodium amylobarbitone is injected into one internal carotid artery, and tests for speech and memory are conducted during contralateral hemiplegia and in the presence of ipsilateral hemispheric, high-amplitude, 1.5- to 3-Hz slowing on the EEG. Hemispheric lateralization of speech or memory is established by appropriate testing.

The decision to perform selective amygdalohippocampectomy in the context of medial temporal epilepsy or anterior temporal lobectomy in the context of combined medial and lateral temporal epilepsy is based on two conditions. First, focal or regional seizures must originate in one hippocampus or anterior temporal lobe, and there must be no evidence of memory impairment originating in the contralateral temporal lobe. When seizures originate from the lateral temporal or extratemporal cortex, it is especially important to outline the precise site and extent of the seizure focus by chronic stereo EEG, subdural or epidural electrode recordings, and intraoperative electrocorticography. Intraoperative evoked potentials mapping the primary motor

cortex and, if necessary, eloquent areas of the hemisphere dominant for language usually precede cortical resection.

BIBLIOGRAPHY

Chauvel P, Delgado-Escueta AV, Halgren E, et al. *Frontal lobe seizures and epilepsies.* New York: Raven Press, 1992. (*Advances in neurology*, vol 57.)

Delgado-Escueta AV. Seizures and epilepsies in adolescents and adults. In: Rakel RE. *Conn's current therapy*, Philadelphia: WB Saunders, 1998.

Delgado-Escueta AV, Janz D, Beck-Mannagetta G. Pregnancy and teratogenesis in epilepsy. *Neurology* 1992;42(suppl 5):xx–xx.

Delgado-Escueta AV, Wilson W, Olsen R, et al. *Jasper's basic mechanisms of the epilepsies.* New York: Lippincott, Williams & Wilkins, 1999. (*Advances in neurology*, vol 94.)

Wyllie E. *The treatment of epilepsy: principles and practice.* Philadelphia: Lea & Febiger, 1997.

Kelley's Textbook of Internal Medicine, fourth edition. Edited by H. David Humes. Lippincott Williams & Wilkins, Philadelphia © 2000.

C H A P T E R
427

APPROACH TO THE PATIENT WITH VISUAL COMPLAINTS

PRESTON C. CALVERT

INTRODUCTION

Visual complaints are frequent among patients evaluated by the internist. Such patients may have important underlying ophthalmologic or neurologic disease. The physician is faced with the problem of making an initial determination of the likely causes of the patient's complaint and deciding on the urgency of referral to an ophthalmologist or neurologist for definitive evaluation. Fortunately, through applying knowledge of the common ophthalmologic disorders and carrying out an elementary ophthalmologic history and examination, this referral decision usually can be made with confidence.

THE ESSENTIAL OPTHAMOLOGIC EXAMINATION

The single most important measurement of visual function is the visual acuity (VA), which is easily determined using a standard wall chart. The patient should be tested using each eye individually, with a properly illuminated chart at the specified distance from the patient and with distance spectacles, if prescribed. The standard Snellen VA chart results in a VA reported as 20/X, where X is the distance in feet at which a person with normal vision would be able to identify the characters. VA should be correctable to 20/20 or better in each eye, and the reason for failing this standard should be sought. The most common cause of diminished VA is uncorrected refractive error. VA also may be checked using a "near card" designed for this purpose. Assessing VA in this way, however, may underestimate impairment at distance in myopic (nearsighted) individuals and must be done with the patient's appropriate refractive correction for the reading distance, to correct for presbyopia (decreased ability to focus close up by persons over 40 to 45) or hyperopia (farsightedness).

The VA is only one of a group of measurements of visual function and depends on the object resolution of the very center of the visual field (VF). The peripheral VF extends more than 90 degrees temporally from the fixation point in each eye and more than 60 degrees nasally. Many ocular and neurologic conditions take the form of impairment of the VFs, sometimes sparing the VA. These conditions include glaucoma, retinitis pigmentosa, and the VF defects due to infarction and other pathologic processes in one cerebral hemisphere. A screening examination of the VF in a patient with visual complaints is very quickly done by having the patient cover one eye and fixate the examiner's nose. The examiner places the hands in upper or lower quadrants of the patient's VF and quickly shows one, two, or three fingers on one hand. The patient reports the number of fingers. This test is repeated until the sensitivity of all four quadrants of the VF in each eye is determined. Consistent failure to report the number of fingers in one or more quadrants correctly is indicative of a defect in the VF in that area. The examiner must make sure that the patient maintains stable fixation on the examiner's nose, since shifting fixation to the presented fingers can obscure a defect.

Special note is taken of defects that appear on the same side of the body in both eyes, called *homonymous* defects, which often also approach but do not cross the vertical line through the patient's fixation point, thus being *hemianopic* in quality (Fig. 427.1). Such a homonymous hemianopia may affect mainly the upper or lower VF and is indicative of a lesion posterior to the optic chiasm in the central visual pathways. The most common cause of an isolated homonymous hemianopia is an infarct in the contralateral occipital lobe, though other processes, such as tumors or demyelinating disease, also can be the source. A unilateral or bilateral temporal hemianopic VF defect may be seen in the context of optic chiasm disease or from compression by a large pituitary adenoma or other suprasellar mass. Optic nerve disease and retinal disease are other typical sources of monocular or binocular VF defects, sometimes with relative sparing of VA. Glaucoma, a special kind of optic neuropathy, is associated mainly with VF loss in its early stages.

The pupil is the opening in the iris through which light reaches the interior of the eye to form images on the retina. The size of the pupil is adjusted automatically by the nervous system based on the amount of ambient light and the desired depth of focus of the eye. Increased ambient light or efforts to focus at near range activate the parasympathetic innervation of the pupil constrictor muscle and result in pupillary constriction. Decreased ambient light or distance fixation after focusing close up result in relaxation of the parasympathetic innervation and activation of the sympathetic innervation to the pupil dilator muscles. This leads to active pupil dilatation. A small amount

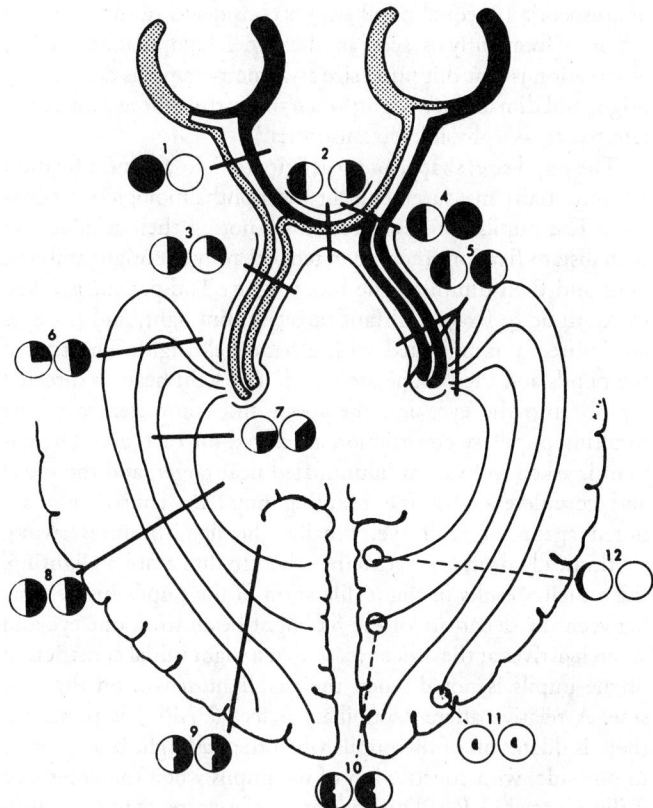

FIGURE 427.1. Abnormal visual field. Schematic representation of visual pathway, showing sites of total interruption of nerve fibers and various abnormal visual fields produced by such interruption.

1. Optic nerve—blindness on side of lesion, with normal contralateral field
2. Chiasm—bitemporal hemianopsia
3. Optic tract—contralateral incongruous homonymous hemianopsia
4. Optic nerve—chiasmal junction: blindness on side of lesion, with contralateral temporal hemianopsia or hemianopic scotoma
5. Posterior optic tract, external geniculate ganglion, posterior limb of internal capsule—complete contralateral homonymous hemianopsia or incomplete incongruous contralateral homonymous hemianopsia
6. Optic radiation in anterior loop in temporal lobe—incongruous contralateral homonymous hemianopsia or superior quadrantanopsia
7. Medial fibers of optic radiation—contralateral incongruous inferior homonymous quadrantanopsia
8. Optic radiation in parietal lobe—contralateral homonymous hemianopsia, sometimes slightly incongruous, with minimal macular sparing
9. Optic radiation in posterior parietal lobe and occipital lobe—contralateral congruous homonymous hemianopsia with macular sparing
10. Midportion of calcarine cortex—contralateral congruous homonymous hemianopsia with wide macular sparing and sparing of contralateral temporal crescent
11. Tip of occipital lobe—contralateral congruous homonymous hemianopic scotomas
12. Anterior tip of calcarine fissure—contralateral loss of temporal crescent with otherwise normal visual fields

(From Harrington DO, Drake MV. *The visual fields*, sixth ed. St. Louis: Mosby, 1990, with permission.)

of anisocoria (unequal pupil size) is considered normal—up to 0.5 mm frequently is seen in the general population. A key observation is that this pupil size asymmetry remains the same in bright and dim ambient light; when this is true, the asymmetry is referred to as "physiologic anisocoria,"

The pupil size, shape, and reactivity to light and near fixation are important measurements in the ophthalmologic examination. The pupils are best assessed by noting their relative size with distant fixation (more than ten feet away) in bright ambient light and then dimming the room lights. The patient is asked to continue to fixate a distant target in dim light, and the eyes are indirectly illuminated with a hand-held light. The size of the pupils and their shape are noted. The light beam is directed rapidly into the eye, and the speed and completeness of the resulting pupillary constriction are noted for each eye. The patient is asked to fixate an illuminated near target, and the speed and completeness of the resulting pupillary constriction are noted again for each eye. Finally, the light beam is swung rhythmically from one eye to the other. In dim ambient lighting, this usually results in slight dilatation of the pupils in the time between the departure of the flashlight beam from one eye and when it arrives at the other eye, so that a slight initial constriction of the pupils is noted when the flashlight arrives on the new side. A relative afferent pupillary defect (RAPD) is present if there is dilatation of the pupils when the flashlight beam comes to one side, with constriction of the pupils when the other side is illuminated. A RAPD is indicative of a decrease in the pupil-constricting drive to the brain stem from one eye compared with the other and is seen most often in unilateral or asymmetric bilateral optic nerve disease, such as optic neuritis, ischemic optic neuropathy, or compressive optic neuropathy. A RAPD also can be seen in retinal disease but is not present in the context of corneal disease or cataracts.

The external examination of the eyes may reveal a number of important signs. The size of the palpebral fissure and the position of the lids should be noted, and the presence of ptosis (drooping of the upper lid) should be recorded. The ability of the lids to open fully with attempted gaze upward should be evaluated. The conjunctivae and sclera must be inspected for redness due to dilatation of their vessels and for the presence of discharge. The character of any discharge is important; if it is purulent, it should be cultured and a smear examined. Proptosis (bulging of the eye from the orbit) should be noted. The clarity of the cornea should be assessed and lesions recorded. Sensation of the skin of the face and the position and mobility of the facial musculature also must be determined.

An assessment of extraocular movements should be made. The patient should be asked about the presence of diplopia and whether it produces mainly horizontal or vertical separation of the two images. By inspection of the patient, note whether there is an obvious turning of one eye inward toward the nose (esotropia), outward (exotropia), or upward (hypertropia). While the patient is attempting to fixate a distant target, look for any spontaneous movements of the eyes, such as the rhythmic to-and-fro movements of nystagmus (Table 427.1). The patient then should be asked to fixate a small, interesting object in the examiner's hand about three feet away. The examiner should test the range of ocular movements for each eye individually in adduc-

TABLE 427.1.	TYPES OF NYSTAGMUS AND THEIR ANATOMIC LOCATION
Type	**Anatomic Location**
Downbeat	Craniocervical junction, cerebellum
Gaze-evoked	Craniocervical junction
Upbeat	Cerebellum, medulla
Seesaw	Diencephalon mesencephalon
Torsional	Central vestibular
Convergence-retraction	Dorsal midbrain
Rebound	Cerebellum

tion (toward the nose), abduction (away from the nose), upward, and downward gaze. This is called *testing of ocular ductions* and is a basic part of determining the cause of misalignment of the eyes.

Patients with congenital esotropia or exotropia usually will not show significant loss of duction in any direction unless there has been previous eye muscle surgery. On the other hand, patients with acquired eye movement problems often will show a limitation of duction that can help in diagnosis. For example, acquired esotropia may be associated with limited abduction on one side and be due to weakness of the lateral rectus muscle on that side (Table 427.2). Hypertropia may be seen in a patient with limitation of downward duction of the eyes on the side of the higher eye, and this condition most likely will be due to superior oblique paresis, as from fourth nerve paresis.

Finally, careful funduscopic examination should be undertaken. Ophthalmologists usually dilate the pupil with pharmacologic agents to evaluate the ocular fundus easily, but this is not often feasible for the internist in a busy office setting. Through a small pupil, it is usually possible to assess the clarity of the ocular media and determine the presence of a significant cataract obstructing the view of the fundus, which may explain a decrease in VA. The optic disk should be looked at and evaluated for swelling, as should associated hemorrhages, exudates, and so on (Table 427.3). The retinal macula should be inspected for evidence of age-related macular degeneration in the form of pigment deposition, bleeding, exudates, or a macular hole, any of which may explain diminished VA. Retinal detachments are very difficult to see with the usual direct ophthalmoscope through

TABLE 427.2.	IMAGE SEPARATION IN DIPLOPIA	
Muscle (Right Eye)	**Type of Deviation**	**Position of Gaze with Most Separation**
Lateral rectus	Esotropia	Right
Medial rectus	Exotropia	Left
Superior rectus	Left hypertropia	Up and right
Inferior rectus	Right hypertropia	Down and right
Inferior oblique	Left hypertropia	Up and left
Superior oblique	Right hypertropia	Down and left

TABLE 427.3.	DIFFERENTIATION OF PAPILLEDEMA AND PSEUDOPAPILLEDEMA	

	Early Papilledema	Pseudopapilledema
Disc color		
Hyperemic		Pink, yellowish pink
Disc margins		
	Indistinct early at superior and inferior poles, later entire margin	Irregularly blurred, may be lumpy
Disc elevation		
Minimal		Minimal to marked, center of disc most elevated
Vessels		
	Normal distribution, slight fullness, spontaneous venous pulsations absent	Emanate from center, frequent anomalous pattern, ± spontaneous venous pulsations
Nerve fiber layer		
	Dull due to edema, which may obscure blood vessels	No edema, may glisten with circumpapillary halo of feathery light reflections
Hemorrhages		
Splinter		Subretinal, retinal, vitreous

a small pupil; if they are suspected, they must be diagnosed immediately by an ophthalmologist. The retinal arterioles should be assessed for localized or generalized narrowing, presence of emboli, and the amount of light reflex.

VISUAL SYMPTOMS THAT DO NOT REQUIRE URGENT EVALUATION

A number of complaints by the patient suggest conditions that should be pursued with the ophthalmologist but do not require emergency referral. A common problem is the gradual onset of visual blur, often associated with halos around lights at night and often with monocular diplopia. This condition may be monocular or binocular and is most suggestive of development of a cataract or other problem in the ocular media. The examination may show normal results or evidence of an opacity in the lens suggesting a cataract. It is important to know that this is usually correctable by surgery, which leads to a good outcome. Partially or poorly corrected refractive errors, such as astigmatism, can produce similar problems and respond to a simple change in refraction. If the patient reports long-standing strabismus (misalignment of the eyes) or nystagmus (repetitive jerking of the eyes), there may be benefit in nonurgent ophthalmologic or neuro-ophthalmologic evaluation, primarily to explain the problem to the patient and to look for associated treatable problems. The internist's examination of such patients may uncover evidence of strabismus, though sometimes finding evidence of this problem requires more detailed ophthalmologic testing. Nystagmus may be noted.

Long-standing abnormalities of pupil appearance or function usually result from intraocular inflammation, trauma, or other disorders, such as the tonic pupil (called Adie's syndrome when it is associated with decreased tendon reflexes in the lower extremities). The underlying condition may require additional treatment, and nonurgent referral to an ophthalmologist should

be considered. A disruption of oculosympathetic innervation may give rise to Horner's syndrome, with miosis and ipsilateral ptosis. Horner's syndrome can be confirmed by testing with cocaine eyedrops and can be classified further by pharmacologic testing of the pupil using 1% hydroxyamphetamine into involvement of the preganglionic sympathetic fibers and damage to postganglionic fibers. Preganglionic Horner's syndrome is sometimes associated with Pancoast's syndrome of carcinoma of the thoracic apex or with cervical mass lesions. Imaging directed at this area can be reserved for this form of the condition.

The onset of typical migrainous visual phenomena in a person younger than 45, with or without headaches, can be a worrisome symptom, but it is associated only rarely with underlying intracranial or ocular pathologic conditions. The typical visual symptoms include a zigzag bright arc or streak in the peripheral VF bilaterally, of acute onset and usually lasting less than 20 minutes. Other common variants include a central VF defect of similar duration, described as a blurred area or fuzzy spot—like water on glass. This may be followed by some kind of headache, not necessarily severe, in which case the term *classic migraine* is used. Identical symptoms may occur with no associated headache and are called *acephalgic migraine*. A history of headaches, not always identified as migraine, should be sought, and the VF should be carefully examined. If the patient has no persistent VF defect and the description and duration of the symptoms are typical, the main focus should be on screening for underlying medical conditions that may have triggered migraine phenomena, such as uncontrolled hypertension, hypothyroidism, or connective tissue disorders. If the symptoms are persistent or otherwise atypical in any way, or if they are monocular, the patient should be evaluated by a neurologist for an underlying cerebrovascular or intracranial problem.

Age-related macular degeneration can take the form of gradual onset of decreased VA or of a distortion of objects that are being fixated. This distortion can make straight lines show a curved segment, and it may be monocular or bilateral. The examination shows a decrease in VA, possibly a central scotoma, but

TABLE 427.4.	DIFFERENTIATION OF OPTIC NERVE AND MACULAR DISEASE	
Optic Nerve		**Macula**
Visual acuity		
Reduced		Reduced
Color vision		
Impaired		Preserved
Visual field		
Central scotoma		Normal or small central scotoma
Pupils		
RAPD present		Absent
Photostress test		
Normal		Abnormal
Light brightness		
Reduced		Normal

RAPD, relative afferent pupillary defect.

no RAPD (Table 427.4). Pigmentary changes or hemorrhage may be seen on direct ophthalmoscopy of the macula. There are treatable complications of age-related macular degeneration, but the disease itself is not treatable at present. Nonurgent referral to a general ophthalmologist or retinal specialist is indicated.

Acute unilateral or bilateral conjunctival irritation, discharge, and redness may indicate the presence of viral or bacterial conjunctivitis. Photophobia may be intense, but VA and VF are not impaired. The pupil should function normally, and the lid and eye movement should be normal. The presence of a foreign body should be sought. If any features of the illness are atypical, the patient should be referred immediately to an ophthalmologist. For typical cases of conjunctivitis, a smear and culture of any discharge is essential, and empiric treatment of presumed bacterial conjunctivitis with topical antibiotics may be considered for 7 to 10 days. If at any time VA becomes impaired or other features become atypical, the patient should be referred to an ophthalmologist immediately.

Isolated sudden onset of unequal pupil size, when not associated with any other new visual symptoms or signs is usually not due to a serious underlying disease process. The most common causes are inadvertent or intentional instillation of an anticholinergic agent into the eye, acute tonic pupil, or the transient pupillary dilatation seen in young people, often in association with migraine. More serious pathologic processes almost always also produce other symptoms, such as decreased VA, ocular redness, ptosis, or diplopia and strabismus. Evaluation by an ophthalmologist or neurologist is appropriate but not usually urgently necessary.

URGENT VISUAL SYMPTOMS DUE TO INTRINSIC OCULAR DISEASE

Sudden onset of monocular flashes and floaters is a worrisome symptom, because it may imply a retinal tear or detachment. In middle-aged people, it is more often due to detachment of the posterior face of the vitreous body from the retinal surface, which produces transient traction on the retina and a burst of flashes in the VF from mechanical irritation. Nevertheless, such a posterior vitreous detachment also may cause a retinal tear or detachment, and all patients with this symptom should be evaluated by an ophthalmologist within a few days. The examination outlined earlier usually shows normal results, since a dilated funduscopic examination with special instruments is necessary to define most retinal pathologic conditions. A retinal detachment in the macular area will limit VA and may produce other VF and pupillary signs, however. Persistent flashes or a marked increase in floaters are of more concern and should be urgently evaluated by an ophthalmologist.

Sudden onset of monocular or binocular decreased VA is a symptom that should always prompt rapid referral to an ophthalmologist. This may be due to acute glaucoma, retinal or vitreous hemorrhage, retinal infarction, or optic nerve disease. The examination may reveal corneal clouding, abnormal pupil reactions, blood in the vitreous cavity, retinal bleeding, retinal infarction or inflammation, or optic nerve swelling. Other conditions, such as retrobulbar optic neuritis, show normal results on examination, except for decreased VA, VF, and the presence of a RAPD. Sudden awareness of a monocular VF defect may indicate the presence of a vision-threatening process, such as retinal detachment, and should prompt immediate referral to an ophthalmologist. Other possible causes include branch retinal artery occlusion by emboli, ischemic optic neuropathy, or retinal infections. The examination may show retinal detachment, pale swollen infarcted retina, or retinal exudates and hemorrhage.

Ocular pain of sudden onset is frightening to the patient and may imply the presence of a serious pathologic condition. Acute glaucoma can produce intense pain and cause corneal clouding, redness, and pupillary dysfunction, along with decreased VA and VF. Iritis characteristically generates ocular pain, photosensitivity, and ocular redness. VA and VF typically are not affected. Scleritis, episcleritis, and orbital inflammatory syndromes may cause acute ocular and orbital pain, with generalized or localized scleral flushing and overlying conjunctival injection. There may be tenderness to palpation of the ocular globe or orbit. A foreign body in the eye is painful and provokes intense tearing. Foreign bodies must be removed promptly to prevent corneal abrasions and infection. All of these conditions necessitate urgent ophthalmologic referral.

URGENT VISUAL SYMPTOMS OF NEUROLOGIC ORIGIN

The patient who experiences sudden onset of diplopia should be questioned about whether one of the two images disappears upon covering either eye, to distinguish true diplopia from monocular diplopia. It is also useful to know whether the two images are separated horizontally or vertically, because this can help in beginning to determine the weak muscles responsible. The examination should focus on the ocular muscle ductions; on whether there is exotropia, esotropia, or hypertropia; and on whether there is associated ptosis, pupillary abnormality, VF or VA loss, or facial sensory disturbance. One common condition that causes acute diplopia is microvascular infarcts of the ocular motor nerves due to vasa nervorum occlusive disease in patients with hypertension and diabetes mellitus. This process may affect cranial nerves III, IV, or VI and may be painful.

When the third nerve is affected by a microvascular infarct, the pupil is almost never affected, distinguishing this condition from the most ominous cause of acute third nerve palsy, compression by an enlarging intracranial saccular aneurysm. Both microvascular third nerve infarction and compressive third nerve paresis produce ptosis and weakness of the third nerve–innervated muscles, classically resulting in exotropia and hypotropia of the affected eye. Early in the course of compressive third nerve palsy, the pupil may not be involved; for this reason, all patients with third nerve palsy should be referred immediately to a neurologist or neuro-ophthalmologist for careful assessment and imaging evaluation to help make this distinction.

Another condition causing acute diplopia is myasthenia gravis, which can mimic any ocular motor nerve paresis and can produce findings that fluctuate during the day or even during the examination. A useful fact is that myasthenia gravis never causes abnormal pupillary function. Because of the tendency of myasthenia gravis, left untreated, to generalize to the somatic muscles in up to 80% of patients, prompt referral to a neurologist or neuro-ophthalmologist is essential. Acute diplopia can result from demyelinating disease of the brain stem, causing internuclear ophthalmoplegia, sixth nerve paresis, or other ocular motor disorders. Neurologic evaluation can lead to treatment that shortens the period of disability and helps prevent future episodes.

When a patient has sudden onset of anisocoria in association with ocular pain, diplopia, ptosis, or sensory disturbance on the face, it is more ominous than when anisocoria is an isolated phenomenon. These combinations of anisocoria and other neuro-ophthalmologic signs usually indicate disease in the posterior orbit, cavernous sinus, or brain stem. Such patients need immediate referral to a neurologist or neuro-ophthalmologist.

Acute onset of ptosis of one or both eyelids associated with diplopia, anisocoria, headache, ocular pain, or facial sensory loss has the same implications as other combinations of such findings, usually indicating disease in the posterior orbit, cavernous sinus, or brain stem. Sudden onset of ptosis of one or both eyelids may be an isolated phenomenon, when it generally indicates an underlying condition, such as myasthenia gravis. Acute Horner's syndrome may produce mild unilateral ptosis, typically associated with miosis of the same eye. While acute Horner's syndrome can develop in the course of cluster headache or in a patient with migraine, it also can indicate injury to the internal carotid artery (ICA) with arterial dissection. Thus, a patient with headache, neck pain, and recent-onset Horner's syndrome should be urgently evaluated by a neurologist for internal carotid artery dissection. This evaluation often includes pharmacologic testing of the pupil function and imaging of the ICA with cervical magnetic resonance imaging and magnetic resonance angiography. The danger of an ICA dissection is primarily a risk of distal thromboembolism, especially in the first week; many such patients need short-term anticoagulation, though the natural history is eventual arterial wall healing.

Sudden onset of a binocular VF defect almost always implies an intracranial disease process. Rare exceptions are the acute onset of bilateral demyelinating optic neuritis as well as onset after an episode of systemic arterial hypotension of bilateral ischemic optic neuropathy. Acute onset of homonymous hemianopia usually is caused by ischemia of the occipital cortex, which may be due to atheroembolism to the posterior cerebral artery from the aorta, vertebral arteries, or basilar artery or to cardiogenic embolism. The underlying source must be determined to properly guide therapy. If the patient is examined by the physician within 3 hours of onset of a severe deficit, thrombolytic therapy may be considered. Urgent neurologic referral is indicated. The acute onset of bilateral temporal hemianopia implies acute dysfunction of the optic chiasm. This syndrome is seen in patients with a known or previously unrecognized pituitary macroadenoma that undergoes spontaneous hemorrhage, causing "pituitary apoplexy," and then exerts pressure on the optic chiasm from below. This is a neurosurgical and endocrinologic emergency and requires immediate evaluation.

BIBLIOGRAPHY

Miller NR, Newman NJ. *Clinical neuro-ophthalmology: the essentials.* Baltimore: Williams and Wilkins, 1999.

Rosen ES, Eustace P, Thompson HS, et al. *Neuro-ophthalmology.* London: CV Mosby, 1998.

Kelley's Textbook of Internal Medicine, fourth edition. Edited by H. David Humes. Lippincott Williams & Wilkins, Philadelphia © 2000.

C H A P T E R
428

APPROACH TO THE PATIENT WITH A GAIT DISORDER

STEPHEN G. REICH

Impaired walking, with its associated risk of falling, is one of the most debilitating and demoralizing aspects of aging. It is an important source of morbidity among seniors, a significant contributor to death, and a common reason for nursing home placement. Numerous physiologic changes affect gait and balance with normal aging, yet many of the conditions that cause or contribute to disorders of gait are pathologic. These conditions, often multifactorial, pose not only a diagnostic challenge to the clinician but also a therapeutic imperative, since identifying and treating the cause(s) of impaired gait enhance quality of life and lessen the risk of serious injury.

PATHOPHYSIOLOGY

Although there are undoubtedly centers in the brain and spinal cord where the many discrete contributors to locomotion and maintenance of an upright posture are integrated, they remain largely unknown and currently inaccessible to formal testing. The assessment of gait is approached in clinical terms, by analyzing its various components; this appraisal can be done almost entirely at the bedside. Given the complexity of walking, any scheme attempting to break it down into its parts runs the risk of oversimplification. Nevertheless, when confronted with an elderly patient with a gait disorder, a workable clinical approach is to evaluate four major areas—structural, sensory, motor, and cognitive—since these cover virtually all of the conditions that cause or contribute to impaired walking and balance.

The structural component of gait refers to bones, joints, and ligaments, all of which are frequently diseased in the elderly. Their impairment leads not only to instability but also to pain—itself a major contributor to gait disorders and one of the causes most amenable to treatment. The sensory components of walking allow for the appropriate assessment and response to environmental and somatic cues. In addition to somatosensory perception (for clinical purposes, largely proprioception), these components also include vision, hearing, and vestibular functioning. The testable motor contributions to gait include strength, coordination, tone, balance, posture, and the presence of bradykinesia, suggesting parkinsonism.

The cognitive contribution to ambulation broadly includes level of alertness, insight into the environment, and judgment. These are all susceptible to medications, orthostatic hypotension, neurodegenerative diseases, and cerebrovascular disease, among other common conditions in the elderly. Last, fear of falling (sometimes for good reason) can be as disabling as physical causes of a gait disorder and contributes to isolation and sometimes causes agoraphobia in the elderly.

HISTORY AND PHYSICAL EXAMINATION

The history and physical examination of an elderly person with a gait disorder should focus on the four areas mentioned earlier that contribute to normal ambulation: structural, sensory, motor, and cognitive. The duration of a gait disorder is best determined by asking the patient to determine the last time his or her walking was normal. Most gait disorders begin and progress insidiously, but an abrupt onset, change, or long periods of stability or even improvement suggest cerebrovascular disease. Patients should be queried about pain in the hips, knees, ankles, neck, or lower back. Inquire about vision, hearing, and vertigo. Previous use of aminoglycoside antibiotics should raise the suspicion of a vestibulopathologic condition. Historical clues suggesting a somatosensory deficit include numbness and tingling in the feet and greater difficulty navigating in the dark.

Motor disorders are suspected when there is a history of weakness. Its distribution provides additional clues: hemiparesis suggests stroke, proximal weakness implies myopathy or a neuromuscular junction defect, and distal weakness usually indicates a neuropathic origin. Weakness confined to the legs, with spasticity, suggests a spinal localization. Motor impairment without weakness denotes parkinsonism or cerebellar disease, though the latter is uncommon in the elderly. Inquire about associated signs

that can aid in determining location, including bladder dysfunction, which raises the possibility of spinal cord disease, or hydrocephalus. Additional historical features of importance include medications, use of alcohol, symptoms of orthostatic hypotension, clues suggesting dementia, the patient's emotional state, and the way in which the gait disorder has affected the activities of daily living.

Like the history, the physical and neurologic examination should focus on the four main components of walking. The joints of the lower extremities should be assessed for range of motion and pain. Visual acuity, fields, and hearing should be checked. Vestibular function is evaluated by observing the intactness and symmetry of the vestibulo-ocular reflex. This evaluation can be carried out by having the patient read a near card with the head stationary and then when gently shaking the head from side to side, at a frequency of about 1 Hz. Normally, visual acuity does not decline by more than two lines with head shaking; more than that suggests a vestibular defect requiring further evaluation. The final component of the sensory examination examines proprioception by checking joint position at the great toe as well as vibratory sensation, since they both tend to be affected by disease of large myelinated fibers, dorsal roots, or the posterior columns. A positive Romberg sign also suggests a sensory ataxic component to a gait disorder.

The motor examination begins by testing strength. Mild weakness is rarely the sole explanation for a gait disorder. The cause of weakness is determined by whether it is of upper or lower motor neuron origin and, as mentioned previously, by its topography. In addition to checking strength, the motor examination also should focus on tone and coordination. The gait itself is often diagnostic. Specific types are discussed in the next section, but general features include the patient's ability to arise from a chair; narrowing or broadening of the base; the length, velocity, and regularity of strides; and the ability to turn, stand on toes or heels, and tandem walk. Check the postural righting reflex by determining whether the patient can correct for a pull backward. Watch for diminished arm swing, suggesting either subtle hemiparesis or early parkinsonism. It is sometimes easier to hear a slight asymmetry of gait, by noting a shoe scuff the floor, than it is to see it; this can be confirmed by looking for asymmetrical wear on the soles of the shoes. Final parts of the physical examination should include an assessment of the patient's mental status and a check of supine and standing blood pressure.

DIFFERENTIAL DIAGNOSIS

Most gait disorders in the elderly are chronic and do not require urgent evaluation. Nevertheless, difficulty walking that develops over days to weeks should be considered an emergency. The diagnosis hinges on the specifics from the history and physical examination, but important considerations in this context include stroke; spinal cord compression; a mass lesion, such as a subdural xxxxxxx; transverse myelitis, or Guillain-Barré syndrome.

A very different differential diagnosis emerges when one is confronted with a chronic gait disorder. Only the most common types are discussed briefly here. It is easiest to begin with those gait disorders primarily due to pain. When this condition involves one or more joints, the focus is on rheumatologic or orthopedic considerations. Pain limited to the lower back is not dealt with here. Lumbar spinal stenosis is characterized by neurogenic claudication: pain in the lower back, buttocks, and thighs with walking. Unlike vascular claudication, patients with lumbar spinal stenosis do not obtain relief by stopping and standing but prefer to sit. Making this diagnosis relies more on symptoms than signs, yet many patients have mild weakness and depressed deep tendon reflexes in the lower extremities.

Cervical spinal stenosis is another common cause of a gait disorder in the older patient. It is typically the result of hypertrophic degenerative arthritis, with or without frank disk herniation, causing myelopathy. The gait is spastic, with stiff, dragging legs, and aptly has been described as looking as though the patient is wading through waist-high water. There is often surprisingly little leg weakness, but the lower extremities are spastic, with brisk tendon reflexes; when there is a clinically meaningful degree of stenosis, the toes are up. There also may be radicular symptoms and signs in the upper limbs. It is imperative that this diagnosis be based on clinical findings, since plain films, computed tomography, and magnetic resonance imaging (MRI) often show degenerative cervical disk disease in the elderly. When these findings are unaccompanied by myelopathic signs, however, they are practically never a significant contributor to a gait disorder.

When lower motor neuron disorders cause a gait disorder, there is always weakness. A complete differential diagnosis of disorders of the motor unit is beyond the scope of this chapter, but there are general considerations that focus on the elderly. If the weakness is paradoxically admixed with upper motor neuron signs, the most likely cause is associated cervical stenosis; if this condition is ruled out, then amyotrophic lateral sclerosis should be considered.

Pure lower motor neuron diseases are differentiated by the topography of the weakness and associated symptoms and signs. Multilevel lumbar root disease, in addition to patchy lower extremity weakness, is accompanied by pain, often paresthesias, early loss of deep tendon reflexes, and impaired sensation. A similar picture, evolving over weeks to months in diabetics, is known as diabetic amyotrophy or radiculoplexopathy, but it may be purely motor. Proximal weakness, unaccompanied by sensory symptoms, suggests myopathy or a myasthenic syndrome. Distal weakness is more characteristic of neuropathy, frequently associated with loss of proprioception causing a sensory ataxic gait reminiscent of cerebellar syndrome. A similar picture results from B_{12} deficiency, an important treatable cause of a gait disorder.

When there is no pain or signs of upper or lower motor neuron disease, consider Parkinson's disease (PD) and related disorders, as discussed in Chapter 434. People with PD are hesitant when arising from a chair; have a narrow base and a flexed posture; take small, shuffling steps; turn en bloc; and evidence decreased arm swing. In the middle to later stages, there is loss of postural righting reflexes. In early PD, the gait is affected only mildly. Therefore, if confronted with a moderate or moderately severe parkinsonian gait in a patient who has not been symptom-

atic for more than a year or two, consider a parkinsonian mimic. The condition most likely to show signs of significant disorder of gait, with impaired balance and falls, is progressive supranuclear palsy.

The patient who has parkinsonian symptoms from the waist down but not from the waist up has *lower-half parkinsonism*, raising two diagnostic possibilities. The first is normal pressure hydrocephalus. The classic triad is gait apraxia, dementia, and urinary bladder instability. The apractic gait of normal pressure hydrocephalus, like parkinsonism, is characterized by small steps, with failure to pick up the feet—as if they are glued or magnetized to the floor. In contrast to parkinsonism, the base is normal to broad, arm swing is typically preserved, and there are few if any other compelling features of PD.

In some cases of normal pressure hydrocephalus, the gait is affected disproportionately, with relative sparing of cognition. The diagnosis is contingent upon a compatible clinical picture; a scan showing unequivocal hydrocephalus, not accounted for by atrophy; and improvement in gait after a large volume spinal tap. Documenting this improvement is aided by videotaping the patient before and several hours after the lumbar puncture as well as by obtaining before and after lumbar puncture quantitative data, such as the time it takes to walk a specified distance and the number of steps required to turn 360 degrees. At this point, it is appropriate to consider a shunt.

If there is no improvement after a spinal tap, with otherwise typical clinical and radiographic findings, another diagnostic option is more extensive spinal fluid drainage, with placement of a temporary lumbar catheter. Given the challenge of making the diagnosis of normal pressure hydrocephalus and planning treatment, neurologic and neurosurgical consultation are mandatory.

Aside from normal pressure hydrocephalus, the picture of lower-half parkinsonism also suggests microvascular cerebrovascular disease, sometimes called Binswanger's disease. In contrast to a more traditional multi-infarct state, with a history of stroke(s) and signs of hemiparesis, microvascular disease often develops insidiously, with a parkinsonian gait, often unaccompanied by corticospinal signs. The diagnosis is supported by the finding of patchy or confluent areas of increased T2 signal in the periventricular region and subcortical white matter. Given that such findings are nearly ubiquitous in the elderly, it is important not to overdiagnose microvascular disease.

A far more typical scenario than pure Binswanger's disease is a multifactorial gait disorder—arguably the most common condition. These patients rarely have a single overriding abnormality to account for their impaired walking. Instead, they have a little of this and a little of that: mild vestibulopathy, slightly diminished visual acuity, a bit of lower extremity weakness, brisk knee reflexes without significant spasticity, mildly painful hips and knees, some loss of proprioception, and only modest orthostatic hypotension. Although each of these abnormalities is mild, they tend to add up geometrically in the elderly, so that the sum is more than its parts.

Last, as described by Nutt et al., is a group of higher-level gait disorders. These poorly understood but relatively well-described syndromes should be considered in cases where there is neither a singular nor a multifactorial explanation for a patient's impaired walking. They are recognized by their distinctive phenomenological characteristics, for example, isolated gait ignition failure. This rare disorder is distinguished by difficulty initiating gait and sudden hesitation (freezing), reminiscent of advanced PD.

DIAGNOSTIC TESTS

The choice of laboratory tests to evaluate a gait disorder is dictated by the history and physical examination. Practice diagnostic restraint and avoid a "rubber stamp" approach. Most patients should receive a brain scan, preferably MRI, unless there is an adequate alternative explanation, such as marked lower extremity weakness referable to the motor unit. As such, an electromyogram and laboratory studies searching for metabolic sources of myopathy or neuropathy would be most appropriate.

As mentioned, B_{12} deficiency always should be considered. Since any metabolic disturbance can interfere with the cognitive component of gait, it is reasonable to check liver, kidney, and thyroid function. Symptoms of lumbar spinal stenosis are best evaluated with MRI of the lumbosacral spine, and myelopathy requires the same test of the cervical and sometimes the thoracic spine. It is important to avoid routine tests, which are likely to show abnormal results but are of little clinical relevance and are often misleading (such as plain films of the cervical or lumbosacral spine). Similarly, avoid attaching too much importance to increased T2 signal changes on MRI, unless the clinical picture indicates a multi-infarct state.

MANAGEMENT

Like the choice of laboratory tests, management of a gait disorder is dictated by the underlying cause(s), though there are general principles that can be applied to almost all cases. There are two types of treatment: specific and symptomatic. The former is tailored to curing or improving a specific diagnosis or condition, such as anti-parkinsonian medications for PD or a decompressive laminectomy for lumbar spinal stenosis. This treatment includes optimizing as many abnormalities as possible, even mild ones, such as impaired visual acuity and hearing, orthostatic hypotension, and relief of painful joints—the geriatric equivalent of a "major tune-up."

Along with specific therapies, patients also should receive symptomatic treatment aimed at improving their general functional status and minimizing the risk of a fall. This is often best accomplished by employing a physical and occupational therapist. Patients should be given an exercise regimen and be cautioned about the deleterious effects of immobility in the context of a gait disorder. Consideration should be given to an assist device, such as a cane or walker, particularly one with wheels. Safety features about the home should be reviewed, including the use of handrails on the stairs, adequate lighting, and removal of throw rugs. The bathroom is a notorious place for falls: aids include a raised toilet seat, shower chair, and, if necessary, supervision in the shower. In anticipation of a fall, patients should have an emergency call device on hand. Finally, medications

should be reviewed critically; where possible, eliminate those with central nervous effects or side effects.

BIBLIOGRAPHY

Nutt JG, Marsden CD, Thompson PD. Human walking and higher-level gait disorders, particularly in the elderly. *Neurology* 1993;43:268–279.
Sudarsky L. Geriatrics: gait disorders in the elderly. *N Engl J Med* 1990; 322:1441–1446.
Sudarsky L, Ronthal M. Gait disorders among elderly patients: a survey study of 50 patients. *Arch Neurol* 1983;40:740–743.
Tinetti ME, Speechley M. Prevention of falls among the elderly. *N Engl J Med* 1989;320:1055–1059.

Kelley's Textbook of Internal Medicine, fourth edition. Edited by H. David Humes. Lippincott Williams & Wilkins, Philadelphia © 2000.

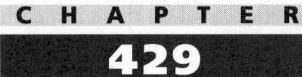

CHAPTER
429

APPROACH TO THE PATIENT WITH ABNORMAL MOVEMENTS AND TREMOR

STEPHEN G. REICH

Movement disorders are a diverse group of neurologic diseases and syndromes characterized by motor dysfunction not attributable to weakness, cerebellar incoordination, changes in tone, cognitive deficits, or impaired sensory feedback. They often are referred to as *extrapyramidal disorders*, emphasizing their anatomic and clinical distinction from the upper motor syndrome characteristic of disease of the pyramidal tract. They manifest as either a paucity of voluntary movement—the hypokinetic (akinetic)/rigid, or parkinsonian, disorders—or excessive involuntary movement—the hyperkinetic disorders.

PATHOPHYSIOLOGY

Movement disorders generally localize to the basal ganglia. These large, paired nuclei at the base of the brain include the caudate nucleus and putamen, known collectively as the striatum, and the globus pallidus, which, when combined with the putamen, is referred to as the lentiform nucleus. Most of the understanding of the basal ganglia comes from observations made in the diseased state. Although movement disorders are the most obvious abnormality, it is now clear that the basal ganglia are involved, either directly or indirectly, through their extensive connections, in myriad other functions. These functions include normal motor planning and execution, behavior, mood, cognition, sensation, and ocular motor functioning, among many others. The basic organization of the basal ganglia is that of a circuit, with functionally and somatotopically segregated parallel pathways connecting the basal ganglia to the thalamus to the cortex and back to the basal ganglia. This complex circuitry is controlled by many neurotransmitters and modulators acting upon a dizzying array of receptors. Lesions anywhere in this circuit, either structural or functional, have the net effect of increasing or decreasing cortical activity, producing a clinical picture of either diminished or excessive motor activity.

HISTORY AND PHYSICAL EXAMINATION

When confronted with a patient with a movement disorder, the diagnostic approach begins with accurate classification of the movement(s) based on clinical phenomenology, thus reversing the usual progression from history to physical examination. Information from the patient's history is most helpful when moving from the type of movement disorder to a specific diagnosis. It should focus on the age and tempo of onset, medication exposure, exacerbating and relieving factors, family history, and the effect of the movement disorder on the activities of daily living.

The physical examination is the cornerstone of the phenomenological diagnosis. As is discussed further later herein, the first step is to determine whether the disorder is hypokinetic (parkinsonian) or hyperkinetic. Between the two, the hyperkinetic disorders typically cause the most confusion. This confusion can be minimized by taking a rather simple and orderly approach to the examination. The key questions include whether the involuntary movements are rhythmic; if they conform to a pattern (stereotyped) or are random and unpredictable from one movement to the next; and their speed and anatomical distribution.

CLASSIFICATION AND DIFFERENTIAL DIAGNOSIS

The prototype *hypokinetic disorder* is Parkinson's disease (PD), characterized by bradykinesia and either tremor at rest or cogwheel rigidity. The latter symptom produces a ratchet-like feeling as a joint is moved and is detected most easily with flexion and extension of the neck or at the elbow or wrist. Additional features seen in the early to middle stages of PD include micrographia, difficulty arising from a low chair, trouble turning in bed, drooling, a stooped posture, decreased blink rate and facial expression (hypomimia), a soft and monotone voice, and decreased arm swing while walking. As the disease advances, bradykinesia often gives way to akinesia in the form of difficulty initiating movement (start hesitation), and freezing—the sudden cessation of movement. There is loss of postural righting reflexes such that the patient cannot correct for even a slight loss of balance, resulting in falls. Because PD and related parkinsonian syndromes are discussed more extensively elsewhere in this volume, the remainder of this chapter focuses on the hyperkinetic disorders.

Tremor is defined as a rhythmical oscillation of a body part. It is the rhythmicity that distinguishes tremor from other hyperkinetic movement disorders. A tremor is classified by its position of maximal activation. A tremor at rest is typical of PD. A postural tremor suggests essential tremor (ET)—enhanced physiologic tremor—and may sometimes accompany PD. Synonyms for ET include benign ET, senile tremor, and familial tremor. A tremor maximally activated with purposeful movement is referred to as a kinetic tremor, replacing the former term *intention tremor*. Although this type traditionally suggests a cerebellar tremor, in clinical practice, cerebellar disease rarely manifests in the form of tremor; instead, an isolated kinetic tremor is usually essential tremor. The frequency of tremor is somewhat helpful in distinguishing different types, but owing to overlap and the challenge of estimating frequency accurately at the bedside, this feature is less reliable than the position of activation. The slowest tremor is seen with cerebellar disease: 3 to 5 Hz. This rate overlaps with the 3 to 6 Hz parkinsonian tremor, and both are slower than ET, at 6 to 12 Hz.

Enhanced physiologic tremor (ET) is a high-frequency, low-amplitude postural tremor encountered in the context of metabolic derangements, drug and alcohol withdrawal, medications, fever, and fatigue. Because it is usually transient, disappearing after the provocation has resolved, it rarely provokes symptoms. There are two exceptions: hyperthyroidism and drug-induced tremor. A list of drugs known to enhance physiologic tremor is included in Table 429.1

In clinical practice, once an enhanced physiologic tremor has been ruled out, the differential diagnosis almost always boils down to either PD or ET. A few key features from the history and physical examination can make this distinction. Most patients with PD are seen within 1 year of onset of tremor, whereas ET is often present for many years, and sometimes decades, before it comes to attention. A small amount of alcohol often transiently suppresses ET but has little effect on PD. At least 60 percent of patients with ET have a positive (autosomal dominant) family history, whereas PD is usually sporadic.

Features from the examination that distinguish ET from PD include the position of activation and frequency, as mentioned earlier. The tremor of PD has a pill-rolling morphologic appearance, whereas ET is typically flexion/extension. Both tremors most commonly affect the upper limbs, but ET sometimes affects the head and voice, which practically never occurs with PD. One of the most helpful differential diagnostic points is whether the tremor begins uni- or bilaterally. Early PD is classically *hemi*-PD, whereas ET is almost always bilateral at onset. A handwriting sample in ET shows the rhythmical oscillation of tremor; in PD the tremor often attenuates with purposeful activities, but there is micrographia. Unlike ET, which is a monosymptomatic disorder (nothing but tremor), PD is characterized not only by tremor but also by the other associated signs mentioned previously. (Note, however, that as many as 30% of PD patients experience no tremor.) Finally, the natural history is different: ET is an insidiously progressive disorder, whereas PD is more noticeably progressive.

There are many other tremor types (see Deuschl), but two deserve brief mention because they are underrecognized. Primary writing tremor is a task-specific movement disorder, meaning that the tremor occurs exclusively or at least disproportionately often with writing. An equally unusual tremor is primary orthostatic tremor, characterized by a fine tremor of the lower extremities upon standing that disappears with walking. Often the diag-

TABLE 429.1.	DRUG-INDUCED MOVEMENT DISORDERS (INCOMPLETE LIST)	
Parkinsonism	Dystonia	Tremor
Antipsychotics	Antipsychotics	Lithium
Metoclopramide	Metoclopramide	Antipsychotics
Aldomet	L-dopa	Valproic acid
Amiodarone	Myoclonus/asterixis	Glucocorticoids
Dopamine depletors	Almost any drug at toxic doses	Tricyclic antidepressants
Chorea	Demerol (especially in the context	β-adrenergic agonists
Phenytoin	of renal insufficiency)	Tics
L-dopa	Tricyclics	Antipsychotics
Antipsychotics	Phenytoin	Amphetamines
Metoclopramide	L-dopa	L-dopa
Estrogens		Carbamazepine

nosis is made from the history alone: the typical patient is an older man or women who complains of the inability to stand still but has no difficulty walking.

Next among the hyperkinetic disorders is dystonia: a syndrome of sustained muscle contractions causing stereotyped, repetitive movements or abnormal postures, generally of a twisting or turning character. Dystonia is distinguished from other hyperkinetic disorders by the sustained and stereotyped nature of the movements. There are several ways to classify dystonia. The first is the age of onset, whether in childhood, adolescence, or adulthood. The younger the age at onset, the more likely dystonia is to be secondary and to spread to other body parts, even becoming generalized. Dystonia is classified as secondary (symptomatic) when there is an identifiable underlying cause and primary (idiopathic) when no cause is found. The majority of adults have primary dystonia. Dystonia can be sporadic or hereditary, and all forms of inheritance have been described. The prototype is seen in Ashkenazic Jews (*DYT1*) on chromosome 9. This is autosomal dominant but has a penetrance of only 30 percent; it typically takes the form of generalized dystonia with onset in childhood, though there is quite a bit of heterogeneity.

The most helpful way to classify the adult-onset dystonias is by their topography. The most common are the focal dystonias, affecting one body part, with a predilection for craniocervical muscles. Segmental dystonia involves two or more contiguous body parts, multifocal dystonia affects two or more noncontiguous body parts, hemidystonia affects an ipsilateral arm and leg, and generalized dystonia involves the lower extremities and another region. As briefly mentioned earlier, dystonia may manifest only during certain tasks, the most common being writing or playing a musical instrument.

The most well-recognized focal dystonia is torticollis, or cervical dystonia, which is characterized by involuntary turning of the head. Similar spasmodic movements involving the orbicularis oculi are known as blepharospasm. The lower portion of the face may be affected (oromandibular dystonia) as well as the vocal cords. The latter condition, known as spasmodic dysphonia, produces a strained quality to the voice, as if being strangled.

Chorea is characterized by brief, nonsustained, nonstereotyped, low-amplitude movements that tend to flow irregularly from one body part to another. It often has a predilection for distal limbs but can affect the trunk and face. The lack of rhythmicity distinguishes chorea from tremor, and the absence of a pattern and its faster frequency separate it from dystonia. Patients with chorea often look fidgety. The prototype choreiform disorder is Huntington's disease (HD), characterized by the clinical triad of chorea, dementia, and an autosomal dominant family history. The gene, located on chromosome 9, causes an expanded trinucleotide repeat (CAG), and there is an inverse correlation between repeat length (over 40 is always pathologic) and age at onset. It typically develops in the third or fourth decade of life, with varying combinations of chorea or psychiatric manifestations, including dementia, impulsively poor judgment, or an affective disorder. Depending on the length of the repeat, it can manifest as early as childhood and well into advanced age.

The differential diagnosis of chorea is long, including other degenerative disorders; such developmental abnormalities as cerebral palsy; drug effects (Table 429.1); metabolic disorders, such as hyperthyroidism; chorea gravidarum; lupus and the antiphospholipid antibody syndrome; and infectious disorders, such as HIV and Sydenham's chorea, among many others. Acute hemichorea is typically due to a stroke or other lesion in or close to the subthalamic nucleus of Luys. Such a lesion also causes acute hemiballismus, which is similar to chorea but is distinguished by its larger-amplitude, more violent, flinging movements, with a tendency to affect proximal muscles. The dramatic picture of acute vascular hemichorea or hemiballismus is contrasted to its usually benign course, with spontaneous resolution in several weeks or months, though there are exceptions.

Similar to chorea in its random spread from one muscle group to another is myoclonus, distinguished from chorea and other hyperkinetic disorders by its lightening-like speed. Myoclonus can be physiologic in origin, such as the jerks many of us experience when falling asleep, or part of a pathologic process. It may be epileptic or part of a degenerative disease (Alzheimer's disease or Creutzfeldt–Jakob disease) but is most commonly encountered in the context of a metabolic, toxic, or hypoxic/ischemic encephalopathy. The same setting causes the related movement, asterixis, sometimes called *negative myoclonus*, in which there is a sudden lapse of posture of the dorsiflexed hands, producing the classic liver flap.

Motor tics are abrupt, focal movements that burst forth on the background of normal motor activity. Tics may be simple and limited to one body region, such as the shrug of a shoulder, or complex, such as touching the nose or clapping the hands. Unlike chorea, patients usually have a limited repertoire of tics. Additional unique features include a buildup of inner tension before the tic and the ability of patients to suppress tics briefly, but they are not otherwise under voluntary control. Tics also may be vocal, ranging from simple sounds, such as sniffing, grunting, throat clearing, or clicking, to complex vocalizations, including the utterance of obscenities, known as coprolalia. The prototype tic disorder is Tourette syndrome, characterized by the combination of motor and vocal tics beginning in childhood or adolescence. Tics may be accompanied by behavioral disturbances, such as obsessive/compulsive disorder. Less severe than Tourette syndrome are transient tics of childhood and chronic mono- or oligo-symptomatic tics.

All of the above-mentioned movement disorders may be induced by drugs (Table 429.1). In most cases, they resolve completely when the offending medication is withdrawn. Drug-induced parkinsonism may take as long as 1 year to disappear, and some drug-induced movement disorders may be permanent. Such is the case with tardive dyskinesia, typically manifested by stereotyped chewing movements. It is now well recognized that the same offending medications also can cause permanent dystonia, akathisia, tics, or myoclonus.

The appearance of any movement disorder, either hypokinetic or hyperkinetic, before the age of 50 should prompt consideration of Wilson's disease. This rare autosomal recessive disorder is due to a defect in copper transport, leading to its toxic accumulation. The workup includes measurement of serum ceruloplasmin, which is usually low, and urinary excretion of copper, which is high. A slit-lamp examination should be performed to search for a Kayser-Fleischer ring in Descemet's membrane of the cornea.

MANAGEMENT

A complete review of the complexities of managing movement disorders is beyond the scope of this chapter, but general guidelines can be provided. Since PD is covered in Chapter xxx, this discussion focuses on the hyperkinetic movement disorders. The presence of a movement disorder by itself does not necessitate treatment; treatment is necessary only when the disorder interferes with the patient's functioning or causes significant embarrassment. Likewise, the benefit of therapy is gauged by its effect on the activities of daily living. Education and reassurance are an essential part of therapy, particularly since many patients with hyperkinetic movement disorders feel freakish and unique and are often labeled as having *psychogenic* problems before the proper diagnosis is reached. There is a large and active network of support and advocacy groups for each of the hyperkinetic movement disorders, and patients should be encouraged to seek them out.

When treatment of ET is required, the first-line medications are propranolol and primidone. Each is started at a low dose and escalated gradually, until there is either sufficient functional improvement or clinical signs of toxicity. For the small percentage of patients with disabling tremor unresponsive to medical therapy, surgical therapy, including either stereotactic thalamotomy or deep brain stimulation of the thalamus, is available.

The treatment of dystonia depends on its cause. Although some secondary dystonias are amenable to specific therapy, such as penicillamine for Wilson's disease, most treatments focus on symptom management. The mainstay of therapy for the focal dystonias is local injection of botulinum toxin, which produces sufficient weakness to suppress the spasms but not so much as to impair functioning. The toxin generally wears off in 3 to 4 months, and repeated injections are required. A variety of oral medications provide some relief for dystonia, including anticholinergics, benzodiazepines, antispasticity agents, and sometimes dopaminergic or antidopaminergic agents, among many others. Lacking an understanding of the pharmacology of dystonia, the use of oral medications has been guided largely by empiricism and serendipity. Surgery is available for some types of dystonia, such as selective denervation for cervical dystonia. There is a resurgence of interest in stereotactic procedures for the treatment of dystonia, including both lesioning and, more recently, deep brain stimulation of the thalamus and globus pallidus.

Like dystonia, the treatment of chorea depends on its underlying cause. It is surprising that many patients with HD are not particularly bothered by chorea; if they are, it responds best to antidopaminergic agents, such as haloperidol. These agents should be used cautiously in light of their potential to provoke additional movement disorders. For acute vascular hemichorea or hemiballismus, a short-term course of haloperidol is the treatment of choice; other options are clonazepam or valproic acid. The latter two agents also can be used to treat myoclonus when the underlying cause cannot be reversed.

When motor and vocal tics necessitate treatment, they occasionally respond to clonidine. If not, antidopaminergic agents are the mainstay of therapy, and the preferred drug is pemozide. The treatment of Wilson's disease is aimed at removing accumulated copper with a chelator, such as penicillamine, or preventing the absorption of copper by zinc. A more extensive discussion of treatment for Wilson's disease and other movement disorders is included in the bibliography.

BIBLIOGRAPHY

Alexander GE, Crutcher MD, DeLong MR. Basal ganglia–thalamocortical circuits: parallel substrates for motor, oculomotor, "pre-frontal" and "limbic" functions. *Prog Brain Res* 1990;85:119–146.

Bain PG. The effectiveness of treatments for essential tremor. *Neurologist* 1997;5:305.

Deuschl G. Differential diagnosis of tremor. *J Neural Transm Suppl* 1999; 56:211–220.

Fink JK, Hedera P, Brewer GJ. Hepatolenticular degeneration (Wilson's disease). *Neurologist* 1999;5:171.

Jankovic J. Tardive syndromes and other drug-induced movement disorders. *Clin Neuropharmacol* 1995;18:197–214.

Jankovic J, Brin M. Therapeutic uses of botulinum toxin. *N Engl J Med* 1991;324:1186–1194.

Lang AE, Lozano AM. Parkinson's disease. *N Engl J Med* 1998;339: 1044–1053;1130–1143.

Marsden CD, Hallett M, Fahn S. The nosology and pathophysiology of myoclonus. In: Marsden CD, Fahn S, eds. *Movement disorders.* xxxxxxxx: Butterworth, 1982:196.

Marsden CD, Quinn NP. The dystonias. *Br Med J* 1990;300:139–144.

Miyawaki E. The pathophysiology and management of ballism. *Neurologist* 1998;4:120.

Ross CA, Margolis RL, Rosenblatt A, et al. Huntington disease and the related disorder, dentatorubral-pallidoluysian atrophy (DRPLA). *Medicine* 1997;76:305–338.

Shoulson I. On chorea. *Clin Neuropharm* 1986;9:S85–S99.

Singer HS, Walkup JT. Tourette syndrome and other tic disorders: diagnosis, pathophysiology, and treatment. *Medicine* 1991;70:15–32.

Kelley's Textbook of Internal Medicine, fourth edition. Edited by H. David Humes.
Lippincott Williams & Wilkins, Philadelphia © 2000.

CHAPTER
430

APPROACH TO THE PATIENT WITH DISORDERS OF SENSATION

JOHN W. GRIFFIN

SENSORY LOSS

PRESENTATION

The healthy sensory system functions so effortlessly and silently that it is invisible. The gibe "He can't walk and chew gum at the same time" is posited on the assumption that ambulation is a commonplace and trivial accomplishment rather than the wonder of sensory and motor integration that is recognized by physiologists. Happily, at present the elegant mechanisms required for both unconscious sensation and perceived sensation are being demonstrated dramatically by new advances in functional imaging, electrophysiology, and psychophysics.

The ubiquitous role of afferent signaling in neurologic function leads to manifold vulnerabilities in disease. For the clinician, disorders of sensation are prevalent and wide ranging in both origin and significance. For example, carpal tunnel syndrome, spinal disease, and stroke may all be accompanied by initial complaints of numbness in one hand. The patient's description of his or her subjective sensory experience may not translate easily into medical terms that have specific physiological or anatomic implications. These difficulties are compounded by the inherent subjectivity of the examination and the poor interinterval and interexaminer reproducibility of findings (one evening's sensory findings often cannot be shown the next morning on rounds). Successful differential diagnosis requires avoiding distraction by small and inconstant sensory findings, understanding the basic pathophysiologic patterns, and using applied neuroanatomy, as outlined herein.

PATHOPHYSIOLOGY

Disorders of both the central and peripheral nervous systems can produce sensory loss. The various anatomic sites that can be affected each generate patterns of clinical findings that allow for localization, which is the first step in differential diagnosis.

Peripheral Transducers

Somatosensory transduction occurs at cutaneous receptors that have specific modalities but whose functional roles often are not related intuitively to these modalities. For example, Merkel cells at the dermal–epidermal junction are slowly adapting receptors of pressure and are necessary to making the distinction between various textures. Nociceptors, which cause painful sensation, include the nonensheathed "free" sensory endings within the epidermis.

Peripheral Nerves

Pain and temperature sensibility is conveyed by small-caliber nerve fibers, termed C and Aδ fibers. The former are not myelinated and conduct a few meters per second, whereas the latter are larger and myelinated, achieving velocities of up to 30 m per second. The distinction in fast Aδ pain and slow C fiber pain is familiar to anyone who has touched a hot stove and reflexively withdrawn the hand before the lingering burning pain was perceived. Joint position sensibility (*proprioception*), the location of the limb in space (*kinesthesia*), and vibratory sensibility are conveyed by larger myelinated fibers (Aα,β) with velocities of 40 to 100 m per second. Similarly, the afferent limb of the tendon reflex utilizes the large muscle stretch receptors designated *Ia fibers*.

Dermatomes

Each spinal segment has a distinctive area of the body for which it provides sensory innervation (Figs. 430.1 and 430.2).

Spinal Pathways

Within the spinal cord the large fibers ascend ipsilaterally within the dorsal column to reach their first synapse near the cranial–cervical junction in the gracile (legs) or cuneate (arms) nuclei (Fig. 430.3). In contrast, the small fibers synapse ipsilaterally in the dorsal horn (substantia gelatinosa) near the segmental level where they enter, and the second-order neuron crosses in front of the central canal of the cord to ascend in the anterior spinothalamic tract.

Intracranial Pathways

The neospinothalamic tract projects directly to the ventral posterior nucleus of the thalamus, with a final relay to somatosensory areas I and II of the neocortex. In contrast, the second-order neurons of the dorsal column pathways project to the thalamus from the cuneate and gracile nuclei and from there are widely projected to the cortex, including the posterior parietal lobe.

HISTORY AND PHYSICAL EXAMINATION

The goal of the sensory history is to understand as precisely as possible the patient's subjective experience. Disorders of the

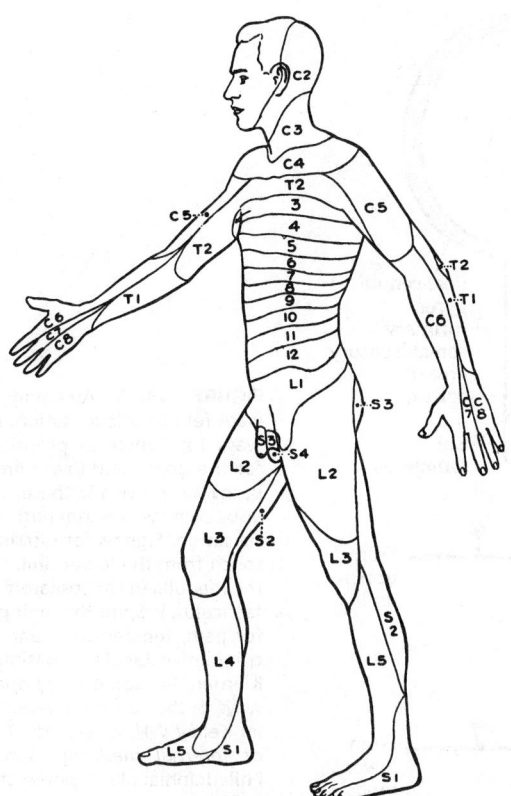

FIGURE 430.1. Anterolateral view of the dermatomes according to Foerster. (From Foerster O, Haymaker W, Woodhall B. *Peripheral nerve injuries*, second ed. Philadelphia: WB Saunders, 1953, with permission.)

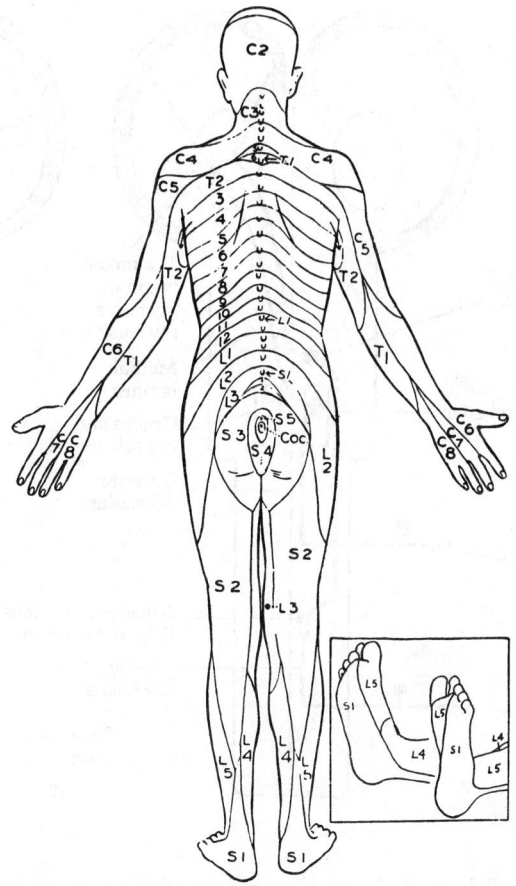

FIGURE 430.2. Posterior view of the dermatomes according to Foerster. (Adapted from Foerster O, Haymaker W, Woodhall B. *Peripheral nerve injuries*, second ed. Philadelphia: WB Saunders, 1953, with permission.)

sensory nervous system often initially show negative symptoms owing to loss of sensibility. Examples include difficulty picking up small objects because of loss of touch and texture perception, gait ataxia due to loss of proprioceptive input, or painless foot ulcers due to loss of protective sensibility. Positive symptoms, such as the pins-and-needles sensations termed *paresthesias*, are common. Many patients volunteer metaphors—for example, "It feels as though I am walking on cotton wool" or "I'm walking on coals." A special type of positive sensory symptom is spontaneous neuropathic pain, discussed later in this chapter.

The examination of the sensory system entails analysis of the primary modalities, as defined clinically—pain perception, thermal sensibility, light touch, vibration (with a 128-cps tuning fork), and joint position sensibility. In no other area of the physical examination is it so easy to be distracted by inconsistent findings. This problem is exaggerated if the patient does not fully understand the task or is trying too hard to please the examiner. Keeping the focus on uncovering consistent large patterns of abnormal sensation—the forest—helps keep the examination from going astray among the trees. The toes, feet, and fingers are always examined. Depending on the hypothesis for localization to be tested, other areas may need to be studied as well. For example, if sensory loss in the legs could be explained by a spinal cord lesion, it is necessary to conduct an examination of touch and pin sensibility on the back, looking for a spinal level.

Localization of a sensory lesion can be done only in the con-

text of the neurologic company the sensory deficit keeps. Are the reflexes decreased, suggesting a segmental spinal, segmental nerve root, or peripheral nerve lesion? Or are they increased, indicating a central nervous system lesion? Is there accompanying motor weakness? If so, is it central upper motor neuron weakness, pointing to lesions in the brain, brain stem, or spinal cord? Or is it lower motor neuron weakness with muscle atrophy, implying involvement of the anterior horn cells, spinal roots, or peripheral nerves?

Sensory ataxia may occur on a peripheral basis with severe loss of large-fiber function. The Romberg sign—the inability to stand with the eyes closed—reflects loss of afferent input from the joint and muscle sensors in the legs, including afferent input from muscle spindles. The Romberg sign and sensory gait ataxia also can result from involvement of the dorsal columns of the spinal cord. The most serious consequence of loss of small-nerve-fiber function is loss of protective sensibility. This can result in nonhealing and usually painless ulcers of the skin or painless bony injuries or fractures. If the fractures of Charcot's foot are suspected, radiographs of the feet are warranted. They often show much more extensive bony injuries and callus formation than suspected by inspection of the feet.

Involvement of the sensory cortex in the posterior parietal

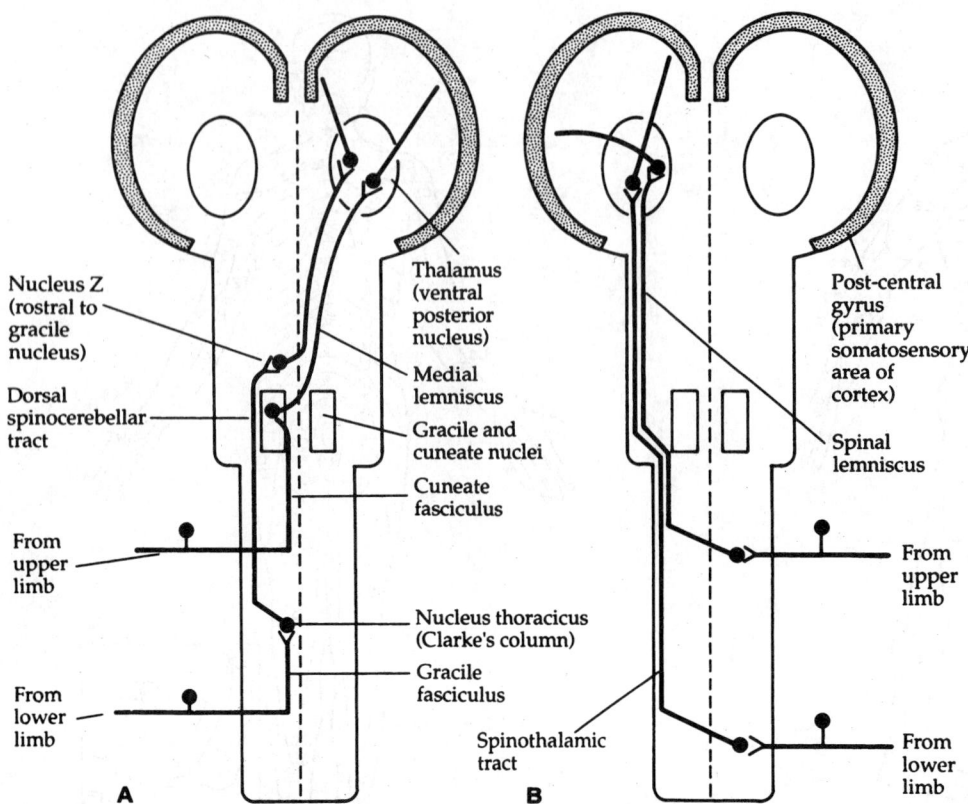

FIGURE 430.3. Ascending pathways for somatic sensation. **A:** Pathways for conscious proprioception for the upper and lower limbs. The pathway shown for the upper limb also conveys discriminative touch sensation. Signals for discriminative touch from the lower limb travel to the medulla in the ipsilateral gracile fasciculus. **B:** Spinothalamic pathway for pain, temperature, and nondiscriminative tactile sensation. (From Kiernan JA. Some functional pathways in the central nervous system. In: Kelley WN, et al., eds. *Textbook of internal medicine*, second ed. Philadelphia: JB Lippincott, 1992: 2142.)

lobe and the underlying white matter often spares the primary systems of sensation but alters discriminative sensory functions. These functions include the patient's ability to discriminate between one- and two-point tactile sensation, distinguish numbers or letters traced on the skin (*graphesthesia*), and identify objects in the hand by their texture, shape, size, and weight (*stereognosis*). The relationship of sensory complaints to alterations of body position is often helpful in diagnosis. Flexion of the neck producing a transient tingling sensation down the back and into the legs and arms (Lhermitte's sign) indicates disease in the cervical portion of the spinal cord. Movements of the neck that result in radiating pain or tingling sensation in the arm are indicative of cervical spinal root compression. The pain of lumbar spinal root compression may be aggravated by coughing, straining, and straight-leg raising. The sensory symptoms of conversion reaction are often of sudden onset and do not relate to anatomic factors. They frequently develop after a patient has undergone a neurologic examination in which testing of sensation has been carried out. Hyperventilation can evoke tingling sensations around the lips and face and in the fingertips. Having the patient hyperventilate may reproduce the sensory symptoms.

LABORATORY STUDIES

Studies Relevant to Peripheral Lesions

Electrodiagnostic studies—nerve conduction studies and electromyography—are integral to the evaluation of patients with peripheral neuropathy. These studies are an extension of the clinical examination and an indicator of the underlying patho-

physiology of the specific neuropathy. Close coordination between the peripheral nerve diagnostician and the neuromuscular electrodiagnostician ensures that the electrodiagnostic studies will have maximal value in differential diagnosis. The basics of nerve conduction studies are summarized in Chapter 450. In interpreting nerve conduction studies, it is important to recall that they test only the largest and fastest 10% to 20% of fibers; smaller fibers are invisible to standard electrodiagnosis.

The clinician should frame a series of questions that can be answered specifically by the electrodiagnostician. These questions parallel the clinical questions described earlier. Is this neuropathy? If so, is it a multiple mononeuropathy or a polyneuropathy? And what is the cellular basis for the nerve disease? If a peripheral neuropathy is confirmed, the other laboratory evaluations required for differential diagnosis are considered in Chapter 445. Relatively pure small-fiber sensory and autonomic neuropathies represent a special diagnostic challenge. Affected patients may have normal strength, proprioception, and tendon reflexes. The recent advent of skin biopsies immunostained for epidermal sensory nerve fibers as well as practical methods of sweat measurement and psychophysical tests of sensation (quantitative sensory tests) are beginning to alter this picture.

Studies Relevant to Central Lesions

If a spinal lesion is suspected, the basic evaluation is imaging, usually magnetic resonance imaging. The technique of somatosensory evoked potentials is occasionally useful in confirming dorsal column involvement and suggesting the level. A catalog of all of the causes of myelopathy is beyond the scope of this chapter, but one that may bring about predominant sensory dysfunction and is treatable early is subacute combined degeneration due to B_{12} deficiency. A serum B_{12} and homocysteine level and methylmevalonic acid determination in the urine are the initial screens for this possibility. Intracranial lesions usually are approached by imaging studies.

DIFFERENTIAL DIAGNOSIS

The differential diagnosis is established in part by the localization of the responsible lesion, distinguishing initially among peripheral and central lesions. If the lesion is central, then is it spinal or intracranial, and if it is intracranial, is it deep or in the parietal lobe? The localization within the nervous system is discovered by analysis of the distribution of the sensory symptoms or signs and the modalities involved. The list of etiologic possibilities is then narrowed from the historical information, including the time course, associated diseases, and so on. With regard to localization (distribution plus modalities affected), several patterns have special localizing value.

Polyneuropathic Patterns

Peripheral neuropathies typically produce loss of sensation in the toes and feet initially; with progression, the level of numbness ascends the leg and comes to affect the fingers (Fig. 430.4) On the trunk, the parasternal region represents the region innervated by the longest intercostal axons (Fig. 430.4). This pattern reflects the tendency of the first nerve fibers affected to be those that are longest in length, with the distal regions degenerating and with progression from distal to proximal with time. Patients may complain of a dead feeling, as with receiving lidocaine. More often they describe a positive sensory symptom—tingling or a pins-and-needles sensation (paresthesia) or painful burning (neuropathic pain), described in detail later in this chapter.

The modalities involved in neuropathies may call into play functions of the large nerve fibers (proprioception and vibration with loss of tendon reflexes, usually occurring first at the ankle) and functions of the small (pain, temperature) nerve fibers, or they may be relatively selective. Prominent involvement of small nerve fibers is, for example, seen in the most prevalent neuropathy, diabetic polyneuropathy. The clinical picture can include both loss of pain sensibility, with consequent predilection to painless injuries, and at the same time spontaneous neuropathic pain, usually most severe in the feet, as considered under the heading Neuropathic Pain. Autonomic functions also are mediated by small fibers, so that impotence, orthostatic hypotension, reduced sinus arrhythmia in response to breathing, and diminished sweating also can be seen.

Individual Nerve Injury Patterns

Single-nerve injury, or mononeuropathy, provokes sensory symptoms related to the cutaneous distribution of the sensory component of that nerve. Such isolated peripheral nerve lesions develop most often as a result of trauma or mechanical compression. For example, compression of the median nerve at the wrist, as in carpal tunnel syndrome, produces paresthesias and sensory loss in the first three fingers of the affected hand, and the loss of pain sensibility lies in the median distribution, typically affecting the medial but not the radial side of the fourth digit. Mononeuropathies also can affect the small vessels, as seen in diabetic third nerve palsies.

Multiple Mononeuropathies

This pattern affects several individual nerves (Fig. 430.4). For example, a patient may have numbness in the median distribution in one hand and in the peroneal distribution in the opposite leg. Multiple mononeuropathies are usually due to small-vessel disease, such as vasculitis or diabetes.

Radicular (Dermatomal) Distributions

Nerve root lesions generate symptoms related to the dermatomal distribution of that nerve root (Fig. 430.2). Mixed spinal root

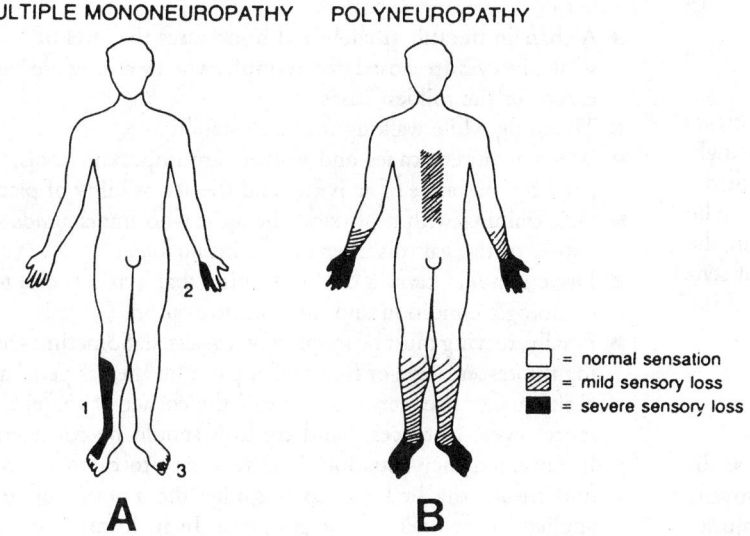

MULTIPLE MONONEUROPATHY   POLYNEUROPATHY

□ = normal sensation
▨ = mild sensory loss
■ = severe sensory loss

A   **B**

FIGURE 430.4. Contrast between mononeuropathy and polyneuropathy. The figure to the left has three individual nerve lesions (multiple mononeuropathies). Number 1 reflects sensory loss in the distribution of the superficial peroneal nerve; number 2, the distribution of the ulnar nerve; and number 3, the distribution of the deep peroneal nerve. These discrete nerve regions contrast with the distally predominant symmetrical sensory loss found in a patient with polyneuropathy. Note that there is mild sensory loss in the sternal and parasternal regions of the chest; these areas represent the sensory fields of the longest axons in the intercostal nerves. (From Griffin J. Diabetic neuropathies. Medical Grand Rounds of the Johns Hopkins Hospital, 1987, with permission)

lesions, such as those caused by herniated intravertebral discs, typically lead to reflex loss and, if severe enough, weakness characteristic of their distribution. One disorder produces a distinctive picture of widespread selective dorsal root degeneration. This disorder, tabes dorsalis due to tertiary syphilis, is seen rarely now, but it remains important to recognize. It provokes sensory ataxia and loss of protective sensibility (Charcot's joints were first described in tabes), but the peripheral nerves are normal in terms of electrodiagnostic and biopsy parameters, because the lesion is confined to degeneration of the dorsal roots.

Intraspinal Lesions

A sensory level below which sensation is altered or lost is most helpful in delineating the level of spinal cord involvement. Lesions of the spinal cord produce sensory signs and symptoms below the level of involvement that are ipsilateral for touch, vibration, and proprioceptive-type sensation and contralateral for pain and temperature. Following segmental transection of one lateral half of the cord, pain and thermal sensibility are lost on the contralateral half of the body below the level of the lesion, whereas proprioception and vibratory sensibility are lost on the side of the lesion. The pattern is the consequence of the crossing of pain and temperature fibers at or near the segment where they enter the spinal cord, as first identified by the French physiologist Eduoard Brown-Séquard.

Dissociated sensation refers to loss of pain and temperature sensibility with preservation of vibration and proprioception. When found to be present over several spinal levels—for example, in the hand and a region of the thorax on one side—dissociated sensation suggests a central intraspinal lesion interrupting the second-order pain and temperature fibers decussating near the central canal. A notorious cause of this picture is syringomyelia, a fluid-filled cavity in the central cord.

Supraspinal Lesions

Central lesions above the spinal cord cause contralateral involvement of limbs and trunk. The disproportionate loss of discriminative abilities suggests involvement of the parietal cortex.

STRATEGIES FOR OPTIMAL CARE

Treatment of sensory loss begins with identification and treatment of the underlying disease. For example, it is increasingly clear that in diabetes, approaching euglycemia lessens both the likelihood and the severity of diabetic polyneuropathy. The management of positive sensory symptoms is discussed in the section Neuropathic Pain. Two aspects of management of sensory loss that require specific comment are management of the insensitive limb and management of sensory ataxia.

Management of the Insensitive Limb

Patients with loss of protective sensibility from disorders as diverse as diabetic neuropathy, leprosy, tabes, and syringomyelia share the need for special education to prevent painless injuries with consequent Charcot joints, ulcers, infections, and amputation. In both the hands and the feet, the keystone is regular careful examination. Because it is important to see both the top and the bottom of the foot, another household member often can perform this task better than the patient. Redness, heat, swelling, calluses, ingrown nails, or redness around the nails are all important warning signs. Development of skin breakage or ulcers should trigger prompt consultation.

Shoes that fit well are essential. Calluses are a sign of long-standing excessive pressure on the skin and thus signal badly fitting shoes. Calluses usually are found on the balls of the feet, the sides of the feet, or the tops of the toes. They should be treated as soon as they begin to form by finding where the shoe is rubbing and removing the pressure from the foot. Patients must avoid using a knife or razor to cut into a callus, because any cut in the skin can result in infection. A persistent or growing callus needs to be examined and treated by a medical professional.

Every time a shoe is put on, the inside of the shoe should be felt with the fingers (assuming they are normally sensitive), and the shoe should be shaken to make sure that there are no protruding nails or stones inside. Similarly, the foot of the socks should be felt to make sure that no foreign objects are within the sock. Shoes must always be worn with socks, and individuals with insensitive feet must *never* walk barefooted.

Management of Sensory Ataxia

In all the ataxic disorders, the most important principle is to avoid falls and injuries. Continued walking provides an important form of physical therapy and continuous relearning. Patients who are in bed for long periods because of broken hips, for example, have a great deal of difficulty returning to walking and regaining their previous level of function. Several strategies are helpful.

- Review safety in the home. The bathroom is the most dangerous room, with many hard surfaces, small space, and sometimes slick footing.
- Handrails placed in the joists of the wall are essential in the bath.
- A chair in the tub or shower also increases the level of safety while the eyes are closed (for example, when washing the hair), except in the mildest cases.
- Touching while walking increases stability.
- When required, canes and walkers are important tools, expanding the range of activities and the accessibility of places.
- Gait training with a physical therapist who understands the nature of the gait disorder can be invaluable.
- Drivers should carry a card indicating that ataxia is due to a neurologic condition and not to intoxication.
- Finally, driving must be frequently reassessed. Sometimes having fluorescent tape or fluorescent paint on the gas pedal and brake makes it easier to see out of the corner of the eye. In more severe instances, hand controls should be considered. In an emergency situation, it is very easy to catch the foot underneath the brake or to misjudge the amount of force applied to the brake or the gas pedal. In such instances, it is

the patient's responsibility to notify the Motor Vehicle Administration about the issue.

NEUROPATHIC PAIN

PRESENTATION

Neuropathic pain represents one of the most prevalent classes of chronic nonmalignant pain. Causes included painful peripheral neuropathies, such as diabetic polyneuropathy; postherpetic neuralgia; neuroma pain from traumatic nerve injury; and the complex problem of causalgia (reflex sympathetic dystrophy or complex regional pain syndrome). Compared with other nonmalignant sources, such as chronic musculoskeletal pain, neuropathic pain is less responsive to nonsteroidal anti-inflammatory agents and to opiate analgesics and thus represents a major challenge in management.

PATHOPHYSIOLOGY

The peripheral nociceptors include the polymodal C nociceptors, which end in the dermis and epidermis. These nociceptors respond to a variety of noxious agents. Among these are capsaicin, a vanilloid extracted from peppers that activates the VR_1 receptor on nociceptors, producing firing and, with sufficient doses, destruction of the fiber. As described earlier, the central processes of Aδ and C fibers extend from the dorsal root ganglia to synapse primarily in the superficial dorsal horn of the spinal cord. The neurotransmitters released at these central synapses include the amino acids glutamate and aspartate and the neuropeptide substance P. The second-order pain neurons in the substantia gelatinosa express the substance P receptor NK1. Most nociceptive dorsal horn neurons ascend in the opposite anterolateral quadrant of the spinal cord, known as the spinothalamic tract. The neospinothalamic tract projects, through a synapse in the ventral posterior nucleus of the thalamus, to the somatosensory areas I and II of the neocortex. The major role of the neospinothalamic projection is to localize pain precisely and gauge its intensity and character. The phylogenetically older paleospinothalamic tract, or spinoreticular tract, projects to the reticular formation of the brain stem and thalamus and then diffusely to the limbic cortex to subserve the arousal and affective components of pain.

The mechanisms of neuropathic pain are manifold, and the relative contributions of the different types are uncertain. The C and Aδ fiber nociceptors are hyperactive in some contexts and can express new sodium channels that may contribute to hyperexcitability. Transmitter release is amplified in the dorsal horn in some models of pain, and the levels of the substance P receptor NK1 are also increased, suggesting that each stimulus produces a heightened response. Finally, there are a series of structural changes in the dorsal root ganglion and dorsal horn that include sprouting of Aβ afferents into the region of the dorsal horn normally occupied by nociceptive afferents, so that stimulation of a hair sensor, for example, triggers a painful sensation.

The brain also contains powerful descending pathways that modulate nociceptive input. The periaqueductal gray region of the midbrain projects to the midline raphe nuclei of the medulla. These nuclei are serotonergic and project in turn to the dorsal horn of the spinal cord, where they suppress nociceptive transmission. Opioid receptors in the region of these brain-stem nuclei allow for the action of opioid analgesics by way of this descending inhibitory pathway, in addition to their direct action on opioid receptors in the dorsal horn. Another major inhibitory pathway is noradrenergic and originates in the pons. Combined with the serotonergic projection from the medulla, these monoaminergic pathways provide one rationale for the analgesic effects of the tricyclic antidepressants that inhibit the reuptake of serotonin and norepinephrine.

HISTORY AND PHYSICAL EXAMINATION

Neuropathic pain often has a burning quality. In painful neuropathies and in tabes, a characteristic description is of lightning pains—sudden stabbing jolts in, for example, one foot. On examination, the threshold to pain may be normal, or there may be sensory loss, even in areas where the perception is of severe pain to a normally non-noxious stimulus once the threshold for perception is reached (allodynia). Hyperesthesia may be reflected in the description of pain produced by the bedsheets touching the feet, for example. As noted previously, painful neuropathies, such as those associated with diabetes, often are accompanied by a predisposition to painless injuries, such as foot ulcers.

DIFFERENTIAL DIAGNOSIS

Painful peripheral neuropathies are seen in most of the disorders listed in Table 430.1. Trigeminal neuralgia, also known as tic douloureux, is the most common cranial neuralgia. This is really an acute recurring pain syndrome in the sense that the patient is seized by episodes of sudden, lightning-like stabs of pain typically involving the second or third divisions of the trigeminal nerve. Each burst of pain lasts a matter of seconds, but they tend to occur in clusters, which are commonly triggered by tactile stimulation in the maxillary or perioral region. Infrequently, the pain is symptomatic of multiple sclerosis or a tumor along the course of the trigeminal nerve. In idiopathic trigeminal neuralgia, the neurologic examination gives negative results. One or more medications provide effective pain relief in 80% of patients with trigeminal neuralgia. Carbamazepine is the drug of choice. Baclofen, in divided doses up to 80 mg daily, may also be effec-

TABLE 430.1.	SOME PAINFUL NEUROPATHIES

Diabetic polyneuropathy
Amyloid
Sensory neuropathy of AIDS
Idiopathic small-fiber sensory neuropathy
Fabry's disease (β-D-glucuronidase deficiency)
Some cases of leprosy
Tabes dorsalis (a dorsal radiculopathy)

tive and sometimes works synergistically with carbamazepine. If medical treatment fails, a percutaneous radiofrequency lesion of the trigeminal ganglion often provides relief, and the procedure can be repeated if necessary. Vascular decompression of the trigeminal sensory root by a posterior fossa craniotomy is also very effective.

Postherpetic neuralgia manifests as severe burning pain, with superimposed shocklike pains along one or more dermatomes after an attack of herpes zoster. Hyperpathic phenomena are common. It tends to be a disease of the elderly, and the pain can be intractable. Tricyclic agents can be helpful. An oral opioid analgesic, such as oxycodone (starting at 5 mg every 3 or 4 hours) or morphine (starting at 10 mg every 3 or 4 hours), can make the difference between bearable and unbearable pain and carries a low risk of psychological dependence or addiction.

Causalgic pain syndromes are characterized by severe burning pain in an extremity after major or minor injury. If the injury involves a peripheral nerve, particularly the sciatic or median nerve, the syndrome is called *causalgia*. If the injury involves soft tissue or bone, the usual term that is applied is *reflex sympathetic dystrophy*. The pain is continuous, is exacerbated by emotional stress, and usually is associated with hyperpathia. The limb becomes glazed and swollen, with vasomotor and sudomotor changes and atrophy of the subcutaneous tissue and muscle. The pain probably is generated by excess sympathetic activity acting on damaged nerves or nerve endings and by deafferentation after nerve transection.

STRATEGIES FOR OPTIMAL MANAGEMENT

Neuropathic pain responds in part to opioid analgesics. The best responses are obtained with the tricyclic antidepressant and anticonvulsant drugs.

Tricyclic Agents

Amitriptyline has been shown in double-blind crossover studies to benefit patients with painful diabetic neuropathy. The mechanism of action remains the subject of controversy; tricyclic agents may affect descending serotonergic pathways or may have direct effects on sodium channels in the peripheral nervous system. In any event, the effect on neuropathic pain appears to be independent of any effect on mood. Amitriptyline, nortriptyline, or desipramine can be started at 25 mg daily and increased, if needed, to 75 to 100 mg daily. The role of serotonin uptake inhibitors has not been defined.

Anticonvulsants

The first anticonvulsant found to have some benefit for neuropathic pain, the sodium channel blocker phenytoin, largely has been supplanted by carbamazepine and gabapentin. Carbamazepine has the advantage of lower cost. Therapy usually is started at 100 mg once or twice daily, with doses gradually increasing to 200 to 400 mg three times daily. In the United States, gabapentin has achieved great popularity for use in the context of painful diabetic neuropathy, in part because of the paucity of

side effects, and its efficacy has been demonstrated in controlled studies. Its superiority over the less-expensive agent carbamazepine has not been established. Gabapentin also is administered in incremental doses, beginning with 100 mg daily and increasing to 900 to 1,200 mg three times a day if required.

Other Agents

In a few patients topical capsaicin preparations may be beneficial, and some patients feel better with topical application of local anesthetic creams, such as lidocaine. Opioids are last resorts, both because of their potential for dependence and because they are less efficacious, in general, than in other pain states.

BIBLIOGRAPHY

Brazis PW, Masdeu JC, Biller J. *Localization in clinical neurology*, third ed. Boston: Little, Brown, 1996.

Devinsky O, Feldman E. *Examination of the cranial and peripheral nerves*. New York: Churchill-Livingstone, 1988.

Holland NR, Crawford TO, Hauer P, et al. Small-fiber sensory neuropathies: clinical course and neuropathology of idiopathic cases. *Ann Neurol* 1998;44:47–59.

Kelley's Textbook of Internal Medicine, fourth edition. Edited by H. David Humes. Lippincott Williams & Wilkins, Philadelphia © 2000.

C H A P T E R

431

APPROACH TO THE PATIENT WITH SUSPECTED INFECTION OF THE CENTRAL NERVOUS SYSTEM

ANTHONY W. CHOW
DONALD W. PATY

Infections of the central nervous system (CNS) continue to have high rates of mortality and morbidity. Early diagnosis and effective therapy are the only means of preventing death and long-term neurologic adverse effects, yet the necessary diagnostic measures and therapeutic interventions often are delayed. This delay may be related in part to the complexity of the clinical problem: a crucial medical history may be unobtainable for a comatose patient, and the differential diagnoses can be numerous. A systematic approach and rapid mobilization and assistance from various specialists (such as neurologist, neurosurgeon, neuroradiologist, infectious disease specialist, microbiologist) are often essential for optimal management. Rapid and irreversible brain damage may occur unless decisive therapeutic measures are implemented quickly.

In approaching the patient with a suspected infection of the

CNS, the first step should be directed at localizing the site of infection. Based on the history, a general examination, and a comprehensive neurologic assessment, the predominant clinical syndrome should be characterized (acute, chronic, or recurrent meningitis; brain abscess or encephalitis; parameningeal infections, such as sphenoid sinusitis, subdural empyema, or epidural abscess—see Chapter 441). In addition, the possibility of a distant source of infection, such as the lungs, heart valve, or pelvis, should be sought rigorously. This first step greatly assists in planning the best strategy for diagnostic procedures and in formulating appropriate initial empiric antimicrobial therapy.

PRESENTATION

The cardinal signs and symptoms of CNS infections include fever, severe or persistent headache, nuchal rigidity, focal neurologic deficit, and changes in mentation, affect, or personality (Table 431.1). Although most patients experience typical symptoms and signs suggesting infection in the CNS, findings in the very young, the elderly, and the immunocompromised host can be quite subtle or varying. Thus, fever and neck stiffness may be absent in such patients, even in the context of overwhelming infection. Absence of such findings should not preclude the diagnosis of meningeal involvement. Likewise, the presence of an unexplained or subtle change in mentation, arousal, or personality may be sufficient to warrant a systematic investigation.

PATHOPHYSIOLOGY

The pathogenesis and clinical manifestations of nervous system infections are critically influenced by the anatomic considera-tions and host responses to injury of the specific affected neural tissues. The brain, spinal cord, and cauda equina are normally quite resistant to infection. Even when cranial bone flaps become infected after surgery, intracranial extension of infection through the dura is relatively rare. Similarly, abscess in the brain is difficult to induce experimentally, even after direct bacterial inoculation. This is because the host defenses of the nervous system in the normal host are extraordinarily effective. Both complement- and antibody-mediated bacteriolysis or opsonophagocytosis, as well as cell-mediated immunity, appear to be important defense mechanisms in the CNS. Specific antibodies, which may be produced locally or transported passively across an impaired blood–brain barrier, are particularly important for opsonic and bactericidal activity against encapsulated bacteria (*Streptococcus pneumoniae*, *Neisseria meningitidis*, and *Haemophilus influenzae*). After splenectomy, patients and people with deficient terminal components of the complement cascade are particularly susceptible to severe and recurrent meningitides associated with these organisms. In contrast, cell-mediated immunity is the major host defense against mycobacterial, fungal, viral, and certain parasitic infections of the CNS. In the absence of immunologic aberrations, infections of the nervous system are often preceded by disruptions of the dural sheath (post-traumatic or postoperative), congenital defects (spina bifida or myelomeningocele), or preexisting ischemic injury (septic emboli, cerebrovascular disease, or tumor necrosis).

Despite the multitude of microorganisms that can infect the nervous system opportunistically, only limited histopathologic responses result from such injury. Thus, acute infections associated with most bacteria tend to elicit a polymorphonuclear inflammatory response associated with infiltration of microglial cells and proliferation of astrocytes. Subacute or chronic infections associated with mycobacteria and fungi usually provoke a

TABLE 431.1.	THE CLINICAL SPECTRUM AND INVESTIGATION OF INTRACRANIAL COMPLICATIONS			
			Computed Tomography	
Complication	**Clinical Signs**	**Cerebrospinal Fluid**	**No Contrast**	**With Contrast**
Meningitis	Headache, fever + +; stiff neck, lethargy + +; rapid course + +	High PMNs and protein, low sugar	Normal	Diffusely enhanced
Brain abscess	Convulsions +, headache +, personality change +	Lymphocytosis, normal sugar	Lucency with mass effect	Capsule
Subdural empyema	Headache + +, convulsions + +, hemiplegia + +, rapid course + +	High PMNs and protein; normal sugar	Lucent area	Crescent-shaped enhancement
Epidural abscess	Headache ±, lever ±	Normal	Lucent area	Biconvex capsule
Venous sinus thrombosis (cavernous)	"Picket-fence" fever + +, rapid course + + (orbital edema + +) (ocular palsies + +)	Normal or high PMNs	Nonspecific	Enhancing lesion
Osteomyelitis	Pott's puffy tumor +	Normal	Bony defect	Bony defect

±, May or may not be seen; +, frequently seen; + +, characteristically seen; PMNs, polymorphonuclear leukocytes.
(From Fairbanks DNF, Milmoe GJ. Complications and sequelae: an otolaryngologist's perspective. In Bluestone CD, ed. *The diagnosis and management of sinusitis in children: Proceedings of a closed conference. Pediatr Infect Dis* 1985;4:575, with permission.)

suppurative, granulomatous response. Intracerebral granulomas, with or without calcification, may develop. Parasitic infections, such as cysticercosis, paragonimiasis, or echinococcosis, may elicit a eosinophilic response in the cerebrospinal fluid (CSF). Abscess formation in the brain is accompanied by encapsulation, which takes place by gliosis rather than by fibrosis. In the CNS, secondary effects of infection, such as cerebral edema, hemorrhage, infarction, and hydrocephalus, often are more dramatic and damaging than the primary effects of microbic invasion. Injury to neural tissue also may occur indirectly, because of an exaggerated immunologic response against basic myelin protein after certain infections, such as the multifocal axonal degeneration and demyelination observed in the course of postinfectious encephalomyelitis or Guillain-Barré syndrome.

Knowledge of the anatomic relationship of the cranium and adjacent structures to the underlying brain and spinal cord also is essential for early recognition and management of infections caused by contiguous spread of a parameningeal focus (see Fig. 441.1). The lower structures of the brain rest within the anterior, middle, and posterior cranial fossae. The anterior fossa forms the roof of the frontal and ethmoidal sinuses; infection within either sinus may cause a frontal epidural abscess, subdural empyema, or a frontal lobe brain abscess. Infection originating in the sphenoid sinus may extend into the anterior fossa to involve the frontal lobe or into the middle fossa to involve the temporal lobe. Infections of the middle ear or mastoid within the petrous bone may extend into the middle fossa to involve the temporal lobe or into the posterior fossa to involve the cerebellum or brain stem. The skull overlying the dura of the cerebrum is covered extracranially by the galea aponeurotica. Pericranial infections, stemming from either head trauma or a craniotomy, may result in subgaleal abscess and cranial osteomyelitis, with possible retrograde spread through the emissary veins to the epidural, subdural, and subarachnoid spaces.

HISTORY AND PHYSICAL EXAMINATION

Because the brain and spinal cord have only limited means of response to different modes of injury, the neurologic manifestations of infection often are indistinguishable from those of other pathologic processes, such as malignancy, autoimmune diseases, or degenerative disorders. For this reason, the complete history, including considerations of age, epidemiologic associations, immunologic status, and precipitating events, is particularly important in raising the suspicion of an infection of the nervous system. A careful history, paying particular attention to epidemiologic considerations, associated disease states, and the specific nature of underlying immunodeficiencies, often provides important clues to the etiologic agents of nervous system infections (Table 431.2). The physical examination should include a careful search for any evidence of a pericranial or parameningeal focus of infection (ear, mastoid, sinuses) or of a systemic infection arising from a distant focus (endocarditis, pneumonia, or pelvic infection).

LABORATORY STUDIES AND DIAGNOSTIC TESTS

LUMBAR PUNCTURE AND CEREBROSPINAL FLUID EXAMINATION

The lumbar puncture (LP) is the most important diagnostic procedure in the evaluation of a patient for suspected CNS infection, particularly bacterial meningitis. Appropriate cytologic, biochemical, and microbiologic studies of CSF are essential. However, the potential risk of brain herniation must be assessed individually before the diagnostic LP. The fundi should be examined carefully for evidence of markedly increased intracranial pressure, such as papilledema or cessation of venous pulsations. The ready availability of computed tomography (CT) scanning should minimize this complication.

The usual CSF profiles in cases of bacterial, fungal, mycobacterial, and viral meningitis are summarized in Table 431.3. Normal CSF contains fewer than five leukocytes per milliliter, a protein content typically less than 40 mg per deciliter, and a CSF/serum glucose ratio greater than 1:2. Measurement of the chloride concentration in CSF is not useful. In the case of acute bacterial meningitis, the cell count is usually greater than 500 per microliter and is frequently polymorphonuclear (more than 90% polymorphonuclear leukocytes). Nevertheless, patients with viral aseptic meningitis also may show signs of polymorphonuclear pleocytosis in the CSF early in the course, falsely suggesting a bacterial or fungal origin. A second LP carried out 12 to 72 hours later often clarifies the diagnosis and obviates unnecessary antimicrobial therapy.

Partially treated bacterial meningitis generally is associated with lymphocytic predominance in the CSF. In bacterial and fungal meningitis, the CSF glucose is low (CSF/serum ratio of less than 1:2). Viral, mycoplasmal, treponemal, rickettsial, and carcinomatous meningitis show a normal or only slightly depressed CSF glucose level. The very lowest levels of CSF glucose are seen in tuberculosis, fulminant bacterial meningitis, primary amoebic meningoencephalitis, and neurocysticercosis. Hypoglycorrhachia (low CSF glucose) is not caused by cells and organisms consuming glucose; instead, it is caused by changes in the transport of glucose between serum and CSF. Thus, the persistence of a relatively low CSF/serum glucose ratio after bacteriologic cure of suppurative meningitis often is associated with evidence of chronic inflammation and neurologic adverse effects. Hypoglycorrhachia also may be caused by subarachnoid bleeding, chemical arachnoiditis (as a complication of radionuclide or metrizamide myelography), sarcoidosis, neoplasms, and certain viral agents (mumps, enteroviruses, herpes simplex, and varicella-zoster).

The CSF should be cultured for both aerobic and anaerobic bacteria as well as mycobacteria and fungi, and the cell pellets should be examined by Gram stain. A Ziehl–Neelsen stain for acid-fast bacilli and an India ink preparation for cryptococci also should be made routinely. Serologic testing for syphilis should be carried out. In very ill patients, a second LP should be made at a different spinal level in 6 to 8 hours if the first LP was inconclusive. Another LP may be considered within the first few days of empiric antimicrobial therapy, to monitor the microbiologic response.

TABLE 431.2.	**EPIDEMIOLOGIC AND CLINICAL CLUES TO ETIOLOGIC AGENTS IN NONVIRAL NERVOUS SYSTEM INFECTIONS**

Clue(s)	Organism(s)
Meningitis and ventriculitis	
Age	
Neonates and infants	*Escherichia coli, Listeria, Streptococcus agalactiae*
Children and young adults	*Haemophilus,* pneumococcus, meningococcus
Elderly	Gram-negative bacilli, pneumococcus, *Listeria*
Geographic area	
San Joaquin Valley	*Coccidioides*
Freshwater lake	*Naegleria*
Animal exposure	
Rodents	*Leptospira*
Pigeons	*Cryptococcus*
Mice and rats	*Spirillum* or *Streptobacillus*
Pork tapeworm	*Cysticercus*
Rat lungworm	*Angiostrongylus*
Ticks	*Borrelia burgdorferi*
Systemic infection	Mycobacteria, *Treponema*
Associated conditions	
Head trauma, craniotomy, and cerebrospinal fluid leak	Pneumococcus, gram-negative bacilli, *Stapylococcus aureus*
Ventricular shunt or pressure catheter	*S. aureus, Staphylococcus epidermidis,* diphtheroids
Cancer chemotherapy or acquired immunodeficiency syndrome	Gram-negative bacilli, *Listeria, Cryptococcus*
Splenectomy	Pneumococcus, *Haemophilus*
Brain abscess and encephalitis	
Contiguous infection	
Sinusitis	*Streptococcus, Peptostreptococcus, Bacteroides*
Otitis media and mastoiditis	*Streptococcus, Peptostreptococcus,* gram-negative bacilli, *Bacteroides*
Distant infection	
Endocarditis	*S. aureus, Streptococcus*
Pneumonia	*Actinomyces, Bacteroides, Streptococcus, Peptostreptococcus, Nocardia, Mycoplasma*
Systemic infection	Rocky Mountain spotted fever, typhus, syphilis
Associated conditions	
Head trauma	Gram-negative bacilli, *s. aureus*
Diabetes	*Mucormyces*
Congenital heart disease	*Streptococcus, Haemophilus*
Cancer chemotherapy or acquired immunodeficiency syndrome	*Listeria,* gram-negative bacilli, Legionella, mycobacteria, *Aspergillus,* Candida, *Toxoplasma, Strongyloides*
Travel	*Plasmodium, Schistosoma, Echinococcus, Paragonimus*
Subdural empyema and epidural abscess	
Contiguous infection	
Sinusitis	*Streptococcus, Peptostreptococcus, Bacteroides*
Otitis media and mastoiditis	*Pseudomonas, Proteus, Streptococcus, Peptostreptococcus, Bacteroides*
Vertebral osteomyelitis	*S. aureus,* gram-negative bacilli
Head trauma or craniotomy	*S. aureus,* gram-negative bacilli
Distant infection	Organisms isolated from primary site

Several rapid methods of CSF examination appear promising for the presumptive diagnosis of infectious and noninfectious causes of meningitis. The acridine orange stain may be more sensitive than Gram stain for rapid identification of microorganisms in the CSF. Use of cytospin centrifugation for examination of cellular elements facilitates the detection of eosinophils, atypical lymphocytes, choroidal and arachnoidal epithelial cells, or neoplastic cells. C-reactive protein, an acute-phase reactant, is elevated markedly in CSF from patients with bacterial meningitis but not in those with viral or noninfectious forms. The CSF lactate and total lactate dehydrogenase isoenzyme levels have a similar correlation. The limulus amebocyte lysate assay, used to detect the presence of endotoxin in the CSF, also appears valuable for the rapid diagnosis of gram-negative bacterial men-

ingitis. Finally, gas–liquid chromatographic analysis of the CSF for microbial metabolic products may aid in the rapid identification of certain bacterial, mycobacterial, and fungal causes of meningitis. These tests are particularly helpful for patients who had been started on empiric antimicrobial therapy before CSF examination.

ANTIGEN AND ANTIBODY DETECTION AND MOLECULAR DIAGNOSIS IN CEREBROSPINAL FLUID

In addition to nonspecific methods, several techniques for rapid detection and quantitation of specific microbial antigens in the CSF are available. These immunologic techniques include coun-

| TABLE 431.3. | CEREBROSPINAL FLUID (CSF) FINDINGS IN BACTERIAL AND NONBACTERIAL MENINGITIS |

CSF Profile	Bacterial	Viral	Mycobacterial or Fungal
Total cells (per μL)	Usually >500	Usually <500	Usually <500
White blood cells	Predominantly polymorphonuclear	Predominantly mononuclear	Predominantly mononuclear
Glucose (% of blood)	≤40%	>40%	≤40%
Protein (mg/dL)	>50	>50	>50
Gram stain	Positive (65–95%)	Negative	Negative

Differential diagnosis of CSF pleocytosis
Brain abscess or subdural empyema with rupture
Central nervous system vasculitis, tumor

Predominantly Polymorphonuclear (>90% PMNs)	Predominantly Mononuclear (<90% PMNs)
Bacterial meningitis	Viral meningitis or encephalitis
Early viral meningitis	Tuberculous or fungal meningitis
Early tuberculous or fungal meningitis	Partially treated bacterial meningitis
Brain abscess or subdural empyema with rupture into subarachnoid space	Brain abscess of subdural empyema
Chemical arachnoiditis	Listeriosis (variable)
Brain abscess of subdural empyema	Neurosyphilis
	Neuroborreliosis (Lyme disease)
	Neurocysticercosis
	Primary amoebic meningoencephalitis
	Guillain–Barré syndrome
	Central nervous system vasculitis, tumor, hemorrhage
	Multiple sclerosis

PMNs, polymorphonuclear leukocytes.
EVIDENCE LEVEL: B. Reference: Lepow ML, et al. Aseptic meningitis: clinical epidemiologic, and laboratory investigation during the four year period 1955–1958. *New Engl J Med* 1962;266:1181–1193.

terimmunoelectrophoresis, latex particle agglutination, staphylococcal protein A coagglutination, and enzyme-linked immunosorbent assays for the detection of microbial polysaccharide antigens of *H. influenzae, S. pneumoniae, N. meningitidis, Streptococcus agalactiae,* and *Cryptococcus neoformans.* An added advantage of these quantitative techniques is that the concentration of microbial antigens detected in the CSF appears to correlate well with the outcome of meningitis and can provide some prognostication of the therapeutic response. A new, rapidly evolving diagnostic technique is the application of DNA probes and polymerase chain reactions to amplify and detect genetic fingerprints of microbial pathogens in the CSF. This powerful technique offers the prospect of rapid diagnosis with improved sensitivity over conventional methods, though the specificity of these assays still requires critical evaluation.

Specific antibody to microbial pathogens is normally excluded from the CNS. During infection, antibody may be detected in the CSF either because of local production or by passive diffusion across an impaired blood–CSF barrier. The serum/CSF antibody ratio in the presence of a normal blood–CSF barrier is usually greater than 200 : 1. This ratio against the causative agent may be significantly diminished after a CNS infection, compared with antibody ratios against other organisms. Apart from viral diseases, detection of specific antibodies in the CSF has been most valuable in the diagnosis of coccidioidomycosis, toxoplasmosis, cysticercosis, schistosomiasis, borreliosis, and mycoplasmal infections involving the CNS.

NEURORADIOLOGY AND NEUROIMAGING

Plain radiographs and tomograms of the paranasal sinuses, skull, and vertebral column may furnish invaluable clues to suppurative foci and contiguous infections of the nervous system. Nevertheless, CT scanning and magnetic resonance imaging (MRI) have improved significantly the diagnostic accuracy of intracranial infections, such as brain abscess, subdural empyema, and epidural abscess. The advent of CT scanning and MRI also has permitted nonoperative treatment of selected patients with cerebritis or early brain abscess. The typical CT finding in brain abscess is an area of decreased attenuation surrounded by a "ring" of enhancement. CT also can detect cerebral edema, hydrocephalus, an associated mass effect, and the presence of extracranial infection. MRI appears to be more sensitive than CT in ascertaining early cerebritis and in identifying abscess fluid, which is isodense relative to CSF on CT but hyperdense by MRI.

In subdural empyema, CT shows inward displacement of cerebral substance due to an extracerebral mass. In epidural abscess, CT shows a thick and circumscribed area of diminished density associated with extracerebral displacement. For both conditions, MRI is the diagnostic procedure of choice, since it can detect empyemas not seen on contrast-enhanced CT and also will identify contiguous cranial osteomyelitis. Radionuclide brain scans and cerebral angiography remain useful as complementary procedures for the localization of certain CNS infections, particularly posterior fossa lesions, and for pinpointing evidence of mycotic aneurysms. Metrizamide or radionuclide ventriculography, cisternography, and myelography are useful for studies of CSF dynamics, hydrocephalus, spinal epidural abscess, and localization of CSF leak. These neuroimaging techniques, however, do not readily distinguish infectious processes from malignancy or vascular lesions. It remains to be seen whether newer techniques, such as positron emission tomography, will improve the diagnostic yield further in the case of early infections (see Chapter 452).

NEUROELECTROPHYSIOLOGY

Electroencephalography may be the earliest laboratory test to show localizing or lateralizing abnormalities in encephalitis. It can detect subclinical seizure activity and provide an early view of the location of cerebral cortical injury. It is neither as specific nor as sensitive as CT, however, in the diagnosis of focal structural disease. Electroencephalography is a useful noninvasive tool to monitor the progress of the disease once the diagnosis is established. Electromyography is appropriate for nerve conduction studies of infectious neuropathies. Slowed conduction is found in the peripheral nerve lesions of Guillain-Barré syndrome, leprosy, and diphtheria. Repetitive nerve stimulation shows an incremental response in muscle contraction, which is characteristic in botulism but not in Guillain-Barré syndrome (see Chapter 451).

HISTOPATHOLOGY

Patients with chronic meningitis, solitary intracranial mass lesions, encephalitis, or puzzling, atypical neurologic syndromes may benefit from histopathologic studies of brain or meningeal biopsy specimens (see Chapter 453). Aspirates of abscess walls should be cultured simultaneously for isolation of aerobic and anaerobic bacteria, fungi, and mycobacteria. Special histochemical and immunofluorescent stains can be prepared to identify various fungal and parasitic agents. Histopathologic studies often are required, to resolve the differential diagnosis between infection and other processes, such as malignancy, demyelination, and connective tissue disorders of the nervous system.

■ DIFFERENTIAL DIAGNOSIS

MENINGITIS

The hallmark of meningitis is a stiff neck that is rigid for forward flexion and subtle to lateral movement. The presence of either Kernig's sign (involuntary flexion at the contralateral knee with hip flexion and knee extension) or Brudzinski's sign (flexion at both hips with passive flexion of the neck) suggests meningeal inflammation. The "aseptic meningitis" syndrome, characterized by lymphocytic pleocytosis and a normal glucose level in the CSF, with negative results on Gram stain and bacterial cultures, typically is associated with viral agents. Nonetheless, it is important to recognize a number of other conditions that may require specific antimicrobial therapy, surgical intervention, or both.

These include partially treated bacterial meningitis, parameningeal suppurative foci, infective endocarditis, and a wide variety of meningitides caused by mycobacteria, fungi, *Mycoplasma* species, *Treponema* species, *Borrelia* species, rickettsiae, and parasites. In recurrent meningitis, the neurologic findings completely subside between acute attacks. The differential diagnosis is broad, but bacterial causes usually are related to post-traumatic or postoperative defects of the cribriform plate, the orbital roof, the paranasal sinuses, or the petrous bone. Infected congenital defects, such as spina bifida, dermoid cyst, and meningocele, are other sources. Noninfectious causes include intracranial tumors, sarcoidosis, Mollaret's and Behçet's syndromes, and Vogt–Koyanagi–Harada syndrome.

BRAIN ABSCESS, SUBDURAL EMPYEMA, AND CRANIAL EPIDURAL ABSCESS

These intracranial or parameningeal infections usually result from a contiguous focus of infection, such as the paranasal sinuses, mastoid, or middle ear; from cranial trauma or surgery; or from hematogenous spread of a distant infection, especially the lung and heart valves. The clinical pictures of brain abscesses vary greatly and appear to be influenced primarily by their anatomic location and proximity to the ventricles, cisterns, or dural sinuses and by major alterations in the intracranial pressure dynamics stemming from the mass effect (Table 431.1). The presence of focal neurologic signs or seizures is particularly suggestive of mass lesions or vascular abnormalities. Papilledema, a finding pathognomonic of increased intracranial pressure, may be present, along with vomiting or impaired consciousness.

Other neurologic findings, such as cranial nerve palsies, may be a manifestation of inflammatory infiltration (third, seventh, and eighth nerves) or increased intracranial pressure (sixth nerve). Sixth cranial nerve palsy developing in the course of bacterial meningitis is considered a false localizing sign, because it is usually the result of increased intracranial pressure rather than a mass lesion and is often bilateral. In subacute cases of brain abscess, a persistent headache and subtle personality changes may be the only clues of CNS infection. Fever is present in only 45% to 50% of patients; therefore, absence of fever should not be used to exclude the diagnosis of brain abscess. Patients with a subdural empyema often complain of an acute flare-up of chronic sinusitis, otitis media, or mastoiditis with an increase in local pain and in purulent nasal or aural discharge.

The onset of generalized headache and high fevers may be the first indications of intracranial spread, followed within days by focal neurologic findings, such as unilateral motor seizures, hemiplegia, hemianesthesia, or aphasia, and signs of increased intracranial pressure with progressive lethargy and coma. The neck is stiff, but CSF examination is more consistent with an aseptic meningitis syndrome. Cranial epidural abscess typically is associated with a postcraniotomy infection or cranial osteomyelitis stemming from chronic sinusitis or middle ear infection. The onset of symptoms may be more insidious and often is overshadowed by the localized inflammatory process. Focal neurologic findings are less common than in subdural empyema. Rarely, fifth and sixth cranial nerve palsy may develop in association with infection of the petrous portion of the temporal bone (Gradenigo's syndrome).

SEPTIC INTRACRANIAL THROMBOPHLEBITIS AND MYCOTIC ANEURYSM

Septic intracranial thrombophlebitis most frequently follows infection of the paranasal sinuses, middle ear, mastoid, or oropharynx. If collateral venous drainage is adequate, septic venous thrombosis may produce only transient neurologic findings or may be silent. If the thrombus outstrips collateral flow, however, progressive neurologic deficits result, with impairment of consciousness, focal or generalized seizures, and increased intracranial pressure. The clinical findings vary with the location of involved cortical veins or dural sinuses. Cavernous sinus thrombosis is characterized by abrupt onset, with diplopia, photophobia, orbital edema, and progressive exophthalmos. Involvement of the third, fourth, fifth, and sixth cranial nerves causes ophthalmoplegia, a midposition fixed pupil, loss of corneal reflex, and diminished sensation over the upper face. Obstruction of venous return from the retina results in papilledema, retinal hemorrhage, and visual loss.

Thrombosis of the superior sagittal sinus leads to bilateral leg weakness and may cause communicating hydrocephalus. Occlusion of the lateral sinus produces pain over the ear and mastoid and may cause edema over the mastoid (Griesinger's sign). Involvement of the fifth and sixth cranial nerves elicits ipsilateral facial pain and lateral rectus weakness (Gradenigo's syndrome). Intracranial mycotic aneurysms usually result from septic embolization as a complication of bacterial endocarditis. They are often multiple and usually are found on distal branches of the middle or anterior cerebral arteries. The early clinical manifestations are similar to those of cerebral emboli and infarction.

ENCEPHALITIS, MYELITIS, AND RADICULITIS

Encephalitis is characterized by diffuse involvement of the brain parenchyma. The most characteristic clinical feature is impairment of mental status, with progression to stupor and coma. Seizures, cranial nerve palsies, and other focal neurologic abnormalities are less common. Because the meninges almost invariably are affected, the term *meningoencephalitis* may be more appropriate for this entity. Although a viral source is most common (see Chapters 442 and 443), nonviral causes of meningoencephalitis are not rare. They are important, because most require specific antimicrobial therapy. These infections include Rocky Mountain spotted fever, typhus, mycoplasmosis, borreliosis (Lyme disease and relapsing fever), leptospirosis, neurosyphilis, invasive mycosis, cerebral malaria, primary amoebic meningoencephalitis, trypanosomiasis, and toxoplasmosis. Nonviral conditions causing meningoencephalitis, including toxoplasmosis, cryptococcosis, and atypical mycobacteriosis, are particularly important complications of the acquired immunodeficiency syndrome.

Myelitis can develop either with or without associated encephalitis. The infectious causes are similar to those of encephalitis, and both can develop as a postinfectious complication due to an exaggerated immunologic response to central myelin (postinfectious encephalomyelitis). In transverse myelitis, the neurologic manifestations resemble those after acute transection of the cord, with rostral limb weakness, decreased sensory level, and loss of bowel and bladder control. In ascending myelitis, there is ascending flaccid paralysis, rising sensory deficit, and early bowel and bladder involvement. As with encephalomyelitis, radiculitis or neuritis also can result from postinfectious sensitization to peripheral myelin (Guillain-Barré syndrome). The patient has clinical symptoms of subjective paresthesias and weakness, progressive flaccid paralysis, and loss of deep tendon reflexes. The onset of poor ventilatory effort and severe autonomic dysfunction with lability of blood pressure may require respiratory support and intensive care monitoring.

PERIPHERAL NEUROPATHY

Leprosy is the only bacterial disease known to result in direct infection of the peripheral nerves, leading to clinical signs of peripheral neuropathy. The cutaneous nerves are destroyed owing to segmental demyelination and axonal degeneration, producing anesthesia. Cranial and peripheral neuropathy also can be caused by bacterial toxins, either directly (diphtheria) or indirectly (tetanus and botulism). Diphtheria toxin provokes noninflammatory demyelination of both cranial and peripheral nerves. The earliest neurologic sign in pharyngeal diphtheria is paralysis of the palate, which imparts a nasal quality to the voice and an increasing tendency to regurgitate fluids through the nose. Other cranial nerves (particularly third, sixth, seventh, ninth, and tenth) may be affected. Later in the course, motor polyneuropathy with symmetrical flaccid paralysis of the distal extremities may evolve. Tetanus toxin binds to the presynaptic endings of motor neurons in the anterior horns of the spinal cord, resulting in uncontrolled motor input and sustained muscle spasms, particularly around the jaw (trismus) and facial muscles (risus sardonicus). Botulinum toxin binds to the presynaptic axon terminal of the neuromuscular junction, preventing release of acetylcholine. The illness manifests within 12 to 36 hours after ingestion of the toxin, with weakness, dizziness, and dryness of the mouth, followed by neurologic symptoms of blurred vision, diplopia, dysphonia, dysphagia, muscle weakness, and flaccid paralysis.

■ STRATEGIES FOR OPTIMAL CARE MANAGEMENT

MANAGEMENT

Antimicrobial Therapy

Early institution of effective antimicrobial therapy is the single most important factor in the favorable outcome of CNS infections. For this reason, establishing the precise etiologic and anatomic diagnosis is of paramount importance in the selection of the most appropriate antimicrobial regimen. Apart from the antimicrobial spectrum, other important considerations for the choice of effective therapeutic agents in CNS infections include penetration into CSF, bactericidal efficacy, mode of antibiotic administration, and the "postantibiotic" effect. All β-lactam antibiotics penetrate into CSF poorly (about 0.5% to 2% of peak serum concentrations) when the blood–brain barrier is normal, but penetration is enhanced in the presence of meningeal inflammation. Penetration also is augmented by high lipid solubility,

TABLE 431.4.	INITIAL EMPIRIC ANTIMICROBIAL THERAPY FOR ACUTE PURULENT MENINGITIS[a]	
Age	**Common Organisms**	**Recommended Therapy**
0–4 wk	*Escherichia coli, Streptococcus agalactiae, Listeria monocytogenes*	Ampicillin plus third-generation cephalosporin[b] or ampicillin plus aminoglycoside
4–12 wk	*E. coli, S. agalactiae, L. monocytogenes, Haemophilus influenzae, Streptococcus pneumoniae*	Ampicillin plus third-generation cephalosporin[b]
3 mo to 18 yr	*Neisseria meningitidis, S. pneumoniae, H. influenzae*	Third-generation cephalosporin or ampicillin plus chloramphenicol
18–50 yr	*S. pneumoniae, N. meningitidis*	Third-generation cephalosporin[a] ± ampicillin
>50 yr	*S. pneumoniae, N. meningitidis, L. monocytogenes, gram-negative bacilli*	Ampicillin plus third-generation cephalosporin[b]

[a] Patients without underlying illness.
[b] Cefotaxime, ceftriaxone—vancomycin should be added if penicillin or cephalosporin-resistant *S. pneumoniae* is suspected.
EVIDENCE LEVEL: A. Reference: Tunkel AR, Wispelweg B, Scheld WM. Bacterial meningitis: recent advances in pathophysiology and treatment. *Ann Intern Med* **1990;122:610.**

a low degree of protein binding in serum, and a low degree of ionization at physiologic pH. Rapid bactericidal activity is clearly desirable for sterilization of the CSF. In general, CSF concentrations of the drug should exceed its minimal bactericidal concentration for the causative organism by five- to tenfold.

Based on the most common causative organisms encountered, the choices for initial empiric antimicrobial therapy for acute purulent meningitis in patients of different age groups are shown in Table 431.4. A third-generation cephalosporin (cefotaxime or ceftriaxone) is recommended as initial empiric therapy for young children and adults, and vancomycin should be added if penicillin-resistant *S. pneumoniae* is suspected. These agents are ineffective against listerial infection. Immunocompromised and elderly patients, who are at increased risk for *L. monocytogenes* infection, should be treated with high-dose ampicillin. The recommended dosages are given in Table 431.5. The final antibiotic selection should be guided by culture results and susceptibility data. The recommended regimens for specific bacterial pathogens in purulent meningitis are outlined in Chapter 441 (see especially Table 441-2). Although the optimal duration of therapy varies with the offending organism, treatment usually is continued for 10 to 14 days for most pathogens, approximately 3 weeks for staphylococci, and 3 to 6 weeks for enteric gram-negative bacilli.

The choices for initial empiric antimicrobial regimens for other suppurative intracranial infections (including brain abscess, subdural empyema, and cranial epidural abscess) are shown in Table 431.6. These regimens are based on the suspected source of infection and the most likely causative organisms. Maximum doses of systemic antimicrobials are required, to optimize penetration of the blood–brain barrier. Therapy should be continued for at least 6 to 8 weeks, and the patient should be carefully monitored both clinically and by repeated CT scans until complete resolution of the infection. Follow-up is necessary for up to 1 year, to ascertain nonrecurrence. Similar regimens with maximum doses and prolonged antimicrobial therapy (6 to 8 weeks of intravenous antibiotics) are recommended for intracranial vascular or bone infections.

Surgical Drainage or Extirpation

The treatment of cerebritis typically does not require surgical drainage if appropriate antibiotic therapy is instituted early. Brain abscesses that are encapsulated are best treated by surgical aspiration. Complete surgical excision or extirpation of the abscess cavity usually is not required. Early surgical evacuation is the cornerstone of therapy for both subdural and cranial epidural empyema. Similarly, because the clinical course of a mycotic aneurysm varies widely and the risk of rupture with catastrophic cerebral hemorrhage cannot be predicted even after successful

TABLE 431.5.	RECOMMENDED DOSES OF ANTIBIOTICS FOR SUPPURATIVE INTRACRANIAL INFECTIONS IN ADULTS	
Antibiotic	**Daily**	**Dosing Interval (h)**
Penicillin G	20–24 million units	4
Ampicillin	12 g	4
Nafcillin, oxacillin	9–12 g	4
Piperacillin	8–12 g	4
Imipenem	4–6 g	6
Cefotaxime	8–12 g	4
Ceftriaxone	4–6 g	12
Ceftizoxime	4–6 g	8
Ceftazidime	6–12 g	8
Chloramphenicol	4–6 g	6
Vancomycin	2 g	12
Gentamicin, tobramycin	3–5 mg/kg	8
Amikacin	15 mg/kg	8
Ciprofloxacin	200–400 mg	12
Metronidazole	30–60 mg/kg	6
Trimethoprim-sulfamethoxazole	5–10 mg/kg 25–50 mg/kg	12 12

EVIDENCE LEVEL: C. Reference: Expert Opinion.

TABLE 431.6.	EMPIRIC ANTIMICROBIAL REGIMENS FOR SUPPURATIVE INTRACRANIAL INFECTIONS[a]		
		Antimicrobial Regimens	
Source of Infection	**Normal Host**		**Compromised Host**
Cranial parameningeal infections			
Otogenic	Penicillin G, 2–4 million units i.v. q4–6 hr, + ciprofloxacin, 0.2 g q12 hr, + metronidazole, 0.5 g i.v. q6 hr		Cefotaxime, 2 g i.v. q6 hr, or ceftizoxime, 4 g i.v. q8 hr, or imipenem, 500 mg i.v. q6 hr
Rhinogenic	Penicillin G, 2–4 million units i.v. q4–6 hr +, metronidazole, 0.5 g i.v. q6 hr		Same as otogenic
Odontogenic	Same as rhinogenic		Same as otogenic
After cranial surgery	Nafcillin, 1.5 g i.v. q4–6 hr, + cefotaxime, 2 g i.v. q6 hr, or ciprofloxacin, 0.2 g i.v. q12 hr		Vancomycin, 0.5 g i.v. q6 hr, + cefotaxim, 2 g i.v. q6 hr, or ceftizoxime, 2 g i.v. q8 hr, or imipenem, 0.5 g i.v.
Hematogenous from distant site	Choice based on suspected organism from primary site		
Spinal epidural abscess	Nafcillin, 1.5 g i.v. q4–6 hr, + tobramycin, 2 mg/kg i.v. q8 hr, or q ciprofloxacin, 0.2 g q12 hr		Vancomycin, 0.5 q i.v. q6 hr, + cefotaxime, 2 g i.v. q6 hr, or ceftizoxime, 2 g i.v. q8 hr, or imipenem, 0.5 g i.v. q6 hr

[a] Includes brain abscess, subdural or cranial epidural abscess and septic venous thrombosis.

therapy of the underlying endocarditis, early surgical intervention is advised in patients with an intracranial mycotic aneurysm.

Other Adjunctive Measures

In addition to antimicrobial therapy, concomitant administration of anti-inflammatory agents, such as dexamethasone, oxindanac, or indomethacin, may be useful in reducing subarachnoid space inflammation. Corticosteroids and osmotic diuretics frequently are used to decrease intracranial pressure and cerebral edema. Use of monoclonal antibodies directed at lipopolysaccharides of gram-negative bacilli and at inflammatory cytokines, such as interleukin-1 and tumor necrosis factor, is being evaluated in animal models and in early clinical trials of sepsis syndrome and purulent meningitis. It remains to be seen whether such measures will improve the outcome substantially and prevent chronic neurologic side effects after these devastating CNS infections.

COMPLICATIONS AND PITFALLS

Brain herniation is the most dreaded complication after LP and in any patient with increased intracranial pressure. CSF is formed by the choroid plexus in the cerebral ventricles (chiefly in the lateral and third ventricles) and flows through the third and fourth ventricles into the subarachnoid space through the foramina of Magendie and Luschka. From the subarachnoid space, CSF is resorbed by arachnoid granulations, primarily in the dural venous sinuses. Any obstruction in the flow of CSF results in increased intracranial pressure, leading to communicating or obstructive hydrocephalus. In communicating hydrocephalus, the increased intracranial pressure usually results from an impairment of CSF reabsorption across the arachnoid villi, such as during basilar meningitis or after occlusion of the superior sagittal or lateral sinuses. In such instances, even though the

intracranial pressure is high, it is transmitted through the entire subarachnoid space around the brain and cord, and unless concomitant abscess or severe cerebral edema is present, there is relatively low risk of brain herniation after LP. Thus, in most patients with acute meningitis who are alert and without papilledema or focal neurologic signs, an LP can be carried out safely without an initial CT scan.

In obstructive hydrocephalus, on the other hand, increased intracranial pressure typically stems from an interruption of CSF circulation within the ventricular system, either directly because of ventriculitis or indirectly because of external compression by an abscess, mass, or hemorrhage. In such instances, the risk of brain herniation after LP is particularly high. For this reason, LP is contraindicated as part of the initial evaluation of a patient with acute head injury, suspected mass lesions in the brain, or increased intracranial pressure, as evidenced by rapid onset of obtundation, papilledema, abducens paresis, split-skull sutures, or an eroded sella turcica. If CSF examination is deemed critical and CT or MRI is unavailable, a cisternal tap undertaken by an experienced neurologist is the preferred alternative. During LP, one must always measure the CSF pressure. If the intracranial pressure is greater than 300 mm H_2O, care must be taken, and the patient must be kept supine. If cerebral edema is suspected, intravenous corticosteroids (1 g methylprednisolone) are indicated, to diminish brain swelling. External or ventriculoperitoneal shunting may be required in the context of hydrocephalus.

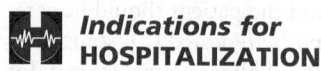

Indications for HOSPITALIZATION

All patients with a suspected infection of the CNS should be hospitalized and appropriate investigations promptly initiated.

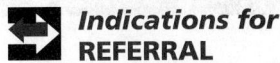

Indications for REFERRAL

A careful and systematic neurologic evaluation is paramount for localizing the site of infection. A multidisciplinary approach with assistance from various specialties, particularly neurology, neuroradiology, neurosurgery, infectious diseases, and microbiology, is often essential for optimal management.

COST-EFFECTIVENESS

By far the most cost-effective strategy for the management of infections of the CNS is prevention of infection. In the case of bacterial meningitis, this can be achieved either by postexposure prophylaxis or by active immunization.

Postexposure Prophylaxis

Household contacts of patients with acute meningitis due to *N. meningitidis* or *H. influenzae* infection should receive prophylaxis with rifampin (600 mg daily for 2 days for contacts with meningococcal meningitis and for 4 days for contacts with *H. influenzae* meningitis). Postexposure prophylaxis also is recommended during epidemic outbreaks and for close contacts, such as the other children in nursery schools, and for medical personnel who have had mouth-to-mouth or other direct contact with infected respiratory aerosols.

Vaccines

Effective vaccines for the prevention of meningococcal disease due to serotypes A, C, Y, and W-135 are available and are recommended for use in potentially epidemic situations, for people with terminal complement component deficiencies, and for those with anatomic or functional asplenia. The pneumococcal polyvalent vaccine should be administered to all people with CSF leak, sickle cell disease, asplenia, and other immunodefi-

ciencies, to prevent recurrent bacteremia and meningitis. Similarly, a safe and effective conjugated polysaccharide vaccine against *H. influenzae* type b is readily available and should be administered to all persons at risk. More recently, a Lyme disease vaccine (LYMErix, SmithKline Beecham) has been released. It contains an immunodominant outer surface protein (OspA) of *B. burgdorferi*. The vaccine has been shown to be safe and effective for the prevention of Lyme disease, but three intramuscular doses, at 0, 1, and 12 months, are required. It is indicated for individuals 15 to 70 years of age who are at high risk for Lyme disease owing to frequent and prolonged exposure to *Ixodes* ticks. Its safety and efficacy in children have not been established.

BIBLIOGRAPHY

Aronin SI, Peduzzi P, Quagliarello VJ. Community-acquired bacterial meningitis: risk stratification for adverse clinical outcome and effect of antibiotic timing. *Ann Intern Med* 1998;129:862–869.

Bradley JS, Scheld WM. The challenge of penicillin-resistant *Streptococcus pneumoniae* meningitis: current antibiotic therapy in the 1990s. *Clin Infect Dis* 1997;24(suppl 2):S213–S221.

Dunbar SA, Eason RA, Musher DM, et al. Microscopic examination and broth culture of cerebrospinal fluid in diagnosis of meningitis. *J Clin Microbiol* 1998;36:1617–1620.

Klugman KP. Impact of antimicrobial resistance and antibiotic choice on the outcome of pneumococcal meningitis. *S Afr Med J* 1997;87:912.

Mackenzie AR, Laing RB, Smith CC, et al. Spinal epidural abscess: the importance of early diagnosis and treatment. *J Neurol Neurosurg Psychiatry* 1998;65:209–212.

McIntyre PB, Berkey CS, King SM, et al. Dexamethasone as adjunctive therapy in bacterial meningitis. A meta-analysis of randomized clinical trials since 1988. *JAMA* 1997;278:925–931.

Quagliarello VJ, Scheld WM. Treatment of bacterial meningitis. *N Engl J Med* 1997;336:708–716.

Sigurdardóttir B, Björnsson OM, Jónsdottir KE, et al. Acute bacterial meningitis in adults. A 20-year overview. *Arch Intern Med* 1997;157:425–430.

Townsend GC, Scheld WM. Microbe-endothelium interactions in blood–brain barrier permeability during bacterial meningitis. *ASM News* 1995;61:294–298.

Kelley's Textbook of Internal Medicine, fourth edition. Edited by H. David Humes.
Lippincott Williams & Wilkins, Philadelphia © 2000.

DISORDERS OF THE NERVOUS SYSTEM

CEREBROVASCULAR DISEASES

JOHN J. CARONNA

Each year in the United States, 500,000 persons suffer a stroke, and 150,000 of them die from the stroke or its complications. The overall mortality rate from stroke is about 25% in the first month and approaches 50% at 5 years. Neurologic complications account for most deaths in the first week; later deaths usually are due to heart disease and intercurrent infection. There are about two million stroke survivors living in the United States today. The sources of stroke in older patients are primary atherosclerosis in 10%, small-vessel occlusion due to lipohyalinosis or vasculitis in 8%, hematologic or cardiac conditions in 48%, and undetermined causes in 34%.

ATHEROSCLEROTIC DISEASE OF CEREBRAL ARTERIES

The importance of atherosclerosis of the major neck vessels (the carotid and vertebral arteries) as a cause of transient ischemic attacks (TIAs) and embolic or thrombotic strokes is well understood. Transient symptoms of cerebral ischemia are often due to microemboli that break off from ulcerated plaques and are carried distally into the brain. Platelet microemboli and cholesterol-lipid emboli that obstruct flow in the ophthalmic artery cause sudden, fleeting ipsilateral monocular blindness; those that lodge in the distal branches of the middle cerebral artery provoke contralateral hemiparesis, hemianesthesia, and homonymous hemianopia. Microemboli carried elsewhere in the carotid and vertebrobasilar distributions cause other symptoms and signs, depending on the vessel obstructed. If a larger thrombus breaks off, embolic stroke results. Occlusion at the site of atherosclerosis results in a thrombotic stroke if the collateral circulation distal to that occlusion is inadequate.

Cerebrovascular syndromes fall into two categories: disorders in which hypertension is one of several possible causes and disorders that occur primarily in the context of hypertension. Atherosclerosis of the large extracranial arteries in the neck and at the base of the brain is the basic pathologic process in the first category. Although hypertension is a prominent risk factor for atherosclerosis, other factors, such as diabetes, elevated serum cholesterol and triglyceride levels, cigarette smoking, hereditary predisposition, and use of oral contraceptives, may be important causes. Extensive atherosclerosis can develop in the absence of hypertension. TIAs and thrombotic and embolic strokes are the clinical syndromes in this category.

Hypertension damages small arteries deep in the brain and produces two clinical syndromes almost exclusive to hypertension: lacunar infarction (small subcortical strokes) and hypertensive hemorrhage (see later discussion). In the Framingham study, the relationship between hypertension and stroke was analyzed epidemiologically. More than 5,000 symptom-free men and women between 30 and 60 years of age were classified according to the initial level of blood pressure. A blood pressure of 160/95 mm Hg during any clinic visit tripled the risk of stroke and justified a decision to begin antihypertensive treatment.

CATEGORIES OF ISCHEMIC OR THROMBOEMBOLIC STROKE

Strokes due to ischemia may be divided clinically into three categories: TIAs, stroke in evolution (also called progressing stroke), and completed stroke. TIAs are ischemic episodes of focal cerebral dysfunction lasting less than 24 hours—typically only a few minutes—followed by complete recovery, with absence of neurologic deficit on neurologic examination. Modern imaging techniques, such as magnetic resonance imaging (MRI), can detect evidence of cerebral infarction in a high percentage of cases of TIA. Therefore, TIAs are small strokes with transient signs and symptoms, especially in patients with symptoms of long duration (hours). TIAs provide a warning of a possible impending permanent neurologic deficit and are a risk factor associated with both stroke and myocardial infarction.

Stroke in evolution describes ischemic signs and symptoms that worsen while the patient is being observed. The pathogenesis of this type of stroke is usually propagation of a thrombus in the carotid or basilar arteries. It is the least common clinical picture. Completed stroke denotes a relatively stable neurologic deficit resulting from a cerebral infarct. The infarcts in patients with completed stroke may vary from tiny necrotic areas that are barely detectable by neurologic testing to massive lesions with secondary edema of the cerebral hemisphere that mimic brain tumors.

TRANSIENT ISCHEMIC ATTACKS

Pathophysiology and Classification

Whenever the cerebral blood flow (CBF) of a region declines to a point low enough to impair neuronal function, clinical symptoms of focal ischemia can appear. If the supply of oxygen and glucose is restored before permanent damage has taken place, the focal neuronal dysfunction is reversible, and the associated clinical symptoms are transient.

TIAs comprise a diverse group of pathologic conditions that result in intermittent focal interruptions of CBF. The causes of TIAs can be divided into three pathophysiologic categories: abnormalities of the blood vessels themselves, including the heart and extracranial and intracranial vessels; alterations in the composition of the circulating blood; and changes in the manner in which the blood circulates (Table 432.1). The major theories advanced to explain TIAs are vasospasm, hemodynamic factors, and thromboembolism. Vasospasm of an intracerebral or extracerebral artery is an unlikely cause of transient ischemia, except in cases of hypertensive encephalopathy, subarachnoid hemorrhage, or migraine. Hemodynamic factors, such as reduced perfusion pressure distal to a severely stenotic or occluded cerebral artery, account for a small proportion of TIAs.

The most common mechanism producing alterations in CBF is probably platelet embolization from atherosclerotic extracranial or intracranial cerebral arteries. The evidence for this action is mainly clinical. In patients with transient monocular blindness, the passage of emboli through the retinal circulation has been witnessed. Cerebral arteriography has shown occlusion of small intracranial arteries in the vascular distribution of diseased carotid arteries of patients with TIAs. Pathologic examination of carotid arteries obtained at the time of endarterectomy from patients with TIAs has found ulcerated atheromatous plaques with an adherent fresh thrombus. TIAs often cease when the source of microemboli is removed by carotid stenosis progressing to complete occlusion. Surgical elimination of carotid stenosis lowers the incidence of TIAs and stroke. TIAs often cease in patients treated with anticoagulants or antiplatelet aggregation drugs.

The history of TIA in the carotid artery territory is generally typical. The most common symptom is sudden onset of weakness, paralysis, or clumsiness in one or both extremities on the same side. Sensory symptoms may be present, including a feeling of numbness or paresthesias involving one or both extremities on the same side. If the TIA involves the hemisphere dominant for language function, dysphasia is present. Another potential component of a carotid system TIA is transient loss of vision in one eye or part of one visual field.

TABLE 432.1.	CONDITIONS PREDISPOSING TO TIA AND STROKE

Arterial stroke
 Abnormalities of blood vessels
  Atherosclerosis of extracranial or intracranial arteries
  Congenital and acquired disorders
   Fibromuscular dysplasia
   Coarctation of the aorta
   Moyamoya syndrome
   Hereditary elastic tissue disorders (Marfan's and Ehlers–Danlos syndromes)
  Dissection of extracranial arteries (spontaneous or traumatic)
  Inflammatory disorders
   Giant cell arteritis
   Systemic lupus erythematosus
   Polyarteritis nodosa
   Granulomatous angiitis
   Takayasu's disease
  Vasospasm
   Migraine
   Post-subarachnoid hemorrhage
   Cocaine and amphetamine use
  Infectious
   Syphilitic aortitis
   Tuberculous meningitis
   Post–herpes zoster angiitis
   Mycotic aneurysm
   Cerebral malaria
 Cardiac abnormalities
  Myocardial infarct with mural thrombus
  Dysrhythmia
  Valvular disease (congenital, rheumatic, prosthetic)
  Infectious and nonbacterial thrombotic endocarditis
  Patent foramen ovale, cyanotic heart disease
  Cardiomyopathy
  Atrial myxoma
 Hypercoagulable states
  Oral contraception, pregnancy and puerperium
  Androgenic steroid use
  Hemoglobinopathies
  Polycythemia
  Thrombocytosis, disseminated intravascular coagulation, and thrombotic thrombocytopenic purpura
  Antiphospholipid antibody syndrome
  Protein C, protein S, and antithrombin III deficiency
 Altered cerebral circulation
  Hypotension
  Cardiac arrest or dysrhythmia
  Orthostatic hypotension
  Abnormal shunting of blood
  Cerebral arteriovenous malformations, carotid cavernous fistula (after repair), subclavian steal syndrome, hereditary hemorrhagic telangiectasia (Rendu-Osler-Weber syndrome with pulmonary arteriovenous shunt)
 Miscellaneous conditions
  Complications of cerebral angiography (embolization of clot and air, multiple cholesterol emboli syndrome)
  Complications of carotid endarterectomy and cardiac bypass surgery
Venous stroke
 Occlusion of cerebral venous sinuses and veins
  Structural occlusion of a cerebral venous sinus by a mass (meningioma or neuroblastoma) or thrombosis (after surgery for AVM or tumor)
  Hypercoagulable states (see earlier)

TIA, transient ischemic attack; AVM, arteriovenous malformation.

In vertebrobasilar TIAs, the most common symptom is a motor defect, such as weakness, clumsiness, or paralysis of any combination of extremities up to quadriplegia. Sensory phenomena include numbness, loss of sensation, and paresthesias in any combination of extremities. The patient may complain of unsteady gait, disequilibrium, and vertigo. There may be loss of vision, varying from complete blindness to partial blindness in homonymous fields. Diplopia is another characteristic visual symptom in vertebrobasilar TIAs.

Diagnostic Evaluation

Rarely does a physician actually observe a patient during a TIA, so he or she must rely on the patient's account of the attack. The examiner should inquire into the patient's lifestyle (cigarette and alcohol use, use of oral contraceptives, illicit drug use), any recent purulent infections or dental work, any neck pain or neck trauma, and family history of cerebrovascular disease. The evaluation is directed toward detecting evidence of vascular disease. Attention should be given to heart rate, rhythm, and size; heart sounds; blood pressure in both upper extremities; and peripheral pulses. There should be a search for audible bruits over various arterial sites.

Cranial arteritis, an unusual cause of TIA, may be detected by palpating the involved temporal artery. Absence of temporal artery pulses also can indicate occlusive disease of the ipsilateral external carotid artery. It is impossible to palpate accurately the internal carotid artery in the neck; what one feels is the common carotid or the bifurcation of the internal carotid. Bruits often can be heard by auscultating over the carotid artery as it passes up the neck; alternatively, they can be heard over the vertebral artery just above the clavicle and sometimes over the back of the neck or head. When present in a patient with TIAs, a bruit strongly suggests that the cerebral vessels are affected by atherosclerosis.

The cause of the TIA generally can be limited to one of three broad categories: vascular, cardiac, or hematologic. Abnormalities in the vascular system can be detected by ultrasonography. Duplex scanning incorporates B-mode scanning, which images the vessel under study, and Doppler techniques, which determine the velocity of blood flow. Extracranial and intracranial vessels can be imaged. Magnetic resonance angiography (MRA) noninvasively delineates the cervical and cerebral circulation. Ultrasonography and MRA have replaced cerebral arteriography in most situations. Nevertheless, transfemoral cerebral arteriography remains the most definitive test for evaluating the cerebral circulation, especially when more qualitative tests, such as ultrasonography and MRA, give conflicting results. The increased availability of new technologies, such as transesophageal echocardiography, has made commonplace the identification of subtle cardiac lesions, such as patent foramen ovale. Routine testing for coagulopathy and blood testing for antiphospholipid antibodies and for deficiency of protein C, protein S, and antithrombin III have widened the diagnostic possibilities in the patient with TIA and minor stroke.

Differential Diagnosis

The differential diagnosis of TIAs includes classic migraine with scintillating scotomas, hemiplegic migraine, focal convulsive events, Ménière's disease, and peripheral vestibulopathy. TIAs can be distinguished from migrainous accompaniments in that TIAs are generally maximal at onset or evolve all at once, whereas migrainous phenomena build up or progress for several minutes. Headache may accompany TIAs, but it is typically brief and not severe. Focal seizures progress from the distal to the proximal portions of an extremity and produce persistent neurologic deficits on physical examination (Todd's postictal paralysis). Isolated vertigo without other motor and sensory phenomena rarely is caused by a TIA.

Management

Control of systemic hypertension that accelerates atherosclerosis is the mainstay of the medical treatment of the stroke-prone patient. Dietary modification by lowering the consumption of cholesterol and saturated fatty acids in younger patients may retard or reverse the atherosclerotic process but is less beneficial in elderly patients. Modification of lifestyle through the elimination of smoking, increasing exercise, and reducing stress may be helpful.

Randomized trials of anticoagulants (heparin given immediately, followed by warfarin) indicate some decrease in the frequency of TIAs and a small decline in the incidence of completed stroke and of stroke-related death in the treated group but no difference in total mortality rates between treated and untreated groups. The latter finding is not unexpected, because the major cause of death among patients with cerebrovascular disease is cardiovascular disease (myocardial infarction). Most of the beneficial effect of anticoagulants is seen in the first 3 months after the first TIA; thereafter, there is little difference between treated groups and untreated groups in terms of the probability of stroke. Anticoagulants must be continued indefinitely in patients with TIAs due to cardiac-origin emboli or in patients with the antiphospholipid antibody syndrome.

The most popular form of therapy for TIAs is treatment with antiplatelet drugs, such as aspirin (one to four 325-mg tablets daily). Several studies have shown a reduced incidence of TIAs and stroke in patients treated with aspirin. The combined use of aspirin and dipyridamole has the theoretical advantage of blocking both platelet aggregation (aspirin) and adhesion to a damaged surface (dipyridamole). One study has shown an enhanced clinical benefit of low-dose aspirin (50 mg) and dipyridamole (400 mg in a delayed-release form) compared with low-dose aspirin alone. Clopidigrel or ticlopidine, antiplatelet agents more potent than aspirin, may be used in patients with recurrent TIAs who are taking aspirin but who are not candidates for anticoagulation or surgery.

Surgery in the form of endarterectomy remains the treatment of choice for patients with TIAs in the carotid arterial territory who have either high-grade stenosis or stenosis and ulcerated plaques but do not have complete occlusion of the carotid artery on the side appropriate to their symptoms. Extracranial–intracranial bypass of an occluded carotid artery did not prove beneficial in a prospective study of patients with TIAs. Balloon angioplasty with stenting of arteries is a promising therapy for carotid stenosis.

CEREBRAL ISCHEMIC INFARCTION

Pathophysiology and Classification

An ischemic cerebral infarct is an area of brain in which blood flow has fallen below the level necessary to maintain the viability of the tissue. Ordinarily, the CBF, which is about 55 mL/100 g per minute, delivers oxygen and glucose in concentrations exceeding the brain's needs. If there is a threat of insufficiency of substrate (hypoxia, anemia, hypotension, hypoglycemia), homeostatic mechanisms induce cerebral vasodilation. Total deprivation of substrate cannot be compensated for, so when occlusive cerebrovascular disease renders a region completely ischemic, infarction occurs.

Cerebral infarcts may enlarge for 4 or 5 days, because of the development of cerebral edema. The degree of edema is roughly proportional to the amount of brain infarcted. Most deaths occurring within a week after massive hemisphere infarction can be attributed to cerebral edema, with swelling of the affected hemisphere causing herniation of the ipsilateral cingulate gyrus across the midline beneath the free edge of the dural falx, followed by downward displacement of brain through the tentorial incisura.

The pathophysiologic picture of ischemic stroke involves several factors that affect, to varying degrees, the extent of brain infarction. These include propagation of thrombus distal and proximal to an arterial occlusion, the effectiveness of collateral circulation, possible vasospasm, development of brain edema, leakage of blood from damaged arterioles, different metabolic requirements in different areas of the brain, and congenital abnormalities in the cerebral arterial system. Systemic factors, such as hypotension, hyperviscosity of blood, and hyperglycemia, also promote more extensive brain infarction. The differential diagnosis of a worsening neurologic deficit includes cerebral hemorrhage, subdural and extradural hematoma, primary or metastatic brain tumor, cerebral abscess, and focal encephalitis. A computed tomographic (CT) scan of the head usually excludes a mass lesion and should be done on an emergency basis before anticoagulation is instituted.

Diagnostic Evaluation

When a stroke patient is seen by a physician, the initial neurologic examination defines the nature and severity of the neurologic deficit. Reexaminations at intervals of 30 to 60 minutes indicate whether the deficit remains the same (completed stroke), is improving (TIA), or is becoming more widespread (progressing stroke). When the area of ischemic infarct is supplied by the carotid arterial system, 48 hours without progression is needed to ensure that further progression is unlikely (less than 5% of patients). Patients who improve and then relapse are considered to have progressing strokes. Patients with hemiplegia due to internal or proximal middle cerebral artery occlusion who are stable for 24 to 48 hours but then become lethargic or comatose have brain swelling and brain herniation rather than progressing stroke.

The evaluation of a patient with an acute ischemic stroke is similar to that described for patients with TIAs. CT scan or MRI of the brain should be carried out as soon as possible after admission, to rule out cerebral hemorrhage and tumor. In many instances, the CT scan shows normal results even when the patient has a severe clinical deficit. For these patients, immediate MRI with diffusion-weighted sequences or another CT scan in 24 to 48 hours will reveal the area of infarction. Cerebral arteriography usually is not required for patients with acute strokes unless vasculitis or a cerebral aneurysm is suspected. Ultrasonography of the cervical and intracranial vessels may be used to define the site of vascular occlusion. In patients without evidence of atherosclerotic disease of the cervical carotid arteries, a thorough search should be made for a cardiac source of emboli.

Management

All patients with acute ischemic strokes and negative results of CT scan who are seen within 3 hours of the time of onset of stroke should be evaluated for treatment with intravenous tissue plasminogen activator, a thrombolytic agent. Thrombolytic therapy in one clinical trial produced a 12% increase in the number of patients with a good clinical outcome when assessed at 3 months after stroke. This improvement was gained at the price of a 6% incidence of cases of cerebral hemorrhage, almost half of which were fatal. While thrombolytic therapy is beneficial in selected patients, it is not a panacea for ischemic stroke, since only a small percentage of patients with ischemic strokes qualify for therapy with this agent.

Anticoagulation with intravenous, unfractionated heparin or with subcutaneous low-molecular-weight heparins and heparinoids may be used to treat un- or under-anticoagulated patients with acute ischemic cardio-embolic strokes. The use of heparin in patients with ischemic strokes, even progressing strokes, remains the subject of controversy, since it is not always effective and can cause serious bleeding. An international stroke trial showed a modest effect from subcutaneously administered heparin in preventing recurrent ischemic stroke within 2 weeks of onset but no improvement in eventual outcome. Nevertheless, there may be a role for intravenous heparin or subcutaneous heparinoids in progressing strokes and perhaps also in acute partial infarcts, to prevent progression. Nevertheless, the use of anticoagulants for acute stroke is associated with an increased risk of intracranial hemorrhage.

Even at present, the mainstay of treatment of patients with acute ischemic stroke is good nursing care to prevent pneumonia and deep venous thromboses in paralyzed or paretic limbs. Medical care is directed at the maintenance of circulation by the judicious treatment of hypertension, dysrhythmias, and cardiac failure. Any seizures should be controlled to avert further cerebral damage from seizure-induced hypoxia and hypertension. Pneumonia and urinary tract infections should receive appropriate antibiotic treatment. Fluid and electrolyte balance should be restored by intravenous fluids.

Recovery and Rehabilitation from Stroke

There is extreme variation in outcomes from stroke. Most patients show some improvement after 14 to 21 days, when the cerebral edema of infarction has resolved. In general, the temporal profile of recovery is that 50% of the potential recovery is attained at 1 month after onset, 75% at 3 months, 90% at 6 months, and almost 100% at 1 year. Rehabilitation after stroke should begin early (days after onset), at first to ensure that paralyzed parts do not develop fixed joints and muscle tendon contractures. After the acute phase, physical and occupational therapy can be used to help the patient regain and sustain independence. Cognitive therapy and speech therapy are also of major importance. Dementia, receptive aphasia, and major impairment in sensory perception are important factors limiting rehabilitation potential.

COMMON CLINICAL SYNDROMES OF ISCHEMIC STROKE ASSOCIATED WITH OCCLUSION OF SPECIFIC VESSELS

Knowledge of individual syndromes associated with occlusion of specific vessels helps the clinician localize a lesion, determine that the deficit is of vascular origin rather than due to a mass lesion, decide on appropriate treatment, and establish a prognosis. Nevertheless, syndromes of specific vessels do not localize the site or nature of the occlusion. For example, infarction in the territory of the middle cerebral artery often is the result of occlusion of the internal carotid artery. Occlusions of individual branches of the middle cerebral artery are usually embolic, but the source of emboli may be either a stenotic internal carotid artery or the heart.

OCCLUSION OF THE INTERNAL CAROTID ARTERY OR PROXIMAL MIDDLE CEREBRAL ARTERY

Sudden occlusion of the internal carotid artery or of the proximal stem of the middle cerebral artery results in devastating infarction of the ipsilateral hemisphere. The area infarcted often is coextensive with the entire cortical and subcortical distribution of the middle cerebral artery. Cortical branches of the middle cerebral artery supply the entire motor and sensory cortex controlling the face, hand, arm, and expressive speech area (Broca's area) of the dominant hemisphere (arterial territory of the superior division of the middle cerebral artery) as well as the visual radiation and macular cortex at the tip of the occipital lobe and the receptive speech area (Wernicke's area) of the dominant hemisphere (arterial territory of the inferior division of the middle cerebral artery). Subcortical or lenticulostriate branches of the most proximal position of the middle cerebral artery supply the basal ganglia and motor fibers to the face, hand, arm, and leg in the genu and posterior limb of the internal capsule.

The presence of paralysis of the face, arm, and leg as part of the syndrome of hemisphere infarction is characteristic of occlusion of the proximal middle cerebral artery. Infarction of the cortex supplied by the superior and inferior divisions of the middle cerebral artery results in contralateral hemiplegia involving the face, hand, and arm, sparing the leg. There is a hemisensory deficit, homonymous hemianopia, and, if the dominant

hemisphere is affected, total (expressive and receptive) aphasia. Infarction of motor fibers of the internal capsule supplied by the lenticulostriate branches of the proximal middle cerebral artery leads to contralateral hemiplegia, including paralysis of the lower extremity. Infarctions of the conjugate gaze area of the frontal lobe result in deviation of the eyes toward the site of damage.

OCCLUSION OF DISTAL BRANCHES OF THE MIDDLE CEREBRAL ARTERY

Occlusion of the superior division of the middle cerebral artery produces infarction of the anterior portions of the cerebral convexity but spares deep structures and the posterior portions of the hemisphere. Weakness and sensory loss are greater in the face and arm than in the leg, and no visual field defect is present. If the dominant hemisphere is involved, Broca's aphasia is present, with impaired speaking, naming, and writing ability but with relative preservation of comprehension.

Occlusion of the inferior division of the middle cerebral artery brings about infarction of the posterior portions of the cerebral cortex, including the visual radiation. In this instance, contralateral sensory loss predominates, and weakness may be minimal or absent. If the dominant hemisphere is involved, Wernicke's aphasia is present, with fluent speech output of jargon and paraphasia. Comprehension, naming, reading, and writing also are affected.

OCCLUSION OF THE ANTERIOR CEREBRAL ARTERY

Infarction of the cortical territory supplied by the anterior cerebral artery causes weakness, clumsiness, and sensory loss affecting mainly the contralateral leg and foot.

OCCLUSION OF THE POSTERIOR CEREBRAL ARTERY

Occlusion of the posterior cerebral artery causes contralateral homonymous hemianopia by infarction of the visual or calcarine cortex. If the lesion affects the dominant hemisphere and includes the posterior corpus callosum, there is alexia without agraphia owing to disconnection of the intact nondominant visual cortex from the dominant hemisphere language area. Unilateral proximal posterior cerebral artery occlusion may cause a transient disturbance of memory as the result of infarction of the medial temporal lobe.

BRAIN-STEM STROKE DUE TO VERTEBROBASILAR OCCLUSIONS

Occlusion of the Basilar Artery

Occlusion of the basilar artery is a serious event that often leads to death. Obstruction of flow in both vertebral arteries or in a lone, unpaired vertebral artery produces a syndrome similar to basilar artery occlusion. The clinical features of basilar artery occlusion differ, depending on whether the cause of occlusion is embolism or thrombosis in situ. Embolism tends to involve the distal portion of the basilar artery; in contrast, atheromatous occlusion affects the proximal and middle portions of the vessel.

Emboli small enough to pass through the vertebral arteries into the larger basilar artery usually are arrested at the top of the basilar artery at its bifurcation into the posterior cerebral arteries. Loss of consciousness occurs immediately because of obstruction of the blood supply to the mesencephalic ascending reticular activating system. Unilateral or bilateral palsies of the third cranial nerve are characteristic. Hemiplegia or quadriplegia ensues, with decerebrate or decorticate posturing. In fact, the "top of the basilar syndrome"—coma, unequal pupils both fixed to light, and bilateral corticospinal tract dysfunction—resembles and may be confused with midbrain failure caused by transtentorial uncal herniation. A history of vertebrobasilar TIAs or coma that came on suddenly accompanied by bilateral oculomotor dysfunction from its onset serves to distinguish acute brain-stem dysfunction from slowly evolving brain-stem compression due to downward transtentorial herniation.

Smaller emboli that occlude the rostral basilar artery only transiently before fragmenting and passing into one or both posterior cerebral arteries either do not result in permanent neurologic deficits or cause infarction of portions of the midbrain, of the thalamus, and of the temporal and occipital lobes. Thrombosis in situ occurs in the proximal and middle portions of the basilar artery. Pontine infarction due to basilar thrombosis is associated with unilateral damage to the sixth cranial nerve or nucleus. Horizontal eye movements are impaired, but vertical nystagmus and ocular bobbing may be present. The pupils are constricted and may be pinpoint, but they remain reactive to light. Hemiplegia or quadriplegia is usual.

In unconscious patients, the syndrome of basilar occlusion can be confused with pontine hemorrhage. A CT scan of the brain can differentiate between ischemic infarction and hematoma. Coma caused by occlusion of the basilar artery carries a poor prognosis for survival. In some cases, the basis pontis is injured permanently, but not the tegmentum of the brain stem. Such patients regain consciousness if they have lost it, but they remain quadriplegic. The term locked-in state has been applied to this condition. Locked-in patients may be able to signify that they are conscious by blinking to command. For patients who lack any clinical signs of consciousness, a conventional electroencephalogram with stimulation or cortical evoked responses may be needed to distinguish the locked-in state from the vegetative state.

Occlusion of the Vertebral Artery

Many syndromes of partial brain-stem infarction have been described after occlusion of the vertebral artery or of branches of the basilar artery. In general, brain-stem infarcts produce bilateral clinical signs. Ipsilateral signs reflect damage to the cranial nerves, their nuclei, and the uncrossed cerebellar pathways. Contralateral signs result from damage to the motor and sensory pathways that cross below the level of the infarct to the opposite side of the body. Occlusion of one vertebral artery when the other is patent causes the relatively benign syndrome of lateral

medullary infarction. This syndrome is the most common of brain-stem infarcts and is prototypical.

Lateral medullary infarction takes the initial form of severe vertigo, nausea, vomiting, and nystagmus as a result of involvement of the lower vestibular nuclei. The descending tract and nucleus of the fifth cranial nerve are affected, with loss of pain and temperature sensation over the face on the side of the lesion. Damage to the inferior cerebellar peduncle causes ataxia of the limbs on the side of the lesion. Ipsilateral Horner's syndrome (miosis, ptosis) and loss of pain and temperature sensation on the contralateral side of the body are found. In addition, if the ninth and tenth cranial nerves are affected, there will be hiccups and difficulty swallowing. In general, ischemic brain-stem syndromes caused by occlusion of individual branches of the vertebral or basilar arteries have a benign prognosis and do not require anticoagulation or vascular surgical intervention. When brain-stem infarction is complicated by extensive cerebellar infarction, however, a life-threatening situation can develop.

CLINICAL SYNDROME OF CEREBELLAR INFARCTION

The symptoms of cerebellar infarction in conscious patients are consistent and resemble those of cerebellar hemorrhage. Common complaints include difficulty standing and walking, headache, nausea, vomiting, dizziness, clumsiness, and slurred speech. The onset of symptoms is abrupt in one-third of patients. With progression of infarction or swelling, most patients show signs of lateral gaze palsy or nystagmus toward the side of infarction. Facial palsies are common, but dysfunction of other cranial nerves and corticospinal and sensory defects typically are absent unless lateral medullary infarction has occurred coincident with cerebellar infarction. As edema develops around the infarct, hydrocephalus and impaired cognitive function or depressed consciousness appear.

When a cerebellar infarct increases in size from edematous swelling, the underlying pons and medulla are compressed against the clivus. The fourth ventricle is distorted, and obstructive hydrocephalus may arise. Brain-stem infarction and hemorrhage may be a late and fatal result of compression of the vessels on the ventral surface of the brain stem. Rapid descent of the cerebellar tonsils and impaction of the medulla cause sudden apnea and circulatory collapse. If tonsillar herniation is not fatal, increasing pressure in the posterior fossa effects upward herniation into and through the incisura or opening of the tentorium. As upward herniation develops, the displaced cerebellum distorts the midbrain. Hemispheric branches of the superior cerebellar arteries may be compressed by upward herniation of the cerebellum against the free edge of the tentorium. In some cases, this results in further infarction of the cerebellar hemispheres. In a review of the literature, my colleagues and I found 39 cases of upward herniation confirmed by postmortem examination. A cerebellar lesion caused upward herniation most frequently (65%) and was most often a hemorrhage (10 cases). Upward herniation followed cerebellar infarction in five patients. Lesions in the cerebellopontine angle (13%), in the pons (11%), and in the fourth ventricle (11%) also were associated with upward herniation.

DIAGNOSIS

An expanding cerebellar mass produces a characteristic syndrome of coma, small reactive pupils, abnormal doll's-eye responses, abnormal ice-water caloric responses, and corticospinal tract dysfunction. These initial signs of pontine compression are followed by signs of midbrain dysfunction, as already described in the context of transtentorial herniation. The gradual caudal-to-rostral progression of brain-stem dysfunction identifies the cause of coma as cerebellar herniation. CT examination of the posterior fossa shows a large area of decreased density in the cerebellum and hydrocephalus.

SURGICAL TREATMENT

Small infarctions of the cerebellum do not lead to coma and can be managed without surgery. Some patients stabilize after ventricular decompression to relieve hydrocephalus. When an extensive cerebellar infarction is recognized, surgical exploration of the posterior fossa and resection of the necrotic cerebellar tissue may be required. The surgical mortality rate is 50% if the patient is operated on while still conscious, but it approaches 80% if the patient becomes comatose or stuporous.

PROGNOSIS

Death from tonsillar herniation and cardiorespiratory failure is a typical outcome of massive, untreated cerebellar infarction. Not all cases of extensive cerebellar infarction are fatal, and patients who remain conscious 1 week after the onset of symptoms are unlikely to deteriorate from brain swelling or to require surgical decompression of the posterior fossa.

◾ VASCULAR SYNDROMES CAUSED BY HYPERTENSION

Lacunar infarction and hypertensive intracerebral hemorrhage differ in clinical characteristics, but the site of the underlying pathologic process uniformly is in the small-resistance cerebral arteries. Before considering the clinical features of hypertensive strokes, we review the normal physiologic responses of the cerebral arteries to changes in systemic blood pressure.

CEREBRAL AUTOREGULATION

Whenever the systemic blood pressure rises too high or falls too low, the cerebral arteries constrict or dilate, respectively, to ensure a constant CBF. Such autoregulation occurs primarily at the small-resistance cerebral arteries. As systemic blood pressure rises, the proportion of pressure dissipated across the small arteries increases; thus, these small-resistance arteries bear the brunt of systemic hypertension. The range of blood pressure over which autoregulatory responses can maintain a normal CBF can be only approximated. In a normotensive young person, the lower limit at which autoregulation occurs is near a mean blood pressure of 60 mm Hg. As the blood pressure falls below this level, even maximal dilatation of the vascular bed of the brain cannot compensate for the decreased perfusion pressure, and the CBF declines. In contrast, when the blood pressure exceeds the upper limit of the range of autoregulation (150 to 200 mm Hg), the CBF rises, and hypertensive encephalopathy may result.

LACUNAR INFARCTIONS

Lacunar infarctions are the most common cerebrovascular lesions, seen in roughly 10% of autopsied brains. They are often multiple, with an average of three per brain and, in some cases, 15 or more. Lacunes ("lakes") are healed ischemic infarctions, with minute cavities ranging from 0.5 to 15 mm in diameter; most are 2 to 4 mm in diameter. They are most common in the deep nuclei of the brain (putamen, 37%; thalamus, 14%; caudate, 10%), the pons (16%), and the posterior limb of the internal capsule (10%). They are found in lesser numbers in the deep cerebral white matter, the anterior limb of the internal capsule, and the cerebellum.

In part because of their small size and location in relatively silent areas of the brain, many lacunar infarctions are not recognized clinically. The onset of lacunar stroke is usually gradual, developing over several hours or days. Headache is absent in almost all cases, and consciousness is unchanged. Recognition of the lacunar stroke syndromes is important because the deficits produced are self-limited and relatively benign. Anticoagulation is not required and actually may be dangerous, because lacunar infarction often is associated with microhemorrhages. The prognosis for almost complete recovery is good, and the likelihood of future lacunar strokes is limited by adequate control of blood pressure.

Syndromes of Lacunar Stroke

Four major syndromes of lacunar stroke have been described. Lacunar stroke with pure motor hemiparesis is characterized by weakness of the face, arm, and leg on one side of the body, with no associated sensory, visual, or cortical deficits. Large deficits limited to the motor system can develop only where the motor fibers to one side of the body run close together, either in the posterior limb of the internal capsule or in the pons.

Pure sensory stroke of the face, arm, and leg is characterized by paresthesias and mild sensory loss involving half the body, with no other neurologic deficit. The affected area is often numb, tingling, itchy, or stiff. Sensory loss may be detectable by touching the patient with a light hair. At the onset of the stroke, the paresthesias spread over the involved side in a period of seconds to hours. The syndrome is caused by a lacune in the posterolateral nucleus of the thalamus, the primary sensory relay nucleus. The outlook for complete recovery is good. This stroke must be distinguished from a cortical sensory stroke due to disease of a large branch artery.

Homolateral ataxia and crural (distal leg) paresis is characterized by weakness of one leg, especially the toes and ankle, with a Babinski's sign and striking lack of coordination of the ipsilateral arm and leg. TIAs precede the stroke in more than half of cases. Transient paresthesias may occur at the onset in half the cases, but they do not recur. The patient often cannot walk without support. The lacune is in the contralateral internal capsule or corona radiata. Ninety percent of patients recover almost completely. The lacunar state is the syndrome of pseudobulbar palsy in which lability of affect, dementia, small-stepped rigid gait, dysarthria, incontinence, and bilateral long tract signs are present. Despite the prevalence of lacunes in the basal ganglia, parkinsonian tremor is not a feature of the lacunar state.

Pathogenesis

Lacunes are not old cavitated hemorrhages but are caused by occlusion of small arteries. The essential pathologic process involves arteries with a diameter of 50 to 200 Em and consists of fibrinoid deposition, mural destruction, and thrombotic occlusion, a process termed *lipohyalinosis* or *segmented arterial disorganization*. This process appears to be a specific result of chronic hypertension.

HYPERTENSIVE INTRACEREBRAL HEMORRHAGE

Hemorrhage is the most lethal complication of chronic hypertension. If cases of trauma and ruptured saccular aneurysm or arteriovenous malformations are excluded, the classic type of intracerebral hemorrhage almost always is caused by hypertension.

Clinical Features

Hypertensive hemorrhage most often occurs in persons older than 50 years. The hemorrhage appears without warning while the patient is awake, often during exertion. Headache may be severe but is absent or trivial in half the cases. Vomiting is common; in the context of thrombotic or embolic strokes, it is rare. The blood pressure almost always remains elevated after onset; if nothing else is known in a particular case, the finding of normal or low blood pressure when a stroke patient is first examined makes the diagnosis of hypertensive hemorrhage unlikely. Once hemorrhage has taken place, the patient's condition worsens steadily over a period of minutes to days, until the neurologic deficit stabilizes or the patient dies. Once the deficit stabilizes, improvement occurs slowly. Because much of the deficit may be caused by an expanding hematoma that compresses rather than destroys the brain, return of neurologic function can be dramatic as the swelling subsides.

Large hypertensive hemorrhages rupture through brain parenchyma into the ventricles. Rupture directly into the subarachnoid space is unusual. When death ensues, it most often is due to herniation caused by the expanding hematoma and surrounding edema. However, hypertensive hemorrhages are not all massive or uniformly fatal, as witnessed by clinical observations, by pathologic studies showing old healed hemorrhages, and by CT, which identifies small, nonfatal hemorrhages.

Pontine Hemorrhage

Hemorrhage into the pons produces a fulminant syndrome in which coma occurs within seconds to minutes and death usually follows within 48 hours. The pupils are pinpoint, and horizontal eye movements are absent or impaired. Vertical eye movements may be preserved, and ocular bobbing, with a distinctive bilateral downbeating, may occur every 5 seconds. Quadriparesis often is present, with bilateral long tract signs and decerebration. Hyperthermia frequently is a feature, because muscular rigidity and shivering increase body heat while interruption of sympathetic pathways in the brain stem prevents sweating. Direct rupture of the hemorrhage into the fourth ventricle is the rule.

Deep Cerebral Hemorrhage

Most hemorrhages above the brain stem develop in the deep nuclear masses of the cerebrum. The two most common sites are the putamen of the basal ganglia and the thalamus, the main sensory relay nucleus. The motor defect is more dense in a putaminal hemorrhage, whereas the sensory defect is more prominent when the hemorrhage occurs in the thalamus. Thalamic hemorrhages often dissect downward and medially, to impinge on the midbrain center for upward gaze; in large thalamic hemorrhages, the eyes look downward and appear to be staring at the tip of the nose. Aphasia may occur if hemorrhage in either nucleus presses laterally on the speech areas. A separate aphasic syndrome has been reported in cases of localized hemorrhage within the thalamus; such patients appear to have an excellent prognosis for full recovery of speech.

Cerebellar Hemorrhage

The onset of cerebellar hemorrhage is sudden, without loss of consciousness. Within several minutes, the patient cannot stand or walk and most vomit repeatedly. Headache and dizziness develop in about half the cases. During the first several hours, most patients are alert, confused, or drowsy. Seventy-five percent become comatose within 12 hours and almost 90% within 24 hours. Conjugate lateral eye movements often are abnormal, with paresis of gaze to the side of the lesion or forced deviation away from the lesion. There may be skew deviation, with depression of the eye ipsilateral to the lesion. The pupils remain small and reactive even with deep stupor. In half the cases, ipsilateral facial weakness of the lower motor neuron type is present. Strength is normal, and appendicular cerebellar function may be intact or minimally impaired. Plantar responses initially are flexor but become extensor as the patient deteriorates. Loss of voluntary or reflex upward gaze is a sign of obstructive hydrocephalus. Rapid diagnosis of cerebellar hemorrhage is crucial. Early surgical decompression is lifesaving and often leads to complete reversal of the neurologic deficit. Surgical results are much better for responsive than for nonresponsive patients. Brain-stem stroke and cerebellar infarction can mimic the picture of cerebellar hemorrhage but are distinguished by CT.

Pathogenesis of Hypertensive Hemorrhage

Multiple microaneurysms arising in small-resistance arteries were found by microangiography by Russell in 1963. These aneurysms were most common in regions of the brain where hypertensive hemorrhages are also most common, and some were surrounded by small leaks of blood. Changes reflective of lipohyalinosis often were present in the aneurysmal walls. Two theories of the underlying cause of hypertensive intracerebral hemorrhage have developed. Russell maintains that these aneurysms are caused by mechanical distention and that lipohyalinosis then occurs as a secondary change. Fisher considers lipohyalinosis to be the initial process and suggests that an affected resistance artery may rupture whether or not an actual aneurysm develops. It is generally agreed that massive cerebral hemorrhage follows the rupture of either an aneurysmal or lipohyalinotic segment of a small-resistance artery and that the basic lesion is caused by chronic hypertension.

Treatment

The importance of surgical decompression for cerebellar hematoma has been mentioned. Surgery is not indicated for pontine or deep cerebral hypertensive hemorrhages. Surgery may be life-saving, however, in the case of a superficial hemorrhage in the white matter large enough to cause shift and herniation. Prognosis is directly related to the level of consciousness before the operation, and surgery usually is fruitless in an already comatose patient.

There is no effective medical treatment for intracerebral hemorrhage. Corticosteroids or dehydrating agents have not been of more than temporary benefit. The use of antihypertensive agents for acute cerebral hemorrhage is the subject of controversy. Attempts to lower systemic blood pressure may compromise CBF and lead to infarction, but continued hypertension may cause cerebral edema. One approach to this problem is derived from measurements of the cerebral autoregulation curve after stroke or trauma. Because of vasomotor paralysis, a damaged brain may lose the ability to autoregulate; CBF then follows blood pressure in a linear fashion. In effect, the "breakthrough point" is lowered, leading to a situation analogous to hypertensive encephalopathy in which elevated blood pressure accelerates the formation of edema. On this basis, it seems reasonable to lower blood pressure to normal levels after cerebral hemorrhage. This must be done with great care because the cerebral vasculature may be unusually sensitive to antihypertensive agents; therefore, smaller doses of the milder agents should be tried initially.

BIBLIOGRAPHY

Antiplatelet Trialists Collaboration. Collaborative overview of randomized trials of antiplatelet therapy (Part 1). *Br Med J* 1994;308:81–106.

Barnett HJ, Eliasziw M, Meldrum HE. Drugs and surgery in prevention of ischemic stroke. *N Engl J Med* 1995;332:238–248.

Barnett HJM, Mohr JP, Stein BM, et al., eds. *Stroke: pathophysiology, diagnosis and management,* second ed. New York: Churchill Livingstone, 1992.

Brown RD Jr, Evans BA, Wiebers DO, et al. Transient ischemic attack and minor ischemic stroke: an algorithm for evaluation and treatment. *Mayo Clin Proc* 1994;69:1027–1039.

CAST (Chinese Acute Stroke Trial) Collaborative Group. CAST: a randomised placebo-controlled trial of early aspirin use in 20,000 patients with acute ischemic stroke. *Lancet* 1997;349:1641–1649.

Cuneo RA, Caronna JJ. The neurologic complications of hypertension. *Med Clin North Am* 1977;61:565–580.

Cuneo RA, Caronna JJ, Pitts L, et al. Upward transtentorial herniation: seven cases and a literature review. *Arch Neurol* 1979;36:618–623.

Fisher CM. Lacunar strokes and infarcts: a review. *Neurology* 1982;32:871–876.

International Stroke Trial Collaborative Group. The International Stroke Trial (IST): a randomised trial of aspirin, subcutaneous heparin, both or neither among 19,435 patients with acute ischemic stroke. *Lancet* 1997;349:1569–1581.

Kannell WB, Dawber TR, Sorlie P, et al. Components of blood pressure and risk of atherothrombotic infarction: the Framingham study. *Stroke* 1976;7:327–331.

Lanska DJ, Kryscio RJ. Endarterectomy for asymptomatic internal carotid artery stenosis. *Neurology* 1997;48:1481–1490.

Kelley's Textbook of Internal Medicine, fourth edition. Edited by H. David Humes. Lippincott Williams & Wilkins, Philadelphia © 2000.

C H A P T E R

433

DEMYELINATING DISEASES

JOHN R. RICHERT

MULTIPLE SCLEROSIS

Multiple sclerosis (MS) is an inflammatory, demyelinating disease of the central nervous system (CNS).

INCIDENCE AND EPIDEMIOLOGY

MS prevalence tends to correlate with distance from the equator, being 70 to 100 per 100,000 population in the northern United States and Canada and less than 5 per 100,000 in the tropics. Onset most commonly occurs between ages 20 and 50 years. Women affected outnumber men by about 2 to 1. Epidemiologic studies suggest that exposure to some as-yet-undetermined environmental agent in the mid-teenage years serves as an inciting event in the disease.

There is a clear hereditary predisposition to MS: the concordance rate among first-degree relatives of MS patients is about 25 to 50 times higher than the prevalence in the general population. Furthermore, the concordance rate among identical twins (255 to 50%) is higher than that for fraternal twins (1% to 2%). In addition, certain ethnic groups (e.g., Inuits) exhibit a strong divergence in prevalence from those in the predominant populations living in the same latitudes.

ETIOLOGY

Speculation has centered on two types of processes: direct infection of the CNS with a neurotropic agent and autoimmunity. Although elevated antibody titers in MS cerebrospinal fluid and serum have been described for several viruses, none of these agents has been reliably detected in the CNS of MS patients.

Recent reports suggesting a causal role of human herpes virus 6 (HHV-6) or *Chlamydia pneumoniae* remain to be substantiated.

Familial cases of MS do not follow mendelian genetics, and current data suggest a polygenic predisposition. Different human leukocyte antigen (HLA) types predominate in different ethnic populations. The most prevalent HLA haplotype in the MS population of northern European origin includes the DR15 subtype of DR2 and DQA1*0102-DQB1*0602. Extensive linkage studies with panels of microsatellite markers are currently under way in several laboratories.

Indirect evidence for an autoimmune component to the disease comes from an animal model of MS, experimental allergic encephalomyelitis, which can be induced by sensitizing laboratory animals to myelin basic protein, proteolipid protein, or myelin oligodendrocyte glycoprotein. Diminished disease activity during pregnancy, which is associated with a state of relative immune suppression, also suggests an autoimmune cause. This is further supported by the tendency for immunosuppressive treatment regimens to be more effective than immunoenhancing ones. Data from several groups have suggested a defect in suppressor cell function. A number of markers associated with immune system activation have been associated with MS disease activity, but these do not distinguish between a primary autoimmune pathogenesis and a viral cause. Current evidence suggests that MS is precipitated by initial exposure of a genetically susceptible host to a relatively common infectious agent in the mid-teenage years and that this ultimately leads to an autoimmune process that pathologically targets CNS myelin.

PATHOGENESIS

The hallmarks of the microscopic examination are multifocal areas (plaques) of mononuclear cell infiltration and demyelination in a perivenular distribution. The mononuclear cell infiltrate consists of lymphocytes (T cells more than B cells) and lipid-laden macrophages. The demyelination results in slowing/blocking of conduction along the axons. At the hemispheric level, plaques tend to occur in a periventricular distribution. With progression of disease, gliotic (fibrotic) scars form, often with secondary axonal loss. Recent evidence suggests that axonal loss or cerebral atrophy or both may occur early in the course of MS.

CLINICAL FINDINGS

Any region of CNS white matter may be affected. For example, involvement of the cerebral hemispheres may produce a hemiparesis or hemisensory deficit or may lead to cognitive dysfunction. Various brain-stem syndromes (e.g., internuclear ophthalmoplegia) and optic neuritis are common. Cerebellar involvement may result in ataxia or intention tremor. Spinal cord disease may produce a spastic paraparesis/paraplegia with neurogenic bowel and bladder and sexual dysfunction. Dysesthetic pain syndromes may result from the involvement of nerve root entry zones in the CNS; trigeminal neuralgia is the classic example.

MS is somewhat arbitrarily divided into four forms. Approximately 15% of patients exhibit the *primary progressive* form, characterized by gradual accumulation of neurologic deficits

without clear-cut exacerbations and remissions. This is seen in many patients with late-onset MS. Approximately 75% of patients begin with a *relapsing-remitting (R-R)* course. These patients tend to return to a somewhat more impaired status after many of their exacerbations, such that the R-R course leads to a progressively worsening baseline. Although most exacerbations have no identifiable precipitating cause, about 30% are preceded by a viral illness. Most patients with R-R MS eventually develop a more gradually progressive course, with or without superimposed exacerbations, referred to as *secondary progressive* MS. A small percentage of patients begin with a gradually progressive course and subsequently experience superimposed exacerbations, hence the term *progressive-relapsing* MS.

The diagnosis rests on well-described criteria for "possible," "probable," and "definite" MS. The hallmark of the disease is "dissemination in time and space" (i.e., multiple episodes of dysfunction and multiple areas of involvement within the CNS). Thus, the diagnosis cannot be made with certainty at the time of initial neurologic symptoms. Similarly, the diagnosis of primary progressive MS is difficult to make.

LABORATORY FINDINGS

No laboratory abnormality is pathognomonic for MS. Therefore, after accumulating information that is consistent with the diagnosis, one must rule out other diseases that may mimic MS.

Magnetic resonance imaging (MRI) has revolutionized our ability to make an early diagnosis of MS. Plaques typically appear as areas of increased signal intensity on T2-weighted (Fig. 433.1)

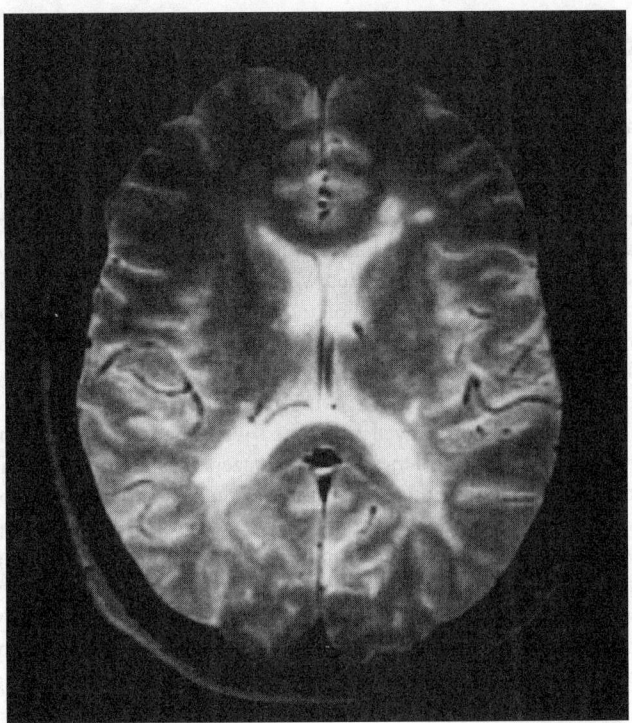

FIGURE 433.1. Magnetic resonance imaging scan of the brain of a 21-year-old patient with isolated spinal cord symptoms showing many deep, white matter lesions.

and proton density images and sometimes as areas of decreased signal intensity on T1-weighted images. Enhancement after gadolinium contrast administration identifies areas of blood–brain barrier breakdown and therefore detects areas of active inflammation in the CNS. Fluid attenuated inversion recovery (FLAIR) images are helpful in distinguishing cerebrospinal fluid from periventricular plaques. Magnetization transfer technology and MR spectroscopy may soon permit more sensitive detection and further information about biochemical abnormalities in MS.

If clinical and MRI evaluations detect only one involved site within the CNS, evoked potential studies (visual, auditory, somatosensory, and motor) may be used to detect an additional, subclinical area of slowed conduction due to demyelination.

Although the cerebrospinal fluid may be normal, a mild mononuclear cell pleocytosis and modest protein elevation are common. Elevated IgG levels and evidence of increased intrathecal IgG synthesis (IgG index, IgG synthesis rate) are often present. Oligoclonal immunoglobulin bands are found in over 90% of patients.

Other diseases that may resemble MS from clinical, imaging, and cerebrospinal fluid standpoints include syphilis, neuroborreliosis, CNS vasculitis, sarcoid, and HTLV (human T-cell lymphotropic virus)-I–associated myelopathy (tropical spastic paraparesis). Multiple infarcts secondary to small-vessel vascular disease must also be considered. Rarely, the inherited dysmyelinating diseases (e.g., metachromatic leukodystrophy, adrenoleukodystrophy) have their onset in adult life, with MRI appearances that resemble MS. Postviral demyelination in a multifocal distribution may occur as a monophasic illness and may mimic the initial episode of MS. Vitamin B_{12} deficiency should also be ruled out.

OPTIMAL MANAGEMENT

Treatment regimens can be categorized as being either symptomatic (to ameliorate various physiologic abnormalities) or directed at suppressing CNS inflammation.

Oxybutynin and other anticholinergic agents are useful in reducing bladder spasticity, thereby reducing urinary frequency and urgency. Large residual bladder volumes (usually due to sphincter spasticity) are treated with intermittent catheterization or (less desirably) chronic Foley drainage. Constipation is also related to autonomic dysfunction and is best treated with stool softeners and adequate fiber intake. More potent laxatives and enemas should be used as sparingly as possible.

Spasticity is often well controlled with the use of baclofen, tizanidine, or dantrolene sodium. Diazepam and various anticonvulsant medications are used less frequently. Some degree of spasticity may be necessary to allow patients with severe leg weakness to maintain a reasonable level of ambulation; reducing spasticity may therefore increase the sense of lower extremity weakness. Patients with otherwise refractory severe spasticity may benefit from continuous intrathecal infusion of baclofen by a subcutaneous pump. Rarely, rhizotomy or a tendon-severing procedure is used to reduce severe spasticity.

Trigeminal neuralgia and neurogenic pain secondary to involvement of dorsal root entry zones in the cord can be treated with anticonvulsants or tricyclic antidepressants. If pharmacologic treatment fails to control the pain of trigeminal neuralgia, neurosurgical ablation of the trigeminal ganglion may be considered, particularly if pain is triggered by peripheral stimulation (e.g., chewing or speaking).

Fatigue, characterized by a global inanition of uncertain pathophysiologic cause, is common. Amantadine, pemoline, and afternoon rest periods may be helpful.

Methods for enhancing nerve conduction velocity in demyelinated nerve are being developed. Because elevated body temperature slows nerve conduction and often aggravates MS symptoms, exposure to cold (e.g., a cooling vest) temporarily increases conduction velocity and, for some patients, provides symptomatic improvement. Aquatic exercise programs in cool water allow aerobic exercise with improved dissipation of heat and provide a buoyant density that permits more vigorous exercise than can be achieved on dry land. Experimental agents that block potassium channels and thereby increase conduction velocity (e.g., 4-aminopyridine) are being developed.

Cerebellar tremor is a notoriously difficult symptom to treat. Modest degrees of success have been reported with the use of clonazepam and with isoniazid, both of which may act through the GABA (γ-aminobutyric acid) system. Very preliminary attempts to use thalamic stimulation to ameliorate tremor appear encouraging.

Of the treatments aimed at reducing inflammation in the CNS, high-dose intravenous methylprednisolone (0.5 to 1.0 g per day for 3 to 7 days) is most effective at rapidly reversing neurologic deficits associated with exacerbation, although it remains unclear whether the eventual level of recovery is improved with its use. A small percentage of patients experience severe hypokalemia during each course of corticosteroids. Therefore, at least during a patient's initial course of treatment, the physician should have access to the results of each day's serum potassium level on the same day. In some locales, this may require hospitalization. Diabetics may also require hospitalization to control glucose homeostasis.

Recombinant interferon-β is effective in the long-term treatment of both R-R and secondary progressive MS. It is unclear whether the beneficial effect is secondary to its antiviral action or its immunomodulatory function. Glatiramer acetate, a random copolymer of four amino acids designed to inhibit the T-cell response to myelin basic protein (but which may actually have a more general immunomodulatory effect), has been shown to reduce the exacerbation rate in R-R MS.

Progressive forms of MS are often more resistant to treatment, and one often resorts to therapy with chemotherapeutic agents. Mitoxantrone (12 mg/m^2 intravenously every 3 months) has recently been reported to be effective in a mixed cohort of secondary progressive and relapsing patients who entered the study with a moderate degree of fixed neurologic disability. There is an unknown degree of risk of vacuolar cardiomyopathy with high cumulative doses of mitoxantrone. Low-dose oral methotrexate (7.5 mg week) produces a mild slowing of progression of MS, but most patients appear to eventually require higher doses. Oral azathioprine has been of minimal proven benefit, although it has not been well studied using modern MS clinical trial designs. Its use is particularly popular in Europe. Varied degrees of success have been reported with high-dose intravenous immunoglobulin. Intravenous cyclophosphamide is a controversial form of therapy used by some neurologists in an initial 8- to 14-day course, followed by monthly intravenous pulses. It appears to be most effective in patients with significant recent worsening of neurologic status that has been refractory to treatment with more conventional agents. Monthly pulses of intravenous methylprednisolone (1 g) are widely used and are well tolerated by most patients with MS, although formal proof of efficacy is currently lacking.

OPTIC NEURITIS

Optic neuritis is an inflammatory, demyelinating disease of the optic nerve. Onset is usually acute or subacute and produces diminished visual acuity, scotomata, or color desaturation. Ocular pain with eye movement is a common concomitant. It usually involves the retrobulbar portion of the nerve and therefore is not associated with abnormal funduscopic findings during the acute stage. A papillitis produces papilledema. Over time, optic atrophy may develop, manifested by disk pallor on ophthalmologic examination. An afferent pupillary defect to light stimulation is a common finding on examination. At least 50% of patients eventually develop frank MS, with the highest risk occurring among those with abnormalities on MRI that are suggestive of MS. In one study, treatment with either intravenous corticosteroid followed by a tapering course of oral corticosteroid, or oral corticosteroid alone, produced more rapid recovery from an acute attack than did placebo, although the eventual level of recovery was similar in all groups. Subjects treated with oral corticosteroids alone tended to have a worse relapse record than that of those in the other two study groups. Treatment with intravenous methylprednisolone appeared to delay the eventual development of clinically definite MS.

ACUTE DISSEMINATED ENCEPHALOMYELITIS

Acute disseminated encephalomyelitis (ADEM) is an acute, monophasic, inflammatory, demyelinating disease of the CNS that is most commonly considered to be a postinfectious process. It is similar to the disseminated encephalomyelitis that occurred secondary to sensitization with CNS antigens found in earlier rabies vaccine preparations. It is the human disease most closely related clinically and pathologically to acute experimental allergic encephalomyelitis, which can be induced in laboratory animals by sensitization with any of several myelin antigens. An elevated T-cell response to myelin basic protein has been reported in those with ADEM.

The clinical manifestations of ADEM may be protean, with involvement of motor, sensory, cerebellar, and cranial nerve function, as well as encephalopathy with mental status changes, sometimes progressing to coma. The mortality rate approaches 30%. Cerebrospinal fluid abnormalities usually include a predominantly mononuclear pleocytosis and elevated protein level. MRI demonstrates extensive areas of increased signal intensity in the white matter on T2-weighted and proton density sequences. Adrenocorticosteroids are often used therapeutically, but their value is uncertain.

ADRENOLEUKODYSTROPHY

Adrenoleukodystrophy is an X-linked recessive disease related to defective peroxisomal β-oxidation of very-long-chain (greater than C_{22}) fatty acids due to either a deficiency of very-long-chain (lignoceric acid) acyl coenzyme A ligase or an abnormality in a peroxisomal membrane protein that is required to transport the ligase into the peroxisome. Childhood and adult forms are recognized; the latter is often referred to as adrenomyeloneuropathy. Both forms occurring within the same kindred suggests that they represent different manifestations of the same mutation. The disease is characterized by CNS demyelination, gliosis, perivascular inflammation, peripheral neuropathy, and adrenal insufficiency. Motor, cognitive, brain-stem, cerebellar, and visual deficits are common. The typical course of adrenoleukodystrophy is one of progressive decline, with death within 5 years. Immunosuppressive therapy has been ineffective. Treatment with a 4:1 mixture of glyceryl trioleate and trierucate oils (Lorenzo's oil) normalized plasma levels of saturated very-long-chain fatty acids but did not prevent progressive loss of neurologic function. There has been a case report of reversal of both neurologic deficits and MRI abnormalities in early disease after bone marrow transplantation.

BIBLIOGRAPHY

Beck RW, Cleary PA, Anderson MM Jr, et al. A randomized, controlled trial of corticosteroids in the treatment of acute optic neuritis. The Optic Neuritis Study Group. *N Engl J Med* 1992;326:581–588.
Ebers GC, Sadovnick AD. The role of genetic factors in multiple sclerosis susceptibility. *J Neuroimmunol* 1994;54:1–17.
Hommes OR, Sandberg M, Silberberg D: Emerging treatments in multiple sclerosis. Proceedings of the European Charcot Foundation Symposium. Brussels, Belgium, 23-24 November 1995. *Mult Scler* 1996;1:305–403.
Lucchinetti CF, Rodriguez M. The controversy surrounding the pathogenesis of the multiple sclerosis lesion. *Mayo Clin Proc* 1997;72:665–678.
Mathews WB, Compston A, Allen IV, et al. *McAlpine's multiple sclerosis.* Edinburgh: Churchill Livingstone, 1991.
Moser HW. Adrenoleukodystrophy: phenotype, genetics, pathogenesis and therapy. *Brain* 1997;120:1485–1508.
Poser CM, Paty DW, Scheinberg L, et al. New diagnostic criteria for multiple sclerosis: guidelines for research protocols. *Ann Neurol* 1983;13:227–231.

Kelley's Textbook of Internal Medicine, fourth edition. Edited by H. David Humes. Lippincott Williams & Wilkins, Philadelphia © 2000.

C H A P T E R
434

PARKINSON'S DISEASE AND RELATED DISORDERS

STEPHEN G. REICH

Extrapyramidal disorders, as discussed in Chapter 429 are divided into hypokinetic/rigid and hyperkinetic disorders. The former includes Parkinson's disease (PD) and related conditions and is the focus of this chapter. PD was described in 1817 by James Parkinson, a general practitioner in London. Little has been added to his description of *The Shaking Palsy*: "Involuntary tremulous motion, with lessened muscular power, in parts not in action and even when supported; with a propensity to bend the trunk forwards, and to pass from a walking to a running pace. . .."

EPIDEMIOLOGY

PD is the second most common degenerative disorder in adults, after Alzheimer's disease. It is estimated that at least 1 million Americans are affected. Both prevalence and incidence rates vary widely, depending on the population surveyed, the methods of case ascertainment, and particularly the definition of PD. A reasonable approximation of incidence, based on studies in the United States, is 20 per 100,000 per year, with a prevalence of at least 100 per 100,000.

ETIOLOGY AND PATHOGENESIS

The pathologic hallmarks of PD are degeneration of the dopaminergic neurons of the substantia nigra and the presence of eosinophilic, cytoplasmic inclusions known as Lewy bodies. What incites the death of nigral neurons is not clear: current hypotheses implicate varying combinations of genetic susceptibility, exogenous or endogenous toxicity, and aging. One of the most important breakthroughs came from identifying MPTP, a meperidine-like drug, as the cause of a small epidemic of parkinsonism in intravenous drug abusers. MPTP is selectively toxic to nigral neurons, producing not only a clinical picture of PD, but also a pathologic picture, and serves as an animal model. Its main effect appears to be on the respiratory chain in mitochondria, particularly complex I, which has been demonstrated to be low in patients with PD. Although it is still not clear what starts the cascade of events leading to the death of nigral neurons, key elements are likely to include energy depletion and oxygen toxicity with the formation of free radicals.

CLINICAL FINDINGS

PD is a clinical diagnosis dependent on recognizing the characteristic features. The sine qua non is bradykinesia—slowness of movements—with either a rest tremor or cogwheel rigidity. Most patients have all three diagnostic signs, but approximately 30% do not have tremor. The signs typically affect one side at presentation (hemiparkinsonism) unrelated to dominant handedness, before eventually becoming bilateral within several years. Additional symptoms and signs encountered early in PD include micrographia; impaired dexterity, especially for rapid repetitive movements such as shampooing or brushing teeth; slowness when arising from a deep chair, the toilet, or car; trouble turning in bed; slight drooling; a soft, monotone voice; diminished facial

expression (hypomimia) and blink rate; and diminished arm swing while walking or dragging a foot. In the middle to latter stages of the disease, other motor problems emerge, including impairment of postural righting reflexes, leading to loss of balance with falls, and bradykinesia gives way to akinesia, with difficulty initiating and maintaining movements.

In addition to the motor findings of PD, there are a number of nonmotor symptoms and signs as well, reflecting the diverse functions of the basal ganglia as reviewed in Chapter 14. PD sometimes begins with pain leading to the diagnosis of arthritis or fibromyalgia. Autonomic problems are common, both from the disease itself and from its treatment. These include constipation, impotence, impaired sexual arousal in women, orthostatic hypotension, impaired thermoregulation—sweating or feeling warm or cold in contrast to the temperature—and urinary bladder instability.

Depression is so common in PD that it is safe to assume that all patients with PD are depressed until proven otherwise. Anxiety, embarrassment, and panic attacks are also encountered. With advancing PD (after 10 years), dementia often appears, but it is important to appreciate that *most* patients with PD *do not develop dementia* and it is not an inevitable consequence of the disease. Therefore, treatable causes need to be ruled out, especially pseudodementia due to depression, and the effects of medications, particularly those with anticholinergic activity.

In most cases, the diagnosis of PD is straightforward, but there are some pitfalls to be aware of. PD may be confused with essential tremor as discussed in Chapter 11. When PD presents in a person younger than age 45, which happens in 5% of cases, the diagnosis is often not considered. Likewise, PD tends to be overdiagnosed in the very elderly because it often merges with features of "normal" aging. Dementing illness, like Alzheimer's, are often accompanied by parkinsonian features. The motor signs, rather than dementia, may prompt medical attention, since the former is often unrecognized because of its insidious onset or mistakenly attributed to normal aging by family members. Parkinsonism may also be drug-induced.

The most common pitfall is failure to recognize *mimickers* of PD (Table 434.1). Up to 25% of diagnoses of PD during life have been shown to be wrong at autopsy; the most common correct diagnoses are parkinsonian syndromes: related degenerative diseases with more extensive clinical and pathologic involvement. The three most reliable clinical features distinguishing PD from related disorders include classic rest tremor, unilateral or asymmetric onset, and a beneficial, sustained response to levodopa. Clues that suggest a cause of parkinsonism other than idiopathic PD include failure to respond to levodopa; symmetric onset; early dementia; early dysphagia; early falls; early and prominent dysautonomia; impaired vertical eye movements; cerebellar, pyramidal, or lower motor neuron signs; and rapid progression, among others. It is not uncommon for features of a parkinsonian syndrome to emerge only after several years; therefore, the diagnosis of PD should be scrutinized at each visit.

In this chapter, the most common parkinsonian syndromes are discussed briefly. All are characterized by a limited or absent response to levodopa and a more rapid course than PD. *Progressive supranuclear palsy* is further distinguished from PD by early falls, vertical ophthalmoparesis, including down gaze, greater

TABLE 434.1.	**DIFFERENTIAL DIAGNOSIS OR PARKINSONISM**

Toxins

Manganese
Carbon monoxide
Carbon disulfide
Cyanide
MPTP

Multisystem Degenerations

Progressive supranuclear palsy
Multi-system atrophy
    Shy–Drager syndrome
    Olivopontocerebellar atrophy
    Striatonigral degeneration
Corticobasal degeneration
Amyotrophic lateral sclerosis–parkinsonism–dementia complex
    of Guam

Heredofamilial Diseases

Wilson's disease
Juvenile Huntington's disease
Hallervorden–Spatz disease
Familial frontotemporal dementia and parkinsonism on chromosome 17

Calcification of the Basal Ganglia

Idiopathic
Hypoparathyroidism
Familial (Fahr's disease)

Trauma

Dementia pugilistica

Drug-Induced

Neuroleptic agents
Metoclopramide (Reglan)
Methyldopa (Aldomet)
Reserpine

Primary Dementing Illness

Alzheimer's disease
Creutzfeldt–Jakob
Lewy body dementia

Multi-Infarct State

Postencephalitic State

Other

Stiff-man syndrome
Normal pressure hydrocephalus

axial (neck and trunk) than appendicular rigidity, and early dysphagia. *Multisystem atrophy*, comes in three overlapping forms, all of which include at least two of the following: pandysautonomia, parkinsonism, cerebellar, or pyramidal signs. Today, the umbrella term multisystem atrophy is preferred, but older names still survive. When parkinsonism dominates, it is referred to as *striatonigral degeneration*; when combined with dysautonomia, it is the *Shy–Drager syndrome*; and *olivopontocerebellar degeneration* is the moniker used when cerebellar and pyramidal signs are dominant.

Corticobasal degeneration is recognized by the onset of unilateral dystonia or a "useless" (alien) limb, combined with parietal signs, parkinsonian features, and myoclonus. *Lewy body dementia* can be considered an overlap between PD and Alzheimer's disease with the more-or-less simultaneous onset of dementia and symmetric parkinsonism, with early hallucinations and delusions. This can be difficult to distinguish from *Alzheimer's disease*, which is often accompanied by parkinsonian features.

■ MANAGEMENT

A full discussion of the complexities of treating PD is beyond the scope of this chapter, but some general guidelines are presented. The pharmacologic treatment of PD follows directly from the pathologic finding of dopamine depletion. Almost all the current therapies are directed at either directly or indirectly increasing dopamine in the striatum.

Before commencing therapy, patients need extensive education about the disease and reassurance that the prognosis is likely to be better than they have imagined. Today, with treatment, most people with PD can have a normal life expectancy and, with some limitation, generally lead a fairly good lifestyle. Some people with PD do have a poor prognosis, but this tends to be the exception rather than the rule. Patients should also be counseled that the goal of treatment is not to alleviate all the symptoms and signs of PD and restore them to a normal level of functioning, but instead to improve the symptoms and allow them to function at an acceptable level.

The initial step in pharmacologic management is to decide whether symptomatic treatment is necessary; this is determined by the level of activities of daily living (ADLs). If little or no compromise exists, for instance, when PD begins with the nondominant hand, there are three possibilities. The first is to withhold treatment and simply follow along until there is compromise in functioning. The second option for the minimally symptomatic patient, is to consider selegiline, a monoamine oxidase-β inhibitor, for its potential, although controversial, neuroprotective effect. Although selegiline has been shown to delay the time before treatment with levodopa is required, it is no longer clear whether this effect is due to an asymptomatic protective effect on the death of nigral neurons, rather than to its ability to improve the symptoms of PD itself. Because selegiline is very safe, some patients may want to use it despite general skepticism today about its role as a neuroprotective agent. The third option is to refer the patient to a center specializing in PD, since most centers are conducting trials of symptomatic and neuroprotective therapies for patients with early PD.

For the patient who is compromised by the symptoms of PD, the next decision is whether to use levodopa, the mainstay of treatment for PD. However, because of its eventual emergence of treatment-related fluctuations and other problems, the general trend today is to withhold levodopa until significant compromise of the activities of daily living exists. Until that point, there are three treatment options. The first is an anticholinergic, such as trihexyphenidyl (Artane) or benztropine (Cogentin). These agents may be slightly more effective for tremor but do help other features of PD as well. Side effects include dry mouth, constipation, blurred vision, urinary retention, and impaired concentration and memory. Because such side effects increase with age, these agents are generally reserved for patients with tremor-predominant PD who are younger than age 65.

Another option is the antiviral agent, amantadine. Given its anticholinergic side effects, it should also be used cautiously in elderly patients. Amantadine may also cause livedo reticularis, which is not a contraindication to continuing therapy. Recent evidence shows that amantadine may also be helpful for reducing dopa-induced dyskinesias and, as such, there is growing, although cautious, enthusiasm for its use as an adjunct in advanced PD.

The general trend today for the mildly symptomatic patient is to begin treatment with a dopamine agonist. These include bromocriptine and pergolide, as well as the newer, nonergot agents, pramipexole and ropinerole. Although their symptomatic effect is somewhat less than levodopa, they have the potential advantage of delaying the use of levodopa. The more traditional and still important role for agonists, is as an adjunct to levodopa in the middle to later stages of PD.

All patients with PD eventually require treatment with levodopa. This is combined with a decarboxylase inhibitor such as carbidopa to increases absorption into the brain and reduce nausea. Since at least 75 mg per day of carbidopa is required to inhibit dopa-decarboxylase, the 25/100 preparation is usually preferred. The first number refers to the milligrams of carbidopa and the second to the milligrams of levodopa. This is started at a low dose of ½ or 1 tablet per day and escalated gradually using the clinical response as a guide. Most patients improve with 300 mg of levodopa per day. The dose is increased gradually to keep the patient functioning at an acceptable level. The usual approach today is to keep the dosage of levodopa at a modest level, between 600 and 1,000 mg per day, with the early introduction of a dopamine agonist. An alternative therapy to enhance the effectiveness of levodopa and specifically to increase its duration of action, is tolcapone, a catechol *O*-methyltransferase inhibitor.

During the first 5 years of therapy, most patients with PD experience only mild compromise in their activities of daily living. Thereafter, management becomes more difficult, although there is tremendous variability from patient to patient. With time, the effectiveness of levodopa wanes, but virtually never completely wears off. Some of the most problematic features that emerge with advanced disease do not respond to levodopa, such as impaired postural righting reflexes, falls, akinesia, and dysphagia. Furthermore, the initial smooth response to levodopa begins to be punctuated by motor fluctuations that are initially predictable, such as the reappearance of parkinsonian signs before the next dose, known as end-of-dose wearing off. With time, however, predictable motor fluctuations become admixed with or give way to unpredictable fluctuations (on-off effect) with the appearance of unwanted involuntary movements, known as *dyskinesias*. At this point, the management of PD should be overseen by a specialist.

In addition to the motor complications and response fluctuations that complicate advanced PD, many patients also experience psychological complications. In addition to dementia, as previously mentioned, this also includes acute confusion, hallucinations, and delusions. These can often be managed with a reduction or discontinuation of antiparkinsonian medications, and when that is ineffective, use of one of the new atypical antipsychotic agents, such as clozapine. Traditional antipsychotic agents should be avoided because of their dopamine-blocking activity with the potential to worsen parkinsonism.

SURGICAL THERAPY

With the advent of levodopa in the 1960s, surgical treatment for PD largely fell out of favor. Yet, it is now experiencing a renaissance as a result of drug-resistant treatment complications seen with advanced disease, a better understanding of the pathophysiology of PD, and refinements in surgical and radiographic techniques. For the small percentage of patients with a disabling, medically refractory tremor, options include either thalamotomy or deep brain stimulation of the motor thalamus. For other features of advanced disease, particularly motor fluctuations and dyskinesias, options include either lesioning or deep brain stimulation of the internal segment of the globus pallidus or subthalamic nucleus. Implantation of fetal nigral tissue has demonstrated promising results but is still considered experimental.

BIBLIOGRAPHY

Koller WC, Pahwa R, Lyons KE, et al. Surgical treatment of Parkinson's disease. *J Neurol Sci* 1999;167:1–10.

Lang AE, Lozano AM. Parkinson's disease (Parts 1 and 2). *N Engl J Med* 1998;339:1044–1053;1130–1143.

LeWitt P, Oertel W. *Parkinson's disease: the treatment options*. Martin Dunits, 1999.

Mendis T, Suchowersky O, Lang A, et al. Management of Parkinson's disease: a review of current and new therapies. *Can J Neurol Sci* 1999; 26:89–103.

Montastruc JL, Rascol O, Senard JM. Treatment of Parkinson's disease should begin with a dopamine agonist. *Mov Disord* 1999;14:725–730.

Parkinson Study Group. Low-dose clozapine for the treatment of drug-induced psychosis in Parkinson's disease. *N Engl J Med* 1999;340: 757–763.

Weiner WJ. The initial treatment of parkinson's disease should begin with levodopa. *Mov Disord* 1999;14:716–724.

Kelley's Textbook of Internal Medicine, fourth edition. Edited by H. David Humes. Lippincott Williams & Wilkins, Philadelphia © 2000.

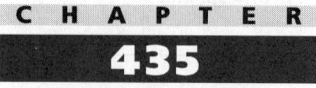

C H A P T E R

435

CHRONIC DEMENTING CONDITIONS

BRUCE L. MILLER

Dementia is an acquired persistent impairment of intellectual function with compromise in at least three of the following mental spheres: language, memory, visuospatial skills, personality, and cognition. Dementia is classified as primary degenerative or nondegenerative in type. Most primary dementias result from Alzheimer's disease (AD), frontotemporal dementia (FTD) and related disorders, or parkinsonian dementia. Nondegenerative dementias are a group of etiologically diverse disorders resulting from vascular, infectious, toxic, metabolic, tumorous, or traumatic causes. Multi-infarct dementia (MID) is the most common of the nondegenerative dementias.

The incidence of dementia is determined by many factors, including age and socioeconomic status. AD, parkinsonian dementia, and MID are most prevalent in the very old, whereas FTD arises in those between the ages of 50 and 65 years. AD accounts for 50% of all dementias, whereas 20% are MID or mixed MID and AD. FTD accounts for about 12% of dementias in presenile populations, whereas at least 10% of all senile cases are parkinsonian in type.

PRIMARY DEGENERATIVE DEMENTIAS

ALZHEIMER'S DISEASE

AD is found in 6% of people older than 65 and in 15% to 20% of those older than 80 years of age. A variety of risk factors predispose a person to AD (Table 435.1). Defects in chromosome 14 or mutations in the amyloid precursor protein on chromosome 21 are seen with early-onset AD. Subtypes of α_2-macroglobulin also predispose to AD. The E4 variant of apolipoprotein E is associated with a higher prevalence of AD in both early- and late-onset cases.

AD is slowly progressive; from onset to death, it takes 7 to 10 years. Early symptoms include memory loss and visuospatial and word-finding deficits. In the middle stages, memory problems become severe, visuospatial skills and language comprehension deteriorate, and delusions and misperceptions are common. Motor, sensory, and primary visual functions are preserved until the end stages of AD, when patients become mute, rigid, and bedridden. Diagnostic accuracy for AD has steadily improved, reaching approximately 90% in most centers. To maximize diagnostic accuracy, a good history accompanied by a mental status evaluation, laboratory studies, and a computed tomography (CT) or magnetic resonance imaging (MRI) scan are needed (Table 435.2). Functional imaging techniques show focal temporoparietal deficits in perfusion or metabolism.

Pathologic changes in AD include amyloid plaques, neurofibrillary tangles, and neuronal and synaptic loss, which is greatest in the hippocampus, entorhinal cortex, and temporoparietal neocortex. Mild to moderate losses of many neurotransmitters are found. Cholinergic cells in basal forebrain are depleted by 50% to 90%; this cholinergic deficit contributes to the amnesia in AD. Boosting brain acetylcholine with anticholinesterases improves symptoms in some patients. However, this does not reverse progression, and anticholinesterases have toxicities. Vitamin E in a 2,000-IU dosage may slow progression of AD.

FRONTOTEMPORAL DEMENTIA

The other major cortical dementia is FTD. Typically, time from onset to death is 7 to 10 years. A strong family history suggesting

---

TABLE 435.1.	**PRIMARY DEGENERATIVE DEMENTIAS**

Cortical
Alzheimer's disease
  Early onset with:
    Amyloid precursor protein mutations (chromosome 21)
    Presenilin 1 and 2 mutations (chromosome 14 and 1)
    Apolipoprotein-ϵ4 homozygosity
    α_2-macroglobulin mutations
  Late onset with:
    Apolipoprotein ϵ4 homozygosity or heterozygosity
Frontotemporal dementia
Tau mutations found in >20 families
  Variants:
    Frontotemporal dementia with motor neuron disease
    Progressive aphasia
    Focal right frontotemporal dementia

Parkinsonian
Diffuse Lewy body dementia
Huntington's disease
Progressive supranuclear palsy
Spatz disease
Idiopathic basal ganglia calcification
Corticobasal degeneration
Azorean disease

Parkinsonian Syndromes Due to Known Abnormalities
Wilson's disease (ceruloplasmim deficiency with excessive copper deposition)
Non-Wilsonian hepatolenticular degeneration (due to liver failure)
Basal ganglia calcification (hyperparathyroidism, hypoparathyroidism, or hypothyroidism)
Vascular (multiple small infarcts of basal ganglia)
Post-traumatic (dementia pugilistica)
Postanoxic (particularly cyanide and carbon monoxide)
Heavy metals (manganese, mercury)
Mitochondrial disorders
Adult-onset Niemann–Pick or Gaucher's disease
Postencephalitic Parkinson's disease
Prion disorders

FTD occurs in 40% of patients, and in some families FTD is associated with motor neuron disease (Table 435.1). Recent work has shown that a series of mutations in the genes coding for the neuronal protein τ, are associated with familial forms of this disorder. An amyotrophic lateral sclerosis–Parkinsonian dementia syndrome is found on the island of Guam for which an environmental cause has been hypothesized (Chapter 437). The clinical and imaging features of FTD are distinct from those of AD, and FTD should be recognized antemortem.

The first FTD symptoms are social withdrawal, behavioral disinhibition, weight gain, and compulsions. Speech output decreases and deficits occur in judgment and insight, whereas visuospatial skills are spared. Focal presentations of FTD occur; patients with left-sided degeneration have progressive aphasia, whereas right-sided degeneration leads to alterations in social skills. MRI shows frontal and anterior temporal atrophy. Functional studies invariably demonstrate focal frontal or temporal deficits. Pathologic study shows neuronal loss and gliosis, great-

---

TABLE 435.2.   ROUTINE EVALUATION OF DEMENTIA

Clinical history, exploring
Progression (rapidity of onset)
Family history
Medications, illicit drugs
Systemic illness
Psychiatric symptoms
Psychosocial issues
Bedside evaluation
Medical examination
Neurologic evaluation
Mental status testing (consider formal neuropsychological testing)
Laboratory tests
Complete blood count
Electrolytes, renal and liver function
Thyroid function
Vitamin B$_{12}$
Computed tomography or magnetic resonance imaging
Optional tests (valuable in selected patients)
Lumbar puncture
Urinalysis for heavy metals or toxicology
Urinalysis for arylsulfatase (metachromatic leukodystrophy)
Syphilis test
Extensive search for systemic illness
Single photon emission computed tomography or position emission tomography
Genetic testing
Other tests suggested by history or examination

---

est in the frontal and anterior temporal regions. In 20% of FTD patients, cellular inclusions, so-called Pick bodies, are found. In some patients, these inclusions consist of abnormal accumulations of τ. A severe presynaptic and postsynaptic deficit in brain serotonin occurs, which may cause the clinical findings of weight gain and compulsions. In some patients, treatment with serotonin-boosting antidepressants alleviates these symptoms.

PARKINSONIAN DEMENTIAS

DIFFUSE LEWY BODY DEMENTIA

Some elderly present with combinations of parkinsonism and dementia. In some, this is a variant of AD, whereas in others, this is a distinctive parkinsonian–dementia syndrome. Some researchers have coined the term "diffuse Lewy body dementia" (DLBD) to describe these patients. With DLBD, the acute onset of delirium with visual hallucinations is a common mode of presentation, and dopamine agonists or anticholinergics can precipitate or exacerbate DLBD. Often, autopsy shows plaques, but few neurofibrillary tangles. Lewy bodies are found throughout the cortex. The substantia nigra loses dopaminergic cells, and basal forebrain cholinergic cells are similarly depleted. Treatment is difficult because dopamine agonists can exacerbate hallucinations. However, recent work suggests that anticholinesterases can ameliorate the psychiatric symptoms associated with this disorder.

HUNTINGTON'S DISEASE

Patients with this autosomal dominantly inherited disease manifest dementia, chorea, and psychiatric symptoms (Chapter 418).

PROGRESSIVE SUPRANUCLEAR PALSY

Progressive supranuclear palsy is an idiopathic disorder characterized by frequent falling, axial rigidity, supranuclear gaze palsy, dysphagia, and frontal deficits. The pathologic process is localized to the midbrain, where gliosis and neurofibrillary tangles occur. Like the frontotemporal dementias, the pathology of this disorder has been increasingly linked to τ.

CORTICOBASAL DEGENERATION

This disorder is associated with a combination of focal parietal and focal basal ganglia deficits. Unlike the other degenerative dementias, focal motor and sensory deficits are common, even early in the course of the illness. Alien hand, severe apraxia, and visuoconstructive deficits are common. Focal dystonias emerge, as does generalized parkinsonism. The pathology overlaps with what is seen in frontotemporal dementia, and marked gliosis, abnormal neuronal inclusions, and accumulations of τ are seen.

NONDEGENERATIVE DEMENTIAS

MULTI-INFARCT DEMENTIA

MID is an etiologically and anatomically diverse group of disorders caused by brain infarction. Hypertension, heart disease, family history, hypercholesterolemia, cocaine abuse, and smoking are risk factors. Carotid and cardiac emboli, arterial or venous thrombosis, and vasculitis cause MID. Patients with multiple cortical embolic infarcts have an abrupt or stepwise deterioration; focal neurologic symptoms and signs are present. Mental slowing, pseudobulbar affect and dysphagia, shuffling gait, urinary incontinence, and bilateral motor abnormalities are hallmark findings of MID. In patients with subcortical white matter or lacunar infarctions, a progressive deterioration in cognition without focal deficits can occur. Infarcts on CT or MRI are necessary for a diagnosis of MID. Typically, patients show at least 100 mL^3 of infarcted tissue, although "critical infarcts" in a single location like the left angular gyrus are more likely to produce a dementia syndrome than are similarly sized strokes in other brain locations. Many patients diagnosed with MID have AD or a mixture of AD and MID at autopsy. With diagnosis, the stroke mechanism must be determined to prevent further injury. Treatment with aspirin or ticlopidine can preserve function.

NORMAL-PRESSURE HYDROCEPHALUS

Normal-pressure hydrocephalus causes the triad of memory loss, gait disturbance, and urinary incontinence. Apathetic frontal syndromes are common. Prior subarachnoid hemorrhage or meningitis predispose to normal-pressure hydrocephalus by altering cerebrospinal fluid absorption; yet most cases are idiopathic. The pathophysiology of normal-pressure hydrocephalus is poorly understood. MRI shows periventricular edema and ventricular enlargement. Some diagnosed with normal-pressure hydrocephalus have MID or AD, and even when patients are well selected for surgery, many do not respond.

METABOLIC/TOXIC CAUSES

Anemia, electrolyte abnormalities, hypothyroidism, vitamin B_{12} deficiency, and medications should be considered potential causes for dementia. Adult-onset variants of metachromatic leukodystrophy should be considered in dementia patients with white matter lesions. Defects in mitochondrial metabolism lead to a group of disorders, *mitochondrial encephalopathies,* in which muscle dysfunction, dementia, myoclonic epilepsy, or parkinsonism occurs. Two variants are MELAS (mitochondrial encephalopathy, lactic acidosis, and stroke) and MERFF (myoclonic epilepsy, ophthalmoplegia, and myopathy [ragged red fibers]).

INFECTIONS/PRION DISEASES

The most common infectious cause of dementia is the AIDS (Chapter 344). Neurosyphilis, now rare, causes dementia with cerebrospinal fluid pleocytosis, or Argyll–Robertson pupils. Dementia is rare with infectious meningitides but does occur with Lyme disease or fungal meningitis. In patients with dementia, diarrhea, or arthritis, Whipple's disease should be considered. It is caused by infection with periodic acid-Schiff–positive organisms and is responsive to antibiotics. Jakob–Creutzfeldt disease, kuru, and Gerstmann–Straussler–Scheinker syndrome are diverse disorders with genetic or infectious transmission modes. Like the animal disease scrapie, infections/prion diseases are caused by the accumulation of prion proteins in the brain (Chapter 446). Jakob–Creutzfeldt disease causes a rapidly progressive dementia, extrapyramidal findings, and myoclonus, although some cases are slowly progressive.

TRAUMA

Multifocal deficits characterize trauma. Frontal and temporal regions are particularly vulnerable and delayed normal-pressure hydrocephalus or subdural hematoma can follow head injury.

TUMOR

Tumors can lead to symptoms suggestive of dementia, which is why an imaging test such as CT or MRI should be performed in the setting of dementia.

BIBLIOGRAPHY

Blessed G, Tomlinson BE, Roth M. The association between quantitative measures of dementia and of senile change in the cerebral grey matter of elderly subjects. *Br J Psychiatr* 1968;114:797–811.
Brun A. Frontal lobe degeneration of non-Alzheimer type: I. neuropathology. *Arch Gerontol Geriatr* 1987;6:193–208.
Cummings JL, Benson DF. *Dementia: a clinical approach.* Boston: Butterworth, 1992.
Hachinski VC, Lassen NA, Marshall J. Multi-infarct dementia: a cause of mental deterioration in the elderly. *Lancet* 1974;2:207–210.
Hong M, Zhukareva V, Vogelsberg-Ragaglia V, et al. Mutation-specific functional impairments in distinct tau isoforms of hereditary FTDP-17. *Science* 1998;282(5395):1914–1917.
Kaufer D, Cummings J. Neuropsychiatric aspects of Alzheimer's disease: The cholinergic hypothesis revisited. *Neurology* 1996;47:871–875.
Mesulam MM. Slowly progressive aphasia without generalized dementia. *Ann Neurol* 1982;11:592–598.
Perry RH, Irving D, Blessed G, et al. Senile dementia of Lewy body type. A clinically and neuropathologically distinct form of Lewy body dementia in the elderly. *J Neurol* Sci 1990;95:119–139.
Schellenberg GD. Genetic dissection of Alzheimer disease: a heterogeneous disorder. *Proc Nat Acad Sci* 1995;92(19):8552–8559.

Kelley's Textbook of Internal Medicine, fourth edition. Edited by H. David Humes. Lippincott Williams & Wilkins, Philadelphia © 2000.

C H A P T E R
436

CEREBELLAR DEGENERATION

GING-YUEK ROBIN HSIUNG
OKSANA SUCHOWERSKY

ANATOMY AND PHYSIOLOGY

The cerebellum and its connections are involved in the maintenance of muscle tone, equilibrium, and coordination of voluntary movement. This is accomplished by receiving inputs from the spinal cord, brain-stem nuclei, and motor cortex and sending efferents back to these structures.

Structurally, the cerebellum is composed of cortex, white matter, and deep nuclei. The cerebellar cortex consists of three layers: molecular, Purkinje, and granular. All afferent fibers, which synapse on one or more of these layers, are of two main types: (1) mossy fibers, originating in the spinocerebellar tracts and brain-stem nuclei and projecting to the granule cell layer, and (2) climbing fibers, originating in the inferior olivary nucleus and projecting to Purkinje's cells. Dopaminergic and serotonergic fibers also arise in brain-stem nuclei and project to Purkinje's and granule cells. Efferents from the cerebellar cortex consist entirely of axons of Purkinje's cells projecting to the deep cerebellar nuclei—the dentate, fastigial, globose, and emboliform (interposed)—and project through the superior cerebellar peduncle to the contralateral motor cortex by way of the thalamus. The fastigial nucleus sends fibers to the vestibular nuclei, other brain-stem nuclei, and spinal cord neurons. All efferent Purkinje fibers are inhibitory, using γ-aminobutyric acid, whereas fibers projecting from the deep nuclei are excitatory. Cortical interneurons consisting of basket cells, stellate cells, and Golgi cells modulate the activity of afferent fibers and Purkinje's cells.

Anatomically, the cerebellum is divided by fissures into anterior, posterior, and flocculonodular lobes. However, a functional division dividing the cerebellum longitudinally is much more useful clinically:

1. The flocculonodular lobe is phylogenetically the oldest structure and is involved in control of equilibrium. It receives afferent impulses from the vestibular nuclei and projects primarily back to the vestibular system.
2. The midline zone, composed of the vermis, is located medially in the cerebellum and projects to the fastigial nuclei. It is involved in control of gait; lesions result in poor balance and wide-based, staggering gait.
3. The intermediate zone, composed of the paravermal area and projecting to the interposed nuclei, controls limb postures and tone.
4. The lateral zone, composed of the cerebellar hemispheres, projects to the dentate nuclei. Dysfunction results in ipsilateral limb incoordination with dysmetria, dysdiadochokinesis, intention tremor, dysarthria, and eye movement abnormalities.

CLINICAL FINDINGS

Signs of cerebellar disease include wide-based gait ataxia, dysarthria, dysphagia, intention tremor, dysmetria, past-pointing, dysdiadochokinesis, and eye movement abnormalities such as nystagmus and ocular dysmetria. The particular combination of signs depends on extent and location of dysfunction (e.g., lesions involving the midline structures result in a disorder of gait, whereas those in the hemisphere result in limb ataxia). It is also important to differentiate ataxia due to noncerebellar disorders, such as sensory ataxia of peripheral neuropathy (Chapter 429) and apraxic gait ataxia of normal-pressure hydrocephalus. A large number of medical conditions can result in cerebellar degeneration (Table 436.1). Only primary genetic or idiopathic forms that result in slowly progressive ataxia are discussed in this chapter. Classification of cerebellar degenerations had been confusing in the past and was predominantly based on pathologic or phenotypic presentations. With advances in molecular research, the genetic classification is becoming clearer. However, it is still convenient to approach the problem with classification by the age of onset (Table 436.2).

PREDOMINANTLY CHILDHOOD ONSET

Friedreich's ataxia is the most common cause of progressive ataxia in childhood with autosomal recessive inheritance. The classic syndrome manifests in prepubertal children with gait ataxia, dysarthria, lower limb areflexia, and proprioceptive sensory loss. Nystagmus and extensor plantar responses are also seen. In later stages, the patient cannot walk and has gross limb ataxia and weakness, head tremor, incomprehensible speech, and ataxic respiration. Cognitive abilities are preserved, but emotional lability may be present. Cardiomyopathy is seen in at least 50% of cases, resulting in arrhythmia or congestive failure. Ten percent have insulin-dependent diabetes. Death usually occurs in the third or

TABLE 436.1.	SOME CAUSES OF SECONDARY CEREBELLAR DEGENERATION

Endocrine/metabolic
  Hypothyroidism
  Hyperparathyroidism
  Wilson's disease
Infection
  Lyme disease
  Legionella
  Mycoplasma
  Prion diseases
  Viral and postinfectious cerebellitis
Paraneoplastic syndrome
Multiple sclerosis
Superficial siderosis
Stroke
Vitamin deficiency (i.e., B_{12}, B_1, folate, zinc)
Toxins/drugs
  Alcohol
  Lithium
  Bismuth subsalicylate
  Heavy metals (e.g., mercury, thallium)
  Antiepileptic agents (e.g., phenytoin)
  Chemotherapy agents (e.g., methotrexate, cytarobine [Ara-C], 5-fluorouricel [5-FU])
  Cyclosporine
  Toluene

fourth decades of life. With genetic testing now available, adult-onset Friedreich's ataxia is not uncommon. These atypical adult cases are usually less severe, may have retained reflexes or hyperreflexia, and progress more slowly. Pathologically, degeneration is seen in the posterior columns, corticospinal tracts, spinocerebellar tracts, peripheral nerves and nuclei of cranial nerves VII, X, XII, and myocardial muscle fibers. The genetic defect is an expanded GAA trinucleotide repeat in the first intron of the X25 gene on chromosome 9. The protein product, named *frataxin,* is believed to be a mitochondrial protein, and its deletion may lead to accumulation of iron in the mitochondria, compromising mitochondrial function.

Abetalipoproteinemia (also known as Bassen–Kornzweig syndrome) is a disorder of lipid metabolism transmitted by autosomal recessive inheritance. Apolipoprotein B, which is essential for synthesis and transport of low-density lipoproteins and very-low-density lipoproteins, is absent from the serum resulting in malabsorption of fat-soluble vitamins. Steatorrhea is present early in life, and cerebellar ataxia develops in the first or second decade of life with loss of tendon reflexes. Proprioceptive loss in hands and feet appear later, whereas pinprick and temperature are mildly reduced. The sensory changes are a result of demyelination in the posterior columns and the peripheral nerves. Diagnosis is made by presence of acanthocytes in the peripheral blood smear and absent serum betalipoprotein. Treatment with vitamin A and E supplementation may slow down the development of neurologic sequelae and reverse the neuropathy.

Ataxia-telangiectasia, xeroderma pigmentosum and *Cockayne syndrome* all may present as cerebellar ataxia and are all thought to result from defective DNA repair.

TABLE 436.2.	CLASSIFICATION OF PRIMARY CEREBELLAR DEGENERATION BY AGE OF ONSET

Condition	Mode of Inheritance
Predominant Childhood Onset	
Friedreich's ataxia	Autosomal recessive
Ataxia-telangiectasia	Autosomal recessive
Xeroderma pigmentosum	Autosomal recessive
Abetalipoproteinemia	Autosomal recessive
Leukodystrophies	Autosomal recessive or X-linked
Refsum's disease	Autosomal recessive
Storage diseases (i.e., GM_2 gangliosidosis, sphingomyelin)	Autosomal recessive
Inborn errors of metabolism (i.e., Hartnup disease, maple syrup urine disease, Niemann–Pick type C)	Most are autosomal recessive
Predominant Adult Onset	
ADCA I (SCA 1,2,3,4,8)	Autosomal dominant
ADCA II (SCA 5,6)	Autosomal dominant
ADCA III (SCA 7)	Autosomal dominant
Dentatrorubropallidoluysian atrophy	Autosomal dominant
Gerstmann–Straussler–Scheinker disease	Autosomal dominant
Gluten-sensitive enteropathy (celiac disease)	Sporadic (not genetic)
Mitochondrial encephalomyopathies	Mitochondrial
Multiple system atrophy	Sporadic (not genetic)

ADCA, autosomal dominant cerebellar ataxia; SCA, spinocerebellar ataxia.

PREDOMINANT ADULT-ONSET ATAXIA

Autosomal dominant cerebellar ataxias (ADCA) are a heterogeneous group of disorders described by Harding based on clinical features. Currently, at least eight genotypes of spinocerebellar ataxias (SCA) have been identified, which fit into this category. SCA 1, 2, 3, 6, and 7 are due to CAG repeat expansions within the protein coding region of the gene that encodes an expanded polyglutamine region in the disease protein. Paternal anticipation is present, resulting in disease being more severe with earlier onset when it is inherited from the father. SCA 8 has recently been identified as a CTG repeat expansion in the noncoding region of the gene.

In ADCA type 1 (SCA 1, 2, 3, 4, 8), there is progressive gait ataxia, dysphagia, dysarthria, and variable degree of ophthalmoplegia, extrapyramidal signs, dementia, optic atrophy, amyotrophy, and peripheral neuropathy. Significant overlap of symptoms is present, making it difficult to distinguish the SCAs clinically. In all the SCAs, cerebellar and brain-stem atrophy may be seen on brain imaging. Pathologically, prominent atrophy of the cerebellum and pons with loss of Purkinje's cells is found.

A variable amount of atrophy is found in the inferior olivary nucleus, brain-stem nuclei, basal ganglia, dorsal columns and pyramidal tracts of the spinal cord, and the peripheral nerves. The cerebral cortex is usually spared.

ADCA type 2 (SCA 7) is characterized by ataxia with retinal degeneration.

ADCA type 3 (SCA 5, 6) is characterized by a pure cerebellar syndrome, although some patients at a late stage may show pyramidal and peripheral signs. The genetic defect of SCA 5 is unknown. SCA 6 is due to a CAG expansion in the gene encoding a voltage-sensitive P/Q type calcium channel on chromosome 19. It is interesting that point mutations in the same gene may lead to episodic ataxia type 2 and familial hemiplegic migraine.

Up to 40% of patients with a clinical syndrome of ADCA type 1 do not have the latter mutations; type 1 probably represents other forms of SCAs yet to be identified. Other sporadic cases may be autosomal recessive cases or may represent new mutations. *Multiple-system atrophy* is a sporadic neurodegenerative disease that may manifest as a predominant olivopontocerebelllar atrophy syndrome.

No satisfactory treatment is available for any of the adult-onset cerebellar ataxias.

BIBLIOGRAPHY

Brice, A. Unstable mutations and neurodegenerative disorders. *J Neurol* 1998;245:505–510.

Dürr A, Cossee M, Agid Y, et al. Clinical and genetic abnormalities in patients with Friedreich's ataxia. *N Engl J Med* 1996;335:1169–1175.

Harding AE. Clinical features and classification of inherited ataxias. *Adv Neurol* 1993;61:1–14.

Koob MD, Moseley ML, Schut LJ, et al. An untranslated CTG expansion causes a novel from of spinocerebellar ataxia (SCA8). *Nat Genet* 1999; 21:379–384.

Thompson PD, Day BL. The anatomy and physiology of cerebellar disease. *Adv Neurol* 1993;61:15–31.

Kelley's Textbook of Internal Medicine, fourth edition. Edited by H. David Humes. Lippincott Williams & Wilkins, Philadelphia © 2000.

CHAPTER 437

AMYOTROPHIC LATERAL SCLEROSIS

ANDREA M. CORSE

Motor neuron diseases are a group of sporadic or, rarely, inherited neurodegenerative disorders characterized by progressive paralysis. *Amyotrophic lateral sclerosis* (ALS), the most common motor neuron disease, involves both upper and lower motor neuron symptoms and signs. Other motor neuron diseases include *primary lateral sclerosis* with symptoms and signs limited to upper motor neuron dysfunction and progressive *spinal muscular atrophy* (SMA), which includes strictly lower motor neuron disorders.

ALS affects primarily adults of all ages with a mean age of onset in the sixth decade. The incidence is 1 or 2 per 100,000. Roughly 35,000 persons have ALS in the United States. It is slightly more common in men with a male to female ratio of 1.5 : 1.

PRESENTATION

The clinical presentation of ALS can be very different among patients, making early diagnosis difficult. Patients can present with upper or lower motor neuron symptoms involving bulbar or limb musculature. Presenting symptoms are as varied as hoarseness, difficulty turning a key or buttoning buttons, or foot drop. Other symptoms might include dysarthria, dysphagia, atrophy in the limbs, fasciculations, cramps, or gait instability. The limb weakness is typically painless and asymmetric. Early involvement of the small muscles of the hand is frequently seen, and atrophy may be apparent before functional loss is recognized. Bulbar onset occurs about 10% of the time, more often in women than men. Rarely, ALS can present as respiratory insufficiency. Control of bladder and bowel function, as well as other autonomic activities, usually is spared, as are the extraocular movements. The presence of any sensory symptoms or signs that cannot be explained on the basis of a coexistent condition, such as unrelated neuropathy, should cast doubt on the diagnosis of ALS.

By far most ALS cases are sporadic, and no definite risk factors have been identified other than age. Age-specific incidence rises with age. Roughly 5% to 10% of ALS cases are inherited as an autosomal dominant trait, so-called familial ALS (FALS). Generally, FALS cases are clinically indistinguishable from sporadic cases.

PATHOPHYSIOLOGY

The pathogenesis of ALS is unknown. However, a mutation in the Cu/Zn superoxide dismutase 1 gene on chromosome 21 has been identified in a small percentage of FALS families. The lack of this gene defect in most FALS families indicates that there is genetic heterogeneity among FALS cases. This has led to increased enthusiasm for multifactorial theories of pathogenesis in familial and sporadic ALS related to oxidative injury and excitotoxicity. Other theories include immune-mediated pathogeneses.

The most prominent neuropathologic change is anterior horn cell loss: the remaining motor neurons appear small and pyknotic. There is degeneration of the lateral corticospinal tract and atrophy of ventral but not dorsal spinal roots. In the brain, the motor and premotor cortex are mildly atrophic, and the number of Betz cells is reduced. Lesser neuron loss also occurs more generally throughout the brain. In the brain stem, motor neuron loss occurs especially in the facial and hypoglossal nuclei. There

may be very late involvement of the oculomotor and sacral motor nuclei only in patients who have survived long-term with ventilation. Studies have also demonstrated ubiquitin-positive inclusions and proximal neurofilamentous axonal swellings in anterior horn motor neurons primarily. Motor nerves show axonal degeneration with reduced numbers of large myelinated fibers, and skeletal muscle reveals neurogenic atrophy.

HISTORY AND PHYSICAL EXAMINATION

The diagnosis is based on the history and examination, which must demonstrate progressive upper and lower motor neuron involvement in at least three body regions (bulbar, cervical, thoracic, or lumbosacral) for definite ALS or in two regions for probable ALS, according to the World Federation of Neurology criteria. Upper motor neuron signs include spasticity, hyperreflexia, and Babinski responses; lower motor neuron signs include weakness, wasting, hyporeflexia, and fasciculations.

ALS is typically a relentlessly progressive disease with a mean survival of 3 to 5 years. Shorter survival correlates with bulbar symptoms, older age, respiratory involvement, and rapid course. The rate of disease progression is, however, highly variable among patients. In an individual patient, the rate of progression tends to be fairly linear such that the course is best predicted by the rate of change over the preceding months.

The relative contribution of upper motor neuron and lower motor neuron involvement is also widely variable among patients with ALS and other motor neuron diseases. At one extreme is primary lateral sclerosis, a rare disorder in which the degenerative process is confined to the upper motor neuron and corticospinal tracts. At the other extreme is progressive SMA, in which the neurodegeneration is limited to the lower motor neurons. In contrast to ALS, both primary lateral sclerosis and progressive SMA are typified by a more chronic, insidiously progressive course, and the limbs are predominantly affected. However, distinguishing these disorders from ALS is not always possible early in their course, since ALS can present with *isolated* upper or lower motor neuron signs for up to 2 years or more. The relation between ALS and these other forms of motor neuron disease remains to be clarified.

In patients who present with bulbar symptoms alone, there is typically a combination of both upper and lower motor neuron involvement. Some patients present with strictly upper motor neuron signs in the bulbar region, a condition termed *pseudobulbar palsy*. Such symptoms include spastic dysarthria, slow and weak tongue movements, and emotional lability (pseudobulbar affect). In contrast, a presentation with strictly lower motor neuron brain-stem signs is termed *progressive bulbar palsy*, manifested clinically by slurred speech, tongue atrophy and fasciculations, and swallowing difficulties. Generally these conditions will progress to ALS within 2 years or, rarely, longer.

LABORATORY STUDIES AND DIAGNOSTIC TESTS

ALS has no specific biochemical features. The serum creatine kinase level can be elevated, although not usually more then

1,000 IU per liter. The cerebrospinal fluid is normocellular with normal or mildly elevated protein levels. A cerebrospinal fluid protein over 70 mg% increases the likelihood of myeloma or lymphoma; more than 100 mg% is virtually unheard of. Electromyographic examination reveals acute denervation potentials (fasciculations, fibrillation potentials, and positive sharp waves) together with chronic reinnervation, as shown by motor units with increased durations and reduced recruitment. Imaging of the neuroaxis is critical to rule out disorders that could mimic ALS.

DIFFERENTIAL DIAGNOSIS

The differential diagnosis can be broad at the time of the initial presentation but becomes increasingly limited as the disease progresses. Magnetic resonance imaging of the brain and spine excludes a number of disorders that could mimic motor neuron disease, that is, spinal arteriovenous malformation, syringomyelia or syringobulbia, ischemic or demyelinating disease, tumor, or spondylotic myelopathy with polyradiculopathies. The finding of a hyperactive jaw jerk on examination is particularly helpful in this regard, suggesting upper motor neuron involvement that cannot be explained by a cervical myelopathy alone.

In cases with predominantly lower motor neuron signs and equivocal upper motor neuron involvement, an acellular cerebrospinal fluid excludes polyradiculopathies due to malignancies or other meningitides. Multifocal motor neuropathy can be investigated with nerve conduction studies directed at identifying partial motor conduction block and features of multifocal demyelination and with serologic testing for antiganglioside antibodies. There are also familial forms of progressive SMA, including autosomal recessive and sex-linked diseases to consider. In addition to *SMA type I* (Werdnig–-Hoffmann disease), the infantile autosomal recessive form in which death occurs before the age of 3 years, both juvenile *SMA type II* and adult-onset *SMA type III* have been described. Some patients with progressive SMA have been found to have a deficiency of hexosaminidase A, which is also inherited as an autosomal recessive trait. A sex-linked form of adult-onset SMA with gynecomastia and reduced fertility (*Kennedy's syndrome*) is associated with abnormalities in the androgen receptor gene, with increased numbers of tandem trinucleotide repeats in the coding region of the gene.

Other diseases that can occasionally mimic a motor neuron disease–like syndrome and cause confusion include autoimmune myopathies (polymyositis, dermatomyositis, or inclusion body myopathy); autoimmune neuropathy (chronic inflammatory demyelinating polyneuropathy); myasthenia gravis; postpolio amyotrophy; endocrinologic disorders (hyperthyroidism or hyperparathyroidism, diabetic amyotrophy); heavy metal intoxications (lead or mercury); postradiation or paraneoplastic motor neuronopathies (most commonly reported with lymphoma); and rare familial spastic paraplegias.

◼ STRATEGIES FOR OPTIMAL CARE

In the absence of a cure, treatment of ALS is directed at slowing disease progression, enhancing muscle strength, and specific multimodality symptom management. Riluzole (Rilutek) is the only medication approved specifically by the Food and Drug Administration for the treatment of ALS. It is an antiglutamate agent proven to prolong survival in ALS to a marginal degree (on the order of months). It appears to be well tolerated and safe. Liver transaminase levels should be checked periodically, since a reversible chemical hepatitis has rarely been reported. A disadvantage of riluzole is its expense; however, the drug manufacturer Rhone-Poulenc Rorer in cooperation with the National Organization for Rare Diseases provides the drug at reduced cost, depending on a financial needs assessment. Gabapentin (Neurontin), originally approved as an anticonvulsant and available by prescription, is another antiglutamate agent that may slow the rate of decline in strength in ALS based on preliminary clinical trial data.

Numerous clinical trials are ongoing for potential new therapies in ALS. A list of trials is available from the Amyotrophic Lateral Sclerosis Association and the Muscular Dystrophy Association. Providing a patient with such clinical trial information gives the patient the added sense of accessibility to the ongoing efforts of clinicians and scientists involved in the search for the cause and a cure for ALS.

Recent data suggest that the over-the-counter bioenergetic supplement creatine monohydrate (5 g daily) enhances creatine phosphate levels and may improve strength to a minor degree in a number of neuromuscular disorders. Many patients combine riluzole, gabapentin, and creatine, although data on combination therapy are lacking.

Symptomatic management is predominantly directed at the dysarthria, dysphagia with sialorrhea, spasticity, and respiratory insufficiency. In patients with dysarthria, consultation with a speech consultant who has expertise in a wide range of communication devices is recommended relatively early because some devices may take months to obtain. Swallowing function can be enhanced with specific dietary recommendations and head positioning technique. Gastrostomy tube (G-tube) placement is particularly beneficial in patients in whom bulbar dysfunction is affected out of proportion to limb function. For sialorrhea, glycopyrrolate (Robinul) is a very effective drying agent without central nervous system side effects. Alternatively, a scopolamine patch may be preferred for its ease of administration. Tricyclic antidepressants can be useful in minimizing the emotional incontinence typical of pseudobulbar affect while also reducing sialorrhea, although their other side effects can be dose-limiting.

As respiratory involvement progresses, periodic discussions regarding long-term ventilatory options and advanced directives are a logical progression and are essential. Many patients appear to benefit from noninvasive respiratory assistance (e.g., nasal BiPAP [bilevel positive ariway pressure] at night) for treatment of dyspnea or as a "bridge" to mechanical ventilation. Only about 4% of patients opt for tracheostomy and invasive mechanical ventilation. Coordinated care with a pulmonologist with expertise in neuromuscular diseases can be very helpful. Finally, hospice services have played an increasing role in the care of the terminal ALS patient in recent years, in many instances providing an invaluable resource and support structure enabling a patient to stay in the comfort of his or her home when it may not have previously been possible.

BIBLIOGRAPHY

Bensimon G, Lacomblez L, Meininger V. A controlled trial of riluzole in amyotrophic lateral sclerosis. ALS/Riluzole Study Group. *N Engl J Med* 1994;330:585–591.

Lowe J. New pathological findings in amyotrophic lateral sclerosis. *J Neurol Sci* 1994;124(suppl):38–51.

Mitsumoto H, Norris FH. *Amyotrophic lateral sclerosis: a comprehensive guide to management*. New York: Demos Publications, 1994.

Rosen DR, Siddique T, Patterson D, et al. Mutations in Cu/Zn superoxide dismutase gene are associated with familial amyotrophic lateral sclerosis. *Nature* 1993;362:59–62.

World Federation of Neurology Research Group on Motor Neuron Diseases. El Escorial revisited: revised criteria for the diagnosis of amyotrophic lateral sclerosis. http://www.wfnals.org/Articles/elescorial1998.htm.

Kelley's Textbook of Internal Medicine, fourth edition. Edited by H. David Humes. Lippincott Williams & Wilkins, Philadelphia © 2000.

C H A P T E R

438

HUNTINGTON'S DISEASE

MICHAEL R. HAYDEN
BLAIR R. LEAVITT

HISTORY

George Huntington was only 8 years old when he first observed patients with Huntington's disease (HD) as he rode with his father on his professional rounds around East Hampton, Long Island, between 1885 and 1870. At age 21, he presented his paper on chorea, which appeared in the *Medical and Surgical Reporter* in Philadelphia on April 13, 1872. The name Huntington quickly gained acceptance as the eponymic designation of the disorder.

EPIDEMIOLOGY

The prevalence of HD in populations of northwestern European ancestry is approximately 1 in 10,000. There is no decrease in the reproductive fitness of people with HD. There is a 10-fold reduced prevalence rate for HD in people of Japanese, Chinese, and African black descent.

NATURAL HISTORY

The mean age at onset is about 40 years, with considerable distribution around this mean. About 5% of affected people have onset of symptoms before age 20, and 5% have onset after age 60 years. Onset of HD symptoms in the 10th decade has been recorded. The likelihood of having inherited the gene for HD in an asymptomatic person at risk decreases from 50% at birth to about 40% at age 40, 25% at 50, 15% at 60, and 2% at 70 years.

The duration of HD varies between 14 and 18 years. Patients whose onset is before age 20 years usually have a more rapidly progressive course, with mean duration around 12 years. The most common cause of death is pneumonia secondary to aspiration after difficulties with swallowing.

CLINICAL FINDINGS

The clinical diagnosis of HD depends on establishing a positive family history for the disorder and on a detailed neurologic assessment. The clinical diagnosis can be confirmed by diagnostic testing for the gene mutation causing HD. The cardinal clinical features of HD are abnormal involuntary movements associated with cognitive impairment, but disorders of voluntary movements often precede the choreiform disorder. Furthermore, affective disorders and frank psychosis may also herald the onset of HD. This broad spectrum of clinical features may result in misdiagnosis in the early stages of the illness.

SIGNS AND SYMPTOMS

Close questioning of the spouse of a patient with HD frequently reveals that the disease presents as subtle mental changes, including irritability, irascibility, impulsiveness, and depression. In the earliest phases, before frank chorea, significant alterations in voluntary movements are common. Impairment of eye movements with impairment of pursuit movements and slow saccades are common. Many people with early signs of HD are unable to keep their tongue protruded for 10 seconds without choreiform movements. Rapid alternating movements of the hands can also be impaired. Some patients also have arrhythmic speech and are unable to repeat sounds such as "la-la-la" with fluency. Tandem walking may evoke mild ataxic movements. Although signs may be minimal, an obvious disturbance of functional ability may be present. As the disease progresses, the single most common complaint is jerkiness, clumsiness, or mild uncoordination. Chorea becomes obviously apparent in most patients and progresses inexorably with eventual ceaseless writhing, jerking, and twisting. Usually, the face, trunk, and extremities are affected, although to varying degrees.

Facial features are common and present a typical appearance with pouting of the lips, together with twitching of the cheeks and irregular elevation of the eyebrows. When sitting, constant movement of the hands and legs is common. The legs are alternatively crossed and uncrossed. In contrast to other choreiform movement disorders, the chorea in HD is usually slower and more athetoid.

Signs of increased muscle tone become more frequent as the disease progresses. In a small number of patients, hypertonicity with minimal choreiform movements may predominate. Pathologically, brisk reflexes occur in at least 50% of patients in the early years. Over the next decade, however, signs of pyramidal dysfunction, including hyperreflexia, extensor plantar responses, and clonus, become more prominent. Bradykinesia with a mask-like facies and a positive glabellar reflex are also more common with longer duration. There is a progressive evolution toward a rigid state. Dystonic posturing is a common sign, usually affecting the hands, head, and trunk.

Slowness of speech occurs early. Eventually, gross disorganization of speech and finally mutism supervene. Dysphagia is a late sign and occurs in patients with predominant chorea or rigidity.

The gait is characteristic. At rest, patients stand on a broad base, and involuntary movements are contained. On walking, the patient has an increasing unsteadiness, and walking is characterized by large lateral deviations from the midline and precipitous advances. Tandem walking becomes difficult. In the terminal years of the illness, incontinence of urine and, later, feces is common.

A striking disparity exists between the features of HD in children and adults, with particular regard to motor abnormalities, rate of progression, and occurrence of epilepsy. Juvenile-onset HD, a rapidly progressive form of the disease sometimes termed the Westphal variant of HD, occurs in about 5% of patients who have a predominantly akinetic-rigid presentation with spasticity, bradykinesia, dystonia, and rapid intellectual decline often complicated by myoclonus and seizures. Chorea occurs early and usually is superseded by rigidity, which is the predominant abnormality in affected people younger than age 20 years. Intellectual deterioration with failure at school is a common presenting finding. Seizures occur in about one third of young people with HD, but with no increased frequency in adults. The earlier the time of onset, the more likely that rigidity will be the major neurologic feature.

In people older than 60 years of age, a milder disease is common, with less obvious chorea and mild intellectual dysfunction.

MENTAL DISTURBANCE

Depression in HD is common, as witnessed by the increased frequency in suicide. In the early phases, a limitation in acquiring new information is evident. With disease progression, spatial and arithmetic functions decrease and memory loss is common. Despite these focal cognitive deficits, perceptive functions remain relatively intact until late in the illness. Occasionally, a schizophreniform psychosis precedes or accompanies the neurologic features of HD. The psychosis is often characterized by paranoid features.

■ THE GENE DEFECT AND PATHOGENESIS OF HUNTINGTON'S DISEASE

The underlying genetic defect in HD is the expansion of a CAG trinucleotide repeat in the first exon of the HD gene that produces a functional protein with an expanded polyglutamine tract. The HD gene (*IT15*) comprises 67 exons and spans a genomic size of approximately 210 kb, with a predicted protein product of 348 kd. The gene product, huntingtin, is ubiquitously expressed in tissues throughout the body. The CAG repeat, located in the 5′ region of the HD gene, is highly polymorphic in the general population, ranging from 8 to 35 copies,

with most (99%) having less than 30 repeats. In contrast, patients with HD have a trinucleotide repeat size ranging from 36 to 121, with a median of 44 repeats. An inverse relation exists between the CAG repeat size and the age of onset of HD (i.e., larger repeat expansions are associated with earlier age of onset).

Molecular analysis of sporadic cases of HD revealed that new mutations for HD are not as rare as previously thought. The length of the CAG repeat is unstable during vertical transmission of the gene from parent to child. Analysis of parental DNA of people who represent new mutations has identified intermediate alleles, which are CAG alleles with repeat size greater than that usually seen in the general population (more than 29), but less than the range seen in patients with HD (less than 36). These intermediate alleles may be unstable in passage through the male germline and, in sporadic cases, expand to the full mutation associated with the clinical phenotype of HD. These findings have significant genetic implications for family members of patients with sporadic HD. Larger CAG repeat sizes exhibit greater instability, and paternal transmission of the CAG repeat allele is more likely to result in expansion rather than contraction of the CAG repeat length. The unstable nature of the CAG expansion in HD provides the molecular basis for the clinical phenomenon of anticipation. Anticipation is defined as increasing severity of disease or decreasing age of onset of disease in successive generations.

These results further support the importance of the CAG repeat in the pathogenesis of HD. Likely, the expanded stretch of polyglutamine residues within huntingtin cause a toxic "gain of function" of the mutated protein, which modulates the selective neuronal cell death seen in this disease. Recent studies have implicated the formation of neuronal intranuclear inclusions (ubiquitinated aggregates containing truncated polyglutamine fragments) in the pathogenesis of HD and other CAG trinucleotide diseases. Transgenic mice expressing a small fragment of huntingtin with a very large CAG expansion develop neuronal intranuclear inclusions. Subsequent immunohistochemical analyses have demonstrated neuronal intranuclear inclusions in postmortem material from HD patients. In vitro models of HD demonstrated that cells transfected with mutant forms of huntingtin undergo cell death and also develop aggregates of truncated huntingtin. Despite the observed correlation of aggregates with neurodegeneration, it appears that aggregates may not play a causal role in the initiation of HD, but rather may be cellular markers for the generation of toxic protein fragments containing the polyglutamine residues.

Truncated huntingtin fragments containing expanded polyglutamine repeats are known to be toxic to neurons and N-terminal htt fragments can be identified in the brains of HD patients. Because small protein fragments containing an expanded polyglutamine are both particularly neurotoxic and prone to aggregation, proteolytic cleavage of the full-length huntingtin protein and generation of a toxic truncated product may be a critical step in neuropathology of HD the other CAG trinucleotide repeat diseases.

■ PREDICTIVE TESTING

The question for people at risk for HD is whether they will manifest signs and symptoms similar to those seen and diagnosed as HD in the parent. If the affected parent has an known expanded CAG repeat in the HD range, this confirms the family history of HD. Therefore, the presence or absence of the CAG expansion in the proband determines whether or not this person has inherited the mutation and whether or not he or she will develop the signs and symptoms of HD. If the affected person in the family does not show CAG expansion in the HD gene, then the disorder in this family, while phenotypically similar, is not HD. Failure to detect a CAG expansion in the proband in this case does not mean that HD-like symptoms will not develop in the future, and the person at risk may still have a 50% chance of developing the same illness as his or her parent.

Current recommendations for predictive testing include the provision of pretest and post-test counseling, the opportunity to withdraw from testing, the need for voluntary participation, and the recognition of the particular vulnerabilities of people presenting to a predictive testing program who are found to be symptomatic.

SPECIAL INVESTIGATIONS

The hallmark neuropathologic feature of HD seen at autopsy is early and selective neuronal loss in the caudate and putamen (striatum). The medium spiny neurons of the striatum are selectively vulnerable to neurodegeneration in HD, and this selective neuronal degeneration leads to loss of caudate volume and ventricular dilation during the course of the illness. Computed tomography often reveals caudate atrophy in patients with well-established signs and symptoms, but can be normal in early disease. Positron emission tomography with fluorodeoxyglucose is often abnormal early in the course of HD, even in patients without any evidence of caudate atrophy on computed tomography.

OPTIMAL MANAGEMENT

No therapy significantly alters the natural progression of HD. Nevertheless, numerous aspects of this disorder may be improved by appropriate intervention. In the early phases of HD, many depressed patients respond to antidepressant medication. As chorea increases, antidepressants with antidopaminergic effects may be helpful. Treatment of the movement disorder is best undertaken once the chorea significantly limits functional activity. Drugs such as halperidol, tetrabenezine, or substituted benzamides such as sulpiride that act functionally to decrease dopaminergic effect can significantly reduce chorea. However, careful balancing of the risks of reduced mental activity versus decreased movements must be determined. Phenothiazines are indicated only in the presence of significant associated mental disturbance.

In the later phases of the illness, as the movements decrease as part of natural progression, it is often possible to reduce or stop medication. In severely handicapped patients, medication may actually exacerbate difficulties in swallowing and may best be discontinued.

The benzodiazepines are useful adjuncts in anxious patients. Rigidity may show mild improvement with administration of drugs such as baclofen, which moderate glutamate release. Most HD patients also benefit from physical, speech, and occupational therapy. Supportive counseling may be helpful. People at risk and the unaffected spouse often have significant problems that require specific interventions and support.

BIBLIOGRAPHY

Brinkman RR, Mezei MM, Thielmann J, et al. The likelihood of being affected with Huntington disease by a particular age, for a specific CAG size. *Am J Hum Genet* 1997;60:1202–1210.

Davies SW, Turmaine M, Cozens BA, et al. Formation of neuronal intranuclear inclusions underlies the neurological dysfunction in mice transgenic for the HD mutation. *Cell* 1997;90:537–548.

DiFiglia M, Sapp E, Chase KO, et al. Aggregation of huntingtin in neuronal intranuclear inclusions and dystrophic neurites in brain. *Science* 1997;277:1990–1993.

Goldberg YP, Kremer B, Andrew SE, et al. Molecular analysis of new mutations for Huntington's disease: intermediate alleles and sex of origin effects. *Nat Genet* 1993;5:174–179.

Goldberg YP, Nicholson DW, Rasper DM, et al. Cleavage of huntingtin by apopain, a proapoptotic cysteine protease, is modulated by the polyglutamine tract. *Nat Genet* 1996;13:442–449.

Gutekunst C-A, Levey AI, Heilman CJ, et al. Identification and localization of huntingtin in brain and human lymphoblastoid cell lines with antifusion protein antibodies. *Proc Nat Acad Sci USA* 1995;92:8710–8714.

Harper PS. *Huntington's disease.* Philadelphia: WB Saunders, 1993.

Hodgson JG, Agopyan N, Gutekunst CA, et al. A YAC mouse model for Huntington's disease wih full-length mutant huntingtin, cytoplasmic toxicity, and selective striatal neurodegeneration. *Neuron* 1999;23:181–192.

Huntington's Disease Collaborative Research Group. A novel gene containing a trinucleotide repeat that is expanded and unstable on Huntington's disease chromosomes. *Cell* 1993;72:971–983.

Kremer B, Goldberg P, Andrew SE, et al. A worldwide study of the Huntington's disease mutation. The sensitivity and specificity of measuring CAG repeats. *N Engl J Med* 1994;330:1401–1406.

Saudou F, Finkbeiner S, Devys D, et al. Huntingtin acts in the nucleus to induce apoptosis but death does not correlate with the formation of intranuclear inclusions. *Cell* 1998;95:55–66.

Kelley's Textbook of Internal Medicine, fourth edition. Edited by H. David Humes. Lippincott Williams & Wilkins, Philadelphia © 2000.

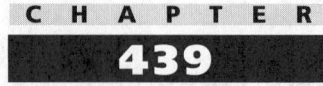

CHAPTER 439

CENTRAL NERVOUS SYSTEM POISONING

J. WILLIAM LANGSTON
IAN IRWIN
SARAH A. JEWELL

True neurotoxins are substances that are biologically elaborated (e.g., botulin and diphtheria toxin), in contrast to neurotoxicants, which are synthetic or naturally occurring substances. In this chapter, neurotoxicants that affect the central nervous system (CNS) as their primary target are discussed.

The clinical presentation after acute exposure to a neurotoxicant often differs from that induced by chronic exposure, and the effects of acute exposure are rarely restricted to the CNS. Although acute poisoning typically occurs as the result of accidental or deliberate (e.g., homicidal or suicidal) exposure to massive amounts of a substance, the abrupt onset of symptoms may also reflect chronic exposure that has finally resulted in sufficient body burden to produce sudden, sometimes life-threatening, symptoms. Chronic exposure to many CNS toxins, however, results in subtle or nonspecific neurobehavioral effects such as mood disorders.

Because neurotoxicants mimic the signs and symptoms of other diseases, they should always be considered in the differential diagnosis. When exposure to a neurotoxicant is suspected, evaluation should include a complete and detailed history and physical examination, along with a careful assessment of the work and home environment and a thorough social history. Laboratory investigations are required and may provide vital diagnostic clues. For example, radiologic evaluation may suggest heavy metal poisoning, as many metals (e.g., lead, mercury, thallium) are radiopaque and can be observed on abdominal radiography after ingestion. Poisons may also be detected in body fluids or in environmental samples. Ultimately, neuropathologic evaluation may be required to characterize the effects of a neurotoxicant. When exposure to unusual neurotoxic agents has occurred, clinical information resources may be inadequate or contradictory. In this case, animal toxicity studies can provide valuable information, although extrapolation to human illness can be difficult.

Many neurotoxicants exist in the environment, and only a few are discussed here. Identifying and eliminating exposure before irreversible damage is the essential theme in the treatment of all types of CNS toxicity.

■ METALS

Because of the importance of mining, metals are the earliest-recognized and most extensively studied of the neurotoxicants. With the advent of organic chemistry, many new metal compounds were created by combination with an organic moiety. The resulting increase in lipophilicity increased their access and hence toxicity to CNS structures.

LEAD

Lead is widely distributed in the environment. Industrial workers in smelting, storage battery, and paint factories have a great risk for exposure. Environmental sources of exposure include older building paints, ceramic cookware glazing, and solder; lead-containing fuels are increasingly restricted.

Absorption, Distribution, and Mechanism of Action

Ingestion and inhalation are the primary routes of absorption of lead. Intestinal lead absorption is influenced by particle size and chemical state and by host factors such as age (children will absorb more than five times more lead than adults) and nutrition (low dietary levels of calcium, iron, zinc, copper, and selenium and increased levels of vitamin D enhance the gastrointestinal absorption of lead). Absorbed lead is initially distributed to soft tissues. Its half-life in blood is 1 to 2 months, and it is excreted in the urine, with small amounts eliminated in sweat, hair, and breast milk. Soft-tissue lead is slowly redistributed to bone, a relatively inert compartment (half-life, 10 to 30 years) that represents more than 90% of the total body burden. Bone lead is nontoxic but is mobilized by low phosphate or high calcium intake. The toxicity derives primarily from lead's ability to bind protein sulfhydryl groups, such as those in heme synthetic enzymes.

Clinical Features and Laboratory Diagnosis

In adults, excessive exposure to lead (blood concentrations more than 50 to 100 μg per deciliter) can be accompanied by pallor, gingival lead line, and gastrointestinal, hematopoietic (anemia), renal, and neurologic symptoms, including peripheral neuropathy (e.g., wrist drop). The gravest CNS disorder is lead encephalopathy, with early signs of irritability, decreased alertness, loss of orientation, and lethargy. With severe intoxication, symptoms progress over hours or weeks to seizures, coma, and death. Signs attributable to increased intracranial pressure include papilledema, blindness, and seizures. Neuropathologic findings include cerebral edema with focal hemorrhages throughout the brain. Massive lymphocytic infiltration and microglial proliferation in cerebral and cerebellar cortices suggest a direct toxic action of lead.

Plumbism is confirmed in the laboratory by showing increased blood lead concentrations (more than 25 μg per deciliter should warn of possible toxic exposure in adults). Blood levels of heme precursors such as zinc protoporphyrin may be elevated. Urinary lead higher than 120 μg per 24 hours also indicates recent exposure. With chronic exposure, urinary levels may be within normal limits. Hair is rich in sulfhydryl groups, so the hair : blood ratios of lead are high. Large amounts of lead (and other metals) can be found in hair, making it possible to reconstruct a chronology of exposure based on a separated analysis of hair. Cerebrospinal fluid findings include an elevated protein level and pleocytosis.

Treatment

Removal from exposure is adequate treatment for mild cases of lead poisoning. Chelation therapy with CaEDTA (or a newer agent, succimer, currently approved for use in children), should be considered for all patients with significant toxicity (usually associated with blood lead levels of more than 80 μg per deciliter in adults). For acute lead encephalopathy, supportive measures such as diazepam for seizures, maintenance of fluid and electrolyte balance, and corticosteroids or osmotic agents to manage cerebral edema are used to treat the acute phase of poisoning.

MERCURY

Occupational exposure to mercury typically occurs in the manufacture of paint and fungicides or in electrical, chemical, mining, and agricultural industries. About 10 million pounds of mercury are used annually, and several disastrous large-scale poisonings have occurred. Inorganic mercury waste disposed of in Minamata Bay, Japan, was converted to methyl mercury by the action of microorganisms and thus gained access to the food chain. Hundreds of humans were poisoned after eating contaminated fish. The inadvertent consumption of seed grain containing methyl mercury as a fungicide has also produced epidemics of poisoning (10,000 cases in Iraq).

Absorption, Distribution, and Mechanism of Action

Absorption of mercury depends on the chemical and physical form; CNS toxicity results primarily from exposure to the elemental and organic forms. When ingested, elemental mercury is poorly absorbed and has low toxicity. However, when inhaled as a vapor, it is completely absorbed and rapidly crosses membranes, reaching the brain with much greater facility (mercury is a liquid at room temperature and has a substantial vapor pressure). Organic mercurials (methyl, ethyl, and aryl derivatives) are absorbed by inhalation, cutaneous absorption, and ingestion. Over 90% of ingested organic mercury compounds are absorbed, and substantial amounts cross into the CNS because of their high lipid solubility. Organic mercury has a half-life of 60 days, is excreted in the urine, and can be found in the hair and nails. Like lead, mercury binds to protein sulfhydryl groups. It also binds to amine and phosphoryl groups, interfering with cellular metabolism.

Clinical Features and Laboratory Diagnosis

Characteristic signs of chronic, low-level exposure to elemental or organic mercury include depression, irritability, forgetfulness, confusion, and tremor (erethism). Methyl mercury is particularly damaging to the CNS, causing sensory disturbances, visual deficits (including blindness), hearing loss, ataxia, movement disorders, and cognitive disturbances. Effects of methyl mercury on the fetus include mental retardation and neuromuscular deficits, and toxicity may occur even when mothers are asymptomatic.

Both organic and elemental mercury concentrates in erythrocytes because of the high lipid solubility; therefore, whole blood should be analyzed. Blood levels above 4 µg per deciliter are considered highly indicative of toxicity and correlate with clinical symptoms after methyl mercury exposure. Urinary mercury determination is less useful, but levels over 50 µg per gram creatinine are significant. Hair:blood ratios may be as high as 300.

Treatment

Elemental mercury poisoning is treated by chelation. In symptomatic patients or those with high blood levels, dimercaprol is the chelator of choice. For low-level exposure, penicillamine can be administered. Poisoning by organic mercurials responds poorly to chelation therapy, and dimercaprol, which may actually increase methyl mercury in brain tissue, is contraindicated. Experience with the Iraqi epidemic suggests that penicillamine

combined with an oral, nonabsorbable thiol resin (which interrupts enterohepatic recirculation of organomercurials) can lower blood levels.

MANGANESE

Manganese is widely distributed in nature and is present in coal and crude oil. Intoxication was first observed in miners and millers of manganese-containing ores. Manganese is used in the making of steel, machinery, electrical equipment (batteries), fertilizers, animal feeds, dyes, wood preservatives, glass, and ceramics.

Absorption, Distribution, and Mechanism of Action

After inhalation or ingestion, manganese rapidly accumulates in the liver, kidney, and brain. It is excreted in the urine, feces, and bile. Manganese is a required trace element and serves as a cofactor for many enzymes. Its role in metabolism and its putative mechanism of toxicity (oxygen radical-mediated) are derived from its ability to assume multiple oxidation states.

Clinical Features and Laboratory Diagnosis

An acute syndrome occurs after exposure to high levels of manganese. Hallucinations, memory impairment, disorientation, and emotional instability ("manganese madness") occur. Symptoms similar to those seen in Parkinson's disease may appear after weeks or years of exposure and include bradykinesia, rigidity, and tremor. Prominent dystonia may help identify manganese toxicity. Extensive changes in the basal ganglia occur, including cell loss and gliosis in the striatum, globus pallidus, and substantia nigra.

There are no specific laboratory tests for chronic manganese intoxication; blood and urine levels do not correlate reliably with exposure nor with clinical manifestations. The diagnosis rests on the history of chronic exposure and the physical examination.

Treatment

Chelating agents such as CaEDTA may have some benefit if used early. However, significant parkinsonism is not reversible. Therapy with levodopa has been reported to be of benefit in some cases.

▓ INDUSTRIAL AND AGRICULTURAL CHEMICALS

Advances in synthetic organic chemistry over the past century have brought an explosion of activity in the chemical, electronics, textile, petroleum, plastics, and agricultural industries. CNS toxicity has been described for many of the compounds used in these industries. Among these chemicals, organophosphorus compounds and organic solvents are some of the more common causes of human poisoning.

ORGANOPHOSPHORUS COMPOUNDS

Organophosphorus compounds comprise one or more hydroxylated organic moieties (e.g., phenol) connected via an ester linkage to a phosphoric acid derivative. Many of these are highly toxic and have been used as war gases and pesticides. They are also used as flame retardants, lubricants, petroleum additives, and plasticizers. Over 50,000 such compounds are known, and many have toxic effects on the CNS and peripheral nervous system. Several outbreaks of poisoning have occurred from the ingestion of these compounds, usually from contaminated food or beverages. The largest exposure, involving as many as 20,000 cases, occurred in the United States in the 1930s and resulted from the consumption of illicit alcohol ("Ginger Jake") flavored with an oil containing triorthocresolphosphate (TOCP).

Absorption, Distribution, and Mechanism of Action

Organophosphorus compounds can be absorbed after respiratory, skin, or gastrointestinal exposure. Lipophilicity and the requirement of some for oxidative activation govern their distribution and the time course of effects. As pesticides, they inactivate acetylcholinesterase. Although this biochemical attribute is responsible for the acute effects of organophosphates, it does not account for the delayed neurotoxic effects, which appear to involve the inhibition of a poorly characterized specific nervous system esterase referred to as neuropathy target esterase (NTE). NTE is found throughout the nervous system and in other tissues, including lymphocytes.

Clinical Features and Laboratory Diagnosis

Acute organophosphorus poisoning can be life-threatening. Effects include a spectrum of muscarinic (salivation, lacrimation, urination, defecation, bradycardia, hypotension), nicotinic (weakness, fatigability, paralysis), and CNS (confusion, ataxia, loss of reflexes, Cheyne—Stokes respiration, confusion, coma) findings. Acute effects can be attributed to the inhibition of acetylcholinesterase and the consequent overstimulation of cholinergic receptors.

Acute or chronic exposure may result in the appearance of a puzzling array of delayed neurologic effects not related to the inhibition of acetylcholinesterase. TOCP is perhaps the most common offender and certainly the best studied. Acute intoxication is followed 1 to 3 weeks later by the development of a myeloneuropathy resembling motor neuron disease. Initial complaints are of cramps and sharp pain in the calves and paresthesias in the hands and feet. Weakness (progressing to paralysis in the lower limbs), loss of balance, and sensory loss develop over a period of up to 2 months. Ankle and knee reflexes are typically depressed or absent. Wrist drop and weakness in the hands may occur. Neuropathologic findings include degeneration of the pyramidal tracts, usually below the cervical level, and reduced numbers of ventral horn cells, particularly in the lower regions of the spinal cord.

Measurement of red blood cell and plasma cholinesterase may be useful in diagnosing acute intoxication. Measurements of NTE activity are not routinely available. Electrophysiologic tests have been suggested as a way to monitor chronic or delayed toxicity.

Treatment

Acute toxicity should be treated by rapid removal of poison, supportive measures, and administration of atropine and the cholinesterase reactivator pralidoxime. There is no known therapy to prevent the delayed effects. The prognosis for recuperation from the central and peripheral nervous system toxicity depends on clinical severity.

ORGANIC SOLVENTS

Organic solvents are hydrocarbon formulations used in a wide variety of industrial and avocational settings (cleaning/stripping, paint and lacquer, manufacturing). Examples of solvents include turpentine, toluene, acetone, and methylene chloride. Nearly 10 million US workers are occupationally exposed to solvents. Together with home use and, in some cases, recreational abuse (e.g., glue sniffing), the potential public health consequences of solvent toxicity are enormous.

Absorption, Distribution, and Mechanism of Action

Organic solvent compounds tend to be lipophilic liquids with significant volatility, characteristics which facilitate systemic uptake via vapor inhalation and dermal absorption, followed by rapid penetration into the lipid-rich tissues of the CNS. Many solvents are metabolized by hepatic enzymes such as cytochrome P450. Excretion occurs via exhalation of the parent compound or urinary disposition of water-soluble metabolites.

The mechanism by which solvents cause CNS toxicity is not well understood. The clinical picture seen after acute exposure mimics that of ethanol intoxication and is attributed to interactions of the agent with nerve cell membranes. Substantial chronic exposures are associated with irreversible structural changes such as cortical atrophy.

Clinical Features and Laboratory Diagnosis

The hypothesis that organic solvents cause CNS toxicity via direct membrane interactions is supported by the similar clinical features after acute exposure to a variety of hydrocarbon compounds: excitation, euphoria, dysequilibrium, slurred speech, light-headedness, delayed reactions, nausea/vomiting, and severe CNS depression. The acute effects resolve as the agent is eliminated (over minutes to hours). As with excessive consumption of alcoholic beverages, tolerance and withdrawal symptoms can develop with repeated exposure.

Epidemiologic studies of workers exposed to chronic, low levels of solvents seem to indicate that subtle neuropsychiatric abnormalities (e.g., depression, memory deficits) can result. The often vague and nonspecific nature of these abnormalities, and the influence of confounding factors such as socioeconomic status and alcohol consumption, make this a challenging area of research.

In addition to assessing neurologic and cognitive function, clinicians should focus their history and physical examination on other common toxicity manifestations, including hepatic damage, contact dermatitis, history of spontaneous abortion, and cardiac arrhythmia. Some solvent compounds have unique toxicity profiles that may facilitate identification of the causative agent (e.g., peripheral neuropathy caused by hexane and aplastic anemia caused by benzene). Although direct measurement of solvents and their metabolites are sometimes used to monitor worker exposure, these tests are generally not available for diagnostic purposes. Laboratory studies should include hepatic transaminases, blood count, and urinalysis.

Treatment

The mainstay of treatment for organic solvent poisoning is avoidance of further exposure to solvents and other CNS depressants, including alcohol.

DRUGS

Many drugs have a direct effect on the CNS. In most cases, these effects are reversible and thus reflect pharmacologic rather than true toxic effects, but frank neurotoxicity has been associated with several therapeutic agents. The long-term persistence of CNS symptoms after the prolonged use of drugs (e.g., tardive dyskinesia with phenothiazine and butyrophenone neuroleptics) leads one to suspect that recognition of persistent structural or functional alterations of the CNS by other drugs is to be anticipated.

Illicit drug abuse has become a major contributor to the field of neurotoxicology. This problem is due, at least in part, to the clandestine manufacture of analogues of controlled substances. Because these new compounds are rarely tested in animals and quality controls are few, novel and unusual clinical sequelae can occur among drug abusers. Although various new compounds have appeared in the past few years with potentially toxic properties (Chapter 55), in this section just one of these compounds, MPTP, is discussed. It has proved to be one of the most selective neurotoxicants described to date.

MPTP

1-Methyl-4-phenyl-1,2,3,6-tetrahydropyridine (MPTP) was first prepared over 40 years ago in the course of pharmaceutical research. In 1982, this compound was present in batches of a synthetic opioid sold as heroin. Its subsequent intravenous use by a group of addicts in northern California produced an outbreak of neurologic illness characterized by severe and permanent parkinsonism. In retrospect, several episodes of human poisoning by MPTP have almost certainly occurred, and current trends in illicit drug abuse make future repetitions likely. In addition, MPTP and similar compounds are also used as intermediates in the preparation of pharmaceuticals and in basic neuroscience research laboratories, thus posing an occupational hazard.

Absorption, Distribution, and Mechanism of Action

Although the toxic properties of MPTP were first recognized after intravenous exposure, other human cases have been reported after intranasal use and probably after cutaneous absorption and vapor inhalation. Studies in nonhuman primates have shown that MPTP is rapidly distributed to all tissues, with substantial amounts reaching the brain.

The expression of MPTP neurotoxicity is intimately associated with factors determining its biodisposition. MPTP is biotransformed to MPP+ by the B form of monoamine oxidase (MAO), an ubiquitous enzyme particularly prevalent in brain tissue. MAO inhibitors completely prevent the development of toxicity. Once formed, MPP+ appears to be accumulated into dopaminergic neurons via their reuptake system; blockers of this system prevent toxicity in some experimental models. The mechanism by which MPP+ damages neurons is attributed to its ability to act as a mitochondrial poison, blocking oxidative phosphorylation at the level of complex I.

Clinical Features and Laboratory Diagnosis

A history of drug abuse or employment in a pharmaceutical or research laboratory should alert the clinician to the possibility of MPTP exposure. Acute signs and symptoms of MPTP exposure include hallucinations, jerking of the extremities, visual blurring, seborrhea, tremors, and, in addicts, a burning sensation at the site of injection. Chronic features that develop within days to weeks include bradykinesia, rigidity, stiffness, and, in some cases, a typical resting tremor. Almost all the motor features of Parkinson's disease may be seen, including masked facies, drooling, fixed stare, shuffling gait, flexed posture, hypophonia, and loss of postural righting reflexes. Even more subtle parkinsonian features, such as micrographia and seborrhea, are present. In a single human case studied neuropathologically, MPTP produced selective cell loss in the zona compacta of the substantia nigra. Studies in young monkeys have revealed similarly selective cell loss. Older monkeys appear to display a broader array of neuropathologic features, including cell loss in the locus ceruleus and the presence of eosinophilic inclusion bodies in the same sites of predilection for Lewy bodies, a characteristic intraneuronal inclusion body seen in Parkinson's disease.

Patients with MPTP-induced neurotoxicity have few laboratory findings. The cerebrospinal fluid protein level may be slightly elevated in some patients. As a group, the mean concentrations of certain neurotransmitters in the cerebrospinal fluid are altered (3-methoxy-4-hydroxyphenethyleneglycol is increased, homovanillic acid is reduced) in MPTP-exposed patients, but many individual values fall within the normal range. With specialized techniques, however, MPTP or MPP+ or both are detectable in blood or urine for several days after exposure.

Treatment

Although no clinical data exist regarding the effects of MAO inhibitors after MPTP exposure in humans, animal studies using pargyline and deprenyl suggest that their use should be considered in cases of recent (within 1 to 12 hours) exposure to MPTP. Because results of primate studies of dopamine-uptake blockade are conflicting, these agents cannot be recommended at this time. The development of full-blown MPTP-induced parkinsonism in humans appears to be irreversible; it is unclear whether milder degrees of exposure eventually lead to a progressive condition. Most patients respond dramatically to treatment with carbidopa/levodopa (Sinemet) and dopamine agonists, but side effects may appear early when compared with the treatment of Parkinson's disease in elderly patients.

BIBLIOGRAPHY

Barbeau A. Manganese and extrapyramidal disorders. *Neurotoxicology* 1984; 5:13–35.

Catsch A, Harmuth-Hoene ARE. Pharmacology and therapeutic applications of agents used in heavy metal poisoning. In: Levine WG, ed. *The chelation of heavy metals.* New York: Pergamon Press, 1979.

Dreisbach RH, Robertson WO. *Handbook of poisoning: prevention, diagnosis and treatment.* Norwalk, CT: Appleton-Lange, 1987.

Goetz GC. *Neurotoxins in clinical practice.* New York: Spectrum Publications, 1985.

Haddad LM, Winchester JF. *Clinical management of poisoning and drug overdose.* Philadelphia: WB Saunders, 1990.

Langston JW, Ballard P. Parkinsonism induced by 1-methyl-4-phenyl-1,2,3,6-tetrahydropyridine (MPTP): implications for treatment and pathogenesis of Parkinson's disease. *Can J Neurol Sci* 1984;11:160–165.

Porru S, Alessio L. The use of chelating agents in occupational lead poisoning. *Occup Med* 1996;46:41–48.

Spencer PS, Schaumberg HH, eds. *Experimental and clinical neurotoxicology.* Baltimore: Williams & Wilkins, 1980.

Wennberg A. Neurotoxic effects of selected metals. *Scand J Work Environ Health* 1994;20:65–71.

White RF, Proctor SP. Solvents and neurotoxicity. *Lancet* 1997;349; 1239–1243.

Kelley's Textbook of Internal Medicine, fourth edition. Edited by H. David Humes. Lippincott Williams & Wilkins, Philadelphia © 2000.

C H A P T E R
440

THE NEUROLOGIC COMPLICATIONS AND CONSEQUENCES OF ETHANOL USE AND ABUSE

STANLEY A. HASHIMOTO
DONALD W. PATY

Ethanol is consumed by about two thirds of the population of North America, but one third of the population is considered to be moderate to heavy drinkers. About 10% of all drinkers become alcoholics and drink more than 50% of all the ethanol consumed. This makes ethanol use and abuse a major health problem. More than 20,000 deaths per year are directly related to alcohol use in the United States; this rate is related in part to motor vehicle accidents and other types of violence. Alcoholism is a major worldwide problem and an increasing one. The development of alcoholism is a complex phenomenon dependent on genetic, cultural, social, and economic factors. Rarely, an underlying problem such as an alcohol-responsive essential tremor may lead to alcohol addiction.

The acute and chronic effects of ethanol are primarily those that relate to its effect on the central nervous system (Table 440.1). Other organs are also involved, including the liver, heart, pancreas, and blood; the involvement of those organs subsequently affects the brain, too. The excessive intake of ethanol is in the form of nonnutritional calories, leading to malnutrition. As such, it becomes impossible to separate the effects of chronic alcoholism from the effects of deficiency of nutritional factors, primarily thiamine.

Ethanol is rapidly absorbed by the gastrointestinal tract, and because of its miscibility in water becomes widely distributed throughout the body. The brain is no exception, and there appears to be no blood–brain barrier to this substance. Ethanol acts on the lipids of the cell membrane and, less likely, directly on the proteins in the cell membrane. Neuronal excitability appears to increase at lower concentrations, and at higher levels neuronal activity progressively decreases. Researchers have studied the impact of ethanol on neurotransmitters, including acetylcholine, serotonin, γ-aminobutyric acid (GABA), and catechola-

TABLE 440.1.	NEUROLOGIC COMPLICATIONS AND CONSEQUENCES OF ETHANOL ABUSE

Acute Intoxication
Acute tolerance
Chronic tolerance
Alcoholic blackouts

Withdrawal Phenomenon
Tremors
Seizures
Hallucinations and auditory hallucinosis
Delerium tremens
Sleep disorders
Movement disorders

Neurologic Complications of Chronic Alcoholism
Wernicke's encephalopathy
Korsakoff's psychosis
Dementia
Marchiafava–Bignami disease
Cerebellar degeneration
Central pontine myelinolysis
Polyneuropathy
Myopathy (acute and chronic)

Fetal Alcohol Syndrome
Indirect Consequences
Head injury, subdural hematoma
Compression mononeuropathy (e.g., radial nerve palsy)
Consequences of liver failure
Impact on stroke

mines; the neurotransmitter most consistently involved may be GABA.

ACUTE INTOXICATION

The intoxicating effect of ethanol depends mainly on the blood level but also on the rate of ingestion and the impact of habitual drinking. Because of the development of acute tolerance, ethanol has less of an impact when the level is reached slowly, and the degree of intoxication is less when the level of ethanol is dropping than at the same level when it is rising. Persons who have achieved chronic tolerance through habitual drinking may tolerate very high levels, ones that may be fatal in a novice drinker.

On average, a blood alcohol level of about 25 to 30 mg per deciliter is associated with mood changes and probably a significant decrease in cognition and coordination. This impairment is sufficient to affect the operation of a motor vehicle; current maximums permitted by law for drivers are 80 to 100 mg per deciliter. At 100 mg per deciliter, alcohol's effect on the brain stem causes diplopia, dysarthria, and nystagmus, with added cerebellar dysfunction. At 200 mg per deciliter, the person has marked confusion; at 400 mg per deciliter, most persons become comatose. A level of 500 mg per deciliter is usually fatal owing to respiratory depression, but with chronic tolerance, drinkers have survived levels up to 1,000 mg per deciliter.

In a patient with a high blood alcohol level, hypotension, and coma, the blood alcohol level must be lowered as rapidly as possible. The rate of metabolism of ethanol remains constant; therefore, hemodialysis should be considered if the level is life-threatening.

A "blackout" is said to occur when, after a large intake of alcohol, a person cannot remember what happened during a circumscribed period of time, although there was no loss of consciousness. It is similar to transient global amnesia and always clears spontaneously. Blackouts occur in persons who would not otherwise be considered alcoholics.

WITHDRAWAL PHENOMENON

Withdrawal symptoms occur when alcohol intake is reduced or stopped after prolonged, excessive intake. These symptoms are more likely to occur with increasing duration of excessive intake and with the amount ingested. The adrenergic system is hyperactive, and β-blockers can reduce some of the signs. The most common finding is tremor, which involves mostly the upper limbs; however, the entire body can be tremulous, including the voice. The tremor, which is present both at rest and with action, starts within the first 12 to 24 hours of withdrawal and gradually recedes on its own. The person is usually anxious and agitated. Treatment is usually not required. One third of these patients develop visual hallucinations and more rarely auditory hallucinosis. Auditory hallucinations are usually not associated with confusion, such as that which occurs with delirium tremens. Visual hallucinations usually disappear within a few days, but auditory hallucinosis is a more unpleasant and prolonged disturbance and may resemble schizophrenia.

One fourth of patients have withdrawal seizures within the first 24 to 48 hours, usually generalized tonic–clonic seizures without focal features. These seizures may be associated with myoclonic jerks, and the patient often has a photomyoclonic response to photic stimulation during an electroencephalogram. Anticonvulsant medication is not indicated unless status epilepticus occurs, which is rare. Prophylactic anticonvulsant medication is ineffective. Seizures that vary from this description should be investigated for another cause, such as subdural hematoma or abscess.

Delirium tremens, the most serious withdrawal manifestation, carries a mortality rate of 20% if untreated. It occurs late, after seizures and tremor, usually 3 to 5 days after the patient stops drinking. It is always preceded by restlessness and anxiety, followed by confusion, hallucinations, and insomnia, with added autonomic dysfunctions of tachycardia, fever, and sweating. Occasionally, circulatory collapse occurs. Treatment is primarily sedation and hydration with appropriate doses of benzodiazepines.

Other possible manifestations of withdrawal include transient parkinsonism, other movement disorders, or sleep disorders. All these phenomena probably relate to the adaptive changes that have occurred in the cell membranes during prolonged and excessive ethanol intake that are suddenly no longer compensated by the presence of alcohol.

EFFECTS OF CHRONIC ALCOHOL ABUSE ON THE NERVOUS SYSTEM

WERNICKE'S ENCEPHALOPATHY

Wernicke's encephalopathy is a disorder related to thiamine deficiency. It is not specific for alcoholism and may occur in persons with hyperemesis gravidarum, gastrointestinal cancer, or any other situation leading to inadequate nutritional intake. Alcoholism, however, is by far the most common cause and reflects poor nutrition. There is a genetic component, probably related to abnormalities of transketolase and other carbohydrate enzymes. The problem may be precipitated by the administration of glucose without thiamine. Although most patients present clinically with incomplete syndromes, the triad of encephalopathy, ophthalmoplegia, and ataxia is seen in about one third of all patients affected. Patients may gradually proceed to coma and die if not treated quickly and adequately with intravenous thiamine. The ataxia is identical with that seen in the cerebellar degeneration of alcoholism. The ophthalmoplegia can consist of gaze palsies, including internuclear ophthalmoplegias, third- and sixth-nerve palsies, and pupillary abnormalities and nystagmus; the latter may persist despite treatment.

The pathologic findings, often visible on computed tomography (CT) scanning and magnetic resonance imaging (MRI), are present within the walls of the third ventricle, the periaqueductal gray matter, the floor of the fourth ventricle, and often both mamillary bodies. There is endothelial proliferation, hemorrhage, gliosis, and demyelination in the areas involved.

The treatment is intravenous thiamine (100 mg per day intravenously) until adequate nutrition is established. Improvement can occur quickly.

KORSAKOFF'S PSYCHOSIS

In Korsakoff's psychosis, which is often associated with Wernicke's encephalopathy, retentive memory, both recent and remote, is absent (or almost so), but other cognitive functions remain relatively intact. Confabulation may be present as a manifestation of impaired recall. The problem may be related to mammillary body destruction and diencephalic lesions and possibly to the involvement of the process within both temporal lobes. The prognosis for recovery to normal function is poor: probably 80% of patients are left with a significant memory deficit.

DEMENTIA SECONDARY TO ALCOHOL ABUSE

Controversy exists about whether dementia is a secondary complication of alcoholism separate from Korsakoff's psychosis and head injury. Dementia is, however, generally accepted as a reversible disorder, and, when combined with Korsakoff's psychosis, alcoholism is probably the third most common cause of dementia (after Alzheimer's disease and vascular disease). Alcoholism as a cause of dementia exceeds head injuries, a group to which alcoholism contributes.

Dementia secondary to alcohol abuse (separate from Korsakoff's disease) is usually a mild, primarily amnestic, and potentially reversible disorder. The major supporting evidence for alcohol-related dementia comes from neuroimaging techniques, which show that the brain volume is less in alcoholics than in normal controls. The reduction in brain volume and dementia appears to improve with cessation of alcohol intake; however, patients free of head injury, malnutrition, poor socioeconomic conditions, and other drug use are unusual and difficult to find, making controlled studies difficult if not impossible to carry out.

MARCHIAFAVA–BIGNAMI DISEASE

Marchiafava–Bignami disease, a rare disorder, was initially described in Italy in young men who were extremely heavy red wine drinkers, but it occurs around the world, involves all races, and is not restricted to wine drinkers. The diagnosis is now made premorbidly through MRI and CT scanning. The demyelinating pathology, similar to that of central pontine myelinosis, affects the middle third of the corpus callosum. Terminally, patients become stuporous and seizures are common; this situation is preceded by dementia and gait disorder. The early manifestations are protean, and the disorder can be acute, subacute, or chronic. Patients are usually very heavy drinkers. The underlying cause again probably relates to malnutrition rather than to the direct impact of alcohol on the brain.

CEREBELLAR DEGENERATION

Cerebellar degeneration secondary to alcoholism affects the midline anterior superior vermis. The clinical presentation is there-

fore that of gait and stance, not functions that relate to the arms. Cerebellar degeneration is similar to the cerebellar ataxia seen in Wernicke's encephalopathy and therefore is probably related to nutritional factors. Alcohol has a direct impact on cerebellar structures, including Purkinje's cells. Cerebellar degeneration occurs in long-term alcoholics, but the problem does not seem to correlate with the amount of alcohol ingested. The problem may recede with abstinence but recurs with drinking and may become irreversible; in rare cases, walking becomes impossible. The treatment is proper nutrition, including thiamine, and cessation of drinking. Genetics probably plays a significant role in the cause of this disorder.

CENTRAL PONTINE MYELINOLYSIS

Central pontine myelinolysis is a disorder consisting of demyelination and at times loss of axons, primarily in the central pons. The disorder also affects both cerebral hemispheres and the cerebellum to a lesser extent. It is usually subacute and often diagnosed after death, but MRI can detect the lesions and brainstem auditory-evoked responses are also helpful. The prognosis for those with central pontine myelinolysis is poor. In the complete form of the disease, patients have quadriparesis or the "locked-in syndrome." The cause can be the rapid correction of hyponatremia, but the disorder has also been seen in hypernatremia, azotemia, and hyperglycemia. Central pontine myelinolysis is more common in alcoholics, but the mechanism is unknown. It can coexist with Wernicke's encephalopathy. The only treatment is prevention by the slow correction of hyponatremia.

MYELOPATHY

Although most cases of myelopathy in alcoholics are due to advanced cirrhosis of the liver, myelopathy may be secondary to alcohol use alone. This is a progressive disorder with dorsal and lateral column dysfunction.

POLYNEUROPATHY

A diffuse polyneuropathy that involves the lower extremities more than the upper extremities is common in alcoholics. This is one cause of a painful neuropathy, with a burning dysesthesia in some cases. The cause is probably related to malnutrition and thiamine deficiency, and treatment consists of thiamine and cessation of alcohol. The disorder is a sensory motor neuropathy, with weakness and distal sensory loss as well as loss of deep tendon reflexes. The gait may be ataxic secondary to proprioceptive loss.

MYOPATHY

Some cases of proximal muscle weakness are due to hypokalemia, often secondary to diarrhea and vomiting, but both acute and chronic myopathies exist secondary to excessive alcohol intake. Acute myopathy always follows a major alcoholic binge and is a serious disorder, with rhabdomyolysis and renal failure resulting from myoglobinuria. The only treatment is abstinence. These patients may be left with a deficit. Chronic myopathy is more indolent and consists of slowly progressive proximal weakness, with a mildly elevated level of creatine phosphokinase in the blood. Abstinence is the only treatment for this disorder as well.

FETAL ALCOHOL SYNDROME

Ethanol and its metabolite acetaldehyde are both probable teratogens. The full fetal alcohol syndrome of mental and physical retardation, with facial and other congenital abnormalities, is uncommon, occurring in about 6% of children born to alcoholic mothers who maintain a high intake throughout the pregnancy. However, partial syndromes are common, especially with exposure in the first trimester. Low IQ and behavioral and physical changes occur. There is probably no safe level of ethanol ingestion in pregnancy, although lower levels have not been shown to be harmful.

MISCELLANEOUS NEUROLOGIC COMPLICATIONS

Because the alcoholic is subject to falls and assault, head injury is common. Owing to cerebral atrophy, the alcoholic is prone to develop subneural hematoma. Recurrent head injuries can lead to dementia, and seizures secondary to this may develop. Pressure while lying in the stuporous state is a common problem and primarily involves the radial nerve ("Saturday night palsy") and the sciatic and peroneal nerves, although any nerve or plexus can be affected. Finally, meningitis and brain abscess secondary to pneumonia should be considered in all alcoholic patients who are ill and who present with either a depressed level of consciousness or seizures.

The other indirect consequences of alcohol abuse consist of central nervous system problems related to liver failure. Moderate use of alcohol has been the focus of several studies in relation to the development of stroke. There appears to be no difference from one type of drink such as wine compared with another such as beer. There appears to be a U- or J-shaped curve with moderate drinking being protective, whereas higher amounts probably increase the chances of stroke. These results had accounted for other risk factors.

BIBLIOGRAPHY

Charness ME, Simon R, Greenberg DA. Medical progress: ethanol and the nervous system. *N Engl J Med* 1989;321:442–454.

Harper CG, Kril JJ. Neuropathology of alcoholism. *Alcohol Alcoholism* 1990;25:207–216.

Lehman LB. Neurologic complications of alcoholism. *Postgrad Med* 1991; 90(5):165–169,172.

Sacco RL, Elkind M, Boden-Albala B, et al. The protective effect of moderate alcohol on ischemic stroke. *JAMA* 1999;281(1):53–60.

Thomas K. Alcohol and disease: central nervous system. *Acta Med Scand* 1985; (suppl 703):251.

Truelsen T, Groenbaek M, Schnohr P, et al. Intake of beer, wine and spirits and risk of stoke. The Copenhagen City Heart Study. *Stroke* 1998;29: 2467–2472.

Weight FF. Cellular and molecular physiology of alcohol actions in the nervous system. *Intl Rev Neurobiol* 1992;33:289–348.

Kelley's Textbook of Internal Medicine, fourth edition. Edited by H. David Humes. Lippincott Williams & Wilkins, Philadelphia © 2000.

BACTERIAL INFECTIONS OF THE NERVOUS SYSTEM

ANTHONY W. CHOW
DONALD W. PATY

Pyogenic bacterial infections of the nervous system can be categorized into distinct entities based on their major anatomical location (i.e., meningitis and ventriculitis, brain abscess and cerebritis, subdural and epidural empyema, septic thrombophlebitis and mycotic aneurysm). In addition to these entities, two other bacterial infections of the nervous system (neurosyphilis and neuroborreliosis [Lyme disease]) deserve special emphasis because of their protean clinical manifestations and the diagnostic challenge that they can represent. In this chapter, the important epidemiologic, anatomical, and etiologic considerations of these conditions are outlined, and their clinical and laboratory findings and optimal management are presented. A more general discussion of the clinical approach to managing the patient with a suspected infection of the nervous system, including specific laboratory investigations and the differential diagnosis, is presented in Chapter 431.

■ MENINGITIS AND VENTRICULITIS

INCIDENCE, EPIDEMIOLOGY, AND ETIOLOGY

The brain and spinal cord are completely encased by three layers of meninges: the pia mater, the arachnoid (leptomeninges), and the dura mater (pachymeninges). Between the pia and arachnoid is the subarachnoid space, which contains cerebrospinal fluid (CSF). Meningitis develops when the subarachnoid space becomes infected, usually because of hematogenous spread and typically involving the entire surface of the leptomeninges surrounding the brain and spinal cord. Ventriculitis occurs either by contiguous spread of infection from the subarachnoid space through the foramina of Magendie and Luschka, or as direct consequence of a ventricular shunt infection.

Community-acquired meningitis is particularly common in children, young adults, and the elderly, and the causative agents vary greatly among the different age groups (Table 431.4). In children and young adults, the most common pathogens are the encapsulated bacteria *Haemophilus influenzae* type b, *Streptococcus pneumoniae*, and *Neisseria meningitidis* (75% of cases). However, the wide use of protein–polysaccharide conjugated vaccines has dramatically reduced the incidence of *H. influenzae* type b infections. Patients with splenectomy or sickle cell traits are particularly susceptible to *S. pneumoniae* and *H. influenzae* infection. Bacterial meningitis secondary to head trauma, craniotomy, CSF leak, or congenital defects such as spina bifida, dermoid cyst, or meningocele is most frequently caused by *Staphylococcus aureus* and *S. pneumoniae* infection and less frequently by *Pseudomonas aeruginosa* or other Enterobacteriaceae (e.g., *Klebsiella pneumoniae,* and *Proteus mirabilis*). Patients undergoing cancer chemotherapy or those with underlying immunodeficiency syndromes are more prone to infection with a variety of pathogens, including *Listeria monocytogenes,* Enterobacteriaceae, as well as mycobacteria and fungi. Ventricular shunt infections are most commonly caused by coagulase-negative staphylococci, *S. aureus,* and diphtheroids. Apart from age and underlying conditions, several other epidemiologic associations such as animal exposure and geographic location may provide important clinical clues to possible causative agents in both bacterial and nonbacterial infections of the nervous system (Table 431.2). An increasing proportion of cases are nosocomially acquired, and approximately one third of such cases are caused by gram-negative bacteria other than *H. influenzae.*

PATHOGENESIS

Purulent meningitis typically occurs after hematogenous dissemination from a distant site of infection, particularly the lung and heart valves. Other sources of purulent meningitis include neurosurgical procedures, basilar skull fractures, congenital neuroectodermal sinus tracts, spontaneous CSF fistulas, and placement of a ventricular shunt for hydrocephalus. In the otherwise healthy host, the subarachnoid space is relatively resistant to microorganisms even during persistent bacteremia. Both complement- and antibody-mediated bacteriolysis and opsonophagocytosis as well as cell-mediated immunity constitute the predominant defense mechanisms in the central nervous system (CNS). Humoral antibodies are particularly important against encapsulated pathogens such as *S. pneumoniae, N. meningitidis,* and *H. influenzae.* Once infection in the subarachnoid space is established, the offending microorganism can rapidly multiply to high levels (more than 10^5 colony-forming units/mm^3 CSF).

This results in the induction and release of several inflammatory and chemotactic cytokines, particularly tumor necrosis factor and interleukin-1, which are responsible for disruption of the blood–brain barrier and the intense inflammatory response in the CNS. These inflammatory changes are directly responsible for various neurologic sequelae, such as hearing impairment, seizure disorders, and hydrocephalus.

CLINICAL FINDINGS

The cardinal manifestations of meningitis are fever, headache, and nuchal rigidity. Other signs of cerebral dysfunction are variable, depending on the onset and clinical course of illness (Table 441.1). In acute purulent meningitis, most commonly caused by infection with *S. pneumoniae, N. meningitidis,* and *H. influenzae,* deterioration in mental status, progressing from confusion and lethargy to coma, may occur rapidly within 24 hours. Weakness, anorexia, shaking chills, profuse sweats, photophobia, vomiting, and myalgias of the lower extremities and back are common presentations. Neck stiffness may be subtle or marked. Cranial nerve palsies (principally third, fourth, sixth, and seventh) occur in 10% to 20% of patients. Seizures are more common in children, whereas focal cerebral signs such as hemiparesis, visual field defects, papilledema, and dysphasia are less frequent (10% to 15%). The presence of focal findings should suggest the coexistence of a brain abscess, subdural empyema, or septic thrombophlebitis. Ventriculitis should be suspected in any patient with an indwelling ventricular shunt or pressure catheter, with an unusual organism, with persistently high intracranial pressure, or with suboptimal response to therapy. In patients with a ventriculoperitoneal shunt, abdominal pain and tenderness may be the initial clinical presentation of a shunt infection.

In subacute or chronic meningitis, the onset is insidious, and neurologic findings may wax and wane. Episodes of acute neurologic deterioration may reflect underlying cerebral edema, cerebrovascular occlusions, hydrocephalus, or seizures. Focal

---

TABLE 441.1.   NEUROLOGIC MANIFESTATIONS OF BACTERIAL MENINGITIS

Condition	Cause	Prevention or Treatment
Acute Phase		
Confusion, depression in level of consciousness	Increased intracranial pressure	Early appropriate antimicrobials
Cerebral edema	Irritation, toxic effects of cerebrospinal fluid reabsorption	Early appropriate antimicrobials, corticosteroids
Stroke, aphasia, cortical blindness	Meningocerebral adhesions	Early appropriate antimicrobials
Cranial nerve palsies	Inflammation, sluggish venous flow	Corticosteroids
Subarachnoid hemorrhage	Mycotic aneurysm	Neurosurgical
Seizure and myoclonus	Cerebritis, vasculitis, venous sinus thrombosis	Anticonvulsants
Late Phase		
Dementia, personality change, gait disturbance, urinary incontinence	Basilar arachnoiditis causing communicating hydrocephalus	Neurosurgical, ventricular shunt
Deafness	Eighth-nerve involvement	Corticosteroids
Optic neuritis	Arachnoiditis, inflammation of optic nerve	Corticosteroids
Seizure	Meningocerebral adhesions, cerebritis	Anticonvulsants

signs are particularly important because they suggest parenchymal mass lesions such as abscess or granuloma. The presence of hydrocephalus in the course of subacute or chronic meningeal inflammation, particularly in association with cranial nerve palsies, is strongly suggestive of basilar leptomeningitis due to tuberculosis, fungi, or parasitic agents. Complications, including cranial neuropathies (ocular, motor, and facial palsies, or deafness), cerebral infarction, and increased intracranial pressure, are common. Myeloradiculitis can occur secondary to inflammatory meningeal exudate involving the spinal roots. Noninfectious causes, such as malignancy, sarcoidosis, and granulomatous angiitis, should be excluded.

LABORATORY FINDINGS

The typical CSF profiles in bacterial and nonbacterial meningitis are shown in Table 431.3. In acute bacterial meningitis, the cell count is usually greater than 300 per microliter and polymorphonuclear (greater than 90% polymorphonuclear leukocytes). Partially treated bacterial meningitis is typically associated with lymphocytic predominance in the CSF. In acute bacterial and tuberculous meningitis, the CSF glucose ordinarily is low (CSF:serum ratio less than 1:2). However, in the very early stages of these infections, the CSF cells and glucose may be normal. Also, the ventricular CSF glucose concentration is 6 to 18 mg per deciliter higher than the lumbar CSF, whereas the protein content is 60% lower under normal conditions. This gradient is maintained even in purulent meningitis. Therefore, the ventricular CSF may show a normal glucose level despite a low concentration in the lumbar CSF. A compartmental cellular response also can occur. For example, the lumbar CSF may be completely normal despite presence of ventriculitis in a patient with shunt infection. Thus, CSF should be sampled from the site most prominently involved even in the absence of an extradural blockage to CSF flow. The CSF Gram's stain is positive in up to 10% of patients with negative CSF cultures and in up to 80% of those with positive cultures. The yield of both Gram's stain and culture is reduced by the prior administration of antimicrobial agents. Blood culture is positive in at least 50% of patients with bacterial meningitis.

OPTIMAL MANAGEMENT

The choice of initial empiric antimicrobial therapy and the recommended dosages for acute purulent meningitis are discussed in Chapter 431 (Tables 431.4 and 431.5). The final antibiotic selection should be guided by culture results and susceptibility data. The recommended regimens for specific bacterial pathogens in purulent meningitis or ventriculitis are shown in Table 441.2. Penicillin G remains the treatment of choice for meningococcal meningitis. A third-generation cephalosporin (ceftriaxone or cefotaxime is the drug of choice for *H. influenzae* type b meningitis, since these strains frequently produce β-lactamase [30% to 50%] in North America) and may be resistant to peni-

---

TABLE 441.2.   ANTIMICROBIAL THERAPY FOR BACTERIAL MENINGITIS OR VENTRICULITIS

Organism	First Choice	Alternate
Streptococcus pneumoniae (penicillin-sensitive, MIC <0.1 µg/mL	Penicillin G or ampicillin	Third-generation cephalosporin[1]; chloramphenicol
Streptococcus pneumoniae (penicillin-intermediate, MIC 0.1–1 µg/mL	Third-generation cephalosporin[1]	Chloramphenicol
Streptococcus pneumoniae (highly penicillin-resistant, MIC >1 µg/mL	Vancomycin plus third-generation cephalosporin[1]	Rifampin plus third-generation cephalosporin; trovafloxacin
Neisseria meningitidis	Penicillin G or ampicillin	Third-generation cephalosporin[1]; chloramphenicol
Haemophilus influenzae (β-lactamase-negative)	Ampicillin	Third-generation cephalosporin[1], chloramphenicol
H. influenzae (β-lactamase-positive)	Third-generation cephalosporin[1]	Chloramphenicol
Enterobacteriaceae	Third-generation cephalosporin[1]	Ureidopenicillin[2] plus aminoglycoside; fluoroquinolone
Pseudomonas aeruginosa	Ceftazidime plus aminoglycoside	Ureidopenicillin or imipenem, each plus aminoglycoside; fluoroquinolone
Streptococcus agalactiae	Penicillin G or ampicillin	Third-generation cephalosporin[1] chloramphenicol
Listeria monocytogenes	Ampicillin or penicillin G plus aminoglycoside	Trimethoprim-sulfamethoxazole
Staphylococcus aureus (methicillin-sensitive)	Nafcillin or oxacillin	Vancomycin
S. aureus (methicillin-resistant)	Vancomycin	Trimethoprim-sulfamethoxazole; fluoroquinolone
Staphylococcus epidermidis	Vancomycin plus rifampin	Fluoroquinolone

MIC, minimum inhibitory concentrations.
[1] Cefotaxime or ceftriaxone.
[2] Piperacillin, mezlocillin, or azlocillin.
Modified with permission from Tunkel AR, Scheld WM. Pathogenesis and pathophysiology of bacterial meningitis. *Clin Microbiol Rev* 1993;6:128.

cillin or ampicillin. Cefuroxime, a second-generation cephalosporin frequently used in pediatric infections, has been associated with suboptimal results for *H. influenzae* meningitis and is not recommended. Although penicillin G or a third-generation cephalosporin has been effective for the treatment of pneumococcal meningitis, the widespread and increasing occurrence of pneumococcal strains resistant to penicillin has raised great concern. Although many third-generation cephalosporins have good in vitro activity against penicillin-intermediate pneumococci, clinical failure has occurred when cephalosporin resistance coexists with penicillin resistance. Accordingly, it is recommended that cefotaxime or ceftriaxone can be used for penicillin-resistant *S. pneumoniae* meningitis if the minimum inhibitory concentration(MIC) for these drugs is less than 0.5 g per milliliter. Vancomycin should be added empirically if there is β-lactam resistance among *S. pneumoniae* isolates locally. Vancomycin should be continued in the presence of high-level penicillin resistance and MIC greater than 0.5 g per milliliter to third-generation cephalosporins. Rifampin may be substituted for vancomycin. The newer fluoroquinolones with enhanced gram-positive activity (e.g., trovafloxacin, clinafloxacin, moxifloxacin) are effective against high-level penicillin-resistant pneumococcal meningitis in experimental models of infection, but clinical experience with these agents is still limited. Gram-negative bacillary meningitis due to enterobacteriaceae infection had a high mortality rate in the past (40% to 90%), but the prognosis is considerably improved when treated with a third-generation cephalosporin or imipenem (cure rates of 78% to 94%).

Meningitis caused by *P. aeruginosa* infection should be treated with the combination of an antipseudomonal β-lactam plus a fluoroquinolone or an aminoglycoside (intrathecal or ventricular administration of the aminoglycoside through an Ommaya reservoir may be necessary). Ampicillin or penicillin G plus an aminoglycoside should be used for the treatment of *L. monocytogenes* meningitis. The extended-spectrum cephalosporins and penicillins usually are ineffective. Trimethoprim-sulfamethoxazole is an alternative for patients allergic to penicillin. Ventricular shunt infections are most commonly caused by coagulase-negative staphylococci or *S. aureus*; initial therapy should consist of intraventricular as well as intravenous vancomycin. Close monitoring of vancomycin CSF concentrations during therapy is required for optimal efficacy. If the patient fails to improve, the addition of rifampin may be warranted and removal of the shunt may be necessary.

Treatment of tuberculous meningitis is with a combination of isoniazid (300 mg per day in adults and 10 mg per kilogram in children), rifampin (600 mg per day in adults and 15 mg per kilogram for children), and pyrazinamide (1,500 mg per day in adults and 20 to 35 mg per kilogram per day in children), each as single daily dose. Pyridoxine (50 mg per day) should be given concurrently to prevent isoniazid induced neuropathy. Treatment is continued for 9 to 12 months.

Dexamethasone as adjunctive therapy has been shown to prevent sensorineural hearing loss and other late sequelae in children but does not improve survival. It is likely to be beneficial in a subset of patients with cerebral edema or raised intracranial pressure or in those who experience profound alterations in consciousness. There is no consensus regarding the usefulness of corticosteroids as adjunctive therapy for acute bacterial meningitis in adults. Whether adjunctive therapy with monoclonal antibodies or other pharmacologic agents directed at blocking the effect of inflammatory cytokines in the CSF can prevent hearing loss, seizure disorders, or other chronic neurologic sequelae of purulent meningitis remains to be determined.

Despite improved antimicrobial therapy, the overall mortality rate of acute bacterial meningitis remains high, ranging from 5% among children to 25% in adults. Both the mortality rate and severe complications are highest for those with *S. pneumoniae*. The presence of hypotension, altered mental status, and seizures are independently associated with an adverse outcome.

BRAIN ABSCESS AND CEREBRITIS

INCIDENCE, EPIDEMIOLOGY, AND ETIOLOGY

Forty percent of brain abscesses result from infection of the paranasal sinuses, middle ear, or mastoid cells, whereas 30% are of hematogenous origin, usually arising from suppurative foci in the lungs or heart valves. Approximately 20% to 30% of cases are identified as "cryptic" brain abscess for which no obvious source can be identified. Of those originating in the middle ear, one third are localized in the cerebellum and two thirds in the temporal lobe. Enterobacteriaceae such as *P. mirabilis*, *K. pneumoniae*, and *P. aeruginosa*, as well as anaerobic organisms, are the most common pathogens (Table 431.2). In rhinogenic brain abscess associated with chronic sinusitis, the frontal and temporal lobes are most commonly involved, and anaerobic or microaerophilic streptococci (*Peptostreptococcus* sp, *Streptococcus anginosus*, and *Streptococcus viridans*) and *Bacteroides* sp are the most common pathogens. Hematogenous brain abscess is predominantly caused by infection with *S. aureus*, streptococci, enterococci, *Nocardia* sp, or the HACEK complex (*Haemophilus aphrophilus*, *Actinobacillus actinomycetem* comitans, Cardiobacterium hominis, Eikenella corrodens, and *Kingella denitrificans*). Brain abscesses secondary to penetrating cranial trauma or postoperative infection are most commonly caused by *S. aureus* and enteric gram-negative bacilli. Brain abscess in cancer or patients with the AIDS can be caused by a wide variety of organisms, including *L. monocytogenes*, enteric gram-negative bacilli, *Legionella* sp, and *Toxoplasma gondii*, as well as mycobacteria and fungi.

PATHOGENESIS

Brain abscess or cerebritis develop either by hematogenous spread from an extracranial focus or by contiguous infection from an adjacent nidus in the dura, meninges, or periosteum (Fig. 441.1). The earliest lesion is a focal area of inflammation and edema in the brain parenchyma ("early cerebritis stage"), which progresses to central necrosis ("late cerebritis stage"). A ring-enhancing capsule can be visualized by computed tomography (CT) scanning with the appearance of peripheral gliosis or fibrosis ("early capsule stage"), ultimately leading to a well-formed abscess ("late capsule stage"). Hematogenous or meta-

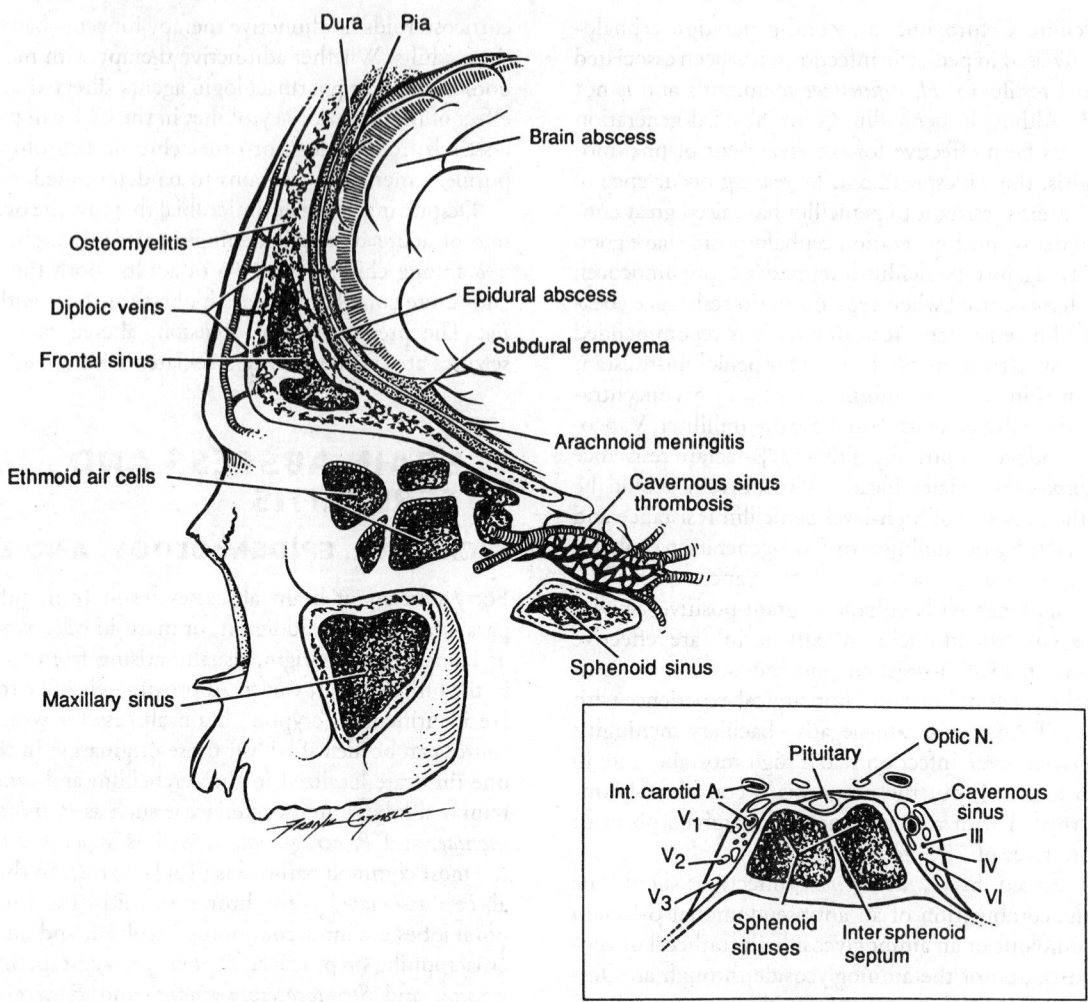

FIGURE 441.1. Intracranial parameningeal infections. The sagittal section shows the major routes of extension either directly or by way of the vascular supply. The coronal section demonstrates the structures adjoining the sphenoid sinus. (Reproduced with permission from Chow AW, Vortel JJ. Infections of the sinuses and parameningeal structures. In: Gorbach SL, Bartlett JG, Blacklow NR, eds. *Infectious diseases.* Philadelphia: WB Saunders, 1992:432.)

static brain abscess usually occurs in the posterior frontal and parietal lobes, which are perfused by the middle cerebral artery. The abscess tends to originate deep in the white matter or gray-white matter junction, where cerebral blood flow is more easily compromised. Inflammation, hemorrhage, edema, and hydrocephalus all may produce displacement of the brain or spinal cord. Displacement of the cerebral hemisphere forces brain tissue beneath the falx cerebri and over the tentorium cerebelli (Fig. 441.2). Herniation beneath the falx is usually asymptomatic, but herniation of the temporal lobe over the tentorium can cause third cranial nerve palsy and ipsilateral corticospinal tract signs due to compression of the contralateral cerebral peduncle against the tentorium. Onset of coma and progressive loss of brain-stem reflexes culminating in respiratory arrest rapidly ensue. Posterior fossa lesions such as a cerebellar abscess or hemorrhage may produce rapid compression of the medulla and pons and herniation of the cerebellar tonsils through the foramen magnum without antecedent midbrain signs.

CLINICAL FINDINGS

The clinical presentations of brain abscesses are variable and are primarily determined by their anatomical location, proximity to the ventricles or cisternal or dural sinuses, and major alterations in the intracranial pressure dynamics secondary to the mass effect. Four distinctive clinical presentations of a brain abscess can be recognized on the basis of the unique pathophysiologic events implicated: rapid focal mass expansion, intracranial hypertension, diffuse brain destruction, and focal neurologic deficit. In the last category, the temporal progression of infection is so slow that it is often misdiagnosed as a neoplasm. Fever is present in only 45% to 50% of patients; therefore, absence of fever should not be used to exclude the diagnosis of brain abscess. An understanding of the alterations in the intracranial pressure dynamics secondary to the mass effect is particularly helpful in correlating the underlying pathophysiologic process with the clinical presentation. Thus, a pontine abscess may bulge posteriorly and block

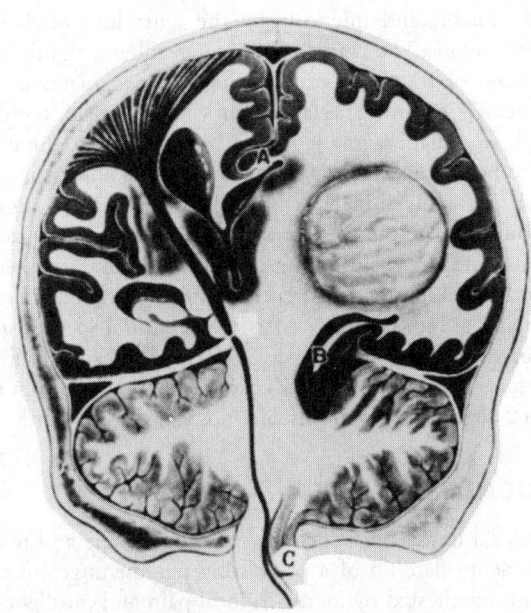

FIGURE 441.2. Herniation of brain tissue (**A**) beneath the falx cerebri; (**B**) over the tentorium cerebelli with compression of the contralateral cerebral peduncle; and (**C**) through the foramen magnum. (Adapted with permission from Greenlee JE. Anatomic considerations in central nervous system infections. In: Mandell GL, Bennett JE, Dolin R, eds. *Principles and practice of infectious diseases,* fourth ed. New York: Churchill Livingstone, 1995:821.)

the aqueduct of Sylvius acutely to cause obstructive hydrocephalus.

An occipital lobe abscess could rupture or leak into the ventricular system, causing ventriculitis, or it could involve the transverse sinus and cause septic thrombophlebitis or a subdural empyema. Both cranial and spinal nerve roots may be involved, either directly because of contiguous infection, or indirectly because of increased intracranial pressure. Of particular importance is the close relation of the third cranial nerve with the tentorium (uncal herniation of the temporal lobe); the third, fourth, fifth, and sixth cranial nerves with the cavernous sinus (septic cavernous sinus thrombosis); the fifth and sixth cranial nerves with the petrous portion of the temporal bone (chronic otitis media and petrous osteomyelitis); and the ninth and eleventh cranial nerves with the jugular foramen (septic jugular thrombophlebitis). Because the second cranial nerve is contained within the subarachnoid space up to its point of entry into the eye, papilledema and optic atrophy may result from a sustained increase in intracranial pressure.

LABORATORY FINDINGS

The diagnosis of brain abscess is no longer difficult with the availability of CT scanning and magnetic resonance imaging (MRI). Such studies should be performed with and without contrast to more easily differentiate early cerebritis from abscess. On a precontrast CT scan, cerebritis is seen as a hypodense area, and abscess is characterized as a low area of density surrounded by a faint ring (capsule). With contrast, both cerebritis and ab-

scess show ring enhancement within 10 minutes of injection, but the ring enhancement does not persist at 60 minutes in cerebritis, in contrast to abscess. In some cases of early cerebritis, the CT may be negative even with contrast. MRI provides more resolution in detecting early cerebritis and the adjacent cerebral edema. MRI is also more accurate than CT in identifying the central liquefactive necrosis of a brain abscess that is hyperintense relative to CSF.

Contrast enhancement with intravenous gadolinium provides even more detail and is the procedure of choice in the evaluation of brain abscesses. Radionuclide brain scans are largely replaced by CT and MRI. Indium-labeled leukocyte scanning may allow differentiation of brain abscess from tumor. A lumbar puncture (LP) is contraindicated if a brain abscess or other mass lesion is suspected. The risk of herniation and death in such patients is high, whereas the potential benefit of obtaining useful information or positive culture from the CSF is relatively low. The CSF cell count is usually normal unless the abscess has ruptured into the subarachnoid space.

OPTIMAL MANAGEMENT

The choice of initial empiric antimicrobial regimens for brain abscess and cerebritis is based on the suspected source of infection, the immunologic status of the patient, and the most likely causative organisms (Tables 431.5 and 431.6). The final antibiotic selection should be guided by culture results and susceptibility data. Where anaerobes are implicated, penicillin G remains the antibiotic of first choice. Chloramphenicol or metronidazole are useful alternatives in the penicillin-allergic patient and have the advantage of more effective coverage against β-lactamase-producing anaerobes. Metronidazole is particularly active against *Bacteroides* sp. Its lack of activity against gram-positive anaerobic cocci such as *Peptostreptococcus* sp and facultative organisms such as streptococci, however, is a disadvantage that precludes monotherapy of otogenic or odontogenic brain abscess with metronidazole alone. Combination of penicillin with metronidazole or chloramphenicol is suitable. Clindamycin penetrates the blood–brain barrier poorly and usually is not recommended in CNS infections. For immunocompromised and critically ill patients, broad coverage with extended-spectrum β-lactams (e.g., cefotaxime, ceftizoxime, imipenem) for aerobic gram-negative rods, *S. aureus*, and anaerobes is indicated.

The fluoroquinolones (ciprofloxacin or trovafloxacin) have excellent CNS penetration and antibacterial activity against gram-negative bacilli. If *S. aureus* is suspected, nafcillin, 2 g every 4 hours, may be added. If the *S. aureus* strain is resistant to methicillin, vancomycin is the agent of choice. Brain abscess caused by infection with *Nocardia* sp is treated with intravenous trimethoprim-sulfamethoxazole (5 to 10 mg per kilogram trimethoprim and 25 to 50 mg per kilogram sulfamethoxazole daily in four divided doses). Maximum doses of systemic antimicrobials are required for the treatment of brain abscess or cerebritis to optimize penetration of the blood–brain barrier. Therapy should usually be continued for at least 6 to 8 weeks. Patients should be carefully monitored both clinically and by repeated

CT scans until complete resolution of the abscess. Follow-up is required for up to 1 year to ascertain nonrecurrence.

Because of the tendency for recurrence, well-encapsulated brain abscesses are best treated by surgical aspiration. If the focal lesion persists, resection of the abscess capsule may be necessary. In contrast, treatment of early cerebritis does not usually require surgical drainage. Indications for nonoperative treatment of brain abscess include poor surgical candidate; multiple abscesses that are remote from one another; abscesses in deep or dominant locations; a relatively small abscess (less than 4 cm); and partial resolution of the abscess attributable to antimicrobial therapy before surgery. The overall mortality of brain abscess remains high and is dictated by the extent of neurologic compromise at the time of presentation and diagnosis. The mortality is highest among patients with symptoms of short duration, severe mental status changes, and rapidly progressing neurologic deterioration. Among survivors, seizures are the the most common complications, occurring in 25% to 50% of cases. Anticonvulsant therapy may be required indefinitely.

■ SUBDURAL EMPYEMA AND EPIDURAL ABSCESS

INCIDENCE, EPIDEMIOLOGY, AND ETIOLOGY

Subdural empyema and epidural abscess are parameningeal infections that most frequently arise by direct extension from a pericranial focus, such as chronic sinusitis, otitis media, mastoiditis, or petrous osteomyelitis. Subdural empyema or cranial epidural abscesses associated with chronic sinusitis are most commonly caused by anaerobic or microaerophilic streptococci (*Peptostreptococcus* sp, *S. viridans*, *S. anginosus*) and *Bacteroides* sp. In otogenic infection associated with chronic otitis media or mastoiditis, enteric gram-negative bacilli, such as *P. aeruginosa* and *P. mirabilis*, as well as anaerobic organisms are most common. Spinal epidural abscess usually arises hematogenously or by contiguous spread from vertebral osteomyelitis, extension of decubitus ulcers, and infection after epidural anesthesia or penetrating injury. Distant sources of infection include infective endocarditis, pneumonia, intra-abdominal or pelvic sepsis, and urinary tract infection with entry of organisms by way of the paravertebral venous plexus. Epidural abscesses secondary to penetrating cranial trauma or postoperative infection are most commonly caused by infection with *S. aureus* and enteric gram-negative bacilli.

PATHOGENESIS

Subdural empyema is characterized by suppuration located between the inner surface of the dura and the outer surface of the arachnoid. The source of infection is usually in the frontal or ethmoid sinuses. The infection gains entry by direct extension or as a result of thrombophlebitis involving the venous sinuses (Fig. 441.1). Because the arachnoid and dura are only loosely attached, subdural infection tends to spread rapidly over the entire surface of the cerebral hemisphere. This infection is usually unilateral because further spread is restricted medially by

the falx cerebri and inferiorly by the tentorium cerebelli. In contrast, because the cranial dura mater adheres tightly to the periosteum of the skull, except where it invaginates into the cranial cavity to form the falx cerebri, falx cerebelli, tentorium cerebelli, and diaphragma selli, infection in the extradural space tends to be more localized. Cranial extradural abscess is associated with osteomyelitis in a cranial bone and usually originates from infection in the middle ear or the paranasal sinuses, or from a neurosurgical procedure. Spinal subdural empyema is rare both in adults and children. The spinal dura mater and the periosteum are separated by a fat-filled epidural space from the foramen magnum to the level of C7. Thus, both spinal subdural empyema and spinal epidural abscess may extend over many vertebral segments and are usually posterior to the cord.

CLINICAL FINDINGS

Generalized headache, associated with high fevers and malaise, and an acute flare-up of a preexisting parameningeal focus of infection manifested by increased local pain and purulent nasal or aural discharge, are the first indications of a subdural empyema. These clinical features are followed within days by the appearance of focal neurologic findings such as unilateral motor seizures, hemiplegia, hemianesthesia, or aphasia, and signs of increased intracranial pressure with progressive lethargy and coma. The neck is stiff, but CSF examination is more consistent with an aseptic meningitis syndrome. In infants and young children, however, an intracranial subdural empyema is almost invariably a complication of bacterial meningitis. Early signs such as irritability, poor feeding, or increased head size are nonspecific, but hemiparesis, convulsions, stupor, and coma may rapidly ensue. Intracranial epidural abscess is usually associated with a postcraniotomy infection, or a cranial osteomyelitis secondary to chronic sinusitis or middle ear infection. The onset of symptoms may be insidious and overshadowed by the localized inflammatory process. Focal neurologic findings are less common than in subdural empyema. Rarely, a fifth and sixth cranial nerve palsy may develop in association with infections of the petrous portion of the temporal bone (Gradenigo's syndrome).

Spinal epidural abscess may span several vertebrae and may be inadvertently entered during an LP. The abscess may develop acutely or follow a more chronic course. Four stages in the clinical presentation can be recognized. The first phase is usually accompanied by fever and back pain. The second phase involves progression to root pain. If symptoms develop in the cervical or lumbar area, it can suggest nerve root compression due to a ruptured disk. The third phase involves progression to motor weakness, sensory changes, and bowel or bladder dysfunction, signaling spinal cord compression. The fourth phase is total paralysis, which may occur within hours after the onset of motor weakness. If the cervical cord is involved, respiratory function may be impaired.

LABORATORY FINDINGS

CT scanning is the procedure of choice for the diagnosis of both subdural empyema and cranial epidural abscess. In subdural empyema, the CT scan usually reveals a crescent-shaped area of low density directly between the inner table of the skull and cerebral cortex or adjacent to the falx cerebri. With contrast, fine, irregular enhancement of the peripheral margins of the subdural empyema is seen. Occasionally, the CT scan may be inconclusive because density of the subdural empyema may be similar to that of cerebral tissue, and the decreased attenuation may not be evident on CT. MRI may provide an advantage over CT in such cases. Angiography is recommended on an emergency basis if the CT scan is negative and facilities for MRI are not available. As with brain abscess, LP should be avoided in patients suspected of having a subdural or epidural empyema.

MRI has replaced myelography as the diagnostic method of choice for spinal epidural abscess because it is positive early in the course of infection and provides the best imaging of the inflammatory changes. MRI is also superior to CT for visualizing the cord and epidural space as well as in identifying an associated vertebral osteomyelitis. CSF is usually nondiagnostic unless the abscess has ruptured into the subarachnoid space, or if the spinal needle has inadvertently entered the epidural abscess during the LP.

OPTIMAL MANAGEMENT

Early surgical evacuation is the cornerstone of therapy for both subdural and cranial epidural empyema. The incidence of mortality and neurologic sequelae varies directly with the time elapsed before surgical drainage. In addition, the primary focus of infection, such as chronic sinusitis, mastoiditis, or petrous osteomyelitis, should be explored and debrided. The choice of initial empiric antimicrobial therapy is similar to that in brain abscess (Table 431.6). Intravenous therapy should be continued for 4 to 6 weeks after surgical drainage.

The initial empiric antimicrobial therapy for spinal epidural abscess should be directed at both *S. aureus* (found in approximately 50% of cases) and enteric gram-negative bacilli. Thus, oxacillin or nafcillin and a third-generation cephalosporin (e.g., cefotaxime, ceftizoxime, ceftriaxone, or ceftazidime) may be suitable. An extended-spectrum penicillin (e.g., piperacillin, ticarcillin-clavulanate, imipenem, mezlocillin, or azlocillin) plus an aminoglycoside is appropriate if *P. aeruginosa* infection is suspected. Intravenous fluoroquinolone (e.g., ciprofloxacin or trovafloxacin) or trimethoprim-sulfamethoxazole may also be considered in the penicillin-allergic patient.

■ SEPTIC INTRACRANIAL THROMBOPHLEBITIS AND MYCOTIC ANEURYSM

INCIDENCE, EPIDEMIOLOGY, AND ETIOLOGY

Intracranial thrombophlebitis most frequently follows infection of the paranasal sinuses, middle ear, mastoid, or oropharynx. These catastrophic complications are fortunately rare in the post-antibiotic era. *Lateral (transverse) sinus thrombophlebitis* usually follows chronic infection of the middle ear, mastoid, or petrous bone. *Cavernous sinus thrombophlebitis* is usually secondary to infection of the ethmoid, sphenoid, or maxillary sinuses. *Superior*

sagittal (longitudinal) sinus thrombophlebitis usually results from head trauma or postneurosurgical complications. The causative organisms depend on the underlying conditions and are similar to those in subdural empyema and cranial epidural abscess (Table 431.1).

PATHOGENESIS

The cranium is drained by a network of superficial veins (external portions of the cerebrum and brain stem), deep veins (central white matter, basal ganglia, and thalamus), and venous sinuses within the dura mater. The superficial veins and venous sinuses also communicate extensively with the extracranial venous system through numerous emissary veins that cross the skull and meninges. The intracranial venous system and sinuses lack valves and allow bidirectional blood flow. Because of extensive anastomosis, cortical venous thrombosis or occlusion of venous sinuses often produces only transient neurologic manifestations and at times may be silent. Because the middle cerebral arteries receive the greatest volume of blood, they are more frequently involved in infectious processes such as septic embolization or mycotic aneurysm, compared with other branches of the anterior and posterior circulation. Intracranial mycotic aneurysm usually results from septic embolization as a complication of bacterial endocarditis. This produces infection and necrosis in the arterial wall, which leads to dilation and possible rupture. Mycotic aneurysms can be multiple and are usually found on distal branches of the middle or anterior cerebral arteries. The spinal arteries are seldom involved in infections.

CLINICAL FINDINGS

The clinical manifestations of septic intracranial thrombophlebitis vary with the location and extent of cortical veins or dural sinuses involved (Fig. 441.1). If collateral venous drainage is adequate, septic venous thrombosis may produce only transient neurologic findings or may be silent. If the thrombus outstrips collateral flow, however, progressive neurologic deficits, including impairment of consciousness, focal or generalized seizures, and increased intracranial pressure, ensues. *Cavernous sinus thrombosis* is characterized by abrupt onset with diplopia, photophobia, orbital edema, and progressive exophthalmos. Involvement of the third, fourth, fifth, and sixth cranial nerves produces ophthalmoplegia, a midposition fixed pupil, loss of corneal reflex, and diminished sensation over the upper face. Obstruction of venous return from the retina results in papilledema, retinal hemorrhage, and visual loss. Thrombosis of the *superior sagittal sinus* usually presents with unilateral convulsions and alternating hemiplegia, monoplegia, or paraplegia due to communicating hydrocephalus. Occlusion of the *lateral sinus* produces pain over the ear and mastoid and may cause edema over the mastoid (Griesinger's sign). Involvement of the fifth and sixth cranial nerves produces ipsilateral facial pain and lateral rectus weakness (Gradenigo's syndrome). The early clinical manifestations of mycotic aneurysms are similar to those of cerebral emboli and infarction. The weakened vessel may be seen to increase in size progressively on serial angiograms. The funduscopic examination is particularly useful for the detection of an embolic source of infection because the ophthalmic artery is a branch of the internal carotid artery, and septic embolization within the anterior circulation may produce characteristic visual field defects and retinal lesions.

LABORATORY FINDINGS

Skull radiographs may also show pineal shift and evidence of sinusitis or mastoiditis. LP reveals increased intracranial pressure, a slight lymphocytic pleocytosis, and slightly elevated protein concentration. The CSF is usually sterile. MRI with angiography is the procedure of choice for the diagnosis of intracranial suppurative thrombophlebitis and mycotic aneurysm because of its ability to distinguish between flowing blood and thrombus. Angiography with close attention to the venous phase for evidence of nonfilling should be considered if venous sinus thrombophlebitis is suspected despite negative CT or MRI. Radionuclide scans may also be helpful. Abscess can be excluded by either CT or MRI. Cavernous sinus thrombosis is readily detected by CT. The definitive diagnosis of mycotic aneurysm requires the combination of both CT or MRI and angiography.

OPTIMAL MANAGEMENT

Treatment of septic cranial thrombophlebitis requires maximum dosages of intravenous antibiotics (Table 431.6) and surgical decompression of the underlying predisposing infection. Anticoagulation is controversial, and glucocorticoids or osmotic diuretics may be required to control intracranial hypertension. Internal jugular vein ligation has been used in lateral sinus thrombosis, and in a few instances thrombectomy has been successful. Antimicrobial therapy of mycotic aneurysm is directed at the causative organism of the underlying endarteritis, often associated with positive blood cultures. Prolonged treatment with high-dose intravenous antibiotics for at least 6 to 8 weeks is required. Because the clinical course of a mycotic aneurysm is variable and the risk of rupture with catastrophic cerebral hemorrhage cannot be predicted even after successful therapy of the underlying endocarditis, early surgical intervention is advised. Fortunately, these vascular lesions tend to occur in the distal branches of the middle or anterior cerebral arteries and hence are relatively accessible for surgical ligation or resection.

■ NEUROSYPHILIS

INCIDENCE, EPIDEMIOLOGY, AND ETIOLOGY

The incidence of syphilis has increased since the mid-1980s. It is the most chronic form of meningitis and has become an increasingly important complication in women with AIDS and in their newborn infants. From a preventive standpoint, asymptomatic neurosyphilis is the most important because it is during this phase of the disease that spread mostly occurs.

PATHOGENESIS

Up to 10% of patients with primary syphilis and 30% to 70% with secondary syphilis have pleocytosis of the CSF with a nor-

mal or slightly elevated CSF protein concentration, probably as the result of meningovasculitis induced by transient treponemia. In a proportion of such patients, meningovasculitis persists as evidenced by elevated treponemal antibodies in the CSF. This condition, without neurologic signs or symptoms, is called *asymptomatic neurosyphilis.* When not adequately treated, 7% to 9% of patients with asymptomatic neurosyphilis go on to have symptomatic neurosyphilis. Invasion of the CNS occurs from 3 to 18 months after initial infection. The early phases of neurosyphilis usually occur within 5 years after initial infection and are caused by treponemal obliterative endarteritis, meningitis or by meningovasculitis at a cerebral or spinal level. These early syndromes can present as transient ischemic attacks, pachymeningitis, or leptomeningitis. The late parenchymatous syndromes occur 5 to 25 years after infection and are primarily caused by neurovascular involvement. Clinically, these syndromes present as tabes dorsalis, general paresis, taboparalysis, syphilitic optic atrophy, and spinal syphilis. Tertiary granulomatous lesions (gummata) are rare today.

CLINICAL FINDINGS

Patients with meningeal syphilis present with headache, stiff neck, cranial nerve palsies, convulsions, and confusion without fever. Meningovascular syphilis may present 6 to 7 years after infection as a stroke (hemiplegia, aphasia, sensory loss, visual disturbance, or mental confusion). Tabes dorsalis is a degeneration of the afferent fibers of the dorsal spinal roots, the cranial nerves, and the sympathetic fibers. Sensory loss, ataxia, muscle hypotonia, and loss of tendon reflexes in the legs are the hallmarks. Impotence, sphincter disturbances, "lightning" pains in the legs, painful functional disorders of the viscera ("tabetic crisis"), and Argyll–Robertson pupils also occur. In general paresis, intellectual deterioration occurs (memory disturbances, poor judgment, delusions), often accompanied by epileptic attacks, slurred speech, Argyll–Robertson pupils, weakness, and fast tic-like movements in the face (*wetterleuchten*). Tabes and general paresis can occur together as taboparalysis. Partial expressions ("formes frustes") of the classic syndromes occur frequently. Syphilitic optic atrophy produces sequential and progressive blindness. Visual fields are constricted. Spinal syphilis manifests as either syphilitic meningomyelitis (Erb's spastic paraplegia, bilateral corticospinal tract signs) or spinal meningovascular syphilis (anterior spinal artery syndrome).

LABORATORY FINDINGS

Active treponemal infection of the CNS is detected by the local production of specific treponemal antibodies (e.g., *Treponema pallidum* hemagglutination assay [TPHA]) in the CSF. This can be measured either by the presence of CSF antitreponemal IgM antibody (TPHA-IgM) or by determining the CSF:serum ratio of TPHA-IgG titers. In the latter instance, the normal range of the CSF:serum TPHA-IgG ratio is between 0.5 and 2.0. In active neurosyphilis, this ratio is increased to 3.0 or higher. The CSF in neurosyphilis may show lymphocytic pleocytosis, normal glucose, and normal or slightly elevated protein concentration. A negative CSF treponemal antibody test (e.g., fluorescent treponemal antibody unabsorbed or TPHA-IgG) virtually rules out neurosyphilis in patients with late disease, but not in those with early disease.

OPTIMAL MANAGEMENT

The treatment of neurosyphilis is aqueous penicillin G, 0.15 million U per kilogram intravenously per day for 15 days in six divided doses. In patients who are allergic to penicillin, tetracycline hydrochloride, or erythromycin, 2 g daily for 30 days is required. Follow-up evaluation by repeating the LP at 6 months is recommended.

LYME DISEASE

INCIDENCE, EPIDEMIOLOGY, AND ETIOLOGY

Lyme disease is caused by the spirochete *Borrelia burgdorferi*. The vector is the common ixodid tick. Although Lyme disease occurs in 43 states and in many countries around the world, in the United States the disease is concentrated along the coastal plains of the Northeast and mid-Atlantic regions, in the upper Midwest, and to a lesser degree along the Pacific coast. Exposure is most common in meadows or woodlands, but infection may also occur in suburban settings.

PATHOGENESIS

The precise pathogenesis of Lyme disease, particularly CNS involvement, is not totally clear. In the early stages of infection, within 3 days to 3 weeks after exposure, a typical skin rash (erythema chronicum migrans [ECM]) occurs in over two thirds of cases. This is accompanied by a flulike illness with fever, headache, stiff neck, arthralgia, myalgia, and regional lymphadenopathy in about 50% of cases. Like neurosyphilis, the early neurologic manifestations of Lyme disease are probably secondary to meningovascular involvement. The late stages of Lyme disease include debilitating arthritis; neurologic manifestations such as fatigue, chronic encephalomyelitis, paraparesis, ataxia, polyradiculopathy, depression, and dementia; and cardiac complications such as heart block, myocarditis, or left ventricular dysfunction. It is suggested that the development and deposition of immune complexes in the skin, synovium, or neural or cardiac tissues is the underlying pathogenesis for the multisystem involvement seen in those with Lyme disease.

CLINICAL FINDINGS

The most distinctive clinical feature of Lyme disease is the large, flat, annular skin lesion of ECM. These skin lesions may be single or multiple and often reach a very large size with a zone of central clearing. Arthritis is the most common complication (45% of cases), followed by neurologic (11%) and cardiac (8%) manifestations. The neurologic presentations are protean, including aseptic meningitis, encephalitis, chorea, cerebellar ataxia, cranial neuritis, motor and sensory radiculoneuritis, mononeuritis multiplex, and myelitis, each in various combinations. The

usual pattern is a fluctuating meningoencephalitis with superimposed cranial and peripheral radiculopathy. These neurologic findings usually appear early in the course, within days to weeks after the antecedent tick bite, often while the ECM is still present or within 1 to 6 weeks after the skin rash has faded.

The onset of meningitis is suggested by intermittent attacks of severe, prostrating headaches with stiff neck, nausea, vomiting, and photophobia, alternating with periods of mild infrequent headache for another several weeks. Symptoms of encephalitis include somnolence, emotional lability, depression, poor memory and concentration, or behavioral changes. The most common manifestation of cranial neuritis is unilateral or bilateral facial palsy. Radiculoneuritis may be motor, sensory, or both. Shoulder girdle neuritis, indistinguishable clinically from neuralgic amyotrophy, is the most common motor radiculopathy. Sensory symptoms include regional or generalized cutaneous hyperesthesia to touch or temperature.

LABORATORY FINDINGS

Lyme disease is diagnosed primarily by the clinical presentation, the classic ECM skin lesions, a history of tick bite or exposure, and the exclusion of other conditions. Confirmation by laboratory diagnosis requires the demonstration of specific serum antibodies to *B. burgdorferi*, either by enzyme-linked immunosorbent assay or by immunoblot techniques. Unfortunately, interpretation of results may be complicated because of poor sensitivity and presence of cross-reactive antibodies to indigenous or other spirochetes. Elevated CSF antibody titer to *B. burgdorferi* compared with serum levels is probably a more sensitive method for making the diagnosis of Lyme neuroborreliosis than serum antibody titers alone. Polymerase chain reaction (PCR) directed at *B. burgdorferi* DNA in the CSF may be helpful. Unfortunately, since PCR does not differentiate between live and dead organisms, it cannot be used to prove active infection. CSF examination in Lyme neuroborreliosis may reveal variable or minimal inflammation. MRI scans may show areas of increased density that are consistent with demyelination. Although such patients often have specific antibody to *B. burgdorferi* in the CSF, a test that unequivocally indicates active infection in the CNS with this organism is lacking. Direct isolation of *B. burgdorferi* from the blood or CSF is difficult and a low-yield procedure.

OPTIMAL MANAGEMENT

Patients in whom frank meningitis, encephalitis, or cranial and peripheral neuropathies develop may be treated with intravenous penicillin G (20 million U per day for 10 to 14 days in four to six divided doses). Headache, stiff neck, and radicular pain usually begin to subside by the second day of therapy and are often completely resolved by 7 to 10 days. Motor deficits, however, frequently require 7 to 8 weeks for complete recovery. Ceftriaxone, 2 g per day in one or two divided doses for 14 days, has also been used successfully in patients with Lyme neuroborreliosis. Patients allergic to penicillin may be treated with tetracycline (2 g per day in four divided doses) or doxycycline (400 mg per day in two divided doses) for 10 to 20 days. There is no established role for the use of corticosteroids in addition to antibiotic treatment in Lyme neuroborreliosis.

BIBLIOGRAPHY

Aronin SI, Peduzzi P, Quagliarello VJ. Community-acquired bacterial meningitis: risk stratification for adverse clinical outcome and effect of antibiotic timing. *Ann Intern Med* 1998;129:862–869.

Bradley JS, Scheld WM. The challenge of penicillin-resistant *Streptococcus pneumoniae* meningitis: current antibiotic therapy in the 1990s. *Clin Infect Dis* 1997;24(suppl 2):S213–S221.

Chow AW. Life-threatening infections of the head and neck. *Clin Infect Dis* 1992;14:991–1002.

Danner RL, Hartman BJ. Update of spinal epidural abscess: 35 cases and review of the literature. *Rev Infect Dis* 1987;9:265–274.

D'Antuono VS, Brown I. Successful treatment of *Enterobacter* meningitis with ciprofloxacin. *Clin Infect Dis* 1998;26:206–207.

Halperin JJ. Nervous system Lyme disease. *J Neurol Sci* 1998;153:182–191.

Kapeller P, Fazekas F, Krametter D, et al. Pyogenic infectious spondylitis: clinical, laboratory and MRI features. *Eur Neurol* 1997;38:94–98.

Kim YS, Liu QX, Chow LL, et al. Trovafloxacin in treatment of rabbits with experimental meningitis caused by high-level penicillin-resistant *Streptococcus pneumoniae*. *Antimicrob Agents Chemother* 1997;41:1186–1189.

Koivunen P, Löppönen H, Syrjälä H. Epidural abscess due to deep-neck infection. *Clin Infect Dis* 1998;26:1461–1462.

Lew D, Southwick FS, Montgomery WW, et al. Sphenoid sinusitis: a review of 30 cases. *N Engl J Med* 1983;309:1149–1154.

Luby JP. Infections of the central nervous system. *Am J Med Sci* 1992;304:379–391.

Mackenzie AR, Laing RBS, Smith CC, et al. Spinal epidural abscess: the importance of early diagnosis and treatment. *J Neurol Neurosurg Psychiatry* 1998;65:209–212.

Mastroianni CM, Lancella L, Mengoni F, et al. Chemokine profiles in the cerebrospinal fluid (CSF) during the course of pyogenic and tuberculous meningitis. *Clin Exp Immunol* 1998;114:210–214.

Mathisen GE, Johnson JP. Brain abscess. *Clin Infect Dis* 1997;25:763–779.

McIntyre PB, Berkey CS, King SM, et al. Dexamethasone as adjunctive therapy in bacterial meningitis. A meta-analysis of randomized clinical trials since 1988. *JAMA* 1997;278:925–931.

Ostergaard C, Sorensen TK, Knudsen JD, et al. Evaluation of moxifloxacin, a new 8-methoxyquinolone, for treatment of meningitis caused by a penicillin-resistant pneumococcus in rabbits. *Antimicrob Agents Chemother* 1998;42:1706–1712.

Quagliarello VJ, Scheld WM. Treatment of bacterial meningitis. *N Engl J Med* 1997;336:708–716.

Satoskar AR. Chemotherapy for tuberculous meningitis in adults. *Clin Infect Dis* 1997;24:743.

Schuchat A, Robinson K, Wenger JD, et al. Bacterial meningitis in the United States in 1995. *N Engl J Med* 1997;337:970–976.

Sigurdardóttir B, Björnsson OM, Jónsdottir KE, et al. Acute bacterial meningitis in adults. A 20-year overview. *Arch Intern Med* 1997;157:425–430.

Steere AC, Sikand VK, Meurice F, et al. Vaccination against Lyme disease with recombinant *Borrelia burgdorferi* outer-surface lipoprotein A with adjuvant. Lyme Disease Vaccine Study Group. *N Engl J Med* 1998;339:209–215.

Townsend GC, Scheld WM. Microbe-endothelium interactions in blood-brain barrier permeability during bacterial meningitis. *ASM News* 1995;61:294–298.

Tunkel AR, Scheld WM. Pathogenesis and pathophysiology of bacterial meningitis. *Clin Microbiol Rev* 1993;6:118–136.

Kelley's Textbook of Internal Medicine, fourth edition. Edited by H. David Humes.
Lippincott Williams & Wilkins, Philadelphia © 2000.

VIRAL INFECTIONS OF THE NERVOUS SYSTEM

JORGE T. GONZALEZ

This chapter deals with four neurologic clinical syndromes that can result from a viral process. The first three syndromes, aseptic meningitis, encephalitis, and poliomyelitis, involve the central nervous system (CNS). The fourth syndrome, herpes zoster ganglionitis, primarily involves the peripheral nervous system. Slow virus infections, HIV infection, and other causes of aseptic meningitis are discussed in separate chapters.

Depending on their ability to infect certain cell populations (i.e., meningeal cells, brain parenchymal cells), many viruses that affect the nervous system have a distinct, although not exclusive, predisposition to manifest as a particular clinical syndrome. For example, enteroviruses are the most common causes of aseptic meningitis, but occasionally cause severe encephalitis. Conversely, arboviruses are common causes of encephalitis but sometimes lead to aseptic meningitis. Specific viruses are discussed in association with the clinical syndromes with which they are most commonly associated.

PATHOGENESIS

As a rule, neurologic manifestations of viral infections represent a small percentage of all infections. Most infective viral agents gain access to the CNS through hematogenous spread. The initial viremia usually is transient and is followed by a phase of viral replication in the reticuloendothelial system and sometimes in muscle tissue. The degree of secondary viremia that follows determines whether successful infection of the CNS will continue.

Viral invasion of the CNS can occur by several mechanisms. The virus may cross the blood–brain barrier directly, or it may infect leukocytes initially, which then cross the disrupted blood–brain barrier. It also may infect endothelial cells, adjacent glial cells, and neurons. On histopathology, this is seen as endothelial inflammation and lymphocytic infiltration of the perivascular areas and surrounding gray matter. Some viruses, such as the mumps virus, cross through the epithelium of the choroid plexus before spreading to the ependyma and parenchyma. Once in the subarachnoid space, the organisms can spread contiguously, through infected leukocytes or along axons, dendrites, and other cell processes. Alternatively, there are three known organisms that can penetrate the CNS through peripheral and olfactory nerves. Herpes simplex virus 1 and *Naegleria fowleri* reach the CNS by extension from the olfactory bulbs. In contrast, the rabies virus spreads from the site of inoculation to the CNS along the motor and sensory fibers.

In acute viral encephalitis, the virus produces parenchymal inflammation by cytotoxicity and lysis of infected cells or by initiation of an immunologic reaction against parenchymal cells. With progression of the disease, histopathologic changes include astrocytosis and gliosis. Cowdry type A and B bodies, which are intranuclear inclusions, are associated with herpesvirus, adenovirus, and the measles virus. Intracytoplasmic inclusions are found in cytomegalovirus encephalitis, and Negri bodies are pathognomonic of the rabies virus. The extent of the pathology depends partly on the type of virus involved. For example, infections with herpes simplex virus 1 and eastern equine virus can lead to severe and widespread neuronal dysfunction, whereas infections with viruses such as the LaCrosse virus usually have milder presentations.

CLINICAL SYNDROMES

VIRAL MENINGITIS

Viral meningitis is inflammation of the meninges due to viral organisms. It is the most common cause of aseptic meningitis, which is characterized by cerebrospinal fluid (CSF) lymphocytic pleiocytosis. By definition, there is no evidence of a bacterial, fungal, protozoal, or parasitic organism.

Incidence and Epidemiology

From 1983 to 1993, the yearly incidence of aseptic meningitis ranged from 8,300 to 12,800 cases. Enteroviruses are most commonly associated with this syndrome, accounting for up to 80% of all cases. The mumps virus has been described as the second most common cause, but its incidence has decreased substantially with vaccination.

Factors that influence the epidemiology of viral meningitis include season, geographic location, and climate. Indirectly, these factors provide significant clues to the identity of the causative agent (Table 442.1). In North America, the enteroviruses and arboviruses are most prevalent in summer and early fall. Between fall and winter, the incidence of lymphocytic choriomeningitis increases, whereas in winter and spring, mumps tends to be more common. In general, viral meningitis is most prevalent during summer, peaking between August and October, which essentially reflects the incidence of the enteroviruses.

Specific Viruses That Cause Meningitis

Enteroviruses

Enteroviruses are RNA viruses that belong to the picornavirus group. They have a worldwide distribution and humans are their only natural hosts. They inhabit the gastrointestinal tract and are spread by the fecal–oral route. Enterovirus infection is most common during summer and fall in temperate countries but has no seasonal prevalence in the tropics. It accounts for 80% to 92% of all cases of aseptic meningitis. Epidemics of aseptic meningitis have been described in young infants.

Because patients with enterovirus infection present with a nonspecific aseptic meningitis picture, evidence of its presence may circumstantially depend on the season, associated signs and

TABLE 442.1.	CLINICAL EPIDEMIOLOGY OF VIRAL MENINGITIS AND ENCEPHALITIS	
Agent	**Characteristic Clinical Findings or History**	**Season/Epidemiology**
Enteroviruses	Myocarditis, pleurodynia, conjunctivitis, rash	Summer/fall; epidemic and sporadic
Lymphocytic choriomeningitis	Contact with rodents; rash, arthralgia, orchitis, myocarditis	Winter; sporadic
Herpes simplex type 2	Primary genital lesions	No seasonality; sporadic
Mumps	Parotitis, orchitis, pancreatitis	Spring/summer; sporadic
Herpes simplex type 1	Focal neurologic deficits	No seasonality; sporadic
Varicella zoster virus	Characteristic rash, cerebellar ataxia	No seasonality; sporadic
Human herpesvirus 6	Focal neurologic presentation	No seasonality
Epstein–Barr virus/ cytomegalovirus	Mononucleosis syndrome, immunosuppression	No seasonality; sporadic
Eastern equine virus	Mosquito-borne; severe encephalopathy	Summer; epidemic, eastern coastal states
Western equine virus	Mosquito-borne; focal seizures	Summer; epidemic western US and Canada
St. Louis virus	Mosquito-borne; dysuria; SIADH; myalgia	Summer; epidemic; southeastern and midwestern US
California virus	Generalized and focal seizures	Summer; epidemic; north central states
Rabies	History of animal bite; dysphagia	No seasonality; sporadic

SIADH syndrome of inappropriate antidiuretic hormone secretion.

symptoms, and knowledge of an ongoing epidemic. The organism may be cultured from any specimen (i.e., CSF, nasopharyngeal swab). However, growth from stool specimens may not be causally related because the organism can stay in the lower gastrointestinal tract for as long as 8 to 12 weeks. Thirty-one serotypes of echovirus, 23 serotypes of coxsackievirus A, six serotypes of coxsackievirus B, and three serotypes of poliovirus have been identified as pathogens in human CNS infections.

Examination of the CSF usually reveals a leukocyte count of less than 500 cells per microliter, with lymphocytic predominance in 48 hours, although up to two thirds of patients have polymorphonuclear predominance initially. The protein level is mildly elevated and the glucose level usually is normal but may be low in up to 18% of cases. Polymerase chain reaction (PCR) techniques are currently available to detect enteroviruses in the CSF with a sensitivity of 85%.

Encephalitis, ataxia, paralysis, and learning disabilities in children are rare complications. In children with agammaglobulinemia, a complication consisting of a dermatomyositis-like syndrome and edema may develop and responds to treatment with intravenous γ-globulin.

Mumps Virus

Mumps is caused by a single-stranded paramyxovirus. Similar to the enteroviruses, the mumps virus has a ubiquitous distribution, but it occurs more commonly during late winter and spring in temperate areas. The mumps virus is spread by respiratory droplet infection or direct contact with saliva and infects primarily the parotids, testes, ovaries, mammary glands, pancreas, and, occasionally, CNS. Involvement of the CNS may be manifested as a meningitis, encephalitis, or meningoencephalitis. Mumps meningitis usually is a benign syndrome with a male:female ratio of 2 to 5. In a few cases, it causes unilateral deafness from cochlear inflammation. Other rare complications include polyradiculitis, cranial nerve palsy, and seizures. The diagnosis is based on the clinical picture of parotitis (50% of cases) or other glandular involvement. This can be confirmed by isolation of the virus from CSF, saliva, or urine. Serologic diagnosis of a recent infection can be established by complement fixation or by documentation of fourfold rise in antibody titers. The CSF leukocyte count is predominantly lymphocytic, ranging from 5 to 500 cells per microliter. The CSF protein level is mildly increased and the glucose level is normal; however, in 5% to 15% of cases, hypoglycorrhachia may be observed. Although 50% to 90% of patients with mumps parotitis have CSF pleocytosis, only 1% to 10% have symptomatic meningitis.

Lymphocytic Choriomeningitis Virus

The virus that causes lymphocytic choriomeningitis is an arenavirus that is transmitted to humans through the inhalation or ingestion of food or particles contaminated with the urine, feces, and other secretions of infected rodents. It does not have any seasonal prevalence, although the incidence is increased slightly during winter, which may reflect increased contact with the common house mouse that typically enters the warmer environment of a household. During the early stages, the patient experiences

a nonspecific viral prodrome with fever, retro-orbital headache, myalgia, arthralgia, rash, and respiratory symptoms. As in mumps, parotitis with or without orchitis may occur. The disease course usually is self-limited, especially if the infection is confined to an aseptic meningitis; however, a severe encephalitis may be part of the clinical picture. Other complications at later stages include orchitis, arthritis, myocarditis, and alopecia.

Examination of the CSF may reveal an unusually high leukocyte count (more than 1,000 cells per microliter) with lymphocytic predominance. Hypoglycorrhachia also may be seen in 25% of cases, and a complete blood count may demonstrate leukopenia and thrombocytopenia.

The virus can be cultured early from blood and CSF and at later stages from urine. Commonly, a fourfold rise of titers in the serum has been used to confirm the diagnosis. The presence of IgM antibody in the blood and CSF may indicate recent infection.

Herpes Simplex Virus

Herpes simplex meningitis usually is caused by herpes simplex virus type 2 that has spread hematogenously from a primary infection, often of the genitourinary tract. Typically, herpes simplex type 2 meningitis is a benign, self-limited disease that affects young, sexually active adults. An active genital lesion often is present. Occasionally, herpes simplex virus type 1 causes aseptic meningitis, but it has a much greater predisposition for meningoencephalitis.

In a few reported cases, a recurrent meningitis has been associated with a sacral radiculitis and low segment myelitis. Similar complications have been observed in patients with AIDS.

Examination of the CSF reveals lymphocytic pleocytosis, which may be as high as 2,600 cells per microliter; a protein level greater than 110 mg per deciliter in more than 50% of cases; and, occasionally, hypoglycorrhachia. A definitive diagnosis can be established by CSF culture, although isolation often is unsuccessful. A fourfold rise in titers can help confirm the diagnosis. If available, use of the PCR test can be sensitive and specific.

Treatment with acyclovir is not necessary unless a primary genital infection is evident.

Mollaret Meningitis

Herpes simplex virus has been detected by PCR in Mollaret meningitis, which is characterized by recurrent benign episodes of meningitic symptoms and fever lasting 1 to 3 days. An initial CSF pleiocytosis with predominance of polymorphonuclear neutrophiles and endothelial leukocytosis on the first day is followed by CSF lymphocytosis. With an active primary genital infection, intravenous acyclovir is recommended. If none, oral acyclovir 200 mg five times per day for 5 days may suffice.

Other Herpesvirus Meningitides

Varicella-zoster virus and Epstein–Barr virus have been associated with aseptic meningitis and have a benign course if the infection remains limited to the meninges. Epstein–Barr virus meningitis usually occurs in the setting of infectious mononucleosis, and also may have features of encephalitis. The CSF profile is characterized by atypical lymphocytes, mononuclear cells, an increased protein level, and heterophile antibodies. Cytomegalovirus meningitis is common in immunocompromised patients.

Clinical Findings

In general, patients with viral meningitis present with a sudden or gradual onset of headache, low- to moderate-grade fever, and mild neck stiffness. Malaise, myalgia, nausea, and vomiting may occur. Photophobia and, occasionally, mental confusion may be present. Although the clinical presentations may be similar, certain findings are associated with specific viral agents (i.e., parotitis with the mumps virus, cutaneous genital lesions with herpesviruses, conjunctivitis with enteroviruses).

The differential diagnosis of viral meningitis includes all other causes of aseptic meningitis (Table 442.2). Nonviral infections, such as partially treated bacterial infections, parameningeal processes, Lyme disease, tuberculosis, and *Mycoplasma*, fungal, parasitic, and protozoal infections, may have similar clinical and CSF presentations. In addition, noninfectious causes, such as neoplastic processes, connective tissue diseases, sarcoidosis, and various drugs, should be included in the differential diagnosis. Appropriate testing should be performed based on the overall assessment to exclude the treatable causes.

Laboratory Findings

The primary objective of the laboratory evaluation is to confirm the clinical diagnosis of a meningitic process and, if possible, identify the causative agent. However, in many cases, the diagnosis of an aseptic meningitis is made, but the agent cannot be identified.

The CSF examination is the most important step in establishing the presence of a viral meningitis. Typically, CSF findings include lymphocytic pleocytosis with a leukocyte count of less than 1,000 cells per microliter, a normal glucose level, and a slightly to moderately elevated total protein level (usually less than 80 to 100 mg per deciliter). Transient polymorphonuclear cell predominance may be seen in the initial stages but soon shifts to a lymphocytic predominance. Up to 14% of all patients with acute bacterial meningitis present with this picture. In addition, some cases of enterovirus meningitis are associated with a persistent polymorphonuclear cell predominance. Certain unique findings also are associated with some virologic agents, such as hypoglycorrhachia in some cases of mumps, herpes virus infection, or lymphocytic choriomeningitis.

Culturing the virus from a reliable source, preferably the CSF, is the most definitive way of identifying the agent involved. The usefulness of this test depends on the rapidity with which results can be obtained and on the sensitivity, which can range from almost nil for herpes simplex virus type 2 to between 40% and 80% for the enteroviruses.

PCR testing, when available, is being used increasingly to identify many organisms, including herpes simplex virus types 1 and 2, varicella-zoster virus, Epstein–Barr virus, cytomegalovirus, enteroviruses, HIV, and JC virus. PCR has been performed on human herpesvirus 6, lymphocytic choriomeningitis virus, measles, mumps, and adenovirus. This technique allows rapid and accurate diagnosis of an organism with results potentially available in a few hours. Moreover, it avoids unnecessary investigation or antibiotic treatment and may lead to early discharge of the patient.

The results of other routine laboratory tests usually are normal. However, these tests still should be performed because some abnormalities may occur that are characteristic of specific viruses, such as thrombocytopenia and leukopenia with the lymphocytic choriomeningitis virus.

Neuroradiologic imaging does not play an important role in meningitis unless there is parenchymal involvement. However, with the improved resolution achieved by modern scanners and with the use of contrast agents, meningeal enhancement sometimes can be seen.

Optimal Management

Please refer to Chapter 431 for information regarding the treatment of viral meningitis.

VIRAL ENCEPHALITIS

Viral encephalitis is an inflammation of the brain parenchyma caused by a virus. It manifests as a syndrome that begins with a viral prodrome of fever, headache, nausea, and vomiting, followed by an encephalopathy characterized by altered mental status, behavioral changes, and convulsions. Focal neurologic deficits may occur in the form of aphasia, hemiparesis, partial seizures, ataxia, or cranial nerve palsy. In severe cases, progression to a fatal coma and death may result.

TABLE 442.2.	NONVIRAL CAUSES OF ASEPTIC MENINGITIS AND ENCEPHALITIS

Leptospirosis (Weil's disease)
Tuberculosis
Toxoplasmosis
Rocky Mountain spotted fever
Mycoplasma infection
Lyme disease
Cryptococcosis
Coccidioidomycosis
Histoplasmosis
Amebic meningoencephalitis
Cysticercosis
Parameningeal processes
Paragonimiasis
Toxocariasis
Schistosomiasis
Systemic lupus erythematosus/Sjögren's syndrome
Uveomeningoencephalitis (Vogt–Koyanagi–Harada syndrome)
Behçet's disease
Whipple's disease
Sarcoidosis
Mollaret's disease
Granulomatous angiitis

It is not always possible to differentiate viral encephalitis from viral meningitis based on the physical examination alone. Moreover, nuchal rigidity and photophobia may be present, giving credence to the term *meningoencephalitis*.

Incidence and Epidemiology

According to the Centers for Disease Control and Prevention, the reported yearly incidence of viral encephalitis in the United States has ranged from 800 to 1,700 cases over the past 10 years. Postinfectious encephalitis accounts for an additional 100 cases per year. However, these figures may represent only 18% to 60% of the actual number of cases. Furthermore, a specific virus is identified in only 25% of the reported cases.

Herpes simplex virus is the most common cause of sporadic encephalitis, accounting for about 10% of all reported cases. Collectively, the arboviruses account for another 10% of cases, and for as many as 50% during epidemics. In the United States, California encephalitis and St. Louis encephalitis are the most common forms of the disease. However, Japanese B encephalitis is the most common epidemic viral encephalitis worldwide. In immunocompetent patients, other viral agents, such as the rabies virus, enteroviruses, the mumps virus, the rubella virus, Epstein–Barr virus, and the measles virus, cause encephalitis much less commonly.

Specific Viruses That Cause Encephalitis

Herpes Simplex Virus

Herpes simplex encephalitis is a potentially devastating and often fatal disease with an estimated incidence of 1 per 250,000 to 500,000 population per year. Most cases in older children and adults are caused by herpes simplex virus type 1, but in neonates, herpes simplex virus type 2 is involved. The initial presentation usually is a nonspecific fever, headache, and lethargy progressing to a more profound altered mental status. In more than 85% of cases, focal neurologic deficits such as cranial nerve palsy,

autonomic dysfunction, hemiparesis, and focal seizures are observed. Untreated, patients quickly deteriorate into a coma and 60% to 80% of them die.

Much of the pathology is in the orbitofrontal and temporal lobes, where localized or widespread hemorrhagic necrosis can be found (Fig. 442.1). Microscopically, neuronal necrosis, polymorphonuclear cells, hemorrhage, and intranuclear Cowdry type A inclusions in neurons and glial cells are evident. Based on animal models, in 30% of cases, primary infection is hypothesized to occur as the virus spreads along olfactory nerve fibers to the CNS after intranasal inoculation. In most cases, it is postulated that latent virus in the trigeminal ganglia from a previous infection is reactivated and spreads anterogradely to involve the temporal and orbitofrontal lobes.

The CSF leukocyte count usually is less than 500 cells per microliter with lymphocytic predominance, and red blood cells are seen in 80% of cases. The protein level commonly is elevated and the glucose level is normal, although hypoglycorrhachia occasionally is observed. However, CSF findings initially are normal in almost 10% of cases. Culture of the virus from the CSF is difficult and other serologic methods, such as immunoblot assay, immunofluorescence, and enzyme-linked immunosorbent assay, usually are not helpful early in the disease course, when a definitive diagnosis is crucial. Neuroimaging studies, particularly magnetic resonance imaging (MRI), can demonstrate the lesions in characteristic areas, but are nonspecific (Fig. 442.2). The finding of focal slowing or epileptiform discharges on electroencephalography is fairly sensitive and has been shown to correlate in 80% of cases.

In current practice, PCR testing for the detection of herpes simplex virus in the CSF is the norm. False-negatives, however, can occur very early in the course; thus, a second lumbar puncture may need to be considered 24 to 48 hours later in suspected cases. PCR is usually negative 2 weeks after onset of symptoms. Determination of herpes simplex virus antibody in serum and CSF may also be helpful in the diagnosis, especially if the PCR result is not convincingly positive. A serum to CSF ratio of less

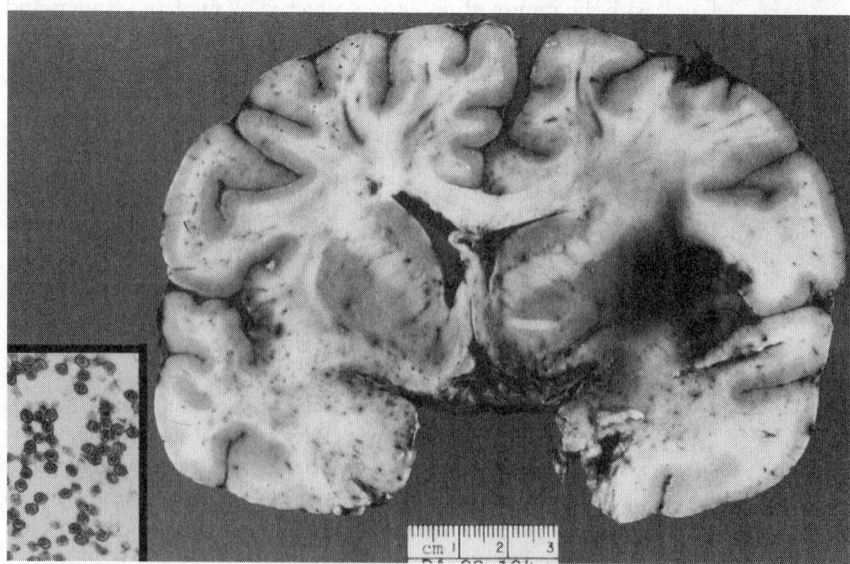

FIGURE 442.1. Gross appearance of a brain infected with herpes simplex virus type I. Note the multiple hemorrhagic encephalomalacia with mass effect involving the temporal and insular lobes on the right. The inset depicts the typical viral nucleocapsid of the herpesvirus.

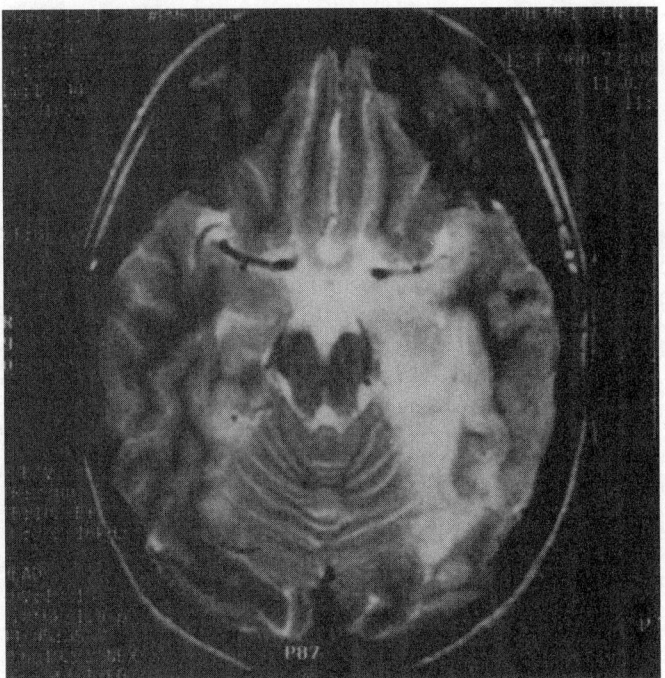

FIGURE 442.2. Herpes encephalitis. The T2-weighted magnetic resonance image shows multiple foci of increased signal primarily in medial aspect of the left temporal lobe with extension to the inferior occipital lobe. There is also some lesser involvement on the right side in similar areas.

than 20:1 of herpes simplex virus antibody implies intrathecal synthesis. This process occurs in the first week of onset of symptoms up to the fourth week. Brain biopsy has been advocated as the gold standard for the diagnosis of herpes encephalitis but is now rarely performed. Specimens should be evaluated by electron microscopy, antigen testing by immunofluorescence, and, most important, viral culture, which is 90% sensitive and 100% specific.

Herpes simplex virus encephalitis is treated with intravenous acyclovir 10 mg per kilogram (ideal body weight) every 8 hours for 10 to 21 days.

Arboviruses

The arboviruses that commonly cause viral encephalitis in humans include the togaviruses (alphavirus), flaviviruses, bunyaviruses, and reoviruses. The most commonly encountered arbovirus infections in the United States are California encephalitis (bunyavirus), St. Louis encephalitis (flavivirus), western equine encephalitis (alphavirus), and eastern equine encephalitis (alphavirus). Venezuelan equine encephalitis, Powassan encephalitis, and Colorado tick fever are reported less often. These viruses are most prevalent during the summer months, just after the mosquito population peaks. In most cases, the clinical and CSF findings are similar and nonspecific. However, serologic testing, especially complement fixation antibodies, is useful in establishing the diagnosis. For some of these viruses, inapparent infection may account for up to 90% of cases.

Western equine encephalitis usually occurs in the western

United States and Canada during the summer months, following the geographic distribution of its vector, the *Culex tarsalis* mosquito. Young children and inhabitants of rural areas are at higher risk for infection with this virus. The incubation period lasts 5 to 20 days and is followed by a prodrome of nonspecific fever, general malaise, vomiting, and myalgia. The severity of the disease ranges from a mild febrile illness to a severe encephalopathy with a mortality rate of 5% to 15% in some series. Full recovery is the rule, although developmental delay, seizure disorder, and paralysis have occurred in children. In adults, postencephalitic parkinsonism after the acute phase has been described.

Eastern equine encephalitis occurs primarily in eastern coastal states, particularly in New England. The virus is transmitted to humans by *Aedes* mosquitoes. Although the disease is not as prevalent, it can cause widespread parenchymal destruction involving whole lobes, similar to herpes simplex virus type 1 encephalitis. This is in contrast to the microscopic lesions caused by other arboviruses. Reportedly, up to one third of patients die and another third have serious morbidity, such as mental retardation, seizures, and hemiplegia.

St. Louis encephalitis has been an important cause of epidemics in the midwestern and southeastern United States. Depending on the region, the virus is transmitted by different *Culex* mosquitoes. The illness is most severe in patients older than 60 years of age. An influenza-like prodrome of fever, headache, and malaise occurs initially, followed by symptoms of encephalitis. Occasionally, severe muscle aches, dysuria, and pyuria are observed. The syndrome of inappropriate antidiuretic hormone secretion also is encountered in up to 25% of cases. More than 90% of patients recover without any sequelae, although some, especially the elderly, are prone to complications such as behavioral disorders, memory loss, and seizures. The elderly also have a higher risk for increased mortality, with rates up to 19.5%.

California encephalitis (LaCrosse virus) is the most common viral encephalitis in the United States. Similar to the other arbovirus infections, it is more common during the summer months and has a propensity for rural areas in which the mosquito vector, *Aedes triseriatus,* inhabits stagnant water. In addition to the usual prodrome and encephalitic picture, generalized and partial seizures occur in 60% of infected children but are less common in adults. Mild variants of the disease are associated with full recovery, but severe infections lead to focal neurologic findings such as aphasia and hemiparesis in up to 25% of cases.

Rabies Virus

The yearly incidence of human rabies in the United States is none to three cases, comparatively much less than the hundreds of cases reported worldwide. This low rate can be attributed to the standardized vaccination of domestic animals. Wild animals such as skunks, foxes, raccoons, bats, and coyotes remain sources of human infection. The incubation period is shorter for bites on areas of increased innervation, such as the face, fingers, and genitalia, than for bites on the arms and legs. After inoculation, the virus ascends along the peripheral nerves by retrograde axonal transport and reaches the CNS. The two presentations of rabies consist of the more well-known rabid form and a less common paralytic form. The prodromal phase of the rabid form starts with fever, headache, malaise, and sore throat. Subsequently, an encephalopathy characterized by severe agitation, anxiety, and confusional psychosis ensues. In about 50% of cases, the patient has severe throat spasm when swallowing liquid, resulting in the appearance of hydrophobia. The dysphagia also makes the patient appear to be frothing with saliva. Death occurs shortly after this overactive phase or after the patient slips into a coma.

In about 20% of rabies cases, the spinal cord is the primary site of involvement. The infection initially presents as paresthesia and pain of the wounded limb, followed by paralysis. A more diffuse weakness with or without bulbar involvement occurs, mimicking Guillain–Barré syndrome. Little treatment is possible once symptoms develop. Most patients succumb within 1 to 2 weeks, although there have been a few reports of survivors.

Varicella-Zoster Virus

Varicella-zoster virus is a herpesvirus that commonly manifests as yearly epidemics of chickenpox. It also can present as several other syndromes, including cerebellitis, encephalitis, herpes zoster ganglionitis, radiculomyelitis, and isolated myelitis. Cerebellitis from varicella-zoster virus has an incidence of 1 per 1,000 cases and usually manifests in childhood during the second week of illness as a result of an immunologic response to the virus. This is a self-limiting disease that lasts for a few days to a few weeks. Varicella-zoster virus encephalitis is less common, with an incidence of 1 per 2,000 cases. Encephalitic symptoms follow the rash after 5 to 6 days and, despite the self-limited nature of the disease, mortality rates can be as high as 15%. Diagnosis can be established by CSF PCR, viral culture, and increase in antibody titer.

Human Herpesvirus 6

Human herpesvirus 6 is the causative agent of roseola infantum, also known as sixth disease or exanthem subitum, which has been associated with meningoencephalitis and recurrent febrile seizures in children. It has also been identified as another cause of focal encephalitis in adults and may present as partial seizures and focal neurologic deficits similar to herpes simplex virus encephalitis. The course of the illness can be mild and self-limiting, but there have been instances of severe neurologic sequelae and death. Laboratory diagnosis is by viral culture, a fourfold or greater rise in IgG titer or by PCR (preferably by RNA detection assay). Gancyclovir or foscarnet are the drugs of choice, although their efficacy has not been proved.

Epstein–Barr Virus

Several neurologic syndromes have been described with Epstein–Barr virus infection, including aseptic meningitis, encephalitis, Guillain–Barré syndrome, Bell's palsy, and transverse myelitis. Epstein–Barr virus encephalitis usually occurs in infectious mononucleosis and manifests as a diffuse or focal involvement. Although most patients recover fully, mortality and morbidity rates of 8% and 12%, respectively, have been reported. The diagnosis can be established by testing for the heterophile antibody, by other Epstein–Barr virus serologic tests, by viral culture, and by PCR.

Clinical Findings

The diagnosis of viral encephalitis rests on clinical findings of a febrile illness as part of a viral prodrome and an encephalopathy. The encephalopathy may be diffuse or focal and may consist of other neurologic deficits, such as altered mental status, behavioral or speech disturbances, seizures, or hemiparesis. In most cases, the presentation is mild. However, severe and sometimes fatal infections do occur.

The encephalopathic presentations of the different viruses are generally similar. However, some viruses have certain patterns of clinical manifestations that may be explained partly by their tropism for specific CNS cell populations or regions. For example, rabies has a strong predisposition for the limbic areas, whereas herpes simplex virus invariably involves the temporal lobe.

The physical examination must distinguish between a generalized encephalopathy and a focal process. Herpes simplex encephalitis is the most common cause of focal encephalitis. However, the differential diagnosis for other organisms that can mimic this entity is considerable. For example, tuberculosis, *Cryptococcus* infections, bacterial abscesses, and some viral infections (e.g., Epstein–Barr virus, several of the arboviruses) present similarly.

Laboratory Findings

As in viral meningitis, CSF findings are nonspecific in most cases of viral encephalitis, with predominantly lymphocytic pleocytosis, a moderately elevated protein level, and a normal glucose level. Predominance of neutrophils is common in the initial stages, especially with eastern equine encephalitis, which may produce CSF findings similar to those of a bacterial infection. However, most of the viral organisms that commonly cause viral encephalitis are more difficult to isolate from the CSF or blood. Serologic methods such as hemagglutination inhibition, neutralizing antibodies, or complement fixation tests have been more successful in identifying the offending agents by demonstrating a fourfold or greater rise in IgG titers. However, these tests take weeks to complete and have limited usefulness from a therapeutic standpoint. In a few viral infections, such as western equine encephalitis, St. Louis encephalitis, and Japanese B encephalitis, acute IgM titers can be obtained a few days after onset. In herpes simplex virus encephalitis, a PCR test using CSF has a sensitivity of 75% to 100% and a specificity of 100%, making it useful for detecting the infection early in its course. PCR has also been used in identifying other agents including varicella-zoster virus, human herpesvirus 6, Epstein–Barr virus, cytomegalovirus, and Jakob–Creutzfeldt virus.

Neuroimaging modalities such as computed tomography (CT) and MRI have become important tools in the evaluation of viral encephalitis. Areas of cerebritis appear as poorly defined regions of lower density on CT. On MRI, they appear as hypointense areas on T1-weighted scans and as hyperintense areas on T2-weighted images. The sensitivity of MRI can be increased with the use of contrast agents. Because of its propensity to cause petechial hemorrhage in the temporal lobe and occasionally along the orbitofrontal lobe, herpes simplex virus type 1 encephalitis lends itself to early detection by CT or MRI.

Electroencephalography has proved to be a sensitive test for an encephalopathic process. Findings include focal or generalized background slowing and epileptiform discharges. Findings of focal activity in or near the temporal regions can be assumed to be herpes simplex virus type 1 encephalitis in the appropriate clinical setting, although patients with conditions such as Epstein–Barr virus infection, eastern equine encephalitis, or human herpesvirus 6 may present similarly. The absence of a focal process does not rule out herpes simplex virus infection.

Optimal Management

Please refer to Chapter 431 for information regarding the treatment of viral encephalitis.

POLIOMYELITIS

Before routine immunization became available, the polioviruses types 1, 2, and 3 were chiefly responsible for the syndrome of poliomyelitis, with serotype 1 accounting for epidemics of the disease. Like the other enteroviruses, polioviruses are single-stranded RNA viruses that are transmitted by the fecal–oral route and reach the CNS by hematogenous spread. The incidence of poliomyelitis in the United States between 1984 and 1993 ranged from three to nine cases per year (average 7.5 cases). Most cases are vaccine-associated after exposure to the live attenuated virus. Other enteroviruses, such as certain serotypes of the echoviruses and coxsackieviruses, have been reported to cause paralytic poliomyelitis.

Most cases of poliomyelitis are inapparent or associated with only a mild viral prodrome. About 1% to 2% of patients have neurologic symptoms, which range from an initial aseptic meningitis to severe asymmetric paralysis of the extremities with or without bulbar involvement resulting from inflammation and central chromatolysis of the lower motor neurons in the brain stem and spinal cord. The lumbar segments more commonly are affected clinically, followed by the cervical segments and, to a lesser extent, the brain stem. Muscle weakness peaks in 2 to 5 days. Treatment is supportive, with special attention paid to respiratory failure and swallowing difficulties.

HERPES ZOSTER

Herpes zoster, commonly referred to as shingles, is caused by varicella-zoster virus, which also is responsible for varicella, or chickenpox. In almost all cases, a history of chickenpox precedes the manifestations of varicella-zoster virus infection, and this initial exposure allows the virus to remain latent within neuronal cells in the sensory ganglia for several years. After spontaneous reactivation, an intense inflammatory process begins in the sensory ganglia and extends to the peripheral nerves.

Most affected patients are elderly. The vesicles usually appear along a single dermatomal distribution on one side and are accompanied by severe pain and dysesthesia that can outlast the vesicles by several months. The thoracic levels are involved in about 70% of cases, but lesions also are common in the distribution of the ophthalmic division of cranial nerve V as a result of

inflammation of the gasserian ganglion. Ramsay Hunt syndrome is encountered less often and has been described as a unilateral facial palsy with herpetic lesions in the external auditory canal. The inflammation of other cranial nerves also has been reported, including cranial nerves III, IV, VI, IX, and X. Encephalitis, cerebral angiitis, and myelitis are other rare complications of this disease.

Treatment of herpes zoster with oral acyclovir (800 mg five times a day for 7 days) shortens the course in immunocompetent persons with uncomplicated cases, although intravenous therapy may be necessary in patients with widespread disease or severe immunosuppression. Symptomatic therapy for postherpetic dysesthesia is approached best with amitriptyline and carbamazepine.

BIBLIOGRAPHY

Aurelius E, Johansson B, Skoldenberg B, et al. Rapid diagnosis of herpes simplex encephalitis by nested polymerase chain reaction assay of cerebrospinal fluid. *Lancet* 1991;337:189–192.
Bale JF Jr. Viral encephalitis. *Med Clin North Am* 1993;77:25–42.
Connolly KJ, Hammer SM. The acute aseptic meningitis syndrome. *Infect Dis Clin North Am* 1990;4:599–622.
Fishman RA. *Cerebrospinal fluid in diseases of the nervous system.* Philadelphia: WB Saunders, 1992.
Johnson RT. *Viral infections of the nervous system.* New York: Raven Press, 1982.
Keating MR. Antiviral agents. *Mayo Clin Proc* 1992;67:160–178.
Latchaw RE, Hirsch WL Jr, Yock D Jr. Imaging of intracranial infection. *Neurosurg Clin North Am* 1992;3:303–322.
Martinez AJ. Free-living amebas: infections of the central nervous system. *Mt Sinai J Med* 1993;60:271–278.
Read SJ, Jeffery KJ, Bangham RM. Aseptic meningitis and encephalitis: the role of PCR in the diagnostic laboratory. *J Clin Microbiol* 1997;35:691–696.
Roos K. Pearls and pitfalls in the diagnosis and management of central nervous system infectious diseases. *Semin Neurol* 1998;18:185–196.
Summary of Notifiable Diseases—United States, 1993. *MMWR* 1994;42:1–73.
Whitley RJ. Viral encephalitis. *N Engl J Med* 1990;323:242–250.

Kelley's Textbook of Internal Medicine, fourth edition. Edited by H. David Humes. Lippincott Williams & Wilkins, Philadelphia © 2000.

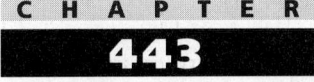

CHAPTER 443

SLOW VIRUS INFECTIONS IN THE NERVOUS SYSTEM, INCLUDING AIDS

JERRY S. WOLINSKY
JUSTIN C. MCARTHUR

Slow viral disease is a recent concept in clinical medicine. As human problems, these disorders have prominent examples

TABLE 443.1.		HUMAN CNS SLOW VIRUS DISEASES		
Pathogen	**Agent Group**	**Disease**	**CSF**[1]	**Pathology**[2]
Measles virus	Paramyxovirus	Subacute sclerosing panencephalitis	+	I, D
Rubella virus	Rubivirus	Progressive rubella panencephalitis	+	I, D
JC virus	Papovavirus	Progressive multifocal leukoencephalopathy	−	N, D
HIV-1	Lentivirus	AIDS dementia	+	I, M
HTLV-I	Oncovirus	Tropical spastic paraparesis	+	I, V
PRP^{CJD}	Prion	Creutzfeldt–Jakob disease, sporadic	−	N, S
PRP^{CJD}	Prion	Kuru	−	N, S, A
PRP^{CJD}	Prion	Creutzfeldt–Jakob disease, familial	−	N, S
PRP^{GSS}	Prion	Gerstumann–Strässler–Scheinker syndrome	−	N, S, A
PRP^{FFI}	Prion	Fatal familial insomnia	−	N, T

HTLV-I, human T-cell lymphotrophic virus type I; PRP, progressive rubella panencephalites.
[1] Typical CSP dominant findings; −, variable mild lymphocytic pleocytosis; elevated IgG index and synthetic rate oligoclonal bands; −, normal in all major constituents.
[2] Typical neuropathologic findings: I, perivascular and parenchymal inflammation; N, no inflammatory change; D, demyelination with relative axonal sparing; M, myelin pallor; V, vacinization of myelin; S, spongiform vacuolization of neuropil; A, amyloid plaques; T, selective thalamic atrophy.

among neurologic diseases. Much of our understanding of slow virus disease rests on observations from veterinary medicine and animal experimentation. Sigurdsson worked with visna and scrapie, two prototype natural slow virus infections of sheep, and found that these illnesses were characterized by long intervals from exposure to onset of clinically recognized disease, presented with symptoms limited to dysfunction of a single organ system and followed a stereotyped, ingravescent, and fatal course. These features are the highlights of slow virus diseases of the central nervous system (CNS). The importance of involvement of the immune system as a reservoir for virus and as an additional target for viral cytopathic effects is increasingly recognized.

Slow virus diseases can be classified as those caused by conventional viruses (e.g., measles and rubella virus), selected human papovaviruses and retroviruses, or unconventional agents whose chemical characteristics distinguish them from viruses. The latter group includes the prions, which are germ line–encoded, protease-resistant, proteinaceous, infectious particles that lack nucleic acids (Table 443.1).

Slow virus diseases caused by conventional viruses have remarkably common laboratory features when they occur in apparently immunocompetent hosts. The cerebrospinal fluid (CSF) often shows a mild lymphocytic pleocytosis, modest protein elevation, increased γ-globulin content, and intrathecal synthesis of oligoclonal immunoglobulins with specificity for the antigens of the causal viral agent. Neuropathologic changes usually include some inflammatory component, suggesting that the disease is at least in part immunologically mediated. Other neurologic diseases with similar features, such as multiple sclerosis, may eventually be shown to be due to conventional viruses. In contrast, slow virus diseases due to unconventional agents show no systemic or intrathecal evidence of host immune recognition of the inciting agent and have neuropathologic features that are noninflammatory and degenerative. Other neurodegenerative

diseases might have a similar cause. A representative disease from each major group is discussed in depth, with brief descriptions of the other slow virus diseases of the CNS.

SUBACUTE SCLEROSING PANENCEPHALITIS

Subacute sclerosing panencephalitis (SSPE) is the prototype human slow virus disease due to a conventional virus. Primarily a disease of childhood, it is characterized by progressive cognitive and motor dysfunction with myoclonus, intrathecal synthesis of extraordinary amounts of measles virus-specific immunoglobulin, and a characteristic inclusion body neuropathology.

INCIDENCE AND EPIDEMIOLOGY

SSPE is an uncommon disease that complicates about 1 in 100,000 patients with measles. The disorder is more common when measles occurs within the first 2 years of life. A rural background also predominates. Males are about three times more frequently affected than females. The disease has declined progressively in the United States with the institution of mandatory attenuated live measles virus vaccination programs. The incidence of SSPE attributable to the use of these vaccines is at worst 1 in 1 million.

ETIOLOGY

SSPE was first recognized in 1933. Based on the characteristic inclusions in glial and neuronal cells, it was believed to be of viral origin. The inclusions are composed of paramyxovirus nucleocapsids. Virus isolation requires the cocultivation of infected brain cells with an indicator cell line to rescue defective variants of measles virus.

PATHOGENESIS

Measles is typically a self-limited childhood disease. Significant complications of the acute disease in the immunocompetent host are generally limited to superimposed bacterial infections or postinfectious measles encephalitis. The latter is believed to be an autoimmune disease that is not dependent on direct viral invasion of the CNS. Persons with defective cell-mediated immunity exposed to measles virus may have acute CNS virus dissemination and develop ongoing defective measles virus replication in the brain, with evolution of a subacute measles encephalitis.

Uncomplicated measles ultimately causes SSPE. Whether virus enters the CNS at the time of the initial infection or remains persistent at systemic sites until it later invades the brain is unknown. Measles virus genome may reside latent in otherwise normal adult human brain and is present in circulating lymphocytes and systemic organs of patients with SSPE. Similarly, it is uncertain whether spread of the virus within the CNS and resultant neuronal dysfunction is continuous but clinically evident only after several years or whether it requires an independent activational event. The role of antiviral antibody in the pathogenesis of SSPE has been emphasized, but well-documented SSPE occurs in children with congenital hypogammaglobulinemia. Nonetheless, antimeasles antibody may contribute to the down-regulation of the tempo of disease through antigenic modulation of viral antigens at the surface of infected cells.

Virus rescued from SSPE brain tissue is uniformly defective. This situation probably reflects attenuated transcription of the 3′ portion of the measles virus genome in brain cells. Consequently, mRNA for virion matrix (M) and surface (fusion [F] and hemagglutinin [H]) proteins are underrepresented and, when transcribed, are poorly translated. Several metabolic and functional alterations of in vitro persistently infected neuronal cells are described, which could readily account for the clinical expression of disease without cell destruction.

CLINICAL FEATURES

Although predominantly a disorder of childhood, well-documented cases of SSPE are described into the seventh decade of life, so the disorder should be considered in the appropriate clinical setting at any age. Initial symptoms are usually limited to subtle cognitive dysfunction. Accompanying behavioral changes and deterioration in school performance are frequently mistaken for emotionally based problems, leading to inappropriate counseling or psychiatric referral. With time, motor disabilities develop and characteristic myoclonic spasms and choreoathetosis appear to reveal the neurologic nature of the illness. Generalized dystonia and spasticity progress, and a decerebrate state evolves as the dementia becomes profound; eventually, a vegetative state ensues. The duration of each stage varies. Half of all patients develop visual symptoms, often attributable to direct retinal in-

volvement by the virus. When present, a characteristic maculopathy and chorioretinitis provide direct evidence for the disease.

LABORATORY FINDINGS

The most useful and specific neurodiagnostic findings are provided by the electroencephalogram (EEG) and by detailed CSF examination. In the early phases of the disease, the EEG may be normal or may show evidence of nonspecific cerebral dysfunction by virtue of slowing or disorganization of the normal background rhythm, occasionally with multifocal paroxysmal sharp wave discharges. Characteristic synchronous high-voltage, slow-wave bursts 2 to 3 seconds in duration that occur at remarkably fixed intervals of 5 to 8 seconds eventually develop. The bursts may be temporally associated with the clinically expressed myoclonic activity. Although not pathognomonic, the presence of these rhythmic periodic complexes in the setting of subacutely evolving childhood dementia strongly suggests SSPE.

With no hypogammaglobulinemia or intensive immunosuppressive chemotherapy, the CSF shows a mild mononuclear pleocytosis, a mildly increased total protein content, and a greatly elevated γ-globulin content. The IgG index and synthetic rate are increased with oligoclonal immunoglobulins, easily shown by electrophoresis of CSF and serum. The serum:CSF ratio of measles virus antibody is greatly reduced (normal, greater than 200), and CSF immunoglobulins generally react with all structural proteins of measles virus except the M protein. Most authorities consider these serologic findings to be diagnostic of the disease without the need for brain biopsy or virus isolation.

Computed tomography (CT) can document evolving cortical atrophy and ventricular enlargement, and it often shows attenuation of the density of the cerebral white matter; however, single examinations do not correlate well with the clinical disease state. Magnetic resonance imaging (MRI) provides similar evidence of the progressive destructive process, but neither CT nor MRI is diagnostically specific.

The brain biopsy shows inflammatory changes in gray and underlying white matter consisting of mononuclear cells, plasma cells, and microglia. Neuronal loss and astrogliosis can be prominent. Eosinophilic intracytoplasmic and intranuclear inclusions are present in neurons and oligodendroglia and can be shown to be measles virus-specific by immunocytochemistry. Virus isolation by sensitive explant and cocultivation techniques is successful in less than 50% of cases. Evidence suggests that more than one variant of measles virus can be isolated from a single patient at once.

OPTIMAL MANAGEMENT

SSPE's disease course is variable. Patients with acute cases progress from first symptoms to death within a few months. The average patient survives for 1.8 years, and up to 5% of patients survive more than 5 years. Well-defined spontaneous disease remissions are reported but uncommon. Treatment is symptomatic and supportive. Myoclonic seizures can often be controlled with clonazepam, with the dosage titrated to suppress seizure activity and avoid undue sedation. Specific therapy is controversial. Several uncontrolled reports suggest that the putative immunomodulatory drug isoprinosine is effective in prolonging the course of the disease for patients with more slowly evolving disease and may have induced symptom remission. Other uncontrolled reports suggest that intrathecal or systemic interferon has beneficial effects.

PROGRESSIVE RUBELLA PANENCEPHALITIS

Progressive rubella panencephalitis (PRP) is a rare slow virus disease of childhood with features similar to those of SSPE. It follows as a late complication of both the congenital rubella syndrome and typical childhood rubella. Intrathecal synthesis of substantial amounts of immunoglobulin specific for the three structural proteins of rubella virus and successful isolation of virus from brain tissue by cocultivation link persistent viral infection with the clinical syndrome. Immune complex deposition in cerebral vasculature suggests an immunopathologic component to the demyelinative disease. Early cerebellar symptoms and absence of myoclonus may clinically distinguish PRP from SSPE. The course is very protracted and usually fatal, but like SSPE, PRP may spontaneously remit. There is no known treatment.

PROGRESSIVE MULTIFOCAL LEUKOENCEPHALOPATHY

Progressive multifocal leukoencephalopathy (PML), first delineated in 1958, is primarily a disease of the immunocompromised host, although several cases have been reported in patients with no known underlying disorder. JC virus, a human papovavirus, is usually the causative agent. Although infection with JC virus is common, PML is not. Whether defective cellular immunity leads to the activation of a long latent B-lymphocyte reservoir of papovavirus infection or precludes clearance of virus during primary infection is uncertain.

PML has a marked predilection for hemispheric white matter. Individual lesions are characterized by plaquelike concentric zones of central necrosis, surrounded by primary demyelination and loss of oligodendroglia. This is bordered by a sector of hypertrophied oligodendroglia containing basophilic intranuclear inclusions consisting of paracrystalline arrays of virions ringed by normal-appearing white matter. Astrocytes within lesions are morphologically bizarre. Once initiated, the pathogenesis of PML appears straightforward. Infected oligodendroglial cells fail to maintain their myelin sheaths, leading to demyelination of adjacent axons. Eventually, the infected cells lyse and progeny virions are released into the microenvironment to infect adjacent oligodendroglia. Macrophages participate in the clearance of cellular debris, but viral specific immune responses are not mounted. Astrocytes in the midst of this activity undergo transformation to a near-malignant state in response either to released substances or more likely to their own infection by virus. Despite the ease of extraction of virions from infected tissue, successful culture of virus from brain requires the presence of immature human glial cells.

Until recently, most patients with PML had an underlying lymphoreticular malignancy such as Hodgkin's disease or chronic lymphocytic leukemia; now AIDS is preeminent. Presenting symptoms vary but often include confusion and disorientation, visual disturbances progressing to cortical blindness, and ataxia. The onset is usually insidious, but may be explosive. The course is generally fatal within 1 year and can be particularly rapid in AIDS patients. Rare spontaneous remission of symptoms with eventual recurrence is well documented; this complicates the interpretation of anecdotal reports of response to antiviral therapy with cytosine arabinoside, interferon, or both. In PML, the CSF is acellular with little alteration of protein content, but polymerase chain reaction amplification of CSF sediments may disclose diagnostically useful JC virus gene sequences. EEG findings are nonspecific. The MRI displays spectacular high-signal-intensity lesions, predominantly restricted to white matter. Despite typical MRI findings, the differential diagnosis can be trying in AIDS patients and may require brain biopsy. Further, the recognition that herpes varicella-zoster virus can produce similar clinical, neurodiagnostic, and gross neuropathologic changes precludes definitive diagnosis without histology and specific immunohistochemical staining in the non-AIDS patient.

AIDS DEMENTIA

Most AIDS patients develop one or more CNS opportunistic infections (Chapter 267). In addition, HIV invades the CNS to cause symptoms of neural dysfunction directly. Initial viral invasion of the CNS can occur very early after exposure to the virus and may be marked by a transient, clinically recognizable aseptic meningitis. Chronic asymptomatic CNS infection follows. After a variable and often protracted interval, the first definite progressive neurologic symptoms unfold.

The early symptoms of AIDS dementia (HIV-associated cognitive motor complex) may precede any systemic manifestations of AIDS, but they become more prevalent late in the course of HIV infection. These are usually heralded by an insidious (rarely abrupt) but generally progressive deterioration of cognitive function with behavioral changes. Severe subcortical dementia ensues over a variable interval of several to many months in association with increasing motor impairment. In the late stages, moderate to profound dementia with psychomotor retardation develops, variably associated with pyramidal weakness and hypertonia, ataxia, incontinence, peripheral neuropathy, seizures, and myoclonus. About 15% of persons with AIDS develop this chronic encephalitis. Symptoms of AIDS dementia may be overshadowed by those of opportunistic CNS infections, lymphoma, or the metabolic consequences of systemic disease.

Diagnosis rests on the clinical features, documentation of HIV infection and exclusion of opportunistic infection or neoplasm. MRI commonly documents cerebral atrophy and ill-defined areas of increased signal intensity deep within the cerebral white matter. from diffuse or multifocal areas of hemispheric white matter correlated with AIDS dementia.

Immunohistochemical and in situ hybridization studies document that macrophages and macrophage-derived multinucleate giant cells harbor virus in neural tissues; these findings are analogous to those in visna. The intensity of the macrophage activation correlates with dementia severity, and it is likely that macrophage secretory products, including proinflammatory cytokines, lead to neuronal dysfunction. There is evidence that these symptoms can be reversed, at least in part, with antiviral therapy, especially since the introduction of combination antiretroviral therapy.

In the spinal cord, spongiform degeneration of the posterior and lateral columns, with vacuoles in the myelin sheaths, can produce progressive spastic paraparesis, a condition termed *vacuolar myelopathy*. The pathogenesis is unknown, and no treatment for this condition has been identified. In the peripheral nerves a dying back axonal degeneration, frequently accompanied by a painful sensory neuropathy clinically, is common late in the course of AIDS. Similar painful neuropathic symptoms are brought out by initiating therapy with some antiretroviral agents, including, ddI, ddC, and d4T. Treatment for these painful neuropathies is symptomatic. Early in the course of HIV infection, usually before immunosuppression, chronic or, less frequently, acute inflammatory polyneuropathy can occur. Immunotherapy for these presumed immune-mediated disorders is the same as in HIV-negative individuals (Chapter).

CREUTZFELDT–JAKOB DISEASE

Creutzfeldt–Jakob (CJD) is the prototype human-transmissible neurodegenerative disorder caused by a prion.

INCIDENCE AND EPIDEMIOLOGY

In its sporadic form, CJD occurs worldwide with an annual incidence of 1 in 1 million. About 10% of CJD cases are familial, autosomal dominant, and due to several well-defined germ line mutations that segregate in families and generally correlate with nuances of disease phenotypes. These cases are also transmissible. Despite the ease of experimental transmission of sporadic CJD, its mode of transmission in nature is unknown. There is no known conjugal or enzootic transmission, and the disease is not more common among medical personnel. There is an increased incidence of prior surgical and particularly neurosurgical procedures for CJD cases compared with matched controls. The disease can occur at nearly any age, with peak incidence in the sixth decade.

ETIOLOGY

In 1921, Jakob differentiated what is now known as CJD from Alzheimer's presenile dementia based on distinctive neuropathologic change. Demonstration of the transmissible nature of scrapie, a disease of sheep, and the subsequent recognition that the clinical course and pathology of kuru, an apparent degenerative disease in an isolated New Guinea tribe, might reflect an analogous disease process culminated in the signal observation that kuru was transmissible to subhuman primates. Classification of CJD among the subacute spongiform encephalopathies

opened the way for transmission of this globally distributed sporadic disorder as well. Kuru, once responsible for ataxia, tremor, and death within a year in 1% of all Fore tribe members, has disappeared with the proscription of ritualistic cannibalism. Sporadic, familial, and iatrogenic CJD, the dominantly inherited Gerstmann–Sträussler–Scheinker syndrome, and fatal familial insomnia are the currently known human prion diseases.

The agents that cause scrapie, "mad cow" or bovine spongiform encephalopathy, and CJD are remarkably similar. Scrapie infectivity copurifies with PrP^{Sc}, a hydrophobic, protease-resistant glycoprotein of 27 to 30 kD. PrP^{Sc} rapidly forms higher-molecular-weight, rodlike, birefringent aggregates. The failure to demonstrate a nucleic acid component associated with purified and infectious PrP^{Sc} is convincing. PrP^{Sc} is an abnormal isoform of the normal PrP gene product PrP^{C}. The *PrP* gene has been cloned and sequenced, is phylogenetically highly conserved, and in humans is localized to chromosome 20. The function of the normal PrP gene product is uncertain, but PrP^{C} may be involved in synaptic inhibition. Introduction of PrP^{Sc} into normal cells is likely to induce conformational change of PrP^{C} into PrP^{Sc} through protein–protein interactions. This results in a cascading conversion of PrP^{C} and accumulating neuropathogenic aggregates of PrP^{Sc}.

PATHOGENESIS

A considerable body of clinical and experimental data is available on the biology of the spongiform encephalopathies. Prions are remarkably resistant to most chemical and physical agents. Transmission can be effected by oral or parenteral inoculation but is most efficient by intracerebral routes. The incubation period depends on the dose and route of inoculation and host genetics and may theoretically exceed the host's life span. Experimentally, replication occurs at many systemic sites; all organs and body fluids from CJD patients must be considered potentially infectious. Symptoms and pathologic change are limited to the CNS. Prion amplification in brain tissue precedes the development of recognizable pathology. Well-developed neuropathologic changes include noninflammatory spongiform degeneration of the neutrophil, neuron loss, and marked astrogliosis. The topography of this change is generally widespread but may show regional variation consistent with the patient's clinical symptoms.

Koch's postulates have been fulfilled for CJD by the inadvertent transfer of disease by corneal transplantation, cadaveric dural grafts and inadequately sterilized depth electrodes, and the administration of contaminated growth hormone preparations. Such incidents can be minimized by avoiding organ transplantation from donors with unexplained neurologic disease and by adequate sterilization of all surgical instruments.

CLINICAL FEATURES

Prodromal manifestations occur in about one third of all cases CJD. These symptoms are subtle and varied and often are initially attributed to neurosis or other psychiatric disorders. As cognitive deficits evolve, the dementing nature of the illness becomes evident. Eventually, myoclonus or startle myoclonus becomes a prominent feature in over 80% of all cases; in contrast, in Alzheimer's disease myoclonus is an infrequent and usually late finding. Because of the widespread nature of the underlying pathology, the dementia is usually accompanied or preceded by other neurologic signs and symptoms. The disease can be subclassified into several subtypes. Pyramidal, extrapyramidal, cerebellar, and cortical visual defects are common in either relatively isolated or mixed patterns. The early development of multisystem neurologic deficits in the presence of dementia suggests the diagnosis of CJD even without myoclonus. Usually, the onset of symptoms is gradual (over weeks or months), but an explosive onset over a matter of hours is well chronicled.

LABORATORY FINDINGS

The EEG can be most helpful. Early in the disease, it can be normal or show only nonspecific slowing or disorganization of the normal cortical patterns. Over 80% of all patients exhibit diffusely slowed background activity with periodic, symmetric, high-voltage biphasic or triphasic sharp waves. Although this periodic complex pattern is not pathognomonic of CJD, it is highly suggestive of the disorder in the appropriate clinical setting. CT and MRI can document rapidly evolving brain atrophy but may be normal in the early phases of the disease. Routine CSF studies are normal. Brain biopsy remains necessary for definitive antemortem diagnosis and may be necessary to distinguish atypical cases of sporadic or iatrogenic CJD from other forms of dementia. Unfortunately, the presence of the characteristic spongiform change in the cortex of the biopsy specimen may be subtle or difficult to differentiate from artifact. Diagnosis by transmission studies is no longer essential, because recently developed techniques to detect the presence of PrP^{CJD} by immunoblot using polyvalent and monoclonal-specific reagents are definitive in difficult cases. Molecular genetic analysis of DNA samples derived from peripheral blood leukocytes provides a powerful means of diagnosis of familial cases of CJD, Gerstmann–Sträussler–Scheinker syndrome, and fatal familial insomnia.

OPTIMAL MANAGEMENT

Typically, the signs and symptoms of CJD evolve dramatically over a matter of months, with death occurring in 90% of patients within 1 year. In some patients, the disease reaches a plateau for protracted intervals at a low level of neurologic function. A slower clinical course may be conferred by heterozygosity at codon 129, a normal human polymorphic allele in the *PrP* gene. The apolipoprotein $\epsilon4$ allele may be an additional risk factor. Attempts at treatment with antiviral chemotherapy have been disappointing.

BIBLIOGRAPHY

Brown P, Gibbs CJ Jr, Rodgers-Johnson P, et al. Human spongiform encephalopathy: the National Institutes of Health series of 300 cases of experimentally transmitted disease. *Ann Neurol* 1994;35:513–529.

Dhib-Jalbut S, Johnson KP. Measles virus diseases. In: McKendall RR, Stroop WG, eds. *Handbook of neurovirology.* New York: Marcel Dekker, 1994.

Gascon G, Yamani S, Crowell J, et al. Combined oral isoprinosine-intraventricular α-interferon therapy for subacute sclerosing panencephalitis. *Brain Dev* 1993;15:346–355.

Major EO, Amemiya K, Tornatore CS, et al. Pathogenesis and molecular biology of progressive multifocal leukoencephalopathy, the JC virus-induced demyelinating disease of the human brain. *Clin Microbiol Rev* 1992;5:49–73.

McArthur JC, Hoover DR, Bacellar H, et al. Dementia in AIDS patients: incidence and risk factors. *Neurology* 1993;43:2245–2252.

Prusiner SB, Hsiao KK. Human prion diseases. *Ann Neurol* 1994;35:385–395.

Weber T, Turner RW, Frye S, et al. Progressive multifocal leukoencephalopathy diagnosed by amplification of JC virus-specific DNA from cerebrospinal fluid. *AIDS* 1994;8:49–57.

Wolinsky JS. Rubella virus. In: Fields BN, Knipe DM, Chanock RM, et al, eds. *Virology,* third ed. New York: Raven Press, 1995.

Worley JM, Price RW. Clinical manifestations of HIV-1 infection of the nervous system. In: McKendall RR, Stroop WG, eds. *Handbook of neurovirology.* New York: Marcel Dekker, 1994.

Kelley's Textbook of Internal Medicine, fourth edition. Edited by H. David Humes. Lippincott Williams & Wilkins, Philadelphia © 2000.

CHAPTER
444

SEIZURES AND EPILEPSIES

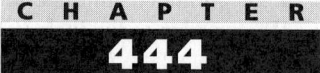

ANTONIO V. DELGADO-ESCUETA

The term "epilepsy" is derived from a Greek word meaning a condition of being overcome or seized. The term is used to describe the brain's innate ability to produce paroxysmal depolarization shifts within neurons and recurrent electroencephalographic (EEG) discharges such as focal spikes or diffuse bilateral 1.5- to 6-Hz spike-and-wave complexes (Chapter 426). Clinically, a person's consciousness and senses may be abruptly suspended, and motor, sensory, or behavioral symptoms result.

An individual seizure is distinguished from epilepsy per se with the latter term being reserved for three or more recurrent seizures. Epileptic seizures should be distinguished from nonepileptic convulsive seizures produced by cerebral ischemia or hypoxia, hypoglycemia, convulsive drugs, such as cocaine, and withdrawal from alcohol, barbiturates, and benzodiazepines. Pseudoepileptic behavior produced by conversion hysteria must not be mistaken for epilepsy.

INCIDENCE AND EPIDEMIOLOGY

Worldwide, the epilepsies, afflicting approximately 40 to 100 million people, are the second most common neurologic disorder, second only to headaches. In developing countries, the epilepsies are the most common serious neurologic disorder, whereas in the United States, the epilepsies are second only to cerebrovascular disease and strokes, affecting at least 2 to 3 million people. Incidences among persons under treatment for recurrent seizures range from approximately 1.5 per 1,000 for Japan, 2.7 per 1,000 in Chile, 4.4 per 1,000 for China, 6 per 1,000 in Rochester, Minnesota, 9 per 1,000 for Sri Lanka and Pakistan, 17 per 1,000 in Ecuador, and up to 16 to 21 per 1,000 in Africa and Panama.

In the United States, at least 105,800 new cases of epilepsy are diagnosed each year. Incidence rates are highest among the very young (especially newborns and infants), drop to a relatively constant rate among those between 10 and 70 years of age, and increase again thereafter. Acquired epilepsies characterized by partial and secondary tonic–clonic seizures are the most common forms. They occur frequently in the first 5 years of life, somewhat less often in persons 5 to 10 years of age, and more often in those older than 20 years. The incidence of genetic epilepsies with grand mal tonic–clonic convulsions peaks during adolescence and early adulthood; juvenile myoclonic epilepsy (JME) is a disease of adolescence. Absence epilepsies are usually childhood disorders and rarely occur before age 3 or after age 20.

CLASSIFICATION: SEIZURES AND EPILEPSIES

Table 444.1 is a classification of epileptic seizures and Table 444.2 is a revised and modern version of the 1989 ILAE Classification of the Epilepsies. It distinguishes genetic epilepsies from acquired epilepsies symptomatic of a neurologic or medical illness.

Genetic epilepsies are divided into (1) genetic epilepsies whose primary and exclusive symptoms are seizures, either generalized (e.g., benign familial neonatal epilepsies, childhood absence epilepsy, and JME) or partial (e.g., autosomal dominant nocturnal frontal lobe epilepsy, familial temporal lobe epilepsy, Rolandic epilepsy), (2) genetic epilepsies associated with severe neurologic deficits or malformations or both (e.g., cortical dysplasias) or associated with progressive degenerations (e.g., progressive myoclonus epilepsies), and (3) idiopathic epilepsies with generalized seizures suspected to be genetic.

Symptomatic epilepsies are divided into symptomatic epilepsies with mainly generalized seizures and symptomatic epilepsies with partial and secondary tonic–clonic seizures, such as those caused by structural lesions.

Thus, the medical practitioner must first identify the type of seizures the patient has and then determine the epilepsy syndrome and cause of the seizures (Table 444.1). Are seizures manifestations of a genetic epilepsy, a cerebral cortical dysplasia, a degenerative disorder, or a structural lesion? Genetic epilepsies most often manifest as generalized seizures but can also manifest mainly as partial seizures. Epilepsies symptomatic of structural disease almost always manifest as partial, complex partial, and secondary generalized tonic–clonic seizures.

GENETIC EPILEPSIES

About 40% of adults and children with epilepsy suffer from genetic epilepsies with primary generalized or partial seizures.

TABLE 444.1. INTERNATIONAL CLASSIFICATION OF EPILEPTIC SEIZURES

I. Partial (focal, local) seizures
  A. Simple partial seizures (consciousness not impaired)
    1. With motor symptoms
    2. With somatosensory or special sensory symptoms
    3. With autonomic symptoms
    4. With psychic symptoms
  B. Complex partial seizures (with impairment of consciousness)
    1. Beginning as simple partial seizures and progressing to impairment of consciousness
      a. With no other features
      b. With features as in I.A.1 to I.A.4.
      c. With automatisms
    2. With impairment of consciousness at onset
      a. With no other features
      b. With features as in I.A.1 to I.A.4
      c. With automatisms
  C. Partial seizures evolving to secondarily generalized seizures
    1. Simple partial seizures evolving to generalized seizures
    2. Complex partial seizures evolving to generalized seizures
    3. Simple partial seizures evolving to complex partial seizures to generalized seizures
II. Generalized seizures (convulsive or nonconvulsive)
  A. Absence seizures
    1. Absence seizures
    2. Atypical absence seizures
  B. Myoclonic seizures
  C. Clonic seizures
  D. Tonic seizures
  E. Tonic–clonic seizures
  F. Atonic seizures (astatic seizures)
III. Unclassified epileptic seizures
  Includes all seizures that cannot be classified because of inadequate or incomplete data and some that defy classification in hitherto described categories. This includes some neonatal seizures, such as rhythmic eye movements, chewing, and swimming movements (From *Epilepsia* 1981;22:489)

Intelligence and neurologic examination results are normal in those with the common genetic epilepsies, whereas they are abnormal in cortical dysplasias and progressive myoclonus epilepsies. Generalized seizures are present when epileptogenic discharges involve both cerebral hemispheres from the onset. Early loss of consciousness is the rule. Generalized seizures may involve only loss of consciousness (absence) or convulsive movements (tonic–clonic, myoclonic, tonic, or clonic). Early childhood myoclonic, myoclonic-astatic, absence, benign JME, and tonic–clonic or clonic–tonic–clonic grand mal epilepsies can be best recognized by their onset in childhood and adolescence. Almost all are genetically transmitted. Structural lesions are rare. The EEG shows bilaterally symmetric and synchronous 2.5- to 3.5-Hz or 3.5- to 6-Hz spike- or polyspike-wave complexes. Genetic partial epilepsies have a localized origin and show any of the partial seizure types described in Table 444.1. Between seizures, the EEG can show localized epileptiform spikes.

TABLE 444.2.   MODERN CLASSIFICATION OF THE EPILEPSIES

I. Genetic epilepsies
  A. Genetic epilepsies whose primary symptoms/signs are main generalized seizures
    1. Benign familial neonatal convulsions in chromosome 20q (EBN1) or 8q24 (EBN2)
    2. Benign familial infantile convulsions in chromosome 19q13
    3. Infantile spasms—X-linked
    4. Benign infantile familial convulsions and paroxysmal choreoathetosis in chromosome 16p12–q12
    5. Childhood absence epilepsy (pyknolepsy) with or without grand mal tonic–clonic seizures in chromosome 8q24
    6. Juvenile myolonic epilepsy in chromosome 6p11 (EJM1) or 15q14
    7. Epilepsy with generalized tonic–clonic seizure on awakening in chromosome 6p21.3
    8. Febrile convulsions in chromosome 8q13-21 or 19p or 2p
    9. Familial adult myoclonus epilepsy in chromosome 8q23-24
    10. Generalized epilepsies with "febrile seizures plus" in chromosome 19q13 or 2q
    11. Idiopathic generalized epilepsy in chromosome 3p14-12.1
  B. Genetic epilepsies whose primary symptoms/signs are mainly partial seizure
    1. Autosomal dominant frontal lobe epilepsy in chromosome 20q or 15q24
    2. Autosomal dominant partial epilepsy with variable foci in chromosomes 2q or 22q12
    3. Rolandic epilepsy or benign epilepsy with centrotemporal spikes in chromosome 15q14
    4. Childhood epilepsy with centrotemporal spikes and writer's cramp/ataxia in chromosome 66p12-q12
    5. Familial temporal lobe epilepsies with auditory symptoms in chromosome 10q
  C. Genetic epilepsy syndromes with severe neurologic deficits and/or progressive degenerations and/or malformations
    1. Cortical dysplasias
      a. Schizencephaly, sporadic with mutation of EMX2 (unknown chromosome lucus)
      b. Aicardi syndrome, X-linked in chromosome Xp22.3 associated with eye abnormalities and agenesis of corpus callosum
      c. Bilateral periventicular nodular heterotopia, X-linked in chromosome Xq28 with 2.25 to 3.25 Mb duplication of Xq28
      d. Isolated lissencephaly, X-linked (males) in chromosome Xq22.3-23 with mutation in double cortin
      e. Subcortical band heterotopia, X-linked (females) in chromosome Xq22.3-23 with mutation in doublecortin
      f. Isolated lissencephaly, autosomal dominant in chromosome 17p13.3; in 30% of cases: deletions or point mutations in lissencephaly 1 or *ILS1* gene, which encodes platelet activating factor acetylhydrolase
      g. Miller–Dieker syndrome, autosomal dominant in chromosome 17p13.3; in 90% of cases: large deletions of *1LS1* gene

    2. Progressive myoclonus epilepsies
      a. Unverricht–Lundborg's disease (EPM1) in chromosome 21q
      b. Lafora's disease in chromosome 6q24
      c. Dentadorubral-pallidoluysian atrophy in chromosome 12p13.31
      d. Infantile neuronal ceroid lipofuscinosis CLN1 (mutation in palmitoyl protein thioesterase) in chromosome 1p32
      e. Late Infantile neuronal ceroid lipofuscinosis
        (1) CLN2 (mutation in carboxyl peptidases) in 11p15
        (2) CLN6 in chromosome 15q21.23
        (3) CLN5 in chromosome 13q21-q23
      f. Juvenile neuronal ceroid lipofuscinosis (CLN3) in chromosome 16p
      g. 2g. Adult neuronal ceroid lipofuscinosis (CLN4) (unknown locus)
      h. Juvenile Gaucher's disease in chromosome 1q
      i. Cherry red spot-myoclonus sydrome or sialidos is type 1 (or Guazzi sydrome) in chromosome 10q
        j. Myoclonus epilepsy and ragged-red fibers, mutation in mitochondrial DNA
  D. Idiopathic epilepsies with generalized seizures with undetermined cause but suspected to be genetic
    1. Benign myoclonic epilepsy in infancy
    2. Idiopathic West syndrome/Lennox–Gastaut–Dravet syndrome with normal psychomotor development
    3. Early childhood primary astatic and myoclonic epilepsy
    4. Severe myoclonic epilepsy of infancy
    5. Juvenile absence epilepsy
    6. Epilepsy with myoclonic absence
    7. Landau–Kleffner syndrome
II. Symptomatic or Acquired Epilepsies
  A. Symptomatic epilepsies with mainly generalized seizures
    1. West Syndrome
    2. Lennox–Gataut–Dravet Syndrome
    3. Epilepsy with myoclonic–astatic seizures
    4. Early myoclonic encephalopathy
    5. Early infantile epileptic encephalopathy with suppression bursts (Ohtahara syndrome)
  B. Symptomatic epilepsies with partial seizures and or secondary generalized seizures
    1. Epilepsia partialis continua of Childhood (Kojewnikow syndrome)
      a. Rasmussen's encephylitis
        b. Benign epilepsia partialis continua
    2. Temporal lobe epilepsies
    3. Frontal lobe epilepsies
    4. Parietal lobe epilepsies
    5. Occipital lobe epilepsies

ACQUIRED OR SYMPTOMATIC PARTIAL, COMPLEX PARTIAL, AND SECONDARY GENERALIZED EPILEPSIES

Symptomatic epilepsies account for 60% of adult and about 40% of childhood epilepsies. The clinical signs of symptomatic partial epilepsies are not different from those of genetic partial epilepsies that have a localized origin. Neurologic signs may be present, and onset can occur at any age. Between seizures, the EEG can show localized epileptiform spikes. During onset of seizures (ictus), the EEG shows epileptogenic discharges related to the lesion. During seizures, the most common EEG pattern consists of localized, rhythmic, low-voltage 16- to 30-Hz rapid potentials, which can propagate and spread.

Partial seizures arise from an anatomical or functional system limited to a part of one or both cerebral hemispheres (Tables 444.2 to 444.4). Localization and preferred routes of spread determine clinical features. Partial seizures are divided into three major subgroups: simple, complex, and secondarily generalized seizures. In simple partial seizures, consciousness is never lost. In complex partial seizures, consciousness is impaired. Synonyms

include psychomotor seizures, fugus epileptique, and Damner atacken. Simple or complex partial seizures can develop into secondary tonic–clonic seizures. Complex partial seizures should be differentiated from absence because the choice of drug for each of these disorders differs. Most absence seizures last 10 seconds or less. Complex partial psychomotor seizures last an average of 3 minutes, and most are not longer than 5 minutes. An aura precedes 44% of complex partial seizures. Full consciousness returns slowly. Absence seizures have no aura and start suddenly; full consciousness returns abruptly.

Automatisms in complex partial seizures are more complex than automatisms of absence. Walking or running, perseverative bilateral arm or leg motions such as kicking and defensive flailing, and bimanual, bipedal movements can appear as stereotyped automatisms at the onset of frontal lobe complex partial seizures. Such complicated motor movements have not been reported in absence. Between seizures (interictus), local spikes or spike-wave formations appear in the EEG. If a circumscribed lesion is present, the term focal or partial epilepsy is most appropriate. If the site and side of seizure onset vary (often the case in benign

---

TABLE 444.3. FRONTAL LOBE EPILEPSIES

Regional/ System Localization	Clinical Seizure Patterns	EEG, Stereo-EEG	Brain Imaging	Psychology[a]	Common Cause
Dorsolateral frontal Dorsolateral frontopolar or premotor or opercular	Psychic intellectual auras with forced thinking, PMT, opercular, aphasia, CPS with initial palilalia, impaired consciousness or somatomotor signs	Dorsolateral frontal interictal and ictal localization	Normal skull radiographs and CTs; MRI and PET usually localize lesion	Perseveration, poor recent judgments, response disinhibition	Trauma, astrocytoma, oligodendroglioma
Medial frontal Supplementary motor	Postural, PMT, vocalization, speech arrest, fencing, CPS, sexual automatisms, urinary incontinence	Flattening rhythmic polyspike (16–24 Hz) and secondary generalization; intracranial electrode exploration mandatory	Normal skull radiographs and CTs; focal atrophic lesion on MRI; PET may be focal	Dominant; impaired verbal fluency Nondominant: impaired design fluency	Focal atrophy, tumor, arteriovenous malformations
Medial frontal Cingular or anterior cingulate	Frequent psychic emotional areas—extreme fear, terror, and autonomic signs; CPS with ambulatory automatisms, bicycling motions with sexual features, vegetative signs, urinary incontinence	Intracranial electrode exploration mandatory	Normal skull radiographs and CT; PET and MRI may be focal	Dominant: impaired verbal fluency Nondominant: impaired design fluency	Focal atrophy, tumor, arteriovenous vascular malformations
Basal frontal Posterior orbitofrontal	Olfactory hallucinations, autonomic signs, CPS with initial vocalization, bimanual, bipedal, or ambulatory and sexual automatisms	Flattening rhythmic polyspike (16–24 Hz) and secondary generalization	Normal skull and CT; signs of trauma, MRI: focal atrophy, PET may be useful	Lability of mood	Trauma, astrocytoma, oligodendroglioma

CT, computed tomography; EEG, electroencephalogram; MRI, magnetic resonance imaging; PET, positron emission tomography; PMT, partial motor tonic including tonic forward or backward elevations of head; CPS, complex partial seizures.
Adapted from Delgado-Escueta AV, et al. New wave of research in the epilepsies. *Adv Neurol* 1990;44:16.
* In this column are listed the neuropsychological tests that most specifically indicate functional damage in the region of the focus. However, functional damage and the seizure focus are not necessarily in the same place. In particular, recent memory deficits, suggestive of hippocampal damage, probably occur in all syndromes of complex partial seizures, especially if there is a history of status epilepticus. A discrepancy of 20 or more points between verbal and nonverbal IQ suggests generalized dysfunction in one hemisphere. If confirmed, this helps to lateralize the focus, although it does not indicate the location of the focus within the hemisphere. Psychomotor slowing is a comon but nonspecific sign of organic brain damage of antiepileptic drug side effects.

TABLE 444.4.	MEDIAL TEMPORAL LOBE EPILEPSIES					
Regional/ System Localization	Aura	Clinical Seizure Patterns	EEG, Stereo-EEG	Brain Imaging	Psychology[a]	Common Causes
Hippocampus and parahippocampal gyrus, amygdala	Strange, indescribable feelings is characteristic; autonomic symptoms/ signs of facial pallor, pupillary dilation, arrest of respiration, tachycardia can also appear	Arrest (motionless stare), chewing, lipsmacking, swallowing and single discrete movements at onset of 50% of attacks, followed by confusion and amnesia averaging 2 minutes; >60% have rare secondary tonic-clonic seizures	Interictal: anterior medial temporal sharp waves and spikes, especially during sleep Ictus: initial unilateral flatting, especially one temporal lobe and background EEG changes or nonlateralizing surface EEG changes or focal or lateralized; 4–6 Hz sharp waves and spikes in one medial temporal area as recorded by sphenoidal electrodes Stereo-EEG: high-frequency 16–28 Hz low-voltage spikes building up in one hippocampus propagating to amygdala, lateral temporal, orbital frontal, and cingulate and parietal regions	Skull radiograph: asymmetry of skull, especially sphenoid fossa CT scan: negative Metrizadmide CT scan: signs of tentorial herniation MRI: increased signal intensity in one hippocampus or hippocampal gyrus with atrophy and decreased volume of hippocampus or entire temporal lobe PET: hypometabolism of one temporal lobe	Impaired recent memory (verbal— dominant hemisphere; visual spatial recent memory— nondominant hemisphere)	More commonly; incisural or hippocampal sclerosis Less frequently: gangliogliomas, hamartomas, arteriovenous malformation, focal gliosis, rarely aneurysms (cicatrix)
Inferotemporal neocortical epilepsy	Prosopagnosia; otherwise no signs or symptoms until spread to superotemporal cortex	Arrest of motion Verbalization, vocalization, hypersalivation, and oral buccal dyskinesias	Interictal EEG: lateral mid temporal and/ or posterior temporal spikes Ictus: high-frequency 16–28 Hz spikes built up in inferior temporal cortex	Normal skull films, but CT, MRI and PET recommended; PET may show lateral more than medial temporal hypometabolism	Dominant: anomia, impaired word sorting Nondominant: tonal memory and timbre tests; lateralizing dichotic auditory detection	Most commonly: trauma, glioma, cavernous angioma, arteriovenous malformations, post cerebral infarctions

CT, computed tomography; EEG, electroencephalogram; MRI, magnetic resonance imaging; PET, positron emission tomography.
[a] In this column are listed the neuropsychological tests that most specifically indicate functional damage in the region of the focus. However, functional damage and the seizure focus are not necessarily in the same place. In particular, recent memory deficits, suggestive of hippocampal damage, probably occur in all syndromes of complex partial seizures, especially if there is a history of status epilepticus. A discrepancy of 20 or more points between verbal and nonverbal IQ suggests generalized dysfunction in one hemisphere. If confirmed, this helps to lateralize the focus, although it does not indicate the location of the focus within the hemisphere. Psychomotor slowing is a comon but nonspecific sign of organic brain damage of antiepileptic drug side effects.

childhood syndromes), the term localization-related is more appropriate.

Acquired generalized epilepsies manifest tonic–clonic seizures, but focal or diffuse cerebral pathology may be recognized by the presence of abnormal neurologic signs, background EEG changes, and brain images. Organic brain disease can also manifest as generalized tonic seizures, myoclonic jerks, infantile spasms, or atonic attacks as in West syndrome of infancy, symptomatic Lennox–Gastaut–Dravet syndrome, and the progressive myoclonus epilepsies.

ETIOLOGY AND PATHOGENESIS

Three factors acting alone or together have long been considered important in the cause and pathogenesis of the epilepsies: (1) an epilepsy gene or gene(s), which predispose persons to recurrent seizures, (2) seizure-generating (epileptogenic) brain lesions; and (3) internal and external stimuli, which affect epilepsy susceptibility genes or epileptogenic lesions and trigger seizures. These three factors contribute to produce the generalized 3- to 6-Hz spike waves of generalized epilepsies or the focal cortical spikes and sharp waves of partial epilepsies.

EPILEPSY GENES

Subvarieties of epilepsies with clear mendelian inheritance such as benign familial neonatal convulsions and forms of epilepsies that are complex genetic diseases such as JME are now being distinguished from multifactorial symptomatic epilepsies. Mutations in potassium channel genes in benign familial neonatal convulsions, in a sodium channel gene in febrile seizures plus, and in a nicotinic ACH β-subunit receptor in autosomal dominant nocturnal frontal lobe epilepsy are examples of monogenic epilepsies. Both 8q24 and 20q loci for benign familial neonatal convulsions are the sites of mutations in two different novel voltage-gated K$^+$ channel genes dubbed *KCNQ2* and *KCNQ3*, channel genes involved in neuronal repolarization. The mutation in the neuronal α4 subunit of the nicotinic acetylcholine receptor in autosomal dominant nocturnal frontal lobe epilepsy in chromosome 20q13.2 renders the receptor to be less efficient and less functional reducing permeability to calcium.

More than 20 separate chromosomal loci of mendelian forms of idiopathic generalized and partial epilepsies have been identified, and their mutations surely will be defined in the next decade with the anticipated completion of the human genome sequence (Table 444.5). Four of these genotypes pertain to common idiopathic generalized epilepsies: (1) JME, which has two chromosomal loci in 6p11 and in 15q14, (2) childhood absence epilepsy, which persists with grand mal seizures in chromosome 8q24; (3) familial febrile seizures, which has three loci in chromosomes 8q13-21, 19p, and 2p. The locus for benign adult familial myo-

| TABLE 444.5. | LATERAL TEMPORAL LOBE EPILEPSIES |

Regional Localization	Aura	Clinical Seizure Patterns	EEG, Stereo-EEG	Brain Imaging	Psychology[a]	Common Causes
Posterior superotemporal–opercular epilepsy	Vestibular hallucinations followed by borborygmal belching, autonomic symptoms, or gustatory hallucinations owing to spread to parietal operculum; psychical seizures containing songs, music, voices, the dreamy state, or experiential hallucinations and affective signs	Initial vestibular hallucinations followed by staring arrest of motions, swallowing, puckering lips, tongue movements, blowing, salivation during confusion and amnesia	Interictal scalp, lateral, midtemporal or posterior temporal spikes Ictal stereo-EEG: isolated opercular rapid spikes (16–20 Hz) with minimal spread	Normal skull films, but CT, MRI, and PET are recommended. PET may show lateral more than medial temporal hypometabolism	Dominant: anomia (Benson); impaired word-sorting (Hiatt) Non-dominant: tonal memory and timbre tests (seashore), McGill picture anomalies Lateralizing: dichotic, auditory detection	Glioma, astrocytoma, arteriovenous malformation, aneurysms, postcerebral infarction
Posterior perisylvian: temporal–parietal opercular epilepsy	Auditory hallucinations, visual perceptual hallucinations, language disorder when lateralized to hemisphere dominant for language; psychical seizures containing songs, music, voices, the dreamy state or experiential hallucinations and affective signs	Fluent dysphasia, disturbed orientation and prolonged auditory hallucinations, head movement to one side; sometimes staring and puckering lips, tongue and mouth movements, salivation, unilateral area automatisms, and amnesia	Interictal scalp: lateral midtemporal or post-temporal spikes Ictal stereo-EEG: high-frequency rapid spikes (16–20 Hz) building up in the supramarginal angular gyrus and posterior temporal regions	Normal skull films, but CT, A/G and MRI recommended; PET may show lateral temporal and parietal hypometabolism.	Dominant: anomia (Benson); impaired word-sorting (Hiatt) Nondominant: tonal memory and timbre tests (seashore), McGill picture anomalies Lateralizing: dichotic, auditory detection	Most common due to trauma with focal gliosis, postinfections, glioma, postcerebral infarction, cavernous angioma
Anterior prisylvian: temporal frontal opercular epilepsy	Silent until discharges spread to Heschl's gyrus or produce experiential hallucinations or dreamy state, psychical seizures with emotions	Nonfluent dysphasia, impaired responsiveness, auditory hallucinations due to spread to posterior superior temporal cortex, oral buccal dyskinetic automatisms, hypersalivation	Interictal scalp, lateral anterior, temporal and/or medial temporal spikes Ictus: high-frequency rapid spikes (16–20 Hz) in lateral anterior aspect of superior temporal cortex	Normal skull films but CT, MRI and PET recommended; PET may show lateral temporal and frontal hypometabolism	Dominant: anomia (Benson); impaired word-sorting (Hiatt) Nondominant: tonal memory and timbre tests (seashore), McGill picture anomalies Lateralizing: dichotic, auditory detection	Most common due to trauma with focal gliosis, postinfections, glioma, postcerebral infarction, cavernous angioma

[a] In this column are listed the neuropsychological tests that most specifically indicate functional damage in the region of the focus. However, functional damage and the seizure focus are not necesarily in the same place. In particular, recent memory deficits, suggestive of hippocampal damage, probably occur in all syndromes of complex partial seizures, especially if there is a history of status epilepticus. A discrepancy of 20 or more points between verbal and nonverbal IQ suggests generalized dysfunction in one hemisphere. If confirmed, this helps to lateralize the focus, although it does not indicate the location of the focus within the hemisphere. Psychomotor slowing is a common but nonspecific sign of organic brain damage of antiepileptic drug side effects.
Modified from Commission on Classification and Terminology of the ILAE, closed workshop for revised clinical and EEG classification of epilepsies, Bethesda, MD 1984. *Epilepsia* 1985;26:268.
CT, computed tomography; EEG, electroencephalography; MRI, magnetic resonance imaging; PET, positron emission tomography.

clonic epilepsy is also in 8q23.3-q24.1. A susceptibility locus for idiopathic generalized epilepsies with generalized spike waves is also present in chromosome 3p. The chromosome locus for childhood absence epilepsy that remits during adolescence has not been defined.

FOCAL EPILEPTOGENIC BRAIN LESIONS

Three factors contribute to focal epileptogenesis in temporal lobe epilepsy with hippocampal scleroses, post-traumatic epilepsy and cerebral cortical dysplasias. These three key elements are (1) the capacity of membranes in some pacemaker neurons to develop intrinsic burst discharges (e.g., pyramidal neurons in the CA3 region of the hippocampus and in layer 4 of the cerebral cortex), (2) the reduction of γ-aminobutyric acid (GABA)ergic inhibition or presence of disinhibition; and (3) the enhancement of synaptic excitation, as in the presence of recurrent excitatory synaptic circuits produced by mossy fiber sprouting. Resected human epileptic hippocampal tissue has consistently shown a pattern of neuronal circuit alteration, namely, neuronal loss, ectopic granule cells, and mossy fiber reorganization and sprouting in the inner molecular layer of the dentate gyrus. These sprouting fibers synapse with proximal apical dendrites of granular cells where more dendritic spines and more branching in apical dendrites are present.

Repeated seizures and prolonged convulsive status epilepticus cause such hippocampal damage that in turn sets up reverberating and recurrent excitatory circuits, focal epileptogenesis, and impaired recent memory. Immunocytochemical studies in human temporal lobe epilepsy also support the notion of reduced GABAergic interneurons as indicated by reduced parvalbumin, calbindin D28k and calretinin, and reduced glutamic acid decarboxylase. Neurotrophin expression, and increased mRNA levels for brain-derived neurotrophic factor, nerve growth factor, and NT-3 also correlate with neuron losses or supragranular mossy fiber sprouting in the chronically damaged and epileptic human hippocampus. These latter growth factors may be the trigger for the structural remodeling of granule cells, their dendritic changes, and axonal sprouting.

Even in epileptogenic cortical dysplasia, reorganization with a reduction of putative GABAergic neurons, increased numbers of balloon cells with NMDAR1 and GluR2-3 subunits of glutamate receptors are present. In the epileptogenic zones adjacent to cortical microgyria and dysplasias, neurofilaments increase in numbers and glutamate staining is more prominent. Furthermore, polysynaptic inhibitory postsynaptic currents are larger in amplitude and their frequency more dependent on glutamatergic input. Mossy fiber sprouting and its recurrent excitatory circuits plus the reduced GABAergic interneurons thus provide the substrate for cortical hyperexcitability and chronic epilepsy.

In post-traumatic neocortical epilepsy, similar mechanisms operate and layer 5 neurons increase input resistance, prolong membrane time constants, reduce slow spike after hyperpolarizations, and fire more rapidly during depolarizations. Axons of injured neurons sprout, double their contacts, and increase recurrent excitation. GABAergic terminals also sprout and increase their innervation of interneurons. Moreover, there is evidence that complex febrile convulsions and status epilepticus in infancy can induce molecular and cellular mechanisms subserving sprouting and reorganization of hippocampal circuits and eventually cause hippocampal scleroses and chronic temporal lobe epilepsy in adolescents and adults. Magnetic resonance imaging (MRI) studies of infants who have complex and prolonged febrile seizures can show acute edematous hippocampi in the hemisphere of seizure origin and the subsequent development of hippocampal atrophy and scleroses.

▇ CLINICAL FEATURES: EPILEPSY SYNDROMES

GENETIC EPILEPSIES WITH BENIGN GENERALIZED SEIZURES

Childhood absence epilepsy, JME, and grand mal epilepsy on awakening are the three most common forms of genetic generalized epilepsies. Together, these three syndromes account for almost half of all epilepsies. Benign familial neonatal convulsions and benign myoclonic epilepsy of infancy and early childhood are rare syndromes with generalized seizures.

Childhood Absence Epilepsy (Petit Mal)

Childhood absence appears in 3% to 4% of all patients with epilepsy. Onset is between 4 and 8 years of age. Absences are the first manifestation. Because seizures occur at least 1 per day or up to several hundred times per day, the absences are called *pyknoleptic* (meaning dense, compact). The child is otherwise neurologically normal. There is sudden interruption of activities, such as walking or talking. Responsiveness is partially or totally lost for a period of less than 10 seconds. A blank stare and a slight upward rotation of the eyeballs is the typical manifestation. Rhythmic clonic movements of eyelids and eyebrows, stereotyped automatisms (lip smacking, chewing movements, blinking), and mild clonic, atonic, or tonic movements may appear. Pupil dilation and changes in facial color, heart rate, and respiration may also occur. The ictal EEG reveals bilateral symmetric and synchronous 3-Hz spike-wave complexes with a normal background. Hyperventilation, photic stimulation, drowsiness, and non-REM sleep activate the 3-Hz spike-wave complexes.

In over 50% of patients with childhood absence epilepsy, absences are the only manifestation. These absences usually resolve during adolescence. Fourteen percent experience both petit mal and tonic–clonic seizures at onset. Tonic–clonic seizures develop after absence in 32% of patients. These forms of absence epilepsy associated with grand mal seizures usually persist longer into adulthood. Another syndrome should be suspected when seizures start as myoclonias or grand mal later to be followed by absences.

A family history of seizures is noted in 40% of patients with absences. Spike-wave complexes of 3 Hz may be inherited as an autosomal dominant trait. Expression declines with age. Siblings and offspring have a lifelong 50% risk for inheriting the spike-wave trait (dominant), a 12% risk for generalized seizures, and an 8% risk for having absence. Diffuse 3-Hz spike-wave complexes are also prevalent in relatives of probands with febrile convulsions or focal seizures.

Other rare forms of absences occur during late childhood

and adolescence (juvenile absence epilepsy). The attacks are infrequent and random (spanioleptic) and are usually associated with tonic–clonic seizures; the electroclinical traits persist into later life. Because closed-circuit television with biotelemetry of the EEG (CCTV-EEG) shows that grand mal seizures are often preceded (as much as 45%) by absences, absence epilepsy with grand mal seizures may account for up to 15% of all epilepsies.

Juvenile Myoclonic Epilepsy

JME occurs in at least 10% to 20% and up to 30% of patients with epilepsy. Patients have normal intelligence and an excellent prognosis. JME is extremely sensitive to valproic acid. The syndrome usually starts at 13 to 15 years of age with mild myoclonic jerks of arms and shoulders. Myoclonic jerks may be mistaken for nervousness. Major tonic–clonic convulsions follow myoclonic seizures—usually in 2 to 3 years. Seizures may be induced by lack of sleep, premature awakening, fatigue, or alcohol. In 10% to 37% of patients JME may be atypical and also have absences. Rapid 4- to 6-Hz diffuse polyspike-wave complexes are characteristic. This 10% to 37% of patients also has 3-Hz spike-wave sequences in addition to the fast 4- to 6-Hz polyspike waves. Patients with JME have a high recurrence rate (90%) on withdrawal of treatment.

The genetic locus of autosomal dominant JME with 3.5- to 6-Hz polyspike-wave complexes is in chromosome 6p11. Segregation analysis agrees with linkage mapping and shows that JME is a heterogeneous syndrome. Autosomal recessive, autosomal dominant, two-loci, and polygenic forms all have been suggested.

Genetic Epilepsy with Clonic–Tonic–Clonic and Tonic–Clonic Seizures (Grand Mal Epilepsy)

Commonly, absences or myoclonic seizures precede grand mal seizures. Hence, pure grand mal epilepsy is rare. Two forms are now recognized: awakening clonic–tonic–clonic grand mal and random tonic–clonic grand mal. Awakening clonic–tonic–clonic grand mal seizures are usually triggered by sleep deprivation, fatigue, and alcohol. The interictal EEG shows the rapid form of diffuse 4- to 6-Hz polyspike-wave complexes. Diffuse 14- to 24-Hz polyspikes fire during brief and violent flexor spasms of the entire body (initial clonic phase). Consciousness is preserved early and, if upright, the patient may fall. Consciousness is abruptly lost with tonic contraction. The tonic phase lasts 10 to 20 seconds, followed by clonic jerks. Sixty-eight percent of cases present at puberty; 85% disappear on treatment with valproic acid. Seizures persist, and 60% to 90% of patients suffer relapse on withdrawal of treatment. Awakening grand mal epilepsy appears to be an allelic form of the chromosome 6p-linked JME syndrome.

Grand mal epilepsy with tonic–clonic seizures is characterized by seizures that occur randomly with no special circadian pattern. Its interictal EEG is more similar to the pattern of childhood absences and consists of diffuse 3-Hz spike-wave complexes or 3-Hz polyspike-wave complexes. Recruiting patterns of 9- to 12-Hz diffuse rhythms herald the tonic phase. Seizures may

appear only nocturnally. Up to 70% of seizures disappear with treatment, and 22% decrease in frequency. Eight to 20% of patients suffer relapse after drug withdrawal.

Benign Familial Neonatal Convulsions

Benign familial neonatal convulsions, a rare cause of neonatal convulsions, is an autosomal dominant disorder with favorable outcome. Psychomotor development proceeds normally. In 80% of patients, partial or generalized clonic seizures, sometimes with apneic spells start on the second and third days of life. Seizures usually stop by 6 months without any neurologic sequelae. Childhood or adult epilepsy subsequently develops in about 10% to 14% of patients.

Two genetic loci are responsible—one on chromosome 20q13.2 and another on chromosome 8q. Cosegregation of a nonsense mutation in the α4 subunit of the nicotinic acetylcholine receptor with the chromosome 20q13.2-linked benign familial neonatal convulsions was recently demonstrated. In 1995, the syndrome of autosomal dominant nocturnal frontal lobe epilepsy was shown to be an allelic form of the chromosome 20q13.2 epilepsy gene.

Benign Myoclonic Epilepsy of Infancy

Benign myoclonic epilepsy of infancy is a rare condition characterized by brief bouts of massive or mild generalized myoclonic seizures without loss of consciousness in normal children during the first 3 years of life. The neurologic examination is normal. During drowsiness, there is an increase in the frequency of the myoclonias and during slow sleep they usually disappear. The EEG always shows diffuse irregular 3-Hz spike-wave or polyspike-wave discharges synchronous with the myoclonic muscle activity in the electromyograph (EMG). No other seizure types are involved, although generalized tonic–clonic attacks may occur later in life. Seizures are easily controlled by valproic acid monotherapy. Prognosis is good if treatment is started early. If left untreated, patients may present impaired psychomotor development and behavioral disturbances. A family history of epilepsy or febrile convulsions is present in 31% of the cases.

Benign Myoclonic Epilepsy of Early Childhood

When familial myoclonic epilepsy starts in early childhood (between 1 and 5 years), a combination of myoclonic-astatic, myoclonic, absence and tonic–clonic or clonic–tonic–clonic seizures may occur. The EEG shows bilateral synchronous 2- to 3-Hz spike-wave and polyspike-wave complexes, 4- to 6-Hz polyspike-wave complexes, and bursts of diffuse 4- to 7-Hz rhythms. No evidence of brain damage is present on neuroimaging; the disease does not progress, and no cognitive deficits emerge on neuropsychological tests. A strong family history is present, since 20% of nonproband family members are affected. Most present a primary generalized epilepsy syndrome. Response to valproate monotherapy is good to excellent.

Benign myoclonic epilepsy in infants and young children may be the infantile and early childhood equivalent of JME.

GENETIC EPILEPSIES WITH BENIGN PARTIAL SEIZURES

Even in partial epilepsy syndromes, genetic linkage studies have been successful. Partial epilepsy with auditory symptoms has been linked to chromosome 10q. Two separate loci have been found in Rolandic epilepsy—Rolandic epilepsy with writer's cramps and ataxia in the pericentromeric region of chromosome 16p and Rolandic epilepsy with centrotemporal spikes on 15q14. First-degree relatives of patients with symptomatic partial seizures have an increased incidence of seizures, and genetic susceptibility is important even in partial epilepsies. An environmental insult such as head trauma might not produce seizures in a person with low susceptibility.

The most common form of genetic epilepsy with partial seizures is autosomal dominant benign rolandic epilepsy, which accounts for 15% of all childhood seizures. Less common is benign occipital epilepsy. Seizures develop between 4 and 8 years of age in benign rolandic epilepsy. Most attacks occur at night as secondary tonic clonic seizures preceded by twitching of one side of the face, tongue or hands. Unilateral or bilateral diphasic or triphasic sharp waves over the rolandic regions increase during sleep. Declining in frequency with age, seizures disappear by age 16 years, and are associated with a normal background EEG, positive family history for seizures or rolandic spikes and normal neurologic examination.

GENETIC EPILEPSIES CHARACTERIZED BY A PROGRESSIVE MYOCLONUS EPILEPSY

The progressive myoclonus epilepsies (PMEs) are a rare, heterogeneous group of debilitating, often fatal epileptic encephalopathies characterized by segmental arrhythmic myoclonus, massive myoclonias, generalized tonic–clonic or clonic seizures, with or without absences, dementia, and other progressive neurologic manifestations, especially cerebellar. Unverricht–Lundborg and Lafora types of PME are the most common, relatively speaking. Specific mutations have also been defined among the more than 12 loci of the PMEs. These include Lafora's disease, Unverricht–Lundborg disease, ceroid lipofuscinoses 3 (Spielmeyer–Vogt syndrome) within Batten disease, or sialidosis, dentadorubropallidoluysian atrophy, and the mitochondrial syndrome, MERRF (myoclonic epilepsy and ragged red fibers).

Unverricht–Lundborg or Baltic–Mediterranean PME

This debilitating but not fatal form of autosomal recessive PME was first described in 1891 and 1895 by Unverricht in Estonia and in 1903 by Lundborg in Sweden. The incidence is at least 1 : 20,000 in Finland. Although rarely seen in North and South America, it is, relatively speaking, the most common form of PME in the Americas. Presenting with severe stimulus-sensitive myoclonias in a person between 6 and 18 years, the disease progresses slowly with cognitive decline and emotional lability. Tendon tapping, or passive joint movements, auditory and light stimuli are common precipitants of myoclonias. Clonic, tonic–clonic, and myoclonic seizures mostly appear on awaken-ing and should be differentiated from JME. Late in the course of illness, motor incoordination, dysmetria, dysdiakinesia, and ataxic gait appear. Valproate, topiramate, and lamotrigine can reduce seizure frequencies, but eventually resistance to antiepileptic drug treatment develops. After a period of approximately 5 years, the patient is usually incapacitated.

Armpit skin biopsy reveals membrane-bound vacuoles in eccrine cells. The genetic mutation for Unverricht–Lundborg Baltic type and Mediterranean type PME are both in chromosome 21q22.3 and consists of a loss of function in cystatin B. Cystatin B is a member of the superfamily of cysteine proteinase inhibitors.

Lafora's Disease

Lafora's disease, a fatal autosomal recessive form of PME, starts with epileptic seizures during early adolescence or as late as 18 years. Patients die 5 to 10 years after the first symptoms—usually by 20 years of age. The disease is relatively common in the Mediterranean countries, the Middle East, India, and other geographical areas where consanguinity occurs. Initial tonic-clonic, partial visual, absence, or drop seizures are followed by myoclonus. Trains of photic-sensitive high-voltage, usually bilaterally synchronous, spike-wave and polyspike-wave complexes interrupt a disorganized slow EEG background. Dementia, apraxia, and visual loss lead to a vegetative state. The hallmark of the disease is a periodic acid-Schiff–positive cytoplasmic inclusion body, originally described by Lafora in 1911. Lafora bodies contain polyglycosans and are found in the brain, striated muscle, liver, and skin. An axillary skin biopsy is the diagnostic procedure of choice.

The mutated gene for Lafora's disease maps to chromosome 20q and encodes protein tyrosine phosphatase. Based on its sequence analyses alone, protein tyrosine phosphatase probably has dual-specific activities catalyzing the dephosphorylation of glycogen synthase kinase-3B. Glycogen synthase forms and extends outer linear chains, and new outer linear branches (a1 to 6 branches) of glycogen. In the presence of mutations in the protein tyrosine phosphatase, the phosphorylated form of glycogen synthase would remain in an activated form, and excessive glycogen could be synthesized and Lafora inclusion bodies form.

Other rare forms of PME can be caused by the neuronal ceroid- lipofuscinoses: juvenile Gaucher's disease, sialidosis type I, and MERRF. PME can be caused by three types of neuronal ceroid- lipofuscinoses: late infantile (Jansky–Bielschowsky disease), juvenile (Batten disease or Spielmeyer–Vogt–Sjögren disease) and adult (Kufs' disease). The late infantile form (CLN-2) is autosomal recessive, starts in early childhood between 2.5 and 4 years, and is fatal. Myoclonic, generalized tonic–clonic seizures, atonic, and atypical absence seizures cause the disease to be mistaken for Lennox–Gastaut–Dravet syndrome. Intellectual loss, blindness, spasticity, and ataxia lead to a decorticate state and death between 6 and 10 years. Slow irregular spikes and polyspike-wave discharges interrupt a slow disorganized EEG background. Photic stimulation induces posterior high-amplitude, polyphasic spikes, and giant visual-evoked potentials. An autosomal recessive juvenile form of ceroid-lipofuscinosis (CLN-3) is also fatal and starts in early childhood or childhood (4 to

10 years) with loss of central vision that progresses to blindness. Absence seizures and generalized tonic–clonic seizures appear 2 years later with ataxia, dysarthria, and mental deterioration. Death occurs in the late teens or early 20s.

Vacuolated lymphocytes in peripheral blood and characteristic fingerprint profiles and curvilinear inclusions in ultrastructural study of skin biopsy or lymphocytes confirm the diagnosis. The gene locus of CLN-3 is 16p.

Only the juvenile type (type 3) of Gaucher's disease presents as PME in childhood or early adulthood. Severe intention myoclonus, abnormal saccadic horizontal eye movements, and supranuclear gaze paralysis are the first symptoms. Cerebellar deficits, generalized and partial seizures, and some degree of dementia are common. Hepatosplenomegaly is present. Death occurs 10 years from the diagnosis. The EEG shows rapid 6- to 10-Hz diffuse polyspike and rhythmical sharp waves most prominent posteriorly, and 6- to 10-Hz photic stimulation induces a photoparoxysmal or photomyoclonic response. The juvenile type of Gaucher's disease is an autosomal recessive disease caused by a deficiency of glucocerebrosidase. The gene for glucocerebrosidase has been mapped to the q21-231 region of chromosome 1.

Sialidosis type I also known as the *cherry-red-spot myoclonus syndrome* was first described by Guazzi and colleagues in 1968. It causes a PME syndrome in childhood and adolescence, appearing between the ages of 8 to 15 years. Macular cherry-red spots are seen in the fundus with visual failure. These are combined with easily controlled seizures and pains of "burning hand and feet." There is usually no dementia. Stimulus-sensitive myoclonic jerks as well as sporadic, stimulus-insensitive facial myoclonus can be triggered by active and passive movements, the thought of movements, and touch, but not by light or sound. An inherited primary deficiency of neuraminidase is observed in those with sialidosis type I.

MERRF is a tRNA^{Lys} mutation in mitochondrial DNA and can cause a childhood or adult form of PME. Cerebellar ataxia, action myoclonus epilepsy, tonic–clonic seizures, and ragged-red fiber myopathy occur with deafness, dementia, dysarthria short stature, optic atrophy, neuropathy, lactic acidosis, hypoventilation, and migraine. Inheritance is consistent with mitochondrial (maternal) transmission. Muscle biopsy reveals subsarcolemmal aggregates of mitochondria, the so-called ragged-red fibers. Giant visual-evoked potentials are recorded in all cases. Several investigators have demonstrated, in a number of patients with MERRF syndrome, the presence of a disease-related A-to-G substitution at nucleotide 8344 in the mitochondrial DNA, which affects the pseudouridine loop of the mitochondrial tRNA^{Lys}. A causal relation between this genetic mutation and MERRF disease is present, and the A-to-G mutation in the mitochondrial tRNA^{Lys} gene is disease-specific for MERRF.

SEVERE ACQUIRED GENERALIZED EPILEPSIES OF INFANCY AND EARLY CHILDHOOD

The West syndrome and the Lennox–Gastaut–Dravet syndrome are the most common acquired generalized epilepsy syndromes in infancy and early childhood.

West Syndrome or Infantile Spasms

Spasms, arrest of psychomotor development, and hypsarrhythmia begin during the first year of life. Spasms may be flexor, extensor, or mixed and are described as jackknife. In salaam spasms, the arms are abducted. The EEG hypsarrhythmia is defined as grossly chaotic diffuse, asymmetric mixtures of very high-amplitude slow waves, sharp waves, and spikes. Evolution from West syndrome to Lennox–Gastaut–Dravet syndrome is common, and both disorders represent a peculiar response of the brain to an insult at different stages of maturation. Affected patients do not respond to most antiepileptic drugs, but corticotropin (ACTH), corticosteroids, or clonazepam control the spasms.

Most cases are symptomatic and related to one of an innumerable list of diseases. An idiopathic and possibly genetic form of West syndrome is characterized by normal psychomotor development and spontaneous recovery. Probably less than 5% of patients with West syndrome have the idiopathic form.

Lennox–Gastaut–Dravet Syndrome

Atypical absences, atonic seizures, and tonic seizures are common, although partial seizures and myoclonic seizures also occur and may be difficult to distinguish clinically from atonic or short tonic seizures. An EMG recording is essential to determine whether a drop attack is an atonic seizure or a true myoclonic seizure, since both are characterized by a sudden fall of the head or body. The EEG shows slow background and the slow form (less than 2 Hz) of spike-wave or polyspike-wave discharges with no EMG activity during atonic seizures. Diffuse rapid 10- to 20-Hz rhythms fire with EMG muscle activity during myolonic seizures. Tonic seizures show either desynchronization of background activity or a recruiting 10- to 20-Hz rhythm of increasing amplitude, or both. Myoclonias are rare in the Lennox–Gastaut–Dravet syndrome. A family history has been reported in 3% to 27% of the patients. In 20% to 30%, no underlying cause is found. A cryptogenic form in which a family history of epilepsy was present in 48% of patients has been described.

Early Myoclonic Encephalopathy

Erratic, fragmentary myoclonus, massive myoclonias, infantile spasms, focal motor seizures, and tonic seizures start in the neonatal period. The EEG shows a burst-suppression. Severe neurologic impairment leads to death in the first year of life in 60% of patients. The remaining 40% survive in vegetative states. No obstetric or perinatal complications have been recognized. Although the high incidence of familial cases suggests a genetic cause, most cases of early myoclonic encephalopathy are considered acquired.

Early Infantile Epileptic Encephalopathy

Also called Ohtahara's syndrome, early infantile epileptic encephalopathy appears during the first weeks of life as a subacute condition that progresses over a period of several days or weeks. Flexor, extensor, or asymmetric spasms and tonic–clonic or unilateral seizures characterize the disease and progressively increase in frequency. Normal at onset, the patient deteriorates soon as mental retardation and neurologic deficits appear. Burst-suppression EEG pattern consists of several seconds of flat periods, alternating with high-amplitude spike-wave complexes. The cause is variable and includes brain malformations and diffuse prenatal lesions. The prognosis is poor, and 50% die in infancy or childhood. The rest survive severely incapacitated. The syndrome has been considered an early variant of the West syndrome.

Epilepsy with Myoclonic Absences

Myoclonic absences, which are the only or main seizure type, start from 2 to 12.5 years, usually at 7 years of age. Rhythmic, bilateral, diffuse 3-Hz myoclonias of severe intensity are accompanied by EEG bilateral, synchronous, and symmetric 3-Hz spike-wave discharges identical with those of classic petit mal. Seizures are longer than petit mal absences, lasting 10 to 60 seconds. Impairment of consciousness can range from a complete to a lesser degree of disruption. Myoclonic absences are frequently provoked by hyperventilation and in some cases by photic stimulation. Patients may have associated generalized tonic–clonic seizures. There is a positive family history in 19% of patients. The prognosis is usually poor because of the lack of response to antiepileptic drugs and frequent mental deterioration. The treatment of choice is valproic acid, but a combination of valproic acid and ethosuximide is often necessary to control the seizures. Epilepsy with myoclonic absences is considered an intermediate syndrome between primary and secondary generalized epilepsies.

Severe Myoclonic Epilepsy of Infancy of Dravet

Severe myoclonic epilepsy of infancy of Dravet, although presently considered an acquired form of epilepsy, presents certain characteristics of a genetic epilepsy: absence of causative factors, high incidence of family history (25%), initial epileptic symptomatology, and photosensitivity. Onset is always during the first year of life as generalized or unilateral febrile clonic seizures. No abnormality in development is apparent before seizure onset. Myoclonic seizures, which develop later in the illness, can induce a fall if severe enough, but subtle, inconspicuous seizures also occur. Consciousness is not disturbed unless the seizures are frequent (one seizure every few seconds). Partial seizures evocative of complex partial and partial motor seizures also form part of this syndrome. Generalized spike-wave or polyspike-wave complexes are seen interictally, and photosensitivity is common. The prognosis for those affected with severe myoclonic epilepsy of infancy of Dravet is poor because of the intractability of the fragmentary and segmental myoclonus seizures, the slow psychomotor development, and progressive neurologic signs.

Acquired Partial Epilepsies with or without Secondarily Generalized Seizures in Children and Adults

Temporal lobe and frontal lobe epilepsies are the most common forms of acquired epilepsies and account for almost half of all epilepsies in children and adults.

Frontal Lobe Epilepsies

In the United States, an estimated 600,000 patients have frontal lobe seizures and epilepsies. Frontal lobe seizures and epilepsies account for 20% to 30% of all partial epilepsies. These seizures are classified according to the dominant region and systems of the frontal lobe involved (Table 444.2):

Dorsolateral region seizures—anterior polar or frontopolar, frontal operculoinsular, and premotor frontal

Medial frontal seizures—supplementary motor and anterior cingulate.

Orbital frontal seizures—anterior mesio-orbital and posterior orbital frontal–temporal.

A combination of various frontal lobe regions involved by seizures

In general, secondary tonic–clonic convulsions and simple partial seizures with somatomotor or postural signs and contraversive head and eye movements are common in those with frontal lobe epilepsies. When psychomotor attacks appear, motor manifestations are prominent. This contrasts to the paucity of motor signs seen in those with temporal lobe seizures in whom arrest of movements, staring, proptosis, and masticatory oroalimentary automatisms are more common, as in amygdalar–hippocampal–parahippocampal epilepsy. Complex partial seizures, which originate from the frontal basal and anterior cingulate cortex, can begin with extreme fear and terror, bizarre vocalization, bilateral motor automatisms, bipedal movements, frenetic arm- and leg-thrusting behavior, sexual automatisms, and running. The latter motor signs are rare in those with temporal lobe seizures, although fear, bizarre vocalization, and sexual automatisms can appear rarely in temporal lobe opercular seizures. Oroalimentary masticatory automatisms combined with a motionless staring phase may also appear in those with frontal lobe seizures but usually in the middle or late stages of the attack.

Certain characteristics or oroalimentary automatisms can be valuable in differentiating frontal from temporal lobe seizures. Mastication, chewing, smacking, and licking lips are characteristic of amygdalar–hippocampal–parahippocampal seizures with its lateral temporal and subcortical connections. Swallowing, orofacial dyskinesia-like movements of mouth and lips are more suggestive of frontal opercular seizures.

Pseudoabsence attacks lasting 10 to 30 seconds with minimal automatisms are also observed in frontal lobe seizures. Such short attacks occur frequently, often in clusters, and may be associated with sphincter incontinence. These seizures can be associated with drop attacks.

Complex partial seizures of frontal lobe origin very commonly evolve to tonic–clonic convulsions or complex partial status epilepticus. When secondary tonic–clonic seizures appear in 40% of temporal lobe epilepsy, such convulsions appear rarely.

Temporal Lobe Epilepsies

Temporal lobe epilepsies account for approximately 40% to 50% of adult and 25% to 30% of childhood epilepsies. Temporal lobe epilepsies are divided into medial temporal (hippocampal–parahippocampal and amygdalar), lateral temporal neocortical (inferotemporal, superotemporal, and perisylvian-opercular), combined medial-lateral temporal lobe epilepsies, and combined temporal–extratemporal lobe epilepsies (Tables 444.3 and 444.4). Hippocampal–parahippocampal epilepsy accounts for 60% of all temporal lobe epilepsies and commonly combines with amygdalar epilepsy.

The classic hippocampal psychomotor attack is preceded by symptoms of an "indescribable strange feeling" and autonomic signs. Fifty-five percent of attacks start with arrest reaction (motionless staring), oroalimentary automatisms, or a single discrete motion. A typical seizure lasts 2 minutes. The motionless stare lasts 5 to 20 seconds and is followed by lip-smacking, chewing, and then lingering confusion for 60 to 90 seconds. Tonic movements, postures, and clonic jerks appear late as a manifestation of seizure spread. The surface interictal EEG commonly shows anterior medial spikes or sharp waves. Sixty percent show hippocampal atrophy on MRI, and 80% show hypometabolic temporal lobe on positron emission tomography. Ninety percent of cases show hippocampal scleroses on pathology; less frequently neuronal migration, hamartoma, ganglioglioma, astrocytoma, and oligodendroglioma are observed.

Rising epigastric discomfort and autonomic symptoms and signs, including borborygmi, belching, pallor, fullness or flushing of face, arrest of respiration, and pupillary dilation, suggest either an amygdalar or a lateral temporal opercular onset. Simple auditory hallucinations, psychical seizures containing illusions or hallucinations of voices, songs, and music, visual perceptual hallucinations, interpretive illusions, the dreamy state and experiential hallucinations (*déjà vu*, *jamais vu*, dream-like sequences, memory recording), and vestibular hallucinations can mean lateral superotemporal seizures, including Heschl's gyrus.

Inferotemporal neocortical seizures are usually silent clinically until discharges spread medially to the hippocampal–amygdalar circuit or laterally to the perisylvian opercular regions. The interictal surface EEG shows midtemporal or posterior temporal spikes. Traumatic encephalomalacia, arteriovenous malformations, or gliomas are observed on pathologic study.

Combined temporal lobe extratemporal lobe seizures manifest clinically with the motor signs of frontal lobe complex partial seizures, such as running, bipedal movements, frenetic arm- and leg- thrusting, and sexual automatisms or parietal lobe seizures with body circling.

Parietal Lobe Epilepsies

Localized parietal seizures do not involve changes in consciousness, although changes in perception are expected. They can rapidly spread to subcortical regions, can impair consciousness, and can be mistaken for temporal and frontal lobe seizures. Gustatory hallucinations, pharyngeal automatisms, feelings of uncontrolled movement, body turning, bilateral arm automatisms, primary sensations, and misperceptions can occur. Unformed visual hallucinations, contralateral numbness, vertigo and tinnitus, and speech arrest have been reported.

Occipital Lobe Epilepsies

Occipital lobe lesions produce simple visual hallucinations. Spread of paroxysms can result in urges to urinate, posturing,

speech arrest, complex vivid hallucinations, confusion, and automatisms. The initial visual aura can be eclipsed by psychomotor automatisms. Blindness, dim vision, field cuts, visual hallucinations, forced blinking, eye deviations, visual agnosia, or abnormal perception can precede or follow complex partial seizures.

■ COMMON LESIONAL EPILEPSIES

Age at onset, birth and developmental history, family history, personal and social drug habits, nature of seizures, neurologic signs, and EEG results are important considerations in looking for epileptogenic brain lesions. In infants, children, and young adults, perinatal lesions, anoxia, neuronal migration disorders, focal cerebral cortical dysplasias, and birth trauma without hemorrhage are observed in 25% of cases. Postnatal trauma causes 20% of simple partial seizures in young adults. Trauma, neoplasm, birth injuries, and arteriovenous malformations are the most common causes when seizures begin in a person between 20 and 35 years of age. Neoplasm, trauma, and infarction or hemorrhages are most common causes when seizures start in a person between 40 and 55 years of age. Cerebrovascular accidents and neoplasms are common causes in seizures starting between 55 and 70 years of age. Neurocysticercosis is a common cause of epilepsy, especially in patients emigrating from Mexico, Central America, Ecuador, Iran, and India.

Asymmetry of extremities and facial and cranial bones may suggest cerebral hemiatrophy and atrophic epileptogenic process. Todd's postictal hemiparesis suggests a focal process.

NEURONAL MIGRATION DISORDERS AND CEREBRAL CORTICAL DYSPLASIAS

In the last decade, a body of evidence, advanced by MRI imaging and neuropathology of surgical specimens, has placed neuronal migration disorders and cerebral cortical dysplasias as crucial in the pathogenesis of familial and sporadic epilepsies. These malformations of cerebral cortical development are classified into two major distinct groups, namely, generalized dysplasias and focal dysplasias. Bilateral and generalized dysplasias include the microlissencephalies, classic and "cobblestone" lissencephalies, heterotopia, periventricular nodular heterotopia, and diffuse polymicrogyria. Focal dysplasias include focal cortical dysplasia of the Taylor type with giant balloon neurons in the temporal lobe, developmental neoplastic lesions, hemimegalencephaly, focal polymicrogyria, and schizencephaly. Dysplasias can also be bilateral and focal, as in the subcortical band heterotopia or "double cortex syndrome," bilateral parasagittal parietooccipital polymicrogyria and, bilateral perisylvian polymicrogyria. Dysplasias can be unilateral and hemispheric, as in hemimegalencephaly. Bilateral generalized dysplasias more often have a genetic basis, whereas environmental causes that impair development are suspected in focal dysplasias.

Seven separate chromosomal loci have now been defined for some of these generalized cortical dysplasias (see Table 2IC1). Three specific mutations have been unraveled, one for X-linked bilateral periventricular nodular heterotopia in the form of a

2.25 to 3.25 Mb duplication in chromosome Xq28, one for lissencephaly 1, a deletion in chromosome 17p13.3, and one mutation in a gene that encodes for the protein "doublecortin" in the syndrome of subcortical band heterotopia. The locus 17p13.3 appears phenotypically as a sporadic disorder but actually represents either an isolated autosomal dominant lissencephaly or an isolated autosomal dominant Miller Dieker syndrome. Duplication of 9p was recently implicated in centrosylvian polymicrogyria.

Although most cases of generalized neuronal migration disorders appear to be sporadic, a genetic cause is actually present. Either sex-linked dominant inheritance with male lethality or severe expression in hemizygous males explains the female preponderance, the high frequency of spontaneous abortions, and the abnormal sex ratios in sibships of subcortical band heterotopia or double cortex syndrome and periventricular nodular heterotopia. These X-linked disorders are allelic human disorders, which map to chromosome Xq22.3-Xq23. It is interesting that families typically have females and daughters with subcortical band heterotopia, mild mental retardation, and seizures, whereas their sons have lissencephaly, seizures, and severe retardation. In 1998, mutations of doublecortin were identified in four families and three sporadic cases of the double cortex syndrome. A novel 10-kb brain-specific cDNA interrupted by a balanced translocation was originally observed in an XLIS patient that encodes the novel 40-kd protein called doublecortin. Mutations in doublecortin impair migration and explain the disruption of the six-layered cortex as a failure of early events associated with neuron dispersion.

In contrast to subcortical band heterotopia, periventricular nodular heterotopia appears in persons with normal intelligence who present clinically with epilepsy, often temporal lobe epilepsy. Bilateral perisylvian polymicrogyria is probably also a genetic disorder, having been reported in monozygotic twins and families.

In the 1970s and 1980s, histopathologic abnormalities, such as abnormal distribution of granule cells, focal cortical dysplasia, and forme fruste of tuberous sclerosis, had already been observed in surgical specimens removed from patients with hippocampal temporal lobe epilepsy, frontal neocortical epilepsy, infantile spasms, and Lennox–Gastaut syndrome. Neuronal migration disorders—specifically microdysgenesis—had originally been recognized as important pathological substrates in the autopsy specimens of genetically determined idiopathic generalized epilepsies and symptomatic partial epilepsies, such as West syndrome and Lennox–Gastaut syndrome. More recently, birth defects, such as cleft lip/palate, spina bifida aperta/occulta, and other forms of rachischisis, have been reported to be increased in infants of mothers with epilepsy with or without antiepileptic drug treatment.

SEIZURES FROM INTRACRANIAL TUMORS

Epileptic seizures that recur in 5 to 20 years may be the only symptom of a slow-growing neoplasm (Chapter 426). Seizures are presenting symptoms in 40% of brain tumors and precede focal neurologic signs and increased intracranial pressure in two thirds of these cases. Seizures occur in 37% of patients with glioblastomas, 70% with astrocytomas, 67% with meningiomas, and 92% with oligodendrogliomas.

Five to 10% of patients who undergo anterior temporal lobectomy or cortectomy because of drug-resistant seizures have a cerebral neoplasm. A cerebral tumor should be suspected when seizures increase in frequency or change patterns or when patients develop status epilepticus or new neurologic signs or symptoms.

POST-TRAUMATIC SEIZURES

Trauma is a common cause of symptomatic or acquired epilepsy and accounts for 10% to 20% of seizures overall and up to 50% in the 15- to 24-year age range. Moderate to severe head injury can increase the risk of epilepsy up to 7% and even 34% in patients injured in combat. Seizures that recur within the first week of head injury are called *early post-traumatic seizures*. They occur in 4% of patients with head injuries. Late traumatic epilepsy (seizures occurring more than 1 week after injury) develop in approximately 5% of nonmissile head injuries and in one third of those with gunshot wounds who are admitted to the hospital. The risk for epilepsy rises to 25% if one early seizure has occurred. About one third of early seizures occur in the first hour after injury, a third occur in the next 23 hours, and the rest occur in the next 6 days. However, the risk for late epilepsy is similar whenever early epilepsy has occurred. Almost 25% of late epilepsy develops more than 4 years after injury. Fifty percent of patients with post-traumatic epilepsy recover spontaneously within 8 years.

Risk factors for post-traumatic seizures include post-traumatic amnesia of more than 24 hours, depressed skull fracture, dural tear, and focal neurologic signs. Brief cerebral concussion in closed-head injuries, which is not associated with loss of consciousness, rarely causes seizures. Treatment should be continued for at least 2 years after the last seizure. Early post-traumatic seizures are not likely to persist. Delayed post-traumatic seizures have a less favorable prognosis. Intractable drug-resistant seizures may be expected in 25% to 30% of cases. Onset of seizures 10 years after head injury is extremely rare.

Phenytoin, phenobarbital, carbamazepine, and valproate have all been futile in preventing chronic epilepsy after head injuries.

At the present time, we have no explanation for the "silent period" between traumatic head injury and the appearance of chronic epilepsy months or years after the injury. Intracellular transduction and gene expressions during head trauma, sprouting of mossy fibers, and granule cell dispersion all may have a role in the silent period between trauma and the induction of chronic epilepsy.

NEUROCYSTICERCOSIS

Neurocysticercosis is a major cause of epileptic seizures in areas of the United States, such as Los Angeles, Chicago, New York, and Miami, which have large populations of immigrants from endemic areas in Asia, Africa, Mexico, and South and Central

America. In Mexico, cerebral cysticercosis is found in 2% to 4% of unselected autopsies.

Neurocysticercosis is the encystment of the larvae of *Taenia solium,* the pork tapeworm in the brain. Infestation is produced by ingestion of the ova through fecally contaminated food, by autoinfection via anal–oral transfer, or by reverse peristalsis of proglottids into the stomach. The larvae are not acquired by eating infected pork; the latter results in adult tapeworm infection. Neurocysticercosis occurs even among vegetarians in endemic areas. Central nervous system invasion occurs in 50% to 70% of all cases of cysticercosis. Epileptic seizures occur in more than 50% of patients with neurocysticercosis. Several clinical subtypes of neurocysticercosis exist and determine whether treatment should be done with anticysticercal drugs. Epileptic seizures should be treated with antiepileptic drugs. These clinical subtypes can occur alone but in 50% of patients, they occur in combinations of two or more subtypes in the same patient. Following are the clinical subtypes of neurocysticercosis:

1. Parenchymal—when the cyst resides in the brain parenchyma. No, minimal, moderate, or severe inflammation can exist around the cyst. A fibrous capsule due to reactive astrogliosis may surround the cyst. Granulomas may form and, over years, be replaced by calcification. The number of cysts vary from one to hundreds.
2. Meningeal—when cysts measuring 0.5 to 1 cm to 10 to 15 cm (giant cysts) reside within the subarachnoid space and cause widespread inflammation and fibrosis of arachnoid membranes. This can lead to hydrocephalus and vasculitis, the most severe and often fatal form of neurocysticercosis syndrome. Severe arachnoiditis at the base of the brain may produce Parinaud's syndrome. Vasculitis and occlusion of vertebral and basilar arteries can lead to death. Multiple vascular occlusion in the cerebral hemispheres causes multi-infarct dementia.
3. Ventricular—when an oncosphere arrives at the choroid plexus of the fourth ventricle through the bloodstream (in 1% of neurocysticercosis), it grows to a size large enough to produce a ball valve that occludes cerebrospinal fluid flow. Hydrocephalus occurs, and episodic intracranial hypertension characterizes the syndrome.

Computed tomography (CT) and MRI, both with contrast enhancement, complement each other in diagnosing the subtypes of neurocysticercosis. When either or both imaging studies suggests neurocysticercosis, cerebrospinal fluid analysis is mandatory to quantify the inflammatory reaction. Enzyme-linked immunoabsorbent assay (ELISA) for anticysticercus antibodies has 94% sensitivity and 98% specificity. The complement fixation test has 84% sensitivity and 94% specificity for anticysticercus antibodies when cerebral spinal fluid shows inflammation.

Simultaneous administration of albendazole and dexamethasone is the suggested treatment for parenchymal cysticercosis and clumps of cysts in the subarachnoid space. Albendazole (15 mg per kilogram per day in two daily doses for 8 days) destroys 85% of parenchymal cysts. Dexamethasone ameliorates the intense inflammation produced by cysticidal therapy. Three months later, a second CT and MRI should be done to determine whether cysts remain. If so, praziquantel (50 mg per kilo-

gram per day in three daily doses for 15 days) should be given as a second course in all patients. When parenchymal cysts respond to cysticidal treatment without leaving granuloma, withdrawal from antiepileptic drug treatment is usually successful. Inactive forms of neurocysticercosis, such as granulomas and calcifications, do not respond to cysticidal treatment but need antiepileptic drugs to stop seizures. Ventricular shunting is performed when hydrocephalus with or without an obstructing cyst in the fourth ventricle is present. Shunting is usually performed before cysticidal treatment is begun. After intracranial hypertension is relieved, cysticidal and corticosteroid treatments are started.

At present, there is one blinded randomized small study that questions the usefulness of albendazole and praziquantel, in (1) ameliorating acute seizures, (2) preventing epileptogenesis, and (3) interrupting the pathologic consequences of central nervous system invasion by cysts. Unfortunately, such a small study had not been able to separate the various clinical subsyndromes of neurocysticercosis, such as the following:

- Active lesions with edema and enhancement after contrast medium
- Inactive lesions with residual calcification and gliosis
- Perisylvian subarachnoidal cysts
- Basilar subarachnoidal cysts
- Intraventricular cysts

This difficulty included their responsiveness or contraindication to cysticidal drugs or surgical treatment. A prospective double-blind controlled study of a large cohort with long-term follow-up is clearly needed.

SEIZURES FROM CEREBROVASCULAR DISEASE

After a person is 50 years of age, cerebrovascular diseases, especially acute embolic cerebrovascular disease, frequently cause seizures (Chapter 426). Cerebrovascular arteriosclerosis without cerebral infarction or hemorrhage rarely causes seizures. Twelve percent of patients have seizures 6 to 12 months after cerebral infarction or hemorrhage. Only 2% of stroke patients experience seizures acutely. These usually present as epilepsia partialis continua or partial status with periodic lateralized epileptiform discharges.

COURSE AND PROGNOSIS

GENETIC EPILEPSIES WITH GENERALIZED OR PARTIAL SEIZURES

Almost all genetic epilepsies with primary generalized seizures have an excellent prognosis. Sixty to 95% are stopped by drug treatment. Genetic partial epilepsies, such as rolandic epilepsy are usually controlled by monotherapy, and clinical features usually disappear by age 16.

ACQUIRED PARTIAL EPILEPSIES

Because partial seizures are often due to atrophic nonprogressive structural changes, they stand a good chance of being controlled and even cured. Seizures from tumors, vascular malformation, and cerebral infarctions are unlikely to be cured. Control of attacks should be the goal. Partial seizures occurring early in life and in newborns have a favorable prognosis. Early treatment in adults also produces a favorable prognosis as long as an underlying progressive structural disease is not present.

BIBLIOGRAPHY

Chauvel P, Delgado-Escueta AV, Halgren E, Bancaud J. *Frontal lobe seizures and epilepsies.* Advances in Neurology, vol. 57. New York: Raven Press, 1992.
Delgado-Escueta AV, Wilson WW, Olsen RW, et al. *Jasper's basic mechanisms of the epilepsies.* Advances in Neurology, vol. 79 New York: Lippincott Williams & Wilkins, 1999.
Wyllie E. *The Treatment of epilepsy: principles and practice.* Philadelphia: Lea & Febiger, 1998.

Kelley's Textbook of Internal Medicine, fourth edition. Edited by H. David Humes. Lippincott Williams & Wilkins, Philadelphia © 2000.

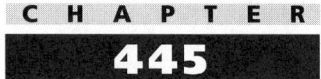

CHAPTER 445

STRUCTURAL DISORDERS OF THE SPINAL COLUMN

JOHN DEAN RYBOCK

Spinal disorders probably account for more physician visits than any other group of medical disorders. One of every five to six adults seek treatment for back problems each year, 85% of the population experiences a significant episode of back dysfunction during his lifetime, and 25% of time lost from work is due to spinal problems. The bulk of neurosurgical practice is devoted to spinal diseases, and a large percentage of orthopedic, chiropractic, and physical therapy practices involve spinal problems. Most patients treated in specialized pain programs have spinal disorders.

It is neither reasonable nor practical to create a comprehensive list of all the disorders of the spine. The standard disease processes require multivolume texts for basic coverage; furthermore, the clearly defined diagnoses explain only a limited portion of the spinal complaints seen in daily practice. Fortunately, most complaints encountered in the office result from definable structural problems with straightforward treatment approaches, or they can be grouped into a nonspecific (and nonserious) class, which can be successfully treated empirically. The goal of this section is to differentiate between potentially serious conditions that require specialty referral and the much more common benign spinal problems that are best treated in the primary care setting.

The key to understanding the basic spinal dysfunctions and their significance is knowledge of the anatomy of the spine and how it changes with aging. The spine is a stack of 24 blocks of bone (vertebral bodies) separated by flexible spacers (intervertebral discs) running from the sacrum to the base of the skull. It provides the central support for the body while allowing for a certain degree of motion, and it provides a housing for the spinal cord and its nerve roots (spinal canal). In some sense, this combination of the flexible supporting structure of the body with the passageway for the spinal cord is unfortunate, because the stresses of the upright posture and the increasing human longevity lead to degenerative changes in the supporting structures that make an impact on the spinal cord and its nerve roots.

Most patient complaints are a result of aging processes that progress at various rates in all human spines. In the simplest case, the muscular and ligamentous structures that labor to keep this stack of blocks from toppling are always near the limits of their strength and even minor events can overwhelm them, leading to mechanical pain. As the patient ages, the intervertebral disc becomes less flexible and the muscular and ligamentous stresses increase. Each disc goes through a fairly well-defined sequence of changes, in which it loses its hydration, flexibility, and cohesiveness.

Tears occur in its outer cover, and nuclear disc substance may escape the confines of the disc. This is most likely to occur posterolaterally where the spinal nerve roots pass over the disc, and so nerve root compression may occur. Tears may also occur centrally, impinging on the spinal cord, or, in the lumbar area, the cauda equina. As time goes on, all discs become more dehydrated and narrower. The adjacent bone reacts by thickening, as if to provide the support the disc no longer gives. The facet joints, bordering the spinal canal, hypertrophy, as does the lining of the posterior lining of the spinal canal. The result is progressive encroachment on the spinal canal, progressively reducing its cross-sectional area and therefore the space for the spinal cord and its roots. Depending on where such bony growth and ligamentous thickening occur, the spinal cord, the cauda equina, or individual nerve roots can become compressed and symptomatic.

Most spinal problems by far can be traced to either mechanical stress on a less-than-robust structural assembly, an extrusion of substance from a degenerative disc, or the chronic changes that are an inevitable part of the aging process.

Structural spinal dysfunction can manifest clinically in one of three patterns: (1) encroachment on the spinal canal, with compression of its contents (myelopathy in the cervical or thoracic regions, neurogenic claudication in the lumbar region), (2) focal intrusion on a single nerve root (radiculopathy), or (3) mechanical and soft-tissue dysfunction causing pain (cervicalgia or lumbalgia). Each of these distinct clinical syndromes has characteristic features.

■ MYELOPATHY

Myelopathy is dysfunction of the spinal cord itself. This can result from intrinsic disease of the spinal cord or extrinsic compression of it. The presentation depends on the rapidity of development, the spinal levels involved, and the portion of the cord (left-right, anterior-posterior) predominantly affected. Intrinsic processes include neural tumors, demyelinating diseases, and syringomyelia; such conditions are beyond the scope of this chapter.

The more common extrinsic compression can occur as an acute event (fracture-dislocation of the spinal column), a subacute event (metastatic carcinoma occupying the epidural space) or an insidious process (gradual compression due to progressive encroachment on the spinal canal by degenerative changes).

The characteristics of myelopathy are long tract signs and motor and sensory loss patterns confined to the regions below a specific segmental level. The most obvious long tract signs are hyperreflexia, including ankle clonus, and "pathologic reflexes" such as Babinski's sign. If the lesion is in the thoracic region, upper extremity function remains intact. As the involvement moves up the spinal cord from C7 to C4, functional loss progresses from hand to arm to shoulder; higher lesions are usually incompatible with survival.

Acute and subacute presentations of myelopathy warrant early neurosurgical referral; diagnosis and treatment are urgent. Insidious onset myelopathy in patients under 50 years of age is uncommon and generally should be evaluated by a neurologist. In older patients, the most common cause of gradual-onset myelopathy is progressive narrowing of the spinal canal (stenosis) due to the chronic degenerative changes (spondylosis) as previously described. This spondylotic stenosis can occur without neck pain; the patient may simply note that his or her sense of steadiness of the legs has declined or that he or she is having increasing difficulty with fine manipulations with the hands. If physical examination reveals signs of long tract dysfunction, cervical spondylotic myelopathy should be suspected. Magnetic resonance imaging (MRI) can confirm the diagnosis. The condition tends to be slowly progressive and can be arrested only by surgery. The appropriateness of surgical evaluation should be based on the patient's level of disability, rate of progression of the impairment, and age and health status.

NEUROGENIC CLAUDICATION

Neurogenic claudication is the primary syndrome resulting from "spondylotic stenosis" at levels of the cauda equina rather than the spinal cord. The spinal cord typically ends at the L1 level, so that stenosis in the lumbar region produces neurogenic claudication rather than myelopathy.

Neurogenic claudication derives its name from its symptomatic similarity to intermittent claudication, the difficulty with walking due to vascular insufficiency. In both conditions, the main symptom is limitation of walking distance by progressive leg fatigue. Whereas intermittent claudication results from ischemia of the leg muscles, neurogenic claudication is probably due to ischemia of the cauda equina as a result of compression. The two syndromes differ in that the neurogenic variety is more quickly relieved by sitting, is not associated with trophic changes in the legs, and can be relieved by lumbar flexion, which reduces the degree of spinal canal narrowing. A report of increased walk-

ing distance while pushing (and leaning on) a shopping cart is typical of neurogenic claudication.

A noteworthy aspect of neurogenic claudication is that pain is rarely a major presenting symptom. The presence of significant back pain suggests that spinal stenosis, to whatever degree it is present, is not the primary source of the patient's complaint.

Spinal stenosis is a slowly evolving compression; there is the rare occurrence of acute compression of the cauda equina, usually by a massive lumbar disc herniation. Acute cauda equina compression may produce significant pain, but the main presentation is that of severe sudden bilateral leg weakness and numbness with loss of bowel and bladder control. This event represents a surgical emergency and requires urgent neurosurgical referral.

Spinal stenosis, presenting as neurogenic claudication, is commonplace; the caricature of the elderly figure, bent forward and leaning on a cane, is symbolic of this condition. The diagnosis of spinal stenosis is established by imaging studies of the lumbar spine. Both computed tomography scans and MRI can confirm the diagnosis. In interpreting either scan, it is important to evaluate the cross-sectional area of the thecal sac at each motion segment. The bony canal may appear adequate, but hypertrophic ligaments lining the posterior canal usually are the main source of thecal compression.

The most effective nonsurgical treatment for neurogenic claudication is regular performance of a specific back exercise program, called *William's exercises*. This program consists of a series of lumbar flexion stretches, which, over time, flatten the degree of lumbar lordosis. In so doing, the hypertrophic ligaments in the posterior canal are stretched out, decreasing their inward buckling, which is a major component of the stenosis. If regular performance of such exercises over a 2- to 3-month period fails to yield an acceptable degree of improvement, surgical intervention should be considered. Removal of hypertrophic bone and ligament yields marked improvement in walking distance in most patients.

RADICULOPATHY

Widespread neural dysfunction (myelopathy or neurogenic claudication) results from major encroachment on the spinal canal by a structural lesion; however, significant focal neural dysfunction can result from small structural lesions in certain critical areas. The critical areas are the far lateral spinal canal and the neural foramina, where the nerve roots pass through confined spaces. The upper portion of this passageway, where the nerve root arises from the thecal sac, overlies the intervertebral disc. Disc protrusion due to bulging as a result of gradual weakening of its outer layers or due to rupture of its inner material (nucleus pulposus) through the outer layers cause nerve root compression (i.e., herniated disc). Degenerative changes causing reactive bone thickening and spur development (osteophytes) can produce root compression in the lower portions of the passageway (lateral recess and neural foramen). Nerve root compression, by either disc herniation or osteophytes, causes radiculopathy, the loss of the root's motor and sensory functions, and pain in its sensory distribution.

There is a characteristic pattern of neurologic deficit for each nerve root (Chapter 429). Since disc herniation and osteophyte formation are uncommon in the thoracic region, we are usually dealing with cervical or lumbar radiculopathy. Persistent radiculopathy is the main indication for spinal surgical intervention.

Disc herniation is the classic cause of radiculopathy, generally affecting patients in the 30- to 55-year age range. The onset is often sudden, evolving from back or neck pain to the full pattern of radiculopathy over hours to a few days. There may be an episode of trauma causing the onset, but spontaneous occurrence is not uncommon.

Nerve root compression due to osteophyte formation is more common past the age of 50. Onset is less often related to trauma and is often insidious, progressing over months to years. Compared with radiculopathy due to disc herniation, the pain tends to be duller, the weakness less marked, and neck or back pain more significant.

In the cervical area, the most common nerve roots affected by either disc herniation or osteophytic compression are C6 and C7. The C6 root innervates the biceps muscle and carries sensation from the thumb and first finger. Therefore, loss of the biceps reflex and radial hand numbness and paresthesias are characteristics of C6 radiculopathy. The C7 root innervates the triceps and carries sensation from the middle digits, so C7 radiculopathy is characterized by loss of triceps jerk and sensory abnormalities in the central portion of the hand.

In the lumbar area, the L5 and S1 roots account for 95% of radicular loss in clinical practice. The L5 root provides sensation from the medial foot and innervates the dorsiflexors of the ankle; its loss is characterized by numbness of the great toe and partial foot drop. The S1 root serves the lateral foot and the gastrocnemius muscles, so an S1 radiculopathy produces small toe numbness and loss of the ankle reflex.

The diagnosis of radiculopathy is made on clinical grounds. Although imaging studies can clarify the structural cause, such clarification is not initially important. Nonsurgical therapy is initiated, with the expectation that at least 75% of cases can be resolved without surgery. The most important treatment modality for cervical radiculopathy is cervical traction. Although physical therapy modalities appears to help reduce the pain level, it is "over-the-door" cervical traction, done twice daily at home, which appears to most effectively promote resolution. Traction works well even when root dysfunction is due to osteophytic compression, suggesting that radiculopathy is due to more complex pathology than simple impingement. Once an episode of radiculopathy has resolved, physical therapy, stressing neck-strengthening exercises, can reduce the risk of recurrence.

With lumbar radiculopathy, initial treatment depends on the rapidity of onset and the severity of the symptoms. Acute onset with severe radicular pain usually requires several days of reduced activity, occasionally bed rest, until the degree of disability decreases. Pain medication, either a nonsteroidal anti-inflammatory or a narcotic-acetaminophen combination, is prescribed. In the more severe cases, the addition of diazepam provides some muscle relaxation and makes reduced activity more easily tolerated. Prolonged periods of marked inactivity should be avoided. As the degree of pain decreases, activity can be gradually increased; in general, the highest level of activity that does not aggravate the radicular pain should be maintained. Aggravation of nonradicular back pain does not delay recovery.

After the acute episode has settled down or with gradual-onset radiculopathy, physical therapy progressing to a home back exercise program is recommended. Particularly in older patients with probable osteophytic compression of a nerve root, a lumbar flexion exercise program (Williams exercises) can gradually open up the neural foramen and resolve the radiculopathy.

Except in cases of major neural dysfunction, such as a complete foot drop, the described should be undertaken before specialty referral. Since most radiculopathies resolve with such treatment, surgical intervention is seldom a valid consideration before 4 to 6 weeks of conservative therapy. Even if some pain or neurologic deficit persists at that point and the patient is showing any evidence of improvement, conservative therapy should be continued. In some cases, it may take 3 months for complete resolution of the radiculopathy.

■ NECK AND BACK PAIN

In classic cases of myelopathy, neurogenic claudication, or radiculopathy, nonradicular pain is not a prominent component. When neck or back pain predominates, the causes are usually not stenosis or nerve root compression. Such pain, constituting the bulk of patient spinal complaints, is not well understood. Most cases appear to be a combination of chronic stress on spinal structures, such as facet joints, and acute stress to the paravertebral muscles. Although the intervertebral disc is not highly pain-sensitive, the facet joints are. Considering the typical forces born by these true diarthrodial joints, chronic injury and pain are probably fairly common. Furthermore, maintaining competent body support about a flexible stack of vertebrae requires significant continual muscle tension; fairly trivial movements, particularly when lifting or bending, can require a level of tension that exceeds the strength of some muscle bands. Acute strain can occur without an identifiable event. Once paraspinal muscles are injured and in spasm, the baseline stress level can delay resolution.

If a patient is experiencing predominantly neck or back pain, even if studies demonstrate some spinal stenosis or disc pathology, surgery is generally not beneficial. The initial approach is standard physical therapy, using modalities to reduce the acute discomfort and exercises to restore normal function and strengthen the muscles to minimize future episodes. If the patient fails to respond to a basic course of therapy, referral to a physiatrist should be considered.

BIBLIOGRAPHY

Bigos SJ, Bowyer OR, Braen GR, et al. Clinical practice guideline number 14 acute low back problems in adults. US Department of Health and Human Services AHCPR 1994; Publication no. 95-0642;1:160.

Porter RW. Spinal Stenosis and neurogenic claudication. *Spine* 1996;21: 2046–2052.

Waddell G, Feder G, Macintosh A, Hutchison A. Low back pain evidence. *Roy Coll Gen Pract* 1996;1:62.

Zdeblick TA. The treatment of degenerative lumbar disorders. A critical review of the literature. *Spine* 1995;20:126S–137S.

Kelley's Textbook of Internal Medicine, fourth edition. Edited by H. David Humes.
Lippincott Williams & Wilkins, Philadelphia © 2000.

C H A P T E R

446

DISORDERS OF THE PERIPHERAL NERVOUS SYSTEM

AHMET HÖKE
THOMAS E. FEASBY

RELEVANT ANATOMY AND PATHOPHYSIOLOGY

ANATOMY

The anatomy of the peripheral nervous system (PNS) is complicated by its diverse array of cell types and broad expanse (Fig. 446.1). The concept of the PNS is itself arbitrary because many of its cells lie in part in the central nervous system (CNS). Cross sections of nerve biopsy specimens reveal only a limited snapshot of the PNS, showing myelinated and unmyelinated fibers of various sizes, but not their orientation or function.

The alpha and gamma motor neurons lie in the anterior horns of the spinal cord but may extend for up to 1 m in length in the PNS. The cell bodies of the primary sensory neurons are in the dorsal root ganglia (DRG), and their central processes extend into the spinal cord segmentally. They project either up the dorsal columns to the gracile and cuneate nuclei or synapse with second-order neurons in the dorsal horn, which form the spinothalamic tracts. The proximal portions of the PNS are the dorsal and ventral spinal nerve roots, which lie in the subarachnoid space and are bathed in cerebrospinal fluid. Only the postganglionic autonomic neurons lie entirely within the PNS. The long length of PNS axons, their dependence on axonal transport for renewal of structural membrane and cytoskeletal components, and other factors make them especially vulnerable. Retrograde transport is essential for trophic function and recycling.

Schwann cells envelop myelinated and unmyelinated axons in the PNS. The signal for myelination comes from the axon, and myelination occurs in axons larger than 1 to 2 μm in diameter. Each segment of a myelinated axon is the territory of a single Schwann cell, the length of the segments correlating with the diameter of the axon. For unmyelinated fibers, single Schwann cells usually surround multiple axons. The myelin sheath is composed of compacted layers of the Schwann cell membrane. It is predominantly lipid but contains several proteins that have key roles in maintaining the structure and compaction of the myelin

and adhesion of the sheath to the axon. Several of these proteins and lipids may be important immunogens in disease.

Peripheral nerves are divided into fascicles surrounded by the perineurium, a connective tissue sheath, and are bound together by the epineurium. The endoneurium surrounding the individual nerve fibers contains collagen, fibroblasts, mast cells, and resident macrophages. The endoneurial arterioles are supplied by a plexus of epineurial blood vessels with multiple systemic feeders. Circulating macromolecules are excluded from the endoneurium by the blood–nerve barrier, which is analogous to the blood–brain barrier and is formed by the endothelial cells and their tight junctions. The blood–nerve barrier is relatively deficient in the DRG and in the preterminal regions of nerves.

PATHOLOGIC FACTORS

The major pathologic reactions of nerve fibers are axonal degeneration and demyelination. Axonal degeneration can be distal, sometimes referred to as dying back or distal axonopathy. This is characteristic of metabolic and toxic neuropathies. Transection of an axon results in complete degeneration of its distal extent, a process known as wallerian degeneration. This occurs in nerve injuries and entrapments. Repair after either of these axonal lesions is by axonal regeneration, a vigorous response that proceeds distally at 1 to 3 μm per day. With distal lesions, regeneration can produce an excellent result, but the likelihood of success is inversely related to the distance to be covered and, in the case of traumatic transection, the timeliness and accuracy of repair. Recovery may be limited in distal axonopathies by the degeneration of the central processes of the DRG cells, which do not effectively regenerate.

Damage to Schwann cells or myelin can result in segmental demyelination or paranodal demyelination. Segmental demyelination results in stripping of the myelin sheath from a complete segment, up to 1 mm in length, whereas paranodal demyelination usually covers less than 50 μm. Macrophages remove myelin debris, and Schwann cells divide after segmental demyelination. Remyelination can begin quickly, within a few days, producing shorter segments of myelin, usually about 300 μm.

PHYSIOLOGY

Conduction in myelinated fibers is saltatory, with the action potential regenerated at successive nodes of Ranvier, the site of sodium channels. During the action potential, sodium flows down its electrical and concentration gradients into the axon through the nodal sodium channels. The action current flows along the core of the axon, confined because of the insulating qualities of the myelin, and depolarizes the next node. The major effect of demyelination is to cause current leakage from the axon, so that not enough current reaches the next node to cause depolarization. This results in conduction block. This failure of transmission produces weakness and sensory loss. However, even minor degrees of remyelination can quickly result in restoration of conduction and recovery of function. The combination of demyelination and remyelination often causes several other characteristic physiologic abnormalities, such as slowed conduction velocity, temporal dispersion of nerve impulses, and reduced

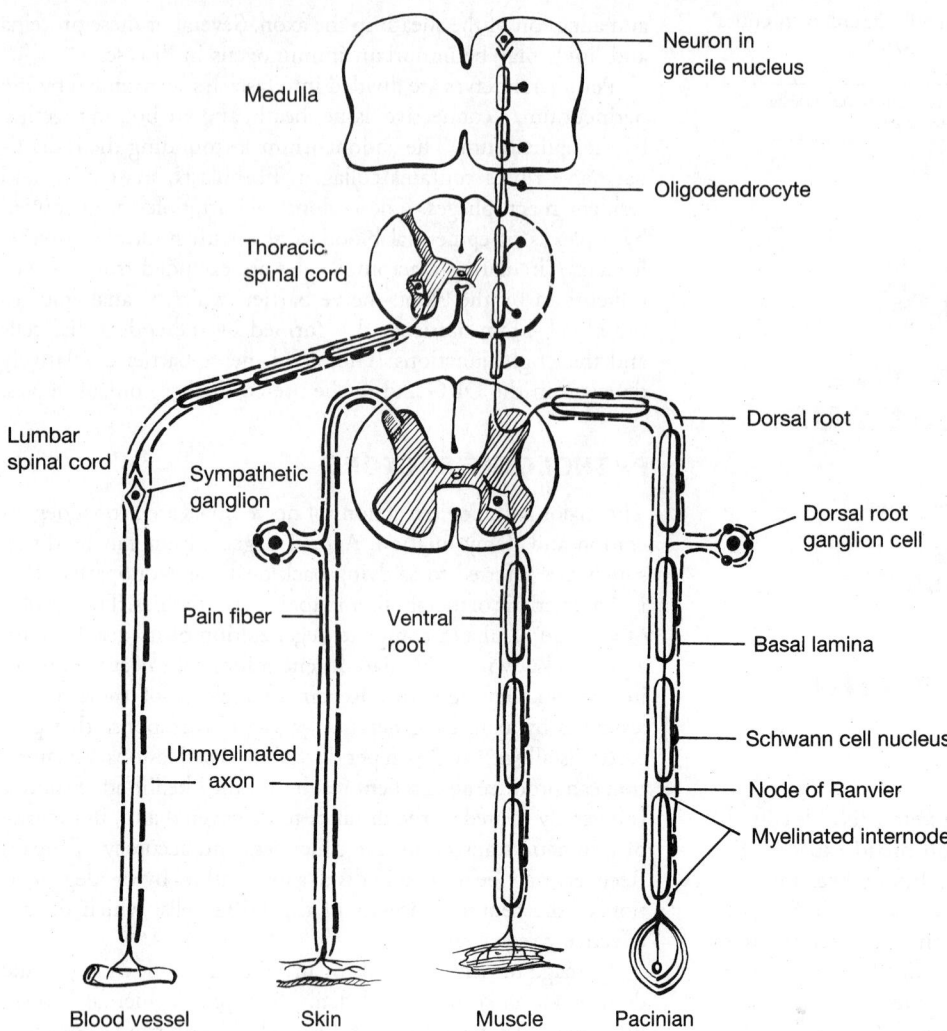

Medulla

Neuron in
gracile nucleus

Oligodendrocyte

Thoracic
spinal cord

Dorsal root

Lumbar
spinal cord

Sympathetic
ganglion

Dorsal root
ganglion cell

Pain fiber

Ventral
root

Basal lamina

Schwann cell nucleus

Unmyelinated
axon

Node of Ranvier

Myelinated internode

Blood vessel   Skin   Muscle   Pacinian
corpuscle

FIGURE 446.1. The principal compo-
nents of the peripheral nervous system.
(Redrawn from Schaumburg HH, Berger
AR, Thomas PK. *Disorders of peripheral
nerves,* second ed. Philadelphia: FA Davis
Company, 1992.)

ability to conduct impulses at high frequency; however, these
defects have only minor clinical effects.

CLINICAL FEATURES OF NEUROPATHY

A thorough history is essential in neuropathy diagnosis. The
onset and progression of symptoms vary tremendously, from
acute over hours to days, to chronic over many years. The progression may be gradual or stepwise, the latter in multiple mononeuropathy. A history of infections, travel, diet, toxic exposure,
alcohol, and medications must be sought. Occupational factors
may be important in causation as well as therapy. The family
history is often critical. A detailed family tree should be drawn
and information sought from key relatives. In cases of doubt,
examination and electrophysiologic or genetic testing of family
members may be necessary.

Negative symptoms predominate in polyneuropathy (usually
weakness and numbness). Positive motor symptoms (cramps and
fasciculations) are uncommon, whereas positive sensory symp-

toms (tingling and pain) occur more frequently. Imbalance, especially at night or in the shower, is a common complaint with
loss of proprioception. Signs found on examination correspond
closely to the symptoms and are predominantly distal and symmetrical. Weakness is common and wasting, if present, signifies
axonal loss. Loss of superficial pain sensation is found with loss
of small myelinated and unmyelinated axons, but loss of vibration sense is more common with large-fiber neuropathies. Sensory loss is usually in a glove-and-stocking distribution. Loss
of tendon reflexes is common with all polyneuropathies. Both
vibration sensation and tendon reflexes are lost early in demyelinating neuropathies, probably because of desynchronization of
afferent nerve impulses produced by the variable slowing of conduction velocities. Automated quantitative sensory testing may
improve the reliability of the sensory examination in neuropathy.
Autonomic neuropathy can cause postural hypotension, urinary
retention and incontinence, constipation, nocturnal diarrhea,
impotence, and sweating abnormalities. Nerve hypertrophy occurs occasionally. Ulnar and peroneal nerves can be palpated,
and several nerves, including the dorsal cutaneous nerve of the
foot, the great auricular nerve, and the distal branch of the super-

ficial radial nerve at the wrist, can be both seen and felt. These nerves must be examined often to establish a sense of normal.

Multiple mononeuropathy differs from polyneuropathy in its distribution. It often affects the territory of individual nerves and is usually asymmetrical. Symptoms are more abrupt in onset. The symptoms may be sensory alone or combined motor and sensory. Pain is often a feature.

LABORATORY INVESTIGATION OF PERIPHERAL NEUROPATHY

Nerve conduction studies and electromyography provide a physiologic nerve "biopsy." The goal is to determine if the predominant pathologic process is demyelination or axonal loss. The pattern of disease can often be discerned, which may be helpful in multiple mononeuropathy.

The major physiologic features are shown in Table 446.1. Demyelination is characterized by slowed conduction velocity, temporal dispersion of the compound muscle action potential, and conduction block. Hereditary demyelinating neuropathies do not usually show the latter two features. Prolonged distal motor and sensory latencies and prolonged F-wave latencies are reflections of slowed conduction velocities in distal and proximal portions of the nerves, respectively. Axonal disease and loss are characterized by modest slowing of velocities, more marked reductions in the amplitudes of the compound muscle action potentials and the sensory nerve action potentials, and evidence of denervation on needle electromyography. The latter includes the presence of fibrillation potentials and positive waves indicative of recent denervation, and enlarged hypercomplex motor unit potentials indicative of chronic denervation with subsequent re-innervation.

Nerve biopsy is reserved for difficult diagnostic and management situations in which the information may yield a specific diagnosis or increase diagnostic security before the use of potentially toxic or expensive treatment. Many diseases formerly diagnosed in part by biopsy can now be diagnosed better by genetic analysis, rendering biopsy unnecessary. Suspicion of vasculitis is

the most important current reason for nerve biopsy. A sample of an adjacent muscle may increase the diagnostic yield. Biopsy is also valuable in the search for neuropathy due to amyloid, sarcoid, or leprosy. Occasionally, when steroid or immunosuppressive therapy is being considered for an acquired demyelinating neuropathy, a biopsy may be helpful to ease diagnostic uncertainty. There are, of course, exceptions to these guidelines and a variety of research indications for biopsy.

The sural nerve is the usual site of biopsy, and fascicular biopsy is adequate except when vasculitis is a consideration, in which case it is essential to take a segment of the whole nerve so that the epineurial vessels can be examined. When a motor nerve is required, the deep peroneal nerve can be sampled just above the ankle along with the sensory superficial peroneal nerve and the peroneus brevis muscle. In the search for vasculitis, it may be useful to examine all of these nerves electrophysiologically and then select an abnormal one for biopsy.

Toluidine blue–stained plastic cross sections of nerve are the most informative, yielding the best morphologic details. Paraffin-embedded sections stained with hematoxylin–eosin are useful in the search for vasculitis, and Congo red stains are positive for amyloid. Teased-fiber analysis may be useful to distinguish demyelinating neuropathies in questionable cases. Electron microscopy is sometimes helpful.

Patients must be told that the biopsy will result in an area of permanent numbness and that there may be tingling and, occasionally, pain. Meticulous surgical technique is required to yield a biopsy specimen free from artifacts and to ensure good wound healing.

Quantitative autonomic testing may be useful in neuropathies with autonomic features; however, it is not widely available.

CLASSIFICATION OF PERIPHERAL NEUROPATHIES

Anatomical and pathologic classifications of peripheral neuropathies facilitate clinical diagnosis. The two common patterns are a symmetrical, usually distal distribution, and an asymmetrical or multifocal distribution. The former is often usefully termed polyneuropathy and can be divided pathologically (physiologically) into distal axonopathies (axonal neuropathies) and myelinopathies (demyelinating neuropathies). Sensory neuronopathies (diseases of the DRG) may have a similar distribution. Asymmetrical neuropathies may be focal (mononeuropathy) or multifocal (mononeuropathy multiplex). In general, the causes of each of these categories of neuropathy differ, although diabetes is a notable exception. These neuropathies may be further subdivided into acute, subacute, and chronic conditions. A differential diagnosis of common neuropathies based on the temporal course of the illness is given in Table 446.2. Causes of multiple mononeuropathy are listed in Table 446.3. Figure 446.2 outlines a schematic approach to diagnosis of specific neuropathies. Despite extensive investigations, cause may be elusive in up to one-third of the patients.

TABLE 446.1.	ELECTROPHYSIOLOGIC FEATURES OF AXONAL AND DEMYELINATING POLYNEUROPATHIES	
Feature	**Axonal**	**Demyelinating**
Distal latency	↑	↑↑↑
Conduction velocity	↓	↓↓↓
F-wave latency	↔	↑↑
Conduction block	No	Yes
Temporal dispersion	No	Yes
CMAP amplitude	↓↓	↓
SNAP amplitude	↓	↓↓
Denervation on EMG	+++	+/–

CMAP, compound muscle action potential; EMG, electromyography; SNAP, sensory nerve action potential.

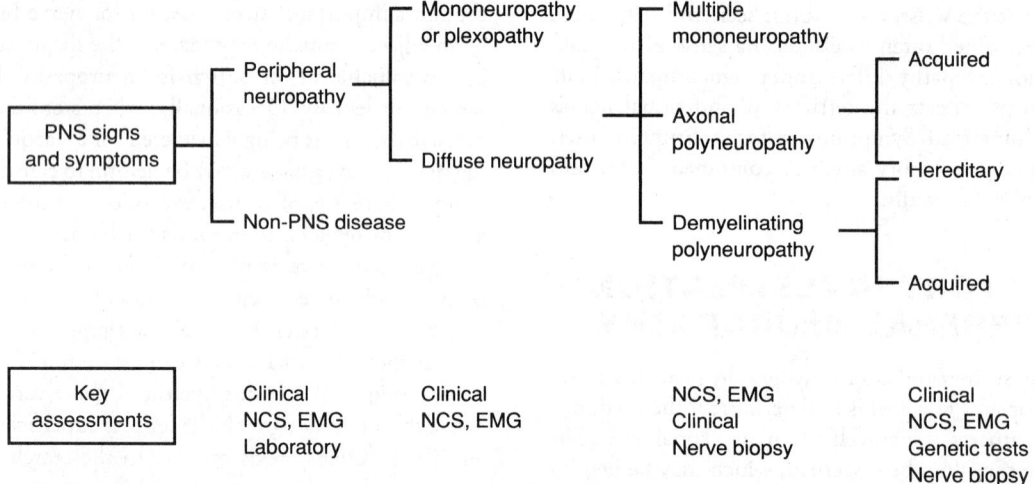

FIGURE 446.2. Stages in the diagnosis of peripheral neuropathy. "Clinical" includes history and physical examination. NCS, nerve conduction studies; EMG, electromyography. (Adapted from Schaumburg HH, Berger AR, Thomas PK. *Disorders of the peripheral nerves,* second ed. Philadelphia: FA Davis Company, 1992.)

SPECIFIC NEUROPATHIES

GUILLAIN–BARRÉ SYNDROME

This dramatic illness is sometimes called Landry's paralysis or acute inflammatory polyneuropathy. It has long been thought to be a classic inflammatory–demyelinating polyneuropathy, but the concept has broadened considerably more recently. The annual incidence is 1 to 2 per 100,000.

The principal symptoms and signs of Guillain–Barré syndrome (GBS) are weakness and sensory loss. The illness typically begins with tingling and numbness in the feet, followed by a gradually progressive, often ascending weakness. Sensory signs are usually minor blunting of distal pain and more marked loss of vibration sensation, but all modalities can be involved. Facial weakness occurs in up to 50% of cases, and bulbar weakness and oculomotor signs in less than 10%. Pain occurs in 70%, usually in the back and upper legs. Respiratory failure requiring mechanical ventilation develops in about 25% of patients. The disease progresses for an average of about 2 weeks, and the arbitrary upper limit for research studies has been set at 4 weeks. The progressive stage is usually followed by a brief plateau; then recovery begins, which may take many months and occasionally 1 to 2 years.

The differential diagnosis includes spinal cord disease and acute motor disorders, such as botulism and myasthenia gravis. Spinal cord disease can usually be excluded on clinical examination by the absence of spasticity, hyperreflexia, and Babinski responses, and often by the presence of facial weakness. Nerve

---

TABLE 446.2. **CLASSIFICATION OF NEUROPATHIES BASED ON TEMPORAL COURSE**

Acute (days–weeks)
  Acute inflammatory polyneuropathies (Guillain–Barré syndrome and variants)
  Diphtheritic neuropathy
  Porhyric neuropathy
  Diabetic amyotrophy
  Some toxic neuropathies
Subacute (weeks–months)
  Vasculitic neuropathy
  Nutritional and alcoholic neuropathy
  Most toxic and infectious neuropathies (e.g., HIV)
Chronic (months–years)
  Diabetic polyneuropathy
  Chronic inflammatory polyneuropathy
  Paraneoplastic and paraproteinemic neuropathies
  Most metabolic neuropathies (e.g., hypothyroidism)
  Idiopathic small-fiber sensory neuropathy
Very chronic (many years, often childhood onset)
  Inherited neuropathies (e.g., Charcot–Marie–Tooth disease)

(Adapted from Griffin JW, Cornblath DR. Peripheral neuropathies. In: Harvey M, et al., eds. *Principles and practice of medicine,* 22nd ed. Norwalk, CT: Appleton and Lange, 1988.)

TABLE 446.3. **CAUSES OF MULTIPLE MONONEUROPATHY**

Vasculitis
Diabetes
Sarcoidosis
Hereditary neuropathy with liability to pressure palsies (tomaculous neuropathy)
Multifocal motor neuropathy with conduction block
HIV infection
Lyme disease
Leprosy
Malignant infiltration of nerves
Lymphomatoid granulomatosis
Neurofibromatosis

conduction studies may be helpful, but in difficult cases spinal cord imaging may be necessary. Acute motor disorders are usually excluded by the presence of sensory signs. Physiologic studies may again be helpful. Unusual disorders, such as poliomyelitis and porphyria, should be kept in mind.

Cerebrospinal fluid examination and nerve conduction studies often yield characteristic findings. The cerebrospinal fluid protein level is usually elevated without a cellular response after the first few days. The major early electrophysiologic finding is conduction block in motor nerves. This may be very distal or proximal, and multiple stimulation sites must be used to detect it. Distal latencies and F-wave latencies may be prolonged early. Conduction velocity reduction is usually most pronounced after a few weeks, likely reflecting early remyelination.

Pathologic examination of nerves from GBS cases usually reveals perivascular lymphocytic infiltration of the endoneurium, although some biopsy studies have failed to find this. The cardinal pathologic finding is segmental demyelination, best seen on teased-fiber studies. Axonal degeneration is also seen, especially in severe cases, and is thought to be a "bystander" effect of inflammation and demyelination. This secondary axonal degeneration, if marked, is likely to cause a poor outcome.

The pathogenesis of GBS is still unclear. GBS is preceded by an infection in up to 70% of cases, including various viruses, *Mycoplasma pneumoniae*, and *Campylobacter jejuni*. The antigenic heterogeneity of these agents suggests that they may act as nonspecific immunologic triggers. *C. jejuni*, a common intestinal pathogen, may be an exception. It shares epitopes with G_{M1} ganglioside, a component of axonal membranes and myelin. Some series have found up to 40% of GBS patients to have anti-G_{M1} antibodies, but their role in demyelination is not certain. The effectiveness of plasma exchange suggests that antinerve antibodies may be significant. There is also evidence of T-cell activation in GBS, although the administration of anti–T-cell antibodies does not seem to stop progression of the disease.

Complete recovery from GBS occurs in about 70%, good functional recovery with minor residua in 10%, moderate disability in 10%, severe disability in 5%, and death in up to 5%. Death is usually caused by pulmonary embolism, sepsis, or cardiac arrhythmias. There are several useful prognostic factors. Older age, rapid onset, and the need for artificial ventilation all indicate a relatively poor prognosis. A more specific indicator of poor outcome is severe reduction of the compound muscle action potential (less than 20% of the lower limit of normal). This usually indicates severe axonal loss, which might be expected to correlate with poor recovery.

Treatment has an important impact on the outcome from GBS. Excellent nursing care and physiotherapy are essential. Subcutaneous heparin is given to prevent deep venous thrombosis. Careful monitoring of the vital capacity during the progressive phase is necessary to detect the onset of respiratory failure. It is important to provide adequate information to patients and families at the time of diagnosis to prepare them for progression of the disease and its implications.

Two specific treatments speed recovery from GBS. Plasma exchange has been shown in several studies to improve outcome at 6 months. It is started as early as possible in patients who cannot walk without assistance. The optimum schedule is not known, but the usual approach is to give four to five exchanges (200 to 250 mL per kilogram) over 7 to 10 days. Intravenous immunoglobulin (IVIG) in a dose of 0.4 g per kilogram per day for 5 days has been shown to have an equivalent beneficial effect in GBS. Combination of plasma exchange and IVIG does not provide further benefit from either one given alone. High-dose methylprednisolone has been shown to be ineffective.

VARIANTS OF GUILLAIN–BARRÉ SYNDROME

An acute axonal form of GBS (acute motor and sensory axonal neuropathy) has been described. It presents more acutely than typical GBS and is clinically more severe. Milder cases may occur, but the clinical spectrum has not been defined. These patients often reach their nadir in less than 5 days and are frequently quadriplegic. Pathologic examination of nerves early in the course has shown severe axonal degeneration without demyelination or inflammation. The motor nerves are often electrically inexcitable. The prognosis is poor; less than half of reported patients have recovered well. Specific treatment has not yet been developed.

Acute motor axonal neuropathy has been described mainly in northern China, where it has a high incidence in spring and summer, especially in children. Marked paralysis and respiratory failure are common, but good recovery often occurs. Physiologic studies show marked motor involvement of the axonal type with sensory sparing. Pathologic studies show axonal degeneration with macrophages clustered at the nodes of Ranvier, perhaps causing axonal damage. Many of these patients have preceding infections with *C. jejuni*. Antibodies against G_{M1} ganglioside have been found in some of these cases. Because G_{M1} and *C. jejuni* have common epitopes, *C. jejuni* may trigger an antibody response that targets G_{M1}, which is localized to the nodes. Macrophages then are attracted to the nodes and produce axonal damage.

The Miller Fisher syndrome is a GBS variant with ophthalmoplegia, ataxia, areflexia, and, often, facial weakness but at most minor limb weakness. The onset is subacute and recovery is usually good. Antibodies to the ganglioside G_{Q1B} are found in most cases. These antibodies are capable of blocking neuromuscular transmission in the mouse nerve–diaphragm preparation, and may be active at ocular motor nerve terminals in humans. Mechanisms of ataxia and areflexia are not clear. No good data exist on the usefulness of specific treatments, but the relatively benign prognosis must be kept in mind.

CHRONIC INFLAMMATORY DEMYELINATING POLYNEUROPATHY

Chronic inflammatory demyelinating polyneuropathy is pathologically similar to GBS but is slower in onset, with the lower limit for progression arbitrarily being 12 weeks; however, some patients progress more quickly. Sensory signs are usually more prominent than in GBS and tremor sometimes occurs. There is seldom a history of preceding infection. Electrophysiologic studies are critical in making the diagnosis and typically show slowed conduction velocities, temporal dispersion of the compound muscle action potentials (CMAPs) and sensory nerve action potentials (SNAPs), and conduction block. The pathogenesis is unclear, but evidence favors an immune mechanism, perhaps antibody-mediated. Antibodies to several neural antigens have been reported in chronic inflammatory demyelinating polyneuropathy (CIDP), most recently to tubulin, but the significance is unclear. Nerve biopsy, which is not usually necessary, shows thinly myelinated and occasionally demyelinated fibers. Cross sections may show "onion bulbs" (myelinated fibers surrounded by concentric layers of Schwann cell cytoplasm and basement membranes), indicative of past cycles of demyelination and remyelination.

Several treatments are available. Prednisone produces improvement in most CIDP patients. It is usually started at 60 to 80 mg per day and then tapered slowly with alternate-day dosing after a significant response occurs. Unfortunately, significant side effects occur with prednisone, a complete response does not always occur, and relapse is common as the dose is reduced. Plasma exchange also is effective in many patients. The optimal treatment schedule has not been determined. It is often given intensively, two or three times weekly at the start, and then progressively less frequently. Its main disadvantages are its cost, the need for good venous access, and the risk of relapse as it is withdrawn. Some patients become dependent on plasma exchange, requiring it weekly. IVIG is the newest treatment and works in about 70% of CIDP patients, especially those whose disease is of fairly recent onset and with typical signs of demyelination. The dosage and maintenance schedules must be individualized. Most patients require some type of long-term treatment.

PARAPROTEINEMIC NEUROPATHIES

Monoclonal gammopathy is found in up to 5% of patients with polyneuropathy, particularly in those older than 60 years, in whom it occurs in 3% of normals. The finding of an M protein should always initiate a search for a plasma cell dyscrasia, such as multiple myeloma. Multiple myeloma and Waldenström's macroglobulinemia are frequently associated with an axonal polyneuropathy. Cryoglobulinemia, which may be associated with either of these or occur independently, may be associated with multiple mononeuropathy, usually distal. The mechanism is thought to be deposits of cryoglobulin in the vasa nervorum causing nerve infarction.

There is a specific neuropathy associated with monoclonal gammopathy, usually IgA or IgG and osteosclerotic plasmacytoma. This is often called the POEMS syndrome, the acronym standing for polyneuropathy, organomegaly, endocrinopathy, M protein, and skin changes. The neuropathy is usually chronic, 1 to 2 years in duration, with motor and sensory involvement. Physiologic and pathologic studies confirm its demyelinating nature. There may be hepatomegaly, hyperpigmentation, gynecomastia, testicular atrophy, and, occasionally, pleural effusions and ascites. An osteosclerotic plasmacytoma is best diagnosed by a skeletal survey. It is usually proximal and may have associated lytic areas. It is presumed that the monoclonal protein is an antinerve antibody of some type, but this is unproven. Radiotherapy, the preferred treatment, is effective in most cases, although improvement may be slow. Excision of accessible lesions

has proved effective. More extensive disease may respond to chemotherapy.

Another chronic demyelinating neuropathy is that associated with IgM monoclonal gammopathy, with the M protein directed against the myelin-associated glycoprotein of peripheral nerve myelin. This predominantly sensory neuropathy is often of many years' duration. Microscopy shows characteristic widened spacing of the myelin lamellae. Long-term plasma exchange may be helpful, but the results are not dramatic.

The most common paraproteinemia is monoclonal gammopathy of uncertain significance (MGUS), which occurs in up to 5% of patients with neuropathy, especially older patients. About half of patients with IgM gammopathy are in this category, as are most patients with IgG and IgA gammopathies. The pathologic process may be demyelinating or axonal. The demyelinating cases are likely variants of CIDP and differ little in clinical features, course, or response to treatment from those without MGUS. The axonal cases are usually chronic and vary in severity. In some cases, the M proteins seem to be antinerve antibodies, but this has been an inconsistent finding. Treatment of the axonal cases has been unrewarding.

MULTIFOCAL MOTOR NEUROPATHY

Multifocal motor neuropathy is a slowly progressive asymmetrical neuropathy usually presenting in the third and fourth decades. Although minor distal sensory signs may be present, the signature of this neuropathy is marked motor involvement of individual nerves that have normal sensory function both clinically and electrophysiologically. The weakness and wasting are usually much greater in the arms than the legs, especially in the forearms and hands. Although the patients usually remain ambulatory, the hand weakness can result in significant disability. Areflexia is common. Physiologic studies often show motor conduction block, but not at sites typical of nerve entrapment. The few pathologic studies available have shown signs of chronic demyelination.

Anti-G_{M1} antibodies are found in some multifocal motor neuropathy patients. In preliminary studies, these antibodies have produced conduction block in an experimental nerve–muscle preparation. The roles of these and other antibodies and of demyelination remain to be clarified.

Multifocal motor neuropathy usually does not respond to steroids or plasma exchange. Cyclophosphamide is sometimes effective but potentially toxic. IVIG produces a positive response in about 70% of patients. The result is often seemingly modest but may be functionally important if it leads to improved intrinsic hand muscle strength or better extension of wrist or fingers. Maintenance treatment at intervals of 2 weeks to 2 months is often necessary to sustain improvement.

DIABETIC NEUROPATHY

Diabetic neuropathy (DN) is the most common specific diagnosis made in neuromuscular clinics. Its prevalence is directly related to the duration of the diabetes, approaching 50% in those who have been diabetic for 25 years. Two general types of DN

TABLE 446.4.	CLASSIFICATION OF DIABETIC NEUROPATHY

Mononeuropathies
   Cranial neuropathies
   Limb and trunk mononeuropathies
   Asymmetrical lower-limb motor neuropathy
Polyneuropathies
   Distal sensorimotor (+ autonomic) polyneuropathy
   Autonomic neuropathy
   Acute painful polyneuropathy

occur—symmetrical polyneuropathies and focal or mononeuropathies—each having several subcategories (Table 446.4).

The pathogenesis is unknown. A metabolic cause is likely for the polyneuropathies, probably secondary to hyperglycemia. The concept of increased sorbitol, reduced myoinositol, and lowered Na^+,K^+-ATPase activity in nerve has been popular but remains unproven. Attempts to treat DN by reducing sorbitol levels with aldose reductase inhibitors or by increasing myoinositol levels by dietary supplementation have been unconvincing. The alternative hypothesis is that endoneurial hypoxia is responsible for DN. The common occurrence of endoneurial vascular thickening supports this, but definitive proof in humans is lacking. The presence of vascular thickening and nerve infarcts in the few autopsy studies available of cranial and limb mononeuropathies, and the usually abrupt onset of these disorders, is strong evidence for a vascular cause in these cases.

SYMMETRICAL POLYNEUROPATHIES

Distal sensory and motor polyneuropathy is the most common form of DN. Its onset is usually insidious, sometimes preceding the diagnosis of diabetes in late-onset cases. All fiber sizes are affected, although large- and small-fiber categories have been noted. The former usually presents with distal tingling and numbness and the latter with foot pain, often burning in quality. Rarely, a distal, very painful neuropathy presents acutely and without much sensory loss, and this may have a different mechanism. Mild autonomic features are common. The symptoms of distal sensory DN may remain mild or may produce moderate disability. Progression to severe disability is uncommon. Motor signs are mild.

Strict control of blood sugar is the standard treatment approach and probably slows progression. Pain control may be the major problem. Amitriptyline is the most effective drug, starting at a dose of 25 mg at bedtime and gradually increasing to as high as 150 mg if tolerated. Drowsiness and xerostomia often limit the dose. Gabapentin at a dosage of 900 to 2,400 mg daily in three divided doses may be used as a second-line agent. Carbemazepine and phenytoin are rarely effective. Capsaicin cream can provide short-term relief.

Autonomic neuropathy is part of the spectrum of distal sensory neuropathy, but at times it predominates. The most common symptom is erectile failure, although this may in part be caused by diabetic vascular disease. Incomplete bladder emptying is less common. Cardiovascular reflex abnormalities can be detected but are usually asymptomatic. Occasionally, postural hypotension is disabling. Nocturnal diarrhea and gastroparesis are well known but uncommon. The most common gastrointestinal problem is constipation. Loss of distal sweating is common.

MONONEUROPATHIES

Diabetic mononeuropathies may affect cranial nerves, limb nerves, truncal nerves, or the lumbosacral plexus. These tend to affect older diabetics and may be the first evidence of diabetes. The third nerve is most commonly affected. The onset is abrupt and associated with periocular pain. All divisions of the nerve may be affected, but the pupil is spared in most cases, which helps to differentiate this from intracranial causes. The sixth nerve is less often affected, and rarely the fourth or the seventh nerve is affected. Spontaneous recovery in 1 to 3 months is usual.

Mononeuropathies can affect most major limb nerves. The deficit usually appears suddenly and is often painful. The clinical features resemble those of other "vascular" neuropathies, such as those caused by vasculitis. Recovery is often satisfactory after distal lesions, but proximal lesions do less well. The affected sites in these painful mononeuropathies are usually not common entrapment sites. However, diabetic nerves are sensitive to compression, and entrapment neuropathies, such as carpal tunnel syndrome, occur frequently. They may respond to decompression, but not as well as those in nondiabetics.

Diabetic truncal neuropathy presents in older patients as radicular thoracic pain, often dysesthetic, in one or more thoracic dermatomes. The sensory loss may be strictly radicular or, more commonly, patchy. Hyperesthesia is common. The symptoms usually improve, but the time course is often more than a year. Pain management is the major problem. Amitriptyline and other tricyclics are the mainstays of treatment.

Diabetic lumbosacral plexus neuropathy has also been called diabetic amyotrophy, a useful descriptive term because muscle wasting and weakness are major symptoms and there is usually minimal sensory loss. Typically, the weakness affects the quadriceps, psoas, thigh adductors, and, occasionally, the glutei. Wasting ensues over a few weeks. The quadriceps reflex is usually absent. The onset is sudden but may evolve over a week or two. There is usually deep, aching proximal leg or hip pain that lasts a few weeks, and occasionally much longer. Moderate recovery often occurs but takes a year or more. There is some recent evidence that some of these conditions may be inflammatory in nature and may respond to immunosuppression.

HEREDITARY NEUROPATHIES

This large group of neuropathies is now much better understood as a result of molecular genetic advances. The major disorders are listed in Table 446.5, along with their genetic loci and gene products. Specific diagnosis is now possible by genetic analysis in appropriate phenotypes, obviating the need for nerve biopsy in many cases. Neurologic assessment and counseling of at-risk family members is necessary.

TABLE 446.5.	GENETIC CLASSIFICATION OF THE HEREDITARY SENSORI MOTOR NEUROPATHIES		
Disease	**Locus**	**Gene**	**Mechanism**
HMSN I			
CMT1A	17p11.2–12	*PMP22*	Duplication or point mutation
CMT1B	1q22–23	*P0*	Point mutation
CMTX	xq13.1	*CX32*	Point mutation
HMSN II			
CMT2A	1p35–p36	Unknown	Unknown
CMT2B	3q13–q22	Unknown	Unknown
CMT2C	Unknown	Unknown	Unknown
CMT2D	7p14	Unknown	Unknown
HMSN III			
DSDA	17p11.2–12	*PMP22*	Point mutation
DSDB	1q22–23	*P0*	Point mutation
HNPP			
HNPPA	17p11.2–12	*PMP22*	Deletion or point mutation
HNPPB	Unknown	Unknown	Unknown

HMSN, hereditary motor and sensory neuropathy; CMT, Charcot–Marie–Tooth disease; DSD, Dejerine–Sottas disease; HNPP, hereditary neuropathy with liability to pressure palsies.

HEREDITARY MOTOR AND SENSORY NEUROPATHIES (FORMERLY CHARCOT–MARIE–TOOTH DISEASE)

Hereditary motor and sensory neuropathy (HMSN) type I is a chronic demyelinating polyneuropathy that presents in the first and second decades with slowly progressive distal weakness, wasting, and sensory loss that is most pronounced in the legs. High arches (pes cavus), hammer toes, ankle instability, and eventually deformity are common. Nerve hypertrophy may be seen. Slowed nerve conduction velocities, usually to 20 to 30 m per second, without conduction block are typical. Biopsies show loss of myelinated fibers, signs of demyelination and remyelination, and onion bulbs. Ankle braces, special shoes, and corrective foot and ankle surgery are often helpful. Most patients remain ambulatory. Types Ia and Ib are similar phenotypically, although they have defects in different myelin proteins (in type Ia the PMP22 protein and in Ib the P0 protein).

Hereditary motor and sensory neuropathy type II is a chronic axonal motor–sensory polyneuropathy, similar phenotypically to HMSN type I. High arches, hammer toes, and a distal predominance of wasting, weakness, and sensory loss are typical. Electrophysiologic studies show signs of chronic distal muscle denervation and minor slowing of nerve conduction velocities. Biopsies show chronic axonal loss without signs of demyelination. The clinical course is quite similar for HMSN I and II. Both conditions are autosomal dominant and common.

Hereditary motor and sensory neuropathy type III (Dejerine–Sottas disease) is a rare and probably genetically heterogeneous group of neuropathies presenting in infancy. There is evidence suggestive of both autosomal dominant and recessive inheritance. Defects in the *PMP22* and *P0* genes have been found. The typical patient shows impaired motor development, weakness, sensory loss, and nerve hypertrophy as well as histologic evidence of chronic demyelination and remyelination. HMSN type IV (Refsum's disease), another hypertrophic neuropathy associated with onion-bulb formation, is caused by phytanic acid accumulation. Other HMSN variants have been associated with spastic paraplegia and optic neuropathy.

Charcot–Marie–Tooth X disease is an X-linked form of HMSN. It is expressed more fully in male subjects who clinically resemble patients with HMSN types I and II. About half of female carriers are mildly affected. There is mild slowing of nerve conduction velocities to 30 to 40 m per second. The pathologic changes suggest an axonal defect, but the abnormal protein, connexin-32, is a gap junction protein found in compacted myelin.

HEREDITARY NEUROPATHY WITH LIABILITY TO PRESSURE PALSIES

Hereditary neuropathy with liability to pressure palsies (HNPP) is a common, dominantly inherited neuropathy that is underdiagnosed. It causes mononeuropathies that usually follow minor compression of a nerve, such as from sleeping awkwardly on a limb. Typical nerves to be affected include the radial nerve in the spiral groove of the humerus, the ulnar nerve at the elbow, the median nerve at the wrist, and the peroneal nerve at the fibular head. Brachial plexus palsies sometimes occur, often after unrelated surgical procedures. The lack of pain in typical cases of this neuropathy helps to distinguish this from inherited brachial plexus neuropathy, which is usually painful. The major symptoms are weakness, tingling, and numbness. Recovery is the rule, but it may take several months and may be incomplete. Major disability is unusual.

Nerve conduction studies reveal focal conduction block at symptomatic sites and slowing across other common entrapment sites. Mild, generalized changes are seen, such as prolonged distal latencies, suggesting that there is also a mild polyneuropathy. Nerve biopsies show sausage-like thickenings of the myelin sheaths, known as tomaculi, produced by redundant wrapping of the sheath around the fiber. The genetic defect is a deletion in the *PMP22* gene, the same gene that is duplicated in HMSN type Ia.

HEREDITARY SENSORY AND AUTONOMIC NEUROPATHIES

These rare conditions are classified into four categories. Hereditary sensory and autonomic neuropathy (HSAN) type I is a dominantly inherited sensory neuropathy with predominantly small-fiber loss, resulting in distal pain insensitivity, especially in the feet. It presents in the second decade and progresses slowly. Excellent foot care is the mainstay of treatment. HSAN type II is autosomally recessive, presents in infancy, and progresses slowly. HSAN type III is another autosomal recessive neuropathy presenting in infancy. It is a severe disorder with loss of pain and temperature sensation and autonomic instability. Nerve biopsy shows a near-absence of unmyelinated fibers and depletion of myelinated sensory fibers. HSAN type IV is another recessive condition presenting in infancy. There is loss of pain and temperature sensation, anhidrosis, and mental retardation.

AMYLOID NEUROPATHIES

Amyloid neuropathies may be acquired or dominantly inherited. The cardinal feature of these conditions is the endoneurial deposition of various amyloid proteins identified on nerve biopsy by positive staining (apple-green birefringence) with Congo red. The acquired forms occur with primary systemic amyloidosis and plasma cell dyscrasias. The protein deposited is immunoglobulin light chain. Identification of the specific proteins deposited in the familial amyloid neuropathies has facilitated classification. The first is transthyretin amyloidosis. Transthyretin, formerly called prealbumin, can be affected by several different amino acid substitutions, leading to phenotypic variations in this group. The second group is apolipoprotein A-I amyloidosis. The least common is gelsolin amyloidosis. The transthyretin and apolipoprotein A-I cases have painful distal sensory loss and autonomic dysfunction, and often carpal tunnel syndrome. Weakness can occur. The gelsolin cases have systemic amyloidosis with late-onset neuropathy.

TOXIC NEUROPATHY

Many therapeutic, environmental, and industrial agents can produce neuropathy. The major culprits are listed in Table 446.6, and the most important are discussed in the following paragraphs. Most produce a distal axonopathy, often after prolonged exposure.

PHARMACEUTICALS

Several antineoplastic agents commonly produce neuropathy. The best known of these, vincristine, causes neuropathy in most patients. Sensory symptoms occur first, followed by weakness, which is the most prominent feature on examination. Early cessation of treatment results in good recovery, but prolonged treatment leads to significant disability. Cisplatin produces a mainly sensory neuropathy at higher doses. Occasionally, the symptoms

TABLE 446.6.	TOXIC NEUROPATHIES
Pharmaceuticals	**Industrial and Environmental Agents**
Amiodarone	Acrylamide
Chloramphenicol	Allyl chloride
Chloroquine	Arsenic
Cisplatin	Buckthorn
Colchicine	Carbon disulfide
Dapsone	Dimethylaminoproprionitrile
Disulfiram	Ethylene oxide
Doxorubicin	Hexacarbons (e.g., *n*-hexane)
Ethambutol	Lead
Gold	Mercury
Hydralazine	Methyl bromide
Isoniazid	Organophosphates
Metronidazole	Polychlorinated biphenyls
Misonidazole	Thallium
Nitrofurantoin	Trichloroethylene
Nitrous oxide	Vacor (pyrinuron)
Nucleosides (ddC, ddI, d4T)	
Phenytoin	
Pyridoxine	
Suramin	
Taxol	
Thalidomide	
Vincristine	

begin and progress after treatment is stopped. There is often gradual improvement. Taxol also causes a sensory neuropathy, often soon after the start of treatment when given in doses higher than 200 mg per square meter of body surface area. Suramin can cause a severe demyelinating neuropathy with bulbar and respiratory involvement in 10% of the patients.

Nitrofurantoin and isoniazid are the most frequent antibiotics to cause neuropathy. Nitrofurantoin neuropathy is more common after prolonged treatment and when there is coexistent renal failure. The symptoms may be rapid in onset, and weakness may be prominent. Recovery is good if the drug is stopped immediately. Isoniazid neuropathy happens most often in those who are slow acetylators and have high blood levels. Isoniazid interferes with the action of vitamin B_6. Peripheral neuropathy can be prevented in most cases with daily administration of 100 mg of pyridoxine.

Amiodarone, an antiarrhythmic drug, causes a mainly motor neuropathy after prolonged treatment at high doses. Recovery occurs with early drug stoppage. Gold, usually used to treat rheumatoid arthritis, rarely causes a subacute neuropathy. Numbness, often with hyperesthesia, is followed by weakness. Gradual recovery can occur. Pyridoxine (B_6), an essential vitamin, is safe in low doses but may cause a sensory neuropathy after prolonged use at high doses, often up to 1 g per day for a year. Gradual recovery occurs when the vitamin is stopped. Intravenous administration can result in the acute onset of an irreversible sensory neuropathy. Thalidomide causes dorsal root ganglion degeneration and selective involvement of large myelinated fibers. Distal painful paresthesias and numbness are common; patients develop palmar erythema and brittle fingernails.

TOXINS

Many environmental and industrial agents can produce neuropathy. Heavy metals have long been implicated but are now uncommon causes. Lead produces a mainly motor neuropathy after chronic low-level exposure, usually in smelters or battery manufacturing facilities. Oral ingestion of lead paint in children was once a common cause. The onset is gradual, with the arms weaker than the legs. The pathologic process in humans is probably a distal axonopathy, although experimentally lead can cause demyelination. Arsenic also causes neuropathy after chronic low-level exposure or acute ingestion. The former is usually seen among miners and the latter as a result of attempted suicide or murder. Chronic exposure results in the gradual onset of a painful distal sensory neuropathy, whereas acute ingestion causes the subacute onset of a painful sensory–motor neuropathy. The pathologic process is distal axonal degeneration. Recovery after chelation may be satisfactory. Mercury is a rare cause of neuropathy; it more commonly causes CNS dysfunction.

Industrial agents have caused several neuropathy "epidemics"; organophosphates, the hexacarbons, and acrylamide are the best known. Many of these exposures occurred in factories, but accidental ingestion has occurred with some, such as triorthocresyl phosphate, an industrial lubricant that has been accidentally added to food or substituted for cooking oil. The hexacarbons are solvents and subject to intentional inhalation by "sniffers." A chronic axonal neuropathy that is mainly motor develops. Acrylamide poisoning has usually come from inhalation or skin exposure in industry. A predominantly motor axonal neuropathy develops slowly and may resolve if caught early.

NEUROPATHY ASSOCIATED WITH METABOLIC DISORDERS AND NUTRITIONAL DEFICIENCY

Deficiency Disorders

Alcoholism is the major cause of neuropathy due to nutritional deficiency in the Western world. There remains some controversy over the role of alcohol as a neurotoxin, but most studies favor a primary role for multiple vitamin deficiency, thiamine in particular. Alcoholic polyneuropathy usually occurs in malnourished alcoholics, often after substantial weight loss. This is a distal axonopathy, as are other nutritional neuropathies. Sensory symptoms appear first, followed by distal weakness. About 25% of patients have distal pain and hypersensitivity ("burning feet" syndrome). There may be signs of alcoholic nutritional deficiency–related CNS disease such as cerebellar truncal ataxia or Wernicke's disease. Treatment requires abstinence from alcohol, multiple vitamin supplements orally, intramuscular thiamine, and good caloric and protein nourishment. The neuropathy responds well to this regimen if treated early.

Dietary vitamin deficiency causing neuropathy occurs in the setting of severe nutritional deficiency. It is unusual for a single vitamin to be missing. The major vitamins involved are thiamine (B_1), riboflavin (B_2), niacin (B_3), and pyridoxine (B_6). The symptoms are similar to those of alcoholic neuropathy and reflect a distal axonopathy, often painful. Pure thiamine deficiency is classically associated with beriberi and niacin deficiency with

pellagra, but these are seldom seen in pure form. Recovery depends on vitamin replacement at an early symptomatic stage. A similar neuropathy and sometimes signs of Wernicke's encephalopathy can occur several months after gastroplasty for morbid obesity, especially if there is prolonged vomiting.

Vitamin B_{12} deficiency has long been considered a cause of neuropathy. Myelopathy also occurs and is usually more prominent, often overshadowing the deficit caused by neuropathy. Distal sensory loss may result from myelopathy, but ankle areflexia likely reflects the neuropathy. There may be minor distal nerve conduction abnormalities. Malabsorption due to pernicious anemia or gastrectomy is the principal cause. Rarely, it can be seen in the setting of a purely vegetarian diet. Hematologic abnormalities are usually prominent. Treatment is parenteral vitamin B_{12}.

Vitamin E malabsorption also produces a neuropathy that may be obscured by CNS abnormalities. It occurs with chronic cholestasis and abetalipoproteinemia. It is a distal axonal neuropathy and responds to treatment only if caught early.

Metabolic Disorders

Uremia is the most common intrinsic metabolic cause of neuropathy, producing typical distal axonal changes and corresponding symptoms and signs. About 50% of chronic hemodialysis patients show signs, but it seldom produces major disability with modern treatment. The specific metabolite causing the neuropathic damage is unknown. The most effective treatment is renal transplantation.

Hypothyroidism is associated with a slowly progressive distal axonopathy. It presents with distal numbness and tingling and eventually includes weakness, which may become marked. This neuropathy responds well to early thyroid replacement therapy. Carpal tunnel syndrome is a common feature of hypothyroidism. The mechanism is different and is presumably related to myxedematous deposits in the carpal tunnel causing compression.

The porphyrias are well known but uncommon causes of neuropathy. They are caused by autosomal dominantly inherited defects in several different enzymes in the synthesis of heme, resulting in accumulation of intermediate products. Acute intermittent porphyria, the most common disorder, is characterized by acute attacks that usually begin after puberty. It remains latent in many carriers. Attacks are often provoked by drugs, including many sedatives, estrogens, various antibiotics, and ethanol. The first symptoms are usually crampy abdominal pain and mental disturbances, which may be severe, and, occasionally, seizures. The neuropathy then develops over days to weeks with weakness, either proximal or distal, limb pain, and paresthesias. The weakness may become severe and may include facial weakness and respiratory failure. Autonomic dysfunction is often present. A peak is usually reached in 6 to 10 weeks, followed by slow but often complete recovery. Death may occur in the acute phase. The neurologic features of variegate porphyria and hereditary coproporphyria are similar.

The differential diagnosis includes acute GBS and toxic neuropathies, such as those caused by organophosphates. A history of brown urine suggests porphyria. The key to diagnosis is the increased urine excretion of δ-aminolevulinic acid and porphobilinogen. The acute attacks often respond to high-dose intravenous glucose or intravenous hematin. Provocative drugs must be avoided. Identification of carriers and education about specific drug avoidance are essential.

Several defects in lipid metabolism cause neuropathy. Metachromatic leukodystrophy, usually caused by an autosomal recessively inherited deficiency of the enzyme arylsulfatase A, causes deposition of sulfatides in the central and peripheral nervous systems. It usually presents in late infancy with spastic weakness, dementia, and eventually blindness. Peripheral neuropathy is present and may produce hypotonia, weakness, and areflexia, but the CNS signs usually predominate. Both magnetic resonance imaging and autopsy demonstrate severe cerebral white matter damage. Nerve biopsies show segmental demyelination and metachromatic inclusions in Schwann cells. Nerve conduction velocities are severely slowed. Other lipid and lipoprotein disorders such as Krabbe's globoid cell leukodystrophy, Tangier disease (high-density lipoprotein deficiency), and Bassen–Kornzweig disease (abetalipoproteinemia) also produce peripheral neuropathy.

CARCINOMATOUS NEUROPATHY

Sensory and motor neuropathy, sensory neuronopathy, and malignant infiltration of peripheral nerves all occur with carcinoma, lymphoma, and leukemia. The sensory and motor neuropathy is associated with many different tumors and seldom precedes tumor diagnosis. It is a distal axonopathy that progresses slowly. Its pathogenesis is unknown, but toxic, nutritional, and immunologic causes have been suggested.

The sensory neuronopathy syndrome is uncommon but is much more specific and better understood. Because it frequently presents months before the neoplasm is evident, a careful search for malignancy is necessary. It is most frequently associated with oat cell carcinoma of the lung and occasionally with other lung tumors and cancers of the breast, ovary, and gastrointestinal tract. The illness presents with distal tingling, numbness, and pain that spreads proximally and worsens over 2 to 3 months. Proprioceptive loss is marked, but all modalities are affected. The coordination and gait are impaired by sensory loss, and there may be pseudoathetosis. Weakness does not occur. The cerebrospinal fluid protein may be raised. Electrophysiologic studies show reduced or absent sensory nerve action potentials. Pathologic studies show degeneration of DRG cells with inflammation and secondary degeneration of sensory axons. In many cases associated with oat cell carcinoma, an IgG antibody specific for a tumor and neuronal antigen is found, which has been termed anti-Hu. Its role in the pathogenesis is not certain, but it might gain access to the DRG through its relatively deficient blood–nerve barrier to damage the DRG neurons.

Several other syndromes have been associated with malignancy. Both acute and chronic demyelinating neuropathies have been seen with cancers, most frequently Hodgkin's disease. A curious transient motor neuropathy is sometimes seen with Hodgkin's disease. Some loss of anterior horn motor neurons occurs, but the syndrome is self-limited. Neuropathies associated with myeloma were discussed earlier.

INFECTIOUS AND GRANULOMATOUS NEUROPATHIES

Infectious Neuropathy

Leprosy has been called the world's most common neuropathy, but it occurs rarely in the West. It is caused by chronic infection with *Mycobacterium leprae*. Schwann cells appear to be targets, especially those investing unmyelinated fibers. Small-fiber sensory loss is prominent, in cutaneous patches in both tuberculoid and lepromatous leprosy, and distally in the digits and other cool areas in the latter. Complete anesthesia of the extremities with ulceration and mutilation occurs in severe cases. Progression occurs over many years. Early treatment of the lepromatous variety with dapsone may result in stabilization.

Lyme disease, caused by the spirochete *Borrelia burgdorferi*, may cause a peripheral neuropathy. The organism is carried by ticks that infest mice and deer. The typical clinical course begins with the characteristic rash, erythema migrans, followed after a few weeks by systemic symptoms, including arthritis, carditis, meningitis, and sometimes radiculitis. In the chronic stage, there are persistent symptoms of skin, joint, and neurologic involvement. Cranial neuropathies are common, especially facial, usually during the meningitic phase. The peripheral nerves are affected in a variety of ways, reflecting what is thought to be a multifocal process. The lesions may involve the brachial or lumbosacral plexus or individual nerves or roots. A distal axonal sensory and motor neuropathy occurs in some cases. A form of GBS has been described. Cerebrospinal fluid pleocytosis distinguishes this from typical GBS. Antibiotic treatment is mandatory and is usually beneficial.

Neuropathy is common in HIV infection. Autopsy studies reveal nerve degeneration in almost all cases, and symptomatic neuropathy likely occurs in 30% to 50% of patients. Several distinct varieties of neuropathy occur and are related to the stage of the illness (Table 446.7). Both GBS and CIDP seem to occur with increased frequency in HIV infection. The clinical features are typical except that cerebrospinal fluid pleocytosis is common. Both neuropathies tend to occur early in the course of HIV infection, with GBS, in particular, often seen in relation to the initial HIV infection. Treatment is the same as for these neuropathies in non–HIV-infected patients.

Multiple mononeuropathies frequently occur later in the course of HIV infection. Major nerves may be affected, often with pain at onset. Nerve biopsies have often shown necrotizing vasculitis. The presumed mechanism is vascular deposition of

---

TABLE 446.7.   HIV-RELATED NEUROPATHIES

Inflammatory demyelinating polyneuropathies
    Guillain–Barré syndrome
    Chronic inflammatory demyelinating polyneuropathy
Multiple mononeuropathy (vasculitic)
Distal sensory (+ autonomic) polyneuropathy
Cytomegalovirus polyradiculoneuropathy
Drug-induced polyneuropathy (ddI, ddC, d4T)

immune complexes. Therapy is uncertain because there is often reluctance to use immunosuppression at that stage of the illness.

A distal, mainly sensory neuropathy is the most common neuropathy of AIDS, usually occurring late in the illness. It is a distal axonal neuropathy with nonspecific pathologic and physiologic features, and is of unknown cause. The legs are much more involved than the arms and pain may be a major feature, causing some disability. The neuropathy may be slowly progressive, and there is no specific treatment.

Cytomegalovirus infection is common in late-stage AIDS and may produce a recognizable and devastating neuropathy. Inflammatory lesions with axonal degeneration are found in the lumbar spinal roots. Cytomegalovirus may be cultured. The illness presents subacutely with a cauda equina syndrome with radiating lower back pain, asymmetrical weakness of the legs, sacral sensory loss, and, often, urinary incontinence. Occasionally, the arms are affected. The illness is progressive. Early recognition and treatment with ganciclovir may result in stabilization.

Iatrogenic dose-dependent neuropathy has been reported with anti-HIV treatment with the dideoxynucleotide analogs zalcitabine (ddC), didanosine (ddI), and stavudine (d4T). It appears to be a distal axonopathy.

Sarcoid Neuropathy

Sarcoidosis, a granulomatous disease of unknown etiology, causes peripheral neuropathy in 5% to 10% of cases. Granulomas are found within the endoneurium, presumably causing compression and possible ischemia of nerve fibers. Multiple mononeuropathy is the usual clinical presentation. Limb or trunk nerves can be affected, and patchy truncal sensory loss with pain is common. Cranial nerves may be involved, particularly the facial nerve, which is affected abruptly and often bilaterally. Rarely, a distal sensory and motor polyneuropathy occurs. Diagnosis is made by nerve muscle biopsies showing the typical granulomas and by the systemic involvement, usually pulmonary or cutaneous. Corticosteroids are often used, but there is no proof of effectiveness for the neuropathy. Individual nerve symptoms often improve spontaneously.

ISCHEMIC NEUROPATHY

Peripheral nerves are much more susceptible to occlusion of small vessels than large vessels. Atherosclerotic or embolic occlusion of major leg arteries often spares nerve function, but a mild sensory neuropathy is common in severe peripheral vascular disease, although it may be obscured by the ischemic features. Small-vessel disease caused by vasculitis commonly causes neuropathy, often with a distinctive pattern.

Multiple mononeuropathy is the classic clinical feature of vasculitic neuropathy. However, other conditions can produce this, as shown in Table 446.3. Also, pathologic studies have shown that vasculitic neuropathy can present as a distal symmetrical sensory and motor polyneuropathy, perhaps in 25% of cases. Classically, individual nerves are affected acutely, with sudden loss of strength and sensation, often painful and dysesthetic. Gradual recovery may occur but can be very slow. At times, only cutaneous nerves are affected. Clinical and electro-

TABLE 446.8.	CAUSES OF VASCULITIC NEUROPATHY

Polyarteritis nodosa
Allergic granulomatosis (Churg–Strauss syndrome)
Rheumatoid arthritis
Sjögren's syndrome
Systemic lupus erythematosus
Wegener's granulomatosis
Hypersensitivity angiitis
Systemic sclerosis
Giant cell arteritis
HIV infection
Nonsystemic vasculitic neuropathy

physiologic examinations may reveal subclinical involvement of other nerves, which helps in diagnosis.

Several conditions (Table 446.8) can cause vasculitic neuropathy. Systemic vasculitis, notably polyarteritis nodosa, is an important cause, involving relatively larger vessels. Multiple organ involvement is usually easily found. Connective tissue diseases, rheumatoid arthritis, systemic lupus erythematosus, and Sjögren's syndrome can all cause vasculitic neuropathy. Another important cause is nonsystemic vasculitic neuropathy, with the vasculitis apparently confined to the PNS. Up to 30% of cases have this diagnosis, despite a search for systemic involvement.

Management involves first a specific diagnosis of nerve vasculitis. Whole-nerve biopsy is necessary to examine the epineurial vessels. Adjacent muscle should be sampled because it often yields a positive diagnosis whereas the segment of nerve sampled shows only nonspecific fiber loss. Fiber loss in sectors of nerve on cross section is suggestive of ischemic neuropathy. Evidence of systemic vasculitis must be sought to make a specific diagnosis. Treatment is difficult for two reasons. First, no trials have established proven therapies. Second, improvement from intervention is unlikely in the short term because recovery depends on axonal regeneration—a slow process. The best that can be expected is that no further lesions will develop. Prednisone and cyclophosphamide are the usual treatments and are required in polyarteritis nodosa and other systemic vasculitides. The prognosis in nonsystemic vasculitic neuropathy is better, and treatment must be judged accordingly.

IDIOPATHIC NEUROPATHIES

Idiopathic Distal Axonal Polyneuropathy

Chronic distal axonal polyneuropathy of uncertain cause is the diagnosis in 10% to 20% of patients who have undergone full evaluations in neuromuscular clinics. This group represents a diminishing proportion of patients as knowledge of disease and diagnostic methods improve. In general, these patients progress very slowly over many years and seldom have major disability. Reexamination on an annual basis is warranted.

Idiopathic Brachial Plexus Neuropathy

Idiopathic brachial plexus neuropathy, often called neuralgic amyotrophy, presents with shoulder pain and arm weakness, usually proximal. The upper brachial plexus is most involved, but occasionally individual nerves, such as the long thoracic nerve, may be affected. Wasting develops over several weeks. The pain subsides in 3 to 6 weeks but recovery of strength, which is usually incomplete, takes a year or more. Wasting persists. Electrophysiologic studies reveal axonal degeneration. The cause is unknown and there is no specific treatment. There is an autosomal dominantly inherited form of this disorder, known as hereditary neuralgic amyotrophy. It is characterized by recurrent episodes and may be bilateral.

CRITICAL-ILLNESS POLYNEUROPATHY

Critical-illness polyneuropathy develops in patients who are critically ill with multiple organ failure and sepsis, usually for more than 30 days. The first sign often is difficulty weaning from a respirator. Variable weakness and sensory loss are found. Physiologic and pathologic studies reveal axonal degeneration. No specific cause has been found, although nutritional factors, drugs, sepsis, and multiple organ failure may all play a role. Recovery is possible.

BIBLIOGRAPHY

Donofrio PD, Albers JW. Polyneuropathy: classification by nerve conduction studies and electromyography. *Muscle Nerve* 1990;13:889–903.

Dyck PJ, Thomas PK, Griffin JW, et al. *Peripheral neuropathy,* third ed. Philadelphia: WB Saunders, 1993.

McLeod JG. Investigation of peripheral neuropathy. *J Neurol Neurosurg Psychiatry* 1995;58(3):274–283.

Ropper AH, Wijdicks EFM, Truax BT. *Guillain–Barré syndrome.* Philadelphia: FA Davis Company, 1991.

Schaumburg HH, Berger AR, Thomas PK. *Disorders of peripheral nerves,* second ed. Philadelphia: FA Davis Company, 1992.

Kelley's Textbook of Internal Medicine, fourth edition. Edited by H. David Humes. Lippincott Williams & Wilkins, Philadelphia © 2000.

CHAPTER

447

MONONEUROPATHIES AND ENTRAPMENT NEUROPATHIES

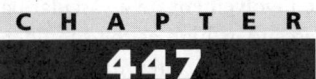

ANDREW A. EISEN

■ NERVE COMPRESSION AND ENTRAPMENT

Compression and *entrapment* of a nerve are not synonymous terms, but they may be difficult to differentiate. In general, entrapment is a slowly progressive chronic process, whereas compression is acute and may be repetitive. Both mechanisms can occur together. Compression and entrapment are the most common physical injuries affecting peripheral nerves. Other injuries, such as cold neuropathy, vibration neuropathy, radiation neuropathy, and electroshock neuropathy, are less common. The history can be helpful. For example, forestry workers who use chain saws are subject to so-called *vibration white finger* and commonly have a carpal tunnel syndrome, but they may be reluctant to disclose the source of the damage for economic reasons.

Entrapment produces a characteristic pathologic process. Internodal myelin is separated and prolapses into the adjacent internode. This is repeated over several segments. The same mechanism occurs in acute compressive neuropathy. Focal demyelination results in a variable degree of conduction block: if it is mild, electrophysiologic changes occur without clinical deficit; if it is severe, paresis or even paralysis results. Reversible myelin dysfunction also accounts for transient tingling, such as of the peroneal nerve when the legs are crossed. In these situations, myelin is not interrupted anatomically but it malfunctions because sodium channels fail to open. The extent of the conduction block is related directly to the force and duration of the compression. Herein lies the importance of prolonged tourniquet application, with its potential for paralysis. There also is a vascular element to most peripheral nerve injuries. However, the vascular component becomes important in several mononeuritides, especially diabetes, collagen vascular diseases, and carcinomas.

Those nerve fibers that have the largest diameters are involved earliest and most prominently with compression injuries. These include the alpha motor fibers, the type Ia muscle afferent fibers, and the type II cutaneous fibers.

The most common symptoms in carpal tunnel syndrome are nocturnal pain and dysesthesia in the absence of objective sensory or motor deficits. These findings are best explained by the involvement of small-diameter pain fibers and autonomic nerve fibers through a vascular mechanism. However, clumsiness may be an early and predominant complaint, and is in keeping with the compression of type Ia muscle afferent fibers.

Accurate localization usually is possible by clinical examination. Electromyography (EMG) can aid in localization; it often reveals the severity of the damage and suggests the prognosis. Computed tomography and magnetic resonance imaging are particularly useful for investigating entrapment of the spinal roots but also can be helpful for other nerves.

Systemic diseases that can underlie entrapment neuropathies are listed in Table 447.1. Other symmetrical polyneuropathies can predispose to entrapment injury.

The treatment of nerve entrapment usually is straightforward but can be difficult. Surgical decompression often is curative. Many cases remit spontaneously, especially if aggravating factors are removed. Autopsy studies in older patients have revealed asymptomatic ulnar and median nerve compression. A local hydrocortisone injection (25 mg) may be the only treatment necessary, as in carpal tunnel syndrome of pregnancy. Many cases of nerve entrapment associated with systemic diseases (Table 447.1) improve with treatment of the underlying disorder. A rare but distinctive cause of multiple compression neuropathies

TABLE 447.1.	SYSTEMIC CONDITIONS ASSOCIATED WITH ENTRAPMENT NEUROPATHY

Myeloidosis
Blood dyscrasias
Cancer
Collagen vascular diseases
Diabetes
Guillain–Barré syndrome
Hunter's syndrome (mucopolysaccharidosis type II)
Hypothyroidism
Leprosy
Mumps
Pregnancy
Rheumatoid arthritis
Sarcoidosis
Tomaculous neuropathy

is hereditary neuropathy with liability to pressure palsies. This disorder is associated with excessively thick myelin sheaths and is a dominantly inherited disorder due to deletion of one copy of the gene for the myelin protein PMP22. These patients are prone to repeated compressive neuropathies and often have associated asymptomatic EMG abnormalities.

BENIGN BRACHIAL PLEXOPATHY

Benign brachial plexopathy usually presents as transient nocturnal numbness and paresis of the arm associated with a particular posture. It is seen more often in alcoholics and can occur as well in hereditary neuropathy with pressure palsies. Reversible brachial plexopathy can be confused with transient cerebral ischemic attacks.

THORACIC OUTLET SYNDROMES

The neurogenic thoracic outlet syndrome is rare. It predominantly affects young women and presents as painless thenar muscle wasting, which can be confused with carpal tunnel syndrome. The neck roentgenogram may reveal rudimentary cervical ribs, commonly on both sides. Compression usually results from a radiologically nonvisible fibrous band attached to a rudimentary rib. If ribs are seen, it is the smaller one that is important. EMG findings include a reduced compound muscle action potential from the thenar muscle as compared with a normal hypothenar muscle; a small or absent ulnar sensory nerve action potential; a small, prolonged, or absent ulnar F wave; and a small or undetectable ulnar sensory evoked potential compared with a normal median study. These findings suggest compression of the lower trunk of the brachial plexus, particularly the first thoracic nerve root. Decompression by removal of the offending fibrous band prevents further deterioration but seldom is curative.

The droopy-shoulder syndrome is a more common condition that also predominantly affects young women. It is characterized by pain or paresthesia in the shoulder, neck, arm, forearm, or hand that is exacerbated by palpation of the brachial plexus or downward traction on the arm. The patient usually has a long, graceful, swanlike neck and low-set shoulders with horizontal or downsloping clavicles. The second thoracic or lower vertebrae are visible above the shoulders on lateral cervical spine roentgenograms. Symptoms are relieved instantly by passive elevation of the shoulders. The physical examination and EMG are normal, and treatment involves educational reposturing of the shoulders.

Physical injury to the brachial plexus also may be associated with cancer by tumor infiltration, compression, or radiation therapy. Radiation injury usually is painless, predominantly affects the upper trunk, and is associated with lymphedema. A painful lower trunk plexopathy associated with Horner's syndrome suggests direct compression from tumor infiltration.

Rucksack paralysis is an occupational hazard of hikers and military personnel. The lower trunk of the brachial plexus commonly is compressed, with weakness of the hand grip and numbness involving the ring and little fingers and extending to the medial aspect of the forearm. Any part of the brachial plexus may be involved. Most patients recover promptly after recognition, but axonal degeneration occasionally occurs.

MEDIAN NERVE LESIONS

CARPAL TUNNEL SYNDROME

Carpal tunnel syndrome is a common nerve entrapment syndrome that affects adults of all ages, women more than men. In women, it usually is idiopathic, but in men, house painting, carpentry, or the use of a power saw are associated activities. It is common in the later months of pregnancy and often remits after childbirth. It is important to recognize and treat diseases associated with carpal tunnel syndrome (Table 447.1).

Symptoms caused by the compression of large-diameter fibers produce median nerve motor weakness and sensory loss. Nocturnal pain and paresthesia probably result from small-fiber and autonomic nerve involvement on a vascular basis. The pain and discomfort can ascend as high as the shoulder. Tinel's sign and Phalen's maneuver are of limited diagnostic value.

The diagnosis can be confirmed by EMG in 85% of patients. Decompressive surgery should be considered on the basis of clinical rather than EMG criteria. Indications for surgery are persistent pain that does not resolve with nocturnal splinting and rapidly developing neurologic motor or sensory deficits. Chronic, painless carpal tunnel syndromes may not improve with surgery.

ANTERIOR INTEROSSEOUS NERVE ENTRAPMENT

The anterior interosseous nerve is a pure motor branch of the median nerve that supplies the flexor pollicis longus, the long flexors to the index and middle fingers, and the pronator quadratus. Entrapment occurs between the heads of the pronator teres under the tendinous arch of the flexor digitorum sublimis. The patient is unable to pinch the thumb and first finger together (the "OK" sign). Thenar muscles and sensation are normal.

EMG shows denervation in the flexor pollicis longus and pronator quadratus in the presence of normal terminal median nerve motor and sensory conduction and normal thenar muscle activity.

PRONATOR TERES SYNDROME

Occasionally, the median nerve is entrapped more proximally, producing weakness of all the muscles it innervates, except the pronator teres. Carpal tunnel symptoms are reported, along with weakness of the flexor pollicis longus and the finger flexors supplied by the median nerve. Pronation of the forearm is spared. If pronation is involved, a more proximal entrapment of the nerve has occurred. The most common cause is a ligament of Struthers (a fibrous extension of the supratrochlear spur at the distal humerus). EMG reveals abnormalities in the pronator teres muscle.

■ ULNAR NERVE ENTRAPMENT SYNDROMES

The ulnar nerve is entrapped commonly at the level of the elbow and rarely at the wrist (Guyon's canal).

CUBITAL TUNNEL SYNDROME

At the elbow, the ulnar nerve passes between the heads of the flexor carpi ulnaris under an aponeurosis (the cubital tunnel). The site of compression is not always discrete. EMG shows restricted slowing of conduction across the elbow. The pathologic signs of typical chronic nerve compression can be found in many asymptomatic patients. Repeated elbow flexion and minor trauma probably are responsible.

A sensory deficit is observed in an ulnar distribution, with little or no motor deficit. Pain in the elbow region may be a problem. Occasionally, there is wasting and weakness of the first dorsal interosseous muscle. Involvement of the hypothenar muscles usually is less pronounced. The more proximal flexor carpi ulnaris is involved only in about 25% of cases, even when motor symptoms are severe.

The results of surgical intervention are not clear. Improvement is considerably less than with surgery for carpal tunnel syndrome. Pain is relieved and further neurologic deficit is prevented. Surgical approaches are simple decompression, transposition of the nerve, and removal of the olecranon. Simple decompression is preferred.

Ulnar neuropathy can occur after surgery (particularly of the gallbladder or heart), coma, or severe burns. These situations produce an acute ulnar deficit with predominant sensory involvement. The mechanism appears to be acute infarction of the nerve at the elbow, and EMG suggests axonal degeneration. Surgery is contraindicated and may be harmful. Most patients recover spontaneously.

ULNAR NERVE ENTRAPMENT IN GUYON'S CANAL

The ulnar nerve enters the hand through an osseofibrous tunnel (Guyon's canal) formed by the pisiform and the hook of the hamate. In most cases, compression occurs at the distal end of the canal at the origin of the deep branch of the ulnar nerve, which is purely motor. Wasting and weakness of the interossei occur, but the hypothenar muscles, supplied by proximal branches, are spared. There are no sensory signs. Compression may occur slightly more proximally when the recurrent sensory branch is involved and may be difficult to distinguish from the cubital tunnel syndrome without EMG.

An easily reversible condition known as *bicycle rider's neuropathy* is caused by compression at the proximal end of Guyon's canal. In this condition, sensory and motor symptoms and signs develop.

■ RADIAL NERVE LESIONS

Lengthy pressure on the radial nerve in the spiral groove of the humerus in patients who are falling asleep or are drunk and have an arm hanging over the back of a chair produces so-called *Saturday night palsy*. The degree of deficit is related directly to the amount and duration of pressure.

Complete wristdrop develops. Examination reveals an inability to extend the fingers and wrist. The brachioradialis muscle is involved, but the triceps is spared. Sensory complaints are few and spontaneous recovery is the rule. If denervation is severe, recovery is protracted and a wrist support is required.

POSTERIOR INTEROSSEOUS SYNDROME

The posterior interosseous branch of the radial nerve is purely motor. Damage results in weakness of extension of the fingers and thumb. Wrist extensors are spared, apart from the extensor carpi ulnaris. Entrapment occurs where the branch passes through the supinator muscle or as a result of pressure from a lipoma or other benign tumor.

Characteristic initial drooping of the ring finger occurs, with subsequent weakness of other fingers. There is no sensory loss. EMG localization shows normal motor unit activity in the extensor digitorum communis, extensor carpi radialis longus, extensor carpi radialis brevis, and brachioradialis, but abnormalities in the extensor carpi ulnaris, extensor digiti proprius, abductor pollicis longus, extensor pollicis brevis, and extensor pollicis longus. Surgical exploration usually is required.

TENNIS ELBOW

The condition known as *tennis elbow* is caused by entrapment of both the deep (posterior interosseous) and the recurrent epicondylar branches of the radial nerve. Pain usually is severe enough to force cessation of the offending activity, which prevents a motor deficit from occurring. Tennis elbow is common with the use of hammers or other tools, or with any activity that requires repeated forceful supination against resistance.

Symptoms usually resolve spontaneously, but a local intra-articular injection of hydrocortisone (25 mg) can help.

HANDCUFF PALSY

So-called *handcuff palsy* results from compression of the superficial radial nerve at the wrist. Handcuffs and tight watch bands or bracelets often are responsible. Numbness is experienced over the dorsum of the thumb and first finger and the web of skin between the two. If the neuropathy is severe, the radial nerve sensory action potential is lost.

PERONEAL NERVE PALSY

Common peroneal nerve palsy arises from compression at the fibular neck. It produces weakness of dorsiflexion and eversion along with sensory loss over the dorsum of the foot and the lateral aspect of the leg. It can be difficult to distinguish from a fifth lumbar root lesion. The resulting footdrop usually is acute and complete, and the ankle jerk is maintained. Pain or tenderness occurs at the fibular neck. In contrast, radiculopathy of the fifth lumbar nerve root commonly results in a partial, slowly developing footdrop along with a depressed or lost ankle jerk. Back pain and sciatica may be predominant. In addition, about 20% of patients with amyotrophic lateral sclerosis (motor neuron disease) have a footdrop.

Distal compression of the deep branch of the peroneal nerve produces weakness of dorsiflexion but normal eversion. Sensory loss is minimal. Compression of the superficial branch of the peroneal nerve results in weakness of eversion from paralysis of the peroneus longus and peroneus brevis, and from a sensory deficit over the dorsum of the foot extending proximally over the lateral aspect of the leg.

The only muscle supplied by the common peroneal nerve above the knee is the short head of the biceps femoris. If the results of needle EMG are normal, the lesion is at or below the fibular neck. This finding rules out a fifth lumbar–first sacral root lesion. In contrast, denervation of the tibialis posterior, which is innervated by a fifth lumbar nonperoneal nerve, points to a fifth lumbar radiculopathy.

Spontaneous recovery can take several weeks, and a foot splint may be required. In such a compressive lesion, there is no justification for surgical decompression. Repeated crossing of the legs should be discouraged.

LATERAL FEMORAL CUTANEOUS NERVE SYNDROME (MERALGIA PARESTHETICA)

The lateral femoral cutaneous nerve is derived predominantly from the second and third lumbar roots. It emerges from the lateral border of the psoas major muscle, runs laterally to cross the iliacus muscle, and passes through the inguinal ligament beneath the deep fascia of the upper thigh, supplying the skin over the lateral thigh. It may be entrapped as it passes under the inguinal ligament, producing chronic pain and paresthesia over the lateral thigh. This syndrome commonly is of sudden onset and probably results from vascular occlusion. It occurs in patients with diabetes accompanied by lumbar radiculoplexopathy, producing weakness of the quadriceps and loss of the knee jerk. It usually remits spontaneously and can be helped with carbamazepine (Tegretol, 200 to 300 mg per day). Rare chronic entrapment requires surgical decompression.

TARSAL TUNNEL SYNDROME

The posterior tibial nerve rarely is entrapped by the flexor retinaculum between the tibial malleolus and the posterior part of the calcaneus. Proximal entrapment involves the medial and lateral plantar nerves, causing painful paresthesia and sensory loss on the sole of the foot and weakness of the intrinsic foot muscles. Distal entrapment produces a medial or lateral plantar syndrome with a restricted sensory deficit. EMG shows a prolonged terminal latency to the abductor hallucis (medial plantar nerve) or the abductor digiti minimi pedis (lateral plantar nerve). Surgical decompression relieves the symptoms. Tarsal tunnel syndrome can be confused with reversible compression of the tibial nerve proximal to the ankle by tight-fitting ski or other boots.

FACIAL NERVE PALSY

Spontaneous and idiopathic Bell's palsy is the most common facial palsy. Accessory serratus anterior palsy and paralytic brachial palsy (neuralgic amyotrophy) probably have a similar pathogenesis.

Bell's palsy can occur at any age, may be unilateral or bilateral, and occasionally is recurrent. The deficit is variable, and 90% of patients recover spontaneously. Excessive tearing, hyperacusis, and loss of taste, which are clinical features indicating a proximal lesion of the facial nerve, are suggestive of a poor prognosis.

If the facial nerve can be stimulated after 4 to 5 days, a good recovery can be anticipated. Inability to stimulate the nerve accompanied by the development of fibrillation and positive sharp waves is suggestive of a poor prognosis. Aberrant reinnervation can occur and produces mass facial movements in the resultant interfacial synkinesis, accompanied by movement of the mouth. So-called *crocodile tears* may result from misdirection of the autonomic fibers subserving taste and lacrimation. Rarely, hemifacial spasm is a late feature.

In an attempt to prevent severe axonal degeneration, a short course (10 days) of corticosteroid therapy can be administered. The use of prednisone (50 to 100 mg per day) is recommended. Treatment must be started within 24 hours of presentation. Surgical decompression is controversial. An eye patch should be used to prevent corneal abrasions.

Mumps, mononucleosis, sarcoidosis, and Ramsay Hunt syndrome are associated diseases. In Ramsay Hunt syndrome, pain develops in and around the ear, with an associated vesicular eruption (herpes zoster). If the gasserian ganglion is involved, there may be sensory loss on the face. Cholesteatomas, acoustic neuromas, and sphenoid ridge meningiomas also may present as an acute or subacute facial palsy and require surgical exploration.

RADICULOPATHY

Cervical and lumbosacral nerve roots are subject to entrapment within the vertebral foramina by osteophyte formation or compression from a disk protrusion. Neck or back pain usually is the predominant symptom, with radiation down the arm or leg in an appropriate dermatomal distribution. Coughing or sneezing raises intraspinal pressure and increases the symptoms. Myotonic weakness and wasting can develop, along with loss of an appropriate deep tendon reflex.

A radiculopathy should be investigated by EMG and magnetic resonance imaging or computed tomography before a contrast myelogram is considered.

The primary dorsal root ramus can be compressed, causing back pain. Paraspinal denervation can be detected on EMG, whereas the results of radiologic investigation usually are normal.

OTHER ENTRAPMENT NEUROPATHIES

ACCESSORY NERVE PALSY

Spontaneous accessory nerve palsy is rare. It may occur after an upper respiratory tract infection or an operation, or be associated with heavy exertion. Neck pain occurs initially, followed within several days by weakness of the trapezius muscle. There is drooping and inability to shrug the shoulders, with scapular winging. The winging is accentuated by lateral extension of the arm. This contrasts with the winging that occurs with serratus anterior palsy, which is brought out by forward extension of the arm. In addition, the inferior angle of the scapula moves upward and outward in accessory nerve palsy but downward and medially in serratus anterior palsy.

Accessory nerve palsy must be differentiated from the more common brachial plexopathy, suprascapular nerve palsy, and circumflex nerve injury. EMG shows slowed conduction along the distal part of the accessory nerve.

Spontaneous recovery over 6 to 9 months is the rule. During recovery, traction on the plexus may produce pain in the shoulder and arm.

SERRATUS ANTERIOR PALSY

Serratus anterior palsy is a common, painless mononeuritis that produces winging of the scapula accentuated by anterior extension of the arm. The tip of the scapula moves downward and medially. Most patients recover spontaneously. Persistence of the condition in young women can become a cosmetic problem.

SUPRASCAPULAR NERVE PALSY

Derived from the upper trunk of the brachial plexus (the fifth and sixth cervical nerve roots), the suprascapular nerve innervates the supraspinatus and infraspinatus muscles. Entrapment of this nerve within the suprascapular notch produces an inability to initiate elevation and extension of the arm. Rarely, the inferior branch is involved in isolation.

SAPHENOUS NERVE ENTRAPMENT

The saphenous nerve is a branch of the femoral nerve. It supplies the skin over the medial aspect of the leg below the knee. The saphenous nerve pierces the adductor canal just above the popliteal fossa, where it occasionally is entrapped. Pain is felt in the knee joint from compression of an articular branch. Paresthesia and sensory loss may be evident down the medial aspect of the leg. Surgical decompression usually is curative.

SURAL NERVE ENTRAPMENT

A purely sensory nerve, the sural nerve supplies the skin over the lateral aspect of the foot. It is derived mainly from the tibial nerve but also from the peroneal nerve (fifth lumbar–first sacral roots). It may be entrapped as it becomes superficial in the midcalf between the two heads of the gastrocnemius, where it pierces the fascia, causing pain over the lateral malleolus and outer aspect of the foot.

BIBLIOGRAPHY

Copell HP, Thompson WAL. *Peripheral entrapment neuropathies.* Baltimore: Williams & Wilkins, 1963.
Dawson DM, Hallett M, Millender LH. *Entrapment neuropathies.* Boston: Little, Brown and Company, 1983.

Kelley's Textbook of Internal Medicine, fourth edition. Edited by H. David Humes. Lippincott Williams & Wilkins, Philadelphia © 2000.

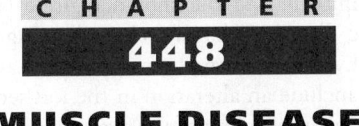

CHAPTER
448

MUSCLE DISEASE

ANDREW A. EISEN
KENNETH BERRY

BENIGN MYOPATHIES OF CHILDREN

The benign myopathies of children often present as floppy-infant syndromes. They usually progress slowly or not at all, but occasionally lead to severe deficits and even death at an early age. Many of these conditions are transmitted genetically, although the patterns of inheritance can be unclear and variable. Most are characterized by specific biopsy findings from which their names are derived (e.g., central core disease, nemaline rod disease, centronuclear myopathy, congenital fiber-type dispro-portion).

MUSCULAR DYSTROPHIES

The muscular dystrophies are primary myopathies of genetic origin that usually have their onset in childhood and are progressive in nature. Although skeletal muscle bears the brunt of the genetic defect, other structures, including the heart and brain, may be involved.

The most common is Duchenne-type muscular dystrophy, a sex-linked recessive disorder that is transmitted by females and expressed only in males. The defective gene on the X chromosome *(Xp21)* is responsible for the gene product, dystrophin, which is localized to the inner surface of the muscle membrane. The absence or reduction of membrane dystrophin leads to the progressive muscle damage that produces the disease. As a result of progressive proximal weakness in the limbs and trunk, affected individuals usually are wheelchair-bound by their early teenage years and seldom live beyond 20 years of age. In a milder variant, Becker's muscular dystrophy, disability progresses more slowly and life expectancy is longer. Mental retardation and cardiomyopathy commonly coexist with muscular dystrophy, particularly the Duchenne type. Both Duchenne's and Becker's muscular dystrophy are characterized by pseudohypertrophy of the calves. Muscle biopsy reveals a myopathic pattern with random variation in fiber diameter, internally situated sarcolemmal nuclei, fiber splitting, "opaque" fibers, and a relatively marked increase in endomysial connective tissue.

Less common types of muscular dystrophy are named according to the primary distribution of muscle weakness. They include facioscapulohumeral muscular dystrophy, a dominant disease that produces facial and shoulder weakness with characteristic winging of the scapulae. The gene is on chromosome 4, but the abnormal gene product is not yet known. Limb-girdle muscular dystrophy is an autosomal recessive disorder that involves the pelvic girdle initially and the shoulder girdle later. There are several genetic disorders that are clinically diagnosed as limb-girdle dystrophy. The abnormal gene products have been defined for some and include an alteration in the ion-sensitive protease calpain. Oculopharyngeal muscular dystrophy is a rare and relatively benign dominantly inherited myopathy that produces bilateral ptosis, weakness of the extraocular muscles, dysphagia, and variable limb weakness.

MYOTONIC SYNDROMES

Myotonia is the persistent contraction of a muscle after the cessation of voluntary contraction or in response to a mechanical or electrical stimulus. Myotonia has a characteristic "dive bomber" sound on electromyography (EMG). It is a nonspecific finding and occurs in many different diseases.

MYOTONIC DYSTROPHY

Myotonic dystrophy is the most common myotonic syndrome. It is a dominantly inherited multisystem disorder attributable to a triplet repeat in a noncoding region of chromosome 17. It usually becomes evident between 15 and 30 years of age. Mild cases may be clinically inapparent. When the disease is fully developed, patients have bilateral ptosis, facial diplegia, frontal balding, and wasting of the temporalis and sternomastoid muscles. There is tapering of the arms and legs, with partial bilateral wristdrop and footdrop. By this stage, tendon reflexes usually are absent. Cataracts, infertility, cardiomyopathy, and mental retardation are part of the syndrome. Some patients, usually children of affected mothers, have a severe infantile form. Muscle biopsy may show a variety of nonspecific myopathic features. Classically, there is a marked increase in endomysial connective tissue, many internally situated sarcolemmal nuclei, ring fibers, and sarcoplasmic pads. There may be a predominance of type 1 muscle fibers.

MYOTONIA CONGENITA

Originally described by Thomsen, who had the disease himself, myotonia congenita has an autosomal dominant pattern of inheritance. It is a benign disorder associated with myotonia, which usually manifests as muscle stiffness at the beginning of or after exercise, and characteristically hypertrophied muscles. The importance of recognizing this syndrome lies in differentiating it from myotonic dystrophy.

PARAMYOTONIA CONGENITA

Paramyotonia congenita is one of the manifestations of hyperkalemic periodic paralysis. The myotonia may be apparent only after exercise or exposure to cold. Families have been described in which there has been overlap between the two manifestations of the disease. The pattern of inheritance is autosomal dominant.

INFLAMMATORY MYOPATHIES

POLYMYOSITIS

Polymyositis, the most common of the inflammatory myopathies, may begin acutely or in a subacute or chronic manner. It may occur in a pure form or be associated with a collagen vascular disease, such as systemic lupus erythematosus, rheumatoid arthritis, or scleroderma. Muscle weakness usually is diffuse and proximal, and involves the pectoral and pelvic girdles and the muscles of the neck. Muscle pain and tenderness also may be present. Systemic features include weight loss, dysphagia, and an elevated erythrocyte sedimentation rate. In addition, the serum creatine kinase level usually is elevated. The electromyogram is nonspecific, with fibrillation and positive sharp waves more evident than in most other myopathies. Muscle biopsy characteristically reveals necrotic and regenerating fibers and foci of autoaggressive inflammatory cells that invade otherwise normal-appearing muscle fiber.

Polymyositis is treated initially with corticosteroid therapy. A therapeutic response is evidenced by clinical improvement and a decreasing creatine kinase level. There is a role for cytotoxic immunosuppressive therapy in some patients. The role of intravenous immunoglobulin remains to be critically studied.

DERMATOMYOSITIS

Originally considered to be a variant of polymyositis with associated skin involvement, dermatomyositis should be regarded as a separate entity. The disease involves immune attack and destruction of small blood vessels in the muscle rather than the muscle fiber itself. For this reason, the muscle biopsy characteristically shows perifascicular atrophy of muscle fibers, as well as scattered muscle fiber neurosis and lymphocytic inflammation. The inflammatory infiltrate tends to be located more in the interstitial connective tissue than in the muscle fiber itself. Malignancy may be associated with this disorder in older patients.

INCLUSION BODY MYOSITIS

Inclusion body myositis characteristically occurs in older individuals. In typical cases the clinical picture is distinctive. There is weakness of wrist flexors and finger flexors, as well as quadriceps. The disease is slowly progressive and often is associated with absent reflexes. Muscle biopsy reveals the changes of an inflammatory myopathy, with cytoplasmic vacuoles and ultrastructural findings of laminated membranous debris and filamentous inclusions measuring 10 to 20 nm. In contrast to polymyositis and dermatomyositis, inclusion body myositis does not improve with corticosteroid therapy.

SARCOIDOSIS

Sarcoidosis may involve muscle and rarely leads to symptomatic muscle disease, including weakness. Muscle biopsy shows sarcoid granulomas and, occasionally, myositis.

PARASITIC INFESTATIONS

Muscle infection results in weakness, tenderness, and pain. The most common parasitic infestations are trichinosis and cysticercosis. The diagnosis may be suggested by clinical findings or by the presence of calcification in the soft tissue on radiography. The diagnosis should be confirmed by muscle biopsy.

FOCAL NODULAR MYOSITIS

Focal nodular myositis is an unusual condition characterized by a progressively increasing lump in the muscle that on biopsy shows a histologic picture of myositis with necrosis, regeneration, and fibrosis. Because generalized polymyositis or some form of neurogenic disorder can develop, patients with focal myositis require careful follow-up.

■ METABOLIC MYOPATHIES

The metabolic myopathies are a large group of uncommon diseases with primarily autosomal recessive patterns of inheritance. They are characterized by fatigability and exercise intolerance, often associated with muscle cramps and pain, occasionally myoglobinuria, and eventually muscle weakness.

GLYCOGENOSES

Only a few of the more than ten recognized varieties of glycogenosis produce clinical myopathy.

MCARDLE'S DISEASE

McArdle's disease (glycogenosis type V, myophosphorylase deficiency) usually is inherited as a recessive trait, although a few autosomal dominant forms have been described. Patients classically complain of exercise intolerance with pain in the muscles on exercise. Myoglobinuria is common and may lead to renal impairment. The diagnosis may be supported by the presence of an abnormal ischemic exercise test in which the normal elevation in serum lactate levels after ischemic exercise fails to occur. Muscle biopsy may reveal abnormal glycogen storage in muscle fibers and the absence of phosphorylase staining.

ACID MALTASE DEFICIENCY

Type II glycogenosis in infants corresponds to Pompe's disease, but it also may occur in adults as an isolated skeletal muscle disorder. It is characterized by weakness, often of the respiratory muscles. Muscle biopsy shows multiple vacuoles containing glycogen in muscle fibers. Some of the glycogen is seen to be within lysosomes, which show striking acid phosphatase reactivity.

PHOSPHOFRUCTOKINASE DEFICIENCY

Type VII glycogenosis presents in a fashion similar to McArdle's disease and produces the same biochemical and electrophysiologic abnormalities. Muscle biopsy usually shows only minimal abnormalities, although a specific stain for phosphofructokinase demonstrates the absence of this enzyme activity. The diagnosis should be confirmed by muscle biochemical analysis.

LIPID STORAGE DISEASES

Carnitine deficiency can occur in a systemic form with widespread manifestations or can be localized to muscle. In the latter case, an autosomal recessive disorder, patients usually have slowly progressive weakness with occasional exacerbations. Muscle biopsy may show excessive lipid deposition, particularly in type I fibers.

Carnitine palmitoyltransferase deficiency usually affects young men, producing attacks of muscle pain and often myoglobinuria after periods of prolonged exercise. The results of muscle biopsy may be normal, and the diagnosis may require biochemical determination of carnitine palmitoyltransferase levels.

MYOADENYLATE DEAMINASE DEFICIENCY

The activity of myoadenylate deaminase can be demonstrated in muscle biopsy by histochemical and biochemical means. Myoadenylate deaminase deficiency may be seen in patients whose only complaints are excessive cramping and pain with exercise intolerance. However, patients with other recognized myopathic and neurogenic disorders have been described with this abnormality, and its significance remains in dispute.

MITOCHONDRIAL MYOPATHIES

The characteristic clinical finding in the mitochondrial myopathies is exercise intolerance, often with markedly elevated serum lactate levels after relatively little exertion. Some patients have fixed myopathic features, sometimes restricted to extraocular muscles. Other systems commonly are involved, particularly the central nervous system. In one group of mitochondrial myopathies, there is a morphologically demonstrable abnormality on muscle biopsy known as *ragged red fibers,* which appear ultrastructurally as abnormal mitochondria, commonly containing unusual crystalloid structures. One of these myopathies is the Kearns–Sayre syndrome, which is characterized by limb muscle weakness, retinitis pigmentosa, myocardial conduction abnormalities, and a positive family history. Others include the MELAS syndrome (mitochondrial encephalopathy, lactic acidosis, and strokes) and the MERRF syndrome (myoclonus epilepsy with ragged red fibers). Both myopathic and central nervous system abnormalities are present in these disorders.

The mitochondrial myopathies also can be characterized by muscle dysfunction without a definite histochemical mitochondrial abnormality. Various biochemical abnormalities of mitochondrial function have been demonstrated in some affected families.

ENDOCRINE DISEASES

Most endocrine disorders can affect muscle function, probably through failed calcium efflux or increased calcium influx into the T-tubular system of muscle. Hyperthyroidism and hypothyroidism, hyperadrenalism and hypoadrenalism, and hyperparathyroidism are associated with muscle weakness. Many of these conditions are reversible with treatment of the endocrinopathy.

MALIGNANT HYPERTHERMIA

Malignant hyperthermia is an unusual genetic disorder that occurs on exposure to certain inhalational anesthetics and results in the excessive release of calcium ions from the sarcoplasmic reticulum. This produces hypercontraction of the muscle with associated severe rigidity and a marked increase in body temperature. Because this disease can be fatal, it is mandatory that a family history be obtained before any patient undergoes general anesthesia. Clinically, there may be no muscle complaints, although some patients with central core myopathy have been shown to have malignant hyperthermia. Diagnosis of the disease is difficult and may require the use of special techniques, including measurement of muscle contractility on exposure to solutions of caffeine and inhalational anesthetics. Patients with family histories of malignant hyperthermia should be considered affected unless proven otherwise, so that appropriate precautionary measures can be taken when general anesthesia is required.

DISEASES OF NEUROMUSCULAR TRANSMISSION

MYASTHENIA GRAVIS

In myasthenia gravis, antibodies against the acetylcholine receptor destroy the receptor site on the postsynaptic membrane. As a result, acetylcholine quantal release from the motor nerve terminals is ineffectual. Miniature end-plate potentials, the electrophysiologic measure of the response of the postsynaptic muscle membrane to quantal acetylcholine release, are reduced in size but not in number, reflecting the decreased availability of receptor sites.

The clinical result is exercise-induced muscle fatigability that resolves with a period of rest. Any skeletal muscle can be involved. Muscle end plates are dynamic structures with a turnover rate of 5 to 7 days, so that at any given moment, various end plates can be in different states of efficiency in response to acetylcholine.

Most patients with myasthenia gravis complain of double vision and ptosis. They also may have dysarthria, dysphagia, dysphonia, and difficulty with chewing and limb weakness. Only skeletal muscles are involved, and the sphincter muscles are spared. Sensory findings are absent and tendon reflexes are normal.

The presence of acetylcholine receptor antibodies in serum is specific for the diagnosis and is found in more than 90% of patients. Electromyograms, especially single-fiber studies, also are sensitive. About 5% of patients with myasthenia gravis have associated thymomas. These are treated by thymectomy, which is curative in about 75% of cases. Treatment otherwise involves the use of anticholinesterase drugs, often in combination with prednisone. Acute exacerbations may be treated by plasmapheresis. Disease that does not respond to conventional therapy can be treated with stronger methods of immunosuppression.

EATON–LAMBERT SYNDROME

Initially described in patients with oat cell carcinoma, Eaton–Lambert syndrome also has been shown to occur spontaneously or in association with conditions such as sarcoidosis, tuberculosis, blood dyscrasia, or penicillamine therapy. It is due to antibodies against a component of the calcium channel on motor axons, which produces failure of release of acetylcholine. As a consequence, miniature end-plate potentials are reduced in number but not in size.

Eaton–Lambert syndrome can mimic myasthenia gravis but also produces dry mouth, vague sensory findings, and sometimes absent reflexes, particularly when it is associated with cancer. Acetylcholine receptor antibodies are not present in the serum, and repetitive transmission studies show an exquisite increment in muscle potential amplitude with stimuli at 10 to 20 Hz. Plasmapheresis and immunosuppressive treatment can produce partial benefit.

BOTULISM

The toxin produced by *Clostridium botulinum* is one of the most potent biologic toxins. In adults, botulism usually results from improper sterilization of home-canned foods, resulting in ingestion of preformed toxin. Symptoms include blurred vision, obstipation, and dry mouth followed by variable degrees of asymmetrical weakness, including severe paralysis with respiratory failure. Midposition unreactive pupils and paresis of eye movements are usually seen. Treatment is with multivalent antitoxin, which must be given early, and patient and prolonged nursing care. Particular attention must be paid to respiratory care, occasionally including tracheostomy and assisted ventilation.

CLINICAL ASSESSMENT

Neuromuscular diseases often can be diagnosed on clinical grounds, but laboratory investigations may provide additional clues when doubt exists.

Features suggestive of primary muscle disease include proximal pelvic or pectoral girdle weakness with normal or only moderately depressed tendon reflexes, and the absence of sensory findings or fasciculation. There may be involvement of the facial musculature, producing a facial diplegia and weakness of the neck and trunk muscles. The weakness may be disproportionate to the minimal degree of muscle wasting that is present. Gowers' sign, in which the patient rises from the floor by "climbing up himself," is a nonspecific sign of pelvic girdle weakness. Muscle hypertrophy is characteristic of some muscle diseases in the early stages, particularly Duchenne-type muscular dystrophy. Muscle pain is not specific to muscle disease but also occurs in neurogenic conditions such as Guillain–Barré syndrome, motor neuron disease, and radiculopathy. However, muscle pain induced by exercise often indicates a metabolic myopathy.

Although many myopathies commonly are inherited, a negative family history may be deceptive. Family photographs can be revealing, uncovering such subtleties as facial diplegia, ptosis, or scapular winging in "normal" family members.

LABORATORY INVESTIGATION

BLOOD TESTS

The creatine kinase level often is elevated in primary myopathies and inflammatory myopathies. The presence of acetylcholine receptor antibodies in the blood is specific and sensitive for myasthenia gravis.

An ischemic exercise test may be helpful in elucidating some metabolic myopathies. The serum lactate dehydrogenase level normally rises after a period of ischemic exercise. This elevation fails to occur when there is a block in the metabolic glycolytic pathway, as in McArdle's disease and several rare glycogenoses.

ELECTROMYOGRAPHY

Needle EMG, although not disease-specific, usually makes it possible to differentiate between a primary myopathy and a neurogenic disease. The characteristic finding in myopathy is hyperrecruitment of motor units that are of reduced amplitude and duration because of the random fallout of muscle fibers within a motor unit.

MUSCLE BIOPSY

Muscle biopsy may be necessary to reach a diagnosis in difficult cases. The biopsy should be limited to mildly or moderately impaired muscle; end-stage muscle should not be sampled. Muscles that have been needled during EMG should be avoided. The variability of muscle involvement in some diseases can produce false-negative results, necessitating a second biopsy from another site.

Combined with clinical assessment and electrophysiologic results, routinely processed sections, frozen sections subjected to enzyme histochemistry, and, occasionally, specimens evaluated by electron microscopy provide useful diagnostic information. However, pathologic findings rarely are pathognomonic for any disease process.

BIBLIOGRAPHY

Brooke H. *A clinician's view of neuromuscular diseases.* second ed. Baltimore: Williams & Wilkins, 1986.

Carpenter S, Karpati G. *Pathology of skeletal muscle.* New York: Churchill Livingstone, 1984.

Engel AG, Franzini-Armstrong C. *Myology,* second ed. New York: McGraw-Hill, 1994.

Layzer RB. *Neuromuscular manifestations of systemic disease.* Philadelphia: FA Davis Company, 1985.

Petty RK, Harding AE, Morgan-Hughes JA. The clinical features of mitochondrial myopathy. *Brain* 1986;109:915–938.

Walton J. *Disorders of voluntary muscle,* fourth ed. Edinburgh: Churchill Livingstone, 1981.

Kelley's Textbook of Internal Medicine, fourth edition. Edited by H. David Humes. Lippincott Williams & Wilkins, Philadelphia © 2000.

DIAGNOSTIC AND THERAPEUTIC MODALITIES IN NEUROLOGIC DISEASES

LUMBAR PUNCTURE AND CEREBROSPINAL FLUID ANALYSIS

GEORGE C. EBERS

Lumbar puncture remains an essential study in the evaluation of meningeal and other diseases of the nervous system and for the instillation of radiographic contrast material and chemotherapy. The physician considering lumbar puncture should ask the following questions:

- Will the procedure yield useful information?
- Are there contraindications to the procedure?
- Do the benefits of the procedure outweigh the risks?
- Which tests maximize information and efficiency?

Lumbar puncture is contraindicated in patients with intracranial mass lesions; where it may introduce infection into the subarachnoid space; and before the correction of significant bleeding diathesis has been accomplished.

TECHNIQUE

The key to successful lumbar puncture is positioning. The patient is reassured and placed in a lateral decubitus position with knees flexed on the abdomen, neck flexed, and unrotated back perpendicular to the bed. After a local anesthetic is injected, a needle is inserted in the midline, perpendicular to the back, usually at the L4–L5 interspace (just below the iliac crest), and directed slightly rostrally. As the needle is advanced, the stylet is frequently removed to indicate whether the subarachnoid space has been reached in order to avoid entering the epidural venous plexus (denser ventrally). If the bevel is parallel to the longitudinal running fibers in the dura, it may lessen the chance of continued cerebrospinal fluid (CSF) leakage. Pressure measurement (usually 80 to 180 mm) is carried out before CSF removal and with the patient relaxed and the legs straightened. The fluid level should rise and fall with the pulse, and more so with deep respiration. The CSF pressure may be falsely elevated by straining (Valsalva's maneuver). Unexpectedly high CSF pressure from mass effect demands a contingency plan in case of deterioration. Lumbar puncture is safe in pseudotumor cerebri, in which CSF pressures may be high. It is more difficult when anatomical landmarks are obscured (e.g., in patients with obesity, spinal deformity), and puncture in the seated position or under fluoroscopic guidance may be necessary. Lateral cervical or cisternal puncture provides alternative routes under special circumstances.

NORMAL CEREBROSPINAL FLUID

Normal CSF (total volume 120 mL) is clear and colorless. It is routinely examined for differential cell count (first and last tube) and protein and glucose values. There are few cells in normal CSF (fewer than 4 mononuclear cells per microliter). A pleocytosis of more than 30 cells per microliter can be identified with the practiced eye by swirling the collecting tube (Tyndall's effect). CSF protein levels are normally in the range of 15 to 45 mg per deciliter for lumbar fluid. Elevation of these levels usually reflects alteration of the blood–CSF barrier. It is commonly seen in persons with diabetes. CSF protein levels above 80 mg per deciliter produce an increasingly yellow tinge (xanthochromia). The relative CSF/serum ratio of serum protein is inversely proportional to the protein's hydrodynamic radius, so that large proteins, such as IgM, are virtually absent from normal CSF. Below a subarachnoid block (e.g., by a lumbar epidural tumor), the CSF protein may exceed 1.5 g per deciliter and clot spontaneously (Froin's syndrome). In 95% of children age 3 months to 13 years, the CSF protein level is below 25 mg per deciliter. CSF glucose concentration is normally 0.6 times that of blood at equilibrium. Changes in the blood are reflected in

CSF after a delay of 1 to 2 hours. Reduction of CSF glucose (hypoglycorrhachia) occurs in bacterial, fungal, and neoplastic meningitis and less often in subarachnoid hemorrhage, but also occasionally in viral, sarcoid, and rheumatic meningitis.

CEREBROSPINAL FLUID IN DISEASE: AN EVALUATION

The sensitivity and specificity of CSF studies in the conditions in which they are most valuable are outlined in Table 449.1.

MENINGITIS

The removal of CSF itself can be diagnostic (improvement in normal-pressure hydrocephaly) or therapeutic in lowering pressure in cerebri pseudotumor.

In bacterial meningitis, CSF is important for a microbial diagnosis and *optimal* antibiotic selection (see Chapters 431, 441, and 442). CSF pressure is often raised and the fluid may be turbid. Pleocytosis, which may exceed 1,000 cells per microliter, usually shows a predominance of polymorphonuclear leukocytes, although in 10% of cases (especially in neonates) it may be lymphocytic. Gram's staining is done on spun sediment, and

---

TABLE 449.1.   SELECTIVE EVALUATION OF LUMBAR PUNCTURE

	Sensitivity (%)	Specificity (%)
Bacterial Meningitis		
Polymorphic pleocytosis	→100	Low
Low glucose (<40 mg/dL)	58	Also seen in many other disorders (eg, 15%–20% of subarachnoid hemorrhage)
CSF/serum glucose <0.31	70	
Gram's stain	60–90	→100
Culture	?80	→100
Antigen detection–CIE, latex agglutination	50–90	→100
Tuberculous meningitis: culture with Ziehl–Nielsen stain	75–90	→100
	25	→100
Viral Meningitis		
Predominantly mononuclear pleocytosis (early cases)	50	Low
Predominantly mononuclear pleocytosis (repeat lumbar puncture)	→100	Low
Viral culture	→40	→100
Subarachnoid Hemorrhage		
Gross blood in CSF	→100	→80
Xanthochromia	90	Seen with high-protein traumatic tap
Reduction in red blood cell count from first tube to last tube in traumatic tap	80	56
Fungal Meningitis		
↑ Mononuclear cell count	→100	Low
India ink preparation (cryptococci)	26–53	→100
Latex agglutination (cryptococci)	50–90	High
Multiple culture (cryptococci)	100	100
Culture *Coccidioides*	76	100
Serology *Coccidioides*	95	Not specific for CNS disease
Neurosyphilis		
FTA serum	→100	Not specific for CNS disease
VDRL CSF	40–60	
Mononuclear pleocytosis	80	Low
Oligoclonal bands	High	Moderate
Neoplastic Meningitis		
Cytology	70	97
Multiple Sclerosis (Clinically Definite)		
Oligoclonal bands	90	85–90

→, approaches; CSF, cerebrospinal fluid; CIE, counterimmunoelectrophoresis; CNS, central nervous system; FTA, fluorescent treponemal antibody; VDRL, Venereal Disease Research Laboratory; CNS, central nervous system.
(Modified from Marton KI, Dean AD. The spinal tap: a new look at an old test. *Ann Intern Med* 1986;104:840)

the organism is seen in 60% to 90% of cases. Culture is diagnostic. Immunosuppressed patients and newborns may be atypical, showing little or no pleocytosis. A parameningeal infection (e.g., subdural empyema) may produce pleocytosis and slightly elevated protein with normal glucose and cultures. Tuberculous meningitis produces a high-protein, low-sugar, and lymphocytic pleocytosis. Acid-fast bacilli are seen with Ziehl–Nielsen staining in only 25% of cases. Viral meningitis is usually associated with mononuclear pleocytosis, but a polymorphonuclear leukocyte predominance may be present in up to 50% of early cases. Repeat puncture in 24 hours shows a mononuclear response predominating or developing. The protein level is often normal or modestly elevated. In sporadic meningoencephalitis (e.g., herpes simplex), an increase in red and white blood cell counts and protein is noted, with occasional reduction in the glucose. Polymerase chain reaction–based diagnosis is available for some organisms, but sensitivity and specificity have not been firmly established. The CSF in fungal meningitis shows mononuclear pleocytosis, low glucose, and elevated protein. In cryptococcal meningitis, the India ink wet mound demonstrates the clear capsule of the organism, and cryptococcal polysaccharide antigen is usually detectable by later agglutination. Multiple cultures of large CSF volumes may be needed to grow cryptococci and other fungi, but still may not grow *Coccidioides*. Serology is helpful in this instance.

NEUROSYPHILIS

Essentially all patients with neurosyphilis have a positive serum fluorescent treponemal antibody test. Confirmation of neurologic involvement is made by CSF examination. Although CSF serologic examination is of little value, active disease is characterized by mononuclear pleocytosis, normal or elevated protein levels, and local IgG antibody production with the presence of oligoclonal IgG bands.

NEOPLASTIC MENINGITIS

A mild pleocytosis, elevated protein level, and reduced glucose level are usual with meningeal infiltration by tumor. Malignant cells are seen in more than two-thirds of patients; detection of these cells is aided by taking large amounts of fluid directly into cytologic preservative. Tumor-specific monoclonal antibodies may also aid in the detection of malignant cells.

SUBARACHNOID HEMORRHAGE

Lumbar puncture almost invariably demonstrates bloody CSF. In true subarachnoid hemorrhage, the red blood cell count should stay the same in the first and last tube, and it should drop (often visibly) in traumatic puncture. The spun supernatant of a traumatic tap should be clear, but a spun supernatant may also be clear for 4 hours or more following subarachnoid hemorrhage before xanthochromia develops. Xanthochromic supernatant can also be seen occasionally in traumatic tap, which also raises the CSF protein level by 1 mg per deciliter for every 1,000 red blood cells per microliter and accounts for 1 white blood cell per microliter for every 7,000 red blood cells per microliter (assuming a normal hemogram). The CSF in subarachnoid hemorrhage can clear completely in 3 or 4 days in young people.

"AUTOIMMUNE" DISORDERS

CSF electrophoresis is used to demonstrate oligoclonal IgG bands. In several inflammatory/infective disorders, enough immunoglobulin product of single B-cell clones is present to show up as multiple single bands. Oligoclonal CSF bands are seen in multiple sclerosis, neurosyphilis, paraneoplastic cerebellar degeneration, and some other inflammatory disorders, and in a small percentage (less than 10%) of patients considered to be "normal" or to have noninflammatory disorders.

◼ COMPLICATIONS

Complications of lumbar puncture include the following:

- Aggravation or precipitation of cerebral or cerebellar herniation in the presence of mass lesions may occur. A computed tomographic scan may be necessary before a lumbar puncture can be performed. Removal of CSF below a spinal block may also precipitate deterioration in cord function.
- Symptomatic epidural or subdural hemorrhage is rare unless coagulation is impaired.
- Postlumbar puncture headache affects 10% to 20% of patients and can be transiently incapacitating. Onset of the headache is often delayed by a few hours or longer. The headache is usually bilaterally occipital and frontotemporal, throbbing, and immediately relieved by lying down, only to return upon standing. It is caused by continued leakage of CSF through the dural puncture hole, with traction on pain-sensitive structures at the base of the brain resulting from low CSF pressure. Leaking may also be spontaneous or pressure-induced. (The removal of 10 mL of CSF is replaced in 30 minutes at the normal rate of CSF production of 0.3 mL per minute.) Risk is reduced by the use of small-gauge, "atraumatic" needles. The headache is managed by rest and analgesics and usually lasts for 1 to 2 days (occasionally several days).
- Back or root pain is transient but common.
- Introduction of infection rarely occurs.
- Spinal epidermoid cyst rarely occurs.
- Cranial neuropathies VI, IV, and VIII rarely occur.

BIBLIOGRAPHY

Health and Public Policy Committee, American College of Physicians. The diagnostic spinal tap. *Ann Intern Med* 1986;104:880–886.
Fishman RA. *Cerebrospinal fluid in diseases of the nervous system.* Philadelphia: WB Saunders, 1980.
Marton KI, Gean AD. The spinal tap: a new look at an old test. *Ann Intern Med* 1986;104:840–848.
Paty DW, Ebers GC. *Multiple sclerosis.* Philadelphia: FA Davis Company, 1998.

ELECTROENCEPHALOGRAPHY AND EVOKED POTENTIALS

DAVID B. MACDONALD

▌ ELECTROENCEPHALOGRAPHY

Clinical electroencephalography is based on the diffuse and regional synchronous postsynaptic potentials of radially oriented cortical pyramidal cell columns. These potentials generate spatiotemporally summated extracellular currents of sufficient voltage to detect at the scalp. Other electrically active cellular elements of the cerebrum with more random geometry contribute little to this summation. Thus, scalp recordings predominantly reflect electrical activity of the cortical pyramidal cells and indirectly their modulation by subcortical structures. Electroencephalography is the discipline of interpreting these recordings in a clinical context.

Electrical potential differences between selected pairs of 21 or more electrodes placed at standard scalp locations are amplified and displayed in anatomically organized multichannel graphs, similar to that done in electrocardiography. The electroencephalogram (EEG) in wakefulness and its appearance in different states (such as drowsiness, hyperventilation, sleep, and photic stimulation) is analyzed, and the findings are correlated with clinical information to form an interpretation. Standards for electroencephalographic training and practice and certifying board examinations exist; these generally require at least 6 months (preferably a year or more) of full-time training in order for an individual to qualify as an electroencephalographer.

Computer technology has replaced traditional analog techniques with digital recordings that augment diagnostic precision through mathematical manipulation, Advanced methods, including source localization, quantitative electroencephalographic brain mapping, and high-resolution electroencephalography are beginning to contribute to clinical medicine.

NORMAL ACTIVITY

Unlike electrocardiograms, EEGs contain rhythmic sinusoidal or sharply contoured patterns intermingled with more irregular waveforms. These patterns vary with age and state of arousal, and are characterized by their voltage, frequency, morphologic characteristics, distribution, symmetry, persistence, and reactivity. There are four clinically useful frequency bands: delta, below 4 Hz; theta, 4 to 7 Hz; alpha, 8 to 13 Hz; and beta, above 13 Hz. An ontogenic progression in the frequency content of the human EEG is seen from infancy, dominated by delta and theta activity, to adulthood, dominated by alpha and beta activity, and finally to senescence, when slower frequencies may reappear. A typical adult record contains the famous posterior "alpha rhythm" that reacts (attenuates or "desynchronizes") to eye opening, a central "mu rhythm" that reacts to hand movements, and variable frontocentral beta activity. These features blend together over the scalp to create the "background." Hyperventilation may induce diffuse paroxysmal slow waves; photic stimulation may induce time-locked occipital waveforms; drowsiness is accompanied by slower frequencies and sometimes paroxysmal events that are easily misinterpreted; sleep is defined and staged by the appearance of characteristic patterns. Many variations, some unusual or even rare, including benign epileptiform patterns, have been identified and shown to have no or uncertain clinical significance. Extreme amplification creates frequent artifacts from eye or tongue movement, scalp muscle, and other sources. Substantial training and experience are required to reliably identify these artifacts and shadings of normal before clinically meaningful interpretations can be expected.

ABNORMALITIES

There are four general categories of abnormality: asymmetry, dysrhythmia, persistent polymorphic delta activity (PPDA), and suppression. Asymmetry is an abnormal difference in background voltage between homologous regions. Nonspecific dysrhythmias are persistent, intermittent, or paroxysmal irregularities that demonstrate diffuse or focal cerebral dysfunction but do not imply any particular etiologic process. Excessive diffuse fast dysrhythmia is a common a side effect of sedative medication. Other dysrhythmias are distinctive patterns with specific names (e.g., spike, burst suppression) and tend to have particular clinical correlations. PPDA—excessive delta activity present throughout the recording—signifies relatively continuous nonspecific brain dysfunction and may be generalized or focal. Focal PPDA is the hallmark of focal structural pathology but may also be seen in focal dysfunction without structural damage. Suppression refers to abnormal voltage depression, the most severe form of which is electrocerebral silence.

CLINICAL UTILITY

Electroencephalography is valuable in the investigation of intermittent or persistent brain dysfunction and remains essential in the evaluation of epilepsy. The recording of a clinical seizure may be diagnostic but occurs infrequently. Unequivocally abnormal interictal spike or sharp wave discharges uniquely reflect epileptic pathophysiologic processes and strongly support a diagnosis of epilepsy. However, caution is required because electroencephalographers vary in their ability to distinguish between epileptiform abnormalities and other apiculate or paroxysmal events, and because epileptiform discharges infrequently occur without a clinical history of epilepsy, especially in children. To detect these intermittent discharges, it may be necessary to repeat the study or to record a sleep EEG (which may activate epileptiform abnormalities). However, electroencephalography cannot exclude epilepsy because up to 10% of persons with epilepsy yield persistently negative interictal findings. Focal epileptiform abnormalities suggest a localization-related epilepsy syndrome, whereas diffuse epileptiform discharges generalized from onset suggest a generalized epilepsy syndrome, refining clinical diagnosis and aiding management.

Patients with impaired consciousness may benefit from electroencephalography. Evidence of nonconvulsive status epilepticus can lead to specific interventions; psychogenic unresponsiveness and the "locked-in syndrome" demonstrate essentially normal findings; encephalopathies produce nonspecific diffuse abnormalities; and marked focal temporal abnormalities in encephalitis may suggest herpesvirus. Some coma patterns have prognostic value, and electrocerebral silence characterizes brain death when hypothermia and suppressant drugs are excluded.

Electroencephalography can help to differentiate dementia from pseudodementia by providing objective evidence of cerebral dysfunction. Periodic sharp wave discharges may suggest Jakob–Creutzfeldt disease in the appropriate clinical setting.

Valuable specialized studies include prolonged video electroencephalographic monitoring with scalp or intracranial electrodes in difficult or surgical epilepsy cases, electrocorticography during epilepsy surgery, and monitoring in the operating room or intensive care unit.

EVOKED POTENTIALS

Evoked potentials are computer-averaged electrical responses of the nervous system elicited by specific stimuli. Random activity unrelated to the stimulus averages toward 0, while time-locked activity is revealed. The short latency sensory evoked potentials mentioned below are the most common in clinical use.

VISUAL EVOKED POTENTIALS

Usually, the occipital response to monocular stimulation with a reversing high-contrast black-and-white checkerboard pattern is recorded. In the absence of retinal or ocular disease, monocular absence or delay of the response suggests an ipsilateral prechiasmal defect. Bilaterally symmetrical abnormality suggests bilateral but unlocalized visual pathway defects.

SOMATOSENSORY EVOKED POTENTIALS

Most commonly, responses to electrical stimulation of the median and tibial nerves are recorded from peripheral nerve, spinal cord, brain stem, and cortex (see Chapter 451). Delay or absence of expected responses may suggest and localize a somatosensory pathway defect. Visual and somatosensory evoked potentials are useful in the detection of subclinical abnormalities in multiple sclerosis and in other neurologic disorders.

BRAIN STEM AUDITORY EVOKED POTENTIALS

Responses to click stimuli from the distal auditory nerve through to the upper pons and midbrain are usually recorded. In neurology, brain stem auditory evoked potentials are useful in retrocochlear or brain stem dysfunction, such as suspected acoustic neuroma.

EVOKED POTENTIAL MONITORING

Brain stem auditory evoked potentials and somatosensory evoked potentials can be monitored intraoperatively or in the intensive care unit, and may help to prevent neurologic deficits. Motor evoked potential monitoring using transcranial electric stimulation and recordings from the spinal cord or distal muscles is emerging as a safe and reliable method to predict the integrity of the corticospinal system intraoperatively.

BIBLIOGRAPHY

American Electroencephalographic Society. Guidelines in electroencephalography, evoked potentials, and polysomnography. *J Clin Neurophysiol* 1994;11:1–147.

Daly DD, Pedley TA, eds. *Current practice of clinical electroencephalography,* second ed. New York: Raven Press, 1990.

Neidermeyer E, Lopes da Silva F. *Electroencephalography: basic principles, clinical applications and related fields,* second ed. Baltimore: Urban & Schwartzenburg, 1987.

Kelley's Textbook of Internal Medicine, fourth edition. Edited by H. David Humes. Lippincott Williams & Wilkins, Philadelphia © 2000.

C H A P T E R
451

NEUROPHYSIOLOGY: NERVE CONDUCTION AND ELECTROMYOGRAPHY

ANDREW A. EISEN

The term *electromyography* (EMG) is generic and includes several electrophysiologic tests that are useful for examining the peripheral and central nervous systems. The different tests used are not mutually exclusive (Table 451.1). They complement each other, and often several are required to reach a logical conclusion. EMG is a sophisticated extension of the neurologic examination and should be designed specifically to evaluate further the clinical problem in each patient. There are no routines in EMG, making it challenging and exciting. Well-designed EMG enables a lesion to be localized, its severity determined, and the probable prognosis offered.

MOTOR AND SENSORY CONDUCTION STUDIES

Nerve conduction studies measure the velocity and the evoked amplitude of the largest, most rapidly conducting nerve fiber. Both motor and sensory studies are obtained. Seventy percent of the fibers in a peripheral nerve are of small diameter, including autonomic (sympathetic and parasympathetic) fibers, pain (C

TABLE 451.1.	APPLICATIONS OF ELECTROMYOGRAPHY
Test	**Application**
Motor conduction velocity	Focal neuropathies and polyneuropathies
Sensory conduction velocity	Focal neuropathies and polyneuropathies
F-wave response	Motor conduction through roots
H reflex	Sensory conduction through roots
Somatosensory evoked potentials	Sensory conduction through roots, sensory conduction through nerves that is not ameniable to routine study, sensory potentials that are absent, and conduction through the spinal cord
Transcranial magnetic stimulation	Central motor conduction and conduction through proximal segments of peripheral nerve
Repetitive stimulation	Neuromuscular transmission failure
Needle electroyography	To document denervation, fasciculation, myotonia, reinnervation, myopathy; to differentiate upper vs. lower motor neuron weakness; and to differentiate true hysterical weakness
Single-fiber electromyography	Same as for needle electromyography, but gives additional information about the motor unit and is a sensitive indicator of neuromuscular failure

and A Δ fibers), and gamma efferent fibers supplying the intrafusal muscle fibers of muscle spindles. These fibers cannot be evaluated directly because the stimulating current required would be intolerable. The autonomic nervous system can be evaluated indirectly using several different techniques, but direct assessment of autonomic nerve fibers is still experimental. Therefore, normal results on conventional conduction studies do not rule out disease of the peripheral nerve but merely reflect normal conduction through the fastest conducting large-diameter nerve fibers. Further, routine conduction studies do not incorporate the proximal parts of the peripheral nervous system: the roots and plexus. Different techniques are required for their evaluation (see below).

Diseases of peripheral nerves may produce demyelination, degeneration of the axon, or both. Marked conduction slowing (velocities of 30 m per second or less) indicates demyelination of nerve. This may be focal [i.e., carpal tunnel syndrome, compressive ulnar neuropathy (cubital tunnel syndrome)] or diffuse and multisegmental (Guillain–Barré syndrome, hereditary neuropathies such as Charcot–Marie–Tooth disease). However, most toxins and deficiency states primarily involve the axon or cell body, with resulting degenerative nerve diseases, including most loss of the nerve fiber. Conduction velocity in these so-called axonal neuropathies may be normal; if slowing occurs, it usually is modest. However, the evoked potential amplitude is usually reduced, reflecting the loss of large nerve fibers.

No direct relation exists between the degree of conduction slowing and the severity of clinical disease. Marked conduction slowing can occur with minimal neurologic deficit, and vice versa. Similarly, improvement in conduction does not invariably follow, for example, decompressive surgery for carpal or cubital tunnel syndrome, even when there has been considerable clinical improvement. A nerve, once diseased, never returns to its normal structure, although it can transmit impulses in a sufficiently accurate manner to allow normal clinical function.

Other conduction characteristics require consideration. An important one is conduction block. The amplitude of the motor or sensory nerve action potential reflects the number of axons activated. The number can be reduced because of axonal destruction, as after trauma with resulting denervation. In addition to slowing of conduction described above in axonal neuropathies, demyelination can produce conduction block, which lowers the evoked amplitude in a fashion similar to functional loss of axons. The latter may be focal or multifocal. Functional conduction block may be seen early in carpal tunnel syndrome, cubital tunnel syndrome, radial nerve or Saturday night palsy, mild cases of Bell's palsy, and some cases of Guillain–Barré syndrome and chronic acquired demyelinating neuropathy, a disorder presumed to be immune-mediated (Fig. 451.1). This type of conduction block usually can be reversed in a short time unless axonal degeneration supersedes. Conduction block occurring in the absence of denervation heralds a good prognosis, but the

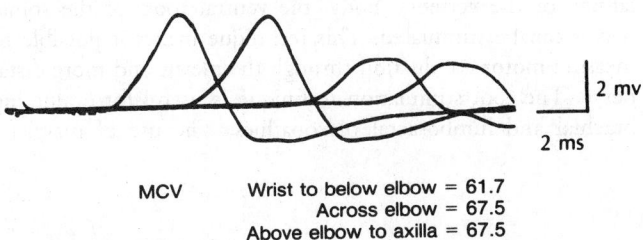

MCV   Wrist to below elbow = 61.7
Across elbow = 67.5
Above elbow to axilla = 67.5

FIGURE 451.1. To localize a focal lesion of nerve, several sites along the nerve must be stimulated. In this example—a cubital tunnel syndrome—conduction velocity below the elbow is normal, as is the size of the distal two-compound motor action potentials, evoked by stimulation of the ulnar nerve below the elbow and at the wrist. Conduction from the axilla to above the elbow is also normal, but the two responses elicited by stimulation in the axilla and above the elbow are less than half the size of the distal responses. This indicates that there is a region of conduction block located at the elbow (cubital tunnel).

recovery period can be protracted. Conduction slowing without conduction block is a useful means of distinguishing between acquired and hereditary demyelinating neuropathies; the latter usually do not demonstrate conduction block.

EVALUATION OF CONDUCTION THROUGH THE PROXIMAL PERIPHERAL NERVOUS SYSTEM

Conventional techniques for measuring motor and sensory conduction velocity cannot measure conduction through the proximal nerve segments, roots, or plexuses. Several techniques have been devised to measure conduction through these structures. They are F-wave measurement, H-reflex measurement, root stimulation, somatosensory evoked potential measurement, and cortical magnetic stimulation.

F-WAVE MEASUREMENT

When a motor nerve is stimulated, pulses travel in two directions: to the muscle supplied by the particular nerve stimulated, and antidromically toward the spinal cord. When they reach the spinal cord, the anterior horn cell is excited, setting up a second discharge that travels back down the nerve to reach and reexcite the same muscle (F wave). The F-wave action potential that can be recorded from muscle is small, but its latency is a measure of motor conduction through the nerve roots.

H-REFLEX MEASUREMENT

The H reflex is the electrical equivalent of the tendon jerk bypassing the muscle spindle. If the type Ia afferent fibers are stimulated selectively, which can be done using a small stimulus of long duration, a monosynaptic reflex is activated in which the anterior horn cells for a given muscle are excited. This can be used indirectly to measure sensory conduction through the nerve roots.

ROOT STIMULATION

By introducing a narrow-gauge needle so that its tip lies on the lamina or the vertebral body, the ventral roots of the spinal nerves can be stimulated. This technique makes it possible to measure motor conduction through the plexus and more distal nerve. The root stimulation technique is useful for evaluating brachial and lumbosacral plexopathies. The use of magnetic stimulation, which is relatively painless, has obviated the need for invasive needle stimulation.

SOMATOSENSORY EVOKED POTENTIAL

The somatosensory evoked potential is a cortically evoked response that is recorded from the scalp in a fashion similar to that of the electroencephalogram. The response is elicited via stimulation of a peripheral nerve. In patients with peripheral neuropathy, the somatosensory evoked potential can be used to measure sensory conduction velocity when this is not possible using conventional techniques. During recovery from nerve injury, the somatosensory evoked potential may be measurable many months before its peripheral counterpart, providing useful evidence of reestablished axonal continuity. The somatosensory evoked potential also may be used to measure conduction through a nerve from which it is difficult or impossible to record action potentials by conventional means because of anatomical inaccessibility.

These methods are better for evaluating plexopathies than radiculopathies because the shortness of the nerve root is diluted by the length of normally conducting nerve, which the F-wave, H-reflex, and somatosensory evoked potential techniques incorporate. Nevertheless, these tests have a place in the study of root lesions.

TRANSCRANIAL MAGNETIC STIMULATION

Transcranial magnetic stimulation enables in vivo painless stimulation of the awake human motor cortex, making it possible to evaluate the central motor pathways. This is particularly useful in amyotrophic lateral sclerosis, multiple sclerosis, and myelopathies resulting from lesions that are not visible on radiographs. Transcranial magnetic stimulation also can provide useful information regarding proximal parts of the peripheral nervous system.

NEEDLE ELECTROMYOGRAPHY

Needle examination of muscle often is the only means of determining the severity of disease and provides important information that cannot be obtained with conduction studies. The detection of myotonia, characterized clinically by delayed muscle relaxation after contraction, exemplifies this phenomenon (Fig. 451.2). There are three essential elements to needle EMG, each

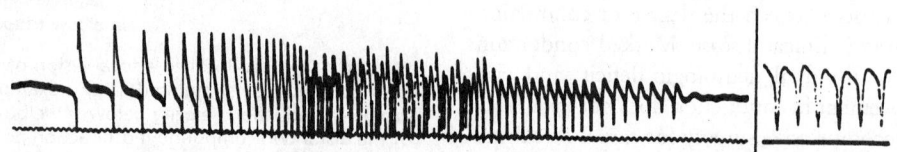

FIGURE 451.2. Myotonia is the clinical phenomenon of delayed muscle relaxation. It is most commonly seen in myotonic dystrophy but is symptomatic of several other hereditary and acquired diseases. Electrically there is a characteristic, high-frequency rhythmic discharge with a "dive bomber" sound. Electrical myotonia may be recorded without clinical counterpart.

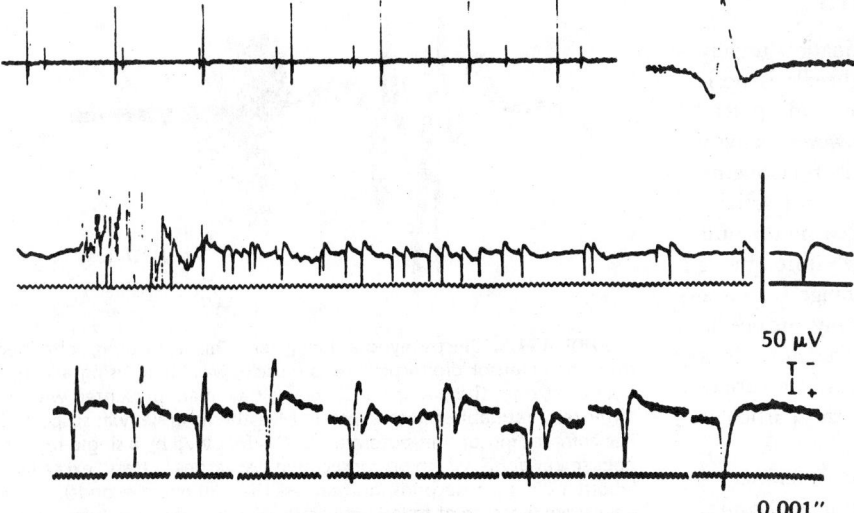

50 μV

0.001"

FIGURE 451.3. These fibrillation and positive sharp-wave potentials were recorded from the relaxed tibialis anterior muscle of a patient who had developed a peroneal palsy 2 weeks previously. Each spike and positive sharp wave reflects spontaneous, nonvisible contraction of a single, denervated muscle fiber. Fibrillation may also be seen in primary muscle disease if the end plate is separated from the nerve terminal.

of which provides different information: analysis of spontaneous activity, the firing pattern of the motor units on voluntary effort, and the morphologic characteristics of the recruited motor units.

SPONTANEOUS ACTIVITY

When the recording needle is inserted into a relaxed muscle, the muscle is electrically silent except for brief "insertional activity." Loss of nerve–muscle continuity (denervation) results in fibrillation, which is the spontaneous firing of individual muscle fibers (Fig. 451.3). This cannot be seen clinically.

The onset of fibrillation is related directly to the length of the nerve segment distal to the site of injury. In radiculopathy, for example, denervation appears first in the paraspinal muscles, then in the proximal limb muscles, and finally in the distal musculature. It may not be seen in the distal muscles of the arms or legs for up to 3 weeks after the injury. Therefore, in the early postinjury period, the absence of fibrillation does not rule out denervation. Once fibrillation has developed, it may persist for many years. After disk surgery, fibrillation often can be recorded for at least a year. This finding makes it difficult to evaluate recurrent symptoms ("failed back surgery") by needle EMG.

Fibrillation does not equate invariably with nerve disease. It also occurs in botulism, a disease of the neuromuscular junction, and in primary myopathies. In myopathies, it results from functional separation of a portion of the muscle fiber from its end plate.

Fasciculation is the spontaneous firing of part or all of a motor unit; all of the muscle fibers are innervated by a single motor neuron. Fasciculations can be clinically visible. When seen in isolation in the absence of clinical muscle wasting, weakness, or other EMG abnormalities, fasciculation usually is benign. Diseases associated with fasciculation invariably are neurogenic, with the most common being those that involve the anterior horn cell, such as motor neuron disease (Fig. 451.4). Myokymia (bursts of discharges) is less disease-specific but is not uncommonly associated with radiation neuropathy. Facial

myokymia, usually resulting from multiple sclerosis, has a characteristic EMG pattern. Neuromyotonia, or Isaac's syndrome, also has a characteristic associated high-frequency spontaneous discharge. Occasionally, an early parkinsonian tremor that is not clinically apparent can be detected on needle EMG.

FIRING FREQUENCY

The earliest, and often the only, needle EMG abnormality is altered (rapid) firing of the motor units. This begins at the onset of the disease and lasts for as long as the disease is present. Normally, motor units seldom exceed firing frequencies of 8 per second; rates faster than 15 per second are abnormal. Increased firing frequency of motor units is compensatory for any lower motor neuron disease (myopathic or neurogenic disorders) but does not occur if effort is withheld voluntarily because of pain, malingering, or the presence of upper motor neuron disease.

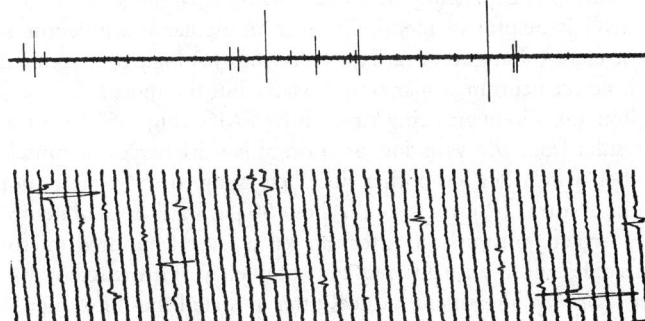

FIGURE 451.4. Fasciculation potentials. The top tracing was recorded at a slow sweep (1 minute). Given potentials occur only every few seconds and correspond to visible spontaneous muscle twitching. The lower tracing shows several (three or four) different fasciculation potentials recorded at a faster (10 millisecond) sweep. It is usually not possible to differentiate a "benign" from a "malignant" fasciculation, but one that is complex and is of increased fiber density is often associated with disease.

MORPHOLOGY OF THE MOTOR UNITS

The motor units recorded on the needle examination usually are biphasic or triphasic. When the recording needle is positioned near the muscle fiber, the spike of the motor unit potential reflects activity in a single muscle fiber. However, activity also is picked up from other surrounding muscle fibers belonging to the same motor unit. It is not possible to record activity from all of the muscle fibers belonging to a given motor unit simultaneously because they are scattered diffusely throughout the muscle and many are outside the "pick-up range" of most of the electrodes used. This limitation means that any one needle site can sample only part of the motor unit. Therefore, it is customary to explore several different needle sites in a variety of muscles. The number sampled depends on the particular problem.

The motor unit changes dramatically in disease. As reinnervation proceeds through terminal or collateral spouting, it becomes larger because the same motor unit now innervates its own muscle fibers and several of those belonging to one or more "foreign" units. The motor unit potential becomes longer in duration and more complex in shape (polyphasic).

These changes in the motor unit potential are appreciated more readily using a single-fiber electrode. Single-fiber EMG makes it possible to measure several aspects of the motor unit. For example, because individual muscle fibers are easily recognized, they can be counted and assigned a fiber density. Fiber density increases as part of the reinnervation process.

FAILURE OF NEUROMUSCULAR TRANSMISSION

Several diseases are characterized by failure of neuromuscular transmission. The most common is myasthenia gravis, but others, such as botulism and Eaton–Lambert syndrome, are not rare. These conditions have specific clinical features but share the hallmark symptom of muscle fatigability on voluntary effort. However, not all muscle fatigue results from a neuromuscular transmission defect; other causes include multiple sclerosis, postviral fatigue syndromes, rare metabolic myopathies, and, most commonly, depression and other forms of psychogenic fatigue. EMG is helpful in identifying neuromuscular transmission as the cause of fatigue. A variety of electrophysiologic tests are used to detect neuromuscular transmission, but the most sensitive is jitter measurement using single-fiber EMG (Fig. 451.5). Jitter results from the variation of consecutive discharges of muscle fiber in relation to another fiber belonging to the same motor unit. Normally, jitter is small, about 50 μs. In diseases of neuromuscular transmission, jitter can reach several hundred microseconds and eventually may fail completely. This is referred to as *blocking*. Treatment reduces jitter and abolishes blocking, so patients must be evaluated when they are not taking medication.

SPINAL CORD CONDUCTION

The scope of EMG has been broadened to include the investigation of central nervous system diseases. One example is the measurement of spinal cord conduction, which is useful in condi-

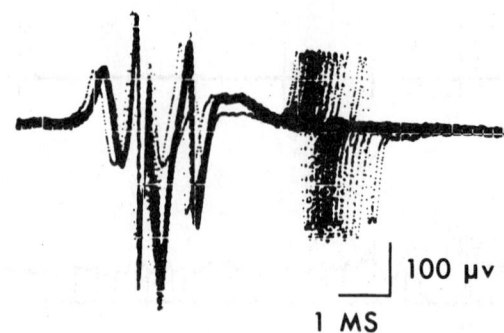

FIGURE 451.5. Electromyographic jitter. This recording, obtained from the extensor digitorum brevis muscle, was made using a single-fiber electrode. The patient, a 32-year-old woman, presented with intermittent, fatigable, bilateral ptosis. Myasthenia gravis was suspected. The complex motor unit potential (*left*) is followed by a single-muscle-fiber spike (*right*), which on consecutive discharges "jitters" excessively (about 1,000 microseconds, normal less than 50 microseconds). This is a sensitive measure of failed neuromuscular transmission. It is not specific for myasthenia gravis, however, because it is also seen in botulism and Eaton–Lambert syndrome.

tions that cannot be visualized by computed tomography or magnetic resonance imaging. In addition, many EMG methods are included under the general term *reflexology*. These are helpful in evaluating disorders of muscle tone (upper motor neuron spasticity, parkinsonian rigidity) and their responses to drug therapy.

BIBLIOGRAPHY

Brown WF, Bolton CF. *Clinical electromyography*. Boston: Butterworth, 1987.
Chu-Andrews J. *Electrodiagnosis: an anatomical and clinical approach*. Philadelphia: JB Lippincott, 1986.
Kimura J. *Electrodiagnosis in diseases of nerve and muscle: principles and practice*. Philadelphia: FA Davis Company, 1983.

Kelley's Textbook of Internal Medicine, fourth edition. Edited by H. David Humes.
Lippincott Williams & Wilkins, Philadelphia © 2000.

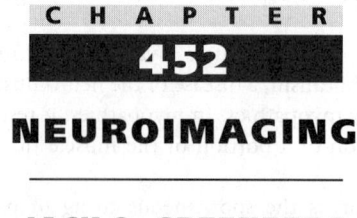

C H A P T E R

452

NEUROIMAGING

JACK O. GREENBERG

The development of methods to image the brain has led to much of the progress in clinical neurology. Many earlier technologies are gone (e.g., pneumoencephalography, ventriculography, epidural venography), and plain skull films are being used less frequently. Spine plain films continue to have limited use in trauma, degenerative disease, and developmental abnormalities.

In the early 1970s, new imaging techniques revealed unprecedented information about structure and disease in living patients. In traditional shadow radiography, introduced in 1896, all shadow-producing structures appear superimposed, making delineation of tissue difficult. Tomography, developed between 1920 and 1940, created a series of slices representing only one plane through the tissue, which allowed the creation of a three-dimensional mental image of the structures.

In 1961, Oldendorf, using a deceptively simple apparatus, demonstrated that the distribution of radiodensities within a plane could be reconstructed. Hounsfield, beginning in 1967, used a computer to calculate an image of the body from x-ray readings taken from many different projections. Further refinement led to a great day in 1972 when a brain cyst was clearly seen in a woman with a suspected brain lesion using computed tomography (CT). CT continues to be an important technique in neuroimaging. It is more accurate than other techniques in defining acute brain hemorrhages (72 hours or less), especially in the subarachnoid space, but also within the brain when compared to magnetic resonance imaging (MRI). Bony abnormalities, including fractures and calcification, are also better defined by CT than MRI. CT historically has been faster than MRI and was more appropriate for the patient who could not cooperate or who had severe claustrophobia. Today, on newer scanners, MRI is as fast as CT. CT revolutionized the practice of neurology and neurosurgery, becoming as important to these specialties as bone roentgenology is to orthopedics. CT provided direct visualization of normal and abnormal soft tissues, unlike previous attempts at body imaging.

Despite its usefulness, however, CT is limited in its ability to characterize tissue. It shows tissues that have an electron density different from that of surrounding tissue. Iodinated contrast material can demonstrate lesions with an abnormal blood–brain barrier. Unlike MRI, it has no great analytical potential to define brain chemistry and function.

MRI is a form of tissue analysis in which radio waves applied in a magnetic field are used as a probe to measure and localize chemical characteristics. A radiofrequency pulse is introduced into tissue and the magnetic resonance is analyzed. Before imaging, the main magnetic field is uniform, strong, and constant. When actually imaging, gradient coils rapidly alter the magnetic field in all three planes to provide spatial localization. Because of the gradients, the protons spin at unique frequencies, allowing them to be encoded and localized in the field. CT can give gray–white contrast because the electron density (the source of detail in CT) of gray matter is 0.2% greater than that of white matter. Magnetic resonance proton imaging emphasizes free water and free fat protons. Even though the actual concentration of protons is similar in gray and white matter, gray matter contains about 15% more water than white (82% vs. 72%). Because the magnetic resonance system is designed to differentiate water protons from nonwater protons, there is considerably more contrast between gray and white matter in MRI than in CT when T2-weighted images are used. Lesions such as infarcts, tumors, and abscesses differ more profoundly in the quality and quantity of their water content than in their specific gravity, thus explaining the greater contrast in these lesions on MRI than on CT. Because cortical bone does not produce artifacts with MRI, the posterior fossa structures, sella, and spinal cord are easily seen. In CT, the x-ray must pass through a great deal of bone, resulting in artifacts (streaking and beam hardening). Medullary bone contains fatty and hematopoietic marrow, and these can be visualized in vivo for the first time and may open a whole new field of regional hematology.

The technologic advantage of MRI is that it can characterize and discriminate among tissues using their biochemical and physical properties. This includes water, fat, and blood and its breakdown products (hemosiderin and ferritin). The velocity of cerebrospinal fluid (CSF) and blood flow can be evaluated. Images can be obtained in three orthogonal planes, as well as obliquely, without moving the patient. Orthogonal imaging has been a boon to surgeons and radiation therapists and is also an excellent aid in learning and relearning neuroanatomy. Paramagnetic contrast agents allow for the safe demonstration of the breakdown of the blood–brain barrier. Unlike the agents used in CT, these are noniodinated and much less hazardous to the patient. Often, contrast is unnecessary in MRI; the use of these expensive agents should be tailored to each patient. MRI is safe, does not use ionizing radiation, requires little patient preparation, is noninvasive (unless contrast is used), and is accepted by all but the most claustrophobic or obese patients. It has become the diagnostic procedure of choice in almost all diseases of the brain and spine, and in many instances it is the only test necessary.

The disadvantages of MRI include the expense of purchasing, operating, and maintaining the equipment. The magnetic field will not allow the standard life-support equipment to be used. Patients with pacemakers and certain ferromagnetic and electronic devices cannot be imaged. Metal, such as clips from previous surgery, causes artifacts, which sometimes obscure the study. Previously, a relatively slow scan acquisition time resulted in motion artifact. Fast scanning, improved coils, chemical shift imaging, and other improvements used in concert have alleviated many of these problems.

SPECTROSCOPY

Particular nuclei, when exposed to an external magnetic field, resonate at a characteristic frequency. For example, a phosphorus 31 nucleus, when placed in an external magnetic field, precesses at a particular frequency, depending on where it is located on the phosphate chain of the ATP molecule. Thus, there is a frequency signature for different molecules containing the same atom. This allows for the study of the distribution and concentration of high-energy phosphate metabolites and phosphocreatine, the intracellular pH of tissue, and tissue temperature. How this will affect the clinical practice of neurology is uncertain, but it could lead to important biochemical information that will help our patients.

ANGIOGRAPHY

The development of MRI has diminished the use of angiography, especially as a screening tool for symptomatic neurology

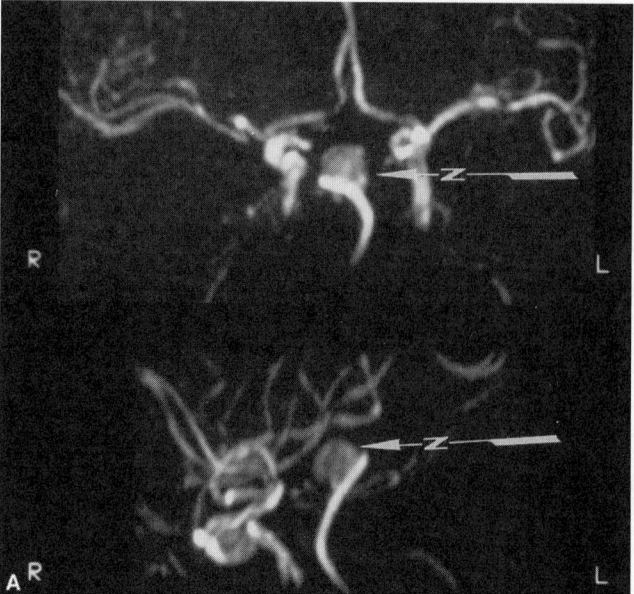

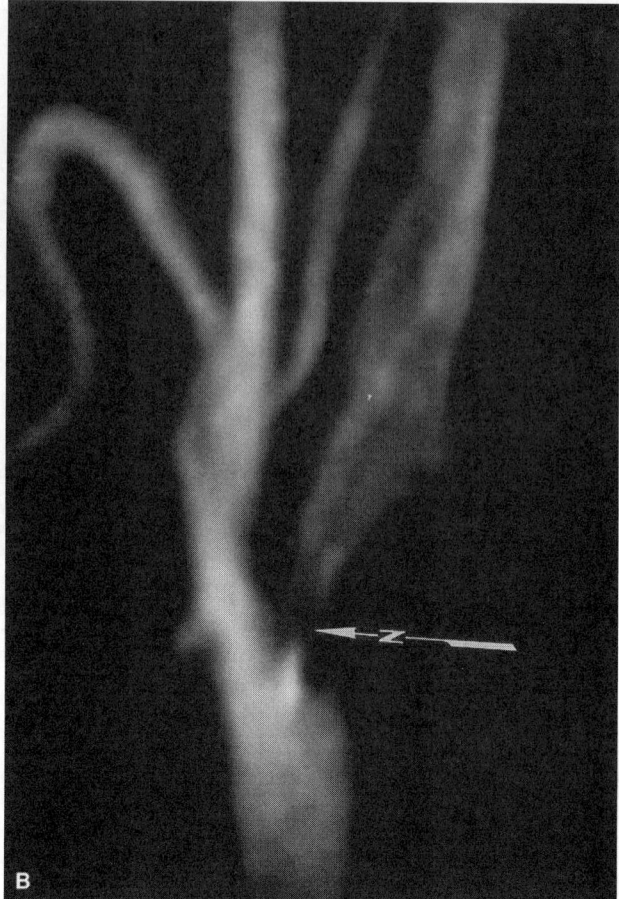

FIGURE 452.1. A: Three-dimensional time-of-flight magnetic resonance angiogram demonstrating an aneurysm at the top of the basilar artery *(arrows).* **B:** Three-dimensional time-of-flight magnetic resonance angiogram demonstrating severe stenosis of the internal carotid artery *(arrow).*

patients. Even more exciting is the development of magnetic resonance angiography (MRA), which in only a few years has become a clinically useful tool. In many instances it can replace routine angiography in the diagnosis of aneurysms, arteriovenous malformations (AVMs), carotid stenoses, dural sinus thrombosis, and other venous disorders (Fig. 452.1). Selective MRA provides information about the origin and direction of flow and circulation in collateral vessels. Flow effects can be seen in routine spin-echo imaging, including the ability to visualize aneurysms and AVMs, which will lead to further study with MRA. Carotid occlusions are often seen as a lack of flow void; this may be an indication for MRA in some stroke patients.

DIFFUSION/PERFUSION IMAGING IN ACUTE ISCHEMIC STROKE

CT and standard T2-weighted MRI images are typically normal in the first few hours after the onset of ischemic stroke. Nonspecific changes, such as tissue swelling, arterial enhancement with contrast, or absent flow voids, may be present early. It takes 6 to 12 hours to detect the presence and extent of ischemic damage. In animal studies, diffusion weighted imaging (DWI) can visualize the ischemic changes within minutes of the stroke (Fig.

452.2). In standard MRI, the results depend on relaxation times, proton density, and flow. By adding short dephasing and rephasing current to the standard pulse sequences, the signal can be sensitized to the acquisition of molecular diffusion. In normal brains, there is an apparent diffusion coefficient (ADC) that is relatively uniform along the direction of axonal flow, but this coefficient declines rapidly in ischemic brains. The water protons have less brownian movement over time, leading to a reduction in ADC. In animal stroke models, DWI is highly predictive of ultimate infarction. When N-methyl-D-asparate antagonists were given to rats 15 minutes after arterial occlusion, DWI studies performed at 30 and 180 minutes after stroke onset revealed hyperintense lesions that were 70% smaller in the treated group than in controls.

Perfusion imaging is another new MRI technique that is promising in the evaluation of the acute stroke patient. The development of ultrafast scanning techniques, such as echo planar imaging and fast-gradient echo imaging, has led to the capability for scanning the entire brain in seconds, or less than a second per slice. This allows evaluation of brain microcirculation and provides quantitative information about localized changes in cerebral blood flow (CBF) and cerebral blood volume (CBV). Contrast agents, such as gadolinium, are injected intravenously. As the agent travels through the brain, it interferes with the acquisition of signal intensity in normally perfused brain tissue; ischemic brain tissue has less reduction of signal.

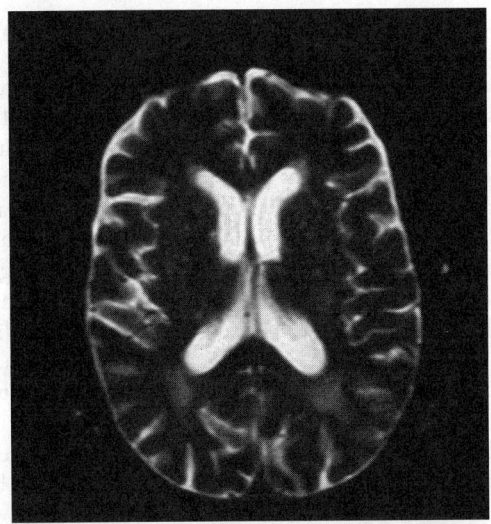

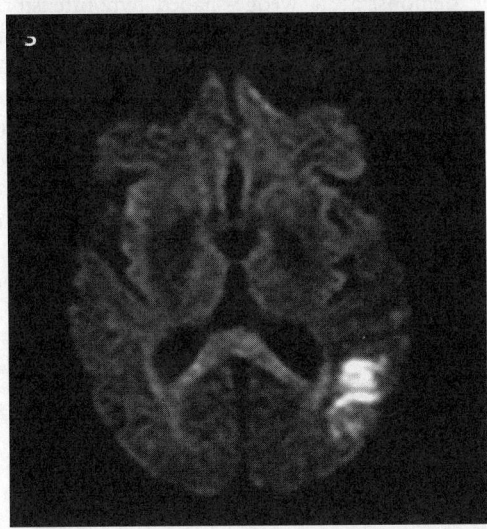

FIGURE 452.2. A: T2 Axial demonstrating some high signals posterior to posterior horns but no evidence of infarction in left parietal area. **B:** Diffusion-weighted study done at the same time (within 2 hours of ictus) demonstrates area of high signal in left parietal lobe, which is an area of ischemia.

Relative CBV can be calculated by evaluating signal intensity changes over time, and an index of CBF can be derived by dividing the relative CBF by vascular transit time. Perfusion imaging should provide easy and quick measurement of impaired CBF in stroke patients.

POSITRON EMISSION TOMOGRAPHY

Positron emission tomography (PET) is a complex, expensive method of brain imaging that depicts physiologic processes. It can supply information about oxygen and glucose metabolic rates, local CBF, blood volume, and oxygen extractions. The three-dimensional images provide real physiologic data regarding brain function. The combination of physical and chemical properties of positron-labeled compounds allows for quantifiable imaging.

Single photon emission computed tomography (SPECT) has recently been introduced. A flow tracer is tagged with a radionuclide and injected into the patient. A three-dimensional image of the distribution of the radionuclide is obtained using a gamma camera and CT techniques. SPECT may be able to predict the likelihood of an early stroke after a transient ischemic attack and can separate lacunar from cortical stroke. It also can differentiate ischemia from epilepsy as the cause of a neurologic symptom: ischemia causes an area of hypoperfusion on SPECT, but epileptic phenomena are often manifested by hyperperfusion.

ULTRASONOGRAPHY

The most important neurologic use of ultrasonography is in stroke. Eighty-five percent of strokes are ischemic, and it is here that ultrasonography plays an important role. At least half of ischemic strokes occur in large vessels, mostly the carotid artery. CT and MRI readily diagnose hemorrhagic strokes but often do not identify the blockage site in the large vessels. Ultrasonography is a noninvasive, accurate, quick, and relatively cost-effective way to visualize the vascular system and identify the cause of ischemic stroke. Recent studies confirm that tight carotid stenoses (greater than 70%) have better outcomes with carotid endarterectomy and medical therapy than with medical therapy alone. Ultrasongraphy is an effective way to identify these patients, who then may have angiography to identify these lesions further. In some centers, ultrasonography and MRA may suffice, although many surgeons are still reluctant to operate without contrast angiography. Ideally, this will not be the case as MRA becomes more widely accepted and improved.

Using duplex sonography, high-resolution B-mode gray-scale images of the vessels can be obtained and selective image-guided Doppler sampling performed. Blood flow velocities can be calculated. This technique should reach 90% to 95% sensitivity and more than 90% specificity for identifying significant carotid stenosis. Color flow imaging provides anatomical and hemodynamic information simultaneously. Transcranial Doppler sonography using low-frequency Doppler sonography can obtain flow velocity data from the basal cerebral arteries; this has opened a new window to the understanding of cerebral hemodynamics. Doppler techniques are allowing the detection of emboli for the first time.

CLINICAL APPLICATIONS

CEREBROVASCULAR DISEASE

The four basic goals in approaching the stroke patient are to identify the cause and mechanism of the stroke, to localize the lesion in the brain and particular blood vessel, to quantify the severity of brain damage to guide management decisions and prognosis, and to identify vascular lesions that may cause another stroke.

Often the clinical distinction among intracerebral hemor-

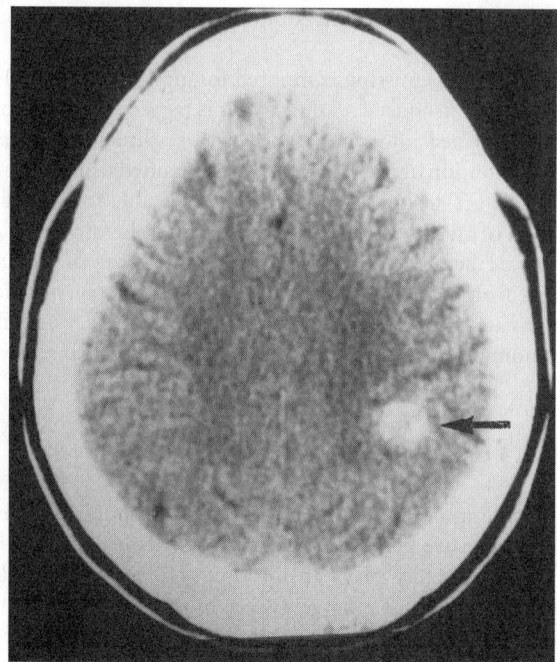

FIGURE 452.3. Computed tomographic scan demonstrating hemorrhagic contusion in the parietal lobe *(arrow).*

rhage, subarachnoid hemorrhage, and cerebral infarction is readily apparent, but sometimes the distinction is unclear. After a careful history and physical examination, an imaging procedure is usually necessary. In the acute bleed, CT is the best first test (Fig. 452.3). It readily demonstrates blood in any of the brain spaces, whereas the changes on MRI are subtle in the acute stage. MRI is especially weak in the diagnosis of subarachnoid hemorrhage, and CT is the imaging modality of choice. However, in the subacute and chronic stage of the hemorrhage, MRI is the test of choice and may demonstrate lesions (parenchymal and subdural) not seen on CT (Fig. 452.4). Sometimes the cause of the hemorrhage is readily seen on MRI (e.g., aneurysm, AVM, neoplasm); this guides the clinician to the next appropriate imaging study (e.g., angiography, MRA).

In the absence of hemorrhage, ischemia may be present. CT often demonstrates a hypodensity in a vascular pattern, but CT may be normal in the presence of a focal neurologic deficit; MRI may demonstrate a wedge-shaped hypointensity on the T1-weighted study and an increased signal in the same distribution on the T2-weighted study. The pattern of the lesion often identifies the offending branch, and the astute imager can often spot it. This is important because most lesions of the brain are of low intensity on T1-weighted studies and bright on T2-weighted studies. By using the clinical history and knowing the branch patterns of the major vessels, it is relatively easy to make a diagnosis or at least to establish a cogent differential.

Other features that can be identified in vascular and other

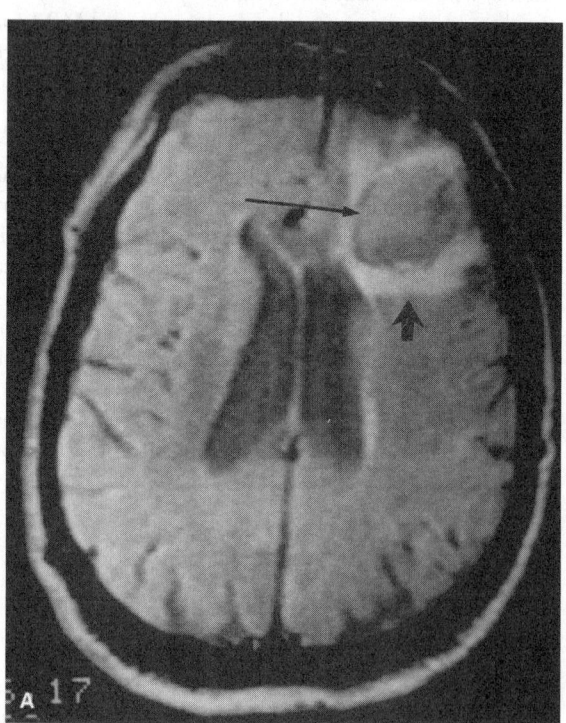
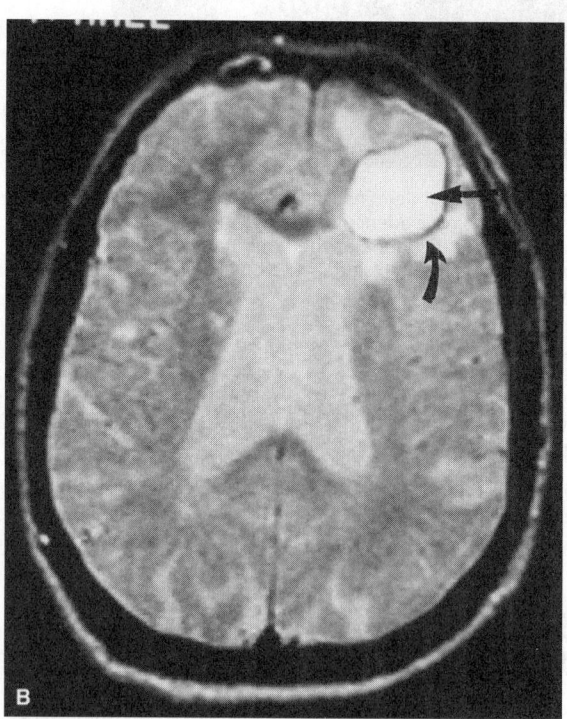

FIGURE 452.4. A: Acute intracerebral hemorrhage in left frontal area (TR 2128, TE 45) imaged in the first 24 hours. Hematoma *(long arrow)* is isointense to brain. The bright signal surrounding it *(short arrow)* is edema. Computed tomography (CT) showed a typical, high-density, easily diagnosed hematoma. **B:** Four weeks later, high-signal methemoglobin *(straight arrow)* is seen in the center surrounded by low-intensity hemosiderin *(curved arrow)*, indicating the beginning of a more chronic phase (TR 2128, TE 90). CT at this time was isodense, and the hemorrhage was not as easily appreciated.

lesions of the brain include surrounding edema, which may help the surgeon decide if the lesion is operable in the case of hematoma or help the neurologist determine the prognosis and medical treatment in the case of ischemic infarction. Hemorrhage may give rise to blockage of CSF pathways, leading to hydrocephalus. CT and MRI readily demonstrate this, allowing for ventricular drainage in the appropriate setting. The location of the lesion is helpful. A hemorrhage in the basal ganglia in a hypertensive patient does not require further studies. A lobar hemorrhage may be due to an AVM and requires angiography. A subarachnoid hemorrhage always requires angiography to identify aneurysms, the most likely source. MRI is superior to CT in the diagnosis of cavernous angiomas, AVMs, and tumors. The presence of other lesions, such as hemosiderin-lined cavities, suggests previous small bleeds, as in hypertensive patients, cocaine addicts, and patients with amyloid angiopathy. The latter would be particularly suspected in the presence of lobar hemorrhages in an elderly patient.

In most ischemic stroke patients, CT and, more often, MRI serve well as the first imaging study. Ultrasonography is often extremely helpful in illuminating the pathophysiology of the ischemic stroke. More complex studies, such as PET and diffusion/perfusion imaging, are not widely available but can be helpful. SPECT is more commonly available and, as mentioned previously, can be quite helpful in the stroke patient.

INTRACRANIAL NEOPLASMS

Of all the imaging modalities, MRI is the best single test in the diagnosis of brain tumor. Multiplanar techniques allow the exact location to be pinpointed. Features of common tumors on MRI have become widely recognized, as have the specific appearances of uncommon tumors. A safe contrast agent (gadolinium) makes possible the distinction between tumor and edema, which is so important to the surgeon in deciding where to biopsy the lesion. The T1-weighted sequence is exquisite for anatomy, and the T2-weighted image readily demonstrates the bright signal of increased water in the lesion. CT may be normal in a tumor and MRI abnormal (Fig. 452.5). Even with the use of contrast, there are differences: more metastases are seen with MRI than with CT, especially using a triple dose. If a patient has one metastasis on contrast-enhanced CT, contrast-enhanced MRI may demonstrate more than one lesion, thus completely changing the treatment and the prognosis. CT is a useful adjunct for identifying tumoral calcification.

Establishing whether a tumor is in the extra-axial or intra-axial space narrows the differential. A meningioma, the typical extra-axial lesion, has a sharp border, with a cleft of CSF between the tumor and brain. It may also cause inward displacement of the brain surface with compression of the white matter layers, the "buckled white matter sign." These findings may all be seen on the initial T1-weighted study. The suggestion of a meningioma should lead to contrast enhancement because small meningiomas may blend into the parenchyma, and many may not be bright on the T2-weighted study, as most other tumors are.

The signal intensity within the same tumor can vary, depending on cystic changes, hemorrhage, necrosis, calcification, fat, and vascularity. Several pulse sequences are necessary for qualitative analysis of signal intensity, including T1- and T2-weighted studies, proton density, and contrast-enhanced T1-weighted studies. Gradient echo (T2*) may identify calcium or hemosiderin not seen on routine spin-echo studies, especially in midfield magnets. It is often possible to infer the degree of malignancy in the contrast-enhanced scan because of more enhancement and other certain patterns. In CT, the iodine is made directly visible by attenuating the x-ray beam; paramagnetic contrast agents of MRI are made indirectly visible by diffusing to the extracellular space, where they enhance the relaxation rates of nearby water protons. In many cases, MRI with contrast is the only study necessary for the neurosurgeon to proceed with removal or biopsy (Fig. 452.6).

INTRACRANIAL INFECTION

CT and MRI demonstrate the gross neuropathologic process of infection of the brain and meninges, but neither is specific for any one disease. Multiple enhancing rings may be due to bacterial or nonbacterial infections or other pathologies, such as metastases, multiple sclerosis (MS), and contusions. As usual, the history and the associated symptoms direct the imager and the clinician to the correct diagnosis. The association of fever, travel in locations endemic to brain infections, and the location of the lesions is helpful. An example of the latter is a lesion in the temporal lobe with fever, headache, altered consciousness, and focal seizures, which should cause the clinician to consider herpes simplex encephalitis as the most likely diagnosis (Fig. 452.7). MRI is more sensitive than CT in revealing temporal and frontal lobe involvement. In the acute phase, MRI demonstrates swelling and edema, which is of low intensity on T1-weighted images and bright on T2-weighted images. When gadolinium is used, there is pial and cortical enhancement. If available, postcontrast T1-weighted images should be made with magnetization transfer, which improves contrast. In the late stages, tissue loss and brain necrosis are seen.

Neurologic involvement occurs in over 80% of patients with AIDS, and autopsy reveals an even higher frequency of CNS involvement in this disorder (90% or more). The illnesses may be the direct result of CNS involvement, such as AIDS dementia complex or HIV-associated myelopathy. They also may be related to immunosuppression, e.g., infections such as cerebral toxoplasmosis (Fig. 452.8) and cryptococcosis, or primary and metastatic neoplasm. Neuroimaging is essential in determining whether there is a focal mass lesion. The most common causes of intracranial mass lesions in HIV infection are toxoplasmosis and lymphoma, in that order of frequency. These patients may have subarachnoid or ventricular blockage. Cardiac-gated cine-flow MRI, which uses gradient-recalled images in various portions of the cardiac cycle, may yield important information about the location of the blockage and the direction of CSF flow. The most common cause of nonmass lesions in this setting is progressive multifocal leukoencephalopathy. This opportunistic infection is caused by the JC virus and is seen in 5% of AIDS patients. Nonenhancing lesions in the parieto-occipital and frontal white matter are present without mass effect. Serial CT or MRI shows a progressive increase in the size and number of lesions, with the focal lesions becoming diffuse and confluent.

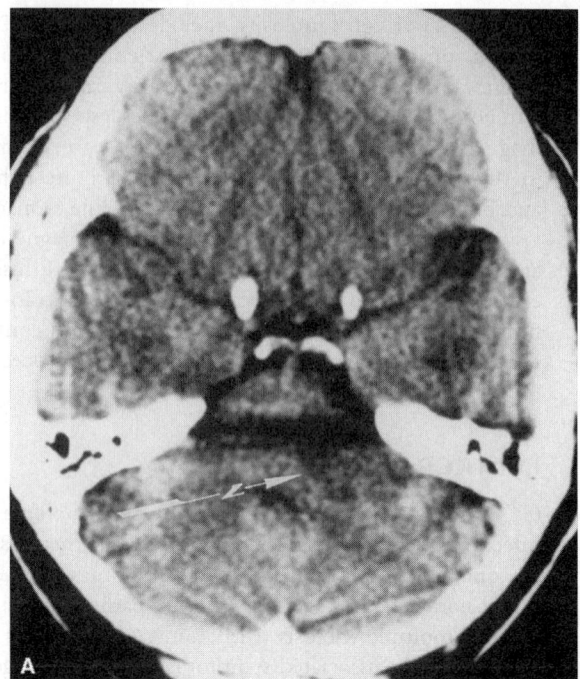

FIGURE 452.5. A: Computed tomographic scan originally read as normal in a patient with left-sided neurosensory hearing loss. In retrospect, low density is noted in the left cerebellopontine angle *(arrow)*, along with much beam hardening artifact. **B:** T1-weighted axial magnetic resonance image in the same patient. Note the low-intensity large lesion in the left cerebellopontine angle compressing the fourth ventricle *(arrow)*. This is much more obvious than on the scan, which also showed compression of the fourth ventricle. **C:** Enhanced T1-weighted magnetic resonance image demonstrating large enhancing lesion with two cysts. Enhancement of the eighth nerve complex confirms that this is a large acoustic neuroma.

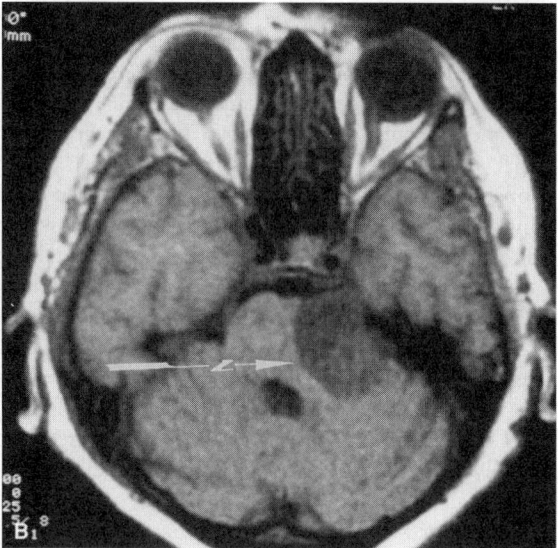

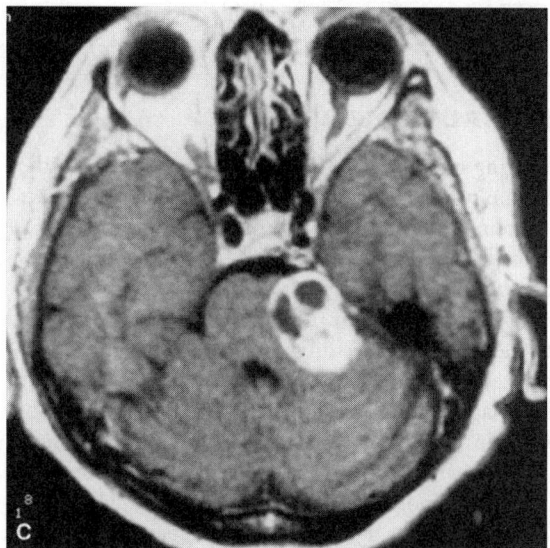

HIV encephalopathy shows nonspecific atrophy with widening of the fissures and cisterns. Periventricular white matter lesions are also seen. A young or middle-aged patient with a positive history of intravenous drug use or other dangerous behaviors with dementia and atrophy of the brain should be considered as a possible HIV suspect, and proper investigations should follow.

MULTIPLE SCLEROSIS

There are about 300,000 to 500,000 MS patients in the United States, and about 200 new cases are diagnosed each week. CT occasionally demonstrates the typical distribution of lesions with dissemination in space, and enhancement patterns may indicate dissemination in time, but MRI has replaced CT in the diagnosis

of MS. MRI has provided a quantum leap in the diagnosis of MS because of its exquisite sensitivity to the changes in water content of MS plaques. MRI may detect MS plaques at early stages, when the disease is often missed by other techniques. MRI has shown that MS is an evolving process in which lesions come and go; no other technique has been as successful in demonstrating this phenomenon. With the use of the latest equipment, MS plaques can be identified in 87% to 95% of cases; in the best hands, CT has been positive in 36% to 44% of cases.

The lesions are dark or isointense on T1-weighted images and bright on proton density and T2-weighted studies. Proton density can be especially helpful because the CSF is gray and the plaques are bright, so there is less difficulty in differentiating one from the other. The lesions are either discrete or confluent.

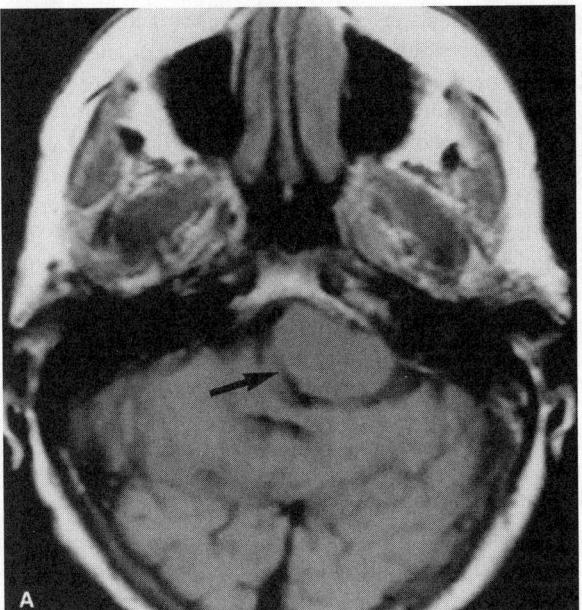
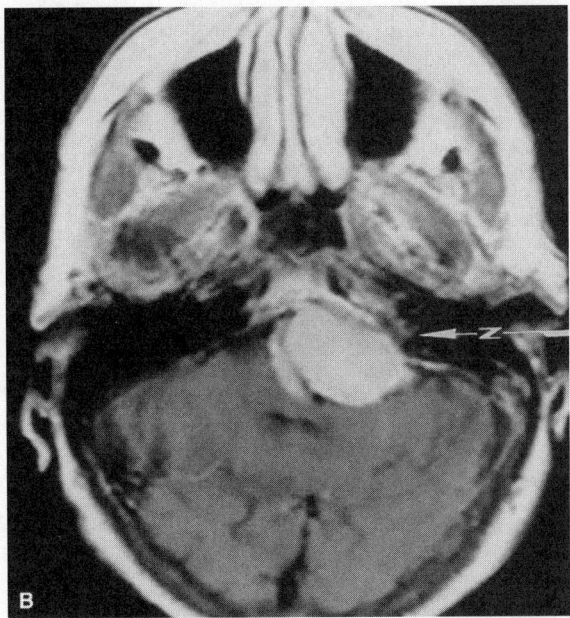

FIGURE 452.6. A: Axial T1-weighted magnetic resonance image in a patient with normal hearing demonstrating a large cerebellopontine angle lesion *(arrow)*. **B:** Post-gadolinium T1 study on the same patient demonstrates that the eighth nerve complex *(arrow)* does not enhance, which confirms that this is a meningioma rather than an acoustic neuroma.

The former are focal, oval or round, and are located near the anterior or posterior horns of the body of the ventricles; they may extend up to the subconvexity area. Confluent lesions are larger and cap the posterior horn of the ventricles with undulating borders. Unlike vascular lesions, MS often involves the corpus callosum and should be considered in all lesions of that structure, especially in the appropriate clinical setting. Lesions are often seen in the cerebellum, especially the peduncles and the brain stem. As with most diseases, the pathologic lesion

is best demonstrated on the more T2-weighted studies. One common pattern is the ovoid lesion at right angle to the ventricles, which may be seen in up to 86% of MS patients (Fig. 452.9).

The breakdown of the blood–brain barrier in the MS lesion allows for enhancement with contrast on both CT and MRI. It is usually unnecessary to enhance these lesions unless using a research protocol. In a young female patient whose lesions are

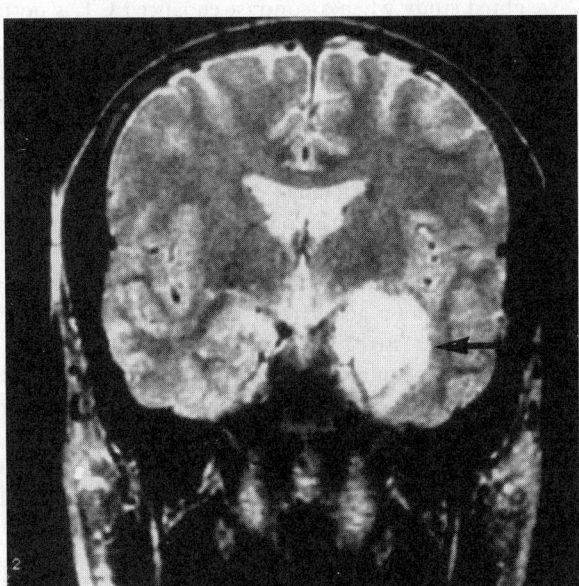

FIGURE 452.7. T2-weighted coronal magnetic resonance image demonstrating herpes simplex encephalitis in the left temporal lobe *(arrow)*.

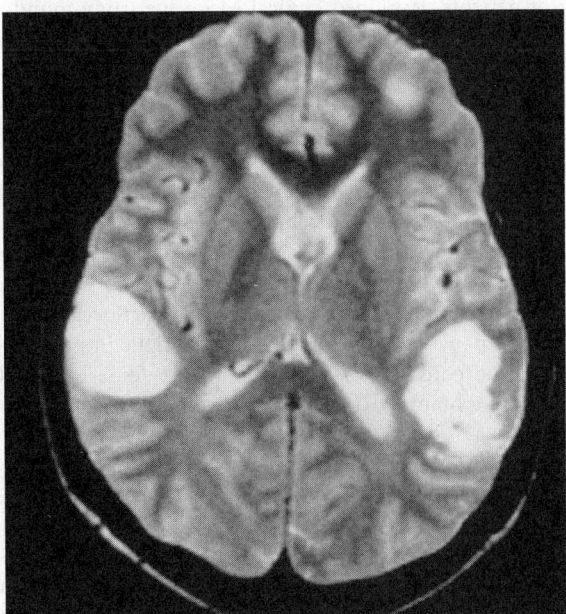

FIGURE 452.8. T2-weighted study in a young man with AIDS. The two high-signal lesions on either side represent toxoplasmosis.

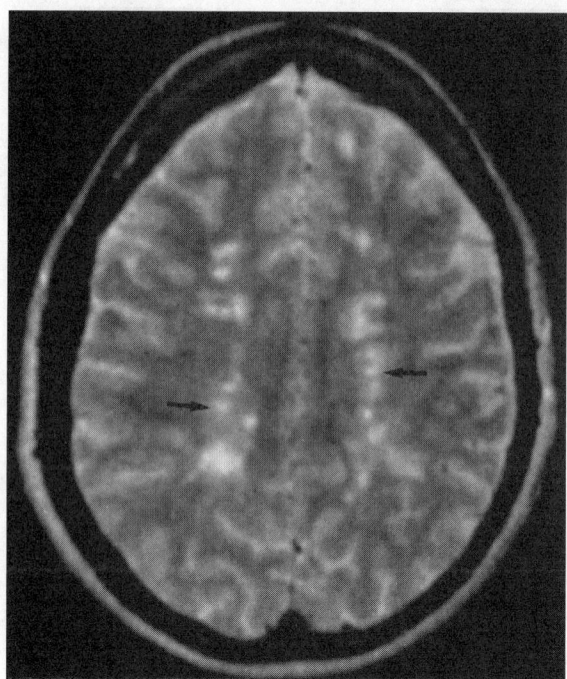

FIGURE 452.9. T2-weighted axial view in a young woman with multiple sclerosis. Note the high signals in a periventricular distribution horizontal to the ventricles *(arrows)*.

clinically disseminated in time and space, and who has a positive MRI with typical horizontal lesions, there is rarely any need to proceed further with other studies (e.g., CSF, evoked potentials). However, these studies should be used when the evidence is not so clear.

What is the relation between an isolated attack of optic neuritis and possible future development of MS? In 31 studies involving optic neuritis followed for variable periods of time, 13% to 85% of patients developed clinical MS. One study found that 48% (23 of 48) of patients with optic neuritis had silent lesions of MS in the white matter. After 5 years, 19% had developed definite clinical MS. Two-thirds of the converting patients had abnormal MRIs, and one-third had normal studies. The authors concluded that an abnormal MRI did not necessarily predict future clinical MS. It is wise not to diagnose MS in the optic neuritis patient, even with an abnormal MRI, unless other clinical symptoms develop. Lesions may be seen in the optic nerve itself if thin T1-weighted sections are used with and without contrast. Lesions of the spinal cord are also seen occasionally. A young patient with a myelopathy and a bright intramedullary lesion of the cord on T2-weighted images (especially at C2) should have a brain MRI; if it is positive, no further studies are necessary.

DEVELOPMENTAL DISEASES OF THE NERVOUS SYSTEM

Because of its lack of ionizing radiation, its capacity to image in multiple planes, its capacity to demonstrate CSF dynamics, and its capacity to show myelination (allowing for the study of brain maturation), MRI is easily the procedure of choice in this area, which affects primarily infants and children. Sedation with close observation is mandatory; a nurse or anesthesiologist must monitor the patient before, during, and after the study when sedation is used.

The lack of myelination and the high water content of the brain in the infant and young child require different sequences in the performance of MRI. For unknown reasons, infarction in infants may be of lower signal intensity in the T2-weighted study, unlike that in older patients. Various insults to the brain, such as trauma, infection, ischemia, systemic disorders, chemotherapy, or radiation therapy, may cause delays in myelination. The latter is a dynamic process that begins before birth and is almost complete by age 24 months. MRI is unique in demonstrating these changes.

The T1-weighted sagittal view can make visible the entire nervous system of an infant or small child, and often demonstrates congenital anomalies in patients with developmental delays. Failure of neural tube closure (e.g., Chiari I and II malformations) is easily diagnosed. Sometimes patients with Chiari I malformations are referred to neurology clinics with the diagnosis of MS. In the past, myelography was necessary to identify this entity, but the use of myelography has dropped by as much as 80% in most neurology centers.

EPILEPSY

Epilepsy may be divided into idiopathic and symptomatic forms of the disease. In the latter, structural abnormalities are found and imaging is most helpful. Functional imaging is of academic interest in idiopathic epilepsy (e.g., CBF, receptor binding, and metabolism).

The common causes of symptomatic epilepsy include scars, atrophic lesions, tumors, vascular anomalies, cortical dysplasias, and stroke. In patients presenting with seizures due to a tumor, the symptoms are often indolent and the neurologic examination may be normal. MRI can detect tumors with a bright signal on a T2-weighted study when a contrast-enhanced CT is normal. Therefore, MRI should be done on all patients with symptomatic epilepsy. Performance of CT in addition is rarely needed, other than to make visible bone or calcifications (e.g., meningioma).

CT and, more recently, MRI are extremely useful in the surgical placement of intracranial electrodes and in stereotactic removal of the epileptogenic lesion. PET with ^{18}F-fluorodeoxyglucose (FDG) is helpful in choosing patients for surgical removal of epileptogenic foci. Interictal unilateral temporal lobe hypometabolism may predict a good result after such surgery. During partial seizures, increased FDG uptake is present because of an increase in energy requirements. Neuroreceptor binding using PET can be useful in demonstrating neuronal loss in brain areas where there is diminished benzodiazepine binding.

In the presence of an equivocal electroencephalogram (EEG), SPECT perfusion scanning may be a less expensive method of determining whether a behavior is epileptic. SPECT and PET add important cognitive and behavioral information to the anatomical and structural information provided by MRI and CT. CT is often obscured by bony artifact in the middle fossa. Tumors presenting as a first seizure typically have no mass effect or edema. The use of contrast does not increase the detection of tumors in epilepsy because they usually are more benign lesions that do not precipitate a breakdown in the blood–brain barrier. Dysplasia, heterotopias, gyral malformations, abnormal clefts (schizencephaly), and migrational anomalies all may cause epilepsy and are readily made visible by MRI. Surgical removal of some of these abnormalities, including tumor, has been greatly enhanced by the use of MRI. Coronal MRI is very helpful in demonstrating focal atrophy in the hippocampus in 70% to 90% of patients with temporal lobe epilepsy.

AGING AND DEMENTIA

The new imaging techniques are useful in the study of brain development, maturation, and myelination, and these procedures are also of use in elderly patients. A primary difficulty is distinguishing a normal old person's scan from a demented person's scan. In both, atrophy is seen, and often it is impossible to make this distinction with routine CT or MRI. The most common—and therefore the most important—dementing illness is Alzheimer's disease. Using special angled cuts, the temporal horn and choroidal–hippocampal fissure can be imaged in a single slice and temporal lobe atrophy can be identified. The absence of temporal lobe atrophy differentiated normal from Alzheimer's patients with a specificity of up to 95% in one study. In another study, hippocampal lucency, probably related to widening of the choroidal fissures, correctly distinguished 80% of Alzheimer's and elderly control patients.

MRI allows the visualization of the temporal lobe with even greater clarity, especially in the coronal view. It has added a new phenomenon, the white matter hyperintensities (WMHs) or "unidentified bright objects" seen so often in normal persons, even in the early decades. WMHs have a definite association with increasing age, vascular risk factors (especially hypertension), and the presence of dementia, either degenerative or (especially) vascular. In one study of 101 normal controls age 31 to 84 years, WMHs were demonstrated in 48% and periventricular hyperintensities (PVHs) in 45%. The WMHs were small and discrete; the PVHs were caps at the ventricular apexes or smooth, bright, thin lines around the ventricles. Subjects with risk factors (hypertension, diabetes, heart disease, or age greater than 60 years) had more WMHs and PVHs. According to this study, the prevalence for WMHs and PVHs by decade is about 20% for the fourth decade, 30% for the fifth decade, 50% for the sixth decade, 60% for the seventh decade, and 70% for those older than 70 years. However, many persons with extensive WMHs have relatively subtle cognitive impairment and may have an otherwise completely normal neurologic examination.

The same researchers also studied the postmortem brain on six patients without clinically significant dementia or cerebrovascular disease who had WMHs incidentally on premortem MRI. They saw an abnormality in only one brain with visual observation. Histologic examination revealed areas of decreased myelination with thinned neuropil around fibrohyalinotic arteries. They speculated that this represented minor perivascular ischemia but not complete infarction as the most likely cause of WMHs.

PET studies suggest that regional metabolic interactions, especially between frontal and parietal association areas, become less tightly linked with normal aging. A decline in frontal metabolism is probably a feature of "usual" aging that corresponds with deterioration of frontal lobe executive functions with age.

Treatable disease (e.g., tumor, subdural hematoma, hydrocephalus, metabolic disease) can be found in only about 15% to 20% of demented patients. Once these diseases are excluded, one is left with either Alzheimer's or multi-infarct dementia in most of the rest. The following guidelines, proposed by Chawluk and associates, are clinically useful:

1. Mild to moderate PVHs on MRI may be seen in normal elderly persons as well as in patients with Alzheimer's or multi-infarct dementia; thus, this is usually not a helpful finding.
2. Scattered small subcortical hyperintensities may be seen in normal persons or demented patients, and are also generally not useful.
3. In patients 65 years or younger, the presence of medial temporal lobe atrophy, especially in the absence of prominent WMHs, strongly supports the diagnosis of Alzheimer's disease.
4. Extensive subcortical (white matter or deep gray nuclei, but no periventricular) high-signal abnormality, in conjunction with a positive Hachinski's ischemia score, suggests multi-infarct dementia.
5. The diagnosis of multi-infarct dementia is more likely if multiple cortical infarcts are seen or if CT demonstrates prominent subcortical lucencies.
6. In patients over age 65 years, the presence of medial temporal lobe atrophy does not necessarily indicate Alzheimer's, nor does the presence of moderate WMHs imply multi-infarct dementia.
7. The diagnosis of vascular dementia does not rule out coexistent Alzheimer's disease.

DISEASES OF THE SPINE

In most centers, the frequency of spine imaging has surpassed that of brain imaging, primarily because of the enormous numbers of persons with back pain. In Britain, every year 2 million adults consult their physicians for back pain, accounting for 6.5% of all visits to the general practitioner. In Britain, more than 19 million working days per year are lost due to back pain, with nearly 1 in 50 persons losing time from work.

One of the major challenges of any imaging modality is to ascertain whether the abnormality seen is causing the clinical symptoms. MRI, more than any other imaging modality to date, reveals "lesions" that are not producing symptoms. Astute clinical evaluation is necessary to decide whether a bright signal or an abnormal structure is of any clinical importance. More than ever, clinicians must be involved in this area to add important clinical input. There have been reports of asymptomatic lumbar disc herniations in patients who have had myelography for cervical problems; more recently, studies of large numbers of asymptomatic persons have revealed the incidence of disc herniations to be as high as 28%, with higher numbers of bulges and disc desiccation, all of which increase with age. Clinical judgment

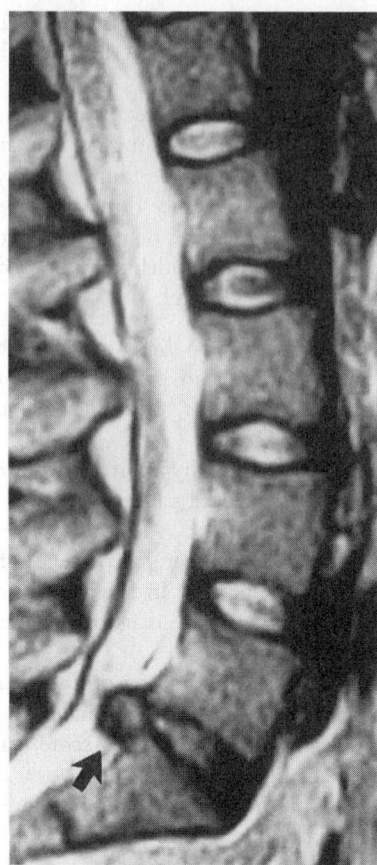

FIGURE 452.10. T2-weighted sagittal magnetic resonance image demonstrating a large disc herniation at L5–S1 *(arrow)*.

should be the major factor in determining whether or not surgery should be performed; a patient with an L2 radiculopathy should not have an L5–S1 disc removed "just because it is there" (Fig. 452.10).

Where high-resolution MRI of the spine is in daily use it is accepted as the diagnostic imaging modality of choice and has replaced other modalities, including myelography, CT, and plain-film radiography. The latter two are still useful in bony diseases and fractures and when the MRI is not diagnostic. In centers where the imagers have earned the trust of the surgeons, spine and cord lesions are removed without invasive myelography with all its discomfort and expense. When a patient with sciatica undergoes plain-film radiography, CT, MRI, electromyography, and, occasionally, evoked potentials followed by myelography, there is a lack of clinical astuteness or worse. Quality standards and practice guidelines should address and correct this.

The argument over field strength is fading as improved software makes low- and midfield imaging quite acceptable. Managed care does not allow every center to have the most expensive equipment when less expensive technology is adequate. The addition of surface coil imaging increases the signal-to-noise ratio by threefold to fivefold, and this one advance has conferred to spine MRI its current effectiveness. Fast scanning and phase-arrayed coils allow quick and excellent visualization of the entire

spine, even in difficult patients. In some cases, tumor patients are being diagnosed and treated with radiation, without a costly hospital stay and all the attendant risks of intrathecal dye and excessive radiation.

MRI is superior to myelography and CT because of the following:

1. The ability to scan in the sagittal plane directly without reformatting
2. High sensitivity to pathologic lesions
3. Excellent tissue contrast, which allows separation of CSF, spinal cord, bone, discs, and other soft tissues
4. The potential for tissue characterization (e.g., blood, fat)
5. Significant additional information with the use of gadolinium

NERVOUS SYSTEM TRAUMA—HEAD INJURY

Before the advent of MRI, neuroradiologic evaluation sometimes failed to demonstrate pathologic processes in head trauma because conventional imaging techniques—based on interfaces and differences in tissue densities—could not provide adequate resolution and definition, particularly in small subdural hematomas and cerebral contusions. MRI has demonstrated the focal cortical lesions that provide the substrate for acute post-traumatic psychosis. The lack of association between these symptoms and the presumed subfrontal and temporal contusions is a known limitation of CT scanning.

CT and MRI both can detect hemorrhagic lesions. CT is best for acute hemorrhages; MRI is more sensitive in subacute or chronic hemorrhages, or nonhemorrhagic lesions such as cortical contusions and diffuse axonal injury. The latter two constitute 91.9% of all traumatic intra-axial lesions. MRI is also more sensitive in detecting brain stem injuries because of the lack of artifact in the posterior fossa that so often obscures the CT scan. As in other diseases, bony abnormalities, such as fractures, are better seen on CT. The advantage of CT in the rapid assessment of unstable patients who may need surgery is widely accepted.

SPINAL TRAUMA

Each year there are about 10,000 new cases of traumatic spinal cord injury. Plain films, tomography, CT, and myelography provide only indirect evidence of spinal cord injury (such as fractures with bony fragments), overall cord size and configuration, and patency of the subarachnoid space. MRI can directly image hemorrhage, edema, syrinx, and all other sequelae of spinal cord trauma. This information, along with observations from the neurologic examination, determines the initial management (medical or surgical) that will determine the ultimate outcome. The presence of cord edema and swelling correlates well with more severe deficits. As the severity of the deficit increases, the underlying cord contusion is likely to be larger and rendered more easily visible by MRI.

BIBLIOGRAPHY

Caplan LR. *Stroke: a clinical approach,* second ed. Boston: Butterworth–Heineman, 1993.

Chawluk JB, Alavi A, Jamieson DG, et al. Changes in local cerebral glucose metabolism with normal aging: the effects of cardiovascular and systemic health factors. *J Cerebr Blood Flow Metab* 1987;7(Suppl 1):S411.

Edelman RR, Warach S. Magnetic resonance imaging (2). *N Engl J Med* 1993;328:708–716.

Fisher M, Sotak CH, Minematsu K, et al. New magnetic resonance techniques for evaluating cerebrovascular disease. *Ann Neurol* 1992;32: 115–122.

Greenberg JO. *Neuroimaging.* New York: McGraw-Hill, 1995.

Oldendorf WH. *The quest for an image of brain.* New York: Raven Press, 1980.

Kelley's Textbook of Internal Medicine, fourth edition. Edited by H. David Humes. Lippincott Williams & Wilkins, Philadelphia © 2000.

C H A P T E R
453

SEROLOGIC AND MOLECULAR GENETIC DIAGNOSES

RUSSEL MARGOLIS
CHRISTOPHER ROSS

The molecular genetic revolution is transforming our understanding of the classification and the pathogenesis of neurologic disorder's. Disorders such as Alzheimer's disease (AD) and Parkinson's disease (PD), which were once thought to be almost entirely sporadic and hence nongenetic, are now known to have subtypes caused by distinct and readily detectable genetic mutations. Specific genetic diagnoses are now possible in a majority of familial spinocerebellar ataxias, ending a century of nosologic confusion. In concert with these advances in diagnosis, molecular genetics has provided numerous clues about the pathogenesis of various neurologic disorders. For instance, at least eight neurodegenerative diseases are caused by a mutation in which the number of CAG repeats in a gene becomes excessive. This repeat expansion is translated into a protein containing an excessively long stretch of consecutive glutamine residues, resulting in abnormal aggregates of the protein accumulating in the neurons of affected individuals. Other neurodegenerative diseases result from abnormalities in a group of proteins, including the amyloid precursor protein alpha synuclein and the microtubule-associated protein tau, which have provided a focus for studies of neuronal injury and death. The puzzling episodic nature of several disorders has become clarified by the discovery of causative mutations in genes encoding ion channels. Here we emphasize the unique issues that arise in genetic testing for neurologic disorders and some of the more widely available genetic tests for specific disorders. We also describe in brief the few serologic tests (excluding those for infectious agents) that may be of clinical value.

Despite the remarkable advances of the last decade, genetic tests provide a definitive diagnosis for a minority of patients with neurologic conditions. For the more common diseases, particularly AD and PD, the known genes account for a very small percentage of the total cases. In addition, genetic testing is expensive and can be misleading if used indiscriminately. Therefore, the major issue is determining the proper indications for obtaining a given genetic test. As a general rule, genetic testing tends to be most useful for patients with a known family history of a similar disorder or for patients with an usually early onset of a normally late-onset disease. On occasion, genetic testing may be helpful in a seemingly sporadic case of common disorder, particularly when the family history is not known or the presentation of the disease is unusual. As genetic variants that constitute risk factors for the late-onset disorders are uncovered, the indications for obtaining genetic tests will likely broaden.

A distinguishing feature of genetic testing is that the results have implications not just for the patient but for other family members as well. The determination that one family member has a genetic disease, particularly if it is a rare disease, implies that other family members with similar signs and symptoms also have that disease. This "diagnosis by proxy" is almost unavoidable, and the information may be viewed by symptomatic but untested family members in many ways. Some family members may regard knowing the "family diagnosis" with great relief; other may be indifferent; and for others, the news may be taken as a devastating invasion of their personal autonomy. Genetic counseling prior to genetic testing is essential in helping members of a family to resolve these issues.

The issues become more complex when a member of a family requests a presymptomatic genetic test (a test performed before the patient has developed any manifestations of the disease). The problem has been termed the "Tiresias complex" by Nancy Wexler in regard to HD (in which it has been most studied) in recognition of the sophoclean aphorism that "it is but sorrow to be wise when wisdom profits not." The primary concern was that learning that one was destined to develop a progressive and fatal disease would lead to severe psychological reactions. In fact, worldwide experience with presymptomatic testing for HD has demonstrated that, with appropriate counseling, most individuals cope remarkably well. The incidence of serious adverse psychological reactions in these individuals has not been substantially different than would be expected had the same individuals not had the testing. More problematic concerns relate to possible discrimination in such matters as employment and insurance. Because of the complexities of consent and the uncertain implications for the future, it is not advisable to offer presymptomatic genetic testing to minors. At present, relatively few at-risk individuals are requesting presymptomatic testing for genetic disorders, such as HD, in which only symptomatic treatment is currently available. As treatments emerge that slow or even stop the fundamental disease process, the criteria for who should receive presymptomatic genetic testing and when they should receive it may change radically. In any case, referral to a genetic counselor or genetic specialist is essential prior to obtaining presymptomatic genetic tests.

Most genetic diagnosis involves methods such as the polymerase chain reaction, DNA sequencing, restriction digest, gel electrophoresis, and Southern blotting. New technologies, such as mass spectroscopy, for obtaining results faster, more accurately, and with less expense are on the horizon. While the technology for genetic diagnosis has become increasingly sophisticated and routine, test interpretation remains complex. For instance, in the triplet-repeat expansion disorders, such as HD and most of the SCAs, there are several different interpretations of test results depending on the length of the repeat (see below). In other situations, test results can only be interpreted in the context of results from other family members. Another issue involves the number of mutations that can cause a particular disease. For some diseases, such as HD, essentially all cases are caused by a single mutation. However, other disorders, such as early-onset AD, may arise from any of a number of different mutations, each requiring a separate genetic test. Furthermore, the interpretation of negative test results is complicated by the likelihood that other mutations causing a given phenotype will be discovered in the future.

For AD, genetic testing is indicated for patients with a family history suggestive of autosomal dominant transmission and early age of disease onset. About half of these cases will be caused by mutations in the *presenilin-1* gene. Rare families have mutations in the *presenilin-2* gene or the *amyloid precursor protein (APP)* gene. However, the great majority of AD patients have late-onset disease, usually without a family history of AD. Three different versions (alleles) of the *apolipoprotein E (ApoE)* gene have been discovered, termed 2, 3, and 4. The ApoE4 allele is a risk factor for AD and appears to predispose to an earlier onset. Individuals homozygotic for ApoE4 (both the maternally and the paternally inherited copies of ApoE are of the ApoE4 allele) have a significantly increased risk for developing AD. However, because the ApoE4 allele is neither necessary nor sufficient for the development of AD and because testing for ApoE only marginally increases the sensitivity and specificity of an AD diagnosis, genetic testing for ApoE is not currently recommended. Mutations causing some cases of frontotemporal dementia, another relatively common cause of late-life cognitive impairment, have been identified in the *tau* gene on chromosome 17.

PD is rather like AD in that most cases appear sporadic, but a few families exist with clear mendelian inheritance. Mutations in alpha synuclein are responsible for disease in a small number of families of Mediterranean origin. All of these have early-onset PD with typical neurologic and neuropathologic features. An early-onset recessive form of PD has also been described caused by mutations in a gene termed *parkin*. The clinical presentation tends to be atypical, and the pathology is remarkable for the loss of neurons in the substantia nigra without Lewy bodies. It is likely that in the future genetic risk factors for more typical cases of PD will be found.

HD illustrates the complexities of interpreting tests for triplet-repeat expansion. In most cases, the result will be relatively clear. Individuals with 27 or fewer CAG triplets in the *huntingtin* gene will not develop HD, whereas individuals with 41 or more CAG triplets will develop the disease. In the affected range, longer repeat lengths tend to lead to an earlier age of disease onset. However, individuals with 36 to 40 CAG triplets may or may not develop the disease, a phenomenon referred to as incomplete penetrance. Within this range, the longer the repeat, the greater the penetrance, such that only about half of the individuals with 36 triplets will develop HD before age 65 while

most, but not all, individuals with 40 triplets will develop the disease. In addition, individuals with between 28 and 35 triplets have never been known to develop HD, but repeats of this length are unstable, and in paternal transmission may expand to a length sufficient to cause disease in the subsequent generation.

Dentatorubral-pallidoluysian atrophy (DRPLA) is a disease that resembles HD but is extremely rare outside of Japan. Like HD, DRPLA is caused by a CAG repeat expansion, though in a different gene *(atrophin-1)*. The expansion mutation can be readily detected with a genetic test. The rarity of the disease in North America and Europe suggests that the test should only be obtained in families with an HD-like disorder after the HD mutation has been excluded.

The mutations that cause Wilson's disease, a disorder of copper metabolism manifested most prominently in the central nervous system and liver, can in principle be diagnosed by molecular genetic tests. However, there are many different mutations which can cause Wilson's disease, and therefore tests for ceruloplasmin levels and other metabolic indexes of copper metabolism are much more useful in initial efforts to establish the diagnosis.

The diagnosis of hereditary ataxia has been greatly improved by recent advances in molecular genetics. Friedreich's ataxia, a recessive disorder and the most common form of hereditary ataxia, results from the presence of long expansions of a GAA triplet repeat in both alleles of the in the *frataxin* gene, or, rarely, a GAA repeat expansion in one allele and a missense mutation on the other allele. Seemingly sporadic or autosomal dominant cases of ataxia not infrequently turn out to be cases of Friedreich's ataxia in which the recessive inheritance has been obscured.

The autosomal dominant ataxias are extremely difficult to separate on clinical grounds, and correct diagnosis is only possible with the assistance of genetic tests. There are now at least eight of these disorders for which a specific genetic test is available, and it is likely that genetic testing for other subtypes will emerge over the next few years. On occasion, it is possible to predict which mutation is present in a given family (spinocerebellar ataxia type 7, for instance, typically involves visual impairment), but the extent of overlap in the clinical presentations makes such diagnoses the exception rather than the rule. Compounding the difficulty, most of the known mutations (including all for which routine genetic testing is available) are triplet-repeat expansions, in which the clinical presentation of a given disease will vary by repeat length. SCA2 and SCA3 are the most common of these disorders, but disease prevalence varies with patient ethnic origin. As with HD, there are complexities in interpreting the results of genetic tests, since the length of the repeat associated with each disease has both normal and abnormal ranges, occasionally with intermediate zones. For SCA8, penetrance appears to be incomplete, for reasons that are not yet clear. From a genetic testing standpoint, it is a reasonable strategy to test for these diseases as a group. It is also reasonable to consider genetic testing of selected ataxia patients with no known family history of a dominant ataxia, since occasionally the family history is obscured by lack of information, early parental death, or false paternity. However, the differential of sporadic cerebellar ataxia is complex (see Chapter 435).

Episodic ataxia type 1 (EA1, intermitent ataxia with persis-

TABLE 453.1.	SELECTED NEUROLOGICAL DISORDERS FOR WHICH GENE TESTING IS CURRENTLY AVAILABLE

Disease	Gene	Mutation	Transmission	Incidence/Comments
Ceberebral Cortex				
Alzheimer's disease	APP	Missense	Dominant	Very rare/early onset
Alzheimer's disease	PS1	Mostly missense	Dominant	50% of early onset Alzheimer's
Alzheimer's disease	PS2	Missense	Dominant	Very rare/early onset
Alzheimer's disease	ApoE	Polymorphism	Dominant	Increases risk, routine testing not indicated
Frontal temporal dementia	Tau	Missense and splice site mutations	Dominant	Possible alleleic disorders, variable phenotype
Basal Ganglia				
Huntington's disease	Huntingtin	CAG repeat expansion	Dominant	New or short expansion may cause seemingly sporadic cases
DRPLA	Atrophin-1	CAG repeat expansion	Dominant	Rate outside of Japan/Huntington like phenotype anticipation
Wilson's disease	Wc1 (ATPase)	Missense, frameshift small deletion	Recessive	Metabolic tests better for initial diagnosis
Parkinson's disease	Alpha synuclein	Missense	Dominant	Rare/early onset
Parkinson's disease	Parkin	Deletions, missense, nonsense, frameshift	Recessive	Rare/no Lewy bodies
Brain Stem and Cerebellum				
Friedreich's ataxia	Frataxin	GAA repeat expansion missense	Recessive	Most common hereditary ataxia
Spinocerebellar ataxia (types 1, 2, 3, 6, 7, 8)	Ataxin 1, 2, 3, 7, CACNA1A, SCA8	CAG repeat exapansions (some untranslated)	Dominant	Account as a group for the majority of dominantly inherited ataxias
Motor System				
Amyotrophic lateral sclerosis	SOD1	Missense	Dominant	10% of familial cases
Spinal and bulbar muscular atrophy	Androgen receptor	CAG repeat expansion	X-linked	Rare/males only
Peripheral Neuropathies				
Charcot–Marie–Tooth disease type Ia	Peripheral myelin protein (PMP) 22	Duplication	Dominant	
Charcot–Marie–Tooth disease type Ib	Po protein	Mutation	Dominant	
Charcot–Marie–Tooth disease type Ix	Connexin-32	Mutation	X-linked	
Hereditary neuropathy with pressure palsies	PMP22	Deletion	Dominant	
Episodic Diseases				
Episodic ataxia type 1	KCNA1	Missense	Dominant	Acetazolamide-responsive
Episodic ataxia type 2/ hereditary familial migraine	CACNA1A	Missense	Dominant	Acetazolamide-responsive
Mitochondrial Disorders				
KSS/CPEO/Pearson syndrome	Variable	Rearrangements	Maternal	
MELAS	tRNA-leu	Missense	Maternal	
MERRF	tRNA-lys, tRNA-leu	Missense	Maternal	
LHON/dystonia	ND1, ND4, ND6, also others	Misense	Maternal	Predominantly in males
NARP/Leigh's syndrome	ATPase6	Misense	Maternal	Same phenotype also associated with mutations in nuclear genes

KSS, Kearns–Sayre syndrome; CPEO, chronic progressive external ophthalmoplegia; MELAS, mitochondrial myopathy, encephalopathy, lactic acidosis, and strokelike episodes; MERFF, myoclonic epilepsy and ragged red fibers; NARP, neurogenic muscle weakness, ataxia, and retinitis pigmentosa.

tent myokymia) and episodic ataxia type 2 (EA2, intermittent ataxia with persistent eye movement abnormalities) are caused by mutations in ion channels. Mutations in the potassium channel gene *KCNA1* result in EA1, while mutations in *CACNA1A*, a gene encoding a subunit of a calcium channel, result in EA2. Other mutations in *CACNA1A* cause familial hemiplegic migraine and SCA6.

In rare cases, sporadic ataxia may be the result of a paraneoplastic syndrome, in which an antibody against a tumor antigen cross-reacts with a neuronal antigen, triggering a destructive cytotoxic T-cell response. In addition to cerebellar damage, other paraneoplastic syndromes include encephalomyelitis, retinal degeneration, and dysfunction of the brain stem or limbic regions. The different antineuronal antibodies associated with paraneoplastic syndromes typically are associated with specific tumors. The presence of these antibodies therefore establishes a potentially treatable cause for the neurologic disease but may also help in the diagnosis and treatment of the underlying cancer. This is particularly important because the neurologic syndrome often presents before the cancer has been discovered or even suspected. Anti-Yo, found with gynecologic neoplasms, is associated with cerebellar degeneration, as is Anti-Ri, Anti-Tr, and Anti-Ma. The latter, as well as Anti-Hu (found with small-cell lung cancer and neuroblastomas) and Anti-Ta, can be associated with dysfunction of other brain regions.

Most cases of amyotrophic lateral sclerosis (ALS) are sporadic. However, about 10% have autosomal dominant transmission. About 10% of these cases are caused by a mutation in the *superoxide dismutase–1* gene *(SOD1)*. Another rare motor neuron disease, spinal and bulbar muscular atrophy, is caused by CAG repeat expansions in the *androgen receptor* gene. Since this gene is located on the X chromosome, only males are affected, and the mode of inheritance is X-linked. A mutation in the gene *DYT1* has recently been shown to cause a form of familial dystonia.

The most well-known mitochondrial diseases are maternally inherited, a consequence of the maternal transmission of mitochodrial DNA. From the standpoint of genetic testing, it is important to recognize that the syndromes caused by mutations in mitochondrial DNA tend to overlap, with clinical features reflecting both the specific mutation and the percentage of mitochondrial DNAs that contain the mutation. Neurologic manifestations may include muscle weakness, ataxia, optic atrophy, seizures, dystonia, neurogenic hearing impairments, strokelike episodes, and mental retardation. Routine genetic testing is now commercially available for six of the mitochondrial syndromes (Table 453.1).

BIBLIOGRAPHY

Durr A, Cossee M, Agid Y, et al. Clinical and genetic abnormalities in patients with Friedreich's ataxia. *N Engl J Med* 1996;335:1169–1175.

Gusella JF, Persichetti F, MacDonald ME. The genetic defect causing Huntington's disease: repeated in other contexts? *Mol Med* 1997;33:238–246.

Hardy J, Gwinn-Hardy K. Genetic classification of primary neurodegenerative disease. *Science* 1998;282:1045–1078.

Jen J, Ptacek LJ. Channelopathies. In: Scriver CR, Beaudet AL, Sly WS, et al., eds. *Metabolic and molecular bases of inherited disease*, eighth ed. New York: McGraw-Hill, 1999 *(in press)*.

Margolis RL, McInnis MG, Rosenblatt A, et al. Trinucleotide repeat expansion and neuropsychiatric disease. *Arch Gen Psychiatry* 1999 *(in press)*.

Martin JB. *Mol Basis Neurodeg Dis* 1999;340:1970–1980.

Nussbaum RL, Polymeropoulos MH. Genetics of Parkinson's disease. *Hum Mol Genet* 1997;6(10):1687–1691.

Ross CA. Intranuclear neuronal inclusions: a common pathogenic mechanism for glutamine-repeat neurodegenerative diseases? *Neuron* 1997;19:1147–1150.

Ross CA, Margolis RL, Rosenblatt A, et al. Huntington disease and the related disorder, dentatorubral-pallidoluysian atrophy (DRPLA). *Medicine* 1997;76(5):305–338.

Wallace DC. Mitochondrial diseases in man and mouse. *Science* 1999;283:1482–1488.

Wexler NS. The Tiresias complex: Huntington's disease as a paradigm of testing for late-onset disorders. *FASEB J* 1992;6:2820–2825.

11

GERIATRICS

William R. Hazzard, Editor

APPROACH TO ASSESSMENT AND MANAGEMENT OF THE ELDERLY PATIENT WITH A MAJOR GERIATRIC PROBLEM COMPLEX

DIAGNOSIS AND MANAGEMENT OF THE ELDERLY PATIENT

MICHELE F. BELLANTONI

Perhaps more than any other discipline in medicine, geriatric medicine (the diagnosis and management of diseases of elderly patients) combines the best aspects of the art and science of medicine. Elderly persons typically have several chronic diseases, have lost sensory function, and have lost considerable homeostatic reserve in a number of organ systems. The result of this constellation of events is a clinical conundrum in a patient whose evaluation is difficult and time consuming and who is very susceptible to environmental or iatrogenic perturbations. The physician, therefore, must have a comprehensive understanding of a vast array of disease processes, diagnostic avenues, and therapeutic possibilities and balance these with great care in developing an optimal and dynamic care plan for each older patient. Indeed, a physician caring for an older patient must be highly selective in applying the ever expanding diagnostic and therapeutic options available in current medical practice. Only by such careful and thoughtful selection can the physician avoid contributing to the initiation and promulgation of a cascade of adverse events. For all of these reasons, the diagnosis and management of disease in older patients is an enormous intellectual challenge, requiring integration of complicated multisystem care with a clear personal knowledge of the patient and his or her family, living situation, and support network. This challenge makes caring for the elderly most rewarding and satisfying on an emotional

basis. Embodied in these concepts are several principles of geriatric medicine that are fundamental in the diagnosis and management of elderly patients, and it is the purpose of this chapter to delineate these.

PRESENCE OF MULTIPLE HEALTH PROBLEMS AND DISABILITIES

An ideal goal for health care in the United States can be stated very simply: for an individual to live an active and healthy life until death occurs at the upper limit of his or her potential life span. While life expectancy increased dramatically in the United States and other developed countries during the twentieth century, improvement in health and vitality has not shown equivalent advances. In fact, national surveys now indicate that most elders develop chronic diseases and typically experience several years of physical dependency before death. These dependencies are in part related to a clustering of chronic health problems, specifically affecting the eyes, ears, nervous system, heart, blood vessels, and joints. Fried and colleagues have proposed a modal pathway of physical frailty that begins with physical impairments, such as the onset of a chronic health problem (e.g., angina pectoris from progressive atherosclerosis) or age-related change in physiologic function (e.g., decrease in oxygen consumption with exercise) (Fig. 454.1). The impairment presents with clinical signs and symptoms (e.g. shortness of breath with exertion) that may at first result in a minimal loss of function, called *preclinical disability*. As the disease progresses or additional physical impairments develop, one becomes unable to perform a physical task such as climbing stairs, termed *disability*. Multisystem disease often associated with disabilities complicates to a great extent the approach to diagnosis and management of disease in older patients. Symptoms of one problem may be accentuated or blunted by the presence of chronic diseases and disabilities, and diagnostic and therapeutic interventions often are limited

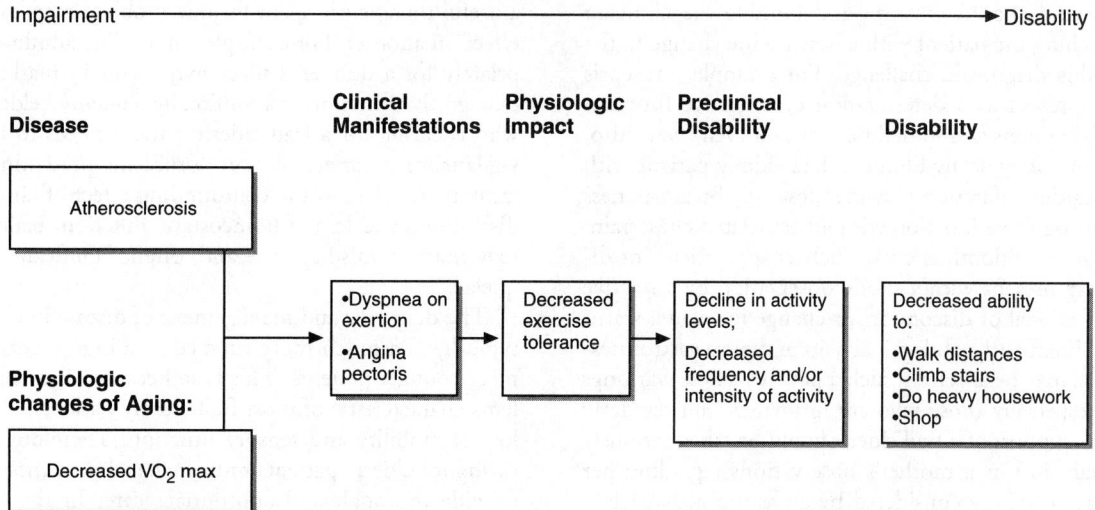

FIGURE 454.1. Model pathway of physical frailty. (From Fried LP, Kronmal RA, Newman AB, et al. Risk factors for 5-year mortality in older adults. The Cardiovascular Health Study. *JAMA* 1998;279:585–592, with permission.)

because of comorbidities. In addition, certain chronic conditions, particularly gait/balance disorders and depression, are associated with significant decline in functional status in community-dwelling older persons.

LOSS OF HOMEOSTATIC FUNCTION

Many physiologic functions deteriorate with aging alone. These physiologic losses result in the increased susceptibility of older individuals to perturbations created by disease, diagnostic undertakings, therapeutic interventions, or environmental stresses. Several examples illustrate this point. The decreases of body water and lean body mass that occur with normal aging result in a diminished volume of distribution of certain drugs, such as phenytoin, resulting in the greater likelihood of toxicity should that agent be prescribed. Drugs cleared by the liver or kidney, such as aminophylline or cimetidine, respectively, may result in higher blood levels should a standard dose be prescribed. Impaired thermoregulatory processes result in a greater risk of cold or heat injury. Impaired glucose metabolism with aging may result in hyperglycemia occurring in the setting of acute infection. These age-related homeostatic losses in organ function are an important cause of iatrogenic problems among the elderly, which are common. Also, because of these homeostatic losses, disease processes may present in complicated or atypical patterns. For example, even moderate salt and water losses such as might occur in higher environmental temperatures or as a result of acute diarrhea in the elderly often result in renal failure, delirium, stroke, or cardiac or gastrointestinal ischemia in an older person unable to withstand the perturbation because of impaired homeostasis in several organs. This results in a blurring of diagnostic pictures and requires that the physician be especially vigilant,

broad thinking, and quick to recognize or anticipate impending catastrophes that could result from mild perturbation.

AGE-RELATED DISEASE: GENETIC AND ENVIRONMENTAL FACTORS

Many of the common diseases associated with aging, such as diabetes mellitus, certain cancers, and osteoarthritis have both genetic and environmental factors that contribute to their development. The genetic influences are thought to be polygenic, in contrast to the inherited diseases that manifest in childhood and young adulthood that result from single-gene defects, such as sickle cell anemia. For example, mutations in several genes coding for β-adrenergic receptors and proteins that regulate glucose metabolism are linked to the development of obesity and type II diabetes mellitus. Similarly, the environmental factors that contribute to the diseases of aging are also multifactorial and include both under- and overnutrition, sedentary lifestyle, tobacco use or exposure, alcohol consumption, radiation from the sun, or environmental pollution. Given the contributions of unhealthy behaviors to the development of the diseases of aging, the successful clinician's treatment plan must address the contributing behaviors and environmental factors.

ATYPICAL DISEASE

In the elderly, especially those who are frail, the loss of homeostatic function in the presence of multiple chronic diseases and disabilities modifies the presentation of an illness, which may appear quite atypically from that same illness in a younger individual. This complicates the approach to the diagnosis of disease in the elderly and should sensitize and humble the clinician who is approaching the patient with a nonspecific change to the subtleties of this diagnostic challenge. For example, urosepsis may typically present as a deterioration of cognitive function without localizing signs and sometimes without even fever. Also, the pain response is typically blunted. The elderly patient with an acute myocardial infarction may manifest only breathlessness or a change in cognitive function without associated chest pain. Similarly, an acute abdominal crisis, such as appendicitis or diverticulitis, may present with a subtle observation by a relative or health professional of discomfort or change in mental status of the patient. Frequently, abdominal pain or typical gastrointestinal symptoms may be absent in such a patient. These warnings by observers, especially those who are intimately and regularly involved in the support of a frail elder, should be taken seriously by the clinician, just as a mother's observations regarding her child are always carefully considered by an astute pediatrician. A careful examination whenever there has been an indication of a change in status should focus on problems that are common and often "atypical" in presentation in the elderly, such as urinary tract infection, pneumonia, abdominal crisis, or drug toxicity.

Even when the clinician finds no clear diagnosis to account for a patient's symptoms, careful ongoing surveillance is mandatory. Serial observation is indeed the clinicians most valuable diagnostic tool. Waiting, watching, and worrying is a valuable diagnostic approach used by experienced geriatricians when an older person presents in a non-diagnostic manner. Often it is the frail homebound elder or nursing home patient who provides the most treacherous of diagnostic situations. Frequent telephone contact is especially important for such individuals. Information obtained in such subsequent contacts over time often provide the clue to the emerging problem or assurance that there is no serious underlying disorder. It is important for a physician to initiate such follow-up contacts. Most often patients or their caretakers after seeing a physician will assume that any serious illness has been ruled out and try not to be a burden by telephoning repeatedly. Further, the physician initiating the phone call demonstrates a great interest in the patient that leads to a better level of trust and communication between patient/caregiver and physician.

THE NARROW LIMIT OF THERAPEUTIC AND DIAGNOSTIC TOLERANCE

Part of the enormous challenge in providing health care to elders is the narrowing of diagnostic and therapeutic tolerance resulting from losses of homeostatic function and the presence of multiple diseases and disabilities. Quite simply, there is much less room for mistakes in judgment when caring for elderly patients than for younger individuals. In the elderly, a diagnostic test for one problem may adversely affect the overall function of a patient because of these losses. For example, dehydration and discomfort resulting from a bowel preparation initiated for colonoscopy may promptly result in reduced renal function, deterioration of mental function, and/or initiation of cardiac ischemia. Likewise

a useful therapeutic agent for one problem may have a negative effect on another. For example, cimetidine administered appropriately for a duodenal ulcer may result in marked worsening of cognitive function in a minimally demented elder. A clinician who is caring for a frail elderly patient needs to be constantly vigilant for a variety of acute problems presenting in atypical fashion and alert to the confounding effect of chronic diseases, disabilities, and loss of homeostatic function. Failure to do this may result in misdiagnoses and, often, significant iatrogenic sequelae.

The diagnosis and management of disease in elderly patients typically is a much more time-consuming process than that in most younger patients. This is so because of the multiple problems characteristic of most frail elderly patients, including their loss of mobility and sensory function. Therefore, the clinician caring for elderly patients must make adjustments in practice to provide thorough and appropriate care. In the current reimbursement climate, this requires relative financial sacrifices because the payment by Medicare for the service provided is often comparatively low, given the relatively great amount of professional time required. Nevertheless, nonfinancial rewards may be greater in providing comprehensive, coordinated, compassionate care to the elderly, who are typically highly grateful. That to many physicians more than compensates for time expended. Finally, especially in geriatric medicine, physician extenders, such as physician's assistants, nurse practitioners, and nurse clinicians, effectively leverage the physician's effort to provide appropriate care to medically complex elders and allow increased time to provide patient and family education and counsel.

THE CONCEPT OF SMALL THERAPEUTIC GAINS

Because of the presence of chronic disease states and disabilities in elderly patients, cure is often not the goal; rather, the preservation or restoration of function is the aim. The physician who does not appreciate this fact will be frustrated by the establishment of unrealistic therapeutic goals. For a patient with a new and disabling problem, even the slightest improvement may be significant. For example, a patient who has had a stroke can improve his or her functional ability significantly if he or she can learn to transfer from a bed to a chair or from a chair to a toilet. Similarly, regaining the ability to self-feed or use a telephone permits the disabled person to function much more independently in a wider variety of environments, including the home. A patient impaired from propelling a wheel chair because of a minor episode of bursitis may become totally dependent from what otherwise might be considered a trivial problem. Also, an individual who is incapacitated socially because of urinary incontinence can achieve a very acceptable level of socialization by even partial control of the incontinent episodes. Similarly, the primary caregiver who is attentive to the adequate control of pain can improve the quality of life of elders with chronic disease or those who are facing the end of life.

Therefore, the physician must work with the patient and other health providers and caregivers to establish and achieve reasonable goals and, indeed, small therapeutic gains often are appreciated far more by elderly than by younger patients. In elderly patients small gains may yield major increases in self-worth and independence as they decrease the patient's personal and environmental support care requirements.

PREVENTION AND SAFETY

Preventive health care practices in medicine may be applied even to the oldest of the old and the younger elderly who may be frail. This includes attention to such vaccinations as influenza and *Streptococcus pneumoniae,* which have been shown to reduce mortality in the elderly. Also, there are now data to support the prescription of physical exercise to improve function, reverse age-related conditions such as diabetes and cardiovascular disease, and reduce pain in osteoarthritis even in the very old. Therefore, in the management of frail patients much can be done to diminish the risks of catastrophe, disease burden, and disability through timely and effective preventive strategies.

Preventive medicine for the elderly includes assessment of an individual's safety in the current living arrangement. Important safety risks are usually self-evident during a home assessment but are often difficult to elicit from a patient or caregiver during an office or hospital visit. Poor lighting, loose throw rugs, absence of handrails, and stairs in poor repair are typical examples of environmental factors that increase the risk of falling and injury. Solutions to some of these problems are simple, such as removing the throw rugs or using brighter light bulbs and night lights. The solution to others, such as installing handrails, may require a contractor. The physician or professionals working with the physician should be aware of the increasing number of home-repair services specifically focused on the health care needs of the elderly. A telephone call to the area agency on aging will help the physician identify such local resources. In the absence of such a service and where an elderly patient has no local family, the physician may want to provide the name of several reliable contractors.

An excellent communication system is vital for the security and safety of a fragile elder living at home. A workable, easily accessible telephone system, usually with extensions in several rooms, is advisable. There should be good lighting in the area of the telephone so that the patient can use the telephone effectively at night. Ideally the patient should have an automated instrument that will dial specified numbers with the press of a single button. Increasingly available in many communities are automated communication systems whereby a patient can contact a central monitoring service, which can respond by phone or send help if necessary. Such systems are offered by many hospitals, as well as government and community agencies that deal with the elderly.

Frequent visitors to an isolated elderly person are also important resources in the stabilization of and communication with a patient in his or her own home. Thus, the creation of an observer network should be part of the physician's plan to manage the homebound elderly patient. For the patient who requires skilled nursing care, a home health care agency may provide regular surveillance. Governmental programs may also be a resource for persons who qualify for state medical assistance. Many

TABLE 454.1.	COMMUNITY RESOURCES FOR THE ELDERLY

Government
  Area agency on aging
    Resource for community-specific public and private programs
    Legal guardianship services
    Senior transportation programs
  Senior citizen centers
    Meals
    Leisure activities, exercise, education
    Socialization
  Health department
    Geriatric medical evaluation
    Government-sponsored home-skilled services
  Adult protective services
    Agency that responds to allegations of elder abuse or neglect
  Community services
    Local government–based programs that serve all ages
Private nonprofit community organizations
  Meals on wheels
    Home-delivered meals
  Medical foundations
    Disease-specific assistance—education, philanthropic funds (e.g, American Cancer Society, Alzheimer's Association, American Diabetes Association)
  Senior Citizen Organizations
    Advocacy, educational programs, relief programs
    American Association of Retired Persons
    Gray Panthers
  Church Organizations
    Senior clubs
    Volunteer-based assistance for transportation and home visits
Home health agencies
  Skilled nursing services
  Personal care
  Rehabilitation services
Durable medical equipment suppliers
  Adaptive equipment—raised commode seats, tub benches, etc.
Private sector
  Telephone company—communication systems
  Home repair companies—installation of handrails, ramps

communities have a wide variety of well-developed resources that are available to help the elderly and their caregivers (Table 454.1). Examples are home-delivered meals, home repair and maintenance services, and domestic assistants supplied by agencies of the city, county, and state government as well as by many private voluntary and church organizations. The combination of resources available in each community is specific to that locale. The physician needs to be aware of these local resources; such knowledge can be gained by contacting the city, county, or state health department; a regional office on aging; or the department of social work at a local hospital. In addition, willing neighbors and friends may be crucial to provide support for the patient at home. Identification of these individuals by the physician is important when no local family is available or willing to provide surveillance.

ADVANCE DIRECTIVES (SEE CHAPTER 473)

The physician caring for elderly patients should make a special effort to determine an individual's wishes should a crisis ever develop. While this principle applies to all adult patients, it is a more immediate and more universal concern among the elderly than among those who are younger. To avoid a precipitous, stressful, and inappropriate decision-making process, it is best to initiate discussions regarding cardiopulmonary resuscitation, prolonged artificial feeding, mechanical ventilation, or, in certain circumstances (e.g., a patient in a nursing home), indications for the appropriateness of hospitalization at a time when the patient and his or her family are able to consider the issues thoughtfully and thoroughly and are able to consult relatives and other counselors when making a decision. Most states have developed laws concerning durable power of attorney for health care or living wills. All patients should be encouraged to develop advance directives consistent with state laws. Of the several advance directives currently available, the naming of a health care agent is generally preferred. The advantages of appointing a health care agent are that (a) such a mechanism is universally applicable and (b) if there is a reliable agent who knows a patient's wishes well, the decisions of that patient in any situation are more likely to be followed. The living will, an advance directive that is often perceived as most important, is valid in most states only in restricted situations such as the presence of a terminal disease, persisting vegetative state, or end-stage medical condition from which there is no expectation of recovery. For example, the situation of a moderately demented patient usually would not meet the criteria for a living will to be applied.

Studies have shown that elderly individuals are not upset when their physicians initiate conversations about advance directives; in fact, they appreciate the opportunity to review these important concerns. Properly executed and honored advance directives may avoid therapy that is inconsistent with a patient's wishes. For the many patients who fear prolonged suffering and disability more than they fear death, care can be properly focused and maximum comfort and dignity provided. Important as is it to help a patient develop advance directives, it is of equal importance to ensure that developed advance directives are widely noted and prominently displayed in a patient's record, so that all involved health care providers can be aware of them and honor them strictly.

CONTINUUM OF HEALTH CARE FOR THE ELDERLY

The physician who cares for the elderly patient is called on to render care in a variety of settings, including the traditional medical office, the patient's home, a senior citizens complex, the hospital, and the nursing home. The most effective medical care of the elderly is provided in the least restrictive environment. A significant number of noninstitutionalized elderly persons are homebound and cannot be transported to a medical office without a specially equipped bus or van, or an ambulance. In spite of this, only a very small number of patient–physician encounters occur in the home. Yet a house call allows first-hand evaluation of the patient's environmental circumstances and interactions with family and other caregivers. The physician can better assess the patient's physical function and need for home services, such as physical therapy and durable medical equipment, which require a physician's order. House calls result in a rapport between physician, patient, and family that can be immensely gratifying.

Whenever possible, an elderly person recovers from an acute illness most comfortably at home, as hospitals are necessary but dangerous environments for elderly patients. This is especially so for elderly patients who are critically ill. Such patients commonly sustain nosocomial complications, which initiate an accelerated cascade of events resulting in death or permanent loss of function, and often long-term institutionalization. The attending physician plays a critical role in minimizing the chance of such a scenario taking place. The attending physician is the "captain" of the health care "team" or the "conductor" of the health care "orchestra," to use two common metaphors. This role is of paramount importance and requires a broad knowledge base, an enormous amount of tact, and a major commitment of time. Figure 454.2 depicts a typical scenario of a seriously ill elderly patient hospitalized for an acute illness. To prevent or minimize the chances of such a sequence requires sustained vigilance and coordination with nurses, therapists, consultants, and all other hospital personnel to preserve a patient's function, to prevent iatrogenic injury, and to provide maximum comfort and human dignity.

Key aims for the physician in providing hospital care to the elderly are to minimize the potential for drug toxicity, ensure mobilization as early as possible, minimize the incidence of pressure sores, and look for infectious complications such as diarrhea, especially that of *Clostridium difficile* infection. A physician must work with nursing personnel to avoid the use of physical restraints, to search for signs of undernutrition, and, where appropriate, to treat it aggressively. Throughout the hospitalization period the physician will need to maintain a dialogue with the patient and the patient's family to minimize misunderstanding or misperceptions. This communication on the part of the attending physician is especially critical because there are many people who will be communicating with the patient and his or her family. Misconceptions and misconstrued plans often lead to severe emotional strife and even destructive adversarial relationships between the patient and his or her family, and health care workers. An important bond of confidence between the attending physician and the patient and family is critical and will result if communication remains open, thorough, and frequent.

In an effort to reduce the financial costs of hospitalization, subacute inpatient care has become part of modern medicine. The acute hospital stay includes an initial period of diagnostic studies and implementation of a treatment plan. However, once an acute illness has been stabilized and a treatment plan established, a patient may be transferred to a subacute care unit in which the inpatient treatment continues in a setting of less intensive nursing surveillance and without expensive equipment for hemodynamic monitoring. There is benefit as well as risk associ-

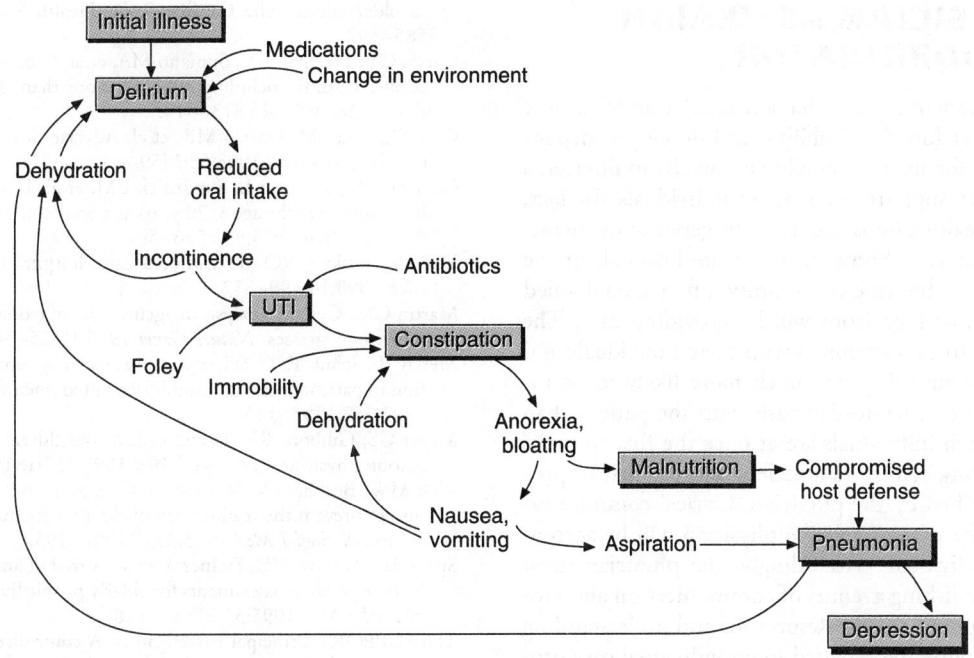

FIGURE 454.2. Typical scenario of a seriously ill elderly patient hospitalized for an acute illness.

ated with the transfer of an elderly patient to a subacute unit. While there is often more attention to nutrition and ambulation in the subacute setting than in the acute hospital, the transfer requires the patient to adjust to the new surroundings and staff—a particular burden for an older person who has suffered delirium or other problems during the acute illness.

The physical deconditioning that occurs following acute hospitalization usually can be effectively managed in an inpatient setting that emphasizes rehabilitation and is staffed by a multidisciplinary team (see Chapter 472). Whether this takes place in a Commission on Accreditation and Rehabilitation Facilities (CARF)–accredited acute rehabilitation unit or a subacute care setting is likely to relate to the patient's level of tolerance for an aggressive rehabilitation program (defined as at least 3 hours of rehabilitation therapy daily), required for CARF level rehabilitation. The physical therapist addresses mobilization and endurance, while the occupational therapist teaches adaptive approaches to personal care. Nurses implement scheduled toileting to correct hospital-acquired incontinence, a commonly seen new problem. The nutritionist assesses dietary preferences and nutritional needs to promote adequate oral intake, enhance wound healing, and improve constipation that occurs during the hospitalization as a result of medications and lack of physical activity. A psychologist assists the patient and family in coping with a new physical or mental disability. The physician's role is to coordinate the services provided by the rehabilitation team and to reassess the medical plan implemented in the hospital setting. For example, as an older man is recovering from a stroke and begins to stand and ambulate with the use of a walker, orthostatic hypotension may become evident, thus necessitating an adjustment in antihypertensive medications.

With increasing physical and cognitive decline, the ability of

a frail elder to live safely in his or her own home may be lost, particularly if there is a lack of family to provide 24-hour supervision. Alternatives to institutionalization include senior assisted-living apartments or assisted-living facilities where more functional seniors can receive minimal nursing services. Continuing care (life care) communities provide a range of services but are often not an option for seniors with ordinary incomes and assets. For elders who prefer to remain at home, in-home services can be purchased as needed, such as home maintenance, meal preparation, and personal care. Physicians must be aware that such services are not provided for the long term by Medicare or most other health insurance programs. While often these services must be purchased individually, there is growing interest in comprehensive, community-based " life care" services provided by a single vendor for a monthly fee. Medical day centers, under physician's order, may provide needed daytime supervision for seniors with dementia or physical disability while family caregivers are employed.

Nursing home placement often is the only option for seniors who are functionally dependent in basic activities of daily living and who lack a social support system to provide such care. There are state and federal regulations that govern the medical care provided to nursing home residents. The Omnibus Budget Reconciliation Act of 1987 set exacting operational standards for nursing homes that participate in the Medicare and Medicaid programs. These regulations, which became effective in 1995, require a safe environment with minimal use of physical and chemical restraints and that provides residents with physical comfort, adequate nutrition, timely medical care, and recreation. Often, family members seek advice from the physician before selecting a nursing home.

THE PHYSICIAN AS HEALTH CARE COORDINATOR

Because an elderly patient typically has a constellation of chronic health problems, lost functional ability, and developed dependencies, health care for such an individual must be multifaceted and usually requires support from many individuals. In fact, multidisciplinary health care is the norm in geriatric medicine. Whether the patient is at home, in the acute hospital, in the nursing home, or in a life care community, often several allied health professionals or laypersons will be providing care. The physician will need to be acquainted with these individuals and their capabilities because they are much more likely to be involved closely and on a day-to-day basis with the patient than is the physician. Such individuals are at once the first to make observations regarding change in a patient and the first to provide the care prescribed by the physician. Critical communication to and from the patient and the physician will be accomplished by such individuals. Accordingly, the physician must take the lead in establishing avenues of communication and rapport with these helping persons. Respect for and understanding of the various disciplines represented in an individual care program are critical for effective communication. This requires the physician to be familiar with the capabilities and contributions of nurses; physician's assistants; nurse practitioners; social workers; physical, occupational, and recreational therapists; home health aides; and case managers. While the coordinating role of physician in a multidisciplinary team is time consuming, it is absolutely crucial. Confounding the problem is that a health care network supporting an elder individual is often quite unconnected and may involve a variety of different organizations that are community-, government-, or hospital-based. In spite of such a maze, it remains the physician's responsibility to work with this diverse group as the physician is responsible for orchestrating, from among the available resources, the best possible care for the patient.

The coordinating role of the physician is never more critical or complex than it is in geriatric medicine. This is so because (a) older individuals have multiple health problems, (b) there is an ever increasing complexity in the health care system, (c) the scientific basis of medical practice is expanding continuously, and (d) there is a wide reliance on subspecialists in current practice patterns. Therefore, initiating and coordinating consultations to specialists and reviewing previous evaluations and records that are often widely scattered are important tasks that are both labor-intense and undercompensated. However, should this coordinating role for physicians not be performed well, the patient may suffer discomfort, disability, and the lack of appropriate resource utilization.

BIBLIOGRAPHY

Birn S, Levenson S. *The OBRA '87 enforcement rule: implications for attending physicians and medical directors.* Publication of the American Medical Directors Association, Columbia, Maryland, 1995.

Cho CY, Alessi CA, Cho M, et al. The association between chronic illness and functional change among participants in a comprehensive geriatric assessment program. *J Am Geriatr Soc* 1998;46:677–682.

Fried LP, Kronmal RA, Newman AB, et al. Risk factors for 5-year mortality in older adults. The Cardiovascular Health Study. *JAMA* 1998;279:585–592.

Garcia GV, Freeman RV, Supiano MA, et al. Glucose metabolism in older adults: a study including subjects more than 80 years of age. *J Am Geriatr Soc* 1997;45:813–817.

Gray SL, Sager M, Lestico MR, et al. Adverse drug events in hospitalized elderly. *J Gerontol* 1998;53:M59–63.

Guarlnik JM, Ferrucci L, Simonsick EM, et al. Lower-extremity function in persons over the age of 70 years as a predictor of subsequent disability. *N Engl J Med* 1995;332:556–561.

Hall WJ, Oskvig RO. Transitional care: hospital to home. *Clin Geriatr Med* 1998;14:799–812.

Martin GM. Genetic analysis of ageing: role of oxidative damage and environmental stresses. *Nature Genet* 1996;13:25–34.

Metlay JP, Schulz R, Li YH, et al. Influence of age on symptoms at presentation in patients with community-acquired pneumonia. *Arch Intern Med* 1997;157:1453–1459.

Meyer GS, Gibbons RV. House calls to the elderly—a vanishing practice among physicians. *N Engl J Med* 1997;337:1815–1820.

Rich MW, Beckham V, Wittenberg C, et al. A multidisciplinary intervention to prevent the readmission of elderly patients with congestive heart failure. *N Engl J Med* 1995;333:1190–1195.

Stuck AE, Aronow HU, Steiner A, et al. A trial of annual in-home comprehensive geriatric assessments for elderly people living in the community. *N Engl J Med* 1995;333:1184–1189.

The SUPPORT Principal Investigators. A controlled trial to improve care for seriously ill hospitalized patients. *JAMA* 1995;274:1591–1598.

Tinetti ME, Williams CS. Falls, injuries due to falls, and the risk of admission to a nursing home. *N Engl J Med* 1997;337:1279–1284.

Kelley's Textbook of Internal Medicine, fourth edition. Edited by H. David Humes. Lippincott Williams & Wilkins, Philadelphia © 2000.

CHAPTER

455

APPROACH TO THE ELDERLY PATIENT WITH HYPERTENSION

WILLIAM B. APPLEGATE

PRESENTATION

Unless previously diagnosed, high blood pressure is usually detected in an asymptomatic older person at a routine office visit or through various programs that offer blood pressure screening examination to older people. However, in about 10% of older people, high blood pressure is first diagnosed when the older person presents with a clinical event that was probably triggered by longstanding high blood pressure, such as stroke, congestive heart failure, or myocardial infarction. On the other hand, at times older patients complain of dizziness or headaches that they believe might be associated with elevations of blood pressure; however, studies have consistently shown that, unless the blood pressure is either extremely high or extremely low, symptoms are usually absent unless the patient presents with a cardiovascular clinical event. However, as blood pressure increases with age, the baroreceptor reflex is diminished, and patients may also present with either postural hypotension or postprandial hypotension.

Elevation of either systolic blood pressure (SBP) or diastolic blood pressure (DBP) is a prevalent problem with major health implications in older patients. In all industrialized countries, average SBP rises throughout the life span, whereas average DBP rises until age 55 to 60 years and then levels off or even declines. Therefore, most of the increase in prevalence of high blood pressure in older persons results from an increase in isolated systolic hypertension (SBP higher than 140 mm Hg, DBP lower than 90 mm Hg).

Although the clinical treatment of hypertension has classically focused more on DBP levels, epidemiologic data indicate that for middle-aged and elderly adults, SBP is more predictive of future cardiovascular disease than DBP.

Estimates of the prevalence of hypertension [both systolic/diastolic hypertension (SDH) and isolated systolic hypertension (ISH)] in persons older than 65 years vary greatly, depending on the age and race of the group studied, the blood pressure cutoff point used for the definition of hypertension, and the number of measurements made. Because levels of DBP tend to stabilize at about 55 years of age, the prevalence of SDH tends to be constant at age 55 and older. Based on estimates from the Hypertension Detection and Follow-up Program, the prevalence of SDH in persons older than 65 years is about 15% in whites and 25% in blacks. In screening for the pilot study of the Systolic Hypertension in the Elderly Program (SHEP), ISH was found in about 10% of persons aged 70 years and 20% of persons older than 80 years (both black and white).

PATHOPHYSIOLOGIC FACTORS

The exact causal mechanisms for development of hypertension in the elderly, as compared with younger persons, remain to be fully determined. Because most cases of SDH occur by age 55 years, it is unlikely that the pathophysiology of SDH is much different in the elderly than it is in the middle-aged. Older persons with hypertension usually have lower renin levels and are more sensitive to sodium repletion or depletion than are younger hypertensive individuals. Structural changes in the large vessels may play a predominant role in the rise of SBP levels with age. Both a decrease in connective tissue elasticity and an increase in the prevalence of atherosclerosis result in an increase in peripheral vascular resistance and aortic impedance with age. There is a strong negative correlation between large-vessel compliance and systolic pressure in older patients. A decrease in aortic compliance results in greater resistance to systolic ejection and disproportionate elevations of SBP. However, the hemodynamic characteristics of ISH are different in patients younger than 40 years compared with patients older than 65 years. Younger patients with ISH usually demonstrate a hyperkinetic circulation manifested by a significantly increased heart rate, elevated left ventricular ejection rate and cardiac indexes, and normal vascular resistance. On the other hand, older patients with ISH tend to have a normal heart rate, significantly reduced cardiac and left

ventricular ejection rate indexes, and increased vascular resistance. Also, plasma volume is reduced in older patients with ISH.

Because renin levels usually are lower in older patients, it is unlikely that the renin–angiotensin system plays a major role in the pathogenesis of ISH. However, functional changes in vascular smooth muscle may have some impact on the increased peripheral resistance seen in elderly patients with ISH. Studies in animals indicate that α-adrenergic responsiveness of vascular smooth muscle is not greatly changed with age. However, β-adrenergic responsiveness of vascular smooth muscle declines with age, with a consequent decrease in the relaxation of vascular smooth muscle. Therefore, it has been postulated that the increase in peripheral resistance in elderly hypertensives with ISH may be caused in part by diminished β-adrenergic-mediated vasodilatation, whereas α-adrenergic-mediated vasoconstriction continues unabated.

HISTORY AND PHYSICAL EXAMINATION

Although most older individuals who present with high blood pressure are asymptomatic, it is important to question patients about potential symptoms related to acute rises in blood pressure as well as symptoms related to the vascular complications of high blood pressure (Table 455.1). For instance, questions regarding syncope, tachycardia, flushing, headaches, chest pain, nocturnal dyspnea, and numbness or localized paralysis of a part of the body are all appropriate. Of course, it is important to question the patient about previous times when blood pressure may have been measured and, if possible, it is important to document the

TABLE 455.1.	SYMPTOMS RELATED TO HIGH BLOOD PRESSURE

Symptoms Related to Pressure Rise
Headache (only with very high pressure)
Clouded sensorium
Syncope
Seizures
Tachycardia
Dyspnea

Symptoms Related to Chronic Effects of High Blood Pressure
Postprandial syncope
Postnatural syncope
Edema
Dyspnea

Symptoms/Conditions Related To Cardiovascular Morbidity
Low energy (low cardiac output)
Symptoms of multi-infarct dementia
Stroke
Myocardial infarction
Congestive heart failure
Renal failure

duration for which the blood pressure has been elevated. Often older persons who present with elevations of blood pressure report having been treated previously with antihypertensive agents. It is important to document the type of antihypertensive agent used, its effectiveness, and any reason for its discontinuation. Finally, older patients frequently take multiple prescription or over-the-counter medicines, some of which can cause an elevation of blood pressure. These include sympathomimetics, nonsteroidal anti-inflammatory drugs, alcohol, caffeine (acutely only), postmenopausal hormone replacement therapy (rarely), and corticosteroids (including heavy topical use).

The physical examination should focus on examining the patient for potential signs of organ damage from high blood pressure and for any potential underlying physical abnormalities that may contribute to the rise in blood pressure. Examination of the retina for signs of arteriolar damage and other funduscopic changes, the heart (particularly heart size), and the peripheral blood vessels is critical. Many older people with longstanding untreated high blood pressure present with a combination of high blood pressure–related funduscopic changes, a diffuse lateral cardiac point of maximum impulse, and diminished peripheral pulses. Auscultation of the major vessels for bruits is important to help assess the degree of atherosclerosis. Of particular importance are the carotid arteries and abdominal aorta. In addition, auscultation should be done over the kidneys because renal artery stenosis is the most common secondary cause of hypertension in older adults. Checking the patient for Osler's sign (a palpable radial or brachial artery after the blood pressure cuff has been inflated above peak SBP) is not advised because it has low sensitivity and specificity for pseudohypertension (discussed in more detail later).

Meticulous and accurate measurement of the blood pressure itself is the most critical component of the physical examination in an elderly person with high blood pressure. This is also the part of the physical examination that may be the most poorly performed in terms of reliability and accuracy. First, blood pressure should only be measured in an older person who is seated, with his or her back supported, and after 5 minutes of rest. The blood pressure cuff should be placed just above the elbow, and the arm should be resting so that the cuff is at the same level as the heart in the chest cavity. Blood pressure should never be taken over clothing, and use of an appropriate cuff size is critical. The width of the cuff should be about 40% of the circumference of the patient's arm. If the clinician is in doubt about the size of cuff to use, use of an oversized cuff introduces very little measurement error, whereas use of an undersized cuff can induce a great deal of measurement error. While the sphygmomanometer cuff is being inflated, the clinician should palpate the radial artery and continue to inflate the cuff until the pulse at the radius is obliterated (this avoids mismeasurement due to an auscultatory gap). A standard mercury sphygmomanometer is the instrument of choice, although aneroid sphygmomanometers are reasonably accurate if standardized every few months against a mercury sphygmomanometer. A common source of measurement error is overly rapid deflation of the cuff. The cuff should be deflated at the rate of 2 mm per second.

The diagnosis of high blood pressure should be based on the average of three measures taken over two or three visits. By doing this, the natural variation in blood pressure is somewhat diminished and a more reliable estimate of the true intra-arterial pressure can be obtained. Once the average of six to nine measures is obtained, the patient can be classified according to the potential severity of high blood pressure. The most recent classification system is shown in Table 455.2. It is important to note that ISH *is covered* by this classification system because the stage for a given patient is determined by the component of blood pressure (SBP or DBP) that is highest. Recent studies of the utility of ambulatory blood pressure monitoring (ABMP) indicate that persons who have stage 1 hypertension can be controlled with less medication or even no medication (e.g., erroneous diagnosis based on office blood pressure) if ABPM is used. Some studies indicate that 24 ABPM measures are more highly correlated with end-organ damage than office blood pressures. Most older people with stage 2 or higher hypertension after an

---

TABLE 455.2.	**RISK STRATIFICATION AND TREATMENT**[a]		
Blood Pressure Stages (mm Hg)	**Risk Group A (No Risk Factors; No TOD/CCD)**[b]	**Risk Group B (At Least One Risk Factor, Not Including Diabetes; No TOD/CCD)**	**Risk Group C (TOD/CCD and/or Diabetes, With or Without Other Risk Factors)**
High-normal (130–139/85–89)	Lifestyle modification	Lifestyle modification	Drug therapy[d]
Stage 1 (140–159/90–99)	Lifestyle modification (up to 12 mo)	Lifestyle modification[c] (up to 6 mo)	Drug therapy
Stages 2 and 3 (≥160/≥100)	Drug therapy	Drug therapy	Drug therapy

[a] Lifestyle modification should be adjunctive therapy for all patients recommended for pharmacologic therapy.
[b] TOD/CCD indictes target organ disease/clinical cardiovascular disease (see Table 4).
[c] For patients with multiple risk factors, clinicians should consider drugs as initial therapy plus lifestyle medifications.
[d] For those with heart failure, renal insufficiency, or diabetes.
For example, a patient with diabetes and a blood pressure of 142/94 mm Hg plus left ventricular hypertrophy should be classified as having stage 1 hypertension with target organ disease (left ventricular hypertrophy) and with another major risk factor (diabetes). This patient would be categorized as stage 1, risk group C, and recommended for immediate initiation of pharmacologic treatment.

average of six to nine office measurements have true high blood pressure. There may be some room for a routine use of ABPM in persons with stage 1 hypertension where diagnosis is in doubt because the blood pressure varies a great deal from visit to visit, or in special instances when circumstances may dictate the relevance of blood pressure to symptoms (e.g., postprandial syncope).

The other concern with regard to accuracy of office blood pressure measurements has to do with "white-coat hypertension." Actually, part of the problem of white-coat hypertension is related to poor measurement technique in the physician's office, including not allowing the patient to rest for 5 minutes before the measurement and not having the patient comfortably seated with the back supported. If the nature of the practice is such that it is too inefficient or cumbersome to follow carefully standard blood pressure measurement techniques, then ABPM probably can be a valuable adjunct to confirming a suspected diagnosis of high blood pressure in an older person.

Because the prevalence of postural hypotension increases as the blood pressure increases, older persons with elevations of blood pressure also should regularly have the blood pressure measured both supine and standing. As much as 10% to 15% of untreated elderly persons with high blood pressure have a decrease in standing SBP of 20 mm Hg or more.

LABORATORY STUDIES AND DIAGNOSTIC TESTS

Current national guidelines for laboratory tests include a urinalysis, complete blood count, fasting serum glucose, and cholesterol with high-density lipoprotein and triglyceride (for estimations of low-density lipoprotein), serum potassium, creatinine, uric acid, and a 12-lead electrocardiogram. Although older persons with high blood pressure have a higher prevalence of cardiac enlargement than younger people, routine echocardiographic screening is not recommended.

DIFFERENTIAL DIAGNOSIS

The diagnosis of high blood pressure is relatively straightforward except for the issues of measurement, misclassification, and stress responses. Measurement has been discussed earlier. There is one major type of misclassification, pseudohypertension, and one major type of stress response, white coat hypertension. Pseudohypertension is thought to occur in elderly people who have very rigid arteries. It is known that the rigidity of arteries on average goes up with age. The indirect sphygmomanometer can overestimate the true intraarterial pressure because increased pressure is required for the blood pressure cuff to compress a stiff artery. Unfortunately, studies of this phenomenon do not contain representative samples of older people, so it is difficult to assess the potential prevalence of this condition in the general population. In addition, the articles on this subject indicate that although there may be some increased estimate of blood pressure by indirect sphygmomanometry in older people, the actual magnitude of misclassification in most patients is not that high and

often does not alter whether an older person would be classified as having hypertension. Ancillary studies associated with SHEP indicate that the prevalence of pseudohypertension is low in an aging cohort. A diagnosis of pseudohypertension should be suspected in older persons who have relatively high blood pressures but have no evidence of end-organ damage, or in older persons who have symptoms of excessive low blood pressure on antihypertensive therapy even though their blood pressures appear to be in the normal range. In other words, pseudohypertension is really only diagnosed based on clinical presentation and is not a common phenomenon.

White-coat hypertension is thought to be a stress response whereby a person in a doctor's office, particularly when confronted with the doctor and/or the impending examination, has a stress response and an increase in blood pressure. Some researchers have indicated that the proportion of patients diagnosed as having high blood pressure in an office practice who actually have normal blood pressure but are classified as hypertensive because they have white-coat hypertension may be as high as 20% to 25%. However, studies of this phenomenon give few details with regard to indirect blood pressure measurement methodology and provide insufficient data to estimate the true prevalence of white-coat hypertension. For years, many physicians have obtained home blood pressure readings to verify their office readings. Having a visiting nurse visit the home once or twice, or having the patient's spouse take the blood pressure with a calibrated device, is cheaper than ABPM and can alert the physician to the possibility that the patient is exhibiting a stress response.

The other aspect of differential diagnosis of primary (essential) systolic or diastolic hypertension in older persons is whether there may be underlying secondary causes that could be treated so that the blood pressure can return to normal. However, probably less than 1% of older persons have a secondary cause of hypertension amenable to targeted therapy. The most common cause of secondary hypertension in older persons is renal vascular hypertension, but this diagnosis is difficult to make, and surgical treatment is often less than curative. Criteria for considering an evaluation for an underlying secondary cause of hypertension are listed in Table 455.3.

TABLE 455.3.	INDICATIONS FOR FURTHER EVALUATION FOR SECONDARY HYPERTENSION

New onset of stage 3 or 4 hypertension in person older than 60 years
Hypertension refractory to three-drug regimen
Clinical or laboratory findings suggesting identifiable causes of hypertension
Spontaneous and refractory hypokalemia while on thiazides
Symptoms suggestive of pheochromocytoma
Continued creatinine rise while on appropriate antihypertensive therapy

(Adapted from Joint National Committee. The fifth report of the Joint National Committee Detection Evaluation and Treatment of High Blood Pressure, *Arch Intern Med* 1993;153:1037.)

STRATEGIES FOR OPTIMAL CARE MANAGEMENT

MANAGEMENT

Once the diagnosis of high blood pressure has been firmly established in an older person, the first step in managing the patient is to assess his or her nutritional habits and lifestyle. Excessive ethanol abuse, high sodium intake, increased body weight, inactivity, and use of certain drugs, such as oral sympathomimetics or nonsteroidal anti-inflammatory drugs, alone or in combination, may actually be the culprit in raising the blood pressure. At present, it would be prudent to advise weight loss, decreased sodium intake, increased physical activity, and a review of over-the-counter and prescription medications for all older persons before prescribing drug treatment for high blood pressure.

Most older individuals who have been diagnosed with high blood pressure ultimately go on to antihypertensive therapy. The goals for blood pressure lowering are shown in Table 455.2. The choice of drugs and their proper usage have been well detailed in the Joint National Committee–6 (JNC-6) recommendations from the National Heart, Lung and Blood Institute. A recommended approach to the management of an elderly person with high blood pressure is as follows:

1. The stage of hypertension (Table 455.2) should be established; this can be based on the SBP alone.
2. Stages 1 and 2 should first be verified by averaging the blood pressure measurements from three visits (three measurements per visit). If confirmed, the patient should first be treated conservatively with nonpharmacologic interventions. If the blood pressure does not drop into the high-normal range in 3 to 6 months, institute pharmacologic therapy. With drug dosage, "start low and go slow."
3. A diuretic is the drug of first choice for the treatment of hypertension in older patients. Diuretic dosages equivalent to 12.5 to 25 mg per day of chlorthalidone (or hydrochlorothiazide) appear to be most effective. The risks associated with toxicity outweigh efficacy once the dosage increases above the equivalent of 25 mg per day. Use of a potassium-sparing agent is indicated if the serum potassium falls in the first 6 months.
4. Mitigating factors such as comorbid disease or persistent lipoprotein disorders may mandate another first choice for monotherapy (Table 455.4).
5. Pharmacologic therapy should not be continued for elderly patients with stage 1 hypertension in whom significant side effects persist despite attempts with a variety of pharmacologic agents.
6. After blood pressure has been controlled for 6 months, the dosage of the drug should be lowered if possible.

Once a plan for management with nondrug and drug therapy is devised for an older patient with high blood pressure, the issue of adherence becomes critical. Unfortunately, self-report of adherence and pill counts have been proved to be less than totally accurate in assessing overall adherence. Research findings

Condition	Preferred	Not Preferred
Coronary artery disease	B	—
Congestive heart failure		
Systolic	D, ACE	B, Ca
Diastolic	Ca, ACE	—
Arrhythmias	B, CA	
Peripheral arterial disease	Ca	B
Obstructive pulmonary disease	Ca	B
Diabetes	ACE, CA	—
Hyperlipidemia	ACE, Ca	—
Gout	—	D

TABLE 455.4. CONCOMITANT CONDITIONS AFFECTING CHOICE OF ANTIHYPERTENSIVE AGENT

D, diuretic; B, β-blocker; Ca, calcium channel blocker; ACE, angiotensin-converting enzyme inhibitor.

indicate that it is important to assess adherence as best the physician can (self-report, pill count, talking with the spouse or significant other), and that if the physician does this on a routine basis, compliance will probably increase or be maintained even though the physician will never have a precise estimate of the actual level of patient adherence.

COMPLICATIONS AND PITFALLS

Complications or problems in the management of high blood pressure in older people range from the subtle to the fatal. More subtle complications of antihypertensive medications include postural hypotension, notably after meals, falls, depression, and mild to moderate clouding of the sensorium.

On every visit, the clinician should include a formal evaluation of mental status and mood, and directly measure postural changes in blood pressure as well as question the patient about symptoms of dizziness. It is also crucial to obtain a history from family members with regard to the patient's relative vitality, cognition, and overall state of health.

Studies indicate that less than half of all persons diagnosed with high blood pressure and on therapy are under good control. These problems are related to nonadherence to therapeutic regimens, use of therapeutic regimens with multiple side effects, cost of therapeutic regimens, and inadequate attention to adherence by physicians. Elderly patients should be given various compliance aids, particularly pill boxes, which give immediate feedback with regard to noncompliance. Families and relatives of older patients should be enlisted in the effort to maintain adherence to the therapeutic regimen. On the other hand, if older individuals adhere rigidly to an antihypertensive regimen, they may encounter problems from side effects of medications. Frequently, older people who experience side effects from prescription medications are more likely to attribute the cause of the side effect to the aging process than the drug itself.

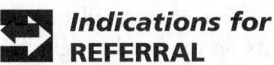

Indications for HOSPITALIZATION

Simply putting an older person in a hospital can have disastrous complications in terms of loss of function and iatrogenic disorders. Therefore, indications for hospitalization must be carefully weighed. In general, older persons with problems related to high blood pressure should be hospitalized only in the most extreme circumstances. Specifically, any older person who presents with a SBP greater than 240 mm Hg or a DBP greater than 125 mm Hg should be hospitalized if the pressure cannot be brought down in the physician's office. If the pressure can be reduced in the physician's office, careful home monitoring on a daily basis can be a substitute for hospitalization. Any older person who has this level of elevation of blood pressure and who has either an altered sensorium, papillary edema, or other signs of central nervous system dysfunction should be hospitalized immediately. In addition, any older person with a dramatically elevated blood pressure who has focal neurologic deficits, signs or symptoms of congestive heart failure, or other ischemic disorders should also be hospitalized.

Indications for REFERRAL

Indications for referral of older persons with high blood pressure are straightforward:

1. An older person who maintains systolic pressures above 179 mm Hg or diastolic pressures above 109 mm Hg despite two-drug therapy should be referred to an expert consultant.
2. An older person with new onset of very high elevations of systolic or DBP should be referred to a consultant.
3. An older person with symptoms suggestive of pheochromocytoma or other secondary causes of hypertension should be referred to a consultant.
4. An older person with repeated episodes of blood pressure escaping from control, possibly with cardiovascular events or side effects, should be referred to a consultant.

COST-EFFECTIVENESS

For persons of any age, drug management of uncomplicated high blood pressure does not clearly result in net cost savings. In other words, it is difficult to predict for any level of SBP or DBP which patients will have a cardiovascular event at a given point in their lives. Treatment of mild to moderate high blood pressure does prevent some suffering and the cost of some future hospitalizations. However, according to one study, these savings are more than offset by the cost of long-term therapy. It appears that only 22% of the cost of treating moderate diastolic hypertension (DBP greater than 105 mm Hg) and only 15% of the costs of treating mild hypertension (DBP 90 to 104 mm Hg)

is recovered. In 1984 U.S. dollars, costs per quality-adjusted life-year saved by treatment for a DBP of 90 to 94, 95 to 104, and 105 or more mm Hg are $45,000, $22,000, and $9,000, respectively. The cost of the medication used has substantial impact on the cost per year of life saved. However, as in all medical therapy, preventive interventions that result in net cost savings are very rare.

If a physician uses an inexpensive generic drug, then the cost per cardiovascular event or cost per year of life saved compares relatively favorably with that for other preventive measurements (e.g., smoking cessation). If physicians choose antihypertensive agents based on concepts of potential drug class benefits (e.g., calcium channel blockers and angiotensin-converting enzyme inhibitors) without a prior trial of a less expensive agent, there is no scenario under which the treatment of hypertension is cost-effective relative to that of other preventive services.

No one would argue against managing high blood pressure in patients who have a variety of concomitant conditions (e.g., angina pectoris, congestive heart failure) with drugs that will both lower the blood pressure and control the concomitant condition. However, more than 60% of older persons with high blood pressure do not have overt end-organ disease. To treat these patients with nongeneric medications increases the cost dramatically and lowers the cost-effectiveness exponentially.

This does not mean that it can never be cost-effective to treat high blood pressure in older patients. In fact, because high blood pressure–related complications are still as preventable in older as in younger persons, and because older persons have a higher absolute number of events, treating high blood pressure in older individuals is actually relatively more cost-effective at the start. Therefore, the issue of whether treatment is cost-effective is driven not by the age of the patient but by the cost of the drug.

BIBLIOGRAPHY

Applegate WB. Hypertension in elderly patients. *Ann Intern Med* 1989; 110:901–915.

Applegate WB, Miller ST, Elam JT, et al. Nonpharmacologic intervention to reduce blood pressure in older patients with mild hypertension. *Arch Intern Med* 1992;152:1162–1166.

Joint National Committee. The sixth report of the Joint National Committee on detection, evaluation, and treatment of high blood pressure. *Arch Intern Med* 1997;157:2413–2446.

Medical Research Council Working Party. Medical Research Council trial of treatment of hypertension in older adults: principal results. *Br Med J* 1992;304:405–412.

National High Blood Pressure Education Program Working Group. Report on hypertension in the elderly. *Hypertension* 1994;23:275–285.

Stason WB. Cost and quality trade-offs in the treatment of hypertension. *Hypertension* 1989;13(Suppl 1):I145–I148.

Taylor JO, Cornoni-Huntley J, Curb JD, et al. Blood pressure and mortality risk in the elderly. *Am J Epidemiol* 1991;134:489–501.

SHEP Cooperative Research Group. Prevention of stroke by antihypertensive drug treatment in older persons with isolated systolic hypertension: final results of the Systolic Hypertension in the Elderly Program (SHEP). *JAMA* 1991;265:3255–3264.

Trial Investigators. Morbidity and mortality in the placebo-controlled European Trial on Isolated Systolic Hypertenstion in the elderly. *Lancet* 1997;360:757–764.

Kelley's Textbook of Internal Medicine, fourth edition. Edited by H. David Humes.
Lippincott Williams & Wilkins, Philadelphia © 2000.

CHAPTER 456

APPROACH TO THE ELDERLY PATIENT WITH DIABETES

JEFFREY B. HALTER

PRESENTATION

Diabetes mellitus is a common health problem affecting elderly people, with a prevalence rate of 15% to 20% in persons over the age of 65 years in the United States. Diabetes mellitus is not a benign condition in older people, as it is associated with substantially increased risk for long-term diabetes complications and associated mortality. Older adults can present with any of the full spectrum of the heterogeneous manifestations of diabetes mellitus. At one end of this spectrum is asymptomatic hyperglycemia of type 2 diabetes mellitus. Indeed, it is estimated that approximately one-third of older adults who meet current American Diabetes Association (ADA) criteria for diabetes mellitus (see Chapter 411) are unaware of the diagnosis.

While type 2 diabetes is by far the most common form in an older adult population, increasing numbers of individuals with type 1 diabetes mellitus are living to old age. Such individuals have the usual metabolic characteristics of type 1 diabetes, with labile hyperglycemia and risk for development of diabetic ketoacidosis. Those with a long history of diabetes may exhibit any of the full range of diabetes complications. Much more rarely, an older individual may present with a new onset of symptomatic hyperglycemia and ketoacidosis.

The usual lag time between diagnosis of diabetes and the development of diabetes-related complications is not well defined in an older adult population. This may reflect some interaction between aging and the mechanisms by which hyperglycemia leads to diabetes complications. In addition, as suggested by the high rate of undiagnosed diabetes in the older adult population, it is possible that some older patients with type 2 diabetes may have had asymptomatic hyperglycemia for a substantial period of time prior to their diagnosis. For this reason, a careful search for evidence of diabetes complications should be carried out in older patients, even when the diagnosis of diabetes is recent. Diabetes mellitus with poor control of hyperglycemia is one cause of an insidious decline in an older patient, with weight loss, muscle weakness, and deterioration of functional status. As control of hyperglycemia can reverse the deterioration in such a patient, appropriate diagnosis and treatment is particularly important.

An extreme form of metabolic decompensation that is of particular concern in older adults is the hyperosmolar coma syndrome, characterized by marked hyperglycemia, hyperosmolality, and severe volume depletion. The associated mortality rate is high, in part because there is often a severe underlying illness, such as pneumonia or cerebrovascular accident. Associated renal insufficiency limits renal excretion of glucose, thereby accelerating the degree of hyperglycemia. Metabolic acidosis may be present but is due to accumulation of lactic acid rather than ketoacids. This condition may occur in an older individual with no prior diagnosis of diabetes or a history of type 2 diabetes not considered severe enough to warrant pharmacologic therapy. Hyperosmolar coma is associated with marked elevations of stress hormones and insulin deficiency. The explanation for lack of mobilization of fatty acids and production of ketoacids under these circumstances remains unclear.

PATHOPHYSIOLOGIC FACTORS

The reasons for the high rates of type 2 diabetes in older populations are not known, but there appears to be a complex interaction among genetic, lifestyle, and aging influences, as illustrated in Fig. 456.1. The heterogeneity of type 2 diabetes likely reflects the varying contributions of each of multiple factors to the development of hyperglycemia in a given individual or family. Many studies have demonstrated age-related glucose intolerance in normal people who do not meet the criteria for diabetes mellitus. One cause of this glucose intolerance is an age-related decline of pancreatic β-cell function. Another factor contributing to age-related glucose intolerance is a decline in sensitivity to the metabolic effects of insulin with age. This age-related impairment of insulin action is due to effects on the insulin-signaling mechanism that limit the mobilization of glucose transporters needed for insulin-mediated glucose uptake and metabolism in insulin-dependent tissues, such as muscle and fat. There is currently little evidence for an age-related impairment of insulin effects on protein or fat metabolism. The age-related decline in insulin action is due in part to age-related changes in body composition (increased adiposity, particularly centrally, and decreased muscle mass) and decreased physical activity.

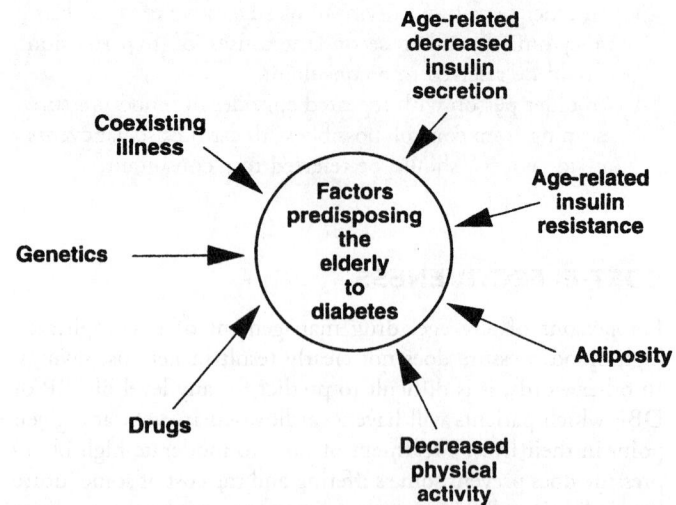

FIGURE 456.1. Summary of factors that may contribute to the high rate of diabetes mellitus and impaired glucose tolerance among elderly persons. (From Halter JB. In Masoro EJ, ed. *Handbook of physiology. Section 11: aging.* New York: Oxford University Press, 1995, with permission.)

TABLE 456.1.	DRUGS THAT MAY INCREASE GLUCOSE LEVELS
Diuretics	Caffeine
Adrenergic agonists	Nicotine
?β-Adrenergic blockers	Alcohol
?Calcium channel blockers	Nicotinic acid
Glucocorticoids	Oral contraceptives
Growth hormone	(estrogen/progesterone)
Nonsteroidal anti-inflammatory	Phenytoin
drugs	Pentamidine

Coexisting illness can be another confounding factor affecting insulin sensitivity in an older person. Both hypertension and hyperlipidemia are common in older people and have been associated with diminished insulin sensitivity. An acute illness can precipitate hyperglycemia because of effects of stress hormones to cause insulin resistance and to inhibit insulin secretion. Finally, drugs that may be used by older people may also contribute to hyperglycemia by causing insulin resistance (Table 456.1). Impaired pancreatic β-cell adaptation to insulin resistance further contributes to age-related glucose intolerance and risk for diabetes mellitus.

The pathophysiology of diabetes complications appears to be similar in older and younger patients. Chronic exposure to hyperglycemia leads to protein glycosylation and subsequent formation of advanced glycosylation end products. The advanced glycosylation end products can accumulate in slow-turnover proteins, such as collagen, potentially leading to tissue damage and injury. Tissue exposure to high concentrations of glucose can also lead to accumulation of metabolic products of the aldose reductase system, including non-metabolized molecules such as sorbitol. Such accumulation can affect cellular energy metabolism and contribute to cell injury and death. The possibility also exists that the genetic complexity of type 2 diabetes may contribute to the risk for one or more long-term complications of diabetes independent from the effects of hyperglycemia.

HISTORY AND PHYSICAL EXAMINATION

An older patient with diabetes should have a thorough history and physical examination at periodic intervals. This medical evaluation should address diabetes self-management activities and skills, diabetes knowledge, medication use, cardiovascular risk factors, health maintenance activities, and microvascular and macrovascular complications of diabetes. Given the uncertainty about the duration of diabetes mellitus for many older patients, the search for evidence of diabetes complications should not be postponed. Thus, the medical evaluation should be complemented by a detailed eye examination by an ophthalmologist, as early signs of diabetic retinopathy can be easily missed. Given the high rate of vascular disease in older people with diabetes mellitus, a careful assessment for evidence of cerebrovascular disease, coronary heart disease, and peripheral vascular disease should be carried out. In addition to a thorough neurologic

exam for evidence of neuropathy, a careful foot examination is needed to identify possible structural abnormalities that might contribute to risk for skin breakdown and damage. The genitourinary system should be a focus for attention, as many older patients may have other factors contributing to bladder or sexual dysfunction that may be exacerbated by the coexistence of diabetes. Because of the high frequency of coexisting health problems in older patients, a thorough review of drug utilization is important. The drug history will help to identify drug therapy that may be contributing to the patient's hyperglycemia (Table 456.1) as well as drug interactions that may affect diabetes management.

The search for and documentation of coexisting illnesses may have a substantial influence on the decision about the intervention chosen for management of diabetes in an older patient. In particular, a coexisting illness that substantially limits remaining life expectancy will affect any decision regarding the goal for control of hyperglycemia. The diet history should address the patient's cultural and historical background, which may have a substantial impact on the efficacy of various types of dietary interventions. Oral health should be assessed, given the frequency of oral health problems in older adults and the importance of oral health to dietary intervention.

Several aspects of the history and physical examination are particularly important for an older patient with diabetes. These include an assessment of the patient's functional status for activities of daily living. Functional status may influence decisions about the choice of therapeutic regimen for the patient in terms of goal setting as well as the patient's ability to adhere to a diabetes treatment program. The patient's cognitive and psychosocial status should also be carefully assessed. Cognitive function may be critical, given the complexity of many diabetes management programs. Cognition is key to recognition and treatment of hypoglycemia and in turn may be worsened by recurrent hypoglycemia. The presence of a psychiatric disorder, such as depression, could have a major impact on diabetes treatment and require a separate intervention. The patient's socioeconomic status can also have an important impact on the diabetes treatment plan and should be assessed. The degree of support available from caregivers can affect treatment plans, as caregivers can compensate for some of the patient's own limitations in self-care capabilities and can play a key role in promoting the effectiveness of lifestyle interventions. The patient's economic status may affect the ability to adhere to a costly medical regimen, and cultural influences may have to be considered as a treatment plan is developed.

LABORATORY STUDIES AND DIAGNOSTIC TESTS

The current criteria for diagnosis of diabetes mellitus (see Chapter 411) are not adjusted by age. Thus, the same diagnostic criteria apply to older persons. The ADA's recommendations focus on the fasting glucose level for clinical purposes. However, it should be recognized that a substantial number of older persons meet the post-glucose challenge criteria for a diagnosis of diabetes mellitus but do not meet criteria based only on the fasting glucose level. Thus follow-up testing and possible use of an oral glucose tolerance test should be considered in some older people with borderline fasting glucose levels. Diagnostic tests for diabetes-related complications should be carried out as in a younger population, based on the findings from a thorough history and physical examination. Given the high rate of asymptomatic or mildly symptomatic cardiovascular disease in this population, a low threshold should be set for a Doppler evaluation for carotid artery stenosis or reduced extremity blood flow and for cardiovascular stress testing. Blood and urine screening for kidney disease should be carried out as in younger patients, but the interpretation may be more difficult in an older patient with other potential causes for kidney disease. Screening for a lipid disorder should also be carried out, as there is growing evidence that both older persons and persons with diabetes can benefit from lipid-lowering therapy to reduced risk for cardiovascular disease.

DIFFERENTIAL DIAGNOSIS

The differential diagnosis of hyperglycemia in an older adult should consider the potential contribution of drug therapy or a coexisting illness to the hyperglycemia and identify individuals in whom hyperglycemia is secondary to an underlying illness. Ideally, it is best to reevaluate glucose levels after discontinuing any of the drugs listed in Table 456.1 to determine if the criteria for diabetes are still being met. Similarly, glucose levels should be reevaluated after resolution of an acute concomitant stressful illness. As in a younger patient, endocrine syndromes with overproduction of stress hormones or conditions resulting in severe damage to the pancreas can lead to significant hyperglycemia and should be considered in the diagnosis.

STRATEGIES FOR OPTIMAL CARE

MANAGEMENT

Hyperglycemia

The first key step in developing a diabetes management program for an elderly patient is to establish the treatment goal. The ADA recommends a goal of a fasting glucose less than 120 mg per deciliter and a hemoglobin AIC within 1 g % of the upper limit of normal to markedly reduce the risk for diabetes complications. The ADA's recommendation is broad and not limited to a specific type of diabetes or to any age group. However, it may be neither feasible nor appropriate to attempt to establish such a goal for some elderly patients. Table 456.2 lists some of the factors to consider in deciding on a treatment goal designed to minimize risk for diabetes complications in an older patient.

A limited remaining life expectancy shortens the time in which long-term complications can develop and progress. However, the life expectancy of older adults is increasing. Thus, for example, it would be hard to justify abandoning the ADA's goal in an otherwise healthy 75-year-old woman with a recent diagnosis of diabetes mellitus, since such a person's remaining life expectancy may be 15 years or more. The commitment on

TABLE 456.2.	FACTORS TO CONSIDER IN SETTING A DIABETES TREATMENT GOAL FOR ELDERLY PATIENTS

Patient's estimated remaining life expectancy
Patient's preference and commitment
Opinion of the primary care provider: control vs. complications
Availability of support services
Economic issues
Coexisting health problems
   Major psychiatric disorder
   Major cognitive disorder
   Diabetes complications
   Major limitation of diabetes functional status
Complexity of medical regimen

the part of an adequately informed patient is clearly critical to achieve tight diabetes control. Availability of a supportive environment, including a strong, committed diabetes treatment team and adequate economic support for an intensive treatment program, are also important issues. Any decision about an intensive treatment program must take into account coexisting conditions and the overall complexity of the patient's medical regimen. The existence of advanced diabetes complications in a patient may provide a rationale for less strict control of hyperglycemia. A significant psychiatric or cognitive disorder may also preclude implementation of an intensive management program. However, many older adults are able to devote a substantial amount of time to their own health care and are able to manage complex multidrug interventions for multiple health problems. The ADA's recommended intensive treatment goal may be appropriate for such individuals.

Regardless of whether a decision is made to try to prevent diabetes complications with intensive diabetes management, the treatment plan for virtually all older patients with diabetes should prevent metabolic decompensation and control other risk factors that may contribute to diabetes complications. Metabolic decompensation with weight loss, muscle wasting, and a catabolic state is unlikely to occur if the average circulating glucose level is in the range of 200 mg per deciliter and the glycosylated hemoglobin value is within 3% to 4% of the upper limit of normal. Thus, this seems a reasonable target goal for basic diabetes care. Coexisting hypertension, hyperlipidemia, and cigarette smoking should be identified and treated, and all elderly patients with diabetes should receive a basic diabetes education, including recognition and treatment of hypoglycemia. Basic diabetes care should include yearly follow-up and reevaluation for the development of diabetes complications, and intervention for those complications as appropriate.

Elderly individuals who are selected for an aggressive treatment program meeting ADA guidelines should receive all aspects of basic diabetes care, including aggressive detection and treatment of hypertension, hyperlipidemia, and cigarette smoking; monitoring for diabetes complications; and institution of complication-specific interventions. Elderly patients participating in an aggressive treatment program should be trained to carry out home blood glucose monitoring on a regular basis and should

TABLE 456.3.	RISK FACTORS FOR HYPOGLYCEMIA IN OLDER DIABETIC PATIENTS

Impaired autonomic nervous system function
Diminished glucagon secretion
Poor or irregular nutrition
Cognitive disorder
Use of alcohol or other sedating agent
Polypharmacy
Kidney or liver failure

participate in a formal diabetes education program that covers various treatment approaches for hyperglycemia, including diet, exercise, and medications. Access to a multidisciplinary diabetes care team should be part of an aggressive treatment program.

The full range of therapeutic options for diabetes management, including diet, exercise, oral agents, and insulin, is available for use in elderly patients (see Chapter 411). There is no absolute contraindication to any of these agents in relation to age. All of the newer oral agents have been tested in older patients, at least in short-term trials, and there is a growing body of information regarding the response of older patients to all diabetes treatment interventions. At this point there is no clear, preferred algorithm to utilize for an older patient with diabetes. Factors to consider include whether the treatment target is for basic care or an aggressive program, the side-effect profile of the various agents that are available (discussed below), the costs of the various agents, and the overall complexity of the medical regimen. For example, combination therapy with different categories of oral agents and/or insulin may be attractive in a patient with few other health problems. However, single-agent therapy may be more attractive for an elderly patient who is already on multiple medications for several coexisting health problems. There is also growing recognition that achievement and maintenance of the ADA's target for hyperglycemia control is difficult for many patients with type 2 diabetes, even on combination drug therapy. Thus, more ongoing, intensive effort may be needed than is the usual standard practice.

Diabetes Complications

As in younger patients with diabetes, identification and management of hypertension and lipid abnormalities should be part of optimal diabetes care. Smoking cessation should also be emphasized. Use of aspirin to reduce cardiovascular risk, angiotensin-converting enzyme inhibitors for diabetic renal disease, and aggressive intervention for diabetic retinopathy should also be provided to elderly people. Since older patients with diabetes are at high risk for amputation, careful attention to peripheral vascular disease, neuropathy, and foot care is also critical.

COMPLICATIONS AND PITFALLS

Hypoglycemia is the primary short-term risk of a diabetes treatment program, particularly one that is targeted at achieving near-normal control of glucose levels. Table 456.3 summarizes a number of risk factors for hypoglycemia in an older patient with diabetes. As counterregulatory hormone responses are important for both symptom recognition and hypoglycemia counterregulation, impairment of autonomic nervous system reflexes can contribute to the risk for hypoglycemia. As in younger patients, this can occur in the setting of previous bouts of hypoglycemia, leading to the hypoglycemia unawareness syndrome. Some older patients may have autonomic neuropathy due to longstanding diabetes or other causes. Other older patients are treated with β-adrenergic blocking drugs or other antiadrenergic agents for cardiovascular diseases.

Some patients with longstanding type 1 diabetes or those with diabetes due to inflammatory disease of the exocrine pancreas may have impaired glucagon secretion as well. Patients who have relatively poor nutrition and an irregular meal pattern can be at increased risk of hypoglycemia, in part because of inadequate maintenance of muscle and liver glycogen stores. Use of alcohol or a sedating agent should be avoided in patients receiving hypoglycemic agents, particularly if an aggressive treatment program is being pursued. A coexisting cognitive disorder will interfere with recognition of hypoglycemia and possibly affect decisions about responding to hypoglycemia. Patients with underlying renal or hepatic insufficiency may have problems related to the elimination of hypoglycemic agents—particularly an issue for sulfonylurea drugs. A patient with severe hepatic insufficiency may have difficulty mobilizing a counterregulatory increase of glucose production. Finally, any complex drug regimen may include agents that influence the pharmacokinetics of hypoglycemic agents, or counterregulatory or behavioral responses to hypoglycemia, and therefore should be an issue when considering risk for hypoglycemia.

Despite all of these issues and concerns, many older patients with diabetes can be treated aggressively with minimal risk for hypoglycemia. By providing a strong educational program focused on hypoglycemia recognition and treatment, and considering the risk factors outlined in Table 456.3, problems with severe hypoglycemia can generally be avoided. Studies of hypoglycemia counterregulatory mechanisms have identified only subtle alterations in healthy older adults, and patients who are hyperglycemic actually have elevated thresholds for counterregulation. Furthermore, patients with type 2 diabetes generally are at less risk for severe hypoglycemia than intensively treated patients with type 1 diabetes. Thus, the rate of severe hypoglycemia in older, type 2 diabetes patients appears to be substantially lower than in patients participating in the Diabetes Control and Complications Trial, for example.

Dietary issues may affect management of older adults with diabetes. Older adults with a significant mobility limitation may be relatively inactive and have low caloric utilization. Thus, caloric intake may have to be limited to rather low levels to achieve significant weight reduction. The potential benefit of caloric restriction and weight reduction under such circumstances has to be balanced against the potential risk for complications related to undernutrition. Elderly patients may have difficulty with access to food in terms of both food preparation and shopping for food. Furthermore, dietary habits established over a lifetime, and often with a cultural background, may be particularly difficult to modify. Older men living alone may have limited food preparation skills. Following a dietary prescription may be particularly difficult for a patient with impaired cognitive function. Any of these issues can be modified if there is sufficient caregiver and/or social service support that can assist with providing meals in the home setting. Problems with taste and oral health, which are common in older people, may further limit adaptation to a prescribed diet. Oral health problems can be exacerbated by diabetes, which may increase the rate of periodontal disease. This may be a growing issue as increasing numbers of older adults are keeping their teeth for longer periods. Xerostomia is also more common in older people owing to decreased salivary gland flow, sometimes exacerbated by coexisting medication use.

Exercise training may be a useful adjunct to drug therapy and may contribute to the enhanced effectiveness of glucose-lowering agents. Given the high prevalence of coronary artery disease in older patients with diabetes mellitus, which may often be asymptomatic or atypical in its symptoms, it is important for such patients to have medically supervised stress testing prior to entering any challenging exercise training program. An additional issue to consider in an older person is the potential for foot and joint injury with upright exercise such as jogging. Thus, particular attention should be given to the foot examination in an older person prior to and during the course of exercise training. Because it may enhance glucose uptake by muscle, exercise training may contribute to the risk for hypoglycemia in patients who are taking hypoglycemic agents.

Sulfonylurea drugs have an established, long record of safety, with hypoglycemia being the main side effect of significance. These agents should not be used in patients with renal insufficiency or with significant liver disease, as they are dependent on the liver for metabolism and on the kidney for excretion. Hyponatremia has also been observed as a complication of sulfonylurea use in some patients. Because of similar risk with the use of thiazide diuretics, the combination of thiazide and sulfonylurea drugs should be avoided.

α-*Glucosidase inhibitors* work by inhibiting the key gastrointestinal enzyme responsible for breakdown of carbohydrates prior to absorption. The major side effect is local to the gastrointestinal tract, as these drugs are not absorbed to any significant degree. However, 20% to 30% of patients may develop diarrhea. To some degree this may be a welcome side effect in some elderly people with chronic constipation, and other patients may tolerate it without much discomfort.

The most common side effect of *metformin* is gastrointestinal discomfort, which in some patients can be associated with decreased appetite and modest weight loss. While some have viewed this as a potential benefit for a patient on a weight reduction program, this effect must be balanced against the degree of symptoms and the appropriateness of decreased caloric intake and weight loss in a specific individual. The biguanide class of drugs can be associated with development of life-threatening lactic acidosis under some circumstances. While this complication appears to be rare in patients with metformin, the drug should not be used in patients with chronic congestive heart failure and should be withheld during acute hospitalization for any major illness that could result in decreased tissue perfusion as a precipitating factor for lactic acidosis. Metformin should also be avoided in patients with significant liver disease or renal insufficiency (a creatinine level greater than 1.5 mg per deciliter).

Thiazolidinediones have largely been well tolerated in initial clinical trials that have included older adults. One disadvantage is their high cost. Because of reports of severe idiocyncratic hepatic toxicity with troglitazone, liver enzymes should be monitored during treatment with one of these drugs, and significant elevation should result in prompt discontinuation.

Insulin can be used for an older patient with type 2 diabetes, either as a primary hyperglycemic agent or to maintain glucose control in the hospital setting during acute stressful illness or when oral agents cannot be ingested. There are virtually no absolute contraindications to the use of insulin. Insulin can effectively lower glucose levels in virtually any patient and in sufficient dosage has at least the potential to normalize circulating glucose levels if the regimen intensity is sufficient. However, the requirement for injection may represent an insurmountable psychological barrier for some patients, and for others insulin injections may not be feasible due to functional limitations or insufficient caregiver support. Hypoglycemia is the major risk associated with the taking of insulin, as discussed previously. It should be kept in mind that achievement of a basic goal for hyperglycemia management can often be accomplished with a fairly simple regimen of one or two injections of intermediate-acting insulin in a patient with type 2 diabetes. Another concern regarding use of a high dose of insulin is the potential for weight gain. However, the largest weight gain often occurs in individuals who have lost a substantial amount of weight prior to insulin therapy due to decompensated diabetes. For other patients, it may be necessary to balance the potential risk of weight gain against the benefit of lowering the circulating glucose level.

INDICATIONS FOR HOSPITALIZATION OR REFERRAL

Diabetes mellitus is one of the most common diagnoses of patients who are hospitalized. However, hospitalization is usually for a diabetes-related complication rather than the metabolic disturbance itself. Hyperglycemia can be managed on an outpatient basis unless there is associated significant metabolic acidosis or the hyperglycemia has been severe enough to lead to volume depletion requiring intravenous fluid therapy. Particular attention should be paid to areas of skin breakdown or apparent infection in the lower extremity of an older patient with diabetes. These lesions may appear indolent due to poor vascular supply that does not support an inflammatory response. Hospital admission may be appropriate for individuals with such lesions if very close outpatient follow-up is not possible and self-care ability is questionable. In an analogous fashion, there should be a low threshold for hospital admission for an older patient with chest pain, as clinical manifestations of coronary artery disease may be atypical or silent in such individuals.

COST-EFFECTIVENESS

There is great potential for cost savings due to the high morbidity associated with diabetes and its complications in older adults, and the associated high rates of utilization of acute hospital and long-term care services. Interventions for hypertension and lipid lowering are likely to be cost-effective, even a primary prevention approach for lipid lowering. There is also strong evidence for support of interventions for diabetic neuropathy and nephropathy in older adults. However, the cost-effectiveness of glucose level lowering in this population has been questioned, given the limited information about the rate of development of microvascular complications in relation to hyperglycemia in older adults and the overall lack of clear evidence of benefit for glucose lowering to reduce the rate of macrovascular disease in any population. Clearly, further study is needed.

BIBLIOGRAPHY

American Diabetes Association: clinical practice recommendations 1999. *Diabetes Care* 1999;22(Suppl 1):S1–S114.

Barzilay JI, Spiekerman CF, Wahl, PW, et al. Cardiovascular disease in older adults with glucose disorders: comparison of American Diabetes Association criteria for diabetes mellitus with WHO criteria. *Lancet* 1999;354:622–625.

Dechenes CJ, Verchere CB, Andrikopoulos S, et al. Human aging is associated with parallel reductions in insulin and amylin release. *Am J Physiol* 1998;275 (*Endocrinol Metab* 38):E785–E791.

The Expert Committee on the Diagnosis and Classification of Diabetes Mellitus. Report of the Expert Committee on the Diagnosis and Classification of Diabetes Mellitus. *Diabetes Care* 1997;20:1183–1197.

Halter JB. Carbohydrate metabolism. In: Masoro EJ, ed. *Handbook of physiology, Section 11: aging,* Oxford University Press, 1995; 119.

Harris MI, Flegal KM, Cowie C, et al. Prevalence of diabetes, impaired fasting glucose and impaired glucose tolerance in U.S. adults: The Third National Health and Nutrition Examination Survey 1988–1994. *Diabetes Care* 1998;21:518–524.

Morisaki N, Watanabe S, Kobayashi J, et al. Diabetic control and progression of retinopathy in elderly patients: five-year follow-up study. *J Am Geriatr Soc* 1994;42:142–145.

National Diabetes Data Group, eds. *Diabetes in America,* second ed. Bethesda, MD: National Institutes of Health, National Institute of Diabetes and Digestive and Kidney Diseases, 1995.

Schleicher ED, Wagner E, Nerlich AG. Increased accumulation of the glycoxidation product N$^{\epsilon}$-(carboxymethyl)lysine in human tissues in diabetes and aging. *J Clin Invest* 1997;99:457–468.

Weiner JP, Parente ST, Garnick DW, et al. Variation in office-based quality: a claims-based profile of care provided to Medicare patients with diabetes. *JAMA* 1995;273:1503–1508.

Kelley's Textbook of Internal Medicine, fourth edition. Edited by H. David Humes.
Lippincott Williams & Wilkins, Philadelphia © 2000.

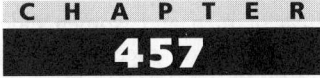

CHAPTER
457

APPROACH TO THE ELDERLY PATIENT WITH DYSLIPIDEMIA

WALTER H. ETTINGER, JR.
WILLIAM R. HAZZARD

Coronary heart disease (CHD) is the leading cause of death and disability in the elderly, and most CHD deaths occur in older persons. Although CHD mortality is declining, even among the very old, the prevalence, yearly incidence rates, and costs of CHD in the elderly will increase dramatically through the first decade of the twenty-first century because of the aging of the population. Therefore, efforts to reduce the premature mortality, disability, and costs associated with CHD in older persons are an important public health priority.

Dyslipoproteinemia is a modifiable risk factor for CHD in young and middle-aged adults. This is dealt with extensively in Chapters 12 and 13. However, the role of lipoprotein lipids as risk factors for CHD in older adults is controversial, as are recommendations for treatment. This chapter addresses this controversy by describing changes in lipoprotein metabolism and blood lipid levels that occur with age, reviewing the evidence linking blood lipid levels with CHD in older persons, and discussing special considerations for treatment of dyslipoproteinemia in older persons.

AGING AND LIPOPROTEIN METABOLISM

Between childhood and midlife (around 50 years of age), increasing age is associated with alterations in average plasma lipid levels principally attributable to age-associated physiologic or normative processes: puberty and subsequent sex steroid secretion patterns and increasing adiposity in both genders. Between infancy and adolescence, average total plasma, low-density lipoprotein (LDL) and high-density lipoprotein (HDL) levels, and LDL/HDL ratios are equivalent between the genders (Fig. 457.1). However, between puberty and age 50 years (around the menopausal age for women), average LDL and hence total plasma cholesterol levels rise in both genders, presumably because of increasing adiposity. However, the rate and amount of increase are lower in women than men, a circumstance that is reversed after the age of menopause. Hence, the difference in lipid levels between men and women is presumably attributable to the effects of endogenous sex hormones, with estrogens in women reducing LDL cholesterol concentrations, an effect lost with cessation of ovarian estrogen secretion in postmenopausal women. Average LDL levels in postmenopausal women exceed those in men of comparable age. Although the cause of this phenomenon remains uncertain, it may be attributable to the conversion of testosterone to estrogens in men. Thus, testosterone, unlike exogenous androgens such as anabolic steroids, which are not metabolized to estrogen, does not raise LDL cholesterol concentrations; however, lack of estrogen clearly does.

Regarding HDL, whereas average concentrations in women do not decline between puberty and menopause (and even beyond menopause), levels decrease in boys across puberty (in parallel with the Tanner adolescent development scale) and, presumably because of continuing testosterone secretion, remain lower in men than women throughout the remainder of life. Because the effects of androgens on HDL appear to be greater than those of the deficiency of estrogen in postmenopausal women on LDL levels, the LDL/HDL ratio (a single index of lipid-related atherogenic risk preferred by many practitioners) remains higher in men than women throughout adult life, al-

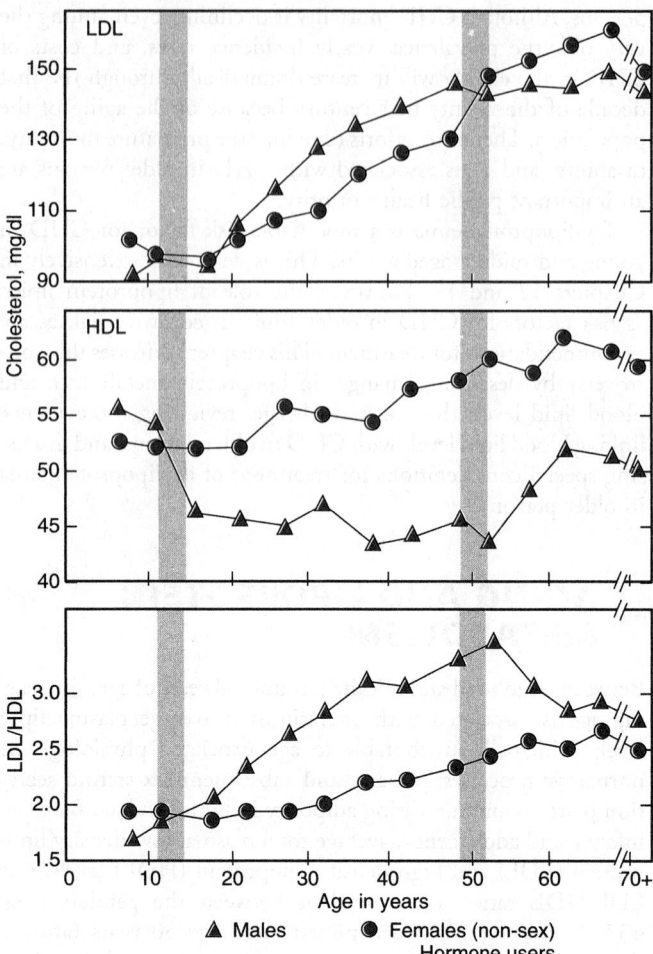

FIGURE 457.1. Median North American population high-density lipoprotein (HDL) cholesterol, low-density lipoprotein (LDL) cholesterol, and the ratio between the two versus age in white subjects. (Data from Lipid Research Clinic Prevalence Survey.)

though the gender differential declines in the postmenopausal era (even as the gender differential in cardiovascular risk narrows, principally attributable to a slower age-related rise in cardiovascular disease deaths in men beyond age 50 than in postmenopausal women). It is of practical significance that because average LDL levels in postmenopausal women exceed those in men of comparable age even as their HDL levels remain higher, the mean total plasma cholesterol levels in postmenopausal women exceed those in men of comparable age (even as their cardiovascular risk remains lower, principally attributable to a lower LDL/HDL ratio). Thus, screening of older adults using total plasma cholesterol levels identifies more hypercholesterolemic women than men. This underscores the National Cholesterol Education Program Adult Treatment Panel II (NCEP-ATP II) recommendation that screening include HDL cholesterol levels so as not only to avoid missing the patient at increased risk by virtue of a low HDL but to be able to reassure those with average or even high HDL cholesterol levels that they may be at acceptable CHD risk because of the probable protective effect of HDL in offsetting the adverse risk associated with an elevated LDL.

The mechanism of the increase in average LDL cholesterol

levels between puberty and midlife remains controversial. Certain investigators have suggested time-related saturation of hepatic and extrahepatic tissue cholesterol levels, down-regulating the LDL receptor. However, increasing average adiposity, especially that in central or upper body distribution, is a more likely explanation because those who remain slender with advancing age have LDL and total cholesterol levels at the lower end of the distribution, and changes in population average cholesterol concentrations are correlated with changes in weight throughout adult life. Although the upper body pattern of that adiposity (reflecting intra-abdominal stores) is more characteristic of men (the "android" pattern), women who do gain weight in the male pattern (as well as those with hyperandrogenism, notably the polycystic ovary syndrome) appear to be at special risk for dyslipoproteinemia, diabetes, hypertension, and coronary heart disease as well ("syndrome X"). However, these age-associated average plasma lipid changes are complete in most people by midlife (men by their sixth and women by their seventh decade), and average cholesterol and triglyceride levels stabilize beyond that point, ultimately declining in advanced old age. Thus, new-onset dyslipidemia is highly uncommon in the elderly, and the prevalence of hyperlipidemia declines in old age.

For this reason, identification of new-onset or exaggerated hyperlipidemia in an elderly patient demands an especially careful search for secondary causes. These include those diseases of increasing incidence with advancing age, notably diabetes mellitus and hypothyroidism, and drug-related causes (see Chapter 31), especially corticosteroids, β-blockers, and thiazides (the latter in combination being a cause of both a low HDL and an increased triglyceride in hypertensive individuals). The decision to discontinue or change these medications must be weighed against the benefits, especially in lowering blood pressure or, in the case of β-blockers, the protective effects conferred when given after a myocardial infarction.

Evidence suggests that, just as in younger people, population average cholesterol levels are decreasing in older people, and their total lipid profiles may be improving. These changes presumably result from secular changes in diet, as well as recognition and treatment of dyslipidemia. Nevertheless, the number of older persons eligible for referral and treatment of dyslipoproteinemia using the NCEP guidelines is substantial. For example, data from the third National Health and Nutrition Examination Study, a population-based study of U.S. adults, indicate that approximately 50% of men and women older than 65 years would require at least dietary therapy for dyslipoproteinemia using the NCEP-ATP II guidelines. Furthermore, even if a 10% reduction in LDL cholesterol were to be achieved from dietary therapy, between 15% to 20% of persons older than 65 years would require pharmacologic therapy for hyperlipidemia, including a substantial number of individuals older than 80 years. The annual cost of such therapy would be in the billions of dollars.

ASSOCIATION OF LIPOPROTEIN LIPIDS WITH CORONARY HEART DISEASE IN OLDER PEOPLE

Given the importance of CHD as a cause of death and disability in the older population and the high prevalence of dyslipoproteinemia in that population, the potential exists to reduce the incidence of CHD by treating dyslipoproteinemia. However, any recommendation to treat dyslipidemia in older people is based on extrapolation of results from clinical trials in middle-aged people. There are no published clinical trials that have examined the effect of therapy for dyslipidemia on incident CHD in the elderly in either primary- or secondary-prevention studies. Moreover, the epidemiologic data linking blood lipid levels to incident CHD in older people are conflicting and controversial.

The strength of the association between lipoprotein lipids and CHD depends on the person's age, gender, and health status. The weight of the evidence suggests that a positive association of LDL cholesterol with incident CHD most clearly exists in the "young-old" (age 55 to 75 years), and the strength of this relation is stronger in men than in women. The inverse relation between HDL cholesterol and CHD also appears to be present among the young-old. However, relative risk of dyslipidemia-related CHD is smaller for an older person than for one of middle age. However, the population-attributable risk of dyslipidemia is larger in the elderly because of the exponential rise in the number of cases of CHD occurring in older people. The implications of the larger population-attributable risk is that treatment of dyslipidemia, if proven useful, would prevent more cases of incident CHD in older people than middle-aged and younger people.

Beyond the age of 75 years, most data suggest that the association of lipid levels with CHD largely disappears. Indeed, several studies have shown that the relation between lipid levels and incident CHD, as well as total mortality, reverses among the "old-old!" That is, persons with higher levels of total and LDL cholesterol have longer survival and less CHD than those with lower levels.

There are several explanations for these seemingly contradictory findings, and above all the data should not be interpreted to suggest a causal relationship between high cholesterol and survival. First, the weakening relationship between lipid levels and incident CHD may reflect what has been called the "harvest effect." That is, persons who are most susceptible to the adverse effects of dyslipidemia contract disease and die prematurely. This results in fewer hypercholesterolemic survivors among older persons and accounts in part for the decline in average cholesterol levels among the elderly in cross-sectional population studies. It also means that elderly populations are enriched with those who have had no ill effects from high cholesterol levels (notably those with high HDL levels).

Second, health status affects the lipid–CHD–survival relation. Poor health status or illness, especially when of an inflammatory nature, often results in a lowering of total serum cholesterol and lipid subfractions. The incidence of chronic and acute diseases increases with age; thus, lipid levels measured in older people may be lower because of such diseases and not reflect usual lifetime levels. Moreover, given emerging evidence that inflammatory diseases (e.g., *Chlymadia* pneumonia) may contribute to CHD, the circumstance may arise whereby cholesterol levels are falling just as the risk of CHD is rising. A person with low cholesterol due to poor health may develop clinical CHD related to his or her previously high cholesterol level, and the lifetime risk of the association between cholesterol and CHD

will be underestimated at the time of its clinical manifestation. Thus, the Framingham study suggested that cholesterol levels measured in middle age were more predictive of CHD in old age than the levels measured nearer the advent of such CHD. Health status may thereby partly explain in turn the inverse relation between high cholesterol and survival. High cholesterol levels in persons who are relatively resistant to the effects of dyslipidemia on the development of heart disease also may reflect the absence of active inflammation and other potentially fatal diseases.

In addition to influencing cholesterol levels, health status appears to affect the direction of the association of cholesterol with CHD, as is most clearly demonstrated in studies by Harris and colleagues. When subjects were stratified either by activity level (a surrogate index of overall health) or prior weight loss, different patterns of the lipid–heart disease association were seen. Among older persons who had not lost weight or who reported a high physical activity level, there was a graded positive response between total cholesterol and CHD. In contrast, among persons who had lost weight or were inactive, the relation between cholesterol and CHD was negative. When these data were combined, no overall association was found between cholesterol and incident CHD. Therefore, the positive association between lipoprotein lipids and heart disease risk may be maintained in elderly persons who are vigorous and otherwise healthy but lost or even inversely related to CHD among the frail and failing. Finally, a distinction should be drawn between CHD (proceeding from coronary atherosclerosis) and cardiovascular disease (CVD) morbidity and mortality in the elderly. Whereas CVD mortality rises exponentially with age, the portion that CHD may contribute as a direct cause of such mortality may actually decline. Thus, congestive heart failure (CHF) as a final common pathway proceeding from the convergence of CHD hypertensive heart disease and age-related decline in left ventricular compliance has already emerged as the commonest reason for hospitalization of Medicare beneficiaries in the United States.

In summary, abnormal lipoprotein lipid levels appear to remain risk factors for coronary heart disease in young-old persons, especially those who are healthy and active. The potential for preventing premature CHD in this group is high because of the greater attributable risk of dyslipidemia in older persons. However, most studies suggest that the relation between lipid levels and incident CHD as well as total mortality does not hold up in advanced old age because of confounding influences of the diseases that are so prevalent in this group, including other, non-CHD causes of CVD morbidity and mortality.

■ TREATMENT OF DYSLIPIDEMIA IN THE ELDERLY PATIENT

The decision to treat dyslipidemia in older people is still based largely on results from middle-aged people. However, several recent studies of lipid-lowering agents in men and women with existing vascular disease (so-called secondary-prevention trials) have found that persons 65 to 75 years of age benefited from treatment. Clinical trials in otherwise healthy older persons with dyslipidemia are ongoing. There is no a priori reason to believe that the young-old would not benefit from treatment, as have

TABLE 457.1.	PHARMACOLOGIC THERAPY FOR DYSLIPIDEMIA IN THE ELDERLY	
Agent	**Effectiveness**	**Comments**
Estrogen	⇊ LDL, ⇈ HDL, ↑ TG	Has benefits on coronary heart disease risk beyond lipid effects; also positive effects on bone density
Human menopausal gonadotropin coenzyme A reductase inhibitors	⇊ LDL, ↑ HDL, ↓ TG	Potent, safe, well tolerated but expensive
Niacin	↓ LDL, ⇈ HDL, ⇊ TG	Inexpensive but high incidence of side effects in clinical practice
Binding resins	↓ LDL, ↑ HDL, ↑ TG	May be used in low doses in combination with other drugs to enhance effects; side effects oftem limiting
Fibric acid derivatives	⇅ LDL, ↑ HDL, ↓ TG	Most effective for people with high TG and low HDL

LDL, low-density lipoprotein; HDL, high-density lipoprotein, TG, triglyceride.

middle-aged individuals. The difficulty comes in the old-old, especially those over age 80.

If treatment for dyslipidemia is to be initiated in an older person, what modalities should be used? Here the advice to clinicians is relatively straightforward. All modalities of therapy for dyslipidemia, both dietary and pharmacologic, that are effective in younger persons have been demonstrated to be equally safe and effective among the elderly.

Nonetheless, there are several factors to consider when treating the elderly patient for dyslipidemia (see Chapters 12 and 31). When instituting dietary therapy, care must be taken not to cause iatrogenic malnutrition, defined as excessive weight loss or inadequate intake of micronutrients. The latter may lead to increased risk for nutrition-related conditions, such as osteoporosis, because weight loss and inadequate calcium intake accelerate bone loss or lead to muscular weakness, both of which contribute to fall-related fractures (see Chapter 462). When considering pharmacologic therapy (Table 457.1), estrogen deserves special consideration for treatment of dyslipidemia in older women not only because of its proven efficacy in both lowering LDL and raising HDL but because CHD incidence is reduced by approximately 50% in women taking estrogen, and other beneficial effects such as decreased fracture risk may accrue. Evidence from the Prospective Estrogen–Progestin Intervention Trial in middle-aged women indicates that both estrogen alone and estrogen combined with progestin are effective agents in reducing LDL cholesterol and raising HDL cholesterol (although combination therapy has less effect on HDL because of the HDL-lowering effects of androgenic progestins) in postmenopausal women. However, both regimens significantly raise triglyceride levels (suggesting caution in prescription of estrogen in those with preexisting hypertriglyceridemia). Moreover, the sobering adverse early results of estrogen treatment of women with established CHD in the recent Heart Estrogen Replacement Study (HERS) trial have reduced enthusiasm for such therapy and underscored the importance of the Women's Health Initiative Primary Prevention Trial to resolve this issue.

Among the other agents for dyslipidemia, the 3-hydroxy-3-methylglutaryl reductase coenzyme A (HMG-CoA) reductase inhibitors ("statins") have several advantages in older people. They are the most potent LDL-lowering agents of any of the hypolipidemic drugs, and low doses of these agents are effective and safe in older people. In addition, HMG-CoA reductase inhibitors have the lowest discontinuation rate of any of the dyslipidemic agents because of the low burden of side effects. The disadvantage of these medications is their high cost (which will become less onerous as competing congeners enter the market). Niacin and bile acid–binding resins also are effective lipid-lowering agents in older persons. Niacin is the most potent agent for raising HDL cholesterol concentrations. However, these medications often are not well tolerated by older patients and are frequently discontinued because of side effects (notably flushing and dyspepsia with niacin and abdominal discomfort and constipation with the binding resins). Fibric acid derivatives are most useful for persons with elevated triglycerides and low HDL.

When more aggressive therapy is needed, combinations of hypolipidemic agents can be used. Low-dose bile acid–binding resin combined with a fibrate or HMG-CoA reductase inhibitor is a potent combination for lowering LDL levels. However, caution is indicated in aggressive combination lipid-lowering therapy in older people (especially HMG-CoA reductase inhibitors and niacin or a fibrate in the presence of renal insufficiency or therapy with immunosuppressives.) The NCEP-ATP II recommendations are to lower LDL cholesterol below 100 mg per deciliter for persons with existing CHD. Given the lack of efficacy data in older persons and the possible need to be aggressive with therapy to achieve this level of LDL cholesterol, special caution should be exerted in pursuing this goal in an elderly patient.

SUMMARY

Although the data suggest that treatment of dyslipidemia can prevent CHD in younger and middle-aged people, the data that address this issue in older people are incomplete and mixed.

There are no published clinical trials that have shown benefit from treating dyslipidemia in older people. The epidemiologic data suggest that lipid levels predict CHD in the young-old but that these relationships do not hold up among persons older than 75 years. Thus, as a general recommendation, hypolipidemic therapy should be reserved for persons younger than 75 years who are in good health. Very aggressive therapy should be avoided because of the cost, side effects, and lack of efficacy data, especially in the old-old (more than 75 years).

BIBLIOGRAPHY

Bowlin SJ, Medalie JH, Pearson TA. Cholesterol and vascular disease in the elderly. *Nutr Health Aging* 1997;1:1–13.

Ettinger WH, Harris T. Causes of hypocholesterolemia. *Coron Artery Dis* 1993;4:854–859.

Ettinger WH, Hazzard WR. Dyslipoproteinemia in older people. In: Rifkind BM, ed. *Lowering cholesterol in high-risk individuals and populations.* New York: Marcel Dekker, 1995:99–117.

Expert Panel on Detection, Evaluation, and Treatment of High Blood Cholesterol in Adults. Summary of the second report of the National Cholesterol Education Program (NCEP). *JAMA* 1993;269:3015–3023.

Harris TB, Makuc DM, Kleinman JC, et al. Is the serum cholesterol–coronary heart disease relationship modified by activity level in older persons? *J Am Geriatr Soc* 1991;39:747–754.

Krumholz HM, Seeman TE, Merrill SS, et al. Lack of association between cholesterol and coronary heart disease mortality and morbidity and all-cause mortality in persons older than 70 years. *JAMA* 1994;272:1335–1340.

LaRosa JC, Applegate WB, Crouse JR, et al. Cholesterol lowering in the elderly: results of the Cholesterol Reduction in Seniors Program (CRISP) pilot study. *Arch Intern Med* 1994;154:529–539.

Manolio T, Pearson T, Wenger N, et al. Cholesterol and heart disease in older persons in women: review of an NHLBI workshop. *Ann Epidemiol* 1992;2:161–176.

Sempos C, Cleeman J, Carroll M, et al. Prevalence of high blood cholesterol among US adults. An update based on guidelines from the second report of the National Cholesterol Education Program Adult Treatment Panel. *JAMA* 1993;269:3009–3014.

Kelley's Textbook of Internal Medicine, fourth edition. Edited by H. David Humes.
Lippincott Williams & Wilkins, Philadelphia © 2000.

CHAPTER
458

APPROACH TO THE ELDERLY PATIENT WITH INCONTINENCE

JOSEPH G. OUSLANDER
THEODORE M. JOHNSON II

PRESENTATION AND SCOPE OF THE PROBLEM

Urinary incontinence, defined as the involuntary loss of urine severe enough to be a social or health problem, is a common, distressing, and costly health problem. Data indicate that as many as one-third of community-dwelling older adults and 50% to 70% of nursing home residents have some degree of urinary incontinence. The prevalence in acute hospitals and among functionally impaired older people living in the community is in the range of 30% to 50%. Urinary incontinence is more common with increasing age and among women, and is associated with impairments of cognitive and physical functioning.

Urinary incontinence can have adverse effects on physical health, psychosocial well being, and the cost of health care. It can contribute to skin irritation and breakdown and to urinary tract infections if managed inappropriately. A precipitant urge to void may contribute to falls in frail older persons with gait instability, especially at night. Incontinent persons are often embarrassed and reluctant to leave home and can thereby become isolated and depressed. Because it is onerous for community-dwelling older individuals and their caregivers to manage and because many residential facilities do not allow incontinent people to enter, incontinence often is an important contributing factor in the placement of an older person in a nursing home. The overall societal cost of incontinence for individuals age 65 and older has been estimated to be as high as $26 billion.

Because incontinence is embarrassing, and many older patients and their families believe it to be an inevitable consequence of old age, it is important to ask specifically about incontinence symptoms. Questions that can be helpful in identifying incontinent patients include: "Do you ever leak or lose urine when you don't want to?"; "Once your bladder feels full, how long can you hold it?"; "Do you ever have difficulty getting to the bathroom on time?"; "Do you ever wear a pad to protect you from wetness?"

Among older patients, the most common presenting symptoms of incontinence are irritative: urinary frequency during the day (voiding more frequently than every 2 hours), nocturia (two or more voids during normal sleeping hours), and a precipitant urge to void. Older women also commonly present with symptoms of stress incontinence (leakage with increases in intra-abdominal pressure caused by coughing, laughing, and bending). Many older women have mixed (irritative and stress) symptoms. Older men often have obstructive symptoms, which include the irritative symptoms already mentioned and hesitancy, a weak or intermittent stream, and straining to void. Some older patients have less specific symptoms, such as constant dribbling. In acute hospital and nursing home settings, incontinence can be identified and characterized by nursing staff caring for the patient on a regular basis.

PATHOPHYSIOLOGIC FACTORS

To maintain continence, the following criteria must be met:

1. Anatomical structures involved in urination must be intact, including the bladder, urethra, pelvic floor musculature, brain, spinal cord, and peripheral nerves that innervate the lower urinary tract.
2. The lower urinary tract must perform properly its two basic functions: urine storage and bladder emptying. Requirements

TABLE 458.1.	**POTENTIALLY REVERSIBLE CONDITIONS THAT CAN CAUSE OR CONTRIBUTE TO GERIATRIC URINARY INCONTINENCE**

Conditions	Management
Impaired ability or willingness to reach a toilet	
Delirium	Diagnosis and treatment of underlying cause(s) of acute confusional state
	Regular toileting assistance
Illness, injury, or restraint that interferes with mobility	Use of toilet substitutes
	Environmental alterations (e.g., bedside commode)
	Appropriate pharmacologic or nonpharmacologic treatment
Depression	
Irritation or inflammation in or around the lower urinary tract	
Urinary tract infection (symptomatic with new onset of frequency, urgency, and dysuria; sudden onset or worsening of incontinence; unexplained fever or functional decline in impaired patients)	Antimicrobial therapy
Atrophic vaginitis/urethritis	Oral or topical estrogen
Stool impaction	Disimpaction
	Appropriate use of stool softeners and laxatives if necessary
	Adequate mobility and fluid intake
Increased urine production	
Metabolic (hyperglycemia, hypercalcemia)	Better control of diabetes mellitus
	Therapy for hypercalcemia depends on underlying cause
Excess fluid intake	Reduction in intake of diuretic fluids (e.g., caffeinated beverages)
Volume overload	
Venous insufficiency with edema	Support stockings
	Leg elevation
	Sodium restriction
	Diuretic therapy
Congestive heart failure	Medical therapy
Drug side effects	
	Discontinuation of the offending medication if possible
Rapidly acting diuretics causing frequency and urgency	Dosage reduction or modification (e.g., flexible scheduling of rapid-acting diuretics)
Anticholinergics, narcotics, calcium channel blockers, α-adrenergic agonists (in men) causing urinary retention	
α-Adrenergic antagonists causing urethral relaxation and stress incontinence	
Psychotropic drugs with sedative or extrapyramidal effects causing sedation and immobility that interfere with toileting	

for storage include a compliant bladder, the absence of involuntary contractions, and appropriate sensation of bladder fullness. Requirements for emptying include a bladder capable of adequate contraction, lack of anatomical obstruction, and coordinated lowering of resistance in the bladder outlet and urethra during urination.

3. Adequate cognitive function must exist to recognize the need to void and to find an appropriate location.
4. Adequate physical function must exist to use a toilet or toilet substitute and manage clothing and hygiene.
5. The patient must have the motivation to be continent.
6. No environmental and iatrogenic factors can interfere with continence.

Thus, numerous factors can cause or contribute to urinary incontinence in an older person, including urologic and gynecologic disorders, neurologic conditions, psychological disorders, mobility and functional problems, and iatrogenic factors.

POTENTIALLY REVERSIBLE FACTORS

Several potentially reversible factors can cause or contribute to urinary incontinence (Table 458.1). The most common of these factors can be remembered by the acronym DRIP (delirium; restricted mobility, retention; infection, inflammation, impaction; polyuria, pharmaceuticals). Delirium and restricted mobility are common among geriatric patients when they become acutely ill; the latter may result directly from the patient's medical condition or from restrictions on mobility imposed by hospital or nursing home personnel. These conditions can produce incontinence by decreasing the patient's awareness of the need to void or ability to get a commode or use a toilet substitute. Unless an indwelling catheter is indicated to relieve an obstruction, this type of incontinence should be managed by environmental manipulations, scheduled toileting, appropriate use of toilet substitutes and pads, and careful attention to skin care until the underlying acute illness has resolved.

Urinary retention with overflow incontinence should be considered in any patient in whom urinary incontinence develops suddenly. Immobility, anticholinergic, narcotic, and α-adrenergic agonist drugs, and fecal impaction can all precipitate overflow incontinence in a geriatric patient. The existence of an underlying process that is causing spinal cord compression should also be considered.

Any inflammatory condition in the lower urinary tract that

causes frequency and urgency, such as cystitis or urethritis, can precipitate incontinence. Bacteriuria, however, should be treated only if it is associated with symptoms of urinary tract infection and not just for chronic stable incontinence (Table 458.1). Fecal impaction is common in acutely ill geriatric patients and has been associated with transient urinary as well as fecal incontinence.

Conditions that can cause polyuria, including hyperglycemia, excessive intake of coffee and tea, and mobilization of lower-extremity edema while supine, can also contribute to incontinence. These factors may be especially important in contributing to frequency and incontinence at night. Similar to many other conditions affecting the geriatric population, a wide variety of medications can play a role in the development of incontinence (Table 458.1). Whenever feasible, stopping the medication, switching to an alternative, or modifying the dosage schedule can be an important component of the treatment for incontinence (and possibly the only one necessary).

BASIC TYPES OF URINARY INCONTINENCE

There are four basic clinical types of urinary incontinence (Table 458.2). These types of incontinence are not mutually exclusive, and many older patients have more than one type. The most common type of incontinence in women younger than 75 years of age is stress incontinence. The most common type of incontinence among men and patients of both sexes older than 75 years is urge with involuntary bladder contractions (detrusor instability, or detrusor hyperreflexia when associated with a neu-

rologic disorder). Older women commonly present with "mixed" incontinence and have symptoms of both stress and urge types. Although involuntary bladder contractions are most often associated with urge incontinence and neurologic disorders such as stroke and dementia, they also occur in about one-third of women with stress incontinence and 50% to 60% of men with prostatic obstruction. Overflow incontinence is less common, but it important to recognize because of the potential for chronic large postvoid residual urine volumes to cause recurrent infections or upper urinary tract damage.

◼ DIAGNOSTIC EVALUATION

GENERAL APPROACH

Components of the diagnostic evaluation of an incontinent patient are shown in Table 458.3. The appropriate extent of the diagnostic evaluation, especially with respect to the need for cystourethroscopy and urodynamic tests, is controversial. These procedures are relatively invasive and expensive, requiring specialized equipment and personnel trained in their use and the interpretation of results. These procedures also are time consuming, are frequently uncomfortable, and put patients at risk of infection. On the other hand, in carefully selected patients, such procedures can be essential for determining an appropriate treatment plan. A general approach to the diagnostic evaluation is illustrated in Fig. 458.1.

TABLE 458.2.	BASIC TYPES AND CAUSES OF URINARY INCONTINENCE	
Type	**Symptoms**	**Common Causes**
Stress	Involuntary loss of urine (usually small amounts) simultaneous with increases in intra-abdominal pressure, such as those caused by coughing, laughing, and changing positions. Severe stress incontinence may be manifested by constant wetting	Weakness and laxity of pelvic floor musculature resulting in hypermobility of the bladder base and proximal urethra Bladder outlet or urethral sphincter weakness (intrinsic sphincter deficiency) related to prior surgery or trauma
Urge	Leakage of urine (usually larger, but often variable volumes) because of inability to delay voiding after sensation of bladder fullness is perceived	Bladder hyperactivity isolated or associated with one or more of the following: Local genitourinary condition, such as cystitis, urethritis, tumors, stones, diverticula, outflow obstruction; impaired bladder contractility Central nervous system disorders, such as stroke, dementia, parkinsonism, spinal cord injury or disease
Overflow	Leakage of urine (usually small amounts) resulting from mechanical forces on an overdistended bladder. May present similar to stress and urge	Anatomical obstruction by prostate, large cystocele that kinks the urethra A contractile bladder associated with diabetes mellitus or low spinal cord injury
Functional[a]	Urinary leakage associated with inability to toilet because of impairment of cognitive or physical functioning, psychological unwillingness, or environmental barriers	Severe dementia Immobility Physical restraints Inaccessible toilets Unavailability of regular toileting assistance Depression

[a] Functional incontinence should be a diagnosis of exclusion. Many frail geriatric patients have functional factors that may contribute to incontinence but may also have reversible and specifically treatable conditions underlying the incontinence.

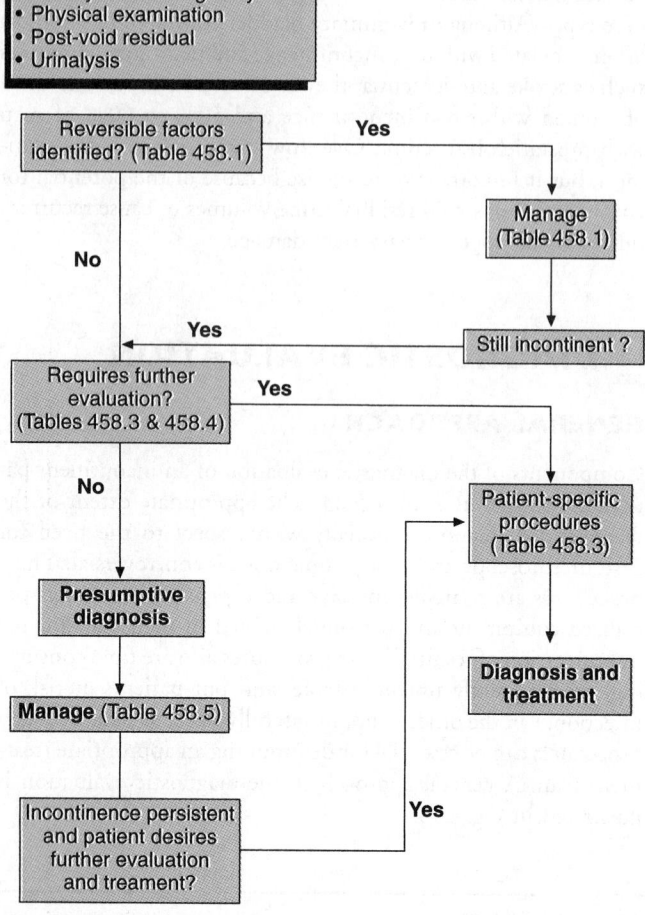

FIGURE 458.1. Basic approach for evaluation of geriatric urinary incontinence.

TABLE 458.3.

COMPONENTS OF THE DIAGNOSTIC EVALUATION OF GERIATRIC URINARY INCONTINENCE

Components	Indications
Basic Evaluation	All patients
History	
Physical examination	
Urinalysis	
Postvoid residual determination by catheterization or ultrasonography	Especially men or diabetics
Further Evaluation	
Urine culture and sensitivity	Patients with the new onset or worsening of incontinence, or symptoms or signs of a urinary tract infection (other than stable incontinence)
Blood urea nitrogen, serum creatinine	Urinary retention
Renal ultrasonography	Urinary retention
Blood glucose, calcium	Polyuria
Urine cytology	Hematuria (sterile) Risk factors for bladder cancer (smoking history, exposure to industrial carcinogens, e.g., aromatic amines contained in aniline dyes)
Prostate-specific antigen	Suspected cancer on digital examination in patients for whom diagnosis will influence management
Cystoscopy	Hematuria Suspected tumor, stone, diverticulum, other lesion
Urodynamic tests	
Cystometry	Suspected obstruction
Pressure flow study	Urinary retention
Urethral or leak point pressure	Uncertain diagnosis Planned surgical intervention

BASIC EVALUATION

All incontinent patients should have a focused history and physical examination, postvoid residual determination, and urinalysis (Table 458.3). The history should focus on a review of active medical problems and all medications; the onset of the incontinence and any precipitating factors; the timing, frequency, and amount of urine loss (voiding diaries, which record the timing and amount of continent and incontinent voids and precipitants of the incontinent episodes, can be helpful if the patient or a caregiver can complete them); and the irritative, stress, obstructive, or other symptoms associated with the incontinence.

The physical examination should include a basic assessment of cognitive function (such as questions about memory and orientation) and mobility (such as watching the patient rise from a chair and ambulate down a hallway). The exam should include a cardiovascular examination to detect signs of volume overload, especially in patients with nighttime symptoms; a neurologic examination focusing on the lumbosacral innervation and the exclusion of an occult neurologic disorder, such as parkinsonism or spinal cord lesion; suprapubic palpation after voiding; and pelvic and rectal examinations. The pelvic examination in

women should include observation of the timing and amount of any urine loss with stress maneuvers (e.g., forceful coughing). This should be done, whenever possible, while the patient's bladder is comfortably full in the supine and standing positions. Many older women have small cystoceles, which may or may not be related to the pathogenesis of their incontinence. Thus, the presence of a small cystocele should not automatically lead to consideration of surgical repair. Most older women who are not taking estrogen have vaginal mucosal atrophy (pale, thin vaginal mucosa with loss of folds); this finding should be differentiated from atrophic vaginitis, in which the preceding findings are present, along with inflammation and friability of the vaginal mucosa.

TABLE 458.4.	EXAMPLES OF CRITERIA FOR FURTHER UROLOGIC, GYNECOLOGIC, OR URODYNAMIC EVALUATION OF INCONTINENT GERIATRIC PATIENTS

Condition	Comments
History	
Recurrent symptomatic urinary tract infections in addition to the incontinence	A structural abnormality or pathologic condition in the urinary tract predisposing to symptomatic infection should be excluded
Physical examination	
Marked pelvic prolapse protruding through the vaginal introitus	Consideration should be given to surgical repair or pessary management to prevent discomfort and tissue erosion, as well as treat the incontinence
Suspicion of prostate cancer	Although surgical intervention to cure the cancer would not be appropriate for many older men, diagnosis of the cancer may be important in managing the incontinence and other complications, such as obstruction and urinary retention.
Urinalysis	
Hematuria (sterile)	Urologic evaluation should be considered to identify urinary tract lesion
Postvoid residual determination	
Residual volumes >200 mL	Although no precise cutoff point can be recommended, residual volumes >200 mL are abnormal and should lead to consideration of further evaluation of the urinary tract to identify complications (e.g., hydronephrosis, renal function impairment) and to determine the cause of the retention (obstruction, impaired bladder contractility, both)
Uncertain diagnosis	A presumptive diagnosis and treatment plan cannot be made based on the basic evaluation
Failure to respond to a therapeutic trial	Failure to respond to an adequate trial of behavioral or pharmacologic treatment in patients who want further treatment

A postvoid residual should be done within a few minutes after the patient voids by catheterization or ultrasonography. If catheterization is performed, the urine obtained should be sent for urinalysis. If not, a clean voided specimen should be collected for urinalysis.

FURTHER EVALUATION

Selected patients should have additional tests or be referred for further gynecologic, urologic, or urodynamic evaluation (Tables 458.3 and 458.4). Women who do not meet any of the criteria for referral can be treated initially for either stress or urge incontinence based on their predominant symptom. Women in whom both types of symptoms are common and bothersome can be treated with a combination of therapies (see next section). Men who do not meet criteria for referral and who have symptoms of urge incontinence can be given a therapeutic trial of behavioral or pharmacologic treatment. Patients who fail to respond adequately to behavioral and pharmacologic interventions or whose symptoms do not clearly fit with either stress, urge, or combined types of incontinence should also be referred for further gynecologic or urologic evaluation.

■ TREATMENT

Table 458.5 outlines the primary treatments for the four basic types of urinary incontinence. Other therapeutic approaches,

TABLE 458.5.	PRIMARY TREATMENTS FOR DIFFERENT TYPES OF GERIATRIC URINARY INCONTINENCE

Type of Incontinence	Primary Treatments
Stress	Behavioral therapy (pelvic muscle exercises, biofeedback)
	α-Adrenergic agonists
	Estrogen (added to α-agonist; topical preferred route of administration)
	Surgical bladder neck suspension
	Periurethral collagen injections
Urge	Behavioral therapy (bladder training, pelvic muscle exercises, biofeedback)
	Bladder relaxants
	Estrogen (if atrophic vaginitis present)
	Surgical removal of obstructing or other irritating pathologic lesions
Overflow	Surgical removal of obstruction
	Intermittent catheterization (if practical)
	Indwelling catheterization
Functional	Prompted voiding
	Environmental manipulations (accessible toilets)
	Incontinence undergarments and pads
	External collection devices
	Bladder relaxants (selected patients with concomitant urge incontinence)
	Indwelling catheters (selected patients)

such as electrical stimulation and the use of artificial sphincters, are also employed to treat urinary incontinence but are rarely used in older patients at present.

STRESS INCONTINENCE

Women whose initial evaluation suggests that stress incontinence is the predominant type should be instructed to perform pelvic muscle (Kegel) exercises and to void regularly to avoid a full bladder. To be effective, pelvic muscle exercises must be taught properly, practiced regularly by the patient, and used in the patient's everyday life to help prevent incontinent episodes. For this approach to be effective, patients must be motivated and capable of performing pelvic muscle exercises and practice them numerous times (e.g., up to 50 times) daily. Biofeedback using rectal or vaginal recordings of pressure or muscle activity may be a helpful adjunct in some patients if it is available. Factors such as obesity and chronic coughing should be addressed if possible. If these techniques are not successful and no contraindications exist, an α-agonist (pseudoephedrine 30 to 60 mg three times a day, phenylpropanolamine 75 mg twice a day, imipramine 10 to 25 mg three times a day) and estrogen (orally or vaginally) can be added. If the patient still has bothersome symptoms after an adequate trial of these treatments, or if she cannot (or is unwilling to) be treated with these approaches, she should be referred for further evaluation and consideration for surgery. Surgical bladder neck suspension procedures are highly effective and usually well tolerated when performed by an experienced surgeon in carefully selected older women with stress incontinence. For both female and male patients with stress incontinence that is primarily related to urethral sphincter weakness (as opposed to hypermobility of the bladder neck in women), periurethral injections of collagen may be effective.

URGE INCONTINENCE

Patients with urge incontinence can be treated with behavioral therapy. Pelvic muscle exercises work because voluntary contraction of pelvic floor muscles inhibits bladder spasticity and contraction. Other behavioral therapies include bladder training for functional and motivated patients, and scheduled toileting or prompted voiding for patients with impaired cognitive or physical functioning. Bladder relaxant drug therapy with an anticholinergic or antispasmodic agent can be added as necessary. All bladder relaxant drugs, including dicyclomine, imipramine, oxybutynin, and propantheline, have some systemic anticholinergic effects, and their use may be limited by bothersome side effects, especially dry mouth. Newer agents, such as tolterodine and extended-release oxybutynin, have fewer side effects, which may result in fewer patients discontinuing the medication. The development of urinary retention is of particular concern, and patients treated with these drugs should be carefully followed for symptoms of retention (and in some cases have periodic postvoid residual determinations). Men with irritative symptoms (urgency, urge incontinence, nocturia) associated with benign prostatic enlargement may benefit from a careful trial of an α-antagonist (e.g., terazosin, tamsulosin) if surgery is neither indicated nor desired for obstruction.

OVERFLOW INCONTINENCE

Patients with overflow incontinence due to anatomical obstruction require surgical intervention unless contraindicated. Patients with overflow incontinence due to an acontractile bladder should be treated with catheter drainage because pharmacologic treatment with a cholinergic agonist or α-adrenergic antagonist usually is not effective on a long-term basis. Although clean (nonsterile) intermittent catheterization may be the treatment of choice for younger patients with urinary retention due to neurologic disorders, this technique may be impractical for older patients who cannot perform it themselves and who do not have a caregiver available. Intermittent catheterization may also be uncomfortable and lead to complications in older men, and it may be unsafe in nursing homes where infection control practices and nosocomial infections are a concern. In these situations, a well-managed chronic indwelling catheter should be considered to relieve the urinary retention, control the incontinence, and prevent upper urinary tract damage and symptomatic infections.

FUNCTIONAL INCONTINENCE

The primary treatment for functional incontinence is a behaviorally oriented approach. The success of behavioral therapies for functionally impaired incontinent patients, such as prompted voiding, is critically dependent on the availability and motivation of caregivers in home and institutional settings. The appropriate use of environmental manipulations and toilet substitutes (e.g., portable commodes) can be helpful to these patients. For patients with functional incontinence who are suspected of also having urge incontinence, based on history and caregiver observations, a trial of a bladder relaxant may help if the patient is attempting to toilet regularly but is still having incontinence episodes. Because many of these patients have substantial impairment of cognitive function, they should be monitored carefully for the development of drug side effects. Nonspecific supportive management techniques, such as incontinence undergarments and pads and external catheters, can be helpful for patient comfort but should not be used as a convenience or in a manner that fosters further dependence. For severely impaired women who are agitated or uncomfortable from pain whenever they are toileted or changed, or who have skin lesions being contaminated by urine, use of an indwelling catheter is a reasonable approach. Chronic indwelling catheters should not, however, be used for functional incontinence unless a specific indication exists because of the risk of recurrent systematic urinary tract infections. When chronic catheters are indicated, careful catheter management may help prevent complications.

BIBLIOGRAPHY

Appell RA. Clinical efficacy and safety of tolterodine in the treatment of overactive bladder: a pooled analysis. *Urology* 1997;50(6A Suppl): 90–99.

Burgio KL, Locher JL, Goode PS, et al. Behavioral vs drug treatment for urge incontinence in older women: a randomized controlled trial. *JAMA* 1998;280(23):1995–2000.

Elbadawi A, Yalla SV, Resnick NM. Structural basis of geriatric voiding dysfunction. I. Methods of a prospective ultrastructural/urodynamic study and an overview of the findings. *J Urol* 1993;150:1650–1656.

Fantl JA, Bump RC, Robinson D, et al. Efficacy of estrogen supplementation in the treatment of urinary incontinence. The Continence Program for Women Research Group. *Obstet Gynecol* 1996;83(5):745–749.

Fantl JA, Newman DK, Colling J, et al. *Urinary incontinence in adults: acute and chronic management.* Clinical Practice Guideline No. 2, 1996 update. Rockville, MD: U.S. Department of Health and Human Services. Public Health Service, Agency for Health Care Policy and Research. AHCPR Publication No. 96-0682; 1996.

Johnson TM 2nd, Kincade JE, Bernard SL, et al. The association of urinary incontinence with poor self-rated health. *J Am Geriatr Soc* 1998;46:693–699.

Naughton MJ, Wyman JF. Quality of life in geriatric patients with lower urinary tract dysfunction. *Am J Med Sci* 1997;314(4):219–227.

Ouslander JG, Schnelle JF. Incontinence in the nursing home. *Ann Intern Med* 1995;122:438–449.

Resnick NM, Yalla SV, Laurino E. The pathophysiology of urinary incontinence among institutionalized elderly persons. *N Engl J Med* 1989;320:1–7.

Skelly J, Flint AJ. Urinary incontinence associated with dementia. *J Am Geriatr Soc* 1995;43:286–294.

CHAPTER
459

APPROACH TO THE ELDERLY PATIENT WITH ALTERED MENTAL STATUS

SHARON K. INOUYE

Acute alteration in mental status represents a leading presenting symptom for acutely ill older persons, accounting for at least 30% of emergency evaluations of older persons. In fact, alterations in mental status serve as a barometer for the underlying health status of elderly persons and are often the only manifestation of serious underlying disease.

Figure 459.1 presents a systematic approach to the evaluation of altered mental status in the older patient. The first step in evaluating altered mental status is to establish the patient's baseline cognitive functioning and the time–course of any cognitive changes. Chronic impairments developing or progressing over months to years are most likely attributable to a dementia, which should be evaluated accordingly (see Chapter 466). Acute alterations occurring over hours to weeks that may be superimposed on an underlying dementia should be further evaluated with cognitive assessment to determine whether delirium is present. If delirium features are not present (see below), then further evaluation for major depression, acute psychotic disorder, or other psychiatric disorders (see Chapters 39 and 460) is indicated. The focus of this chapter is delirium, or acute confusional

state, which is the most common and serious cause of acutely altered mental status in older persons.

DEFINITION OF DELIRIUM

The definition of and diagnostic criteria for delirium continue to evolve (Table 459.1). The standardized criteria for delirium appearing in the *Diagnostic and Statistical Manual Version IV (DSM-IV)* of the American Psychiatric Association are being used as the current diagnostic standard. However, these criteria were based on expert opinion, and their diagnostic sensitivity and specificity have not been tested. The Confusion Assessment Method (CAM) provides a simple, validated tool that is currently in widespread use for identification of delirium. The CAM algorithm, which is based on the presence of the features of acute onset and fluctuating course, inattentiveness, and either disorganized speech or altered level of consciousness, has a sensitivity of 94% to 100%, specificity of 90% to 95%, and negative predictive value of 90% to 100% for delirium.

INCIDENCE AND EPIDEMIOLOGY

The prevalence of delirium—that is, cases present at the time of hospital admission—ranges from 14% to 24%, and the incidence of delirium—that is, new cases arising during hospitalization—ranges from 6% to 56%. The rates of postoperative delirium are estimated at 10% to 52%. Higher delirium rates are found when more frequent and sensitive surveillance methods are used in populations that include older, surgical, and intensive care patients. Hospital mortality rates associated with delirium range from 25% to 33%, analogous to rates associated with acute myocardial infarction or sepsis. Based on extrapolations from U.S. vital health statistics, each year delirium complicates hospital stays for over 2.3 million older persons, involving in excess of 17.5 million inpatient days and accounting for more than $4 billion (1994 U.S. dollars) of Medicare expenditures. Moreover, substantial additional costs associated with delirium accrue after hospital discharge because of the increased need for institutionalization, rehabilitation services, home health care, and other health care services.

ETIOLOGIC FACTORS

MULTIFACTORIAL MODEL

Similar to other common geriatric syndromes (e.g., falls, incontinence, and pressure sores), delirium represents an intrinsically multifactorial syndrome. Thus, the development of delirium usually involves a complex interrelationship between a vulnerable patient with pertinent predisposing factors and noxious insults or precipitating factors. For example, patients who are highly vulnerable to delirium at baseline (e.g., such as cognitively

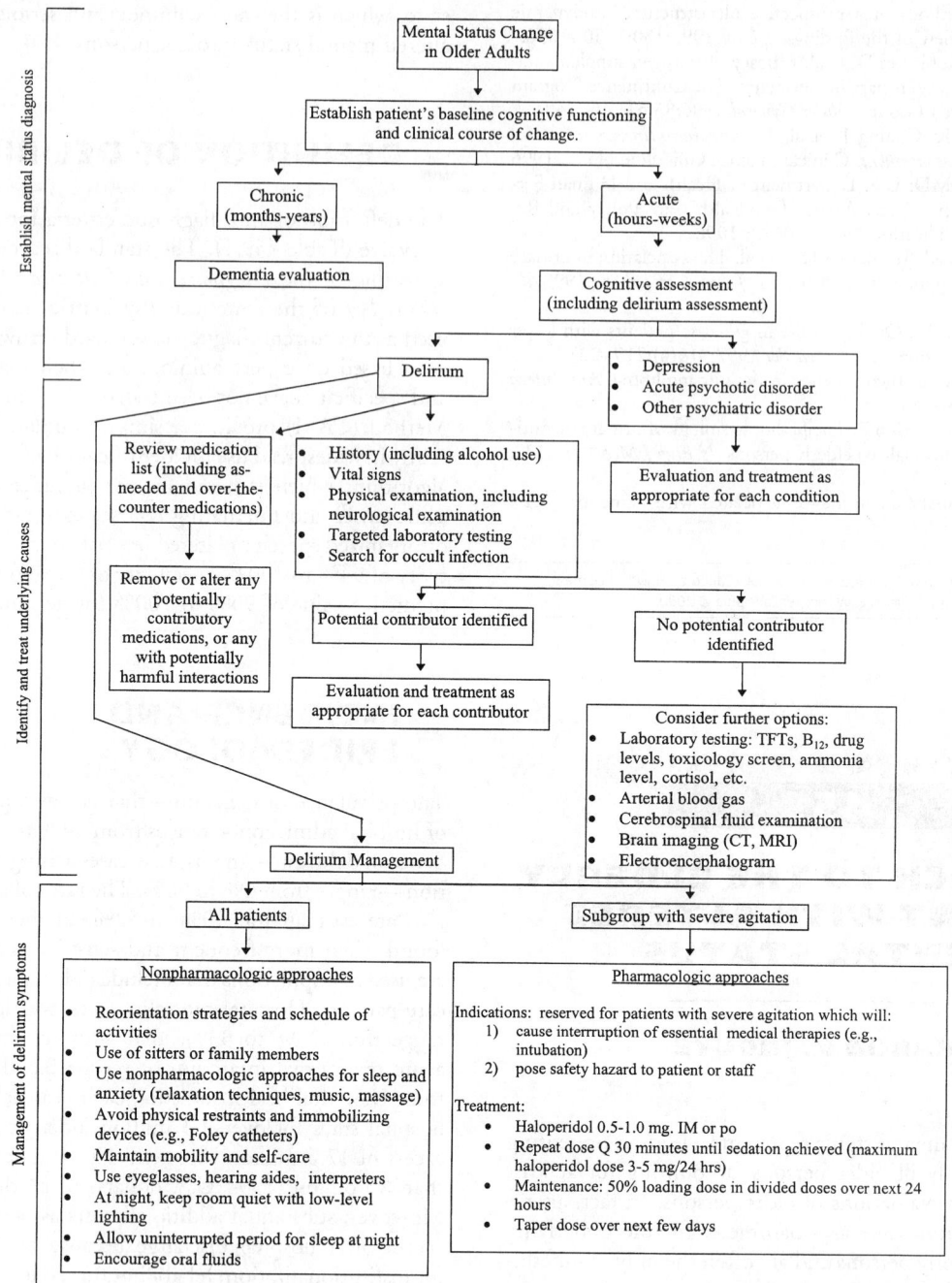

FIGURE 459.1. A systematic approach to the evaluation of mental status change in the older adult. TFT, thyroid function tests; B_{12}, vitamin B_{12} assay; CT, computed tomography; MRI, magnetic resonance imaging; IM, intramuscular injection; PO, oral administration.
EVIDENCE LEVEL: A: Inouye SK, Van Dyck CH, Alessi CA, et al. Clarigying confusion: the confusion assessment method. A new method for detection of delirium. *Ann Intern Med* 1990;113:941–948.

impaired or severely ill patients) may develop delirium with even relatively benign insults, such as a single dose of a sedative medication (e.g., diphenhydramine). Conversely, patients who are not vulnerable would be relatively resistant, with delirium resulting only after exposure to multiple noxious insults. The effects of multiple risk factors appears to be cumulative. To the clinician, the importance of this multifactorial etiologic process is that removal or treatment of one factor alone is usually insufficient to resolve the delirium. Instead, the full spectrum of predisposing and precipitating factors must be addressed.

TABLE 459.1.	**DIAGNOSTIC CRITERIA FOR DELIRIUM**

The Confusion Assessment Method (CAM) Diagnostic Algorithm[a]

Feature 1. Acute Onset and Fluctuating Course
This feature is usually obtained from a family member or nurse and is shown by positive responses to the following questions: Is there evidence of an acute change in mental status from the patient's baseline? Did the (abnormal) behavior fluctuate during the day, that is, tend to come and go, or increase and decrease in severity?

Feature 2. Inattention
This feature is shown by a positive response to the following question: Did the patient have difficulty focusing attention, for example, being easily distractible, or having difficulty keeping track of what was being said?

Feature 3. Disorganized Thinking
This feature is shown by a positive response to the following question: Was the patient's thinking disorganized or incoherent, such as rambling or irrelevant conversation, unclear or illogical flow of ideas, or unpredictable switching from subject to subject?

Feature 4. Altered Level of Consciousness
This feature is shown by any answer other than "alert" to the following question: Overall, how would you rate this patient's level of consciousness? [alert (normal), vigilant (hyperalert), lethargic (drowsy, easily aroused), stupor (difficult to arouse), or coma (unarousable)].

The diagnosis of delirium by CAM requires the presence of features 1 and 2 and either 3 or 4.

Diagnostic and Statistical Manual (DSM-IV) Diagnostic Criteria

A. There is a disturbance of consciousness (reduced clarity of awareness of the environment) with reduced ability to focus, sustain, or shift attention.

B. There is a change in cognition (such as memory deficit, disorientation, language disturbance) or the development of a perceptual disturbance that is not better accounted for by a preexisting, established, or evolving dementia.

C. The disturbance develops over a short period of time (usually hours to days) and tends to fluctuate during the course of the day.

D. There is evidence from the history, physical examination, or laboratory findings that the disturbance is caused by the direct physiologic consequences of a general medical condition.

[a] These ratings should be completed after brief cognitive assessment, such as the Mini-Mental State Examination.

PREDISPOSING FACTORS

Predisposing factors for delirium include preexisting cognitive impairment or dementia, severe underlying illness and comorbidity, functional impairment, advanced age, chronic renal insufficiency, dehydration, malnutrition, and vision or hearing impairment. Dementia is an important and consistent risk factor for delirium, and patients with dementia have a twofold to fivefold increased risk for delirium. Moreover, one-third to one-half of delirious patients have an underlying dementia. Nearly any chronic medical illness can predispose to delirium, including diseases involving the central nervous system (e.g., Parkinson's disease, cerebrovascular disease, mass lesions, trauma, infection, collagen vascular disease), as well as diseases outside the central nervous system, such as infectious, metabolic, cardiac, pulmonary, endocrine, and neoplastic diseases. A validated predictive model, developed to determine delirium risk at the time of hospital admission, identified the following independent predisposing factors: severe underlying illness, vision impairment, baseline cognitive impairment, and high blood urea nitrogen/creatinine ratio (used as an index of dehydration).

PRECIPITATING FACTORS

Leading precipitating factors identified in previous studies have included medications (see below), immobilization, use of indwelling bladder catheters, use of physical restraints, dehydration, malnutrition, iatrogenic events, medical illnesses, infections, metabolic derangement, alcohol or drug intoxication or withdrawal, environmental influences, and psychosocial factors. Immobilization can lead to delirium and functional decline within a few days, yet physicians routinely order bed rest or minimal activity in 57% of patient-days of hospitalization, often without medical justification. Moreover, medical devices (e.g., indwelling bladder catheters and physical restraints) can further contribute to immobilization. Iatrogenic events, occurring in 29% to 38% of older patients, include complications of diagnostic or therapeutic procedures, transfusion reactions, bleeding due to over-anticoagulation, and the like. Insufficiency of any major organ system can precipitate delirium, particularly renal or hepatic failure. Occult respiratory failure has emerged as an increasing problem in elderly patients, often lacking the typical signs and symptoms of dyspnea and tachypnea, and easily overlooked by measuring oxygen saturation alone. Acute myocardial infarction or congestive heart failure commonly presents as delirium or "failure to thrive" in an elderly patient, without the usual symptoms of chest pain or dyspnea. Occult infection is a particularly noteworthy cause of delirium, since older patients frequently fail to mount the expected febrile or leukocytic response to infections, such as pneumonia, urinary tract infection, endocarditis, abdominal abscess, or infected joint. Metabolic disorders may contribute to delirium, such as hyper- or hyponatremia, hypercalcemia, acid–base disorder, hypo- and hyperglycemia, thyroid or adrenal disorders. A validated predictive model, developed to determine delirium risk based on exposure to precipitating factors during the course of hospitalization, identified the following independent precipitating factors: use of physical restraints, malnutrition, more than three medications added during the previous day, indwelling bladder catheter, and any iatrogenic event.

DRUG USE AND DELIRIUM

Medications, the most common remediable cause of delirium, contribute to at least 40% of delirium cases. Many medications can cause delirium; the most common are those with known psychoactive effects, such as sedative-hypnotics, narcotics, H_2-blockers, and medicines with anticholinergic effects. In previous studies, use of any psychoactive medication was associated with a 4-fold increased risk of delirium, whereas use of two or more psychoactive medications was associated with a 5-fold risk. Sedative-hypnotic drugs have been associated with a 3- to 12-fold increased risk of delirium; narcotics with a 3-fold risk; and anticholinergic drugs with a 5- to 12-fold risk. Delirium increases in direct proportion to the number of medications prescribed due to adverse effects of the medications themselves, as well as the increased risk of drug–drug and drug–disease interactions. Recent studies provide strong evidence that inappropriate use and overuse of psychoactive medications are common in older patients, and that many cases of delirium and related adverse drug events may be preventable.

PATHOGENESIS

The pathogenetic mechanisms of delirium remain obscure. Delirium appears to be a functional rather than a structural lesion, with electroencephalographic studies demonstrating global functional derangements and generalized slowing of cortical background (alpha) activity. The leading hypothesis considers delirium to be the final common pathway of many different pathogenetic mechanisms, culminating in widespread reduction of cerebral oxidative metabolism with resultant impairment of cholinergic transmission. Proposed mediators examined have included β-endorphin, somatostatin, lymphokines, tryptophan, phenylalanine metabolites, and cortisol. Although delirium has been considered a transient syndrome, several of these basic mechanisms may not be reversible, particularly those resulting in hypoxic tissue injury. Moreover, the dose and duration of the insult may impact greatly on the reversibility of the delirium.

CLINICAL FINDINGS

KEY FEATURES

The cardinal features of delirium are acute onset and inattentiveness. Determining the acuity of onset requires accurate knowledge of the patients' baseline cognitive functioning. Extra effort may be required to ascertain this information, such as pursuing a reliable informant (e.g., family member, caregiver, or nurse). Another key feature is the fluctuating course of delirium, with symptoms tending to come and go or increase and decrease in severity over a 24 hour period. Lucid intervals are characteristic, which can sometimes be misleading. Inattentiveness is recognized as difficulty with focusing, maintaining, and shifting attention. Delirious patients appear easily distracted, have difficulty following commands, and often perseverate with an answer to a previous question. On cognitive testing, patients may manifest difficulty with simple repetition tasks, digit spans, or backward recitation of months. Other key features include a disorganization of thought, a manifestation of underlying cognitive or perceptual disturbances, and altered level of consciousness (typically lethargy, with reduced awareness of the environment). Although not cardinal elements, features commonly associated with delirium include disorientation, cognitive deficits (e.g., memory impairment, aphasia), psychomotor agitation or retardation, perceptual disturbances (e.g., hallucinations, illusions), paranoid delusions, emotional lability, and sleep–wake cycle disruption.

FORMS OF DELIRIUM

Delirium can present in either hypoactive or hyperactive forms. The hypoactive form of delirium—characterized by lethargy and reduced psychomotor activity—is the most common form in older patients. This form of delirium is often unrecognized and is associated with a poorer overall prognosis. The hyperactive form of delirium, in which the patient is agitated, vigilant, and often hallucinating, is rarely missed. Importantly, patients can fluctuate between the hypoactive and hyperactive forms. Moreover, partial or incomplete forms of delirium have been recognized to be common, particularly during the resolution stages of delirium.

DIFFERENTIAL DIAGNOSIS

The leading differential diagnoses for delirium (Fig. 459.1) are dementia, depression, and nonorganic psychotic disorders. The most difficult challenge in differential diagnosis is distinguishing dementia, a longstanding confusional state, from delirium alone or delirium superimposed on dementia. The differential diagnosis is crucial, however, because delirium often represents a medical emergency; obtaining the history is critical to making this distinction. These two conditions are differentiated both by the acuity of symptom onset in delirium (dementia is much more insidious), and the impaired attention and altered level of consciousness associated with delirium. It is important to note that disorientation and memory impairment are not useful in differential diagnosis because these features may be present with both conditions and may be absent in delirium. Other conditions for differential diagnoses include depression and nonorganic psychotic disorders. Although paranoia, hallucinations, and affective changes can occur with delirium, the key delirium features of acute onset, inattentiveness, altered level of consciousness, and global cognitive impairment will assist with the recognition of delirium. In cases involving an uncooperative patient or where an accurate history is unavailable, it may not be possible to establish the diagnosis with certainty. In these cases, because of the potentially life-threatening nature of delirium and its high occurrence rate in the older hospitalized population, it is prudent to manage the symptoms as a delirium and search for reversible insults (e.g., intercurrent illness, metabolic derangements, drug toxicity) until further information can be obtained.

CLINICAL ASSESSMENT AND LABORATORY FINDINGS

Delirium is a clinical diagnosis, relying on careful observation and history taking from reliable informants. Identification of the multifactorial contributors to the delirium is of critical importance because many of these factors are treatable; if left untreated, they may result in substantial morbidity and mortality. Because the potential contributors are innumerable, the search requires astute clinical judgment combined with a thorough medical evaluation. The challenge is enhanced by the frequently nonspecific, atypical, or muted presentation of the underlying illness in older persons. In fact, delirium may be the *only* sign of underlying life-threatening illness, such as pneumonia, urosepsis, or myocardial infarction, in the geriatric population.

The first step in evaluation should include cognitive assessment and determining any acute change from the patient's baseline level of cognitive functioning. Because cognitive impairment can be easily missed during routine conversation, a brief cognitive screening test, such as the Mini-Mental Status Examination, is recommended. Attention should be assessed with simple tests, such as a forward digit span (inattentiveness indicated by inability to repeat five digits forward) or a backward recitation of the months. The comprehensive history and physical examination remains the cornerstone of the evaluation of delirium. The history should be targeted to establishing the patient's baseline cognitive functioning and the course of any mental status changes, as well as obtaining clues about potential precipitating factors, such as recent medication changes, intercurrent infections, or medical illnesses. The physical examination should include a detailed neurologic examination for focal deficits and a careful search for signs of head trauma, infection, or other acute medical process.

Review of the medication list, including over-the-counter medications, should be carried out for every patient. Medications with psychoactive effects should be removed or minimized whenever possible. In older patients, psychoactive medications may cause adverse effects even at dosages and measured drug levels that are within the "therapeutic range." When these medications cannot be removed, dosage reduction or substitution of less toxic alternatives is recommended. The side effects and potential interactions of all current drugs should be reviewed. Finally, chronic medication and alcohol use should be carefully reviewed to evaluate for any potential withdrawal effects; often high-risk substance use is unrecognized or overlooked during the initial phase of the acute illness and hospitalization.

For the laboratory assessment, the evaluation must be tailored to the individual situation, requiring substantial clinical judgment. An astute history and physical examination, review of medications, targeted laboratory testing, and search for occult infection should be adequate to identify the majority of potential contributors to the delirium. Further testing should be tailored to the clinical picture (e.g., further laboratory testing might include thyroid function tests, vitamin B_{12} level, drug levels or toxicology screen, ammonia level). In patients with cardiac or respiratory diseases, or with related symptoms, an electrocardiogram and/or arterial blood gas determination may be indicated. The indications for cerebrospinal fluid examination, brain imaging, or electroencephalography remains controversial. Overall, these tests are probably indicated in less than 10% of delirium cases, and the diagnostic yield for these procedures is low. Clearly, cerebrospinal fluid examination is indicated for febrile delirious patients where meningitis or encephalitis is suspected. Brain imaging (computed tomography and magnetic resonance imaging) should be reserved for patients with new focal neurologic signs, with history or signs of head trauma, or without another identifiable cause of delirium. Electroencephalography, with a false-negative rate of 17% and a false-positive rate of 22% for distinguishing delirious and nondelirious patients, has a limited role. It is most useful in the detection of occult seizure disorders and in the differentiation of delirium from nonorganic psychiatric disorders.

STRATEGIES FOR OPTIMAL MANAGEMENT

PREVENTION OF DELIRIUM

Preventing delirium before it occurs, or primary prevention, is the most effective strategy to reduce delirium and its attendant complications. Preventive strategies addressing delirium risk factors have been shown to be effective in a controlled clinical trial. Ideally, preventive strategies should address both predisposing and precipitating factors for delirium. Table 459.2 indicates well-documented delirium risk factors and tested preventive interventions for each risk factor. These risk factors were selected since current evidence supports both the clinical relevance and the remediable nature of each risk factor with practical interventions. Implementation of these preventive interventions resulted

TABLE 459.2.	**DELIRIUM RISK FACTORS AND RECOMMENDED INTERVENTIONS**
Risk Factor	**Recommended Intervention**
Cognitive impairment	▪ Orientation protocol: includes orientation board with name of care team members and day's schedule; reorienting communication. ▪ Therapeutic activities protocol: provides cognitively stimulating activities three times daily, such as current events, structured reminiscence, and word games.
Sleep deprivation	▪ Nonpharmacologic sleep protocol: at bedtime, provides warm drink (milk or herbal tea), relaxation tapes or music, and back massage. ▪ Sleep enhancement protocol: reinforces unti-wide noise reduction strategies (e.g., silent pill crushers, vibrating beepers, reduced hallway noise) and adjusting schedule to allow sleep (e.g., rescheduling medications, vital signs, procedures).
Immobility	▪ Early-mobilization protocol: provides ambulation or active range-of-motion exercises three times daily; minimizes use of immobilizing equipment (e.g., bladder catheters, physical restraints).
Visual impairment	▪ Vision protocol: offers visual aids (e.g., eyeglasses, magnifying lenses) and adaptive equipment (e.g., large illuminated phone dials, large-print books, fluorescent tape on call bell). Daily reinforcement of use of adaptations.
Hearing impairment	▪ Hearing protocol: supplies portable amplifying devices, ear wax disimpaction, and special communication techniques. Daily reinforcement of use of adaptations.
Dehydration	▪ Dehydration protocol: provides early recognition and volume repletion measures (i.e., encouraging oral fluids).

in a 40% risk reduction for delirium in hospitalized older patients.

NONPHARMACOLOGIC MANAGEMENT

For management of delirium symptoms, nonpharmacologic approaches should be used for every delirious patient and are beneficial in most patients. These approaches include presence of family members, orienting influences, use of sitters, transferring a disruptive patient to a private room or closer to the nurse's station (for increased supervision). Personal contact and communication are of vital importance, using reorientation strategies, simple instructions, and frequent eye contact. Patients should be allowed to participate in decision making about their care as much as possible. Eyeglasses and hearing aids should be worn to reduce sensory deficits. Mobility, self-care, and independence should be encouraged; physical restraints should be avoided because of their adverse effects on mobility and emotional state, their questionable efficacy, and their potential to increase patient agitation and cause injury. Clocks, calendars, and the day's schedule should be provided to assist with orientation. Room and staff changes should be kept to a minimum. A quiet environment with low-level lighting is optimal for the delirious patient. Provision of an uninterrupted period for sleep at night is of critical importance in the management of the delirious patient. This requires coordination of nursing and medical procedures, such as medications, vital signs, intravenous fluids, and treatments. System-wide changes may be needed to ensure a low level of noise at night, including hallway noise and conversations. Nonpharmacologic approaches for relaxation, including music, relaxation tapes, and massage, can be highly effective in the management of agitation in patients with delirium.

DRUG THERAPY

Pharmacologic approaches should be reserved for patients with severe agitation, which may result in the interruption of essential medical therapies (e.g., intubation, intra-aortic balloon pumps, dialysis catheters) or may endanger the safety of the patient or staff. However, any drug used for the treatment of delirium will have psychoactive effects, which may further cloud the patient's mental status and obscure efforts to follow his or her mental status. Thus, the drug should be given in the lowest dose for the shortest time possible. Neuroleptics are the preferred agents of treatment, with haloperidol representing the most widely used treatment for delirium. If parenteral administration is required, intravenous use results in rapid onset of action with short duration of effect, whereas intramuscular use has a more optimal duration of action. The recommended starting dose of haloperidol is 0.5 to 1.0 mg orally or parenterally, followed by a repeated dose every 20 to 30 minutes after vital signs have been checked until sedation has been achieved. The end point should be an awake but manageable patient. The average elderly patient who has not previously been treated with neuroleptics should require a total loading dose of no more than 3 to 5 mg of haloperidol. Subsequently, a maintenance dose of one-half of the loading dose should be administered in divided doses over the next 24 hours, with tapering doses over the next few days. The leading

side effects of haloperidol include sedation, hypotension, acute dystonias and extrapyramidal side effects, and anticholinergic effects (e.g., dry mouth, constipation, urinary retention).

Benzodiazepines are not recommended for treatment of delirium because of their tendency to cause oversedation and exacerbation of the confusional state. However, they remain the drugs of choice for treatment of withdrawal syndromes from alcohol and sedative drugs. For geriatric patients, lorazepam is the recommended agent of this class because of its favorable half-life (10 to 15 hours), lack of active metabolites, and availability of a parenteral form.

HOSPITAL-WIDE CHANGES

The optimal management of delirium requires system-wide changes to improve the quality of hospital care for older patients. Interventions needed to reduce delirium rates include education of physicians and nurses to improve recognition and heighten awareness of the clinical implications of delirium; encouragement of cognitive assessment of all elderly hospitalized patients; provision of incentives to change practice patterns that lead to delirium (e.g., immobilization, overuse of psychoactive medications, bladder catheters, and physical restraint); and creation of systems that enhance high-quality geriatric care (e.g., geriatric expertise, case management, clinical pathways, and quality monitoring for delirium). With its common occurrence, its frequently iatrogenic nature, and its close linkage to the processes of care, incident delirium serves as an invaluable marker for the quality of hospital care and provides an opportunity for overall improvement.

Acknowledgments

Supported in part by grants from the National Institute on Aging (No. RO1AG12551 and K24AG00949) and the Patrick and Catherine Weldon Donaghue Medical Research Foundation (No. DF98-105). The author thanks Ms. Robbin Bonanno for invaluable assistance in this work.

BIBLIOGRAPHY

American Psychiatric Association. *Diagnostic and statistical manual of mental disorders (DSM-IV)*, fourth ed. Washington, DC, 1994.

Elie M, Cole MG, Primeau FJ, et al. Delirium risk factors in elderly hospitalized patients. *J Gen Intern Med* 1998;13:204–212.

Francis J. Delirium in older patients. *J Am Geriatr Soc* 1992;40:829–838.

Inouye SK. The dilemma of delirium: clinical and research controversies regarding diagnosis and evaluation of delirium in hospitalized elderly medical patients. *Am J Med* 1994;97:278–288.

Inouye SK, Bogardus ST Jr, Charpentier PA, et al. A multicomponent intervention to prevent delirium in hospitalized older patients. *N Engl J Med* 1999;340:669–676.

Inouye SK, Charpentier PA. Precipitating factors for delirium in hospitalized elderly patients: predictive model and interrelationship with baseline vulnerability. *JAMA* 1996;275:852–857.

Inouye SK, van Dyck CH, Alessi CA, et al. Clarifying confusion: The Confusion Assessment Method. A new method for detection of delirium. *Ann Intern Med* 1990;113:941–948.

Rummans TA, Evans JM, Krahn LE, et al. Delirium in elderly patients: evaluation and management. *Mayo Clin Proc* 1995;70:989–998.

Kelley's Textbook of Internal Medicine, fourth edition. Edited by H. David Humes. Lippincott Williams & Wilkins, Philadelphia © 2000.

CHAPTER
460
APPROACH TO THE ELDERLY PATIENT WITH DEPRESSION

DAN G. BLAZER

Depression is a common syndrome among elderly patients that is caused by a number of different diseases and psychosocial stressors that can afflict older adults. The causes of depression range from carcinoma of the pancreas to bereavement. Although most elderly people are satisfied with their lives and experience only episodic or mild symptoms of depression, persistent and severe depression must not be overlooked in diagnostic workups and therapeutic interventions prescribed by physicians caring for older adults.

The symptomatic presentations of depression in late life are by and large similar to the presentations throughout adulthood. The differences in symptom presentation that often are attributed to increased age, such as pseudodementia and depression masked as physical illness, are usually secondary to comorbidity (i.e., depression associated with dementia or physical illness and therefore not related to age). However, depressed older adults may differ from the depressed in middle age in that they more often experience weight loss and less often report feelings of worthlessness and guilt. Although elderly people suffering from major depression perform less well on objective tests of cognitive functioning, they are no more likely to complain of memory problems and concentration than middle-aged depressives.

PATHOPHYSIOLOGIC FACTORS

Biologic, psychological, and social factors contribute to the etiologic process of depression. Even in the so-called biologic depressions, psychological and social factors contribute to the onset and progression of the depressive syndrome. The relative contribution of the various factors to depression may vary with age. Among the biologic factors, structural changes (subcortical white matter lesions now designated as vascular depression) are found more frequently in the brains of older adults suffering from major depression when studied with magnetic resonance imaging. These changes are more prevalent in the depressed elderly than in age-matched older adults diagnosed with dementia of the Alzheimer's disease type, as well as in age-matched controls.

Recent studies suggest that persons with vascular depression present with a different symptom profile, such as more frequent anhedonia and with fewer psychological symptoms.

Dysregulation of the neurotransmitter system has been the most frequently implicated biologic factor contributing to depression at all ages. Studies have documented differences in neuronal transmission in depression. For example, platelets, a derivative of tissue of neural origin, contain natural binding sites for the antidepressant imipramine. When imipramine is radioactively labeled, persons diagnosed with major depression exhibit a decrease in binding sites compared with control subjects. By this technique, depressed elderly individuals exhibit a decreased number of binding sites (they are down-regulated) compared with persons of similar age who are not depressed.

Dysregulation of the hypothalamic–pituitary–adrenal axis has also been implicated as a biologic cause of depression. Depressed patients usually exhibit elevated cortisol levels and are less likely to suppress cortisol secretion when given dexamethasone (the dexamethasone suppression test). Older adults less than 75 years of age usually exhibit hypothalamic–pituitary–adrenal function similar to that of middle-aged adults. However, in persons older than 75 years, elevated dexamethasone cortical levels are commonly seen. Older adults may therefore also be more biologically predisposed to depression secondary to a breakdown of hypothalamic–pituitary–adrenal regulation.

Some investigators have suggested that the elderly are psychologically predisposed to depression because they experience losses of family and friends more often than younger people. In most cases, however, the elderly appear to tolerate loss of significant others better than those who are younger. One reason for this increased adaptation to loss is that loss in late life is an "on-time" event; that is, older adults anticipate that they will lose spouses, siblings, and lifelong companions. They often mentally rehearse their adjustment to the loss, even though they may not discuss an anticipated loss openly. Older adults also appear somewhat more protected from the adverse consequences of a breakdown in their social support system. Therefore, even though the elderly may be more biologically vulnerable to the onset and progression of depression than middle-aged people, they also may be more psychologically protected.

LABORATORY STUDIES AND DIAGNOSTIC TESTS

The evaluation of the symptoms and history of the depressive syndrome remains the cornerstone of the diagnostic workup of the depressed older adult. The history and physical examination should be accompanied by a review of all current medications, both those prescribed and those bought over the counter. Many drugs, such as sedative-hypnotic and antihypertensive agents, can precipitate a depressive episode. Laboratory tests inform the clinician of systemic illnesses that cause depressive symptoms (Table 460.1). Measurement of vitamin B_{12} levels can uncover pernicious anemia, and thyroid function studies can disclose hypothyroidism. Thyroid dysfunction during an episode of late-life depression is usually minimal, however, and returns to normal with recovery from the depressive episode.

TABLE 460.1.	ABNORMALITIES ON LABORATORY TESTS ASSOCIATED WITH SEVERE MAJOR DEPRESSION IN THE ELDERLY

Abnormality	Incidence (%)
Hyperintensities in subcortical regions of the brain on magnetic resonance imaging	30–50
Nonsuppression of cortisol after dexamethasone administration	50–70
Decreased RFM latency and decreased stage 4 sleep on polysomnography	70
Mild lowering of thyroxine and elevation of thyroid-stimulating hormone on thyroid function studies	>50

Given the increased evidence of vascular lesions among the depressed elderly, there is reason to order magnetic resonance imaging to further refine the diagnosis of late-life depression and predict the prognosis. Nevertheless, the test is expensive and it does not inform the clinician regarding therapy. Sleep abnormalities in people suffering from depression in late life and in normal elderly people are similar and include decreased rapid-eye-movement latency, increased awakenings during the night, and early morning awakening; however, depressed elderly patients exhibit these changes more than age-matched controls. Polysomnography is not of value in the routine workup of major depression.

DIFFERENTIAL DIAGNOSIS

Most older adults who complain of depression to a primary care physician suffer from minor or subsyndromal depression (a depression that does not meet criteria for either major depression or dysthymic disorder). Many of these depressed elders may suffer from adjustment disorder with depressed mood or adjustment disorder with mixed depressed and anxious mood. Others, however, suffer intermittent mood swings that are not associated with environmental stressors. Still others are either entering a major depressive episode or are recovering from an episode. Some investigators have suggested that subsyndromal depression can be effectively treated with low doses of antidepressant medication. However, no studies to date have conclusively demonstrated the efficacy of pharmacologic therapy for minor, intermittent depressive symptoms in late life.

Although less common, major depression is the most severe of the depressive syndromes in late life. The disorder is diagnosed when the elderly person reports a 2-week history of a depressed mood or loss of interest or pleasure in usual activities, plus four of the following symptoms: poor appetite or weight loss; insomnia; psychomotor agitation or retardation; lethargy; feelings of worthlessness or self-reproach; difficulty concentrating; and suicidal thoughts. The clinician can usefully disaggregate the symptoms into biologic (such as sleep disturbance, decreased appetite, psychomotor agitation or retardation, diurnal variation in severity of symptoms, and previous response to a biologic therapy) versus psychological symptoms (such as guilt and worry). When

major depression is severe, a psychotic episode (presence of mood-congruent delusions and auditory hallucinations) must be distinguished from a nonpsychotic depression. Between 10% and 20% of elderly persons suffering from major depression report a history of manic episodes. Other elderly persons suffer episodes of mania but never experience an episode of major depression. In both cases, the elderly patients are diagnosed with bipolar disorder.

Dysthymic disorder is a less severe but more chronic depressive syndrome. The elderly person must have suffered persistent depression for all or most of 2 years to meet diagnostic criteria for this disorder. Dysthymic disorder rarely begins in late life and is usually a residual disorder from middle age. Nevertheless, this chronic disorder can be exacerbated by psychosocial stressors of physical disability. Dysthymic disorder and major depression often coexist (an elder with dysthymic disorder falling into a more severe depressive episode), but many elders experience dysthymic disorder without ever experiencing an episode of major depression.

Major depression accompanies dementia of the Alzheimer's disease type and vascular dementia in about 20% of cases. Therefore, a most important diagnostic task is not the differentiation of depression from dementia per se but rather the recognition of a treatable depression in the midst of dementia. Other age-related disorders can mimic depressive disorders. Idiopathic insomnia is a common and disturbing disorder for many elderly people. The combination of significant sleep problems and mood changes that accompany loss of sleep must be differentiated from a major depression that presents with significant sleep abnormalities. Idiopathic insomnia is more likely to be insidious in onset, whereas the sleep problems that accompany major depression are more acute in onset. Physical illnesses, such as chronic congestive heart failure, cause the older adult to lose energy and report less pleasure from life. A depressed mood may be a reaction to the physical disability.

STRATEGIES FOR OPTIMAL CARE MANAGEMENT

The treatment of late-life depression includes four essential components: removal of causative factors, such as medications; pharmacotherapy; psychotherapy; and electroconvulsive therapy (ECT). Each of these interventions requires close coordination with the family of the depressed elderly patient. Families often are the first to insist that the depressed person seek professional consultation, and families are essential allies in the process of implementing a therapeutic plan.

Once potentially harmful medications have been discontinued, the clinician should prescribe antidepressant medications to those who suffer from major depression, especially with melancholia or psychotic features. The selective serotonin reuptake inhibitors are the drugs of choice because they have fewer side effects; however, tricyclic antidepressants are just as effective. Nortriptyline and desipramine are the preferred tricyclics because they have relatively mild anticholinergic effects and a low frequency of cardiotoxicity. Fluoxetine, sertraline, and paroxetine and nefazodone have all been useful as selective serotonin

TABLE 460.2. ANTIDEPRESSANT THERAPY FOR MAJOR DEPRESSION IN OLDER ADULTS

Class and Agent	Recommended Starting Dose	Side Effects of Class
Tricyclic antidepressants		
Notriptyline	50 mg qhs	Anticholinergic effects
Desipramine	50 mg ghs	Postural hypotension, potential for fatal overdose
Selective serotonin Reuptake inhibitors		
Fluoxetine	10 mg in the a.m.	Agitation, insomnia weight loss
Sertraline	50 mg in the a.m.	Persistence of side effects
Paroxetine	20 mg in the a.m.	because of long half-life
Nefazodone	100 mg b.i.d.	

reuptake inhibitors. Dosage and side effects are presented in Table 460.2.

If an elderly patient suffers from a severe depression with many biologic symptoms that do not respond to a traditional antidepressant or exhibit a propensity to rapidly relapse, antidepressant therapy can be augmented with drugs such as lithium carbonate or carbamazepine. Doses of lithium can be much lower than at earlier stages of life, and therapeutic blood levels of 0.3 to 0.6 mEq per deciliter are usually adequate. Psychostimulants, such as methylphenidate, 5 to 10 mg in the morning, are widely prescribed to lethargic elders but have not been proved effective in the treatment of more severe depressive disorders.

Drug therapy alone is not sufficient treatment for depressed older adults, even when the depression appears to be predominantly of biologic origin. Psychotherapy, especially the cognitive and behavioral therapies, augments drugs in treating melancholic depressions. Perhaps the most beneficial result of psychotherapy is that it may reduce the likelihood of a recurrence of the depressive episode and enable the depressed elder to reintegrate into his or her social network.

The elderly are less likely than younger persons to respond to antidepressant medications during a severe depressive episode. However, late-life depressive episodes respond exceptionally well to ECT. Refined techniques in the administration of ECT have improved the tolerance of it; pulse-unilateral stimuli to the non-dominant hemisphere and the advent of multiple methods of physiologic monitoring during treatment (electroencephalography, electrocardiography, and strain gauge monitoring of respirations) have reduced morbidity during treatment. Even with the use of nondominant ECT, however, memory impairment is a common side effect.

PROGNOSIS

The depressive disorders, especially major depression and dysthymic disorder, are chronic disorders characterized by relapse and presence of residual symptoms. Among those elderly who recover from an episode of depression within a year of onset, about one-third suffer a relapse during the year after recovery. Older persons are just as likely to recover from an episode of

major depression and no more likely to suffer a relapse than younger persons. However, the elderly may be more vulnerable to residual symptoms of depression for months and even years following an acute depressive episode.

BIBLIOGRAPHY

Blazer D. Depression in the elderly. *N Engl J Med* 1989;320:164–166.
Blazer D. *Depression in Late Life*, second ed. St. Louis: Mosby, 1993.
Koenig HG, Meador KG, Shelp F, et al. Major depressive disorder in hospitalized medically ill patients: an examination of young and elderly male veterans. *J Am Geriatr Soc* 1991;39:881–890.
Krishnan KR, Hays JC, Blazer DG. MRI-defined vascular depression. *Am J Psychiatry* 1997;154:497–501.
Meechan P, Salsman L, Satin R. Suicide among older United States residents: epidemiologic characteristics and trends. *Am J Public Health* 1991;81:1198–1200.
Reynolds C, Frank E, Parel J, et al. Nortriptylene and interpersonal psychotherapy as maintenance therapies of recurrent major depression: a randomized controlled trial in patients older than 59 years. *JAMA* 1999; 281:39–45.

Kelley's Textbook of Internal Medicine, fourth edition. Edited by H. David Humes. Lippincott Williams & Wilkins, Philadelphia © 2000.

CHAPTER 461

APPROACH TO THE ELDERLY PATIENT WITH DISORDERS OF FLUID AND OSMOLALITY REGULATION

JO WIGGINS

The kidney is responsible for the maintenance of fluid and electrolyte homeostasis. One-fifth of the body's circulating volume passes through the kidney every minute. This is such an important function that nature has endowed the kidney with a huge reserve capacity. Data are now becoming available from individuals who donated a kidney earlier in life. To date, no long-term decline in fluid or electrolyte homeostasis has been demonstrated. There are, however, aging-related changes in the kidney, which over time do compromise the kidney's ability to cope with large and rapid changes in fluid or electrolyte load. These changes are not manifest under normal conditions, but the challenges presented by disease, medications, or iatrogenic interventions can overwhelm the aging kidney's ability to maintain the normal volume and osmolality of the extracellular fluid compartment.

NORMAL AGING CHANGES IN THE KIDNEY

The basic functional unit of the kidney is the nephron. Nephrons differentiate during fetal development and finish their maturation during the first year of life. After this time no new nephrons are made. Renal mass declines with age due primarily to cortical atrophy. Starting in the fourth decade of life, nephrons are lost in a process known as glomerular sclerosis. There is roughly a 10% decline in nephron number per decade. This has been shown both in cross-sectional studies and in an ongoing longitudinal study that is part of the Baltimore Longitudinal Study of Aging. There is also progressive sclerosis of the afferent arteriole, which does not then filter its load through the glomerular tuft, but in effect "shunts" unfiltered blood from afferent to efferent arteriole. This sclerosis happens independent of systemic vascular disease, and the changes of hypertension and atherosclerosis are superimposed on this aging process. There is a parallel loss of tubules, resulting in the development of interstitial fibrosis. There is also significant increase in mesangial matrix and thickening of the basement membrane. Although these changes represent "normal aging" in the population as a whole, there are huge individual variations, with some otherwise healthy people showing declines in nephron mass at twice the predicted rate, and others showing no demonstrable decline at all. At the present time, we do not understand the reasons behind these aging-related changes and have no insight into why some aging persons do not appear to experience any decline in renal function over time.

PHYSIOLOGIC CHANGES WITH AGING

RENAL BLOOD FLOW

Average renal blood flow decreases about 10% per decade, dropping from 600 mL per minute per 1.73 m^2 to 300 mL per minute to 1.73 m^2 by the ninth decade. This is accompanied by increasing resistance in both afferent and efferent arterioles. These changes occur independent of cardiac output and reductions in renal mass. This decline in renal blood flow is thought to contribute to the decline in efficiency with which the aging kidney responds to fluid and electrolyte load and loss.

GLOMERULAR FILTRATION RATE

In concert with the decline in nephron numbers, glomerular filtration rate (GFR) falls with aging. Starting in the fourth decade, GFR declines at about 10% per decade. Serum creatinine, however, tends to remain stable. This is because muscle mass, the source of creatinine, also declines as lean body mass is replaced by fat. This maintenance of serum creatinine can be very misleading in older persons, who can lose significant filtration capacity without demonstrating a marked rise in creatinine. GFR can be estimated using the Cockcroft Gault equation:

$$\text{Creatinine clearance} = (140 - \text{age, years})(\text{weight, kg}) \, 72 \times (\text{serum creatinine concentration, mg/dL})$$

For women, multiply by 0.85.

Use of this equation to estimate GFR for a 230-lb, 25-year-old football player with a serum creatinine of 1.8 mg per deciliter gives an estimated creatinine clearance of 93 mL per minute. Use of the same calculation for an 85-year-old woman weighing 110 lb with the same serum creatinine gives an estimated GFR of 18 mL per minute. Thus, high-normal or minimally elevated serum creatinines in frail elderly patients reflects a large drop in their GFR. The physiologic consequences of this are seen frequently in medical practice, where older patients have a compromised ability to excrete a salt and water load, and develop extracellular fluid overload when given intravenous fluids. Careful use of fluids and renal dosing can thus prevent many of the complications that the frail elderly experience in hospital.

TUBULAR FUNCTION

Homeostasis of electrolytes and water is maintained by the transport systems of the tubule. The decline in the number of nephrons with aging results in a decrease in the ability of the tubule to respond to challenges. The decline in filtration volume as a result of sclerosis in the glomerulus and afferent arteriole results in a diminished volume of filtrate to the tubule. This reduces the kidney's ability to regulate sodium and potassium concentrations, decreases the ability to excrete an electrolyte or acid load, and diminishes the urinary concentrating ability. There are also changes in hormonal responses to salt load and salt deprivation. Older individuals have a much lower renin response to reductions in circulating volume, salt deprivation, or upright position. This results in diminished aldosterone release, with a failure to conserve sodium. Studies have also shown that elderly people have elevated levels of atrial natriuretic peptide, further blunting their renin response. This reduced capacity to conserve sodium renders older patients with fever, diarrhea, and other causes of fluid loss particularly vulnerable to hypovolemia and dehydration. Common disorders of water and electrolyte balance will be addressed individually below.

WATER HOMEOSTASIS

Maintaining the composition and volume of the extracellular fluid compartment is central to the well-being of an individual. Disturbances of osmolality or water and electrolyte balance are common and, often, life threatening in the elderly. The presenting symptoms tend to be nonspecific and include malaise, weakness, apathy, disorientation, agitation, loss of appetite, and cognitive decline. Careful assessment of water intake, electrolytes, renal function, and circulating volume should be made in any older patient who presents with a change in functional status, cognitive status, or behavioral change.

Total body water decreases with normal aging. Young adults have a body composition that is about 60% water, and this drops to around 50% in older persons, and may drop a further 5% in the frailest elderly. This drop is greater in women, as they generally have more fat and less lean body mass. Thus gains and losses of water have more effect in older people, particularly in older women. Superimposed on this underlying vulnerability are age-related functional changes in the ability of the kidneys to handle water deprivation or a water load. Studies have shown that older persons experience less thirst than younger persons when deprived of water for 24 hours and are much slower to correct their increased osmolality when given free access to water. This makes the elderly especially vulnerable to dehydration. Maximal concentrating ability of the urine declines with age, resulting in a mild chronic diuresis that probably has a role in the nocturia that is so common in older adults. The maximum concentrating power of the kidney falls to around 400 to 500 mOsm per kilogram in the over 80-year-old person, compared to 1,100 to 1,200 mOsm per kilogram in a young adult. Since antidiuretic hormone (ADH) levels are usually elevated in older people, this is thought to reflect a decline in tubular function with a diminished capacity to reabsorb water. These factors all contribute to the older patient's susceptibility to dehydration and low intravascular volume. Careful attention should be paid to maintaining fluid volume in the acute hospital setting where losses related to various diseases or their treatments can result in a hyperosmolar state. Institutionalized elders are particularly vulnerable to dehydration, since they are dependent on others for access to fluids. Even the healthy independent senior is vulnerable to dehydration as intercurrent illness limits his or her drive and ability to replace free-water loss.

Older people also exhibit a decline in their ability to excrete a fluid load. Studies comparing older individuals with younger adults show that older subjects took 2-4 times longer to excrete a water load. Renal diluting ability is impaired with age, and during water diuresis older subjects are unable to reduce urine osmolality to levels comparable to younger subjects. This results in vulnerability to fluid overload with attendant pulmonary and peripheral edema, and special care is advised when giving i.v. fluids to older patients.

SODIUM HOMEOSTASIS

Sodium levels are normally maintained across a fairly wide range from 137 to 150 mEq per liter and are important for maintaining the intravascular volume. Older patients have an impaired ability to conserve sodium due to reduced levels of renin release in response to sodium loss or sodium deprivation. They also have high circulating levels of atrial natriuretic peptide with suppression of the renin–angiotensin–aldosterone axis. Older people suffer from a mild and chronic form of salt wasting. Both hyper- and hyponatremia are common in the elderly.

TABLE 461.1.	CAUSES OF HYPERNATREMIA

Infections (pneumonia, urinary track infection, urosepsis, sepsis)
Diuretic use or solute diuresis
Uncontrolled diabetes mellitus
Enternal losses
Lack of free access to water
Impaired mental status (delirium, dementia)
Malignancy
Impaired renal concentrating ability
Diabetes insipdus
Hypercalcemia
Loss of thirst drive
Enteral feeding with high osmotic load
Gastrointestinal bleed
Diuresis following acute renal failure or relief of obstruction

HYPERNATREMIA

Hypernatremia is defined as a plasma sodium ≥150 mEq per liter and occurs in about 3% of hospital admissions. It is associated with a mortality rate of around 50%. The incidence of hypernatremia is higher in woman than in men because woman have lower total body water. Hypernatremia may be present on admission or occur during the hospital stay. Although the causes of hypernatremia are similar in elderly patients to those seen in younger people (see Chapter 145), the frequency with which these are found is quite different. Primary hyperaldosteronism and Cushing's disease are extremely rare in the over-80 age group, whereas dehydration is quite common. The causes of hypernatremia are somewhat different for those patients who are found to be hypernatremic on admission as compared to those who become hypernatremic while in hospital (Table 461.1). Patients who are hypernatremic on admission are likely to be older, more likely to reside in a nursing home, and are more likely to exhibit cognitive impairment. The most common underlying cause of their hypernatremia is dehydration secondary to increased insensible loss associated with infection. In contrast, those patients who become hypernatremic in hospital are younger, more likely to have uncontrolled diabetes mellitus or to have undergone aggressive diuresis with inadequate free-fluid replacement. About 50% of inpatients who develop hypernatremia do so in an intensive care unit while being intubated.

A patient with hypernatremia will show signs of dehydration. Skin turgor can be hard to assess in the frail elderly, and a better assessment can be made by using the skin on the trunk rather than the limbs. Mucosal surfaces will be dry. Neck veins will fail to fill when the patient is lying down. Blood pressure will be lower than normal for the patient with an orthostatic drop. Daily measurement of orthostatic pressures and taking of fall precautions are necessary when working with these patients. The best guide to fluid balance is through accurate daily weights. Patients typically show signs of impaired consciousness, ranging from delirium with mild degrees of hypernatremia to profound coma when the sodium concentration is significantly elevated.

Treatment of these patients should focus on prompt normalization of fluid balance and sodium concentrations, as well as correction of the precipitating cause of the dehydration. Careful reversal of the hypernatremia is associated with better outcomes and improved chances for returning mental function to baseline. The free-water deficit should be calculated to guide the physician in appropriate volumes and rates of replacement. It is calculated by multiplying the patient's weight (in kilograms) by 0.6. This gives the current total body water.

$$\text{Water deficit} = \text{desired total body water} - \text{current total body water}$$

Desired body water is calculated using the following formula:

Measured serum sodium $\times$ (weight in kilograms $\times$ 0.6)
Normal serum sodium or 145 mEq per liter

Approximately one-third of the deficit should be replaced in the first 24 hours, as overly rapid normalization of osmolality can cause swelling in the brain and irreversible brain damage. The remaining two-thirds should be replaced over an additional 24 to 48 hours. If the patient's dehydration is so severe as to cause imminent circulatory collapse, initial rehydration can be given as volume expanders or normal (isotonic) saline. Otherwise water should be replaced with 5% dextrose, supplemented by oral intake. Allowance should be made for insensible loss, keeping in mind that tachypnea, fever, and enteral losses all increase the volume of replacement required. Once the hypernatremia has been corrected, steps must be taken to prevent its recurrence. Adequate access to sufficient water requires more than placing a full jug of water in a patient's room. Elderly persons with impaired levels of consciousness have reduced awareness of thirst and a limited ability to fend for themselves. Patients who are anchored to the bed by multiple tubes, drains, and catheters are restrained just as effectively as those wearing a posey or lap belt. Patients with physical impairments may be unable to open fluids presented in cartons, bottles, or cans. Hospital and nursing home staff are unlikely to be as willing to help a patient who is belligerent, aggressive, combative, or uncooperative with access to adequate fluid intake, so the physician must be alert to the possibility that oral intake may fail again when the intravenous line is removed.

Correction of the precipitating cause for the hypernatremia will depend on the individual circumstances presented by each patient. Hospital-acquired hypernatremia is an iatrogenic problem, and as such it is preventable by careful monitoring of patient weights and adequate replacement of free water. Mortality for a given diagnosis is higher when accompanied by hypernatremia than without it. It is difficult to know how much of this is directly attributable to the hypernatremia itself. Patients who develop hypernatremia may be sicker with a more severe underlying complaint or frailer with more impaired homeostatic functions. Studies have shown that higher serum sodium levels and prolonged periods without correction are both correlated with poorer outcomes.

HYPONATREMIA

Hyponatremia occurs when the serum sodium falls below 137 mEq per liter. Several aging changes in the kidney increase the older patient's susceptibility to hyponatremia. The decreased renal conservation of sodium combined with a decline in the ability to secrete water renders the older patient vulnerable to hyponatremia. Hyponatremia can be found in about 7% of healthy community-dwelling older persons. In nursing homes this figure rises significantly, and longitudinal studies suggest that over the period of a year about 50% of institutionalized older persons have at least one episode of hyponatremia. Hyponatremia is also common in the hospitalized older patient. Most cases of hyponatremia in the elderly are dilutional, resulting from the volume-stimulated retention of water due to a decrease in intravascular volume. Intense salt and water reabsorption in the proximal tubule to maintain circulating volume results in the decreased delivery of solute to the distal tubule and leads to the retention of water. Low circulating volume may be caused by excess loss secondary to aggressive diuretic therapy, gastrointestinal losses, or congestive heart failure where the effective intravascular volume is depleted. Thiazide diuretics are especially prone to causing hyponatremia since they not only cause a diuresis but also decrease the renal dilution capacity.

Nonosmotic release of ADH also occurs when the circulating volume is decreased, further promoting the retention of water. Studies suggest that older persons have increased ADH responses to physiologic or pharmacologic stimuli, compared to younger persons given the same stimulus. This predisposes the older patient to dilutional hyponatremia. Postoperative hyponatremia occurs in more than 4% of older patients undergoing surgery, as a result of high postoperative ADH levels. Older patients may also have the syndrome of inappropriate ADH secretion (SIADH). This may be secondary to a tumor, central nervous system (CNS) lesion, pulmonary disease, or drugs. Many older patients have an idiopathic SIADH, where no underlying cause can be identified. Before the diagnosis of idiopathic SIADH is made, a very careful review of the patient's medications should be carried out. Common culprits include CNS drugs, such as antipsychotics, anticonvulsants, and antidepressants. Sulfonyl ureas and clofibrate have also been shown to cause hyponatremia. More rarely, chemotherapeutic agents have been implicated.

Dilutional hyponatremia can also occur from the movement of water out of cells into the intravascular compartment. This occurs in hyperosmolar states, the most common of which is uncontrolled diabetes mellitus. As the blood sugar rises, water is pulled from the intracellular compartment to offset the osmotic load. There is a dilutional decrease in sodium concentration of 1.6 mEq per liter for each 100 mg per deciliter rise in glucose concentration.

Far more rarely, hypernatremia in an older patient represents true sodium depletion. This happens most often in nursing home residents who are tube-fed. Most tube feeding preparations have a low salt content, and this, combined with the older patient's decline in salt conservation, can lead to a true depletional hyponatremia. Studies suggest that more than 50% of older adults receiving long-term tube feeding become hyponatremic. Institutionalized patients on low-salt diets can also become sodium-depleted. This depletional state can be very simply corrected by the addition of a little salt to the dietary preparations offered.

Older patients with hyponatremia may present with nonspecific complaints, and changes in mental status are common. Severe hyponatremia can cause swelling of brain cells, with seizures and lasting brain damage. Patients with dilutional hyponatremia may show signs of a reduced circulating volume, such as orthostatic hypotension and dehydration. Management depends on the severity of the hyponatremia, the speed of its onset, and the underlying cause. If a medication appears to be responsible, stopping that agent may be sufficient to address the problem. With uncontrolled diabetes, correcting the hyperglycemia may be all that is required, without the necessity of salt supplements. In cases of profound hyponatremia of acute onset, hypertonic saline should be given intravenously, with care taken not to overload the older person with fluid. Replacement of no more than 12 mEq per liter in any 24-hour period is recommended. In cases of idiopathic SIADH or congestive heart failure, where correction of the underlying abnormality is not possible, patients may be treated with fluid restriction or, in more severe cases, with demeclocycline.

POTASSIUM HOMEOSTASIS

The body normally maintains the serum potassium concentration between very narrow limits of 3.5 to 5 mEq per liter. There is great reserve capacity within the system for maintaining potassium levels, since disorders of potassium can be life threatening. Because of diminished renal function, the older patient is particularly susceptible to disorders of potassium homeostasis.

HYPERKALEMIA

Excluding those patients with end-stage renal disease, hyperkalemia is almost exclusively a disease of the elderly. It is also primarily an iatrogenic condition. Age-related declines in GFR, renal blood flow, and the reduction in distal renal tubular function all combine to make the elderly patient particularly vulnerable to hyperkalemia. Impaired tubular response to acidosis and reduced ability to conserve sodium interfere with potassium exchange. Poor renal perfusion, leading to decreased sodium delivery to the distal tubule as seen in heart failure, will also reduce potassium exchange. Extrarenal changes in the elderly also increase their susceptibility to hyperkalemia. Declines in the renin–angiotensin–aldosterone system with age result in the blunting of the renal tubular response to rising potassium concentrations. The age-related rise of atrial natriuretic peptide, a potent suppressor of aldosterone, may also contribute to the impairment of potassium homeostasis. While none of these changes by itself is sufficient to cause hyperkalemia, they all underlie the predisposition of older patients, particularly those with impaired renal function, to develop hyperkalemia.

Hyperkalemia occurs in up to 10% of elderly hospitalized admissions. After renal failure, the two most common causes are medications and hyperglycemia. In most patients the cause of hyperkalemia is multifactorial and cannot be attributed to a lone factor. The major causes of hyperkalemia are summarized in Table 461.2. As can be seen from the list, the common practice of combining β-blockers or angiotensin-converting enzyme (ACE) inhibitors with potassium-sparing diuretics requires careful monitoring in older patients, especially those with even mild

TABLE 461.2.	CAUSES OF HYPERKALEMIA

Pre-renal

Increased potassium load
  Excess Supplementation
  Total Parenteral nutrition
  RBC Transfusion
  Penicillin G potassium
Increased potassium release
  Hyperglycemia
  Rhabdomyolysis
  Metabolic acidosis
  β-blockers
  Digitalis

Renal

Primary:
  Renal failure
  Hypoaldosteronism
Secondary:
Drugs reducing renin–angiotensin activity
  Anpiotensin-converting enzyme inhibitors
  β-blockers
  NSAIDS including the new COX2 inhibitors
  Heparin
Drugs reducing potassium excretion
  Spironolactone
  Amiloride
  Trimethoprim
  Triamterene
  Pentamidine
  Cyclosporine
  Tacrolimus

renal impairment. Small increments in serum creatinine in patients with low body mass can signal profound impairment of renal glomerular filtration rates (see "Aging Kidney," above), and special caution is advised in these patients.

Patients with hyperkalemia usually present with nonspecific complaints, such as weakness, fatigue, and nausea. More frequently, hyperkalemia is a chance finding at the time of routine laboratory testing. Patients may present with cardiac arrhythmias or syncope. Once significant hyperkalemia (potassium levels higher than 6 mEq per liter) is established patients should undergo 12-lead electrocardiography (ECG) to rule out cardiac dysrhythmias. Patients with potassium levels higher than 7 mEq per liter should be on continuous cardiac monitoring. ECG abnormalities include peaked T waves, prolongation of the PR interval, first-degree atrioventricular block, junctional rhythm, widening of the QRS complex, and lengthening of the QT interval. There does not appear to be any relationship between the potassium level and the type or frequency of ECG abnormalities. If ECG abnormalities are found, excitable membranes should be stabilized by the administration of intravenous calcium. An estimate of renal function should be made by measuring the blood urea nitrogen and serum creatinine, and a serum glucose should be obtained. Potassium can be moved intracellularly by the administration of intravenous insulin, together with glucose if the patient is not hyperglycemic. Recently, it was shown that 10 to 20 mg of albuterol administered by nebulizer is also effective at reducing potassium concentrations and has an additive effect when administered with insulin. Sodium bicarbonate has also been used in patients with acidosis but has not been found to be particularly efficacious in patients with advanced renal failure. Potassium can be removed from the body by the administration of exchange resins, either by mouth or by enema. In emergencies, dialysis may be indicated. Once the acute situation has been dealt with, serious attention should be paid to precipitating causes. The medication list should be reviewed and adjusted to match the patient's underlying renal and cardiac function. In the outpatient setting, physicians should obtain frequent potassium levels in older patients on combinations of medications that interfere with potassium excretion, such as potassium-sparing diuretics in combination with ACE inhibitors.

HYPOKALEMIA

Hypokalemia is defined as a serum potassium of less than 3.5 mEq per liter. As with hyperkalemia, the elderly patient is particularly susceptible both to developing hypokalemia and to its consequences. Reductions in GFR and declines in tubular function impair the ability of the older patient to maintain potassium concentrations when the system is challenged. The causes of hypokalemia are no different in older patients than in the general population and have been dealt with at some length in Chapter 146. Extrarenal causes of hypokalemia that are prominent in the elderly include the intracellular movement of potassium that accompanies alkalosis and the hypokalemic response to catecholamine release that accompanies medical emergencies. The older patient frequently develops a mild hypokalemia in response to major surgery, myocardial infarct, stroke, or other medical emergencies. This hypokalemia is usually self-limiting and corrects with supportive therapy. Elderly patients are also somewhat more sensitive to β-agonists and may develop hypokalemia when treated with broncho-dilators.

Low total body potassium is usually caused by renal loss. However, in the elderly patient, poor dietary intake combined with poor renal conservation can result in hypokalemia. Older patients are also susceptible to other causes of loss, such as severe diarrhea and laxative abuse, because of their impaired ability to conserve potassium. By far the most common cause of hypokalemia is the use of diuretics. Careful and regular monitoring of potassium levels is necessary in every older person on diuretics, as even small doses of these agents may result in hypokalemia. Renal potassium loss, such as that of the hereditary conditions associated with renal tubular acidosis, very rarely presents for the first time in the older patients; however, acquired salt-wasting conditions seen after the relief of renal obstruction may present a similar picture in the older patient. Primary excess of mineralo-corticoids and glucocorticoids as a cause of hypokalemia is again rare in the older patient. However, tumors that secrete active peptides, leading to secondary increases in these hormones, should be considered. A recent increase in hypokalemic alkalosis has been related to the surge in popularity of herbal teas. Preparations containing licorice have been shown to cause hypokalemia, and the elderly are particularly vulnerable. A careful assessment of over-the-counter remedies and dietary supplements, including herbal teas, should be made in an older person who presents with unexplained hypokalemia.

The clinical presentation of the patient with hypokalemia is usually nonspecific, with complaints of tiredness, weakness, malaise, and cramps. Tissues that are electrically active are very sensitive to potassium levels, so that muscle, nerve, and cardiac complaints are often part of the picture. Since patients with underlying heart disease or being treated with digoxin are far more likely to develop cardiac arrhythmias, older patients are at far higher risk of adverse consequences from hypokalemia than are younger patients. Ventricular ectopic rhythms are common in hypokalemia. ECG changes include low-voltage complexes with depression of the ST segment and reduced-amplitude T waves and a prominent U wave. If ECG changes are noted, prompt potassium replacement therapy should be initiated, with potassium chloride given either orally or intravenously, to correct the hypokalemia. Very close potassium monitoring of older patients on diuretics should be routine, particularly when there is underlying cardiac disease or the patient is also taking digoxin.

BIBLIOGRAPHY

Acker CG, Johnson JP, Palevsky PM, et al. Hyperkalemia in hospitalized patients: causes, adequacy of treatment, and results of an attempt to improve physician compliance with published therapy guidelines. *Arch Intern Med* 1998;158:917–924.

Ayus JC, Arieff AI. Abnormalities of water metabolism in the elderly. *Nephrol* 31996;16(4):277–288.

Beck LH. Changes in renal function with aging. *Clin Geriatr Med* 1998; 14(2):199–209.

Biswas K, Mulkerrin EC. Potassium homeostasis in the elderly. *QJM* 1997; 90:487–492.

Hirshberg B, Ben-Yehuda A. The syndrome of inappropriate antidiuretic hormone secretion in the elderly. *Am J Med* 1997;103:270–273.

Miller M. Hyponatremia: age related risk factors and therapy decisions. *Geriatrics* 1998;53(7):32–33,37–38,41–42.

Palevsky PM. Hypernatremia. *Semin Nephrol* 1998;18(1):20–30.

Rodriguez-Puyol D. The aging kidney. *Kidney Int* 1998;54:2247–2265.

Siamopoulos K, Elisaf M, Katopodis K. Iatrogenic hyperkalaemia—points to consider in diagnosis and management. *Nephrol Dial Transplant* 1998;13:2402–2406.

Solomon LR, Lye M. Hypernatremia in the elderly patient. *Gerontology* 1990;36:171–179.

Kelley's Textbook of Internal Medicine, fourth edition. Edited by H. David Humes. Lippincott Williams & Wilkins, Philadelphia © 2000.

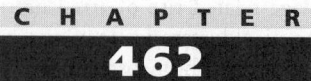

CHAPTER 462

APPROACH TO THE ELDERLY PATIENT WITH FALLS AND IMPAIRED MOBILITY

MARY E. TINETTI

A nonsyncopal fall, the topic of this chapter, refers to an event that results in a person coming to rest inadvertently on the ground or other lower level, for reasons other than as a consequence of sustaining a violent blow, loss of consciousness, stroke, or epileptic seizure.

INCIDENCE AND EPIDEMIOLOGIC FACTORS

About one-third of community persons older than 65 years fall each year; this percentage increases to 50% by age 80 years. Most fallers experience multiple episodes; the frequency of falling is similar in older men and women, at least after age 75 years. Women, however, are about twice as likely to suffer a serious injury during a fall. More than half of ambulatory nursing home residents fall each year. The annual incidence of falling among nursing home residents is 1.5 falls per bed per year.

Falling is a major health problem because of its associated morbidity. Unintentional injury is the sixth leading cause of death in persons older than 65 years. Complications related to falls account for most of these deaths. Moreover, those who survive a fall experience greater decline in activities of daily living and higher level physical and social functioning than nonfallers. This decline is thought to result from several factors, including physical injury, pain, fear of recurrent falls and injuries, and loss of confidence. Almost 10% of persons over age 75 are seen in an emergency department for a fall-related injury each year; 40% of these individuals are hospitalized. Approximately 5% of falls by older persons result in a fracture, most commonly of the humerus, wrist, pelvis, hip, or foot. Serious soft-tissue injuries, including cerebral contusions, subdural hematomas, hemarthroses, joint dislocations, or severe sprain, occur in an additional 5% of falls. Another common fall-related complication is the inability to get up without the help of another person. A small percentage, 2% to 5%, of persons who are unable to get up without help experience a long lying down, which in turn can lead to pressure sores, dehydration, pneumonia, rhabdomyolysis, and renal failure. Falling also increases the likelihood of skilled nursing facility admission, independent of other known risk factors such as age, gender, cognitive impairment, functional disability, and immobility.

PATHOPHYSIOLOGIC FACTORS

Nonsyncopal falls occur when environmental hazards or demands exceed the individual's ability to maintain postural stability. Specific diseases, such as Parkinson's disease, normal-pressure hydrocephalus, Binswanger's disease, and high cervical myelopathy, may result in severe postural instability. Some authors also describe a gait disturbance of unknown central nervous system (CNS) etiology, referred to as senile or essential gait disorder. However, these CNS diseases account for a relatively small percentage of falls by older people.

The pathophysiologic process of nonsyncopal falls can perhaps best be understood by considering falling to be a geriatric syndrome and hence of complex, multifactorial etiology. A fall occurs when an older person who is predisposed because diseases and impairments impede his or her postural stability is exposed to an acute insult or challenge that he or she is unable to withstand. Postural stability requires input from sensory, central integrative, and effector components in a highly integrated manner. These components are overlapping and compensatory. Further, cardiac, circulatory, respiratory, metabolic, and other conditions may influence the functioning of these three primary components. Postural instability and predisposition to falling may not be evident until several of the components are impaired. Indeed, several studies have shown that the risk of falling increases as the number of diseases and impairments increases.

The major sensory modalities responsible for orienting a person in space and identifying hazards include the visual, auditory, vestibular, and proprioceptive systems. These modalities mutually interact and have multiple interconnections. Age-related visual changes include decreased visual acuity, dark adaptation, and accommodation. In addition, ocular diseases, including macular degeneration, glaucoma, and cataracts, are commonplace. Hearing also contributes directly to stability through the detection and interpretation of auditory stimuli, which help to localize and orient the person in space, particularly when other modalities are impaired. More than 50% of elderly individuals have some hearing loss.

The vestibular system contributes to spatial orientation at rest as well as during acceleration and is responsible for visual fixation during head and body movements. Age-related decline in vestibular function has been attributed to changes in the otoconia. Predisposing factors include past aminoglycoside use as well as current use of aspirin, furosemide, quinine, quinidine, and, perhaps, tobacco and alcohol. Head trauma, mastoid or ear surgery, and middle-ear infections are other possible predisposing factors.

The proprioceptive system orients the person in space during position changes, while walking on uneven ground, or when other modalities are impaired. The components of the proprioceptive system include the peripheral nerves, mechanoreceptors located in apophysial joints, the posterior columns, as well as multiple CNS connections. Whether age-related changes occur in peripheral nerves remains unknown. Peripheral neuropathy, however, is common among elderly people. The contribution of cervical mechanoreceptors to proprioception is not widely appreciated. The loss of normal afferent input from mechanoreceptors may result in disturbances of postural sensation (sense of balance) and of kinesthesis (awareness of head and neck movement), on which precise control of voluntary movements, such as walking, depends. Predisposing factors include whiplash injuries and cervical degenerative diseases, such as rheumatoid arthritis or spondylosis.

The CNS channels input from the sensory modalities to the appropriate efferents in the musculoskeletal system. Given the multiple connections and their complexity, essentially any CNS disorder can and will contribute to instability and falling. CNS processes that adversely affect cognition further impede stability because problem solving and judgment are needed to interpret and respond appropriately to environmental stimuli. Dementia is a well-recognized risk factor for falls, even among persons without a clinical gait disorder.

The effector components of mobility include the efferent peripheral nervous system as well as muscles, joints, and bones.

Therefore, all orthopedic and neuromuscular conditions predispose to falling. In addition, foot disorders, including calluses, bunions, toe deformities, and large, thick, deformed toenails, may alter gait patterns and/or impair proprioception.

A wide range of acute host, activity-related, and environmental factors may precipitate a fall, particularly among older persons predisposed by the chronic diseases and impairments described above. Any systemic disorder can transiently or chronically contribute to instability and falling through adverse effects on the sensory, central, or effector components. In addition, systemic disorders may result in decreased cerebral blood flow, fatigue, confusion, or shortness of breath. Common examples include anemia, electrolyte disturbances, hypoglycemia or hyperglycemia, acid–base disturbances, hypothyroidism, or hypercapnia associated with chronic lung disease. Falling may be a nonspecific presentation of many acute illnesses, including pneumonia or urinary tract infection. Cardiac dysrhythmias may obviously precipitate a fall associated with loss of consciousness and absence of cerebral blood flow. However, chronic cardiac conditions, such as congestive heart failure, may also predispose to instability and falling both directly, by compromising cerebral blood flow and activity tolerance (endurance), and indirectly, by medication side effects such as dehydration, postural hypotension, or confusion. Carotid baroreceptor hypersensitivity may cause or contribute to both syncopal and nonsyncopal falls.

Postural hypotension may result in transient instability through compromised cerebral blood flow. Prevalence ranges from 10% to 30% in persons older than 65 years. Causes include volume depletion; decreased venous return from lower extremity disorders, such as varicosities; autonomic dysfunction from aging or disorders such as diabetes or Parkinson's disease; deconditioning; age-related physiologic changes, such as decreased functioning of the renin–angiotensin system or decreased baroreceptor sensitivity; and medications. Symptoms may occur on position change or after a few minutes of activity. Not all persons who experience a drop in blood pressure upon standing experience symptoms such as dizziness. Although a systolic drop of 20 mm Hg is often used to define postural hypotension, the degree of drop required to cause a fall is unknown and likely depends both on the abruptness of the drop and on the presence of other contributing factors.

Another, more recently identified abnormality in blood pressure homeostasis is postprandial hypotension. The mechanisms and mediators of postprandial hypotension remain unknown, although inability to compensate for splanchnic blood pooling after ingestion of a meal has been postulated as a possible cause.

Medications may result in instability and falling through many mechanisms, including impaired cognitive functioning, postural hypotension, fatigue, dehydration, or electrolyte disturbance. Centrally acting medications, including sedative hypnotics (particularly barbiturates and benzodiazepines), neuroleptic medications, and antidepressants, have repeatedly been associated with an increased risk of falling. Recent studies suggest that tricyclic and selective serotonin reuptake inhibitor antidepressants impart a comparable risk of postural instability and falling. Other classes of medications implicated, at least in some studies, include diuretics, antiarrhythmics, anticonvulsants, nonsteroidal anti-inflammatory agents, digoxin, and narcotic analgesics. In addition to specific medications, recent changes in dose and total number of medications have been associated with an increased risk of falling.

Activity-related and environmental factors present challenges to postural stability that must be withstood to avoid falling. The degree to which these factors pose a threat depends on the person's vulnerability. Challenges to stability may be posed by the external environment through hazards (e.g., poor lighting, slippery floors); ordinary activities (e.g., stair climbing or walking on even surfaces); or by movements that place the person's center of mass outside the base of support, such as turning or transferring. Only a small percentage of falls occur during clearly hazardous activities, such as climbing on chairs or ladders or participating in sports. About 10% of falls occur on stairs—well out of proportion to the time spent on them, with descending being more hazardous than ascending. The most commonly mentioned environmental hazards include tripping over objects, slippery floors, and carrying of heavy objects. Slippery or improperly fitting shoes constitutes another potential hazard.

Environmental hazards are thought to be less important among nursing home residents than among community-dwelling older persons. Nursing homes typically are safer environments than the community because many hazards have been removed and the adverse challenges to the elderly person—such as stairs—are fewer. However, even among nursing home residents, environmental contributors, described in the section on management, do exist.

Interest has focused on factors that increase the risk of serious injury, particularly fractures, during a fall. Characteristics of fallers shown to be independently associated with serious injury include white race, older age, female sex, cognitive impairment, more frequent falls, previous fall injury, presence of chronic conditions such as diabetes mellitus or stroke, poor visual acuity, reduced proprioception, impaired balance, impaired muscle strength, decreased body mass index, and reduced bone density. Circumstances of the fall that increase likelihood of serious injuries such as fractures include the direction and impact of the fall, the height of the fall, and the hardness of the landing surface.

■ HISTORY AND PHYSICAL EXAMINATION

Historical and examination findings among older persons who have experienced, or are at risk for experiencing, a fall are listed in Table 462.1. The specific features seen in individual patients depend on which impairments and diseases are present. However, because several conditions often are present simultaneously in older persons, the signs and symptoms of specific impairments or diseases may be obscured or nonspecific. For example, vertigo may occur with nonvestibular problems, whereas patients with vestibular dysfunction may present only with dizziness or instability. Therefore, patients should undergo screening by history and examination for all of the contributing factors listed in Table 462.1.

The neurologic diseases that predispose to falls can be diagnosed from a thorough neurologic history and examination. Although most neurologic diseases associated with falling result in

TABLE 462.1.	CONTRIBUTORS TO INSTABILITY AND FALLING: CLINICAL FINDING AND POTENTIAL INTERVENTIONS

Contributor	History	Examination	Laboratory Evaluation	Potential Interventions
Sensory: Vision	Decreased night vision; unsteady walking with bifocals	Near; distant; contrast sensitivity; dark adaptation	Referral to ophthalmologist or optometrist	Appropriate refraction; surgery; consider avoiding bifocals while walking; good lighting
Vestibular–auditory	Vertigo; decreased hearing; worse in dark or with specific head positions; predisposing factors (see text)	Nystagmus; findings depend on central vs. peripheral etiologies; + hearing screen; + Barany maneuver; + headshaking visual acuity test; balance/gait findings	Referral to audiologist; consider referral to otolaryngologist for vestibular testing	Avoid toxic drugs; surgery; balance or habituation exercises; good lighting
Proprioceptive: Peripheral nerves	Worse in dark, on uneven ground, on thick rugs, or with thick-soled shoes	Decreased position sense and vibration (latter is more sensitive test); gait worsens with eyes closed and improves with support of examiner or cane	Vitamin B_{12}, folate, glucose, VDRL	Treatment of underlying disease (e.g., Vitamin B_{12}, glucose, avoid alcohol); good lighting; gait training; appropriate walking aid and footwear[a]
Cervical	Same as for peripheral nerves; worse with head turning; vertigo; predisposing factors (see text)	Signs of radiculopathy or myelopathy; clumsiness with fine motor tasks; mild spastic quadriparesis	Consider radiography; MRI	Balance exercises; surgery; gait training and appropriate walking aid
Central neurologic: Any central nervous system disease	Variable, depends on disease	Complete neurologic examination; cognitive examination	Consider computed tomography scan or MRI (if localized findings)	Treatment of underlying disease; supervised, structured, safe environment; occupational therapy; gait training; appropriate walking aid
Musculoskeletal: Arthritides, especially lower extremities	"Knee gave out"; pain; stiffness; decreased range of motion	Periarticular muscle atrophy; joint deformity, decreased range of motion; other findings depend on disease	Consider radiographs; workup for inflammatory arthritides	Medical and surgical treatment of underlying disease; strengthening exercise program
Muscle weakness, contractures of upper or lower extremities	Variable, depends on disease	Variable, findings depend on disease	Workup for proximal myopathy if history or examination suggestive	Strengthening and range-of-motion exercises; balance and gait training; appropriate adaptive devices; raised seats
Foot disorders	Foot pain with walking	Bunions, calluses, deformities		Podiatry; orthotics; appropriate footwear[a]

(continued)

TABLE 462.1.	*Continued*			

Contributor	History	Examination	Laboratory Evaluation	Potential Interventions
Systemic diseases:				
Postural hypotension	Light-headed; worse with position change or walking; complaints consistent with predisposing (e.g., Parkinson's disease, diabetes)	Blood pressure and heart rate; signs of predisposing diseases	Glucose; blood urea nitrogen; electrolytes	Hydration; lowest effective dosage of necessary medications; reconditioning exercises; elevate head of bed; stockings; increased salt; dorsiflexion/hand clenching exercises before arising; consider florinef or midodrine if other treatments fail
Cardiac, respiratory, metabolic diseases	Depends on disease	Depends on disease	Electrocardiography, thyroid function tests; glucose; others depending on history or examination	Depends on disease
Depression	Vegetative complaints; poor concentration; apathy	Depression screen		Consideration of risk–benefit ratio of antidepressants; referral to psychiatrist
Medications, all[b]	Confusion; light-headedness; vertigo; fatigue; weakness	Postural hypotension; postural instability	Blood levels for anticonvulsants, antiarrhythmics, antidepressants, aspirin	Lowest effecive dose of essential medications; reevaluate continued need; taper or discontinue as indicated; avoid long-term use of sedative–hypnotics

[a] Optimal footwear: thin firm soles with low heel, completely enclosed foot, and adequate size toebox.
[b] Use of three or more drugs associated with increased risk. Classes of drugs with strongest evidence of risk are listed in text.
MRI, magnetic resonance imaging; VDRL, Venereal Disease Research Laboratory Test

postural instability and pathologic gait patterns, these findings are not disease-specific. Common features of gait seen in persons with central neurologic diseases include difficulty with gait initiation, flexed posture, step-to-step variability, path deviation, legs crossing the midline, step length asymmetry, decreased step height that results in shuffling if severe, instability on turning, and easy backward displacement. Some of these findings (e.g., decreased step height, flexed posture) can be seen in individuals with sensory abnormalities as well.

A careful screen and/or assessment of balance and gait is helpful not only for detecting the possibility of central neurologic disease but for identifying sensory or musculoskeletal contributors to falling. All older persons should undergo a simple screen for postural stability. If the individual can stand on one leg or tandem-stand for 30 seconds, or can walk with a tandem gait accurately for 10 feet, postural stability is likely intact and no further evaluation is warranted. For persons failing the screen,

several quick and reliable assessments of balance and gait, such as that shown in Table 462.2, are available. In addition to identifying sensory or musculoskeletal impairments, a careful assessment of balance and gait may help to identify conditions under which falls are likely to occur and can be used to determine rehabilitative and environmental interventions that may decrease a person's risk of falling.

Carotid hypersensitivity should be suspected if the patient gives a history of "just going down" or falling with head turning or upon looking up. Carotid sinus massage should be performed on these patients if there is no evidence of cerebrovascular disease or cardiac conduction abnormalities, and if the procedure is judged safe. The carotid sinus syndrome is defined as greater than a 3-second sinus pause or more than a 50 mm Hg drop in systolic blood pressure during carotid stimulation. If carotid hypersensitivity is suspected or diagnosed, precipitating actions, such as wearing of tight collars or looking up, should be avoided.

TABLE 462.2.	ASSESSMENT OF BALANCE AND GAIT

Abnormality	Possible Diagnosis	Rehabilitative or Environmental Interventions
Balance[a]		
Difficulty in getting up from and sitting down in chair	Proximal muscle weakness; arthritis; Parkinson's disease; postural hypotension; deconditioning	Exercises to strengthen lower extremities; transfer training; high, firm chairs with arms; raised toilet seats
Unsteadiness during neck turning and extension	Cervical degenerative disorder (e.g., arthritis, spondylosis); vestibular dysfunction; carotid hypersensitivity; vertebral–basilar insuffiency	Neck exercises; cervical collar; appropriate storage of items in kitchen and bedroom; treatment of specific disease(s)
Unable to one-leg or tandem-stand		Balance training; appropriate walking aid
Gait[b]		
Decreased step height (shuffling seen only with central nervous system processes)	Central nervous system disease; compensatory for multiple sensory deficits (visual, vestibular, proprioceptive); fear of falling	Careful sensory evaluation; gait training; proper footwear; appropriate walking aid; low-pile carpet or nonskid floor without throw rugs
Unsteadiness on uneven surfaces	Decreased proprioception; ankle weakness	Gait and balance training; appropriate footwear; appropriate walking aid; avoidance of thick carpet; good lighting
Unsteadiness while turning	Parkinson's disease; multiple sensory deficits; cerebellar disease; hemiparesis; loss of visual field	Gait training; proprioceptive exercises; appropriate walking aid; obstacle-free environment
Increased path deviation	Cerebellar disease; multiple sensory deficits; sensory or motor ataxia	Gait training; appropriate walking aid

[a] Other potential balance and transfer observations include bed transfers; withstanding nudge on sternum or pull at waist.
[b] Other potential gait observations include gait initiation; truncal sway; walking stance; step length and symmetry; heel–toe sequencing; arm swing; and ability to pick up walking pace.

Cardioinhibitory drugs, such as digoxin, β-blockers, methyldopa, or calcium channel blockers should also be avoided, if possible, or used in the lowest possible dose.

LABORATORY STUDIES AND DIAGNOSTIC TESTS

The laboratory findings that may be helpful in identifying potential contributors to fall risk are listed in Table 462.1. Because of prevalence, nonspecific presentation, and potential for modification, all older persons at risk for falling should undergo routine laboratory screening, including complete blood count, thyroid function tests, serum glucose, electrolytes (including blood urea nitrogen and creatinine), and assay of folate and vitamin B$_{12}$ levels. Measurement of drug levels may be useful for patients taking antiarrhythmics, anticonvulsants, or tricyclic antidepressants.

Brain imaging with computed tomography or magnetic resonance imaging is indicated only if there are focal abnormalities on the neurologic examination. Cervical spine films may be useful in the patient with impaired gait, lower extremity spasticity, and hyperreflexia, which together are suggestive of cervical spondylosis. Lateral dimension of the spinal canal of less than 12 mm suggests a significant encroachment on the cervical cord. This finding can be confirmed with magnetic resonance imag-

ing, which should be considered only if the patient is deemed a candidate for neurosurgery.

Ambulatory electrocardiographic monitoring is not warranted for the evaluation of nonsyncopal falls. Results are difficult to interpret in older persons because of the high prevalence of asymptomatic arrhythmias that rarely coincide with falling.

The role of computerized posturography in the clinical evaluation and treatment of balance and falling disorders remains to be determined. Posturography may be helpful in determining the relative contribution of visual, vestibular, and proprioceptive abnormalities to postural instability and may reveal how the older person responds to postural perturbations. These findings may help in the development of effective rehabilitative interventions. Finally, as safer and more effective treatments, such as estrogen, bisphosphonates, calcitonin, and exercise, for enhancing bone mineral content are becoming available, assessment of bone mineral density through a variety of techniques is indicated, particularly for postmenopausal women.

STRATEGIES FOR OPTIMAL CARE MANAGEMENT

The clinician's goal should be to minimize a patient's risk of experiencing falls, particularly injurious falls, while maintaining or improving the patient's mobility and functioning. The optimal strategy for reducing the risk of falling depends on the functional level and living situation of the patient. Among very healthy, community-dwelling older persons with no or few diseases or impairments, individual or group activity or exercise programs that improve balance and muscle strength are the most cost-effective strategy. Examples include tai chi, dancing, walking, and resistive muscle-strengthening activities.

Among community-dwelling older persons who have more than one chronic disease or impairment, who have any functional limitations, or who take prescription medications, a multifactorial approach to reducing the risk of falling has proven effective in several recent studies. Because of the overlapping, compensatory nature of the systems affecting stability as described earlier, simple interventions may result in major improvements, even if the interventions are not aimed at the modalities believed to be the most impaired. The risk of falling has been shown to decrease with reduction in the number of contributing factors, such as medications, postural hypotension, muscle weakness, foot disorders, imbalance, and gait abnormalities. Therefore, the optimal management strategy is the identification and modification of as many of the factors listed in Table 462.1 as possible. Even if the person suffers from a known neurologic disease associated with falling, such as Parkinson's disease, the elimination or amelioration of other impairments may decrease the frequency of falls and fall-related injuries.

As shown in Table 462.1, treatment involves standard medical or surgical interventions, as well as rehabilitative interventions and environmental adaptations. The results from balance and gait assessment can help guide the selection of rehabilitative and environmental interventions. Examples are shown in Table 462.2.

Because most falls occur at home and because environmental factors contribute to many falls, a home safety evaluation by the patient, family, physical therapist, or home health nurse or aide is an important component of the treatment strategy. Hazards to be assessed include lighting; tripping hazards such as cords, loose rugs, or small objects in the walking path; low, soft chairs that are difficult to get out of; slippery floors; and stairs in poor repair or without bilateral handrails. Because individual impairments influence whether a particular environmental factor is a hazard, combining physical therapy assessment with a home safety evaluation may be the optimal approach.

A careful review of previous falls may provide clues to preventing recurrences. The presence of environmental hazards, such as those described, should be elicited. A description of the patient's activity at the time of the fall is important as well. If the fall occurred during routine, nonhazardous activities, the goal should be to improve the safety and effectiveness of these maneuvers. If the fall occurred during more hazardous activities, such as climbing on chairs or carrying heavy objects on stairs, the substitution of safer activities and better organization of the home to render the activity unnecessary should be advised.

Physical therapy, aimed at increasing muscle strength and improving balance and gait performance, has been shown effective in reducing the rate of falls. The optimal intensity and duration of muscle strengthening and balance exercises remain to be determined. Physical therapists can also help in managing the consequences of falls by teaching the patient strategies for getting up from the floor and by fostering the patient's confidence regarding performing activities of daily living without falling. This multifactorial approach to fall prevention among at-risk community-dwelling older persons has been proved cost-effective, indeed cost-saving. Not only has this strategy been shown to reduce the rate of falls; it has also been associated with lower subsequent health care costs (hospital plus home care plus skilled nursing facility), even after accounting for the cost of the interventions.

Contrary to experience in the community setting, intensive physical therapy programs targeting strengthening and balance have not proven effective at reducing the fall rate among frail nursing home residents. On the other hand, comprehensive programs that address the environment, assistive devices, and staff interactions with patients have been effective. The minimal essential use of psychotropic medication is a key component of fall reduction programs in nursing homes. Another important component includes careful assessment for residents using wheelchairs to avoid use of poorly maintained or poorly fitted wheelchairs. Instruction of all staff in safe and appropriate transfer and ambulatory assistance techniques is needed, as problems with transfers and ambulation are commonly associated with falls among nursing home residents. Although institutions may offer a safer environment than the community, the residents also tend to be more frail than elderly persons living in the community. Therefore, more subtle hazards, such as ill-fitting shoes, pants that are too long, slippery floors, beds that are too high or too low, or movable bedside tables that residents may lean against, should all be considered. Fall prevention efforts in institutions should also be aimed at reducing the use of restraints through alternatives, such as alarms that are activated when residents try to get out of bed or move unassisted, adjustable side rails and bed heights for residents who climb out of bed, and increased staff/resident ratios.

Treatment and prevention of osteoporosis, a significant risk factor for fall-related fractures, are discussed in Chapter 465. Providing extra padding, through the use of various types of hip protectors, appears to be a promising approach to the prevention of hip fractures.

BIBLIOGRAPHY

Alexander NB. Gait disorders in older adults. *J Am Geriatr Soc* 1996;44:434–451.

King MB, Tinetti ME. Falls in community-dwelling older persons. *J Am Geriatr Soc* 1995;43:1146–1154.

Leipzig RM, Cumming RG, Tinetti ME. Drugs and falls in older people: a systematic review and meta-analysis: I. Psychotropic drugs. *J Am Geriatr Soc* 1999;47:30–39.

Leipzig RM, Cumming RG, Tinetti ME. Drugs and falls in older people: a systematic review and meta-analysis: II. Cardiac and analgesic drugs. *J Am Geriatr Soc* 1999;47:40–50.

Province MA, Hadley EC, Hornbrook MC, et al. The effects of exercise on falls in elderly patients: a preplanned meta-analysis of the FICSIT trials. *JAMA* 1995; 273:1341–1347.

Tinetti ME. Performance-oriented assessment of mobility problems in elderly patients. *J Am Geriatr Soc* 1986;34:119–126.

Tinetti ME, Baker DI, McAvay G, et al. Multifactorial intervention to reduce the risk of falling among elderly people living in the community. *N Engl J Med* 1994;331:821–824(b).

Wayne AR, Taylor JA, Meador KG, et al. A randomized trial of a consultation service to reduce falls in nursing homes. *JAMA* 1997; 278:557–562.

Kelley's Textbook of Internal Medicine, fourth edition. Edited by H. David Humes. Lippincott Williams & Wilkins, Philadelphia © 2000.

C H A P T E R
463

APPROACH TO THE ELDERLY PATIENT WITH PRESSURE ULCERS

RICHARD M. ALLMAN

A pressure ulcer is any skin lesion caused by unrelieved pressure resulting in damage of underlying tissue. Pressure ulcers usually occur over bony prominences and are staged to classify the degree of tissue damage observed. Stage I is nonblanchable erythema of intact skin. In stage II lesions, skin loss is limited to the epidermis or dermis. Stage III ulcers manifest as full-thickness skin loss involving subcutaneous tissue. The ulcer may extend down to, but not through, underlying fascia. Stage IV lesions extend into muscle or bone or supporting structures.

INCIDENCE AND EPIDEMIOLOGIC FACTORS

Many patients are at risk for pressure ulcers, with 12% or more of adult hospitalized patients being confined to bed or chair. Such activity limitation is even more common in nursing homes, but most patients with pressure ulcers develop the ulcer during a stay at an acute care hospital. More than half of those with pressure ulcers are older than age 70.

The incidence of stage II and higher ulcers during hospitalization is 1% to 3% of all admissions but can be as much as eight times higher for those with activity limitations. Development of a stage I ulcer is associated with the subsequent occurrence of a stage II or higher ulcer in nearly 60% of cases. In nursing homes, the 3-month incidence of stage II and higher ulcers is about 5%; the figure increases to 13.2% after 1 year.

ETIOLOGIC FACTORS AND PATHOGENESIS

Low-level pressure for long periods or high-contact pressure for short periods leads to skin ulceration. Subcutaneous tissues and muscle are more sensitive to pressure-induced necrosis than the epidermis. The effect of pressure on all tissue layers can be augmented by exposure to shearing forces, friction, and moisture. Shearing forces, which are tangential forces generated in deep sacrococcygeal tissues, can cause occlusion of gluteal vessels or mechanical damage to subcutaneous tissues when the patient is sitting in bed or in a chair. Friction-induced epithelial loss can result from being pulled across a bed sheet, or when similar movements result from spasticity. Urinary and fecal incontinence may lead to maceration or irritation of the epidermis.

When bony prominences are exposed to adequate pressure, blood and lymphatic vessels are occluded. As a consequence, endothelial cell swelling occurs, and plasma, proteins, and blood ultimately leak into interstitial tissues. Cellular metabolites and inflammatory cells accumulate, and intravascular thrombosis and fibrin deposition occur. Muscle and subcutaneous tissue necroses ensue, ultimately leading to dermal and epidermal death.

CLINICAL AND LABORATORY FINDINGS

Identification of at-risk patients should involve the systematic assessment of bed- and chairbound persons for risk factors such as mobility impairment, incontinence, nutritional status, and level of consciousness. This can be accomplished by using a validated risk-assessment tool such as the Braden Scale or the Norton Scale. Among bed- and chairbound patients admitted to an acute care hospital, inability to reposition, dry skin, lymphocyte count 1.5×10^9 or less, body weight less than 58 kg, and nonblanchable erythema of intact skin may help identify those at highest risk. After 3 weeks of follow-up, the cumulative incidence of stage II and higher pressure ulcers is 0% among bed- and chair-bound patients without one of these factors. The incidence with one, two, or three factors is significantly higher (11.4%, 39.6%, and 67.9%, respectively).

Evaluation of a patient with a pressure ulcer should include a complete history and physical examination, identification of complications and comorbid conditions, and assessment of nutritional status, pain, psychosocial factors, and risk of additional ulcers. Table 463.1 lists the characteristics of pressure ulcers that should be evaluated and documented weekly. Within 2 to 4 weeks, the clinician can expect a clean pressure ulcer to show

TABLE 463.1.	PRESSURE ULCER ASSESSMENT
Location	
Tunneling	Sinus tracts
Stage	Granulation tissue
Exudate	Undermining
Size	Epithelialization
Necrotic tissue	Surrounding tissue status

TABLE 463.2.	RECOMMENDATIONS FOR ULCER CARE

- Remove devitalized tissue from the ulcer. Dry heel eschar may be left in place.
- When there is no urgency, select appropriate method of debridement: sharp (using a scalpel or scissors); mechanical (wet-to-dry dressings, hydrotherapy, irrigation, or dextranomers); enzymatic (collagenase); or autolytic techniques (using a synthetic dressing cover and permitting wound fluids to destroy necrotic tissues; contraindicated in infected ulcers).
- When cellulitis or sepsis is present, use sharp debridement for quick removal of necrotic tissue.
- Consider the need for subacute bacterial endocarditis prophylaxis when using sharp debridement.
- Use clean, dry dressings for 8–24 hours after sharp debridement associated with bleeding; then reinstitute moist dressings.
- Prevent or manage pain associated with debridement.
- Use normal saline to cleanse wounds at each dressing change using minimal mechanical force.
- Do not use povidone–iodine, iodophor, sodium hypochlorite, hydrogen peroxide, or acetic acid in ulcers.
- Use enough irrigation pressure to enhance wound cleansing without causing trauma to the ulcer bed. This can be accomplished using a 35-mL syringe with a 19-gauge needle or angiocatheter.
- Consider whirlpool for ulcers that contain thick exudate, slough, or necrotic tissue. Discontinue whirlpool when ulcer is clean.
- Use a dressing that will keep a clean ulcer bed continuously moist and the surrounding intact periulcer skin dry. Fill all cavities loosely with dressing material, but avoid overpacking the wound. Use wet-to-dry dressings for mechanical debridement only.
- Consider electrotherapy for recalcitrant stage III and IV ulcers.
- Consider a 2-week trial of topical antibiotics for clean pressure ulcers that are not healing or are continuing to produce exudate after 2–4 weeks of optimal management.
- Use systemic antibiotic therapy only for patients with bacteremia, sepsis, advancing cellulitis, or osteomyelitis.
- Protect ulcers from exogenous sources of contamination (e.g., feces).

evidence of healing manifested by improvements in such parameters.

All stage II, III, and IV ulcers are colonized with bacteria, so that swab cultures have no diagnostic value and should not be used. When signs of advancing cellulitis or systemic infection accompany a pressure ulcer, a culture of fluid obtained by needle aspiration or of tissue obtained by ulcer biopsy may be helpful. If evidence of local infection (purulent exudate, odor, necrotic tissue) persists after ulcer care measures (Table 463.2) have been in place for 4 weeks or longer, then quantitative bacterial cultures of the ulcer base and bone biopsy for culture and histologic examination should be considered. Osteomyelitis should be suspected when an elevated leukocyte count or erythrocyte sedimentation rate or an abnormal bone radiograph is documented.

OPTIMAL MANAGEMENT

PREVENTION

After identifying a patient at risk for developing pressure ulcers, a systematic skin inspection should be performed daily. At the time of soiling and at routine intervals, the skin should be cleansed with a mild agent, avoiding hot water and minimizing the force and friction applied to the skin. Moisturizers should be used for dry skin. Skin exposure to moisture due to incontinence, perspiration, or wound drainage should be minimized. If incontinence cannot be controlled after appropriate assessment and treatment, an absorptive brief or underpad should be used. Topical agents that act as barriers to moisture can also be tried.

Skin injury due to friction and shear can be minimized by using proper positioning; appropriate transferring and turning techniques; as well as lubricants such as cornstarch and creams, protective films, dressings, and pads over bony prominences. Rehabilitation efforts should be instituted if consistent with the overall goals of therapy. Massage over bony prominences should be avoided, as it may reduce blood flow and cause deep-tissue injury.

Adequate dietary intake should be provided to prevent malnutrition, and nutritional deficiencies should be corrected in a way consistent with the overall goals of therapy. For malnourished patients with pressure ulcers, nutritional support providing 30 to 35 calories per kilogram per day and 1.25 to 1.5 g protein per kilogram per day may be needed to achieve a positive nitrogen balance. A daily high-potency vitamin and mineral supplement is recommended for all patients suspected of having vitamin deficiencies.

At-risk patients in bed should be repositioned every 2 hours if consistent with overall patient goals. In addition, a pressure-reducing device, such as a foam, static air, alternating air, gel, or a water mattress, should be used. Although pressure-reducing support surfaces may decrease the frequency of intermittent repositioning required, patients should be carefully monitored for evidence of erythema over bony prominences. Such evidence would indicate the need for more frequent repositioning or a more effective pressure-reducing device.

When repositioned, patients should be alternately turned from the supine position to the side-lying position at 30 degrees to the support surface. When positioned on the side at this angle, direct pressure on the trochanter and lateral malleolus is avoided. Placement of soft pillows between the knees and ankles is also helpful during repositioning. Pillows should be placed under the legs, or another device should be used to relieve heel pressure totally for completely immobile patients.

Because of the shearing forces generated while sitting, at-risk patients should be repositioned at least every hour while in a chair or should be put back to bed. Patients who can move should be taught to shift their weight every 15 minutes while sitting. The use of a pressure-reducing cushion made of foam, gel, air, or a combination is indicated for at-risk patients while sitting. To minimize the impact of shear on patients in bed, the head of the bed should be kept at the lowest degree of elevation and for the shortest amount of time consistent with other medical requirements.

TREATMENT

Pressure ulcer treatment includes the preventive strategies recommended above. During repositioning, no pressure should be put on the ulcer. A static pressure-reducing support surface may be used if the patient can assume a variety of positions without bearing weight on the ulcer and without compressing the support surface or "bottoming out." Positioning devices may be used to raise a pressure ulcer off the support surface. A dynamic support surface, such as an alternating-air mattress, low-air-loss bed, or air-fluidized bed, is indicated if the patient cannot assume a variety of positions without bearing weight on the ulcer, if the patient fully compresses a static support surface, or if the ulcer does not show evidence of healing.

Recommendations for local ulcer care, debridement, wound cleansing, dressings, adjunctive care, and the management of infection are listed in Table 463.2. Once an ulcer is clean and granulating, dressings that provide a moist wound environment should be used to promote healing. Evidence suggests that continuously moist saline gauze, film, and hydrocolloid dressings are similarly effective in achieving this goal, but saline gauze dressings require significantly more caregiver time than film and hydrocolloid dressings because the latter types of dressings need to be changed less frequently than do moist gauze dressings.

Surgical repair can be considered when clean stage III or IV pressure ulcers do not respond to the recommended treatments. Possible candidates are medically stable and adequately nourished patients who can tolerate operative blood loss and postoperative immobility.

Even after 6 months of treatment, as many as 26% of stage II ulcers and 41% of stage III or IV ulcers may fail to heal. These outcomes for pressure ulcer treatment suggest that clinicians should increase the emphasis on preventive interventions while also seeking improvements in ulcer care.

BIBLIOGRAPHY

Allman RM. Pressure ulcers among the elderly. *N Engl J Med* 1989;320: 850–853.

Allman RM. Pressure ulcer prevalence, incidence, risk factors, and impact. *Clin Geriatr Med* 1997;13:421–436.

Allman RM, Goode PS, Patrick MM, et al. Pressure ulcer risk factors among hospitalized patients with activity limitation. *JAMA* 1995;273: 865–870.

Bergstrom N, Bennett MA, Carlson CE, et al. *Treatment of pressure ulcers.* Clinical Practice Guideline No. 15. US Department of Health and Human Services. Public Health Service, Agency for Health Care Policy and Research. AHCPR Publication No. 95-0652, December 1994.

Panel for the Prediction and Prevention of Pressure Ulcers in Adults. *Pressure ulcers in adults: prediction and prevention.* Clinical Practice Guideline No. 3. US Department of Health and Human Services. Public Health Service, Agency for Health Care Policy and Research. AHCPR Publication No. 92-0047, May 1992.

Kelley's Textbook of Internal Medicine, fourth edition. Edited by H. David Humes. Lippincott Williams & Wilkins, Philadelphia © 2000.

APPROACH TO THE FRAIL ELDERLY PATIENT

LINDA P. FRIED
JEREMY WALSTON

CLINICAL IMPORT OF FRAILTY

Frailty is a clinical status whose incidence increases with age. It is estimated that 10% to 25% of older adults are frail. After the age of 85, according to the American Medical Association's White Paper on Elderly Health, "46% of those living in the community fall into this group of frail elderly." Frailty is of particular clinical interest because frail individuals are thought to constitute those older adults at highest risk for a number of adverse health outcomes, including dependency, institutionalization, falls, injuries, acute illness, hospitalization, and mortality. Frail individuals are also thought to be at risk for slow or blocked recovery from illness. Although a clinical "sense" of frailty exists, there is still no explicit consensus or standard clinical definition of frailty that would assist identification of this high-risk subset prior to the onset of these adverse outcomes. However, some early work characterized the clinical presentation of this high-risk state, along with interventions that might be useful in prevention of progression. Effective interventions would minimize adverse outcomes in this high-risk group. In addition, clinical evaluations suggest that the later stages of frailty may not be modifiable and in fact presage death, whereas the earlier stages might have greater potential for modification. Given these observations, those with earlier frailty may be a subset of older adults who are most likely to benefit from evaluation and preventive interventions.

Despite the difficulty of defining who is frail, it is important to translate clinical instinct into explicit definitions of frailty. These permit development of useful clinical screening methods and definition of underlying etiologic processes and opportunities for intervention. The purpose of this chapter is to briefly summarize the potential definitions of frailty and to highlight evidence regarding cause and treatment.

PRESENTATION AND PATHOPHYSIOLOGIC FACTORS

The literature suggests that frailty and failure to thrive constitute a continuum of a clinical syndrome, with failure to thrive being the most extreme manifestation that is associated with a low rate of recovery. The manifestations of frailty that are most widely agreed upon in the literature are a constellation of symptoms including unintentional weight loss and/or loss of muscle mass,

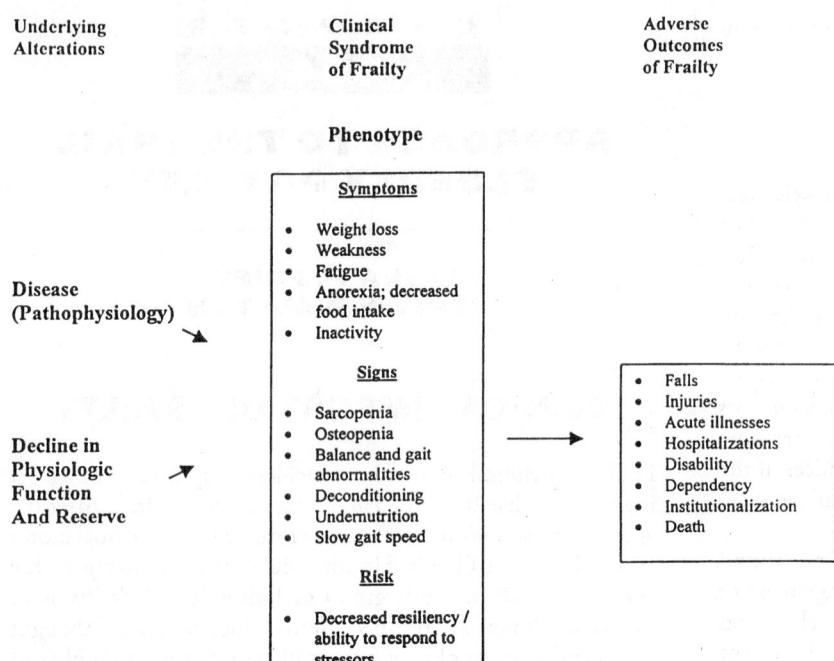

| Underlying Alterations | Clinical Syndrome of Frailty | Adverse Outcomes of Frailty |

FIGURE 464.1. Modal pathway of frailty. The clinical phenotype of frailty is associated with adverse health outcomes and appears to result from declines in physiologic function and reserve, as well as disease precipitants.

weakness, fatigue, inactivity, and decreased dietary intake (Fig. 464.1). In addition, signs of frailty are frequently cited as components of the syndrome; these include sarcopenia (decreased muscle mass), balance and gait abnormalities, deconditioning, and decreased bone mass (osteopenia) (Fig. 464.1). Undernutrition and malnutrition are also cited as characteristics. Each of these clinical characteristics has been shown to be highly predictive of the adverse outcomes clinically associated with frailty, including decline in function, institutionalization, and mortality. Consistent with the definition of a syndrome, the phenotype of frailty appears to include a critical mass of these symptoms and signs, rather than any one being necessarily present or sufficient to define the condition.

It is well established that undernutrition in older adults, including inadequate protein and micronutrient intake, is a contributor to loss of lean body mass, even in the absence of weight loss. It is also clear that decline in lean body mass leads to declines in strength and exercise tolerance, along with decreased walking speed and overall activity levels, and decreased resting metabolic rate. These latter changes contribute to an overall decrease in total energy expenditure. These established connections suggest, potentially, a vicious cycle involving altered energetics that is consistent with the phenotypic presentation of frailty, described above. Based on preliminary studies, Poehlman et al. have suggested that a subset of older adults manifests dysregulation of energy intake, such that it is inadequate relative to energy output, even at low levels of caloric expenditure. If so, this could complete the hypothesized adverse feedback loop, further exacerbating undernutrition and propelling decrements in this energetics cycle. This clinical conceptualization is displayed in Fig. 464.2.

In addition to the clinical manifestations of frailty based on this cycle of adverse energetics, other potential biologic characteristics should be considered. The most widely agreed-upon geriatric definition of frailty from an etiologic perspective is that

it represents a state of age-related physiologic vulnerability resulting from impaired homeostatic reserve and a reduced capacity of the organism to tolerate stressors. This could result in the well-recognized decreased ability to tolerate temperature extremes, increased susceptibility to infections, and relatively poor recovery from injuries and infections clinically associated with frailty. It has been suggested that a decline in reserve occurs with aging across multiple physiologic systems. Those systems whose declines are central to the syndrome of frailty appear to be (a) neuromuscular changes, which result in sarcopenia and thus link this underlying biology to the cycle of energetics and the clinical presentation above; (b) neuroendocrine dysregulation, and (c) immunologic dysfunction. The biologic changes observed in these systems with aging are summarized in Table 464.1. Declines in each of these realms, singly or in combination, can leave the frail older adult especially vulnerable to stressors.

In fact, age-related declines have been described in a number of organ systems (see Chapter 16), indexes of which include reduced creatinine clearance, forced expiratory volume, nerve conduction velocity, insulin sensitivity, heart rate variability, lean body mass, $\dot{V}O_2$ max and strength. Some theorize that there are declines in the basic complexity of biologic responses to alterations in the environment that occur with aging and render the organism more vulnerable to internal or external perturbation. It is theorized that when such age-related declines occur in parallel across multiple systems, beyond an aggregate threshold of severity, they may lead to compromised physiologic reserves and ability to maintain homeostasis. This may, in turn, underlie the organism's decreased ability to tolerate stressors. Frailty appears especially to involve age-related compromise in one's ability to respond appropriately in dynamic situations.

Many definitions of frailty are in use. In particular, it is common to consider frailty to be synonymous with comorbidity or disability. However, there is increasing evidence that frailty is a

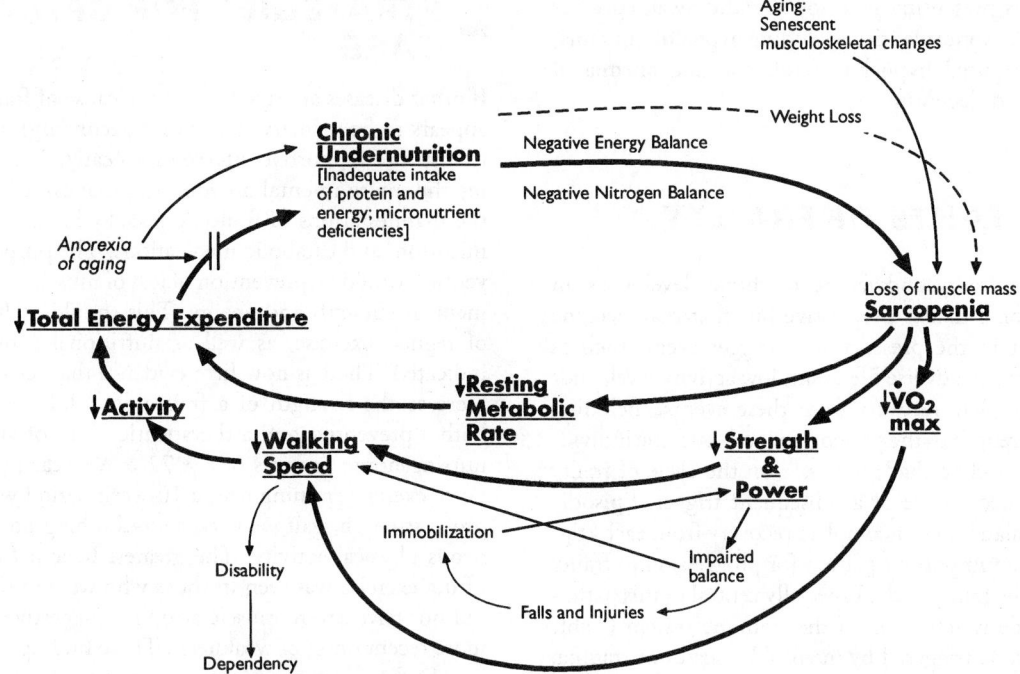

FIGURE 464.2. The cycle of frailty. Key components of frailty that appear to underlie its phenotypic manifestations in a negative feedback cycle are chronic undernutrition; sarcopenia; declines in physical strength, power, and exercise tolerance; and declines in activity and total energy expenditure. Factors that could precipitate or exacerbate this core cycle are indicated with dashed lines. Factors in which a relationship is hypothesized are indicated in italics. (Fried CP, Walston J. Frailty and failure to thrive. In Hazzard WR, Blass JR, Ettinger WH, et al, eds. *Principles of geriatric medicine and gerontology,* fourth ed. New York: McGraw-Hill, 1999: chapter 109, with permission.)

syndrome in and of itself, as described above. It is potentially a cause of mobility- and exercise tolerance–related disability, but it is distinct from (through commonly interacting with) comorbidity as defined by coexisting diseases. Similarly, end-stage disease(s) may lead to frailty, but comorbidity itself is not the same as frailty.

Finally, frailty may itself have an end stage, sometimes termed "failure to thrive." This stage is reached after the occurrence of

many of the adverse outcomes of frailty described above. It is thought to be a time of irreversible decline that progresses to death (sometimes called "predeath")—a final, common end-stage process of both the frailty of extreme old age and severe chronic diseases (e.g., congestive heart failure, malignancy, HIV, and dementia). The hallmarks of failure to thrive are unexplained and include progressive weight loss, with malnutrition and resulting loss of fat as well as muscle mass. This syndrome

TABLE 464.1.	CLINICAL SIGNS AND SYMPTOMS OF AGE-RELATED CHANGES IN PHYSIOLOGIC SYSTEM DECLINES CENTRAL TO THE SYNDROME OF FRAILTY		
	Sarcopenia	**Immune Dysfunction**	**Neuroendocrine Dysregulation**
	↓ Skeletal muscle mass	↑ Memory cells	↓ Growth hormone
	↓ Vo_2 max	↓ Naive cells	↓ Estrogen
	↓ Strength and exercise tolerance	↓ IL-2	↓ Testosterone
	↓ Thermoregulation	↓ IgG, IgA	Cortisol dysregulation
	↓ Energy expenditure	↑ IL-6, IL-1B	↑ Sympathetic tone
	↑ Insulin resistance	↓ Mitogen response	

IL, interleukin.
(From Hazzard W, et al., eds. *Principles of geriatric medicine and gerontology,* fourth ed. New York: McGraw-Hill, 1999, Chapter 109, with permission.)

is also described as presenting with social withdrawal; episodes of falling; metabolic abnormalities, including hypoalbuminemia, low creatinine, acquired hypocholesterolemia, and anemia of chronic disease; and decubitus ulcers.

PRECIPITANTS OF FRAILTY

It is thought that frailty and failure to thrive develop as an age-related syndrome that is progressive but that may become clinically manifest in the presence of a trigger event, such as acute illness, injury, an adverse life event, low activity level, and/ or bed rest. Incomplete recovery from these events, including failure to regain strength to the premorbid level, puts the individual on a stepwise decline that progresses on the cycle of frailty and/or upon the occurrence of a subsequent trigger. Episodic negative energy balance and incomplete recovery from each trigger event may be an important pattern for progression to frailty and initiation of the frailty cycle. Especially central in this pathophysiologic cascade is activation of the immune system (Table 464.1), which can be triggered by manifold diseases or trauma, and with release of catabolic (and anorexogenic) cytokines initiate a final common pathway of decline.

HISTORY, PHYSICAL EXAMINATION, AND DIFFERENTIAL DIAGNOSIS

The first goal in clinical care is to identify vulnerable individuals with latent frailty before the occurrence of the adverse outcomes for which they are at high risk. Such a clinical approach includes early identification of declines in weight, strength, dietary intake, or activity, each of which might precipitate the cycle of frailty. A number of diseases that are responsive to therapy can cause wasting, including congestive heart failure, diabetes, thyroid disease, tuberculosis and other chronic infections, undiagnosed cancer, and inflammatory conditions such as temporal arteritis. Psychological conditions, such as depression, psychosis, and grief, as well as dementia, can also present in this manner. Whether or not frailty is due to a specific underlying disease, focus should also be placed on prevention of related adverse outcomes, including falls and disability. Evaluation should also include screening for factors that may exacerbate vulnerability to these outcomes, such as medications, with intervention as indicated. Another reality enters the diagnostic picture as well: an underlying disease-specific etiologic process of frailty (e.g., occult malignancy) may not be evident when the syndrome first manifests, and each diagnostic effort in search of such an etiologic process carries its own risk and cost, which may be especially high in the frail patient (who is especially vulnerable to iatrogenic misadventures). Hence, constant subsequent vigilance must be exerted for the emergence of clues to, especially, treatable conditions if appropriate initial diagnostic maneuvers fail to disclose a specific cause of the syndrome.

STRATEGIES FOR OPTIMAL CARE

If other diseases are ruled out as the cause of frailty (if the frailty appears to be primary rather than secondary), a goal should be to institute supportive interventions early. These include targeting the environmental provocations that can trigger or accelerate the manifestations of frailty, especially low activity, inadequate nutrition, and catabolic medications. The purpose of this intervention would be prevention of loss of muscle mass and improvement in strength and energy. This should include prescription of regular exercise, as well as nutritional supplementation, if indicated. There is now firm evidence that resistance exercise to increase the strength of a frail older adult has potential from both a preventive and a therapeutic point of view. In very frail nursing home patients of age 72 to 98 years, progressive resistance exercise training over a 10-week period was shown to improve strength, gait velocity, stair-climbing power, and spontaneous physical activity. The greatest benefit from this weight-lifting exercise was seen in those who were initially weakest but did not have severe muscle atrophy (suggestive of a group with more recent onset of weakness). These findings thus suggest that benefit from exercise can accrue to even the most frail but that improvement is greatest if declines in strength are caught early. At the other end of the spectrum, primary prevention of frailty through regular strength training also has therapeutic potential due to both direct effects on muscle strength and indirect effects resulting from increased overall activity levels in people who are getting stronger. Evans has reported that high-intensity strength training appears to have highly anabolic effects in older adults. He reported a 10% to 15% decrease in nitrogen excretion after initiation of such training, which persisted for the 12-week duration of training. In other words, progressive resistance exercise improved nitrogen balance. As a result, older patients performing resistance training had a lower mean protein intake requirement than did sedentary subjects.

It is notable that such increases in strength from high-intensity training are substantially greater than those seen with growth hormone without concurrent training. Studies to date that have evaluated replacement therapies for prevention or treatment of declines in growth hormone have shown some efficacy in increasing lean body mass, decreasing fat mass, and slowing the catabolic effects of acute and chronic diseases or injuries, such as hip fracture and infections. However, it is not clear that such changes from growth hormone can be sustained, and there is no evidence that supplementation improves the functional status of growth hormone–deficient men. In addition, the long-term risks of growth hormone replacement on tumor development remain unclear. Therefore, there is currently no clear indication for the use of growth hormone in relation to the loss of lean body mass with age.

The role of nutritional supplementation in the treatment of frailty is less well defined than that of exercise. In Fiatarone and colleagues' trial of resistance exercise and nutritional supplementation in frail nursing home patients, total energy intake did not increase spontaneously in those exercising (without nutritional supplementation) or in those receiving nutritional supplementation but not exercising, in comparison with controls. This was the case even though this population had a marginal nutritional intake at baseline. Only with both exercise and nutritional supplementation did energy intake increase to a noticeable extent; these people gained weight but not measurably fat-free mass. Additionally, the research of Poehlman et al. indicates that older men and women have to increase energy expenditure by 1,000 kcal per week to get compensatory increases in energy (food) intake and increases in resting metabolic rate.

Preservation of fat-free mass and prevention of sarcopenia appear key in preventing the decrease in metabolic rate and dysregulation of energetics described in association with frailty. Maintenance of strength should also maintain exercise tolerance, both directly and indirectly because those with improved strength appear to engage more spontaneously in other activities. In the prevention of frailty, this appears to be a critical stage in terms of both the prevention of disability and the downward spiral to failure to thrive and death.

BIBLIOGRAPHY

Berkman B, Foster LW, Campion E. Failure to thrive: paradigm for the frail elder. *The Gerontologist* 1989;2: 654–659.

Bortz WM. The physics of frailty. *J Am Geriatr Soc* 1993;41:1004–1008.

Buchner DM, Wagner EH. Preventing frail health. *Clin Geriatr Med* 1992; 8:1–16.

Evans WJ. Exercise, nutrition and aging. *Clin Geriatr Med* 1995; 11: 725–734.

Ferrucci L, Harris TB, Guralurle JM, et al. Serum IL-6 level and the development of disability in older persons. *J Am Geriatr Soc* 1999,47: 639–646.

Fiatarone MA, O'Neill EF, Ryan ND, et al. Exercise training and nutritional supplementation for physical frailty in very elderly people. *N Engl J Med* 1994;330:1769–1775.

Fried LP, Walston J. Frailty and failure to thrive. In: Hazzard WR, Blass JR, Ettinger WH, et al., eds. *Principles of geriatric medicine and gerontology*, fourth ed. New York: McGraw-Hill, 1999: chapter 109.

Lipsitz LA, Goldberger AL. Loss of "complexity" and aging. Potential applications of fractals and chaos theory to senescence. *JAMA* 1992;267: 1806–1809.

Nelson ME, Fiatarone MA, Morganti CM, et al. Effects of high-intensity strength training on multiple risk factors for osteoporotic fractures. *JAMA* 1994;272: 1909–1914.

Poehlman ET, Toth MJ, Fishman PS, et al. Sarcopenia in aging humans: the impact of menopause and disease. *J Gerontol* (Special Issue) 1995; 50A:73–77.

Verdery RB. Failure to thrive in older people. *J Am Geriatr Soc* 1996;44: 465–466.

Kelley's Textbook of Internal Medicine, fourth edition. Edited by H. David Humes.
Lippincott Williams & Wilkins, Philadelphia © 2000.

CHAPTER
465

DIAGNOSIS AND MANAGEMENT OF OSTEOPOROSIS IN OLDER ADULTS

KAREN M. PRESTWOOD

Osteoporosis is a common disease in older adults. In women, the incidence of vertebral fractures begins to increase near the time of menopause; hip fracture incidence accelerates approximately 10 years later. Hip fractures in women are twice as common as in men at age 75 years, but men still suffer more than 75,000 femur fractures annually; the gender ratio of vertebral fractures is 8:1. The direct health care costs related to osteoporosis are estimated to be $38 million per day, or $14 billion per year. The number of older adults in this country is increasing rapidly, and the disability and mortality associated with hip and vertebral crush fractures are concentrated in older Americans. Thus, prevention of osteoporotic fractures is a major public health concern.

DEFINITION OF OSTEOPOROSIS

Osteoporosis is a "disease characterized by low bone mass and microarchitectural deterioration of bone tissue leading to enhanced bone fragility and a consequent increase in fracture incidence." Clinically, osteoporosis can be defined either by the presence of a fragility-related fracture or by bone mineral density (BMD) measurement. In defining BMD criteria for osteoporosis, the World Health Organization (WHO) established the standard as BMD of young adult women who are at the age of peak bone mass. For each standard deviation below peak bone mass (or one-unit decrease in t score), a woman's risk of fracture approximately doubles. For example, a woman with a t score of

-3 at the hip would be eight times more likely to suffer a hip fracture than a woman with a t score of zero. As seen in Table 465.1, a t score of less than -2.5 defines osteoporosis; osteopenia (low bone mass) and normal bone mass are also defined. The advantage to diagnosing osteoporosis by BMD is that the disease can be detected prior to incident fracture. In addition, women with osteopenia can be placed on a preventive regimen and followed carefully for additional bone loss. Similar standards for definitions of osteoporosis have not been established for men or for racial and ethnic groups other than whites, although recent data indicate that the standards for Hispanic women are probably similar to those of white women.

EPIDEMIOLOGIC FACTORS

In the United States, the estimated numbers of hip and vertebral fractures in women are greater than 250,000 and 500,000, respectively, per year. To this number must be added fragility fractures in men, which occur at about one-third the age-specific rate seen in women. Thus, approximately 1 million Americans suffer fragility fractures each year. The consequences of osteoporotic fracture include diminished quality of life, decreased functional independence, and increased morbidity and mortality. Pain and kyphosis, height loss, and other changes in body habitus of vertebral compression fractures diminish quality of life in women and men. Declines in functional status may result in the inability to bathe, to dress, or to ambulate independently; approximately 50% of women do not recover full function after hip fracture. Finally, a 20% excess mortality occurs in older persons in the year following hip fracture.

REVIEW OF BONE REMODELING

Bone remodeling, the coupled process of bone formation and bone resorption, is the process by which bone repairs microfractures and maintains bone health. Bone remodeling is a normal process that occurs in all adults after peak bone mass is reached. Osteoblasts and osteoclasts are the primary cells involved in bone formation and resorption, respectively. As indicated in Fig.

TABLE 465.1.	WORLD HEALTH CRITERIA FOR OSTEOPOROSIS AND RECOMMENDATIONS FOR INTERVENTION IN OLDER ADULTS	
	BMC or BMD *t* score	**Recommended Intervention**
Normal	> -1	Assure adequate Ca + D intake for age; smoking cessation; regular exercise
Osteopenia	≤ -1 but > -2.5	Use preventive measures (Fig. 465.3)
Osteoporosis	≤ -2.5	Use treatment measures (Fig. 465.4)
Severe osteoporosis	≤ -2.5 + fragility fracture	Use treatment measures (Fig. 465.4)

BMC, bone mineral content; BMD, bone mineral density.

465.1, the bone-remodeling cycle begins with "activation." This process may be initiated either by local changes, such as mechanical force and micro-fractures, or by systemic hormones or local factors that influence overall bone turnover. Activation is initiated when factors such as parathyroid hormone (PTH), interleukin-1 (IL-1), prostaglandin E_2 (PGE_2), and 1,25-dihydroxyvitamin D_3, which are known to stimulate bone resorption, alter molecules on the surface of osteoblast precursors or stromal cells. These surface molecules are variably called osteoclast differentiation factor (ODF), osteoprotegerin ligand (OPGL), and receptor activator of NF Kappa B (RANK) ligand (Fig. 465.2). The surface molecule on the osteoblast then interacts with a receptor molecule on osteoclast precursors, presumably a form of RANK, and signals are then likely transmitted to both osteoblast and osteoclast precursors. The osteoblast also makes osteoprotegerin (OPG), which can bind to OPGL and block the interaction between the responsor cells (osteoblast precursors) and osteoclast precursors. Other cell–cell interactions between osteoblast and osteoclast may also be important in the initial steps of activation and osteoclastogenesis. Furthermore, the interaction between

RANK and OPGL is necessary, but not sufficient, for the formation of active functional osteoclasts. At least one other factor, macrophage colony-stimulating factor (M-CSF or CSF-1), which is also produced by osteoblasts, is also important in osteoclastogenesis. M-CSF appears to play a role in the initial replication and activation of the osteoclast precursors, as well as in the subsequent steps of differentiation and fusion that lead to the fully activated osteoclast.

Once the osteoclasts are fully differentiated, bone resorption occurs. One important question in control of bone remodeling is how the depth and breadth of osteoclastic resorption are regulated. The limited extent of osteoclast resorption may be due to the finite life span of osteoclasts, whose nuclei undergo apoptosis. Hormones can regulate the life span and mortality of the osteoclast, but the details of this regulation are not fully understood. Following osteoclastic resorption, the reversal phase of remodeling occurs, during which mononuclear cells are present on the bone surface. The function of these cells is not understood; however, they may be involved in further degradation of bone matrix, in the formation of the so-called cement line that

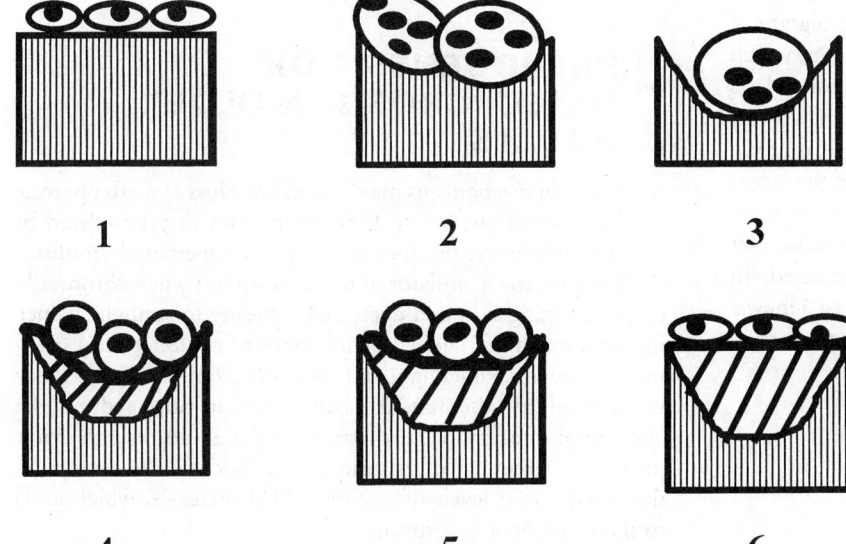

FIGURE 465.1. The bone remodeling cycle. (1) Resting phase. (2) Osteoclast activation. (3) Active resorption by mature osteoclasts. (4) Osteoblasts lay down osteoid. (5) Osteoblasts calcify new bone. (6) Resting phase.

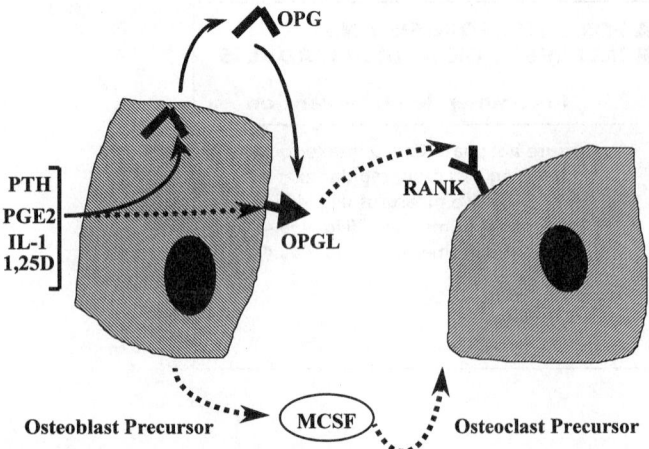

FIGURE 465.2. Schematic illustration of the interaction of osteoblast and osteoclast precursor. On the surface of osteoblast precursors are molecules called osteoprotegerin ligands (OPGLs) (also known as osteo-clast-differentiating factors, TRANCE, or RANK-L). These molecules interact with RANK on the surface of osteoclast precursors, resulting in activation of osteoclasts. Parathyroid hormone (PTH), prostaglandin E_2 (PGE$_2$), interleukin-1 (IL-1), and 1,25-hydroxyvitamin D (1,25D) have a positive effect on OPGL, resulting in increased activation of osteoclasts and, thus, bone resorption. Osteoblasts also make osteoprotegerin (OPG), which can bind to OPGL and block the interaction of osteoblast and osteoclast precursors. PTH, PGE$_2$, IL-1, and 1,25D have a negative effect on OPG production, resulting in increased bone resorption. Osteoblast precursors also produce macrophage colony-stimulating factor (M-CSF), which acts by another pathway to activate osteoclasts. It appears that both types of osteoblast–osteoclast interactions are necessary for activation of the bone remodeling cycle to take place. Solid lines represent negative effects and dotted lines represent positive effects.

is present between old and new bone, or in signaling of osteoblasts to migrate and differentiate and begin new-bone formation at the resorption site. The initiation of the formation phase is probably dependent not on cell–cell interactions but on local release of growth factors either from the matrix or from the various cells involved in the resorption and reversal phases. These growth factors stimulate the subsequent replication, migration, and differentiation of new osteoblasts in successive waves, which may also depend on signals from the differentiated osteoblasts themselves. In younger individuals, the amount of new bone formed during the coupled phase of bone remodeling is approximately equal to that resorbed; however, the capacity of the osteoblast population to multiply and to lay down new bone decreases with aging. Therefore, the amount of new bone on a trabecular surface, as measured by mean wall thickness, is decreased. In cortical bone, the consequence of impaired osteoblast renewal is incomplete filling in of the haversian canal, resulting in formation of a porotic cortex.

BONE LOSS WITH AGING

Bone mass changes over the life span of an individual. In women, bone mass increases rapidly from the time of puberty until ap-

proximately the mid-twenties to mid-thirties, at which time peak bone mass is reached. Once women reach peak bone mass, a few years of stability are followed by a slow rate of bone loss beginning well before the onset of menopause. After menopause, the rate of bone loss is quite high—from 3% to 7% per year—for up to 7 years, due to estrogen deficiency. In later life, bone loss continues, albeit at a slower rate, perhaps 1% to 2% per year; the data strongly suggest that terminating bone loss at any time will decrease fracture risk. Further, investigators estimate that a 14% increase in bone density in 80-year-old women would halve hip fracture risk. This 14% increase would also be realized if bone loss were prevented in 70-year-old women.

Men also lose bone with increasing age. Cross-sectional studies have detected a slower rate of bone loss in men than in women, but in longitudinal studies, rates of bone loss in men equaled those of older women. In spite of similar rates of bone loss in older men and women, vertebral fracture rates are lower in men. Both men and women lose predominantly cancellous bone, which is concentrated in the vertebral spine. Cortical bone accounts for 45% to 75% of the mechanical resistance to compression of the vertebral spine, and men actually gain cortical bone through periosteal bone deposition. Men also undergo an increase in the cross-sectional area of their vertebrae by 15% to 20%, increasing maximum load levels until the age of 75 years. The increased bone strength seems to be reversed by thinning of the cortical ring by age 75, the age at which men begin to present with vertebral fractures. Bone loss at the hip has not been extensively studied in men, but cross-sectional studies indicate that healthy men lose 30% to 40% of femoral neck BMD between the ages of 20 and 90 years. On iliac crest biopsies men demonstrate trabecular thinning, but they perforate the trabeculae less often than women, thereby preserving strength and providing greater potential for repair. In both femur and tibia, men and women showed endosteal resorption of bone and medullary expansion with aging; but only men had concurrent periosteal bone apposition and expansion, potentially compensating for the loss of endosteal bone.

PATHOGENESIS OF OSTEOPOROSIS IN OLDER ADULTS

A number of mechanisms may lead to bone loss and osteoporosis in older women and men. One mechanism may be related to calcium deficiency, producing secondary hyperparathyroidism. PTH is a potent stimulator of bone resorption when chronically elevated. Aging skin and decreased exposure to sunlight reduce the conversion of 7-dehydrocholesterol to cholecalciferol (vitamin D_3) by ultraviolet light and result in vitamin D insufficiency in older adults. Vitamin D insufficiency, in turn, reduces the absorption of calcium. Furthermore, older adults tend to ingest inadequate amounts of vitamin D and calcium. As a result of decreased serum levels of calcium, PTH increases, which leads to increased bone resorption.

The pathogenesis of osteoporosis in women is complex. Factors that affect the level of peak bone mass, the rate of bone resorption, and the rate of bone formation need to be considered. Peak bone mass appears to be 75% to 80% genetically determined, although the genes involved are not clearly known. At this time, candidate genes include vitamin D receptor, estrogen receptor, transforming growth factor, IL-6, IL-1 receptor 2, type I collagen genes, and collagenases.

After menopause, and with estrogen deficiency, a variety of factors that act locally on bone may lead to increased bone resorption. Factors thought to play a role in the postmenopausal bone include IL-1, IL-1 receptor antagonist, IL-6, and tumor necrosis factor, as well as their binding proteins and receptors. The exact mechanism by which estrogen deficiency leads to increased bone resorption and bone loss is not fully understood.

Androgens are important determinants for peak bone mass in men. Bone accretion is closely related to sexual maturity, and men who have abnormal puberty or delayed puberty have reduced bone mass. In addition, men with estrogen deficiency or resistance have decreased bone mass and failure of epiphysial closure. Late-onset hypogonadism may also play a role in osteoporosis in men, although further study is required to determine the exact mechanism.

Osteoblast activity appears to decrease with aging, compounding the bone loss that results from increased resorption seen with aging and menopause. Growth factors such as transforming growth factor β and insulin-like growth factor I may be impaired with estrogen deficiency or with aging, resulting in decreased osteoblast function.

■ DIAGNOSIS OF OSTEOPOROSIS AND PREDICTION OF FRACTURE

RISK FACTORS

Risk factors for osteoporosis and osteoporotic fracture have been identified and have been used to determine who should be placed

TABLE 465.2.	RISK FACTORS FOR OSTEOPOROTIC FRACTURE	
Potentially Modifiable	**Nonmodifiable**
Current cigarette smoking	Personal history of fracture
Low body weight (<127 lb)	History of fracture in first-
Estrogen deficiency:	degree relative
Early menopause (<45 y)	Advanced age
Prolonged premenopuasal	Female sex
amenorrhea (>1 y)	Dementia
Low calcium intake	Poor health/frailty
(lifelong)	
Alcoholism	
Impaired eyesight despite	
adequate correction	
Recurrent falls	
Inadequate physical activity	
Poor health/frailty	

(Modified from National Osteoporosis Foundation. Physician's Guide to Prevention and Treatment of Osteoporosis.)

TABLE 465.3.	RECOMMENDATIONS FOR EVALUATION OF SECONDARY CAUSES OF OSTEOPOROSIS	
Disease	**Laboratory Tests**
Primary hyperparathyroidism	Ionized calcium
Multiple myeloma	Serum and urine protein electrophoresis
Paget's disease	Alkaline phosphatase
Osteomalacia	Alkaline phosphatase, 25(OH)D$_3$
Hyperthyroidism	T$_4$, TSH
Hypogonadism (men only)	Bioavailable testosterone, prolactin

T$_4$, thyroxine; TSH, thyroid-stimulating hormone; 25(OH)D$_3$ 25-hydroxycholecalciferol.

on preventive or therapeutic regimens. Risk factors, however, are mediocre predictors of low bone density and fractures, and it is more useful to identify modifiable risk factors and to implement change as part of a treatment or prevention program (Table 465.2).

SECONDARY CAUSES OF OSTEOPOROSIS

The diagnosis of idiopathic or primary osteoporosis is made by bone density measurement prior to fracture or by incident fracture. Exclusion of diseases that may present as fracture or with low bone mass is important in the evaluation of women and men with osteoporosis. The major secondary causes of osteoporosis are listed in Table 465.3, along with laboratory tests used to exclude each disease. These laboratory tests should be considered in persons who present with acute compression fracture or who present with a diagnosis of osteoporosis by BMD measurement. Men are more likely to have a secondary cause of osteoporosis than women. The most commonly reported secondary causes of osteoporosis in men include hypogonadism and malabsorption syndromes. Some medications may have a detrimental effect on bone and should be identified to allow dose adjustment or discontinuation of the medications. Medications that have been shown to adversely affect BMD include glucocorticoids, excess thyroid supplement, anticonvulsants, methotrexate, cyclosporine, and heparin. In older adults, glucocorticoids and thyroid hormone are used quite commonly; accordingly, clinicians should consider the effects these medications may have on the already increased risk of fracture when prescribing them to older adults.

BONE DENSITY MEASUREMENT

Bone mineral density (BMD), or bone mass measurement, is the best predictor of fracture. BMD of the hip, spine, wrist, or calcaneus may be measured by a variety of techniques. The preferred method of BMD measurement is dual-energy x-ray absorptiometry (DXA). BMD of the hip, anteroposterior spine, lateral spine, calcaneus, and wrist can be measured using this technology. Quantitative computed tomography (QCT) is also used to measure BMD of the spine. Specific software can adapt CT scanners for BMD measurement. The advantages of DXA over QCT include lower cost, lower radiation exposure, and better reproducibility over time. Newer techniques, such as peripheral DXA (measures wrist BMD) or ultrasonography of the calcaneus, may be useful for general osteoporosis screening, and they have the advantage of reduced cost and portability. The cost of DXA is approximately $200, and Medicare covers approximately two-thirds of the cost. Current recommendations for measurement of BMD are as follows: (a) all postmenopausal women under the age of 65 years with one or more additional risk factors (other than menopause); (b) all women over 65 years, regardless of additional risk factors; (c) all postmenopausal women who present with fracture (to confirm diagnosis and determine severity); (d) women considering therapy for osteoporosis, if BMD testing would facilitate the decision; and (e) women who have been on hormone replacement therapy for prolonged periods of time (even with long-term hormone replacement therapy, women may have low BMD).

BMD may also be used to establish the diagnosis and severity of osteoporosis in men, and should be considered in men with low-trauma fracture, radiographic criteria consistent with low bone mass, or diseases known to place an individual at risk for osteoporosis. Data relating to fracture risk are derived from studies completed in women, but data also suggest that similar associations may be valid in men as well.

BIOCHEMICAL MARKERS OF BONE TURNOVER

Serum and urine biochemical markers of bone turnover have been used successfully to assess rapid turnover states, such as Paget's disease and primary hyperparathyroidism. Bone turnover changes in osteoporosis are generally smaller and require more sensitive methods. Over the last few years, new markers have been developed that reflect collagen breakdown (or bone resorption) and bone formation. Some markers are associated with increased risk of hip fracture, decreased bone density, and excess bone loss in older adults. In addition, markers of bone resorption and formation decrease in response to antiresorptive treatment. However, the use of markers in clinical practice is controversial because of the substantial overlap of marker values in women with high and low bone density or rate of bone loss. Furthermore, few studies have compared the response of a particular marker (or combination of markers) and bone density to therapy to determine the magnitude of decrease of a biochemical marker necessary to prevent bone loss or, more importantly, fracture. Urinary deoxypyridinoline cross-links and N-telopeptides of type I collagen and serum N-telopeptides of type I collagen are commercially available markers of bone resorption that may be useful in monitoring response to treatment in older women. The advantage of the serum versus urinary markers is that the intrapatient variability tends to be lower with serum markers,

thus reducing error. Further evaluation of the clinical use of markers in older women is ongoing.

◼ PREVENTION AND TREATMENT OF OSTEOPOROSIS

Osteoporosis develops in older adults when the normal processes of bone formation and resorption become uncoupled or unbalanced, resulting in bone loss. Therefore, osteoporosis prevention and treatment programs should focus on strategies that minimize bone resorption and maximize bone formation, as well as strategies that reduce falls. A number of nonpharmacologic and pharmacologic options are available to health care providers. Modification of risk factors (Table 465.2) is an important first step in preventing osteoporotic fractures in older adults.

ROLE OF EXERCISE

Exercise is an important component of osteoporosis treatment and prevention programs. Data in older men and women suggest a positive association between current exercise and hip BMD. Among regular exercisers, those who reported strenuous or moderate exercise had higher BMD at the hip than those who reported mild or less than mild exercise. Similar associations were seen for lifelong regular exercisers and hip BMD. In a randomized study of women at least 10 years past menopause, the group receiving calcium supplementation plus exercise had less bone loss at the hip than those assigned to calcium alone. Furthermore, high-intensity strength training effectively maintains femoral neck BMD and improves muscle mass, strength, and balance in postmenopausal women, in comparison with unexercised controls, suggesting that resistance training would be useful to help maintain BMD and to reduce the risk of falls in older adults.

Marked decrease in physical activity or immobilization results in a decline in bone mass; accordingly, it is important to encourage older adults to be as active as possible. Weight-bearing exercise, such as walking, can be recommended for older adults, who should be encouraged to start slowly and gradually increase both the number of days and the actual time devoted to walking. Physical therapy is an important part of osteoporosis treatment programs, especially after acute vertebral compression fracture. The physical therapist can provide postural exercises, alternative modalities for pain reduction, as well as information on changes in body mechanics that may help prevent future fracture.

CALCIUM AND VITAMIN D

Calcium and vitamin D are required for bone health at all ages. A consensus conference recommended 1,500 mg per day of elemental calcium for postmenopausal women and men over age 65 in order to maintain a positive calcium balance. The amount of vitamin D required is between 400 and 800 IU per day.

Calcium plus vitamin D at different doses has been shown to increase or maintain bone density in pre- and postmenopausal women and to prevent hip as well as all nonvertebral fractures in older adults. Adequate calcium and vitamin D intake should be recommended to all older adults, regardless of BMD, in order to maximize bone health.

PHARMACOLOGIC OPTIONS (FIGS. 465.3 AND 465.4)

Estrogen Replacement Therapy

Estrogen replacement therapy remains an important choice for the treatment and prevention of osteoporosis. In case-control and cohort studies, estrogen replacement therapy is associated with 30% to 70% reduction in the incidence of hip fracture. Multiple studies have demonstrated that postmenopausal estrogen use prevents bone loss at the hip and spine when initiated within 10 years of menopause, and other studies suggest that older women with low initial bone mass gain more bone than younger women.

Few studies have evaluated the use of estrogen in truly older women (women in their seventies, eighties, and nineties); however, small short-term studies suggest that older women are responsive to estrogen treatment. Other studies suggest that low-dose estrogen, in combination with calcium and vitamin D, has an additive effect on bone turnover in women over 70 years of age. Data from the Study of Osteoporotic Fractures support current estrogen use as protective against hip fracture, even in the oldest women. Furthermore, more and more data are accumulating to suggest that lower doses of estrogen are effective in reducing bone resorption and bone loss in older women; the lower doses also result in fewer side effects than the usual replacement doses typically used by clinicians. Although estrogen confers benefits to several organ systems, side effects and concerns about increased cancer risk associated with estrogen therapy have limited its use by postmenopausal women. Unopposed estrogen replacement therapy in women with a uterus has been associated with endometrial hyperplasia at a rate of about 30% per year, with endometrial cancer at a lower rate; concurrent progesterone therapy greatly reduces the incidence of both conditions. Hormone replacement therapy also has been associated, in some studies, with an increased incidence of breast cancer. Multiple case-control and cohort studies have variously suggested both increased and decreased breast cancer risk with estrogen replacement. Prospective data regarding the relationship between hormone replacement therapy and the incidence of breast cancer are not currently available; however, the Women's Health Initiative is addressing this issue. The various preparations of estrogen are listed, along with dosing regimens, in Table 465.4. Estrogen may be given in either continuous or cyclical fashion, depending on the preference of the woman. Because of other potential health benefits (cardiovascular, cognitive, genitourinary), hormone replacement therapy remains a primary consideration in women in whom estrogen is not contraindicated.

Bisphosphonates

Alendronate sodium is a bisphosphonate that was approved for osteoporosis treatment several years ago. When compared with placebo, alendronate increased bone density of the spine and

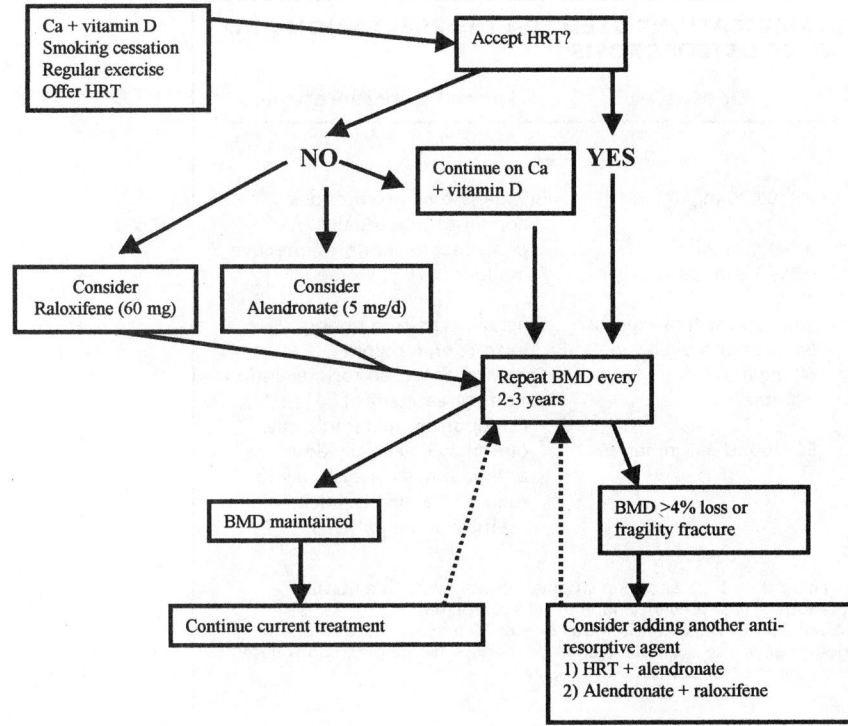

FIGURE 465.3. Algorithm for prevention of osteoporosis in postmenopausal women.
EVIDENCE LEVEL: B. Reference: National Osteoporosis Foundation. Physicians guide to prevention and treatment of osteoporosis. Belle Meade, NJ: Excerpta Medica, 1998.

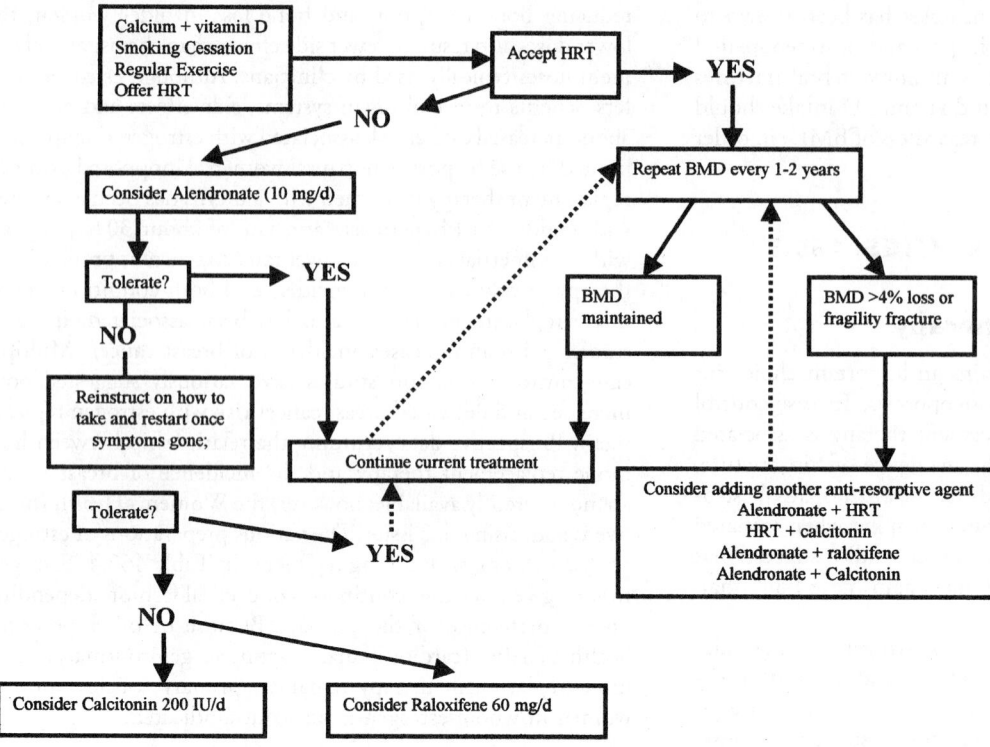

FIGURE 465.4. Algorithm for treatment of osteoporosis in post-menopausal women.
EVIDENCE LEVEL: B. Reference: National Osteoporosis Foundation. Physicians guide to prevention and treatment of osteoporosis. Belle Meade, NJ: Excerpta Medica, 1998.

hip, and decreased the vertebral fracture rate in women with osteoporosis. In women with low hip bone density and prevalent vertebral fractures, a decrease in both vertebral and hip fracture was seen with alendronate, in comparison with placebo. Women with two or more vertebral fractures at baseline had the best

response to alendronate therapy, suggesting that alendronate is effective in preventing fractures in women at highest risk for fracture. In women with low hip bone mass without previous vertebral fracture, bone density of the spine and hip also increased, and the vertebral fracture rate decreased by 51% with

TABLE 465.4.	APPROVED MEDICATIONS USED FOR THE PREVENTION AND TREATMENT OF OSTEOPOROSIS	
Medication	**Dosage**	**Special Considerations**
Estrogen replacement therapy:		
1) Conjugated equine estrogen (Premarin)	0.3–0.625 mg/d[a]	In older women continuous administration usually
2) 17β-Estradiol (Estrace)	0.5–1.0 mg/d	preferred; lower doses effective
3) Transdermal estrogen (Estraderm)	0.05–0.1 mg biweekly	in older (>70 y) women
Alendronate (Fosamax)	10 mg/d for treatment 5 mg/d for prevention	Strict adherence to dosing instruction required
Raloxifene (Evista)	60 mg/d	Currently approved for prevention
Calcitonin, nasal spray (Miacalcin)	200 IU/d	Used for treatment of osteoporosis; metered spray;
Calcitonin, injection (SC or IM) (Miacalcin, Calcimar)	50–100 IU 3–5 times/wk	one spray gives daily dose; alternate nostrils each day to reduce side effects; injectable useful in some patients

[a] For cyclical therapy, estrogen is given on days 1–25 and then stopped. In women with a uterus, progesterone must be given with the estrogen to prevent endometrial hyperplasia. Medroxyprogesterone (Provera) is given 2.5–5.0 mg/d continuously or 5 or 10 mg/d on days 16–25 for cyclical treatment. Micronized progesterone is also available (200 mg/d on days 16–25; continuous dose probably lower but no studies have so demonstrated).

alendronate, in comparison with placebo. Another study in women 60 to 85 years of age indicated that an even lower dose of alendronate may be effective in older women. Recently, alendronate was also approved for prevention of osteoporosis in early postmenopausal women. The dose for prevention is a lower dose than that given for the treatment of osteoporosis (Table 465.4). Alendronate should be considered in women with osteoporosis, either by bone density or by the presence of a fragility-related fracture, who are unwilling or unable to take hormone replacement therapy. Alendronate is also effective in prevention of bone loss and fractures in men and women with glucocorticoid-induced osteoporosis.

The major side effects of alendronate are gastrointestinal, including abdominal pain, dyspepsia, esophagitis, nausea, vomiting, and diarrhea; musculoskeletal pain may also occur. Esophagitis, particularly erosive esophagitis, may be seen most frequently in patients who do not take the medication properly. For this reason, it is extremely important to provide specific and detailed instructions for patients receiving alendronate therapy.

Intermittent etidronate therapy was shown to increase spinal bone mass and decrease vertebral fractures in women with osteoporosis. However, etidronate is not approved for use in osteoporosis treatment or prevention and should be considered only if all other options have been exhausted. A recent study indicated that etidronate was also effective in preventing bone loss in patients requiring long-term glucocorticoids.

Calcitonin

Calcitonin is a peptide hormone that is used to treat osteoporosis. It is available as a subcutaneous injection and as a nasal spray. The advantages of a nasal spray over injectable calcitonin are fewer reported side effects and greater patient acceptance. Calcitonin has been shown to increase bone density in the spine and to reduce vertebral fractures. In epidemiologic studies calcitonin has been shown to reduce hip fractures, although in clinical trials hip bone density does not increase. A recent 5-year study demonstrated a decrease in vertebral fracture in women on nasal spray calcitonin (200 IU per day), in comparison with those on placebo. Calcitonin, however, does not appear to be as effective in preventing fractures as estrogen replacement therapy or alendronate; therefore, its use should be limited to those women who are unable to tolerate other treatments. In some studies, calcitonin therapy has also been associated with an analgesic effect in acute compression fractures, in Paget's disease of bone, and in bone pain attributable to metastatic disease.

Selective Estrogen Receptor Agonists

The selective estrogen receptor modulators (SERMs) are agents that act as estrogen agonists in bone and heart but act as estrogen antagonists in breast and uterine tissue. These medications have the potential to prevent osteoporosis or heart disease without the increased risk of breast or uterine cancer. Tamoxifen, an agent used in breast cancer treatment, has been shown to have beneficial effects on bone in several studies but has stimulatory effects on the uterus; it is not approved for treatment or prevention of osteoporosis. Postmenopausal osteoporotic women

treated with raloxifene had decreased bone turnover and maintenance of proximal femur and total body bone density as well as fewer vertebral fractures, in comparison with women who received placebo. There were no differences among groups in breast abnormalities or endometrial thickness. In a short-term study, raloxifene had effects on bone histomorphometry and bone turnover that were similar in direction to conjugated equine estrogen (CEE) but were lower in magnitude than CEE. Raloxifene is currently approved for prevention of osteoporosis. Its use for treatment of osteoporosis is still being evaluated, although recent data suggest that raloxifene is effective in preventing vertebral fractures in postmenopausal women with osteoporosis.

THERAPEUTIC APPROACHES IN MEN

Very little is known about successful treatment or prevention of osteoporosis in men. Although the data are scarce, reasonable therapeutic approaches, based on successful outcomes in women or understanding of the differences in pathophysiologic factors, can be undertaken until more information is available. Thus, adequate calcium and vitamin D intake and exercise would be part of a prevention and treatment program in older men. Calcium intake is less than 800 mg per day in 60% of adult men in the United States, and approximately 900 mg per day is required to ensure calcium balance in men. Antiresorptive agents, which are effective in women, hold promise but have not been investigated in men. Treatment of osteoporosis due to secondary causes should focus on treatment of the underlying cause.

INVESTIGATIONAL AGENTS FOR OSTEOPOROSIS TREATMENT AND PREVENTION

A number of medications are currently under investigation for use in osteoporosis treatment and prevention, including additional bisphosphonates and SERMs, as well as PTH and fluoride. Other bisphosphonates under investigation for osteoporosis include risedronate, tiludronate, pamidronate, and ibandronate. Additional SERMs currently under evaluation include idoxifene and droloxifene.

PTH, while leading to increased bone resorption when chronically elevated, increases bone mass, trabecular connectivity, and mechanical strength in rodents when administered intermittently; in uncontrolled studies, it has been shown to increase spinal BMD in osteoporotic men and women. In a 3-year randomized study of postmenopausal women with osteoporosis, the group receiving estrogen plus intermittent PTH had a continuous increase in spinal bone mass over the study period, as well as a decreased rate of vertebral fracture. Bone mass of the hip and total body also increased significantly in the estrogen plus PTH group, in comparison with estrogen alone.

The use of fluoride to treat osteoporosis is appealing, since fluoride results in a large increase in spine BMD; however, the increase in BMD was not associated with a decrease in vertebral fractures. In fact, the group receiving fluoride had a higher rate of appendicular fractures. Recently, slow-release intermittent fluoride administration has been associated with an increase in spine BMD, as well as decreased incidence of vertebral fractures. Additional studies are required before slow-release fluoride can be recommended for the treatment of osteoporosis.

BIBLIOGRAPHY

Black DM, Cummings SR, Karpf DB, et al. Randomised trial of effect of alendronate on risk of fracture in women with existing vertebral fractures. Fracture Intervention Trial Research Group. *Lancet* 1996; 348(9041):1535–1541.

Cummings SR, Nevitt MC, Browner WS, et al. Risk factors for hip fracture in white women. Study of Osteoporotic Fractures Research Group. *N Engl J Med* 1995;332(12):767–773.

Dawson-Hughes B, Harris SS, Krall EA, et al. Effect of calcium and vitamin D supplementation on bone density in men and women 65 years of age or older. *N Engl J Med* 1997;337(10):670–676.

Greendale GA, Barrett-Connor E, Edelstein S, et al. Lifetime leisure exercise and osteoporosis. The Rancho Bernardo study. *Am J Epidemiol* 1995; 141(10):951–959.

Lindsay R, Bush TL, Grady D, et al. Therapeutic controvesy: estrogen replacement in menopause. *J Clin Endocrinol Metab* 1996;81(11): 3829–3838.

Manolagas SC, Jilka RL. Bone marrow, cytokines, and bone remodeling. Emerging insights into the pathophysiology of osteoporosis. *N Engl J Med* 1995;332(5):305–311.

NIH Consensus Conference. Optimal calcium intake. NIH consensus development panel on optimal calcium intake. *JAMA* 1994;272(24): 1942–1948.

Riggs BL, Khosla S, Melton LJ III. A unitary model for involutional osteoporosis: estrogen deficiency causes both type I and type II osteoporosis in postmenopausal women and contributes to bone loss in aging men. *J Bone Miner Res* 1998;13(5) 3–773.

Seeman E. Osteoporosis in men: epidemiology, pathophysiology, and treatment possibilities. *Am J Med* 1993;95(5A):22S–28S.

World Health Organization Technical Report Series No. 843. *Assessment of fracture risk and its application to screening for postmenopausal osteoporosis.* Geneva, 1994.

Kelley's Textbook of Internal Medicine, fourth edition. Edited by H. David Humes. Lippincott Williams & Wilkins, Philadelphia © 2000.

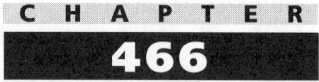

CHAPTER 466

DEMENTIA, INCLUDING ALZHEIMER'S DISEASE

CHRISTOPHER M. CLARK

ALZHEIMER'S DISEASE

Alzheimer's disease (AD) is the most common form of late-life brain failure. It is a heterogeneous, neurodegenerative, dementing illness that produces progressive memory loss, changes in behavior and personality, psychotic symptoms, and impairments in insight, judgment, and executive abilities as well as the ability to perform complex motor and visual tasks (e.g., apraxia).

Pathologically it is defined by extensive neuron loss, numerous amyloid plaques, and abundant neurofibrillary tangles (NFTs) in selectively vulnerable regions of the brain, including the hippocampus, entorhinal cortex, and association areas of the neocortex. The hallmark clinical features of memory loss, behavioral changes, and confused thinking are a direct consequence of these pathologic changes. While there has been considerable progress in understanding the pathologic mechanisms responsible for this late-life neurodegenerative disorder, at present the specific factors responsible for producing these changes in the brain remain obscure. Only a few risk factors have been well established. These include age, presence of an ApoE ϵ4 allele, female gender, history of head trauma, and having a first-degree blood relative with an AD-like dementia.

A small number of patients have an autosomal dominant form of AD. To date, more than 59 mutations have been identified that are capable of causing AD in this group. Twelve are on the *amyloid precursor* gene on chromosome 21, forty-five are on the *presenilin-1* gene on chromosome 14, and two are on the *presenilin-2* gene on chromosome 1. How these mutations produce the pathologic changes of AD has not been definitively established.

Most patients will have either a "sporadic" or "familial" (non–autosomal dominant) form of AD. For these individuals, the conditions capable of initiating and contributing to the pathologic changes in the brain are even more obscure, but they are certain to be multiple and to involve complex biological and environmental interactions.

PREVALENCE

Epidemiologic studies document the relationship between AD and advancing age. For individuals whose age is between 65 to 74 years, the prevalence is about 3%. This climbs to 47% for individuals over age 85. Because of the debilitating nature of the illness, its prolonged duration (6 to 12 years on average, with a range of 4 to 23 years), the high cost associated with care during its terminal stages, and the fact that individuals at highest risk are among the most rapidly growing segment of the United States population, AD is now recognized as a serious and escalating public health problem.

CLINICAL DESCRIPTION AND DIAGNOSTIC EVALUATION

AD is characterized by the insidious onset of memory failure. Symptoms most commonly begin between the ages of 70 and 85, but can occur as early as 40 and as late as 90. During the first several years, patients may also have difficulty with problem solving and word finding. They often exhibit subtle personality and behavioral changes. Frequently, they develop symptoms that mimic mild depression as they withdraw from social situations and lose enthusiasm for participating in activities that they find confusing and/or anxiety provoking. While they may be aware that their memory is failing, they usually do not appreciate the extent of the problem and rarely seek medical help. Thus, it is almost always a family member (spouse or adult child) who brings them to medical attention.

TABLE 466.1.	DIAGNOSTIC CRITERIA FOR ALZHEIMER'S DISEASE BASED ON THE 1984 NINCDS–ADRDA CONSENSUS CRITERIA

Probable Alzheimer's disease

    Dementia with onset between ages 40 and 90
    Cognitive deficits in two or more areas
    Progressive memory and cognitive deterioration
    No other illness that could account for the dementia
    No disturbance of consciousness

Possible Alzheimer's disease

    Variations in the onset or clinical course
    Presence of a secondary disorder sufficient to produce dementia but not felt to be the primary cause

Definite Alzheimer's disease

    Clinical criteria for probable Alzheimer's disease
    Neuropathologic evidence sufficient for the diagnosis

NINDS, National Institute of Neurological and Communicative Disorders and Stroke; ADRDA, Alzheimer's Disease and Related Disorders Association.

A clinical diagnosis of AD is best made using the consensus criteria developed in 1994. The main elements are listed in Table 466.1.

A key feature is the documentation of memory loss as the earliest manifestation of the illness. Elements that strengthen the diagnosis but do not confirm or, in their absence, refute a diagnosis of AD include a family history of one or more first-degree relatives with a similar late-life dementia (especially if autopsy-proven AD), normal routine blood studies (including those for thyroid disease and B_{12} deficiency), presence of one or more ApoE $\epsilon 4$ alleles, elevated cerebrospinal fluid tau level, and a magnetic resonance image that either is "normal for age" or shows mild generalized cortical atrophy.

Findings that cast doubt on the diagnosis include the following: parkinsonism (slow gait, decreased arm swing, en-bloc turning), presence early in the course of the illness of a language impairment and/or mental confusion that is more prominent than the patient's memory impairment, prominent symptoms or signs of frontal lobe dysfunction (e.g., disinhibition, perseveration, delusions, psychosis and/or hallucinations) within the first several years of illness, the finding of any focal neurologic signs on examination, and seizures or myoclonus early in course.

TREATMENT

There are several components of treatment. First and foremost is the education of the primary caregiver about the illness, the need for long-range planning, how to maintain a living environment that will maximize the patient's ability to function, how to avoid precipitating behavior problems, and how to handle the problems that do occur despite the efforts of all concerned. Over the past several years, donepazil (Aricept) has become the standard symptomatic treatment. Its benefits are modest and are not seen in all patients. High-dose vitamin E (α-tocopherol) has also been adopted as the standard disease-slowing treatment.

Treatment for the behavioral, psychotic, anxiety, and mood changes that occur with AD is generally accomplished through the gentle and short-term use of psychotropic, antianxiety, and hypnotic medications.

OTHER COMMON CONDITIONS THAT PRODUCE LATE-LIFE DEMENTIA

FRONTAL DEMENTIA

The diagnostic category of frontal dementia (Table 466.2) includes several pathologically defined conditions that cannot be distinguished with certainty during life. These include Pick's disease, frontotemporal dementia, and dementia lacking definitive histopathology. In general, the presentation of a neurodegenerative frontal dementia takes one of two forms. In each case the onset is gradual, with the first symptoms often beginning before age 65 years.

The most common presentation involves early changes in social behavior. Patients in this grouping undergo the insidious onset of personality and behavioral changes that are clearly out of character. These include impaired interpersonal conduct, as manifest by a disregard for manners, social graces, and decorum; as well as disinhibited verbal, physical, or sexual behaviors. They may demonstrate difficulty with goal-directed behavior as manifest by apathy, passivity, inertia, or, alternatively, hyperactivity without clear purpose. Frequently, they exhibit emotional blunting, with indifference and lack of empathy. In general, they are unconcerned about or unaware of these mental changes. These changes usually begin at a time when there is relative preservation of memory.

The next most common presentation involves the early development of language impairment, characterized by one or more of the following: nonfluent, hesitant, and effortful speech; sentences with missing words; mispronunciation of words; and word-finding difficulties, impaired repetition of phrase, decreased fluency, and impaired reading and writing.

TABLE 466.2.	CLINICAL DIAGNOSIS IN PATIENTS EVALUATED BY A UNIVERSITY-BASED MEMORY DISORDERS CLINIC (N = 1,072)

Diagnosis	Frequency (%)
Alzheimer's disease	58
Mild cognitive impairment	9
Frontal dementia	5
Dementia with Lewy bodies	3
Parkinson's dementia	3
Ischemic vascular dementia	3
Depression	3
Miscellaneous[a]	16

---

[a] Includes undefined dementia, Creutzfeldt–Jakob disease, corticobasilar degeneration, multisystem atrophy, and other uncommon conditions.

A diagnosis of frontal dementia is supported by a family history of a similar disorder; a decline in personal hygiene and grooming; the presence of mental rigidity and inflexibility; easy distractibility; hyperorality, such as binge eating; perseverative or stereotyped speech, including a tendency to repeat utterances; incontinence without concern early in the course of the illness; and an imaging study result showing focal frontal and/or temporal atrophy.

There is no disease-specific treatment. Behavioral difficulties are common, and management often requires a combination of caregiver education and the gentle use of psychotropic medication.

DEMENTIA WITH LEWY BODIES

The neurodegenerative dementia known as dementia with Lewy bodies shares clinical and pathologic features with AD and Parkinson's disease. Despite the symptom overlap, it is pathologically distinct from AD in that there are no cortical neurofibrillary tangles. It differs from routine Parkinson's disease in that patients have psychotic symptoms (hallucinations, delusions, paranoia) early in the course of their illness. The response to standard antiparkinsonian medication is often poor, and patients have a low threshold for the psychosis-inducing side effects of these drugs The clinical distinction between the Lewy body variant of AD, dementia with Lewy bodies, and Parkinson's dementia is difficult. However, the distinction is important as the primary treatment strategy differs among these three conditions.

The typical clinical picture includes the insidious onset of confusion with psychosis (hallucinations, delusions, and paranoia). The patient's level of alertness and degree of confusion may seem to fluctuate from hour to hour or be episodic. Hallucinations (when present) are often visual, well formed, detailed, and typically involve people. They are often most evident during periods of marked confusion. Parkinsonian features (rigidity, resting tremor, slow movements, and changes in gait and postural balance) usually develop in concert with the cognitive and psychotic features. Memory impairments may not be present in the early stages but are usually evident with progression.

The diagnosis is supported by the presence of repeated falls due to impairments of gait and postural balance, syncope-like episodes, and exquisite sensitivity to the parkinsonism-inducing effects of typical antipsychotic medication.

There is no uniformly satisfactory treatment. The symptoms of parkinsonism may respond to gentle use of carbidopa or other dopamine agonists. The psychotic symptoms may respond to low doses of atypical neuroleptic medications, but these drugs often exacerbate the parkinsonian symptoms. When present, depression may respond to selective serotonin reuptake inhibitor antidepressant.

ISCHEMIC VASCULAR DEMENTIA (MULTI-INFARCT DEMENTIA)

Although cerebrovascular disease is common, autopsy studies on patients with dementia indicate that it is the primary cause in only 3% to 5% of cases. Thus, only rarely will it be the principal diagnosis for patients with insidious progressive cognitive im-

pairment. Nevertheless, ischemic cerebrovascular disease may contribute to symptoms of dementia that are primarily due to other causes (e.g., AD).

The typical clinical picture of vascular dementia involves an abrupt onset of focal cognitive impairment associated with motor and/or sensory signs of stroke. The episodes may be repetitive, and if there is concordance between the location of the infarction and the patient's cognitive deficits, thee patient should be treated for cerebrovascular disease with an emphasis on the use of antiplatelet medication, control of stroke risk factors, and adequate treatment of hypertension.

■ SUMMARY

Neurodegenerative dementia represents a common affliction of late life and is one of the leading causes of severe disability and death in individuals older than 75 years. Clinical diagnostic criteria have recently become available for the more common disorders. Modestly effective treatment is now available for AD. It is important for clinicians to recognize these disorders when the symptoms are at their earliest stage so they can educate family members and begin treatment to reduce the symptoms and slow the progression. Ideally, planning for long-term care should begin at a stage when the patient can still participate in the discussions. From a medical management, public health, and patient benefit standpoint, the most effective treatment strategy will be to identify individuals at high risk who are still free of symptoms and initiate therapy that will delay the onset of clinical manifestations of dementia and slow its rate of progression so that they can live their natural lives free of severe cognitive disability.

BIBLIOGRAPHY

Evans DA, Funkenstein HH, Albert MS, et al. Prevalence of Alzheimer's disease in a community population of older persons. Higher than previously reported. *JAMA* 1989;262:2551–2556.

McKeith IG, Galasko D, Kosaka K, et al. Consensus guidelines for the clinical and pathologic diagnosis of dementia with Lewy bodies (DLB): report of the consortium on DLB international workshop. *Neurology* 1996;47:1113–1124.

McKhann G, Drachman D, Folstein M, et al. Clinical diagnosis of Alzheimer's disease: report of the NINCDS–ADRDA Work Group under the auspices of Department of Health and Human Services Task Force on Alzheimer's disease. *Neurology* 1984;34:939–944.

The National Institute on Aging, and Reagan Institute Working Group on Diagnostic Criteria for the Neuropathological Assessment of Alzheimer's Disease. Consensus Recommendations for the Postmortem Diagnosis of Alzheimer's disease. *Neurobiol Aging* 1997;18(S4):1–2.

Neary D, Snowden JS, Gustafson L, et al. Frontotemporal lobar degeneration. A consensus on clinical diagnostic criteria. *Neurology* 1998;51:1546–1554.

Rogers SL, Farlow MR, Doody RS, et al. A 24-week, double-blind, placebo-controlled trial of donepezil in patients with Alzheimer's disease. Donepezil Study Group. *Neurology* 1998;50:136–145.

Roman GC, Tatemichi TK, Erkinjuntti T, et al. Vascular dementia: diagnostic criteria for research studies. Report of the NINDS–AIREN International Workshop. *Neurology* 1993;43:250–260.

Sano M, Ernesto C, Thomas RG, et al. A controlled trial of selegiline, alpha-tocopherol, or both as treatment for Alzheimer's disease. The Alzheimer's Disease Cooperative Study. *N Engl J Med* 1997;336: 1216–1222.

Kelley's Textbook of Internal Medicine, fourth edition. Edited by H. David Humes. Lippincott Williams & Wilkins, Philadelphia © 2000.

C H A P T E R
467

BENIGN PROSTATIC HYPERPLASIA/URINARY OBSTRUCTION

J. LISA TENOVER

BACKGROUND AND PATHOGENESIS

Benign prostatic hyperplasia (BPH; historically, incorrectly often called hypertrophy) is a histopathologic entity characterized by stromal and epithelial prostatic cell hyperplasia of the transitional and periurethral zones of the prostate. As a histopathologic diagnosis, the process is nearly universal in the aging human male; greater than 95% of men will demonstrate this prostate pathologic lesion if they live long enough. The prevalence of histologic BPH is comparable across ethnic groups and locales. Progression of histologic BPH to benign prostatic enlargement (detectable by digital rectal examination, or DRE, or by imaging techniques such as ultrasonography) is somewhat selective and occurs in about half of men with histologic BPH. Environmental and genetic factors may play a role. However, since increased prostate size alone does not produce clinical symptoms, not all men who develop an enlarged prostate experience symptoms of urinary tract outlet obstruction. Nonetheless, clinical BPH is a condition that affects the majority of older men, having an impact on morbidity and well-being.

The pathogenesis of histologic BPH is poorly understood. The two major risk factors are aging and the presence of androgens. Thus far, epidemiologic studies have produced no evidence for any association between development of BPH and diet, smoking, caffeine, frequency of sexual intercourse, medications, or other diseases. Androgens are important in prostate development and growth. The fetal surge of testosterone production is needed for prostate imprinting for later development; adolescent growth of the prostate coincides with the increase in testosterone secretion; and the growth of the prostate that begins in the fourth and fifth decades of life is not seen in the setting of castration or profound hypogonadism. The predominant androgen in the prostate is dihydrotestosterone (DHT), a more potent androgen than testosterone and one that is derived primarily at the target organ tissue by conversion of testosterone to DHT by the 5α-reductase enzyme. While DHT plays a permissive role in the development of BPH, there clearly are other factors involved.

The major histologic growth of BPH occurs in a man aged 40 to 70 years, a time when prostatic DHT levels do not change. Other pathogenetic factors that are probably involved include intraprostatic estrogens, intraprostatic growth factors, and stromal–epithelial interactions.

Prostate enlargement due to BPH may lead to varying degrees of symptomatology related to urinary outlet obstruction. Clinically diagnosed BPH, formerly called prostatism, currently is more aptly described as lower urinary tract symptoms (LUTS) due to BPH. It should be noted, however, that not all LUTS in men are due to prostate enlargement (BPH). Urethral stricture is a notable alternative cause. However, there is a steady increase in the age-specific prevalence of LUTS due to BPH; community-based epidemiologic studies estimate the prevalence of LUTS due to BPH to be about 40% to 50% for men in their seventies.

The development of LUTS as a result of BPH is influenced by a number of factors. Increase in prostate size can result in a decreased functional urethral diameter and an increased urinary outflow resistance; the strength of bladder detrusor muscle contractions is important in overcoming urethral resistance and impacts on the degree of bladder outlet obstruction necessary to result in symptoms; the elasticity of the prostatic capsule can also affect the degree to which prostate growth will cause urethral constriction; and the smooth-muscle tone of the prostate can dynamically affect urethral diameter. There is still disagreement about the relative roles of these factors in the development of LUTS, but clearly enlarged prostate size alone does not necessarily lead to development of symptoms.

CLINICAL PRESENTATION

Urinary symptoms related to BPH can be divided into two categories: obstructive and irritative (Table 467.1). The obstructive symptoms are directly related to the process of partial urinary outlet obstruction, whereas the irritative symptoms have a more complicated etiologic process. For example, some of the daytime urinary frequency and urgency may be due to incomplete bladder emptying, leading to shortened time intervals until the bladder is again "full" and there is a need to void; however, detrusor irritability also occurs in BPH. Nocturia may be a continuation of the daytime urinary frequency process, but it may also be a result of heightened urine production at night. Most evaluations

TABLE 467.1.	LOWER URINARY TRACT SYMPTOMS DUE TO BENIGN PROSTATIC HYPERPLASIA

Obstructive symptoms:
  Decreased caliber and force of urine stream
  Hesitancy and straining to void
  Dribbling at termination of voiding
  Feeling of incomplete emptying
Irritative symptoms:
  Urgency
  Frequency
  Nocturia
Urinary incontinence

of therapy for LUTS due to BPH have emphasized the effects of treatment on obstructive symptoms, since these are easier to quantitate objectively (measuring urine flow rates, urine flow patterns, and postvoid urine residual volumes), and because irritative symptoms may be multifactorial, often responding less well to therapeutic interventions. Nonetheless, it is clear that the irritative symptoms are most bothersome to patients.

Urinary incontinence, which may have both obstructive and irritative components, also is very disruptive to the patient.

It is usually irritative LUTS that bring patients to the attention of the physician. Although LUTS are rarely life threatening, they are associated with significant morbidity (self-reported bother, interference with common daily activities, decreased psy-

chological well-being, worry, and embarrassment). Occasionally, the presence of symptomatic BPH can come to the attention of the physician in a more dramatic presentation. These presentations include (a) acute complete urinary retention; (b) gross hematuria; (c) finding of bladder stones; (d) discovery of large bladder diverticuli and/or bladder wall hypertrophy; (e) recurrent urinary infections; or (f) renal failure.

EVALUATION

The primary goals of initial evaluation, especially for the nonurologist, are (a) to ascertain the presence or absence of LUTS

Prostate Test

FOR YOUR URINARY ACTIVITIES

NAME _____   DATE _____

Circle your numerical score for each question below.

	None	1 time	2 times	3 times	4 times	5 or more times
1 Over the last month or so, how many times did you most typically get up to urinate from the time you went to bed at night until the time you got up in the morning?	0	1	2	3	4	5

	Not at all	Less than 1 time in 5	Less than half the time	About half the time	More than half the time	Almost always
2 Over the past month or so, how often have you had a sensation of not emptying your bladder completely after you finished urinating?	0	1	2	3	4	5
3 Over the past month or so, how often have you had to urinate again less than two hours after you finished urinating?	0	1	2	3	4	5
4 Over the past month or so, how often have you found that you stopped and started again several times when you urinated?	0	1	2	3	4	5
5 Over the past month or so, how often have you found it difficult to postpone urination?	0	1	2	3	4	5
6 Over the past month or so, how often have you had a weak urinary stream?	0	1	2	3	4	5
7 Over the past month or so, how often have you had to push or strain to begin urination?	0	1	2	3	4	5

From the American Urological Association (AUA) Symptom Index for BPH.

Total your score here.
Total Symptom Score = Sum of Questions 1 to 7 = ▢

FIGURE 467.1. American Urological Association symptom score sheet for lower urinary tract symptoms (also known as I-PSS).

in the male patient, (b) to determine the likelihood that LUTS are due to BPH, (c) to screen for imperative indicators for rapid (usually surgical) intervention, and (d) to establish the degree to which the LUTS are bothersome to the patient. This fourth goal is especially important, since LUTS affect quality of life and the same symptoms may impact different men in different ways. Most treatment recommendations are based on the degree of symptom "bothersomeness," weighing this against the possible benefits and risks of treatment.

In an attempt to quantify LUTS, the American Urological Association (AUA), in combination with the U.S. Public Health Service, has designed a patient self-administered symptom score sheet (Fig. 467.1). Also known as the I-PSS (International Prostate Symptom Score), this sheet is in the public domain, may be reproduced without permission, and is used worldwide. This questionnaire is not specific for LUTS due to BPH, but in the correct clinical setting it may be helpful in suggesting who may

need treatment and in monitoring therapy. Patients with total scores of 7 or less have "mild" symptoms and rarely need therapy. Scores from 8 to 19 denote "moderate" symptoms, and these patients may or may not need therapy, depending on the impact of the symptoms on their quality of life. Patients with scores of 20 to 35 are felt to have "severe" symptoms, and most, but not all, of these patients will require some form of treatment.

Both national and international clinical practice guidelines for the diagnosis and treatment of symptomatic BPH have been published. The two guidelines are very similar in both the diagnostic and treatment realms. Figure 467.2 is the diagnosis and treatment guidelines algorithm for BPH from the U.S. Agency of Health Care Policy and Research (AHCPR). In the initial evaluation of possible clinical BPH, a medical history is very important. Not only should the history ascertain the presence and degree of LUTS symptoms (using I-PSS or similar questions), it should also gather information to assist in the evalua-

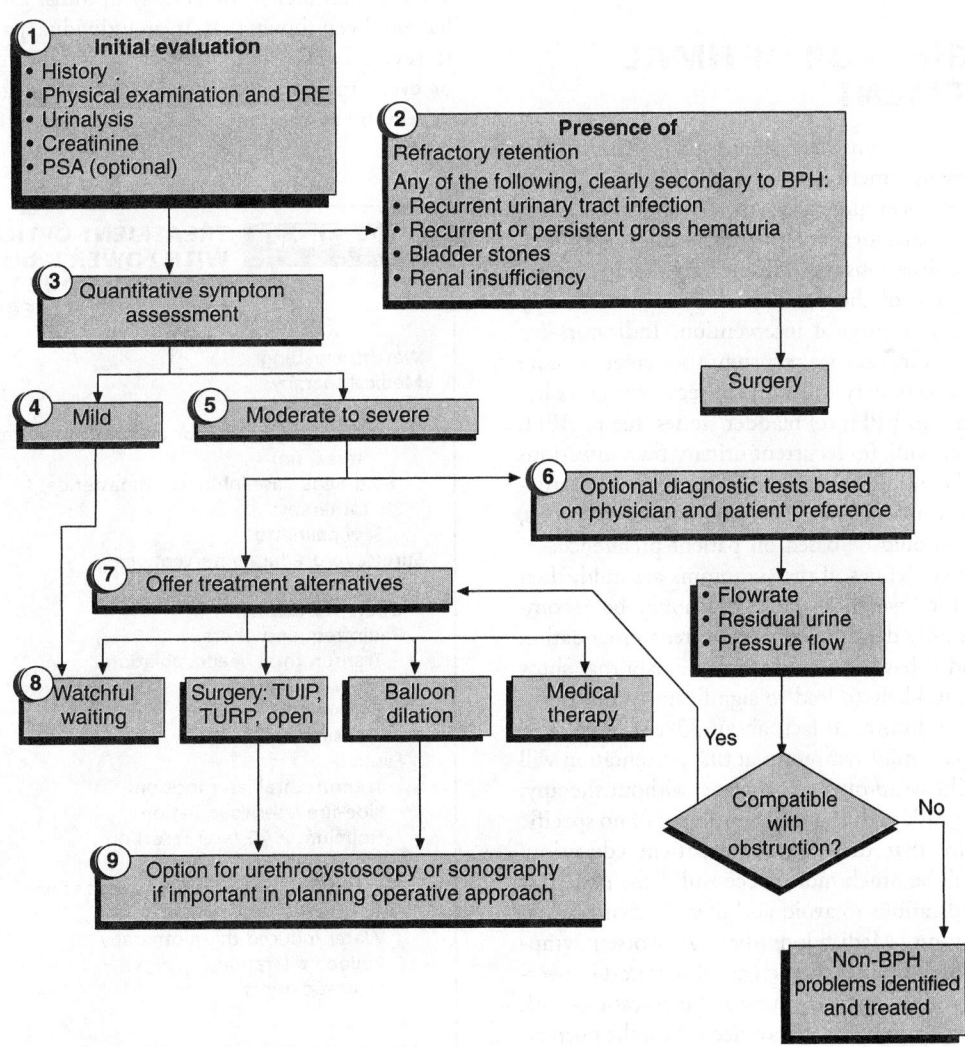

FIGURE 467.2. Benign prostatic hyperplasia diagnosis and treatment guidelines issued by the U.S. Agency of Health Care Policy and Research. DRE, digital rectal examination; PSA, prostate-specific antigen; TUIP, transurethral incision of the prostate; TURP, transurethral resection of the prostate.

tion of diagnoses for LUTS other than BPH. Alternative diagnoses for LUTS in men include concurrent urinary infection; detrusor muscle dysfunction due to pelvic nerve damage from trauma, infections, diabetes mellitus, or neurologic disease; bladder cancer; urethral stricture; or use of medications that can worsen detrusor function or heighten bladder outlet obstruction.

In addition to the medical history, other evaluation recommendations include physical examination, including DRE of the prostate (to evaluate anal sphincter tone, prostate gland size, consistency, and abnormalities suggestive of prostate cancer), urinalysis (to evaluate for hematuria, proteinuria, pyuria, and glucosuria), and serum creatinine level. These evaluations are carried out to assist in discriminating between the differential diagnoses of LUTS, to evaluate whether BPH may have already led to renal insufficiency, and to ascertain if there is a likelihood that concurrent prostate cancer is present. Although the presence of BPH is not a risk factor for prostate cancer and prostate cancer rarely causes LUTS, the two can coexist in the same prostate. The use of prostate-specific antigen (PSA) in the evaluation process is optional and is for the purpose of prostate cancer screening.

STRATEGIES FOR OPTIMAL MANAGEMENT

If from the evaluation it seems likely that a patient has LUTS due to BPH, then management decisions will arise as noted in Fig. 467.2. If there is uncertainty as to the cause of the LUTS, then a referral to a urologist for other diagnostic tests is appropriate. There are certain situations when immediate therapy is warranted. Usually, because of the urgency of treatment, therapy consists of some type of surgical intervention. Indicators for immediate intervention include (a) recurrent spontaneous acute urinary retention felt secondary to BPH; (b) recurrent gross hematuria felt secondary to BPH; (c) bladder stones due to BPH; (d) large bladder diverticuli; (e) recurrent urinary tract infections felt secondary to BPH; and (f) renal failure due to outlet obstruction from BPH. In the absence of these complicating situations, the decision to treat should be based on patient preference.

According to the guidelines, if the symptoms are mild, then no therapy except for "watchful waiting" should be recommended. This is the only definitive treatment recommendation in the guidelines and is based on epidemiologic data that show that mild LUTS are unlikely to lead to significant health problems in the immediate future. In fact, about 75% of men aged 40 to 79 years who have mild symptoms at first presentation will continue to have mild symptoms 4 years later without therapy.

Watchful waiting, although it implies initiation of no specific therapy, does require that there be some patient education. Watchful waiting will be much more successful if the patient is counseled about medications to avoid and lifestyle changes that may improve symptoms. Medications that can worsen symptoms include α-sympathomimetics, such as those found in over-the-counter cold remedies; antihistamines; and medications with anticholinergic effects. If diuretics are not needed for the purpose of fluid management, the patient may also benefit by avoiding their use (alternative treatments for hypertension should be con-

sidered). Consideration of the amount, timing, and type of fluid ingested is also important; caffeine-containing products and alcohol can worsen BPH symptoms, and large amounts of any type of fluid should be avoided within hours of bedtime. In addition, avoiding long intervals between voiding may be helpful, as a large, full, and nearly optimally stretched bladder contracts with less force than a less full bladder. If watchful waiting is the management approach taken for symptomatic BPH, yearly evaluations that mimic the initial evaluation should be done to confirm that symptoms are still not bothersome and that no complications have developed.

If patient symptoms are moderate or severe but there are no complicating situations, then patient treatment preference, obtained after counseling on the alternatives, should be the deciding factor. Table 467.2 lists the treatment options for these men. Again, watchful waiting is one of the possible treatment approaches. Data from community-based epidemiologic studies and from the placebo treatment arms of drug trials have shown that men with more severe symptoms at first presentation are more likely to need medical or surgical therapy within the next 4 years than men with mild symptoms. On the other hand, it has also been shown that, in an individual patient with moderate to severe LUTS symptoms, these symptoms can remain stable or even improve over that same time period. In terms of the development of spontaneous acute urinary retention (retention

---

TABLE 467.2. **TREATMENT OPTIONS FOR MEN WITH LOWER URINARY TRACT SYMPTOMS DUE TO BENIGN PROSTATIC HYPERPLASIA**

Watchful waiting
Medical therapy
  Pharmacologic:
    α-Adrenergic receptor antagonists (doxazosin, tamsulosin, terazosin)
    5 α-Reductase inhibitors (finasteride)
  Phytotherapy:
    Saw palmetto
Surgical/procedural interventions
  Transurethral prostatectomy
  Open prostatectomy
  Radiofrequency therapy:
    Transurethral needle ablation
  Microwave therapy:
    Transrectal
    Transurethral
  Laser:
    Transurethral laser incision
    Side-fire laser coagulation
    Holmium: YAG laser resection
  Electroresection:
    Transurethral incision or vaporization
  Other:
    Water-induced thermotherapy
    Balloon dilatation
    Prostatic stents

YAG, yttrium–aluminum–garnett.

not precipitated by surgery, anesthesia, medications, or alcohol), having moderate to severe BPH symptoms does not predict occurrence, although the prevalence of acute urinary retention in men with LUTS due to BPH increases dramatically with age after the age of 60 years, with an incidence of 8 to 14 events per 1,000 person-years.

In the last decade, medical (pharmacologic) management has become the principal initial therapy for most men with LUTS due to BPH. In general, medical management results in less change in symptom scores and urine flow rates than do the surgical interventions, but pharmacologic therapy is noninvasive, results in long-term sustained improvements, and is satisfactory to a large number of patients. At the current time, there are two classes of medications for the treatment of symptomatic BPH: α-adrenergic receptor antagonists and 5α-reductase inhibitors. There are a number of factors to consider when selecting medical therapy, including mode of action, prostate size, and adverse-effect profiles of the medications.

Prostatic smooth-muscle tone contributes to outlet obstruction, and contraction of the prostate and urethral smooth muscle is mediated by α-adrenergic receptors. There are several subtypes of α-adrenergic receptors present in varying amounts at the bladder neck, prostatic urethra, prostatic capsule, and in the prostatic stroma; the majority of these are of the alpha-1A subtype. It has been shown that men taking α-adrenergic receptor antagonists experience smooth-muscle relaxation in these areas and, in addition, have a down regulation of expression of the myosin heavy chain gene in smooth-muscle cells. Currently, three selective α-adrenergic receptor blockers have been approved for the treatment of BPH in the United States. These agents are the two $α_1$-selective long-acting agents terazosin and doxazosin, and the more $α_{-1A}$ selective agent, tamsulosin. The "uroselectivity" of α-blockers is important from the perspective of trying to avoid side effects, such as orthostatic hypotension, which are due to interactions with vascular smooth muscle.

α-Adrenergic receptor antagonists have a relatively rapid onset of action (agents can be titrated to effectiveness within days) and have been shown to remain effective in the treatment of LUTS due to BPH for at least 4 years. The most common adverse effects from these agents include postural hypotension (4% to 8%), fatigue (1% to 12%), dizziness (3% to 10%), flulike syndrome (2% to 6%), and headache (2% to 12%). All three of the α-adrenergic receptor antagonists approved for the treatment of BPH have been shown to be efficacious in improving symptoms, urine flow rates, and quality of life. Differences between the agents, such as the claimed decreased occurrence of orthostatic hypotension with the more $α_{1A}$-selective agent, tamsulosin, have not yet been tested in head-to-head studies.

Finasteride is the 5α-reductase inhibitor currently available for the treatment of BPH, and it blocks the conversion of testosterone to DHT, thus decreasing intraprostatic DHT levels by about 90%. Associated with this decline in intraprostatic DHT is a marked decrease in epithelial cell size and function, and a decrease in prostate size by about 20% to 25%. With the decline in prostate size there is an improvement in urine flow rate, symptom score, and quality of life. The onset of clinical symptom improvement with finasteride is slower than with the α-adrener-

gic receptor antagonists, taking 3 to 6 months for improvement to begin, and reaching maximum improvement at about 24 months. Both symptom improvement and prostate size have been maintained with finasteride for at least 5 years of treatment. Prostate size is important in selecting medical therapy because finasteride is less effective than the α-adrenergic antagonists in those prostates that are smaller. On the other hand, finasteride has been shown to reduce the risk of development of acute urinary retention and the need for prostate surgery, especially in men with larger prostates.

Adverse effects of finasteride include impotence (3.7%), decreased libido (3.3%), and gynecomastia (0.4%). In addition, it should be noted that the medication leads to about a 50% reduction in serum total PSA, but does not change the percentage of free PSA. Estimation of the "true" PSA for men taking finasteride should be done by multiplying the obtained value by a factor of two. To date there is no evidence that finasteride masks detection or progression of prostate cancer.

There are currently about 80 plant extracts available as phytotherapeutic compounds for the treatment of BPH. These are nonprescription unlicensed dietary supplements. The most widely used is an extract from the dried ripe fruit of the American dwarf saw palmetto plant. The mechanism of action of saw palmetto is uncertain, but is said to include antiestrogenic, antiandrogenic, and anticholinergic effects. Studies on the use of saw palmetto in the treatment of symptomatic BPH are limited by short duration (4 to 48 weeks), the different preparations evaluated, and the outcomes measured. Nonetheless, a 1998 published meta-analysis of the literature on the use of saw palmetto for BPH concluded that saw palmetto, at least in the short term, seemed to produce similar improvement in symptom scores and urine flow rates as compared to the licensed pharmaceuticals for BPH.

Surgical intervention for BPH is the treatment of choice for refractory urinary retention, renal failure secondary to outlet obstruction, or recurrent hematuria due to BPH. In addition, surgery for symptoms would be necessary in men who fail, or cannot tolerate, pharmacological therapy. Transurethral resection of the prostate (TURP) has been the gold standard surgical treatment for BPH. Although its use has declined dramatically in this decade due to the availability of pharmacologic agents and the development of alternative surgical interventions, it is the procedure of comparison for treatment outcomes. It is very effective in improving LUTS symptoms due to BPH and improving urine flow but is associated with a 3% to 18% morbidity. The most common complications are blood loss, retrograde ejaculation, urinary incontinence, epididymitis, urinary tract infection, urethral stricture, and sexual dysfunction. Other surgical/procedural approaches, many of which can be done in the outpatient setting using local anesthesia, are listed in Table 467.2. As with pharmacologic management, prostate size is an important determinant in the selection of surgical therapy. TURP does not work optimally for small prostates, as it can lead to bladder neck contractures in that setting. Transurethral microwave thermotherapy (heating the prostate to cause coagulation necrosis) and transurethral needle ablation do not work well if there is medial lobe enlargement, and transurethral incision does not work well in large prostates.

BIBLIOGRAPHY

Arrighi HM, Metter EJ, Guess HA, et al. Natural history of benign prostatic hyperplasia and risk of prostatectomy. The Baltimore Longitudinal Study of Aging. *Urology* 1991; 38(Suppl 1):4–8.

Goldenberg SL, Ramsey E, Trachtenberg J. Alpha-blocker therapy for benign prostatic hyperplasia: a comparative review. *Can J Urol* 1998;5: 551–557.

Jacobsen SJ, Girman CJ, Guess HA, et al. Natural history of prostatism: longitudinal changes in voiding symptoms in community dwelling men. *J Urol* 1996;155:595–600.

McConnell JD, Bruskewitz R, Walsh P, et al. The effect of finasteride on the risk of acute urinary retention and the need for surgical treatment among men with benign prostatic hyperplasia. Finasteride Long-term Efficacy and Safety Study Group. *N Engl J Med* 1998;338:557–563.

US Department of Health and Human Services, Clinical Practice Guideline No. 8: *Benign prostatic hyperplasia: diagnosis and treatment.* Public Health Service, Agency for Health Care Policy and Research, Rockville MD. AHCPR Publication No. 94-0582, 1994.

Wilt TJ, Ishani A, Stark G, et al. Saw palmetto extracts for treatment of benign prostatic hyperplasia: a systematic review. *JAMA* 1998;280: 1604–1609.

Kelley's Textbook of Internal Medicine, fourth edition. Edited by H. David Humes. Lippincott Williams & Wilkins, Philadelphia © 2000.

DIAGNOSTIC AND THERAPEUTIC MODALITIES IN THE ELDERLY: SPECIAL ASPECTS AND CONSIDERATIONS

CHAPTER

468

GERIATRIC ASSESSMENT

DAVID B. REUBEN

■ PRINCIPLES OF GERIATRIC ASSESSMENT

Geriatric assessment differs from the more traditional medical assessment by recognizing that the health status of older persons is dependent on influences beyond the manifestations of their medical conditions. Among these are social, psychological and mental health, and environmental factors. Geriatric assessment also places high value on functional status, both as a dimension to be evaluated and as an outcome to be improved or maintained.

Although in the strictest sense geriatric assessment is a diagnostic process, many use the term to include both evaluation and management. Moreover, geriatric assessment is sometimes used to refer to evaluation by the individual clinician and at other times to refer to a more intensive interdisciplinary process, i.e., comprehensive geriatric assessment (CGA). In fact, as geriatric assessment has evolved, the multidimensional principles of CGA are increasingly being incorporated into routine practices of individual clinicians.

When caring for older patients who are younger and are in good health or have few chronic conditions, the emphasis is placed on preventive geriatrics (lifestyle modifications, chemoprophylaxis, immunizations, and screening for diseases, including potential geriatric syndromes). In contrast, for those older than 85 years and those with multiple complex health and social problems, a more extensive assessment is indicated. This assessment extends beyond the traditional medical evaluation of older persons' health to include assessment of cognitive, affective, functional, social, economic, environmental, and spiritual status,

as well as a discussion of patient preferences regarding advance directives.

Assessment instruments can be used to guide these evaluations but must be interpreted in the context of their limitations. They are rarely, if ever, diagnostic tests. Rather, they indicate the need for further evaluation. Nor do they substitute for good clinical skills and judgment, including the skill of eliciting important information from the patient's history and physical examination. Nevertheless, information obtained from assessment instruments can be used to quickly direct the clinician's attention to issues that are particularly relevant to an individual patient.

Geriatric assessment differs according to the setting in which the patient is being evaluated. In the hospital setting, the initial assessment is usually directed at the acute medical problem that precipitated the hospitalization. As the patient begins to recover and plans are initiated for discharge, other components (e.g., social support, environment) assume increasing importance in the assessment. The inpatient setting can also be problematic for geriatric assessment because of the rapidly changing status of several key dimensions. For example, a patient's functional status may temporarily be "dependent in all tasks" when the patient is acutely ill and gradually improve prior to discharge. Because patients may overestimate their functional status based on their previous level of functioning, alternative sources (e.g., by nurses or physical or occupational therapists) may be necessary for an accurate assessment. Similarly, the patient's full potential to participate in rehabilitation may not be ascertained until near the time of discharge.

Nursing home geriatric assessment requires that closer attention be directed to some aspects of assessment (e.g., risk of falling, nutritional status), whereas others, such as functional status at the level of the instrumental activities of daily living, are less relevant. In contrast, geriatric assessment conducted in the patient's home provides an opportunity for a substantially different type of assessment, where environmental (often including social) factors can be directly assessed but other aspects of the traditional examination (e.g., the gynecologic examination) are much more difficult to assess.

Since the primary site of most clinicians' practices is the office, assessment techniques utilized in this setting are emphasized in this chapter. When appropriate, differing or particularly important information about assessment in other settings is included.

MEDICAL ASSESSMENT

In addition to the standard medical history and physical examination, the clinician should systematically search for specific conditions that are common among older persons and might have considerable impact on function. These disorders include impairments of vision, hearing, and mobility, as well as the geriatric syndromes of malnutrition and urinary incontinence. Assessment instruments or simple screening questions have been developed and validated for each of these disorders (Table 468.1). Polypharmacy and inappropriate prescribing may be assessed by several methods. Because older persons often receive care from multiple providers who may not communicate with each other and because prescriptions might be filled at several pharmacies, each patient should be instructed to bring all current medications to each office visit. Office personnel can check these against the medication list in the medical record and discrepancies can be brought to the clinician's attention at the time of the patient's visit. Several drug interaction programs are commercially available to check for potential drug–drug interactions.

COGNITIVE ASSESSMENT

Because the prevalence of Alzheimer's disease and other forms of dementia rises considerably with advancing age, the yield of screening for cognitive impairment is highest in the 85 and older group. The most commonly used screen is the Mini-Mental State Examination, a 30-item interviewer-administered assessment of several dimensions of cognitive function. Several shorter screens have also been validated, including recall of three items at 1 minute, the clock drawing test, the serial 7's test (patients are asked to subtract 7 from 100 five times), and the Time and Change Test. Although normal results on these tests vastly reduce the probability of dementia and abnormal results increase

the likelihood that the patient has dementia, these tests are neither diagnostic for dementia, nor do normal results exclude the possibility of this disorder. Shortcomings of mental status screens include their lack of relevance to functional activities of daily life and their failure to account for educational level, languages other than English, and cultural differences.

Among hospitalized patients, mental status should be assessed at the time of hospital admission and then again periodically because older persons are especially prone to develop delirium during the hospital stay. Abnormal findings on the mental status examination in hospitalized patients must be interpreted in the context of change from baseline and the clinical situation. The Confusion Assessment Method provides a guide to interpreting such changes. Other valuable tests when evaluating for delirium include those that measure attention (e.g., the "A" test and physical examination for asterixis).

AFFECTIVE ASSESSMENT

Although major depression is no more common in the elderly population than in younger cohorts (see Chapter 460), symptoms of depression and other affective disorders are common and cause considerable morbidity. A simple inquiry such as, "Do you often feel sad or depressed?" can be used as a screen. This single question, however, tends to be overly sensitive and may be better used in tandem with a second screen, such as the Geriatric Depression Scale, which has 15- and 30-item versions.

ASSESSMENT OF FUNCTION

Measurement of functional status is an essential component of the assessment of older persons. The patient's ability to function can be viewed as a summary measure of the overall impact of medical conditions in the context of his or her environment and social support system. Moreover, for each older person, the ability to function consistently within the context of his or her personal lifestyle should be an important consideration in all care planning. Therefore, changes in functional status frequently

TABLE 468.1. COMMONLY USED ASSESSMENT INSTRUMENTS AND APPROXIMATE PERFORMANCE TIME

Problem	Instrument	Average Time to Perform (min)	For More Information (First Author, Year)
Vision impairment	Snellen chart	2	
Hearing impairment	Whisper test	1	
	Audioscope	2	Mulrow, 1991
	Hearing Handicap Inventory for the Elderly	2	Mulrow, 1991
	National Health and Nutrition Examination Battery	2	Reuben, 1998
Mobility/balance	Performance-Oriented Assessment of Mobility	3	Tinetti, 1986
	Timed "Up and Go"	1	Podsiadlo, 1991
Malnutrition	Height/weight	2	
	Nutrition Screening Initiative Checklist	3	White, 1992
Urinary incontinence	Specific questions	1	Moore, 1996
Cognitive impairment	Mini-Mental State Examination	9	Tombough, 1992
	Clock drawing	2	Siu, 1991
Depression	Geriatric Depression Scale	5	Sheikh, 1986

prompt further diagnostic evaluation and intervention. Measurement of functional status can also be valuable in monitoring response to treatment and may provide prognostic information that will be helpful in the planning for long-term care.

Functional status can be assessed at three levels: basic activities of daily living (BADLs), instrumental or intermediate activities of daily living (IADLs), and advanced activities of daily living (AADLs). BADLs assess the ability of the patient to complete basic self-care tasks (bathing, dressing, toileting, continence, feeding, and transferring). IADLs measure the patient's ability to maintain an independent household (shopping for groceries, driving or using public transportation, using the telephone, preparing meals, doing housework, doing handyman work, doing laundry, taking medications, and handling finances). AADLs measure the patient's ability to fulfill societal, community, and family roles as well as participate in recreational or occupational tasks. These advanced activities vary considerably from individual to individual, but may be exceptionally valuable in monitoring functional status prior to the development of disability.

Questions about specific BADL and IADL function have also been incorporated into a variety of more generic health-related quality-of-life instruments (e.g., the Medical Outcomes Study, Short Form 36).

ASSESSMENT OF SOCIAL SUPPORT

The older patient's family structure can be assessed by a few questions during the social history; however, the quality of these relationships should also be determined. For very frail older persons, the availability of assistance from family and friends is frequently the determining factor as to whether a functionally dependent older person remains at home or is institutionalized. If dependency is noted during functional assessment, the clinician should inquire as to who provides help for specific BADL and IADL functions and whether these persons are paid or voluntary help, and whether such help is available only periodically or is sustainable over the long term.

ECONOMIC ASSESSMENT

Although some clinicians may feel uncomfortable in assessing the economic status of their patients, insurance status is routinely collected by office staff. The patient's income can also be assessed and eligibility for state or local benefits to provide services for the functionally impaired can be determined. For the frail and functionally impaired, physicians may need to begin discussions of planning to mobilize savings and other resources to provide personal-attendant care. Referral to a social worker can be exceptionally valuable in such planning.

ENVIRONMENTAL ASSESSMENT

Environmental assessment encompasses two dimensions: the safety of the home environment and the adequacy of the patient's access to needed personal and medical services. Particularly among the frail and those with mobility and balance problems, the home environment should be assessed for safety. The National Safety Council has developed a Home Safety Checklist that patients and their families can complete. For those receiving home health services, in-home safety inspections can be performed, including recommendations for installation of adaptive devices (e.g., shower bars, raised toilet seats).

Older persons who begin to develop IADL dependencies should be evaluated for the geographic proximity of necessary services (e.g., grocery shopping, banking), their need for such services, and their ability to utilize such services in their current living situation.

SPIRITUALITY

Spirituality, whether expressed through affiliation with a formal religious denomination or nonreligious intangible elements, has increasingly been recognized as an important dimension that can affect health. Formal instruments assessing spirituality have not yet been developed, but asking older persons whether religion or spirituality is important to them may provide insights that will facilitate their care. Especially in hospital settings, involvement of pastoral or professional care may be valuable in supporting the patient and in framing medical decisions in the context of the patient's personal belief system.

ADVANCE DIRECTIVES

Discussions of advance directives are important for all patients and should be initiated early on (though usually not on the initial office visit) to elucidate patients' goals and preferences for care should they become unable to speak for themselves due to progressive cognitive impairment or acute illness. A particularly important time in which to discuss such preferences is prior to surgery because of the possibility of surgical complications or postoperative delirium, which may preclude discussions following the procedure. The durable power of attorney for health care, which asks the patient to designate a surrogate to make medical decisions if the patient loses decision-making capacity, is often less emotionally laden than the specifying of treatments that the patient may or may not want. Such discussions should also be revisited any time there are significant changes in a patient's medical condition or a better understanding about prognosis becomes available; patients may revise their thoughts about the benefits and burdens of treatment.

■ PUTTING GERIATRIC ASSESSMENT INTO PRACTICE

In an attempt to improve clinician efficiency without sacrificing comprehensiveness in geriatric assessment, many clinical practices have begun to use previsit questionnaires that can be completed by the patient or a family member (or other proxy) in advance of the clinical encounter. These questionnaires typically gather information on medical history, medications, preventive measures, and functional status (including information on who helps when the patient is functionally dependent). As a result, they can markedly reduce the time needed to conduct an initial assessment and can ensure a consistent level of comprehensive-

| TABLE 468.2. | MULTIDIMENSIONAL SCREENING INSTRUMENT |

	Screening Package Characteristics			
Problem	Screening Measure	Positive Screen	Positive Predictive Value	Negative Predictive Value
Vision	2 Parts: Ask: "Do you have difficulty driving, or watching television, or reading, or doing any of your daily activities because of your eyesight?" If yes, then: Test each eye with Snellen chart while patent wears corrective lenses (if applicable).	Yes to question and inability to read greater than 20/40 on Snellen chart	0.75	0.89
Hearing	Use audioscope set at 40 dB. Test hearing using 1,000 and 2,000 Hz.	Inability to hear 1,000 or 2,000 Hz in both ears or either of these frequencies in one ear	0.75	0.91
Leg mobility	Time the patient after asking: "Rise from the chair. Walk 20 feet briskly, turn, walk back to the chair and sit down."	Unable to complete task in 15 s	0.91	0.92
Urinary incontinence	2 Parts: Ask: "In the last year, have you ever lost your urine and gotten wet?" If yes, then ask: "Have you lost urine on at least six separate days?"	Yes to both questions	0.86	0.96
Nutrition/weight loss	2 Parts: Ask: "Have you lost 10 lb over the past 6 months without trying to do so?" Weight the patient.	Yes to the question or weight <100 lb	0.62	0.92
Memory	Three-item recall.	Unable to remember all three items after 1 min	0.60	0.92
Depression	Ask: "Do you often feel sad or depressed?"	Yes to the question	0.71	0.90
Physical disability	Six questions: "Are you able to . . .: " . . . do strenuous activities like fast walking or bicycling?" " . . . do heavy work around the house like washing windows, walls, or floors?" " . . . go shopping for groceries or clothes?" " . . . get to places out of walking distance?" "bathe, either by sponge bath, tub bath, or shower?" " . . . dress, like putting on a shirt, buttoning and zipping, or putting on shoes?"	Yes to any of the questions	0.88	0.77

(Adapted from Moore AA, Siu AL. Screening for common problems in ambulatory elderly; clinical confirmation of a screening instrument. *Am J Med* 1996;100:438.)

ness for every patient. By including validated screening instruments, previsit questionnaires can also be used to detect geriatric syndromes.

A second method of streamlining the office visit is by delegating the administration of screening instruments for many of the important geriatric problems to trained office staff. Thus, the clinician may spend a short time reviewing the results of these screens and then decide which dimensions, if any, need greater evaluation. Recently, researchers have demonstrated the feasibility and yield of utilizing office staff to administer case-finding and screening instruments (Table 468.2) that assess many of the dimensions described above.

COMPREHENSIVE GERIATRIC ASSESSMENT

Comprehensive geriatric assessment (CGA) began with the notion that a systematic evaluation of frail older persons by a team of health professionals could uncover treatable health problems and lead to improved health outcomes. Early randomized clinical trials provided convincing evidence that such programs conducted in hospital-based and rehabilitation units, which typically required several weeks of treatment, could lead to better survival rates, improved functional status, and more desirable placement (e.g., home rather than nursing home) following discharge from the hospital. Conceptually, comprehensive geriatric assessment is a three-step process: (a) screening to target appropriate patients, (b) assessment and development of recommendations, and (c) implementation of recommendations, including monitoring physician and patient adherence with recommendations. Each of these steps is essential if the process is to be successful in achieving health and functional benefits.

Within this broad conceptualization, CGA has been implemented using many different models in various health care settings. Because of changes in length of hospital stays, an increasing number of CGA programs are relying on postdischarge and community-based assessment. Furthermore, most of the early programs focused on restorative or rehabilitative goals (tertiary prevention), whereas many newer programs are aimed at primary and secondary prevention. These new models of CGA have assumed responsibility for primary care temporarily or permanently or have utilized consultative programs that have included patient empowerment and physician education methods. Most have used some type of identification of high risk (targeting) as a criterion for inclusion in the program. Such targeting criteria have included conditions such as functional impairment, falls, depressive symptoms, urinary incontinence, and expected high health care utilization.

The principles of comprehensive geriatric assessment have also been incorporated into programs that have applied CGA approaches, such as standardized assessment and interdisciplinary teams, to individual conditions (e.g., falls and congestive heart failure) and to improving the care of hospitalized patients (e.g., acute care for the elderly units). Undoubtedly, additional generations of CGA-like interventions will be forthcoming.

BIBLIOGRAPHY

Inouye SK, van Dyck CH, Alessi CA, et al. Clarifying confusion: the confusion assessment method. A new method for detection of delirium. *Ann Intern Med* 1990;113:941–948.

Moore AA, Siu AL. Screening for common problems in ambulatory elderly: clinical confirmation of a screening instrument. *Am J Med* 1996;100: 438–443.

Mulrow CD, Lichtenstein MJ. Screening for hearing impairment in the elderly. *J Gen Intern Med* 1991;6:249–258.

Podsiadlo D, Richardson S. The timed "Up and Go": a test of basic functional mobility for frail elderly persons. *J Am Geriatr Soc* 1991;39: 142–148.

Reuben DB, Walsh K, Moore AA, et al. Hearing loss in community-dwelling older persons: national prevalence data and identification using simple questions. *J Am Geriatr Soc* 1998;46:1008–1011.

Sheikh JI, Yesavage JA. Geriatric Depression Scale: recent evidence and development of a shorter version. *Clin Gerontol* 1986;5:165–172.

Siu AL. Screening for dementia and investigating its causes. *Ann Intern Med* 1991;115:122–132.

Tinetti ME. Performance-oriented assessment of mobility problems in elderly patients. *J Am Geriatr Soc* 1986;34:119–126.

Tombaugh TN, McIntyre NJ. The Mini-Mental State Examination: a comprehensive review. *J Am Geriatr Soc* 1992;40:922–935.

White JV, Dwyer JT, Posner BM, et al. Nutrition Screening Initiative: development and implementation of the public awareness checklist and screening tools. *J Am Diet Assoc* 1992;92:163–167.

Kelley's Textbook of Internal Medicine, fourth edition. Edited by H. David Humes. Lippincott Williams & Wilkins, Philadelphia © 2000.

C H A P T E R
469

GERIATRIC CLINICAL PHARMACOLOGY

JANICE B. SCHWARTZ

Although representing only slightly more than 12% of the population, older patients consume more than 25% of therapeutic drug prescriptions in the United States. In the older patient, altered pharmacokinetics, pharmacodynamics, and multiple disease states with multiple drugs consumed combine to increase the complexities of optimal medication prescribing and the risk of adverse drug-related events. The purpose of this chapter is to review general principles of clinical pharmacology and age-related changes in pharmacokinetic and pharmacodynamic parameters as they relate to optimizing drug therapy for older patients.

PHARMACOKINETICS

Pharmacokinetic processes determine the rate of appearance, distribution throughout tissues, and elimination of drug from the body. As shown in Fig. 469.1, the major pharmacokinetic terms that describe these processes are (a) bioavailability, (b) distribution, and (c) clearance.

BIOAVAILABILITY

Bioavailability is defined as the fraction of drug reaching the circulation after administration. Intravascular (i.v.) administra-

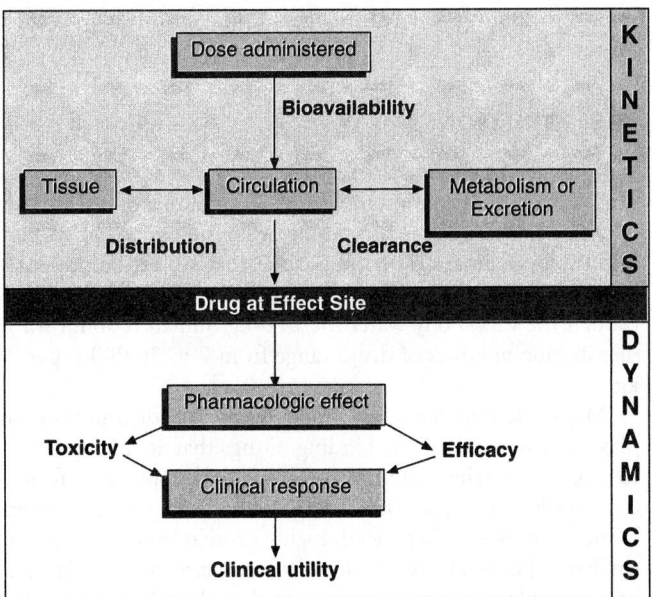

FIGURE 469.1. Schematic representation of the pharmacokinetic and pharmacodynamic processes that relate a drug to its effects.

tion of a drug results in a bioavailability of 1 or 100%. Bioavailability for extravascular routes of drug administration is estimated by comparing the area under the curve (AUC) of drug concentration vs. time after extravascular administration divided by the AUC vs. time data after intravascular dosage (AUC extravascular/AUC intravascular). The result is often expressed as a fraction or a percentage. Bioavailability defines the dose adjustment between intravascular and extravascular drug administration. Low-bioavailability drugs require much greater extravascular, as compared to intravascular, doses. Low bioavailability is frequently found for drugs that undergo oxidative metabolism by the cytochrome P450 system, which has recently been identified in the intestine as well as the liver. Both hepatic and intestinal metabolism can decrease the amount reaching the circulation after oral dosing. Examples of drugs with low bioavailability include cyclosporine, nifedipine, metoprolol, midazolam, propranolol, and verapamil. Interactions with nutrients and dietary factors also are most common for drugs that undergo intestinal metabolism by the same cytochrome P450 isoform. Examples include the increased bioavailability of felodipine when administered with grapefruit juice.

Age-related changes in bioavailability depend on route of drug administration, age-related changes in the organ of absorption (bowel vs. skin), and changes in hepatic drug metabolism during the first pass of the drug through the liver after oral drug administration. Gastric pH, gastrointestinal (GI) motility, blood flow, and active membrane transport processes are altered to a variable extent by aging. There is decreased acid secretion, decreased perfusion of the GI tract, and possibly decreased membrane transport activity. These changes are, however, counterbalanced by longer GI transit time, providing longer times for drug absorption to take place. Studies of traditional oral formulations suggest little clinically significant age-related changes in the rate or extent of drug absorption from the GI tract. Data regarding slow-release preparations, transdermal, transbuccal, and transbronchial drug administration are too limited to allow conclusions regarding age-related changes in drug absorption via those routes.

DISTRIBUTION

Volume of distribution terms relate the amount of drug in the body to the concentration measured. The volume of distribution does not represent a "real" volume or physiologic compartment but an approximation of the volume that would be present if drug were distributed equally throughout the body. Thus, although the total body water for a 70-kg human is about 42 L, distribution volumes of drugs range from 7 to 30,000 L per 70 kg.

Major determinants of drug volume of distribution are plasma protein and tissue binding. Drugs that are highly bound to plasma proteins (albumin or α_1-acid glycoprotein) form a drug–protein complex that is large and less able to cross membranes into tissues. In general, highly protein-bound drugs have smaller volumes of distribution that are more closely related to vascular volumes. An example of such a drug is warfarin. If a drug is highly bound to tissue proteins, distribution volumes will be large. An example of such a drug is digoxin, which distributes into and binds to muscle. Volume of distribution is an

important concept for drugs administered with loading doses. Clinically, the volume of distribution defines the loading dose of a drug since:

Loading dose = (concentration desired)

$\times$ (volume of distribution of the drug)

This simplification assumes immediate and uniform distribution of drug in the total drug volume of distribution. Clinically, it is often more desirable to administer a loading dose over a period of time or by infusion to avoid toxicity due to high concentrations before distribution is complete.

Age-related changes in volume of drug distribution result from body composition changes with senescence. Important gender-related differences in body composition also exist. Lean body muscle mass decreases with aging, and this decrease results in less creatinine production. Total body water is also somewhat decreased with aging, leading to decreased volumes of distribution for some drugs (Table 469.1). The clinical consequence of a reduction in distribution volume is a higher drug concentration for any given dose of drug. An illustrative example is the calculation of loading doses of antibiotics (polar drugs that usually distribute only in body water). For aminoglycosides, much of the toxicity is related to peak concentrations, and age and weight adjustments of loading doses are necessary to avoid toxicity. Another example of the impact of distribution volume changes is that seen with alcohol. Increased effects of alcohol (or decreased tolerance) seen in older individuals, and in women compared to men, are attributable to reduced distribution volumes leading to higher alcohol concentrations for an amount consumed.

An important determinant of drug distribution is plasma protein binding. Total protein binding of drugs usually is not altered by aging in healthy individuals. In the presence of disease, serum albumin concentration may decrease, but the decrease in albumin is usually counterbalanced by an increase in α_1-acid glycoprotein with acute illnesses. The net result is that clinically important age-related changes in total drug protein binding are largely absent and, in general, not a clinical consideration. Protein binding can, however, be altered by competition for binding by coadministered drugs. Since administration of multiple drugs is more common in the elderly, this becomes a clinical issue. It is especially important during administration of warfarin, which is about 99% protein-bound. Displacement of warfarin from albumin by other highly bound drugs, such as amiodarone, phenytoin, sulfonamides, fluoroquinolones, or azole antifungal agents, among others, can also cause marked increases in anticoagulation. The influence of drug transporters, such as P-glycoprotein, in determining tissue drug distribution and concentrations is currently being investigated but potential age-related changes are largely unexplored at this time.

CLEARANCE

Total Body Drug Clearance

Total body drug clearance is the net rate of removal of drug from the body. It is usually described as a unit of volume cleared of drug per unit time. To maintain a constant drug concentration, input must equal output or clearance. Clinically, clearance defines the drug dosing rate. For most currently prescribed

TABLE 469.1.	CYTOCHROME P450 (CYP) SUBSTRATES AND DRUG INTERACTIONS[a]			
Enzyme Isoform	**Model Compound**	**Drug Substrates**	**Inducers[b]**	**Inhibitors[b]**
CYP1A2	Caffeine Nicotine	Acetaminophen Clozapine Tacrine Theophylline	Rifampin Cigarette smoke Charbroiled meat Lansoprazole, omeprazole	Cimetidine Grapefruit juice Fluoroquinolones Omeprazole
CYP2C Polymorphic	Dapsone S-Mephenytoin	Diazepam S-Mephenytoin S-warfarin	Dexamethasone Phenobarbital Phenytoin	Amiodarone Cimetidine

CYP2D6
Polymorphic
	Debrisoquine
	Dextromethorphan
		β-blockers
		  Metoprolol
		  Propranolol
		DHEA
		Omeprazole
		Haloperidol
		SSRI antidepressants
		Tolterodine
		Tricyclic antidepressants
		Testosterone
			None known	Cimetidine
				Desipramine
				Quinidine
				SSRI antidepressants,
				  ex. fluoxetine

CYP3A	Dapsone (hydroxylation index) Erythromycin breath test 6-β-OH-cortisol/cortisol ratio Lidocaine/MEGX ratio Midazolam clearance	Astemizole β-blockers Carbamazepine Cisapride Clozapine Diazepam Dihydropyridines Diltiazem Erythromycin Estrogen HMG-CoA reductase inhibitors Itraconazole Ketoconazole Lidocaine Quinidine Rifampin Verapamil Tamoxifen Terfenadine Theophylline Triazolam Troglitazone	Rifampin St. John's Wort	Ketoconazole Itraconazole Protease inhibitors Amiodarone Cimetidine Grapefruit juice Cyclosporine Erythromycin Verapamil

[a] Examples of drug (and diet) interactions for cytochrome P450 substrates.
[b] In order of potency.
6-β-OH, 6-beta-hydroxy; MEGX, monoethylglycine xylidide; DHEA, dehydroepiandrosterone; SSRI, selective serotonin reuptake inhibitor; HMG-CoA, 3-hydroxy-3-methylglutaryl coenzyme A.

drugs, the major organs of clearance are the kidney and liver. As newer drugs come to more closely resemble hormones, receptor antagonists and agonists, peptides, and intracellular messengers, routes of biotransformation at other sites will assume more importance. For now, knowledge of renal and hepatic elimination provides sufficient background for understanding clearance of most drugs administered to the older patient.

Renal Drug Clearance

Drugs can undergo three processes of elimination in the kidney: (a) glomerular filtration, (b) tubular secretion, and (c) tubular reabsorption. Glomerular filtration can be approximated by estimates of creatinine clearance. Protein binding can influence renal drug clearance because only unbound drug can be filtered. Renal tubular secretion is detected in vivo when renal clearance of a substance exceeds clearance by filtration. Secretion is an active process, with separate processes for acids and bases. Secretion efficiently eliminates protein-bound drugs. Tubular reabsorption is detected when urinary excretion of a compound is less than filtration rates. For most drugs, reabsorption is passive and can be affected by both urine flow and changes in pH.

Alterations in renal function are the most consistent and well-described changes associated with aging. Renal blood flow is decreased, resulting in delivery of less drug to the kidney for clearance. Renal blood flow may also be more dependent on prostaglandin regulation in older individuals than in younger individuals, and renal mass is decreased. These changes lead to an average decrease in creatinine clearance of about 10% per decade after age 20 years. Algorithms designed to estimate creatinine clearance based on subject's age, gender, and serum creatinine level have widespread clinical applications, especially for dosing of renally eliminated drugs, such as digitalis glycosides, aminoglycosides, and lithium, which have narrow therapeutic ranges and toxicities that are closely related to concentration. One commonly used formula is as follows:

$$\text{Creatinine clearance} = \frac{140 - \text{age (y)} \times \text{lean body weight (kg)}^*}{72 \times \text{serum creatinine}}$$

It is important to note that serum creatinine concentrations alone do not accurately reflect creatinine clearance in the elderly and that the serum creatinine may be normal when significant reduction of creatinine clearance or glomerular filtration is present.

Age-related changes in the sensitivity to drugs that further impair renal function warrant mention. Nonsteroidal anti-inflammatory drugs (NSAIDs) can decrease production of vasodilating renal prostaglandins, and NSAID inhibition of cyclooxygenase has been postulated to be the mechanism for the variable azotemia seen during administration of NSAIDs in older patients. NSAIDs may also decrease potassium excretion and can cause hyperkalemia when administered to older patients, especially when given in combination with other drugs which decrease potassium excretion. Angiotensin-converting enzyme (ACE) inhibitors may reduce renal perfusion that can lead to significant reductions in renal clearance in the presence of renal artery disease. ACE inhibitors also block production of angiotensin II, which is responsible for dilatation of the efferent arteriole, and alter the balance between afferent and efferent arteriolar resistance such that glomerular perfusion decreases. These effects of ACE inhibitors can result in clinically significant decreases in glomerular filtration and increases in serum potassium in the elderly patient.

Hepatic Drug Clearance

The rate and extent of hepatic drug metabolism depends on both extrahepatic and intrahepatic factors. Hepatic blood flow determines the delivery of drug to the liver, and hepatic enzyme type, numbers, affinity, and activity rate determine hepatic drug metabolism. A simplified view of hepatic drug clearance divides drugs into "high" clearance or "low" clearance drugs. A high-clearance drug is rapidly metabolized by the liver such that the clearance rate is limited only by the rate of drug presentation to the liver (hepatic blood flow). Examples of high-clearance drugs are lidocaine, morphine, propranolol, and verapamil. For a low-clearance drug, the rate of removal is limited by hepatic enzymatic processes. Hepatic disease leading to decreased liver enzyme content, damage, or fibrosis will have a major impact on hepatic metabolism of low-clearance drugs. Examples of low-clearance drugs are amlodipine and phenytoin.

Most hepatic drug clearance results not in removal of drug from the body but in drug metabolism to a more polar compound for renal excretion or to an inactive compound by oxidative biotransformation, largely via cytochrome P450 pathways (Table 469.1). The supergene family of enzymes, responsible for the majority of oxidative metabolism of drugs, environmental chemicals, a number of hormones, foods, and toxins, is called the cytochrome P450 (CYP) family. Approximately 100 variations of the cytochrome P450 protein have been identified in plant and animal species, yet human liver CYP protein content is largely from three major groups—the CYP1, CYP2, and CYP3A families. It is estimated that 50% to 55% of hepatically cleared drugs undergo metabolism by the CYP3 family, and CYP3 proteins compose about 25% of protein in the liver. CYP3 metabolizes amiodarone, astemizole, many β-blockers, most benzodiazepines, carbamazepine, cisapride, clarithromycin, cortisol, most dihydropyridine calcium channel blockers, dapsone, diltiazem, erythromycin, estrogens, 3-hydroxy-3-methylglutaryl reductase coenzyme A (HMG-CoA) inhibitors, itraconazole, ketoconazole, lidocaine, nefazodone, quinidine, rifampin, tamoxifen, terfenadine, troglitazone, verapamil, and warfarin, among others. CYP2D6 is estimated to be responsible for metabolism of 25% of hepatically metabolized drugs, including debrisoquine, dextromethorphan, dehydroepiandrosterone, haloperidol, mexiletine, propafenone, most selective serotonin reuptake inhibitors (SSRIs), testosterone, and tricyclic antidepressants. Five percent to ten percent of whites and 1% of Asians are deficient in 2D6. CYP2C9 accounts for another 20% of hepatic drug metabolism, and substrates are losartan, phenytoin, S-warfarin (the active enantiomer), and many NSAIDs. CYP1 in humans is designated as CYP1A2 and accounts for 5% of human hepatic drug metabolism. Acetaminophen, caffeine, nicotine, tacrine, and theophylline are metabolized via this pathway.

Genetic polymorphisms have been described for CYP 2D6, 2C9, and 2C19, whereas no functional ones have been described for CYP3A4. It appears that 7% to 10% of whites are phenotypically deficient in the CYP2D6 isoform, whereas only 1% to 3% of Asians are deficient. Genetic probes do not exist for all pathways, and in vitro investigations of liver content and substrate affinities do not always correlate with in vivo drug metabolism. Validated in vivo probes for the phenotyping of CYP2D6 are debrisoquine and dextromethorphan. Sparteine and dapsone are in vivo probes for CYP2C. Mephenytoin is a CYP2C19 substrate, and caffeine and nicotine have been used as probes for CYP1A2. There remains disagreement regarding the best in vivo probes for the CYP3A4 pathway. Endogenous cortisol to 17-hydroxycortisol urinary ratios, erythromycin clearance as estimated by the ^{14}C-erythromycin breath test, and midazolam clearance have all been used for this purpose.

Genetic polymorphisms have also been described for conjugation by acetylation, sulfotransferases, and hepatic uridine diphosphonate glucuronosyltransferases (UGTs). The first widely recognized genetic polymorphism for drug biotransformation appeared with the description of slow- or rapid-acetylator status for isoniazid. Additional drugs that undergo acetylation for which clinically important polymorphisms have been identified are procainamide and hydralazine. A clinical example of accumulation of an endogenous substrate due to low UGT(1A) activity is bilirubin in individuals with Gilbert's syndrome. It has been

---

* For females, multiply by 0.85.

suggested that individuals with low UGT(1A) activity have an increased risk for toxicity of a cancer agent metabolized by UGT(1A). Model substrates of glucuronidation that have been administered to humans include paracetamol, menthol, lorazepam, oxazepam, clofibrate, and fenofibric acids.

While definitive evidence for genetic polymorphisms for CYP3A has not emerged, Asians have been reported to have slower clearance of several CYP3A-metabolized drugs, and women have variably been reported to have faster CYP3A-mediated clearance than men. It also appears that CYP1A clearance is higher in men than in women; and conjugative biotransformation is more rapid in men than in women.

Hepatic drug metabolism is far more variable than renal drug clearance, and reliable algorithms to estimate hepatic drug clearance are not available. The marked variability of factors influencing hepatic clearance, such as hepatic blood flow, hepatic size, enzyme inducibility and inhibition, genetic polymorphisms in cytochrome P450 isoforms, and cumulative and differential exposures to modulating environmental influences, contributes to the wide variability in hepatic drug clearance between individuals and with aging.

Age-related Changes in Hepatic Drug Clearance

Although conclusions from studies of potential age-related changes in hepatic drug metabolism vary, there is agreement regarding extrahepatic changes. In general, hepatic blood flow decreases with aging. Decreased hepatic blood flow usually results in decreased hepatic clearance of high-clearance drugs. In most studies, reduced clearance of high-clearance drugs has been seen with increasing age. Variability is marked, however, and gender and smoking history may influence results.

There is agreement on several age-related changes in hepatic factors. Hepatic size decreases with aging. Data from in vitro experiments with tissues from male rodent models of aging also show marked and consistent declines in hepatic enzyme affinity and oxidative metabolic rates, whereas in vitro experiments with human liver biopsy tissues from men fail to demonstrate age-related declines. Differences in hepatic enzyme content and cytochrome P450 isoforms in the male rodent versus human potentially explain discrepancies related to in vitro measures of hepatic enzyme activity. Most in vivo studies of aging effects in humans show decreases in oxidative drug metabolism by the cytochrome P450 system. Examples include α-blockers (doxazosin, prazosin, terazosin), anti-infectious drugs (clarithromycin, erythromycin, itraconazole, ketoconazole), antihistamines (terfenadine), most benzodiazepines, some β-blockers (metoprolol, propranolol, timolol), the calcium channel blockers (dihydropyridines, diltiazem, and verapamil), several HMG-CoA inhibitors (atorvastatin, fluvastatin), sex hormones (estrogen, progesterone, testosterone), several H$_2$ blockers (cimetidine), and proton pump inhibitors (lansoprazole, omeprazole). In contrast, in vivo studies of drugs metabolized by the conjugative reactions of glucuronidation (e.g., acetaminophen, morphine, diazepam), sulfation (e.g., steroids, methyldopa), and acetylation (e.g., sulfonamides, isonia-

zid, dapsone, clonazepam) have not found significant effects of aging.

Hepatic enzyme activity induction and inhibition form the basis for many drug–drug interactions. Drugs metabolized by a common CYP isoform often compete for biotransformation and interact, but drugs may also affect pathways that do not appear to be their primary route of metabolism. Inducibility of hepatic enzyme activity is relevant to the use of several drugs that may be prescribed for the very elderly or the nursing home population. The antituberculous drug rifampin has recently been shown to be the most potent inducer of the microsomal oxidase system activity (CYP1A and CYP3A). It is far more potent in this effect than phenobarbital. When rifampin is administered to patients, profound increases in drug clearance occur, and concentrations of coadministered drugs may become negligible. Dosages of drugs cleared by CYP1A and CYP3A that are coadministered with rifampin may need to be increased, and then decreased upon discontinuation of rifampin. Other potent hepatic enzyme inducers include dexamethasone and phenytoin (CYP2C), caffeine, cigarette smoke, lanzoprazole, and omeprazole (CYP1A), and St. John's Wort (CYP3A). Considerations regarding hepatic drug enzyme inhibitors are also pertinent. One of the first drugs to be shown to influence hepatic clearance of drugs, cimetidine, both decreases hepatic blood flow and inhibits microsomal oxidase system activity (CYP1A2, CYP2C, and CYP3A) and can profoundly decrease hepatic drug clearance. Marked elevations of serum lidocaine and propranolol concentrations occurred in elderly patients receiving these drugs in combination with cimetidine. Newer antihistaminergic blocking drugs, such as ranitidine, famotidine, and nizatidine, have little or no inhibition of hepatic drug metabolism. More recently, clinically significant decreases in drug clearance accompanying the use of amiodarone (all CYP isoforms), the antifungal drugs itraconazole and ketoconazole (CYP3A), erythromycin (CYP3A), protease inhibitors (CYP3A), and terfenadine (CYP3A) have been reported.

Nonrenal, Nonhepatic Drug Metabolism

Although the liver and kidney are the major sites for clearance of currently available therapeutic drugs, metabolism by both non-CYP processes and CYP-mediated metabolism can occur at other sites. Cloning of the genes for the CYP isoforms and use of cDNA probes has led to the discovery of CYP in organs other than liver, including the mucosa of the GI tract, kidney, lung, brain, or skin. CYP3A intestinal metabolism following oral drug administration probably contributes to the low bioavailability of CYP3A substrates, such as cyclosporine, lorazepam, midazolam, propranolol, verapamil, and other highly metabolized drugs (alcohol, clozapine, ergotamine, fluorouracil, isosorbide dinitrate). CYP1A1 has also been detected in the duodenum, and the CYP2B family has been found in the brain. Hydrolyzing enzymes, glutathione S-transferases (GSTs), UDP-glucuronosyltransferases, N-acetyltransferases, and methyltransferases are also found extrahepatically. Nonspecific esterases are widely distributed in tissues of the body (including blood, liver, and GI tract). Adenosine is an example of a drug that has a very rapid inactivation/clearance because it is metabolized and inactivated by an esterase present in blood. Pentoxifylline, hydralazine, and fluorouracil are metabolized to some extent in blood. Other circulating esterases include acetylcholinesterase and carbonic anhydrase. GSTs and UDP-glucuronosyltransferases are found in the kidney and lung, as well as in the liver. Protease and peptidase enzymes are found in many tissues and cause biotransformation of polypeptides. Potential age-related changes in nonrenal, nonhepatic drug metabolism have not been elucidated.

Elimination Half-life

A half-life ($t_{1/2}$) of a drug is described as the time it takes for the amount of drug in the body to decrease by half. This term is used clinically to refer to the time for drug concentrations to decrease by half after drug distribution has occurred throughout the body. This terminal drug elimination $t_{1/2}$ is described by:

$$t_{1/2} = 0.693 \text{ (volume)/clearance}$$

Half-life, therefore, is a dependent variable, and changes in drug $t_{1/2}$ can occur secondary to changes in drug distribution volume, drug clearance, or combined changes in distribution and clearance.

The $t_{1/2}$ defines the time required to reach steady-state drug concentrations in the body during both drug initiation and after drug discontinuation. It takes approximately 3.3 drug half-lives to eliminate 90% of drug from the body or to reach 90% of steady-state concentrations after drug initiation. Therefore, the $t_{1/2}$ provides information necessary for determination of the time between dosage adjustments or the time necessary for stabilization or reduction in effects of the drug related to drug concentrations. Sustained-release preparations do not alter the drug half-life or the time necessary for stabilization or for reduction of drug concentrations.

Age-related Effects on Elimination Half-lives

The elimination $t_{1/2}$ has been reported to increase with age for a number of drugs (Table 469.1). When age-related increases in terminal elimination $t_{1/2}$ occur, it is important that the time between dosage adjustments be increased to allow evaluation of the full effect of a given drug dosage. It is also important to allow increased time for complete drug elimination before concluding possible adverse effects to be irreversible or non–drug-related.

A summary of the literature available on drugs commonly prescribed in older patients with suggested dosage adjustments are found in Table 469.2.

▪ PHARMACODYNAMICS

Pharmacodynamic models relate drug dose or concentration to the intensity of response or "effect." The most commonly used models have evolved from drug receptor theory and assume steady-state conditions.

E$_\text{MAX}$ MODELS

The maximum effect model (E_max) is one of the simplest which describes drug (or agonist or antagonist) effect over a range of concentrations. It predicts no effect when there is no drug and maximum effect when "infinite" drug is present. It is based on the premise that drug combines reversibly with a receptor to form a drug receptor complex which then produces an effect and by the equation:

Effect

$$= \frac{(E_\text{max})\,(\text{drug concentration})}{(\text{drug concentration}) + (\text{concentration at } 50\%\ E_\text{max}\ \text{or}\ C_{50})}$$

The measured effect is proportional to the fraction of occupied receptors. Graphically, this relationship is a hyperbola. A minor modification of the E_max model creates the sigmoidal E_max model, where

$$\text{Effect} = (E_\text{max}) \text{ concentration}^n / C_{50}{}^n + \text{drug concentration}^n$$

The sigmoidal E_max model predicts a sigmoidal response curve whereby no effect is seen at zero drug concentration or at lower concentrations until a concentration is reached at which a steep rise in the effect vs. response curve is seen. The steeply rising portion of the response curve is approximately linear throughout the 20% to 80% response range and then slowly approaches maximal effect. This model is qualitatively similar to physiologic or clinical circumstances wherein a threshold concentration must be reached to produce an appreciable effect, with increasing concentrations then producing increasing effects; however, as near-maximal effect is reached, increasing concentrations produce only slight changes in effect. The derived parameters have clinical applications. The E_max can estimate maximal effects for comparisons between drugs or between individuals. The concentration for half-maximal effect (C_{50}) can be an estimate or representation of the sensitivity of an individual or group to a drug (or affinity for a receptor). The slope factor describes the steepness of responses and amount of change anticipated due to changes in drug concentration and, to some extent, the wideness or narrowness of a drug's therapeutic range. These models can take more complex forms for the known physiologic conditions of tolerance, nonproportionality of response, multiple drugs and multiple receptors, and non–steady-state conditions.

Administration of drugs at dosages that produce maximal effects are often impractical in humans because of potential toxicity or undesired effects. In pharmacodynamic studies not attaining maximal effect, the linear portion of the relationship is often approximated using simple linear regression, where effect = (slope)(concentration) + basal value or $y = mx + b$. This model estimates the steepness of response (slope) and can be used as an index of sensitivity to the drug for between group and between drug comparisons and desired concentration guidelines.

For many compounds found in nature, such as quinidine (cinchona bark) or digitalis (foxglove), and local anesthetics (cocaine), a linear concentration vs. response relationship with toxicity at increased concentrations is frequently observed. For receptor agonist and antagonist drugs (α- and β-adrenergic and calcium receptor–blocking drugs) and enzyme-inhibiting drugs

TABLE 469.2. COMMONLY PRESCRIBED DRUGS BY THERAPEUTIC CLASS AND REPORTED ALTERATIONS IN PHARMACOKINETICS, AND SUGGESTED DOSE ADJUSTMENTS IN OLDER PATIENTS

	Route of Elimination	Aging Effects			Dose Adjustment
		Clearance	Volume	$t_{1/2}$	
ANTIARTHRITICS					
Acetaminophen	Hepatic (CYP1A2)	↔, ↓	↓, ↔	↔	↔
Aspirin	Hepatic	↑, ↔	↑	↑	↓, ↔
Diclofenac	Hepatic	↓	N.A.	↑	↓
Etodolac	Hepatic	N.A.	N.A.	↔	↔
Fenoprofen	Hepatic	N.A.	N.A.	N.A.	N.A.
Flurbiprofen	Hepatic	N.A.	N.A.	↔	↔
Ibuprofen	Hepatic (CYP2C)	↔, or ↓ in men	N.A.	↔ in men	↔ or ↓ in men
Indomethacin	Hepatin	↓	↔	↔, ↑	↔, ↓ (25%)
Ketoprofen	Hepatic	↓, ↔	N.A.	↑, ↔	↓, ↔
Naproxen	Hepatic (CYP1A, 2C), renal	↓	N.A.	↑	↓
Oxaprozin	Hepatic (CYP,>conjug)	↔	↔	↔	↔
Piroxicam	Hepatic	↔	N.A.	↔	↔
Prednisone	Hepatic	N.A.	N.A.	N.A.	?, ↔
Salicylic acid	Hepatic	↔	N.A.	↔ or ↑	↔
Sulfasalazine	Hepatic	N.A.	N.A.	↑	↔, ↓
Sulindac[a]	Hepatic, renal	↓	N.A.	↑	↓
ANTI-INFECTIOUS					
Amantidine	Renal	↓	N.A.	↑	↓, by CrCL
Amikacin	Renal	↓	↔, ↓	↑	↓, by CrCL
Amoxicillin	Renal	sl. ↓	↓	sl. ↑	↓, ↔
Ampicillin	Renal	↓	↔	↑	↓
Azithromycin	Biliary (and CYP3A)	↔	↔	↔	↔
Aztreonam	Renal	↓	↔	↑	↓
Carbenicillin	Renal	N.A.	N.A.	N.A.	↓
Cephalosporins[d]	Renal	↓	?	↑	↓
Ciprofloxacin	Renal	↓	?	↑	↓
Clarithromycin	Hepatic (CYP3A)	↓	↔	↑	↓
Cloxacillin	Renal	N.A., ↓ with renal ↓	N.A.	N.A, ↑ with renal ↓	↓
Erythromycin	Hepatic (CYP3A)	↓	↔	↑	↓
Ethambutol	Renal	N.A.	N.A.	N.A., ↑ with renal ↓	↔, ↓ with renal ↓
Fluconazole	Renal	↓, ↔	N.A.	↑, ↔	↓
Gentamicin	Renal	↓, ↔	↑, ↔	↑, ↔	↓, by CrCL
Isoniazid (INH)					
Slow acetylators	Hepatic	↔	↔	↔	↔
Rapid acetylators	Hepatic	↓, ↔	↔	↑	↓
Itraconazole	Hepatic (CYP3A)	?, ↓	N.A.	?, ↑	?, ↓
Ketoconazole	Hepatic (CYP3A)	?, ↓	N.A.	?, ↑	?, ↓
Methicillin	Renal	N.A., ↓ with renal ↓	N.A.	N.A., ↑ with renal ↓	↓
Metronidazole	Hepatic (CYP + gluc)	?, ↔	sl. ↓	?, ↔	?, ↔, ↓
Nafcillin	Hepatic	N.A.	N.A.	N.A.	?, ↔
Penicillin	Renal	N.A.	N.A.	N.A.	↔ [e]
Piperacillin	Renal	N.A.	N.A.	N.A.	N.A, by CrCL
Rifampin	Hepatic (CYP1A)	N.A.	N.A.	N.A.	?
Tetracyclines	Renal, hepatic	N.A.	N.A.	N.A.	↓
Tobramycin	Renal	↓, ↔	N.A.	↑, ↔	↓, by CrCL
Trimethoprim	Renal (acetylation)	↓	↔	↑	↓
Vancomycin	Renal	↓	N.A.	↑	↓, by CrCL
CARDIOVASCULAR					
Adenosine	Circulating esterase	N.A.	N.A.	N.A.	↓, [c]
Amiloride	Hepatic, renal	↓	↔	↑	↓
Amiodarone	Hepatic (CYP2C, 3A)	↔	N.A.	↔	↓, [c]
Chlorthalidone	Renal	N.A.	N.A.	N.A.	↓ [c]
Digoxin	Renal	↓	↓, ↔	↑	↓based on CrCL
Furosemide	Hepatic, renal	↓	? ↓	? ↑	↓ [c]
Hydrochlorothiazide	Renal	? N.A.	N.A.	N.A.	↓ [c]
Lidocaine	Hepatic (CYP3A)	↓, ↔	↔, ↑	↑	↓
Mexiletine	Hepatic (CYP2D6)	↔, (sl. ↓)	N.A.	↔	↔, (sl. ↓)
Procainamide + NAPA	Renal	↓	N.A.	↑	↓
Propafenone	Hepatic (CYP2D6)	↔	↔	↔	↔
Quinidine	Hepatic (CYP3A)	↓	?	↑	↓
Spironolactone	Hepatic	↓	↔	↑	↓
Beta Blockers					
Acebutolol[a]	Hepatic, renal	↔	N.A.	↑	↓
Atenolol	Renal	sl. ↓	N.A.	sl. ↑	↔

(continued)

TABLE 469.2.   *Continued*

		Aging Effects			
	Route of Elimination	Clearance	Volume	$t_{1/2}$	Dose Adjustment
Carvedilol	Hepatic	↔	N.A.	↔	↔
Metoprolol	Hepatic (2D6)	↑, ↔	N.A.	↑, ↔	↓, ↔
Nadolol	Renal	N.A.	N.A.	N.A.	↓
Pindolol	Renal, hepatic	N.A.	N.A.	N.A.	↓
Propranolol	Hepatic (2D6, 1A)	↓ (men)	↔	↑	↓
Sotalol	Renal	↓	↓	↑	↓
Timolol	Hepatic (2D6)	↔	N.A.	N.A.	↔
Calcium Antagonists					
Amlodipine (DHP)	Hepatic (CYP3A)	↓	↔	↑	↓
Diltiazem	Hepatic (CYP3A)	↓, ↔	↔	↑, ↔	↓
Felodipine (DHP)	Hepatic (CYP3A)	↓	N.A.	↑	↓
Isradipine (DHP)	Hepatic (CYP3A)	↓	N.A.	↑	↓
Nicardipine (DHP)	Hepatic (CYP3A)	↔, ↑	↔	↔	↓, c
Nifedipine (DHP)	Hepatic (CYP3A)	↓	↔	↑	↓
Nisoldipine (DHP)	Hepatic (CYP3A)	↓, ↔	N.A.	↑, ↔	↓, ↔
Nitrendipine (DHP)	Hepatic (CYP3A)	↓	N.A.	↑	↓
Verapamil	Hepatic (CYP3A)	↓, ↔	↔	↑, ↔	↓
α-Blockers					
α-Methyldopa	Hepatic, renal	↓	N.A.	?, ↑	↓
Clonidine	Renal, hepatic	↓	N.A.	N.A.	↓ c
Doxazosin	Hepatic	↑	↑, ↔	↔	↔, ↓ c
Labetalol	Hepatic	↓, ↔	N.A.	↑, ↔	? ↓
Prazosin	Hepatic	↔	↔	↑	↓, ↔ c
Terazosin	Hepatic	↓, ↔	N.A.	↔, ↓	↔, ↓ c
Nitrates					
Isosorbide dinitrate	Hepatic	N.A.	N.A.	N.A.	↓ c
Isosorbide 5-mononitrate	Hepatic	↔	↔	↔	↓ c
Lipid-Lowering Drugs					
Atorvastatin	Hepatic (CYP3A)	↓	↓	↑	↔, ↓ e
Clofibrate a	Renal	N.A.	N.A.	N.A.	↔, (↓ for renal ↓)
Fluvastatin	Hepatic (CYP3A)	↔	N.A.	↔	↔
Gemfibrozil	Hepatic	N.A.	N.A.	N.A.	↔
Lovastatin a	Renal (CYP3A)	N.A.	N.A.	N.A.	↔, (↓ for renal ↓)
Pravastatin a	Renal (CYP3A)	↔	N.A.	↔	↔
Simvastatin a	Renal (CYP3A)	N.A.	N.A.	N.A.	↔, (↓ for renal ↓)
Angiotensin-Converting Enzyme Inhibitors					
Benazepril a	Renal	↔	↔	↔	↓, esp. initial dose c
Captopril	Renal	↓	N.A.	↑	↓ c
Enalapril a	Renal	↓, ↔	N.A.	↑, ↔	↓ c
Fosinipril a	Renal	↔	N.A.	↔	↓ c
Lisinopril	Renal	↓	N.A.	↑	↓ c
Quinapril a	Renal	↓	N.A.	↑	↓ c
Ramipril a	Renal	↓	N.A.	↑	↓ c
ARB (angiotensin II receptor blockers)					
Irbesartan	Biliary, renal	↓, ↔	N.A.	↑, ↔	↔, ↓
Losartin (am)	Biliary a (CYP3A, 2C9)	↔	↔	↔	↔
Valsartan	Biliary	↓	N.A.	↑	↔ (initial dose)
Miscellaneous					
Pentoxifylline	Hepatic	↓	N.A.	↑	↓
Warfarin	Hepatic (CYP3A)	↔	↔	↔	↓, b,c
CENTRAL NERVOUS SYSTEM					
Anticonvulsants					
Carbamazepine	Hepatic (CYP3A)	? ↓	N.A.	↑	↓, ↔
Phenytoin	Hepatic (CYP2C)	↔, N.A.	N.A.	↔	↔, ↓ c
Valproic acid	Hepatic (mixed)	N.A.	N.A.	N.A.	? ↓, ↔
Antidepressants					
Amitriptyline a	Hepatic	↔	↑	↑	(prob) ↓
Buproprion	Hepatic	↔, sl. ↓	N.A.	↔, sl. ↑	↓, ↔, e
Desipramine	Hepatic (2D6)	↓	N.A.	↑	sl. ↓
Doxepin a	Hepatic	N.A.	N.A.	N.A.	sl. ↓
Fluoxetine a (SSRI)	Hepatic (2D6), renal	↓	N.A.	↔	↓, χ
Imipramine a	Hepatic (2D6)	↓	↔	↑	↓
Lithium	Renal	↓	?	↑	↓
Mirtazapine	Hepatic	↓	N.A.	↑	↓

(continued)

TABLE 469.2. *Continued*

	Route of Elimination	Aging Effects			Dose Adjustment
		Clearance	Volume	t_{1/2}	
Nefazadone	Hepatic (CYP3A)	↓	N.A.	↑	↓
Nortriptyline	Hepatic (2D6)	↓	N.A.	↑	↓
Paroxetine (SSRI)	Hepatic (2D6)	↓	N.A.	↑	↓
Sertraline (SSRI)	Hepatic (2D6)	↓	N.A.	↑	↓
Trazodone[a]	Hepatic	↓	↓	↑	
Venlafaxine	Hepatic	↓	N.A.	↑	↓, + by CrCL
Cognitive Enhancers					
Donezepil	Hepatic (CYP2D6, 3A)	↔, ?M = W	N.A.	↔, ?M = W	↔, tested in elderly
Tacrine	Hepatic (CYP1A)	↔, M > W	N.A.	↔, W > M	↔, ↓ in W
Neuroleptics					
Clozapine	Hepatic (CYP1A2)	↔, M > W	?, ↔	?, ↔	?, ↔
Haloperidol	Hepatic (CYP2D6)	↓	N.A.	↑	↓
Olanzapine	Hepatic (CYP1A2, ± 2D6)	?, ↔	N.A.	N.A.	?, ↔
Risperidone	Hepatic (CYP2D6)	N.A.	↓	?, ↑	↓
Parkinson's disease					
L-dopa	Hepatic + other	↓	↓	↔	↓
ENDOCRINE					
Antidiabetic agents					
Biguanides					
Acarbose	Intestinal	sl. ↓	N.A.	sl. ↑	↔
Metformin	Renal	↓	↓	↑	↓
Sulfonylureas**					
Glibenclamide	Renal	↓	N.A.	↑	↓
Glimepiride	Hepatic	↔	↔	↔	↔
Glipizide	Hepatic, renal	↔	N.A.	↔	↔, ?
Glyburide	Hepatic, renal	↔	↑	↑	↔
Thiazolidinediones					
Troglitazone	Hepatic (CYP3A)	↔	↔	↔	↔ [e]
Hormonal					
Estrogen	Hepatic (CYP3A)	↔, ↓	↓	↑	↓
Progesterone	Hepatic	N.A.	N.A.	N.A.	N.A.
Raloxifene	Hepatic	N.A.	N.A.	N.A.	N.A.
Testosterone	Hepatic (CYP2)	↔, ↓	?, ↓	?, ↑	↓ [c]
Levothyroxine	Hepatic	N.A.	N.A.	N.A.	[c]
GASTROINTESTINAL					
Cimetidine	Hepatic (CYP1–3), renal	↓	N.A.	↑	↓
Famotidine	Renal, hepatic	↓	N.A.	↑	↓
Lansoprazole	Hepatic (CYP3A, 2C)	↓	N.A.	↑	↓, ↔
Misoprostil	Renal?	↔	N.A.	sl. ↑	↔
Nizatidine	Renal	↓	N.A.	↑	↓
Omeprazole	Hepatic (CYP2C, 3A)	↓	↓	↑	↓, ↔, [e]
Pantoprazole	Hepatic (mixed)	↓	N.A.	↑	↓, ↔
Ranitidine	Renal, hepatic	↓	N.A.	↑	↓
SEDATIVE/HYPNOTICS					
Alprazolam	Hepatic (CYP3A)	↓	↔	↑	↓
Diazepam	Hepatic (CYP3A)	↓, M > W	↑	↑	↓ [c]
Lorazepam	Hepatic	↔	N.A.	↔	↓ [c]
Midazolam	Hepatic (CYP3A)	↓, M > W	↔	↑	↓, X
Triazolam	Hepatic (CYP3A)	↓	N.A.	↔	↓
OTHER					
Alendronate	Renal	↔	↔	↔	↔, by CrCL
Tolterodine (am)	Hepatic	?, N.A.	?, N.A.	?, N.A.	?, N.A.
Terfenadine	Hepatic	?, T	N.A.	↑	↓

N.A., not available; W, women; M, men; sl., slight; DHP, dehydropyridine; SSRI, selective serotonin reuptake inhibitor.
[a] Active drug is metabolite produced by hepatic metabolism. Elimination route is for active metabolite. am = active metabolite.
[b] Decreased plasma binding → ↑ effect.
[c] Aging effects on specific pharmacokinetic parameters have not been well studied or may show no change, but clinical efficacy has been observed with reduced doses in the elderly.
[d] All cephalosporins undergo renal elimination.
[e] Efficacy studies report similar dose requirements in the young and the elderly.
* Acetylator status most important factor.
** Only second-generation sulfonylureas are listed as these are preferred over first-generation sulfonylureas in the elderly.

(ACE inhibitors), the E_{max} type of models better approximate the concentration vs. response relationship. New concepts in drug design based on targeted organ delivery or inhibition of intracellular phenomena will require new pharmacodynamic models.

INDIRECT DRUG EFFECTS/REFLEX RESPONSES

The pharmacodynamic models described above assume that effects are directly related to the drug concentration alone. This assumption is valid in vitro, but in vivo homeostatic or reflex mechanisms often counter "direct" drug effects. Reflex responses can be considered "indirect" drug effects. A more realistic representation of effects produced after drug dosing in humans is as follows:

$$\text{Total or net effect} = \text{direct effect} + \text{indirect effect}$$

The contribution or lack of contribution of reflex responses to net drug effect is of especial importance in understanding responses to drugs, such as potent vasodilators, in the older patient. Few tools are available to measure reflex responses, but studies of variability of heart rate, blood pressure, or respiration may provide a measure of vagal or baroreceptor activation.

AGE-RELATED CHANGES IN RECEPTOR SYSTEMS

Dynamic responses to autonomic stimuli have been a focus of investigation and have documented age-related changes. One of the most consistent age-related findings in all species and tissues is the decline in β-adrenergic responsiveness. Decreased responses of white blood cells, platelets, heart rate, atrioventricular conduction, cardiac contractility, and vasodilatation are seen following isoproterenol or other β₁-adrenergic stimuli in animal and human models of aging. Decreased β₁-adrenergic responsiveness with aging results in a shift of the concentration vs. response relationship to the right; higher concentrations are necessary for any given effect and the C_{50} (concentration for half-maximal effect) is higher. The maximum effect is also reduced. The mechanism for the age-related decrease in β-adrenergic responsiveness results from both decreased receptor numbers and altered G-protein coupling to the β-adrenergic receptor and G-protein–mediated signal transduction. Physiologically this results in decreased heart rate responses to β-adrenergic stimulation, such as exercise or stress, and a decrease in the maximal heart rate, which is directly related to age. This decreased β₁-adrenergic responsiveness contributes to the blunted baroreflex responses seen with aging.

Age-related changes of other adrenergic receptor systems are less uniform. For the α receptor, data from humans support the lack of age-related α-adrenergic mediated changes in human hand vein responses. Data from humans also support the presence of age-related decreases in α-adrenergic platelet receptors and decreased α-adrenergic-mediated arterial vasoreactivity of forearm blood vessels in healthy men that are similar to the decreased β-adrenergic-mediated blunting of responses seen

with aging. For dopaminergic receptors, there are convincing data for decreased dopaminergic receptor content and dopaminergic transporters with healthy aging in humans. In brain tissue from animals, dopaminergic mRNA, as well as receptor and transporter content, decreases with aging. Cardiac responses to dopaminergic stimulation vary by the effect end point. Contractile responses may be blunted with aging, whereas chronotropic and dromotropic responses are preserved or enhanced in models of aging.

Disparity in age-related changes in peripheral versus central dynamic responses to muscarinic parasympathetic stimulation or blockade also exist. Decreased sensitivity and responses to parasympathetic stimulation are commonly seen in cardiac and vascular tissues, whereas increased central nervous system effects are frequently seen in the elderly. The physiologic consequences are blunted heart rate responses to atropine but increased anticholinergic central nervous system effects, including delirium, in older subjects. Greater sensitivity may also explain the increased incidence of adverse effects, such as urinary retention, constipation, and fecal impaction in the elderly who receive drugs with anticholinergic properties.

The vascular wall has become a target for pharmacologic manipulation of blood pressure and blood flow. Age-related decreases in vasodilatation in response to acetylcholine have been shown in both normal and diseased coronary and peripheral arteries. Coronary vascular responses to endothelin are also blunted with aging. Vasodilatation in response to non–endothelium-dependent agents, such as nitrates or nitroprusside, do not appear to be altered by aging.

BAROREFLEX RESPONSES

In intact humans, age-related alterations in stimulation and suppression tests of baroreceptor function have been well documented. Blunted responses to vasodilators, vasoconstrictors, postural maneuvers, and the Valsalva maneuver have been shown with aging in the absence of detectable disease. Diseases and deconditioning further decrease responses. Pharmacodynamic alterations at many levels (sensing, signal transmission, central processing, autonomic β-adrenergic and parasympathetic pathways, and vessel receptor content and responsiveness) contribute to the blunted baroreceptor responses seen with aging in humans.

Blunted baroreflex responses help to explain the greater postural hypotension and even syncope after potent nitrate or vasodilator administration to older patients. The lack of evidence for increased vascular responses suggests the mechanism for the greater hypotension following vasodilator drug administration in older individuals is primarily due to blunted baroreflex responses to the hypotension. A similar mechanism can be postulated for greater postural hypotension with tricyclic antidepressant drugs in older versus younger patients.

ADVERSE DRUG EFFECTS AND DRUG INTERACTIONS

The prevalence of chronic and multiple diseases increases with age and contributes to polypharmacy. The most common chronic diseases or conditions are arthritis, hypertension, hearing impairments, heart disease, orthopedic impairments, cataracts, sinusitis, and diabetes. The categories of drugs most frequently prescribed in both hospitalized and community-dwelling older patients are cardiovascular and antiarthritis drugs. Therapeutic classes cited in ≥2% of outpatient encounters involving older patients are antihypertensives, β- and α,β-blockers, coronary vasodilators, calcium channel blockers, digitalis preparations, diuretics, anti-infectives, ophthalmics, analgesics, antiarthritics, antidiabetics (oral therapy and insulin), psychotherapeutics, bronchial therapeutics, corticoids, antispasmodics, nutrients/supplements, and cough/cold products. It has been estimated that older community-dwelling North Americans take an average of 4.5 medications at any one time and that most patients use both prescription and over-the-counter drugs. The institutionalized elderly are prescribed from three to eight drugs daily, with a somewhat higher use of psychotropics than older outpatients.

Although the frequency of adverse drug reactions had often been thought to correlate with the age of the patient, consistent observations demonstrate that age is not the major determinant of adverse drug effects. Rather, it is the number of drugs administered that is directly related to the risk of adverse drug-related events. Studies have correlated increasing numbers of medications consumed with increased rates of adverse drug effects and hospital admissions, as well as a decrease in the incidence of adverse drug reactions with reductions in the number of medications consumed. Most studies suggest that the chronic administration of two drugs is associated with a risk of adverse effects of about 15%. The risk of interactions rises to 50% to 60% with the administration of five drugs per day. While drug interactions can be minimized by reducing the number of drugs prescribed, multidrug regimens for single diseases and the presence of multiple diseases may make this an unrealistic goal in many older patients. Therefore, a framework for understanding and preventing adverse drug interactions is necessary.

Drug interactions can result from a pharmacokinetic or pharmacodynamic interaction. Interactions of drugs that are metabolized by a similar route can be anticipated. Routes of elimination are discussed in the renal and hepatic clearance sections, as are pharmacokinetic drug interactions that both increase and decrease drug clearance and concentrations. Pharmacodynamic drug interactions have been less well studied. Pharmacodynamic interactions can lead to either potentiation of drug action or decreased drug effects. In the elderly, common types of pharmacodynamic interactions include those that lead to postural hypotension (direct vasodilators or nitrates combined with α-blockers, β-blockers, calcium channel blockers, ACE inhibitors, diuretics, or sildenafil) or bradycardia (β-blockers combined with digoxin, verapamil, or amiodarone).

The highest probability of problems in the older patient will be in connection with drugs that have narrow therapeutic ranges, and these should be particularly closely monitored (i.e., digitalis, theophylline, warfarin, lithium, lidocaine, quinidine, aminoglycoside antibiotics, tricyclic antidepressants). Central nervous system effects or side effects may be more common in older patients and may significantly affect quality of life, mentation, and functional status (i.e., long-acting hypnotics, histaminergic and α-

blocking drugs, and drugs with anticholinergic effects, such as disopyramide and antihistamines). Adverse drug effects may present "atypically" as a change in mental status in the older patient, and a high index of suspicion must always be present (i.e., digitalis excess presenting as altered mental status).

OVER-THE-COUNTER DRUGS AND NUTRACEUTICALS

A number of drugs are currently available without prescription or over the counter. Although patients may not report using them, such drugs may produce significant pharmacologic effects and can interact with prescription drugs. A common example is the use of NSAIDs and GI bleeding. Aluminum-containing antacids interfere with the absorption of drugs and calcium. Ingestion of mineral oil inhibits absorption of fat-soluble vitamins. Vitamin K intake can reverse warfarin effects.

The term "nutraceuticals" has been coined for a diverse group of substances, such as dietary supplements, vitamins, herbs, and herbal teas, that are becoming increasingly popular with older populations for the self-treatment of depression, memory impairment, sleep disorders, and other common disorders. Two that appear to have widespread use are St. John's wort and ginkgo biloba. St. John's wort is taken for mild depression. It is similar in action to SSRIs, produces additive effects, and should not be combined with SSRIs. It also produces photosensitivity and should not be used in combination with other photosensitizing drugs. Ginkgo biloba has long been advocated for memory loss and as a vasodilator. It inhibits coagulation, can cause bleeding, and interacts with warfarin. Vitamin E also interacts with warfarin to increase anticoagulant effects. Nutraceuticals are not regulated as to purity, health claims, labeling, or bioequivalency, and limited efficacy data are available. Rigorous evaluation of these and other alternative therapies is just beginning.

Dietary exposure can also influence drug concentrations or effects. Alcohol interferes with the absorption of calcium, folate, and thiamine. Ingestion of char-broiled meat has been shown to induce CYP1A2, leading to increased clearance of substrates metabolized by this pathway. High-salt diets increase clearance of quinidine; and cabbage and Brussels sprouts have been shown to increase hepatic clearance of antipyrine. Recently, grapefruit juice has been shown to be a selective and potent inhibitor of intestinal CYP3A. Ingestion of 150 ml of reconstituted grapefruit juice in combination with a number of dihydropyridines leads to markedly increased drug concentrations and increased antihypertensive effects. The role of diet and nutrients in drug metabolism is only now being recognized, and there are no data on potential age-related changes in these processes.

PHARMACOEPIDEMIOLOGY AND PHARMACOECONOMICS

The challenges of evaluating drug utilization and outcomes associated with therapeutic drug use has stimulated the development of new models and fields for pharmacologic study. Two such fields are pharmacoepidemiology and pharmacoeconomics.

PHARMACOEPIDEMIOLOGY

Pharmacoepidemiology applies epidemiologic methods to the study of drug utilization and effects (both beneficial and adverse) in the clinical setting. Basic tools include survey methods for epidemiologic database review, case-control and cohort studies to address the effects of patient variables on clinical outcomes, unexpected drug effects, drug utilization, and individualization of therapy. Examples of these types of analyses in older subgroups are Medicaid database reviews that identified an increased risk of hip fractures in elderly subjects receiving sedative drugs and increased risk of peptic ulcer disease in elderly patients receiving NSAIDs. The pharmacoepidemiologic factors involved in urinary tract infections in patients in long-term care facilities has also been addressed with Medicaid database analysis. Although the field is not fully developed, it is evolving rapidly, with efforts focused on standardization of methodology, development of methods to deal with confounding of effects by indication, and development of the capacity to adjust accurately for disease severity.

PHARMACOECONOMICS

Pharmacoeconomics incorporates cost considerations into the analyses of drug utilization, benefits, and outcomes. The purpose is to define methods or therapies that accomplish an objective in the least costly manner. Cost/benefit analyses compare the cost of a therapy to its benefit. Cost-effectiveness analyses compare the cost of a therapy in monetary terms with its effectiveness, measured in clinical units—either outcomes or surrogate markers—and are usually reported as a ratio of cost to benefit. Cost/utility analyses estimate cost in monetary units and outcomes in terms of the value patients gain from the therapy. Cost/identification analysis estimates the cost of therapy. Results are expressed in cost per unit of service provided and do not calculate clinical outcomes. This field is newer than pharmacoepidemiology, and few studies of cost-effectiveness have stratified by age. One such study found the cost-effectiveness benefit for thrombolytic therapy with streptokinase to be greater in elderly patients than in younger patients with myocardial infarction. A subsequent study of tissue plasminogen activator in patients after acute myocardial infarction reached the same conclusion. Analyses to date have largely focused on costs per day or costs per year of life saved, and have not typically incorporated multidimensional outcomes that include social function, employment, rehospitalization, paid and unpaid assistance in the home for management of health care problems, symptoms, quality-of-life measures, or drug-related morbidity and mortality.

■ SUMMARY

Age-related changes have been reliably found and estimated for renal drug clearance; however, changes in hepatic drug clearance, half-life, bioavailability, and volume of distribution are less predictable. In general, one should reduce drug dosages in elderly

TABLE 469.3.	**DRUG PRESCRIBING GUIDELINES FOR OLDER PATIENTS**

- Introduce drug at low dosage
- Increase dosages slowly
- Use as few drugs as possible
- Avoid interacting drugs if possible
- Monitor for adverse effects
- Consider effects of over-the-counter drugs, diet, and dietary supplements

individuals and titrate drug dosages slowly (Table 469.3, Fig. 469.2). The current state of knowledge is limited by the paucity of investigations in women, minority groups, the old-old, and patient populations with multiple diseases. Age-related changes in responses have been less extensively studied than changes in drug metabolism and clearance but contribute to clinical effects following drug administration. The increasing use of drugs that act as receptor agonists and antagonists will render investigations of age-related changes in the dynamics of receptor-based systems of growing importance to drug therapy in the elderly. Because the co-administration of multiple medications is the single most important factor in the risk for adverse drug effects, the fewest number of drugs possible should be used in patients. When multiple-drug regimens are necessary, drug interactions should be anticipated based on metabolic route or mechanism of effect and adjustments in drug administration made to avoid adverse drug interactions. Newer tools of pharmacoepidemiology and pharmacoeconomics may help to identify drug efficacy and adverse effects in larger clinical populations.

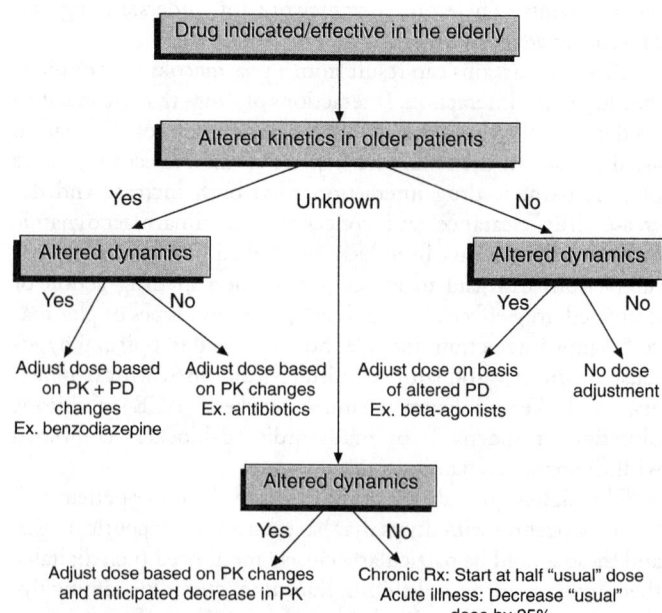

FIGURE 469.2. Schematic representation of the steps involved in choosing a therapeutic dosage regimen for an older patient.
EVIDENCE LEVEL: C. Expert Opinion.

BIBLIOGRAPHY

Abernethy DR, Azarnoff DL. Pharmacokinetic investigations in elderly patients: clinical and ethical considerations. *Clin Pharmacokinet* 1990;19: 89–93.

Chrischilles EA, Foley DJ, Wallace RB, et al. Use of medications by persons 65 and over: data from the Established Populations for Epidemiologic Studies of the Elderly. *Gerontol Med Sci* 1992;47:M137–144.

Department of Health and Human Services. Public Health Service. Food and Drug Administration. Center for Drug Evaluation and Research. *Guidelines for the study of drugs likely to be used in the elderly.* November 1989.

Feely J, Coakley D. Altered pharmacodynamics in the elderly. *Clin Geriatr Med* 1990;6:269–283.

Harris RZ, Benet LZ, Schwartz JB. Gender effects in pharmacokinetics and pharmacodynamics. *Drugs* 1995;50:222–239.

Institute of Medicine (IOM). *Pharmacokinetics and drug interactions in the elderly and special issues in elderly African–American populations.* Washington, DC: National Academy Press, 1997.

Oie S, Schwartz JB, Benet LZ. Design and optimization of dosage regimens: pharmacokinetic data. Appendix II. In Hardman JG, Limbird LE, eds.: *Goodman and Gilman's The Pharmacological Basis of Therapeutics,* ninth ed. New York: McGraw-Hill 1996:1707–1792.

Rowland M, Tozer TN. *Clinical pharmacokinetics: concepts and applications,* third ed. Philadelphia: Lea & Febiger, 1995.

Schwartz JB. Clinical pharmacology. In: Hazzard WR, Bierman EL, Blass JP, et al., eds. *Principles of geriatric medicine and gerontology,* fourth ed. New York: McGraw-Hill 1999:303–331.

Strom BL. *Pharmacoepidemiology.* New York: John Wiley and Sons, 1994.

Walker J, Wynne H. Review: the frequency and severity of adverse drug reactions in elderly people. *Age Ageing* 1994;23(3):255–259.

Walley T, Haycox A. Pharmacoeconomics: basic concepts and terminology. *Br J Clin Pharmacol* 1997;43(4):343.

Yuen GJ. Altered pharmacokinetics in the elderly. *Clin Geriatr Med* 1990; 6:257–267.

Kelley's Textbook of Internal Medicine, fourth edition. Edited by H. David Humes. Lippincott Williams & Wilkins, Philadelphia © 2000.

CHAPTER

470

GERIATRIC CLINICAL NUTRITION, INCLUDING MALNUTRITION, OBESITY, AND WEIGHT LOSS

JEFFREY I. WALLACE
ROBERT S. SCHWARTZ

Much of the intense scientific interest in the field of nutrition stems from the hope that an ideal diet, while not necessarily increasing maximal life span, may prolong the active and useful life expectancy within the genetically determined maximal life span. Defining nutritional adequacy, much less an ideal diet, is a formidable task in the elderly because aging can affect each of the processes that together make up good nutrition: the procurement, consumption, assimilation, and use of the substrates necessary to sustain life. In addition, the wide physiologic variation found within this age group greatly influences the nutritional requirements of the elderly.

NUTRITIONAL REQUIREMENTS AND RECOMMENDED DAILY DIETARY ALLOWANCES

The recommended daily dietary allowances (RDAs) are standards for good nutrition that are set to be safe and to meet or exceed the nutritional requirements of all but the 2.5% of the population considered whose needs are the highest. The majority of current RDAs have not been updated since 1989 and are inadequate with regard to the elderly because they divide physiologically mature adults into one group 19 to 24 years old, a second group 25 to 50 years old, and a third group that includes all those older than 51 years. Further, it should be noted that the RDAs were established to prevent dietary deficiencies rather than to prevent or control chronic conditions (including those that may stem from dietary excesses, notably obesity). Moreover, they have been extrapolated from research conducted primarily in younger, healthier populations. Hence, judgments regarding dietary intake in the elderly must be tempered by recognition of the inadequacy of present RDAs for this group. However, recently updated recommendations (referred to as dietary reference intake, or DRI) from the Food and Nutrition Board of the National Academy of Sciences–Institute of Medicine have attempted to address some of these shortcomings for selected vitamins and minerals (B-complex vitamins, vitamin D, calcium, phosphorus, magnesium, and fluoride) and are considered in greater detail below.

ENERGY INTAKE

Energy intake declines significantly with aging. Of the 600-kcal disparity in daily intake between 30- and 80-year-old men noted in the Baltimore Longitudinal Study of Aging, about one-third could be accounted for by a reduction in basal energy expenditure, attributed to a decrement in lean body mass. The remaining two-thirds was associated with a decline in physical activity with aging. A still greater reduction in caloric intake below the RDA, particularly among persons of low socioeconomic status, has been one of the most consistent findings in surveys of nutritional status in the elderly. The first National Health and Nutrition Examination Survey (NHANES I) found that over 50% of older adults with incomes below the poverty level consumed less than two-thirds of the RDA for energy intake and that 15% of the elderly consumed fewer than 1,000 kcal per day. In the NHANES II study, the mean energy intake for the study population 65 to 74 years old was about 1,600 kcal for men (70% of the RDA) and 1,200 kcal for women (63% of the RDA). Smaller studies using superior assessment methods have generally found higher energy intakes, pointing out potential problems with the use of the NHANES dietary recall methodology, but most studies confirm that caloric intake decreases with age.

The observed fall in energy intake with aging may be an important predisposing factor for malnutrition because if noncaloric ("micronutrient") requirements remain constant or increase with age, then the elderly would be required to consume essentially the same amounts of noncaloric nutrients within the constraint of a reduced overall energy intake. Thus, the inactive elderly are compelled to choose a more nutrient-dense diet if nutritional deficiency is to be avoided. This task is especially difficult because the elderly as a group are the least knowledgeable about nutritional matters, and social, psychological, and biologic forces frequently conspire to inhibit adequate food intake in those of advanced age. Accordingly, many experts recommend multivitamins to help supplement micronutrient intake in older adults, a practice supported by a number of randomized trials whose results indicate that multivitamins can improve nutritional parameters, enhance immunity, and, in one study, reduce episodes of clinical infection. Moreover, the ingestion of one or more over-the-counter vitamin or mineral preparations is very common, especially among generally healthy older adults of middle- and upper-income status in the belief that their health and longevity will be further enhanced, confounding scientific assessment of the rationale for "megavitamin" intake.

PROTEIN INTAKE

Absolute protein intake is closely linked to energy intake and, thus, declines with age. Nonetheless, most adults in Western societies normally consume more than twice the RDA for protein (0.8 g per kilogram), and diminished protein intake alone is unlikely to account for the large reduction in total body protein in the elderly. Studies reveal a mean 40% decline in muscle mass in elderly men compared with young controls, the cause of which is most likely related to excessive muscle catabolism and in the extreme produces sarcopenia and related weakness (see Chapter 464). Visceral protein is also affected by aging, as evidenced by a small reduction in albumin concentration and a defective regulation of albumin synthesis in response to changes in dietary protein intake. However, an albumin concentration below 3.5 mg per deciliter should not be considered a normal finding in an elderly person.

Different studies that attempt to determine the minimal protein intake necessary for protein balance in the elderly are contradictory, variously supporting protein needs less than, equal to, or greater than the RDA. These discordant findings are not surprising, considering the number of possible factors that affect nitrogen balance (acute and chronic illness, energy balance, and exercise) and the methodologic problems of the nitrogen balance technique. Some studies indicate that increased protein intake can enhance healing of pressure ulcers, and recently published guidelines recommend protein intakes of 1.0 to 1.5 g per kilogram per day for these patients. Similarly, acutely ill or injured patients may benefit from increased protein intakes of up to 1.2 to 1.8 g per kilogram per day, depending on the severity of the stressor. Still other studies suggest that higher than normal RDA intakes of protein (1.0 to 1.2 g per kilogram) may be required for older subjects to accrue significant lean body mass during a strength training program.

CARBOHYDRATE, FAT, AND FIBER INTAKE

Carbohydrate and fat intake are usually inversely related (in the caloric steady state), and the increase in fat consumption in the American diet this century has been paralleled by a reduced consumption of carbohydrates, especially complex carbohydrates. Epidemiologic data have demonstrated that excessive dietary fat intake is associated with increased risks for obesity, coronary heart disease, and certain cancers. Although data indicate that fat consumption has declined in recent years from nearly 40% to around 34% of total energy intake in the face of widespread public education on the risks of high-fat diets, the prevalence of obesity has continued to rise, with more than 40% of persons age 60 to 74 being classified as overweight in the NHANES III study. Dietary fiber has been another area of intense interest because high intakes of dietary fiber have been associated with reduced risks for coronary heart disease, and high-fiber diets may have positive effects on lipids, glucose tolerance, and blood pressure. However, a recent, randomized, double-blind study noted no difference in the parameters in individuals receiving diets supplemented with high- or low-fiber foods. The observed small reduction in cholesterol in the high-fiber group was thought to be secondary to a reduction in the intake of cholesterol and saturated fatty acids. Although high-fiber diets can be recommended for treatment of constipation and diverticulosis, a recent large trial did not find an inverse association between fiber intake and the risk for colorectal cancer, casting doubt on the purported protective role of fiber in colon cancer. Despite these and other areas of controversy, there is general agreement that healthy diets for adults should include adequate dietary fiber (20 to 30 g per day) and more than five daily servings of fruits and vegetables, and should restrict total and saturated fat intake to less than 30% and more 10% of energy intake, respectively.

VITAMIN AND MINERAL INTAKE

Numerous studies have examined vitamin and mineral nutriture in the elderly. Most of these studies have been cross-sectional and have estimated nutrient adequacy by the level of dietary intake of specific nutrients in comparison to the RDA, direct or indirect measurements of blood nutrient concentrations, or cell or tissue nutrient concentrations. Despite frequent dietary or laboratory evidence for inadequacy, clinical evidence for classic vitamin deficiency syndromes in the absence of general malnutrition is rarely documented in the elderly in America.

Water-Soluble Vitamins

Thiamine (Vitamin B₁)

Thiamine is a key coenzyme in the metabolism of sugars by the pentose phosphate pathway; thus, its requirement depends on the caloric intake. A mandatory enrichment of food with vitamin B_1 (especially flour) ensures that the RDA is met in most elderly persons in the United States. In alcoholics, however, interference with active absorption in combination with poor dietary intake can induce the classic clinical triad of thiamine deficiency that defines the Wernicke–Korsakoff syndrome: confusion (acute and chronic), ataxia, and ophthalmoplegia. Heart failure and peripheral neuropathy are also occasionally seen in patients suffering from beriberi. At least 3% to 4% of the population older than 65 years suffers from alcoholism, with higher rates observed in widowers, hospitalized elderly, and nursing home patients. Accordingly, a high level of suspicion for thiamine deficiency in the elderly must be maintained, especially among those at risk for alcohol abuse or with diseases that produce anorexia. Because of the danger of acutely precipitating sequelae of thiamine deficiency, alcoholic and malnourished elderly patients receiving intravenous glucose solutions should also receive thiamine.

Ascorbic Acid (Vitamin C)

Vitamin C is necessary for the hydroxylation of proline and the formation of collagen, and it is a major antioxidant of dietary origin. Although the overt clinical syndrome of scurvy (weakening of collagenous structures, poor wound healing, and hemorrhage) is seldom seen in the United States today, the NHANES I survey found that 23% to 42% of the population studied have intakes of vitamin C that are less than half of the RDA. The lowest intake was found in the poorest socioeconomic group. Other studies have found much lower rates of dietary deficiency, a difference explained mainly by the higher socioeconomic status of the subjects studied. Vitamin C in blood and tissue is diminished in the elderly, and although low levels in hospitalized elderly are enhanced by vitamin C supplementation, little or no clinical improvement has been detected after this intervention. The potential utility of vitamin C in patients with wounds and pressure ulcers has been an area of particular clinical interest, perhaps due to an older, small, placebo-controlled study that found that ascorbic acid 500 mg twice daily improved pressure sore healing rates among surgical patients, many of whom were vitamin C–deficient. However, a recent, much larger, randomized trial of ascorbic acid (500 mg vs. 10 mg, twice daily) in nursing home patients found that higher intakes of vitamin C did not enhance pressure ulcer healing, even among patients with lower baseline vitamin C levels. This result is consistent with extensive evidence that 10 to 20 mg of ascorbic acid per day is sufficient to correct scurvy-related delayed wound healing and that additional supplementation does not appear to further accelerate healing. Thus, although vitamin C in doses of 500 mg twice daily is nontoxic and inexpensive, there is no evidence that such supplements accelerate wound healing among patients who are not vitamin C–deficient.

The ingestion of megadoses of vitamin C has been suggested to reduce the incidence of viral upper respiratory infection, but double-blind studies have repeatedly failed to support this contention. Similarly, although epidemiologic data suggest that vitamin C may protect against atherosclerosis, malignancy, and cataracts (perhaps related to antioxidant properties of ascorbic acid), prospective and randomized studies have not consistently supported these associations. Despite all of the negative or inconclusive studies, vitamin C remains the most common dietary supplement in adults (with up to 60% of some retirement populations taking vitamin C supplements), and it is often taken in megadoses. Megadose vitamin C (more than 10,000 mg per day) may be associated with significant risks: oxalic acid renal calculi, malabsorption of vitamin B$_{12}$, increased absorption of iron, false-negative tests for occult blood in the stool, rebound

scurvy, and possibly bone calcium loss secondary to buffering of the added acid load. In addition, the increment in plasma concentration is only 0.2 mg for a dietary intake of 1,000 mg of ascorbic acid, with up to 90% of the vitamin being excreted unchanged in the urine. Therefore, massive supplementation should not be endorsed. However, several common conditions, such as smoking and stress, negatively affect vitamin C nutriture, and additional intake (250 mg per day) may be warranted under these conditions.

Folate

Folate is essential for the synthesis of nucleic acids and the metabolism of certain amino acids, and a deficiency state is associated with impaired cell division and protein synthesis. It is most abundant in liver, leafy green vegetables, fruit, and yeast. Although a large percentage of older adults do not consume even half of the current DRI for folate, low serum folate levels are unusual in nonalcoholic elderly people. Nonetheless, there is currently a great deal of interest in increasing the folate intake of all adults, in part due to this vitamin's pivotal role in the metabolism of homocysteine, a purportedly important independent risk factor for atherosclerotic cardiovascular disease. Strong epidemiologic evidence indicates that elevated homocysteine levels are associated with cardiovascular disease and that increasing folate intake to at least 400 µg per day can reduce serum homocysteine levels. However, to date no randomized trials have demonstrated that lowering homocysteine by increasing folate intake reduces cardiovascular events.

A folate fortification program for grain products started in 1998 (140 µg of folate per 100 g) increased folate intake by 100 µg per day on average. However, the main impetus for this program was the prevention of neural tube defects in fetuses in pregnant women, and it appears that further increases in folate intake are necessary to optimally reduce serum homocysteine levels. Other evidence that increased folate intake might be beneficial includes prospective data indicating that folate might be protective against colon cancer. Although further study is clearly needed in these areas, the Food and Nutrition Board recently increased the RDA for folate from 200 to 400 µg per day based on many of the above potential benefits of higher folate intakes.

Vitamin B$_{12}$

Vitamin B$_{12}$ functions as a coenzyme for methyl transfer reactions [converting homocysteine to methionine and methylmalonyl coenzyme A (Coa) to succinyl-CoA], and deficiency states cause hematologic and neurologic abnormalities. Although the classic presentation of vitamin B$_{12}$ deficiency includes macrocytic anemia, it has been well documented that patients can develop significant irreversible neurologic complications, including dementia, in the absence of anemia or macrocytosis. Vitamin B$_{12}$ is found in foods of animal origin, and despite median intakes in the United States (4 µg for older men, 2.5 µg for women) that exceed the recently revised RDA for B$_{12}$ (2.4 µg per day), studies of community-dwelling elderly individuals demonstrate that 10% to 15% of older adults have metabolic evidence of vitamin B$_{12}$ deficiency. The high prevalence of vitamin B_{12} deficiency in older adults appears to be attributable, in large part, to a reduced ability to absorb food-bound vitamin B_{12} (food–cobalamin malabsorption). Because 10% to 30% of older adults may be unable to absorb naturally occurring food-bound vitamin B_{12}, the recently updated RDAs for B-complex vitamins advised that persons over the age of 50 meet their B_{12} requirement by taking foods fortified with B_{12} or by taking B_{12}-containing supplements. Individuals with B_{12} deficiency caused by a lack of intrinsic factor (e.g., pernicious anemia) require medical treatment with pharmacologic doses of vitamin B_{12}. However, it appears that pernicious anemia is a very uncommon cause of vitamin B_{12} deficiency in older adults. Because of its high prevalence and potential for irreversible neurologic sequelae that can occur without hematologic warning signs, routine screening of older adults for vitamin B_{12} deficiency is recommended.

Fat-Soluble Vitamins

Retinol (Vitamin A)

Vitamin A is important in the maintenance of normal dark-adapted vision and mucosal membranes, and deficiency can cause night blindness, dry skin, and dry mucous membranes. The prevalence of dietary deficiency of vitamin A varies from 12% in study of a healthy white population to 60% in the NHANES I survey. However, even in the NHANES study, serum concentrations were normal in more than 99% of the subjects tested. Epidemiologic data support an inverse relationship between dietary vitamin A consumption and cancers of the lung, bladder, upper gastrointestinal tract, and breast. Possible protective effects of vitamin A and its precursors on age-related macular degeneration and coronary heart disease have also been observed, perhaps related to their antioxidant properties. It is unclear, however, whether these potential protective effects are caused by retinol itself or by carotenoid precursors (e.g., beta carotene) in the diet that are capable of quenching free oxygen radicals (or by other substances and effects associated with diets rich in fruits and vegetables). The possible protective effects of vitamin A and its precursors have spurred the frequent use of these vitamins in megadoses. However, four recent randomized controlled trials failed to demonstrate beneficial effects (or even found detrimental effects) of beta carotene (with and without vitamin A) on cancer or cardiovascular outcome events. Furthermore, recent studies suggest that preformed vitamin A in doses as low as 5,000 to 10,000 IU per day may have adverse effects, including reduced bone mineral density and higher hip fracture rates among women consuming more than 5,000 IU per day and teratogenic effects of doses exceeding 10,000 IU per day. In contrast, several studies have shown that beta carotene is safe for humans and that carotenoids do not cause hypervitaminosis A even when ingested in large amounts (but, as noted above, beneficial effects of carotenoids have not been demonstrated).

α-Tocopherol (Vitamin E)

α-Tocopherol comes mainly from vegetable and seed oils. Clinical deficiency of vitamin E in human beings is limited to cases of severe, longstanding fat malabsorption. The amount of vitamin E in the diet of most elderly people in the United States is probably adequate to meet the RDA of 30 IU, but vitamin E supplements are needed to achieve the high levels of vitamin E intake that have been studied in most randomized trials. The major contemporary interest in vitamin E concerns its antioxidant properties, particularly its potential role in decreasing atherogenesis by decreasing oxidized low-density lipoprotein particles. Adding support to this biologic hypothesis, two epidemiologic studies and two randomized controlled trials have found that high doses of vitamin E (from 50 to 800 IU per day) are associated with reduced risks of primary and recurrent coronary heart disease events. Other randomized trials indicate that vitamin E supplements may slow the progression of Alzheimer's disease (2,000 IU per day) and can enhance immune function (200 to 800 IU per day). Most randomized trials concerning the relationship of vitamin E to cancer have produced negative results, except for some encouraging data indicating that vitamin E (50 IU per day) may reduce the incidence of clinically relevant prostatic cancer. Little toxicity has been noted in adults taking pharmacologic doses of vitamin E; however, there is some concern that vitamin E may increase bleeding risks through its antiplatelet effects, and caution has been suggested for patients taking warfarin. While recommendation of widespread supplementation should await further trials of sufficient size and duration to more fully assess risks and benefits, evidence is mounting that vitamin E supplements are safe and may offer important clinical benefits.

Vitamin D

Hypovitaminosis D is common among older adults and is an important, and remediable, risk factor for osteopenia and bone fractures. Prevalence rates of low vitamin D levels in older adults range from 5% to 15% in the Framingham cohort to over 50% of hospitalized and institutionalized elderly. Reasons for these high prevalence rates include poor dietary intake, inadequate sun exposure, chronic liver and renal diseases, and therapy with drugs that can impair vitamin D activity (e.g., phenytoin, corticosteroids). A recent U.S. trial involving healthy older men and women demonstrated that supplemental vitamin D and calcium (700 IU and 500 mg, respectively) can reduce bone loss and decrease fracture rates. Other data suggest that vitamin D may also play an important role in muscle function, immune function, and osteoarthritis progression, and a recent trial demonstrated functional improvements after vitamin D replenishment in frail vitamin D–deficient older adults. The Food and Nutrition Board recently recommended a doubling of the previous RDA for vitamin D to 10 μg per day (400 IU) for adults age 51 to 70 and a tripling to 15 μg per day (600 IU) for adults over age 70. Because mean intake in community-dwelling elderly is approximately 2.5 μg per day, low-dose supplementation (10 μg per day) should be considered for all older adults. However, in one study of hospitalized patients, hypovitaminosis D was still highly prevalent despite the common daily use of vitamins that contained, on average, 10 μg vitamin D. Accordingly, some experts recommend that higher doses of supplements (15 to 20 μg) be considered, particularly for chronically ill, homebound, or institutionalized people with infrequent exposure to sunlight. Such doses appear to have a considerable margin of safety.

Minerals

Calcium

Osteopenia is a very common and costly disorder in the United States that affects 25% of elderly women and, at a given age, half as many men as well. The cause is multifactorial, with several nutritional factors playing important roles in calcium balance. Almost all nutritional surveys indicate that calcium intake in the elderly is far less than the RDA (which was recently increased from 800 mg to a DRI of 1,200 mg for persons over age 50). Still higher intakes of 1,500 mg per day were recommended for men and women over age 65 by a 1994 National Institutes of Health consensus panel on optimal calcium intake. The NHANES II study found mean calcium intakes of 596 and 475 mg per day in older men and women, respectively, and NHANES III found that virtually all elderly had intakes below 800 mg per day. Calcium intake is also inadequate in younger women, with 66% of women 18 to 30 years old and 75% older than 35 years similarly consuming less than 800 mg per day. Reduced consumption at these early ages may be critical because peak bone mass is attained during early adulthood. Of interest, a recent large randomized trial found that supplemental calcium (1,200 mg per day) also decreased the risk of colorectal adenomas, providing another potential rationale for calcium supplementation beyond its beneficial effects on bone. Absorption of calcium supplements appears to be most efficient at individual elemental calcium doses of 500 mg or less and when taken between meals (except for persons with reduced gastric acid production, in whom calcium citrate may be preferable to more commonly used calcium carbonate supplements).

Zinc

Estimates of zinc intake from large surveys reveal that the elderly consume about 10 mg per day of zinc (zinc RDA for women is 12 mg per day, men 15 mg per day). The lowest intakes were in poor elderly women, who consumed less than half the RDA. There appears to be only a small decline, if any, in blood zinc concentration with aging, but the relationship between blood and tissue levels is poor. Zinc nutriture is especially meaningful in the elderly because of its relationship in animal models with immune function, wound healing, and taste perception. A number of small studies suggest that zinc supplementation in doses of 15 to 25 mg may increase the number of circulating T lymphocytes, improve delayed hypersensitivity in elderly subjects, and decrease clinically relevant infections. Interest in the potential role of zinc in wound healing was spurred in part by a small older study whose results indicated that zinc supplements in higher dose (220 mg zinc sulfate t.i.d.) accelerated the healing of excised pilonidal–sinus tracts in young healthy airmen. However, subsequent studies indicate that the benefits of zinc supplementation on wound healing appear limited to patients with baseline zinc deficiencies. Zinc supplementation (zinc sulfate 220 mg t.i.d.) has been demonstrated to promote healing of

venous stasis leg ulcers in older subjects with documented low serum zinc levels in double-blind studies. Although clinical zinc deficiency is unquestionably associated with anorexia, the appetite response to zinc supplementation in the elderly has been unimpressive. One double-blind, placebo-controlled study demonstrated that zinc supplementation (zinc sulfate 100 mg twice daily) reduced the progression of macular degeneration, but this intriguing result was not confirmed in a subsequent study. Zinc supplements can cause side effects that include gastrointestinal irritation; paradoxically, high serum zinc levels may inhibit healing and impair immune function, as well as interfere with copper metabolism.

Multivitamins

Most older adults do not consume fruits and vegetables in recommended quantities (more than five servings per day), and their frequently reduced energy intakes often result in diets that are deficient in one or more micronutrients. Studies show that 30% to 60% of older adults already take multivitamins, and there is some evidence that even healthy elderly persons may benefit from such supplements. Most standard multivitamins contain quantities of vitamins and minerals in the RDA range, and such doses appear to have little to no toxicity. Although supplementation is not a substitute for a healthy balanced diet (which may contain beneficial nutrients that remain to be identified), the use of a standard multivitamin appears to be a safe and reasonable approach to ensure adequate micronutrition in the elderly.

■ MALNUTRITION AND WEIGHT LOSS

BARRIERS TO ADEQUATE NUTRITION

The socioeconomic, psychological, and physiologic variation found in the elderly has a profound influence on the risk for malnutrition in any given person. Further, although undernutrition has been frequently observed in virtually all older-adult populations studied, prevalence rates and the implications of malnutrition vary considerably across the spectrum of health, from well community-dwelling to frail hospitalized or institutionalized elders. Many of the common and often interacting factors that can act as barriers to adequate nutrition in the elderly are listed in Table 470.1. These, along with the drugs listed in Table 470.2, must be considered and addressed in any effort to assess and reduce the risk of malnutrition in older adults.

INVOLUNTARY WEIGHT LOSS IN THE ELDERLY

Definition and Clinical Significance

Although no clear consensus exists on the degree of unintentional weight loss that should prompt concern and investigation, most studies on weight loss have used decrements in the range of 5% of body weight, over 6 to 12 months, to signify clinically important weight loss. Available data indicate that this degree

TABLE 470.1.	**BARRIERS TO ADEQUATE NUTRITION IN THE ELDERLY**

Socioeconomic
  Fixed income/poverty
  Access to food
    Isolation or lack of transportation
    Lack of storage facilities (refrigerator, freezer)
    Lack of adequate cooking facilities (oven, microwave)
  Poor knowledge of nutrition
  Dependence on others (institutions, caretakers)
  Elder abuse and neglect
Psychologic
  Depression
  Dementia
  Loss of mealtime companions
  Anxiety, fear, paranoia
Physiologic
  Reduced mobility or dexterity producing decreased ability to
    prepare food or feed oneself
    Arthritis
    Stroke or other neurologic impairment
  Decreased metabolic requirements and reduced food intake
    Inactivity
    Reduced lean body mass
  Impaired sensory input (sight, smell, taste)
  Poor or no dentition
  Alcohol and other drugs (Table 470.2)
  Gastrointestinal disorders (e.g., dysphagia, malabsorption)
  Chronic illnesses that affect nutrient intake, appetite, or utilization

TABLE 470.2.	**DRUGS THAT FREQUENTLY AFFECT NUTRITIONAL STATUS**

Enhance catabolism
  Corticosteroids
  Cancer chemotherapeutic agents
Impair taste
  Clofibrate
  Griseofulvin
Cause dry mouth/impair gastrointestinal motility
  Anticholinergics
  Antihistamines
  Tricyclic antidepressants
  Antipsychotics
Cause nausea/anorexia
  Narcotics
  Xanthines
  Digoxin
  Antibiotics
  Serotonin reuptake inhibitors
  Dopaminergics (L-dopa)
  Nonsteroidal anti-inflammatory agents
  Reserpine
  Cancer chemotherapeutic agents
Cause malabsorption of nutrients
  Corticosteroids (calcium)
  Proton pump inhibitors, metformin (vitamin B_{12})
  Laxatives (energy)
  Bile acid binders (fat-soluble vitamins)
  Antibiotics (fat, calcium)
  Aluminum-containing antacids (calcium)
  Alcohol (folate, thiamine, calcium)
Cause abnormal nutrient metabolism
  Diphenylhydantoin, phenobarbital, corticosteroids (vitamin D)
  Isoniazid (vitamin D, vitamin B_6, niacin)
  Cimetidine (vitamin D)

of weight loss occurs not infrequently (prevalence (5%) among community-dwelling elderly, commonly ($\geq$20%) in institutionalized elderly, and is associated with increased morbidity and mortality.

Etiologic Factors

Explanations for weight loss in the elderly have ranged from physiologic changes associated with aging to an increased prevalence of poverty, psychosocial problems, chronic disease, and medication use (Tables 470.1 and 470.2). Although limited, current data provide some insight into the causes of involuntary weight loss in older adults (Table 470.3).

Pathogenesis

Anorexia with diminished caloric intake is often the pathway through which disease, dysfunction, and psychosocial problems lead to weight loss. Possible common underlying pathophysiologic mechanisms that might account for changes in intake and metabolism in the elderly include alterations in neurohumoral regulators of feeding drive and satiety (e.g., endogenous opioids and cholecystokinin); increases in cytokines [e.g., cachectin (tumor necrosis factor), interleukin-6 and other interleukins]; decreases in anabolic factors (e.g., growth hormone, androgens, and insulin-like growth factors); and diminished senses of taste and smell.

Diagnostic Evaluation of Weight Loss

Losses of 5% or more of body weight over 6 to 12 months should prompt clinical evaluation. Actual weight loss should be verified (e.g., medical record, observer corroboration) because in one study almost half of the patients claiming significant weight loss had stable weights, as recorded in their charts. Careful clinical evaluation, with special attention paid to factors listed in Table 470.1, reveals the cause in most cases. Whether the patient has adequate caloric intake may help focus the investigation further (Fig. 470.1). If the basic initial evaluation is unrevealing, it is probably best to enter a period of "watchful waiting" rather than continue extensive testing. If a serious physical disease is present, the diagnosis usually becomes evident within 6 months.

Management and Prognosis

Treatment should be directed at the specific cause (albeit often complex or multifactorial) and hence may require multidisciplinary assessment and longitudinal case management (Fig. 470.1). The availability of adequate food supply, meal preparation, and appropriate assistance for dependent patients needs to be ensured. Depression and nonmalignant gastrointestinal disorders

TABLE 470.3.　　DIAGNOSTIC SPECTRUM OF INVOLUNTARY WEIGHT LOSS

	Study (Study Size)				
	Marton et al. (*N* = 91)	Rabinovitz et al. (*N* = 154)	Huerta et al. (*N* = 50)	Thompson et al. (*N* = 45)	Levine (*N* = 107)
Study population	70% Inpatient	Inpatient	Inpatient	Outpatient	Outpatient
Mean age (range)	59 ± 17	64 (27–88)	59 (18–83)	72 (63–83)	62 (17–91)
Diagnosis (*n*, %)					
Cancer	18 (19%)	56 (36%)	5 (10%)	7 (16%)	6 (6%)
Gastrointestinal	13 (14%)	26 (17%)	9 (18%)	5 (11%)	6 (6%)
Psychiatric	8 (9%)	16 (10%)	21 (42%)	8 (18%)	24 (22%)
Endocrine	4 (4%)	6 (4%)	5 (10%)	4 (9%)	5 (5%)
Cardiopulmonary	13 (14%)	—	1 (2%)	—	9 (9%)
Other med dx[a]	16 (18%)	14 (9%)	4 (8%)	10 (22%)	17 (16%)
Unknown	24 (26%)	36 (23%)	5 (10%)	11 (24%)	38 (36%)

[a] Other medical diagnoses: neurologic, infectious, alcohol, medication, renal, inflammatory disease, multifactorial.
(Modified from Wallace JI, Schwartz RS. *Clin Geriatr Med* 1997;13:717.)

appear to be the most common, specific, remediable causes of weight loss.

Strategies to overcome anorexia and improve oral intake include assessing and meeting food preferences to the highest degree possible and providing frequent small meals and high-calorie snacks. Anecdotally, the use of favorite high-calorie foods (e.g., sweets) has proved useful in helping to overcome anorexia in some hospitalized patients, and a few controlled studies suggest that flavor enhancement of foods can improve food intake. Multivitamins and protein-calorie supplements are generally recommended to improve nutritional status, but there are no widely available diets to promote weight gain. When nutritional supplements are used, those with higher caloric density (1.5 to 2.0 kcal per milliliter) should be favored over standard (1 kcal per

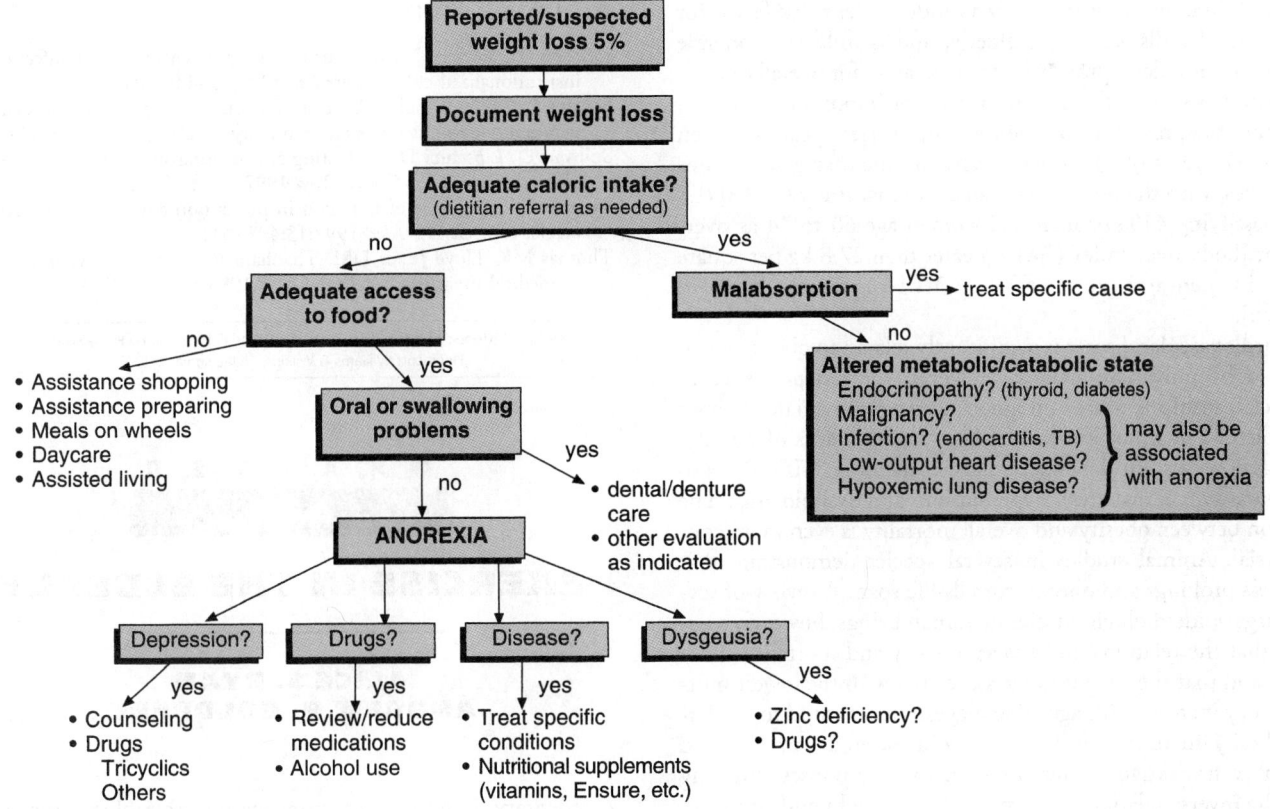

FIGURE 470.1. Weight loss algorithm.

milliliter) formulas. Costs are only slightly higher, and as these supplements deliver higher caloric content per milliliter ingested, patients need not drink as much volume to improve caloric intake. Also, supplements should be provided between, rather than with, meals to minimize their potential for reducing usual mealtime intakes. Pharmacologic approaches to stimulate appetite may also be considered, but the few agents (megestrol acetate, dronabinol, cyproheptadine) that have been shown to improve intake in some patient populations (e.g., cancer, HIV, anorexia) have the potential to cause important side effects and are virtually unstudied in the elderly. Cyproheptadine, a serotonin antagonist, has anticholinergic and antihistaminic properties, and thus its use in the elderly may be problematic. Megestrol acetate can cause fluid retention, thromboembolic phenomena, and impotence, and dronabinol can cause confusion and hallucinations. Although a trial of an appetite stimulant might be considered in selected cases where other approaches have failed, in general their use should await clarification of safety and efficacy in studies of older adults. In patients unable to increase their oral intake despite attention to the preceding measures, tube feedings may be considered if deemed appropriate by the physician and patient. Long-term goals should be specified before tube feeding is begun, and periodic reassessment and reconsideration are essential.

OBESITY IN THE ELDERLY

There is no more hotly debated issue in all nutrition than the consequences of obesity in the elderly. There are two separate issues of disagreement: is obesity an independent risk factor for cardiovascular disease in the elderly, and is mild to moderate obesity in the elderly protective or a risk factor for overall mortality? The answers to these questions are of importance because, although the prevalence of obesity in our society peaks between 55 and 65 years of age, obesity rates are increasing in persons of all ages, with the most recent large national study (NHANES III) classifying 41% of men and women age 60 to 74 as overweight [body mass index (BMI) greater than 27.8 kg per square meter in men and greater than 27.3 kg per square meter in women].

Cardiovascular disease is significantly related to obesity when assessed by univariate analysis; however, the independence of this relationship is more ambiguous using multivariate analyses that factor out other known medical concomitants of obesity, such as non–insulin-dependent diabetes mellitus (NIDDM, also known as type 2 diabetes), hypertension, and dyslipidemia. The relation between obesity and overall mortality is even more controversial. Animal studies in several species demonstrate that leanness prolongs and obesity curtails life span. A review of several large epidemiologic studies in human beings, however, indicates that the relationship between obesity and mortality is not linear and that the weight range associated with the lowest mortality may increase with age. The suggestion that mild to moderate obesity in older adults might be associated with reduced mortality has provoked intense dissenting responses, stressing that the inverse relationship between body weight and smoking, not considered in many of the epidemiologic studies, accounts

for the apparent increased mortality at lower weight ranges; low-weight nonsmokers as a group have a reduced mortality risk in all age groups from 30 to 62 years; the independent association between obesity and mortality occurs only after a latency period of up to 16 years and would be missed in short-term follow-up studies; and obesity is known to be correlated to several important morbid conditions in human beings (NIDDM, hypertension, dyslipidemia, and cancer), whereas few, if any, protective effects of obesity have been defined (osteoporosis being one notable exception). A recent national study of white nonsmokers found that thinness (BMI 19.0 to 21.9 kg per square meter) was associated with the lowest rates of cardiovascular and all-cause mortality up to age 75. However, the relationship between increasing BMI and increased mortality diminished with age, and after age 75 the BMI range associated with the lowest mortality risk was much higher at 27.0 to 28.9 kg per square meter. Thus, protective effects of mild to moderate obesity in the elderly are possible. For instance, the increases in both energy reserves and lean body mass associated with obesity might benefit the elderly during an acute illness. Increased body weight might also reduce osteoporosis and subsequent fractures, a condition associated with significant mortality (and morbidity) in the elderly. The role of adipose tissue in prevention of pressure sores seems clear. It is unclear, however, as to whether these or any other proposed benefits of obesity in the elderly could outweigh its well-known deleterious effects, perhaps most notably osteoarthritis and problems with mobility, and most experts agree that weight maintenance and avoidance of obesity are appropriate goals in adults of all ages.

BIBLIOGRAPHY

Johnson M, Porter K. Micronutrient supplementation and infection in institutionalized elders. *Nutr Rev* 1997;55:400–404.
Stevens J, Cai J, Pamuk ER, et al. The effect of age on the association between body-mass index and mortality. *N Engl J Med* 1998;338:1–7.
Sullivan D, Lipschitz D. Evaluating and treating nutritional problems in older patients. *Clin Geriatr Med* 1997;13(4):753–768.
Thomas DR. The role of nutrition in prevention and healing of pressure ulcers. *Clin Geriatr Med* 1997;13:497–511.
Thomas MK, Lloyd-Jones DM, Thadhani RI, et al. Hypovitaminosis D in medical inpatients. *N Engl J Med* 1998;338:777–783.

Kelley's Textbook of Internal Medicine, fourth edition. Edited by H. David Humes.
Lippincott Williams & Wilkins, Philadelphia © 2000.

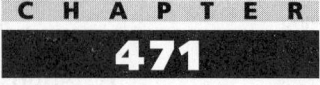

CHAPTER 471

EXERCISE IN THE ELDERLY

ALICE S. RYAN
ANDREW P. GOLDBERG

A sedentary lifestyle results in numerous physiologic and functional declines with aging that increase the risk for disease. Obesity and the special propensity for weight gain in the abdominal region with aging in sedentary older people are strongly associated with the development of hypertension, dyslipidemia, and insulin resistance—all risk factors for cardiovascular disease (CVD). There is increasing evidence that exercise training benefits the health of older persons. The reduced risk for age-related CVD with regular physical activity suggests that people should sustain activity habits as they age. Evidence is emerging that, in addition to its preventive benefits, regular aerobic exercise effectively rehabilitates older people with chronic cardiovascular and musculoskeletal diseases. The focus of this chapter is to provide a clinical framework to guide the clinician in prescribing regular exercise to prevent and treat common diseases in the elderly, as well as to increase functional capacity and independence in older persons disabled by cardiovascular and musculoskeletal complications. Understanding the potential for physical activity to provide health benefits and functional gains not only can enhance the quality of life in older adults but also carries substantial impact for the health care system, considering the rapid growth in the elderly population projected over the next 20 years.

EXERCISE PHYSIOLOGY/BODY COMPOSITION AND AGING

EXERCISE AND THE CARDIOVASCULAR SYSTEM

Aging is associated with numerous changes in the cardiovascular system. As detailed by Lakatta (and reviewed in Chapter 16), these include a decrease in β-adrenergic stimulation of myocardial contractility, an increase in arterial stiffness and total peripheral vascular resistance, a rise in systolic blood pressure (BP), moderate hypertrophy of the left ventricle, and prolongation of myocardial contraction. These changes in cardiac function are accompanied by a decline in maximal oxygen uptake (VO_2max) and maximal heart rate with age in men and women. VO_2max, the highest rate of oxygen consumption attained during maximal exercise, is a function of maximal cardiac output and maximal tissue oxygen extraction, measured as the arteriovenous oxygen difference. In healthy people, VO_2max is generally believed to be not limited by pulmonary function, blood flow, or oxygen uptake by skeletal muscle. Although stroke volume during exercise does not decline with aging in healthy individuals, there is a smaller increase in left ventricular ejection fraction during exercise in older individuals. Changes in cardiac structure and vascular properties also contribute to the reduction in left ventricular reserve in the elderly.

Cross-sectional data suggest that in healthy subjects the decline in VO_2max is 8% per decade in men and 10% per decade in women. However, longitudinal studies performed in healthy sedentary individuals confirm that VO_2max declines with aging at a rate of 10% to 13% per decade in men and 7% to 11% per decade in women. In older athletes who maintain their physical activity levels and do not change their body composition, the decline is somewhat smaller (5% to 9%) per decade, suggesting that maintenance of exercise training programs attenuates the age-related decline in VO_2max. These older endurance-trained athletes have VO_2max values nearly twice those of sedentary age-matched peers, and similar to those of 30-year-old sedentary individuals. Endurance exercise training can increase VO_2max between 10% and 30% in older individuals, primarily due to an increase in the ability of skeletal muscle to extract oxygen and a rise in cardiac index and left ventricular ejection fraction measured at peak exercise. Older women do not appear to undergo an increase in central cardiac function similar to that of older men; this is possibly related to estrogen deficiency associated with the menopause.

EXERCISE AND BODY COMPOSITION

Body weight and the components of body composition are altered in the aging process (Fig. 471.1). Body weight is the combined weight of a variety of tissues; the largest component is body water, which composes approximately 60% of body weight. Body water can be further divided into intracellular (40%) and extracellular (20%) components. The remaining cellular components of the body are lipid, proteins, glycogen, and minerals. At the tissue level, these body components are adipose tissue, skeletal muscle, visceral organs, and bone. In healthy people, body weight and fat mass increase gradually from early adulthood until the fifth to sixth decade, after which weight tends to plateau even as fat mass continues to rise, at least until advanced old age. Aging is especially associated with body fat accumulation in the abdominal region, with increases in both subcutaneous and visceral fat. This change is somewhat greater in men than women. In contrast to the increase in fat mass during the aging process, skeletal muscle, body water, and bone mass decline. A number of studies have demonstrated an average loss of fat-free mass (FFM) of approximately 16% between the ages of 25 and 70 years peak. FFM in men is reached in the midthirties and then progressively declines. In females, FFM remains relatively stable until approximately age 50 years, at which point

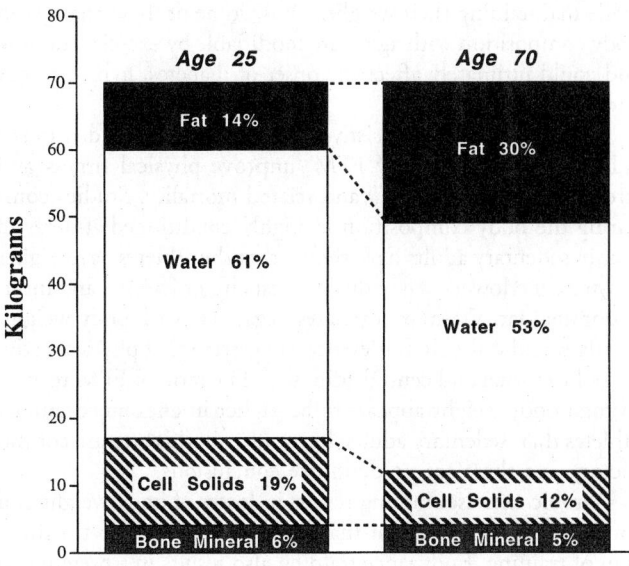

FIGURE 471.1. Age and body composition in adults.

the decline in FFM occurs, but at a slower rate than in men. The muscle mass loss, muscle fiber loss, and decline in motor units with aging are referred to as sarcopenia. The loss of muscle mass is strongly associated with a loss of total body water, which begins to occur after age 70 in women and somewhat earlier in men, with a nadir in the eighth decade of life.

In addition to the losses of FFM and total body water with age, a loss of bone mass is consistently documented. Peak bone mineral mass is reached at age 30 to 35 years in both sexes, followed by a progressive decline. Menopause is a period of more dramatic loss of bone mass in women. By age 70, spinal bone mineral density (BMD) is diminished by approximately 20% in women, slightly less than the 25% loss observed in the femoral neck. Men lose BMD at a rate two-thirds that of women in the spine and one-fourth in the femur, which may explain the reduced fracture risk and rate in males (see Chapter 465). The loss of muscle mass and muscular strength with age may influence both falls and disability in the elderly, and thus increase fracture risk, especially in women.

The significant changes in body weight and composition that occur during the aging process affect health and can increase the propensity for disease. Chronic morbidity is related to these changes, and accelerated weight loss in the elderly predicts death. The health implications of overweight and obesity generally support a higher relative risk with aging, at least until age 70. Specifically, the increase in obesity is associated with increased prevalence of CVD, dyslipidemia, hypertension, insulin resistance, and diabetes. Moreover, the loss of muscle mass with age results in reductions in muscular strength and aerobic fitness in older individuals. These age-associated declines in VO_2max, FFM, and leisure time physical activity, as well as age itself, contribute to the declines in both resting metabolic rate and energy expenditure seen with aging. Results of cross-sectional as well as longitudinal studies suggest that older subjects can modify their daily energy requirements by increasing physical activity habits to raise total daily energy expenditure. This would counter the age-related tendency for weight gain and obesity-associated cardiovascular risk by allowing older subjects to consume more calories while maintaining their weight. Thus, some of these changes in body composition with aging are modifiable by exercise training and could ultimately affect the onset of diabetes, hypertension, and CVD.

Regular aerobic and resistive exercise is recommended in the elderly to prevent loss of FFM, improve physical fitness and strength, and reduce CVD and related mortality. Studies comparing the body composition in highly conditioned athletes to that in sedentary adults have shown that the athletes have higher VO_2max and lower total body fat, waist circumference, and intra-abdominal fat. VO_2max correlates negatively with body weight, fat mass, and waist circumference, suggesting that physical activity reduces total and central adiposity. The ratio of FFM relative to total body weight appears to be higher in endurance-trained athletes than sedentary adults, but studies in this area are contradictory and there are no definitive conclusions.

Aerobic exercise training results in losses of body weight and total and regional body fat that are directly related to the duration of training. Endurance training also results in a preferential loss of fat in the central visceral fat and depots, with little or no change in FFM in older individuals. However, aerobic exercise seems to increase thigh muscle mass in older men, suggesting that specific muscle groups may be altered with aerobic exercise. In general, resistive training does not result in a loss of body weight or total body fat, although one study showed a decrease in visceral fat after resistive training in older women. However, total body FFM and muscle area, measured in the thigh, increase after resistive training in postmenopausal women and middle-aged and older men. Thus, in contrast to aerobic exercise that results in minimal changes in FFM, resistive training increases total body and regional muscle mass.

The changes in muscle mass with exercise training in the elderly are accompanied by alterations in muscle structure and function. Older individuals have lower skeletal muscle oxidative enzymes and capillary density than young sedentary persons, whereas there is some controversy regarding whether type II muscle fiber area decreases with age. These changes in muscle characteristics with aging are modified by aerobic exercise and raise mitochondrial enzyme levels, type II muscle area, and capillary densities to levels comparable to that in young athletes. This increases both the oxidative capacity of the muscle and the muscle glycogen and triglyceride stores. Resistive training increases type I and II muscle fiber area, resulting in an increase in muscle size, and may also increase capillary density and citrate synthase activity.

Regular aerobic weight-bearing exercise has a positive impact on bone density such that physically active men and women have higher BMD than those who are sedentary. Female athletes have higher BMDs of the femoral neck and a tendency toward higher lumbar spine bone densities than sedentary women. Nevertheless, older women athletes have lower lumbar spine and femoral BMD than young women athletes with normal menstrual function. The presence of amenorrhea in female athletes, however, is associated with reduced BMD. Longitudinal training studies show improvements in BMD with aerobic exercise training, but these changes are not as dramatic as those observed between active and sedentary individuals. Some studies suggest that the addition of aerobic exercise training to weight loss programs in older women may prevent the loss in regional BMD seen with weight loss alone. There is a lack of consensus on the effects of resistive training on BMD, but in some studies there were increases or maintenance of BMD. Cross-sectional studies also reveal that weight-lifters have greater BMD than inactive control subjects. However, this does not detract from the increase in muscular strength and muscle mass that comes with resistive training. These adaptations may translate into a reduction in risk of falls, disability, and fracture. Many of these studies were not randomized trials; thus, the recent meta-analysis of randomized trials by Kelley, which reported that both aerobic and resistive training enhanced regional BMD, supports the notion that physical activity has positive effects on BMD and may reduce risk for fracture with aging.

In summary, exercise training has the potential to significantly alter body composition by reducing total and central adiposity, and by increasing muscle mass and bone density. These changes could have a positive impact on the prevention and management of age-related disease, especially those strongly associated with obesity, such as diabetes, hypertension, and dyslipidemia, and with losses in BMD and muscle that predispose to weakness, fractures, falls, and decreased musculoskeletal function.

EXERCISE IN THE PREVENTION AND TREATMENT OF DISEASE

TYPE 2 DIABETES MELLITUS

The prevalence of diabetes approaches 20% in persons over age 70, with an additional 14% meeting criteria for impaired glucose tolerance (IGT). This is three times the prevalence in 40-year-olds and nearly twice that observed in 50-year-olds. Higher rates are observed in African Americans and Mexican Americans. Furthermore, the risk of diabetes is approximately twice as high in overweight than non-overweight adults. It is also affected by physical inactivity, coexisting illness, medications often used in older persons, and dietary intake of fiber and fat. Upper body obesity, which increases with age, augments the risk for glucose intolerance and associated metabolic abnormalities of hyperinsulinemia, which predispose to hypertension, dyslipidemia, and dysfibrinolysis, all components of the insulin resistance syndrome. Moreover, the level of intra-abdominal fat is directly correlated with glucose intolerance and severity of insulin resistance, even after controlling for obesity. Glucose disposal rate and endogenous glucose production are correlated with total body fat, truncal, subcutaneous, and intraperitoneal fat. Thus, total and abdominal obesity are associated with insulin resistance and increase the risk for the development of type 2 diabetes and CVD in the elderly.

As summarized by Ivey, physical deconditioning contributes to insulin resistance (Fig. 471.2) by increasing fat storage and

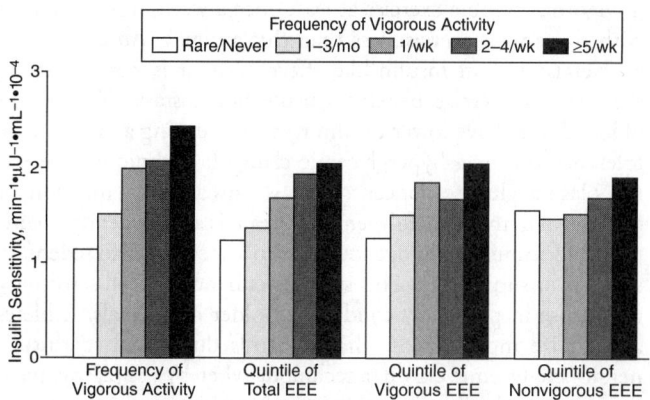

FIGURE 471.3. The Insulin Resistance Atherosclerosis Study. Average, unadjusted values of insulin sensitivity, according to reported participation in physical activity. EEE, estimated energy expenditure.

adipocyte hypertrophy, which reduces free fatty acid clearance and muscle sensitivity to insulin action. Also, physical inactivity in those so predisposed unmasks a genetic defect in the skeletal muscle, which results in insulin resistance and a compensatory increase in β-cell secretion and hyperinsulinemia, which, however, is insufficient to completely overcome the resistance. These defects in insulin secretion and action increase the risk for the development of diabetes. As reported by Mayer-Davis et al., regular participation in nonvigorous and vigorous activities was associated with higher insulin sensitivity in a large sample of normal glucose tolerant, IGT, and diabetic individuals in the Insulin Resistance Atherosclerosis Study (IRAS) (Fig. 471.3). Although this study was cross-sectional, other longitudinal studies suggest that the risk of diabetes is lower in individuals engaged

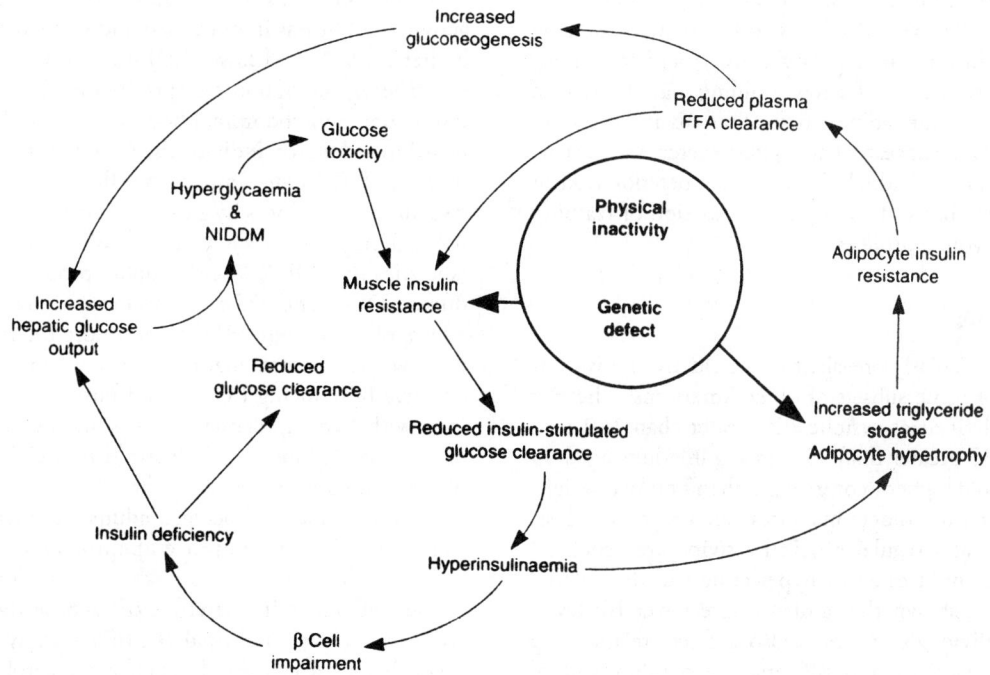

FIGURE 471.2. Mechanisms by which physical inactivity may lead to insulin resistance.

in vigorous aerobic exercise at least once a week, in comparison with those who exercise less than this amount. An acute bout of exercise has an insulin-like effect; thus, it is not surprising that regular exercise benefits glucose homeostasis. Young and older athletes have lower insulin responses during a oral glucose tolerance test or a hyperglycemic clamp (a technique whereby the plasma glucose concentration is raised by an infusion of glucose and the hyperglycemic plateau is subsequently maintained to stimulate endogenous insulin secretion) than sedentary subjects of similar age. This suggests enhanced β-cell sensitivity to glucose in physically conditioned older individuals. Athletes also utilize more glucose than controls during a hyperinsulinemic–euglycemic clamp (a technique whereby the plasma insulin concentration is raised above basal level and maintained concurrently with the plasma glucose concentration by a variable glucose infusion), indicating there is enhanced peripheral tissue sensitivity to insulin with exercise training in highly trained athletes, in comparison with sedentary adults. Moreover, there is no decline in glucose metabolism in comparably fit athletes across a wide age span, which has been interpreted to suggest that a high level of exercise training and its associated adaptations in body composition greatly benefit glucose homeostasis in the elderly.

In longitudinal aerobic exercise training studies, glucose metabolism in healthy older individuals was shown to improve by approximately 20% (13% to 36%). Resistive training also increases glucose uptake and improves insulin action in healthy older men and women. Intensive aerobic exercise normalizes glucose and insulin levels in patients with IGT and mild type 2 diabetes, and increases insulin-mediated glucose disposal and glucose transporter (GLUT-4) levels in glucose-intolerant older men and women. The mechanisms for improvements in glucose metabolism after exercise training include (a) reductions in body fat; (b) increases in muscle mass, GLUT-4, and the enzymes responsible for the phosphorylation, storage, and oxidation of glucose; (c) changes in muscle morphology (increase in conversion of fast-twitch glycolytic IIb fibers to fast-twitch oxidative IIa fibers); (d) an increase in capillary density; and (e) an enhanced blood flow to muscles. Exercise training may also reduce hepatic glucose production, adipose tissue lipolysis and free fatty acid production. This suggests that regular exercise should be an integral part of an individual's lifestyle, as a deterioration in glucose tolerance is observed shortly after cessation of training in older as well as young athletes.

HYPERTENSION

Hypertension is particularly prevalent in the elderly and is present in over 50% of some subsets of older Americans. The risk of hypertension, defined as systolic BP greater than 160 mm Hg and diastolic BP greater than 95 mm Hg in adults aged 45 to 75 years, is twofold higher in overweight than non-overweight individuals. Nonpharmacologic measures, such as weight loss, sodium restriction, and regular physical activity, are beneficial in the treatment of mild essential hypertension in the elderly. Several studies have shown that athletes have lower BP levels than sedentary individuals. There is also a direct relationship between physical inactivity and BP, and the development of hypertension among Harvard male alumni was independently

related to the lack of regular strenuous exercise. A regular aerobic endurance exercise training program is recommended for persons with hypertension and results in a decrease in systolic and diastolic BP of 5 to 10 mm Hg in hypertensive individuals. These improvements may be independent of weight loss, but the addition of weight loss to aerobic training further lowers BP in older men. In contrast, resistive training does not generally result in improvements in BP in normotensive individuals, though it can lower both systolic and diastolic BP in mildly hypertensive individuals. There are no studies of the effects of resistive training and weight loss, or on the combined effects of aerobic and resistive training, on BP in normal or hypertensive older subjects.

DYSLIPIDEMIA

The risk of CVD is higher in the elderly and even more so in the overweight and obese. Regional obesity with preferential deposition of body fat in the truncal region is independently associated with CVD and related mortality. Numerous studies have shown that increased body weight associated with aging, as well as the abdominal fat distribution, is associated with abnormal lipid concentrations, thus increasing the risk for CVD in the elderly. Total cholesterol, low-density lipoprotein cholesterol (LDL-C), and triglyceride (TG) levels all rise across the age span through middle age, while high-density lipoprotein cholesterol (HDL-C) remains stable. In addition to abdominal obesity, the sedentary habits and physical inactivity associated with aging, along with such age-associated common diseases as diabetes, hypothyroidism, renal failure, and medications often taken by older people (e.g., thiazide diuretics, β-blockers, corticosteroids), have a detrimental effect on lipid profiles. Thus, dyslipidemia is an important contributing factor to the development of atherosclerosis in the elderly.

Cross-sectional studies indicate that higher levels of physical activity and fitness in both men and women are associated with higher HDL-C and lower LDL-C and plasma TG levels. This less atherogenic lipoprotein profile may be partially due to the lower total and abdominal body fat observed in trained, as opposed to sedentary, individuals. Although acute aerobic exercise increases HDL-C in women, the effects of chronic aerobic exercise on lipoproteins is of greater clinical importance. Longitudinal training studies show that aerobic training raises HDL-C (specifically HDL-2 levels), apolipoprotein A-I levels, and reduces LDL-C and TG concentrations. However, the beneficial effects of exercise on HDL-C are more dramatic in leaner subjects, whereas a combination of exercise and weight loss is most effective in reducing LDL-C and raising HDL-C in obese subjects with hyperlipidemia. Thus, some of the beneficial effects of exercise on lipids are influenced by weight loss and the loss of total and abdominal body fat.

In young and middle-aged adults, resistive training without weight loss does not improve lipoprotein levels; however, there are no longitudinal studies in the elderly. Some studies show a gender difference in the effect of exercise training on HDL-C and LDL-C levels in the elderly. In one study, hormone replacement therapy accentuated the effects of aerobic exercise by raising HDL-C and lowering LDL-C and TG levels more than exercise or hormone replacement alone. Collectively, these findings indicate that exercise benefits lipoprotein lipids in the elderly. Special populations, such as obese subjects, diabetics, or patients on medications or those with chronic diseases, may require additional treatments to maximize these effects.

OSTEOPOROSIS

Osteoporosis (see Chapter 465) is one of the most prevalent chronic health conditions among the elderly. A reduction in physical activity that occurs in aging may also contribute to osteoporosis. The few longitudinal exercise studies in osteoporotic women that report increases in regional BMD suggest that weight-bearing exercise is not only a beneficial treatment for osteoporosis but also an effective preventive measure.

EXERCISE REHABILITATION IN CHRONIC DISEASE

OSTEOARTHRITIS

Osteoarthritis (OA) afflicts the elderly and is present in more than 60% of individuals 65 years and older. It is characterized by progressive loss of cartilage and bony overgrowth, joint distention, and stretching of periosteal nerve endings, all of which contribute to the pain, stiffness, and reduced range of motion observed in persons with OA. OA of the knee is linked to obesity and inactivity, which in turn are associated with CVD, type 2 diabetes, dyslipidemia, and stroke. As of yet, there is no cure for OA. However, pharmacologic strategies to alleviate pain and disability could improve the quality of life in individuals with this disease. Weight loss, as well as aerobic and resistive exercise, are recommended in the treatment of OA. Preliminary studies showed that both aerobic and resistive exercise reduce pain and disability in this population and also improve physical fitness and reduce depression. In the Fitness Arthritis and Seniors Trial (FAST) randomized control trial conducted by Ettinger's group, an 18-month regimen of either aerobic or resistance exercise training resulted in greater improvements in self-reported pain and disability, as well as physical performance (6-minute walk, stair climb, lift-and-carry task, peak VO_2, and knee flexion strength), than health education in older men and women with knee osteoarthritis. Although there is some evidence to suggest that exercise may accelerate the progression of OA, the results of the FAST indicate that moderate exercise does not worsen the disease, as there was no change in the x-ray scores.

STROKE

Cerebrovascular accidents, or strokes, occur in more than 700,000 persons each year in the United States; the vast majority are reported in persons older than 55 years. A stroke leads to persistent neurologic deficits that impair functional ability, balance, and mobility, and promotes physical inactivity and, ultimately, disuse muscle atrophy. The increase in body fat and a loss of FFM that occurs in normal aging accelerates functional disability in stroke patients, where a sedentary habitus due to

functional immobility compounds sarcopenia. The low endurance, muscular weakness, and impaired functional mobility in stroke patients are potentially modifiable with treadmill exercise training. Improvements in peak aerobic capacity, gait, strength, and functional mobility were seen in selected studies of hemiparetic stroke patients following 6 months of this training. Cycle ergometry also increases VO_2max, and in wheelchair-bound stroke patients, myocardial oxygen demand decreased and peak exercise left ventricular ejection fraction and fractional shortening improved after wheelchair ergometry training.

Treadmill exercise training reduced the energy expenditure and cardiovascular demands of walking and increased quadriceps strength in older (65 years and up) stroke patients in both the paretic and non-affected limb. In addition to the use of treadmill and cycle exercise training programs designed to promote functional improvements in stroke patients, other programs have used Proprioceptive Neuromuscular Facilitation Patterns (PNFs) and Therabands (elastic bands of varying elasticity that provide resistance) with success. Home-based exercise programs also improved lower extremity motor function and gait speed in individuals with stroke. None of these programs reported excessive injuries, morbidity, or patient intolerance to the exercise training. In general, patients were enthusiastic, and compliance rates were greater than 80% in most reports. Thus, aerobic exercise in the stroke patient not only reduces disability but may also reduce the risk of a second stroke and provide such psychological benefits as improving self-esteem and depression, and reducing caregiver burden.

CONGESTIVE HEART FAILURE

Congestive heart failure (CHF) secondary to reduced left ventricular systolic function is common in the elderly, and as such the most frequently assigned Medicare diagnosis-related group (DRG) in older beneficiaries. The prevalence of CHF increases nearly 50-fold from age 40 to age 65 due to the increasing prevalence of coronary artery disease and hypertension in older people. Furthermore, age- and disease-related declines in cardiovascular, renal, and musculoskeletal function make the elderly particularly susceptible to the functional declines associated with left ventricular dysfunction. Many physicians limit the physical activity of older patients with CHF out of concern for precipitating myocardial ischemia, worsening heart failure, or eliciting serious arrhythmias in these disabled, high-risk patients.

Recent studies, however, show that young and middle-aged New York Heart Association/American Heart Association class II and III heart failure patients derive substantial physiologic, functional, and lifestyle benefits from aerobic exercise training. Significant increases in systemic arteriovenous oxygen difference, peak exercise limb blood flow, neuroendocrine hormones, and muscle capillary density and oxidative capacity were associated with increased maximal treadmill exercise time and peak VO_2. These functional changes translate into increased free-living activity, improved quality of life, reduced hospitalizations, and lower mortality in middle-aged patients. Few studies have examined these effects in older CHF patients, but some show significant improvements in 6-minute walk distance, submaximal treadmill exercise duration, and peak VO_2. However, longitudinal follow-up of exercise training outcomes is not yet available in older heart failure patients.

PERIPHERAL ARTERIAL OCCLUSIVE DISEASE

Peripheral arterial occlusive disease (PAOD) is present in approximately 6% of persons older than 65 years. It is a major disabling medical problem because it frequently coexists with coronary and cerebrovascular disease in these patients and severely limits their functional mobility and independence. Patients with PAOD often experience intermittent claudication that impairs their walking ability and curtails physical activities. These patients have an approximately 60% lower functional capacity, measured as maximal attainable oxygen consumption, than age-matched individuals without the disease. This reduced aerobic capacity may be a function of disease severity, sarcopenia, smoking status, general health, and other comorbidities. Thus, exercise rehabilitation is recommended for patients in Fontaine stage II with intermittent claudication, or even those with less severe PAOD.

Aerobic exercise training increases physical fitness, increases the time and distance to onset and maximal claudication pain, and improves exercise economy in PAOD patients. Resistance training increased muscular strength but did not change onset of claudication pain, peak walking time, or peak Vo_2 in these patients. The mechanisms for the improvement in physical conditioning after aerobic exercise training are both hemodynamic and peripheral adaptations. Some studies report that exercise rehabilitation increases calf blood flow, reduces blood viscosity, red cell aggregation, and fibrinogen levels in PAOD patients. More research is needed to elucidate the structural and enzymatic adaptations in muscle and the vascular changes associated with exercise training in this population. At the present time, exercise seems to be the most cost-effective, efficacious treatment for reduction of the progressive disability associated with this disease in the elderly.

EXERCISE GUIDELINES FOR THE ELDERLY

EXERCISE PRESCRIPTION

An exercise test with BP and heart rate monitoring is recommended for men over age 40 and women over age 50, as well as for older patients with and without CVD, prior to commencement of an exercise program. Whether a maximal, submaximal, intermittent, or continuous exercise test is used, the mode of testing (treadmill, cycle, step test, field test) employed depends on the purpose of the test. The test could be performed for the development of an exercise prescription, an evaluation of baseline cardiovascular data and progress of an exercise participant, motivation purposes, education regarding the individual's fitness status, risk stratification, and for clinical applications (e.g., predischarge exercise testing after myocardial infarction, or postdischarge testing after myocardial infarction, coronary artery bypass grafting, and percutaneous transluminal coronary angioplasty, for diagnostic testing, functional testing, and testing for disease

TABLE 471.1.	CONTRAINDICATIONS TO EXERCISE TESTING

Absolute Contraindications

1. A recent significant change in the resting ECG suggesting infarction or other acute cardiac event
2. Recent complicated myocardial infarction (unless patient is stable and pain-free)
3. Unstable angina
4. Uncontrolled ventricular arrhythmia
5. Uncontrolled atrial arrhythmia that compromises cardiac function
6. Third degree atrioventricular heart block without pacemaker
7. Acute congestive heart failure
8. Severe aortic stenosis
9. Suspected or known dissecting aneurysm
10. Active or suspected myocarditis or pericarditis
11. Thrombophlebitis or intracardiac thrombi
12. Recent systemic or pulmonary embolus
13. Acute infections
14. Significant emotional distress (psychosis)

Relative Contraindications

1. Resting diastolic blood pressure >115 mm Hg or resting systolic blood pressure >200 mm Hg
2. Moderate valvular heart disease
3. Known electrolyte abnormalities (hypokalemia, hypomagnesemia)
4. Fixed-rate pacemaker (rarely used)
5. Frequent or complex ventricular ectopy
6. Ventricular aneurysm
7. Uncontrolled metabolic disease (e.g., diabetes, thyrotoxicosis, or myxedema)
8. Chronic infectious disease (e.g., mononucleosis, hepatitis, AIDS)
9. Neuromuscular, musculoskeletal, or rheumatoid disorders that are exacerbated by exercise
10. Advanced or complicated pregnancy

severity and prognosis). In addition, depending on the medical history of the individual being tested, a medical evaluation carried out prior to the fitness test could include a physical examination as well as measurement of BP, serum cholesterol and lipoproteins, blood chemistry profiles, and pulmonary function. There are numerous contraindications to exercise testing (Table 471.1). Patients with absolute contraindications should not undergo an exercise test until those conditions have been stabilized, whereas patients with relative contraindications may be tested after careful assessment of the risk/benefit ratio of exercise training.

The exercise prescription is composed of the intensity, duration, frequency, mode of exercise, and progression of physical activity. Both an appropriate warm-up to stretch the muscles and tendons and a cool-down to return the body to its resting level are necessary precautions to avoid injury and muscle soreness and are integral to every exercise session. The exercise prescription should be individualized to meet personal goals and integrated into each individual's lifestyle to enhance and maintain compliance. Maximal oxygen uptake or Vo_2max improves with aerobic exercise that involves large muscle groups and is continuous and rhythmic in nature (e.g., running, walking, swimming, bicycling, rowing, cross-country skiing). To improve cardiorespiratory fitness, the heart rate during exercise should be raised by 60% of the heart rate reserve (HRR), or the difference between the maximal and resting heart rate ($HR_{max} - HR_{rest}$). The training or target rate is calculated by multiplying the difference between the maximal and resting rates by 0.60 and adding the result to the resting heart rate. An exercise intensity between 50% and 70% of HRR is safe and effective for developing cardiorespiratory fitness in older adults. Recently, it was shown that the HRR method is not recommended in older women because it results in an inappropriately high exercise intensity (higher % VO_2max than expected). Rather, the exercise intensity prescription, which includes heart rate expressed as a percentage of maximal heart rate, was more appropriate for older women. Several studies show that high-intensity training for more than 6 months at a frequency of three times a week is necessary to increase VO_2max by more than 15% in older individuals. It should be emphasized that moderate levels of physical activity can be used to attain cardiorespiratory fitness and high-intensity exercise is not necessarily appropriate for all individuals. Exercise prescriptions may need to be modified for patients on medications that could affect heart rate (e.g., β-blockers) or BP responses to exercise. If persons are on medications that contribute to postural hypotension, they need to be advised to be well hydrated and learn to return gradually to the upright position from supine posture to avoid an episode of postural hypotension. The final components of the exercise prescription are the duration and frequency of exercise. The sedentary beginner should initially start a gradual program of 5- to 10-minute exercise bouts interspersed with 3- to 5-minute rest periods for 2 weeks. Every 2 weeks thereafter, an additional 5 minutes of exercise could be added to reach the final goal. The American College of Sports Medicine (ACSM) and the U.S. Centers for Disease Control recent recommendation published suggested that persons engage in moderate physical activity for 30 minutes or more most, if not all, days of the week to gain important health benefits.

In contrast to aerobic exercise, resistive training does not typically improve VO_2max, but it enhances muscular strength and muscular endurance. A resistive training program for the elderly should begin with minimal resistance and with proper supervision. The first two or three training sessions should be performed without any weight or load to ensure proper lifting technique and avoidance of breath holding during lifting. An individual can begin with one set of eight to ten exercises that train all the major muscle groups, including quadriceps, gluteals, hamstrings, latissimus dorsi, pectorals, deltoids, biceps, triceps, and abdominals, and then progress to two sets of exercises. Use of alternating arm and leg exercises is advantageous for older individuals beginning resistance training programs because this allows for some recovery of the muscles between exercises. As an individual progresses, the number of repetitions should first be increased, followed by an increase in the resistance. Each set should involve 8 to 15 repetitions, with the entire training session completed within 30 minutes. Lastly, resistance training should be conducted at least twice a week, with at least 48 hours of rest between exercise sessions.

Increasing flexibility is another important goal of an exercise program although it is often overlooked. Ten to twenty minutes of stretching before or after aerobic or resistive exercise increases range of motion and flexibility. Furthermore, abdominal exercises are important to include in any exercise program because weak abdominal muscles can contribute to poor posture and lower back pain. Chair stands are recommended to build coordination, strength, balance, and trunk stability. For these exercises, individuals can progress from supporting their body weight with their hands to crossing their arms to stand and eventually holding their hands out in front as they stand from the chair. Ankle strength and flexibility are also important for reducing fall risk.

DISEASE-SPECIFIC RECOMMENDATIONS
Diabetes

Specific guidelines exist for the evaluation of a diabetic patient before enrollment in an exercise program, with special considerations for symptoms of the disease and other comorbidities. We recommend exercise testing with cardiac monitoring prior to training due to the greater risk for arrhythmias and silent ischemia in this patient population. Some types of exercise are not recommended for diabetic patients with moderate or severe retinopathy, including high-impact running and aerobics, racquet sports, boxing, and resistive training. Non–weight-bearing exercise (e.g., swimming, cycling, arm ergometry) is advocated for patients with loss of protective sensation. Patients with proliferative retinopathy are at risk for hemorrhage and retinal detachment during isometric exercise. Older diabetic individuals or those with a long history of the disease should avoid high-intensity resistive training, although light-weight lifting with high repetitions may be performed in most patients with diabetes. Hydration status must be carefully monitored to avoid dehydration, which affects blood glucose and BP levels. Diabetics should drink isotonic or hypotonic fluids (preferably water) prior to exercise and take precautions when exercising in very hot or very cold temperatures. To avoid a hypoglycemic reaction during exercise in patients treated by insulin, such individuals should eat a meal containing complex carbohydrate 1 to 3 hours before exercise, consider a complex carbohydrate snack at least every 30 minutes during exercise of long duration, carry a source of monosaccharide during exercise, and increase food intake during the 4 to 6 hours following exercise. Special care and attention to the feet is especially important to prevent blisters and other foot injury in diabetic individuals. Recommendations include the use of silica gel or air midsoles and polyester or cotton–polyester socks. Feet should be dried carefully and moisturizer used as needed to maintain skin turgor.

Stroke

Exercise programs should be individualized. They should begin slowly and gradually increase in intensity and duration for patients disabled by stroke. Stretching, range-of-motion exercises, and muscle-strengthening exercises should also be incorporated into the stroke patient's exercise prescription. Depending on the severity of each individual's stroke and the use of assisted devices, swimming, aqua-aerobics, and cross-country skiing may be other aerobic options. Resistance training is currently not recommended for stroke patients without medical supervision and guidance. Additional information as to how to start an exercise program and how to safely exercise for stroke survivors is available in *Stroke: Your Complete Exercise Guide* as part of the Cooper Clinic and Research Institute Fitness Series. Treadmill aerobic exercise is effective in improving ambulatory function, but careful screening is necessary before the appropriate prescription can be designed.

Cardiovascular Disease

Cardiac rehabilitation is important for the patient who has suffered a myocardial infarction or undergone coronary artery bypass graft surgery to decrease overall and cardiovascular mortality. In addition to the peripheral and cardiac adaptations that occur after exercise training, maximal work capacity increases and the intensity of work increases at the ischemic threshold for those who achieve a higher workload or VO_2max after training. Preexisting cardiac conditions must be considered before patients embark on an exercise regimen. Guidelines for both inpatient and outpatient programs for cardiac patients is available in the ACSM's *Handbook for Exercise Testing and Prescription*. For patients with hypertension, BP should be monitored before, during, and after the exercise session. As there are no longitudinal studies in moderate/severe hypertension, exercise should be low intensity, with regular BP monitoring as the intensity and duration of exercise are increased.

Peripheral Arterial Occlusive Disease

Exercise programs developed for the patient with intermittent claudication and PAOD have relatively specific guidelines. Patients should walk on a level surface or hill, or use a treadmill to walk intermittently beyond the onset of claudication as long as they can safely tolerate near-maximal claudication pain for an initial duration of 15 minutes, and progress to 40 to 50 minutes at least three times per week. The walking should be intermittent to a claudication pain score of 3 using a 4-point pain scale at an initial intensity of 50% of peak exercise capacity and progressing to 80% by the end of 6 months, as suggested by Gardner. Stair climbing could also be used as the main mode of exercise training, whereas cycling could be used for the warm-up and cool-down periods. There are no specific exercise guidelines for resistance training in this population because aerobic training may be the best option for conferring improvements in daily activities with little or no claudication pain.

Osteoporosis

Exercise programs designed to enhance BMD should involve weight bearing and be of moderately high intensity since the loading forces are a considerable component of the osteogenic response. Animal studies suggest that loading should be high with minimal repetitions. There is some evidence that the effects of exercise may be site-specific such that particular exercises designed to load a specific skeletal site result in improvements in BMD at that site. In general, the aerobic or resistive exercise prescriptions in the prevention or treatment of osteoporosis are similar to that prescribed to improve cardiovascular function and/or to improve muscular strength in the elderly. For older women, hormone replacement therapy when combined with weight-bearing exercise could have additive and independent effects on BMD. The benefits of exercise, such as increased physical fitness, strength, and muscle mass, as well as improvements in balance and coordination, may be just as important as increases in BMD in the prevention of fracture.

Osteoarthritis

The goal of an exercise program for persons with OA is to reduce pain and improve the quality of life. Therefore, it should be enjoyable and as such incorporated into the individual's lifestyle so as to be maintained. As always, appropriate warm-up and cool-down are necessary with range-of-motion and flexibility exercises. However, no specific modifications to an exercise prescription of moderate intensity aerobic or resistive training programs appear to be necessary for individuals with OA. In addition to cycling and walking, swimming is another excellent aerobic exercise that persons with OA can enjoy. Lastly, application of ice after exercise is recommended to control postexercise inflammation. Individuals who have OA and are overweight or obese should be strongly encouraged to lose weight to enhance their health.

SUMMARY

We recommend the large-scale implementation of combined aerobic and resistive exercise programs with flexibility training for the elderly. Although there are some contraindications to exercise that should be addressed in a thorough medical evaluation and exercise test in older patients, as well as possible complications during exercise training, such as tendonitis, falls, sprained joints, broken bones, muscle soreness, and even sudden death, we strongly advocate exercise as being of vital importance to the well-being and health of the elderly. The elderly should be encouraged to exercise, and practitioners should advise their patients of the benefits of exercise. The public should be made aware of the positive health benefits of regular exercise programs for the elderly and be urged to develop pleasant, easily accessible, comfortable environments in which older adults can exercise. The elderly should be given every opportunity to incorporate both aerobic and resistive exercise into their lives, and the maintenance of regular activity should be a priority for our society. It is likely that regular exercise training can improve the quality of life in older persons, and that preventive and rehabilitative exercise training programs could reduce health care expenditures and chronic morbidity and mortality in high-risk as well as disabled older patients.

BIBLIOGRAPHY

American College of Sports Medicine. *Guidelines for exercise testing and prescription,* fifth ed. Philadelphia: Lea & Febiger, 1995.
Belardinelli R, Georgiou D, Cianci G, et al. Randomized, controlled trial of

long-term moderate exercise training in chronic heart failure. *Circulation* 1999;99:1173–1182.

Ettinger WH, Burns R, Messier SP, et al. A randomized trial comparing aerobic exercise and resistance exercise with a health education program in older adults with knee osteoarthritis. *JAMA* 1997;277:25–31.

Gardner AW. Peripheral vascular disease. In: Hazzard WR, Blass JR, Ettinger WH, et al., eds. *Principles of geriatric medicine and gerontology*, fourth ed. New York: McGraw-Hill, 1999:705–712.

Ivey JL. Role of exercise training in the prevention and treatment of insulin resistance and non–insulin-dependent diabetes mellitus. *Sports Med* 1997;24:321–336.

Kelley GA. Exercise and regional bone mineral density in postmenopausal women. *Am J Phys Med Rehab* 1998;77:76–87.

Lakatta EG. Cardiovascular regulatory mechanism in advanced age. *Physiol Rev* 1993;73:413–467.

Mayer-Davis EJ, D'Agostino R, Karter AJ, et al., for the IRAS Investigators. Intensity and amount of physical activity in relation to insulin sensitivity. *JAMA* 1998;279:669–674.

Pate RR, Pratt M, Blair SN, et al. Physical activity and public health: a recommendation from the Centers for Disease Control and Prevention and the American College of Sports Medicine. *JAMA* 1995; 273: 402–407.

Ryan AS, Nicklas BJ, Elahi D. A cross-sectional study on body composition and energy expenditure in women athletes during aging. *Am J Physiol* 1996;271:E916–E921.

Kelley's Textbook of Internal Medicine, fourth edition. Edited by H. David Humes. Lippincott Williams & Wilkins, Philadelphia © 2000.

CHAPTER
472

GERIATRIC REHABILITATION

KENNETH BRUMMEL-SMITH

Rehabilitation is a basic component of geriatric care. While there may be few diseases that can be cured in geriatrics, there is almost always something that can be done to enhance an older person's ability to function more safely and live more independently. Functional assessment and rehabilitation are inextricably linked. Through functional assessment we determine what sort of rehabilitation the patient needs. All primary physicians should have an understanding of the role of rehabilitation interventions when dealing with older persons.

Rehabilitation links the traditional biomedical model of disease to the functional orientation used in geriatrics. That link is illustrated in the definitions promoted by the World Health Organization (Table 472.1). Disability is very common in the older age group. Approximately 40% of all disabled persons are over age 65 years. The rate of disability increases markedly with age. While 14% of all ages are disabled, the prevalence increases to 47% for those over 65 and 53% for those over 75. Twenty-two percent of those over 75 years of age cannot carry out at

---

TABLE 472.1.	WORLD HEALTH ORGANIZATION CLASSIFICATIONS

Disease: An intrinsic pathology or disorder.
Impairment: Loss or abnormality of structure or function at the organ system level. At this stage the person becomes aware that she or he is unhealthy.
Disability: A restriction or lack of ability to perform an activity in a normal manner; a disturbance in the performance of daily tasks.
Handicap: A disadvantage resulting from impairment or disability that limits or prevents fulfillment of a role that is normal.

---

least one basic activity of daily living, such as dressing, feeding, or toileting.

EVALUATION OF REHABILITATION POTENTIAL

Though the basic principles of rehabilitation are the same regardless of age, the application of those principles may change when one is dealing with an older person (Table 472.2). The first step in providing rehabilitation is recognizing who needs it. There have been no randomized trials to establish the best method for assessing rehabilitation potential, regardless of the cause of disability. The proper clinical approach is to consider rehabilitation in *any* patient who has had a recent significant loss of functional abilities, who has enough cognitive capacity to follow two-step commands, and who can retain information from day to day. A strong social support system is perhaps the most important factor determining good outcome. Those with better functioning prior to development of the disabling condition also do best in rehabilitation. A comprehensive geriatric assessment clarifies underlying medical, psychological, and socioeconomic conditions that may affect the course of rehabilitation.

Often it is necessary to provide a trial of rehabilitation to determine whether the patient will benefit. If the primary care provider is asked to approve rehabilitation therapies, he or she should expect the therapist to provide very specific goals and outcomes that will be measured and reported. The proper duration of a trial is dependent on the condition being treated and the outcome expected, and so it must be individualized. The provider should carefully review the progress of the patient, and

---

TABLE 472.2.	PRINCIPLES OF REHABILITATION

1. Stabilize the primary disorder.
2. Prevent secondary disabilities (e.g., pressure sores, contractures, shoulder subluxation, or depression).
3. Restore lost functional capabilities.
4. Promote adaptation—the patient to his or her disability, the family to the patient, and the environment to the patient's needs.

if none is seen, the cost-effective and ethical approach would be to discontinue the intervention.

SITES FOR REHABILITATION

Rehabilitation can be provided in the hospital, home, skilled nursing facility, or outpatient center. Inpatient rehabilitation is usually reserved for those who can tolerate 3 hours of therapy per day and requires close physician supervision. The use of this modality has declined with the advent of managed care. Recent studies of rehabilitation in skilled nursing facilities have shown excellent outcomes in stroke and hip fracture rehabilitation. There it can be provided 5 to 7 days per week and can be less intense than that provided in hospital settings. Some managed care programs have promoted the use of short-stay, subacute units in the hospital for rehabilitation. Outpatient rehabilitation is helpful for those with good cognition and available transportation. Home rehabilitation is especially useful with frail patients, but such patients must have a good support system to assist with his or her practice of newly learned activities.

REHABILITATION OF PATIENTS WITH COMMON GERIATRIC CONDITIONS

STROKE

Stroke is the most common diagnosis for which older persons receive rehabilitation. Early rehabilitation interventions are important in the acute care setting as they can prevent secondary disabilities and set the stage for functional recovery. Proper bed positioning, turning, range-of-motion exercises, and attentiveness to hydration, nutrition, and maintenance of an appropriate blood pressure (higher than 135/85) is emphasized in the acute hospital.

The patient and family need information about outcomes and plans (Table 472.3). Overall, about 85% of persons survive (90% with the more common infarction and 50% with hemorrhage). Certain features allow further prognostication. Those with less severe paralysis, less perceptual neglect, no (or only receptive) aphasia, less sensory loss, no pseudobulbar palsy, and good cognition usually have better outcomes and can often return home. Most gains in motor function are seen in the first month. Virtually all motor recovery is completed by 6 months.

TABLE 472.3.	FUNCTIONAL OUTCOMES OF STROKE	
Outcome		**Incidence (%)**
Complete recovery		10
Minor disability		40
Major disability		40
Total dependency		10

Speech, swallowing, and sensory return may be seen up to 2 years after the stroke. Guidelines have been developed for selecting the appropriate site of care (Fig. 472.1).

The Interdisciplinary Team

The appropriate approach to rehabilitation of the geriatric patient is inherently interdisciplinary. Each member of the team must not only understand and appreciate the roles and contributions of every other member but must also collaborate and communicate effectively to promote an optimal outcome.

Physical therapy (PT) is devoted to promoting both static and dynamic balance, first while the patient is sitting on the bed, then during transfers, and finally during ambulation. In bed mobility, transfers from bed to wheelchair and from chair to toilet are taught. Gait training can begin when the person can maintain standing balance, support his or her weight on the unaffected side, and advance the affected limb somewhat. Depending on the person's strength and balance, some sort of walking aid is usually provided.

Straight canes are rarely used because they are not stable. A hemiwalker is used when more assistance of the upper extremities is needed. A four-pronged cane is used when less support is required. Regular walkers may be very difficult to use because the arm is often weak. Any assistive device is often resigned to the closet once the patient goes home if training has been inadequate or the emotional response to these devices has not been addressed. Wheelchairs are often provided for negotiating longer distances even to those who can walk. A wheelchair, when provided, should be fitted by a physical therapist, who can ensure that it is the right height and width. Steering the chair with the unaffected leg allows propulsion with one arm. Braces are commonly used and the PT is helpful in choosing appropriate types. Two main types are used. A metal ankle–foot orthosis (AFO) is heavy, unattractive, and difficult to don, but it is the brace of choice for those with muscle spasticity or ankle instability. The plastic posterior AFO is often more acceptable to older persons. It supports those with muscle weakness but has limited use in the presence of spastic muscles.

The occupational therapist provides training in the activities of daily living. New methods of dressing, feeding, and grooming are addressed early. Attention is given to the improvement of sensory, perceptual, and cognitive deficits. A wide variety of adaptive equipment may be offered, such as rocker knives for one-handed cutting, dressing sticks, or buttonhooks (Table 472.4). Grooming adaptations include the use of special bathroom equipment, such as bath benches, shower hoses, and raised toilet seats.

Speech and language pathologists provide much more than retraining in communication. Cognitive reorganization, training in the use of alternative communication techniques (such as picture boards), and evaluation and retraining for swallowing problems are all pursued. With a recreational therapist the patient may experience skill advancement during play that could not have occurred in the more task-oriented gym setting. The rehabilitation nurse is the coordinator of care. Besides regular nursing duties, she or he provides reinforcement of techniques learned in therapy, teaches families caregiving skills, and observes

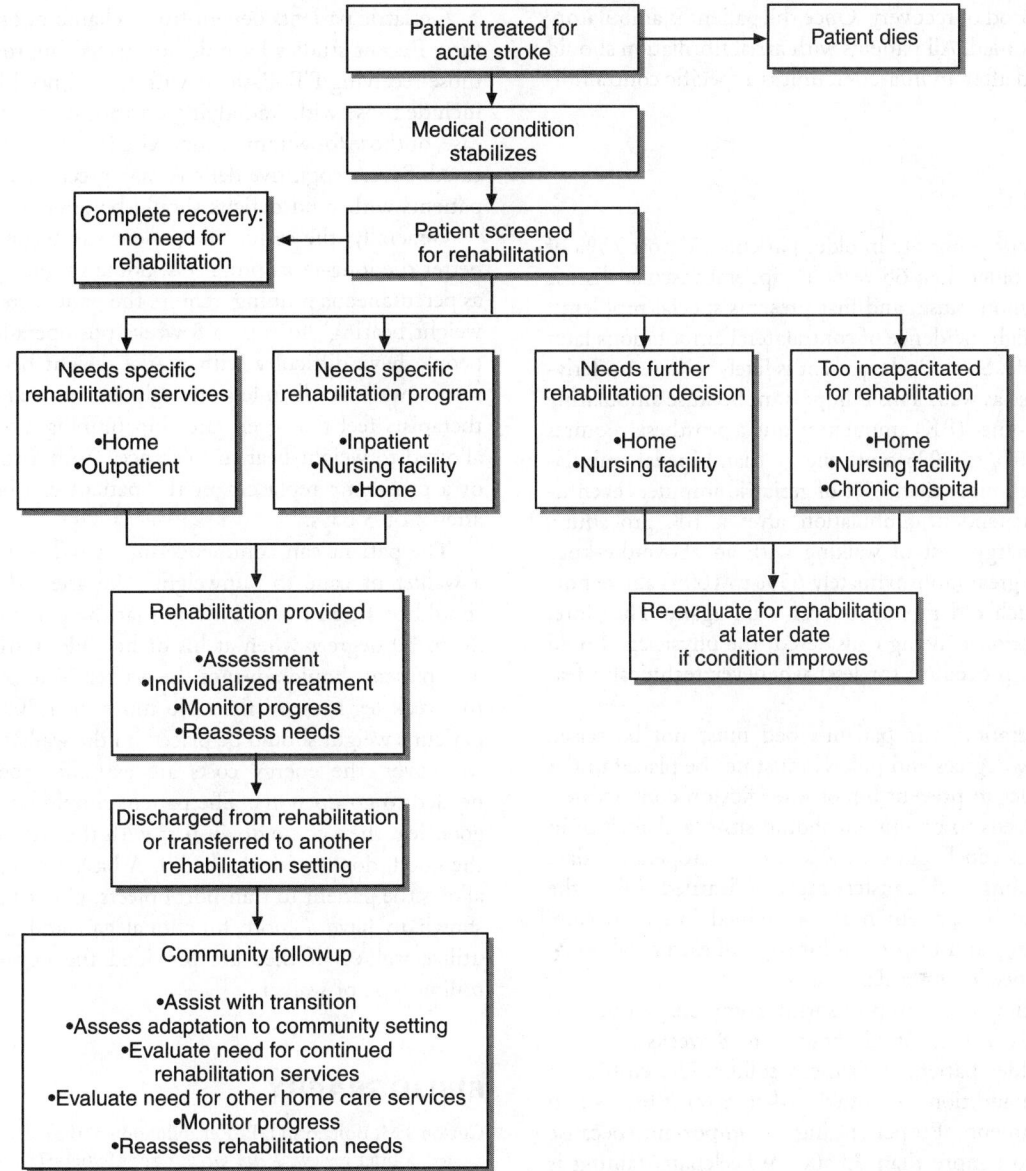

FIGURE 472.1. Choosing a site to provide rehabilitation. (See Gresham GE, Duncan PW, Stason WB, et al. *Post-stroke rehabilitation: assessment, referral, and patient management.* Clinical Practice Guideline No. 16: Quick Reference Guide for Clinicians. Rockville, MD: US Department of Health and Human Services, Public Health Service, Agency for Health Care and Policy Research. AHCPR Publication No. 95-0663, May 1995.

TABLE 472.4.	AIDS FOR ACTIVITIES OF DAILY LIVING

Feeding—rocker knives, cutting boards, plate retainers
Dressing—button hooks, Velcro closures, tilted mirrors, reachers
Toileting—grab bars, arm frames, raised seats
Bathing—tub bench, shower hose, grab bars, long-handled brush
Grooming—tilt mirror, built-up handles
Safety—"Lifeline" service, remote control lights, telephone dialers, stair rails, removal of throw rugs

for signs of complications or problems. In skilled nursing facilities and home settings, the nurse plays a crucial role in providing most of the care.

The role of the primary physician varies with the site of care. In the inpatient setting he or she usually works with a physiatrist and is responsible for medical management and patient advocacy. All drugs that may cause confusion or depression must be removed or reduced. Depression must be recognized early to provide optimum results. Malnutrition due to swallowing dysfunction may require temporary tube placement, though it must be remembered that neither nasogastric tubes nor gastrostomy tubes significantly reduce the risk of aspiration over oral feeding. Anticoagulation for deep venous thrombosis is controversial. Many authorities recommend it for those with infarctions during the immobile period of recovery. Once the patient is ambulatory it can be discontinued. All patients with atrial fibrillation should be anticoagulated after an infarction unless a specific contraindication is present.

AMPUTATION

Amputations occur primarily in older patients. Almost 75% of all amputees are older than 65 years. Peripheral vascular disease is the most common cause, and that presents special problems. First, there is a high incidence of contralateral amputations later in the patient's life. Second, the patient is likely to have underlying cardiac disease as well. This is important because ambulating with a below-the-knee (BK) amputation and a prosthesis requires approximately 10% to 40% more energy than bipedal ambulation. Nevertheless, more than 75% of geriatric amputees eventually achieve independent ambulation after a BK procedure. However, the energy cost of walking with an above-the-knee amputation is so great (approximately 65% to 100% above normal) that few such older patients ever walk again. Therefore, when an amputation is being considered, the physician should advocate for BK procedure (or less) whenever technically feasible.

After the operation, the patient's bed must not be raised higher than a few degrees and pillows must not be placed under the knees, in order to prevent hip or knee flexion contractures. A patient who needs to be upright should sit in a chair, not in the bed. Exercises can begin on the second postoperative day. Single-limb standing and transfers must be learned. Once the stump has healed the patient must be trained in stump care. Massage, wrapping, and inspection for signs of skin breakdown or irritation are needed on a daily basis.

In order to allow the stump to shrink completely, a permanent prosthesis is usually fitted about 6 to 8 weeks after the surgery. Most older patients will use a solid-ankle, cushioned heel (SACH). In addition to a fitted socket, a waist belt is also used for attachment. Proper fitting is important because prostheses can cost more than $2,500. Wheelchair training is also important. Most older patients also make use of a wheelchair for long distances. The patient for whom a functioning prosthesis is inappropriate (e.g., moderate cognitive deficits, severe contralateral vascular disease or weakness, or joint disease) may nevertheless desire a cosmetic prosthesis.

Although phantom limb sensation occurs frequently, pain is uncommon. Such pain is best treated with a combination of analgesic drugs, massage, and, sometimes, local anesthetic injections. Skin breakdown is usually attributable to poor stump care and an improperly fitting prosthesis.

HIP FRACTURES

All patients should be medically stabilized before surgery. The uninvolved limb can be exercised while the patient awaits surgery. On the day after surgery, the patient can sit up and begin quadriceps exercises. With a total hip arthrosis the joint should not be flexed more than 90 degrees or excessively adducted. Good pain management is required.

Geriatric patients benefit from rehabilitation after a hip fracture. Recent studies have demonstrated improved outcomes in those receiving PT. Patients with special need for rehabilitation include those with underlying arthritis or cardiopulmonary disease, or those for whom unsupervised exercise may be contraindicated. Severe cognitive deficits may preclude rehabilitation, but patients with mild deficits should be offered a trial.

Generally, the earlier the patient can begin ambulation, the better the long-term prognosis. Some surgical procedures, such as percutaneous pinning, require the patient to only use "partial weight bearing" for up to 8 weeks postoperatively. Most older people have difficulty with partial weight bearing and choose not to walk at all unless strongly encouraged to do so. Many therapists feel that even after hip pinning a patient should be allowed to weight-bear to tolerance. With a compression screw or a prosthetic replacement the patient can begin ambulation after 2 or 3 days.

The patient can commence supervised ambulation by using a walker or cane to "unweight" the affected leg. The walker should be fitted in such a way that the patient's arms are bent 20 to 30 degrees when at his or her side, resting on the grips. The patient should advance the walker 20 to 30 cm, then move the weak leg forward first. No more than 20% to 25% of the patient's weight should be placed on the walker or a fall is likely. Moreover, the energy costs are extreme. Special walkers are needed to go up stairs. The patient should go up first with the good leg, then come down first with the affected leg ("up with the good, down with the bad"). A basket or bag on the walker allows the patient to transport objects. Older patients have been shown to have a more functional gait and more consistently utilize walkers if they are provided the newer, four-wheeled, rolling type of walker.

BIBLIOGRAPHY

Cutson TM, Bongiorni DR. Rehabilitation of the elderly lower limb amputee: a brief review. *J Am Geriatr Soc* 1996;44:1388–1393.

Dobkin BH. The rehabilitation of elderly stroke patients. *Clin Geriatr Med* 1991;7:507–523.

Goldstein FC, Strasser DC, Woodard J, et al. Functional outcome of cognitively impaired hip fracture patients on a geriatric rehabilitation unit. *J Am Geriatr Soc* 1997;45:35–42.

Gresham GE, Duncan PW, Stason WB, et al. *Post-stroke rehabilitation: assessment, referral, and patient management.* Clinical Practice Guideline No. 16: Quick Reference Guide for Clinicians. Rockville, MD: US Department of Health and Human Services, Public Health Service, Agency for Health Care and Policy Research. AHCPR Publication No. 95-0663, May 1995.

Guccioni AA, Fagerson TL, Anderson JJ. Regaining functional independence in the acute care setting following hip fracture. *Phys Ther* 1996;76:818–826.

Hoenig H, Nusbaum N, Brummel-Smith K. Geriatric rehabilitation: state of the art. *J Am Geriatr Soc* 1997;45:1371–1381.

Kemp B, Brummel-Smith K, Ramsdell JW. eds. *Geriatric rehabilitation.* Austin, TX: Pro-Ed Press, 1990.

Portnow J, Kline T, Daly MA, et al. Multidisciplinary home rehabilitation: a practical model. *Clin Geriatr Med* 1991;7:695–706.

Von-Sternberg T, Hepburn K, Cibuzar P, et al. Post-hospital sub-acute care: an example of a managed care model. *J Am Geriatr Soc* 1997;45:87–91.

World Health Organization. International classification of impairments, disabilities, and handicaps: a manual of classifications relating to the consequences of disease. Geneva, 1990.

Kelley's Textbook of Internal Medicine, fourth edition. Edited by H. David Humes.
Lippincott Williams & Wilkins, Philadelphia © 2000.

CHAPTER

473

PHILOSOPHICAL AND ETHICAL ISSUES IN GERIATRICS

CHRISTINE K. CASSEL

The special ethical issues facing physicians as they care for aged patients and the moral challenges for health policy in our aging society stem from the increase in life expectancy in this century, which is unprecedented in human history. It presents dramatic challenges to existing models of social structure, expectations of life events and family relationships, and the fundamental meaning of the life cycle.

Before the middle of the twentieth century and throughout the previous existence of the human race, only a small, biologically and socially privileged group of people could expect to survive into old age. However, currently close to 80% of persons born in the United States can expect to live past their sixty-fifth birthday, and a large fraction of those can expect to live into their ninth and tenth decades. This shift, which is largely attributable to decreased mortality in childhood and adulthood before old age, has coincided with advances in medical science that make it possible to treat diseases that are common in old age, some of which are intrinsically linked with the degenerative senescent processes. For example, atherosclerotic heart disease is the number one cause of death in the United States, yet death from heart disease for most people has been postponed by decades. In the first part of this century, death by cardiac disease was unusual in older people, who died primarily from pneumonia, other infectious diseases, and renal failure. The rise in cancer deaths, which is the second leading cause of death, is also linked to increased life expectancy. As one escapes premature death from infectious disease and other causes, the likelihood of the occurrence of cancer increases—particularly breast cancer, prostate cancer, and colon cancer, all of which are linked to aging. As deaths cluster at later and later ages, how are "premature" and "natural" deaths to be distinguished?

Because older persons are susceptible to many more illnesses, it is not surprising that the costs of medical care are much higher for this group (approximately three times greater per year, on average, for those older than 65 years than those younger than

65 years). This high use has led to ethical questions at the societal level and at the individual clinical level. At the societal level, we wonder if it is right to be spending so much money on health care for one sector of the population. At the individual level, should we continue to delay and prevent death in people of advanced age, and how will we know when to stop?

JUSTICE AND THE ALLOCATION OF RESOURCES

Ethicists have long been examining questions pertaining to the values that underlie the allocation of health care resources in society because there have always been inequities in this allocation. The ethical principle of justice is the major one under consideration when we examine the allocation of resources. In the past, some have argued that physicians should not be involved in rationing decisions at the bedside or in their dealings with individual patients, but rather that society should make these decisions and physicians should operate within social guidelines. However, in a diverse and politically complex society such as our own, with a market-driven health system, this fairly straightforward approach has not succeeded. For that reason, physicians have an increasingly important voice in the decision-making process in terms of allocation of resources. Some would argue that it is better to have physicians who understand clinical efficacy involved in allocation decisions, whereas others are concerned that to be so involved conflicts with the physician's Hippocratic responsibility to do everything that is possible for individual patients. Because both perspectives are valid, a balance must be sought.

As many health care systems in the United States are transformed into variations of managed care structures, physicians become critical decision makers about the rationing of care. Indeed, in full-risk capitation systems they are the ones who must decide which clinical expenditures are warranted and which are not. This situation creates important new and challenging ethical problems for physicians and demands more explicit moral guidelines if they are to avoid frank financial conflict of interest. It must be remembered that fee-for-service models also have inherent financial conflicts, often in the direction of overtreatment rather than undertreatment. Both require that serious attention be paid to ethics and professionalism.

Health care has become the subject of much scrutiny as a result of the cost-containment efforts of government, insurance companies, and businesses during the last 20 to 30 years, as health care costs have outstripped inflation for more than three decades. There are three underlying reasons for this dramatic increase in costs: one is advances in medical technology, which are continuing to explode as modern biologic science progresses with exciting new approaches to illnesses that previously were thought untreatable; the second is the patterns of payment of health professionals and prices charged by hospitals and medical technology providers for their services under cost-based, fee-for-service structures common since the beginning of Medicare; the third is the aging of the population. This third reality, which we should acknowledge as a success story, is also of major concern because there are more and more older people who can benefit from the expanding medical armamentarium; in addition, the elderly are the only sector of society enjoying universal publicly funded health insurance, however incomplete the coverage.

When Medicare was established in 1965 as a public system to create health care insurance for older people, it was originally designed as a "safety net," a catastrophic insurance system that would cover only the very high costs, such as hospitalization, that older individuals and their families could not afford. As health care became more and more complex, as well as less and less affordable, Medicare continually expanded to cover physician payments, outpatient care, and, to some extent, home care. Thus, the combination of increasing numbers of older people and the preexisting societal commitment to insure them through a public system increased the proportion of health care costs paid through general taxation.

This reality has led to concern among some that we are spending too much of the resources of society and of families on the elderly at the cost of other social goods and, in particular, undermining the well-being of the younger generation. This tension has been framed by policymakers and philosophers as the intergenerational equity debate. Demographers in the 1980s noted that at the time Medicare was instituted there were more impoverished elderly people than impoverished children, whereas at the present time, the numbers of impoverished elderly have declined and the numbers of children living in poverty have increased dramatically. In addition, children are dramatically overrepresented among the uninsured and those covered by inadequate public insurance, such as Medicaid. This observation has led to an obvious debate about justice, framed as follows: "Is it fair that society expends so much of its resources on the older generation and is unable, therefore, to support children?" Indeed, at its most stark, this reality has been described as the "wealthy elderly stealing from needy children."

To evaluate this argument adequately, the following observations must be made:

First, would cutting the funding for Medicare and social security improve the situation of poor children? To fulfill the moral intent of such an exchange, one would have to be confident that the political process will put money into the support of children in poverty—a social commitment that has not been clearly articulated over the decades in which those inequities developed.

Second, the well-being of children is in many ways linked to the well-being of elderly people. It is rarely the case that generations exist in isolation from one another. Indeed, transfer of financial assets is predominantly from the older generation to the younger generation until well into very advanced old age. Thus, it is often the case in multigenerational families that financial support from grandparents helps a young couple to finance their first home or a grandchild to attend college. Even in families that do not have substantial financial resources, it is often the older generation who help with child care and who make possible multigenerational families supporting children of single parents so that the parents can work.

Looking at Medicare specifically as a target for spending reductions does not recognize the overall need for a systematic approach to allocation of resources in health care. Elderly people pay more out of pocket for medical care now than they did before Medicare was instituted, suggesting that rising costs will continue to be a problem and that cuts in Medicare would lead to significant loss of access to care.

It also often is not remembered that a very small percentage of older people, less than 5%, actually have incomes above $50,000 a year, and that there are still 12% to 15% of elderly people living below the poverty level. Most of these are women, many of whom are widows. One of the unique realities of the continued disparity in life expectancy between the sexes is that women often have inadequate pensions and are subject to greater disability related to advanced old age. Old-age policy is thus reflective of the historical role of women in our society during an era in which women were at significant financial disadvantage, especially in widowhood.

One must also consider the role of the fabric of society between families and generations. There is a great deal of concern that young people exist in a kind of "futurelessness," wherein they have little confidence in the stability of the world they are facing. They are concerned about global warfare, about the economy, about environmental degradation, and about declining opportunity for themselves. If they were to see older people devalued within society, this would be another measure of loss of confidence in their own future. These are all reasons why a simple age-based rationing approach to the question of fairness and intergenerational equity is not adequate.

Nonetheless, unprecedented changes in the age structure of our society will require new ways of thinking about resource allocation. The relationship between the generations may indeed be an argument for greater concern about the plight of poor children in our society. The major policy concern for the financing of benefits for the elderly has been in looking ahead to the aging of the baby boomers, expected to begin approximately in the year 2010. This is a group many of whom have benefited from the expanding economy of the 1970s and 1980s. Those who are well off have done well by their children, enabling them often to attend private schools or to live in suburbs where there are good public schools, and to prepare themselves to be productive citizens.

The future for the baby-boomer generation depends in a major way on the strength of the economy in the year 2010 and beyond. No matter what public policies are enacted between now and then, an aging society requires a strong economy to support the inevitably large numbers of frail people and those in need of medical care during those years. In addition, the economy must be strong enough that pension arrangements remain stable and funded. This strength of the economy, however, depends not only on the children and grandchildren of the baby boomers but, perhaps more importantly, on "other people's children." The 20% of children in poverty are not randomly distributed throughout the population. They are largely children of minority families, many of whom are trapped in the cycle of poverty within inner cities. These children do not have an opportunity to receive the benefits of education, which would allow them to become productive members of society and to contribute to the economy necessary to support those who are elderly in the years 2010, 2020, and 2030. Thus, it would be prudent, as well as fair, for the current baby-boomer generation to consider more actively their responsibility to the support of other people's children who are currently struggling in poverty with poor prospects for the future. The intergenerational equity argument, if framed in this way, could be a way of allocating resources and responsibilities between generations that acknowledges not only the link between the welfare of generations across the life span, but the link in society between the better off and the less well off.

CLINICAL DECISIONS TO LIMIT THERAPY

No one would deny that the responsibility of the physician is to do whatever is reasonably possible to help patients. What is now under scrutiny is how to define those reasonable expectations. Two fundamental principles outline a large gray area. One principle is that the patient always has the right to refuse medical treatment, regardless of its chances of benefit or lack thereof. The other is that the physician is never required to provide futile treatment or treatment that is not medically indicated. The large gray area in the middle comes into play when a patient's preference is not clear or has not been made clear; or when treatment is likely to be virtually, but not necessarily 100%, futile; or when individuals disagree about the futility of treatment or have different definitions of futility.

PATIENT CHOICE

The patient is always the most important one to decide whether to use extensive life-saving or life-sustaining medical measures. Although many older people have given a great deal of thought to this matter and have firm, well-informed views on the subject, others may not have given the issues much attention or may not have specific opinions regarding medical treatments. However, they may have very clear values in terms of which they can clarify a description, sometimes called a *values history,* of the framework within which their life is meaningful to them and the point at which death is acceptable and medical intervention unwarranted. The sorting of these issues requires the physician's willingness to spend time in discussion with the patient and with the family, and to do so periodically over time, because the patient's views may change with accumulated life experience and with personal experience of illness or disability. These discussions are referred to broadly as *advance care planning.* They are best implemented in the ambulatory setting or with a patient in the nursing home, as the physician gets to know that patient in the primary care relationship. This way, discussions can be held in an unhurried way, allowing for reflection and for the bringing out of questions and answers, and providing the opportunity for family members to be involved when the patient feels it is appropriate. The least desirable time for these discussions to occur is during an acute illness or on admission to the hospital, when the patient may be too sick to think clearly or too frightened to process information. Paradoxically, however, because many physicians and patients have not had these advance care planning discussions, decisions about end-of-life care choices often occur at the point of acute illness. In 1990, a federal law, called the Patient Self-Determination Act, was passed, requiring all hospitals and nursing homes to inform patients upon admission of their right to execute an advance directive. This has led to a much broader awareness of the need for more advance care planning.

An advance directive is a document that demonstrates and records the patient's views on advance care planning. The two most common forms of advance directives are living wills, which usually stipulate that some limits be set to heroic medical measures taken in the event of critical or terminal illness, and durable powers of attorney for health care, which specify one or more individuals who are responsible for those decisions in the event of a patient's incapacity. These are discussed in greater detail in Chapter 2. In the event that neither such document exists and that there is no record of advance care planning discussion with a physician, many states now have legislated next-of-kin authority for proxy decision making. Although the purpose of advance directives and advance care planning is, as much as possible, to elicit and respect the autonomous wishes of the patient with regard to end-of-life decisions, the recognition by the states of the role of families reflects what research has shown about the views of many elderly people. Older people often refer to family members as key decision makers or support their reasons for a decision to limit therapy by asserting that they do not want to be a burden on the family. Elderly persons should be afforded the same respect for their individuality as younger persons, but autonomy is not the only—or even the preeminent—value for many people. In seeking respect for autonomy, we must not forget that the connectedness to a family network, be it large or small, is often as important as, or more important than, individual self-determination.

Physicians sometimes are reluctant to bring up discussions of advance care planning with their patients, especially in the absence of an acute life-threatening illness, because they are afraid it will upset the patient. However, most studies show that most elderly people are quite open to such discussions and feel relieved when the physician initiates such a discussion. Indeed, consideration of the finality, expectability, and proximity of death is an attitude of old age that makes such conversations easier and more natural than with a younger patient. At the age of 70, 80, or 90 years, most people have experienced the death of a number of family members and close friends, and undoubtedly have had the stimulus to consider what they would want for themselves as they face the end of their lives. Although these discussions should always occur with appropriate sensitivity and compassion, in most cases it is not unduly upsetting to the patient to have such a discussion, and may indeed empower the patient to raise other questions with the physician.

When describing the risks of medical treatment to a patient, the physician should be able to discuss possible outcomes of intermediate success as well as the chances—if known—of survival or of death. Older people may be more concerned about the risks of survival with major impairment (such as in the event of an intraoperative stroke during cardiac surgery) than about mortality rates. When facing the last stages of one's life, quality of life can become a much more vivid concern than extending the number of years of life if those years entail living with major disabilities.

FUTILITY

Because of society's emphasis on respecting a patient's autonomy, some experts believe that we have gone too far in offering all medical interventions, even to patients of very advanced age, when the chances of their being used with success are extremely slim. This creates a situation where the patient is presented with a menu of options, with no values placed on any of them; often this occurs when the patient is critically ill and, as a result, the family are made to feel that it is their burden to decide whether to attempt to save the person's life or to refuse life-saving medical intervention and allow death to occur. Ethicists and policy makers have begun to articulate an area where life-saving medical treatment may be considered futile and therefore is not offered. An example of this is cardiopulmonary resuscitation in long-term care settings, where the staff are not well trained and the patients are extremely frail and unlikely to survive. Most studies show that there are virtually no survivors of such interventions. When the data show that the outcomes are almost uniformly fatal, then it is acceptable for the physician not to offer the intervention to the family, and to simply write an order not to resuscitate or to make a decision to withhold that treatment.

Unfortunately, in most situations where life-sustaining treatment decisions must be made, there are not such conclusive data. Physicians have the clinical impression that there are patients for whom intensive care, intubation, cardiopulmonary resuscitation, chemotherapy, major surgery, and similar interventions have an exceedingly small chance of promoting meaningful survival. The ethical dilemma is how to weigh the extremely small chance of success. This is a controversial area, but many experts argue that the physician is obligated to tell the patient his or her own opinion about the chances of success and advise, in a way that is comforting, when such interventions should not be instituted. Of course, these discussions are always easier on and more beneficial to the family if there is a preexisting relationship, but even if there is not, the physician can provide great comfort to the family by clearly expressing his or her own views about the expected chances of success or failure. Here is an opportunity to regain some of the paternalistic aspect of the physician's role and its potential to comfort a family that is facing the loss of an elderly relative.

However, this comforting role can be an empty one if there is no positive alternative to intrusive life-sustaining therapy. Many of our hospitals have not developed the teamwork and skills among physicians, nurses, and others to deliver excellent palliative care with control of symptoms, care during the grieving process, spiritual counseling, and sophisticated approaches to problems such as pain, nausea, vomiting, dyspnea, and other such symptoms that are likely to occur in the face of critical or terminal illness. Patients, families, and physicians alike may find it more difficult to accept the withholding or withdrawal of life-sustaining measures if they believe that the only alternative is abandonment. It is thus the physician's responsibility to ensure that there is a more caring and clinically appropriate alternative.

For many people, the best alternative is home hospice care, if there are family members at home who are able to care for the patient and if the patient's illness is one that can be appropriately cared for in that setting. It is still true, however, that 80% of people die in hospitals or in nursing homes, and that for many people, either because of the lack of someone in the home full time or because of other factors, this ideal of home hospice care is not always possible. Thus, we must create within our hospitals and nursing homes the option of aggressive comfort care. This is an important area for training and research, as is health care financing.

The traditional hospice patient has been one with widespread metastatic cancer for whom expectation of survival can be confidently considered quite short. It is now widely accepted that such patients should be treated with extensive pain medication and attention to other symptoms. It is necessary to expand this concept of hospice care, however, and not demand that there be such a demonstrably short survival prognosis to provide extensive comfort care for patients. For example, some demonstrations have now been done with hospice care for patients with advanced Alzheimer's disease. One must make the same conceptual shift that the goal of treatment is not to prolong survival but to enhance comfort, and orient the treatment toward that goal. If treatment of pain or dyspnea by narcotics or sedation unintentionally shortens life when given for the purpose of comfort, then such an outcome is acceptable. The distinction that the goal of treatment is to relieve suffering rather than to prolong life should be applied in the evaluation of any intervention being considered in patients for whom comfort care is the appropriate mode of therapy.

HOW DEATH OCCURS

The fundamental principles that guide the physician and patient through decisions to withdraw or withhold life-sustaining treatments and to provide comfort care in patients facing the end of life are substantively no different if the patient is 58 years old or 98 years old. Specifically, the physician's responsibility is to respect the wishes of the patient, always to relieve suffering, and to not abandon the patient even though the search for ways to prolong life may be foregone. However, there is no doubt that our feelings about decisions and care at the end of life might be quite different for a person of very advanced age, regardless of quality of life. Physicians often acquiesce more easily to withholding life-sustaining treatment in a patient who has far advanced physical or cognitive impairment and for whom life no longer holds any personal meaning, and perhaps especially if the patient is of advanced old age. We must caution the physician to observe the distinction between his or her own values about meaningful further life and those of the patient or family. But beyond this, we must recognize that there is a sense in which human survival and the meaning of it is related to a connectedness to other people and to one's own identity. Within a broad range of personal spiritual perspectives, these realities seem to hold.

It is also logical to most that a person who is 95 or 100 years old is ready for the end of life in a way that a person who is 50 years old is not. We have a sense of the naturalness of the human life span and that it is unseemly to push the frontiers of human life beyond that span. The challenge in our aging society, and with the success of increasing life expectancy, is to find the right definition for that natural human life span. The best definition, as always, reverts back to the patient and the history of his own life and its meaning to him. Writers have described the sense of a "closing biography" for person's who are ready for the end of life, even though they may not be actively seeking it. Patients, too, describe this feeling of being "finished" or "almost finished" with their life's tasks. Physicians who have the privilege to treat patients in advanced old age should make use of the opportunity to explore with them these philosophical viewpoints about the human life span and the sense of meaning and closure that a long life can bring.

In this context, then, a decision to withhold heroic measures may take on a very different meaning than it does in a younger person. In a person who no longer looks forward to his future life or for whom cognitive impairment has erased the ability to identify self or relate to other people, measures such as tube feeding, intravenous fluids, and antibiotics for infections all may be viewed as unnecessarily heroic, and within the framework of ethics may be withheld or withdrawn, if done so in accordance with the values history of the patient. Ideally, these values are ones that have been clearly and explicitly articulated by the patient and the family, but the ability to be explicit may vary enormously depending on the specific situation of the doctor–patient relationship and the level of sophistication of the family. It should not rest on the family to insist on each specific medical treatment that they wish to have withheld or withdrawn. The physician, as advocate for the patient, should work with the family to establish the values framework but may need to act on these values in terms of specific medical treatments without getting "releases" or specific permission from the family for each separate decision.

■ CONCLUSION

In summary, the ethical principles that apply to other aspects of medical care apply equally strongly and convincingly to the care of elderly patients. In addition, there are perspectives to be gained by understanding the concept of a personal life biography and the role of advance planning as it empowers the older person and his or her family to gain strength in their awareness of facing mortality, a universal human characteristic that younger people can more easily avoid. In addition, the social implications of the aging society will continue to put great pressure on the profession of medicine to demonstrate wisdom in the allocation of resources. Here it is important that we take seriously the physician's part in making sensible use of the resources of society and understanding the importance of the concept of futility, even in situations where it cannot be conclusively proven. It is equally important for the physician not to assume that because someone is old medical care is not indicated and to realize that aiming for functional goals, such as hip or knee replacements in an 85-year-old person who would then be able to walk again, is an entirely justifiable use of medical technology. As our ability to use these techniques advances, we will need to hone further our moral conversations with one another and with our patients to establish the appropriateness of their use. Finally, important clinical skills are necessary to fully meet the requirements of ethics, especially in facing end-of-life care. The first of these is communication skills and the second is palliative care. The secret of patient care, as Peabody said, is in caring for the patient. In addition, it requires attentiveness to the advances in biomedical science that present us with ever more useful and challenging ways to improve the lives of patients well into advanced old age.

BIBLIOGRAPHY

Callahan D. Setting limits: a response. *Gerontologist* 1994;34:393–398.

Cassel CK, Neugarten BL. The goals of medicine in an aging society. In: Binstock RH, Post SG, eds. *Too old for health care? Controversies in medicine, law, economics, and ethics.* Baltimore: Johns Hopkins University Press, 1991:75–91.

Cassel CK, Rudberg MA, Olshansky SJ. The price of success: health care in an aging society. *Health Aff (Millwood)* 1992;11(2):87–99.

Cole T. *The journey of life: a cultural history of aging in America.* Cambridge, UK: Cambridge University Press, 1992.

Emanuel EJ, Emanuel LL. The economics of dying: the illusion of cost savings at the end of life. *N Engl J Med* 1994;330:540–544.

Hanrahan P, Luchins DJ. Access to hospice programs in end-stage dementia: a national survey of hospice programs. *J Am Geriatr Soc* 1995;43:56–59.

High DM. Surrogate decision making: who will make decisions for me when I can't? *Clin Geriatr Med* 1994;10:445–462.

Jecker NS. Age-based rationing and women. *JAMA* 1991;266:3012–3015.

Kapp MB. Futile medical treatment: a review of the ethical arguments and legal holdings. *J Gen Intern Med* 1994;9:170–177.

McCue JD. The naturalness of dying. *JAMA* 1995;273:1039–1043.

Quill TE, Cassel CK. Nonabandonment: a central obligation for physicians. *Ann Intern Med* 1995;122:368–374.

Rodwin M. *Money, medicine and morals.* New York: Oxford University Press, 1992.

Zirker M, Zirker H. *Medical futility.* Cambridge, UK: Cambridge University Press, 1997.

Kelley's Textbook of Internal Medicine, fourth edition. Edited by H. David Humes.
Lippincott Williams & Wilkins, Philadelphia © 2000.

Index

Page numbers followed by t indicate tables.